PDR GENERICS · 1995

FIRST EDITION

PDR
Generics™

MEDICAL ECONOMICS

MONTVALE, NEW JERSEY

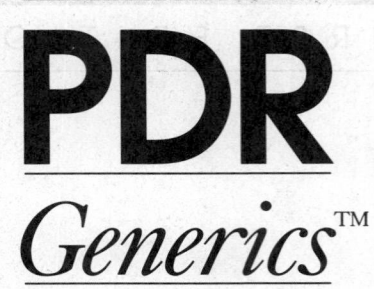

PDR
Generics™

MEDICAL CONSULTANT
Ronald Arky, MD
Charles S. Davidson Professor of Medicine
Master, Francis Weld Peabody Society
Harvard Medical School, Boston, Mass.

PHARMACEUTICAL DIRECTOR
Mukesh Mehta, R Ph

SENIOR PHARMACEUTICAL EDITOR
Bruce Weiner, MS, R Ph, FASHP
St. Elisabeth's Medical Center, Boston, Mass.
Tufts University School of Medicine
Bouve College of Pharmacy, Northeastern
University
Massachusetts College of Pharmacy

PHARMACEUTICAL EDITORS
Paula R. Ajmera, R Ph

Denise A. Arena, R Ph
Beth Israel Hospital, Boston, Mass.

Cheryl A. Avedissian, R Ph
St. Elizabeth's Medical Center, Boston, Mass.

Keith Vaughan Belken, R Ph
Beth Israel Hospital, Boston, Mass.

Edward R. Bezzaro, R Ph
Faulkner Hospital, Boston, Mass.

Marie Cohen, R Ph
Beth Israel Hospital, Boston, Mass.

Linda D' Amore, R Ph
MetroWest Medical Center, Framingham, Mass.

Michael J. D'Amore, R Ph
St. Elizabeth's Medical Center, Boston, Mass.

Amy DeBesse, R Ph
Beth Israel Hospital, Boston, Mass.

Serenella R. Donahue, R Ph
St. Elizabeth's Medical Center, Boston, Mass.

Thomas L. Fleming, R Ph

Marion Gray, R Ph

Christopher Hughes, R Ph
South Shore Hospital, South Weymouth, Mass.

Nancy Jacoby, R Ph

Michael Lee, R Ph
St. Elizabeth's Medical Center, Boston, Mass.

Carolyn Ann Maroun, R Ph
St. Elizabeth's Medical Center, Boston, Mass.

Christopher McCoy, R Ph
St. Elizabeth's Medical Center, Boston, Mass.

Leila A. Noueihed, R Ph

Donna S. Parker, R Ph
South Shore Hospital, South Weymouth, Mass.

Jennifer Salvon, R Ph
Beth Israel Hospital, Boston, Mass.

Amy L. Shafer, R Ph, Pharm D
Beth Israel Hospital, Boston, Mass.

Catherine L. Simonian, R Ph
Value Pharmacy, Leominster, Mass.

Jon D. Swetzoff, R Ph Pharm D
St. Elizabeth's Medical Center, Boston, Mass.

Felicia Wessenberg, R PH
Beth Israel Hospital, Boston, Mass.

In addition, we gratefully acknowledge
the assistance of the entire staff and board of
pharmaceutical consultants of MICROMEDEX, INC.

PUBLISHING STAFF
President and Chief Operating Officer,
Drug Information Services Group:
William J. Gole

Senior Vice President and General Manager:
Thomas F. Rice

Product Manager: Stephen B. Greenberg

Associate Product Manager: Cy S. Caine

Editor: David W. Sifton

Design Director: Robert Hartman

Manager, Database Administration:
Lynne Handler

Vice President of Production:
Steven R. Andreazza

Director of Contracts and Special Services:
Marjorie A. Duffy

Director of Production: Carrie Williams

Production Managers: Kimberly Hiller-Vivas,
Tara Walsh

Production Coodinator: Dawn McCall

Assistant Editors: Ann Ben Larbi,
Beret Erway, Sarah G. Terzides

Format Editor: Gregory J. Westley

Art Associate: Joan K. Akerlind

Production Editors: Catherine Akerlind,
Paula Benus, Dick Burnon, George Dickstein,
Joan Frawley, Michael Holmes, Jayne Jacobson,
Thomas Johnson, Gwynned Kelly, Barbara Klink,
Leslie Kolvek, David Marinelli, Thelma Perin

Production Assistants: Annette Gharabegie,
Lisa Lotti, Martina Murtagh

Information Systems: Reginald Davis, David Levy,
Norma Musciotto, Erez Wolf

Director of Corporate Communications:
Gregory J. Thomas

Digital Photography:
Shawn W. Cahill, Frank J. McElroy, III

Digital Prepress Processing:
Joanne Pearson, Richard Weinstock,
Kevin J. Leckner, Ron Scalici

Special Acknowledgements: Korey Halsch,
Barry Krelitz, Krelitz Industries, Inc.;
Sony Corporation of America

OFFICERS OF MEDICAL ECONOMICS:
President and Chief Executive Officer: Norman R. Snesil; *Executive Vice President and Chief Financial Officer:* J. Crispin Ashworth; *Senior Vice President of Corporate Operations Group:* John R. Ware; *Senior Vice President of Corporate Business Development:* Raymond M. Zoeller; *Vice President of Information Services and Chief Information Officer:* Edward J. Zecchini

ISBN: 1-56363-118-0

Contents

Foreword

Decision-makers in today's cost-driven healthcare arena know that—for better or worse—clinical considerations are no longer the sole determinant of treatment. These days it's not sufficient to simply identify the best therapeutic modality. Now it's incumbent on clinicians to select the most cost-effective source as well.

In this lean, new environment, healthcare providers need more information than ever—and they need to find it fast. When choosing drug therapy, they require a reference that presents not only all the therapeutic alternatives, but every source of supply—a resource that provides both a thorough clinical overview and a meaningful perspective on cost, a book that quickly and conveniently establishes a comprehensive basis of comparison.

It is to fulfill precisely this need that *Physicians' Desk Reference®* proudly introduces *PDR Generics,* a comprehensive compendium of nearly all single- and multi-source prescription drugs in general use today, covering a total of nearly 24,000 products in all. In this single handy volume you'll find all the information you need to quickly select the optimum drug at the most advantageous price. Carefully crafted indices will guide you to all available alternatives for any indication—both labeled and unlabeled—or to a complete roster of drugs in any therapeutic class. And when you've located the ideal candidate, you'll find not only complete prescribing information, but detailed pricing data as well.

The prescribing information found in *PDR Generics* is a complete, unbiased synthesis of relevant FDA-approved labeling supplemented with peer-reviewed data on off-label uses drawn from the extensive DRUGDEX® Drug Information System maintained by the *PDR®* affiliate, MICROMEDEX, INC. The prescribing information is neither sponsored nor approved by the products' manufacturers. It has been selected, integrated, and reviewed solely by *PDR Generics'* board of pharmaceutical editors. Information on suppliers and prices comes from the *Red Book Database,* the nation's premier drug price directory and another affiliate of *PDR.* (If you require the very latest pricing information, *Red Book®* offers a monthly update service. Call 1-800-232-7399 for details.)

The prescribing information in *PDR Generics* has been compiled to reflect all major forms and sources of each generic entity.

For information specific to a particular brand, please refer to *PDR* itself, or to one of its companion volumes. The *PDR* library of drug references includes:

- *Physicians' Desk Reference®* and its supplements
- *PDR For Nonprescription Drugs®*
- *PDR For Ophthalmology®*
- *PDR Guide to Drug Interactions•Side Effects•Indications™*

Data from these printed references is also available in a variety of electronic formats:

- *Pocket PDR™* A handheld personal database of key sections from each prescription-drug listing in *PDR.*
- *PDR Library on CD-ROM™* Complete prescribing information from *PDR* and the companion volumes listed above—with the full contents of *The Merck Manual* and *Stedman's Medical Dictionary* as optional enhancements—all on one convenient disc for use on PC networks and individual PCs.
- *PDR Drug Interactions/Side Effects/Indications Diskettes™* A powerful screening program for patient regimens of up to 20 drugs.
- *PDR Database Services* A preformatted text file suitable for integration in large mainframe-based information systems.

For more information on any of these products, please call, toll-free, 1-800-232-7379 or fax 201-573-4956.

While every effort has been made to provide comprehensive information on each of the generic entities described in *PDR Generics,* the publisher can guarantee neither the accuracy nor the completeness of the entries herein. The publisher has conducted no independent analysis of the information, and disclaims all liability in connection with its use. The publisher also does not warrant or guarantee any product listed herein: Inclusion of a product should not be construed as endorsement or recommendation by the publisher; and absence of a product should not be regarded as a criticism or rejection.

This first edition of *PDR Generics* represents a completely new kind of drug reference. As we begin preparation of the second edition, we welcome your comments and suggestions. Is there additional information we should include? Is there a better way of presenting it? Please let us know. Call us, toll-free, 1-800-232-7379 or fax 201-573-4956.

How to Use *PDR Generics*

Locating Product Information

PDR Generics is designed to make look-ups as quick and easy as possible. The entries are organized alphabetically by generic name and cross-referenced by leading brand names. For consistency, ingredients of combination products are also listed alphabetically. So, for example, you will find product information under "Hydrochlorothiazide and Lisinopril," but not the reverse.

To help speed your research, *PDR Generics* also provides you with three specialized indices.

Brand and Generic Name Index

This index helps you zero in on a product—by either brand or generic name— without thumbing through the book. All names are listed alphabetically, and are followed by the page number of the entry in which they appear. Generic names are underlined; brand names are not. Under each generic name, brand names covered by that monograph are repeated.

Product Category Index

This index enables you to identify and compare all generic entities in a given therapeutic or pharmacologic category. Listings are alphabetical by major category and sub-category. For instance, beta-blocking drugs can be found under the "Beta Blockers" subhead in the "Cardiovascular Agents" section.

Indications Index

If you are seeking alternative medications for a specific diagnosis, this is the index to turn to. It lists over 2,300 specific indications and the drugs used for each. All FDA-approved uses are included, along with all generally accepted off-label uses documented in the peer-reviewed literature. The entries are listed alphabetically. An italic entry indicates an off-label use.

The Product Information Listings

Each entry in the Product Information Section provides you with complete prescribing information plus comprehensive data on available forms and strengths, their suppliers and prices, and applicable reimbursement codes.

PRESCRIBING INFORMATION

A monograph containing full prescribing information leads off each entry. The monographs are a synthesis of FDA-approved labeling for the various forms in which the generic ingredient is available. In them you will find information on all standard topics, including:

Description	*Precautions*
Clinical Pharmacology	*Adverse Reactions*
Indications and Usage	*Overdosage*
Contraindications	*Dosage and Administration*
Warnings	

Structural Formulas

The chemical structure of single-entity products is depicted in the "Description" section of the monograph. Structural formulas for combination products do not appear.

Off-label Indications

In the "Indications and Usage" section of many monographs you will find a paragraph entitled "Unlabeled Uses." This information is drawn from the *Computerized Clinical Information System* (CCIS) maintained by MICROMEDEX, INC., an affiliate of PDR and the world leader in evaluative clinical drug information. All information is drawn from peer-reviewed literature. Additional information on these uses, including dosage and adverse reactions, can be found in MICROMEDEX Healthcare Systems, which is available in most hospital pharmacies. (For information on subscribing, call MICROMEDEX at 1-800-525-9083.)

Use-in-Pregnancy Ratings

A rating indicating the degree of risk in pregnancy can be found in the "Precautions" section of most monographs. The rating system, established by the U.S. Food and Drug Administration, weighs the degree to which available information has ruled out risk to the fetus against the drug's potential benefit to the patient. The ratings, and their interpretation, are as follows:

A: Controlled studies show no risk.
Adequate, well-controlled studies in pregnant women have failed to demonstrate risk to the fetus.

B: No evidence of risk in humans.
Either animal finding show risk while human findings do not, or, if no adequate human studies have been done, animal findings are negative.

C: Risk cannot be ruled out.
Human studies are lacking, and animal studies are either positive for risk or are lacking as well. However, potential benefits may justify any potential risk.

D: Positive evidence of risk.
Investigational or postmarketing data show risk to the fetus. Nevertheless, potential benefits may outweigh the potential risk.

X: Contraindicated in pregnancy.
Studies in animals or humans, or investigational or post-marketing reports, have demonstrated fetal risk which clearly outweighs any possible benefit to the patient.

A listing of drugs in these categories can be found near the end of the book.

Reimbursement Codes

When applicable, Health Care Common Procedure Coding System (HCPCS) Level II "J codes" appear at the end of the monograph. Shown first is the amount of drug to be administered, then the reimbursable routes of administration, and finally the J code itself. The amount is expressed as a range up to a given maximum or, in some cases, as a specific dose. Routes are abbreviated as follows:

IA	Intra-arterial
IV	Intravenous
IM	Intramuscular
SC	Subcutaneous
INH	Inhaled solution
VAR	Various routes
OTH	Other routes
ORAL	Oral

Level II HCPCS codes were established by the Health Care Finance Administration to supplement the CPT codes used in reporting professional services, procedures, and supplies on Medicare claims. The codes are also required by many state Medicaid programs.

INFORMATION ON AVAILABLE SUPPLIES

This section, entitled "How Supplied," provides you with pricing data on a broad range of available supplies. (Selected additional alternatives can be found at the end of the book.) With this information, you can quickly reach a judgment on the comparative cost of a given brand or generic selection. Products that are therapeutically equivalent are listed first, followed by those for which equivalence is unconfirmed, and finally those which have never been rated.

Within these broad equivalency categories, supplies are organized by form and strength. Under each form/strength heading, brands appear first, followed by their generic counterparts. Products are listed in ascending order of package size. To permit quick identification of the most economical generic substitutes, within each size category the products appear in ascending order of average wholesale price (AWP).

Therapeutic Equivalency Indicators

Equivalency is determined from codes assigned by the Food and Drug Administration and published in the guide entitled "Approved Drug Products with Therapeutic Equivalence Evaluations," commonly known as the "Orange Book." A product's therapeutic-equivalence status is indicated by a symbol appearing in the left-hand margin of the price listings.

- A BLACK DIAMOND [◆] denotes products carrying a code of "A" in the Orange Book, signifying that they are considered therapeutically equivalent.
- An OPEN DIAMOND [◇] denotes products carrying a "B" code in the Orange Book, signifying that they have not been proven equivalent. (Note however, that B-rated products have not necessarily been proven *inequivalent* either).
- An OPEN CIRCLE [○] denotes products that do not carry an Orange Book rating.

Controlled Substances Categories

When applicable, a product's controlled substance status is indicated in the form/strength heading immediately following the form. Any product subject to the Controlled Substances Act of 1970 is assigned a category according to its potential for abuse. The greater the danger, the more severe the limitations on prescriptions for the drug. The categories are as follows:

CII: High potential for abuse.

Use may lead to severe physical or psychological dependence. Prescriptions must be written in ink, or typewritten and signed by the practitioner. Verbal prescriptions must be confirmed in writing within 72 hours, and may be given only in a genuine emergency. No renewals are permitted.

CIII: Some potential for abuse.

Use may lead to low-to-moderate physical dependence or high psychological dependence. Prescriptions may be oral or written. Up to 5 renewals are permitted within 6 months.

CIV: Low potential for abuse.

Use may lead to limited physical or psychological dependence. Prescriptions may be oral or written. Up to 5 renewals are permitted within 6 months.

CV: Subject to state and local regulation.

Abuse potential is low; a prescription may not be required.

Average Unit Prices

Whenever applicable, two small tables head the list of products available in a particular form and strength. The first provides you with a comparison between the average unit price of the leading brand versus the typical unit cost of a generic alternative. As an additional benchmark, the Health Care Finance Administration's Federal Upper Limit price is shown as well.

The averages are based on unit costs of all package sizes from all suppliers of therapeutically equivalent products. Such global averages are, of course, only suggestive. Actual unit costs will depend on the quantities in which the drug is purchased.

Federal Upper Limit prices determine Medicaid reimbursement for multiple-source drugs. The prices shown here were effective as of July 1, 1994. They are designated in the table by the abbreviation HCFA FUL. The package size to which the price applies is also given.

The table appears whenever there is more than one alternative source of a given generic entity or the product is available in more than one package size.

Generic A-Rated Average Prices

At the right of the Average Unit Price table is a second table that provides a more specific basis for judging a particular supplier's price. This table shows the average cost of each package size offered by generic suppliers. Only products rated therapeutically equivalent are included in the averages, which appear for any package size available from more than one supplier.

PRICES

The price table lists all package sizes of supplies bearing a therapeutic equivalency rating or, if the drug is unrated, all currently available supplies.

- The BRAND/MANUFACTURER column gives the product's brand name, if any, and the name of the supplier.
- The NDC column supplies the item's National Drug Code number in standardized 5-4-2 format.
- The SIZE column gives each item's package, grouping like sizes together in ascending order. Items packaged in unit-dose form are flagged with the abbreviation "UD" and grouped separately.
- The AWP column provides the item's Average Wholesale Price, again in ascending order.

A small arrow at the left of an entry means that a photo of the product appears in the Visual Identification Guide.

All prices are drawn from *Red Book,* the nation's premier drug price database. The Average Wholesale Prices published by *Red Book* are based on data obtained from manufacturers, distributors, and other suppliers. Prices shown are those in effect as *PDR Generics* went to press. Because actual prices paid by retailers may vary and are subject to frequent change, these prices should be used only as a basis for comparison. Be sure to check with the supplier before making a final decision.

A TYPICAL PRICE TABLE

TABLETS: 250 MG

AVERAGE UNIT PRICE (AVAILABLE SIZES)		GENERIC A-RATED AVERAGE PRICE (GAAP)	
BRAND	0.402	**GAAP 100s**	$11.66
GENERIC	0.104	**GAAP 500s**	$40.55
HCFA FUL (5s)	$0.084	**GAAP 1000s**	$83.98

BRAND/MANUFACTURER	NDC	SIZE	AWP
BRAND			
➤ DIAMOX: Storz/Lederle	57706-0755-23	100s	$38.78
	57706-0755-60	100s ud	$44.89
	57706-0755-34	1000s	$368.24
◆ **GENERICS**			
Harber	51432-0002-03	100s	$8.50
Moore,H.L.	00839-5953-06	100s	$9.17
Major	00904-0350-60	100s	$9.40
CMC-Cons	00223-0039-01	100s	$9.75
Qualitest	00603-2070-21	100s	$9.80
Mutual	53489-0167-01	100s	$9.85
URL	00677-0577-01	100s	$11.40
Schein	00364-0400-01	100s	$11.45

The Product Identification Guide

PDR Generics provides you with two ways of identifying an unknown tablet or capsule: by comparing it with the photos in the Visual Identification Guide, or by matching its imprint with those listed in the Imprint Identification Guide. Here's additional information on each of these convenient identification aids, both of which appear in the section immediately preceding the Product Information.

THE VISUAL IDENTIFICATION GUIDE

Products shown in this section are organized alphabetically by generic name. More than 1,000 of the most frequently dispensed brand and generic products are included. All items are reproduced in actual size and color. Each product is labeled with its brand name, if applicable, and the name of its supplier.

THE IMPRINT IDENTIFICATION GUIDE

For quick comparison, all entries in this table are organized by key identification number. For example, the imprint "LL A2" can be found under Identification Number 2, while "25 LL A13," which also includes a reference to the product's 25 mg strength, appears under 13.

In addition to the full identification code as imprinted on the product, the table includes the product's generic name and, to confirm its identification, its strength, color, form, and shape. For tablets, indicators show whether the product is scored or coated (for capsules, only a dash appears). The product's supplier and primary use round out each listing.

This convenient table is reprinted with permission from *The Med-Scan Manual®*, Fifth Edition, copyright © 1994 and published by Med-Scan International, Inc.

Additional Features

Near the end of the book, you'll find several convenient, ready-reference sections.

- USE-IN-PREGNANCY RATINGS lists all drugs in *PDR Generics* that fall into each of the U.S. Food and Drug Administration's five pregnancy risk categories. A quick check of these listings may be all that's needed to verify the status of a particular drug.
- CERTIFIED POISON CONTROL CENTERS provides you with a comprehensive national directory of the largest 24-hours-a-day facilities.
- DRUG INFORMATION CENTERS presents a nationwide list of centers organized alphabetically by state and city.
- NEW MOLECULAR ENTITIES presents a list of the completely original compounds released for marketing during the previous year. It serves as a handy summary of the most important new products now available for general use.

Finally, *PDR Generics* cooperates with the Food and Drug Administration to provide health care professionals with a master copy of the form used in reporting vaccine adverse events. Together with instructions for completion, it can be found at the close of the book.

Brand and Generic Name Index

Listed in this index are all generic products profiled in the Product Information section, along with the leading brand names cited in the profiles. Generic names are underlined; brand names are not. Under each generic name, the names of all associated brands are repeated in smaller type. All listings are alphabetical.

This arrangement allows you to find any product by either of its names. For instance, the ACE inhibitor quinapril is listed under the brand name Accupril and again under the generic name Quinapril Hydrochloride. Both listings direct you to the quinapril product profile.

UNDERLINE DENOTES GENERIC NAME

UNDERLINE DENOTES GENERIC NAME

Product Category Index

Entries in this index are organized by therapeutic or pharmacologic category, enabling you to quickly identify and compare agents with similar properties. Listings are alphabetical by major category and subcategory. For example, all medications for acne can be found under the "Acne Preparations" subhead under the major heading "Dermatologicals."

Indications Index

Listed in this index are over 1,700 specific medical problems and the drugs indicated for each, enabling you to quickly review all the alternatives for a particular diagnosis. The listings include all drugs specifically approved for each condition by the Food and Drug Administration, plus all those with generally accepted off-label uses documented in the peer-reviewed literature. Products used off-label are shown in italics. All entries are alphabetical.

ITALIC LISTING INDICATES UNLABELED USE

ITALIC LISTING INDICATES UNLABELED USE

Phenoxybenzamine
Hydrochloride 2225

URINARY RETENTION, NEUROGENIC ATONY OF THE URINARY BLADDER
Phenoxybenzamine
Hydrochloride 2225

URINARY RETENTION, POSTPARTUM NONOBSTRUCTIVE
Bethanechol Chloride 342

URINARY TRACT, BURNING, SYMPTOMATIC RELIEF OF
Phenazopyridine
Hydrochloride 2211

URINARY TRACT, HYPERMOTILITY, CONTROL OF SYMPTOMS
Hyoscyamine Sulfate 1485

URINARY TRACT, LOWER, HYPERMOTILITY DISORDERS
Atropine Sulfate/Benzoic
Acid/Hyoscyamine/
Methenamine/Methylene
Blue/Phenylsalicylate 251

URINARY URGENCY, SYMPTOMATIC RELIEF OF
Flavoxate Hydrochloride 1195
Phenazopyridine
Hydrochloride 2211

URINARY VOIDING, IRRITABLE, SYMPTOMATIC RELIEF OF
Oxybutynin Chloride 2134

URINE, ACIDIFICATION OF
Potassium Acid
Phosphate 2286
Potassium Acid Phosphate
and Sodium Acid
Phosphate 2286
Racemethionine 2424

URINE, ALKALINIZATION OF
Citric Acid and Potassium
Citrate 635
Citric Acid and Sodium
Citrate 636
Citric Acid/Potassium
Citrate/Sodium Citrate 639
Potassium Citrate and
Sodium Citrate 2298
Sodium Bicarbonate 2505

UROGRAPHY, DIAGNOSTIC AID IN
Diatrizoate Meglumine 844
Diatrizoate Sodium 851
Hyaluronidase 1401
Indigotindisulfonate
Sodium 1507
Iodamide Meglumine 1544
Iohexol 1548
Iothalamate 1566
Iothalamate Meglumine 1572
Iothalamate Meglumine and
Iothalamate Sodium 1576
Ioversol 1579
Ioxaglate Meglumine and
Ioxaglate Sodium 1584

UROLITHIASIS, MANAGEMENT OF
Citric Acid/Magnesium
Oxide/Sodium Carbonate ...638
Sodium Lactate 2513

URTICARIA PIGMENTOSA
Betamethasone, Topical 334

Manufacturer Directory

Listed below are all pharmaceutical manufacturing companies, subsidiaries, and divisions currently monitored by *PDR Generics* and its *Red Book* affiliate. The address and principal telephone number are included for each organization. The entries are alphabetical by company name.

3M COMPANY,
CONSUMER HEALTH CARE
3M CENTER 223-4N-10
ST.PAUL, MN 551441000
612-736-0894

3M COMPANY
MEDICAL-SURGICAL DIVISON
3M CENTER 275-4W-02
ST. PAUL, MN 55144-1000
612-736-4860

3M PHARMACEUTICALS
3M CENTER 275-3W-01
ST. PAUL, MN 55133
800-447-4537

A-A SPECTRUM
DIV. OF
SPECTRUM CHEM. MFG. CORP.
14422 SO. SAN PEDRO STREET
GARDENA, CA 90248
800-772-8796

A-T SURGICAL MFG. CO., INC.
115 PARK STREET
HOLYOKE, MA 01040
413-532-4551

ABANA PHARMACEUTICALS, INC.
P. O. BOX 360388
BIRMINGHAM, AL 35236
800-828-1969

ABBOTT DIAGNOSTIC
DIV. OF ABBOTT LABS.
1 ABBOTT PARK ROAD
ABBOTT PARK, IL 60064
800-323-9100

ABBOTT HOSPITAL PRODUCTS
DIV. OF ABBOTT LABS.
1 ABBOTT PARK RD. D-R10
ABBOTT PARK IL 60064-3500
800-222-6883

ABBOTT PHARMACEUTICAL
DIV. OF ABBOTT LABS
1 ABBOTT PARK ROAD
ABBOTT PARK, IL 60064-3500
800-255-5162

ABLE LABORATORIES
177 RYAN STREET
SOUTH PLAINFIELD, NJ 07080
908-754-2253

ACME UNITED CORPORATION
MEDICAL PRODUCTS DIVISION
75 KINGS HIGHWAY CUTOFF
FAIRFIELD, CT 06430
203-332-7330

ACTION LABS, INC.
2851 VIA MARTENS
ANAHEIM, CA 92806
714-630-5941

ADAMS LABORATORIES INC.
14801 SOVEREIGN ROAD
FORT WORTH, TX 76155
800-932-1950

ADH HEALTH PRODUCTS INC.
215 NORTH ROUTE 303
CONGERS, NY 10920-1726
914-268-0027

ADVANCE PHARMACEUTICAL INC.
2201-F 5TH AVENUE
RONKONKOMA, NY 11779
516-981-4600

ADVANCED NUTRITIONAL
TECHNOLOGY, INC.
1111 JEFFERSON AVENUE
P. O. BOX 3225
ELIZABETH, NJ 07207-3225
800-624-6543

AEROSEPTICS PA
2800 WEST 21ST STREET
EBCO BUSINESS PARK
ERIE, PA 16506-2980
814-838-4944

AKORN, INC.
100 AKORN DRIVE
ABITA SPRINGS, LA 70420
800-535-7155

AKPHARMA
P. O. BOX 111
PLEASANTVILLE, NJ 08232
800-732-6441

ALCON LABORATORIES
6201 S. FREEWAY, T5-19
FT. WORTH, TX 76134-2099
817-293-0450

ALCON SURGICAL PROD. DIV.
6201 S. FREEWAY
I.L. 34
FT. WORTH, TX 76134
800-862-5266

ALEXANDER, JAMES, CORP.
R.D. 3, BOX 192, RT. 94
BLAIRSTOWN, NJ 07825
908-362-9266

ALHAMBRA CHEMICAL CO.
34501 ESPINOZA
CAPISTRANO BEACH, CA 92624
714-496-3055

ALIGEN INDEPENDENT LABS, INC.
MEDTECH BLDG. AT THE ASPENS
P. O. BOX 1861
JACKSON HOLE, WY 83001
307-733-0570

ALK LABORATORIES, INC.
RESEARCH CENTER
27 VILLAGE LANE
WALLINGFORD, CT 06492
800-325-7354

ALLEN & HANBURYS
5 MOORE DRIVE
RESEARCH TRIANGLE PK, NC
27709 919-248-2100

ALLERGAN HERBERT, SKIN CARE
DIV. ALLERGAN
PHARMACEUTICALS
2525 DU PONT DRIVE
IRVINE, CA 92715
714-752-4500

ALLERGAN OPTICAL
DIV. OF ALLERGAN INC.
2525 DUPONT DRIVE
IRVINE, CA 92715
714-752-4500

ALLERGAN PHARMACEUTICALS, INC.
DIV. OF ALLERGAN, INC.
2525 DUPONT DRIVE
IRVINE, CA 92715
714-752-4500

ALLIED-MED
DIVISION OF PHARMED GROUP
7350-7356 N.W. PHARMED WAY
MIAMI, FL 33122-1261
800-683-7342

ALLSCRIPS PHARMACEUTICAL INC.
1033 BUTTERFIELD ROAD
VERNON HILLS, IL 60061
800-654-0889

ALPERN LABORATORIES
691 MELROSE AVENUE
CHULA VISTA, CA 91910
619-425-4100

ALPHA THERAPEUTIC CORP.
5555 VALLEY BLVD.
LOS ANGELES, CA 90032
800-421-0008

ALPHAGEN LABORATORIES, INC.
11515 N. FULTON INDUSTRIAL BLVD.
ALPHARETTA, GA 30201
404-475-8976

ALRA LABORATORIES, INC.
3850 CLEARVIEW COURT
GURNEE, IL 60031
800-248-2572

ALTAIRE PHARMACEUTICALS, INC.
91-1 COLIN DRIVE
HOLBROOK, NY 11741
516-472-8186

ALTO PHARMACEUTICALS, INC.
P. O. BOX 1910
LAND O'LAKES, FL 34639
800-330-2891

ALVA/AMCO PHARMACAL COS. INC.
6625 N. AVONDALE
CHICAGO, IL 60631
312-792-0200

ALZA PHARMACEUTICALS
950 PAGE MILL RD.
P. O. BOX 10950
PALO ALTO, CA 94303-0802
800-634-8977

**AMEND DRUG &
CHEMICAL COMPANY**
83 CORDIER STREET
IRVINGTON, NJ 07111
800-274-2636

AMERICAN CHICLE GROUP
WARNER-LAMBERT CO.
201 TABOR RD.
MORRIS PLAINS, NJ 07950
201-540-6760

AMERICAN DRUG INDUSTRIES, INC.
5810-20 SOUTH PERRY AVENUE
CHICAGO, IL 60621
312-667-7070

AMERICAN DRUG STORES
1818 SWIFT DRIVE
OAK BROOK, IL 60521
708-572-5205

AMERICAN GENERICS INC.
48 WOODSTEAD ROAD
BALLSTON LAKE, NY 12019
518-762-5692

AMERICAN HYGIENIC LABS., INC.
4041 ROYAL PALM AVENUE
MIAMI BEACH, FL 33140
305-673-8805

**AMERICAN INTERNATIONAL MEDICAL
SUPPLY CO.**
3762 SOUTH 150 EAST
SALT LAKE CITY, UT 84115
800-426-0244

AMERICAN PHARMACEUTICAL CO.
245 FOURTH STREET
P. O. BOX 448
PASSAIC, NJ 07055
201-779-5300

**AMERICAN RED CROSS,
BLOOD SERVICES**
PLASMA OPERATIONS
1730 E. STREET
WASHINGTON, DC 20006
202-639-3261

**AMERICAN RED CROSS,
BLOOD SERVICES**
N.E. REGIONAL HEADQUARTERS
180 RUSTCRAFT ROAD
DEDHAM, MA 02026
800-851-4313

**AMERICAN REGENT
LABORATORIES, INC.**
SUB. OF LUITPOLD PHARM. INC.
ONE LUITPOLD DRIVE
SHIRLEY, NY 11967
800-645-1706

AMERICAN THERMOMETER CO.
6212 EXECUTIVE BOULEVARD
HUBER HEIGHTS, OH 45424
513-233-5080

AMERICAN UROLOGICALS, INC.
7881 HOLLYWOOD BLVD., SUITE 4
PEMBROKE PINES, FL 33024
305-438-5070

AMERSHAM HEALTHCARE
2636 SOUTH CLEARBROOK DRIVE
ARLINGTON HEIGHTS, IL 60005
800-633-4123

AMGEN INC.
1900 OAK TERRACE LANE
THOUSAND OAKS, CA 91320-1789
800-282-6436

AMIDE PHARMACEUTICALS, INC.
101 E. MAIN STREET
LITTLE FALLS, NJ 07424
201-890-1440

AMKAS LABORATORIES, INC.
4008 DENICE COURT
GLENVIEW, IL 60025
312-481-2089

**AMPHARCO INC.
INTERNATIONAL PHARM.
DISTRIB. CO.**
9549 A. BOLSA AVENUE
WESTMINSTER, CA 92683
714-531-3560

ANDERSEN LABORATORIES, INC.
P.O. BOX 848
NORWICH, NY 13815
800-441-0619

APOTEX USA, INC.
3 BOULDEN CIRCLE
NEW CASTLE, DE 19720
800-627-6839

APOTHECARY PRODUCTS
11531 RUPP DRIVE
BURNSVILLE, MN 55337
800-328-2742

APOTHECON PRODUCTS
A BRISTOL-MYERS
SQUIBB COMPANY
P. O. BOX 4500
PRINCETON, NJ 08543-4500
800-631-5244

ARCO PHARMACEUTICALS, INC.
90 ORVILLE DRIVE
DEPT. DT
BOHEMIA, NY 11716
800-645-5412

ARCOLA LABORATORIES
A DIVISION OF
RHONE-POULENC RORER
P.O. BOX 1200
COLLEGEVILLE, PA 19426-0107
800-727-6737

ARMAN DRUG CO., INC.
1005 WEST 11TH STREET
SIOUX FALLS, SD 57104
605-336-0445

ARMOUR PHARMACEUTICAL CO.
500 ARCOLA ROAD
BOX 1200, MAIL STOP 3B22
COLLEGEVILLE, PA 19426-0107
610-454-8523

ARZOL CHEMICAL COMPANY
208 BENTON ROAD
P.O. BOX 91
NORTH HAVERHILL, NH 03774
603-787-6889

ASCHER, B. F. & CO., INC.
15501 WEST 109TH
LENEXA, KS 66219
913-888-1880

ASTRA USA, INC.
50 OTIS STREET
WESTBOROUGH, MA 01581
800-225-4803

ATHENA NEUROSCIENCES, INC.
800F GATEWAY BOULEVARD
SO. SAN FRANCISCO, CA 94080
415-877-0900

ATLEY PHARMACEUTICALS
340 S. RICHARDSON RD.
ASHLAND, VA 23005
804-550-1979

AURO PHARMACEUTICALS, INC.
80 EARHART DRIVE
BLDG. 20
WILLIAMSVILLE, NY 14221
800-447-6801

**AUTOMATIC LIQUID
PACKAGING, INC.**
2200 W. LAKE SHORE DRIVE
WOODSTOCK, IL 60098
815-338-9500

BAJAMAR CHEMICAL CO.
9609 DIELMAN ROCK ISLAND
P. O. BOX 12411
ST. LOUIS, MO 63132
314-997-3414

**BAKER NORTON
PHARMACEUTICALS INC**
8800 NORTHWEST 36TH ST
MIAMI, FL 33178-2404
800-735-2315

BAKER, J.T., INC.
222 RED SCHOOL LANE
PHILLIPSBURG, NJ 08865
908-859-2151

**BAKER/CUMMINS
DERMATOLOGICALS, INC.**
1950 SWARTHMORE AVENUE
P O BOX 3009
LAKEWOOD, NJ 08701
800-735-2315

BALAN, J.J. INC.
5725 FOSTER AVE.
BROOKLYN, NY 11234
718-251-8663

BALASSA LABORATORIES, INC.
P. O. BOX 291161
PORT ORANGE, FL 32129
904-761-8039

BARD PATIENT CARE DIVISION
111 SPRING STREET
MURRAY HILL, NJ 07974
800-526-4930

BARD UROLOGICAL DIVISION
C.R. BARD, INC
8195 INDUSTRIAL BLVD
COVINGTON, CA 30209
800-526-4455

**BARLAN PHARMACAL
COMPANY, INC.**
3 SPIELMAN ROAD
FAIRFIELD, NJ 07006
201-882-3790

BARON PHARMACEUTICALS, INC.
4503 N.W. 103 AVENUE
SUITE 103
SUNRISE, FL 33351
305-749-8008

BARR LABS., INC.
2 QUAKER ROAD
BOX D2900
POMONA, NY 10970-0519
800-222-4043

BARRE-NATIONAL, INC.
7205 WINDSOR BLVD.
BALTIMORE, MD 21244-2654
800-638-9096

BASEL PHARMACEUTICALS
DIV. OF CIBA-GEIGY CORP.
556 MORRIS AVE.
SUMMIT, NJ 07901
908-277-5000

BASIC VITAMINS
P.P. BOX 412
VANDALIA, OH 45377
800-782-2742

BAUSCH & LOMB EYE CARE
1400 N. GOODMAN STREET
ROCHESTER, NY 14692
800-828-6974

**BAUSCH & LOMB
PHARMACEUTICALS, INC.**
8500 HIDDEN RIVER PARKWAY
TAMPA, FL 33637
800-227-1427

BAXTER BIOTECH NORTH AMERICA
HYLAND DIVISION
1425 LAKE COOK ROAD, LCIV-2
DEERFIELD, IL 60015
800-423-2090

BAXTER HEALTHCARE CORP.
RTL-10,
ROUTE 120 & WILSON ROAD
ROUND LAKE, IL 60073
800-933-0303

BEACH PRODUCTS, INC.
5220 S. MANHATTAN AVENUE
BOX 13447
TAMPA, FL 33681
800-845-8210

**BECTON DICKINSON
CONSUMER PROD.**
ONE BECTON DRIVE
FRANKLIN LAKES, NJ 07417
201-847-7100

**BECTON DICKINSON
MICROBIOLOGY SYSTEMS**
P. O. BOX 243
COCKEYSVILLE, MD 21030
800-854-4477

BEIERSDORF, INC.
P. O. BOX 5529
NORWALK, CT 06856-5529
203-853-8008

BELL-HORN
WM. H. HORN & BRO.
451 N. 3RD ST.
PHILADELPHIA, PA 19123
215-627-2773

BERGEN BRUNSWIG DRUG COMPANY
4000 METROPOLITAN DRIVE
ORANGE, CA 92668
714-385-4000

BERKELEY BIOLOGICALS
2840 EIGHTH STREET
BERKELEY, CA 94710
800-544-6656

BERLEX LABORATORIES
300 FAIRFIELD ROAD
WAYNE, NJ 07470-7358
800-2375391

BERNA PRODUCTS, CORP.
4216 PONCE DE LEON BLVD.
CORAL GABLES, FL 33146
305-443-2900

BETA DERMACEUTICALS, INC.
P. O. BOX 691106
SAN ANTONIO, TX 78269-1106
210-349-9326

BEUTLICH, LP.
1541 SHIELDS DRIVE
WAUKEGAN, IL 60085
800-238-8542

BIO-PHARM INC
10 H RUNWAY ROAD
LEVITTOWN, PA 19057
215-949-3711

BIO-TECH
P. O. BOX 1992
FAYETTEVILLE, AR 72702
800-345-1199

BIOCHEMICAL LABORATORIES, INC.
SEE ALSO A-A SPECTRUM
14422 S. SAN PEDRO STREET
GARDENA, CA 90248
800-772-8796

BIOCRAFT LABS, INC.
18-01 RIVER ROAD
FAIR LAWN, NJ 07410
201-703-0400

BIOMERICA, INC.
1533 MONROVIA AVENUE
NEWPORT BEACH, CA 92663
800-8543002

BIOPRACTIC GROUP II INC.
99 BROAD STREET
P.O. BOX 5300
PHILLIPSBURG, NJ 08865
908-859-4060

BLAINE CO., INC.
1465 JAMIKE LANE
ERLANGER, KY 41018
606-283-9437

BLAIR LABS., INC.
100 CONNECTICUT AVE.
NORWALK, CT 06856
203-853-0123

BLAIREX LABS., INC.
3240 NORTH INDIANAOPLIS ROAD
COLUMBUS, IN 47202
800-252-4739

BLANSETT PHARMACAL CO. INC.
3304 PIKE AVE.
NO. LITTLE ROCK, AR 72118
501-758-8635

BLISTEX, INC.
1800 SWIFT DRIVE
OAK BROOK, IL 60521
708-571-2870

BLOCK DRUG CO., INC.
257 CORNELISON AVE.
JERSEY CITY, NJ 07307
201-434-3000

BOCK PHARMACAL CO.
P.O.BOX 419056
ST. LOUIS, MO 63141-9056
800-727-2625

BOEHRINGER INGELHEIM PHARMACEUTICALS,INC.
900 RIDGEBURY ROAD
P. O. BOX 368
RIDGEFIELD, CT 06877-0368
203-798-9988

BOEHRINGER MANNHEIM DIAGNOSTICS
9115 HAGUE ROAD
P. O. BOX 50100
INDIANAPOLIS, IN 46250
800-428-5074

BOEHRINGER MANNHEIM PHARMACEUTICALS
15204 OMEGA DRIVE
ROCKVILLE, MD 20850-3241
301-216-3900

BOLAN PHARMACEUTICAL, INC.
SUITE A 204
BEDFORD AULESS ROAD
HURST, TX 76053
800-526-5369

BOOTS LABORATORIES, INC.
300 TRI-STATE INTERNATIONAL CTR.
SUITE 200
LINCOLNSHIRE, IL 60069-4415
800-323-1817

BOOTS PHARMACEUTICALS, INC.
300 TRI-STATE INTERNATIONAL CTR.
SUITE 200
LINCOLNSHIRE, IL 60069-4415
800-323-1817

BRACCO DIAGNOSTICS INC.
777 SCUDDERS MILL ROAD
PLAINSBORO, NJ 08536
800-631-5245

BRADLEY PHARMACEUTICALS, INC.
383 ROUTE 46, WEST
FAIRFIELD, NJ 07004-2402
201-882-1505

BRAINTREE LABORATORIES, INC.
60 COLUMBIAN STREET
P. O. BOX 361
BRAINTREE, MA 02184
617-843-2202

BREATHEASY CO.
2929 N. E. NORTHRUP WAY
P. O. BOX 1478
BELLEVUE, WA 98009
206-827-4694

BRECKENRIDGE PHARMACEUTICAL INC.
P.O. BOX 206
BOCA RATON, FL 33429
407-367-8512

BRENNER PHARMACAL CO.
3560 ARBORCREST COURT
CINCINNATI, OH 45236
513-793-7428

BRIOSCHI, INC.
19-01 POLLITT DRIVE
P. O. BOX 427
FAIR LAWN, NJ 07410
201-796-4226

BRISTOL LABORATORIES
A BRISTOL-MYERS SQUIBB CO.
P. O. BOX 4500
PRINCETON, NJ 08543-4500
800-631-5244

BRISTOL-MYERS ONCOLOGY DIV/HIV PRODUCTS
A BRISTOL-MYERS SQUIBB COMPANY
P. O. BOX 4500
PRINCETON, NJ 08543-4500
800 6315244

BRISTOL-MYERS PRODUCTS DIV. OF BRISTOL-MEYERS CO.
345 PARK AVENUE
NEW YORK, NY 10154
212-546-5000

BRITISH AMERICAN MEDICAL INC.
27111 ALISO CREEK RD #115
ALISO VIEJO, CA 92656-3366
800-866-1187

BTG PHARMACEUTICALS CORP C/O LIVINGSTON HEALTHCARE SVCS INC.
3195 LANIER PARKWAY
DECATUR, GA 30034
800-424-9639

BUFFINGTON DIVISION OTIS CLAPP & SON INC.
143 ALBANY ST.
CAMBRIDGE, MA 02139
617-821-5400

BURROUGHS WELLCOME CO.
3030 CORNWALLIS ROAD
RESEARCH TRIANGLE PA, NC 27709
800-722-9292

BYFIELD SNUFF CO.
44 MAIN ST.
BYFIELD, MA 01922
508-465-7531

C & M PHARMACAL, INC.
24047 DEQUINDRE
HAZEL PARK, MI 48030-1215
800-423-5173

C.R.C. UNIT FORMULAS, INC.
914 18TH STREET, N.W., SUITE 101
CANTON, OH 44703
216-452-0151

CAL-WHITE MINERAL COMPANY
P.O. BOX 7890
KLAMATH FALLS, OR 97602
503-884-0687

CALEB LABORATORIES, INC.
529 S. 7TH STREET
MINNEAPOLIS, MN 55415
612-338-8355

CALGON VESTAL LABORATORIES SUB. OF MERCK & CO., INC.
P. O. BOX 147
ST. LOUIS, MO 631660147
800-243-5799

CAMALL COMPANY
P.O. BOX 307
ROMEO, MI 48065
810-752-9683

CAMPBELL LABORATORIES, INC.
P.O. BOX 639 700
W HILLSBORO BVLD
DEERFIELD BEACH, FL 33443
800-458-2681

CAN-AM SURGICAL CORP.
3068 STONEWOOD STREET
SIMI VALLEY, CA 93063
800-328-3818

CARACO PHARMACEUTICAL LABS., LTD.
1150 ELIJAH MCCOY DRIVE
DETROIT, MI 48202
313-871-8400

CARE TECHNOLOGIES, INC.
55 HOLLY HILL LANE
GREENWICH, CT 06830
203-661-3161

CARE-TECH LABORATORIES DIV. CONSOLIDATED CHEMICAL INC.
3224 SO. KINGS HIGHWAY
ST. LOUIS, MO 631391183
800-325-9681

CAREMARK PRESCRIPTION SERVICE DIV BAXTER HEALTHCARE CORPORATION
111 BARCLAY BOULEVARD
LINCOLNSHIRE IL 60069
708-634-7900

CARLSON, J. R., LABS. INC.
15 COLLEGE DRIVE
ARLINGTON HEIGHTS, IL 60004-1985
800-323-4141

CARMA LABORATORIES, INC.
5801 W. AIRWAYS AVENUE
FRANKLIN, WI 53132
414-421-7707

CARNRICK LABORATORIES, INC.
65 HORSE HILL ROAD
CEDAR KNOLLS, NJ 07927
201-267-2670

CAROLINA MEDICAL PRODUCTS CO.
P. O. BOX 147
FARMVILLE. NC 27828
800-227-6637

CARRINGTON LABORATORIES, INC.
P. O. BOX 569500
DALLAS, TX 75356
800-527-5216

CARTER PRODUCTS DIVISION OF CARTER-WALLACE, INC.
P.O. BOX 1001,
HALF ACRE ROAD
CRANBURY, NJ 085120181
609-655-6000

CASCADE MEDICAL, INC.
10180 VIKING DRIVE
EDEN PRAIRIE, MN 55344
800-525-6718

CEMCO PHARMACAL INC.
6121 PEBBLE BEACH
MEMPHIS, TN 38115
901-363-8782

CENCI, H.R. LABS. INC.
P. O. BOX 12524
FRESNO, CA 937782524
800-232-3624

CENTER LABORATORIES, INC.
35 CHANNEL DRIVE
PORT WASHINGTON. NY 11050
800-223-6837

CENTRAL PHARMACEUTICALS, INC.
120 E. THIRD STREET
SEYMOUR, IN 47274
812-522-3915

CENTURY PHARMACEUTICALS, INC.
10377 HAGUE ROAD
INDIANAPOLIS, IN 46256
317-849-4210

CERENEX PHARMACEUTICALS
P. O. BOX 13438
RESEARCH TRIANGLE PK, NC 27709
919-248-2100

CETYLITE INDUSTRIES, INC.
9051 RIVER ROAD
P. O. BOX CN6
PENNSAUKEN, NJ 08110-3293
800-257-7740

CHALLENGE PRODUCTS INC.
LAKE ROAD 54-22
P. O. BOX 468
OSAGE BEACH, MO 65065
800-322-9800

CHASE LABORATORIES
280 CHESTNUT STREET
NEWARK, NJ 07105
201-465-7014

CHATTEM CONSUMER PRODUCTS
1715 W. 38TH STREET
CHATTANOOGA, TN 37409
800-366-6833

CHESEBROUGH-POND'S USA CO.
33 BENEDICT PLACE
P.O. BOX 6000
GREENWICH, CT 068366000
800-242-0203

CHESHIRE DRUGS
2280 CHESHIRE BRIDGE RD, NE
ATLANTA, GA 30324
404-634-7210

**CHEW-RITE COMPANY DIV. OF
MAGNESIA PRODUCTS INC.**
265 PIONEER BLVD.
SPRINGBORO, OH 45066
513-746-5509

CHILTON LABORATORIES, INC.
23 FAIRFIELD PLACE
WEST CALDWELL, NJ 07006
201-575-1990

CHIRON THERAPEUTICS
4560 HORTON STREET
EMERYVILLE, CA 94608-2916
800-244-7668

**CHREN LABORATORIES DIV. OF DYNA-
PEDIC COMPANY**
P. O. BOX 44
HOPKINS, MN 55343
612-935-3565

**CIBA CONSUMER PHARMACEUTICALS
DIV. CIBA-GEIGY CORP.**
MACK WOODBRIDGE II
581 MAIN ST.
WOODBRIDGE, NJ 07095
908-602-6600

**CIBA PHARMACEUTICAL COMPANY DIV.
CIBA-GEIGY CORP.**
556 MORRIS AVE.
SUMMIT, NJ 07901
908-277-5000

CIBA VISION CORPORATION
2910 AMWILER COURT
ATLANTA, GA 30360
404-418-3282

CIBA VISION OPHTHALMICS
P. O. BOX 100024
DULUTH, GA 30136-0024
800-845-6585

CINCINNATI PHARMACAL CO.
P.O. BOX 12885
CINCINNATI, OH 45212-0885
513-861-8340

CIRCA PHARMACEUTICALS, INC.
P.O. BOX 30
33 RALPH AVENUE
COPAIGUE, NY 117260030
516-842-8383

CIRCLE PHARMACEUTICALS, INC.
6320 RUCKER ROAD
INDIANAPOLIS, IN 46220
317-475-1921

CITY CHEMICAL CORP.
100 HOBOKEN AVENUE
JERSEY CITY, NJ 07310
201-653-6900

CLAY-PARK LABORATORIES, INC.
BATHGATE INDUSTRIAL PARK 1700
BATHGATE AVENUE
BRONX, NY 10457
800-933-5550

CLINIPAD CORP.
P. O. BOX 387 66
HIGH STREET
GUILFORD, CT 06437
800-243-6548

CLINT PHARMACEUTICALS, INC.
1451 ELM HILL PIKE - SUITE 252
NASHVILLE, TN 37210
615-366-0086

**CLINTEC NUTRITION CO., AFFIL OF
BAXTER HEALTHCARE CORP & NESTLE S A**
3 PARKWAY N., SUITE 500
BOX 760
DEERFIELD, IL 60015-0760
800-388-0300

CMC-CONSOLIDATED MIDLAND CORP
195 E. MAIN STREET
BREWSTER, NY 10509
914-2796-108

COLGATE ORAL PHARMACEUTICALS
1 COLGATE WAY
CANTON, MA 02021
800-2253756

COLOPLAST, INC.
5610 W. SLIGHT AVENUE SUITE 100-C
TAMPA, FL 33634-4468
800-237-4555

COLORADO CHEMICAL CO.
1 ANDERSON AVENUE
MOONACHIE, NJ 07074
201-460-7713

COLUMBIA DRUG CO., INC.
P. O. BOX 210515
COLUMBIA, SC 29221
803-356-2766

COLUMBIA LABORATORIES, INC.
4000 HOLLYWOOD BLVD., THIRD FLOOR
SOUTH HOLLYWOOD, FL 33021
305-964-6666

CONCORD SHEAR CORP.
38 LEUNING STREET
SO. HACKENSACK, NJ 07606
201-489-2400

**CONNAUGHT LABORATORIES, INC.
A PASTEUR MERIEUX COMPANY**

RT. 611. BOX 187
SWIFTWATER, PA 18370
800-822-2463

**CONVATEC
A BRISTOL-MYERS SQUIBB COMPANY**
P.O. BOX 5254
PRINCETON, NJ 08543-5254
800-422-8811

COOPER DRUG CO. INC.
1151 ALLEN DRIVE,
TROY, MI 48083
313-583-6300

COPLEY PHARMACEUTICAL, INC.
CANTON COMMERCE CENTER
25 JOHN ROAD
CANTON, MA 02021
617-821-6111

COWLEY, B. C.,
CO. 24 MAPLE CIRCLE
SHREWSBURY, MA 01545
508-845-8141

CRANDALL ASSOCIATE, INC.
32529 MOUND ROAD
WARREN, MI 48092
810-939-2310

CREIGHTON PRODUCTS CORPORATION
59 ROUTE 10, C.S. 1980
EAST HANOVER, NJ 07936
800-472-4467

**CREOMULSION/LANTISEPTIC DIV. SUM-
MIT INDUSTRIES, INC.**
P. O. BOX 7529
MARIETTA GA 30065
800-241-6996

CUMBERLAND-SWAN, INC.
ONE SWAN DRIVE
P. O. BOX 129
SMYRNA, TN 37167-0129
800-251-3068

CURATEK PHARMACEUTICALS, LTD.
1965 PRATT BOULEVARD
ELK GROVE, VILLAGE IL 60007
800-332-7680

CYCLIN PHARMACEUTICALS, INC.
429 GAMMON PLACE
P.O. BOX 9651
MADISON, WI 53715
800-558-7046

CYTOSOL LABORATORIES, INC.
55 MESSINA DRIVE
BRAINTREE, MA 02184
800-288-3858

D'FRANSSIA CORP.
4505 W. FIRST STREET
LOS ANGELES, CA 90004
213-461-3444

DAKRYON PHARMACEUTICALS
2579 SOUTH LOOP 289, SUITE 008
LUBBOCK, TX 79423
800-658-2024

DANIELS PHARMACEUTICALS, INC.
2517 25TH AVENUE, N.
ST. PETERSBURG, FL 33713-3999
800-237-7427

DARTMOUTH PHARMACEUTICALS, INC.
37 PINE HILL LANE
MARION, MA 02738-1149
508-748-3209

DAWN PHARMACEUTICALS
4555 WEST ADDISON
CHICAGO, IL 60641
800-745-3296

DAYTON LABORATORIES, INC.
3307 N.W. 74TH AVENUE
MIAMI, FL 33122
305-594-0988

DAYWELL LABORATORIES, CORP.
78 UNQUOWA PLACE
P. O. BOX 490
FAIRFIELD, CT 06430
800-243-4141

DE WITT USA, INC.
1604 STOCKTON STREET
JACKSONVILLE, FL 32236
800-735-0666

**DEL PHARMACEUTICALS, INC.
SUB. DEL LABORATORIES, INC.**
565 BROAD HOLLOW ROAD
FARMINGDALE, NY 11735
516-293-7070

DEL-RAY LAB., INC.
22- 20TH AVENUE, N.W.
BIRMINGHAM, AL 35215
205-853-8247

**DELASCO DERMATOLOGIC LAB
& SUPPLY INC.**
608 13TH AVENUE
COUNCIL BLUFFS, IA 51501
800-831-6273

**DELMONT LABORATORIES, INC.
IMMUNO THERAPEUTICS**
P. O. BOX 269
SWARTHMORE, PA 19081
800-562-5541

DENISON PHARMACEUTICALS, INC.
60 DUNNELL LANE
P. O. BOX 1305
PAWTUCKET, RI 02860
401-723-5500

**DENT, C. S., & CO.,
DIV. OF THE GRANDPA BRANDS**
317-321 E. 8TH STREET
CINCINNATI, OH 45202
513-241-1677

DENTAL CONCEPTS INC.
9 NORTH GOODWIN AVENUE
ELMSFORD, NY 10523
914-592-1860

DERMALAB, LTD.
3800 NORTH ACORN LANE
FRANKLIN PARK, IL 60131
800-545-4858

DERMASCIENCES, INC.
121 WEST GRACE STREET
OLD FORGE, PA 18518
717-457-1232

DERMATONE LABORATORIES, INC.
80 KING SPRING ROAD
P.O. BOX 3536
WINDSOR LOCKS, CT 06096
800-225-7546

DERMIK LABORATORIES, INC.
500 ARCOLA ROAD P.O. BOX 1200
COLLEGEVILLE, PA 1942-60107
800-727-6737

DERMOL PHARMACEUTICALS, INC.
3807 ROSWELL ROAD
MARIETTA, GA 30062
800-344-7779

DEWITT INTERNATIONAL CORP.
P. O. BOX 6827
GREENVILLE, SC 29606
800-962-8599

DEY LABORATORIES, INC.
2751 NAPA VALLEY CORP. DRIVE
NAPA, CA 94558
800-755-5560

DIANE PHARMACEUTICALS, LTD.
131 W. GLENVIEW COURT
MEQUON, WI 53092
414-241-9600

DIAPREX MARKETING INC.
P.O. BOX 3186
CARMEL, IN 46032
317-573-0161

DICKINSON, E. E., CO., THE
2 ENTERPRISE DRIVE
SHELTON, CT 06484
203-929-1197

DICKINSON, T. N., CO., THE
36-44 WEST POINT ROAD
P. O. BOX 319
EAST HAMPTON, CT 06424
203-267-2279

DISTA PROD. CO. DIV. ELI LILLY & CO.
LILLY CORPORATE CENTER
INDIANAPOLIS, IN 46285
317-276-4000

DIXON-SHANE INC.
256 GEIGER ROAD
PHILADELPHIA, PA 19115
800-262-7770

DOAK DERMATOLOGICS
383 ROUTE 46 WEST
FAIRFIELD, NJ 07004-2402
201-882-1505

DOLISOS AMERICA INC.
3014 RIGEL AVENUE
LAS VEGAS, NV 89102
800-365-4767

DOME INDUSTRIES, INC.
TEN NEW ENGLAND WAY
WARWICK, RI 02886
401-738-7900

DONELL, INC.
342 MADISON AVENUE SUITE 1422
NEW YORK, NY 10173
800-526-3461

DOVER PHARMACEUTICAL, INC.
P. O. BOX 809
ISLINGTON, MA 02090-9942
617-821-5400

DOW HICKAM PHARMACEUTICALS INC.
P. O. BOX 2006
SUGAR LAND, TX 77478
800-231-3052

DRUG GUILD DISTRIBUTORS, INC.
350 MEADOWLANDS PARKWAY
SECAUCUS, NJ 07096
201-348-3700

DSC LABORATORIES
1979 LATIMER DRIVE
MUSKEGON, MI 49442
616-777-3012

DU PONT MULTI-SOURCE PRODUCTS DIV. OF DU PONT PHARMA
1000 STEWART AVENUE
GARDEN CITY, NY 11530
800-462-3636

DU PONT PHARMACEUTICALS DIV. OF DU PONT PHARMA
BARLEY MILL PLAZA,
BOX 80026
WILMINGTON, DE 19880-0026
800-474-2762

DUNHALL PHARMACEUTICALS, INC.
HIGHWAY 59N
P. O. BOX 100
GRAVETTE, AR 72736
501-787-5232

DURA PHARMACEUTICALS, INC.
5880 PACIFIC CENTER BLVD.
SAN DIEGO, CA 92121
800-859-8586

DURAMED PHARMACEUTICALS, INC.
5040 LESTER ROAD
CINCINNATI, OH 45213
800-543-8338

DURHAM PHARMACAL CORP.
ROUTE 145
OAK HILL, NY 12460
518-239-4195

DYNAPHARM, INC.
P. O. BOX 2141
DEL MAR, CA 92014
619-453-5818

E.T. BROWNE DRUG COMPANY
140 SYLVAN AVENUE
P.O. BOX 1613
ENGLEWOOD CLIFFS, NJ 07632
201-947-3050

ECONOLAB
P. O. BOX 850543
WESTLAND, MI 48185-0543
303-532-4462

ECONOMED PHARMACEUTICALS, INC.
4305 SARTIN ROAD
BURLINGTON, NC 27217
800-327-6007

ECR PHARMACEUTICALS
3911 DEEP ROCK ROAD
RICHMOND, VA 23233
804-527-1950

EDWARDS PHARMACEUTICALS, INC.
111 MULBERRY STREET
RIPLEY, MS 38663
800-543-9560

EFFCON LABS
P.O BOX 7509
MARIETTA, GA 30065
800-722-2428

ELAN PHARMA
2 THURBER BOULEVARD
SMITHFIELD, RI 02917
401-233-3526

ELECTROLYTE LABORATORIES, INC.
6803 E. BUCKNELL PLACE
DENVER, CO 80224
303-757-8767

ELKINS-SINN, INC.
2 ESTERBROOK LANE
CHERRY HIL,L NJ 08034
800-257-8349

EMERSON LABORATORIES
1008 WHITAKER
P. O. BOX 1996
TEXARKANA, TX 75504
903-792-5848

ENDO LABORATORIES,
L.L.C. BARLEY MILL PLAZA
P. O. BOX 80390
WILMINGTON, DE 19880-0026
800-462-3636

ENERGY FACTORS INC.
10720 72ND STREET, NO. SUITE 305
LARGO, FL 34647
813-544-8866

ENZON, INC.
40 KINGSBRIDGE RD.
PISCATAWAY. NJ 08854
908-9804-500

EON LABS MANUFACTURING, INC.
227-15 NORTH CONDUIT AVE.
LAURELTON, NY 11413
800-526-0225

EQUIPHARM
P. O. BOX 8
POMONA, NY 10970
914-354-7077

ESCALON OPHTHALMICS, INC.
182 TAMARACK CIRCLE
SKILLMAN, NJ 08558
800-486-4848

ESI PHARMA, INC. DIVISION OF WYETH/AYERST
P.O. BOX 41502
PHILADELPHIA, PA 19101
800-964-6374

ETHEX CORPORATION
10888 METRO COURT
ST. LOUIS, MO 63043-2413
800-321-1705

ETHITEK PHARMACEUTICALS COMPANY
7701 N. HUSTIN AVENUE
SKOKIE. IL 60077
708-675-6611

EVER READY FIRST AID MEDICAL SUPPLY CORP.
5 E. 17TH STREET
NEW YORK, NY 10003
800-325-4655

EVEREADY DRUGS LTD. D/B/A PRESCRIPTIONS EXCLUSIVE
1229 THIRD AVENUE
NEW YORK, NY 10021
800-424-3378

EVERETT LABORATORIES, INC.
71 GLENWOOD PLACE
E. ORANGE, NJ 07017
201-674-8455

FAHRNEY, DR. PETER, & SONS CO.
3000 HEMPSTEAD TPKE.
LEVITTOWN, NY 11756
516-731-5380

FAMILY PHARMACY
P.O. BOX 1027
SOUTHEASTERN, PA 19398-1027
800-333-7347

FERNDALE LABORATORIES, INC.
780 W. EIGHT MILE ROAD
FERNDALE, MI 48220
810-548-0900

FERRING LABORATORIES
400 RELLA BLVD. SUITE 201
SUFFERN, NY 10901-4249
800-445-3690

FERRIS MFG. CORP.
16 WEST 300 83RD STREET
BURR RIDGE, IL 60521
708-887-9797

FIBERTONE
14851 NORTH SCOTSDALE ROAD
SCOTSDALE, AZ 85254
800-848-2633

FIELDING CO., THE
94 WELDON PARKWAY
ST. LOUIS. MO 63043
314-567-5462

FISCHER PHARMACEUTICALS, INC.
165 GIBRALTER COURT
SUNNYVALE, CA 94089
800-782-0222

FISONS PRESCRIPTION PRODUCTS FISONS PHARMACEUTICALS
P. O. BOX 1766
ROCHESTER, NY 14603-1766
800-334-6433

FLAHERTY, BRYAN J., CO., INC.
780 EAST 138TH STREET
BRONX, NY 10454
212 -993-2007

FLANDERS, INC.
P. O. BOX 391
43 NORTHBRIDGE STATION
CHARLESTON, SC 29407
803-571-3363

FLEET, C. B., CO., INC.
4615 MURRAY PLACE
LYNCHBURG, VA 24506
804-528-4000

FLEETWOOD CO., THE
1500 BROOK DRIVE
DOWNERS GROVE, IL 60515
708-495-9300

FLEMING & CO.
1600 FENPARK DRIVE
FENTON, MO 63026
314-343-8200

FLEMMING PHARMACEUTICALS, INC.
11 GREENWAY PLAZA, 11TH FLOOR
HOUSTON, TX 77046
713-621-1985

FLUORITAB CORP.
P. O. BOX 507
TEMPERANCE, MI 48182
313-847-3985

FOREST PHARMACEUTICALS, INC. SUB.
FOREST LABORATORIES, INC.
13622 LAKEFRONT DRIVE
ST. LOUIS, MO 63045
800-678-1605

FOUGERA E. & CO. DIV. ALTANA INC.
60 BAYLIS ROAD
MELVILLE, NY 11747
800-645-9833

FOX PHARMACAL, INC.
6420 NW 5TH WAY
FT. LAUDERDALE, FL 33310
305-772-7487

FREEDA VITAMINS, INC.
36 E. 41ST STREET
NEW YORK, NY 10017
212-685-4980

FRUIT OF THE EARTH, INC.
P. O. BOX 152044
IRVING, TX 750152044
800-527-7731

FUJISAWA USA INC
PARKWAY NORTH CENTER
3 PARKWAY NORTH
DEERFIELD, IL 60015-2548
800-888-7704

FUTURO CO., THE DIV. OF JUNG CORP.
5801 MARIEMONT AVE.
CINCINNATI, OH 45227
513-576-8000

G & W LABORATORIES, INC.
111 COOLIDGE STREET
SO. PLAINFIELD, NJ 07080
800-922-1038

GAINOR MEDICAL USA, INC.
P. O. BOX 93127
LONG BEACH, CA 90809-3127
800-825-8282

GALDERMA LABORATORIES, INC.
3000 ALTA MESA BLVD
P.O. BOX 331329
FT. WORTH, TX 76115
817-263-2600

GALLIPOT, INC.
2020 SILVER BELL ROAD
ST. PAUL, MN 55122
800-423-6967

GATE PHARMACEUTICALS
650 CATHILL ROAD
SELLERSVILLE, PA 18960
800-292-4283

GEBAUER COMPANY, INC.
9410 ST. CATHERINE AVENUE
CLEVELAND, OH 44104
800-321-9348

GEIGY PHARMACEUTICALS
DIV. CIBA-GEIGY CORP.
556 MORRIS AVENUE
SUMMIT, NJ 07901-1398
908-277-5000

GENDERM CORPORATION
600 KNIGHTSBRIDGE PKWY.
LINCOLNSHIRE, IL 60069
708-634-7373

GENENTECH, INC.
460 POINT SAN BRUNO BLVD.
SO. SAN FRANCISCO, CA 94080-4990
415-225-1000

GENERAL INJECTABLES & VACCINES, INC.
U. S. HIGHWAY 52
P. O. BOX 9
BASTIAN, VA 24314-0009
800-521-7468

GENESIS BIO-PHARMACEUTICALS. INC.
9 BRICK COURT
TENAFLY, NJ 07670
800-828-6941

GENETCO, INC.
711 UNION PARKWAY
RONKONKOMA, NY 11779
800-969-8007

GENEVA PHARMACEUTICALS, INC.
2555 W. MIDWAY BLVD.
P. O. BOX 446
BROOMFIELD, CO 80038-0446
800-525-8747

GENSIA LABORATORIES LTD.
11025 ROSELLE ST.
SAN DIEGO, CA 92121-1204
800-729-9991

GENZYME CORP.
ONE KENDALL SQUARE
CAMBRIDGE, MA 02139
800-332-1042

GERI-CARE PHARMACEUTICALS
840 MCDONALD AVENUE
BROOKLYN, NY 11218
718-382-5000

GERIATRIC PHARMACEUTICAL, CORP.
DIV. OF ROBERTS LABS
4 INDUSTRIAL WAY
WEST EATONTOWN, NJ 07724
908-389-1182

GERITREX CORPORATION
2 E. SANDFORD BLVD.
MOUNT VERNON, NY 10550
914-668-4003

GLADES PHARMACEUTICALS
255 ALHAMBRA CIRCLE, SUITE 1000
CORAL GABLES, FL 331347412
800-452-3371

GLASGOW PHARMACEUTICAL CORPORATION
890 NORTH L ROGERS WELLS BLVD
P. O. BOX 1209
GLASGOW, KY 42141
800-825-2369

GLAXO DERMATOLOGY
5 MOORE DRIVE
RESEARCH TRIANGLE PK, NC 27709
800-545-2965

GLAXO PHARMACEUTICALS
5 MOORE DRIVE
RESEARCH TRIANGLE PK, NC 27709
919-248-2100

GLENWOOD INC.
83 N. SUMMIT STREET
P. O. BOX
518 TENAFLY, NJ 07670
201-569-0050

**GLOBAL SOURCE MANAGEMENT & CON-
SULTING, INC.**
3001 NORTH 29TH STREET
HOLLYWOOD, FL 33020
305-921-0006

GM PHARMACEUTICALS
P. O. BOX 150312
ARLINGTON, TX 76015
800-866-7281

GOLDLINE LABORATORIES, INC.
1900 W. COMMERCIAL BLVD.
FT. LAUDERDALE, FL 33309
800-327-4114

GOOD SAMARITAN LABORATORIES, INC.
P. O. BOX 2138
DOYLESTOWN, PA 18901-0649
215-345-4106

GOODY'S PHARMACEUTICALS, INC.
436 SALT STREET
P. O. BOX 10518
WINSTON-SALEM, NC 27108-0518
800-322-6639

GORDON LABORATORIES
6801 LUDLOW STREET
UPPER DARBY, PA 19082
800-356-7870

GORDSHELL SALVE CO., THE
3927 FALLS ROAD
BALTIMORE, MD 21211
410-889-2960

GRACE, A. C., CO.
1100 QUITMAN ROAD
P.O. BOX 570
BIG SANDY, TX 75755
903-636-4368

GRAY PHARMACEUTICAL CO.
100 CONNECTICUT AVENUE
NORWALK, CT 06856
203-853-0123

GREAT SOUTHERN LABS
10863 ROCKLEY ROAD
HOUSTON, TX 77099
800-238-7511

GREENSTONE LIMITED
8225 MOORS BRIDGE ROAD
PORTAGE, MI 49002
800-447-3360

GREENTREE LABORATORIES
P. O. BOX 425
TUSTIN, CA 92680
714-546-9520

GRIFFITH, JIM, CO.
P. O. BOX 590036
SAN FRANCISCO, CA 94159
415-668-8586

GUARDIAN LABORATORIES
DIV. UNITED-GUARDIAN, INC.
P. O. BOX 2500
SMITHTOWN, NY 11787
800-645-5566

GYNOPHARMA, INC.
50 DIVISION STREET
SOMERVILLE, NJ 08876
800-322-4966

HALLMARK ORTHOPEDIC SPECIALTIES
20 LAPORTE STREET
P.O. BOX 661060
ARCADIA, CA 91006
800-446-8668

HALSEY PHARMACEUTICAL
1827 PACIFIC STREET
BROOKLYN, NY 11233-3599
800-237-9939

HAMILTON PHARMA, INC.
3401 HILLVIEW AVENUE
P.O. BOX 10850
PALO ALTO, CA 94303
800-472-4467

HARMONY LABORATORIES, INC.
P.O. BOX 39 1109
SOUTH MAIN STREET
LANDIS, NC 28023
704-857-0707

HART HEALTH AND SAFETY
P. O. BOX 94044
SEATTLE, WA 98124
800-234-4278

HAUSER, A. F., INC. PHARMACEUTICALS
4401 EAST US HIGHWAY 30
VALPARAISO, IN 46383-9573
219-464-2300

HEALTH & MEDICAL TECHNIQUES
400 RABRO DRIVE EAST
HAUPPAUGE, NY 11788
516-582-5900

HEALTH VITAMIN COMPANY, INC.
1060 NEPPERHAN AVENUE
YONKERS, NY 107031413
914-423-2900

HEPP INDUSTRIES
687 KILDARE CRESCENT
SEAFORD, NY 11783
516-796-1924

HERALD PHARMACAL INC.
6503 WARWICK ROAD
RICHMOND, VA 23225
800-253-9499

HERAN PHARMACEUTICAL, INC
7215 ECKHERT ROAD
SAN ANTONIO, TX 78238
210-680-2969

HERMAL PHARMACEUTICAL LABS., INC.
163 DELAWARE AVENUE
DELMAR, NY 12054
800-437-6251

HERMELL PRODS. INC.
23 BRITTON DRIVE
BLOOMFIELD, CT 06002
800-233-2342

HEXOL, INC.
1500 17TH STREET
SAN FRANCISCO, CA 94107
416-621-2562

HI-TECH PHARMACAL COMPANY, INC.
369 BAYVIEW AVENUE
AMITYVILLE, NY 11701
516-789-8228

HIGH CHEMICAL COMPANY
3901A NEBRASKA STREET
LEVITTOWN, PA 19056
800-447-8792

HILL DERMACEUTICALS INC.
P. O. BOX 149283
ORLANDO, FL 32814
407-896-8280

HILLMAN PHARMACEUTICAL CO.
P. O. BOX 30093
SANTA BARBARA, CA 93130
805-687-2585

HIRSCH INDUSTRIES, INC.
4912 W. BROAD STREET, SUITE 201
RICHMOND, VA 23230
804-355-4500

HOBART LABORATORIES, INC.
2226 W. WABANSIA AVENUE
CHICAGO, IL 60647
312-235-4000

HOECHST-ROUSSEL DERMATOLOGICAL
P. O. BOX 2500
SOMERVILLE, NJ 08876-1258
908-231-2000

HOECHST-ROUSSEL PHARMACEUTICALS INC.
ROUTE 202-206
P.O. BOX 2500
SOMERVILLE, NJ 08876-1258
908-231-2000

HOLLISTER INCORPORATED
2000 HOLLISTER DRIVE
LIBERTYVILLE, IL 60048
708-680-1000

HOME DIAGNOSTICS, INC.
51 JAMES WAY
EATONTOWN, NJ 07724
800-342-7226

HOME HEALTH PRODUCTS, INC.
P.O. BOX 3130
VIRGINIA BEACH, VA 23454
800-468-7313

HOPE PHARMACEUTICALS
2961 W. MAC ARTHUR BLVD, STE.130
SANTA ANA, CA 92704
714-556-4673

HORIZON PHARMACEUTICAL CORPORATION
POST OFFICE BOX 486
ROSWELL, GA 30077-0486
404-442-9707

HORIZON PHARMACEUTICALS, INC.
1833-W PLANTSIDE DRIVE
LOUISVILLE, KY 40299
502-495-0142

HORIZON PRODUCTS COMPANY
2339 MOUNT ROYAL DRIVE
CASTLE ROCK, CO 80104
303-688-9694

HORUS THERAPEUTICS, INC.
2320 BRIGHTON-HENRIETTA TOWN LINE
ROCHESTER, NY 14623
716-292-4820

HOUSE OF SCHOMBURG
2021 N. SHERMAN STREET
FT. WAYNE, IN 46808
219-426-7487

HTD PHARMACEUTICAL
(DIV. OF HTD MEDICAL)
1904 WINEWOOD ROAD
BIRMINGHAM, AL 35215
205-856-1291

HUCKABY PHARMACAL, INC.
104 EAST MAIN
LA GRANGE, KY 40031
502-222-4700

HUDSON CORPORATION
90 ORVILLE DRIVE
BOHEMIA, NY 11716
516-567-9500

HUFFMAN LABORATORIES
77350-7356 PHARMED WAY N.W.
35TH TERRACE
MIAMI, FL 33122
800-683-7342

HUMCO LABORATORIES
1008 WHITAKER STREET
P. O. DRAWER 2550
TEXARKANA, TX 75501
903-793-3174

HUMPHREYS PHARMACAL, INC.
63 MEADOW ROAD
RUTHERFORD, NJ 07070
201-933-7744

HYREX PHARMACEUTICALS
3494 DEMOCRAT ROAD
P. O. BOX 18385
MEMPHIS, TN 38118
901-794-9050

ICN PHARMACEUTICALS, INC.
ICN PLAZA
3300 HYLAND AVE.
COSTA MESA, CA 92626
800-548-5100

IMMUNEX CORPORATION
51 UNIVERSITY STREET
SEATTLE, WA 98101
206-587-0430

IMMUNO-U.S., INC.
MARKETING & SALES DIV.
1200 PARKDALE ROAD
ROCHESTER, MI 483071744
810-652-7872

INLAND ALKALOID CO.
4200 LACLEDE ST.
ST. LOUIS, MO 63108
314-533-9600

INNO VISIONS, INC.
4889 SINCLAIR ROAD, SUITE 201
COLUMBUS, OH 43229
800-525-1908

INSOURCE WILLIAMS
P.O. BOX 39
BLAND, VA 24315-0039
800-366-3829

INTEGRA CHEMICAL COMPANY
710 THOMAS AVENUE, S.W.
RENTON, WA 98055
800-322-6646

INTERNATIONAL ETHICAL LABS.
AVENUE AMERICO MIRANDA #1021
REPTO. METROPOLITANO
SAN JUAN, PR 00921
809-765-3510

INTERNATIONAL LABORATORIES
901 SAWYER ROAD
MARIETTA, GA 30062
404-578-9000

INTERNATIONAL MEDICATION SYSTEMS LTD.
1886 SANTA ANITA AVE.
SO. EL MONTE, CA 91733
800-423-4136

INTERNATIONAL TECHNIDYNE CORP.
23 NEVSKY STREET
EDISON, NJ 08820
800-631-5945

INTERNATIONAL YOGURT CO.
628 N. DOHENY DRIVE
LOS ANGELES, CA 90069
800-962-7326

INTERPHARM INC.
3 FAIRCHILD AVENUE
PLAINVIEW, NY 11803
516-349-1730

INTERSTATE DRUG EXCHANGE INC.
1500 NEW HORIZONS BLVD.
AMITYVILLE, NY 11701-1130
516-957-8300

INVAMED, INC.
12 DWIGHT PLACE
FAIRFIELD, NJ 07004
201-575-3303

INWOOD LABORATORIES, INC.
300 PROSPECT STREET
INWOOD, NY 11696
800-876-5227

IOLAB PHARMACEUTICALS
500 IOLAB DRIVE
CLAREMONT, CA 91711
800-443-6440

ION LABORATORIES, INC.
7431 PEBBLE DRIVE
FT. WORTH, TX 76118
817-589-7257

IPR PHARMACEUTICALS
P. O. BOX 6000
CAROLINA, PR 00984
800-472-4467

IVO OF CALIFORNIA
8533 S. SERENATA DRIVE
P. O. BOX 1936
WHITTIER, CA 90609
310-947-4100

IVY CORPORATION
23 FAIRFIELD PLACE
W. CALDWELL, NJ 07006
201-575-1990

JACOBUS PHARMACEUTICAL
COMPANY, INC.
37 CLEVELAND LANE
P. O. BOX 5290
PRINCETON, NJ 08540
609-921-7447

JAMOL LABORATORIES, INC.
13 ACKERMAN AVENUE
EMERSON, NJ 07630
201-262-6363

JANSSEN PHARMACEUTICALS
1125 TRENTON-HARBOURTON RD
P.O. BOX 200
TITUSVILLE, NJ 08560-0200
609-730-2000

JEROME STEVENS PHARMACEUTICALS, INC.
60 DA VINCI DRIVE
BOHEMIA, NY 11716
800-635-3359

JMI PHARMACEUTICAL DIVISION
P. O. BOX 46903
ST. LOUIS, MO 63146
314-432-7557

JOHNSON & JOHNSON CONSUMER
PRODUCTS INC.
410 GEORGE STREET
NEW BRUNSWICK, NJ 08901-2023
908-524-0400

JOHNSON & JOHNSON MEDICAL, INC.
2500 ARBROOK BOULEVARD
P.O. BOX 130
ARLINGTON, TX 76004
800-433-5170

JOHNSON & JOHNSON/MERCK
CAMP HILL ROAD
FORT WASHINGTON, PA 19034
215-233-7654

JOHNSON LABORATORIES
P.O. BOX 2184
EDEN, NC 27289

JONES MEDICAL INDUSTRIES, INC.
P. O. BOX 46903
ST. LOUIS, MO 63146
800-525-8466

JONES MEDICAL-WESTERN RESEARCH
P. O. BOX 46903
ST. LOUIS, MO 63146
314-432-7530

KEENE PHARMACEUTICALS, INC.
333 S. MOCKINGBIRD
P.O. BOX 7
KEENE, TX 76059
800-541-0530

KENDALL COMPANY
15 HAMPSHIRE STREET
MANSFIELD, MA 02048
800-962-988

KENDALL-FUTURO COMPANY
5405 DUPONT CIRCLE SUITE A
MILFORD, OH 45150
800-933-0210

KENWOOD LABORATORIES, INC. DIV. OF
BRADLEY PHARM. INC.
383 ROUTE 46 WEST
FAIRFIELD, NJ 07004-2402
201-882-1505

KENYON DRUG CO., INC.
207 2ND AVENUE S.W.
P.O. BOX 1546
CEDAR RAPIDS, IA 52406
800-553-7907

KERR, FRANK W., CHEMICAL COMPANY
43155 W. NINE MILE ROAD
NOVI, MI 48376-8026
810-349-5510

KEY PHARMACEUTICALS, INC.
2000 GALLOPING HILL ROAD
KENILWORTH, NJ 07033-0530
800-222-7579

KING PHARMACEUTICALS, INC.
501 FIFTH STREET
BRISTOL, TN 37620
800-336-7783

KINGSWOOD LABORATORIES, INC.
10375 HAGUE ROAD
INDIANAPOLIS, IN 46256
317-849-9513

KIRKMAN LABORATORIES, INC.
P. O. BOX 3929
PORTLAND, OR 97208
503-245-4551

KLI CORP
1119 THIRD AVENUE S.W.
P.O. BOX 567
CARMEL, IN 46032
317-846-7452

KNIGHT INDUSTRIES, INC.
750 EAST SAMPLE ROAD
POMPANO, BEACH FL 33064
305-942-8708

KNOLL PHARMACEUTICAL COMPANY
30 NORTH JEFFERSON ROAD
WHIPPANY, NJ 07981
201-887-8300

KONSYL PHARMACEUTICALS, INC.
4200 S. HULEN STREET
FORT WORTH, TX 76109
800-356-6795

KRAMER DISTRIBUTORS
P.O. BOX 191775
SAN JUAN, PR 00919
809-767-2072

KRAMER LABORATORIES, INC.
8778 S.W. 8TH STREET
MIAMI, FL 33174-9990
800-824-4894

LA HAYE LABORATORIES
2205 152ND AVENUE N.E.
REDMOND, WA 98052
800-344-2020

LAKE MEDICAL PRODUCTS
11445 MOOG DRIVE
ST. LOUIS, MO 63146
314-872-2973

LAKE PHARMACEUTICAL
625 FOREST EDGE DRIVE
THE CORPORATE WOODS
VERNON HILLS, IL 60061
708-793-0230

LANNETT CO. INC., THE
9000 STATE ROAD
PHILADELPHIA, PA 19136
215-333-9000

LANSINOH LABORATORIES
1670 OAK RIDGE TURNPIKE
OAK RIDGE, TN 37830
800-292-4794

LARKOTEX CO., THE
1002 OLIVE STREET
P. O. BOX 449
TEXARKANA, TX 75501
800-972-3037

LARKSPUR GROUP, INC., THE
19 CONCORD STREET
S. NORWALK, CT 06854
203-853-7856

LASER, INC.
2200 WEST 97TH PLACE
P. O. BOX 905
CROWN POINT, IN 46307
219-663-1165

LAST, ALVIN, INC.
19 BABCOCK PLACE
YONKERS, NY 10701
914-376-1000

LAVOPTIK CO., INC.
661 WESTERN AVENUE N.
ST. PAUL, MN 55103
612-489-1351

LEDERLE LABS DIV.
AMERICAN CYANAMID CO.
ONE CYANAMID PLAZA
WAYNE, NJ 074708426
800-533-3753

LEDERLE STANDARD PRODUCTS DIV.
AMERICAN CYANAMID CO.
ONE CYANAMID PLAZA
WAYNE, NJ 07470
201-831-2000

LEE PHARMACEUTICALS
1444 SANTA ANITA AVENUE
SOUTH EL MONTE, CA 91733-3312
800-950-5337

LEGERE PHARMACEUTICALS, INC.
7326 EAST EVANS ROAD
SCOTTSDALE, AZ 85260
800-528-3144

LEHN & FINK CONSUMER PRODUCTS
DIV. STERLING DRUG INC.
225 SUMMIT AVENUE
MONTVALE, NJ 07645
201-573-5300

LEMAX PHARMACEUTICAL CORP.
6915 S.W. 92 CT.
MIAMI, FL 33173
305-598-2333

LEMMON COMPANY
1510 DELP DR.
P.O. BOX 904
KULPSVILLE, PA 19443
215-256-8400

LEPAGE'S, INC.
P. O. BOX 111303
PITTSBURGH, PA 15238
800-628-5702

LETTEAU, FRANK & ASSOC., LTD.
22 WEST 32ND STREET 10TH FLOOR
NEW YORK, NY 10001
212-268-3400

LEX PHARMACEUTICAL MFG. & PKGING.
7155 N. W. 77TH TERRACE
MEDLEY, FL 33166
305-888-7375

LEXIS PHARMACEUTICALS, INC.
P.O. BOX 202887
AUSTIN, TX 78720
512-328-8484

LIBBY LABORATORIES, INC.
1700 SIXTH STREET
BERKLEY, CA 94710
510-527-5400

LIDE LABORATORIES, INC.
15422 COUSTEAU
FLORISSANT, MO 63034
314-831-2933

LIFESCAN, INC.
1000 GIBRALTAR DRIVE
MILPITAS, CA 95035-6312
800-227-8862

LILLY, ELI & CO.
LILLY CORPORATE CENTER
INDIANAPOLIS, IN 46285
800-545-5979

LIQUIPHARM, INC.
10716 MC CUNE AVENUE
LOS ANGELES, CA 90034
310-558-3344

LMA, LTD.
3 DUKE PLACE
SO. NORWALK, CT 06854
203-852-0807

LOBOB LABORATORIES
1440 ATTEBERRY LANE
SAN JOSE, CA 95131
800-835-6262

LOGEN PHARMACEUTICAL, INC.
60 PIERCES ROAD
NEWBURGH, NY 12550
800-252-8890

LONGS DRUG STORES, INC.
141 NORTH CIVIC DRIVE
P.O. BOX 5222
WALNUT CREEK, CA 94596-9878
510-937-1170

LONGSTREET PHARMACAL CORP.
1224 FIFTIETH STREET
BROOKLYN, NY 11219
800-633-7878

LORVIC CORP., THE
8810 FROST AVENUE
ST. LOUI,S MO 63134
314-524-7444

LOTUS BIOCHEMICAL CORPORATION
7335 LEE HIGHWAY
P.O. BOX 3587
RADFORD, VA 24143
800-355-6556

LUMISCOPE CO., INC.
400 RARITAN CENTER PKWY.
EDISON, NJ 08837
800-422-5864

LUNSCO, INC.
ROUTE 2
P. O. BOX 62
PULASKI, VA 24301
800-624-8614

LUYTIES PHARMACAL CO.
4200 LACLEDE AVE.
ST. LOUIS, MO 63108
314-533-9600

LYNE LABORATORIES
260 TOSCA DRIVE
STOUGHTON, MA 02072
617-344-4676

MAJOR PHARMACEUTICAL CORP.
1640 WEST FULTON STREET
CHICAGO, IL 60612
800-688-9696

MALLARD PHARMACEUTICALS
6 INDUSTRIAL WAY WEST
EATONTOWN, NJ 07724
800-442-5532

MALLINCKRODT CHEMICAL, INC.
PERFORMANCE & LABORATORY
CHEM. DIV.
16305 SWINGLEY RIDGE DRIVE
CHESTERFIELD, MO 63017-1777
314-530-2000

MALLINCKRODT MEDICAL INC.
675 MCDONNELL BLVD.
P. O. BOX 5840
ST. LOUIS, MO 63134
314-895-2000

MALLINCKRODT SPECIALTY CHEMICAL
CO. PHARMACEUTICAL SPECIALTIES
GROUP
16305 SWINGLEY RIDGE DRIVE
CHESTERFIELD, MO 63017
314-530-2000

MANN CHEMICAL CORP.
520 W. MAIN STREET
LOUISVILLE, KY 40202
502-585-2001

MANNE, KENNETH A., CO.
P.O. BOX 825
JOHNS ISLAND, SC 29457
800-517-0228

MANUFACTURING CHEMISTS INC.
5767 THUNDERBIRD RD
INDIANAPOLIS, IN 46236
317-823-6878

MARIN PHARMACEUTICAL
P. O. BOX 174
MIAMI, FL 33144
305-593-5333

MARION MERRELL DOW INC.
9300 WARD PARKWAY
P. O. BOX 8480
KANSAS CITY, MO 64114-0480
816-966-4000

MARLEN MFG. & DEVELOP. CO.
5150 RICHMOND ROAD
BEDFORD, OH 44146
216-292-7060

MARLEX PHARMACEUTICALS
875 PULASKI HIGHWAY
BEAR, DE 19701
302-328-3355

MARLOP PHARMACEUTICAL, INC.
5704 MOSHOLU AVENUE
P. O. BOX 536
BRONX, NY 10471
800-345-7192

MARLYN CO., INC.
14851 N. SCOTTSDALE ROAD
SCOTTSDALE, AZ 85254
800-462-7596

MARNEL PHARMACEUTICALS, INC.
206 LUKE DRIVE
LAFAYETTE, LA 70506
318-232-1396

MARSAM PHARMACEUTICALS
BUILDING 31, OLNEY AVE.
P. O. BOX 1022
CHERRY HILL. NJ 08034
609-424-5600

MARSHALLAN PRODUCTS, INC.
1971 WEST 85TH STREET
CLEVELAND, OH 44102
216-631-2400

MARTEC PHARMACEUTICAL, INC.
1800 N. TOPPING
P. O. BOX 33510
KANSAS CITY, MO 64120-3510
800-822-6782

MAS LABORATORIES, INC.
50 LAKE DRIVE
EAST WINDSOR, NJ 08520
609-443-4402

MASON DISTRIBUTORS, INC.
5105 N.W. 159TH STREET
HIALEAH, FL 33014
800-327-6005

MASON PHARMACEUTICALS, INC.
4425 JAMBORE SUITE 250
NEWPORT BEACH, CA 92660
714-851-6860

MAXIM CHEMICALS, LTD.
116 BELLINGHAM STREET
CHELSEA, MA 02150
617-884-2824

MAYER LABORATORIES
231 FALLON STREET
OAKLAND, CA 94607
510-452-5555

MAYRAND PHARMACEUTICALS
P.O. BOX 10518
WINSTON-SALEM, NC 27108
800-334-0514

MCCOY'S PRODUCTS, INC.
1075 CENTRAL PARK AVENUE
SCARSDALE, NY 10583
914-472-2737

MCGAW INC.
P. O. BOX 19791
IRVINE, CA 92713-9791
714-660-2000

MCGREGOR PHARMACEUTICALS
8420 ULMERTON ROAD SUITE 408
LARGO, FL 34641
813-530-4361

MCGUFF CO.
3617 W. MAC ARTHUR BLVD. SUITE 507
SANTA ANA, CA 92704
800-854-7220

MCKEON PRODUCTS CO.
P. O. BOX 69009
PLEASANT RIDGE, MI 48069
313-548-7560

MCKESSON DRUG COMPANY
ONE POST STREET, 12TH FL.
SAN FRANCISCO, CA 94104-5296
415-983-8300

MCLEAN, DR., J. H., MEDICINE CO.
3000 HEMPSTEAD TURNPIKE
LEVITTOWN, NY 11756
516-731-5380

MCNEIL CONSUMER PRODUCTS CO.
CAMP HILL ROAD
FORT WASHINGTON, PA 19034
800-225-8263

MCNEIL INSTITUTIONAL PRODUCTS
WELCH & MC KEAN ROAD
SPRING HOUSE, PA 19477
215-628-5090

MCNEIL PHARMACEUTICAL
1000 U.S. HIGHWAY ROUTE 202
P.O. BOX 300
RARITAN, NJ 08869-0602
908-218-6000

MCNEIL, R.A., CO.
1210 E. DALLAS ROAD
CHATTANOOGA, TN 37405
615-265-8240

MCR/AMERICAN PHARMACEUTICALS, INC.
120 SUMMIT PARKWAY, #101
BIRMINGHAM, AL 35209
205-942-6415

MD PHARMACEUTCAL INC.
3501 W. GARRY AVENUE
SANTA ANA, CA 92704
800-854-6161

ME PHARMACEUTICALS DIV. OF VESCO, INC.
2200 S.E. PKWY.,
BOX 565
RICHMOND. IN 47375
317-962-4410

**MEAD JOHNSON LABORATORIES
BRISTOL-MYERS SQUIBB COMPANY**
P. O. BOX 4500
PRINCETON, NJ 085434500
800-631-5244

**MEAD JOHNSON NUTRITIONALS
DIV. MEAD JOHNSON & CO.**
2400 W. LLOYD EXPRESSWAY
EVANSVILLE, IN 477210001
800-457-3550

**MEAD JOHNSON PHARMACEUTICALS
DIV. MEAD JOHNSON & CO.**
P. O. BOX 4500
PRINCETON, NJ 08543-4500
800-631-5244

MED-DERM PHARMACEUTICALS, INC.
P. O. BOX 5193
KINGSPORT, TN 37663
800-334-4286

MED-PRO, INC.
210 EAST FOURTH ST.
LEXINGTON, NE 68850
800-447-6060

**MED-TEK PHARMACEUTICALS OF
AMERICA, INC.**
721 CHANEY COVE
COLLIERVILLE, TN 38017
901-853-5333

MEDCHEM PRODUCTS, INC.
232 WEST CUMMINGS PARK
WOBURN, MA 01801
617-938-9328

MEDCO LAB INC.
P. O. BOX 864
SIOUX CITY, IA 51102
712-255-8770

MEDI-JECT CORPORATION
1840 BERKSHIRE LANE
MINNEAPOLIS, MN 55441
800-328-3074

MEDICAL PRODUCTS PANAMERICANA INC.
P. O. BOX 771
CORAL GABLES, FL 33134
305-545-6524

**MEDICIS DERMATOLOGICS, INC.
MEDICIS PHARMACEUTICAL CORP.**
100 E. 42ND ST, 15TH FL.
NEW YORK, NY 10017
212-599-2000

MEDICRAT, INC.
287 EAST SIXTH STREET
ST. PAUL, MN 55101
612-291-7909

MEDIMMUNE, INC.
35 WEST WATKINS MILL ROAD
GAITHERSBURG, MD 20878
301-417-0770

MEDIQUE PRODUCTS
7855 GROSS POINT ROAD
SKOKIE, IL 60077
800-634-7680

MEDIREX, INC.
20 CHAPIN ROAD,
UNIT H P. O.
BOX 731
PINE BROOK, NJ 07058
800-343-3848

MEDISENSE, INC.
266 SECOND AVENUE
WALTHAM, MA 02154
800-527-3339

MEDTECH LABORATORIES, INC.
P. O. BOX 1108
JACKSON, WY 83001
800-443-4908

**MEDTRONIC, INC. NEUROLOGICAL
DIVISION**
800 53RD AVENUE NE
MINNEAPOLIS, MN 55421
800-328-0810

**MELVILLE BIOLOGICS
DIV. OF N.Y. BLOOD CTR.,INC.**
155 DURYEA ROAD
MELVILLE, NY 11747
516-752-7360

MENLEY & JAMES LABORATORIES, INC.
COMMONWEALTH CORP. CENTER
100 TOURNAMENT DRIVE
HORSHAM, PA 19044
800-523-1910

MENTHOLATUM CO., THE
1360 NIAGARA STREET
BUFFALO, NY 14213
716-882-7660

MENTOR CORP.
600 PINE AVENUE
GOLETA, CA 93117
800-338-7908

**MERCK & CO., INC.
HUMAN HEALTH DIVISION**
SUMNEYTOWN PIKE
WEST POINT, PA 19486
215-652-5000

MERICON INDUSTRIES
8819 N. PIONEER ROAD
PEORIA, IL 61615
309-693-2150

MERIT PHARMACEUTICALS
2611 SAN FERNANDO ROAD
LOS ANGELES, CA 90065
213-227-4831

MERRICK MEDICINE CO., INC.
P. O. BOX 1489
WACO, TX 76703
817-753-3461

MGI PHARMA
SUITE 300E,
OPUS CENTER
9900 BREN ROAD
EAST MINNEAPOLIS, MN 55343-9667
800-562-5580

MIKART, INC.
2090 MARIETTA BOULEVARD, N.W.
ATLANTA, GA 30318
404-351-4510

MILANCE LABORATORIES, INC.
P. O. BOX 368
MILLINGTON, NJ 07946
908-580-1591

MILES ALLERGY DIV. OF MILES, INC.
P.O. BOX 3145
SPOKANE, WA 99220
800-992-1120

**MILES BIOLOGICAL PRODUCTS
DIV. OF MILES, INC.**
400 MORGAN LANE
WEST HAVEN, CT 065164175
800-468-0894

**MILES CONSUMER HEALTHCARE
DIV. OF MILES, INC.**
1127 MYRTLE STREET
ELKHART, IN 46514
219-262-6722

**MILES DIAGNOSTICS
DIV. OF MILES, INC.**
1127 MYRTLE STREET
ELKHART, IN 46515
800-248-2637

**MILES PHARMACEUTICALS
DIV. OF MILES, INC.**
400 MORGAN LANE
WEST HAVEN, CT 06516-4175
800-468-0894

MILEX PRODUCTS, INC.
5915 NORTHWEST HIGHWAY
CHICAGO, IL 60631
800-621-1278

MILLER PHARMACAL GROUP INC.
4563 PRIME PARKWAY DR.
P.O. BOX 1297
MCHENRY, IL 60050-1297
800-323-2935

MILLERS FORGE INC.
1411 CAPITAL AVENUE
PLANO, TX 75074
800-527-3474

MILLGOOD LABORATORIES, INC.
250 D ARIZONA AVENUE
P. O. BOX 170159
ATLANTA, GA 30317
404-377-6538

MISEMER PHARMACEUTICALS, INC.
4553 S. CAMPBELL
SPRINGFIELD, MO 65807
417-881-0660

MISSION PHARMACAL CO.
1325 E. DURANGO STREET
P. O. BOX 1676
SAN ANTONIO, TX 78296
800-531-3333

MITCHELL, F.A., CO. INC.
15 CHURCHILL TERRACE
NEWTONVILLE, MA 02160
617-244-1523

MODERN AIDS, INC.
201 BOND STREET
ELK GROVE VILLAGE, IL 60007
312-437-8600

MODERN OFFICE DEVICES, INC.
731 HEMPSTEAD TPKE.
FRANKLIN SQ, NY 11010
516-483-9410

MODERN PRODUCTS, INC.
3015 W. VERA AVENUE
MILWAUKEE, WI 53209
800-543-8076

MONTICELLO DRUG CO.
1604 STOCKTON STREET
P.O. BOX 61749
JACKSONVILLE, FL 32236
800-735-0666

MOORE, H.L. DRUG EXCHANGE INC.
389 JOHN DOWNEY DRIVE
P.O. BOX 1500
NEW BRITAIN, CT 06050
800-444-8765

MORGAN, FRANK E. & SONS, INC.
AT STRAWBRIDGES, 4TH FLR.
PHILADELPHIA, PA 19107
215-563-1811

MORTON PHARMACEUTICALS, INC
1625 N. HIGHLAND STREET
MEMPHIS, TN 38018
901-386-8840

MOVA PHARMACEUTICAL CORPORATION
P.O. BOX 8639
CAGUAS, PR 00626
800-468-5201

MOYCO INDUSTRIES, INC.
21ST & CLEARFIELD
PHILADELPHIA, PA 19132
800-523-3676

MURA REMEDIES INC.
94 NASSAU AVE.
BROOKLYN, NY 11222
718-383-0236

MURO PHARMACEUTICAL, INC.
890 EAST STREET
TEWKSBURY, MA 01876-1496
800-225-0974

**MUTUAL PHARMACEUTICAL
COMPANY, INC.**
1100 ORTHODOX STREET
PHILADELPHIA, PA 19124
215-288-6500

MYLAN PHARMACEUTICALS, INC.
781 CHESTNUT RIDGE ROAD
P.O. BOX 4310
MORGANTOWN, WV 26505-4310
800-796-9526

**NABI (NORTH AMERICAN
BIOLOGICALS, INC.)**
16500 NW 15TH AVE
MIAMI, FL 33169
800-458-4244

NARD LABORATORIES, INC.
P.O. BOX 3514
BOARDMAN, OH 44512
216-726-9623

NATIONAL AEROSOL LABORATORIES
340 W. IVY LANE
ENGLEWOOD, NJ 07631
201-569-7878

NATIONAL MEDICAL SEMINARS, INC.
1224 COLOMA WAY
ROSEVILLE, CA 95661-4602
916-784-6200

NATIONAL VITAMIN COMPANY, INC.
2075 WEST SCRANTON AVENUE
PORTERVILLE, CA 93257-8358
800-538-5828

NATREN
3105 WILLOW LANE
WESTLAKE VILLAGE, CA 91361
800-992-3323

**NATURAL NUTRITIONALS CO. DIV.
AMERICAN PHARMACEUTICAL CO.**
245 FOURTH ST.,
BOX 448
PASSAIC, NJ 07055
201-779-5300

NATURE DISTRIBUTORS
P.O. BOX 11423
ATLANTA, GA 30310
404-755-4178

NATURE MADE VITAMINS
15451 SAN FERNANDO MISSION BLVD.
MISSION HILLS, CA 91345
800-423-2405

NATURE'S BOUNTY, INC.
90 ORVILLE DRIVE
BOHEMIA, NY 11716
800-645-5412

NCI MEDICAL FOODS
5801 AYALA AVENUE
IRWINDALE, CA 91706
818-815-3393

NELKIN
400 RARITAN CENTER PARKWAY
EDISON, NJ 08837-3908
908-225-5533

NEPHRO-TECH, INC.
P.O. BOX 14703
LENAXA, KS 66285
800-879-4755

NEPHRON PHARMACEUTICAL CORP.
4121 34TH STREET
ORLANDO, FL 32811-6458
800-443-4313

NEUE COSMETIC COMPANY, INC.
711 SOUTH MAIN STREET
BURBANK, CA 91506
800-832-8311

NEUE MEDICAL PRODUCTS
711 SOUTH MAIN STREET
BURBANK, CA 91506
800-832-8311

NEUROVITES, INC. C/O FLANDERS PHCY.
2330 N.W. FLANDERS
PORTLAND, OR 97210
503-228-4119

NEUTROGENA CORP.
5760 W. 96TH STREET
LOS ANGELES, CA 90045
310-642-1150

NEW LIFE HEALTH PRODUCTS CORP
P O BOX 9157
MORRIS PLAINS, NJ 07950-9157
201-989-7500

NEW WORLD TRADING CORP., THE
P.O. BOX 952
DE BARY, FL 32713
407-668-7520

NEWTON INDUSTRIES
1 HICKS AVENUE
NEWTON, NJ 07860
201-383-2332

NICHE PHARMACEUTICALS, INC.
300 TROPHY CLUB DRIVE SUITE-400
ROANOKE, TX 76262
800-677-0355

NILODOR CO., INC.
10966 INDUSTRIAL PARKWAY NW
P.O. BOX 660
BOLIVAR, OH 44612
800-443-4321

NION LABORATORIES
15501 FIRST STREET
IRWINDALE, CA 91706
800-227-852

NMC LABORATORIES, INC.
70-36 83RD STREET
GLENDALE, NY 11385
800-431-5014

NOBLE PINE PRODUCTS CO.
BOX 41, CENTUCK STA.
YONKERS, NY 10710
914-664-5877

NOMAX, INC.
40 N. ROCK HILL ROAD
ST. LOUIS, MO 63119
314-961-2500

NORSTAR CPC INC.
206 PEGASUS AVENUE
NORTHVALE, NJ 07647
201-784-8155

NORTECH LABORATORIES
4 MIDLAND AVENUE
HICKSVILLE, NY 11801
516-935-2040

NORTHAMPTON MEDICAL, INC.
3039 AMWILER ROAD SUITE 122
ATLANTA, GA 30360
404-416-8889

NORTON, H N & CO.
8910 LINWOOD AVENUE
P.O. BOX 6038
SHREVEPORT, LA 71106
318-688-4800

NOVO-NORDISK PHARMACEUTICALS INC.
100 OVERLOOK CTR. #200
PRINCETON, NJ 085407810
609-987-5800

NOVOPHARM USA INC.
165 EAST COMMERCE DRIVE
SUITE 100-200
SCHAUMBURG, IL 60173-5326
800-635-5067

NOXELL CORP.
11050 YORK ROAD
HUNT VALLEY, MD 21030-2098
301-628-7300

NOYES, P. J., CO., INC.
BRIDGE STREET
P.O. BOX 381
LANCASTER, NH 03584
800-522-2469

NU-TEK LABORATORIES
P O BOX 166
PALMYRA, PA 17078
800-532-1494

NUMARK LABORATORIES, INC.
P.O. BOX 6321
EDISON, NJ 08818
800-338-8079

NUTRALORIC
350 N. LANTANA DIV. CHARTER
OAK PHARMACY
CAMARILLO, CA 93010
805-388-2811

NUTRAMAX PRODUCTS INC.
9 BLACKBURN DRIVE
GLOUCESTER, MA 01930
508-283-1800

NUTRICIA, INC.
13246 WOOSTER ROAD
MOUNT VERNON, OH 43050
800-936-5525

NUTRIPHARM LABORATORIES, INC.
8 BARTLES CORNER ROAD
SUITE 101
FLEMINGTON, NJ 08822
908-806-8954

NUTRITIONAL RESEARCH ASSOC., INC.
407 E. BROAD
P.O. BOX 354
SO. WHITLEY, IN 46787
219-723-4931

OAKHURST CO.
3000 HEMPSTEAD TURNPIKE
LEVITTOWN, NY 11756
516-731-5380

OAKTREE PRODUCTS, INC.
2134 HEATHER GLEN DRIVE
CHESTERFIELD, MO 63017
800-347-1960

OCLASSEN PHARMACEUTICALS, INC.
100 PELICAN WAY
SAN RAFAEL, CA 94901
800-288-4508

OCTOGEN PHARMACAL COMPANY, INC.
P.O. BOX 52595
ATLANTA, GA 30355
404-266-2220

OCUMED, INC.
119 HARRISON AVENUE
ROSELAND, NJ 07068
201-226-2330

OCUSOFT
P.O. BOX 429
RICHMOND, TX 77406-0429
800-233-5469

OHM LABORATORIES, INC.
P.O. BOX 7397
NORTH BRUNSWICK, NJ 08902
800-527-6481

**OHMEDA SUBS. OF BOC HEALTH
CARE INC.**
P.O. BOX 804
LIBERTY CORNER, NJ 07938-0804
800-262-3784

OLAN LABORATORIES, INC.
36 GRAND BLVD.
BRENTWOOD, NY 11717
800-882-6526

OMICRON INTERNATIONAL
P.O. BOX 270465
TAMPA, FL 33688
813-264-7155

OMNII INTERNATIONAL
P.O. BOX 100
GRAVETTE, AR 72736
800-643-3639

OMRON HEALTHCARE, INC.
300 LAKEVIEW PARKWAY
VERNON HILLS, IL 60061
708-680-6200

OPTIMOX CORPORATION
2720 MONTEREY STREET, SUITE 406
TORRANCE, CA 90503
800-223-1601

OPTOPICS LABORATORIES CORP.
DIV OF NUTRAMAX CO.
32 MAIN ST.
P.O. BOX 210
FAIRTON, NJ 08320-0210
508-283-1800

ORACHEM PHARMACEUTICALS
DIV. OF MEDICAL PRODUCTS LABS.
9990 GLOBAL ROAD
PHILADELPHIA, PA 19115
800-654-3997

ORAL B LABORATORIES
DIV. GILLETTE COMPANY
1 LAGOON DRIVE
REDWOOD CITY, CA 94065-1561
800-446-7252

ORAL-IVY, INC.
104 GUY'S LANE
BLOOMSBURG, PA 17815
717-389-1814

ORGANON PHARMACEUTICALS
375 MT. PLEASANT AVENUE
WEST ORANGE, NJ 07052
201-325-4500

ORTHO BIOTECH
P.O. BOX 300, RT. 202
RARITAN, NJ 08869-0602
908-704-5000

ORTHO DIAGNOSTIC SYSTEMS, INC.
100 U.S. HIGHWAY 202
RARITAN, NJ 08869
800-322-6374

ORTHO PHARMACEUTICAL CORPORATION
ROUTE 202
RARITAN, NJ 08869-0602
908-218-6000

**ORTHO PHARMACEUTICAL CORPORATION-
ADVANCED CARE**
ROUTE 202
RARITAN, NJ 08869
908-218-1300

ORTHO-MCNEIL PHARMACEUTICAL
U.S. ROUTE 202
RARITAN, NJ 08869-0602
908-218-6000

OTIS CLAPP & SON, INC.
P.O. BOX 9160
115 SHAWMUT RD
CANTON, MA 02021
617-821-5400

**OTSUKA AMERICA PHARMACEUTICALS,
INC.**
2440 RESEARCH BOULEVARD
ROCKVILLE, MD 20850
800-336-8817

**OWENS-BROCKWAY PRESCRIPTION PROD-
UCTS UNIT OF OWENS-ILLINOIS**
ONE SEAGATE
TOLEDO, OH 43666
419-247-5000

P & S LABORATORIES, INC.
210 W. 131ST STREET
P.O. BOX 61067
LOS ANGELES, CA 90061
213-321-4284

PACO PHARMACEUTICAL SERVICES, INC.
1200 PACO WAY
LAKEWOOD, NJ 08701
201-367-9000

PADDOCK LABORATORIES, INC.
3940 QUEBEC AVENUE NORTH
P.O. BOX 27286
MINNEAPOLIS, MN 55427
800-328-5113

PAL MIDWEST LTD.
1030 S. MAIN STREET
P.O. BOX 624
ROCKFORD, IL 61105
815-399-2689

PAL-PAK, INC.
1201 LIBERTY STREET
ALLENTOWN, PA 18102
215-433-7579

PALISADES PHARMACEUTICALS, INC.
219 COUNTY ROAD
TENAFLY, NJ 07670
800-237-9083

PAN AMERICAN LABORATORIES, INC.
P.O. BOX 2649
COVINGTON, LA 70434-2649
504-893-4097

PAR PHARMACEUTICAL, INC.
ONE RAM RIDGE ROAD
SPRING VALLEY, NY 10977
800-828-9393

PARAEUSAL CO., THE
1809 BELMONT AVENUE
YOUNGSTOWN, OH 44504
216-744-4544

PARAGON VISION SCIENCES
1100 E. BELL ROAD
PHOENIX, AZ 85022
800-800-0369

PARK SURGICAL CO., INC.
5001 NEW UTRECHT AVENUE
BROOKLYN, NY 11219
800-633-7878

**PARKE-DAVIS DIV.
WARNER LAMBERT CO.**
201 TABOR ROAD
MORRIS PLAINS, NJ 07950
800-223-0432

PARKER LABORATORIES, INC.
307 WASHINGTON STREET
ORANGE, NJ 07050
800-631-8888

PARMED PHARMACEUTICALS, INC.
4220 HYDE PARK BLVD.
NIAGARA FALLS, NY 14305
716-284-5666

PARNELL PHARMACEUTICALS, INC.
100 LARKSPUR LANDING
LARKSPUR, CA 94939
800-457-4276

PARTHENON CO., INC., THE
3311 W. 2400 SOUTH
SALT LAKE CITY, UT 84119
801-972-5184

**PASADENA RESEARCH LABORATORIES,
INC.**
P.O. BOX 5136
SAN CLEMENTE, CA 92674-5136
800-223-9851

PASCAL CO.
2929 N.E. NORTHRUP WAY
P.O. BOX 1478
BELLEVUE, WA 98009-1478
800-426-8051

PECOS PHARMACEUTICAL
25301 CABOT ROAD SUITE 212-213
LAGUNA HILLS, CA 92653
714-770-5431

PEDIFIX
P.O. DRAWER B
ARMONK, NY 10504
800-356-8185

PEDINOL PHARMACAL, INC.
30 BANFI PLAZA NORTH
FARMINGDALE, NY 11735
800-733-4665

PEGASUS MEDICAL, INC.
ONE TECHNOLOGY DR. BLDG.1C
SUITE 527
IRVINE, CA 92718
714-753-9055

PENDLETON, PENNY
10526 OLD OLIVE ST. RD.
ST. LOUIS, MO 63141
314-432-5200

PENN HERB CO., LTD.
603 N. 2ND ST.
PHILADELPHIA, PA 19123
215-925-3336

PENNEX LABORATORIES
ONE PENNEX DRIVE
VERONA, PA 15147
800-245-6110

PENNEX PHARMACEUTICALS, INC.
6451 MAIN STREET
MORTON GROVE, IL 60053
800-346-6854

PENOX TECHNOLOGIES, INC.
ONE PENOX PLAZA
COMMERCE ROAD
PITTSTON, PA 18640
800-233-3029

PERRY LABORATORIES, INC.
P.O. BOX 66066
ROSEVILLE, MI 48066
810-294-1539

PERRY MEDICAL PRODUCTS, INC.
3580 N.W. BROADWAY
PORTLAND, OR 97232
503-288-7071

PERRY PRODUCTS
3803 E. LAKE ST.
MINNEAPOLIS, MN 55406
612-722-4783

PERSON & COVEY
616 ALLEN AVENUE
P.O. BOX 25018
GLENDALE, CA 91221-5018
800-423-2341

PFEIFFER PHARMACEUTICALS, INC.
43-45 N. WASHINGTON AVE.
P.O. BOX 100
WILKES BARRE, PA 18773
800-342-6450

PFIZER CONSUMER PRODUCTS
235 EAST 42ND STREET
NEW YORK, NY 10017-5755
212-573-3139

PFIZER LABORATORIES
DIV. PFIZER, INC.
235 E. 42ND STREET
NEW YORK, NY 10017
800-533-4535

PHARM-TECH PACKAGING CORP.
P.O. BOX 163
HOBART, NY 13788
704-788-4495

PHARMA-PLAST (USA) INC.
ENTERPRISE CENTER, SUITE 412
26133 U.S. 19
NORTH CLEARWATER, FL 34623
813-791-8303

PHARMA-TEK, INC.
P.O. BOX 1148
ELMIRA, NY 14902
516-757-5522

PHARMACEUTICAL ASSOCIATES, INC.
SUB. BEACH PRODUCTS INC.
5220 S. MANHATTAN AVENUE
TAMPA, FL 33611
813-839-6565

PHARMACEUTICAL CORP. OF AMERICA
12348 HANCOCK ST
CARMEL, IN 46032
800-722-0772

PHARMACEUTICAL INNOVATIONS, INC.
897 FRELINGHUYSEN AVENUE
NEWARK, NJ 07114
201-242-2900

PHARMACEUTICAL SPECIALTIES, INC.
P.O. BOX 6298
ROCHESTER, MN 55903-6298
800-325-8232

PHARMACEUTICS CO. C/O NYCO DRUG
425 MADISON AVENUE
NEW YORK, NY 10017
800-237-2124

PHARMACHEM CORP.
719 STEFKO BLVD.
P.O. BOX 1035
BETHLEHEM, PA 18016-1035
215-867-4654

PHARMACIA ADRIA LABORATORIES INC.
P.O. BOX 16529
COLUMBUS, OH 43216-6529
800-729-2902

PHARMACIST'S CHOICE
2444 RANCH DRIVE
SPRINGFIELD, OR 97477
503-747-5223

PHARMAKRAFT, INC.
606 NORTH MAIN STREET
MISHAWAKA, IN 46545
800-726-5774

PHARMICS, INC.
2350 S. REDWOOD ROAD
P.O. BOX 27554
SALT LAKE CITY, UT 84127
800-456-4138

PHYSICIANS FORMULARY SERVICES, INC.
4506 L B MCLEOD ROAD, SUITE F
ORLANDO, FL 32811
407-425-2139

PHYSICIANS TOTAL CARE
5415 SOUTH 125TH EAST AVENUE
TULSA, OK 74146-6214
918-254-2273

PIC CORP.
23 S. ESSEX AVE.
ORANGE, NJ 07050
201-678-7300

PIONEER PHARMACEUTICALS, INC.
209 40TH STREET
IRVINGTON, NJ 07111
800-631-7992

PLOUGH SALES CORP.
P. O. BOX 377
MEMPHIS, TN 38151
901-320-2201

POLAMER DRUG CO., INC.
54 MAIN ST.
SOUTH RIVER, NJ 08882
908-257-5296

POLY PHARMACEUTICALS, INC.
 P. O. BOX 93
QUITMAN, MS 39355
601-776-3497

POLYMEDICA PHARMACEUTICALS (U.S.A.)
11 STATE STREET
WOBURN, MA 01801
617-933-2020

POLYMER TECHNOLOGY CORPORATION
100 RESEARCH DRIVE
WILMINGTON, MA 01887
800-343-1445

POLYMER TECHNOLOGY INTERNATIONAL
1871 GILMAN BLVD.
ISSAQUAH, WA 98027
800-877-4449

POPPER & SONS, INC.
300 DENTON AVE.
NEW HYDE PARK, NY 11040
516-248-0300

PORTER'S PRODUCTS
8525 W. COVINGTON-BRADFORD BLVD.
P. O. BOX 142
COVINGTON, OH 45318
513-473-2157

PORTO-LIFT CORPORATION
P. O. BOX 5
HIGGINS LAKE, MI 48627
517-821-6688

PORTON PRODUCTS, LTD.
30401 AGOURA ROAD, SUITE 102
AGOURA HILLS. CA 91301
818-879-2200

POUND INTERNATIONAL CORPORATION
1221 BRICKELL AVENUE
SUITE 1480
MIAMI, FL 33131
305-530-8702

POYTHRESS, WILLIAM P.
3911 DEEP ROCK ROAD
RICHMOND, VA 23233
804-527-1950

PRESS CHEM. & PHARM. LABS.
P. O. BOX 09103
COLUMBUS, OH 43209
614-239-7620

PRESTON PHARMACEUTICS DIVISION PRESTON BUSINESS CONSULTANTS INC.
568A PEPPERIDGE TREE LANE
KINNELON, NJ 07405
201-838-4873

PRIMA PHARMACEUTICALS, INC.
3443 TRIPP COURT, STE. A
SAN FRANSISCO, CA 92121
619-259-8876

PRIMATEC PHARMACEUTICALS, INC.
P.O. BOX 778
567 LIBERTY LANE WEST
KINGSTON, RI 02892
800-368-5254

PRIMEDICS LABORATORIES ETHICAL DIV., IRENDA CORP.
15524 SOUTH BROADWAY
GARDENIA, CA 90248
800-533-0173

PRIMUS PHARMACEUTICAL, INC.
P. O. BOX 123
MACON, GA 31202-0123
912-743-2123

PRINCESS PHARMACEUTICALS PHYTO-THERAPEUTIC & BIOCHEMICAL LABS
4343 COLONIAL AVENUE
JACKSONVILLE, FL 32210
904-388-1564

PRINCETON PHARMACEUTICAL PRODUCTS A BRISTOL-MYERS SQUIBB COMPANY
P. O. BOX 4500
PRINCETON, NJ 08543-4500
800-631-5244

PRIVATE FORMULATIONS, INC.
460 PLAINFIELD AVENUE
EDISON, NJ 08818
908-985-7100

PROCTER & GAMBLE COMPANY
2 PROCTER & GAMBLE PLAZA
CINCINNATI, OH 45202-3315
800-621-5516

PROCTER & GAMBLE DISTRIBUTING CO.
6TH & SYCAMORE STREETS
BOX 599
CINCINNAT,I OH 45201
513-983-1100

PROCTER & GAMBLE PHARMACEUTICALS INC. MANAGED CARE ADMINISTRATION
11520 REED HARTMAN HIGHWAY
CINCINNATI, OH 45241
800-621-5516

PROFESSIONAL PRODUCTS MART
P. O. BOX 321
BURBANK, CA 91503-0321
818-842-9041

PROTEIN RESEARCH PRODUCTS
1999 PIKE AVENUE
SAN LIANDRO, CA 94577
510-614-7716

PURDUE FREDERICK COMPANY INC.
100 CONNECTICUT AVENUE
NORWALK, CT 06850-3590
800-877-5666

PUREPAC PHARMACEUTICAL CO.
200 ELMORA AVENUE
ELIZABETH, NJ 07207
800-526-6978

PUTNAM, I.
P.O. BOX 444
BIG FLATS, NY 14814
607-732-6251

QUAKER HOUSE PRODUCTS INC.
P. O. BOX 21088
HOUSTON, TX 77226
713-526-1248

QUAKER INDUSTRIES
1971 WEST 85TH STREET
CLEVELAND, OH 44102
216-631-2400

QUALITEST PRODUCTS, INC.
1025 JORDAN ROAD
HUNTSVILLE, AL 35811
205-859-4011

QUALITY CARE PHARMACEUTICALS
17911 SAMPSON LANE
HUNTINGTON BEACH, CA 92647
800-533-8745

QUALITY FORMULATIONS, INC. PHARMACEUTICAL COMPANY
P.O. BOX 827
ZACHARY, LA 70791
800-259-3376

QUALITY RESEARCH PHARM., INC.
1117 THIRD AVE., S.W.
CARMEL, IN 46032
800-842-2022

R & D LABORATORIES, INC.
4094 GLENCOE AVENUE
MARINA DEL REY, CA 90292
800-338-9066

R & R DRUGS, INC.
506 N. 12TH STREET
MURRAY, KY 42071
502-753-7565

R-A PHARMACEUTICALS
4625 WARM SPRINGS ROAD
P. O. BOX 8229
COLUMBUS, GA 31908
404-568-1881

R.I.D. INC., DISTRIBUTOR
525 N. MEDNIK AVENUE
LOS ANGELES, CA 90022
213-268-0635

R.I.J. PHARMACEUTICAL CORP.
BLACKMEADOW ROAD
CHESTER, NY 10918
914-692-5799

RANDOB LABORATORIES, LTD.
P. O. BOX 345
MT. VERNON, NY 10551
914-534-2197

RAWAY PHARMACAL INC.
15 GRANIT ROAD
ACCORD, NY 12404
914-626-8133

RAWSON, INC.
13595 SE 177TH ST.
BORING, OR 97009
503-228-4119

RECKITT & COLMAN PHARMACEUTICALS, INC.
1901 HUGUENOT ROAD - 110
RICHMOND, VA 23235
800-444-7599

RECREO COMPANY
7845 MALTLAGE DRIVE
LIVERPOOL, NY 13090
315-652-4570

RECSEI LABORATORIES
330 S. KELLOGG, BUILDING M
GOLETA, CA 93117
805-964-2912

REDI-PRODUCTS
8741 LANDMARK ROAD
RICHMOND, VA 23228
800-955-6782

REED & CARNRICK DIV. OF BLOCK DRUG CO.,INC.
257 CORNELISON AVENUE
JERSEY CITY, NJ 07302
201-434-4000

REESE CHEMICAL CO., THE
10617 FRANK AVE.
CLEVELAND, OH 44106
800-321-7178

REGENT LABORATORIES
700 W. HILLSBORO BLVD.
BLDG. 2-206
DEERFIELD BEACH, FL 33441
800-872-1525

REGIONAL SERVICE CENTER
17A EVERBERG ROAD
WOBURN, MA 01801-1019
800-447-1006

REPUBLIC DRUG COMPANY, INC.
175 GREAT ARROW
BUFFALO, NY 14207
800-242-8655

REQUA, INC.
1 SENECA PLACE
P. O. BOX 4008
GREENWICH, CT 06830
800-321-1085

RESEARCH INDUSTRIES CORP.
6864 SOUTH, 300 WEST
MIDVALE, UT 84047
800-453-8432

RESPA PHARMACEUTICALS, INC.
P.O. BOX 88222
CAROL STREAM, IL 60188
708-462-9986

REXALL GROUP, THE
4031 N.E.,12TH TERRACE
FT. LAUDERDALE, FL 33334
800-255-7399

REXALL MANAGED CARE
ONE PENNEX DRIVE
VERONA, PA 15147
800-700-0065

REXAR PHARMACAL CORP.
396 ROCKAWAY AVENUE
P. O. BOX 397
VALLEY STREAM, NY 11582
516-561-7662

RHODE, J. G., CO., INC., THE
302 S. CENTRAL AVENUE
BALTIMORE, MD 21202
410-675-5525

RHONE-POULENC RORER PHARMACEUTICAL INC.
500 ARCOLA ROAD
P.O. BOX 1200
COLLEGEVILLE. PA 19426-0107
215-454-8000

RICHLYN LABORATORIES
CASTOR AVE. & KENSINGTON ,
PHILADELPHIA, PA 19124
215-289-2220

RICHWOOD PHARMACEUTICAL CO., INC.
7900 TANNER'S GATE LANE
SUITE 200
FLORENCE, KY 41042
606-282-2100

ROBERTS PHARMACEUTICAL CORP.
DIV. OF ROBERTS LABS
4 INDUSTRIAL WAY
WEST EATONTOWN, NJ 07724
908-389-1182

ROBERTS/HAUCK PHARMACEUTICAL
CORP. DIV. OF ROBERTS LABS
4 INDUSTRIAL WAY
WEST EATONTOWN, NJ 07724
908-389-1182

ROBINS, A.H.,
CONSUMER PRODUCTS DIVISION
1405 CUMMINGS DRIVE
RICHMOND, VA 23220
804-226-6700

ROBINS, A.H.,
PHARMACEUTICAL DIVSION
1407 SHERWOOD AVENUE
BOX 26609
RICHMOND, VA 23261
800-666-7248

ROCHE LABORATORIES
DIV. HOFFMANN-LA ROCHE INC.
340 KINGSLAND STREET
NUTLEY, NJ 071101199
201-235-5000

ROCHE PRODUCTS, INC.
CARRETERA ESTATAL
#670 KM. 2.7
MANATI, PR 00674
809-854-3020

ROERIG, J. B. & CO. DIV. PFIZER, INC.
235 E. 42ND STREET
NEW YORK, NY 10017
212-573-2323

ROMAN LABS, INC. ADVANCED MEDICAL
SOLUTIONS
7325 SO. REVERE PARKWAY,
UNIT 503
ENGLEWOOD, CO 80112
800-255-0514

ROMNICO BY FILIPO
1114 N. COURT STREET #161
MEDINA, OH 44256-1522

RONSON CONSUMER PRODUCTS CORP.
CORPORATE PARK III
P. O. BOX 6709
SOMERSET, NJ 08875-6709
800-526-4281

ROOSA & RATLIFF DRUG CO., THE
P.O. BOX 12885
CINCINNATI, OH 45212-0885
513-242-6661

ROSE LABORATORIES DIVISION
168 COTTAGE ROAD
MADISON, CT 06443
203-245-1210

ROSEMONT PHARMACEUTICAL
CORPORATION
301 SO. CHEROKEE STREET
DENVER, CO 80223
800-445-8091

ROSS LABORATORIES,
CONSUMER PRODUCTS
DIV. ABBOTT LABORATORIES
625 CLEVELAND AVENUE
COLUMBUS, OH 43215
614-624-5619

ROSS LABORATORIES,
NUTRITIONAL PRODUCTS
DIV. ABBOTT LABORATORIES
625 CLEVELAND AVENUE
COLUMBUS, OH 43215-1724 }
800-367-7677

ROSS PHARMACEUTICALS
DIV. ABBOTT LABORATORIES
625 CLEVELAND AVENUE
COLUMBUS, OH 43215
614-227-3333

ROXANE LABORATORIES, INC.
1809 WILSON ROAD
COLUMBUS, OH 43228
614-276-4000

ROYCE LABORATORIES, INC.
16600 N.W. 54 AVENUE
MIAMI, FL 33014
305-624-1500

RUGBY LABORATORIES, INC.
898 ORLANDO AVENUE
WEST HEMPSTEAD, NY 11552
800-645-2158

RYSTAN COMPANY, INC.
47 CENTER AVENUE
P. O. BOX 214
LITTLE FALLS, NJ 07424-0214
201-256-3737

S.B.S.
302 WALLER STREET
P. O. BOX 1387
SAGINAW, MI 48605
800-248-7190

S.S.S. CO., THE
71 UNIVERSITY AVENUE, S.W.
P. O. BOX 4447
ATLANTA, GA 30302
800-237-3843

SAGAMI, INC.
8725 W. HIGGINS ROAD SUITE 481
CHICAGO, IL 60631
800-551-1888

SANALINE MICROBIOLOGICAL TESTING
PRODUCTS
2 CENTER PLAZA
BOSTON, MA 02108-1906
800-332-0449

SANDOCARE DIVISION SANDOZ
CORPORATION
59 ROUTE 10
EAST HANOVER, NJ 07936-1951
800-526-0175

SANDOZ CONSUMER HEALTH CARE GROUP
59 ROUTE 10, BLDG. 701-3
EAST HANOVER, NJ 07936-1080
201-503-7500

SANDOZ NUTRITIONAL CORPORATION
5320 W. 23RD STREET
P.O.BOX 370
MINNEAPOLIS, MN 55440
800-777-8103

SANDOZ PHARMACEUTICALS CORP.
59 ROUTE 10
EAST HANOVER, NJ 07936-1080
800-526-0175

SANITUBE CO., THE
19 CONCORD ST.
S. NORWALK, CT 06854
203-853-7856

SANOFI WINTHROP PHARMACEUTICALS
90 PARK AVENUE
NEW YORK, NY 10016
212-907-2000

SARON PHARMACAL CORP.
1640 CENTRAL AVENUE
ST. PETERSBURG, FL 33712
813-384-2323

SAVAGE LABORATORIES
60 BAYLIS ROAD
P. O. BOX 2006
MELVILLE, NY 11747
800-231-0206

SAVOL CO., THE
201 W. VENANGO STREET
MERCER, PA 16137
412-662-4064

SCANDIPHARM, INC.
22 INVERNESS CTR. PKWY.
SUITE 310
BIRMINGHAM, AL 35242
800-950-8085

SCHEIN PHARMACEUTICAL, INC.
100 CAMPUS DRIVE
FLORHAM PARK, NJ 07932
800-553-4044

SCHERER LABORATORIES, INC.
315 GILMER FERRY ROAD
BALL GROUND, GA 30107
800-858-9888

SCHERING CORPORATION
2000 GALLOPING HILL ROAD
KENILWORTH, NJ 07033
800-222-7579

SCHERING-PLOUGH HEALTHCARE
PRODUCTS INC.
110 ALLEN ROAD
P. O. BOX 276
LIBERTY CORNER, NJ 07938
908-604-1640

SCHMID LABORATORIES, INC.
CITY CENTER
1819 MAIN STREET
SARASOTA, FL 34236
800-827-0987

SCHUCO
DIV. AMERICAN CADUCEUS IND.
1419 EXPRESSWAY DRIVE NORTH
TOLEDO, OH 43608
800-645-2500

SCHWARZ PHARMA
P. O. BOX 2038
MILWAUKEE, WI 53201
800-472-9309

SCLAVO, INC.
5 MANSORD COURT
WAYNE, NJ 07470
800-526-5260

SCOT-TUSSIN PHARM. CO., INC.
50 CLEMENCE STREET
P. O. BOX 8217
CRANSTON, RI 02920-0217
800-638-7268

SCOTT SPECIALTIES, INC.
512 M STREET
P. O. BOX 0508
BELLVILLE, KS 66935-0508
800-255-7136

SCS PHARMACEUTICALS
P. O. BOX 5110
CHICAGO, IL 60680
800-323-1603

SDI LABORATORIES, INC.
1825 HOLSTE ROAD
NORTHBROOK, IL 60062
708-564-5775

SE PRO HEALTHCARE, INC.
1272 NO. CHURCH STREET
MOORESTOWN, NJ 08057
800-523-3660

SEARLE, G.D., & CO.
PO BOX 5110
CHICAGO, IL 606
800-323-1603

SEATRACE PHARMACEUTICALS, INC.
P. O. BOX 363
GADSDEN, AL 35902
205-442-5023

SENECA PHARMACEUTICALS
P. O BOX 25021
RALEIGH, NC 27611
919-783-6936

SENTINEL CONSUMER PRODUCTS, INC.
7750 TYLER BOULEVARD
MENTOR, OH 44060
216-974-8144

SERES LABORATORIES, INC.
3331 INDUSTRIAL DRIVE
P. O. BOX 470
SANTA ROSA, CA 95402
707-526-4526

SERONO LABS., INC.
100 LONGWATER CIRCLE
NORWELL, MA 02061
800-283-8088

SETON PHARMACEUTICAL CO., INC.
2717 NIRA AVENUE
EAST MEADOW, NY 11554
516-785-5763

SHERWOOD MEDICAL
1915 OLIVE STREET
ST. LOUIS, MO 63103-1642
800-325-7030

SHIELD HEALTHCARE CENTERS, INC.
P. O. BOX 916
SANTA CLARITA, CA 91380-9016
800-525-8049

SHIONOGI USA, INC.
3848 CARSON STREET SUITE 206
TORRANCE, CA 90503
310-540-1161

SIDMAK LABORATORIES INC.
17 WEST STREET
P. O. BOX 371
EAST HANOVER, NJ 07936
800-922-0547

SIERRA LABORATORIES, INC.
3520 S. CAMPBELL AVENUE
P.O. BOX 27005
TUCSON, AZ 85726
800-726-2904

SIGMA-TAU PHARMACEUTICALS, INC.
200 ORCHARD RIDGE DRIVE
SUITE 300
GAITHERSBURG, MD 20878
800-447-0169

SILARX PHARMACEUTICALS, INC.
15 WEST STREET
P.O. BOX 449
SPRING VALLEY, NY 10977
914-352-4020

SILVER'S PHARMACEUTICALS
1100 HAGLER DRIVE WEST
NEPTUNE BEACH, FL 32266
904-241-5171

SIMILASAN CORPORATION
1321 S. CENTRAL AVENUE
SUITE D
KENT, WA 98032
800-426-1644

SINCLAIR PHARMACAL CO., INC.
ORIENTAL AVENUE
P. O. DRAWER D
FISHERS ISLAND, NY 06390
516-788-7210

SKIN CULTURE CO.
38 WEST 32ND STREET
NEW YORK, NY 10001
212-564-8060

SMITH & NEPHEW UNITED, INC.
P.O. BOX 1970
11775 STARKEY ROAD
LARGO, FL 34649-1970
800-876-1261

SMITH, B. W., LAB. 210
ALCORN AVENUE
P. O. BOX 1408
HATTIESBURG, MS 39401
800-844-6721

SMITHKLINE BEECHAM CONSUMER PRODUCTS
100 BEECHAM DRIVE
P.O. BOX 1467
PITTSBURGH, PA 15230
412-928-1000

SMITHKLINE BEECHAM PHARMACEUTICALS
ONE FRANKLIN PLAZA
P.O. BOX 7929
PHILADELPHIA, PA 19101
215-751-400

SNUGFIT EYE PATCH CO., THE
BOX 264
YUCAIPA, CA 92399
909-797-3169

SNUVA, INC. MEDICAL INNOVATORS
715 SOUTH BOULEVARD
OAK PARK, IL 60302
708-848-4783

SOLAR OINTMENT CO.
36 W. BROAD STREET
HAZLETON, PA 18201
717-454-0051

SOLAR SUNTAN PRODS. CORP.
16361 NW 49 AVENUE
HIALEAH, FL 33014
305-621-5551

SOLO PAK LABORATORIES
DIV. OF SOLO PAK PHARMACEUTICALS
1845 TONNE ROAD
ELK GROVE VILLAGE, IL 60007-5125
800-654-0870

SOLO PAK MEDICAL PRODUCTS INC.
DIV. OF SOLO PAK PHARMACEUTICALS
1845 TONNE ROAD
ELK GROVE VILLAGE, IL 60007-5125
800-654-0870

SOLVAY PHARMACEUTICALS
901 SAWYER ROAD
MARIETTA, GA 30062
800-241-1643

SOMERSET PHARMACEUTICALS, INC.
777 S. HARBOUR ISLAND BLVD.
SUITE 880
TAMPA, FL 33602
813-223-7677

SORBOL COMPANY
39 S. MAIN STREET
MECHANICSBURG, OH 43044
513-834-2973

SOUTHWEST TECHNOLOGIES, INC.
2018 BALTIMORE
KANSAS CITY, MO 64108
800-247-9951

SOUTHWOOD PHARMACEUTICALS, INC.
SUITE 404
3860 DEL AMO BOULEVARD
TORRANCE, CA 90503
310-370-5233

SPECTRA PHARMACEUTICALS, INC.
HANOVER BUSINESS PARK
155 WEBSTER STREET
HANOVER, MA 02339
800-225-2578

SPECTRUM CHEMICAL MFG. CORP.
SEE ALSO A-A SPECTRUM
14422 S. SAN PEDRO STREET
GARDENA, CA 90248
800-772-8786

SPECTRUM CONSUMER PRODUCTS COMPANY
ONE RIVERWAY SUITE 1700
HOUSTON, TX 77056
713-621-0381

SPENCER-MEAD INC.
900 ORLANDO AVENUE
WEST HEMPSTEAD, NY 11552
800-645-3737

SQUIBB DIAGNOSTICS A BRISTOL-MYERS SQUIBB COMPANY
P. O. BOX 4500
PRINCETON, NJ 08543-4500
609-243-7000

SQUIBB, E.R. & SONS A BRISTOL-MYERS SQUIBB COMPANY
P. O. BOX 4500
PRINCETON, NJ 08543-4500
800-631-5244

SQUIBB, E.R. & SONS INSTITUTIONAL A BRISTOL-MYERS SQUIBB COMPANY
P. O. BOX 4500
PRINCETON, NJ 08543-4500
800-631-5244

STAFFORD-MILLER
DIV. OF BLOCK DRUG
257 CORNELISON AVENUE
JERSEY CITY, NJ 07302
201-434-3000

STANBACK COMPANY
P. O. BOX 1669
SALISBURY, NC 28145
800-338-5428

STANDARD HOMEOPATHIC COMPANY
210 WEST 131 STREET
P. O. BOX 61067
LOS ANGELES, CA 90061
213-321-4284

STANSBURY CHEMICAL CO.
21003 N.E. 67TH
REDMOND, WA 98052
206-868-5300

STAR PHARMACEUTICALS, INC.
1990 N.W. 44TH STREET
POMPANO BEACH, FL 33064
305-971-9704

STELLAR PHARMACAL CORP.
1990 N.W. 44TH STREET
POMPANO BEACH, FL 33064
305-971-9704

STERIS LABORATORIES, INC.
620 NORTH 51ST AVENUE
PO BOX 23160
PHOENIX, AZ 85063-3160
800-692-9995

STERLING HEALTH U.S.A.
90 PARK AVENUE
NEW YORK, NY 10016
800-331-4536

STEWART JACKSON PHARMACAL, INC.
4200 LAMAR #103
MEMPHIS, TN 38118
800-367-1395

STIEFEL LABORATORIES, INC.
255 ALHAMBRA CIRCLE
CORAL GABLES, FL 33134
800-327-3858

STORZ/LEDERLE OPHTHALMIC PHARMACEUTICALS
DIV. AMERICAN CYANAMID CO.
ONE CYANAMID PLAZA
WAYNE, NJ 07470
201-831-2000

STRATUS PHARMACEUTICALS, INC.
14377 SOUTHWEST 142ND ST
P O BOX 4632
MIAMI, FL 33186
800-442-7882

STUART PHARMACEUTICALS
CONCORD PIKE & MURPHY ROAD
WILMINGTON, DE 19897
800-441-7758

STURTEVANT, F. C., CO., THE
P. O. BOX 471
W. HARTFORD, CT 06107
203-634-3334

SUMMERS LABORATORIES, INC.
1276 CRESSMAN ROAD
P.O. BOX 144
SKIPPACK, PA 19474
800-533-7546

SUMMIT PHARMACEUTICALS
556 MORRIS AVENUE
SUMMIT, NJ 07901
908-277-5000

SUNDOWN VITAMINS, INC.
4031 N.E. 12TH TERRACE
FT. LAUDERDALE, FL 33334
305-565-3566

SUPERIOR PHARMACEUTICAL COMPANY
858 E. CRESCENTVILLE ROAD
CINCINNATI, OH 45246-4843
513-346-7100

SUPPOSITORIA LABORATORIES, INC.
1700 BATHGATE AVENUE
BRONX, NY 10457
212-901-2800

SURGICAL APPLIANCE INDUSTRIES, INC.
ERIE AVENUE & PENN. R.R.
CINCINNATI, OH 45209
513-271-4594

SWEEN CORP.
1940 COMMERCE DRIVE
P. O. BOX 8300
N. MANKATO, MN 56001
800-533-0464

SYNTEX LABORATORIES, INC.
3401 HILLVIEW AVENUE
PALO ALTO, CA 94304
800-227-7311

SYOSSET LABORATORIES
150 EILEEN WAY
SYOSSET, NY 11791
800-645-7577

TAP PHARMACEUTICALS
2355 WAUKEGAN ROAD
DEERFIELD, IL 60015
800-621-1020

TARMAC PRODS., INC.
13295 N.W. 107TH AVENUE
HIALEAH GARDENS, FL 33016
800-457-7728

TARO PHARMACEUTICALS U.S.A., INC.
SIX SKYLINE DRIVE
HAWTHORNE, NY 10532
800-544-1449

TEC LABORATORIES
P. O. BOX 1958
ALBANY, OR 97321-0512
503-926-4577

TERUMO CORPORATION
2100 COTTONTAIL LANE
SOMERSET, NJ 08873
800-283-7866

THAMES PHARMACAL CO. INC.
2100 FIFTH AVENUE
RONKONKOMA, NY 11779
800-225-1003

THOMAS & THOMPSON CO., INC.
THOMAS BUILDING
3927 FALLS ROAD
BALTIMORE, MD 21211
410-889-2960

THOMPSON MEDICAL CO., INC.
222 LAKEVIEW AVENUE
17TH FLOOR
WEST PALM BEACH, FL 33401
407-820-9900

THRIFT DRUG INC.
615 ALPHA DRIVE
PITTSBURGH, PA 15238-2876
412-963-6600

THRIFT DRUG SERVICES, INC.
615 ALPHA DR
PITTSBURGH, PA 15238
412-967-8815

TIME-CAP LABORATORIES, INC.
7 MICHAEL AVENUE
FARMINGDALE, NY 11735
516-753-9090

TMK PHARMACEUTICALS
1505 WEST REYNOLDS
PLANT CITY, FL 33567
800-554-8399

TOPI-CANA SPECIALTY PRODUCTS
P.O. BOX 636408
MARGATE, FL 33063
800-829-6610

TORBOT GROUP INC.
1185 JEFFERSON BLVD.
PO BOX 6008
WARWICK, RI 02887
401-739-2241

TORRANCE COMPANY, THE
800 LENOX AVENUE
PORTAGE, MI 49002
800-327-0722

TRASK INDUSTRIES
163 FARRELL STREET
SOMERSET, NJ 08873
908-214-9267

TRI-MED LABORATORIES, INC.
68 VERONICA AVENUE
SOMERSET, NJ 08873
908-249-6363

TRINITY TECHNOLOGIES CORP.
28510 HAYES
ROSEVILLE, MI 48066
313-778-5630

TRUXTON, CO., INC.
P.O. BOX 1081
BELLMAWR, NJ 08099
609-933-2333

TSUMURA MEDICAL
1000 VALLEY PARK DRIVE
SHAKOPEE, MN 55379
612-945-9400

TYSON AND ASSOCIATES, INC.
12832 CHADRON AVENUE
HAWTHORNE, CA 90250
800-367-7744

U-TRI PRODUCTS INC.
P. O. BOX 2152
GARDENA, CA 90247
213-321-5241

U.S. BIOSCIENCE
ONE TOWER BRIDGE
100 FRONT STREET
WEST CONSHOHOCKEN, PA 19428
215-832-0570

U.S. DENTEK CORP.
1320 INDUSTRIAL AVE.
PETALUMA, CA 94952
707-762-4646

U.S. PHARMACEUTICAL CORP.
2401 C. MELLON COURT
DECATUR, GA 30035
404-987-4745

UDL LABORATORIES
P.O. BOX 10319
ROCKFORD, IL 61131-3019
815-282-1201

ULMER PHARMACAL
2440 FERNBROOK LANE
PLYMOUTH, MN 55447
800-8485-637

ULSTER SCIENTIFIC, INC.
P.O. BOX 819
NEW PALTZ, NY 12561-0819
800-431-8233

UNIMED
3 BOULDEN CIRCLE
NEW CASTLE, DE 19720
800-756-6056

UNITED RESEARCH LABORATORIES, INC.
3600 MEADOW LANE
P.O. BOX 8546
BENSALEM, PA 19020-8546
800-523-3684

UNITED STATES TRADING CORP.
10718 MC CUNE AVENUE
LOS ANGELES, CA 90034-6292
800-382-9201

UPJOHN CO., THE
7000 PORTAGE ROAD
KALAMAZOO, MI 49001-0199
800-253-8600

UPSHER-SMITH LABORATORIES, INC.
14905 23RD AVENUE NORTH
MINNEAPOLIS, MN 55447
800-328-3344

UROCARE PRODUCTS, INC.
2735 MELBOURNE AVENUE
POMONA, CA 91767
714-621-6013

V.I.P. PHARMACEUTICAL
3000 ALP BLVD.
GRAND ISLAND, NY 14072
800-847-3784

VALMED INC.
203 SOUTHWEST CUTOFF
NORTHBORO, MA 01532
800-487-0487

VANCO CO.
P. O. BOX 227
GOTHENBURG, NE 69138
308-537-2619

VANGARD LABS.
890 N.L. ROGER WELLS BLVD
GLASGOW, KY 42141
800-825-4123

VENTURE PHARMACEUTICALS
3115 NORTHINGTON COURT
FLORENCE, AL 35630
205-740-5528

VENTURI, INC.
1757 PARK DRIVE
TRAVERSE CITY, MI 49684
616-929-7732

VERATEX CORP.
1304 E. MAPLE ROAD
P. O. BOX 4031
TROY, MI 48084
800-552-8387

VERAZIL PHARMACEUTICALS
P. O. BOX 360854
SAN JUAN, PR 00936
809-727-1763

VERNON LABORATORIES, INC.
508 FRANKLIN AVENUE
MT. VERNON, NY 10551
914-699-3131

VINTAGE PHARMACEUTICALS, INC.
1236 JORDAN ROAD
HUNTSVILLE, AL 35811
205-859-4011

VISION PHARMACEUTICALS
P.O. BOX 400
MITCHELL, SD 57301
800-325-6789

VITA ELIXIR CO., INC.
P. O. BOX 92026
ATLANTA, GA 30314
404-522-5399

VITA PHARM
2835 KEW DRIVE
WINDSOR, ON 00000
519-944-1007

VITA-FOOD CO.
PO BOX 5439
TRENTON, NJ 08638
609-392-3127

VITA-RX CORP.
P. O. BOX 8229
COLUMBUS, GA 31908
800-241-8276

VITALIFE CO.
1573 FIRST AVE., S.E.
CEDAR RAPIDS, IA 52402
319-362-2271

VITALINE CORPORATION
385 WILLIAMSON WAY
ASHLAND, OR 97520
800-648-4755

VITAMED LABORATORIES
3935 GROVE AVENUE
GURNEE, IL 60031
708-623-8839

VOLUNTARY HOSPITALS OF AMERICA SUPPLY COMPANY
300 DECKER DRIVE
IRVING, TX 75016
214-650-4444

VOLUNTARY HOSPITALS OF AMERICA, INC.
300 DECKER DRIVE
IRVING, TX 75062
214-650-4328

WAKEFIELD PHARMACEUTICALS, INC.
1050 CAMBRIDGE SQUARE SUITE C
ALPHARETTA, GA 30201
404-664-1661

WALKER PHARMACAL CO.
4200 LACLEDE AVENUE
ST. LOUIS, MO 63108
314-533-9600

WALKER, CORP & CO., INC.
EASTHAMPTON PL./N.
COLLINGWOOD AVE.
P. O. BOX 1320
SYRACUSE, NY 13201
315-463-4511

**WALLACE LABORATORIES DIV.
CARTER-WALLACE, INC. H**
ALF ACRE ROAD
CRANBURY, NJ 08512
609-655-6000

WALTMAN PHARMACEUTICALS INC.
P. O. BOX 12442
JACKSON, MS 39236
601-939-0833

**WARNER CHILCOTT LABORATORIES DIV.
WARNER-LAMBERT CO.**
182 TABOR ROAD
MORRIS PLAINS, NJ 07950
201-540-2000

WARNER WELLCOME
201 TABOR ROAD
MORRIS PLAINS, NJ 07950
201-540-2000

WARNER-LAMBERT CONSUMER HEALTH PRODUCTS DIV.
201 TABOR ROAD
MORRIS PLAINS, NJ 07950
201-540-2000

WARNER-LAMBERT PERSONAL CARE
201 TABOR ROAD
MORRIS PLAINS, NJ 07950
201-540-2000

WARRICK PHARMACEUTICALS
7500 NORTH NATCHEZ AVENUE
NILES. IL 60648
800-547-3869

WASHINGTON HOMEOPATHIC PHARMACY
4914 DEL RAY AVENUE
BETHESDA, MD 20814
301-656-1695

WATSON LABORATORIES, INC.
311 BONNIE CIRCLE
CORONA, CA 91720
909-270-1400

WE PHARMACEUTICALS, INC.
P. O. BOX 1142
RAMONA, CA 92065
800-262-9555

WEEKS & LEO CO., INC.
4000 N.W. 100TH STREET
P. O. BOX 3570
DES MOINES, IA 50322
515-276-1586

WELEDA, INC.
175 NORTH RT. 9W
P.O.BOX 249
CONGERS, NY 10920
914-268-8572

WESLEY PHARMACAL CO., INC.
114 RAILROAD DRIVE
IVYLAND, PA 18974
215-953-1680

WEST POINT PHARMA
MAIL STOP WP39-223
SUMNEYTOWN & BROAD STS
WEST POINT, PA 19486
800-472-4467

WEST-WARD PHARMACEUTICAL CORP.
465 INDUSTRIAL WAY WEST
EATONTOWN, NJ 07724
800-631-2174

WESTWOOD-SQUIBB PHARMACEUTICALS, INC.
100 FOREST AVENUE
BUFFALO, NY 14213
800-333-0950

WEYMOUTH LABORATORIES
DIV. CONNOR PRODS. CORP.
P. O. BOX 2121
MORRISTOWN, NJ 07960
201-538-1023

WHITBY PHARMACEUTICALS, INC.
1211 SHERWOOD AVENUE
P.O. BOX 85054
RICHMOND, VA 23261-5054
800-477-7877

WHITEHALL LABORATORIES
DIV. AMERICAN HOME PRODS. CORP.
5 GIRALDA FARMS
MADISON, NJ 07940
201-660-5000

WILCOLE PHARMACEUTICALS, INC.
508 HARLEY STREET
SCOTTSBORO, AL 35768
205-259-1236

WILLIAMS GENERICS, INC.
1871 THOMAS ROAD
MEMPHIS, TN 38134
800-869-9869

WILLIAMS LABORATORY
P. O. BOX 101
ORADELL, NJ 07649
201-489-3183

WILLIAMS, T. E., PHARM. INC.
PO BOX 312
DIVIDE, CO 80814
719-687-3092

WINSOR PHARMACEUTICALS
1211 SHERWOOD AVENUE
BOX 85054
RICHMOND, VA 232615054
804-254-4400

WITHROW PHARM. & HEALTH SPECIALTIES LAB.
5729 MAYWOOD AVENUE
MAYWOOD, CA 90270
213-587-8453

WONDERFUL DREAM SALVE CORP.
18546 OLD HOMESTEAD
HARPER WOODS, MI 48225
313-521-4233

WUNDERLICH-DIEZ CORP.
361 STATE HIGHWAY 17
P. O. BOX 126
HASBROUCK HEIGHTS, NJ 07604
201-288-8887

WYETH-AYERST LABS.
DIV. AMERICAN HOME PRODS. CORP.
P. O. BOX 8299
PHILADELPHIA, PA 19101-8299
800-666-7248

XACTDOSE, INC.
722 PROGRESSIVE LANE
SOUTH BELOIT, IL 61080
815-624-8523

YERBA PRIMA
740 JEFFERSON AVENUE
ASHLAND, OR 97520-3743
800-488-4339

YORK, L. T., COMPANY
P.O. BOX 50
BUCKLIN, MO 64631
816-258-2291

YOUNG, W. F., INC.
111 LYMAN STREET
SPRINGFIELD, MA 01103
413-737-0201

Z M O CO., THE
4188 ALKIRE ROAD
GROVE CITY, OH 43123
614-882-2005

ZENECA PHARMACEUTICALS
CONCORD PIKE & MURPHY ROAD
WILMINGTON, DE 19897
800-842-9920

ZENITH LABORATORIES, INC.
140 LEGRAND AVE.
NORTHVALE, NJ 07647
800-631-1583

ZILA PHARMACEUTICALS, INC.
5227 N. 7TH STREET
PHOENIX, AZ 85014
602-266-6700

ZYGIENE MEDICAL TECHNOLOGY
855 VIRGINIA AVENUE
P.O.BOX 1376
PALM HARBOR, FL 34683
813-786-6703

ZYTRON SPORTS INJURY PRODUCTS INC.
P. O. BOX 693
CORAM, NY 11727
800-424-2677

Product Identification Guide

This section gives you two ways of identifying an unknown tablet or capsule: by matching its imprint with those listed in the Imprint Identification Guide below, or comparing it with the photos in the Visual Identification Guide that begins on page G-73.

Imprint Identification Guide

This convenient table enables you to quickly identify any of 6,000 drugs from the imprint alone. For quick comparison, all entries are organized by key identification number. For example, the imprint "LL A2" can be found under Identification Number 2, while "25 LL A13," appears under 13 (the "25" in this imprint being an indicator of strength, rather than an identifier).

Identification numbers are organized by number of digits, so that "1" appears near the beginning of the list, while "001" appears after "99." Identifiers with decimal extensions are inserted numerically according to the number of digits to the left of the decimal. The few imprints that include no number are listed alphabetically at the end of the section.

In addition to the full identification code as imprinted on the product, the table includes the product's generic name and, to confirm its identification, its strength, color, form, and shape. For tablets, indicators show whether the product is scored or coated (for capsules, only a dash appears). The product's supplier and primary use round out each listing.

This guide is reprinted with permission from The Med-Scan Manual®, Fifth Edition, copyright © 1994 and published by Med-Scan International, Inc.

ID NO.	ID CODE	GENERIC NAME	STRENGTH	COLOR	FORM	SHAPE	SCORED	COATED	MFG.	USE
0	Central 1/0	Vitamin Combination	n/a	White	Tab	Capsule	Y	Y	Central	Vitamin
0.25	AL/0.25mg G	Alprazolam	0.25mg	Yellow	Tab	Oval	N	N	Par	Antianxiety
0.5	AL/0.5mg G	Alprazolam	0.5mg	Yellow	Tab	Oval	N	N	Par	Antianxiety
1	1	Detrothyroxine Sodium	1mg	Orange	Tab	Oval	Y	N	Boots	Hypolipidemic
	1	Nitroglycerine CR Buccal	1mg	White	Tab	Round	N	N	PD	Antianginal
	5mg Lederle L1	Loxapine	5mg	Green	Cap	–	–	–	Lederle	Tranquilizer
	832/BM1	Benztropine Mesylate	1mg	White	Tab	Round	–	–	PBI	Antiparkinson
	832/LR1C	Lorazepam	1mg	White	Tab	Round	Y	N	PBI	Antianxiety
	AL/1mg G	Alprazolam	1.0mg	White	Tab	Oval	N	N	Par	Antianxiety
	AP 1	Phenazopyradine	100mg	–	Tab	Round	N	Y	Able Labs	Urinary Tract Agent
	AP 1	Phenazopyridine HCl	100mg	Maroon	Tab	Round	Y	N	Able	Urinary Antiseptic
	BL C1	Cefadroxil	1gm	White	Tab	Oblong	Y	N	Bristol	Anti–Infective
	BL S1	Hydroflumethiazide & Reserpine	50mg/0.125mg	Green	Tab	Round	Y	N	Bristol	Antihypertensive
	BL V1	Penicillin V Potassium	250mg	White	Tab	Round	–	N	BMS	Anti–Infective
	bp 1	Thioridazine HCl	10mg	Green	Tab	Capsule	N	Y	Bolar	Tranquilizer
	C 1	Atenolol	25mg	White	Tab	Round	N	N	IPR	Antihypertensive
	C1	Rauwolfia Serpentina & Bendroflumethiazide	50mg/100mg	Blue	Tab	Round	N	Y	Econolab	Antihypertensive
	Central 1/0	Vitamin Combination	n/a	White	Tab	Capsule	Y	Y	Central	Vitamin
	CL/1	Isosorbide Dinitrate SL	2.5mg	Yellow	Tab	Round	N	N	Geneva	Antianginal
	G1–LL	Vitamin/Mineral	n/a	Brown	Tab	Oblong	N	Y	Lederle	Vitamin
	GG 1	Isosorbide Dinitrate SL	2.5mg	Yellow	Tab	Round	N	N	Geneva	Antianginal
	K 1	Hydromorphone HCl	1mg	Green	Tab	Round	N	N	Knoll	Analgesic
	KU 1	Ergocalciferol	1.25mg	Yellow	Tab	Oval	N	N	KV	Vitamin D
	LL A1	Triamcinolone	1mg	Yellow	Tab	Oblong	Y	N	Lederle	Steroid
	LL F1	Folic Acid	1mg	Orange	Tab	Round	Y	N	Lederle	Antianemic
	LL H1	Quinethazone	50mg	White	Tab	Round	Y	N	Lederle	Diuretic
	LL K1	Ketoprofen	25mg	Green	Cap	–	–	–	Lederle	Anti–Inflammatory
	LL M1	Methotrexate	2.5mg	Yellow	Tab	Round	Y	N	Lederle	Antineoplastic
	LL N1	Methazolamide	50mg	White	Tab	Round	Y	N	Lederle	Antiglaucoma
	LL S 1	Vitamin	n/a	Orange	Tab	Oblong	–	–	Lederle	Vitamin
	LL T1	Vitamin comb.	n/a.	Red	Tab	Capsule	N	Y	Lederle	Vitamin
	M 1	Clonidine HCl & Chlorthalidone	0.1mg/15mg	Yellow	Tab	Round	Y	N	Mylan	Antihypertensive
	M 1	Methenamine Mandelate	1Gm	Purple	Tab	Oval	N	Y	Able Labs	Urinary Antiseptic
	Mylan G1	Glipizide	5mg	White	Tab	Round	Y	N	Mylan	Hypoglycemic
	Ortho 1	Norethindrone & Mestranol	1mg/0.08mg	White	Tab	Round	N	N	Ortho	Hormone
	R 1	Risperidone	1mg	White	Tab	Oblong	N	N	Janssen	Antipsychotic
	RR 1	Prednisone	1mg	Pink	Tab	Round	Y	N	RR	Steroid
	SKF 1	Isopropamide Iodide/Trifluoperazine HCl	5mg/1mg	Yellow	Tab	Round	–	Y	SKB	Tranquilizer
	SKF 1	Trifluoperazine HCl	1mg	Blue	Tab	Round	–	Y	SKB	Tranquilizer
	SYNTEX 1	Norethindrone & Mestranol	1mg/0.05mg	White	Tab	Round	–	N	Syntex	Contraceptive
	W 1	Isosorbide Dinitrate Sublingual	2.5mg	Yellow	Tab	Round	N	N	West–ward	Antianginal

ID NO.	ID CODE	GENERIC NAME	STRENGTH	COLOR	FORM	SHAPE	SCORED	COATED	MFG.	USE
2	Wyeth 1	Meprobamate	400mg	White	Tab	Round	Y	N	Wyeth	Antianxiety
	10mg Lederle L2	Loxapine	10mg	Green/Yellow	Cap	–	–	–	Lederle	Tranquilizer
	2	Detrothyroxine Sodium	2mg	Yellow	Tab	Oval	Y	N	Boots	Hypolipidemic
	2	Nitroglycerine CR Buccal	2mg	White	Tab	Round	N	N	PD	Antianginal
	50mg Lederle M2	Minocycline HCl	50mg	Orange	Cap	–	–	–	Lederle	Anti-Infective
	832/2C	Diazepam	2mg	White	Tab	Round	Y	N	PBI	Antianxiety
	832/BM2	Benztropine Mesylate	2mg	White	Tab	Round	–	–	PBI	Antiparkinson
	832/LR2C	Lorazepam	2mg	White	Tab	Round	Y	N	PBI	Antianxiety
	A2C	Digoxin	0.05mg	Red	Cap	–	–	–	BW	Cardiac Glycoside
	AF 2	Sodium Fluoride	2.2mg	–	Tab	Round	–	N	Able Labs	Mineral
	AP 2	Phenazopyradine	200mg	–	Tab	Round	N	Y	Able Labs	Urinary Tract Agent
	B2C	Digoxin	0.1mg	Yellow	Cap	–	–	–	BW	Cardiac Glycoside
	BL S2	Hydroflumethiazide	50mg	White	Tab	Round	Y	N	Bristol	Diuretic
	BL V2	Penicillin V Potassium	500mg	White	Tab	Round	–	N	BMS	Anti-Infective
	bp 2	Lorazepam	0.5mg	White	Tab	Round	–	–	Bolar	Antianxiety
	C2C	Digoxin	0.2mg	Green	Cap	–	–	–	BW.	Cardiac Glycoside
	DPI 2	Acetaminophen & Codeine Phosphate	300mg/15mg	White	Tab	Round	N	N	Duramed	Analgesic
	FL W/2 Hearts	Chlorpheniramine Maleate/Pseudoephedrine HCl	8mg/120mg	Blue/Clear	Cap	–	–	–	Econolabs	Decongestant Comb.
	G2–LL	Vitamin/Mineral	n/a	Maroon	Tab	Oblong	N	Y	Lederle	Vitamin
	GG/2	Isosorbide Dinitrate SL	5mg	Pink	Tab	Round	Y	N	Geneva	Antianginal
	K 2	Hydromorphone HCl	2mg	Orange	Tab	Round	N	N	Knoll	Analgesic
	L 2	Loperamide	2mg	Green	Tab	Oblong	Y	N	L'Perrigo	Antidiarrheal
	LL A2	Triamcinolone	2mg	Pink	Tab	Oblong	Y	N	Lederle	Steroid
	LL E2	Erythromycin Sterate	250mg	Pink	Tab	Round	N	Y	Lederle	Anti-Infective
	LL H2	Quinethazone & Reserpine	50mg/0.125mg	Yellow	Tab	Round	Y	N	Lederle	Antihypertensive
	LL K2	Ketoprofen	50mg	Green	Cap	–	–	–	Lederle	Anti-Inflammatory
	LL S 2	Vitamin/Mineral	n/a	Red	Tab	Oblong	–	–	Lederle	Vitamin
	LL–F2	Vitamin/Mineral	n/a	Green	Tab	Oblong	N	Y	Lederle	Vitamin
	M 2	Furosemide	20mg	White	Tab	Round	Y	N	Mylan	Diuretic
	M–2	Furosemide	20mg	White	Tab	Round	Y	N	Martec	Diuretic
	Mylan G2	Glipizide	10mg	White	Tab	Round	Y	N	Mylan	Hypoglycemic
	N N2	Methazolamide	25mg	White	Tab	Square	Y	N	Lederle	Antiglaucoma
	Ortho 2	Norethindrone & Mestranol	2mg/0.1mg	White	Tab	Round	N	N	Ortho	Hormone
	R 2	Risperidone	2mg	Peach	Tab	Oblong	N	N	Janssen	Antipsychotic
	Rugby 2	Isorsorbide SL	2.5mg	–	Tab	Round	–	–	Rugby	Vasodilator
	S 78–2	Thioridazine HCl	10mg	Green	Tab	Round	N	Y	Sandoz	Tranquilizer
	SKF 2	Trifluoperazine HCl	2mg	Blue	Tab	Round	–	Y	SKB	Tranquilizer
2.5	Wyeth 2	Meprobamate	200mg	White	Tab	Pentagonal	N	N	Wyeth	Antianxiety
3	W/2.5	Isosorbide Dinitrate SL	2.5mg	Yellow	Tab	Round	–	–	Wyeth	Vasodilator
	25mg Lederle L3	Loxapine	25mg	Green	Cap	–	–	–	Lederle	Tranquilizer
	3	Nitroglycerine CR Buccal	3mg	White	Tab	Round	N	N	PD	Antianginal
	A 3	Indapamide	2.5mg	White	Tab	Round	N	N	Arcola Labs	Antihypertensive
	BL S3	Hydroflumethiazide & Reserpine	25mg/0.125mg	Yellow	Tab	Round	Y	N	Bristol	Antihypertensive
	Ciba 3	Methylphenidate HCl	10mg	Green	Tab	Round	Y	N	Ciba	Psychostimulant
	DPI 3	Acetaminophen & Codeine Phosphate	300mg/30mg	White	Tab	Round	N	N	Duramed	Analgesic
	K 3	Hydromorphone HCl	3mg	Pink	Tab	Round	N	N	Knoll	Analgesic
	Lederle A3	Tetracycline HCl	250mg	Blue/Yellow	Cap	–	–	–	Lederle	Anti-Infective
	Lederle D3	Acetazolamide	500mg	Orange	Cap	–	–	–	Lederle	Antiglaucoma
	LL E3	Ergoloid Mesylates Oral	1mg	White	Tab	Round	N	N	Lederle	Vasodilator
	LL K3	Ketoprofen	75mg	White	Cap	–	–	–	Lederle	Anti-Inflammatory
	LL M3	Minocycline HCl	50mg.	Orange	Tab	Round	N	Y	Lederle	Anti-Infective
	LL S 3	Vitamin/Mineral	n/a	Peach	Tab	Oblong	–	–	Lederle	Vitamin
	MP 3	Hydroxyzine HCl	10mg	Purple	Tab	Round	N	Y	Mutual	Antipruritic
	PP–3	Dipyridamole	25mg	White	Tab	Round	N	Y	Eon	Antiplatelet
	R 3	Risperidone	3mg	Yellow	Tab	Oblong	N	N	Janssen	Antipsychotic
	SYNTEX 3	Norethindrone & Mestranol	1mg/0.08mg	Yellow	Tab	Round	–	N	Syntex	Contraceptive
	W 3	Isosorbide Dinitrate Sublingual	5mg	White	Tab	Round	N	N	West–ward	Antianginal
	WELLCOME U3B	Thioguanine	40mg	Green	Tab	Round	Y	N	BW	Antineoplastic
4	100mg Lederle M4	Minocycline HCl	100mg	Purple/Orange	Cap	–	–	–	Lederle	Anti-Infective
	4	Detrothyroxine Sodium	4mg	White	Tab	Oval	Y	N	Boots	Hypolipidemic
	4	Ibuprofen	400mg	White	Tab	Round	N	Y	Norton	Anti-Inflammatory
	50mg Lederle L4	Loxapine	50mg	Green/Blue	Cap	–	–	–	Lederle	Tranquilizer
	Central 60/4	Chlorpheniramine Maleate/Pseudoephedrine	4mg/60mg	Clear	Cap	–	–	–	Central	Decongestant
	DPI 4	Acetaminophen & Codeine Phosphate	300mg/60mg	White	Tab	Round	N	N	Duramed	Analgesic
	GG4	Diphenoxylate & Atropine	2.5mg/0.025mg	White	Tab	Round	N	N	Geneva	Antidiarrheal
	HD 4	Meperidine HCl	50mg	White	Tab	Round	N	N	Halsey	Analgesic
	K 4	Hydromorphone HCl	4mg	Yellow	Tab	Round	N	N	Knoll	Analgesic
	LL A4	Triamcinolone	4mg	White	Tab	Oblong	Y	N	Lederle	Steroid
	LL O 4 Lederle	Vitamin/Mineral	n/a	Red/White	Tab	Oval	–	–	Lederle	Vitamin
	LL P4	Tridihexethyl Chloride	25mg	Pink	Tab	Round	N	Y	Lederle	Antispasmodic
	LL U4	Aminophylline	100mg	White	Tab	Round	Y	N	Lederle	Bronchodilator
	LL V4	Verapamil HCl	80mg	White	Tab	Round	Y	N	Lederle	Antihypertensive
	LL–F4	Prenatal Vitamin/Mineral	n/a	Pink	Tab	Oblong	N	Y	Lederle	Vitamin
	M/4	Fluphenazine HCl	1mg	Pink	Tab	Triangle	N	Y	Mylan	Tranquilizer
	M/4	Fluphenazine HCl	1mg	White	Tab	Triangle	N	Y	Mylan	Tranquilizer
	MP 4	Imipramine Hydrochloride	10mg	Yellow	Tab	Round	N	Y	Mutual	Antidepressant
	Par/4	Dexchlorpheniramine Maleate	4mg	Yellow	Tab	Oval	N	Y	Par	Antihistamine
	R 4	Risperidone	4mg	Green	Tab	Oblong	N	N	Janssen	Antipsychotic
5	0822/5	Diphenoxylate & Atropine	2.5mg/0.025mg	White	Tab	Round	N	N	Pharmafair	Antidiarrheal
	832 A5	Amiloride HCl	5mg	–	Tab		–	–	PBI	Antihypertensive
	832 C5C	Chlordiazepoxide HCl with Clidinum Bromide	5mg/2.5mg	–	Cap	–	–	–	PBI	Antispasmodic
	832 M5	Methyclothiazide	5mg	Orange	Tab	Round	Y	N	PBI	Diuretic
	832/5	Chlordiazepoxide HCl	5mg	Green/Yellow	Cap	–	–	–	PBI	Antianxiety
	832/5C	Diazepam	5mg	Yellow	Tab	Round	Y	N	PBI	Antianxiety
	832/C5C	Chlordiazepoxide HCl with Clidinum Bromide	5mg/2.5mg	Green/Blue	Cap	–	–	–	PBI	Antispasmodic
	832/P5C	Prazepam	5mg	Green/White	Cap	–	–	–	PBI	Antianxiety
	832/T5	Timolol Maleate	5mg	Green	Tab	Round	–	–	PBI	Antihypertensive
	C5	Chlordiazepoxide	5mg	Yellow/Green	Cap	–	–	–	Geneva	Antianxiety
	Central 500/5	Hydrocodone & Acetaminophen	5mg/500mg	White	Tab	Oval	Y	N	Central	Analgesic
	G/P 5	Pindolol	5mg	White	Tab	Round	Y	N	Par	Anti-Hypertensive
	HD 5	Meperidine HCl	100mg	White	Tab	Round	N	N	Halsey	Analgesic
	Lederle 500 A5	Tetracycline HCl	500mg	Blue/Yellow	Cap	–	–	–	Lederle	Anti-Infective
	Lederle S 5	Vitamin/Mineral	n/a	Brown	Cap	–	–	–	Lederle	Vitamin
	LL E5	Erythromycin Sterate	500mg	Yellow	Tab	Oval	N	Y	Lederle	Anti-Infective
	LL F5	Prenatal Vitamin Combination	n/a	Pink	Tab	Capsule	Y	Y	Lederle	Vitamin

ID NO.	ID CODE	GENERIC NAME	STRENGTH	COLOR	FORM	SHAPE	SCORED	COATED	MFG.	USE
	LL H 5	Diethylcarbamazine Citrate	50mg	White	Tab	Round	Y	N	Lederle	Antiparasitic
	LL M5	Minocycline HCl	100mg.	Orange	Tab	Round	Y	Y	Lederle	Anti–Infective
	LL N5	Nystatin Oral	500,000 Units	Pink	Tab	Round	N	Y	Lederle	Anti–Infective
	LL U5	Aminophylline	200mg	White	Tab	Round	Y	N	Lederle	Bronchodilator
	LL V5	Verapamil HCl	120mg	White	Tab	Round	Y	N	Lederle	Antihypertensive
	LUCHEM 5	Hydrocodone Bitartrate with Acetaminophen	5mg/500mg	White	Tab	Oblong	Y	N	LuChem	Analgesic
	RR 5	Prednisone	5mg	White	Tab	Round	Y	N	RR	Steroid
	Rugby 5	Isosorbide SL	5mg	–	Tab	Round	–	–	Rugby	Vasodilator
	SKF 5	Trifluoperazine HCl	5mg	Blue	Tab	Round	–	Y	SKB	Tranquilizer
	W/5	Isosorbide Dinitrate SL	5mg	Pink	Tab	Round	N	N	Wyeth	Vasodilator
6	6	Detrothyroxine Sodium	6mg	Green	Tab	Oval	Y	N	Boots	Hypolipidemic
	6	Ibuprofen	600mg	White	Tab	Oval	Y	Y	Norton	Anti–Inflammatory
	BI/6	Clonidine HCl	0.1mg	Tan	Tab	Oval	Y	N	BI	Antihypertensive
	bp 6	Methocarbamol	750mg	White	Tab	Capsule	Y	N	Bolar	Muscle Relaxant
	LL F6	Prenatal Vitamin Combination	n/a.	Pink	Tab	Capsule	Y	Y	Lederle	Vitamin
	LL M6	Ethambutol HCl	100mg.	White	Tab	Round	N	Y	Lederle	Antituberculosis
	LL N6	Nystatin Vaginal	100,000 Units	Yellow	Tab	Oval	N	N	Lederle	Anti–Infective
	LL/L6	Vitamin	n/a	Brown	Cap	–	N	Y	Lederle	Vitamin
	M 6	Erythromycin Stearate	250mg	Pink	Tab	Round	N	Y	Mylan	Anti–Infective
	M 6	Erythromycin Stearate	250mg	Yellow	Tab	Round	N	Y	Mylan	Anti–Infective
	MP 6	Lorazepam	0.5mg	White	Tab	Round	Y	N	Mutual	Antianxiety
	Par/6	Dexchlorpheniramine Maleate	6mg	White	Tab	Oval	N	Y	Par	Antihistamine
	Rufen 6	Ibuprofen	600mg	White	Tab	Elongated	N	Y	Boots	Anti–Inflammatory
7	68–7	Desipramine HCl	10mg	Blue	Tab	Round	N	Y	Merrell	Antidepressant
	7/41 LuChem	Phenylpropanolamine HCl & Guaifenesin LA	75mg/400mg	Blue/White Speks	Tab	Oblong	Y	N	LuChem	Decongestant Comb.
	93 7	Chlorpropamide	250mg	Blue	Tab	Round	Y	N	Lemmon	Hypoglycemic
	BI/7	Clonidine HCl	0.2mg	Orange	Tab	Oval	Y	N	BI	Antihypertensive
	Ciba 7	Methylphenidate HCl	5mg	Yellow	Tab	Round	Y	N	Ciba	Psychostimulant
	GG L7	Atenolol	25mg	White	Tab	Round	Y	N	Geneva	Antihypertensive
	LL A 7	Atenolol	25mg	White	Tab	Round	Y	N	Lederle	Antihypertensive
	LL C7	Chlorthalidone	25mg	Orange	Tab	Round	Y	N	Lederle	Diuretic
	LL M7	Ethambutol HCl	400mg.	White	Tab	Round	Y	Y	Lederle	Antituberculous
	LL P7	Vitamin comb./ Stool Softener	n/a	Red	Cap	–	–	–	Lederle	Vitamin
	LL–F7	Prenatal Vitamin/Mineral	n/a	Pink	Tab	Oblong	N	Y	Lederle	Vitamin
	M 7	Erythromycin Stearate	500mg	Pink	Tab	Oval	N	Y	Mylan	Anti–Infective
	M 7	Erythromycin Stearate	500mg	Yellow	Tab	Oval	N	Y	Mylan	Anti–Infective
	MP 7	Hydroxyzine HCl	25mg	Purple	Tab	Round	N	Y	Mutual	Antipruritic
	R 7	Indapamide	1.25mg	Orange	Tab	Hexagonal	N	N	Arcola Labs	Antihypertensive
7.5	7.5	Phenylpropanolamine/Guaifenesin	75mg/600mg	White	Tab	Round	Y	N	Dura	Decongestant Comb.
8	8	Ibuprofen	800mg	White	Tab	Oval	Y	Y	Norton	Anti–Inflammatory
	BI/8	Clonidine HCl & Chlorthalidone	0.1mg/15mg	Pink	Tab	Oval	Y	N	BI	Antihypertensive
	GG8	Nylidrin	6mg	White	Tab	Round	N	Y	Geneva	Vasodilator
	K 8	Potassium Chloride SA	600mg (8mEq)	Orange	Tab	Round	N	Y	Alra	Potassium Supp.
	LL A8	Triamcinolone	8mg	Yellow	Tab	Oblong	Y	N	Lederle	Steroid
	LL P 8	Vitamin/Mineral	n/a	Maroon	Tab	Oblong	–	–	Lederle	Vitamin
	MP 8	Imipramine Hydrochloride	25mg	Brown	Tab	Round	N	Y	Mutual	Antidepressant
	PP 8	Imipramine HCl	10mg	Yellow	Tab	Round	N	Y	Eon	Antidepressant
	R 8	Indapamide	2.5mg	White	Tab	Hexagonal	N	N	Rorer	Antihypertensive
	Rufen 8	Ibuprofen	800mg	White	Tab	Elongated	N	Y	Boots	Anti–Inflammatory
	S 78–8	Thioridazine HCl	15mg	Rose	Tab	Round	N	Y	Sandoz	Tranquilizer
	USL 8	Potassium SR	600mg	Blue	Tab	Round	N	N	Upsher	Potassium Supp.
9	A9L	Trihexyphenidyl HCl	5mg	Blue	Cap	–	–	–	Lederle	Antiparkinson
	BI/9	Clonidine HCl & Chlorthalidone	0.2mg/15mg	Blue	Tab	Oval	Y	N	BI	Antihypertensive
	BL–LL–D9	Demeclocycline HCl	150mg	Coral	Cap	–	–	–	Lederle	Anti–Infective
	Lederle C9	Chlordiazepoxide HCl	5mg	Green/Yellow	Cap	–	–	–	Lederle	Antianxiety
	Lemmon 9	Phentermine HCl	37.5mg	Blue & White	Tab	Oblong	Y	N	Lemmon	Anorectic
	LL L9	Penicillin V Potassium	500mg	White	Tab	Round	Y	N	Lederle	Anti–Infective
	LL P9	Vitamin comb.	n/a	Red	Cap	–	–	–	Lederle	Vitamin
	M/9	Fluphenazine HCl	2.5mg	Yellow	Tab	Triangle	N	Y	Mylan	Tranquilizer
	P–9	Imipramine HCl	25mg	Brown	Tab	Round	N	Y	Eon	Antidepressant
	Wellcome Y9C/ 100	Zidovudine	100mg	White/Blue Band	Cap	–	–	–	BW	Antiviral
01	832 L01	L–Thyroxine Sodium	0.1mg	Yellow	Tab	Round	Y	N	PBI	Hormone
	biocraft 01	Amoxicillin	250mg	Caramel\Buff	Cap	–	N	N	Biocraft	Anti–Infective
	dp 01	Clonidine HCl	0.1mg	Tan	Tab	Round	Y	N	Duramed	Antihypertensive
	FO1/CPI	Folic Acid	1mg	Yellow	Tab	Round	–	–	Charlotte/Phoe	Antianemic
	SP 01	Furosemide	40mg	White	Tab	Round	Y	N	Superpharm	Diuretic
	U01	Paramethasone Acetate	2mg	Orange	Tab	Round	Y	N	Lilly	Steroid
02	832 L02	L–Thyroxine Sodium	0.2mg	White	Tab	Round	Y	N	PBI	Hormone
	biocraft 02	Dicloxacillin Sodium	250mg	Green\Lt.Green	Cap	–	N	N	Biocraft	Anti–Infective
	dp 02	Clonidine HCl	0.2mg	Orange	Tab	Round	Y	N	Duramed	Antihypertensive
	J02	Atropine Sulfate	0.4mg	White	Tab	Round	N	N	Lilly	Antispasmodic
	Lilly H02	Propoxyphene HCl	32mg	Pink	Cap	–	–	–	Lilly	Analgesic
	SP 02	Furosemide	20mg	White	Tab	Oval	N	N	Superpharm	Diuretic
03	832 L03	L–Thyroxine Sodium	0.3mg	Green	Tab	Round	Y	N	PBI	Hormone
	biocraft 03	Amoxicillin	500mg	Buff	Cap	–	N	N	Biocraft	Anti–Infective
	dp 03	Clonidine HCl	0.3mg	Peach	Tab	Round	Y	N	Duramed	Antihypertensive
	SKF S03	Trifluoperazine HCl	1mg	Blue	Tab	Round	N	Y	SKB	Tranquilizer
	U03	Acetohexamide	250mg	White	Tab	Capsule	Y	Y	Lilly	Antiglaucoma
04	biocraft 04	Dicloxacillin Sodium	500mg	Green\Lt.Green	Cap	–	–	–	Biocraft	Anti–Infective
	F04	Cycloserine	250mg	Red/Gray	Cap	–	–	–	Lilly	Anti–Infective
05	SKF S04	Trifluoperazine HCl	2mg	Blue	Tab	Round	N	Y	SKB	Tranquilizer
	832/05	Oxybutynin Chloride	5mg	Pink	Tab	Round	Y	N	PBI	Antispasmodic
	832/BM05	Benztropine Mesylate	0.5mg	White	Tab	Round	–	–	PBI	Antiparkinson
	A05	Potassium Chloride	300mg	Red	Tab	Round	N	Y	Lilly	Potassium Supp.
	biocraft 05	Ampicillin	250mg	Scarlet\Gray	Cap	–	–	–	Biocraft	Anti–Infective
	Central 131/05	Vitamin Combination	n/a	Blue	Tab	Oval	N	Y	Central	Vitamin
	U05	Erythromycin Estolate Chewable	125mg	Pink	Tab	Square	N	N	Lilly	Anti–Infective
06	A06	Potassium Iodide	300mg	Red	Tab	Round	N	Y	Lilly	Mineral Supp.
	biocraft 06	Ampicillin	500mg	Scarlet\Gray	Cap	–	–	–	Biocraft	Anti–Infective
	Par 06	Dexchlorpheniramine Maleate TD	6mg	White	Tab	Oval	N	Y	Par	Antihistamine
07	SKF S06	Trifluoperazine HCl	5mg	Blue	Tab	Round	N	Y	SKB	Tranquilizer
	A07/pB	Hydrocodone Bitartrate with Acetaminophen	5mg/500mg	White	Tab	Capsule	N	N	Martec	Analgesic
	BL\07	Penicillin G Potassium	200,000 Units	White	Tab	Round	N	N	Biocraft	Anti–Infective
	Central 131/07	Prednisone	5mg	Red	Tab	Round	N	Y	Central	Steroid
	SKF S07	Trifluoperazine HCl	10mg	Blue	Tab	Round	N	Y	SKB	Tranquilizer

ID NO.	ID CODE	GENERIC NAME	STRENGTH	COLOR	FORM	SHAPE	SCORED	COATED	MFG.	USE
	SL 07	Hydroxyzine HCl	10mg	White	Tab	Round	N	Y	Sidmak	Antipruritic
	SL 07	Hydroxyzine HCl	10mg	White	Tab	Round	N	Y	Sidmak	Antipruritic
	U07	Acetohexamide	500mg	Yellow	Tab	Capsule	Y	Y	Lilly	Antiglaucoma
08	0131 20/08	Ghlorpheniramine/Pseudoephedrine/APAP	2mg/30mg/325mg	Peach	Tab	Capsule	N	Y	Central	Antihistamine
	SL 08	Hydroxyzine HCl	25mg	White	Tab	Round	N	Y	Sidmak	Antipruritic
09	BL\09	Penicillin G Potassium	250,000 Units	White	Tab	Round	N	N	Biocraft	Anti–Infective
	H09	Erythromycin Estolate	250mg	Brown/Orange	Cap	–	–	–	Lilly	Anti–Infective
	J09	Codeine Sulfate	15mg	White	Tab	Round	N	N	Lilly	Analgesic
	SKF J09	Lithium Carbonate	300mg	Gray	Tab	Round	Y	N	SKB	Tranquilizer
	U09	Cyclothiazide	2mg	Blue	Tab	Capsule	Y	N	Lilly	Diuretic
10	832/10	Chlordiazepoxide HCl	10mg	Green/Black	Cap	–	–	–	PBI	Antianxiety
	832/10	Chlorpromazine	10mg	Tan	Tab	Round	N	Y	PBI	Tranquilizer
	832/10C	Diazepam	10mg	Blue	Tab	Round	Y	N	PBI	Antianxiety
	832/BC10	Baclofen	10mg	White	Tab	Round	–	–	PBI	Muscle Relaxant
	832/MS10	Metaproterenol Sulfate	10mg	White	Tab	Round	Y	N	PBI	Bronchodilator
	832/P10C	Prazepam	10mg	Green/White	Cap	–	–	–	PBI	Antianxiety
	832/T10	Timolol Maleate	10mg	Green	Tab	Round	–	–	PBI	Antihypertensive
	879 G10C 2	Acetaminophen with Codeine Phosphate	300mg/15mg	White	Tab	Round	N	N	Halsey	Analgesic
	93 10	Chlorpropamide	100mg	Blue	Tab	Round	Y	N	Lemmon	Hypoglycemic
	A 10	Nifedipine	10mg	Greyish Pink	Tab	Round	–	–	Miles	Antihypertensive
	BI/10	Clonidine HCl & Chlorthalidone	0.3mg/15mg	White	Tab	Oval	Y	N	BI	Antihypertensive
	BI/10	Mesoridazine Besylate	10mg	Red	Tab	Round	N	Y	BI	Tranquilizer
	BL\10	Penicillin G Potassium	400,000 Units	White	Tab	Round	N	N	Biocraft	Anti–Infective
	C10	Chlordiazepoxide	10mg	Black/Green	Cap	–	–	–	Geneva	Antianxiety
	dp 10	Propranolol	10mg	Peach	Tab	Round	Y	N	Duramed	Antihypertensive
	G BN/10	Baclofen	10mg	White	Tab	Round	Y	N	Genpharm	Muscle Relaxant
	G TN/10	Tamoxifen Citrate	10mg	White	Tab	Round	N	N	Genpharm	Antineoplastic
	G/P 10	Pindolol	10mg	White	Tab	Round	Y	N	Par	Antihypertensive
	H10	Vitamin Combination	n/a	Pink/Blue	Cap	–	–	–	Lilly	Vitamin
	J10	Codeine Sulfate	30mg	White	Tab	Round	N	N	Lilly	Analgesic
	JANSSEN AST/10	Astemizole	10mg	White	Tab	Round	Y	N	Janssen	Antihistamine
	JANSSEN P 10	Cisapride	10mg	White	Tab	Round	Y	N	Janssen	Antireflux
	K 10	Potassium Chloride SA	750mg (10mEq)	Peach	Tab	Capsule	N	Y	Alra	Potassium Supp.
	KCl 10/Bolar/KV	Potassium Chloride	10mEq	Clear	Cap	–	–	–	Bolar	Potassuim Supp.
	Key 10	Potassium Chloride SR	10mEq	White	Tab	Oblong	N	N	Key	Potassium Supp.
	Lederle C10	Chlordiazepoxide HCl	10mg	Green/Black	Cap	–	–	–	Lederle	Antianxiety
	LL A10	Aminocaproic Acid	500mg	White	Tab	Round	Y	N	Lederle	Antifibrinolytic
	LL B10	Benztropine Mesylate	1mg	White	Tab	Oval	Y	N	Lederle	Antiparkinson
	LL E10	Erythromycin Ethylsuccinate	400mg	Beige	Tab	Capsule	Y	Y	Lederle	Anti–Infective
	LL L10	Penicillin V Potassium	250mg	White	Tab	Round	Y	N	Lederle	Anti–Infective
	LL N10	Neomycin Sulfate	500mg	White	Tab	Round	N	N	Lederle	Anti–Infective
	LL T10	Thioridazine HCl	10mg	Orange	Tab	Round	N	Y	Lederle	Tranquilizer
	M 10	Propranolol	10mg	Orange	Tab	Round	Y	N	Martec	Antihypertensive
	MET–10/832	Metoclopramide HCl	10mg	White	Tab	Round	Y	N	PBI	Antireflux
	MP 10	Amitriptyline HCl	10mg	Pink	Tab	Round	N	Y	Mutual	Antidepressant
	RR 10	Prednisone	10mg	Blue	Tab	Round	Y	N	RR	Steroid
	Rugby 10	Isoxsuprine HCl	10mg	–	Tab	Round	–	–	Rugby	Vasodilator
	SKF J10	Lithium Carbonate	450mg	Buff	Tab	Round	Y	N	SKB	Tranquilizer
	SKF/ H10	Triamterene	100mg	Yellow	Tab	Round	Y	N	SKB	Diuretic
	USL 10	Potassium SR	750mg	Orange	Tab	Round	N	N	Upsher	Potassium Supp.
11	W/10	Isosorbide Dinitrate SL	10mg	White	Tab	Round	N	N	Wyeth	Vasodilator
	(triangle) 11	Biperiden HCl & Biperiden Lactate	2mg	White	Tab	Round	Y	N	Knoll	Antiparkinson
	1 LL L11	Levothyroxine Sodium	0.1mg	Yellow	Tab	Round	N	N	Lederle	Hormone
	879 G11C 3	Acetaminophen with Codeine Phosphate	300mg/30mg	White	Tab	Round	N	N	Halsey	Analgesic
	93 11 / 2	Aspirin & Codeine	325mg/15mg	White	Tab	Round	N	N	Lemmon	Analgesic
	B 11	Inert Tablets	n/a	Green	Tab	Round	N	N	Berlex	Inert Tablets
	BI/11	Clonidine HCl	0.3mg	Peach	Tab	Oval	Y	N	BI	Antihypertensive
	CS 11 – Silver	Multivitamin/Minerals	n/a	Gray	Tab	Oblong	–	–	Lederle	Vitamin
	dp 11	Trifluoperazine HCl	1mg	Lavender	Tab	Round	N	Y	Duramed	Tranquilizer
	GG11	Chlorthalidone	25mg	Yellow	Tab	Round	Y	N	Geneva	Diuretic
	GL 535–11	Acetaminophen/Caffeine/Butalbital	325/40/50mg	White	Tab	Round	–	–	Gilbert	Analgesic
	IKA 11	Clomiphene Citrate	50mg	White	Tab	Round	Y	N	Serono	Hormone
	J11	Codeine Sulfate	60mg	White	Tab	Round	N	N	Lilly	Analgesic
	Lederle C11	Chlordiazepoxide HCl	25mg	Green/White	Cap	–	–	–	Lederle	Antianxiety
	Lederle P11	Papaverine HCl TD	150mg	Natural/Brown	Cap	–	–	–	Lederle	Vasodilator
	LL B11	Benztropine Mesylate	2mg	White	Tab	Round	Y	N	Lederle	Antiparkinson
	LL D11	Demeclocycline HCl	150mg	Red	Tab	Round	N	Y	Lederle	Anti–Infective
	LL F11	Furosemide	20mg	White	Tab	Round	N	N	Lederle	Diuretic
	LL H11	Hydralazine	25mg	Red	Tab	Round	N	Y	Lederle	Antihypertensive
	LL I11	Imipramine HCl	10mg	Yellow	Tab	Round	N	N	Lederle	Antidepressant
	LL N11	Naproxen	250mg	Green	Tab	Round	–	Y	Lederle	Anti–Inflammatory
	LL Q11	Quinidine Sulfate	200mg	White	Tab	Round	Y	N	Lederle	Antiarrhythmic
	LL T11	Thiamine HCl	50mg	White	Tab	Round	N	N	Lederle	Vitamin
	LL\A11	Trihexyphenidyl HCL	2mg	White	TAB	Round	–	–	Lederle	Antispasmodic
	M/11	Penicillin VK	250mg	White	Tab	Oval	N	N	Mylan	Anti–Infective
	MP 11	Dipyridamole	25mg	White	Tab	Round	N	Y	Mutual	Antiplatelet
	P–11	Butabarbital Sodium	15mg	Purple	Tab	Round	Y	N	Eon	Sedative
	R 11	Verapamil	40mg	–	Tab	Round	–	–	Rugby	Antihypertensive
	SKF/ H11	Triamterene	50mg	Yellow	Tab	Round	Y	N	SKB	Diuretic
	SL 11	Dipyridamole	25mg	White	Tab	Round	N	Y	Sidmak	Antiplatelet
12	10 LL C12	Leucovorin Calcium	10mg	Yellow	Tab	Square	Y	N	Lederle	Antineoplastic
	2 LL L12	Levothyroxine Sodium	0.2mg	Pink	Tab	Round	N	N	Lederle	Hormone
	879 G12C 4	Acetaminophen with Codeine Phosphate	300mg/60mg	White	Tab	Round	N	N	Halsey	Analgesic
	93 12 / 3	Aspirin & Codeine	325mg/30mg	White	Tab	Round	N	N	Lemmon	Analgesic
	BI/12	Bisacodyl	5mg	Yellow	Tab	Round	N	Y	BI	Laxative
	biocraft 12	Oxacillin	250mg	Blue Opaque	Cap	–	–	N	Biocraft	Anti–Infective
	dp 12	Trifluoperazine HCl	2mg	Lavender	Tab	Round	N	Y	Duramed	Tranquilizer
	GG 12	Medroxyprogesterone Acetate	10mg	White	Tab	Round	N	N	Solvay	Steroid
	GG12	Medroxyprogesterone Acetate	10mg	White	Tab	Round	N	N	PBI	Hormone
	GL 535–12	Acetaminophen/Caffeine/Butalbital	325/40/50mg	White	Cap	–	–	–	Gilbert	Analgesic
	LL D12	Demeclocycline HCl	300mg	Red	Tab	Round	N	Y	Lederle	Anti–Infective
	LL F12	Furosemide	40mg	White	Tab	Round	Y	N	Lederle	Diuretic
	LL H12	Hydralazine	50mg	Red	Tab	Round	N	Y	Lederle	Antihypertensive
	LL I12	Imipramine HCl	25mg	Salmon	Tab	Round	N	Y	Lederle	Antidepressant
	LL M12	Meclizine HCl	12.5mg	Blue/White	Tab	Oval	N	N	Lederle	Antivertigo

ID NO.	ID CODE	GENERIC NAME	STRENGTH	COLOR	FORM	SHAPE	SCORED	COATED	MFG.	USE
	LL S12	Spironolactone & Hydrochlorothiazide	25mg/25mg	White	Tab	Round	Y	N	Lederle	Diuretic
	LL T12	Thiamine HCl	100mg	White	Tab	Round	N	N	Lederle	Vitamin
	LL A12	Trihexyphenidyl HCL	5mg	White	TAB	Round	–	–	Lederle	Antispasmodic
	M/12	Penicillin VK	500mg	White	Tab	Round	Y	N	Mylan	Anti-Infective
	MP 12	Thioridazine HCl	10mg	Yellow	Tab	Round	N	Y	Mutual	Tranquilizer
	PP–12	Ferrous Sulfate	325mg	Red	Tab	Round	N	Y	Eon	Iron Supp.
	SKF E12	Dextroamphetamine Sulfate	5mg	Brown/Natural	Cap	–	–	Y	SKB	Psychostimulant
	SKF T 12	Cimetidine	200mg	Green	Tab	Round	–	Y	SKB	Anti-ulcer
13	25 LL A13	Amoxapine	25mg	White	Tab	Heptagonal	Y	N	Lederle	Antidepressant
	3 LL L13	Levothyroxine Sodium	0.3mg	Green	Tab	Round	N	N	Lederle	Hormone
	93 13 / 4	Aspirin & Codeine	325mg/60mg	White	Tab	Round	N	N	Lemmon	Analgesic
	bp 13	Chlorothiazide	500mg	White	Tab	Round	Y	N	Bolar	Diuretic
	Ciba 13	Reserpine & Hydrochlorothiazide	0.1mg/25mg	Orange	Tab	Round	N	N	Ciba	Antihypertensive
	dp 13	Trifluoperazine HCl	5mg	Lavender	Tab	Round	N	Y	Duramed	Tranquilizer
	GG13	Chlorthalidone	50mg	Green	Tab	Round	Y	N	Geneva	Diuretic
	J13	Colchicine	0.6mg	White	Tab	Round	N	N	Lilly	Antigout
	LL C13	Chlorothiazide	250mg	White	Tab	Round	Y	N	Lederle	Diuretic
	LL F13	Furosemide	80mg	White	Tab	Round	Y	N	Lederle	Diuretic
	LL I13	Imipramine HCl	50mg	Green	Tab	Round	N	Y	Lederle	Antidepressant
	LL M13	Meclizine HCl	25mg	Yellow/White	Tab	Oval	N	N	Lederle	Antivertigo
	LL P13	Papaverine HCl	100mg	White	Tab	Round	N	N	Lederle	Vasodilator
	LL Q13	Quinidine Gluconate SR	324mg	White	Tab	Round	Y	N	Lederle	Antiarrhythmic
	LL S13	Spironolactone	25mg	White	Tab	Round	Y	N	Lederle	Diuretic
	LL T13	Sulfamethoxazole & Trimethoprim	400mg/80mg	White	Tab	Round	Y	N	Lederle	Anti-Infective
	M 13	Tolbutamide	500mg	White	Tab	Round	Y	N	Mylan	Hypoglycemic
	MP 13	Hydroxyzine HCl	50mg	Purple	Tab	Round	N	Y	Mutual	Antipruritic
	PP–13	Ferrous Sulfate	325mg	Green	Tab	Round	N	Y	Eon	Iron Supp.
	SKF E13	Dextroamphetamine Sulfate	10mg	Brown/Natural	Cap	–	–	–	SKB	Psychostimulant
	SKF T 13	Cimetidine	300mg	Green	Tab	Round	–	Y	SKB	Antiulcer
14	(triangle) 14	Ephedrine,Pb,Theophylline,Potassium Iodide	24/24/65/320mg	White	Tab	Round	Y	N	Knoll	Bronchodilator Comb.
	25mg LL H14	Hydrochlorothiazide	25mg	Peach	Tab	Round	Y	N	Lederle	Diuretic
	A14	Thyroid	30mg	Red	Tab	Round	N	Y	Lilly	Hormone
	biocraft 14	Oxacillin	500mg	Blue Opaque	Cap	–	N	N	Biocraft	Anti-Infective
	dp 14	Trifluoperazine HCl	10mg	Lavender	Tab	Round	N	Y	Duramed	Tranquilizer
	F14	Ephedrine Sulfate & Amobarbital	25mg/50mg	Yellow	Cap	–	–	–	Lilly	Antiasthmatic
	Geigy 14	Phenylbutazone	100mg	Red	Tab	Round	N	Y	Geigy	Anti-Inflammatory
	GG14	Prednisolone	5mg	Peach	Tab	Round	Y	N	Geneva	Steroid
	LL C14	Chlorothiazide	500mg	White	Tab	Round	Y	N	Lederle	Diuretic
	LL S14	Sulfasalazine	500mg	Brown	Tab	Round	Y	N	Lederle	Anti-Inflammatory
	LL T14	Thyroid	65mg	Tan	Tab	Round	N	N	Lederle	Hormone
	LL–A14	Amiloride HCl & Hydrochlorothiazide	5mg/50mg	Yellow	Tab	Round	Y	N	Lederle	Antihypertensive
	M 14	Methotrexate	2.5mg	Orange	Tab	Round	Y	N	Mylan	Antineoplastic
	MP 14	Thioridazine HCl	25mg	Yellow	Tab	Round	N	Y	Mutual	Tranquilizer
	PP 14	Chlorpheniramine	4mg	Yellow	Tab	Round	Y	N	Eon	Antihistamine
	SKF D14	Liothyronine Sodium	5mcg	White	Tab	Round	Y	N	SKB	Hormone
	SKF E14	Dextroamphetamine Sulfate	15mg	Brown/Natural	Cap	–	–	–	SKB	Psychostimulant
	SP 14	Diazepam	2mg	White	Tab	Round	Y	N	Superpharm	Antianxiety
15	50 LL A15	Amoxapine	50mg	Orange	Tab	Heptagonal	Y	N	Lederle	Antidepressant
	50mg LL H15	Hydrochlorothiazide	50mg	Peach	Tab	Round	Y	N	Lederle	Diuretic
	832 L15	L–Thyroxine Sodium	0.15mg	Blue	Tab	Round	Y	N	PBI	Hormone
	832/ TEM15	Temazepam	15mg	Green/White	Cap	–	–	–	PBI	Hypnotic
	A15	Thyroid	60mg	Red	Tab	Round	N	Y	Lilly	Hormone
	BL\15	Penicillin V Potassium	250mg	White	Tab	Round	N	N	Biocraft	Anti-Infective
	CL15	Nylidrin	12mg	White	Tab	Round	Y	N	Geneva	Vasodilator
	DAN–P 15	Phenobarbital	15mg	White	Tab	Round	Y	N	Danbury	Sedative
	dp 15	Diazepam	2mg	White	Tab	Round	Y	N	Duramed	Antianxiety
	F15	Comb. Liver Stomach Conc./Iron/B Vitamins	n/a	Red	Cap	–	–	–	Lilly	Hematinic
	GG15	Nylidrin	12mg	White	Tab	Round	Y	N	Geneva	Vasodilator
	Lederle F15	Flurazepam	15mg	Blue/White	Cap	–	–	–	Lederle	Hypnotic
	Lederle Q15	Quinine Sulfate	325mg	Transparent	Cap	–	–	–	Lederle	Muscle Relaxant
	LL C15	Chlorthalidone	50mg	Blue	Tab	Round	Y	N	Lederle	Diuretic
	LL I15	Isosorbide Dinitrate	5mg	Pink	Tab	Round	Y	N	Lederle	Antianginal
	M 15	Diphenoxylate HCl and Atropine Sulfate	2.5mg/0.025mg	White	Tab	Round	N	N	Mylan	Antidiarrheal
	M 15	Diphenoxylate/Atropine	2.5mg/0.025mg	–	Tab	–	–	–	Roxane	Antidiarrheal
	MP 15	Dipyridamole	50mg	White	Tab	Round	N	Y	Mutual	Antiplatelet
	P–15	Phenobarbital	15mg	White	Tab	Round	Y	N	Eon	Sedative
	PF M 15	Morphine Sulfate	15mg	White	Tab	Round	Y	N	PF	Analgesic
	PF M 15	Morphine Sulfate	15mg	Blue	Tab	Round	N	Y	PF	Analgesic
	SP 15	Diazepam	5mg	Yellow	Tab	Round	Y	N	Superpharm	Antianxiety
	UPJOHN 15	Cortisone Acetate	5mg	White	Tab	Round	Y	N	Upjohn	Steroid
16	BIOCRAFT/16	Penicillin V Potassium	250mg	White	Tab	Oval	–	N	Biocraft	Anti-Infective
	BL/16	Penicillin V Potassium	250mg	White	Tab	Oval	–	N	Biocraft	Anti-Infective
	Ciba 16	Methylphenidate HCl SR	20mg	White	Tab	Round	N	Y	Ciba	Psychostimulant
	F16	Comb. Liver Stomach Conc./Iron/B Vitamins	n/a.	Red	Cap	–	–	–	Lilly	Hematinic
	Lederle D16	Dicloxacillin Sodium	250mg	Green	Cap	–	–	–	Lederle	Anti-Infective
	LL A 16	Triamcinolone	16mg	White	Tab	Oglong	Y	N	Lederle	Steroid
	LL C16	Chlorpheniramine Maleate	4mg	Yellow	Tab	Round	Y	N	Lederle	Antihistamine
	LL I16	Isosorbide Dinitrate	10mg	White	Tab	Round	Y	N	Lederle	Antianginal
	LL S 16	Sulindac	150mg	Yellow	Tab	Round	Y	N	Lederle	Anti-Inflammatory
	LL T16	Sulfamethoxazole & Trimethoprim	800mg/160mg	White	Tab	Oval	Y	N	Lederle	Anti-Infective
	PP–16	Triprolidine & Pseudoephedrine	2.5mg/60mg	White	Tab	Round	Y	N	Eon	Decongestant Comb.
	SKF D16	Liothyronine Sodium	25mcg	White	Tab	Round	Y	N	SKB	Hormone
	SP 16	Diazepam	10mg	Blue	Tab	Round	Y	N	Superpharm	Antianxiety
17	100 LL A17	Amoxapine	100mg	Blue	Tab	Heptagonal	Y	N	Lederle	Antidepressant
	400/000 LL P17	Penicillin G Potassium	400,000 Units	White	Tab	Round	Y	N	Lederle	Anti-Infective
	BI/17	Dipyridamole	25mg	Orange	Tab	Round	N	Y	BI	Antiplatelet
	BL\17	Penicillin V Potassium	500mg	White	Tab	Round	Y	N	Biocraft	Anti-Infective
	H17	Nortriptyline Hydrochloride	10mg	Yellow/White	Cap	–	–	–	Lilly	Antidepressant
	ICN A17	Diphenhydramine HCl	25mg	Blue/Pink	Cap	–	–	–	ICN	Antihistamine
	Lederle C17	Chlorpheniramine Maleate TD	8mg	Green/Natural	Cap	–	–	–	Lederle	Antihistamine
	Lederle D17	Dicloxacillin Sodium	500mg	Green	Cap	–	–	–	Lederle	Anti-Infective
	LL G17	Gemfibrozil	600mg	White	Tab	Oval	N	Y	Lederle	Antihyperlipidemic
	LL H17	Hydroxyzine HCl	10mg	Lavender	Tab	Round	N	Y	Lederle	Antipruritic
	LL L17	Levothyroxine Sodium	0.15mg	Blue	Tab	Round	Y	N	Lederle	Hormone
	LL N17	Naproxen	375mg	Lavender	Tab	Capsule	–	Y	Lederle	Anti-Inflammatory

ID NO.	ID CODE	GENERIC NAME	STRENGTH	COLOR	FORM	SHAPE	SCORED	COATED	MFG.	USE
	LL S 17	Sulindac	200mg	Yellow	Tab	Round	Y	N	Lederle	Anti–Inflammatory
	LL T17	Tolbutamide	500mg	White	Tab	Round	Y	N	Lederle	Hypoglycemic
	MP 17	Thioridazine HCl	50mg	Yellow	Tab	Round	N	Y	Mutual	Tranquilizer
	PP–17	Baclofen	10mg	White	Tab	Round	Y	N	Eon	Muscle Relaxant
	SKF D17	Liothyronine Sodium	50mcg	White	Tab	Round	Y	N	SKB	Hormone
18	150 LL A18	Amoxapine	150mg	Peach	Tab	Heptagonal	Y	N	Lederle	Antidepressant
	18–0010	Potassium Chloride CR	750mg	Clear	Cap	–	–	–	Penwalt	Potassium Supp.
	BI/18	Dipyridamole	50mg	Orange	Tab	Round	N	Y	BI	Antiplatelet
	BL\18	Neomycin Sulfate	500mg	White	Tab	Round	Y	N	Biocraft	Anti–Infective
	GG 18	Perphenazine	2mg	White	Tab	Round	N	Y	Geneva	Tranquilizer
	ICN A18	Diphenhydramine HCl	50mg	Pink/White	Cap	–	–	–	ICN	Antihistamine
	Lederle C18	Chlorpheniramine Maleate TD	12mg	Green/Natural	Cap	–	–	–	Lederle	Antihistamine
	LL H18	Hydroxyzine HCl	25mg	Fuchsia	Tab	Round	N	Y	Lederle	Antipruritic
	MP 18	Dipyridamole	75mg	White	Tab	Round	N	Y	Mutual	Antiplatelet
	PP–18	Baclofen	20mg	White	Tab	Round	Y	N	Eon	Muscle Relaxant
19	UPJOHN 18	Benzphetamine HCl	25mg	Yellow	Tab	Round	N	N	Upjohn	Appetite Suppresant
	555/19	Hydrochlorothiazide HCl	25mg	Peach	Tab	Round	Y	N	Barr	Diuretic
	832/P19C	Hydrocodone Bitartrate / Acetaminophen	5mg/500mg	White	Tab	Capsule	Y	N	PBI	Analgesic
	A/19–LL	Acetaminophen	500mg	White	Tab	Round	Y	N	Lederle	Analgesic
	A19	Diethylstilbestrol	0.1mg	Red	Tab	Round	N	Y	Lilly	Hormone
	BI/19	Dipyridamole	75mg	Orange	Tab	Round	N	Y	BI	Antiplatelet
	BL\19	Imipramine Hydrochloride	10mg	Yellow	Tab	Round	N	Y	Biocraft	Antidepressant
	E 19	Disipramine	25mg	Blue	Tab	Round	N	Y	Eon	Antidepressant
	F19	Liver Stomach Concentrate	n/a	Brown	Cap	–	–	–	Lilly	Hematinic
	H19	Nortriptyline Hydrochloride	25mg	Yellow/White	Cap	–	–	–	Lilly	Antidepressant
	Lederle I19	Indomethacin	25mg	Pink/White	Cap	–	–	–	Lederle	Anti–Inflammatory
	LL C19	Chlorzoxazone & Acetaminophen	250mg/300mg	Yellow	Tab	Round	Y	N	Lederle	Muscle Relaxant
	LL M19	Methocarbamol	500mg	White	Tab	Round	Y	N	Lederle	Muscle Relaxant
	LL T19	Tolazamdie	100mg	White	Tab	Round	Y	N	Lederle	Hypoglycemic
	PP 19	Desipramine HCl	25mg	Blue	Tab	Round	N	Y	Eon	Antidepressant
	SKF E19	Dextroamphetamine Sulfate	5mg	Orange	Tab	Triangular	Y	N	SKB	Psychostimulant
20	Wyeth 19	Promethazine	12.5mg	Orange	Tab	Round	Y	N	Wyeth	Antiemetic
	0131 20/08	Ghlorpheniramine/Pseudoephedrine/APAP	2mg/30mg/325mg	Peach	Tab	Capsule	N	Y	Central	Antihistamine
	20/20	Caffeine	175mg	White/Speckled	Tab	Oblong	Y	N	B & M Labs	Stimulant
	555/20	Hydrochlorothiazide HCl	50mg	Peach	Tab	Round	Y	N	Barr	Diuretic
	832/BC20	Baclofen	20mg	White	Tab	Round	–	–	PBI	Muscle Relaxant
	832/MS20	Metaproterenol Sulfate	20mg	White	Tab	Round	Y	N	PBI	Bronchodilator
	832/T20	Timolol Maleate	20mg	Green	Tab	Round	–	–	PBI	Antihypertensive
	879 G20C	Oxycodone HCl & Acetaminophen	5mg/325mg	White	Tab	Round	Y	N	Halsey	Analgesic
	A20/A20	Orciprenaline Sulfate	20mg	White	Tab	Round	–	n	BI	Bronchodilator
	BL\20	Imipramine Hydrochloride	25mg	Rust	Tab	Round	N	Y	Biocraft	Antidepressant
	Central 20	Vitamin/Mineral Supp.	–	Lavender	Tab	Round	N	Y	Central	Vitamin Supp.
	dp 20	Propranolol	20mg	Blue	Tab	Round	Y	N	Duramed	Antihypertensive
	G BN/20	Baclofen	20mg	White	Tab	Round	Y	N	Genpharm	Muscle Relaxant
	G TN/20	Tamoxifen Citrate	20mg	White	Tab	Octagonal	N	N	Genpharm	Antineoplastic
	Geigy 20	Imipramine Pamoate	75mg	Coral	Cap	–	–	–	Geigy	Antidepressant
	H 20	Chlorthalidone	50mg	Aqua	Tab	Square	–	N	Rorer	Diuretic
	J20	Quinidine Sulfate	200mg	White	Tab	Round	Y	N	Lilly	Antiarrhythmic
	JANSSEN P 20	Cisapride	20mg	White	Tab	Round	Y	N	Janssen	Antireflux
	Key 20	Potassium Chloride SR	20mEq	White	Tab	Oblong	Y	N	Key	Potassium Supp.
	Lederle I20	Indomethacin	50mg	Pink/White	Cap	–	–	–	Lederle	Anti–Inflammatory
	Lederle N20	Nitroglycerin SR	2.5mg	Purple/Natural	Cap	–	–	–	Lederle	Antianginal
	LEDERLE/A20	Acetaminophen	500mg	Blue	Cap	–	–	–	Lederle	Analgesic
	LL M20	Methocarbamol	750mg	White	Tab	Capsule	Y	N	Lederle	Muscle Relaxant
	LL T20	Tolazamide	250mg	White	Tab	Round	Y	N	Lederle	Hypoglycemic
	LL/F20	Ferrous Sulfate	300mg	Red	Tab	Round	N	Y	Lederle	Mineral
	M 20	Propranolol	20mg	Blue	Tab	Round	Y	N	Martec	Antihypertensive
	MILES 20	Nifedipine	20mg	Greyish Pink	Tab	Round	–	–	Miles	Antihypertensive
	MP 20	Ergoloid Mesylates	1mg	White	Tab	–	N	N	Mutual	Vasodilator
	RR 20	Prednisone	20mg	Yellow	Tab	Round	Y	N	RR	Steroid
21	Rugby 20	Isoxsuprine HCl	20mg	–	Tab	Round	–	–	Rugby	Vasodilator
	SP 20	Pseudoephedrine HCl	60mg	White	Tab	Round	Y	N	Superpharm	Decongestant
	21	Chlorthalidone	100mg	White	Tab	Round	N	N	Rorer	Diuretic
	555/153 LL P21	Phenobarbital	30mg	White	Tab	Round	N	N	Lederle	Sedative
	93 21	Diltiazem HCl ER	60mg	White/Pink	Cap	–	–	–	Lemmon	Antianginal
	A/21–LL	Acetaminophen	325mg	White	Tab	Round	Y	N	Lederle	Analgesic
	B 21	Levonorgestrel/Ethinyl Estradiol	0.15mg/0.03mg	Orange	Tab	Round	N	N	Berlex	Hormone
	BL\21	Imipramine Hydrochloride	50mg	Green	Tab	Round	N	Y	Biocraft	Antidepressant
	C 21	Hydrocodone Bitartrate/Aspirin	5mg/500mg	White/Pink Specks	Tab	Oval	Y	N	Central	Analgesic
	C 21	Hydrocodone Bitartrate with Acetaminophen	5mg/500mg	Pink(mottled)	Tab	Unique	N	N	Central	Analgesic
	GG21	Furosemide	20mg	White	Tab	Round	Y	N	Geneva	Diuretic
	ICN A21	Allopurinol	100mg	White	Tab	Round	Y	N	ICN	Antigout
	Lederle N21	Nitroglycerin SR	6.5mg	Blue/Yellow	Cap	–	–	–	Lederle	Antianginal
	LL H21	Hydroxyzine HCl	50mg	Purple	Tab	Round	N	Y	Lederle	Antipruritic
	LL I21	Isoxsuprine HCl	10mg	White	Tab	Round	N	N	Lederle	Vasodilator
	LL M21	Methyldopa	125mg	Peach	Tab	Round	N	Y	Lederle	Antihypertensive
	LL/F21	Ferrous Gluconate	300mg	Gree	Tab	Round	N	Y	Lederle	Mineral
	M21	Penicillin G Potassium	250,000 Units	White	Tab	Round	Y	N	Mylan	Anti–Infective
	P–21	Imipramine HCL	50mg	Green	Tab	Round	Y	N	Eon	Antidepressant
22	W N21	Nalidixic Acid	250mg	Yellow	Tab	Oblong	N	N	Winthrop	Anti–Infective
	93 22	Diltiazem HCl ER	90mg	Pink/Yellow	Cap	–	–	–	Lemmon	Antianginal
	A22	Diethylstilbestrol	1mg	Red	Tab	Round	N	Y	Lilly	Hormone
	A22–LL	Acetaminophen	500mg	White	Tab	Capsule	N	N	Lederle	Analgesic
	BL\22	Amitriptyline Hydrochloride	10mg	Pink	Tab	Round	N	Y	Biocraft	Antidepressant
	Ciba 22	Hydrochlorothiazide	25mg	Pink	Tab	Round	Y	N	Ciba	Diuretic
	Geigy 22	Imipramine Pamoate	150mg	Coral	Cap	–	–	–	Geigy	Antidepressant
	GG22	Pseudoephedrine	60mg	White	Tab	Round	Y	N	Geneva	Decongestant
	H 22	Chlorthalidone	25mg	Peach	Tab	Square	–	N	Rorer	Diuretic
	ICN A22	Allopurinol	200mg	Orange	Tab	Rectangular	Y	N	ICN	Antigout
	Lederle D22	Doxycycline Hyclate	50mg	Green/Brown	Cap	–	–	–	Lederle	Anti-Infective
	Lederle N22	Nitroglycerin SR	9mg	Amber/Green	Cap	–	–	–	Lederle	Antianginal
	LL C22	Chlorpromazine	25mg	Tan	Tab	Round	N	Y	Lederle	Tranquilizer
	LL F22	Fenoprophen Calcium	600mg	White	Tab	Oblong	N	Y	Lederle	Anti–Inflammatory
	LL H22	Reserpine/Hydralazine HCl/Hydrochlorothiazide	0.1mg/25mg/15mg	Brown	Tab	Round	N	N	Lederle	Antihypertensive
	LL I22	Isoxsuprine HCl	20mg	White	Tab	Round	Y	N	Lederle	Vasodilator

ID NO.	ID CODE	GENERIC NAME	STRENGTH	COLOR	FORM	SHAPE	SCORED	COATED	MFG.	USE
	LL M22	Methyldopa	250mg	Peach	Tab	Round	N	Y	Lederle	Antihypertensive
	LL T22	Tolazamide	500mg	White	Tab	Round	Y	N	Lederle	Hypoglycemic
	MP 22	Hydralazine HCl	10mg	White	Tab	Round	N	N	Mutual	Antihypertensive
	RC 22	Penbutolol Sulfate	20mg	Yellow	Tab	Capsule	Y	–	R &C	Antihypertension
	W N22	Nalidixic Acid	500mg	Yellow	Tab	Oblong	Y	N	Winthrop	Anti–Infective
	W V22	Stanozolol	2mg	Speckled Buff	Tab	Oblong	N	N	Winthrop	Steroid
23	93 23	Diltiazem HCl ER	120mg	Pink/Orange	Cap	–	–	–	Lemmon	Antianginal
	BL\23	Amitriptyline Hydrochloride	25mg	Green	Tab	Round	N	Y	Biocraft	Antidepressant
	F23	Amobarbital Sodium	60mg	Blue/Blue	Cap	–	–	–	Lilly	Hypnotic
	Geigy 23	Baclofen	10mg	White	Tab	Oval	Y	N	Geigy	Muscle Relaxant
	ICN A23	Allopurinol	300mg	Orange	Tab	Round	Y	N	ICN	Antigout
	Lederle D23	Dicyclomine HCl	10mg	Blue	Cap	–	–	–	Lederle	Antispasmodic
	LL A23	Acetaminophen with Codeine	300mg/30mg	White	Tab	Round	N	N	Lederle	Analgesic
	LL C23	Chlorpromazine	50mg	Tan	Tab	Round	N	Y	Lederle	Tranquilizer
	LL I23	Isosorbide Dinitrate SA	40mg	Green	Tab	Round	Y	N	Lederle	Antianginal
	LL M23	Methyldopa	500mg	Peach	Tab	Round	N	Y	Lederle	Antihypertensive
	LL N23	Nylidrin HCl	6mg	White	Tab	Round	Y	N	Lederle	Vasodilator
	LL T23	Triprolidine HCl & Pseudoephedrine HCl	2.5mg/60mg	White	Tab	Round	Y	N	Lederle	Decongestant Comb.
	M 23	Diltiazem HCl	30mg	White	Tab	Round	N	Y	Mylan	Antianginal
	SP 23	Chlorthalidone	25mg	Peach	Tab	Round	N	N	Superpharm	Diuretic
	U23	Isoniazid	300mg	White	Tab	Round	Y	N	Lilly	Anti–Infective
	UPJOHN 23	Cortisone Acetate	10mg	White	Tab	Round	Y	N	Upjohn	Steroid
	W N23	Nalidixic Acid	1000mg	Yellow	Tab	Oval	Y	N	Winthrop	Anti–Infective
	93 23	Diltiazem HCl ER	120mg	Pink/Orange	Cap	–	–	–	Lemmon	Antianginal
	BL\23	Amitriptyline Hydrochloride	25mg	Green	Tab	Round	N	Y	Biocraft	Antidepressant
	F23	Amobarbital Sodium	60mg	Blue/Blue	Cap	–	–	–	Lilly	Hypnotic
	Geigy 23	Baclofen	10mg	White	Tab	Oval	Y	N	Geigy	Muscle Relaxant
	ICN A23	Allopurinol	300mg	Orange	Tab	Round	Y	N	ICN	Antigout
	Lederle D23	Dicyclomine HCl	10mg	Blue	Cap	–	–	–	Lederle	Antispasmodic
	LL A23	Acetaminophen with Codeine	300mg/30mg	White	Tab	Round	N	N	Lederle	Analgesic
	LL C23	Chlorpromazine	50mg	Tan	Tab	Round	N	Y	Lederle	Tranquilizer
	LL I23	Isosorbide Dinitrate SA	40mg	Green	Tab	Round	Y	N	Lederle	Antianginal
	LL M23	Methyldopa	500mg	Peach	Tab	Round	N	Y	Lederle	Antihypertensive
	LL N23	Nylidrin HCl	6mg	White	Tab	Round	Y	N	Lederle	Vasodilator
	LL T23	Triprolidine HCl & Pseudoephedrine HCl	2.5mg/60mg	White	Tab	Round	Y	N	Lederle	Decongestant Comb.
	M 23	Diltiazem HCl	30mg	White	Tab	Round	N	Y	Mylan	Antianginal
	SP 23	Chlorthalidone	25mg	Peach	Tab	Round	N	N	Superpharm	Diuretic
	U23	Isoniazid	300mg	White	Tab	Round	Y	N	Lilly	Anti–Infective
	UPJOHN 23	Cortisone Acetate	10mg	White	Tab	Round	Y	N	Upjohn	Steroid
	W N23	Nalidixic Acid	1000mg	Yellow	Tab	Oval	Y	N	Winthrop	Anti–Infective
24	BL\24	Amitriptyline Hydrochloride	50mg	Brown	Tab	Round	N	Y	Biocraft	Antidepressant
	Ciba 24	Aminoglutethimide	250mg	White	Tab	Round	Y	N	Ciba	Adrenal Suppressant
	GG24	Theophylline/Ephedrine Sulfate/Hydroxyzine HCl	130mg/25mg/10mg	White	Tab	Round	Y	N	Geneva	Antiasthmatic
	GG24	Theophylline/Ephedrine Sulfate/Hydroxyzine HCl	130mg/25mg/10mg	White	Tab	Round	Y	N	Geneva	Antiasthmatic
	LL A24	Amitriptyline HCl	10mg	Pink	Tab	Round	N	N	Lederle	Antidepressant
	LL C24	Chlorpromazine	100mg	Tan	Tab	Round	N	Y	Lederle	Tranquilizer
	LL D24	Dicyclomine HCl	20mg	Blue	Tab	Round	N	N	Lederle	Antispasmodic
	LL I24	Isosorbide Dinitrate	20mg	Green	Tab	Round	Y	N	Lederle	Antianginal
	LL N24	Nylidrin HCl	12mg	White	Tab	Round	Y	N	Lederle	Vasodilator
	LL P24	Prednisone	5mg	White	Tab	Round	Y	N	Lederle	Steroid
25	SP 24	Chlorthalidone	50mg	Blue	Tab	Round	N	N	Superpharm	Diuretic
	832/25	Chlordiazepoxide HCl	25mg	Green/White	Cap	–	–	–	PBI	Antianxiety
	832/25	Chlorpromazine HCl	25mg	Butterscotch	Tab	Round	N	Y	PBI	Tranquilizer
	832/D25	Dipyridamole	25mg	White	Tab	Round	N	Y	PBI	Antiplatelet
	832/TM25	Trimipramine Maleate	25mg	Purple/Orange	Cap	–	–	–	PBI	Antidepressant
	832/X25	Minoxidil	2.5mg	White	Tab	Round	–	–	PBI	Antihypertensive
	BI/25	Mesoridazine Besylate	25mg	Red	Tab	Round	N	Y	BI	Tranquilizer
	BL\25	Amitriptyline Hydrochloride	75mg	Purple	Tab	Round	N	Y	Biocraft	Antidepressant
	C25	Chlordiazepoxide	25mg	White/Green	Cap	–	–	–	Geneva	Antianxiety
	dp 25	Levothyroxine Sodium	0.025mg	Orange	Tab	Oval	Y	N	Daniels	Hormone
	dp 25	Dipyridamole	25mg	White	Tab	Round	N	Y	Duramed	Antiplatelet
	F25	Ephedrine Sulfate	50mg	Pink	Cap	–	–	–	Lilly	Antiasthmatic
	Flint 25	Levothyroxine Sodium	25mcg	Orange	Tab	Round	Y	N	Boots	Hormone
	GG 25	Triprolidine HCl/Pseudoephedrine HCl	2.5mg/60mg	White	Tab	Round	Y	N	Geneva	Decongestant Comb.
	GG 25	Triprolidine HCl & Pseudoephedrine HCl	2.5mg/60mg	White	Tab	Round	Y	N	Geneva	Decongestant Comb.
	J25	Thyroid	60mg	Brown	Tab	Round	N	N	Lilly	Hormone
	Lederle D25	Doxycycline Hyclate	100mg	Brown	Cap	–	–	–	Lederle	Anti–Infective
	LL A25	Amitriptyline HCl	25mg	Green	Tab	Round	N	N	Lederle	Antidepressant
	LL C25	Chlorpromazine	200mg	Tan	Tab	Round	N	Y	Lederle	Tranquilizer
	LL H25	Haloperidol	0.5mg	Orange	Tab	Round	Y	N	Lederle	Tranquilizer
	LL M25	Methyclothiazide	5mg	Blue	Tab	Round	Y	N	Lederle	Diuretic
	LL P25	Probenecid	500mg	Orange	Tab	Capsule	Y	Y	Lederle	Antigout
	LL T25	Thioridazine HCl	25mg	Orange	Tab	Round	N	Y	Lederle	Tranquilizer
	LNK 25	Diphenhydramine HCl	25mg	White/Pink	Cap	–	–	–	Pioneer	Antihistamine
	M 25	Levothyroxine Sodium	0.025mg	Peach	Tab	Round	Y	N	Duramed	Hormone
	MP 25	Amitriptyline HCl	25mg	Green	Tab	Round	N	Y	Mutual	Antidepressant
	P–25	Hydrochlorothiazide	25mg	Peach	Tab	Round	Y	N	Eon	Diruretic
	Par/25	Dipyridamole	25mg	White	Tab	Round	N	N	Par	Antiplatelet
	SKF 25	Diphenidol	25mg	Yellow	Tab	Round	N	N	SKB	Antivertigo
	SKF T25	Diphenidol HCl	25mg	Orange	Tab	Round	–	–	SKB	Antiemetic
26	U25	Erythromycin Estolate Chewable	250mg	Pink	Tab	Square	N	N	Lilly	Anti–Infective
	555/26	Prednisone	5mg	White	Tab	Round	Y	N	Barr	Steroid
	BL\26	Amitriptyline Hydrochloride	100mg	Orange	Tab	Round	N	Y	Biocraft	Antidepressant
	Ciba 26	Maprotiline HCl	50mg	Orange	Tab	Round	N	Y	Ciba	Antidepressant
	E–26	Docusate Calcium	240mg	Red	Cap	–	–	–	Chase	Stool Softener
	GG26	Isosorbide Dinitrate	10mg	White	Tab	Round	Y	N	Geneva	Antianginal
	J26	Thyroid	120mg	Brown	Tab	Round	N	N	Lilly	Hormone
	LL A26	Amitriptyline HCl	50mg	Brown	Tab	Round	N	N	Lederle	Antidepressant
	LL H26	Haloperidol	1mg	Orange	Tab	Round	Y	N	Lederle	Tranquilizer
	LL M26	Metronidazole	250mg	White	Tab	Round	N	Y	Lederle	Anti–Infective
	LL P26	Probenecid & Colchicine	500mg/0.5mg	White	Tab	Capsule	Y	Y	Lederle	Antigout
	MP 26	Amitriptyline HCl	50mg	Brown	Tab	Round	N	Y	Mutual	Antidepressant
	RO26	Phenobarbital	15mg	White	Tab	Round	Y	N	Rondex	Sedative
	SP 26	Methocarbamol	500mg	White	Tab	Round	Y	N	Superpharm	Muscle Relaxant
	U26	Erythromycin Estolate	500mg	Salmon–Pink	Tab	Capsule	Y	N	Lilly	Anti–Infective

ID NO.	ID CODE	GENERIC NAME	STRENGTH	COLOR	FORM	SHAPE	SCORED	COATED	MFG.	USE
27	50 LL T27	Thioridazine HCl	50mg	Orange	Tab	Round	N	Y	Lederle	Tranquilizer
	78–27	Bellafoline & Phenobarbital	0.25mg/50mg	Green/Orange/White	Tab	Round	Y	N	Sandoz	Antispasmodic
	E–27	Docusate Sodium	100mg	Orange/Red	Cap	–	–	–	Chase	Stool Softener
	GG27	Hydrochlorothiazide	50mg	Peach	Tab	Round	Y	N	Geneva	Diuretic
	LL A27	Amitriptyline HCl	75mg	Purple	Tab	Round	N	Y	Lederle	Antidepressant
	LL D27	Ergoloid Mesylates Sublingual	0.5mg	White	Tab	Round	N	N	Lederle	Vasodilator
	LL E27	Ergoloid Mesylates SL	0.5mg	White	Tab	Round	N	N	Lederle	Vasodilator
	LL H27	Haloperidol	2mg	Orange	Tab	Round	Y	N	Lederle	Tranquilizer
	LL I27	Ibuprofen	200mg	Orange	Tab	Round	N	Y	Lederle	Analgesic
	LL M27	Metronidazole	500mg	White	Tab	Oval	N	Y	Lederle	Anti–Infective
	M 27	Clonidine HCl & Chlorthalidone	0.2mg/15mg	Yellow	Tab	Round	Y	N	Mylan	Antihypertensive
	MP 27	Amitriptyline HCl	75mg	Purple	Tab	Round	N	Y	Mutual	Antidepressant
	R 27	Propranolol HCl	10mg	Peach	Tab	Round	–	N	Rondex	Antihypertensive
	R 27	Propranolol	10mg	Orange	Tab	Round	Y	N	Purepac	Antihypertensive
	SP 27	Methocarbamol	750mg	White	Tab	Capsule	N	N	Superpharm	Muscle Relaxant
	Winthrop T 27	Pentazocine HCl/Aspirin	12.5mg/325mg	White	Tab	Capsule	N	Y	Winthrop	Analgesic
	Wyeth 27	Promethazine	25mg	White	Tab	Round	Y	N	Wyeth	Antiemetic
28	100 LL T28	Thioridazine HCl	100mg	Orange	Tab	Round	N	Y	Lederle	Tranquilizer
	78–28	Bellafoline & Phenobarbital	0.25mg/50mg	White	Tab	Round	Y	N	Sandoz	Antispasmodic
	B 28	Inert Tablets	n/a	Pink	Tab	Round	N	N	Berlex	Inert Tablets
	BI/28	Thiethylperazine Maleate	10mg	Yellow	Tab	Round	N	Y	BI	Antiemetic
	biocraft 28	Cloxacillin	250mg	Green\Scarlet	Cap	–	N	N	Biocraft	Anti–Infective
	bp 28	Imipramine HCl	25mg	Brown	Tab	Round	N	Y	Bolar	Antidepressant
	GG28	Hydrochlorothiazide	25mg	Peach	Tab	Round	Y	N	Geneva	Diuretic
	LL A28	Amitriptyline HCl	100mg	Orange	Tab	Round	N	Y	Lederle	Antidepressant
	LL E28	Ergoloid Mesylates SL	1mg	White	Tab	Oval	N	N	Lederle	Vasodilator
	LL H28	Haloperidol	5mg	Orange	Tab	Round	Y	N	Lederle	Tranquilizer
	LL I28	Ibuprofen	400mg	White	Tab	Round	N	Y	Lederle	Anti–Inflammatory
	LL M28	Metoclopramide	10mg	White	Tab	Round	Y	N	Lederle	Antireflux
	MP 28	Amitriptyline HCl	100mg	Orange	Tab	Round	N	Y	Mutual	Antidepressant
	RO28	Phenobarbital	30mg	White	Tab	Round	Y	N	Rondex	Sedative
	Wyeth 28	Promazine	50mg	Red	Tab	Round	N	Y	Wyeth	Tranquilizer
29	C 29	Docusate Sodium	250mg	Red	Cap	–	–	–	Chase	Stool Softner
	E–29	Docusate Sodium	250mg	Orange/Red	Cap	–	–	–	Chase	Stool Softener
	J29	Thyroid	30mg	Brown	Tab	Round	N	N	Lilly	Hormone
	Lederle P29	Procainamide HCl	250mg	Yellow	Cap	–	–	–	Lederle	Antiarrhythmic
	LL H29	Haloperidol	10mg	Green	Tab	Round	Y	N	Lederle	Tranquilizer
	LL I29	Ibuprofen	600mg	White	Tab	Oval	N	Y	Lederle	Anti–Inflammatory
	LL T29	Trazodone HCl	50mg	White	Tab	Round	Y	N	Lederle	Antidepressant
	M29	Methyclothiazide	5mg	Blue	Tab	Round	N	N	Mylan	Diuretic
	MP 29	Amitriptyline HCl	150mg	Peach	Tab	Capsule	N	Y	Mutual	Antidepressant
	PP–29	Desipramine HCl	10mg	White	Tab	Round	N	Y	Eon	Antidepressant
	R 29	Propranolol HCl	20mg	Blue	Tab	Round	–	N	Rondex	Antihypertensive
	R 29	Propranolol	20mg	Blue	Tab	Round	Y	N	Purepac	Antihypertensive
	U29	Reserpine	0.25mg	Green	Tab	Round	Y	N	Lilly	Antihypertensive
	Wyeth 29	Promazine	25mg	Yellow	Tab	Round	N	Y	Wyeth	Tranquilizer
30	30/30	Caffeine	200mg	Blue	Tab	Oblong	Y	N	B & M Labs	Stimulant
	832/ TEM30	Temazepam	30mg	White	Cap	–	–	–	PBI	Hypnotic
	biocraft 30	Cloxacillin	500mg	Green\Scarlet	Cap	–	N	N	Biocraft	Anti–Infective
	Ciba 30	Methyltestosterone	10mg	White	Tab	Round	Y	N	Ciba	Hormone
	DAN–P 30	Phenobarbital	30mg	White	Tab	Round	Y	N	Danbury	Sedative
	dp 30	Conjugated Estrogens	0.3mg	White	Tab	Round	N	Y	Duramed	Hormone
	GG30	Thioridazine	10mg	Orange	Tab	Round	N	Y	Geneva	Tranquilizer
	Lederle F30	Flurazepam	30mg	Blue	Cap	–	–	–	Lederle	Hypnotic
	Lederle P30	Procainamide HCl	375mg	Orange/White	Cap	–	–	–	Lederle	Antiarrhythmic
	LEMMON 30	Dyphylline	200mg	White	Tab	Round	Y	N	Lemmon	Bronchodilator
	LL I30	Ibuprofen	800mg	White	Tab	Capsule	Y	Y	Lederle	Anti–Inflammatory
	LL L30	Lorazepam	0.5mg	White	Tab	Round	N	N	Lederle	Antianxiety
	LL T30	Trazodone HCl	100mg	White	Tab	Round	Y	N	Lederle	Antidepressant
	M 30	Clorazepate Dipotassium	3.75mg	Blue	Tab	Round	Y	N	Mylan	Antianxiety
	MP 30	Chlorthalidone	25mg	Yellow	Tab	Round	N	N	Mutual	Diuretic
	P–30	Phenobarbital	30mg	White	Tab	Round	Y	N	Eon	Sedative
	PF M 30	Morphine Sulfate	30mg	White	Tab	Oblong	Y	N	PF	Analgesic
	PF M30	Morphine Sulfate CR	30mg	Lavender	Tab	Round	N	N	PF	Analgesic
	S 78–30	Belladonna Alkaloids	0.25mg	White	Tab	Round	Y	N	Sandoz	Antispasmodic
31	SKF/ N 30	Phenylpropanolamine & Chlorpheniramine Maleate	75mg/8mg	Blue/Clear	Cap	–	–	–	SKB	Decongestant Comb.
	78–31	Bellafoline/Phenobarbital/Ergotamine Tartrate	0.2mg/40mg/.6mg	Green/Orange/Yellow	Tab	Round	Y	N	Sandoz	Vasodilator
	832/G31	Acetohexamide	250mg	White	Tab	Capsule	Y	N	PBI	Antiglaucoma
	A31	Potassium Chloride	1000mg	Red	Tab	Round	N	Y	Lilly	Potassium Supp.
	bp 31	Thioridazine HCl	15mg	Pink	Tab	Capsule	N	Y	Bolar	Tranquilizer
	D31	Meperidine HCl & Acetaminophen	50mg/300mg	Pink	Tab	Round	Y	N	Winthrop	Analgesic
	dp 31	Conjugated Estrogens	0.625mg	White	Tab	Round	N	Y	Duramed	Hormone
	GG31/15	Thioridazine	15mg	Orange	Tab	Round	N	Y	Geneva	Tranquilizer
	J31	Phenobarbital	15mg	White	Tab	Round	N	N	Lilly	Sedative
	Lederle 250 A31	Ampicillin Trihydrate	250mg	Green/White	Cap	–	–	–	Lederle	Anti–Infective
	Lederle P31	Procainamide HCl	500mg	Orange/Yellow	Cap	–	–	–	Lederle	Antiarrhythmic
	LL D31	Diphenoxylate HCl & Atropine Sulfate	2.5mg/0.025mg	White	Tab	Round	Y	N	Lederle	Antidiarrheal
	LL L31	Lorazepam	1mg	White	Tab	Round	Y	N	Lederle	Antianxiety
	LL T31–50/100	Trazodone HCl	150mg	White	Tab	Rectangular	Y	N	Lederle	Antidepressant
	M 31	Allopurinol	100mg	White	Tab	Round	Y	N	Mylan	Antigout
	R 31	Chlorthalidone & Reserpine	50mg/0.25mg	Pink	Tab	–	–	N	Rorer	Antihypertensive
	R 31	Amitriptyline Hydrochloride	10mg	Pink	Tab	Round	N	Y	Purepac	Antidepressant
	SKF/ N 31	Phenylpropanolamine & Chlorpheniramine Maleate	75mg/12mg	Orange/Clear	Cap	–	–	–	SKB	Decongestant Comb.
	W M31	Mephobarbital	32mg	White	Tab	Round	–	N	Winthrop	Sedative
	W T31	Iopanoic Acid	500mg	Yellow	Tab	Round	Y	N	Winthrop	Diagnostic
32	832/G32	Acetohexamide	500mg	White	Tab	Capsule	Y	N	PBI	Antiglaucoma
	BL/32	Sulfamethoxazole and Trimethoprim	400mg/80mg	White	Tab	Round	Y	N	Biocraft	Anti–Infective
	bp 32	Dexamethasone	0.75mg	Blue	Tab	Pentagon	–	–	Bolar	Steroid
	Ciba 32	Methyltestosterone	25mg	Yellow	Tab	Round	Y	N	Ciba	Hormone
	dp 32	Conjugated Estrogens	1.25mg	White	Tab	Round	N	Y	Duramed	Hormone
	Geigy 32	Imipramine HCl	10mg	Coral	Tab	Round	N	Y	Geigy	Antidepressant
	GG32/25	Thioridazine	25mg	Orange	Tab	Round	N	Y	Geneva	Tranquilizer
	J32	Phenobarbital	30mg	White	Tab	Round	N	N	Lilly	Sedative
	Lederle 500 A32	Ampicillin Trihydrate	500mg	Green/White	Cap	–	–	–	Lederle	Anti–Infective
	Lederle T32	Temazepam	15mg	Peach	Cap	–	–	–	Lederle	Hypnotic

ID NO.	ID CODE	GENERIC NAME	STRENGTH	COLOR	FORM	SHAPE	SCORED	COATED	MFG.	USE
	LL D32	DSS	100mg	Red	Cap	–	–	–	Lederle	Stool Softener
	LL L32	Lorazepam	2mg	White	Tab	Round	Y	N	Lederle	Antianxiety
	M 32	Metoprolol Tartrate	50mg	Pink	Tab	Round	Y	Y	Mylan	Antihypertensive
	P–32	Reserpine	0.1mg	White	Tab	Round	Y	N	Eon	Antihypertensive
	R 32	Chlorthalidone & Reserpine	25mg/0.125mg	White	Tab	–	–	N	Rorer	Antihypertensive
	R 32	Amitriptyline Hydrochloride	25mg	Green	Tab	Round	N	Y	Purepac	Antidepressant
	T32	Amobarbital	100mg	Pink	Tab	Round	Y	N	Lilly	Hypnotic
	W M32	Mephobarbital	50mg	White	Tab	Round	–	N	Winthrop	Sedative
33	5 C33	Leucovorin Calcium	5mg	Yellow	Tab	Round	Y	N	Lederle	Antineoplastic
	A33	Diethylstilbestrol	5mg	Red	Tab	Round	N	Y	Lilly	Hormone
	biocraft 33	Sulfamethoxazole and Trimethoprim DS	800mg/160mg	White	Tab	Oval	Y	N	Biocraft	Anti–Infective
	bock HS 33	Ferrous Fumarate/Vitamin C/Docusate Na	335/200/20mgs	Tan	Tab	Capsule	Y	Y	KV	Hematinic
	bp 33	Chlorthalidone	25mg	Peach	Tab	Round	–	–	Bolar	Diuretic
	F33	Amobarbital Sodium	200mg	Blue/Blue	Cap	–	–	–	Lilly	Hypnotic
	Geigy 33	Baclofen	20mg	White	Tab	Capsule	Y	N	Geigy	Muscle Relaxant
	GG33/50	Thioridazine	50mg	Orange	Tab	Round	N	Y	Geneva	Tranquilizer
	J33	Phenobarbital	100mg	White	Tab	Round	N	N	Lilly	Sedative
	L 33	Aspirin / Codeine	325mg/30mg	White	Tab	Round	N	N	Lee	Analgesic
	L 33	Aspirin / Codeine	325mg/60mg	White	Tab	Round	N	N	Lee	Analgesic
	Lederle A33	Amoxicillin	250mg	Gray/White	Cap	–	–	–	Lederle	Anti–Infective
	Lederle T33	Temazepam	30mg	Yellow	Cap	–	–	–	Lederle	Hypnotic
	LL P33	Propylthiouracil	50mg	White	Tab	Round	Y	N	Lederle	Antithyriod
	M33	Chlorothiazide & Reserpine	250mg/0.125mg	Orange	Tab	Round	Y	N	Mylan	Antihypertensive
	SKF E33	Phenoxybenzamine HCl	10mg	Red	Cap	–	–	–	SKB	Antihypertensive
	W M33	Mephobarbital	100mg	White	Tab	Round	–	N	Winthrop	Sedative
	Wyeth 33	Meprobamate	400mg	Yellow	Tab	Round	Y	Y	Wyeth	Antianxiety
34	biocraft/34	Trimethoprim	100mg	White	Tab	Round	N	N	Biocraft	Anti–Infective
	bp 34	Chlorthalidone	50mg	Blue	Tab	Round	–	–	Bolar	Diuretic
	Ciba 34	Methylphenidate HCl	20mg	Yellow	Tab	Round	Y	N	Ciba	Psychostimulant
	dp 34	Conjugated Estrogens	2.5mg	White	Tab	Round	N	Y	Duramed	Hormone
	F34	Arsenic Extract	250mg	Pink	Cap	–	–	–	Lilly	–
	GG34/100	Thioridazine	100mg	Orange	Tab	Round	N	Y	Geneva	Tranquilizer
	Lederle A34	Amoxicillin	500mg	Gray	Cap	–	–	–	Lederle	Anti–Infective
	LL D 34	DSS/Casanth	100mg/30mg	Maroon	Cap	–	–	–	Lederle	Laxative
	LL P34	Pseudoephedrine HCl	60mg	White	Tab	Round	Y	N	Lederle	Decongestant
	LL T 34	Theophylline CR	100mg	White	Tab	Round	Y	N	Lederle	Bronchodilator
	UPJOHN 34	Cortisone Acetate	25mg	White	Tab	Round	Y	N	Upjohn	Steroid
	W B34	Tyropanoate	750mg	Tan/Cream	Cap	–	–	–	Winthrop	Diagnostic
35	555/35	Meprobamate	200mg	White	Tab	Round	Y	N	Barr	Antianxiety
	BL/35	Trimethoprim	200mg	White	Tab	Round	N	N	Biocraft	Anti–Infective
	bp 35	Chlorthalidone	100mg	White	Tab	Round	–	–	Bolar	Diuretic
	Ciba 35	Reserpine	0.1mg	White	Tab	Round	N	N	Ciba	Antihypertensive
	Geigy 35/35	Metoprolol Tartrate & Hydrochlorothiazide	50mg/25mg	Blue/White	Tab	Capsule	Y	N	Geigy	Antihypertensive
	GG35	Thioridazine	150mg	Orange	Tab	Round	N	Y	Geneva	Tranquilizer
	Laser 35	Phendimetrazine Tartrate	35mg	Orange	Tab	Round	–	–	Laser	Anoretic
	Lederle D35	Propoxyphene HCL & Acetaminophen	65mg/650mg	Pink	Tab	Oval	N	N	Lederle	Analgesic
	LL A 35–3	Aspirin with Codeine	325mg/30mg	White	Tab	Round	N	N	Lederle	Analgesic
	LL M35	Medroxyprogesterone Acetate	10mg	White	Tab	Round	Y	N	Lederle	Hormone
	LL P35	Pseudoephedrine HCl	30mg	Red	Tab	Round	N	Y	Lederle	Decongestant
	LL T 35	Theophylline CR	200mg	White	Tab	Oval	Y	N	Lederle	Bronchodilator
	LL15 C35	Leucovorin Calcium	15mg	Yellow	Tab	Oval	Y	N	Lederle	Antineoplastic
	M 35	Chlorthalidone	25mg	Yellow	Tab	Round	Y	N	Mylan	Diuretic
	MP 35	Spironolactone	25mg	White	Tab	Round	Y	N	Mutual	Diuretic
	W D35	Meperidine HCl	50mg	White	Tab	Round	–	N	Winthrop	Analgesic
36	555/36	Meprobamate	400mg	White	Tab	Round	Y	N	Barr	Antianxiety
	Ciba 36	Reserpine	0.25mg	White	Tab	Round	Y	N	Ciba	Antihypertensive
	F36	Papaverine/Codeine	15mg/15mg	Clear	Cap	–	–	–	Lilly	Antitussive
	GG36	Thioridazine	200mg	Orange	Tab	Round	N	Y	Geneva	Tranquilizer
	J36	Ergonovine Maleate	0.2mg	White	Tab	Round	N	N	Lilly	Antimigraine
	Lederle D36	Propoxyphene HCL	65mg	Pink	Cap	–	–	–	Lederle	Analgesic
	LL M36	Methyldopa & Hydrochlorothiazide	250mg/15mg	Chartreuse	Tab	Round	N	Y	Lederle	Antihypertensive
	LL P36	Pyrazinamide	500mg	White	Tab	Round	Y	N	Lederle	Anti–Infective
	LL T 36	Theophylline CR	300mg	White	Tab	Oblong	Y	N	Lederle	Bronchodilator
	LL–A36	Ascorbic Acid	250mg	White	Tab	Round	N	N	Lederle	Vitamin
	M36	Amitriptyline HCl	50mg	Brown	Tab	Round	N	Y	Mylan	Antidepressant
	MP 36	Metoclopramide	10mg	White	Tab	Round	Y	N	Mutual	Antireflux
	S 78–36	Ergotamine/Caffeine/Bellafoline/Pentobarbital	1/100/.125/30mg	Green	Tab	Round	N	Y	Sandoz	Antimigraine
	SKF V 36	Phenylpropanolamine/Caraminphen/Chlorpheniramine	50mg/20mg/8mg	White	Cap	–	–	–	SKB	Cold/Cough Comb.
	SL 36	Desipramine HCl	25mg	Yellow	Tab	Round	N	Y	Sidmak	Antidepressant
37	252/37	Sodium Fluoride	2.2mg	Pink	Tab	Round	N	N	Jones	Mineral Supp.
	37–4401	Penicillamine Titratable	250mg	White	Tab	Oval	Y	N	Wallace	Antiarthritic
	37/37	Dyphylline	400mg	White	Tab	Oblong	Y	N	Lemmon	Bronchodilator
	Ciba 37	Hydralazine HCl	10mg	Yellow	Tab	Round	N	N	Ciba	Antihypertensive
	GG37	Hydroxyzine HCl	10mg	Lavender	Tab	Round	N	Y	Geneva	Antipruritic
	J37	Phenobarbital	60mg	White	Tab	Round	N	N	Lilly	Sedative
	LEMMON 37	Dyphylline	400mg	White	Tab	Oblong	Y	N	Lemmon	Bronchodilator
	LL C37	Chlorpropamide	100mg	Green	Tab	Round	Y	N	Lederle	Hypoglycemic
	LL M37	Methyldopa & Hydrochlorothiazide	250mg/25mg	Pink	Tab	Round	N	Y	Lederle	Antihypertensive
	LL–A37	Ascorbic Acid	500mg	White	Tab	Round	N	N	Lederle	Vitamin
	LL–P37	Pyridoxine HCl	25mg	White	Tab	Round	Y	N	Lederle	Vitamin
	M37	Amitriptyline HCl	75mg	Blue	Tab	Round	N	Y	Mylan	Antidepressant
	MERRELL 37	Metenzolate Bromide	25mg	Yellow	Tab	Round	N	N	Merrell	Antispasmodic
	MP 37	Doxycycline Hyclate	100mg	Orange	Tab	Round	N	Y	Mutual	Anti–Infective
	T37	Amobarbital	50mg	Orange	Tab	Round	Y	N	Lilly	Hypnotic
	W/D37	Meperidine HCl	100mg	White	Tab	Round	–	N	Winthrop	Analgesic
38	Winthrop T37	Pentazocine HCl & Acetaminophen	25mg/500mg	Blue	Tab	Capsule	–	N	Winthrop	Analgesic
	BL38	Chloroquine	250mg	White	Tab	Round	Y	N	Biocraft	Antimalarial
	GG38	Hydroxyzine HCl	25mg	Lavender	Tab	Round	N	Y	Geneva	Antipruritic
	LL C38	Chlorpropamide	250mg	Green	Tab	Round	N	N	Lederle	Hypoglycemic
	LL–A38	Ascorbic Acid	1000mg	White	Tab	Round	N	N	Lederle	Vitamin
	LL–P38	Pyridoxine HCl	50mg	White	Tab	Round	Y	N	Lederle	Vitamin
	M38	Amitriptyline HCl	100mg	Orange	Tab	Round	N	Y	Mylan	Antidepressant
	SP 38	Hydralazine & Hydrochlorothiazide	25mg/25mg	Green	Cap	–	–	–	Superpharm	Antihypertensive
39	4 LL A39	Acetaminophen with Codeine	300mg/60mg	White	Tab	Round	N	N	Lederle	Analgesic
	bp 39	Imipramine HCl	10mg	Yellow	Tab	Triangular	N	Y	Bolar	Antidepressant

ID NO.	ID CODE	GENERIC NAME	STRENGTH	COLOR	FORM	SHAPE	SCORED	COATED	MFG.	USE
	Ciba 39	Hydralazine HCl	25mg	Blue	Tab	Round	N	N	Ciba	Antihypertensive
	F39	Quinidine Sulfate	200mg	Pink	Cap	–	–	–	Lilly	Antiarrhythmic
	GG39	Hydroxyzine HCl	50mg	Purple	Tab	Round	N	Y	Geneva	Antipruritic
	LL P39	Propoxyphene Napsylate & Acetaminophen	100mg/650mg	White	Tab	Capsule	N	Y	Lederle	Analgesic
	M39	Amitriptyline	150mg	Flesh	Tab	Round	N	Y	Mylan	Antidepressant
	MP 39	Lorazepam	1mg	White	Tab	Round	Y	N	Mutual	Antianxiety
	SP 39	Hydralazine & Hydrochlorothiazide	50mg/50mg	Lt.Green/Dk.Green	Cap	–	–	–	Superpharm	Antihypertensive
40	(triangle) 40	Verapamil HCl	40mg	Blue	Tab	Round	Y	Y	Knoll	Antianginal
	biocraft 40	Disopyramide Phosphate	100mg	Scarlet\Blue	Cap	–	N	N	Biocraft	Antiarrhythmic
	bp 40	Imipramine HCl	50mg	Green	Tab	Round	N	Y	Bolar	Antidepressant
	C/40 LL	Calcium/Vitamin D	600mg	Brown	Tab	Oblong	Y	Y	Lederle	Vitamin
	Central 40	Chlorpheniramine/Pseudoephedrine	8mg/120mg	Red/Clear	Cap	–	–	–	Central	Decongestant Comb.
	Ciba 40	Reserpine & Hydralazine HCl	0.1mg/25mg	Yellow	Tab	Round	N	N	Ciba	Antihypertensive
	dp 40	Propranolol	40mg	Green	Tab	Round	Y	N	Duramed	Antihypertensive
	F40	Secobarbital Sodium	100mg	Orange	Cap	–	–	–	Lilly	Hypnotic
	Geigy 40	Imipramine Pamoate	100mg	Coral/Yellow	Cap	–	–	–	Geigy	Antidepressant
	GG40	Amitriptyline	10mg	Pink	Tab	Round	N	Y	Geneva	Antidepressant
	M 40	Propranolol	40mg	Green	Tab	Round	Y	N	Martec	Antihypertensive
	M 40	Clorazepate Dipotassium	7.5mg	White	Tab	Round	Y	N	Mylan	Antianxiety
	MP 40	Spironolactone/Hydrochlorothiazide	25mg/25mg	Buff	Tab	Round	Y	N	Mutual	Diuretic
41	7/41 LuChem	Phenylpropanolamine HCl & Guaifenesin LA	75mg/400mg	Blue/White Specks	Tab	Oblong	Y	N	LuChem	Decongestant Comb.
	879 G41	Aminophylline	100mg	White	Tab	Round	Y	N	Halsey	Bronchodilator
	93–41	Clomiphene Citrate	50mg	White	Tab	Round	Y	N	Lemmon	Hormone
	biocraft 41	Disopyramide Phosphate	150mg	Buff\Scarlet	Cap	–	N	N	Biocraft	Antiarrhythmic
	bp 41	Ergoloid Mesylates Oral	1mg	White	Tab	Round	N	N	Bolar	Vasodilator
	Ciba 41	Sulfinpyrazone	100mg	White	Tab	Round	Y	N	Ciba	Antigout
	GG41	Imipramine	10mg	Yellow	Tab	Round	N	Y	Geneva	Antidepressant
	HL T41	Trimeprazine Tartrate	2.5mg	Gray	Tab	Round	N	Y	Forest	Antipruretic
	Lederle M41	Meclofenamate Sodium	50mg	Coral	Cap	–	–	–	Lederle	Anti–Inflammatory
	LL D41	Doxycycline Hyclate	100mg	Green	Tab	Round	N	Y	Lederle	Anti–Infective
	Mylan 41	Spironolactone w/Hydrochlorothiazide	25mg/25mg	Ivory	Tab	Round	Y	N	Mylan	Diuretic
	SP 41	Cyproheptadine HCl	4mg	White	Tab	Round	Y	N	Superpharm	Antipruritic
	T 41	Phenazopyridine HCl	100mg	Burgundy	Tab	Round	N	Y	Trinity	Urinary Antiseptic
42	BL/42	Thioridazine Hydrochloride	10mg	Green	Tab	Oval	N	Y	Biocraft	Tranquilizer
	bp 42	Acetazolamide	250mg	White	Tab	Round	Y	N	Bolar	Antiglaucoma
	F42	Secobarbital Sodium	50mg	Orange	Cap	–	–	–	Lilly	Hypnotic
	Geigy 42	Theophylline Anhydrous	200mg	Pink	Tab	Oval	Y	N	Geigy	Bronchodilator
	GG42	Imipramine	50mg	Green	Tab	Round	N	Y	Geneva	Antidepressant
	Lederle M42	Meclofenamate Sodium	100mg	Coral/White	Cap	–	–	–	Lederle	Anti–Inflammatory
	LL C42	Clonidine HCl	0.1mg	Brown	Tab	Round	Y	N	Lederle	Antihypertensive
43	SKF X 42	Diphenidol	25mg	Yellow	Tab	Round	N	N	SKB	Antivertigo
	Lederle D43	Disopyramide	150mg	Buff/Red	Cap	–	–	–	Lederle	Antiarrhythmic
	LL A43	Allopurinol	100mg	White	Tab	Round	Y	N	Lederle	Antigout
	LL C43	Clonidine HCl	0.2mg	Yellow	Tab	Round	Y	N	Lederle	Antihypertensive
	M43	Chlorothiazide & Reserpine	500mg/0.125mg	Orange	Tab	Round	Y	N	Mylan	Antihypertensive
	MP 43	Chlorthalidone	50mg	Green	Tab	Round	Y	N	Mutual	Diuretic
	SP 43	Dipyridamole	25mg	White	Tab	Round	N	Y	Superpharm	Antiplatelet
44	bp 44	Warfarin Sodium	2.5mg	Orange	Tab	Round	–	N	Bolar	Anticoagulant
	Central 44	Vitamin Combination	n/a	Red/Brown	Cap	–	–	–	Central	Vitamin
	EL 44	Trimethobenzamide	250mg	Blue/Blue	Cap	–	–	–	Econolab	Antinausea
	GG44	Amitriptyline	25mg	Green	Tab	Round	N	Y	Geneva	Antidepressant
	LL A44	Allopurinol	300mg	White	Tab	Round	Y	N	Lederle	Antigout
	LL C44	Clonidine HCl	0.3mg	Green	Tab	Round	Y	N	Lederle	Antihypertensive
	LL D44	Dipyridamole	25mg	Lavender	Tab	Round	N	Y	Lederle	Antiplatelet
	LL P44	Propranolol HCl	10mg	Gray	Tab	Round	Y	N	Lederle	Antihypertensive
	M 44	Cyproheptadine HCl	4mg	White	Tab	Round	Y	N	Mylan	Antihistamine
	MP 44	Benztropine Mesylate	1.0mg	White	Tab	Round	Y	N	Mutual	Antiparkinson
	SKF C44	Prochlorperazine	10mg	Black/Natural	Cap	–	–	–	SKB	Antiemetic
45	SP 44	Dipyridamole	50mg	White	Tab	Round	N	Y	Superpharm	Antiplatelet
	C 45	Atenolol	50mg	White	Tab	Round	Y	N	IPR	Antihypertensive
	C/45 LL	Calcium/Iron	600mg	Red	Tab	Oblong	Y	Y	Lederle	Vitamin
	Geigy 45	Imipramine Pamoate	125mg	Coral/Yellow	Cap	–	–	–	Geigy	Antidepressant
	GG45	Dipyridamole	50mg	White	Tab	Round	N	Y	Geneva	Antiplatelet
	Lederle M 45 50mg	Minocycline	50mg	Yellow/Green	Cap	–	–	–	Lederle	Anti–Infective
	LL D45	Dipyridamole	50mg	Lavender	Tab	Round	N	Y	Lederle	Antiplatelet
	LL P45	Propranolol HCl	20mg	Lavender	Tab	Round	Y	N	Lederle	Antihypertensive
	LL–A45	Albuterol Sulfate	2mg	White	Tab	Round	Y	N	Lederle	Bronchodilator
	M 45	Diltiazem HCl	60mg	White	Tab	Round	N	Y	Mylan	Antianginal
	MP 45	Metronidazole	250mg	White	Tab	Round	N	N	Mutual	Anti–Infective
46	SP 45	Dipyridamole	75mg	White	Tab	Round	N	Y	Superpharm	Antiplatelet
	BL/46	Thioridazine Hydrochloride	100mg	Lt. Green	Tab	Oval	N	Y	Biocraft	Tranquilizer
	bp 46	Warfarin Sodium	7.5mg	Yellow	Tab	Round	–	N	Bolar	Anticoagulant
	Ciba 46	Hydrochlorothiazide	50mg	Yellow	Tab	Round	Y	N	Ciba	Diuretic
	Lederle M 46 100mg	Minocycline	100mg	Green	Cap	–	–	–	Lederle	Anti–Infective
	LL D46	Dipyridamole	75mg	Lavender	Tab	Round	N	Y	Lederle	Antiplatelet
	LL P46	Propranolol HCl	40mg	Brown	Tab	Round	Y	N	Lederle	Antihypertensive
	LL–A46	Albuterol Sulfate	4mg	White	Tab	Round	Y	N	Lederle	Bronchodilator
	MP 46	Metronidazole	500mg	White	Tab	Capsule	N	N	Mutual	Anti–Infective
	SKF C46	Prochlorperazine	15mg	Black/Natural	Cap	–	–	–	SKB	Antiemetic
47	T46	Sulfapyridine	500mg	White	Tab	Round	N	N	Lilly	Anti–Infective
	bp 47	Warfarin Sodium	10mg	White	Tab	Round	–	N	Bolar	Anticoagulant
	Ciba 47	Guanethidine Monosulfate & Hydrochlorothiazide	10mg/25mg	White	Tab	Round	Y	N	Ciba	Antihypertensive
	Geigy 47	Carbamazepine Chewable	100mg	White/Red Specks	Tab	Round	Y	N	Geigy	Anticonvulsant
	GG47	Imipramine	25mg	Beige	Tab	Round	N	Y	Geneva	Antidepressant
	Lederle D47	Doxepin	25mg	Ivory/White	Cap	–	–	–	Lederle	Antidepressant
	Lilly F 47	Aminophylline/Ephedrine/Amobarbital	130mg/25mg/25mg	Orange/Blue	Cap	–	–	–	Lilly	Antiasthmatic
	LL P47	Propranolol HCl	80mg	Blue	Tab	Round	Y	N	Lederle	Antihypertensive
	M 47	Metoprolol Tartrate	100mg	Blue	Tab	Round	Y	Y	Mylan	Antihypertensive
	MP 47	Albuterol Sulfate	2mg	White	Tab	Round	Y	N	Mutual	Bronchodilator
48	SKF C47	Prochlorperazine	30mg	Black/Natural	Cap	–	–	–	SKB	Antiemetic
	BI/48	Theophylline SR	250mg	White	Tab	Round	Y	N	BI	Bronchodilator
	Geigy 48	Tripelennamine Hydrochloride SR	100mg	Lavender	Tab	Round	N	N	Geigy	Antihistamine
	GG48	Pseudoephedrine	30mg	Red	Tab	Round	N	Y	Geneva	Decongestant
	Lederle D48	Doxepin	50mg	Ivory	Cap	–	–	–	Lederle	Antidepressant
	LL P48	Procainamide HCl SR	250mg	Blue	Tab	Oval	N	Y	Lederle	Antiarrhythmic

ID NO.	ID CODE	GENERIC NAME	STRENGTH	COLOR	FORM	SHAPE	SCORED	COATED	MFG.	USE
49	BI/49	Theophylline SR	500mg	White	Tab	Capsule	Y	N	BI	Bronchodilator
	BIOCRAFT 49	Penicillin V Potassium	500mg	White	Tab	Oval	–	N	Biocraft	Anti–Infective
	Ciba 49	Guanethidine Monosulfate	10mg	Yellow	Tab	Round	Y	N	Ciba	Antihypertensive
	GG49	Dipyridamole	25mg	White	Tab	Round	N	Y	Geneva	Antiplatelet
	Lederle D49	Doxepin	75mg	Green	Cap	–	–	–	Lederle	Antidepressant
	LL A49	Atenolol	50mg	White	Tab	Round	Y	N	Lederle	Antihypertensive
	LL P49	Procainamide HCl SR	500mg	Pink	Tab	Oval	Y	Y	Lederle	Antiarrhythmic
	SP 49	Tripolidine & Pseudoephedrine	2.5mg/60mg	White	Tab	Round	Y	N	Superpharm	Decongestant Comb.
	W 49	Aluminum & Magnesium Hydroxide	180mg/160mg	Pink	Tab	Round	N	N	Winthrop	Antacid
50	3M/TR50	Flecainide Acetate	50mg	White	TAB	Round	–	–	3M	Antiarrhythmic
	832/50	Chlorpromazine	50mg	Tan	Tab	Round	N	Y	PBI	Tranquilizer
	832/D50	Dipyridamole	50mg	White	Tab	Round	N	Y	PBI	Antiplatelet
	832/MC50	Meclofenamate Sodium	50mg	Maroon/Pink	Cap	–	–	–	PBI	Anti–Inflammatory
	832/TM50	Trimipramine Maleate	50mg	Pink/White	Cap	–	–	–	PBI	Antidepressant
	93 50 / 2	Acetaminophen & Codeine	300mg/15mg	White	Tab	Round	N	N	Lemmon	Analgesic
	AC 50	Choline Magnesium Trisalicylate	500mg	White	Tab	Oblong	Y	Y	Able Labs	Antiarthritic
	BI/50	Mesoridazine Besylate	50mg	Red	Tab	Round	N	Y	BI	Tranquilizer
	bp 50	Warfarin Sodium	2mg	Lavender	Tab	Round	–	N	Bolar	Anticoagulant
	dp 50	Levothyroxine Sodium	0.05mg	White	Tab	Oval	Y	N	Daniels	Hormone
	dp 50	Dipyridamole	50mg	White	Tab	Round	N	Y	Duramed	Antiplatelet
	Flint 50	Levothyroxine Sodium	50mcg	White	Tab	Round	Y	N	Boots	Hormone
	GG407/50	Chlorpromazine HCl	50mg	Butterscotch	Tab	Round	N	Y	Geneva	Tranquilizer
	HL T50	Trimeprazine Tartrate	5mg	Gray/Natural	Cap	–	–	–	Forest	Antipruretic
	JANSSEN L 50	Levamisole HCl	50mg	White	Tab	Round	–	Y	Janssen	–
	Lederle D50	Doxepin	10mg	Buff	Cap	–	–	–	Lederle	Antidepressant
	LL P50	Procainamide HCl SR	750mg	Tan	Tab	Oval	Y	Y	Lederle	Antiarrhythmic
	LNK 50	Diphenhydramine HCl	50mg	Pink	Cap	–	–	–	Pioneer	Antihistamine
	M 50	Levothyroxine Sodium	0.05mg	White	Tab	Round	Y	N	Duramed	Hormone
	M 50 LEVO T	Levothyroxine Sodium	0.05mg	White	Tab	Round	–	N	Mova	Hormone
	M50	Chlorothiazide	250mg	White	Tab	Round	Y	N	Mylan	Diuretic
	MP 50	Tolmetin Sodium	200mg	–	Tab	–	–	–	Mutual	Anti–Inflammatory
	Par/50	Dipyridamole	50mg	White	Tab	Round	N	Y	Par	Antiplatelet
	PP–50	Hydrochlorothiazide	50mg	Peach	Tab	Round	Y	N	Eon	Diuretic
	RR 50	Prednisone	50mg	Whhite	Tab	Round	Y	N	RR	Steroid
	Syntex 50	Oxymetholone	50mg	White	Tab	Round	Y	N	Syntex	Antianemia
	TZD50 832	Trazodone HCl	50mg	White	Tab	Round	Y	Y	PBI	Antidepressant
	WHR 50mg	Theophylline	50mg	White/Clear	Cap	–	–	–	Rorer	Bronchodilator
51	C 51	Atenolol/Chlorthalidone	50mg/25mg	White	Tab	Round	–	N	IPR	Antihypertensive
	Ciba 51	Methyltestosterone Sublingual	5mg	White	Tab	Oval	N	N	Ciba	Hormone
	Geigy 51/51	Metoprolol Tartrate	50mg	Pink	Tab	Capsule	Y	N	Geigy	Antihypertensive
	GG51/1	Trifluoperazine HCl	1mg	Lavender	Tab	Round	N	Y	Geneva	Tranquilizer
	GG51/1	Trifluoperazine HCl	1mg	Lavendar	Tab	Round	N	Y	Geneva	Tranquilizer
	LL A51	Alprazolam	0.25mg	White	Tab	Oval	Y	N	Lederle	Antianxiety
	LL D51	Diazepam	2mg	White	Tab	Round	Y	N	Lederle	Antianxiety
	M51	Amitriptyline HCl	25mg	Green	Tab	Round	N	Y	Mylan	Antidepressant
	MP 51	Prednisone	5mg	White	Tab	Round	Y	N	Mutual	Steroid
	SEARLE 51	Norethynodrel & Mestranol	5mg/75mcg	Tan	Tab	Round	N	N	Searle	Hormone
	W T51	Pentazocine HCl & Naloxone HCl	50mg/0.5mg	Yellow	Tab	Capsule	Y	N	Winthrop	Analgesic
52	B52	Vitamin A	50,000 Units	Red	Cap	–	–	–	Lilly	Vitamin A
	BL/52	Amiloride HCl & Hydrochlorothiazide	5mg/50mg	Yellow	Tab	Round	Y	N	Biocraft	Antihypertensive
	Geigy 52	Carbamazepine Chewable	100mg	White/Red Specks	Tab	Round	Y	N	Geigy	Anticonvulsant
	GG52	L–Thyroxine	0.1mg	Yellow	Tab	Round	Y	N	PBI	Hormone
	J52	Diethylstilbestrol	1mg	White	Tab	Round	N	N	Lilly	Hormone
	LL A52	Alprazolam	0.5mg	Yellow	Tab	Oval	Y	N	Lederle	Antianxiety
	LL D52	Diazepam	5mg	Tan	Tab	Round	Y	N	Lederle	Antianxiety
	M 52	Pindolol	5mg	White	Tab	Round	Y	N	Mylan	Anti–Hypertensive
	MP 52	Prednisone	10mg	White	Tab	Round	Y	N	Mutual	Steroid
	MP 52	Prednisone	10mg	White	Tab	Round	Y	N	Mutual	Steroid
	S Sandoz 78–52	Mephenytoin	100mg	White	Tab	Round	Y	N	Sandoz	Anticonvulsant
	SP 52	Isosorbide Dinitrate	5mg	Pink	Tab	Round	Y	N	Superpharm	Antianginal
53	BL/53	Furosemide (Veterinary)	12.5mg	White	Tab	Capsule	–	N	Biocraft	Diuretic
	Geigy 53/53	Metoprolol Tartrate & Hydrochlorothiazide	100mg/25mg	Pink/White	Tab	Capsule	Y	N	Geigy	Antihypertensive
	GG53/2	Trifluoperazine HCl	2mg	Lavender	Tab	Round	N	Y	Geneva	Tranquilizer
	GG53/2	Trifluoperazine HCl	2mg	Lavendar	Tab	Round	N	Y	Geneva	Tranquilizer
	Lederle P53	Phenytoin Sodium Extended	100mg	Transparent	Cap	–	–	–	Lederle	Anticonvulsant
	LL A53	Alprazolam	1mg	Green	Tab	Oval	Y	N	Lederle	Antianxiety
	LL D53	Diazepam	10mg	Green	Tab	Round	Y	N	Lederle	Antianxiety
	MP 53	Prednisone	20mg	Peach	Tab	Round	Y	N	Mutual	Steroid
	MP 53	Prednisone	20mg	Peach	Tab	Round	Y	N	Mutual	Steroid
	PP–53	Prenatal Vitamin with Folic Acid	n/a	Pink	Tab	Capsule	N	Y	Eon	Vitamin
	SP 53	Isosorbide Dinitrate	10mg	White	Tab	Round	Y	N	Superpharm	Antianginal
	U53	Methadone HCl Chewable	40mg	Peach	Tab	Square	Y	N	Lilly	Analgesic
	W L53	Talbutal	120mg	White	Tab	Round	–	–	Winthrop	Hypnotic
	W W53	Stanozolol	2mg	White	Tab	Round	N	N	Winthrop	Steroid
	Wyeth 53	Ampicillin	250mg	Pink/Purple	Cap	–	–	–	Wyeth	Anti–Infective
54	BL/54	Furosemide (Veterinary)	50mg	White	Tab	Capsule	–	N	Biocraft	Diuretic
	GG54	L–Thyroxine	0.2mg	White	Tab	Round	Y	N	PBI	Hormone
	J54	Diethylstilbestrol	5mg	White	Tab	Round	N	N	Lilly	Hormone
	Lederle D54	Doxepin	100mg	Green/White	Cap	–	–	–	Lederle	Antidepressant
	LL A54	Alprazolam	2mg	Green	Tab	Rectangular	Y	N	Lederle	Antianxiety
	M 54 / 10	Thioridazine	10mg	Orange	Tab	Round	N	Y	Mylan	Tranquilizer
	Par/54	Imipramine HCl	10mg	Yellow	Tab	Triangular	N	Y	Par	Antidepressant
	PP–54	Triamterene & Hydrochlorothiazide	75mg/50mg	Yellow	Tab	Round	–	N	Eon	Diuretic
	PPL 54	Triamterene & Hydrochlorothiazide	75mg/10mg	Yellow	Tab	Round	–	N	Eon	Diuretic
	SANDOZ 78–54	Methylergonovine Maleate	0.2mg	Rose	Tab	Round	N	N	Sandoz	–
	SP 54	Isosorbide Dinitrate	20mg	Green	Tab	Round	Y	N	Superpharm	Antianginal
	T54	Sulfadiazine	500mg	White	Tab	Round	Y	N	Lilly	Anti–Infective
55	832/G55C	Chlordiazepoxide & Amitriptyline	5mg/12.5mg	White	Tab	Round	N	Y	PBI	Antianxiety
	CL55/5	Trifluoperazine HCl	5mg	Lavender	Tab	Round	N	Y	Cord	Tranquilizer
	GG55/5	Trifluoperazine HCl	5mg	Lavender	Tab	Round	N	Y	Geneva	Tranquilizer
	GG55/5	Trifluoperazine HCl	5mg	Lavendar	Tab	Round	N	Y	Geneva	Tranquilizer
	Lederle C55	Clorazepate Dipotassium	3.75mg	Lavender/White	Cap	–	–	–	Lederle	Antianxiety
	Lederle D55	Doxepin	150mg	Orange/Gray	Cap	–	–	–	Lederle	Antidepressant
	M 55	Timolol	5mg	Green	Tab	Round	N	N	Mylan	Antihypertensive
	MP 55	Hydralazine HCl	50mg	Orange	Tab	Round	N	N	Mutual	Antihypertensive

ID NO.	ID CODE	GENERIC NAME	STRENGTH	COLOR	FORM	SHAPE	SCORED	COATED	MFG.	USE
56	Par/55	Imipramine HCl	25mg	Brown	Tab	Round	N	Y	Par	Antidepressant
	T55	Papaverine HCl	100mg	White	Tab	Round	N	N	Lilly	Vasodilator
	832/G56C	Chlordiazepoxide & Amitriptyline	10mg/25mg	Green	Tab	Round	N	Y	PBI	Antianxiety
	bp 56	Chlorothiazide & Reserpine	250mg/0.125mg	Pink	Tab	Round	–	–	Bolar	Antihypertensive
	GG 56	Disopyramide Phosphate	100mg	Orange	Cap		–	–	Geneva	Antiarrhythmic
	Lederle C56	Clorazepate Dipotassium	7.5mg	Lavender/Maroon	Cap	–	–	–	Lederle	Antianxiety
	Par/56	Imipramine HCl	50mg	Green	Tab	Round	N	Y	Par	Antidepressant
	T56	Amobarbital	30mg	Yellow	Tab	Round	Y	N	Lilly	Hypnotic
	U56	Folic Acid	1mg	Yellow	Tab	Round	N	N	Lilly	Antianemic
	Wyeth 56	Norgestrel & Ethinyl Estradiol	0.5mg/0.05mg	White	Tab	Round	N	N	Wyeth	Contraceptive
57	B 57	Aspirin	800mg	White	Tab	Capsule	Y	N	Boots	Analgesic
	Geigy 57	Theophylline Anhydrous	300mg	Blue	Tab	Oval	Y	N	Geigy	Bronchodilator
	GG 57	Disopyramide Phosphate	150mg	Brown	Cap		–	–	Geneva	Antiarrhythmic
	Lederle C57	Clorazepate Dipotassium	15mg	Lavender	Cap	–	–	–	Lederle	Antianxiety
	R 57	Lorazepam	0.5mg	White	Tab	Round	Y	N	Purepac	Antianxiety
	R 57	Lorazepam	1mg	–	Tab	Round	–	–	Rugby	Antianxiety
	Rugby Logo R 57	Lorazepam	1mg	–	Tab		–	–	Rugby	Antianxiety
	SP 57	Tolazamide	250mg	White	Tab	Round	Y	N	Superpharm	Hypoglycemic
	T 57	Phenyleph/Phenylpro/Chlorphen/Hyosc/Atro/Scop	25/50/8/.19/.04	Green	Tab	Elongated	Y	–	Anabolic	Decongestant Comb.
	Wyeth 57	Nafcillin Sodium	250mg	Green/Yellow	Cap		–	–	Wyeth	Anti–Infective
58	Boots logo 58	Phenyleph/Phenylpro/Chlorphen/Hyosc/Atro/Scop	25/50/8/.19/.04	Green	Tab	Elongated	Y	–	Eon	Decongestant Comb.
	GG58/10	Trifluoperazine HCl	10mg	Lavender	Tab	Round	N	Y	Geneva	Tranquilizer
	M 58 / 25	Thioridazine	25mg	Orange	Tab	Round	N	Y	Mylan	Tranquilizer
	MP 58	Carisoprodol	350mg	White	Tab	Round	N	Y	Mutual	Muscle Relaxant
	PP–58	Hydroxyzine HCl	50mg	Yellow	Tab	Round	N	Y	Eon	Antipruritic
	SANDOZ 78–58	Methysergide	2mg	Yellow	Tab	Round	N	Y	Sandoz	Antimigraine
	SP 58	Tolazamide	500mg	White	Tab	Round	Y	N	Superpharm	Hypoglycemic
59	GG59	Allopurinol	100mg	White	Tab	Round	Y	N	Geneva	Antigout
	M 59 / 50	Thioridazine	50mg	Orange	Tab	Round	N	Y	Mylan	Tranquilizer
	PP–59	Hydroxyzine HCl	25mg	Green	Tab	Round	N	Y	Eon	Antipruritic
	R 59	Lorazepam	0.5mg	–	Tab	–	–	–	Rugby	Antianxiety
	R 59	Lorazepam	1mg	White	Tab	Round	Y	N	Purepac	Antianxiety
	Rugby Logo R 59	Lorazepam	0.5mg	–	Tab	–	–	–	Rugby	Antianxiety
	Wyeth 59	Penicillin V Potassium	250mg	White	Tab	Round	Y	N	Wyeth	Anti–Infective
60	B60	Ergocalciterol	50,000 Units	Brown	Cap	–	–	–	Lilly	Vitamin
	bp 60	Liothyronine Sodium	25mcg	White	Tab	Round	N	N	Bolar	Hormone
	Central 60/4	Chlorpheniramine Maleate/Pseudoephedrine	4mg/60mg	Clear	Cap	–	–	–	Central	Decongestant
	DAN–P 60	Phenobarbital	60mg	White	Tab	Round	Y	N	Danbury	Sedative
	dp 60	Propranolol	60mg	Pink	Tab	Round	Y	N	Duramed	Antihypertensive
	GG60	Allopurinol	300mg	Peach	Tab	Round	Y	N	Geneva	Antigout
	J60	Digitoxin	0.1mg	Pink	Tab	Round	Y	N	Lilly	Cardiac Agent
	M/60	Maprotiline HCl	25mg	White	Tab	Round	N	Y	Mylan	Antidepressant
	Muro 400/60	Pseudoephedrine HCl/Guaifenesin	60mg/400mg	Purple Layered	Tab	–	Y	–	Central	Decongestant
	PF M 60	Morphine Sulfate	60mg	Orange	Tab	Round	N	Y	PF	Analgesic
	PP–60	Hydroxyzine HCl	10mg	Orange	Tab	Round	N	Y	Eon	Antipruritic
	R 60	Phendimetrazine	35mg	–	Tab	Round	Y	–	Rugby	Anorectic
	U60	Cephalexin	1 g	Green	Tab	Capsule	N	N	Lilly	Anti–Infective
61	GG61	Chlorpropamide	100mg	White	Tab	Round	Y	N	Geneva	Hypoglycemic
	J61	Papaverine HCl	30mg	White	Tab	Round	N	N	Lilly	Vasodilator
	Lederle C61	Cephradine	250mg	Green/Pink	Cap	–	–	–	Lederle	Anti–Infective
	M 61 / 100	Thioridazine	100mg	Orange	Tab	Round	N	Y	Mylan	Tranquilizer
	SEARLE 61	Diphenoxylate & Atropine	2.5mg/0.025mg	White	Tab	Round	N	N	Searle	Antidiarrheal
	W P61	Hydroxychloroquine Sulfate	200mg	White	Tab	Round	Y	N	Winthrop	Antimalarial
62	BI/62	Phenmetrazine HCl	75mg	Pink	Tab	Round	N	N	BI	Anorectic
	bp 62	Methyclothiazide	2.5mg	Orange	Tab	Round	Y	N	Bolar	Diuretic
	C 86/62	Metaxalone	400mg	Rose	Tab	Round	Y	N	Carnrick	Muscle Relaxant
	GG 62	Sodium Fluoride	2.2mg	Pink	Tab	Round	Y	N	Trinity	Mineral
	J62	Papaverine HCl	60mg	White	Tab	Round	N	N	Lilly	Vasodilator
	Lederle C62	Cephradine	500mg	Green	Cap	–	–	–	Lederle	Anti–Infective
	Lederle D62	Disopyramide	100mg	Blue/Red	Cap	–	–	–	Lederle	Antiarrhythmic
	M 62	Chlorothiazide	500mg	White	Tab	Round	Y	N	Mylan	Diuretic
	MERRELL 62	Trichlormethiazide	2mg	Pink	Tab	Round	–	N	Merrell	Diuretic
	SKF D62	Isopropamide Iodide	5mg	Pink	Tab	Round	–	–	SKB	Antispasmodic
	SP 62	Acetaminophen & Codeine Phosphate	300mg/60mg	White	Tab	Round	N	N	Superpharm	Analgesic
	Wyeth 62	Norgestrel	0.075mg	Yellow	Tab	Round	N	N	Wyeth	Contraceptive
63	bp 63	Methyclothiazide	5mg	Reddish Orange	Tab	Round	Y	N	Bolar	Diuretic
	GG 63	Desipramine HCl	10mg	White	Tab	Round	N	Y	Geneva	Antidepressant
	MERRELL 63	Trichlormethiazide	4mg	Blue	Tab	Round	–	N	Merrell	Diuretic
	SKF T63	Chlorpromazine HCl	30mg	Orange/Natural	Cap	–	–	–	SKB	Tranquilizer
	SP 63	Acetaminophen & Codeine Phosphate	300mg/30mg	White	Tab	Round	N	N	Superpharm	Analgesic
64	A/Wyeth 64	Lorazepam	1mg	White	Tab	Pentagonal	N	N	Wyeth	Antianxiety
	BI/64	Phendimetrazine HCl	105mg	Celery/Green	Cap	–	–	–	BI	Anorectic
	bp 64	Hydralazine HCl & Hydrochlorothiazide	100mg/50mg	Blue/Blue	Cap	–	–	–	Bolar	Antihypertensive
	Ciba 64	Methyltestosterone Sublingual	10mg	Yellow	Tab	Oval	N	N	Ciba	Hormone
	F64	Amobarbital Sodium & Secobarbital Sodium	25mg/25mg	Blue/Orange	Cap	–	–	–	Lilly	Hypnotic
	GG 64	Desipramine HCl	25mg	White	Tab	Round	N	Y	Geneva	Antidepressant
	J64	Methadone HCl	5mg	White	Tab	Round	N	N	Lilly	Analgesic
	Lederle C64	Cephalexin	250mg	Red/Gray	Cap	–	–	–	Lederle	Anti–Infective
	MERRELL 64	Trichlormethiazide & Reserpine	2mg/0.1mg	Yellow	Tab	Round	–	N	Merrell	Antihypertensive
	MP 64	Hydralazine HCl	25mg	Orange	Tab	Round	N	N	Mutual	Antihypertensive
	SKF T64	Chlorpromazine HCl	75mg	Orange/Natural	Cap	–	–	–	SKB	Tranquilizer
	SP 64	Acetaminophen & Codeine	300mg/15mg	White	Tab	Round	N	N	Superpharm	Analgesic
	SP 64	Acetaminophen & Codeine Phosphate	300mg/15mg	White	Tab	Round	N	N	Superpharm	Analgesic
65	A/Wyeth 65	Lorazepam	2mg	White	Tab	Pentagonal	N	N	Wyeth	Antianxiety
	Ciba 65	Lithium Carbonate	300mg	Peach	Tab	Round	N	N	Ciba	Tranquilizer
	F65	Amobarbital Sodium & Secobarbital Sodium	50mg/50mg	Blue/Orange	Cap	–	–	–	Lilly	Hypnotic
	GG 65	Desipramine HCl	50mg	White	Tab	Round	N	Y	Geneva	Antidepressant
	Lederle C65	Cephalexin	500mg	Red	Cap	–	–	–	Lederle	Anti–Infective
	LL P65	Propranolol HCl	60mg	White	Tab	Round	Y	N	Lederle	Antihypertensive
	M 65	Propoxyphene HCl and Acetaminophen.	65/650 mg	Orange	Tab	Capsule	N	Y	Mylan	Analgesic
	MERRELL 65	Trichlormethiazide & Reserpine	4mg/0.1mg	Lavendar	Tab	Round	–	N	Merrell	Antihypertensive
	MP 65	Acetazolamide	125mg	White	Tab	Round	Y	N	Mutual	Antiglaucoma Agent
66	BI 66	Mexiletine HCl	150mg	Red/Caramel	Cap	–	–	–	BI	Antiarrhythmic
	F/66–LL	Fibercon	n/a	Beige	Tab	Oblong	Y	Y	Lederle	Laxative
	F66	Amobarbital Sodium & Secobarbital Sodium	100mg/100mg	Blue/Orange	Cap	–	–	–	Lilly	Hypnotic

ID NO.	ID CODE	GENERIC NAME	STRENGTH	COLOR	FORM	SHAPE	SCORED	COATED	MFG.	USE
	GG66	Diazepam	2mg	White	Tab	Round	Y	N	Geneva	Antianxiety
	LL C66	Carbamazepine	200mg	White	Tab	Round	Y	N	Lederle	Anticonvulsant
	MP 66	Quinidine Gluconate SA	324mg	White	Tab	Round	N	N	Mutual	Antiarrhythmic
	SANDOZ 78–66	Mazindol	2mg	White	Tab	Round	Y	N	Sandoz	Anorectic
	SKF C66	Prochlorperazine	5mg	Yellow	Tab	Round	N	Y	SKB	Antiemetic
	SKF T66	Chlorpromazine HCl	150mg	Orange/Natural	Cap	–	–	–	SKB	Tranquilizer
	SL 66	Amitriptyline HCl	10mg	Pink	Tab	Round	N	Y	Sidmak	Antidepressant
67	BI 67	Mexiletine HCl	200mg	Red	Cap	–	–	–	BI	Antiarrhythmic
	GG67	Diazepam	5mg	Orange	Tab	Round	Y	N	Geneva	Antianxiety
	LL C67	Chlordiazepoxide HCl & Amitriptyline	5mg/12.5mg	Green	Tab	Round	N	Y	Lederle	Antidepressant
	LL P67	Propranolol HCl & Hydrochlorthiazide	40mg/25mg	White	Tab	Round	Y	N	Lederle	Antihypertensive
	SKF C67	Prochlorperazine	10mg	Yellow	Tab	Round	N	Y	SKB	Antiemetic
	SKF T67	Chlorpromazine HCl	200mg	Orange/Natural	Cap	–	–	–	SKB	Tranquilizer
	SL 67	Amitriptyline HCl	25mg	Green	Tab	Round	N	Y	Sidmak	Antidepressant
	T 67	Carbinoxamine Maleate & Pseudoephedrine	8mg/120mg	Purple	Tab	Oval	N	N	Econolab	Decongestant Comb.
68	BI 68	Mexiletine HCl	250mg	Red/Aqua Green	Cap	–	–	–	BI	Antiarrhythmic
	GG68	Diazepam	10mg	Green	Tab	Round	Y	N	Geneva	Antianxiety
	LL C68	Chlordiazepoxide HCl & Amitriptyline	10mg/25mg	White	Tab	Round	N	Y	Lederle	Antidepressant
	LL P68	Propranolol HCl & Hydrochlorthiazide	80mg/25mg	White	Tab	Round	Y	N	Lederle	Antihypertensive
	MP 68	Tolazamide	100mg	White	Tab	Round	Y	N	Mutual	Hypoglycemic
69	H69	Cephalexin	250mg	White/green	Cap	–	–	–	Lilly	Anti–Infective
	J69	Propylthiouracil	50mg	White	Tab	Round	Y	N	Lilly	Antithyroid
	Lederle P69	Prazosin HCl	1mg	Pink	Cap	–	–	–	Lederle	Antihypertensive
	LL C69	Clorazepate Dipotassium	3.75mg	Blue	Tab	Round	Y	N	Lederle	Antianxiety
	MP 69	Verapamil HCl	80mg	White	Tab	Round	Y	Y	Mutual	Antihypertensive
	RPC 69	Phentermine	30mg	Yellow	Cap	–	–	–	Rexar	Anorexiant
	SKF C69	Prochlorperazine	25mg	Yellow	Tab	Round	N	Y	SKB	Antiemetic
	SKF T69	Chlorpromazine HCl	300mg	Orange/Natural	Cap	–	–	–	SKB	Tranquilizer
70	Lederle P70	Prazosin HCl	2mg	Pink	Cap	–	–	–	Lederle	Antihypertensive
	LL C70	Clorazepate Dipotassium	7.5mg	Peach	Tab	Round	Y	N	Lederle	Antianxiety
	M 70	Clorazepate Dipotassium	15mg	White	Tab	Round	Y	N	Mylan	Antianxiety
	MP 70	Tolazamide	250mg	White	Tab	Round	Y	N	Mutual	Hypoglycemic
	R 70	Dipyridamole	25mg	White	Tab	Round	N	Y	Rugby	Antiplatelet
71	BL\71	Clonidine	0.1mg	Brown	Tab	Round	Y	N	Biocraft	Antihypertensive
	C 71	Atenolol/Chlorthalidone	100mg/25mg	White	Tab	Round	–	N	IPR	Antihypertensive
	Ciba 71	Reserpine, Hydralazine HCl, Hydrochlorothiazide	0.1mg/25mg/15mg	Pink	Tab	Round	N	N	Ciba	Antihypertensive
	Geigy 71/71	Metoprolol Tartrate	100mg	Blue	Tab	Capsule	Y	N	Geigy	Antihypertensive
	GG71	Propranolol	10mg	Peach	Tab	Round	Y	N	Geneva	Antihypertensive
	H71	Cephalexin	500mg	Green/Green	Cap	–	–	–	Lilly	Anti–Infective
	Lederle P71	Prazosin HCl	5mg	Blue	Cap	–	–	–	Lederle	Antihypertensive
	LEMMON 71	Phendimetrazine tartrate	35mg	Green/White Specs	Tab	Oblong	Y	N	Lemmon	Anorectic
	LL A71	Atenolol	100mg	White	Tab	Round	Y	N	Lederle	Antihypertensive
	LL C71	Clorazepate Dipotassium	15mg	Lavender	Tab	Round	Y	N	Lederle	Antianxiety
	LL D 71	Diltiazem HCl	30mg	Blue	Tab	Round	N	Y	Lederle	Antianginal
	LL D71	Diltiazem HCl	30mg	Green	Tab	Round	N	–	Lederle	Antianginal
	M 71	Allopurinol	300mg	White	Tab	Round	Y	N	Mylan	Antigout
	MP 71	Allopurinol	100mg	White	Tab	Round	Y	N	Mutual	Antigout
	SEARLE 71	Ethynodiol Diacetate & Ethinyl Estradiol	1mg/50mcg	White	Tab	Round	N	N	Searle	Hormone
	SKF N 71	Tranylcypromine Sulfate	10mg	Rose	Tab	Round	–	Y	SKB	Antidepressant
	Wyeth 71	Mazindol	1mg	White	Tab	Round	Y	N	Wyeth	Anorectic
72	BI/72	Metaproterenol Sulfate	20mg	White	Tab	Round	N	N	BI	Bronchodilator
	BL\72	Clonidine	0.2mg	Purple	Tab	Round	Y	N	Biocraft	Antihypertensive
	bp 72	Hydroflumethiazide	50mg	White	Tab	Round	–	N	Bolar	Diuretic
	Geigy 72	Terbutaline Sulfate	2.5mg	White	Tab	Oval	Y	N	Geigy	Bronchodilator
	GG72	Propranolol	20mg	Blue	Tab	Round	Y	N	Geneva	Antihypertensive
	H72	Vitamin Combination	n/a	Black	Cap	–	–	–	Lilly	Vitamin
	Hoescht 72	Digestive Enzymes	n/a	White	Tab	Round	N	Y	Hoechst	Digestant
	J72	Methadone HCl	10mg	White	Tab	Round	N	N	Lilly	Analgesic
	LL D 72	Diltiazem HCl	60mg	Blue	Tab	Round	N	Y	Lederle	Antianginal
	LL D72	Diltiazem HCl	60mg	Yellow	Tab	Round	N	–	Lederle	Antianginal
	LL P72	Perphenazine & Amitriptyline HCl	2mg/10mg	Blue	Tab	Round	N	Y	Lederle	Antidepressant
	M 72	Clonidine HCl & Chlorthalidone	0.3mg/15mg	Yellow	Tab	Round	Y	N	Mylan	Antihypertensive
	MP 72	Tolazamide	500mg	White	Tab	Round	Y	N	Mutual	Hypoglycemic
73	BL\73	Clonidine	0.3mg	Pink	Tab	Round	Y	N	Biocraft	Antihypertensive
	Ciba 73	Hydralazine HCl	50mg	Blue	Tab	Round	N	N	Ciba	Antihypertensive
	Geigy 73/73	Metoprolol Tartrate & Hydrochlorothiazide	100mg/50mg	Yellow/White	Tab	Capsule	Y	N	Geigy	Antihypertensive
	GG73	Propranolol	40mg	Green	Tab	Round	Y	N	Geneva	Antihypertensive
	Hoescht 73	Digestive Enzymes & Atropine Methyl Nitrate	n/a	Orange	Tab	Round	N	Y	Hoechst	Digestant
	J73	Methyltestosterone	10mg	White	Tab	Oblong	Y	N	Lilly	Hormone
	LL P73	Perphenazine & Amitriptyline HCl	2mg/25mg	Orange	Tab	Round	N	Y	Lederle	Antidepressant
	MYLAN/73	Perphenazine & Amitriptyline	4mg/50mg	Purple	Tab	Round	N	Y	Mylan	Antidepressant
	SKF T73	Chlorpromazine HCl	10mg	Orange	Tab	Round	N	Y	SKB	Tranquilizer
	T73	Papaverine HCl	200mg	White	Tab	Round	N	N	Lilly	Vasodilator
	W4/Wyeth 73	Guanabenz Acetate	4mg	White	Tab	Pentagonal	N	N	Wyeth	Antihypertensive
74	BI/74	Metaproterenol Sulfate	10mg	White	Tab	Round	N	N	BI	Bronchodilator
	Dista H74	Ethinamate	500mg	Blue/Blue	Cap	–	–	–	Dista	Hypnotic
	F74	Vitamin Combination	n/a	Red	Cap	–	–	–	Lilly	Vitamin
	GG74	Propranolol	60mg	Salmon	Tab	Round	Y	N	Geneva	Antihypertensive
	H74	Ethinamate	500mg	Blue	Cap	–	–	–	Lilly	Hypnotic
	J74	Methyltestosterone	25mg	White	Tab	Round	N	N	Lilly	Hormone
	LL P74	Perphenazine & Amitriptyline HCl	4mg/10mg	Salmon	Tab	Round	N	Y	Lederle	Antidepressant
	M/74	Fluphenazine HCl	5mg	Green	Tab	Triangle	N	Y	Mylan	Tranquilizer
	MP 74	Chlorzoxazone	500mg	Green	Tab	Oval	Y	N	Mutual	Muscle Relaxant
	SKF T74	Chlorpromazine HCl	25mg	Orange	Tab	Round	N	Y	SKB	Tranquilizer
	SP 74	Chlordiazepoxide HCl & Clidinium	5mg/2.5mg	Green/Clear	Cap	–	–	–	Superpharm	Antispasmodic
	W8/Wyeth 74	Guanabenz Acetate	8mg	White	Tab	Pentagonal	N	N	Wyeth	Antihypertensive
75	832/D75	Dipyridamole	75mg	White	Tab	Round	N	Y	PBI	Antiplatelet
	AC 75	Choline Magnesium Trisalicylate	750mg	White	Tab	Oblong	Y	Y	Able Labs	Antiarthritic
	CC 75P	Phenylpropanolamine	75mg	Yellow	Cap	–	–	–	Camall	Appetite Suppressant
	CC 75P	Phenylpropanolamine	75mg	Black	Cap	–	–	–	Camall	Appetite Suppressant
	CC 75P	Phenylpropanolamine	75mg	Blue/Clear	Cap	–	–	–	Camall	Appetite Suppressant
	CC 75P	Phenylpropanolamine	75mg	Yellow/Black	Cap	–	–	–	Camall	Appetite Suppressant
	dp 75	Levothyroxine Sodium	0.075mg	Lavender	Tab	Oval	Y	N	Daniels	Hormone
	dp 75	Dipyridamole	75mg	White	Tab	Round	N	Y	Duramed	Antiplatelet
	Flint 75	Levothyroxine Sodium	75mcg	Violet	Tab	Round	Y	N	Boots	Hormone

ID NO.	ID CODE	GENERIC NAME	STRENGTH	COLOR	FORM	SHAPE	SCORED	COATED	MFG.	USE
	GG75	Propranolol	80mg	Yellow	Tab	Round	Y	N	Geneva	Antihypertensive
	J 75	Isoproterenol HCl	10mg	White	Tab	Round	Y	N	Winthrop	Bronchodilator
	J75	Digitoxin	0.05mg	Orange	Tab	Round	Y	N	Lilly	Cardiac Agent
	LL D 75	Diltiazem HCl	90mg	Blue	Tab	Round	N	Y	Lederle	Antianginal
	LL D75	Diltiazem HCl	90mg	Green	Tab	Oblong	N	–	Lederle	Antianginal
	LL P75	Perphenazine & Amitriptyline HCl	4mg/25mg	Yellow	Tab	Round	N	Y	Lederle	Antidepressant
	M 75	Chlorthalidone	50mg	Green	Tab	Round	Y	N	Mylan	Diuretic
	M 75	Levothyroxine Sodium	0.075mg	Purple	Tab	Round	Y	N	Duramed	Hormone
	Ortho 75	Norethindrone & Ethinyl Estradiol	0.75mg/0.035mg	Lt. Peach	Tab	Round	N	N	Ortho	Hormone
	Par/75	Dipyridamole	75mg	White	Tab	Round	N	N	Par	Antiplatelet
	PP–75	Phendimetrazine Tartrate	35mg	Pink/White/Blue	Tab	Capsule	Y	N	Eon	Anorectic
	WHR 75mg	Theophylline	75mg	White/Clear	Cap	–	–	–	Rorer	Bronchodilator
	Wyeth 75	Levonorgestrel & Ethinyl Estradiol	0.15mg/0.03mg	Orange	Tab	Round	N	N	Wyeth	Contraceptive
76	BI/76	Chlorthalidone	25mg	White	Tab	Kidney	N	N	BI	Diuretic
	bp 76	Oxtriphylline Enteric coated	100mg	Red	Tab	Round	N	Y	Bolar	Bronchodilator
	GG76	L–Thyroxine	0.3mg	Green	Tab	Round	Y	N	PBI	Hormone
	H76	Fenoprofen Calcium	200mg	Yellow/White	Cap	–	–	–	Lilly	Analgesic
	J76	Digitoxin	0.15mg	Yellow	Tab	Round	Y	N	Lilly	Cardiac Agent
	LL P76	Perphenazine & Amitriptyline HCl	4mg/50mg	Orange	Tab	Round	N	Y	Lederle	Antidepressant
	M 76	Flurbiprofen	50mg	Beige	Tab	Round	N	N	Mylan	Analgesic
	MP 76	Verapamil HCl	120mg	White	Tab	Round	Y	Y	Mutual	Antihypertensive
	SKF T76	Chlorpromazine HCl	50mg	Orange	Tab	Round	N	Y	SKB	Tranquilizer
	VT 76	Phendimetrazine Tartrate	35mg	Yellow	Tab	Round	Y	N	Eon	Anorectic
77	BI/77	Chlorthalidone	15mg	White	Tab	Kidney	N	N	BI	Diuretic
	bp 77	Oxtriphylline Enteric coated	200mg	Yellow	Tab	Round	N	Y	Bolar	Bronchodilator
	GG77	L–Thyroxine	0.15mg	Blue	Tab	Round	Y	N	PBI	Hormone
	H77	Fenoprofen Calcium	300mg	Yellow	Cap	–	–	–	Lilly	Analgesic
	J 77	Isoproterenol HCl	15mg	White	Tab	Round	Y	N	Winthrop	Bronchodilator
	LEMMON 77	Phendimetrazine tartrate	35mg	Green	Tab	Oblong	Y	N	Lemmon	Anorectic
	LL D77	Diltiazem HCl	120mg	Yellow	Tab	Oblong	N	–	Lederle	Antianginal
	LL N77	Naproxen	500mg	Green	Tab	Capsule	–	Y	Lederle	Anti–Inflammatory
	M77	Amitriptyline HCl	10mg	Pink	Tab	Round	N	Y	Mylan	Antidepressant
	M77	Amitriptyline HCl	10mg	White	Tab	Round	N	Y	Mylan	Antidepressant
	MP 77	Ibuprofen	200mg	White	Tab	Round	N	Y	Mutual	Analgesic
	SKF T77	Chlorpromazine HCl	100mg	Orange	Tab	Round	N	Y	SKB	Tranquilizer
	T 77	Carbinoxamine Maleate & Pseudoephedrine	4mg/60mg	White	Tab	Oval	N	N	Econolab	Decongestant Comb.
	VT–77	Phendimetrazine Tartrate	35mg	Pink	Tab	Capsule	Y	N	Eon	Anorectic
	W A77	Chloroquine Phosphate	500mg	Pink	Tab	Round	N	Y	Winthrop	Antimalarial
78	bp 78	Cyproheptadine HCL	4mg	White	Tab	Round	Y	–	Bolar	Antipruritic
	GG 78	Methazolamide	25mg	White	Tab	Round	Y	N	Geneva	Antiglaucoma
	SP 78	Ergoloid Mesylates Oral	1mg	White	Tab	Round	N	N	Superpharm	Vasodilator
	Wyeth 78	Norgestrel & Ethinyl Estradiol	0.3mg/0.03mg	White	Tab	Round	N	N	Wyeth	Contraceptive
79	bp 79	Clonidine HCL	0.1mg	White	Tab	Round	–	–	Bolar	Antihypertensive
	GG79	Prednisone	5mg	White	Tab	Round	Y	N	Geneva	Steroid
	MP 79	Imipramine Hydrochloride	50mg	Green	Tab	Round	N	Y	Mutual	Antidepressant
	SKF T79	Chlorpromazine HCl	200mg	Orange	Tab	Round	N	Y	SKB	Tranquilizer
	W A 79	Chloroquin Phosphate/Primaquine Phosphate	500mg/79mg	Orange	Tab	Round	N	Y	Winthrop	Antimalarial
80	bp 80	Clonidine HCL	0.2mg	Orange	Tab	Round	–	–	Bolar	Antihypertensive
	dp/80	Propranolol	80mg	Yellow	Tab	Round	Y	N	Duramed	Antihypertensive
	GG80	Furosemide	80mg	White	Tab	Round	Y	N	Geneva	Diuretic
	M 80	Propranolol	80mg	Yellow	Tab	Round	Y	N	Martec	Antihypertensive
	MP 80	Allopurinol	300mg	Orange	Tab	Round	Y	N	Mutual	Antigout
	USL 80	Zinc Sulfate	220mg	Pink	Cap	–	–	–	Upsher	Mineral Supp.
81	A/Wyeth 81	Lorazepam	0.5mg	White	Tab	Pentagonal	N	–	Wyeth	Antianxiety
	bp 81	Clonidine HCL	0.3mg	Peach	Tab	Round	–	–	Bolar	Antihypertensive
	GG81	Clonidine	0.1mg	Green	Tab	Round	Y	N	Geneva	Antihypertensive
	Lederle LL C81	Cephalexin	250mg	White	Cap	–	–	–	Lederle	Anti–Infective
	MP 81	Sulfamethoxazole & Trimethoprim	400mg/80mg	White	Tab	Round	Y	N	Mutual	Anti–Infective
82	82	Indapamide	2.5mg	White	Tab	Round	N	Y	Rorer	Antihypertensive
	GG82	Clonidine	0.2mg	Yellow	Tab	Round	Y	N	Geneva	Antihypertensive
	Lederle LL C82	Cephalexin	500mg	White	Cap	–	–	–	Lederle	Anti–Infective
	W A82	Quinacrine HCl	100mg	Yellow	Tab	Round	N	Y	Winthrop	Antimalarial
83	GG83	Clonidine	0.3mg	Blue	Tab	Round	Y	N	Geneva	Antihypertensive
	MP 83	Nystatin	500,000 Units	Brown	Tab	Round	Y	Y	Mutual	Anti–Infective
84	GG 84	Timolol Maleate	5mg	White	Tab	Round	–	–	Geneva	Antihypertensive
	PP 84	Iodinated Glycerol	30mg	Orange	Tab	Round	Y	N	Eon	Expectorant
	SP 84	Quinine Sulfate	260mg	White	Tab	Round	N	N	Superpharm	Muscle Relaxant
85	85–WMH	Dexbrompheniramine Maleate & Pseudoephedrine Sulf	6mg/120mg	Red	Tab	Round	N	Y	Schering	Decongestant Comb.
	879 G85C 2	Aspirin with Codeine Phosphate	325mg/15mg	White	Tab	Round	N	N	Halsey	Analgesic
	GG85	Spironolactone	25mg	White	Tab	Round	Y	Y	Geneva	Diuretic
	MP 85	Sulfamethoxazole & Trimethoprim	800mg/160mg	White	Tab	Oval	Y	N	Mutual	Anti–Infective
86	Wyeth 85	Propoxyphene HCl & Acetaminophen	65mg/650mg	Green	Tab	Capsule	Y	Y	Wyeth	Analgesic
	879 G86C 3	Aspirin with Codeine Phosphate	325mg/30mg	White	Tab	Round	N	N	Halsey	Analgesic
87	LEMMON 86	Secobarbital/Butabarbital/Phenobarbital	50mg/30mg/15mg	White	Tab	Round	Y	N	Lemmon	Hypnotic
	879 G87C 4	Aspirin with Codeine Phosphate	325mg/60mg	White	Tab	Round	N	N	Halsey	Analgesic
	bp 87	Sulfamethoxazole	500mg	Green	Tab	Round	–	N	Bolar	Anti–Infective
	M/87	Maprotiline HCl	50mg	Blue	Tab	Round	N	Y	Mylan	Antidepressant
	W M 87	Ambenonium	10mg	White	Tab	Capsule	N	N	Winthrop	Muscle Stimulant
88	879 G88C	Diphenoxylate HCl & Atropine Sulfate	2.5mg/0.025mg	White	Tab	Round	N	N	Halsey	Antidiarrheal
	bp 88	Primidone (Veterinary)	250mg	White	Tab	Round	N	N	Bolar	Anticonvulsant
	dp 88	Levothyroxine Sodium	0.088mg	Green	Tab	Oval	Y	N	Daniels	Hormone
	Flint 88	Levothyroxine Sodium	0.088mg	Olive	Tab	Oval	Y	N	Boots	Hormone
89	MP 88	Albuterol Sulfate	4mg	White	Tab	Round	Y	N	Mutual	Bronchodilator
	GG 89	Amoxapine	25mg	–	Tab	Round	Y	N	Geneva	Antidepressant
	SP 89	Ergoloid Mesylates SL	1mg	White	Tab	Oval	N	N	Superpharm	Vasodilator
90	879 G90C	Phenobarbital with Belladonna Alkaloids	16.2mg	White	Tab	Round	Y	N	Halsey	Antispasmodic
	Bock PN 90	Prenatal Vitamin	n/a	White	Tab	Oval	N	Y	Bock	Prenatal Vitamin
	BOOTS logo 90	Guaifenesin/Pseudoephedrine HCl	600mg/120mg	Blue	Tab	Elongated	Y	Y	Boots	Decongestant Comb.
	C 90	Atenolol	100mg	White	Tab	Round	Y	N	IPR	Antihypertensive
	dp 90	Propranolol	90mg	Lavender	Tab	Round	Y	N	Duramed	Antihypertensive
	GG 90	Amoxapine	50mg	–	Tab	Round	Y	N	Geneva	Antidepressant
	Marion 90mg	Diltiazem HCl	90mg	Green	Tab	Oblong	N	Y	Marion	Antianginal
	SKF P 90	Isopropamide Iodide	5mg	Yellow	Tab	Round	–	Y	SKB	Anticholinergic
	SKF P 90	Isopropamide Iodide/Trifluoperazine HCl	5mg/1mg	Yellow	Tab	Round	–	Y	SKB	Tranquilizer
	SP 90	Ergoloid Mesylates SL	0.5mg	White	Tab	Round	N	N	Superpharm	Vasodilator

ID NO.	ID CODE	GENERIC NAME	STRENGTH	COLOR	FORM	SHAPE	SCORED	COATED	MFG.	USE
	W M–90 60mg	Trilostane	60mg	Pink/Black	Cap	–	–	–	Winthrop	
91	GG 91	Lorazepam	0.5mg	White	Tab	Round	N	N	Geneva	Antianxiety
	MP 91	Sulfasalazine	500mg	Gold	Tab	Round	Y	N	Mutual	Anti–Inflammatory
	SKF P 91	Isopropamide Iodide/Trifluoperazine HCl	5mg/2mg	Yellow	Tab	Round	–	Y	SKB	Tranquilizer
	W M–91 30mg	Trilostane	30mg	Pink	Cap	–	–	–	Winthrop	
92	Wyeth 91	Meprobamate & Aspirin	200mg/325mg	Pink/Yellow	Tab	Round	Y	N	Wyeth	Analgesic
	BL/92	Metoclopramide	5mg	White	Tab	Round	Y	N	Biocraft	Antireflux
	GG 92	Lorazepam	1mg	White	Tab	Round	Y	N	Geneva	Antianxiety
	M 92	Maprotiline HCl	75mg	White	Tab	Round	N	Y	Mylan	Antidepressant
	SKF P 92	Isopropamide Iodide/Trifluoperazine HCl	7.5mg/2mg	Yellow	Tab	Round	–	Y	SKB	Tranquilizer
93	W D 92	Ergocalciferol	1.25mg	Green	Cap	–	–	–	Winthrop	Vitamin
	W16/Wyeth 92	Guanabenz Acetate	16mg	White	Tab	Pentagonal	N	N	Wyeth	Antihypertensive
	93 DOXY	Doxycycline Hyclate	100mg	Orange	Tab	Round	N	Y	Lemmon	Anti–Infective
	BL\93	Metoclopramide HCl	10mg	White	Tab	Round	Y	N	Biocraft	Antireflux
	bp 93	Prochlorperazine	10mg	Chartreuse	Tab	Round	N	Y	Bolar	Antiemetic
	GG 93	Lorazepam	2mg	White	Tab	Round	Y	N	Geneva	Antianxiety
	M 93	Flurbiprofen	100mg	Beige	Tab	Round	N	N	Mylan	Analgesic
	SKF P 93	Isopropamide Iodide/Trifluoperazine HCl	10mg/2mg	Yellow	Tab	Round	–	Y	SKB	Tranquilizer
	SKF/ E93	Triamterene & Hydrochlorothiazide	50mg/25mg	Peach	Tab	Round	Y	N	SKB	Diuretic
	T93	Isoniazid	100mg	White	Tab	Round	Y	N	Lilly	Anti–Infective
94	Biocraft/94	Cyclacillin	250mg	White	Tab	Capsule	–	–	Biocraft	Anti–Infective
	GG 94	Albuterol	2mg	White	Tab	Round	Y	N	Geneva	Broncodilator
	J94	Methimazole	5mg	White	Tab	Round	Y	N	Lilly	Antithyroid
	MP 94	Ibuprofen	300mg	White	Tab	Round	N	Y	Mutual	Anti–Inflammatory
95	B 95	Levonorgestrel/Ethinyl Estradiol	0.05mg/0.03mg	Brown	Tab	Round	N	N	Berlex	Hormone
	Biocraft/95	Cyclacillin	500mg	White	Tab	Capsule	–	–	Biocraft	Anti–Infective
	GG95	Spironolactone & Hydrochlorothiazide	25mg/25mg	White	Tab	Round	Y	Y	Geneva	Diuretic
	J95	Methimazole	10mg	White	Tab	Round	Y	N	Lilly	Antithyroid
	M 95	Penicillin V Potassium	250mg	White	Tab	Round	Y	N	Mylan	Anti–Infective
	MP 95	Ibuprofen	400mg	White	Tab	Round	N	Y	Mutual	Anti–Inflammatory
96	T95	Sulfadiazine/Sulfamerazine/Sulfamethazine	167/167/167mg	White	Tab	Round	Y	N	Lilly	Anti–Infective
	B 96	Levonorgestrel/Ethinyl Estradiol	0.075mg/0.04mg	White	Tab	Round	N	N	Berlex	Hormone
	F96	Liver Stomach Conc./Vitamin Comb.	n/a	Brown	Cap	–	–	–	Lilly	Hematinic
	J96	Methyltestosterone & Diethylstilbestrol	5mg/0.25mg	White	Tab	Round	Y	N	Lilly	Hormone
	MP 96	Lorazepam	2mg	White	Tab	Round	Y	N	Mutual	Antianxiety
	Par/96	Thioridazine HCl	10mg	Orange	Tab	Round	N	N	Par	Tranquilizer
97	T96	Neomycin Sulfate	500mg	White	Tab	Round	N	N	Lilly	Anti–Infective
	B 97	Levonorgestrel/Ethinyl Estradiol	0.125mg/0.03mg	Yellow	Tab	Round	N	N	Berlex	Hormone
	Ciba 97	Reserpine & Hydrochlorothiazide	0.1mg/50mg	Orange	Tab	Round	N	N	Ciba	Antihypertensive
	GG97	Fluphenazine HCl	1mg	Rust	Tab	Round	N	Y	Geneva	Tranquilizer
	M/97	Fluphenazine HCl	10mg	Orange	Tab	Triangle	N	Y	Mylan	Tranquilizer
	Par/97	Thioridazine HCl	15mg	Orange	Tab	Round	N	N	Par	Tranquilizer
	SP 97	Metronidazole	500mg	White	Tab	Round	N	N	Superpharm	Anti–Infective
98	W P 97	Primaquine Phosphate	26.3mg	White	Tab	Round	N	Y	Winthrop	Antimalarial
	IP 98	Guaifenesin & Pseudoephedrine	600mg/60mg	Blue	Tab	Oval	Y	N	Rugby	Antitussive comb.
	M 98	Penicillin V Potassium	500mg	White	Tab	Oval	N	N	Mylan	Anti–Infective
	MP 98	Ibuprofen	600mg	White	Tab	Oval	N	Y	Mutual	Anti–Inflammatory
	Par/98	Thioridazine HCl	25mg	Orange	Tab	Round	N	N	Par	Tranquilizer
99	SP 98	Chlorthalidone	100mg	White	Tab	Round	N	N	Superpharm	Diuretic
	MP 99/800	Ibuprofen	800mg	White	Tab	Capsule	N	Y	Mutual	Anti–Inflammatory
	Par/99	Thioridazine HCl	50mg	Orange	Tab	Round	N	N	Par	Tranquilizer
001	T99	Paramethasone Acetate	1mg	Yellow	Tab	Round	Y	N	Lilly	Steroid
	AMIDE 001	Multivitamin with Fluoride	1mg	Orange/Pink/Purple	Tab	Round	N	N	Amide	Vitamin
	ETHEX 001	Potassium Chloride ER	10 mEq	Clear/Clear	Cap	–	–	–	Ethex	Potassium Supp.
	P–D 001	Pentaerythritol Tetranitrate	20mg	Green	Tab	Round	N	N	PD	Antianginal
002	R 001/3	Acetaminophen & Codeine	300mg/30mg	White	Tab	Round	Y	N	Purepac	Analgesic
	59743 002	Guaifenesin & Pseudoephedrine	600mg/60mg	White	Cap	–	–	–	Qualitest	Antitussive Comb.
	ETHEX 002	Disopyramide Phosphate Ext. Release	150mg	Orange/Purple	Cap	–	–	–	Ethex	Antiarrhythmic
003	AMIDE 003	Phenazopyridine HCl	100mg	Maroon	Tab	Round	N	Y	Amide	Urinary Analgesic
	ETHEX 003	Disopyramide Phosphate Ext. Release	100mg	Yellow/Purple	Cap	–	–	–	Ethex	Antiarrhythmic
004	R 003/4	Acetaminophen & Codeine	300mg/60mg	White	Tab	Round	Y	N	Purepac	Analgesic
	AMIDE 004	Phenazopyridine HCl	200mg	Maroon	Tab	Round	N	Y	Amide	Urinary Analgesic
	ETHEX 004	Nitroglycerin TD	2.5mg	Purple/Clear	Cap	–	–	–	Ethex	Antianginal
	P–D 004	Pentaerythritol Tetranitrate SA	80mg	Green/Green	Tab	Round	N	N	PD	Antianginal
	West–ward 004	Acetaminophen & Codeine Phosphate	300mg/30mg	White	Tab	Round	N	N	West–ward	Analgesic
005	ETHEX 005	Nitroglycerin TD	6.5mg	Dark Blue/Yellow	Cap	–	–	–	Ethex	Antianginal
	West–ward 005	Acetaminophen & Codeine Phosphate	300mg/60mg	White	Tab	Round	N	N	West–ward	Analgesic
006	ETHEX 006	Nitroglycerin TD	9.0mg	Clear/Clear	Cap	–	–	–	Ethex	Antianginal
	Hoyt 006	Sodium Fluoride	1mg	Pink	Tab	Round	N	N	Colgate	Mineral Supp.
	SP 006	Chlorzoxazone & Acetaminophen	250mg/300mg	Green	Tab	Hexagonal	N	N	Superpharm	Muscle Relaxant
007	43797–007	Hyoscyamine Sulfate	0.125mg	Green	Tab	Hexagonal	Y	N	Hauck	Antispasmodic
	Hoyt 007	Sodium Fluoride	1mg	White	Tab	Round	N	N	Colgate	Mineral Supp.
008	P–D 007	Phenytoin	50mg	Off White	Tab	Triangular	N	N	PD	Anticonvulsant
009	P–D 008	Pentaerythritol Tetranitrate	40mg	Coral	Tab	Round	N	N	PD	Antianginal
	54–009	Propranolol HCl	20mg	White	Tab	Round	N	N	Roxane	Antihypertensive
	DURA 009	Guaifenesin	600mg	Blue	Tab	–		Y	N	Dura	Expectorant
010	Par/009	Isosorbide Dinitrate	30mg	Blue	Tab	Round	Y	N	Par	Antianginal
	54 010	Diflunisal	250 mg	Orange	Tab	Capsule	N	Y	Roxane	Anti–inflammatory
	barr/ 010	Tetracycline HCl	500mg	Black/Yellow	Cap	–	–	–	Barr	Anti–Infective
	OHM 010	Acetaminophen	325mg	White	Tab	Round	Y	N	OHM	Analgesic
011	West–ward 010	Allopurinol	100mg	White	Tab	Round	Y	N	West–ward	Antigout
	barr/ 011	Tetracycline HCl	500mg	Orange/Yellow	Cap	–	–	–	Barr	Anti–Infective
	OHM 011	Acetaminophen	500mg	White	Tab	Round	Y	N	OHM	Analgesic
	Sch. Logo 011	Betamethasone	0.6mg	Pink	Tab	Round	Y	N	Schering	Steroid
012	012	Chlorzoxazone With Acetaminophen	250mg/300mg	Green	Tab	Round	Y	N	Amide	Muscle Relaxant
	54–012	Amitriptyline	25mg	White	Tab	Round	N	N	Roxane	Antidepressant
	Par/012	Hydroxyzine HCl	10mg	Lavender	Tab	Round	N	Y	Par	Antipruritic
	R 012	Chloral Hydrate	500mg	Green	Cap	–	–	–	Rondex	Hypnotic
013	R 012	Meprobamate	200mg	White	Tab	Round	N	N	Rondex	Antianxiety
	54–013	Leucovorin Calcium	25mg	–	Tab	Round	–	–	Roxane	Antineoplastic
	555/013,bar	Erythromycin Stearate	250mg	Red	Tab	Round	N	Y	Barr	Anti–Infective
	Amide 013	Ephedrine, Theophylline, Hydroxyzine HCl	25/130/10mg	White	Tab	Round	N	N	Amide	Bronchodilator
	Hoyt 013	Sodium Fluoride	0.5mg	Blue	Tab	Round	N	N	Colgate	Mineral Supp.
	P–D 013	Pentaerythritol Tetranitrate	10mg	Green	Tab	Round	N	N	PD	Antianginal
	Par/013	Hydroxyzine HCl	25mg	Lavender	Tab	Round	N	Y	Par	Antipruritic

ID NO.	ID CODE	GENERIC NAME	STRENGTH	COLOR	FORM	SHAPE	SCORED	COATED	MFG.	USE
014	West–ward 013	Allopurinol	300mg	Orange	Tab	Round	Y	N	West–ward	Antigout
	Amide 014	Dexchlorpheniramine TR	4mg	–	Tab	Pumpkin Seed	Y	n	Amide	Antihistamine
	Hoyt 014	Sodium Fluoride	0.5mg	Purple	Tab	Round	N	N	Colgate	Mineral Supp.
	Hoyt 014	Sodium Fluoride	0.5mg	Purple	Tab	Round	N	N	Colgate	Mineral Supp.
	Par/014	Hydroxyzine HCI	50mg	White	Tab	Round	N	Y	Par	Antipruritic
	WC 014	Propranolol & Hydrochlorothiazide	40mg/25mg	White	Tab	Round	Y	N	WC	Antihypertensive
015	Amide 015	Dexchlorpheniramine TR	6mg	–	Tab	Oval	Y	N	Amide	Antihistamine
	Par/015	Meclizine HCl	50mg	Yellow/Blue	Tab	Pumpkin Seed	N	N	Par	Antinauseant
	WC 015	Propranolol & Hydrochlorothiazide	80mg/25mg	White	Tab	Round	Y	N	WC	Antihypertensive
016	Par/016	Chlorzoxazone	250mg	Orange	Tab	Round	Y	N	Par	Muscle relaxant
	R 016	Meprobamate	200mg	White	Tab	Round	Y	N	Purepac	Antianxiety
018	Par/018	Doxycycline Hyclate	50mg	Blue/White	Cap	–	–	–	Par	Anti–Infective
	R 018	Meprobamate	400mg	White	Tab	Round	Y	N	Purepac	Antianxiety
019	54–019	Chlorpheniramine Maleate	4mg	–	Tab	Round	–	–	Roxane	Antihistamine
	93 019	Phentermine HCI	37.5mg	Blue/White	Cap	–	–	–	Lemmon	Anorectic
	AMIDE 019	Salsalate	500mg	Yellow	Tab	Round	N	Y	Amide	Analgesic
	DMSP 019	Cimetidine	200mg	White	Tab	Oval	–	Y	Dupont	Antiulcer
	Par/019	Doxycycline Hyclate	100mg	Blue	Cap	–	–	–	Par	Anti–Infective
020	AMIDE 020	Salsalate	750mg	Yellow	Tab	Capsule	N	Y	Amide	Analgesic
	N 020/2	Loperamide	2mg	White	Cap	–	–	–	Novopharm	Antidiarrheal
	Par/020	Isosorbide Dinitrate	5mg	White	Tab	Round	Y	N	Par	Antianginal
	West–ward 020	Aminophylline	100mg	White	Tab	Round	N	N	West–ward	Bronchodilator
021	Par/021	Isosorbide Dinitrate	10mg	White	Tab	Round	Y	N	Par	Antianginal
	R 021	Flurazepam Hydrochloride	15mg	Blue/White	Cap	–	–	–	Purepac	Hypnotic
	STUART 021	Multivitamin/Multimineral combination	n/a	Yellow	Tab	Capsule	N	Y	Stuart	Vitamin
022	AMIDE 022	Prenatal Vitamins w/Beta–Carotene	–	Yellow	Tab	Oval	N	Y	Amide	Vitamin
	Par/022	Isosorbide Dinitrate	20mg	Green	Tab	Round	Y	N	Par	Antianginal
	R 022	Flurazepam Hydrochloride	30mg	Blue	Cap	–	–	–	Purepac	Hypnotic
023	R 023	Butalbital, Aspirin and Caffeine	50/40/325mg	White	Tab	Round	N	N	Purepac	Analgesic
025	Par/025	Isosorbide Dinitrate Sustained Action	40mg	Green	Tab	Round	Y	N	Par	Antianginal
	West–ward 025	Aminophylline	200mg	White	Tab	Round	Y	N	West–ward	Bronchodilator
026	Amide 026	Multivitamin with Fluoride DF	1mg	Orange/Pink/Purple	Tab	Round	N	N	Amide	Vitamin
	G–026	Piroxicam	10mg	Olive/Green	Cap	–	–	–	Par	Anti–inflammatory
	R 026	Phenobarbital	15mg	White	Tab	Round	Y	N	Purepac	Sedative
027	879 027	Pentobarbital Sodium	100mg	Yellow	Cap	–	–	–	Halsey	Hypnotic
	G–027	Piroxicam	20mg	Green/Green	Cap	–	–	–	Par	Anti–inflammatory
	Par/027	Hydralazine HCl	25mg	Peach	Tab	Round	N	N	Par	Antihypertensive
	R 027	Alprazolam	0.25mg	White	Tab	Round	Y	N	Purepac	Antianxiety
028	Par/028	Hydralazine HCl	50mg	Peach	Tab	Round	N	N	Par	Antihypertensive
	R 028	Phenobarbital	30mg	White	Tab	Round	Y	N	Purepac	Sedative
029	IP 029	Aspirin CR	800mg	White	Tab	Capsule	N	Y	Interpharm	Analgesic
	Par/029	Hydralazine HCl	10mg	Lt. Pink	Tab	Round	N	N	Par	Antihypertensive
	R 029	Alprazolam	0.5mg	Peach	Tab	Round	Y	N	Purepac	Antianxiety
030	Par/030	Phenylprop.,phenyleph.,phenyltolox.,chlorphenir.	40,10,15,5mg	White w blue/green	Tab	Round	N	N	Par	Decongestant comb.
	WC 030	Methyldopa & Hydrochlorothiazide	250mg/15mg	Green	Tab	Round	N	Y	WC	Antihypertensive
031	AMIDE/031	Multivitamin with Fluoride Chewable	0.5mg	Multicolor	Tab	Pillow	N	N	Amide	Vitamin
	R 031	Alprazolam	1mg	Blue	Tab	Round	Y	N	Purepac	Antianxiety
	WC 031	Methyldopa & Hydrochlorothiazide	250mg/25mg	White	Tab	Capsule	N	Y	WC	Antihypertensive
032	WC 032	Methyldopa & Hydrochlorothiazide	500mg/30mg	Maroon	Tab	–	N	Y	WC	Antihypertensive
	Barr 033	Chlordiazepoxide HCI	10mg	Green/Black	Cap	–	–	–	Barr	Antianxiety
	WC 033	Methyldopa & Hydrochlorothiazide	500mg/50mg	Gray	Tab	–	–	Y	WC	Antihypertensive
034	Par/034	Meclizine HCl	12.5mg	White/Blue	Tab	Oval	N	N	Par	Antinauseant
	AMIDE 035	Theophylline/Ephedrine HCI/Phenobarbital	130mg/24mg/8mg	White	Tab	Round	Y	N	Amide	Bronchodilator
	Ortho 0.35	Norethindrone	0.35mg	Lime	Tab	Round	N	N	Ortho	Hormone
	Par/035	Meclizine HCl	25mg	White/Yellow	Tab	Oval	N	N	Par	Antinauseant
036	Eaton 036	Nitrofurantoin	50mg	Yellow	Tab	Round	Y	N	Norwich	Anti–Infective
037	Eaton 037	Nitrofurantoin	100mg	Yellow	Tab	Round	Y	N	Norwich	Anti–Infective
038	Par/038	Trichlormethiazide	2mg	Pink	Tab	Round	N	N	Par	Diuretic
	WC 038	Amoxicillin Chewable	250mg	Cherry	Tab	–	–	Y	WC	Antibiotic
039	54–039	Naproxen	500mg	–	Tab	–	–	–	Roxane	Anti–Inflammatory
	AMIDE 039	Isometheptene Mucate, Dichloralphenazone, APAP	65mg/100mg/325	Red/White	Cap	–	–	–	Amide	Vasodilator
	N 039/50	Atenolol	50mg	White	Tab	Round	Y	N	Novopharm	Antihypertensive
	Par/039	Trichlormethiazide	4mg	Blue	Tab	Round	N	N	Par	Diuretic
	R 039	Alprazolam	2mg	Yellow	Tab	Rectangular	Y	N	Purepac	Antianxiety
040	A 040	Dimenhydrinate	50mg	White	Tab	Round	Y	N	Amide	Antiemetic
	EL 040	Guaifenesin	600mg	Green	Tab	Oval	Y	N	Rugby	Expectorant
	PP–040	Furosemide	40mg	White	Tab	Round	Y	N	Eon	Diuretic
043	Par/043	Cyproheptadine HCl	4mg	White	Tab	Round	Y	N	Par	Antipruritic
044	044 HD	Meprobamate	400mg	White	Tab	Round	Y	N	Halsey	Antianxiety
045	West–ward 045	Amitriptyline Hydrochloride	10mg	Pink	Tab	Round	N	Y	West–ward	Antidepressant
046	West–ward 046	Amitriptyline Hydrochloride	25mg	Green	Tab	Round	N	Y	West–ward	Antidepressant
047	West–ward 047	Amitriptyline Hydrochloride	50mg	Brown	Tab	Round	N	Y	West–ward	Antidepressant
048	WC 048	Benzonatate	100mg	Yellow	Cap	–	–	–	WC	Antitussive
	West–ward 048	Amitriptyline Hydrochloride	75mg	Purple	Tab	Round	N	Y	West–ward	Antidepressant
049	WC 049	Butalbital, Aspirin and Caffeine	50/325/40mg	White	Tab	Round	Y	N	WC	Analgesic
	West–ward 049	Amitriptyline Hydrochloride	100mg	Orange	Tab	Round	N	Y	West–ward	Antidepressant
050	54–050 1	Haloperidol	1mg	White	Tab	Round	Y	N	Roxane	Tranquilizer
	DMSP 050	Cimetidine	300mg	White	Tab	Oval	–	Y	Dupont	Antiulcer
	KU 050	Pseudoephedrine HCl & Chlorpheniramine	60mg/4mg	White	Tab	Oval	Y	N	K–U	Decongestant Comb.
	West–ward 050	Amitriptyline Hydrochloride	150mg	Peach	Tab	Round	N	Y	West–ward	Antidepressant
051	R 051	Diazepam	2mg	White	Tab	Round	Y	N	Purepac	Antianxiety
052	R 052	Diazepam	5mg	Yellow	Tab	Round	Y	N	Purepac	Antianxiety
053	54–053 300	Quinidine Sulfate	300mg	White	Tab	Round	Y	N	Roxane	Antiarrhythmic
	AT 053	Clorazepate Dipotassium	3.75mg	White/White	Cap	–	–	–	ATI	Antianxiety
	HAUCK logo 053	Phendimetrazine Tartrate	35mg	Maroon/Pink	Cap	–	–	–	W.E.Hauck	Anorectic
	Kremers Urban 053	Pseudoephedrine HCl & Chlorpheniramine	65mg/10mg	White/Yellow	Cap	–	–	–	Central	Decongestant Comb
	KREMERS URBAN 053	Pseudoephedrine HCI/Chlorpheniramine Maleate	65mg/10mg	White/Yellow	Cap	–	–	–	K–U	Decongestant Comb.
	Par 053	B–Complex w/Folic Acid	–	Orange	Tab	Capsule	N	Y	Par	Vitamin
	R 053	Diazepam	10mg	Blue	Tab	Round	Y	N	Purepac	Antianxiety
054	AT 054	Clorazepate Dipotassium	7.5mg	Orange/Orange	Cap	–	–	–	ATI	Antianxiety
055	AT 055	Clorazepate Dipotassium	15mg	Red/Red	Cap	–	–	–	ATI	Antianxiety
	Kremers Urban 055	Pseudoephedrine HCl & Chlorpheniramine	120mg/8mg	Clear	Cap	–	–	–	Central	Decongestant Comb.
	KREMERS URBAN 055	Pseudoephedrine HCl/Chlorpheniramine Maleate	120mg/8mg	Clear	Cap	–	–	–	K–U	Decongestant Comb.
056	A 056	Chlorpheniramine Maleate	4mg	–	Tab	Round	Y	N	Amide	Antihistamine
	AT 0.5/056	Lorazepam	0.5mg	White	Tab	Round	Y	N	ATI	Antianxiety

ID NO.	ID CODE	GENERIC NAME	STRENGTH	COLOR	FORM	SHAPE	SCORED	COATED	MFG.	USE
057	WC 057	Cyclobenzaprine HCl	10mg	White	Tab	Round	N	Y	WC	Muscle Relaxant
058	058	Chewable Vitamin with Fluoride	1mg	Cr./orange specks	Tab	Round	N	N	Amide	Vitamin
	AT 1.0/058	Lorazepam	1.0mg	White	Tab	Round	Y	N	ATI	Antianxiety
	barr, 058	Diphenhydramine HCl	25mg	Pink/Clear	Cap	–	–	–	Barr	Antihistamine
059	barr, 059	Diphenhydramine HCl	50mg	Pink/Pink	Cap	–	–	–	Barr	Antihistamine
060	AT 2.0/060	Lorazepam	2.0mg	White	Tab	Round	Y	N	ATI	Antianxiety
	West–ward 060	Ascorbic Acid	500mg	White	Tab	Round	–	–	West–ward	Vitamin
061	PAR 061	Fluphenazine HCl	1mg	White	Tab	Round	N	Y	Par	Tranquilizer
062	54–062	Propranolol HCl	60mg	–	Tab	Round	–	–	Roxane	Antihypertensive
	PAR 062	Fluphenazine HCl	2.5mg	Blue	Tab	Round	N	Y	Par	Tranquilizer
	SP 062	Acetaminophen with Codeine Phosphate	300mg/60mg	White	Tab	Round	N	N	Superpharm	Analgesic
063	54–063	Acetaminophen	325mg	White	Tab	Round	–	–	Roxane	Anaglesic
	R 063	Lorazepam	2mg	White	Tab	Round	Y	N	Purepac	Antianxiety
	SP 063	Acetaminophen with Codeine Phosphate	300mg/30mg	White	Tab	Round	N	N	Superpharm	Analgesic
064	555/064	Hydralazine HCl	25mg	Orange	Tab	Round	N	N	Barr	Antihypertensive
	93–064	Tetracycline HCl	250mg	Yellow/Orange	Cap	–	–	–	Lemmon	Anti–Infective
	PAR 064	Fluphenazine HCl	10mg	Orange	Tab	Round	N	Y	Par	Tranquilizer
065	555/065	Hydralazine HCl	50mg	Orange	Tab	Round	N	N	Barr	Antihypertensive
066	barr/066, 100	Isoniazid	100mg	White	Tab	Round	–	–	Barr	Anti–Infective
	Par 066	Doxylamine Succinate	25mg	–	Tab	Round	–	–	Par	Sleep Aid
067	Par/067	Indomethacin	25mg	Green	Cap	–	–	–	Par	Anti–Inflammatory
	R 067	Oxazepam	10mg	Pink	Cap	–	–	–	Purepac	Antianxiety
068	Par/068	Indomethacin	50mg	Green	Cap	–	–	–	Par	Anti–Inflammatory
069	Par/069	Hydroxyzine Pamoate	25mg	Green/Green	Cap	–	–	–	Par	Antianxiety
	R 069	Oxazepam	15mg	Red	Cap	–	–	–	Purepac	Antianxiety
070	P–D 070	Propranolol	10mg	White	Tab	Round	–	–	PD	Antihypertensive
	Par/070	Hydroxyzine Pamoate	50mg	White/Green	Cap	–	–	–	Par	Antianxiety
	Sch. Logo 070	Ethinyl Estradiol	0.05mg	Pink	Tab	Round	N	Y	Schering	Hormone
	WC 070	Propranolol	10mg	Orange	Tab	Round	–	–	WC	Antihypertensive
071	barr/071, 300	Isoniazid	300mg	White	Tab	Round	Y	N	Barr	Anti–Infective
	P–D 071	Propranolol	20mg	White	Tab	Round	–	–	PD	Antihypertensive
	Par/071	Hydroxyzine Pamoate	100mg	Grey/Green	Cap	–	–	–	Par	Antianxiety
	PP–071	Chlorthalidone	50mg	Blue	Tab	Round	N	N	Eon	Diuretic
	STUART 071	Multivitamin/Multimineral combination	n/a	Pink	Tab	Capsule	N	Y	Stuart	Vitamin
	WC 071	Propranolol	20mg	Blue	Tab	Round	–	–	WC	Antihypertensive
072	Eaton 072	Furazolidone	100mg	Brown	Tab	Round	N	Y	Norwich	Anti–Infective
	P–D 072	Propranolol	40mg	White	Tab	Round	–	–	PD	Antihypertensive
	WC 072	Propranolol	40mg	Green	Tab	Round	–	–	WC	Antihypertensive
073	P–D 073	Propranolol	60mg	White	Tab	Round	–	–	PD	Antihypertensive
	PP/073	Chlorthalidone	100mg	White	Tab	Round	Y	N	Eon	Diuretic
	R 073	Oxazepam	30mg	Maroon	Cap	–	–	–	Purepac	Antianxiety
	WC 073	Propranolol	60mg	Pink	Tab	Round	–	–	WC	Antihypertensive
074	P–D 074	Propranolol	80mg	White	Tab	Round	–	–	PD	Antihypertensive
	WC 074	Propranolol	80mg	Yellow	Tab	Round	–	–	WC	Antihypertensive
	West–ward 074	Bro–Phen Time Release	n/a	Blue	Tab	Round	N	Y	West–ward	Antihistamine Comb.
076	AMIDE 076	Vitamin B Comp. with Folic Acid	n/a	Orange	Tab	Olbong	N	Y	Amide	Vitamin
	ATI 076	Chlordiazepoxide HCl with Clidinum Bromide	5mg/2.5mg	White/White	Cap	–	–	–	ATI	Antispasmodic
	PAR 076	Fluphenazine HCl	5mg	Pink	Tab	Round	N	Y	Par	Tranquilizer
	R 076	Temazepam	15mg	Green/White	Cap	–	–	–	Purepac	Hypnotic
077	AMIDE 077	Vitamin B Comp. with Folic Acid Plus	n/a	–	Tab	Oval	N	Y	Amide	Vitamin
	AMIDE/077	Vitamin B–C with Folic Acid Plus	n/a	Mustard	Tab	Capsule	N	Y	Amide	Vitamin
	Par/077	Chlorpropamide	100mg	Blue	Tab	Round	Y	N	Par	Hypoglycemic
	R 077	Temazepam	30mg	White/White	Cap	–	–	–	Purepac	Hypnotic
	Sch. Logo 077	Perphenazine	16mg	Gray	Tab	Round	N	Y	Schering	Tranquilizer
	WC 077	Fenoprofen	600mg	Peach	Tab	Oval	Y	Y	WC	Anti–Inflammatory
078	Par/078	Chlorpropamide	250mg	Blue	Tab	Round	Y	N	Par	Hypoglycemic
	R 078	Clorazepate Dipotassium	3.75mg	Blue	Tab	Round	Y	N	Purepac	Antianxiety
	WC 078	Nifedipine	10mg	White	Cap	–	–	–	WC	Antihypertensive
079	079	Aspirin SR	800mg	White	Tab	Capsule	N	Y	Amide	Analgesic
	WC 079	Nifedipine	20mg	White	Cap	–	–	–	WC	Antihypertensive
080	54 080	Prednisone	25mg	White	Tab	Round	Y	N	Roxane	Steroid
081	PP–081	Folic Acid	1mg	Yellow	Tab	Round	N	N	Eon	Antianemic
	R 081	Clorazepate Dipotassium	7.5mg	Peach	Tab	Round	Y	N	Purepac	Antianxiety
	WC 081	Fenoprofen	300mg	Yellow	Cap	–	–	–	WC	Anti–Inflammatory
082	dp 082	Hydrocodone / Homatropine	5mg/1.5mg	Blue	Tab	Round	Y	N	Daniels	Antitussive
	R 082	Propoxyphene Hydrochloride	65mg	Pink/Pink	Cap	–	–	–	Purepac	Analgesic
083	AT 083	Danozol	200mg	Orange/Orange	Cap	–	–	–	ATI	Hormone
	Par/083	Dexamethasone	0.25mg	Pale Orange	Tab	Pentagonal	Y	N	Par	Steroid
	R 083	Clorazepate Dipotassium	15mg	Pink	Tab	Round	Y	N	Purepac	Antianxiety
084	L/N 084–250	Cephalexin	250mg	Gray/Orange	Cap	–	–	–	Novopharm	Anti–Infective
	Par/084	Dexamethasone	0.5mg	Pale Yellow	Tab	Pentagonal	Y	N	Par	Steroid
	WC 084	Gemfibrozil	600mg	White	Tab	Oblong	N	Y	WC	Antihyperlipidemic
085	Par/085	Dexamethasone	0.75mg	Pale Blue	Tab	Pentagonal	Y	N	Par	Steroid
	R 085	Propoxyphene Napsylate and Acetaminophen	100mg/650mg	Pink	Tab	Capsule	N	Y	Purepac	Analgesic
086	Par/086	Dexamethasone	1.5mg	Pale Pink	Tab	Pentagonal	Y	N	Par	Steroid
087	DMSP 087	Cimetidine	400mg	White	Tab	Oval	–	Y	Dupont	Antiulcer
	HAUCK 087	Hydrocodone Bitartrate/Guaifenesin	5mg/300mg	Orange	Tab	–	–	–	W.E.Hauck	Antitussive
	Par/087	Dexamethasone	4mg	White	Tab	Pentagonal	Y	N	Par	Steroid
	West–ward 087	Chlorpromazine Hydrochloride	100mg	Butterscotch	Tab	Round	N	Y	West–ward	Tranquilizer
088	93 088	Sulfamethoxazole & Trimethoprim	400mg/80mg	White	Tab	Round	Y	N	Lemmon	Anti–Infective
	DMSP 088	Cimetidine	800mg	White	Tab	Oval	–	Y	Dupont	Antiulcer
	N 088/5	Pindolol	5mg	White	Tab	Round	Y	N	Novopharm	Antihypertensive
089	555/089	Propylthiouracil	50mg	White	Tab	Round	Y	N	Barr	Antithyroid
	93 089	Sulfamethoxazole & Trimethoprim	800mg/160mg	White	Tab	Oval	Y	N	Lemmon	Anti–Infective
090	54 090 30	Morphine Sulfate SR	30mg	White	Tab	Round	Y	N	Roxane	Analgesic
	93–090	Carbamazepine	200mg	White	Tab	Round	Y	N	Lemmon	Anticonvulsant
	West–ward 090	Chlordiazepoxide Hydrochloride	5mg	Yellow/Green	Cap	–	–	–	West–ward	Antianxiety
	West–ward 090	Chlorpromazine Hydrochloride	200mg	Butterscotch	Tab	Round	N	Y	West–ward	Tranquilizer
091	SP 091	Allopurinol	100mg	White	Tab	Round	N	N	Superpharm	Antigout
	WC 091	Doxycycline Hyclate Coated Pellets	100mg	Yellow/Blue/Clear	Cap	–	–	–	WC	Anti–Infective
092	54 092	Prednisone	1mg	White	Tab	Round	Y	N	Roxane	Steroid
	Pfizer 092	Oxytetracycline,Sulfamethizole,Phenazopyridine	250/250/50 mg	Aqua/White	Cap	–	–	–	Pfizer	Anti–Infective
	SP 092	Allopurinol	300mg	Peach	Tab	Round	Y	N	Superpharm	Antigout
093	54 093	Diflunisal	500 mg	Orange	Tab	Capsule	N	Y	Roxane	Anti–inflammatory
	MILES 093	Clotrimazole	100mg	White	Tab	Bullet	–	–	Miles	Anti–Infective

ID NO.	ID CODE	GENERIC NAME	STRENGTH	COLOR	FORM	SHAPE	SCORED	COATED	MFG.	USE
	N 093/10	Pindolol	10mg	White	Tab	Round	Y	N	Novopharm	Antihypertensive
	West–ward 093	Chlordiazepoxide Hydrochloride	10mg	Green/Black	Cap	–	–	–	West–ward	Antianxiety
094	SP 094	Chlorpropamide	100mg	White	Tab	Round	Y	N	Superpharm	Hypoglycemic
095	bp 095	Carisoprodol & Aspirin	200mg/325mg	Lavender/White	Tab	Round	–	–	Bolar	Muscle Relaxant
	MILES 095	Clotrimazole	10mg	White	Tab	Round	N	N	Miles	Anti–Infective
	Par/095	Metronidazole	250mg	White	Tab	Round	N	N	Par	Anti–Infective
	Sch. Logo 095	Dexchlorpheniramine ER	4mg	Red	Tab	Oval	N	Y	Schering	Antihistamine
	SP 095	Chlorpropamide	250mg	White	Tab	Round	Y	N	Superpharm	Hypoglycemic
	West–ward 095	Chlordiazepoxide Hydrochloride	25mg	White/Green	Cap	–	–	–	West–ward	Antianxiety
096	AT 096	Chlorzoxazone With Acetaminophen	250mg/300mg	Green	Tab	Hexagon	N	N	ATI	Muscle Relaxant
097	MILES 097	Clotrimazole	500mg	White	Tab	Bullet	N	N	Miles	Anti–Infective
098	AT 098	Theranatal Plus One	n/a	Yellow	Tab	Capsule	N	Y	ATI	Prenatal Vitamin
099	54–099	Amitriptyline	50mg	White	Tab	Round	–	–	Roxane	Antidepressant
100	832/100	Chlorpromazine	100mg	Tan	Tab	Round	N	Y	PBI	Tranquilizer
	832/GC100	Chlorthalidone	100mg	White	Tab	Round	N	N	PBI	Diuretic
	832/MC100	Meclofenamate Sodium	100mg	Maroon/White	Cap	–	–	–	PBI	Anti–Inflammatory
	832/TM100	Trimipramine Maleate	100mg	Green/Brown	Cap	–	–	–	PBI	Antidepressant
	AT 100	Therapeutic Vitamin Plus	n/a	Golden Yellow	Tab	Capsule	N	Y	ATI	Vitamin
	BI/100	Mesoridazine Besylate	100mg	Red	Tab	Round	N	Y	BI	Tranquilizer
	bp 100	Hydroxyzine Pamoate	25mg	Green/Green	Cap	–	–	–	Bolar	Antihistamine
	Breon 100	Theophylline Anhydrous	100mg	Brown/White	Cap	–	–	–	Winthrop	Bronchodilator
	BREON T 100	Chlormezanone	100mg	Peach	Tab	Capsule	Y	N	Winthrop	Antianxiety
	DAN–P 100	Phenobarbital	100mg	White	Tab	Round	Y	N	Danbury	Sedative
	dp 100	Levothyroxine Sodium	0.1mg	Yellow	Tab	Oval	Y	N	Daniels	Hormone
	Flint 100	Levothyroxine Sodium	100mcg	Yellow	Tab	Round	Y	N	Boots	Hormone
	Forest 100	Theophylline SR	100mg	White	Tab	Round	–	N	Forest	Bronchodilator
	GG100	Propoxyphene Napsylate & Acetaminophen	100mg/650mg	White	Tab	Capsule	N	Y	Geneva	Analgesic
	M 100	Levothyroxine Sodium	0.1mg	Yellow	Tab	Round	Y	N	Duramed	Hormone
	MUTUAL 100	Doxycycline Hyclate	50mg	White/Blue	Cap	–	–	–	Mutual	Anti–Infective
	Mylan 100 / 4	Cyproheptadine HCl	4mg	White	Tab	Round	Y	N	Mylan	Antipruritic
	PF M 100	Morphine Sulfate	100mg	Gray	Tab	Round	N	Y	PF	Analgesic
	RIKER/TR 100	Flecainide Acetate	100mg	White	Tab	Round	N	N	3M	Antiarrhythmic
	SP 100	Doxycycline	100mg	Yellow	Tab	Round	N	N	Superpharm	Anti–Infective
	TZD100 832	Trazodone HCl	100mg	White	Tab	Round	Y	Y	PBI	Antidepressant
	Wellcome Y9C/ 100	Zidovudine	100mg	White/Blue Band	Cap	–	–	–	BW	Antiviral
	WHR 100	Theophylline	100mg	White/Clear	Cap	–	–	–	Rorer	Bronchodilator
101	101	Sulfasalazine	500mg	Gold	Tab	Round	Y	N	Pharmacia	Antiarrthritic
	AT 101	Meclofenamate Sodium	50mg	Orange/Orange	Cap	–	–	–	ATI	Anti–Inflammatory
	bp 101	Hydroxyzine Pamoate	50mg	White/Green	Cap	–	–	–	Bolar	Antihistamine
	Ciba 101	Hydralazine HCl	100mg	Peach	Tab	Round	N	N	Ciba	Antihypertensive
	GG101	Methocarbamol	750mg	White	Tab	Oblong	N	N	Geneva	Muscle Relaxant
	ICI 101	Atenolol	50mg	White	Tab	Round	Y	N	Stuart	Antihypertensive
	Jacobus 25–101	Dapsone	100mg	White	Tab	Round	Y	N	Jacobus	Anti–Infective
	KP 101	Sulfasalazine	500mg	Yellow	Tab	Round	N	Y	Kabi	Anti–Inflammatory
	MUTUAL 101	Indomethacin	25mg	Green/Green	Cap	–	–	–	Mutual	Anti–Inflammatory
	Mylan 101	Tetracycline HCl	250mg	Orange/Yellow	Cap	–	–	–	Mylan	Anti–Infective
	Par/101	Thioridazine HCl	100mg	Orange	Tab	Round	N	N	Par	Tranquilizer
	SEARLE 101	Norethynodrel & Mestranol	10mg/75mcg	Brown	Tab	Round	N	N	Searle	Hormone
	SP 101	Doxycycline	50mg	Blue/White	Cap	–	–	–	Superpharm	Anti–Infective
102	102	Sulfasalazine	500mg	Gold	Tab	Oval	N	Y	Pharmacia	Antiarrthritic
	AT 102	Meclofenamate Sodium	100mg	Orange/Orange	Cap	–	–	–	ATI	Anti–Inflammatory
	bp 102	Hydroxyzine Pamoate	100mg	Grey/Green	Cap	–	–	–	Bolar	Antihistamine
	CC 102	Phentermine HCl	8mg	Green	Tab	Round	Y	N	Camall	Anorectic
	Jacobus 100–102	Dapsone	25mg	White	Tab	Round	Y	N	Jacobus	Anti–Infective
	KP 102	Sulfasalazine	500mg	Yellow	Tab	Elliptical	N	Y	Kabi	Anti–Inflammatory
	MUTUAL 102	Quinine Sulfate	5gr	Clear	Cap	–	–	–	Mutual	Muscle Relaxant
	Mylan 102	Tetracycline HCl	500mg	Black/Yellow	Cap	–	N	N	Mylan	Anti–Infective
	Par 102	Thioridazine HCl	150mg	Orange	Tab	Round	N	Y	Par	Tranquilizer
	R 102	Allopurinol	100mg	White	Tab	Round	Y	N	Purepac	Antigout
	SP 102	Doxycycline	100mg	Blue/Blue	Cap	–	–	–	Superpharm	Anti–Infective
103	54–103	Bisacodyl	5mg	–	Tab	Round	N	Y	Roxane	Laxative
	Ciba 103	Guanethidine Monosulfate	25mg	White	Tab	Round	Y	N	Ciba	Antihypertensive
	GG103	Metronidazole	250mg	White	Tab	Round	Y	N	Geneva	Anti–Infective
	MUTUAL 103	Diphenhydramine HCl	25mg	Pink/Clear	Cap	–	–	–	Mutual	Antihistamine
	Par 103	Thioridazine HCl	200mg	Orange	Tab	Round	N	Y	Par	Tranquilizer
	R 103	Allopurinol	300mg	Peach	Tab	Round	Y	N	Purepac	Antigout
	S–103	Chlorpheniramine/Phenylephrine/Methscopolamine	8mg/20mg/2.5mg	Brown	Tab	Round	Y	N	Dura	Decongestant Comb.
	SP 103	Hydralazine	10mg	Peach	Tab	Round	N	Y	Superpharm	Antihypertensive
104	Ciba 104	Reserpine & Hydralazine HCl	0.2mg/50mg	Yellow	Tab	Round	N	Y	Ciba	Antihypertensive
	GG 104	Methyldopa	125mg	White	Tab	Round	N	Y	Geneva	Antihypertensive
	Par/104	Allopurinol	100mg	White	Tab	Round	Y	N	Par	Antigout
	SP 104	Hydralazine	25mg	Peach	Tab	Round	N	Y	Superpharm	Antihypertensive
105	225/105	Ferrous Fumarate/Cyanocobalamin/Ascorbic Acid	600mg/25mcg/100	Brown	Tab	Round	N	Y	B.F.Ascher	Vitamin
	CC 105	Phendimetrazine Tartrate	35mg	White	Tab	Round	Y	N	Camall	Anorectic
	CC 105	Phendimetrazine Tartrate	35mg	Gray	Tab	Round	Y	N	Camall	Anorectic
	CC 105	Phendimetrazine Tartrate	35mg	Pink	Tab	Round	Y	N	Camall	Anorectic
	CC 105	Phendimetrazine Tartrate	35mg	Yellow	Tab	Round	Y	N	Camall	Anorectic
	F–C#1 Sandoz 78–105	Codeine/Butalbital/Caffeine/Aspirin	7.5/50/40/325mg	Red/Yellow	Cap	–	–	–	Sandoz	Analgesic
	Geigy 105	Terbutaline Sulfate	5mg	White	Tab	Round	Y	N	Geigy	Bronchodilator
	GG 105	Haloperidol	0.5mg	White	Tab	Round	Y	N	Geneva	Tranquilizer
	ICI 105	Atenolol	50mg	White	Tab	Round	Y	N	Stuart	Antihypertensive
	MUTUAL 105	Doxycycline Hyclate	100mg	Blue/Blue	Cap	–	–	–	Mutual	Anti–Infective
	Par/105	Allopurinol	300mg	Orange	Tab	Round	Y	N	Par	Antigout
	SP 105	Hydralazine	50mg	Peach	Tab	Round	N	Y	Superpharm	Antihypertensive
106	F–C#2 Sandoz 78–106	Codeine/Butalbital/Caffeine/Aspirin	15/50/40/325mg	Gray/Yellow	Cap	–	–	–	Sandoz	Analgesic
	MUTUAL 106	Indomethacin	50mg	Green/Green	Cap	–	–	–	Mutual	Anti–Inflammatory
	MYLAN 106/250	Erythromycin Stearate	250mg	Yellow	Tab	Round	N	Y	Mylan	Anti–Infective
	Par/106	Propranolol HCl	10mg	Orange	Tab	Round	Y	N	Par	Antihypertensive
	SP 106	Hydroxyzine HCl	10mg	Lavender	Tab	Round	N	Y	Superpharm	Antipruritic
107	3M/107	Aluminum Hydroxide	600mg	Green	Tab	Capsule	N	N	3M	Antacid
	CC 107	Phendimetrazine Tartrate	35mg	Pink	Tab	Round	Y	N	Camall	Anorectic
	CC 107	Phendimetrazine Tartrate	35mg	Yellow	Tab	Round	Y	N	Camall	Anorectic
	F–C#3 Sandoz 78–107	Codeine/Butalbital/Caffeine/Aspirin	30/50/40/325mg	Blue/Yellow	Cap	–	–	–	Sandoz	Analgesic
	GG 107	Perphenazine	4mg	White	Tab	Round	N	Y	Geneva	Tranquilizer
	MUTUAL 107	Diphenhydramine HCl	50mg	Pink/Pink	Cap	–	–	–	Mutual	Antihistamine

ID NO.	ID CODE	GENERIC NAME	STRENGTH	COLOR	FORM	SHAPE	SCORED	COATED	MFG.	USE
	MYLAN 107/500	Erythromycin Stearate	500mg	Yellow	Tab	Oval	N	Y	Mylan	Anti–Infective
	Par/107	Propranolol HCl	20mg	Blue	Tab	Round	Y	N	Par	Antihypertensive
	SP 107	Hydroxyzine HCl	25mg	Violet	Tab	Round	N	Y	Superpharm	Antipruritic
	West–ward 107	Dipyridamole	25mg	White	Tab	Round	N	Y	West–ward	Antiplatelet
108	CC 108	Hydrochlorothiazide	50mg	Peach	Tab	Round	Y	N	Camall	Diuretic
	Geigy 108	Clofazimine	50mg	Brown	Cap	–	–	–	Geigy	Antileprosy
	GG 108	Perphenazine	8mg	White	Tab	Round	N	Y	Geneva	Tranquilizer
	MP 108	Quinidine Sulfate	200mg	White	Tab	Round	Y	N	Mutual	Antiarrhythmic
	Par/108	Propranolol HCl	40mg	Green	Tab	Round	Y	N	Par	Antihypertensive
	SP 108	Hydroxyzine HCl	50mg	Purple	Tab	Round	N	Y	Superpharm	Antipruritic
109	AT-109	Oxazepam	10mg	Pink/Clear	Cap	–	–	–	ATI	Antianxiety
	CC 109	Diethylpropion HCl	25mg	Blue	Tab	Round	N	N	Camall	Anorectic
	CC 109	Diethylpropion HCl	25mg	White	Tab	Round	N	N	Camall	Anorectic
	Geigy 109	Clofazimine	100mg	Brown	Cap	–	–	–	Geigy	Antileprosy
	GG 109	Perphenazine	16mg	White	Tab	Round	N	Y	Geneva	Tranquilizer
	Par/109	Propranolol HCl	80mg	Yellow	Tab	Round	Y	N	Par	Antihypertensive
	SP 109	Tetracycline HCl	250mg	Orange/Yellow	Cap	–	–	–	Superpharm	Anti–Infective
	Star logo 109	Ortho–Phosphate Formula	1GM	Peach	Tab	Capsule	–	–	Star	–
	T 109	Carbamazepine	200mg	White	Tab	Round	Y	N	Lemmon	Anticonvulsant
	West–ward 109	Dipyridamole	50mg	White	Tab	Round	N	Y	West–ward	Antiplatelet
110	AT–110	Oxazepam	15mg	Orange/Clear	Cap	–	–	–	ATI	Antianxiety
	Ciba 110	Maprotiline HCl	25mg	Orange	Tab	Oval	N	Y	Ciba	Antidepressant
	GG110	Chlorzoxazone & Acetaminophen	250mg/300mg	Green	Tab	Round	Y	N	Geneva	Muscle Relaxant
	LEMMON 110	APAP/Salicylamide/Phenylpropanol/Chlorpheniramine	300/300/60/4mg	White	Tab	Round	Y	N	Lemmon	Decongestant Comb.
	LuChem logo 110	Yohimbine HCl	5.4mg	White/Pink Specks	Tab	Oblong	Y	N	LuChem	Sympatholytic
	MIA 110	Butalbital, APAP, & Caffeine	50/325/40mg	White	Tab	Oval	N	N	Mikart	Analgesic
	Par/110	Clonidine HCl	0.1mg	Green	Tab	Round	Y	N	Par	Antihypertensive
	SP 110	Tetracycline HCl	500mg	Black/Yellow	Cap	–	–	–	Superpharm	Anti–Infective
	SYNTEX 110	Norethindrone & Ethinyl Estradiol	0.5mg/0.035mg	Blue	Tab	Round	–	N	Syntex	Contraceptive
	West–ward 110	Chloral Hydrate	500mg	Green	Cap	Oval	–	–	West–ward	Hypnotic
111	52273–111/Q	Nystatin Vaginal	100,000 Units	Yellow	Tab	Diamond	N	N	Quantum	Anti–Infective
	52273–111/Q	Nystatin Vaginal	100,000 Units	Yellow	Tab	Diamond	N	N	Quantum	Anti–Infective
	bp 111	Prochlorperazine	5mg	Chartreuse	Tab	Round	N	Y	Bolar	Antiemetic
	C111	Clofibrate	500mg	Yellow	Cap	–	–	–	PBI	Hypolipidemic
	Copley 111	Prenatal Vitamin	n/a	Yellow	Tab	Oblong	N	Y	Copley	Prenatal Vitamin
	Geigy 111	Tripelennamine Hydrochloride	25mg	White	Tab	Round	Y	N	Geigy	Antihistamine
	GG111	Methyldopa	250mg	White	Tab	Round	N	Y	Geneva	Antihypertensive
	MP 111/2	Acetaminophen & Codeine	300mg/15mg	White	Tab	Round	Y	N	Mutual	Analgesic
	Mylan 111/250	Penicillin V Potassium	250mg	White	Tab	Oval	N	N	Mylan	Anti–Infective
	P–D 111	Ergotamine Tartrate SL	2mg	Orange	Tab	Round	N	N	PD	Antimigraine
	Par/111	Clonidine HCl	0.2mg	Yellow	Tab	Round	Y	N	Par	Antihypertensive
	PP–111	Sulfamethoxazole & Trimethoprim	400mg/80mg	White	Tab	Round	Y	N	Eon	Anti–Infective
	R 111	Ibuprofen	800mg	White	Tab	Oval	N	Y	Purepac	Anti–Inflammatory
	SP 111	Tolbutamide	500mg	White	Tab	Round	Y	N	Superpharm	Hypoglycemic
	SYNTEX 111	Norethindrone & Ethinyl Estradiol	1mg/0.035mg	Green	Tab	Round	–	N	Syntex	Contraceptive
	West–ward 111	Dipyridamole	75mg	White	Tab	Round	N	Y	West–ward	Antiplatelet
112	112	Theophylline/Guaifenesin/Pseudoephedrine	n/a	Purple	Tab	–	Y	N	Marlop	Antiasthmatic
	biocraft 112	Cephradine	250mg	Green\Pink	Cap	–	N	N	Biocraft	Anti–Infective
	BMP 112	Atropine/ASA/Caffeine/Ipecac/Camphor	0.13/130/8/3/15	Yellow	Cap	–	–	–	Beecham	Analgesic
	bp 112	Prochlorperazine	25mg	Chartreuse	Tab	Round	N	Y	Bolar	Antiemetic
	dp 112	Levothyroxine Sodium	0.112mg	Rose	Tab	Oval	Y	N	Daniels	Hormone
	Flint 112	Levothyroxine Sodium	112mcg	Rose	Tab	Round	Y	N	Boots	Hormone
	GG 112	Propoxyphene HCl and Acetaminophen	65mg/650 mg	Orange	Tab	Oblong	Y	Y	Geneva	Analgesic
	MP 112	Sulindac	150mg	Yellow	Tab	Round	Y	N	Mutual	Anti–Inflammatory
	Mylan 112/500	Penicillin V Potassium	500mg	White	Tab	Round	Y	N	Mylan	Anti–Infective
	Par/112	Clonidine HCl	0.3mg	Blue	Tab	Round	Y	N	Par	Antihypertensive
	PP–112	Sulfamethoxazole & Trimethoprim	800mg/160mg	White	Tab	Oval	Y	N	Eon	Anti–Infective
	SP 112	Amitriptyline HCl	10mg	Pink	Tab	Round	N	Y	Superpharm	Antidepressant
113	879 113	Isoniazid	100mg	White	Tab	Round	Y	N	Halsey	Anti–Infective
	AT–113	Oxazepam	30mg	White/Clear	Cap	–	–	–	ATI	Antianxiety
	biocraft 113	Cephradine	500mg	Green	Cap	–	N	N	Biocraft	Anti–Infective
	Copley 113	Phenylephrine/Chlorpheniramine/Pyrilamine	25mg/8mg/25mg	Tan	Tab	Capsule	Y	Y	Copley	Decongestant Comb.
	GG113	Metoclopramide	10mg	White	Tab	Round	N	N	Geneva	Antireflux
	Par/113	Clonidine HCl/Chlorthalidone	0.1mg/15mg	White	Tab	Round	Y	N	Par	Antihypertensive
	SP 113	Amitriptyline HCl	25mg	Green	Tab	Round	N	Y	Superpharm	Antidepressant
	SQUIBB 113	Cephradine	250mg	Orange/Blue	Cap	–	–	–	Squibb	Anti–Infective
114	BIOCRAFT 114	Cefadroxil	500mg	Yellow	Cap	–	–	–	Biocraft	Anti Infective
	Copley 114	Procainamide HCl SR	750mg	Tan	Tab	Oval	–	Y	Copley	Antiarrhythmic
	GG114	Ergoloid Mesylates	1mg	White	Tab	Round	N	N	Danbury	Vasodilator
	L/N 114–500	Cephalexin	250mg	Swedish Orange	Cap	–	–	–	Novopharm	Anti–Infective
	MP 114	Trazodone HCl	100mg	White	Tab	Round	Y	N	Mutual	Antidepressant
	Par/114	Metronidazole	500mg	White	Tab	Round	N	N	Par	Anti–Infective
	QPL–114	Nystatin Oral	500,000 Units	Brown	Tab	Round	N	Y	Quantum	Anti–Infective
	SP 114	Amitriptyline HCl	50mg	Brown	Tab	Round	N	Y	Superpharm	Antidepressant
	SQUIBB 114	Cephradine	500mg	Blue	Cap	–	–	–	Squibb	Anti–Infective
115	barr,115	Reserpine, Hydralazine HCl, Hydrochlorothiazide	0.1mg/25mg/15mg	Salmon	Tab	Round	N	N	Barr	Antihypertensive
	biocraft 115	Cephalexin	250mg	Gray\Swed.Orange	Cap	–	N	N	Biocraft	Anti–Infective
	GG115	Ergoloid Mesylates SL	1mg	White	Tab	Oval	N	N	Danbury	Vasodilator
	ICI 115	Atenolol & Chlorthalidone	50mg/25mg	White	Tab	Round	Y	N	Stuart	Antihypertensive
	Mylan 115	Ampicillin	250mg	Scarlet/Gray	Cap	–	–	–	Mylan	Anti–Infective
	Par/115	Clonidine HCl/Chlorthalidone	0.2mg/15mg	Blue	Tab	Round	Y	N	Par	Antihypertensive
	QPL 115 Q	Benztropine Mesylate	2mg	White	Tab	Round	Y	N	Quantum	Antiparkinson
	SP 115	Amitriptyline HCl	75mg	Purple	Tab	Round	N	Y	Superpharm	Antidepressant
116	CC 116	Hydrochlorothiazide	25mg	Peach	Tab	Round	Y	N	Camall	Diuretic
	GG116	Ergoloid Mesylates SL	0.5mg	White	Tab	Round	N	N	Danbury	Vasodilator
	MP 116	Sulindac	200mg	Yellow	Tab	Round	Y	N	Mutual	Anti–Inflammatory
	Mylan 116	Ampicillin	500mg	Scarlet/Gray	Cap	–	–	–	Mylan	Anti–Infective
	Par/116	Clonidine HCl/Chlorthalidone	0.3mg/15mg	White	Tab	Round	Y	N	Par	Antihypertensive
	QPL–116 Q	Benztropine Mesylate	0.5mg	White	Tab	Round	–	–	Quantum	Antiparkinson
	SP 116	Amitriptyline HCl	100mg	Orange	Tab	Round	N	Y	Superpharm	Antidepressant
117	117	Vitamin B Complex with C	n/a	Green/Yellow	Cap	–	–	–	Fresh	Vitamin
	biocraft 117	Cephalexin	500mg	Swedish\Orange	Cap	–	N	N	Biocraft	Anti–Infective
	bp 117	Trifluoperazine HCl	5mg	Red	Tab	Round	N	Y	Bolar	Tranquilizer
	Geigy 117	Tripelennamine Hydrochloride	50mg	White	Tab	Round	Y	N	Geigy	Antihistamine
	ICI 117	Atenolol & Chlorthalidone	100mg/25mg	White	Tab	Round	Y	N	Stuart	Antihypertensive

ID NO.	ID CODE	GENERIC NAME	STRENGTH	COLOR	FORM	SHAPE	SCORED	COATED	MFG.	USE
	Par/117	Amiloride HCl	5mg	Yellow	Tab	Round	N	N	Par	Diuretic
118	QPL 117 Q	Benztropine Mesylate	1mg	White	Tab	Oval	Y	N	Quantum	Antiparkinson
	bp 118	Thioridazine HCl	25mg	Buff	Tab	Capsule	N	Y	Bolar	Tranquilizer
	GG118	Decongestant S.R.	–	White/Blue specks	Tab	Round	Y	N	Geneva	Decongestant Comb.
	MP 118	Trazodone HCl	50mg	White	Tab	Round	Y	N	Mutual	Antidepressant
	Par/118	Propantheline Bromide	15mg	Peach	Tab	Round	N	Y	Par	Antispasmodic
	R 118	Belladonna Alkaloids & Phenobarbital	n/a	White	Tab	Round	Y	N	Purepac	Antispasmodic
	SP 118	Hydroxyzine Pamoate	25mg	Dk.Green/Lt.Green	Cap	–	–	–	Sidmak	Antianxiety
119	bp 119	Thioridazine HCl	50mg	White	Tab	Capsule	N	Y	Bolar	Tranquilizer
	GG119	Butalbital, Aspirin and Caffeine	50/40/325mg	White	Tab	Round	N	N	Geneva	Analgesic
	Par/119	Nystatin	500,000 Units	Brown	Tab	Round	N	N	Par	Anti–Infective
	Sch. Logo 119	Perphenazine & Amitriptyline HCl	4mg/10mg	Orange	Tab	Round	N	Y	Schering	Antidepressant
	SP 119	Hydroxyzine Pamoate	50mg	Dk.Green/White	Cap	–	–	–	Superpharm	Antianxiety
120	13 120	Aspirin/Phenacetin/Phenobarbital	250/120/15mg	Orange	Tab	Round	N	N	Adria	Analgesic
	bp 120	Thioridazine HCl	100mg	Yellow	Tab	Capsule	N	Y	Bolar	Tranquilizer
	Marion 120mg	Diltiazem HCl	120mg	Yellow	Tab	Oblong	N	Y	Marion	Antianginal
	SP 120	Hydroxyzine Pamoate	100mg	Dk.Green/Gray	Cap	–	–	–	Superpharm	Antianxiety
121	AT 121	Trazodone HCl	50mg	White	Tab	Round	Y	N	ATI	Antidepressant
	BMP 121	Multivitamin Combination	n/a	Pink	Cap	–	–	–	Beecham	Vitamin
	bp 121	Thioridazine HCl	150mg	Yellow	Tab	Capsule	N	Y	Bolar	Tranquilizer
	GG121/4	Acetaminophen & Codeine	300mg/60mg	White	Tab	Round	Y	N	Geneva	Analgesic
	MILES 121	Dehydrocholic Acid	250mg	White	Tab	Round	–	N	Miles	Stool Softener
	Mylan 121	Penicillin G Potassium	250,000 Units	White	Tab	Round	Y	N	Mylan	Anti–Infective
	P–D 121	Chlorthalidone	50mg	Blue	Tab	Round	–	N	PD	Diuretic
	Par/121	Hydralazine HCl	100mg	Peach	Tab	Round	N	N	Par	Antihypertensive
	SP 121	Prednisolone	5mg	Salmon	Tab	Round	N	N	Superpharm	Steroid
	U/121 2.5	Minoxidil	2.5mg	White	Tab	Round	Y	N	Upjohn	Antihypertensive
	WC 121	Chlorthalidone	50mg	Blue	Tab	Round	–	N	WC	Diuretic
122	879 G122C	Butabarbital Sodium	30mg	Green	Tab	Round	Y	N	Halsey	Hypnotic
	BMP 122	Multivitamin Combination	n/a	Green	Cap	–	–	–	Beecham	Vitamin
	bp 122	Thioridazine HCl	200mg	pink	Tab	Capsule	N	Y	Bolar	Tranquilizer
	C 122	Amantadine	100mg	Yellow	Cap	–	–	–	Chase	Antiviral
	GG122	Sulfasalazine	500mg	Brownish Yellow	Tab	Round	Y	N	Bolar	Anti–Inflammatory
	MP 122/3	Acetaminophen & Codeine	300mg/30mg	White	Tab	Round	Y	N	Mutual	Analgesic
	Mylan 122	Penicillin G Potassium	400,000 Units	White	Tab	Round	Y	N	Mylan	Anti–Infective
	Par/122	Tolazamide	100mg	White	Tab	Round	Y	N	Par	Hypoglycemic
	SP 122	Prednisone	5mg	White	Tab	Round	N	N	Superpharm	Steroid
123	BMP 123	Multivitamin	n/a	Orange	Tab	–	–	–	Beecham	Vitamin
	bp 123	Propranolol HCl	10mg	Peach	Tab	Round	–	N	Bolar	Antihypertensive
	CC 123	Hydrochlorothiazide	50mg	Yellow	Tab	Round	Y	N	Camall	Diuretic
	Copley 123	Sodium Fluoride	0.5mg	Purple	Tab	Round	N	N	Copley	Mineral
	GG 123	Haloperidol	1mg	Yellow	Tab	Round	Y	N	Geneva	Tranquilizer
	P–D 123	Chlorthalidone	25mg	Orange	Tab	Round	–	N	PD	Diuretic
	Par/123	Tolazamide	250mg	White	Tab	Round	Y	N	Par	Hypoglycemic
	SP 123	Prednisone	10mg	White	Tab	Round	Y	N	Superpharm	Steroid
124	WC 123	Chlorthalidone	25mg	Orange	Tab	Round	–	N	WC	Diuretic
	bp 124	Propranolol HCl	20mg	Blue	Tab	Round	–	N	Bolar	Antihypertensive
	CC 124	Hydralazine/Hydrochlorothiazide/Reserpine	25mg/15mg/0.1mg	Salmon	Tab	Round	Y	N	Camall	Antihypertensive
	GG 124	Haloperidol	2mg	Pink	Tab	Round	Y	N	Geneva	Tranquilizer
	H 124	Hydrochlorothiazide	50mg	Peach	Tab	Round	N	N	Heather	Diuretic
	MP 124	Quinidine Sulfate	300mg	White	Tab	Round	Y	N	Mutual	Antiarrhythmic
	Par/124	Tolazamide	500mg	White	Tab	Round	Y	N	Par	Hypoglycemic
	R 124	Ibuprofen	400mg	White	Tab	Round	N	Y	Purepac	Anti–Inflammatory
	SP 124	Prednisone	20mg	Peach	Tab	Round	Y	N	Superpharm	Steroid
125	WC 124	Estropipate	0.75mg	Yellow	Tab	Round	–	N	WC	Hormone
	AT 125	Trazodone Hydrochloride	100mg	White	Tab	Round	Y	N	ATI	Antidepressant
	BMP 125	Esterified Estrogens	0.3mg	Yellow	Tab	Oblong	N	Y	Beecham	Hormone
	bp 125	Propranolol HCl	40mg	Green	Tab	Round	–	N	Bolar	Antihypertensive
	CC 125	Hydrochlorothiazide/Reserpine	50mg/0.125mg	Green	Tab	Round	–	–	Camall	Antihypertensive
	dp 125	Levothyroxine Sodium	0.125mg	Brown	Tab	Oval	Y	N	Daniels	Hormone
	DPI 125	Estropipate	1.5mg	White	Tab	Diamond	–	N	Duramed	Hormone
	Flint 125	Levothyroxine Sodium	125mcg	Brown	Tab	Round	Y	N	Boots	Hormone
	GG 125	Haloperidol	5mg	Green	Tab	Round	Y	N	Geneva	Tranquilizer
	HD 125	Digoxin	0.125mg	White	Tab	Round	–	N	Halsey	Cardiac Glycoside
	M 125	Levothyroxine Sodium	0.125mg	Tan	Tab	Round	–	N	Duramed	Hormone
	M 125 LEVO T	Levothyroxine Sodium	0.125mg	Brown	Tab	Round	Y	N	Mova	Hormone
	Par/125	Valproic Acid	250mg	Off White	Cap	–	–	–	Par	Anticonvulsant
	PP–125	Methylprednisolone	4mg	White	Tab	Oval	Y	N	Eon	Steroid
	R 125	Ibuprofen	600mg	White	Tab	Oval	N	Y	Purepac	Anti–Inflammatory
	RIKER/125 Plus	Theophylline & Guaifenesin	125mg/100mg	White	Tab	Round	N	N	Riker	Bronchodilator
	TR/125 G	Triazolam	0.125mg	White	Tab	Oval	N	N	Par	Sedative/Hypnotic
126	WHR 125	Theophylline	125mg	White	Cap	–	–	–	Rorer	Bronchodilator
	555/126	Dicyclomine HCl	20mg	Blue	Tab	Round	Y	N	Barr	Antispasmodic
	BMP 126	Esterified Estrogens	0.625mg	Orange	Tab	Oblong	N	Y	Beecham	Hormone
	bp 126	Propranolol HCl	80mg	Yellow	Tab	Round	–	N	Bolar	Antihypertensive
	Copley 126	Multivitamin with Folic Acid 500	n/a	Pink	Tab	Capsule	N	Y	Copley	Vitamin
	Copley 126	Multibret–Folic–500	n/a	Fuchsia	Tab	–	N	Y	Copley	Vitamin
	GG 126	Haloperidol	10mg	Green	Tab	Round	Y	N	Geneva	Tranquilizer
	N 126	Alprazolam	0.25mg	White	Tab	Round	Y	N	Novopharm	Antianxiety
	SP 126	Chlordiazepoxide HCl	5mg	Green/Yellow	Cap	–	–	–	Superpharm	Antianxiety
127	WC 126	Estropipate	1.5mg	Peach	Tab	Round	–	N	WC	Hormone
	BMP 127	Esterified Estrogens	1.25mg	Pink	Tab	Oblong	N	Y	Beecham	Hormone
	bp 127	Hydroflumethiazide & Reserpine	25mg/0.125mg	Yellow	Tab	Round	–	N	Bolar	Antihypertensive
	GG127	Quinine Sulfate	260mg	White	Tab	Round	N	N	Geneva	Muscle Relaxant
	M 127	Pindolol	10mg	White	Tab	Round	Y	N	Mylan	Antihypertensive
	MP 127/4	Acetaminophen & Codeine	300mg/60mg	White	Tab	Round	Y	N	Mutual	Analgesic
	N 127	Alprazolam	0.5mg	Orange	Tab	Round	Y	N	Novopharm	Antianxiety
	Par/127	Propranolol HCl	60mg	Pink	Tab	Round	Y	N	Par	Antihypertensive
	R 127	Clonidine Hydrochloride	0.1mg	Orange	Tab	Round	N	N	Purepac	Antihypertensive
128	SP 127	Chlordiazepoxide HCl	10mg	Green/Black	Cap	–	–	–	Superpharm	Antianxiety
	A 128	Sodium Fluoride Chewable	2.2mg	Pink	Tab	Round	N	N	Amide	Mineral
	barr 128	Dicyclomine HCl	10mg	Blue/Blue	Cap	–	–	–	Barr	Antispasmodic
	BMP 128	Esterified Estrogens	2.5mg	Pink	Tab	Oblong	N	Y	Beecham	Hormone
	bp 128	Hydroflumethiazide & Reserpine	50mg/0.125mg	Green	Tab	Round	Y	N	Bolar	Antihypertensive
	LEMMON 128	Dyphylline & Guaifenesin	200mg/200mg	White	Tab	Round	Y	N	Lemmon	Bronchodilator

ID NO.	ID CODE	GENERIC NAME	STRENGTH	COLOR	FORM	SHAPE	SCORED	COATED	MFG.	USE
	Par 128	Amiloride HCl/Hydrochlorothiazide	5mg/50mg	Peach	Tab	Round	–	–	Par	Antihypertensive
	R 128	Clonidine Hydrochloride	0.2mg	Orange	Tab	Round	Y	N	Purepac	Antihypertensive
	SP 128	Chlordiazepoxide HCl	25mg	Green/White	Cap	–	–	–	Superpharm	Antianxiety
	WC 128	Estropipate	3mg	Blue	Tab	Round	–	N	WC	Hormone
129	879 129	Prednisone	5mg	White	Tab	Round	Y	N	Halsey	Steroid
	Ciba 129	Hydralazine HCl & Hydrochlorothiazide	25mg/15mg	Orange	Tab	Round	N	N	Ciba	Antihypertensive
	Par/129	Dexamethasone	6mg	Green	Tab	Pentagonal	Y	N	Par	Steroid
	R 129	Clonidine Hydrochloride	0.3mg	Orange	Tab	Round	Y	N	Purepac	Antihypertensive
	SP 129	Hydrochlorothiazide	25mg	Peach	Tab	Round	Y	N	Superpharm	Diuretic
130	879 130	Propylthiouracil	50mg	White	Tab	Round	Y	N	Halsey	Antithyroid
	Adria/130	Butalbital, Aspirin	50mg/650mg	White	Tab	Capsule	N	N	Adria	Analgesic
	B 130	Hyoscyamine Sulfate	0.125 mg	White	Tab	Round	Y	N	Econolab	Antispasmodic
	BL 130	Albuterol	2mg	White	Tab	Round	Y	N	Biocraft	Bronchodilator
	Central 130mg	Theophylline Anhydrous	130mg	Clear	Cap	–	–	–	Central	Bronchodilator
	Ciba 130	Metyrapone	250mg	White	Tab	Round	Y	N	Ciba	Diagnostic
	GG130	Aminophylline	100mg	White	Tab	Round	Y	N	Geneva	Bronchodilator
	M 130	Propoxyphene HCl and Acetaminophen	65mg/650 mg	Orange	Tab	Capsule	Y	Y	Mylan	Analgesic
	Mylan 130	Propoxyphene HCl and Acetaminophen	65mg/650 mg	Orange	Tab	Capsule	Y	Y	Mylan	Analgesic
	Par/130	Metronidazole	250mg	White	Tab	Round	N	Y	Par	Anti-Infective
	SP 130	Hydrochlorothiazide	50mg	Peach	Tab	Round	Y	N	Superpharm	Diuretic
131	BL 131	Albuterol	4mg	White	Tab	Round	Y	N	Biocraft	Bronchodilator
	bp 131	Sulfasalazine Enteric Coated	500mg	Brownish Orange	Tab	Round	–	N	Bolar	Anti-Inflammatory
	Central 131/05	Vitamin Combination	n/a	Blue	Tab	Oval	N	Y	Central	Vitamin
	Copley 131	Sodium Fluoride	2.2mg	Pink	Tab	Round	N	N	Copley	Mineral
	IP 131/400	Ibuprofen	400mg	White	Tab	Round	N	Y	Interpharm	Anti-Inflammatory
	N 131	Alprazolam	1mg	Blue	Tab	Round	Y	N	Novopharm	Antianxiety
	Par/131	Metronidazole	500mg	White	Tab	Capsule	N	Y	Par	Anti-Infective
	SEARLE 131	Norethynodrel & Mestranol	2.5mg/0.1mg	Peach	Tab	Round	N	N	Searle	Hormone
	SP 131	Hydrochlorothiazide	100mg	Peach	Tab	Round	Y	N	Superpharm	Diuretic
132	93 132	Acetaminophen & Codeine	300mg/15mg	Caramel/White	Cap	–	–	–	Lemmon	Analgesic
	BL 132	Metaproterenol	10mg	White	Tab	Round	Y	N	Biocraft	Bronchodilator
	bp 132	Chlorothiazide & Reserpine	500mg/0.125mg	Pink	Tab	Round	–	–	Bolar	Antihypertensive
	GG132	Verapamil	80mg	White	Tab	Round	N	Y	Geneva	Antihypertensive
	MILES 132	Diethylstilbestrol Diphosphate	50mg	White/Gray specks	Tab	Round	Y	N	Miles	Hormone
	Par/132	Metoclopramide HCl	10mg	White	Tab	Round	Y	N	Par	Antireflux
	SP 132	Quinidine Sulfate	200mg	White	Tab	Round	Y	N	Superpharm	Antiarrhythmic
133	832/G133	Carbamazepine	200mg	White	Tab	Round	Y	N	PBI	Anticonvulsant
	AT 133	Therapeutic Vitamin	n/a	Yellow	Tab	Capsule	N	Y	ATI	Vitamin
	BL 133	Metaproterenol	20mg	White	Tab	Round	Y	N	Biocraft	Bronchodilator
	bp 133	Allopurinol	100mg	White	Tab	Round	Y	N	Bolar	Antigout
	C 133	Valproic Acid	250mg	Yellow	Cap	–	–	–	Chase	Anticonvulsant
	GG133	Verapamil	120mg	White	Tab	Round	N	Y	Geneva	Antihypertensive
	LEMMON 133	Dextroamphetamine Sulfate	15mg	Green/Clear	Cap	–	–	–	Lemmon	Anorectic
	Par/133	Amitriptyline HCl	10mg	Pink	Tab	Round	N	N	Par	Antidepressant
	R 133	Amitriptyline Hydrochloride	50mg	Brown	Tab	Round	N	Y	Purepac	Antidepressant
134	Biocraft 134	Minocycline	50mg	Pink	Cap	–	–	–	Biocraft	Anti-Infective
	bp 134	Allopurinol	300mg	Peach	Tab	Round	Y	N	Bolar	Antigout
	GG 134	Haloperidol	20mg	Coral	Tab	Round	Y	N	Geneva	Tranquilizer
	Par/134	Amitriptyline HCl	25mg	Green	Tab	Round	N	N	Par	Antidepressant
	PP–134	Reserpine	0.25mg	White	Tab	Round	Y	N	Eon	Antihypertensive
135	R 134	Amitriptyline Hydrochloride	75mg	Purple	Tab	Round	N	Y	Purepac	Antidepressant
	AT 135	Methocarbamol	500mg	White	Tab	Round	Y	N	ATI	Muscle Relaxant
	Biocraft 135	Minocycline	100mg	Pink/Maroon	Cap	–	–	–	Biocraft	Anti-Infective
	bp 135	Guanethidine Monosulfate	10mg	Orange	Tab	Round	–	N	Bolar	Antihypertensive
	CC 135	Phendimetrazine Tartrate	35mg	Lavender	Tab	Oblong	Y	N	Camall	Anorectic
	CC 135	Phendimetrazine Tartrate	35mg	Wh./Green Specks	Tab	Oblong	Y	N	Camall	Anorectic
	Ciba 135	Maprotiline HCl	75mg	White	Tab	Oval	N	Y	Ciba	Antidepressant
	M 135	Diltiazem HCl	90mg	White	Tab	Capsule	Y	Y	Mylan	Antianginal
	MP 135	Acetaminophen	325mg	White	Tab	Round	–	N	Mutual	Analgesic
	Ortho 135	Norethindrone & Ethinyl Estradiol	1mg/0.035mg	Peach	Tab	Round	N	N	Ortho	Hormone
	Par/135	Amitriptyline HCl	50mg	Brown	Tab	Round	N	N	Par	Antidepressant
136	R 135	Amitriptyline Hydrochloride	100mg	Orange	Tab	Round	N	Y	Purepac	Antidepressant
	BL 136	Cephalexin	250mg	White	Tab	Capsule	N	Y	Biocraft	Anti-Infective
	bp 136	Guanethidine Monosulfate	25mg	White	Tab	Round	–	N	Bolar	Antihypertensive
	CC 136	Phentermine HCl	8mg	Orange/Peach	Tab	Round	Y	N	Camall	Anorectic
	COPLEY 136	Metoprolol Tartrate	50mg	Pink	Tab	Capsule	Y	N	Copley	Antihypertensive
	Geigy 136	Imipramine HCl	50mg	Coral	Tab	Round	N	Y	Geigy	Antidepressant
	IP 136	Isometheptene Mucate & Dichloralphenazone & APAP	65/100/325mg	Red/White	Cap	–	–	–	Interpharm	Antimigraine
	Par/136	Amitriptyline HCl	75mg	Purple	Tab	Round	N	N	Par	Antidepressant
	SP 136	Thioridazine	10mg	Orange	Tab	Round	N	Y	Superpharm	Tranquilizer
137	West–ward 136	Diphenhydramine HCl	25mg	Pink/Clear	Cap	–	–	–	West–ward	Antihistamine
	AT 137	Methocarbamol	750mg	White	Tab	Capsule	Y	N	ATI	Muscle Relaxant
	BL 137	Cephalexin	500mg	White	Tab	Capsule	N	Y	Biocraft	Anti-Infective
	bp 137	Fluoxymesterone	2mg	Peach	Tab	Round	–	–	Bolar	Hormone
	Par/137	Amitriptyline HCl	100mg	Orange	Tab	Round	N	N	Par	Antidepressant
	SP 137	Thioridazine	25mg	Orange	Tab	Round	N	Y	Superpharm	Tranquilizer
	West–ward 137	Diphenhydramine HCl	50mg	Pink/Pink	Cap	–	–	–	West–ward	Antihistamine
138	93 138	Diphenhydramine HCl	25mg	Pink/Clear	Cap	–	–	–	Lemmon	Antihistamine
	bp 138	Fluoxymesterone	5mg	Green	Tab	Round	–	–	Bolar	Hormone
	Par/138	Amitriptyline HCl	150mg	Peach	Tab	Round	N	N	Par	Antidepressant
	SP 138	Thioridazine	50mg	Orange	Tab	Round	N	Y	Superpharm	Tranquilizer
139	SQUIBB 138	Sulfamethoxazole & Trimethoprim	400mg/80mg	–	Tab	–	–	–	Squibb	Anti-Infective
	93 139	Diphenhydramine HCl	50mg	Pink/Pink	Cap	–	–	–	Lemmon	Antihistamine
	M–139	Sulfamethoxazole & Trimethoprim	400mg/80mg	White	Tab	Round	N	N	Mylan	Anti-Infective
	Par/139	Sulfamethoxazole & Trimethoprim	400mg/80mg	White	Tab	Round	Y	N	Par	Anti-Infective
140	140	Multivitamin with Fluoride Chewables	n/a	–	Tab	–	–	–	Marlop	Vitamin
	BMP 140	Ampicillin	250mg	Brown/Orange	Cap	–	N	–	Beecham	Anti-Infective
	Geigy 140	Imipramine HCl	25mg	Coral	Tab	Round	N	Y	Geigy	Antidepressant
	Hoyt 140	Sodium Fluoride	1mg	Green	Tab	Round	N	N	Colgate	Mineral Supp.
	M–140	Sulfamethoxazole & Trimethoprim	800mg/160mg	White	Tab	Round	N	N	Mylan	Anti-Infective
	Par/140	Sulfamethoxazole & Trimethoprim	800mg/160mg	White	Tab	Capsule	Y	N	Par	Anti-Infective
141	SP 140	Quinidine Gluconate SR	324mg	White	Tab	Round	N	N	Superpharm	Antiarrhythmic
	AT 141	Prednisone	5mg	White	Tab	Round	Y	N	ATI	Steroid
	BL/141	Baclofen	10mg	White	Tab	Round	Y	N	Biocraft	Muscle Relaxant
	BMP 141	Ampicillin	500mg	Brown/Orange	Cap	–	N	–	Beecham	Anti-Infective

ID NO.	ID CODE	GENERIC NAME	STRENGTH	COLOR	FORM	SHAPE	SCORED	COATED	MFG.	USE
	GG141	Meclizine HCl	12.5mg	Blue	Tab	Oval	N	N	Geneva	Antivertigo
	GG141	Meclizine HCl	12.5mg	Blue/White	Tab	Oval	N	N	Geneva	Antivertigo
	Hoyt 141	Sodium Fluoride	1mg	Yellow	Tab	Round	N	N	Colgate	Mineral Supp
	MP 141	Acetazolamide	250mg	White	Tab	Round	Y	N	Mutual	Antiglaucoma Agent
	Mylan 141	Spironolactone w/Hydrochlorothiazide	25mg/25mg	Ivory	Tab	Round	Y	N	Mylan	Diuretic
	P–D 141/2	Diazepam	2mg	White	Tab	Oval	Y	N	PD	Antianxiety
	SP 141	Diphenoxylate HCl, Atropine	2.5mg/.025mg	White	Tab	Round	N	N	Superpharm	Antidiarrheal
	WC 141	Diazepam	2mg	White	Tab	Oval	Y	N	WC	Antianxiety
	West–ward 141	Doxycycline Hyclate	50mg	Blue/White	Cap	–	–	–	West–ward	Anti–Infective
142	142	Acetaminophen	325mg	White	Tab	Round	Y	N	Granutec	Analgesic
	2 Rorer 142	Aspirin/Codeine Phosphate/Maalox	325/15/150mg	White	Tab	Round	–	N	Rorer	Analgesic
	54/142	Methadone HCl	10mg	White	Tab	Round	Y	N	Roxane	Analgesic
	AT 142	Prednisone	10mg	White	Tab	Round	Y	N	ATI	Steroid
	BL/142	Baclofen	20mg	White	Tab	Round	Y	N	Biocraft	Muscle Relaxant
	GG142	Tolbutamide	500mg	White	Tab	Round	Y	N	Geneva	Hypoglycemic
	Hoyt 142	Sodium Fluoride	1mg	Orange	Tab	Round	N	N	Colgate	Mineral Supp.
	MP 142	Benztropine Mesylate	2.0mg	White	Tab	Round	Y	N	Mutual	Antiparkinson
	P–D 142/5	Diazepam	5mg	White	Tab	Triangular	Y	N	PD	Antianxiety
	SP 142	Diphenhydramine HCl	25mg	Pink/Clear	Cap	–	–	–	Superpharm	Antihistamine
	T 142	Phenazopyridine HCl	200mg	Burgundy	Tab	Round	N	Y	Trinity	Urinary Antiseptic
	WC 142	Diazepam	5mg	White	Tab	Triangular	Y	N	WC	Antianxiety
	West–ward 142	Doxycycline Hyclate	100mg	Blue/Blue	Cap	–	–	–	West–ward	Anti–Infective
143	3 Rorer 143	Aspirin/Codeine Phosphate/Maalox	325/30/150mg	White	Tab	Round	–	N	Rorer	Analgesic
	54–143	Amitriptyline	100mg	White	Tab	Round	–	Y	Roxane	Antidepressant
	93–143	Warfarin Sodium	2mg	Lavender	Tab	Round	Y	N	Lemmon	Anticoagulant
	AT 143	Prednisone	20mg	White	Tab	Round	Y	N	ATI	Steroid
	BMP 143	Oxacillin Sodium	250mg	Brown/Yellow	Cap	–	–	–	Beecham	Anti–Infective
	CC 143	Trichlormethiazide	4mg	Aqua	Tab	Round	N	N	Camall	Diuretic
	Copley 143	Salsalate	500mg	Aqua	Tab	Capsule	–	Y	Copley	Analgesic
	Mylan 143	Indomethacin	25mg	Green/Green	Cap	–	–	–	Mylan	Anti–Inflammatory
	P–D 143/10	Diazepam	10mg	White	Tab	Round	Y	N	PD	Antianxiety
	Par/143	Hydralazine HCl & Hydrochlorothiazide	25mg/25mg	White	Cap	–	–	–	Par	Antihypertensive
	R 143	Carbamazepine	200mg	White	Tab	Round	Y	N	Purepac	Anticonvulsant
	Roerig 143	Carbenicillin Indanyl	382mg	Yellow	Tab	Capsule	Y	Y	Pfizer	Anti–infective
	SP 143	Diphenhydramine HCl	50mg	Pink/Pink	Cap	–	–	–	Superpharm	Antihistamine
	WC 143	Diazepam	10mg	White	Tab	Round	Y	N	WC	Antianxiety
	West–ward 143	Benztropine Mesylate	1mg	White	Tab	Round	Y	N	West–ward	Antiparkinson
144	93–144	Warfarin Sodium	2.5mg	Orange	Tab	Round	Y	N	Lemmon	Anticoagulant
	BMP 144	Oxacillin Sodium	500mg	Brown/Yellow	Cap	–	–	–	Beecham	Anti–Infective
	bp 144	Carisoprodol Compound (Aspirin & Carisoprodol)	200mg/325mg	White/Lavender	Tab	Round	N	N	Bolar	Muscle Relaxant
	Copley 144	Salsalate	750mg	Aqua	Tab	Capsule	–	Y	Copley	Analgesic
	GG144	Chlorpropamide	250mg	White	Tab	Round	Y	N	Geneva	Hypoglycemic
	Par/144	Hydralazine HCl & Hydrochlorothiazide	50mg/50mg	White/Black	Cap	–	–	–	Par	Antihypertensive
	SP 144	Meclizine HCl	12.5mg	Blue/White	Tab	Oval	N	N	Superpharm	Antivertigo
	West–ward 144	Benztropine Mesylate	2mg	White	Tab	Round	Y	N	West–ward	Antiparkinson
145	93–145	Warfarin Sodium	5mg	Pink	Tab	Round	Y	N	Lemmon	Anticoagulant
	AT 145	Quinine Sulfate	260mg	White	Tab	Round	Y	N	ATI	Muscle Relaxant
	BMP 145	Oxyphencyclimine Hydrochloride	10mg	White	Tab	Round	Y	N	Beecham	Antispasmodic
	bp 145	Indomethacin	25mg	Green/Green	Cap	–	–	–	Bolar	Anti–Inflammatory
	GG145	Dimenhydrinate	50mg	Yellow	Tab	Round	Y	N	Geneva	Antiemetic
	Mylan 145	Doxycycline Hyclate	50mg	Blue/White	Cap	–	–	–	Mylan	Anti–Infective
	Par/145	Hydralazine HCl & Hydrochlorothiazide	100mg/50mg	Blue/Blue	Cap	–	–	–	Par	Antihypertensive
	SP 145	Meclizine HCl	25mg	Yellow/White	Tab	Oval	N	N	Superpharm	Antivertigo
146	AT 146	Quinine Sulfate	325mg	White	Tab	Round	N	N	ATI	Muscle Relaxant
	bp 146	Indomethacin	50mg	Green/Green	Cap	–	–	–	Bolar	Anti–Inflammatory
	COPLEY 146	Naproxen	250mg	Off White	Tab	Round	N	Y	Copley	Anti–Inflammatory
	MP 146	Atenolol	50mg	White	Tab	Round	Y	N	Mutual	Antihypertensive
	Mylan 146/25	Spironolactone	25mg	White	Tab	Round	Y	N	Mylan	Diuretic
	SP 146	Sulfamethoxazole/Trimethoprim	400mg/80mg	White	Tab	Round	Y	N	Superpharm	Anti–Infective
147	93–147	Naproxen Sodium	250mg	Mottled Red	Tab	Round	N	N	Lemmon	Anti–Inflammatory
	AT 147	Fenoprofen Calcium	600mg	Peach	Tab	Capsule	–	Y	ATI	Anti Inflammatory
	MP 147	Atenolol	100mg	White	Tab	Round	Y	N	Mutual	Antihypertensive
	Mylan 147	Indomethacin	50mg	Green/Green	Cap	–	–	–	Mylan	Anti–Inflammatory
	Par/147	Hydroflumethiazide	50mg	White	Tab	Round	Y	N	Par	Diuretic
	R 147	Prenatal Vitamins	n/a	Blue	Tab	Oblong	N	Y	Ross	Vitamin
	SP 147	Sulfamethoxazole/Trimethoprim DS	800mg/160mg	White	Tab	Oval	Y	N	Superpharm	Anti–Infective
	T 147	Phenazopyridine HCl	200mg	Burgundy	Tab	Round	N	Y	Trinity	Urinary Antiseptic
	West–ward 147	Imipramine Hydrochloride	25mg	Rust	Tab	Round	N	Y	West–ward	Antidepressant
148	93–148	Naproxen Sodium	375mg	Mottled Peach	Tab	Oval	N	N	Lemmon	Anti–Inflammatory
	AT 148	Clonidine Hydrochloride	0.1mg	Orange	Tab	Round	Y	N	ATI	Antihypertensive
	biocraft 148	Clindamycin HCl	75mg	Red	Cap	–	–	–	Biocraft	Anti–Infective
	Mylan 148	Doxycycline Hyclate	100mg	Blue/Blue	Cap	–	–	–	Mylan	Anti–Infective
	Par/148	Hydroflumethiazide & Reserpine	50mg/0.125mg	Green	Tab	Round	Y	N	Par	Antihypertensive
	Sch. Logo 148	Dexchlorpheniramine ER	6mg	Red	Tab	Oval	N	Y	Schering	Antihistamine
	SP 148	Sulfasalazine	500mg	Yellow	Tab	Round	Y	N	Superpharm	Anti–Inflammatory
149	93–149	Naproxen Sodium	500mg	Mottled Red	Tab	Oval	N	N	Lemmon	Anti–Inflammatory
	AT 149	Clonidine Hydrochloride	0.2mg	White	Tab	Round	Y	N	ATI	Antihypertensive
	biocraft 149	Clindamycin HCl	150mg	Red/Blue	Cap	–	–	–	Biocraft	Anti–Infective
150	3M/TR150	Flecainide Acetate	150mg	White	Tab	Oval	y	–	3M	Antiarrhythmic
	93 150 / 3	Acetaminophen & Codeine	300mg/30mg	White	Tab	Round	N	N	Lemmon	Analgesic
	AT 150	Clonidine Hydrochloride	0.3mg	White	Tab	Round	Y	N	ATI	Antihypertensive
	COPLEY 150	Naproxen	500mg	Off White	Tab	Capsule	N	Y	Copley	Anti–Inflammatory
	dp 150	Levothyroxine Sodium	0.15mg	Blue	Tab	Oval	Y	N	Daniels	Hormone
	Flint 150	Levothyroxine Sodium	150mcg	Blue	Tab	Round	Y	N	Boots	Hormone
	Forest 150	Guaifenesin	200mg	Burgundy	Tab	Round	–	Y	Forest	Expectorant
	GG150	Meprobamate	400mg	White	Tab	Round	N	N	Geneva	Antianxiety
	M 150	Levothyroxine Sodium	0.15mg	Blue	Tab	Round	Y	N	Duramed	Hormone
	M 150 LEVO T	Levothyroxine Sodium	0.15mg	Blue	Tab	Round	Y	N	Mova	Hormone
	MYLAN 150/250	Chlorothiazide	250mg	White	Tab	Round	Y	N	Mylan	Diuretic
	Ortho 150	Norethindrone & Mestranol	1mg/0.05mg	Yellow	Tab	Round	N	N	Ortho	Hormone
	Par/150	Methyldopa	125mg	White	Tab	Round	N	Y	Par	Antihypertensive
	Sch. Logo 150	Ethinyl Estradiol	0.5mg	Peach	Tab	Round	N	Y	Schering	Hormone
	Triangle 150	Propafenone HCl	150mg	White	Tab	Round	Y	Y	Knoll	Antiarrhythmic
	West–ward 150	Imipramine Hydrochloride	50mg	Green	Tab	Round	N	Y	West–ward	Antidepressant
151	AT 151	Thiothixene	1mg	Orange/Yellow	Cap	–	–	–	ATI	Tranquilizer

ID NO.	ID CODE	GENERIC NAME	STRENGTH	COLOR	FORM	SHAPE	SCORED	COATED	MFG.	USE
	bp 151	Trifluoperazine HCl	10mg	Red	Tab	Round	N	Y	Bolar	Tranquilizer
	Copley 151	B Complex Vitamins	n/a	Green	Tab	–	N	Y	Copley	Vitamin
	GG151/3	Aspirin & Codeine	325mg/30mg	White	Tab	Round	N	N	Geneva	Analgesic
	MP 151	Prednisone	5mg	White	Tab	Round	Y	N	Mutual	Steroid
	Par/151	Methyldopa	250mg	White	Tab	Round	N	Y	Par	Antihypertensive
	SEARLE 151	Ethynodiol Diacetate & Ethinyl Estradiol	1mg/35mcg	White	Tab	Round	N	N	Searle	Hormone
152	93 152	Acetaminophen & Codeine	300mg/30mg	Coral/Scarlet	Cap	–	–	–	Lemmon	Analgesic
	AT 152	Thiothixene	2mg	Green/Yellow	Cap	–	–	–	ATI	Tranquilizer
	bp 152	Procainamide HCl SR	250mg	Blue	Tab	Oval	N	Y	Bolar	Antiarrhythmic
	Copley 152	B Complex Vitamin Plus	n/a	Yellow	Tab	Capsule	N	Y	Copley	Vitamin
	MP 152	Atenolol/Chlorthalidone	100mg/25mg	–	Tab	Round	–	–	Mutual	Antihypertensive
	MP 152	Atenolol & Chlorthalidone	100mg/25mg	White	Tab	Round	Y	N	Mutual	Antihypertensive
	Mylan 152	Clonidine HCl	0.1mg	White	Tab	Round	Y	N	Mylan	Antihypertensive
	Par/152	Methyldopa	500mg	White	Tab	Round	N	Y	Par	Antihypertensive
	SP 152	Indomethacin	25mg	Green	Cap	–	–	–	Superpharm	Anti–Inflammatory
153	WPPh 152	Methyldopa	250mg	Yellow	Tab	Round	N	Y	West Point Pharma	Antihypertensive
	AT 153	Thiothixene	5mg	Orange/White	Cap	–	–	–	ATI	Tranquilizer
	bp 153	Procainamide HCl SR	500mg	Pink	Tab	Oval	Y	Y	Bolar	Antiarrhythmic
	GG153	Propranolol/Hydrochlorothiazide	40mg/25mg	White	Tab	Round	Y	Y	Geneva	Antihypertensive
	MP 153	Atenolol/Chlorthalidone	50mg/25mg	–	Tab	Round	–	–	Mutual	Antihypertensive
	MP 153	Atenolol & Chlorthalidone	50mg/25mg	White	Tab	Round	Y	N	Mutual	Antihypertensive
	Par/153	Disulfiram	250mg	Off White	Tab	Round	Y	N	Par	Alcohol Deterrent
	SP 153	Indomethacin	50mg	Green	Cap	–	–	–	Superpharm	Anti–Inflammatory
	WALLACE 153	Methyclothiazide	5mg	Peach	Tab	Rectangular	Y	N	Wallace	Diuretic
	West–ward 153	Methyldopa	250mg	White	Tab	Round	Y	Y	West–ward	Antihypertensive
154	WPPh 153	Methyldopa & Hydrochlorothiazide	250mg/25mg	White	Tab	Round	N	Y	West Point Pharma	Antihypertensive
	AT 154	Thiothixene	10mg	Green/White	Cap	–	–	–	ATI	Tranquilizer
	bp 154	Procainamide HCl SR	750mg	Buff	Tab	Oval	Y	Y	Bolar	Antiarrhythmic
	bp 154	Procainamide HCl SR	750mg	Tan	Tab	–	–	Y	Bolar	Antiarrhythmic
	Ciba 154	Rifampin	300mg	Scarlet/Carmel	Cap	–	–	–	Ciba	Anti–Infective
	GG154	Propranolol/Hydrochlorothiazide	80mg/25mg	White	Tab	Round	Y	Y	Geneva	Antihypertensive
	Par/154	Disulfiram	500mg	Off White	Tab	Round	Y	N	Par	Alcohol Deterrent
	QPL 154	Phenazopyridine HCl	100mg	Maroon	Tab	Round	N	Y	Quantum	Urinary Antiseptic
	SP 154	Spironolactone & Hydrochlorothiazide	25mg/25mg	White	Tab	Round	Y	N	Superpharm	Diuretic
	SQUIBB 154	Pravastatin Sodium	10mg	White	Tab	Round	–	–	Squibb	Hypolipidemic
155	WPPh 154	Sulindac	200mg	Yellow	Tab	Hexagonal	–	–	West Point Pharma	Anti–Inflammatory
	AT 155	Thiothixene	20mg	White/Blue	Cap	–	–	–	ATI	Tranquilizer
	GG155	Prednisone	20mg	Peach	Tab	Round	Y	N	Geneva	Steroid
	MP 155	Quinine Sulfate	260mg	White	Tab	Round	Y	N	Mutual	Muscle Relaxant
	Mylan 155	Propoxyphene Napsylate and Acetaminophen	100mg/650mg	Pink	Tab	Capsule	N	Y	Mylan	Analgesic
	QPL 155	Phenazopyridine HCl	200mg	Maroon	Tab	Round	N	Y	Quantum	Urinary Antiseptic
	West–ward 155	Butabarbital Sodium	15mg	Lavender	Tab	Round	Y	N	West–ward	Sedative
156	West–ward 155	Methyldopa	500mg	White	Tab	Oblong	Y	Y	West–ward	Antihypertensive
	AT 156	Clorazepate Dipotassium	3.75mg	Blue	Tab	Round	Y	N	ATI	Antianxiety
	GG 156	Prednisone	10mg	White	Tab	Round	Y	N	Geneva	Steroid
	Mylan 156/500	Probenecid	500mg	Yellow	Tab	Capsule	N	Y	Mylan	Antigout
	QPL/156 Q	Lorazepam	0.5mg	White	Tab	Round	N	N	Quantum	Antianxiety
157	WPPh 156	Cyclobenzaprine HCl	10mg	Yellow	Tab	D–shaped	N	Y	West Point Pharma	Muscle Relaxant
	555/157, barr	Prednisone	20mg	Peach	Tab	Round	Y	N	Barr	Steroid
	93 157	Diethylpropion HCl	25mg	White	Tab	Round	N	N	Lemmon	Anorectic
	AT 157	Clorazepate Dipotassium	7.5mg	Peach	Tab	Round	Y	N	ATI	Antianxiety
	bp 157	Methyclothiazide & Deserpidine	5mg/0.5mg	Grey	Tab	Round	Y	N	Bolar	Antihypertensive
	GG 157	Prednisone	50mg	White	Tab	Round	Y	N	Geneva	Steroid
	HD 157	Quinine Sulfate	325mg	Clear	Cap	–	–	–	Halsey	Muscle Relaxant
	QPL/157 Q	Lorazepam	1mg	White	Tab	Round	N	N	Quantum	Antianxiety
	West–ward 157	Butabarbital Sodium	30mg	Lavender	Tab	Round	Y	N	West–ward	Sedative
158	WPPh 157	Indomethacin ER	75mg	Blue/Clear	Cap	–	–	–	West Point Pharma	Anti–Inflammatory
	AT 158	Clorazepate Dipotassium	15mg	Pink	Tab	Round	Y	N	ATI	Antianxiety
	Barr 158	Chlordiazepoxide HCl	5mg	Green/Yellow	Cap	–	–	–	Barr	Antianxiety
	bp 158	Methyclothiazide & Deserpidine	5mg/0.25mg	Yellow	Tab	Round	Y	N	Bolar	Antihypertensive
	Copley 158	Multivitamins/Fluoride	0.5mg	Orange/Pink/Purple	Tab	Square	–	N	Copley	Vitamin
	GG158	Sulfisoxazole	500mg	White	Tab	Round	N	N	Geneva	Anti–Infective
	MJ 158	Fosinopril Sodium	10mg	White	Tab	Diamond	Y	N	MJ	Anti–hypertensive
	Par/158	Methylprednisolone	16mg	White	Tab	Round	Y	Y	Par	Steroid
	QPL/158 Q	Lorazepam	2mg	White	Tab	Round	N	N	Quantum	Antianxiety
159	Squibb 158 M	Fosinopril Sodium	10mg	White	Tab	Diamond	N	N	Squibb	Antihypertensive
	879 159	Tetracycline HCl	500mg	Yellow/Black	Cap	–	–	–	Halsey	Anti–Infective
	Barr 159	Chlordiazepoxide HCl	25mg	Green/White	Cap	–	–	–	Barr	Antianxiety
	barr 159	Chlordiazepoxide Hydrochloride	25mg	White/Green	Cap	–	–	–	Barr	Antianxiety
	Copley 159	Multivitamins/Fluoride + Iron	1mg	Purple	Tab	Square	–	–	Copley	Vitamin
	GG 159	Clemastine Fumarate	1.34mg	White	Tab	Capsule	–	–	Geneva	Antihistamine
	Mylan 159	Disopyramide Phosphate	100mg	Maroon/White	Cap	–	–	–	Mylan	Antiarrhythmic
	Par 159	Methylprednisolone	24mg	White	Tab	Round	N	N	Par	Steroid
160	WPPh 159	Indomethacin	50mg	Blue/White	Cap	–	–	–	West Point Pharma	Anti–Inflammatory
	GG 160	Clemastine Fumarate	2.68mg	White	Tab	Round	Y	N	Geneva	Antihistamine
	MP 160	Thioridazine Hydrochloride	100mg	Yellow	Tab	Round	N	Y	Mutual	Tranquilizer
	Par 160	Methylprednisolone	32mg	White	Tab	Round	N	N	Par	Steroid
	Sch. Logo 160	Carisoprodol	350mg	Pink	Tab	Round	N	Y	Schering	Muscle Relaxant
161	SQUIBB 160	Erythromycin Stearate	500mg	White	Tab	Round	–	N	Squibb	Anti–Infective
	Forest 161	Powdered Opium/Bismuth Subcarbonate/Calcium carb.	1.23/125/125mg	White	Tab	Round	–	N	Forest	Antidiarrheal
	GG161/4	Aspirin & Codeine	325mg/60mg	White	Tab	Round	N	N	Geneva	Analgesic
	Mylan 161	Disopyramide Phosphate	150mg	Maroon/Maroon	Cap	–	–	–	Mylan	Antiarrhythmic
	Par/161 300	Ibuprofen	300mg	White	Tab	Round	N	N	Par	Anti–Inflammatory
	R 161	Chlorthalidone	25mg	Yellow	Tab	Round	Y	N	Purepac	Diuretic
	RIKER/161	Orphenadrine HCl	50mg	Green	Tab	Round	N	N	3M	Muscle Relaxant
	SP 161	Metoclopramide	10mg	White	Tab	Round	Y	N	Superpharm	Antireflux
162	SQUIBB 161	Erythromycin Stearate	500mg	–	Tab	–	–	–	Squibb	Anti–Infective
	EVERETT 162	Butalbital/Caffeine/Acetaminophen	50mg/40mg/325mg	–	Tab	–	–	–	Everett	Analgesic
	GG 162	Triazolam	0.125mg	White	Tab	–	N	N	Upjohn	Sedative/Hypnotic
	Mylan 162	Chlorothiazide	500mg	White	Tab	Round	Y	N	Mylan	Diuretic
	Par/162 400	Ibuprofen	400mg	White	Tab	Round	N	Y	Par	Anti–Inflammatory
163	WPPh 162	Amiloride HCl & Hydrochlorothiazide	5mg/50mg	Peach	Tab	Diamond	–	–	West Point Pharma	Antihypertensive
	barr,555/163	Diazepam	2mg	White	Tab	Round	Y	N	Barr	Antianxiety
	biocraft 163	Cinoxacin	250mg	Blue/Yellow	CAP	–	–	N	Biocraft	Anti–Infective
	bp 163	Fluphenazine HCl	1mg	White	Tab	Round	N	Y	Bolar	Tranquilizer

ID NO.	ID CODE	GENERIC NAME	STRENGTH	COLOR	FORM	SHAPE	SCORED	COATED	MFG.	USE
	GG 163	Triazolam	0.25mg	Blue	Tab	–	Y	N	Upjohn	Sedative/Hypnotic
	Par/163 600	Ibuprofen	600mg	White	Tab	Oval	N	Y	Par	Anti-Inflammatory
164	R 163	Chlorthalidone	50mg	Green	Tab	Round	Y	N	Purepac	Diuretic
	AT 164	Triamterene & Hydrochlorothiazide	75mg/50mg	Yellow	Tab	Round	Y	N	ATI	Diuretic
	AT–164	Triamterene & Hydrochlorothiazide	75mg/50mg	Yellow	Tab	Round	Y	N	ATI	Antihypertensive
	barr,555/164	Diazepam	10mg	Blue	Tab	Round	Y	N	Barr	Antianxiety
	biocraft 164	Cinoxacin	500mg	Blue/Yellow	CAP	–	N	–	Biocraft	Anti-Infective
	bp 164	Fluphenazine HCl	2.5mg	Beige	Tab	Round	N	Y	Bolar	Tranquilizer
	Par/164	Benztropine Mesylate	0.5mg	White	Tab	Round	Y	N	Par	Antiparkinson
	SP 164	Disopyramide Phosphate	100mg	Scarlet/Blue	Cap	–	–	–	Superpharm	Antiarrhythmic
	SQUIBB 164	Penicillin G Potassium	125mg	–	Tab	–	Y	N	Squibb	Anti-Infective
165	AT 165	Metaproterenol Sulfate	10mg	White	Tab	Round	Y	N	ATI	Bronchodilator
	BMP 165	Dicloxacillin Sodium	250mg	Blue/Cream	Cap	–	–	–	Beecham	Anti-Infective
	bp 165	Fluphenazine HCl	5mg	Blue	Tab	Round	N	Y	Bolar	Tranquilizer
	Ciba 165	Potassium Chloride	600mg (8mEq)	Orange	Tab	Round	N	Y	Ciba	Potassium Supp.
	GG 165	Triamterene & Hydrochlorothiazide	37.5mg/25mg	Green	Tab	Round	Y	N	Geneva	Diuretic
	MUTUAL 165	Piroxicam	10mg	–	Cap	–	–	–	Mutual	Anti-inflammatory
	Par/165	Benztropine Mesylate	1.0mg	White	Tab	Oval	Y	N	Par	Antiparkinson
	SP 165	Disopyramide Phosphate	150mg	Buff/Scarlet	Cap	–	–	–	Superpharm	Antiarrhythmic
	SQUIBB 165	Penicillin G Potassium	250mg	–	Tab	–	Y	N	Squibb	Anti-Infective
166	AT 166	Metaproterenol Sulfate	20mg	White	Tab	Round	Y	N	ATI	Bronchodilator
	BMP 166	Dicloxacillin Sodium	500mg	Blue/Cream	Cap	–	–	–	Beecham	Anti-Infective
	bp 166	Fluphenazine HCl	10mg	Red	Tab	Round	N	Y	Bolar	Tranquilizer
	CC 166	Phendimetrazine Tartrate	35mg	Green	Tab	Round	Y	N	Camall	Anorectic
	Copley 166	Multivitamins/Fluoride	1mg	Orange,Pink,Purple	Tab	Square	–	N	Copley	Vitamin
	GG 166	Desipramine HCl	75mg	White	Tab	Round	N	Y	Geneva	Antidepressant
	MUTUAL 166	Piroxicam	20mg	–	Cap	–	–	–	Mutual	Anti-inflammatory
	P–D 166	Methenamine Mandelate	500mg	Brown	Tab	Oval	N	Y	PD	Anti-Infective
	Par/166	Benztropine Mesylate	2.0mg	White	Tab	Round	Y	N	Par	Antiparkinson
	SP 166	Spironolactone	25mg	White	Tab	Round	–	–	Superpharm	Diuretic
167	AT 167	Maprotiline	25mg	Orange	Tab	Round	Y	Y	ATI	Antidepressant
	bp 167	Chlorpropamide	100mg	Blue	Tab	Round	Y	N	Bolar	Hypoglycemic
	GG 167	Desipramine HCl	100mg	White	Tab	Round	N	Y	Geneva	Antidepressant
	MP 167	Fenoprofen Calcium	600mg	Yellow	Tab	Capsule	Y	Y	Mutual	Anti-Inflammatory
	Mylan 167 / 100	Doxycycline Hyclate	100mg	Beige	Tab	Round	N	Y	Mylan	Anti-Infective
	P–D 167	Methenamine Mandelate	1000mg	Purple	Tab	Oval	N	Y	PD	Anti-Infective
168	AT 168	Maprotiline	50mg	Orange	Tab	Round	Y	Y	ATI	Antidepressant
	bp 168	Chlorpropamide	250mg	Blue	Tab	Round	Y	N	Bolar	Hypoglycemic
	GG 168	Desipramine HCl	150mg	White	Tab	Round	N	Y	Geneva	Antidepressant
	SQUIBB 168	Penicillin G Potassium	500mg	–	Tab	–	Y	N	Squibb	Anti-Infective
169	54–169 1/2	Haloperidol	0.5mg	White	Tab	Round	N	N	Roxane	Tranquilizer
	555/169, barr	Furosemide	40mg	White	Tab	Round	N	N	Barr	Diuretic
	AT 169	Maprotiline	75mg	White	Tab	Round	Y	Y	ATI	Antidepressant
	BMP 169	Cloxacillin Sodium	250mg	Lime/Beige	Cap	–	N	N	Beecham	Anti-Infective
	Copley 169	Prenatal Vitamin RX	n/a	Coral	Tab	Oblong	N	Y	Copley	Prenatal Vitamin
	LEMMON 169	Opium/Bismuth Sulgal/Pectin/Kaolin/Zinc Phenolsulf	n/a	Yellow	Tab	Round	N	N	Lemmon	Antidiarrheal
170	Barr, 170	Furosemide	20mg	White	Tab	Oval	N	N	Barr	Diuretic
	BL 170	Amoxicillin Veterinary	50mg	White	Tab	Round	N	N	Biocraft	Anti-Infective
	BMP 170	Cloxacillin Sodium	500mg	Lime/Beige	Cap	–	N	N	Beecham	Anti-Infective
	Copley 170	Prenatal Vitamin with Folic Acid	n/a	Blue	Tab	Oblong	N	Y	Copley	Prenatal Vitamin
	Par/170	Sulfinpyrazone	100mg	White	Tab	Round	Y	N	Par	Antigout
	SP 170	Ibuprofen	400mg	White	Tab	Round	N	Y	Superpharm	Anti-Inflammatory
	WPPh 170	Sulindac	150mg	Yellow	Tab	Hexagonal	–	–	West Point Pharma	Anti-Inflammatory
171	BL 171	Amoxicillin Veterinary	100mg	White	Tab	Round	N	N	Biocraft	Anti-Infective
	bp 171	Trifluoperazine HCl	1mg	Red	Tab	Round	N	Y	Bolar	Tranquilizer
	KU 171	Aspirin/Acetaminophen	325mg/325mg	White	Tab	Oval	Y	N	Schwarz	Analgesic
	N 171	Nifedipine	10mg	Brown	Cap	–	–	–	Novopharm	Antianginal
	Par/171	Sulfinpyrazone	200mg	Orange	Cap	–	–	–	Par	Antigout
	QPL 171	Meprobamate & Aspirin	200mg/325mg	Green/Yellow	Tab	Round	N	N	Quantum	Analgesic
	SP 171	Ibuprofen	600mg	White	Tab	Oval	N	Y	Superpharm	Anti-Inflammatory
172	SQUIBB 171	Sulfamethoxazole & Trimethoprim	800mg/160mg	–	Tab	–	–	–	Squibb	Anti-Infective
	93 172	Acetaminophen & Codeine	300mg/60mg	Brown/Gray	Cap	–	–	–	Lemmon	Analgesic
	AT 172	Albuterol Sulfate	2mg	White	Tab	Round	Y	N	ATI	Bronchodilator
	b 172	Isosorbide Dinitrate Sublingual	2.5mg	Yellow	Tab	Round	N	N	Barr	Antianginal
	BL 172	Amoxicillin Veterinary	200mg	White	Tab	Round	N	N	Biocraft	Anti-Infective
	bp 172	Trifluoperazine HCl	2mg	Red	Tab	Round	N	Y	Bolar	Tranquilizer
	GG 172	Triamterene/Hydrochlorothiazide	75mg/50mg	Yellow	Tab	Round	Y	N	Geneva	Diuretic
173	WPPh 172	Indomethacin	25mg	Blue/White	Cap	–	–	–	West Point Pharma	Anti-Inflammatory
	b 173	Isosorbide Dinitrate Sublingual	5.0mg	Pink	Tab	Round	N	N	Barr	Antianginal
	BL 173	Amoxicillin Veterinary	400mg	White	Tab	Round	N	N	Biocraft	Anti-Infective
174	LASER 173	Multivitamin with Minerals	–	White	TAb	Oval	N	Y	Central	Prenatal Supp.
	555/174	Isosorbide Dinitrate	5mg	Pink	Tab	Round	Y	N	Barr	Antianginal
	AT 174	Chlorzoxazone	500mg	Green	Tab	Capsule	Y	N	ATI	Muscle Relaxant
	GG174	Sulfamethoxazole & Trimethoprim	400mg/80mg	White	Tab	Round	Y	N	Geneva	Anti-Infective
	MP 174	Salsalate	500mg	Yellow	Tab	Round	N	Y	Mutual	Analgesic
175	WPPh 174	Methyldopa	125mg	Yellow	Tab	Round	N	Y	West Point Pharma	Antihypertensive
	175	Hexavitamin	n/a	Red	Cap	–	–	–	West-ward	Vitamin
	555/175	Isosorbide Dinitrate	10mg	White	Tab	Round	Y	N	Barr	Antianginal
	COPLEY 175	Quinidine Sulfate ER	300mg	White	Tab	Round	N	Y	Copley	Antiarrhythmic
	dp 175	Levothyroxine Sodium	0.175mg	Aqua	Tab	Oval	Y	N	Daniels	Hormone
	Flint 175	Levothyroxine Sodium	175mcg	Lilac	Tab	Round	Y	N	Boots	Hormone
	GG175	Sulfamethoxazole & Trimethoprim	800mg/160mg	White	Tab	Oval	Y	N	Geneva	Anti-Infective
	Mylan 175	Chlorothiazide with Reserpine	250mg/0.125mg	Orange	Tab	Round	N	Y	Mylan	Antihypertensive
176	SP 175	Propoxyphene Napsylate & Acetaminophen	100mg/650mg	Pink	Tab	Capsule	N	Y	Superpharm	Analgesic
	Copley 176	Triple Vitamins/Fluoride	1mg	Orange,Pink,Purple	Tab	Pillow	N	N	Copley	Vitamin
	Mylan 176	Chlorothiazide with Reserpine	500mg/0.125mg	Orange	Tab	Round	N	Y	Mylan	Antihypertensive
	Par/176	Meprobamate & Aspirin	200mg/325mg	Green/Orange	Tab	Round	N	N	Par	Analgesic
	R 176	Digitoxin	0.1mg	Pink	Tab	Round	N	N	Purepac	Cardiac Agent
177	WPPh 176	Methyldopa	500mg	Yellow	Tab	Round	N	Y	West Point Pharma	Antihypertensive
	AT 177	Albuterol Sulfate	4mg	White	Tab	Round	Y	N	ATI	Bronchodilator
	COPLEY 177	Bromatapp E.R.	n/a	Blue	Tab	Round	N	Y	Copley	Decongestant Comb.
	MP 177	Salsalate	750mg	Yellow	Tab	Capsule	N	Y	Mutual	Analgesic
	P–D 177	Phenylpropanolamine/Phenyltoloxamine/APAP	100/66/600mg	Pink	Tab	Oval	Y	N	PD	Decongestant comb.
178	Par/177	Methyclothiazide	2.5mg	Orange	Tab	Round	N	N	Par	Diuretic
	AT 178	Fenoprofen Calcium	200mg	Light Brown	Cap	–	–	–	ATI	Anti Inflammatory

ID NO.	ID CODE	GENERIC NAME	STRENGTH	COLOR	FORM	SHAPE	SCORED	COATED	MFG.	USE
	LEMMON 178	Methamphetamine HCl	10mg	Pink	Tab	Oblong	Y	N	Lemmon	Anorectic
	MP 178	Pindolol	5mg	White	Tab	Round	Y	N	Mylan	Anti–Hypertensive
	Par/178	Methyclothiazide	5mg	Salmon	Tab	Round	Y	N	Par	Diuretic
	R 178	Digitoxin	0.2mg	White	Tab	Round	Y	N	Purepac	Cardiac Agent
	SQUIBB 178	Pravastatin Sodium	20mg	White	Tab	Round	–	–	Squibb	Hypolipidemic
	West–ward 178	Propoxyphene Napsylate and Acetaminophen	50mg/325mg	White	Tab	Round	N	Y	West–ward	Analgesic
179	54–179	Chloral Hydrate	500mg	Reddish–Orange	Cap	–	–	–	Roxane	Hypnotic
	LEMMON 179	Dextroamphetamine Sulfate	5mg	Blue	Tab	Oblong	N	N	Lemmon	Anorectic
	MUTUAL 179	Tolmetin Sodium	400mg	–	Cap	–	–	–	Mutual	Anti–Inflammatory
	QPL–179	Phentermine Resin Complex	–	Blue/Clear	Cap	–	–	–	Quantum	Anorectic
	West–ward 179	Propoxyphene Napsylate and Acetaminophen	100mg/650mg	White	Tab	Capsule	N	Y	West–ward	Analgesic
	WPPh 179	Methyldopa & Hydrochlorothiazide	250mg/15mg	Salmon	Tab	Round	N	Y	West Point Pharma	Antihypertensive
180	54–180	Naproxen Sodium	275mg	–	Tab	–	–	–	Roxane	Anti–Inflammatory
	879 G180	Chlorpheniramine Maleate	4mg	Green	Tab	Round	Y	N	Halsey	Antihistamine
	GG180	Aminophylline	200mg	White	Tab	Round	Y	N	Geneva	Bronchodilator
	LEMMON 180	Dextroamphetamine Sulfate	10mg	Pink	Tab	Oblong	N	N	Lemmon	Anorectic
	P–D 180	Phenazopyridine HCl	100mg	Maroon	Tab	Round	N	Y	PD	Urinary Analgesic
181	Berlex 181	Chlorpheniramine Maleate/Pseudoephedrine HCl	8mg/120mg	Yellow/Blue	Cap	–	–	–	Berlex	Decongestant Comb.
	bp 181	Lorazepam	1mg	White	Tab	Round	–	N	Bolar	Antianxiety
	GG 181	Methazolamide	50mg	White	Tab	Round	Y	N	Geneva	Antiglaucoma
	N 181/200	Cimetidine	200mg	Green	Tab	Oval	N	Y	Novopharm	Anti–Ulcer
	P–D 181	Phenazopyridine HCl	200mg	Maroon	Tab	Round	N	Y	PD	Urinary Analgesic
	Par/181	Perphenazine & Amitriptyline	2mg/10mg	Blue	Tab	Round	N	Y	Par	Antidepressant
	QPL/2/181 Q	Diazepam	2mg	White	Tab	Round	–	–	Quantum	Antianxiety
	SP 181	Lorazepam	0.5mg	White	Tab	Round	N	N	Superpharm	Antianxiety
	SQUIBB 181	Cephalexin	250mg	–	Cap	–	–	–	Squibb	Anti–Infective
	West–ward 181	Carbamazepine	200mg	White	Tab	Round	N	N	West–ward	Anticonvulsant
182	AT 182	Prazosin HCl	1mg	White	Cap	–	–	–	ATI	Antihypertensive
	BMP 182	Codeine and Pseudoephedrine HCl	20mg/60mg	Green/White	Cap	–	N	–	Beecham	Antitussive
	bp 182	Lorazepam	2mg	White	Tab	Round	–	N	Bolar	Antianxiety
	GG 182	Timolol Maleate	10mg	White	Tab	Round	Y	N	Geneva	Antihypertensive
	Mylan 182/10	Propranolol HCl	10 mg	Orange	Tab	Round	Y	N	Mylan	Antihypertensive
	P–D 182	Phenazopyridine HCl/Hyoscyamine HBr/Butabarbital	150mg/.3mg/15mg	Maroon	Tab	Square	N	Y	PD	Urinary Analgesic
	Par/182	Perphenazine & Amitriptyline	2mg/25mg	Orange	Tab	Round	N	Y	Par	Antidepressant
	Quantum/5/182	Diazepam	5mg	Yellow	Tab	Round	–	–	Quantum	Antianxiety
	SP 182	Lorazepam	1mg	White	Tab	Round	N	N	Superpharm	Antianxiety
183	54–183	Prenisolone	5mg	White	Tab	Round	Y	N	Roxane	Steroid
	GG 183	Timolol Maleate	20mg	Blue	Tab	Round	Y	N	Geneva	Antihypertensive
	MP 183	Pindolol	10mg	White	Tab	Round	Y	N	Mylan	Anti–Hypertensive
	Mylan 183/20	Propranolol HCl	20 mg	Blue	Tab	Round	Y	N	Mylan	Antihypertensive
	Par/183	Perphenazine & Amitriptyline	4mg/10mg	Salmon	Tab	Round	N	Y	Par	Antidepressant
	Quantum/10/183	Diazepam	10mg	Blue	Tab	Round	–	–	Quantum	Antianxiety
	R 183	Dipyridamole	50mg	White	Tab	Round	N	Y	Purepac	Antiplatelet
	SP 183	Lorazepam	2mg	White	Tab	Round	N	N	Superpharm	Antianxiety
	West–ward 183	Chlorpropamide	100mg	Blue	Tab	Round	Y	N	West–ward	Hypoglycemic
184	184/Q	Doxepin HCl	10mg	Buff/Buff	Cap	–	–	–	Quantum	Antidepressant
	AT 184	Prazosin HCl	2mg	Pink	Cap	–	–	–	ATI	Antihypertensive
	Berlex 184	Chlorpheniramine Maleate/Pseudoephedrine HCl	4mg/60mg	White	Tab	Round	Y	N	Berlex	Decongestant Comb.
	MP 184	Metoprolol Tartrate	50mg	–	Tab	–	Y	N	Mutual	Antihypertensive
	Mylan 184/40	Propranolol HCl	40 mg	Green	Tab	Round	Y	N	Mylan	Antihypertensive
	Par/184	Perphenazine & Amitriptyline	4mg/25mg	Yellow	Tab	Round	N	Y	Par	Antidepressant
	SP 184	Flurazepam Hydrochloride	15mg	Blue/White	Cap	–	–	–	Superpharm	Hypnotic
185	185/Q	Doxepin HCl	25mg	Ivory/White	Cap	–	–	–	Quantum	Antidepressant
	Beecham 185	Penicillin V Potassium	250mg	White	Tab	Oval	N	N	Beecham	Anti–Infective
	BIOCRAFT 185	Ketoprofen	25mg	White/White	Cap	–	–	–	Biocraft	Anti–Inflammatory
	GG185	Glutethimide	500mg	White	Tab	Round	N	N	Geneva	Hypnotic
	MP 185	Metoprolol Tartrate	100mg	–	Tab	–	Y	N	Mutual	Antihypertensive
	Mylan 185/80	Propranolol HCl	80 mg	Yellow	Tab	Round	Y	N	Mylan	Antihypertensive
	Par/185	Perphenazine & Amitriptyline	4mg/50mg	Orange	Tab	Round	N	Y	Par	Antidepressant
	R 185	Dipyridamole	75mg	White	Tab	Round	N	Y	Purepac	Antiplatelet
	SP 185	Flurazepam Hydrochloride	30mg	Blue/Blue	Cap	–	–	–	Superpharm	Hypnotic
	West–ward 185	Chlorpropamide	250mg	Blue	Tab	Round	Y	N	West–ward	Hypoglycemic
186	186/QPL	Doxepin HCl	50mg	Ivory/Ivory	Cap	–	–	–	Quantum	Antidepressant
	555/186	Isosorbide Dinitrate	20mg	Green	Tab	Round	Y	N	Barr	Antianginal
	Beecham 186	Penicillin V Potassium	500mg	White	Tab	Oval	N	N	Beecham	Anti–Infective
	Hoyt 186	Sodium Fluoride	0.25mg	Beige	Tab	Round	N	N	Colgate	Mineral Supp.
	Mylan 186	Clonidine HCl	0.2mg	White	Tab	Round	Y	N	Mylan	Antihypertensive
	Par/186	Methyldopa & Hydrochlorothiazide	250mg/15mg	Green	Tab	Round	N	N	Par	Antihypertensive
	West–ward 186	Clonidine Hydrochloride	0.1mg	Yellow	Tab	Round	–	N	West–ward	Antihypertensive
187	187/Q	Doxepin HCl	75mg	Green/Green	Cap	–	–	–	Quantum	Antidepressant
	AT 187	Prazosin HCl	5mg	Blue	Cap	–	–	–	ATI	Antihypertensive
	BIOCRAFT 187	Ketoprofen	50mg	Blue/Blue	Cap	–	–	–	Biocraft	Anti–Inflammatory
	bp 187	Procainamide HCl SR	1000mg	Pink	Tab	Capsule	Y	Y	Bolar	Antiarrhythmic
	H 187	Prednisolone	5mg	Salmon	Tab	Round	N	N	Heather	Steroid
	P–D 187	Tetrachloroethylene	1.0ml	–	Cap	–	–	–	PD	Anthelmintic
	Par/187	Methyldopa & Hydrochlorothiazide	250mg/25mg	White	Tab	Capsule	N	N	Par	Antihypertensive
	West–ward 187	Clonidine Hydrochloride	0.2mg	White	Tab	Round	–	N	West–ward	Antihypertensive
188	555/188, barr	Quinidine Sulfate	200mg	White	Tab	Round	Y	N	Barr	Antiarrhythmic
	93 188	Sulfamethoxazole & Trimethoprim	400mg/80mg	White	Tab	Round	Y	N	Lemmon	Anti–Infective
	BMP 188	Hydrocodone Bitartrate & Acetaminophen	7.5mg/650mg	Pink	Tab	Oblong	Y	N	Beecham	Analgesic
	Copley 188	Procainamide HCl SR	500mg	Pink	Tab	Oval	–	Y	Copley	Antiarrhythmic
	P–D 188	Tetrachloroethylene	0.2ml	–	Cap	–	–	–	PD	Anthelmintic
	Par/188	Methyldopa & Hydrochlorothiazide	500mg/30mg	Yellow	Tab	Oval	N	N	Par	Antihypertensive
189	93 189	Sulfamethoxazole & Trimethoprim	800mg/160mg	White	Tab	Oval	Y	N	Lemmon	Anti–Infective
	BPM 189	Amoxicillin/Clavulanate Potassium Chewable	125mg/31.25mg	Yellow	Tab	Round	N	N	Beecham	Anti–infective
	Par/189	Methyldopa & Hydrochlorothiazide	500mg/50mg	Pink	Tab	Oval	N	N	Par	Antihypertensive
	SP 189	Propranolol HCl	10mg	Orange	Tab	Round	Y	N	Superpharm	Antihypertensive
190	AT 190	Fenoprofen Calcium	300mg	Yellow	Cap	–	–	–	ATI	Anti Inflammatory
	BPM 190	Amoxicillin/Clavulanate Potassium Chewable	250mg/62.5mg	Yellow	Tab	Round	N	N	Beecham	Anti–infective
	GG190	Methocarbamol	500mg	White	Tab	Round	Y	N	Geneva	Muscle Relaxant
	P–D 190	Tetrachloroethylene	5.0ml	–	Cap	–	–	–	PD	Anthelmintic
	Par/190	Diazepam	2mg	White	Tab	Round	Y	N	Par	Antianxiety
	SP 190	Propranolol HCl	20mg	Blue	Tab	Round	Y	N	Superpharm	Antihypertensive
191	GG 191	Amoxapine	100mg	–	Tab	Round	Y	N	Geneva	Antidepressant
	P–D 191	Tetrachloroethylene	0.5ml	–	Cap	–	–	–	PD	Anthelmintic

ID NO.	ID CODE	GENERIC NAME	STRENGTH	COLOR	FORM	SHAPE	SCORED	COATED	MFG.	USE
	Par/191	Diazepam	5mg	Yellow	Tab	Round	Y	N	Par	Antianxiety
	R 191	Diphenhydramine HCl	25mg	Pink/Clear	Cap	–	–	–	Purepac	Antihistamine
	SP 191	Propranolol HCl	40mg	Green	Tab	Round	Y	N	Superpharm	Antihypertensive
192	192–Q	Temazepam	15mg	Green/White	Cap	–	–	–	Quantum	Hypnotic
	555/192, barr	Hydrochlorothiazide HCl	100mg	Peach	Tab	Round	Y	N	Barr	Diuretic
	BIOCRAFT 192	Ketoprofen	75mg	Blue/White	Cap	–	–	–	Biocraft	Anti–Inflammatory
	BMP 192	Metoclopramide	10mg	Blue	Tab	Round	Y	N	Beecham	Antireflux
	Ciba 192	Hydrochlorothiazide	100mg	Blue	Tab	Round	Y	N	Ciba	Diuretic
	Copley 192	Prenatal Vitamins w/Zinc	n/a	Blue	Tab	Capsule	N	Y	Copley	Vitamin
	GG 192	Amoxapine	150mg	–	Tab	–	–	–	Geneva	Antidepressant
	N 192/300	Cimetidine	300mg	Green	Tab	Oval	N	Y	Novopharm	Anti–Ulcer
	Par/192	Diazepam	10mg	Blue	Tab	Round	Y	N	Par	Antianxiety
	R 192	Diphenhydramine HCl	50mg	Pink	Cap	–	–	–	Purepac	Antihistamine
	SP 192	Propranolol HCl	80mg	Yellow	Tab	Round	Y	N	Superpharm	Antihypertensive
	WPPh 192	Timolol Maleate	5mg	Blue	Tab	Round	–	N	West Point Pharma	Antihypertensive
193	193–Q	Temazepam	30mg	White	Cap	–	–	–	Quantum	Hypnotic
	H 193	Methocarbamol	500mg	White	Tab	Round	Y	N	Heather	Muscle Relaxant
	Par/193	Flurazepam HCl	15mg	Blue/White	Cap	–	–	–	Par	Hypnotic
	R 193	Dipyridamole	25mg	White	Tab	Round	N	Y	Purepac	Antiplatelet
	SQUIBB 193	Perphenazine & Amitriptyline HCl	2mg/10mg	–	Tab	–	–	–	Squibb	Antidepressant
194	Par/194	Flurazepam HCl	30mg	Blue	Cap	–	–	–	Par	Hypnotic
	QPL–194/Q	Haloperidol	0.5mg	White	Tab	Round	–	N	Quantum	Tranquilizer
	R 194	Doxycycline Hyclate	50mg	Blue/White	Cap	–	–	–	Purepac	Anti–Infective
	WPPh 194	Timolol Maleate	10mg	Blue	Tab	Round	–	N	West Point Pharma	Antihypertensive
195	GG195	Metronidazole	500mg	White	Tab	Oblong	Y	N	Geneva	Anti–Infective
	Mylan 195/250	Penicillin V Potassium	250mg	White	Tab	Round	Y	N	Mylan	Anti–Infective
	QPL–195/Q	Haloperidol	1mg	Yellow	Tab	Round	–	N	Quantum	Tranquilizer
	R 195	Doxycycline Hyclate	100mg	Blue	Cap	–	–	–	Purepac	Antibiotic
	SQUIBB 195	Tolazamide	100mg	–	Tab	–	–	–	Squibb	Hypoglycemic
	West–ward 195	Chloroquine Phosphate	250mg	White	Tab	Round	Y	N	West–ward	Antimalarial
	WPPh 195	Diflunisal	250 mg	Peach	Tab	Oblong	N	Y	West Point Pharma	Anti–inflammatory
196	barr, 555/196	Furosemide	80mg	White	Tab	Round	Y	N	Barr	Diuretic
	GG196	Chlorpheniramine Maleate	4mg	Yellow	Tab	Round	Y	N	Geneva	Antihistamine
	H 196	Methenamine Mandelate	500mg	Brown	Tab	Oblong	N	Y	Heather	Urinary Antiseptic
	QPL–196/Q	Haloperidol	2mg	Lavender	Tab	Round	–	N	Quantum	Tranquilizer
	WC 196	Theophylline Controlled Release	100mg	White/Clear	Cap	–	–	–	WC	Bronchodilator
	WPPh 196	Diflunisal	500 mg	Orange	Tab	Oblong	N	Y	West Point Pharma	Anti–inflammatory
197	832 G197	Chlorpropamide	250mg	Blue	Tab	Round	Y	N	PBI	Hypoglycemic
	Copley 197	Multivitamins/Fluoride + Iron	0.5mg	Pink	Tab	Square	–	N	Copley	Vitamin
	GG 197	Acetohexamide	250mg	White	Tab	Oval	Y	N	PBI	Antiglaucoma
	Mylan 197 / 100	Chlorpropamide	100mg	Green	Tab	Round	Y	N	Mylan	Hypoglycemic
	QPL–197/Q	Haloperidol	5mg	Green	Tab	Round	–	N	Quantum	Tranquilizer
	WC 197	Theophylline Controlled Release	125mg	Clear/Clear	Cap	–	–	–	WC	Bronchodilator
198	832/G198	Chlorpropamide	100mg	Blue	Tab	Round	Y	N	PBI	Hypoglycemic
	Barr/198,3	Acetaminophen with Codeine	300mg/30mg	White	Tab	Round	Y	N	Barr	Analgesic
	GG 198	Acetohexamide.	500mg	White	Tab	Capsule	Y	N	PBI	Antiglaucoma
	Mylan 198/500	Penicillin V Potassium	500mg	White	Tab	Oval	N	N	Mylan	Anti–Infective
	WC 198	Theophylline Controlled Release	200mg	White/Clear	Cap	–	–	–	WC	Bronchodilator
199	GG 199	Acetaminophen	325mg	White	Tab	Round	Y	N	Geneva	Analgesic
	Mylan 199	Clonidine HCl	0:3mg	White	Tab	Round	Y	N	Mylan	Antihypertensive
200	WC 199	Theophylline Controlled Release	300mg	White/Clear	Cap	–	–	–	WC	Bronchodilator
	200 ZPP	Phenylpropanolamine HCl / Caramiphen Edisylate	75mg/40mg	Clear/White	Cap	–	–	–	Pioneer	Antitussive Comb.
	3M/SR 200	Theophylline SR	200mg	White	Tab	Round	Y	N	3M	Bronchodilator
	555/200	Diphenoxylate HCl with Atropine Sulfate	2.5mg/0.025mg	White	Tab	Round	N	N	Barr	Antidiarrheal
	832/200	Chlorpromazine	200mg	Tan	Tab	Round	N	Y	PBI	Tranquilizer
	A 200	Ibuprofen	200mg	White	Tab	Oblong	N	Y	Sterling	Analgesic
	Adria/200	Pancrelipase,Lipase,Protease NLT,Amylase NLT	400mg	Beige	Tab	Round	N	N	Adria	Digestant
	b 200	Ibuprofen	200mg	White	Tab	Round	N	Y	Barr	Anti–Inflammatory
	Breon 200	Theophylline Anhydrous	200mg	Green/White	Cap	–	–	–	Winthrop	Bronchodilator
	Breon 200	Guaifenesin	200mg	Red	Cap	–	–	Y	Winthrop	Expectorant
	BREON T 200	Chlormezanone	200mg	Green	Tab	Capsule	Y	N	Winthrop	Antianxiety
	dp 200	Levothyroxine Sodium	0.2mg	Pink	Tab	Oval	Y	N	Daniels	Hormone
	Flint 200	Levothyroxine Sodium	200mcg	Pink	Tab	Round	Y	N	Boots	Hormone
	Forest 200	Theophylline SR	200mg	White	Tab	Capsule	–	N	Forest	Bronchodilator
	GG200	Propoxyphene Napsylate and Acetaminophen	100mg/650mg	Pink	Tab	Capsule	N	Y	Bolar	Analgesic
	Horner 200mg	Ibuprofen	200mg	White	Cap	–	–	–	Horner	Anti–Inflammatory
	M 200	Levothyroxine Sodium	0.2mg	Pink	Tab	Round	Y	N	Duramed	Hormone
	M 200 LEVO T	Levothyroxine Sodium	0.2mg	Pink	Tab	Round	Y	N	Mova	Hormone
	P–D 200	Oxytriphylline & Guaifenesin	200mg/100mg	Salmon	Tab	Round	N	N	PD	Bronchodilator
	PD 200	Oxtriphylline & Guaifenesin	–	Salmon	Tab	Round	N	Y	PD	Bronchodilator
	PF U200	Theophylline	200mg	White	Tab	Round	Y	N	PF	Bronchodilator
	West–ward 200	Chlorpheniramine Maleate	4mg	Yellow	Tab	Round	Y	N	West–ward	Antihistamine
	WHR 200	Theophylline	200mg	White/Clear	Cap	–	–	–	Rorer	Bronchodilator
	Wyeth 200	Promazine	100mg	Pink	Tab	Round	N	Y	Wyeth	Tranquilizer
201	AT 201/2	Acetaminophen & Codeine Phosphate	300mg/15mg	White	Tab	Round	N	N	ATI	Analgesic
	CL 201	Furosemide	40mg	White	Tab	Round	Y	N	Geneva	Diuretic
	GG201	Furosemide	40mg	White	Tab	Round	Y	N	Geneva	Diuretic
	INV 201	Procainamide HCl SR	500mg	Pink	Tab	Oval	N	Y	Duramed	Antiarrhythmic
	SEARLE 201	Spironolactone with Hydrochlorothiazide	25mg/25mg	White	Tab	Round	Y	N	Searle	Diuretic
	U 201	Hydrocodone Bitartrate & Acetaminophen	7.5mg/650mg	White	Tab	Capsule	–	N	UAD	Analgesic
	U 201	Hydrocodone Bitartrate & Acetaminophen	7.5mg/650mg	White	Tab	Capsule	–	N	UAD	Analgesic
202	West–ward 201	Colchicine	0.6mg	White	Tab	Round	N	N	West–ward	Antigout
	AT 202/3	Acetaminophen & Codeine Phosphate	300mg/30mg	White	Tab	Round	N	N	ATI	Analgesic
	H 202	Sulfisoxazole	500mg	White	Tab	Round	Y	N	Heather	Anti–Infective
	HAUCK 202 & BESTA	Vitamin Combination	n/a	Orange/Orange	Cap	–	–	–	W.E.Hauck	Vitamin
	KU 202	Belladona Extract & Phenobarbital	15mg/15mg	Gray	Tab	Round	N	N	K–U	Antispasmodic
	P–D 202	Procainamide HCl SR	250mg	Green	Tab	Oval	N	Y	PD	Antiarrhythmic
	Par/202	Methyldopa & Chlorothiazide	250mg/150mg	Beige	Tab	Round	N	Y	Par	Antihypertensive
	SQUIBB 202	Dicloxacillin Sodium	250mg	–	Cap	–	–	–	Squibb	Anti–Infective
	West–ward 202	Cortisone Acetate	25mg	White	Tab	Round	Y	N	West–ward	Steroid
203	203, b	Amitriptyline HCl	25mg	Green	Tab	Round	N	Y	Barr	Antidepressant
	832/G203	Chlorthalidone	25mg	Orange	Tab	Round	N	N	PBI	Diuretic
	AT 203/4	Acetaminophen & Codeine Phosphate	300mg/60mg	White	Tab	Round	N	N	ATI	Analgesic
	H 203	Tetracycline HCl	500mg	Black/Yellow	Cap	–	–	–	Heather	Anti–Infective
	Par/203	Methyldopa & Chlorothiazide	250mg/250mg	Green	Tab	Round	N	Y	Par	Antihypertensive

ID NO.	ID CODE	GENERIC NAME	STRENGTH	COLOR	FORM	SHAPE	SCORED	COATED	MFG.	USE
	SQUIBB 203	Dicloxacillin Sodium	500mg	–	Cap	–	–	–	Squibb	Anti–Infective
204	832/G204	Chlorthalidone	50mg	Blue	Tab	Round	N	N	PBI	Diuretic
	Mylan 204	Amoxicillin	250mg	Buff/Caramel	Cap	–	–	–	Mylan	Anti–Infective
	N 204/400	Cimetidine	400mg	Green	Tab	Oval	N	Y	Novopharm	Anti–Ulcer
	P–D 204	Procainamide HCl SR	500mg	Yellow	Tab	Oval	Y	Y	PD	Antiarrhythmic
	R 204	Erythromycin Stearate	250mg	Pink	Tab	Round	N	Y	Purepac	Anti–Infective
	T 204	Colchicine	0.6mg	White	Tab	Round	N	N	Trinity	Antigout
205	INV 205	Methyldopa & Hydrochlorothiazide	250mg/15mg	White	Tab	Round	N	Y	Duramed	Antihypertensive
	LEMMON 93 205	Phenobarbital/Hyoscyamine/Atropine/Scopolamine	–	Pink	Tab	Round	Y	N	Lemmon	Antispasmodic
	Mylan 205	Amoxicillin	500mg	Buff/Buff	Cap	–	–	–	Mylan	Anti–Infective
	P–D 205	Procainamide HCl SR	750mg	Orange	Tab	Oval	Y	Y	PD	Antiarrhythmic
	SEARLE 205	Spironolactone	25mg	White	Tab	Round	Y	N	Searle	Diuretic
	West–ward 205	Chlorpromazine Hydrochloride	25mg	Butterscotch	Tab	Round	N	Y	West–ward	Tranquilizer
206	Copley 206	Amitriptyline HCl	10mg	Blue	Tab	Round	N	Y	Copley	Antidepressant
	INV 206	Methyldopa & Hydrochlorothiazide	250mg/25mg	White	Tab	Round	N	Y	Duramed	Antihypertensive
	Par/206	Lorazepam	0.5mg	White	Tab	Round	Y	N	Par	Antianxiety
207	BMP 207	Hydrocodone Bitartrate & Acetaminophen	5mg/500mg	White	Tab	Round	Y	N	Beecham	Analgesic
	Copley 207	Amitriptyline HCl	25mg	Yellow	Tab	Round	N	Y	Copley	Antidepressant
	INV 207	Metoclopramide	10mg	White	Tab	Round	Y	N	Duramed	Antireflux
	P–D 207	Procainamide HCl SR	1000mg	Red	Tab	Oblong	Y	Y	PD	Antiarrhythmic
	Par/207	Lorazepam	1.0mg	White	Tab	Round	Y	N	Par	Antianxiety
	PPP 207	Nadolol	40mg	Blue	Tab	Round	Y	N	Bristol	Antihypertensive
	QPL–207	Oxazepam	30mg	Green/Yellow	Cap	–	–	–	Quantum	Antianxiety
	SQUIBB 207	Nadolol	40mg	Blue	Tab	Round	Y	N	Princeton	Antihypertensive
	West–ward 207	Chlorpromazine Hydrochloride	50mg	Butterscotch	Tab	Round	N	Y	West–ward	Tranquilizer
208	Copley 208	Amitriptyline HCl	50mg	Beige	Tab	Round	N	Y	Copley	Antidepressant
	INV 208	Benztropine Mesylate	0.5mg	White	Tab	Round	Y	N	Invamed	Antiparkinson
	INV 208	Benztropine Mesylate	0.5mg	White	Tab	Round	Y	N	Par	Antiparkinson
	Mylan 208/20	Furosemide	20mg	White	Tab	Round	N	N	Mylan	Diuretic
	Par/208	Lorazepam	2.0mg	White	Tab	Round	Y	N	Par	Antianxiety
	PPP 208	Nadolol	120mg	Blue	Tab	Oblong	Y	N	Bristol	Antihypertensive
	QPL–208	Oxazepam	15mg	Green/White	Cap	–	–	–	Quantum	Antianxiety
	SQUIBB 208	Nadolol	120mg	Blue	Tab	Oblong	Y	N	Princeton	Antihypertensive
209	209, b	Amitriptyline HCl	10mg	Pink	Tab	Round	N	Y	Barr	Antidepressant
	COPLEY 209	Amitriptyline Hydrochloride	75mg	Orange	Tab	Round	N	Y	Copley	Antidepressant
	INV 209	Benztropine Mesylate	1mg	White	Tab	Oval	Y	N	Invamed	Antiparkinson
	INV 209	Benztropine Mesylate	1mg	White	Tab	Oval	Y	N	Par	Antiparkinson
	QPL–209	Oxazepam	10mg	Green/Black	Cap	–	–	–	Quantum	Antianxiety
	West–ward 209	Chlorothiazide	250mg	White	Tab	Round	Y	N	West–ward	Diuretic
210	12 210	D–Alpha Tocopheryl Acetate	100 Units	Yellow	Cap	–	–	–	Adria	Vitamin
	210/40	Furosemide	40mg	White	Tab	Round	Y	N	Martec	Diuretic
	54/210	Methadone HCl	5mg	White	Tab	Round	Y	N	Roxane	Analgesic
	555/210	Amitriptyline HCl	50mg	Brown	Tab	Round	N	Y	Barr	Antidepressant
	BMP 210	Phenylephrine/Guaifenesin/DM/Acetaminophen	10/100/15/300mg	White	Tab	Oblong	N	N	Beecham	Decongestant Comb.
	COPLEY 210	Amitriptyline Hydrochloride	100mg	Pink	Tab	Round	N	Y	Copley	Antidepressant
	INV 210	Benztropine Mesylate	2mg	White	Tab	Round	Y	N	Invamed	Antiparkinson
	INV 210	Benztropine Mesylate	2mg	White	Tab	Round	Y	N	Par	Antiparkinson
	MCG 210	Phenylpropanolamine/Chlorpheniramine SR	75mg/8mg	–	Cap	–	–	–	McGregor	Decongestant Comb.
	Mylan 210 / 250	Chlorpropamide	250mg	Green	Tab	Round	N	N	Mylan	Hypoglycemic
	P–D 210	Oxtriphylline	100mg	Red	Tab	Round	N	Y	PD	Bronchodilator
	R 210	Folic Acid	1mg	Yellow	Tab	Round	–	–	Purepac	Antianemic
	SEARLE 210	Spironolactone	100mg	White	Tab	Round	Y	N	Searle	Diuretic
	West–ward 210	Chlorothiazide	500mg	White	Tab	Round	Y	N	West–ward	Diuretic
	West–ward 210	Oxytetracycline Hydrochloride	250mg	Yellow/Yellow	Cap	–	–	–	West–ward	Anti–Infective
211	555/211	Amitriptyline HCl	75mg	Purple	Tab	Round	N	Y	Barr	Antidepressant
	AT 211	Theralins RX	n/a	White	Tab	Oval	N	Y	ATI	Prenatal Vitamin
	bp 211	Maprotiline HCL	25mg	Blue	Tab	Round	Y	Y	Bolar	Antidepressant
	COPLEY 211	Amitriptyline Hydrochloride	150mg	Blue	Tab	Capsule	N	Y	Copley	Antidepressant
	INV 211	Amantadine	100mg	Red	Cap	Capsule	–	–	Duramed	Antiviral
	MCG 211	Phenylpropanolamine/Chlorpheniramine SR	75mg/12mg	–	Cap	–	–	–	McGregor	Decongestant Comb.
	Mylan 211	Chlordiazepoxide/Amitriptyline HCl	5mg/12.5mg	Green	Tab	Round	N	Y	Mylan	Antidepressant
	Ortho 211	Griseofulvin Microsize	250mg	White	Tab	Round	Y	N	Ortho	Antifungal
	P–D 211	Oxtriphylline	200mg	Yellow	Tab	Round	N	Y	PD	Bronchodilator
	SQUIBB 211	Cloxacillin Sodium	250mg	–	Cap	–	–	–	Squibb	Anti–Infective
212	10 78–212	Metaproterenol	10mg	White	Tab	Round	Y	N	Sandoz	Bronchodilator
	54–212	Neomycin Sulfate	500mg	White	Tab	Round	–	–	Roxane	Anti–Infective
	555/212	Amitriptyline HCl	100mg	Red/Orange	Tab	Round	N	Y	Barr	Antidepressant
	bp 212	Maprotiline HCL	50mg	Yellow	Tab	Round	Y	Y	Bolar	Antidepressant
	ETHEX 212	Prenatal Vitamin	–	White	Tab	Oval	N	Y	Ethex	Vitamin
	PP–212	Butabarbital Sodium	30mg	Blue	Tab	Round	Y	N	Eon	Sedative
	QPL 212	Meprobamate & Aspirin	200mg/325mg	Green/Yellow	Tab	Round	N	N	Quantum	Analgesic
	R 212	Hydrocortisone	10mg	White	Tab	Round	Y	N	Purepac	Steroid
	R/212	Hydrocortisone	10mg	White	Tab	Round	Y	N	Rondex	Steroid
	SQUIBB 212	Cloxacillin Sodium	500mg	–	Cap	–	–	–	Squibb	Anti–Infective
213	20 78–213	Metaproterenol	20mg	White	Tab	Round	Y	N	Sandoz	Bronchodilator
	213	Acetaminophen	500mg	White	Tab	Round	N	N	Granutec	Analgesic
	54 213	Lithium Carbonate	150mg	Opaque	Cap	–	–	–	Roxane	Tranquilizer
	93 213	Tolmetin Sodium	400mg	Blue	Cap	–	–	–	Lemmon	Anti–Inflammatory
	bp 213	Maprotiline HCL	75mg	White	Tab	Round	Y	Y	Bolar	Antidepressant
	GG 213	Perphenazine & Amitriptyline	2mg/10mg	Blue	Tab	Round	N	Y	Geneva	Antidepressant
	Mylan 213/50	Chlorthalidone	50mg	Green	Tab	Round	Y	N	Mylan	Antihypertensive
	Par/213	Orphenadrine, Aspirin, Caffeine	25mg/325mg/30mg	White/Green	Tab	Round	N	N	Par	Muscle Relaxant
	QPL/213 Q	Trazodone HCl	50mg	White	Tab	Round	Y	N	Quantum	Antidepressant
214	Barr 214	Chlordiazepoxide HCl with Clidinum Bromide	5mg/2.5mg	Green/White	Cap	–	–	–	Barr	Antispasmodic
	GG 214	Perphenazine & Amitriptyline	2mg/25mg	Orange	Tab	Round	N	Y	Geneva	Antidepressant
	H 214	Tetracycline HCl	250mg	Blue/Yellow	Cap	–	–	–	Heather	Anti–Infective
	H 214	Tetracycline HCl	250mg	Orange/Yellow	Cap	–	–	–	Heather	Anti–Infective
	H 214	Tetracycline HCl	250mg	Orange/Yellow	Cap	–	–	–	Heather	Anti–Infective
	Mylan 214	Haloperidol	2mg	Orange	Tab	Round	Y	N	Mylan	Tranquilizer
	Ortho 214	Griseofulvin Microsize	500mg	White	Tab	Round	Y	N	Ortho	Antifungal
	Par/214	Orphenadrine, Aspirin, Caffeine	50mg/770mg/60mg	White/Green	Tab	Capsule	N	N	Par	Muscle Relaxant
	PD 214	Oxtriphylline	400mg	Pink	Tab	Round	N	Y	PD	Bronchodilator
	QPL/214 Q	Trazodone HCl	100mg	White	Tab	Round	Y	N	Quantum	Antidepressant
	R 214	Hydrocortisone	20mg	White	Tab	Round	Y	N	Purepac	Steroid
	R/214	Hydrocortisone	20mg	White	Tab	Round	Y	N	Rondex	Steroid

ID NO.	ID CODE	GENERIC NAME	STRENGTH	COLOR	FORM	SHAPE	SCORED	COATED	MFG.	USE
215	215/Q	Meclofenamate Sodium	50mg	Ivory	Cap	–	–	–	Quantum	Anti–Inflammatory
	ALRA 215	Ibuprofen	200mg	Orange	Tab	Round	N	Y	Alra	Anti–Inflammatory
	GG 215	Perphenazine & Amitriptyline	4mg/10mg	Salmon	Tab	Round	N	Y	Geneva	Antidepressant
	MCG 215	Phenylpropanolamine SR	75mg	–	Cap	–	–	–	McGregor	Decongestant
	Mylan 215	Tolbutamide	500mg	White	Tab	Round	Y	N	Mylan	Hypoglycemic
216	216/Q	Meclofenamate Sodium	100mg	Yellow	Cap	–	–	–	Quantum	Anti–Inflammatory
	GG 216	Perphenazine & Amitriptyline	4mg/25mg	Yellow	Tab	Round	N	Y	Geneva	Antidepressant
	Mylan 216/40	Furosemide	40mg	White	Tab	Round	Y	N	Mylan	Diuretic
	Par/216 800	Ibuprofen	800mg	White	Tab	Capsule	N	Y	Par	Anti–Inflammatory
217	Adria 217	Phenolphthalein	130mg	Red	Tab	Round	N	Y	Adria	Laxative
	Barr/217,2	Acetaminophen with Codeine	300mg/15mg	White	Tab	Round	N	N	Barr	Analgesic
	GG 217	Perphenazine & Amitriptyline	4mg/50mg	Orange	Tab	Round	N	Y	Geneva	Antidepressant
	Mylan 217 / 250	Tolazamide	250mg	White	Tab	Round	Y	N	Mylan	Hypoglycemic
	Par 217	Doxepin HCl	10mg	Buff/Buff	Cap	–	–	–	Par	Antidepressant
	QPL 217/Q	Metoclopramide	10mg	White	Tab	Round	Y	N	Quantum	Antireflux
218	West–ward 217	Reserpine and Chlorothiazide	0.125mg/250mg	Pink	Tab	Round	Y	N	West–ward	Antihypertensive
	218, barr	Ergoloid Mesylates Sublingual	0.5mg	White	Tab	Round	N	N	Barr	Vasodilator
	93 218	Phenobarbital	30mg	White	Tab	Round	Y	N	Lemmon	Sedative
	GG218/2	Acetaminophen & Codeine	300mg/15mg	White	Tab	Round	N	N	KV	Analgesic
	Par 218	Doxepin HCl	25mg	White/Ivory	Cap	–	–	–	Par	Antidepressant
219	West–ward 218	Reserpine and Chlorothiazide	0.125mg/500mg	Pink	Tab	Round	Y	N	West–ward	Antihypertensive
	barr 219	Erythromycin Stearate	500mg	Pink	Tab	Capsule	N	Y	Barr	Anti–Infective
	GG219	Methyldopa & Hydrochlorothiazide	250mg/15mg	Green	Tab	Round	N	Y	Geneva	Antihypertensive
	MCG 219	Phenylpropanolamine/Chlorpheniramine/Methscop.	75mg/8mg/2.5mg	–	Cap	–	–	–	McGregor	Decongestant Comb.
	Par 219	Doxepin HCl	50mg	Ivory/Ivory	Cap	–	–	–	Par	Antidepressant
220	R 219	Hydralazine Hydrochloride	25mg	Green	Tab	Round	N	Y	Purepac	Antihypertensive
	832/G220C	Clorazepate Dipotassium	3.75mg	White	Cap	–	–	–	PBI	Antianxiety
	GG220	Propoxyphene Napsylate & Acetaminophen	100mg/650mg.	Pink	Tab	Capsule	–	Y	Bolar	Analgesic
	GG220/3	Acetaminophen & Codeine	300mg/30mg	White	Tab	Round	Y	N	Geneva	Analgesic
	INV 220	Aspirin Delayed Release (E.C.)	15gr.	Yellow	Tab	Round	N	Y	Duramed	Analgesic
	Par 220	Doxepin HCl	75mg	Green/Green	Cap	–	–	–	Par	Antidepressant
	PP–220	Urinary Antiseptic #2	–	Blue	Tab	Round	N	Y	Eon	Urinary Antiseptic
	QPL–220/Q	Triamterene & Hydrochlorothiazide	75mg/50mg	Yellow	Tab	Round	–	–	Quantum	Diuretic
	R 220	Hydralazine Hydrochloride	50mg	Green	Tab	Round	N	Y	Purepac	Antihypertensive
	STUART 220	Belladonna Alkaloids & Phenobarbital	n/a	White	Tab	Oval	Y	N	Stuart	Antispasmodic
221	West–ward 220	Diazepam	2mg	White	Tab	Round	Y	N	West–ward	Antianxiety
	3M/221	Orphenadrine HCl SA	100mg	White	Tab	Round	N	N	3M	Muscle Relaxant
	832/G221C	Clorazepate Dipotassium	7.5mg	White	Cap	–	–	–	PBI	Antianxiety
	M 221	Timolol	10mg	Green	Tab	Round	Y	Y	Mylan	Antihypertensive
	P–D 221	Oxtriphylline	600mg	Salmon	Tab	Oval	Y	Y	PD	Bronchodilator
	Par 221	Doxepin HCl	100mg	White/Green	Cap	–	–	–	Par	Antidepressant
	R 221	Hydrochlorothiazide	25mg	Peach	Tab	Round	Y	N	Purepac	Diuretic
	SCS 221	Norethindrone/Ethinyl Estradiol	1mg/35mcg	White	Tab	Round	–	N	Searle	Contraceptive
	SEARLE 221	Norethindrone/Ethinyl Estradiol	1mg/35mcg	White	Tab	Round	–	N	Searle	Contraceptive
222	832/G222C	Clorazepate Dipotassium	15mg	White	Cap	–	–	–	PBI	Antianxiety
	B/L 222	Amoxicillin Chewable	250mg	White	Tab	Capsule	Y	N	Biocraft	Anti–Infective
	Mylan 222 / 25	Chlorthalidone	25mg	Yellow	Tab	Round	N	N	Mylan	Antihypertensive
	Par 222	Doxepin HCl	150mg	White/Blue	Cap	–	–	–	Par	Antidepressant
	R 222	Hydrochlorothiazide	50mg	Peach	Tab	Round	Y	N	Purepac	Diuretic
223	West–ward 222	Diazepam	5mg	Yellow	Tab	Round	Y	N	West–ward	Antianxiety
	54–223	Diphenhydramine HCl	50mg	–	Cap	–	–	–	Roxane	Antihistamine
	dp 223	Aminophylline	100mg	White	Tab	Round	Y	N	Duramed	Brochodilator
	INV 223	Ibuprofen	400mg	White	Tab	Round	N	Y	Duramed	Anti–Inflammatory
	Par/223	Haloperidol	0.5mg	White	Tab	Round	Y	N	Par	Tranquilizer
224	224 / 2.5	Minoxidil	2.5mg	White	Tab	Round	–	N	Royce	Antihypertensive
	dp 224	Aminophylline	200mg	White	Tab	Round	Y	N	Duramed	Bronchodilator
	GG 224	Phenylpropanolamine HCl & Guaifenesin LA	75mg/400mg	White	Tab	Oblonge	Y	N	Amide	Decongestant Comb.
	GG224	Phenylpropanolamine HCl / Guaifenesin	75mg/400mg	White	Tab	Capsule	Y	N	Amide	Decongestant Comb.
	INV 224	Ibuprofen	600mg	White	Tab	Oval	N	Y	Duramed	Anti–Inflammatory
	Par/224	Haloperidol	1mg	Yellow	Tab	Round	Y	N	Par	Tranquilizer
225	225 / 10	Minoxidil	10mg	White	Tab	Round	–	N	Royce	Antihypertensive
	Copley 225	Potassium Chloride SA	600mg (8mEq)	Dark Peach	Tab	Round	N	Y	Copley	Potassium Supp.
	dp 225	Haloperidol	0.5mg	White	Tab	Round	Y	N	Duramed	Tranquilizer
	GG225	Promethazine	25mg	White	Tab	Round	N	N	Geneva	Antiemetic
	INV 225	Ibuprofen	800mg	White	Tab	Capsule	N	Y	Duramed	Anti–Inflammatory
	Par/225	Haloperidol	2mg	Pink	Tab	Round	Y	N	Par	Tranquilizer
	QPL–225 Q	Clorazepate Dipotassium	3.75mg	Blue	Tab	Round	–	–	Quantum	Antianxiety
	West–ward 225	Diazepam	10mg	Blue	Tab	Round	Y	N	West–ward	Antianxiety
226	dp 226	Haloperidol	1mg	Yellow	Tab	Round	Y	N	Duramed	Tranquilizer
	Par/226	Haloperidol	5mg	Green	Tab	Round	Y	N	Par	Tranquilizer
	PP–226	Chlorzoxazone & Acetaminophen	250mg/300mg	Green	Tab	Round	N	N	Eon	Muscle Relaxant
	QPL–226 Q	Clorazepate Dipotassium	7.5mg	Peach	Tab	Round	–	–	Quantum	Antianxiety
227	227, 555	Ergoloid Mesylates Sublingual	1mg	White	Tab	Oval	N	N	Barr	Vasodilator
	Bolar 227	Triamterene & Hydrochlorothiazide	50mg/25mg	Maroon	Cap	–	–	–	Bolar	Diuretic
	CC 227	Thyroid	3gr.	Tan	Tab	Round	N	N	Camall	Hormone
	dp 227	Haloperidol	2mg	Lavender	Tab	Round	Y	N	Duramed	Tranquilizer
	GG 227	Isosorbide Dinitrate	20mg	Green	Tab	Round	Y	N	Geneva	Antianginal
	INV 227	Metoclopramide	5mg	White	Tab	Round	N	N	Duramed	Antireflux
	Par/227	Haloperidol	10mg	Aqua	Tab	Round	Y	N	Par	Tranquilizer
	QPL–227 Q	Clorazepate Dipotassium	15mg	Lavender	Tab	Round	–	–	Quantum	Antianxiety
	R 227	Hydrochlorothiazide, Reserpine, Hydralazine	15mg/0.1mg/25mg	Salmon	Tab	Round	–	N	Rondex	Antihypertensive
	West–ward 227	Prazosin HCl	1mg	White	Cap	–	–	–	West–ward	Antihypertensive
	Wyeth 227	Promethazine	50mg	Pink	Tab	Round	Y	N	Wyeth	Antiemetic
228	228/QPL/10	Minoxidil	10mg	White	Tab	Round	Y	N	Quantum	Antihypertensive
	dp 228	Haloperidol	5mg	Green	Tab	Round	Y	N	Duramed	Tranquilizer
	Par/228	Haloperidol	20mg	Salmon	Tab	Round	Y	N	Par	Tranquilizer
	Sch. Logo 228	Griseofulvin Ultramicrosize	125mg	White	Tab	Round	Y	N	Schering	Antifungal
	West–ward 228	Prazosin HCl	2mg	Pink	Cap	–	–	–	West–ward	Antihypertensive
229	229/0.5	Haloperidol	0.5mg	White	Tab	Round	N	N	Royce	Tranquilizer
	Barr/229,4	Acetaminophen with Codeine	300mg/60mg	White	Tab	Round	N	N	Barr	Analgesic
	dp 229	Haloperidol	10mg	Aqua	Tab	Round	Y	U	Duramed	Tranquilizer
	GG229	Isosorbide Dinitrate ER	40mg	Yellow	Tab	Round	Y	N	Geneva	Antianginal
	West–ward 229	Prazosin HCl	5mg	Blue	Cap	–	–	–	West–ward	Antihypertensive
230	230/1	Haloperidol	1mg	Yellow	Tab	Round	N	N	Royce	Tranquilizer
	Adria/230	Metoclopramide	10mg	Yellow	Tab	Octagonal	Y	N	Adria	Antireflux

ID NO.	ID CODE	GENERIC NAME	STRENGTH	COLOR	FORM	SHAPE	SCORED	COATED	MFG.	USE
	barr, 230	Erythromycin Estolate	250mg	Orange/Buff	Cap	–	–	–	Barr	Anti–Infective
	dp 230	Haloperidol	20mg	Salmon	Tab	Round	N	N	Duramed	Tranquilizer
	E 230	Urinary Antiseptic #2	–	Blue	Tab	Round	N	Y	Eon	Urinary Antiseptic
	PD 230	Phenobarbital,Theophylline,Ephedrine	8mg/130mg/24mg	White	Tab	Round	Y	N	PD	Bronchodilator
	SQUIBB 230	Amoxicillin	250mg	Green	Cap	–	–	–	Squibb	Anti–Infective
231	231/2	Haloperidol	2mg	Purple	Tab	Round	N	N	Royce	Tranquilizer
	Adria/231	Dexpanthenol, Choline Bitartrate	50mg/25mg	White	Tab	Round	N	N	Adria	Antiflatulent
	Copley 231	Choline Magnesium Trisalicylate	500mg	Peach	Tab	Capsule	–	–	Copley	Antiarthritic
	M 231	Atenolol	50mg	White	Tab	Round	Y	N	Mylan	Antihypertensive
	P–D 231	Theophylline/Ephedrine/Phenobarbital SA	180/48/25mg	Coral/White	Tab	Round	–	N	PD	Antiasthmatic
	Sch. Logo 231	Dexbrompheniramine Maleate & Pseudoephedrine Sulf	6mg/120mg	Red	Tab	Round	N	Y	Schering	Decongestant Comb.
	SQUIBB 231	Amoxicillin	500mg	Green/Lt.Green	Cap	–	–	–	Squibb	Anti–Infective
232	232/5	Haloperidol	5mg	Green	Tab	Round	N	N	Royce	Tranquilizer
	232/80	Furosemide	80mg	White	Tab	Round	Y	N	Martec	Diuretic
	CC 232	Phentermine HCl	37.5mg	Yellow	Tab	Oblong	Y	N	Camall	Anorectic
	CC 232	Phentermine HCl	37.5mg	White/Blue Specks	Tab	Oblong	Y	N	Camall	Anorectic
	CC 232	Phentermine HCl	37.5mg	Green Speckled	Tab	–	–	–	Camall	Anorectic
	GG 232	Hydrocodone/APAP	5mg/500mg	White	Tab	Capsule	Y	N	PBI	Analgesic
	INV 232	Aspirin SR	800mg	White	Tab	Capsule	N	Y	Duramed	Analgesic
	Mylan 232/80	Furosemide	80mg	White	Tab	Round	Y	N	Mylan	Diuretic
	PPP 232	Nadolol	20mg	Blue	Tab	Round	Y	N	Bristol	Antihypertensive
	SQUIBB 232	Nadolol	20mg	Blue	Tab	Round	Y	N	Princeton	Antihypertensive
233	233/10	Haloperidol	10mg	Green–Blue	Tab	Round	N	N	Royce	Tranquilizer
	555/233	Prednisone	10mg	White	Tab	Round	Y	N	Barr	Steroid
	Copley 233	Choline Magnesium Trisalicylate	750mg	White	Tab	Capsule	–	–	Copley	Antiarthritic
234	234/20	Haloperidol	20mg	Salmon	Tab	Round	N	N	Royce	Tranquilizer
	GG234	Methylprednisolone	4mg	White	Tab	Oval	Y	N	Duramed	Steroid
	INV 234	Triotann	–	Buff	Tab	Capsule	Y	N	Duramed	Decongestant comb.
235	GG235	Promethazine	50mg	Pink	Tab	Round	N	N	Geneva	Antiemetic
	N 235/800	Cimetidine	800mg	Green	Tab	Oval	N	Y	Novopharm	Anti–Ulcer
	West–ward 235	Propoxyphene Hydrochloride	65mg	Pink/Pink	Cap	–	–	–	West–ward	Analgesic
236	CC 236	Cyproheptadine HCl	4mg	White	Tab	Round	Y	N	Camall	Antipruritic
	GG 236	Sulindac	150mg	Yellow	Tab	Round	Y	N	Geneva	Anti–Inflammatory
	QPL–236/Q	Fenoprofen Calcium	200mg	Lavender/Flesh	Cap	–	–	–	Quantum	Anti–Inflammatory
	SL 236	Pseudoephedrine HCl	300mg	Red	Tab	Round	N	Y	Sidmak	Decongestant
237	b, 237	Perphenazine & Amitriptyline	2mg/25mg	Pink	Tab	Triangle	N	Y	Barr	Antidepressant
	G 237	Chloral Hydrate	500mg	Green	Cap	–	–	–	R. P. Scherer	Hypnotic
	GG 237	Sulindac	200mg	Yellow	Tab	Round	Y	N	Geneva	Anti–Inflammatory
	P–D 237	Ethosuximide	250mg	Orange	Cap	–	–	–	PD	Anticonvulsant
	Par/237	Leucovorin Calcium	5mg	Off White	Tab	Round	Y	N	Par	Antineoplastic
	QPL–237/Q	Fenoprofen Calcium	300mg	Orange/Flesh	Cap	–	–	–	Quantum	Anti–Inflammatory
238	b, 238	Perphenazine & Amitriptyline	4mg/25mg	Lt.Green	Tab	Round	N	Y	Barr	Antidepressant
	GG 238	Glyburide	1.25mg	White	Tab	Round	Y	N	Greenstone	Hypoglycemic
	Par/238	Leucovorin Calcium	25mg	Green	Tab	Round	Y	N	Par	Antineoplastic
	QPL–238/Q	Fenoprofen Calcium	600mg	Peach	Tab	–	–	Y	Quantum	Anti–Inflammatory
239	GG 239	Glyburide	2.5mg	Pink	Tab	Round	Y	N	Greenstone	Hypoglycemic
	Par/239	Propranolol HCl	90mg	Lavender	Tab	Round	Y	N	Par	Antihypertensive
	Royce logo 239	Chlorzoxazone	500mg	Green	Tab	Capsule	Y	N	Royce	Muscle relaxant
	SQUIBB 239	Cephalexin	500mg	–	Cap	–	–	–	Squibb	Anti–Infective
	West–ward 239	Dimenhydrinate	50mg	White	Tab	Round	Y	N	West–ward	Antiemetic
240	GG 240	Glyburide	5mg	Blue	Tab	Round	Y	N	Greenstone	Hypoglycemic
	Par/240	Temazepam	15mg	White/Green	Cap	–	–	–	Par	Hypnotic
	Royce logo 240 / 0.5	Lorazepam	0.5mg	White	Tab	Round	N	N	Royce	Antianxiety
	WPPh 240	Chlorothiazide	250mg	White	Tab	Round	–	N	West Point Pharma	Diuretic
241	555/241, barr	Allopurinol	100mg	White	Tab	Round	Y	N	Barr	Antigout
	93 241	Phenobarbital	15mg	White	Tab	Round	Y	N	Lemmon	Sedative
	dp 241	Choline Magnesium Trisalate	500mg	Yellow	Tab	Oval	Y	N	Duramed	Anti–Inflammatory
	INV 241	Choline Magnesium Trisalate	500mg	White	Tab	Oval	Y	N	Duramed	Anti–Inflammatory
	Par/241	Temazepam	30mg	White/White	Cap	–	–	–	Par	Hypnotic
	PPP 241	Nadolol	80mg	Blue	Tab	Round	Y	N	Bristol	Antihypertensive
	R 241	Lorazepam	1mg	White	Tab	Round	Y	N	Royce	Antianxiety
	R 241,1	Lorazepam	1.0mg	White	Tab	Round	Y	N	Royce	Antianxiety
	SQUIBB 241	Nadolol	80mg	Blue	Tab	Round	Y	N	Princeton	Antihypertensive
	WPPh 241	Hydrochlorothiazide	25mg	Peach	Tab	Round	–	N	West Point Pharma	Diuretic
242	555/242	Allopurinol	300mg	Peach	Tab	Round	Y	N	Barr	Antigout
	CC 242	Thyroid	1/2gr.	Tan	Tab	Round	N	N	Camall	Hormone
	dp 242	Choline Magnesium Trisalate	750mg	Blue	Tab	Oval	Y	N	Duramed	Anti–Inflammatory
	GG 242	Methylclothiazide	5mg	Salmon	Tab	Round	Y	N	Geneva	Diuretic
	INV 242	Choline Magnesium Trisalate	750mg	White	Tab	Oval	Y	N	Duramed	Anti–Inflammatory
	QPL 242/Q	Meprobamate & Aspirin	400mg/325mg	Green/Yellow	Tab	Round	N	N	Quantum	Antianxiety
	R 242	Lorazepam	2mg	White	Tab	Round	Y	N	Royce	Antianxiety
	R 242,2	Lorazepam	2.0mg	White	Tab	Round	Y	N	Royce	Antianxiety
	WC 242	Carbamazepine Chewable	100mg	Pink	Tab	–	–	N	WC	Anticonvulsant
243	Barr, 243	Chlordiazepoxide HCl with Amitriptyline	10mg/25mg	White	Tab	Round	N	Y	Barr	Antidepressant
	CC 243	Thyroid	1gr.	Tan	Tab	Round	N	N	Camall	Hormone
	GG243	Methyldopa & Hydrochlorothiazide	500mg/30mg	Green	Tab	Round	N	Y	Geneva	Antihypertensive
	QPL–243/2.5	Minoxidil	2.5mg	White	Tab	Round	–	–	Quantum	Antihypertensive
	WC 243	Carbamazepine	200mg	White	Tab	–	–	N	WC	Anticonvulsant
	WPPh 243	Hydrochlorothiazide	50mg	Peach	Tab	Round	–	N	West Point Pharma	Diuretic
244	Barr, 244	Chlordiazepoxide HCl with Amitriptyline	5mg/12.5mg	Peach	Tab	Round	N	Y	Barr	Antidepressant
	CC 244	Thyroid	2gr.	Tan	Tab	Round	N	N	Camall	Hormone
	GG 244	Methylclothiazide	2.5mg	Orange	Tab	Round	Y	N	Geneva	Diuretic
	SEARLE 244	Spironolactone with Hydrochlorothiazide	50mg/50mg	White	Tab	Round	N	N	Searle	Diuretic
245	b, 245	Perphenazine & Amitriptyline	2mg/10mg	White	Tab	Triangle	N	Y	Barr	Antidepressant
	Forest 245	Aminoacetic Acid/Calcium Carbonate	150mg/300mg	Green	Tab	Round	–	N	Forest	–
	GG245	Minoxidil	10mg.	White	Tab	Round	N	N	Quantum	Antihypertensive
	QPL/245–Q	Oxybutynin Chloride	5mg	White	Tab	Round	Y	N	Quantum	Antispasmodic
	West–ward 245	Diphenoxylate HCl and Atropine Sulfate	2.5mg/0.025mg	White	Tab	Round	N	N	West–ward	Antidiarrheal
	WPPh 245	Chlorothiazide	500mg	White	Tab	Round	–	N	West Point Pharma	Diuretic
246	b, 246	Perphenazine & Amitriptyline	4mg/10mg	Salmon	Tab	Triangle	N	Y	Barr	Antidepressant
	dp 246	Cyproheptadine HCl	4mg	White	Tab	Round	N	N	Duramed	Antipruritic
	Par/246	Carisoprodol / Aspirin	200mg/325mg	White/Lavender	Tab	Round	N	N	Par	Muscle Relaxant
	PPP 246	Nadolol	160mg	Blue	Tab	Oblong	Y	N	Bristol	Antihypertensive
	SQUIBB 246	Nadolol	160mg	Blue	Tab	Oblong	Y	N	Princeton	Antihypertensive
247	Par–247	Salsalate	500mg	Yellow	Tab	Round	N	Y	Par	Analgesic

ID NO.	ID CODE	GENERIC NAME	STRENGTH	COLOR	FORM	SHAPE	SCORED	COATED	MFG.	USE
	R 247	Methocarbamol	500mg	White	Tab	Round	Y	N	Purepac	Muscle Relaxant
	Royce logo 247, 2–10	Perphenazine & Amitriptyline	2mg/10mg	Blue	Tab	Round	N	Y	Royce	Antidepressant
	West–ward 247	Ergoloid Mesylates	1mg	White	Tab	Round	Y	N	West–ward	Vasodilator
248	barr/248	Methyldopa	500mg	White	Tab	Round	N	Y	Barr	Antihypertensive
	Par–248	Salsalate	750mg	Yellow	Tab	Round	N	Y	Par	Analgesic
	Royce logo 248,2–25	Perphenazine & Amitriptyline	2mg/25mg	Orange	Tab	Round	N	Y	Royce	Antidepressant
	West–ward 248	Folic Acid	1mg	Yellow	Tab	Round	Y	N	West–ward	Antianemic
249	54–249	Propranolol HCl	80mg	White	Tab	Round	Y	n	Roxane	Antihypertensive
	GG 249	Alprazolam	2mg	White	Tab	Oblong	Y	N	Upjohn	Antianxiety
	Par/249	Methocarbamol/Aspirin	400mg/325mg	Pink/White	Tab	Round	N	N	Par	Muscle Relaxant
	R 249	Methocarbamol	750mg	White	Tab	Oblong	Y	N	Purepac	Muscle Relaxant
	Royce logo 249,4–10	Perphenazine & Amitriptyline	4mg/10mg	Salmon	Tab	Round	N	Y	Royce	Antidepressant
	West–ward 249	Furosemide	20mg	White	Tab	Round	Y	N	West–ward	Diuretic
250	225–250	Ethaverine HCl	100mg	White	Tab	–	–	–	B.F.Ascher	Vasodilator
	250	Niacin SR	250mg	Pink	Tab	Capsule	Y	N	Upsher	Vasodilator
	3M/SR 250	Theophylline SR	250mg	White	Tab	Round	Y	N	3M	Bronchodilator
	Abana 250	Guaifenesin & Pseudoephedrine	250mg/90mg	Yellow	Cap	–	–	–	Abana	Antitussive comb.
	Atral 250mg	Amoxicillin	250mg	Pink	Cap	–	–	–	Lab A	Anti–Infective
	Atral 250mg	Cephalexin	250mg	Lt. Green	Cap	–	–	–	Lab A	Anti–Infective
	Ayerst 250	Amoxicillin	250mg	Caramel\Red	Cap	–	–	–	Ayerst	Anti–Infective
	CC 250	Vitamin Combination	n/a	White	Tab	Oblong	Y	N	Camall	Vitamin
	CP250	Nortriptyline Hydrochloride	10mg	Green/White	Cap	–	–	–	Creighton Prod. Corp	Antidepressant
	GG250	Quinidine Gluconate	324mg	White	Tab	Round	N	N	Geneva	Antiarrhythmic
	HD 250	Digoxin	0.25mg	White	Tab	Round	–	N	Halsey	Cardiac Glycoside
	Par/250	Cephalexin	250mg	Grey/Orange	Cap	–	–	–	Par	Anti–Infective
	PP–250	Mefenamic Acid	250mg	Blue/Yellow	Cap	–	–	–	Eon	Analgesic
	RIKER/250 Plus	Theophylline & Guaifenesin	250mg/200mg	White	Tab	–	–	–	Riker	Bronchodilator
	Royce logo 250,4–25	Perphenazine & Amitriptyline	4mg/25mg	Yellow	Tab	Round	N	Y	Royce	Antidepressant
	TR/250 G	Triazolam	0.25mg	Yellow	Tab	Oval	N	N	Par	Sedative/Hypnotic
	West–ward 250	Furosemide	40mg	White	Tab	Round	Y	N	West–ward	Diuretic
251	555/251	Tolbutamide	500mg	White	Tab	Round	Y	N	Barr	Hypoglycemic
	CP251	Nortriptyline Hydrochloride	25mg	Green/White	Cap	–	–	–	Creighton Prod. Corp	Antidepressant
	DMSP 251	Carbidopa/Levodopa	25mg/250mg	Dapple Blue	Tab	Oval	–	–	Dupont	Antiparkinson
	dp 251	Chlorpropamide	250mg	Blue	Tab	Round	Y	N	Duramed	Hypoglycemic
	Forest 251	Sulfamethazole	500mg	Blue	Tab	Capsule	–	Y	Forest	Anti–Infective
	IP 251	Quinine Sulfate	260mg	White	Tab	Round	–	N	Interpharm	Muscle Relaxant
	MYLAN 251	Trazodone HCl	50mg	White	Tab	Round	N	N	Mylan	Antidepressant
	P–D 251	Thyroglobulin	32mg	Gray	Tab	Round	N	N	PD	Hormone
	Sch. Logo 251	Halazepam	20mg	Orange	Tab	Round	Y	N	Schering	Antianxiety
252	252, b	Dipyridamole	25mg	White	Tab	Round	N	Y	Barr	Antiplatelet
	54–252	Acetaminophen	500mg	White	Tab	–	–	–	Roxane	Analgesic
	AYERST 252	Vitamin Combination	n/a	Black	Cap	–	–	–	Ayerst	Vitamin Comb.
	CP252	Nortriptyline Hydrochloride	50mg	Green/Yellow	Cap	–	–	–	Creighton Prod. Corp	Antidepressant
	dp–252	Chlorpropamide	100mg	Blue	Tab	Round	Y	N	Duramed	Hypoglycemic
	INV 252	Cyclobenzaprine HCl	10mg	White	Tab	Round	N	Y	Duramed	Muscle Relaxant
	MYLAN 252	Trazodone HCl	100mg	White	Tab	Round	N	N	Mylan	Antidepressant
	P–D 252	Thyroglobulin	65mg	Gray	Tab	Round	N	N	PD	Hormone
253	54 253	Sulfamethoxazole & Trimethoprim	400mg/80mg	White	Tab	Capsule	Y	N	Roxane	Anti–Infective
	CP253	Nortriptyline Hydrochloride	75mg	Green	Cap	–	–	–	Creighton Prod. Corp	Antidepressant
	P–D 253	Thyroglobulin	100mg	Gray	Tab	Round	N	N	PD	Hormone
	R 253	Methyldopa	250mg	White	Tab	Round	–	–	Purepac	Antihypertensive
	R 253	Methyldopa	250mg	Beige	Tab	Round	–	Y	Rondex	Antihypertensive
	West–ward 253	Furosemide	80mg	White	Tab	Round	Y	N	West–ward	Diuretic
254	832/G254	Desipramine HCl	25mg	Lavender	Tab	Round	N	Y	PBI	Antidepressant
	GG 254	Fenoprofen Calcium	600mg	White	Tab	Oval	Y	Y	Geneva	Anti–Inflammatory
	P–D 254	Thyroglobulin	200mg	Gray	Tab	Round	N	N	PD	Hormone
	West–ward 254	Hydrocortisone	20mg	White	Tab	Round	Y	N	West–ward	Steroid
255	555/255	Chlorzoxazone With Acetaminophen	250mg/300mg	Green	Tab	Round	N	N	Barr	Muscle Relaxant
	832/G255	Desipramine HCl	50mg	Blue	Tab	Round	N	Y	PBI	Antidepressant
	CC 255	Hydralazine HCl	10mg	Orange	Tab	Round	N	N	Camall	Antihypertensive
	GG255	Pseudoephedrine & Dexbrompheniramine SA	120mg/6mg	White	Tab	Round	N	Y	Geneva	Decongestant Comb.
	M 255	Albuterol Sulfate	2mg	White	Tab	Round	Y	N	Mylan	Bronchodilator
	R 255	Methyldopa	500mg	White	Tab	Round	–	–	Purepac	Antihypertensive
	R 255	Methyldopa	500mg	Beige	Tab	Capsule	N	Y	Rondex	Antihypertensive
	Royce logo 255/10	Baclofen	10mg	White	Tab	Oval	Y	N	Royce	Muscle Relaxant
256	832/G256	Desipramine HCl	75mg	White	Tab	Round	N	Y	PBI	Antidepressant
	CC 256	Hydralazine HCl	25mg	Orange	Tab	Round	N	N	Camall	Antihypertensive
	GG 256	Alprazolam	0.25mg	White	Tab	Oval	Y	N	Upjohn	Antianxiety
	INV 256	Atenolol	50mg	White	Tab	Round	Y	N	Duramed	Antihypertensive
	Par/256	Minoxidil	2.5mg	White	Tab	Round	Y	N	Par	Antihypertensive
	PP–256	Chlorpheniramine Maleate & Phenylpropanolamine HCl	12mg/75mg	Blue/Clear	Cap	–	–	–	Eon	Decongestant Comb.
	Royce logo 256/10	Baclofen	20mg	White	Tab	Round	Y	N	Royce	Muscle Relaxant
	West–ward 256	Hydrochlorothiazide	25mg	Peach	Tab	Round	Y	N	West–ward	Diuretic
257	832/G257	Desipramine HCl	100mg	Butterscotch	Tab	Round	N	Y	PBI	Antidepressant
	CC 257	Hydralazine HCl	50mg	Orange	Tab	Round	N	N	Camall	Antihypertensive
	GG 257	Alprazolam	0.5mg	Peach	Tab	Oval	Y	N	Upjohn	Antianxiety
	INV 257	Atenolol	100mg	White	Tab	Round	Y	N	Duramed	Antihypertensive
	Mylan 257	Haloperidol	1mg	Orange	Tab	Round	Y	N	Mylan	Tranquilizer
	P–D 257	Thyroglobulin	130mg	Gray	Tab	Round	N	N	PD	Hormone
	Par/257	Minoxidil	10mg	White	Tab	Round	Y	N	Par	Antihypertensive
	PP–257	Prenatal Vitamin	n/a	Yellow	Tab	Capsule	N	Y	Eon	Vitamin
	West–ward 257	Hydrochlorothiazide	50mg	Peach	Tab	Round	Y	N	West–ward	Diuretic
258	CC 258	Hydralazine HCl	100mg	Orange	Tab	Round	N	N	Camall	Antihypertensive
	GG 258	Alprazolam	1mg	Blue	Tab	Oval	Y	N	Upjohn	Antianxiety
	HAUCK 258	Hydrocodone Bitartrate/Guaifenesin/Pseudoephedrine	5mg/300mg/30mg	White	Tab	–	–	–	W.E.Hauck	Antitussive
	Par/258	Metaproterenol Sulfate	10mg	White	Tab	Round	Y	N	Par	Bronchodilator
	Sch. Logo 258	Pseudoephedrine Sulfate	120mg	Blue	Tab	Round	N	Y	Schering	Decongestant
	West–ward 258	Isoxsuprine Hydrochloride	10mg	White	Tab	Round	N	N	West–ward	Vasodilator
259	259, barr	Erythromycin Ethylsuccinate	400mg	Beige	Tab	Capsule	N	Y	Barr	Anti–Infective
	GG259	Isosorbide Dinitrate	5mg	Pink	Tab	Round	Y	N	Geneva	Antianginal
	INV 259	Atenolol	25mg	White	Tab	Round	Y	N	Duramed	Antihypertensive
	Par/259	Metaproterenol Sulfate	20mg	White	Tab	Round	Y	N	Par	Bronchodilator
	PP 259	Prenatal Vitamin	–	Yellow	Tab	Capsule	N	Y	Eon	Prenatal Vitamin
	SQUIBB 259	Perphenazine & Amitriptyline HCl	2mg/25mg	–	Tab	–	–	–	Squibb	Antidepressant
	West–ward 259	Isoxsuprine Hydrochloride	20mg	White	Tab	Round	Y	N	West–ward	Vasodilator

ID NO.	ID CODE	GENERIC NAME	STRENGTH	COLOR	FORM	SHAPE	SCORED	COATED	MFG.	USE
260	b, 260	Thioridazine HCl	10mg	Beige	Tab	Round	N	Y	Barr	Tranquilizer
	Central 260mg	Theophylline Anhydrous	260mg	Clear	Cap	–	–	–	Central	Bronchodilator
	P–D 260	Liotrix	30mcg/7.5mcg	Peach	Tab	Square	Y	N	PD	Hormone
	West–ward 260	Isoniazid	100mg	White	Tab	Round	Y	N	West–ward	Anti-Infective
261	b, 261	Thioridazine HCl	25mg	Yellow	Tab	Round	N	Y	Barr	Tranquilizer
	GG261	Meclizine HCl	25mg	White/Yellow	Tab	Oval	N	N	Geneva	Antivertigo
	GG261	Meclizine HCl	25mg	Yellow	Tab	Oval	N	N	Geneva	Antivertigo
	P–D 261	Liotrix	60mcg/15mcg	Tan	Tab	Square	Y	N	PD	Hormone
	R 261	Methyldopa & Hydrochlorothiazide	250mg/15mg	Tan	Tab	Round	N	Y	Purepac	Antihypertensive
	West–ward 261	Isoniazid	300mg	White	Tab	Round	Y	N	West–ward	Anti-Infective
	Wyeth 261	Meperidine HCl & Promethazine HCl	50mg/25mg	Red	Cap	–	–	–	Wyeth	Analgesic
262	54/262	Morphine Sulfate	30mg	White	Tab	Round	Y	N	Roxane	Analgesic
	barr, 262	Thioridazine HCl	50mg	Pink	Tab	Round	N	Y	Barr	Tranquilizer
	P–D 262	Liotrix	120mcg/30mcg	Lavender	Tab	Square	Y	N	PD	Hormone
263	54–263	Phenobarbital	100mg	White	Tab	Round	Y	N	Roxane	Hypnotic
	barr, 263	Thioridazine HCl	100mg	White	Tab	Round	N	Y	Barr	Tranquilizer
	GG263	Atenolol	50mg	White	Tab	Round	Y	Y	Geneva	Antihypertensive
	P–D 263	Liotrix	180mcg/45mcg	Gray	Tab	Square	Y	N	PD	Hormone
	Par/263	Meclofenamate Sodium	50mg	Maroon/Pink	Cap	–	–	–	Par	Antiinflammatory
	R 263	Methyldopa & Hydrochlorothiazide	250mg/25mg	White	Tab	Round	N	Y	Purepac	Antihypertensive
264	Barr/264,3	Aspirin with Codeine	325mg/30mg	White	Tab	Round	N	N	Barr	Analgesic
	GG264	Atenolol	100mg	White	Tab	Round	–	Y	Geneva	Antihypertensive
	Par/264	Meclofenamate Sodium	100mg	Maroon/White	Cap	–	–	–	Par	Antiinflammatory
265	555/265	Spironolactone with Hydrochlorothiazide	25mg/25mg	White	Tab	Round	Y	N	Barr	Diuretic
	dp 265	Hydroxyzine Pamoate	25mg	Green	Cap	Capsule	–	–	Duramed	Antianxiety
	GG265	Methyldopa & Hydrochlorothiazide	250mg/25mg	White	Tab	Round	N	Y	Geneva	Antihypertensive
	Par/265	Chlordiazepoxide/Amitriptyline	5mg/12.5mg	Peach	Tab	Round	N	Y	Par	Antianxiety
	R 265	Methyldopa & Hydrochlorothiazide	500mg/30mg	Tan	Tab	Oval	N	Y	Purepac	Antihypertensive
	RIKER/265	Rauwolfia serpentina	2mg	Brown	Tab	Round	N	N	3M	Antihypertensive
	West–ward 265	Reserpine and Hydrochlorothiazide	0.125mg/50mg	Green	Tab	Round	Y	N	West–ward	Antihypertensive
266	555/266	Spironolactone	25mg	White	Tab	Round	Y	N	Barr	Diuretic
	dp 266	Hydroxyzine Pamoate	50mg	White/Green	Cap	Capsule	–	–	Duramed	Antianxiety
	Par/266	Chlordiazepoxide/Amitriptyline	10mg/25mg	White	Tab	Round	N	Y	Par	Antianxiety
267	barr, 267	Chlorthalidone	25mg	Yellow	Tab	Round	N	N	Barr	Diuretic
	dp 267	Hydroxyzine Pamoate	100mg	Gray/Green	Cap	Capsule	–	–	Duramed	Antianxiety
	R 267	Methyldopa & Hydrochlorothiazide	500mg/50mg	White	Tab	Oval	N	Y	Purepac	Antihypertensive
	SQUIBB 267	Perphenazine & Amitriptyline HCl	4mg/10mg	–	Tab	–	–	–	Squibb	Antidepressant
268	barr, 268	Chlorthalidone	50mg	Green	Tab	Round	N	N	Barr	Diuretic
	GLAXO 268	Theophylline SR	260mg	Blue/Clear	Cap	–	–	–	Glaxo	Bronchodilator
269	R 269	Metoclopramide	10mg	White	Tab	Round	Y	N	Purepac	Antireflux
	West–ward 269	Hydralazine Hydrochloride	25mg	Orange	Tab	Round	N	Y	West–ward	Antihypertensive
270	CC 270	Phenylpropanolamine HCl	37.5mg	White	Tab	Oval	N	N	Camall	Appetite Supp.
	CC 270	Phenylpropanolamine HCl	37.5mg	Pink	Tab	Oval	N	N	Camall	Appetite Supp.
	CC 270	Phenylpropanolamine HCl	37.5mg	Gray	Tab	Oval	N	N	Camall	Appetite Supp.
	CC 270	Phenylpropanolamine HCl	37.5mg	Green	Tab	Oval	N	N	Camall	Appetite Supp.
	CC 270	Phenylpropanolamine HCl	37.5mg	Peach	Tab	Oval	N	N	Camall	Appetite Supp.
	CC 270	Phenylpropanolamine HCl	37.5mg	Blue	Tab	Oval	N	N	Camall	Appetite Supp.
	CC 270	Phenylpropanolamine HCl	37.5mg	Yellow	Tab	Oval	N	N	Camall	Appetite Supp.
	GG270	Tolazamide	100mg	White	Tab	Round	N	Y	Geneva	Hypoglycemic
	P–D 270	Phenelzine Sulfate	15mg	Orange	Tab	Round	N	Y	PD	Antidepressant
	QPL–270/Q	Metoclopramide HCl	5mg	Pink	Tab	Round	–	–	Quantum	Antireflux
271	555/271, barr	Sulfinpyrazone	100mg	White	Tab	Round	Y	N	Barr	Antigout
	DMSP 271	Carbidopa/Levodopa	10mg/100mg	Dapple Blue	Tab	Oval	–	–	Dupont	Antiparkinson
	GG271	Tolazamide	250mg	White	Tab	Round	Y	Y	Geneva	Hypoglycemic
	Mylan 271	Diazepam	2mg	White	Tab	Round	Y	N	Mylan	Antianxiety
	P–D 271	Amitriptyline	100mg	Mustard	Tab	Round	N	Y	PD	Antidepressant
	SQUIBB 271	Perphenazine & Amitriptyline HCl	4mg/25mg	–	Tab	–	–	–	Squibb	Antidepressant
	WC 271	Amitriptyline	100mg	Mustard	Tab	Round	N	Y	WC	Antidepressant
	West–ward 271	Hydralazine Hydrochloride	50mg	Orange	Tab	Round	N	Y	West–ward	Antihypertensive
272	barr/272	Sulfinpyrazone	200mg	Orange/Orange	Cap	–	–	–	Barr	Antigout
	DMSP 272	Carbidopa/Levodopa	25mg/100mg	Yellow	Tab	Oval	–	–	Dupont	Antiparkinson
	GG272	Tolazamide	500mg	White	Tab	Round	Y	N	Geneva	Hypoglycemic
	P–D 272	Amitriptyline	10mg	Tan	Tab	Round	N	Y	PD	Antidepressant
	SYNTEX 272	Naproxen	250mg	Yellow	Tab	Round	N	Y	Syntex	Anti-Inflammatory
	W–C 272	Amitriptyline	10mg	Tan	Tab	Round	N	Y	WC	Antidepressant
	WALLACE 272	Cryptenamine & Methyclothiazide	2mg/2.5mg	White–Blue	Tab	Round	–	N	Wallace	Antihypertensive
	West–ward 272	Lorazepam	0.5mg	White	Tab	Round	N	N	West–ward	Antianxiety
273	P–D 273	Amitriptyline	25mg	Coral	Tab	Round	N	Y	PD	Antidepressant
	QPL–273/Q	Timolol Maleate	5mg	Green	Tab	Round	–	–	Quantum	Antihypertensive
	SYNTEX 273	Naproxen	375mg	Peach	Tab	Oblong	–	Y	Syntex	Anti-Inflammatory
	W–C 273	Amitriptyline	25mg	Coral	Tab	Round	N	Y	WC	Antidepressant
	West–ward 273	Lorazepam	1mg	White	Tab	Round	Y	N	West–ward	Antianxiety
274	dp 274	Isoniazid	100mg	White	Tab	Round	Y	N	Duramed	Anti-Infective
	GG274	Isoxsuprine	10mg	White	Tab	Round	Y	N	Geneva	Vasodilator
	P–D 274	Amitriptyline	50mg	Blue/Purple	Tab	Round	N	Y	PD	Antidepressant
	QPL–274/Q	Timolol Maleate	10mg	Green	Tab	Round	–	N	Quantum	Antihypertensive
	SYNTEX 274	Naproxen Sodium	275mg	Blue	Tab	Oval	N	Y	Syntex	Anti-Inflammatory
	W–C 274	Amitriptyline	50mg	Blue	Tab	Round	N	Y	WC	Antidepressant
	WALLACE 274	Methyclothiazide & Reserpine	2.5mg/0.1mg	White–Pink	Tab	Round	–	N	Wallace	Antihypertensive
	West–ward 274	Lorazepam	2mg	White	Tab	Round	N	N	West–ward	Antianxiety
275	dp 275	Indomethacin	25mg	Green	Cap	Capsule	–	–	Duramed	Anti-Inflammatory
	P–D 275	Amitriptyline	75mg	Green	Tab	Round	N	Y	PD	Antidepressant
	PF C 275	Quinidine Polygalacturonate	275mg	White	Tab	Round	Y	N	PF	Antiarrhythmic
	QPL–275/Q	Timolol Maleate	20mg	Green	Tab	Round	–	N	Quantum	Antihypertensive
	W–C 275	Amitriptyline	75mg	Green	Tab	Round	N	Y	WC	Antidepressant
276	barr/276	Chlorpropamide	250mg	White	Tab	Round	Y	N	Barr	Hypoglycemic
	dp 276	Indomethacin	50mg	Green	Cap	–	–	–	Duramed	Anti-Inflammatory
	P–D 276	Prazepam	10mg	Blue	Tab	Round	Y	N	PD	Antianxiety
	R 276	Reserpine	0.25mg	White	Tab	Round	N	Y	Rondex	Antihypertensive
277	b,277	Isosorbide Dinitrate Sublingual	10mg	White	Tab	Round	N	N	Barr	Antianginal
	Bolar 277	Triamterene & Hydrochlorothiazide	50mg/25mg	Red	Cap	–	–	–	Bolar	Diuretic
	dp 277	Isoniazid	300mg	White	Tab	Round	Y	N	Duramed	Anti-Infective
	LEMMON 277	Phendimetrazine Tartrate	35mg	Green/White	Cap	–	–	–	Lemmon	Anorectic
	MERRELL 277	Methenamine Hippurate	1GM	Yellow	Tab	Capsule	Y	N	Merrell	Anti-Infective
	Mylan 277	Chlordiazepoxide/Amitriptyline HCl	10mg/25mg	White	Tab	Round	N	Y	Mylan	Antidepressant

ID NO.	ID CODE	GENERIC NAME	STRENGTH	COLOR	FORM	SHAPE	SCORED	COATED	MFG.	USE
	SQUIBB 277	Tolazamide	250mg	–	Tab	–	–	–	Squibb	Hypoglycemic
	SYNTEX 277	Naproxen	500mg	Yellow	Tab	Oblong	–	Y	Syntex	Anti–Inflammatory
278	555/278	Oxycodone HCl with Acetaminophen	5mg/325mg	White	Tab	Round	Y	N	Barr	Analgesic
	P–D 278	Amitriptyline	150mg	Orange	Tab	Oval	N	Y	PD	Antidepressant
	R 278	Oxytetracycline Hydrochloride	250mg	Yellow/Yellow	Cap	–	–	–	Purepac	Anti–Infective
	R278	Oxytetracycline	250mg	Yellow	Cap	–	–	–	Rondex	Anti–Infective
	Rondex 278	Oxytetracylcine	250mg	Yellow	Cap	–	–	–	Rondex	Anti–Infective
	WC 278	Amitriptyline	150mg	Orange	Tab	Round	N	Y	WC	Antidepressant
279	555/279	Isosorbide Dinitrate	30mg	Blue	Tab	Round	Y	N	Barr	Antianginal
	Par/279	Triamterene/Hydrochlorothiazide	75mg/50mg	Yellow	Tab	Round	Y	N	Par	Antihypertensive
	SQUIBB 279	Isosorbide Dinitrate SA	40mg	–	Tab	–	–	–	Squibb	Vasodilator
	West–ward 279	Phenylprop.,phenyleph.,phenyltolox.,chlorphenir.	40,10,15,5mg	White/red specks	Tab	Round	N	N	West–ward	Decongestant comb.
280	54–280	Dihydrotachysterol	0.125mg	White	Tab	Round	N	N	Roxane	Blood Ca++ Regulator
	Barr/280,4	Aspirin with Codeine	325mg/60mg	White	Tab	Round	N	N	Barr	Analgesic
	R 280	Haloperidol	1mg	Yellow	Tab	Round	N	N	Purepac	Tranquilizer
281	281	Acetaminophen	500mg	White	Tab	Oblong	N	N	Granutec	Analgesic
	Forest 281	Dehydrochloric Acid/Pb/Homatropine Methylbromide	125mg/8mg/2.5mg	Green	Tab	Round	–	Y	Forest	Antispasmodic
	GLAXO 281	Ethaverine HCl	100mg	Yellow	Tab	Oval	N	N	Glaxo	Vasodilator
	R 281	Haloperidol	2mg	Pink	Tab	Round	N	N	Purepac	Tranquilizer
282	P–D 282	Prenatal Vitamin Combination	n/a	Yellow	Tab	Capsule	N	Y	PD	Vitamin
	R 282	Haloperidol	5mg	Green	Tab	Round	N	N	Purepac	Tranquilizer
	Sch. Logo 282	Azatadine Maleate	1mg	White	Tab	Round	Y	N	Schering	Antihistamine
283	PPP 283	Nadolol & Bendroflumethiazide	40mg/5mg	White/Blue Specks	Tab	Round	Y	N	Bristol	Antihypertensive
	SQUIBB 283	Nadolol & Bendroflumethiazide	40mg/5mg	White/Blue Specks	Tab	Round	Y	N	Princeton	Antihypertensive
284	CL284	Isoxsuprine	20mg	White	Tab	Round	Y	N	Geneva	Vasodilator
	GG284	Isoxsuprine	20mg	White	Tab	Round	Y	N	Geneva	Vasodilator
	PPP 284	Nadolol & Bendroflumethiazide	80mg/5mg	White/Blue Specks	Tab	Round	Y	N	Bristol	Antihypertensive
	SQUIBB 284	Nadolol & Bendroflumethiazide	80mg/5mg	White/Blue Specks	Tab	Round	Y	N	Princeton	Antihypertensive
285	285, b	Dipyridamole	50mg	White	Tab	Round	N	Y	Barr	Antiplatelet
	GG285	Quinidine Sulfate	200mg	White	Tab	Round	Y	N	Geneva	Antiarrhythmic
	West–ward 285	Sulfinpyrazone	200mg	Orange/Orange	Cap	–	–	–	West–ward	Antigout
	West–ward 285	Hydrocodone Bitartrate/Acetaminophen	5mg/500mg	White	Tab	Capsule	Y	N	West–ward	Analgesic
286	286, barr	Dipyridamole	75mg	White	Tab	Round	N	Y	Barr	Antiplatelet
	GG 286	Quinidine Sulfate	300mg	White	Tab	Round	Y	N	Geneva	Antiarrhythmic
	Par/286	Fenoprofen Calcium	600mg	White	Tab	Capsule	Y	Y	Par	Antiinflamatory
	R 286	Haloperidol	10mg	Aqua	Tab	Round	N	N	Purepac	Tranquilizer
	SQUIBB 286	Quinidine Gluconate	324mg	–	Tab	–	–	–	Squibb	Antiarrhythmic
287	Par/287	Fenoprofen Calcium	200mg	Flesh/Lavender	Cap	–	–	–	Par	Antiinflamatory
	R 287	Haloperidol	20mg	Salmon	Tab	Round	N	N	Purepac	Tranquilizer
	Sch. Logo 287	Perphenazine & Amitriptyline HCl	2mg/10mg	Yellow	Tab	Round	N	Y	Schering	Antidepressant
288	555/288	Isosorbide Dinitrate Oral	40mg	Green	Tab	Round	Y	N	Barr	Antianginal
	barr 288	Isosorbide Dinitrate	40mg	Yellow	Tab	Round	N	N	Barr	Antianginal
	GG 288	Cyclobenzaprine HCl	10mg	Yellow	Tab	Round	N	Y	Geneva	Muscle Relaxant
	Par/288	Fenoprofen Calcium	300mg	Flesh/Orange	Cap	–	–	–	Par	Antiinflamatory
	SQUIBB 288	Allopurinol	300mg	–	Tab	Round	–	–	Squibb	Antigout
289	GG 289	Methyldopa/Hydrochlorothiazide	500mg/50mg	White	Tab	Round	N	Y	Geneva	Antihypertensive
	Par/289	Megestrol Acetate	20mg	White	Tab	Round	Y	N	Par	Hormone
	R 289	Haloperidol	0.5mg	White	Tab	Round	Y	N	Purepac	Tranquilizer
290	D & E	Caffeine	325mg	Black	Cap	–	–	–	D & E	Stimulant
	Par/290	Megestrol Acetate	40mg	White	Tab	Round	Y	N	Par	Hormone
	West–ward 290	Methocarbamol	500mg	White	Tab	Round	Y	N	West–ward	Muscle Relaxant
291	291, barr	Metronidazole	250mg	Off White	Tab	Round	N	N	Barr	Anti–Infective
	GG291	Ibuprofen	400mg	White	Tab	Round	N	Y	Ciba	Anti–Inflammatory
292	292, barr	Metronidazole	500mg	Off White	Tab	Oblong	N	N	Barr	Anti–Infective
	93–292	Carbidopa/Levodopa	10mg/100mg	Mottled Blue	Tab	Round	Y	N	Lemmon	Antiparkinson
	GG292	Ibuprofen	600mg	White	Tab	Oval	N	Y	Interpharm	Anti–Inflammatory
	R 292	Papaverine HCl SR	150mg	Brown/Clear	Cap	–	–	–	Purepac	Vasodilator
	West–ward 292	Methocarbamol	750mg	White	Tab	Capsule	Y	N	West–ward	Muscle Relaxant
293	54–293	Leucovorin Calcium	5mg	–	Tab	Round	Y	N	Roxane	Antineoplastic
	555/293, Barr	Oxycodone HCl, Oxycodone Terephthalate, Aspirin	4.5/.38mg/325	Yellow	Tab	Round	Y	N	Barr	Analgesic
	93–293	Carbidopa/Levodopa	25mg/100mg	Mottled Yellow	Tab	Round	Y	N	Lemmon	Antiparkinson
	dp 293	Phenylpropanolamine/PE/Guaifenesin	45mg/5mg/200mg	Orange/Beige	Cap	Capsule	–	–	Duramed	Decongestant Comb.
	GG293	Ibuprofen	200mg	White	Tab	Round	N	Y	Geneva	Anti–Inflammatory
294	93–294	Carbidopa/Levodopa	25mg/250mg	Mottled Blue	Tab	Round	Y	N	Lemmon	Antiparkinson
	Barr/294,2	Aspirin with Codeine	325mg/15mg	White	Tab	Round	N	N	Barr	Analgesic
	GG 294	Ibuprofen	800mg	White	Tab	Capsule	N	Y	Geneva	Anti–Inflammatory
295	225/295	Hyoscyamine Sulfate	0.125 mg	Yellow	Tab	Round	Y	N	B.F.Ascher	Antispasmodic
	barr/295,Doxytab	Doxycycline Hyclate	100mg	Beige	Tab	Round	N	Y	Barr	Anti–Infective
	dp 295	Phenylpropanolamine HCl & Guaifenesin LA	75mg/400mg	Blue	Tab	Oval	Y	N	Duramed	Decongestant Comb.
	Forest 295	Potassium Iodide/Niacinamide Hydroiodide	135mg/25mg	Pink	Tab	Round	–	Y	Forest	
	GG 295	Albuterol	4mg	White	Tab	Round	Y	N	Geneva	Broncodilator
	GLAXO 295	Theophylline SR	130mg	Blue/Clear	Cap	–	–	–	Glaxo	Bronchodilator
	West–ward 295	Metronidazole	250mg	White	Tab	Round	Y	N	West–ward	Anti–Infective
	West–ward 295	Tetracycline Hydrochloride	250mg	Orange/Yellow	Cap	–	–	–	West–ward	Anti–Infective
296	barr/296,Doxycap	Doxycycline Hyclate	50mg	White/White	Cap	–	–	–	Barr	Anti–Infective
	dp 296	Salsalate	500mg	Blue	Tab	Round	N	Y	Duramed	Antiinflammatory
	INV 296	Salsalate	500mg	Blue	Tab	Round	N	Y	Duramed	Antiinflammatory
	R 296	Penicillin G Potassium	200,000 Units	White	Tab	Round	N	N	Rondex	Anti–Infective
	West–ward 296	Thioridazine Hydrochloride	10mg	Beige	Tab	Round	N	Y	West–ward	Tranquilizer
297	barr/297,Doxycap	Doxycycline Hyclate	100mg	White/White	Cap	–	–	–	Barr	Anti–Infective
	dp 297	Salsalate	750mg	Blue	Tab	Capsule	Y	Y	Duramed	Antiinflammatory
	G 297	Chloral Hydrate	500mg	Red	Cap	–	–	–	R. P. Scherer	Hypnotic
	G 297	Chloral Hydrate	500mg	Green	Cap	–	–	–	R. P. Scherer	Hypnotic
	INV 297	Salsalate	750mg	Blue	Tab	Capsule	Y	Y	Duramed	Anti–Inflammatory
	West–ward 297	Metronidazole	500mg	White	Tab	Capsule	Y	N	West–ward	Anti–Infective
298	West–ward 297	Thioridazine Hydrochloride	15mg	Blue	Tab	Round	N	Y	West–ward	Tranquilizer
	298, b	Hydroxyzine HCl	25mg	Orange	Tab	Round	N	Y	Barr	Antipruritic
	dp 298	Salsalate	500mg	Yellow	Tab	Round	N	Y	Duramed	Antiinflammatory
	Sch. Logo 298	Ethinyl Estradiol	0.02mg	Beige	Tab	Round	N	Y	Schering	Hormone
	West–ward 298	Thioridazine Hydrochloride	25mg	Yellow	Tab	Round	N	Y	West–ward	Tranquilizer
299	299, barr	Hydroxyzine HCl	50mg	Orange	Tab	Round	N	Y	Barr	Antipruritic
	54–299	Dexamethasone	0.5mg	Yellow	Tab	Round	Y	N	Roxane	Steroid
	dp 299	Salsalate	750mg	Yellow	Tab	Capsule	N	Y	Duramed	Antiinflammatory
	West–ward 299	Thioridazine Hydrochloride	50mg	Pink	Tab	Round	N	Y	West–ward	Tranquilizer
300	300	Cimetidine	300mg	Green	Tab	Round	–	Y	SKB	Anti–ulcer

ID NO.	ID CODE	GENERIC NAME	STRENGTH	COLOR	FORM	SHAPE	SCORED	COATED	MFG.	USE
	300, barr	Hydroxyzine HCl	100mg	Orange	Tab	Round	N	Y	Barr	Antipruritic
	3M/SR 300	Theophylline SR	300mg	White	Tab	Oval	Y	N	3M	Bronchodilator
	832/L–300	Lithium Carbonate	300mg	White	Cap	–	–	–	PBI	Tranquilizer
	dp 300	Levothyroxine Sodium	0.3mg	Green	Tab	Oval	Y	N	Daniels	Hormone
	Flint 300	Levothyroxine Sodium	300mcg	Green	Tab	Round	Y	N	Boots	Hormone
	Forest 300	Theophylline SR	300mg	White	Tab	Capsule	–	N	Forest	Bronchodilator
	Horner 300mg	Ibuprofen	300mg	Yellow	Cap	–	–	–	Horner	Anti–Inflammatory
	M 300	Levothyroxine Sodium	0.3mg	Green	Tab	Round	Y	N	Duramed	Hormone
	M 300 LEVO T	Levothyroxine Sodium	0.3mg	Green	Tab	Round	Y	N	Mova	Hormone
	Triangle 300	Propafenone HCl	300mg	White	Tab	Round	Y	Y	Knoll	Antiarrhythmic
	Watson 300	Furosemide	20mg	White	Tab	Round	N	N	Watson	Diuretic
	West–ward 300	Ibuprofen	400mg	White	Tab	Round	N	Y	West–ward	Anti–Inflammatory
	WHR 300	Theophylline	300mg	White/Clear	Cap	–	–	–	Rorer	Bronchodilator
301	301, b	Hydroxyzine HCl	10mg	Yellow	Tab	Round	N	Y	Barr	Antipruritic
	dp 301	Methylprednisolone	4mg	White	Tab	Oval	Y	N	Duramed	Steroid
	SL 301	Nitroglycerin TD	2.5mg	Lavender/Clear	Cap	–	–	–	Sidmak	Antianginal
	Watson 301	Furosemide	40mg	White	Tab	Round	Y	N	Watson	Diuretic
302	54–302	Calcium Carbonate	1250mg	White	Tab	Capsule	Y	Y	Roxane	Antacid
	879 G302	Diphenhydramine HCl	25mg	Pink/Clear	Cap	–	–	–	Halsey	Antihistamine
	barr/302, 50	Hydroxyzine Pamoate	50mg	Ivory/Maroon	Cap	–	–	–	Barr	Antianxiety
	SL 302	Nitroglycerin TD	6.5mg	Blue/Clear	Cap	–	–	–	Sidmak	Antianginal
	Watson 302	Furosemide	80mg	White	Tab	Round	Y	N	Watson	Diuretic
	West–ward 302	Thioridazine Hydrochloride	100mg	White	Tab	Round	N	Y	West–ward	Tranquilizer
	West–ward 302	Ibuprofen	600mg	White	Tab	Oblong	N	Y	West–ward	Anti–Inflammatory
303	54–303	Propantheline Bromide	15mg	White	Tab	Round	N	Y	Roxane	Antispasmodic
	879 G303	Diphenhydramine HCl	50mg	Pink	Cap	–	–	–	Halsey	Antihistamine
	Royce logo 303/325	Quinine Sulfate	324mg	White	Cap	–	–	–	Royce	Muscle Relaxant
	SL 303	Nitroglycerin TD	9mg	Green/Yellow	Cap	–	–	–	Sidmak	Antianginal
	Watson 303	Indomethacin	25mg	Green	Cap	–	–	–	Watson	Anti–Inflammatory
	West–ward 303	Thioridazine Hydrochloride	150mg	Green	Tab	Round	N	Y	West–ward	Tranquilizer
304	Adria/304	Potassium Chloride	10 mEq	Green	Tab	Capsule	N	Y	Adria	Potassium Supp.
	Par 304	Divalproex sodium	250mg	Peach	Tab	Round	N	N	Par	Anticonvulsant
	Watson 304	Indomethacin	50mg	Green	Cap	–	–	–	Watson	Anti–Inflammatory
	West–ward 304	Thioridazine Hydrochloride	200mg	Orange	Tab	Round	N	Y	West–ward	Tranquilizer
	West–ward 304	Ibuprofen	800mg	White	Tab	Oblong	N	Y	West–ward	Anti–Inflammatory
305	305	Hematinic Concentrate with IF	n/a	–	Cap	–	–	–	Marlop	Vitamin
	Par 305	Divalproex sodium	500mg	Lavender	Tab	Round	N	N	Par	Anticonvulsant
	PFIZER 305	Azithromycin	250mg	Red	Cap	–	–	–	Pfizer	Anti–Infective
	TP305	Colchicine	648mcg	White	Tab	Round	N	N	Towne Paulsen	Antigout
	Watson 305	Propranolol	10mg	Orange	Tab	Round	–	–	Watson	Antihypertensive
306	Watson 306	Propranolol	20mg	Blue	Tab	Round	–	–	Watson	Antihypertensive
	West–ward	Metoclopramide	10mg	White	Tab	Round	N	N	West–ward	Anit–Reflux
307	93 307	Clemastine Fumarate	1.34mg	White	Tab	Round	Y	N	Lemmon	Antihistamine
	Adria/307	Potassium Chloride	6.7mEq	Yellow	Tab	Round	N	Y	Adria	Potassium Supp.
	Watson 307	Propranolol	40mg	Green	Tab	Round	–	–	Watson	Antihypertensive
	West–ward 307	Trifluoperazine Hydrochloride	1mg	Lavender	Tab	Round	N	Y	West–ward	Tranquilizer
308	13/308	Potassium Chloride	10mEq	Green	Cap	–	–	–	Adria	Potassium Supp.
	93 308	Clemastine Fumarate	2.68mg	White	Tab	Round	Y	N	Lemmon	Antihistamine
	Watson 308	Propranolol	80mg	Yellow	Tab	Round	–	–	Watson	Antihypertensive
309	GLAXO 309	Phenylpropanolamine/Chlorpheniramine	75mg/8mg	Pink/Clear	Cap	–	–	–	Glaxo	Decongestant Comb.
	Royce logo 309/10	Doxepin HCl	10mg	Scarlet/Pink	Cap	–	–	–	Royce	Antidepressant
	SL 309	Hydroxyzine HCl	50mg	White	Tab	Round	N	Y	Sidmak	Antipruritic
	SL 309	Hydroxyzine HCl	50mg	White	Tab	Round	N	Y	Sidmak	Antipruritic
	West–ward 309	Trifluoperazine Hydrochloride	2mg	Lavender	Tab	Round	N	Y	West–ward	Tranquilizer
	Wyeth 309	Ampicillin	500mg	Pink/Purple	Cap	–	–	–	Wyeth	Anti–Infective
310	310	Hematinic	n/a	–	Tab	–	–	–	Marlop	Vitamin
	Royce logo 310/25	Doxepin HCl	25mg	Blue/Pink	Cap	–	–	–	Royce	Antidepressant
311	311	Hematinic	n/a	Brown	Tab	–	–	–	Marlop	Vitamin
	93 311	Loperamide	2mg	Brown	Cap	–	–	–	Lemmon	Antidiarrheal
	dp 311	Prednisone	5mg	White	Tab	Round	Y	N	Duramed	Steroid
	Royce logo 311/50	Doxepin HCl	50mg	Flesh/Pink	Cap	–	–	–	Royce	Antidepressant
	Sch. Logo 311	Methyltestosterone	10mg	White	Tab	Round	N	N	Schering	Hormone
	Watson 311	Furosemide	20mg	White	Tab	Oval	N	N	Watson	Diuretic
	West–ward 311	Trifluoperazine Hydrochloride	5mg	Lavender	Tab	Round	N	Y	West–ward	Tranquilizer
312	312	Therapeutic Multivitamin	n/a	–	Tab	–	–	–	Marlop	Vitamin
	Adria/312	Potassium Gluconate	5mEq	Purple	Tab	Capsule	N	Y	Adria	Potassium Supp.
	dp 312	Prednisone	10mg	White	Tab	Round	Y	N	Duramed	Steroid
	SL 312	Dipyridamole	50mg	White	Tab	Round	N	Y	Sidmak	Antiplatelet
	Watson 312	Metoclopramide	10mg	White	Tab	Round	N	N	Watson	Antireflux
313	313	Therapeutic Multivitamin with Minerals	n/a	–	Tab	–	–	–	Marlop	Vitamin
	dp 313	Prednisone	20mg	Orange	Tab	Round	Y	N	Duramed	Steroid
	Sch. Logo 313	Perphenazine	8mg	Gray	Tab	Round	N	Y	Schering	Tranquilizer
	SL 313	Dipyridamole	75mg	White	Tab	Round	N	Y	Sidmak	Antiplatelet
	West–ward 313	Trifluoperazine Hydrochloride	10mg	Lavender	Tab	Round	N	Y	West–ward	Tranquilizer
314	dp 314	Prochlorperazine	5mg	Yellow	Tab	Round	N	Y	Duramed	Antiemetic
	SL 314	Cyproheptadine	4mg	White	Tab	Round	Y	N	Sidmak	Antipruritic
	WC 314	Amoxapine	25mg	White	Tab	Round	N	N	WC	Antidepressant
315	315	Hematinic	n/a	Red	Cap	–	–	–	Marlop	Vitamin
	dp 315	Prochlorperazine	10mg	Yellow	Tab	Round	N	Y	Duramed	Antiemetic
	WC 315	Amoxapine	50mg	Salmon	Tab	Round	N	N	WC	Antidepressant
316	dp 316	Prochlorperazine	25mg	Yellow	Tab	Round	N	Y	Duramed	Antiemetic
	GLAXO 316	Vitamin Combination	n/a	Black/Orange	Cap	–	–	–	Glaxo	Vitamin
	Russ 316	Vitamin/Mineral Comb.	n/a	Orange/Black	Cap	–	–	–	Eon	Vitamin/Mineral
	Sch. Logo 316	Fluphenazine HCL	10mg	Red	Tab	Oval	Y	N	Schering	Tranquilizer
	WC 316	Amoxapine	100mg	Blue	Tab	Round	N	N	WC	Antidepressant
317	317, b	Propoxyphene Napsylate & Acetaminophen	50mg/325mg	White	Tab	Capsule	N	Y	Barr	Analgesic
	879 317	Dextroamphetamine Sulfate	10mg	Yellow	Tab	Round	Y	N	Halsey	Psychostimulant
	M 317	Cimetidine	300mg	Green	Tab	Pentagonal	N	Y	Mylan	Antiulcer
	R 317	Fenoprofen Calcium	600mg	Yellow	Tab	Capsule	Y	Y	Purepac	Anti–Inflammatory
	S15/Wyeth 317	Oxazepam	15mg	Yellow	Tab	Pentagonal	N	N	Wyeth	Antianxiety
	WC 317	Amoxapine	150mg	Peach	Tab	Round	N	N	WC	Antidepressant
318	318, barr	Propoxyphene Napsylate & Acetaminophen	100mg/650mg	White	Tab	Capsule	N	Y	Barr	Analgesic
	318, barr	Propoxyphene Napsylate & Acetaminophen	100mg/650mg	Orange	Tab	Capsule	N	Y	Barr	Analgesic
	SL 318	Papaverine HCl TD	150mg	Brown/Clear	Cap	–	–	–	Sidmak	
319	WC 319	Hydrocodone Bitartrate with Acetaminophen	7.5mg/500mg	White	Tab	Capsule	Y	N	WC	Analgesic

ID NO.	ID CODE	GENERIC NAME	STRENGTH	COLOR	FORM	SHAPE	SCORED	COATED	MFG.	USE
320	320	Pancrelipase	8mg/30mg/30mg	Off White	Tab	Round	Y	N	Econolab	Enzyme
	KREMERS–URBAN 320	Nitroglycerin SR	2.5mg	Violet/Clear	Cap	–	–	–	KV	Antianginal
	P–D 320	Ethopropazine	10mg	White	Tab	Round	N	N	PD	Antiparkinson
	SL 320	Florvite Chewable	n/a	Wh./Orange fleck	Tab	Round	N	N	Sidmak	Vitamin
	West–ward 320	Hydroxyzine Pamoate	25mg	Ivory/Fuchsia	Cap	–	–	–	West–ward	Antianxiety
321	barr/321	Sulfamethoxazole & Trimethoprim	400mg/80mg	White	Tab	Capsule	Y	N	Barr	Anti–Infective
	M/321	Lorazepam	0.5mg	White	Tab	Round	N	N	Mylan	Antianxiety
	P–D 321	Ethopropazine	50mg	White	Tab	Round	Y	N	PD	Antiparkinson
	R 321	Propranolol	60mg	Pink	Tab	Round	Y	N	Purepac	Antihypertensive
	SL 321 10	Isoxsuprine HCl	10mg	White	Tab	Round	N	N	Sidmak	Vasodilator
322	barr/322	Sulfamethoxazole & Trimethoprim	800mg/160mg	White	Tab	Oval	Y	N	Barr	Anti–Infective
	SL 322 20	Isoxsuprine HCl	20mg	White	Tab	Round	Y	N	Sidmak	Vasodilator
323	barr/323, 25	Hydroxyzine Pamoate	25mg	Ivory/Fushia	Cap	–	–	–	Barr	Antianxiety
	EL 323	Pancreatic Enzyme	n/a	–	Cap	–	–	–	Anabolic	Enzyme
	SL 323	Bethanechol Chloride	5mg	White	Tab	Round	Y	N	Sidmak	Urinary Tract Agent
	WC 323	Methyldopa	250mg	White	Tab	Round	N	Y	WC	Antihypertensive
324	barr/324, 100	Hydroxyzine Pamoate	100mg	Ivory/Fushia	Cap	–	–	–	Barr	Antianxiety
	G 324	Chloral Hydrate	500mg	Red	Cap	–	–	–	R. P. Scherer	Hypnotic
	SL 324	Bethanechol Chloride	10mg	White	Tab	Round	Y	N	Sidmak	Urinary Tract Agent
	SL 324	Bethanechol Chloride	10mg	White	Tab	Round	Y	N	Sidmak	Urinary Tract Agent
	WC 324	Methyldopa	500mg	White	Tab	Round	N	Y	WC	Antihypertensive
325	93–325	Desipramine HCl	25mg	Lavender	Tab	Round	N	Y	Lemmon	Antidepressant
	barr – 325	Hydrocodone Bitartrate with Acetaminophen	5mg/500mg	White	Tab	Capsule	Y	N	Barr	Analgesic
	dp 325	Tolazamide	100mg	White	Tab	Round	Y	N	Duramed	Hypoglycemic
	Royce logo 303/325	Quinine Sulfate	324mg	White	Cap	–	–	–	Royce	Muscle Relaxant
	SL 325	Bethanechol Chloride	25mg	Yellow	Tab	Round	Y	N	Sidmak	Urinary Tract Agent
	West–ward 325	Hydroxyzine Pamoate	50mg	Ivory/Red	Cap	–	–	–	West–ward	Antianxiety
	West–ward 325	Temazepam	15mg	Green/White	Cap	–	–	–	West–ward	Hypnotic
326	93–326	Desipramine HCl	50mg	Blue	Tab	Round	N	Y	Lemmon	Antidepressant
	dp 326	Tolazamide	250mg	White	Tab	Round	Y	N	Duramed	Hypoglycemic
	SL 326	Bethanechol Chloride	50mg	Yellow	Tab	Round	Y	N	Sidmak	Urinary Tract Agent
327	93–327	Desipramine HCl	75mg	White	Tab	Round	N	Y	Lemmon	Antidepressant
	barr, 327	Thioridazine HCl	150mg	Green	Tab	Round	N	Y	Barr	Tranquilizer
	dp 327	Tolazamide	500mg	White	Tab	Round	Y	N	Duramed	Hypoglycemic
	Mylan 327	Haloperidol	5mg	Orange	Tab	Round	Y	N	Mylan	Tranquilizer
	SL 327	Hydralazine HCl	25mg	Orange	Tab	Round	N	N	Sidmak	Antihypertensive
	West–ward 327	Temazepam	30mg	White/White	Cap	–	–	–	West–ward	Hypnotic
328	93–328	Desipramine HCl	100mg	Butterscotch	Tab	Round	N	Y	Lemmon	Antidepressant
	barr, 328	Thioridazine HCl	200mg	Orange	Tab	Round	N	Y	Barr	Tranquilizer
	SL 328	Hydralazine HCl	50mg	Orange	Tab	Round	N	N	Sidmak	Antihypertensive
	WC 328	Verapamil HCl	80mg	White	Tab	Round	–	–	WC	Antiarrhythmic
329	54–329	Indomethacin	50mg	–	Cap	–	–	–	Roxane	Anti–Inflammatory
	b, 329	Thioridazine HCl	15mg	Blue	Tab	Round	N	Y	Barr	Tranquilizer
	SL 329	Cyclandelate	200mg	Orange/Orange	Cap	–	–	–	Sidmak	Vasodilator
	WC 329	Verapamil HCl	120mg	White	Tab	Round	–	–	WC	Antiarrhythmic
330	West–ward 329	Triamterene & Hydrochlorothiazide	50mg/25mg	Maroon	Cap	–	–	–	West–ward	Diuretic
	BOCK 330	Ferrous Fumarate/Docusate Na/Vitamin C	110/20/200mg	Beige	Tab	Round	N	Y	Bock	Hematinic Agent
	KREMERS–URBAN 330	Nitroglycerin SR	6.5mg	Blue/Orange	Cap	–	–	–	KV	Antianginal
	MYLAN/330	Perphenazine & Amitriptyline	2mg/10mg	White	Tab	Round	N	Y	Mylan	Antidepressant
	R 330	Penicillin V Potassium	500mg	White	Tab	Round	Y	N	Rondex	Anti–Infective
	SL 330	Cyclandelate	400mg	Green/White	Cap	–	–	–	Sidmak	Vasodilator
	West–ward 330	Hydroxyzine Pamoate	100mg	Ivory/Fuchsia	Cap	–	–	–	West–ward	Antianxiety
	West–ward 330	Methyltestosterone	25mg	Yellow	Tab	Round	Y	N	West–ward	Hormone
331	barr,331	Disopyramide Phosphate	100mg	Blue/Red	Cap	–	–	–	Barr	Antiarrhythmic
	R 331	Propranolol	40mg	Green	Tab	Round	Y	N	Purepac	Antihypertensive
	SL 331	Disulfiram	250mg	White	Tab	Round	N	N	Sidmak	Alcohol Deterrent
332	barr,332	Disopyramide Phosphate	150mg	Red/Ivory	Cap	–	–	–	Barr	Antiarrhythmic
	dp 332	Propranolol & Hydrochlorothiazide	40mg/25mg	Yellow	Tab	Round	Y	N	Duramed	Antihypertensive
	SL 332	Disulfiram	500mg	White	Tab	Round	N	N	Sidmak	Alcohol Deterrent
	Watson 332 /0.5	Lorazepam	0.5mg	White	Tab	Round	Y	N	Watson	Antianxiety
	West–ward 332	Vitamin B Complex	n/a	Yellow	Tab	Capsule	N	Y	West–ward	Vitamin
333	54–333	Propranolol HCl	40mg	White	Tab	Round	N	N	Roxane	Antihypertensive
	barr, E–BASE 333mg	Erythromycin Delayed–Release	333mg	White	Tab	Capsule	N	Y	Barr	Anti–Infective
	barr, E–BASE 333mg	Erythromycin Delayed–Release	333mg	White	Tab	Round	N	Y	Barr	Anti–Infective
	dp 333	Propranolol & Hydrochlorothiazide	80mg/25mg	Yellow	Tab	Round	Y	N	Duramed	Antihypertensive
	PP–333	Meprobamate & Aspirin	200mg/325mg	White/Green	Tab	Round	Y	N	Eon	Analgesic
	R 333	Propranolol HCl	80mg	Yellow	Tab	Round	–	N	Rondex	Antihypertensive
	R 333	Propranolol	80mg	Yellow	Tab	Round	Y	N	Purepac	Antihypertensive
	SL 333	Metronidazole	250mg	White	Tab	Round	N	N	Sidmak	Anti–Infective
	Watson 333/1.0	Lorazepam	1mg	White	Tab	Round	Y	N	Watson	Antianxiety
334	SL 334	Metronidazole	500mg	White	Tab	Oblong	N	N	Sidmak	Anti–Infective
	Watson 334/2.0	Lorazepam	2mg	White	Tab	Round	Y	Y	Watson	Antianxiety
	WC 334	Levothyroxine Sodium	0.25mg	Orange	Tab	Round	–	N	WC	Hormone
335	Royce logo 335/10	Piroxicam	10mg	Blue/White	Cap	–	–	–	Royce	Anti–inflammatory
	SL 335	Ethaverine HCl TD	100mg	Blue/Clear	Cap	–	–	–	Sidmak	Vasodilator
336	barr/336	Indomethacin	25mg	Green/Green	Cap	–	–	–	Barr	Anti–Inflammatory
	R 336	Prednisone	5mg	White	Tab	Round	Y	N	Purepac	Steroid
	Royce logo 336/20	Piroxicam	20mg	Blue	Cap	–	–	–	Royce	Anti–inflammatory
	SL 336	Ethaverine HCl	100mg	Yellow	Tab	Oval	N	N	Sidmak	Vasodilator
	WC 336	Levothyroxine Sodium	0.5mg	White	Tab	Round	–	N	WC	Hormone
337	West–ward 336	Acetaminophen	325mg	White	Tab	Round	Y	N	West–ward	Analgesic
	barr/337	Indomethacin	50mg	Green/Green	Cap	–	–	–	Barr	Anti–Inflammatory
	P–D 337	Vitamin Combination	n/a	Blue/Blue Band	Cap	–	–	–	PD	Vitamin
	R 337	Prednisone	20mg	Peach	Tab	Round	Y	N	Purepac	Steroid
	SL 337	Nylidrin HCl	6mg	White	Tab	Round	Y	N	Sidmak	Vasodilator
338	R 338	Prednisone	10mg	White	Tab	Round	Y	N	Purepac	Steroid
	SL 338	Nylidrin HCl	12mg	White	Tab	Round	Y	N	Sidmak	Vasodilator
	WC 338	Levothyroxine Sodium	0.075mg	Violet	Tab	Round	–	N	WC	Hormone
339	54 339	Prednisone	2.5mg	White	Tab	Round	Y	N	Roxane	Steroid
	SL 339	Procainamide HCl TD	250mg	Blue	Tab	Oval	N	Y	Sidmak	Antiarrhythmic
340	West–ward 339	Acetaminophen	500mg	White	Tab	Round	Y	N	West–ward	Analgesic
	KREMERS–URBAN 340	Nitroglycerin SR	9mg	Clear	Cap	–	–	–	KV	Antianginal
	SL 340	Procainamide HCl TD	500mg	Pink	Tab	Oval	N	Y	Sidmak	Antiarrhythmic
341	879 341	Isoniazid	300mg	White	Tab	Round	N	N	Halsey	Anti–Infective
	SL 341	Sulfamethoxazole & Trimethoprim	400mg/80mg	White	Tab	Round	Y	N	Sidmak	Anti–Infective

ID NO.	ID CODE	GENERIC NAME	STRENGTH	COLOR	FORM	SHAPE	SCORED	COATED	MFG.	USE
342	WC 341	Levothyroxine Sodium	0.1mg	Yellow	Tab	Round	–	N	WC	Hormone
	RIKER/342	Theophylline	125mg	White	Tab	Round	Y	N	3M	Bronchodilator
	SL 342	Sulfamethoxazole & Trimethoprim	800mg/160mg	White	Tab	Oval	Y	N	Sidmak	Anti–Infective
343	54 343	Prednisone	50mg	White	Tab	Round	Y	N	Roxane	Steroid
	SL 343	Papaverine HCl HP	300mg	Peach	Tab	Oval	Y	N	Sidmak	–
	Watson 343	Verapamil	80mg	White	Tab	Round	Y	N	Watson	Antihypertensive
	WC 343	Levothyroxine Sodium	0.125mg	Brown	Tab	Round	–	N	WC	Hormone
344	Watson 344	Verapamil	80mg	Peach	Tab	Round	–	N	Watson	Antihypertensive
	WC 344	Levothyroxine Sodium	0.15mg	Blue	Tab	Round	–	N	WC	Hormone
345	E 345	Caramiphen Edisylate/Phenylpropanolamine	40mg/75mg	White/Clear	Cap	–	–	–	Eon	Decongestant Comb.
	Mylan 345	Diazepam	5mg	Orange	Tab	Round	Y	N	Mylan	Antianxiety
	PP 345	Phenylpropanolamine HCl / Caramiphen Edisylate	75mg/40mg	White/Clear	Cap	–	–	–	Eon	Antitussive Comb.
	Royce logo 345/10	Hydroxyzine HCl	10mg	Orange	Tab	Round	N	Y	Royce	Antipruritic
	Watson 345	Verapamil	120mg	White	Tab	Round	N	N	Watson	Antihypertensive
346	Forest 346	Rauwolfia Serpentina	50mg	Blue	Tab	Round	–	Y	Forest	Antihypertensive
	R 346	Procainamide HCl	500mg	Orange	Cap	–	–	–	Rondex	Antiarrhythmic
	Royce logo 346/25	Hydroxyzine HCl	25mg	Green	Tab	Round	N	Y	Royce	Antipruritic
	SL 346	Isosorbide Dinitrate SL	10mg	White	Tab	Round	N	N	Sidmak	Antianginal
	Watson 346	Verapamil	120mg	Peach	Tab	Round	–	–	Watson	Antihypertensive
347	347, barr	Chlorpropamide	100mg	White	Tab	Round	N	N	Barr	Hypoglycemic
	Mylan 347	Propranolol HCl and Hydrochlorothiazide	80mg/25 mg	White	Tab	Round	Y	N	Mylan	Antihypertensive
	Royce logo 347/50	Hydroxyzine HCl	50mg	Yellow	Tab	Round	N	Y	Royce	Antipruritic
	SL 347	Isosorbide Dinitrate	5mg	Pink	Tab	Round	Y	N	Sidmak	Antianginal
	WC 347	Levothyroxine Sodium	0.2mg	Pink	Tab	Round	–	N	WC	Hormone
348	R 348	Propylthiouracil	50mg	White	Tab	Round	Y	N	Purepac	Antithyroid
	R/348	Propylthiouracil	50mg	White	Tab	Round	Y	N	Rondex	Antithyroid
	SL 348	Isosorbide Dinitrate	10mg	White	Tab	Round	Y	N	Sidmak	Antianginal
	Watson 348	Triamterene & Hydrochlorothiazide	75mg/50mg	Yellow	Tab	Round	–	–	Watson	Diuretic
	WC 348	Levothyroxine Sodium	0.3mg	Green	Tab	Round	–	N	WC	Hormone
349	barr, 349	Chlorpropamide	100mg	Blue	Tab	Round	N	N	Barr	Hypoglycemic
	SL 349	Isosorbide Dinitrate	20mg	Green	Tab	Round	Y	N	Sidmak	Antianginal
	Watson 349	Hydrocodone Bitartrate with Acetaminophen	5mg/500mg	White	Tab	Capsule	Y	N	Watson	Analgesic
350	93 350 / 4	Acetaminophen & Codeine	300mg/60mg	White	Tab	Round	N	N	Lemmon	Analgesic
	barr, 350	Chlorpropamide	250mg	Blue	Tab	Round	N	N	Barr	Hypoglycemic
	SL 350	Isosorbide Dinitrate	30mg	Blue	Tab	Round	N	N	Sidmak	Antianginal
351	Mylan 351	Haloperidol	0.5mg	Orange	Tab	Round	Y	N	Mylan	Tranquilizer
	SL 351	Isosorbide Dinitrate SR	40mg	Yellow	Tab	Round	Y	N	Sidmak	Antianginal
	WHR 351	Theophylline	100mg	White	Tab	Round	Y	N	Rorer	Bronchodilator
352	TP352	Zinc Sulfate	220mg	Pink	Cap	–	–	–	Towne Paulsen	Mineral
	Watson 352	Propranolol	60mg	Pink	Tab	Round	–	–	Watson	Antihypertensive
	WHR 352	Theophylline	200mg	White	Tab	Round	Y	N	Rorer	Bronchodilator
353	SL 353	Meclizine HCl	12.5mg	Blue/White	Tab	Oval	N	N	Sidmak	Antinauseant
	Watson 353	Propranolol	90mg	Lavender	Tab	Round	–	–	Watson	Antihypertensive
354	SL 354	Meclizine HCl	25mg	Yellow/White	Tab	Oval	N	N	Sidmak	Antinauseant
355	Forest 355	Racemethionine	200mg	Pink/Blue	Cap	–	–	–	Forest	–
	SL 355	Meclizine HCl Chewable	25mg	Pink	Tab	Round	N	N	Sidmak	Antinauseant
356	Ascher logo 225/356	Magnesium salicate/Phenyltoloxamine citrate	600mg/30mg	White	Tab	Capsule	Y	N	B.F.Ascher	Analgesic
	R 356	Quinidine Sulfate	200mg	White	Tab	Round	Y	N	Purepac	Antiarrhythmic
357	357 Magnum	Caffeine	200mg	Pink	Tab	Bullet	Y	N	B & M Labs	Stimulant
	barr, 357	Methyldopa	125mg	White	Tab	Round	N	Y	Barr	Antihypertensive
358	Watson 357	Methyldopa & Hydrochlorothiazide	250mg/15mg	White	Tab	Round	N	N	Watson	Antihypertensive
	879 358	Quinidine Sulfate	200mg	White	Tab	Round	Y	N	Halsey	Antiarrhythmic
	barr, 358	Methyldopa	250mg	White	Tab	Round	N	Y	Barr	Antihypertensive
	R 358	Propranolol HCl & Hydrochlorothiazide	40mg/25mg	White	Tab	Round	Y	N	Purepac	Antihypertensive
	R/358	Propranolol HCl & Hydrochlorothiazide	40mg/25mg	White	Tab	Round	Y	N	Rondex	Antihypertensive
	Royce logo 358 5–50	Amiloride HCl & Hydrochlorothiazide	5mg/50mg	Peach	Tab	Round	Y	N	Royce	Antihypertensive
	Watson 358	Methyldopa & Hydrochlorothiazide	250mg/25mg	White	Tab	Round	N	N	Watson	Antihypertensive
359	832/G359	Fluoxmesterone	10mg	Green	Tab	Round	–	N	PBI	Hormone
	SL 359	Dexchlorpheniramine Maleate	2mg	Pink	Tab	Oval	N	N	Sidmak	Antihistamine
	Watson 359	Methyldopa & Hydrochlorothiazide	500mg/30mg	White	Tab	Round	N	N	Watson	Antihypertensive
360	54–360	Amitriptyline	75mg	White	Tab	Round	–	–	Roxane	Antidepressant
	879 360	Triprolidine HCl & Pseudoephedrine HCl	2.5mg/60mg	White	Tab	Round	Y	N	Halsey	Decongestant Comb.
	C/360–LL	Calcium/Vitamin D	–	Orange	Tab	Oblong	N	N	Lederle	Vitamin
	PP–360 & 2	Acetaminophen & Codeine	300mg/15mg	White	Tab	Round	N	N	Eon	Analgesic
	R 360	Propranolol HCl & Hydrochlorothiazide	80mg/25mg	White	Tab	Round	Y	N	Purepac	Antihypertensive
	R/360	Propranolol HCl & Hydrochlorothiazide	80mg/25mg	White	Tab	Round	Y	N	Rondex	Antihypertensive
	Watson 360	Methyldopa & Hydrochlorothiazide	500mg/50mg	White	Tab	Round	N	N	Watson	Antihypertensive
	Wyeth 360	Dicloxacillin Sodium Monohydrate	250mg	Purple/White	Cap	–	–	–	Wyeth	Anti–Infective
361	361	Yohimbine HCl	5.4mg	White	Tab	Round	Y	N	Royce	Sympathicolytic
	Royce loge 361,5.4	Yohimbine HCl	5.4mg	White	Tab	Round	Y	N	Royce	Sympathicolytic
362	P–D 362	Extended Phenytoin Sodium	100mg	White/Orange Band	Cap	–	–	–	PD	Anticonvulsant
	SL 362	Chlorthalidone	25mg	Peach	Tab	Round	N	N	Sidmak	Diuretic
363	barr,555/363	Diazepam	5mg	Yellow	Tab	Round	Y	N	Barr	Antianxiety
	SL 363	Chlorthalidone	50mg	Blue	Tab	Round	Y	N	Sidmak	Diuretic
	Watson 363	Clorazepate Dipotassium	3.75mg	Blue	Tab	Round	N	N	Watson	Antianxiety
364	879 364	Chlordiazepoxide Hydrochloride	5mg	Yellow/Green	Cap	–	–	–	Halsey	Antianxiety
	dp 364	Isometheptene Mucate, Dichloralphenazone, APAP	65mg/100mg/325	Scarlet/White	Cap	–	–	–	Duramed	Vasodilator
	GLYBUR 364	Glyburide	5mg	Blue	Tab	Oblong	–	N	Copley	Hypoglycemic
	SL 364	Chlorthalidone	100mg	White	Tab	Round	Y	N	Sidmak	Diuretic
	Watson 364	Clorazepate Dipotassium	7.5mg	Biege	Tab	Round	N	N	Watson	Antianxiety
365	555/365	Propranolol	10mg	Peach	Tab	Round	Y	N	Barr	Antihypertensive
	879 365	Chlordiazepoxide	10mg	Green/Black	Cap	–	–	–	Halsey	Antianxiety
	879 365	Chlordiazepoxide Hydrochloride	10mg	Black/Green	Cap	–	–	–	Halsey	Antianxiety
	P–D 365	Extended Phenytoin Sodium	30mg	White/Pink Band	Cap	–	–	–	PD	Anticonvulsant
	PP–365 & 3	Acetaminophen & Codeine	300mg/30mg	White	Tab	Round	N	N	Eon	Analgesic
	Watson 365	Clorazepate Dipotassium	15mg	Pink	Tab	Round	N	N	Watson	Antianxiety
366	555/366	Propranolol	20mg	Blue	Tab	Round	Y	N	Barr	Antihypertensive
	832/G366C	Flurazepam Hydrochloride	15mg	Blue/White	Cap	–	–	–	PBI	Hypnotic
	879 366	Chlordiazepoxide	25mg	Green/White	Cap	–	–	–	Halsey	Antianxiety
	879 366	Chlordiazepoxide Hydrochloride	25mg	White/Green	Cap	–	–	–	Halsey	Antianxiety
367	Watson 366	Fenoprofen Calcium	600mg	Peach	Tab	Tablet	–	N	Watson	Antiinflammatory
	555/367	Propranolol	40mg	Green	Tab	Round	Y	N	Barr	Antihypertensive
	832/G367C	Flurazepam Hydrochloride	30mg	Blue/Blue	Cap	–	–	–	PBI	Hypnotic
	Watson 367	Fenoprofen Calcium	200mg	Yellow/White	Cap	–	–	–	Watson	Antiinflammatory
	West–ward 367	Flurazepam Hydrochloride	15mg	Blue/White	Cap	–	–	–	West–ward	Hypnotic

ID NO.	ID CODE	GENERIC NAME	STRENGTH	COLOR	FORM	SHAPE	SCORED	COATED	MFG.	USE
368	555/368	Propranolol	60mg	Pink	Tab	Round	Y	N	Barr	Antihypertensive
	832 G368	Folic Acid	1mg	–	Tab	–	–	–	PBI	Vitamin
	879 G368	Folic Acid	1mg	Yellow	Tab	Round	Y	N	Halsey	Antianemic
	LEMMON 368	Pheniramine/Pyrilamine/Phenylpropan/Phenylephrine	12.5/12.5/25/2.	Blue/Blue	Cap	–	–	–	Lemmon	Decongestant Comb.
	R 368	Rauwolfia Serpentina	50mg	Red	Tab	Round	N	Y	Rondex	Antihypertensive
	R 368	Rauwolfia Serpentina	50mg	Red	Tab	Round	N	Y	Purepac	Antihypertensive
	SL 368	Amitriptyline HCl	50mg	Brown	Tab	Round	N	Y	Sidmak	Antidepressant
	Watson 368	Fenoprofen Calcium	300mg	Yellow	Cap	–	–	–	Watson	Antiinflammatory
369	54 369	Loperamide	2mg	Green	Cap	–	–	–	Roxane	Antidiarrheal
	555/369	Propranolol	80mg	Yellow	Tab	Round	Y	N	Barr	Antihypertensive
	SL 369	Amitriptyline HCl	75mg	Lavender	Tab	Round	N	Y	Sidmak	Antidepressant
	Watson 369	Loxapine	5mg	White	Cap	–	–	–	Watson	Tranquilizer
370	370, b	Lorazepam	0.5mg	White	Tab	Round	N	N	Barr	Antianxiety
	PP–370 & 4	Acetaminophen & Codeine	300mg/60mg	White	Tab	Round	N	N	Eon	Analgesic
	R 370	Rauwolfia Serpentina	100mg	Red	Tab	Round	N	Y	Purepac	Antihypertensive
	SL 370	Amitriptyline HCl	100mg	Orange	Tab	Round	N	Y	Sidmak	Antidepressant
	Watson 370	Loxapine	10mg	Yellow/White	Cap	–	–	–	Watson	Tranquilizer
	West–ward 370	Flurazepam Hydrochloride	30mg	Blue/Blue	Cap	–	–	–	West–ward	Hypnotic
371	371, b	Lorazepam	1mg	White	Tab	Round	Y	N	Barr	Antianxiety
	dp 371	Methyldopa	250mg	White	Tab	Round	N	Y	Duramed	Antihypertensive
	Glaxo 371	Labetalol HCl/Hydrochlorothiazide	100mg/25mg	Peach	Tab	Oval	N	Y	Glaxo	Antihypertensive
	SL 371	Amitriptyline HCl	150mg	Peach	Tab	Round	N	Y	Sidmak	Antidepressant
	Watson 371	Loxapine	25mg	Green/White	Cap	–	–	–	Watson	Tranquilizer
372	372, barr	Lorazepam	2mg	White	Tab	Round	Y	N	Barr	Antianxiety
	54–372	Calcium Gluconate	500mg	White	Tab	Capsule	–	–	Roxane	Mineral Supplement
	dp 372	Methyldopa	500mg	White	Tab	Round	N	Y	Duramed	Antihypertensive
	FOREST 372	Ferrous Fumarate	33.3mg (Fe)	Brown	Tab	Round	N	Y	Forest	Mineral
	Glaxo 372	Labetalol HCl/Hydrochlorothiazide	200mg/25mg	White	Tab	Oval	N	Y	Glaxo	Antihypertensive
	M 372	Cimetidine	400mg	Green	Tab	Pentagonal	Y	Y	Mylan	Anti-ulcer
	SL 372	Chlorpropamide	100mg	Blue	Tab	Round	Y	N	Sidmak	Hypoglycemic
373	Watson 372	Loxapine	50mg	Blue/White	Cap	–	–	–	Watson	Tranquilizer
	373,barr	Oxazepam	15mg	Yellow	Tab	Round	N	N	Barr	Antianxiety
	Glaxo 373	Labetalol HCl/Hydrochlorothiazide	300mg/25mg	Peach	Tab	Oval	N	Y	Glaxo	Antihypertensive
	P–D 373	Diphenhydramine HCl	50mg	Pink	Cap	–	–	–	PD	Antihistamine
	SL 373	Chlorpropamide	250mg	Blue	Tab	Round	Y	N	Sidmak	Hypoglycemic
374	Watson 373	Maprotiline HCl	25mg	Peach	Tab	Oval	N	N	Watson	Antidepressant
	Barr, 374	Oxazepam	10mg	White/White	Cap	–	–	–	Barr	Antianxiety
	R 374	Reserpine	0.1mg	White	Tab	Round	N	N	Purepac	Antihypertensive
	Watson 374	Maprotiline HCl	50mg	Peach	Tab	Round	N	N	Watson	Antidepressant
375	832/P37.5C	Phentermine HCl	37.5mg	Yellow	Tab	Round	–	–	PBI	Anorectic
	832/P37.5C	Phentermine HCl	37.5mg	White/Blue	Tab	Round	–	–	PBI	Anorectic
	Barr, 375	Oxazepam	15mg	Red/Red	Cap	–	–	–	Barr	Antianxiety
	CC 37.5	Phentermine HCl	37.5mg	Red/Black	Cap	–	–	–	Camall	Anorectic
	CC 37.5	Phentermine HCl	37.5mg	Black/Yellow	Cap	–	–	–	Camall	Anorectic
	CC 37.5	Phentermine HCl	37.5mg	Yellow/Yellow	Cap	–	–	–	Camall	Anorectic
	CC 37.5	Phentermine HCl	37.5mg	Black/Black	Cap	–	–	–	Camall	Anorectic
	CC 37.5	Phentermine HCl	37.5mg	Brown/Clear	Cap	–	–	–	Camall	Anorectic
	CC 37.5	Phentermine HCl	37.5mg	Green/Clear	Cap	–	–	–	Camall	Anorectic
	CC 37.5P	Phenylpropanolamine	37.5mg	Yellow	Tab	Round	–	–	Camall	Appetite Suppressant
	CC 37.5P	Phenylpropanolamine	37.5mg	White	Tab	Round	–	–	Camall	Appetite Suppressant
	CC 37.5P	Phenylpropanolamine	37.5mg	Pink	Tab	Round	–	–	Camall	Appetite Suppressant
	CC 37.5P	Phenylpropanolamine	37.5mg	Gray	Tab	Round	–	–	Camall	Appetite Suppressant
	CC 37.5P	Phenylpropanolamine	37.5mg	Peach	Tab	Round	–	–	Camall	Appetite Suppressant
	CC 37.5P	Phenylpropanolamine	37.5mg	Green	Tab	Round	–	–	Camall	Appetite Suppressant
	CC 37.5P	Phenylpropanolamine	37.5mg	White/Green Specks	Tab	Round	–	–	Camall	Appetite Suppressant
	P–D 375	Phenytoin Sodium & Phenobarbital	100mg/16mg	White/Red Band	Cap	–	–	–	PD	Anticonvulsant
	PFIZER 375	Polythiazide	1mg	White	Tab	Round	Y	N	Pfizer	Diuretic
	SIDMAK 375	Nystatin Vaginal	100,000 Units	White	Tab	Oval	N	N	Sidmak	Anti–Infective
	Watson 375	Maprotiline HCl	75mg	White	Tab	Oval	N	N	Watson	Antidepressant
376	Barr, 376	Oxazepam	30mg	Maroon/Maroon	Cap	–	–	–	Barr	Antianxiety
	PFIZER 376	Polythiazide	2mg	Yellow	Tab	Round	Y	N	Pfizer	Diuretic
	R 376	Reserpine	0.25mg	White	Tab	Round	Y	N	Purepac	Antihypertensive
	R/376	Reserpine	0.25mg	White	Tab	Round	Y	N	Rondex	Antihypertensive
377	Barr/377	Flurazepam HCl	15mg	White/Blue	Cap	–	–	–	Barr	Hypnotic
	PFIZER 377	Polythiazide	4mg	White	Tab	Round	Y	N	Pfizer	Diuretic
	SL 377	Doxycycline Hyclate DR	100mg	Opaque/Blue	Cap	–	–	–	Sidmak	Anti–Infective
378	Barr/378	Flurazepam HCl	30mg	Blue/Blue	Cap	–	–	–	Barr	Hypnotic
379	P–D 379	Chloramphenicol	250mg	White/Gray Band	Cap	–	–	–	PD	Anti–Infective
	Watson 379	Amoxapine	25mg	White	Tab	Round	Y	N	Watson	Antidepressant
380	STUART 380	Docusate Potassium	240mg	Brown	Cap	–	–	–	Stuart	Stool Softener
381	Watson 380	Amoxapine	50mg	Salmon	Tab	Round	Y	N	Watson	Antidepressant
	b 381	Meperidine HCl	50mg	White	Tab	Round	N	N	Barr	Analgesic
	Organon 381	Pancrelipase	n/a.	Green	Cap	–	–	–	Organon	Digestant
	SL 381	Phenylprop.,phenyleph.,phenyltolox.,chlorphenir.	40,10,15,5mg	Blue w blue specks	Tab	Round	N	N	Sidmak	Decongestant comb.
	Watson 381	Amoxapine	100mg	Blue	Tab	Round	Y	N	Watson	Antidepressant
382	54–382 10	Haloperidol	10mg	White	Tab	Round	Y	N	Roxane	Tranquilizer
	barr 382	Meperidine HCl	100mg	White	Tab	Round	N	N	Barr	Analgesic
	L/N 382 / 500	Clofibrate	500mg	Golden	Cap	–	–	–	Novopharm	Hyperlipidemia
	Watson 382	Amoxapine	150mg	Peach	Tab	Round	Y	N	Watson	Antidepressant
383	54–383	Methyldopa	500mg	–	Tab	Round	N	Y	Roxane	Antihypertensive
	barr, 383	Ergoloid Mesylates	1mg	White	Tab	Round	N	N	Barr	Vasodilator
	SL 383	Sidcon TD	n/a	White	Tab	Round	N	Y	Sidmak	Decongestant comb.
384	SL 384	Isosorbide Dinitrate SR	20mg	Pink	Tab	Round	Y	N	Sidmak	Antianginal
385	SL 385	Phenylpropanolamine HCl & Guaifenesin LA	75mg/400mg	Blue	Tab	Oval	Y	N	Sidmak	Decongestant Comb.
	Watson 385	Hydrocodone Bitartrate with Acetaminophen	7.5mg/500mg	White	Tab	Capsule	Y	N	Watson	Analgesic
386	R 386	Sulfisoxazole	500mg	White	Tab	Round	Y	N	Purepac	Anti–Infective
387	GLAXO 387	Cefuroxime Axetil	250mg	Green	Tab	Capsule	N	Y	Glaxo	Anti–Infective
	SL 387	Ibuprofen	400mg	White	Tab	Round	N	Y	Sidmak	Anti–Inflammatory
	Watson 387	Hydrocodone Bitartrate with Acetaminophen	7.5mg/750mg	White	Tab	Capsule	Y	N	Watson	Analgesic
388	barr, 388	Hydralazine HCl	10mg	Orange	Tab	Round	N	N	Barr	Antihypertensive
	Organon 388	Pancrelipase	n/a	Clear	Cap	–	–	–	Organon	Digestant
	R 388	Spironolactone	25mg	White	Tab	Round	Y	N	Purepac	Diuretic
	SL 388	Ibuprofen	600mg	White	Tab	Oval	N	Y	Sidmak	Anti–Inflammatory
389	252–389	Phenobarbital	100mg	White	Tab	Round	–	N	Bowman	Sedative
	barr/389	Hydralazine HCl	100mg	Orange	Tab	Round	N	N	Barr	Antihypertensive

ID NO.	ID CODE	GENERIC NAME	STRENGTH	COLOR	FORM	SHAPE	SCORED	COATED	MFG.	USE
	P–D 389	Bromodiphenhydramine	25mg	—	Cap	—	—	—	PD	Antihistamine
	Wyeth 389	Tetracycline HCl	250mg	Yellow/Blue	Cap	—	—	—	Wyeth	Anti–Infective
390	PD 390	Vitamin/Mineral Combination	n/a	Pink/Blue	Cap	—	—	—	PD	Prenatal Vitamin
	R 390	Spironolactone with Hydrochlorothiazide	25mg/25mg	White	Tab	Round	Y	N	Purepac	Diuretic
	SL 390	Salgesic–500	500mg	Yellow	Tab	Round	N	Y	Sidmak	Antiarthritic
391	Wyeth 390	Penicillin V Potassium	500mg	White	Tab	Round	Y	N	Wyeth	Anti–Infective
	SL 391	Salgesic–750	750mg	Yellow	Tab	Oblong	N	Y	Sidmak	Antiarthritic
393	Organon 393	Lipase/Protease/Amylase	n/a	Green/Clear	Cap	—	—	—	Organon	Digestive Enzyme
	P–D 393	Phensuximide	500mg	Orange	Cap	—	—	—	PD	Anticonvulsant
	PFIZER 393	Chlorpropamide	100mg	Blue	Tab	D–Shaped	Y	N	Pfizer	Hypoglycemic
	SL 393	Benztropine Mesylate	0.5mg	White	Tab	Round	Y	N	Sidmak	Antiparkinson
394	GLAXO 394	Cefuroxime Axetil	500mg	Blue	Tab	Capsule	N	Y	Glaxo	Anti–Infective
	PFIZER 394	Chlorpropamide	250mg	Blue	Tab	D–Shaped	Y	N	Pfizer	Hypoglycemic
	Sch. Logo 394	Reserpine & Trichlormethiazide	0.1mg/4mg	Peach	Tab	Round	Y	N	Schering	Antihypertensive
	SL 394	Benztropine Mesylate	1.0mg	White	Tab	Oval	Y	N	Sidmak	Antiparkinson
395	barr, 395	Phenylbutazone	100mg	Orange/Red	Tab	Round	N	Y	Barr	Anti–Inflammatory
	GLAXO 395	Cefuroxime Axetil	125mg	White	Tab	Capsule	N	Y	Glaxo	Anti–Infective
	SL 395	Benztropine Mesylate	2.0mg	White	Tab	Round	Y	N	Sidmak	Antiparkinson
396	b 396	Phenylbutazone	100mg	Blue	Cap	—	—	—	Barr	Anti–Inflammatory
	barr, 396	Phenylbutazone	100mg	Green/White	Cap	—	—	—	Barr	Anti–Inflammatory
	Schering 396	Clotrimazole Vaginal	500mg	White	Tab	Bullet shaped		N	N	Schering Antifungal
	SL 396	Procainamide HCl SR	750mg	Peach	Tab	Oval	Y	Y	Sidmak	Antiarrhythmic
397	b , 397	Clonidine	0.1mg	Yellow	Tab	Round	N	N	Barr	Antihypertensive
	R 397	Doxepin HCl	75mg	Green	Cap	—	—	—	Purepac	Antidepressant
	SL 397	Hydralazine HCl	100mg	Orange	Tab	Round	N	N	Sidmak	Antihypertensive
398	b , 398	Clonidine	0.2mg	White	Tab	Round	N	N	Barr	Antihypertensive
	R 398	Doxepin HCl	100mg	Green/White	Cap	—	—	—	Purepac	Antidepressant
	SL 398	Hydralazine HCl	10mg	Orange	Tab	Round	N	N	Sidmak	Antihypertensive
399	b , 399	Clonidine	0.3mg	Green	Tab	Round	N	N	Barr	Antihypertensive
400	832/M400	Tridihexethyl Chloride & Meprobamate	25mg/400mg	Yellow	Tab	Round	N	N	PBI	Antispasmodic
	ALRA IF 400	Ibuprofen	400mg	Orange	Tab	Round	N	Y	Alra	Anti–Inflammatory
	CL400	Ergotamine Tartrate & Caffeine	1mg/100mg	Beige	Tab	Round	N	Y	Geneva	Antimigraine
	Horner 400mg	Ibuprofen	400mg	Scarlet	Cap	—	—	—	Horner	Anti–Inflammatory
	IBU 400	Ibuprofen	400mg	White	Tab	Elongated	N	Y	Boots	Anti–Inflammatory
	M 400	Erythromycin Ethylsuccinate	400mg	Beige	Tab	Capsule	N	Y	Mylan	Anti–Infective
	Muro 400/60	Pseudoephedrine HCl/Guaifenesin	60mg/400mg	Purple Layered	Tab	—	Y	—	Central	Decongestant
	N 815 400	Tolmetin Sodium	400mg	Red	Cap	—	—	—	Novopharm	Anti–Inflammatory
	PF U400	Theophylline	400mg	White	Tab	Round	Y	N	PF	Bronchodilator
	R 400	Doxepin HCl	150mg	White	Cap	—	—	—	Purepac	Antidepressant
	Rufen 400	Ibuprofen	400mg	Magenta	Tab	Round	N	Y	Boots	Anti–Inflammatory
401	dp 401	Pseudoephedrine HCl & Guaifenesin	120mg/600mg	Yellow	Tab	Capsule	Y	Y	Duramed	Decongestant Comb.
	Mylan 401	Ibuprofen	400mg	White	Tab	Round	N	Y	Mylan	Anti–Inflammatory
	N 401/50	Atenolol	100mg	White	Tab	Round	N	N	Novopharm	Antihypertensive
	SEARLE 401	Ethynodiol Diacetate & Mestranol	1mg/0.1mg	White	Tab	Five–sided	N	N	Searle	Hormone
402	P&G 402	Etidronate Disodium	200mg	White	Tab	Rectangular	N	N	Norwich	Ca Metabolism Regul
	P–D 402	Ampicillin	250mg	Blue/Gray	Cap	—	—	—	PD	Anti–Infective
	Sch. Logo 402	Theophylline LA	125mg	Green/Yellow	Cap	—	—	—	Schering	Bronchodilator
	WC 402	Ampicillin	250mg	Blue/Gray	Cap	—	—	—	WC	Anti–Infective
403	H 403	Sulfamethoxazole	500mg	Green	Tab	Round	Y	N	Heather	Anti–Infective
	TP403	Hydrochlorothiazide	100mg	Peach	Tab	Round	N	N	Towne Paulsen	Diuretic
404	barr 404	Doxepin HCl	25mg	Ivory	Cap	—	—	—	Barr	Antidepressant
	P–D 404	Ampicillin	500mg	Blue/Gray	Cap	—	—	—	PD	Anti–Infective
	R 404	Tetracycline Hydrochloride	250mg	Orange/Yellow	Cap	—	—	—	Purepac	Anti–Infective
	SL 404	Extended Phenytoin Sodium	100mg	White	Cap	—	—	—	Sidmak	Anticonvulsant
	TP404	Hydrochlorothiazide	25mg	Peach	Tab	Round	N	N	Towne Paulsen	Diuretic
	Watson 404	Verapamil	40mg	Peach	Tab	Round	—	N	Watson	Antihypertensive
	WC 404	Ampicillin	500mg	Blue/Gray	Cap	—	—	—	WC	Anti–Infective
405	225/405	Chlorpheniramine Maleate/Phenylpropranolamine	12/75 mg	Clear	Cap	—	—	—	B.F.Ascher	Decongestant Comb.
	405 HD	Amitriptyline HCl	10mg	Pink	Tab	Round	N	Y	Halsey	Antidepressant
	barr 405	Doxepin HCl	50mg	Ivory	Cap	—	—	—	Barr	Antidepressant
	GG 405	Acetaminophen	500mg	White	Tab	Round	Y	N	Geneva	Analgesic
	TP405	Hydrochlorothiazide	50mg	Peach	Tab	Round	Y	N	Towne Paulsen	Diuretic
406	406 HD	Amitriptyline HCl	25mg	Green	Tab	Round	N	Y	Halsey	Antidepressant
	879 G406	Hydrochlorothiazide	25mg	Peach	Tab	Round	Y	N	Halsey	Diuretic
	barr 406	Doxepin HCl	75mg	Green	Cap	—	—	—	Barr	Antidepressant
	N E 406	Etidronate Disodium	400mg	White	Tab	Capsule	Y	N	Norwich	Ca Metabolism Regul
	R 406	Tetracycline Hydrochloride	500mg	Black/Yellow	Cap	—	—	—	Purepac	Anti–Infective
	R/406	Tetracycline HCl	500mg	Black/Yellow	Cap	—	—	—	Rondex	Anti–Infective
	SL 406	Indomethacin	25mg	Green/Green	Cap	—	—	—	Sidmak	Anti–Inflammatory
407	407 HD	Amitriptyline HCl	50mg	Brown	Tab	Round	N	Y	Halsey	Antidepressant
	879 G407	Hydrochlorothiazide	50mg	Peach	Tab	Round	Y	N	Halsey	Diuretic
	barr 407	Doxepin HCl	100mg	Green/White	Cap	—	—	—	Barr	Antidepressant
	GG 407/50	Chlorpromazine HCl	50mg	Butterscotch	Tab	Round	N	Y	Geneva	Tranquilizer
	P–D 407	Tetracycline HCl	250mg	Red/White	Cap	—	—	—	PD	Anti–Infective
	SL 407	Indomethacin	50mg	Green/Green	Cap	—	—	—	Sidmak	Anti–Inflammatory
408	WC 407	Tetracycline HCl	250mg	Red/White	Cap	—	—	—	WC	Anti–Infective
409	408 HD	Amitriptyline HCl	75mg	Purple	Tab	Round	N	Y	Halsey	Antidepressant
	409 HD	Amitriptyline HCl	100mg	Orange	Tab	Round	N	Y	Halsey	Antidepressant
	54–409 30	Morphine SR	30mg	White	Tab	Round	N	N	Roxane	Analgesic
	R 409	Cephalexin	250mg	Gray/Orange	Cap	—	—	—	Rondex	Anti–Infective
410	54–410	Levorphanol	2mg	White	Tab	Round	Y	N	Roxane	Analgesic
	SL 410	Carbamazepine	200mg	White	Tab	Round	Y	N	Sidmak	Anticonvulsant
411	13 411	Magnesium Salicylate	650mg	Pink	Tab	Capsule	N	N	Adria	Analgesic
	COPLEY 411	Methazolamide	25mg	White	Tab	Square	N	N	Copley	Antiglaucoma
	GG 411	Carisoprodol	350mg	White	Tab	Round	N	Y	Geneva	Muscle Relaxant
	MILES 411	Aluminum Sulfate & Calcium Acetate	n/a	White	Tab	Round	N	N	Miles	Astringent
	Pfizer 411	Glipizide	5mg	White	Tab	—	Y	N	Pfizer	Hypoglycemic
412	54–412	Codeine Sulfate	60mg	White	Tab	Round	Y	N	Roxane	Analgesic
	Adria/412	Magnesium Salicylate	545mg	Pink	Tab	Capsule	N	Y	Adria	Analgesic
	Pfizer 412	Glipizide	10mg	White	Tab	—	Y	N	Pfizer	Hypoglycemic
413	54–413	Aluminum Hydroxide	500mg	White	Tab	Round	—	—	Roxane	Antacid
414	GG 414	Metoprolol Tartrate	50mg	White	Tab	Oblong	—	N	Ciba	Antihypertensive
	Watson 414	Estropipate	0.75mg	Yellow	Tab	Round	—	N	Watson	Hormone
415	A 415	Ergoloid Mesylates	1mg	White	Tab	Oval	N	N	B.F.Ascher	Vasodilator
	barr, 415	Tolazamide	100mg	White	Tab	Round	Y	N	Barr	Hypoglycemic

ID NO.	ID CODE	GENERIC NAME	STRENGTH	COLOR	FORM	SHAPE	SCORED	COATED	MFG.	USE
	GG 415	Metoprolol Tartrate	100mg	White	Tab	Oblong	Y	N	Ciba	Antihypertensive
	MYLAN 415	Diphenoxylate HCl and Atropine Sulfate	2.5mg/0.025mg	White	Tab	Round	N	N	Mylan	Antidiarrheal
	SL 415	Griseofulvin w/PEG (ultramicrosize)	165mg	White	Tab	Oval	N	N	Sidmak	Antifungal
	Watson 415	Estropipate	1.5mg	Peach	Tab	Round	–	N	Watson	Hormone
416	barr, 416	Tolazamide	250mg	White	Tab	Round	Y	N	Barr	Hypoglycemic
	Forest 416	Hydrocodone & Acetaminophen	5mg/300mg	Green	Tab	Round	Y	N	Forest	Analgesic
	Forest 416	Hydrocodone & Acetaminophen	5mg/500mg	Green	Tab	Round	–	N	Forest	Analgesic
	GG416	Hydralazine HCl	50mg	Green	Tab	Round	N	Y	Geneva	Antihypertensive
	SL 416	Griseofulvin w/PEG (ultramicrosize)	330mg	White	Tab	Oval	N	N	Sidmak	Antifungal
	Watson 416	Estropipate	3mg	Blue	Tab	Round	–	N	Watson	Hormone
417	barr, 417	Tolazamide	500mg	White	Tab	Oval	Y	N	Barr	Hypoglycemic
	COPLEY 417	Metoprolol Tartrate	100mg	Blue	Tab	Capsule	Y	N	Copley	Antihypertensive
	GG 417	Naproxen Sodium	275mg	White	Tab	Oval	N	Y	Geneva	Anti–Inflammatory
	Watson 417	Estropipate	6mg	Green	Tab	Round	–	N	Watson	Hormone
418	GG 418	Naproxen Sodium	550mg	White	Tab	Oval	N	Y	Geneva	Anti–Inflammatory
	R 418	Cephalexin	500mg	Orange/Orange	Cap	–	–	–	Rondex	Anti–Infective
	Watson 418	Cyclobenzaprine HCl	10mg	White	Tab	Round	N	Y	Watson	Muscle Relaxant
419	barr/419	Ibuprofen	400mg	White	Tab	Round	N	Y	Barr	Anti–Inflammatory
	GG419	Trazodone	50mg	White	Tab	Round	Y	Y	Geneva	Antidepressant
420	420, barr	Ibuprofen	600mg	White	Tab	Oval	N	Y	Barr	Anti–Inflammatory
	832/G420	Hydroflumethiazide & Reserpine	50mg/0.125mg	Green	Tab	Round	–	–	PBI	Antihypertensive
	Adria/420	Magnesium Lactate	7mEq	Yellow	Tab	Capsule	–	–	Adria	Magnesium Supp.
	GG420	Trazodone	100mg	White	Tab	Round	Y	Y	Geneva	Antidepressant
	L/N 420–25	Indomethacin	25mg	Green	Cap	–	–	–	MP	Anti–Inflammatory
	N 420–25	Indomethacin	25mg	Green	Cap	–	–	–	Novopharm	Antiinflammatory
	WC 420	Quinine Sulfate	325mg	White	Tab	Round	–	–	WC	Muscle Relaxant
421	GG 421	Chlorzoxazone	250mg	Orange	Tab	Round	N	N	Geneva	Muscle Relaxant
	Mylan 421	Methyldopa	500mg	Beige	Tab	Capsule	N	Y	Mylan	Antihypertensive
	TP421/4	Aspirin with Codeine	325mg/60mg	White	Tab	Round	N	N	Towne Paulsen	Analgesic
422	54–422	Indomethacin	25mg	–	Cap	–	–	–	Roxane	Anti–Inflammatory
	GG 422	Chlorzoxazone	500mg	Orange	Tab	Round	N	N	Geneva	Muscle Relaxant
423	832/G423	Hydroxyzine HCl	10mg	Purple	Tab	Round	N	Y	PBI	Antipruritic
424	555/424 b	Metoclopramide	10mg	White	Tab	Round	Y	N	Barr	Antireflux
	832/G424	Hydroxyzine HCl	25mg	Purple	Tab	Round	N	Y	PBI	Antipruritic
	COPLEY 424	Methazolamide	50mg	White	Tab	Round	–	N	Copley	Antiglaucoma
	NPL 51081/424	Isometheptene/Dichloralphenzaone/APAP	65/100/325mg	White	Cap	–	–	–	Nutripharm Labs	Analgesic
	TP424/3	Aspirin with Codeine	325mg/30mg	White	Tab	Round	N	N	Towne Paulsen	Analgesic
	Watson 424	Triamterene & Hydrochlorothiazide	37.5mg/25mg	Green	Tab	Round	–	N	Watson	Diuretic
425	832/G425	Hydroxyzine HCl	50mg	Lavender	Tab	Round	N	Y	PBI	Antipruritic
	barr/425	Verapamil HCl	80mg	Beige	Tab	Round	Y	Y	Barr	Antiarrhythmic
	SL/425	Aspirin Enteric Coated	975mg	Pink	Tab	Capsule	N	Y	Sidmak	Analgesic
427	555/427,barr	Propranolol HCl & Hydrochlorothiazide	40mg/25mg	White	Tab	Round	N	N	Barr	Antihypertensive
	MYLAN 427	Sulindac	150mg	Yellow	Tab	Round	N	N	Mylan	Anti–Inflammatory
	SL 427	Phenylpropanolamine/PE/Guaifenesin	45mg/5mg/200mg	Orange/Beige	Cap	Capsule	–	–	Sidmak	Decongestant Comb.
428	555/428,barr	Propranolol HCl & Hydrochlorothiazide	80mg/25mg	White	Tab	Round	Y	N	Barr	Antihypertensive
429	555/429	Trimethoprim	100mg	White	Tab	Round	Y	N	Barr	Anti–Infective
	Forest 429	Phenobarbital/Sodium Nitrate	16mg/65mg	White	Tab	Round	–	Y	Forest	–
	SQUIBB 429	Fludrocortisone Acetate	0.1mg	–	Tab	–	–	–	Squibb	Steroid
430	555/430	Trimethoprim	200mg	White	Tab	Round	Y	N	Barr	Anti–Infective
	SL 430	Metoclopramide HCl	10mg	White	Tab	Round	Y	N	Sidmak	Antireflux
431	Watson 430	Carbidopa/Levodopa	10mg/100mg	Blue	Tab	Round	Y	N	Watson	Antiparkinson
	93 431	Chlorthalidone	50mg	Blue	Tab	Round	N	N	Lemmon	Diuretic
	GG431	Amitriptyline	50mg	Brown	Tab	Round	N	Y	Geneva	Antidepressant
	Sch. Logo 431	Albuterol Sulfate ER	4mg	White	Tab	Round	N	Y	Schering	Bronchodilator
	SCS 431	Norethindrone/Mestranol	1mg/50mcg	White	Tab	Round	–	N	Searle	Contraceptive
	SEARLE 431	Norethindrone/Mestranol	1mg/50mcg	White	Tab	Round	–	N	Searle	Contraceptive
	SQUIBB 431	Procainamide HCl	250mg	Yellow	Tab	Oblong	N	Y	Princeton	Antiarrhythmic
	Watson 431	Carbidopa/Levodopa	25mg/100mg	Tan	Tab	Round	N	N	Watson	Antiparkinson
	WC 431	Lorazepam	0.5mg	White	Tab	Round	Y	N	WC	Antianxiety
432	GG432	Conjugated Estrogens	0.3mg	White	Tab	Round	N	Y	Duramed	Hormone
	Watson 432	Carbidopa/Levodopa	25mg/250mg	Blue	Tab	Round	Y	N	Watson	Antiparkinson
	WC 432	Lorazepam	1mg	White	Tab	Round	–	N	WC	Antianxiety
433	93 433	Chlorthalidone	100mg	White	Tab	Round	Y	N	Lemmon	Diuretic
	GG433	Conjugated Estrogens	0.625mg	White	Tab	Round	N	Y	Duramed	Hormone
	GLYBUR 433	Glyburide	2.5mg	Pink	Tab	Oblong	–	N	Copley	Hypoglycemic
	SL 433	Trazodone HCl	50mg	White	Tab	Round	N	N	Sidmak	Antidepressant
	WC 433	Lorazepam	2mg	White	Tab	Round	N	N	WC	Antianxiety
434	GG434	Conjugated Estrogens	1.25mg	White	Tab	Round	N	Y	Duramed	Hormone
	SL 434	Trazodone HCl	100mg	White	Tab	Round	Y	N	Sidmak	Antidepressant
	SQUIBB 434	Procainamide HCl	375mg	Gold	Tab	Oblong	N	Y	Princeton	Antiarrhythmic
435	Wyeth 434	Promethazine & Pseudoephedrine	6.25mg/60mg	Orange/White	Tab	Round	Y	N	Wyeth	Decongestant Comb.
436	GG435	Conjugated Estrogens	2.5mg	White	Tab	Round	N	Y	Duramed	Hormone
437	GG 436	Nystatin Oral	500,000 Units	Brown	Tab	Round	N	Y	Eon	Anti–Infective
	GG437/100	Chlorpromazine HCl	100mg	Butterscotch	Tab	Round	N	Y	Geneva	Tranquilizer
	P–D 437	Quinestrol	100mcg	Blue	Tab	Round	–	–	PD	Hormone
438	SL 437	Desipramine HCl	50mg	Green	Tab	Round	N	Y	Sidmak	Antidepressant
	GG 438	Pindolol	5mg	White	Tab	Round	Y	N	Geneva	Anti–Hypertensive
	SL 438	Desipramine HCl	75mg	Orange	Tab	Round	N	Y	Sidmak	Antidepressant
	SQUIBB 438	Procainamide HCl	500mg	Orange	Tab	Oblong	N	Y	Princeton	Antiarrhythmic
439	GG 439	Pindolol	10mg	White	Tab	Round	Y	N	Geneva	Anti–Hypertensive
	L/N 439–50	Indomethacin	50mg	Green	Cap	–	–	–	MP	Anti–Inflammatory
	N 439–50	Indomethacin	50mg	Green	CAP	–	–	–	Novopharm	Antiinflammatory
	R 439	Trazodone HCl	50mg	White	Tab	Round	N	Y	Purepac	Antidepressant
	SL 439	Desipramine HCl	100mg	Peach	Tab	Round	N	Y	Sidmak	Antidepressant
440	P–D 440	Furosemide	20mg	White	Tab	Oval	N	N	PD	Diuretic
	R 440	Tolbutamide	500mg	White	Tab	Round	–	–	Purepac	Hypoglycemic
	RR 440	Amantidine	100mg	Red	Cap	–	–	–	Reid–Rowell	Antiparkinson
	SL 440	Desipramine HCl	150mg	White	Tab	Round	N	Y	Sidmak	Antidepressant
	WC 440	Furosemide	20mg	White	Tab	Oval	N	N	WC	Diuretic
	West–ward 440	Phenobarbital	30mg	White	Tab	Round	Y	N	West–ward	Sedative
441	GG441	Chewable Vitimins with Flu	0.5mg	Cr./Orange specks	Tab	Round	N	N	Amide	Vitamin
	P–D 441	Furosemide	40mg	White	Tab	Round	Y	N	PD	Diuretic
	PFIZER 441	Rescinnamine	0.25mg	Yellow	Tab	Oval	Y	N	Pfizer	Antihypertensive
	R 441	Trazodone HCl	100mg	White	Tab	Round	N	Y	Purepac	Antidepressant
	SL 441 50/100	Trazodone HCl	150mg	White	Tab	Unique	N	N	Sidmak	Antidepressant

ID NO.	ID CODE	GENERIC NAME	STRENGTH	COLOR	FORM	SHAPE	SCORED	COATED	MFG.	USE
	WC 441	Furosemide	40mg	White	Tab	Round	Y	N	WC	Diuretic
442	barr/442	Acetohexamide	250mg	White	Tab	Oval	Y	N	Barr	Antiglaucoma
	MYLAN/442	Perphenazine & Amitriptyline	2mg/25mg	Purple	Tab	Round	N	Y	Mylan	Antidepressant
	P–D 442	Furosemide	80mg	White	Tab	Round	N	N	PD	Diuretic
	PFIZER 442	Rescinnamine	0.5mg	Salmon	Tab	Oval	Y	N	Pfizer	Antihypertensive
	Sch. Logo 442	Fluphenazine HCL	2.5mg	Orange	Tab	Oval	Y	N	Schering	Tranquilizer
	WC 442	Furosemide	80mg	White	Tab	Round	N	N	WC	Diuretic
443	barr/443	Acetohexamide	500mg	White	Tab	Capsule	Y	N	Barr	Antiglaucoma
	COPLEY 443	Naproxen	375mg	Off White	Tab	Capsule	N	Y	Copley	Anti–Inflammatory
	P–D 443	Clonidine HCl	0.1mg	Pink	Tab	Round	–	N	PD	Antihypertensive
	WC 443	Clonidine HCl	0.1mg	Pink	Tab	Round	–	N	WC	Antihypertensive
444	barr 555/444	Triamterene & Hydrochlorothiazide	75mg/50mg	Yellow	Tab	Oval	Y	N	Barr	Diuretic
	GG444	Pseudoephedrine & Dexbrompheniramine SA	120mg/6mg	White	Tab	Round	N	Y	Geneva	Decongestant Comb.
	P–D 444	Clonidine HCl	0.2mg	White	Tab	Round	–	N	PD	Antihypertensive
	WC 444	Clonidine HCl	0.2mg	White	Tab	Round	–	N	WC	Antihypertensive
445	P–D 445	Clonidine HCl	0.3mg	White	Tab	Round	–	N	PD	Antihypertensive
	WC 445	Clonidine HCl	0.3mg	White	Tab	Round	–	N	WC	Antihypertensive
	West–ward 445	Phenobarbital	15mg	White	Tab	Round	N	N	West–ward	Sedative
	Wyeth 445	Inert tablets	n/a	Pink	Tab	Round	N	N	Wyeth	Contraceptive
446	barr/ 446	Tamoxifen Citrate	10mg	White	Tab	Round	N	N	Barr	Antineoplastic
	PFIZER 446	Polythiazide & Reserpine	2mg/0.25mg	Blue	Tab	Round	Y	N	Pfizer	Antihypertensive
447	Copley 447	Iodinated Glycerol	30mg	Orange	Tab	Round	Y	N	Copley	Expectorant
	GG447	Phenylpropanolamine HCl & Brompheniramine Sulfate	75mg/12mg	Blue	Tab	Round	N	Y	Geneva	Decongestant Comb.
448	WC 448	Hydrocodone Bitartrate with Acetaminophen	5mg/500mg	White	Tab	Capsule	Y	N	WC	Analgesic
450	225/450	Hydrocodone Bitartrate/Acetaminophen	5mg/500mg	White	Tab	Capsule	Y	N	B.F.Ascher	Analgesic
	450 MD	Diethylpropion HCl SA	75mg	White	Tab	Oval	N	N	MD	Anorectic
	GG450	Amitriptyline	150mg	Green	Tab	Oblong	N	Y	Geneva	Antidepressant
	SQUIBB 450	Captopril	12.5mg	White	Tab	Oblong	Y	N	Squibb	Antihypertensive
	STUART 450	Simethicone	40mg	White	Tab	Round	Y	N	Stuart	Antiflatulent
	West–ward 450	Phenobarbital	30mg	White	Tab	Round	Y	N	West–ward	Sedative
451	GG451	Amitriptyline	75mg	Purple	Tab	Round	N	Y	Geneva	Antidepressant
	MD/451	Guaifenesin & Pseudoephedrine HCl	600mg/120mg	Blue	Tab	Capsule	Y	N	MD	Antitussive Comb.
	MYLAN 451	Naproxen Sodium	500mg	Blue	Tab	Oval	N	N	Mylan	Anti–Inflammatory
	SL 451	Ibuprofen	800mg	White	Tab	Capsule	N	Y	Sidmak	Anti–Inflammatory
	WC 451	Clorazepate	3.75mg	Blue	Tab	Round	–	N	WC	Antianxiety
452	54 452	Lithium Carbonate	300mg	White	Tab	Round	Y	N	Roxane	Tranquilizer
	879 452	Acetaminophen	500mg	Red/White	Cap	–	–	–	Halsey	Analgesic
	Forest 452	Tetracycline HCl	250mg	Orange/Yellow	Cap	–	–	–	Forest	Anti–Infective
	SQUIBB 452	Captopril	25mg	White	Tab	Square	Y	N	Squibb	Antihypertensive
	WC 452	Clorazepate	7.5mg	Beige	Tab	Round	–	N	WC	Antianxiety
453	879 453	Acetaminophen	500mg	White	Tab	–	Y	N	Halsey	Analgesic
	WC 453	Clorazepate	15mg	Pink	Tab	Round	–	N	WC	Antianxiety
454	SL 454	Ethchlorvynol	500mg	Red	Cap	–	–	–	PBI	Hypnotic
455	b/b 455	Verapamil HCl	120mg	Orange	Tab	Oval	N	Y	Barr	Antiarrhythmic
	GG455/10	Chlorpromazine HCl	10mg	Butterscotch	Tab	Round	N	Y	Geneva	Tranquilizer
	SL 455	Ethchlorvynol	750mg	Green	Cap	–	–	–	PBI	Hypnotic
	SQUIBB 455	Ipodate Sodium	500mg	–	Cap	–	–	–	Squibb	Diagnostic
	STUART 455	Simethicone	125mg	Pink	Tab	Round	Y	N	Stuart	Antiflatulent
	West–ward 455	Phenobarbital	60mg	White	Tab	Round	N	N	West–ward	Sedative
456	SL 456	Oxybutynin Chloride	5mg	Blue	Tab	Round	Y	N	Sidmak	Antispasmodic
457	Copley 457	Magnesium Gluconate	–	Orange	Tab	Capsule	–	–	Copley	Mineral Supp.
	GG457/200	Chlorpromazine HCl	200mg	Butterscotch	Tab	Round	N	Y	Geneva	Tranquilizer
	MYLAN 457	Lorazepam	1mg	White	Tab	Round	Y	N	Mylan	Antianxiety
	SQUIBB 457	Nystatin	100,000 Units	Beige	Tab	Oval	N	N	Squibb	Anti–Infective
458	458 b	Amitriptyline HCl	150mg	White	Tab	Capsule	Y	Y	Barr	Antidepressant
	GG 458	Acetaminophen	500mg	White	Tab	Capsule	–	–	Geneva	Analgesic
	SL 458	Theophylline TD	300mg	White	Tab	Capsule	Y	N	Sidmak	Bronchodilator
459	GG 459	Acetaminophen	325mg	White	Tab	Capsule	–	–	Geneva	Analgesic
	SL 459	Theophylline TD	300mg	White	Tab	Capsule	Y	N	Sidmak	Bronchodilator
460	bock 460	Pseudoephedrine/Guaifenesin	60mg/400mg	Blue	Tab	Oval	Y	Y	Chase	Decongestant/Exp.
	SL 460	Clonidine HCl	0.1mg	Green	Tab	Round	N	N	Sidmak	Antihypertensive
461	GG461	Amitriptyline	100mg	Orange	Tab	Round	N	Y	Geneva	Antidepressant
	SL 461	Clonidine HCl	0.2mg	Yellow	Tab	Round	Y	N	Sidmak	Antihypertensive
462	SL 462	Clonidine HCl	0.3mg	Blue	Tab	Round	N	N	Sidmak	Antihypertensive
463	54 463	Lithium Carbonate	300mg	Flesh	Cap	–	–	–	Roxane	Tranquilizer
	832/G463	Medroxyprogesterone Acetate	10mg	White	Tab	Round	Y	N	PBI	Hormone
	N/463	Methyldopa	125mg	White	Tab	Round	N	Y	Novopharm	Antihypertensive
	SL 463	Clonidine HCl & Chlorthalidone	0.1mg/15mg	Pink	Tab	Round	Y	N	Sidmak	Antihypertensive
464	CPC 464	Multivitamin/Mineral	n/a	Brown/Red	Cap	–	–	–	Moore	Vitamin
	GG464	Dipyridamole	75mg	White	Tab	Round	N	Y	Geneva	Antiplatelet
	HD 464	Oxycodone HCl, Oxycodone Terephthalate, Aspirin	4.5mg/.38mg/325	Yellow	Tab	Round	Y	N	Halsey	Analgesic
	SL 464	Clonidine HCl & Chlorthalidone	0.2mg/15mg	Blue	Tab	Round	Y	N	Sidmak	Antihypertensive
	Wyeth 464	Nafcillin Sodium	500mg	White	Tab	Capsule	Y	N	Wyeth	Anti–Infective
465	G465/832	Megesterol Acetate	20mg	White	Tab	Round	Y	N	PBI	Hormone
	SL 465	Clonidine HCl & Chlorthalidone	0.3mg/15mg	White	Tab	Round	Y	N	Sidmak	Antihypertensive
	TP465/3	Acetaminophen with Codeine	300mg/30mg	White	Tab	Round	N	N	Towne Paulsen	Analgesic
466	G466/832	Megesterol Acetate	40mg	White	Tab	Round	Y	N	PBI	Hormone
	TP466/4	Acetaminophen with Codeine	300mg/60mg	White	Tab	Round	N	N	Towne Paulsen	Analgesic
467	467 HD	Dipyridamole	75mg	White	Tab	Round	N	Y	Halsey	Antiplatelet
	SL 467	Propranolol HCl	10mg	Orange	Tab	Round	Y	N	Sidmak	Antihypertensive
468	879 G468C	Meperidine HCl	50mg	White	Tab	Round	N	N	Halsey	Analgesic
	MJ 468	Vitamin Combination Chewable	n/a	Orange/Purple/Rose	Tab	Oval Rect.	N	N	Mead Johnson	Vitamin
	SL 468	Propranolol HCl	20mg	Blue	Tab	Round	Y	N	Sidmak	Antihypertensive
469	879 G469C	Meperidine HCl	100mg	White	Tab	Round	Y	N	Halsey	Analgesic
	SL 469	Propranolol HCl	40mg	Green	Tab	Round	Y	N	Sidmak	Antihypertensive
470	225/470	Phendimetrazine Tartrate	105mg	White/Clear	Cap	–	–	–	B.F.Ascher	Anorectic
	470/barr	Propoxyphene Napsylate & Acetaminophen	100mg/650mg	Pink	Tab	Capsule	N	Y	Barr	Analgesic
	SL 470	Propranolol HCl	60mg	Pink	Tab	Round	Y	N	Sidmak	Antihypertensive
	STUART 470	Docusate Potassium	100mg	Pink	Cap	–	–	–	Stuart	Stool Softener
471	879 /G471C	Meprobamate	400mg	White	Tab	Round	Y	N	Halsey	Antianxiety
	GG 471	Methyldopa	500mg	White	Tab	Round	N	Y	Geneva	Antihypertensive
	M 471	Fenoprofen Calcium	600mg	Orange	Tab	Capsule	N	Y	Mylan	Analgesic
	N/471	Methyldopa	250mg	White	Tab	Round	N	Y	Novopharm	Antihypertensive
	P–D 471	Diphenhydramine HCl	25mg	Pink/White	Cap	–	–	–	PD	Antihistamine
	SL 471	Propranolol HCl	80mg	Yellow	Tab	Round	Y	N	Sidmak	Antihypertensive

ID NO.	ID CODE	GENERIC NAME	STRENGTH	COLOR	FORM	SHAPE	SCORED	COATED	MFG.	USE
	Wyeth 471	Tetracycline HCl	500mg	Yellow/Blue	Cap	–	–	–	Wyeth	Anti–Infective
472	54–472	Piroxicam	10mg	–	Cap	–	–	–	Roxane	Anti–inflammatory
	GG472	Procainamide HCl SR	250mg	White	Tab	Capsule	Y	Y	Geneva	Antiarrhythmic
	ORG 472	Calcifediol	20mcg	White	Cap	–	–	–	Organon	Vitamin D
	SL 472	Propranolol HCl	90mg	Lavender	Tab	Round	Y	N	Sidmak	Antihypertensive
473	GG473	Procainamide HCl SR	500mg	White	Tab	Capsule	Y	Y	Geneva	Antiarrhythmic
	R 473	Verapamil HCl	80mg	White	Tab	Round	N	N	Purepac	Antiarrhythmic
	SL 473	Propranolol HCl & Hydrochlorothiazide	40mg/25mg	White	Tab	Round	N	N	Sidmak	Antihypertensive
	West–ward 473	Prednisone	10mg	White	Tab	Round	Y	N	West–ward	Steroid
474	GG474	Procainamide HCl SR	750mg	White	Tab	Capsule	Y	Y	Danbury	Antiarrhythmic
	MJ 474	Vitamin Combination Chewable	n/a	Orange/Purple/Rose	Tab	Oval Square	N	N	Mead Johnson	Vitamin
	ORG 474	Calcifediol	50mcg	Orange	Cap	–	–	–	Organon	Vitamin D
	SL 474	Propranolol HCl & Hydrochlorothiazide	80mg/25mg	White	Tab	Round	N	N	Sidmak	Antihypertensive
475	GG475	Hydralazine HCl	10mg	White	Tab	Round	N	Y	Geneva	Antihypertensive
	Kremers Urban 475	Enzyme Combination	n/a	Green/White	Cap	–	–	–	K–U	Digestant
	R 475	Verapamil HCl	120mg	White	Tab	Round	N	N	Purepac	Antiarrhythmic
	SL 475	Methyldopa	125mg	Off White	Tab	Round	N	Y	Sidmak	Antihypertensive
	STUART 475	Docusate Potassium & Casanthranol	100mg/30mg	Yellow	Cap	–	–	–	Stuart	Laxative Comb.
	West–ward 475	Prednisone	5mg	White	Tab	Round	Y	N	West–ward	Steroid
476	GG476/25	Chlorpromazine HCl	25mg	Butterscotch	Tab	Round	N	Y	Geneva	Tranquilizer
	MJ 476	Vitamin Combination Chewable	n/a	Rose	Tab	Oval Square	N	N	Mead Johnson	Vitamin
	SL 476	Methyldopa	250mg	Off White	Tab	Round	N	Y	Sidmak	Antihypertensive
477	b 477	Haloperidol	0.5mg	White	Tab	Round	N	N	Barr	Tranquilizer
	GG 477	Brompheniramine,Phenylephrine,Phenylpropanolamine	12mg/15mg/15mg	Blue	Tab	Round	N	Y	Geneva	Decongestant Comb.
	GLYBUR 477	Glyburide	1.25mg	White	Tab	Oblong	–	N	Copley	Hypoglycemic
	Mylan 477	Diazepam	10mg	Green	Tab	Round	Y	N	Mylan	Antianxiety
	SL 477	Methyldopa	500mg	Off White	Tab	Round	N	Y	Sidmak	Antihypertensive
	West–ward 477	Prednisone	20mg	Peach	Tab	Round	Y	N	West–ward	Steroid
478	b 478	Haloperidol	1mg	Yellow	Tab	Round	N	N	Barr	Tranquilizer
	SL 478	Methyldopa & Hydrochlorothiazide	250mg/15mg	Brown	Tab	Round	N	Y	Sidmak	Antihypertensive
479	479 HD	Dipyridamole	50mg	White	Tab	Round	N	Y	Halsey	Antiplatelet
	54–479	Piroxicam	20mg	–	Cap	–	–	–	Roxane	Anti–inflammatory
	b 479	Haloperidol	2mg	White	Tab	Round	N	N	Barr	Tranquilizer
	SL 479	Methyldopa & Hydrochlorothiazide	250mg/25mg	White	Tab	Round	N	Y	Sidmak	Antihypertensive
480	225–480	Brompheniramine Maleate/Pseudoephedrine	12mg/120mg	Clear	Cap	–	–	–	B.F.Ascher	Decongestant Comb.
	b 480	Haloperidol	5mg	Green	Tab	Round	N	N	Barr	Tranquilizer
	GG480	Prenatal Vitamins w/Zinc	–	White	Tab	Capsule	N	Y	Amide	Vitamin
	N 480/2	Albuterol Sulfate	2mg	White	Tab	Round	–	N	Novopharm	Bronchodilator
	R 480	Tolmetin Sodium	600mg	White	Tab	Oval	N	Y	Purepac	Anti–Inflammatory
	SL 480	Methyldopa & Hydrochlorothiazide	500mg/30mg	Brown	Tab	Oval	N	Y	Sidmak	Antihypertensive
	W480	Propylthiouracil	50mg	White	Tab	Round	Y	N	Rondex	Antithyroid
	West–ward 480	Propylthiouracil	50mg	White	Tab	Round	Y	N	West–ward	Antithyroid
481	481, barr	Haloperidol	10mg	Aqua	Tab	Round	N	N	Barr	Tranquilizer
	GG 481	Prenatal Vitamin with Zinc Improved	n/a	Tan	Tab	Capsule	N	Y	Amide	Prenatal Vitamin
	SL 481	Methyldopa & Hydrochlorothiazide	500mg/50mg	White	Tab	Oval	N	Y	Sidmak	Antihypertensive
	West–ward 481	Prednisone	50mg	White	Tab	Round	Y	N	West–ward	Steroid
482	482, barr	Haloperidol	20mg	Salmon	Tab	Round	N	N	Barr	Tranquilizer
	MJ 482	Vitamin Combination Chewable	n/a.	Rose	Tab	Oval Rect.	N	N	Mead Johnson	Vitamin
	SL 482	Theophylline TD	200mg	White	Tab	Oval	Y	N	Sidmak	Bronchodilator
	SQUIBB 482	Captopril	50mg	White	Tab	Oval	Y	N	Squibb	Antihypertensive
483	barr 483	Amiloride/Hydrochlorothiazide	5mg/50mg	Yellow	Tab	Round	–	–	Barr	Diuretic
	SL 483	Theophylline TD	100mg	White	Tab	Round	Y	N	Sidmak	Bronchodilator
484	484,b	Leucovorin	5mg	White	Tab	Round	N	N	Barr	Antineoplastic
	93 484	Doxycycline Hyclate	100mg	Orange	Tab	Round	N	Y	Lemmon	Anti–Infective
	SL 484	Sulindac	150mg	Yellow	Tab	Round	N	Y	Sidmak	Anti–Inflammatory
485	485,b	Leucovorin	25mg	Green	Tab	Round	N	N	Barr	Antineoplastic
	GG485	Hydralazine HCl	25mg	Green	Tab	Round	N	Y	Geneva	Antihypertensive
	SL 485	Sulindac	200mg	Yellow	Tab	Round	Y	N	Sidmak	Anti–Inflammatory
	SQUIBB 485	Captopril	100mg	White	Tab	Oval	Y	N	Squibb	Antihypertensive
	West–ward 485	Pseudoephedrine HCl	60mg	White	Tab	Round	Y	N	West–ward	Decongestant
486	93 486	Ibuprofen	200mg	White	Tab	Round	N	Y	Lemmon	Anti–Inflammatory
	Barr, 486	Chlorthalidone	50mg	Blue	Tab	Round	N	N	Barr	Diuretic
	SL 486	Verapamil	80mg	White	Tab	Round	N	Y	Sidmak	Antihypertensive
	WC 486	Hydrocodone Bitartrate with Acetaminophen	7.5mg/750mg	White	Tab	Oblong	Y	N	WC	Analgesic
	Wyeth 486	Inert tablets	–	Pink	Tab	Round	N	N	Wyeth	Placebo
487	barr/ 487	Temazepam	15mg	Green/White	Cap	–	–	–	Barr	Hypnotic
	GG487	Probenecid & Colchicine	500mg/0.5mg	White	Tab	Capsule	N	N	Danbury	Antigout
	SL 487	Verapamil	120mg	White	Tab	Round	Y	Y	Sidmak	Antihypertensive
488	barr/ 488	Temazepam	30mg	White/White	Cap	–	–	–	Barr	Hypnotic
	GG488	Fluphenazine HCl	2.5mg	Beige	Tab	Round	N	Y	Geneva	Tranquilizer
489	54–489	Dexamethasone	1mg	Yellow	Tab	Round	Y	N	Roxane	Steroid
	555/489, barr	Trazodone HCl	50mg	Yellow	Tab	Round	Y	N	Barr	Antidepressant
	GG489	Fluphenazine HCl	5mg	Rust	Tab	Round	N	Y	Geneva	Tranquilizer
490	225/490	Docusate Na/Phenolphthalein	230mg/130mg	–	Cap	–	–	–	B.F.Ascher	Laxative
	555/490, barr	Trazodone HCl	100mg	White	Tab	Round	N	N	Barr	Antidepressant
	93 490	Propoxyphene Napsylate & Acetaminophen	100mg/650mg	White	Tab	Oblong	N	Y	Lemmon	Analgesic
	GG490	Fluphenazine HCl	10mg	Rust	Tab	Round	N	Y	Geneva	Tranquilizer
	PD 490	Aspirin Delayed Release	975mg	Rose	Tab	Elliptical	N	Y	PD	Analgesic
491	93–491	Ibuprofen	400mg	White	Tab	Round	N	Y	Lemmon	Anti–Inflammatory
	SL 491	Albuterol Sulfate	2mg	White	Tab	Round	N	N	Sidmak	Bronchodilator
492	54–492	Amitriptyline	150mg	–	Tab	Round	–	–	Roxane	Antidepressant
	93–492	Ibuprofen	600mg	White	Tab	Oval	N	Y	Lemmon	Anti–Inflammatory
	SL 492	Albuterol Sulfate	4mg	White	Tab	Round	Y	N	Sidmak	Bronchodilator
493	SL 493	Aspirin Controlled Release	800mg	White	Tab	Oval	N	Y	Sidmak	Analgesic
494	494 HD	Dipyridamole	25mg	White	Tab	Round	N	Y	Halsey	Antiplatelet
495	Sch. Logo 496	Griseofulvin	500mg	White	Tab	Round	Y	N	Schering	Antifungal
497	497	Nifedipine	10mg	Yellow	CAP	–	–	–	Novopharm	Antihypertensive
	PP–497	Diphenoxylate HCl & Atropine Sulfate	2.5mg/0.025mg	White	Tab	Round	N	N	Eon	Antidiarrheal
	R 497	Nifedipine	10mg	Yellow	Cap	–	–	–	Purepac	Antianginal
	SL 497	Fenoprofen Calcium	600mg	Yellow	Tab	Capsule	N	Y	Sidmak	Anti–Inflammatory
498	93–498	Ibuprofen	800mg	White	Tab	Capsule	N	Y	Lemmon	Anti–Inflammatory
	N/498	Methyldopa	500mg	White	Tab	Round	N	Y	Novopharm	Antihypertensive
499	54–499	Hydrochlorothiazide	50mg	–	Tab	Round	–	–	Roxane	Diuretic
	barr, 499	Ibuprofen	800mg	White	Tab	Capsule	N	Y	Barr	Anti–Inflammatory
	N 499/4	Albuterol Sulfate	4mg	White	Tab	Round	–	N	Novopharm	Bronchodilator

ID NO.	ID CODE	GENERIC NAME	STRENGTH	COLOR	FORM	SHAPE	SCORED	COATED	MFG.	USE
500	Sch. Logo 499	Methyltestosterone	25mg	Peach	Tab	Round	N	N	Schering	Hormone
	239/500	Chlorzoxazone	500mg	Green	Tab	Oblong	Y	N	Royce	Muscle relaxant
	3M/SR 500	Theophylline SR	500mg	White	Tab	Capsule	Y	N	3M	Bronchodilator
	500	Niacin SR	500mg	Pink	Tab	Capsule	Y	N	Upsher	Vasodilator
	832 S500	Salsalate	500mg	Blue	Tab	Round	N	Y	PBI	Analgesic
	832 S500	Salsalate	500mg	Yellow	Tab	Round	N	Y	PBI	Analgesic
	832/FC500	Fenoprofen Calcium	600mg	Peach	Tab	Capsule	N	Y	PBI	Anti-Inflammatory
	Atral 500mg	Amoxicillin	500mg	Pink	Cap	–	–	–	Lab A	Anti-Infective
	Atral 500mg	Cephalexin	500mg	Orange/Gray	Cap	–	–	–	Lab A	Anti-Infective
	Ayerst 500	Amoxicillin	500mg	Caramel\Red	Cap	–	–	–	Ayerst	Anti-Infective
	Central 500/5	Hydrocodone & Acetaminophen	5mg/500mg	White	Tab	Oval	Y	N	Central	Analgesic
	Central 500mg	Salsalate	500mg	Pink	Tab	Round	Y	Y	Central	Antiarthritic
	E-Base/500mg barr	Erythromycin Delayed-Release	500mg	White	Tab	Capsule	–	–	Barr	Anti-Infective
	Par/500	Cephalexin	500mg	Orange/Orange	Cap	–	–	–	Par	Anti-Infective
	PF T 500	Choline Magnesium Trisalicylate	500mg	Peach	Tab	Oblong	Y	Y	PF	Analgesic
	R 500	Prazosin HCl	1mg	White	Cap	–	–	–	Purepac	Antihypertensive
	Russ 500	Hydrocodone Bitartrate/Aspirin	5mg/500mg	Pink	Tab	Oblong	Y	N	Russ	Analgesic
	US 500	Salsalate	500mg	Blue	Tab	Round	N	Y	Upsher	Analgesic
501	879 501	Chlordiazepoxide HCl & Clidinium Bromide	5mg/2.5mg	White	Cap	–	–	–	Halsey	Antispasmodic
	GG501	Nitroglycerine SR	6.5mg	Blue/Yellow	Cap	–	–	–	Geneva	Antianginal
	H 501	Methocarbamol	750mg	White	Tab	Capsule	N	N	Heather	Muscle Relaxant
	R 501	Prazosin HCl	2mg	Pink	Cap	–	–	–	Purepac	Antihypertensive
	SEARLE 501	Metolazone	2.5mg	Rose	Tab	Round	N	N	Searle	Diuretic
502	GG502	Phenylpropanolamine & Chlorpheniramine Maleate	75mg/12mg	Blue/Clear	Cap	–	–	–	Geneva	Decongestant Comb.
	R 502	Prazosin HCl	5mg	Blue	Cap	–	–	–	Purepac	Antihypertensive
503	West-ward 502	Propranolol	10mg	Peach	Tab	Round	Y	N	West-ward	Antihypertensive
	503 HD	Chlorpropamide	250mg	Blue	Tab	Round	Y	N	Halsey	Hypoglycemic
	54-503	Phenobarbital	15mg	White	Tab	Round	Y	N	Roxane	Hypnotic
	GG503	Papaverine TD	150mg	Clear/Brown	Cap	–	–	–	Geneva	Vasodilator
	H 503	Methenamine Mandelate	1Gm	Purple	Tab	Oval	N	Y	Heather	Urinary Antiseptic
504	MJ 503	Cyclophosphamide	50mg	White/Blue flecks	Tab	Round	–	–	BM	Antineoplastic
	West-ward 503	Propranolol	20mg	Blue	Tab	Round	Y	N	West-ward	Antihypertensive
	MJ 504	Cyclophosphamide	25mg	White/Blue flecks	Tab	Round	–	–	BM	Antineoplastic
	West-ward 504	Propranolol	40mg	Green	Tab	Round	Y	N	West-ward	Antihypertensive
505	GG 505	Oxazepam	10mg	White	Cap	–	–	–	Geneva	Antianxiety
	KREMERS-URBAN 505	Lactase Enzyme	125mg	Brown/White	Cap	–	–	–	K-U	Digestant
	SL 505	Triamterene & Hydrochlorothiazide	75mg/50mg	Yellow	Tab	Rectangular	Y	N	Sidmak	Antihypertensive
	West-ward 505	Propranolol	60mg	Pink	Tab	Round	Y	N	West-ward	Antihypertensive
506	506 HD	Metronidazole	250mg	White	Tab	Round	N	N	Halsey	Anti-Infective
	832/G506	Nystatin	500,000 Units	Brown	Tab	Round	–	Y	PBI	Antifungal
	GG 506	Oxazepam	15mg	White	Cap	–	–	–	Geneva	Antianxiety
	West-ward 506	Propranolol	80mg	Yellow	Tab	Round	Y	N	West-ward	Antihypertensive
507	507 HD	Indomethacin	25mg	Green	Cap	–	–	–	Halsey	Anti-Inflammatory
	GG 507	Oxazepam	30mg	White	Cap	–	–	–	Geneva	Antianxiety
	JSP 507	Butalbital, Aspirin, Caffeine, Codeine	50/325/40/30mg	Blue/Yellow	Cap	–	N	N	Halsey	Analgesic
	Mylan 507	Methyldopa & Hydrochlorothiazide	250mg/15mg	Green	Tab	Round	N	Y	Mylan	Antihypertensive
	Sch. Logo 507	Griseofulvin Ultramicrosize	250mg	White	Tab	Round	Y	N	Schering	Antifungal
508	508 HD	Indomethacin	50mg	Green	Cap	–	–	–	Halsey	Anti-Inflammatory
	527/508	Pentobarbital Sodium	1 1/2gr	Yellow	Cap	–	–	–	Lannett	Hypnotic
	WC 508	Cimetidine	800mg	Green	Tab	Oval	–	Y	WC	Anti-ulcer
510	West-ward 508	Quinidine Gluconate	324mg	White	Tab	Round	N	N	West-ward	Antiarrhythmic
	527/510	Phendimetrazine Tartrate 8	35mg	Black	Tab	–	–	–	Lannett	Anorectic
	832/M 510	Metoproterenol	10mg	White	Tab	Round	Y	N	PBI	Bronchodilator
	H 510	Methylprednisolone	4mg	White	Tab	Oval	Y	N	Heather	Steroid
	West-ward 510	Quinidine Sulfate	200mg	Clear/Clear	Cap	–	–	–	West-ward	Antiarrhythmic
511	13 511	Docusate Sodium	100mg	Green	Cap	Oval	–	–	Adria	Stool Softener
	527/511	Pentobarbital Sodium	3/4gr	Yellow/Clear	Cap	–	–	–	Lannett	Hypnotic
	E 511	Quinidine Sulfate	200mg	White	Tab	Round	Y	N	Eon	Antiarrhythmic
	GG511	Nitroglycerine SR	2.5mg	Clear/Lavender	Cap	–	–	–	Geneva	Antianginal
	PP-511	Quinidine Sulfate	200mg	White	Tab	Round	Y	N	Eon	Antiarrhythmic
512	SEARLE 511	Metolazone	5mg	Blue	Tab	Round	N	N	Searle	Diuretic
	54-512	Alprazolam	0.25mg	–	Tab	–	N	–	Roxane	Antianxiety
	A 512	Phenolphthalein	60mg	Pink	Tab	Round	N	Y	Adria	Laxative
	BL 512	Theophylline Anhydrous	300mg	Ivory	Tab	Rectangular	Y	N	Bristol	Bronchodilator
	CL512	Nitroglycerine SR	9mg	Green/Yellow	Cap	–	–	–	Geneva	Antianginal
	E 512	Quinidine Sulfate	300mg	White	Tab	Round	Y	N	Eon	Antiarrhythmic
	GG512	Nitroglycerin SR	9mg	Green/Yellow	Cap	–	–	–	Geneva	Antianginal
	HD 512	Oxycodone HCl & Acetaminophen	5mg/325mg	White	Tab	Round	Y	N	Halsey	Analgesic
	MILES 512	Ciprofloxacin	250mg	White	Tab	Round	N	N	Miles	Anti-Infective
	MYLAN 512	Verapamil HCl	80mg	White	Tab	Round	N	Y	Mylan	Antiarrhythmic
513	PP-512	Quinidine Sulfate	300mg	White	Tab	Round	N	N	Eon	Antiarrhythmic
	SQUIBB 512	Triamcinolone	4mg	–	Tab	–	–	–	Squibb	Steroid
	A 513	Phenolphthalein	130mg	Red	Tab	Round	N	Y	Adria	Laxative
	H 513	Cortisone Acetate	25mg	White	Tab	Round	Y	N	Heather	Steroid
	JSP 513	Levothyroxine Sodium	25mcg	Peach	Tab	Round	Y	N	Jerome Stevens	Hormone
514	MILES 513	Ciprofloxacin	500mg	White	Tab	Oblong	Y	N	Miles	Anti-Infective
	Barr 514	Cephalexin	250mg	Red/Gray	Cap	–	–	–	Barr	Anti-Infective
	JSP 514	Levothyroxine Sodium	50mcg	White	Tab	Round	Y	N	Jerome Stevens	Hormone
	MILES 514	Ciprofloxacin	750mg	White	Tab	Oblong	Y	N	Miles	Anti-Infective
	SL 514	Meclizine HCl	50mg	Blue/Yellow	Tab	Round	Y	N	Sidmak	Antinauseant
515	527/515	Amobarbital Sodium	3 gr	Blue	Cap	–	–	–	Lannett	Hypnotic
	A 515	Phenolphthalein/Docusate Sodium	65mg/100mg	Orange	Tab	Round	N	Y	Adria	Laxative
	Barr 515	Cephalexin	500mg	Orange/Orange	Cap	–	–	–	Barr	Anti-Infective
	Bristol 515	Theophylline & Guaifenesin	300mg/180mg	Yellow/White	Cap	–	–	–	Bristol	Bronchodilator
	GG515	Quinine Sulfate	5gr	Clear	Cap	–	–	–	Geneva	Muscle Relaxant
	JSP 515	Levothyroxine Sodium	75mcg	Purple	Tab	Round	Y	N	Jerome Stevens	Hormone
	SL 515	Hydroxyzine HCl	100mg	White	Tab	Round	N	Y	Sidmak	Antipruritic
	WC 515	Allopurinol	100mg	White	Tab	Round	–	N	WC	Anti-Gout
516	Bristol 516	Theophylline & Guaifenesin	150mg/90mg	Yellow	Cap	–	–	–	Bristol	Bronchodilator
	Forest 516	Phendimetrazine	35mg	Green	Tab	Round	–	–	Forest	Anorectic
517	WC 516	Ibuprofen	400mg	White	Tab	Elongated	N	Y	WC	Anti-Inflammatory
	GG517	Indomethacin	25mg	Green	Cap	–	–	–	Geneva	Anti-Inflammatory
	N 517/250	Naproxen	250mg	Yellow/Peach	Tab	Oval	N	N	Novopharm	Anti-Inflammatory
	SL 517	Metoclopramide	5mg	Green	Tab	Round	N	N	Sidmak	Antireflux
	WC 517	Allopurinol	300mg	Peach	Tab	Round	–	N	WC	Anti-Gout

ID NO.	ID CODE	GENERIC NAME	STRENGTH	COLOR	FORM	SHAPE	SCORED	COATED	MFG.	USE
518	518 MD	Diethylpropion HCl	25mg	Blue	Tab	Round	N	N	MD	Anorectic
	GG518	Indomethacin	50mg	Green	Cap	–	–	–	Geneva	Anti–Inflammatory
	N 518/375	Naproxen	375mg	Pink	Tab	Oval	N	N	Novopharm	Anti–Inflammatory
	SL 518	Theophylline T.D.	450mg	White	Tab	Capsule	Y	N	Sidmak	Bronchodilator
	SQUIBB 518	Triamcinolone	8mg	–	Tab	–	–	–	Squibb	Steroid
519	BL 519	Theophylline Anhydrous SR	300mg	White	Tab	Rectangular	Y	N	Bristol	Bronchodilator
520	832/M 520	Metoproterenol	20mg	White	Tab	Round	Y	N	PBI	Bronchodilator
	N 520/500	Naproxen	500mg	Yellow/Peach	Tab	Oval	N	N	Novopharm	Anti–Inflammatory
	R 520	Tolmetin Sodium	400mg	Orange/White	Cap	–	–	–	Purepac	Anti–Inflammatory
	SL 520	Phenylephrine/Chlorpheniramine/Pyrilamine	25mg/8mg/25mg	Orange	Tab	Capsule	Y	N	Sidmak	Decongestant Comb.
521	TP 520	Meprobamate	400mg	White	Tab	Round	Y	N	Towne Paulsen	Antianxiety
	MILES 521	Praziquantel	600mg	White	Tab	Oblong	Y	N	Miles	Anti–Infective
	Mylan 521	Propoxyphene Napsylate and Acetaminophen	100mg/650mg	White	Tab	Capsule	N	Y	Mylan	Analgesic
	R 521	Naproxen	250mg	White	Tab	Round	N	N	Purepac	Anti–Inflammatory
	SEARLE 521	Metolazone	10mg	Yellow	Tab	Round	N	N	Searle	Diuretic
	SL 521	Carbetapentane/Chlorpheniramine/Ephedrine/PhenEph.	60/5/10/10mg	Pink	Tab	Capsule	Y	N	Sidmak	Antitussive Comb.
	WALLACE 521	Diphylline	200mg	White	Tab	Rectangular	–	N	Wallace	Antiasthmatic
522	522 HD	Chlorpropamide	100mg	Blue	Tab	Round	Y	N	Halsey	Hypoglycemic
	GG522	Flurazepam	15mg	Blue/White	Cap	–	–	–	Par	Hypnotic
	Kremers Urban 522	Amylase,Protease,Lipase,Cellulase	30/6/75/2mg	Yellow/White	Cap	–	–	–	K–U	Digestant
	R 522	Naproxen	375mg	White	Tab	Capsule	N	N	Purepac	Anti–Inflammatory
	SL 522	Phenylpropanolamine HCl & Guaifenesin LA	75mg/400mg	Green	Tab	Oval	Y	N	Sidmak	Decongestant Comb.
	TP 522	Meprobamate	200mg	White	Tab	Round	Y	N	Towne Paulsen	Antianxiety
523	GG523	Flurazepam	30mg	Blue	Cap	–	–	–	Par	Hypnotic
	R 523	Naproxen	500mg	White	Tab	Capsule	N	N	Purepac	Anti–Inflammatory
524	524 HD	Cyproheptadine HCl	4mg	White	Tab	Round	N	N	Halsey	Antipruritic
	GG524	Meclofenamate Sodium	50mg	Maroon/Pink	Cap	–	–	–	Geneva	Anti–Inflammatory
	LH 524	Chlorphen/Phenyltolox/Phenylephrine	4mg/20mg/50mg	Yellow/Clear	Cap	–	–	–	Econolab	Antihistamine/Dec.
525	879 525	Doxycycline Hyclate	50mg	Blue/White	Cap	–	–	–	Halsey	Anti–Infective
	93 525	Amitriptyline HCl	10mg	Pink	Tab	Round	N	Y	Lemmon	Antidepressant
	GG525	Meclofenamate Sodium	100mg	Maroon/White	Cap	–	–	–	Geneva	Anti–Inflammatory
	Kremers Urban 525	Pancrelipase	n/a	White/White	Cap	–	–	–	K–U	Digestant
	M 525	Diltiazem HCl	120mg	White	Cap	Capsule	Y	Y	Mylan	Antianginal
	P–D 525	Methsuximide	300mg	Cream/Orange Band	Cap	–	–	–	PD	Anticonvulsant
	Schering 525	Flutamide	125mg	Opaque Brown	Cap	–	–	–	Schering	Antiandrogen
526	879 526	Doxycycline Hyclate	100mg	Blue	Cap	–	–	–	Halsey	Anti–Infective
	DAN 526	Isoniazid	300mg	White	Tab	Round	Y	N	Danbury	Anti–Infective
	GG 526	Clorazepate	3.75mg	White/bnds	Cap	–	–	–	Geneva	Antianxiety
	JSP 526	Bromophen/Pseudoephedrine	6mg/60mg	Green/Clear	Cap	–	–	–	Jerome Stevens	Antihistamine/Dec
527	93 527	Amitriptyline HCl	25mg	Green	Tab	Round	N	Y	Lemmon	Antidepressant
	B 527	Doxycycline Hyclate	100mg	Off White	Tab	Round	N	Y	Martec	Anti–Infective
	GG 527	Clorazepate	7.5mg	White/bnds	Cap	–	–	–	Geneva	Antianxiety
	GG 527	Prednisone	50mg	White	Tab	Round	Y	N	Geneva	Steroid
	H527	Prednisone	50mg	White	Tab	Round	Y	N	Heather	Steroid
	JSP 527	Bromophen/Pseudoephedrine	12mg/120mg	Green/Clear	Cap	–	–	–	Jerome Stevens	Antihistamine/Dec
	PD 527 5	Quinapril HCl	5mg	Brown	Tab	Elliptical	Y	Y	PD	Antihypertensive
	PD527	Quinapril HCl	5mg	Brown	TAB	Elliptical	y	y	PD	antihypertensive
528	832/G528C	Phendimetrazine HCl	35mg	Yellow	Tab	Round	–	–	PBI	Anorectic
	832/G528C	Phendimetrazine HCl	35mg	Green	Tab	Round	–	–	PBI	Anorectic
	832/G528C	Phendimetrazine HCl	35mg	Orange	Tab	Round	–	–	PBI	Anorectic
	GG 528	Clorazepate	15mg	White/bnds	Cap	–	–	–	Geneva	Antianxiety
	SL 528	Choline Magnesium Trisalicylate	500mg	Yellow	Tab	Oblong	Y	N	Sidmak	Analgesic
	WC 528	Ketoprofen	50mg	Blue/Blue	Cap	–	–	–	WC	Anti–Inflammatory
529	529 MD	Glutethimide	500mg	White	Tab	Round	Y	N	MD	Hypnotic
	54 529	Thiethylperazine Maleate	10mg	Yellow	Tab	Round	N	Y	Roxane	Antiemetic
	93 529	Amitriptyline HCl	50mg	Brown	Tab	Round	N	Y	Lemmon	Antidepressant
	P–D 529	Paromomycin Sulfate	250mg	Brown/Yellow	Cap	–	–	–	PD	Anti–Infective
	SL 529	Choline Magnesium Trisalicylate	750mg	Blue	Tab	Oblong	Y	N	Sidmak	Analgesic
530	530	Nifedipine	20mg	Reddish/Brown	Cap	–	–	–	Novopharm	Antianginal
	E 530	Isoxsuprine Hydrochloride	10mg	White	Tab	Round	Y	N	Eon	Vasodilator
	GG 530	Loperamide	2mg	White	Cap	–	–	–	Geneva	Antidiarrheal
	MD/530	Methylphenidate HCl	10mg	Blue–Green	Tab	Round	Y	N	MD	Psychostimulant
	PD 530 10	Quinapril HCl	10mg	Brown	Tab	Triagular	Y	Y	PD	Antihypertensive
	PP–530 & 10	Isoxsuprine HCl	10mg	White	Tab	Round	Y	N	Eon	Vasodilator
	R 530	Nifedipine	20mg	Reddish Brown	Cap	–	–	–	Purepac	Antianginal
	SL 530	Choline Magnesium Trisalicylate	1000mg	Pink	Tab	Oblong	Y	N	Sidmak	Analgesic
	West–ward 530	Reserpine	0.1mg	White	Tab	Round	N	N	West–ward	Antihypertensive
531	832 / G531C	Phenobarbital	15mg	White	Tab	Round	Y	N	PBI	Sedative
	93 531	Amitriptyline HCl	75mg	Purple	Tab	Round	N	Y	Lemmon	Antidepressant
	E 531	Isoxsuprine Hydrochloride	20mg	White	Tab	Round	Y	N	Eon	Vasodilator
	GG 531	Temazepam	15mg	Green/White	Cap	–	–	–	Geneva	Sedative
	K–U 531	Hyoscyamine Sulfate	0.125mg	White	Tab	Round	N	N	K–U	Antispasmodic
	MD/531	Methylphenidate HCl	5mg	Yellow	Tab	Round	N	N	MD	Psyhcostimulant
	MYLAN 531	Sulindac	200mg	Yellow	Tab	Round	Y	N	Mylan	Anti–Inflammatory
	N 531/275	Naproxen Sodium	275mg	Blue	Tab	Round	N	Y	Novopharm	Anti–Inflammatory
	P–D 531	Phenytoin Sodium & Phenobarbital	100mg/32mg	White/Black Band	Cap	–	–	–	PD	Anticonvulsant
	PP–531 & 20	Isoxsuprine HCl	20mg	White	Tab	Round	Y	N	Eon	Vasodilator
	SEARLE 531	Chlorthalidone	25mg	Yellow	Tab	Round	–	N	Searle	Diuretic
532	532 HD	Oxycodone & Acetaminophen	5mg/500mg	Red/Buff	Cap	–	–	–'	Halsey	Analgesic
	54–532	Pseudoephedrine	60mg	White	Tab	Round	N	N	Roxane	Decongestant
	832 / G532C	Phenobarbital	30mg	White	Tab	Round	Y	N	PBI	Sedative
	GG 532	Temazepam	30mg	White/White	Cap	–	–	–	Geneva	Sedative
	MD/532	Methylphenidate HCl	20mg	Orange	Tab	Round	Y	N	MD	Psychostimulant
	PD 532 20	Quinapril HCl	20mg	Brown	Tab	Round	Y	Y	PD	Antihypertensive
	SCHWARTZ 532	Hyoscyamine Sulfate	0.125mg	Blue/Green	Tab	–	N	N	Schwartz	Antispasmodic
533	533 HD	Flurazepam HCl	30mg	Blue	Cap	–	–	–	Halsey	Hypnotic
	54–533	Furosemide	80mg	White	Tab	Round	–	–	Roxane	Diuretic
	832/G533C	Phenobarbital	60mg	White	Tab	Round	N	N	PBI	Sedative
	93 533	Amitriptyline HCl	100mg	Orange	Tab	Round	N	Y	Lemmon	Antidepressant
	GG533	Diphenhydramine	25mg	Pink/Clear	Cap	–	–	–	Geneva	Antihistamine
534	N 533/550	Naproxen Sodium	550mg	Blue	Tab	Oval	N	Y	Novopharm	Anti–Inflammatory
	534 HD	Flurazepam HCl	15mg	Blue/white	Cap	–	–	–	Halsey	Hypnotic
	K–U 534	Hyoscyamine Sulfate & Phenobarbital	0.125mg/15mg	Pink	Tab	Round	Y	N	K–U	Antispasmodic
	P–D 534	Prenatal Vitamin Combination with Fluoride	n/a	Pink/Purple Band	Cap	–	–	–	PD	Vitamin
	PD 534	Vitamin/Mineral Combination	n/a	Pink/Red Band	Cap	–	–	–	PD	Prenatal Vitamin

ID NO.	ID CODE	GENERIC NAME	STRENGTH	COLOR	FORM	SHAPE	SCORED	COATED	MFG.	USE
535	R 534	Pindolol	5mg	White	Tab	Round	N	N	Purepac	Antihypertensive
	527/535	Secobarbital Sodium/Butalbital Sodium/Pb	0.5/0.5/0.5gr	–	Cap	–	–	–	Lannett	Hypnotic
	535 HD	Hydralazine HCl	10mg	Pink	Tab	Round	N	N	Halsey	Antihypertensive
	535 MD	Diphenoxylate HCl/Atropine Sulfate	2.5mg/0.025mg	White	Tab	Round	N	N	MD	Antidiarrhea
	93 535	Amitriptyline HCl	150mg	Peach	Tab	Round	N	Y	Lemmon	Antidepressant
	E 535	Tolbutamide	500mg	White	Tab	Round	Y	N	Eon	Hypoglycemic
	GG535	Nitrofurantoin	50mg	Yellow/White	Cap	–	–	–	Proctor	Anti-Infective
	Ortho 535	Norethindrone & Ethinyl Estradiol	0.5mg/0.035mg	White	Tab	Round	N	N	Ortho	Hormone
	PD 535 40	Quinapril HCl	40mg	Brown	Tab	Elliptical	Y	Y	PD	Antihypertensive
	PP–535	Tolbutamide	500mg	White	Tab	Round	N	N	Eon	Hypoglycemic
	R 535	Pindolol	10mg	White	Tab	Round	N	N	Purepac	Antihypertensive
	SQUIBB 535	Vitamin Combination with Hematinic	n/a	Pink	Tab	Capsule	N	Y	Squibb	Vitamin
	West–ward 535	Reserpine	0.25mg	White	Tab	Round	Y	N	West–ward	Antihypertensive
536	536 HD	Hydralazine HCl	25mg	Peach	Tab	Round	N	N	Halsey	Antihypertensive
	832/G536C	Phentermine HCl	30mg	Blue/Clear	Cap	–	–	–	PBI	Anorectic
	832/G536C	Phentermine HCl	30mg	Yellow	Cap	–	–	–	PBI	Anorectic
	832/G536C	Phentermine HCl	30mg	Black	Cap	–	–	–	PBI	Anorectic
	93–536	Naproxen Sodium	275mg	White	Tab	Oval	N	Y	Lemmon	Anti-Inflammatory
	Forest 536	Rauwolfia Serpentina	100mg	Orange	Tab	Round	–	Y	Forest	Antihypertensive
	GG536	Nitrofurantoin	100mg	Yellow	Cap	–	–	–	Proctor	Anti-Infective
537	537 HD	Hydralazine HCl	50mg	Orange	Tab	Round	N	N	Halsey	Antihypertensive
	93–537	Naproxen Sodium	550mg	White	Tab	Oval	N	Y	Lemmon	Anti-Inflammatory
	KREMERS URBAN 537	Hyoscyamine Sulfate	0.375mg	Brown/Clear	Cap	–	–	–	Schwartz	Antispasmodic
	KREMERS–URBAN 537	Hyoscyamine Sulfate SR	0.375mg	Brown/Clear	Cap	–	–	–	KV	Antispasmodic
	KREMERS–URBAN 537	Hyoscyamine Sulfate & Phenobarbital	0.375mg/45mg	Pink/Clear	Cap	–	–	–	KV	Antispasmodic
	P–D 537	Methsuximide	150mg	Cream/Gray Band	Cap	–	–	–	PD	Anticonvulsant
	SQUIBB 537	Niacin	500mg	White	Tab	–	–	–	Squibb	Vitamin
538	538 HD	Hydralazine HCl	100mg	Orange	Tab	Round	N	N	Halsey	Antihypertensive
	GG538	Nitrofurantoin	25mg	White	Cap	–	–	–	Proctor	Anti-Infective
	MD 538	Amitriptyline HCl	10mg	Pink	Tab	Round	N	Y	MD	Antidepressant
	R 538	Carbidopa/Levodopa	10mg/100mg	Blue	Tab	Round	Y	N	Purepac	Antiparkinson
	Sch. Logo 538	Halazepam	40mg	White	Tab	Round	Y	N	Schering	Antianxiety
	WC 538	Cefadroxil	500mg	Yellow/Blue	Cap	–	–	–	WC	Anti-Infective
539	MD 539	Amitriptyline HCl	25mg	Green	Tab	Round	N	Y	MD	Antidepressant
	R 539	Carbidopa/Levodopa	25mg/100mg	Yellow	Tab	Round	Y	N	Purepac	Antiparkinson
540	540 HD	Metronidazole	500mg	White	Tab	Round	Y	N	Halsey	Anti-Infective
	MD 540	Amitriptyline HCl	50mg	Brown	Tab	Round	N	Y	MD	Antidepressant
	P–D 540	Mefenamic Acid	250mg	Cream/Blue	Cap	–	–	–	PD	Analgesic
	R 540	Carbidopa/Levodopa	25mg/250mg	Blue	Tab	Round	Y	N	Purepac	Antiparkinson
541	93–541	Cephalexin	250mg	Orange/Gray	Cap	–	–	–	Lemmon	Anti-Infective
	GG541	Diphenhydramine	50mg	Pink	Cap	–	–	–	Geneva	Antihistamine
	M 541	Cimetidine	800mg	Green	Tab	Oval	Y	Y	Mylan	Anti-ulcer
	MD 541	Amitriptyline HCl	75mg	Purple	Tab	Round	N	Y	MD	Antidepressant
	PD 541	Vitamin/Mineral Combination	n/a	Pink/White Band	Cap	–	–	–	PD	Prenatal Vitamin
	SEARLE 541	Chlorthalidone	50mg	Green	Tab	Round	–	N	Searle	Diuretic
	WALLACE 541	Diphylline & Guaifenesin	200mg/200mg	Yellow	Tab	Round	Y	N	Wallace	Antiasthmatic
542	93–542	Chlorzoxazone	500mg	White	Tab	Oblong	N	Y	Lemmon	Muscle Relaxant
	MD 542	Amitriptyline HCl	100mg	Orange	Tab	Round	N	Y	MD	Antidepressant
	ORGANON 542	Ergotamine Tartrate & Caffeine	1mg/100mg	White	Tab	Round	–	N	Organon	Antimigraine
543	54 543	Oxycodone HCl/Acetaminophen	5mg/325mg	White	Tab	Round	Y	N	Roxane	Analgesic
	543 HD	Butalbital & APAP	50mg/325mg	White	Tab	Round	Y	N	Halsey	Analgesic
	93–543	Cephalexin	500mg	Orange/Orange	Cap	–	–	–	Lemmon	Anti-Infective
544	527/544	Secobarbital Sodium	1 1/2gr	Reddish–Orange	Cap	–	–	–	Lannett	Hypnotic
	544 HD 5	Diazepam	5mg	Yellow	Tab	Round	Y	N	Halsey	Antianxiety
	PD 544	Vitamin/Mineral Combination	n/a	Blue/Yellow	Cap	–	–	–	PD	Vitamin
545	879 G545	Prednisolone	5mg	Orange	Tab	Round	Y	N	Halsey	Steroid
	93 545	Chlorzoxazone & Acetaminophen	250mg/300mg	Green	Tab	Round	Y	N	Lemmon	Muscle Relaxant
	Barr 545	Cephalexin	250mg	Orange	Cap	Capsule	N	Y	Barr	Anti-Infective
546	527/546	Secobarbital Sodium	3/4gr	Reddish–Orange	Cap	–	–	–	Lannett	Hypnotic
	546 HD 2	Diazepam	2mg	White	Tab	Round	Y	N	Halsey	Antianxiety
	Barr 546	Cephalexin	500mg	Orange	Cap	Capsule	N	Y	Barr	Anti-Infective
	Forest 546	Butalbital & Acetaminophen	50mg/325mg	Red/White	Cap	–	–	–	Forest	Analgesic
547	P–D 547	Prenatal Vitamin Combination	n/a	Blue/White Band	Cap	–	–	–	PD	Vitamin
	S 547	Trichlormethiazide	4mg	Aqua	Tab	Clover	Y	N	Schering	Diuretic
	W MERRELL 547	Quinine Sulfate	260mg	White	Tab	Round	Y	N	Merrell	Muscle Relaxant
548	93–548	Amantadine HCl	100mg	Yellow	Cap	–	–	–	Lemmon	Antiviral
	WC 548	Cephalexin	250mg	White	Tab	Round	–	–	WC	Anti-Infective
549	527/549	Phentermine HCl	30mg	Yellow	Cap	–	–	N	Lannett	Anorectic
	527/549	Phentermine HCl	30mg	Black	Cap	–	–	N	Lannett	Anorectic
	527/549	Phentermine HCl	30mg	Green/Clear	Cap	–	–	N	Lannett	Anorectic
	527/549	Phentermine HCl	30mg	Brown/Clear	Cap	–	–	N	Lannett	Anorectic
	527/549	Phentermine HCl	30mg	Blue/Clear	Cap	–	–	N	Lannett	Anorectic
	527/549	Phentermine HCl	30mg	Red/Yellow	Cap	–	–	N	Lannett	Anorectic
	549 HD 10	Diazepam	10mg	Blue	Tab	Round	Y	N	Halsey	Antianxiety
	879 G549	Prednisone	20mg	Peach	Tab	Round	Y	N	Halsey	Steroid
	WC 549	Cephalexin	500mg	White	Tab	Round	–	–	WC	Anti-Infective
550	550 HD	Glutethimide	500mg	White	Tab	Round	Y	N	Halsey	Hypnotic
	barr 550	Cephradine	250mg	Green\Pink	Cap	–	–	–	Barr	Anti-Infective
	Sch. Logo 550	Fluphenazine HCL	5mg	Purple–Pink	Tab	Oval	Y	N	Schering	Tranquilizer
551	barr 551	Cephradine	500mg	Green\Green	Cap	–	–	–	Barr	Anti-Infective
	E 551	Metronidazole	250mg	White	Tab	Round	Y	N	Eon	Anti-Infective
	GG551	Procainamide HCl	250mg	Yellow	Cap	–	–	–	Geneva	Antiarrhythmic
	Mylan 551 / 500	Tolazamide	500mg	White	Tab	Round	Y	N	Mylan	Hypoglycemic
	PP–551	Metronidazole	250mg	White	Tab	Round	N	N	Eon	Anti-Infective
	WC 551	Oxazepam	15mg	Yellow	Tab	Round	–	–	WC	Antianxiety
552	0527/1552	Isobutylallylbarbituric Acid/Caff./ASA/Phenacetin	50/40/200/130mg	Green	Cap	–	–	–	Lannett	Analgesic
	GG552	Procainamide HCl	375mg	Orange/White	Cap	–	–	–	Geneva	Antiarrhythmic
	PD 552	Prazepam	5mg	Celery	Cap	–	–	–	PD	Antianxiety
553	GG553	Procainamide HCl	500mg	Orange/Yellow	Cap	–	–	–	Geneva	Antiarrhythmic
	PD 553	Prazepam	10mg	Aqua	Cap	–	–	–	PD	Antianxiety
	R 553	Erythromycin Delayed Release	250mg	Natural	Cap	–	–	–	Faulding	Anti-Infective
	R 553	Erythromycin Delayed Release	250mg	Natural	Cap	–	–	–	Purepac	Antiinfective
554	A 554	Carbamazepine	200mg	White	Tab	Round	Y	N	Lemmon	Anticonvulsant
	barr 554	Meclofenamate Sodium	50mg	Pink/Maroon	Cap	–	–	–	Barr	Anti-Inflammatory
	GG554	Niacin SR	125mg	Black/Clear	Cap	–	–	–	Eon	Vitamin

ID NO.	ID CODE	GENERIC NAME	STRENGTH	COLOR	FORM	SHAPE	SCORED	COATED	MFG.	USE
555	PD 554	Prazepam	20mg	Ivory	Cap	–	–	–	PD	Antianxiety
	barr 555	Meclofenamate Sodium	100mg	White/Maroon	Cap	–	–	–	Barr	Anti–Inflammatory
	E 555	Metronidazole	500mg	White	Tab	Oblong	Y	N	Eon	Anti–Infective
	GG555	Cephalexin	500mg	Orange	Cap	–	–	–	Novopharm	Anti–Infective
	PP–555	Metronidazole	500mg	White	Tab	Oblong	Y	N	Eon	Anti–Infective
556	GG556	Cephalexin	250mg	Orange/Gray	Cap	–	–	–	Novopharm	Anti–Infective
557	527/557	Chloral Hydrate	500mg	Green	Cap	–	–	–	Lannett	Hypnotic
	557 HD	Ibuprofen 200mg	200mg	White	Tab	Round	N	Y	Halsey	Analgesic
	P–D 557	Verapamil	80mg	White	Tab	Round	–	–	PD	Antihypertensive
	WC 557	Verapamil	80mg	White	Tab	Round	–	–	WC	Antihypertensive
558	527/558	Glutethimide	500mg	Blue/White	Cap	–	–	–	Lannett	Hypnotic
	GG 558	Fenoprofen Calcium	200mg	White/Gold & Black	Cap	–	–	–	Geneva	Anti–Inflammatory
	WC 558	Disopyramide Phosphate CR	100mg	Yellow/Purple	Cap	–	–	–	WC	Antiarrhythmic
559	559 HD	Ibuprofen	400mg	White	Tab	Round	N	Y	Halsey	Anti–Inflammatory
	GG 559	Fenoprofen Calcium	300mg	White/Gold Bands	Cap	–	–	–	Geneva	Anti–Inflammatory
	Wyeth 559	Amoxicillin	250mg	Gray/Green	Cap	–	–	–	Wyeth	Anti–Infective
560	560 HD	Ibuprofen	600mg	White	Tab	Oval	N	Y	Halsey	Anti–Inflammatory
	Wyeth 560	Amoxicillin	500mg	Gray/Green	Cap	–	–	–	Wyeth	Anti–Infective
561	527/561	Dover's Pwd./Phenacetin/ASA/Camphor/Caff./Atropine	n/a	Pink/White	Cap	–	–	–	Lannett	–
	561 HD	Metoclopramide HCl	10mg	White	Tab	Capsule	N	N	Halsey	Antireflux
562	562 HD	Brompheniramine Maleate	4mg	Peach	Tab	Round	Y	N	Halsey	Antihistamine
	MD/562	Methylphenidate HCl ER	20mg	White	Tab	Round	Y	N	MD	Psychostimulant
563	0832/G563C	Phentermine HCl	30mg	Blue/Clear	Cap	–	–	–	PBI	Anorectic
564	GG564	Niacin SR	250mg	Green/Clear	Cap	–	–	–	Eon	Vitamin
565	565 HD 0.5	Lorazepam	0.5mg	White	Tab	Round	Y	N	Halsey	Antianxiety
	GG 565	Nortriptyline Hydrochloride	10mg	Wht. org/blk bd	Cap	–	–	–	Geneva	Antidepressant
566	527/566	Amobarbital Sodium/Secobarbital Sodium	3/4gr/3/4gr	Orange/Blue	Cap	–	–	–	Lannett	Hypnotic
	566 HD	Butalbital, Aspirin, Caffeine	50/325/40mg	White	Tab	Round	N	N	Halsey	Analgesic
	GG 566	Nortriptyline Hydrochloride	25mg	Wht. org/blk bd	Cap	–	–	–	Geneva	Antidepressant
	WC 566	Ketoprofen	75mg	Blue/White	Cap	–	–	–	WC	Anti–Inflammatory
567	527/567	Amobarbital Sodium/Secobarbital Sodium	1.5gr/1.5gr	Orange/Blue	Cap	–	–	–	Lannett	Hypnotic
	567 HD	Butalbital, APAP, & Caffeine	50/325/40mg	White	Tab	Round	N	N	Halsey	Analgesic
	GG 567	Nortriptyline Hydrochloride	50mg	Wht./blk bd	Cap	–	–	–	Geneva	Antidepressant
568	527/568	Dover's Pwd./Phenacetin/ASA/Camphor/Caff./Atropine	n/a	Blue/Gold	Cap	–	–	–	Lannett	–
	GG 568	Nortriptyline Hydrochloride	75mg	Wht./org bd	Cap	–	–	–	Geneva	Antidepressant
570	54–570 2	Haloperidol	2mg	White	Tab	Round	Y	N	Roxane	Tranquilizer
	GG570	Chlorpheniramine Maleate TD	8mg	Clear/Green	Cap	–	N	N	Geneva	Antihistamine
571	GG571	Chlordiazepoxide HCl & Clidinium Bromide	5mg/2.5mg	White	Cap	–	–	–	Geneva	Antispasmodic
	SEARLE 571	Furosemide	20mg	White	Tab	Round	–	N	Searle	Diuretic
572	54–572	Phenobarbital	30mg	White	Tab	Round	Y	N	Roxane	Hypnotic
	572 HD 1	Lorazepam	1mg	White	Tab	Round	Y	N	Halsey	Antianxiety
	b 572	Methotrexate	2.5mg	Yellow	Tab	Oval	Y	Y	Barr	Antineoplastic
	GG572	Doxepin HCl	25mg	White/Pink&Gold Bnd	Cap	–	–	–	Geneva	Antidepressant
	M 572	Albuterol Sulfate	4mg	White	Tab	Round	Y	N	Mylan	Bronchodilator
573	573 HD 2	Lorazepam	2mg	White	Tab	Round	Y	N	Halsey	Antianxiety
	Forest 573	Opium/Bismuth Subcarbonate/Kaolin	3/60/350mg	Brown/Red	Cap	–	–	–	Forest	Antidiarrheal
	GG573	Doxepin HCl	50mg	Wh./Pink&Green Bnd	Cap	–	–	–	Geneva	Antidepressant
	P–D 573	Verapamil	120mg	White	Tab	Round	–	–	PD	Antihypertensive
	SQUIBB 573	Fluoxymesterone	5mg	–	Tab	–	–	–	Squibb	Hormone
	WC 573	Verapamil	120mg	White	Tab	Round	–	–	WC	Antihypertensive
574	574 HD	Hydrocodone Bitartrate & Acetaminophen	5mg/500mg	White	Tab	Capsule	Y	N	Halsey	Analgesic
	GG574	Doxepin HCl	75mg	Wh./Blk&Gold Bnd	Cap	–	–	–	Geneva	Antidepressant
	MYLAN/574	Perphenazine & Amitriptyline	4mg/25mg	Orange	Tab	Round	N	Y	Mylan	Antidepressant
575	WC 575	Danozol	200mg	Orange/Clear	Cap	–	–	–	WC	Hormone
576	GG576	Doxepin HCl	10mg	Wh./Red&Gold Bnd	Cap	–	–	–	Geneva	Antidepressant
	Wyeth 576	Erythromycin Ethylsuccinate	250mg	Pink	Tab	Round	N	Y	Wyeth	Anti–Infective
577	GG577	Doxepin HCl	100mg	Wh./Blue&Green Bnd	Cap	–	–	–	Geneva	Antidepressant
	M577	Amiloride HCL/Hydrochlorothiazide	5/50	Orange	Tab	–	Y	–	Mylan	Antihypertensive
	WC 577	Trazodone	50mg	White	Tab	Round	–	–	WC	Antidepressant
578	WC 578	Trazodone	100mg	White	Tab	Round	–	–	WC	Antidepressant
	Wyeth 578	Erythromycin Ethylsuccinate	500mg	Pink	Tab	Oval	N	Y	Wyeth	Anti–Infective
580	GG 580	Triamterene/Hydrochlorothiazide	50mg/25mg	Red	Cap	–	–	–	Geneva	Diuretic
	GG 580	Triamterene/Hydrochlorothiazide	50mg/25mg	White	Cap	–	–	–	Geneva	Diuretic
	SQUIBB 580	Nystatin	500,000 Units	Brown	Tab	Round	N	Y	Squibb	Anti–Infective
581	581 HD	Acetaminophen	500mg	White	Tab	Capsule	N	Y	Halsey	Analgesic
	GG581	Propoxyphene/Aspirin/Caffeine	65/389/32.4mg	Red/Gray	Cap	–	–	–	Geneva	Analgesic
	SEARLE 581	Furosemide	40mg	White	Tab	Round	–	N	Searle	Diuretic
582	54/582	Oxycodone HCl	5mg	White	Tab	Round	Y	N	Roxane	Analgesic
	582 HD	Quinidine Gluconate	324mg	White	Tab	Round	Y	N	Halsey	Antiarrhthymic
	GG582	Hydroxyzine Pamoate	25mg	Green/Green	Cap	–	–	–	Eon	Antihistamine
583	54 583	Furosemide	40mg	White	Tab	Round	Y	N	Roxane	Diuretic
	GG 583	Hydroxyzine Pamoate	50mg	White/Green	Cap	–	–	–	Eon	Antianxiety
	MJ 583	Norethindrone & Ethinyl Estradiol	1mg/0.035mg	Peach	Tab	Round	N	N	Mead Johnson	Hormone
584	527/584	Propoxyphene Compound 65	n/a	Red/Grey	Cap	–	–	–	Lannett	Analgesic
	barr 584	Erythromycin Delayed Release	250mg	Green/Clear	Cap	–	–	–	Barr	Anti–Infective
	GG 584	Hydroxyzine Pamoate	100mg	Dark Green	Cap	–	–	–	Geneva	Antianxiety
	MJ 584	Norethindrone & Ethinyl Estradiol	1mg/0.05mg	Yellow	Tab	Round	N	N	Mead Johnson	Hormone
585	93 585	Indomethacin	25mg	Green/Green	Cap	–	–	–	Lemmon	Anti–Inflammatory
	A 585	Carbidopa/Levodopa	25mg/100mg	Mottled Yellow	Tab	Round	Y	N	Lemmon	Antiparkinson
	barr, 555/585	Chlorzoxazone	500mg	Green	Tab	Round	Y	N	Barr	Muscle relaxant
586	PP 585	Methocarbamol	500mg	White	Tab	Round	Y	N	Eon	Muscle Relaxant
	RR 586	Fluoxymesterone	10mg	Green	Tab	Octagonal	N	N	RR	Steroid
587	879 G587	Rauwolfia Serpentina	100mg	Red	Tab	Round	N	Y	Halsey	Antihypertensive
	93 587	Indomethacin	50mg	Green/Green	Cap	–	–	–	Lemmon	Anti–Inflammatory
	A 587	Carbidopa/Levodopa	25mg/250mg	Mottled Blue	Tab	Round	Y	N	Lemmon	Antiparkinson
	PP 587	Methocarbamol	750mg	White	Tab	Capsule	N	N	Eon	Muscle Relaxant
589	GG 589	Thiothixene	1mg	White	Cap	–	–	–	Geneva	Tranquilizer
590	93 590	Propoxyphene Napsylate with APAP	100mg/650mg	White	Tab	Oblong	N	Y	Lemmon	Analgesic
	GG590	Chlorpheniramine Maleate TD	12mg	Clear/Green	Cap	–	–	–	Geneva	Antihistamine
591	527/591	Chlordiazepoxide HCl	5mg	Green/Yellow	Cap	–	–	–	Lannett	Antianxiety
	591 – C	Phenobarbital	15mg	White	Tab	Round	Y	N	Danbury	Sedative
	591 – D	Phenobarbital	30mg	White	Tab	Round	Y	N	Danbury	Sedative
	591 – O	Phenobarbital	100mg	White	Tab	Round	Y	N	Danbury	Sedative
	591 – V	Phenobarbital	60mg	White	Tab	Round	Y	N	Danbury	Sedative
	591 A	Meprobamate	200mg	White	Tab	Round	N	N	Danbury	Antianxiety

ID NO.	ID CODE	GENERIC NAME	STRENGTH	COLOR	FORM	SHAPE	SCORED	COATED	MFG.	USE
	591–F	Butalbital & Acetaminophen	50mg/325mg	White	Tab	Round	N	N	Danbury	Analgesic
	DAN 591–A	Meprobamate	400mg	White	Tab	Round	Y	N	Danbury	Antianxiety
	Forest 591	Dextromethorphan Hydrobromide/Guaifenesin	15mg/100mg	Orange	Tab	Round	–	N	Forest	Antitussive
	GG 591	Propoxyphene Hydrochloride	65mg	Pink/Pink	Cap	–	–	–	Geneva	Analgesic
	GG591	Propoxyphene Hydrochloride	65mg	Pink	Cap	–	–	–	Geneva	Analgesic
592	527/592	Chlordiazepoxide HCl	10mg	Green/Black	Cap	–	–	–	Lannett	Antianxiety
	GG 592	Prazosin	1mg	White/Black bands	Cap	–	–	–	Geneva	Antihypertensive
	WC 592	Theophylline CR	300mg	White	Tab	Capsule	Y	N	WC	Bronchodilator
593	527/593	Chlordiazepoxide HCl	25mg	Green/White	Cap	–	–	–	Lannett	Antianxiety
	GG 593	Prazosin	2mg	White/Black&Pink Bd	Cap	–	–	–	Geneva	Antihypertensive
	WC 593	Theophylline Controlled Release	450mg	White	Tab	Oval	Y	N	WC	Bronchodilator
	Wyeth 593	Dicloxacillin Sodium Monohydrate	500mg	Purple/White	Cap	–	–	–	Wyeth	Anti–Infective
594	879 G594C	Secobarbital Sodium	100mg	Reddish–Orange	Cap	–	–	–	Halsey	Hypnotic
	GG 594	Prazosin	5mg	White/Black&Blue Bd	Cap	–	–	–	Geneva	Antihypertensive
	WC 594	Desipramine	25mg	Green	Tab	Round	N	Y	WC	Antidepressant
595	527/595	Propoxyphene HCl	65mg	Pink	Cap	–	–	–	Lannett	Analgesic
	MJ 595	Megestrol Acetate	20mg	Blue	Tab	Round	Y	N	BM	Hormone
	WC 595	Desipramine	50mg	Green	Tab	Round	N	Y	WC	Antidepressant
596	GG 596	Thiothixene	2mg	White	Cap	–	–	–	Geneva	Tranquilizer
	MJ 596	Megestrol Acetate	40mg	Blue	Tab	Round	Y	N	BM	Hormone
	WC 596	Desipramine	75mg	Orange	Tab	Round	N	Y	WC	Antidepressant
597	GG 597	Thiothixene	5mg	White	Cap	–	–	–	Geneva	Tranquilizer
598	GG 598	Thiothixene	10mg	White	Cap	–	–	–	Geneva	Tranquilizer
	Sch. Logo 598	Perphenazine & Amitriptyline HCl	2mg/25mg	Pink	Tab	Round	N	Y	Schering	Antidepressant
599	54–599	Alprazolam	0.5mg	–	Tab	–	–	–	Roxane	Antianxiety
600	ALRA IF 600	Ibuprofen	600mg	Orange	Tab	Oval	N	Y	Alra	Anti–Inflammatory
	C/600–LL	Calcium	600mg	White	Tab	Oblong	Y	Y	Lederle	Vitamin
	G–600	Guaifenesin	600mg	Green	Tab	Oval	Y	N	Trinity	Expectorant
	IBU 600	Ibuprofen	600mg	White	Tab	Oblong	N	Y	Boots	Anti–Inflammatory
	MPC 600	Potassium Citrate	5mEq	Tan	Tab	Round	Y	N	Mission	Potassium Supp.
601	Mylan 601	Ibuprofen	600mg	White	Tab	Capsule	N	Y	Mylan	Anti–Inflammatory
	SEARLE 601	Propantheline Bromide	15mg	Peach	Tab	Round	N	Y	Searle	Antispasmodic
	TP601	Colchicine	540mcg	White	Tab	Round	N	N	Towne Paulsen	Antigout
602	832/G602	Sulfamethoxazole & Trimethoprim	400mg/80mg	White	Tab	Capsule	Y	N	PBI	Anti–Infective
603	54–603	Naproxen Sodium	550mg	–	Tab	–	–	–	Roxane	Anti–Inflammatory
	832/G603	Sulfamethoxazole & Trimethoprim	800mg/160mg	White	Tab	Capsule	Y	N	PBI	Anti–Infective
	ENDO 603	Carbidopa/Levodopa	10mg/100mg	Blue	Tab	Oval	Y	N	Endo	Antiparkinson
	SQUIBB 603	Tetracycline	500mg	Pink	Tab	Oblong	N	Y	Squibb	Anti–Infective
604	TP604	Cortisone Acetate	25mg	White	Tab	Round	N	N	Towne Paulsen	Steroid
605	ENDO 605	Carbidopa/Levodopa	25mg/100mg	Yellow	Tab	Oval	Y	N	Endo	Antiparkinson
	PP–605	Chlordiazepoxide HCl	5mg	Green/Yellow	Cap	–	–	–	Eon	Antianxiety
606	606HD	Methyldopa	125mg	White	Tab	Round	N	Y	Halsey	Antihypertensive
	Forest 606	Phentermine HCl	30mg	Black	Cap	–	–	–	Forest	Anorectic
	GG 606	Triamterene & Hydrochlorothiazide	37.5mg/25mg	White	Cap	–	–	–	Penn	Diuretic
	SQUIBB 606	Bendroflumethiazide	5mg	Green	Tab	Round	Y	N	Princeton	Diuretic
	TP. 606	Hydrocortisone	20mg	White	Tab	Round	N	Y	Towne Paulsen	Steroid
	WC 606	Aspirin	325mg	White	Tab	Round	N	N	WC	Analgesic
607	607HD	Methyldopa	250mg	White	Tab	Round	N	Y	Halsey	Antihypertensive
	ENDO 607	Carbidopa/Levodopa	25mg/250mg	Blue	Tab	Oval	Y	N	Endo	Antiparkinson
	P–D 607	Phenobarbital	60mg	White	Tab	Round	–	N	PD	Sedative
	WC 607	Phenobarbital	60mg	White	Tab	Round	–	N	WC	Sedative/Hypnotic
608	608HD	Methyldopa	500mg	White	Tab	Round	N	Y	Halsey	Antihypertensive
	TP608	Hydrocortisone	10mg	White	Tab	Round	N	N	Towne Paulsen	Steroid
609	54–609 4	Hydromorphone HCl	4mg	White	Tab	Round	N	N	Roxane	Analgesic
	L 609	Phenyleph/Phenylpro/Chlorphen/Hyosc/Atro/Scop	25/50/8/.19/.04	Green	Tab	Oblong	Y	N	LuChem	Decongestant Comb.
	Squibb 609 M	Fosinopril Sodium	20mg	White	Tab	Oval	N	N	Squibb	Anti–hypertensive
610	610HD	Propoxyphene Napsylate and Acetaminophen	50mg/325mg	White	Tab	Capsule	N	Y	Halsey	Analgesic
	Forest 610	Hydrocodone & Acetaminophen	5mg/500mg	Black/Red	Cap	–	–	–	Forest	Analgesic
	PP–610	Chlordiaepoxide HCl	10mg	Green/Black	Cap	–	–	–	Eon	Antianxiety
	SCHWARZ 610	Isosorbide Mononitrate	10mg	White	Tab	Round	Y	N	Schwarz	Antianginal
611	Mylan 611	Methyldopa	250mg	Beige	Tab	Round	N	Y	Mylan	Antihypertensive
	SEARLE 611	Propantheline Bromide	7.5mg	White	Tab	Round	N	Y	Searle	Antispasmodic
	SQUIBB 611	Niacin	50mg	White	Tab	–	–	–	Squibb	Vitamin
	WC 611	Baclofen	10mg	White	Tab	Round	–	N	WC	Anticonvulsant
612	54 612	Prednisone	5mg	White	Tab	Round	Y	N	Roxane	Steroid
	SQUIBB 612	Niacin	100mg	White	Tab	–	–	–	Squibb	Vitamin
	WC 612	Baclofen	20mg	White	Tab	Round	–	N	WC	Anticonvulsant
	WHITBY 612	Guaifenesin & Pseudoephedrine	600mg/120mg	White	Tab	Oblong	Y	N	Whitby	Antitussive comb.
613	54–613	Codeine Sulfate	15mg	White	Tab	Round	Y	N	Roxane	Analgesic
	832/G613	Thyroid	30mg	Tan	Tab	Round	N	N	PBI	Hormone
	93–613	Amoxicillin	250mg	Ivory/Caramel	Cap	–	–	–	Lemmon	Anti–Infective
	E 613	Hydroxyzine Pamoate	25mg	Green/Green	Cap	–	–	–	Eon	Antianxiety
	PP–613	Hydroxyzine Pamoate	25mg	Green/Green	Cap	–	–	–	Eon	Antianxiety
614	832/G614	Thyroid	60mg	Tan	Tab	Round	N	N	PBI	Hormone
	832/G614	Thyroid	1gr	Wh./Brown specks	Tab	Round	Y	N	PBI	Hormone
	HB 93 614	Phenobarbital & Belladonna Extract	16.2mg/10.8mg	Green	Tab	Round	N	N	Lemmon	Antispasmodic
	Wyeth 614	Cyclacillin	250mg	Yellow	Tab	Capsule	Y	N	Wyeth	Anti–Infective
615	832/G615	Thyroid	120mg	Tan	Tab	Round	N	N	PBI	Hormone
	93–615	Amoxicillin	500mg	Ivory/Ivory	Cap	–	–	–	Lemmon	Anti–Infective
	E 615	Hydroxyzine Pamoate	50mg	Green/White	Cap	–	–	–	Eon	Antianxiety
	PP–615	Hydroxyzine Pamoate	50mg	Green/White	Cap	–	–	–	Eon	Antianxiety
	WC 615	Minocycline HCl	50mg	Olive/Brown	Cap	–	–	–	WC	Anti–Infective
	Wyeth 615	Cyclacillin	500mg	Yellow	Tab	Capsule	Y	N	Wyeth	Anti–Infective
616	832/G616	Thyroid	180mg	Tan	Tab	Round	N	N	PBI	Hormone
	WC 616	Minocycline HCl	100mg	Olive/White	Cap	–	–	–	WC	Anti–Infective
	WC 616	Minocycline	100mg	White/Green	Cap	–	–	–	WC	Anti–Infective
617	93 617	Chlordiazepoxide HCl/Clidinium	5mg/2.5mg	White/White	Cap	–	–	–	Lemmon	Antianxiety
	E 617	Chlordiazepoxide HCl with Clidinum Bromide	5mg/2.5mg	White/White	Cap	–	–	–	Eon	Antispasmodic
	f 617 1mg	Tacrolimus	1mg	White/Red Band	Cap	–	–	–	Fujisawa	
	f 617 1mg	Tacrolimus	1mg	White/Red Band	Cap	–	–	–	Fujisawa	Immunosuppressant
	Forest 617	Chlorpheniramine/APAP/Phenylpropanolamine/PwdOpium	4/325/25/2mg	Red	Cap	–	–	–	Forest	Decongestant Comb.
	N 617/10	Piroxicam	10mg	Green/Grey	Cap	–	–	–	Novopharm	Anti–inflammatory
	PP–617	Chlordiazepoxide HCl & Clindinium Bromide	5mg/2.5mg.	White	Cap	–	–	–	Eon	Antispasmodic
	WC 617	Quinidine Gluconate	324mg	White	Tab	Round	Y	N	WC	Antiarrhythmic
618	832/G618	Tolazamide	100mg	White	Tab	Round	Y	N	PBI	Hypoglycemic

ID NO.	ID CODE	GENERIC NAME	STRENGTH	COLOR	FORM	SHAPE	SCORED	COATED	MFG.	USE
	P–D 618	Placebo	n/a	White	Tab	Round	N	N	PD	Placebo
	SQUIBB 618	Bendroflumethiazide	10mg	Peach	Tab	Round	Y	N	Princeton	Diuretic
620	93 620	Propranolol	20mg	Blue	Tab	Round	Y	N	Lemmon	Antihypertensive
	SCHWARZ 620	Isosorbide Mononitrate	20mg	White	Tab	Round	Y	N	Schwarz	Antianginal
	Stuart 620	Aluminum/Magnesium Hydroxide/Simethicone	200/200/20 mg	Yellow/White	Tab	Round	N	N	Stuart	Antacid
621	832/G621	Tolazamide	500mg	White	Tab	Round	Y	N	PBI	Hypoglycemic
	Forest 621	Hyoscyamine Sulfate	0.125mg	White	Tab	Capsule	–	N	Forest	Antispasmodic
	WC 621	Loxapine	5mg	White	Cap	–	–	–	WC	Antidepressant
622	54 622	Methyldopa	250mg	Beige	Tab	Round	N	Y	Roxane	Antihypertensive
	622HD	Ibuprofen	800mg	White	Tab	Capsule	N	Y	Halsey	Anti–Inflammatory
	832/G622	Tolazamide	250mg	White	Tab	Round	Y	N	PBI	Hypoglycemic
	dp 622	Diazepam	5mg	Yellow	Tab	Round	Y	N	Duramed	Antianxiety
	P–D 622	Ferrous Fumarate	75mg	Brown	Tab	Round	N	N	PD	Iron Supp.
	SQUIBB 622	Meclofenamate	50mg	–	Cap	–	–	–	Squibb	Anti–Inflammatory
623	54–623	Acetaminophen/Codeine	300mg/30mg	White	Tab	Round	–	–	Roxane	Analgesic
	dp 623	Diazepam	10mg	Blue	Tab	Round	Y	N	Duramed	Antianxiety
	SQUIBB 623	Chloral Hydrate	250mg	–	Cap	–	–	–	Squibb	Hypnotic
624	Forest 624	Phenylpropanolamine/Chlorpheniramine/APAP	25mg/4mg/325mg	Green	Tab	Capsule	–	Y	Forest	Decongestant Comb.
625	527/625	Phendimetrazine Tartrate 5	35mg	Yellow	Cap	–	–	–	Lannett	Anorectic
	DPI 625	Estropipate	0.75mg	Orange	Tab	Diamond	–	N	Duramed	Hormone
	PP–625	Chlordiazepoxide	25mg	Green/White	Cap	–	–	–	Eon	Antianxiety
	West–ward 625	Sulfamethoxazole & Trimethoprim	800mg/160mg	White	Tab	Oval	N	Y	West–ward	Anti–Infective
626	527/626	Phendimetrazine Tartrate 6	35mg	Blue/Clear	Cap	–	–	–	Lannett	Anorectic
	SQUIBB 626	Chloral Hydrate	500mg	–	Cap	–	–	–	Squibb	Hypnotic
627	527/627	Phendimetrazine Tartrate 7	35mg	Brown/Clear	Cap	–	–	–	Lannett	Anorectic
	Forest 627	Phenylpropanolamine/Chlorpheniramine	37.5mg/4mg	Chartreuse	Tab	Round	–	Y	Forest	Decontestant Comb.
628	527/628	Phendimetrazine Tartrate 9	35mg	Green/Clear	Cap	–	–	–	Lannett	Anorectic
	93–628	Indomethacin ER	75mg	Lavender/Clear	Cap	–	–	–	Lemmon	Anti–Inflammatory
	Forest 628	Phenylpropanolamine/Chlorpheniramine	75mg/8mg	Yellow/Clear	Cap	–	–	–	Forest	Decongestant Comb.
629	SQUIBB 629	Meclofenamate	100mg	–	Cap	–	–	–	Squibb	Anti–Inflammatory
630	630HD	Propoxyphene Napsylate and Acetaminophen	100mg/650mg	Pink	Tab	Capsule	N	Y	Halsey	Analgesic
	ENDO 630	Cimetidine	200mg	White	Tab	Oval	N	Y	Endo	Anti–Ulcer
	FOREST 630	Acetaminophen/Caffeine/Butalbital	325/40/50mg	White	Tab	Round	–	–	Forest	Analgesic
	PP–630	Propoxyphene HCl	65mg	Pink	Cap	–	–	–	Eon	Analgesic
	WC 630	Pindolol	5mg	White	Tab	Round	Y	N	WC	Antihypertensive
631	COPLEY 631	Diltiazem HCl	30mg	Blue	Tab	Round	N	Y	Copley	Antianginal
	ENDO 631	Cimetidine	300mg	White	Tab	Oval	N	Y	Endo	Antiulcer
	FOREST 631	Acetaminophen/Caffeine/Butalbital	325/40/50mg	White	Cap	–	–	–	Forest	Analgesic
	WC 631	Pindolol	10mg	White	Tab	Round	Y	N	WC	Antihypertensive
632	632 HD	Fenoprofen Calcium	200mg	Flesh/Lavender	Cap	–	–	–	Halsey	Anti–Inflammatory
	ENDO 632	Cimetidine	400mg	White	Tab	Oval	Y	Y	Endo	Antiulcer
	WC 632	Loxapine	10mg	Yellow/White	Cap	–	–	–	WC	Antidepressant
633	633 HD	Fenoprofen Calcium	300mg	Flesh/Orange	Cap	–	–	–	Halsey	Anti Inflammatory
	ENDO 633	Cimetidine	800mg	White	Tab	Oval	Y	Y	Endo	Antiulcer
634	634 HD	Fenoprofen Calcium	600mg	Peach	Tab	Capsule	–	–	Halsey	Anti–Inflammatory
	K–634	Nitroglycerin T.D.	2.5 mg	Lavender/Clear	Cap	–	–	–	KV	Antianginal
	N/634	Methyldopa/Hydrochlorothiazide	250mg/15mg	Green	Tab	Round	N	Y	Novopharm	Antihypertensive
	P–D 634	Acetaminophen & Codeine	300mg/15mg	White	Tab	Round	–	N	PD	Analgesic
	W–C 634	Acetaminophen & Codeine	300mg/15mg	White	Tab	Round	–	N	WC	Analgesic
635	K–635	Nitroglycerin T.D.	6.5 mg	Blue/Yellow	Cap	–	–	–	KV	Antianginal
	N/635	Methyldopa/Hydrochlorothiazide	500mg/30mg	Green	TAB	Round	N	Y	Novopharm	Antihypertensive
	P–D 635	Acetaminophen & Codeine	300mg/30mg	White	Tab	Round	–	N	PD	Analgesic
	PP–635	Phentermine HCl	30mg	Red/Black	Cap	–	–	–	Eon	Anorectic
	W–C 635	Acetaminophen & Codeine	300mg/30mg	White	Tab	Round	–	N	WC	Analgesic
637	527/637	Phendimetrazine Tartrate 1	35mg	Brown/Clear	Cap	–	–	–	Lannett	Anorectic
	93–637	Trazodone HCl	50mg	White	Tab	Round	Y	Y	Lemmon	Antidepressant
	P–D 637	Acetaminophen & Codeine	300mg/60mg	White	Tab	Round	–	N	PD	Analgesic
	SQUIBB 637	Isoniazid	100mg	–	Tab	–	–	–	Squibb	Anti–Infective
	W–C 637	Acetaminophen & Codeine	300mg/60mg	White	Tab	Round	–	N	WC	Analgesic
638	527/638	Phendimetrazine Tartrate 2	35mg	Red/Yellow	Cap	–	–	–	Lannett	Anorectic
	93–638	Trazodone HCl	100mg	White	Tab	Round	Y	Y	Lemmon	Antidepressant
	P–D 638	Vitamin Combination	n/a	Brown	Tab	Oval	N	Y	PD	Vitamin
639	527/639	Phendimetrazine Tartrate 3	35mg	Green/Clear	Cap	–	–	–	Lannett	Anorectic
640	93 640	Propranolol	40mg	Green	Tab	Round	Y	N	Lemmon	Antihypertensive
	N 640/20	Piroxicam	20mg	Green/Green	Cap	–	–	–	Novopharm	Anti–inflammatory
	PP–640	Phentermine HCl	30mg	Black	Cap	–	–	–	Eon	Anorectic
	WC 640	Acetaminophen	325mg	White	Tab	Round	Y	N	WC	Analgesic
641	Forest 641	Hydrocodone & Acetaminophen	5mg/500mg	Green	Tab	Round	–	N	Forest	Analgesic
	Pfizer 641	Oxamniquine	250mg	Green/Yellow	Cap	–	–	–	Pfizer	Anthelminitics
	Wyeth 641	Levonorestrel & Ethinyl Estradiol	0.05mg/0.03mg	Brown	Tab	Round	N	Y	Wyeth	Contraceptive
642	FOREST 642	Theophylline	100mg	White	Cap	–	–	–	Forest	Bronchial Dilator
	N/642	Methyldopa/Hydrochlorothiazide	250mg/25mg	White	Tab	Round	N	Y	Novopharm	Antihypertensive
	Wyeth 642	Levonorestrel & Ethinyl Estradiol	0.075mg/0.04mg	White	Tab	Round	N	Y	Wyeth	Contraceptive
643	54–643	Naproxen	250mg	–	Tab	–	–	–	Roxane	Anti–Inflammatory
	FOREST 643	Theophylline	200mg	White	Cap	–	–	–	Forest	Bronchial Dilator
	N/643	Methyldopa/Hydrochlorothiazide	500mg/50mg	White	TAB	Round	N	Y	Novopharm	Antihypertensive
	Wyeth 643	Levonorestrel & Ethinyl Estradiol	0.125mg/0.03mg	Yellow	Tab	Round	N	Y	Wyeth	Contraceptive
644	DPI 644	Oxycodone & Acetaminophen	5mg/500mg	Red/White	Cap	–	–	–	Duramed	Analgesic
	E 644	Phentermine HCl	15mg	Gray/Yellow	Cap	–	–	–	Eon	Anorectic
646	FOREST 646	Theophylline	125mg	White	Cap	–	–	–	Forest	Bronchial Dilator
647	647 HD	Codeine/Butalbital/Caffeine/Aspirin	30/50/40/325mg	Blue/White	Cap	–	–	–	Halsey	Analgesic
	E 647	Phentermine HCl	30mg	Yellow	Cap	–	–	–	Eon	Anorectic
	FOREST 647	Theophylline	250mg	White	Cap	–	–	–	Forest	Bronchial Dilator
	PP–647	Phentermine HCl	30mg	Yellow/Yellow	Cap	–	–	–	Eon	Anorectic
648	648 HD	Codeine/Butalbital/Caffeine/Aspirin	15/50/40/325mg	Gray/White	Cap	–	–	–	Halsey	Analgesic
	Adria 648	Cyclothiazide	2mg	Peach	Tab	Oval	–	N	Adria	Diuretic
	E 648	Diphenhydramine HCl	25mg	Pink/Clear	Cap	–	–	–	Eon	Antihistamine
	P–D 648	Penicillin V Potassium	250mg	White	Tab	Oval	–	–	PD	Anti–Infective
	PP 648	Diphenhydramine HCl	25mg	Pink/Clear	Cap	–	–	–	Eon	Antihistamine
	SQUIBB 648	Penicillin V Potassium	500mg	White	Tab	Oblong	N	Y	Squibb	Anti–Infective
	WC 648	Penicillin V Potassium	250mg	White	Tab	Oval	–	–	WC	Anti–Infective
649	E 649	Diphenhydramine HCl	50mg	Pink/Pink	Cap	–	–	–	Eon	Antihistamine
	PP 649	Diphenhydramine HCl	50mg	Pink	Cap	–	–	–	Eon	Antihistamine
650	54–650	Leucovorin Calcium	15mg	–	Tab	Round	–	–	Roxane	Antineoplastic
	879 G650C	Oxycodone HCl, Oxycodone Terephthalate, Aspirin	4.5mg/.38mg/325	Yellow	Tab	Round	Y	–	Halsey	Analgesic

ID NO.	ID CODE	GENERIC NAME	STRENGTH	COLOR	FORM	SHAPE	SCORED	COATED	MFG.	USE
	STUART 650	Chewable Hematinic	–	Brown/Yellow	Tab	Round	N	N	Stuart	Vitamin
	WC 650	Loxapine	25mg	Green/White	Cap	–	–	–	WC	Antidepressant
	Wyeth 650	Inert tablet	n/a	Blue	Tab	Round	N	Y	Wyeth	Placebo
651	dp 651	Phentermine HCl	30mg	Blue/Clear	Cap	Capsule	–	–	Duramed	Anorectic
	Stuart 651	Aluminum/Magnesium Hydroxide/Simethicone	400/400/40 mg	Green/White	Tab	Round	N	N	Stuart	Antacid
	WC 651	Loxapine	50mg	Blue/White	Cap	–	–	–	WC	Antidepressant
653	93–653	Doxycycline Hyclate	100mg	Blue/Blue	Cap	–	–	–	Lemmon	Anti–Infective
655	SQUIBB 655	Tetracycline	250mg	Pink	Cap	–	–	–	Squibb	Anti–Infective
656	656 HD	Chlordiazepoxide HCl with Clidinum Bromide	5mg/2.5mg	Green	Cap	–	–	–	Halsey	Antispasmodic
657	f 657 5mg	Tacrolimus	5mg	Grayish Red/wt. bnd	Cap	–	–	–	Fujisawa	Immunosuppressant
	WC 657	Theophylline CR	100mg	White	Tab	Round	Y	N	WC	Bronchodilator
659	WC 659	Theophylline CR	200mg	White	Tab	Oval	Y	N	WC	Bronchodilator
660	dp 660	Temazepam	15mg	Green/White	Cap	–	–	–	Duramed	Hypnotic
661	dp 661	Temazepam	30mg	White	Cap	–	–	–	Duramed	Hypnotic
662	54–662	Dexamethasone	2mg	White	Tab	Round	Y	N	Roxane	Steroid
	COPLEY 662	Diltiazem HCl	60mg	White	Tab	Round	N	Y	Copley	Antianginal
663	LUCHEM 663	Hydrocodone Bitartrate with Acetaminophen	5mg/500mg	Red/Black	Cap	–	–	–	LuChem	Analgesic
	PD 663	Erythromycin Delayed Release	125mg	Clear/Orange	Cap	–	–	–	PD	Anti–Infective
	SQUIBB 663	Tetracycline	250mg	Pink	Tab	Oblong	N	Y	Squibb	Anti–Infective
665	93–665	Albuterol Sulfate	2mg	White	Tab	Round	Y	N	Lemmon	Bronchodilator
	WC 665	Oxazepam	15mg	Natural	Cap	–	–	–	WC	Antianxiety
666	93–666	Albuterol Sulfate	4mg	White	Tab	Round	Y	N	Lemmon	Bronchodilator
667	WC 667	Oxazepam	30mg	Orange/White	Cap	–	–	–	WC	Antianxiety
670	93–670	Gemfibrozil	600mg	White	Tab	Oval	Y	Y	Lemmon	Antihyperlipidemic
	93/670	Gemfibrozil	600mg	White	Tab	Oblong	N	N	Upsher	Antihyperlipidemic
	E 670	Tetracycline Hydrochloride	250mg	Orange/Yellow	Cap	–	–	–	Eon	Anti–Infective
	L & 670	Quinine Sulfate	260mg	White	Tab	Round	Y	N	LuChem	Muscle Relaxant
	PP–670	Tetracycline	250mg	Yellow/Orange	Cap	–	–	–	Eon	Anti–Infective
671	PP–671	Tetracycline	500mg	Black/Yellow	Cap	–	–	–	Eon	Anti–Infective
672	P–D 672	Erythromycin Stearate	250mg	Yellow	Tab	Round	N	Y	PD	Anti–Infective
	WC 672	Erythromycin Stearate	250mg	Yellow	Tab	Round	N	Y	WC	Anti–Infective
673	P–D 673	Penicillin V Potassium	500mg	White	Tab	Oval	–	–	PD	Anti–Infective
	WC 673	Penicillin V Potassium	500mg	White	Tab	Oval	–	–	WC	Anti–Infective
674	SQUIBB 674	Doxycycline Hyclate	50mg	–	Cap	–	–	–	Squibb	Anti–Infective
677	Forest 677	Acetaminophen/Caffeine/Butalbital/Codeine	325/40/50/30mg	Black/Blue	Cap	–	–	–	Forest	Analgesic
678	FOREST 678	Butalbital/Acetaminophen/Caffeine	50mg/500mg/40mg	White	Tab	Capsule	Y	N	Forest	Analgesic
680	54 680	Vitamin C	500mg	White	Tab	Round	Y	N	Roxane	Vitamin
	West–ward 680	Sulfinpyrazone	100mg	White	Tab	Round	Y	N	West–ward	Antigout
683	West–ward 683	Sulfisoxazole	500mg	White	Tab	Round	Y	N	West–ward	Anti–Infective
684	SQUIBB 684	Penicillin V Potassium	250mg	Peach	Tab	Oblong	N	Y	Squibb	Anti–Infective
686	93 686	Propoxyphene W/Aspirin & Caffeine	65/389/32.4mg	Red/Gray	Cap	–	–	–	Lemmon	Analgesic
	L 686	Thyroid	60mg	Tan	Tab	Round	N	N	LuChem	Hormone
	PP–686	Propoxyphene HCl/Aspirin/Caffeine	65/389/32.4mg	Red/Gray	Cap	–	–	–	Eon	Analgesic
687	L 687	Thyroid	120mg	Tan	Tab	Round	N	N	LuChem	Hormone
689	West–ward 689	Theophylline (Anhydrous) Controlled Release	200mg	White	Tab	Oval	Y	N	West–ward	Bronchodilator
690	54–690 20	Haloperidol	20mg	White	Tab	Round	Y	N	Roxane	Tranquilizer
	MERRELL 690	Chlorotrianisene	12mg	Green	Cap	–	–	–	Merrell	Hormone
	SQUIBB 690	Testolactone	50mg	–	Tab	–	–	–	Squibb	Antineoplastic
	WC 690	Oxazepam	10mg	Blue/White	Cap	–	–	–	WC	Antianxiety
	West–ward 690	Theophylline (Anhydrous) Controlled Release	300mg	White	Tab	Capsule	Y	N	West–ward	Bronchodilator
691	93–691	Propranolol HCl ER	60mg	Brown/Clear	Cap	–	–	–	Lemmon	Antihypertensive
	COPLEY 691	Diltiazem HCl	90mg	Blue	Tab	Oblong	N	Y	Copley	Antianginal
	MERRELL 691	Chlorotrianisene	25mg	Green	Cap	–	–	–	Merrell Dow	Hormone
	MERRELL 691	Chlorotrianisene	25mg	Green/Green	Cap	–	–	–	Merrell	Hormone
692	93–692	Propranolol HCl ER	80mg	Blue/Clear	Cap	–	–	–	Lemmon	Antihypertensive
	MERRELL 692	Chlorotrianisene	72mg	Green/Yellow	Cap	–	–	–	Merrell	Hormone
	P–D 692	Propoxyphene HCL	65mg	–	Cap	–	–	–	PD	Analgesic
693	93–693	Propranolol HCl ER	120mg	Blue/Clear	Cap	–	–	–	Lemmon	Antihypertensive
694	93–694	Propranolol HCl ER	160mg	Blue/Clear	Cap	–	–	–	Lemmon	Antihypertensive
695	West–ward 695	Theophylline/Ephedrine HCl/Phenobarbital	118mg/24mg/8mg	White	Tab	Round	Y	N	West–ward	Bronchodilator
696	PD 696	Erythromycin Delayed Release	250mg	Clear/Orange	Cap	–	–	–	PD	Anti–Infective
697	P–D 697	Tetracycline HCl	500mg	Orange/White	Cap	–	–	–	PD	Anti–Infective
	WC 697	Tetracycline HCl	500mg	Orange/White	Cap	–	–	–	WC	Anti–Infective
698	P–D 698	Phenobarbital	100mg	White	Tab	Round	–	N	PD	Sedative
	PP–698	Doxycycline Hyclate	50mg	Blue/White	Cap	–	–	–	Eon	Anti–Infective
	WC 698	Phenobarbital	100mg	White	Tab	Round	–	N	WC	Sedative/Hypnotic
699	P–D 699	Phenobarbital	15mg	White	Tab	Round	N	N	PD	Sedative
	PP–699	Doxycycline Hyclate	100mg	Blue	Cap	–	–	–	Eon	Anti–Infective
	WC 699	Phenobarbital	15mg	White	Tab	Round	N	N	WC	Sedative/Hypnotic
700	P–D 700	Phenobarbital	30mg	White	Tab	Round	–	N	PD	Sedative
	WC 700	Phenobarbital	30mg	White	Tab	Round	–	N	WC	Sedative/Hypnotic
702	54 702	Lithium Carbonate	600mg	White/Flesh	Tab	–	–	–	Roxane	Tranquilizer
	MJ 702	Prenatal Vitamins	n/a	White	Tab	Oval	N	Y	Mead Johnson	Vitamin
	P–D 702	Hydrochlorothiazide	25mg	White	Tab	Round	Y	N	PD	Diuretic
	WC 702	Hydrochlorothiazide	25mg	White	Tab	Round	Y	N	WC	Diuretic
703	54–703	Imipramine HCl	50mg	Coral	Tab	Round	N	Y	Roxane	Antidepressant
705	Sch. Logo 705	Perphenazine	2mg	Gray	Tab	Round	N	Y	Schering	Tranquilizer
707	Forest 707	Sucrose & Starch	n/a	Blue/Clear	Cap	–	–	–	Forest	Placebo
708	Forest 708	Sucrose & Starch	n/a	Green/Clear	Cap	–	–	–	Forest	Placebo
709	Forest 709	Sucrose & Starch	n/a	Orange/Clear	Cap	–	–	–	Forest	Placebo
710	P–D 710	Hydrochlorothiazide	50mg	White	Tab	Round	Y	N	PD	Diuretic
	STUART 710	Fluoride & Multivitamins	n/a	Orange	Tab	Round	Y	N	Stuart	Vitamin
	WC 710	Hydrochlorothiazide	50mg	White	Tab	Round	Y	N	WC	Diuretic
711	COPLEY 711	Guanabenz Acetate	8mg	Peach	Tab	Square	–	N	Copley	Antihypertensive
	HD 711	Propoxyphene/Acetaminophen	100mg/650mg	White	Tab	–	–	–	Halsey	Analgesic
	Mylan 711	Methyldopa & Hydrochlorothiazide	250mg/25mg	White	Tab	Capsule	N	Y	Mylan	Antihypertensive
	PP711	Salsalate	500mg	Green	Tab	Round	N	Y	Eon	Antiarthritic
712	P–D 712	Spironolactone with Hydrochlorothiazide	25mg/25mg	White	Tab	Round	Y	N	PD	Diuretic
	PP712	Salsalate	750mg	Green	Tab	Capsule	N	Y	Eon	Antiarthritic
	WC 712	Spironolactone with Hydrochlorothiazide	25mg/25mg	White	Tab	Round	Y	N	WC	Diuretic
713	P–D 713	Spironolactone	25mg	White	Tab	Round	Y	N	PD	Diuretic
	PP–713	Orphenadrine/Aspirin/Caffeine	25mg/385mg/60mg	Green/White	Tab	Round	N	Y	Eon	Muscle Relaxant
	SQUIBB 713	Rauwolfia Serpentina	50mg	Red	Tab	Round	N	Y	Princeton	Antihypertensive
	WALLACE 713	Phenylephrine/Chlorpheniramine/Pyrilamine	25mg/8mg/25mg	Buff	Tab	Capsule	Y	N	Wallace	Decongestant Comb.
	WC 713	Spironolactone	25mg	White	Tab	Round	Y	N	WC	Diuretic

ID NO.	ID CODE	GENERIC NAME	STRENGTH	COLOR	FORM	SHAPE	SCORED	COATED	MFG.	USE
714	LEMMON 714	Methaqualone HCl	300mg	White	Tab	Round	Y	N	Lemmon	Hypnotic
	PP–714	Orphenadrine/Aspirin/Caffeine	50mg/770mg/60mg	Green/White	Tab	Round	Y	N	Eon	Muscle Relaxant
715	HD 715/#2	Hydromorphone HCl	2mg	White	Tab	Round	N	N	Halsey	Analgesic
	M 715	Timolol	20mg	Green	Tab	Oblong	Y	Y	Mylan	Antihypertensive
716	E 716	Meprobamate	200mg	White	Tab	Round	N	N	Eon	Antianxiety
	N 716–500	Amoxicillin	500mg	Buff/Buff	Cap	–	–	–	Novopharm	Anti–Infective
	PP–716	Meprobamate	200mg	White	Tab	Round	N	N	Eon	Antianxiety
	WC 716	Trazodone	150mg	White	Tab	Trape.	–	–	WC	Antidepressant
717	COPLEY 717	Guanabenz Acetate	4mg	Peach	Tab	Square	–	N	Copley	Antihypertensive
	E 717	Meprobamate	400mg	White	Tab	Round	Y	N	Eon	Antianxiety
	HD 717/#4	Hydromorphone HCl	4mg	White	Tab	Round	N	N	Halsey	Analgesic
	PP–717	Meprobamate	400mg	White	Tab	Round	Y	N	Eon	Antianxiety
	WALLACE 717	Carbetapentane/Chlorpheniramine/Ephedrine/PhenEph.	60/5/10/10mg	Black	Tab	Capsule	Y	N	Wallace	Antitussive Comb.
718	PP–718	Indomethacin	25mg	Green/Opaque	Cap	–	–	–	Eon	Anti–Inflammatory
719	PP–719	Indomethacin	50mg	Green/Opaque	Cap	–	–	–	Eon	Anti–Inflammatory
720	COPLEY 720	Diltiazem HCl	120mg	White	Tab	Oblong	N	Y	Copley	Antianginal
	PP–720	Indomethacin SR	75mg	Green/Clear	Cap	–	–	–	Eon	Anti–Inflammatory
	Sch. Logo 720	Perphenazine & Amitriptyline HCl	4mg/25mg	Red	Tab	Round	N	Y	Schering	Antidepressant
	WC 720	Disopyramide Phosphate CR	150mg	Orange/Purple	Cap	–	–	–	WC	Antiarrhythmic
721	E 721	Disipramine	50mg	Blue	Tab	Round	N	Y	Eon	Antidepressant
	MILES 721	Niclosamide Chewable	500mg	Yellow	Tab	Round	Y	N	Miles	Antihelmintic
	PP 721	Desipramine HCl	50mg	Blue	Tab	Round	N	Y	Eon	Antidepressant
722	E 722	Disipramine	75mg	Blue	Tab	Round	N	Y	Eon	Antidepressant
	PP–722	Desipramine HCl	75mg	Blue	Tab	Round	N	N	Eon	Antidepressant
723	PP–723	Carisoprodol	350mg	White	Tab	Round	–	–	Eon	Muscle Relaxant
	SQUIBB 723	Phenytoin	100mg	–	Cap	–	–	–	Squibb	Anticonvulsant
724	GG 724	Naproxen	250mg	Yellow	Tab	Round	N	Y	Geneva	Anti–Inflammatory
	HD 724	Doxycycline Hyclate	50mg	Beige	Tab	Round	N	Y	Halsey	Anti–Infective
	N 724–250	Amoxicillin	250mg	Caramel/Buff	Cap	–	–	–	Novopharm	Anti–Infective
	WC 724	Timolol Maleate	20mg	White	Tab	Oblong	–	–	WC	Antihypertensive
725	GG 725	Naproxen	375mg	Orange	Tab	Capsule	N	Y	Geneva	Anti–Inflammatory
	HD 725	Doxycycline Hyclate	100mg	Beige	Tab	Round	N	Y	Halsey	Anti–Infective
	Merrell 725	Terbutaline Sulfate	2.5mg	White	Tab	Round	–	N	Merrell	Bronchodilator
	P–D 725	Aspirin With Codeine Phosphate	325mg/15mg	White	Tab	Round	–	N	PD	Analgesic
	PP–725	Meclofenamate Sodium	50mg	Rust	Cap	–	–	–	Eon	Anti–Inflammatory
	WC 725	Aspirin With Codeine Phosphate	325mg/15mg	White	Tab	Round	–	N	WC	Analgesic
726	GG 726	Naproxen	500mg	Yellow	Tab	Capsule	N	Y	Geneva	Anti–Inflammatory
	P–D 726	Aspirin With Codeine Phosphate	325mg/30mg	White	Tab	Round	–	N	PD	Analgesic
	PP–726	Meclofenamate Sodium	100mg	Rust/White	Cap	–	–	–	Eon	Anti–Inflammatory
	SQUIBB 726	Procainamide HCl SR	250mg	–	Tab	–	–	–	Squibb	Antiarrhythmic
	WC 726	Aspirin With Codeine Phosphate	325mg/30mg	White	Tab	Round	–	N	WC	Analgesic
727	93 727	Papaverine HCl	150mg	Brown/Clear	Cap	–	–	–	Lemmon	Vasodilator
	MYLAN/727	Perphenazine & Amitriptyline	4mg/10mg	Blue	Tab	Round	N	Y	Mylan	Antidepressant
	P–D 727	Aspirin With Codeine Phosphate	325mg/60mg	White	Tab	Round	–	N	PD	Analgesic
	WC 727	Aspirin With Codeine Phosphate	325mg/60mg	White	Tab	Round	–	N	WC	Analgesic
728	93 728	Sulindac	150mg	Yellow	Tab	Round	N	N	Lemmon	Anti–Inflammatory
	WC 728	Timolol Maleate	10mg	White	Tab	Round	–	–	WC	Antihypertensive
729	93 729	Sulindac	200mg	Yellow	Tab	Round	N	N	Lemmon	Anti–Inflammatory
	WC 729	Timolol Maleate	5mg	White	Tab	Round	–	–	WC	Antihypertensive
730	54–730	Oxycodone & Acetaminophen	5mg/500mg	White	Tab	Capsule	Y	N	Roxane	Analgesic
	MSD 730	Lovastatin	10mg	Peach	Tab	Octagonal	–	–	MSD	Hypolipidemic
	P–D 730	Amoxicillin	250mg	Pink/Red	Cap	–	–	–	PD	Anti–Infective
	WC 730	Amoxicillin	250mg	Pink/Red	Cap	–	–	–	WC	Anti–Infective
731	MSD 731	Lovastatin	20mg	Blue	Tab	Octagonal	–	–	MSD	Hypolipidemic
	Mylan 731	Propranolol HCl and Hydrochlorothiazide	40mg/25 mg	White	Tab	Round	Y	N	Mylan	Antihypertensive
	P–D 731	Amoxicillin	500mg	Pink/Red	Cap	–	–	–	PD	Anti–Infective
	WALLACE 731	Diphylline	400mg	White	Tab	Capsule	–	N	Wallace	Antiasthmatic
	WC 731	Amoxicillin	500mg	Pink/Red	Cap	–	–	–	WC	Anti–Infective
732	54–732	Diphenoxylate/Atropine	2.5mg/0.025mg	–	Tab	–	–	–	Roxane	Antidiarrheal
	MSD 732	Lovastatin	40mg	Green	Tab	Octagonal	–	–	MSD	Hypolipidemic
733	54/733	Morphine Sulfate	15mg	White	Tab	Round	Y	N	Roxane	Analgesic
	GG 733	Salsalate	500mg	Green	Tab	Round	N	Y	Geneva	Anti–Inflammatory
734	GG 734	Salsalate	750mg	Green	Tab	Capsule	Y	Y	Geneva	Anti–Inflammatory
735	GG 735	Flurbiprofen	50mg	White	Tab	Oval	N	Y	Greenstone	Analgesic
	Sch. Logo 735	Theophylline LA	250mg	Green/Clear	Cap	–	–	–	Schering	Bronchodilator
736	E 736	Disipramine	100mg	Blue	Tab	Round	N	Y	Eon	Antidepressant
	GG 736	Flurbiprofen	100mg	White	Tab	Oval	N	Y	Greenstone	Analgesic
	PP–736	Desipramine HCl	100mg	Blue	Tab	Round	N	N	Eon	Antidepressant
737	PP–737	Cephradine	250mg	Green/Pink	Cap	–	–	–	Eon	Anti–Infective
738	LC/738	Propranolol HCl	10mg	–	Tab	–	–	–	Rugby	Antihypertensive
	PP–738	Cephradine	500mg	Green	Cap	–	–	–	Eon	Anti–Infective
	SQUIBB 738	Temazepam	15mg	–	Cap	–	–	–	Squibb	Hypnotic
739	LC/739	Propranolol HCl	20mg	–	Tab	–	–	–	Rugby	Antihypertensive
	PP739	Trimipramine Maleate	25mg	Yellow/White	Cap	–	–	–	Eon	Antidepressant
740	LC/740	Propranolol HCl	40mg	–	Tab	–	–	–	Rugby	Antihypertensive
	PP740	Trimipramine Maleate	50mg	Orange/White	Cap	–	–	–	Eon	Antidepressant
741	93 741	Propoxyphene	65mg	Pink	Cap	–	–	–	Lemmon	Analgesic
	COPLEY 741	Naproxen Sodium	275mg	Blue	Tab	Capsule	N	Y	Copley	Anti–Inflammatory
	LC/741	Propranolol HCl	80mg	–	Tab	–	–	–	Rugby	Antihypertensive
	LUCHEM 741	Phenylpropanolamine HCl & Guaifenesin LA	75mg/400mg	Blue	Tab	Oval	Y	N	LuChem	Decongestant Comb.
	PP–741	Trimipramine Maleate	100mg	White	Cap	–	–	–	Eon	Antidepressant
742	93 742	Doxycycline Hyclate	50mg	Blue/White	Cap	–	–	–	Lemmon	Anti–Infective
	SQUIBB 742	Procainamide HCl SR	500mg	–	Tab	–	–	–	Squibb	Antiarrhythmic
743	54 743 2	Hydromorphone HCl	2mg	White	Tab	Round	Y	N	Roxane	Analgesic
	93 743	Doxycycline Hyclate	100mg	Blue/Blue	Cap	–	–	–	Lemmon	Anti–Infective
	LUCHEM 743	Phenylephrine/Chlorpheniramine/Pyrilamine	25mg/8mg/25mg	Tan	Tab	Oblong	Y	N	LuChem	Decongestant Comb.
	PP 743	Niacin SR	250mg	Green/Clear	Cap	–	–	–	Eon	Vitamin
744	COPLEY 744	Naproxen Sodium	550mg	Blue	Tab	Capsule	N	Y	Copley	Anti–Inflammatory
745	E 745	Phenylpropanolamine HCl & Guaifenesin LA	75mg/400mg	Blue	Tab	–	Y	N	Eon	Decongestant Comb.
	PP–745	Phenylpropanolamine & Guiafenesin	75mg/400mg	Blue	Tab	Oval	Y	N	Eon	Decongestant Comb.
747	SQUIBB 747	Temazepam	30mg	–	Cap	–	–	–	Squibb	Hypnotic
749	SQUIBB 749	Cephalexin	250mg	–	Cap	–	–	–	Squibb	Anti–Infective
750	750	Niacin SR	750mg	Pink	Tab	Capsule	Y	N	Upsher	Vasodilator
	832 S750	Salsalate	750mg	Yellow	Tab	Oblong	N	Y	PBI	Analgesic
	832 S750	Salsalate	750mg	Blue	Tab	Oblong	N	Y	PBI	Analgesic

ID NO.	ID CODE	GENERIC NAME	STRENGTH	COLOR	FORM	SHAPE	SCORED	COATED	MFG.	USE
	Central 750mg	Salsalate	750mg	Pink	Tab	Oval	Y	Y	Central	Antiarthritic
	E 750	Nystatin	500,000 Units	Brown	Tab	Round	N	Y	Eon	Anti–Infective
	PF T 750	Choline Magnesium Trisalicylate	750mg	White	Tab	Oblong	Y	Y	PF	Analgesic
	PF T750	Choline Magnesium Trisalicylate	750mg	White	Tab	Oblong	Y	Y	PF	Antiarrthritic
	PP/750	Nystatin Oral	500,000	Brown	Tab	Round	N	Y	Eon	Anti–Infective
	US 750	Salsalate	750mg	Blue	Tab	Capsule	N	Y	Upsher	Analgesic
	West–ward 750	Triamterene & Hydrochlorothiazide	75mg/50mg	Yellow	Tab	Round	Y	N	West–ward	Diuretic
751	M 751	Cyclobenzaprine HCl	10mg	Yellow	Tab	Round	N	Y	Mylan	Muscle Relaxant
	PP–751 2	Aspirin/Codeine	325mg/15mg	White	Tab	Round	N	N	Eon	Analgesic
752	AYERST 752	Vitamin Combination	n/a	Orange	Tab	Oblong	N	Y	Ayerst	Vitamin Comb.
	PP–752 3	Aspirin/Codeine	325mg/30mg	White	Tab	Round	N	N	Eon	Analgesic
753	PP–753 4	Aspirin/Codeine	325mg/60mg	White	Tab	Round	N	N	Eon	Analgesic
754	93 754	Diflunisal	250 mg	Blue/Lavender	Tab	Caplet	N	Y	Lemmon	Anti–inflammatory
	PP 754	Clindamycin HCl	75mg	Flesh/Flesh	Cap	–	–	–	Eon	Anti–Infective
755	93 755	Diflunisal	500 mg	Blue/Lavender	Tab	Caplet	N	Y	Lemmon	Anti–inflammatory
	MJ 755	Estradiol	1mg	Lavender	Tab	Round	Y	N	MJ	Hormone
	PP 755	Clindamycin HCl	150mg	Flesh/Lavender	Cap	–	–	–	Eon	Anti–Infective
756	93–756	Piroxicam	10mg	Green/Olive	Cap	–	–	–	Lemmon	Anti–inflammatory
	MJ 756	Estradiol	2mg	Turquoise	Tab	Round	Y	N	MJ	Hormone
	PP–756	Triamterene & Hydrochlorothiazide	50mg/25mg	Red	Cap	–	–	–	Eon	Diuretic
	SQUIBB 756	Procainamide HCl	375mg	White/Orange	Cap	–	–	–	Princeton	Antiarrhythmic
757	93–757	Piroxicam	20mg	Green/Green	Cap	–	–	–	Lemmon	Anti–inflammatory
	M 757	Atenolol	100mg	White	Tab	Round	N	N	Mylan	Antihypertensive
	SQUIBB 757	Procainamide HCl	500mg	Yellow/Orange	Cap	–	–	–	Princeton	Antiarrhythmic
758	SQUIBB 758	Procainamide HCl	250mg	Yellow	Cap	–	–	–	Princeton	Antiarrhythmic
	TP–758	Acetaminophen	325mg	White	Tab	Round	Y	N	PBI	Analgesic
759	WC 759	Acetaminophen	500mg	White	Tab	Round	Y	N	WC	Analgesic
760	54 760	Prednisone	20mg	White	Tab	Round	Y	N	Roxane	Steroid
	PP–760	Desipramine HCL	150mg	White	Tab	Round	N	Y	Eon	Antidepressant
	S 760	Isosorbide Dinitrate SL	5mg	Pink	Tab	Round	N	N	Stuart	Antianginal
761	E 761	Salsalate	500mg	Yellow	Tab	Capsule	N	–	Eon	Analgesic
	PP 761	Salsalate	500mg	Yellow	Tab	Round	N	Y	Eon	Analgesic
	S 761	Isosorbide Dinitrate SL	10mg	Yellow	Tab	Round	N	N	Stuart	Antianginal
762	E 762	Salsalate	750mg	Yellow	Tab	Capsule	N	–	Eon	Analgesic
	PP 762	Salsalate	750mg	Yellow	Tab	Capsule	N	Y	Eon	Analgesic
763	SQUIBB 763	Tetracycline	500mg	Pink/White	Cap	–	–	–	Squibb	Anti–Infective
765	WC 765	Cimetidine	400mg	Green	Tab	Oval	–	Y	WC	Anti–ulcer
	West–ward 765	Isosorbide Dinitrate Sublingual	2.5mg	Yellow	Tab	Round	N	N	West–ward	Antianginal
766	Forest 766	Phentermine HCl	30mg	Yellow	Cap	–	–	–	Forest	Anorectic
767	West–ward 767	Isosorbide Dinitrate Sublingual	5mg	Pink	Tab	Round	N	N	West–ward	Antianginal
768	WC 768	Cimetidine	300mg	Green	Tab	Oval	–	Y	WC	Anti–ulcer
769	54–769	Dexamethasone	6mg	Aqua	Tab	Round	Y	N	Roxane	Steroid
	SQUIBB 769	Rauwolfia Serpentina & Bendroflumethiazide	50mg/4mg	Green	Tab	Round	N	Y	Princeton	Antihypertensive
	West–ward 769	Isosorbide Dinitrate Oral	5mg	White	Tab	Round	N	N	West–ward	Antianginal
770	LG/770	Phenytoin Sodium Prompt	100mg	–	Cap	–	–	–	Rugby	Anticonvulsant
	S 770	Isosorbide Dinitrate Oral	5mg	Green	Tab	Oval	Y	N	Stuart	Antianginal
771	West–ward 771	Isosorbide Dinitrate Oral	10mg	White	Tab	Round	Y	N	West–ward	Antianginal
772	54–772	Dihydrotachysterol	0.4mg	White	Tab	Round	N	N	Roxane	Blood Ca++ Regulator
	MYLAN 772	Verapamil HCl	120mg	White	Tab	Round	N	Y	Mylan	Antiarrhythmic
	West–ward 772	Isosorbide Dinitrate Oral	20mg	Green	Tab	Round	Y	N	West–ward	Antianginal
773	54–773 5	Haloperidol	5mg	White	Tab	Round	Y	N	Roxane	Tranquilizer
	773	Hyoscyamine Sulfate	0.125mg	White	Tab	Round	–	–	Marlop	Antispasmodic
	S 773	Isosorbide Dinitrate Oral	30mg	White	Tab	Oval	Y	N	Stuart	Antianginal
	WC 773	Sulindac	150mg	Yellow	Tab	Round	Y	N	WC	Anti–Inflammatory
774	S 774	Isosorbide Dinitrate Oral	40mg	Blue	Tab	Oval	Y	N	Stuart	Antianginal
	WC 774	Sulindac	200mg	Yellow	Tab	Eliptical	Y	N	WC	Anti–Inflammatory
775	SQUIBB 775	Procainamide HCl SR	500mg	Yellow	Tab	Oval	N	Y	Princeton	Antirrhythmic
776	SQUIBB 776	Rauwolfia Serpentina	100mg	Red	Tab	Round	N	Y	Princeton	Antihypertensive
777	93 777	Hydrochlorothiazide	25mg	Peach	Tab	Round	Y	N	Lemmon	Diuretic
	MYLAN 777	Lorazepam	2mg	White	Tab	Round	Y	N	Mylan	Antianxiety
	PP–777	Nystatin Vaginal	100,000 Units	Yellow	Tab	Diamond	N	N	Eon	Anti–Infective
	SQUIBB 777	Procainamide HCl SR	750mg	–	Tab	–	–	–	Squibb	Antiarrhythmic
778	93/93 778	Carbamazepine Chewable	100mg	Pink/Red Specks	Tab	Round	N	N	Lemmon	Anticonvulsant
779	54–779	Phenobarbital	60mg	White	Tab	Round	Y	N	Roxane	Hypnotic
	93 779	Hydrochlorothiazide	50mg	Peach	Tab	Round	Y	N	Lemmon	Diuretic
	SQUIBB 779	Tetracycline & Amphotericin B	250mg/50mg	–	Cap	–	–	–	Squibb	Anti–Infective
780	S 780	Isosorbide Dinitrate Oral	10mg	Yellow	Tab	Oval	Y	N	Stuart	Antianginal
783	54–783	Codeine Sulfate	30mg	White	Tab	Round	Y	N	Roxane	Analgesic
	93 783	Propoxyphene	65mg	Pink/Pink	Cap	–	–	–	Lemmon	Analgesic
	AYERST 783	Sulfamethizole & Phenazopyridine	500mg/50mg	Yellow	Tab	Round	–	–	Ayerst	Anti–Infective
	TP783	Butabarbital	30mg	Blue Green	Tab	Round	N	N	Towne Paulsen	Antianxiety
784	AYERST 784	Sulfamethizole & Phenazopyridine	250mg/50mg	Red	Tab	Round	N	Y	Ayerst	Anti–Infective
	MJ 784	Cefadroxil	500mg	Red/White	Cap	–	–	–	MJ	Anti–Infective
	WC 784	Potassium Chloride ER	10mEq	Yellow	Tab	Oval	N	Y	WC	Potassium Supp.
785	MJ 785	Cefadroxil	1gm	White	Tab	Oval	Y	N	MJ	Anti–Infective
	WC 785	Alprazolam	1mg	White	Tab	Oval	Y	N	WC	Antianxiety
	West–ward 785	Butalbital, Aspirin and Caffeine	50/325/40mg	White	Tab	Round	Y	N	West–ward	Analgesic
786	AYERST 786	Sulfamethizole	500mg	White	Tab	Oval	Y	N	Ayerst	Anti–Infective
	WC 786	Alprazolam	0.5mg	Yellow	Tab	Oval	Y	N	WC	Antianxiety
787	WC 787	Alprazolam	0.25mg	Yellow	Tab	Oval	Y	N	WC	Antianxiety
	West–ward 787	Butalbital/Acetaminophen/Caffeine	50/325/40mg	White	Tab	Round	Y	N	West–ward	Analgesic
788	SQUIBB 788	Allopurinol	300mg		Tab	Round	–	–	Squibb	Antigout
	WC 788	Nitrofurantoin	50mg	Pink/Yellow	Cap	–	–	–	WC	Anti–Infective
789	93–789	Perphenazine	2mg	Gray	Tab	Round	N	Y	Lemmon	Antidepressant
	WC 789	Nitrofurantoin	100mg	Pink/Pink	Cap	–	–	–	WC	Anti–Infective
790	93–790	Perphenazine	4mg	Gray	Tab	Round	N	Y	Lemmon	Antidepressant
	ORGANON 790	Dexamethasone	1.5mg	Peach	Tab	Round	Y	N	Organon	Steroid
	WC 790	Maprotiline	25mg	Peach	Tab	Round	–	–	WC	Antidepressant
791	93–791	Perphenazine	8mg	Gray	Tab	Round	N	Y	Lemmon	Antidepressant
	ORGANON 791	Dexamethasone	0.75mg	White	Tab	Round	Y	N	Organon	Steroid
	W 791	Allopurinol Sulphate	4mg	–	Tab	–	–	–	Squibb	Antigout
	WC 791	Maprotiline	50mg	Peach	Tab	Round	–	–	WC	Antidepressant
792	93–792	Perphenazine	16mg	Gray	Tab	Round	N	Y	Lemmon	Antidepressant
	ORGANON 792	Dexamethasone	0.5mg	Yellow	Tab	Round	Y	N	Organon	Steroid
795	Sch. Logo 795	Anisindione	50mg	Pink	Tab	Round	Y	N	Schering	Anticoagulant

ID NO.	ID CODE	GENERIC NAME	STRENGTH	COLOR	FORM	SHAPE	SCORED	COATED	MFG.	USE
796	WC 795	Maprotiline	75mg	White	Tab	Round	–	–	WC	Antidepressant
796	WC 796	Fluphenazine	1mg	White	Tab	Round	–	–	WC	Tranquilizer
797	WC 797	Fluphenazine	2.5mg	Beige	Tab	Round	–	–	WC	Tranquilizer
798	93–798	Indomethacin	25mg	Green	Cap	–	–	–	Lemmon	Anti-Inflammatory
	ORGANON 798	Dexamethasone	4mg	Green	Tab	Round	Y	N	Organon	Steroid
	WC 798	Fluphenazine	5mg	Blue	Tab	Round	–	–	WC	Tranquilizer
799	93–799	Indomethacin	50mg	Green	Cap	–	–	–	Lemmon	Anti-Inflammatory
	WC 799	Fluphenazine	10mg	Red	Tab	Round	–	–	WC	Tranquilizer
800	ALRA IF 800	Ibuprofen	800mg	Light Peach	Tab	Oval	N	Y	Alra	Anti-Inflammatory
	IBU 800	Ibuprofen	800mg	White	Tab	Elongated	N	Y	Boots	Anti-Inflammatory
801	MYLAN 801	Ibuprofen	800mg	White	Tab	Oval	N	Y	Mylan	Anti-Inflammatory
802	93 802	Phenobarbital/Hyoscyamine/Atropine/Scopolamine	n/a	Green/Clear	Cap	–	–	–	Lemmon	Antispasmodic
804	93 804	Phentermine HCl	30mg	Black/Scarlet	Cap	–	–	–	Lemmon	Anorectic
807	GG 807	Phenylpropanolamine/PE/Guaifenesin	45mg/5mg/200mg	Orange	Cap	Capsule	–	–	Amide	Decongestant Comb.
808	WC 808	Cephradine	250mg	Green/Pink	Cap	–	–	–	WC	Anti-Infective
809	WC 809	Cephradine	500mg	Green/Green	Cap	–	–	–	WC	Anti-Infective
810	54–810	Propranolol HCl	90mg	–	Tab	Round	–	–	Roxane	Antihypertensive
	S 810	Isosorbide Dinitrate Chewable	5mg	Green	Tab	Round	Y	N	Stuart	Antianginal
812	812	Butalbital/Acetaminophen/Caffeine	50mg/325mg/40mg	White/Blue	Cap	–	–	–	Marlop	Analgesic
	SQUIBB 812	Doxycycline Hyclate	100mg	–	Tab	–	–	–	Squibb	Anti-Infective
813	P–D 813	Doxycycline Hyclate	100mg	Orange	Tab	Round	N	Y	PD	Anti-Infective
	WC 813	Doxycycline Hyclate	100mg	Beige	Tab	Round	N	Y	WC	Anti-Infective
814	814	Ibuprofen	400mg	–	Tab	–	N	Y	Marlop	Anti-Inflammatory
815	N 815 400	Tolmetin Sodium	400mg	Red	Tab	–	–	–	Novopharm	Anti-Inflammatory
	S 815	Isosorbide Dinitrate Chewable	10mg	Yellow	Tab	Round	Y	N	Stuart	Antianginal
816	93 816	Belladonna Alkaloids & Phenobarbital	n/a	White	Tab	Round	Y	N	Lemmon	Antispasmodic
	93/816	Belladonna Alkaloids with Phenobarbital	–	White	Tab	Round	Y	N	Rondex	Antispasmodic
	TP816	Chlorpheniramine Maleate	4mg	Yellow	Tab	Round	N	N	Towne Paulsen	Antihistamine
819	54–819	Acetaminophen	650mg	White	Tab	–	–	–	Roxane	Analgesic
	Watson 819	Indomethacin	50mg	Green	Cap	Capsule	–	–	Watson	Anti-Inflammatory
820	S 820	Isosorbide Dinitrate Oral	20mg	Blue	Tab	Oval	Y	N	Stuart	Antianginal
	Sch. Logo 820	Dexchlorpheniramine	2mg	Red	Tab	Oval	N	N	Schering	Antihistamine
821	93 821	Reserpine	0.25mg	White	Tab	Round	Y	N	Lemmon	Antihypertensive
822	54 822	Sulfamethoxazole & Trimethoprim	800mg/160mg	White	Tab	Capsule	Y	N	Roxane	Anti-Infective
	S 822	Trichlormethiazide	2mg	Pink	Tab	Clover	Y	N	Schering	Diuretic
823	54–823	Pseudoephedrine	30mg	White	Tab	Round	–	–	Roxane	Decongestant
824	93 824	Pseudoephedrine HCl	60mg	White	Tab	Round	Y	N	Lemmon	Decongestant
827	93 827	Reserpine	0.1mg	White	Tab	Round	Y	N	Lemmon	Antihypertensive
	TP827	Diphenhydramine	50mg	Pink	Cap	–	–	–	Towne Paulsen	Antihistamine
828	93 828	Urinary Antiseptic Comb.	n/a	Blue	Tab	Round	N	Y	Lemmon	Urinary Tract Agent
829	P–D 829	Doxycycline Hyclate	50mg	Aqua/Cream	Cap	–	–	–	PD	Anti-Infective
	WC 829	Doxycycline Hyclate	50mg	Aqua/Cream	Cap	–	–	–	WC	Anti-Infective
830	MMS 830	Diazoxide	50mg	Orange/Clear	Cap	–	–	–	MMS	Antihypertensive
	P–D 830	Doxycycline Hyclate	100mg	Aqua/Aqua	Cap	–	–	–	PD	Anti-Infective
	SQUIBB 830	Hydroxyurea	500mg	Pink/Green	Cap	–	–	–	Squibb	Antineoplastic
	WC 830	Doxycycline Hyclate	100mg	Aqua/Aqua	Cap	–	–	–	WC	Antianxiety
831	SEARLE 831	Haloperidol	0.5mg	White	Tab	Round	–	–	Searle	Tranquilizer
832	Met–10 832	Metoclopramide HCl	10mg	White	Tab	Round	–	N	PBI	Antireflux
	W–C 832	Amiloride & Hydrochlorothiazide	5mg/50mg	Yellow	Tab	–	–	N	WC	Diuretic
833	TP833	Diphenhydramine	25mg	Pink/White	Cap	–	–	–	Towne Paulsen	Antihistamine
	WC 833	Triamterene & Hydrochlorothiazide	75mg/50mg	Yellow	Tab	–	–	–	WC	Diuretic
834	SQUIBB 834	Multivitamin with Iron & Biotin	n/a	–	Tab	–	–	–	Squibb	Vitamin
	WC 834	Triamterene & Hydrochlorothiazide	50mg/25mg	Red/Red	Cap	–	–	–	WC	Diuretic
835	93 835	Urinary Antiseptic Comb. (Veterinary)	n/a	Purple	Tab	Round	N	Y	Lemmon	Urinary Tract Agent
839	E–839	Docusate Sodium/Casanthranol	100mg	Red	Cap	–	–	–	Chase	Stool Softener
840	54 840	Furosemide	20mg	White	Tab	Round	Y	N	Roxane	Diuretic
841	93 841	Dicyclomine HCl	10mg	Blue	Cap	–	–	–	Lemmon	Antispasmodic
	SEARLE 841	Haloperidol	1mg	White	Tab	Round	Y	N	Searle	Tranquilizer
842	SQUIBB 842	Multivitamin	n/a	–	Tab	–	–	–	Squibb	Vitamin
843	Sch. Logo 843	Prednisone	1mg	White	Tab	Round	N	N	Schering	Steroid
	WC 843	Prazosin	1mg	Ivory/Opaque	Cap	–	–	–	WC	Antihypertensive
844	WC 844	Prazosin	2mg	Pink/Opaque	Cap	–	–	–	WC	Antihypertensive
845	93 845	Urinary Antiseptic Combination	n/a	Purple	Tab	Round	N	Y	Lemmon	Urinary Tract Agent
	93/845	Atrosept (Combination)	–	Blue	Tab	Round	N	Y	Eon	Urinary Antiseptic
	SQUIBB 845	Allopurinol	100mg	–	Tab	Round	–	–	Squibb	Antigout
	WC 845	Prazosin	5mg	Blue/Opaque	Cap	–	–	–	WC	Antihypertensive
848	93 848	Triprolidine HCl & Pseudoephedrine HCl	2.5mg/60mg	White	Tab	Round	Y	N	Lemmon	Decongestant Comb.
849	P–D 849	Quinidine Sulfate	200mg	White	Tab	Round	–	N	PD	Antiarrhythmic
	SQUIBB 849	Multivitamin/Minerals	n/a	–	Tab	–	–	N	Squibb	Vitamin
	WC 849	Quinidine Sulfate	200mg	White	Tab	Round	–	N	WC	Antiarrhythmic
850	MJ 850	Inert tablets	n/a	Green	Tab	Round	N	N	Mead Johnson	Placebo
	P–D 850	Quinidine Gluconate	330mg	White	Tab	Round	–	N	PD	Antiarrhythmic
	WC 850	Quinidine Gluconate	330mg	White	Tab	Round	–	N	WC	Antiarrhythmic
851	93/851	Metronidazole	250mg	White	Tab	Round	N	N	Lemmon	Anti-Infective
	SEARLE 851	Haloperidol	2mg	White	Tab	Round	Y	N	Searle	Tranquilizer
852	93–852	Metronidazole	500mg	White	Tab	Oblong	Y	N	Lemmon	Anti-Infective
853	54–853	Methyldopa	125mg	–	Tab	Round	N	Y	Roxane	Antihypertensive
	S 853	Isosorbide Dinitrate SL	2.5mg	White	Tab	Round	N	N	Stuart	Antianginal
	W–C 853	Amantadine	100mg	Yellow	Cap	–	–	–	WC	Antiviral
855	Miles 855	Nimodipine	30mg	Ivory	Cap	–	–	–	Miles	Calcium Channel Bloc
856	E 856	Salsalate	500mg	Blue	Tab	Capsule	N	–	Eon	Analgesic
	PP 856	Salsalate	500mg	Blue	Tab	Round	N	Y	Eon	Analgesic
857	E 857	Salsalate	750mg	Blue	Tab	Capsule	N	Y	Eon	Analgesic
	PP 857	Salsalate	750mg	Blue	Tab	Capsule	N	Y	Eon	Analgesic
858	STUART 858	Simethicone	80mg	Pink	Tab	Round	Y	N	Stuart	Antiflatulent
859	54–859	Aminophylline	100mg	–	Tab	Round	–	–	Roxane	Bronchodilator
860	54–860	Alprazolam	1mg	–	Tab	–	–	–	Roxane	Antianxiety
	93 860	Phentermine HCl	30mg	Yellow/Yellow	Cap	–	–	–	Lemmon	Anorectic
861	SEARLE 861	Haloperidol	5mg	White	Tab	Round	Y	N	Searle	Tranquilizer
863	SQUIBB 863	Fluphenazine HCl	1mg	Pink	Tab	Round	N	Y	Princeton	Tranquilizer
864	SQUIBB 864	Fluphenazine HCl	2.5mg	Yellow	Tab	Round	N	Y	Princeton	Tranquilizer
	STUART 864	Buclizine HCl	50mg	Yellow	Tab	Round	Y	N	Stuart	Antiemetic
865	P–D 865	Methyldopa	250mg	Blue	Tab	Round	N	Y	PD	Antihypertensive
	TP865	Isoniazide	100mg	Yellow	Tab	Round	N	N	Towne Paulsen	Anti-Infective
	WC 865	Methyldopa	250mg	Blue	Tab	Round	N	Y	WC	Antihypertensive

ID NO.	ID CODE	GENERIC NAME	STRENGTH	COLOR	FORM	SHAPE	SCORED	COATED	MFG.	USE
866	P–D 866	Methyldopa	500mg	Blue	Tab	Round	N	Y	PD	Antihypertensive
	Sch. Logo 866	Dexbrompheniramine Maleate & Pseudoephedrine Sulf	2mg/60mg	White with Blue	Tab	Round	Y	N	Schering	Decongestant Comb.
	WC 866	Methyldopa	500mg	Blue	Tab	Round	N	Y	WC	Antihypertensive
868	WC 868	Hydralazine & Hydrochlorothiazide	25mg/25mg	Green/Green	Cap	–	–	–	WC	Antihypertensive
871	SEARLE 871	Haloperidol	10mg	White	Tab	Round	Y	N	Searle	Tranquilizer
	WC 871	Hydralazine & Hydrochlorothiazide	50mg/50mg	Green/Green	Cap	–	–	–	WC	Antihypertensive
872	93 872	Butabarbital Sodium	15mg	Purple	Tab	Round	Y	N	Lemmon	Antianxiety
	CARACO 872	Nifedipine	10mg	Yellow	Cap	–	–	–	Caraco	Antianginal
	WC 872	Fluoxymesterone	10mg	Green	Tab	Round	–	–	WC	Hormone
873	93 873	Butabarbital Sodium	30mg	Green	Tab	Round	Y	N	Lemmon	Antianxiety
	TP873	Folic Acid	1mg	Yellow	Tab	Round	N	N	PBI	Antianemic
874	SQUIBB 874	Cephalexin	500mg	–	Cap	–	–	–	Squibb	Anti-Infective
	WC 874	Medroxyprogesterone	10mg	White	Tab	Round	–	–	WC	Hormone
875	WC 875	Indomethacin SR	75mg	Lavender/Clear	Cap	–	–	–	WC	Anti-Inflammatory
877	SQUIBB 877	Fluphenazine HCl	5mg	Green	Tab	Round	N	Y	Princeton	Antihypertensive
878	AYERST 878	Conjugated Estrogens & Methyltestosterone	0.625mg/5mg	Maroon	Tab	Round	N	Y	Ayerst	Hormone
	WC 878	Metoclopramide	10mg	White	Tab	Round	–	–	WC	Antireflux
879	./879	Codeine Sulfate	30mg	White	Tab	Round	N	N	Halsey	Analgesic
	AYERST 879	Conjugated Estrogens & Methyltestosterone	1.25mg/10mg	Yellow	Tab	Round	N	Y	Ayerst	Hormone
888	54–880	Imipramine HCl	25mg	Coral	Tab	Round	N	Y	Roxane	Antidepressant
	AYERST 880	Conjugated Estrogens/Meprobamate	0.45/200mg	Green	Tab	Oblong	N	Y	Ayerst	Hormone
	S 880	Isosorbide Dinitrate SR Oral	40mg	Yellow	Tab	Round	N	N	Stuart	Antianginal
881	AYERST 881	Conjugated Estrogens/Meprobamate	0.45/400mg	Pink	Tab	Oblong	N	Y	Ayerst	Hormone
	SEARLE 881	Haloperidol	20mg	White	Tab	Round	Y	N	Searle	Tranquilizer
882	P–D 882	Norethindrone	5mg	White	Tab	Round	N	N	PD	Hormone
	PP–882	Phentermine HCl	15mg	Gray/Yellow	Cap	–	–	–	Eon	Anorectic
884	Miles 30 884	Nifedipine ER	30mg	Pink	Tab	Round	N	Y	Miles	Antihypertensive
885	Miles 60 885	Nifedipine ER	60mg	Brown	Tab	Round	N	Y	Miles	Antihypertensive
886	Miles 90 886	Nifedipine ER	90mg	Brown	Tab	Round	N	Y	Miles	Antihypertensive
887	P–D 887	Indomethacin	25mg	Blue/Aqua	Cap	–	–	–	PD	Anti-Inflammatory
	WC 887	Indomethacin	25mg	Blue/Aqua	Cap	–	–	–	WC	Anti-Inflammatory
888	93 888	Phentermine HCl	30mg	Black/Black	Cap	–	–	–	Lemmon	Anorectic
	P–D 888	Indomethacin	50mg	Blue/Aqua	Cap	–	–	–	PD	Anti-Inflammatory
	WC 888	Indomethacin	50mg	Blue/Aqua	Cap	–	–	–	WC	Anti-Inflammatory
889	889	Phentermine HCl	30mg	Red/Yellow	Cap	–	–	–	Marlop	Anorectic
890	890	Phendimetrazine Tartrate	105mg	Black	Cap	–	–	–	Marlop	Anorectic
	93 890	Propoxyphene Napsylate with APAP	100mg/650mg	Pink	Tab	Oblong	N	Y	Lemmon	Analgesic
891	93 891	Dicyclomine HCl	20mg	Blue	Tab	Round	N	N	Lemmon	Antispasmodic
	W 891	Allopurinol Sulphate	2mg	–	Tab	–	–	–	Squibb	Antigout
892	54–892	Dexamethasone	4mg	Green	Tab	Round	Y	n	Roxane	Steroid
898	K 898	Nitroglycerin TD	9mg	Clear/Clear	Cap	–	–	–	KV	Antianginal
899	54 899	Prednisone	10mg	White	Tab	Round	Y	N	Roxane	Steroid
900	527/900	Acetaminophen with Codeine	300mg/30mg	White	Tab	Round	–	N	Lannett	Analgesic
	TP 900	Quinidine Sulfate	200mg	White	Tab	Octagonal	Y	N	Towne Paulsen	Antiarrhythmic
901	P–D 901	Norethindrone Acetate & Ethinyl Estradiol	2.5mg/50mcg	Pink	Tab	Round	N	N	PD	Hormone
	Russ 901	Hydrocodone Bitartrate/Acetaminophen	2.5mg/500mg	White/Pink Specks	Tab	Oblong	Y	N	Russ	Analgesic
	WHITBY 901	Hydrocodone Bitartrate with Acetaminophen	2.5mg/500mg	White/Pink specks	Tab	Capsule	Y	N	Whitby	Analgesic
902	54–902	Oxycodone HCl, Oxycodone Terephthalate, Aspirin	4.5mg/.38mg/325	–	Tab	Round	Y	N	Roxane	Analgesic
	Russ 902	Hydrocodone Bitartrate/Acetaminophen	5mg/500mg	White/Blue Specks	Tab	Oblong	Y	N	Russ	Analgesic
	WHITBY 902	Hydrocodone Bitartrate with Acetaminophen	5mg/500mg	White/Blue specks	Tab	Capsule	Y	N	Whitby	Analgesic
903	527/903	Codeine/Salicylamide/Acetaminophen/Caffeine	8/230/150/30mg	Orange	Tab	Round	–	N	Lannett	Analgesic
	54–903	Dihydrotachysterol	0.2mg	Pink	Tab	Round	N	N	Roxane	Blood Ca++ Regulator
	Russ 903	Hydrocodone Bitartrate/APAP	7.5mg/500mg	White/Green Specks	Tab	Oblong	Y	N	Russ	Analgesic
	WHITBY 903	Hydrocodone Bitartrate with Acetaminophen	7.5mg/500mg	White/Green specks	Tab	Capsule	Y	N	Whitby	Analgesic
904	527/904	Codeine/Salicylamide/Acetaminophen/Caffeine	15/230/150/30mg	White	Tab	Round	–	N	Lannett	Analgesic
	P–D 904	Norethindrone Acetate & Ethinyl Estradiol	1mg/50mcg	Yellow	Tab	Round	N	N	PD	Hormone
905	527/905	Codeine/Salicylamide/Acetaminophen/Caffeine	30/230/150/30mg	Green	Tab	Round	–	N	Lannett	Analgesic
906	Russ 906	Hydrocodone Bitartrate/Acetaminophen	7.5mg/500mg	White/Green Specks	Tab	Oblong	Y	N	Russ	Analgesic
910	S/T SS 910	Sulfamethoxazole & Trimethoprim	400mg/80mg	White	Tab	Round	Y	N	Lemmon	Anti-Infective
911	93 911/10	Isoxsuprine HCl	10mg	White	Tab	Round	N	N	Lemmon	Vasodilator
	S/T DS 911	Sulfamethoxazole & Trimethoprim	800mg/160mg	White	Tab	Oval	Y	N	Lemmon	Anti-Infective
913	93 913/20	Isoxsuprine HCl	20mg	White	Tab	Round	N	N	Lemmon	Vasodilator
	TP913	Prednisone	10mg	White	Tab	Round	Y	N	Towne Paulsen	Steroid
914	WC 914	Ibuprofen	800mg	White	Tab	Elongated	N	Y	WC	Anti-Inflammatory
915	P–D 915	Norethindrone Acetate & Ethinyl Estradiol	1mg/20mcg	White	Tab	Round	N	N	PD	Hormone
916	P–D 916	Norethindrone Acetate & Ethinyl Estradiol	1.5mg/30mcg	Green	Tab	Round	N	N	PD	Hormone
917	MSD 917	Amiloride HCl & Hydrochlorothiazide	5mg/50mg	Peach	Tab	Diamond	Y	N	MSD	Antihypertensive
918	P–D 918	Norethindrone Acetate	5mg	Pink	Tab	Round	N	N	PD	Hormone
919	P–D 919	Erythromycin Stearate	500mg	Yellow	Tab	Oval	N	Y	PD	Anti-Infective
	WC 919	Erythromycin Stearate	500mg	Yellow	Tab	Oval	N	Y	WC	Anti-Infective
922	TP922	Prednisolone	5mg	Orange	Tab	Round	N	N	Towne Paulsen	Steroid
	WC 922	Ibuprofen	600mg	White	Tab	Elongated	N	Y	WC	Anti-Inflammatory
924	TP924	Prednisone	5mg	White	Tab	Round	Y	N	Towne Paulsen	Steroid
925	TP925	Prednisone	20mg	Peach	Tab	Round	Y	N	Towne Paulsen	Steroid
926	TP926	Prednisone	2.5mg	Peach	Tab	Round	N	N	Towne Paulsen	Steroid
930	54–930	Aminophylline	200mg	–	Tab	Round	–	–	Roxane	Bronchodilator
	WC 930	Norethindrone & Ethinyl Estradiol	1mg/35mcg	Yellow	Tab	Round	–	–	WC	Contraceptive
932	54–932	Acetaminophen/Codeine	300mg/60mg	White	Tab	Round	–	–	Roxane	Analgesic
937	CT 937	Calcium Lactate	10gr	White	Tab	Round	N	N	Fresh	Mineral Supp.
	DAN 937	Papaverine HCl	60mg	White	Tab	Round	N	N	Danbury	Vasodilator
938	DAN 938	Papaverine HCl	100mg	White	Tab	Round	Y	N	Danbury	Vasodilator
	WC 938	Cephalexin	250mg	Gray/Orange	Cap	–	–	–	WC	Anti-Infective
939	54–939	Imipramine HCl	10mg	Coral	Tab	Round	N	Y	Roxane	Antidepressant
	WC 939	Cephalexin	500mg	Swedish/Orange	Cap	–	–	–	WC	Anti-Infective
940	Sch. Logo 940	Perphenazine	4mg	Gray	Tab	Round	N	Y	Schering	Tranquilizer
	SQUIBB 940	Doxycycline Hyclate	100mg	White	Cap	–	–	–	Squibb	Anti-Infective
	WC 940	Phenylephrine/Chlorpheniramine/Pyrilamine	25mg/8mg/25mg	Beige	Tab	Capsule	Y	N	WC	Decongestant Comb.
941	WC 941	Norethindrone & Ethinyl Estradiol	.5mg/35mcg	White	Tab	Round	–	–	WC	Contraceptive
942	54–942	Leucovorin Calcium	10mg	–	Tab	Round	–	–	Roxane	Antineoplastic
	WC 942	Norethindrone & Mestranol	1mg/50mcg	Blue	Tab	Round	–	–	WC	Contraceptive
943	54–943	Dexamethasone	1.5mg	Pink	Tab	Round	U	N	Roxane	Steroid
	93–943	Nystatin Vaginal	100,000 Units	Yellow	Tab	Diamond	N	N	Lemmon	Antifungal
944	DAN 944	Colchicine	0.6mg	White	Tab	Round	N	N	Danbury	Antigout
	WC 944	Nelova 10/11	–	Yellow	Tab	Round	N	N	WC	Hormone
945	WC 945	Dicloxacillin	250mg	Green/Green	Cap	–	–	–	WC	Antianxiety

ID NO.	ID CODE	GENERIC NAME	STRENGTH	COLOR	FORM	SHAPE	SCORED	COATED	MFG.	USE
946	WC 946	Dicloxacillin	500mg	Green/Green	Cap	–	–	–	WC	Antianxiety
948	Sch. Logo 948	Griseofulvin	250mg	White	Tab	Round	Y	N	Schering	Antifungal
949	UPJOHN 949	Uracil Mustard	1mg	Yellow/Blue	Cap	–	–	–	Upjohn	Antineoplastic
	WC 949	Cloxacillin	250mg	Green/Red	Cap	–	–	–	WC	Anti–Infective
950	WC 950	Cloxacillin	500mg	Green/Red	Cap	–	–	–	WC	Anti–Infective
951	MILES 951	Lithium Carbonate	300mg	Green	Tab	Round	Y	N	Miles	Tranquilizer
	WC 951	Potassium Chloride Extended Release	8mEq	Peach	Tab	Round	N	Y	WC	Potassium Supp.
954	WC 954	Metoprolol Tartrate	50mg	White	Tab	Oblong	Y	N	WC	Antihypertensive
955	WC 955	Metoprolol Tartrate	100mg	White	Tab	Oblong	Y	N	WC	Antihypertensive
956	BP 956	Methyltestosterone Buccal	5mg	White	Tab	Oblong	N	N	Heather	Hormone
	BP 956	Methyltestosterone	5mg	White	Tab	Oblong	N	N	ICN	Steroid
	SQUIBB 956	Fluphenazine HCl	10mg	Dark Pink	Tab	Round	N	Y	Princeton	Tranquilizer
	WC 956	Albuterol Sulfate	2mg	White	Tab	Round	Y	N	WC	Bronchodilator
957	93 957	Chlordiazepoxide HCl	5mg	Green/Yellow	Cap	–	–	–	Lemmon	Antianxiety
	WC 957	Albuterol Sulfate	4mg	White	Tab	Round	Y	N	WC	Bronchodilator
958	BP 958	Methyltestosterone	10mg	Green	Tab	Square	N	N	Heather	Hormone
	BP 958	Methyltestosterone	10mg	Green	Tab	Square	N	N	ICN	Steroid
959	93 959	Chlordiazepoxide HCl	10mg	Green/Black	Cap	–	–	–	Lemmon	Antianxiety
960	54–960	Dexamethasone	0.75mg	Blue	Tab	Round	Y	N	Roxane	Steroid
961	93 961	Chlordiazepoxide HCl	25mg	Green/White	Cap	–	–	–	Lemmon	Antianxiety
966	WC 966	Thioridazine HCl	10mg	Orange	Tab	Round	–	–	WC	Tranquilizer
967	WC 967	Thioridazine HCl	25mg	Orange	Tab	Round	–	–	WC	Tranquilizer
968	E 968	Chlordiazepoxide HCl with Clidinium Bromide	5mg/2.5mg	Green	Cap	–	–	–	Eon	Antispasmodic
	PP 968	Chlordiazepoxide HCl & Clindinium Bromide	5mg/2.5mg.	Green	Cap	–	–	–	Eon	Antispasmodic
	Sch. Logo 968	Acetophenazine Maleate	20mg	Salmon	Tab	Round	N	Y	Schering	Antipsycotic
	WC 968	Thioridazine HCl	50mg	Orange	Tab	Round	–	–	WC	Tranquilizer
969	54–969	Diazepam	2mg	–	Tab	Round	–	–	Roxane	Antianxiety
	WC 969	Thioridazine HCl	100mg	Orange	Tab	Round	–	–	WC	Tranquilizer
970	54–970	Propranolol HCl	10mg	White	Tab	Round	Y	N	Roxane	Antihypertensive
	PP–970	Cephalexin	250mg.	Red/Gray	Cap	–	–	–	Eon	Anti–Infective
	Sch. Logo 970	Methyltestosterone Buccal	10mg	Lavender	Tab	Oval	N	N	Schering	Hormone
	WC 970	Thiothixene	1mg	–	Cap	–	–	–	WC	Tranquilizer
971	PP–971	Cephalexin	500mg.	Red	Cap	–	–	–	Eon	Anti–Infective
	SQUIBB 971	Ampicillin	250mg	Gray	Cap	–	–	–	Squibb	Anti–Infective
	WC 971	Thiothixene	2mg	Caramel/Yellow	Cap	–	–	–	WC	Tranquilizer
972	54–972	Propoxyphene HCl	65mg		Cap	–	–	–	Roxane	Analgesic
	WC 972	Thiothixene	5mg	Caramel/White	Cap	–	–	–	WC	Tranquilizer
973	54–973 5	Diazepam	5mg	Peach	Tab	Round	Y	N	Roxane	Antianxiety
974	SQUIBB 974	Ampicillin	500mg	Gray/Dark Gray	Cap	–	–	–	Squibb	Anti–Infective
975	WC 975	Thiothixene	10mg	Caramel/Peach	Cap	–	–	–	WC	Tranquilizer
977	WC 977	Temazepam	15mg	Green/White	Cap	–	–	–	WC	Sedative/Hypnotic
978	WC 978	Temazepam	30mg	White	Cap	–	–	–	WC	Sedative/Hypnotic
979	54–979 200	Quinidine Sulfate	200mg	White	Tab	Round	Y	N	Roxane	Antiarrhythmic
	WC 979	Propoxyphene & APAP	65mg/650mg	Orange	Tab	Capsule	N	Y	WC	Analgesic
980	WC 980	Propoxyphene Napsylate & APAP	100mg/650mg	Pink	Tab	–	N	Y	WC	Analgesic
981	WC 981	Haloperidol	0.5mg	Orange	Tab	Round	–	N	WC	Tranquilizer
982	54 982 10	Diazepam		Peach	Tab	Round	Y	N	Roxane	Antianxiety
	WC 982	Haloperidol	1mg	Orange	Tab	Round	–	N	WC	Tranquilizer
983	54–983	Amitriptyline	10mg	White	Tab	Round	–	N	Roxane	Antidepressant
	93 983	Nystatin Oral	500,000 Units	Brown	Tab	Round	N	Y	Lemmon	Antifungal
	WC 983	Haloperidol	2mg	Orange	Tab	Round	–	N	WC	Tranquilizer
984	WC 984	Haloperidol	5mg	Orange	Tab	Round	–	N	WC	Tranquilizer
985	WC 985	Clonidine HCl & Chlorthalidone	0.1mg/15mg	Yellow	Tab	Round	–	N	WC	Antihypertensive
986	WC 986	Clonidine HCl & Chlorthalidone	0.2mg/15mg	Yellow	Tab	Round	–	N	WC	Antihypertensive
987	WC 987	Clonidine HCl & Chlorthalidone	0.3mg/15mg	Yellow	Tab	Round	–	N	WC	Antihypertensive
988	E 988	Quinine Sulfate	260mg	White	Tab	Round	Y	N	Eon	Muscle Relaxant
	PP 988	Quinine Sulfate	260mg	White	Tab	Round	Y	N	Eon	Muscle Relaxant
	WC 988	Flurazepam	15mg	Peach/Orange	Cap	–	–	–	WC	Hypnotic
989	WC 989	Flurazepam	30mg	Peach/Red	Cap	–	–	–	WC	Hypnotic
992	54–992	Naproxen	375mg	–	Tab	–	–	–	Roxane	Anti–Inflammatory
	LUCHEM 992	Chlorpheniramine Maleate	12mg	Green/Clear	Cap	–	–	–	LuChem	Antihistamine
995	PP 995	Choline Magnesium Trisalicylate	500mg	Yellow	Tab	Capsule	–	–	Eon	Antiarthritic
996	BP 996	Methyltestosterone	25mg	Orange	Tab	Square	N	N	Heather	Hormone
	BP 996	Methyltestosterone	25mg	Yellow	Tab	Square	N	N	ICN	Steroid
	PP 996	Choline Magnesium Trisalicylate	750mg	Blue	Tab	Capsule	–	–	Eon	Antiarthritic
997	PP 997	Choline Magnesium Trisalicylate	1000mg	Pink	Tab	Capsule	–	–	Eon	Antiarthritic
998	BP 998	Fluoxymesterone	10mg	White	Tab	Round	Y	N	Heather	Hormone
	E 998	Yohimbine HCl	5.4mg	White	Tab	Round	Y	N	Eon	Sympatholytic
0004	bp 0004	Primidone Human	250mg	White	Tab	Round	Y	N	Bolar	Anticonvulsant
0005	bp 0005	Methocarbamol	500mg	White	Tab	Round	Y	N	Bolar	Muscle Relaxant
0007	bp 0007	Trihexyphenidyl HCl	2mg	White	Tab	Round	–	N	Bolar	Antiparkinson
0008	377–0008	Aminophylline	100mg	White	Tab	Round	–	N	Vale	Bronchodilator
0010	18–0010	Potassium Chloride CR	750mg	Clear	Cap	–	–	–	Penwalt	Potassium Supp.
0011	bp 0011	Furosemide (Veterinary)	12.5mg	Yellow	Tab	Round	N	N	Bolar	Diuretic
0012	Adams/0012	Guaifenesin	600mg	Green	Tab	Oblong	Y	N	Adams	Expectorant
	bp 0012	Furosemide (Veterinary)	50mg	Yellow	Tab	Capsule	N	N	Bolar	Diuretic
0016	Adams/0016	Phenylephrine /Guaifenesin	10mg/200mg	Clear/Blue	Cap	–	–	–	Adams	Decongestant Comb.
0017	Adams 0017	Guaifenesin/Pseudoephedrine	600mg/60mg	Blue	Tab	–	Y	N	Adams	Cough/Congestion
	bp 0017	Pentaerythritol Tetranitrate SR	80mg	Green/Green	Tab	Round	N	N	Bolar	Antianginal
0018	Adams/0018	Guaifenesin	300mg	Green/Clear	Cap	–	–	–	Adams	Expectorant
0022	Adams/0022	Brompheniramine/Phenyltoloxamine/Phenylephrine	2mg/25mg/10mg	Clear/Yellow	Cap	–	–	–	Adams	Decongestant Comb.
0024	bp 0024	Trihexyphenidyl HCl	5mg	White	Tab	Round	N	N	Bolar	Antiparkinson
0026	bp 0026	Isosorbide Dinitrate SA	40mg	Green	Tab	Round	Y	N	Bolar	Antianginal
0030	Adams 0030	Guaifenesin/Dextromethorphan Hydrobromide	600mg/30mg	Green	Tab	–	Y	N	Adams	Cough Preparation
0036	bp 0036	Chlorothiazide	250mg	White	Tab	Round	Y	N	Bolar	Diuretic
0037	bp 0037	Orphenadrine Citrate SR	100mg	White	Tab	Round	N	N	Bolar	Muscle Relaxant
0045	bp 0045	Warfarin Sodium	5mg	Pink	Tab	Round	Y	N	Bolar	Anticoagulant
0049	bp 0049	Isosorbide Dinitrate Oral	20mg	Green	Tab	Round	Y	N	Bolar	Antianginal
0051	Boots 0051	Allopurinol	100mg	White	Tab	Round	Y	N	Boots	Antigout
0052	Boots 0052	Allopurinol	300mg	Orange	Tab	Round	Y	N	Boots	Antigout
	bp 0052	Ergoloid Mesylates Sublingual	0.5mg	White	Tab	Round	–	–	Bolar	Vasodilator
0057	0057	Docusate Na/Casanthranol	–	Maroon	Cap	–	–	–	Scherer	Laxative
0058	bp 0058	Hydrochlorothiazide	100mg	Orange	Tab	Round	–	N	Bolar	Diuretic
0059	bp 0059	Sulfasalazine	500mg	Brownish Yellow	Tab	Round	Y	N	Bolar	Anti–Inflammatory
0065	bp 0065	Hydralazine HCl & Hydrochlorothiazide	25mg/25mg	White/White	Cap	–	–	–	Bolar	Antihypertensive

ID NO.	ID CODE	GENERIC NAME	STRENGTH	COLOR	FORM	SHAPE	SCORED	COATED	MFG.	USE
0066	bp 0066	Hydralazine HCl & Hydrochlorothiazide	50mg/50mg	White/Black	Cap	–	–	–	Bolar	Antihypertensive
0069	bp 0069	Ergoloid Mesylates Sublingual	1mg	White	Tab	Oval	–	–	Bolar	Vasodilator
0070	Rugby 0070	Amoxicillin	250mg	–	Cap	–	–	–	Rugby	Anti–infective
0072	EVERETT 0072	Multivitamin/Iron/Folic Acid	n/a	–	Tab	–	–	–	Everett	Multivitamin
0073	bp 0073	Bethanechol Chloride	5mg	White	Tab	Round	Y	N	Bolar	Urinary Tract Agent
	bp 0073	Bethanechol Chloride	5mg	White	Tab	Round	Y	N	Bolar	Urinary Tract Agent
0074	bp 0074	Bethanechol Chloride	10mg	pink	Tab	Round	Y	N	Bolar	Urinary Tract Agent
0075	bp 0075	Bethanechol Chloride	25mg	Yellow	Tab	Round	Y	N	Bolar	Urinary Tract Agent
0080	Rugby 0080	Amoxicillin	500mg	–	Cap	–	–	–	Rugby	Anti–infective
0083	bp 0083	Hydralazine HCl & Hydrochlorothiazide	25mg/15mg	Orange	Cap	Round	–	N	Bolar	Antihypertensive
0084	bp 0084	Phenytoin Sodium Extended Release	100mg	White/White	Cap	–	–	–	Bolar	Anticonvulsant
0093	bp 0093	Prochlorperazine	10mg	Chartreuse	Tab	Round	N	Y	Bolar	Antiemetic
0094	bp 0094	Carisoprodol	350mg	White	Tab	Round	N	N	Bolar	Muscle Relaxant
0100	0100	Vitamin A Palmitate	25,000 Units	Yellow	Cap	–	–	–	Richlyn	Vitamin
0101	0101	Vitamin A Natural	25,000 Units	Yellow	Cap	–	–	–	Richlyn	Vitamin
0102	0102	Vitamin A Palmitate	50,000 Units	Red	Cap	–	–	–	Richlyn	Vitamin
0104	0104	Vitamin A Solubilized	25,000 Units	Yellow	Cap	–	–	–	Richlyn	Vitamin
	G-0104	Phenylpropanolamine HCl / Caramiphen Edisylate	75mg/40mg	Purple/Black	Cap	–	–	–	Pioneer	Antitussive Comb.
0105	0105	Vitamin A Natural	50,000 Units	Red	Cap	–	–	–	Richlyn	Vitamin
0106	377–0106	Chlorpheniramine,Pyrilamine,Phenylephrine	1mg/12.5mg/5mg	Yellow	Tab	Round	–	Y	Vale	Decongestant Comb.
0109	0109	Vitamin A Solubilized	50,000 Units	Yellow	Cap	–	–	–	Richlyn	Vitamin
	377–0109	Ephedrine & Sodium Phenobarbital	16.2mg/24.3mg	Yellow	Tab	Round	–	N	Vale	Antiasthmatic
0111	0111	Butalbital, Acetaminophen, Caffeine	50mg/325mg/40mg	White	Tab	Round	–	–	D.M. Graham	Analgesic
	bp 0111	Prochlorperazine	5mg	Chartreuse	Tab	Round	N	Y	Bolar	Antiemetic
0120	Rugby 0120	Cephalexin	250mg	–	Cap	–	–	–	Rugby	Anti–infective
0125	377–0125	Guaifenesin	100mg	White	Tab	Round	–	N	Vale	Expectorant
0129	bp 0129	Spironolactone & Hydrochlorothiazide	25mg/25mg	White	Tab	Round	Y	N	Bolar	Antihypertensive
0130	Rugby 0130	Cephalexin	500mg	–	Cap	–	–	–	Rugby	Anti–infective
0131	0131 20/08	Ghlorpheniramine/Pseudoephedrine/APAP	2mg/30mg/325mg	Peach	Tab	Capsule	N	Y	Central	Antihistamine
0139	bp 0139	Fluoxymesterone	10mg	Green	Tab	Round	–	–	Bolar	Hormone
0140	0140	Vitamin D	50,000 Units	Green	Cap	–	–	–	Richlyn	Vitamin
0147	CC 0147	Phentermine HCl	15mg	Gray/Yellow	Cap	–	–	–	Camall	Anorectic
	CC 0147	Phentermine HCl	30mg	Blue/Clear	Cap	–	–	–	Camall	Anorectic
	CC 0147	Phentermine HCl	30mg	Black/Black	Cap	–	–	–	Camall	Anorectic
	CC 0147	Phentermine HCl	30mg	Black/Yellow	Cap	–	–	–	Camall	Anorectic
	CC 0147	Phentermine HCl	30mg	Brown/Clear	Cap	–	–	–	Camall	Anorectic
	CC 0147	Phentermine HCl	30mg	Green/Clear	Cap	–	–	–	Camall	Anorectic
	CC 0147	Phentermine HCl	30mg	Yellow/Yellow	Cap	–	–	–	Camall	Anorectic
	CC 0147	Phentermine HCl	30mg	Red/Black	Cap	–	–	–	Camall	Anorectic
0149	bp 0149	Acepromazine Maleate (Veterinary)	10mg	White	Tab	Round	N	Y	Bolar	–
0150	bp 0150	Acepromazine Maleate (Veterinary)	25mg	Yellow	Tab	Round	N	Y	Bolar	–
0155	879 0155	Propoxyphene HCl	65mg	Pink	Cap	–	–	–	Halsey	Analgesic
0158	879 0158	Tetracycline HCl	250mg	Yellow/Orange	Cap	–	–	–	Halsey	Anti–Infective
0167	377–0167	Pyrilamine Maleate	25mg	White	Tab	Round	–	N	Vale	Antihistamine
0169	LASER 0169	Pseudoephedrine HCl/Guaifenesin	120mg/250mg	Orange/Clear	Cap	–	–	–	Central	Decongestant
0174	LASER 0174	Pseudoephedrine HCl/Guaifenesin	60mg/200mg	Green/Clear	Cap	–	–	–	Central	Decongestant
0187	377–0187	Phenobarbital	15mg	Pink	Tab	Round	–	N	Vale	Sedative
	bp 0187	Procainamide HCl SR	1000mg	Pink	Tab	Capsule	Y	Y	Bolar	Antiarrhythmic
0188	377–0188	Phenobarbital	15mg	White	Tab	Round	–	N	Vale	Sedative
0189	377–0189	Phenobarbital	15mg	Green	Tab	Round	–	N	Vale	Sedative
0192	377–0192	Phenobarbital	30mg	White	Tab	Round	–	N	Vale	Sedative
0193	377–0193	Phenobarbital	30mg	Pink	Tab	Round	–	N	Vale	Sedative
0196	377–0196	Phenobarbital	90mg	White	Tab	Round	–	N	Vale	Sedative
0201	EVERETT 0201	Multivitamin/Minerals	n/a	–	Tab	–	–	–	Everett	Multivitamin
0211	bp 0211	Maprotiline HCl	25mg	Blue	Tab	Round	N	Y	Bolar	Antidepressant
0212	bp 0212	Maprotiline HCl	50mg	Yellow	Tab	Round	N	Y	Bolar	Antidepressant
0213	bp 0213	Maprotiline HCl	75mg	White	Tab	Round	N	Y	Bolar	Antidepressant
0214	377–0214	Rauwolfia Serpentina	50mg	Red	Tab	Round	–	Y	Vale	Antihypertensive
0215	377–0215	Rauwolfia Serpentina	100mg	Pink	Tab	Round	–	Y	Vale	Antihypertensive
0216	377–0216	Phenylephrine,Chlorpheniramine,Salicylamide,APAP	5/2/250/150mg	Green/White mottled	Tab	Round	–	N	Vale	Decongestant Comb.
0217	377–0217	Phenylephrine,Chlorpheniramine,Salicylamide,APAP	2/1/90mg/60mg	Green/White mottled	Tab	Round	–	N	Vale	Decongestant Comb.
0220	252/0220	Thyroid	130mg	Natural	Tab	Round	–	N	Jones	Hormone
0230	Rugby 0230	Doxycycline Hyclate	100mg	–	Cap	–	–	–	Rugby	Anti–Infective
0232	377–0232	Sodium Butabarbital	15mg	Pink	Tab	Round	–	N	Vale	Sedative
0233	377–0233	Sodium Butabarbital	30mg	Green	Tab	Round	–	N	Vale	Sedative
0238	377–0238	Sodium Salicylate	324mg	Pink	Tab	Round	–	N	Vale	Analgesic
0240	377–0240	Sodium Salicylate	324mg	Red	Tab	Round	–	Y	Vale	Analgesic
0242	377–0242	Sodium Salicylate	324mg	Purple	Tab	Round	–	Y	Vale	Anti–Infective
0250	Rugby 0250	Erythromycin Stearate	250mg	–	Tab	–	–	–	Rugby	Antihypertensive
0251	rPr 0251 180mg	Diltiazem HCl	180mg	–	Cap	–	–	–	Rorer	Antihypertensive
0252	rPr 0252 240mg	Diltiazem HCl	240mg	–	Cap	–	–	–	Rorer	Anti–Infective
0265	Rugby 0265	Erythromycin Stearate	500mg	–	Tab	–	–	–	Rugby	Hormone
0272	377–0272	Thyroid	30mg	Tan	Tab	Round	–	N	Vale	Anti–Infective
0277	377–0277	Sulfadiazine,Sulfamerazine,Sulfamethazine	167/167/167mg	Pink	Tab	Round	–	N	Vale	Anti–Infective
0280	Rugby 0280	Doxycycline Hyclate	50mg	–	Cap	–	–	–	Rugby	Antihistamine
0290	377–0290	Diphenhydramine HCl	50mg	Orange	Tab	Round	Y	N	Vale	Analgesic
0310	Ascher logo 0310	Magnesium salicilate	600mg	White	Tab	Capsule	Y	N	B.F.Ascher	Decongestant Comb.
0311	377–0311	Phenyleph.,Chlorphenir,Salicylamide,APAP,Guaifen	5/2/250/150/100	Pink,Green/White	Tab	Round	–	N	Vale	Vitamin Comb.
0331	M/P 0331	Vitamin/Mineral Comb.	–	Maroon	Tab	–	Y	Y	Central	Digestant
0332	377–0332	Pepsin,Pancreatin,Diastase	259/32/2mg	Tan	Tab	Round	–	N	Vale	Anti–Infective
0340	Rugby 0340	Doxycycline Hyclate	100mg	–	Tab	–	–	–	Rugby	Antiarthritic
0349	377–0349	Magnesium Trisilicate	500mg	Yellow	Tab	Oval	–	N	Vale	Anorectic
0351	377–0351	Phendimetrazine Tartrate	35mg	Yellow	Tab	Round	–	N	Vale	Decongestant
0358	377–0358	Pseudoephedrine	60mg	Green	Tab	Round	–	N	Vale	Antitussive Comb.
0359	377–0359	Guaifenesin & Pseudoephedrine HCl	100mg/30mg	Pink/White mottled	Tab	Round	–	N	Vale	Antianxiety
0364	879 0364	Chlordiazepoxide	5mg	Green/Yellow	Cap	–	–	–	Halsey	Antispasmodic
0365	377–0365	Pb,Hyoscyamine,Scopolamine,Atropine	n/a	Green	Tab	Round	–	N	Vale	Antianxiety
	879 0365	Chlordiazepoxide	10mg	Green/Black	Cap	–	–	–	Halsey	Antianxiety
0366	879 0366	Chlordiazepoxide	25mg	Green/White	Cap	–	–	–	Halsey	Decongestant Comb.
0379	M R 0379	Guaifenesin/Pseudoephedrine	400mg/120mg	White	Tab	Oval	Y	N	Mayrand	Decongestant/Exp.
	M/R 0379	Guaifenesin/Pseudoephedrine	400mg/120mg	Off White	Tab	Oblong	Y	Y	KV	Decongestant/Exp.
0382	M/R 0382	Guaifenesin/Dextromethorphan/Pseudoephedrine	400/20/60mg	Orange	Tab	–	Y	Y	Vintage	Vitamin Comb.
0384	MP 0384	Vitamin E/Vitamin C/Beta–Carotene	100I.U/120/25mg	Brown	Cap	Oval	–	–	Scherer	Anti–Infective
0390	Rugby 0390	Doxycycline Hyclate	50mg	–	Tab	–	–	–	Rugby	Hormone
0396	377–0396	Thyroid	65mg	Green	Tab	Round	–	Y	Vale	Hormone

ID NO.	ID CODE	GENERIC NAME	STRENGTH	COLOR	FORM	SHAPE	SCORED	COATED	MFG.	USE
0400	252/0400	Phenobarbital	15mg	White	Tab	Round	N	N	Jones	Sedative
0401	252/0401	Phenobarbital	30mg	White	Tab	Round	N	N	Jones	Sedative
0405	0822/0405	Allopurinol	100mg	White	Tab	Round	Y	N	Boots	Antigout
0409	DUNHALL 0409	Pseudoephedrine HCl & Chlorpheniramine	120mg/12mg	Gray/Aqua	Cap	–	–	–	Dunhall	Decongestant Comb.
0410	0822/0410	Allopurinol	300mg	Peach	Tab	Round	Y	N	Boots	Antigout
0420	832-0420	Hydroflumethiazide & Reserpine	50mg/0.125mg	Green	Tab	Round	N	N	PBI	Antihypertensive
0430	0822/0430	Butalbital, Aspirin, Caffeine	50/325/40mg	White	Tab	Round	N	N	Halsey	Analgesic
0431	Wallace 0431	Felbamate	600mg	Peach	Tab	Oval	Y	N	Wallace	Antiepileptic
0494	252/0494	Thyroid	32mg	Natural	Tab	Round	–	N	Jones	Hormone
0495	252/0495	Thyroid	65mg	Natural	Tab	Round	–	N	Jones	Hormone
0496	FL0496	Phenylephrine/Chlorpheniramine/Pyrilamine	25mg/8mg/25mg	Tan	Tab	Round	Y	N	Econolabs	Decongestant Comb.
0498	377-0498	Pb,Hyoscyamine,Scopolamine,Atropine	n/a	Yellow	Tab	Round	–	N	Vale	Antispasmodic
0506	G-0506	Reserpine,Hydralazine HCl,Hydrochlorothiazide.	0.1mg/25mg/15mg	White	Tab	Round	Y	N	–	Antihypertensive
0519	COPLEY 0519	Vitamin/Flor (Chewable)	1mg	–	Tab	Square	N	N	Copley	Vitamin
0576	0822/0576	Meclizine HCl Chewable	25mg	Pink	Tab	Round	N	N	Boots	Antiemetic
0630	377-0630	Dover's Pwd,Aspirin,Caffeine	24mg/324mg/32mg	Blue/White	Cap	–	–	–	Vale	Analgesic
0636	377-0636	Dover Pwd,Aspirin,Caffeine	15/162/8.1mg	Red	Tab	Round	N	Y	Vale	Analgesic
0642	377-0642	Pb,Hyoscyamine,Scopolamine,Camphor,Valerian, Passif	n/a	Yellow	Tab	Round	–	Y	Vale	Antispasmodic
0650	377-0650	Barbital,Hyoscyamine,Scopolamine,Passiflora,Valeri	n/a	Blue	Tab	Round	–	Y	Vale	Antispasmodic
0656	HD 0656	Chlordiazepoxide HCl & Clidinium Bromide	5mg/2.5mg	Green	Cap	–	–	–	Halsey	Antispasmodic
0659	K 0659	Ergoloid Mesylate SL	1mg	White	Tab	Oval	N	N	KV	Vasodilator
0665	0665	Lithium Carbonate	300mg	White	Cap	–	–	–	RR	Antipsychotic
0677	AHR 0677	B Complex/Ascorbic Acid/Vitamin E	n/a	Orange	Tab	Elliptical	N	Y	Robins	Vitamin
0678	AHR 0678	B Complex/Ascorbic Acid/Vitamin E/Iron	n/a	Red	Tab	Elliptical	N	Y	Robins	Vitamin
0765	SCHEIN 0765/400	Ibuprofen	400mg	White	Tab	Round	N	Y	Schein	Anti-Inflammatory
0766	SCHEIN 0766/600	Ibuprofen	600mg	White	Tab	Oval	N	Y	Schein	Anti-Inflammatory
0805	DUNHALL 0805	Doxycycline Hyclate	100mg	Red	Cap	–	–	–	Dunhall	Anti-Infective
0822	0822	Souduim Fluoride Chewable	2.2mg	Pink	Tab	Round	N	N	Pharmafair	Mineral
0840	RR-0840	Acetaminophen,Codeine,Phenephrine,Chlorpheniramine	325/16/10/2 mg	Yellow	Cap	–	–	–	RR	Cold/Cough
	SOLVAY 0840	Acetaminophen,Codeine,Phenephrine,Chlorpheniramine	325/16/10/2 mg	Yellow	Cap	–	–	–	Solvay	Cold/Cough
0841	0822/0841	Sodium Fluoride Chewable	2.2mg	Pink	Tab	Round	N	N	Boots	Mineral
0849	K 0849	Papaverine HCl SR	150mg	Brown/Clear	Cap	–	–	–	KV	Sm.Musc. Relaxer
0897	0897	Docusate Na	–	Red	Cap	–	–	–	Scherer	Stool Softener
0898	0898	Docusate Na	–	Red	Cap	–	–	–	Scherer	Stool Softener
0901	ICN 0901	Methyltestosterone	10mg	Red	Cap	–	–	–	ICN	Hormone
0920	R&C Logo 0920	Isosorbide Dinitrate SR	40mg	Pink/Clear	Cap	–	–	–	R & C	Antianginal
1000	PF T 1000	Choline Magnesium Trisalicylate	1000mg	Red	Tab	Oblong	Y	Y	PF	Analgesic
	PF T1000	Choline Magnesium Trisalicylate	1000mg	Red	Tab	Oblong	Y	Y	PF	Antiarrthritic
1001	01001	Pancreatin	425mg	Beige	Tab	Round	N	N	Viobin Corp.	Enzyme Supplement
	1001	Aminophylline	100mg	White	Tab	Round	–	–	Vortech	Bronchodilator
	Mylan 1001	Thiothixene	1mg	Caramel/Blue	Cap	–	–	–	Mylan	Tranquilizer
	WALLACE 37 1001	Meprobamate	400mg	White	Tab	Round	Y	N	Wallace	Tranquilizer
1007	bp 1007	Trazodone HCl	50mg	White	Tab	Round	Y	N	Bolar	Antianxiety
	RR 1007	Medroxyprogestrone Acetate	10mg	White	Tab	Round	Y	N	RR	Antidepressnt
	SOLVAY 1007	Medroxyprogestrone Acetate	10mg	White	Tab	Round	Y	N	Solvay	Hormone
1008	1008	Dextro–Amphetamine Sulfate	5mg	–	Tab	Round	–	–	Vortech	Hormone
	bp 1008	Trazodone HCl	100mg	White	Tab	Round	Y	N	Bolar	Anorectic
1009	1009	Digitoxin	0.2mg	–	Tab	Round	–	–	Vortech	Antidepressant
1010	MYLAN 1010	Piroxicam	10mg	Green/Olive	Cap	–	–	–	Mylan	Cardiac Agent
1014	RR 1014	Esterified Estrogens	0.3mg	Blue	Tab	Round	N	Y	RR	Anti–inflammatory
	SOLVAY 1014	Esterified Estrogens	0.3mg	Blue	Tab	Round	N	Y	Solvay	Hormone
1015	bp 1015	Nitrofurantoin	100mg	Yellow/Yellow	Cap	–	–	–	Bolar	Hormone
1016	bp 1016	Nitrofurantoin	50mg	White/Yellow	Cap	–	–	–	Bolar	Anti–Infective
1022	RR 1022	Esterified Estrogens	0.625mg	Yellow	Tab	Round	N	Y	RR	Anti–Infective
	SOLVAY 1022	Esterified Estrogens	0.625mg	Yellow	Tab	Round	N	Y	Solvay	Hormone
1023	RR 1023	Esterified Estrogens with Methyltestosterone	0.625mg/2.5mg	Green	Tab	Capsule	N	Y	RR	Hormone
	SOLVAY 1023	Esterified Estrogens with Methyltestosterone	0.625mg/2.5mg	Green	Tab	Oblong	N	Y	Solvay	Hormone
1024	RR 1024	Esterified Estrogens	1.25mg	Red	Tab	Round	N	Y	RR	Hormone
	SOLVAY 1024	Esterified Estrogens	1.25mg	Red	Tab	Round	N	Y	Solvay	Hormone
1025	RR 1025	Esterified Estrogens	2.5mg	Pink	Tab	Round	N	Y	RR	Hormone
	SOLVAY 1025	Esterified Estrogens	2.5mg	Purple	Tab	Round	N	Y	Solvay	Hormone
1026	RR 1026	Esterified Estrogens with Methyltestosterone	1.25mg/2.5mg	Green	Tab	Capsule	N	Y	RR	Hormone
	SOLVAY 1026	Esterified Estrogens with Methyltestosterone	1.25mg/2.5mg	Green	Tab	Oblong	N	Y	Solvay	Hormone
1027	bp 1027	Amantadine HCl	100mg	Pink	Cap	–	–	–	Bolar	Antiviral
1031	1031	Carbetapentane/Chlorpheniramine/Ephedrine/PhenEph.	60/5/10/10mg	Pink	Tab	Oblong	Y	N	Econolabs	Antitussive Comb.
1032	0345 1032	Propoxyphene W/Aspirin & Caffeine	65/389/32.4mg	Red/Gray	Cap	–	–	–	Lemmon	Analgesic
	1032	Reserpine	0.25mg	White	Tab	Round	–	–	Vortech	Antihypertensive
1033	1033	Rauwolfia Serpentina	100mg	–	Tab	Round	–	–	Vortech	Antihypertensive
	1033/FL	Ergotamine/Phenobarbital/belladonna	0.6mg/40mg/0.2	Blue	Tab	Round	Y	N	Econolabs	Antispasmodic
	FL 1033	Bel–Phen–Ergot	n/a	Aqua	Tab	Round	Y	N	Ferndale	Vasodilator
1039	RR 1039	Phenylpropanolamine/pyrilamine/chlorophen/phenylep	50/25/4/10mg	White/Blue specks	Tab	Oblong	Y	N	RR	Decongestant Comb.
	SOLVAY 1039	Phenylpropanolamine/pyrilamine/chlorophen/phenylep	50/25/4/10mg	White/Blue specks	Tab	Oblong	Y	N	Solvay	Decongestant Comb.
1043	1043	Thyroid	2gr	Tan	Tab	Round	–	N	Vortech	Hormone
	527/1043	Isobutylallylbarbituric Acid/Caff./ASA/Phenacetin	50/40/200/130mg	–	Tab	Round	–	N	Lannett	Analgesic
1044	1044	Thyroid	1gr	Tan	Tab	Round	–	N	Vortech	Hormone
1045	1045	Thyroid	1gr	Red	Tab	Round	N	Y	Vortech	Hormone
1049	Mylan 1049	Doxepin HCl	10mg	Buff/Buff	Cap	–	–	–	Mylan	Antidepressant
1050	RPL 1050	Pseudoephedrine HCl/Guaifenesin	120mg/400mg	White/Green specks	Tab	Round	Y	–	RR	Decongestant Comb.
	SOLVAY 1050	Pseudoephedrine HCl/Guaifenesin	120mg/400mg	White/Green specks	Tab	Round	Y	–	Solvay	Decongestant Comb.
1052	VT–1052	Theophylline SR	260mg	Brown/Clear	Cap	–	–	–	Eon	Bronchodilator
1053	527/1053	Phenobarbital	1/4gr	White	Tab	Round	–	N	Lannett	Sedative
	527/1053	Phenobarbital	1/4gr	Pink	Tab	Round	–	N	Lannett	Sedative
	527/1053	Phenobarbital	1/4gr	Green	Tab	Round	–	N	Lannett	Sedative
1054	527/1054	Phenobarbital	1/2gr	Green	Tab	Round	–	N	Lannett	Sedative
	527/1054	Phenobarbital	1/2gr	Pink	Tab	Round	–	N	Lannett	Sedative
	527/1054	Phenobarbital	1/2gr	White	Tab	Round	–	N	Lannett	Sedative
	Forest 1054	Racemethionine	200mg	Pink/Blue	Cap	–	–	–	Forest	–
1055	527/1055	Phenobarbital	1 1/2gr	White	Tab	Round	–	N	Lannett	Sedative
	527/1055	Phenobarbital	1 1/2gr	Pink	Tab	Round	–	N	Lannett	Sedative
1057	527/1057	Phenobarbital	1gr	White	Tab	Round	–	N	Lannett	Sedative
1060	527/1060	Glutethimide	500mg	White	Tab	Round	Y	N	Lannett	Hypnotic
1077	1077	Chlorpheniramine Maleate	8mg	–	Tab	Round	–	N	Vortech	Antihistamine
1078	1078	Phenobarbital & Belladonna	15mg/10mg	–	Tab	Round	–	N	Vortech	Antispasmodic
1079	1079	Digitoxin	0.1mg	–	Tab	Round	–	–	Vortech	Cardiac Agent
1082	RPL 1082	Phendimetrazine tartrate	105mg	Orange/Clear	Cap	–	–	–	RR	Anorectic

ID NO.	ID CODE	GENERIC NAME	STRENGTH	COLOR	FORM	SHAPE	SCORED	COATED	MFG.	USE
	SOLVAY 1082	Phendimetrazine tartrate	105mg	Orange/Clear	Cap	–	–	–	Solvay	Anorectic
1088	527/1088	Glutethimide	250mg	White	Tab	Round	Y	N	Lannett	Hypnotic
	RR 1088	Hydrocodone Bitartrate/Phenindamine/Guaifenesin	5mg/25mg/200mg	Brown	Tab	Rectangular	Y	N	RR	Antitussive Comb.
	SOLVAY 1088	Hydrocodone Bitartrate/Phenindamine/Guaifenesin	5mg/25mg/200mg	Peach	Tab	Capsule	Y	N	Solvay	Antitussive Comb.
1093	1093	Thyroid	2gr	Red	Tab	Round	–	Y	Vortech	Hormone
1094	1094	Penicillin G	250,000 Units	–	Tab	Round	–	–	Vortech	Anti–Infective
1098	1098	Prednisone	5mg	–	Tab	Round	–	–	Vortech	Steroid
1101	MYLAN 1101	Prazosin HCl	1mg	Green/Brown	Cap	–	–	–	Mylan	Antihypertensive
	WALLACE 37 1101	Meprobamate	200mg	White	Tab	Round	N	Y	Wallace	Antianxiety
1103	R 1103	Acetaminophen	325mg	White	Tab	Round	–	N	Purepac	Analgesic
1110	0115 1110	Diphenhydramine HCl	25mg	Pink/Clear	Cap	–	–	–	Richlyn	Antihistamine
1111	0115 1111	Diphenhydramine HCl	50mg	Pink	Cap	–	–	–	Richlyn	Antihistamine
	Beach 1111	Potassium Acid Phosphate	500mg	White	Tab	Round	Y	N	Beach	Urinary Tract Agent
1112	Beach 1112	Methenamine Mandelate/Sodium Acid Phosphate	350mg/200mg	Yellow	Tab	Round	N	Y	Beach	Urinary Tract Agent
1114	Beach 1114	Methenamine Mandelate/Sodium Acid Phosphate	500mg/500mg	Yellow	Tab	Capsule	Y	Y	Beach	Urinary Tract Agent
1115	Beach 1115	Methenamine Mandelate/Potassium Acid Phosphate	500mg/250mg	Green	Tab	Capsule	Y	N	Beach	Urinary Tract Agent
	Sav. Logo 1115	Diphylline	200mg	Blue	Tab	Round	Y	N	Savage	Bronchodilator
1116	Sav. Logo 1116	Diphylline	400mg	White	Tab	Round	Y	N	Savage	Bronchodilator
1120	UAD logo 1120	Hydrocodone Bitartrate & Acetaminophen	5mg/500mg	Maroon	Cap	–	–	N	UAD	Analgesic
1123	527/1123	Dextro–Amphetamine Sulfate	15mg	Green	Tab	Round	Y	N	Lannett	CNS Stimulant
1124	Sav. Logo 1124	Diphylline & Guaifenesin	200mg/200mg	Pink	Tab	Round	Y	N	Savage	Bronchodilator
1125	Beach 1125	Phosphate Combination	–	White	Tab	Capsule	N	Y	Beach	Urinary Tract Agent
1132	Beach 1132	Magnesium/Vitamin B-6	600mg/25mg	Tan	Tab	Round	N	Y	Beach	Vitamin
	RR 1132	Hydralazine, Reserpine, Hydrochlorothiazide	25/0.1/15mg	Yellow	Tab	Round	Y	N	RR	Antihypertensive
	SOLVAY 1132	Hydralazine, Reserpine, Hydrochlorothiazide	25/0.1/15mg	Yellow	Tab	Round	Y	N	Solvay	Antihypertensive
1134	Beach 1134	Potassium Acid Phosphate/Sodium Acid Phosphate	305mg/700mg	Brown	Cap	–	–	–	Beach	Urinary Tract Agent
1135	Beach 1135	Potassium Acid Phosphate/Sodium Acid Phosphate	155mg/350mg	White	Tab	Round	Y	N	Beach	Urinary Tract Agent
1138	527/1138	Amphetamine Sulfate	5mg	–	Tab	Round	–	–	Lannett	CNS Stimulant
1139	527/1139	Amphetamine Sulfate	10mg	–	Tab	Round	–	–	MD	Antidepressant
1140	G1140	Amitriptyline HCl	150mg	Flesh	Tab	Oblong	N	N	Richlyn	Antiasthmatic
1142	0115 1142	Ephedrine Sulfate	3/4gr	Pink	Cap	–	–	–	Richlyn	Antiasthmatic
1143	527/1143	Dextro–Amphetamine Sulfate	5mg	Yellow	Tab	Round	Y	N	Lannett	CNS Stimulant
1146	RR 1146	Prenatal Vitamin	n/a	Blue	Tab	Oblong	N	Y	RR	Vitamin
	SOLVAY 1146	Prenatal Vitamin	n/a	Blue	Tab	Oblong	N	Y	Solvay	Vitamin
1151	527/1151	Acetaminophen with Phenobarbital	325mg/16mg	White	Tab	Round	–	N	Lannett	Analgesic
1153	DAN 1153	Carisoprodol	350mg	White	Tab	Round	N	N	Danbury	Muscle Relaxant
1170	527/1170	Diphenoxylate HCl/Atropine Sulfate	2.5mg/0.025mg	White	Tab	Round	–	N	Lannett	Antidiarrheal
1179	527/1179	Butabarbital Sodium	1/4 gr	Lavender	Tab	Round	–	N	Lannett	Sedative
1180	527/1180	Butabarbital Sodium	1/2 gr	Green	Tab	Round	Y	N	Lannett	Sedative
1184	527/1184	Butabarbital Sodium	1 1/2 gr	Pink	Tab	Round	Y	N	Lannett	Sedative
1189	G 1189 500	Chlorzoxazone	500mg	Green	Tab	Capsule	Y	N	Royce	Muscle relaxant
1200	SOLVAY 1200	Pancreatin/Lipase/Protease/Amylase	n/a	Brown/Clear	Cap	–	–	–	Solvay	Digestive Enzyme
1204	0032–1204	Multivitamins	n/a	Brown	Cap	–	–	–	Solvay	Vitamin Comb.
1210	SOLVAY 1210	Pancreatin/Lipase/Protease/Amylase	n/a	Brown/Clear	Cap	–	–	–	Solvay	Digestive Enzyme
1216	RR 1216	Vitamin Comb.	n/a	Brown	Cap	–	–	–	RR	Vitamin
	SOLVAY 1216	Vitamin Comb.	n/a	Brown	Cap	–	–	–	Solvay	Vitamin
1217	E 1217	Nitroglycerin SR	9mg	Green/Yellow	Cap	–	–	–	Eon	Antianginal
	PP–1217	Nitroglycerin	9mg	Green/Yellow	Cap	–	–	–	Eon	Antianginal
1218	RR 1218	Vitamin Comb.	n/a	Brown	Tab	Capsule	–	–	RR	Vitamin
1219	527/1219	Dextro–Amphetamine Sulfate	10mg	Orange	Tab	Round	Y	N	Lannett	CNS Stimulant
1221	TCL 1221	Nitroglycerin TD	2.5mg	Lavender/Clear	Cap	–	–	–	Time–Caps	Antianginal
1222	TCL 1222	Nitroglycerin TD	6.5mg	Black/Yellow	Cap	–	–	–	Time–Caps	Antianginal
1223	TCL 1223	Nitroglycerin T.D.	9mg	Green/Yellow	Cap	–	–	–	Time–Caps	Antianginal
1224	527/1224	Meprobamate	400mg	White	Tab	Round	Y	N	Lannett	Antianxiety
1225	SOLVAY 1225	Pancreatin/Lipase/Protease/Amylase	n/a	Orange/Yellow	Cap	–	–	–	Solvay	Digestive Enzyme
1231	SEARLE 1231	Aminophylline	100mg	White	Tab	Round	Y	N	Searle	Bronchodilator
1235	E 1235	Nitroglycerin SR	6.5mg	Blue/Yellow	Cap	–	–	–	Eon	Antianginal
	PP–1235	Nitroglycerin	6.5mg	Blue/Yellow	Cap	–	–	–	Eon	Antianginal
1237	1237	Pentaerythritol Tetranitrate	20mg	–	Tab	Round	–	N	Vortech	Antianginal
1242	1242	Prednisolone	5mg	–	Tab	Round	–	–	Vortech	Steroid
1250	527/1250	Meprobamate	200mg	White	Tab	Round	Y	N	Lannett	Antianxiety
1251	SEARLE 1251	Aminophylline	200mg	White	Tab	Oval	Y	N	Searle	Bronchodilator
1252	527/1252	Phendimetrazine Tartrate 4	35mg	Green	Tab	Round	Y	N	Lannett	Anorectic
1269	527/1269	Phendimetrazine Tartrate 10	35mg	Speckled	Tab	Oval	–	N	Lannett	Anorectic
1270	527/1270	Phendimetrazine Tartrate 11	35mg	Pink	Tab	Round	–	N	Lannett	Anorectic
1271	527/1271	Phendimetrazine Tartrate 12	35mg	Yellow	Tab	Round	–	N	Lannett	Anorectic
1272	527/1272	Phendimetrazine Tartrate 13	35mg	Grey	Tab	Round	–	N	Lannett	Anorectic
1273	527/1273	Phendimetrazine Tartrate 14	35mg	White	Tab	Round	–	N	Lannett	Anorectic
1274	527/1274	Phendimetrazine Tartrate 15	35mg	Green/White Specks	Tab	Round	–	N	Lannett	Anorectic
1276	1276	Thyroid	1/2gr	Tan	Tab	Round	–	–	Vortech	Hormone
1278	M/R 1278	Butalbital/Acetaminohen	50mg/650mg	White	Tab	Capsule	Y	N	Mayrand	Analgesic
1300	0115 1300	Oxytetracycline	250mg	Yellow	Cap	–	–	–	Richlyn	Anti–Infective
1303	E 1303	Quinine Sulfate	325mg	Clear	Cap	–	–	–	Eon	Muscle Relaxant
	PP 1303	Quinine Sulfate	325mg	Clear	Cap	–	–	–	Eon	Muscle Relaxant
1304	E 1304	Chlorpheniramine Maleate/Pseudoephedrine HCl	8mg/120mg	Blue/Clear	Cap	–	–	–	Eon	Decongestant Comb.
	PP 1304	Chlorpheniramine Maleate/Pseudoephedrine HCl	8mg/120mg	Blue/Clear	Cap	–	–	–	Eon	Decongestant Comb.
1332	1332	Chlorpheniramine Maleate	4mg	–	Tab	Round	–	N	Vortech	Antihistamine
1339	1339	Phenylprop,Phenyleph,Phentoloxamine,Chlorphenirami	40/10/15/5mg	–	Tab	Round	–	–	Vortech	Decongestant Comb.
1342	1342	Penicillin G	400,000 Units	–	Tab	Round	–	–	Vortech	Anti–Infective
1343	GG1343	Reserpine, Hydralazine, Hydrochlorothiazide	0.1/25/15mg	White	Tab	Round	N	N	Danbury	Antihypertensive
1354	WHR 1354	Theophylline	60mg	White	Cap	–	–	–	Rorer	Bronchodilator
1355	WHR 1355	Theophylline	125mg	Brown	Cap	–	–	–	Rorer	Bronchodilator
1356	WHR 1356	Theophylline	250mg	Purple	Cap	–	–	–	Rorer	Bronchodilator
1375	Marion 1375	Oxybutynin	5mg	Blue	Tab	Round	N	N	Marion	Urin. Antispasmodic
1388	1388	Urinary Tract Combination	n/a	Blue	Tab	Round	–	Y	Vortech	Urinary Tract Agent
1390	0063 /1390	Hydralazine/Hydrochlorothiazide/Reserpine	25/15/0.1mg	Peach	Tab	Round	Y	N	Reid–Rowell	Antihypertensive
	1390	Sodium Levothyroxine	0.2mg	–	Tab	Round	–	–	Vortech	Hormone
1393	0665–1393	Reserpine,Hydralazine HCl,Hydrochlorothiazide	0.1/25/15mg	White	Tab	Round	Y	N	RR	Antihypertensive
1398	0115 1398	Tetracycline	100mg	Orange/Yellow	Cap	–	–	–	Richlyn	Anti–Infective
1400	0115/1400	Tetracycline HCl	250mg	Orange/Yellow	Cap	–	–	–	Richlyn	Anti–Infective
1401	SEARLE 1401	Oxandrolone	2.5mg	White	Tab	Oval	Y	N	Searle	Steroid
1402	0115/1402	Tetracycline HCl	500mg	Black/Yellow	Cap	–	–	–	Richlyn	Anti–Infective
1405	0115 1405	Tetracycline	250mg	Blue/Yellow	Cap	–	–	–	Richlyn	Anti–Infective
	0115/1405	Tetracycline HCl	250mg	Blue/Yellow	Cap	–	–	–	Richlyn	Anti–Infective
1451	Searle 1451	Misoprostol	100mcg	White	Tab	Round	Y	N	Searle	Anti–ulcer

ID NO.	ID CODE	GENERIC NAME	STRENGTH	COLOR	FORM	SHAPE	SCORED	COATED	MFG.	USE
1458	1458	Allylbutylbarbituric Acid with A.P.C.	50/200/130/40mg	–	Tab	Round	–	N	Vortech	Analgesic
1461	Searle 1461	Misoprostol	200mcg	White	Tab	Hexagonal	Y	N	Searle	Anti–ulcer
1463	1463	Conjugated Estrogens	0.625mg	–	Tab	Round	–	–	Vortech	Hormone
1501	SEARLE 1501	Methantheline Bromide	50mg	Peach	Tab	Round	Y	N	Searle	Antispasmodic
1507	R 1507	Quinine Sulfate	200mg	White	Tab	Round	–	N	Purepac	Muscle Relaxant
1511	R 1511	Quinine Sulfate	325mg	White	Tab	Round	–	N	Purepac	Muscle Relaxant
1530	0822/1530	Levothyroxine Sodium.	300mcg	Pink	Tab	Round	Y	N	Boots	Hormone
1531	0822/1531	Levothyroxine Sodium.	300mcg	Green	Tab	Round	Y	N	Boots	Hormone
	1531	Sulfasoxazole	500mg	–	Tab	Round	–	–	Vortech	Anti–Infective
1533	1533	Digoxin	0.25mg	–	Tab	Round	–	–	Vortech	Cardiac Agent
1535	AHR 1535	Calcium Polycarbophil	500mg	Yellow	Tab	Round	N	N	A.H.Robins	Stool Normalizer
1554	1554	Dextro–Amphetamine Sulfate	10mg	–	Tab	Round	–	–	Vortech	Anorectic
1555	Marion 1555	Papaverine HCl	150mg	Brown/Clear	Cap	–	–	–	Marion	Sm. Muscle Relaxant
1570	Ortho 1570	Metronidazole	250mg	White	Tab	Capsule	Y	N	Ortho	Anti–Infective
1571	Ortho 1571	Metronidazole	500mg	White	Tab	Capsule	Y	N	Ortho	Anti–Infective
1601	WALLACE 37 1601	Meprobamate	600mg	White	Tab	Capsule	–	N	Wallace	Antianxiety
1611	RR 1611	Vitamin/Mineral Comb.	n/a	Peach	Tab	Oval	N	Y	RR	Vitamin/Mineral Comb
	SOLVAY 1611	Vitamin/Mineral Comb.	n/a	Peach	Tab	Oval	N	Y	Solvay	Vitamin/Mineral Comb
1701	SEARLE 1701	Dimenhydrinate	50mg	White	Tab	Round	Y	N	Searle	Antiemetic
1705	1705	Diphenoxylate & Atropine	2.5mg/0.025mg	White	Tab	Round	–	–	Vortech	Antidiarrheal
1712	Marion/1712	Sucralfate	1Gm	Pink	Tab	Capsule	Y	N	Marion	Antiulcer
1739	1739	Butabarbital Sodium	30mg	–	Tab	Round	–	N	Vortech	Antianxiety
1757	1757	Phenobarbital	15mg	Pink	Tab	Round	–	–	Vortech	Sedative
1758	1758	Phenobarbital	15mg	White	Tab	Round	–	–	Vortech	Sedative
1759	1759	Phenobarbital	30mg	Pink	Tab	Round	–	–	Vortech	Sedative
1761	1761	Phenobarbital	30mg	White	Tab	Round	–	–	Vortech	Sedative
1771	Marion 1771	Diltiazem HCl	30mg	Green	Tab	Round	N	Y	Marion	Antianginal
1772	1772	Phenobarbital	16mg	White	Tab	Round	–	N	Vortech	Sedative
	Marion 1772	Diltiazem HCl	60mg	Yellow	Tab	Round	N	Y	Marion	Antianginal
1778	1778	Pb/Hyoscine/Atropine/Hyoscyamine	n/a	–	Tab	Round	–	–	Vortech	Antispasmodic
1779	1779	Colchicine	0.65mg	–	Tab	Round	–	–	Vortech	Antigout
1796	1796 180mg	Diltiazem HCl CD	180mg	Blue/Lt. Blue	Cap	–	–	–	Marion	Antihypertensive
1797	1797 240mg	Diltiazem HCl CD	240mg	Blue	Cap	–	–	–	Marion	Antihypertensive
1798	1798 300mg	Diltiazem HCl CD	300mg	Blue/Gray	Cap	–	–	–	Marion	Antihypertensive
1806	G 1806 / 0.5	Lorazepam	0.5mg	White	Tab	Round	N	N	Royce	Antianxiety
1807	G 1807 / 1	Lorazepam	1mg	White	Tab	Round	N	N	Royce	Antianxiety
1807	G 1808 / 2	Lorazepam	2mg	White	Tab	Round	N	N	Royce	Antianxiety
1812	1812	Benzthiazide	50mg	–	Tab	Round	–	–	Vortech	Diuretic
1820	Rugby 1820	Tetracycline HCl	250mg	Orange/Yellow	Cap	–	–	–	Rugby	Anti–Infective
1830	Rugby 1830	Tetracycline HCl	250mg	Black/Yellow	Cap	–	–	–	Rugby	Anti–Infective
1840	1840	Nitrofurantoin	50mg	–	Tab	Round	–	–	Vortech	Anti–Infective
1843	AHR 1843	Brompheniramine Maleate	12mg	–	Tab	Round	N	Y	A.H.Robins	Antihistamine
1857	AHR 1857	Brompheniramine Maleate	4mg	–	Tab	Round	Y	N	A.H.Robins	Antihistamine
1868	AHR 1868	Brompheniramine Maleate	8mg	–	Tab	Round	N	Y	A.H.Robins	Antihistamine
1870	Rugby 1870	Tetracycline HCl	500mg	Black/Yellow	Cap	–	–	–	Rugby	Anti–Infective
1875	CC 18.75	Phentermine HCl	18.75mg	Gray/Yellow	Cap	–	–	–	Camall	Anorectic
1876	1876	Phentermine	8mg	–	Tab	Round	–	–	Vortech	Anorectic
1879	1879	Phendimetrazine	35mg	Yellow	Tab	Round	–	–	Vortech	Anorectic
1886	1886	Propantheline Bromide	15mg	–	Tab	Round	–	–	Vortech	Antispasmodic
1908	1908	Orphenadrine Citrate	100mg	White	Tab	Round	–	N	Vortech	Muscle Relaxant
1915	1915	Hydrochlorothiazide	50mg	–	Tab	Round	–	–	Vortech	Diuretic
1922	1922	Brompheniramine/Phenyleph/Phenylpropanolamine	12/15/15mg	–	Tab	Round	–	N	Vortech	Decongestant Comb.
1934	Sav. Logo 1934	Chlorpheniramine Maleate/Pseudoephedrine HCl	8mg/120mg	Red/Clear	Cap	–	–	–	Savage	Decongestant Comb.
1945	1945	Trichlormethiazide	4mg	–	Tab	Round	–	–	Vortech	Diuretic
1975	1975	Triprolidine HCl & Pseudoephedrine	2.5mg/60mg	–	Tab	Round	–	N	Vortech	Decongestant Comb.
1998	1998	Methocarbamol	750mg	–	Tab	Oblong	–	N	Vortech	Muscle Relaxant
2000	PAN/2000	Pancrelipase EC	n/a	White	Cap	–	–	–	Jones	Digestive Enzyme
2001	WALLACE 37 2001	Carisoprodol	350mg	White	Tab	Round	–	N	Wallace	Muscle Relaxant
2002	2002 PP	Phenylpropanolamine & Caraminphen Edisylate	75mg/40mg	Clear	Cap	–	–	N	Pioneer	Antitussive Comb.
	Mylan 2002	Thiothixene	2mg	Caramel/Yellow	Cap	–	N	N	Mylan	Tranquilizer
2005	bp 2005	Disopyramide Phosphate	100mg	White/Orange	Cap	–	–	–	Bolar	Antiarrhythmic
2006	bp 2006	Disopyramide Phosphate	150mg	Orange/Brown	Cap	–	–	–	Bolar	Antiarrhythmic
2007	PP 2007	Papaverine HCl	150mg	Brown/Clear	Cap	–	–	–	Pioneer	Vasodilator
2013	2013	Chlorpheniramine Maleate	4mg	Yellow	Tab	Round	Y	N	Bolar	Antihistamine
2014	bp 2014	Methyldopa	125mg	White	Tab	Round	–	Y	Bolar	Antihypertensive
2015	bp 2015	Methyldopa	250mg	White	Tab	Round	–	Y	Bolar	Antihypertensive
2016	bp 2016	Methyldopa	500mg	White	Tab	Round	–	Y	Bolar	Antihypertensive
2020	2020	Caffeine	175mg	White/Specks	Tab	Oblong	Y	N	B & M Labs	Stimulant
	MYLAN 2020	Piroxicam	20mg	Green	Cap	–	–	–	Mylan	Anti–inflammatory
2023	bp 2023	Dicyclomine HCl	10mg	Blue/Blue	Cap	–	–	–	Bolar	Antispasmodic
2024	bp 2024	Meclofenamate Sodium	50mg	Maroon/Pink	Cap	–	–	–	Bolar	Anti–Inflammatory
2025	bp 2025	Meclofenamate Sodium	100mg	Maroon/White	Cap	–	–	–	Bolar	Anti–Inflammatory
2026	bp 2026	Dicyclomine HCl	20mg	Blue	Tab	Round	Y	N	Bolar	Antispasmodic
2027	bp 2027	Metoclopramide HCl	10mg	White	Tab	Round	–	N	Bolar	Antireflux
2035	2035	Chlordiazepoxide	10mg	–	Cap	–	–	–	Vortech	Antianxiety
2036	bp 2036	Methyldopa & Hydrochlorothiazide	250mg/15mg	Chartreuse	Tab	Round	N	Y	Bolar	Antihypertensive
2037	bp 2037	Methyldopa & Hydrochlorothiazide	250mg/25mg	Pink	Tab	Round	N	Y	Bolar	Antihypertensive
2038	bp 2038	Methyldopa & Hydrochlorothiazide	500mg/30mg	Chartreuse	Tab	Oval	N	Y	Bolar	Antihypertensive
2039	bp 2039	Methyldopa & Hydrochlorothiazide	500mg/50mg	Pink	Tab	Oval	N	Y	Bolar	Antihypertensive
2042	.625 Z/2042	Conjugated Estrogens	0.625mg	White	Tab	Round	–	Y	Zenith	Hormone
	bp 2042	Verapamil HCl	80mg	White	Tab	Round	–	Y	Bolar	Antihypertensive
2043	bp 2043	Verapamil HCl	120mg	White	Tab	Round	–	Y	Bolar	Antihypertensive
2045	1.25 Z/2045	Conjugated Estrogens	1.25mg	White	Tab	Round	–	Y	Zenith	Hormone
2047	bp 2047	Hydrochlorothiazide & Reserpine	25mg/0.125mg	Green	Tab	Round	N	N	Bolar	Antihypertensive
	Z 2047	Colchicine	0.6mg	White	Tab	Round	–	N	Zenith	Antigout
2048	bp 2048	Hydrochlorothiazide & Reserpine	50mg/0.125mg	Green	Tab	Round	N	N	Bolar	Antihypertensive
2049	bp 2049	Hydrochlorothiazide, Reserpine, Hydralazine	15/0.1/25mg	White	Tab	Round	N	N	Bolar	Antihypertensive
2053	bp 2053	Perphenazine & Amitriptyline	2mg/25mg	Orange	Tab	Round	N	Y	Bolar	Antidepressant
2054	bp 2054	Perphenazine & Amitriptyline	4mg/25mg	Yellow	Tab	Round	N	Y	Bolar	Antidepressant
2055	bp 2055	Perphenazine & Amitriptyline	4mg/50mg	Orange	Tab	Round	N	Y	Bolar	Antidepressant
	Z 2055	Diphenhydramine HCl	25mg	Pink/Clear	Cap	–	–	–	Zenith	Antihistamine
2056	bp 2056	Perphenazine & Amitriptyline	2mg/10mg	Blue	Tab	Round	N	Y	Bolar	Antidepressant
	Z 2056	Diphenhydramine HCl	50mg	Pink/pink	Cap	–	–	–	Zenith	Antihistamine
2057	bp 2057	Perphenazine & Amitriptyline	4mg/10mg	Salmon	Tab	Round	N	Y	Bolar	Antidepressant
	Z 2057	Phenytoin Sodium Prompt	100mg	Natural/Natural	Cap	–	–	–	Zenith	Anticonvulsant

ID NO.	ID CODE	GENERIC NAME	STRENGTH	COLOR	FORM	SHAPE	SCORED	COATED	MFG.	USE
2058	Z 2058	Digoxin	0.25mg	White	Tab	Round	–	N	Zenith	Cardiac Glycoside
2060	bp 2060	Propranolol HCl	60mg	Pink	Tab	Round	–	N	Bolar	Antihypertensive
2062	bp 2062	Tolbutamide	250mg	White	Tab	Round	–	N	Bolar	Hypoglycemic
2063	bp 2063	Tolbutamide	500mg	White	Tab	Round	–	N	Bolar	Hypoglycemic
2064	bp 2064	Pentaerythritol Tetranitrate	10mg	Green	Tab	Round	–	N	Bolar	Antianginal
2066	bp 2066	Lithium Carbonate	300mg	White/Pink	Cap	–	–	–	Bolar	Tranquilier
2067	bp 2067	Pentaerythritol Tetranitrate	20mg	Green	Tab	Round	–	N	Bolar	Antianginal
2068	bp 2068	Tolazamide	100mg	White	Tab	Round	–	N	Bolar	Hypoglycemic
2069	bp 2069	Tolazamide	250mg	White	Tab	Round	–	N	Bolar	Hypoglycemic
2070	bp 2070	Tolazamide	500mg	White	Tab	Round	–	N	Bolar	Hypoglycemic
2074	bp 2074	Probenecid & Colchicine	0.5GM/0.5mg	White	Tab	Capsule	–	N	Bolar	Antigout
2075	bp 2075	Nitrofurantoin	50mg	Yellow	Tab	Round	–	N	Bolar	Anti–Infective
2076	bp 2076	Procainamide HCl	250mg	Yellow/Yellow	Cap	–	–	–	Bolar	Antiarrhythmic
2078	bp 2078	Procainamide HCl	500mg	Yellow/Orange	Cap	–	–	–	Bolar	Antiarrhythmic
2080	bp 2080	Nitrofurantoin	100mg	Yellow	Tab	Round	–	N	Bolar	Anti–Infective
2081	bp 2081	Flurazepam HCl	15mg	White/Green	Cap	–	–	–	Bolar	Hypnotic
2082	bp 2082	Flurazepam HCl	30mg	White/Green	Cap	–	–	–	Bolar	Hypnotic
2083	Z 2083	Hydrochlorothiazide	25mg	Orange	Tab	Round	–	N	Zenith	Diuretic
2085	bp 2085	Propoxyphene Napsylate & Acetaminophen	50mg/325mg	Pink	Tab	Capsule	N	Y	Bolar	Analgesic
2086	bp 2086	Propoxyphene Napsylate & Acetaminophen	100mg/650mg	Pink	Tab	Capsule	N	Y	Bolar	Analgesic
2087	bp 2087	Temazepam	15mg	Pink/Pink	Cap	–	–	–	Bolar	Hypnotic
2088	bp 2088	Temazepam	30mg	Yellow/Pink	Cap	–	–	–	Bolar	Hypnotic
2089	Z 2089	Hydrochlorothiazide	50mg	Orange	Tab	Round	–	N	Zenith	Diuretic
2092	bp 2092	Trichlormethiazide & Reserpine	4mg/0.1mg	Lavender	Tab	Round	–	N	Bolar	Antihypertensive
2093	bp 2093	Hydrochlorothiazide	25mg	Orange	Tab	Round	–	N	Bolar	Diuretic
2094	bp 2094	Hydrochlorothiazide	50mg	Orange	Tab	Round	–	N	Bolar	Diuretic
2095	2095	Dioctyl Sodium Sulfosuccinate	100mg	–	Cap	–	–	–	Vortech	Laxative
2100	MYLAN 2100	Loperamide Hydrochloride	2mg	Brown/Brown	Cap	–	–	–	Mylan	Antidiarrheal
2103	WALLACE 2103	Carisoprodol & Aspirin	200mg/325mg	Peach	Tab	Round	–	N	Wallace	Muscle Relaxant
2118	bp 2118	Disopyramide Phosphate CR	100mg	Yellow/Purple	Cap	–	–	–	Bolar	Antiarrhythmic
2119	bp 2119	Disopyramide Phosphate CR	150mg	Orange/Purple	Cap	–	–	–	Bolar	Antiarrhythmic
2126	bp 2126	Potassium Chloride	750mg	White/White	Cap	–	–	–	Bolar	Potassium Supp.
2130	Zenith 2130	Nitrofurantoin Macrocrystals	50mg	Pink/White	Cap	–	–	–	Zenith	Anti–Infective
2131	Zenith 2131	Nitrofurantoin Macrocrystals	100mg	Pink/Pink	Cap	–	–	–	Zenith	Anti–Infective
2137	SCHEIN 2137/800	Ibuprofen	800mg	White	Tab	Capsule	N	Y	Schein	Anti–Inflammatory
2150	0115 2150	Aminophylline	100mg	White	Tab	Round	N	N	Richlyn	Bronchodilator
	bp 2150	Isoniazid	100mg	White	Tab	Round	N	N	Bolar	Anti–Infective
	Mylan 2150	Meclofenamate Sodium	50mg	Coral/Coral	Cap	–	–	–	Mylan	Anti–Inflammatory
2151	0115 2151	Aminophylline	100mg	Beige	Tab	Round	N	N	Richlyn	Bronchodilator
2155	bp 2155	Isoniazid	300mg	White	Tab	Round	Y	N	Bolar	Anti–Infective
2158	0115 2158	Aminophylline	200mg	White	Tab	Round	N	N	Richlyn	Bronchodilator
2160	2.5 Z/2160	Conjugated Estrogens	2.5mg	White	Tab	Round	N	Y	Zenith	Hormone
2162	0115 2162	Aminophylline	200mg	White	Tab	Round	N	Y	Richlyn	Bronchodilator
2168	Z 2168	Hydrochlorothiazide/Reserpine (Hydroserpine #2)	50mg/0.125mg	Green	Tab	Round	–	N	Zenith	Antihypertensive
2169	Z 2169	Hydrochlorothiazide/Reserpine (Hydroserpine #1)	25mg/0.125mg	Green	Tab	Round	–	N	Zenith	Antihypertensive
2183	W 2183	Atro,Hyoscy,Methenamine,M.Blue,Phenyl Sali,Benz. A	–	Purple	Tab	Round	N	Y	Webcon	Urinary Antiseptic
2184	Z 2184	Quinine Sulfate	325mg	Natural/Natural	Cap	–	–	–	Zenith	Muscle Relaxant
2186	Z 2186	Propoxyphene HCl	65mg	Pink/Pink	Cap	–	–	–	Zenith	Analgesic
2190	Z 2190	Probenecid	500mg	Yellow	Tab	Capsule	Y	Y	Zenith	Antigout
2193	Z 2193	Probenecid & Colchicine	500mg/0.5mg	White	Tab	Capsule	Y	N	Zenith	Antigout
2200	CENTRAL 2200	Vitamin/Mineral Supp.	–	Brown	Tab	Round	N	Y	Central	Vitamin Supp.
2201	Z 2201	Quinidine Sulfate	200mg	White	Tab	Round	–	N	Zenith	Antiarrhythmic
2218	Z 2218	Sulfisoxazole	500mg	White	Tab	round	–	N	Zenith	Anti–Infective
2225	W 2225	Hyoscyamine	0.15mg	Blue	Tab	Round	–	N	Webcon	Antispasmodic
2245	Z 2245	Tolbutamide	500mg	White	Tab	round	–	N	Zenith	Hypoglycemic
2260	W 2260	Hyoscyamine	0.375mg	Blue	Cap	–	–	–	Webcon	Antispasmodic
2302	MYLAN 2302	Prazosin HCl	2mg	Brown/Brown	Cap	–	–	–	Mylan	Antihypertensive
2335	Z 2335	HCTZ/Hydralazine/Reserpine (Hydroserpine Plus)	15mg/25mg/0.1mg	White	Tab	Round	–	N	Zenith	Antihypertensive
2338	Z 2338	Hydralazine HCl	10mg	Orange	Tab	Round	–	N	Zenith	Antihypertensive
2339	Z 2339	Hydralazine HCl	25mg	Orange	Tab	Round	–	N	Zenith	Antihypertensive
2345	Z Z–2345	Procainamide HCl	250mg	Yellow/Yellow	Cap	–	–	–	Zenith	Antiarrhythmic
2346	Z–2346	Procainamide HCl	375mg	Orange/White	Cap	–	–	–	Zenith	Antiarrhythmic
2347	Z 2347	Procainamide HCl	500mg	Orange/Yellow	Cap	–	–	–	Zenith	Antiarrhythemic
2348	Z 2348	Nylidrin HCl	6mg	White	Tab	Round	Y	N	Zenith	Vasodilator
2349	Z 2349	Nylidrin HCl	12mg	White	Tab	Round	Y	N	Zenith	Vasodilator
2350	Z 2350	Meclizine HCl	25mg	Yellow/White	Tab	Oval	–	N	Zenith	Antivertigo
2359	Z 2359	Quinine Sulfate	200mg	Natural/Natural	Cap	–	–	–	Zenith	Muscle relaxant
2384	2384	Hematinic Combination	n/a	–	Cap	–	–	–	Vortech	Hematinic
	Z 2384	Meclizine HCl	12.5mg	Blue/White	Tab	Oval	–	N	Zenith	Antivertigo
2387	Z 2387	Isoxsuprine HCl	10mg	White	Tab	Round	–	N	Zenith	Vasodilator
2388	Z 2388	Isoxsuprine HCl	20mg	White	Tab	Round	–	N	Zenith	Vasodilator
2390	0115 2390	Sulfasoxazole & Phenazopyridine HCl	500mg/50mg	Maroon	Tab	Round	N	Y	Richlyn	Anti–Infective
2400	0115 2400	Phenobarbital & Belladonna	16.2mg/10.8mg	Green	Tab	Round	N	N	Richlyn	Antispasmodic
2403	WALLACE 2403	Carisoprodol & Aspirin & Codeine Phosphate	200/325/16mg	Yellow/White	Tab	Oval	–	N	Wallace	Analgesic
2407	Z 2407	Tetracycline HCL	500mg	Black/Yellow	Cap	–	–	–	Zenith	Antihypertensive
2416	Z 2416	Tetracycline HCL	250mg	Orange/Yellow	Cap	–	–	–	Zenith	Anti–Infective
2428	2428	Diphenylhydantoin Sodium	100mg	–	Cap	–	–	–	Vortech	Anticonvulsant
2430	Z 2430	Tetracycline HCL	250mg	Purple/Yellow	Cap	–	–	–	Zenith	Anti–Infective
2458	Z 2458	Erythromycin Stearate	250mg	Pink	Tab	Round	–	Y	Zenith	Anti–Infective
2472	2472	Diphenhydramine HCl	25mg	–	Cap	–	–	–	Vortech	Antihistamine
2473	2473	Diphenhydramine HCl	50mg	–	Cap	–	–	–	Vortech	Antihistamine
2485	Z 2485	Hydrochlorothiazide	100mg	Orange	Tab	Roung	Y	N	Zenith	Diuretic
2493	Z 2493	Hydralazine HCl	50mg	Orange	Tab	Round	–	N	Zenith	Antihypertensive
2507	Z 2507	Reserpine & Hydroflumethiazide	0.125mg/50mg	Green	Tab	Round	–	N	Zenith	Antihypertensive
2525	2525	Butalbital/Aspirin/Phenacetin/Caffeine	50/200/130/40mg	–	Cap	–	–	–	Vortech	Analgesic
2715	2715	Nitroglycerine SA	6.5mg	–	Cap	–	–	–	Vortech	Antianginal
2718	2718	Nitroglycerine SA	2.5mg	–	Cap	–	–	–	Vortech	Antianginal
2758	0115 2758	Chlordiazepoxide HCl	5mg	Green/Yellow	Cap	–	–	–	Richlyn	Antianxiety
2760	0115 2760	Chlordiazepoxide HCl	10mg	Green/Black	Cap	–	–	–	Richlyn	Antianxiety
2762	0115 2762	Chlordiazepoxide HCl	25mg	Green/White	Cap	–	–	–	Richlyn	Antianxiety
2768	2768	Tetracycline HCl	250mg	–	Cap	–	–	–	Vortech	Anti–Infective
2790	0115 2790	Chloroquin Phosphate	250mg	White	Tab	Round	Y	N	Richlyn	Antimalarial
2808	SOLVAY 2808	Prednisone	1mg	Pink	Tab	Round	Y	N	Solvay	Steroid
2810	0115 2810	Chlorpheniramine Maleate	4mg	Yellow	Tab	Round	Y	N	Richlyn	Antihistamine
	SOLVAY 2810	Prednisone	5mg	White	Tab	Round	Y	N	Solvay	Steroid

ID NO.	ID CODE	GENERIC NAME	STRENGTH	COLOR	FORM	SHAPE	SCORED	COATED	MFG.	USE
2811	DUNHALL 2811	Acetaminophen & Butalbital	325mg/50mg	Orange/White	Cap	–	–	–	Dunhall	Analgesic
2812	SOLVAY 2812	Prednisone	10mg	Blue	Tab	Round	Y	N	Solvay	Steroid
2813	Z 2813	Methocarbamol & Aspirin	400mg/325mg	Pink/White	Tab	Round	–	N	Zenith	Muscle Relaxant
2814	SOLVAY 2814	Prednisone	20mg	Yellow	Tab	Round	Y	N	Solvay	Steroid
	Z 2814	Cyclandelate	200mg	Orange/Orange	Cap	–	–	–	Zenith	Vasodilator
2815	Z 2815	Cyclandelate	400mg	Green/White	Cap	–	–	–	Zenith	Vasodilator
2816	SOLVAY 2816	Prednisone	50mg	White	Tab	Round	Y	N	Solvay	Steroid
2823	Z 2823	Erythromycin Stearate	500mg	Pink	Tab	Oval	–	Y	Zenith	Anti–Infective
2829	DUNHALL 2829	Combination	n/a	Red/Yellow	Cap	–	–	–	Dunhall	Decongestant Comb.
2835	USV 2835	Nicotinic Acid Time Release	125mg	Black/Clear	Cap	–	–	–	Rorer	Vitamin
2840	USV 2840	Nicotinic Acid Time Release	250mg	Green/Clear	Cap	–	–	–	Rorer	Vitamin
2841	USV 2841	Nicotinic Acid Time Release	500mg	Blue/White	Cap	–	–	–	Rorer	Vitamin
2867	2867	Tetracycline HCI	500mg	–	Cap	–	–	–	Vortech	Anti–Infective
2869	2869	Propoxyphene HCI	65mg	–	Cap	–	–	–	Vortech	Analgesic
2874	2874	Dicyclomine HCI	10mg	–	Cap	–	–	–	Vortech	Antispasmodic
2902	SYNTEX 2902	Oxymetholone	50mg	White	Tab	Round	Y	N	Syntex	Steroid
	Z 2902	Chlorpropamide	250mg	Blue	Tab	Round	–	N	Zenith	Hypoglycemic
2903	Z 2903	Spironolactone	25mg	White	Tab	Round	–	N	Zenith	Diuretic
2904	Z 2904	Chlorthalidone	100mg	White	Tab	Round	–	N	Zenith	Diuretic
2907	Z 2907	Furosemide	40mg	White	Tab	Round	–	N	Zenith	Diuretic
2908	Z 2908	Furosemide	20mg	White	Tab	Oval	–	N	Zenith	Diuretic
2909	Z 2909	Hydroxyzine Pamoate	50mg	Green/White	Cap	–	–	–	Zenith	Antihistamine
2911	Z 2911	Hydroxyzine Pamoate	25mg	Green/Green	Cap	–	–	–	Zenith	Antihistamine
2916	Z–1 2916	Trifluoperazine HCL	1mg	Lavender	Tab	Round	–	Y	Zenith	Tranquilizer
2920	0115 2920	Cortisone Acetate	25mg	White	Tab	Round	Y	N	Richlyn	Steroid
2929	Z 2929	Cyproheptadine	4mg	White	Tab	Round	–	N	Zenith	Antipruritic
2931	Z 2931	Methyldopa	250mg	White	Tab	Round	–	Y	Zenith	Antihypertensive
2932	Z 2932	Methyldopa	500mg	White	Tab	Round	–	Y	Zenith	Antihypertensive
2936	Z 2936	Perphenazine & Amitriptyline HCL	2mg/10mg	Blue	Tab	Round	–	Y	Zenith	Antidepressant
2937	Z 2937	Perphenazine & Amitriptyline HCL	2mg/25mg	Orange	Tab	Round	–	Y	Zenith	Antidepressant
2938	Z 2938	Perphenazine & Amitriptyline HCL	4mg/10mg	Salmon	Tab	Round	–	Y	Zenith	Antidepressant
2939	Z 2939	Perphenazine & Amitriptyline HCL	4mg/25mg	Yellow	Tab	Round	–	Y	Zenith	Antidepressant
2940	Z–2 2940	Trifluoperazine HCL	2mg	Lavender	Tab	Round	–	Y	Zenith	Tranquilizer
2941	Z–5 2941	Trifluoperazine HCL	5mg	Lavender	Tab	Round	–	Y	Zenith	Tranquilizer
2942	Z 2942	Trifluoperazine HCL	10mg	Lavender	Tab	Round	–	Y	Zenith	Tranquilizer
2958	Z 2958	Ergoloid Mesylates sublingual	0.5mg	White	Tab	Round	–	N	Zenith	Vasodilator
2959	Z 2959	Ergoloid Mesylates sublingual	1mg	White	Tab	Oval	–	N	Zenith	Vasodilator
2960	Z 2960	Chloramphenicol	250mg	White/White	Cap	–	–	–	Zenith	Anti–Infective
2962	Z 2962	Ephedrine, Theophylline, Hydroxyzine HCI	25/130/10mg	White	Tab	Round	–	N	Zenith	Bronchodilator
2963	Z 2963	Nitroglycerin TD	2.5mg	Amethyst/Natural	Cap	–	–	–	Zenith	Antianginal
2964	Z 2964	Nitroglycerin TD	6.5mg	Blue/Yellow	Cap	–	–	–	Zenith	Antianginal
2969	Z 2969	Sulfinpyrazone	200mg	Orange/Orange	Cap	–	–	–	Zenith	Antigout
2970	Z 2970	Sulfinpyrazone	100mg	White	Tab	Round	–	–	Zenith	Antigout
2971	Z 2971	Metronidazole	250mg	White	Tab	Round	–	N	Zenith	Anti–Infective
2974	Z 2974	Chlorthalidone	25mg	Yellow	Tab	Round	–	N	Zenith	Diuretic
2975	2975	Propoxyphene HCI,Aspirin,Phenacetin,Caffeine	65/227/162/32mg	–	Cap	–	–	–	Vortech	Analgesic
2976	Z 2976	Dipyridamole	50mg	White	Tab	Round	–	Y	Zenith	Antiplatelet
2977	Z 2977	Dipyridamole	75mg	White	Tab	Round	–	Y	Zenith	Antiplatelet
2978	Z–2978	Tolazamide	100mg	White	Tab	Round	Y	N	Zenith	Hypoglycemic
2979	Z–2979	Tolazamide	250mg	White	Tab	Round	Y	N	Zenith	Hypoglycemic
2980	Z–2980	Tolazamide	500mg	White	Tab	Round	Y	N	Zenith	Hypoglycemic
2982	Z 2982	Chlordiazepoxide and Clindinium	5mg/2.5mg	White/White	Cap	–	–	–	Zenith	Antispasmodic
2984	Z 2984	Doxycycline Hyclate	50mg	Blue/White	Cap	–	–	–	Zenith	Anti–Infective
2985	Z 2985	Doxycycline Hyclate	100mg	Blue/Blue	Cap	–	–	–	Zenith	Anti–Infective
2986	Z 2986	Methyclothiazide	2.5mg	Orange	Tab	Round	Y	N	Zenith	Diuretic
2987	Z 2987	Methyclothiazide	5mg	Salmon	Tab	Round	–	N	Zenith	Diuretic
2994	Z 2994	Dipyridamole	25mg	White	Tab	Round	–	Y	Zenith	Antiplatelet
2999	Z 2999	Chlorthalidone	50mg	Green	Tab	Round	–	N	Zenith	Diuretic
3000	3000	Quinidine Gluconate	324mg	–	Tab	Round	–	–	Roxane	Antiarrhythmic
	bp 3000	Quinidine Gluconate SR	324mg	White	Tab	Round	N	N	Bolar	Antiarrhythmic
	Mylan 3000	Meclofenamate Sodium	100mg	Coral/White	Cap	–	–	–	Mylan	Anti–Inflammatory
3001	PP 3001	Phenylprop.,phenyleph.,phenyltolox.,chlorphenir.	40,10,15,5mg	White w red specks	Tab	Round	N	N	Pioneer	Decongestant comb.
	WALLACE 3001	Meprobamate & Benactyzine HCI	400mg/1mg	Pink	Tab	Round	Y	N	Wallace	Antidepressant
	Z 3001	Quinine Sulfate	260mg	White	Tab	Round	–	–	Zenith	Muscle Relaxant
3005	Mylan 3005	Thiothixene	5mg	Caramel/White	Cap	–	N	N	Mylan	Tranquilizer
3007	Rugby logo 3007	Acetazolamide	250mg	–	Tab	Round	Y	N	Rugby	Antiglaucoma
	Z 3007	Metronidazole	500mg	White	Tab	Oblong	–	N	Zenith	Anti–Infective
3008	PP 3008	Brompheniramine,Phenylephrine,Phenylpropanolamine	12mg/15mg/15mg	Blue	Tab	Round	N	Y	Pioneer	Decongestant Comb.
	Rugby 3018	Triprolidine HCI & Pseudoephedrine HCI	2.5mg/60mg	–	Tab	–	–	–	Rugby	Decongestant Comb.
3020	bp 3020	Trichlormethiazide	4mg	Blue	Tab	Round	–	N	Bolar	Diuretic
3021	Rugby Logo 3021	Triprolidine HCI & Pseudoephedrine HCI	2.5mg/60mg	White	Tab	Round	Y	N	Rugby	Decongestant Comb.
3027	Rugby 100/3027	Allopurinol	100mg	White	Tab	Round	Y	N	Rugby	Antigout
3028	Rugby 300/3028	Allopurinol	300mg	Peach	Tab	Round	Y	N	Rugby	Antigout
3030	0115 3030	Dehydrocholic Acid	250mg	White	Tab	Round	N	N	Richlyn	Digestant
	Bristol 3030/10mg	Lomustine	10mg	White	Cap	–	–	–	BM	Antineoplastic
3031	Bristol 3031/40mg	Lomustine	40mg	White/Green	Cap	–	–	–	BM	Antineoplastic
3032	Bristol 3032/100mg	Lomustine	100mg	Green/Green	Cap	–	–	–	BM	Antineoplastic
3044	Rugby 3044	Amiloride/Hydrochlorothiazide	5mg/50mg	–	Tab	–	–	–	Rugby	Antihypertensive
3046	Rugby 3046	Aminophylline	100mg	–	Tab	–	–	–	Rugby	Bronchodilator
3060	Rugby 3060	Aminophylline	200mg	–	Tab	–	–	–	Rugby	Bronchodilator
3061	3061	Cefaclor	250mg	Purple/White	Cap	–	–	–	Lilly	Anti–Infective
3062	3062	Cefaclor	500mg	Purple/Gray	Cap	–	–	–	Lilly	Anti–Infective
3071	Rugby 3071	Amitriptyline	10mg	–	Tab	–	–	–	Rugby	Antidepressant
3072	Rugby 3072	Amitriptyline	25mg	–	Tab	–	–	–	Rugby	Antidepressant
3073	Rugby 3073	Amitriptyline	50mg	–	Tab	–	–	–	Rugby	Antidepressant
3074	Rugby 3074	Amitriptyline	75mg	–	Tab	–	–	–	Rugby	Antidepressant
3075	Rugby 3075	Amitriptyline	100mg	–	Tab	–	–	–	Rugby	Antidepressant
3076	Rugby 3076	Amitriptyline	150mg	–	Tab	–	–	–	Rugby	Antidepressant
3077	Rugby 3077	Amitriptyline HCI & Perphenazine	10mg/2mg	–	Tab	–	–	–	Rugby	Antidepressant
3078	Rugby 3078	Amitriptyline HCI & Perphenazine	10mg/4mg	–	Tab	–	–	–	Rugby	Antidepressant
3082	Rugby 3082	Amitriptyline HCI & Perphenazine	25mg/2mg	–	Tab	–	–	–	Rugby	Antidepressant
3083	Rugby 3083	Amitriptyline HCI & Perphenazine	25mg/4mg	–	Tab	–	–	–	Rugby	Antidepressant
3084	Rugby 3084	Amitriptyline HCI & Perphenazine	50mg/4mg	–	Tab	–	–	–	Rugby	Antidepressant
3089	252/3089	Phenobarbital	100mg	White	Tab	Round	N	N	Jones	Sedative
3091	Bristol 3091	Etoposide	50mg	Pink	Cap	–	–	–	BM	Antineoplastic

ID NO.	ID CODE	GENERIC NAME	STRENGTH	COLOR	FORM	SHAPE	SCORED	COATED	MFG.	USE
3100	0115 3100	Dexamethasone	0.75mg	Blue	Tab	Pentagonal	Y	N	Richlyn	Steroid
	3100	Phentermine	30mg	Yellow	Cap	–	–	–	Vortech	Anorectic
3113	3113	Codeine Phosphate, Aspirin, Caffeine	30/380/30mg	White/Gray	Cap	–	–	–	Lilly	Analgesic
3115	3115	Phentermine	30mg	Black	Cap	–	–	–	Vortech	Anorectic
3125	3125	Vancomycin HCl	125mg	Blue/Brown	Cap	–	–	–	Lilly	Anti–Infective
	Mylan 3125	Doxepin HCl	25mg	Ivory/White	Cap	–	–	–	Mylan	Antidepressant
3126	3126	Vancomycin HCl	250mg	Blue/Gray	Cap	–	–	–	Lilly	Anti–Infective
3136	West–ward 3136	Diphenhydramine HCl	25mg	Pink/Clear	Cap	–	–	–	West–ward	Antihistamine
3141	West–ward 3141	Doxycycline Hyclate	50mg	Blue/White	Cap	–	–	–	West–ward	Anti–Infective
3142	West–ward 3142	Doxycycline Hyclate	100mg	Blue/Blue	Cap	–	–	–	West–ward	Anti–Infective
3145	West–ward 3145	Ephedrine Sulfate	25mg	Pink	Cap	–	–	–	West–ward	Antiasthmatic
3148	C 3148	Clofibrate	500mg	Yellow	Cap	–	–	–	Chase	Antilipidemic
3200	0115 3200	Dicyclomine HCl	10mg	Blue	Cap	–	–	–	Richlyn	Antispasmodic
3205	MYLAN 3205	Prazosin HCl	5mg	Blue/Brown	Cap		–	–	Mylan	Antihypertensive
	RR 3205	Dexamethasone	0.5mg	Yellow	Tab	Round	Y	N	RR	Steroid
	SOLVAY 3205	Dexamethasone	0.5mg	Yellow	Tab	Round	Y	N	Solvay	Steroid
3210	0115 3210	Dicyclomine HCl & Phenobarbital	10mg/15mg	Blue/Clear	Cap	–	–	–	Richlyn	Antispasmodic
	RR 3210	Dexamethasone	0.75mg	Green	Tab	Round	Y	N	RR	Steroid
	SOLVAY 3210	Dexamethasone	0.75mg	Green	Tab	Round	Y	N	Solvay	Steroid
3215	RR 3215	Dexamethasone	1.5mg	Pink	Tab	Round	Y	N	RR	Steroid
	Rugby 4/3215	Acetaminophen & Codeine	300mg/60mg	–	Tab	Round	–	–	Rugby	Analgesic
	SOLVAY 3215	Dexamethasone	1.5mg	Pink	Tab	Round	Y	N	Solvay	Steroid
3220	0115 3220	Dicyclomine HCl	20mg	Blue	Tab	–	N	N	Richlyn	Antispasmodic
	RR 3220	Dexamethasone	4mg	White	Tab	Round	Y	N	RR	Steroid
	SOLVAY 3220	Dexamethasone	4mg	White	Tab	Round	Y	N	Solvay	Steroid
3222	Rugby Logo 3222	Acetaminophen	325mg	–	Tab	–	–	–	Rugby	Analgesic
3225	0115 3225	Dicyclomine HCl & Phenobarbital	20mg/15mg	White	Tab	–	N	N	Richlyn	Antispasmodic
3227	C–3227	Nifedipine	10mg	White	Cap	–	–	–	Chase	Antihypertensive
	Rugby 3/3227	Acetaminophen & Codeine	300mg/30mg	–	Tab	Round	–	–	Rugby	Analgesic
3228	Rugby 2/3228	Acetaminophen & Codeine	300mg/15mg	–	Tab	Round	–	–	Rugby	Analgesic
3231	Rugby Logo 3231	Acetaminophen	500mg	–	Tab	–	–	–	Rugby	Analgesic
3250	0115 3250	Pepsin, Pancreatin, Dehydrocholic Acid	250mg/300mg/150	White	Tab	Round	N	Y	Richlyn	Digestant
3279	Rugby 3279	Hydralazine & Hydrochlorothiazide	25mg/15mg	–	Tab	–	–	–	Rugby	Antihypertensive
3329	Rugby 3329	Aspirin & Codeine	325mg/60mg	–	Tab	–	–	–	Rugby	Analgesic
3360	Rugby 3360	Belladonna & Phenobarbital	–	–	Tab	–	–	–	Rugby	Antispasmodic
3364	Rugby 3364	Bethanechol Chloride	5mg	–	Tab	–	–	–	Rugby	Urinary Tract Agent
3365	Rugby 3365	Bethanechol Chloride	10mg	–	Tab	–	–	–	Rugby	Urinary Tract Agent
3367	Rugby 3367	Dicyclomine HCl	10mg	–	Cap	–	–	–	Rugby	Antispasmodic
3369	Rugby 3369	Bethanechol Chloride	25mg	–	Tab	–	–	–	Rugby	Urinary Tract Agent
3370	Rugby 3370	Benztropine Mesylates	0.5mg	White	Tab	–	–	–	Rugby	Antiparkinson
3371	Rugby 3371	Benztropine Mesylates	1mg	White	Tab	–	–	–	Rugby	Antiparkinson
3372	Rugby 3372	Benztropine Mesylates	2mg	White	Tab	–	–	–	Rugby	Antiparkinson
3377	Rugby 3377	Dicyclomine HCl	20mg	–	Tab	–	–	–	Rugby	Antispasmodic
3399	3399	Chlorpheniramine/Phenylpropanolamine HCl	12mg/75mg	–	Cap	–	–	–	Vortech	Decongestant Comb.
3406	Rugby 3406	Clorazepate Dipotassium	3.75mg	–	Cap	–	–	–	Rugby	Antianxiety
3407	Rugby 3407	Clorazepate Dipotassium	7.5mg	–	Cap	–	–	–	Rugby	Antianxiety
3408	Rugby 3408	Clorazepate Dipotassium	15mg	–	Cap	–	–	–	Rugby	Antianxiety
3415	Rugby 3415	Carbamazepine	200mg	–	Tab	–	–	–	PBI	Anticonvulsant
	Rugby 3415	Carbamazepine	200mg	–	Tab	–	–	–	Rugby	Anticonvulsant
3420	Rugby 3420	Pseudoephedrine HCl/Chlorpheniramine	120mg/8mg	–	Cap	–	–	–	Rugby	Decongestant
3435	Rugby 3435	Carisoprodol	350mg	–	Tab	–	–	–	Rugby	Muscle Relaxant
3444	Rugby 3444	Chlorzoxazone	500mg	–	Tab	–	–	–	Rugby	Muscle Relaxant
3450	Rugby 3450	Chlorzoxazone & Acetaminophen	250mg/300mg	–	Tab	–	–	–	Rugby	Muscle Relaxant
3453	C–3453	Nifedipine	20mg	White	Cap	–	–	–	Chase	Antihypertensive
3454	Rugby 3454	Chlorpromazine	10mg	–	Tab	–	–	–	Rugby	Tranquilizer
3455	Rugby 3455	Chlorpromazine	25mg	–	Tab	–	–	–	Rugby	Tranquilizer
3456	Rugby 3456	Chlorpromazine	50mg	–	Tab	–	–	–	Rugby	Tranquilizer
3457	Rugby 3457	Chlorpromazine	100mg	–	Tab	–	–	–	Rugby	Tranquilizer
3458	Rugby 3458	Chlorpromazine	200mg	–	Tab	–	–	–	Rugby	Tranquilizer
3460	Rugby 3460	Chlorothiazide	250mg	White	Tab	Round	Y	N	Rugby	Diuretic
3461	Rugby 3461	Chlorothiazide	500mg	White	Tab	Round	Y	N	Rugby	Diuretic
3462	Rugby 3462	Chlorpropamide	100mg	Blue	Tab	Round	Y	N	Rugby	Hypoglycemic
3465	Rugby 3465	Chlorpropamide	250mg	Blue	Tab	Round	Y	N	Rugby	Hypoglycemic
3466	Rugby 3466	Clofibrate	500mg	–	Cap	–	–	–	Rugby	Hypolipidemic
3468	Rugby 3468	Chlorthalidone	50mg	–	Tab	–	–	–	Rugby	Diuretic
3469	Rugby 3469	Chlorthalidone	100mg	–	Tab	–	–	–	Rugby	Diuretic
3473	Rugby 3473	Chloral Hydrate	500mg	Red	Cap	–	–	–	Rugby	Hypnotic
3477	Rugby 3477	Chloral Hydrate	500mg	Green	Cap	–	–	–	Rugby	Hypnotic
3485	Rugby 3485	Chlorthalidone	25mg	–	Tab	–	–	–	Rugby	Diuretic
3487	R 3487	Chlordiazepoxide HCl	5mg	Green/Yellow	Cap	–	–	–	Rugby	Antianxiety
3488	R 3488	Chlordiazepoxide HCl	10mg	Green/Black	Cap	–	–	–	Rugby	Antianxiety
3489	R 3489	Chlordiazepoxide HCl	25mg	Green/White	Cap	–	–	–	Rugby	Antianxiety
3490	Rugby 3490	Chlordiazepoxide & Clidinium Bromide	5mg/2.5mg	–	Cap	–	–	–	Rugby	Antispasmodic
3494	Rugby 3494	Colchicine	0.6mg.	White	Tab	Round	N	N	West–ward	Antigout
3496	Rugby Logo 3496	Conjugated Estrogens	0.3mg	–	Tab	–	–	–	Rugby	Hormone
3497	Rugby Logo 3497	Conjugated Estrogens	0.625mg	–	Tab	–	–	–	Rugby	Hormone
3498	Rugby Logo 3498	Conjugated Estrogens	1.25mg	–	Tab	–	–	–	Rugby	Hormone
3501	Rugby Logo 3501	Conjugated Estrogens	2.5mg	–	Tab	–	–	–	Rugby	Hormone
3506	Bristol 3506	Kanamycin Sulfate	500mg	White	Cap	–	–	–	Bristol	Anti–Infective
3512	SFC–3512	Docusate Calcium/Phenolphthaline	60mg/65mg	Maroon	Cap	–	–	–	Chase	Laxative
3515	Rugby 3515	Cyproheptadine	4mg	–	Tab	–	–	–	Rugby	Antipruritic
3516	Rugby 3516	Conjugated Estrogens	0.625mg	–	Tab	–	–	–	Rugby	Hormone
3517	Rugby 3517	Conjugated Estrogens	0.3mg	–	Tab	–	–	–	Rugby	Hormone
3522	Rugby 3522	Conjugated Estrogens	1.25mg	–	Tab	–	–	–	Rugby	Hormone
3523	Rugby 3523	Clonidine HCl	0.1mg	–	Tab	–	–	–	Par	Antihypertensive
	Rugby 3523	Clonidine HCl	0.1mg	–	Tab	–	–	–	Rugby	Antihypertensive
3524	Rugby 3524	Clonidine HCl	0.2mg	–	Tab	–	–	–	Par	Antihypertensive
	Rugby 3524	Clonidine HCl	0.2mg	–	Tab	–	–	–	Rugby	Antihypertensive
3526	Rugby 3526	Clonidine HCl	0.3mg	–	Tab	–	–	–	Par	Antihypertensive
	Rugby 3526	Clonidine HCl	0.3mg	–	Tab	–	–	–	Rugby	Antihypertensive
3528	Rugby 3528	Conjugated Estrogens	2.5mg	–	Tab	–	–	–	Rugby	Hormone
3529	Rugby 3529	Cyclandelate	400mg	–	Cap	–	–	–	Rugby	Vasodilator
3530	Rugby 3530	Cortisone Acetate	25mg	–	Tab	–	–	–	Rugby	Steroid
3531	Rugby 3531	Cyclandelate	200mg	–	Cap	–	–	–	Rugby	Vasodilator
3549	IL/3549	Isosorbide Dinitrate C.R.	40mg	Peach	Tab	Round	Y	N	Inwood	Antianginal

ID NO.	ID CODE	GENERIC NAME	STRENGTH	COLOR	FORM	SHAPE	SCORED	COATED	MFG.	USE
3571	Rugby 3571	Dipyridamole	50mg	White	Tab	Round	N	Y	Rugby	Antiplatelet
3572	Rugby 3572	Dipyridamole	75mg	White	Tab	Round	N	Y	Rugby	Antiplatelet
3575	IL/3575	Isosorbide Dinitrate C.R.	40mg	White/Clear	Cap	–	–	–	Inwood	Antianginal
3577	IL/3577	Pentaerythritol Tetranitrate C.R.	80mg	White/Clear	Cap	–	–	–	Inwood	Antianginal
3581	IL/3581	Theophylline (Anhydrous) C.R.	300mg	White	Tab	Capsule	Y	N	Inwood	Bronchodilator
3583	IL/3583	Theophylline (Anhydrous) C.R.	200mg	White	Tab	Oval	Y	N	Inwood	Bronchodilator
	Rugby 3583	Dexamethasone	0.75mg	–	Tab	–	–	–	Rugby	Steroid
3584	IL/3584	Theophylline (Anhydrous) C.R.	100mg	White	Tab	Round	Y	N	Inwood	Bronchodilator
3585	0115 3585	Folic Acid	1mg	Yellow	Tab	Round	Y	N	Richlyn	Antianemic
3587	IL/3587	Carbamazepine	200mg	White	Tab	Round	Y	N	Inwood	Anticonvulsant
3591	Rugby 3591	Diazepam	2mg	White	Tab	Round	Y	N	Rugby	Antianxiety
3592	Rugby 3592	Diazepam	5mg	Orange	Tab	Round	Y	N	Rugby	Antianxiety
3593	Rugby 3593	Diazepam	10mg	Green	Tab	Round	Y	N	Rugby	Antianxiety
3595	Rugby 3595	Disopyramide Phosphate	100mg	–	Cap	–	–	–	Rugby	Antiarrhythmic
3596	Rugby 3596	Disopyramide Phosphate	150mg	–	Cap	–	–	–	Rugby	Antiarrhythmic
3597	Rugby 3597	Diphenhydramine	25mg	–	Cap	–	–	–	Rugby	Antihistamine
3606	Z 3606	Thioridazine HCL	10mg	Orange	Tab	Round	–	Y	Zenith	Tranquilizer
3607	IL-3607	Indomethacin ER	75mg	Lavender/Clear	Cap	–	–	–	Inwood	Anti-Inflammatory
	Z 3607	Thioridazine HCL	15mg	Orange	Tab	Round	–	Y	Zenith	Tranquilizer
3608	Z 3608	Thioridazine HCL	25mg	Orange	Tab	Round	–	Y	Zenith	Tranquilizer
3609	IL-3609	Propranolol ER	60mg	Brown/Clear	Cap	–	–	–	Inwood	Antihypertensive
	Z 3609	Thioridazine HCL	50mg	Orange	Tab	Round	–	Y	Zenith	Tranquilizer
3610	IL-3610	Propranolol ER	80mg	Blue/Clear	Cap	–	–	–	Inwood	Antihypertensive
	Z 3610	Thioridazine HCL	100mg	White	Tab	Round	–	Y	Zenith	Tranquilizer
3611	IL-3611	Propranolol ER	120mg	Blue/Clear	Cap	–	–	–	Inwood	Antihypertensive
3612	IL-3612	Propranolol ER	160mg	Blue/Clear	Cap	–	–	–	Inwood	Antihypertensive
3614	Z 3614	Propranolol HCL	10mg	Orange	Tab	Round	–	N	Zenith	Antihypertensive
3615	Z 3615	Propranolol HCL	20mg	Blue	Tab	Round	–	N	Zenith	Antihypertensive
3616	Z 3616	Propranolol HCL	40mg	Green	Tab	Round	–	N	Zenith	Antihypertensive
3617	Z 3617	Propranolol HCL	80mg	Yellow	Tab	Round	–	N	Zenith	Antihypertensive
3618	U 3618	Ceftodoxime Proxetil	200mg	Orange	Tab	Oval	N	Y	Upjohn	Anti-infective
3626	Z 3626	Doxycycline Hyclate	100mg	Orange	Tab	Round	–	Y	Zenith	Anti-Infective
3636	.3/Z 3636	Conjugated Estrogens	0.3mg	White	Tab	Round	N	Y	Zenith	Hormone
3638	Z 3638	Propranolol HCL	60mg	Red	Tab	Round	–	N	Zenith	Antihypertensive
3642	3642	Papaverine HCl	150mg	–	Cap	–	–	–	Vortech	Vasodilator
3643	Z 3643	Nitroglycerin TD	9mg	Green/Yellow	Cap	–	–	–	Zenith	Antianginal
3657	Z 3657	Chlorpropamide	100mg	Blue	Tab	Round	–	N	Zenith	Hypoglycemic
3660	0115 3660	Hydralazine HCl	25mg	Blue	Tab	Round	N	N	Richlyn	Antihypertensive
3662	0115 3662	Hydralazine HCl	50mg	Blue	Tab	Round	N	N	Richlyn	Antihypertensive
3667	Z 3667 2	Perphenazine	2mg	Gray	Tab	–	N	Y	Zenith	Antidepressant
3668	Z 3668 4	Perphenazine	4mg	Gray	Tab	–	N	Y	Zenith	Antidepressant
3669	Z 3669 8	Perphenazine	8mg	Gray	Tab	–	N	Y	Zenith	Antidepressant
3670	0115 3670	Hydrochlorothiazide	25mg	Peach	Tab	Round	Y	N	Richlyn	Diuretic
	Z 3670	Perphenazine	16mg	Gray	Tab	–	N	Y	Zenith	Antidepressant
3671	Z 3671	Perphenazine & Amitriptyline HCL	4mg/50mg	Orange	Tab	Round	–	Y	Zenith	Antidepressant
3675	0115 3675	Hydrochlorothiazide	50mg	Peach	Tab	Round	Y	N	Richlyn	Diuretic
3677	0115 3677	Hydrochlorothiazide	100mg	Peach	Tab	Round	Y	N	Richlyn	Diuretic
3678	3678	Phentermine	30mg	–	Cap	–	–	–	Vortech	Anorectic
3685	0115 3685	Hydrocortisone	20mg	White	Tab	Round	Y	N	Richlyn	Steroid
3702	Rugby logo R 3702	Diethylpropion	25mg	–	Tab	–	–	–	Rugby	Anorectic
3706	0115 3706	Isoniazid	100mg	White	Tab	Round	Y	N	Richlyn	Anti-Infective
3717	G 3717	Triazolam	0.125mg	White	Tab	Oval	N	N	Greenstone	Sedative/Hypnotic
3718	G 3718	Triazolam	0.25mg	Blue	Tab	Oval	N	N	Greenstone	Sedative/Hypnotic
3719	G 3719	Alprazolam	0.25mg	White	Tab	Eliptical	Y	N	Greenstone	Antianxiety
3720	G 3720	Alprazolam	0.5mg	Peach	Tab	Eliptical	Y	N	Greenstone	Antianxiety
3721	G 3721	Alprazolam	1mg	Blue	Tab	Eliptical	Y	N	Greenstone	Antianxiety
3722	G 3722	Alprazolam	2mg	White	Tab	Rectangular	Y	N	Greenstone	Antianxiety
3723	G 3723	Flurbiprofen	50mg	White	Tab	Oval	N	Y	Greenstone	Analgesic
3724	G 3724	Flurbiprofen	100mg	Blue	Tab	Oval	N	Y	Greenstone	Analgesic
3725	G 3725	Glyburide	1.25mg	White	Tab	Round	Y	N	Greenstone	Hypoglycemic
3726	G 3726	Glyburide	2.5mg	Pink	Tab	Round	Y	N	Greenstone	Hypoglycemic
3727	G 3727	Glyburide	5mg	Blue	Tab	Round	Y	N	Greenstone	Hypoglycemic
3728	Rugby 3728	Doxepin	25mg	–	Cap	–	–	–	Rugby	Antidepressant
3729	Rugby 3729	Doxepin	50mg	–	Cap	–	–	–	Rugby	Antidepressant
3730	Rugby 3730	Doxepin	100mg	–	Cap	–	–	–	Rugby	Antidepressant
3736	Rugby 3736	Doxepin	10mg	–	Cap	–	–	–	Rugby	Antidepressant
3737	Rugby 3737	Doxepin HCl	75mg	Green	Cap	–	–	–	Rugby	Antidepressant
3738	Rugby 3738	Doxepin	150mg	Blue/White	Cap	–	–	–	Rugby	Antidepressant
3740	G 3740	Medroxyprogesterone Acetate	2.5mg	Orange	Tab	Oval	Y	N	Greenstone	Steroid
3741	G 3741	Medroxyprogesterone Acetate	5mg	White	Tab	Hexagon	Y	N	Greenstone	Steroid
3742	G 3742	Medroxyprogesterone Acetate	10mg	White	Tab	Oval	Y	N	Greenstone	Steroid
3747	Z 3747	Phenobarbital,Theophylline,Ephedrine (Azpan)	8mg/130mg/24mg	White	Tab	Round	–	N	Zenith	Bronchodilator
3758	Rugby 3758	Diphenhydramine HCl	25mg	–	Cap	–	–	–	Rugby	Antihistamine
3762	Rugby 3762	Diphenhydramine HCl	50mg	–	Cap	–	–	–	Rugby	Antihistamine
3763	Rugby Logo R 3763	Diphenoxylate HCl & Atropine Sulfate	2.5mg/0.025mg	–	Tab	–	–	–	Rugby	Antidiarrheal
3764	Rugby 3764	Prompt Phenytoin Sodium	100mg	–	Cap	–	–	–	Rugby	Anticonvulsant
	Rugby 3764	Prompt Phenytoin Sodium	100mg	–	Cap	–	–	–	Rugby	Anticonvulsant
3767	Rugby 3767	Disulfiram	250mg	–	Tab	–	–	–	Rugby	Alcohol Deterrent
3768	Rugby 3768	Disulfiram	500mg	–	Tab	–	–	–	Rugby	Alcohol Deterrent
3770	Rugby 3770	Trichlormethiazide	4mg	Blue/Green	Tab	–	–	–	Par	Diuretic
	Rugby 3770	Trichlormethiazide	4mg	–	Tab	–	–	–	Rugby	Diuretic
3778	Rugby 3778	Ephedrine Sulfate	50mg	–	Cap	–	–	–	Rugby	Antiasthmatic
3780	Rugby 3780	Ephedrine Sulfate	25mg	–	Cap	–	–	–	Rugby	Antiasthmatic
3795	Rugby 3795	Flurazepam HCl	15mg	–	Cap	–	–	–	Par	Sedative
	Rugby 3795	Flurazepam	15mg	–	Cap	–	–	–	Rugby	Hypnotic
3796	3796	Dextro-Amphetamine Sulfate	15mg	–	Cap	–	–	–	Vortech	Anorectic
	Rugby 3796	Flurazepam HCl	30mg	–	Cap	–	–	–	Par	Sedative
	Rugby 3796	Flurazepam	30mg	–	Cap	–	–	–	Rugby	Hypnotic
3798	Rugby 3798	Meprobamate & Aspirin	400mg/325mg	Salmon/Blue Green	Tab	Round	N	N	Quantum	Antianxiety
	Rugby 3798	Meprobamate & Aspirin	200mg/325mg	–	Tab	Round	–	–	Rugby	Analgesic
3804	Rugby 3804	Vitamin Combination	n/a	–	Cap	–	–	–	Rugby	Vitamin Comb.
3813	Rugby 3813	Fenoprofen	600mg	–	Tab	–	–	–	Rugby	Anti-Inflammatory
3835	Rugby 3835	Furosemide	80mg	–	Tab	–	–	–	Rugby	Diuretic
3840	Rugby 3840	Furosemide	20mg	–	Tab	–	–	–	Rugby	Diuretic
3841	Rugby 3841	Furosemide	40mg	–	Tab	–	–	–	Rugby	Diuretic

ID NO.	ID CODE	GENERIC NAME	STRENGTH	COLOR	FORM	SHAPE	SCORED	COATED	MFG.	USE
3845	Rugby 3845	Folic Acid	1mg	–	Tab	–	–	–	Rugby	Antianemia
3856	Rugby 3856	Ergoloid Mesylates Oral	1mg	White	Tab	Round	N	N	Rugby	Vasodilator
3857	Rugby 3857	Ergoloid Mesylates SL	1mg	White	Tab	Round	N	N	Rugby	Vasodilator
3859	Rugby 3859	Ergoloid Mesylates SL	0.5mg	White	Tab	Oval	N	N	Rugby	Vasodilator
3862	Rugby 3862	Hydralazine HCl	25mg	Peach	Tab	Round	–	–	Par	Antihypertensive
3863	Rugby 3863	Hydralazine HCl	50mg	Peach	Tab	Round	–	–	Par	Antihypertensive
3870	Rugby logo R 3870	Glutethimide	500mg	–	Tab	–	–	–	Rugby	Hypnotic
3871	Rugby 3871	Phenylpropanolamine HCl / Guaifenesin	75mg/400mg	–	Tab	–	–	–	Rugby	Decongestant Comb.
3874	Rugby 3874	Hydroxyzine HCl	10mg	–	Tab	–	–	Y	Rugby	Antipruritic
3875	Rugby 3875	Hydroxyzine HCl	25mg	Maroon	Tab	Round	N	Y	Rugby	Antipruritic
3876	Rugby 3876	Hydroxyzine HCl	50mg	Purple	Tab	Round	N	Y	Rugby	Antipruritic
3882	Rugby 3882	Hydroflumethiazide	50mg	Peach	Tab	Round	Y	N	Rugby	Diuretic
3888	0115 3888	Meprobamate	200mg	White	Tab	Round	N	N	Richlyn	Antianxiety
3890	0115 3890	Meprobamate	400mg	White	Tab	Round	Y	N	Richlyn	Antianxiety
3893	Rugby 3893	Hydroxyzine Pamoate	25mg	–	Cap	–	–	–	Rugby	Antianxiety
3894	Rugby 3894	Hydroxyzine Pamoate	50mg	–	Cap	–	–	–	Rugby	Antianxiety
3895	Rugby 3895	Hydroxyzine Pamoate	100mg	–	Cap	–	–	–	Rugby	Antianxiety
3900	0115 3900	Methocarbamol	500mg	White	Tab	Round	Y	N	Richlyn	Muscle Relaxant
	P 3900	Theophylline & Guaifenesin	150mg/90mg	Yellow	Cap	–	–	–	Pharmacaps	Bronchodilator
	P/3900	Theophylline / Guaifenesin	150mg/90mg	Yellow	Cap	–	–	–	Pharmafair	Bronchodilator
3902	0115 3902	Methocarbamol	750mg	White	Tab	Capsule	Y	N	Richlyn	Muscle Relaxant
3904	Z 3904	Meprobamate	400mg	White	Tab	Round	–	N	Zenith	Antianxiety
3905	Z 3905	Meprobamate	200mg	White	Tab	Round	–	N	Zenith	Antianxiety
3906	Rugby 3906	Theophylline/Ephedrine Sulfate/Hydroxyzine HCl	130/25/10mg	–	Tab	–	–	–	Rugby	Antiasthmatic
	Rugby 3906	Ephedrine, Theophylline, Hydroxyzine HCl	25/130/10mg	–	Tab	Round	–	–	Rugby	Bronchodilator
3914	Rugby 3914	Hydrocodone Bitartrate with Acetaminophen	5mg/500mg	–	Tab	–	–	–	Rugby	Analgesic
3915	Rugby 3915	Reserpine & Hydrochlorothiazide	0.125mg/25mg	–	Tab	–	–	–	Rugby	Antihypertensive
	Z 3915	Acetaminophen and Codeine	300mg/30mg	White	Tab	Round	Y	N	Zenith	Analgesic
3916	Rugby 3916	Reserpine & Hydrochlorothiazide	0.125mg/50mg	–	Tab	–	–	–	Rugby	Antihypertensive
	Z 3916	Acetaminophen and Codeine	300mg/60mg	White	Tab	Round	Y	N	Zenith	Analgesic
3919	Rugby 3919	Hydrochlorothiazide	50mg	Peach	Tab	Round	Y	N	Rugby	Diuretic
3920	Rugby 3920	Belladonna Alkaloids with Phenobarbital	n/a	White	Tab	Round	Y	N	Rugby	Antispasmodic
3921	Rugby 3921	Hydrochlorothiazide	50mg	Yellow	Tab	Round	Y	N	Rugby	Diuretic
3922	Rugby 3922	Hydrochlorothiazide	25mg	Peach	Tab	Round	Y	N	Rugby	Diuretic
3923	Rugby 3923	Hydrochlorothiazide	100mg	Peach	Tab	Round	Y	N	Rugby	Diuretic
3924	R 3924	Butalbital, Aspirin and Caffeine	50/40/325mg	–	Cap	–	–	–	Rugby	Analgesic
3925	3925	Phentermine	30mg	Blue/Clear	Cap	–	–	–	Vortech	Anorectic
	Z 3925	Diazepam	2mg	White	Tab	Round	–	N	Zenith	Antianxiety
3926	Z 3926	Diazepam	5mg	Yellow	Tab	Round	–	N	Zenith	Antianxiety
3927	Rugby 3927	Isosorbide Dinitrate Oral	20mg	Green	Tab	–	–	–	Rugby	Vasodilator
	Z 3927	Diazepam	10mg	Blue	Tab	Round	–	N	Zenith	Antianxiety
3929	Rugby 3929	Imipramine HCl	10mg	Yellow	Tab	–	–	–	Rugby	Antidepressant
3930	Rugby 3930	Imipramine HCl	25mg	Orange	Tab	–	–	–	Rugby	Antidepressant
3931	Rugby 3931	Imipramine HCl	50mg	Green	Tab	–	–	–	Rugby	Antidepressant
3933	Rugby Logo R 3933	Butalbital/Aspirin/Caffeine	50/40/325mg	–	Cap	–	–	–	Rugby	Analgesic
3934	Rugby 3934	Ibuprofen	200mg	–	Tab	–	–	–	Rugby	Analgesic
3935	Rugby 3935	Isoxsuprine	10mg	–	Tab	–	–	–	Rugby	Vasodilator
3936	Rugby 3936	Isoxsuprine	20mg	–	Tab	–	–	–	Rugby	Vasodilator
3937	Rugby 3937	Butalbital/Aspirin/Caffeine	50/40/325mg	–	Tab	–	–	–	Rugby	Analgesic
3938	3938	Phentermine	15mg	Pink/Blue	Cap	–	–	–	Vortech	Anorectic
	Rugby 3938	Isosorbide Dinitrate Oral	30mg	Blue	Tab	–	–	–	Rugby	Vasodilator
3940	Rugby 3940	Isosorbide Dinitrate TR	40mg	–	Tab	–	–	–	Rugby	Vasodilator
3941	Rugby 3941	Isoniazide	300mg	White	Tab	Round	Y	N	Rugby	Anti–Infective
3943	Rugby 3943	Isosorbide Dinitrate Oral	10mg	White	Tab	–	–	–	Rugby	Vasodilator
3946	Rugby 3946	Isosorbide Dinitrate Oral	5mg	Pink	Tab	Round	–	–	Par	Antianginal
3947	Rugby 3947	Isosorbide Dinitrate Oral	5mg	–	Tab	–	–	–	Rugby	Vasodilator
	Rugby logo 3947	Levothyroxine Sodium	25mcg	–	Tab	Round	Y	N	Rugby	Hormone
3948	Rugby 3948	Isoniazid	100mg	–	Tab	–	–	–	Rugby	Anti–Infective
3950	Rugby 3950	Isosorbide Dinitrate SL	10mg	White	Tab	Round	–	–	Rugby	Vasodilator
	Rugby 3950	Levothyroxine Sodium	50mcg	Pink	Tab	Round	Y	N	Rugby	Hormone
	Rugby logo 3950	Levothyroxine Sodium	50mcg	Pink	Tab	Round	Y	N	Rugby	Hormone
3951	Rugby logo 3951	Levothyroxine Sodium	75mcg	–	Tab	Round	Y	N	Rugby	Hormone
3952	Rugby 3952	L–Thyroxine Sodium	0.1mg	–	Tab	–	–	–	Rugby	Hormone
3953	Rugby 3953	L–Thyroxine Sodium	0.15mg	–	Tab	–	–	–	Rugby	Hormone
3954	Rugby 3954	L–Thyroxine Sodium	0.2mg	–	Tab	–	–	–	Rugby	Hormone
3956	Rugby 3956	Lithium Carbonate	300mg	–	Cap	–	–	–	Rugby	Antipsychotic
3957	Rugby 3957	Prochlorperazine Maleate/Isopropamide Iodide	10mg/5mg	–	Cap	–	–	–	Rugby	Antispasmodic
3958	Rugby 3958	L–Thyroxine Sodium	0.3mg	–	Tab	–	–	–	Rugby	Hormone
3961	Rugby 3961	Lorazepam	2mg	–	Tab	–	–	–	Rugby	Antianxiety
3963	Rugby logo 3963	Levothyroxine Sodium	125mcg	–	Tab	Round	Y	N	Rugby	Hormone
3966	Z 3966	Diphenoxylate HCl & Atropine Sulfate	2.5mg/0.025mg	White	Tab	Round	–	N	Zenith	Antidiarrheal
3975	0115 3975	Methenamine Mandelate	250mg	Brown	Tab	Round	N	Y	Richlyn	Urinary Antiseptic
3976	0115 3976	Methenamine Mandelate	500mg	Brown	Tab	Capsule	N	Y	Richlyn	Urinary Antiseptic
	Rugby 3976	Ibuprofen	300mg	–	Tab	–	–	–	Rugby	Anti–Inflammatory
3977	0115 3977	Methenamine Mandelate	1 Gm	Lavender	Tab	Oval	N	Y	Richlyn	Urinary Antiseptic
	Rugby 3977	Ibuprofen	400mg	Orange	Tab	Round	N	Y	Rugby	Analgesic
3978	Rugby 3978	Ibuprofen	600mg	Orange	Tab	Oval	N	Y	Rugby	Analgesic
3979	Rugby 3979	Ibuprofen	800mg	–	Tab	–	–	–	Rugby	Anti–Inflammatory
3980	Rugby 3980	Indomethacin SR	75mg	Purple/White	Cap	–	–	–	Rugby	Anti–Inflammatory
3981	Rugby 3981	Indomethacin	25mg	Green/Green	Cap	–	–	–	Rugby	Anti–Inflammatory
	Z 3981	Propoxyphene Napsylate & Acetaminophen	100mg/650mg	White	Tab	Oblong	–	Y	Zenith	Analgesic
3982	0115 3982	Methyltestosterone SL	10mg	Yellow	Tab	Capsule	Y	N	Richlyn	Hormone
	Rugby 3982	Indomethacin	50mg	Green/Green	Cap	–	–	–	Rugby	Anti–Inflammatory
3984	0115 3984	Methyltestosterone Oral	10mg	White	Tab	Round	Y	N	Richlyn	Hormone
	Z 3984	Aspirin and Codeine	325mg/30mg	White	Tab	Round	Y	N	Zenith	Analgesic
3985	Rugby 3985	Meclizine HCl	12.5mg	White	Tab	–	–	–	Rugby	Antivertigo
	Z 3985	Aspirin and Codeine	325mg/60mg	White	Tab	Round	Y	N	Zenith	Analgesic
3986	0115 3986	Methyltestosterone Oral	25mg	Yellow	Tab	Round	Y	N	Richlyn	Hormone
	Rugby 3986	Meclizine HCl	12.5mg	Blue/White	Tab	Oval	–	–	Rugby	Antivertigo
3988	Rugby 3988	Meclizine HCl	25mg	Yellow/White	Tab	Oval	–	–	Rugby	Antivertigo
3990	Rugby 3990	Meclizine HCl Chewable	25mg	–	Tab	–	–	–	Rugby	Antivertigo
3995	Rugby 3995	Medroxyprogesterone Acetate	10mg	–	Tab	–	–	–	Rugby	Hormone
3996	Rugby 3996	Methyldopa & Hydrochlorothiazide	250mg/15mg	–	Tab	–	–	–	Bolar	Antihypertensive
	Z 3996	Butalbital,Aspirin,Caffeine (Butalbital Compound)	50/325/40mg	White	Tab	Round	Y	N	Zenith	Analgesic
3997	Rugby 3997	Methyldopa & Hydrochlorothiazide	250mg/25mg	–	Tab	–	–	–	Bolar	Antihypertensive

ID NO.	ID CODE	GENERIC NAME	STRENGTH	COLOR	FORM	SHAPE	SCORED	COATED	MFG.	USE
4001	0665–4001	Medroxyprogesterone Acetate	10mg	White	Tab	Round	N	N	Reid–Rowell	Steroid
	150 WALLACE 37–4001	Methacycline HCl	150mg	Blue/White	Cap	–	–	–	Wallace	Anti–Infective
	PP 4001	Cyclandelate	200mg	Blue	Cap	–	–	–	Pioneer	Vasodilator
4002	PP 4002	Cyclandelate	400mg	Blue/Red	Cap	–	–	–	Pioneer	Vasodilator
	Rugby 4002	Meclofenamate Sodium	50mg	–	Cap	–	–	–	Rugby	Anti–Inflammatory
4003	Rugby 4003	Meclofenamate Sodium	100mg	–	Cap	–	–	–	Rugby	Anti–Inflammatory
4005	PP 4005	Indomethacin	25mg	Green	Cap	–	–	–	Pioneer	Anti–Inflammatory
	Rugby logo R 4005	Meprobamate	200mg	–	Tab	–	–	–	Rugby	Antianxiety
4006	PP 4006	Indomethacin	50mg	Green	Cap	–	–	–	Pioneer	Anti–Inflammatory
	Rugby logo R 4006	Meprobamate	400mg	–	Tab	–	–	–	Rugby	Antianxiety
4008	PP 4008	Diphenhydramine	50mg	Pink	Cap	–	–	–	Pioneer	Antihistamine
4009	PP 4009	Chlordiazepoxide & Clidinium	5mg/2.5mg	Green	Cap	–	–	–	Pioneer	Antispasmodic
4010	Mylan 4010	Temazepam	15mg	Peach/Peach	Cap	–	N	N	Mylan	Sedative
	PP 4010	Chlordiazepoxide Hydrochloride	5mg	Yellow/Green	Cap	–	–	–	Pioneer	Antianxiety
	Rugby 4010	Methyldopa	250mg	White	Tab	Round	N	Y	Rugby	Antihypertensive
4011	PP 4011	Chlordiazepoxide Hydrochloride	10mg	Black/Green	Cap	–	–	–	Pioneer	Antianxiety
	Rugby 4011	Methyldopa	500mg	White	Tab	Round	N	Y	Rugby	Antihypertensive
4012	PP 4012	Chlordiazepoxide Hydrochloride	25mg	White/Green	Cap	–	–	–	Pioneer	Antianxiety
	Rugby 4012	Methyldopa	125mg	White	Tab	Round	N	Y	Rugby	Antihypertensive
4013	PP 4013	Diphenhydramine	25mg	Pink/Clear	Cap	–	–	–	Pioneer	Antihistamine
4017	PP 4017	Dicyclomine HCl	10mg	Blue/Blue	Cap	–	–	–	Pioneer	Antispasmodic
4018	Rugby 4018	Metronidazole	250mg	White	Tab	Round	N	Y	Rugby	Anti–Infective
4019	Rugby 4019	Metronidazole	500mg	White	Tab	Oval	N	Y	Rugby	Anti–Infective
4020	RR 4020	Quinidine Sulfate	300mg	Clear	Cap	–	–	–	RR	Antiarrhythmic
	Rugby 4020	Methyldopa	125mg	Peach	Tab	Round	N	Y	Rugby	Antihypertensive
	SOLVAY 4020	Quinidine Sulfate	300mg	Clear	Cap	–	–	–	Solvay	Antiarrhythmic
4021	Rugby 4021	Methyldopa	250mg	Peach	Tab	Round	N	Y	Rugby	Antihypertensive
4023	Rugby 4023	Methyldopa	500mg	Peach	Tab	Round	N	Y	Rugby	Antihypertensive
4024	RR 4024	Quinidine Sulfate	100mg	White	Tab	Round	Y	N	RR	Antiarrhythmic
4025	Rugby logo 4025	Methyclothiazide	5mg	–	Tab	Round	Y	N	Rugby	Diuretic
4026	Rugby 4026	Methocarbamol	500mg	–	Tab	–	–	–	Rugby	Muscle Relaxant
4027	Rugby 4027	Methocarbamol	750mg	–	Tab	–	–	–	Rugby	Muscle Relaxant
4028	RR 4028	Quinidine Sulfate	200mg	White	Tab	Round	Y	N	RR	Antiarrhythmic
	Rugby 4028	Methocarbamol/Aspirin	500mg/325mg	–	Tab	–	–	–	Rugby	Muscle Relaxant
	SOLVAY 4028	Quinidine Sulfate	200mg	White	Tab	Round	Y	N	Solvay	Antiarrhythmic
4029	Z 4029	Indomethacin	25mg	Green/Green	Cap	–	–	–	Zenith	Anti–Inflammatory
4030	Z 4030	Indomethacin	50mg	Green/Green	Cap	–	–	–	Zenith	Anti–Inflammatory
4032	RR 4032	Quinidine Sulfate	300mg	White	Tab	Round	Y	N	RR	Antiarrhythmic
	SOLVAY 4032	Quinidine Sulfate	300mg	White	Tab	Round	Y	N	Solvay	Antiarrhythmic
4036	Rugby 4036	Methylprednisolone	4mg	–	Tab	–	–	–	Rugby	Steroid
4040	Rugby 4040	Methyclothiazide	2.5mg	Peach	Tab	Round	Y	N	Rugby	Diuretic
4041	Rugby 4041	Methyclothiazide	5mg	Pinkish–Orange	Tab	Round	Y	N	Rugby	Diuretic
4042	Rugby 4042	Metoclopramide HCl	10mg	–	Tab	–	–	–	Rugby	Antireflux
4043	Rugby 4043	Minoxidil	10mg	–	Tab	–	–	–	Rugby	Antihypertensive
4051	Z 4051	Disopyramide Phosphate	100mg	Blue/Clear	Cap	–	–	–	Zenith	Antiarrhythmic
4052	Rugby 4052	Methyldopa/Chlorothiazide	250mg/150mg	–	Tab	–	–	Y	Rugby	Antihypertensive
	Z 4052	Disopyramide Phosphate	150mg	Blue/Clear	Cap	–	–	–	Zenith	Antiarrhythmic
4053	Rugby 4053	Methyldopa/Chlorothiazide	250mg/250mg	–	Tab	–	–	Y	Rugby	Antihypertensive
4058	Z 4058	Cefadroxil	500mg	Red/White	Cap	–	–	–	Zenith	Anti–Infective
	Z 4058	Cefadroxil	500mg	Clear/White	Cap	–	–	–	Zenith	Antiinfective
4059	Z 4059	Cefadroxil	1000mg	White	Tab	Oval	–	–	Zenith	Anti–Infective
4060	Muro 4060	Brompheniramine/Pseudoephedrine	4mg/60mg	White	Tab	Round	Y	N	Central	Decongestant
4063	Z 4063	Cephradine	250mg	Maroon/Maroon	Cap	–	–	–	Zenith	Anti–Infective
4064	Z 4064	Cephradine	500mg	Pink/Pink	Cap	–	–	–	Zenith	Anti–Infective
4067	4067	Codeine Phosphate, Aspirin, Caffeine	30/380/30mg	White	Tab	Round	N	N	Lilly	Analgesic
	Z 4067	Prazosin HCl	1mg	Ivory/Opaque	Cap	–	–	–	Zenith	Antihypertensive
4068	Z 4068	Prazosin HCl	2mg	Pink/Opaque	Cap	–	–	–	Zenith	Antihypertensive
4069	Z 4069	Prazosin HCl	5mg	Blue/Opaque	Cap	–	–	–	Zenith	Antihypertensive
4073	Z 4073	Cephalexin	250mg	Gray/Red	Cap	–	–	–	Zenith	Anti–Infective
4074	Z 4074	Cephalexin	500mg	Red	Cap	–	–	–	Zenith	Anti–Infective
4081	Rugby 4081	Nitrofurantoin	50mg	–	Tab	–	–	–	Rugby	Anti–Infective
4082	Rugby 4082	Nitrofurantoin	100mg	–	Tab	–	–	–	Rugby	Anti–Infective
4083	Rugby 4083	Nitroglycerin TD	2.5mg	Lavender/Clear	Cap	–	–	–	Rugby	Antianginal
4084	Rugby 4084	Nitroglycerin TD	6.5mg	Black/Yellow	Cap	–	–	–	Rugby	Antianginal
4086	0115 4086	Nicotinic Acid	500mg	White	Tab	Round	Y	N	Richlyn	Vitamin
4090	Rugby 4090	Nitroglycerin TD	9mg	Green/Yellow	Cap	–	–	–	Rugby	Antianginal
4091	Rugby 4091	Nystatin Vaginal	100,000 Units	–	Tab	–	–	–	Rugby	Anti–Infective
4094	Rugby 4094	Nystatin	500,000 Units	Brown	Tab	Round	N	Y	Rugby	Anti–Infective
4096	Z 4096	Baclofen	10mg	White	Tab	Round	–	–	Zenith	Muscle Relaxant
4097	Z 4097	Baclofen	20mg	White	Tab	Round	–	–	Zenith	Muscle Relaxant
4101	300 WALLACE 37–4101	Methacycline HCl	300mg	Blue/White	Cap	–	–	–	Wallace	Anti–Infective
4111	W–T 4111	Magnesium Salicylate	500mg	White	Tab	Capsule	N	N	Adria	Analgesic
4114	Rugby 4114	Oxazepam	10mg	–	Cap	–	–	–	Rugby	Antianxiety
4115	Rugby 4115	Oxazepam	15mg	–	Cap	–	–	–	Rugby	Antianxiety
4116	Rugby 4116	Oxazepam	30mg	–	Cap	–	–	–	Rugby	Antianxiety
4120	0665 4120	Valproic Acid	250mg	Orange	Cap	Oval	–	–	Scherer	Anticonvulsant
	0665 4120	Valproic Acid	250mg	Orange	Cap	Oval	–	–	Solvay	Anticonvulsant
	RR 4120	Valproic Acid	250mg	Orange	Cap	Oval	–	–	Reid–Rowell	Anticonvulsant
	SOLVAY 4120	Valproic Acid	250mg	Orange	Cap	Oval	–	–	Solvay	Anticonvulsant
4124	Rugby 4124	Papaverine HCl T.D.	150mg	–	Cap	–	–	–	Rugby	Vasodilator
4125	Wyeth 4125	Isosorbide Dinitrate SA	40mg	Green	Tab	Round	Y	N	Wyeth	Vasodilator
4130	Rugby 4130	Pentaerythritol Tetranitrate	10mg	–	Tab	–	–	–	Rugby	Antianginal
	Wyeth 4130	Ethionamide	250mg	Orange	Tab	Round	N	Y	Wyeth	Antituberculous
4131	Lilly 4131	Pergolide Mesylate	0.05mg	Ivory	Tab	Rectangular	Y	N	Lilly	Antiparkinson
	Rugby 4131	Perphenazine	2mg	–	Tab	Round	N	Y	Rugby	Tranquilizer
4132	Rugby 4132	Perphenazine	4mg	–	Tab	Round	N	Y	Rugby	Tranquilizer
	Wyeth 4132	Trimipramine Maleate	25mg	Blue/Yellow	Cap	–	–	–	Wyeth	Antidepressant
4133	Lilly 4133	Pergolide Mesylate	0.25mg	Green	Tab	Rectangular	Y	N	Lilly	Antiparkinson
	Rugby 4133	Perphenazine	8mg	–	Tab	Round	N	Y	Rugby	Tranquilizer
	Wyeth 4133	Trimipramine Maleate	50mg	Blue/Yellow	Cap	–	–	–	Wyeth	Antidepressant
4134	Rugby 4134	Perphenazine	16mg	–	Tab	Round	N	Y	Rugby	Tranquilizer
4135	Lilly 4135	Pergolide Mesylate	1mg	Pink	Tab	Rectangular	Y	N	Lilly	Antiparkinson
4138	Rugby 4138	Pentaerythritol Tetranitrate	20mg	–	Tab	–	–	–	Rugby	Antianginal
4140	RR 4140	Amantadine HCl	100mg	Red	Cap	Oval	–	–	Reid–Rowell	Antiviral
	S 4140	Amantadine HCl	100mg	Red	Cap	Oval	–	–	Solvay	Antiviral

ID NO.	ID CODE	GENERIC NAME	STRENGTH	COLOR	FORM	SHAPE	SCORED	COATED	MFG.	USE
4140	Wyeth 4140	Isosorbide Dinitrate SA	40mg	Blue/Clear	Cap	–	–	–	Wyeth	Vasodilator
4141	Z 4141	Fenoprofen	600mg	Peach	Tab	Oval	–	Y	Zenith	Anti–Inflammatory
4147	Rugby 4147	Perphenazine	8mg	–	Tab	–	–	–	Rugby	Antidepressant
4148	Rugby 4148	Leucovorin	5mg	–	Tab	–	–	–	Rugby	Antineoplastic
4149	Rugby 4149	Leucovorin	25mg	–	Tab	–	–	–	Rugby	Antineoplastic
4152	Wyeth 4152	Isosorbide Dinitrate Oral	5mg	Pink	Tab	Round	Y	N	Wyeth	Vasodilator
4153	Wyeth 4153	Isosorbide Dinitrate Oral	10mg	White	Tab	Round	Y	N	Wyeth	Vasodilator
4154	Wyeth 4154	Isosorbide Dinitrate Oral	20mg	Green	Tab	Round	Y	N	Wyeth	Vasodilator
4158	Wyeth 4158	Trimipramine Maleate	100mg	Blue/Yellow	Cap	–	–	–	Wyeth	Antidepressant
4159	Wyeth 4159	Isosorbide Dinitrate Oral	30mg	Blue	Tab	Round	Y	N	Wyeth	Vasodilator
4160	0665–4160	Lithium Carbonate	300mg	White	Cap	–	–	–	Reid–Rowell	Tranquilizer
	Rugby 4160	Phendimetrazine Tartrate	35mg	Yellow	Tab	–	–	–	Rugby	Anorectic
4161	Rugby 4161	Phendimetrazine Tartrate	35mg	Gray	Tab	–	–	–	Rugby	Anorectic
4162	Rugby 4162	Phendimetrazine Tartrate	35mg	Pink	Tab	–	–	–	Rugby	Anorectic
4167	Rugby 4167	Phendimetrazine Tartrate	35mg	White	Tab	–	–	–	Rugby	Anorectic
4188	Wyeth 4188 200	Amiodarone HCl	200mg	Pink	Tab	Round	Y	N	Wyeth	Antiarrhythmic
4191	Wyeth 4191	Dihydrocodeine bitartrate/Aspirin/Caffeine	16/356.4/30mg	Blue/Gray	Cap	–	–	–	Wyeth	Analgesic
4192	Wyeth 4192	Isosorbide Dinitrate Oral	40mg	Green	Tab	Round	Y	N	Wyeth	Vasodilator
4207	AHR 4207	Phenobarbital,Hyoscyamine,Atropine,Scopolamine	n/a	Green/White	Cap	–	–	–	A.H.Robins	Antispasmodic
4214	0115 4214	Phenobarbital	15mg	Green	Tab	Round	N	N	Richlyn	Hypnotic
	0115 4214	Phenobarbital	15mg	Pink	Tab	Round	N	N	Richlyn	Hypnotic
	0115 4214	Phenobarbital	15mg	White	Tab	Round	N	N	Richlyn	Hypnotic
4217	Z 4217	Pindolol	5mg	White	Tab	Round	Y	N	Zenith	Anti–Hypertensive
4218	Z 4218	Pindolol	10mg	White	Tab	Round	Y	N	Zenith	Anti–Hypertensive
4224	Rugby 4224	Phenobarbital	20mg	–	Tab	–	–	–	West–ward	Sedative
	WALLACE 37 4224	Iodinated Glycerol	30mg	Rose	Tab	Round	Y	N	Wallace	Expectorant
4229	Z 4229	Triamterene/Hydrochlorothiazide	50mg/25mg	Red	Cap	–	–	–	Zenith	Diuretic
4233	0115 4233	Phenobarbital	30mg	Green	Tab	Round	Y	N	Richlyn	Hypnotic
	0115 4233	Phenobarbital	30mg	Pink	Tab	Round	Y	N	Richlyn	Hypnotic
	0115 4233	Phenobarbital	30mg	White	Tab	Round	Y	N	Richlyn	Hypnotic
4234	Rugby 4234	Ergotamine/Phenobarbital/belladonna	0.6mg/40mg/0.2	–	Tab	–	–	–	Rugby	Antispasmodic
4235	Rugby 4235	Phentermine HCl	30mg	–	Cap	–	–	–	Rugby	Anorectic
4250	Mylan 4250	Doxepin HCl	50mg	Ivory/Ivory	Cap	–	–	–	Mylan	Antidepressant
	R 4250	Phenobarbital,Hyoscyamine,Atropine,Scopolamine	n/a	White	Tab	Round	Y	N	A.H.Robins	Antispasmodic
4252	0115 4252	Piperazine Citrate	250mg	White	Tab	Round	Y	N	Richlyn	–
4264	R 4264	Phenobarbital,Hyoscyamine,Atropine,Scopolamine	n/a	–	Tab	Round	Y	N	A.H.Robins	Antispasmodic
4280	0115 4280	Prednisolone	5mg	Orange	Tab	Round	Y	N	Richlyn	Steroid
	377–4280	Prednisolone	5mg	Orange	Tab	Round	–	N	Vale	Steroid
	Z 4280 SR 240	Verapamil SR	240mg	Off White	Tab	Capsule	Y	Y	Zenith	Antiarrhythmic
	Z 4280/SR240	Verapamil SR	240mg	Off White	Tab	Capsule	Y	Y	Zenith	Antiarrhythmic
	Zenith 4280	Verapamil SR	240mg	Off White	Tab	Capsule	Y	Y	Zenith	Antiarrhythmic
4285	Sav. Logo 4285	Vitamin & Iron	n/a	Maroon	Cap	–	–	–	Savage	Vitamin + Iron
4286	Z 4286 SR 180	Verapamil SR	180mg	Off White	Tab	Oval	Y	Y	Zenith	Antiarrhythmic
	Z 4286/SR180	Verapamil SR	180mg	Off White	Tab	Oval	Y	Y	Zenith	Antiarrhythmic
	Zenith 4286	Verapamil SR	180mg	Off White	Tab	Oval	Y	Y	Zenith	Antiarrhythmic
4288	Rugby 4288	Phentermine HCl	8mg	–	Tab	–	–	–	Rugby	Anorectic
4290	Rugby 4290	Phenylpropanolamine	25mg	–	Tab	–	–	–	Rugby	Decongestant
4294	0115 4294	Prednisone	5mg	White	Tab	Round	Y	N	Richlyn	Steroid
	377–4294	Prednisone	5mg	White	Tab	Round	–	N	Vale	Steroid
4295	Rugby 4295	Phenylbutazone	100mg	–	Cap	–	–	–	Rugby	Anti–Inflammatory
4298	Rugby 4298	Phenylbutazone	100mg	–	Tab	–	–	–	Rugby	Anti–Inflammatory
4299	Rugby 4299	Phenylbutazone	100mg	–	Tab	–	–	–	Rugby	Anti–Inflammatory
4302	0115–4302	Colchicine & Probenecid	0.5mg/500mg	White	Tab	Capsule	Y	N	Richlyn	Antigout
4305	Rugby 4305	Phenylbutazone	100mg	–	Cap	–	–	–	Rugby	Anti–Inflammatory
4306	0115/4306	Promethazine	25mg	White	Tab	Round	N	N	Richlyn	Antiemetic
4307	Rugby 4307	Poly Vitamins with Fluoride	1mg	Orange,Pink,Purple	Tab	Round	–	–	Rugby	Vitamin
4308	0115 4308	Propantheline Bromide	15mg	Peach	Tab	Round	N	Y	Richlyn	Antispasmodic
	Rugby 4308	Poly Vitamins / Fluoride / Iron	1mg	Orange,Pink,Purple	Tab	Round	–	–	Rugby	Vitamin
4309	Rugby 4309	Propranolol HCl	10mg	Orange	Tab	Round	Y	N	Rugby	Antihypertensive
4312	AT–4312	Poly Vitamins with Fluoride	0.5mg	Orange/Pink/Purple	Tab	Round	N	N	ATI	Vitamin
	Rugby 4312	Poly Vitamins with Fluoride	0.5mg	Pink/Orange/Purple	Tab	Round	N	N	Rugby	Vitamin
4313	Rugby 4313	Propranolol HCl	20mg	Blue	Tab	Round	Y	N	Rugby	Antihypertensive
4314	Rugby 4314	Propranolol HCl	40mg	Yellow	Tab	Round	Y	N	Rugby	Antihypertensive
4315	Rugby 4315	Propranolol HCl	60mg	–	Tab	–	Y	N	Rugby	Antihypertensive
4316	Rugby 4316	Propranolol HCl	80mg	Green	Tab	Round	Y	N	Rugby	Antihypertensive
4322	0115 4322	Propylthiouracil	50mg	White	Tab	Round	Y	N	Richlyn	Antithyroid
	Rugby 4322	Potassium Chloride	600mg (8mEq)	–	Tab	Round	N	Y	Rugby	Potassium Supp.
4324	Rugby 4324	Prednisone	5mg	–	Tab	–	–	–	Rugby	Steroid
4325	Rugby 4325	Prednisone	10mg	–	Tab	–	–	–	Rugby	Steroid
4326	Rugby 4326	Prednisone	20mg	–	Tab	–	–	–	Rugby	Steroid
4328	Rugby 4328	Prednisone	50mg	–	Tab	–	–	–	Rugby	Steroid
4331	0115 4331	Pseudoephedrine & Triprolidine	60mg/2.5mg	White	Tab	Round	Y	N	Richlyn	Decongestant Comb.
4332	0115 4332	Pseudoephedrine HCl	60mg	White	Tab	Round	Y	N	Richlyn	Decongestant
4334	0115 4334	Phenazopyridine HCl	100mg	Dark Red	Tab	Round	N	Y	Richlyn	Urinary Antiseptic
4335	Rugby 4335	Prenatal W/Folic Acid & Iron Improved	n/a	–	Tab	–	–	–	Rugby	Vitamin
4336	0115 4336	Phenazopyridine HCl	200mg	Dark Red	Tab	Round	N	Y	Richlyn	Urinary Antiseptic
4339	Rugby 4339	Prenatal W/Folic Acid & Iron Plus	n/a	–	Tab	–	–	–	Rugby	Vitamin
4340	Rugby 4340	Prednisolone	5mg	White	Tab	–	–	–	Rugby	Steroid
4346	Rugby 4346	Prednisolone	5mg	Salmon	Tab	–	–	–	Rugby	Steroid
4350	4350	Isoniazid	300mg	White	Tab	Round	Y	N	Eon	Anti–Infective
	E 4350	Isoniazid	300mg	White	Tab	Round	Y	N	Eon	Anti–Infective
4351	E 4351	Isoniazid	100mg	White	Tab	Round	Y	N	Eon	Anti–Infective
4352	Rugby 4352	Prednisolone	5mg	Green	Tab	–	–	–	Rugby	Steroid
4354	4354	Isoniazid	100mg	White	Tab	Round	Y	N	Eon	Anti–Infective
4360	0115 4360	Pyrilamine Maleate	25mg	Yellow	Tab	Round	N	N	Richlyn	Antihistamine
	Rugby 4360	Propoxyphene Napsylate with APAP	50mg/325mg	–	Tab	–	–	–	Rugby	Analgesic
4361	Rugby 4361	Propoxyphene Napsylate with APAP	100mg/650mg	Pink	Tab	Oblong	N	Y	Rugby	Analgesic
4365	Rugby 4365	Probenecid & Colchicine	500mg/0.5	–	Tab	–	–	–	Rugby	Antigout
4366	Rugby 4366	Probenecid	500mg	–	Tab	–	–	–	Rugby	Antigout
4367	Rugby 4367	Procainamide HCl	250mg	Yellow/Yellow	Cap	–	–	–	Rugby	Antiarrhythmic
4368	Rugby 4368	Procainamide HCl	500mg	Lt. Orange/White	Cap	–	–	–	Rugby	Antiarrhythmic
4369	Rugby 4369	Promethazine	50mg	–	Tab	–	–	–	Rugby	Antiemetic
4374	Rugby logo R 4374	Propoxyphene /Aspirin/ Caffeine	65/389/32.4mg	Red/Gray	Cap	–	–	–	Rugby	Analgesic
4377	Rugby 4377	Procainamide HCl	375mg	Orange/White	Cap	–	–	–	Rugby	Antiarrhythmic
4378	Rugby 4378	Promethazine	12.5mg	–	Tab	–	–	–	Rugby	Antiemetic

ID NO.	ID CODE	GENERIC NAME	STRENGTH	COLOR	FORM	SHAPE	SCORED	COATED	MFG.	USE
4379	Rugby 4379	Promethazine	25mg	–	Tab	–	–	–	Rugby	Antiemetic
4380	0115 4380	Quinidine Sulfate	200mg	White	Tab	Round	Y	N	Richlyn	Antiarrhythmic
	Rugby 4380	Levothyroxine Sodium	0.15mg	–	Tab	–	–	–	Rugby	Hormone
4381	Rugby 4381	Levothyroxine Sodium	0.2mg	–	Tab	–	–	–	Rugby	Hormone
4382	Rugby logo R 4382	Propoxyphene HCl	65mg	Pink	Cap	–	–	–	Rugby	Analgesic
4383	Rugby Logo R 4383	Propoxyphene/Aspirin/Caffeine	65/389/32.4mg	–	Cap	–	–	–	Rugby	Analgesic
4384	Rugby 4384	Propylthiouracil	50mg	–	Tab	–	–	–	Rugby	Antithyroid
4387	Rugby 4387	Propoxyphene and Acetaminophen	65mg/650mg	–	Tab	–	N	Y	Rugby	Analgesic
4388	R 4388	Phenazopyridine HCl	100mg	–	Tab	Round	N	Y	Rugby	Urinary Antiseptic
4390	Rugby 4390	Pseudoephedrine HCl	60mg	–	Tab	–	–	–	Rugby	Decongestant
4391	Rugby 4391	Pseudoephedrine HCl	30mg	–	Tab	–	–	–	Rugby	Decongestant
4392	R 4392	Phenazopyridine HCl	200mg	–	Tab	Round	N	Y	Rugby	Urinary Antiseptic
4399	Rugby 4399	Pseudoephedrine HCl	60mg	–	Tab	Round	–	–	Rugby	Decongestant
4400	0115 4400	Rauwolfia Serpentina	50mg	Orange	Tab	Round	N	Y	Richlyn	Antihypertensive
4401	37–4401	Penicillamine	250mg	White	Tab	Oval	–	–	Wallace	Antiarthritic
	37–4401	Penicillamine Titratable	250mg	White	Tab	Oval	Y	N	Wallace	Antiarthritic
4402	Rugby 4402	Propranolol HCl/Hydrochlorothiazide	40mg/25mg	–	Tab	–	–	–	Rugby	Antihypertensive
4403	Rugby 4403	Propranolol HCl/Hydrochlorothiazide	80mg/25mg	–	Tab	–	–	–	Rugby	Antihypertensive
4404	0115 4404	Rauwolfia Serpentina	100mg	Orange	Tab	Round	N	Y	Richlyn	Antihypertensive
4410	0063–4410 25/25	Hydralazine HCl & Hydrochlorothiazide	25mg/25mg	Green	Cap	–	–	–	Reid–Rowell	Antihypertensive
	0665–4410 25/25	Hydralazine HCl & Hydrochlorothiazide	25mg/25mg	Green	Cap	–	–	–	Reid–Rowell	Antihypertensive
4411	Rugby 4411	Pyrilamine	25mg	–	Tab	–	–	–	Rugby	Antihistamine
4415	Mylan 4415	Flurazepam HCl	15mg	Blue/White	Cap	–	–	–	Mylan	Hypnotic
4420	0063–4420 50/50	Hydralazine HCl & Hydrochlorothiazide	50mg/50mg	Lt. Green/Green	Cap	–	–	–	Reid–Rowell	Antihypertensive
	0665–4420 50/50	Hydralazine HCl & Hydrochlorothiazide	50mg/50mg	Lt. Green/Green	Cap	–	–	–	Reid–Rowell	Antihypertensive
4423	0115–4423	Reserpine	0.25mg	White	Tab	Round	Y	N	Qualitest	Antihypertensive
4426	0115 4426	Reserpine	0.1mg	White	Tab	Round	N	N	Richlyn	Antihypertensive
	Rugby 4426	Quinine Sulfate	260mg	–	Tab	–	–	–	Rugby	Muscle Relaxant
4428	0115 4428	Reserpine	0.25mg	White	Tab	Round	Y	N	Richlyn	Antihypertensive
4429	R/4429	Quinidine Sulfate	300mg	–	Tab	–	–	–	Eon	Antiarrhythmic
	Rugby 4429	Quinine Sulfate	5gr	–	Cap	–	–	–	Rugby	Muscle Relaxant
4430	Mylan 4430	Flurazepam HCl	30mg	Blue/Blue	Cap	–	–	–	Mylan	Hypnotic
4432	Rugby 4432	Quinidine Sulfate	200mg	–	Tab	–	–	–	Rugby	Antiarrthymic
4433	Rugby 4433	Quinine Sulfate	325mg	–	Cap	–	–	–	Rugby	Muscle Relaxant
4434	Rugby 4434	Quinidine Gluconate SR	324mg	White	Tab	Round	N	N	Rugby	Antiarrhythmic
4454	Rugby 4454	Reserpine	0.1mg	–	Tab	–	–	–	Rugby	Antihypertensive
4458	Rugby 4458	Reserpine	0.25mg	–	Tab	–	–	–	Rugby	Antihypertensive
4494	Rugby 4494	Nylidrin	6mg	–	Tab	–	–	–	Rugby	Vasodilator
4495	Rugby 4495	Nylidrin	12mg	–	Tab	–	–	–	Rugby	Vasodilator
4515	Rugby 4515	Thiothixene	2mg	–	Cap	–	–	–	Rugby	Tranquilizer
4516	Rugby 4516	Thiothixene	5mg	–	Cap	–	–	–	Rugby	Tranquilizer
4517	Rugby 4517	Thiothixene	10mg	–	Cap	–	–	–	Rugby	Tranquilizer
4522	Rugby 4522	Salicylic Acid	500mg	–	Tab	–	–	–	PBI	Antiarthritic
4523	Rugby 4523	Salicylic Acid	750mg	–	Tab	–	–	–	PBI	Antiarthritic
4547	Rugby 4547	Sodium Fluoride	2.2mg	Pink	Tab	Round	–	–	Copley	Mineral
4548	Rugby 4548	Sodium Fluoride	2.2mg	–	Tab	–	–	–	Rugby	Mineral
4549	Rugby 4549	Sodium Fluoride Chewables	2.2mg	–	Tab	–	–	–	Rugby	Mineral
4556	4556	Phenylpropanolamine/Pheniramine/Pyrilamine	50mg/25mg/25mg	Yellow	Tab	Round	N	Y	Eon	Decongestant Comb.
4563	Rugby Logo 4563	Doxepin HCl	10mg	Buff	Cap	–	–	–	Rugby	Antidepressant
4564	Rugby Logo 4564	Doxepin HCl	25mg	White/Ivory	Cap	–	–	–	Rugby	Antidepressant
4565	Rugby Logo 4565	Doxepin HCl	50mg	Ivory	Cap	–	–	–	Rugby	Antidepressant
4566	Rugby Logo 4566	Doxepin HCl	100mg	White/Green	Cap	–	–	–	Rugby	Antidepressant
4575	Rugby 4575	Spironolactone	25mg	Tan	Tab	Round	Y	N	Rugby	Diuretic
4576	Rugby 4576	Spironolactone & Hydrochlorothiazide	25mg/25mg	–	Tab	–	–	–	Rugby	Diuretic
4600	P 4600	Benzonatate	100mg	Yellow	Cap	–	–	–	Sidmak	Antitussive
4604	Rugby Logo 4604	Ibuprofen	400mg	–	Tab	–	N	Y	Rugby	Anti–Inflammatory
4605	Rugby Logo 4605	Ibuprofen	600mg	–	Tab	–	N	Y	Rugby	Anti–Inflammatory
4606	Rugby Logo 4606	Ibuprofen	800mg	–	Tab	–	N	Y	Rugby	Anti–Inflammatory
4617	Rugby 4617	Sulfasalazine	500mg	–	Tab	–	–	–	Rugby	Anti–Inflammatory
4618	Rugby 4618	Sulfisoxazole	500mg	–	Tab	–	–	–	Rugby	Anti–Inflammatory
4628	Rugby 4628	Temazepam	15mg	–	Cap	–	–	–	Quantum	Hypnotic
4629	Rugby 4629	Temazepam	30mg	–	Cap	–	–	–	Quantum	Hypnotic
4631	0115 4631	Sodium Fluoride	2.2mg	Pink	Tab	Round	Y	N	Richlyn	Mineral
4640	Rugby 4640	Thioridazine HCl	15mg	Orange	Tab	Round	N	Y	Rugby	Tranquilizer
4641	Rugby 4641	Thioridazine HCl	10mg	Orange	Tab	Round	N	Y	Rugby	Tranquilizer
4642	Rugby 4642	Thioridazine HCl	25mg	Orange	Tab	Round	N	Y	Rugby	Tranquilizer
4643	Rugby 4643	Thioridazine HCl	50mg	Orange	Tab	Round	N	Y	Rugby	Tranquilizer
4644	Rugby 4644	Thioridazine HCl	100mg	Orange	Tab	Round	N	Y	Rugby	Tranquilizer
4648	Rugby 4648	Phenobarbital,Theophylline,Ephedrine (Azpan)	8mg/130mg/24mg	–	Tab	–	–	–	Rugby	Antiasthmatic
4649	AHR 4649	Combination Enzyme / Antispasmodic	n/a	Green	Tab	Round	N	Y	A.H.Robins	Digestant/Antispas
	Rugby 4649	Theophylline CR	250mg	–	Cap	–	–	–	Rugby	Bronchodilator
4652	0115 4652	Hyoscyamine,Atropine,Scopolamine,Phenobarbital	n/a	White	Tab	Round	Y	N	Richlyn	Antispasmodic
4657	Rugby 4657	Theophylline CR	300mg	–	Cap	–	–	–	Rugby	Bronchodilator
4668	Rugby 4668	Tolbutamide	500mg	White	Tab	Round	–	N	Bolar	Hypoglycemic
4687	Rugby 4687	Trazodone	50mg	–	Tab	–	–	–	Rugby	Antidepressant
4688	Rugby 4688	Trazodone	100mg	–	Tab	–	–	–	Rugby	Antidepressant
4692	Rugby 4692	Sulfamethoxazole and Trimethoprim	400mg/80mg	–	Tab	–	–	–	Rugby	Anti–Infective
4693	Rugby 4693	Sulfamethoxazole and Trimethoprim	800mg/160mg	White	Tab	Oval	Y	N	Rugby	Anti–Infective
4694	Rugby 4694	Thyroid	30mg	–	Tab	–	–	–	Rugby	Hormone
4698	Rugby 4698	Thyroid	30mg	–	Tab	–	–	–	Rugby	Hormone
4700	MYLAN 4700	Gemfibrozil	300mg	Orange	Cap	–	–	–	Mylan	Antihyperlipidemic
4702	Rugby 4702	Thyroid	60mg	–	Tab	–	–	–	Rugby	Hormone
4706	Rugby 4706	Thyroid	60mg	–	Tab	–	–	–	Rugby	Hormone
4710	Rugby 4710	Thyroid	125mg	–	Tab	–	–	–	Rugby	Hormone
4711	0115 4711	Sulfadiazine,Sulfamerazine,Sulfamethazine	2.5/2.5/2.5gr	White	Tab	Round	Y	N	Richlyn	Anti–Infective
4714	0115 4714	Sulfadiazine	500mg	White	Tab	Round	Y	N	Richlyn	Anti–Infective
	Rugby 4714	Thyroid	125mg	–	Tab	–	–	–	Rugby	Hormone
4717	Rugby 4717	Triamcinolone	4mg	–	Tab	–	–	–	Rugby	Steroid
4720	Rugby 4720	HCTZ/Hydralazine/Reserpine (Hydroserpine Plus)	15mg/25mg/0.1mg	–	Tab	–	–	–	Rugby	Antihypertensive
4721	Rugby 4721	HCTZ/Hydralazine/Reserpine	15mg/25mg/0.1mg	–	Tab	–	–	–	Rugby	Antihypertensive
4725	Rugby 4725	Phenylprop.,phenyleph.,phenyltolox.,chlorphenir.	40,10,15,5mg	–	Tab	–	–	–	Rugby	Decongestant Comb.
4736	Rugby 4736	Tripelennamine	50mg	–	Tab	–	–	–	Rugby	Antihistamine
4737	Rugby 4737	Multivitamin/Fluoride	n/a	–	Tab	–	–	–	Rugby	Vitamin
4738	Rugby 4738	Tolazamide	100mg	–	Tab	–	–	–	Rugby	Hypoglycemic
4739	Rugby 4739	Tolazamide	250mg	–	Tab	–	–	–	Rugby	Hypoglycemic

ID NO.	ID CODE	GENERIC NAME	STRENGTH	COLOR	FORM	SHAPE	SCORED	COATED	MFG.	USE
4744	Rugby 4744	Tolazamide	500mg	–	Tab	–	Y	N	Rugby	Hypoglycemic
4747	0115 4747	Sulfasoxazole	500mg	White	Tab	Round	Y	N	Richlyn	Anti–Infective
4759	Rugby 4759	Therapeutic Vitamins	n/a	–	Tab	–	–	–	Amide	Vitamin
4760	Z 4760	Cefaclor	250mg	Purple	Cap	–	–	–	Zenith	Antiinfective
4761	Z 4761	Cefaclor	500mg	White/Gray	Cap	–	–	–	Zenith	Antiinfective
4804	Z 4804	Oxazepam	10mg	Blue/White	Cap	–	–	–	Zenith	Antianxiety
4805	Z 4805	Oxazepam	15mg	Clear	Cap	–	–	–	Zenith	Antianxiety
4806	Z 4806	Oxazepam	30mg	Orange/White	Cap	–	–	–	Zenith	Antianxiety
4811	Z 4811	Propoxyphene/Aspirin/Caffeine	65/389/32.4mg	Red/Gray	Cap	–	–	–	Zenith	Analgesic
4812	0115 4812	Thyroglobulin	1gr	Beige	Tab	Round	Y	N	Richlyn	Hormone
	Rugby 4812	Verapamil HCl	80mg	Aqua	Tab	Round	Y	N	Rugby	Antihypertensive
4813	Rugby 4813	Verapamil HCl	120mg	Blue	Tab	Round	Y	N	Rugby	Antihypertensive
4824	0115 4824	Thyroid	1gr	Beige	Tab	Round	N	N	Richlyn	Hormone
4825	0115 4825	Thyroid	1gr	Red	Tab	Round	N	Y	Richlyn	Hormone
4826	0115 4826	Thyroid	2gr	Beige	Tab	Round	N	N	Richlyn	Hormone
4827	0115 4827	Thyroid	2gr	Red	Tab	Round	N	Y	Richlyn	Hormone
4840	0115/4840	Triamcinolone	4mg	White	Tab	Round	Y	N	Richlyn	Steroid
	Rugby Logo 4840	Cyclobenzaprine HCl	10mg	–	Tab	–	–	–	Rugby	Muscle Relaxant
4841	4841	Neomycin Sulfate	500mg	White	Tab	Round	–	N	Eon	Anti–Infective
4860	0115/4860	Trichlormethiazide	4mg	Aqua	Tab	Round	Y	N	Richlyn	Diuretic
4861	Rugby 4861	Desipramine HCl	25mg	–	Tab	–	–	–	Rugby	Antidepressant
4862	Rugby 4862	Desipramine HCl	50mg	–	Tab	–	–	–	Rugby	Antidepressant
4863	Rugby 4863	Desipramine HCl	75mg	–	Tab	–	–	–	Rugby	Antidepressant
4864	Rugby 4864	Desipramine HCl	100mg	–	Tab	–	–	–	Rugby	Antidepressant
4871	0115 4871	Tripelennamine HCl	50mg	Blue	Tab	Round	Y	N	Richlyn	Antihistamine
4895	0115 4895	Benzoic A.,Methenamine,Phenyl Sal.,Atropine,Hyoscy	n/a	Purple	Tab	Round	N	Y	Richlyn	Urinary Anti–Infect
4900	0115 4900	Benzoic A.,Methen,Phenyl Sal.,Atropine,Hyosc,M.Blu	n/a	Blue	Tab	Round	N	Y	Richlyn	Urinary Anti–Infect
4902	0115 4902	Benzoic A.,Methen,Phenyl Sal.,Atropine,Hyosc,M.Blu	n/a	Purple	Tab	Round	N	Y	Richlyn	Urinary Anti–Infect
4903	Rugby 4903	Chlorpromazine	10 mg	Tan	Tab	Round	N	Y	PBI	Tranquilizer
4906	Rugby 4906	Chlorpromazine	25mg	Tan	Tab	Round	N	Y	PBI	Tranquilizer
4909	Rugby logo 4909	Reserpine, Hydralazine HCl, Hydrochlorothiazide	0.1mg/25mg/15mg	–	Tab	–	N	N	Rugby	Antihypertensive
4915	Rugby 4915	Chlorpromazine	50mg	Tan	Tab	Round	N	Y	PBI	Tranquilizer
4916	Rugby 4916	Chlorpromazine	100mg	Tan	Tab	Round	N	Y	PBI	Tranquilizer
4918	Rugby 4918	Chlorpromazine	200mg	Tan	Tab	Round	N	Y	PBI	Tranquilizer
4926	Rugby 4926	Triamterene & Hydrochlorothiazide	50mg/25mg	–	Cap	–	–	–	Rugby	Diuretic
4930	Rugby 4930	Triamterene/Hydrochlorothiazide	50mg/25mg	–	Cap	–	–	–	Rugby	Diuretic
4931	Rugby logo 4931	Verapamil HCl	80mg	–	Tab	–	–	–	Rugby	Antiarrhythmic
4932	Rugby logo 4932	Verapamil HCl	120mg	–	Tab	–	–	–	Rugby	Antiarrhythmic
4939	Rugby 4939	Indomethacin SR	75mg	Purple/White	Cap	–	–	–	Rugby	Anti–Inflammatory
4940	Rugby 4940	Clorazepate Dipotassium	3.75mg	–	Tab	–	–	–	Rugby	Antianxiety
4941	Rugby 4941	Clorazepate Dipotassium	7.5mg	–	Tab	–	–	–	Rugby	Antianxiety
4942	Rugby 4942	Clorazepate Dipotassium	15mg	–	Tab	–	–	–	Rugby	Antianxiety
4948	Rugby 4948	Disipramine	25mg	–	Tab	Round	N	Y	Rugby	Antidepressant
4949	Rugby 4949	Disipramine	50mg	–	Tab	Round	N	Y	Rugby	Antidepressant
4950	Rugby logo 4950	Theophylline (Anhydrous) Controlled Release	100mg	White	Tab	–	–	–	Rugby	Bronchodilator
4951	Rugby logo 4951	Theophylline (Anhydrous) Controlled Release	200mg	White	Tab	–	–	–	Rugby	Bronchodilator
4952	Rugby logo 4952	Theophylline (Anhydrous) Controlled Release	300mg	White	Tab	–	–	–	Rugby	Bronchodilator
4956	Rugby 4956	Triamterene/Hydrochlorothiazide	75mg/50mg	Yellow	Tab	Round	Y	N	Rugby	Diuretic
4957	Rugby 4957	Disipramine	75mg	–	Tab	Round	N	Y	Rugby	Antidepressant
4958	Rugby 4958	Disipramine	100mg	–	Tab	Round	N	Y	Rugby	Antidepressant
4959	Rugby 4959	Baclofen	10mg	–	Tab	–	–	–	Rugby	Anticonvulsive
4960	Rugby 4960	Baclofen	20mg	–	Tab	–	–	–	Rugby	Anticonvulsive
4963	Rugby 4963	Danazol	200mg	–	Cap	–	–	–	Rugby	Hormone
4972	V 4972	Phenazopyridine HCl	200mg	Red	Tab	Round	Y	Y	–	Urinary Antiseptic
4989	Rugby 4989	Yohimbine HCl	5.4mg	–	Tab	–	–	–	Rugby	Sympathicolytic
4996	Rugby logo 4996	Theophylline (Anhydrous) Controlled Release	100mg	White	Tab	–	–	–	Rugby	Bronchodilator
4997	Rugby logo 4997	Theophylline (Anhydrous) Controlled Release	200mg	White	Tab	–	–	–	Rugby	Bronchodilator
4998	Rugby logo 4998	Theophylline (Anhydrous) Controlled Release	300mg	White	Tab	–	–	–	Rugby	Bronchodilator
5000	bp 5000	Spironolactone	25mg	White	Tab	Round	Y	N	Bolar	Diuretic
	E 5000	Phentermine HCl	30mg	Blue/Clear	Cap	–	–	–	Eon	Anorectic
	PP 5000	Phentermine HCl	30mg	Blue/Natural	Cap	–	–	–	Eon	Anorectic
5002	DAN 5002	Diphenhydramine HCl	25mg	Pink/Clear	Cap	–	–	–	Danbury	Antihistamine
5003	DAN 5003	Diphenhydramine HCl	50mg	Pink/Pink	Cap	–	–	–	Danbury	Antihistamine
5010	bp 5010	Bethanechol Chloride	50mg	Yellow	Tab	Round	–	–	Bolar	Urinary Tract Agent
	Mylan 5010	Thiothixene	10mg	Caramel/Peach	Cap	–	N	N	Mylan	Tranquilizer
5023	PP 5023	Vitamin Combination	n/a	Yellow	Tab	Capsule	N	Y	Pioneer	Vitamin
5026	DAN 5026	Procainamide HCl	250mg	Yellow	Cap	–	–	–	Danbury	Antiarrhythmic
5028	DAN 5028	Quinine	5gr.	Clear/Clear	Cap	–	–	–	Danbury	Muscle Relaxant
	DAN 5028	Quinine Sulfate	325mg	White	Cap	–	–	–	Danbury	Muscle Relaxant
5040	BMS 5040	Atenolol	50mg	White	Tab	Round	–	–	BMS	Antihypertensive
5049	AHR 5049	Pancreatin/Pepsin/Bile Salts	300/250/150mg	White	Tab	Round	N	Y	A.H.Robins	Digestant
5050	DAN 5050	Hydralazine HCl	25mg	Orange	Tab	Round	N	Y	Danbury	Antihypertensive
	Mylan 5050	Temazepam	30mg	Yellow/Yellow	Cap	–	N	N	Mylan	Sedative
5052	DAN 5052	Prednisone	5mg	White	Tab	Round	Y	N	Danbury	Steroid
5055	DAN 5055	Hydralazine HCl	50mg	Orange	Tab	Round	N	Y	Danbury	Antihypertensive
5058	DAN/5058	Tripelennamine HCl	50mg	Bluish Green	Tab	Round	Y	N	Danbury	Antihistamine
5059	DAN 5059	Prednisolone	5mg	Peach	Tab	Round	Y	N	Danbury	Steroid
5156	E 5156	Papaverine HCl SR	150mg	Brown/Clear	Cap	–	–	–	Eon	Vasodilator
	PP–5156	Papaverine HCl	150mg	Brown/Clear	Cap	–	–	–	Eon	Vasodilator
5162	DAN 5162	Tetracylcine HCl	250mg	Orange/Yellow	Cap	–	–	–	Danbury	Anti–Infective
5174	E 5174	Nitroglycerin SR	2.5mg	Amethyst/Clear	Cap	–	–	–	Eon	Antianginal
	PP–5174	Nitroglycerin	2.5mg	Amethyst/Clear	Cap	–	–	–	Eon	Antianginal
5183	DAN 5183	Hydrocortisone	20mg	White	Tab	Round	Y	N	Danbury	Steroid
5196	DAN 5196	Papaverine HCl	150mg	Brown/Clear	Cap	–	–	–	Danbury	Vasodilator
5200	MYLAN 5200	Tolmetin Sodium	400mg	Blue	Cap	–	–	–	Mylan	Anti–Inflammatory
5204	DAN 5204	Pseudoephedrine HCl	60mg	White	Tab	Round	Y	N	Danbury	Decongestant
5216	DAN/5216	Folic Acid	1mg	Yellow	Tab	Round	N	N	Danbury	Antianemic
5240	BMS 5240	Atenolol	100mg	White	Tab	Round	–	–	BMS	Antihypertensive
5254	PP–5254	Phendimetrazine Tartrate TR	105mg	Brown/Clear	Cap	–	–	–	Eon	Anorectic
5304	DAN 5304	Promethazine HCl	12.5mg	Gray	Tab	Round	Y	N	Danbury	Antiemetic
5307	DAN 5307	Promethazine HCl	25mg	White	Tab	Round	Y	N	Danbury	Antiemetic
5316	DAN 5316	Phenylbutazone (Veterinary)	100mg	White	Tab	Round	N	Y	Danbury	Anti–Inflammatory
5319	DAN 5319	Promethazine HCl	50mg	Pink	Tab	Round	Y	N	Danbury	Antiemetic
5321	DAN/5321	Primidone	250mg	White	Tab	Round	N	N	Danbury	Anticonvulsant
5325	DAN 5325	Colchicine & Probenecid	0.5mg/500mg	White	Tab	Capsule	Y	N	Danbury	Antigout

ID NO.	ID CODE	GENERIC NAME	STRENGTH	COLOR	FORM	SHAPE	SCORED	COATED	MFG.	USE
5326	DAN 5326	Probenecid & Colchicine	500mg/0.5mg	White	Tab	Capsule	Y	N	Danbury	Antigout
5333	DAN 5333	Procainamide HCl	500mg	Orange/Yellow	Cap	–	–	–	Danbury	Antiarrhythmic
5335	DAN/5335	Trihexyphenidyl	2mg	White	Tab	Round	N	N	Danbury	Antiparkinson
5337	DAN/5337	Trihexyphenidyl	5mg	White	Tab	Round	N	N	Danbury	Antiparkinson
5342	DAN 5342	Nylidrin HCl	6mg	White	Tab	Round	Y	N	Danbury	Vasodilator
5345	DAN 5345	Hydrochlorothiazide	50mg	Peach	Tab	Round	Y	N	Danbury	Diuretic
5347	DAN/5347	Probenecid	500mg	Yellow	Tab	Capsule	Y	Y	Danbury	Antigout
	U:DAN L:5347	Minoxidil	10mg	White	Tab	Round	Y	N	Danbury	Antihypertensive
5350	DAN/5350	Procainamide HCl	375mg	Orange/White	Cap	–	–	–	Danbury	Antiarrhythmic
5361	DAN 5361 0.75	Dexamethasone	0.75mg	Blue	Tab	Pentagonal	Y	N	Danbury	Steroid
5368	Dan/5368	Disulfiram	500mg	White	Tab	Round	N	N	Danbury	Alcohol Deterrent
5369	DAN/5369	Bethanechol	10mg	White	Tab	Round	Y	N	Danbury	Urinary Tract Agent
5373	DAN 5373	Isosorbide Dinitrate	10mg	White	Tab	Round	Y	N	Danbury	Antianginal
5374	DAN 5374	Isosorbide Dinitrate	5mg	Pink	Tab	Round	Y	N	Danbury	Antianginal
5375	Mylan 5375	Doxepin HCl	75mg	Green/Green	Cap	–	–	–	Mylan	Antidepressant
5376	Dan/5376	Disulfiram	250mg	White	Tab	Round	N	N	Danbury	Alcohol Deterrent
5380	E 5380	Foltrin	–	Red/Scarlet	Cap	–	–	–	Eon	Iron Supplement
	PP 5380	Multivitamin/Mineral	n/a	Red/Maroon	Cap	–	–	–	Eon	Vitamin
5381	DAN 5381	Methocarbamol	500mg	White	Tab	Round	Y	N	Danbury	Muscle Relaxant
5382	DAN 5382	Methocarbamol	750mg	White	Tab	Capsule	Y	N	Danbury	Muscle Relaxant
5385	DAN 5385	Isosorbide Dinitrate Sublingual	5mg	White	Tab	Round	N	N	Danbury	Antianginal
	E 5385	Ferrous Sulfate SR	250mg	Red/Clear	Cap	–	–	–	Eon	Iron Supp.
5387	DAN 5387	Isosorbide Dinitrate Sublingual	2.5mg	Yellow	Tab	Round	N	N	Danbury	Antianginal
5388	DAN/5388	Triamcinolone	4mg	White	Tab	Oglong	Y	N	Danbury	Steroid
5390	DAN 5390	Nylidrin HCl	12mg	White	Tab	Round	Y	N	Danbury	Vasodilator
5402	DAN/5402	Bethanechol	25mg	Yellow	Tab	Round	N	N	Danbury	Urinary Tract Agent
5406	DAN/5406	Hydrochlorothiazide & Reserpine	25mg/0.125mg	Green	Tab	Round	N	N	Danbury	Antihypertensive
5407	DAN/5407	Hydrochlorothiazide & Reserpine	50mg/0.125mg	Green	Tab	Round	N	N	Danbury	Antihypertensive
5428	DAN 5428	Hydrochlorothiazide/Hydralazine HCl/Reserpine	15mg/25mg/.1mg	Yellow	Tab	Round	N	N	Danbury	Antihypertensive
5430	DAN/DAN 5430	Acetazolamide	250mg	White	Tab	Round	Y	N	Danbury	Antiglaucoma
5432	5432	Amphetamine/Dextroamphetamine Combination	n/a	Blue	Tab	Round	–	–	Rexar	Anoretic
5434	DAN 5434	Triprolidine HCl & Pseudoephedrine HCl	2.5mg/60mg	White	Tab	Round	Y	N	Danbury	Decongestant Comb.
5438	DAN 5438	Quinidine Sulfate	200mg	White	Tab	Round	Y	N	Danbury	Antiarrhythmic
5440	Dan 5440	Doxycycline	100mg	Blue	Cap	–	–	–	Danbury	Anti–Infective
5442	DAN 5442	Prednisone	10mg	White	Tab	Round	Y	N	Danbury	Steroid
	DAN/5442	Prednisone	10mg	White	Tab	Round	N	N	Geneva	Steroid
5443	DAN 5443	Prednisone	20mg	Peach	Tab	Round	Y	N	Danbury	Steroid
5444	DAN 5444	Chlorothiazide	250mg	White	Tab	Round	Y	N	Danbury	Diuretic
5449	AHR 5449	Benzthiazide	50mg	Yellow	Tab	Round	Y	N	A.H.Robins	Diuretic
	DAN 5449 0.25	Dexamethasone	0.25mg	Orange	Tab	Pentagonal	Y	N	Danbury	Steroid
5450	DAN 5450 0.5	Dexamethasone	0.5mg	Yellow	Tab	Pentagonal	Y	N	Danbury	Steroid
5451	5451	Dextroamphetamine Sulfate	10mg	Yellow	Tab	Round	Y	N	Rexar	Psychostimulant
	DAN 5451 1.5	Dexamethasone	1.5mg	White	Tab	Pentagonal	Y	N	Danbury	Steroid
5452	5452	Dextroamphetamine Sulfate	5mg	Yellow	Tab	Round	Y	N	Rexar	Psychostimulant
5453	DAN 5453	Quinidine Sulfate	100mg	White	Tab	Round	Y	N	Danbury	Antiarrhythmic
5454	DAN/5454	Quinidine Sulfate	300mg	White	Tab	Round	Y	N	Danbury	Antiarrhythmic
5455	5455	Methamphetamine HCl	5mg	Pink	Tab	Round	Y	N	Rexar	Psychostimulant
	DAN 5455	Chlorpropamide	250mg	Blue	Tab	Round	Y	N	Danbury	Hypoglycemic
5456	5456	Methamphetamine HCl	10mg	Pink	Tab	Round	Y	N	Rexar	Psychostimulant
5457	5457	Phendimetrazine Tartrate	35mg	Blue	Tab	Round	–	–	Rexar	Anoretic
	5457	Phendimetrazine Tartrate	35mg	Green	Tab	Round	–	–	Rexar	Anoretic
	5457	Phendimetrazine Tartrate	35mg	Pink	Tab	Round	–	–	Rexar	Anoretic
	5457	Phendimetrazine Tartrate	35mg	Yellow	Tab	Round	–	–	Rexar	Anoretic
5460	5460	Phendimetrazine Tartrate	35mg	Yellow	Tab	Round	–	–	Rexar	Anoretic
5462	5462	Phendimetrazine Tartrate	105mg	Brown/Clear	Cap	–	–	–	Rexar	Anoretic
5463	5463	Phendimetrazine Tartrate	35mg	Blue	Cap	–	–	–	Rexar	Anoretic
	5463	Phendimetrazine Tartrate	35mg	Blue	Cap	–	–	–	Rexar	Anoretic
	5463	Phendimetrazine Tartrate	35mg	Red/White	Cap	–	–	–	Rexar	Anoretic
5468	5468	Phentermine HCl	30mg	Black	Cap	–	–	–	Rexar	Anoretic
	5468	Phentermine HCl	30mg	Black	Cap	–	–	–	Rexar	Anoretic
	5468	Phentermine HCl	30mg	Yellow	Tab	Round	–	–	Rexar	Anoretic
5479	DAN/5479	Erythromycin Estolate	250mg	Orange/Ivory	Cap	–	–	–	Danbury	Anti–Infective
5484	DAN 5484	Cyproheptadine HCl	4mg	White	Tab	Round	Y	N	Danbury	Antipruretic
5490	DAN 5490	Prednisone	50mg	White	Tab	Round	Y	N	Danbury	Steroid
5495	DAN 5495	Chlorzoxazone	250mg	Peach	Tab	Round	Y	N	Danbury	Muscle Relaxant
5496	DAN 5496	Spironolactone & Hydrochlorothiazide	25mg/25mg	Buff	Tab	Round	Y	N	Danbury	Diuretic
5501	DAN 5501	Ergoloid Mesylates S.L.	1mg	White	Tab	Round	N	N	Danbury	Vasodilator
5502	DAN 5502	Ergoloid Mesylates S.L.	0.5mg	White	Tab	Round	N	N	Danbury	Vasodilator
5503	DAN/5503	Sulfasalazine	500mg	Butterscotch	Tab	Round	N	N	Danbury	Anti–Inflammatory
5504	DAN 5504	Ergoloid Mesylates Oral	1mg	White	Tab	Round	N	N	Danbury	Vasodilator
5506	DAN 5506	Pseudoephedrine HCl	30mg	Red	Tab	Round	N	Y	Danbury	Decongestant
5507	DAN 5507	Chlorthalidone	25mg	Yellow	Tab	Round	N	N	Danbury	Diuretic
5508	DAN 5508	Tolbutamide	500mg	White	Tab	Round	Y	N	Danbury	Hypoglycemic
5510	DAN 5510	Dipyridamole	25mg	White	Tab	Round	N	Y	Danbury	Antiplatelet
5511	DAN 5511	Dipyridamole	50mg	White	Tab	Round	N	Y	Danbury	Antiplatelet
	PP-5511	Chlorpheniramine Maleate SR	8mg	Green/Clear	Cap	–	–	–	Eon	Antihistamine
5512	DAN 5512	Dipyridamole	75mg	White	Tab	Round	N	Y	Danbury	Antiplatelet
	PP-5512	Chlorpheniramine Maleate SR	12mg	Green/Clear	Cap	–	–	–	Eon	Antihistamine
5513	DAN/5513	Carisoprodol	350mg	White	Tab	Round	N	N	Danbury	Muscle Relaxant
5514	DAN 5514	Sulfinpyrazone	100mg	White	Tab	Round	N	N	Danbury	Anti–Inflammatory
5515	Dan 5515	Bethanechol Chloride	50mg	Yellow	Tab	Round	Y	N	Danbury	Urinary Tract Agent
5516	DAN 5516	Quinine Sulfate	260mg	White	Tab	Round	Y	N	Danbury	Muscle Relaxant
5518	DAN 5518	Chlorthalidone	50mg	Green	Tab	Round	N	N	Danbury	Diuretic
5520	DAN 5520	Tetracycline HCl	500mg	Black/Yellow	Cap	–	–	–	Danbury	Anti–Infective
5522	DAN 5522	Hydroxyzine HCl	10mg	Orange	Tab	Round	N	Y	Danbury	Antipruritic
5523	DAN 5523	Hydroxyzine HCl	25mg	Green	Tab	Round	N	Y	Danbury	Antipruritic
5535	Dan 5535	Doxycycline	50mg	Blue/White	Cap	–	–	–	Danbury	Anti–Infective
5538	DAN 5538	Quinidine Gluconate	324mg	White	Tab	Round	N	N	Danbury	Antiarrhythmic
5540	DAN 5540	Metronidazole	250mg	White	Tab	Round	N	N	Danbury	Anti–Infective
5542	25/DAN 5542	Thioridazine HCl	25mg	Beige	Tab	Triangular	N	Y	Danbury	Tranquilizer
5543	DAN 5543	Allopurinol	100mg	White	Tab	Round	Y	N	Danbury	Antigout
5544	DAN 5544	Allopurinol	300mg	Orange	Tab	Round	Y	N	Danbury	Antigout
5546	DAN/5546	Sulfamethoxazole & Trimethoprim	400mg/80mg	White	Tab	Round	N	N	Danbury	Anti–Infective
5547	DAN/5547	Sulfamethoxazole & Trimethoprim	800mg/160mg	White	Tab	Oval	Y	N	Danbury	Anti–Infective
5548	DAN 5548	Chloroquine Phosphate	250mg	White	Tab	Round	Y	N	Danbury	Antimalarial

ID NO.	ID CODE	GENERIC NAME	STRENGTH	COLOR	FORM	SHAPE	SCORED	COATED	MFG.	USE
	DAN/5548	Chloroquine Phosphate	250mg	White	Tab	Round	Y	N	Danbury	Antimalarial
5549	DAN 5549	Chloroquine Phosphate	500mg	White	Tab	Round	N	Y	Danbury	Antimalarial
5552	DAN 5552	Metronidazole	500mg	White	Tab	Round	Y	N	Danbury	Anti-Infective
5553	Dan 5553	Doxycycline	100mg	Salmon	Tab	Round	–	–	Danbury	Anti-Infective
	DAN 5553	Doxyclcline Hyclate	100mg	Orange	Tab	Round	N	Y	Danbury	Anti-Infective
5554	DAN 5554 / 10	Propranolol HCI	10mg	Orange	Tab	Round	Y	N	Danbury	Antihypertensive
5555	DAN 5555 / 20	Propranolol HCI	20mg	Blue	Tab	Round	Y	N	Danbury	Antihypertensive
5556	DAN 5556 / 40	Propranolol HCI	40mg	Green	Tab	Round	Y	N	Danbury	Antihypertensive
5557	DAN 5557 / 80	Propranolol HCI	80mg	Yellow	Tab	Round	Y	N	Danbury	Antihypertensive
5560	DAN 5560	Disopyramide Phosphate	100mg	Orange/Orange	Cap	–	–	–	Danbury	Antiarrhythmic
5561	DAN 5561	Disopyramide Phosphate	150mg	Brown/Brown	Cap	–	–	–	Danbury	Antiarrhythmic
5562	DAN/DAN 5562	Procainamide HCI SR	250mg	White	Tab	Oval	N	Y	Danbury	Antiarrhythmic
5563	DAN/DAN 5563	Procainamide HCI SR	500mg	White	Tab	Oval	Y	Y	Danbury	Antiarrhythmic
5564	DAN/DAN 5564	Procainamide HCI SR	750mg	White	Tab	Oval	Y	Y	Danbury	Antiarrhythmic
5565	DAN 5565	Hydroxyzine HCI	50mg	Yellow	Tab	Round	N	Y	Danbury	Antipruritic
5566	10/DAN 5566	Thioridazine HCI	10mg	Yellowish green	Tab	Triangular	N	Y	Danbury	Tranquilizer
5568	50/DAN 5568	Thioridazine HCI	50mg	White	Tab	Triangular	N	Y	Danbury	Tranquilizer
5569	DAN 5569	Thioridazine HCI	100mg	Orange	Tab	Round	N	Y	Danbury	Tranquilizer
5571	DAN 5571	Trimethoprim	100mg	White	Tab	Oval	Y	N	Danbury	Anti-Infective
5572	DAN 5572	Thioridazine HCI	15mg	White	Tab	Round	N	Y	Danbury	Tranquilizer
5575	DAN 5575	Furosemide	40mg	White	Tab	Round	Y	N	Danbury	Diuretic
5576	DAN 5576	Furosemide	20mg	White	Tab	Round	N	N	Danbury	Diuretic
5579	DAN 5579	Chlorpropamide	100mg	Blue	Tab	Round	Y	N	Danbury	Hypoglycemic
5580	DAN 5580	Thioridazine HCI	150mg	Orange	Tab	Round	N	Y	Danbury	Tranquilizer
5581	DAN/5581	Thioridazine	200mg	Orange	Tab	Round	N	Y	Danbury	Tranquilizer
5582	DAN 5582	Tolazamide	250mg	White	Tab	Round	Y	N	Danbury	Hypoglycemic
5584	DAN 5584	Ibuprofen	400mg	White	Tab	Round	N	Y	Danbury	Anti-Inflammatory
5585	DAN 5585	Ibuprofen	200mg	White	Tab	Round	N	Y	Danbury	Analgesic
5586	DAN 5586	Ibuprofen	600mg	White	Tab	Oval	N	Y	Danbury	Anti-Inflammatory
5587	DAN–5587	Methyldopa	500mg	White	Tab	Round	N	Y	Danbury	Antihypertensive
5588	DAN–5588	Methyldopa	250mg	White	Tab	Round	N	Y	Danbury	Antihypertensive
5589	DAN 5589	Metoclopramide HCI	10mg	White	Tab	Round	Y	N	Danbury	Antireflux
5590	DAN 5590	Tolazamide	500mg	White	Tab	Round	Y	N	Danbury	Hypoglycemic
5591	DAN 5591	Tolazamide	100mg	White	Tab	Round	Y	N	Danbury	Hypoglycemic
5592	DAN/5592	Thiothixene	2mg	Green	Cap	–	–	–	Danbury	Tranquilizer
5593	DAN/5593	Thiothixene	1mg	Yellow	Cap	–	–	–	Danbury	Tranquilizer
5594	DAN/5594	Thiothixene	10mg	White	Cap	–	–	–	Danbury	Tranquilizer
5595	DAN/5595	Thiothixene	5mg	Orange	Cap	–	–	–	Danbury	Tranquilizer
5597	Dan/Dan 5597	Acetohexamide	500mg	White	Tab	Capsule	N	N	Danbury	Antiglaucoma
5598	Dan/Dan 5598	Acetohexamide	250mg	White	Tab	Capsule	N	N	Danbury	Antiglaucoma
5599	DAN 5599	Trazodone	100mg	White	Tab	Round	Y	Y	Danbury	Antidepressant
5600	DAN 5600	Trazodone	50mg	White	Tab	Round	Y	Y	Danbury	Antidepressant
	Z 5600	Lorazepam	0.5mg	White	Tab	Round	–	N	Zenith	Antianxiety
5601	DAN 5601	Verapamil HCI	80mg	White	Tab	Round	Y	Y	Danbury	Antihypertensive
5602	DAN 5602	Verapamil HCI	120mg	White	Tab	Round	Y	Y	Danbury	Antihypertensive
5603	DAN 5603/2	Haloperidol	2mg	Peach	Tab	Round	Y	N	Danbury	Tranquilizer
5604	DAN 5604/1	Haloperidol	1mg	Orange	Tab	Round	Y	N	Danbury	Tranquilizer
5605	DAN 5605 0.5	Haloperidol	0.5mg	White	Tab	Round	Y	N	Danbury	Tranquilizer
5606	DAN 5606/5	Haloperidol	5mg	Blue	Tab	Round	Y	N	Danbury	Tranquilizer
5607	DAN 5607 15	Methyldopa & Hydrochlorothiazide	250mg/15mg	White	Tab	Round	N	Y	Danbury	Antihypertensive
5608	DAN 5608 25	Methyldopa & Hydrochlorothiazide	250mg/25mg	White	Tab	Round	N	Y	Danbury	Antihypertensive
5609	DAN 5609/0.1	Clonidine	0.1mg	White	Tab	Pentagonal	Y	N	Danbury	Antihypertensive
5610	DAN 5610 50	Methyldopa & Hydrochlorothiazide	500mg/50mg	White	Tab	Round	N	Y	Danbury	Antihypertensive
5611	DAN 5611 30	Methyldopa & Hydrochlorothiazide	500mg/30mg	Yellow	Tab	Round	N	Y	Danbury	Antihypertensive
5612	DAN 5612/0.2	Clonidine	0.2mg	Yellow	Tab	Pentagonal	Y	N	Danbury	Antihypertensive
5613	DAN 5613/0.3	Clonidine	0.3mg	Blue	Tab	Pentagonal	Y	N	Danbury	Antihypertensive
5614	DAN 5614	Flurazepam HCI	15mg	Blue/White	Cap	–	–	–	Danbury	Hypnotic
5615	DAN 5615	Flurazepam HCI	30mg	Blue/Blue	Cap	–	–	–	Danbury	Hypnotic
5616	DAN 5616	Oxazepam	15mg	Red/Red	Cap	–	–	–	Danbury	Antianxiety
5617	DAN 5617	Oxazepam	10mg	White/White	Cap	–	–	–	Danbury	Antianxiety
5618	DAN 5618	Oxazepam	30mg	Maroon/Maroon	Cap	–	–	–	Danbury	Antianxiety
5619	DAN 5619/5	Diazepam	5mg	Yellow	Tab	Round	Y	N	Danbury	Antianxiety
5620	DAN 5620/10	Diazepam	10mg	Blue	Tab	Round	Y	N	Danbury	Antianxiety
5621	DAN 5621/2	Diazepam	2mg	White	Tab	Round	Y	N	Danbury	Antianxiety
5622	DAN 5622 / 2	Lorazepam	2mg	White	Tab	Round	Y	N	Danbury	Antianxiety
5623	DAN 5623 / 60	Propranolol HCI	60mg	Red	Tab	Round	Y	N	Danbury	Antihypertensive
5624	DAN 5624 / 1	Lorazepam	1mg	White	Tab	Round	Y	N	Danbury	Antianxiety
5625	DAN 5625 / 0.5	Lorazepam	0.5mg	White	Tab	Round	Y	N	Danbury	Antianxiety
5629	DAN 5629	Doxepin HCI	10mg	Buff/Buff	Cap	–	–	–	Danbury	Antidepressant
5630	DAN 5630	Doxepin HCI	25mg	Ivory/White	Cap	–	–	–	Danbury	Antidepressant
5631	DAN 5631	Doxepin HCI	50mg	Ivory/Ivory	Cap	–	–	–	Danbury	Antidepressant
5632	DAN 5632	Doxepin HCI	75mg	Green/Green	Cap	–	–	–	Danbury	Antidepressant
5633	DAN 5633	Doxepin HCI	100mg	Green/White	Cap	–	–	–	Danbury	Antidepressant
5635	DAN 5635 / 90	Propranolol HCI	90mg	Lavender	Tab	Round	Y	N	Danbury	Antihypertensive
5636	DAN 5636	Meclofenamate	50mg	Coral/Coral	Cap	–	–	–	Danbury	Anti-Inflammatory
5637	DAN 5637	Meclofenamate	100mg	Coral/White	Cap	–	–	–	Danbury	Anti-Inflammatory
5642	DAN 5642 /2.5	Minoxidil	2.5mg	White	Tab	Round	Y	N	Danbury	Antihypertensive
5643	DAN 5643 /10	Minoxidil	10mg	White	Tab	Round	Y	N	Danbury	Antihypertensive
5644	DAN 5644	Ibuprofen	800mg	White	Tab	Oval	N	Y	Danbury	Anti-Inflammatory
5658	DAN 5658	Cyclobenzaprine HCI	10mg	White	Tab	Round	N	Y	Danbury	Muscle Relaxant
5659	DAN 5659	Furosemide	80mg	White	Tab	Round	Y	N	Danbury	Diuretic
5660	DAN 5660	Sulindac	200mg	Yellow	Tab	Round	Y	N	Danbury	Anti-Inflammatory
5661	DAN 5661	Sulindac	150mg	Yellow	Tab	Round	Y	N	Danbury	Anti-Inflammatory
5662	DAN/5662	Nalidixic Acid	1GM	White	Tab	Oval	N	N	Danbury	Anti-Infective
5677	DAN/5677	Nalidixic Acid	500mg	White	Tab	Round	N	N	Danbury	Anti-Infective
5678	DAN 5678	Chlordiazepoxide/Amitriptyline HCI	10mg/25mg	White	Tab	Round	N	Y	Danbury	Antianxiety
5679	DAN 5679	Chlordiazepoxide/Amitriptyline HCI	5mg/12.5mg	Green	Tab	Round	N	Y	Danbury	Antianxiety
5682	DAN 5682	Triamterene & Hydrochlorothiazide	75mg/50mg	Yellow	Tab	Round	Y	N	Danbury	Antihypertensive
5693	DAN 5693	Prazosin HCI	5mg	Orange	Cap	–	–	–	Danbury	Antihypertensive
5696	DAN 5696	Prazosin HCI	2mg	Gray	Cap	–	–	–	Danbury	Antihypertensive
5697	DAN 5697	Prazosin HCI	1mg	Yellow	Cap	–	–	–	Danbury	Antihypertensive
5704	DAN/DAN 5704	Fenoprofen Calcium	600mg	White	Tab	Tablet	Y	Y	Danbury	Antiinflammatory
5706	DAN-500, 5706	Chlorzoxazone	500mg	Green	Tab	Round	Y	N	Danbury	Muscle Relaxant
5708	DAN 5708	Clindamycin	150mg	Gray/Pink	Cap	–	N	N	Danbury	Anti-Infective
5710	DAN-5710, 2	Albuterol Sulfate	2mg	White	Tab	Round	Y	N	Danbury	Antiasthmatic

ID NO.	ID CODE	GENERIC NAME	STRENGTH	COLOR	FORM	SHAPE	SCORED	COATED	MFG.	USE
5711	DAN–5711, 4	Albuterol Sulfate	4mg	White	Tab	Round	Y	N	Danbury	Antiasthmatic
5713	DAN 5713 25	Amoxapine	25mg	White	Tab	Round	Y	N	Danbury	Antidepressant
5714	DAN 5714 50	Amoxapine	50mg	Orange	Tab	Round	Y	N	Danbury	Antidepressant
5715	DAN 5715 100	Amoxapine	100mg	White	Tab	Round	Y	N	Danbury	Antidepressant
5716	DAN 5716 150	Amoxapine	150mg	Orange	Tab	Round	Y	N	Danbury	Antidepressant
5720	VT–5720	Phendimetrazine Tartrate	35mg	Red/Clear	Cap	–	–	–	Eon	Anorectic
5724	DAN 10 5724	Metaproterenol Sulfate	10mg	White	Tab	Round	N	N	Danbury	Bronchodilator
5725	DAN 20 5725	Metaproterenol Sulfate	20mg	White	Tab	Round	N	N	Danbury	Bronchodilator
5726	DAN 5726	Hydroxyzine Pamoate	25mg	Green/Lt.Green	Cap	–	–	–	Danbury	Antianxiety
	R 5726	Carbinoxamine Maleate & Pseudoephedrine	4mg/60mg	Tan	Tab	Oblong	N	N	Ross	Decongestant Comb.
5730	DAN–10, 5730	Baclofen	10mg	White	Tab	Round	Y	N	Danbury	Muscle Relaxant
	PP–5730	Phendimetrazine Tartrate	35mg	Blue/Clear	Cap	–	–	–	Eon	Anorectic
5731	DAN–20, 5731	Baclofen	20mg	White	Tab	Round	Y	N	Danbury	Muscle Relaxant
5736	DAN 5736 5	Timolol Maleate	5mg	White	Tab	Round	N	N	Danbury	Antihypertensive
5737	DAN 5737 10	Timolol Maleate	10mg	White	Tab	Round	Y	N	Danbury	Antihypertensive
5738	DAN/20 5738	Timolol Maleate	20mg	White	Tab	Capsule	Y	N	Danbury	Antihypertensive
5740	PP–5740	Phendimetrazine Tartrate	35mg	Orange/Clear	Cap	–	–	–	Eon	Anorectic
5752	SCS 5752	Piroxicam	10mg	Blue/Orange	Cap	–	N	N	Searle	Anti–Inflammatory
5762	SCS 5762	Piroxicam	20mg	Orange/Opaque	Cap	–	N	N	Searle	Anti–Inflammatory
5777	DAN–5777, 50	Atenolol	50mg	White	Tab	Round	Y	N	Danbury	Antihypertensive
5778	DAN–5778, 100	Atenolol	100mg	White	Tab	Round	Y	N	Danbury	Antihypertensive
5782	DAN 5782	Atenolol/Chlorthalidone	50mg/25mg	White	Tab	Round	Y	N	Danbury	Antihypertensive
5783	DAN 5783	Atenolol/Chlorthalidone	100mg/25mg	White	Tab	Round	Y	N	Danbury	Antihypertensive
5800	Z 5800	Lorazepam	1mg	White	Tab	Round	–	N	Zenith	Antianxiety
5816	AHR 5816	Sodium Salicylate & Sodium Aminobenzoate	300mg/300mg	Yellow	Tab	Round	N	Y	A.H.Robins	Analgesic
5825	M 5825	Thioridazine HCl	25mg	–	Tab	Round	N	Y	Roxane	Antipsychotic
5883	AHR 5883	Potassium Salicylate & Potassium Aminobenzoate	300mg/300mg	Rose	Tab	Round	N	Y	A.H.Robins	Analgesic
5950	M 5950	Thioridazine HCl	50mg	–	Tab	Round	N	Y	Roxane	Antipsychotic
6000	Z 6000	Lorazepam	2mg	White	Tab	Round	–	N	Zenith	Antianxiety
6001	PP 6001	Ephedrine,Hydroxyzine,Theophylline	25mg/10mg/130mg	Blue	Tab	Round	N	N	Pioneer	Antiasthmatic
6004	PP 6004	Folic Acid	1mg	Yellow	Tab	Round	Y	N	Pioneer	Antianemic
6007	PP 6007	Diazepam	2mg	White	Tab	Round	Y	N	Pioneer	Antianxiety
6008	PP 6008	Diazepam	5mg	Yellow	Tab	Round	Y	N	Pioneer	Antianxiety
6009	PP 6009	Diazepam	10mg	Blue	Tab	Round	Y	N	Pioneer	Antianxiety
6012	PP 6012	Chlorzoxazone	250mg	Peach	Tab	Round	Y	N	Pioneer	Muscle relaxant
6013	PP 6013	Dicyclomine HCl	20mg	Blue	Tab	Round	Y	N	Pioneer	Antispasmodic
6015	PP 6015	Cyproheptadine HCl	4mg	White	Tab	Round	N	N	Pioneer	Antipruritic
6017	PP 6017	Chlorzoxazone & APAP	250mg/300mg	Green	Tab	Round	N	N	Pioneer	Muscle Relaxant
6018	PP 6018	Carisoprodol	350mg	White	Tab	Round	–	–	Pioneer	Muscle Relaxant
6026	PP 6026	Chlorpheniramine Maleate	4mg	Yellow	Tab	Round	Y	N	Pioneer	Antihistamine
6031	PP 6031	Brompheniramine Maleate	4mg	Orange	Tab	Round	Y	N	Pioneer	Antihistamine
6036	PP 6036	Methocarbamol	500mg	White	Tab	Round	Y	N	Pioneer	Muscle Relaxant
6038	PP 6038	Methocarbamol	750mg	White	Tab	Oblong	N	N	Pioneer	Muscle Relaxant
6048	PP 6048	Chlorzoxazone	500mg	Green	Tab	Capsule	N	N	Pioneer	Muscle relaxant
6062	PP 6062	Chlorthalidone	25mg	Peach	Tab	Round	–	–	Pioneer	Diuretic
6063	PP 6063	Chlorthalidone	50mg	Blue	Tab	Round	–	–	Pioneer	Diuretic
6100	Z 6100	Hydroxyzine HCl	10mg	Lavender	Tab	Round	–	Y	Zenith	Antipruritic
6110	M 6110	Thioridazine HCl	100mg	–	Tab	Round	N	Y	Roxane	Antipsychotic
6113	832/6113	Carbamazepine	200mg	White	Tab	Round	Y	N	PBI	Anticonvulsant
6120	C 86120	Isometheptene Mucate/Dichloralphenazone/APAP	65mg/100mg/325	Red with Pink Band	Cap	–	–	–	Carnrick	Antimigraine
6200	Z 6200	Hydroxyzine HCl	25mg	Magenta	Tab	Round	–	Y	Zenith	Antipruritic
6204	C 86204	Phenindamine/Chlorpheniramine/Phenylpropanolamine	24mg/4mg/50mg	Pink	Tab	Round	N	Y	Carnrick	Decongestant Comb.
6240	R 6240	Carbinoxamine Maleate & Pseudoephedrine	8mg/120mg	Blue	Tab	Oblong	N	Y	Ross	Decongestant Comb.
6242	AHR 6242	Acetaminophen & Codeine	325mg/15mg	Black/Yellow	Cap	–	–	–	A.H.Robins	Analgesic
6251	AHR 6251	Acetaminophen & Codeine	650mg/30mg	White	Tab	Capsule	Y	N	A.H.Robins	Analgesic
6257	AHR 6257	Acetaminophen & Codeine	325mg/30mg	Black/Green	Cap	–	–	–	A.H.Robins	Analgesic
6265	PP–6265	Phendimetrazine Tartrate	35mg	Black/Orange	Cap	–	–	–	Eon	Anorectic
6274	AHR 6274	Acetaminophen & Codeine	325mg/60mg	Green/White	Cap	–	–	–	A.H.Robins	Analgesic
6300	Z 6300	Hydroxyzine HCl	50mg	Purple	Tab	Round	–	Y	Zenith	Antipruritic
6350	UAD 6350	Hydrocodone Bitartrate with Acetaminophen	10mg/650mg	Blue	Tab	Oblong	Y	N	UAD	Analgesic
6410	Mylan 6410	Doxepin HCl	100mg	Green/White	Cap	–	–	–	Mylan	Antidepressant
6447	AHR 6447	Fenfluramine HCl	20mg	Orange	Tab	Round	Y	N	A.H.Robins	Anorectic
7025	RR 7025	Meclizine HCl	20mg	Red	Tab	Round	N	Y	RR	Antivertigo
7131	AHR/50 7131	Amoxicillin Veterinary Tablets	50mg	White	Tab	Round	–	–	Biocraft	Anti–Infective
7141	AHR/100 7141	Amoxicillin Veterinary Tablets	100mg	White	Tab	Round	–	–	Biocraft	Anti–Infective
7151	AHR/200 7151	Amoxicillin Veterinary Tablets	200mg	White	Tab	Round	–	–	Biocraft	Anti–Infective
7171	AHR/400 7171	Amoxicillin Veterinary Tablets	400mg	White	Tab	Round	–	–	Biocraft	Anti–Infective
7271	BRISTOL 7271 500mg	Cefadroxil	500mg	Blue/Black	Cap	–	–	–	Bristol	Anti–Infective
7278	Bristol 7278	Amoxicillin	250mg	Pink/Maroon	Cap	–	–	–	Bristol	Anti–Infective
7279	Bristol 7279	Amoxicillin	500mg	Pink/Maroon	Cap	–	–	–	Bristol	Anti–Infective
7300	W 7300	Methdilazine	3.6mg	Pink	Tab	Round	N	N	Westwood	Antihistamine
	X 7300	Verapamil HCl ER	240mg	White	Tab	Oblong	Y	Y	Baker	Antihypertensive
7301	X 7301	Verapamil HCl ER	180mg	Orange	Tab	Capsule	Y	Y	Baker	Antihypertensive
7400	BCP 7400	Tolmetin Sodium	400mg	Orange	Cap	–	–	–	Baker	Anti–Inflammatory
	W 7400	Methdilazine HCl	8mg	Peach	Tab	Round	Y	N	Westwood	Antihistamine
7496	Bristol 7496	Cloxacillin	500mg	Orange/Black	Cap	–	–	–	Bristol	Anti–Infective
7512	RR 7512	Lithium Carbonate	300mg	Peach	Cap	–	–	–	RR	Tranquilizer
	SOLVAY 7512	Lithium Carbonate	300mg	Peach	Cap	–	–	–	Solvay	Tranquilizer
7516	RR 7516	Lithium Carbonate	300mg	White	Tab	Round	Y	N	RR	Tranquilizer
	SOLVAY 7516	Lithium Carbonate	300mg	White	Tab	Round	Y	Y	Solvay	Tranquilizer
7621	R 7621	Multivitamin with Fluoride & Iron	n/a	Maroon	Tab	Oval	Y	N	Ross	Vitamin
7626	R 7626	Multivitamin with Fluoride	n/a	Yellow	Tab	Oval	Y	N	Ross	Vitamin
7658	Bristol 7658/500	Dicloxacillin Sodium	500mg	Blue/White	Cap	–	–	–	Bristol	Anti–Infective
7720	Rowell 7720	Chenodiol	250mg	White	Tab	Round	N	Y	RR	Gallstone agent
	S 7720	Chenodiol	250mg	White	Tab	Round	N	Y	Solvay	Gallstone agent
7824	AHR 7824	Glycopyrrolate	1mg	Pink	Tab	Round	Y	N	A.H.Robins	Antiulcer
7840	AHR 2/ 7840	Glycopyrrolate	2mg	Pink	Tab	Round	Y	N	A.H.Robins	Antiulcer
7892	Bristol 7892/125	Dicloxacillin Sodium	125mg	Blue/White	Cap	–	–	–	Bristol	Anti–Infective
7893	Bristol 7893/250	Dicloxacillin Sodium	250mg	Blue/White	Cap	–	–	–	Bristol	Anti–Infective
7895	Bristol 7935	Cloxacillin	250mg	Orange/Black	Cap	–	–	–	Bristol	Anti–Infective
7977	Bristol 7977	Oxacillin Sodium	250mg	Pink	Cap	–	–	–	Bristol	Anti–Infective
7982	Bristol 7982	Oxacillin Sodium	500mg	Pink	Cap	–	–	–	Bristol	Anti–Infective
7992	Bristol 7992	Ampicillin	250mg	Gray/Maroon	Cap	–	–	–	Bristol	Anti–Infective
7993	Bristol 7993	Ampicillin	500mg	Gray/Maroon	Cap	–	–	–	Bristol	Anti–Infective
8217	ROBITAB 8217	Penicillin VK	250mg	White	Tab	Round	Y	N	A.H.Robins	Anti–Infective

ID NO.	ID CODE	GENERIC NAME	STRENGTH	COLOR	FORM	SHAPE	SCORED	COATED	MFG.	USE
8227	ROBITAB 8227	Penicillin VK	500mg	White	Tab	Round	Y	N	A.H.Robins	Anti-Infective
8375	832/8375C	Phentermine HCl	37.5mg	Yellow	Tab	Round	N	N	PBI	Anorectic
8417	AHR ROBICAP 8417	Tetracycline	250mg	–	Cap	–	–	–	A.H.Robins	Anti-Infective
8427	AHR ROBICAP 8427	Tetracycline	500mg	–	Cap	–	–	–	A.H.Robins	Anti-Infective
8647	C 8647	Phendimetrazine Tartrate SR	105mg	Green/Yellow	Cap	–	–	–	Carnrick	Anorectic
8648	C 8648	Phendimetrazine Tartrate	35mg	Green/White/Yellow	Tab	Round	Y	N	Carnrick	Anorectic
8650	C 8650	Butalbital & Acetaminophen	50mg/325mg	Violet	Tab	Round	Y	N	Carnrick	Analgesic
8652	C 8652	Phenindamine Tartrate	25mg	White	Tab	Capsule	Y	N	Carnrick	Antihistamine
8655	C 8655	Butalbital & Acetaminophen with Codeine	50mg/650mg/30mg	Amethyst/White	Cap	–	–	–	Carnrick	Analgesic
8656	C 8656	Butalbital & Acetaminophen	50mg/650mg	Amethyst	Cap	–	–	–	Carnrick	Analgesic
8657	C 8657	Hydrocodone & Acetaminophen	5mg/500mg	Blue/White	Cap	–	–	–	Carnrick	Analgesic
8666	C 8666	Acetaminophen/Chlorpheniramine/Phenylpropanolamine	650mg/4mg/25mg	Peach	Tab	Round	Y	N	Carnrick	Decongestant Comb.
8671	C 8671	Salsalate	500mg	White	Tab	Round	N	Y	Carnrick	Antiarthritic
8672	C 8672	Salsalate	750mg	White	Tab	Oval	Y	Y	Carnrick	Antiarthritic
8673	C 8673	Phenylpropanolamine HCL/Guaifenesin	75mg/400mg	White/Blue Specks	Tab	Oval	Y	N	Carnrick	Decongestant Comb.
8674	C 8674	Difenoxin HCl/Atropine Sulfate	1mg/0.25mg	White	Tab	Pentagonal	Y	N	Carnrick	Antidiarrheal
9000	bp 9000	Quinine Sulfate	260mg	White	Tab	Round	–	N	Bolar	Muscle Relaxant
9007	51479007	Chlorpheniramine/Pseudoephedrine HCl	4mg/60mg	Blue/Clear	Cap	–	–	–	Dura	Decongestant Comb.
9523	P 9523	Phenobarbital	16mg	White	Tab	Round	N	N	Poythress	Sedative
9525	WmP 9525	Phenobarbital	16mg	Brown/Yellow	Cap	–	–	–	Poythress	Sedative
9531	9531	Methenamine/ Sodium Biphosphate	300mg/500mg	White	Tab	Round	N	Y	Poythress	Urinary Tract Agent
9532	9532	Potassium Iodide/Aminophylline	195mg/130mg	White	Tab	Round	Y	N	Poythress	Bronchodilator Comb.
9533	9533	Aminophylline/Guaifenesin	130/100mg	Green	Tab	Round	N	N	Poythress	Bronchodilator Comb.
9540	9540	Atropine Sulfate/Phenobarbital	0.195mg/16mg	Yellow	Tab	Round	–	N	Poythress	Antispasmodic
9550	9550	Potassium Iodide/Aminophylline/Pb/Ephedrine	195/130/8/16mg	Yellow	Tab	Round	Y	N	Poythress	Bronchodilator Comb.
9551	9551	Aminophylline/Ephedrine/Pb/Guaifenesin	130/16/8/100mg	Yellow molted	Tab	Round	N	N	Poythress	Bronchodilator Comb.
C	(Clock) C	Quinidine Gluconate	324mg	White	Tab	Round	N	N	Berlex	Antiarrhythmic
L	L	Iodinated Glycerol	30mg	Orange	Tab	Round	Y	N	LuChem	Expectorant
P	SEARLE	Placebo	n/a	Blue	Tab	Round	–	–	Searle	Placebo
T	T	Iodinated Glycerol	30mg	Orange	Tab	Round	Y	N	Trinity	Mucolytic
	T	Benzonatate	100mg	Yellow	Cap	–	–	–	Inwood	Antitussive
Z	bock Z LA	Pseudoephedrine/Guaifenesin	120mg/600mg	Orange	Tab	Oval	Y	Y	Midland	Decongestant/Exp.
AA	AA	Aspirin SR	800mg	White	Tab	Oblong	N	N	Able Labs	Analgesic
	Abb. Logo AA	Chlorthalidone	25mg	Peach	Tab	Round	Y	N	Abbott	Diuretic
AB	Abb. Logo AB	Chlorthalidone	50mg	Lavender	Tab	Round	Y	N	Abbott	Diuretic
AD	Abb. Logo AD	Ethotoin	250mg	White	Tab	Round	Y	N	Abbott	Anticonvulsant
AE	Abb. Logo AE	Ethotoin	500mg	White	Tab	Round	Y	N	Abbott	Anticonvulsant
AF	AF	Colchicine	0.6mg	White	Tab	Round	N	N	Abbott	Antigout
AH	Abb. Logo AH	Hydrochlorothiazide & Deserpidine	25mg/0.125mg	Rose	Tab	Round	Y	N	Abbott	Antihypertensive
AI	Abb. Logo AI	Hydrochlorothiazide & Deserpidine	50mg/0.125mg	Rose	Tab	Round	Y	N	Abbott	Antihypertensive
AJ	Abb. Logo AJ	Ferrous Sulfate/Folic Acid/Vitamin C	525/80/500mg	Red	Tab	Oval	N	Y	Abbott	Antianemic
AK	Abb. Logo AK	Ferrous Sulfate/Vitamin C/B-Complex/Folic Acid	N/A	Red	Tab	Oval	N	N	Abbott	Antianemic
AL	AL	Clorazepate	3.75mg	Blue	Tab	Round	Y	N	Able Labs	Antianxiety
AM	Abb. Logo AM	Trimethadione	300mg	White	Cap	–	–	–	Abbott	Anticonvulsant
	AM	Clorazepate	7.5mg	Peach	Tab	Round	Y	N	Able Labs	Antianxiety
AN	Abb. Logo AN	Dicumarol	25mg	White	Tab	Round	N	N	Abbott	Anticoagulant
	AN	Clorazepate	15mg	White	Tab	Round	Y	N	Able Labs	Antianxiety
AO	Abb. Logo AO	Dicumarol	50mg	Pink	Tab	Round	N	N	Abbott	Anticoagulant
AT	Abb. Logo AT	Pipobroman	25mg	–	Tab	Round	–	–	Abbott	
BE	Sch. Logo BE	Methyltestosterone Buccal	10mg	Lavender	Tab	Oval	N	N	Schering	Hormone
BV	BV	Cyproterone Acetate	50mg	White	Tab	Round	Y	N	Berlex Canada	Antiandrogen
CF	Abb. Logo CF	Pentobarbital Sodium	50mg	Transparent/Orange	Cap	–	–	–	Abbott	Hypnotic
CH	Abb. Logo CH	Pentobarbital Sodium	100mg	Yellow	Cap	–	–	–	Abbott	Hypnotic
DA	DURA DA JR	Chlorpheniramine/Phenylephrine/Methscopolamine	2/10/1.25 mg	Orange	Tab	–	N	N	Dura	Antihistamine Comb.
DC	M D-C	Hydrocodone Bitartrate/Acetaminophen	5mg/500mg	Blue	Tab	Round	N	N	Mason	Analgesic
DF	Abb. Logo DF	Terazosin HCl	1mg	White	Tab	Round	Y	N	Abbott	Antihypertensive
DH	Abb. Logo DH	Terazosin HCl	2mg	Orange	Tab	Round	Y	N	Abbott	Antihypertensive
DI	Abb. Logo DI	Terazosin HCl	10mg	Green	Tab	Round	Y	N	Abbott	Antihypertensive
DJ	Abb. Logo DJ	Terazosin HCl	5mg	Tan	Tab	Round	Y	N	Abbott	Antihypertensive
DK	GEIGY DK	Clomipramine HCl	10mg	Cream	Tab	Triangular	N	Y	Geigy	Antidepressant
DP	M D-P	Hydrocodone Bitartrate/Aspirin/Caffeine	5mg/224mg/32mg	Pink	Tab	Round	N	N	Mason	Analgesic
DT	MILES DT	Nifedipine	10mg	Greyish Pink	Tab	Round	–	–	Miles	Antihypertensive
EA	Abb. Logo EA	Erythromycin	500mg	Pink	Tab	Oval	N	Y	Abbott	Anti-Infective
EB	Abb. Logo EB	Erythromycin	250mg	Pink	Tab	Oval	N	Y	Abbott	Anti-Infective
EC	Abb. Logo EC	Erythromycin Delayed Release	250mg	Pink	Tab	Oval	N	Y	Abbott	Anti-Infective
ED	Abb. Logo ED	Erythromycin Delayed Release	500mg	Pink	Tab	Oval	N	Y	Abbott	Anti-Infective
EE	Abb. Logo EE	Erythromycin Ethylsuccinate	400mg	Pink	Tab	Round	N	N	Abbott	Anti-Infective
EF	Abb. Logo EF	Erythromycin Ethylsuccinate	200mg	White	Tab	Round	N	N	Abbott	Anti-Infective
EH	Abb. Logo EH	Erythromycin Delayed Release	333mg	White	Tab	Round	N	Y	Abbott	Anti-Infective
EK	Abb. Logo EK	Erythromycin	500mg	White	Tab	Oval	N	–	Abbott	Anti-Infective
EM	EM	Dyphylline	200mg	White	Tab	Round	Y	N	Lemmon	Bronchodilator
	Sch. Logo EM	Ethinyl Estradiol	0.05mg	Pink	Tab	Round	N	Y	Schering	Hormone
EP	Sch. Logo EP	Ethinyl Estradiol	0.5mg	Peach	Tab	Round	Y	N	Schering	Hormone
ER	Abb. Logo ER	Erythromycin Delayed Release	250mg	Clear/Maroon	Cap	–	–	–	Abbott	Anti-Infective
	Sch. Logo ER	Ethinyl Estradiol	0.02mg	Beige	Tab	Round	N	Y	Schering	Hormone
ES	Abb. Logo ES	Erythromycin Stearate	250mg	Pink	Tab	Round	N	Y	Abbott	Anti-Infective
ET	Abb. Logo ET	Erythromycin Stearate	500mg	Pink	Tab	Oval	N	Y	Abbott	Anti-Infective
EZ	Abbott logo EZ	Erythromycin Chewable	200mg	White	Tab	Round	–	N	Abbott	Anti-Infective
FC	Abbott logo FC	Temafloxacin Hydrochloride	400mg	White	Tab	Oval	N	Y	Abbott	Anti-Infective
FH	GEIGY FH	Clomipramine HCl	25mg	Cream	Tab	Round	N	Y	Geigy	Antidepressant
FL	FL	Isometheptene Mucate, Dichloralphenazone, APAP	65mg/100mg/325	Red/White	Cap	–	–	–	Ferndale	Vasodilator
	FL (black ink)	Pseudoephedrine HCl/Chlorpheniramine Maleate	120mg/8mg	White/Clear	Cap	–	–	–	Ferndale	Decongestant Comb.
	FL (red ink)	Pseudoephedrine HCl/Chlorpheniramine Maleate	60mg/4mg	White/Clear	Cap	–	–	–	Ferndale	Decongestant Comb.
FP	Geigy FP	Phenylbutazone	100mg	White	Tab	Round	N	Y	Geigy	Anti-Inflammatory
FS	Abbott logo FS	Temafloxacin Hydrochloride	600mg	White	Tab	Oval	N	Y	Abbott	Anti-Infective
GM	Geigy GM	Clofazimine	100mg	Brown	Cap	–	–	–	Geigy	Antileprosy
GN	ALRA GN	Chlorazepate Dipotassium	15mg	Green	Tab	Round	Y	N	Alra	Antianxiety
GT	ALRA GT	Chlorazepate Dipotassium	7.5mg	Yellow	Tab	Round	Y	N	Alra	Antianxiety
GX	ALRA GX	Chlorazepate Dipotassium	3.75mg	Gray	Tab	Round	Y	N	Alra	Antianxiety
HH	Abb. Logo HH	Valproic Acid	250mg	Orange	Cap	–	–	–	Abbott	Anticonvulsant
IA	Abbott logo IA	Carteolol HCl	2.5mg	Gray	Tab	Round	–	–	Abbott	Antihypertensive
IC	Abbott logo IC	Carteolol HCl	5mg	White	Tab	Round	–	–	Abbott	Antihypertensive
II	Abb. Logo II	Phenacemide	500mg	White	Tab	–	Y	N	Abbott	Anticonvulsant
JD	Sch. Logo JD	Methyltestosterone	10mg	White	Tab	Round	N	N	Schering	Hormone
JE	Sch. Logo JE	Methyltestosterone	25mg	Peach	Tab	Round	N	N	Schering	Hormone

ID NO.	ID CODE	GENERIC NAME	STRENGTH	COLOR	FORM	SHAPE	SCORED	COATED	MFG.	USE
JR	DURA DA JR	Chlorpheniramine/Phenylephrine/Methscopolamine	2/10/1.25 mg	Orange	Tab	–	N	N	Dura	Antihistamine Comb.
	F (in triangle) JR	Anhydrous Theophylline	130mg	Red/Clear	Cap	–	–	–	Fleming	Bronchodilator
	F (in triangle) JR	Guaifenesin & Pseudoephedrine	125mg/60mg	Blue/Clear	Cap	–	–	–	Fleming	Antitussive comb.
	F (in triangle) JR	Chlorpheniramine/Phenylephrine/Methscopolamine	4/10/1.25mg	Green/Red	Cap	–	–	–	Fleming	Decongestant comb.
KH	Abb. Logo KH	Ethchlorvynol	500mg	Red	Cap	–	–	–	Abbott	Hypnotic
KL	Abbott Logo KL	Clarithromycin	500mg	Off White	Tab	Oval	N	Y	Abbott	Anti-Infective
KN	Abb. Logo KN	Ethchlorvynol	750mg	Green	Cap	–	–	–	Abbott	Hypnotic
KT	Abbott Logo KT	Clarithromycin	250mg	Off White	Tab	Oval	N	Y	Abbott	Anti-Infective
LA	bock Z LA	Pseudoephedrine/Guaifenesin	120mg/600mg	Orange	Tab	Oval	Y	Y	Midland	Decongestant/Exp.
LE	Abb. Logo LE	Trimethadione	150mg	White	Tab	Square	–	N	Abbott	Anticonvulsant
LF	Abb. Logo LF	Warfarin Sodium	10mg	White	Tab	Round	Y	N	Abbott	Anticoagulant
LH	USV logo LH	Levothyroxine Sodium	125mcg	Purple	Tab	Round	–	N	USV	Hormone
LK	Abb. Logo LK	Deserpidine	0.25mg	Salmon–Pink	Tab	Round	Y	N	Abbott	Antihypertensive
	USV logo LK	Levothyroxine Sodium	25mcg	Orange	Tab	Round	–	N	USV	Hormone
LL	Abb. Logo LL	Hydrochlorothiazide & Deserpidine	25mg/0.25mg	Gray	Tab	Round	Y	N	Abbott	Antihypertensive
	USV logo LL	Levothyroxine Sodium	50mcg	White	Tab	Round	–	N	USV	Hormone
LM	Abb. Logo LM	Warfarin Sodium	2mg	Lavender	Tab	Round	Y	N	Abbott	Anticoagulant
	USV logo LM	Levothyroxine Sodium	100mcg	Yellow	Tab	Round	–	N	USV	Hormone
LN	Abb. Logo LN	Warfarin Sodium	2.5mg	Orange	Tab	Round	Y	N	Abbott	Anticoagulant
	USV logo LN	Levothyroxine Sodium	150mcg	Blue	Tab	Round	–	N	USV	Hormone
LO	Abb. Logo LO	Warfarin Sodium	5mg	Peach	Tab	Round	Y	N	Abbott	Anticoagulant
lp	GEIGY LP	Clomipramine HCl	50mg	Cream	Tab	Round	N	Y	Geigy	Antidepressant
LP	USV logo LP	Levothyroxine Sodium	175mcg	Turquoise	Tab	Round	–	N	USV	Hormone
LR	Abb. Logo LR	Warfarin Sodium	7.5mg	Yellow	Tab	Round	Y	N	Abbott	Anticoagulant
	USV logo LR	Levothyroxine Sodium	200mcg	Pink	Tab	Round	–	N	USV	Hormone
LS	Abb. Logo LS	Methyclothiazide & Deserpidine	5mg/0.25mg	Yellow	Tab	Square	Y	N	Abbott	Antihypertensive
	USV logo LS	Levothyroxine Sodium	300mcg	Green	Tab	Round	–	N	USV	Hormone
LT	Abb. Logo LT	Methyclothiazide & Deserpidine	5mg/0.5mg	Gray	Tab	Square	Y	N	Abbott	Antihypertensive
	USV logo LT	Levothyroxine Sodium	75mcg	Grey	Tab	Round	–	N	USV	Hormone
LU	Abb. Logo LU	Estropipate	0.625mg	Yellow	Tab	Oblong	Y	N	Abbott	Hormone
LV	Abb. Logo LV	Estropipate	1.25mg	Peach	Tab	Oblong	Y	N	Abbott	Hormone
LX	Abb. Logo LX	Estropipate	2.5mg	Blue	Tab	Oblong	Y	N	Abbott	Hormone
LY	Abb. Logo LY	Estropipate	5mg	Green	Tab	Oblong	Y	N	Abbott	Hormone
MC	Abb. Logo MC	Methamphetamine HCl	5mg	White	Tab	Round	N	N	Abbott	Psychostimulant
ME	Abb. Logo ME	Methamphetamine HCl	10mg	Orange	Tab	Round	N	N	Abbott	Psychostimulant
MF	Abb. Logo MF	Methamphetamine HCl	15mg	Yellow	Tab	Round	N	N	Abbott	Psychostimulant
mo	A/mo	Metoprolol	50mg	White	Tab	Round	Y	Y	Astra	Antihypertensive
MR	M/R	Butalbital/Aspirin/Caffeine	50mg/650mg/40mg	Yellow/White	Tab	Capsule	Y	N	Mayrand	Analgesic
	M/R	APAP/Guaifenesin/Dextromethorphan/Phenylpropanol	325/100/15/25mg	Green	Tab	Oblong	Y	Y	Central	Antihistamine/Dec.
	M/s	Guaifenesin	200mg	White	Tab	Oblong	Y	Y	Central	Expectorant
ms	A/ms	Metoprolol	100mg	White	Tab	Round	Y	Y	Astra	Antihypertensive
my	A/my	Metoprolol	200mg	White	Tab	Oval	Y	Y	Astra	Antihypertensive
NA	Abb. Logo NA	Pargyline HCl	10mg	Pink	Tab	Round	–	Y	Abbott	Antihypertensive
NB	Abb. Logo NB	Pargyline HCl	25mg	Apricot	Tab	Round	–	Y	Abbott	Antihypertensive
ND	Abb. Logo ND	Imipramine	10mg	Orange	Tab	Round	N	Y	Abbott	Antidepressant
NE	A NE	Niacin	500mg	Yellow	Tab	Oblong	Y	N	Rorer	Vitamin
	Abb. Logo NE	Imipramine	25mg	Yellow	Tab	Round	N	Y	Abbott	Antidepressant
NF	Abb. Logo NF	Hexocyclium Methylsulfate	25mg	Green	Tab	–	N	Y	Abbott	Antispasmodic
NJ	Abb. Logo NJ	Vitamin Combination	n/a	Green	Tab	Oval	N	Y	Abbott	Vitamin
NK	Abb. Logo NK	Pargyline HCl & Methyclothiazide	25mg/5mg	Purple	Tab	Oval	Y	Y	Abbott	Antihypertensive
NL	Abb. Logo NL	Imipramine	50mg	Peach	Tab	Oval	N	Y	Abbott	Antidepressant
NM	Abb. Logo NM	Potassium Chloride Extended Release	750mg	Yellow	Tab	Oval	N	Y	Abbott	Potassium Supp.
NR	Abb. Logo NR	Divalproex Sodium	250mg	Peach	Tab	Oval	N	Y	Abbott	Anticonvulsant
NS	Abb. Logo NS	Divalproex Sodium	500mg	Lavender	Tab	Oval	N	Y	Abbott	Anticonvulsant
NT	Abb. Logo NT	Divalproex Sodium	125mg	Salmon–Pink	Tab	Oval	N	Y	Abbott	Anticonvulsant
Nz	PF Nz	Thiethylperazine Maleate	10mg	Yellow	Tab	Round	N	Y	PF	Antinausea
pH	pH pH	pHos–pHaid	500mg	Blue	Tab	Round	–	Y	Guardian	Urinary Acidifier
	pH pH	pHos–pHaid	500mg	Orange	Tab	Round	–	Y	Guardian	Urinary Acidifier
	pH pH	pHos–pHaid	250mg	Green	Tab	Round	–	Y	Guardian	Urinary Acidifier
RL	RL	Dronabinol	2.5mg	White	Cap	–	–	–	Roxane	Antiemetic
	RL	Dronabinol	5mg	Brown	Cap	–	–	–	Roxane	Antiemetic
	RL	Dronabinol	10mg	Orange	Cap	–	–	–	Roxane	Antiemetic
SR	F (in triangle) SR	Anhydrous Theophylline	260mg	Red/Clear	Cap	–	–	–	Fleming	Bronchodilator
	F (in triangle) SR	Guaifenesin & Pseudoephedrine	250mg/120mg	Blue/Clear	Cap	–	–	–	Fleming	Antitussive Comb.
	F (in triangle) SR	Chlorpheniramine/Phenylephrine/Methscopolamine	8mg/20mg/2.5mg	Green/Red	Cap	–	–	–	Fleming	Decongestant Comb.
TC	A TC	Levothyroxine/Liothyronine	1/4 gr.	Tan	Tab	Round	N	N	Rorer	Hormone
	Abb. Logo TC	Methamphetamine HCl	2.5mg	White	Tab	Round	N	N	Abbott	Psychostimulant
TD	A TD	Levothyroxine/Liothyronine	1/2 gr.	Tan	Tab	Round	N	N	Rorer	Hormone
TE	A TE	Levothyroxine/Liothyronine	1 gr.	Tan	Tab	Round	N	N	Rorer	Hormone
	Abb. Logo TE	Methamphetamine HCl	5mg	White	Tab	Round	N	N	Abbott	Psychostimulant
TF	A TF	Levothyroxine/Liothyronine	2 gr.	Tan	Tab	Round	N	N	Rorer	Hormone
	Abb. Logo TF	Metharbital	100mg	–	Tab	–	Y	N	Abbott	Sedative
TG	A TG	Levothyroxine/Liothyronine	3 gr.	Tan	Tab	Round	Y	N	Rorer	Hormone
TH	A TH	Levothyroxine/Liothyronine	4 gr.	Tan	Tab	Round	–	N	Rorer	Hormone
	Abb. Logo TH	Pemoline	18.75mg	White	Tab	Round	N	N	Abbott	Psychostimulant
TI	A TI	Levothyroxine/Liothyronine	5 gr.	Tan	Tab	Round	Y	N	Rorer	Hormone
	Abb. Logo TI	Pemoline	37.5mg	Orange	Tab	Round	N	N	Abbott	Psychostimulant
TJ	A TJ	Levothyroxine/Liothyronine	1 1/2 gr.	Tan	Tab	Round	N	N	Rorer	Hormone
	Abb. Logo TJ	Pemoline	75mg	Tan	Tab	Round	N	N	Abbott	Psycostimulant
TK	Abb. Logo TK	Pemoline	37.5mg	Orange	Tab	Square	N	N	Abbott	Psychostimulant
TL	Abb. Logo TL	Clorazepate Dipotassium	3.75mg	Blue	Tab	T–Tab	N	N	Abbott	Antianxiety
TM	Abb. Logo TM	Clorazepate Dipotassium	7.5mg	Peach	Tab	T–Tab	N	N	Abbott	Antianxiety
TN	Abb. Logo TN	Clorazepate Dipotassium	15mg	Lavender	Tab	T–Tab	N	N	Abbott	Antianxiety
TT	TT	Pseudoephedrine/Chlorpheniramine/APAP	60mg/4mg/650mg	Pink	Tab	Oblong	N	Y	Trinity	Antihistamine/Dec.
TX	Abb. Logo TX	Clorazepate Dipotassium	11.25mg	Blue	Tab	Round	Y	N	Abbott	Antianxiety
TY	Abb. Logo TY	Clorazepate Dipotassium	22.5mg	Tan	Tab	Round	Y	N	Abbott	Antianxiety
UC	Abbott logo UC	Estazolam	1mg	White	Tab	Round	Y	N	Abbott	Hypnotic
UD	Abbott logo UD	Estazolam	2mg	Coral	Tab	Round	Y	N	Abbott	Hypnotic
TC	A YC	Levothyroxine/Liothyronine	3.1mcg/12.5mcg	Violet/White	Tab	Round	–	N	Rorer	Hormone
YD	A YD	Levothyroxine/Liothyronine	6.25mcg/25mcg	Peach/White	Tab	Round	–	N	Rorer	Hormone
YE	A YE	Levothyroxine/Liothyronine	12.5mcg/50mcg	Pink/White	Tab	Round	–	N	Rorer	Hormone
YF	A YF	Levothyroxine/Liothyronine	25mcg/100mcg	Green/White	Tab	Round	–	N	Rorer	Hormone
YH	A YH	Levothyroxine/Liothyronine	37.5/150mcg	Yellow/White	Tab	Round	–	N	Rorer	Hormone
	A YH	Levothyroxine/Liothyronine	37.5/150mcg	Yellow/White	Tab	Round	–	N	Rorer	Hormone
ADH	Sch. Logo ADH	Perphenazine	2mg	Gray	Tab	Round	N	Y	Schering	Tranquilizer

ID NO.	ID CODE	GENERIC NAME	STRENGTH	COLOR	FORM	SHAPE	SCORED	COATED	MFG.	USE
ADJ	Sch. Logo ADJ	Perphenazine	8mg	Gray	Tab	Round	N	Y	Schering	Tranquilizer
ADK	Sch. Logo ADK	Perphenazine	4mg	Gray	Tab	Round	N	Y	Schering	Tranquilizer
ADM	Sch. Logo ADM	Perphenazine	16mg	Gray	Tab	Round	N	Y	Schering	Tranquilizer
AGA	Sch. Logo AGA	Dexchlorpheniramine ER	4mg	Red	Tab	Oval	N	Y	Schering	Antihistamine
AGB	Sch. Logo AGB	Dexchlorpheniramine ER	6mg	Red	Tab	Oval	N	Y	Schering	Antihistamine
AGT	Sch. Logo AGT	Dexchlorpheniramine	2mg	Red	Tab	Oval	N	N	Schering	Antihistamine
AHG	S AHG	Trichlormethiazide	2mg	Pink	Tab	Clover	Y	N	Schering	Diuretic
AHH	S AHH	Trichlormethiazide	4mg	Aqua	Tab	Clover	Y	N	Schering	Diuretic
AHR	Sch. Logo AHR	Carisoprodol	350mg	Pink	Tab	Round	N	Y	Schering	Muscle Relaxant
AHT	Sch. Logo AHT	Reserpine & Trichlormethiazide	0.1mg/4mg	Peach	Tab	Round	Y	N	Schering	Antihypertensive
ANA	Sch. Logo ANA	Perphenazine & Amitriptyline HCl	2mg/10mg	Yellow	Tab	Round	N	Y	Schering	Antidepressant
ANB	Sch. Logo ANB	Perphenazine & Amitriptyline HCl	4mg/10mg	Orange	Tab	Round	N	Y -	Schering	Antidepressant
ANC	Sch. Logo ANC	Perphenazine & Amitriptyline HCl	2mg/25mg	Pink	Tab	Round	N	Y	Schering	Antidepressant
ANE	Sch. Logo ANE	Perphenazine & Amitriptyline HCl	4mg/25mg	Red	Tab	Round	N	Y	Schering	Antidepressant
ANK	Sch. Logo ANK	Anisindione	50mg	Pink	Tab	Round	Y	N	Schering	Anticoagulant
AUF	Sch. Logo AUF	Griseofulvin	250mg	White	Tab	Round	Y	N	Schering	Antifungal
AUG	Sch. Logo AUG	Griseofulvin	500mg	White	Tab	Round	Y	N	Schering	Antifungal
BBA	Sch. Logo BBA	Acetophenazine Maleate	20mg	Salmon	Tab	Round	N	Y	Schering	Antipsycotic
BDA	Sch. Logo BDA	Betamethasone	0.6mg	Pink	Tab	Round	Y	N	Schering	Steroid
KEM	Sch. Logo KEM	Prednisone	1mg	White	Tab	Round	N	N	Schering	Steroid
nmi	nmi	Prenatal Vitamins	n/a	Orange	Tab	Capsule	Y	Y	—	Vitamin
PBA	MMS PBA	Diazoxide	50mg	Orange/Clear	Cap	–	–	–	MMS	Antihypertensive
PCE	Abb. Logo PCE	Erythromycin	333mg	Pink-Speckled	Tab	Oval	N	–	Abbott	Anti-Infective
WBS	Sch. Logo WBS	Dexbrompheniramine Maleate & Pseudoephedrine Sulf	2mg/60mg	White with Blue	Tab	Round	Y	N	Schering	Decongestant Comb
WDR	Sch. Logo WDR	Fluphenazine HCL	2.5mg	Orange	Tab	Oval	Y	N	Schering	Tranquilizer
WFF	Sch. Logo WFF	Fluphenazine HCL	5mg	Purple-Pink	Tab	Oval	Y	N	Schering	Tranquilizer
WFG	Sch. Logo WFG	Fluphenazine HCL	10mg	Red	Tab	Oval	Y	N	Schering	Tranquilizer
WMP	WMP	Atropine Sulfate/Phenobarbital	0.195mg/16mg	Green	Cap	–	–	–	Poythress	Antispasmodic
ZLA	bock Z LA	Pseudoephedrine/Guaifenesin	120mg/600mg	Orange	Tab	Oval	Y	Y	Midland	Decongestant/Exp.
ERVA	ERVA, 5.4	Yohimbine HCl	5.4mg	White	Tab	Round	Y	N	Royce	Sympatholytic
MOLE	Mole	Caffeine	200mg	White	Cap	–	–	–	B & M Labs	Stimulant
PPPC	832/PPPC	Nalspan SR	n/a	White/Red Mottles	Tab	–	–	N	PBI	–
n/a	LEMMON	Hydralazine HCl	25mg	Yellow	Tab	Oblong	N	N	Lemmon	Antihypertensive
	LEMMON	Promethazine HCl	25mg	Blue	Tab	Round	Y	N	Lemmon	Antiemetic
none	none	Isosorbide Dinitrate SL	2.5mg	Yellow	Tab	Round	N	N	Sidmak	Antianginal
	none	Isosorbide Dinitrate SL	5mg	Pink	Tab	Round	N	N	Sidmak	Antianginal

Visual Identification Guide

Products shown in this section are organized alphabetically by generic name. Included are more than 1,600 photographs of tablets, capsules, and other solid dosage forms, covering leading brands and the most frequently dispensed doses from generic manufacturers. All items are reproduced in actual size and color. For products with distinguishing features on both sides, the front view is supplemented with a picture of the back. Each product is labeled with its brand name, if applicable, as well as its strength and the name of the supplier.

ACEBUTOLOL HCL

SECTRAL
WYETH-AYERST

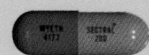

200 mg

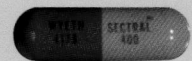

400 mg

ACETAMINOPHEN / BUTALBITAL / CAFFEINE

ESGIC
FOREST

325 mg / 50 mg / 40 mg

ESGIC-PLUS
FOREST

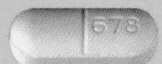 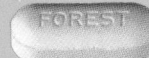

500 mg / 50 mg / 40 mg

FIORICET
SANDOZ

325 mg / 50 mg / 40 mg

GENERIC
HALSEY

325 mg / 50 mg / 40 mg

ACETAMINOPHEN / BUTALBITAL CAFFEINE / CODEINE PHOSPHATE

FIORICET W/CODEINE
SANDOZ

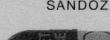 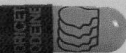

325 mg / 50 mg / 40 mg / 30 mg

ACETAMINOPHEN / CODEINE PHOSPHATE

GENERIC
GENEVA

300 mg / 60 mg

GENERIC
GOLDLINE

300 mg / 30 mg

GENERIC
LEMMON

300 mg / 30 mg

GENERIC
RUGBY

300 mg / 30 mg

GENERIC
UNITED RESEARCH

300 mg / 30 mg

PHENAPHEN-650 W/CODEINE
A. H. ROBINS

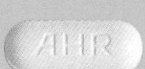

650 mg / 30 mg

TYLENOL W/CODEINE NO.2
MCNEIL

300 mg / 15 mg

TYLENOL W/CODEINE NO.3
MCNEIL

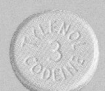 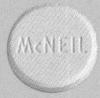

300 mg / 30 mg

TYLENOL W/CODEINE NO.4
MCNEIL

 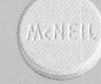

300 mg / 60 mg

ACETAMINOPHEN / DICHLORALPHENAZONE / ISOMETHEPTENE MUCATE

MIDRIN
CARNRICK

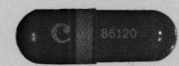

325 mg / 100 mg / 65 mg

ACETAMINOPHEN / HYDROCODONE BITARTRATE

ANEXSIA 5/500
BOEHRINGER MANNHEIM

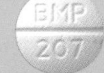

500 mg / 5 mg

ANEXSIA 7.5/650
BOEHRINGER MANNHEIM

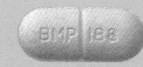

650 mg / 7.5 mg

CO-GESIC
CENTRAL

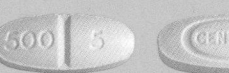

500 mg / 5 mg

GENERIC
HALSEY

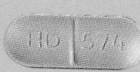

500 mg / 5 mg

GENERIC
QUALITEST

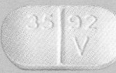

500 mg / 5 mg

GENERIC
RUGBY

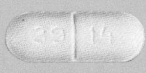

500 mg / 5 mg

GENERIC
WATSON

500 mg / 5 mg

GENERIC
WATSON

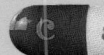

750 mg / 7.5 mg

HYDROCET
CARNRICK

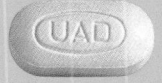 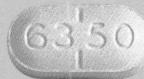

500 mg / 5 mg

LORCET 10/650
UAD

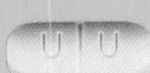

650 mg / 10 mg

LORCET PLUS
UAD

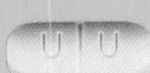

650 mg / 7.5 mg

LORTAB 2.5/500
WHITBY

650 mg / 7.5 mg

500 mg / 2.5 mg

LORTAB 5/500
WHITBY

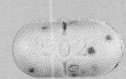

500 mg / 5 mg

LORTAB 7.5/500
WHITBY

500 mg / 7.5 mg

VICODIN
KNOLL

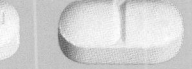

500 mg / 5 mg

VICODIN ES
KNOLL

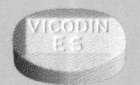 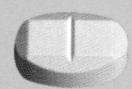

750 mg / 7.5 mg

ACETAMINOPHEN / OXYCODONE HCL
PERCOCET
DUPONT

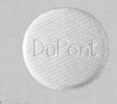

325 mg / 5 mg

ROXICET
ROXANE

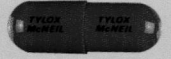

325 mg / 5 mg

TYLOX
MCNEIL

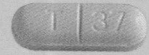 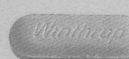

500 mg / 5 mg

ACETAMINOPHEN / PENTAZOCINE HCL
TALACEN
SANOFI WINTHROP

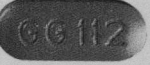

650 mg / 25 mg

ACETAMINOPHEN / PROPOXYPHENE HCL
GENERIC
GENEVA

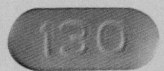

650 mg / 65 mg

GENERIC
MYLAN

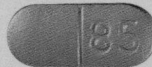

650 mg / 65 mg

WYGESIC
WYETH-AYERST

85

650 mg / 65 mg

ACETAMINOPHEN / PROPOXYPHENE NAPSYLATE
DARVOCET-N 100
ELI LILLY

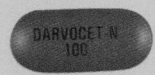

650 mg / 100 mg

GENERIC
GENEVA

650 mg / 100 mg

GENERIC
GOLDLINE

650 mg / 100 mg

GENERIC
MAJOR

650 mg / 100 mg

GENERIC
MYLAN

650 mg / 100 mg

GENERIC
RUGBY

650 mg / 100 mg

PROPACET 100
LEMMON

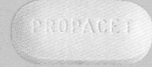

650 mg / 100 mg

ACETAZOLAMIDE
DIAMOX
LEDERLE

125 mg

DIAMOX
LEDERLE

250 mg

DIAMOX SEQUELS
LEDERLE

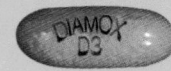

500 mg

ACRIVASTINE / PSEUDOEPHEDRINE HCL
SEMPREX-D
BURROUGHS WELLCOME

8 mg / 60 mg

ACYCLOVIR
ZOVIRAX
BURROUGHS WELLCOME

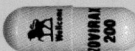

200 mg

400 mg

800 mg

ALBUTEROL SULFATE
GENERIC
LEMMON

2 MG

PROVENTIL
SCHERING

2 mg

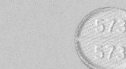

4 mg

PROVENTIL REPETABS
SCHERING

431

4 mg

VENTOLIN
ALLEN & HANBURYS

2 mg

4 mg

ALLOPURINOL
GENERIC
MYLAN

300 mg

GENERIC
SCHEIN

300 mg

GENERIC
RUGBY

100 mg   300 mg

LOPURIN
BOOTS

100 mg   300 mg

ZYLOPRIM
BURROUGHS WELLCOME

100 mg   300 mg

ALPRAZOLAM

GENERIC
GENEVA

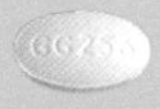

0.25 mg

GENERIC
LEDERLE STANDARD

0.25 mg

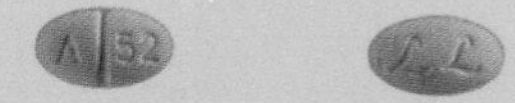

0.50 mg

1 mg

XANAX
UPJOHN

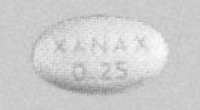

0.25 mg

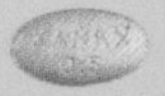

0.5 mg

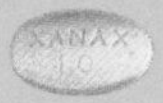

1 mg

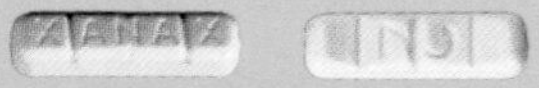

2 mg

AMANTADINE HCL

SYMMETREL
DUPONT

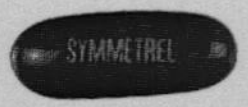

100 mg

AMILORIDE HCL / HYDROCHLOROTHIAZIDE

GENERIC
WEST POINT

5 mg / 50 mg

MODURETIC
MERCK

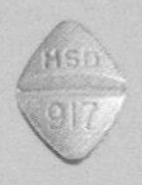

5 mg / 50 mg

AMITRIPTYLINE HCL

ELAVIL
STUART

10 mg

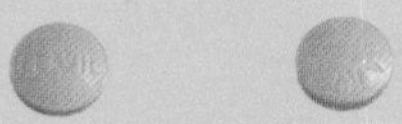

25 mg

50 mg

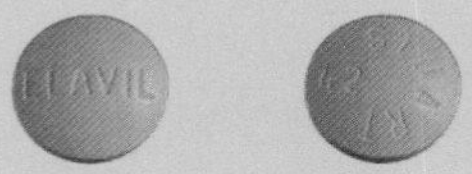

75 mg

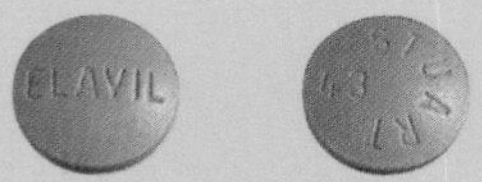

100 mg

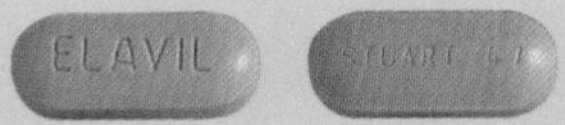

150 mg

GENERIC
GENEVA

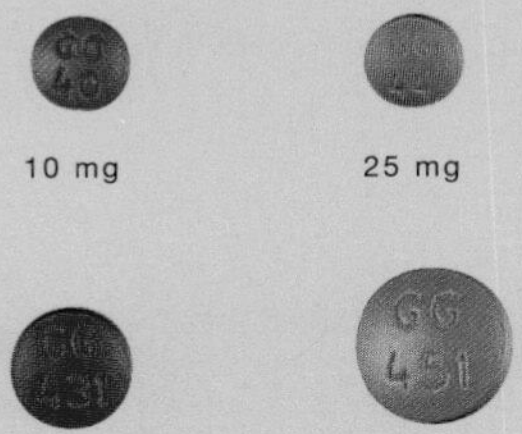

10 mg   25 mg

50 mg   75 mg

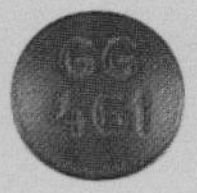

100 mg

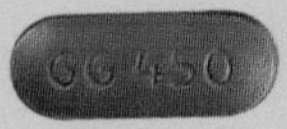

150 mg

GENERIC
MYLAN

25 mg

GENERIC
RUGBY

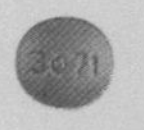

10 mg

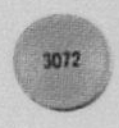

25 mg

50 mg

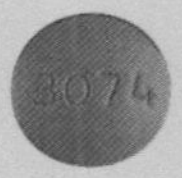

75 mg

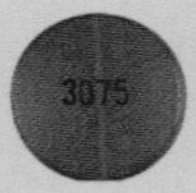

100 mg

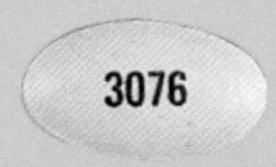

150 mg

AMITRIPTYLINE HCL / PERPHENAZINE

ETRAFON
SCHERING

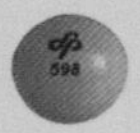

25 mg / 2 mg

ETRAFON 2-10
SCHERING

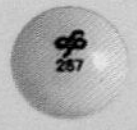

10 mg / 2 mg

ETRAFON-FORTE
SCHERING

25 mg / 4 mg

GENERIC
MYLAN

25 mg / 2 mg

TRIAVIL 2-10
MERCK

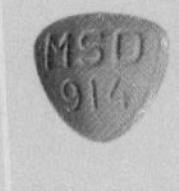

10 mg / 2 mg

TRIAVIL 2-25
MERCK

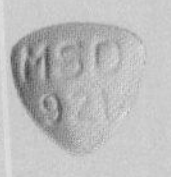

25 mg / 2 mg

TRIAVIL 4-10
MERCK

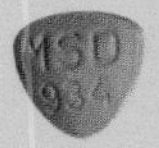

10 mg / 4 mg

TRIAVIL 4-25
MERCK

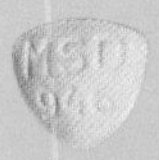

25 mg / 4 mg

TRIAVIL 4-50
MERCK

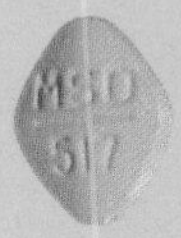

50 mg / 4 mg

AMLODIPINE BESYLATE

NORVASC
PFIZER

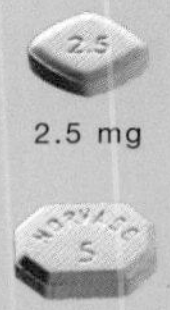

2.5 mg

5 mg

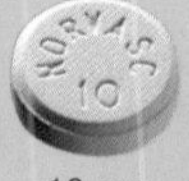

10 mg

AMOXICILLIN

AMOXIL
SMITHKLINE BEECHAM

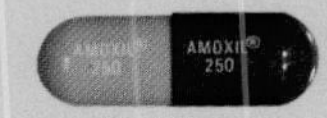

250 mg

AMOXIL
SMITHKLINE BEECHAM

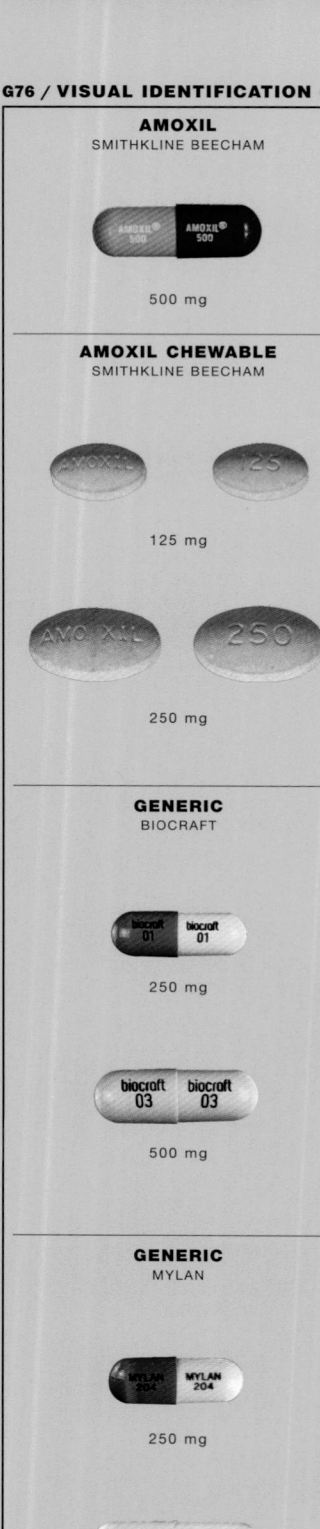

500 mg

AMOXIL CHEWABLE
SMITHKLINE BEECHAM

125 mg

250 mg

GENERIC
BIOCRAFT

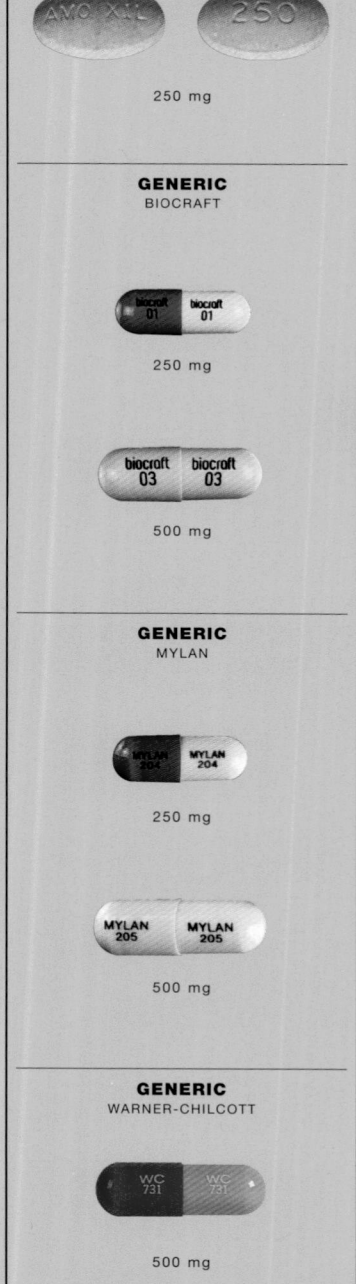

250 mg

500 mg

GENERIC
MYLAN

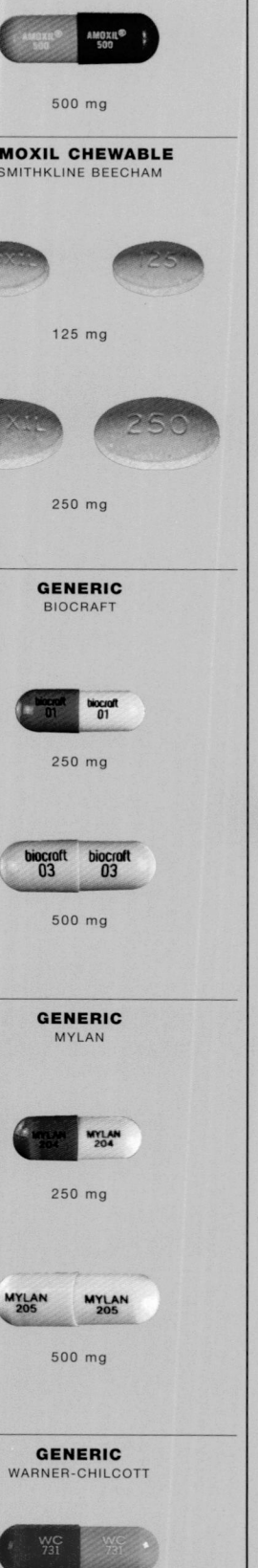

250 mg

500 mg

GENERIC
WARNER-CHILCOTT

500 mg

TRIMOX
APOTHECON

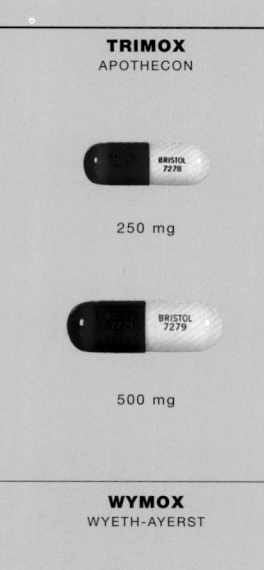

250 mg

500 mg

WYMOX
WYETH-AYERST

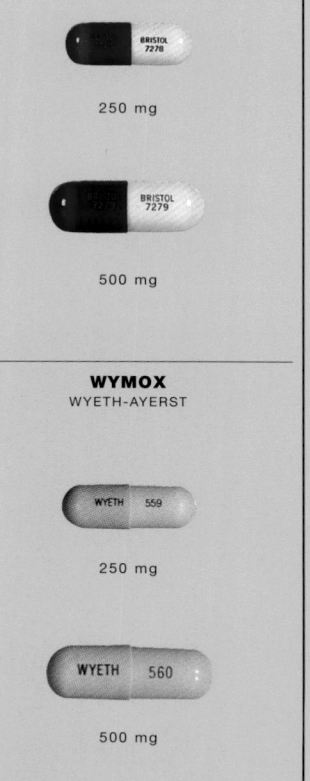

250 mg

500 mg

AMOXICILLIN / CLAVULANATE POTASSIUM
AUGMENTIN
SMITHKLINE BEECHAM

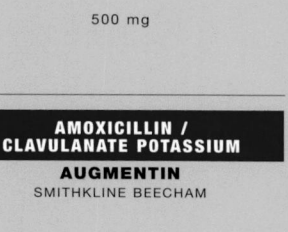

250 mg / 125 mg

500 mg / 125 mg

AUGMENTIN CHEWABLE
SMITHKLINE BEECHAM

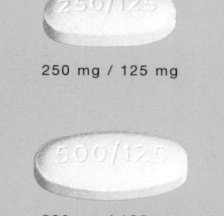

125 mg / 31.25 mg

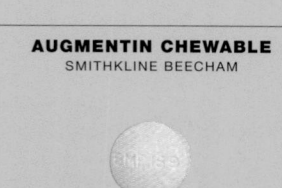

250 mg / 62.5 mg

AMPICILLIN
GENERIC
MYLAN

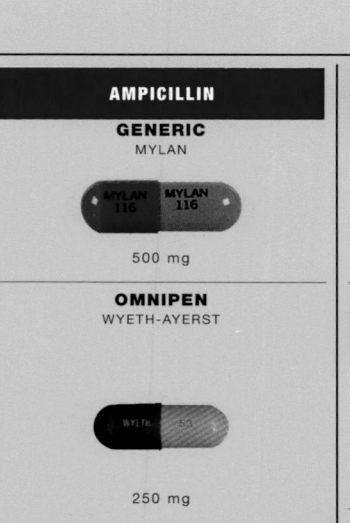

500 mg

OMNIPEN
WYETH-AYERST

250 mg

500 mg

PRINCIPEN
APOTHECON

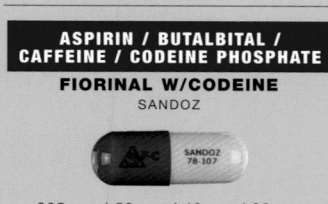

250 mg

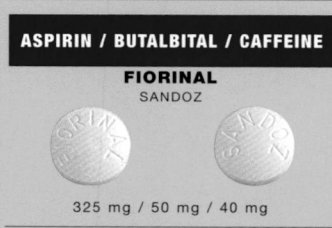

500 mg

ASPIRIN / BUTALBITAL / CAFFEINE / CODEINE PHOSPHATE
FIORINAL W/CODEINE
SANDOZ

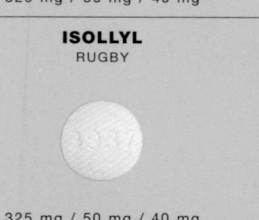

325 mg / 50 mg / 40 mg / 30 mg

ASPIRIN / BUTALBITAL / CAFFEINE
FIORINAL
SANDOZ

325 mg / 50 mg / 40 mg

ISOLLYL
RUGBY

325 mg / 50 mg / 40 mg

ASPIRIN / CARISOPRODOL
SOMA COMPOUND
WALLACE

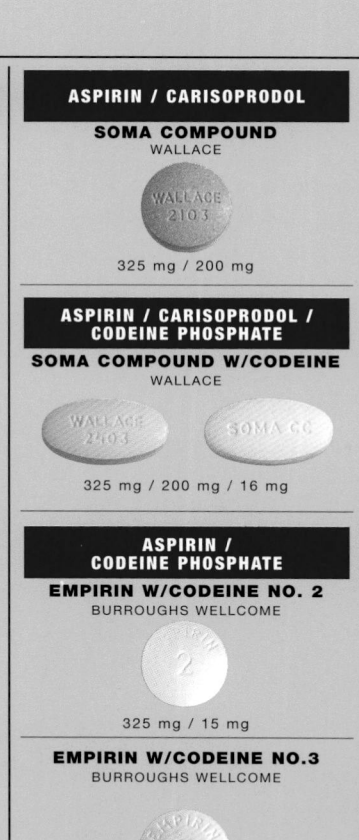

325 mg / 200 mg

ASPIRIN / CARISOPRODOL / CODEINE PHOSPHATE
SOMA COMPOUND W/CODEINE
WALLACE

325 mg / 200 mg / 16 mg

ASPIRIN / CODEINE PHOSPHATE
EMPIRIN W/CODEINE NO. 2
BURROUGHS WELLCOME

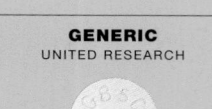

325 mg / 15 mg

EMPIRIN W/CODEINE NO.3
BURROUGHS WELLCOME

325 mg / 30 mg

EMPIRIN W/CODEINE NO.4
BURROUGHS WELLCOME

325 mg / 60 mg

GENERIC
UNITED RESEARCH

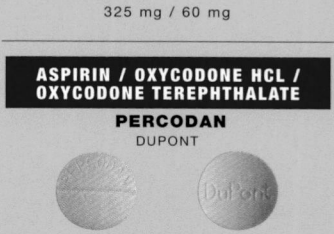

325 mg / 15 mg

325 mg / 30 mg

325 mg / 60 mg

ASPIRIN / OXYCODONE HCL / OXYCODONE TEREPHTHALATE
PERCODAN
DUPONT

325 mg / 4.5 mg / 0.38 mg

ROXIPRIN
ROXANE

325 mg / 4.5 mg / 0.38 mg

ASTEMIZOLE

HISMANAL
JANSSEN

10 mg

ATENOLOL

GENERIC
APOTHECON

50 mg

GENERIC
GENEVA

50 mg

GENERIC
IPR

50 mg

GENERIC
LEDERLE STANDARD

50 mg

GENERIC
MYLAN

50 mg

GENERIC
SCHEIN

50 mg

TENORMIN
ZENECA

25 mg

50 mg

100 mg

**ATENOLOL /
CHLORTHALIDONE**

TENORETIC
ZENECA

50 mg / 25 mg

100 mg / 25 mg

**ATROPINE SULFATE / HYOSCYAMINE /
PHENOBARBITAL / SCOPOLAMINE**

DONNATAL
A. H. ROBINS

0.0194 mg / 0.1037 mg / 16.2 mg / 0.0065 mg

0.0194 mg / 0.1037 mg / 16.2 mg / 0.0065 mg

DONNATAL EXTENTABS
A. H. ROBINS

0.0582 mg / 0.3111 mg / 48.6 mg / 0.0195 mg

**AZATADINE MALEATE /
PSEUDOEPHEDRINE SULFATE**

TRINALIN REPETABS
SCHERING

1 mg / 120 mg

AZATHIOPRINE

IMURAN
BURROUGHS WELLCOME

50 mg

AZITHROMYCIN DIHYDRATE

ZITHROMAX
PFIZER

250 mg

BACLOFEN

LIORESAL
GEIGY

10 mg

20 mg

BENAZEPRIL HCL

LOTENSIN
CIBA

5 mg

10 mg

20 mg

40 mg

**BENAZEPRIL HCL /
HYDROCHLOROTHIAZIDE**

LOTENSIN HCT
CIBA

5 mg / 6.25 mg

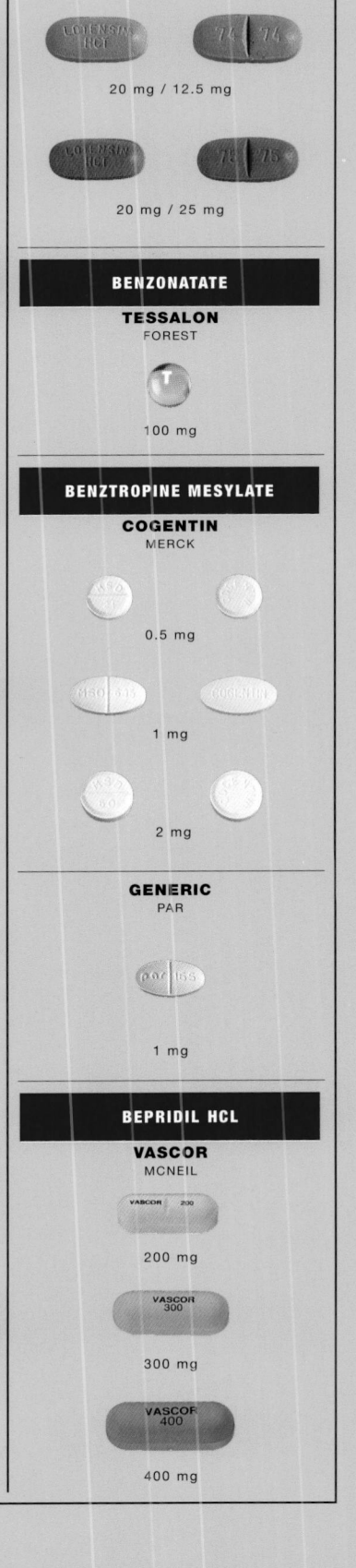

LOTENSIN HCT
CIBA

10 mg / 12.5 mg

20 mg / 12.5 mg

20 mg / 25 mg

BENZONATATE

TESSALON
FOREST

100 mg

BENZTROPINE MESYLATE

COGENTIN
MERCK

0.5 mg

1 mg

2 mg

GENERIC
PAR

1 mg

BEPRIDIL HCL

VASCOR
MCNEIL

200 mg

300 mg

400 mg

BETAXOLOL HCL

KERLONE
G. D. SEARLE

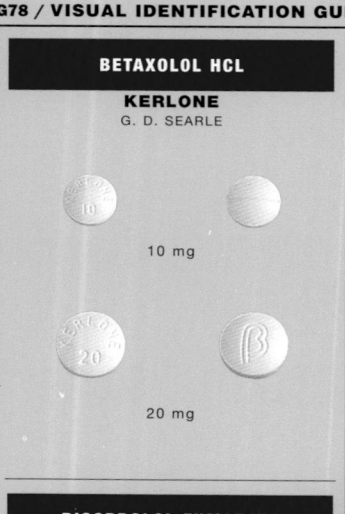

10 mg

20 mg

BISOPROLOL FUMARATE

ZEBETA
LEDERLE

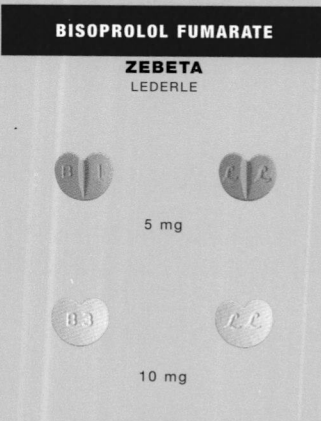

5 mg

10 mg

BISOPROLOL FUMARATE / HYDROCHLOROTHIAZIDE

ZIAC
LEDERLE

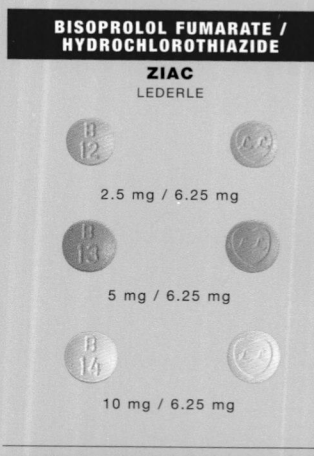

2.5 mg / 6.25 mg

5 mg / 6.25 mg

10 mg / 6.25 mg

BROMOCRIPTINE MESYLATE

PARLODEL
SANDOZ

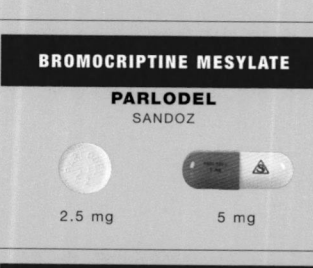

2.5 mg   5 mg

BUMETANIDE

BUMEX
ROCHE

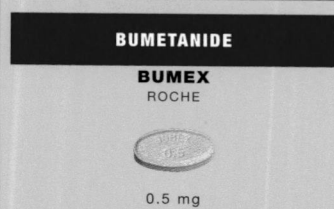

0.5 mg

BUMEX
ROCHE

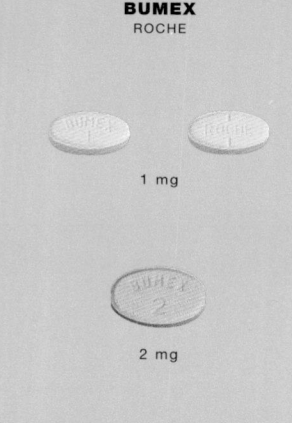

1 mg

2 mg

BUPROPION HCL

WELLBUTRIN
BURROUGHS WELLCOME

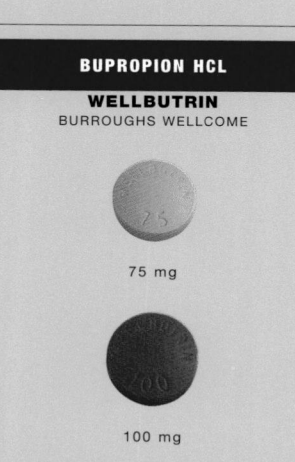

75 mg

100 mg

BUSPIRONE HCL

BUSPAR
BRISTOL-MYERS SQUIBB

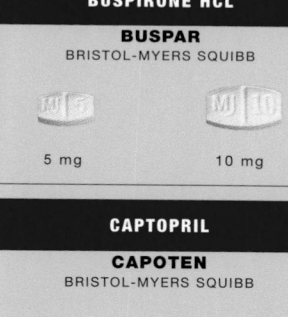

5 mg   10 mg

CAPTOPRIL

CAPOTEN
BRISTOL-MYERS SQUIBB

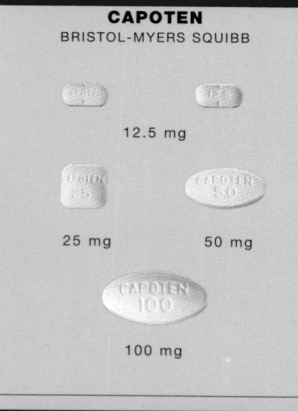

12.5 mg

25 mg   50 mg

100 mg

CAPTOPRIL / HYDROCHLOROTHIAZIDE

CAPOZIDE
BRISTOL-MYERS SQUIBB

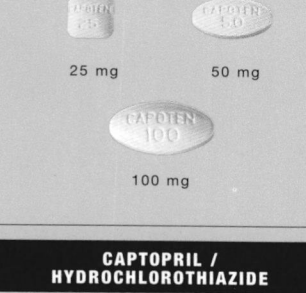
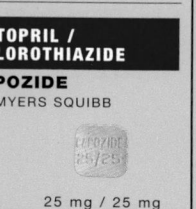

25 mg / 15 mg   25 mg / 25 mg

CAPOZIDE
BRISTOL-MYERS SQUIBB

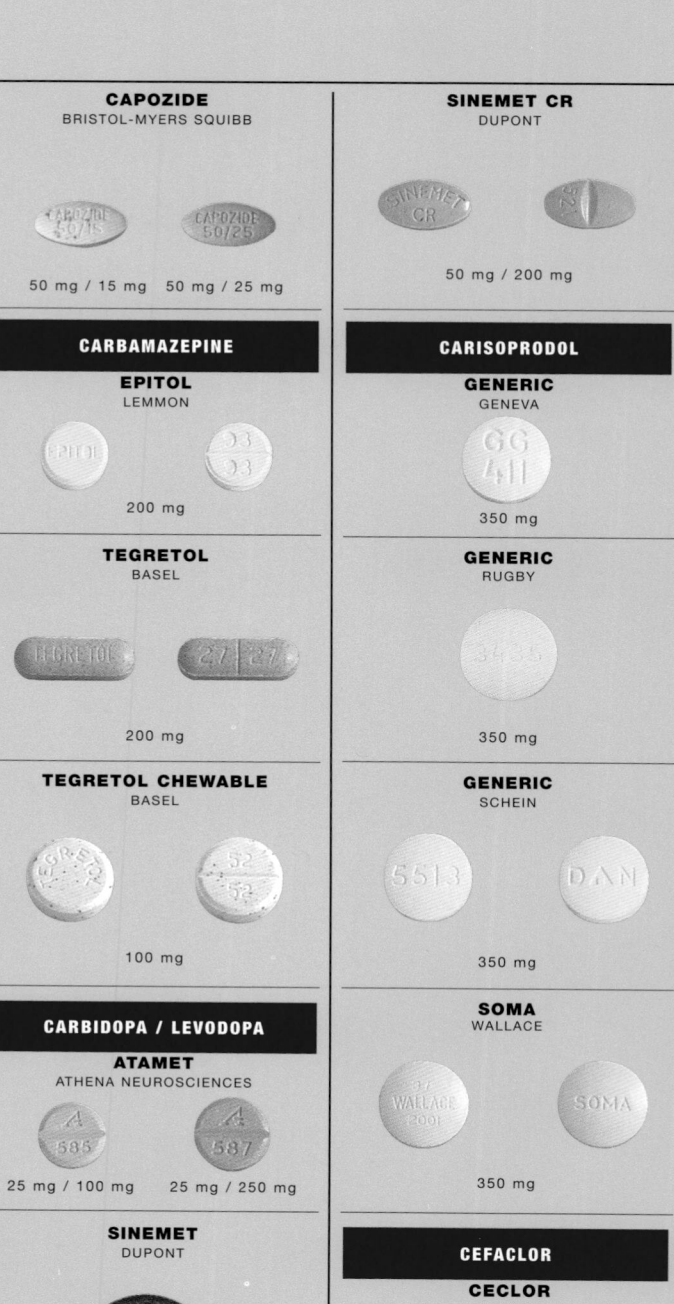

50 mg / 15 mg   50 mg / 25 mg

CARBAMAZEPINE

EPITOL
LEMMON

200 mg

TEGRETOL
BASEL

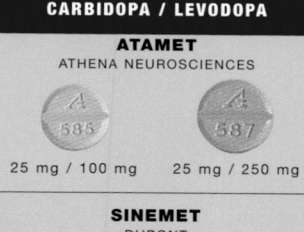

200 mg

TEGRETOL CHEWABLE
BASEL

100 mg

CARBIDOPA / LEVODOPA

ATAMET
ATHENA NEUROSCIENCES

25 mg / 100 mg   25 mg / 250 mg

SINEMET
DUPONT

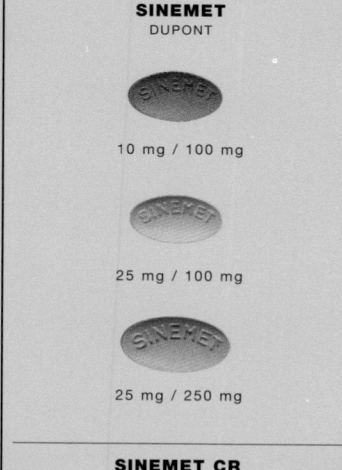

10 mg / 100 mg

25 mg / 100 mg

25 mg / 250 mg

SINEMET CR
DUPONT

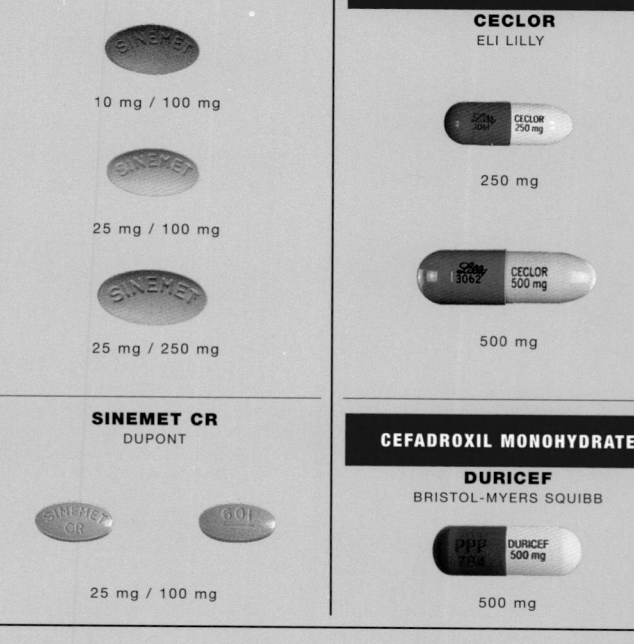

25 mg / 100 mg

SINEMET CR
DUPONT

50 mg / 200 mg

CARISOPRODOL

GENERIC
GENEVA

350 mg

GENERIC
RUGBY

350 mg

GENERIC
SCHEIN

350 mg

SOMA
WALLACE

350 mg

CEFACLOR

CECLOR
ELI LILLY

250 mg

500 mg

CEFADROXIL MONOHYDRATE

DURICEF
BRISTOL-MYERS SQUIBB

500 mg

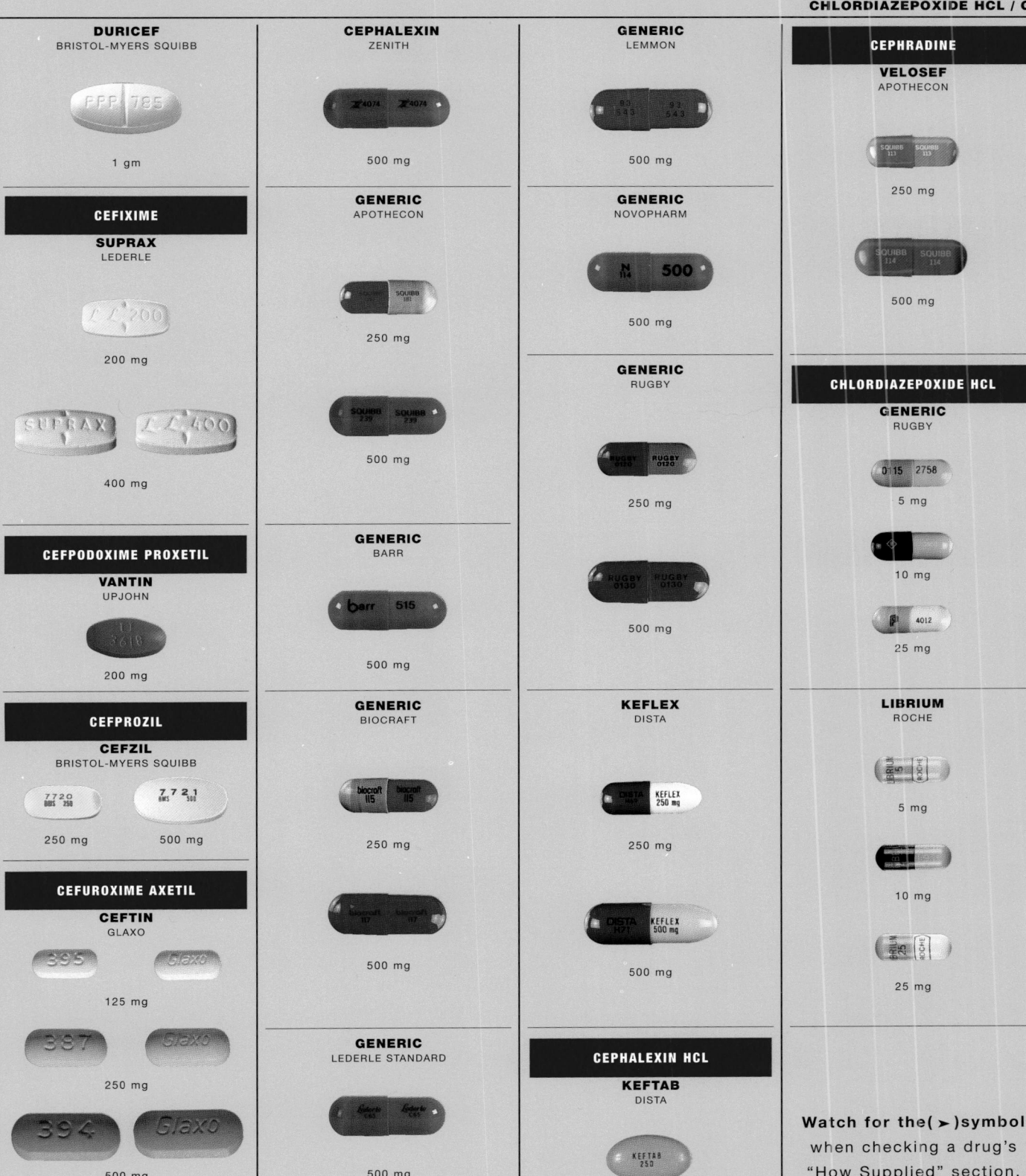

DURICEF
BRISTOL-MYERS SQUIBB

1 gm

CEFIXIME

SUPRAX
LEDERLE

200 mg

400 mg

CEFPODOXIME PROXETIL

VANTIN
UPJOHN

200 mg

CEFPROZIL

CEFZIL
BRISTOL-MYERS SQUIBB

250 mg   500 mg

CEFUROXIME AXETIL

CEFTIN
GLAXO

125 mg

250 mg

500 mg

CEPHALEXIN

CEPHALEXIN
ZENITH

250 mg

CEPHALEXIN
ZENITH

500 mg

GENERIC
APOTHECON

250 mg

500 mg

GENERIC
BARR

500 mg

GENERIC
BIOCRAFT

250 mg

500 mg

GENERIC
LEDERLE STANDARD

500 mg

GENERIC
LEMMON

250 mg

GENERIC
LEMMON

500 mg

GENERIC
NOVOPHARM

500 mg

GENERIC
RUGBY

250 mg

500 mg

KEFLEX
DISTA

250 mg

500 mg

CEPHALEXIN HCL

KEFTAB
DISTA

250 mg

500 mg

CEPHRADINE

VELOSEF
APOTHECON

250 mg

500 mg

CHLORDIAZEPOXIDE HCL

GENERIC
RUGBY

5 mg

10 mg

25 mg

LIBRIUM
ROCHE

5 mg

10 mg

25 mg

Watch for the (➤) symbol when checking a drug's "How Supplied" section. It means that a color photo of the product appears here in *PDR Generics'* Visual Identification Guide.

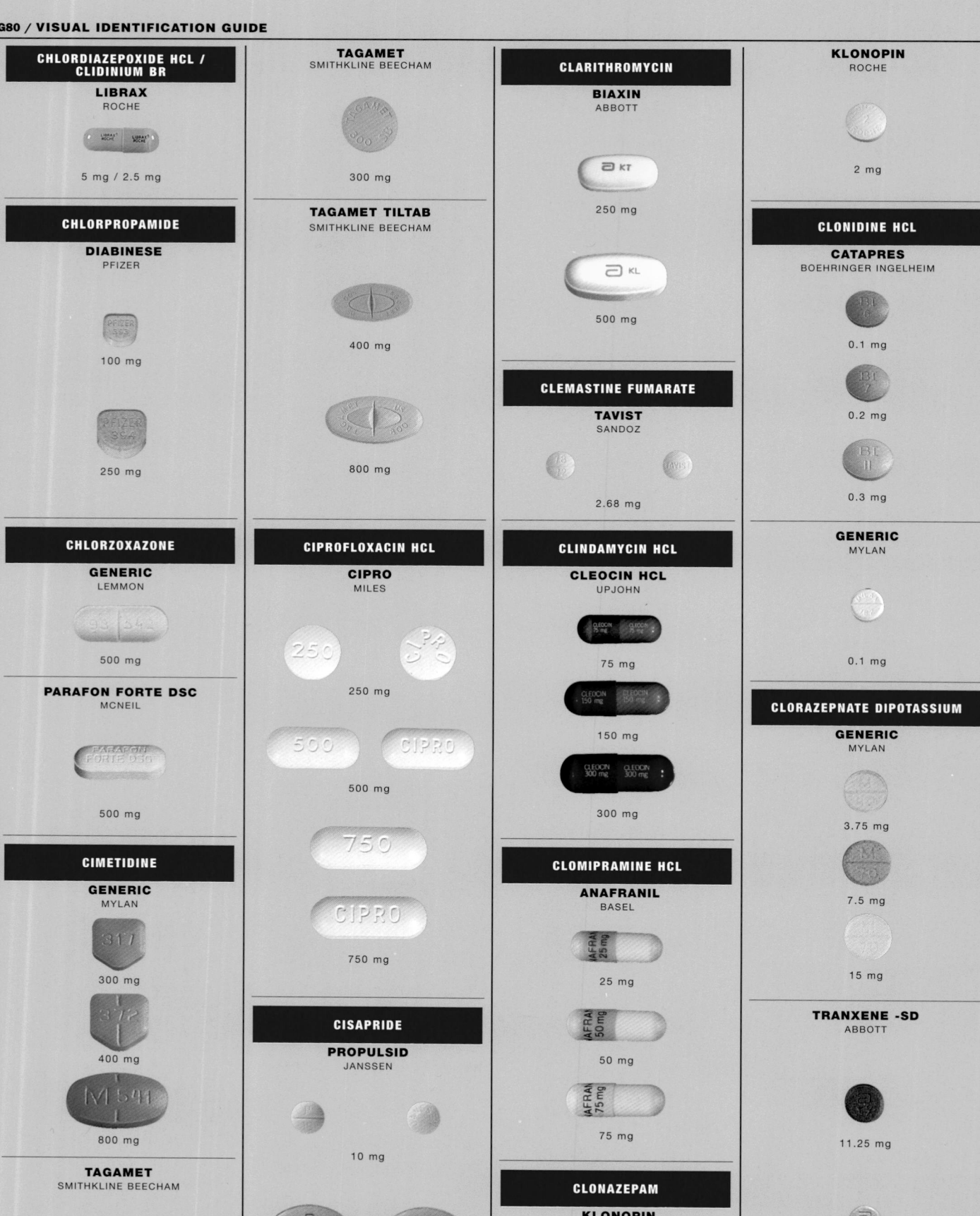

CHLORDIAZEPOXIDE HCL / CLIDINIUM BR

LIBRAX
ROCHE

5 mg / 2.5 mg

CHLORPROPAMIDE

DIABINESE
PFIZER

100 mg

250 mg

CHLORZOXAZONE

GENERIC
LEMMON

500 mg

PARAFON FORTE DSC
MCNEIL

500 mg

CIMETIDINE

GENERIC
MYLAN

300 mg

400 mg

800 mg

TAGAMET
SMITHKLINE BEECHAM

200 mg

TAGAMET
SMITHKLINE BEECHAM

300 mg

TAGAMET TILTAB
SMITHKLINE BEECHAM

400 mg

800 mg

CIPROFLOXACIN HCL

CIPRO
MILES

250 mg

500 mg

750 mg

CISAPRIDE

PROPULSID
JANSSEN

10 mg

20 mg

CLARITHROMYCIN

BIAXIN
ABBOTT

250 mg

500 mg

CLEMASTINE FUMARATE

TAVIST
SANDOZ

2.68 mg

CLINDAMYCIN HCL

CLEOCIN HCL
UPJOHN

75 mg

150 mg

300 mg

CLOMIPRAMINE HCL

ANAFRANIL
BASEL

25 mg

50 mg

75 mg

CLONAZEPAM

KLONOPIN
ROCHE

0.5 mg   1 mg

KLONOPIN
ROCHE

2 mg

CLONIDINE HCL

CATAPRES
BOEHRINGER INGELHEIM

0.1 mg

0.2 mg

0.3 mg

GENERIC
MYLAN

0.1 mg

CLORAZEPNATE DIPOTASSIUM

GENERIC
MYLAN

3.75 mg

7.5 mg

15 mg

TRANXENE -SD
ABBOTT

11.25 mg

22.5 mg

TRANXENE T-TAB
ABBOTT

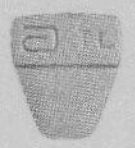

3.75 mg

7.5 mg

15 mg

CLOZAPINE
CLOZARIL
SANDOZ

25 mg

100 mg

CYCLOBENZAPRINE HCL
GENERIC
DANBURY

10 mg

GENERIC
MYLAN

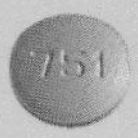

10 mg

GENERIC
WEST POINT

10 mg

FLEXERIL
MERCK

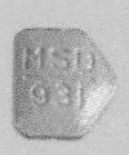

10 mg

CYCLOPHOSPHAMIDE
CYTOXAN
BRISTOL-MYERS ONCOLOGY

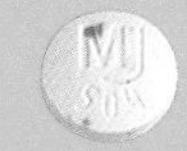

25 mg

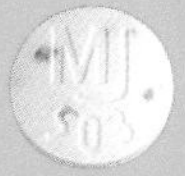

50 mg

DESOGESTREL / ETHINYL ESTRADIOL
ORTHO-CEPT
ORTHO

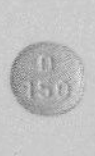

0.15 mg / 0.03 mg

DEXAMETHASONE
DECADRON
MERCK

0.25 mg

0.5 mg

0.75 mg

1.5 mg

4 mg

6 mg

DIAZEPAM
GENERIC
LEDERLE STANDARD

5 mg

GENERIC
MYLAN

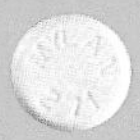

2 mg

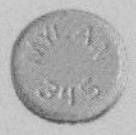

5 mg

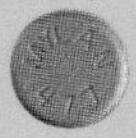

10 mg

GENERIC
RUGBY

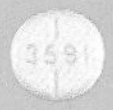

2 mg

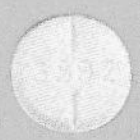

5 mg

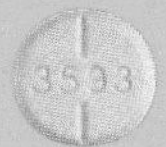

10 mg

GENERIC
SCHEIN

5 mg

GENERIC
ZENITH

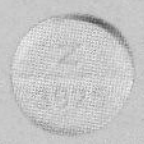

2 mg

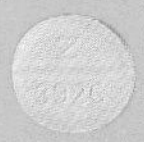

5 mg

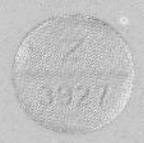

10 mg

VALIUM
ROCHE

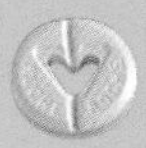

2 mg

VALIUM
ROCHE

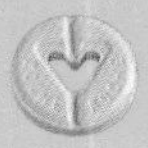

5 mg

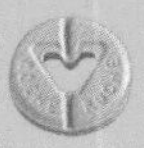

10 mg

VALRELEASE
ROCHE

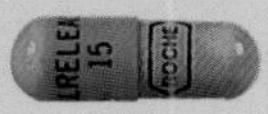

15 mg

DICLOFENAC POTASSIUM
CATAFLAM
GEIGY

50 mg

DICLOFENAC SODIUM
VOLTAREN
GEIGY

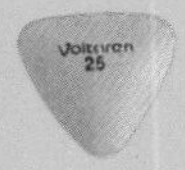

25 mg

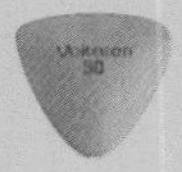

50 mg

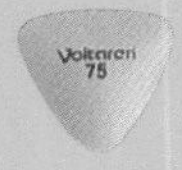

75 mg

DICYCLOMINE HCL
GENERIC
RUGBY

20 mg

BENTYL
MARION MERRELL DOW

10 mg

20 mg

DIDANOSINE

VIDEX
BRISTOL-MYERS ONCOLOGY

100 mg

DIGOXIN

LANOXICAPS
BURROUGHS WELLCOME

0.05 mg

0.1 mg

0.2 mg

LANOXIN
BURROUGHS WELLCOME

0.125 mg

0.25 mg

0.5 mg

DILTIAZEM HCL

CARDIZEM
MARION MERRELL DOW

30 mg

60 mg

CARDIZEM
MARION MERRELL DOW

90 mg

120 mg

CARDIZEM CD
MARION MERRELL DOW

120 mg

180 mg

240 mg

300 mg

CARDIZEM SR
MARION MERRELL DOW

60 mg

90 mg

120 mg

DILACOR XR
RHONE-POULENC RORER

120 mg

180 mg

240 mg

GENERIC
COPLEY

30 mg

60 mg

90 mg

120 mg

GENERIC
RUGBY

30 mg

DIPHENOXYLATE HCL / ATROPINE SULFATE

LOMOTIL
G. D. SEARLE

2.5 mg / 0.025 mg

LONOX
GENEVA

2.5 mg / 0.025 mg

DIPYRIDAMOLE

GENERIC
BARR

50 mg · 75 mg

GENERIC
GENEVA

25 mg · 50 mg

GENERIC
GENEVA

GG 464

75 mg

GENERIC
LEDERLE STANDARD

50 mg

PERSANTINE
BOEHRINGER INGELHEIM

25 mg

50 mg

75 mg

DIVALPROEX SODIUM

DEPAKOTE
ABBOTT

125 mg

250 mg

500 mg

DEPAKOTE SPRINKLE
ABBOTT

125 mg

DOXAZOSIN MESYLATE

CARDURA
ROERIG

1 mg

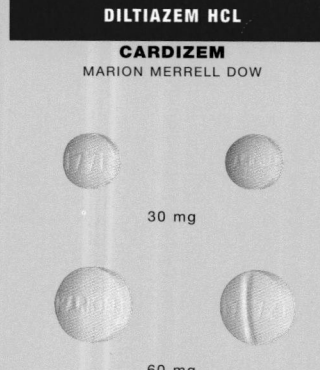
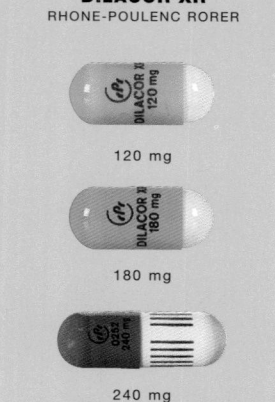
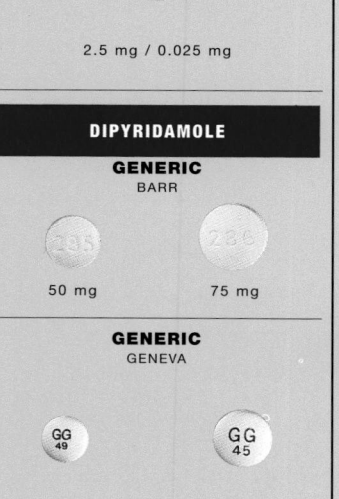
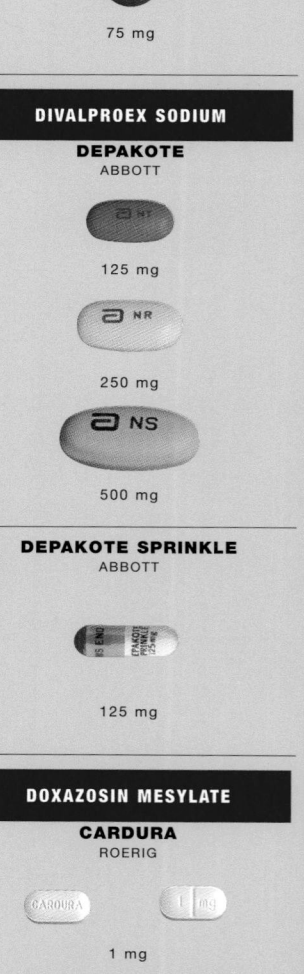

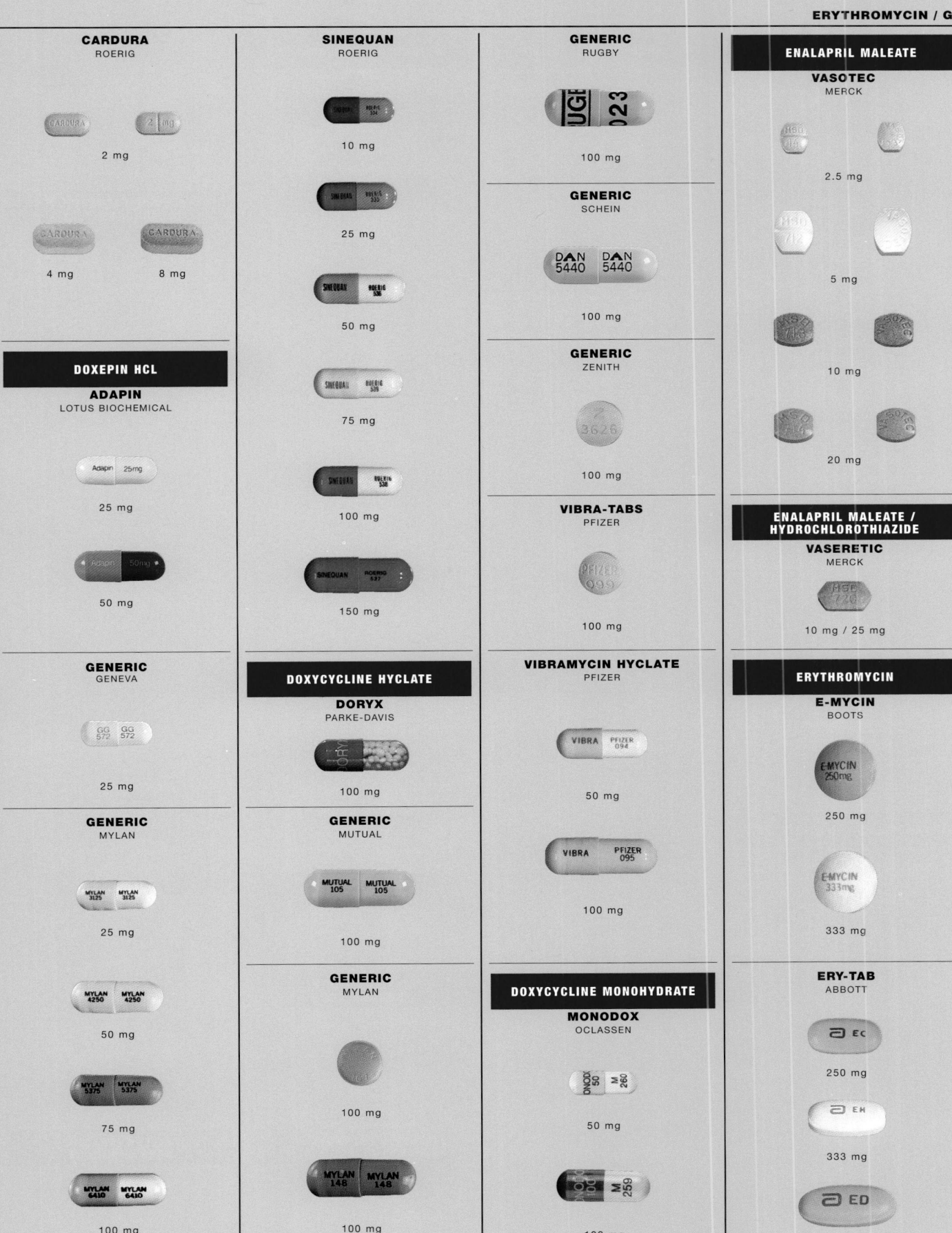

CARDURA
ROERIG

2 mg

4 mg   8 mg

DOXEPIN HCL

ADAPIN
LOTUS BIOCHEMICAL

25 mg

50 mg

GENERIC
GENEVA

25 mg

GENERIC
MYLAN

25 mg

50 mg

75 mg

100 mg

SINEQUAN
ROERIG

10 mg

25 mg

50 mg

75 mg

100 mg

150 mg

DOXYCYCLINE HYCLATE

DORYX
PARKE-DAVIS

100 mg

GENERIC
MUTUAL

100 mg

GENERIC
MYLAN

100 mg

100 mg

GENERIC
RUGBY

100 mg

GENERIC
SCHEIN

100 mg

GENERIC
ZENITH

100 mg

VIBRA-TABS
PFIZER

100 mg

VIBRAMYCIN HYCLATE
PFIZER

50 mg

100 mg

DOXYCYCLINE MONOHYDRATE

MONODOX
OCLASSEN

50 mg

100 mg

ENALAPRIL MALEATE

VASOTEC
MERCK

2.5 mg

5 mg

10 mg

20 mg

ENALAPRIL MALEATE / HYDROCHLOROTHIAZIDE

VASERETIC
MERCK

10 mg / 25 mg

ERYTHROMYCIN

E-MYCIN
BOOTS

250 mg

333 mg

ERY-TAB
ABBOTT

250 mg

333 mg

500 mg

ERYC
PARKE-DAVIS

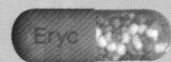

250 mg

ERYTHROMYCIN BASE FILMTAB
ABBOTT

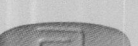

500 mg

ERYTHROMYCIN DELAYED-RELEASE
ABBOTT

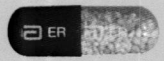

250 mg

PCE
ABBOTT

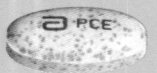

333 mg

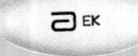

500 mg

ERYTHROMYCIN ETHYLSUCCINATE

E.E.S. 400 FILMTAB
ABBOTT

400 mg

ERYPED CHEWABLE
ABBOTT

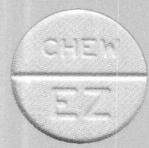

200 mg

ERYTHROMYCIN STEARATE

ERYTHROCIN STEARATE FILMTAB
ABBOTT

250 mg

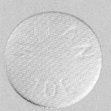

500 mg

GENERIC
MYLAN

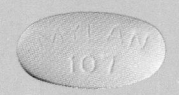

250 mg

500 mg

ESTAZOLAM

PROSOM
ABBOTT

1 mg

2 mg

ESTRADIOL

ESTRACE
BRISTOL-MYERS SQUIBB

0.5 mg

1 mg

2 mg

ESTROGENS, CONJUGATED

PREMARIN
WYETH-AYERST

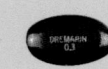

0.3 mg

0.625 mg

0.9 mg

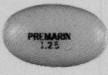

1.25 mg

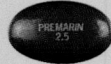

2.5 mg

ESTROPIPATE

ORTHO-EST .625
ORTHO

0.75 mg

ORTHO-EST 1.25
ORTHO

1.5 mg

ETHINYL ESTRADIOL / NORGESTREL

LO/OVRAL
WYETH-AYERST

0.03 mg / 0.3 mg

ETHINYL ESTRADIOL / ETHYNODIOL DIACETATE

DEMULEN 1/35
G. D. SEARLE

0.035 mg / 1 mg

DEMULEN 1/50
G. D. SEARLE

0.05 mg / 1 mg

ETHINYL ESTRADIOL / LEVONORGESTREL

LEVLEN
BERLEX

0.03 mg / 0.15 mg

NORDETTE
WYETH-AYERST

0.03 mg / 0.15 mg

TRI-LEVLEN
BERLEX

0.03 mg / 0.05 mg

0.03 mg / 0.125 mg

0.04 mg / 0.075 mg

TRIPHASIL
WYETH-AYERST

0.03 mg / 0.05 mg

0.03 mg / 0.125 mg

0.04 mg / 0.075 mg

ETHINYL ESTRADIOL / NORETHINDRONE

GENORA 1/35
RUGBY

0.035 mg / 1 mg

JENEST
ORGANON

0.035 mg / 0.5 mg

0.035 mg / 1 mg

NORINYL 1+35
SYNTEX

0.035 mg / 1 mg

ORTHO-NOVUM 1/35
ORTHO

0.035 mg / 1 mg

ORTHO-NOVUM 7/7/7
ORTHO

0.035 mg / 0.5 mg

0.035 mg / 0.75 mg

0.035 mg / 1 mg

ORTHO-NOVUM 10/11
ORTHO

0.035 mg / 0.5 mg

0.035 mg / 1 mg

OVCON-35
BRISTOL-MYERS SQUIBB

0.035 mg / 0.4 mg

OVCON-50
BRISTOL-MYERS SQUIBB

0.05 mg / 1 mg

TRI-NORINYL
SYNTEX

0.035 mg / 0.5 mg

0.035 mg / 1 mg

**ETHINYL ESTRADIOL /
NORETHINDRONE ACETATE**
LOESTRIN-21 1/20
PARKE-DAVIS

0.02 mg / 1 mg

LOESTRIN-21 1.5/30
PARKE-DAVIS

0.03 mg / 1.5 mg

**ETHINYL ESTRADIOL /
NORGESTIMATE**
ORTHO-CYCLEN
ORTHO

0.035 mg / 0.25 mg

ORTHO TRI-CYCLEN
ORTHO

0.035 mg / 0.18 mg

ORTHO TRI-CYCLEN
ORTHO

0.035 mg / 0.215 mg

0.035 mg / 0.25 mg

**ETHINYL ESTRADIOL /
NORGESTREL**
LO/OVRAL
WYETH-AYERST

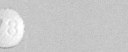

0.03 mg / 0.3 mg

OVRAL
WYETH-AYERST

0.05 mg / 0.5 mg

ETHOSUXIMIDE
ZARONTIN
PARKE-DAVIS

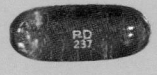

250 mg

ETODOLAC
LODINE
WYETH-AYERST

200 mg

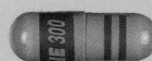

300 mg

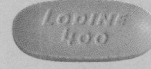

400 mg

FAMCICLOVIR
FAMVIR
SMITHKLINE BEECHAM

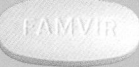 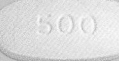

500 mg

FAMOTIDINE
PEPCID
MERCK

20 mg   40 mg

FELBAMATE
FELBATOL
WALLACE

400 mg

 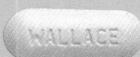

600 mg

FELODIPINE
PLENDIL
ASTRA MERCK

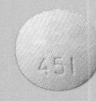

5 mg

10 mg

FENOPROFEN CALCIUM
NALFON
DISTA

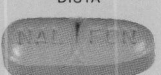

600 mg

FINASTERIDE
PROSCAR
MERCK

5 mg

FLUCONAZOLE
DIFLUCAN
ROERIG

50 mg

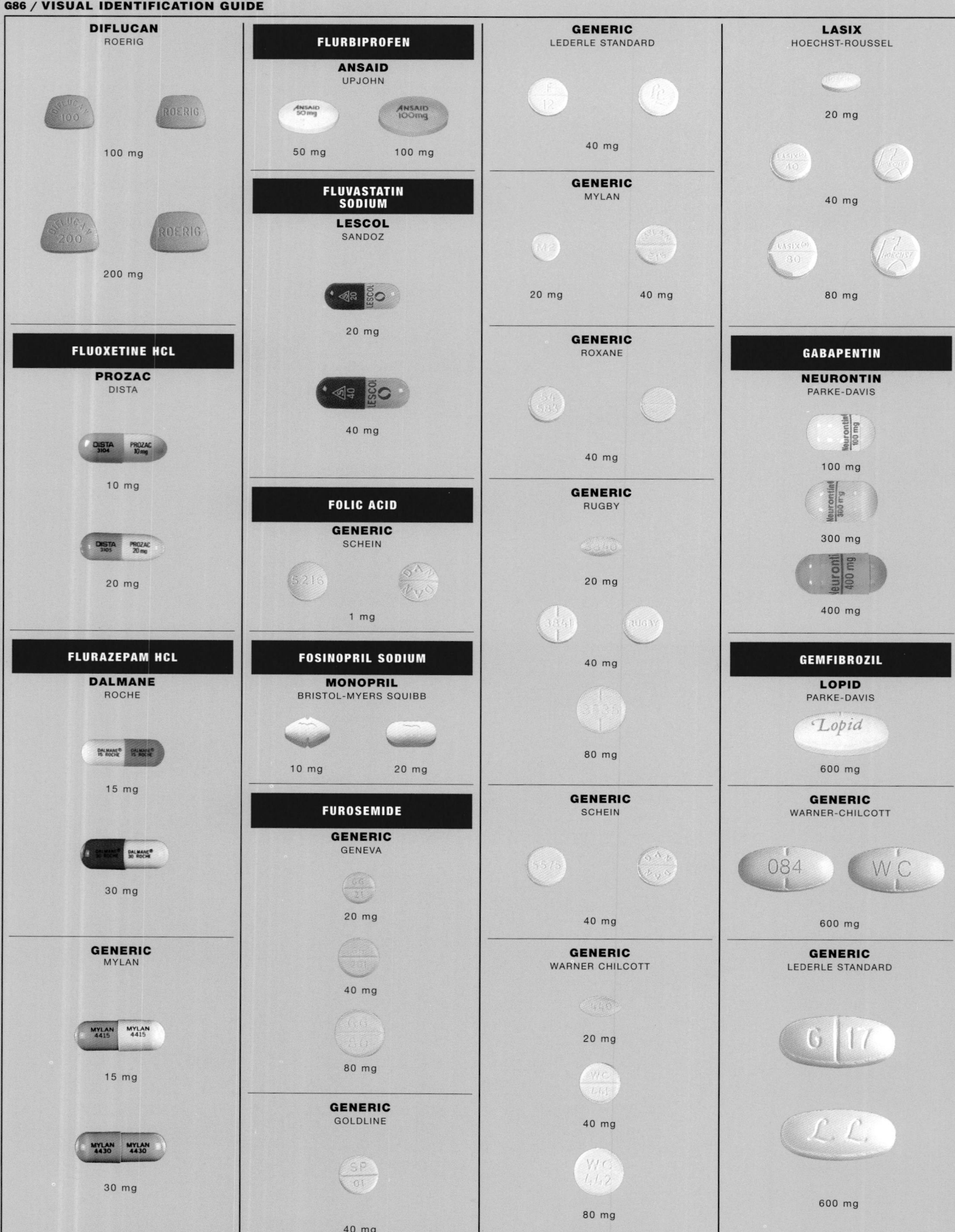

DIFLUCAN
ROERIG

100 mg

200 mg

FLUOXETINE HCL

PROZAC
DISTA

10 mg

20 mg

FLURAZEPAM HCL

DALMANE
ROCHE

15 mg

30 mg

GENERIC
MYLAN

15 mg

30 mg

FLURBIPROFEN

ANSAID
UPJOHN

50 mg   100 mg

FLUVASTATIN SODIUM

LESCOL
SANDOZ

20 mg

40 mg

FOLIC ACID

GENERIC
SCHEIN

1 mg

FOSINOPRIL SODIUM

MONOPRIL
BRISTOL-MYERS SQUIBB

10 mg   20 mg

FUROSEMIDE

GENERIC
GENEVA

20 mg

40 mg

80 mg

GENERIC
GOLDLINE

40 mg

GENERIC
LEDERLE STANDARD

40 mg

GENERIC
MYLAN

20 mg   40 mg

GENERIC
ROXANE

40 mg

GENERIC
RUGBY

20 mg

40 mg

80 mg

GENERIC
SCHEIN

40 mg

GENERIC
WARNER CHILCOTT

20 mg

40 mg

80 mg

LASIX
HOECHST-ROUSSEL

20 mg

40 mg

80 mg

GABAPENTIN

NEURONTIN
PARKE-DAVIS

100 mg

300 mg

400 mg

GEMFIBROZIL

LOPID
PARKE-DAVIS

600 mg

GENERIC
WARNER-CHILCOTT

600 mg

GENERIC
LEDERLE STANDARD

600 mg

GLIPIZIDE

GLUCOTROL
PRATT

 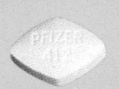

5 mg   10 mg

GLUCOTROL XL
PRATT

5 mg   10 mg

GLYBURIDE

DIABETA
HOECHST-ROUSSEL

1.25 mg

2.5 mg

5 mg

GLYNASE PRESTAB
UPJOHN

1.5 mg

3 mg

MICRONASE
UPJOHN

1.25 mg

2.5 mg

5 mg

GUAIFENESIN

HUMIBID LA
ADAMS

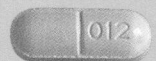 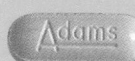

600 mg

GUAIFENESIN / PHENYLPROPANOLAMINE HCL

ENTEX LA
PROCTER & GAMBLE

 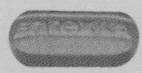

400 mg / 75 mg

EXGEST LA
CARNRICK

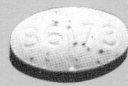

400 mg / 75 mg

GENERIC
DURAMED

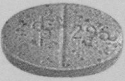

400 mg / 75 mg

GUAIFENESIN / PSEUDOEPHEDRINE HCL

DECONSAL-II
ADAMS

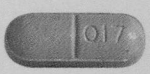 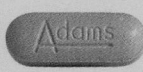

600 mg / 60 mg

DURATUSS
WHITBY

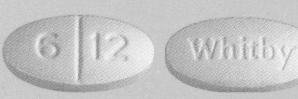

600 mg / 120 mg

ENTEX PSE
PROCTER & GAMBLE

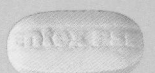 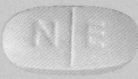

600 mg / 120 mg

GUAIMAX-D
CENTRAL

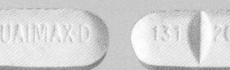

600 mg / 120 mg

RU-TUSS DE
BOOTS

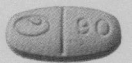 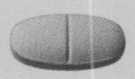

600 mg / 120 mg

ZEPHREX LA
BOCK

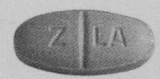 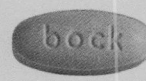

600 mg / 120 mg

GUANFACINE HCL

TENEX
A. H. ROBINS

1 mg

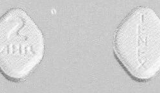

2 mg

HALOPERIDOL

HALDOL
MCNEIL

0.5 mg   1 mg

2 mg   5 mg

10 mg   20 mg

HYDROCHLOROTHIAZIDE

ESIDRIX
CIBA

25 mg

50 mg

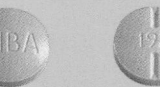

100 mg

GENERIC
GENEVA

25 mg   50 mg

GENERIC
SCHEIN

50 mg

GENERIC
PUREPAC

25 mg

GENERIC
RUGBY

25 mg   50 mg

GENERIC
WEST POINT

25 mg

50 mg

GENERIC
ZENITH

25 mg

50 mg

100 mg

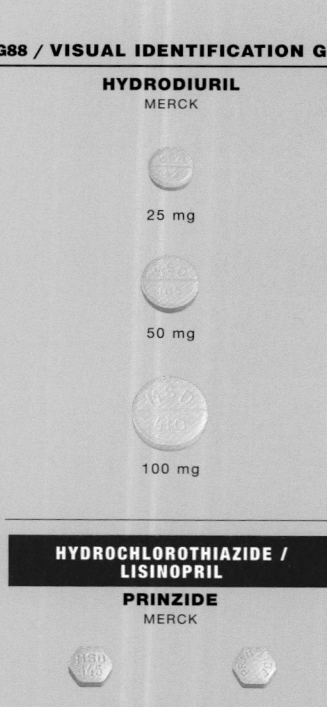

HYDRODIURIL
MERCK

25 mg

50 mg

100 mg

HYDROCHLOROTHIAZIDE / LISINOPRIL

PRINZIDE
MERCK

12.5 mg / 10 mg

12.5 mg / 20 mg

25 mg / 20 mg

ZESTORETIC
STUART

12.5 mg / 20 mg

25 mg / 20 mg

HYDROCHLOROTHIAZIDE / METOPROLOL TARTRATE

LOPRESSOR HCT
GEIGY

25 mg / 50 mg

25 mg / 100 mg

50 mg / 100 mg

HYDROCHLOROTHIAZIDE / PROPRANOLOL HCL

INDERIDE
WYETH-AYERST

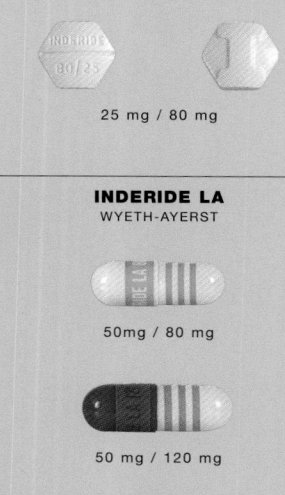

25 mg / 40 mg

25 mg / 80 mg

INDERIDE LA
WYETH-AYERST

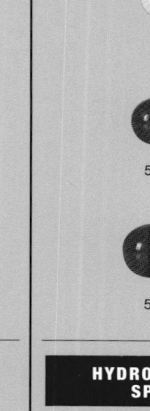

50mg / 80 mg

50 mg / 120 mg

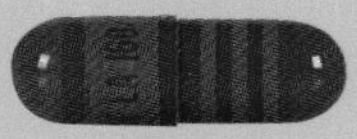

50 mg / 160 mg

HYDROCHLOROTHIAZIDE / SPIRONOLACTONE

ALDACTAZIDE
G. D. SEARLE

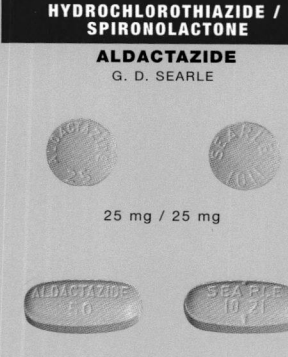

25 mg / 25 mg

50 mg / 50 mg

HYDROCHLOROTHIAZIDE / TRIAMTERENE

DYAZIDE
SMITHKLINE BEECHAM

25 mg / 37.5 mg

GENERIC
GENEVA

25 mg / 50 mg

GENERIC
RUGBY

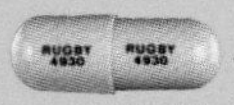

25 mg / 50 mg

50 mg / 75 mg

GENERIC
SCHEIN

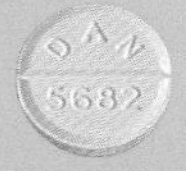

50 mg / 75 mg

MAXZIDE
LEDERLE

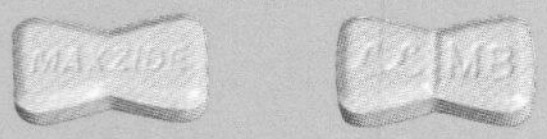

50 mg / 75 mg

MAXZIDE 25 MG
LEDERLE

25 mg / 37.5 mg

HYDROMORPHONE HCL

DILAUDID
KNOLL

2 mg

4 mg

GENERIC
ROXANE

2 mg   4 mg

HYDROXYCHLOROQUINE SULFATE

PLAQUENIL
SANOFI WINTHROP

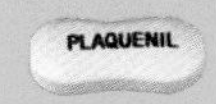

200 mg

HYDROXYZINE HCL

ATARAX
ROERIG

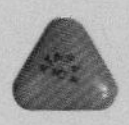

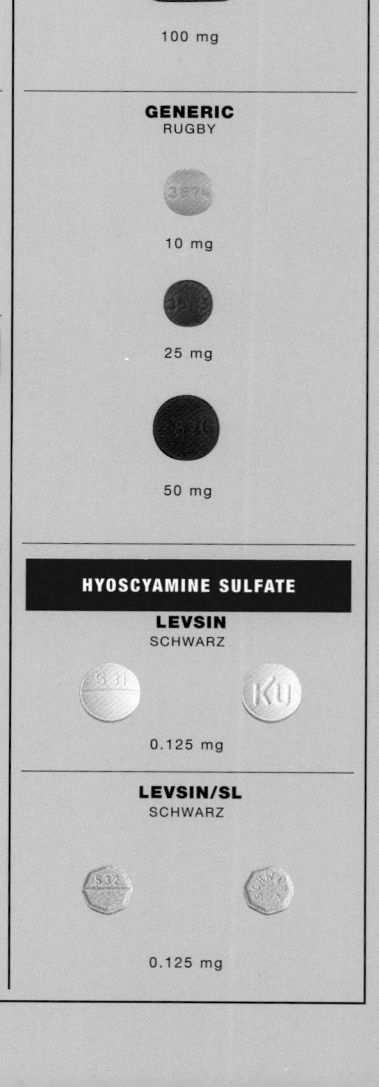

10 mg

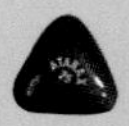

25 mg

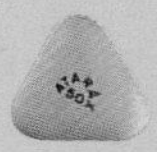

50 mg

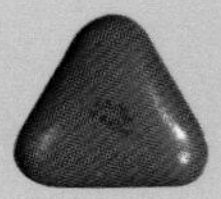

100 mg

GENERIC
RUGBY

10 mg

25 mg

50 mg

HYOSCYAMINE SULFATE

LEVSIN
SCHWARZ

0.125 mg

LEVSIN/SL
SCHWARZ

0.125 mg

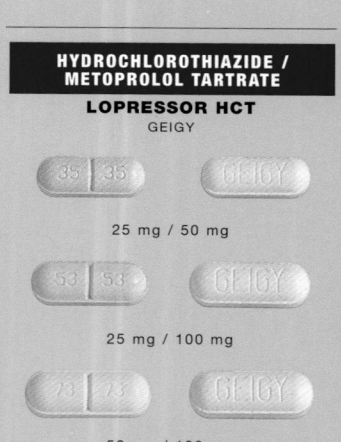

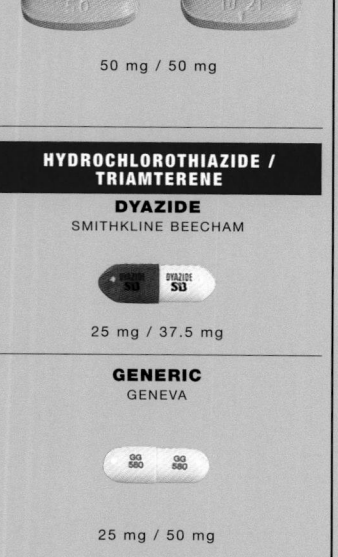

LEVSINEX TIMECAPS
SCHWARZ

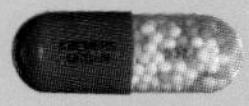

0.375 mg

IBUPROFEN
GENERIC
PAR

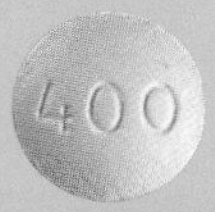

400
400 mg

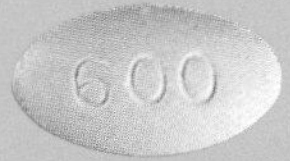

600
600 mg

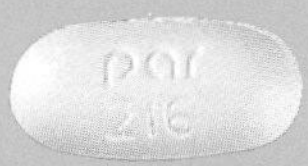

par 216
800 mg

GENERIC
RUGBY

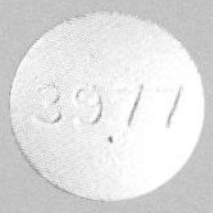

3977
400 mg

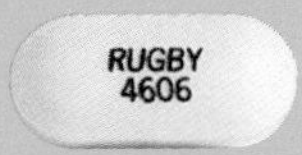

RUGBY 4606
800 mg

GENERIC
SCHEIN

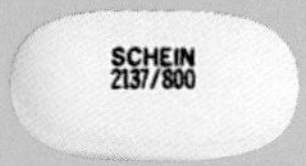

SCHEIN 2137/800
800 mg

MOTRIN
UPJOHN

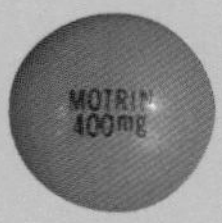

MOTRIN 400mg
400 mg

MOTRIN
UPJOHN

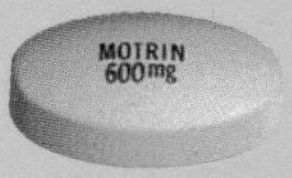

MOTRIN 600mg
600 mg

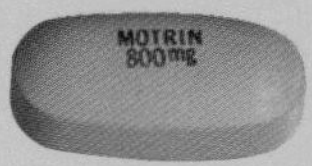

MOTRIN 800mg
800 mg

RUFEN
BOOTS

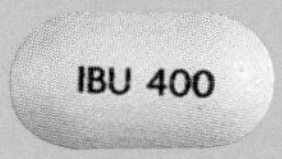

IBU 400
400 mg

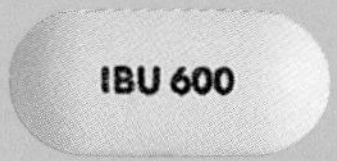

IBU 600
600 mg

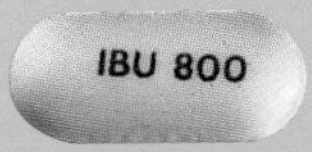

IBU 800
800 mg

IMIPRAMINE HCL
GENERIC
BIOCRAFT

BL   21
50 mg

GENERIC
GENEVA

47   GG
25 mg

JANIMINE
ABBOTT

10 mg

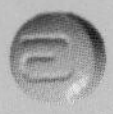

25 mg

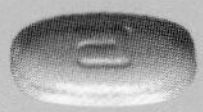

50 mg

TOFRANIL
GEIGY

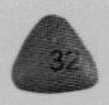

32
10 mg

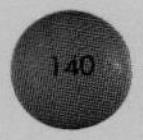

140
25 mg

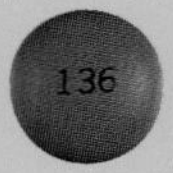

136
50 mg

INDAPAMIDE
LOZOL
RHONE-POULENC RORER

7   R
1.25 mg

8   R
2.5 mg

INDOMETHACIN
GENERIC
MYLAN

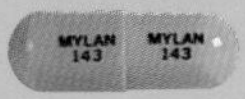

MYLAN 143   MYLAN 143
25 mg

GENERIC
WEST POINT

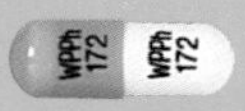

WPPh 172   WPPh 172
25 mg

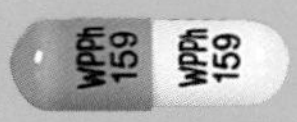

WPPh 159   WPPh 159
50 mg

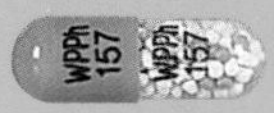

WPPh 157   WPPh 157
75 mg
SUSTAINED RELEASE

INDOCIN
MERCK

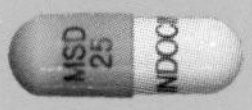

MSD 25   INDOCIN
25 mg

INDOCIN
MERCK

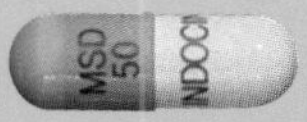

MSD 50   INDOCIN
50 mg

INDOCIN-SR
MERCK

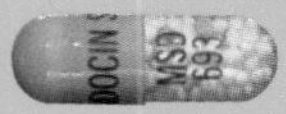

INDOCIN S   693 GSVI
75 mg

ISONIAZID
GENERIC
BARR

Barr 066   100
100 mg

ISONIAZID / PYRAZINAMIDE / RIFAMPIN
RIFATER
MARION MERRELL DOW

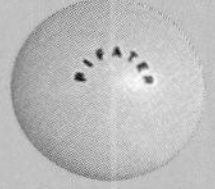

RIFATER
50 mg / 300 mg / 120 mg

ISOSORBIDE DINITRATE
GENERIC
GENEVA

1   2
2.5 mg   5 mg
SUBLINGUAL   SUBLINGUAL

GG 259   GG 26
5 mg   10 mg

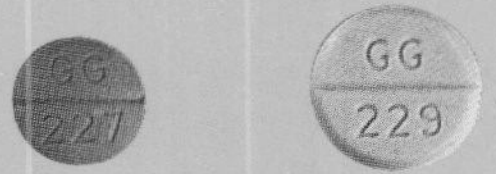

GG 227   GG 229
20 mg   40 mg

GENERIC
RUGBY

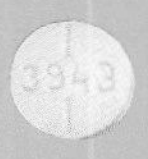

3943
10 mg

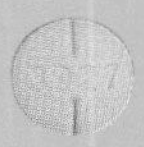

3947
20 mg

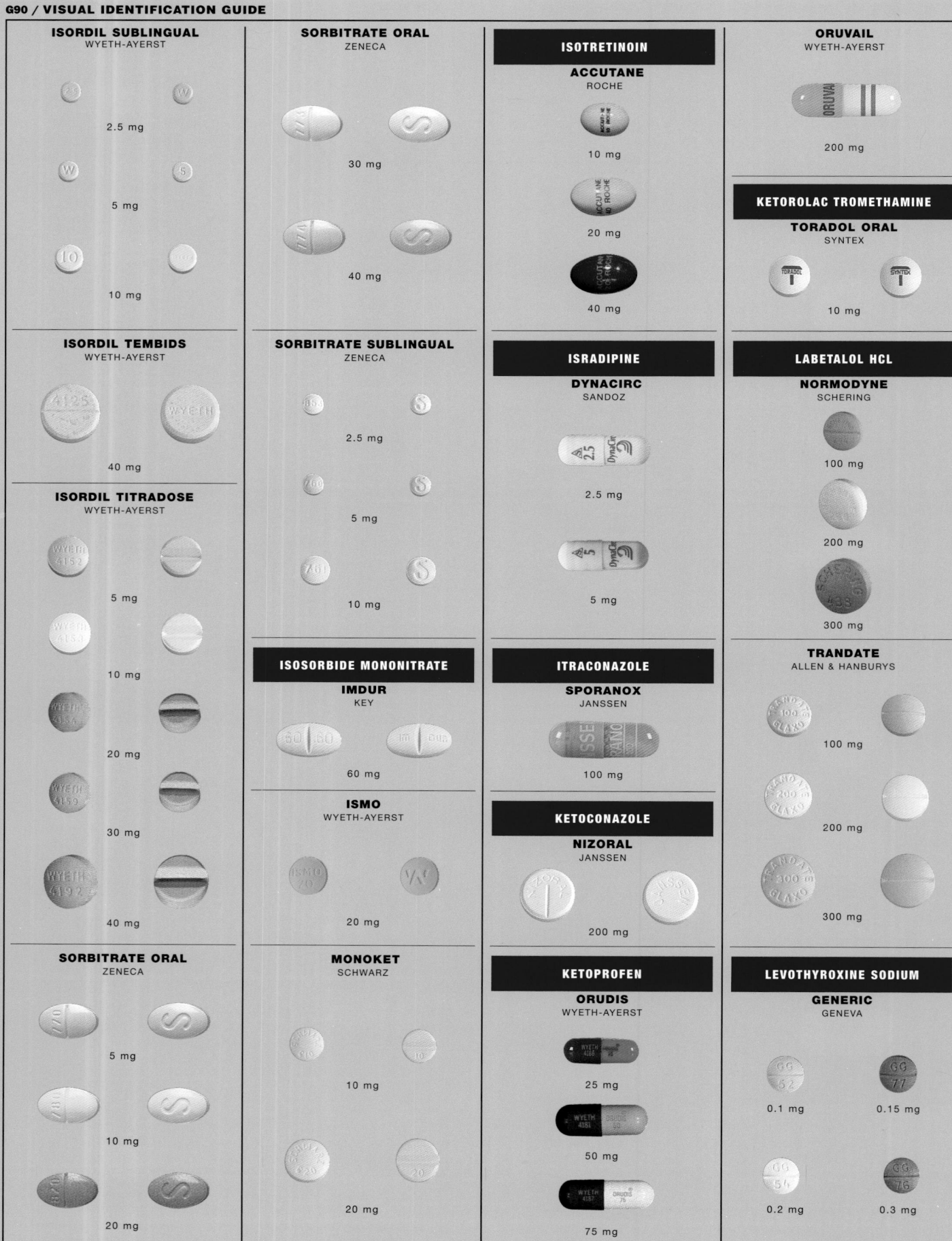

ISORDIL SUBLINGUAL
WYETH-AYERST

2.5 mg

5 mg

10 mg

ISORDIL TEMBIDS
WYETH-AYERST

40 mg

ISORDIL TITRADOSE
WYETH-AYERST

5 mg

10 mg

20 mg

30 mg

40 mg

SORBITRATE ORAL
ZENECA

5 mg

10 mg

20 mg

SORBITRATE ORAL
ZENECA

30 mg

40 mg

SORBITRATE SUBLINGUAL
ZENECA

2.5 mg

5 mg

10 mg

ISOSORBIDE MONONITRATE

IMDUR
KEY

60 mg

ISMO
WYETH-AYERST

20 mg

MONOKET
SCHWARZ

10 mg

20 mg

ISOTRETINOIN

ACCUTANE
ROCHE

10 mg

20 mg

40 mg

ISRADIPINE

DYNACIRC
SANDOZ

2.5 mg

5 mg

ITRACONAZOLE

SPORANOX
JANSSEN

100 mg

KETOCONAZOLE

NIZORAL
JANSSEN

200 mg

KETOPROFEN

ORUDIS
WYETH-AYERST

25 mg

50 mg

75 mg

ORUVAIL
WYETH-AYERST

200 mg

KETOROLAC TROMETHAMINE

TORADOL ORAL
SYNTEX

10 mg

LABETALOL HCL

NORMODYNE
SCHERING

100 mg

200 mg

300 mg

TRANDATE
ALLEN & HANBURYS

100 mg

200 mg

300 mg

LEVOTHYROXINE SODIUM

GENERIC
GENEVA

0.1 mg

0.15 mg

0.2 mg

0.3 mg

GENERIC
RUGBY

0.1 mg   0.15 mg

0.2 mg   0.3 mg

LEVO-T
LEDERLE STANDARD

0.025 mg   0.05 mg

0.075 mg   0.1 mg

0.125 mg   0.15 mg

0.2 mg   0.3 mg

LEVOTHROID
FOREST

0.025 mg

0.05 mg

0.075 mg

0.088 mg

0.1 mg

LEVOTHROID
FOREST

0.112 mg

0.125 mg

0.137 mg

0.150 mg

0.175 mg

0.2 mg

0.3 mg

LEVOXYL
DANIELS

0.025 mg   0.05 mg

0.075 mg   0.088 mg

0.1 mg   0.112 mg

0.125 mg   0.15 mg

0.175 mg   0.2 mg

0.3 mg

SYNTHROID
BOOTS

0.025 mg   0.05 mg

SYNTHROID
BOOTS

0.075 mg   0.088 mg

0.1 mg   0.112 mg

0.125 mg   0.15 mg

0.175 mg   0.2 mg

0.3 mg

LIOTRIX
THYROLAR-1/4
FOREST

15 mg

THYROLAR-1/2
FOREST

30 mg

THYROLAR-1
FOREST

60 mg

THYROLAR-2
FOREST

120 mg

THYROLAR-3
FOREST

180 mg

LISINOPRIL
PRINIVIL
MERCK

2.5 mg

5 mg

10 mg

20 mg

40 mg

ZESTRIL
STUART

5 mg

10 mg

20 mg

40 mg

LITHIUM CARBONATE
ESKALITH
SMITHKLINE BEECHAM

300 mg

ESKALITH CR
SMITHKLINE BEECHAM

450 mg

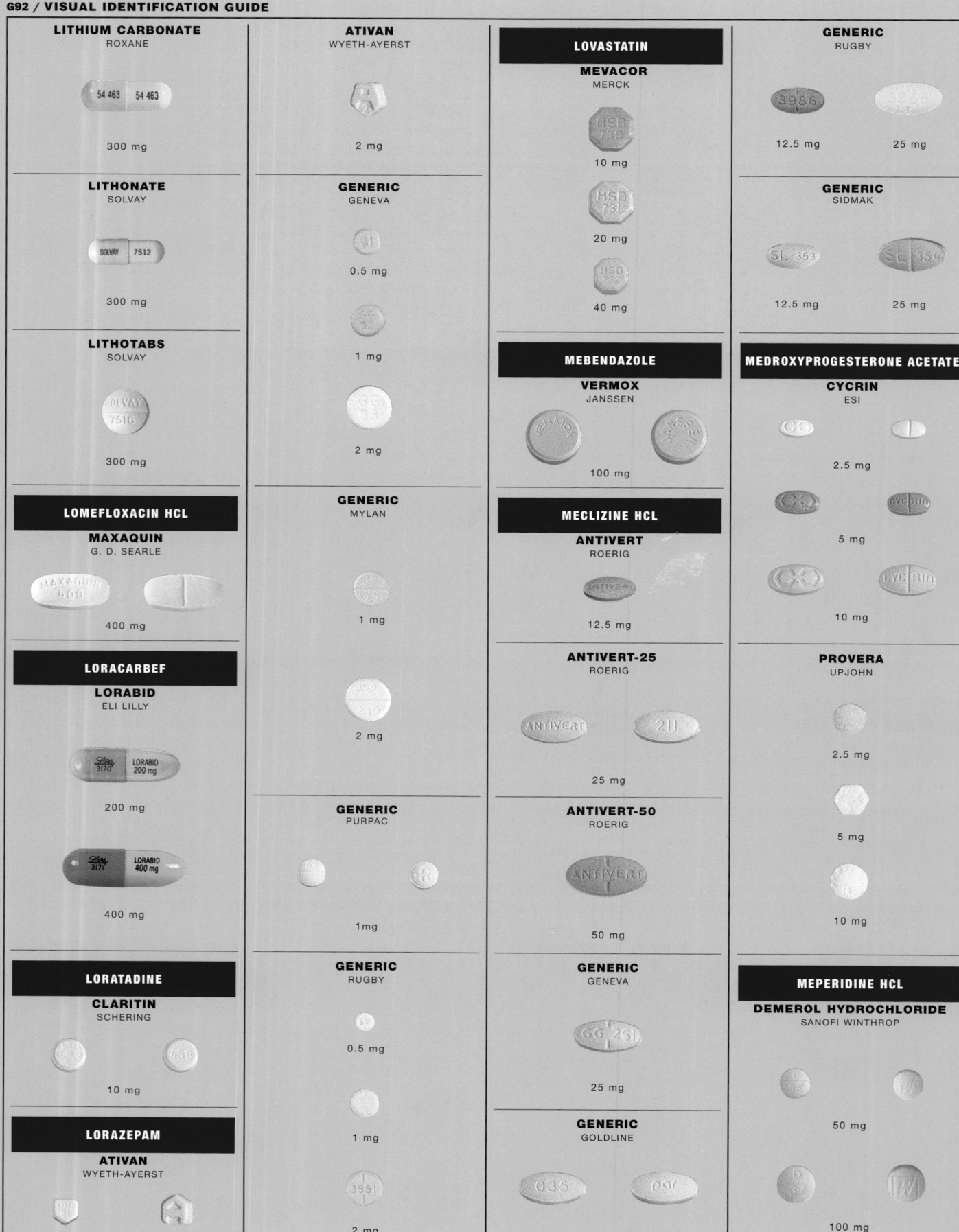

LITHIUM CARBONATE
ROXANE

300 mg

LITHONATE
SOLVAY

300 mg

LITHOTABS
SOLVAY

300 mg

LOMEFLOXACIN HCL

MAXAQUIN
G. D. SEARLE

400 mg

LORACARBEF

LORABID
ELI LILLY

200 mg

400 mg

LORATADINE

CLARITIN
SCHERING

10 mg

LORAZEPAM

ATIVAN
WYETH-AYERST

0.5 mg   1 mg

ATIVAN
WYETH-AYERST

2 mg

GENERIC
GENEVA

0.5 mg

1 mg

2 mg

GENERIC
MYLAN

1 mg

2 mg

GENERIC
PURPAC

1mg

GENERIC
RUGBY

0.5 mg

1 mg

2 mg

LOVASTATIN

MEVACOR
MERCK

10 mg

20 mg

40 mg

MEBENDAZOLE

VERMOX
JANSSEN

100 mg

MECLIZINE HCL

ANTIVERT
ROERIG

12.5 mg

ANTIVERT-25
ROERIG

25 mg

ANTIVERT-50
ROERIG

50 mg

GENERIC
GENEVA

25 mg

GENERIC
GOLDLINE

25 mg

GENERIC
RUGBY

12.5 mg   25 mg

GENERIC
SIDMAK

12.5 mg   25 mg

MEDROXYPROGESTERONE ACETATE

CYCRIN
ESI

2.5 mg

5 mg

10 mg

PROVERA
UPJOHN

2.5 mg

5 mg

10 mg

MEPERIDINE HCL

DEMEROL HYDROCHLORIDE
SANOFI WINTHROP

50 mg

100 mg

MESTRANOL / NORETHINDRONE

NORINYL 1+50
SYNTEX

0.05 mg / 1 mg

ORTHO-NOVUM 1/50
ORTHO

0.05 mg / 1 mg

METAPROTERENOL SULFATE

ALUPENT
BOEHRINGER INGELHEIM

10 mg

METHAZOLAMIDE

NEPTAZANE
STORZ

25 mg

50 mg

METHOCARBAMOL

GENERIC
SCHEIN

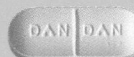

750 mg

ROBAXIN
A. H. ROBINS

500 mg

ROBAXIN -750
A. H. ROBINS

750 mg

METHYLDOPA

ALDOMET
MERCK

125 mg

250 mg

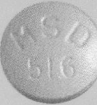

500 mg

GENERIC
WEST POINT

125 mg

250 mg

 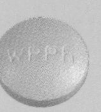

500 mg

METHYLPHENIDATE HCL

GENERIC
MD

5 mg

10 mg

20 mg

20 mg
SUSTAINED RELEASE

RITALIN
CIBA

5 mg

10 mg

20 mg

RITALIN-SR
CIBA

20 mg

METHYLPREDNISOLONE

GENERIC
DURAMED

4 mg

MEDROL
UPJOHN

2 mg   4 mg

8 mg   16 mg

24 mg   32 mg

METOCLOPRAMIDE HCL

GENERIC
INVAMED

5 mg

GENERIC
PUREPAC

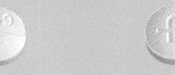

10 mg

REGLAN
A. H. ROBINS

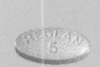 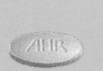

5 mg

 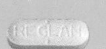

10 mg

METOLAZONE

ZAROXOLYN
FISONS

2.5 mg

5 mg

10 mg

METOPROLOL SUCCINATE

TOPROL-XL
ASTRA

50 mg

METOPROLOL TARTRATE

GENERIC
MUTUAL

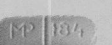 

50 mg   100 mg

LOPRESSOR
GEIGY

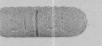

50 mg   100 mg

METRONIDAZOLE

FLAGYL
G. D. SEARLE

 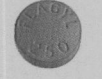

250 mg

FLAGYL
G. D. SEARLE

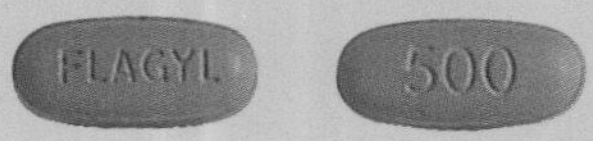

500 mg

GENERIC
SCHEIN

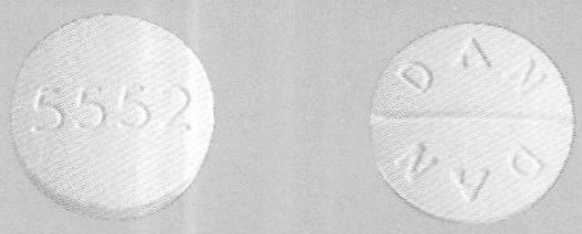

500mg

PROTOSTAT
ORTHO

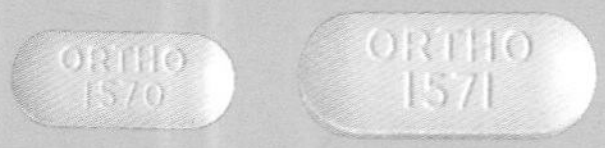

250 mg   500 mg

MINOCYCLINE HCL

GENERIC
LEDERLE STANDARD

50 mg   100 mg

GENERIC
WARNER-CHILCOTT

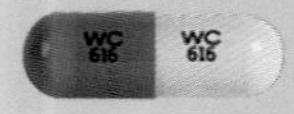

100 mg

MINOCIN
LEDERLE

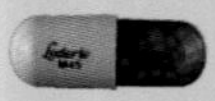

50 mg

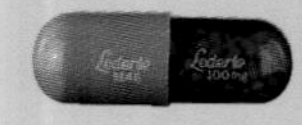

100 mg

MISOPROSTOL

CYTOTEC
G. D. SEARLE

100 mcg

CYTOTEC
G. D. SEARLE

200 mcg

MULTIVITAMINS

BEROCCA
ROCHE

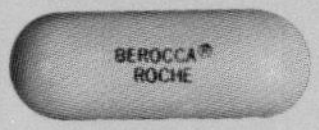

MULTIVITAMINS / MINERALS

BEROCCA PLUS
ROCHE

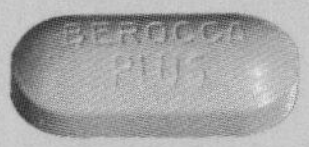

VICON FORTE
WHITBY

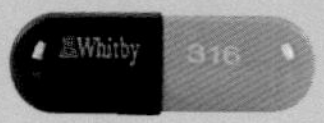

MULTIVITAMINS / SODIUM FLUORIDE

GENERIC
COPLEY

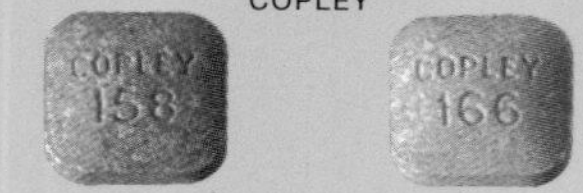

0.5 mg   1 mg

POLY-VI-FLOR
MEAD JOHNSON NUTRITIONALS

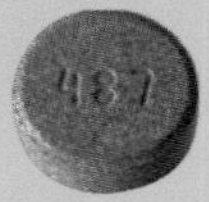

0.25 mg

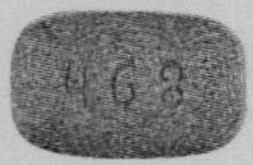

0.5 mg

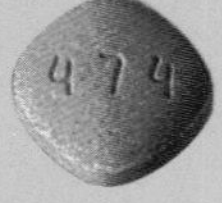

1.0 mg

NABUMETONE

RELAFEN
SMITHKLINE BEECHAM

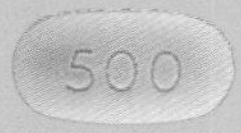

500 mg

RELAFEN
SMITHKLINE BEECHAM

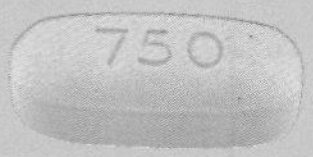

750 mg

NADOLOL

CORGARD
BRISTOL-MYERS SQUIBB

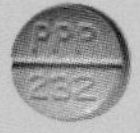

20 mg

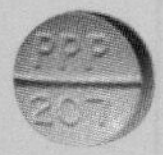

40 mg

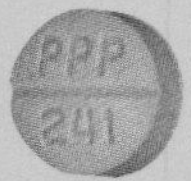

80 mg

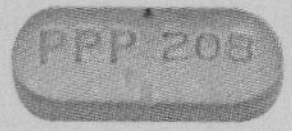

120 mg

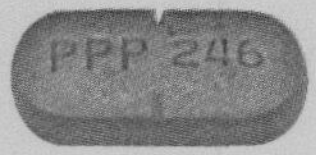

160 mg

**NALOXONE HCL /
PENTAZOCINE HCL**

TALWIN NX
SANOFI WINTHROP

0.5 mg / 50 mg

NAPROXEN

GENERIC
HAMILTON

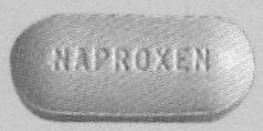

500 mg

GENERIC
LEDERLE STANDARD

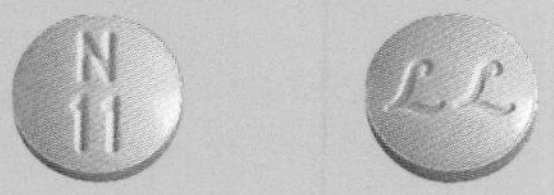

250 mg

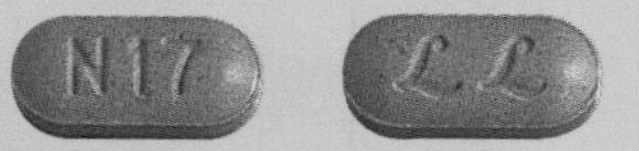

375 mg

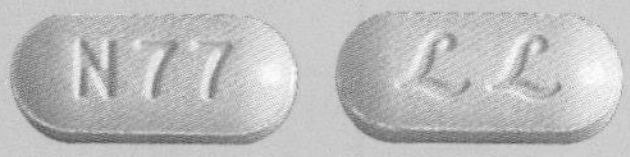

500 mg

NAPROSYN
SYNTEX

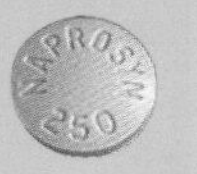

250 mg

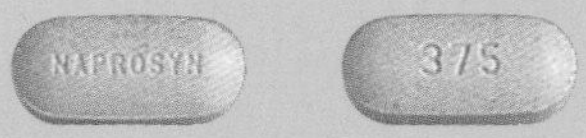

375 mg

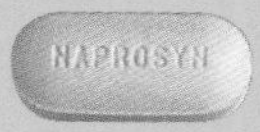

500 mg

NAPROXEN SODIUM

ANAPROX
SYNTEX

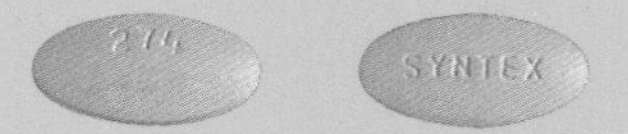

275 mg

ANAPROX DS
SYNTEX

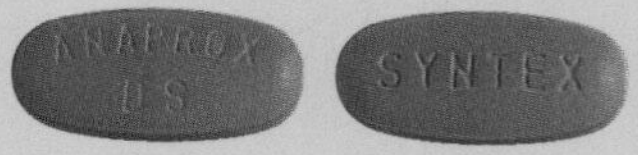

550 mg

NICARDIPINE HCL

CARDENE
SYNTEX

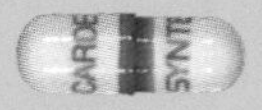

20 mg

30 mg

CARDENE SR
SYNTEX

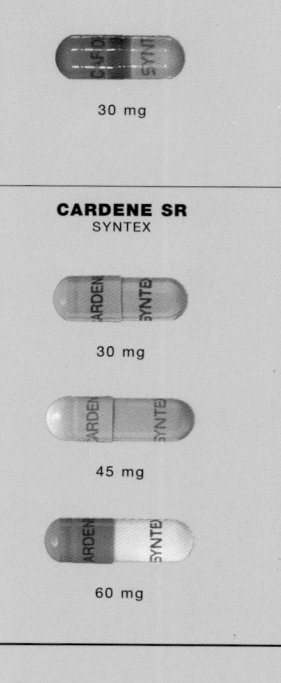

30 mg

45 mg

60 mg

NIFEDIPINE
ADALAT
MILES

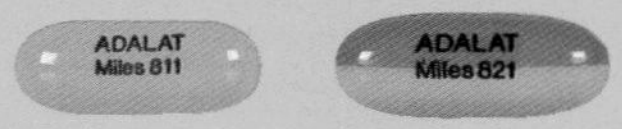

10 mg   20 mg

ADALAT CC
MILES

30 mg

60 mg

90 mg

PROCARDIA
PRATT

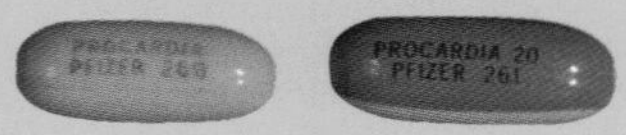

10 mg   20 mg

PROCARDIA XL
PRATT

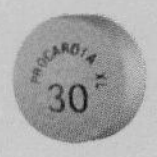

30 mg

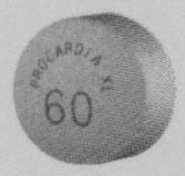

60 mg

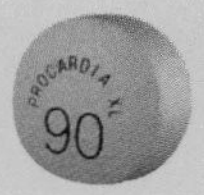

90 mg

NITROFURANTOIN MACROCRYSTALS
GENERIC
GENEVA

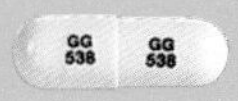

25 mg

MACRODANTIN
PROCTER & GAMBLE

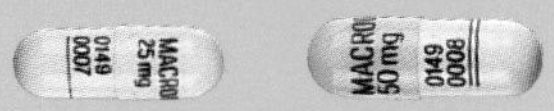

25 mg   50 mg

MACRODANTIN
PROCTER & GAMBLE

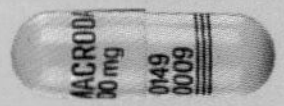

100 mg

NITROFURANTOIN MACROCRYSTALS / NITROFURANTOIN MONOHYDRATE
MACROBID
PROCTER & GAMBLE

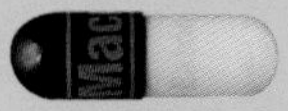

25 mg / 75 mg

NITROGLYCERIN
GENERIC
ETHEX

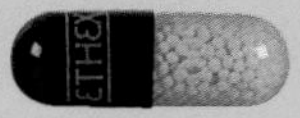

6.5 mg

NITROGARD
FOREST

2 mg

NIZATIDINE
AXID
ELI LILLY

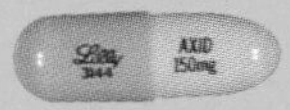

150 mg

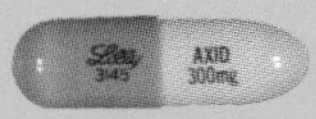

300 mg

NORFLOXACIN
NOROXIN
MERCK

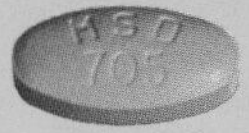

400 mg

NORGESTREL
OVERETTE
WYETH-AYERST

0.075 mg

NORTRIPTYLINE HCL
GENERIC
SCHEIN

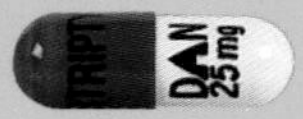

25 mg

PAMELOR
SANDOZ

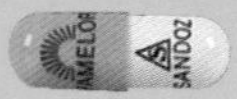

10 mg

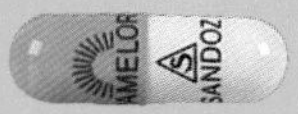

25 mg

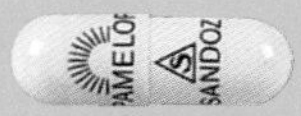

50 mg

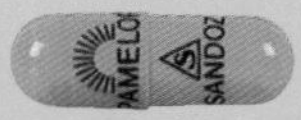

75 mg

NYSTATIN
GENERIC
RUGBY

500,000 units

MYCOSTATIN
APOTHECON

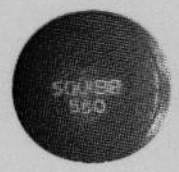

500,000 units

OFLOXACIN
FLOXIN
MCNEIL

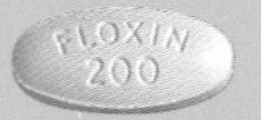

200 mg

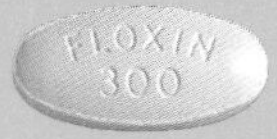

300 mg

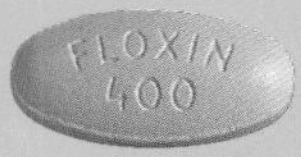

400 mg

OMEPRAZOLE
PRILOSEC
ASTRA MERCK

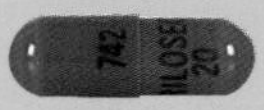

20 mg

ONDANSETRON HCL
ZOFRAN
CERENEX

4 mg

8 mg

ORPHENADRINE CITRATE
NORFLEX
3M

100 mg

OXAPROZIN
DAYPRO
G. D. SEARLE

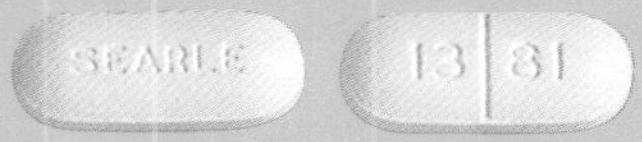

600 mg

OXYBUTYNIN CHLORIDE
DITROPAN
MARION MERRELL DOW

5 mg

GENERIC
SIDMAK

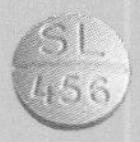

5 mg

PAROXETINE HCL
PAXIL
SMITHKLINE BEECHAM

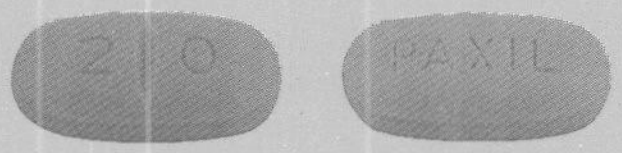

20 mg

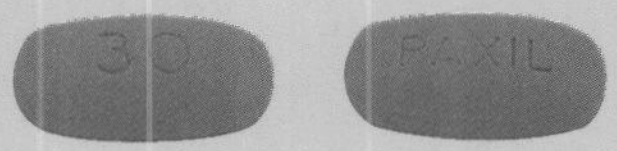

30 mg

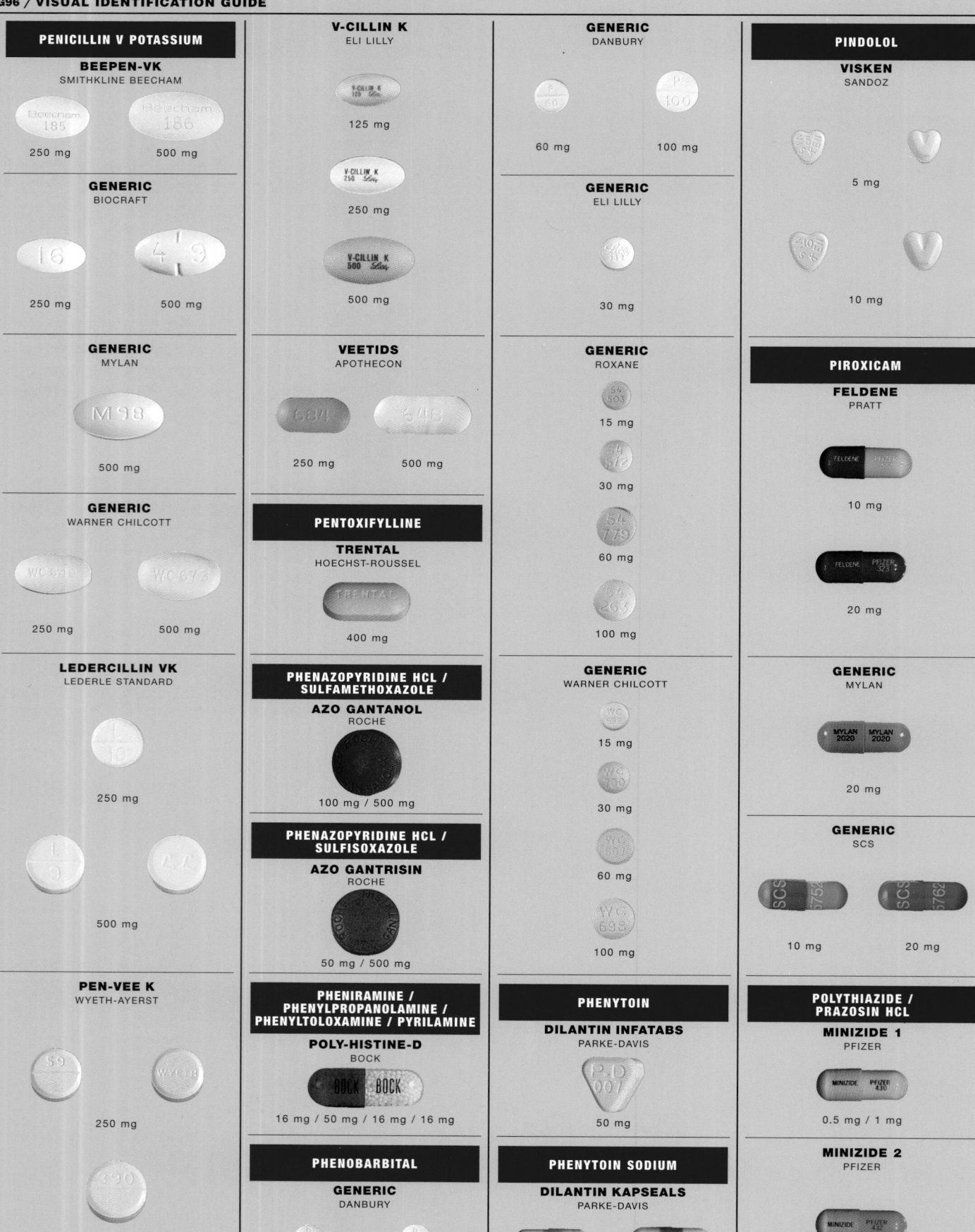

PENICILLIN V POTASSIUM

BEEPEN-VK
SMITHKLINE BEECHAM

250 mg   500 mg

GENERIC
BIOCRAFT

250 mg   500 mg

GENERIC
MYLAN

500 mg

GENERIC
WARNER CHILCOTT

250 mg   500 mg

LEDERCILLIN VK
LEDERLE STANDARD

250 mg

500 mg

PEN-VEE K
WYETH-AYERST

250 mg

500 mg

V-CILLIN K
ELI LILLY

125 mg

250 mg

500 mg

VEETIDS
APOTHECON

250 mg   500 mg

PENTOXIFYLLINE

TRENTAL
HOECHST-ROUSSEL

400 mg

PHENAZOPYRIDINE HCL / SULFAMETHOXAZOLE

AZO GANTANOL
ROCHE

100 mg / 500 mg

PHENAZOPYRIDINE HCL / SULFISOXAZOLE

AZO GANTRISIN
ROCHE

50 mg / 500 mg

PHENIRAMINE / PHENYLPROPANOLAMINE / PHENYLTOLOXAMINE / PYRILAMINE

POLY-HISTINE-D
BOCK

16 mg / 50 mg / 16 mg / 16 mg

PHENOBARBITAL

GENERIC
DANBURY

15 mg   30 mg

GENERIC
DANBURY

60 mg   100 mg

GENERIC
ELI LILLY

30 mg

GENERIC
ROXANE

15 mg

30 mg

60 mg

100 mg

GENERIC
WARNER CHILCOTT

15 mg

30 mg

60 mg

100 mg

PHENYTOIN

DILANTIN INFATABS
PARKE-DAVIS

50 mg

PHENYTOIN SODIUM

DILANTIN KAPSEALS
PARKE-DAVIS

30 mg   100 mg

PINDOLOL

VISKEN
SANDOZ

5 mg

10 mg

PIROXICAM

FELDENE
PRATT

10 mg

20 mg

GENERIC
MYLAN

20 mg

GENERIC
SCS

10 mg   20 mg

POLYTHIAZIDE / PRAZOSIN HCL

MINIZIDE 1
PFIZER

0.5 mg / 1 mg

MINIZIDE 2
PFIZER

0.5 mg / 2 mg

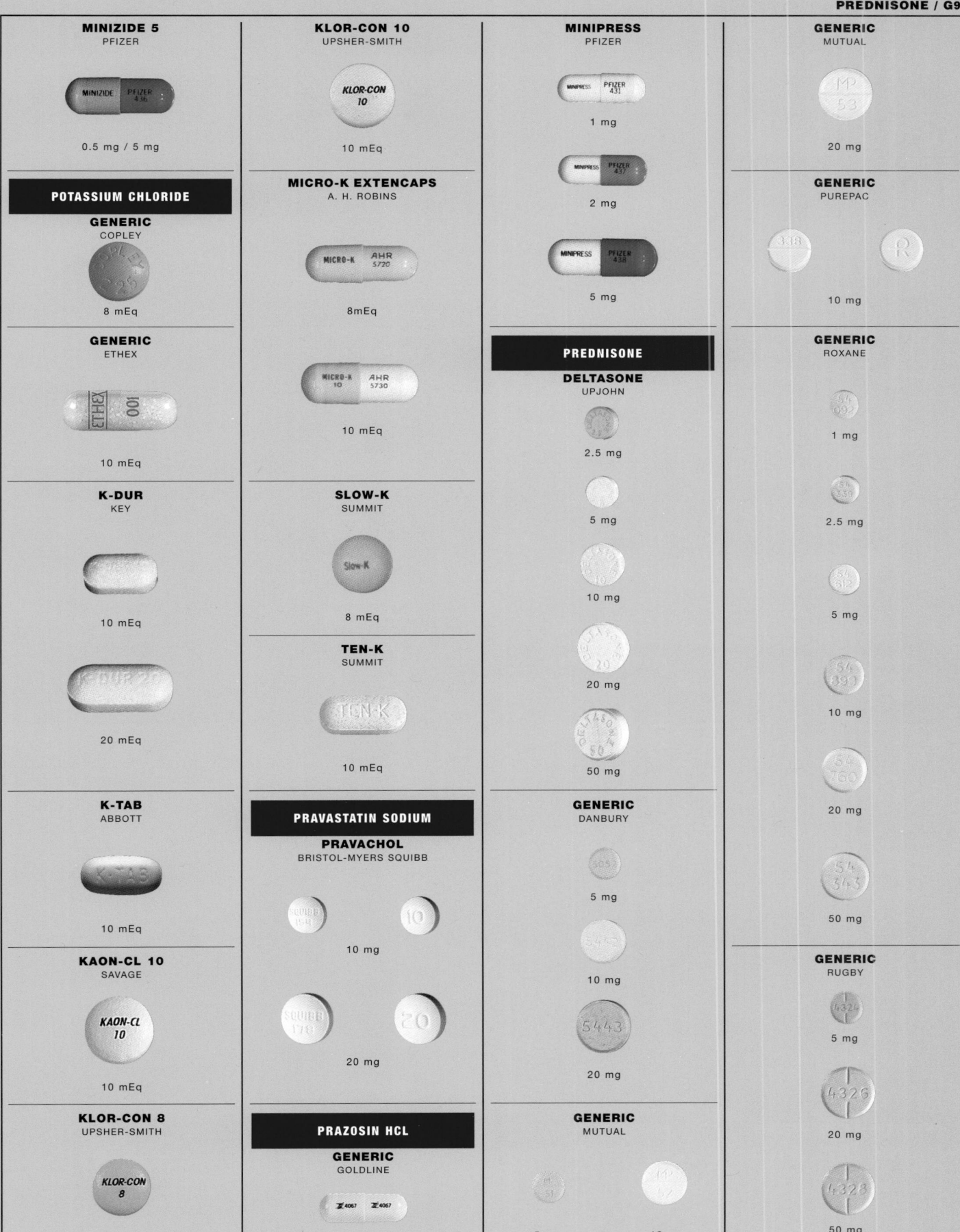

MINIZIDE 5
PFIZER

0.5 mg / 5 mg

POTASSIUM CHLORIDE

GENERIC
COPLEY

8 mEq

GENERIC
ETHEX

10 mEq

K-DUR
KEY

10 mEq

20 mEq

K-TAB
ABBOTT

10 mEq

KAON-CL 10
SAVAGE

10 mEq

KLOR-CON 8
UPSHER-SMITH

8 mEq

KLOR-CON 10
UPSHER-SMITH

10 mEq

MICRO-K EXTENCAPS
A. H. ROBINS

8mEq

10 mEq

SLOW-K
SUMMIT

8 mEq

TEN-K
SUMMIT

10 mEq

PRAVASTATIN SODIUM

PRAVACHOL
BRISTOL-MYERS SQUIBB

10 mg

20 mg

PRAZOSIN HCL

GENERIC
GOLDLINE

1 mg

MINIPRESS
PFIZER

1 mg

2 mg

5 mg

PREDNISONE

DELTASONE
UPJOHN

2.5 mg

5 mg

10 mg

20 mg

50 mg

GENERIC
DANBURY

5 mg

10 mg

20 mg

GENERIC
MUTUAL

5 mg   10 mg

GENERIC
MUTUAL

20 mg

GENERIC
PUREPAC

10 mg

GENERIC
ROXANE

1 mg

2.5 mg

5 mg

10 mg

20 mg

50 mg

GENERIC
RUGBY

5 mg

20 mg

50 mg

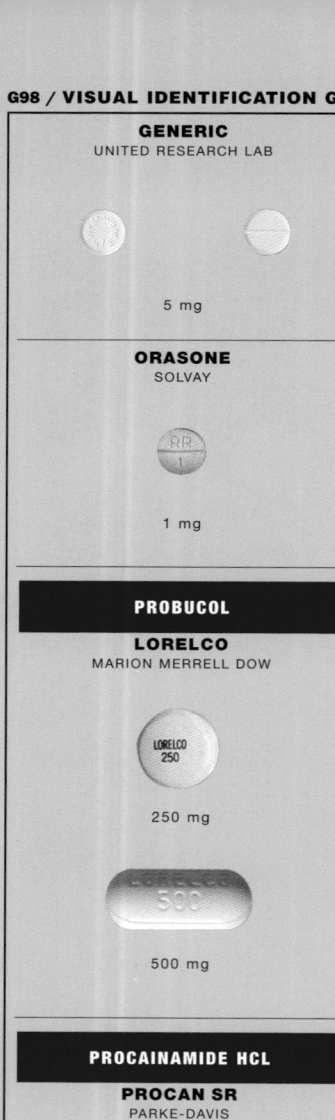

GENERIC
UNITED RESEARCH LAB

5 mg

ORASONE
SOLVAY

1 mg

PROBUCOL

LORELCO
MARION MERRELL DOW

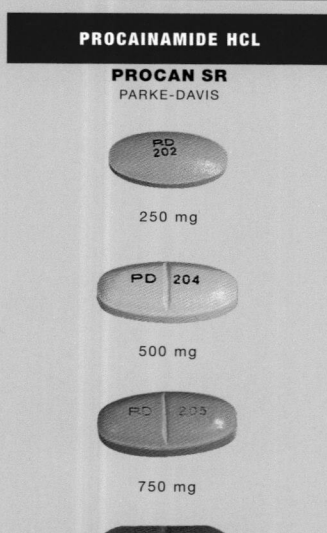

250 mg

500 mg

PROCAINAMIDE HCL

PROCAN SR
PARKE-DAVIS

250 mg

500 mg

750 mg

1000 mg

PROCHLORPERAZINE MALEATE

COMPAZINE
SMITHKLINE BEECHAM

5 mg

COMPAZINE
SMITHKLINE BEECHAM

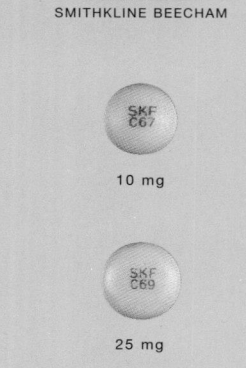

10 mg

25 mg

COMPAZINE SPANSULE
SMITHKLINE BEECHAM

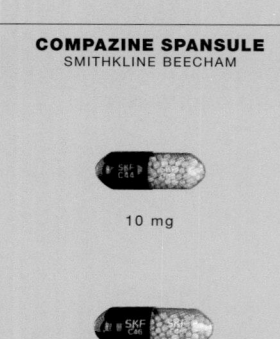

10 mg

15 mg

PROMETHAZINE HCL

GENERIC
SCHEIN

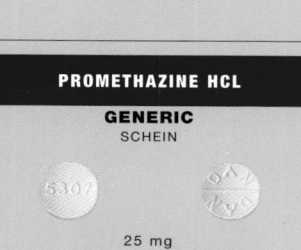

25 mg

PHENERGAN
WYETH-AYERST

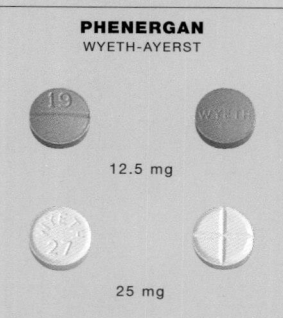

12.5 mg

25 mg

50 mg

PROPOXYPHENE HCL

DARVON
ELI LILLY

65 mg

GENERIC
LEMMON

65 mg

PROPOXYPHENE NAPSYLATE

DARVON-N
ELI LILLY

100 mg

PROPRANOLOL HCL

BETACHRON E-R
INWOOD

60 mg

80 mg

120 mg

160 mg

GENERIC
LEDERLE STANDARD

10 mg

20 mg

40 mg

60 mg   80 mg

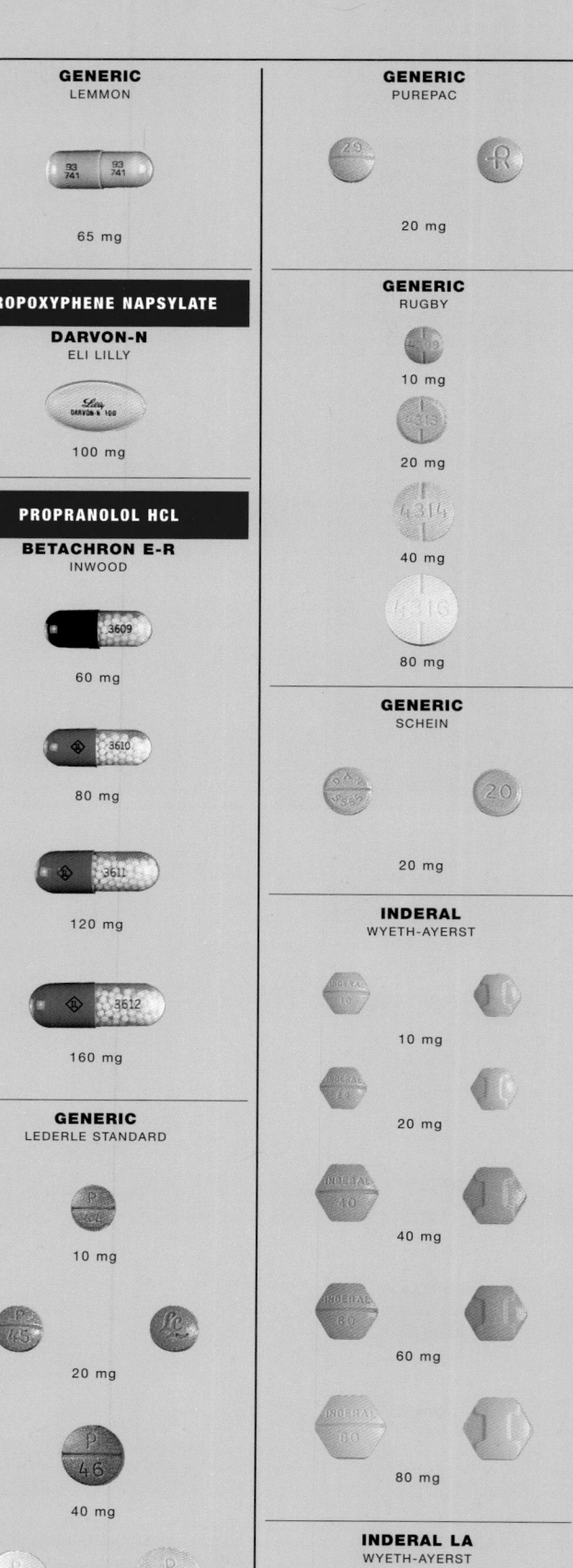

GENERIC
PUREPAC

20 mg

GENERIC
RUGBY

10 mg

20 mg

40 mg

80 mg

GENERIC
SCHEIN

20 mg

INDERAL
WYETH-AYERST

10 mg

20 mg

40 mg

60 mg

80 mg

INDERAL LA
WYETH-AYERST

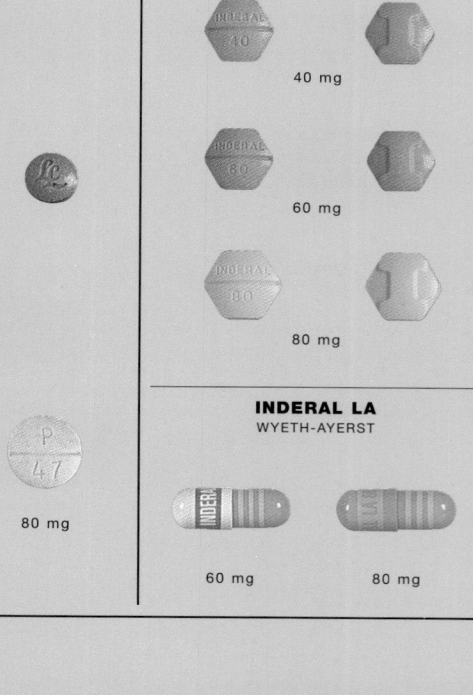

60 mg   80 mg

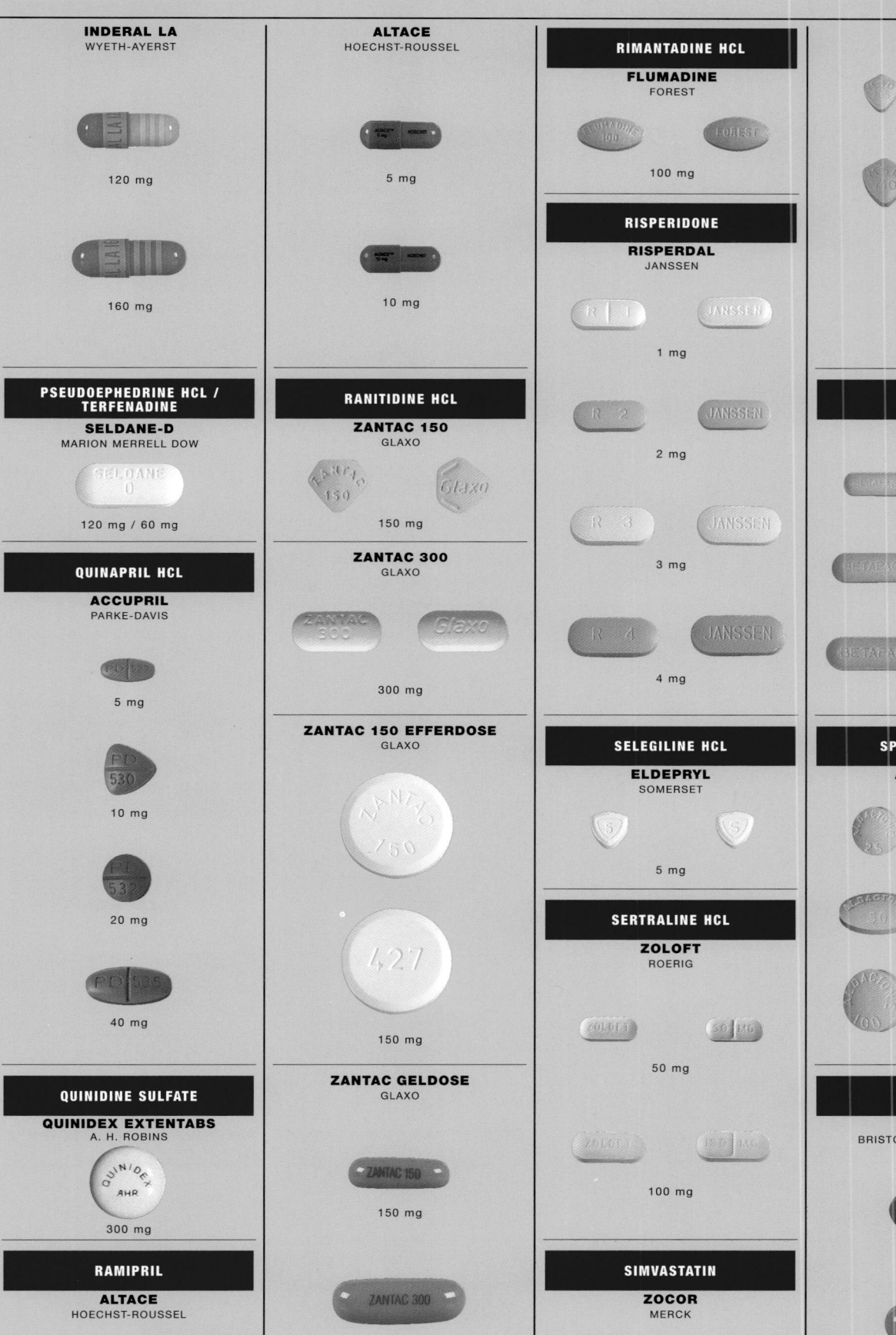

INDERAL LA
WYETH-AYERST

120 mg

160 mg

PSEUDOEPHEDRINE HCL / TERFENADINE
SELDANE-D
MARION MERRELL DOW

120 mg / 60 mg

QUINAPRIL HCL
ACCUPRIL
PARKE-DAVIS

5 mg

10 mg

20 mg

40 mg

QUINIDINE SULFATE
QUINIDEX EXTENTABS
A. H. ROBINS

300 mg

RAMIPRIL
ALTACE
HOECHST-ROUSSEL

1.25 mg   2.5 mg

ALTACE
HOECHST-ROUSSEL

5 mg

10 mg

RANITIDINE HCL
ZANTAC 150
GLAXO

150 mg

ZANTAC 300
GLAXO

300 mg

ZANTAC 150 EFFERDOSE
GLAXO

150 mg

ZANTAC GELDOSE
GLAXO

150 mg

300 mg

RIMANTADINE HCL
FLUMADINE
FOREST

100 mg

RISPERIDONE
RISPERDAL
JANSSEN

1 mg

2 mg

3 mg

4 mg

SELEGILINE HCL
ELDEPRYL
SOMERSET

5 mg

SERTRALINE HCL
ZOLOFT
ROERIG

50 mg

100 mg

SIMVASTATIN
ZOCOR
MERCK

5 mg

ZOCOR
MERCK

10 mg

20 mg

40 mg

SOTALOL HCL
BETAPACE
BERLEX

80 mg

160 mg

240 mg

SPIRONOLACTONE
ALDACTONE
G. D. SEARLE

25 mg

50 mg

100 mg

STAVUDINE
ZERIT
BRISTOL-MYERS ONCOLOGY

15 mg

20 mg

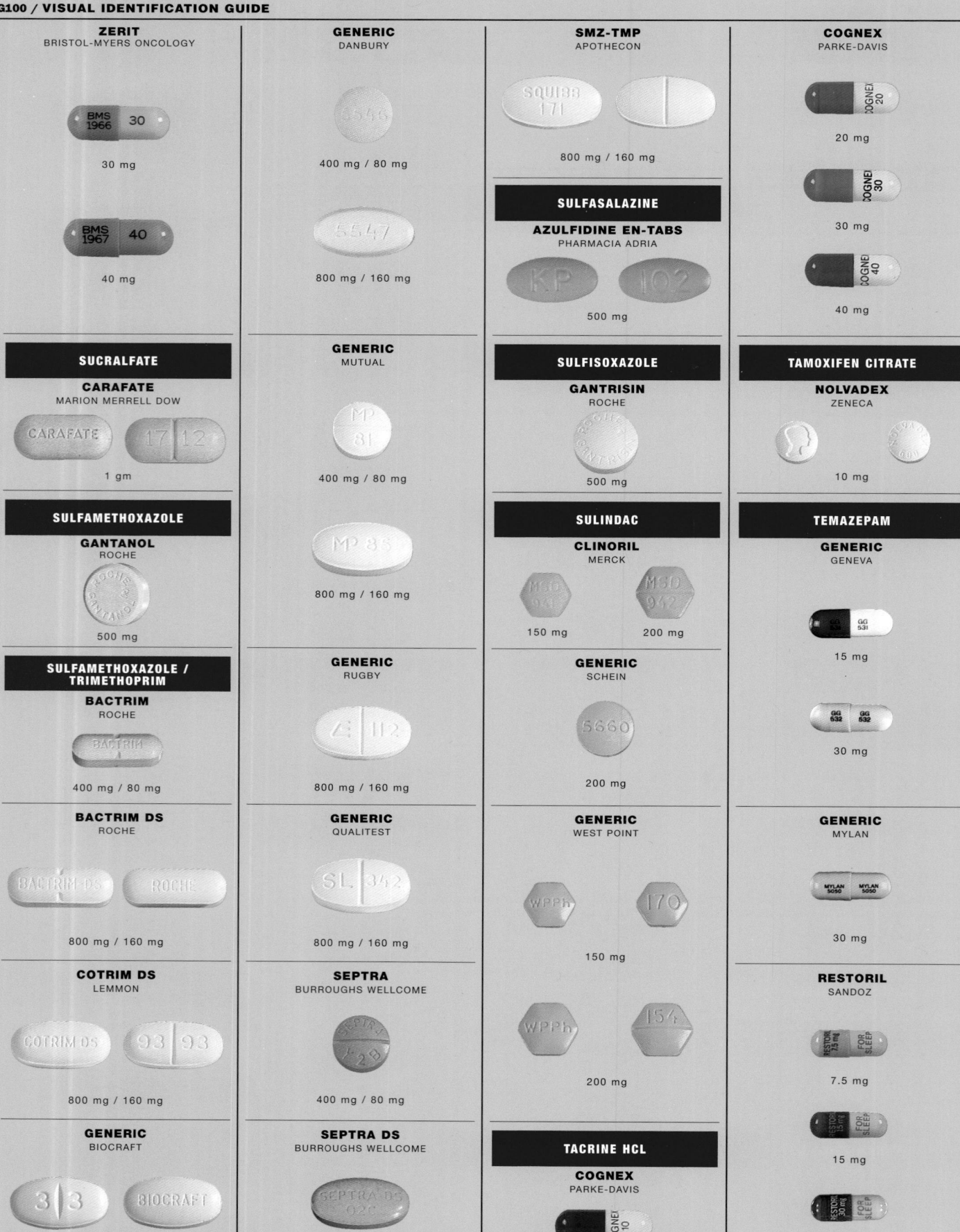

ZERIT
BRISTOL-MYERS ONCOLOGY

BMS 1966 30

30 mg

BMS 1967 40

40 mg

SUCRALFATE

CARAFATE
MARION MERRELL DOW

1 gm

SULFAMETHOXAZOLE

GANTANOL
ROCHE

500 mg

SULFAMETHOXAZOLE / TRIMETHOPRIM

BACTRIM
ROCHE

400 mg / 80 mg

BACTRIM DS
ROCHE

800 mg / 160 mg

COTRIM DS
LEMMON

800 mg / 160 mg

GENERIC
BIOCRAFT

800 mg / 160 mg

GENERIC
DANBURY

400 mg / 80 mg

800 mg / 160 mg

GENERIC
MUTUAL

400 mg / 80 mg

800 mg / 160 mg

GENERIC
RUGBY

800 mg / 160 mg

GENERIC
QUALITEST

800 mg / 160 mg

SEPTRA
BURROUGHS WELLCOME

400 mg / 80 mg

SEPTRA DS
BURROUGHS WELLCOME

800 mg / 160 mg

SMZ-TMP
APOTHECON

800 mg / 160 mg

SULFASALAZINE

AZULFIDINE EN-TABS
PHARMACIA ADRIA

500 mg

SULFISOXAZOLE

GANTRISIN
ROCHE

500 mg

SULINDAC

CLINORIL
MERCK

150 mg   200 mg

GENERIC
SCHEIN

200 mg

GENERIC
WEST POINT

150 mg

200 mg

TACRINE HCL

COGNEX
PARKE-DAVIS

10 mg

COGNEX
PARKE-DAVIS

20 mg

30 mg

40 mg

TAMOXIFEN CITRATE

NOLVADEX
ZENECA

10 mg

TEMAZEPAM

GENERIC
GENEVA

15 mg

30 mg

GENERIC
MYLAN

30 mg

RESTORIL
SANDOZ

7.5 mg

15 mg

30 mg

TERAZOSIN HCL

HYTRIN
ABBOTT

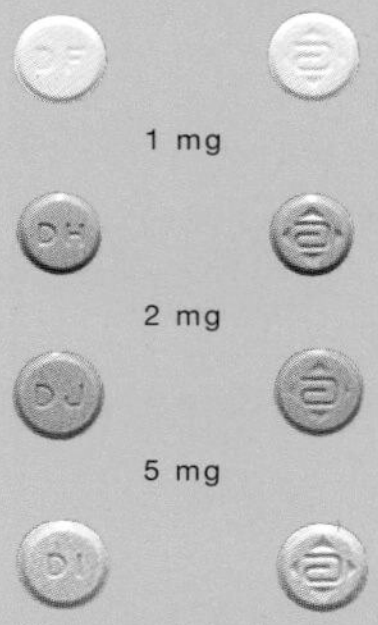

1 mg

2 mg

5 mg

10 mg

TERBUTALINE SULFATE

BRETHINE
GEIGY

2.5 mg   5 mg

BRICANYL
MARION MERRELL DOW

2.5 mg   5 mg

TERFENADINE

SELDANE
MARION MERRELL DOW

60 mg

TETRACYCLINE HCL

ACHROMYCIN V
LEDERLE STANDARD

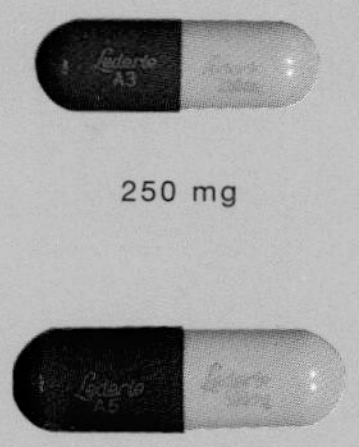

250 mg

500 mg

GENERIC
MYLAN

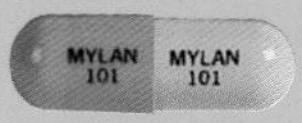

250 mg

SUMYCIN
APOTHECON

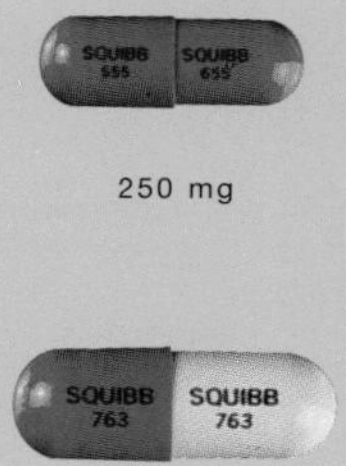

250 mg

500 mg

GENERIC
WYETH-AYERST

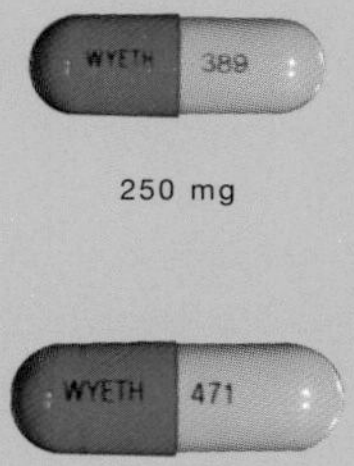

250 mg

500 mg

THEOPHYLLINE

GENERIC
SIDMAK

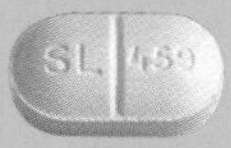

300 mg

RESPBID
BOEHRINGER INGELHEIM

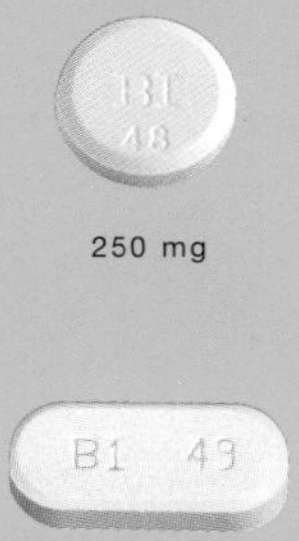

250 mg

500 mg

SLO-BID GYROCAPS
RHONE-POULENC RORER

50 mg   75 mg

SLO-BID GYROCAPS
RHONE-POULENC RORER

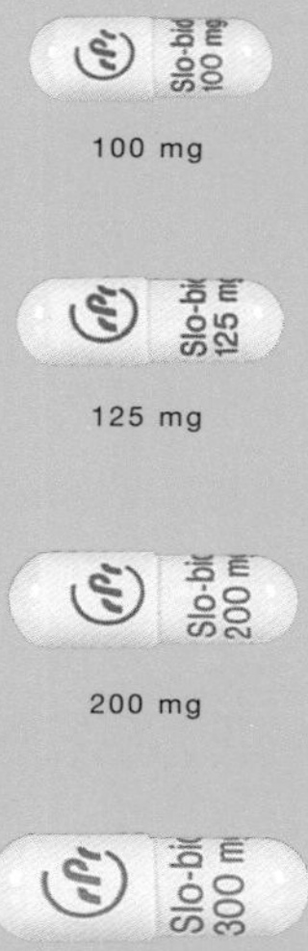

100 mg

125 mg

200 mg

300 mg

SLO-PHYLLIN
RHONE-POULENC RORER

100 mg   200 mg

SLO-PHYLLIN GYROCAPS
RHONE-POULENC RORER

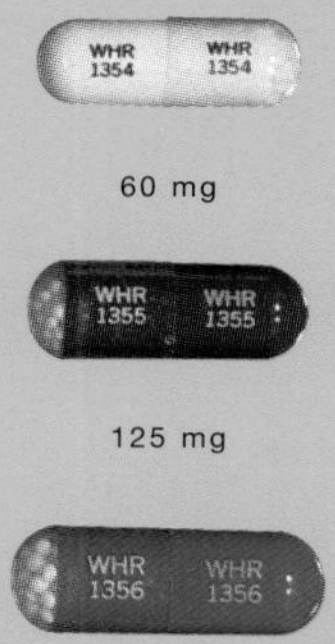

60 mg

125 mg

250 mg

T-PHYL
PURDUE FREDERICK

200 mg

THEO-DUR
KEY

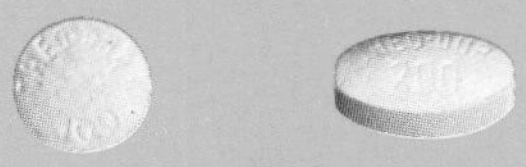

100 mg   200 mg

THEO-DUR
KEY

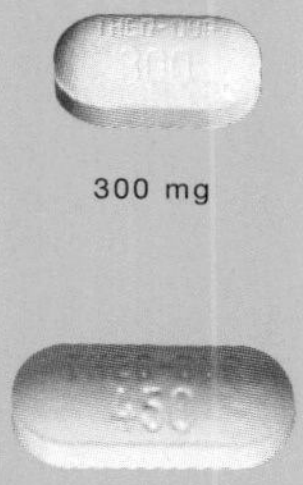

300 mg

450 mg

THEO-DUR SPRINKLE
KEY

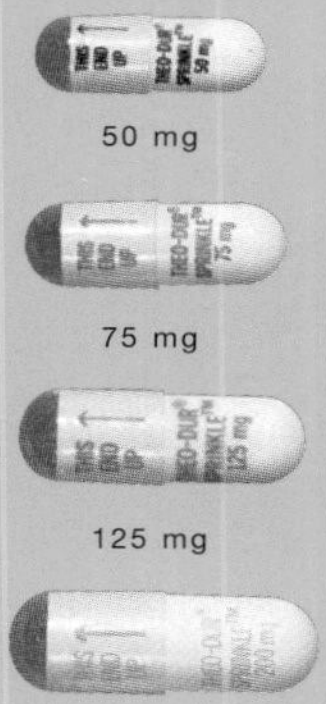

50 mg

75 mg

125 mg

200 mg

THEO-X
CARNRICK

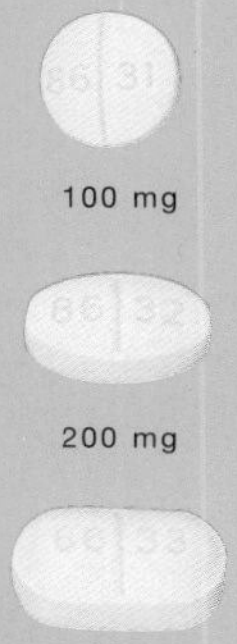

100 mg

200 mg

300 mg

THEO-24
WHITBY

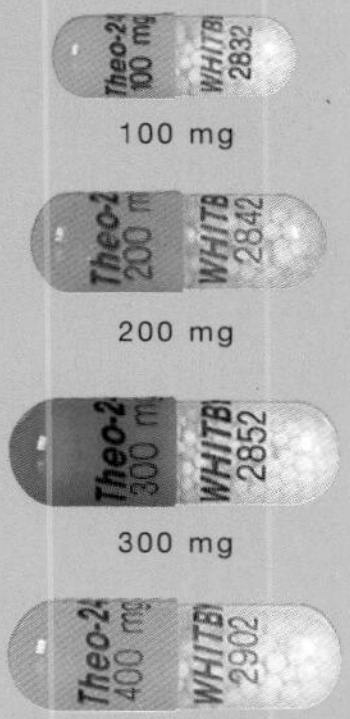

100 mg

200 mg

300 mg

400 mg

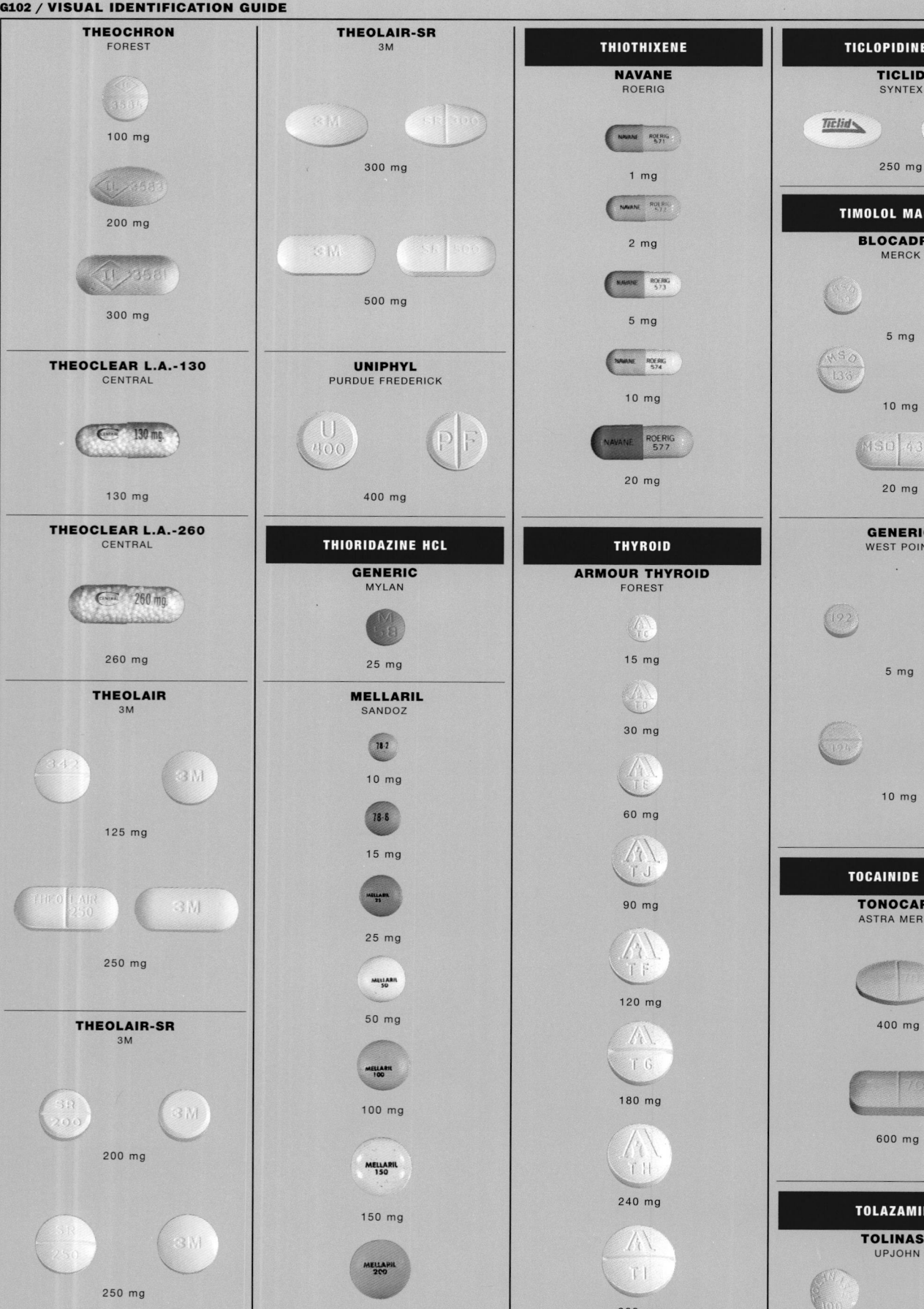

THEOCHRON
FOREST

100 mg

200 mg

300 mg

THEOCLEAR L.A.-130
CENTRAL

130 mg

THEOCLEAR L.A.-260
CENTRAL

260 mg

THEOLAIR
3M

125 mg

250 mg

THEOLAIR-SR
3M

200 mg

250 mg

THEOLAIR-SR
3M

300 mg

500 mg

UNIPHYL
PURDUE FREDERICK

400 mg

THIORIDAZINE HCL

GENERIC
MYLAN

25 mg

MELLARIL
SANDOZ

10 mg

15 mg

25 mg

50 mg

100 mg

150 mg

200 mg

THIOTHIXENE

NAVANE
ROERIG

1 mg

2 mg

5 mg

10 mg

20 mg

THYROID

ARMOUR THYROID
FOREST

15 mg

30 mg

60 mg

90 mg

120 mg

180 mg

240 mg

300 mg

TICLOPIDINE HCL

TICLID
SYNTEX

250 mg

TIMOLOL MALEATE

BLOCADREN
MERCK

5 mg

10 mg

20 mg

GENERIC
WEST POINT

5 mg

10 mg

TOCAINIDE HCL

TONOCARD
ASTRA MERCK

400 mg

600 mg

TOLAZAMIDE

TOLINASE
UPJOHN

100 mg

250 mg

TOLINASE
UPJOHN

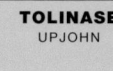

500 mg

TOLBUTAMIDE

ORINASE
UPJOHN

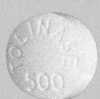

250 mg

500 mg

TOLMETIN SODIUM

TOLECTIN 200
MCNEIL

200 mg

TOLECTIN DS
MCNEIL

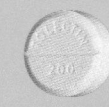

400 mg

TOLECTIN 600
MCNEIL

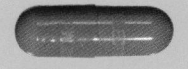

600 mg

TORSEMIDE

DEMADEX
BOEHRINGER MANNHEIM

5 mg

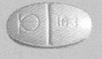

10 mg

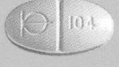   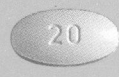

20 mg

DEMADEX
BOEHRINGER MANNHEIM

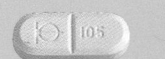   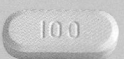

100 mg

TRAZODONE HCL

DESYREL
MEAD JOHNSON

50 mg

100 mg

DESYREL DIVIDOSE
MEAD JOHNSON

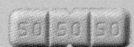   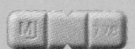

150 mg

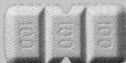   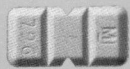

300 mg

GENERIC
SCHEIN

50 mg

GENERIC
SIDMAK

50 mg

100 mg

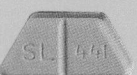

150 mg

TRIAZOLAM

HALCION
UPJOHN

0.125 mg

0.25 mg

TRIMETHOBENZAMIDE HCL

TIGAN
SMITHKLINE BEECHAM

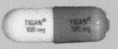

100 mg

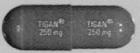

250 mg

VENLAFAXINE HCL

EFFEXOR
WYETH-AYERST

25 mg

37.5 mg

50 mg

75 mg

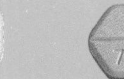

100 mg

VERAPAMIL HCL

CALAN
G. D. SEARLE

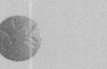

40 mg

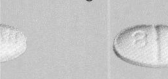

80 mg

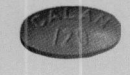   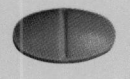

120 mg

CALAN SR
G. D. SEARLE

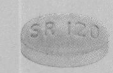

120 mg

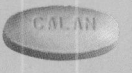   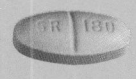

180 mg

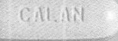   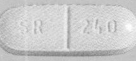

240 mg

GENERIC
GOLDLINE

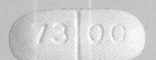   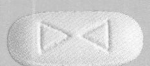

240 mg

ISOPTIN
KNOLL

40 mg

80 mg

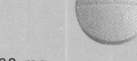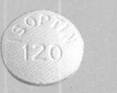

120 mg

ISOPTIN SR
KNOLL

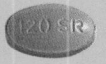   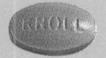

120 mg

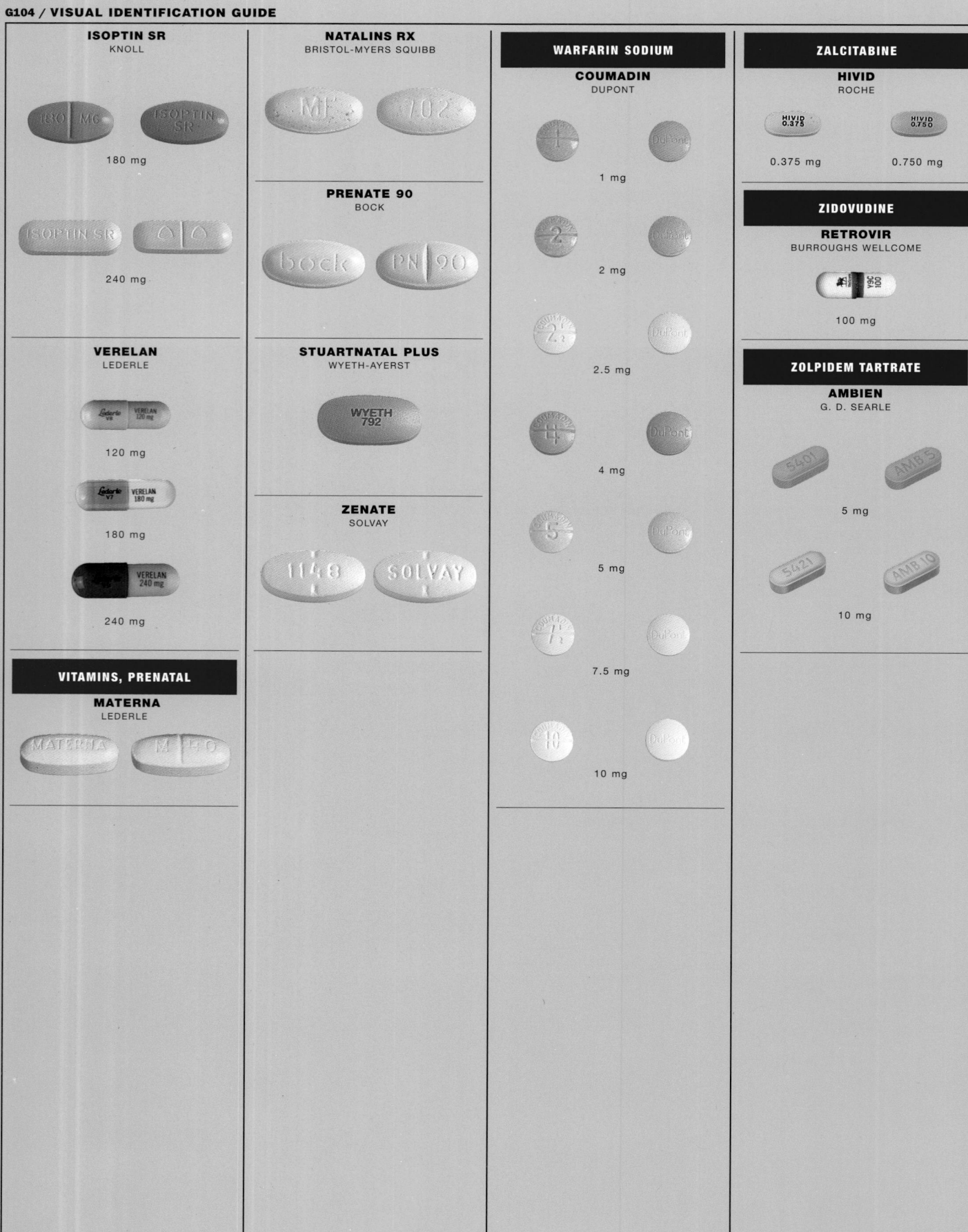

ISOPTIN SR
KNOLL

180 mg

240 mg

VERELAN
LEDERLE

120 mg

180 mg

240 mg

VITAMINS, PRENATAL

MATERNA
LEDERLE

NATALINS RX
BRISTOL-MYERS SQUIBB

PRENATE 90
BOCK

STUARTNATAL PLUS
WYETH-AYERST

ZENATE
SOLVAY

WARFARIN SODIUM

COUMADIN
DUPONT

1 mg

2 mg

2.5 mg

4 mg

5 mg

7.5 mg

10 mg

ZALCITABINE

HIVID
ROCHE

0.375 mg   0.750 mg

ZIDOVUDINE

RETROVIR
BURROUGHS WELLCOME

100 mg

ZOLPIDEM TARTRATE

AMBIEN
G. D. SEARLE

5 mg

10 mg

Product Information

This section contains comprehensive profiles of virtually every prescription drug currently on the market. The profiles are organized alphabetically by generic name and cross-referenced by leading brand names. If a product contains multiple generic ingredients, they are listed alphabetically in the profile's name. For example, you will find product information on "Hydrochlorothiazide and Lisinopril" in the H's rather than the L's.

PRESCRIBING INFORMATION

Each profile begins with a monograph containing complete clinical guidelines. They are a synthesis of FDA-approved labeling for the various forms in which the generic ingredient is available. Compiled by *PDR Generics* consultants, these monographs have not been reviewed, edited or approved by the products' manufacturers.

The chemical structure of single-entity products is depicted in the "Description" section of the monograph. Structural formulas for combination products do not appear.

In the "Indications and Usage" section of many monographs you will find a paragraph entitled "Unlabeled Uses." This information is drawn from peer-reviewed literature summarized in the DRUGDEX® System and related drug databases maintained by MICROMEDEX, INC.

When applicable, Health Care Common Procedures Coding System (HCPCS) Level II "J codes" appear at the end of the monograph. Shown first is the amount of drug to be administered, then the reimbursable routes of administration, and finally the J code itself. The amount is expressed as a range up to a given maximum or, in some cases, as a specific dose. A key to the abbreviations used for routes of administration can be found in the "How to Use *PDR Generics*" section near the beginning of the book.

INFORMATION ON AVAILABLE SUPPLIES

This section, entitled "How Supplied," provides you with comprehensive data on all supplies of the drug currently on the market. Products that are therapeutically equivalent are listed first, followed by those for which equivalence is unconfirmed,

and finally those which have never been rated.

Within these broad equivalency categories, supplies are organized by form and strength. Under each form/strength heading, the leading brand appears first, followed by its generic counterparts. Products are listed in ascending order of package size. To permit quick identification of the most economical generic substitutes, within each size category the products appear in ascending order of average wholesale price (AWP).

Therapeutic equivalency is determined from codes assigned by the Food and Drug Administration and published in the "Orange Book." A product's therapeutic-equivalence status is indicated by a symbol appearing in the left-hand margin of the price listings.

- A BLACK DIAMOND [◆] denotes products carrying a code of "A" in the Orange Book, signifying that they are considered therapeutically equivalent.
- An OPEN DIAMOND [◇] denotes products carrying a "B" code in the Orange Book, signifying that they have not been proven equivalent. (Note, however, that B-rated products have not necessarily been proven *inequivalent* either).
- An OPEN CIRCLE [○] denotes products that do not carry an Orange Book Rating.

When applicable, a product's controlled substance status is indicated immediately following its form in the form/strength heading. Any product subject to the Controlled Substances Act of 1970 is assigned a category according to its potential for abuse. Turn to "How to Use *PDR Generics*" for a key to these categories.

Heading the list of products available in a particular form and strength are two small tables. The first provides you with a comparison between the average unit price of the leading brand versus the typical unit cost of a generic alternative. As an additional benchmark, the Healthcare Finance Administration's Federal Upper Limit price is shown as well. The table appears whenever there is more than one alternative source of a given generic entity or the product is available in more than one package size.

At the right of the Average Unit Price table is a second that provides a more specific basis for judging a particular supplier's price. This table shows the average cost of each package size offered by generic suppliers. Only products rated therapeutically equivalent are included in the averages, which appear for any package size available from more than one supplier.

The price table lists all package sizes available from all suppliers.

- The BRAND/MANUFACTURER column gives the product's brand name, if any, and the name of the supplier.
- The NDC column supplies the item's National Drug Code number in standardized 5-4-2 format.
- The SIZE column gives each item's package, grouping like sizes together in ascending order. Items packaged in unit-dose form are flagged with the abbreviation "UD" and grouped separately.
- The AWP column provides the item's Average Wholesale Price, again in ascending order.

A small arrow at the left of an entry means that a photo of the product appears in the Product Identification Guide.

All prices are drawn from *Red Book*, the nation's premier drug price database. Because actual prices paid by retailers may vary and are subject to frequent change, these prices should be used only as a basis for comparison. Be sure to check with the supplier before making a final decision.

Abbokinase *SEE* UROKINASE

Accupril *SEE* QUINAPRIL HYDROCHLORIDE

Accutane *SEE* ISOTRETINOIN

Acebutolol Hydrochloride

DESCRIPTION

Acebutolol HCl is a selective, hydrophilic beta-adrenoreceptor blocking agent with mild intrinsic sympathomimetic activity for use in treating patients with hypertension and ventricular arrhythmias. It is marketed in capsule form for oral administration. Acebutolol capsules are provided in two dosage strengths which contain 200 or 400 mg.

Acebutolol HCl is a white or slightly off-white powder freely soluble in water, and less soluble in alcohol. Chemically it is defined as the hydrochloride salt of Butanamide, N-[3-acetyl-4-[2-hydroxy-3-[(1-methylethyl)amino]prepoxy]phenyl]-, (±)- or (±)-3'-Acetyl-4'-[2-hydroxy-3-(isopropylamino)propoxy] butyranilide. Its molecular formula is $C_{18}H_{28}N_2O_4 \cdot HCl$ and its molecular weight is 372.9.

Following is its chemical structure:

CH₃CH₂CH₂CONH

CCH₃

OCH₂CHCH₂NHCH(CH₃)₂

OH

CLINICAL PHARMACOLOGY

Acebutolol is a cardioselective, β-adrenoreceptor blocking agent, which possesses mild intrinsic sympathomimetic activity (ISA) in its therapeutically effective dose range.

PHARMACODYNAMICS

$β_1$-cardioselectivity has been demonstrated in experimental animal studies. In anesthetized dogs and cats, Acebutolol is more potent in antagonizing isoproterenol-induced tachycardia ($β_1$) than in antagonizing isoproterenol-induced vasodilatation ($β_2$). In guinea pigs and cats, it is more potent in antagonizing this tachycardia than in antagonizing isoproterenol-induced bronchodilatation ($β_2$). ISA of Acebutolol has been demonstrated in catecholamine-depleted rats by tachycardia induced by intravenous administration of this agent. A membrane-stabilizing effect has been detected in animals, but only with high concentrations of Acebutolol.

Clinical studies have demonstrated $β_1$-blocking activity at the recommended doses by: a) reduction in the resting heart rate and decrease in exercise-induced tachycardia; b) reduction in cardiac output at rest and after exercise; c) reduction of systolic and diastolic blood pressures at rest and postexercise; d) inhibition of isoproterenol-induced tachycardia.

The $β_1$-selectivity of Acebutolol has also been demonstrated on the basis of the following vascular and bronchial effects: Vascular Effects: Acebutolol has less antagonistic effects on peripheral vascular $β_2$-receptors at rest and after epinephrine stimulation than nonselective β-antagonists.

Bronchial Effects: In single-dose studies in asthmatics examining effects of various beta-blockers on pulmonary function, low doses of acebutolol produce less evidence of bronchoconstriction and less reduction of beta₂ agonist, bronchodilating effects, than nonselective agents like propranolol but more than atenolol.

ISA has been observed with Acebutolol in man, as shown by a slightly smaller (about 3 beats per minute) decrease in resting heart rate when compared to equivalent β-blocking doses of propranolol, metoprolol or atenolol. Chronic therapy with Acebutolol induced no significant alteration in the blood lipid profile.

Acebutolol has been shown to delay AV conduction time and to increase the refractoriness of the AV node without significantly affecting sinus node recovery time, atrial refractory period, or the HV conduction time. The membrane-stabilizing effect of Acebutolol is not manifest at the doses used clinically.

Significant reductions in resting and exercise heart rates and systolic blood pressures have been observed 1.5 hours after Acebutolol administration with maximal effects occurring between 3 and 8 hours postdosing in normal volunteers. Acebutolol has demonstrated a significant effect on exercise-induced tachycardia 24 to 30 hours after drug administration.

There are significant correlations between plasma levels of Acebutolol and both the reduction in resting heart rate and the percent of β-blockade of exercise-induced tachycardia. The antihypertensive effect of Acebutolol has been shown in double-blind controlled studies to be superior to placebo and similar to propranol and hydrochlorothiazide. In addition, patients responding to Acebutolol administered twice daily had a similar response whether the dosage regimen was changed to once daily administration or continued on a b.i.d. regimen. Most patients responded to 400 to 800 mg per day in divided doses.

The antiarrhythmic effect of Acebutolol was compared with placebo, propranolol, and quinidine. Compared with placebo, Acebutolol significantly reduced mean total ventricular ectopic beats (VEB), paired VEB, multiform VEB, R-on-T beats, and ventricular tachycardia (VT). Both Acebutolol and propranolol significantly reduced mean total and paired VEB and VT. Acebutolol and quinidine significantly reduced resting total and complex VEB; the antiarrhythmic efficacy of Acebutolol was also observed during exercise.

PHARMACOKINETICS AND METABOLISM

Acebutolol is well absorbed from the GI tract. It is subject to extensive first-pass hepatic biotransformation, with an absolute bioavailability of approximately 40% for the parent compound. The major metabolite, an N-acetyl derivative (diacetolol), is pharmacologically active. This metabolite is equipotent to Acebutolol and in cats is more cardioselective than Acebutolol, therefore, this first-pass phenomenon does not attenuate the therapeutic effect of Acebutolol. Food intake does not have a significant effect on the area under the plasma concentration-time curve (AUC) of Acebutolol although the rate of absorption and peak concentration decreased slightly.

The plasma elimination half-life of Acebutolol is approximately 3 to 4 hours, while that of its metabolite, diacetolol, is 8 to 13 hours. The time to reach peak concentration for Acebutolol is 2.5 hours and for diacetolol, after oral administration of Acebutolol 3.5 hours.

Within the single oral dose range of 200 to 400 mg, the kinetics are dose proportional. However, this linearity is not seen at higher doses, probably due to saturation of hepatic biotransformation sites. In addition, after multiple dosing the lack of linearity is also seen by AUC increases of approximately 100% as compared to single oral dosing. Elimination via renal excretion is approximately 30% to 40% and by non-renal mechanisms 50% to 60%, which includes excretion into the bile and direct passage through the intestinal wall. Acebutolol has a low binding affinity for plasma proteins (about 26%). Acebutolol and its metabolite, diacetolol, are relatively hydrophilic and, therefore, only minimal quantities have been detected in the cerebrospinal fluid (CSF).

Drug interaction studies with tolbutamide and warfarin indicated no influence on the therapeutic effects of these compounds. Digoxin and hydrochlorothiazide plasma levels were not affected by concomitant Acebutolol administration. The kinetics of Acebutolol were not significantly altered by concomitant administration of hydrochlorothiazide, hydralazine, sulfinpyrazone, or oral contraceptives.

In patients with renal impairment, there is no effect on the elimination half-life of Acebutolol, but there is decreased elimination of the metabolite, diacetolol, resulting in a two- to three-fold increase in its half-life. For this reason, the drug should be administered with caution in patients with renal insufficiency (see *"Precautions"*). Acebutolol and its major metabolite are dialyzable.

Acebutolol crosses the placental barrier and is secreted in breast milk.

In geriatric patients, the bioavailability of Acebutolol and its metabolite is increased, approximately two-fold, probably due to decreases in the first-pass metabolism and renal function in the elderly.

INDICATIONS AND USAGE

HYPERTENSION

Acebutolol is indicated for the management of hypertension in adults. It may be used alone or in combination with other antihypertensive agents, especially thiazide-type diuretics.

VENTRICULAR ARRHYTHMIAS

Acebutolol is indicated in the management of ventricular premature beats; it reduces the total number of premature beats, as well as the number of paired and multiform ventricular ectopic beats, and R-on-T beats.

UNLABELED USES

Acebutolol is used alone or as an adjunct in the treatment of angina pectoris.

CONTRAINDICATIONS

Acebutolol is contraindicated in: 1) persistently severe bradycardia; 2) second- and third-degree heart block; 3) overt cardiac failure; and 4) cardiogenic shock. (See *"Warnings."*)

WARNINGS

CARDIAC FAILURE

Sympathetic stimulation may be essential for support of the circulation in individuals with diminished myocardial contractility, and its inhibition by β-adrenergic receptor blockade may precipitate more severe failure. Although β-blockers should be avoided in overt cardiac failure, Acebutolol can be used with caution in patients with a history of heart failure who are controlled with digitalis and/or diuretics. Both digitalis and Acebutolol impair AV conduction. If cardiac failure persists, therapy with Acebutolol should be withdrawn.

IN PATIENTS WITHOUT A HISTORY OF CARDIAC FAILURE

In patients with aortic or mitral valve disease or compromised left ventricular function, continued depression of the myocardium with β-blocking agents over a period of time may lead to cardiac failure. At the first signs of failure, patients should be digitalized and/or be given a diuretic and the response observed closely. If cardiac failure continues despite adequate digitalization and/or diuretic, Acebutolol therapy should be withdrawn.

EXACERBATION OF ISCHEMIC HEART DISEASE
FOLLOWING ABRUPT WITHDRAWAL

Following abrupt cessation of therapy with certain β-blocking agents in patients with coronary artery disease, exacerbation of angina pectoris and, in some cases, myocardial infarction and death have been reported. Therefore, such patients should be cautioned against interruption of therapy without a physician's advice. Even in the absence of overt ischemic heart disease, when discontinuation of Acebutolol is planned, the patient should be carefully observed, and should be advised to limit physical activity to a minimum while Acebutolol is gradually withdrawn over a period of about two weeks. (If therapy with an alternative β-blocker is desired, the patient may be transferred directly to comparable doses of another agent without interruption of β-blocking therapy.) If an exacerbation of angina pectoris occurs, antianginal therapy should be restarted immediately in full doses and the patient hospitalized until his condition stabilizes.

PERIPHERAL VASCULAR DISEASE

Treatment with β-antagonists reduces cardiac output and can precipitate or aggravate the symptoms of arterial insufficiency in patients with peripheral or mesenteric vascular disease. Caution should be exercised with such patients, and they should be observed closely for evidence of progression of arterial obstruction.

BRONCHOSPASTIC DISEASES

PATIENTS WITH BRONCHOSPASTIC DISEASE SHOULD, IN GENERAL, NOT RECEIVE A β-BLOCKER. Because of its relative β_1-selectivity, however, low doses of Acebutolol may be used with caution in patients with bronchospastic disease who do not respond to, or who cannot tolerate, alternative treatment. Since β_1-selectivity is not absolute and is dose-dependent, the lowest possible dose of Acebutolol should be used initially, preferably in divided doses to avoid the higher plasma levels associated with the longer dose-interval. A bronchodilator, such as a theophylline or a β_2-stimulant, should be made available in advance with instructions concerning its use.

ANESTHESIA AND MAJOR SURGERY

The necessity, or desirability, of withdrawal of a β-blocking therapy prior to major surgery is controversial. β-adrenergic receptor blockade impairs the ability of the heart to respond to β-adrenergically mediated reflex stimuli. While this might be of benefit in preventing arrhythmic response, the risk of excessive myocardial depression during general anesthesia may be enhanced and difficulty in restarting and maintaining the heart beat has been reported with beta-blockers. If treatment is continued, particular care should be taken when using anesthetic agents which depress the myocardium, such as ether, cyclopropane and trichlorethylene, and it is prudent to use the lowest possible dose of Acebutolol. Acebutolol like other β-blockers, is a competitive inhibitor of β-receptor agonists, and its effect on the heart can be reversed by cautious administration of such agents (e.g., dobutamine or isoproterenol—see *"Overdose"*).

Manifestations of excessive vagal tone (e.g., profound bradycardia, hypotension) may be corrected with atropine 1 to 3 mg IV in divided doses.

DIABETES AND HYPOGLYCEMIA

β-blockers may potentiate insulin-induced hypoglycemia and mask some of its manifestations such as tachycardia; however, dizziness and sweating are usually not significantly affected. Diabetic patients should be warned of the possibility of masked hypoglycemia.

THYROTOXICOSIS

β-adrenergic blockade may mask certain clinical signs (tachycardia) of hyperthyroidism. Abrupt withdrawal of β-blockade may precipitate a thyroid storm; therefore, patients suspected of developing thyrotoxicosis from whom Acebutolol therapy is to be withdrawn should be monitored closely.

PRECAUTIONS

IMPAIRED RENAL OR HEPATIC FUNCTION

Studies on the effect of Acebutolol in patients with renal insufficiency have not been performed in the U.S. Foreign published experience shows that Acebutolol has been used successfully in chronic renal insufficiency. Acebutolol is excreted through the GI tract, but the active metabolite, diacetolol, is eliminated predominantly by the kidney. There is a linear relationship between renal clearance of diacetolol and creatinine clearance. Therefore, the daily dose of Acebutolol should be reduced by 50% when the creatinine clearance is less than 50 mL/min and by 75% when it is less than 25 mL/min. Acebutolol should be used cautiously in patients with impaired hepatic function.

Acebutolol has been used successfully and without problems in elderly patients in the U.S. clinical trials without specific adjustment of dosage. However, elderly patients may require lower maintenance doses because the bioavailability of both Acebutolol and its metabolite are approximately doubled in this age group.

INFORMATION FOR PATIENTS

Patients, especially those with evidence of coronary artery disease, should be warned against interruption or discontinuation of Acebutolol therapy without a physician's supervision. Although cardiac failure rarely occurs in properly selected patients, those being treated with β-adrenergic blocking agents should be advised to consult a physician if they develop signs or symptoms suggestive of impending CHF, or unexplained respiratory symptoms.

Patients should also be warned of possible severe hypertensive reactions from concomitant use of α-adrenergic stimulants, such as the nasal decongestants commonly used in OTC cold preparations and nasal drops.

CLINICAL LABORATORY FINDINGS

Acebutolol, like other β-blockers, has been associated with the development of antinuclear antibodies (ANA). In prospective clinical trials, patients receiving Acebutolol had a dose-dependent increase in the development of positive ANA titers, and the overall incidence was higher than that observed with propranolol.

Symptoms (generally persistent arthralgias and myalgias) related to this laboratory abnormality were infrequent (less than 1% with both drugs). Symptoms and ANA titers were reversible upon discontinuation of treatment.

DRUG INTERACTIONS

Catecholamine-depleting drugs, such as reserpine, may have an additive effect when given with β-blocking agents. Patients treated with Acebutolol plus catecholamine depletors should, therefore, be observed closely for evidence of marked bradycardia or hypotension which may present as vertigo, syncope/presyncope, or orthostatic changes in blood pressure without compensatory tachycardia. Exaggerated hypertensive responses have been reported from the combined use of β-adrenergic antagonists and α-adrenergic stimulants, including those contained in proprietary cold remedies and vasoconstrictive nasal drops. Patients receiving β-blockers should be warned of this potential hazard.

Blunting of the antihypertensive effect of beta-adrenoceptor blocking agents by nonsteroidal anti-inflammatory drugs has been reported.

No significant interactions with digoxin, hydrochlorothiazide, hydralazine, sulfinpyrazone, oral contraceptives, tolbutamide, or warfarin have been observed.

CARCINOGENESIS, MUTAGENESIS, IMPAIRMENT OF FERTILITY

Chronic oral toxicity studies in rats and mice, employing dose levels as high as 300 mg/kg/day, which is equivalent to 15 times the maximum recommended (60 kg) human dose, did not indicate a carcinogenic potential for Acebutolol. Diacetolol, the major metabolite of Acebutolol in man, was without carcinogenic potential in rats when tested at doses as high as 1800 mg/kg/day. Acebutolol and diacetolol were also shown to be devoid of mutagenic potential in the Ames Test. Acebutolol administered orally to two generations of male and female rats at doses of up to 240 mg/kg/day (equivalent to 12 times the maximum recommended therapeutic dose in a 60-kg human) and diacetolol, administered to two generations of male and female rats at doses of up to 1000 mg/kg/day, had no significant impact on reproductive performance or fertility.

PREGNANCY

Teratogenic Effects: Pregnancy Category B: Reproduction studies have been performed with Acebutolol in rats (up to 630 mg/kg/day) and rabbits (up to 135 mg/kg/day). These doses are equivalent to approximately 31.5 and 6.8 times the maximum recommended therapeutic dose in a 60-kg human, respectively. The compound was not teratogenic in either species. In the rabbit, however, doses of 135 mg/kg/day caused slight fetal growth retardation; this effect was considered to be a result of maternal toxicity, as evidenced by reduced food intake, a lowered rate of body weight gain, and mortality. Studies have also been performed in these species with diacetolol (at doses of up to 450 mg/kg/day in rabbits and up to 1800 mg/kg/day in rats.) Other than a significant elevation in postimplantation loss with 450 mg/kg/day diacetolol, a level at which food consumption and body weight gain were reduced in rabbit dams and a nonstatistically significant increase in incidence of bilateral cataract in rat fetuses from dams treated with 1800 mg/kg/day diacetolol, there was no evidence of harm to the fetus. There are no adequate and well-controlled trials in pregnant women. Because animal teratology studies are not always predictive of the human response, Acebutolol should be used during pregnancy only if the potential benefit justifies the risk to the fetus.

Nonteratogenic Effects: Studies in humans have shown that both Acebutolol and diacetolol cross the placenta. Neonates of mothers who have received Acebutolol during pregnancy have reduced birth weight, decreased blood pressure, and decreased heart rate. In the newborn the elimination half-life of Acebutolol was 6 to 14 hours, while the half-life of diacetolol was 24 to 30 hours for the first 24 hours after birth, followed by a half-life of 12 to 16 hours. Adequate facilities for monitoring these infants at birth should be available.

LABOR AND DELIVERY

The effect of Acebutolol on labor and delivery in pregnant women is unknown. Studies in animals have not shown any effect of Acebutolol on the usual course of labor and delivery.

NURSING MOTHERS

Acebutolol and diacetolol also appear in breast milk with a milk:plasma ratio of 7.1 and 12.2, respectively. Use in nursing mothers is not recommended.

PEDIATRIC USE

Safety and effectiveness in children have not been established.

ADVERSE REACTIONS

Acebutolol is well tolerated in properly selected patients. Most adverse reactions have been mild, not required discontinuation of therapy, and tended to decrease as duration of treatment increases.

The following table shows the frequency of treatment-related side effects derived from controlled clinical trials in patients with hypertension, angina pectoris, and arrhythmia. These patients received Acebutolol, propranolol, or hydrochlorothiazide as monotherapy, or placebo. (See related table).

The following selected (potentially important) side effects were seen in up to 2% of Acebutolol patients:

Cardiovascular: hypotension, bradycardia, heart failure.

Central Nervous System: anxiety, hyper/hypoesthesia, impotence.

Dermatological: pruritus.

Gastrointestinal: vomiting, abdominal pain.

Genitourinary: dysuria, nocturia.

Liver and Biliary System: A small number of cases of liver abnormalities (increased SGOT, SGPT, LDH) have been reported in association with Acebutolol therapy. In some cases increased bilirubin or alkaline phosphatase, fever, malaise, dark urine, anorexia, nausea, headache, and/or other symptoms have been reported. In some of the reported cases, the symptoms and signs were confirmed by rechallenge with Acebutolol. The abnormalities were reversible upon cessation of Acebutolol therapy.

Musculoskeletal: back pain, joint pain.

Respiratory: pharyngitis, wheezing.

Special Senses: conjunctivitis, dry eye, eye pain.

Autoimmune: In extremely rare instances, systemic lupus erythematosus has been reported.

The incidence of drug-related adverse effects (volunteered and solicited) according to Acebutolol dose is shown below. (Data from 266 hypertensive patients treated for 3 months on a constant dose.)

Body System	400 mg/day (N = 132)	800 mg/day (N = 63)	1200 mg/day (N = 71)
Cardiovascular	5%	2%	1%
Gastrointestinal	3%	3%	7%
Musculoskeletal	2%	3%	4%
Central Nervous System	9%	13%	17%
Respiratory	1%	5%	6%
Skin	1%	2%	1%
Special Senses	2%	2%	6%
Genitourinary	2%	3%	1%

POTENTIAL ADVERSE EFFECTS

In addition, certain adverse effects not listed above have been reported with other β-blocking agents and should also be considered as potential adverse effects of Acebutolol.

Central Nervous System: Reversible mental depression progressing to catatonia (an acute syndrome characterized by disorientation for time and place), short-term memory loss, emotional lability, slightly clouded sensorium, and decreased performance (neuropsychometrics).

Cardiovascular: Intensification of AV block (see *"Contraindications"*).

Allergic: Erythematous rash, fever combined with aching and sore throat, laryngospasm, and respiratory distress.

Hematologic: Agranulocytosis, nonthrombocytopenic, and thrombocytopenic purpura.

Gastrointestinal: Mesenteric arterial thrombosis and ischemic colitis.

Miscellaneous: Reversible alopecia and Peyronie's disease. The oculomucocutaneous syndrome associated with the β-blocker practolol has not been reported with Acebutolol during investigational use and extensive foreign clinical experience.

OVERDOSAGE

No specific information on emergency treatment of overdose is available for Acebutolol. However, overdosage with other β-blocking agents has been accompanied by extreme bradycardia, advanced atrioventricular block, intraventricular conduction defects, hypotension, severe congestive heart failure, seizures, and in susceptible patients, bronchospasm and hypoglycemia. Although specific information on the emergency treatment of Acebutolol overdose is not available, on the basis of the pharmacological actions and the observations in treating overdoses with other β-blockers, the following general measures should be considered:

1. Empty stomach by emesis or lavage.
2. Bradycardia: IV atropine (1 to 3 mg in divided doses). If antivagal response is inadequate, administer isoproterenol cautiously since larger than usual doses of isoproterenol may be required.
3. Persistent hypotension in spite of correction of bradycardia: Administer vasopressor (e.g., epinephrine, levarterenol, dopamine, or dobutamine) with frequent monitoring of blood pressure and pulse rate.
4. Bronchospasm: A theophylline derivative, such as aminophylline and/or parenteral β2-stimulant, such as terbutaline.
5. Cardiac failure: Digitalize the patient and/or administer a diuretic. It has been reported that glucagon is useful in this situation.

Sectral is dialyzable.

DOSAGE AND ADMINISTRATION

HYPERTENSION

The initial dosage of Acebutolol in uncomplicated mild-to-moderate hypertension is 400 mg. This can be given as a single daily dose, but in occasional patients twice daily dosing may be required for adequate 24-hour blood-pressure control. An optimal response is usually achieved with dosages of 400 to 800 mg per day, although some patients have been maintained on as little as 200 mg per day. Patients with more severe hypertension or who have demonstrated inadequate control may respond to a total of 1200 mg daily (administered b.i.d.), or to the addition of a second antihypertensive agent. Beta-1 selectivity diminishes as dosage is increased.

VENTRICULAR ARRHYTHMIA

The usual initial dose of Acebutolol is 400 mg daily given as 200 mg b.i.d. Dosage should be increased gradually until an optimal clinical response is obtained, generally at 600 to 1200 mg per day. If treatment is to be discontinued, the dosage should be reduced gradually over a period of about two weeks.

USE IN OLDER PATIENTS

Older patients have an approximately 2-fold increase in bioavailability and may require lower maintenance doses. Doses above 800 mg/day should be avoided in the elderly.

STORAGE

Keep tightly closed. Store at room temperature, approximately 25°C (77°F). Protect from light. Dispense in light-resistant, tight container. Use carton to protect contents from light.

TOTAL VOLUNTEERED AND ELICITED (U.S. STUDIES)

Body System/Adverse Reaction	Acebutolol (N = 1002) %	Propranolol (N = 424) %	Hydrochlorothiazide (N = 178) %	Placebo (N = 314) %
Cardiovascular				
Chest Pain	2	4	4	1
Edema	2	2	4	1
Central Nervous System				
Depression	2	1	3	1
Dizziness	6	7	12	2
Fatigue	11	17	10	4
Headache	6	9	13	4
Insomnia	3	6	5	1
Abnormal dreams	2	3	0	1
Dermatologic				
Rash	2	2	4	1
Gastrointestinal				
Constipation	4	2	7	0
Diarrhea	4	5	5	1
Dyspepsia	4	6	3	1
Flatulence	3	4	7	1
Nausea	4	6	3	0
Genitourinary				
Micturition (frequency)	3	1	9	< 1
Musculoskeletal				
Arthralgia	2	1	3	2
Myalgia	2	1	4	0
Respiratory				
Cough	1	1	2	0
Dyspnea	4	6	4	2
Rhinitis	2	1	4	< 1
Special Senses				
Abnormal Vision	2	2	3	0

HOW SUPPLIED
CAPSULE: 200 MG

BRAND/MANUFACTURER	NDC	SIZE	AWP
○ BRAND			
▶ SECTRAL: Wyeth-Ayerst	00008-4177-01	100s	$87.96
	00008-4177-04	100s ud	$94.86

CAPSULE: 400 MG

BRAND/MANUFACTURER	NDC	SIZE	AWP
○ BRAND			
▶ SECTRAL: Wyeth-Ayerst	00008-4179-01	100s	$116.94

Acel-Imune SEE DIPHTHERIA/PERTUSSIS/TETANUS

Acetaminophen and Oxycodone Hydrochloride

DESCRIPTION

Each tablet of Acetaminophen/Oxycodone Hydrochloride contains:

Oxycodone Hydrochloride ....5 mg*
   WARNING: May be habit forming
Acetaminophen, USP ....325 mg

Each capsule of Acetaminophen/Oxycodone Hydrochloride contains:

Oxycodone Hydrochloride USP 5mg*
   WARNING—May be habit forming.
Acetaminophen USP ....500 mg
* 5 mg Oxycodone Hydrochloride is equivalent to 4.4815 mg Oxycodone.

Certain brands of Acetaminophen/Oxycodone Hydrochloride (APAP/Oxycodone) capsules contain sulfite (see *"Warnings"*).
   Acetaminophen occurs as a white, odorless, crystalline powder, possessing a slightly bitter taste.
   The Oxycodone component is 14-hydroxydihydrocodeinone, a white, odorless, crystalline powder having a saline, bitter taste. It is derived from the opium alkaloid thebaine.

CLINICAL PHARMACOLOGY
The principal ingredient, Oxycodone, is a semisynthetic narcotic analgesic with multiple actions qualitatively similar to those of morphine; the most prominent of these involve the central nervous system and organs composed of smooth muscle. The principal actions of therapeutic value of the Oxycodone in APAP/Oxycodone are analgesia and sedation.
   Oxycodone is similar to codeine and methadone in that it retains at least one-half of its analgesic activity when administered orally.
   Acetaminophen is a nonopiate, nonsalicylate analgesic and antipyretic.

INDICATIONS AND USAGE
APAP/Oxycodone is indicated for the relief of moderate to moderately severe pain.

CONTRAINDICATIONS
APAP/Oxycodone should not be administered to patients who are hypersensitive to Oxycodone or Acetaminophen.

WARNINGS
Contains sodium metabisulfite, a sulfite that may cause allergic-type reactions including anaphylactic symptoms and life-threatening or less severe asthmatic episodes in certain susceptible people. The overall prevalence of sulfite sensitivity in the general population is unknown and probably low. Sulfite sensitivity is seen more frequently in asthmatic than in nonasthmatic people.

Drug Dependence: Oxycodone can produce drug dependence of the morphine type and, therefore, has the potential for being abused. Psychic dependence, physical dependence and tolerance may develop upon repeated administration of APAP/Oxycodone, and it should be prescribed and administered with the same degree of caution appropriate to the use of other oral narcotic-containing medications. Like other narcotic-containing medications APAP/Oxycodone is subject to the Federal Controlled Substances Act (Schedule II).

PRECAUTIONS
GENERAL
Head Injury and Increased Intracranial Pressure: The respiratory depressant effects of narcotics and their capacity to elevate cerebrospinal fluid pressure may be markedly exaggerated in the presence of head injury, other intracranial lesions or a pre-existing increase in intracranial pressure. Furthermore, narcotics produce adverse reactions which may obscure the clinical course of patients with head injuries.

Acute Abdominal Conditions: The administration of APAP/Oxycodone or other narcotics may obscure the diagnosis or clinical course in patients with acute abdominal conditions.

Special Risk Patients: APAP/Oxycodon should be given with caution to certain patients such as the elderly or debilitated, and those with severe impairment of hepatic or renal function, hypothyroidism, Addison's disease, and prostatic hypertrophy or urethral stricture.

Information for Patients: Oxycodone may impair the mental and/or physical abilities required for the performance of potentially hazardous tasks such as driving a car or operating machinery. The patient using APAP/Oxycodone should be cautioned accordingly.

Drug Interaction: Patients receiving other narcotic analgesics, general anesthetics, phenothiazines, other tranquilizers, sedative-hypnotics or other CNS depressants (including alcohol) concomitantly with APAP/Oxycodone may exhibit an additive CNS depression. When such combined therapy is contemplated, the dose of one or both agents should be reduced.
   The use of MAO inhibitors or tricyclic antidepressants with Oxycodone preparations may increase the effect of either the antidepressant or Oxycodone.
   The concurrent use of anticholinergics with narcotics may produce paralytic ileus.

Usage In Pregnancy Pregnancy Category C: Animal reproductive studies have not been conducted with APAP/Oxycodone. It is also not known whether APAP/Oxycodone can cause fetal harm when administered to a pregnant woman or can affect reproductive capacity. APAP/Oxycodone should not be given to a pregnant woman unless in the judgment of the physician, the potential benefits outweigh the possible hazards.

Nonteratogenic Effects: Use of narcotics during pregnancy may produce physical dependence in the neonate.

Labor and Delivery: As with all narcotics, administration of APAP/Oxycodone to the mother shortly before delivery may result in some degree of respiratory depression in the newborn and the mother, especially if higher doses are used.

Nursing Mothers: It is not known whether APAP/Oxycodone is excreted in human milk. Because many drugs are excreted in human milk, caution should be exercised when APAP/Oxycodone is administered to a nursing woman.

Pediatric Use: Safety and effectiveness in children have not been established.

ADVERSE REACTIONS
The most frequently observed adverse reactions include lightheadedness, dizziness, sedation, nausea and vomiting. These effects seem to be more prominent in ambulatory than in nonambulatory patients, and some of these adverse reactions may be alleviated if the patient lies down.
   Other adverse reactions include euphoria, dysphoria, constipation, skin rash and pruritus. At higher doses, Oxycodone has most of the disadvantages of morphine including respiratory depression.

DRUG ABUSE AND DEPENDENCE
APAP/Oxycodone tablets and capsules are a Schedule II controlled substance. Oxycodone can produce drug dependence and has the potential for being abused. (see *"Warnings"*.)

OVERDOSAGE
ACETAMINOPHEN
Signs and Symptoms: In acute Acetaminophen overdosage, dose-dependent, potentially fatal hepatic necrosis is the most serious adverse effect. Renal tubular necrosis, hypoglycemic coma and thrombocytopenia may also occur.
   In adults, hepatic toxicity has rarely been reported with acute overdoses of less than 10 grams and fatalities with less than 15 grams. Importantly, young children seem to be more resistant than adults to the hepatotoxic effect of an Acetaminophen overdose. Despite this, the measures outlined below should be initiated in any adult or child suspected of having ingested an Acetaminophen overdose.
   Early symptoms following a potentially hepatotoxic overdose may include: nausea, vomiting, diaphoresis and general malaise. Clinical and laboratory evidence of hepatic toxicity may not be apparent until 48 to 72 hours post-ingestion.

Treatment: The stomach should be emptied promptly by lavage or by induction of emesis with syrup of ipecac. Patient's estimates of the quantity of a drug ingested are notoriously unreliable. Therefore, if an Acetaminophen overdose is suspected, a serum Acetaminophen assay should be obtained as early as possible, but no sooner than four hours following ingestion. Liver function studies should be obtained initially and repeated at 24-hour intervals.
   The antidote, N-acetylcysteine, should be administered as early as possible, preferably within 16 hours of the overdose ingestion for optimal results, but in any case, within 24 hours. Following recovery, there are no residual, structural, or functional hepatic abnormalities.

OXYCODONE
Signs and Symptoms: Serious overdosage with Oxycodone is characterized by respiratory depression (a decrease in respiratory rate and or tidal volume, Cheyne-Stokes respiration, cyanosis), extreme somnolence progressing to stupor or coma, skeletal muscle flaccidity, cold and clammy skin, and sometimes bradycardia and hypotension. In severe overdosage, apnea, circulatory collapse, cardiac arrest and death may occur.

◆ RATED THERAPEUTICALLY EQUIVALENT; ◇ THERAPEUTIC EQUIVALENCE UNCONFIRMED; ○ UNRATED

Treatment: Primary attention should be given to the re-establishment of adequate respiratory exchange through provision of a patent airway and the institution of assisted or controlled ventilation. The narcotic antagonist naloxone hydrochloride is a specific antidote against respiratory depression which may result from overdosage or unusual sensitivity to narcotics, including Oxycodone. Therefore, an appropriate dose of naloxone hydrochloride (usual initial adult dose 0.4 mg to 2 mg) should be administered preferably by the intravenous route, and simultaneously with efforts at respiratory resuscitation (see package insert) Since the duration of action of Oxycodone may exceed that of the antagonist, the patient should be kept under continued surveillance and repeated doses of the antagonist should be administered as needed to maintain adequate respiration.

An antagonist should not be administered in the absence of clinically significant respiratory or cardiovascular depression. Oxygen, intravenous fluids, vasopressors and other supportive measures should be employed as indicated.

Gastric emptying may be useful in removing unabsorbed drug.

DOSAGE AND ADMINISTRATION

Dosage should be adjusted according to the severity of the pain and the response of the patient. It may occasionally be necessary to exceed the usual dosage recommended below in cases of more severe pain or in those patients who have become tolerant to the analgesic effect of narcotics.

APAP/Oxycodone are give orally. The usual adult dosage is one tablet or capsule every 6 hours as needed for pain.

TABLETS AND CAPSULES

Store at controlled room temperature (15°-30°C, 59°-86°F).

Dispense in tight, light-resistant container as defined in the official compendium.

HOW SUPPLIED
CAPSULE: 500 MG-5 MG

AVERAGE UNIT PRICE (AVAILABLE SIZES)		GENERIC A-RATED AVERAGE PRICE (GAAP)	
BRAND	$0.78	100s	$49.35
GENERIC	$0.49		
HCFA FUL (100s ea)	$0.37		

BRAND/MANUFACTURER	NDC	SIZE	AWP
◆ BRAND			
➤ TYLOX: McNeil Pharm	00045-0526-60	100s	$67.72
	00045-0526-79	100s ud	$89.04
◆ GENERICS			
ROXILOX: Roxane	00054-2795-25	100s	$38.94
Qualitest	00603-4997-21	100s	$41.67
Aligen	00405-0140-01	100s	$46.61
Halsey Pharm	00879-0532-01	100s	$48.75
Duramed	51285-0644-02	100s	$49.50
Parmed	00349-8659-01	100s	$51.95
Schein	00364-2395-01	100s	$54.38
Goldline	00182-9175-01	100s	$54.75
Rugby	00536-3219-01	100s	$57.59
Halsey Pharm	00879-0532-05	500s	$226.65

CAPSULE (C-II): 500 MG-5 MG

AVERAGE UNIT PRICE (AVAILABLE SIZES)		GENERIC A-RATED AVERAGE PRICE (GAAP)	
BRAND	$0.78	100s	$49.35
GENERIC	$0.49		
HCFA FUL (100s ea)	$0.37		

BRAND/MANUFACTURER	NDC	SIZE	AWP
◆ BRAND			
➤ TYLOX: McNeil Pharm	00045-0526-60	100s	$67.72
	00045-0526-79	100s ud	$89.04
◆ GENERICS			
ROXILOX: Roxane	00054-2795-25	100s	$38.94
Qualitest	00603-4997-21	100s	$41.67
Aligen	00405-0140-01	100s	$46.61
Halsey Pharm	00879-0532-01	100s	$48.75
Duramed	51285-0644-02	100s	$49.50
Parmed	00349-8659-01	100s	$51.95
Schein	00364-2395-01	100s	$54.38
Goldline	00182-9175-01	100s	$54.75
Rugby	00536-3219-01	100s	$57.59
Halsey Pharm	00879-0532-05	500s	$226.65

TABLETS (C-II): 325 MG-5 MG

AVERAGE UNIT PRICE (AVAILABLE SIZES)		GENERIC A-RATED AVERAGE PRICE (GAAP)	
BRAND	$0.63	100s	$22.46
GENERIC	$0.21	500s	$96.23
HCFA FUL (100s ea)	$0.13		

BRAND/MANUFACTURER	NDC	SIZE	AWP
◆ BRAND			
➤ PERCOCET: Du Pont Pharma	00590-0127-70	100s	$63.18
	00590-0127-65	250s ud	$161.75
	00590-0127-85	500s	$300.00

BRAND/MANUFACTURER	NDC	SIZE	AWP
◆ GENERICS			
Halsey Pharm	00879-0512-01	100s	$18.65
Qualitest	00603-4998-21	100s	$19.33
Major	00904-0465-60	100s	$19.55
Rugby	00536-5670-01	100s	$20.73
Rugby	00536-3217-01	100s	$21.12
ENDOCET: Endo	60951-0602-70	100s	$22.50
Parmed	00349-8859-01	100s	$22.50
➤ ROXICET: Roxane	00054-4650-25	100s	$22.55
Goldline	00182-1465-01	100s	$22.95
Aligen	00405-0139-01	100s	$25.32
Schein	00364-0605-01	100s	$25.69
ROXICET: Roxane	00054-8650-24	100s ud	$28.68
Major	00904-0465-40	500s	$79.45
➤ ROXICET: Roxane	00054-4650-29	500s	$83.75
Halsey Pharm	00879-0512-05	500s	$86.75
Parmed	00349-8859-05	500s	$91.95
ENDOCET: Endo	60951-0602-25	500s	$98.45
Rugby	00536-5670-05	500s	$98.46
Goldline	00182-1465-05	500s	$108.00
Schein	00364-0605-05	500s	$123.00

TABLETS (C-II): 500 MG-5 MG

BRAND/MANUFACTURER	NDC	SIZE	AWP
◆ GENERICS			
Major	00904-1973-60	100s	$46.50

Acetaminophen and Pentazocine Hydrochloride

DESCRIPTION
Each scored caplet for oral administration contains Acetaminophen, USP, 650 mg and Pentazocine Hydrochloride, USP, equivalent to 25 mg base.

Pentazocine is a member of the benzazocine series (also known as the benzomorphan series). Chemically, Pentazocine is 1,2,3,4,5,6-hexahydro-6,11-dimethyl-3-(3-methyl-2-butenyl)-2,6-methano-3- benzazocin-8-ol, a white, crystal-line substance soluble in acidic aqueous solutions.

Chemically, Acetaminophen is acetamide, *N*- (4-hydroxyphenyl)-.

Pentazocine is an analgesic and Acetaminophen is an analgesic and antipyretic.

CLINICAL PHARMACOLOGY
Acetaminophen/Pentazocine HCl is an analgesic possessing antipyretic actions. Pentazocine is an analgesic with agonist/antagonist action which when administered orally is approximately equivalent on a mg for mg basis in analgesic effect to codeine. Acetaminophen is an analgesic and antipyretic.

Onset of significant analgesia with Pentazocine usually occurs between 15 and 30 minutes after oral administration, and duration of action is usually three hour or longer. Onset and duration of action and the degree of pain relief are related both to dose and the severity of pretreatment pain. Pentazocine weakly antagonizes the analgesic effects of morphine, meperidine, and phenazocine; in addition, it produces incomplete reversal of cardiovascular, respiratory, and behavioral depression induced by morphine and meperidine. Pentazocine has about 1/50 the antagonistic activity of nalorphine. It also has sedative activity.

Pentazocine is well absorbed from the gastrointestinal tract. Plasma levels closely correspond to the onset, duration, and intensity of analgesia. The mean peak concentration in 24 normal volunteers was 1.7 hours (range 0.5 to 4 hours) after oral administration and the mean plasma elimination half-life was 3.6 hours (range 0.5 to 10 hours).

The action of Pentazocine is terminated for the most part by biotransformation in the liver with some free Pentazocine excreted in the urine. The products of the oxidation of the terminal methyl groups and glucuronide conjugates are excreted by the kidney. Elimination of approximately 60% of the total dose occurs within 24 hours. Pentazocine passes the placental barrier.

Onset of significant analgesic and antipyretic activity of Acetaminophen when administered orally occurs within 30 minutes and is maximal at approximately 2 ½ hours. The pharmacological mode of action of Acetaminophen is unknown at this time.

Acetaminophen is rapidly and almost completely absorbed from the gastrointestinal tract. In 24 normal volunteers the mean peak plasma concentration was 1 hour (range 0.25 to 3 hours) after oral administration and the mean plasma elimination half-life was 2.8 hours (range 2 to 4 hours).

The effect of Pentazocine on Acetaminophen plasma protein binding or vice versa has not been established. For Acetaminophen there is little or no plasma protein binding at normal therapeutic doses. When toxic doses of Acetaminophen are ingested and drug plasma levels exceed 90 µg/mL, plasma binding may vary from 8% to 43%.

Acetaminophen is conjugated in the liver with glucuronic acid and to a lesser extent with sulfuric acid. Approximately 80% of Acetaminophen is excreted in the urine after conjugation and about 3% is excreted unchanged. The drug is also conjugated to a lesser extent with cysteine and additionally metabolized by hydroxylation.

If Acetaminophen/Pentazocine HCl is taken every 4 hours over an extended period of time, accumulation of Pentazocine and to a lesser extent, Acetaminophen, may occur.

INDICATIONS AND USAGE
Acetaminophen/Pentazocine HCl is indicated for the relief of mild to moderate pain.

CONTRAINDICATIONS
Acetaminophen/Pentazocine HCl should not be administered to patients who are hypersensitive to either Pentazocine or Acetaminophen.

WARNINGS
Contains sodium metabisulfite, a sulfite that may cause allergic-type reactions including anaphylactic symptoms and life-threatening or less severe asthmatic episodes in certain susceptible people. The overall prevalence of sulfite sensitivity in the general population is unknown and probably low. Sulfite sensitivity is seen more frequently in asthmatic than in nonasthmatic people.

Head Injury and Increased Intracranial Pressure: As in the case of other potent analgesics, the potential of Pentazocine for elevating cerebrospinal fluid pressure may be attributed to CO_2 retention due to the respiratory depressant effects of the drug. These effects may be markedly exaggerated in the presence of head injury, other intracranial lesions, or a preexisting increase in intracranial pressure. Furthermore, Pentazocine can produce effects which may obscure the clinical course of patients with head injuries. In such patients, Acetaminophen/Pentazocine HCl must be used with extreme caution and only if its use is deemed essential.

Acute CNS Manifestations: Patients receiving therapeutic doses of Pentazocine have experienced hallucinations (usually visual), disorientation, and confusion which have cleared spontaneously within a period of hours. The mechanism of this reaction is not known. Such patients should be closely observed and vital signs checked. If the drug is reinstituted, it should be done with caution since these acute CNS manifestations may recur.

There have been instances of psychological and physical dependence on parenteral Pentazocine in patients with a history of drug abuse, and rarely, in patients without such a history. (See *"Drug Abuse and Dependence"*.)

Due to the potential for increased CNS depressant effects, alcohol should be used with caution in patients who are currently receiving Pentazocine.

Pentazocine may precipitate opioid abstinence symptoms in patients receiving courses of opiates for pain relief.

PRECAUTIONS
In prescribing Acetaminophen/Pentazocine HCl for chronic use, the physician should take precautions to avoid increases in dose by the patient.

Myocardial Infarction: As with all drugs, Acetaminophen/Pentazocine HCl should be used with caution in patients with myocardial infarction who have nausea or vomiting.

Certain Respiratory Conditions: Although respiratory depression has rarely been reported after oral administration of Pentazocine, the drug should be administered with caution to patients with respiratory depression from any cause, severely limited respiratory reserve, severe bronchial asthma and other obstructive respiratory conditions, or cyanosis.

Impaired Renal or Hepatic Function: Decreased metabolism of the drug by the liver in extensive liver disease may predispose to accentuation of side effects. Although laboratory tests have not indicated that Pentazocine causes or increases renal or hepatic impairment, the drug should be administered with caution to patients with such impairment. Since Acetaminophen is metabolized by the liver, the question of the safety of its use in the presence of liver disease should be considered.

Biliary Surgery: Narcotic drug products are generally considered to elevate biliary tract pressure for varying periods following their administration. Some evidence suggests that Pentazocine may differ from other marketed narcotics in this respect (ie, it causes little or no elevation in biliary tract pressures). The clinical significance of these findings, however, is not yet known.

CNS Effect: Caution should be used when Acetaminophen/Pentazocine HCl is administered to patients prone to seizures; seizures have occurred in a few such patients in association with the use of Pentazocine although no cause and effect relationship has been established.

Information for Patients: Since sedation, dizziness, and occasional euphoria have been noted, ambulatory patients should be warned not to operate machinery, drive cars, or unnecessarily expose themselves to hazards. Pentazocine may cause physical and psychological dependence when taken alone and may have additive CNS depressant properties when taken in combination with alcohol or other CNS depressants.

Drug Interactions: Pentazocine is a mild narcotic antagonist. Some patients previously given narcotics, including methadone for the daily treatment of narcotic dependence, have experienced withdrawal symptoms after receiving Pentazocine.

Carcinogenesis, Mutagenesis, Impairment of Fertility: Carcinogenesis, mutagenesis, and impairment of fertility studies have not been done with this combination product.

Pentazocine, when administered orally or parenterally, had no adverse effect on either the reproductive capabilities or the course of pregnancy in rabbits and rats. Embryotoxic effects on the fetuses were not shown.

The daily administration of 4 mg/kg to 20 mg/kg Pentazocine subcutaneously to female rats during a 14 day pre-mating period and until the 13th day of pregnancy did not have any adverse effects on the fertility rate.

There is no evidence in long-term animal studies to demonstrate that Pentazocine is carcinogenic.

Pregnancy Category C: Animal reproduction studies have not been conducted with Acetaminophen/Pentazocine HCL. It is also not known whether Acetaminophen/Pentazocine HCl can cause fetal harm when administered to pregnant women or can affect reproduction capacity. Acetaminophen/Pentazocine HCl should be given to pregnant women only if clearly needed. However, animal reproduction studies with Pentazocine have not demonstrated teratogenic or embryotoxic effects.

Nonteratogenic Effects: There has been no experience in this regard with the combination Pentazocine and Acetaminophen. However, there have been rare reports of possible abstinence syndromes in newborns after prolonged use of Pentazocine during pregnancy.

Labor and Delivery: Patients receiving Pentazocine during labor have experienced no adverse effects other than those that occur with commonly used analgesics. Acetaminophen/Pentazocine HCl should be used with caution in women delivering premature infants. The effect of Acetaminophen/Pentazocine HCl on the mother and fetus, the duration of labor or delivery, the possibility that forceps delivery or other intervention or resuscitation of the newborn may be necessary, or the effect of Acetaminophen/Pentazocine HCl, on the later growth, development, and functional maturation of the child are unknown at the present time.

Nursing Mothers: It is not known whether this drug is excreted in human milk. Because many drugs are excreted in human milk, caution should be exercised when Acetaminophen/Pentazocine HCl is administered to a nursing woman.

Pediatric Use: Safety and effectiveness in children below the age of 12 have not been established.

ADVERSE REACTIONS
Clinical experience with Acetaminophen/Pentazocine HCl has been insufficient to define all possible adverse reactions with this combination. However, reactions reported after oral administration of Pentazocine Hydrochloride in 50 mg dosage include:

Gastrointestinal: nausea, vomiting, infrequently constipation; and rarely abdominal distress, anorexia, diarrhea.

CNS effects: dizziness, light-headedness, hallucinations, sedation, euphoria, headache, confusion, disorientation; infrequently weakness, disturbed dreams, insomnia, syncope, visual blurring and focusing difficulty, depression; and rarely tremor, irritability, excitement, tinnitus.

Autonomic: sweating; infrequently flushing; and rarely chills.

Allergic: infrequently rash; and rarely urticaria, edema of the face.

Cardiovascular: infrequently decrease in blood pressure, tachycardia.

Hematologic: rarely depression of white blood cells (especially granulocytes), which is usually reversible, moderate transient eosinophilia.

Other: rarely respiratory depression, urinary retention, paresthesia, toxic epidermal necrolysis, and in one instance, an apparent anaphylactic reaction has been reported.

Numerous clinical studies have shown that acetaminophen, when taken in recommended doses, is relatively free of adverse effects in most age groups, even in the presence of a variety of disease states.

A few cases of hypersensitivity to Acetaminophen have been reported, as manifested by skin rashes, thrombocytopenic purpura, rarely hemolytic anemia and agranulocytosis. Occasional individuals respond to ordinary doses with nausea and vomiting and diarrhea.

DRUG ABUSE AND DEPENDENCE
Controlled Substance: Acetaminophen/Pentazocine HCl is a Schedule IV controlled substance.

Abuse and Dependence: There have been some reports of dependence and of withdrawal symptoms with orally administered Pentazocine. There have been recorded instances of psychological and physical dependence in patients using parenteral Pentazocine. Abrupt discontinuance following the extended use of parenteral Pentazocine has resulted in withdrawal symptoms. Patients with a history of drug dependence should be under close supervision while receiving Acetaminophen/Pentazocine HCl. There have been rare reports of possible abstinence syndromes in newborns after prolonged use of Pentazocine during pregnancy.

Some tolerance to the analgesic and subjective effects of Pentazocine develops with frequent and repeated use.

Drug addicts who are given closely spaced doses of Pentazocine (eg, 60 mg to 90 mg every 4 hours) develop physical dependence which is demonstrated by abrupt withdrawal or by administration of naloxone. The withdrawal symptoms exhibited after chronic doses of more than 500 mg of Pentazocine per day have similar characteristics, but to a lesser degree, of opioid withdrawal and may be associated with drug seeking behavior.

◆ RATED THERAPEUTICALLY EQUIVALENT; ◇ THERAPEUTIC EQUIVALENCE UNCONFIRMED; ○ UNRATED

OVERDOSAGE

Manifestations: Clinical experience with Acetaminophen/Pentazocine HCl has been insufficient to define the signs of overdosage with this product. It may be assumed that signs and symptoms of Acetaminophen/Pentazocine HCl overdose would be a combination of those observed with Pentazocine overdose and Acetaminophen over-dose.

For Pentazocine alone in single doses above 60 mg there have been reports of the occurrence of nalorphine-like psychotomimetic effects such as anxiety, nightmares, strange thoughts, and hallucinations. Marked respiratory depression associated with increased blood pressure and tachycardia have also resulted from excessive doses as have dizziness, nausea, vomiting, lethargy, and paresthesias. The respiratory depression is antagonized by naloxone (see *"Treatment"*). In acute Acetaminophen overdosage, dose-dependent, potentially fatal hepatic necrosis is the most serious adverse effect. Renal tubular necrosis, hypoglycemic coma, and thrombocytopenia may also occur.

In adults, a single dose of 10 g to 15 g (200 mg/kg to 250 mg/kg) of Acetaminophen may cause hepatotoxicity. A dose of 25 g or more is potentially fatal. The potential seriousness of the intoxication may not be evident during the first two days of acute Acetaminophen poisoning. During the first 24 hours, nausea, vomiting, anorexia, and abdominal pain occur. These may persist for a week or more. Liver injury may become evident the second day, initial signs being elevation of serum transaminase and lactic dehydrogenase activity, increased serum bilirubin concentration, and prolongation of prothrombin time. Serum albumin concentration and alkaline phosphatase activity may remain normal. The hepatotoxicity may lead to encephalopathy, coma, and death. Transient azotemia is evident in a majority of patients and acute renal failure occurs in some.

There have been reports of glycosuria and impaired glucose tolerance, but hypoglycemia may also occur. Metabolic acidosis and metabolic alkalosis have been reported. Cerebral edema and nonspecific myocardial depression have also been noted. Biopsy reveals centrolobular necrosis with sparing of the periportal area. The hepatic lesions are reversible over a period of weeks or months in nonfatal cases.

The severity of the liver injury can be determined by measurement of the plasma half-time of acetaminophen during the first day of acute poisoning. If the half-time exceeds 4 hours, hepatic necrosis is likely and if the half-time is greater than 12 hours, hepatic coma will probably occur. Only minimal liver damage has developed when the serum concentration was below 120 µg/mL at 12 hours after ingestion of the drug. If serum bilirubin concentration is greater than 4 mg/100 mL during the first 5 days, encephalopathy may occur.

The seven day oral LD_{50} value for Acetaminophen/Pentazocine HCl in mice is 3570 mg/kg.

Treatment: Oxygen, intravenous fluids, vasopressors, and other supportive measures should be employed as indicated. Assisted or controlled ventilation should also be considered. For respiratory depression due to overdosage or unusual sensitivity to Acetaminophen/Pentazocine HCl, parenteral naloxone is a specific and effective antagonist.

The toxic effects of Acetaminophen may be prevented or minimized by antidotal therapy with N-acetylcysteine. In order to obtain the best possible results, N-acetylcysteine should be administered within approximately 16 hours of ingestion of the overdose.

For complete guidelines for the approved use of acetylcysteine in the treatment of Acetaminophen overdose, see the product information on acetylcysteine.

Vigorous supportive therapy is required in severe intoxication. Procedures to limit the continuing absorption of the drug must be readily performed since the hepatic injury is dose dependent and occurs early in the course of intoxication. Induction of vomiting or gastric lavage, followed by oral administration of activated charcoal should be done in all cases.

If hemodialysis can be initiated within the first 12 hours, it is advocated for patients with a plasma Acetaminophen concentration exceeding 120 µg/mL at 4 hours after ingestion of the drug.

DOSAGE AND ADMINISTRATION

Adult: The usual adult dose is 1 tablet every 4 hours as needed for pain relief, up to a maximum of 6 tablets per day. The usual duration of therapy is dependent upon the condition being treated but in any case should be reviewed regularly by the physician. The effect of meals on the rate and extent of bioavailability of both Pentazocine and Acetaminophen has not been documented.

HOW SUPPLIED
TABLETS (C-IV): 650 MG-25 MG

BRAND/MANUFACTURER	NDC	SIZE	AWP
○ BRAND			
▶ TALACEN: Sanofi Winthrop	00024-1937-04	100s	$69.14
	00024-1937-14	250s ud	$190.45

Acetaminophen and Propoxyphene Hydrochloride

DESCRIPTION
Acetaminophen/Propoxyphene Hydrochloride tablets contain 65 mg Propoxyphene Hydrochloride and 650 mg Acetaminophen. Propoxyphene Hydrochloride is an odorless white crystalline powder with a bitter taste. It is freely soluble in water. Chemically, it is [S-(R*,S*)]-α[2-(dimethylamino)-1-methylethyl]-α-phenylbenzeneethanol, propanoate (ester), hydrochloride.

Acetaminophen is a white, crystalline powder, possessing a slightly bitter taste. It is soluble in boiling water and freely soluble in alcohol. Chemically, it is N-Acetyl-p-aminophenol.

CLINICAL PHARMACOLOGY
Propoxyphene is a centrally acting narcotic analgesic agent. Equimolar doses of Propoxyphene Hydrochloride provide similar plasma concentrations. Following administration of 65, 130, or 195 mg of Propoxyphene Hydrochloride, the bioavailability of Propoxyphene is equivalent to that of 100, 200, or 300 mg respectively of Propoxyphene napsylate. Peak plasma concentrations of Propoxyphene are reached in 2 to 2 ½ hours. After a 65 mg oral dose of Propoxyphene Hydrochloride, peak plasma levels of 0.05 to 0.1 mcg/mL are achieved.

Repeated doses of Propoxyphene at 6-hour intervals lead to increasing plasma concentrations, with a plateau after the ninth dose at 48 hours.

Propoxyphene is metabolized in the liver to yield norpropoxyphene. Propoxyphene has a half-life of 6 to 12 hours, whereas that of norpropoxyphene is 30 to 36 hours.

Norpropoxyphene has substantially less central nervous system depressant effect than Propoxyphene, but a greater local anesthetic effect, which is similar to that of amitriptyline antiarrhythmic agents, such as lidocaine and quinidine.

In animal studies in which Propoxyphene and norpropoxyphene were continuously infused in large amounts, intracardiac conduction time (P-R and QRS intervals) was prolonged. Any intracardiac conduction delay attributable to high concentrations of norpropoxyphene may be of relatively long duration.

ACTIONS
Propoxyphene is a mild narcotic analgesic structurally related to methadone. The potency of Propoxyphene Hydrochloride is from two-thirds to equal that of codeine.

Propoxyphene Hydrochloride and Acetaminophen provide the analgesic activity of Propoxyphene napsylate and the antipyretic-analgesic activity of Acetaminophen.

The combination of Propoxyphene and Acetaminophen produces greater analgesia than that produced by either Propoxyphene or Acetaminophen alone.

INDICATIONS
Acetaminophen/Propoxyphene Hydrochloride is indicated for the relief of mild-to-moderate pain, either when pain is present alone or when it is accompanied by fever.

CONTRAINDICATIONS
Hypersensitivity to Propoxyphene or to Acetaminophen.

WARNINGS

DO NOT PRESCRIBE PROPOXYPHENE FOR PATIENTS WHO ARE SUICIDAL OR ADDICTION-PRONE.

PRESCRIBE PROPOXYPHENE WITH CAUTION FOR PATIENTS TAKING TRANQUILIZERS OR ANTIDEPRESSANT DRUGS AND PATIENTS WHO USE ALCOHOL IN EXCESS.

TELL YOUR PATIENTS NOT TO EXCEED THE RECOMMENDED DOSE AND TO LIMIT THEIR INTAKE OF ALCOHOL.

PROPOXYPHENE PRODUCTS IN EXCESSIVE DOSES, EITHER ALONE OR IN COMBINATION WITH OTHER CNS DEPRESSANTS, INCLUDING ALCOHOL, ARE A MAJOR CAUSE OF DRUG-RELATED DEATHS. FATALITIES WITHIN THE FIRST HOUR OF OVERDOSAGE ARE NOT UNCOMMON. IN A SURVEY OF DEATHS DUE TO OVERDOSAGE CONDUCTED IN 1975, IN APPROXIMATELY 20% OF THE FATAL CASES, DEATH OCCURRED WITHIN THE FIRST HOUR (5% OCCURRED WITHIN 15 MINUTES). PROPOXYPHENE SHOULD NOT BE TAKEN IN DOSES HIGHER THAN THOSE RECOMMENDED BY THE PHYSICIAN. THE JUDICIOUS PRESCRIBING OF PROPOXYPHENE IS ESSENTIAL TO THE SAFE USE OF THIS DRUG. WITH PATIENTS WHO ARE DEPRESSED OR SUICIDAL, CONSIDERATION SHOULD BE GIVEN TO THE USE OF NONNARCOTIC ANALGESICS. PATIENTS SHOULD BE CAUTIONED ABOUT THE CONCOMITANT USE OF PROPOXYPHENE PRODUCTS AND ALCOHOL BECAUSE OF POTENTIALLY SERIOUS CNS-ADDITIVE EFFECTS OF THESE AGENTS. BECAUSE OF ITS ADDED DEPRESSANT EFFECTS, PROPOXYPHENE SHOULD BE PRESCRIBED WITH CAUTION FOR THOSE PATIENTS WHOSE MEDICAL CONDITION REQUIRES THE CONCOMITANT ADMINISTRATION OF SEDATIVES, TRANQUILIZERS, MUSCLE RELAXANTS, ANTIDEPRESSANTS, OR OTHER CNS-DEPRESSANT DRUGS. PATIENTS SHOULD BE ADVISED OF THE ADDITIVE DEPRESSANT EFFECTS OF THESE COMBINATIONS.

MANY OF THE PROPOXYPHENE-RELATED DEATHS HAVE OCCURRED IN PATIENTS WITH PREVIOUS HISTORIES OF EMOTIONAL DISTURBANCES OR SUICIDAL IDEATION OR ATTEMPTS AS WELL AS HISTORIES OF MISUSE OF TRANQUILIZERS, ALCOHOL, AND OTHER CNS-ACTIVE DRUGS. SOME DEATHS HAVE OCCURRED AS A CONSEQUENCE OF THE ACCIDENTAL INGESTION OF EXCESSIVE QUANTITIES OF

PROPOXYPHENE ALONE OR IN COMBINATION WITH OTHER DRUGS. PATIENTS TAKING PROPOXYPHENE SHOULD BE WARNED NOT TO EXCEED THE DOSAGE RECOMMENDED BY THE PHYSICIAN.

DRUG DEPENDENCE
Propoxyphene, when taken in higher-than-recommended doses over long periods of time, can produce drug dependence characterized by psychic dependence and, less frequently, physical dependence and tolerance. Propoxyphene will only partially suppress the withdrawal syndrome in individuals physically dependent on morphine or other narcotics. The abuse liability of Propoxyphene is qualitatively similar to that of codeine although quantitatively less, and Propoxyphene should be prescribed with the same degree of caution appropriate to the use of codeine.

USAGE IN AMBULATORY PATIENTS
Propoxyphene may impair the mental and/or physical abilities required for the performance of potentially hazardous tasks, such as driving a car or operating machinery. The patient should be cautioned accordingly.

PRECAUTIONS
GENERAL
Propoxyphene should be administered with caution to patients with hepatic or renal impairment since higher serum concentrations or delayed elimination may occur.

DRUG INTERACTIONS
The CNS-depressant effect of Propoxyphene is additive with that of other CNS depressants, including alcohol.

As is the case with many medicinal agents, Propoxyphene may slow the metabolism of a concomitantly administered drug. Should this occur, the higher serum concentrations of that drug may result in increased pharmacologic or adverse effects of that drug. Such occurrences have been reported when Propoxyphene was administered to patients on antidepressants, anticonvulsants, or warfarin-like drugs.

USAGE IN PREGNANCY
Safe use in pregnancy has not been established relative to possible adverse effects on fetal development. Instances of withdrawal symptoms in the neonate have been reported following usage during pregnancy. Therefore, Propoxyphene should not be used in pregnant women unless, in the judgment of the physician, the potential benefits outweigh the possible hazards.

USAGE IN NURSING MOTHERS
Low levels of Propoxyphene have been detected in human milk. In postpartum studies involving nursing mothers who were given Propoxyphene, no adverse effects were noted in infants receiving mother's milk.

USAGE IN CHILDREN
Propoxyphene is not recommended for use in children, because documented clinical experience has been insufficient to establish safety and a suitable dosage regimen in the pediatric age group.

A Patient Information Sheet is available for this product. See text following *"Dosage and Administration"* section below.

ADVERSE REACTIONS
In a survey conducted in hospitalized patients, less than 1% of patients taking Propoxyphene Hydrochloride at recommended doses experienced side effects. The most frequently reported have been dizziness, sedation, nausea, and vomiting. Some of these adverse reactions may be alleviated if the patient lies down.

Other adverse reactions include constipation, abdominal pain, skin rashes, light-headedness, headache, weakness, euphoria, dysphoria, and minor visual disturbances.

Liver dysfunction has been reported in association with both active components of Propoxyphene and Acetaminophen tablets.

Propoxyphene therapy has been associated with abnormal liver-function tests and, more rarely, with instances of reversible jaundice.

Hepatic necrosis may result from acute overdoses of Acetaminophen (see *"Management of Overdosage"*). In chronic ethanol abusers, this has been reported rarely with short-term use of Acetaminophen doses of 2.5 to 10 g/day. Fatalities have occurred.

MANAGEMENT OF OVERDOSAGE
In all cases of suspected overdosage, call your regional poison control center to obtain the most up-to-date information about the treatment of overdosage. This recommendation is made because, in general, information regarding the treatment of overdosage may change more rapidly than do package inserts.

Initial consideration should be given to the management of the CNS effects of Propoxyphene overdosage. Resuscitative measures should be initiated promptly.

SYMPTOMS OF PROPOXYPHENE OVERDOSAGE
The manifestations of acute overdosage with Propoxyphene are those of narcotic overdosage. The patient is usually somnolent, but may be stuporous or comatose and convulsing. Respiratory depression is characteristic. The ventilatory rate and/or tidal volume is decreased, which results in cyanosis and hypoxia. Pupils, initially pinpoint, may become dilated as hypoxia increases. Cheyne-Stokes respiration and apnea may occur. Blood pressure and heart rate are usually normal initially, but blood pressure falls and cardiac performance deteriorates, which ultimately results in pulmonary edema and circulatory collapse unless the respiratory depression is corrected and adequate ventilation is restored promptly. Cardiac arrhythmias and conduction delay may be present. A combined respiratory-metabolic acidosis occurs, owing to retained CO_2 (hypercapnea) and to lactic acid formed during anaerobic glycolysis. Acidosis may be severe if large amounts of salicylates have also been ingested. Death may occur.

TREATMENT OF PROPOXYPHENE OVERDOSAGE
Attention should be directed first to establishing a patent airway and to restoring ventilation. Mechanically assisted ventilation, with or without oxygen, may be required, and positive-pressure respiration may be desirable if pulmonary edema is present.

The narcotic antagonist naloxone hydrochloride will markedly reduce the degree of respiratory depression, and 0.4 to 2 mg should be administered promptly, preferably intravenously. If the desired degree of counteraction with improvement in respiratory function is not obtained, naloxone should be repeated at 2- to 3-minute intervals. The duration of action of the antagonist may be brief. If no response is observed after 10 mg of naloxone have been administered, the diagnosis of Propoxyphene toxicity should be questioned. Naloxone hydrochloride may also be administered by continuous intravenous infusion.

TREATMENT OF PROPOXYPHENE OVERDOSAGE IN CHILDREN
The usual initial dose of naloxone in children is 0.01 mg/kg body weight given intravenously. If this dose does not result in the desired degree of clinical improvement, a subsequent increased dose of 0.1 mg/kg body weight may be administered. If an IV route of administration is not available, naloxone may be administered IM or subcutaneously in divided doses. If necessary, naloxone can be diluted with sterile water for injection.

Blood gases, pH, and electrolytes should be monitored in order that acidosis and any electrolyte disturbance present may be corrected promptly. Acidosis, hypoxia, and generalized CNS depression predispose to the development of cardiac arrhythmias. Ventricular fibrillation or cardiac arrest may occur and necessitate the full complement of cardiopulmonary resuscitation (CPR) measures. Respiratory acidosis rapidly subsides as ventilation is restored and hypercapnea eliminated, but lactic acidosis may require intravenous bicarbonate for prompt correction.

Electrocardiographic monitoring is essential. Prompt correction of hypoxia, acidosis, and electrolyte disturbance (when present) will help prevent these cardiac complications and will increase the effectiveness of agents administered to restore normal cardiac function.

In addition to the use of a narcotic antagonist, the patient may require careful titration with an anticonvulsant to control convulsions. Analeptic drugs (for example, caffeine or amphetamine) should not be used because of their tendency to precipitate convulsions.

General supportive measures, in addition to oxygen, include, when necessary, intravenous fluids, vasopressor-inotropic compounds, and, when infection is likely, anti-infective agents. Gastric lavage may be useful, and activated charcoal can adsorb a significant amount of ingested Propoxyphene. Dialysis is of little value in poisoning due to Propoxyphene. Efforts should be made to determine whether other agents, such as alcohol, barbiturates, tranquilizers, or other CNS depressants, were also ingested, since these increase CNS depression as well as cause specific toxic effects.

SYMPTOMS OF ACETAMINOPHEN OVERDOSAGE
Shortly after oral ingestion of an overdosage of Acetaminophen and for the next 24 hours, anorexia, nausea, vomiting, and abdominal pain have been noted. The patient may then present no symptoms, but evidence of liver dysfunction may be apparent during the next 24 to 48 hours, with elevated serum transaminase and lactic dehydrogenase levels, an increase in serum bilirubin concentrations, and a prolonged prothrombin time. Death from hepatic failure may result 3 to 7 days after overdosage.

Acute renal failure may accompany the hepatic dysfunction and has been noted in patients who do not exhibit signs of fulminant hepatic failure. Typically, renal impairment is more apparent 6 to 9 days after ingestion of the overdose.

TREATMENT OF ACETAMINOPHEN OVERDOSAGE
Acetaminophen in massive overdosage may cause hepatic toxicity in some patients. In all cases of suspected overdose, you may wish to call your regional poison center for assistance in diagnosis and for directions in the use of N-acetylcysteine as an antidote.

In adults, hepatic toxicity has rarely been reported with acute overdoses of less than 10 g and fatalities with less than 15 g. Importantly, young children seem to be more resistant than adults to the hepatotoxic effect of an Acetaminophen overdose. Despite this, the measures outlined below should be initiated in any adult or child suspected of having ingested an Acetaminophen overdose. Clinical and laboratory evidence of hepatic toxicity may not be apparent until 48 to 72 hours postingestion. Early symptoms following a potentially hepatotoxic overdose may include: nausea, vomiting, diaphoresis, and general malaise.

The stomach should be emptied promptly by lavage or by induction of emesis with syrup of ipecac. Patients' estimates of the quantity of a drug ingested are notoriously unreliable. Therefore, if an Acetaminophen overdose is suspected, a serum Acetaminophen assay should be obtained as early as possible, but no sooner than four hours following ingestion. Liver-function studies should be obtained initially and repeated at 24-hour intervals.

The antidote, N-acetylcysteine, should be administered as early as possible, preferably within 16 hours of the overdose ingestion for optimal results, but in any case, within 24 hours. Following recovery, there are no residual, structural or functional hepatic abnormalities.

ANIMAL TOXICOLOGY

The acute lethal doses of the Hydrochloride and napsylate salts of Propoxyphene were determined in 4 species. The results shown in Figure 1 indicate that on a molar basis, the napsylate salt is less toxic than the Hydrochloride. This may be due to the relative insolubility and retarded absorption of Propoxyphene napsylate.

Figure 1
ACUTE ORAL TOXICITY OF PROPOXYPHENE

Species	LD50 (mg/kg) = SE LD50 (mMole/kg) Propoxyphene Hydrochloride	Propoxyphene Napsylate
Mouse	282 ± 39	915 ± 163
	0.75	1.62
Rat	230 ± 44	647 ± 95
	0.61	1.14
Rabbit	ca. 82	≥183
	0.22	>0.32
Dog	ca 100	≥183
	0.27	>0.32

Some indication of the relative insolubility and retarded absorption of Propoxyphene napsylate was obtained by measuring plasma Propoxyphene levels in 2 groups of 4 dogs following oral administration of equimolar doses of the 2 salts. Although none of the animals in this experiment died, 3 of the 4 dogs given Propoxyphene Hydrochloride exhibited convulsive seizures during the time interval corresponding to the peak plasma levels. The 4 animals receiving the napsylate salt were ataxic but not acutely ill.

DOSAGE AND ADMINISTRATION

The product is given orally. The usual dose is 65 mg Propoxyphene Hydrochloride and 650 mg Acetaminophen every 4 hours as needed for pain. The maximum recommended dose of Propoxyphene Hydrochloride is 390 mg per day.

Consideration should be given to a reduced total daily dosage in patients with hepatic or renal impairment.

Keep tightly closed.

Protect from light.

Store at controlled room temperature, 20°—25°C (68°—77°F)

Dispense in tight, light-resistant container as defined in the USP.

HOW SUPPLIED
TABLETS (C-IV): 650 MG-65 MG

AVERAGE UNIT PRICE (AVAILABLE SIZES)

BRAND	$0.42	GENERIC A-RATED AVERAGE PRICE (GAAP)		
GENERIC	$0.23	100s		$25.60
HCFA FUL (100s ea)	$0.15	500s		$98.47

BRAND/MANUFACTURER	NDC	SIZE	AWP
◆ **BRAND**			
➤ WYGESIC: Wyeth-Ayerst	00008-0085-01	100s	$42.44
	00008-0085-04	100s ud	$42.44
	00008-0085-02	500s	$198.19
◆ **GENERICS**			
Schein	00364-0396-01	100s	$16.50
Parmed	00349-2187-01	100s	$18.99
Qualitest	00603-5463-21	100s	$19.40
Goldline	00182-0800-01	100s	$20.40
➤ Geneva	00781-1378-01	100s	$21.50
➤ Mylan	00378-0130-01	100s	$21.95
E-LOR: Forest Pharm	00785-1117-01	100s	$45.59
Geneva	00781-1378-13	100s ud	$31.30
UDL	51079-0741-20	100s ud	$34.78
Schein	00364-0396-05	500s	$77.75
Qualitest	00603-5463-28	500s	$94.60
Goldline	00182-0800-05	500s	$95.25
➤ Geneva	00781-1378-05	500s	$96.75
➤ Mylan	00378-0130-05	500s	$97.95
Moore,H.L.	00839-1566-12	500s	$98.62
Parmed	00349-2187-05	500s	$128.35

Acetaminophen and Propoxyphene Napsylate

DESCRIPTION

Propoxyphene Napsylate, USP is an odorless, white crystalline powder with a bitter taste. It is very slightly soluble in water and soluble in methanol, ethanol, chloroform, and acetone. Chemically, it is (αS,1R)-α-[2-(Di-methylamino)-1-me-thylethyl]-α-phenylphenethyl propionate compound with 2-naphthalenesulfonic acid (1:1) monohydrate. Its molecular weight is 565.72.

Each tablet of Acetaminophen and Propoxyphene Napsylate contains:

Propoxyphene Napsylate	50 mg or 100 mg
Acetaminophen	325 mg or 650 mg

Propoxyphene Napsylate differs from propoxyphene hydrochloride in that it allows more stable liquid dosage forms and tablet formulations. Because of differences in molecular weight, a dose of 100 mg (176.8 µmol) of propoxyphene napsylate is required to supply an amount of Propoxyphene equivalent to that present in 65 mg (172.9 µmol) of propoxyphene hydrochloride.

CLINICAL PHARMACOLOGY

Propoxyphene is a centrally acting narcotic analgesic agent. Equimolar doses of propoxyphene hydrochloride or napsylate provide similar plasma concentrations. Following administration of 65, 130, or 195 mg of propoxyphene hydrochloride, the bioavailability of Propoxyphene is equivalent to that of 100, 200, or 300 mg respectively of propoxyphene napsylate. Peak plasma concentrations of propoxyphene are reached in 2 to 2 ½ hours. After a 100-mg oral dose of Propoxyphene Napsylate, peak plasma levels of 0.05 to 0.1 µg/mL are achieved. As shown in Figure 1, the Napsylate salt tends to be absorbed more slowly than the hydrochloride. At or near therapeutic doses, this absorption difference is small when compared with that among subjects and among doses. (See figure 1).

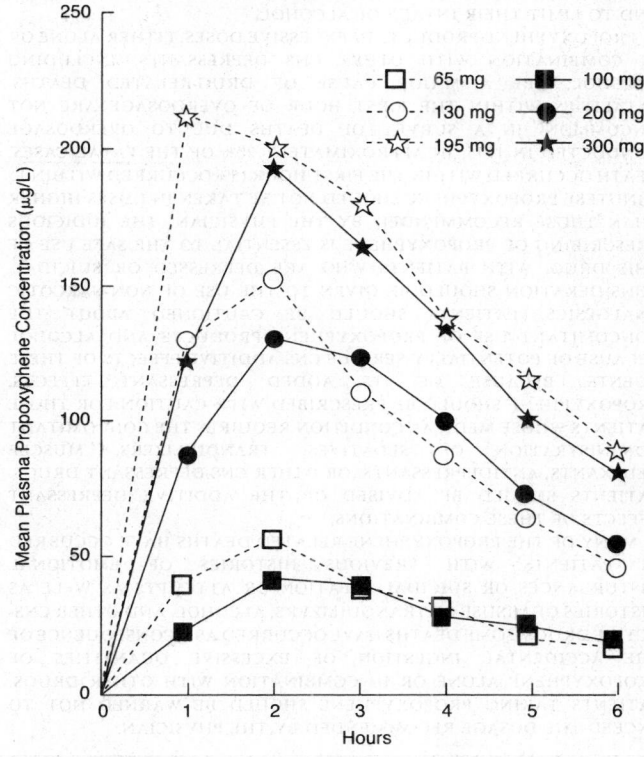

Figure 1. Mean plasma concentrations of propoxyphene in 8 human subjects following oral administration of 65 and 130 mg of the hydrochloride salt and 100 and 200 mg of the Napsylate salt and in 7 given 195 mg of the hydrochloride and 300 mg of the Napsylate salt.

Because of this several hundredfold difference in solubility, the absorption rate of very large doses of the Napsylate salt is significantly lower than that of equimolar doses of the hydrochloride.

Repeated doses of Propoxyphene at 6-hour intervals lead to increasing plasma concentrations, with a plateau after the ninth dose at 48 hours.

Propoxyphene is metabolized in the liver to yield norpropoxyphene. Propoxyphene has a half-life of 6 to 12 hours, whereas that of norpropoxyphene is 30 to 36 hours.

Norpropoxyphene has substantially less central-nervous-system-depressant effect than propoxyphene but a greater local anesthetic effect, which is similar to that of amitriptyline and antiarrhythmic agents, such as lidocaine and quinidine.

In animal studies in which propoxyphene and norpropoxyphene were continuously infused in large amounts, intracardiac conduction time (PR and QRS intervals) was prolonged. Any intracardiac conduction delay attributable to high concentrations of norpropoxyphene may be of relatively long duration.

ACTIONS

Propoxyphene is a mild narcotic analgesic structurally related to methadone. The potency of Propoxyphene Napsylate is from two-thirds to equal that of codeine.

Acetaminophen/Propoxyphene Napsylate provide the analgesic activity of Propoxyphene Napsylate and the antipyretic-analgesic activity of Acetaminophen.

The combination of Propoxyphene and Acetaminophen produces greater analgesia than that produced by either Propoxyphene or Acetaminophen administered alone.

INDICATIONS

Acetaminophen/Propoxyphene Napsylate tablets, USP are indicated for the relief of mild to moderate pain, either when pain is present alone or when it is accompanied by fever.

CONTRAINDICATIONS

Hypersensitivity to Propoxyphene or Acetaminophen.

WARNINGS

■ DO NOT PRESCRIBE PROPOXYPHENE FOR PATIENTS WHO ARE SUICIDAL OR ADDICTION-PRONE.

■ PRESCRIBE PROPOXYPHENE WITH CAUTION FOR PATIENTS TAKING TRANQUILIZERS OR ANTIDEPRESSANT DRUGS AND PATIENTS WHO USE ALCOHOL IN EXCESS.

■ TELL YOUR PATIENTS NOT TO EXCEED THE RECOMMENDED DOSE AND TO LIMIT THEIR INTAKE OF ALCOHOL.

PROPOXYPHENE PRODUCTS IN EXCESSIVE DOSES, EITHER ALONE OR IN COMBINATION WITH OTHER CNS DEPRESSANTS, INCLUDING ALCOHOL, ARE A MAJOR CAUSE OF DRUG-RELATED DEATHS. FATALITIES WITHIN THE FIRST HOUR OF OVERDOSAGE ARE NOT UNCOMMON. IN A SURVEY OF DEATHS DUE TO OVERDOSE CONDUCTED IN 1975, IN APPROXIMATELY 20% OF THE FATAL CASES, DEATH OCCURRED WITHIN THE FIRST HOUR (5% OCCURRED WITHIN 15 MINUTES). PROPOXYPHENE SHOULD NOT BE TAKEN IN DOSES HIGHER THAN THOSE RECOMMENDED BY THE PHYSICIAN. THE JUDICIOUS PRESCRIBING OF PROPOXYPHENE IS ESSENTIAL TO THE SAFE USE OF THIS DRUG. WITH PATIENTS WHO ARE DEPRESSED OR SUICIDAL, CONSIDERATION SHOULD BE GIVEN TO THE USE OF NON-NARCOTIC ANALGESICS. PATIENTS SHOULD BE CAUTIONED ABOUT THE CONCOMITANT USE OF PROPOXYPHENE PRODUCTS AND ALCOHOL BECAUSE OF POTENTIALLY SERIOUS CNS-ADDITIVE EFFECTS OF THESE AGENTS. BECAUSE OF ITS ADDED DEPRESSANT EFFECTS, PROPOXYPHENE SHOULD BE PRESCRIBED WITH CAUTION FOR THOSE PATIENTS WHOSE MEDICAL CONDITION REQUIRES THE CONCOMITANT ADMINISTRATION OF SEDATIVES, TRANQUILIZERS, MUSCLE RELAXANTS, ANTIDEPRESSANTS, OR OTHER CNS-DEPRESSANT DRUGS. PATIENTS SHOULD BE ADVISED OF THE ADDITIVE DEPRESSANT EFFECTS OF THESE COMBINATIONS.

MANY OF THE PROPOXYPHENE-RELATED DEATHS HAVE OCCURRED IN PATIENTS WITH PREVIOUS HISTORIES OF EMOTIONAL DISTURBANCES OR SUICIDAL IDEATION OR ATTEMPTS AS WELL AS HISTORIES OF MISUSE OF TRANQUILIZERS, ALCOHOL, AND OTHER CNS-ACTIVE DRUGS. SOME DEATHS HAVE OCCURRED AS A CONSEQUENCE OF THE ACCIDENTAL INGESTION OF EXCESSIVE QUANTITIES OF PROPOXYPHENE ALONE OR IN COMBINATION WITH OTHER DRUGS. PATIENTS TAKING PROPOXYPHENE SHOULD BE WARNED NOT TO EXCEED THE DOSAGE RECOMMENDED BY THE PHYSICIAN.

Drug Dependence: Propoxyphene, when taken in higher-than-recommended doses over long periods of time, can produce drug dependence characterized by psychic dependence and, less frequently, physical dependence and tolerance. Propoxyphene will only partially suppress the withdrawal syndrome in individuals physically dependent on morphine or other narcotics. The abuse liability of Propoxyphene is qualitatively similar to that of codeine although quantitatively less, and Propoxyphene should be prescribed with the same degree of caution appropriate to the use of codeine.

Usage in Ambulatory Patients: Propoxyphene may impair the mental and/or physical abilities required for the performance of potentially hazardous tasks, such as driving a car or operating machinery. The patient should be cautioned accordingly.

PRECAUTIONS

General: Propoxyphene should be administered with caution to patients with hepatic or renal impairment, since higher serum concentrations or delayed elimination may occur.

Drug Interactions: The CNS-depressant effect of Propoxyphene is additive with that of other CNS depressants, including alcohol.

As is the case with many medicinal agents, Propoxyphene may slow the metabolism of a concomitantly administered drug. Should this occur, the higher serum concentrations of that drug may result in increased pharmacologic or adverse effects of that drug. Such occurrences have been reported when Propoxyphene was administered to patients on antidepressants, anticonvulsants, or warfarin-like drugs. Severe neurologic signs, including coma, have occurred with concurrent use of carbamazepine.

Usage in Pregnancy: Safe use in pregnancy has not been established relative to possible adverse effects on fetal development. Instances of withdrawal symptoms in the neonate have been reported following usage during pregnancy. Therefore, Propoxyphene should not be used in pregnant women unless, in the judgment of the physician, the potential benefits outweigh the possible hazards.

Usage in Nursing Mothers: Low levels of Propoxyphene have been detected in human milk. In postpartum studies involving nursing mothers who were given Propoxyphene, no adverse effects were noted in infants receiving mother's milk.

Usage in Children: Propoxyphene is not recommended for use in children, because documented clinical experience has been insufficient to establish safety and a suitable dosage regimen in the pediatric age group.

Usage in the Elderly: The rate of Propoxyphene metabolism may be reduced in some patients. Increased dosing interval should be considered.

ADVERSE REACTIONS

In a survey conducted in hospitalized patients, less than 1% of patients taking Propoxyphene Hydrochloride at recommended doses experienced side effects. The most frequently reported were dizziness, sedation, nausea, and vomiting. Some of these adverse reactions may be alleviated if the patient lies down.

Other adverse reactions include constipation, abdominal pain, skin rashes, light-headedness, headache, weakness, euphoria, dysphoria, hallucinations, and minor visual disturbances.

Liver dysfunction has been reported in association with both active components of Acetaminophen/Propoxyphene Napsylate tablets, USP.

Propoxyphene therapy has been associated with abnormal liver function tests and, more rarely, with instances of reversible jaundice (including cholestatic jaundice). Hepatic necrosis may result from acute overdose of acetaminophen. (see "Management of Overdosage"). In chronic ethanol abusers, this has been reported rarely with short-term use of acetaminophen doses of 2.5 to 10 g/day. Fatalities have occurred.

Renal papillary necrosis may result from chronic acetaminophen use, particularly when the dosage is greater than recommended and when combined with aspirin.

Subacute painful myopathy has occurred following chronic Propoxyphene overdosage.

MANAGEMENT OF OVERDOSAGE

In all cases of suspected overdosage, call your regional poison control center to obtain the most up-to-date information about the treatment of overdosage. This recommendation is made because, in general, information regarding the treatment of overdosage may change more rapidly than do package inserts.

Initial consideration should be given to the management of the CNS effects of Propoxyphene overdosage. Resuscitative measures should be initiated promptly.

Symptoms of Propoxyphene Overdosage: The manifestations of acute overdosage with Propoxyphene are those of narcotic overdosage. The patient is usually somnolent but may be stuporous or comatose and convulsing. Respiratory depression is characteristic. The ventilatory rate and/or tidal volume is decreased, which results in cyanosis and hypoxia. Pupils, initially pinpoint, may become dilated as hypoxia increases. Cheyne-Stokes respiration and apnea may occur. Blood pressure and heart rate are usually normal initially, but blood pressure falls and cardiac performance deteriorates, which ultimately results in pulmonary edema and circulatory collapse, unless the respiratory depression is corrected and adequate ventilation is restored promptly. Cardiac arrhythmias and conduction delay may be present. A combined respiratory-metabolic acidosis occurs owing to retained CO_2 (hypercapnia) and to lactic acid formed during anaerobic glycolysis. Acidosis may be severe if large amounts of salicylates have also been ingested. Death may occur.

Treatment of Propoxyphene Overdosage: Attention should be directed first to establishing a patent airway and to restoring ventilation. Mechanically assisted ventilation, with or without oxygen, may be required, and positive pressure respiration may be desirable if pulmonary edema is present. The narcotic antagonist naloxone will markedly reduce the degree of respiratory depression, and 0.4 to 2 mg should be administered promptly, preferably intravenously. If the desired degree of counteraction with improvement in respiratory functions is not obtained, naloxone should be repeated at 2- to 3-minute intervals. The duration of action of the antagonist may be brief. If no response is observed after 10 mg of naloxone have been administered, the diagnosis of propoxyphene toxicity should be questioned. Naloxone may also be administered by continuous intravenous infusion.

Treatment of Propoxyphene Overdosage in Children: The usual initial dose of naloxone in children is 0.01 mg/kg body weight given intravenously. If this dose does not result in the desired degree of clinical improvement, a subsequent increased dose of 0.1 mg/kg body weight may be administered. If an IV route of administration is not available, naloxone may be administered IM or subcutaneously in divided doses. If necessary, naloxone can be diluted with Sterile Water for Injection.

Blood gases, pH, and electrolytes should be monitored in order that acidosis and any electrolyte disturbance present may be corrected promptly. Acidosis, hypoxia, and generalized CNS depression predispose to the development of cardiac arrhythmias. Ventricular fibrillation or cardiac arrest may occur and necessitate the full complement of cardiopulmonary resuscitation (CPR) measures. Respiratory acidosis rapidly subsides as ventilation is restored and hypercapnia eliminated, but lactic acidosis may require intravenous bicarbonate for prompt correction.

Electrocardiographic monitoring is essential. Prompt correction of hypoxia, acidosis, and electrolyte disturbance (when present) will help prevent these cardiac complications and will increase the effectiveness of agents administered to restore normal cardiac function.

In addition to the use of a narcotic antagonist, the patient may require careful titration with an anticonvulsant to control convulsions. Analeptic drugs (for example, caffeine or amphetamine) should not be used because of their tendency to precipitate convulsions.

General supportive measures, in addition to oxygen, include, when necessary, intravenous fluids, vasopressor-inotropic compounds, and, when infection is likely, anti-infective agents. Gastric lavage may be useful, and activated charcoal can adsorb a significant amount of ingested Propoxyphene. Dialysis is of little value in poisoning due to Propoxyphene. Efforts should be made to determine whether other agents, such as alcohol, barbiturates, tranquilizers, or other CNS depressants, were also ingested, since these increase CNS depression as well as cause specific toxic effects.

Symptoms of Acetaminophen Overdosage: Shortly after oral ingestion of an overdose of Acetaminophen and for the next 24 hours, anorexia, nausea, vomiting, diaphoresis, general malaise, and abdominal pain have been noted. The patient may then present no symptoms, but evidence of liver dysfunction may become apparent up to 72 hours after ingestion, with elevated serum transaminase and lactic dehydrogenase levels, an increase in serum bilirubin concentrations, and a prolonged prothrombin time. Death from hepatic failure may result 3 to 7 days after overdosage.

Acute renal failure may accompany the hepatic dysfunction and has been noted in patients who do not exhibit signs of fulminant hepatic failure. Typically, renal impairment is more apparent 6 to 9 days after ingestion of the overdose.

Treatment of Acetaminophen Overdosage: Acetaminophen in massive overdosage may cause hepatic toxicity in some patients. *In all cases of suspected overdose, immediately call your regional poison center or the Rocky Mountain Poison Center's toll-free number* (800-525-6115) for assistance in diagnosis and for directions in the use of N-acetylcysteine as an antidote.

In adults, hepatic toxicity has rarely been reported with acute overdoses of less than 10 g and fatalities with less than 15 g. Importantly, young children seem to be more resistant than adults to the hepatotoxic effect of an acetaminophen overdose. Despite this, the measures outlined below should be initiated in any adult or child suspected of having ingested an acetaminophen overdose.

Because clinical and laboratory evidence of hepatic toxicity may not be apparent until 48 to 72 hours postingestion, liver function studies should be obtained initially and repeated at 24-hour intervals.

Consider emptying the stomach promptly by lavage or by induction of emesis with syrup of ipecac. Patients' estimates of the quantity of a drug ingested are notoriously unreliable. Therefore, if an acetaminophen overdose is suspected, a serum acetaminophen assay should be obtained as early as possible, but no sooner than 4 hours following ingestion. The antidote, N-acetylcysteine, should be administered as early as possible, and within 16 hours of the overdose ingestion for optimal results. Following recovery, there are no residual, structural, or functional hepatic abnormalities.

DOSAGE AND ADMINISTRATION

These products are given orally. The usual dosage of Acetaminophen/Propoxyphene Napsylate tablets, USP is 100 mg Propoxyphene Napsylate and 650 mg Acetaminophen every 4 hours as needed for pain.

The maximum recommended dose of Propoxyphene Napsylate is 600 mg/day.

Consideration should be given to a reduced total daily dosage in patients with hepatic or renal impairment.

Store at controlled room temperature, 59° to 86°F (15° to 30°C).

ANIMAL TOXICOLOGY

The acute lethal doses of the hydrochloride and Napsylate salts of Propoxyphene were determined in 4 species. The results shown in Figure 2 indicate that on a molar basis, the Napsylate salt is less toxic than the hydrochloride. This may be due to the relative insolubility and retarded absorption of Propoxyphene Napsylate.

Figure 2
ACUTE ORAL TOXICITY OF PROPOXYPHENE

Species	LD_{50} (mg/kg) $\pm$ SE LD_{50} (mmole/kg) Propoxyphene Hydrochloride	Propoxyphene Napsylate
Mouse	282 ± 39 0.75	915 ± 163 1.62
Rat	230 ± 44 0.61	647 ± 95 1.14
Rabbit	*ca.* 82 0.22	$\geq$183 $>$0.32
Dog	*ca.* 100 0.27	$\geq$183 $>$0.32

Some indication of the relative insolubility and retarded absorption of Propoxyphene Napsylate was obtained by measuring plasma propoxyphene levels in 2

groups of 4 dogs following oral administration of equimolar doses of the 2 salts. As shown in Figure 3, the peak plasma concentration observed with propoxyphene hydrochloride was much higher than that obtained after administration of the Napsylate salt.

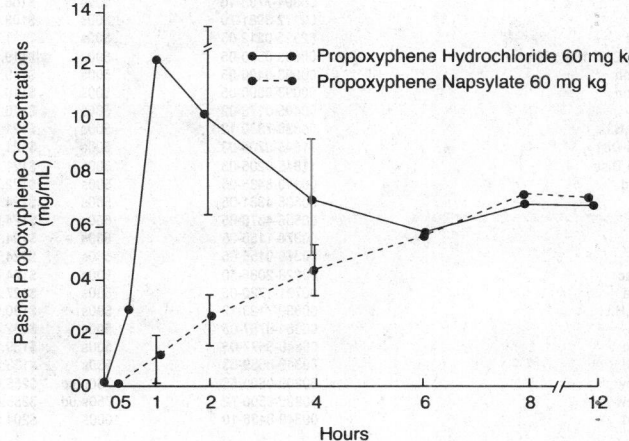

Figure 3. Plasma propoxyphene concentrations in dogs following large doses of the hydrochloride and napsylate salts.

Although none of the animals in this experiment died, 3 of the 4 dogs given propoxyphene hydrochloride exhibited convulsive seizures during the time interval corresponding to the peak plasma levels. The 4 animals receiving the napsylate salt were mildly ataxic but not acutely ill.

HOW SUPPLIED
TABLETS (C-IV): 325 MG-50 MG

AVERAGE UNIT PRICE (AVAILABLE SIZES)	
BRAND	$0.28
GENERIC	$0.16

BRAND/MANUFACTURER	NDC	SIZE	AWP
◆ **BRAND**			
DARVOCET-N 50: Lilly	00002-0351-02	100s	$27.85
◆ **GENERICS**			
Parmed	00349-8814-01	100s	$17.88
Parmed	00349-8814-05	500s	$72.91

TABLETS (C-IV): 650 MG-100 MG

AVERAGE UNIT PRICE (AVAILABLE SIZES)		GENERIC A-RATED AVERAGE PRICE (GAAP)	
BRAND	$0.54	100s	$28.03
GENERIC	$0.27	500s	$118.22
HCFA FUL (100s ea)	$0.12	750s	$255.60

BRAND/MANUFACTURER	NDC	SIZE	AWP
◆ **BRAND**			
► DARVOCET-N 100: Lilly	00002-0363-02	100s	$52.53
	00002-0363-33	100s ud	$56.91
	00002-0363-03	500s	$249.52
	00002-0363-46	500s	$277.39
	00002-0363-43	500s ud	$268.31
◆ **GENERICS**			
Allscrips	54569-0015-05	12s	$3.03
Medirex	57480-0507-06	30s	$11.30
UDL	51079-0322-99	90s	$60.00
Goldline	00182-1266-01	100s	$16.50
► Goldline	00182-0317-01	100s	$22.50
Zenith	00172-3981-60	100s	$23.30
► PROPACET 100: Lemmon	00093-0590-01	100s	$23.95
Lemmon	00093-0890-01	100s	$23.95
Aligen	00405-0178-01	100s	$24.53
Schein	00364-0767-01	100s	$25.46
Rugby	00536-4361-01	100s	$25.50
► Rugby	00536-4370-01	100s	$25.50
► Mylan	00378-0155-01	100s	$26.25
► Geneva	00781-1720-01	100s	$26.79
Parmed	00349-8436-01	100s	$26.98
URL	00677-1034-01	100s	$27.11
Purepac	00228-2085-10	100s	$29.06
Moore,H.L.	00839-7330-06	100s	$31.66
► Goldline	00182-0317-89	100s ud	$15.00
► Geneva	00781-1720-13	100s ud	$33.00
Vangard	00615-0455-13	100s ud	$34.08
Vangard	00615-0455-47	100s ud	$34.08
UDL	51079-0322-20	100s ud	$36.49
UDL	51079-0322-21	100s ud	$36.49
Medirex	57480-0507-01	100s ud	$37.50
Auro	55829-0866-10	100s ud	$38.97
Goldline	00182-1266-05	500s	$75.00

BRAND/MANUFACTURER	NDC	SIZE	AWP
Qualitest	00603-5466-28	500s	$101.90
➤ Goldline	00182-0317-05	500s	$102.50
Major	00904-7702-40	500s	$108.30
➤ Major	00904-7703-40	500s	$108.30
Zenith	00172-3981-70	500s	$109.34
Martec	52555-0212-05	500s	$111.55
➤ PROPACET 100: Lemmon	00093-0590-05	500s	$119.75
Lemmon	00093-0490-05	500s	$119.75
Lemmon	00093-0890-05	500s	$119.75
Aligen	00405-0178-02	500s	$119.75
Moore,H.L.	00839-7330-12	500s	$121.49
Mason Dist	11845-0204-03	500s	$121.91
Mason Dist	11845-0205-03	500s	$121.91
Parmed	00349-8436-05	500s	$122.98
Rugby	00536-4361-05	500s	$124.50
➤ Rugby	00536-4370-05	500s	$124.50
Mylan	00378-1155-05	500s	$124.72
➤ Mylan	00378-0155-05	500s	$124.72
Purepac	00228-2085-50	500s	$124.86
○ Geneva	00781-1720-05	500s	$127.26
Moore,H.L.	00839-7123-12	500s	$130.95
Schein	00364-0767-05	500s	$132.43
Parmed	00349-8577-05	500s	$139.10
Parmed	00349-8889-53	550s	$133.27
Glasgow	60809-0500-55	750s ud	$255.60
Glasgow	60809-0500-72	750s ud	$255.60
Parmed	00349-8436-10	1000s	$204.98

Acetaminophen with Butalbital

DESCRIPTION

Each Acetaminophen/Butalbital tablet, for oral administration, contains Acetaminophen, USP 325 mg or 650 mg, Butalbital*, USP 50 mg *(WARNING - may be habit forming).

Each Acetaminophen/Butalbital capsule, for oral administration, contains Acetaminophen, USP 650 mg, Butalbital*, USP 50 mg *(WARNING—May be habit forming).

Acetaminophen, (4'-hydroxyacetanilide), a slightly bitter, white, odorless, crystalline powder, is a non-opiate, non-salicylate analgesic and antipyretic. Its molecular formula is $C_8H_9NO_2$ and molecular weight is 151.16.

Butalbital (5-allyl-5-isobutylbarbituric acid), a slightly bitter, white, odorless, crystalline powder, is a short to intermediate-acting barbiturate. Its molecular formula in $C_{11}H_{16}N_2O_3$ and molecular weight is 224.26.

CLINICAL PHARMACOLOGY

This combination drug product is intended as a treatment for tension headache.

It consists of a fixed combination of Acetaminophen and Butalbital. The role each component plays in the relief of the complex of symptoms known as tension headache is incompletely understood.

Pharmacokinetics: The behavior of the individual components is described below.

Acetaminophen: Acetaminophen is rapidly absorbed from the gastrointestinal tract and is distributed throughout most body tissues. The plasma half-life is 1.25 to 3 hours, but may be increased by liver damage and following overdosage. Elimination of Acetaminophen is principally by liver metabolism (conjugation) and subsequent renal excretion of metabolites. Approximately 85% of an oral dose appears in the urine within 24 hours of administration, most as the glucuronide conjugate, with small amounts of other conjugates and unchanged drug.

See "Overdosage" for toxicity information.

Butalbital: Butalbital is well absorbed from the gastrointestinal tract and is expected to distribute to most tissues in the body. Barbiturates in general may appear in breast milk and readily cross the placental barrier. They are bound to plasma and tissue proteins to a varying degree and binding increases directly as a function of lipid solubility.

Elimination of Butalbital is primarily via the kidney (59% to 88% of the dose) as unchanged drug or metabolites. The plasma half-life is about 35 hours. Urinary excretion products include parent drug (about 3.6% of the dose), 5-isobutyl-5-(2,3-dihydroxypropyl) barbituric acid (about 24% of the dose), 5-allyl-5(3-hydroxy-2-methyl-1-propyl) barbituric acid (about 4.8% of the dose), products with the barbituric acid ring hydrolyzed with excretion of urea (about 14% of the dose), as well as unidentified materials. Of the material excreted in the urine, 32% is conjugated.

See "Overdosage" for toxicity information.

INDICATIONS AND USAGE

Acetaminophen/Butalbital tablets and capsules are indicated for the relief of the symptom complex of tension (or muscle contraction) headache.

Evidence supporting the efficacy and safety of this combination product in the treatment of multiple recurrent headaches is unavailable. Caution in this regard is required because Butalbital is habit-forming and potentially abusable.

CONTRAINDICATIONS

This product is contraindicated under the following conditions:

- Hypersensitivity or intolerance to any component of this product.
- Patients with porphyria.

WARNINGS

Butalbital is habit-forming and potentially abusable. Consequently, the extended use of this product is not recommended.

PRECAUTIONS

General: Acetaminophen/Butalbital tablets and capsules should be prescribed with caution in certain special-risk patients, such as the elderly or debilitated, and those with severe impairment of renal or hepatic function, or acute abdominal conditions.

Information for Patients: This product may impair mental and/or physical abilities required for the performance of potentially hazardous tasks such as driving a car or operating machinery. Such tasks should be avoided while taking this product.

Alcohol and other CNS depressants may produce an additive CNS depression, when take with this combination product, and should be avoided.

Butalbital may be habit-forming. Patients should take the drug only for as long as it is prescribed, in the amounts prescribed, and no more frequently than prescribed.

Laboratory Tests: In patients with severe hepatic or renal disease, effects of therapy should be monitored with serial liver and/or renal function tests.

Drug Interactions: The CNS effects of Butalbital may be enhanced by monoamine oxidase (MAO) inhibitors.

Acetaminophen and Butalbital may enhance the effects of: other narcotic analgesics, alcohol, general anesthetics, transguilizers such as chlordiazepoxide, sedative-hypnotics, or other CNS depressants, causing increased CNS depression.

Drug/Laboratory Test Interactions: Acetaminophen may produce false-positive test results for urinary 5-hydroxyindoleacetic acid.

Carcinogenesis, Mutagenesis, Impairment of Fertility: No adequate studies have been conducted in animals to determine whether Acetaminophen or Butalbital have a potential for carcinogenesis, mutagenesis or impairment of fertility.

Pregnancy: Teratogenic Effects: Pregnancy Category C: Animal reproduction studies have not been conducted with this combination product. It is also not known whether Acetaminophen and Butalbitol can cause fetal harm when administered to a pregnant woman or can affect reproduction capacity. These products should be given to a pregnant woman only when clearly needed.

Nonteratogenic Effects: Withdrawal seizures were reported in a two-day-old male infant whose mother had taken a Butalbital-containing drug during the last two months of pregnancy. Butalbital was found in the infant's serum. The infant was given phenobarbital 5 mg/kg, which was tapered without further seizure or other withdrawal symptoms.

Nursing Mothers: Acetaminophen and barbiturates are excreted in breast milk in small amounts, but the significance of their effects on nursing infants is not known. Because of potential for serious adverse reactions in nursing infants from Acetaminophen and Butalbital, a decision should be made whether to discontinue nursing or to discontinue the drug, taking into account the importance of the drug to the mother.

Pediatric Use: Safety and effectiveness in children below the age of 12 have not been established.

ADVERSE REACTIONS

Frequently Observed: The most frequently reported adverse reactions are drowsiness, lightheadedness, dizziness, sedation, shortness of breath, nausea, vomiting, abdominal pain, and intoxicated feeling.

Infrequently Observed: All adverse events tabulated below are classified as infrequent.

Central Nervous: headache, shaky feeling, tingling, agitation, fainting, fatigue, heavy eyelids, high energy, hot spells, numbness, sluggishness, seizure. Mental confusion, excitement or depression can also occur due to intolerance, particularly in elderly or debilitated patients, or due to overdosage of Butalbital.

Autonomic Nervous: dry mouth, hyperhidrosis.

Gastrointestinal: difficulty swallowing, heartburn, flatulence, constipation.

Cardiovascular: tachycardia.

Musculoskeletal: leg pain, muscle fatigue.

Genitourinary: diuresis.

Miscellaneous: pruritus, fever, earache, nasal congestion, tinnitus, euphoria, allergic reactions.

Several cases of dermatological reactions, including toxic epidermal necrolysis and erythema multiforme, have been reported.

The following adverse drug events may be borne in mind as potential effects of the components of this product. Potential effects of high dosage are listed in the "Overdosage" section.

Acetaminophen: allergic reactions, rash, thrombocytopenia, agranulocytosis.

DRUG ABUSE AND DEPENDENCE

Abuse and Dependence: Butalbital: Barbiturates may be habit forming. Tolerance, psychological dependence, and physical dependence may occur especially following prolonged use of high doses of barbiturates. The average daily dose for the barbiturate addict is usually about 1500 mg. As tolerance to barbiturates develops, the amount needed to maintain the same level of intoxication increases; tolerance to a fatal dosage, however, does not increase more than two-fold. As this

---

◆ RATED THERAPEUTICALLY EQUIVALENT; ◇ THERAPEUTIC EQUIVALENCE UNCONFIRMED; ○ UNRATED

occurs, the margin between an intoxication dosage and fatal dosage becomes smaller. The lethal dose of a barbiturate is far less if alcohol is also ingested. Major withdrawal symptoms (convulsions and delirium) may occur within 16 hours and last up to 5 days after abrupt cessation of these drugs. Intensity of withdrawal symptoms gradually declines over a period of approximately 15 days. Treatment of barbiturate dependence consists of cautious and gradual withdrawal of the drug. Barbiturate-dependent patients can be withdrawn by using a number of different withdrawal regimens. One method involves initiating treatment at the patient's regular dosage level and gradually decreasing the daily dosage as tolerated by the patient.

OVERDOSAGE

Following an acute overdosage of Acetaminophen and Butalbital, toxicity may result from Acetaminophen or the barbiturate.

Signs and Symptoms: Toxicity from *barbiturate* poisoning include drowsiness, confusion, and coma; respiratory depression; hypotension; and hypovolemic shock.

In *Acetaminophen* overdosage: dose-dependent, potentially fatal hepatic necrosis is the most serious adverse effect. Renal tubular necroses, hypoglycemic coma and thrombocytopenia may also occur. Early symptoms following a potentially hepatotoxic overdose may include: nausea, vomiting, diaphoresis and general malaise. Clinical and laboratory evidence of hepatic toxicity may not be apparent until 48 to 72 hours post-ingestion. In adults hepatic toxicity has rarely been reported with acute overdoses of less than 10 grams, or fatalities with less than 15 grams.

Treatment: A single or multiple overdose with these combination products is a potentially lethal polydrug overdose, and consultation with a regional poison control center is recommended.

Immediate treatment includes support of cardiorespiratory function and measures to reduce drug absorption. Vomiting should be induced mechanically, or with syrup of ipecac, if the patient is alert (adequate pharyngeal and laryngeal reflexes). Oral activated charcoal (1 g/kg) should follow gastric emptying. The first dose should be accompanied by an appropriate cathartic. If repeated doses are used, the cathartic might be included with alternate doses as required. Hypotension is usually hypovolemic and should respond to fluids. Pressors should be avoided. A cuffed endotracheal tube should be inserted before gastric lavage of the unconscious patient and, when necessary, to provide assisted respiration. If renal function is normal, forced diuresis may aid in the elimination of the barbiturate. Alkalinization of the urine increases renal excretion of some barbiturates, especially phenobarbital.

Meticulous attention should be given to maintaining adequate pulmonary ventilation. In severe cases of intoxication, peritoneal dialysis, or preferably hemodialysis may be considered. If hypoprothrombinemia occurs due to Acetaminophen overdose, vitamin K should be administered intravenously.

If the dose of Acetaminophen may have exceeded 140 mg/kg, acetylcysteine should be administered as early as possible. Serum Acetaminophen levels should be obtained, since levels four or more hours following ingestion help predict Acetaminophen toxicity. Do not await Acetaminophen assay results before initiating treatment. Hepatic enzymes should be obtained initially, and repeated at 24-hour intervals.

Methemoglobinemia over 30% should be treated with methylene blue by slow intravenous administration.

TOXIC DOSES (FOR ADULTS)

Acetaminophen/Butalbital tablets (Acetaminophen 325 or 650 mg and Butalbital 50 mg tablets)
Acetaminophen: toxic dose 10 g (15 or 30 tablets)
Butalbital: toxic dose 1 g (20 tablets)
Acetaminophen/Butalbital capsules (Acetaminophen 650 mg and Butalbital 50 mg capsules)
Acetaminophen: toxic dose 10 g (15 capsules)
Butalbital: toxic dose 1 g (20 capsules)

DOSAGE AND ADMINISTRATION

Acetaminophen/Butalbital: Tablets: One or two 325 mg Acetaminophen or one 650 mg Acetaminophen tablet every four hours. Total daily dosage should not exceed 6 tablets.

Acetaminophen/Butalbital: Capsules: One capsule every four hours. Total daily dosage should not exceed 6 capsules.

Extended and repeated use of these products is not recommended because of the potential for physical dependence.

Store Acetaminophen/Butalbital tablets and capsules at controlled room temperature, 15°-30°C (59°-86°F). Dispense in a tight container as defined in the usp.

HOW SUPPLIED
CAPSULE: 325 MG-50 MG

AVERAGE UNIT PRICE (AVAILABLE SIZES)			
GENERIC	$0.17		

BRAND/MANUFACTURER	NDC	SIZE	AWP
◆ GENERICS			
TRIAPRIN: Dunhall	00217-2811-01	100s	$18.00
TRIAPRIN: Dunhall	00217-2811-03	500s	$80.00

CAPSULE: 650 MG-50 MG

BRAND/MANUFACTURER	NDC	SIZE	AWP
◆ BRAND			
PHRENILIN FORTE: Carnrick	00086-0056-10	100s	$22.20
◆ GENERICS			
AXOCET: Savage	00281-0198-17	100s	$45.05

TABLETS: 325 MG-50 MG

BRAND/MANUFACTURER	NDC	SIZE	AWP
◆ BRAND			
PHRENILIN: Carnrick	00086-0050-10	100s	$18.65

TABLETS: 650 MG-50 MG

AVERAGE UNIT PRICE (AVAILABLE SIZES)		GENERIC A-RATED AVERAGE PRICE (GAAP)	
GENERIC	$0.30	100s	$30.10

BRAND/MANUFACTURER	NDC	SIZE	AWP
◆ GENERICS			
REPAN CF: Everett	00642-0166-10	100s	$29.25
SEDAPAP: Mayrand	00259-1278-01	100s	$30.95

Acetaminophen with Codeine Phosphate

DESCRIPTION

Each capsule contains:

No. 3 Codeine Phosphate*	.30 mg
Acetaminophen	.325 mg
No. 4 Codeine Phosphate*	.60 mg
Acetaminophen	.325 mg

Each 5 mL. of elixir contains:

Codeine phosphate*	.12 mg
Acetaminophen	.120 mg
Alcohol	.7%

Each tablet contains:

No. 2 Codeine Phosphate*	.15 mg
Acetaminophen	.300 mg
No. 3 Codeine Phosphate*	.30 mg
Acetaminophen	.300 mg
No. 4 Codeine Phosphate*	.60 mg
Acetaminophen	.300 mg

Each Acetaminophen 650 with codeine tablet contains:

Acetaminophen, USP	.650 mg
Codeine Phosphate*, USP	.30 mg

Warning—May be habit forming.

Certain brands of Acetaminophen with Codeine Phosphate tablets contain sodium metabisulfite as an inactive ingredient. (See *"Warnings"*.)

Acetaminophen, 4'-hydroxyacetanilide, is a non-opiate, non-salicylate analgesic and antipyretic which occurs as a white, odorless, crystalline powder, possessing a slightly bitter taste.

Codeine is an alkaloid, obtained from opium or prepared from morphine by methylation. Codeine Phosphate occurs as fine, white, needle-shaped crystals, or white, crystalline powder. It is affected by light. Its chemical name is 7,8-didehydro-4,5α-epoxy-3-methoxy-17-methylmorphinan-6α-ol phosphate (1:1) (salt) hemihydrate.

CLINICAL PHARMACOLOGY

Acetaminophen with Codeine Phosphate tablets, capsules and oral solution USP combine the analgesic effects of a centrally acting analgesic, Codeine, with a peripherally acting analgesic, Acetaminophen. Both ingredients are well absorbed orally. The plasma elimination half-life ranges from 1 to 4 hours for Acetaminophen, and from 2.5 to 3 hours for Codeine.

Codeine retains at least one-half of its analgesic activity when administered orally. A reduced first-pass metabolism of Codeine by the liver accounts for the greater oral efficacy of codeine when compared to most other morphine-like narcotics. Following absorption, Codeine is metabolized by the liver and metabolic products are excreted in the urine. Approximately 10 percent of the administered Codeine is demethylated to morphine, which may account for its analgesic activity.

Acetaminophen is distributed throughout most fluids of the body, and is metabolized primarily in the liver. Little unchanged drug is excreted in the urine, but most metabolic products appear in the urine within 24 hours.

INDICATIONS AND USAGE

Acetaminophen with Codeine Phosphate tablets and capsules are indicated for the relief of mild to moderately severe pain.

➤ SHOWN IN PRODUCT IDENTIFICATION GUIDE

Acetaminophen with Codeine Phosphate elixir solution USP is indicated for the relief of mild to moderate pain.

CONTRAINDICATIONS
Acetaminophen with Codeine Phosphate tablets and oral solution USP should not be administered to patients who have previously exhibited hypersensitivity to any component.

WARNINGS
Certain brands of Acetaminophen with Codeine Phosphate contain sodium metabisulfite, a sulfite that may cause allergic-type reactions including anaphylactic symptoms and life-threatening or less severe asthmatic episodes in certain susceptible people. The overall prevalence of sulfite sensitivity in the general population is unknown and probably low. Sulfite sensitivity is seen more frequently in asthmatic than in nonasthmatic people.

PRECAUTIONS
GENERAL
Head Injury and Increased Intracranial Pressure: The respiratory depressant effects of narcotics and their capacity to elevate cerebrospinal fluid pressure may be markedly exaggerated in the presence of head injury, other intracranial lesions or a pre-existing increase in intracranial pressure. Furthermore, narcotics produce adverse reactions which may obscure the clinical course of patients with head injuries.

Acute Abdominal Conditions: The administration of this product or other narcotics may obscure the diagnosis or clinical course of patients with acute abdominal conditions.

Special Risk Patients: This drug should be given with caution to certain patients such as the elderly or debilitated, and those with severe impairment of hepatic or renal function, hypothyroidism, Addison's disease, and prostatic hypertrophy or urethral stricture.

INFORMATION FOR PATIENTS
Codeine may impair the mental and/or physical abilities required for the performance of potentially hazardous tasks such as driving a car or operating machinery. The patient using this drug should be cautioned accordingly.

The patient should understand the single-dose and 24 hour dose limits, and the time interval between doses.

DRUG INTERACTIONS
Patients receiving other narcotic analgesics, antipsychotics, antianxiety agents, or other CNS depressants (including alcohol) concomitantly with this drug may exhibit an additive CNS depression. When such combined therapy is contemplated, the dose of one or both agents should be reduced. The concurrent use of anticholinergics with codeine may produce paralytic ileus.

CARCINOGENESIS, MUTAGENESIS, IMPAIRMENT OF FERTILITY
No long-term studies in animals have been performed with Acetaminophen or Codeine to determine carcinogenic potential or effects on fertility.

Acetaminophen and Codeine have been found to have no mutagenic potential using the Ames Salmonella-Microsomal Activation test, the Basc test on Drosophila germ cells, and the Micronucleus test on mouse bone marrow.

PREGNANCY
Teratogenic Effects: Pregnancy Category C.

Codeine: A study in rats and rabbits reported no teratogenic effect of codeine administered during the period of organogenesis in doses ranging from 5 to 120 mg/kg. In the rat, doses at the 120 mg/kg level, in the toxic range for the adult animal, were associated with an increase in embryo resorption at the time of implantation. In another study a single 100 mg/kg dose of Codeine administered to pregnant mice reportedly resulted in delayed ossification in the offspring. There are no studies in humans, and the significance of these findings to humans, if any, is not known.

Acetaminophen with Codeine Phosphate tablets, capsules and oral solution USP should be used during pregnancy only if the potential benefit justifies the potential risk to the fetus.

Nonteratogenic Effects: Dependence has been reported in newborns whose mothers took opiates regularly during pregnancy. Withdrawal signs include irritability, excessive crying, tremors, hyperreflexia, fever, vomiting, and diarrhea. These signs usually appear during the first few days of life.

LABOR AND DELIVERY
Narcotic analgesics cross the placental barrier. The closer to delivery and the larger the dose used, the greater the possibility of respiratory depression in the newborn. Narcotic analgesics should be avoided during labor if delivery of a premature infant is anticipated. If the mother has received narcotic analgesics during labor, newborn infants should be observed closely for signs of respiratory depression. Resuscitation may be required (see *"Overdosage"*). The effect of Codeine, if any, on the later growth, development, and functional maturation of the child is unknown.

NURSING MOTHERS
Some studies, but not others, have reported detectable amounts of codeine in breast milk. The levels are probably not clinically significant after usual therapeutic dosage. The possibility of clinically important amounts being excreted in breast milk in individuals abusing codeine should be considered.

PEDIATRIC USE
Safe dosage of Acetaminophen with Codeine Phosphate oral solution USP has not been established in children below the age of three years.

ADVERSE REACTIONS
The most frequently observed adverse reactions include light-headedness, dizziness, sedation, shortness of breath, nausea and vomiting. These effects seem to be more prominent in ambulatory than in non-ambulatory patients, and some of these adverse reactions may be alleviated if the patient lies down. Other adverse reactions include allergic reactions, euphoria, dysphoria, constipation, abdominal pain and pruritus.

At higher doses, codeine has most of the disadvantages of morphine including respiratory depression.

DRUG ABUSE AND DEPENDENCE
Acetaminophen with Codeine Phosphate tablets and capsules are a Schedule III controlled substance.

Acetaminophen with Codeine Phosphate oral solution USP is a Schedule V controlled substance.

Codeine can produce drug dependence of the morphine type and, therefore, has the potential for being abused. Psychic dependence, physical dependence and tolerance may develop upon repeated administration of this drug, and it should be prescribed and administered with the same degree of caution appropriate to the use of other oral narcotic-containing medications.

OVERDOSAGE
ACETAMINOPHEN
Signs and Symptoms: In acute acetaminophen overdosage, dose-dependent, potentially fatal hepatic necrosis is the most serious adverse effect. Renal tubular necrosis, hypoglycemic coma and thrombocytopenia may also occur.

In adults, hepatic toxicity has rarely been reported with acute overdoses of less than 10 grams and fatalities with less than 15 grams. Importantly, young children seem to be more resistant than adults to the hepatotoxic effect of an acetaminophen overdose. Despite this, the measures outlined below should be initiated in any adult or child suspected of having ingested an acetaminophen overdose.

Early symptoms following a potentially hepatotoxic overdose may include: nausea, vomiting, diaphoresis and general malaise. Clinical and laboratory evidence of hepatic toxicity may not be apparent until 48 to 72 hours post-ingestion.

Treatment: The stomach should be emptied promptly by lavage or by induction of emesis with syrup of ipecac. Patients' estimates of the quantity of a drug ingested are notoriously unreliable. Therefore, if an acetaminophen overdose is suspected, a serum acetaminophen assay should be obtained as early as possible, but no sooner than four hours following ingestion. Liver function studies should be obtained initially and repeated at 24-hour intervals.

The antidote, N-acetylcysteine, should be administered as early as possible, preferably within 16 hours of the overdose ingestion for optimal results, but in any case, within 24 hours. Following recovery, there are no residual, structural or functional hepatic abnormalities.

CODEINE
Signs and Symptoms: Serious overdose with Codeine is characterized by respiratory depression (a decrease in respiratory rate and/or tidal volume, Cheyne-Stokes respiration, cyanosis), extreme somnolence progressing to stupor or coma, skeletal muscle flaccidity, cold and clammy skin, and sometimes bradycardia and hypotension. In severe overdosage, apnea, circulatory collapse, cardiac arrest and death may occur.

Treatment: Primary attention should be given to the reestablishment of adequate respiratory exchange through provision of a patent airway and the institution of assisted or controlled ventilation. The narcotic antagonist naloxone is a specific antidote against respiratory depression which may result from overdosage or unusual sensitivity to narcotics, including codeine. Therefore, an appropriate dose of naloxone hydrochloride (see package insert) should be administered, preferably by the intravenous route, and simultaneously with efforts at respiratory resuscitation. Since the duration of action of codeine may exceed that of the antagonist, the patient should be kept under continued surveillance and repeated doses of the antagonist should be administered as needed to maintain adequate respiration.

An antagonist should not be administered in the absence of clinically significant respiratory or cardiovascular depression. Oxygen, intravenous fluids, vasopressors and other supportive measures should be employed as indicated.

Gastric emptying may be useful in removing unabsorbed drug.

DOSAGE AND ADMINISTRATION
Dosage should be adjusted according to severity of pain and response of the patient.

It should be kept in mind, however, that tolerance to codeine can develop with continued use and that the incidence of untoward effects is dose related. Adult doses of codeine higher than 60 mg fail to give commensurate relief of pain but merely prolong analgesia and are associated with an appreciably increased incidence of undesirable side effects. Equivalently high doses in children would have similar effects.

The usual adult dosage for tablets is:

	Single Doses (Range)	Maximum 24 Hour Dose
Codeine Phosphate	15mg-60mg	360mg
Acetaminophen	300mg-1000mg	4000mg

Doses may be repeated up to every 4 hours.

The prescriber must determine the number of tablets per dose, and the maximum number of tablets per 24 hours, based upon the above dosage guidance. This information should be conveyed in the prescription.

For children, the dose of codeine phosphate is 0.5 mg/kg.

Acetaminophen with Codeine Phosphate oral solution USP contains 120 mg of Acetaminophen and 12 mg of Codeine Phosphate/5 mL and is given orally.

The usual doses are:

Children:	(7 to 12 years): 10 mL (2 teaspoonfuls) 3 or 4 times daily.
	(3 to 6 years): 5 mL (1 teaspoonful) 3 or 4 times daily.
	(under 3 years): safe dosage has not been established.
Adults:	15 mL (1 tablespoonful) every 4 hours as needed.

Dispense in a tight, light-resistant container as defined in the official compendium.

HOW SUPPLIED
CAPSULE (C-III): 325 MG-30 MG

AVERAGE UNIT PRICE (AVAILABLE SIZES)	
BRAND	$0.30

BRAND/MANUFACTURER	NDC	SIZE	AWP
◆ BRAND			
PHENAPHEN W/CODEINE: Robins Pharm	00031-6257-63	100s	$30.66
	00031-6257-70	500s	$145.28

CAPSULE (C-III): 325 MG-60 MG

BRAND/MANUFACTURER	NDC	SIZE	AWP
◆ BRAND			
PHENAPHEN W/CODEINE: Robins Pharm	00031-6274-63	100s	$52.63

ELIXIR (C-V): 120 MG/5 ML-12 MG/5 ML

AVERAGE UNIT PRICE (AVAILABLE SIZES)		GENERIC A-RATED AVERAGE PRICE (GAAP)	
BRAND	$0.10	120 ml	$4.04
GENERIC	$0.04	480 ml	$12.63
		3840 ml	$84.27
		5 ml 100s	$50.27
		12.5 ml 100s	$53.32
		15 ml 100s	$55.00

BRAND/MANUFACTURER	NDC	SIZE	AWP
◆ BRAND			
TYLENOL ELIXIR W/CODEINE: McNeil Pharm	00045-0508-16	480 ml	$47.57
◆ GENERICS			
Pennex	00426-8245-04	120 ml	$3.74
Pennex	00832-8245-04	120 ml	$3.74
Barre	00472-1419-04	120 ml	$3.80
Pharm Assoc	00121-0504-04	120 ml	$4.41
Goldline	00182-1078-37	120 ml	$4.50
Pennex	00426-8245-16	480 ml	$10.10
Pennex	00832-8245-16	480 ml	$10.10
Schein	00364-7207-16	480 ml	$11.25
Qualitest	00603-1020-58	480 ml	$12.06
Geneva	00781-6052-16	480 ml	$12.95
Rugby	00536-0082-85	480 ml	$13.13
Major	00904-7775-16	480 ml	$13.25
URL	00677-0996-33	480 ml	$13.50
Goldline	00182-1078-40	480 ml	$13.50
Pharm Assoc	00121-0504-16	480 ml	$13.72
Barre	00472-1419-16	480 ml	$14.00
Roxane	00054-3005-63	500 ml	$20.77
Barre	00472-1419-28	3840 ml	$83.60
Major	00904-0173-28	3840 ml	$84.60
Major	00904-7775-28	3840 ml	$84.60
Pharm Assoc	00121-0504-05	5 ml 100s ud	$45.66
Roxane	00054-8013-04	5 ml 100s ud	$54.87
Pharm Assoc	00121-0504-10	10 ml 100s ud	$47.10
Pharm Assoc	00121-0504-12	12.5 ml 100s ud	$49.55
Roxane	00054-8002-04	12.5 ml 100s ud	$57.08
Pharm Assoc	00121-0504-15	15 ml 100s ud	$52.17
Roxane	00054-8017-04	15 ml 100s ud	$57.83

SUSPENSION (C-V): 120 MG/5 ML-12 MG/5 ML

BRAND/MANUFACTURER	NDC	SIZE	AWP
◆ GENERICS			
CAPITAL W/CODEINE SUSPENSION: Carnrick	00086-0046-16	480 ml	$17.85

TABLETS (C-III): 300 MG-7.5 MG

BRAND/MANUFACTURER	NDC	SIZE	AWP
◆ BRAND			
TYLENOL W/CODEINE: McNeil Pharm	00045-0510-60	100s	$18.40

TABLETS (C-III): 300 MG-15 MG

AVERAGE UNIT PRICE (AVAILABLE SIZES)		GENERIC A-RATED AVERAGE PRICE (GAAP)	
BRAND	$0.26	100s	$7.84
GENERIC	$0.07	500s	$32.80
HCFA FUL (100s ea)	$0.04	1000s	$55.72

BRAND/MANUFACTURER	NDC	SIZE	AWP
◆ BRAND			
▶ TYLENOL W/CODEINE: McNeil Pharm	00045-0511-60	100s	$27.55
	00045-0511-70	500s	$110.35
	00045-0511-72	500s ud	$138.35
◆ GENERICS			
Lemmon	00093-0050-01	100s	$6.50
Rugby	00536-3228-01	100s	$6.65
Major	00904-0571-60	100s	$7.50
Qualitest	00603-2337-21	100s	$7.56
Vintage	00254-2063-28	100s	$7.85
Goldline	00182-1268-01	100s	$7.85
Parmed	00349-2118-01	100s	$7.95
Schein	00364-0323-01	100s	$8.13
URL	00677-0611-01	100s	$8.20
Mutual	53489-0159-01	100s	$8.20
Moore,H.L.	00839-6717-06	100s	$8.22
Aligen	00405-0007-01	100s	$9.43
URL	00677-0611-05	500s	$32.80
Mutual	53489-0159-05	500s	$32.80
Lemmon	00093-0050-10	1000s	$52.50
Major	00904-0571-80	1000s	$55.20
Parmed	00349-2118-10	1000s	$59.45

TABLETS (C-III): 300 MG-30 MG

AVERAGE UNIT PRICE (AVAILABLE SIZES)		GENERIC A-RATED AVERAGE PRICE (GAAP)	
BRAND	$0.27	100s	$12.75
GENERIC	$0.12	500s	$40.05
HCFA FUL (100s ea)	$0.06	1000s	$79.96

BRAND/MANUFACTURER	NDC	SIZE	AWP
◆ BRAND			
▶ TYLENOL W/CODEINE: McNeil Pharm	00045-0513-60	100s	$29.95
	00045-0513-70	500s	$129.59
	00045-0513-72	500s ud	$142.67
	00045-0513-80	1000s	$235.55
◆ GENERICS			
Medirex	57480-0500-06	30s	$4.99
UDL	51079-0161-99	90s	$60.00
Geneva	00781-1752-01	100s	$8.45
▶ Lemmon	00093-0150-01	100s	$8.50
Qualitest	00603-2338-21	100s	$8.96
Moore,H.L.	00839-6245-06	100s	$9.57
▶ Rugby	00536-3227-01	100s	$9.82
Vintage	00254-2064-28	100s	$9.90
Major	00904-0175-60	100s	$9.90
▶ URL	00677-0612-01	100s	$10.00
Mutual	53489-0160-01	100s	$10.00
Aligen	00405-0008-01	100s	$10.59
Purepac	00228-2001-10	100s	$10.81
▶ Goldline	00182-0948-01	100s	$10.81
Parmed	00349-2322-01	100s	$10.95
Schein	00364-0324-01	100s	$13.71
UDL	51079-0161-21	100s	$17.51
Geneva	00781-1752-13	100s ud	$11.75
Roxane	00054-8022-25	100s ud	$14.67
Auro	55829-0801-10	100s ud	$14.76
▶ Goldline	00182-0948-89	100s ud	$15.70
Vangard	00615-0430-13	100s ud	$16.08
Vangard	00615-0430-47	100s ud	$16.08
UDL	51079-0161-20	100s ud	$17.51
Medirex	57480-0500-01	100s ud	$17.95
Roxane	00054-8022-24	100s ud	$22.13
▶ URL	00677-0612-05	500s	$40.05
Mutual	53489-0160-05	500s	$40.05
Sandocare	58345-0800-65	640s ud	$103.55
Major	00904-0175-80	1000s	$66.40
Aligen	00405-0008-03	1000s	$66.88
Geneva	00781-1752-10	1000s	$67.50
Mason Dist	11845-0367-04	1000s	$70.46
Qualitest	00603-2338-32	1000s	$70.88
▶ Rugby	00536-3227-10	1000s	$73.88
▶ Lemmon	00093-0150-10	1000s	$74.30
Vintage	00254-2064-38	1000s	$74.40
▶ URL	00677-0612-10	1000s	$74.90
Mutual	53489-0160-10	1000s	$74.90
Moore,H.L.	00839-6245-10	1000s	$74.99
Purepac	00228-2001-96	1000s	$82.05
▶ Goldline	00182-0948-10	1000s	$82.05

BRAND/MANUFACTURER	NDC	SIZE	AWP
Schein	00364-0324-02	1000s	$88.74
Parmed	00349-2322-10	1000s	$98.95
Parmed	00349-8861-10	1000s	$98.95
Roxane	00054-4022-31	1000s	$119.14

TABLETS (C-III): 300 MG-60 MG

AVERAGE UNIT PRICE (AVAILABLE SIZES)		GENERIC A-RATED AVERAGE PRICE (GAAP)	
BRAND	$0.50	100s	$20.21
GENERIC	$0.18	500s	$78.10
HCFA FUL (100s ea)	$0.10	1000s	$143.45

BRAND/MANUFACTURER	NDC	SIZE	AWP
◆ **BRAND**			
➤ TYLENOL W/CODEINE: McNeil Pharm	00045-0515-60	100s	$52.91
	00045-0515-70	500s	$228.56
	00045-0515-72	500s ud	$254.20
◆ **GENERICS**			
Lemmon	00093-0350-01	100s	$14.50
Aligen	00405-0009-01	100s	$16.76
Mutual	53489-0161-01	100s	$17.50
Vintage	00254-2065-28	100s	$17.55
Qualitest	00603-2339-21	100s	$17.70
Major	00904-3916-60	100s	$17.90
Rugby	00536-3215-01	100s	$17.93
URL	00677-0632-01	100s	$18.50
➤ Geneva	00781-1654-01	100s	$19.10
Purepac	00228-2003-10	100s	$19.14
Goldline	00182-1338-01	100s	$19.14
Moore,H.L.	00839-6499-06	100s	$19.29
Parmed	00349-2324-01	100s	$21.75
Schein	00364-0526-01	100s	$21.87
UDL	51079-0106-21	100s	$25.68
UDL	51079-0106-20	100s ud	$25.68
Goldline	00182-1338-89	100s ud	$25.75
Auro	55829-0802-10	100s ud	$26.96
Lemmon	00093-0350-05	500s	$66.75
Parmed	00349-2324-05	500s	$67.70
Qualitest	00603-2339-28	500s	$71.70
Major	00904-3916-40	500s	$75.70
Vintage	00254-2065-35	500s	$78.80
URL	00677-0632-05	500s	$80.65
Mutual	53489-0161-05	500s	$80.65
Rugby	00536-3215-05	500s	$80.70
➤ Geneva	00781-1654-05	500s	$82.51
Moore,H.L.	00839-6499-12	500s	$85.39
Purepac	00228-2003-50	500s	$85.55
Goldline	00182-1338-05	500s	$85.55
Mason Dist	11845-0368-04	1000s	$105.25
Lemmon	00093-0350-10	1000s	$133.50
Parmed	00349-2324-10	1000s	$143.33
Schein	00364-0526-02	1000s	$191.72

TABLETS (C-III): 650 MG-30 MG

BRAND/MANUFACTURER	NDC	SIZE	AWP
◆ **BRAND**			
EZ III: Stewart Jackson	45985-0625-01	100s	$28.56
◆ **GENERICS**			
MARGESIC #3: Marnel	00682-0806-01	100s	$25.60

Acetaminophen with Hydrocodone Bitartrate

DESCRIPTION

Each Acetaminophen/Hydrocodone Bitartrate tablet contains:

Hydrocodone Bitartrate*	...5	mg
Acetaminophen	...500	mg
Hydrocodone Bitartrate*	...7.5	mg
Acetaminophen	...650	mg
Hydrocodone Bitartrate*	...7.5	mg
Acetaminophen	...750	mg
Hydrocodone Bitartrate*	...10	mg
Acetaminophen	...650	mg

***(WARNING**: May be habit forming)*

Hydrocodone Bitartrate is an opioid analgesic and antitussive and occurs as fine, white crystals or as a crystalline powder. It is affected by light. The chemical name is: 4,5α epoxy-3-methoxy-17- methylmorphinan-6-one tartrate (1:1) hydrate (2:5). Hydrocodone has the chemical formula $C_{18}H_{21}NO_3C_4H_6O_6 \cdot 2\ \frac{1}{2}H_2O$ and molecular weight 494.50, 4'-hydroxyacetanilide, is a non-opiate, nonsalicylate analgesic and antipyretic which occurs as a white, odorless crystalline powder possessing a slightly bitter taste. Acetaminophen has the chemical formula $C_8H_9NO_2$ and molecular weight 151.16.

CLINICAL PHARMACOLOGY

Hydrocodone is a semisynthetic narcotic analgesic and antitussive with multiple actions qualitatively similar to those of codeine. Most of these involve the central nervous system and smooth muscle. The precise mechanism of action of Hydrocodone and other opiates is not known, although it is believed to relate to the existence of opiate receptors in the central nervous system. In addition to analgesia, narcotics may produce drowsiness, changes in mood and mental clouding.

Radioimmunoassay techniques have recently been developed for the analysis of Hydrocodone in human plasma. After a 10 mg oral dose of Hydrocodone Bitartrate, a mean peak serum drug level of 23.6 ng/mL and an elimination half-life of 3.8 hours were found.

The analgesic action of Acetaminophen (APAP) involves peripheral and central influences, but the specific mechanism is as yet undetermined. Antipyretic activity is mediated through hypothalamic heat regulating centers. APAP inhibits prostaglandin synthetase. Therapeutic doses of APAP have negligible effects on the cardiovascular or respiratory systems; however, toxic doses may cause circulatory failure and rapid, shallow breathing. APAP is rapidly and almostly completely absorbed from the gastrointestinal tract, producing maximum serum concentrations within 30 minutes to one hour. The plasma half-life in adults and children ranges from 0.90 hours to 3.25 hours with an average of approximately 2 hours. The drug distributes uniformly in most body fluids and is approximately 25% protein bound. APAP is conjugated in the liver, with less than 3% of the dose excreted unchanged in 24 hours. The primary metabolic pathway is conjugation to sulfate and glucuronide by-products. A minor oxidative pathway forms cysteine and mercapturic acid. These compounds are subsequently excreted by the kidneys into the urine.

INDICATIONS AND USAGE
For the relief of moderate to moderately severe pain.

CONTRAINDICATIONS
Hypersensitivity to APAP or Hydrocodone.

WARNINGS
Respiratory Depression: At high doses or in sensitive patients, Hydrocodone may produce dose-related respiratory depression by acting directly on the brain stem respiratory center. Hydrocodone also affects the center that controls respiratory rhythm, and may produce irregular and periodic breathing.

Head Injury and Increased Intracranial Pressure: The respiratory depressant effects of narcoticsa and their capacity to elevate cerebrospinal fluid pressure may be markedly exaggerated in the presence of head injury, other intracranial lesions or a preexisting increase in intracranial pressure. Furthermore, narcotics produce adverse reactions which may obscure the clinical course of patients with head injuries.

Acute Abdominal Conditions: The administration of narcotics may obscure the diagnosis or clinical course of patients with acute abdominal conditions.

PRECAUTIONS
Special Risk Patients: As with any narcotic analgesic agent, APAP/Hydrocodone should be used with caution in elderly or debilitated patients and those with severe impairment of hepatic or renal function, hypothyroidism, Addison's disease, prostatic hypertrophy or urethral stricture. The usual precautions should be observed and the possibility of respiratory depression should be kept in mind.

Information for Patients: APAP/Hydrocodone, like all narcotics, may impair the mental and/or physical abilities required for the performance of potentially hazardous tasks such as driving a car or operating machinery; patients should be cautioned accordingly.

Cough Reflex: Hydrocodone suppresses the cough reflex; as with all narcotics, caution should be exercised when APAP/Hydrocodone is used postoperatively and in patients with pulmonary disease.

Drug Interactions: Patients receiving other narcotic analgesics, antipsychotics, antianxiety agents, or other CNS depressants (including alcohol) concomitantly with APAP/Hydrocodone may exhibit an additive CNS depression. When combined therapy is contemplated, the dose of one or both agents should be reduced.

The use of MAO inhibitors or tricyclic antidepressants with Hydrocodone preparations may increase the effect of either the antidepressant or Hydrocodone.

The concurrent use of anticholinergics with Hydrocodone may produce paralytic ileus.

Usage in Pregnancy

Teratogenic Effects: Pregnancy Category C. Hydrocodone has been shown to be teratogenic in hamsters when given in doses 700 times the human dose. There are no adequate and well-controlled studies in pregnant women. APAP/Hydrocodone should be used during pregnancy only if the potential benefit justifies the potential risk to the fetus.

Nonteratogenic Effects: Babies born to mothers who have been taking opioids regularly prior to delivery will be physically dependent. The withdrawal signs include irritability and excessive crying, tremors, hyperactive reflexes, increased respiratory rate, increased stools, sneezing, yawning, vomiting, and fever. The intensity of the syndrome does not always correlate with the duration of maternal opioid use or dose. There is no consensus on the best method of managing withdrawal. Chlorpromazine 0.7 to 1.0 mg/kg q6h, and paregoric 2 to 4 drops/kg q4h, have been used to treat withdrawal symptoms in infants. The duration of therapy is 4 to 28 days, with the dosage decreased as tolerated.

◆ RATED THERAPEUTICALLY EQUIVALENT; ◇ THERAPEUTIC EQUIVALENCE UNCONFIRMED; ○ UNRATED

Labor and Delivery: As with all narcotics, administration of APAP/Hydrocodone to the mother shortly before delivery may result in some degree of respiratory depression in the newborn, especially if higher doses are used.

Nursing Mothers: It is not known whether this drug is excreted in human milk. Because many drugs are excreted in human milk and because of the potential for serious adverse reactions in nursing infants from APAP/Hydrocodone, a decision should be made whether to discontinue nursing or to discontinue the drug, taking into account the importance of the drug to the mother.

Pediatric Use: Safety and effectiveness in children have not been established.

ADVERSE REACTIONS
The most frequently observed adverse reactions include light-headedness, dizziness, sedation, nausea and vomiting. These effects seem to be more prominent in ambulatory than in nonambulatory patients and some of these adverse reactions may be alleviated if the patient lies down.

Other adverse reactions include:

Central Nervous System: Drowsiness, mental clouding, lethargy, impairment of mental and physical performance, anxiety, fear, dysphoria, psychic dependence, mood changes.

Gastrointestinal System: The antiemetic phenothiazines are useful in suppressing the nausea and vomiting which may occur (see above); however, some phenothiazine derivatives seem to be antianalgesic and to increase the amount of narcotic required to produce pain relief, while other phenothiazines reduce the amount of narcotic required to produce a given level of analgesia. Prolonged administration of APAP/Hydrocodone may produce constipation.

Genitourinary System: Ureteral spasm, spasm of vesical sphincters and urinary retention have been reported.

Respiratory Depression: Hydrocodone Bitartrate may produce dose-related respiratory depression by acting directly on the brain stem respiratory center. Hydrocodone also affects the center that controls respiratory rhythm, and may produce irregular and periodic breathing. If significant respiratory depression occurs, it may be antagonized by the use of naloxone hydrochloride. Apply other supportive measures when indicated.

DRUG ABUSE AND DEPENDENCE
APAP/Hydrocodone is subject to the Federal Controlled Substance Act (Schedule C III).

Psychic dependence, physical dependence, and tolerance may develop upon repeated administration of narcotics; therefore, APAP/Hydrocodone should be prescribed and administered with caution. However, psychic dependence is unlikely to develop when APAP/Hydrocodone is used for a short time for the treatment of pain.

Physical dependence, the condition in which continued administration of the drug is required to prevent the appearance of a withdrawal syndrome, assumes clinically significant proportions only after several weeks of continued narcotic use, although some mild degree of physical dependence may develop after a few days of narcotic therapy. Tolerance, in which increasingly large doses are required in order to produce the same degree of analgesia, is manifested initially by a shortened duration of analgesic effect, and subsequently by decreases in the intensity of analgesia. The rate of development of tolerance varies among patients.

OVERDOSAGE
APAP
Signs and Symptoms: In acute APAP overdosage, dose-dependent, potentially fatal hepatic necrosis is the most serious adverse effect. Renal tubular necrosis, hypoglycemic coma, and thrombocytopenia may also occur.

In adults, hepatic toxicity has rarely been reported with acute overdoses of less than 10 grams and fatalities with less than 15 grams. Importantly, young children seem to be more resistant than adults to the hepatotoxic effect of an APAP overdose. Despite this, the measures outlined below should be initiated in any adult or child suspected of having ingested an APAP overdose.

Early symptoms following a potentially hepatotoxic overdose may include: nausea, vomiting, diaphoresis and general malaise. Clinical and laboratory evidence of hepatic toxicity may not be apparent until 48 to 72 hours post-ingestion.

Treatment: The stomach should be emptied promptly by lavage or by induction of emesis with syrup of ipecac. Patients' estimates of the quantity of a drug ingested are notoriously unreliable. Therefore, if an APAP overdose is suspected, a serum APAP assay should be obtained as early as possible, but no sooner than four hours following ingestion. Liver function studies should be obtained initially and repeated at 24-hour intervals.

The antidote, N-acetylcysteine, should be administered as early as possible, preferably within 16 hours of the overdose ingestion for optimal results, but in any case, within 24 hours. Following recovery, there are no residual, structural or functional hepatic abnormalities.

HYDROCODONE
Signs and Symptoms: Serious overdose with Hydrocodone is characterized by respiratory depression (a decrease in respiratory rate and/or tidal volume, Cheyne-Stokes respiration, cyanosis), extreme somnolence progressing to stupor or coma, skeletal muscle flaccidity, cold and clammy skin, and sometimes bradycardia and hypotension. In severe overdosage, apnea, circulatory collapse, cardiac arrest and death may occur.

Treatment: Primary attention should be given to the reestablishment of adequate respiratory exchange through provision of a patent airway and the institution of assisted or controlled ventilation. The narcotic antagonist naloxone is a specific antidote against respiratory depression which may result from overdosage or unusual sensitivity to narcotics, including Hydrocodone. Therefore, an appropriate dose of naloxone hydrochloride (see package insert) should be administered, preferably by the intravenous route, and simultaneously with efforts at respiratory resuscitation.

Since the duration of action of Hydrocodone may exceed that of the antagonist, the patient should be kept under continued surveillance and repeated doses of the antagonist should be administered as needed to maintain adequate respiration. An antagonist should not be administered in the absence of clinically significant respiratory or cardiovascular depression. Oxygen, intravenous fluids, vasopressors and other supportive measures should be employed as indicated.

Gastric emptying may be useful in removing unabsorbed drug.

DOSAGE AND ADMINISTRATION
Dosage should be adjusted according to the severity of the pain and the response of the patient. However, it should be kept in mind that tolerance to Hydrocodone can develop with continued use and that the incidence of untoward effects is dose related.

The usual adult dosage is: for APAP 500 mg/Hydrocodone Bitartrate 5 mg: one or two tablets every four to six hours as needed for pain. The total 24 hour dose should not exceed 8 tablets; for APAP 650 mg/Hydrocodone Bitartrate 10 mg: one tablet every four to six hours as needed for pain. The total 24 hour dose should not exceed 6 tablets; for APAP 650 mg/Hydrocodone Bitartrate 7.5 mg: one tablet every four to six hours as needed for pain. The total 24 hour dose should not exceed 6 tablets; for APAP 750 mg/Hydrocodone Bitartrate 7.5 mg: one tablet every four to six hours as needed for pain. The total 24 hour dose should not exceed 5 tablets.

Store at controlled room temperature 15°-30°C (59°-86°F).

Dispense in a tight, light-resistant container with a child-resistant closure as defined in the USP.

HOW SUPPLIED
CAPSULE (C-III): 500 MG-5 MG

AVERAGE UNIT PRICE (AVAILABLE SIZES)		GENERIC A-RATED AVERAGE PRICE (GAAP)	
BRAND	$0.38	100s	$31.19
GENERIC	$0.34	500s	$248.13
HCFA FUL (100s ea)	$0.18		

BRAND/MANUFACTURER	NDC	SIZE	AWP
◆ **BRAND**			
ZYDONE: Du Pont Multi	00056-0091-70	100s	$38.40
◆ **GENERICS**			
Goldline	00182-0156-01	100s	$18.00
Rugby	00536-3964-01	100s	$20.25
➤ HYDROCET: Carnrick	00086-0057-10	100s	$21.70
Major	00904-3442-60	100s	$23.95
MARGESIC-H: Marnel	00682-0808-01	100s	$24.40
Norton,HN	50732-0786-01	100s	$25.15
DOLAGESIC: Alphagen	59743-0011-01	100s	$26.05
ANOLOR DH 5: Blansett	51674-0010-01	100s	$26.95
UGESIC: Stewart Jackson	45985-0630-01	100s	$28.05
HYCOMED: Med-Tek	52349-0300-10	100s	$28.50
PANLOR: Pan Amer	00525-9301-01	100s	$30.90
LORCET-HD: Forest Pharm	00785-1120-01	100s	$34.01
ALLAY: Norton,HN	50732-0128-01	100s	$39.05
BANCAP H.C.: Forest Pharm	00456-0601-01	100s	$89.76
Norton,HN	50732-0786-05	500s	$117.37
BANCAP H.C.: Forest Pharm	00456-0601-02	500s	$378.89

ELIXIR (C-III): 500 MG-7.5 MG/15 ML

BRAND/MANUFACTURER	NDC	SIZE	AWP
○ **BRAND**			
LORTAB ELIXIR: Whitby	50474-0909-16	480 ml	$43.59

TABLETS (C-III): 500 MG-2.5 MG

AVERAGE UNIT PRICE (AVAILABLE SIZES)		GENERIC A-RATED AVERAGE PRICE (GAAP)	
GENERIC	$0.31	100s	$30.71

BRAND/MANUFACTURER	NDC	SIZE	AWP
◆ **GENERICS**			
Major	00904-7630-60	100s	$29.95
Watson	52544-0388-01	100s	$31.46

TABLETS (C-III): 500 MG-2.5 MG

BRAND/MANUFACTURER	NDC	SIZE	AWP
○ **BRAND**			
➤ LORTAB: Whitby	50474-0925-01	100s	$39.24

➤ SHOWN IN PRODUCT IDENTIFICATION GUIDE

TABLETS (C-III): 500 MG-5 MG

AVERAGE UNIT PRICE (AVAILABLE SIZES)		GENERIC A-RATED AVERAGE PRICE (GAAP)	
BRAND	$0.38	100s	$22.21
GENERIC	$0.20	500s	$78.41
HCFA FUL (100s ea)	$0.07	1000s	$145.70

BRAND/MANUFACTURER	NDC	SIZE	AWP
◆ BRAND			
➤ ANEXSIA: Boehr Mann Pharm	53169-0109-01	100s	$28.65
➤ VICODIN: Knoll	00044-0727-02	100s	$37.81
➤ LORTAB 5/500: Whitby	50474-0902-01	100s	$39.95
	50474-0902-60	100s ud	$42.70
➤ VICODIN: Knoll	00044-0727-41	100s ud	$44.98
	00044-0727-03	500s	$175.84
➤ LORTAB 5/500: Whitby	50474-0902-50	500s	$188.38
◆ GENERICS			
UDL	51079-0420-99	90s	$60.00
Geneva	00781-1606-01	100s	$14.50
Mason Dist	11845-0136-01	100s	$14.60
➤ Rugby	00536-3914-01	100s	$14.85
Goldline	00182-1765-01	100s	$15.00
Norton,HN	50732-0785-01	100s	$16.50
Mikart	46672-0052-10	100s	$16.65
Vintage	00254-3592-28	100s	$16.95
Martec	52555-0076-01	100s	$17.45
Moore,H.L.	00839-7176-06	100s	$17.54
Warner Chilcott	00047-0448-24	100s	$17.64
Major	00904-3440-60	100s	$18.50
Pharmics	00813-2500-01	100s	$18.52
➤ Watson	52544-0349-01	100s	$19.75
URL	00677-1184-01	100s	$20.24
➤ Qualitest	00603-3881-21	100s	$20.25
Parmed	00349-8494-01	100s	$20.76
Aligen	00405-0015-01	100s	$21.21
Schein	00364-0744-01	100s	$23.65
ONCET: Wakefield	59310-0103-10	100s	$26.56
PANACET 5/500: ECR	00095-0141-01	100s	$27.00
HY-PHEN: Ascher	00225-0450-15	100s	$27.54
➤ CO-GESIC: Central	00131-2104-37	100s	$29.95
UDL	51079-0420-21	100s	$39.10
Auro	55829-0849-10	100s ud	$22.89
Major	00904-3440-61	100s ud	$25.98
Goldline	00182-1765-89	100s ud	$37.00
UDL	51079-0420-20	100s ud	$39.10
Goldline	00182-1765-05	500s	$36.00
Geneva	00781-1606-05	500s	$60.50
Mason Dist	11845-0136-03	500s	$64.84
➤ Rugby	00536-3914-05	500s	$68.25
Moore,H.L.	00839-7176-12	500s	$69.59
Warner Chilcott	00047-0448-30	500s	$70.35
Vintage	00254-3592-35	500s	$71.48
Martec	52555-0076-05	500s	$73.62
Major	00904-3440-40	500s	$73.90
URL	00677-1184-05	500s	$79.95
Schein	00364-0744-05	500s	$80.00
Norton,HN	50732-0785-05	500s	$80.00
➤ Qualitest	00603-3881-28	500s	$80.15
Mikart	46672-0052-50	500s	$80.75
➤ Watson	52544-0349-05	500s	$97.75
Parmed	00349-8494-05	500s	$100.33
➤ CO-GESIC: Central	00131-2104-41	500s	$145.50
Parmed	00349-8494-53	550s	$104.18
Vintage	00254-3592-38	1000s	$121.44
Parmed	00349-8494-10	1000s	$169.95

TABLETS (C-III): 500 MG-7.5 MG

AVERAGE UNIT PRICE (AVAILABLE SIZES)		GENERIC A-RATED AVERAGE PRICE (GAAP)	
BRAND	$0.43	100s	$34.41
GENERIC	$0.33	500s	$152.13
HCFA FUL (100s ea)	$0.28		

BRAND/MANUFACTURER	NDC	SIZE	AWP
◆ BRAND			
➤ LORTAB 7.5/500: Whitby	50474-0907-01	100s	$44.67
	50474-0907-60	100s ud	$45.12
	50474-0907-50	500s	$197.33
◆ GENERICS			
Warner Chilcott	00047-0319-24	100s	$26.40
Goldline	00182-0691-01	100s	$29.00
Geneva	00781-1513-01	100s	$31.98
Qualitest	00603-3882-21	100s	$33.80
Rugby	00536-5507-01	100s	$33.85
Aligen	00405-0016-01	100s	$37.62
Watson	52544-0385-01	100s	$37.97
Moore,H.L.	00839-7781-06	100s	$39.29
Major	00904-7631-60	100s	$39.75
Warner Chilcott	00047-0319-30	500s	$116.59
Geneva	00781-1513-05	500s	$139.90
Qualitest	00603-3882-28	500s	$146.30
Goldline	00182-0691-05	500s	$156.00
Major	00904-7631-40	500s	$162.00
Watson	52544-0385-05	500s	$167.73
Moore,H.L.	00839-7781-12	500s	$176.38

TABLETS (C-III): 650 MG-7.5 MG

AVERAGE UNIT PRICE (AVAILABLE SIZES)	
BRAND	$0.40

BRAND/MANUFACTURER	NDC	SIZE	AWP
◆ BRAND			
➤ ANEXSIA: Boehr Mann Pharm	53169-0110-05	100s	$40.20
➤ LORCET PLUS: Forest Pharm	00785-1122-01	100s	$42.60
	00785-1122-63	100s ud	$46.51
➤ ANEXSIA: Boehr Mann Pharm	53169-0110-07	500s	$175.08
➤ LORCET PLUS: Forest Pharm	00785-1122-50	500s	$182.75

TABLETS (C-III): 650 MG-10 MG

BRAND/MANUFACTURER	NDC	SIZE	AWP
○ BRAND			
➤ LORCET 10/650: Forest Pharm	00785-6350-01	100s	$52.68
	00785-6350-63	100s ud	$56.68
	00785-6350-50	500s	$244.96

TABLETS (C-III): 750 MG-7.5 MG

AVERAGE UNIT PRICE (AVAILABLE SIZES)		GENERIC A-RATED AVERAGE PRICE (GAAP)	
BRAND	$0.43	100s	$37.07
GENERIC	$0.35	500s	$158.25
HCFA FUL (100s ea)	$0.32		

BRAND/MANUFACTURER	NDC	SIZE	AWP
◆ BRAND			
➤ VICODIN ES: Knoll	00044-0728-02	100s	$41.69
	00044-0728-41	100s ud	$49.61
	00044-0728-03	500s	$194.78
◆ GENERICS			
Warner Chilcott	00047-0486-24	100s	$30.83
Goldline	00182-0681-01	100s	$32.00
Schein	00364-2505-01	100s	$32.50
Geneva	00781-1532-01	100s	$32.76
Moore,H.L.	00839-7728-06	100s	$32.93
Qualitest	00603-3883-21	100s	$34.40
Rugby	00536-5508-01	100s	$34.69
➤ Watson	52544-0387-01	100s	$35.44
Major	00904-7632-60	100s	$37.55
Aligen	00405-0017-01	100s	$41.66
UDL	51079-0748-21	100s	$48.10
URL	00677-1504-01	100s	$52.00
Warner Chilcott	00047-0486-30	500s	$126.07
Goldline	00182-0681-05	500s	$150.00
Geneva	00781-1532-05	500s	$153.09
Qualitest	00603-3883-28	500s	$160.74
Rugby	00536-5508-05	500s	$162.00
➤ Watson	52544-0387-05	500s	$165.56
Major	00904-7632-40	500s	$165.95
Moore,H.L.	00839-7728-12	500s	$166.58
Aligen	00405-0017-02	500s	$174.27

Acetaminophen/Butalbital/Caffeine

DESCRIPTION

Acetaminophen/Butalbital/Caffeine is available as both tablets and capsules for oral administration.

The tablets are available as:

Acetaminophen	325 mg
Butalbital,* USP	50 mg
*WARNING: May be habit forming.	
Caffeine, USP	40 mg

and

Acetaminophen	500 mg
Butalbital, *USP	50 mg
*WARNING: May be habit forming.	
Caffeine, USP	40 mg

The capsules are available as:

Acetaminophen	325 mg
Butalbital, *USP	50 mg
*WARNING: May be habit forming.	
Caffeine, USP	40 mg

Butalbital, 5-allyl-5-isobutylbarbituric acid, a white, odorless, crystalline powder having a slightly bitter taste, is a short to intermediate-acting barbiturate.

The molecular formula is $C_{11}H_{16}N_2O_3$. The molecular weight is 224.26

Acetaminophen, 4'-hydroxyacetanilide, is a non-opiate, non-salicylate analgesic and antipyretic which occurs as a white, odorless, crystalline powder possessing a slightly bitter taste.

◆ RATED THERAPEUTICALLY EQUIVALENT; ◇ THERAPEUTIC EQUIVALENCE UNCONFIRMED; ○ UNRATED

The molecular formula is $C_8H_9NO_2$ The molecular weight is 151.16

Caffeine, 1,3,7-trimethylxanthine, is a central nervous system stimulant which occurs as a white powder or white glistening needles. It also has a bitter taste.

The molecular formula is $C_8H_{10}N_4O_2$. The molecular weight is 194.19

CLINICAL PHARMACOLOGY

Pharmacologically Acetaminophen/Butalbital/Caffeine combines the analgesic properties of Acetaminophen-Caffeine with the anxiolytic and muscle relaxant properties of Butalbital.

INDICATIONS AND USAGE

Acetaminophen/Butalbital/Caffeine is indicated for the relief of the symptom complex of tension (or muscle contraction) headache.

CONTRAINDICATIONS

Hypersensitivity to acetaminophen, barbiturates, or caffeine. Patients with porphyria.

PRECAUTIONS

GENERAL

Barbiturates should be administered with caution, if at all, to patients who are mentally depressed, have suicidal tendencies, or a history of drug abuse.

Elderly or debilitated patients may react to barbiturates with marked excitement, depression, and confusion. In some persons, barbiturates repeatedly produce excitement rather than depression.

INFORMATION FOR PATIENTS

Practitioners should give the following information and instructions to patients receiving barbiturates:

A. The use of barbiturates carries with it an associated risk of psychological and/or physical dependence. The patient should be warned against increasing the dose of the drug without consulting a physician.

B. Barbiturates may impair mental and/or physical abilities required for the performance of potentially hazardous tasks (e.g., driving, operating machinery, etc.).

C. Alcohol should not be consumed while taking barbiturates. Concurrent use of the barbiturates with other CNS depressants (e.g., alcohol, narcotics, tranquilizers, and antihistamines) may result in additional CNS depressant effects.

DRUG INTERACTIONS

Patients receiving narcotic analgesics, antipsychotics, anti-anxiety agents, or other CNS depressants (including alcohol) concomitantly with Acetaminophen/Butalbital/Caffeine may exhibit additive CNS depressant effects.

Drugs	Effect
Butalbital w/coumarin anticoagulants	Decreased effect of anticoagulant because of increased metabolism resulting from enzyme induction.
Butalbital w/tricyclic antidepressants	Decreased blood levels of the antidepressant.

USAGE IN PREGNANCY

Adequate studies have not been performed in animals to determine whether this drug affects fertility in males or females, has teratogenic potential or has other adverse effects on the fetus. There are no well-controlled studies in pregnant women. Although there is no clearly defined risk, one cannot exclude the possibility of infrequent or subtle damage to the human fetus. Acetaminophen/Butalbital/Caffeine should be used in pregnant women only when clearly needed.

NURSING MOTHERS

The effects of Acetaminophen/Butalbital/Caffeine on infants of nursing mothers are not known. Barbiturates are excreted in the breast milk of nursing mothers. The serum levels in infants are believed to be insignificant with therapeutic doses.

PEDIATRIC USE

Safety and effectiveness in children below the age of 12 have not been established.

ADVERSE REACTIONS

The most frequent adverse reactions are drowsiness and dizziness. Less frequent adverse reactions are light-headedness and gastrointestinal disturbances including nausea, vomiting, and flatulence. Mental confusion or depression can occur due to intolerance or overdosage of Butalbital. Several cases of dermatological reactions including toxic epidermal necrolysis and erythema multiforme have been reported.

DRUG ABUSE AND DEPENDENCE

Prolonged use of barbiturates can produce drug dependence, characterized by psychic dependence and tolerance. The abuse liability of Acetaminophen/Butalbital/Caffeine is similar to that of other barbiturate-containing drug combinations. Caution should be exercised when prescribing medication for patients with a known propensity for taking excessive quantities of drugs, which is not uncommon in patients with chronic tension headache.

OVERDOSAGE

The toxic effects of acute overdosage of Acetaminophen/Butalbital/Caffeine are attributable mainly to its barbiturate component, and, to a lesser extent, acetaminophen. Because toxic effects of caffeine occur in very high dosages only, the possibility of significant caffeine toxicity from Acetaminophen/Butalbital/Caffeine overdosage is unlikely.

BARBITURATE

Signs and Symptoms: Drowsiness, confusion, coma; respiratory depression; hypotension; shock.

Treatment: 1. Maintenance of an adequate airway, with assisted respiration oxygen administration as necessary.

2. Monitoring of vital signs and fluid balance.

3. If the patient is conscious and has not lost the gag reflex, emesis may be induced with ipecac. Care should be taken to prevent pulmonary aspiration of vomitus. After completion of vomiting, 30 grams of activated charcoal in a glass of water may be administered.

4. If emesis is contraindicated, gastric lavage may be performed with a cuffed endotracheal tube in place with the patient in the facedown position. Activated charcoal may be left in the emptied stomach and a saline cathartic administered.

5. Fluid therapy and other standard treatment of shock, if needed.

6. If renal function is normal, forced diuresis may aid in the elimination of the barbiturate. Alkalinization of the urine increases renal excretion of some barbiturates, especially phenobarbital.

7. Although not recommended as a routine procedure, hemodialysis may be used in severe barbiturate intoxication or if the patient is anuric or in shock.

ACETAMINOPHEN

Signs and Symptoms: In acute Acetaminophen overdosage, dose-dependent, potentially fatal hepatic necrosis is the most serious adverse effect. Renal tubular necrosis, hypoglycemic coma, and thrombocytopenia may also occur.

In adults, hepatic toxicity has rarely been reported with acute overdoses of less than 10 grams and fatalities with less than 15 grams. Importantly, young children seem to be more resistant than adults to the hepatotoxic effect of an Acetaminophen overdose.

Early Symptoms following a Potentially Hepatotoxic Overdosage may include: nausea, vomiting, diaphoresis, and general malaise. Clinical and laboratory evidence of hepatic toxicity may not be apparent until 48-72 hours post-ingestion.

Treatment: The stomach should be emptied promptly by lavage or by induction of emesis with syrup of ipecac. Patients' estimates of the quantity of a drug ingested are notoriously unreliable. Therefore, if an Acetaminophen overdose is suspected, a serum Acetaminophen assay should be obtained as early as possible, but no sooner than four hours following ingestion. Liver function studies should be obtained initially and repeated at 24-hour intervals.

The antidote, N-acetylcysteine, should be administered as early as possible, preferably within 16 hours of the overdose ingestion for optimal results, but in any case, within 24 hours. Following recovery, there are no residual, structural or functional hepatic abnormalities.

DOSAGE AND ADMINISTRATION

One or 2 tablets every 4 hours as needed. Do not exceed 6 tablets per day.

Store at room temperature, below 86°F (30°C); dispense in a tight, light-resistant container. Protect from moisture.

HOW SUPPLIED
CAPSULE: 325 MG-50 MG-40 MG

AVERAGE UNIT PRICE (AVAILABLE SIZES)		GENERIC A-RATED AVERAGE PRICE (GAAP)	
BRAND	$0.23	100s	$27.28
GENERIC	$0.25		
HCFA FUL (100s ea)	$0.12		

BRAND/MANUFACTURER	NDC	SIZE	AWP
◆ BRAND			
TWO-DYNE: Hyrex	00314-2229-01	100s	$16.70
EZOL: Stewart Jackson	45985-0578-01	100s	$29.70
◆ GENERICS			
ANOQUAN: Mallard	59441-0178-01	100s	$7.95
TENAKE: Seatrace	00551-0181-01	100s	$19.85
ARCET: EconoMed	38130-0325-01	100s	$19.98
MARGESIC: Marnel	00682-0804-01	100s	$21.10
FEMCET: Northampton	58436-0703-01	100s	$22.19
ANOLOR 300: Blansett	51674-0009-01	100s	$22.85
Qualitest	00603-2546-21	100s	$23.70
GEONE: Alphagen	59743-0004-01	100s	$23.75
TENCET: Roberts/Hauck	59441-0153-01	100s	$25.56
MEDIGESIC: U.S. Pharm	52747-0600-60	100s	$40.38
▶ ESGIC: Forest Pharm	00535-0012-01	100s	$72.73
ANOQUAN: Mallard	59441-0178-05	500s	$22.90

TABLET: 325 MG-50 MG-40 MG

AVERAGE UNIT PRICE (AVAILABLE SIZES)		GENERIC A-RATED AVERAGE PRICE (GAAP)	
BRAND	$0.49	100s	$18.40
GENERIC	$0.18	500s	$83.41
HCFA FUL (100s ea)	$0.06	1000s	$104.14

➤ SHOWN IN PRODUCT IDENTIFICATION GUIDE

BRAND/MANUFACTURER	NDC	SIZE	AWP
◆ **BRAND**			
➤ FIORICET: Sandoz Pharm	00078-0084-05	100s	$47.76
	00078-0084-06	100s ud	$52.20
	00078-0084-08	500s	$228.24
◆ **GENERICS**			
Southwood	58016-0995-15	15s	$5.07
Southwood	58016-0995-20	20s	$6.14
Southwood	58016-0995-30	30s	$6.81
Southwood	58016-0995-50	50s	$9.28
Major	00904-3280-60	100s	$10.60
ISOCET: Rugby	00536-5567-01	100s	$11.48
Schein	00364-2297-01	100s	$11.50
Qualitest	00603-2547-21	100s	$12.00
Geneva	00781-1901-01	100s	$12.90
➤ Halsey Pharm	00879-0567-01	100s	$13.75
URL	00677-1242-01	100s	$13.85
Parmed	00349-8793-01	100s	$13.89
ARCET: EconoMed	38130-0111-01	100s	$13.96
Martec	52555-0079-01	100s	$14.28
Lemmon	00093-0854-01	100s	$15.00
Mikart	46672-0053-10	100s	$15.25
Goldline	00182-1274-01	100s	$15.25
Caremark	00339-5843-12	100s	$15.46
Moore,H.L.	00839-7480-06	100s	$15.92
Moore,H.L.	00839-7831-06	100s	$15.92
DOLMAR: Marlop	12939-0811-12	100s	$21.35
REPAN: Everett	00642-0162-10	100s	$26.00
ESGIC: Forest Pharm	00456-0630-01	100s	$77.14
Schein	00364-2297-05	500s	$33.75
Moore,H.L.	00839-7480-12	500s	$38.81
➤ Halsey Pharm	00879-0567-05	500s	$42.39
ISOCET: Rugby	00536-5567-05	500s	$43.32
Parmed	00349-8793-05	500s	$49.88
Qualitest	00603-2547-28	500s	$52.51
Major	00904-3280-40	500s	$52.90
Mikart	46672-0053-50	500s	$74.95
Goldline	00182-1274-05	500s	$74.95
DOLMAR: Marlop	12939-0811-50	500s	$101.40
ESGIC: Forest Pharm	00456-0630-02	500s	$352.60
Parmed	00349-8793-10	1000s	$89.77
➤ Halsey Pharm	00879-0567-10	1000s	$118.50

TABLET: 500 MG-50 MG-40 MG

BRAND/MANUFACTURER	NDC	SIZE	AWP
○ **BRAND**			
➤ ESGIC-PLUS: Forest Pharm	00456-0678-01	100s	$62.59
	00456-0678-02	500s	$291.02

Acetaminophen/Butalbital/ Caffeine/Codeine Phosphate

DESCRIPTION
Acetaminophen/Butalbital/Caffeine/Codeine Phosphate is supplied in capsule form for oral administration.

Each capsule contains:

Codeine Phosphate, USP . . . . .30 mg (½ gr)
   Warning: May be habit-forming.
Butalbital, USP . . . . .50 mg
   Warning: May be habit-forming.
Caffeine, USP . . . . .40 mg
Acetaminophen, USP . . . . 325 mg

Codeine Phosphate [morphine-3-methyl ether Phosphate (1:1) (salt) hemihydrate, $C_{18}H_{24}NO_7P$, anhydrous mw 397.37], a white crystalline powder, is a narcotic analgesic and antitussive.

Butalbital (5-allyl-5-isobutylbarbituric acid, $C_{11}H_{16}N_2O_3$, mw 224.26), a slightly bitter, white crystalline powder, is a short-to intermediate-acting barbiturate.

Caffeine (1,3,7-trimethylxanthine, $C_8H_{10}N_4O_2$, mw 194.19), a bitter, white crystalline powder, is a central nervous system stimulant.

Acetaminophen (4′-hydroxyacetanilide, $C_8H_9NO_2$, mw 151.16), a slightly bitter white crystalline powder, is a nonopiate, non-salicylate analgesic and antipyretic.

Active Ingredients: Codeine Phosphate, USP, Butalbital, USP, Caffeine, USP, and Acetaminophen, USP.

CLINICAL PHARMACOLOGY
Acetaminophen/Butalbital/Caffeine/Codeine Phosphate (APAP/Butalbital/Caff/Cod) is a combination drug product intended as a treatment for tension headache.

APAP/Butalbital/Caff consists of a fixed combination of Butalbital 50 mg, Acetaminophen 325 mg and Caffeine 40 mg. The role each component plays in the relief of the complex of symptoms known as tension headache is incompletely understood.

PHARMACOKINETICS
The behavior of the individual components is described below.

CODEINE
Codeine is readily absorbed from the gastrointestinal tract. It is rapidly distributed from the intravascular spaces to the various body tissues, with preferential uptake by parenchymatous organs such as the liver, spleen and kidney. Codeine crosses the blood-brain barrier, and is found in fetal tissue and breast milk. The plasma concentration does not correlate with brain concentration or relief of pain; however, Codeine is not bound to plasma proteins and does not accumulate in body tissues.

The plasma half-life is about 2.9 hours. The elimination of Codeine is primarily via the kidneys, and about 90% of an oral dose is excreted by the kidneys within 24 hours of dosing. The urinary secretion products consist of free and glucuronide conjugated Codeine (about 70%), free and conjugated norCodeine (about 10%), free and conjugated morphine (about 10%), normorphine (4%), and hydrocodone (1%). The remainder of the dose is excreted in the feces.

At therapeutic doses, the analgesic effect reaches a peak within 2 hours and persists between 4 and 6 hours. See *"Overdosage"* for toxicity information.

BUTALBITAL
Butalbital is well absorbed from the gastrointestinal tract and is expected to distribute to most tissues in the body. Barbiturates in general may appear in breast milk and readily cross the placental barrier. They are bound to plasma and tissue proteins to a varying degree and binding increases directly as a function of lipid solubility.

Elimination of Butalbital is primarily via the kidney (59%-88% of the dose) as unchanged drug or metabolites. The plasma half-life is about 35 hours. Urinary excretion products include parent drug (about 3.6% of the dose), 5-isobutyl-5-(2,3-dihydroxypropyl) barbituric acid (about 24% of the dose), 5-allyl-5(3-hydroxy-2-methyl-1-propyl) barbituric acid (about 4.8% of the dose), products with the barbituric acid ring hydrolyzed with excretion of urea (about 14% of the dose), as well as unidentified materials. Of the material excreted in the urine, 32% is conjugated.

See *"Overdosage"* for toxicity information.

CAFFEINE
Like most xanthines, Caffeine is rapidly absorbed and distributed in all body tissues and fluids, including the CNS, fetal tissues, and breast milk.

Caffeine is cleared through metabolism and excretion in the urine. The plasma half-life is about 3 hours. Hepatic biotransformation prior to excretion results in about equal amounts of 1-methyl-xanthine and 1-methyluric acid. Of the 70% of the dose that is recovered in the urine, only 3% is unchanged drug.

See *"Overdosage"* for toxicity information.

ACETAMINOPHEN
Acetaminophen is rapidly absorbed from the gastrointestinal tract and is distributed throughout most body tissues. The plasma half-life is 1.25-3 hours, but may be increased by liver damage and following overdosage. Elimination of Acetaminophen is principally by liver metabolism (conjugation) and subsequent renal excretion of metabolites. Approximately 85% of an oral dose appears in the urine within 24 hours of administration, most as the glucuronide conjugate, with small amounts of other conjugates and unchanged drug.

See *"Overdosage"* for toxicity information.

INDICATIONS
APAP/Butalbital/Caff/Cod is indicated for the relief of the symptom complex of tension (or muscle contraction) headache.

Evidence supporting the efficacy and safety of APAP/Butalbital/Caff/Cod in the treatment of multiple recurrent headaches is unavailable. Caution in this regard is required because Codeine and Butalbital are habit-forming and potentially abusable.

CONTRAINDICATIONS
APAP/Butalbital/Caff/Cod is contraindicated under the following conditions.
   —Hypersensitivity or intolerance to Acetaminophen, Caffeine, Butalbital, or Codeine.
   —Patients with porphyria.

WARNINGS
In the presence of head injury or other intracranial lesions, the respiratory depressant effects of Codeine and other narcotics may be markedly enhanced, as well as their capacity for elevating cerebrospinal fluid pressure. Narcotics also produce other CNS depressant effects, such as drowsiness, that may further obscure the clinical course of the patients with head injuries.

Codeine or other narcotics may obscure signs on which to judge the diagnosis or clinical course of patients with acute abdominal conditions.

Butalbital and Codeine are both habit-forming and potentially abusable. Consequently, the extended use of APAP/Butalbital/Caff/Cod is not recommended.

PRECAUTIONS
GENERAL
APAP/Butalbital/Caff/Cod should be prescribed with caution in certain special-risk patients such as the elderly or debilitated, and those with severe impairment of renal or hepatic function, head injuries, elevated intracranial pressure, acute abdominal conditions, hypothyroidism, urethral stricture. Addison's disease, or prostatic hypertrophy

---

◆ **RATED THERAPEUTICALLY EQUIVALENT;** ◇ **THERAPEUTIC EQUIVALENCE UNCONFIRMED;** ○ **UNRATED**

INFORMATION FOR PATIENTS
APAP/Butalbital/Caff/Cod may impair mental and/or physical abilities required for the performance of potentially hazardous tasks such as driving a car or operating machinery. Such tasks should be avoided while taking APAP/Butalbital/Caff/Cod.

Alcohol and other CNS depressants may produce an additive CNS depression, when taken with APAP/Butalbital/Caff/Cod and should be avoided.

Codeine and Butalbital may be habit-forming. Patients should take the drug only for as long as it is prescribed, in the amounts prescribed, and no more frequently than prescribed.

LABORATORY TESTS
In patients with severe hepatic or renal disease, effects of therapy should be monitored with serial liver and/or renal function tests.

DRUG INTERACTIONS
The CNS effects of Butalbital may be enhanced by monoamine oxidase (MAO) inhibitors.

APAP/Butalbital/Caff/Cod may enhance the effects of:
—Other narcotic analgesics, alcohol, general anesthetics, tranquilizers such as chlordiazepoxide, sedative-hypnotics, or other CNS depressants, causing increased CNS depression.

DRUG/LABORATORY TEST INTERACTIONS
CODEINE
Codeine may increase serum amylase levels.

ACETAMINOPHEN
Acetaminophen may produce false-positive test results for urinary 5-hydroxyindoleacetic acid.

CARCINOGENESIS, MUTAGENESIS, IMPAIRMENT OF FERTILITY
No adequate studies have been conducted in animals to determine whether Acetaminophen, Codeine and Butalbital have a potential for carcinogenesis or mutagenesis. No adequate studies have been conducted in animals to determine whether Acetaminophen and Butalbital have a potential for impairment of fertility.

PREGNANCY
TERATOGENIC EFFECTS
Pregnancy category C: Animal reproduction studies have not been conducted with APAP/Butalbital/Caff/Cod. It is also not known whether APAP/Butalbital/Caff/Cod can cause fetal harm when administered to a pregnant woman or can affect reproduction capacity. APAP/Butalbital/Caff/Cod should be given to a pregnant woman only when clearly needed.

NONTERATOGENIC EFFECTS
Withdrawal seizures were reported in a two-day-old male infant whose mother had taken a Butalbital-containing drug during the last 2 months of pregnancy. Butalbital was found in the infant's serum. The infant was given phenobarbital 5 mg/kg, which was tapered without further seizure or other withdrawal symptoms.

LABOR AND DELIVERY
Use of Codeine during labor may lead to respiratory depression in the neonate.

NURSING MOTHERS
Caffeine, barbiturates, Acetaminophen and Codeine are excreted in breast milk in small amounts, but the significance of their effects on nursing infants is not known. Because of potential for serious adverse reactions in nursing infants from APAP/Butalbital/Caff/Cod, a decision should be made whether to discontinue nursing or to discontinue the drug, taking into account the importance of the drug to the mother.

PEDIATRIC USE
Safety and effectiveness in children below the age of 12 have not been established.

ADVERSE REACTIONS
FREQUENTLY OBSERVED
The most frequently reported adverse reactions are drowsiness, light-headedness, dizziness, sedation, shortness of breath, nausea, vomiting, abdominal pain, and intoxicated feeling.

INFREQUENTLY OBSERVED
All adverse events tabulated below are classified as infrequent.

Central Nervous: headache, shaky feeling, tingling, agitation, fainting, fatigue, heavy eyelids, high energy, hot spells, numbness, sluggishness, seizure. Mental confusion, excitement or depression can also occur due to intolerance, particularly in elderly or debilitated patients, or due to overdosage of Butalbital.

Autonomic Nervous: dry mouth, hyperhidrosis.

Gastrointestinal: difficulty swallowing, heartburn, flatulence, constipation.

Cardiovascular: tachycardia.

Musculoskeletal: leg pain, muscle fatigue.

Genitourinary: diuresis.

Miscellaneous: pruritus, fever, earache, nasal congestion, tinnitus, euphoria, allergic reactions.

The following adverse reactions have been voluntarily reported as temporally associated with ASA/Butalbital/Caff/Cod, a related product containing Aspirin, Butalbital, Caffeine, and Codeine.

Central Nervous: abuse, addiction, anxiety, disorientation, hallucination, hyperactivity, insomnia, libido decrease, nervousness, neuropathy, psychosis, sexual activity increase, slurred speech, twitching, unconsciousness, vertigo.

Autonomic Nervous: epistaxis, flushing, miosis, salivation.

Gastrointestinal: anorexia, appetite increased, diarrhea, esophagitis, gastroenteritis, gastrointestinal spasms, hiccup, mouth burning, pyloric ulcer.

Cardiovascular: chest pain, hypotensive reaction, palpitations, syncope.

Skin: erythema, erythema multiforme, exfoliative dermatitis, hives, rash, toxic epidermal necrolysis.

Urinary: kidney impairment, urinary difficulty.

Miscellaneous: allergic reaction, anaphylactic shock, cholangiocarcinoma, drug interaction with erythromycin (stomach upset), edema.

The following adverse drug events may be borne in mind as potential effects of the components of APAP/Butalbital/Caff/Cod. Potential effects of high dosage are listed in the "Overdosage" section.

Acetaminophen: allergic reactions, rash, thrombocytopenia, agranulocytosis.

Caffeine: cardiac stimulation, irritability, tremor, dependence, nephrotoxicity, hyperglycemia.

Codeine: nausea, vomiting, drowsiness, light-headedness, constipation, pruritus.
Several cases of dermatological reactions, including toxic epidermal necrolysis and erythema multiforme, have been reported for APAP/Butalbital/Caff.

DRUG ABUSE AND DEPENDENCE
CONTROLLED SUBSTANCE
APAP/Butalbital/Caff/Cod is controlled by the Drug Enforcement Administration and is classified under Schedule III.

ABUSE AND DEPENDENCE
CODEINE
Codeine can produce drug dependence of the morphine type and, therefore, has the potential for being abused. Psychological dependence, physical dependence, and tolerance may develop upon repeated administration and it should be prescribed and administered with the same degree of caution appropriate for the use of other oral narcotic medications.

BUTALBITAL
Barbiturates may be habit-forming: Tolerance, psychological dependence, and physical dependence may occur especially following prolonged use of high doses of barbiturates. The average daily dose for the barbiturate addict is usually about 1,500 mg. As tolerance to barbiturates develops, the amount needed to maintain the same level of intoxication increases; tolerance to a fatal dosage, however, does not increase more than two-fold. As this occurs, the margin between an intoxication dosage and fatal dosage becomes smaller. The lethal dose of a barbiturate is far less if alcohol is also ingested. Major withdrawal symptoms (convulsions and delirium) may occur within 16 hours and last up to 5 days after abrupt cessation of these drugs. Intensity of withdrawal symptoms gradually declines over a period of approximately 15 days. Treatment of barbiturate dependence consists of cautious and gradual withdrawal of the drug. Barbiturate-dependent patients can be withdrawn by using a number of different withdrawal regimens. One method involves initiating treatment at the patient's regular dosage level and gradually decreasing the daily dosage as tolerated by the patient.

OVERDOSAGE
Following an acute overdosage of APAP/Butalbital/Caff/Cod toxicity may result from the barbiturate, the Codeine, or the Acetaminophen. Toxicity due to the Caffeine is less likely, due to the relatively small amounts in this formulation.

SIGNS AND SYMPTOMS
Toxicity from *barbiturate* poisoning include drowsiness, confusion, and coma; respiratory depression; hypotension; and hypovolemic shock. Toxicity from *Codeine* poisoning includes the opioid triad of: pinpoint pupils, depression of respiration, and loss of consciousnes. Convulsions may occur. In *Acetaminophen* overdosage: dose-dependent, potentially fatal hepatic necrosis is the most serious adverse effect. Renal tubular necroses, hypoglycemic coma, and thrombocytopenia may also occur. Early symptoms following a potentially hepatotoxic overdose may include: nausea, vomiting, diaphoresis, and general malaise. Clinical and laboratory evidence of hepatic toxicity may not be apparent until 48-72 hours postingestion. In adults hepatic toxicity has rarely been reported with acute overdoses of less than 10 grams, or fatalities with less than 15 grams. Acute *Caffeine* poisoning may cause insomnia, restlessness, tremor, and delirium, tachycardia, and extrasystoles.

TREATMENT
A single or multiple overdose with APAP/Butalbital/Caff/Cod is a potentially lethal polydrug overdose, and consultation with a regional poison control center is recommended. Immediate treatment includes support of cardiorespiratory function and measures to reduce drug absorption. Vomiting should be induced mechanically, or with syrup of ipecac, if the patient is alert (adequate pharyngeal and laryngeal reflexes). Oral activated charcoal (1 g/kg) should follow gastric emptying. The first dose should be accompanied by an appropriate cathartic. If repeated doses are used, the cathartic might be included with alternate doses as

required. Hypotension is usually hypovolemic and should respond to fluids. Pressors should be avoided. A cuffed endotracheal tube should be inserted before gastric lavage of the unconscious patient and, when necessary, to provide assisted respiration. If renal function is normal, forced diuresis may aid in the elimination of the barbiturate. Alkalinization of the urine increases renal excretion of some barbiturates, especially phenobarbital.

Meticulous attention should be given to maintaining adequate pulmonary ventilation. In severe cases of intoxication, peritoneal dialysis, or preferably hemodialysis may be considered. If hypoprothrombinemia occurs due to Acetaminophen overdose, vitamin K should be administered intravenously.

Naloxone, a narcotic antagonist, can reverse respiratory depression and coma associated with opioid overdose. Naloxone 0.4-2 mg is given parenterally. Since the duration of action of Codeine may exceed that of the naloxone, the patient should be kept under continuous surveillance and repeated doses of the antagonist should be administered as needed to maintain adequate respiration. A narcotic antagonist should not be administered in the absence of clinically significant respiratory or cardiovascular depression.

If the dose of Acetaminophen may have exceeded 140 mg/kg, N-acetyl-cysteine should be administered as early as possible. Serum Acetaminophen levels should be obtained, since levels 4 or more hours following ingestion help predict Acetaminophen toxicity. Do not await Acetaminophen assay results before initiating treatment. Hepatic enzymes should be obtained initially, and repeated at 24-hour intervals.

Methemoglobinemia over 30% should be treated with methylene blue by slow intravenous administration.

TOXIC DOSES (FOR ADULTS)
Butalbital: toxic dose 1.0 g (20 capsules of APAP/Butalbital/Caff/Cod)

Acetaminophen: toxic dose of 10 g (30 capsules of APAP/Butalbital/Caff/Cod)

Caffeine: toxic dose 1.0 g (25 capsules of APAP/Butalbital/Caff/Cod)

Codeine: toxic dose 240 mg (8 capsules of APAP/Butalbital/Caff/Cod)

DOSAGE AND ADMINISTRATION
One or 2 capsules every 4 hours. Total daily dosage should not exceed 6 capsules.
Extended and repeated use of this product is not recommended because of the potential for physical dependence.

Store and dispense below 86°F (30°C); tight container.

HOW SUPPLIED
CAPSULE (C-III): 325 MG-50 MG-40 MG-30 MG

BRAND/MANUFACTURER	NDC	SIZE	AWP
○ BRAND			
➤ FIORICET W/CODEINE: Sandoz Pharm	00078-0243-05	100s	$94.56

Acetaminophen/Caffeine/ Chlorpheniramine/Hydrocodone/ Phenylephrine

DESCRIPTION
Acetaminophen/Caffeine/Chlorpheniramine/Hydrocodone/Phenylephrine (APAP/Caff/CPM/Hydrocod/PE) contains Hydrocodone (dihydrocodeinone) Bitartrate, a semi-synthetic centrally-acting narcotic antitussive; Chlorpheniramine Maleate, an antihistamine; Phenylephrine Hydrochloride, a sympathomimetic amine decongestant; Acetaminophen, an analgesic/antipyretic; and Caffeine, a centrally-acting stimulant; for oral administration.

Each APAP/Caff/CPM/Hydrocod/PE tablet contains:

Hydrocodone Bitartrate, USP	5 mg
WARNING: May be habit forming	
Chlorpheniramine Maleate, USP	2 mg
Phenylephrine Hydrochloride, USP	10 mg
Acetaminophen, USP	250 mg
Caffeine anhydrous, USP	30 mg

CLINICAL PHARMACOLOGY
Clinical trials have proven Hydrocodone Bitartrate to be an effective antitussive agent which is pharmacologically 2 to 8 times as potent as codeine. At equi-effective doses, its sedative action is greater than codeine. The precise mechanism of action of Hydrocodone and other opiates is not known, however, Hydrocodone is believed to act by directly depressing the cough center. In excessive doses Hydrocodone, like other opium derivatives, will depress respiration. The effects of Hydrocodone in therapeutic doses on the cardiovascular system is insignificant. The constipation effects of Hydrocodone are much weaker than that of morphine and no stronger than that of codeine. Hydrocodone can produce miosis, euphoria, physical and psychological dependence. At therapeutic antitussive doses, it does exert analgesic effects. Following a 10 mg oral dose of Hydrocodone administered to five adult male human subjects, the mean peak concentration was 23.6 ± 5.2 ng/mL. Maximum serum levels were achieved at 1.3 ± 0.3 hours and the half-life was determined to be 3.8 ± 0.3 hours. Hydrocodone exhibits a complex pattern of metabolism including O-demethylation. N-demethylation and 6-keto reduction to the corresponding 6-α- and 6-β-hydroxymetabolites.

Chlorpheniramine Maleate is a competitive H_1-receptor histamine blocking drug, thereby counteracting the effects of histamine release associated with allergic manifestations of upper respiratory tract inflammatory disorders. H_1-blocking drugs inhibit the actions of histamine on smooth muscle, capillary permeability, and can both stimulate and depress the central nervous system. Phenylephrine Hydrochloride effects its vasconstrictor activity by releasing noradrenaline from sympathetic nerve endings, and from direct stimulation of α-adrenoreceptors in blood vessels. Acetaminophen is an antipyretic and peripherally acting analgesic. Caffeine is a central nervous system stimulant.

INDICATIONS AND USAGE
APAP/Caff/CPM/Hydrocod/PE is indicated for the symptomatic relief of cough, nasal congestion, and discomfort associated with upper respiratory tract infections.

CONTRAINDICATIONS
APAP/Caff/CPM/Hydrocod/PE is contraindicated in patients hypersensitive to any component of the drug, and concurrent MAO inhibitor therapy. Patients known to be hypersensitive to other opioids, antihistamines, or sympathomimetic amines may exhibit cross sensitivity with APAP/Caff/CPM/Hydrocod/PE. Phenylephrine is contraindicated in patients with heart disease, hypertension, diabetes or hyperthyroidism. Hydrocodone is contraindicated in the presence of an intracranial lesion associated with increased intracranial pressure, and whenever ventilatory function is depressed.

WARNINGS
May be habit forming. Hydrocodone can produce drug dependence of the morphine type and therefore has the potential for being abused. Psychic dependence, physical dependence and tolerance may develop upon repeated administration of APAP/Caff/CPM/Hydrocod/PE and it should be prescribed and administered with the same degree of caution appropriate to the use of other narcotic drugs (See *"Drug Abuse and Dependence"*).

Respiratory Depression: APAP/Caff/CPM/Hydrocod/PE produces dose-related respiratory depression by directly acting on brain stem respiratory centers. If respiratory depression occurs, it may be antagonized by the use of naloxone and other supportive measures when indicated.

Head Injury and Increased Intracranial Pressure: The respiratory depressant properties of narcotics and their capacity to elevate cerebrospinal fluid pressure may be markedly exaggerated in the presence of head injury, other intracranial lesions or a pre-existing increase in intracranial pressure. Furthermore, narcotics produce adverse reactions which may obscure the clinical course of patients with head injuries.

Acute Abdominal Conditions: The administration of APAP/Caff/CPM/Hydrocod/PE or other narcotics may obscure the diagnosis or clinical course of patients with acute abdominal conditions.

Phenylephrine: Hypertensive crises can occur with concurrent use of Phenylephrine and monoamine oxidase (MAO) inhibitors, indomethacin or with beta-blockers and methyldopa.

If a hypertensive crisis occurs these drugs should be discontinued immediately and therapy to lower blood pressure should be instituted immediately. Fever should be managed by means of external cooling.

Chlorpheniramine: Antihistamines may produce drowsiness or excitation, particularly in children and elderly patients.

PRECAUTIONS
Before prescribing medication to suppress or modify cough, it is important to ascertain that the underlying cause of cough is identified, that modification of cough does not increase the risk of clinical or physiologic complications, and that appropriate therapy for the primary disease is provided.

Usage in Ambulatory Patients: Hydrocodone, like all narcotics, and antihistamines such as Chlorpheniramine Maleate, may impair the mental and/or physical abilities required for the performance of potentially hazardous tasks such as driving a car or operating machinery; Phenylephrine may produce a rapid pulse, dizziness or palpitations; patients should be cautioned accordingly.

Drug Interactions: Patients receiving other narcotic analgesics, general anesthetics, phenothiazines, other tranquilizers, sedative-hypnotics or other CNS depressants (including alcohol) concomitantly with Hydrocodone may exhibit an additive CNS depression. When such combined therapy is contemplated, the dose of one or both agents should be reduced. The use of Phenylephrine with other sympathomimetic amines and MAO inhibitors may produce an additive elevation of blood pressure. MAO inhibitors may prolong the anticholinergic effects of antihistamines. (See *"Warnings"*.)

Carcinogenesis, Mutagenesis, Impairment of Fertility: Carcinogenicity, mutagenicity, and reproduction studies have not been conducted with APAP/Caff/CPM/Hydrocod/PE.

Usage in Pregnancy: Pregnancy Category C. Animal reproduction studies have not been conducted with APAP/Caff/CPM/Hydrocod/PE. It is also not known whether APAP/Caff/CPM/Hydrocod/PE can cause fetal harm when administered to a pregnant woman or can affect reproductive capacity. APAP/Caff/CPM/Hydrocod/PE should be given to a pregnant woman only if clearly needed.

Nonteratogenic Effects: Babies born to mothers who have been taking opioids regularly prior to delivery will be physically dependent. The withdrawal signs include irritability and excessive crying, tremors, hyperactive reflexes, increased respiratory rate, increased stools, sneezing, yawning, vomiting and fever. The intensity of the syndrome does not always correlate with the duration of maternal opioid use or dose. Chlorpromazine 0.7-1.0 mg/kg q 6 h, phenobarbital 2 mg/kg q 6 h, and paregoric 2-4 drops/kg q 4 h, have been used to treat withdrawal symptoms in infants. The duration of therapy is 4 to 28 days, with the dosages decreased as tolerated.

Nursing Mothers: It is not known whether this drug is excreted in human milk. Because many drugs are excreted in human milk and because of the potential for serious adverse reactions in nursing infants from APAP/Caff/CPM/Hydrocod/PE, a decision should be made whether to discontinue nursing or discontinue the drug, taking into account the importance of the drug to the mother.

Pediatric Use: Safety and effectiveness in children below the age of 2 years have not been established.

ADVERSE REACTIONS
Respiratory System: Hydrocodone produces dose-related respiratory depression by acting directly on brain stem respiratory centers.

Cardiovascular System: Hypertension, postural hypotension, tachycardia and palpitations.

Genitourinary System: Ureteral spasm, spasm of vesical sphincters and urinary retention have been reported with opiates.

Central Nervous System: Sedation, drowsiness, mental clouding, lethargy, impairment of mental and physical performance, anxiety, fear, dysphoria, dizziness, psychic dependence, mood changes, and blurred vision.

Gastrointestinal System: Nausea and vomiting occur more frequently in ambulatory than in recumbent patients.

DRUG ABUSE AND DEPENDENCE
Special care should be exercised in prescribing Hydrocodone for emotionally unstable patients and for those with a history of drug misuse. Such patients should be closely supervised when long term therapy is contemplated.

APAP/Caff/CPM/Hydrocod/PE is a Schedule III narcotic. Psychic dependence, physical dependence, and tolerance may develop upon repeated administration of narcotics; therefore, APAP/Caff/CPM/Hydrocod/PE should always be prescribed and administered with caution. Physical dependence is the condition in which continued administration of the drug is required to prevent the appearance of a withdrawal syndrome. Patients physically dependent on opioids will develop an abstinence syndrome upon abrupt discontinuation of the opioid or following the administration of a narcotic antagonist. The character and severity of the withdrawal symptoms are related to the degree of physical dependence. Manifestations of opioid withdrawal are similar to but milder than that of morphine and include lacrimation, rhinorrhea, yawning, sweating, restlessness, dilated pupils, anorexia, goose-flesh, irritability and tremor. In more severe forms, nausea, vomiting, intestinal spasm and diarrhea, increased heart rate and blood pressure, chills, and pains in bones and muscles of the back and extremities may occur. Peak effects will usually be apparent at 48 to 72 hours.

Treatment of withdrawal is usually managed by providing sufficient quantities of an opioid to suppress **severe** withdrawal symptoms and then gradually reducing the dose of opioid over a period of several days.

OVERDOSAGE
The signs and symptoms of overdosage of the individual components of APAP/Caff/CPM/Hydrocod/PE may be modified in varying degrees by the presence of other active ingredients. Overdosage with Phenylephrine alone may result in tremor, restlessness, increased motor activity, agitation and hallucinations.

ACETAMINOPHEN
Signs and Symptoms: In acute Acetominophen overdosage, dose-dependent, potentially fatal hepatic necrosis in the most serious adverse effect. Renal tubular necrosis, hypoglycemic coma and thrombocytopenia may also occur.

Acetaminophen in massive overdosage may cause hepatic toxicity in some patients. In cases of suspected overdose, you may wish to call your regional poison center for assistance in diagnosis and for directions in the use of N-acetylcysteine as an antidote.

In adults, hepatic toxicity has rarely been reported with acute overdoses of less than 10 grams and fatalities with less than 15 grams. Importantly, young children seem to be more resistant than adults to the hepatotoxic effect of an Acetominophen overdose. Despite this, the measures outlined below should be initiated in any adult or child suspected of having ingested an Acetominophen overdose.

Early symptoms following a potentially hepatotoxic overdose may include nausea, vomiting, diaphoresis and general malaise. Clinical and laboratory evidence of hepatic toxicity may not be apparent until 48 to 72 hours post-ingestion.

Treatment: The stomach should be emptied promptly by lavage or by induction of emesis with syrup of ipecac. Patient's estimates of the quantity of a drug ingested are notoriously unreliable. Therefore, if an Acetominophen overdose is suspected, a serum Acetominophen assay should be obtained as early as possible, but no sooner than four hours following ingestion. Liver function studies should be obtained initially and repeated at 24-hour intervals.

The antidote, N-acetylcysteine should be administered as early as possible, preferably within 16 hours of the overdose ingestions for optimal results, but in any case, within 24 hours. Following recovery, there are no residual structural or functional hepatic abnormalities.

HYDROCODONE
Signs and Symptoms: Serious overdosage with Hydrocodone is characterized by respiratory depression (a decrease in respiratory rate and/or tidal volume, Cheyne-Stokes respiration, cyanosis), extreme somnolence progressing to stupor or coma, skeletal muscle flaccidity, cold and clammy skin, and sometimes bradycardia and hypotension. In severe overdosage apnea, circulatory collapse, cardiac arrest and death may occur.

Treatment: Primary attention should be given to the reestablishment of adequate respiratory exchange through provision of a patent airway and the institution of assisted or controlled ventilation. The narcotic antagonist naloxone hydrochloride is a specific antidote for respiratory depression which may result from overdosage or unusual sensitivity to narcotics including Hydrocodone. Therefore, an appropriate dose of naloxone hydrochloride should be administered, preferably by the intravenous route, simultaneously with efforts at respiratory resuscitation. For further information, see full prescribing information for naloxone hydrochloride. An antagonist should not be administered in the absence of clinically significant respiratory depression. Oxygen, intravenous fluids, vasopressors and other supportive measures should be employed as indicated. Gastric emptying may be useful in removing unabsorbed drug. Activated charcoal may be of benefit.

DOSAGE AND ADMINISTRATION
Usual dosage, not less than 4 hours apart:
  Adults: 1 tablet 4 times a day.
  Children: 6 to 12 years: 1/2 tablet 4 times a day.
  Store at controlled room temperature (59° -86° F, 15° -30° C).
  Oral prescription where permitted by State Law.

HOW SUPPLIED
TABLETS (C-III):

AVERAGE UNIT PRICE (AVAILABLE SIZES)			
BRAND		$0.69	
BRAND/MANUFACTURER	NDC	SIZE	AWP
◆ **BRAND**			
HYCOMINE COMPOUND: Du Pont Multi	00056-0048-70	100s	$73.68
	00056-0048-85	500s	$325.02

Acetaminophen/Caffeine/ Dihydrocodeine Bitartrate

DESCRIPTION
Each capsule contains:

Dihydrocodeine bitartrate	16 mg
(Warning: May be habit forming)	
Acetaminophen	356.4 mg
Caffeine	30 mg

Dihydrocodeine bitartrate is 6-hydroxy-3-methoxy-N-methyl-4,5-epoxy-morphinan bitartrate. Its molecular formula is $C_{18}H_{23}NO_3 \cdot C_4H_6O_6$ and its molecular weight is 451.46.

Acetaminophen is N-(4-Hydroxyphenyl)acetamide. Its molecular formula is $C_8H_9NO_2$ and its molecular weight is 151.16.

Caffeine is 3,7-Dihydro-1,3,7-trimethyl-1H-purine-2,6-dione. Its molecular formula is $C_8H_{10}N_4O_2$ (anhydrous) and its molecular weight is 194.19.

CLINICAL PHARMACOLOGY
Acetaminophen/Caffeine/Dihydrocodeine Bitartrate capsules contain Dihydrocodeine which is a semi-synthetic narcotic analgesic related to Codeine, with multiple actions qualitatively similar to those of Codeine; the most prominent of these involve the central nervous system and organs with smooth muscle components. The principal action of therapeutic value is analgesia.

Acetaminophen/Caffeine/Dihydrocodeine Bitartrate capsules also contain Acetaminophen, a non-opiate, non-salicylate analgesic, and antipyretic.

Acetaminophen/Caffeine/Dihydrocodeine Bitartrate capsules contain Caffeine as an analgesic adjuvant. Caffeine is also a CNS and cardiovascular stimulant.

INDICATIONS AND USAGE
Acetaminophen/Caffeine/Dihydrocodeine Bitartrate capsules are indicated for the relief of moderate to moderately severe pain.

CONTRAINDICATIONS
Hypersensitivity to Dihydrocodeine, Codeine, Acetaminophen, Caffeine, or the other components noted above.

WARNINGS
DihydroCodeine may impair the mental and/or physical abilities required for the performance of potentially hazardous tasks such as driving a car or operating machinery.

PRECAUTIONS

GENERAL

Acetaminophen/Caffeine/Dihydrocodeine Bitartrate capsules should be given with caution to certain patients such as the elderly or debilitated.

Acetaminophen is relatively non-toxic at therapeutic doses, but should be used with caution in patients with severe renal or hepatic disease.

Caffeine in high doses may produce CNS and cardiovascular stimulation and GI irritation.

INFORMATION FOR PATIENTS

DihydroCodeine may impair the mental and/or physical abilities required for the performance of potentially hazardous tasks such as driving a car or operating machinery. The patient using Acetaminophen/Caffeine/Dihydrocodeine Bitartrate capsules should be cautioned accordingly.

DRUG INTERACTIONS

DihydroCodeine Patients receiving other narcotic analgesics, general anesthetics, tranquilizers, sedative-hypnotics, or other CNS depressants (including alcohol) concomitantly with Acetaminophen/Caffeine/Dihydrocodeine Bitartrate capsules may exhibit an additive CNS depression. When such combined therapy is contemplated, the dose of one or both agents should be reduced.

Caffeine Caffeine may enhance the cardiac inotropic effects of beta-adrenergic stimulating agents. Co-administration of Caffeine and disulfiram may lead to a substantial decrease in Caffeine clearance. Caffeine may increase the metabolism of other drugs such as phenobarbital and aspirin. Caffeine accumulation may occur when products or foods containing Caffeine are consumed concomitantly with quinolones such as ciprofloxacin.

PREGNANCY

Teratogenic Effects—Pregnancy Category C. Animal reproduction studies have not been conducted with Acetaminophen/Caffeine/Dihydrocodeine Bitartrate capsules. It is also not known whether Acetaminophen/Caffeine/Dihydrocodeine Bitartrate capsules can cause fetal harm when administered to pregnant women or can affect reproduction capacity in males and females. Acetaminophen/Caffeine/Dihydrocodeine Bitartrate capsules should be given to a pregnant woman only if clearly needed.

NURSING MOTHERS

Because of the potential for serious adverse reactions in nursing infants from Acetaminophen/Caffeine/Dihydrocodeine Bitartrate capsules, a decision should be made whether to discontinue nursing or to discontinue the drug, taking into account the importance of the drug to the mother.

PEDIATRIC USE

Since there is no experience in children who have received this drug, safety and efficacy in children have not been established.

ADVERSE REACTIONS

The most frequently observed reactions include light-headedness, dizziness, drowsiness, sedation, nausea, vomiting, constipation, pruritus, and skin reactions.

DRUG ABUSE AND DEPENDENCE

Acetaminophen/Caffeine/Dihydrocodeine Bitartrate capsules are subject to the provisions of the Controlled Substance Act, and has been placed in Schedule III.

Dihydrocodeine can produce drug dependence of the Codeine type and therefore has the potential of being abused. Psychic dependence, physical dependence, and tolerance may develop upon repeated administration of Dihydrocodeine, and it should be prescribed and administered with the same degree of caution appropriate to the use of other oral narcotic-containing medications.

Prolonged, high intake of Caffeine may produce tolerance, and habituation. Physical signs of withdrawal, such as headaches, irritation, nervousness, anxiety, and dizziness, may occur upon abrupt discontinuation.

OVERDOSAGE

Following an acute overdosage with Acetaminophen/Caffeine/Dihydrocodeine Bitartrate capsules, toxicity may result from the Dihydrocodeine, Acetaminophen, or, less likely, Caffeine component. An overdose is a potentially lethal polydrug overdose situation, and consultation with a regional poison control center is recommended.

SIGNS AND SYMPTOMS AND LABORATORY FINDINGS

Toxicity from *Dihydrocodeine* is typical of opiates and includes pinpoint pupils, respiratory depression, and loss of consciousness. Convulsions, cardiovascular collapse, and death may occur. With *Acetaminophen*, dose-dependent hepatic necrosis is the most serious adverse effect. Renal tubular necrosis, hypoglycemic coma, thrombocytopenia may occur. Early symptoms of hepatotoxicity include nausea, vomiting, diaphoresis, and general malaise. Clinical and laboratory evidence of hepatic toxicity may not be apparent until 48 to 72 hours post-ingestion. In adults, hepatic toxicity has rarely been reported with acute overdoses of less than 10 grams or fatalities with less than 15 grams. Acute *Caffeine* poisoning may cause insomnia, restlessness, tremor, delirium, tachycardia, extrasystoles, and seizures.

Because overdose information on Acetaminophen/Caffeine/Dihydrocodeine Bitartrate capsules is limited, it is unclear which of the signs and symptoms of toxicity would manifest in any particular overdose situation.

TREATMENT

Immediate treatment includes support of cardiorespiratory function and measures to reduce drug absorption. Vomiting should be induced with syrup of ipecac, if the patient is alert and has adequate laryngeal reflexes. Oral activated charcoal should follow. The first dose should be accompanied by an appropriate cathartic. Gastric lavage may be necessary. Hypotension is usual and should be treated with fluids. Endotracheal intubation and artificial respiration may be necessary. Peritoneal or hemodialysis may be necessary. If hypoprothrombinemia occurs, Vitamin K should be administered.

The pure opioid antagonist, naloxone, is a specific antidote against respiratory depression which results from opioid overdose. Naloxone (usually 0.4 to 2.0 mg) should be administered intravenously; however, because its duration of action is relatively short, the patient must be carefully monitored until spontaneous respiration is reliably re-established. Readministration may be necessary. Naloxone should not be given in the absence of clinically significant respiratory or circulatory depression secondary to opioid overdose.

In adults and adolescents, regardless of the quantity of Acetaminophen reported to have been ingested, administer acetylcysteine immediately if 24 hours or less have elapsed from the reported time since ingestion. Do not await the plasma concentration determination of Acetaminophen before administisitering acetylcysteine. Serum liver enzyme levels should be quantitated. Therapy in children involves a similar treatment scheme; however, a regional poison control center should be contacted.

No specific antidote is available for Caffeine. In addition to the supportive measures above, administration of demulcents such as aluminum hydroxide gel may diminish GI irritation. Seizures may be treated with intravenous diazepam or a barbiturate.

DOSAGE AND ADMINISTRATION

The usual adult dose is two (2) Acetaminophen/Caffeine/Dihydroycodeine Bitartrate capsules orally every four (4) hours. Dosage should be adjusted according to the severity of the pain and the response of the patient. No more than twelve (12) capsules should be taken in a 24-hour period.

Store at controlled room temperature, 15°–30°C (59°–86°F).

Protect from moisture.

Dispense in a tight, light-resistant container as defined in the USP.

HOW SUPPLIED

CAPSULE (C-III): 356.4 MG-30 MG-16 MG

BRAND/MANUFACTURER	NDC	SIZE	AWP
○ BRAND			
DHC PLUS: Purdue Frederick	00034-8000-80	100s	$40.82

Acetaminophen/ Chlorpheniramine Maleate/ Codeine Phosphate/ Phenylephrine Hydrochloride

DESCRIPTION

Acetaminophen/Chlorpheniramine Maleate/Codeine Phosphate/Phenylephrine Hydrochloride capsules are formulated to provide symptomatic relief of the common cold and other acute respiratory conditions. The product combines antitussive, antihistaminic, decongestant, analgesic and antipyretic actions.

Each capsule contains:

Codeine Phosphate	16 mg
(Warning: May be habit forming)	
Acetaminophen	325 mg
Chlorpheniramine Maleate	2 mg
Phenylephrine Hydrochloride	10 mg

INDICATIONS

Adjunct for temporary relief of cough, congestion, headache and muscle soreness of common colds and upper respiratory infections. Infections should be identified and, if bacterial, given appropriate antimicrobial therapy.

SIDE EFFECTS AND PRECAUTIONS

Codeine may cause constipation, and an occasional patient may display idiosyncratic response to it. Chlorpheniramine, especially with codeine, may cause drowsiness; use with caution in patients who operate machinery. Phenylephrine may cause gastric upset and, because of its sympathominetic effect, should be used with caution in cardiovascular disease, thyrotoxicosis and diabetes.

DOSAGE

Adults, 1 or 2 capsules three or four times daily. For children 6 to 12, 1 capsule three or four times daily. Not recommended for children under 6.

◆ RATED THERAPEUTICALLY EQUIVALENT; ◇ THERAPEUTIC EQUIVALENCE UNCONFIRMED; ○ UNRATED

HOW SUPPLIED
CAPSULE (C-III):

BRAND/MANUFACTURER	NDC	SIZE	AWP
○ BRAND			
COLREX COMPOUND: Numark	00032-0840-01	100s	$31.51

Acetaminophen/ Chlorpheniramine Maleate/ Phenylpropanolamine Hydrochloride

DESCRIPTION
Acetaminophen 500mg, Chlorpheniramine Maleate 4mg, and Phenylpropanolamine HCl 25mg.

INDICATIONS
In the reduction of fever or relief of pain in common upper respiratory infections; grippe; allergic rhinitis; vasomotor rhinitis; and mild, uncomplicated allergic skin reactions of urticara and angioedema.

PRECAUTION
Withdraw medication if drowsiness, restlessness or nervousness occurs. Do not drive or operate machinery. Heart, blood pressure and diabetes patients should use with caution.

CONTRAINDICATIONS
If cardiac diseases, high blood pressure, and thyroid disease, or if high fever persists.

DOSAGE
Adult: two tablets initially, then one tablet every four hours.

Children 6-12 years old: one tablet initially, then one-half tablet every four hours.

HOW SUPPLIED
TABLETS:

BRAND/MANUFACTURER	NDC	SIZE	AWP
○ GENERICS			
ALUMADRINE: Fleming	00256-0107-01	100s	$14.00
ALUMADRINE: Fleming	00256-0107-02	1000s	$128.25

Acetaminophen/ Chlorpheniramine Maleate/ Phenylpropanolamine Hydrochloride/Phenyltoloxamine Citrate

DESCRIPTION
Each capsule for oral administration contains:

Acetaminophen	325 mg
Phenyltoloxamine Dihydrogen Citrate	25 mg
Phenylpropanolamine Hydrochloride	25 mg
Chlorpheniramine Maleate	4 mg

Acetaminophen: N-(4-hydroxyphenyl)-acetamide, $C_1H_1NO_2$, is a non-opiate, nonsalicylate analgesic and antipyretic which occurs as a white, odorless, crystalline powder possessing a slightly bitter taste.

Phenyltoloxamine Dihydrogen Citrate: N, N-Dimethyl-2 (alpha-phenyl-o-tolyl-oxy), ethylamine dihydrogen citrate is an antihistamine that forms crystals from water or methanol, and is soluble in water.

Phenylpropanolamine Hydrochloride: Benzenemethanol, alpha (1-aminoethyl)hydrochloride, (R*,S*) —, (+)•$C_9H_{13}NO$•HCl. It is a white, crystalline powder, having a slight aromatic odor. It is affected by light. It is freely soluble in water and alcohol and insoluble in ether.

Chlorpheniramine Maleate: 2-pyridinepropanamine, lambda(4-chlorophenyl)-N, N,-dimethyl-, (Z)-2-butenedioate (1:1), $C_{16}H_{19}CLN_2$,• $C_4H_4O_4$, is an antihistaminic that exists as a white, odorless, crystalline powder. It is freely soluble in water, soluble in alcohol and chloroform, and slightly soluble in ether and benzene.

CLINICAL PHARMACOLOGY
Acetaminophen. The analgesic action of Acetaminophen involves peripheral and central influences, but the specific mechanism is as yet undetermined. Antipyretic activity is mediated through hypothalamic heat regulating centers. Acetaminophen inhibits prostaglandin synthetase. Therapeutic doses of Acetaminophen have negligible effects on the cardiovascular or respiratory systems; however, toxic doses may cause circulatory failure and rapid, shallow breathing. Acetaminophen is rapidly and almost completely absorbed from the gastrointestinal tract, producing maximum serum concentrations within 30 minutes to one hour. The plasma half-life in adults and children ranges from 0.90 hours to 3.25 hours with an average of approximately 2 hours. The drug distributes uniformly in most body fluids and is approximately 25% protein bound. Acetaminophen is conjugated in the liver, with less than 3% of the dose excreted unchanged in 24 hours. The primary metabolic pathway is conjugation to sulfate and glucuronide by-products. A minor oxidative pathway forms cysteine and mercapturic acid. These compounds are subsequently excreted by the kidneys into the urine.

Phenyltoloxamine Dihydrogen Citrate: Phenyltoloxamine Citrate is an antihistamine which acts on the H1 receptors as an antagonist and interferes in the action of histamine, primarily in capillaries surrounding mucous tissues and sensory nerves of nasal and adjacent areas. It is rapidly and almost completely absorbed from the gastrointestinal tract and distributed throughout the body, including the central nervous system (CNS). Little, if any of the drug is excreted into the urine; most is apparently metabolized by the liver and excreted as degradation products within 24 hours. Phenyltoloxamine Citrate is an ethanolamine-type antihistamine and it is an effective H1 blocker that possesses significant antimuscarinic activity and a pronounced tendency to induce sedation.

Phenylpropanolamine Hydrochloride: This is a sympathomimetic (vasoconstrictor) which may directly stimulate adrenergic receptors, but probably indirectly stimulates both alpha and beta adrenergic receptors by releasing norepinephrine from its storage sites. It increases heart rate, force of contraction, cardiac output and excitability. It acts on alpha receptors in the mucosa of the respiratory tract, producing vasoconstriction which results in shrinkage of swollen mucous membranes, reduction of tissue, hyperemia, edema and nasal congestion, and an increase in nasal airway patency. Phenylpropanolamine causes CNS stimulation and reportedly has an anorexigenic effect.

Chlorpheniramine Maleate: Chlorpheniramine is an antihistamine belonging to the alkylamine class. It possesses antichloinergic and sedative effects. Antihistamines appear to compete with histamine for H1 cell receptor sites on effector cells, thereby counteracting the effects of histamine release associated with allergic manifestations of upper respiratory tract inflammatory disorders. Chlorpheniramine Maleate does not prevent the release of histamine in response to injury, drugs, or antigens. Antihistamines effectively block most smooth muscle responses to histamine and act as an antagonist of the constrictor action of histamine on respiratory smooth muscle. Antihistamines counteract edema formation and whealing in response to injury, antigens, or histamine-liberating drugs. Chlorpheniramine is readily absorbed from the gastrointestinal tract and has a duration of 4 to 6 hours. Plasma half-life is approximately 22 hours. Degradation products of Chlorpheniramine's metabolic transformation by the liver are almost completely excreted in 24 hours via the kidney. The alkylamines of which Chlorpheniramine is the prototype, are among the most potent H1 blockers. Although not so prone as others to cause drowsiness, a significant proportion of patients do experience this effect. CNS stimulation is more common in Chlorpheniramine than in other groups of H1 blockers.

INDICATIONS AND USAGE
For the symptomatic relief of headache, facial pain, malaise, fever, nasal and sinus congestion associated with acute and chronic sinusitis, allergic rhinitis, and vasomotor rhinitis.

CONTRAINDICATIONS
Severe hypertension, hyperthyroidism, organic heart disease, severe diabetes mellitus. This combination is contraindicated in any patient exhibiting hypersensitivity to any of its ingredients. Antihistamines should not be administered to premature or newborn infants or be used to treat lower respiratory tract symptoms. Phenylpropanolamine Hydrochloride is contraindicated in patients sensitive to sympathomimetics or those receiving monoamine oxidase inhibitors.

WARNINGS
Keep this and all drugs out of the reach of children. Antihistamines may impair mental and physical abilities required for the performance of potentially hazardous tasks such as driving a vehicle or operating machinery and may impair mental alertness in children. Chlorpheniramine has an atropinelike action and should be used with caution in patients with increased intraocular pressure, cardiovascular disease, hypertension or in patients with a history of bronchial asthma. Sympathomimetic amines should be used with caution in patients with hypertension, diabetes mellitus, heart disease, peripheral vascular disease, increased intraocular pressure, hyperthyroidism, or prostatic hypertrophy. If symptoms do not improve within 7 days or are accompanied by fever, rash or persistent headache, consult a physician before continuing use. Do not exceed recommended dosage because at higher doses nervousness, dizziness, or sleeplessness are more likely to occur.

PRECAUTIONS
Information for Patients: Antihistamines may impair mental and physical abilities required for the performance of potentially hazardous tasks such as driving a vehicle or operating machinery. Patients should also be warned about possible

additive effects with alcohol and other central nervous system depressants (hypnotics, sedatives, and tranquilizers).

Drugs/Laboratory Test Interactions: Acetaminophen may increase the effects of oral anticoagulants and this may result in abnormal bleeding. The effect of Acetaminophen may be decreased by phenobarbital which hastens its elimination from the body. Concomitant use of antihistamines with alcohol, tricyclic depressants, barbiturates and other CNS depressants may have an additive effect. MAO inhibitors and beta adrenergic blockers increase the effects of sympathomimetics. Sympathomimetics may reduce the antihypertensive effects of methyldopa, mecamylamine, reserpine, and veratrum alkaloids. Phenylpropanolamine should not be taken concurrently with digitalis or ergot preparations or with guanethidine.

Carcinogenesis, Mutagenesis, and Impairment of Fertility: No long term studies have been performed using this combination to determine the long-term potential for carcinogenesis, mutagenesis, or impairment of fertility.

Usage in Pregnancy: Pregnancy Category C: Animal reproduction studies have not been conducted with this combination. It is also not known whether this combination can cause fetal harm when administered to a pregnant woman or can affect reproduction capacity. Therefore, this combination should be given to a pregnant woman only if the potential benefit justifies the possible risk to the fetus.

Nursing Mothers: Acetaminophen and Phenylpropanolamine Hydrochloride are known to be excreted in human milk. Because many drugs are excreted in human milk and because of the potential for serious adverse reactions in nursing infants, a decision should be made whether to discontinue nursing or discontinue the product, taking into account the important of the drug to the mother.

Pediatric Use: In infants and children, especially, antihistamines in overdosage can cause hallucinations, convulsions or death. As in adults, antihistamines may diminish mental alertness in children. In the young child particularly they may produce excitation. As in adults, sympathomimetic amines can elicit either mild stimulation or mild sedation. Safety and effectiveness in children below the age of 12 have not been established.

Geriatric Use: Antihistamines are more likely to cause dizziness, sedation and hypertension in elderly patients. The elderly are also more likely to exhibit adverse reactions to sympathomimetics. At doses higher than the recommended dose, nervousness, dizziness, and sleeplessness may occur.

ADVERSE REACTIONS

Acetaminophen: Dizziness, drowsiness, and occasionally gastrointestinal irritation are seen with high doses. Other possible adverse reactions include allergic reactions such as skin rash, impaired thinking and concentration. In rare cases, an anaphylactic reaction or hemolytic anemia may be observed. If any of these develop, discontinue use and notify your physician as soon as possible.

Phenyltoloxamine Dihydrogen Citrate and Chlorpheniramine Maleate: Antihistamines may cause slight to moderate drowsiness. Less frequent side effects include: urticaria, drug rash, anaphylactic shock, photosensitivity, excessive perspiration, chills, dryness of mouth, nose, and throat; cardiovascular effects (hypotension, headache, palpitation, tachycardia, extrasystoles); hematological effects (hemolytic anemia, thrombocytopenia, agranulocytosis); CNS disturbances; sedation, dizziness, disturbed coordination, fatigue, confusion, restlessness, excitation, nervousness, tremor, irritability, insomnia, euphoria, paresthesia, blurred vision, diplopia, vertigo, tinnitis, hysteria, neuritis, convulsions); gastrointestinal effects (epigastric distress, anorexia, nausea, vomiting, diarrhea, constipation); genitourinary effects (urinary frequency, difficult urination, urinary retention, early menses); and respiratory effects (thickening of bronchial secretions, tightening of chest, wheezing and nasal stuffiness).

Phenylpropanolamine Hydrochloride: Possible adverse reactions include nervousness, insomnia, restlessness, headache, nausea, or gastric irritation. These reactions seldom, if ever, require discontinuation of therapy. Urinary retention may occur in patients with prostatic hypertrophy.

OVERDOSE

ACETAMINOPHEN

Signs and Symptoms: Acetaminophen in massive overdosage may cause hepatic toxicity in some patients. In all cases of suspected overdose, you may wish to call your regional poison center for assistance in diagnosis and for directions in the use of N-acetylcysteine as an antidote. In adults, hepatic toxicity has rarely been reported with acute overdoses of less than 10 grams and fatalities with less than 15 grams. Importantly, young children seem to be more resistant than adults to the hepatotoxic effect of an Acetaminophen overdose. Despite this, the measures outlined below should be initiated in any adult or child suspected of having ingested an Acetaminophen overdose. Early symptoms following a potentially hepatotoxic overdose may include nausea, vomiting, diaphoresis and general malaise. Clinical and laboratory evidence of hepatic toxicity may not be apparent until 48 to 72 hours postingestion.

Treatment: The stomach should be emptied promptly by lavage or by induction of emesis with syrup of ipecac. Patients' estimates of the quantity of a drug ingested are notoriously unreliable. Therefore, if an Acetaminophen overdose is suspected, a serum Acetaminophen assay should be obtained as early as possible, but no sooner than four hours following ingestion. Liver function studies should be obtained initially and repeated at 24-hour intervals. The antidote N-acetylcysteine should be administered as early as possible, preferably within 16 hours of the overdose ingestion for optimal results, but in any case within 24 hours. Following recovery, there are no residual, structural or function hepatic abnormalities.

PHENYLTOLOXAMINE DIHYDROGEN CITRATE AND CHLORPHENIRAMINE MALEATE

Signs and Symptoms: Manifestations of antihistamine overdosage may vary from central nervous system depression (sedation, apnea, cardiovascular collapse) to stimulation (insomnia, hallucinations, tremors or convulsions). Other signs and symptoms may be dizziness, tinnitis, ataxia, blurred vision and hypotension. Stimulation is particularly likely in children, as are atropine-like signs and symptoms (dry mouth; fixed, dilated pupils; flushing, hyperthermia and gastrointestinal symptoms). Treatment: The patient should be induced to vomit, even if emesis has occurred spontaneously. Pharmacologic vomiting by the administration of ipecac syrup is the preferred method. However, vomiting should not be induced in patients with impaired consciousness. The action of ipecac is facilitated by physical activity and by the administration of eight to twelve fluid ounces of water. If emesis does not occur within fifteen minutes, the dose of ipecac should be repeated. Precautions against aspiration must be taken, especially in infants and children. Following emesis, any drug remaining in the stomach may be absorbed by activated charcoal administered as a slurry with water. If vomiting is unsuccessful or contraindicated, gastric lavage should be performed. Isotonic and one-half isotonic saline are the lavage solutions of choice. Saline cathartics, such as milk of magnesia, draw water into the bowel by osmosis and therefore, may be valuable for their action in rapid dilution of bowel content. After emergency treatment the patient should continue to be medically monitored. Treatment of the signs and symptoms of overdosage is symptomatic and supportive. Only in cases of extreme overdosage or individual sensitivity do vital signs including respiration, pulse, blood pressure, temperature and EKG need to be monitored.

PHENYLPROPANOLAMINE HYDROCHLORIDE

Signs and Symptoms: Moderate overdose may be marked by excessive nervousness, restlessness, headache, heart palpitation, sweating, nausea, or vomiting. More serious overdose of Phenylpropanolamine is characterized by anxiety, confusion, delirium, muscular tremors, and a rapid and irregular pulse.

Treatment: The treatment should provide symptomatic and supportive care (see treatment for antihistamine overdose).

DOSAGE AND ADMINISTRATION

The usual adult dose is one capsule taken orally every 3-4 hours. Do not exceed 6 capsules in any 24 hour period.

Dispense in a tight, light-resistant closure as defined in the USP/NF, with a child-resistant closure. Store at controlled room temperature, 15-30°C (59-86°F).

HOW SUPPLIED
CAPSULE:

BRAND/MANUFACTURER	NDC	SIZE	AWP
○ GENERICS			
NOREL PLUS: U.S. Pharm	52747-0128-60	100s	$36.00

Acetaminophen/ Dichloralphenazone/ Isometheptene Mucate

DESCRIPTION

Each capsule contains:

Acetaminophen	325 mg
Dichloralphenazone	100 mg
Isometheptene Mucate	65 mg

Acetaminophen, a nonsalicylate, occurs as a white, odorless, crystalline powder possessing a slightly bitter taste.

Dichloralphenazone is a white, microcrystalline powder, with slight odor and a saline taste that becomes acrid. It is a mild sedative.

Isometheptene Mucate is a white crystalline powder having a characteristic aromatic odor and bitter taste. It is an unsaturated aliphatic amine with sympathomimetic properties.

ACTIONS

Acetaminophen raises the threshold to painful stimuli, thus exerting an analgesic effect against all types of headaches.

Dichloralphenazone, a mild sedative, reduces the patient's emotional reaction to the pain of both vascular and tension headaches.

Isometheptene Mucate, a sympathomimetic amine, acts by constricting dilated cranial and cerebral arterioles, thus reducing the stimuli that lead to vascular headaches.

INDICATIONS

For relief of tension and vascular headaches.*

---

* BASED ON A REVIEW OF THIS DRUG (ISOMETHEPTENE MUCATE) BY THE NATIONAL ACADEMY OF SCIENCES-NATIONAL RESEARCH COUNCIL AND/OR OTHER INFORMATION, FDA HAS CLASSIFIED THE OTHER INDI-

---

◆ RATED THERAPEUTICALLY EQUIVALENT; ◇ THERAPEUTIC EQUIVALENCE UNCONFIRMED; ○ UNRATED

CATION AS "POSSIBLY" EFFECTIVE IN THE TREATMENT OF MIGRAINE HEADACHE.

FINAL CLASSIFICATION OF THE LESS-THAN-EFFECTIVE INDICATION REQUIRES FURTHER INVESTIGATION.

CONTRAINDICATIONS
Contraindicated in glaucoma and/or severe cases of renal disease, hypertension, organic heart disease, hepatic disease and in those patients who are on monoamine-oxidase (MAO) inhibitor therapy.

PRECAUTIONS
Caution should be observed in hypertension, peripheral vascular disease and after recent cardiovascular attacks.

ADVERSE REACTIONS
Transient dizziness and skin rash may appear in hypersensitive patients. This can usually be eliminated by reducing the dose.

DOSAGE AND ADMINISTRATION
For Relief of Migraine Headache: The usual adult dosage is two capsules at once, followed by one capsule every hour until relieved, up to 5 capsules within a twelve-hour period.

For Relief of Tension Headache: The usual adult dosage is one or two capsules every four hours up to 8 capsules a day.

Storage: Store at controlled room temperature 15—30°C (59-86°F) in a dry place.

HOW SUPPLIED
CAPSULE: 325 MG-100 MG-65 MG

BRAND/MANUFACTURER	NDC	SIZE	AWP
○ BRAND			
► MIDRIN: Carrnick	00086-0120-05	50s	$20.30
	00086-0120-10	100s	$35.55
○ GENERICS			
Southwood	58016-0288-40	40s	$16.22
ISOCOM: Nutripharm	51081-0424-05	50s	$8.20
MIGRAZONE: Moore,H.L.	00839-7561-04	50s	$9.38
ISOPAP: Columbia Drug	11735-0999-11	100s	$12.00
MIGRAZONE: Moore,H.L.	00839-7561-06	100s	$14.84
ISOCOM: Nutripharm	51081-0424-10	100s	$15.35
AMIDRINE: Amide	52152-0039-02	100s	$16.55
MIGREND: Econolab	55053-0420-01	100s	$16.75
MIGRAZONE: Econolab	55053-0512-01	100s	$16.75
MIGRAZONE: Pharmacist's Choice	54979-0144-01	100s	$16.75
Pecos	59879-0222-01	100s	$16.95
Jerome Stevens	50564-0508-01	100s	$16.95
MIGRAPAP: Mikart	46672-0253-10	100s	$17.95
MIGRATINE: Major	00904-1588-60	100s	$19.00
MIGRATINE: Major	00904-7622-60	100s	$19.00
MITRIDE: Interstate	00814-4860-14	100s	$19.43
MIGQUIN: Vintage	00254-4270-28	100s	$19.71
DURADRIN: Duramed	51285-0364-02	100s	$19.95
I.D.A.: Goldline	00182-1234-01	100s	$20.00
URL	00677-1125-01	100s	$20.45
MIDCHLOR: Schein	00364-2342-01	100s	$20.50
MIGQUIN: Qualitest	00603-4664-21	100s	$20.80
MIGREX: Parmed	00349-8783-01	100s	$20.95
ALIDRIN: Aligen	00405-4039-01	100s	$21.45
ISO-ACETAZONE: Rugby	00536-3932-01	100s	$22.11
MIGREX: Parmed	00349-8914-01	100s	$24.61
ISOCOM: Nutripharm	51081-0424-25	250s	$29.40
MIGRAPAP: Mikart	46672-0253-25	250s	$31.75
AMIDRINE: Amide	52152-0039-03	250s	$36.41
MIGQUIN: Vintage	00254-4270-33	250s	$37.75
MIGQUIN: Qualitest	00603-4664-24	250s	$37.75
MIGRATINE: Major	00904-1588-70	250s	$46.45
MIGRATINE: Major	00904-7622-70	250s	$46.45
MIGRAZONE: Pharmacist's Choice	54979-0144-05	500s	$79.56
MIGREX: Parmed	00349-8783-05	500s	$99.95
ISO-ACETAZONE: Rugby	00536-3932-05	500s	$107.75

Acetaminophen/ Phenyltoloxamine Citrate/ Salicylamide

DESCRIPTION
Each capsule for oral administration contains: Acetaminophen, USP, 300 mg; Salicylamide, 200 mg and Phenyltoloxamine, 20 mg.

Acetaminophen, 4'-hydroxyacetanilide, is a nonopiate, nonsalicylate analgesic and antipyretic which occurs as a white, odorless, crystalline powder possessing a slightly bitter taste.

Salicylamide, 2-Hydroxybenzamide, is a white or slightly pink, crystalline powder with a somewhat bitter taste. It gives the sensation of warmth on the tongue.

Phenyltoloxamine Citrate, N, N-dimethyl-2 (alpha phenyl-ortho-toloxy)-ethylamine citrate, is a white, practically odorless powder with a bitter taste.

CLINICAL PHARMACOLOGY
This product is designed to combine the analgesic, antipyretic properties of Acetaminophen and Salicylamide with mild antihistamine properties of Phenyltoloxamine.

INDICATIONS AND USAGE
This combination is indicated for the temporary relief of mild to moderate pain and discomfort due to simple headache, for temporary relief of such pain associated with muscle and joint soreness, neuralgia, sinusitis, minor menstrual cramps, the common cold or grippe, toothache, and minor aches and pains of rheumatism and arthritis.

CONTRAINDICATIONS
Hypersensitivity to Acetaminophen, salicylates or Phenyltoloxamine.

WARNINGS
Caution: If pain persists for more than 10 days, or redness is present, or in conditions affecting children under 12 years of age, consult a physician immediately.

Acetaminophen in massive overdosage may cause hepatotoxicity in some patients (see *"Overdosage"*).

Salicylates should be used with extreme caution in the presence of peptic ulcer or coagulation abnormalities. In rare instances, the use of Salicylamide in persons allergic to salicylates can result in life-threatening allergic episodes.

PRECAUTIONS
Use in Ambulatory Patients: Instruct patients not to drive or use or operate machinery if drowsiness occurs.

Usage in Pregnancy: Since there is no adequate experience in pregnant women who have received this drug, safety in pregnancy has not been established. Therefore, this product should not be used in pregnant women unless in the judgment of the physician, the potential benefits outweigh the possible hazards.

NURSING MOTHERS
The effects on infants of nursing mothers are not known. This drug should not be used in nursing mothers.

PEDIATRIC USE
Safety and effectiveness in children below the age of 6 have not been established.

ADVERSE REACTIONS
The following adverse reactions have been reported for each of the individual or combinations of ingredients:

Acetaminophen: urticaria, epigastric distress, dizziness and palpitation;

Salicylamide: nausea, epigastric distress, mild salicylism;

Phenyltoloxamine: urticaria, drowsiness, disturbed coordination, inability to concentrate, dizziness, insomnia, tremors, nervousness, palpitation, convulsions, muscular weakness, gastric distress, diarrhea, intestinal cramps, blurred vision, hypotension, urinary retention, dryness of mouth, throat and nose.

OVERDOSAGE
Acetaminophen in massive overdosage may cause heptatic toxicity. Since clinical and laboratory evidence may be delayed up to 1 week, close clinical monitoring and serial hepatic enzyme determinations are recommended. The toxic effects of Salicylamide and Phenyltoloxamine may occur to a lesser extent. Early symptoms following a potentially hepatotoxic overdose of Acetaminophen include nausea, vomiting, diaphoresis and general malaise. Mild salicylate toxicity may produce symptoms of dizziness, tinnitus, difficulty in hearing, nausea, vomiting, diarrhea and mental confusion. These symptoms will usually disappear after the medication is discontinued and blook levels of the salicylate drops.

DOSAGE AND ADMINISTRATION
Adults: 1 or 2 capsules every 4 hours: maximum daily dose, 8 capsules.

Children: 6-12 years—one-half adult dose; maximum daily dose, 4 capsules.
Do not use for more than 10 days unless directed by physician.
Store at controlled room temperature, 15°-30°C (59°-86°F).

HOW SUPPLIED
CAPSULE: 300 MG-20 MG-200 MG

BRAND/MANUFACTURER	NDC	SIZE	AWP
○ GENERICS			
LOBAC: Seatrace	00551-0176-01	100s	$24.90

Acetazolamide

DESCRIPTION

Each tablet contains:	
Acetazolamide	125 mg or 250 mg
Each vial for intravenous use contains:	
Acetazolamide	500 mg

Each sustained-release capsule contains:

Acetazolamide .... 500 mg

Acetazolamide, an inhibitor of the enzyme carbonic anhydrase, is a white to faintly yellowish white crystalline, odorless powder, weakly acidic, very slightly soluble in water and slightly soluble in alcohol. The chemical name for Acetazolamide is *N*-(5-Sulfamoyl-1,3,4-thiadiazol-2yl)-acetamide. Its molecular weight is 222.24. Its chemical formula is $C_4H_6N_4O_3S_2$.

Following is its chemical structure:

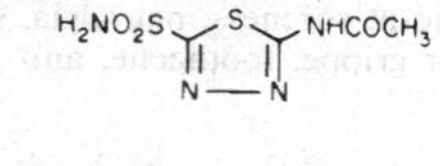

CLINICAL PHARMACOLOGY

Acetazolamide is a potent carbonic anhydrase inhibitor, effective in the control of fluid secretion (eg, some types of glaucoma), in the treatment of certain convulsive disorders (eg, epilepsy) and in the promotion of diuresis in instances of abnormal fluid retention (eg, cardiac edema).

Acetazolamide is not a mercurial diuretic. Rather, it is a nonbacteriostatic sulfonamide possessing a chemical structure and pharmacological activity distinctly different from the bacteriostatic sulfonamides.

Acetazolamide is an enzyme inhibitor that acts specifically on carbonic anhydrase, the enzyme that catalyzes the reversible reaction involving the hydration of carbon dioxide and the dehydration of carbonic acid. In the eye, this inhibitory action of acetazolamide decreases the secretion of aqueous humor and results in a drop in intraocular pressure, a reaction considered desirable in cases of glaucoma and even in certain nonglaucomatous conditions. Evidence seems to indicate that Acetazolamide has utility as an adjuvant in the treatment of certain dysfunctions of the central nervous system (eg, epilepsy). Inhibition of carbonic anhydrase in this area appears to retard abnormal, paroxysmal, excessive discharge from central nervous system neurons. The diuretic effect of Acetazolamide is due to its action in the kidney on the reversible reaction involving hydration of carbon dioxide and dehydration of carbonic acid. The result is renal loss of HCO_3 ion, which carries out sodium, water, and potassium. Alkalinization of the urine and promotion of diuresis are thus effected. Alteration in ammonia metabolism occurs due to increased reabsorption of ammonia by the renal tubules as a result of urinary alkalinization.

Acetazolamide sustained-release capsules provide prolonged action to inhibit aqueous humor secretion for 18 to 24 hours after each dose, whereas tablets act for only 8 to 12 hours. The prolonged continuous effect of the sustained-release capsules permits a reduction in dosage frequency.

Plasma concentrations of acetazolamide peak between 3 to 6 hours after administration of the sustained-release capsules, compared to 1 to 4 hours with tablets.

Placebo-controlled clinical trials have shown that prophylactic administration of Acetazolamide at a dose of 250 mg every 8 to 12 hours (or a 500 mg controlled-release capsule once daily) before and during rapid ascent to altitude results in fewer and/or less severe symptoms (such as headache, nausea, shortness of breath, dizziness, drowsiness, and fatigue) of acute mountain sickness (AMS). Pulmonary function (eg, minute ventilation, expired vital capacity, and peak flow) is greater in the Acetazolamide treated group, both in subjects with AMS and asymptomatic subjects. The Acetazolamide treated climbers also had less difficulty in sleeping.

INDICATIONS AND USAGE

Acetazolamide tablets and intravenous are indicated for adjunctive treatment of: edema due to congestive heart failure: drug-induced edema; centrencephalic epilepsies (petit mal, unlocalized seizures). All forms of Acetazolamide are indicated in chronic simple (open-angle) glaucoma, secondary glaucoma, and preoperatively in acute angle-closure glaucoma where delay of surgery is desired in order to lower intraocular pressure. Acetazolamide is also indicated for the prevention or amelioration of symptoms associated with acute mountain sickness in climbers attempting rapid ascent and in those who are very susceptible to acute mountain sickness despite gradual ascent.

UNLABELED USES

Acetazolamide is used alone or as an adjunct in the treatment of cystinuria and hydrocephalus.

CONTRAINDICATIONS

Acetazolamide therapy is contraindicated in situations in which sodium and/or potassium blood serum levels are depressed, in cases of marked kidney and liver disease or dysfunction, in suprarenal gland failure, and in hyperchloremic acidosis. It is contraindicated in patients with cirrhosis because of the risk of development of hepatic encephalopathy.

Long-term administration of Acetazolamide is contraindicated in patients with chronic noncongestive angle-closure glaucoma since it may permit organic closure of the angle to occur while the worsening glaucoma is masked by lowered intraocular pressure.

WARNINGS

Fatalities have occurred, although rarely, due to severe reactions to sulfonamides including Stevens-Johnson syndrome, toxic epidermal necrolysis, fulminant hepatic necrosis, agranulocytosis, aplastic anemia, and other blood dyscrasias. Sensitizations may recur when a sulfonamide is readministered irrespective of the route of administration. If signs of hypersensitivity or other serious reactions occur, discontinue use of this drug.

Caution is advised for patients receiving concomitant high-dose aspirin and Acetazolamide as anorexia, tachypnea, lethargy, coma and death have been reported.

PRECAUTIONS

General: Increasing the dose does not increase the diuresis and may increase the incidence of drowsiness and/or paresthesia. Increasing the dose often results in a decrease in diuresis. Under certain circumstances, however, very large doses have been given in conjunction with other diuretics in order to secure diuresis in complete refractory failure.

Information for Patients: Adverse reactions common to all sulfonamide derivatives may occur: anaphylaxis, fever, rash (including erythema multiforme, Stevens-Johnson syndrome, toxic epidermal necrolysis), crystalluria, renal calculus, bone marrow depression, thrombocytopenic purpura, hemolytic anemia, leukopenia, pancytopenia and agranulocytosis. Precaution is advised for early detection of such reactions and the drug should be discontinued and appropriate therapy instituted. In patients with pulmonary obstruction or emphysema where alveolar ventilation may be impaired, Acetazolamide which may precipitate or aggravate acidosis, should be used with caution.

Gradual ascent is desirable to try to avoid acute mountain sickness. If rapid ascent is undertaken and Acetazolamide is used, it should be noted that such use does not obviate the need for prompt descent if severe forms of high altitude sickness occur, ie, high altitude pulmonary edema (HAPE) or high-altitude cerebral edema.

Caution is advised for patients receiving concomitant high-dose aspirin and Acetazolamide, as anorexia, tachypnea, lethargy, coma and death have been reported (see *"Warnings"*).

Laboratory Tests: To monitor for hematologic reactions common to all sulfonamides, it is recommended that a baseline CBC and platelet count be obtained on patients prior to initiating Acetazolamide therapy and at regular intervals during therapy. If significant changes occur, early discontinuance and institution of appropriate therapy are important. Periodic monitoring of serum electrolytes is recommended.

Carcinogenesis, Mutagenesis, Impairment of Fertility: Long-term studies in animals to evaluate the carcinogenic potential of Acetazolamide have not been conducted. In a bacterial mutagenicity assay Acetazolamide was not mutagenic when evaluated with and without metabolic activation.

The drug had no effect on fertility when administered in the diet to male and female rats at a daily intake of up to 4 times the maximum recommended human dose of 1000 mg in a 50 kg individual.

Pregnancy: Pregnancy Category C. Acetazolamide, administered orally or parenterally, has been shown to be teratogenic (defects of the limbs) in mice, rats, hamsters, and rabbits. There are no adequate and well-controlled studies in pregnant women. Acetazolamide should be used in pregnancy only if the potential benefit justifies the potential risk to the fetus.

Nursing Mothers: Because of the potential for serious adverse reactions in nursing infants from Acetazolamide, a decision should be made whether to discontinue nursing or to discontinue the drug, taking into account the importance of the drug to the mother.

Pediatric Use: The safety and effectiveness of Acetazolamide in children have not been established.

ADVERSE REACTIONS

Adverse reactions, occurring most often early in therapy, include paresthesias, particularly a "tingling" feeling in the extremities, hearing dysfunction or tinnitus, loss of appetite, taste alteration and gastrointestinal disturbances such as nausea, vomiting and diarrhea; polyuria, and occasional instances of drowsiness and confusion.

Metabolic acidosis and electrolyte imbalance may occur. Transient myopia has been reported. This condition invariably subsides upon diminution or discontinuance of the medication.

Other occasional adverse reactions include urticaria, melena, hematuria, glycosuria, hepatic insufficiency, flaccid paralysis, photosensitivity and convulsions. Also see *"Precautions: Information for Patients"* for possible reactions common to sulfonamide derivatives. Fatalities have occurred although rarely, due to severe reactions to sulfonamides including Stevens-Johnson syndrome, toxic epidermal necrolysis, fulminant hepatic necrosis, agranulocytosis, aplastic anemia and other blood dyscrasias (see *"Warnings"*).

OVERDOSAGE

No data are available regarding Acetazolamide overdosage in humans as no cases of acute poisoning with this drug have been reported. Animal data suggest that Acetazolamide is remarkably nontoxic. No specific antidote is known. Treatment should be symptomatic and supportive. Electrolyte imbalance, development of an acidotic state, and central nervous system effects might be expected to occur. Serum electrolyte levels (particularly potassium) and blood pH levels should be monitored.

Supportive measures are required to restore electrolyte and pH balance. The acidotic state can usually be corrected by the administration of bicarbonate.

Despite its high intraerythrocytic distribution and plasma protein binding properties, Acetazolamide may be dialyzable. This may be particularly important in the management of Acetazolamide overdosage when complicated by the presence of renal failure.

DOSAGE AND ADMINISTRATION

Preparation and Storage of Parenteral Solution: Each 500 mg vial containing sterile Acetazolamide sodium parenteral should be reconstituted with at least 5 mL of Sterile Water for Injection prior to use. Reconstituted solutions retain potency for 1 week if refrigerated. Since this product contains no perservative, use within 24 hours of reconstitution is strongly recommended. The direct intravenous route of administration is preferred. Intramuscular administration is not recommended.

Glaucoma: Tablets and Intravenous: Acetazolamide should be used as an adjunct to the usual therapy. The dosage employed in the treatment of *chronic simple (open-angle) glaucoma* ranges from 250 mg to 1 g of Acetazolamide per 24 hours, usually in divided doses for amounts over 250 mg. It has usually been found that a dosage in excess of 1 g per 24 hours does not produce an increased effect. In all cases, the dosage should be adjusted with careful individual attention both to symptomatology and ocular tension. Continuous supervision by a physician is advisable.

In treatment of secondary glaucoma and in the preoperative treatment of some cases of *acute congestive (closed-angle) glaucoma,* the preferred dosage is 250 mg every 4 hours, although some cases have responded to 250 mg twice daily on short-term therapy. In some acute cases, it may be more satisfactory to administer an initial dose of 500 mg followed by 125 or 250 mg every 4 hours depending on the individual case. Intravenous therapy may be used for rapid relief of ocular tension in acute cases. A complementary effect has been noted when Acetazolamide has been used in conjunction with miotics or mydriatics as the case demanded.

Sustained-Release Capsules: The recommended dosage is one capsule (500 mg) two times a day. Usually one capsule is administered in the morning and one capsule in the evening. It may be necessary to adjust the dose, but it has usually been found that dosage in excess of two capsules (1 g) does not produce an increased effect. The dosage should be adjusted with careful individual attention both to symptomatology and intraocular tension. In all cases, continuous supervision by a physician is advisable.

Epilepsy: It is not clearly known whether the beneficial effects observed in epilepsy are due to direct inhibition of carbonic anhydrase in the central nervous system or whether they are due to the slight degree of acidosis produced by the divided dosage. The best results to date have been seen in petit mal in children. Good results, however, have been seen in patients, both children and adult, in other types of seizures such as grand mal, mixed seizure patterns, myoclonic jerk patterns, etc. The suggested total daily dose is 8 to 30 mg per kg in divided doses. Although some patients respond to a low dose, the optimum range appears to be from 375 to 1000 mg daily. However, some investigators feel that daily doses in excess of 1 g do not produce any better results than a 1 g dose. When Acetazolamide is given in combination with other anticonvulsants, it is suggested that the starting dose should be 250 mg once daily in addition to the existing medications. This can be increased to levels as indicated above. The change from other medications to Acetazolamide should be gradual and in accordance with usual practice in epilepsy therapy.

Congestive Heart Failure: For diuresis in congestive heart failure, the starting dose is usually 250 to 375 mg once daily in the morning (5 mg/kg). If, after an initial response, the patient fails to continue to lose edema fluid, do not increase the dose but allow for kidney recovery by skipping medication for a day. Acetazolamide yields best diuretic results when given on alternate days, or for 2 days alternating with a day of rest.

Failures in therapy may be due to overdosage or too frequent dosage. The use of Acetazolamide does not eliminate the need for other therapy such as digitalis, bed rest, and salt restriction.

Drug-Induced Edema: Recommended dosage is 250 to 375 mg of Acetazolamide once a day for 1 or 2 days, alternating with a day of rest.

Acute Mountain Sickness: Dosage is 500 mg to 1000 mg daily, in divided doses using tablets or sustained-release capsules as appropriate. In circumstances of rapid ascent, such as in rescue or military operations, the higher dose level of 1000 mg is recommended. It is preferable to initiate dosing 24 to 48 hours before ascent and to continue for 48 hours while at high altitude, or longer as necessary to control symptoms.

Note: The dosage recommendations for glaucoma and epilepsy differ considerably from those for congestive heart failure, since the first two conditions are not dependent upon carbonic anhydrase inhibition in the kidney which requires intermittent dosage if it is to recover from the inhibitory effect of the therapeutic agent.

Parenteral drug products should be inspected visually for particulate matter and discoloration prior to administration, whenever solution and container permit.

Store at controlled room temperature 15°-30°C (59°-86°F).

J CODES
Up to 500 mg IM,IV—J1120

HOW SUPPLIED
CAPSULE, EXTENDED RELEASE: 500 MG

BRAND/MANUFACTURER	NDC	SIZE	AWP
○ BRAND			
➤ DIAMOX SEQUELS: Storz/Lederle	57706-0753-23	100s	$96.30

POWDER FOR INJECTION: 500 MG

BRAND/MANUFACTURER	NDC	SIZE	AWP
◆ BRAND			
DIAMOX SODIUM: Storz/Lederle	57706-0762-96	1s	$36.59

TABLETS: 125 MG

AVERAGE UNIT PRICE (AVAILABLE SIZES)		GENERIC A-RATED AVERAGE PRICE (GAAP)	
BRAND	$0.30	100s	$7.50
GENERIC	$0.07		
HCFA FUL (100s ea)	$0.08		

BRAND/MANUFACTURER	NDC	SIZE	AWP
◆ BRAND			
➤ DIAMOX: Storz/Lederle	57706-0754-23	100s	$30.06
◆ GENERICS			
Mutual	53489-0166-01	100s	$6.70
Moore,H.L.	00839-7687-06	100s	$7.55
URL	00677-1248-01	100s	$8.25
Mutual	53489-0166-05	500s	$27.00
Mutual	53489-0166-10	1000s	$51.00

TABLETS: 250 MG

AVERAGE UNIT PRICE (AVAILABLE SIZES)		GENERIC A-RATED AVERAGE PRICE (GAAP)	
BRAND	$0.40	100s	$11.20
GENERIC	$0.10	500s	$40.55
HCFA FUL (100s ea)	$0.08	1000s	$83.98

BRAND/MANUFACTURER	NDC	SIZE	AWP
◆ BRAND			
➤ DIAMOX: Storz/Lederle	57706-0755-23	100s	$38.78
	57706-0755-60	100s ud	$44.89
	57706-0755-34	1000s	$368.24
◆ GENERICS			
Moore,H.L.	00839-5953-06	100s	$9.17
Major	00904-0350-60	100s	$9.40
CMC-Cons	00223-0039-01	100s	$9.75
Qualitest	00603-2070-21	100s	$9.80
Mutual	53489-0167-01	100s	$9.85
URL	00677-0577-01	100s	$11.40
Schein	00364-0400-01	100s	$11.45
Rugby	00536-3007-01	100s	$11.95
Raway	00686-0052-20	100s	$12.15
Aligen	00405-4019-01	100s	$13.80
U.S. Trading	56126-0203-11	100s ud	$7.26
UDL	51079-0052-20	100s ud	$18.40
Mutual	53489-0167-05	500s	$38.75
URL	00677-0577-05	500s	$42.35
Mutual	53489-0167-10	1000s	$72.00
Moore,H.L.	00839-5953-16	1000s	$80.99
Major	00904-0350-80	1000s	$83.50
CMC-Cons	00223-0039-02	1000s	$87.50
Rugby	00536-3007-10	1000s	$89.35
Aligen	00405-4019-03	1000s	$90.55

Acetic Acid and Desonide

DESCRIPTION
Acetic Acid/Desonide Otic solution contains Desonide 0.05% and Acetic Acid 2% (the active ingredients) in a compatible vehicle buffered to the pH range of the normal ear. Otic Desonide 0.05%/Acetic Acid 2% solution is instilled into the external auditory canal.

Desonide is a nonfluorinated corticosteroid. Chemically, Desonide is Pregna-1,4-diene-3,20-dione,11,21-dihydroxy-16,17-[(1-methylethylidene) bis(oxy)]-,(11β,16α). Its empirical formula is $C_{24}H_{32}O_6$, its molecular weight is 416.51, and CAS Registry number is 638-94-8.

Acetic Acid is an astringent and antimicrobial agent. Chemically, it is $C_2H_4O_2$.

The base is composed of purified water, propylene glycol, sodium acetate, and citric acid.

CLINICAL PHARMACOLOGY
Topical corticosteroids share anti-inflammatory, antipruritic and vasoconstrictive actions.

The mechanism of anti-inflammatory activity of the topical corticosteroids is unclear. Various laboratory methods, including vasoconstrictor assays, are used to compare and predict potencies and/or clinical efficacies of the topical corticosteroids. There is some evidence to suggest that a recognizable correlation exists between vasoconstrictor potency and therapeutic efficacy in man.

Pharmacokinetics: The extent of percutaneous absorption of topical corticosteroids is determined by many factors including the vehicle, the integrity of the epidermal barrier, and the use of occlusive dressings.

Topical corticosteroids can be absorbed from normal intact skin. Inflammation and/or other disease processes in the skin increase percutaneous absorption. Occlusive dressings substantially increase the percutaneous absorption of topical corticosteroids.

Once absorbed through the skin, topical corticosteroids are handled through pharmacokinetic pathways similar to systemically administered corticosteroids. Corticosteroids are bound to plasma proteins in varying degrees. Corticosteroids are metabolized primarily in the liver and are then excreted by the kidneys. Some of the topical corticosteroids and their metabolites are also excreted into the bile.

INDICATIONS AND USAGE

Otic Acetic Acid/Desonide Solution is indicated for the treatment of superficial infections of the external auditory canal caused by organisms susceptible to the action of the antimicrobial and accompanied by inflammation.

CONTRAINDICATIONS

Otic Acetic Acid/Desonide Solution is contraindicated in those patients who have shown hypersensitivity to any of the components of the preparation. Perforated tympanic membranes are frequently considered a contraindication to the use of external ear canal medication.

PRECAUTIONS

General: Systemic absorption of topical corticosteroids has produced reversible hypothalamic-pituitary-adrenal (HPA) axis suppression, manifestations of Cushing's syndrome, hyperglycemia, and glucosuria in some patients.

Conditions which augment systemic absorption include the application of the more potent steroids, use over large surface areas, prolonged use, and the addition of occlusive dressings.

Children may absorb proportionally larger amounts of topical corticosteroids and thus be more susceptible to systemic toxicity (See *"Precautions—Prediatric Use"*).

If irritation develops, the product should be discontinued and appropriate therapy instituted.

If infection persists or new infection appears, appropriate therapy should be instituted. If a favorable response does not occur promptly, the corticosteroid should be discontinued until the infection has been adequately controlled.

Information for the Patient: Patients using topical corticosteroids should receive the following information and instructions:

1. This medication is to be used as directed by the physician. It is for external use only. Avoid contact with eyes.

2. Patients should be advised not to use this medication for any disorder other than for which it was prescribed.

Laboratory Tests: The following tests may be helpful in evaluating the HPA axis suppression:
   Urinary free cortisol test
   ACTH stimulation test

Carcinogenesis, Mutagenesis, and Impairment of Fertility: Long-term animal studies have not been performed to evaluate the carcinogenic potential or the effect on fertility of topical corticosteroids. Studies to determine mutagenicity with prednisolone and hydrocortisone have revealed negative results.

Pregnancy Category C: Corticosteroids are generally teratogenic in laboratory animals when administered systemically at relatively low dosage levels. The more potent corticosteroids have been shown to be teratogenic after dermal application in laboratory animals. There are no adequate and well-controlled studies in pregnant women on teratogenic effects from topically applied corticosteroids. Therefore, topical corticosteroids should be used during pregnancy only if the potential benefit justifies the potential risk to the fetus. Drugs of this class should not be used extensively on pregnant patients, in large amounts, or for prolonged periods of time.

Nursing Mothers: It is not known whether topical administration of corticosteroids could result in sufficient systemic absorption to produce detectable quantities in breast milk. Systemically administered corticosteroids are secreted into breast milk in quantities not likely to have a deleterious effect on the infant. Nevertheless, caution should be exercised when topical corticosteroids are administered to a nursing woman.

Pediatric Use: Pediatric patients may demonstrate greater susceptibility to topical corticosteroid-induced HPA axis suppression and Cushing's syndrome than mature patients because of a larger skin surface area to body weight ratio.

Hypothalamic-pituitary-adrenal (HPA) axis suppression, Cushing's syndrome, and intracranial hypertension have been reported in children receiving topical corticosteroids. Manifestations of adrenal suppression in children include linear growth retardation, delayed weight gain, low plasma cortisol levels, and absence of response to ACTH stimulation. Manifestations of intracranial hypertension include bulging fontanelles, headaches, and bilateral papilledema.

Administration of topical corticosteroids to children should be limited to the least amount compatible with an effective therapeutic regimen. Chronic corticosteroid therapy may interfere with the growth and development of children.

ADVERSE REACTIONS

The following local adverse reactions may occur infrequently with otic use of topical corticosteroids. These reactions are listed in an approximate decreasing order of occurrence.

Burning
Itching
Irritation
Dryness
Folliculitis
Hypertrichosis
Hypopigmentation
Allergic contact dermatitis
Maceration of the skin
Secondary infection
Skin atrophy

OVERDOSAGE

Topically applied corticosteroids can be absorbed in sufficient amounts to produce systemic effects (see *"Precautions"*).

DOSAGE AND ADMINISTRATION

All ceruminous material and debris should be carefully removed to permit Otic Acetic Acid/Desonide Solution to contact the infected surfaces. Instill 3 to 4 drops into the ear 3 to 4 times daily. If preferred, a gauze or cotton wick saturated with the solution may be inserted in the ear canal and allowed to remain in situ. It should be kept moist by further addition of the solution, as required.

Store below 86°F (30°C), avoid freezing.

HOW SUPPLIED
DROP: 2%-0.05%

BRAND/MANUFACTURER	NDC	SIZE	AWP
○ **BRAND**			
OTIC TRIDESILON: Miles Pharm	00026-7210-10	10 ml	$16.18

Acetic Acid with Hydrocortisone Otic Solution

DESCRIPTION

Acetic Acid/Hydrocortisone Otic Solution, USP contains Hydrocortisone (1%) and citric acid (0.05%). The empirical formulas for Acetic Acid and Hydrocortisone are CH_3COOH and $C_{21}H_{30}O_5$, with a molecular weight of 60.05 and 362.46, respectively.

Chemically, Hydrocortisone is: Pregn-4-ene-3,20-dione, 11,17,21-trihydroxy-(11β).

Acetic Acid/Hydrocortisone Otic Solution is available as nonaqueous otic solution buffered at pH 3 for use in the external ear canal.

CLINICAL PHARMACOLOGY

Acetic Acid is antibacterial and antifungal; propylene glycol is hydrophilic and provides a low surface tension; benzethonium chloride is a surface active agent that promotes contact of the solution with tissues; Hydrocortisone is anti-inflammatory, antiallergic and antipruritic.

INDICATIONS AND USAGE

Acetic Acid/Hydrocortisone Otic Solution—For the treatment of superficial infections of the external auditory canal caused by organisms susceptible to the action of the antimicrobial, complicated by inflammation.

CONTRAINDICATIONS

Hypersensitivity to any of the ingredients. Acetic Acid/Hydrocortisone Otic Solution is contraindicated in vaccinia and varicella. Perforated tympanic membrane is considered a contraindication to the use of any medication in the external ear canal.

WARNINGS

Discontinue promptly if sensitization or irritation occurs.

PRECAUTIONS

Transient stinging or burning may be noted occasionally when the solution is first instilled into the acutely inflamed ear.

ADVERSE REACTIONS

Stinging or burning may be noted occasionally: local irritation has occurred very rarely.

DOSAGE AND ADMINISTRATION

Carefully remove all cerumen and debris to allow Acetic Acid/ Hydrocortisone Otic Solution to contact infected surfaces directly. To promote continuous contact, insert a wick saturated with Acetic Acid/Hydrocortisone Otic Solution into the ear canal; the wick may also be saturated after insertion. Instruct the patient to keep the wick in for at least 24 hours and to keep it moist by adding 3 to 5 drops of Acetic Acid/Hydrocortisone Otic Solution every 4 to 6 hours. The wick may be removed after 24 hours.

Store at controlled room temperature 15°C—30°C (59°F—86°F).

HOW SUPPLIED
DROP: 2%-1%

AVERAGE UNIT PRICE (AVAILABLE SIZES)		GENERIC A-RATED AVERAGE PRICE (GAAP)	
BRAND	$3.70	10 ml	$5.57
GENERIC	$0.57		

BRAND/MANUFACTURER	NDC	SIZE	AWP
◆ **BRAND**			
VOSOL HC: Wallace	00037-3811-12	10 ml 3s	$111.11

◆ RATED THERAPEUTICALLY EQUIVALENT; ◇ THERAPEUTIC EQUIVALENCE UNCONFIRMED; ○ UNRATED

BRAND/MANUFACTURER	NDC	SIZE	AWP
◆ GENERICS			
Thames	49158-0197-43	10 ml	$3.98
VASOTATE HC: Major	00904-0316-10	10 ml	$5.15
Goldline	00182-1776-63	10 ml	$5.25
ACETASOL HC: Moore,H.L.	00839-6645-90	10 ml	$5.47
URL	00677-1408-21	10 ml	$5.50
Qualitest	00603-7036-39	10 ml	$5.68
ACETASOL HC: Barre	00472-0882-82	10 ml	$5.72
Raway	00686-0882-82	10 ml	$5.95
Geneva	00781-6311-70	10 ml	$6.04
Rugby	00536-2110-70	10 ml	$6.94
Schein	00364-0751-54	10 ml	$7.15

Acetic Acid, Otic

DESCRIPTION
Acetic Acid, Otic Solution contains 2% acetic acid as the active ingredient, in modified Burow's solution (water, aluminum acetate, and sodium acetate) with boric acid as a stabilizer. Acetic Acid, Otic Solution is instilled in the external auditory canal. Acetic acid is an astringent and antimicrobial agent. The pH range is from 4.5 to 6.0.
Chemically, acetic acid is $C_2H_4O_2$.

CLINICAL PHARMACOLOGY
Acetic acid is antibacterial and antifungal; and is effective against microorganisms (bacteria and fungi) that infect the ears of patients with acute diffuse external otitis. In *in vitro* tests, minimum lethal-time was less than 0.25 minutes when bacteria and fungi isolated from patients with otitis externa were exposed to 2% acetic acid. Quantitative absorption of acetic acid 2% from external auditory canal is not known.

INDICATIONS AND USAGE
Acetic Acid, Otic Solution is indicated for the treatment of superficial infections of the external auditory canal caused by organisms susceptible to the action of the antimicrobial.

CONTRAINDICATIONS
Hypersensitivity to acetic acid or any of the ingredients of this product. Perforated tympanic membrane is considered a contraindication to the use of any medication in the external ear canal.

WARNINGS
Avoid use or use with caution in patients with perforated tympanic membrane (see "Contraindications").

PRECAUTIONS
General: Care should be taken to assure that the Acetic Acid, Otic Solution gets into the ear canal and stays in contact with the affected area long enough for the drug to act.
Discontinue promptly if sensitization or irritation occurs.

Carcinogenesis, Mutagenesis, Impairment of Fertility: No long term studies in animals have been performed to evaluate the carcinogenic potential of Acetic Acid, Otic Solution.

ADVERSE REACTIONS
Irritation may occur.

OVERDOSAGE
No toxic effect has been reported with overdosage of Acetic Acid, Otic Solution.

DOSAGE AND ADMINISTRATION
Patient should lie on his side with affected ear uppermost. Instill 4 to 6 drops into the external auditory canal and maintain this position for five minutes. Repeat the procedure every 2 to 3 hours.
Store below 86°F (30°C), avoid freezing.
Acetic Acid, Otic Solution is a clear colorless liquid.

HOW SUPPLIED
DROP: 2%

AVERAGE UNIT PRICE (AVAILABLE SIZES)		GENERIC A-RATED AVERAGE PRICE (GAAP)	
BRAND	$1.31	15 ml	$3.68
GENERIC	$0.22	60 ml	$8.55

BRAND/MANUFACTURER	NDC	SIZE	AWP
◆ BRAND			
DOMEBORO: Miles Pharm	00026-4312-02	60 ml	$15.24
VOSOL: Wallace	00037-3611-10	15 ml 3s	$91.46
	00037-3611-30	30 ml 3s	$147.25
◆ GENERICS			
Thames	49158-0195-42	15 ml	$2.60
Qualitest	00603-7035-41	15 ml	$3.32
UDL	51079-0262-15	15 ml	$3.48
Schein	00364-0732-72	15 ml	$3.60
ACETASOL: Moore,H.L.	00839-6644-61	15 ml	$3.63
VASOTATE: Major	00904-0315-35	15 ml	$3.75

BRAND/MANUFACTURER	NDC	SIZE	AWP
Goldline	00182-1775-64	15 ml	$3.75
Geneva	00781-6310-85	15 ml	$4.19
Rugby	00536-2102-72	15 ml	$4.20
ACETASOL: Barre	00472-0880-99	15 ml	$4.29
Thames	49158-0195-41	30 ml	$4.00
Moore,H.L.	00839-7383-64	60 ml	$7.95
BUROW'S SOLUTION: Rugby	00536-0252-96	60 ml	$9.15

Acetic Acid/Oxyquinoline Sulfate/ Ricinoleic Acid

DESCRIPTION
Acetic Acid/Oxyquinoline Sulfate/Ricinoleic Acid Vaginal Jelly is a bland, nonirritating, waterdispersible, buffered acid jelly for intravaginal use. Acetic Acid/Oxyquinoline Sulfate/Ricinoleic Acid (Acetic/Oxyquinoline/Ricinoleic) is classified as a Vaginal Therapeutic Jelly. Acetic/Oxyquinoline/Ricinoleic contains 0.921% Acetic Acid ($C_2H_4O_2$), 0.025% Oxyquinoline Sulfate ($C_{18}H_{16}N_2O_6S$), 0.7% Ricinoleic Acid ($C_{18}H_{34}O_3$). Acetic/Oxyquinoline/Ricinoleic is formulated to pH 3.9-4.1.

CLINICAL PHARMACOLOGY
Acetic/Oxyquinoline/Ricinoleic acts to restore and maintain normal vaginal acidity through its buffer action.

INDICATIONS AND USAGE
Acetic/Oxyquinoline/Ricinoleic is indicated as adjunctive therapy in those cases where restoration and maintenance of vaginal acidity are desirable.

CONTRAINDICATIONS
None known.

WARNINGS
No serious adverse reactions or potential safety hazards have been reported with the use of Acetic/Oxyquinoline/Ricinoleic.

PRECAUTIONS
General: No special care is required for the safe and effective use of Acetic/Oxyquinoline/Ricinoleic.

Drug Interactions: No incidence of drug interactions have been reported with concomitant use of Acetic/Oxyquinoline/Ricinoleic and any other medications.

Laboratory Tests: The monitoring of vaginal acidity (pH) may be helpful in following the patient's response. (The normal vaginal pH has been shown to be in the range of 4.0 to 5.0.)

Carcinogenesis: No long-term studies in animals have been performed to evaluate carcinogenic potential.

Pregnancy: Pregnancy Category C. Animal reproduction studies have not been conducted with Acetic/Oxyquinoline/Ricinoleic. It is also not known whether Acetic/Oxyquinoline/Ricinoleic can cause fetal harm when administered to a pregnant woman or can affect reproduction capacity Acetic/Oxyquinoline/Ricinoleic should be given to a pregnant woman only if clearly needed.

Nursing Mothers: It is not known whether this drug is excreted in human milk. Because many drugs are excreted in human milk, caution should be exercised when Acetic/Oxyquinoline/Ricinoleic is administered to a nursing woman.

ADVERSE REACTIONS
Occasional cases of local stinging and burning have been reported.

DOSAGE AND ADMINISTRATION
The usual dose is one applicatorful, administered intravaginally, morning and evening. Duration of treatment may be determined by the patient's reponse to therapy.

HOW SUPPLIED
GEL:

BRAND/MANUFACTURER	NDC	SIZE	AWP
○ BRAND			
ACI-JEL: Ortho Pharm	00062-5421-01	85 gm	$23.88

Acetohexamide

DESCRIPTION
Acetohexamide USP is an oral blood-glucose lowering drug of the sulfonylurea class. Acetohexamide is a white to off-white, crystalline, practically odorless powder. It is practically insoluble in water and ether, soluble in pyridine and dilute solutions of alkali hydroxides, and slightly soluble in alcohol and chloroform. Chemically, it is benzenesulfonamide, 4-acetyl-N-[[cyclohexylamino]amino]carbonyl]- or 1-[(p-acetylphenyl) sulfonyl]-3-cyclohexylurea. The empirical formula for Acetohexamide is $C_{15}H_{20}N_2O_4S$. Its molecular weight is 324.39.

Acetohexamide is supplied in 250-mg (770 µmol) and 500-mg (1,540 µmol) tablets.

Following is its chemical structure:

$$CH_3CO \text{---} \bigcirc \text{---} SO_2NHCONH \text{---} \bigcirc$$

CLINICAL PHARMACOLOGY

Acetohexamide appears to lower the blood glucose acutely by stimulating the release of insulin from the pancreas, an effect that is dependent on functioning β cells in the pancreatic islets. The mechanism by which Acetohexamide lowers blood glucose during long-term administration has not been clearly established.

Acetohexamide is rapidly absorbed from the gastrointestinal tract, and maximum hypoglycemic activity is observed about 3 hours after ingestion. The total duration of action is 12 to 24 hours. Much of the activity is ascribable to a metabolite, hydroxyhexamide, which has a plasma half-life of approximately 6 hours; the parent compound, Acetohexamide, has a plasma half-life of 1.3 hours. In persons with normal renal and hepatic function, more than 80% is excreted, largely as metabolites, in 24 hours.

INDICATIONS AND USAGE

Acetohexomide is indicated as an adjunct to diet for lowering the blood glucose in patients with non-insulin-dependent diabetes mellitus (type II) whose hyperglycemia cannot be controlled by diet alone.

In initiating treatment for non-insulin-dependent diabetes, diet should be emphasized as the primary form of treatment. Caloric restriction and weight loss are essential in the obese diabetic patient. Proper dietary management alone may be effective in controlling the blood glucose and symptoms of hyperglycemia. The importance of regular physical activity should also be stressed, and cardiovascular risk factors should be identified and corrective measures taken when possible.

If this treatment program fails to reduce symptoms and/or blood glucose, the use of an oral sulfonylurea or insulin should be considered. The use of Acetohexamide must be viewed by both the physician and patient as a treatment in addition to diet, and not as a substitute for diet or as a convenient mechanism for avoiding dietary restraint. Furthermore, loss of blood glucose control with diet alone may be transient, thus requiring only short-term administration of Acetohexamide.

During maintenance programs, Acetohexomide should be discontinued if satisfactory lowering of blood glucose is no longer achieved. Judgments should be based on regular clinical and laboratory evaluations.

In considering the use of Acetohexamide in asymptomatic patients, it should be recognized that controlling the blood glucose in non-insulin-dependent diabetes has not been definitely established as being effective in preventing the long-term cardiovascular or neural complications of diabetes.

CONTRAINDICATIONS

Acetohexamide is contraindicated in patients with:

1. known hypersensitivity to the drug
2. diabetic ketoacidosis, with or without coma. This condition should be treated with insulin
3. insulin-dependent (type I) diabetes mellitus, as sole therapy
4. diabetes when complicated by pregnancy (see *"Pregnancy"* under *"Precautions"*)

WARNINGS
SPECIAL WARNING ON INCREASED RISK OF CARDIOVASCULAR MORTALITY

The administration of oral hypoglycemic drugs has been reported to be associated with increased cardiovascular mortality as compared to treatment with diet alone or diet plus insulin. This warning is based on the study conducted by the University Group Diabetes Program (UGDP), a long-term prospective clinical trial designed to evaluate the effectiveness of glucose-lowering drugs in preventing or delaying vascular complications in patients with non-insulin-dependent diabetes. The study involved 823 patients who were randomly assigned to 1 of 4 treatment groups (*Diabetes* 1970; 19 [suppl 2]:747-830).

UGDP reported that patients treated for 5 to 8 years with diet plus a fixed dose of tolbutamide (1.5 g/day) had a rate of cardiovascular mortality approximately 2 ½ times that of patients treated with diet alone. A significant increase in total mortality was not observed, but the use of tolbutamide was discontinued based on the increase in cardiovascular mortality, thus limiting the opportunity for the study to show an increase in overall mortality. Despite controversy regarding the interpretation of these results, the findings of the UGDP study provide an adequate basis for this warning. The patient should be informed of the potential risks and advantages of Acetohexamide and of alternative modes of therapy.

Although only 1 drug in the sulfonylurea class (tolbutamide) was included in this study, it is prudent from a safety standpoint to consider that this warning may also apply to other oral hypoglycemic drugs in this class, in view of their close similarities in mode of action and chemical structure.

PRECAUTIONS
GENERAL

Hypoglycemia: All sulfonylurea drugs are capable of producing severe hypoglycemia. Proper patient selection, dosage, and instructions are important for avoiding hypoglycemic episodes. Renal or hepatic insufficiency may cause elevated blood levels of Acetohexamide, and the latter may also diminish gluconeogenic capacity, both of which increase the risk of serious hypoglycemic reactions. Elderly, debilitated or malnourished patients, and those with adrenal or pituitary insufficiency are particularly susceptible to the hypoglycemic action of glucose-

lowering drugs. Hypoglycemia may be difficult to recognize in the elderly and in people who are taking β-adrenergic blocking drugs. Hypoglycemia is more likely to occur when caloric intake is deficient, after severe or prolonged exercise, when alcohol is ingested, or when more than 1 glucose-lowering drug is used.

Loss of Control of Blood Glucose: When a patient stabilized on any diabetic regimen is exposed to stress, such as fever, trauma, infection, or surgery, a loss of control may occur. At such times, it may be necessary to discontinue Acetohexamide and administer insulin.

The effectiveness of any oral hypoglycemic drug, including Acetohexamide in lowering blood glucose to a desired level decreases in many patients over a period of time; this decrease in effectiveness may be due to progression of the severity of the diabetes or to diminished responsiveness to the drug. This phenomenon is known as secondary failure, to distinguish it from primary failure in which the drug is ineffective in an individual patient when first given.

Information for Patients: Patients should be informed of the potential risks and advantages of Acetohexamide and of alternative modes of therapy. They should also be informed about the importance of adherence to dietary instructions, of a regular exercise program, and of regular testing of urine and/or blood glucose.

The risks of hypoglycemia, its symptoms and treatment, and conditions that predispose to its development should be explained to patients and responsible family members. Primary and secondary failure should also be explained.

Laboratory Tests: Blood and urine glucose should be monitored periodically. Measurement of glycosylated hemoglobin may be useful.

Drug Interactions: The hypoglycemic action of sulfonylurea agents may be potentiated by certain drugs, including nonsteroidal anti-inflammatory agents and other drugs that are highly protein bound, salicylates, sulfonamides, chloramphenicol, probenecid, coumarins, monoamine oxidase inhibitors, and β-adrenergic blocking agents. When such drugs are administered to a patient receiving Acetohexamide the patient should be observed closely for hypoglycemia. When such drugs are withdrawn from a patient receiving Acetohexamide the patient should be observed closely for loss of control.

Certain drugs tend to produce hyperglycemia and may lead to loss of control. These drugs include the thiazides and other diuretics, corticosteroids, phenothiazines, thyroid products, estrogens, oral contraceptives, phenytoin, nicotinic acid, sympathomimetics, calcium channel blocking drugs, and isoniazid. When such drugs are administered to a patient receiving Acetohexamide the patient should be closely observed for loss of control. When such drugs are withdrawn from a patient receiving Acetohexamide the patient should be observed closely for hypoglycemia.

A potential interaction between oral miconazole and oral hypoglycemic agents leading to severe hypoglycemia has been reported. Whether this interaction also occurs with the intravenous, topical, or vaginal preparations of miconazole is not known.

Carcinogenesis, Mutagenesis, and Impairment of Fertility: Long-term studies in rats and mice revealed no evidence of carcinogenicity of Acetohexamide. A sister chromatid exchange study performed with Acetohexamide showed no evidence of mutagenicity. No animal studies have been conducted to determine whether Acetohexamide has the potential to impair fertility.

Pregnancy—Teratogenic Effects—Pregnancy Category C: Acetohexamide has not been shown to be teratogenic in animals. However, teratogenesis in animals has been observed following administration of high doses of other sulfonylurea agents. There are no adequate and well-controlled studies in pregnant women. Therefore, Acetohexamide is not recommended for the management of diabetes when complicated by pregnancy.

Because recent information suggests that abnormal blood glucose levels during pregnancy are associated with a higher incidence of congenital abnormalities, many experts recommend that insulin be used during pregnancy to maintain blood glucose levels as close to normal as possible.

Nonteratogenic Effects: Prolonged severe hypoglycemia (4 to 10 days) has been reported in neonates born to mothers who were receiving a sulfonylurea drug at the time of delivery. This has been reported more frequently with the use of agents with prolonged half-lives. The use of Acetohexamide is not recommended for the management of diabetes when complicated by pregnancy.

Nursing Mothers: It is not known whether this drug is excreted in human milk. Because some sulfonylurea drugs are excreted in human milk and because of the potential for serious adverse reactions in nursing infants from Acetohexamide a decision should be made whether to discontinue nursing or to discontinue the drug, taking into account the importance of the drug to the mother.

ADVERSE REACTIONS

Hypoglycemia: See *"Precautions"* and *"Overdosage"*.

Gastrointestinal Reactions: Cholestatic jaundice may occur rarely; Acetohexamide should be discontinued if this occurs. Gastrointestinal disturbances, eg, nausea, epigastric fullness, and heartburn, are the most common reactions and occur in 1 in 40 patients. These reactions tend to be dose related and may disappear when dosage is reduced.

Dermatologic Reactions: Allergic skin reactions, eg, pruritus, erythema, urticaria, and morbilliform or maculopapular eruptions, occur in less than 1 in 100 patients. These may be transient and may disappear despite continued use of Acetohexamide; if skin reactions persist, the drug should be discontinued.

Porphyria cutanea tarda and photosensitivity reactions have been reported with sulfonylurea agents.

Endocrine Reactions: Cases of hyponatremia and the syndrome of inappropriate antidiuretic hormone (SIADH) secretion have been reported with this and other sulfonylurea agents.

Hematologic Reactions: Leukopenia, agranulocytosis, thrombocytopenia, hemolytic anemia, aplastic anemia, and pancytopenia have been reported with sulfonylurea agents.

Metabolic Reactions: Hepatic porphyria and disulfiram-like reactions have been reported with sulfonylurea agents.

OVERDOSAGE

Signs and Symptoms: Hypoglycemia is the predominant finding in cases of sulfonylurea overdose (including overdose with Acetohexamide but this condition may be preceded by nausea, vomiting, and mild epigastric pain. Symptoms of hypoglycemia may include headache, weakness, confusion, dizziness, lethargy, convulsions, coma, and death. Patients may be especially susceptible to hypoglycemia if they are elderly, if they have had restricted carbohydrate intake (especially during periods of exercise), or if they have kidney or liver dysfunction.

Treatment: To obtain up-to-date information about the treatment of overdose, a good resource is your certified Regional Poison Control Center. Telephone numbers of certified poison control centers are listed in the *Physicians' Desk Reference (PDR).* In managing overdosage, consider the possibility of multiple drug overdoses, interaction among drugs, and unusual drug kinetics in your patient.

Overdosage of sulfonylureas, including Acetohexamide, can produce hypoglycemia. Mild hypoglycemic symptoms without loss of consciousness or neurologic findings should be treated aggressively with oral glucose and adjustments in drug dosage and/or meal patterns. Close monitoring should continue until the physician is assured that the patient is out of danger. Severe hypoglycemic reactions with coma, seizure, or other neurologic impairment occur infrequently but constitute medical emergencies requiring immediate hospitalization. If hypoglycemic coma is diagnosed or suspected, the patient should be given a rapid intravenous injection of concentrated (50%) glucose solution. This should be followed by a continuous infusion of a more dilute (10%) glucose solution at a rate that will maintain the blood glucose at a level of about 100 mg/dL. Patients should be closely monitored for a minimum of 24 to 48 hours, since hypoglycemia may recur after apparent clinical recovery.

Monitor the patient's vital signs, blood gases, glucose, serum electrolytes, etc. Absorption of drugs from the gastrointestinal tract may be decreased by giving activated charcoal, which, in many cases, is more effective than emesis or lavage; consider charcoal instead of or in addition to gastric emptying. Repeated doses of charcoal over time may hasten elimination of some drugs that have been absorbed. Safeguard the patient's airway when employing gastric emptying or charcoal.

DOSAGE AND ADMINISTRATION

There is no fixed dosage regimen for the management of diabetes mellitus with Acetohexamide or any other hypoglycemic agent. In addition to the usual monitoring of urinary glucose, the patient's blood glucose must also be monitored periodically to determine the minimum effective dose for a patient; to detect primary failure, ie, inadequate lowering of blood glucose with the recommended dose of medication; and to detect secondary failure, ie, loss of an adequate blood-glucose lowering response after an initial period of effectiveness. Glycosylated hemoglobin levels may also be of value in monitoring the patient's response to therapy.

Short-term administration of Acetohexamide may be sufficient during periods of transient loss of control in patients usually well controlled on diet.

Daily oral dosage of Acetohexamide may range between 250 mg and 1.5 g. No loading dose is required. Patients who do not respond to 1.5 g daily usually will not respond to a higher dose. For this reason, doses in excess of 1.5 g daily are not recommended.

The majority of patients receiving 1 g or less/day can be controlled on a convenient once-daily dosage. Patients who need 1.5 g/day usually benefit from twice-daily dosage, given before the morning and evening meals.

Various measures have been employed to establish patients on Acetohexamide, and the following procedures are suggested.

Patients Not Previously Receiving Insulin or Drug Therapy: In mild, stable diabetes (after dietary regulation), therapy may be initiated with 250 mg daily before breakfast; subsequent adjustment of the dosage may be made by increments of 250 to 500 mg every 5 to 7 days as necessary. The 250-mg or 500-mg tablet (scored and easily broken in half) may be used.

Because of reports of hyperresponsiveness to Acetohexamide of some elderly patients with diabetes, patients in this group should be started with a single dose of 250 mg before breakfast, and their blood and urine sugars should be checked during the first 24 hours of therapy. If control appears to be satisfactory, this dose may be continued on a daily basis or, if necessary, gradually increased. If, however, there appears to be a tendency toward hypoglycemia, this dose should be reduced or the drug should be discontinued.

Patients Receiving Other Oral Agents: When transfer is made from tolbutamide, the initial dose of Acetohexamide should be about half the tolbutamide dose (eg, 250 mg of Acetohexamide in place of 500 mg of tolbutamide), up to a maximum of 1.5 g of Acetohexamide.

When transfer is made from chlorpropamide, the initial dose of Acetohexamide should be about double the chlorpropamide dose (eg, 500 mg of Acetohexamide in place of 250 mg of chlorpropamide).

A transition period usually is required because of the long half-life of chlorpropamide. Subsequent adjustment of dosage should be made according to clinical response. The maximum recommended dose of Acetohexamide is 1.5 g.

Clinical reports on the efficacy of once-daily dosage of Acetohexamide indicate that its effect on the blood sugar is better sustained than that of tolbutamide. However, patients requiring more than 1 g of Acetohexamide daily should be treated with divided doses.

Patients Receiving Insulin: In general, patients who were previously maintained on insulin in small dosage (eg, up to 20 units/day) may be placed on Acetohexamide directly and their insulin administration abruptly discontinued. Patients receiving larger doses of insulin, such as 20 to 40 units or more/day, should have an initial reduction of insulin dosage by 25% to 30% daily or every other day and subsequent further reduction depending on the response to Acetohexamide. An initial dose of 250 mg of Acetohexamide can be used, with readjustment depending on response to therapy. Because of the potential hazards of hypoglycemia in the elderly, patients in this age group should be carefully observed during the transition from insulin to Acetohexamide.

During the period of insulin withdrawal, the patient should test his/her blood or urine for sugar and urine for acetone at least 3 times a day and report the results frequently to his/her physician so that appropriate adjustments of therapy may be made. In some cases, it may be advisable to consider hospitalization during the transition period from insulin to Acetohexamide.

It should be noted that, as with other sulfonylureas, primary and secondary failures may occur with Acetohexamide.

In elderly, debilitated, or malnourished patients and patients with impaired renal or hepatic function, the initial and maintenance doses should be conservative to avoid hypoglycemic reactions (see *"Precautions"*).

Store at controlled room temperature, 59° to 86°F (15° to 30°C).

HOW SUPPLIED
TABLETS: 250 MG

AVERAGE UNIT PRICE (AVAILABLE SIZES)		GENERIC A-RATED AVERAGE PRICE (GAAP)	
BRAND	$0.24	100s	$22.52
GENERIC	$0.23		
HCFA FUL (100s ea)	$0.24		

BRAND/MANUFACTURER	NDC	SIZE	AWP
◆ BRAND			
DYMELOR: Lilly	00002-2103-22	200s	$47.89
◆ GENERICS			
Raway	00686-0442-02	100s	$13.00
Moore,H.L.	00839-7386-06	100s	$23.07
Schein	00364-2232-01	100s	$26.42
Aligen	00405-4024-01	100s	$27.60

TABLETS: 500 MG

AVERAGE UNIT PRICE (AVAILABLE SIZES)		GENERIC A-RATED AVERAGE PRICE (GAAP)	
BRAND	$0.44	100s	$38.31
GENERIC	$0.38		
HCFA FUL (100s ea)	$0.32		

BRAND/MANUFACTURER	NDC	SIZE	AWP
◆ BRAND			
DYMELOR: Lilly	00002-2107-50	50s	$22.53
	00002-2107-22	200s	$86.52
◆ GENERICS			
Moore,H.L.	00839-7387-06	100s	$29.03
Schein	00364-2233-01	100s	$37.69
Aligen	00405-4025-01	100s	$48.20

Acetohydroxamic Acid

DESCRIPTION

Acetohydroxamic Acid is a stable, synthetic compound derived from hydroxylamine and ethyl acetate.

Acetohydroxamic Acid is weakly acidic, highly soluble in water, and chelates metals — notably iron. The molecular weight is 75.068. Acetohydroxamic Acid has a pKa of 9.32 and a melting point of 89-91° C. Acetohydroxamic Acid is a urease inhibitor. Available as 250 mg tablets.

Following is its chemical structure:

$$CH_3-\overset{\overset{\displaystyle O}{\|}}{C}-\underset{\underset{\displaystyle H}{|}}{N}-OH$$

CLINICAL PHARMACOLOGY

Acetohydroxamic Acid (AHA) reversibly inhibits the bacterial enzyme urease, thereby inhibiting the hydrolysis of urea and production of ammonia in urine infected with urea-splitting organisms. The reduced ammonia levels and decreased pH enhance the effectiveness of antimicrobial agents and allow an increased cure rate of these infections.

AHA is well absorbed from the gastrointestinal tract after oral administration; peak blood levels occur from 0.25 to 1 hour after dosing. The compound is distributed throughout body water, and there is no known binding to any tissue.

AHA chelates with dietary iron within the gut. This reaction may interfere with absorption of AHA and with iron. Concomitant hypochromic anemia should be treated with intramuscular iron.

In rodents, the metabolic fate of AHA is well known; 55% is excreted unchanged in urine, 25% is excreted as acetamide or acetate and 7% is excreted by the lungs as carbon dioxide. Less than 1% is excreted in the feces. Approximately 5% of the administered dose is unaccounted for. In rodents, AHA shows a dose-related change in pharmacokinetics; with increasing dose, there is an increase in the half-life and an increase in the percent of the administered dose recovered in urine as unchanged AHA.

Pharmacokinetics in man are generally similar to rodents including the dose-related increase in half-life, but they are not as well characterized as in the rodent. Thirty-six to sixty-five percent (36-65%) of the oral dosage is excreted unchanged in the urine. It is unaltered AHA in the urine that provides the therapeutic effect, but the precise concentration of AHA in urine that is necessary to inhibit urease is incompletely delineated. Therapeutic benefit may be obtained from concentrations as low as 8 mcg/ml; higher concentrations (i.e., 30 mcg/ml) are expected to provide more complete inhibition of urease. The plasma half-life of AHA is approximately 5-10 hours in subjects with normal renal function and is prolonged in patients with reduced renal function.

Acetohydroxamic Acid has been evaluated clinically in patients with urea-splitting urinary infections, often accompanied by struvite stone disease, that were recalcitrant to other forms of medical and surgical management. In these clinical trials, AHA reduced the pathologically elevated urinary ammonia and pH levels that result from the hydrolysis of urea by the enzyme, urease.

AHA does not acidify urine directly nor does it have a direct anti-bacterial effect. The usefulness of reducing ammonia levels and decreasing urinary pH is suggested by single (not yet replicated) clinical trials in which urease inhibition 1) allowed successful antibiotic treatment of urea-splitting Proteus infections after surgical removal of struvite stones in patients not cured by 3 months of antibacterial treatment alone, and 2) reduced the rate of stone growth in patients who were not candidates for surgical removal of stones.

INDICATIONS AND USAGE

Acetohydroxamic Acid is indicated as adjunctive therapy in patients with chronic urea-splitting urinary infection. AHA is intended to decrease urinary ammonia and alkalinity, but it should not be used in lieu of curative surgical treatment (for patients with stones) or antimicrobial treatment. Long-term treatment with AHA may be warranted to maintain urease inhibition as long as urea-splitting infection is present. Experience with AHA does not go beyond 7 years. A patient package insert should be distributed to each patient who receives AHA.

CONTRAINDICATIONS

Acetohydroxamic Acid should not be used in:
  a. patients whose physical state and disease are amenable to definitive surgery and appropriate antimicrobial agents
  b. patients whose urine is infected by non-urease producing organisms
  c. patients whose urinary infections can be controlled by culture-specific oral antimicrobial agents.
  d. patients whose renal function is poor (i.e., serum creatinine more than 2.5 mg/dl and/or creatinine clearance less than 20 ml/min)
  e. female patients who do not evidence a satisfactory method of contraception
  f. patients who are pregnant
  Acetohydroxamic Acid may cause fetal harm when administered to a pregnant woman. AHA was teratogenic (retarded and/or clubbed rear leg at 750 mg/kg and above and exencephaly and encephalocele at 1,500 mg/kg) when given intraperitoneally to rats. AHA is contraindicated in women who are or may become pregnant. If this drug is used during pregnancy, or if the patient becomes pregnant while taking this drug, the patient should be informed of the potential hazard to the fetus.

WARNINGS

A Coombs negative hemolytic anemia has occurred in patients receiving AHA. Gastrointestinal upset characterized by nausea, vomiting, anorexia and generalized malaise have accompanied the most severe forms of hemolytic anemia. Approximately 15% of patients receiving AHA have had only laboratory findings of an anemia. However, most patients developed a mild reticulocytosis. The untoward reactions have reverted to normal following cessation of treatment. A complete blood count, including a reticulocyte count, is recommended after two weeks of treatment. If the reticulocyte count exceeds 6%, a reduced dosage should be entertained. A CBC and reticulocyte count are recommended at 3-month intervals for the duration of treatment.

PRECAUTIONS
GENERAL
Hematologic Effects: Bone marrow depression (leukopenia, anemia, and thrombocytopenia) has occurred in experimental animals receiving large doses of AHA, but has not been seen in man to date. AHA is a known inhibitor of DNA synthesis and also chelates metals - notably iron. Its bone marrow suppressant effect is probably related to its ability to inhibit DNA synthesis, but anemia could also be related to depletion of iron stores. To date, the only clinical effect noted has been hemolysis, with a decrease in the circulating red blood cells, hemoglobin and hematocrit. Abnormalities in platelet or white blood cell count have not been noted. However, clinical monitoring of the platelet and white cell count is recommended.

Monitoring Liver Function: Abnormalities of liver function have not been reported to date. However, a chloro-benzene derivative of Acetohydroxamic Acid

caused significant liver dysfunction in an unrelated study. Therefore, close monitoring of liver function is recommended. (See *"Carcinogenesis"* for discussion of possible hepatic carcinogenesis.)

Use in Patients With Renal Impairment: Since AHA is eliminated primarily by the kidneys, patients with significantly impaired renal function should be closely monitored, and a reduction of daily dose may be needed to avoid excessive drug accumulation. (See *"Dosage and Administration"*.)

DRUG INTERACTIONS: AHA has been used concomitantly with insulin, oral and parenteral antibiotics, and progestational agents. No clinically significant interactions have been noted, but until wider clinical experience is obtained, AHA should be used with caution in patients receiving other therapeutic agents.

AHA taken in association with alcoholic beverages has resulted in a rash. (See *"Adverse Reactions"*.)

AHA chelates heavy metals — notably iron. The absorption of iron and AHA from the intestinal lumen may be reduced when both drugs are taken concomitantly. When iron administration is indicated, intramuscular iron is probably the product of choice.

Carcinogenesis, Mutagenesis, Impairment of Fertility: Well controlled, long-term animal studies that identify the carcinogenic potential of AHA treatment have not been conducted. Acetamide, a metabolite of AHA, has been shown to cause hepatocellular carcinoma in rats at oral doses 1,500 times the human dose. AHA is cytotoxic and was positive for mutagenicity in the Ames test.

Pregnancy: Pregnancy Category X. (See *"Contraindications"*.)

Nursing Mothers: It is not known whether AHA is secreted in human milk. Because many drugs are excreted in human milk, and because of the potential for serious adverse reactions in nursing infants from AHA, a decision should be made to discontinue nursing or the drug, taking into account the significance of the drug to the mother's well being.

Pediatric Use: Children with chronic, recalcitrant, urea-splitting urinary infection may benefit from treatment with AHA. However, detailed studies involving dosage and dose intervals in children have not been established. Children have tolerated a dose of 10 mg/kg/day, taken in two or three divided doses, satisfactorily for periods up to one year. Close monitoring of such patients is mandatory.

ADVERSE REACTIONS

Experience with AHA is limited. About 150 patients have been treated, most for periods of more than a year.

Adverse reactions have occurred in up to thirty percent (30%) of the patients receiving AHA. In some instances the reactions were symptomatic; in others only changes in laboratory parameters were noted. Adverse reactions seem to be more prevalent in patients with preexisting thrombophlebitis or phlebothrombosis and/or in patients with advanced degrees of renal insufficiency. The risk of adverse reactions is highest during the first year of treatment. Chronic treatment does not seem to increase the risk nor the severity of adverse reactions.

The following reactions have been reported:

Neurological: Mild headaches are commonly reported (about 30%) during the first 48 hours of treatment. These headaches are mild, responsive to oral salicylate-type analgesics, and usually disappear spontaneously. The headaches have not been associated with vertigo, tinnitus, or visual or auditory abnormalities. Tremulousness and nervousness have also been reported.

Gastrointestinal: Gastrointestinal symptoms, nausea, vomiting, anorexia, and malaise have occurred in 20-25% of patients. In most patients the symptoms were mild, transitory, and did not result in interruption of treatment. Approximately 3% of patients developed a hemolytic anemia of sufficient magnitude to warrant interruption in treatment; several of these patients also had symptoms of gastrointestinal upset.

Hematological: Approximately 15% of patients have had laboratory findings characteristic of a hemolytic anemia. A mild reticulocytosis (5-6%) without anemia, is even more prevalent. The laboratory findings are occasionally accompanied by systemic symptoms such as malaise, lethargy and fatigue, and gastrointestinal symptoms. Symptoms and laboratory findings have invariably improved following cessation of treatment with AHA. The hematological abnormalities are more prevalent in patients with advanced renal failure.

Dermatological: A nonpruritic, macular skin rash has occurred in the upper extremities and on the face of several patients taking AHA on a long-term basis, usually when AHA has been taken concomitantly with alcoholic beverages, but in a few patients in the absence of alcohol consumption. The rash commonly appears 30-45 minutes after ingestion of alcoholic beverages; it characteristically disappears spontaneously in 30-60 minutes. The rash may be associated with a general sensation of warmth. In some patients the rash is sufficiently severe to warrant discontinuation of treatment, but most patients have continued treatment, avoiding alcohol or using smaller quantities of it. Alopecia has also been reported in patients taking AHA.

Cardiovascular: Superficial phlebitis involving the lower extremities has occurred in several patients on AHA during the early (Phase II) clinical trials. Several of the affected patients had had phlebitic episodes prior to treatment. One patient developed deep vein thrombosis of the lower extremities. The patient with phlebothrombosis had an associated traumatic injury to the groin. It is unclear whether the phlebitis was related to or exacerbated by treatment with AHA. No patient in the three (3) year controlled (Phase III) clinical trial developed phlebitis. In all instances these vascular abnormalities returned to normal

---

following appropriate medical therapy. Embolic phenomena have been reported in three patients taking AHA in the Phase II trial. The phlebitis and emboli resolved following discontinuation of AHA and implementation of appropriate medical therapy. Several patients have resumed treatment with AHA without ill effect. Palpitations have also been reported in patients taking AHA.

Respiratory: No symptoms have been reported. Radiographic evidence of small pulmonary emboli has been seen in three patients with phlebitis in their lower legs.

Psychiatric: Depression, anxiety, nervousness, and tremulousness have been observed in approximately 20% of patients taking AHA. In most patients the symptoms were mild and transitory, but in about 6% of patients the symptoms were sufficiently distressing to warrant interruption or discontinuation of treatment.

OVERDOSAGE
Acute deliberate overdosage in man has not occurred, but would be expected to induce the following symptoms: anorexia, malaise, lethargy, diminished sense of well being, tremulousness, anxiety, nausea and vomiting. Laboratory findings are likely to include an elevated reticulocyte count and a severe hemolytic reaction requiring hospitalization, symptomatic treatment, and possibly blood transfusions. Concomitant reduction in platelets and/or white blood cells should be anticipated.

Milder overdosages resulting in hemolysis have occurred in an occasional patient with reduced renal function after several weeks or months of continuous treatment.

The acute LD 50 of AHA in animals (rats) is 4.8 gm/kg.

Recommended treatment for an overdosage reaction consists of (1) cessation of treatment, (2) close monitoring of hematologic status, (3) symptomatic treatment, and (4) blood transfusions as required by the clinical circumstances. The drug is probably dialyzable, but this property has not been tested clinically.

DOSAGE AND ADMINISTRATION
AHA should be administered orally, one tablet 3-4 times a day in a total daily dose of 10-15 mg/kg/day. The recommended starting dose is 12 mg/kg/day, administered at 6-8 hour intervals at a time when the stomach is empty. The maximum daily dose should be no more than 1.5 grams, regardless of body weight.

The dosage should be reduced in patients with reduced renal function. Patients whose serum creatinine is greater than 1.8 mg/dl should take no more than 1.0 gm/day; such patients should be dosed at q-12-h intervals. Further reductions in dosage to prevent the accumulation of toxic concentrations in the blood may also be desirable. Insufficient data exists to accurately characterize the optimum dose and/or dose interval in patients with moderate degrees of renal insufficiency.

Patients with advanced renal insufficiency (i.e., serum creatinine more than 2.5 mg/dl) should not be treated with AHA. The risk of accumulation of toxic blood levels of AHA seems to be greater than the chances for a beneficial effect in such patients.

In children an initial dose of 10 mg/kg/day is recommended. Close monitoring of the patient's clinical condition and hematologic status is recommended. Titration of the dose to higher or lower levels may be required to obtain an optimum therapeutic effect and/or to reduce the risk of side effects.

Acetohydroxamic Acid should be stored in a dry place at room temperature, 15°-30°C (59°-86°F). Container should be closed tightly.

HOW SUPPLIED
TABLETS: 250 MG

BRAND/MANUFACTURER	NDC	SIZE	AWP
○ BRAND			
LITHOSTAT: Mission	00178-0500-01	100s	$93.75

Acetylcholine Chloride

DESCRIPTION
Acetylcholine Chloride is a parasympathomimetic preparation for intraocular use. When reconstituted, the liquid will be a sterile isotonic solution containing 20 mg acetylcholine chloride (1:100 solution).

The chemical name for Acetylcholine Chloride, $C_7H_{16}CINO_2$, is 2-acetoxyethyltrimethylammonium chloride.

Following is its chemical structure:

$$CH_3CO(CH_2)_2N^+(CH_3)_3 \quad Cl^-$$

CLINICAL PHARMACOLOGY
Acetylcholine, is a naturally occurring neurohormone which mediates nerve impulse transmission at all cholinergic sites involving somatic and autonomic nerves. After release from the nerve ending, Acetylcholine is rapidly inactivated by the enzyme acetylcholinesterase by hydrolysis to acetic acid and choline.

Direct application of Acetylcholine Chloride to the iris will cause rapid miosis of short duration. Topical ocular instillation of Acetylcholine Chloride to the intact eye causes no discernible response as cholinesterase destroys the molecule more rapidly than it can penetrate the cornea.

INDICATIONS AND USAGE
To obtain complete miosis of the iris in seconds after delivery of the lens in cataract surgery, in penetrating keratoplasty, iridectomy and other anterior segment surgery where rapid, complete miosis may be required.

CONTRAINDICATIONS
There are presently no known contraindications to the use of intraocular Acetylcholine Chloride.

WARNINGS
If blister or peelable backing is damaged or broken, sterility of the enclosed bottle cannot be assured. Open under aseptic conditions only.

WARNING: DO NOT GAS STERILIZE

PRECAUTIONS
General: In the reconstitution of the solution, as described under *"Directions for Using"*, if the center rubber plug seal in the vial does not go down or is down, do not use the vial.

If miosis is to be obtained quickly and completely with Acetylcholine Chloride, obstructions to miosis, such as anterior or posterior synechiae, may require surgery prior to administration of Acetylcholine Chloride. In cataract surgery, use Acetylcholine Chloride only after delivery of the lens.

Note: Aqueous solutions of Acetylcholine Chloride are unstable. Prepare solution immediately before use. Do not use solution which is not clear and colorless. Discard any solution that has not been used.

Drug Interactions: Although clinical studies with Acetylcholine Chloride and animal studies with Acetylcholine or carbachol revealed no interference, and there is no known pharmacological basis for an interaction, there have been reports that Acetylcholine Chloride and carbachol have been ineffective when used in patients treated with topical nonsteroidal anti-inflammatory agents.

Pediatric Use: Safety and effectiveness in children have not been established.

ADVERSE REACTIONS
Infrequent cases of corneal edema, corneal clouding, and corneal decompensation have been reported with the use of Acetylcholine Chloride.

Adverse reactions have been reported rarely which are indicative of systemic absorption. These include bradycardia, hypotension, flushing, breathing difficulties and sweating.

OVERDOSAGE
Atropine sulfate (0.5 to 1 mg) should be given intramuscularly or intravenously and should be readily available to counteract possible overdosage. Epinephrine (0.1 to 1 mg subcutaneously) is also of value in overcoming severe cardiovascular or bronchoconstrictor responses.

DOSAGE AND ADMINISTRATION
With a new needle of sturdy gauge, 18-20, draw all of the solution into a dry, sterile syringe. Replace needle with a suitable atraumatic cannula for intraocular irrigation.

The Acetylcholine Chloride solution is instilled into the anterior chamber before or after securing one or more sutures. Instillation should be gentle and parallel to the iris face and tangential to pupil border.

If there are no mechanical hindrances, the pupil is rapidly constricted and the peripheral iris drawn away from the angle of the anterior chamber. Any anatomical hindrance to miosis may require surgery to permit the desired effect of the drug. In most cases, ½ to 2 mL produces satisfactory miosis. The Acetylcholine Chloride solution need not be flushed from the chamber after miosis occurs. Since the action of Acetylcholine is of short duration, pilocarpine may be applied topically before dressing to maintain miosis.

In cataract surgery, use Acetylcholine Chloride only after delivery of the lens.

Note: Aqueous solutions of Acetylcholine Chloride are unstable. Prepare solution immediately before use. Do not use solution which is not clear and colorless. Discard any solution that has not been used.

DIRECTIONS FOR USING VIALS (STERILE UNLESS PACKAGE OPEN OR BROKEN)
1. Inspect vial while inside unopened blister. Diluent must be in upper chamber.
   2. Peel open blister.
   3. Aseptically transfer vial to sterile field. Maintain sterility of outer container during preparation of solution.
   4. Immediately before use, give plunger-stopper a quarter turn and press to force diluent and center plug into lower chamber.
   5. Shake gently to dissolve drug.
   6. Discard vial and any unused solution.

STORAGE
Keep from freezing; store at 15°-30°C (59°-86°F).

HOW SUPPLIED
POWDER FOR RECONSTITUTION: 1:100

BRAND/MANUFACTURER	NDC	SIZE	AWP
○ **BRAND**			
MIOCHOL: Iolab	00058-2757-52	2 ml	$21.36
MIOCHOL-E/IOCARE: Iolab	00058-2772-52	2 ml	$21.36
MIOCHOL SYSTEM-PAK: Iolab	00058-2763-53	2 ml	$23.52
MIOCHOL-E SYSTEM PAK: Iolab	00058-2775-53	2 ml	$23.52
MIOCHOL SYSTEM-PAK PLUS: Iolab	00058-2764-54	2 ml	$33.72

Acetylcysteine

DESCRIPTION
Acetylcysteine is a mucolytic agent available as sterile, unpreserved solutions (not for injection). The solutions contain 20% or 10% Acetylcysteine. Each vial contains 4, 10, or 30 ml. Acetylcysteine is the N-acetyl derivative of the naturally-occurring amino acid, cysteine. The compound is a white crystalline powder with the molecular formula $C_5H_9NO_3S$, a molecular weight of 163.2, and chemical name of N-acetyl-L-cysteine.

Following is its chemical structure:

$$HSCH_2 - \overset{\overset{\displaystyle NHCOCH_3}{|}}{\underset{\underset{\displaystyle H}{|}}{C}} - COOH$$

ACETYLCYSTEINE AS A MUCOLYTIC AGENT

CLINICAL PHARMACOLOGY
The viscosity of pulmonary mucous secretions depends on the concentrations of mucoprotein and, to a lesser extent, deoxyribonucleic acid (DNA). The latter increases with increasing purulence owing to the presence of cellular debris. The mucolytic action of Acetylcysteine is related to the sulfhydryl group in the molecule. This group probably "opens" disulfide linkages in mucus thereby lowering the viscosity. The mucolytic activity of Acetylcysteine is unaltered by the presence of DNA, and increases with increasing pH. Significant mucolysis occurs between pH 7 and 9.

Acetylcysteine undergoes rapid deacetylation *in vivo* to yield cysteine or oxidation to yield diacetylcysteine.

Occasionally, patients exposed to the inhalation of an Acetylcysteine aerosol respond with the development of increased airway obstruction of varying and unpredictable severity. Those patients who are reactors cannot be identified a *priori* from a random patient population. Even when patients are known to have reacted previously to the inhalation of an Acetylcysteine aerosol, they may not react during a subsequent treatment. The converse is also true; patients who have had inhalation treatments of Acetylcysteine without incident may still react to a subsequent inhalation with increased airway obstruction. Most patients with bronchospasm are quickly relieved by the use of a bronchodilator given by nebulization. If bronchospasm progresses, the medication should be discontinued immediately.

INDICATIONS AND USAGE
Acetylcysteine is indicated as adjuvant therapy for patients with abnormal, viscid, or inspissated mucous secretions in such conditions as:

Chronic bronchopulmonary disease (chronic emphysema, emphysema with bronchitis, chronic asthmatic bronchitis, tuberculosis, bronchiectasis and primary amyloidosis of the lung).

Acute bronchopulmonary disease (pneumonia, bronchitis, tracheobronchitis)
Pulmonary complications of cystic fibrosis
Tracheostomy care
Pulmonary complications associated with surgery
Use during anesthesia
Post-traumatic chest conditions
Atelectasis due to mucous obstruction
Diagnostic bronchial studies (bronchograms, bronchospirometry, and bronchial wedge catheterization)

UNLABELED USES
Acetylcysteine is used as an adjunct in the treatment of patients with severe unstable angina pectoris and in the carbon monoxide toxicity.

CONTRAINDICATIONS
Acetylcysteine is contraindicated in those patients who are sensitive to it.

WARNINGS
After proper administration of Acetylcysteine, an increased volume of liquefied bronchial secretions may occur. When cough is inadequate, the airway must be maintained open by mechanical suction if necessary. When there is a mechanical block due to foreign body or local accumulation, the airway should be cleared by endotracheal aspiration, with or without bronchoscopy. Asthmatics under treatment with Acetylcysteine should be watched carefully. Most patients with bronchospasm are quickly relieved by the use of a bronchodilator given by nebulization. If bronchospasm progresses, the medication should be discontinued immediately.

PRECAUTIONS
With the administration of Acetylcysteine, the patient may observe initially a slight disagreeable odor that is soon not noticeable. With a face mask there may be stickiness on the face after nebulization. This is easily removed by washing with water.

Under certain conditions, a color change may occur in Acetylcysteine in the opened bottle. The light purple color is the result of a chemical reaction which does not significantly affect safety or mucolytic effectiveness of Acetylcysteine.

Continued nebulization of Acetylcysteine solution with a dry gas will result in an increased concentration of the drug in the nebulizer because of evaporation of the solvent. Extreme concentration may impede nebulization and efficient delivery of the drug. Dilution of the nebulizing solution with appropriate amounts of Sterile Water for Injection, USP, as concentration occurs, will obviate this problem.

CARCINOGENESIS, MUTAGENESIS, AND IMPAIRMENT OF FERTILITY
Carcinogenesis: Carcinogenicity studies in laboratory animals have not been performed with Acetylcysteine alone, nor with Acetylcysteine in combination with isoproterenol.

Long-term oral studies of Acetylcysteine alone in rats (12 months of treatment followed by 6 months of observation) at doses up to 1,000 mg/kg/day (5.2 times the human dose) provided no evidence of oncogenic activity.

Mutagenesis: Published data[*] indicate that Acetylcysteine is not mutagenic in the Ames test, both with and without metabolic activation.

Impairment of Fertility: A reproductive toxicity test to assess potential impairment of fertility was performed with Acetylcysteine (10%) combined with isoproterenol (0.05%) and administered as an aerosol into a chamber of 12.43 cubic meters. The combination was administered for 25, 30, or 35 minutes twice a day for 68 days before mating, to 200 male and 150 female rats; no adverse effects were noted in dams or pups. Females after mating were continued on treatment for the next 42 days.

Reproductive toxicity studies of Acetylcysteine in the rat given oral doses of Acetylcysteine up to 1,000 mg/kg (5.2 times the human dose) have also been reported in the literature.[*] The only adverse effect observed was a slight non-dose-related reduction in fertility at dose levels of 500 or 1,000 mg/kg/day (2.6 or 5.2 times the human dose) in the Segment I study.

PREGNANCY
Teratology: In a teratology study of Acetylcysteine in the rabbit, oral doses of 500 mg/kg/day (2.6 times the human dose) were administered to pregnant does by intubation on days 6 through 16 of gestation. Acetylcysteine was found to be nonteratogenic under the conditions of study.

In the rabbit, two groups (one of 14 and one of 16 pregnant females) were exposed to an aerosol of 10% Acetylcysteine and 0.05% isoproterenol hydrochloride for 30 or 35 minutes twice a day from the 6th through the 18th day of pregnancy. No teratogenic effects were observed among the offspring.

Teratology and a perinatal and postnatal toxicity study in rats were performed with a combination of Acetylcysteine and isoproterenol administered by the inhalation route. In the rat, two groups of 25 pregnant females each were exposed to the aerosol for 30 and 35 minutes, respectively, twice a day from the 6th through the 15th day of gestation. No teratogenic effects were observed among the offspring.

In the pregnant rat (30 rats per group), twice-daily exposure to an aerosol Acetylcysteine and isoproterenol for 30 or 35 minutes from the 15th day of gestation through the 21st day postpartum was without adverse effect on dams or newborns.

Pregnancy Category: Pregnancy Category B. Reproduction studies of Acetylcysteine with isoproterenol have been performed in rats and of Acetylcysteine alone in rabbits at doses up to 2.6 times the human dose. These have revealed no evidence of impaired fertility or harm to the fetus due to Acetylcysteine. There are, however, no adequate and well-controlled studies in pregnant women. Because animal reproduction studies may not always be predictive of human responses, this drug should be used during pregnancy only if clearly needed.

NURSING MOTHERS
It is not known whether this drug is excreted in human milk. Because many drugs are excreted in human milk, caution should be exercised when Acetylcysteine is administered to a nursing woman.

ADVERSE REACTIONS
Adverse effects have included stomatitis, nausea, vomiting, fever, rhinorrhea, drowsiness, clamminess, chest tightness, and bronchoconstriction. Clinically overt Acetylcysteine induced bronchospasm occurs infrequently and unpredictably even in patients with asthmatic bronchitis or bronchitis complicating bronchial asthma. Acquired sensitization to Acetylcysteine has been reported rarely. Reports of sensitization in patients have not been confirmed by patch testing. Sensitization has been confirmed in several inhalation therapists who reported a history of dermal eruptions after frequent and extended exposure to Acetylcysteine. Reports of irritation to the tracheal and bronchial tracts have been received and although hemoptysis has occurred in patients receiving Acetylcysteine such findings are not uncommon in patients with bronchopulmonary disease and a causal relationship has not been established.

---

* Bonanomi L, Gazzaniga A. Toxicological pharmacokinetic and metabolic studies on acetylcysteine. *Eur J Respir Dis* 1981;61(suppl III): 45-51.

◆ RATED THERAPEUTICALLY EQUIVALENT; ◇ THERAPEUTIC EQUIVALENCE UNCONFIRMED; ○ UNRATED

ing Acetylcysteine treatment. Activated charcoal adsorbs Acetylcysteine *in vitro* and may do so in patients and thereby may reduce its effectiveness.

3. Draw blood for acetaminophen plasma assay and for baseline SGOT, SGPT, bilirubin, prothrombin time, creatinine, BUN, blood sugar and electrolytes. The acetaminophen assay provides a basis for determining the need for continuing with the maintenance doses of Acetylcysteine treatment. If an assay cannot be obtained or if the acetaminophen level is clearly in the toxic range (above the dashed line of the nomogram) dosing with Acetylcysteine should be continued for the full course of therapy. The laboratory measurements are used to monitor hepatic and renal function and electrolyte and fluid balance.

4. Administer the loading dose of Acetylcysteine, 140 mg per kg of body weight. (Prepare Acetylcysteine for oral administration as described in the Dosage Guide and Preparation table.)

5. Four hours after the loading dose, administer the first maintenance dose. (70 mg of Acetylcysteine per kg of body weight.) The maintenance dose is then repeated at 4-hour intervals for a total of 17 doses unless the acetaminophen assay reveals a nontoxic level as discussed below.

6. If the patient vomits the loading dose or any maintenance dose within 1 hour of administration, repeat that dose.

7. In the occasional instances where the patient is persistently unable to retain the orally administered Acetylcysteine, the antidote may be administered by duodenal intubation.

8. Repeat SGOT, SGPT, bilirubin, prothrombin time, creatinine, BUN, blood sugar and electrolytes daily if the acetaminophen plasma level is in the potentially toxic range as discussed below.

PREPARATION OF ACETYLCYSTEINE FOR ORAL ADMINISTRATION
Oral administration requires dilution of the 20% solution with diet cola or other diet soft drinks, to a final concentration of 5% (see Dosage and Preparation table). If administered via gastric tube or Miller-Abbott tube, water may be used as the diluent. The dilutions should be freshly prepared and utilized within one hour. Remaining undiluted solutions in opened vials can be stored in the refrigerator up to 96 hours. ACETYLCYSTEINE IS NOT APPROVED FOR PARENTERAL INJECTION.

ACETAMINOPHEN ASSAYS — INTERPRETATION AND METHODOLOGY
The acute ingestion of acetaminophen in quantities of 150 mg/kg or greater may result in hepatic toxicity. However, the reported history of the quantity of a drug ingested as an overdose is often inaccurate and is not a reliable guide to therapy of the overdose. **THEREFORE, PLASMA OR SERUM ACETAMINOPHEN CONCENTRATIONS, DETERMINED AS EARLY AS POSSIBLE, BUT NO SOONER THAN 4 HOURS FOLLOWING AN ACUTE OVERDOSE, ARE ESSENTIAL IN ASSESSING THE POTENTIAL RISK OF HEPATOTOXICITY. IF AN ASSAY FOR ACETAMINOPHEN CANNOT BE OBTAINED, IT IS NECESSARY TO ASSUME THAT THE OVERDOSE IS POTENTIALLY TOXIC.**

Interpretation of Acetaminophen Assays: 1. When results of the plasma acetaminophen assay are available refer to the nomogram below to determine if plasma concentration is in the potentially toxic range. Values above the solid line connecting 200 µ/mL at 4 hours with 50 µ/mL at 12 hours are associated with a possibility of hepatic toxicity if an antidote is not administered. (Do not wait for assay results to begin Acetylcysteine treatment.)

2. If the plasma level is above the broken line, continue with maintenance doses of Acetylcysteine. It is better to err on the safe side and thus the broken line is plotted 25% below the solid line which defines possible toxicity.

3. If the initial plasma level is below the broken line described above, there is minimal risk of hepatic toxicity and Acetylcysteine treatment can be discontinued.

Acetaminophen Assay Methodology: Assay procedures most suitable for determining acetaminophen concentrations utilize high pressure liquid chromatography (HPLC) or gas liquid chromatography (GLC). The assay should measure only parent acetaminophen and not conjugated. The assay procedures listed below fulfill this requirement:

HPLC: Selected techniques (noninclusive):
1. Blair D, Rumack BH. *Clin Chem* 1977;23(4):743-745.

2. Howie D, Andriaenssens PI, Prescott LF, *J Pharm Pharmacol* 1977;29(4):235-237.

GLC:
3. Prescott LF. *J Pharm Pharmacol* 1971;23(10):807-808.

Colorimetric:
4. Glynn JP, Kendal SE. *Lancet* 1975;1(May 17):1147-1148.

Supportive Treatment of Acetaminophen Overdose:
1. Maintain fluid and electrolyte balance based on clinical evaluation of state of hydration and serum electrolytes.
2. Treat as necessary for hypoglycemia.
3. Administer vitamin K_1 if prothrombin time ratio exceeds 1.5 or fresh frozen plasma if the prothrombin time ratio exceeds 3.0. (See related table).
4. Diuretics and forced diuresis should be avoided. (See related table).

Estimating Potential for Hepatotoxicity: The following nomogram has been developed to estimate the probability that plasma levels in relation to intervals post ingestion will result in hepatotoxicity.

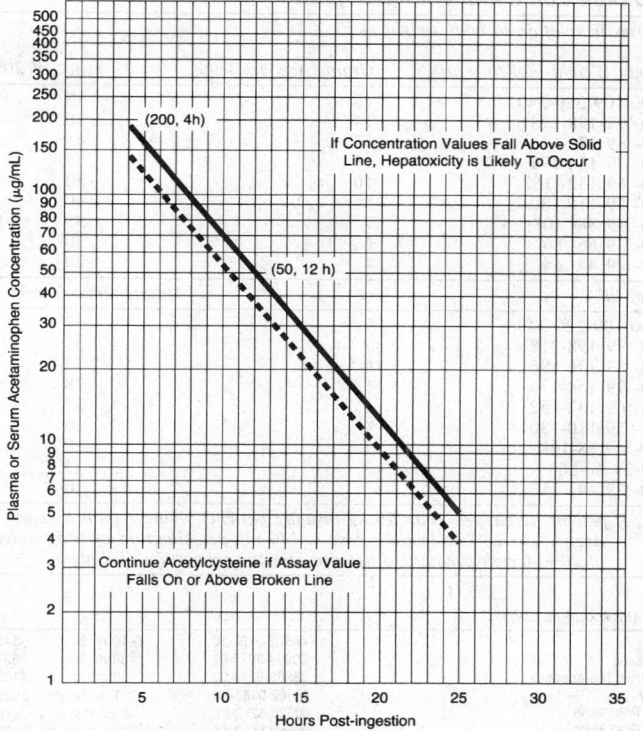

*Adapted from Rumack and Matthews, Pediatrics 1975;55:871-876.

STORAGE
Store unopened vials at controlled room temperature, 59° to 86°F (15° to 30°C).

J CODES
10%, per ml INH—J7610
20%, per ml INH—J7615

HOW SUPPLIED
SOLUTION: 10%

AVERAGE UNIT PRICE (AVAILABLE SIZES)		GENERIC A-RATED AVERAGE PRICE (GAAP)		
		10 ml 3s		$33.30
BRAND	$1.94	30 ml 3s		$85.25
GENERIC	$1.001	4 ml 12s		$49.27
BRAND/MANUFACTURER		NDC	SIZE	AWP
◆ **BRAND**				
MUCOMYST-10: Apothecon		00087-0572-01	10 ml 3s	$59.39
		00087-0572-02	30 ml 3s	$161.12
		00087-0572-03	4 ml 12s ud	$98.84
◆ **GENERICS**				
Roxane		00054-3027-02	10 ml 3s	$19.56
Chiron Therapeutics		53905-0211-03	10 ml 3s	$40.08
Dey		49502-0181-10	10 ml 3s	$40.26
Roxane		00054-3025-02	30 ml 3s	$34.94
Chiron Therapeutics		53905-0212-03	30 ml 3s	$110.34
Dey		49502-0181-30	30 ml 3s	$110.48
Du Pont Multi		00590-5214-61	4 ml 10s	$49.88
Du Pont Multi		00590-5214-85	30 ml 10s	$161.88
Dey		49502-0181-04	4 ml 12s	$67.80
Roxane		00054-8059-05	4 ml 12s ud	$30.74

SOLUTION: 20%

AVERAGE UNIT PRICE (AVAILABLE SIZES)		GENERIC A-RATED AVERAGE PRICE (GAAP)		
		10 ml 3s		$40.55
BRAND	$2.33	30 ml 3s		$101.97
GENERIC	$1.15	4 ml 12s		$57.45
BRAND/MANUFACTURER		NDC	SIZE	AWP
◆ **BRAND**				
MUCOMYST: Apothecon		00087-0570-03	10 ml 3s	$71.03
		00087-0570-09	30 ml 3s	$194.60
		00087-0570-07	4 ml 12s ud	$118.64
◆ **GENERICS**				
Dey		49502-0182-00	100 ml	$92.21
Roxane		00054-3028-02	10 ml 3s	$24.45
Chiron Therapeutics		53905-0213-03	10 ml 3s	$48.54

DOSAGE GUIDE AND PREPARATION

Doses in relation to body weight are:

Body Weight (kg) (lb)	Grams Acetylcysteine	Loading Dose of Acetylcysteine mL of 20% Acetylcysteine	mL of Diluent	Total mL of 5% Solution
100-109 220-240	15	75	225	300
90- 99 198-218	14	70	210	280
80- 89 176-196	13	65	195	260
70- 79 154-174	11	55	165	220
60- 69 132- 152	10	50	150	200
50- 59 110-130	8	40	120	160
40- 49 88- 108	7	35	105	140
30- 39 66- 86	6	30	90	120
20- 29 44- 64	4	20	60	80

(kg) (lb)		Maintenance Dose**		
100-109 220-240	7.5	37	113	150
90- 99 198-218	7	35	105	140
80- 89 176-196	6.5	33	97	130
70- 79 154-174	5.5	28	82	110
60- 69 132-152	5	25	75	100
50- 59 110-130	4	20	60	80
40- 49 88-108	3.5	18	52	70
30-39 66-86	3	15	45	60
20- 29 44- 64	2	10	30	40

** *If patient weighs less than 20 kg (usually patients younger than 6 years), calculate the dose of Acetyleysteine. Each mL of 20% solution contains 200 mg of Acetylcysteine. The loading dose is 140 mg per kilogram of body weight. The maintenance dose is 70 mg/kg. Three (3) mL of diluent are added to each mL of 20% Acetylcysteine. Do not decrease the proportion of diluent.*

BRAND/MANUFACTURER	NDC	SIZE	AWP
Dey	49502-0182-10	10 ml 3s	$48.66
Roxane	00054-3026-02	30 ml 3s	$39.13
Chiron Therapeutics	53905-0214-03	30 ml 3s	$133.35
Dey	49502-0182-30	30 ml 3s	$133.43
Du Pont Multi	00590-5212-61	4 ml 10s	$51.63
Du Pont Multi	00590-5212-85	30 ml 10s	$186.38
Dey	49502-0182-04	4 ml 12s	$81.36
Roxane	00054-8060-05	4 ml 12s ud	$33.54

Achromycin SEE TETRACYCLINE HYDROCHLORIDE, OPHTHALMIC *AND* TETRACYCLINE HYDROCHLORIDE, ORAL

Aci-Jel SEE ACETIC ACID/OXYQUINOLINE SULFATE/ RICINOLEIC ACID

Aclovate SEE ALCLOMETASONE DIPROPIONATE

Acrivastine and Pseudoephedrine Hydrochloride

DESCRIPTION
Acrivastine/Pseudoephedrine Hydrochloride is a fixed combination product formulated for oral administration. Acrivastine is an antihistamine and Pseudoephedrine is a decongestant. Each capsule contains 8 mg Acrivastine and 60 mg Pseudoephedrine HCl.

The chemical name of Acrivastine is (E,E)-3-[6-[1-4 methylphenyl)-3-(1-pyrrolidinyl)-1-propenyl]-2-pyridinyl]-2-propenoic acid; the molecular formula is $C_{22}H_{24}N_2O_2$. As an analog of triprolidine hydrochloride, Acrivastine is classified as an alkylamine antihistamine. Acrivastine is an odorless, white to pale cream crystalline powder that is soluble in chloroform and alcohol and slightly soluble in water.

The chemical name of Pseudoephedrine Hydrochloride is [S-(R*, R*)]-α-[1-(methylamino)ethyl]benzenemethanol hydrochloride; the molecular formula is $C_{10}H_{15}NO \cdot HCl$. Pseudoephedrine is one of the naturally occurring dextrorotatory diastereoisomers of ephedrine and is classified as an indirect sympathomimetic amine. Pseudoephedrine Hydrochloride occurs as odorless, fine white to off-white crystals or powder; the drug is soluble in water, alcohol and chloroform.

CLINICAL PHARMACOLOGY
Acrivastine, a structural analog of triprolidine hydrochloride, exhibits H_1-antihistaminic activity in isolated tissues, animals, and humans, and has sedative effects in humans (see *"Precautions"*). The propionic acid derivative of Acrivastine is a metabolite in several animal species (as well as in man) and also exhibits H_1-antihistaminic activity.

Pseudoephedrine hydrochloride is an indirect sympathomimetic agent; that is, it releases norepinephrine from adrenergic nerves.

In vitro tests and in vivo studies in animals of Acrivastine and pseudoephedrine in combination failed to demonstrate evidence of any beneficial or deleterious pharmacologic interaction between the two agents.

PHARMACOKINETICS AND METABOLISM
Acrivastine was absorbed rapidly from the combination capsule following oral administration and was as bioavailable as a solution of Acrivastine. After administration of Acrivastine Pseudoephedrine Hydrochloride Capsules, maximum plasma Acrivastine concentrations were achieved at 1.14 ± 0.23 hour. A mass balance study in 7 healthy volunteers showed that Acrivastine is primarily eliminated by the kidneys. Over a 72-hour collection period, about 84% of the administered total radioactivity was recovered in urine and about 13% in feces, for a combined recovery of about 97%. Further, 67% of the administered radioactive dose was recovered in urine as the unchanged drug, 11% as the propionic acid metabolite, and 6% as other unknown metabolites.

Acrivastine exhibits linear kinetics over dosages ranging from 2 to 32 mg t.i.d. The mean ± SD terminal half-life for Acrivastine was 1.9 ± 0.3 hours following single oral doses and increased to 3.5 ± 1.9 hours at steady state. The terminal half-life for the propionic acid metabolite was 3.8 ± 1.4 hours. Because of the short half-lives of both Acrivastine and its metabolites, accumulation in the plasma following multiple dosing is not expected.

The steady-state maximum Acrivastine plasma concentration was 227 ± 47 ng/mL. The oral clearance and apparent volume of distribution were 2.9 ± 0.7 mL/min/kg and 0.46 ± 0.05 L/kg, respectively, following a single oral dose; oral clearance did not change at steady state (2.86 ± 0.75 mL/min/kg). The apparent volume of distribution increased to 0.82 ± 0.6 L/kg to parallel the increase in the elimination half-life of the drug.

Acrivastine binding to human plasma proteins was 50 ± 2.0% and was concentration-independent over the range of 5 to 1000 ng/mL. The main binding protein was serum albumin although the drug was slightly bound to α1-acid glycoprotein. No displacement interaction was observed between Acrivastine and either phenytoin or theophylline. The binding of Acrivastine was not affected by the presence of Pseudoephedrine.

Pseudoephedrine Hydrochloride was also rapidly absorbed from the combination capsule, and the capsule was as bioavailable as a solution of Pseudoephedrine. Steady state maximum plasma concentration for Pseudoephedrine was 498 ± 129 ng/mL. The terminal half-life, oral clearance and apparent volume of distribution were 6.2 ± 1.8 hour, 5.9 ± 1.7 mL/min/kg, and 30 ± 0.4 L/kg, respectively. Elimination of Pseudoephedrine is primarily through the renal route as 55% to 75% of an administered dose appears unchanged in the urine. Pseudoephedrine elimination, however, is highly dependent upon urine pH; the plasma half-life decreased to about 4 hours at pH 5 and increased to 13 hours at pH 8. Pseudoephedrine did not bind to human plasma proteins over the concentration range of 50 to 2000 ng/mL.

Acrivastine and Pseudoephedrine do not influence the pharmacokinetics of the other drug when administered concomitantly.

SPECIAL POPULATIONS
A single dose pharmacokinetic study showed that the elimination half-lives of Acrivastine, the propionic acid metabolite of Acrivastine, and Pseudoephedrine were prolonged in patients with chronic renal insufficiency. Compared to normal volunteers, the elimination half-life of Acrivastine was about 50% increased in patients with mild renal insufficiency (creatinine clearance = 26 to 48 mL/min) and was increased by about 130% in patients with moderate (creatinine clearance = 12 to 17 mL/min) or severe (creatinine clearance 6 to 10 mL/min) renal insufficiency. Oral clearance of Acrivastine was diminished by the same

magnitude as the half-life was prolonged in each of the three renally impaired groups. The elimination half-life of the propionic acid metabolite of Acrivastine was about 140% increased in patients with mild renal insufficiency and about 5 times increased in patients with moderate or severe renal insufficiency. Compared to normal volunteers, the elimination half-life of Pseudoephedrine was about 3 times increased in patients with mild renal insufficiency, about 7 times increased in patients with moderate renal insufficiency, and about 10 times increased in patients with severe renal insufficiency. Oral clearance of Pseudoephedrine was diminished by about the same magnitude as the half-life was prolonged in each of the three renally impaired groups (see *"Precautions, Use in Patients with Diminished Renal Function"*).

The total body load removed by dialysis is approximately 20%, 27% and 38% for Acrivastine, the propionic acid metabolite of Acrivastine, and Pseudoephedrine, respectively, and therefore, a supplemental dose after a dialysis session is not required.

Based on a multiple dose cross study comparison, the apparent volume of distribution for Acrivastine was 44% lower in elderly (n = 36, 65-75 yr) than in young volunteers (n = 16, 19-33 yr). This difference could be attributed to the decrease in total body water that occurs with aging. Despite this difference, no appreciable differences in plasma Acrivastine concentrations were seen in the elderly compared to the young, and no appreciable accumulation of Acrivastine occurred in plasma at steady-state. The elimination half-life for Pseudoephedrine was 18% longer in elderly (7.9 hours) than in younger subjects (6.7 hours), presumably due to the decline in average renal function that occurs with aging. Despite this difference, clearance of Pseudoephedrine was not appreciably different in elderly and younger subjects. Elderly patients should therefore be given the same dosage as younger patients. Acrivastine/Pseudoephedrine Hydrochloride Capsules are not recommended, however, in patients with renal impairment (see *"Precautions, Use in Patients with Diminished Renal Function"*).

The effect of age and sex on the pharmacokinetic parameters of Acrivastine and Pseudoephedrine was determined in 93 healthy volunteers who participated in various studies. All of the 93 volunteers were Caucasian (81 males and 12 females); 57 were between the ages of 18 and 38 years and 36 were between the ages of 65 and 75 years. There were no age- or sex-related differences in the pharmacokinetic parameters of either Acrivastine or Pseudoephedrine.

The effect of race on Acrivastine and Pseudoephedrine pharmacokinetics was examined by screening data obtained from 1035 patients, age 12 to 71 years, who participated in the 8 safety and efficacy studies. No race-related differences were observed in the pharmacokinetics of either Acrivastine or Pseudoephedrine.

CLINICAL STUDIES

In healthy volunteers, histamine-induced wheal and flare areas were significantly reduced relative to placebo at 30 minutes after administration of a single dose of Acrivastine 8 mg. Maximum reductions of wheal and flare occurred by 1 to 2 hours and significant reductions relative to placebo persisted for up to 6 hours after a single oral dose of Acrivastine 8 mg. No additional reductions of wheal and flare were observed following single doses of Acrivastine up to 24 mg. The exact correlation between responses on skin testing and clinical efficacy is not established.

Five randomized placebo- and/or active-controlled trials compared Acrivastine and Pseudoephedrine Hydrochloride with its Acrivastine and Pseudoephedrine components for the symptomatic relief of seasonal allergic rhinitis. In these studies, 696 patients received four daily doses of Acrivastine 8 mg plus Pseudoephedrine Hydrochloride 60 mg (i.e., Acrivastine/Pseudoephedrine Hydrochloride Capsules or bioequivalent formulations administered concurrently) or the same doses of the components for 14 days. The combination reduced the intensity of sneezing, rhinorrhea, pruritus, and lacrimation more than Pseudoephedrine and reduced the intensity of nasal congestion more than Acrivastine, demonstrating a contribution of each of the components. The onset of antihistaminic and nasal decongestant actions occurred within one or two hours after the first dose of Acrivastine/Pseudoephedrine Hydrochloride capsules. Somnolence occurred in about 12% of patients given Acrivastine/Pseudoephedrine Hydrochloride compared with about 6% on placebo.

INDICATIONS AND USAGE

Acrivastine/Pseudoephedrine Hydrochloride capsules are indicated for relief of symptoms associated with seasonal allergic rhinitis such as sneezing, rhinorrhea, pruritus, lacrimation, and nasal congestion. Acrivastine/Pseudoephedrine Hydrochloride capsules should be administered when both the antihistaminic activity of Acrivastine and the nasal decongestant activity of Pseudoephedrine are desired (see *"Clinical Pharmacology"*). The efficacy of Acrivastine/Pseudoephedrine Hydrochloride capsules beyond 14 days of continuous treatment in patients with seasonal allergic rhinitis has not been adequately investigated in clinical trials.

Acrivastine/Pseudoephedrine Hydrochloride capsules have not been adequately studied for effectiveness in relieving the symptoms of the common cold.

CONTRAINDICATIONS

Acrivastine/Pseudoephedrine Hydrochloride capsules are contraindicated in patients with a known sensitivity to Acrivastine, other alkylamine antihistamines (e.g., triprolidine), Pseudoephedrine, other sympathomimetic amines (e.g., phenylpropanolamine) or to any other components of the formulation. Acrivastine/Pseudoephedrine Hydrochloride capsules are contraindicated in patients with severe hypertension or severe coronary artery disease. Acrivastine/Pseudoephedrine Hydrochloride capsules are contraindicated in patients taking monoamine oxidase (MAO) inhibitors and for two weeks after stopping use of an MAO inhibitor (see *"Drug Interactions"*).

WARNINGS

Acrivastine/Pseudoephedrine Hydrochloride capsules should be used with caution in patients with hypertension, diabetes mellitus, ischemic heart disease, increased intraocular pressure, hyperthyroidism, prostatic hypertrophy, stenosing peptic ulcer, or pyloroduodenal obstruction. Overdose of sympathomimetic amines may produce CNS stimulation with convulsions or cardiovascular collapse with accompanying hypotension. The elderly are more likely to have adverse reactions to sympathomimetic amines.

PRECAUTIONS

General: Acrivastine is sedating in some patients. In controlled clinical trials, somnolence (i.e., drowsiness, sedation, sleepiness) was more common with Acrivastine/Pseudoephedrine Hydrochloride Capsules (by an average of 6%) than with placebo (see *"Adverse Experiences"*).

Patients should be advised to assess their individual responses to Acrivastine/Pseudoephedrine Hydrochloride capsules before engaging in any activity requiring mental alertness, such as driving a motor vehicle or operating machinery. Concurrent use of Acrivastine/Pseudoephedrine Hydrochloride capsules with alcohol or other CNS depressants may cause additional reductions in alertness and impairment of CNS performance and should be avoided (see *"Drug Interactions"*).

Use in Patients with Diminished Renal Function: Acrivastine and Pseudoephedrine are excreted primarily through the kidney. Both compounds therefore accumulate in patients with impaired renal function. Due to the differential effects of renal failure on the serum half-life and clearance of acrivastine and Pseudoephedrine, use of Acrivastine/Pseudoephedrine Hydrochloride capsules, a fixed combination product, in patients with renal impairment (creatinine clearance ≤ 48 mL/min) is not recommended (see *"Overdosage"* and *"Clinical Pharmacology"*).

Information to Patients: Patients taking Acrivastine/Pseudoephedrine Hydrochloride Capsules should receive the following information. Acrivastine/Pseudoephedrine Hydrochloride capsules are prescribed to reduce symptoms associated with seasonal allergic rhinitis. Patients should be instructed to take Acrivastine/Pseudoephedrine Hydrochloride Capsules only as prescribed and not to exceed the prescribed dose. Patients should be advised against the concurrent use of Acrivastine/Pseudoephedrine Hydrochloride with over-the-counter antihistamines and decongestants. Patients who are or may become pregnant should be told that this product should be used in pregnancy or during lactation only if the potential benefit justifies the potential risks to the fetus or nursing infant. Due to the risk of hypertensive crisis, patients should be instructed not to take Acrivastine/Pseudoephedrine Hydrochloride capsules if they are presently taking a monoamine oxidase inhibitor or for two weeks after stopping use of a MAO inhibitor. Patients should be advised to assess their individual responses to Acrivastine/Pseudoephedrine Hydrochloride capsules before engaging in any activity requiring mental alertness, such as driving a car or operating machinery. Patients should be advised that the concurrent use of Acrivastine/Pseudoephedrine Hydrochloride capsules with alcohol and other CNS depressants may lead to additional reductions in alertness and impairment of CNS performance and should be avoided.

Use in the Elderly (Approximately 60 Years or Older): Elderly patients who participated in clinical trials did not differ in effectiveness or adverse effects from younger patients. Antihistamines, however, as a pharmaceutical class, are more likely to cause dizziness, sedation, bladder-neck obstruction, and hypotension in elderly patients. The elderly are also more likely to have adverse reactions to sympathomimetics such as Pseudoephedrine (see *"Clinical Pharmacology"* and *"Warnings"*).

Drug Interactions: MAO inhibitors and beta-adrenergic agonists increase the effects of sympathomimetic amines. Concomitant use of sympathomimetic amines with MAO inhibitors can result in a hypertensive crisis (see *"Contraindications"*). Because MAO inhibitors are long-acting, Acrivastine/Pseudoephedrine Hydrochloride capsules should not be taken with a MAO inhibitor or for two weeks after stopping use of a MAO inhibitor.

Because of their Pseudoephedrine content, Acrivastine/Pseudoephedrine Hydrochloride capsules may reduce the antihypertensive effects of drugs that interfere with sympathetic activity. Care should be taken in the administration of Acrivastine/Pseudoephedrine Hydrochloride capsules concomitantly with other sympathomimetic amines because the combined effects on the cardiovascular system may be harmful to the patient.

Concomitant administration of Acrivastine/Pseudoephedrine Hydrochloride capsules with alcohol and other CNS depressants may result in additional reductions in alertness and impairment of CNS performance and should be avoided.

No formal drug interaction studies between Acrivastine/Pseudoephedrine Hydrochloride capsules and other possibly co-administered drugs have been performed.

Carcinogenesis, Mutagenesis, and Impairment of Fertility: Carcinogenicity studies with the combination of Acrivastine and Pseudoephedrine have not been performed. Oral doses of Acrivastine alone at levels up to 40 mg/kg/day (236 mg/m^2/day or 10 times the recommended human daily dose) for 20 to 22 months in rats and up to 250 mg/kg/day (750 mg/m^2/day or 32 times the recommended human daily dose) for 20 to 24 months in mice revealed no evidence of carcinogenic potential. No evidence of mutagenicity (with or without metabolic activation) was observed in the Ames Salmonella mutagenicity assay or in the L5178Y/tk$^{+/-}$ mouse lymphoma assay. In an *in vitro* cytogenetic study performed in cultured human lymphocytes, Acrivastine induced structural chromosomal abnormalities in the absence of metabolic activation, but not in its presence. In an *in vivo* cytogenetic study in rats given single oral doses of Acrivastine up to 1000 mg/kg (5900 mg/m^2 or 249 times the recommended human daily dose) there were no structural chromosomal alterations.

Reproduction-fertility studies in rats given Acrivastine alone at levels up to 200 mg/kg/day (1180 mg/m^2/day or 50 times the recommended human daily dose) had no effect on male or female fertility. Similarly, no effect on fertility was seen in male rats given Acrivastine 20 mg/kg/day and Pseudoephedrine 100 mg/kg/day (118 and 590 mg/m^2/day or 5 and 3 times the recommended human daily doses, respectively) or in female rats given Acrivastine 4 mg/kg/day and Pseudoephedrine 20 mg/kg/day (23.6 and 118 mg/m^2/day or 1 and 0.7 times the recommended human daily doses, respectively).

Pregnancy: Pregnancy Category B: Teratogenic Effects: No evidence of teratogenicity was seen in rats and rabbits given Acrivastine 1000 and 400 mg/kg/day, respectively (5900 and 4720 mg/m^2/day or 249 and 200 times the recommended human daily dose). No evidence of teratogenicity was seen in rats given a combination of Acrivastine 30 mg/kg/day and Pseudoephedrine 150 mg/kg/day (177 and 885 mg/m^2/day or 8 and 5 times the recommended human daily dose, respectively). Similarly, no evidence of teratogenicity was observed in rabbits given Acrivastine 20 mg/kg/day and Pseudoephedrine 100 mg/kg/day (236 and 1180 mg/m^2/day or 10 and 7 times the recommended human daily doses, respectively). There are, however, no adequate and well-controlled studies in pregnant women. Because animal teratology studies are not always predictive of human responses, Acrivastine/Pseudoephedrine Hydrochloride Capsules should be used during pregnancy only if the potential benefit justifies the potential risks to the fetus.

Nonteratogenic Effects: In a perinatal-postnatal study in rats. Acrivastine given alone at levels up to 500 mg/kg/day (2950 mg/m^2/day or 124 times the recommended human daily dose) was associated with maternal and neonatal mortality at the maximum dose level. Neonatal survival was decreased in rats given a combination of Acrivastine 20 mg/kg/day kg/day and pseudoephedrine 100 mg/kg/day (118 and 590 mg/m^2/day or 5 and 3 times the human dose, respectively).

Nursing Mothers: It is not known whether acrivastine is excreted in human milk: pseudoephedrine is excreted in human milk. Acrivastine/Pseudoephedrine Hydrochloride capsules should only be used in nursing mothers when the potential benefit justifies the potential risks to the nursing infant.

Pediatric Use: Safety and effectiveness of Acrivastine/Pseudoephedrine capsules in children under the age of 12 years have not been established.

ADVERSE EXPERIENCES

Information on the incidence of adverse events in clinical investigations conducted in the U.S. was obtained from 33 controlled and 15 uncontrolled clinical studies in which 2499 patients received Acrivastine and 2631 received Acrivastine plus Pseudoephedrine Hydrochloride for treatment periods ranging from one day to one year. The majority of patients in clinical trials were exposed to Acrivastine or Acrivastine plus Pseudoephedrine for less than 90 days. Acrivastine dosages ranged from 3 to 96 mg/day; 1336 patients received dosages equal to or greater than Acrivastine 24 mg/day. Acrivastine plus Pseudoephedrine Hydrochloride dosages ranged from Acrivastine 8 to 48 mg/day plus Pseudoephedrine Hydrochloride 60 to 240 mg/day. A total of 2335 patients received three or four daily doses of Acrivastine 8 mg plus Pseudoephedrine hydrochloride 60 mg.

In controlled clinical trials, only 12 spontaneously elicited adverse events were reported with frequencies greater than 1% in the Acrivastine plus Pseudoephedrine Hydrochloride treatment group (see table).

The nature and overall frequencies of adverse events from international clinical trials (35 studies involving approximately 1600 patients) were similar to the results obtained in the U.S. studies.

Post-marketing clinical experience reports with Acrivastine and Acrivastine plus Pseudoephedrine have included rare serious hypersensitivity reactions manifested by anaphylaxis, angioedema, bronchospasm, and erythema multiforme. No deaths associated with use of Acrivastine or Acrivastine plus Pseudoephedrine have been reported.

Pseudoephedrine may cause ephedrine-like reactions such as tachycardia, palpitations, headache, dizziness, or nausea (see *"Warnings"* and *"Overdosage"*).

OVERDOSAGE

There have been no reports of overdosage with Acrivastine/Pseudoephedrine Hydrochloride capsules. In the clinical trial program and international post-marketing experience, there have been two reported overdoses with Acrivastine. Doses were 72 mg and 322 mg. Both patients recovered without sequelae. Adverse events included trembling, stridor, loss of consciousness and possible convulsions in the first patient and somnolence in the second.

Since Acrivastine/Pseudoephedrine have pharmacologically different actions, it is difficult to predict how an individual will respond to overdosage with Acrivastine/Pseudoephedrine Hydrochloride capsules. However, acute overdosage with Acrivastine/Pseudoephedrine Hydrochloride capsules may produce clinical signs of either CNS stimulation or depression. Overdosage of sympathomimetics has been associated with the following events: fear, anxiety, tenseness, restlessness, tremor, weakness, pallor, respiratory difficulty, dysuria, insomnia, hallucinations, convulsions. CNS depression, arrhythmias, and cardiovascular collapse with hypotension. Treatment for overdosage with Acrivastine/Pseudoephedrine Hydrochloride capsules should follow general symptomatic and supportive principles.

In a placebo-controlled, double-blind clinical trial in 18 healthy male subjects, single doses of Acrivastine up to 400 mg (50 times the recommended antihistaminic dose) produced only a weak vagolytic effect, manifested as an increase in heart rate, and did not cause cardiac repolarization delays (i.e., increased QTc). Daily doses of Acrivastine up to 2400 mg 75 times the recommended antihistamine dose) in an uncontrolled study in 38 cancer patients produced a 15 beats per minute increase in mean heart rate and occasional episodes of nausea and vomiting. The effects of Acrivastine plus Pseudoephedrine at single or multiple doses higher than the recommended daily dose of Acrivastine/Pseudoephedrine Hydrochloride Capsules (i.e., 32 mg Acrivastine plus 240 mg Pseudoephedrine) on heart rate and cardiac repolarization have not been investigated in clinical trials.

The mean LD$_{50}$ (single, oral dose) of Acrivastine is greater than 4000 mg/kg (23600 mg/m^2 or 1000 times the recommended human daily doses) in rats and greater than 1200 mg/kg (3600 mg/m^2 or 153 times the recommended human daily dose in mice. The mean LD$_{50}$ (single, oral dose) of Pseudoephedrine Hydrochloride is 2206 mg/kg (13015 mg/m^2 or 73 times the recommended human daily dose) in rats and 726 mg/kg (2178 mg/m^2 or 12 times the recommended human daily dose) in mice. The toxic and lethal concentrations of Acrivastine and Pseudoephedrine in human biologic fluids are not known. Based upon pharmacokinetic screening data from clinical trials, the maximum plasma Acrivastine concentration after dosing with Acrivastine 8 mg was 393 ng/mL and the maximum plasma Pseudoephedrine concentration after dosing with Pseudoephedrine Hydrochloride 60 mg was 1308 ng/mL.

DOSAGE AND ADMINISTRATION

The recommended dosage for adults and children 12 years and older is one capsule administered orally, every 4 to 6 hours four times a day.

The capsules should be stored at 15° to 25°C (59° to 77°F) in a dry place and protected from light.

ADVERSE EVENTS REPORTED IN CLINICAL TRIALS* (PERCENT OF PATIENTS REPORTING)†

		Controlled Studies		
	Placebo (N = 1767)	Acrivastine (N = 1935)	Pseudoephedrine (N=887)	Acrivastine plus Pseudoephedrine (N= 1650)
CNS				
Somnolence‡	6	12	8	12
Headache	18	19	19	19
Dizziness	2	3	3	3
Nervousness‡	1	2	4	3
Insomnia‡	1	1	6	4
Miscellaneous				
Nausea	2	3	3	2
Dry Mouth‡	2	3	5	7
Asthenia	2	3	2	2
Dyspepsia	1	2	2	2
Pharyngitis	2	1	1	3
Cough Increase	1	2	1	2
Dysmenorrhea	1	2	3	2

* *Includes all events regardless of causal relationship to treatment.*
† *Includes all adverse events with a reported frequency of > 1% for the Acrivastine plus Pseudoephedrine treatment group.*
‡ *Acrivastine/Pseudoephedrine Hydrochloride demonstrates a statistically higher frequency of events than placebo, p < 0.05.*

◆ RATED THERAPEUTICALLY EQUIVALENT; ◇ THERAPEUTIC EQUIVALENCE UNCONFIRMED; ○ UNRATED

HOW SUPPLIED
CAPSULE: 8 MG-60 MG

BRAND/MANUFACTURER	NDC	SIZE	AWP
○ BRAND			
➤ SEMPREX-D: Burr Wellcome	00081-0280-55	100s	$45.60

Acthar *SEE* CORTICOTROPIN

Acthar Gel, H.P. *SEE* CORTICOTROPIN

Actifed with Codeine *SEE* CODEINE PHOSPHATE/
PSEUDOEPHEDRINE HYDROCHLORIDE/TRIPROLIDINE
HYDROCHLORIDE

Actigall *SEE* URSODIOL

Actimmune *SEE* INTERFERON GAMMA-1B

Actinex *SEE* MASOPROCOL

Activase *SEE* ALTEPLASE, RECOMBINANT

Acular *SEE* KETOROLAC TROMETHAMINE, OPHTHALMIC

Acyclovir

DESCRIPTION
Acyclovir is an antiviral drug active against herpes viruses. Acyclovir Capsules, Tablets, and Suspension are formulations for oral administration; Acyclovir Ointment is a formulation for topical administration; Acyclovir Sterile Powder is a formulation for intravenous administration.

Each capsule contains:	
Acyclovir	200 mg

Each gram of 5% ointment contains:	
Acyclovir	50 mg

Each teaspoonful (5 mL) suspension contains:	
Acyclovir	200 mg

Each tablet contains:	
Acyclovir	400 mg
or	
Acyclovir	800 mg

Each vial for intravenous use contains:	
Acyclovir 10 mL	50 mg/mL
Acyclovir 20 mL	50 mg/mL

The chemical name of Acyclovir is 9-[(2-hydroxyethoxy)methyl]guanine.

Following is its chemical structure:

(chemical structure: H_2N-substituted purine with $CH_2OCH_2CH_2OH$ side chain)

CLINICAL PHARMACOLOGY
Mechanism of Antiviral Effects: Acyclovir is a synthetic purine nucleoside analogue with *in vitro* and *in vivo* inhibitory activity against human herpes viruses including herpes simplex types 1 (HSV-1) and 2 (HSV-2), varicella-zoster virus (VZV), Epstein-Barr virus (EBV) and cytomegalovirus (CMV). In cell culture, Acyclovir has the highest antiviral activity against HSV-1, followed in decreasing order of potency against HSV-2, VZV, EBV and CMV.[1]

The inhibitory activity of Acyclovir for HSV-1, HSV-2, VZV, and EBV is highly selective. The enzyme thymidine kinase (TK) of normal uninfected cells does not effectively use Acyclovir as a substrate. However, TK encoded by HSV, VZV, and EBV[2] converts Acyclovir into Acyclovir monophosphate, a nucleotide analogue. The monophosphate is further converted into diphosphate by cellular guanylate kinase and into triphosphate by a number of cellular enzymes.[3] Acyclovir triphosphate interferes with herpes simplex virus DNA polymerase and inhibits viral DNA replication. Acyclovir triphosphate also inhibits cellular α-DNA polymerase, but to a lesser degree. *In vitro*, Acyclovir triphosphate can be incorporated into growing chains of DNA by viral DNA polymerase and to a much smaller extent by cellular α-DNA polymerase.[4] When incorporation occurs, the DNA chain is terminated.[5,6] Acyclovir is preferentially taken up and selectively converted to the active triphosphate form by herpesvirus-infected cells. Thus, Acyclovir is much less toxic *in vitro* for normal uninfected cells because: 1) less is taken up; 2) less is converted to the active form; 3) cellular α-DNA polymerase is less sensitive to the effects of the active form. The mode of Acyclovir phosphorylation in cytomegalovirus-infected cells is not clearly established, but may involve virally induced cell kinases or an unidentified viral enzyme. Acyclovir is not efficiently activated in cytomegalovirus infected cells, which may account for the reduced susceptibility of cytomegalovirus to Acyclovir *in vitro.*

Microbiology: The quantitative relationship between the *in vitro* susceptibility of herpes simplex and varicella-zoster viruses to Acyclovir and the clinical response to therapy has not been established in man, and virus sensitivity testing has not been standardized. Sensitivity testing results, expressed as the concentration of drug required to inhibit by 50% the growth of virus in cell culture (ID_{50}), vary greatly depending upon the particular assay used,[7] the cell type employed,[8] and the laboratory performing the test.[1] The ID_{50} of Acyclovir against HSV-1 isolates may range from 0.02 µg/mL (plaque reduction in Vero cells) to 5.9 to 13.5 µg/mL (plaque reduction in green monkey kidney [GMK] cells).[1] The ID_{50} against HSV-2 ranges from 0.01 µg/mL to 9.9 µg/mL (plaque reduction in Vero and GMK cells, respectively).

Using a dye-uptake method in Vero cells,[9] which gives ID_{50} values approximately 5- to 10-fold higher than plaque reduction assays, 1417 HSV isolates (553 HSV-1 and 864 HSV-2) from approximately 500 patients were examined over a 5-year period.[10] These assays found that 90% of HSV-1 isolates were sensitive to ≤ 0.9 µg/mL Acyclovir and 50% of all isolates were sensitive to ≤ 0.2 µg/mL Acyclovir. For HSV-2 isolates, 90% were sensitive to ≤ 2.2 µg/mL and 50% of all isolates were sensitive to ≤ 0.7 µg/mL of Acyclovir. Isolates with significantly diminished sensitivity were found in 44 patients. It must be emphasized that neither the patients nor the isolates were randomly selected and, therefore, do not represent the general population.

Most of the less sensitive HSV clinical isolates have been relatively deficient in the viral TK.[11-19] Strains with alterations in viral TK[20] or viral DNA polymerase[21] have also been reported. Prolonged exposure to low concentrations (0.1 µg/mL) of Acyclovir in cell culture has resulted in the emergence of a variety of Acyclovir-resistant strains.[22]

The ID_{50} against VZV ranges from 0.17 to 1.53 µg/mL (yield reduction, human foreskin fibroblasts) to 1.85 to 3.98 µg/mL (foci reduction, human embryo fibroblasts [HEF]). Reproduction of EBV genome is suppressed by 50% in superinfected Raji cells or P3HR-1 lymphoblastoid cells by 1.5 µg/mL Acyclovir. CMV is relatively resistant to Acyclovir with ID_{50} values ranging from 2.3 to 17.6 µg/mL (plaque reduction, HEF cells) to 1.82 to 56.8 µg/mL (DNA hybridization, HEF cells). The latent state of the genome of any of the human herpesviruses is not known to be sensitive to Acyclovir.[1]

Two clinical pharmacology studies were performed with Acyclovir Ointment 5% in adult immunocompromised patients, at risk of developing mucocutaneous Herpes simplex virus infections or with localized varicella-zoster infections. These studies were designed to evaluate the dermal tolerance, systemic toxicity and percutaneous absorption of Acyclovir.

In one of these studies, which included 16 inpatients, the complete ointment or its vehicle were randomly administered in a dose of 1 cm strips (25 mg Acyclovir) four times a day for seven days to an intact skin surface area of 4.5 square inches. No local intolerance, systemic toxicity or contact dermatitis were observed. In addition, no drug was detected in blood and urine by radioimmunoassay (sensitivity, 0.01 µg/mL).

The other study included eleven patients with localized varicella-zoster. In this uncontrolled study, Acyclovir was detected in the blood of 9 patients and in the urine of all patients tested. Acyclovir levels in plasma ranged from < 0.01 to 0.28 µg/mL in eight patients with normal renal function, and from < 0.01 to 0.78 µg/mL in one patient with impaired renal function. Acyclovir excreted in the urine ranged from < 0.02 to 9.4 percent of the daily dose. Therefore, systemic absorption of Acyclovir after topical application is minimal.

Pharmacokinetics: The pharmacokinetics of Acyclovir after oral administration have been evaluated in 6 clinical studies involving 110 adult patients. In one uncontrolled study of 35 immunocompromised patients with herpes simplex or varicella-zoster infection, Acyclovir Capsules were administered in doses of 200 to 1000 mg every 4 hours, 6 times daily for 5 days, and steady-state plasma levels were reached by the second day of dosing. Mean steady-state peak and trough concentrations following the final 200 mg dose were 0.49 µg/mL (0.47 to 0.54 µg/mL) and 0.31 µg/mL (0.18 to 0.41 µg/mL), respectively, and following the final 800 mg dose were 2.8 µg/mL (2.3 to 3.1 µg/mL) and 1.8 µg/mL (1.3 to 2.5 µg/mL), respectively. In another uncontrolled study of 20 younger immunocompetent patients with recurrent genital herpes simplex infections Acyclovir Capsules were administered in doses of 800 mg every 6 hours, 4 times daily for 5 days; the mean steady-state peak and trough concentrations were 1.4 µg/mL (0.66 to 1.8 µg/mL) and 0.55 µg/mL (0.14 to 1.1 µg/mL), respectively.

In general, the pharmacokinetics of Acyclovir in children is similar to adults. Mean half-life after oral doses of 300 mg/m^2 and 600 mg/m^2, in children ages 7 months to 7 years, was 2.6 hours (range 1.59 to 3.74 hours).

A single oral dose bioavailability study in 23 normal volunteers showed that Acyclovir Capsules 200 mg are bioequivalent to 200 mg Acyclovir in aqueous solution; and in a separate study in 20 volunteers, it was shown that Acyclovir Suspension is bioequivalent to Acyclovir Capsules. In a different single-dose bioavailability/bioequivalence study in 24 volunteers, one Acyclovir 800 mg Tablet was demonstrated to be bioequivalent to four Acyclovir 200 mg Capsules.

In a multiple-dose crossover study where 23 volunteers received Acyclovir as one 200 mg capsule, one 400 mg tablet and one 800 mg tablet 6 times daily, absorption decreased with increasing dose and the estimated bioavailabilities of Acyclovir were 20%, 15%, and 10%, respectively. The decrease in bioavailability is believed to be a function of the dose and not the dosage form. It was demonstrated that Acyclovir is not dose proportional over the dosing range 200 mg to 800 mg. In this study, steady-state peak and trough concentrations of Acyclovir were 0.83 and 0.46 µg/mL, 1.21 and 0.63 µg/mL, and 1.61 and 0.83 µg/mL for the 200, 400, and 800 mg dosage regimens, respectively.

In another study in 6 volunteers, the influence of food on the absorption of Acyclovir was not apparent.

Following oral administration, the mean plasma half-life of Acyclovir in volunteers and patients with normal renal function ranged from 2.5 to 3.3 hours. The mean renal excretion of unchanged drug accounts for 14.4% (8.6% to 19.8%) of the orally administered dose. The only urinary metabolite (identified by high performance liquid chromatography) is 9-[(carboxymethoxy)methyl]guanine. The half-life and total body clearance of Acyclovir are dependent on renal function. A dosage adjustment is recommended for patients with reduced renal function (see "Dosage and Administration").

Orally administered Acyclovir in children less than 2 years of age has not yet been fully studied.

The pharmacokinetics of Intravenous Acyclovir has been evaluated in 95 patients (9 studies). Results were obtained in adult patients with normal renal function during Phase 1/2 studies after single doses ranging from 0.5 to 15 mg/kg and after multiple doses ranging from 2.5 to 15 mg/kg every 8 hours. Pharmacokinetics was also determined in pediatric patients with normal renal function ranging in age from 1 to 17 years at doses of 250 mg/m^2 or 500 mg/m^2 every 8 hours. In these studies, dose-independent pharmacokinetics is observed in the range of 0.5 to 15 mg/kg. Proportionality between dose and plasma levels is seen after single doses or at steady state after multiple dosing. When Acyclovir was administered to adults at 5 mg/kg (approximately 250 mg/m^2) by 1-hr infusions every 8 hours, mean steady-state peak and trough concentrations of 9.8 µg/mL (5.5 to 13.8 µg/mL) and 0.7 µg/mL (0.2 to 1.0 µg/mL), respectively, were achieved. Similar concentrations are achieved in children over 1 year of age when doses of 250 mg/m^2 are given by 1-hr infusions every 8 hours. At a dose to 10 mg/kg given by 1-hr infusion every 8 hours, mean steady-state peak and trough concentrations were 22.9 µg/mL (14.1 to 44.1 µg/mL) and 1.9 µg/mL (0.5 to 2.9 µg/mL). Similar concentrations were achieved in children dosed at 500 mg/m^2 given by 1-hr infusion every 8 hours. Concentrations achieved in the cerebrospinal fluid are approximately 50% of plasma values.

Plasma protein binding is relatively low (9% to 33%) and drug interactions involving binding site displacement are not anticipated.

Renal excretion of unchanged drug by glomerular filtration and tubular secretion is the major route of Acyclovir elimination accounting for 62% to 91% of the dose as determined by ^{14}C-labelled drug. The only major urinary metabolite detected is 9-carboxymethoxymethylguanine. This may account for up to 14.1% of the dose in patients with normal renal function. An insignificant amount of drug is recovered in feces and expired CO_2 and there is no evidence to suggest tissue retention. However, postmortem examinations have shown that Acyclovir is widely distributed in tissues and body fluids including brain, kidney, lung, liver, muscle, spleen, uterus, vaginal mucosa, vaginal secretions, cerebrospinal fluid and herpetic vesicular fluid.

The half-life and total body clearance of Acyclovir is dependent on renal function as shown below.

Creatinine Clearance (mL/min/1.73m^2)	Half-Life (hour)	Total Body Clearance (mL/min/1.73m^2)
> 80	2.5	327
50-80	3.0	248
15-50	3.5	190
0 (Anuric)	19.5	29

Acyclovir intravenous was administered at a dose of 2.5 mg/kg to 6 adult patients with severe renal failure. The peak and trough plasma levels during the 47 hours preceding hemodialysis were 8.5 µg/mL and 0.7 µg/mL, respectively.

Consult "Dosage and Administration" section for recommended adjustments in dosing based upon creatinine clearance.

The half-life and total body clearance of Acyclovir intravenous in pediatric patients over 1 year of age is similar to those in adults with normal renal function (see "Dosage and Administration").

INDICATIONS AND USAGE

Acyclovir Capsules, Tablets, and Suspension are indicated for the treatment of initial episodes and the management of recurrent episodes of genital herpes in certain patients.

Acyclovir Capsules, Tablets, and Suspension are indicated for the acute treatment of herpes zoster (shingles) and chicken-pox (varicella).

Acyclovir Sterile Powder is indicated for the treatment of initial and recurrent mucosal and cutaneous Herpes simplex (HSV-1 and HSV-2) and varicella-zoster (shingles) infections in immunocompromised patients. It is also indicated for herpes simplex encephalitis in patients over 6 months of age and for severe initial clinical episodes of herpes genitalis in patients who are not immunocompromised.

Acyclovir Ointment 5% is indicated in the management of initial herpes genitalis and in limited nonlife-threatening mucocutaneous Herpes simplex virus infections in immunocompromised patients.

Genital Herpes Infections: The severity of disease is variable depending upon the immune status of the patient, the frequency and duration of episodes, and the degree of cutaneous or systemic involvement. These factors should determine patient management, which may include symptomatic support and counseling only, or the institution of specific therapy. The physical, emotional, and psycho-social difficulties posed by herpes infections as well as the degree of debilitation, particularly in immunocompromised patients, are unique for each patient, and the physician should determine therapeutic alternatives based on his or her understanding of the individual patient's needs. Thus, orally administered Acyclovir is not appropriate in treating all genital herpes infections. The following guidelines may be useful in weighing the benefit/risk considerations in specific disease categories.

First Episodes:[23,24,25] (primary and nonprimary infections—commonly known as initial genital herpes): Double-blind, placebo-controlled studies have demonstrated that orally administered Acyclovir significantly reduced the duration of acute infection (detection of virus in lesions by tissue culture) and lesion healing. The duration of pain and new lesion formation was decreased in some patient groups. The promptness of initiation of therapy and/or the patient's prior exposure to herpes simplex virus may influence the degree of benefit from therapy. Patients with mild disease may derive less benefit than those with more severe episodes. In patients with extremely severe episodes, in which prostration, central nervous system involvement, urinary retention, or inability to take oral medication require hospitalization and more aggressive management, therapy may be best initiated with intravenous Acyclovir.

Recurrent Episodes: Double-blind, placebo-controlled studies[16,26,32] in patients with frequent recurrences (6 or more episodes per year) have shown that orally administered Acyclovir given daily for 4 months to 3 years prevented or reduced the frequency and/or severity of recurrences in greater than 95% of patients.

In a study of 283 patients who received 400 mg (two 200 mg capsules) twice daily for 3 years, 45%, 52% and 63% of patients remained free of recurrences in the first, second, and third years, respectively. Serial analyses of the 3-month recurrence rates for the 283 patients showed that 71% to 87% were recurrence-free in each quarter, indicating that the effects are consistent over time.

The frequency and severity of episodes of untreated genital herpes may change over time. After 1 year of therapy, the frequency and severity of the patient's genital herpes infection should be re-evaluated to assess the need for continuation of Acyclovir therapy. Re-evaluation will usually require a trial off Acyclovir to assess the need for reinstitution of suppressive therapy. Some patients, such as those with very frequent or severe episodes before treatment, may warrant uninterrupted suppression for more than a year.

Chronic suppressive therapy is most appropriate when, in the judgement of the physician, the benefits of such a regimen outweigh known or potential adverse effects. In general, orally administered Acyclovir should not be used for the suppression of recurrent disease in mildly affected patients. Unanswered questions concerning the relevance to humans of *in vitro* mutagenicity studies and reproductive toxicity studies in animals given high parenteral doses of Acyclovir for short periods (see *Carcinogenesis, Mutagenesis, Impairment of Fertility*) should be borne in mind when designing long-term management for individual patients. Discussion of these issues with patients will provide them the opportunity to weigh the potential for toxicity against the severity of their disease. Thus, this regimen should be considered only for appropriate patients with annual re-evaluation.

Limited studies[31,32] have shown that there are certain patients for whom intermittent short-term treatment of recurrent episodes is effective. This approach may be more appropriate than a suppressive regimen in patients with infrequent recurrences.

Immunocompromised patients with recurrent herpes infections can be treated with either intermittent or chronic suppressive therapy. Clinically significant resistance, although rare, is more likely to be seen with prolonged or repeated therapy in severely immunocompromised patients with active lesions.

In placebo-controlled trials, 58 patients with initial genital herpes were treated with intravenous Acyclovir 5 mg/kg or placebo (27 patients treated with Acyclovir and 31 treated with placebo) every eight hours for 5 days. Acyclovir decreased the duration of viral excretion, new lesion formation, and duration of vesicles and promoted healing of lesions.

In clinical trials of initial herpes genitalis, Acyclovir Ointment 5% has shown a decrease in healing time and in some cases a decrease in duration of viral shedding and duration of pain. In studies in immunocompromised patients with mainly herpes labialis, there was a decrease in duration of viral shedding and a slight decrease in duration of pain.

By contrast, in studies of recurrent herpes genitalis and of herpes labialis in nonimmunocompromised patients, there was no evidence of clinical benefit: there was some decrease in duration of viral shedding.

Herpes Zoster Infections: In a double-blind, placebo-controlled study of 187 normal patients with localized cutaneous zoster infection (93 randomized to Acyclovir and 94 to placebo), Acyclovir (800 mg 5 times daily for 10 days) shortened the times to lesion scabbing, healing, and complete cessation of pain, and reduced the duration of viral shedding and the duration of new lesion formation.[33]

In a similar double-blind, placebo-controlled study in 83 normal patients with herpes zoster (40 randomized to Acyclovir and 43 to placebo), Acyclovir (800 mg 5 times daily for 7 days) shortened the times to complete lesion scabbing, healing, and cessation of pain, reduced the duration of new lesion formation, and reduced the prevalence of localized zoster-associated neurologic symptoms (paresthesia, dysesthesia, or hyperesthesia).[34]

Chickenpox: In a double-blind, placebo-controlled efficacy study in 110 normal patients, ages 5 to 16 years, who presented **within 24 hours** of the onset of a typical chickenpox rash, Acyclovir was administered orally 4 times daily for 5 to 7 days at doses of 10, 15, or 20 mg/kg depending on the age group. Acyclovir treatment reduced the maximum number of lesions (336 vs. greater than 500; lesions beyond 500 were not counted). Acyclovir treatment also shortened the mean time to 50% healing (7.1 days vs. 8.7 days), reduced the number of vesicular lesions by the second day of treatment (49 vs. 113), and decreased the proportion of patients with fever (temperature greater than 100°F) by the second day (19% vs. 57%). Acyclovir treatment did not affect the antibody response to varicella-zoster virus measured one month and one year following the treatment.[35]

In two concurrent double-blind, placebo-controlled studies, a total of 883 normal patients, ages 2 to 18 years, were enrolled *within 24 hours* of the onset of a typical chickenpox rash, and Acyclovir was administered at 20 mg/kg orally up to 800 mg 4 times daily for 5 days. In the larger study of 815 children ages 2 to 12 years, Acyclovir treatment reduced the median maximum number of lesions (277 vs. 386), reduced the median number of vesicular lesions by the second day of treatment (26 vs. 40), and reduced the proportion of patients with moderate to severe itching by the third day of treatment (15% vs 34%).[36] In addition, in both studies (883 patients ages 2 to 18 years), Acyclovir treatment also decreased the proportion of patients with fever (temperature greater than 100°F), anorexia, and lethargy by the second day of treatment, and decreased the mean number of residual lesions on Day 28.[36,37] There were no substantial differences in VZV-specific humoral or cellular immune responses measured at one month following treatment in patients receiving Acyclovir compared to patients receiving placebo.[38]

Herpes Simplex Infections in Immunocompromised Patients: A multicenter trial of Acyclovir Sterile Powder at a dose of 250 mg/m^2 every 8 hours (750 mg/m^2/day) for 7 days was conducted in 98 immunocompromised patients (73 adults and 25 children) with oro-facial, esophageal, genital and other localized infections (52 treated with Acyclovir and 46 with placebo). Acyclovir significantly decreased virus excretion, reduced pain, and promoted scabbing and rapid healing of lesions.

Herpes Simplex Encephalitis: Sixty-two patients ages 6 months to 79 years with brain biopsy-proven herpes simplex encephalitis were randomized to receive either Acyclovir (30 mg/kg/day) or adenine arabinoside (15 mg/kg/day) for 10 days (28 were treated with Acyclovir and 34 with adenine arabinoside. Overall mortality for Acyclovir recipients at 6 months was 18% compared to 59% for adenine arabinoside treated patients ($P = 0.003$). The proportion of Acyclovir recipients functioning normally or with only mild sequelae (e.g., decreased attention span) was 39% compared to 9% of adenine arabinoside treated patients ($P = 0.01$). The remaining patients in both groups had moderate (e.g., hemiparesis, speech impediment or seizure) or severe (continuous supportive care required) neurologic sequelae.

After 12 months of follow-up, two additional Acyclovir recipients had died, resulting in an overall mortality of 25% compared to 59% for adenine arabinoside treated patients ($P = 0.02$). Morbidity assessments at that time indicated that 32% of Acyclovir recipients were functioning normally, or with only mild sequelae compared to 12% adenine arabinoside patients ($P = 0.06$). Moderate to severe impairment was noted in all remaining patients in both groups who were available for evaluation. Patients less than 30 years of age and those who had the least severe neurologic involvement at time of entry into study had the best outcome with Acyclovir treatment. An additional controlled study performed in Europe demonstrated similar findings. The superiority of Acyclovir over adenine arabinoside for neonatal herpes encephalitis has not been demonstrated.

Varicella-Zoster Infections in Immunocompromised Patients: A multicenter trial of Acyclovir Sterile Powder at a dose of 500 mg/m^2 every 8 hours for 7 days was conducted in immunocompromised patients with zoster infections (shingles).

Ninety-four (94) patients were evaluated (52 patients were treated with Acyclovir and 42 with placebo). Acyclovir halted progression of infection as determined by significant reductions in cutaneous dissemination, visceral dissemination, or the proportion of patients deemed treatment failures.

A comparative trial of Acyclovir and vidarabine was conducted in 22 severely immunocompromised patients with zoster infections. Acyclovir was shown to be superior to vidarabine as demonstrated by significant differences in the time of new lesion formation, the time to pain reduction, the time to lesion crusting, the time to complete healing, the incidence of fever and the duration of positive viral cultures. In addition, cutaneous dissemination occurred in none of the 10 Acyclovir recipients compared to 5 of the 10 vidarabine recipients who presented with localized dermatomal disease.

Diagnosis: Diagnosis is confirmed by virus isolation. Accelerated viral culture assays or immunocytology allow more rapid diagnosis than standard viral culture. For patients with initial episodes of genital herpes, appropriate examinations should be performed to rule out other sexually transmitted diseases. While cutaneous lesions associated with herpes simplex and varicella-zoster infections are often characteristic, the finding of multinucleated giant cells in smears prepared from lesion exudate or scrapings may provide additional support to the clinical diagnosis.[35] Positive cultures for Herpes simplex virus offer a reliable means for confirmation of the diagnosis.

The Tzanck smear or multinucleated giant cells in smears do not distinguish varicella-zoster from herpes simplex infections.

Herpes encephalitis should be confirmed by brain biopsy to obtain tissue for histologic examination and viral culture and to exclude other causes of neurologic disease. A presumptive diagnosis of herpes encephalitis may be made on the basis of focal changes in the temporal lobe visualized with various diagnostic methods including magnetic resonance imaging, computerized tomography, radionuclide scans or electroencephalography. Culture of the cerebrospinal fluid for Herpes simplex virus is unreliable.

UNLABELED USES
Acyclovir is used alone or as an adjunct in the treatment of acquired immunodeficiency syndrome (AIDS) and AIDS-related complex, herpeticum eczema, and chronic hepatitis B.

CONTRAINDICATIONS
Acyclovir is contraindicated for patients who develop hypersensitivity or intolerance to the components of the formulations.

WARNINGS
Acyclovir Capsules, Tablets, and Suspension are intended for oral ingestion only.

Acyclovir Sterile Powder is intended for intravenous infusion only, and should not be administered topically, intramuscularly, orally, subcutaneously, or in the eye. Intravenous infusions must be given over a period of at least 1 (one) hour to reduce the risk of renal tubular damage (see *"Precautions"* and *"Dosage and Administration"*).

Acyclovir Ointment 5% is intended for cutaneous use only and should not be used in the eye.

PRECAUTIONS
GENERAL
Acyclovir Capsules, Tablets, and Suspension:
Acyclovir has caused decreased spermatogenesis at high parenteral doses in some animals and mutagenesis in some acute studies at high concentrations of drug (see *"Precautions—Carcinogenesis, Mutagenesis, Impairment of Fertility"*). The recommended dosage should not be exceeded (see *"Dosage and Administration"*). Exposure of Herpes simplex and varicella-zoster isolates to Acyclovir *in vitro* can lead to the emergence of less sensitive viruses. The possibility of the appearance of less sensitive viruses in humans must be borne in mind when treating patients. The relationship between the *in vitro* sensitivity of herpes simplex or varicella-zoster virus to Acyclovir and clinical response to therapy has yet to be established (see *"Clinical Pharmacology-Microbiology"*).

Because of the possibility that less sensitive virus may be selected in patients who are receiving Acyclovir, all patients should be advised to take particular care to avoid potential transmission of virus if active lesions are present while they are on therapy. In severely immunocompromised patients, the physician should be aware that prolonged or repeated courses of Acyclovir may result in selection of resistant viruses which may not fully respond to continued Acyclovir therapy.

Caution should be exercised when administering Acyclovir to patients receiving potentially nephrotoxic agents since this may increase the risk of renal dysfunction.

Information for Patients: Patients are instructed to consult with their physician if they experience severe or troublesome adverse reactions, they become pregnant or intend to become pregnant, they intend to breastfeed while taking orally administered Acyclovir or they have any other questions.

Genital Herpes Infections: Genital herpes is a sexually transmitted disease and patients should avoid intercourse when visible lesions are present because of the risk of infecting intimate partners. Acyclovir Capsules, Tablets, and Suspension are for oral ingestion only. Medication should not be shared with others. The prescribed dosage should not be exceeded. Acyclovir does not eliminate latent viruses. Patients are instructed to consult with their physician if they do not receive sufficient relief in the frequency and severity of their genital herpes recurrences.

There are still unanswered questions concerning reproductive/gonadal toxicity and mutagenesis: long-term studies are continuing. Decreased sperm production has been seen at high doses in some animals; a placebo-controlled clinical study using 400 mg or 1000 mg of Acyclovir per day for six months in humans did not show similar findings.[40] Chromosomal breaks were seen *in vitro* after brief exposure to high concentrations. Some other currently marketed medications also cause chromosomal breaks, and the significance of this finding is unknown. A placebo-controlled clinical study using 800 mg of Acyclovir per day for one year in humans did not show any abnormalities in structure or number of chromosomes.[28]

Herpes Zoster Infections: Adults age 50 or older tend to have more severe shingles, and Acyclovir treatment showed more significant benefit for older patients.

Treatment was begun within 72 hours of rash onset in these studies, and was more useful if started within the first 48 hours.

Chickenpox: Although chickenpox in otherwise healthy children is usually a self-limited disease of mild to moderate severity, adolescents and adults tend to have more severe disease. Treatment was initiated within 24 hours of the typical chickenpox rash in the controlled studies, and there is no information regarding the effects of treatment begun later in the disease course. It is unknown whether the treatment of chickenpox in childhood has any effect on long-term immunity. However, there is no evidence to indicate that Acyclovir treatment of chickenpox would have any effect on either decreasing or increasing the incidence or severity of subsequent recurrences of herpes zoster (shingles) later in life. Intravenous Acyclovir is indicated for the treatment of varicella-zoster infections in immuno-compromised patients.

Acyclovir Sterile Powder for Intravenous Infusion:
The recommended dosage, frequency and length of treatment should not be exceeded (see *"Dosage and Administration"*).
Although the aqueous solubility of Acyclovir Sodium (for infusion) is > 100 mg/mL, precipitation of Acyclovir crystals in renal tubules can occur if the maximum solubility of free Acyclovir (2.5 mg/mL at 37°C in water) is exceeded or if the drug is administered by bolus injection. This complication causes a rise in serum creatinine and blood urea nitrogen (BUN), and a decrease in renal creatinine clearance. Ensuing renal tubular damage can produce acute renal failure.

Abnormal renal function (decreased creatinine clearance) can occur as a result of Acyclovir administration and depends on the state of the patient's hydration, other treatments, and the rate of drug administration. Bolus administration of the drug leads to a 10% incidence of renal dysfunction, while in controlled studies, infusion of 5 mg/kg (250 mg/m^2) and 10 mg/kg (500 mg/m^2) over an hour was associated with a lower frequency—3.8%. Concomitant use of other nephrotoxic drugs, pre-existing renal disease, and dehydration make further renal impairment with Acyclovir more likely. In most instances, alterations of renal function were transient and resolved spontaneously or with improvement of water and electrolyte balance, drug dosage adjustment or discontinuation of drug administration. However, in some instances, these changes may progress to acute renal failure.

Administration of Acyclovir by intravenous infusion must be accompanied by adequate hydration. Since maximum urine concentration occurs within the first 2 hours following infusion, particular attention should be given to establishing sufficient urine flow during that period in order to prevent precipitation in renal tubules. Recommended urine output is ≥ 500 mL per gram of drug infused. In patients with encephalitis, the recommended hydration should be balanced by the risk of cerebral edema.

When dosage adjustments are required they should be based on estimated creatinine clearance (see *"Dosage and Administration"*).

Approximately 1% of patients receiving intravenous Acyclovir have manifested encephalopathic changes characterized by either lethargy, obtundation, tremors, confusion, hallucinations, agitation, seizures or coma. Acyclovir should be used with caution in those patients who have underlying neurologic abnormalities and those with serious renal, hepatic, or electrolyte abnormalities or significant hypoxia. It should also be used with caution in patients who have manifested prior neurologic reactions to cytotoxic drugs or those receiving concomitant intrathecal methotrexate or interferon.

Exposure of HSV isolates to Acyclovir *in vitro* can lead to the emergence of less sensitive viruses. These viruses usually are deficient in thymidine kinase (required for Acyclovir activation) and are less pathogenic in animals. Similar isolates have been observed in severely immunocompromised patients during the course of controlled and uncontrolled studies of intravenously administered Acyclovir. These occurred in patients with severe combined immunodeficiencies or following bone marrow transplantation. The presence of these viruses was not associated with a worsening of clinical illness and, in some instances, the virus disappeared spontaneously. The possibility of the appearance of less sensitive viruses must be recognized when treating such patients. The relationship between the *in vitro* sensitivity of herpes simplex or varicella-zoster virus to Acyclovir and clinical response to therapy has not been established.

Acyclovir Ointment:
The recommended dosage, frequency of applications, and length of treatment should not be exceeded (see *"Dosage and Administration"*). There exist no data which demonstrate that the use of Acyclovir Ointment 5% will either prevent transmission of infection to other persons or prevent recurrent infections when applied in the absence of signs and symptoms. Acyclovir Ointment 5% should not be used for the prevention of recurrent HSV infections. Although clinically significant viral resistance associated with the use of Acyclovir Ointment 5% has not been observed, this possibility exists.

DRUG INTERACTIONS
Co-administration of probenecid with intravenous Acyclovir has been shown to increase the mean half-life and the area under the concentration-time curve. Urinary excretion and renal clearance were correspondingly reduced.[41] The clinical effects of this combination have not been studied.

Clinical experience has identified no interactions resulting from topical or systemic administration of other drugs concomitantly with Acyclovir Ointment 5%.

CARCINOGENESIS, MUTAGENESIS, IMPAIRMENT OF FERTILITY
The data presented below include references to peak steady-state plasma Acyclovir concentrations observed in humans treated with 800 mg given orally 6

times a day (dosing appropriate for treatment of herpes zoster) or 200 mg given orally 6 times a day (dosing appropriate for treatment of genital herpes).

Plasma drug concentrations in animal studies are expressed as multiples of human exposure to Acyclovir at the higher and lower dosing schedules (see *"Pharmacokinetics"*).

Acyclovir was tested in lifetime bioassays in rats and mice at single daily doses of up to 450 mg/kg administered by gavage. There was no statistically significant difference in the incidence of tumors between treated and control animals, nor did Acyclovir shorten the latency of tumors. At 450 mg/kg/day, plasma concentrations were 3 to 6 times human levels in the mouse bioassay and 1 to 2 times human levels in the rat bioassay.

Acyclovir was tested in two *in vitro* cell transformation assays. Positive results were observed at the highest concentration tested (31 to 63 times human levels) in one system and the resulting morphologically transformed cells formed tumors when inoculated into immunosuppressed, syngeneic, weanling mice. Acyclovir was negative (40 to 80 times human levels) in the other, possibly less sensitive, transformation assay.

In acute cytogenetic studies, there was an increase, though not statistically significant, in the incidence of chromosomal damage at maximum tolerated parenteral doses of Acyclovir (100 mg/kg) in rats (62 to 125 times human levels) but not in Chinese hamsters; higher doses of 500 and 1000 mg/kg were clastogenic in Chinese hamsters (380 to 760 times human levels). In addition, no activity was found after 5 days dosing in a dominant lethal study in mice (36 to 73 times human levels). In all 4 microbial assays, no evidence of mutagenicity was observed. Positive results were obtained in 2 of 7 genetic toxicity assays using mammalian cells *in vitro*. In human lymphocytes, a positive response for chromosomal damage was seen at concentrations 150 to 300 times the Acyclovir plasma levels achieved in humans. At one locus in mouse lymphoma cells, mutagenicity was observed at concentrations 250 to 500 times human plasma levels. Results in the other five mammalian cell loci follow: at 3 loci in a Chinese hamster ovary cell line, the results were inconclusive at concentrations at least 1850 times human levels; at 2 other loci in mouse lymphoma cells, no evidence of mutagenicity was observed at concentrations at least 1500 times human levels.

Acyclovir has not been shown to impair fertility or reproduction in mice (450 mg/kg/day, p.o.) or in rats (25 mg/kg/day, s.c.). In the mouse study plasma levels were 9 to 18 times human levels, while in the rat study they were 8 to 15 times human levels. At a higher dose in the rat (50 mg/kg/day, s.c.), there was a statistically significant increase in post-implantation loss, but no concomitant decrease in litter size. In female rabbits treated subcutaneously with Acyclovir subsequent to mating, there was a statistically significant decrease in implantation efficiency but no concomitant decrease in litter size at a dose of 50 mg/kg/day (16 to 31 times human levels). No effect upon implantation efficiency was observed when the same dose was administered intravenously (53 to 106 times humans levels). In a rat peri- and postnatal study at 50 mg/kg/day s.c. (11 to 22 times human levels), there was a statistically significant decrease in the group mean numbers of corpora lutea, total implantation sites and live fetuses in the F_1 generation. Although not statistically significant, there was also a dose-related decrease in group mean numbers of live fetuses and implantation sites at 12.5 mg/kg/day and 25 mg/kg/day, s.c. The intravenous administration of 100 mg/kg/day, a dose known to cause obstructive nephropathy in rabbits, caused a significant increase in fetal resorptions and a corresponding decrease in litter size (plasma levels were not measured). However, at a maximum tolerated intravenous dose of 50 mg/kg/day in rabbits (53 to 106 times human levels), no drug-related reproductive effects were observed.

Intraperitoneal doses of 80 or 320 mg/kg/day Acyclovir given to rats for 6 and 1 months, respectively, caused testicular atrophy. Plasma levels were not measured in the one month study and were 24 to 48 times human levels in the six-month study. Testicular atrophy was persistent through the 4-week postdose recovery phase after 320 mg/kg/day; some evidence of recovery of sperm production was evident 30 days post-dose. Intravenous doses of 100 and 200 mg/kg/day Acyclovir given to dogs for 31 days caused aspermatogenesis. At 100 mg/kg/day plasma levels were 47 to 94 times human levels, while at 200 mg/kg/day they were 159 to 317 times human levels. No testicular abnormalities were seen in dogs given 50 mg/kg/day i.v. for one month (21 to 41 times human levels) and in dogs given 60 mg/kg/day orally for one year (6 to 12 times human levels).

PREGNANCY
Teratogenic Effects: Pregnancy Category C. Acyclovir was not teratogenic in the mouse (450 mg/kg/day, p.o.), rabbit (50 mg/kg/day, s.c. and i.v.), or in standard tests in the rat (50 mg/kg/day, s.c.). These exposures resulted in plasma levels 9 and 18, 16 and 106, and 11 and 22 times, respectively, human levels. In a non-standard test in rats, there were fetal abnormalities, such as head and tail anomalies, and maternal toxicity.[42] In this test, rats were given 3 s.c. doses of 100 mg/kg Acyclovir on gestation day 10, resulting in plasma levels 63 and 125 times human levels. There are no adequate and well-controlled studies in pregnant women. Acyclovir should not be used during pregnancy unless the potential benefit justifies the potential risk to the fetus. Although Acyclovir was not teratogenic in standard animal studies, the drug's potential for causing chromosome breaks at high concentration should be taken into consideration in making this determination.

NURSING MOTHERS
It is not known whether topically applied Acyclovir is excreted in breast milk. Acyclovir concentrations have been documented in breast milk in two women following oral administration of Acyclovir and ranged from 0.6 to 4.1 times corresponding plasma levels.[43,44] These concentrations would potentially expose

the nursing infant to a dose of Acyclovir up to 0.3 mg/kg/day. Caution should be exercised when Acyclovir is administered to a nursing woman.

PEDIATRIC USE
Safety and effectiveness in children less than 2 years of age have not been adequately studied.

ADVERSE REACTIONS

Herpes Simplex: Short-Term Administration: The most frequent adverse events reported during clinical trials of treatment of genital herpes with orally administered Acyclovir were nausea and/or vomiting in 8 of 298 patient treatments (2.7%) and headache in 2 of 298 (0.6%). Nausea and/or vomiting occurred in 2 of 287 (0.7%) patients who received placebo.

Less frequent adverse events, each of which occurred in 1 of 298 patient treatments with orally administered Acyclovir (0.3%), included diarrhea, dizziness, anorexia, fatigue, edema, skin rash, leg pain, inguinal adenopathy, medication taste, and sore throat.

Long-Term Administration: The most frequent adverse events reported in a clinical trial for the prevention of recurrences with continuous administration of 400 mg (two 200 mg capsules) 2 times daily for 1 year in 586 patients treated with orally administered Acyclovir were: nausea (4.8%), diarrhea (2.4%), headache (1.9%), and rash (1.7%). The 589 control patients receiving intermittent treatment of recurrences with orally administered Acyclovir for 1 year reported diarrhea (2.7%), nausea (2.4%), headache (2.2%), and rash (1.5%).

The most frequent adverse events reported during the second year by 390 patients who elected to continue daily administration of 400 mg (two 200 mg capsules) 2 times daily for 2 years were headache (1.5%), rash (1.3%), and paresthesia (0.8%). Adverse events reported by 329 patients during the third year include asthenia (1.2%), paresthesia (1.2%), and headache (0.9%).

Herpes Zoster: The most frequent adverse events reported during three clinical trials of treatment of herpes zoster (shingles) with 800 mg of oral Acyclovir 5 times daily for 7 to 10 days in 323 patients were: malaise (11.5%), nausea (8.0%), headache (5.9%), vomiting (2.5%), diarrhea (1.5%), and constipation (0.9%). The 323 placebo recipients reported malaise (11.1%), nausea (11.5%), headache (11.1%), vomiting (2.5%), diarrhea (0.3%), and constipation (2.4%).

Chickenpox: The most frequent adverse events reported during three clinical trials of treatment of chickenpox with oral Acyclovir in 495 patients were: diarrhea (3.2%), abdominal pain (0.6%), rash (0.6%), vomiting (0.6%), and flatulence (0.4%). The 498 patients receiving placebo reported: diarrhea (2.2%), flatulence (0.8%), and insomnia (0.4%).

The adverse reactions listed below have been observed in controlled and uncontrolled clinical trials in approximately 700 patients who received Intravenous Acyclovir at ~ 5 mg/kg (250 mg/m^2) three times daily, and approximately 300 patients who received ~ 10 mg/kg (500 mg/m^2) three times daily.

The most frequent adverse reactions reported during Intravenous Acyclovir administration were inflammation or phlebitis at the injection site in approximately 9% of the patients, and transient elevations of serum creatinine or BUN in 5% to 10% (the higher incidence occurred usually following rapid [less than 10 minutes] intravenous infusion). Nausea and/or vomiting occurred in approximately 7% of the patients (the majority occurring in nonhospitalized patients who received 10 mg/kg). Itching, rash or hives occurred in approximately 2% of patients. Elevation of transaminases occurred in 1% to 2% of patients.

Approximately 1% of patients receiving Intravenous Acyclovir have manifested encephalopathic changes characterized by either lethargy, obtundation, tremors, confusion, hallucinations, agitation, seizures or coma (see *"Precautions"*).

Adverse reactions which occurred at a frequency of less than 1% and which were probably or possibly related to intravenous Acyclovir administration were: anemia, anuria, hematuria, hypotension, edema, anorexia, light-headedness, thirst, headache, diaphoresis, fever, neutropenia, thrombocytopenia, abnormal urinalysis (characterized by an increase in formed elements in urine sediment) and pain on urination. Other reactions have been reported with a frequency of less than 1% in patients receiving Intravenous Acyclovir, but a causal relationship between Intravenous Acyclovir and the reaction could not be determined. These include pulmonary edema with cardiac tamponade, abdominal pain, chest pain, thrombocytosis, leukocytosis, neutrophilia, ischemia of digits, hypokalemia, purpura fulminans, pressure on urination, hemoglobinemia and rigors.

Because ulcerated genital lesions are characteristically tender and sensitive to any contact or manipulation, patients may experience discomfort upon application of ointment. In the controlled clinical trials, mild pain (including transient burning and stinging) was reported by 103 (28.3%) of 364 patients treated with Acyclovir and by 115 (31.1%) of 370 patients treated with placebo; treatment was discontinued in 2 of these patients. Other local reactions among Acyclovir-treated patients included pruritus in 15 (4.1%), rash in 1 (0.3%) and vulvitis in 1 (0.3%). Among the placebo-treated patients, pruritus was reported by 17 (4.6%) and rash by 1 (0.3%).

In all studies, there was no significant difference between the drug and placebo group in the rate or type of reported adverse reactions nor were there any differences in abnormal clinical laboratory findings.

Observed During Clinical Practice: Based on clinical practice experience in patients treated with oral or intravenous Acyclovir or Acyclovir Ointment in the U.S., spontaneously reported adverse events are uncommon. Data are insufficient to support an estimate of their incidence or to establish causation. These events may also occur as part of the underlying disease process. Voluntary reports of adverse events which have been received since market introduction include:

General: fever, headache, pain, peripheral edema, and rarely, anaphylaxis (With ointment: edema and/or pain at application site)

Nervous: confusion, dizziness, hallucinations, paresthesia, somnolence (These symptoms may be marked, particularly in older adults.) (*Intravenously:* also agitation, coma, convulsions, delirium, obtundation, psychosis)

Digestive: diarrhea, elevated liver function tests, gastrointestinal distress, nausea

Hemic and Lymphatic: leukopenia, lymphadenopathy

Musculoskeletal: myalgia

Skin: alopecia, pruritus, rash, urticaria

Special Senses: visual abnormalities

Urogenital: elevated creatinine (*Intravenously:* also elevated BUN, renal failure)

OVERDOSAGE

Patients have ingested intentional overdoses of up to 100 capsules (20 g) of Acyclovir, with no unexpected adverse effects.

Overdosage has been reported following administration of bolus injections, or inappropriately high doses, and in patients whose fluid and electrolyte balance was not properly monitored. This has resulted in elevations in BUN, serum creatinine and subsequent renal failure. Lethargy, convulsions and coma have been reported rarely.

Precipitation of Acyclovir in renal tubules may occur when the solubility (2.5 mg/mL) in the intratubular fluid is exceeded. Renal lesions considered to be related to obstruction of renal tubules by precipitated drug crystals occurred in the following species: rats treated with i.v. and i.p. doses of 20 mg/kg/day for 21 and 31 days, respectively, and at s.c. doses of 100 mg/kg/day for 10 days; rabbits at s.c. and i.v. doses of 50 mg/kg/day for 13 days; and dogs at i.v. doses of 100 mg/kg/day for 31 days. In the event of overdosage, sufficient urine flow must be maintained to prevent precipitation of drug in renal tubules. Recommended urine output is ≥ 500 mL per gram of drug infused. A 6-hour hemodialysis results in a 60% decrease in plasma Acyclovir concentration. Data concerning peritoneal dialysis are incomplete but indicate that this method may be significantly less efficient in removing Acyclovir from the blood. In the event of acute renal failure and anuria, the patient may benefit from hemodialysis until renal function is restored (see *"Dosage and Administration"*).

Overdosage by topical application of Acyclovir Ointment 5% is unlikely because of limited transcutaneous absorption (see *"Clinical Pharmacology"*).

DOSAGE AND ADMINISTRATION
ACYCLOVIR CAPSULES, TABLETS, AND SUSPENSION
Treatment of Initial Genital Herpes: 200 mg (one 200 mg capsule or one teaspoonful [5 mL] suspension) every 4 hours, 5 times daily for 10 days.

Chronic Suppressive Therapy for Recurrent Disease: 400 mg (two 200 mg capsules, one 400 mg tablet, or two teaspoonfuls [10 mL] suspension) 2 times daily for up to 12 months, followed by re-evaluation. See *"Indications and Usage"* and *"Precautions"* for considerations on continuation of suppressive therapy beyond 12 months. Alternative regimens have included doses ranging from 200 mg 3 times daily to 200 mg 5 times daily.

Intermittent Therapy: 200 mg (one 200 mg capsule or one teaspoonful [5 mL] suspension) every 4 hours, 5 times daily for 5 days. Therapy should be initiated at the earliest sign or symptom (prodrome) of recurrence.

Acute Treatment of Herpes Zoster: 800 mg (four 200 mg capsules, two 400 mg tablets, one 800 mg tablet, or four teaspoonfuls [20 mL] suspension) every 4 hours orally 5 times daily for 7 to 10 days.

Treatment of Chickenpox: 20 mg/kg (not to exceed 800 mg) orally, 4 times daily for 5 days. Therapy should be initiated at the earliest sign or symptom.

Patients With Acute or Chronic Renal Impairment: Comprehensive pharmacokinetic studies have been completed following intravenous Acyclovir infusions in patients with renal impairment. Based on these studies, dosage adjustments are recommended in the following chart for genital herpes and herpes zoster indications:

Normal Dosage Regimen	Creatinine Clearance (mL/min/1.73m^2)	Adjusted Dosage Regimen	
		Dose (mg)	Dosing Interval
200 mg every 4 hours	> 10	200	every 4 hours, 5x daily
	0-10	200	every 12 hours
400 mg every 12 hours	> 10	400	every 12 hours
	0-10	200	every 12 hours
800 mg every 4 hours	> 25	800	every 4 hours, 5x daily
	10-25	800	every 8 hours
	0-10	800	every 12 hours

Hemodialysis: For patients who require hemodialysis, the mean plasma half-life of Acyclovir during hemodialysis is approximately 5 hours. This results in a 60% decrease in plasma concentrations following a six-hour dialysis period. Therefore, the patient's dosing schedule should be adjusted so that an additional dose is administered after each dialysis.[45,46]

Peritoneal Dialysis: No supplemental dose appears to be necessary after adjustment of the dosing interval.[47,48]

ACYCLOVIR STERILE POWDER FOR INTRAVENOUS INFUSION

Caution—Rapid or Bolus Intravenous and Intramuscular or Subcutaneous Injection Must be Avoided. Therapy should be initiated as early as possible following onset of signs and symptoms. For diagnosis— see *"Indications"*.

Herpes Simplex Infections: Mucosal And Cutaneous Herpes Simplex (HSV-1 and HSV-2) Infections In Immunocompromised Patients—5 mg/kg infused at a constant rate over 1 hour, every 8 hours (15 mg/kg/day) for 7 days in adult patients with normal renal function. In children under 12 years of age, more accurate dosing can be attained by infusing 250 mg/m^2 at a constant rate over 1 hour, every 8 hours (750 mg/m^2/day) for 7 days.

Severe Initial Clinical Episodes of Herpes Genitalis—The same dose given above—administered for 5 days.

Herpes Simplex Encephalitis—10 mg/kg infused at a constant rate over at least 1 hour, every 8 hours for 10 days. In children between 6 months and 12 years of age, more accurate dosing is achieved by infusing 500 mg/m^2, at a constant rate over at least one hour, every 8 hours for 10 days.

Varicella Zoster Infections: Zoster in Immunocompromised Patients—10 mg/kg infused at a constant rate over 1 hour, every 8 hours for 7 days in adult patients with normal renal function. In children under 12 years of age, equivalent plasma concentrations are attained by infusing 500 mg/m^2 at a constant rate over at least 1 hour, every 8 hours for 7 days. Obese patients should be dosed at 10 mg/kg (Ideal Body Weight). A maximum dose equivalent to 500 mg/m^2 every 8 hours should not be exceeded for any patient.

Patients With Acute Or Chronic Renal Impairment: Refer to *"Dosage and Administration"* section for recommended doses, and adjust the dosing interval as indicated in the table below.

Creatinine Clearance (mL/min/1.73m^2)	Percent of Recommended Dose	Dosing Interval (hours)
> 50	100%	8
25-50	100%	12
10-25	100%	24
0-10	50%	24

Hemodialysis: For patients who require dialysis, the mean plasma half-life of Acyclovir during hemodialysis is approximately 5 hours. This results in a 60% decrease in plasma concentrations following a six-hour dialysis period. Therefore, the patient's dosing schedule should be adjusted so that an additional dose is administered after each dialysis.

Peritoneal Dialysis: No supplemental dose appears to be necessary after adjustment of the dosing interval.

Method of Preparation: Each 10 mL vial contains Acyclovir Sodium equivalent to 500 mg of Acyclovir. Each 20 mL vial contains Acyclovir Sodium equivalent to 1000 mg of Acyclovir. The contents of the vial should be dissolved in Sterile Water for Injection as follows:

Contents of Vial	Amount of Diluent
500 mg	10 mL
1000 mg	20 mL

The resulting solution in each case contains 50 mg Acyclovir per mL (pH approximately 11). Shake the vial well to assure complete dissolution before measuring and transferring each individual dose. DO NOT USE BACTERIOSTATIC WATER FOR INJECTION CONTAINING BENZYL ALCOHOL OR PARABENS.

Administration: The calculated dose should then be removed and added to any appropriate intravenous solution at a volume selected for administration during each 1 hour infusion. Infusion concentrations of approximately 7 mg/mL or lower are recommended. In clinical studies, the average 70 kg adult received between 60 and 150 mL of fluid per dose. Higher concentrations (e.g., 10 mg/mL) may produce phlebitis or inflammation at the injection site upon inadvertent extravasation. Standard, commercially available electrolyte and glucose solutions are suitable for intravenous administration; biologic or colloidal fluids (e.g., blood products, protein solutions, etc.) are not recommended.

Once in solution in the vial at a concentration of 50 mg/mL, the drug should be used within 12 hours. Once diluted for administration, each dose should be used within 24 hours. Refrigeration of reconstituted solutions may result in formation of a precipitate which will redissolve at room temperature.

Acyclovir Ointment:
Apply sufficient quantity to adequately cover all lesions every 3 hours 6 times per day for 7 days. The dose size per application will vary depending upon the total lesion area but should approximate a one-half inch ribbon of ointment per 4 square inches of surface area. A finger cot or rubber glove should be used when applying Acyclovir Ointment to prevent autoinoculation of other body sites and transmission of infection to other persons. *Therapy should be initiated as early as possible following onset of signs and symptoms.*

STORAGE:
Acyclovir Capsules, Tablets
Store at 15° to 25°C (59° to 77°F) and protect from light and moisture.

Acyclovir Suspension and Sterile Powder
Store at 15° to 25°C (59° to 77°F)

Acyclovir Ointment
Store at 15° to 25°C (59° to 77°F) in a dry place.

ANIMAL PHARMACOLOGY AND ANIMAL TOXICOLOGY
Topical treatment of guinea pigs with 10% Acyclovir in polyethylene glycol ointment for three weeks did not result in cutaneous irritation or systemic toxicity. Also, a wide variety of animal tests by parenteral routes demonstrated that Acyclovir has a low order of toxicity.

Acyclovir did not cause dermal sensitization in guinea pigs.

REFERENCES
1. O'Brien JJ, Campoli-Richards DM. Acyclovir—an updated review of its antiviral activity, pharmacokinetic properties, and therapeutic efficacy. *Drugs.* 1989;37: 233-309. 2. Little E, Zeuthen J, McBride AA, et al. Identification of an Epstein-Barr virus-coded thymidine kinase. *EMBO J.* 1986;5(8):1959-1966. 3. Miller WH, Miller RL. Phosphorylation of Acyclovir (acycloguanosine) monophosphate by GMP kinase. *J Biol Chem.* 1980;255:7204-7207. 4. Furman PA, St Clair MH, Fyfe JA, et al. Inhibition of herpes simplex virus-induced DNA polymerase activity and viral DNA replication by 9-(2-hydroxyethoxymethyl)guanine and its triphosphate. *J Virol.* 1979;32:72-77. 5. Derse D, Cheng YC, Furman PA, et al. Inhibition of purified human and herpes simplex virus-induced DNA polymerases by 9-(2-hydroxyethoxymethyl)guanine triphosphate: effects on primer-template function. *J Biol Chem.* 1981;256:11447-11451. 6. McGuirt PV, Shaw JE, Elion GB, et al. Identification of small DNA fragments synthesized in herpes simplex virus-infected cells in the presence of Acyclovir. *Antimicrob Agents Chemother.* 1984;25:507-509. 7. Barry DW, Blum MR. Antiviral drugs: Acyclovir. In Turner P, Shand DG, (eds). *Recent Advances in Clinical Pharmacology,* ed 3. New York, Churchill Livingstone, 1983, chap 4. 8. DeClercq E. Comparative efficacy of antiherpes drugs in different cell lines. *Antimicrob Agents Chemother.* 1982; 21:661-663. 9. McLaren C, Ellis MN, Hunter GA. A colorimetric assay for the measurement of the sensitivity of herpes simplex viruses to antiviral agents. *Antiviral Res.* 1983;3:223-234. 10. Barry DW, Nusinoff-Lehrman S. Viral resistance in clinical practice: summary of five years experience with Acyclovir. In Kono R, Nakajima A (eds): *Herpes Viruses and Virus Chemotherapy (Ex Med Int Congr Ser 667).* New York, Excerpta Medica, 1985;269-270. 11. Dekker C. Ellis MN, McLaren C, et al. Virus resistance in clinical practice. *J Antimicrob Chemother.* 1983;12 (suppl B);137-152. 12. Sibrack CD, Gutman LT, Wilfert CM, et al. Pathogenicity of Acyclovir-resistant herpes simplex virus type 1 from an immunodeficient child. *J Infect Dis.* 1982;146: 673-682. 13. Crumpacker CS, Schnipper LE, Marlowe SI, et al. Resistance to antiviral drugs of herpes simplex virus isolated from a patient treated with Acyclovir. *N Engl J Med.* 1982;306:343-346. 14. Wade JC, Newton B, McLaren C, et al. Intravenous Acyclovir to treat mucocutaneous herpes simplex virus infection after marrow transplantation, a double-blind trial. *Ann Intern Med.* 1982;96:265-269. 15. Burns WH, Saral R, Santos GW, et al. Isolation and characterization of resistant herpes simplex virus after Acyclovir therapy. *Lancet.* 1982;1:421-423. 16. Straus SE, Takiff HE, Seidlin M, et al. Suppression of frequently recurring genital herpes; a placebo-controlled double-blind trial of oral Acyclovir. *N Engl J Med.* 1984;310:1545-1550. 17. Collins, P. Viral sensitivity following the introduction of Acyclovir. *Am J Med.* 1988;85(2A):129-134. 18. Erlich KS, Mills J, Chatis P, et al. Acyclovir-resistant herpes simplex virus infections in patients with the acquired immunodeficiency syndrome. *N Engl J Med.* 1989;320(5):293-296. 19. Hill EL, Ellis MN, Barry DW. In: *28th Intersci Conf on Antimicrob Agents Chemother.* Los Angeles 1988, Abst. No. 0840:260. 20. Ellis MN, Keller PM, Fyfe JA, et al. Clinical isolates of herpes simplex virus type 2 that induces thymidine kinase with altered substrate specificity. *Antimicrob Agents Chemother.* 1987;31(7):1117-1125. 21. Collins P, Larder BA, Oliver NM. et al. Characterization of a DNA polymerase mutant of herpes simplex virus from a severely immunocompromised patient receiving Acyclovir. *J gen Virol.* 1989;(70):375-382. 22. Field HJ, Darby G, Wildy P. Isolation and characterization of Acyclovir-resistant mutants of herpes simplex virus. *J gen Virol.* 1980;49:115-124. 23. Bryson YJ, Dillon M, Lovett M, et al. Treatment of first episodes of genital herpes simplex virus infection with oral Acyclovir: a randomized double-blind controlled trial in normal subjects. *N Engl J Med.* 1983;308:916-921. 24. Mertz GJ, Critchlow CW, Benedetti J, et al. Double-blind placebo-controlled trial of oral Acyclovir in first-episode genital herpes simplex virus infection. *JAMA.* 1984;252:1147-1151. 25. Nilsen AE, Aasen T, Halsos AM, et al. Efficacy of oral Acyclovir in the treatment of initial and recurrent genital herpes. *Lancet.* 1982;2:571-573. 26. Douglas JM, Critchlow C, Benedetti J, et al. A double-blind study of oral Acyclovir for suppression of recurrences of genital herpes simplex virus infection. *N Engl J Med.* 1984;310:1551-1556. 27. Mindel A, Weller IV, Faherty A, et al. Prophylactic oral Acyclovir in recurrent genital herpes. *Lancet.* 1984;2:57-59. 28. Mattison HR, Reichman RC, Benedetti J, et al. Double-blind, placebo-controlled trial comparing long-term suppressive with short-term oral Acyclovir therapy for management of recurrent genital herpes. *Am J Med.* 1988;85(suppl 2A):20-25. 29. Straus SE, Croen KD, Sawyer MH, et al. Acyclovir suppression of frequently recurring genital herpes. *JAMA.* 1988;260:2227-2230. 30. Mertz GJ, Eron L, Kaufman R, et al. The Acyclovir Study Group. Prolonged continuous versus intermittent oral Acyclovir treatment in normal adults with frequently recurring genital herpes simplex virus infection. *Amer J Med.* 1988;85(suppl 2A):14-19. 31. Data on file, Burroughs Wellcome Co. 32. Reichman RC, Badger GJ, Mertz GJ, et al. Treatment of recurrent genital herpes simplex infections with oral Acyclovir: a controlled trial. *JAMA.* 1984;251:2103-2107. 33. Huff JC, Bean B; Balfour HH, Jr. et al. Therapy of herpes zoster with oral Acyclovir. *Am J Med.* 1988;85(2A):85-89. 34. Morton P, Thompson AN. Oral Acyclovir in the treatment of herpes zoster in general practice. *NZ Med J.* 1989;102:93-95. 35. Balfour HH Jr. Kelly JM, Suarez, CS, et al. Acyclovir treatment of varicella in otherwise healthy children. *J Pediatr.* 1990;116:633-639. 36. Dunkle LM, Arvin AM, Whitley RJ, et al. A controlled trial of Acyclovir for chickenpox in normal children. *N Engl J Med.* 1991;325:1539-1544. 37. Balfour HH Jr, Rotbart HA, Feldman S, et al. Acyclovir treatment of varicella in otherwise healthy adolescents. *J Pediatr.* 1992. In press. 38. Data on file, Burroughs Wellcome Co. 39. Naib ZM, Nahmias AJ, Josey WE, et al. Relation of cytohistopathology of genital herpesvirus infection to cervical anaplasia. *Cancer Res* 1973;33:1452-1463. 40. Douglas JM, David LG, Remington ML, et al. A double-blind, placebo-controlled trial of the effect of chronically administered oral Acyclovir on sperm production in man with frequently recurrent genital herpes. *J Infect Dis.* 1988;157:588-593. 41. Laskin OL, deMiranda P, King DH, et al. Effects of probenecid on the pharmacokinetics and elimination of Acyclovir, in humans. *Antimicrob Agents Chemother.* 1982;21:804-807. 42. Stahlmann R, Klug S, Lewandowski C, et al. Teratogenicity of Acyclovir in rats. *Infection.* 1987;15:261-262. 43. Lau RJ, Emery MG, Galinsky

RE, et al. Unexpected accumulation of Acyclovir in breast milk with estimate of infant exposure. *Obstet Gynecol.* 1987;69(3):468-471. 44. Meyer LJ, deMiranda P, Sheth N, et al. Acyclovir in human breast milk. *Am J Obstet Gynecol.* 1988;158(3):586-588. 45. Laskin OL, Longstreth JA, Whelton A, et al. Effect of renal failure on the pharmacokinetics of Acyclovir. *Am J Med.* 1982;73:197-201. 46. Krasny HC, Liao SH, deMiranda P, et al. Influence of hemodialysis on Acyclovir pharmacokinetics in patients with chronic renal failure. *Am J Med.* 1982;73:202-204. 47. Boelart J, Schurgers M, Daneels R, et al. Multiple dose pharmacokinetics of intravenous Acyclovir in patients on continuous ambulatory peritoneal dialysis. *J Antimicrob Chemother.* 1987; 20:69-76. 48. Shah GM, Winer RL, Krasny HC. Acyclovir pharmacokinetics in a patient on continuous ambulatory peritoneal dialysis. *Am J Kidney Dis.* 1986;7:507-510.

HOW SUPPLIED

ACYCLOVIR
CAPSULE: 200 MG

BRAND/MANUFACTURER	NDC	SIZE	AWP
○ **BRAND**			
➤ ZOVIRAX: Burr Wellcome	00081-0991-55	100s	$93.88
	00081-0991-56	100s ud	$106.93

OINTMENT: 5%

BRAND/MANUFACTURER	NDC	SIZE	AWP
○ **BRAND**			
ZOVIRAX: Burr Wellcome	00081-0993-41	3 gm	$14.86
	00081-0993-94	15 gm	$34.36

SUSPENSION: 200 MG/5 ML

BRAND/MANUFACTURER	NDC	SIZE	AWP
○ **BRAND**			
ZOVIRAX: Burr Wellcome	00081-0953-96	473 ml	$80.89

TABLETS: 400 MG

BRAND/MANUFACTURER	NDC	SIZE	AWP
○ **BRAND**			
➤ ZOVIRAX: Burr Wellcome	00081-0949-55	100s	$182.18

TABLETS: 800 MG

BRAND/MANUFACTURER	NDC	SIZE	AWP
○ **BRAND**			
➤ ZOVIRAX: Burr Wellcome	00081-0945-01	35s	$123.98
	00081-0945-55	100s	$354.26
	00081-0945-56	100s ud	$361.34

ACYCLOVIR SODIUM
POWDER FOR INJECTION: 500 MG

BRAND/MANUFACTURER	NDC	SIZE	AWP
○ **BRAND**			
ZOVIRAX: Burr Wellcome	00081-0995-01	10s	$489.46

POWDER FOR INJECTION: 1000 MG

BRAND/MANUFACTURER	NDC	SIZE	AWP
○ **BRAND**			
ZOVIRAX: Burr Wellcome	00081-0952-01	10s	$978.92

Adagen *SEE* PEGADEMASE BOVINE

Adalat *SEE* NIFEDIPINE

Adapin *SEE* DOXEPIN HYDROCHLORIDE

Adderall *SEE* AMPHETAMINE

Adeflor M *SEE* SODIUM FLUORIDE AND VITAMINS, MULTI

Adenocard IV *SEE* ADENOSINE

Adenosine

DESCRIPTION

Adenosine is an endogenous nucleoside occurring in all cells of the body. It is chemically 6-amino-9-β-D-ribofuranosyl-9-H-purine.

Its molecular formula is $C_{10}H_{13}N_5O_4$ and its molecular weight is 267.24.

Adenosine is a white crystalline powder. It is soluble in water and practically insoluble in alcohol. Solubility increases by warming and lowering the pH. Adenosine is not chemically related to other antiarrhythmic drugs.

Adenosine is a sterile solution for rapid bolus intravenous injection and is available in 6mg/2 mL vials. Each mL contains 3 mg adenosine and 9 mg sodium chloride in Water for Injection. The pH of the solution is between 5.5 and 7.5.

Following is its chemical structure:

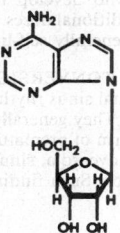

CLINICAL PHARMACOLOGY
MECHANISM OF ACTION

Adenosine slows conduction time through the A-V node, can interrupt the reentry pathways through the A-V node and can restore normal sinus rhythm in patients with paroxysmal supraventricular tachycardia (PSVT), including PSVT associated with Wolff-Parkinson-White Syndrome.

Adenosine is antagonized competitively by methylxanthines such as caffeine and theophylline and potentiated by blockers of nucleoside transport such as dipyridamole. Adenosine is not blocked by atropine.

HEMODYNAMICS

The usual intravenous bolus dose of 6 or 12 mg Adenosine will have no systemic hemodynamic effects. When larger doses are given by infusion, Adenosine decreases blood pressure by decreasing peripheral resistance.

PHARMACOKINETICS

Intravenously administered Adenosine is removed from the circulation very rapidly. Following an intravenous bolus, Adenosine is taken up by erythrocytes and vascular endothelial cells. The half-life of intravenous Adenosine is estimated to be less than 10 seconds. Adenosine enters the body pool and is primarily metabolized to inosine and adenosine monophosphate (AMP).

HEPATIC AND RENAL FAILURE

Hepatic and renal failure should have no effect on the activity of a bolus Adenosine injection. Since Adenosine has a direct action, hepatic and renal function are not required for the activity or metabolism of a bolus Adenosine injection.

CLINICAL TRIAL RESULTS

In controlled studies in the United States, bolus doses of 3, 6, 9, and 12 mg were studied. A cumulative 60% of patients with paroxysmal supraventricular tachycardia had converted to normal sinus rhythm within one minute after an intravenous bolus dose of 6 mg Adenosine (some converted on 3 mg and failures were given 6 mg), and a cumulative 92% converted after a bolus dose of 12 mg. Seven to sixteen percent of patients converted after 1-4 placebo bolus injections. Similar responses were seen in a variety of patient subsets, including those using or not using digoxin, those with Wolff-Parkinson-White Syndrome, males, females, Caucasians, and Hispanics.

Adenosine is not effective in converting rhythms other than PSVT, such as atrial flutter, atrial fibrillation, or ventricular tachycardia to normal sinus rhythm. To date, such patients have not had adverse consequences following administration of Adenosine.

INDICATIONS AND USAGE

Intravenous Adenosine is indicated for the following:

Conversion to sinus rhythm of paroxysmal supraventricular tachycardia (PSVT), including that associated with accessory bypass tracts (Wolff-Parkinson-White Syndrome). When clinically advisable, appropriate vagal maneuvers (e.g., Valsalva maneuver), should be attempted prior to Adenosine administration.

It is important to be sure that Adenosine solution actually reaches the systemic circulation (see *"Dosage and Administration"*).

Adenosine does not convert atrial flutter, atrial fibrillation, or ventricular tachycardia to normal sinus rhythm. In the presence of atrial flutter or atrial fibrillation, a transient modest slowing of ventricular response may occur immediately following Adenosine administration.

UNLABELED USES
Adenosine has been used alone or as an adjunct in the diagnosis of tachycardia.

➤ SHOWN IN PRODUCT IDENTIFICATION GUIDE

CONTRAINDICATIONS

Intravenous Adenosine is contraindicated in:

1. Second- or third-degree A-V block (except in patients with a functioning artificial pacemaker).
2. Sick sinus syndrome (except in patients with a functioning artificial pacemaker).
3. Known hypersensitivity to Adenosine.

WARNINGS

HEART BLOCK

Adenosine exerts its effect by decreasing conduction through the A-V node and may produce a short-lasting first-, second- or third-degree heart block. In extreme cases, transient asystole may result (one case has been reported in a patient with atrial flutter who was receiving carbamazepine). Appropriate therapy should be instituted as needed. Patients who develop high-level block on one dose of Adenosine should not be given additional doses. Because of the very short half-life of Adenosine, these effects are generally self-limiting.

ARRHYTHMIAS AT TIME OF CONVERSION

At the time of conversion to normal sinus rhythm, a variety of new rhythms may appear on the electrocardiogram. They generally last only a few seconds without intervention, and may take the form of premature ventricular contractions, atrial premature contractions, sinus bradycardia, sinus tachycardia, skipped beats, and varying degrees of A-V nodal block. Such findings were seen in 55% of patients.

PRECAUTIONS

DRUG INTERACTIONS

Intravenous Adenosine has been effectively administered in the presence of other cardioactive drugs, such as digitalis, quinidine, beta-adrenergic blocking agents, calcium-channel blocking agents, and angiotensin-converting enzyme inhibitors, without any change in the adverse reaction profile.

The effects of Adenosine are antagonized by methylxanthines such as caffeine and theophylline. In the presence of methylxanthines, larger doses of Adenosine may be required or Adenosine may not be effective.

Adenosine effects are potentiated by dipyridamole. Thus, smaller doses of Adenosine may be effective in the presence of dipyridamole. Carbamazepine has been reported to increase the degree of heart block produced by other agents. As the primary effect of Adenosine is to decrease conduction through the A-V node, higher degrees of heart block may be produced in the presence of carbamazepine.

ASTHMA

Most patients with asthma who have received intravenous Adenosine have not experienced exacerbation of their asthma. Cases of bronchospasm have been reported rarely in both asthmatic and non-asthmatic patients. Inhaled Adenosine has been reported to induce broncho-constriction in asthmatic patients but not in normal individuals.

CARCINOGENESIS, MUTAGENESIS

Studies in animals have not been performed to evaluate the carcinogenic potential of Adenosine. Adenosine tested negative for mutagenic potential in the Salmonella/Mammalian Microsome Assay (Ames Test).

Adenosine, like other nucleosides at millimolar concentrations present for several doubling times of cells in culture, is known to produce a variety of chromosomal alterations. In rats and mice, Adenosine administered intraperitoneally once a day for 5 days at 50, 100, and 150 mg/kg caused decreased spermatogenesis and increased numbers of abnormal sperm, a reflection of the ability of Adenosine to produce chromosomal damage.

PREGNANCY CATEGORY C

Animal reproduction studies have not been conducted with Adenosine; nor have studies been performed in pregnant women. As Adenosine is a naturally occurring material, widely dispersed throughout the body, no fetal effects would be anticipated. However, since it is not known whether Adenosine can cause fetal harm when administered to pregnant women, Adenosine should be used during pregnancy only if clearly needed.

PEDIATRICS

No controlled studies have been conducted in pediatric patients.

ADVERSE REACTIONS

The following reactions were reported with intravenous Adenosine used in controlled U.S. clinical trials. The placebo group had a *less than* 1% rate of all of these reactions.

Cardiovascular: Facial flushing (18%), headache (2%), sweating, palpitations, chest pain, hypotension (less than 1%)

Respiratory: Shortness of breath/dyspnea (12%), chest pressure (7%), hyperventilation, head pressure (less than 1%)

Central Nervous System: Light-headedness (2%), dizziness, tingling in arms, numbness (1%), apprehension, blurred vision, burning sensation, heaviness in arms, neck and back pain (less than 1%)

Gastrointestinal: Nausea (3%), metallic taste, tightness in throat, pressure in groin (less than 1%)

In postmarket clinical experience with Adenosine, cases of prolonged asystole, ventricular tachycardia, ventricular fibrillation, transient increase in blood pressure, and bronchospasm, in association with Adenosine use, have been reported.

OVERDOSAGE

The half-life of Adenosine is less than 10 seconds. Thus, adverse effects are generally rapidly self-limiting. Treatment of any prolonged adverse effects should be individualized and be directed toward the specific effect. Methylxanthines, such as caffeine and theophylline, are competitive antagonists of adenosine.

DOSAGE AND ADMINISTRATION

For rapid bolus intravenous use only.

Adenosine injection should be given as a rapid bolus by the peripheral intravenous route. To be certain the solution reaches the systemic circulation, it should be administered either directly into a vein or, if given into an IV line, it should be given as close to the patient as possible and followed by a rapid saline flush.

The dose recommendation is based on clinical studies with peripheral venous bolus dosing. Central venous (CVP or other) administration of Adenosine has not been systematically studied.

The recommended intravenous doses for adults are as follows:

Initial Dose: 6 mg given as a rapid intravenous bolus (administered over a 1-2 second period).

Repeat Administration: If the first dose does not result in elimination of the supraventricular tachycardia within 1-2 minutes, 12 mg should be given as a rapid intravenous bolus. This 12 mg dose may be repeated a second time if required.

Doses greater than 12 mg are not recommended.

Note: Parenteral drug products should be inspected visually for particulate matter and discoloration prior to administration.

Store at controlled room temperature 15°-30°C (59°-86°F). *Do not refrigerate* as crystallization may occur. If crystallization has occurred, dissolve crystals by warming to room temperature. The solution must be clear at the time of use. Discard unused portion.

J CODES

6 mg IV—J0150

HOW SUPPLIED

INJECTION: 3 MG/ML

BRAND/MANUFACTURER	NDC	SIZE	AWP
○ BRAND			
ADENOCARD IV: Fujisawa	57317-0232-10	2 ml	$26.97

Adenosine Phosphate

DESCRIPTION

Adenosine Phosphate injection is a sterile solution of adenosine-5-monophosphate available for intramuscular use. Adenosine Phosphate (AMP) has the molecular formula $C_{19}H_{16}N_6O_7P$ with a molecular weight of 347.22. It is Adenosine-5-Monophosphoric Acid and occurs as white crystals with a melting point of 196°–200°C. It is readily soluble in boiling water.

Each mL contains:
Adenosine-5-Monophosphate . . . . .25 mg

CLINICAL PHARMACOLOGY

It is not yet understood by what exact mechanism Adenosine Phosphate provides certain therapeutic benefits. Perhaps correction of deficiencies or underlying biochemical imbalances at the cellular level provides this clinical benefit. However, the rationale for the therapeutic use of Adenosine Phosphate must rely essentially upon clinical evidence until more is known about cellular biochemistry and its relation to normal and disturbed physiological processes.

INDICATION AND USAGE

The symptomatic relief of varicose vein complications with stasis dermatitis.

CONTRAINDICATIONS

Adenosine Phosphate injection is contraindicated in patients with a history of myocardial infarction; cerebral hemorrhage.

WARNINGS

Adenosine Phosphate and Adenosine are not interchangeable drugs. Therefore, extreme care should be utilized to avoid possible inadvertent interchange, since such use could result in serious toxicity and/or therapeutic failure, which may potentially be fatal.

Anaphylactoid reactions following administration of Adenosine Phosphate injection have been reported. If patient complains of dyspnea and tightness in the chest following an injection, further injections should not be made. Prompt treatment for the allergic reaction should be immediately instituted when and if they occur.

Usage in Pregnancy: Safe use of Adenosine Phosphate has not been established with respect to adverse effects upon fetal development. Therefore, this drug should not be used in women of child-bearing potential and particularly during early pregnancy unless in the judgement of the physician the benefits outweigh the potential hazards.

◆ RATED THERAPEUTICALLY EQUIVALENT; ◇ THERAPEUTIC EQUIVALENCE UNCONFIRMED; ○ UNRATED

Usage in Children: Adenosine Phosphate is not recommended for use in children because documented clinical experience has been insufficient to establish safety and a suitable dosage regimen in the pediatric age group.

PRECAUTION
Do not inject intravenously.

ADVERSE REACTIONS
Flushing, dizziness, and palpitation may occur. Hypotension, dyspnea, epigastric discomfort, and nausea. Occasional local rash and diuresis. Increase in symptoms of bursitis and tendinitis.

DOSAGE AND ADMINISTRATION
For Intramuscular Use Only.

Adults: Usually 1 mL (25 mg) once or twice daily until relief is obtained, and then 1 mL (25 mg) two or three times weekly for maintenance.

Parenteral drug products should be inspected visually for particulate matter and discoloration prior to administration, whenever the solution and container permit.

Store at controlled room temperature 15°–30°C (59°–86°F).

REFERENCES
3. Boller, R., Rottino, A., and Pratt, G.H.: Angiology 3:260-266 (June), 1952. 4. Bozonnet, G.E.: Concours med. 78:1775 (April 14), 1956. 5. Gugel-Frank, M.: Med. Klin. 52:2004-2005 (November 15), 1957. 6. Harth, V.: Med. Klin 53:1309-1311, 1958. 7. Hess, H., Deut. mod. Wschr. 81:1308-1324 (August 17), 1956. 8. Karcher, K.H., and Thelen, C.: Fortsehr Med. 72:167-168 (April 15), 1954. 9. Lawrence, E.D.: Am. J. Surg. 95:434-437 (March), 1958. 10. Lawrence, E.D.: Doktor, D., and Sall, J.: Angiology 2:405-411 (October), 1951. 11. Mattucks, I.L.: J. Am. Osteopath. Assn. 65:256-258 (December), 1955. 12. Michel, D.: Nocker, J., and Hartleb, O.: Klrn. Wschr. 34:701-704 (July 1), 1956. 13. O'Brien, F.L., Tosi, G.A., and Brunelle, A.R.: J. Nat. Assn. Chiropod. 46:376-382 (June), 1956. 14. Pratt, G.H.: J.A.M.A. 147:1121-1126 (November 17), 1951. 15. Pratt, G.H.: Surg. Clin. N. Amer. 1229-1244 (October), 1953. 16. Pratt, G.H.: Am. J. Surg. 97:696-697 (June), 1959. 17. Quintera, R.V.: Rev. Inst. Venez. Saguros Soc. 1:115-122 (October), 1952. 18. Rice, J.: Rev. Podiat. Res. 1:1-8 (June), 1954. 19. Ronina, A., Boller, R., and Pratt, G.H.: Angiology 1:194-200 (April), 1950. 20. Shapiro, A.: Ann. New York Acad Sc. 58:633-644 (July 28), 1954. 21. Steinberg, M.H.: Angiology 9:154-161 (June), 1958.

HOW SUPPLIED
INJECTION: 25 MG/ML

BRAND/MANUFACTURER	NDC	SIZE	AWP
○ GENERICS			
McGuff	49072-0011-10	10 ml	$5.55
ADENO-JEC: Hauser,A.F.	52637-0690-10	10 ml	$6.95
Steris	00402-0087-10	10 ml	$7.20
Pasadena	00418-6420-10	10 ml	$9.35
CMC-Cons	00223-7717-10	10 ml	$11.95
Merit	30727-0382-70	10 ml	$17.85
ADENIC: Intl Ethical	11584-1006-01	10 ml	$18.50
Legere	25332-0043-10	10 ml	$18.95

Adipex-P *SEE* PHENTERMINE

Adrenalin *SEE* EPINEPHRINE, SYSTEMIC

Adriamycin *SEE* DOXORUBICIN HYDROCHLORIDE

Adsorbocarpine *SEE* PILOCARPINE, OPHTHALMIC

AeroBid *SEE* FLUNISOLIDE

Aeroseb-Dex *SEE* DEXAMETHASONE, TOPICAL

A-Hydrocort *SEE* HYDROCORTISONE, SYSTEMIC

Akineton HCl *SEE* BIPERIDEN

AK-Neo-Dex *SEE* DEXAMETHASONE SODIUM
PHOSPHATE WITH NEOMYCIN SULFATE, OPHTHALMIC

Albalon *SEE* NAPHAZOLINE HYDROCHLORIDE

Albamycin *SEE* NOVOBIOCIN SODIUM

Albay Venomil *SEE* ALLERGENIC EXTRACTS

Albumin, Normal Serum, Human

DESCRIPTION
Albumin, Normal Serum, Human, 5% Solution, contains in each 100 mL, 5 g of Albumin prepared from pooled human venous plasma; Albumin Human 25% contains in each 100 mL 25 g of Albumin. This product was prepared using the Cohn cold ethanol fractionation process.[1,2] It has been adjusted to physiological pH with sodium bicarbonate and/or sodium hydroxide and has been stabilized with 0.004 M sodium caprylate (0.02 M for 25%) and 0.004 M sodium acetyltryptophanate (0.02 M for 25%). The solution contains 145 ± 15 mEq of sodium per liter. Albumin Human contains no preservative and none of the coagulation factors of fresh whole blood or fresh plasma.

In addition to sterilization by filtration, this product has been heated for 10 hours at 60°C in the final container. This procedure has been shown to be an effective method of inactivating hepatitis viruses in 25% solutions of Albumin even when prepared from plasma known to contain transmissible hepatitis viruses.[3]

The processing of Albumin Human has removed blood group isoagglutinins to permit its administration without regard to the recipient's blood group. The absence of cellular elements removes the danger of sensitization with repeated infusions. Albumin Human must be administered INTRAVENOUSLY.

CLINICAL PHARMACOLOGY
Albumin is a highly soluble, ellipsoidal protein (MW 66,500), accounting for 70-80% of the colloid osmotic pressure of plasma. It is, therefore, important in regulating the volume of circulating blood.[4,5,6] This solution supplies the oncotic equivalent of approximately its volume of normal human plasma. When injected intravenously, 5% Albumin will increase the circulating plasma volume by an amount approximately equal to the volume infused; 50 mL of 25% Albumin draws approximately 175 mL of additional fluid into the circulation within 15 minutes, except in the presence of marked dehydration. This extra fluid reduces hemoconcentration and decreases blood viscosity. The degree and duration of volume expansion depend upon the initial blood volume. When treating patients with diminished blood volume, the effect of infused Albumin may persist for many hours. In individuals with normal blood volumes, the hemodilution lasts for a much shorter time.

Albumin is also a transport protein and binds naturally occurring, therapeutic, and toxic materials in the circulation.[4,5]

Albumin is distributed throughout the extracellular water and more than 60% of the body Albumin pool is located in the extravascular fluid compartment. The total body Albumin in a 70 kg man is approximately 320 g; it has a circulating life span of 15-20 days, with a turnover of approximately 15 g per day.[5]

The minimum serum Albumin level necessary to prevent or reverse peripheral edema is unknown. Although it undoubtedly varies from patient to patient, there is some evidence that it falls near 2.5 g per deciliter. This concentration provides a plasma oncotic pressure of 20 mm Hg (the equivalent of a total protein concentration of 5.2 g/dL).[6,7]

INDICATIONS AND USAGE
1. HYPOVOLEMIA (WITH OR WITHOUT SHOCK)
Hypovolemia is a possible indication for Albumin administration. The effectiveness of 5% Albumin in reversing hypovolemia depends largely upon its colloid osmotic pressure.

Although crystalloid solutions or colloid-containing plasma substitutes may be used in the emergency treatment of shock, Albumin Human has a longer intravascular half-life.[7,8,9]

When the hypovolemia is long-standing and hypoalbuminemia exists in the presence of adequate hydration or edema, 25% Albumin is preferable to 5% protein solutions.[4,6]

When the blood volume deficit is the result of hemorrhage, replacement with compatible red blood cells or whole blood should be undertaken as quickly as is possible.

Shock: Albumin 5% and 25% are indicated in the emergency treatment of shock due to burns, trauma, operations and infections, in the treatment of severe injuries, and in other similar conditions where the restoration of blood volume is urgent. The primary function is maintenance of colloid osmotic pressure. If there has been considerable loss of red blood cells, transfusion with whole blood is indicated.

2. HYPOALBUMINEMIA

A. GENERAL
Hypoalbuminemia is another possible indication for Albumin administration. Hypoalbuminemia may result from one or more of the following:[5]

1. *Inadequate production* (malnutrition, burns, major injury, congenital analbuminemia, liver disease, infection, malignancy, endocrine disorders).

2. *Excessive catabolism* (burns, major injury, pancreatitis, thyrotoxicosis, pemphigus, nephrosis).

3. *Loss from the body* (hemorrhage, excessive renal excretion, burn exudates, exudative enteropathy, exfoliative dermatoses).

4. *Redistribution within the body* (major surgery, cirrhosis with ascites, various inflammatory conditions).

In almost every instance, treatment of the underlying disorder and emphasis on increased nutritional replacement of amino acids and/or protein will be more likely to restore normal plasma Albumin levels than will the transfusion of Albumin-containing solutions.[4,6]

Whenever hypoalbuminemia results from excessive protein loss, the effect of Albumin administration will be temporary unless the underlying disorder is reversed.

There are occasional patients with hypoproteinemia accompanying major infections or injuries, or severe pancreatitis, for whom reversal of the disorder cannot be accomplished quickly. In these situations, supplementation of nutritional protein intake with amino acid infusions may fail to restore serum Albumin to adequate levels, and 5% Albumin may be a useful therapeutic adjuvant.

B. BURNS
The optimal mix of crystalloid and colloid solutions which should be administered following extensive burns remains the subject of continuing discussion.[4,7] During the initial 24 hours of therapy, large volumes of crystalloids are infused to restore the depleted extracellular fluid volume—proteins, electrolytes, and water. Beyond 24 hours. Albumin is indicated to replace the protein loss which accompanies any severe burn.[4,6,7]

C. CIRRHOSIS
When repeated paracenteses are being performed for ascites and the fluid is not being reinfused, supplementary Albumin infusion may be needed.[7]

3. MISCELLANEOUS INDICATIONS FOR ALBUMIN HUMAN, 5% SOLUTION
A. The administration of Albumin prior to or during cardiopulmonary bypass surgery has been recommended although there are no clear data indicating its advantages over crystalloid solutions. Which is the most propitious time to infuse Albumin is also unclear.[4,7,10]

B. When large volumes of packed red blood cells have been transfused to correct blood loss, 5% Albumin may be administered in order to avoid the development of hypoalbuminemia.

Albumin 5% may be used in acutely hypoproteinemic patients, provided sodium restriction is not a problem.

4. HYPOPROTEINEMIA
Albumin 5% may be used in acutely hypoproteinemic patients, provided sodium restriction is not a problem.

Hypoproteinemia with or without edema: Albumin is indicated in those clinical situations usually associated with a low concentration of plasma protein and a resulting decreased circulating blood volume. Although diuresis may occur soon after Albumin administration has been instituted, best results are obtained if Albumin is continued until the normal serum protein level is regained.

CIRCUMSTANCES IN WHICH ALBUMIN ADMINISTRATION IS USUALLY NOT INDICATED
The internal redistribution of plasma Albumin which accompanies major surgery only occasionally causes clinical evidence of hypovolemia or insufficient plasma oncotic pressure. Moreover, there is no evidence that this temporary redistribution adversely affects wound healing. Therefore, the administration of 5% Albumin to such post-surgical patients is not usually indicated.

The sequestration of protein-rich fluid during the course of acute inflammatory conditions (peritonitis, pancreatitis, cellulitis) rarely causes significant morbidity due to hypovolemia and treatment with Albumin is rarely indicated.

Rarely does a valid reason exist for administering Albumin to treat the stabilized hypoproteinemias accompanying chronic cirrhosis, chronic nephrosis, protein-losing enteropathy, malabsorption, or pancreatic insufficiency.[4,6,7] However, when a patient in this category has to cope with a superimposed acute stress (e.g., anesthesia, major injection, etc.) his hemodynamic state, oncotic deficit and fluid balance should be carefully assessed and appropriate measure taken, as indicated by the individual circumstances.[6,7]

There is no valid reason for the use of Albumin as an intravenous nutrient.

UNLABELED USES
Albumin, Normal Serum, Human, is used alone or as an adjunct in the treatment of adult respiratory distress syndrome.

CONTRAINDICATIONS
The history of an allergic reaction to Albumin is a specific contraindication to the use of this product.

Albumin may be contraindicated in patients with severe anemia or cardiac failure.

WARNINGS
This solution should be administered with great caution to patients with hypertension, cardiac disease, severe pulmonary infection, or severe chronic anemia. For the treatment of patients with hypoalbuminemia accompanied by peripheral edema, 25% Albumin solution should be used.

Although the volume administered and the speed of infusion should be adapted to the patient, 5% Albumin solution usually can be administered safely to older children and adults at the rate of 100 mL per hour. Patients should always be carefully monitored in order to guard against the possibility of circulatory overload.

DO NOT USE IF TURBID OR IF THERE IS SEDIMENT IN THE BOTTLE. DO NOT BEGIN ADMINISTRATION MORE THAN 4 HOURS AFTER THE CONTAINER HAS BEEN ENTERED. DISCARD PARTIALLY USED BOTTLES.

PRECAUTIONS
A) GENERAL
The rise in blood pressure following Albumin infusion necessitates careful observation of the injured or post-operative patient in order to detect and treat severed blood vessels that may not have bled at the lower blood pressure. The increase in blood volume which follows the administration of 5% Albumin may cause a significant fall in hemoglobin concentration and red blood cell transfusion may become appropriate.

If dehydration is present additional fluids must accompany or follow the administration of Albumin. Administration of large quantities of Albumin should be supplemented with or replaced by whole blood to combat the relative anemia which would follow such use. Albumin should be administered with caution to patients with low cardiac reserve or with no Albumin deficiency because a rapid increase in plasma volume may cause circulatory embarrassment or pulmonary edema. In cases of hypertension, a slower rate of administration—200 mL of Albumin solution may be mixed with 300 mL of 10% glucose solution and administered at a rate of 10 grams of Albumin (100 mL) per hour.

B) LABORATORY TESTS
Although laboratory testing is not necessary in order to monitor the treatment of shock or moderate hypoproteinemia, when Albumin is being administered for treatment of severe hypoproteinemia, periodic measurement of Serum Albumin levels is advisable.

C) PREGNANCY — CATEGORY C
Animal reproduction studies have not been conducted with Albumin. It is not known if Albumin can cause fetal harm when given to a pregnant woman, or can affect reproductive capacity. Albumin, should be given to a pregnant woman only if clearly needed.

D) PEDIATRIC USE
Safety of this product has been demonstrated in children. Use in children is not associated with special or specific hazards, if dose is appropriate for body weight.

ADVERSE REACTIONS
Untoward reactions to Albumin are extremely rare, although nausea, vomiting, fever, chills, increased salivation, skin rash, or urticaria may occasionally occur. Such symptoms usually disappear when the infusion is slowed or stopped for a short period of time.

DOSAGE AND ADMINISTRATION
Albumin 5% Solution, must be administered INTRAVENOUSLY. It may be given without dilution, or it may be given in conjunction with, or combined with other parenteral solutions, such as whole blood, plasma, saline, glucose, or sodium lactate.

HYPOVOLEMIC SHOCK
Although the volume of administered 5% Albumin and the rate of infusion must be individualized, the initial treatment of acute hypovolemia should be in the range of 500 to 750 mL of 5% Albumin (25-37.5 g) for adults or 12 to 20 mL of 5% Albumin per kilogram body weight (0.6-1.0 g/kg) for infants and children. The initial dose may be repeated after 15 to 30 minutes, if the response is not adequate.

HYPOPROTEINEMIA WITH OR WITHOUT EDEMA
Hypoalbuminemia is usually accompanied by a hidden extravascular Albumin deficiency of equal magnitude. This total body Albumin deficit must be considered when determining the amount of Albumin necessary to reverse the hypoproteinemia. When using the patient's serum Albumin concentration to estimate Albumin deficit, the body Albumin space should be calculated to be 80-100 mL per kilogram body weight.[4,5,7] Daily doses should not exceed 2 g of Albumin per kilogram body weight.

When the hypovolemia is long-standing and hypoalbuminemia exists in the presence of adequate hydration or edema, 25% Albumin is usually preferable to 5% protein.[4]

In the treatment of hypoproteinemia, 200 to 300 mL of 25% Albumin may be required to reduce edema and to bring serum protein values to normal. Since such patients usually have approximately normal blood volume, doses of more than 100 mL of 25% Albumin, should not be given faster than 100 mL in 30 to 45 minutes to avoid circulatory embarrassment. If slower rate of administration is desired, 200 mL of 25% Albumin may be mixed with 300 mL of 10% glucose solution and administered by continuous drip at a rate of 100 mL of this glucose solution an hour.

In severe burns, immediate therapy should include large volumes of crystalloid with lesser amounts of 5% Albumin solution to maintain an adequate plasma volume. After the first 24 hours, the ratio of Albumin to crystalloid may be increased to establish and maintain a plasma Albumin level of about 2.5 g/100mL or a total serum protein level of about 5.2 g/100mL. However, an optimal regimen for the use of colloids, electrolytes and water after severe burns has not been established.

Duration of treatment varies depending upon the extent of protein loss through renal excretion, denuded areas of skin and decreased Albumin synthesis. Attempts to raise the Albumin level above 4.0 g/100 mL may only result in an increased rate of catabolism.

PREPARATION FOR ADMINISTRATION
1. Remove cap from bottle to expose central portion of rubber stopper.
2. Clean stopper with germicidal solution.
3. Parenteral drug products should be inspected visually for particulate matter and discoloration prior to administration, whenever solution and container permit.

ADMINISTRATION
Follow directions for use printed on the administration set container. Make certain that the administration set contains an adequate filter.

Parenteral drug products should be inspected visually for particulate matter and discoloration prior to administration, whenever solution and container permit.

Store Albumin, 5% Solution, at room temperature between 15° and 30°C (59° and 86°F). Avoid freezing to prevent damage to the bottle. Do not use after expiration date.

REFERENCES
1. Cohn EJ, Strong LE, Hughes WL, et al: Preparation and properties of serum and plasma proteins. IV. A system for the separation into fractions of the protein and lipoprotein components of biological tissue and fluids. J Am Chem Soc 68;459-475, 1946. 2. Janeway CA: Human serum Albumin: Historical review, in Proceedings of the Workshop on Albumin. Sgouris JT and René A (eds), Bethesda, MD, DHEW Publication NIH 76-1975, pp 3-21 3. Gerety RJ, Aronson DL: Plasma derivatives and viral hepatitis. Transfusion 22:347-351, 1982 4. Finlayson JS: Albumin products. Sem Thromb Hemostasis 6:85-120, 1980 5. Peters T Jr: Serum Albumin, in The Plasma Proteins, 2nd Edition, Vol 1.Putnam FW (ed), New York, Academic Press, 1975, pp 133-181 6. Tullis JL: Albumin 1. Background and use. 2. Guidelines for clinical use. JAMA 237:355-360, 460-463, 1977. 7. O'Riordan JP, Aebischer M, Darnborough J, et al: The indications for the use of Albumin, plasma protein solutions and plasma substitutes. Strasbourg (67006), France. Council of Europe — Public Health Committee Report,1976 Programme. Coordinated Research in Blood Transfusion, 1978 8. Heyl JT, Gibson JG II, Janeway CA: Studies on the plasma proteins. V. The effect of concentrated solutions of human and bovine serum Albumin of blood volume after acute blood loss in man. J Clin Invest 22:763-773, 1943 9. Shoemaker WC, Hauser CJ: Critique of crystalloid versus colloid therapy in shock and shock lung. Crit Care Med 7:117-124, 1979 10. Lowenstein E: Blood conversation in open heart surgery. Cleve Clin Q 48:112-125, 1981.

J CODES
5%, 500 ml vial IV—J7080
25%, 50 ml vial IV—J7090

HOW SUPPLIED
INJECTION: 5%

BRAND/MANUFACTURER	NDC	SIZE	AWP
○ BRAND			
ALBUMINAR-5: Armour	00053-7670-06	50 ml	$36.00
	00053-7670-01	250 ml	$90.00
	00053-7670-02	500 ml	$180.00
	00053-7670-03	1000 ml	$360.00
○ GENERICS			
Miles Biol	00192-0685-20	50 ml	$28.13
Immuno-U.S.	54129-0218-05	50 ml	$32.00
BUMINATE: Baxter Biotech	00944-0491-01	250 ml	$56.00
ALBUMARC: Amer Red Cross	52769-0450-25	250 ml	$65.00
Miles Biol	00192-0685-25	250 ml	$66.56
ALBUTEIN: Alpha Therapeutic	49669-5211-01	250 ml	$75.00
Immuno-U.S.	54129-0218-25	250 ml	$75.00
BUMINATE: Baxter Biotech	00944-0491-02	500 ml	$112.00
ALBUMARC: Amer Red Cross	52769-0450-50	500 ml	$130.00
Miles Biol	00192-0685-27	500 ml	$133.13
ALBUTEIN: Alpha Therapeutic	49669-5211-02	500 ml	$150.00
Immuno-U.S.	54129-0218-50	500 ml	$150.00

INJECTION: 25%

BRAND/MANUFACTURER	NDC	SIZE	AWP
○ BRAND			
ALBUMINAR-25: Armour	00053-7680-01	20 ml	$36.00
	00053-7680-02	50 ml	$90.00
	00053-7680-03	100 ml	$180.00
○ GENERICS			
BUMINATE: Baxter Biotech	00944-0490-01	20 ml	$23.50
Miles Biol	00192-0684-16	20 ml	$24.38
ALBUTEIN: Alpha Therapeutic	49669-5213-01	20 ml	$30.00
Immuno-U.S.	54129-0228-02	20 ml	$32.00
BUMINATE: Baxter Biotech	00944-0490-02	50 ml	$56.00
Miles Biol	00192-0684-20	50 ml	$59.75

BRAND/MANUFACTURER	NDC	SIZE	AWP
ALBUMARC: Amer Red Cross	52769-0451-05	50 ml	$65.00
Amer Red Cross	52769-0251-05	50 ml	$65.00
ALBUTEIN: Alpha Therapeutic	49669-5213-02	50 ml	$75.00
Immuno-U.S.	54129-0228-05	50 ml	$75.00
Miles Allergy	00118-9996-12	100 ml	$6.79
BUMINATE: Baxter Biotech	00944-0490-03	100 ml	$112.00
Miles Biol	00192-0684-71	100 ml	$118.50
ALBUMARC: Amer Red Cross	52769-0451-10	100 ml	$130.00
Amer Red Cross	52769-0251-10	100 ml	$130.00
ALBUTEIN: Alpha Therapeutic	49669-5213-03	100 ml	$150.00
Immuno-U.S.	54129-0228-10	100 ml	$150.00

Albuminar SEE ALBUMIN, NORMAL SERUM, HUMAN

Albuterol

DESCRIPTION
The active component of Albuterol Inhalation Aerosol is Albuterol, USP, racemic (α^1-[tert-butylamino)methyl]-4-hydroxy-m-xylene- α, α'-diol) and a relatively selective beta$_2$-adrenergic bronchodilator.

Albuterol is the official generic name in the United States. The World Health Organization recommended name for the drug is salbutamol. The molecular weight of Albuterol is 239.3, and the empirical formula is $C_{13}H_{21}NO_3$.

The active component of Albuterol Inhalation Solution, Albuterol Inhalation Solution in Unit Dose, Albuterol Capsules for Inhalation, Albuterol Syrup, Albuterol Tablets and Albuterol Extended-Release Tablets is Albuterol Sulfate, the racemic form of Albuterol and a relatively selective beta$_2$-adrenergic bronchodilator with the chemical name α^1-[tert-butylamino)methyl]-4-hydroxy-m-xylene- α, α'-diol Sulfate (2:1) (salt).

Albuterol Sulfate has a molecular weight of 576.7, and the empirical formula is $(C_{13}H_{21}NO_3)_2 \cdot H_2SO_4$. Albuterol Sulfate is a white crystalline powder, soluble in water and slightly soluble in ethanol.

The World Health Organization recommended name for Albuterol base is salbutamol.

Each capsule for inhalation contains:	
Albuterol	200 mcg
Each actuation of inhalation aerosol contains:	
Albuterol	90 mcg
Each mL inhalation solution contains:	
Albuterol	5 mg
Each mL inhalation solution in unit dose contains:	
Albuterol	0.83 mg
Each 5 mL of syrup contains:	
Albuterol	2 mg
Each tablet contains:	
Albuterol	2 mg
or	
Albuterol	4 mg
Each extended-release tablet contains:	
Albuterol	4 mg
or	
Albuterol	8 mg

Following is its chemical structure:

$$HOCH_2 - \underset{OH}{\underset{|}{C}}H - CH_2NHC(CH_3)_3$$

CLINICAL PHARMACOLOGY
In vitro and in vivo pharmacologic studies have demonstrated that Albuterol has a preferential effect on beta$_2$-adrenergic receptors compared with isoproterenol. While it is recognized that beta$_2$-adrenergic receptors are the predominant receptors in bronchial smooth muscle, recent data indicate that there is a population of beta$_2$-receptors in the human heart existing in a concentration between 10% and 50%. The precise function of these, however, is not yet established (see "Warnings").

The pharmacologic effects of beta-adrenergic agonist drugs, including Albuterol, are at least in part attributable to stimulation through beta-adrenergic receptors of intracellular adenyl cyclase, the enzyme that catalyzes the conversion of adenosine triphosphate (ATP) to cyclic-3',5'-adenosine monophosphate (cyclic

AMP). Increased cyclic AMP levels are associated with relaxation of bronchial smooth muscle and inhibition of release of mediators of immediate hypersensivity from cells, especially from mast cells.

Albuterol has been shown in most controlled clinical trials to have more effect on the respiratory tract, in the form of bronchial smooth muscle relaxation, than isoproterenol at comparable doses while producing fewer cardiovascular effects. Controlled clinical studies and other clinical experience have shown that inhaled Albuterol, like other beta-adrenergic agonist drugs, can produce a significant cardiovascular effect in some patients, as measured by pulse rate, blood pressure, symptoms, and/or electrocardiographic changes. Albuterol is longer acting than isoproterenol in most patients by any route of administration because it is not a substrate for the cellular uptake processes for catecholamines nor for catechol-*O*-methyl transferase.

Because of its gradual absorption from the bronchi, systemic levels of Albuterol are low after inhalation of recommended doses. Studies undertaken with four subjects administered tritiated Albuterol from a metered-dose aerosol inhaler resulted in maximum plasma concentrations occurring within 2-4 hours. Due to the sensitivity of the assay method, the metabolic rate and half-life of elimination of Albuterol in plasma could not be determined. However, urinary excretion provided data indicating that Albuterol has an elimination half-life of 3.8 hours. Approximately 72% of the inhaled dose is excreted within 24 hours in the urine, and consists of 28% as unchanged drug and 44% as metabolite.

Studies in asthmatic patients have shown that less than 20% of a single Albuterol dose was absorbed following either IPPB (intermittent positive-pressure breathing) or nebulizer administration; the remaining amount was recovered from the nebulizer and apparatus and expired air. Most of the absorbed dose was recovered in the urine 24 hours after drug administration. Following a 3-mg dose of nebulized Albuterol, the maximum Albuterol plasma levels at 0.5 hours were 2.1 ng/mL (range, 1.4-3.2 ng/mL). There was a significant dose-related response in FEV_1 (forced expiratory volume in 1 second) and peak flow rate. It has been demonstrated that following oral administration of 4 mg of Albuterol, the elimination half-life was 5-6 hours.

Albuterol is rapidly absorbed after oral administration of 10 mL of Albuterol Sulfate Syrup (4 mg of Albuterol) and 4-mg Albuterol Sulfate Tablets in normal volunteers. Maximum plasma concentrations of about 18 ng/mL of Albuterol are achieved within 2 hours, and the drug is eliminated with a half-life of about 5 hours. In other studies, the analysis of urine samples of patients given 8 mg of tritiated Albuterol orally showed that 76% of the dose was excreted over 3 days, with the majority of the dose being excreted within the first 24 hours. Sixty percent of this radioactivity was shown to be the metabolite. Feces collected over this period contained 4% of the administered dose.

Animal studies show that Albuterol dose not pass the blood-brain barrier.

Recent studies in laboratory animals (minipigs, rodents, and dogs) recorded the occurrence of cardiac arrhythmias and sudden death (with histologic evidence of myocardial necrosis) when beta-agonists and methylxanthines were administered concurrently. The significance of these findings when applied to humans is currently unknown.

The effects of rising doses of Albuterol and isoproterenol aerosols were studied in volunteers and asthmatic patients. Results in normal volunteers indicated that Albuterol is one half to one quarter as active as isoproterenol in producing increases in heart rate. In asthmatic patients similar cardiovascular differentiation between the two drugs was also seen.

In controlled clinical trials with Albuterol Inhalation Aerosol involving adults with asthma, the onset of improvement in pulmonary function was within 15 minutes, as determined by both MMEF (maximum midexpiratory flow rate) and FEV_1. MMEF measurements also showed that near maximum improvement in pulmonary function generally occurs within 60-90 minutes following two inhalations of Albuterol and that clinically significant improvement generally continues for 3-4 hours in most patients. Some patients showed a therapeutic response (defined as maintaining FEV_1 values 15% or more above baseline) that was still apparent at 6 hours. Continued effectiveness of Albuterol was demonstrated over a 13-week period in these same trials. In controlled clinical trials involving children 4-12 years of age, FEV_1 measurements showed that maximum improvement in pulmonary function occurs within 30-60 minutes. The onset of clinically significant (≥15%) improvement in FEV_1 was observed as soon as 5 minutes following 180 mcg of Albuterol in 18 of 30 (60%) children in a controlled dose-ranging study. Clinically significant improvement in FEV_1 continued in the majority of patients for 2 hours and in 33%-47% for 4 hours among 56 patients receiving inhalation aerosol in one pediatric study. In a second study among 48 patients receiving inhalation aerosol, clinically significant improvement continued in the majority for up to 1 hour and in 23%-40% for 4 hours. In addition, at least 50% of the patients in both studies achieved an improvement in $FEF_{25\%-75\%}$ (forced expiratory flow rate between 25% and 75% of the forced vital capacity) of at least 20% for 2-5 hours. Continued effectiveness of Albuterol was demonstrated over the 12-week study period.

In other clinical studies, two inhalations of Albuterol taken approximately 15 minutes before exercise prevented exercise-induced bronchospasm, as demonstrated by the maintenance of FEV_1 within 80% of baseline values in the majority of patients. One of these studies also evaluated the duration of the prophylactic effect to repeated exercise challenges, which was evident at 4 hours in the majority of patients and at 6 hours in approximately one third of the patients.

In controlled clinical trials with Albuterol Sulfate Inhalation Solution, most patients exhibited an onset of improvement in pulmonary function within 5 minutes as determined by FEV_1. FEV_1 measurements also showed that the maximum average improvement in pulmonary function usually occurred at approximately 1 hour following inhalation of 2.5 mg of Albuterol by compressor-nebulizer and remained close to peak for 2 hours. Clinically significant improvement in pulmonary function (defined as maintenance of a 15% or more increase in FEV_1 over baseline values) continued for 3-4 hours in most patients, with some patients continuing up to 6 hours. In repetitive dose studies, continued effectiveness was demonstrated throughout the 3-month period of treatment in some patients.

In single, dose-range, crossover trials with Albuterol Sulfate Capsules for Inhalation in patients 12 years of age and older, the onset of improvement in pulmonary function was within 5 minutes, as determined by a 15% increase in FEV_1 following administration of either a 200-or 400-mcg dose. Maximum increases in FEV_1 occurred within 60 minutes following inhalation of either dose. The duration of effect (defined as an increase in FEV_1 of 15% or greater in a single-dose study) was 1-2 hours after the 200-mcg dose and 3-4 hours after the 400-mcg dose. In a single-dose study, an increase in $FEF_{25\%-75\%}$ of 20% or greater continued for 3-4 hours after the 200-mcg dose and for 3-6 hours following the 400-mcg dose. A therapeutic response continued for 4 hours in the majority of patients and for 6 hours in 38% of the patients following the 400-mcg dose. Twenty-two percent of the patients receiving the 200-mcg dose had a duration of effect of 8 hours.

In 12-week, double-blind, comparative evaluations in patients 12 years of age and older of one 200-mcg Albuterol Sulfate Capsule for Inhalation versus two inhalations of Albuterol Inhalation Aerosol, the two dosage regimens were found to be equivalent. Based on a 15% or more increase in FEV_1 determinations, both provided a therapeutic response that persisted for 2 or 3 hours in 50% of 231 patients aged 12 years and older. Similar results were found in two controlled, 12-week clinical trials involving 204 children aged 4-11 years. Both formulations produced a therapeutic response (defined as maintenance of mean increase over baseline of at least 15% in FEV_1 or 20% in $FEF_{25\%-75\%}$). Therapeutic improvement of $FEF_{25\%-75\%}$ persisted for 3-5 hours in over 50% of the children throughout the study. Continued effectiveness and safety of Albuterol Sulfate Capsules for Inhalation were demonstrated over the 12-week study periods in both adults and children.

In controlled clinical trials with Albuterol Sulfate Syrup and Albuterol Sulfate Tablets in patients with asthma, the onset of improvement in pulmonary function, as measured by MMEF and FEV_1 and by MMEF, respectively, was within 30 minutes, with peak improvement occurring between 2 and 3 hours.

In a controlled clinical trial with Albuterol Sulfate Syrup involving 55 children, clinically significant improvement (defined as maintenance of mean values over baseline of 15%-20% or more in the FEV_1 and MMEF, respectively) continued to be recorded up to 6 hours. No decrease in the effectiveness was reported in one uncontrolled study of 32 children who took Albuterol Sulfate Syrup for a 3-month period.

In controlled clinical trials with Albuterol Sulfate Tablets in which measurements were conducted for 6 hours, clinically significant improvement (defined as maintaining a 15% or more increase in FEV_1 and a 20% or more increase in MMEF over baseline values) was observed in 60% of patients at 4 hours and in 40% at 6 hours. In other single-dose, controlled clinical trials, clinically significant improvement was observed in at least 40% of the patients at 8 hours. No decrease in the effectiveness of Albuterol Sulfate Tablets has been reported in patients who received long-term treatment with the drug in uncontrolled studies for periods up to 6 months.

In a single-dose study comparing one 8-mg Albuterol Sulfate Extended-Release Tablet with two 4-mg immediate-release Albuterol Sulfate Tablets in 17 normal volunteers, the extent of availability of Albuterol Sulfate Extended-Release Tablets was shown to be about 80% of Albuterol Sulfate Tablets with or without food. In addition, lower mean peak plasma concentration and longer time to reach the peak level were observed with Albuterol Sulfate Extended-Release Tablets as compared with Albuterol Sulfate Tablets. (However, bioequivalence between Albuterol Sulfate Tablets [4 mg q6h] and Albuterol Sulfate Extended-Release Tablets [8 mg b.i.d.] was shown in a multiple-dose, steady-state study in fed condition.) The single-dose study results also showed that food decreases the rate of absorption of Albuterol from Albuterol Sulfate Extended-Release Tablets without altering the extent of bioavailability. In addition, the study indicated that food causes a more gradual increase in the fraction of the available dose absorbed from the extended-release formulation as compared with the fasting condition.

In another single-dose study, 8- and 4-mg Albuterol Sulfate Extended-Release Tablets were shown to be bioequivalent in the fasting state. Definitive studies for the effect of food on 4-mg Albuterol Sulfate Extended-Release Tablets have not been conducted. However, since food lowers the rate of absorption of 8-mg Albuterol Sulfate Extended-Release Tablets, it is expected that food reduces the rate of absorption of 4-mg Albuterol Sulfate Extended-Release Tablets also.

Albuterol Sulfate Extended-Release Tablets have been formulated to provide duration of action of up to 12 hours. In an 8-day, multiple-dose, crossover study, 15 normal male volunteers were given 8-mg Albuterol Sulfate Extended-Release Tablets every 12 hours or 4-mg Albuterol Sulfate Tablets every 6 hours. Each dose of Albuterol Sulfate Extended-Release Tablets and the corresponding doses of Albuterol Sulfate Tablets were administered in the postprandial state. Steady-state plasma concentrations were reached within 2 days for both formulations. Fluctuations (C_{max}-C_{min}/$C_{average}$) in plasma concentrations were similar for Albuterol Sulfate Extended-Release Tablets administered at 12-hour intervals and Albuterol Sulfate Tablets administered every 6 hours. In addition, the relative bioavailability of Albuterol Sulfate Extended-Release Tablets was approximately 100% of the immediate-release tablet at steady state.

A summary of these results is shown in the following table:

MEAN VALUES AT STEADY STATE

	C_{max} (ng/mL)	C_{min} (ng/mL)	T_{max} (h)	$T_{1/2}$ (h)	AUC (ng-h/mL)
Albuterol Sulfate Extended-Release Tablets	14.3	8.1	6.0	9.3	134
Albuterol Sulfate Tablets	14.5	8.1	2.6	7.2	132

The mean plasma Albuterol concentration versus time data at steady state after the administration of Albuterol Sulfate Extended-Release Tablets 8 mg q12h are displayed in the following graph.

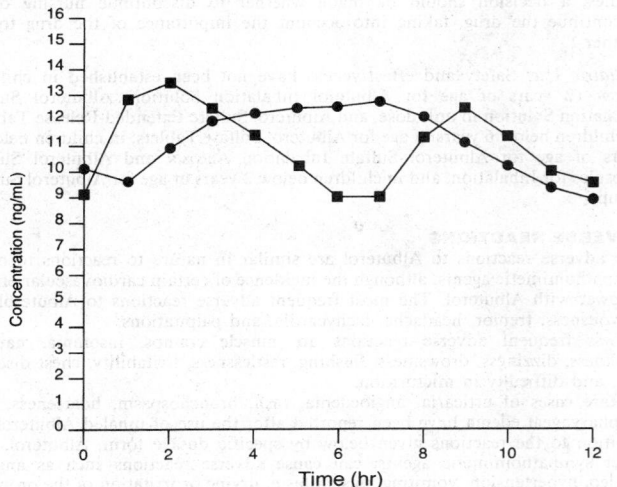

- Albuterol Sulfate Tablets 4 mg q6h
- Albuterol Sulfate Extended-Release Tablets 8 mg q12h

INDICATIONS AND USAGE
Albuterol Sulfate Inhalation Aerosol is indicated for the prevention and relief of bronchospasm in patients 4 years of age and older with reversible obstructive airway disease and for the prevention of exercise-induced bronchospasm in patients 12 years of age and older. Albuterol Inhalation Aerosol can be used with or without concomitant steroid therapy.

Albuterol Sulfate Inhalation Solution is indicated for the relief of bronchospasm in patients with reversible obstructive airway disease and acute attacks of bronchospasm.

Albuterol Sulfate in Unit Dose Inhalation Solution is indicated for the relief of bronchospasm in patients with reversible obstructive airway disease and acute attacks of bronchospasm.

Albuterol Sulfate Capsules for Inhalation are indicated for the prevention and relief of bronchospasm in patients 4 years of age and older with reversible obstructive airway disease and for the prevention of exercise-induced bronchospasm in patients 12 years of age and older. This formulation is particularly useful in patients who are unable to properly use the pressurized aerosol form of Albuterol or who prefer an alternative formulation. Albuterol Sulfate Capsules for Inhalation can be used with or without concomitant steroid therapy.

Albuterol Sulfate Syrup is indicated for the relief of bronchospasm in adults and children 2 years of age and older with reversible obstructive airway disease.

Albuterol Sulfate Tablets and **Extended-Release Tablets** are indicated for the relief of bronchospasm in patients with reversible obstructive airway disease.

UNLABELED USES
Albuterol is used alone or as an adjunct in the treatment of premature labor.

CONTRAINDICATIONS
The Albuterol/Albuterol Sulfate preparations are contraindicated in patients with a history of hypersensitivity to any of the components.

WARNINGS
As with other inhaled beta-adrenergic agonists, Albuterol Inhalation Aerosol, Albuterol Sulfate Inhalation Solution, Albuterol Sulfate Inhalation Solution in unit dose, and Albuterol Sulfate for Inhalation can produce paradoxical bronchospasm that can be life-threatening. If it occurs, the preparation should be discontinued immediately and alternative therapy instituted.

Fatalities have been reported in association with excessive use of inhaled sympathomimetic drugs and with the home use of nebulizers. The exact cause of death is unknown, but cardiac arrest following the unexpected development of a severe acute asthmatic crisis and subsequent hypoxia is suspected. It is therefore essential that the physician instruct the patient in the need for further evaluation if his/her asthma becomes worse. In individual patients, any beta2-adrenergic agonist, including Albuterol Sulfate Inhalation Solution, may have a clinically significant cardiac effect.

Immediate hypersensitivity reactions may occur after administration of Albuterol, as demonstrated by rare cases of urticaria, angioedema, rash, bronchospasm, anaphylaxis, and oropharyngeal edema. Albuterol, like other beta-adrenergic agonists, can produce a significant cardiovascular effect in some patients, as measured by pulse rate, blood pressure, symptoms, and/or electrocardiographic changes.

As with other beta-agonists, cardiac arrhythmias and sudden death have been reported in patients receiving Albuterol Sulfate Extended-Release Tablets. Whether these adverse events are directly related to Albuterol Sulfate Extended-Release Tablet administration is unclear.

The contents of Albuterol Inhalation Aerosol are under pressure. Do not puncture. Do not use or store near heat or open flame. Exposure to temperatures above 120 °F may cause bursting. Never throw container into fire or incinerator. Keep out of reach of children.

PRECAUTIONS
General: Although no effect on the cardiovascular system is usually seen after the administration of inhaled Albuterol at recommended doses, cardiovascular and central nervous system effects seen with all sympathomimetic drugs can occur after use of inhaled Albuterol and may require discontinuation of the drug. As with all sympathomimetic amines, Albuterol should be used with caution in patients with cardiovascular disorders, especially coronary insufficiency, cardiac arrhythmias, and hypertension; in patients with convulsive disorders, hyperthyroidism, or diabetes mellitus; and in patients who are unusually responsive to sympathomimetic amines. Clinically significant changes in systolic and diastolic blood pressure have been seen in individual patients and could be expected to occur in some patients after use of any beta-adrenergic bronchodilator.

In controlled clinical trials, increases in SGPT were more frequent among patients treated with Albuterol Sulfate Extended-Release Tablets (12 of 247 patients, 4.9%) than among the theophylline (6 to 188 patients, 3.2%) and placebo (1 of 138 patients, 0.7%) groups. Increases in serum glucose concentration were also more frequent among patients treated with Albuterol Sulfate Extended-Release Tablets (23 of 234 patients, 9.8%) than among the theophylline (11 of 173 patients 6.45%) and placebo (3 of 129 patients, 2.3%) groups. Increases in SGOT were also more frequent among patients treated with Albuterol Sulfate Extended-Release Tablets (10 of 248 patients, 4%) and theophylline (5 of 193, 2.6%) than among patients treated with placebo. Decreases in white blood cell counts were more frequent in patients treated with Albuterol Sulfate Extended-Release Tablets (10 of 247 patients, 4%) compared with patients receiving theophylline (2 of 185 patients, 1.1%) and patients receiving placebo (1 of 141 patients, 0.7%). Decreases in hemoglobin and hematocrit were more frequent in patients receiving Albuterol Sulfate Extended-Release Tablets (16 of 228 patients, 7.0%, and 17 of 230 patients, 7.4%, respectively) than in patients receiving theophylline (5 of 171 patients, 2.9%, and 9 of 173 patients, 5.2%, respectively) and patients receiving placebo (5 of 129 patients, 3.9%, and 3 of 132 patients, 2.3%, respectively). The clinical significance of these results is unknown.

Large doses of intravenous Albuterol have been reported to aggravate preexisting diabetes mellitus and ketoacidosis. As with other beta-agonists, inhaled and intravenous Albuterol may produce significant hypokalemia in some patients, possibly through intracellular shunting, which has the potential to produce adverse cardiovascular effects. The decrease is usually transient, not requiring supplementation.

Although there have been no reports concerning the use of Albuterol Inhalation Aerosol or Albuterol Sulfate Capsules for Inhalation during labor and delivery, it has been reported that high doses of Albuterol administered intravenously inhibit uterine contractions. Although this effect is extremely unlikely as a consequence of Albuterol Inhalation Aerosol or Albuterol Sulfate Capsules for Inhalation use, it should be kept in mind.

Information for Patients: The action of Albuterol Inhalation Aerosol, Albuterol Sulfate Inhalation Solution, Albuterol Sulfate Inhalation Solution in Unit Dose, and Albuterol Sulfate Syrup may last up to 6 hours; the action of Albuterol Sulfate Capsules for Inhalation may last for 6 hours or longer; and the action of Albuterol Sulfate Tablets may last for 8 hours or longer. Therefore, they should not be used more frequently than recommended. Do not increase the dose or frequency of medication without medical consultation. If the recommended dosage does not provide relief of symptoms or symptoms become worse, seek immediate medical attention.

While using Albuterol Inhalation Aerosol or Albuterol Sulfate Capsules for Inhalation, other inhaled drugs should not be used unless prescribed. While taking Albuterol Inhalation Solution or Albuterol Sulfate Inhalation Solution in Unit Dose, other antiasthma medicines should not be used unless prescribed. In general, the technique for administering Albuterol Inhalation Aerosol to children is similar to that for adults, since children's smaller ventilatory exchange capacity automatically provides proportionally smaller aerosol intake. Children should use Albuterol Inhalation Aerosol and Albuterol Sulfate Capsules for Inhalation under adult supervision, as instructed by the patient's physician.

See package inserts for Albuterol Inhalation Aerosol, Albuterol Sulfate Inhalation Solution, Albuterol Sulfate Inhalation Solution in Unit Dose, and Albuterol Sulfate Capsules for Inhalation for illustrated *"Patient's Instructions for Use."*

As with any other nondeformable material, caution should be used when administering Albuterol Sulfate Extended-Release Tablets to patients with preexisting gastrointestinal narrowing from any cause. There have been rare reports of gastrointestinal obstruction in such patients occurring in association with ingestion of products containing delivery systems similar to that contained in Albuterol Sulfate Extended-Release Tablets.

Each Albuterol Sulfate Extended-Release Tablet contains a small hole that is part of the unique extended-release system. Albuterol Sulfate Extended-Release Tablets must be swallowed whole with the aid of liquids. DO NOT CHEW OR CRUSH THESE TABLETS.
The outer coating of the tablet is not absorbed and is excreted in the feces; in some instances the empty outer coating may be noticeable in the stool.

Drug Interactions: Other sympathomimetic aerosol bronchodilators or epinephrine should not be used concomitantly with Albuterol. If additional adrenergic drugs are to be administered by any route to patients using Albuterol Inhalation Aerosol or Albuterol Sulfate Capsules for Inhalation, they should be used with caution to avoid deleterious cardiovascular effects.

In addition, the concomitant use of Albuterol Sulfate Syrup, Albuterol Sulfate Tablets, or Extended-Release Tablets and other oral sympathomimetic agents is not recommended since such combined use may lead to deleterious cardiovascular effects. This recommendation does not preclude the judicious use of an aerosol bronchodilator of the adrenergic stimulant type in patients receiving Albuterol Sulfate Syrup or Albuterol Sulfate Tablets or Extended-Release Tablets. Such concomitant use, however, should be individualized and not given on a routine basis. If regular coadministration is required, then alternative therapy should be considered.

Albuterol should be administered with extreme caution to patients being treated with monoamine oxidase inhibitors or tricyclic antidepressants because the action of Albuterol on the vascular system may be potentiated.

Beta-receptor blocking agents and Albuterol inhibit the effect of each other.

Carcinogenesis, Mutagenesis, Impairment of Fertility: Albuterol Sulfate, like other agents in its class, caused a significant dose-related increase in the incidence of benign leiomyomas of the mesovarium in a 2-year study in the rat at doses corresponding to 93, 463, and 2,315 times, the maximum inhalational dose for a 50-kg human; to 10, 50, and 250 times the maximum nebulization dose for a 50-kg human; to 42, 208, and 1,042 times the maximum inhalational dose for a 50-kg human (Albuterol Sulfate Capsules for Inhalation); to 2, 9, and 46 times the maximum human (child weighing 21 kg) oral dose (syrup); and to 3, 16, and 78 times the maximum oral dose for a 50-kg human (tablets). In another study this effect was blocked by the coadministration of propranolol. The relevance of these findings to humans is not known. An 18-month oral study in mice, at doses corresponding to 10,417 times the human inhalational dose, and a lifetime oral study in hamsters, at doses corresponding to 1,042 times the human inhalational dose, revealed no evidence of tumorigenicity. Studies with Albuterol revealed no evidence of mutagenesis. Oral reproduction studies in rats, at doses corresponding to 1,042 times the human inhalational dose, revealed no evidence of impaired fertility.

Albuterol Sulfate Extended-Release Tablets: Safety margins are adjusted to take account of differences in surface area to body weight ratio between test species and man. Albuterol Sulfate, like other agents in its class, caused a significant dose-related increased incidence of mesovarian leiomyomas in a 24-month dietary study in Sprague-Dawley rats. Doses of 2, 10, and 50 mg/kg, corresponding to 1, 4, and 18 times the maximum oral dose for a 50-kg human, were associated with incidences of mesovarian leiomyomas of 2.4%, 18.6%, and 27.0%, respectively. In a second 24-month dietary study in the same strain, no leiomyomas occurred at 2 mg/kg, and those induced at 20 mg/kg were blocked by coadministration of 33 mg/kg of propranolol. The relevance of these findings to man is not known. There was no evidence of tumorigenicity after dietary administration to CD-1 mice for 18 months or to hamsters for 23 months at doses of 500 and 50 mg/kg, 89 and 14 times the maximum oral dose for a 50-kg human, respectively. *In vitro* studies with Albuterol revealed no evidence of mutagenicity at concentrations between 0.5 and 8 mg/plate. A reproduction study in Wistar rats revealed no evidence of impaired fertility in either of two successive generations treated orally with doses up to 50 mg/kg (15 times the maximum oral dose for a 50-kg human) throughout the periods of gametogenesis, mating, pregnancy, and lactation.

Pregnancy: Teratogenic Effects: Pregnancy Category C: Albuterol has been shown to be teratogenic in mice when given subcutaneously in doses corresponding to 14 times the human aerosol dose; to 1.25 times the human nebulization dose (based on a 50-kg human); to five times the human inhalational dose (Albuterol Sulfate Capsules for Inhalation); to 0.2 times the maximum human (child weighing 21 kg) oral dose (syrup); to 0.4 times the maximum human oral dose (tablets). There are no adequate and well-controlled studies in pregnant women. Albuterol should be used during pregnancy only if the potential benefit justifies the potential risk to the fetus.

A reproduction study in CD-1 mice given Albuterol subcutaneously (0.025, 0.25, and 2.5 mg/kg, corresponding to 1.15, 11.5, and 115 times, respectively, the maximum inhalational dose for a 50-kg human; to 0.125, 1.25, and 12.5 times, respectively, the maximum human nebulization dose for a 50-kg human; to 0.52, 5.2, and 52 times, respectively, the maximum inhalational dose for a 50-kg human (Albuterol Sulfate Capsules for Inhalation); and to 0.04, 0.4, and 3.9 times, respectively, the maximum oral dose for a 50-kg human (tablets) showed cleft palate formation in 5 of 111 (4.5%) fetuses at 0.25 mg/kg and in 10 of 108 (9.3%) fetuses at 2.5 mg/kg. None was observed at 0.025 mg/kg. Cleft palate also occurred in 22 of 72 (30.5%) fetuses treated with 2.5 mg/kg of isoproterenol (positive control). A reproduction study with oral Albuterol in Stride Dutch rabbits revealed cranioschisis in 7 of 19 (37%) fetuses at 50 mg/kg, corresponding to 2,315 times the maximum inhalational dose for a 50-kg human; to 250 times the

maximum human nebulization dose; to 1,042 times the maximum inhalational dose for a 50-kg human (Albuterol Sulfate Capsules for Inhalation); to 46 times the maximum human (child weighing 21 kg) oral dose (Syrup) of Albuterol Sulfate; to 78 times the maximum oral dose for a 50-kg human (Tablets); and to 31 times the maximum oral dose for a 50-kg human (Extended-Release Tablets).

Labor and Delivery: Oral Albuterol has been shown to delay preterm labor in some reports. There are presently no well-controlled studies that demonstrate that it will stop preterm labor or prevent labor at term. Therefore, cautious use of Albuterol Inhalation Solution, Albuterol Sulfate Inhalation Solution in unit dose, Albuterol Sulfate Capsules for Inhalation, Albuterol Sulfate Syrup, and Albuterol Sulfate Tablets or Extended-Release Tablets is required in pregnant patients when given for relief of bronchospasm so as to avoid interference with uterine contractility. Use in such patients should be restricted to those patients in whom the benefits clearly outweigh the risks.

Nursing Mothers: It is not known whether Albuterol is excreted in human milk. Because of the potential for tumorigenicity shown for Albuterol in some animal studies, a decision should be made whether to discontinue nursing or to discontinue the drug, taking into account the importance of the drug to the mother.

Pediatric Use: Safety and effectiveness have not been established in children below 12 years of age for Albuterol Inhalation Solution, Albuterol Sulfate Inhalation Solution in unit dose, and Albuterol Sulfate Extended-Release Tablets; in children below 6 years of age for Albuterol Sulfate Tablets; in children below 4 years of age for Albuterol Sulfate Inhalation Aerosol and Albuterol Sulfate Capsules for Inhalation; and in children below 2 years of age for Albuterol Sulfate Syrup.

ADVERSE REACTIONS
The adverse reactions to Albuterol are similar in nature to reactions to other sympathomimetic agents, although the incidence of certain cardiovascular effects is lower with Albuterol. The most frequent adverse reactions to Albuterol are nervousness, tremor, headache, tachycardia, and palpitations.

Less frequent adverse reactions are muscle cramps, insomnia, nausea, weakness, dizziness, drowsiness, flushing, restlessness, irritability, chest discomfort, and difficulty in micturition.

Rare cases of urticaria, angioedema, rash, bronchospasm, hoarseness, and oropharyngeal edema have been reported after the use of inhaled Albuterol. In addition to the reactions given below by specific dosage form, Albuterol, like other sympathomimetic agents, can cause adverse reactions such as angina, vertigo, hypertension, vomiting, unusal taste, drying or irritation of the oropharynx, and CNS stimulation.

Albuterol Inhalation Aerosol: A 13-week, double-blind study compared Albuterol and isoproterenol aerosols in 147 asthmatic patients aged 12 years and older. The results of this study showed that the incidence of cardiovascular effects was: palpitations, fewer than 10 per 100 with Albuterol and fewer than 15 per 100 with isoproterenol; tachycardia, 10 per 100 with both Albuterol and isoproterenol; and increased blood pressure, fewer than 5 per 100 with both Albuterol and isoproterenol. In the same study, both drugs caused tremor or nausea in fewer than 15 patients per 100, and dizziness or heartburn in fewer than 5 per 100 patients. Nervousness occurred in fewer than 10 per 100 patients receiving Albuterol and in fewer than 15 per 100 patients receiving isoproterenol.

Twelve-week, double-blind studies involving the use of Albuterol Inhalation Aerosol 180 mcg q.i.d. by 104 asthmatic children aged 4-11 years showed the following side effects:

Central Nervous System: Headache, 3 of 104 patients (3%); nervousness, lightheadedness, agitation, nightmares, hyperactivity, and aggressive behavior, each in 1%.

Gastrointestinal: Nausea and/or vomiting, 6 of 104 (6%); stomachache, 3 of 104 (3%); diarrhea in 1%.

Oropharyngeal: Throat irritation, 6 of 104 (6%); discoloration of teeth in 1%.

Respiratory: Epistaxis, 3 of 104 (3%); coughing, 2 of 104 (2%).

Musculoskeletal: Tremor and muscle cramp, each in 1%.

Albuterol Sulfate Inhalation Solution: The results of clinical trials in 135 patients showed the following side effects that were considered probably or possibly drug related:

Central Nervous System: Tremors (20%), dizziness (7%), nervousness (4%), headache (3%), insomnia (1%).

Gastrointestinal: Nausea (4%), dyspepsia (1%).

Ear, Nose, and Throat: Pharyngitis (< 1%), nasal congestion (1%).

Cardiovascular: Tachycardia (1%), hypertension (1%).

Respiratory: Bronchospasm (8%), cough (4%), bronchitis (4%), wheezing (1%).

No clinically relevant laboratory abnormalities related to Albuterol Inhalation Solution administration were determined in these studies.

In comparing the adverse reactions reported for patients treated with Albuterol Inhalation Solution with those of patients treated with isoproterenol during clinical trials of 3 months, the following moderate to severe reactions, as judged by the investigators, were reported. This table does not include mild reactions.

◆ RATED THERAPEUTICALLY EQUIVALENT; ◇ THERAPEUTIC EQUIVALENCE UNCONFIRMED; ○ UNRATED

PERCENT INCIDENCE OF MODERATE TO SEVERE ADVERSE REACTIONS

Reaction	Albuterol n = 65	Isoproterenol n = 65
Central nervous system		
Tremor	10.7%	13.8%
Headache	3.1%	1.5%
Insomnia	3.1%	1.5%
Cardiovascular		
Hypertension	3.1%	3.1%
Arrhythmias	0%	3.0%
Palpitation*	0%	22.0%
Respiratory		
Bronchospasm†	15.4%	18.0%
Cough	3.1%	5.0%
Bronchitis	1.5%	5.0%
Wheezing	1.5%	1.5%
Sputum increase	1.5%	1.5%
Dyspnea	1.5%	1.5%
Gastrointestinal		
Nausea	3.1%	0%
Dyspepsia	1.5%	0%
Systemic		
Malaise	1.5%	0%

* *The finding of no arrhythmias and no palpitations after Albuterol administration in this clinical study should not be interpreted as indicating that these adverse effects cannot occur after the administration of inhaled Albuterol.*

† *In the most cases of bronchospasm, this term was generally used to describe exacerbations in the underlying pulmonary disease.*

Albuterol Sulfate Capsules for Inhalation: Results of clinical trials with Albuterol Sulfate Capsules for Inhalation 200 mcg in 172 patients aged 12 years and older (adults) and 129 patients aged 4-12 years (children) showed the following side effects:

Central Nervous System: Adults: Headache, 4 of 172 patients (2%); nervousness, 2 of 172 (1%); dizziness, insomnia, lightheadedness, each in <1%. *Children*: Headache, 6 of 129 (5%), dizziness and hyperactivity, each in <1%.

Gastrointestinal: Adults: Burning in stomach in <1%. *Children:* Nausea and/or vomiting in 5 of 129 (4%), stomachache in 2 of 129 (2%), diarrhea in <1%.

Oropharyngeal: Adults: Throat irritation in 3 of 172 (2%); dry mouth and voice changes, each in <1%. *Children*: Throat irritation in 3 of 129 (2%), unusual taste in 2 of 129 (2%).

Respiratory: Adults: Cough in 8 of 172 (5%), bronchospasm in 2 of 172 (1%). *Children*: Cough and nasal congestion, each in 3 of 129 (2%); hoarseness and epistaxis, each in 2 of 129 (2%).

Musculoskeletal: Adults: Tremor in 2 of 172 (1%). *Children*: None reported.

Albuterol Sulfate Syrup: The most frequent adverse reactions to Albuterol Sulfate Syrup in adults and older children were tremor, 10 of 100 patients, and nervousness and shakiness, each in 9 of 100 patients. Other reported adverse reactions were headache, 4 of 100 patients; dizziness and increased appetite, each in 3 of 100 patients; hyperactivity and excitement, each in 2 of 100 patients; and tachycardia, epistaxis, and sleeplessness, each in 1 of 100 patients. The following adverse effects each occurred in fewer than 1 of 100 patients: muscle spasm, disturbed sleep, epigastric pain, cough, palpitations, stomachache, irritable behavior, dilated pupils, sweating, chest pain, and weakness.

In young children 2-6 years of age, some adverse reactions were noted more frequently than in adults and older children. Excitement was noted in approximately 20% of patients and nervousness in 15%. Hyperkinesia occurred in 4% of patients, with insomnia, tachycardia, and gastrointestinal symptoms in 2% each. Anorexia, emotional lability, pallor, fatigue, and conjunctivitis were seen in 1%.

Albuterol Sulfate Tablets: The most frequent adverse reactions to Albuterol Sulfate Tablets were nervousness and tremor, with each occurring in approximately 20 of 100 patients. Other reported reactions were headache, 7 of 100 patients; tachycardia and palpitations, 5 of 100 patients; muscle cramps, 3 of 100 patients; and insomnia, nausea, weakness, and dizziness, each in 2 of 100 patients. Drowsiness, flushing, restlessness, irritability, chest discomfort, and difficulty in micturition each occurred in fewer than 1 of 100 patients.

The reactions to Albuterol Sulfate Syrup and Albuterol Sulfate Tablets are generally transient in nature, and it is usually not necessary to discontinue treatment. In selected cases, however, dosage may be reduced temporarily; after the reaction has subsided, dosage should be increased in small increments to the optimal dosage.

Event	Albuterol Sulfate Extended-Release Tablets (n = 330)	Theophylline (n = 197)	Other β-Agonists (n = 20)	Placebo (n = 178)
Nervousness	8.5%	5.1%	10.0%	2.8%
Tremor	24.2%	6.1%	35.0%	1.1%

Event	Albuterol Sulfate Extended-Release Tablets (n = 330)	Theophylline (n = 197)	Other β-Agonists (n = 20)	Placebo (n = 178)
Headache	18.8%	26.9%	35.0%	20.8%
Tachycardia	2.7%	0.5%	5.0%	0%
Palpitations	2.4%	0.5%	0%	1.1%
Muscle cramps	2.7%	0.5%	0%	0.6%
Insomnia	2.4%	6.1%	0%	1.7%
Nausea/vomiting	4.2%	19.8%	5.0%	3.9%
Dizziness	1.5%	2.0%	0%	5.1%
Somnolence	0.3%	1.0%	0%	0.6%

A trend was observed among patients treated with Albuterol Sulfate Extended-Release Tablets toward increasing frequency of muscle cramps with increasing patient age (12-20 years, 1.2%; 21-30 years, 2.6%; 31-40 years, 6.9%; 41-50 years, 6.9%), compared with no such events in the placebo group. Also observed was an increasing frequency of tremor with increasing patient age (12-20 years, 29.4%; 21-30 years, 29.9%; 31-40 years, 27.6%; 41-50 years, 37.9%), compared to 2.9% or less in the placebo group.

The reactions are generally transient in nature, and it is usually not necessary to discontinue treatment with Albuterol Sulfate Extended-Release Tablets.

OVERDOSAGE

The expected symptoms with overdosage are those of excessive beta-stimulation and/or occurrence or exaggeration of any of the symptoms listed under "*Adverse Reactions*", e.g., seizures, angina, hypertension or hypotension, tachycardia with rates up to 200 beats per minute, arrhythmias, nervousness, headache, tremor, dry mouth, palpitation, nausea, dizziness, fatigue, malaise, and insomnia. Hypokalemia may also occur.

Treatment consists of discontinuation of Albuterol together with appropriate symptomatic therapy.

As with all sympathomimetic aerosol medications, cardiac arrest and even death may be associated with abuse of aerosol Albuterol.

The oral LD_{50} in male and female rats and mice was greater than 2,000 mg/kg. The inhalational LD_{50} could not be determined.

Intravenous administration to male and female mice and rats caused significant lethality at 60-70 mg/kg.

Dialysis is not appropriate treatment for overdosage of Albuterol Inhalation Aerosol, Albuterol Sulfate Capsules for Inhalation, or Albuterol Sulfate Syrup. The judicious use of a cardioselective beta-receptor blocker, such as metoprolol tartrate, is suggested, bearing in mind the danger of inducing an asthmatic attack. There is insufficient evidence to determine if dialysis is beneficial for overdosage of Albuterol Sulfate Inhalation Solution, Albuterol Sulfate Inhalation Solution in unit dose, Albuterol Sulfate Tablets, or Albuterol Sulfate Extended Release Tablets.

DOSAGE AND ADMINISTRATION

Albuterol Inhalation Aerosol: For treatment of acute episodes of bronchospasm or prevention of asthmatic symptoms, the usual dosage for adults and children 4 years and older is two inhalations repeated every 4-6 hours; in some patients, one inhalation every 4 hours may be sufficient. More frequent administration or a larger number of inhalations are not recommended.

The use of Albuterol Inhalation Aerosol can be continued as medically indicated to control recurring bouts of bronchospasm. During this time most patients gain optimal benefit from regular use of the inhaler. Safe usage for periods extending over several years has been documented.

If a previously effective dosage regimen fails to provide the usual relief, medical advice should be sought immediately as this is often a sign of seriously worsening asthma that would require reassessment of therapy.

Exercise-induced Bronchospasm Prevention: The usual dosage for adults and children 12 years and older is two inhalations 15 minutes before exercise. For treatment, see above.

Albuterol Sulfate Inhalation Solution: The usual dosage for adults and children 12 years of age and older is 2.5 mg of Albuterol administered three to four times daily by nebulization. More frequent administration or higher doses are not recommended. To administer 2.5 mg of Albuterol, dilute 0.5 mL of the 0.5% inhalation solution with 2.5 mL of sterile normal saline solution. The flow rate is regulated to suit the particular nebulizer so that Albuterol Sulfate Inhalation Solution will be delivered over approximately 5-15 minutes.

The use of Albuterol Sulfate Inhalation Solution can be continued as medically indicated to control recurring bouts of bronchospasm. During this time most patients gain optimal benefit from regular use of the inhalation solution.

If a previously effective dosage regimen fails to provide the usual relief, medical advice should be sought immediately as this is often a sign of seriously worsening asthma that would require reassessment of therapy.

Albuterol Sulfate Inhalation Solution in unit dose: The usual dosage for adults and children 12 years and older is 2.5 mg of Albuterol administered three to four times daily by nebulization. More frequent administration or higher doses are not recommended. To administer 2.5 mg of Albuterol, administer the contents of one sterile unit dose nebule (3 mL of 0.083% inhalation solution) by nebulization. The flow rate is regulated to suit the particular nebulizer so that Albuterol Sulfate Inhalation Solution in unit dose will be delivered over approximately 5-15 minutes.

The use of Albuterol Sulfate Inhalation Solution in unit dose can be continued as medically indicated to control recurring bouts of bronchospasm. During this time most patients gain optimal benefit from regular use of the inhalation solution.

If a previously effective dosage regimen fails to provide the usual relief, medical advice should be sought immediately as this is often a sign of seriously worsening asthma that would require reassessment of therapy.

Albuterol Sulfate Capsules for Inhalation: The usual dosage for adults and children 4 years of age and older is the contents of one 200-mcg capsule inhaled every 4-6 hours using an inhalation device. In some patients, the contents of two 200-mcg capsules inhaled every 4-6 hours may be required. Larger doses or more frequent administration are not recommended.

The use of Albuterol Sulfate Capsules for Inhalation can be continued as medically indicated to control recurring bouts of bronchospasm. During this time most patients gain optimal benefit from regular use of the Albuterol Sulfate Capsules for Inhalation formulation.

If a previously effective dosage regimen fails to provide the usual relief, medical advice should be sought immediately as this is often a sign of seriously worsening asthma that would require reassessment of therapy.

Exercise-induced Bronchospasm Prevention: The usual dosage of Albuterol Sulfate Capsules for Inhalation for adults and children 12 years of age and older is the contents of one 200-mcg capsule inhaled using an inhalation device 15 minutes before exercise.

Albuterol Sulfate Syrup: The following dosages of Albuterol Sulfate Syrup are expressed in terms of Albuterol base.

Usual Dosage: The usual starting dosage for adults and children over age 14 is 2 mg (1 teaspoonful) or 4 mg (2 teaspoonfuls) three or four times a day.

The usual starting dosage for children 6-14 years of age is 2 mg (1 teaspoonful) three or four times a day.

For children 2-6 years of age, dosing should be initiated at 0.1 mg/kg of body weight three times a day. This starting dosage should not exceed 2 mg (1 teaspoonful) three times a day.

Dosage Adjustment: For adults and children over age 14, a dosage above 4 mg four times a day should be used *only* when the patient fails to respond. If a favorable response does not occur, the dosage may be cautiously increased stepwise, but not to exceed 8 mg four times a day.

For children 6-14 years of age who fail to respond to the initial starting dosage of 2 mg four times a day, the dosage may be cautiously increased stepwise, but not to exceed 24 mg per day (given in divided doses).

For children 2-6 years of age who do not respond satisfactorily to the initial dosage, the dosage may be increased stepwise to 0.2 mg/kg of body weight three times a day, but not to exceed a maximum of 4 mg (2 teaspoonfuls) given three times a day.

Elderly Patients and Those Sensitive to Beta-adrenergic Stimulators: The initial dosage should be restricted to 2 mg three or four times a day and individually adjusted thereafter.

Albuterol Sulfate Tablets: The following dosages of Albuterol Sulfate Tablets are expressed in terms of Albuterol base.

Usual Dosage: The usual starting dosage for adults and children 12 years of age and older is 2 or 4 mg three or four times a day.

The usual starting dosage for children 6-12 years of age is 2 mg three or four times a day.

Dosage Adjustment: For adults and children 12 years of age and older, a dosage above 4 mg four times a day should be used *only* when the patient fails to respond. If a favorable response does not occur with the 4-mg initial dosage, it should be cautiously increased stepwise up to a maximum of 8 mg four times a day as tolerated.

For children 6-12 years of age who fail to respond to the initial starting dosage of 2 mg four times a day, the dosage may be cautiously increased stepwise, but not to exceed 24 mg per day (given in divided doses).

Elderly Patients and Those Sensitive to Beta-adrenergic Stimulators: An initial dosage of 2 mg three or four times a day is recommended for elderly patients and for those with a history of unusual sensitivity to beta-adrenergic stimulators. If adequate bronchodilatation is not obtained, dosage may be increased gradually to as much as 8 mg three or four times a day.

The total daily dose should not exceed 32 mg in adults and children 12 years of age and older.

Albuterol Sulfate Extended-Release Tablets: The following dosages of Albuterol Sulfate Extended-Release Tablets are expressed in terms of Albuterol base.

Usual Dosage: The usual recommended dosage for adults and adolescents 12 years of age and older is 8 mg every 12 hours. In some patients, 4 mg every 12 hours may be sufficient.

Alternatively, patients currently maintained on Albuterol Sulfate Tablets or Albuterol Sulfate Syrup can be switched to Albuterol Sulfate Extended-Release Tablets. For example, the administration of one 4-mg Albuterol Sulfate Extended-Release Tablet every 12 hours is equivalent to one 2-mg Albuterol Sulfate Tablet every 6 hours. Multiples of this regimen up to the maximum recommended daily dose also apply.

Dosage Adjustment: In unusual circumstances, such as adults of low body weight, it may be desirable to use a starting dosage of 4 mg every 12 hours and progress to 8 mg every 12 hours according to response.

Where control of airway obstruction is not achieved with the recommended doses, the doses may be cautiously increased under the control of the supervising physician to a maximum dose of 32 mg per day in divided doses (i.e., q12h) in adults.

Each Albuterol Sulfate Extended-Release Tablet contains a small hole that is part of the unique extended-release system. Albuterol Sulfate Extended-Release Tablets must be swallowed whole with the aid of liquids. DO NOT CHEW OR CRUSH THESE TABLETS.

Store Albuterol Inhalation Aerosol between 15 and 30°C (59° and 86°F). As with most inhaled medications in aerosol canisters, the therapeutic effect of this medication may decrease when the canister is cold. Shake well before using.

Store Albuterol Sulfate Inhalation Solution between 2° and 25°C (36° and 77°F). Protect Albuterol Sulfate Inhalation Solution in unit dose from light. Store in a refrigerator between 2° and 8°C (36° and 46°F). Albuterol Sulfate Inhalation Solution in unit dose may be held at room temperature for up to 2 weeks before use. (Must be used within 2 weeks of removal from refrigerator; record date removed from the refrigerator on the product carton.) Discard if solution becomes discolored. (Note: Albuterol Sulfate Inhalation Solution in unit dose is colorless.)

Store Albuterol Sulfate Capsules, Syrup, and Extended-Release Tablets between 2° and 30°C (36° and 86°F).

Store Albuterol Sulfate Tablets between 2° and 25°C (36° and 77°F). Replace cap securely after each opening.

J CODES
.083%, per ml INH—J7620
0.5%, per ml INH—J7625

HOW SUPPLIED

ALBUTEROL
AEROSOL SOLID INGREDIENTS: 0.09 MG/INH

BRAND/MANUFACTURER	NDC	SIZE	AWP
◇ **BRAND**			
VENTOLIN: Allen & Hanburys	00173-0463-00	6.8 gm	$13.24
PROVENTIL: Schering	00085-0614-03	17 gm	$21.24
VENTOLIN: Allen & Hanburys	00173-0321-98	17 gm	$21.24

AEROSOL SOLID W/ADAPTER: 0.09 MG/INH

BRAND/MANUFACTURER	NDC	SIZE	AWP
◇ **BRAND**			
PROVENTIL: Schering	00085-0614-02	17 gm	$23.05
VENTOLIN: Allen & Hanburys	00173-0321-88	17 gm	$23.05

ALBUTEROL SULFATE
CAPSULE: 200 MCG

BRAND/MANUFACTURER	NDC	SIZE	AWP
○ **BRAND**			
VENTOLIN ROTACAPS: Allen & Hanburys	00173-0389-03	24s	$18.67
	00173-0389-02	100s	$23.05
	00173-0389-01	100s	$27.19

SOLUTION: 0.083%

AVERAGE UNIT PRICE (AVAILABLE SIZES)		GENERIC A-RATED AVERAGE PRICE (GAAP)	
BRAND	$0.45	3 ml	$16.31
GENERIC	$1.09	3 ml 25s	$31.70
		3 ml 60s	$73.71

BRAND/MANUFACTURER	NDC	SIZE	AWP
◆ **BRAND**			
VENTOLIN NEBULES: Allen & Hanburys	00173-0419-00	3 ml 25s	$32.40
PROVENTIL: Schering	00085-0209-01	3 ml 25s	$35.39
◆ **GENERICS**			
Major	00904-7731-17	3 ml	$1.25
Geneva	00781-9150-93	3 ml	$31.37
Dey	49502-0697-03	3 ml 25s	$30.25
Qualitest	00603-1005-40	3 ml 25s	$30.42
URL	00677-1522-72	3 ml 25s	$32.00
Aligen	00405-2131-25	3 ml 25s	$32.20
Rugby	00536-2677-04	3 ml 25s	$32.50
AIRET: Adams	53014-0075-25	3 ml 25s	$35.72
Astra	00186-1491-04	3 ml 25s ud	$30.25
Goldline	00182-8010-24	3 ml 25s ud	$30.25
Dey	49502-0697-33	3 ml 30s	$36.30
URL	00677-1522-73	3 ml 60s	$72.50
Dey	49502-0697-60	3 ml 60s	$72.60
AIRET: Adams	53014-0075-60	3 ml 60s	$77.15
Astra	00186-1491-17	3 ml 60s ud	$72.60

◆ RATED THERAPEUTICALLY EQUIVALENT; ◇ THERAPEUTIC EQUIVALENCE UNCONFIRMED; ○ UNRATED

SOLUTION: 0.5%

AVERAGE UNIT PRICE (AVAILABLE SIZES)		GENERIC A-RATED AVERAGE PRICE (GAAP)	
BRAND	$0.78	20 ml	$13.34
GENERIC	$0.67		

BRAND/MANUFACTURER	NDC	SIZE	AWP
◆ BRAND			
PROVENTIL: Schering	00085-0208-02	20 ml	$15.53
VENTOLIN: Allen & Hanburys	00173-0385-58	20 ml	$15.53
◆ GENERICS			
URL	00677-1521-22	20 ml	$12.45
Astra	00186-1490-01	20 ml	$12.50
Aligen	00405-2130-52	20 ml	$12.50
Copley	38245-0640-09	20 ml	$12.50
Qualitest	00603-1006-43	20 ml	$12.50
Rugby	00536-2675-73	20 ml	$13.50
Schein	00364-2530-55	20 ml	$13.91
Goldline	00182-6014-65	20 ml	$13.95
Moore,H.L.	00839-7730-97	20 ml	$14.16
Moore,H.L.	00839-7861-97	20 ml	$14.16
Major	00904-7658-55	20 ml	$14.65

SYRUP: 2 MG/5 ML

AVERAGE UNIT PRICE (AVAILABLE SIZES)		GENERIC A-RATED AVERAGE PRICE (GAAP)	
BRAND	$0.06	473 ml	$26.13
GENERIC	$0.06	480 ml	$26.29

BRAND/MANUFACTURER	NDC	SIZE	AWP
◆ BRAND			
VENTOLIN: Allen & Hanburys	00173-0351-54	480 ml	$29.14
PROVENTIL: Schering	00085-0315-02	480 ml	$32.42
◆ GENERICS			
Allscrips	54569-3700-01	118.25 ml	$6.88
Aligen	00405-2135-16	473 ml	$24.75
Allscrips	54569-3700-00	473 ml	$27.51
URL	00677-1505-33	480 ml	$24.70
Qualitest	00603-1007-58	480 ml	$24.75
Schein	00364-2522-16	480 ml	$24.96
Warner Chilcott	00047-1006-23	480 ml	$25.50
Rugby	00536-0415-85	480 ml	$26.00
Goldline	00182-6015-40	480 ml	$26.00
Mova	55370-0315-48	480 ml	$26.23
Moore,H.L.	00839-7746-69	480 ml	$26.26
Geneva	00781-6067-16	480 ml	$26.38
Du Pont Multi	00056-0197-16	480 ml	$27.23
Major	00904-7681-16	480 ml	$27.90
Lemmon	00093-0661-16	480 ml	$27.92
UDL	51079-0760-10	5 ml 50s ud	$36.40
UDL	51079-0761-10	10 ml 50s ud	$62.60

TABLET, EXTENDED RELEASE: 4 MG

BRAND/MANUFACTURER	NDC	SIZE	AWP
◇ BRAND			
VOLMAX: Muro	00451-0398-00	60s	$34.13
▶ PROVENTIL REPETABS: Schering	00085-0431-02	100s	$60.58
	00085-0431-04	100s ud	$75.86
	00085-0431-03	500s	$293.88

TABLET, EXTENDED RELEASE: 8 MG

BRAND/MANUFACTURER	NDC	SIZE	AWP
○ BRAND			
VOLMAX: Muro	00451-0399-00	60s	$60.86

TABLETS: 2 MG

AVERAGE UNIT PRICE (AVAILABLE SIZES)		GENERIC A-RATED AVERAGE PRICE (GAAP)	
BRAND	$0.34	100s	$23.55
GENERIC	$0.23	500s	$108.78
HCFA FUL (100s ea)	$0.04		

BRAND/MANUFACTURER	NDC	SIZE	AWP
◆ BRAND			
▶ VENTOLIN: Allen & Hanburys	00173-0341-43	100s	$32.50
▶ PROVENTIL: Schering	00085-0252-02	100s	$36.17
▶ VENTOLIN: Allen & Hanburys	00173-0341-44	500s	$154.28
▶ PROVENTIL: Schering	00085-0252-03	500s	$171.71
◆ GENERICS			
Medirex	57480-0422-06	30s ud	$9.00
Rugby	00536-3008-01	100s	$11.24
Warner Chilcott	00047-0956-24	100s	$18.80
▶ Lemmon	00093-0665-01	100s	$18.99
Geneva	00781-1671-01	100s	$22.25
Mason Dist	11845-0400-01	100s	$22.45
Martec	52555-0491-01	100s	$22.50
Schein	00364-2438-01	100s	$22.80
Moore,H.L.	00839-7611-06	100s	$23.07
Moore,H.L.	00839-7867-06	100s	$23.07
Novopharm	55953-0480-40	100s	$23.50
Qualitest	00603-2093-21	100s	$23.60

BRAND/MANUFACTURER	NDC	SIZE	AWP
URL	00677-1359-01	100s	$23.64
Mutual	53489-0176-01	100s	$23.64
Mylan	00378-0255-01	100s	$23.65
Warrick	59930-1520-01	100s	$23.65
Aligen	00405-4030-01	100s	$24.00
Major	00904-2876-60	100s	$24.90
Copley	38245-0132-10	100s	$25.00
Goldline	00182-1011-01	100s	$25.00
Biocraft	00332-2226-09	100s	$25.00
Sidmak	50111-0491-01	100s	$25.50
Lederle Std Prod	00005-3062-43	100s	$26.29
Parmed	00349-8713-01	100s	$27.29
Parmed	00349-8994-01	100s	$27.29
Du Pont Multi	00056-0198-70	100s	$28.05
Raway	00686-0657-20	100s ud	$16.00
Vangard	00615-3517-13	100s ud	$22.57
Major	00904-2876-61	100s ud	$25.38
UDL	51079-0657-20	100s ud	$28.32
Medirex	57480-0422-01	100s ud	$29.00
Parmed	00349-8713-25	250s	$63.12
Rugby	00536-3008-05	500s	$46.34
Moore,H.L.	00839-7611-12	500s	$89.44
▶ Lemmon	00093-0665-05	500s	$91.15
Qualitest	00603-2093-28	500s	$96.85
Martec	52555-0491-05	500s	$100.52
Novopharm	55953-0480-70	500s	$112.00
URL	00677-1359-05	500s	$112.22
Mutual	53489-0176-05	500s	$112.22
Mylan	00378-0255-05	500s	$112.25
Warrick	59930-1520-02	500s	$112.25
Major	00904-2876-40	500s	$112.90
Mason Dist	11845-0400-03	500s	$115.69
Copley	38245-0132-50	500s	$120.00
Biocraft	00332-2226-13	500s	$120.00
Sidmak	50111-0491-02	500s	$122.00
Parmed	00349-8994-05	500s	$123.20
Lederle Std Prod	00005-3062-31	500s	$124.86
Du Pont Multi	00056-0198-85	500s	$134.20

TABLETS: 4 MG

AVERAGE UNIT PRICE (AVAILABLE SIZES)		GENERIC A-RATED AVERAGE PRICE (GAAP)	
BRAND	$0.50	100s	$35.09
GENERIC	$0.34	500s	$159.68
HCFA FUL (100s ea)	$0.08		

BRAND/MANUFACTURER	NDC	SIZE	AWP
◆ BRAND			
▶ VENTOLIN: Allen & Hanburys	00173-0342-43	100s	$48.47
▶ PROVENTIL: Schering	00085-0573-02	100s	$53.95
▶ VENTOLIN: Allen & Hanburys	00173-0342-44	500s	$230.38
▶ PROVENTIL: Schering	00085-0573-03	500s	$256.39
◆ GENERICS			
Rugby	00536-3009-01	100s	$22.20
Warner Chilcott	00047-0957-24	100s	$27.63
Lemmon	00093-0666-01	100s	$27.91
Moore,H.L.	00839-7612-06	100s	$32.20
Mason Dist	11845-0401-01	100s	$32.60
Geneva	00781-1672-01	100s	$33.25
Schein	00364-2439-01	100s	$34.00
Novopharm	55953-0499-40	100s	$35.00
Qualitest	00603-2094-21	100s	$35.16
Mutual	53489-0177-01	100s	$35.18
Mylan	00378-0572-01	100s	$35.20
Warrick	59930-1530-01	100s	$35.20
Martec	52555-0492-01	100s	$35.25
Major	00904-2877-60	100s	$35.30
Copley	38245-0134-10	100s	$37.50
Goldline	00182-1012-01	100s	$37.50
Biocraft	00332-2228-09	100s	$37.50
Sidmak	50111-0492-01	100s	$38.00
Aligen	00405-4031-01	100s	$38.05
Lederle Std Prod	00005-3063-43	100s	$39.46
Parmed	00349-8714-01	100s	$41.30
Parmed	00349-8995-01	100s	$41.30
Du Pont Multi	00056-0199-70	100s	$41.80
Raway	00686-0658-20	100s ud	$16.00
Vangard	00615-3518-13	100s ud	$34.66
Major	00904-2877-61	100s ud	$36.38
UDL	51079-0658-20	100s ud	$43.08
Medirex	57480-0423-01	100s ud	$43.95
Parmed	00349-8714-25	250s	$93.89
Rugby	00536-3009-05	500s	$92.70
Mason Dist	11845-0401-03	500s	$125.90
Lemmon	00093-0666-05	500s	$128.39
Martec	52555-0492-05	500s	$132.68
Moore,H.L.	00839-7612-12	500s	$139.71
Qualitest	00603-2094-28	500s	$144.00
Major	00904-2877-40	500s	$164.60
Novopharm	55953-0499-70	500s	$168.00
Warrick	59930-1530-02	500s	$168.25
Mutual	53489-0177-05	500s	$168.32

BRAND/MANUFACTURER	NDC	SIZE	AWP
Mylan	00378-0572-05	500s	$168.35
Copley	38245-0134-50	500s	$180.00
Biocraft	00332-2228-13	500s	$180.00
Sidmak	50111-0492-02	500s	$182.00
Parmed	00349-8995-05	500s	$184.80
Lederle Std Prod	00005-3063-31	500s	$186.69
Du Pont Multi	00056-0199-85	500s	$200.20

TABLETS: 5 MG

AVERAGE UNIT PRICE (AVAILABLE SIZES)

GENERIC	$0.34

BRAND/MANUFACTURER	NDC	SIZE	AWP
◆ GENERICS			
URL	00677-1360-01	100s	$35.18
URL	00677-1360-05	500s	$168.32

Alcaine SEE PROPARACAINE HYDROCHLORIDE

Alclometasone Dipropionate

DESCRIPTION

Alclometasone Dipropionate Cream and Ointment contain Alclometasone Dipropionate for dermatologic use. Alclometasone Dipropionate is a synthetic corticosteroid with anti-inflammatory activity.

Chemically, Alclometasone Dipropionate is 7α-chloro-11β,17,21-trihydroxy-16α-methylpregna-1,4-diene-3,20-dione 17,21-Dipropionate.

Alclometasone Dipropionate has a molecular weight of 521. It is a white powder, insoluble in water, slightly soluble in propylene glycol, and moderately soluble in hexylene glycol.

Following is its chemical structure:

CLINICAL PHARMACOLOGY

The corticosteroids are a class of compounds comprising steroid hormones secreted by the adrenal cortex and their synthetic analogs. In pharmacologic doses, corticosteroids are used primarily for their anti-inflammatory and/or immunosuppressive effects. Topical corticosteroids such as Alclometasone Dipropionate are effective in the treatment of corticosteroid-responsive dermatoses primarily because of their anti-inflammatory, antipruritic, and vasoconstrictive actions. However, while the physiologic, pharmacologic, and clinical effects of the corticosteroids are well known, the exact mechanisms of their actions in each disease are uncertain.

Alclometasone Dipropionate, a corticosteroid, has been shown to have topical (dermatologic) and systemic pharmacologic and metabolic effects characteristic of this class of drugs.

Pharmacokinetics: The extent of percutaneous absorption of topical corticosteroids, including Alclometasone Dipropionate, is determined by many factors, including the vehicle, the integrity of the epidermal barrier, and the use of occlusive dressings (see *"Dosage and Administration"*).

Topical corticosteroids can be absorbed from normal intact skin. A study utilizing a radio-labelled Alclometasone Dipropionate *ointment* formulation was performed to measure systemic absorption and excretion. Results indicated that approximately 3% of the steroid was absorbed during 8 hours of contact with intact skin of normal volunteers.

Inflammation and/or other disease processes in the skin may increase percutaneous absorption. Occlusive dressings substantially increase the percutaneous absorption of topical corticosteroids. Thus, occlusive dressings may be a valuable therapeutic adjunct for treatment of resistant dermatoses (see *"Dosage and Administration"*).

The effects of Alclometasone Dipropionate Cream and Ointment on the hypothalamic-pituitary-adrenal (HPA) axis were studied under exaggerated conditions. In one study, Alclometasone Dipropionate Ointment was applied to 30% of the body twice daily for 7 days, and occlusive dressings were used in selected patients either 12 hours or 24 hours daily. In another study, Alclometasone Dipropionate Cream was applied to 80% of the body surface of normal subjects twice daily for 21 days with daily 12-hour periods of whole body occlusion. Average plasma and urinary free cortisol levels and urinary levels of

17-hydroxysteroids were slightly decreased (about 10%), suggesting slight suppression of the HPA axis under the exaggerated conditions of these studies.

Once absorbed through the skin, topical corticosteroids enter pharmacokinetic pathways similarly to systemically administered corticosteroids. Corticosteroids are bound to plasma proteins in varying degrees. Corticosteroids are metabolized primarily in the liver and are then excreted by the kidneys. Some of the topical corticosteroids, including Alclometasone Dipropionate and its metabolites, are also excreted into the bile.

INDICATIONS AND USAGE

Alclometasone Dipropionate Cream and Ointment are indicated for relief of the inflammatory and pruritic manifestations of corticosteroid-responsive dermatoses.

CONTRAINDICATIONS

Alclometasone Dipropionate Cream and Ointment are contraindicated in patients who are hypersensitive to Alclometasone Dipropionate, to other corticosteroids, or to any ingredient in these preparations.

PRECAUTIONS

General: Systemic absorption of topical corticosteroids has resulted in reversible HPA axis suppression, manifestations of Cushing's syndrome, hyperglycemia, and glucosuria in some patients.

Conditions that augment systemic absorption include the application of the more potent steroids, use over large surface areas, prolonged use, and the addition of occlusive dressings.

Children may absorb proportionally larger amounts of topical corticosteroids and thus be more susceptible to systemic toxicity (see *"Precautions: Pediatric Use"*).

If irritation develops, topical corticosteroids should be discontinued and appropriate therapy instituted.

In the presence of dermatologic infections, the use of an appropriate antifungal or antibacterial agent should be instituted. If a favorable response does not occur promptly, the corticosteroid should be discontinued until the infection has been adequately controlled.

Information for Patients: Patients using Alclometasone Dipropionate Cream and Ointment should receive the following information and instructions:

1. This medication is to be used as directed by the physician. It is for external use only. Avoid contact with the eyes.
2. This medication should not be used for any disorder other than that for which it was prescribed.
3. The treated skin area should not be bandaged or otherwise covered or wrapped as to be occlusive unless directed by the physician.
4. Patients should report any signs of local adverse reactions, especially under occlusive dressings, to the physician.
5. Parents of pediatric patients should be advised not to use tight-fitting diapers or plastic pants on a child being treated in the diaper area, as these garments may constitute occlusive dressings.

Laboratory Tests: Although Alclometasone Dipropionate Cream and Ointment were shown not to produce HPA axis suppression, the following tests may be helpful in evaluating if HPA axis suppression does occur: Urinary free cortisol test and ACTH stimulation test.

Carcinogenesis, Mutagenesis, Impairment of Fertility: Long-term animal studies have not been performed to evaluate the carcinogenic potential or the effect on fertility of topical corticosteroids.

Studies to determine mutagenicity with prednisolone have revealed negative results.

Pregnancy: Teratogenic Effects: Pregnancy Category C: Corticosteroids are generally teratogenic in laboratory animals when administered systemically at relatively low dosage levels. The more potent corticosteroids have been shown to be teratogenic in animals after dermal application. There are no adequate and well-controlled studies of the teratogenic effects of topically applied corticosteroids in pregnant women. Therefore, topical corticosteroids should be used during pregnancy only if the potential benefit justifies the potential risk to the fetus. Drugs of this class should not be used extensively on pregnant patients, in large amounts, or for prolonged periods of time.

Nursing Mothers: It is not known whether topical administration of corticosteroids could result in sufficient systemic absorption to produce detectable quantities in breast milk. Systemically administered corticosteroids are secreted into breast milk in quantities not likely to have a deleterious effect on the infant. Nevertheless, caution should be exercised when topical corticosteroids are prescribed for a nursing woman.

Pediatric Use: **Pediatric patients may demonstrate greater susceptibility to topical corticosteroid-induced HPA axis suppression and Cushing's syndrome than mature patients because of a larger skin surface area to body weight ratio.**

HPA axis suppression, Cushing's syndrome, and intracranial hypertension have been reported in children receiving topical corticosteroids. Manifestations of adrenal suppression in children include linear growth retardation, delayed weight gain, low plasma cortisol levels, and absence of response to ACTH stimulation. Manifestations of intracranial hypertension include bulging fontanelles, headaches, and bilateral papilledema.

Administration of topical corticosteroids to children should be limited to the least amount compatible with an effective therapeutic regimen. Chronic corticosteroid therapy may interfere with the growth and development of children.

ADVERSE REACTIONS

The following local adverse reactions have been reported with Alclometasone Dipropionate Cream: itching occurred in about 2 per 100 patients; burning, erythema, dryness, irritation, and papular rashes occurred in about 1 per 100 patients.

The following local adverse reactions have been reported with Alclometasone Dipropionate Ointment: itching or burning, 1 per 200 patients; erythema, 2 per 1,000 patients.

The following local adverse reactions are reported infrequently with the use of topical corticosteroids, but may occur more frequently with the use of occlusive dressings. These reactions are listed in an approximately decreasing order of occurrence: burning, itching, irritation, dryness, folliculitis, hypertrichosis, acneiform eruptions, hypopigmentation, perioral dermatitis, allergic contact dermatitis, maceration of the skin, secondary infection, skin atrophy, striae, and miliaria.

OVERDOSAGE

Topically applied Alclometasone Dipropionate Cream and Ointment can be absorbed in sufficient amounts to produce systemic effects (see "Precautions").

DOSAGE AND ADMINISTRATION

Apply a thin film of Alclometasone Dipropionate Cream or Ointment to the affected skin areas two or three times daily; massage gently until the medication disappears. Occlusive dressings may be used for the management of refractory lesions of psoriasis and other deep-seated dermatoses, such as localized neurodermatitis (lichen simplex chronicus).

Evaporation from the skin is reduced by use of the hydration technique with occlusive dressing as follows:

1. Cover the lesion with a thick layer of Alclometasone Dipropionate Cream or Ointment and a light gauze dressing, then cover the area with a pliable plastic film.
2. Seal the edges to the normal skin by adhesive tape or other means.
3. Leave the dressing in place 1-4 days and repeat the procedure three or four times as needed.

With this method of treatment, marked improvement is often seen in a few days.

If an infection develops, the use of occlusive dressings should be discontinued and appropriate antimicrobial therapy instituted.

Store between 2° and 30°C (36° and 86°F).

HOW SUPPLIED
CREAM: 0.05%

BRAND/MANUFACTURER	NDC	SIZE	AWP
○ BRAND			
ACLOVATE: Glaxo Derm	00173-0401-00	15 gm	$10.31
	00173-0401-01	45 gm	$21.49
	00173-0401-06	60 gm	$27.23

OINTMENT: 0.05%

BRAND/MANUFACTURER	NDC	SIZE	AWP
○ BRAND			
ACLOVATE: Glaxo Derm	00173-0402-00	15 gm	$10.31
	00173-0402-01	45 gm	$21.49
	00173-0402-06	60 gm	$27.23

Alcohol, Dehydrated

DESCRIPTION

Alcohol, Dehydrated Injection consists of not less than 98% by volume of ethanol (ethyl Alcohol). Alcohol, Dehydrated is hypobaric in relation to the cerebrospinal fluid. It is injected proximate to nerve tissues and into spinal subarachnoid spaces to produce degeneration of nerve function (neurolysis) for control of chronic pain.

The product contains no bacteriostat or antimicrobial agent (other than ethanol) and no added buffer.

Alcohol, Dehydrated is chemically designated C_2H_5OH (ethanol), a clear, colorless liquid miscible with water.

CLINICAL PHARMACOLOGY

Alcohol produces injury to tissue cells by dehydration and precipitation of protoplasm. When Alcohol is injected in close proximity to nerve tissues, it produces neuritis and nerve degeneration (neurolysis). Deliberate injury to selected spinal nerves, peripheral nerves, or ganglia by injection of Alcohol results in more or less enduring block of sensory, motor and autonomic function.

The injection of Alcohol used for therapeutic neurolysis involves amounts too small to produce significant systemic effects of ethanol.

Ninety to 98% of ethyl Alcohol that enters the body is completely oxidized.

INDICATIONS AND USAGE

Alcohol, Dehydrated Injection is indicated for therapeutic neurolysis of nerves or ganglia for the relief of intractable chronic pain in such conditions as inoperable cancer and trigeminal neuralgia (tic douloureux), in patients for whom neurosurgical procedures are contraindicated. Relief of trigeminal neuralgia usually is only temporary. Other conditions for which injection of Alcohol has been reported include glossopharyngeal neuralgia, angina pectoris, and severe claudication due to peripheral vascular insufficiency.

Alcohol concentrations of 40 to 50% (prepared by appropriate dilution of Alcohol, Dehydrated) have been used for epidural or individual motor nerve injections to control certain manifestations of cerebral palsy and spastic paraplegia. Similar concentrations also have been injected for celiac plexus block to relieve pain of inoperable upper abdominal cancer, and have been injected intra- and subcutaneously for relief of intractable pruritus ani.

CONTRAINDICATIONS

Subarachnoid injection of Alcohol, Dehydrated is contraindicated in patients receiving anticoagulants because of the danger of bleeding.

WARNINGS

Alcohol is a flammable liquid and should be kept cool and away from flame. Alcohol injections should be made with care to avoid unwanted tissue necrosis. Proper positioning of the patient is essential to control localization of injections of Alcohol, Dehydrated (which is hypobaric) into the subarachnoid space.

PRECAUTIONS

Do not adminster unless solution is clear and container is intact. Discard unused portion.

It is sometimes advisable to make a trial injection of procaine or other local anesthetic prior to Alcohol injection as a means of confirming accurate placement of the needle, and to decrease pain experienced during the procedure. X-ray visualization for precise placement also may be advisable.

When used for selective sensory block within the subarachnoid space, it is essential to avoid contact of the Alcohol with the anterior (motor) roots of the spinal nerve to be treated if motor paralysis is not desired. When peripheral nerves are injected, care should be taken that residual Alcohol is not deposited along the needle track or in any other location where tissue destruction is not wanted. Instances have been reported in which the pain resulting from post-injection neuritis was more severe than that existing before the injection.

Pregnancy Category C. Animal reproduction studies have not been conducted with Alcohol, Dehydrated. It is also not known whether Alcohol, Dehydrated can cause fetal harm when given to a pregnant woman or can affect reproduction capacity. Alcohol, Dehydrated should be given to a pregnant woman only if clearly needed.

ADVERSE REACTIONS

The most commonly encountered side effects are postinjection neuritis with persistent pain hyperesthesia and paresthesia. Subarachnoid neurolysis and lumbar sympathetic block may be followed by motor paralysis, bladder or rectal incontinence, and impotence. Severe hypotension may follow celiac ganglion injection. Corneal anesthesia meningitis or cranial nerve palsy may follow injection of the gasserian ganglion.

DRUG ABUSE AND DEPENDENCE

None known with this size and manner of presentation.

OVERDOSAGE

Excessive or faulty localization of injections may result in unwanted postinjection neuritis and/or tissue necrosis. In such cases, efforts should be directed toward dilution of deposited Alcohol when feasible, relief of pain with analgesics and surgical intervention if indicated.

Hypotension following celiac ganglion injection may be controlled with appropriate vasopressor agents (see "Precautions" and "Adverse Reactions".)

DOSAGE AND ADMINISTRATION

The dosage of Alcohol, Dehydrated Injection for therapeutic nerve or ganglion block varies from as little as 0.05 to 0.5 mL in trigeminal neuralgia to 0.5 to 1.0 mL per interspace for subarachnoid injections. Doses larger than 1.5 mL are seldom required. All injections should be made slowly and only after all steps have been taken to insure precise placement of the alcohol. A 1.0 mL tuberculin syringe is desirable to facilitate accurate measurement of the dose. Separate needles should be used for injection of successive interspaces or other sites. Since Alcohol, Dehydrated Injection is hypobaric as compared to spinal fluid, proper positioning of the patient is essential to control localization of injections into the subarachnoid space.

When lesser concentrations of Alcohol are used, larger volumes are usually injected. A dose of 2 mL of 45% Alcohol has been used for injecting individual motor nerves, or from 1.5 to 4.0 mL for epidural injection in children with spastic cerebral palsy; 50 mL of 50% Alcohol has been used for celiac plexus blockade.

The LD_{50} oral dose in rats is 13.7 g/kg.

Parenteral drug products should be inspected visually for particulate matter and discoloration prior to administration.

See "Precautions".

Store in a cool place away from flame.

HOW SUPPLIED
INJECTION: 98%

BRAND/MANUFACTURER	NDC	SIZE	AWP
◆ GENERICS			
Abbott Hosp	00074-3772-04	1 ml 25s	$299.84

Aldactazide *SEE* HYDROCHLOROTHIAZIDE WITH SPIRONOLACTONE

Aldactone *SEE* SPIRONOLACTONE

Aldesleukin

DESCRIPTION

Aldesleukin, a human recombinant interleukin-2 product, is a highly purified protein with a molecular weight of approximately 15,300 daltons. The chemical name is des-alanyl-1, serine-125 human interleukin-2. Aldesleukin lymphokine, is produced by recombinant DNA technology using a genetically engineered *E. coli* strain containing an analog of the human interleukin-2 gene. Genetic engineering techniques were used to modify the human IL-2 gene, and the resulting expression clone encodes a modified human interleukin-2. This recombinant form differs from native interleukin-2 in the following ways: a) Aldesleukin is not glycosylated because it is derived from *E. coli*.; b) The molecule has no N-terminal alanine; the codon for this amino acid was deleted during the genetic engineering procedure; c) The molecule has serine substituted for cysteine at amino acid position 125; this was accomplished by site specific manipulation during the genetic engineering procedure; and d) The aggregation state of Aldesleukin is likely to be different from that of native interleukin-2.

Biological activities tested *in vitro* for the native non-recombinant molecule have been reproduced with Aldesleukin.[1,2] Aldesleukin for Injection is supplied as a sterile, white to off-white, lyophilized cake in single-use vials intended for intravenous (IV) administration. When reconstituted with 1.2 mL Sterile Water for Injection, USP, each mL contains 18 million IU (1.1 mg) Aldesleukin, 50 mg mannitol, and 0.18 mg sodium dodecyl sulfate, buffered with approximately 0.17 mg, monobasic and 0.89 mg dibasic sodium phosphate to a pH of 7.5 (range 7.2 to 7.8). The manufacturing process for Aldesleukin involves fermentation in a defined medium containing tetracycline hydrochloride. The presence of the antibiotic is not detectable in the final product. Aldesleukin contains no preservatives in the final product.

Aldesleukin biological potency is determined by a lymphocyte proliferation bioassay and is expressed in International Units (IU) as established by the World Health Organization 1ST International Standard for interleukin 2 (human). The relationship between potency and protein mass is as follows: 18 million (18×10^6) IU Aldesleukin = 1.1 mg protein.

CLINICAL PHARMACOLOGY

Aldesleukin has been shown to possess the biological activity of human native interleukin-2.[1,2] *In vitro* studies performed on human cell lines demonstrate the immunoregulatory properties of Aldesleukin, including: a) enhancement of lymphocyte mitogenesis and stimulation of long-term growth of human interleukin-2 dependent cell lines; b) enhancement of lymphocyte cytotoxicity; c) induction of killer cell [lymphokine-activated (LAK) and natural (NK)] activity; and d) induction of interferon-gamma production.

The *in vivo* administration of Aldesleukin in select murine tumor models and in the clinic produces multiple immunological effects in a dose dependent manner. These effects include activation of cellular immunity with profound lymphocytosis, eosinophilia, and thrombocytopenia, and the production of cytokines including tumor necrosis factor, IL-1 and gamma interferon.[3] *In vivo* experiments in murine tumor models have shown inhibition of tumor growth.[4] The exact mechanism by which Aldesleukin mediates its antitumor activity in animals and humans is unknown.

Pharmacokinetics: Aldesleukin exists as biologically active, non-covalently bound microaggregates with an average size of 27 recombinant interleukin-2 molecules. The solubilizing agent, sodium dodecyl sulfate, may have an effect on the kinetic properties of this product. The pharmacokinetic profile of Aldesleukin is characterized by high plasma concentrations following a short IV infusion, rapid distribution to extravascular, extracellular space and elimination from the body by metabolism in the kidneys with little or no bioactive protein excreted in the urine.

Studies of IV Aldesleukin in sheep and humans indicated that approximately 30% of the administered dose initially distributes to the plasma.

This is consistent with studies in rats that demonstrate a rapid (< 1 minute) and preferential uptake of approximately 70% of an administered dose into the liver, kidney and lung. The serum half-life (T ½) curves of Aldesleukin remaining in the plasma are derived from studies done in 52 cancer patients following a 5 minute IV infusion.[5] These patients were shown to have a distribution and elimination T ½ of 13 and 85 minutes, respectively.

The relatively rapid clearance rate of Aldesleukin has led to dosage schedules characterized by frequent, short infusions. Observed serum levels are proportional to the dose of Aldesleukin.

Following the initial rapid organ distribution described above, the primary route of clearance of circulating Aldesleukin is the kidney. In humans and animals, Aldesleukin is cleared from the circulation by both glomerular filtration and peritubular extraction in the kidney.[6-9] This dual mechanism for delivery of Aldesleukin to the proximal tubule may account for the preservation of clearance in patients with rising serum creatinine values. Greater than 80% of the amount of Aldesleukin distributed to plasma, cleared from the circulation and presented to the kidney is metabolized to amino acids in the cells lining the proximal convoluted tubules. In humans, the mean clearance rate in cancer patients is 268 mL/min.[9]

Immunogenicity: Fifty-seven of 77 renal cancer patients (74%) treated with the every 8 hour Aldesleukin regimen developed low titers of non-neutralizing anti-interleukin-2 antibodies. Neutralizing antibodies were not detected in this group of patients, but have been detected in 1/106 (< 1%) patients with IV Aldesleukin using a wide variety of schedules and doses. The clinical significance of anti-interleukin-2 antibodies is unknown.

Clinical Experience: Two hundred and fifty-five patients with metastatic renal cell cancer were treated with single agent Aldesleukin. Treatment was given by the every 8 hour regimen in 7 clinical studies conducted at 21 institutions. To be eligible for study, patients were required to have bidimensionally measurable disease; Eastern Cooperative Oncology Group (ECOG) Performance Status (PS) of 0 or 1 (see Table 1); and normal organ function, including normal cardiac stress test and pulmonary function tests. Patients with brain metastases, active infections, organ allografts and diseases requiring steroid treatment were excluded. In addition, it was noted that 218 of the 255 (85%) patients had undergone nephrectomy prior to treatment with Aldesleukin.

Aldesleukin was given by 15 minute IV infusion every 8 hours for up to 5 days (maximum of 14 doses). No treatment was given on days 6 to 14 and then dosing was repeated for up to 5 days on days 15 to 19 (maximum of 14 doses). These 2 cycles constituted 1 course of therapy. All patients were treated with 28 doses or until dose-limiting toxicity occurred requiring ICU-level support. Patients received a median of 20 of 28 scheduled doses of Aldesleukin. Doses were held for specific toxicities (see *"Dosage and Administration"* section, *"Dose Modification"* subsection). A variety of serious adverse events were encountered including: hypotension; oliguria/anuria; mental status changes including coma; pulmonary congestion and dyspnea; GI bleeding; respiratory failure leading to intubation; ventricular arrhythmias; myocardial ischemia and/or infarction; ileus or intestinal perforation, renal failure requiring dialysis; gangrene; seizures; sepsis and death (see *"Adverse Reactions"* section). Due to the toxicities encountered during the clinical trials, investigators used the following concomitant medications. Acetaminophen and indomethacin were started immediately prior to Aldesleukin to reduce fever. Renal function was particularly monitored because indomethacin may cause synergistic nephrotoxicity. Meperidine was added to control the rigors associated with fever. Ranitidine or cimetidine were given for prophylaxis of gastrointestinal irritation and bleeding. Antiemetics and antidiarrheals were used as needed to treat other gastrointestinal side effects. These medications were discontinued 12 hours after the last dose of Aldesleukin. Hydroxyzine or diphenhydramine was used to control symptoms from pruritic rashes and continued until resolution of pruritus. *Note: Prior to the use of any product mentioned in this paragraph, the physician should refer to the package insert for the respective product.*

For the 255 patients in the Aldesleukin database, objective response was seen in 15% or 37 patients with nine (4%) complete and 28 (11%) partial responders. The 95% confidence interval for response was 11 to 20%. Onset of tumor regression has been observed as early as 4 weeks after completion of the first course of treatment and tumor regression may continue for up to 12 months after the start of treatment. Durable responses were achieved with a median duration of objective (partial or complete) response by Kaplan-Meier projection of 23.2 months (1 to 50 months). The median duration of objective partial response was 18.8 months. The proportion of responding patients who will have response durations of 12 months or greater is projected to be 85% for all responders and 79% for patients with partial responses (Kaplan-Meier).

Complete Responders	Partial Responders	Response Rate	Onset of Response	Median Duration of Response
9 (4%)	28 (11%)	15%	1 to 12 mos.	23.2 months (range 1-50)

Response was observed in both lung and non-lung sites (e.g. liver, lymph node, renal bed recurrences, soft tissue). Patients with individual bulky lesions

($> 5 \times 5$ cm) as well as large cumulative tumor burden (> 25 cm^2 tumor area) achieved durable responses.

An analysis of prognostic factors showed that performance status as defined by the ECOG (see Table I) was a significant predictor of response. PS 0 patients had an 18% overall rate of objective response, which included all 9 complete response patients and 21 of 28 partial response patients. PS 1 patients had a lower rate of response (9%), all of which were partial responses. In this group it was notable that 6 of the 7 responders had resolution of tumor related symptoms and improved performance status to PS 0. All seven patients were fully functional and 4 of the 7 returned to work, suggesting that responses among the PS 1 patients were clinically meaningful as well (see Table 2).

In addition, the frequency of toxicity was related to the performance status. As a group, PS 0 patients, when compared with PS 1 patients, had lower rates of adverse events with fewer on-study deaths (4% vs. 6%), less frequent intubations (8% vs. 25%), gangrene (0% vs. 6%), coma (1% vs. 6%), GI bleeding (4% vs. 8%), and sepsis (6% vs. 18%). These differences in toxicity are reflected in the shorter mean time to hospital discharge for PS 0 patients (2 vs. 3 days) as well as the smaller percentage of PS 0 patients experiencing a delayed (> 7 days) discharge from the hospital (8% vs. 19%).

Table 1
PERFORMANCE STATUS SCALE

Performance Status Equivalent		Performance Status Definitions
ECOG*	Karnofsky	
0	100	Asymptomatic
1	80-90	Symptomatic; fully ambulatory
2	60-70	Symptomatic; in bed less than 50% of day
3	40-50	Symptomatic; in bed more than 50% of day
4	20-30	Bedridden

Zubrod, CG, et al. J Chron Dis 11:7-33, 1960

Table 2
ALDESLEUKIN RESPONSE ANALYZED BY ECOG* PERFORMANCE STATUS (PS)

Pre-Treatment ECOG PS	No. of Patients Treated (n = 255)	Response		% of Patients Responding	On-Study Death Rate
		CR	PR		
0	166	9	21	18%	4%
1	80	0	7	9%	6%
≥ 2	9	0	0	0%	0%

* *Eastern Cooperative Oncology Group*

INDICATIONS AND USAGE
Aldesleukin is indicated for the treatment of adults (≥ 18 years of age) with metastatic renal cell carcinoma.

Careful patient selection is mandatory prior to the administration of Aldesleukin. See "Contraindications", "Warnings" and "Precautions" sections regarding patient screening, including recommended cardiac and pulmonary function tests and laboratory tests.

Evaluation of clinical studies to date reveals that patients with more favorable ECOG performance status (ECOG PS 0) at treatment initiation respond better to Aldesleukin, with a higher response rate and lower toxicity (see "Clinical Pharmacology" section, "Clinical Experience" subsection). Therefore, selection of patients for treatment should include assessment of performance status, as described in Table 1.

Experience in patients with PS > 1 is extremely limited.

UNLABELED USES
Aldesleukin is used as an adjunct in the treatment of melanoma.

CONTRAINDICATIONS
Aldesleukin is contraindicated in patients with a known history of hypersensitivity to interleukin-2 or any component of the Aldesleukin formulation.

Patients with an abnormal thallium stress test or pulmonary function tests are excluded from treatment with Aldesleukin. Patients with organ allografts should be excluded as well. In addition, retreatment with Aldesleukin is contraindicated in patients who experienced the following toxicities while receiving an earlier course of therapy:

- Sustained ventricular tachycardia (≥ 5 beats)
- Cardiac rhythm disturbances not controlled or unresponsive to management
- Recurrent chest pain with ECG changes, consistent with angina or myocardial infarction
- Intubation required > 72 hours
- Pericardial tamponade
- Renal dysfunction requiring dialysis > 72 hours
- Coma or toxic psychosis lasting > 48 hours
- Repetitive or difficult to control seizures

- Bowel ischemia/perforation
- GI bleeding requiring surgery

WARNINGS
See boxed "Warnings".

Aldesleukin administration has been associated with capillary leak syndrome (CLS) which results from extravasation of plasma proteins and fluid into the extravascular space and loss of vascular tone. CLS results in hypotension and reduced organ perfusion which may be severe and can result in death. The CLS may be associated with cardiac arrhythmias (supraventricular and ventricular), angina, myocardial infarction, respiratory insufficiency requiring intubation, gastrointestinal bleeding or infarction, renal insufficiency, and mental status changes.

Because of the severe adverse events which generally accompany Aldesleukin therapy at the recommended dosages, thorough clinical evaluation should be performed to exclude from treatment patients with significant cardiac, pulmonary, renal, hepatic or CNS impairment.

Should adverse events occur, which require dose modification, dosage should be withheld rather than reduced. (See "Dosage and Administration" section, "Dose Modification" subsection.)

Aldesleukin may exacerbate disease symptoms in patients with clinically unrecognized or untreated CNS metastases. All patients should have thorough evaluation and treatment of CNS metastases prior to receiving Aldesleukin therapy. They should be neurologically stable with a negative CT scan. In addition, extreme caution should be exercised in treating patients with a history of seizure disorder because Aldesleukin may cause seizures.

Intensive Aldesleukin treatment is associated with impaired neutrophil function (reduced chemotaxis) and with an increased risk of disseminated infection, including sepsis and bacterial endocarditis, in treated patients. Consequently, pre-existing bacterial infections should be adequately treated prior to initiation of Aldesleukin therapy. Additionally, all patients with indwelling central lines should receive antibiotic prophylaxis effective against *S. aureus*.[10-12] Antibiotic prophylaxis which has been associated with a reduced incidence of staphylococcal infections in Aldesleukin studies includes the use of: oxacillin, nafcillin, ciprofloxacin, or vancomycin. Disseminated infections acquired in the course of Aldesleukin treatment are a major contributor to treatment morbidity and use of antibiotic prophylaxis and aggressive treatment of suspected and documented infections may reduce the morbidity of Aldesleukin treatment. *Note: Prior to the use of any product mentioned in this paragraph, the physician should refer to the package insert for the respective product.*

PRECAUTIONS
General: Patients should have normal cardiac, pulmonary, hepatic and CNS function at the start of therapy. Patients who had had a nephrectomy are still eligible for treatment if they have serum creatinine levels ≤ 1.5 mg/dL.

Adverse events are frequent, often serious, and sometimes fatal.

Capillary leak syndrome (CLS) begins immediately after Aldesleukin treatment starts and is marked by increased capillary permeability to protein and fluids and reduced vascular tone. In most patients, this results in a concomitant drop in mean arterial blood pressure within 2 to 12 hours after the start of treatment. With continued therapy, clinically significant hypotension (defined as systolic blood pressure below 90 mm Hg or a 20 mm Hg drop from baseline systolic pressure) and hypoperfusion will occur. In addition, extravasation of protein and fluids into the extravascular space will lead to edema formation and creation of effusions.

Medical management of CLS begins with careful monitoring of the patient's fluid and organ perfusion status. This is achieved by frequent determination of blood pressure and pulse, and by monitoring organ function, which includes assessment of mental status and urine output. Hypovolemia is assessed by catheterization and central pressure monitoring.

Flexibility in fluid and pressor management is essential for maintaining organ perfusion and blood pressure. Consequently, extreme caution should be used in treating patients with fixed requirements for large volumes of fluid (e.g. patients with hypercalcemia).

Patients with hypovolemia are managed by administering IV fluids, either colloids or crystalloids. IV fluids are usually given when the central venous pressure (CVP) is below 3 to 4 mm H$_2$O. Correction of hypovolemia may require large volumes of IV fluids but caution is required because unrestrained fluid administration may exacerbate problems associated with edema formation or effusions.

With extravascular fluid accumulation, edema is common and some patients may develop ascites or pleural effusions. Management of these events depends on a careful balancing of the effects of fluid shifts so that neither the consequences of hypovolemia (e.g. impaired organ perfusion) nor the consequences of fluid accumulations (e.g. pulmonary edema) exceeds the patient's tolerance.

Clinical experience has shown that early administration of dopamine (1 to 5 μg/kg/min) to patients manifesting capillary leak syndrome, before the onset of hypotension, can help to maintain organ perfusion particularly to the kidney and thus preserve urine output. Weight and urine output should be carefully monitored. If organ perfusion and blood pressure are not sustained by dopamine therapy, clinical investigators have increased the dose of dopamine to 6 to 10 μg/kg/min or have added phenylephrine hydrochloride (1 to 5 μg/kg/min) to low dose dopamine. (See "Clinical Pharmacology" section, "Clinical Experience" subsection.) Prolonged use of pressors, either in combination or as individual agents, at relatively high doses, may be associated with cardiac rhythm disturbances. *Note: Prior to the use of any product mentioned in this paragraph, the physician should refer to the package insert for the respective product.*

Failure to maintain organ perfusion, demonstrated by altered mental status, reduced urine output, a fall in the systolic blood pressure below 90 mm Hg or onset of cardiac arrhythmias, should lead to holding the subsequent doses until recovery of organ perfusion and a return of systolic blood pressure above 90 mm Hg are observed. (See *"Dosage and Administration"* section, *"Dose Modification"* subsection.)

Recovery from CLS begins soon after cessation of Aldesleukin therapy. Usually, within a few hours, the blood pressure rises, organ perfusion is restored and resorption of extravasated fluid and protein begins. If there has been excessive weight gain or edema formation, particularly if associated with shortness of breath from pulmonary congestion, use of diuretics, once blood pressure has normalized, has been shown to hasten recovery.

Oxygen is given to the patient if pulmonary function monitoring confirms that P_aO_2 is decreased.

Aldesleukin administration may cause anemia and/or thrombocytopenia. Packed red blood cell transfusions have been given both for relief of anemia and to insure maximal oxygen carrying capacity. Platelet transfusions have been given to resolve absolute thrombocytopenia and to reduce the risk of GI bleeding. In addition, leukopenia and neutropenia are observed.

Aldesleukin administration results in fever, chills, rigors, pruritus and gastrointestinal side effects in most patients treated at recommended doses. These side effects have been aggressively managed as described in the *"Clinical Pharmacology"* section, *"Clinical Experience"* subsection.

Renal and hepatic function are impaired during Aldesleukin treatment. Use of concomitant medications known to be nephrotoxic or hepatotoxic may further increase toxicity to the kidney or liver. In addition, reduced kidney and liver function secondary to Aldesleukin treatment may delay elimination of concomitant medications and increase the risk of adverse events from those drugs.

Patients may experience mental status changes including irritability, confusion, or depression while receiving Aldesleukin. These mental status changes may be indicators of bacteremia or early bacterial sepsis. Mental status changes due solely to Aldesleukin are generally reversible when drug administration is discontinued. However, alterations in mental status may progress for several days before recovery begins. Impairment of thyroid function has been reported following Aldesleukin treatment. A small number of treated patients went on to require thyroid replacement therapy. This impairment of thyroid function may be a manifestation of autoimmunity, consequently, extra caution should be exercised when treating patients with known autoimmune disease.

Aldesleukin enhancement of cellular immune function may increase the risk of allograft rejection in transplant patients.

Laboratory Tests: The following clinical evaluations are recommended for all patients, prior to beginning treatment and then daily during drug administration.

■ Standard hematologic tests—including CBC, differential and platelet counts
■ Blood chemistries—including electrolytes, renal and hepatic function tests
■ Chest x-rays

All patients should have baseline pulmonary function tests with arterial blood gases. Adequate pulmonary function should be documented ($FEV_1 > 2$ liters or $\geq$ 75% of predicted for height and age) prior to initiating therapy. All patients should be screened with a stress thallium study. Normal ejection fraction and unimpaired wall motion should be documented. If a thallium stress test suggests minor wall motion abnormalities of questionable significance, a stress echocardiogram to document normal wall motion may be useful to exclude significant coronary artery disease.

Daily monitoring during therapy with Aldesleukin should include vital signs (temperature, pulse, blood pressure and respiration rate) and weight. In a patient with a decreased blood pressure, especially less than 90 mm Hg, constant cardiac monitoring for rhythm should be conducted. If an abnormal complex or rhythm is seen, an ECG should be performed. Vital signs in these hypotensive patients should be taken hourly and central venous pressure (CVP) checked.

During treatment, pulmonary function should be monitored on a regular basis by clinical examination, assessment of vital signs and pulse oximetry. Patients with dyspnea or clinical signs of respiratory impairment (tachypnea or rales) should be further assessed with arterial blood gas determination. These tests are to be repeated as often as clinically indicated.

Cardiac function is assessed daily by clinical examination and assessment of vital signs. Patients with signs or symptoms of chest pain, murmurs, gallops, irregular rhythm or palpitations should be further assessed with an ECG examination and CPK evaluation. If there is evidence of cardiac ischemia or congestive heart failure, a repeat thallium study should be done.

Drug Interactions: Aldesleukin may affect central nervous function. Therefore, interactions could occur following concomitant administration of psychotropic drugs (e.g., narcotics, analgesics, antiemetics, sedatives, tranquilizers).

Concurrent administration of drugs possessing nephrotoxic (e.g. aminoglycosides, indomethacin), myelotoxic (e.g. cytotoxic chemotherapy), cardiotoxic (e.g. doxorubicin) or hepatotoxic (e.g. methotrexate, asparaginase) effects with Aldesleukin may increase toxicity in these organ systems. The safety and efficacy of Aldesleukin in combination with chemotherapies have not been established.

Although glucocorticoids have been shown to reduce Aldesleukin-induced side effects including fever, renal insufficiency, hyperbilirubinemia, confusion and dyspnea,[13] concomitant administration of these agents with Aldesleukin may reduce the antitumor effectiveness of Aldesleukin and thus should be avoided.

Beta-blockers and other antihypertensives may potentiate the hypotension seen with Aldesleukin.

Carcinogenesis, Mutagenesis, Impairment of Fertility: There have been no studies conducted assessing the carcinogenic or mutagenic potential of Aldesleukin.

There have been no studies conducted assessing the effect of Aldesleukin on fertility. It is recommended that this drug not be administered to fertile persons of either sex not practicing effective contraception.

Pregnancy: Pregnancy Category C. Animal reproduction studies have not been conducted with Aldesleukin. It is also not known whether Aldesleukin can cause fetal harm when administered to a pregnant woman or can affect reproduction capacity. In view of the known adverse effects of Aldesleukin, it should only be given to a pregnant woman with extreme caution, weighing the potential benefit with the risks associated with therapy.

Nursing Mothers: It is not known whether this drug is excreted in human milk. Because many drugs are excreted in human milk and because of the potential for serious adverse reactions in nursing infants from Aldesleukin, a decision should be made whether to discontinue nursing or to discontinue the drug, taking into account the importance of the drug to the mother.

Pediatric Use: Safety and effectiveness in children under 18 years of age have not been established.

ADVERSE REACTIONS

The rate of drug related deaths in the 255 metastatic renal cell carcinoma patients on study who received single-agent Aldesleukin was 4% (11/255).

Frequency and severity of adverse reactions to Aldesleukin have generally been shown to be dose-related and schedule-dependent. Most adverse reactions are self-limiting and are usually, but not invariably, reversible within 2 or 3 days of discontinuation of therapy.

Examples of adverse reactions with permanent sequelae include: myocardial infarction, bowel perforation/infarction, and gangrene.

The most frequently reported serious adverse reactions include hypotension, renal dysfunction with oliguria/anuria, dyspnea or pulmonary congestion, and mental status changes (i.e., lethargy, somnolence, confusion and agitation). Other serious toxicities have included: myocardial ischemia, myocarditis, gangrene, respiratory failure leading to intubation, GI bleeding requiring surgery, intestinal perforation/ileus, coma, seizure, sepsis and renal impairment requiring dialysis. The incidence of these events has been higher in PS 1 patients than in PS 0 patients (See *"Clinical Pharmacology"* Section, *"Clinical Experience"* Subsection).

The following data on adverse reactions are based on 373 patients (255 with renal cell cancer and 118 with other tumors) treated with the recommended every 8 hour 15-minute infusion dosing regimen. These patients had metastatic or recurrent carcinoma and were enrolled in investigational trials in the United States.

Organ systems in which reactions occurred in a significant number of the patients treated are found in the following table:

Table 3
INCIDENCE OF ADVERSE EVENTS

Events by Body System	% of Patients
CARDIOVASCULAR	
Hypotension	85
(requiring pressors)	71
Sinus Tachycardia	70
Arrhythmias	22
Atrial	8
Supraventricular	5
Ventricular	3
Junctional	1
Bradycardia	7
Premature Ventricular Contractions	5
Premature Atrial Contractions	4
Myocardial Ischemia	3
Myocardial Infarction	2
Cardiac Arrest	2
Congestive Heart Failure	1
Myocarditis	1
Stroke	1
Gangrene	1
Pericardial Effusion	1
Endocarditis	1
Thrombosis	1
PULMONARY	
Pulmonary Congestion	54
Dyspnea	52
Pulmonary Edema	10
Respiratory Failure (leading to intubation)	9
Tachypnea	8
Pleural Effusion	7
Wheezing	6
Apnea	1
Pneumothorax	1
Hemoptysis	1

Events by Body System	% of Patients
HEPATIC	
Elevated Bilirubin	64
Elevated Transaminase	56
Elevated Alkaline Phosphatase	56
Jaundice	11
Ascites	4
Hepatomegaly	1
HEMATOLOGIC	
Anemia	77
Thrombocytopenia	64
Leukopenia	34
Coagulation Disorders	10
Leukocytosis	9
Eosinophilia	6
ABNORMAL LABORATORY FINDINGS	
Hypomagnesemia	16
Acidosis	16
Hypocalcemia	15
Hypophosphatemia	11
Hypokalemia	9
Hyperuricemia	9
Hypoalbuminemia	8
Hypoproteinemia	7
Hyponatremia	5
Hyperkalemia	4
Alkalosis	4
Hypoglycemia	3
Hyperglycemia	2
Hypocholesterolemia	2
Hypercalcemia	1
Hypernatremia	1
Hyperphosphatemia	1
GASTROINTESINAL	
Nausea and Vomiting	87
Diarrhea	76
Stomatitis	32
Anorexia	27
GI Bleeding	13
(requiring surgery)	2
Dyspepsia	2
Constipation	2
Intestinal Perforation/Ileus	2
Pancreatitis	< 1
NEUROLOGIC	
Mental Status Changes	73
Dizziness	17
Sensory Dysfunction	10
Special Sensory Disorders (vision, speech, taste)	7
Syncope	3
Motor Dysfunction	2
Coma	1
Seizure (grand mal)	1
RENAL	
Oliguria/Anuria	76
BUN Elevation	63
Serum Creatinine Elevation	61
Proteinuria	12
Hematuria	9
Dysuria	3
Renal Impairment Requiring Dialysis	2
Urinary Retention	1
Urinary Frequency	1
DERMATOLOGIC	
Pruritus	48
Erythema	41
Rash	26
Dry Skin	15
Exfoliative Dermatitis	14
Purpura/Petechiae	4
Urticaria	2
Alopecia	1
MUSCULOSKELETAL	
Arthralgia	6
Myalgia	6
Arthritis	1
Muscle Spasm	1
ENDOCRINE	
Hypothyroidism	< 1
GENERAL	
Fever and/or Chills	89
Pain (all sites)	54
Abdominal	15

Events by Body System	% of Patients
Chest	12
Back	9
Fatigue/Weakness/Malaise	53
Edema	47
Infection (including urinary tract, injection site, catheter tip, phlebitis, sepsis)	23
Weight Gain (≥ 10%)	23
Headache	12
Weight Loss (≥ 10%)	5
Conjunctivitis	4
Injection Site Reactions	3
Allergic Reactions (non-anaphylactic)	1

Other serious adverse events were derived from trials involving more than 1,800 patients treated with Aldesleukin-based regimens using a variety of doses and schedules. These events each occurred with a frequency of < 1% and included: liver or renal failure resulting in death; duodenal ulceration; fatal intestinal perforation; bowel necrosis; fatal cardiac arrest, myocarditis, and supraventricular tachycardia; permanent or transient blindness secondary to optic neuritis; fatal malignant hyperthermia; pulmonary edema resulting in death; respiratory arrest; fatal respiratory failure; fatal stroke; transient ischemic attack; meningitis; cerebral edema; pericarditis; allergic interstitial nephritis; tracheoesophageal fistula; fatal pulmonary emboli; severe depression leading to suicide.

OVERDOSAGE
Side effects following the use of Aldesleukin are dose-related. Administration of more than the recommended dose has been associated with a more rapid onset of expected dose limiting toxicities. Adverse reactions generally will reverse when the drug is stopped, particularly because its serum half-life is short (see *"Clinical Pharmacology"* section, *"Pharmacokinetics"* subsection). Any continuing symptoms should be treated supportively. Life threatening toxicities have been ameliorated by the intravenous administration of dexamethasone,[13] which may result in loss of therapeutic effect from Aldesleukin. *Note:* **Prior to the use of dexamethasone, the physician should refer to the package insert for this product.**

DOSAGE AND ADMINISTRATION
Aldesleukin for injection should be administered by a 15-minute IV infusion every 8 hours. Before initiating treatment, carefully review the *"Indications and Usage"*, *"Contraindications"*, *"Warnings"*, *"Precautions"*, and *"Adverse Reactions"* sections, particularly regarding patient selection, possible serious adverse events, patient monitoring and withholding dosage.

The following schedule has been used to treat adult patients with metastatic renal cell carcinoma. Each course of treatment consists of two 5-day treatment cycles separated by a rest period.

600,000 IU/kg (0.037 mg/kg) dose administered every 8 hours by a 15-minute IV infusion for a total of 14 doses. Following 9 days of rest, the schedule is repeated for another 14 doses, for a maximum of 28 doses per course.

During clinical trials, doses were frequently held for toxicity (see *"Dose Modification"* subsection). Patients treated with this schedule received a median of 20 of the 28 doses during the first course of therapy.

Retreatment: Patients should be evaluated for response approximately 4 weeks after completion of a course of therapy and again immediately prior to the scheduled start of the next treatment course. Additional courses of treatment may be given to patients only if there is some tumor shrinkage following the last course and retreatment is not contraindicated (see *"Contraindications"* section). Each treatment course should be separated by a rest period of at least 7 weeks from the date of hospital discharge. Tumors have continued to regress up to 12 months following the initiation of Aldesleukin therapy.

Dose Modification: Dose modification for toxicity should be accomplished by holding or interrupting a dose rather than reducing the dose to be given. Decisions to stop, hold, or restart Aldesleukin therapy must be made after a global assessment of the patient. With this in mind, the following guidelines should be used:

Treatment with Aldesleukin should be permanently discontinued for:

Organ System	Permanently discontinue treatment for the following toxicities
Cardiovascular	Sustained ventricular tachycardia (≥ 5 beats)
	Cardiac rhythm disturbances not controlled or unresponsive to management
	Recurrent chest pain with ECG changes, documented angina or myocardial infarction
	Pericardial tamponade
Pulmonary	Intubation required > 72 hours
Renal	Renal dysfunction requiring dialysis > 72 hours

The hemodynamic effects of a particular muscle relaxant and the degree of skeletal muscle relaxation required should be considered in the selection of a neuromuscular blocking agent.

Following an anesthetic induction dose of Alfentanil Hydrochloride, requirements for volatile inhalation anesthetics or Alfentanil Hydrochloride infusion are reduced by 30 to 50% for the first hour of maintenance.

Administration of Alfentanil Hydrochloride infusion should be discontinued at least 10-15 minutes prior to the end of surgery.

Respiratory depression caused by opioid analgesics can be reversed by opioid antagonists such as naloxone. Because the duration of respiratory depression produced by Alfentanil Hydrochloride may last longer than the duration of the opioid antagonist action, appropriate surveillance should be maintained. As with all potent opioids, profound analgesia is accompanied by respiratory depression and diminished sensitivity to CO_2 stimulation which may persist into or recur in the postoperative period. Intraoperative hyperventilation may further alter postoperative response to CO_2. Appropriate postoperative monitoring should be employed, particularly after infusions and large doses of Alfentanil Hydrochloride, to ensure that adequate spontaneous breathing is established and maintained in the absence of stimulation prior to discharging the patient from the recovery area.

Head Injuries: Alfentanil Hydrochloride may obscure the clinical course of patients with head injuries.

Impaired Respiration: Alfentanil Hydrochloride should be used with caution in patients with pulmonary disease, decreased respiratory reserve or potentially compromised respiration. In such patients, opioids may additionally decrease respiratory drive and increase airway resistance. During anesthesia, this can be managed by assisted or controlled respiration.

Impaired Hepatic or Renal Fuction: In patients with liver or kidney dysfunction Alfentanil Hydrochloride should be administered with caution due to the importance of these organs in the metabolism and excretion of Alfentanil Hydrochloride.

Drug Interactions: Both the magnitude and duration of central nervous system and cardiovascular effects may be enhanced when Alfentanil Hydrochloride is administered in combination with other CNS depressants such as barbiturates, tranquilizers, opioids, or inhalation general anesthetics. Postoperative respiratory depression may be enhanced or prolonged by these agents. In such cases of combined treatment, the dose of one or both agents should be reduced. Limited clinical experience indicates that requirements for volatile inhalation anesthetics are reduced by 30 to 50% for the first sixty (60) minutes following Alfentanil Hydrochloride induction.

The concomitant use of erythromycin with Alfentanil Hydrochloride can significantly inhibit Alfentanil Hydrochloride clearance and may increase the risk of prolonged or delayed respiratory depression. Perioperative administration of drugs affecting hepatic blood flow or enzyme function may reduce plasma clearance and prolong recovery.

Carcinogenesis, Mutagenesis and Impairment of Fertility: No long-term animal studies of Alfentanil Hydrochloride have been performed to evaluate carcinogenic potential. The micronucleus test in female rats and the dominant lethal test in female and male mice revealed that single intravenous doses of Alfentanil Hydrochloride as high as 20 mg/kg (approximately 40 times the upper human dose) produced no structural chromosome mutations or induction of dominant lethal mutations. The Ames *Salmonella typhimurium* metabolic activating test also revealed no mutagenic activity.

Pregnancy Category C: Alfentanil Hydrochloride has been shown to have an embryocidal effect in rats and rabbits when given in doses 2.5 times the upper human dose for a period of 10 days to over 30 days. These effects could have been due to maternal toxicity (decreased food consumption with increased mortality) following prolonged administration of the drug.

No evidence of teratogenic effects has been observed after administration of Alfentanil Hydrochloride in rats or rabbits.

There are no adequate and well-controlled studies in pregnant women. Alfentanil Hydrochloride should be used during pregnancy only if the potential benefit justifies the potential risk to the fetus.

Labor and Delivery: There are insufficient data to support the use of Alfentanil Hydrochloride in labor and delivery. Placental transfer of the drug has been reported; therefore, use in labor and delivery is not recommended.

Nursing Mothers: In one study of nine women undergoing post-partum tubal ligation, significant levels of Alfentanil Hydrochloride were detected in colostrum four hours after administration of 60 μg/kg of Alfentanil Hydrochloride with no detectable levels present after 28 hours. Caution should be exercised when Alfentanil Hydrochloride is administered to a nursing woman.

Pediatric Use: Adequate data to support the use of Alfentanil Hydrochloride in children under 12 years of age are not presently available.

ADVERSE REACTIONS

The most common adverse reactions, respiratory depression and skeletal muscle rigidity, are extensions of known pharmacological effects of opioids. See *"Clinical Pharmacology"*, *"Warnings"* and *"Precautions"* on the management of respiratory depression and skeletal muscle rigidity.

Delayed respiratory depression, respiratory arrest, bradycardia, asystole arrhythmias and hypotension have also been reported.

The reported incidences of adverse reactions listed in the following table are derived from controlled and open clinical trials involving 1183 patients, of whom

785 received Alfentanil Hydrochloride. The controlled trials involved treatment comparisons with fentanyl, thiopental sodium, enflurane, saline placebo and halothane. Incidences are based on disturbing and nondisturbing adverse reactions reported. The comparative incidence of certain side effects is influenced by the type of use, e.g., chest wall rigidity has a higher reported incidence in clinical trials of alfentanil induction, and by the type of surgery, e.g., nausea and vomiting have a higher incidence in patients undergoing gynecologic surgery. (See related table.)

In addition, other adverse reactions less frequently reported (1% or less) were:
Laryngospasm, bronchospasm, postoperative confusion, headache, shivering, postoperative euphoria, hypercarbia, pain on injection, urticaria, and itching.

Some degree of skeletal muscle rigidity should be expected with induction doses of Alfentanil Hydrochloride.

DRUG ABUSE AND DEPENDENCE

Alfentanil Hydrochloride is a Schedule II controlled drug substance that can produce drug dependence of the morphine type and therefore has the potential for being abused.

OVERDOSAGE

Overdosage would be manifested by extension of the pharmacological actions of Alfentanil Hydrochloride (see *"Clinical Pharmacology"*) as with other potent opioid analgesics. No experience of overdosage with Alfentanil Hydrochloride was reported during clinical trials. The intravenous LD_{50} of Alfentanil Hydrochloride is 43.0-50.9 mg/kg in rats, 72.2-73.6 mg/kg in mice, 71.8-81.9 mg/kg in guinea pigs and 59.5-87.5 mg/kg in dogs. Intravenous administration of an opioid antagonist such as naloxone should be employed as a specific antidote to manage respiratory depression.

The duration of respiratory depression following overdosage with Alfentanil Hydrochloride may be longer than the duration of action of the opioid antagonist. Administration of an opioid antagonist should not preclude immediate establishment of a patent airway, administration of oxygen, and assisted or controlled ventilation as indicated for hypoventilation or apnea. If respiratory depression is associated with muscular rigidity, a neuromuscular blocking agent may be required to facilitate assisted or controlled ventilation. Intravenous fluids and vasoactive agents may be required to manage hemodynamic instability.

DOSAGE AND ADMINISTRATION

The dosage of Alfentanil Hydrochloride should be individualized in each patient according to body weight, physical status, underlying pathological condition, use of other drugs, and type and duration of surgical procedure and anesthesia. In obese patients (more than 20% above ideal total body weight), the dosage of Alfentanil Hydrochloride should be determined on the basis of lean body weight. The dose of Alfentanil Hydrochloride should be reduced in elderly or debilitated patients (see *"Precautions"*).

Vital signs should be monitored routinely.

See Dosage Chart for the use of Alfentanil Hydrochloride; 1) by incremental injection as an analgesic adjunct to anesthesia with barbiturate/nitrous oxide/oxygen for short surgical procedures (expected duration of less than one hour); 2) by continuous infusion as a maintenance analgesic with nitrous oxide/oxygen for general surgical procedures; and 3) by intravenous injection in anesthetic doses for the induction of anesthesia for general surgical procedures with a minimum expected duration of 45 minutes.

Usage in Children: Clinical data to support the use of Alfentanil Hydrochloride in patients under 12 years of age are not presently available. Therefore, such use is not recommended.

Premedication: The selection of preanesthetic medications should be based upon the needs of the individual patient.

Neuromuscular Blocking Agents: The neuromuscular blocking agent selected should be compatible with the patient's condition, taking into account the hemodynamic effects of a particular muscle relaxant and the degree of skeletal muscle relaxation required (see *"Clinical Pharmacology"*, *"Warnings"* and *"Precautions"* sections).

In patients administered anesthetic (induction) dosages of Alfentanil Hydrochloride, it is essential that qualified personnel and adequate facilities are available for the management of intraoperative and postoperative respiratory depression.

Also see *"Warnings"* and *"Precautions"* sections.

For purposes of administering small volumes of Alfentanil Hydrochloride accurately, the use of a tuberculin syringe or equivalent is recommended.

The physical and chemical compatibility of Alfentanil Hydrochloride have been demonstrated in solution with normal saline, 5% dextrose in normal saline, 5% dextrose in water and Lactated Ringers. Clinical studies of Alfentanil Hydrochloride infusion have been conducted with Alfentanil Hydrochloride diluted to a concentration range of 25 μg/mL to 80 μg/mL.

As an example of the preparation of Alfentanil Hydrochloride for infusion, 20 mL of Alfentanil Hydrochloride added to 230 mL of diluent provides a 40 μg/mL solution of Alfentanil Hydrochloride.

Parenteral drug products should be inspected visually for particulate matter and discoloration prior to administration, whenever solution and container permit. (See related table.)

	Alfentanil Hydrochloride (N = 785) %	Fentanyl (N = 243) %	Thiopental Sodium (N = 66) %	Enflurane (N = 55) %	Halothane (N = 18) %	Saline Placebo* (N = 18) %
Gastrointestinal						
Nausea	28	44	14	5	0	22
Vomiting	18	31	11	9	13	17
Cardiovascular						
Bradycardia	14	7	8	0	0	0
Tachycardia	12	12	39	36	31	11
Hypotension	10	8	7	7	0	0
Hypertension	18	13	30	20	6	0
Arrhythmia	2	6	5	4	6	0
Musculoskeletal						
Chest Wall Rigidity	17	12	0	0	0	0
Skeletal Muscle Movements	6	2	6	0	0	0
Respiratory						
Apnea	7	0	0	0	0	0
Postoperative Respiratory Depression	2	2	0	0	0	0
CNS						
Dizziness	3	5	0	0	0	0
Sleepiness/ Postoperative Sedation	2	8	2	0	0	6
Blurred Vision	2	0	0	0	0	0

* *From two clinical trials, one involving supplemented balanced barbiturate/nitrous oxide anesthesia and one in healthy volunteers who did not undergo surgery.*

DOSAGE RANGE CHART

Indication	Approximate Duration of Anesthesia	Induction Period (Initial Dose)	Maintenance Period (Increments/Infusion)	Total Dose	Effects
Incremental Injection	≤ 30 mins	8-20 µg/kg	3-5 µg/kg or 0.5-1 µg/kg/min	8-40 µg/kg	Spontaneously breathing or assisted ventilation when required.
Incremental Injection	30-60 mins	20-50 µg/kg	5-15 µg/kg	up to 75 µg/kg	Assisted or controlled ventilation required. Attenuation of response to laryngoscopy and intubation.
Continuous Infusion	> 45 mins	50-75 µg/kg	0.5-3.0 µg/kg/min Average Infusion Rate 1-1.5 µg/kg/min	dependent on duration of procedure	Assisted or controlled ventilation required. Some attenuation of response to intubation and incision, with intraoperative stability.
See Guidelines Below					
Anesthetic Induction	> 45 mins	130-245 µg/kg	0.5 to 1.5 µg/kg/min or general anesthetic	dependent on duration of procedure	Assisted or controlled ventilation required. Administer slowly (over three minutes). Concentration of inhalation agents reduced by 30-50% for initial hour.

INFUSION DOSAGE
CONTINUOUS INFUSION: 0.5-3.0 µG/KG/MIN ADMINISTERED WITH NITROUS OXIDE/OXYGEN IN PATIENTS UNDERGOING GENERAL SURGERY. FOLLOWING AN ANESTHETIC INDUCTION DOSE OF ALFENTANIL HYDROCHLORIDE, INFUSION RATE REQUIREMENTS ARE REDUCED BY 30-50% FOR THE FIRST HOUR OF MAINTENANCE.

CHANGES IN VITAL SIGNS THAT INDICATE A RESPONSE TO SURGICAL STRESS OR LIGHTENING OF ANESTHESIA MAY BE CONTROLLED BY INCREASING THE RATE UP TO A MAXIMUM OF 4.0 µG/KG/MIN AND/OR ADMINISTRATION OF BOLUS DOSES OF 7 µG/KG. IF CHANGES ARE NOT CONTROLLED AFTER THREE BOLUS DOSES GIVEN OVER A FIVE MINUTE PERIOD, A BARBITURATE, VASODILATOR, AND/OR INHALATION AGENT SHOULD BE USED. INFUSION RATES SHOULD ALWAYS BE ADJUSTED DOWNWARD IN THE ABSENCE OF THESE SIGNS UNTIL THERE IS SOME RESPONSE TO SURGICAL STIMULATION.

RATHER THAN AN INCREASE IN INFUSION RATE, 7 µG/KG BOLUS DOSES OF ALFENTANIL HYDROCHLORIDE OR A POTENT INHALATION AGENT SHOULD BE ADMINISTERED IN RESPONSE TO SIGNS OF

LIGHTENING OF ANESTHESIA WITHIN THE LAST 15 MINUTES OF SURGERY. ADMINISTRATION OF ALFENTANIL HYDROCHLORIDE INFUSION SHOULD BE DISCONTINUED AT LEAST 10-15 MINUTES PRIOR TO THE END OF SURGERY.

Protect from light. Store at room temperature 15°-30°C (59°-86°F).

HOW SUPPLIED
INJECTION (C-II): 500 MCG/5 ML

BRAND/MANUFACTURER	NDC	SIZE	AWP
○ **BRAND**			
ALFENTA: Janssen	50458-0060-10	10 ml 5s	$103.84
	50458-0060-20	20 ml 5s	$181.73
	50458-0060-02	2 ml 10s	$71.75
	50458-0060-05	5 ml 10s	$128.60

Alferon N *SEE* INTERFERON ALFA-N3

➤ SHOWN IN PRODUCT IDENTIFICATION GUIDE

Alglucerase

DESCRIPTION

Alglucerase is a modified form of the enzyme, β-glucocerebrosidase (β-D-glucosyl-N-acylsphingosine glucohydrolase, EC 3.2.1.45). Alglucerase is a monomeric glycoprotein of 497 amino acids with carbohydrates making up approximately 6% of the molecule (M_r = 59,300 as determined by SDS-PAGE). The unmodified enzyme (β-glucocerebrosidase) also contains 497 amino acids and contains approximately 12% carbohydrate (M_r = 67,000). The carbohydrates on the unmodified enzyme consist of N-linked carbohydrate chains of the complex and high mannose type. Glucocerebrosidase and Alglucerase catalyze the hydrolysis of the glycolipid, glucocerebroside, within the lysosomes of the reticuloendothelial system.

Alglucerase is prepared by modification of the oligosaccharide chains of human β-glucocerebrosidase. The modification alters the sugar residues at the non-reducing ends of the oligosaccharide chains of the glycoprotein so that they are predominantly terminated with mannose residues which are specifically recognized by carbohydrate receptors on macrophage cells. Alglucerase is supplied as a clear sterile non-pyrogenic solution of Alglucerase in a citrate buffered solution (53 mM citrate, 143 mM sodium) containing 1% albumin human USP. The enzyme is supplied in two strengths, 400 international units per bottle (80 U/mL) and 50 international units per bottle (10 U/mL) with a fill volume of 5 mL per bottle. An international enzyme unit (U) is defined as the amount of enzyme required to hydrolyze in one minute one micromole of the synthetic substrate, 4 methylumbelliferyl-β-glucoside.

Alglucerase is purified from a large pool of human placental tissue collected from selected donors. Steps have been introduced into the manufacturing process to reduce further the risk of viral contamination. However, no procedure has been shown to be totally effective in removing viral infectivity. (See "Precautions"). Each lot of product has been tested and found negative for hepatitis B surface antigen (HBsAg) and for antigens of the human immunodeficiency virus (HIV-1).

CLINICAL PHARMACOLOGY

Alglucerase catalyzes the hydrolysis of the glycolipid, glucocerebroside, to glucose and ceramide as part of the normal degradation pathway for membrane lipids. Glucocerebroside is primarily derived from hematologic cell turnover. Gaucher disease is characterized by a functional deficiency in β-glucocerebrosidase enzymatic activity and the resultant accumulation of lipid glucocerebroside in tissue macrophages which become engorged and are termed Gaucher cells. Gaucher cells are typically found in liver, spleen and bone marrow and occasionally, as well, in lung, kidney and intestine. Secondary hematologic sequelae include severe anemia and thrombocytopenia in addition to the characteristic progressive hepatosplenomegaly. Skeletal complications, including osteonecrosis and osteopenia with secondary pathological fractures, are a common feature of Gaucher disease.

PHARMACOKINETICS

Following an intravenous infusion of different doses (between 0.6 and 234 U/kg) of Alglucerase injection over a 4-hour period, steady-state enzymatic activity was achieved by 60 minutes. Individual steady-state enzymatic activity and area under the curve of the activity increased linearly with the infused dose (0.6 to 121 U/kg). Following infusion termination, plasma enzymatic activity declined rapidly with elimination half-life ranging between 3.6 and 10.4 minutes. Plasma clearance of Alglucerase, calculated from its plasma enzymatic activity, was variable and ranged between 6.34 and 25.39 mL/min/kg, whereas the volume of distribution ranged from 49.4 to 282.1 mL/kg. Within the dosage range of 0.6 and 121 U/kg, elimination half-life, plasma clearance, and volume of distribution values appear to be independent of the infused dose.

PHARMACOLOGIC ACTIONS

Chronic administration of Alglucerase injection in 13 patients with Type 1 Gaucher disease induced the following effects:

1. *Splenomegaly and hepatomegaly* were significantly reduced, presumably by disruption of the lysosomal storage sites and metabolism of glucocerebroside in Gaucher cells. This effect was demonstrated within 6 months of initiation of therapy.
2. *Hematologic deficiencies* in hemoglobin, hematocrit, erythrocyte and platelet counts were significantly improved. In most patients a change in hemoglobin was the first observable effect. In some patients hemoglobin levels were normalized after six months of therapy.
3. *Improved mineralization* occurred in four patients after prolonged treatment as a result of a reduction in the osteolytic actions of lipid-laden Gaucher cells in the marrow.
4. *Cachexia and wasting* in children were reduced.

INDICATIONS AND USAGE

Alglucerase injection is indicated for use as long-term enzyme replacement therapy for patients with a confirmed diagnosis of Type 1 Gaucher disease who exhibit signs and symptoms that are severe enough to result in one or more of the following conditions:

a) moderate-to-severe anemia;
b) thrombocytopenia with bleeding tendency;
c) bone disease;
d) significant hepatomegaly or splenomegaly.

CONTRAINDICATIONS

There are no known contraindications to the use of Alglucerase injection. Treatment with Alglucerase should be discontinued if there is significant clinical evidence of hypersensitivity to the product.

PRECAUTIONS

GENERAL

Therapy with Alglucerase injection should be directed by physicians knowledgeable in the management of patients with Gaucher disease.

Alglucerase is prepared from pooled human placental tissue that may contain the causative agents of some viral diseases. Manufacturing steps have been designed to reduce the risk of transmitting viral infectious agents. These steps have demonstrated *in vitro* inactivation of a panel of model viruses, including human immunodeficiency virus (HIV-1). The risk of contamination from slowly acting or latent viruses, including the Creutzfeldt-Jacob disease agent, is believed to be remote but has not been tested. Accordingly, the benefits and the risks of treatment with this product should be assessed prior to use.

CARCINOGENESIS, MUTAGENESIS, IMPAIRMENT OF FERTILITY

Studies have not been conducted to assess the potential effects of Alglucerase on carcinogenesis, mutagenesis, or impairment of fertility in animals or man.

PREGNANCY CATEGORY C

Animal reproductive studies have not been conducted with Alglucerase. It is also not known whether Alglucerase can cause fetal harm when administered to a pregnant woman, or can affect reproductive capacity. Alglucerase should be given to a pregnant woman only if clearly needed.

NURSING MOTHERS

It is not known whether this drug is excreted in human milk. Because many drugs are excreted in human milk, caution should be exercised when Alglucerase is administered to a nursing woman.

ADVERSE REACTIONS

During clinical studies, involving 31 patients, 28 adverse experiences occurred that were possibly related to Alglucerase injection. Seven of these related to the route of administration and were claims of discomfort, burning and swelling at the site of venipuncture. The remaining 21 experiences (of which approximately 75% were reported by 2 patients) consisted of slight fever, chills, abdominal discomfort, nausea or vomiting. None of these events were judged to require medical intervention.

Most patients treated with Alglucerase on a chronic basis have not formed detectable antibodies. A 72 year old patient was found to demonstrate a positive response in testing procedures designed to detect antibodies to Alglucerase, 6 months after initiation of therapy. Close monitoring of this patient indicated no diminution of clinical response, and therapy has been continued. The clinical significance of this finding and its relationship to Alglucerase is unknown.

OVERDOSE

No obvious toxicity was detected after single doses up to 234 U/kg. There is no experience with higher doses.

DOSAGE AND ADMINISTRATION

Alglucerase injection is administered by intravenous infusion over 1–2 hours. Dosage should be individualized for each patient. An initial dosage up to 60 U/kg of body weight per infusion may be used. The usual frequency of infusion is once every two weeks, but disease severity and patient convenience may dictate administration as often as once every other day or as infrequently as once every four weeks. After patient response is well-established, dosage may be adjusted downward for maintenance therapy. Dosage can be progressively lowered at intervals of 3–6 months while closely monitoring response parameters. Ultrastructural evidence suggests that glucocerebroside lipid storage may respond to doses as low as 1 U/kg.

Alglucerase should not be shaken. Alglucerase should be stored at 2–8°C. Each bottle should be inspected visually for particulate matter and discoloration before use. Any bottles exhibiting particulate matter or discoloration should not be used. DO NOT USE Alglucerase after the expiration date on the bottle.

On the day of use, the appropriate amount of Alglucerase for each patient is diluted with normal saline to a final volume not to exceed 100 mL. Aseptic techniques should be used when diluting the dose. Alglucerase when diluted to 100 mL has been shown to be stable for up to 18 hours when stored at 2–8°C. The use of an in-line particulate filter is recommended for the infusion apparatus. Since Alglucerase does not contain any preservative, after opening, bottles should not be stored for subsequent use.

Relatively low toxicity, combined with the extended time course of response, allows small dosage adjustments to be made occasionally to avoid discarding partially used bottles. Thus, the dosage administered in individual infusions may be slightly increased or decreased to utilize fully each bottle as long as the monthly administered dosage remains substantially unaltered.

J CODES

Per 10 units IV—J0205

HOW SUPPLIED

INJECTION: 10 U/ML

BRAND/MANUFACTURER	NDC	SIZE	AWP
○ **BRAND**			
CEREDASE: Genzyme	58468-1781-01	5 ml	$185.00

◆ RATED THERAPEUTICALLY EQUIVALENT; ◇ THERAPEUTIC EQUIVALENCE UNCONFIRMED; ○ UNRATED

INJECTION: 80 U/ML

BRAND/MANUFACTURER	NDC	SIZE	AWP
○ **BRAND**			
CEREDASE: Genzyme	58468-1060-01	5 ml	$1480.00

Alkeran SEE MELPHALAN

Allent SEE BROMPHENIRAMINE MALEATE AND PSEUDOEPHEDRINE HYDROCHLORIDE

Allergenic Extracts

WARNING

HYPERSENSITIVITY TO INSECT STINGS MAY BE EXTREMELY SEVERE. SINCE THE POTENTIAL FOR SEVERE SYSTEMIC REACTIONS EXISTS IN THE USE OF THESE PRODUCTS, THE HYMENOPTERA VENOM PREPARATIONS SHOULD BE USED ONLY BY PHYSICIANS EXPERIENCED IN ADMINISTERING IMMUNOTHERAPY TO THE MAXIMUM TOLERATED DOSE AND/OR UNDER THE GUIDANCE OF AN ALLERGIST, AND ONLY WHERE ADEQUATE MEANS FOR TREATING SYSTEMIC REACTIONS ARE IMMEDIATELY AVAILABLE. THE PATIENT SHOULD BE FULLY INFORMED OF POSSIBLE RISKS AND SHOULD BE CLOSELY OBSERVED.

ALLERGENIC EXTRACTS MAY POTENTIALLY ELICIT A SEVERE LIFE-THREATENING SYSTEMIC REACTION, RARELY RESULTING IN DEATH.[12] THEREFORE, EMERGENCY MEASURES AND PERSONNEL TRAINED IN THEIR USE SHOULD BE AVAILABLE IMMEDIATELY IN THE EVENT OF SUCH A REACTION. PATIENTS SHOULD BE INSTRUCTED TO RECOGNIZE ADVERSE REACTION SYMPTOMS AND CAUTIONED TO CONTACT THE PHYSICIAN'S OFFICE IF SYMPTOMS OCCUR.

ALL PATIENTS SHOULD HAVE AVAILABLE AN EMERGENCY ANAPHYLAXIS KIT (SUCH AS THE ANA-KIT®) CONTAINING EPINEPHRINE AND BE INSTRUCTED IN ITS USE FOR EMERGENCY TREATMENT OF POSSIBLE SYSTEMIC REACTIONS OCCURRING AT TIMES AFTER THE PATIENT HAS DEPARTED THE TESTING OR TREATMENT PREMISES.

HYPOSENSITIZATION FOR INSECT STING ALLERGY SHOULD BE GIVEN TO THOSE PATIENTS WHO HAVE EXPERIENCED SIGNIFICANT SYSTEMIC REACTIONS (FOR DETAILED DESCRIPTION OF SYMPTOMS SEE "INDICATIONS" AND "ADVERSE REACTIONS") FROM INSECT STINGS AND WHO DEMONSTRATE HYPERSENSITIVITY BY SKIN TESTING WITH THESE PRODUCTS. THE ONLY APPROVED METHOD FOR DIAGNOSING INSECT STING ALLERGIC PATIENTS FOR IMMUNIZATION IS BY SKIN TESTING.

PATIENTS CURRENTLY ON WHOLE BODY HYMENOPTERA INSECT IMMUNOTHERAPY SHOULD BE COMPLETELY RE-EVALUATED BY BOTH HISTORY AND VENOM SKIN TESTING BEFORE TREATMENT WITH THESE VENOM PRODUCTS IS INITIATED.

BEFORE TESTING OR TREATMENT OF PATIENTS WITH THESE PRODUCTS THE PHYSICIAN SHOULD BE THOROUGHLY FAMILIAR WITH ALL ASPECTS OF USE OF THESE PRODUCTS INCLUDING INDICATIONS, RISKS, CONTRAINDICATIONS AND TREATMENT OF ADVERSE REACTIONS.

DESCRIPTION

For diagnosis and immunotherapy of allergic reactions to insect stings, freeze-dried venom of honey bees (**Apis mellifera**) and venom protein of yellow jackets (**Vespula sp.**), yellow hornets (**Dolichovespula arenaria**), white-faced hornets (**Dolichovespula maculata**) and wasps (**Polistes sp.**). A Mixed Vespid Venom Protein (Yellow Jacket, Yellow Hornet and White-Faced Hornet) is for treatment only—not for diagnosis.

Because of the difficulty in collecting all species of yellow jackets and wasps, the venom raw materials for these two insects may vary in species composition from lot to lot. A listing of the exact species content for any particular lot of Yellow Jacket Venom Protein or Wasp Venom Protein may be obtained by calling Technical Services at Miles Inc., 1-800-992-1120.

Venom or venom protein is supplied in 1 mL vials for diagnosis, in 2 mL vials for treatment maintenance, and in 10 mL vials as bulks. The chart below lists for each vial size the content of lyophilized venom protein and for the reconstituted product, the mannitol and venom protein concentrations. Trace amounts of sodium chloride, potassium chloride, acetic acid and beta-alanine, as well as the constituents of the reconstituting fluid, will also be present. (See related table).

Maintenance freeze-dried products can be reconstituted in Sterile Albumin Saline with Phenol (which contains 0.9% NaCl, 0.4% phenol and 0.03% normal human serum albumin). The diagnostic product should be reconstituted only with Sterile Albumin Saline with Phenol. (See "Precautions" and "Dose and Administration") for details of dilutions for diagnosis and treatment.)

Space is provided on the container label to record the date (month, day, year) venom is reconstituted. Refer to dating periods shown under "Precautions". At the time of reconstitution, write the calculated reconstituted product expiration date (month, day, year) on the label in the space provided.

CLINICAL PHARMACOLOGY

The single venom products may be used for both diagnosis and immunotherapy. The Mixed Vespid Venom Protein is for immunotherapy only.

DIAGNOSIS

Diluted solutions of stinging insect venoms injected intradermally will produce wheal and erythema reactions in patients who have significant IgE-mediated, Type 1 immediate hypersensitivity to stings of these insects.

TREATMENT

Repeated injections of increasing doses of insect venom extracts have been shown to ameliorate the intensity of allergic symptoms upon subsequent insect stings.[2,4]

The mechanism by which hyposensitization is achieved is not known completely. IgG antibodies (blocking antibodies) appear in the serum of patients treated with injected venom. No direct relationship has been identified between the level of blocking antibody (or the ratio of blocking antibody to IgE antibody directed to the same venom antigens) and the degree of hyposensitization. However, patients who show protection from symptoms after stings have been found to have significant levels of specific blocking antibody.[2,4]

Initially, after a period of immunotherapy with specific venom antigens, levels of IgE antibody may increase.[4] However, from studies carried out with other venom preparations, these levels are reported to decline after a time.[9] After maintenance level has been reached and maintained, symptoms after stings have been shown to decrease considerably.[2,4]

It is not known if skin-sensitizing antibody can be eradicated or if the patient can be entirely cured, nor is it known how long immunotherapy must be continued.

INDICATIONS

Insect stings may induce a wide range of allergic symptoms in sensitive patients. A normal sting response is initial burning or stinging pain, that may be intense and last several minutes to an hour or more. There is usually some immediate swelling persisting for several days. The location of the sting has considerable influence on the intensity of the pain and extent of swelling. Stings on the fingers or feet produce much pain, but less swelling; whereas a sting on the head or face produces extensive swelling with variable pain.

Local reactions coming on rapidly and larger than the usual local reaction, particularly if the swelling spans both adjacent joints on the extremities, can indicate hypersensitivity. Systemic symptoms appear shortly after the sting, often within seconds to minutes. Symptoms may range from generalized flushing, itching, redness, diffuse swelling of the skin or urticarial wheals, abdominal cramps, nausea, vomiting, or incontinence of urine or stool, to faintness, blurring or loss of vision, unconsciousness, seizures, respiratory or cardiac arrest, or death. Later reactions may consist of fever, achiness, malaise, joint swelling, urticaria or other signs of vascular damage typical of serum sickness, a Type III reaction. Typical delayed Type IV reactions may also occur.[1]

DIAGNOSIS

Skin testing with insect venoms is useful to demonstrate the presence of IgE antibodies which account for the patient's symptoms.[2] Since patients seldom are able to identify the insect which stung them, skin testing is used to determine the insect culprit. Dilutions of these venom products will help judge the sensitivity of the patient and whether the patient should be treated. It is not absolutely known what levels (micrograms) of venom eliciting positive skin tests are diagnostic of clinical sensitivity. However, patients with a history of reactions (any of three types: generalized urticaria or angioedema; respiratory difficulty due either to laryngeal edema or to bronchospasm; or vascular collapse, with or without loss of consciousness) to previous stings and a positive skin test to a venom intradermal injection of approximately 1 microgram (µg) per mL had about a 60% chance of reacting again when stung by the same insect. These patients should receive venom immunotherapy.[2]

Patients with a history of reaction (any of the three reaction types described above) to previous stings, but who did not demonstrate a positive skin test reaction to venom, were considered in a previous study not to be clinically sensitive, and were not treated.[2] We cannot recommend treatment for such patients.

Another study[5] demonstrated false positive reactions when skin testing with venom concentrations of 10 µg/mL and 100 µg/mL was carried out. Thus there can be a nonspecific skin test reaction potentially due to the pharmacological action of the venom at concentrations greater than 1 µg/mL.

The best statement that can be made, at present, is that patients with significant positive history (reactions of the three types described above) following an insect sting, and who do react with a positive skin test to a venom concentration of 1 µg/mL or less, are recommended for treatment. Patients who have the history described above, but who do not react to a 1 µg/mL intradermal venom skin test, cannot be recommended for treatment. The data does not exist, at present, to determine whether a patient who might react to a higher concentration, e.g., 2-10 µg/mL is at risk from a subsequent sting or not. Since it is not known if sting-sensitive patients who subsequently lose their IgE anti-venom

	Vial Size	µg Venom Protein	Reconstitution	mg/mL Mannitol	Venom Protein Concentration
Diagnostics:	1 mL	12	1.2 mL	42 mg/mL	10 µg/mL
Treatment:					
Maintenance					
Single Venom	2 mL	120	1.2 mL	4 mg/mL	100 µg/mL
Mixed Vespid	2 mL	360	1.2 mL	8.3 mg/mL	300 µg/mL

antibody can be resensitized by further stings, it is advisable to retest these patients after any subsequent stings.[2] However, since the level of venom-specific IgE may fall to low levels briefly after a sting, patients should not be re-tested until 2 to 4 weeks after any sting.

TREATMENT

Immunotherapy is indicated for those patients diagnosed as sensitive (see "Diagnosis" above) and is accomplished by using graduated dilutions of the appropriate insect venom or venoms to control the severity of the patient's symptoms from subsequent stings.

Increasing doses of venom are given at intervals, dependent on the patient's ability to tolerate the venoms, until a maintenance dosage (100 µg per venom is recommended — 300 µg in the case of the Mixed Vespid Venom Protein) is reached and maintained. It is considered important that the patient be able to reach this dosage since the efficacy of lower maintenance dosages has not been established.

In a clinical trial, 97% of patients at the maintenance dosage (100 µg per venom) showed no systemic reaction following an insect sting challenge. The remaining 3% had a milder reaction than noted prior to treatment. The patients in this study reached maintenance (100 µg per venom) usually within 2½-3½ months after beginning therapy.[4] Whether efficacy of therapy is influenced by the time required to reach maintenance has not yet been determined.

Venom sensitivity differs for individual patients, thus it is not possible to provide a dosage schedule that is universally suited to all patients. The dosage schedule shown under "Dose and Administration" is a summary of the schedule used in clinical trials of our product and found suitable for the majority of patients.

In highly sensitive patients, the physician may be required to use a modified dose schedule, based on the patient's sensitivity to and tolerance of the injections. Lower initial doses and smaller dosage increments than shown under "Dose and Administration" may be necessary.

CONTRAINDICATIONS

There are no known absolute contraindications to immunotherapy using Hymenoptera Venom Products. However, see "Precautions" for pregnancy risks.

Patients showing negative intradermal skin tests to specific venoms at 1 µg/mL are not recommended for venom treatment.

Any injections, including immunotherapy, should be avoided in patients with a bleeding tendency.

Since routine immunizations have been suspected of exacerbating autoimmune diseases, immunotherapy should be given cautiously to patients with other immunologic diseases and only if the risk from insect stings is greater than the risk of exacerbating the underlying disorder.

WARNINGS

See additional warnings given in box at the beginning of this instruction sheet.

Immunotherapy Injections should never be given intravenously: Subcutaneous injection is recommended. Intracutaneous or intramuscular injections may produce large local reactions or be excessively painful.

After inserting needle, but before injecting, always withdraw the plunger slightly. If blood appears in the syringe, change needles and give the injection in another site: Proper selection of the dose and careful injection should prevent most systemic reactions.

PRECAUTIONS

(1) GENERAL

Reconstitute the single freeze-dried venoms by adding 1.2 mL of diluent (Sterile Albumin Saline with Phenol) to the vial using a sterile syringe. (See chart under "Description".) Swirl or rock the container to dissolve the venom completely. DO NOT SHAKE, since foaming leads to denaturation (inactivation) of protein.

Record date of reconstitution and expiration date of reconstituted product in the space provided on the product label. Date of expiration after reconstitution must not exceed the Final Expiration Date indicated on the container label. (See table below for expiration dates, including dilutions.)

Venom Concentration	Diluent	Recommended Expiration Date*
100 µg/mL	Albumin Saline with Phenol	6 months
10 µg/mL	Albumin Saline with Phenol	1 months
1 µg/mL	Albumin Saline with Phenol	1 months
0.1 µg/mL	Albumin Saline with Phenol	14 days

Venom Concentration	Diluent	Recommended Expiration Date*
Less than 0.1 µg/mL	Albumin Saline with Phenol	Prepare fresh daily

* But not to exceed Final Expiration Date indicated on the container label.

Dilutions: (see table below) must be made in Sterile Albumin Saline with Phenol. They should be made accurately and aseptically, using sterile solution, vials, syringes, etc., and thoroughly mixed by rocking or swirling. DO NOT SHAKE. Maintain stock solutions and dilutions constantly at 2° to 8°C. (See related table).

As an example of the above dilution table: (See related table).

Note: Mixed Vespid Venom Protein concentrations will be three times that shown above.

A sterile tuberculin syringe, with a needle at least ⅝ of an inch long and graduated in 0.01 mL units, should be used to measure each dose from the prescribed dilution. *A separate autoclave sterilized or disposable needle and syringe should be used for each patient to prevent transmission of serum hepatitis and other infectious agents from one person to another.*

Do not re-insert a needle, into a diluent or into a vial containing a different venom, which has been previously inserted into a venom vial. Aseptic techniques should always be employed when administering skin tests and/or treatment injections.

Severe local or systemic reactions to venom administration can occur immediately (within one hour) or as delayed reactions (see "Warning" box at the beginning of this monograph. Patients should be kept under direct observation for at least one hour following skin testing and/or therapeutic injections, and should be instructed to contact the physician promptly if symptoms of an allergic reaction or shock occur. For measures to be taken if the patient exhibits an anaphylactic reaction, see "Adverse Reactions". Patients should be instructed in the use of, and have available, an emergency anaphylaxis kit for self-administration of epinephrine.

(2) CARCINOGENESIS, MUTAGENESIS, IMPAIRMENT OF FERTILITY

Long-term studies in animals have not been conducted with Allergenic Extracts to determine their potential for carcinogenicity, mutagenicity, or impairment of fertility.

(3) PREGNANCY

Pregnancy Category C: Animal reproduction studies have not been conducted with Hymenoptera Venom Products. It is also not known whether Hymenoptera Venom Products can cause fetal harm when administered to a pregnant woman or can affect reproduction capacity. Hymenoptera Venom Products should be given to a pregnant woman only if clearly needed. Specific studies addressing risk to mother and fetus have not been done with venom products. On the basis of histamine's known ability to contract uterine muscle, theoretically, a systemic reaction, whether occurring from allergen exposure or immunotherapy overdose, should be avoided.[3] Therefore, the physician must carefully consider the benefit-to-risk ratio, to both patient and fetus, of continuing a treatment program during pregnancy, and especially the initiation of such a program where there is a possibility that the patient may not be able to reach the recommended maintenance dose without significant risk of a systemic reaction.

(4) NURSING MOTHERS

There are no current studies on secretion of the allergenic extract components in human milk or effect on the nursing infant. Because many drugs are excreted in human milk, caution should be exercised when allergic extracts are administered to a nursing woman.

(5) PEDIATRIC USE

The dosage for children is the same as for adults. Because of the smaller size of the child, the larger volumes of solution may produce excessive discomfort. Therefore, in order to achieve the total dose required, the volume of the dose may need to be divided into more than one injection per visit. A study done in children aged 4 to 17 showed no special problems with immunotherapy in this population.[11]

(6) BETA BLOCKERS[10]

Patients on non-selective beta blockers may be more reactive to allergens given for testing or treatment and may be unresponsive to the usual doses of epinephrine used to treat allergic reactions.

(7) DRUG INTERACTIONS

Certain medications may lessen the skin test wheal and erythema responses elicited by allergens and histamine for varying time periods. Conventional antihistamines should be discontinued at least 5 days before skin testing. Long acting antihistamines (e.g., Astemizole) should be discontinued for at least 3

Extract Volume	Extract Concentration		Diluent Volume		Dilution Concentration
1 part of	100 µg/mL	+	9 parts	=	10 µg/mL
1 part of	10 µg/mL	+	9 parts	=	1 µg/mL
1 part of	1 µg/mL	+	9 parts	=	0.1 µg/mL
1 part of	0.1 µg/mL	+	9 parts	=	0.01 µg/mL
1 part of	0.01 µg/mL	+	9 parts	=	0.001 µg/mL
1 part of	0.001 µg/mL	+	9 parts	=	0.0001 µg/mL

Extract Volume	Extract Concentration		Diluent Volume		Dilution Concentration
0.2 mL of	100 µg/mL	+	1.8 mL	=	10 µg/mL
0.2 mL of	10 µg/mL	+	1.8 mL	=	1 µg/mL
0.2 mL of	1 µg/mL	+	1.8 mL	=	0.1 µg/mL
0.2 mL of	0.1 µg/mL	+	1.8 mL	=	0.01 µg/mL
0.2 mL of	0.01 µg/mL	+	1.8 mL	=	0.001 µg/mL
0.2 mL of	0.001 µg/mL	+	1.8 mL	=	0.0001 µg/mL

weeks prior to skin testing.[13] Topical steroids should be discontinued at the skin test site for at least 2-3 weeks before skin testing.[13,14]

Tricyclic antidepressants such as Doxepin should be withheld for at least 7 days before skin testing.[15] Topical local anesthetics may suppress the flare responses and should be avoided in skin test sites.[16]

ADVERSE REACTIONS

Physicians administering venom testing or treatment materials should be experienced in the treatment of severe systemic reactions (see *"Warning"* box at the beginning of this monograph).

Excessively large, painful or persistent local reactions can occur from skin tests or immunotherapy. Large local reactions occurred in approximately 60% of the patients given immunotherapy. None of the local reactions required specific treatment; however, subsequent injections in many instances were held to the previous dose or a reduced dose. Some patients had repeated large local reactions that slowed the increase in the immunotherapy dose.[4] Frequent application of cold to the area will ameliorate the discomfort. Reactions usually subside in 24-36 hours. Adrenal corticosteroids can be used to hasten clearing of the local reaction.

Systemic reactions may occur at any time after skin tests or immunotherapy. Symptoms may range from mild to life-threatening from anaphylaxis as described under *"Indications"*. In a clinical study some form of systemic response occurred, often repeatedly, in one-third of the patients treated. Only one systemic response occurred on the first dose given. The rest occurred at various times in the course of immunotherapy. Some systemic manifestations may have occurred because of the patient's apprehension, and did not require treatment. Approximately one-fourth of the patients experiencing systemic responses were given some form of specific therapy (epinephrine, theophylline, or metaproterenol), some on several occasions.[4]

If a systemic or anaphylactic reaction does occur, apply a tourniquet above the site of injection and inject 1:1000 epinephrine-hydrochloride intramuscularly or subcutaneously into the opposite arm. Loosen the tourniquet at least every 10 minutes. Do not obstruct arterial blood flow with the tourniquet.

EPINEPHRINE DOSAGE

Adult Dosage: 0.3 to 0.5 mL should be injected. Repeat in 5 to 10 minutes if necessary.

Pediatric Dosage: The usual initial dose is 0.01 mg (mL) per kg body weight or 0.3 mg (mL) per square meter of body surface area. Suggested dosage for infants to 2 years of age is 0.05 mL to 0.1 mL; for children 2 to 6 years, 0.15 mL; and children 6 to 12 years, 0.2 mL. Single pediatric doses should not exceed 0.3 mg (mL). Doses may be repeated as frequently as every 20 minutes, depending on the severity of the condition and the response of the patient.

If epinephrine injection is ineffective, intravenous fluids and vasoactive drugs may be needed to reverse lowered blood pressure.

Oxygen should be given by mask.

Intravenous antihistamine, theophylline ethylene diamine or adrenal corticosteroids may be used if necessary after adequate epinephrine and circulatory support has been given. Patients should have available an emergency anaphylaxis kit (such as the Ana-Kit®) containing epinephrine and be instructed in its use for emergency treatment of possible systemic reactions occurring at times after the patient has departed the treatment premises.

Rarely, severe reactions to insect stings have been reported.[1] These include serum sickness, hematologic abnormalities, and neurological disorders commencing some time after a sting, and not associated with anaphylactoid reactions.

These patients are not candidates for immunotherapy using insect venoms as administration of venoms to such patients is contraindicated.

DOSE AND ADMINISTRATION

Skin Testing: Skin testing should be carried out with all five individual venoms, since many patients have multiple sensitivities.[4] Mixed Vespid Venom Protein should be used only for therapy—not for diagnosis.

Prick testing should be done *before* intradermal testing. In *both* the prick and intradermal tests, a negative control test with diluent alone must be performed.

The flexor surface of the forearm is the usual location for skin testing. It is important that a separate sterile syringe and needle be used for each extract and each patient.

Prick tests are accomplished using a solution of 1 µg venom protein/mL. See *"Precautions"* for instructions on reconstituting and diluting the venom. One drop of the 1 µg/mL venom protein solution is applied to the forearm, and the skin is pricked through the surface of the drop with a sterile 27 gauge needle. The prick is superficial and should not draw blood.

For prick tests, a positive reaction (reaction greater than diluent control) at the 1 µg/mL concentration indicates a high level of sensitivity to the test venom. Patients showing a positive reaction to the prick test at this concentration should begin intradermal tests at concentrations of not more than 0.0001 to 0.001 µg/mL. Patients with negative prick tests may begin intradermal tests at a concentration of 0.001 µg/mL.

Intradermal test dilutions must be made in Sterile Albumin Saline with Phenol, following instructions for reconstitution and dilution of the venom as shown under *"Precautions"*.

A volume of 0.05 mL should be used for intradermal testing. Introduce the needle into the superficial skin layers until the bevel is completely buried, then slowly inject a 0.05 mL aliquot of the venom dilution, making a small bleb.

Start intradermal tests with the most dilute solution. If after 20 minutes no skin reaction is obtained, continue the intradermal testing using ten-fold increments in the concentration until a reaction of 5-10 mm wheal and 11-20 mm erythema is obtained, or until a concentration of 1 µg/mL has been tested, whichever occurs first.

A patient should be considered sensitive to the test venom when a skin response of 5-10 mm wheal, 11-20 mm erythema (or greater) occurs at a concentration of 1 µg/mL or less[5], providing that this reaction is greater than that of the diluent control.

Since the level of insect venom specific IgE may fall to low levels briefly after a reaction to a sting, patients should not be tested until 2 to 4 weeks after any sting.

Immunotherapy: Patients who have multiple venom sensitivities should be given each specific venom injection in a separate site. (Except, if the patient has sensitivities to Yellow Jacket, Yellow Hornet, and White-Faced Hornet venoms concurrently, he can be injected with Mixed Vespid Venom Protein, an equal mixture of these three vespid venoms.) Note which venom preparation is injected at a specific site, so that dosage of that venom preparation can be adjusted if an excessive local reaction occurs. In patients receiving more than one venom, there is theoretically a greater risk of systemic reactions.

Reconstitute and dilute the freeze-dried venom as directed under *"Precautions"*.

Caution: Sensitivity to venom differs from patient to patient. Thus, it is not possible to provide a dosage schedule suitable for all patients. The Suggested Dose Schedule shown below was used in clinical trials[4] and should be suitable for a majority of patients.

In Extremely Sensitive Patients, however, an individualized dose schedule must be employed which will be dicated by the patient's sensitivity. This individualized schedule will probably include weaker dilutions and smaller increments between doses in progressing to the maintenance level (100 µg per venom).

In identifying those patients to be classified as extremely sensitive, individuals reacting with significant skin test (wheal greater than 5 mm and erythema greater than 20 mm) at intradermal skin test concentrations of 0.01 µg/mL or less, or those patients experiencing a systemic reaction to any venom skin test concentration, should be considered highly sensitive.

Suggested Dose Schedule for a single venom: (See related table).

ALTERNATE MAINTENANCE DOSE SCHEDULE

IF THE ABOVE SUGGESTED DOSAGE SCHEDULE HAS BEEN FOLLOWED, DOSE #15 WILL HAVE EMPTIED THE THIRD VIAL OF VENOM. THERE SHOULD NOW BE THREE VIALS OF FREEZE-DRIED VENOM REMAINING IN THE MAINTENANCE SET. IF A SMALLER VOLUME MAINTENANCE DOSE IS DESIRED, THEN THE REMAINING VIALS OF VENOM MAY BE

➤ SHOWN IN PRODUCT IDENTIFICATION GUIDE

RECONSTITUTED WITH 0.6 ML OF STERILE ALBUMIN SALINE WITH PHENOL INSTEAD OF THE PREVIOUSLY RECOMMENDED 1.2 ML. WHEN 0.6 ML IS USED FOR RECONSTITUTION, THE MAINTENANCE DOSE VOLUME THEN BECOMES 0.5 ML INSTEAD OF 1.0 ML. THE 0.5 ML INJECTION WILL STILL CONTAIN 100 MICROGRAMS OF VENOM OR VENOM PROTEIN.

PRECAUTIONS SHOULD BE TAKEN TO ENSURE THAT MAINTENANCE LEVEL INJECTIONS OF 0.5 ML ARE GIVEN ONLY FROM THOSE VIALS OF VENOM THAT HAVE BEEN RECONSTITUTED WITH 0.6 ML OF DILUTING FLUID. ANY OTHER VOLUME USED FOR RECONSTITUTION WILL NOT GIVE 100 MICROGRAMS OF VENOM OR VENOM PROTEIN AT A DOSAGE OF 0.5 ML.

Sterile Albumin Saline with Phenol must be used to make treatment dilutions.

In a previous clinical study with Hollister-Stier venom products, injections (using this Suggested Dose Schedule) were given once per week at one study center, and twice or more per week at another center. (For further discussion, see below.)[4] It must be considered important to achieve the 100 µg per venom maintenance dose (the maintenance dose for Mixed Vespid Venom Protein is 300 µg), since there is no data on effectiveness of maintenance levels below 100 µg per venom.

In deciding the criteria for proceeding from dose to dose of the Suggested Dose Schedule (see below), the results of a recent clinical study[4] should be considered. A study center "A" reporting the least number of systemic reactions during pre-maintenance treatment held the dose constant in most of the cases where significant local reactions occurred. With the systemic reactions reported, this center held the dose the same in approximately 80% of the incidences. The treatment injections were given at this center usually once per week, and if a patient missed an appointment, the next dose was often the same as the preceding dose (depending on the previous reactivity of the patient). Patients treated at this center reached maintenance in an average of 17-19 visits.

Another study center "B" reporting a higher incidence of systemic reactions, was more regimented in following the Suggested Dose Schedule. This center reduced or held the dose the same in less than 10% of the cases reporting significant local reactions. With the systemic reactions reported, this center held the dose the same or reduced the dosage in approximately 20% of the cases. This center gave more than one injection per week at the outset as circumstances and sensitivity allowed. Patients treated at this center reached maintenance in an average of 14 visits.

Therefore, in proceeding with the Suggested Dose Schedule, or modified (for highly sensitive patients) schedules, it is suggested that if a systemic, extremely large local (10 cm or more induration, or other severe local symptoms), or persistent and severe delayed local reaction occurs, the dose at the next visit should be held constant (or reduced, depending on judgment of the severity of the reaction) as was done at study center "A" which reported the least number of systemic reactions during the course of therapy.

Following the achievement of maintenance level (100 µg per venom), approximately 80% or more patients were given a second maintenance injection at a 1-week interval. The third maintenance injection was usually (in approximately 60% of the patients) at a 2-week interval. The next injection was usually within 3 weeks, and the patients were then injected for ongoing maintenance at approximately monthly intervals.[4] It is suggested that if a systemic, extremely large local (10 cm or more induration, or other severe local symptoms), or persistent and severe delayed local reaction occurs following a maintenance injection, the dose at the next visit should still remain constant.

The optimum duration for immunotherapy is not known, so current recommendations are that maintenance injections be continued indefinitely, year around, particularly in patients experiencing life-threatening anaphylaxis after insect stings.

OVERDOSE

In the event that an anaphylactic reaction occurs from overdose or inadvertent injection into the blood stream, treat with epinephrine as directed under "Adverse Reactions".

Local reactions at the site of injection in the form of a wheal or swelling occur frequently and are not cause for alarm, but if they persist are indication that dosage may need adjustment.

Prolonged pain, or pain radiating up the arm usually means the injection has been given intramuscularly. The increased pain from this route of injection is undesirable. For best results, be sure to inject subcutaneously.

REFERENCES

1. Reisman, R. E., *Allergy Principles and Practice.* Middleton, E., Reed, C. E., and Ellis, E. F., editors. C. V. Mosby Co., 1978. 2. Hunt, K. J., Valentine, M.D., Sobotka, A. K., Benton, A. W., Amodio, F. J., and Lichtenstein, L. M. A controlled trial of immunotherapy in insect hypersensitivity. *New Eng. J. Med.* 299: 157-161. July 27, 1978. 3. Metzger, W. J., Turner, E., and Patterson, R. The safety of immunotherapy during pregnancy, *J. Allergy Clin. Immunol.* 61 (4): 268-272, 1978. 4. Summary of data from BB-IND 1292 clinical studies, 1978-79, on Hollister-Stier products. 5. Hunt, K. J., Valentine, M.D., Sobotka, A. K., Lichtenstein, L. M. Diagnosis of allergy to stinging insects by skin testing with hymenoptera venoms. *Annals Int. Med.* 85: 56-59, 1976. 6. Kern, F., Sobotka, A. K., Valentine, M.D., Benton, A. W., Lichtenstein, L. M. Allergy to insect sting. *J. Allergy Clin. Immunol.* 57 (6): 554-559, 1976. 7. Claude, C., Shulman, S., Arbesman, C. E. The allergic response to stinging insects. *J Allergy.* 36 (1): 12-22, 1965. 8. Sobotka, A. K., Adkinson, N. F., Jr., Valentine, M. D., and Lichtenstein, L. M. Allergy to insect stings. IV. Diagnosis by R.A.S.T. *J. Immunol.* 121 (6): 2477-2484, 1978. 9. Amodio, F., Markedly, L., Valentine, M.D., Sobotka, A. K., Lichtenstein, L. M. Maintenance immunotherapy for hymenoptera sensitivity. *J. Allergy Clin. Immunol.* 61 (3): 134, 1978. 10. Jacobs, Robert L., Goeffrey W. Rake, Jr., et. al. Potentiated anaphylaxis in patients with drug-induced beta-adrenergic blockade. *J. Allergy and Clin. Immunol.* 68 (2): 125-127, August 1981. 11. Graft, D., Schuberth, K., Kagey-Sobotka, A., Kwiterovich, K., Niv, Y., Lichtenstein, L., Valentine, M. Assessment of prolonged venom immunotherapy in children. *J. Allergy Clin. Immunol.* 80 (2): 162-169, August 1987. 12. Lockey, Richard F., Linda M. Benedict, Paul C. Turkeltaub, Samuel C. Bukantz. Fatalities from immunotherapy (IT) and skin testing (ST). *J. Allergy Clin. Immunol.* 79 (4): 660-677, 1987. 13. Pipkorn, U. Pharmacological influence of anti-allergic medication on *in Vivo* allergen testing. *Allergy.* 43: 81-86, 1988. 14. Andersson, M. and U. Pipkorn. Inhibition of the dermal immediate allergic reaction through prolonged treatment with topical glucol corical steroids. *J. Allergy Clinical Immunology.* 79 (2): 345-349, February 1987. 15. Rao, Kamineni S., et al. Duration of suppressive effect of tricyclic antidepressants on histamine induced wheal and flare reactions on human skin. *Allergy Clinical Immunology.* 82: 752-757, November 1988. 16. Pipkorn, Ulf, and M. Andersson. Topical dermal anesthesia inhibits the flare but not the wheal response to allergen and histamine in the skin prick test. *Clinical Allergy.* 17:307-311, 1987.

J CODES

SC,IM—J0240
SC,IM—J0220
Single dose—J7010
SC,IM—J0230
Multiple dose—J7020

HOW SUPPLIED
INJECTION:

BRAND/MANUFACTURER	NDC	SIZE	AWP
○ **BRAND**			
VENOMIL: Miles Allergy	00118-9940-12	6s	$45.39
	00118-9943-12	6s	$66.18
	00118-9945-12	6s	$115.53
ALBAY VENOMIL: Miles Allergy	00118-9940-05	5.5 ml	$36.35
	00118-9945-05	5.5 ml	$88.26

INJECTION: 10,000 PNU/ML

BRAND/MANUFACTURER	NDC	SIZE	AWP
○ **BRAND**			
ALLPYRAL SPECIAL MIX BULK POLLENS: Miles Allergy	00118-6685-10	10 ml	$74.15
ALLPYRAL SPECIAL MIX BULK EPIDERMAL: Miles Allergy	00118-6687-10	10 ml	$74.15
ALLPYRAL SPECIAL MIX BULK INHALANTS: Miles Allergy	00118-6689-10	10 ml	$74.15
ALLPYRAL SPECIAL MIX BULK MOLDS: Miles Allergy	00118-6691-10	10 ml	$91.55
ALLPYRAL SPECIAL MIX BULK POLLENS: Miles Allergy	00118-6685-30	30 ml	$200.52
ALLPYRAL SPECIAL MIX BULK EPIDERMAL: Miles Allergy	00118-6687-30	30 ml	$200.52
ALLPYRAL SPECIAL MIX BULK INHALANTS: Miles Allergy	00118-6689-30	30 ml	$200.52
ALLPYRAL SPECIAL MIX BULK MOLDS: Miles Allergy	00118-6691-30	30 ml	$249.69

Dose No.	*Volume of 1 µg/mL	Dose No.	Volume of 10 µg/mL	Dose No.	Volume of 100 µg/mL
1	0.05 mL	5	0.05 mL	9	0.05 mL
2	0.10 mL	6	0.10 mL	10	0.10 mL
3	0.20 mL	7	0.20 mL	11	0.20 mL
4	0.40 mL	8	0.40 mL	12	0.40 mL
				13	0.60 mL
				14	0.80 mL
				15	1.00 mL

Mixed Vespid Venom will contain three times the venom protein per mL shown in this table.
*See preceeding "Caution" section.

INJECTION: 20,000 PNU/ML

BRAND/MANUFACTURER	NDC	SIZE	AWP
○ **BRAND**			
ALLPYRAL SPECIAL MIX BULK POLLENS: Miles Allergy	00118-6686-10	10 ml	$86.66
ALLPYRAL SPECIAL MIX BULK EPIDERMAL: Miles Allergy	00118-6688-10	10 ml	$86.66
ALLPYRAL SPECIAL MIX BULK INHALANTS: Miles Allergy	00118-6690-10	10 ml	$86.66
ALLPYRAL SPECIAL MIX BULK POLLENS: Miles Allergy	00118-6686-30	30 ml	$233.07
ALLPYRAL SPECIAL MIX BULK EPIDERMAL: Miles Allergy	00118-6688-30	30 ml	$233.07
ALLPYRAL SPECIAL MIX BULK INHALANTS: Miles Allergy	00118-6690-30	30 ml	$233.07

KIT:

BRAND/MANUFACTURER	NDC	SIZE	AWP
○ **GENERICS**			
DIAGNOSTIC KIT: Alk	53298-1401-01	1s	$.00

SET:

BRAND/MANUFACTURER	NDC	SIZE	AWP
○ **BRAND**			
HOUSE DUST TREATMENT SET: Miles Allergy	00118-6770-01	1s	$49.97
7 GRASS MIX TREATMENT SET: Miles Allergy	00118-6701-01	1s	$49.97
9 SO. GRASS GROUP TREATMENT SET: Miles Allergy	00118-6700-01	1s	$49.97
ALLPYRAL SPECIAL MIX TREATMENT SET: Miles Allergy	00118-6684-01	1s	$109.72

Allopurinol

DESCRIPTION

Allopurinol is known chemically as 1,5-dihydro-4H-pyrazolo[3,4-d]pyrimidin-4-one. It is a xanthine oxidase inhibitor which is administered orally. Its solubility in water at 37°C is 80.0 mg/dL and is greater in an alkaline solution.

Following is its chemical structure:

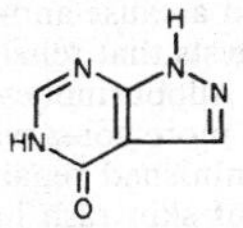

CLINICAL PHARMACOLOGY

Allopurinol acts on purine catabolism, without disrupting the biosynthesis of purines. It reduces the production of uric acid by inhibiting the biochemical reactions immediately preceding its formation.

Allopurinol is a structural analogue of the natural purine base, hypoxanthine. It is an inhibitor of xanthine oxidase, the enzyme responsible for the conversion of hypoxanthine to xanthine and of xanthine to uric acid, the end product of purine metabolism in man. Allopurinol is metabolized to the corresponding xanthine analogue, oxipurinol (alloxanthine), which also is an inhibitor of xanthine oxidase.

It has been shown that reutilization of both hypoxanthine and xanthine for nucleotide and nucleic acid synthesis is markedly enhanced when their oxidations are inhibited by Allopurinol and oxipurinol. This reutilization does not disrupt normal nucleic acid anabolism, however, because feedback inhibition is an integral part of purine biosynthesis. As a result of xanthine oxidase inhibition, the serum concentration of hypoxanthine plus xanthine in patients receiving Allopurinol for treatment of hyperuricemia is usually in the range of 0.3 to 0.4 mg/dL compared to a normal level of approximately 0.15 mg/dL. A maximum of 0.9 mg/dL of these oxypurines has been reported when the serum urate was lowered to less than 2 mg/dL by high doses of Allopurinol. These values are far below the saturation levels at which point their precipitation would be expected to occur (above 7 mg/dL).

The renal clearance of hypoxanthine and xanthine is at least 10 times greater than that of uric acid. The increased xanthine and hypoxanthine in the urine have not been accompanied by problems of nephrolithiasis. Xanthine crystalluria has been reported in only three patients. Two of the patients had Lesch-Nyhan syndrome, which is characterized by excessive uric acid production combined with a deficiency of the enzyme, hypoxanthineguanine phosphoribosyltransferase (HGPRTase). This enzyme is required for the conversion of hypoxanthine, xanthine, and guanine to their respective nucleotides. The third patient had lymphosarcoma and produced an extremely large amount of uric acid because of rapid cell lysis during chemotherapy.

Allopurinol is approximately 90% absorbed from the gastrointestinal tract. Peak plasma levels generally occur at 1.5 hours and 4.5 hours for Allopurinol and oxipurinol respectively, and after a single oral dose of 300 mg Allopurinol, maximum plasma levels of about 3 μg/mL of Allopurinol and 6.5 μg/mL of oxipurinol are produced.

Approximately 20% of the ingested Allopurinol is excreted in the feces. Because of its rapid oxidation to oxipurinol and a renal clearance rate approximately that of glomerular filtration rate, Allopurinol has a plasma half-life of about 1-2 hours. Oxipurinol, however, has a longer plasma half-life (approximately 15.0 hours) and therefore effective xanthine oxidase inhibition is maintained over a 24-hour period with single daily doses of Allopurinol. Whereas Allopurinol is cleared essentially by glomerular filtration, oxipurinol is reabsorbed in the kidney tubules in a manner similar to the reabsorption of uric acid.

The clearance of oxipurinol is increased by uricosuric drugs, and as a consequence, the addition of a uricosuric agent reduces to some degree the inhibition of xanthine oxidase by oxipurinol and increases to some degree the urinary excretion of uric acid. In practice, the net effect of such combined therapy may be useful in some patients in achieving minimum serum uric acid levels provided the total urinary uric acid load does not exceed the competence of the patient's renal function.

Hyperuricemia may be primary, as in gout, or secondary to diseases such as acute and chronic leukemia, polycythemia vera, multiple myeloma, and psoriasis. It may occur with the use of diuretic agents, during renal dialysis, in the presence of renal damage, during starvation or reducing diets and in the treatment of neoplastic disease where rapid resolution of tissue masses may occur. Asymptomatic hyperuricemia is not an indication for Allopurinol treatment (see *"Indications and Usage"*).

Gout is a metabolic disorder which is characterized by hyperuricemia and resultant deposition of monosodium urate in the tissues, particularly the joints and kidneys. The etiology of this hyperuricemia is the overproduction of uric acid in relation to the patient's ability to excrete it. If progressive deposition of urates is to be arrested or reversed, it is necessary to reduce the serum uric acid level below the saturation point to suppress urate precipitation.

Administration of Allopurinol generally results in a fall in both serum and urinary uric acid within two to three days. The degree of this decrease can be manipulated almost at will since it is dose-dependent. A week or more of treatment with Allopurinol may be required before its full effects are manifested; likewise, uric acid may return to pretreatment levels slowly (usually after a period of seven to ten days following cessation of therapy). This reflects primarily the accumulation and slow clearance of oxipurinol. In some patients a dramatic fall in urinary uric acid excretion may not occur, particularly in those with severe tophaceous gout. It has been postulated that this may be due to the mobilization of urate from tissue deposits as the serum uric acid level begins to fall.

Allopurinol's action differs from that of uricosuric agents, which lower the serum uric acid level by increasing urinary excretion of uric acid. Allopurinol reduces both the serum and urinary uric acid levels by inhibiting the formation of uric acid. The use of Allopurinol to block the formation of urates avoids the hazard of increased renal excretion of uric acid posed by uricosuric drugs.

Allopurinol can substantially reduce serum and urinary uric acid levels in previously refractory patients even in the presence of renal damage serious enough to render uricosuric drugs virtually ineffective. Salicylates may be given conjointly for their antirheumatic effect without compromising the action of Allopurinol. This is in contrast to the nullifying effect of salicylates on uricosuric drugs.

Allopurinol also inhibits the enzymatic oxidation of mercaptopurine, the sulfur-containing analogue of hypoxanthine, to 6-thiouric acid. This oxidation, which is catalyzed by xanthine oxidase, inactivates mercaptopurine. Hence, the inhibition of such oxidation by Allopurinol may result in as much as a 75% reduction in the therapeutic dose requirement of mercaptopurine when the two compounds are given together.

INDICATIONS AND USAGE

THIS IS NOT AN INNOCUOUS DRUG. IT IS NOT RECOMMENDED FOR THE TREATMENT OF ASYMPTOMATIC HYPER- URICEMIA.

Allopurinol reduces serum and urinary uric acid concentrations. Its use should be individualized for each patient and requires an understanding of its mode of action and pharmacokinetics (see *"Clinical Pharmacology"*, *"Contraindications"*, *"Warnings"* and *"Precautions"*).

Allopurinol is indicated in:

(1) the management of patients with signs and symptoms of primary or secondary gout (acute attacks, tophi, joint destruction, uric acid lithiasis and/or nephropathy).
(2) the management of patients with leukemia, lymphoma and malignancies who are receiving cancer therapy which causes elevations of serum and urinary uric acid levels Allopurinol treatment should be discontinued when the potential for overproduction of uric acid is no longer present.
(3) the management of patients with recurrent calcium oxalate calculi whose daily uric acid excretion exceeds 800 mg/day in male patients and 750 mg/day in female patients. Therapy in such patients should be carefully assessed initially and reassessed periodically to determine in each case that treatment is beneficial and that the benefits outweigh the risks.

CONTRAINDICATIONS

Patients who have developed a severe reaction to Allopurinol should not be restarted on the drug.

WARNINGS

ALLOPURINOL SHOULD BE DISCONTINUED AT THE FIRST APPEARANCE OF SKIN RASH OR OTHER SIGNS WHICH MAY INDICATE AN ALLERGIC REACTION. In some instances a skin rash may be followed by more severe hypersensitivity reactions such as exfoliative, urticarial and purpuric lesions as well as Stevens-Johnson syndrome (erythema multiforme exudativum), and/or generalized vasculitis, irreversible hepatotoxicity and on rare occasions death.

In patients receiving Purinethol® (mercaptopurine) or Imuran® (azathioprine), the concomitant administration of 300-600 mg of Allopurinol per day will require a reduction in dose to approximately one-third to one-fourth of the usual dose of mercaptopurine or azathioprine. Subsequent adjustment of doses of mercaptopurine or azathioprine should be made on the basis of therapeutic response and the appearance of toxic effects (see *"Clinical Pharmacology"*).

A few cases of reversible clinical hepatotoxicity have been noted in patients taking Allopurinol, and in some patients asymptomatic rises in serum alkaline phosphatase or serum transaminase have been observed. If anorexia, weight loss or pruritus develop in patients on Allopurinol, evaluation of liver function should be part of their diagnostic workup. In patients with pre-existing liver disease, periodic liver function tests are recommended during the early stages of therapy. Due to the occasional occurrence of drowsiness, patients should be alerted to the need for due precaution when engaging in activities where alertness is mandatory.

The occurrence of hypersensitivity reactions to Allopurinol may be increased in patients with decreased renal function receiving thiazides and Allopurinol concurrently. For this reason, in this clinical setting, such combinations should be administered with caution and patients should be observed closely.

PRECAUTIONS

General: An increase in acute attacks of gout has been reported during the early stages of Allopurinol administration, even when normal or subnormal serum uric acid levels have been attained. Accordingly, maintenance doses of colchicine generally should be given prophylactically when Allopurinol is begun. In addition, it is recommended that the patient start with a low dose of Allopurinol (100 mg daily) and increase at weekly intervals by 100 mg until a serum uric acid level of 6 mg/dL or less is attained but without exceeding the maximum recommended dose (800 mg per day). The use of colchicine or anti-inflammatory agents may be required to suppress gouty attacks in some cases. The attacks usually become shorter and less severe after several months of therapy. The mobilization of urates from tissue deposits which cause fluctuations in the serum uric acid levels may be a possible explanation for these episodes. Even with adequate Allopurinol therapy, it may require several months to deplete the uric acid pool sufficiently to achieve control of the acute attacks.

A fluid intake sufficient to yield a daily urinary output of at least two liters and the maintenance of a neutral or, preferably, slightly alkaline urine are desirable to (1) avoid the theoretical possibility of formation of xanthine calculi under the influence of Allopurinol therapy and (2) help prevent renal precipitation of urates in patients receiving concomitant uricosuric agents.

Some patients with pre-existing renal disease or poor urate clearance have shown a rise in BUN during Allopurinol administration. Although the mechanism responsible for this has not been established, patients with impaired renal function should be carefully observed during the early stages of Allopurinol administration and dosage decreased or the drug withdrawn if increased abnormalities in renal function appear and persist.

Renal failure in association with Allopurinol administration has been observed among patients with hyperuricemia secondary to neoplastic diseases. Concurrent conditions such as multiple myeloma and congestive myocardial disease were present among those patients whose renal dysfunction increased after Allopurinol was begun. Renal failure is also frequently associated with gouty nephropathy and rarely with Allopurinol-associated hypersensitivity reactions. Albuminuria has been observed among patients who developed clinical gout following chronic glomerulonephritis and chronic pyelonephritis.

Patients with decreased renal function require lower doses of Allopurinol than those with normal renal function. Lower than recommended doses should be used to initiate therapy in any patients with decreased renal function and they should be observed closely during the early stages of Allopurinol administration. In patients with severely impaired renal function or decreased urate clearance, the half-life of oxipurinol in the plasma is greatly prolonged. Therefore, a dose of 100 mg per day or 300 mg twice a week, or perhaps less, may be sufficient to maintain adequate xanthine oxidase inhibition to reduce serum urate levels.

Bone marrow depression has been reported in patients receiving Allopurinol, most of whom received concomitant drugs with the potential for causing this reaction. This has occurred as early as six weeks to as long as six years after the initiation of Allopurinol therapy. Rarely a patient may develop varying degrees of bone marrow depression, affecting one or more cell lines, while receiving Allopurinol alone.

Information for Patients: Patients should be informed of the following:

(1) They should be cautioned to discontinue Allopurinol and to consult their physician immediately at the first sign of a skin rash, painful urination, blood in the urine, irritation of the eyes, or swelling of the lips or mouth. (2) They should be reminded to continue drug therapy prescribed for gouty attacks since optimal benefit of Allopurinol may be delayed for two to six weeks. (3) They should be encouraged to increase fluid intake during therapy to prevent renal stones. (4) If a single dose of Allopurinol is occasionally forgotten, there is no need to double the dose at the next scheduled time. (5) There may be certain risks associated with the concomitant use of Allopurinol and dicumarol, sulfinpyrazone, mercaptopurine, azathioprine, ampicillin, amoxicillin and thiazide diuretics, and they should follow the instructions of their physician. (6) Due to the occasional occurrence of drowsiness, patients should take precautions when engaging in activities where alertness is mandatory. (7) Patients may wish to take Allopurinol after meals to minimize gastric irritation.

Laboratory Tests: The correct dosage and schedule for maintaining the serum uric acid within the normal range is best determined by using the serum uric acid as an index. In patients with pre-existing liver disease, periodic liver function tests are recommended during the early stages of therapy (see *"Warnings"*).

Allopurinol and its primary active metabolite oxipurinol are eliminated by the kidneys; therefore, changes in renal function have a profound effect on dosage. In patients with decreased renal function or who have concurrent illnesses which can affect renal function such as hypertension and diabetes mellitus, periodic laboratory parameters of renal function, particularly BUN and serum creatinine or creatinine clearance, should be performed and the patient's Allopurinol dosage reassessed.

The prothrombin time should be reassessed periodically in the patients receiving dicumarol who are given Allopurinol.

Drug Interactions: In patients receiving Purinethol (mercaptopurine) or Imuran (azathioprine), the concomitant administration of 300-600 mg of Allopurinol will require a reduction in dose to approximately one-third to one-fourth of the usual dose of mercaptopurine or azathioprine. Subsequent adjustment of doses of mercaptopurine or azathioprine should be made on the basis of therapeutic response and the appearance of toxic effects (see *"Clinical Pharmacology"*).

It has been reported that Allopurinol prolongs the half-life of the anticoagulant, dicumarol. The clinical basis of this drug interaction has not been established but should be noted when Allopurinol is given to patients already on dicumarol therapy.

Since the excretion of oxipurinol is similar to that of urate, uricosuric agents, which increase the excretion of urate, are also likely to increase the excretion of oxipurinol and thus lower the degree of inhibition of xanthine oxidase. The concomitant administration of uricosuric agents and Allopurinol has been associated with a decrease in the excretion of oxypurines (hypoxanthine and xanthine) and an increase in urinary uric acid excretion compared with that observed with Allopurinol alone. Although clinical evidence to date has not demonstrated renal precipitation of oxypurines in patients either on Allopurinol alone or in combination with uricosuric agents, the possibility should be kept in mind.

The reports that the concomitant use of Allopurinol and thiazide diuretics may contribute to the enhancement of Allopurinol toxicity in some patients have been reviewed in an attempt to establish a cause-and-effect relationship and a mechanism of causation. Review of these case reports indicates that the patients were mainly receiving thiazide diuretics for hypertension and that tests to rule out decreased renal function secondary to hypertensive nephropathy were not often performed. In those patients in whom renal insufficiency was documented, however, the recommendation to lower the dose of Allopurinol was not followed. Although a causal mechanism and a cause-and-effect relationship have not been established, current evidence suggests that renal function should be monitored in patients on thiazide diuretics and Allopurinol even in the absence of renal failure, and dosage levels should be even more conservatively adjusted in those patients on such combined therapy if diminished renal function is detected.

An increase in the frequency of skin rash has been reported among patients receiving ampicillin or amoxicillin concurrently with Allopurinol compared to patients who are not receiving both drugs. The cause of the reported association has not been established.

Enhanced bone marrow suppression by cyclophosphamide and other cytotoxic agents has been reported among patients with neoplastic disease, except leukemia, in the presence of Allopurinol. However, in a well-controlled study of patients with lymphoma on combination therapy, Allopurinol did not increase the marrow toxicity of patients treated with cyclophosphamide, doxorubicin, bleomycin, procarbazine and/or mechlorethamine.

Tolbutamide's conversion to inactive metabolites has been shown to be catalyzed by xanthine oxidase from rat liver. The clinical significance, if any, of these observations is unknown.

Chlorpropamide's plasma half-life may be prolonged by Allopurinol, since Allopurinol and chlorpropamide may compete for excretion in the renal tubule. The risk of hypoglycemia secondary to this mechanism may be increased if Allopurinol and chlorpropamide are given concomitantly in the presence of renal insufficiency.

Drug/Laboratory Test Interactions: Allopurinol is not known to alter the accuracy of laboratory tests.

Pregnancy: Teratogenic Effects: Pregnancy Category C. Reproductive studies have been performed in rats and rabbits at doses up to twenty times the usual human dose (5 mg/kg/day), and it was concluded that there was no impaired fertility or harm to the fetus due to Allopurinol. There is a published report of a study in pregnant mice given 50 or 100 mg/kg Allopurinol intraperitoneally on gestation days 10 or 13. There were increased numbers of dead fetuses in dams given 100 mg/kg Allopurinol but not in those given 50 mg/kg. There were increased numbers of external malformations in fetuses at both doses of Allopurinol on gestation day 10 and increased numbers of skeletal malformations in fetuses at both doses on gestation day 13. It cannot be determined whether this represented a fetal effect or an effect secondary to maternal toxicity. There are, however, no adequate or well-controlled studies in pregnant women. Because animal reproduction studies are not always predictive of human response, this drug should be used during pregnancy only if clearly needed.

Experience with Allopurinol during human pregnancy has been limited partly because women of reproductive age rarely require treatment with Allopurinol. There are two unpublished reports and one published paper of women giving birth to normal offspring after receiving Allopurinol during pregnancy.

Nursing Mothers: Allopurinol and oxipurinol have been found in the milk of a mother who was receiving Allopurinol. Since the effect of Allopurinol on the nursing infant is unknown, caution should be exercised when Allopurinol is administered to a nursing woman.

Pediatric Use: Allopurinol is rarely indicated for use in children with the exception of those with hyperuricemia secondary to malignancy or to certain rare inborn errors of purine metabolism (see *"Indications"* and *"Dosage and Administration"*).

ADVERSE REACTIONS

Data upon which the following estimates of incidence of adverse reactions are made are derived from experiences reported in the literature, unpublished clinical trials and voluntary reports since marketing of Allopurinol began. Past experience suggested that the most frequent event following the initiation of Allopurinol treatment was an increase in acute attacks of gout (average 6% in early studies). An analysis of current usage suggests that the incidence of acute gouty attacks has diminished to less than 1%. The explanation for this decrease has not been determined but may be due in part to initiating therapy more gradually (see *"Precautions"* and *"Dosage and Administration"*).

The most frequent adverse reaction to Allopurinol is skin rash. Skin reactions can be severe and sometimes fatal. Therefore, treatment with Allopurinol should be discontinued immediately if a rash develops (see *"Warnings"*). Some patients with the most severe reaction also had fever, chills, arthralgias, cholestatic jaundice, eosinophilia and mild leukocytosis or leukopenia. Among 55 patients with gout treated with Allopurinol for 3 to 34 months (average greater than 1 year) and followed prospectively, Rundles observed that 3% of patients developed a type of drug reaction which was predominantly a pruritic maculopapular skin eruption, sometimes scaly or exfoliative. However, with current usage, skin reactions have been observed less frequently than 1%. The explanation for this decrease is not obvious. The incidence of skin rash may be increased in the presence of renal insufficiency. The frequency of skin rash among patients receiving ampicillin or amoxicillin concurrently with Allopurinol has been reported to be increased (see *"Precautions"*).

MOST COMMON REACTIONS* PROBABLY CAUSALLY RELATED

Gastrointestinal: diarrhea, nausea, alkaline phosphatase increase, SGOT/SGPT increase

Metabolic and Nutritional: acute attacks of gout

Skin and Appendages: rash, maculopapular rash

*Early clinical studies and incidence rates from early clinical experience with Allopurinol suggested that these adverse reactions were found to occur at a rate of greater than 1%. The most frequent event observed was acute attacks of gout following the initiation of therapy. Analyses of current usage suggest that the incidence of these adverse reactions is now less than 1%. The explanation for this decrease has not been determined, but it may be due to following recommended usage (see *"Adverse Reactions"* introduction, *"Indications"*, *"Precautions"* and *"Dosage and Administration"*).

INCIDENCE LESS THAN 1% PROBABLY CAUSALLY RELATED

Body as a Whole: ecchymosis, fever, headache

Cardiovascular: necrotizing angiitis, vasculitis

Gastrointestinal: hepatic necrosis, granulomatous hepatitis, hepatomegaly, hyperbilirubinemia, cholestatic jaundice, vomiting, intermittent abdominal pain, gastritis, dyspepsia

Hemic and Lymphatic: thrombocytopenia, eosinophilia, leukocytosis, leukopenia

Musculoskeletal: myopathy, arthralgias

Nervous: peripheral neuropathy, neuritis, paresthesia, somnolence

Respiratory: epistaxis

Skin and Appendages: erythema multiforme exudativum (Stevens-Johnson syndrome), toxic epidermal necrolysis (Lyell's syndrome), hypersensitivity vasculitis, purpura, vesicular bullous dermatitis, exfoliative dermatitis, eczematoid dermatitis, pruritus, urticaria, alopecia, onycholysis, lichen planus

Special Senses: taste loss/perversion

Urogenital: renal failure, uremia (see *"Precautions"*)

INCIDENCE LESS THAN 1% CAUSAL RELATIONSHIP UNKNOWN

Body as a Whole: malaise

Cardiovascular: pericarditis, peripheral vascular disease, thrombophlebitis, bradycardia, vasodilation

Endocrine: infertility (male), hypercalcemia, gynecomastia (male)

Gastrointestinal: hemorrhagic pancreatitis, gastrointestinal bleeding, stomatitis, salivary gland swelling, hyperlipidemia, tongue edema, anorexia

Hemic and Lymphatic: aplastic anemia, agranulocytosis, eosinophilic fibrohistiocytic lesion of bone marrow, pancytopenia, prothrombin decrease, anemia, hemolytic anemia, reticulocytosis, lymphadenopathy, lymphocytosis

Musculoskeletal: myalgia

Nervous: optic neuritis, confusion, dizziness, vertigo, foot drop, decrease in libido, depression, amnesia, tinnitus, asthenia, insomnia

Respiratory: bronchospasm, asthma, pharyngitis, rhinitis

Skin and Appendages: furunculosis, facial edema, sweating, skin edema

Special Senses: cataracts, macular retinitis, iritis, conjunctivitis, amblyopia

Urogenital: nephritis, impotence, primary hematuria, albuminuria

OVERDOSAGE

Massive overdosing or acute poisoning by Allopurinol has not been reported.

In mice the 50% lethal dose (LD_{50}) is 160 mg/kg given intraperitoneally (i.p.) with deaths delayed up to five days and 700 mg/kg orally (p.o.) (approximately 140 times the usual human dose) with deaths delayed up to three days. In rats the acute LD_{50} is 750 mg/kg i.p. and 6000 mg/kg p.o. (approximately 1200 times the human dose).

In the management of overdosage there is no specific antidote for Allopurinol. There has been no clinical experience in the management of a patient who has taken massive amounts of Allopurinol.

Both Allopurinol and oxipurinol are dialyzable; however, the usefulness of hemodialysis or peritoneal dialysis in the management of a Allopurinol overdose is unknown.

DOSAGE AND ADMINISTRATION

The dosage of Allopurinol to accomplish full control of gout and to lower serum uric acid to normal or near-normal levels varies with the severity of the disease. The average is 200 to 300 mg per day for patients with mild gout and 400 to 600 mg per day for those with moderately severe tophaceous gout. The appropriate dosage may be administered in divided doses or as a single equivalent dose with the 300 mg tablet. Dosage requirements in excess of 300 mg should be administered in divided doses. The minimal effective dosage is 100 to 200 mg daily and the maximal recommended dosage is 800 mg daily. To reduce the possibility of flare-up of acute gouty attacks, it is recommended that the patient start with a low dose of Allopurinol (100 mg daily) and increase at weekly intervals by 100 mg until a serum uric acid level of 6 mg/dL or less is attained but without exceeding the maximal recommended dosage.

Normal serum urate levels are usually achieved in one to three weeks. The upper limit of normal is about 7 mg/dL for men and postmenopausal women and 6 mg/dL for premenopausal women. Too much reliance should not be placed on a single serum uric acid determination since, for technical reasons, estimation of uric acid may be difficult. By selecting the appropriate dosage and, in certain patients, using uricosuric agents concurrently, it is possible to reduce serum uric acid to normal or, if desired, to as low as 2 to 3 mg/dL and keep it there indefinitely.

While adjusting the dosage of Allopurinol in patients who are being treated with colchicine and/or anti-inflammatory agents, it is wise to continue the latter therapy until serum uric acid has been normalized and there has been freedom from acute gouty attacks for several months.

In transferring a patient from a uricosuric agent to Allopurinol, the dose of the uricosuric agent should be gradually reduced over a period of several weeks and the dose of Allopurinol gradually increased to the required dose needed to maintain a normal serum uric acid level.

It should also be noted that Allopurinol is generally better tolerated if taken following meals. A fluid intake sufficient to yield a daily urinary output of at least two liters and the maintenance of a neutral or, preferably, slightly alkaline urine are desirable.

Since Allopurinol and its metabolites are primarily eliminated only by the kidney, accumulation of the drug can occur in renal failure, and the dose of Allopurinol should consequently be reduced. With a creatinine clearance of 10 to 20 mL/min, a daily dosage of 200 mg of Allopurinol is suitable. When the creatinine clearance is less than 10 mL/min the daily dosage should not exceed 100 mg. With extreme renal impairment (creatinine clearance is less than 3 mL/min) the interval between doses may also need to be lengthened.

The correct size and frequency of dosage for maintaining the serum uric acid just within the normal range is best determined by using the serum uric acid level as an index.

For the prevention of uric acid nephropathy during the vigorous therapy of neoplastic disease, treatment with 600 to 800 mg daily for two or three days is advisable together with a high fluid intake. Otherwise similar considerations to the above recommendations for treating patients with gout govern the regulation of dosage for maintenance purposes in secondary hyperuricemia.

The dose of Allopurinol recommended for management of recurrent calcium oxalate stones in hyperuricosuric patients is 200 to 300 mg/day in divided doses or as the single equivalent. This dose may be adjusted up or down depending upon the resultant control of the hyperuricosuria based upon subsequent 24 hour urinary urate determinations. Clinical experience suggests that patients with recurrent calcium oxalate stones may also benefit from dietary changes such as the reduction of animal protein, sodium, refined sugars, oxalate-rich foods, and excessive calcium intake as well as an increase in oral fluids and dietary fiber.

Children, 6 to 10 years of age, with secondary hyperuricemia associated with malignancies may be given 300 mg Allopurinol daily while those under 6 years are generally given 150 mg daily. The response is evaluated after approximately 48 hours of therapy and a dosage adjustment is made if necessary.

Store at 15° to 25°C (59° to 77°F) in a dry place and protect from light.

HOW SUPPLIED
TABLETS: 100 MG

AVERAGE UNIT PRICE (AVAILABLE SIZES)		GENERIC A-RATED AVERAGE PRICE (GAAP)	
BRAND	$0.19	100s	$10.13
GENERIC	$0.09	500s	$39.45
HCFA FUL (100s ea)	$0.03	750s	$93.23
		1000s	$76.44

BRAND/MANUFACTURER	NDC	SIZE	AWP
◆ BRAND			
➤ ZYLOPRIM: Burr Wellcome	00081-0996-55	100s	$18.71
	00081-0996-75	1000s	$182.80
◆ GENERICS			
Medirex	57480-0800-06	30s	$4.26
Allscrips	54569-8564-01	90s	$8.05
➤ Rugby	00536-3027-01	100s	$8.06
Qualitest	00603-2117-21	100s	$8.07
Warner Chilcott	00047-0515-24	100s	$8.23
Mylan	00378-0137-01	100s	$8.40
Geneva	00781-1080-01	100s	$8.55
Boots Labs	00524-0405-01	100s	$8.80
URL	00677-0870-01	100s	$8.95
Par	49884-0104-01	100s	$8.95
Mutual	53489-0156-01	100s	$8.95
Goldline	00182-1481-01	100s	$8.95
Purepac	00228-2102-10	100s	$8.97
Schein	00364-0632-01	100s	$9.15
Aligen	00405-4036-01	100s	$9.20
Martec	52555-0209-01	100s	$9.20
Major	00904-2613-60	100s	$9.25
Parmed	00349-2332-01	100s	$9.69
Parmed	00349-8911-01	100s	$9.69
Moore,H.L.	00839-7713-06	100s	$9.79
➤ LOPURIN: Boots Pharm	00048-0051-01	100s	$16.35
Goldline	00182-1481-89	100s ud	$8.95
Schein	00364-0632-90	100s ud	$9.60
Auro	55829-0121-10	100s ud	$11.24
Geneva	00781-1080-13	100s ud	$12.40
Vangard	00615-1592-13	100s ud	$12.43
Major	00904-2613-61	100s ud	$13.27
UDL	51079-0205-20	100s ud	$14.20
Medirex	57480-0800-01	100s ud	$14.20
Allscrips	54569-8564-00	180s	$15.73
Mutual	53489-0156-05	500s	$36.00
Geneva	00781-1080-05	500s	$38.95
Par	49884-0104-05	500s	$43.41
Glasgow	60809-0106-55	750s ud	$93.23
Glasgow	60809-0106-72	750s ud	$93.23
Warner Chilcott	00047-0515-32	1000s	$63.78
Boots Labs	00524-0405-10	1000s	$66.85
Major	00904-2613-80	1000s	$67.70
➤ Rugby	00536-3027-10	1000s	$68.69
Qualitest	00603-2117-32	1000s	$69.65
URL	00677-0870-10	1000s	$70.00
Schein	00364-0632-02	1000s	$70.00
Mutual	53489-0156-10	1000s	$70.00
Martec	52555-0209-10	1000s	$71.40
Aligen	00405-4036-03	1000s	$72.70
Mylan	00378-0137-10	1000s	$73.60
Parmed	00349-2332-10	1000s	$83.48
Parmed	00349-8911-10	1000s	$89.20
Par	49884-0104-10	1000s	$89.50
Goldline	00182-1481-10	1000s	$89.50
Mason Dist	11845-0459-04	1000s	$89.50
Moore,H.L.	00839-7713-16	1000s	$93.96

TABLETS: 300 MG

AVERAGE UNIT PRICE (AVAILABLE SIZES)		GENERIC A-RATED AVERAGE PRICE (GAAP)	
BRAND	$0.51	100s	$25.42
GENERIC	$0.23	500s	$101.80
HCFA FUL (100s ea)	$0.07	1000s	$195.46

BRAND/MANUFACTURER	NDC	SIZE	AWP
◆ BRAND			
➤ ZYLOPRIM: Burr Wellcome	00081-0998-55	100s	$51.22
	00081-0998-56	100s ud	$51.22
	00081-0998-70	500s	$251.94
◆ GENERICS			
Medirex	57480-0801-06	30s	$10.03
Allscrips	54569-8514-00	90s	$19.55
➤ Rugby	00536-3028-01	100s	$20.50
Warner Chilcott	00047-0517-24	100s	$20.55
Qualitest	00603-2118-21	100s	$20.94
➤ Schein	00364-0633-01	100s	$21.00
Major	00904-2614-60	100s	$21.20
Boots Labs	00524-0410-01	100s	$21.80
Aligen	00405-4037-01	100s	$22.30
URL	00677-0871-01	100s	$22.58
Par	49884-0105-01	100s	$22.60
Purepac	00228-2103-10	100s	$22.60
Goldline	00182-1482-01	100s	$22.60
Mason Dist	11845-0460-01	100s	$22.60
Martec	52555-0210-01	100s	$22.75

BRAND/MANUFACTURER	NDC	SIZE	AWP
Mutual	53489-0157-01	100s	$23.00
Geneva	00781-1082-01	100s	$23.23
➤ Mylan	00378-0181-01	100s	$23.30
Moore,H.L.	00839-7714-06	100s	$23.69
Parmed	00349-2331-01	100s	$25.94
Parmed	00349-8912-01	100s	$25.94
➤ LOPURIN: Boots Pharm	00048-0052-01	100s	$43.15
➤ Schein	00364-0633-90	100s ud	$23.00
Goldline	00182-1482-89	100s ud	$23.00
Auro	55829-0122-10	100s ud	$29.44
Geneva	00781-1082-13	100s ud	$30.37
Vangard	00615-1593-13	100s ud	$30.47
UDL	51079-0206-20	100s ud	$33.23
Major	00904-2614-61	100s ud	$34.94
Medirex	57480-0801-01	100s ud	$34.95
Major	00904-2614-40	500s	$78.35
Aligen	00405-4037-02	500s	$80.68
Qualitest	00603-2118-28	500s	$85.50
➤ Schein	00364-0633-05	500s	$85.75
➤ Rugby	00536-3028-05	500s	$85.94
Boots Labs	00524-0410-05	500s	$88.20
Warner Chilcott	00047-0517-30	500s	$88.44
➤ Mylan	00378-0181-05	500s	$90.30
Martec	52555-0210-05	500s	$92.00
Geneva	00781-1082-05	500s	$92.50
URL	00677-0871-05	500s	$95.00
Mutual	53489-0157-05	500s	$95.00
Par	49884-0105-05	500s	$109.60
Goldline	00182-1482-05	500s	$112.50
Purepac	00228-2103-50	500s	$113.00
Parmed	00349-2331-05	500s	$116.86
Parmed	00349-8912-05	500s	$116.86
➤ LOPURIN: Boots Pharm	00048-0052-05	500s	$206.00
URL	00677-0871-10	1000s	$149.00

Allpyral SEE ALLERGENIC EXTRACTS

Alomide SEE LODOXAMIDE TROMETHAMINE

Alphanine Sd SEE FACTOR IX (HUMAN)

Alprazolam

DESCRIPTION
Alprazolam is a triazolo analog of the 1,4 benzodiazepine class of central nervous system-active compounds.

The chemical name of Alprazolam is 8-Chloro-1-methyl-6-phenyl-4H-s-triazolo[4,3-α] [1,4] benzodiazepine. Its molecular formula is $C_{17}H_{18}ClN_4$.

Alprazolam is a white crystalline powder, which is soluble in methanol or ethanol but which has no appreciable solubility in water at physiological pH.

Each Alprazolam tablet, for oral administration, contains 0.25, 0.5, 1 or 2 mg of Alprazolam.

Each ml for oral administration contains 1 mg Alprazolam.

Following is its chemical structure:

CLINICAL PHARMACOLOGY
CNS agents of the 1,4 benzodiazepine class presumably exert their effects by binding at stereo specific receptors at several sites within the central nervous system. Their exact mechanism of action is unknown. Clinically, all benzodiazepines cause a dose-related central nervous system depressant activity varying from mild impairment of task performance to hypnosis.

Following oral administration, Alprazolam is readily absorbed. Peak concentrations in the plasma occur in one to two hours following administration. Plasma levels are proportionate to the dose given; over the dose range of 0.5 to 3.0 mg, peak levels of 8.0 to 37 ng/ml were observed. Using a specific assay methodology, the mean plasma elimination half-life of Alprazolam has been found to be about 11.2 hours (range: 6.3-26.9 hours) in healthy adults.

The predominant metabolites are α-hydroxy-alprazolam and a benzophenone derived from Alprazolam. The biological activity of α-hydroxy-alprazolam is approximately one-half that of Alprazolam. The benzophenone metabolite is essentially inactive. Plasma levels of these metabolites are extremely low, thus

---

◆ RATED THERAPEUTICALLY EQUIVALENT; ◇ THERAPEUTIC EQUIVALENCE UNCONFIRMED; ○ UNRATED

precluding precise pharmacokinetic description. However, their half-lives appear to be of the same order of magnitude as that of Alprazolam. Alprazolam and its metabolites are excreted primarily in the urine.

The ability of Alprazolam to induce human hepatic enzyme systems has not yet been determined. However, this is not a property of benzodiazepines in general. Further, Alprazolam did not affect the prothrombin or plasma warfarin levels in male volunteers administered sodium warfarin orally.

In vitro, Alprazolam is bound (80 percent) to human serum protein.

Changes in the absorption, distribution, metabolism and excretion of benzodiazepines have been reported in a variety of disease states including alcoholism, impaired hepatic function and impaired renal function. Changes have also been demonstrated in geriatric patients. A mean half-life of Alprazolam of 16.3 hours has been observed in healthy elderly subjects (range: 9.0-26.9 hours, n = 16) compared to 11.0 hours (range: 6.3-15.8 hours, n = 16) in healthy adult subjects. The co-administration of oral contraceptives to healthy women increased the half-life of Alprazolam as compared to that in healthy control women (mean: 12.4 hours, n = 11 versus 9.6 hours, n = 9). There was a prolongation in the mean half-life of Alprazolam from 12.4 hours (range: 7.2-18.4 hours, n = 9) to 16.6 hours (range: 10.0-24.3 hours, n = 9) by the co-administration of cimetidine to the same healthy adults. In patients with alcoholic liver disease the half-life of Alprazolam ranged between 5.8 and 65.3 hours (mean: 19.7 hours, n = 17) as compared to between 6.3 and 26.9 hours (mean = 11.4 hours, n = 17) in healthy subjects. In an obese group of subjects the half-life of Alprazolam ranged between 9.9 and 40.4 hours (mean = 21.8 hours, n = 12) as compared to between 6.3 and 15.8 hours (mean = 10.6 hours, n = 12) in healthy subjects.

Because of its similarity to other benzodiazepines, it is assumed that Alprazolam undergoes transplacental passage and that it is excreted in human milk.

INDICATIONS AND USAGE

Alprazolam Tablets and Oral Solution are indicated for the management of anxiety disorder (a condition corresponding most closely to the APA Diagnostic and Statistical Manual [DSM-III-R] diagnosis of generalized anxiety disorder) or the short-term relief of symptoms of anxiety. Anxiety or tension associated with the stress of everyday life usually does not require treatment with an anxiolytic.

Generalized anxiety disorder is characterized by unrealistic or excessive anxiety and worry (apprehensive expectation) about two or more life circumstances, for a period of six months or longer, during which the person has been bothered more days than not by these concerns. At least 6 of the following 18 symptoms are often present in these patients:

Motor Tension (trembling, twitching, or feeling shaky; muscle tension, aches, or soreness; restlessness; easy fatigability)

Autonomic Hyperactivity: (shortness of breath or smothering sensations; palpitations or accelerated heart rate; sweating, or cold clammy hands; dry mouth; dizziness or light-headedness; nausea, diarrhea, or other abdominal distress; flushes or chills; frequent urination; trouble swallowing or "lump in throat")

Vigilance and Scanning (feeling keyed up on edge; exaggerated startle response; difficulty concentrating or "mind going blank" because of anxiety; trouble falling or staying asleep; irritability). These symptoms must not be secondary to another psychiatric disorder or caused by some organic factor.

Anxiety associated with depression is responsive to Alprazolam. Alprazolam Tablets are also indicated for the treatment of panic disorder, with or without agoraphobia.

Studies supporting this claim were conducted in patients whose diagnoses corresponded closely to the DSM-III-R criteria for panic disorder (see *"Clinical Studies"*).

Panic disorder is an illness characterized by recurrent panic attacks. The panic attacks, at least initially, are unexpected. Later in the course of this disturbance certain situations, e.g. driving a car or being in a crowded place, may become associated with having a panic attack. These panic attacks are not triggered by situations in which the person is the focus of others' attention (as in social phobia). The diagnosis requires four such attacks within a four week period, or one or more attacks followed by at least a month of persistent fear of having another attack. The panic attacks must be characterized by at least four of the following symptoms: dyspnea or smothering sensations; dizziness, unsteady feelings, or faintness; palpitations or tachycardia; trembling or shaking; sweating; choking; nausea or abdominal distress; depersonalization or derealization; paresthesias; hot flashes or chills; chest pain or discomfort; fear of dying; fear of going crazy or of doing something uncontrolled. At least some of the panic attack symptoms must develop suddenly, and the panic attack symptoms must not be attributable to some known organic factors. Panic disorder is frequently associated with some symptoms of agoraphobia.

Demonstrations of the effectiveness of Alprazolam by systematic clinical study are limited to four months duration for anxiety disorder and four to ten weeks duration for panic disorder; however, patients with panic disorder have been treated on an open basis for up to eight months without apparent loss of benefit. The physician should periodically reassess the usefulness of the drug for the individual patient.

UNLABELED USES

Alprazolem is used alone or as an adjunct in the treatment of agoraphobia, depression, and premenstrual syndrome.

CONTRAINDICATIONS

Alprazolam is contraindicated in patients with known, sensitivity to this drug or other benzodiazepines. Alprazolam may be used in patients with open angle glaucoma who are receiving appropriate therapy, but is contraindicated in patients with acute narrow angle glaucoma.

WARNINGS

Dependence and Withdrawal Reactions, Including Seizures: Certain adverse clinical events, some life-threatening, are a direct consequence of physical dependence on Alprazolam. These include a spectrum of withdrawal symptoms; the most important is seizure (see *"Drug Abuse and Dependence"*). Even after relatively short-term use at the doses recommended for the treatment of transient anxiety and anxiety disorder (ie, 0.75 to 4.0 mg per day), there is some risk of dependence. Post-marketing surveillance data suggest that the risk of dependence and its severity appear to be greater in patients treated with relatively high doses (above 4 mg per day) and for long periods (more than 8-12 weeks).

The Importance of Dose and the Risks of Alprazolam Tablets as a Treatment for Panic Disorder: Because the management of panic disorder often requires the use of average daily doses of Alprazolam above 4 mg, the risk of dependence among panic disorder patients may be higher than that among those treated for less severe anxiety. Experience in randomized placebo-controlled discontinuation studies of patients with panic disorder showed a high rate of rebound and withdrawal symptoms in patients treated with Alprazolam compared to placebo treated patients.

Relapse or return of illness was defined as a return of symptoms characteristic of panic disorder (primarily panic attacks) to levels approximately equal to those seen at baseline before active treatment was initiated. Rebound refers to a return of symptoms of panic disorder to a level substantially greater in frequency, or more severe in intensity than seen at baseline. Withdrawal symptoms were identified as those which were generally not characteristic of panic disorder and which occurred for the first time more frequently during discontinuation than at baseline.

In a controlled clinical trial in which 63 patients were randomized to Alprazolam and where withdrawal symptoms were specifically sought, the following were identified as symptoms of withdrawal: heightened sensory perception, impaired concentration, dysosmia, clouded sensorium, paresthesias, muscle cramps, muscle twitch, diarrhea, blurred vision, appetite decrease and weight loss. Other symptoms, such as anxiety and insomnia, were frequently seen during discontinuation, but it could not be determined if they were due to return of illness, rebound or withdrawal.

In a larger database comprised of both controlled and uncontrolled studies in which 641 patients received Alprazolam, discontinuation-emergent symptoms which occurred at a rate of over 5% in patients treated with Alprazolam and at a greater rate than the placebo treated group were as follows:

DISCONTINUATION-EMERGENT SYMPTOM INCIDENCE

Percentage of 641 XANAX-Treated Panic Disorder Patients Reporting Events Body System/Event

Neurologic		Gastrointestinal	
Insomnia	29.5	Nausea/Vomiting	16.5
Light-headedness	19.3	Diarrhea	13.6
Abnormal involuntary movement	17.3	Decreased salivation	10.6
Headache	17.0	**Metabolic-Nutritional**	
Muscular twitching	6.9	Weight loss	13.3
Impaired Coordination	6.6	Decreased appetite	12.8
Muscle tone disorders	5.9		
Weakness	5.8	**Dermatological**	
Psychiatric		Sweating	14.4
Anxiety	19.2		
Fatigue and Tiredness	18.4	**Cardiovascular**	
Irritability	10.5	Tachycardia	12.2
Cognitive disorder	10.3		
Memory impairment	5.5	**Special Senses**	
Depression	5.1	Blurred vision	10.0
Confusional state	5.0		

From the studies cited, it has not been determined whether these symptoms are clearly related to the dose and duration of therapy with Alprazolam in patients with panic disorder.

In two controlled trials of six to eight weeks duration where the ability of patients to discontinue medication was measured, 71%-93% of patients treated with Alprazolam tapered completely off therapy compared to 89%-96% of placebo treated patients. The ability of patients to completely discontinue therapy with Alprazolam after long-term therapy has not been reliably determined.

Seizures attributable to Alprazolam were seen after drug discontinuance or dose reduction in 8 of 1980 patients with panic disorder or in patients participating in clinical trials where doses of Alprazolam greater than 4 mg daily for over 3 months were permitted. Five of these cases clearly occurred during abrupt dose reduction, or discontinuation from daily doses of 2 to 10 mg. Three cases occurred in situations where there was not a clear relationship to abrupt dose reduction or discontinuation. In one instance, seizure occurred after discontinuation from a single dose of 1 mg after tapering at a rate of 1 mg every three days from 6 mg daily. In two other instances, the relationship to taper is indeterminate; in both of these cases the patients had been receiving doses of 3 mg daily prior to seizure. The duration of use in the above 8 cases ranged from 4 to 22 weeks. There have been occasional voluntary reports of patients developing seizures while apparently tapering gradually from Alprazolam. The risk of seizure seems to be greatest 24-72 hours after discontinuation (see *"Dosage and Administration"* for recommended tapering and discontinuation schedule).

Status Epilepticus and Its Treatment: The medical event voluntary reporting system shows that withdrawal seizures have been reported in association with the discontinuation of Alprazolam Tablets and Oral Solution. In most cases, only a single seizure was reported; however, multiple seizures and status epilepticus were reported as well. Ordinarily, the treatment of status epilepticus of any etiology involves use of intravenous benzodiazepines plus phenytoin or barbiturates, maintenance of a patent airway and adequate hydration. For additional details regarding therapy, consultation with an appropriate specialist may be considered.

Interdose Symptoms: Early morning anxiety and emergence of anxiety symptoms between doses of Alprazolam Tablets have been reported in patients with panic disorder taking prescribed maintenance doses of Alprazolam. These symptoms may reflect the development of tolerance or a time interval between doses which is longer than the duration of clinical action of the administered dose.

In either case, it is presumed that the prescribed dose is not sufficient to maintain plasma levels above those needed to prevent relapse, rebound or withdrawal symptoms over the entire course of the interdosing interval. In these situations, it is recommended that the same total daily dose be given divided as more frequent administrations (see *"Dosage and Administration"*).

Risk of Dose Reduction: Withdrawal reactions may occur when dosage reduction occurs for any reason. This includes purposeful tapering, but also inadvertent reduction of dose (e.g., the patient forgets, the patient is admitted to a hospital, etc.). Therefore, the dosage of Alprazolam Tablets or Oral Solution should be reduced or discontinued gradually (see *"Dosage and Administration"*).

Alprazolam Tablets and Oral Solution are not of value in the treatment of psychotic patients and should not be employed in lieu of appropriate treatment for psychosis. Because of its CNS depressant effects, patients receiving Alprazolam should be cautioned against engaging in hazardous occupations or activities requiring complete mental alertness such as operating machinery or driving a motor vehicle. For the same reason, patients should be cautioned about the simultaneous ingestion of alcohol and other CNS depressant drugs during treatment with Alprazolam.

Benzodiazepines can potentially cause fetal harm when administered to pregnant women. If Alprazolam is used during pregnancy, or if the patient becomes pregnant while taking this drug, the patient should be apprised of the potential hazard to the fetus. Because of experience with other members of the benzodiazepine class, Alprazolam is assumed to be capable of causing an increased risk of congenital abnormalities when administered to a pregnant woman during the first trimester. Because use of these drugs is rarely a matter of urgency, their use during the first trimester should almost always be avoided. The possibility that a woman of childbearing potential may be pregnant at the time of institution of therapy should be considered. Patients should be advised that if they become pregnant during therapy or intend to become pregnant they should communicate with their physicians about the desirability of discontinuing the drug.

PRECAUTIONS

General: If Alprazolam is to be combined with other psychotropic agents or anticonvulsant drugs, careful consideration should be given to the pharmacology of the agents to be employed, particularly with compounds which might potentiate the action of benzodiazepines (see *"Drug Interactions"*).

As with other psychotropic medications, the usual precautions with respect to administration of the drug and size of the prescription are indicated for severely depressed patients or those in whom there is reason to expect concealed suicidal ideation or plans.

It is recommended that the dosage be limited to the smallest effective dose to preclude the development of ataxia or oversedation which may be a particular problem in elderly or debilitated patients. (See *"Dosage and Administration"*.) The precautions in treating patients with impaired renal, hepatic or pulmonary function should be observed. There have been rare reports of death in patients with severe pulmonary disease shortly after the initiation of treatment with Alprazolam. A decreased systemic Alprazolam elimination rate (e.g., increased plasma half-life) has been observed in both alcoholic liver disease patients and obese patients receiving Alprazolam. (See *"Clinical Pharmacology"*.)

Episodes of hypomania and mania have been reported in association with the use of Alprazolam in patients with depression.

Alprazolam has a weak uricosuric effect. Although other medications with weak uricosuric effect have been reported to cause acute renal failure, there have been no reported instances of acute renal failure attributable to therapy with Alprazolam.

INFORMATION FOR PATIENTS

For All Users of Alprazolam: To assure safe and effective use of benzodiazepines, all patients prescribed Alprazolam should be provided with the following guidance. In addition, panic disorder patients, for whom higher doses are typically prescribed, should be advised about the risks associated with the use of higher doses.

1. Inform your physician about any alcohol consumption and medicine you are taking now, including medication you may buy without a prescription. Alcohol should generally not be used during treatment with benzodiazepines.

2. Not recommended for use in pregnancy. Therefore, inform your physician if you are pregnant, if you are planning to have a child, or if you become pregnant while you are taking this medication.
3. Inform your physician if you are nursing.
4. Until you experience how this medication affects you, do not drive a car or operate potentially dangerous machinery, etc.
5. Do not increase the dose even if you think the medication "does not work anymore" without consulting your physician. Benzodiazepines, even when used as recommended, may produce emotional and/or physical dependence.
6. Do not stop taking the drug abruptly or decrease the dose without consulting your physician since withdrawal symptoms can occur.

Additional Advice for Panic Disorder Patients: The use of Alprozolam Tablets at the high doses (above 4 mg per day), often necessary to treat panic disorder, is accompanied by risks that you may need to carefully consider. When used at high doses for long intervals, which may or may not be required for your treatment, Alprozolam has the potential to cause severe emotional and physical dependence in some patients and these patients may find it exceedingly difficult to terminate treatment. In two controlled trials of six to eight weeks duration where the ability of patients to discontinue medication was measured, 7 to 29% of patients treated with Alprazolam did not completely taper off therapy. The ability of patients to completely discontinue therapy with Alprazolam after long-term therapy has not been reliably determined. In all cases, it is important that your physician help you discontinue this medication in a careful and safe manner to avoid overly extended use of Alprazolam.

In addition, the extended use at high doses appears to increase the incidence and severity of withdrawal reactions when Alprazolam is discontinued. These are generally minor but seizure can occur, especially if you reduce the dose too rapidly or discontinue the medication abruptly. Seizure can be life-threatening.

LABORATORY TESTS
Laboratory tests are not ordinarily required in otherwise healthy patients.

DRUG INTERACTIONS
The benzodiazepines, including Alprazolam, produce additive CNS depressant effects when coadministered with other psychotropic medications, anticonvulsants, antihistaminics, ethanol and other drugs which themselves produce CNS depression.

The steady state plasma concentrations of imipramine and desipramine have been reported to be increased an average of 31% and 20%, respectively, by the concomitant administration of Alprazolam in doses up to 4 mg/day. The clinical significance of these changes is unknown.

Pharmacokinetic interactions of benzodiazepines with other drugs have been reported. For example, the clearance of Alprazolam and certain other benzodiazepines can be delayed by the co-administration of cimetidine. The clearance of Alprazolam can also be delayed by the co-administration of oral contraceptives (see *"Clinical Pharmacology"*). The clinical significance of these interactions is unclear.

DRUG/LABORATORY TEST INTERACTIONS
Although interactions between benzodiazpines and commonly employed clinical laboratory tests have occasionally been reported, there is no consistent pattern for a specific drug or specific test.

CARCINOGENESIS, MUTAGENESIS, IMPAIRMENT OF FERTILITY
No evidence of carcinogenic potential was observed during 2-year bioassay studies of Alprazolam in rats at doses up to 30 mg/kg/day (150 times the maximum recommended daily human dose of 10 mg/day) and in mice at doses up to 10 mg/kg/day (50 times the maximum recommended daily human dose).

Alprazolam was not mutagenic in the rat micronucleus test at doses up to 100 mg/kg, which is 500 times the maximum recommended daily human dose of 10 mg/day. Alprazolam also was not mutagenic *in vitro* in the DNA Damage/Alkaline Elution Assay or the Ames Assay.

Alprazolam produced no impairment of fertility in rats at doses up to 5 mg/kg/day, which is 25 times the maximum recommended daily human dose of 10 mg/day.

PREGNANCY
Teratogenic Effects: Pregnancy Category D: (See *"Warnings Section"*)

Nonteratogenic Effects: It should be considered that the child born of a mother who is receiving benzodiazepines may be at some risk for withdrawal symptoms from the drug during the postnatal period. Also, neonatal flaccidity and respiratory problems have been reported in children born of mothers who have been receiving benzodiazepines.

LABOR AND DELIVERY
Alprazolam has no established use in labor or delivery.

NURSING MOTHERS
Benzodiazepines are known to be excreted in human milk. It should be assumed that Alprazolam is as well. Chronic administration of diazepam to nursing mothers has been reported to cause their infants to become lethargic and to lose weight. As a general rule, nursing should not be undertaken by mothers who must use Alprazolam.

PEDIATRIC USE
Safety and effectiveness in children below the age of 18 years have not been established.

◆ RATED THERAPEUTICALLY EQUIVALENT; ◇ THERAPEUTIC EQUIVALENCE UNCONFIRMED; ○ UNRATED

ADVERSE REACTIONS

Side effects to Alprazolam, if they occur, are generally observed at the beginning of therapy and usually disappear upon continued medication. In the usual patient, the most frequent side effects are likely to be an extension of the pharmacological activity of Alprazolam, e.g., drowsiness or light-headedness.

The data cited in the two tables below are estimates of untoward clinical event incidence among patients who participated under the following clinical conditions: relatively short duration (i.e., four weeks) placebo-controlled clinical studies with dosages up to 4 mg/day of Alprazolam (for the management of anxiety disorders or for the short-term relief of the symptoms of anxiety) and short-term (up to ten weeks) placebo-controlled clinical studies with dosages up to 10 mg/day of Alprazolam Tablets in patients with panic disorder, with or without agoraphobia.

These data cannot be used to predict precisely the incidence of untoward events in the course of usual medical practice where patient characteristics, and other factors often differ from those in clinical trials. These figures cannot be compared with those obtained from other clinical studies involving related drug products and placebo as each group of drug trials are conducted under a different set of conditions.

Comparison of the cited figures, however, can provide the prescriber with some basis for estimating the relative contributions of drug and non-drug factors to the untoward event incidence in the population studied. Even this use must be approached cautiously, as a drug may relieve a symptom in one patient but induce it in others. (For example, an anxiolytic drug may relieve dry mouth [a symptom of anxiety] in some subjects but induce it [an untoward event] in others.)

Additionally, for anxiety disorders the cited figures can provide the prescriber with an indication as to the frequency with which physician intervention (e.g., increased surveillance, decreased dosage or discontinuation of drug therapy) may be necessary because of the untoward clinical event.

ANXIETY DISORDERS

| | Treatment-Emergent Symptom Incidence† | | Incidence of Intervention Because of Symptom |
	Alprazolam	Placebo	Alprazolam
Number of Patients	565	505	565
% of Patients Reporting:			
Central Nervous System			
Drowsiness	41.0	21.6	15.1
Light-headedness	20.8	19.3	1.2
Depression	13.9	18.1	2.4
Headache	12.9	19.6	1.1
Confusion	9.9	10.0	0.9
Insomnia	8.9	18.4	1.3
Nervousness	4.1	10.3	1.1
Syncope	3.1	4.0	*
Dizziness	1.8	0.8	2.5
Akathisia	1.6	1.2	*
Tiredness/Sleepiness	*	*	1.8
Gastrointestinal			
Dry Mouth	14.7	13.3	0.7
Constipation	10.4	11.4	0.9
Diarrhea	10.1	10.3	1.2
Nausea/Vomiting	9.6	12.8	1.7
Increased Salivation	4.2	2.4	*
Cardiovascular			
Tachycardia/Palpitations	7.7	15.6	0.4
Hypotension	4.7	2.2	*
Sensory			
Blurred Vision	6.2	6.2	0.4
Musculoskeletal			
Rigidity	4.2	5.3	*
Tremor	4.0	8.8	0.4
Cutaneous			
Dermatitis/Allergy	3.8	3.1	0.6
Other			
Nasal Congestion	7.3	9.3	*
Weight Gain	2.7	2.7	*
Weight Loss	2.3	3.0	*

* None reported
† Events reported by 1% or more of patients on Alprazolam are included.

In addition to the relatively common (i.e., greater than 1%) untoward events enumerated above, the following adverse events have been reported in association with the use of benzodiazepines: dystonia, irritability, concentration difficulties, anorexia, transient amnesia or memory impairment, loss of coordination, fatigue, seizures, sedation, slurred speech, jaundice, musculoskeletal weakness, pruritus, diplopia, dysarthria, changes in libido, menstrual irregularities, incontinence and urinary retention.

PANIC DISORDER

| | Treatment-Emergent Symptom Incidence* | |
	Alprazolam Tablets	Placebo
Number of Patients	1388	1231
% of Patients Reporting:		
Central Nervous System		
Drowsiness	76.8	42.7
Fatigue and Tiredness	48.6	42.3
Impaired Coordination	40.1	17.9
Irritability	33.1	30.1
Memory Impairment	33.1	22.1
Light-headedness/Dizziness	29.8	36.9
Insomnia	29.4	41.8
Headache	29.2	35.6
Cognitive Disorder	28.8	20.5
Dysarthria	23.3	6.3
Anxiety	16.6	24.9
Abnormal Involuntary Movement	14.8	21.0
Decreased Libido	14.4	8.0
Depression	13.8	14.0
Confusional State	10.4	8.2
Muscular Twitching	7.9	11.8
Increased Libido	7.7	4.1
Change in Libido (Not Specified)	7.1	5.6
Weakness	7.1	8.4
Muscle Tone Disorders	6.3	7.5
Syncope	3.8	4.8
Akathisia	3.0	4.3
Agitation	2.9	2.6
Disinhibition	2.7	1.5
Paresthesia	2.4	3.2
Talkativeness	2.2	1.0
Vasomotor Disturbances	2.0	2.6
Derealization	1.9	1.2
Dream Abnormalities	1.8	1.5
Fear	1.4	1.0
Feeling Warm	1.3	0.5
Gastrointestinal		
Decreased Salivation	32.8	34.2
Constipation	26.2	15.4
Nausea/Vomiting	22.0	31.8
Diarrhea	20.6	22.8
Abdominal Distress	18.3	21.5
Increased Salivation	5.6	4.4
Cardio-Respiratory		
Nasal Congestion	17.4	16.5
Tachycardia	15.4	26.8
Chest Pain	10.6	18.1
Hyperventilation	9.7	14.5
Upper Respiratory Infection	4.3	3.7
Sensory		
Blurred Vision	21.0	21.4
Tinnitus	6.6	10.4
Musculoskeletal		
Muscular Cramps	2.4	2.4
Muscle Stiffness	2.2	3.3
Cutaneous		
Sweating	15.1	23.5
Rash	10.8	8.1
Other		
Increased Appetite	32.7	22.8
Decreased Appetite	27.8	24.1
Weight Gain	27.2	17.9
Weight Loss	22.6	16.5
Micturition Difficulties	12.2	8.6
Menstrual Disorders	10.4	8.7
Sexual Dysfunction	7.4	3.7
Edema	4.9	5.6
Incontinence	1.5	0.6
Infection	1.3	1.7

* Events reported by 1% or more of patients on Alprazolam Tablets are included.

► SHOWN IN PRODUCT IDENTIFICATION GUIDE

In addition to the relatively common (i.e., greater than 1%) untoward events enumerated in the table above, the following adverse events have been reported in association with the use of Alprazolam Tablets: seizures, hallucinations, depersonalization, taste alterations, diplopia, elevated bilirubin, elevated hepatic enzymes, and jaundice.

There have also been reports of withdrawal seizures upon rapid decrease or abrupt discontinuation of Alprazolam (see *"Warnings"*).

To discontinue treatment in patients taking Alprazolam, the dosage should be reduced slowly in keeping with good medical practice. It is suggested that the daily dosage of Alprazolam be decreased by no more than 0.5 mg every three days (see *"Dosage and Administration"*). Some patients may require an even slower dosage reduction.

Panic disorder has been associated with primary and secondary major depressive disorders and increased reports of suicide among untreated patients. Therefore, the same precaution must be exercised when using the higher doses of Alprazolam Tablets in treating patients with panic disorder as is exercised with the use of any psychotropic drug in treating depressed patients or those in whom there is reason to expect concealed suicidal ideation or plans.

As with all benzodiazepines, paradoxical reactions such as stimulation, increased muscle spasticity, sleep disturbances, hallucinations and other adverse behavioral effects such as agitation, rage, irritability, and aggressive or hostile behavior have been reported rarely. In many of the spontaneous case reports of adverse behavioral effects, patients were receiving other CNS drugs concomitantly and/or were described as having underlying psychiatric conditions. Should any of the above events occur, Alprazolam should be discontinued. Isolated published reports involving small numbers of patients have suggested that patients who have borderline personality disorder, a prior history of violent or aggressive behavior, alcohol or substance abuse, may be at risk for such events. Instances of irritability, hostility, and intrusive thoughts have been reported during discontinuation of Alprazolam in patients with posttraumatic stress disorder.

Laboratory analyses were performed on all patients participating in the clinical program for Alprazolam. The following incidences of abnormalities shown below were observed in patients receiving Alprazolam and in patients in the corresponding placebo group. Few of these abnormalities were considered to be of physiological significance.

	Alprazolam		Placebo	
	Low	High	Low	High
Hematology				
Hematocrit	*	*	*	*
Hemoglobin	*	*	*	*
Total WBC Count	1.4	2.3	1.0	2.0
Neutrophil Count	2.3	3.0	4.2	1.7
Lymphocyte Count	5.5	7.4	5.4	9.5
Monocyte Count	5.3	2.8	6.4	*
Eosinophil Count	3.2	9.5	3.3	7.2
Basophil Count	*	*	*	*
Urinalysis				
Albumin	—	*	—	*
Sugar	—	*	—	*
RBC/HPF	—	3.4	—	5.0
WBC/HPF	—	25.7	—	25.9
Blood Chemistry				
Creatinine	2.2	1.9	3.5	1.0
Bilirubin	*	1.6	*	*
SGOT	*	3.2	1.0	1.8
Alkaline				
Phosphatase	*	1.7	*	1.8

* *Less than 1%*

When treatment with Alprazolam is protracted, periodic blood counts, urinalysis and blood chemistry analyses are advisable.

Minor changes in EEG patterns, usually low-voltage fast activity have been observed in patients during therapy with Alprazolam and are of no known significance.

POST INTRODUCTION REPORTS
Various adverse drug reactions have been reported in association with the use of Alprazolam since market introduction. The majority of these reactions were reported through the medical event voluntary reporting system. Because of the spontaneous nature of the reporting of medical events and the lack of controls, a causal relationship to the use of Alprazolam cannot be readily determined. Reported events include: liver enzyme elevations, gynecomastia and galactorrhea.

DRUG ABUSE AND DEPENDENCE
PHYSICAL AND PSYCHOLOGICAL DEPENDENCE
Withdrawal symptoms similar in character to those noted with sedative/hypnotics and alcohol have occurred following abrupt discontinuance of benzodiazepines, including Alprazolam. The symptoms can range from mild dysphoria and insomnia to a major syndrome that may include abdominal and muscle cramps, vomiting, sweating, tremors and convulsions. Distinguishing between withdrawal emergent signs and symptoms and the recurrence of illness is often difficult in patients undergoing dose reduction. The long term strategy for treatment of these phenomena will vary with their cause and the therapeutic goal. When necessary, immediate management of withdrawal symptoms requires re-institution of treatment at doses of Alprazolam sufficient to suppress symptoms. There have been reports of failure of other benzodiazephines to fully suppress these withdrawal symptoms. These failures have been attributed to incompete cross-tolerance but may also reflect the use of an inadequate dosage regimen of the substituted benzodiazepine or the effects of concomitant medications.

While it is difficult to distinguish withdrawal and recurrence for certain patients, the time course and the nature of the symptoms may be helpful. A withdrawal syndrome typically includes the occurrence of new symptoms, tends to appear toward the end of the taper or shortly after discontinuation, and will decrease with time. In recurring panic disorder, symptoms similar to those observed before treatment may recur either early or late, and they will persist.

While the severity and incidence of withdrawal phenomena appear to be related to dose and duration of treatment, withdrawal symptoms, including seizures, have been reported after only brief therapy with Alprazolam at doses within the recommended range for the treatment of anxiety (e.g., 0.75 to 4 mg/day). Signs and symptoms of withdrawal are often more prominent after rapid decrease of dosage or abrupt discontinuance. The risk of withdrawal seizures may be increased at doses above 4 mg/day (see *"Warnings"*).

Patients, especially individuals with a history of seizures or epilepsy, should not be abruptly discontinued from any CNS depressant agent, including Alprazolam. It is recommended that all patients on Alprazolam who require a dosage reduction be gradually tapered under close supervision (see *"Warnings"* and *"Dosage and Administration"*).

Psychological dependence is a risk with all benzodiazepines, including Alprazolam. The risk of psychological dependence may also be increased at higher doses and with longer term use, and this risk is further increased in patient with a history of alcohol or drug abuse. Some patients have experienced considerable difficulty in tapering and discontinuing from Alprazolam, especially those receiving higher doses for extended periods. Addiction-prone individuals should be under careful surveillance when receiving Alprazolam. As with all anxiolytics, repeat prescriptions should be limited to those who are under medical supervision.

CONTROLLED SUBSTANCE CLASS
Alprazolam is a controlled substance under the Controlled Substance Act by the Drug Enforcement Administration and Alprazolam Tablets have been assigned to Schedule IV.

OVERDOSAGE
Manifestations of Alprazolam overdosage include somnolence, confusion, impaired coordination, diminished reflexes and coma. Death has been reported in association with overdoses of Alprazolam by itself, as it has with other benzodiazepines. In addition, fatalities have been reported in patients who have overdosed with a combination of a single benzodiazepine, including Alprazolam, and alcohol; alcohol levels seen in some of these patients have been lower than those usually associated with alcohol-induced fatality.

The acute oral LD_{50} in rats is 331-2171 mg/kg. Other experiments in animals have indicated that cardiopulmonary collapse can occur following massive intravenous doses of Alprazolam (over 195 mg/kg; 975 times the maximum recommended daily human dose of 10 mg/day). Animals could be resuscitated with positive mechanical ventilation and the intravenous infusion of norepinephrine bitartrate.

Animal experiments have suggested that forced diuresis or hemodialysis are probably of little value in treating overdosage.

GENERAL TREATMENT OF OVERDOSE
Overdosage reports with Alprazolam are limited. As in all cases of drug overdosage, respiration, pulse rate, and blood pressure should be monitored. General supportive measures should be employed, along with immediate gastric lavage. Intravenous fluids should be administered and an adequate airway maintained. If hypotension occurs, it may be combated by the use of vasopressors. Dialysis is of limited value. As with the management of intentional overdosing with any drug, it should be borne in mind that multiple agents may have been ingested.

Flumazenil, a specific benzodiazepine receptor antagonist, is indicated for the complete or partial reversal of the sedative effects of benzodiazepines and may be used in situations when an overdose with a benzodiazepine is known or suspected. Prior to the administration of flumazenil, necessary measures should be instituted to secure airway, ventilation and intravenous access. Flumazenil is intended as an adjunct to, not as a substitute for, proper management of benzodiazepine overdose. Patients treated with flumazenil should be monitored for re-sedation, respiratory depression, and other residual benzodiazepine effects for an appropriate period after treatment. **The prescriber should be aware of a risk of seizure in association with flumazenil treatment, particularly in long-term benzodiazepine users and in cyclic antidepresent overdose.** The complete flumzenil package insert including *"Contraindications," "Warnings"* and *"Precautions"* should be consulted prior to use.

DOSAGE AND ADMINISTRATION
Dosage should be individualized for maximum beneficial effect. While the usual daily dosages given below will meet the needs of most patients, there will be some who require higher doses. In such cases, dosage should be increased cautiously to avoid adverse effects.

◆ RATED THERAPEUTICALLY EQUIVALENT; ◇ THERAPEUTIC EQUIVALENCE UNCONFIRMED; ○ UNRATED

ANXIETY DISORDERS AND TRANSIENT SYMPTOMS OF ANXIETY

Treatment for patients with anxiety should be initiated with a dose of 0.25 to 0.5 mg given three times daily. The dose may be increased to achieve a maximum therapeutic effect, at intervals of 3 to 4 days, to a maximum daily dose of 4 mg, given in divided doses. The lowest possible effective dose should be employed and the need for continued treatment reassessed frequently. The risk of dependence may increase with dose and duration of treatment.

In elderly patients, in patients with advanced liver disease or in patients with debilitating disease, the usual starting dose is 0.25 mg, given two or three times daily. This may be gradually increased if needed and tolerated. The elderly may be especially sensitive to the effects of benzodiazepines.

If side effects occur at the recommended starting dose, the dose may be lowered.

In all patients, dosage should be reduced gradually when discontinuing therapy or when decreasing the daily dosage. Although there are no systematically collected data to support a specific discontinuation schedule, it is suggested that the daily dosage be decreased by no more than 0.5 mg every three days. Some patients may require an even slower dosage reduction.

PANIC DISORDER

The successful treatment of many panic disorder patients has required the use of Alprazolam Tablets at doses greater than 4 mg daily. In controlled trials conducted to establish the efficacy of Alprazolam Tablets in panic disorder, doses in the range of 1 to 10 mg daily were used. The mean dosage employed was approximately 5 to 6 mg daily. Among the approximately 1700 patients participating in the panic disorder development program, about 300 received maximum Alprazolam Tablets dosages of greater than 7 mg/day, including approximately 100 patients who received maximum dosages of greater than 9 mg/day. Occasional patients required as much as 10 mg a day to achieve a successful response.

However, in the absence of systematic studies evaluating the dose response relationship, the dosing regimen for the administration of Alprazolam Tablets to patients with panic disorder must be based on generic principles. Generally, therapy should be initiated at a low dose to minimize the risk of adverse responses in patients especially sensitive to the drug. Thereafter, the dose can be increased at intervals equal to at least 5 times the elimination half-life (about 11 hours in young patients, about 16 hours in elderly patients). Longer titration intervals should probably be used because the maximum therapeutic response may not occur until after the plasma levels achieve steady state. Dose should be advanced until an acceptable therapeutic response (i.e., a substantial reduction in or total elimination of panic attacks) is achieved, intolerance occurs, or the maximum recommended dose is attained. Because of the danger of withdrawal, abrupt discontinuation of treatment should be avoided (see "Warnings," "Precautions," "Drug Abuse and Dependence").

THE FOLLOWING REGIMEN IS ONE THAT FOLLOWS THE PRINCIPLES OUTLINED ABOVE

Treatment may be initiated with a dose of 0.5 mg three times daily. Depending on the response, the dose may be increased at intervals of 3 to 4 days in increments of no more than 1 mg per day. Slower titration to the higher dose levels may be advisable to allow full expression of the pharmacodynamic effect of Alprazolam Tablets. To lessen the possibility of interdose symptoms, the times of administration should be distributed as evenly as possible throughout the waking hours, that is, on a three or four times per day schedule.

The necessary duration of treatment for panic disorder patients responding to Alprazolam Tablets is unknown. After a period of extended freedom from attacks, a carefully supervised tapered discontinuation may be attempted, but there is evidence that this may often be difficult to accomplish without recurrence of symptoms and/or the manifestation of withdrawal phenomena.

In any case, reduction of dose must be undertaken under close supervision and must be gradual. If significant withdrawal symptoms develop, the previous dosing schedule should be reinstituted and, only after stabilization, should a less rapid schedule of discontinuation be attempted. Although no experimental studies have been conducted to assess the comparative benefits of various discontinuation regimens, a possible approach is to reduce the dose by no more than 0.5 mg every three days, with the understanding that some patients may require an even more gradual discontinuation. Some patients may prove resistant to all discontinuation regimens.

PROPER USE OF ALPRAZOLAM ORAL SOLUTION

Alprazolam Oral Solution is a concentrated oral solution as compared to standard oral liquid medications. It is recommended that Alprazolam Oral Solution be mixed with liquid or semi-solid food such as water, jucies, soda or soda-like beverages, applesauce and puddings.

Use only the calibrated dropper provided with this product. Draw into the dropper the amount prescribed for a single dose. Then squeeze the dropper contents into a liquid or semi-solid food. Stir the liquid or food gently for a few seconds. The Alprazolam Oral Solution formulation blends quickly and completely. The entire amount of the mixture, of drug and liquid or drug and food, should be consumed immediately. Do not store for future use.

Store at controlled room temperature 15°-30°C (59°-86°F). Protect Oral Solution from light; dispense in a tight, light-resistant container.

ANIMAL STUDIES

When rats were treated with Alprazolam at 3, 10, and 30 mg/kg/day (15 to 150 times the maximum recommended human dose) orally for 2 years, a tendency for a dose related increase in the number of cataracts was observed in females and a tendency for a dose related increase in corneal vascularization was observed in males. These lesions did not appear until after 11 months of treatment.

CLINICAL STUDIES

ANXIETY DISORDERS

Alprazolam was compared to placebo in double blind clinical studies (doses up to 4 mg/day) in patients with a diagnosis of anxiety or anxiety with associated depressive symptomatology. Alprazolam was significantly better than placebo at each of the evaluation periods of these four week studies as judged by the following psychometric instruments: Physician's Global Impressions, Hamilton Anxiety Rating Scale Target Symptoms, Patient's Global Impressions and Self-Rating Symptom Scale.

PANIC DISORDER

Support for the effectiveness of Alprazolam Tablets in the treatment of panic disorder came from three short-term, placebo controlled studies (up to 10 weeks) in patients with diagnoses closely corresponding to DSM-III-R criteria for panic disorder.

The average dose of Alprazolam was 5-6 mg/day in two of the studies, and the doses of Alprazolam were fixed at 2 and 6 mg/day in the third study. In all three studies Alprazolam was superior to placebo on a variable defined as "the number of patients with zero panic attacks" (range, 37-83% met this criterion), as well as on a global improvement score. In two of the three studies, Alprazolam was superior to placebo on a variable defined as "change from baseline on the number of panic attacks per week" (range, 3.3-5.2), and also on a phobia rating scale. A subgroup of patients who were improved on Alprazolam during short-term treatment in one of these trials was continued on an open basis up to eight months, without apparent loss of benefit.

HOW SUPPLIED
TABLET (C-IV): 0.25 MG

AVERAGE UNIT PRICE (AVAILABLE SIZES)		GENERIC A-RATED AVERAGE PRICE (GAAP)	
BRAND	$0.60	30s	$16.15
GENERIC	$0.51	100s	$52.46
HCFA FUL (100s ea)	$0.07	500s	$248.10
		1000s	$478.94

BRAND/MANUFACTURER	NDC	SIZE	AWP
◆ BRAND			
➤ XANAX: Upjohn	00009-0029-01	100s	$56.63
	00009-0029-20	100s	$72.80
	00009-0029-46	100s ud	$62.68
	00009-0029-02	500s	$274.63
	00009-0029-14	1000s	$537.38
◆ GENERICS			
Allscrips	54569-3755-00	30s	$15.15
Medirex	57480-0520-06	30s	$17.15
Major	00904-7791-60	100s	$46.40
Major	00904-7918-60	100s	$46.40
West Point	59591-0051-68	100s	$48.23
Mylan	00378-4001-01	100s	$50.40
Qualitest	00603-2346-21	100s	$50.55
➤ Geneva	00781-1326-01	100s	$50.95
Roxane	00054-4104-25	100s	$51.00
Warner Chilcott	00047-0787-24	100s	$51.49
Schein	00364-2582-01	100s	$51.52
Novopharm	55953-0126-40	100s	$51.95
Aligen	00405-4043-01	100s	$52.06
Purepac	00228-2027-10	100s	$52.22
Martec	52555-0503-01	100s	$52.50
Goldline	00182-0027-01	100s	$52.80
➤ Lederle Std Prod	00005-3340-43	100s	$52.80
Moore,H.L.	00839-7851-06	100s	$55.08
UDL	51079-0788-21	100s	$63.64
Greenstone	59762-3719-01	100s ud	$48.23
Roxane	00054-8104-25	100s ud	$53.00
UDL	51079-0788-20	100s ud	$54.77
➤ Geneva	00781-1326-13	100s ud	$56.35
Roxane	00054-8104-24	100s ud	$57.00
Medirex	57480-0520-01	100s ud	$57.15
Major	00904-7791-40	500s	$224.90
Major	00904-7918-40	500s	$224.90
Greenstone	59762-3719-03	500s	$233.89
Mylan	00378-4001-05	500s	$244.82
➤ Geneva	00781-1326-05	500s	$247.08
Roxane	00054-4104-29	500s	$248.00
Qualitest	00603-2346-28	500s	$249.60
Warner Chilcott	00047-0787-30	500s	$249.85
Schein	00364-2582-05	500s	$249.86
Novopharm	55953-0126-70	500s	$252.80
Purepac	00228-2027-50	500s	$253.20
Aligen	00405-4043-02	500s	$254.20
Goldline	00182-0027-05	500s	$256.13
➤ Lederle Std Prod	00005-3340-31	500s	$256.13
Martec	52555-0503-05	500s	$256.90
Moore,H.L.	00839-7851-12	500s	$267.37
Greenstone	59762-3719-04	1000s	$457.67
Novopharm	55953-0126-80	1000s	$480.35
➤ Geneva	00781-1326-10	1000s	$483.48
Purepac	00228-2027-96	1000s	$494.24

TABLET (C-IV): 0.5 MG

AVERAGE UNIT PRICE (AVAILABLE SIZES)		GENERIC A-RATED AVERAGE PRICE (GAAP)	
BRAND	$0.71	30s	$19.84
GENERIC	$0.63	100s	$62.85
HCFA FUL (100s ea)	$0.09	500s	$310.59
		1000s	$610.87

BRAND/MANUFACTURER	NDC	SIZE	AWP
◆ BRAND			
➤ XANAX: Upjohn	00009-0055-01	100s	$70.54
	00009-0055-46	100s ud	$76.38
	00009-0055-03	500s	$341.88
	00009-0055-15	1000s	$669.40
◆ GENERICS			
Allscrips	54569-3756-01	20s	$12.52
Allscrips	54569-3756-00	30s	$18.78
Medirex	57480-0521-06	30s	$20.90
Major	00904-7792-60	100s	$57.75
Major	00904-7919-60	100s	$57.75
West Point	59591-0052-68	100s	$60.08
Mylan	00378-4003-01	100s	$62.78
Roxane	00054-4105-25	100s	$63.00
Geneva	00781-1327-01	100s	$63.46
Qualitest	00603-2347-21	100s	$63.50
Warner Chilcott	00047-0786-24	100s	$63.95
Schein	00364-2583-01	100s	$64.17
Novopharm	55953-0127-40	100s	$64.88
Purepac	00228-2029-10	100s	$65.07
Aligen	00405-4044-01	100s	$65.21
Martec	52555-0507-01	100s	$65.80
Goldline	00182-0028-01	100s	$65.81
➤ Lederle Std Prod	00005-3341-43	100s	$65.81
Moore,H.L.	00839-7852-06	100s	$68.51
UDL	51079-0789-01	100s	$75.46
Vangard	00615-0401-13	100s ud	$14.27
Greenstone	59762-3720-01	100s ud	$60.08
Roxane	00054-8105-25	100s ud	$66.00
UDL	51079-0789-20	100s ud	$66.76
Geneva	00781-1327-13	100s ud	$68.67
Medirex	57480-0521-01	100s ud	$69.65
Roxane	00054-8105-24	100s ud	$70.00
Major	00904-7792-40	500s	$279.95
Major	00904-7919-40	500s	$279.95
Greenstone	59762-3720-03	500s	$291.16
Mylan	00378-4003-05	500s	$304.27
Geneva	00781-1327-05	500s	$307.59
Qualitest	00603-2347-28	500s	$308.50
Roxane	00054-4105-29	500s	$310.00
Warner Chilcott	00047-0786-30	500s	$310.25
Schein	00364-2583-05	500s	$311.04
Purepac	00228-2029-50	500s	$315.32
Aligen	00405-4044-02	500s	$316.82
Goldline	00182-0028-05	500s	$318.83
➤ Lederle Std Prod	00005-3341-31	500s	$318.83
Martec	52555-0507-05	500s	$319.55
Moore,H.L.	00839-7852-12	500s	$332.24
Novopharm	55953-0127-50	500s	$345.09
Greenstone	59762-3720-04	1000s	$570.11
Geneva	00781-1327-10	1000s	$602.27
Purepac	00228-2029-96	1000s	$615.40
Novopharm	55953-0127-80	1000s	$655.70

For additional alternatives, turn to the section beginning on page 2859.

Alprostadil

WARNING
APNEA IS EXPERIENCED BY ABOUT 10 TO 12% OF NEONATES WITH CONGENITAL HEART DEFECTS TREATED WITH ALPROSTADIL. APNEA IS MOST OFTEN SEEN IN NEONATES WEIGHING LESS THAN 2 KG AT BIRTH AND USUALLY APPEARS DURING THE FIRST HOUR OF DRUG INFUSION. THEREFORE, RESPIRATORY STATUS SHOULD BE MONITORED THROUGHOUT TREATMENT, AND ALPROSTADIL SHOULD BE USED WHERE VENTILATORY ASSISTANCE IS IMMEDIATELY AVAILABLE.

DESCRIPTION
Alprostadil Sterile Solution for intravascular infusion contains 500 micrograms Alprostadil, more commonly known as prostaglandin E_1, in 1.0 ml dehydrated alcohol.

The chemical name for Alprostadil is (11α, 13E, 15S)-11,15 dihydroxy-9-oxoprost-13-en-1-oic acid, and the molecular weight is 354.49.

Alprostadil is a white to off-white crystalline powder with a melting point between 110° and 116°C. Its solubility at 35°C is 8000 micrograms per 100 mL double distilled water.

Following is its chemical structure:

CLINICAL PHARMACOLOGY
Alprostadil (prostaglandin E_1) is one of a family of naturally occurring acidic lipids with various pharmacologic effects. Vasodilation, inhibition of platelet aggregation, and stimulation of intestinal and uterine smooth muscle are among the most notable of these effects. Intravenous doses of 1 to 10 micrograms of Alprostadil per kilogram of body weight lower the blood pressure in mammals by decreasing peripheral resistance. Reflex increases in cardiac output and rate accompany the reduction in blood pressure.

Smooth muscle of the ductus arteriosus is especially sensitive to Alprostadil, and strips of lamb ductus markedly relax in the presence of the drug. In addition, administration of Alprostadil reopened the closing ductus of newborn rats, rabbits, and lambs. These observations led to the investigation of Alprostadil in infants who had congenital defects which restricted the pulmonary or systemic blood flow and who depended on a patent ductus arteriosus for adequate blood oxygenation and lower body perfusion.

In infants with restricted pulmonary blood flow, about 50% responded to Alprostadil infusion with at least a 10 torr increase in blood pO_2 (mean increase about 14 torr and mean increase in oxygen saturation about 23%). In general, patients who responded best had low pretreatment blood pO_2 and were 4 days old or less.

In infants with restricted systemic blood flow, Alprostadil often increased pH in those having acidosis, increased systemic blood pressure, and decreased the ratio of pulmonary artery pressure to aortic pressure.

Alprostadil must be infused continuously because it is very rapidly metabolized. As much as 80% of the circulating Alprostadil may be metabolized in one pass through the lungs, primarily by β- and ω- oxidation. The metabolites are excreted primarily by the kidney, and excretion is essentially complete within 24 hours after administration. No unchanged Alprostadil has been found in the urine, and there is no evidence of tissue retention of Alprostadil or its metabolites.

INDICATIONS AND USAGE
Alprostadil Sterile Solution is indicated for palliative, not definitive, therapy to temporarily maintain the patency of the ductus arteriosus until corrective or palliative surgery can be performed in neonates who have congenital heart defects and who depend upon the patent ductus for survival. Such congenital heart defects include pulmonary atresia, pulmonary stenosis, tricuspid atresia, tetralogy of Fallot, interruption of the aortic arch, coarctation of the aorta, or transposition of the great vessels with or without other defects.

In infants with restricted pulmonary blood flow, the increase in blood oxygenation is inversely proportional to pretreatment pO_2 values; that is, patients with low pO_2 values respond best, and patients with pO_2 values of 40 torr or more usually have little response.

Alprostadil should be administered only by trained personnel in facilities that provide pediatric intensive care.

UNLABELED USES
Alprostadil is used as an adjunct in the treatment of pulmonary hypertension in patients undergoing mitral valve replacement.

CONTRAINDICATIONS
None.

WARNINGS
See "Warning" box.

Note: Alprostadil Sterile Solution must be diluted before it is administered. See dilution instructions in "Dosage and Administration" section. The administration of Alprostadil to neonates may result in gastric outlet obstruction secondary to antral hyperplasia. This effect appears to be related to duration of therapy and cumulative dose of the drug. Neonates receiving Alprostadil at recommended doses for more than 120 hours should be closely monitored for evidence of antral hyperplasia and gastric outlet obstruction. Alprostadil should be infused for the shortest time and at the lowest dose that will produce the desired effects. The risks of long-term infusion of Alprostadil should be weighed against the possible benefits that critically ill infants may derive from its administration.

PRECAUTIONS
GENERAL PRECAUTIONS
Cortical proliferation of the long bones, first observed in dogs, has also been observed in infants during long-term infusions of Alprostadil. The cortical proliferation in infants regressed after withdrawal of the drug.

In infants treated with Alprostadil at the usual doses for 10 hours to 12 days and who died of causes unrelated to ductus structural weakness, tissue sections of the ductus and pulmonary arteries have shown intimal lacerations, a decrease in medial muscularity and disruption of the medial and internal elastic lamina. Localized and aneurysmal dilatations and vessel wall edema also were seen compared to a series of pathological specimens from infants not treated with Alprostadil. The incidence of such structural alterations has not been defined.

Because Alprostadil inhibits platelet aggregation, use Alprostadil cautiously in neonates with bleeding tendencies.

Alprostadil should not be used in neonates with respiratory distress syndrome. A differential diagnosis should be made between respiratory distress syndrome (hyaline membrane disease) and cyanotic heart disease (restricted pulmonary blood flow). If full diagnostic facilities are not immediately available, cyanosis (pO$_2$ less than 40 torr) and restricted pulmonary blood flow apparent on an x-ray are appropriate indicators of congenital heart defects.

Necessary Monitoring: In all neonates, arterial pressure should be monitored intermittently by umbilical artery catheter, auscultation, or with a Doppler transducer. *Should arterial pressure fall significantly, decrease the rate of infusion immediately.*

In infants with restricted pulmonary blood flow, measure efficacy of Alprostadil by monitoring improvement in blood oxygenation. In infants with restricted systemic blood flow, measure efficacy by monitoring improvement of systemic blood pressure and blood pH.

Drug Interactions: No drug interactions have been reported between Alprostadil and the therapy standard in neonates with restricted pulmonary or systemic blood flow. Standard therapy includes antibiotics, such as penicillin and gentamicin; vasopressors, such as dopamine and isoproterenol; cardiac glycosides; and diuretics, such as furosemide.

Carcinogenesis, Mutagenesis, and Impairment of Fertility: Long-term carcinogenicity studies and fertility studies have not been done. The Ames and Alkaline Elution assays reveal no potential for mutagenesis.

ADVERSE REACTIONS

Central Nervous System: Apnea has been reported in about 12% of the neonates treated. (See *"Warning" box.*) Other common adverse reactions reported have been fever in about 14% of the patients treated and seizures in about 4%. The following reactions have been reported in less than 1% of the patients: cerebral bleeding, hyperextension of the neck, hyperirritability, hypothermia, jitteriness, lethargy, and stiffness.

Cardiovascular System: The most common adverse reactions reported have been flushing in about 10% of patients (more common after intraarterial dosing), bradycardia in about 7%, hypotension in about 4%, tachycardia in about 3%, cardiac arrest in about 1%, and edema in about 1%. The following reactions have been reported in less than 1% of the patients: congestive heart failure, hyperemia, second degree heart block, shock, spasm of the right ventricle infundibulum, supraventricular tachycardia, and ventricular fibrillation.

Respiratory System: The following reactions have been reported in less than 1% of the patients: bradypnea, bronchial wheezing, hypercapnia, respiratory depression, respiratory distress, and tachypnea.

Gastrointestinal System: See *"Warnings"*.

The most common adverse reaction reported has been diarrhea in about 2% of the patients. The following reactions have been reported in less than 1% of the patients; gastric regurgitation, and hyperbilirubinemia.

Hematologic System: The most common hematologic event reported has been disseminated intravascular coagulation in about 1% of the patients. The following events have been reported in less than 1% of the patients: anemia, bleeding, and thrombocytopenia.

Excretory System: Anuria and hematuria have been reported in less than 1% of the patients.

Skeletal System: Cortical proliferation of the long bones has been reported. See *"Precautions"*.

Miscellaneous: Sepsis has been reported in about 2% of the patients. Peritonitis has been reported in less than 1% of the patients. Hypokalemia has been reported in about 1%, and hypoglycemia and hyperkalemia have been reported in less than 1% of the patients.

OVERDOSAGE

Apnea, bradycardia, pyrexia, hypotension, and flushing may be signs of drug overdosage. If apnea or bradycardia occurs, discontinue the infusion, and provide appropriate medical treatment. Caution should be used in restarting the infusion. If pyrexia or hypotension occurs, reduce the infusion rate until these symptoms subside. Flushing is usually a result of incorrect intraarterial catheter placement, and the catheter should be repositioned.

DOSAGE AND ADMINISTRATION

The preferred route of administration for Alprostadil Sterile Solution is continuous intravenous infusion into a large vein. Alternatively, Alprostadil may be administered through an umbilical artery catheter placed at the ductal opening. Increases in blood pO$_2$ (torr) have been the same in neonates who received the drug by either route of administration.

Begin infusion with 0.05 to 0.1 micrograms Alprostadil per kilogram of body weight per minute. A starting dose of 0.1 micrograms per kilogram of body weight per minute is the recommended starting dose based on clinical studies; however, adequate clinical response has been reported using a starting dose of 0.05 micrograms per kilogram of body weight per minute. After a therapeutic response is achieved (increased pO$_2$ in infants with restricted pulmonary blood flow or increased systemic blood pressure and blood pH in infants with restricted systemic blood flow), reduce the infusion rate to provide the lowest possible dosage that maintains the response. This may be accomplished by reducing the dosage from 0.1 to 0.05 to 0.025 to 0.01 micrograms per kilogram of body weight per minute. If response to 0.05 micrograms per kilogram of body weight per minute is inadequate, dosage can be increased up to 0.4 micrograms of body weight per minute although, in general, higher infusion rates do not produce greater effects.

Dilution Instructions: To prepare infusion solutions, dilute 1 mL of Alprostadil Sterile Solution with Sodium Chloride Injection USP or Dextrose Injection USP. Dilute to volumes appropriate for the pump delivery system available. Prepare fresh infusion solutions every 24 hours. *Discard any solution more than 24 hours old.*

SAMPLE DILUTIONS AND INFUSION RATES TO PROVIDE A DOSAGE OF 0.1 MICROGRAMS PER KILOGRAM OF BODY WEIGHT PER MINUTE

Add 1 ampoule (500 micrograms) Alprostadil to:	Approximate concentration of resulting solution (micrograms/mL)	Infusion rate (mL/min per kg of body weight)
250 mL	2	0.05
100 mL	5	0.02
50 mL	10	0.01
25 mL	20	0.005

Example: To provide 0.1 micrograms/kilogram of body weight per minute to an infant weighing 2.8 kilograms using a solution of 1 ampoule Alprostadil in 100 mL of saline or dextrose: INFUSION RATE = 0.02 mL/min per kg × 2.8 kg = 0.056 mL/min or 3.36 mL/hr.

Store in a refrigerator at 2°-8°C (36°-46°F).

HOW SUPPLIED
INJECTION: 0.5 MG/ML

BRAND/MANUFACTURER	NDC	SIZE	AWP
BRAND			
PROSTIN VR PEDIATRIC: Upjohn	00009-3169-01	1 ml	$163.76

Altace *SEE* RAMIPRIL

Alteplase, Recombinant

DESCRIPTION

Alteplase is a tissue plasminogen activator produced by recombinant DNA technology. It is a sterile, purified glycoprotein of 527 amino acids. It is synthesized using the complementary DNA (cDNA) for natural human tissue-type plasminogen activator obtained from a human melanoma cell line. The manufacturing process involves the secretion of the enzyme, Alteplase, into the culture medium by an established mammalian cell line (Chinese Hamster Ovary cells) into which the cDNA for Alteplase has been genetically inserted.

Phosphoric acid and/or sodium hydroxide may be used prior to lyophilization for pH adjustment.

Alteplase, Recombinant is a sterile, white to off-white, lyophilized powder for intravenous administration after reconstitution with Sterile Water for Injection, USP.

Quantitative Composition of the Lyophilized Product

	100 mg Vial	50 mg Vial	20 mg Vial
Alteplase	100 mg (58 million IU)	50 mg (29 million IU)	20 mg (11.6 million IU)
L-Arginine	3.5 g	1.7 g	0.7 g
Phosphoric Acid	1 g	0.5 g	0.2 g
Polysorbate 80	less than or equal to 11 mg	less than 4 mg	less than or equal to 1.6 mg
Vacuum	No	Yes	Yes

Biological potency is determined by an *in vitro* clot lysis assay and is expressed in International Units as tested against the WHO standard. The specific activity of Alteplase, Recombinant is 580,000 IU/mg.

CLINICAL PHARMACOLOGY

Alteplase, Recombinant is an enzyme (serine protease) which has the property of fibrin-enhanced conversion of plasminogen to plasmin. It produces limited conversion of plasminogen in the absence of fibrin. When introduced into the systemic circulation at pharmacologic concentration, Alteplase, Recombinant binds to fibrin in a thrombus and converts the entrapped plasminogen to plasmin. This initiates local fibrinolysis with limited systemic proteolysis. Following administration of 100 mg Alteplase, Recombinant, there is a decrease (16-36%) in circulating fibrinogen.[1,2] In a controlled trial, 8 of 73 patients (11%) receiving Alteplase, Recombinant (1.25 mg/kg body weight over 3 hours) experienced a decrease in fibrinogen to below 100 mg/dL.[2]

Alteplase, Recombinant is cleared rapidly from circulating plasma at a rate of 550-680 mL/min. Alteplase, Recombinant is cleared primarily by the liver. More than 50% of Alteplase, Recombinant present in plasma is cleared within 5 minutes after the infusion has been terminated, and approximately 80% is cleared within 10 minutes. Coronary occlusion due to a thrombus is present in the infarct-related coronary artery in approximately 80% of patients experiencing a transmural myocardial infarction evaluated within four hours of onset of symptoms.[3,4]

In patients studied in a controlled trial with coronary angiography at 90 and 120 minutes following infusion of Alteplase, Recombinant, infarct artery patency was observed in 71% and 85% of patients (n = 85), respectively.[2] In a second study, where patients received coronary angiography prior to and following infusion of Alteplase, Recombinant within six hours of the onset of symptoms, reperfusion of the obstructed vessel occurred within 90 minutes after the commencement of therapy in 71% of 83 patients.[1]

In a double-blind, randomized trial (138 patients) comparing Alteplase, Recombinant to placebo, patients infused with Alteplase, Recombinant within 4 hours of onset of symptoms experienced improved left ventricular function at Day 10 compared to the placebo group, when ejection fraction was measured by gated blood pool scan (53.2% versus 46.4%, p = 0.018). Relative to baseline (Day 1) values, the net changes in ejection fraction were +3.6% and −4.7% for the treated and placebo group, respectively (p = 0.0001). Also documented was a reduced incidence of clinical congestive heart failure in the treated group (14%) compared to the placebo group (33%) (p = 0.009).[5]

In a second double-blind, randomized trial (145 patients) comparing Alteplase, Recombinant to placebo, patients infused with Alteplase, Recombinant within 2.5 hours of onset of symptoms experienced improved left ventricular function at a mean of 21 days compared to the placebo group, when ejection fraction was measured by gated blood pool scan (52% versus 48%, p = 0.08) and by contrast ventriculogram (61% versus 54%, p = 0.006). Although the contribution of Alteplase, Recombinant alone is unclear, the incidence of nonischemic cardiac complications when taken as a group (i.e., congestive heart failure, pericarditis, atrial fibrillation, conduction disturbance) was reduced when compared to those patients treated with placebo (p < 0.01).[6]

In a double-blind, randomized trial (5013 patients) comparing Alteplase, Recombinant to placebo (ASSET study), patients infused with Alteplase, Recombinant within four hours of the onset of symptoms of acute myocardial infarction experienced improved 30-day survival compared to those treated with placebo. At one month the overall mortality rates were 7.2% for the Alteplase, Recombinant treated group and 9.8% for the placebo treated group (p = 0.001).[7,8] This benefit was maintained at 6 months for Alteplase, Recombinant treated patients (10.4%) compared to those treated with placebo (13.1%) (p = 0.008).[8]

In a second double-blind, randomized trial (721 patients) comparing Alteplase, Recombinant to placebo, patients infused with Alteplase, Recombinant within five hours of the onset of symptoms experienced improved ventricular function 10-22 days after treatment compared to the placebo group, when global ejection fraction was measured by contrast ventriculography (50.7% versus 48.5%, p = 0.01). Patients treated with Alteplase, Recombinant had a 19% reduction in infarct size, as measured by cumulative release of HBDH (α-hydroxybutyrate dehydrogenase) activity compared to placebo treated patients (p = 0.001). Patients treated with Alteplase, Recombinant had significantly fewer episodes of cardiogenic shock (p = 0.02), ventricular fibrillation (p < 0.04) and pericarditis (p = 0.01) compared to patients treated with placebo. Mortality at 21 days in Alteplase, Recombinant treated patients was reduced to 3.7% compared to 6.3% in placebo treated patients (1p = 0.05).[9] Although these data do not demonstrate unequivocally a significant reduction in mortality for this study, they do indicate a trend that is supported by the results of the ASSET study. In a comparative randomized trial (n = 45),[10] 59% of patients (n = 22) treated with Alteplase, Recombinant (100 mg over two hours) experienced moderate or marked lysis of pulmonary emboli when assessed by pulmonary angiography two hours after treatment initiation. Alteplase, Recombinant treated patients also experienced a significant reduction in pulmonary embolism-induced pulmonary hypertension within two hours of treatment (p = 0.003). Pulmonary perfusion at 24 hours, as assessed by radionuclide scan, was significantly improved (p = 0.002).

INDICATIONS AND USAGE

ACUTE MYOCARDIAL INFARCTION

Alteplase, Recombinant is indicated for use in the management of acute myocardial infarction (AMI) in adults for the lysis of thrombi obstructing coronary arteries, the reduction of infarct size, the improvement of ventricular function following AMI, the reduction of the incidence of congestive heart failure and the reduction of mortality associated with AMI. Treatment should be initiated as soon as possible after the onset of AMI symptoms (see *"Clinical Pharmacology"*).

PULMONARY EMBOLISM

Alteplase, Recombinant, is indicated in the management of acute massive pulmonary embolism (PE) in adults:

for the lysis of acute pulmonary emboli, defined as obstruction of blood flow to a lobe or multiple segments of the lungs, and

for the lysis of pulmonary emboli accompanied by unstable hemodynamics, e.g., failure to maintain blood pressure without supportive measures.

The diagnosis should be confirmed by objective means, such as pulmonary angiography or noninvasive procedures such as lung scanning.

UNLABELED USES

Alteplase, Recombinant, has been used alone or as an adjunct in the treatment of unstable angina.

CONTRAINDICATIONS

Because thrombolytic therapy increases the risk of bleeding, Alteplase, Recombinant is contraindicated in the following situations:

- Active internal bleeding
- History of cerebrovascular accident
- Recent (within two months) intracranial or intraspinal, surgery or trauma (see *"Warnings"*)
- Intracranial neoplasm, arteriovenous malformation, or aneurysm
- Known bleeding diathesis
- Severe uncontrolled hypertension

WARNINGS

BLEEDING

The most common complication encountered during Alteplase, Recombinant therapy is bleeding. The type of bleeding associated with thrombolytic therapy can be divided into two broad categories:

- Internal bleeding, involving the gastrointestinal tract, genitourinary tract, retroperitoneal or intracranial sites.
- Superficial or surface bleeding, observed mainly at invaded or disturbed sites (e.g., venous cutdowns, arterial punctures, sites of recent surgical intervention).

The concomitant use of heparin anticoagulation may contribute to bleeding. Some of the hemorrhagic episodes occurred one or more days after the effects of Alteplase, Recombinant had dissipated, but while heparin therapy was continuing.

As fibrin is lysed during Alteplase, Recombinant therapy, bleeding from recent puncture sites may occur. Therefore, thrombolytic therapy requires careful attention to all potential bleeding sites (including catheter insertion sites, arterial and venous puncture sites, cutdown sites and needle puncture sites).

Intramuscular injections and nonessential handling of the patient should be avoided during treatment with Alteplase, Recombinant. Venipunctures should be performed carefully and only as required.

Should an arterial puncture be necessary during an infusion of Alteplase, Recombinant, it is preferable to use an upper extremity vessel that is accessible to manual compression. Pressure should be applied for at least 30 minutes, a pressure dressing applied and the puncture site checked frequently for evidence of bleeding.

Should serious bleeding (not controllable by local pressure) occur, the infusion of Alteplase, Recombinant and any concomitant heparin should be terminated immediately.

Each patient being considered for therapy with Alteplase, Recombinant should be carefully evaluated and anticipated benefits weighed against potential risks associated with therapy.

In the following conditions, the risks of Alteplase, Recombinant therapy may be increased and should be weighted against the anticipated benefits:

- Recent (within 10 days) major surgery, e.g., coronary artery bypass graft, obstetrical delivery, organ biopsy, previous puncture of noncompressible vessels
- Cerebrovascular disease
- Recent gastrointestinal or genitourinary bleeding (within 10 days)
- Recent trauma (within 10 days)
- Hypertension: systolic BP ≥ 180 mm Hg and/or diastolic BP ≥ 110 mm Hg
- High likelihood of left heart thrombus, e.g., mitral stenosis with atrial fibrillation
- Acute pericarditis
- Subacute bacterial endocarditis
- Hemostatic defects including those secondary to severe hepatic or renal disease
- Significant liver dysfunction
- Pregnancy
- Diabetic hemorrhagic retinopathy, or other hemorrhagic ophthalmic conditions
- Septic thrombophlebitis or occluded AV cannula at seriously infected site
- Advanced age, i.e., over 75 years old
- Patients currently receiving oral anticoagulants, e.g., warfarin sodium
- Any other condition in which bleeding constitutes a significant hazard or would be particularly difficult to manage because of its location

ARRHYTHMIAS

Coronary thrombolysis may result in arrhythmias associated with reperfusion. These arrhythmias (such as sinus bradycardia, accelerated idioventricular rhythm, ventricular premature depolarizations, ventricular tachycardia) are not different from those often seen in the ordinary course of acute myocardial infarction and may be managed with standard antiarrhythmic measures. It is recommended that anti-arrhythmic therapy for bradycardia and/or ventricular irritability be available when infusions of Alteplase, Recombinant, are administered.

PULMONARY EMBOLISM

It should be recognized that the treatment of pulmonary embolism with Alteplase, Recombinant has not been shown to constitute adequate clinical treatment of underlying deep vein thrombosis. Furthermore, the possible risk of reembolization due to the lysis of underlying deep venous thrombi should be considered.

PRECAUTIONS
GENERAL

Standard management of myocardial infarction or pulmonary embolism should be implemented concomitantly with Alteplase, Recombinant treatment. Noncompressible arterial puncture must be avoided (i.e., internal jugular and subclavian punctures should be avoided to minimize bleeding from noncompressible sites). Arterial and venous punctures should be minimized. In the event of serious bleeding Alteplase, Recombinant and heparin should be discontinued immediately. Heparin effects can be reversed by protamine.

READMINISTRATION

There is no experience with readministration of Alteplase, Recombinant. If an anaphylactoid reaction occurs, the infusion should be discontinued immediately and appropriate therapy initiated.

Although sustained antibody formation in patients receiving one dose of Alteplase, Recombinant, has not been documented, readministration should be undertaken with caution. Detectable levels of antibody (a single point measurement) were reported in one patient but subsequent antibody test results were negative.

LABORATORY TESTS

During Alteplase, Recombinant, therapy, if coagulation tests and/or measures of fibrinolytic activity are performed, the results may be unreliable unless specific precautions are taken to prevent *in vitro* artifacts. Alteplase, Recombinant is an enzyme that when present in blood in pharmacologic concentrations remains active under *in vitro* conditions. This can lead to degradation of fibrinogen in blood samples removed for analysis. Collection of blood samples in the presence of aprotinin (150-200 units/mL) can to some extent mitigate this phenomenon.

DRUG INTERACTIONS

The interaction of Alteplase, Recombinant with other cardioactive drugs has not been studied. In addition to bleeding associated with heparin and vitamin K antagonists, drugs that alter platelet function (such as acetylsalicylic acid, dipyridamole) may increase the risk of bleeding if administered prior to, during or after Alteplase, Recombinant therapy.

USE OF ANTICOAGULANTS

Heparin has been administered concomitantly with and following infusions of Alteplase, Recombinant to reduce the risk of rethrombosis. Because either heparin or Alteplase, Recombinant alone may cause bleeding complications, careful monitoring for bleeding is advised, especially at arterial puncture sites.

CARCINOGENESIS, MUTAGENESIS, IMPAIRMENT OF FERTILITY

Long-term studies in animals have not been performed to evaluate the carcinogenic potential or the effect on fertility.

Short-term studies, which evaluated tumorigenicity of Alteplase, Recombinant and effect on tumor metastases in rodents, were negative.

Studies to determine mutagenicity (Ames test) and chromosomal aberration assays in human lymphocytes were negative at all concentrations tested. Cytotoxicity, as reflected by a decrease in mitotic index, was evidenced only after prolonged exposure and only at the highest concentrations tested.

PREGNANCY (CATEGORY C)

Animal reproduction studies have not been conducted with Alteplase, Recombinant. It is also not known whether Alteplase, Recombinant can cause fetal harm when administered to a pregnant woman or can affect reproduction capacity. Alteplase, Recombinant should be given to a pregnant woman only if clearly needed.

NURSING MOTHERS

It is not known whether Alteplase, Recombinant is excreted in human milk. Because many drugs are excreted in human milk, caution should be exercised when Alteplase, Recombinant, is administered to a nursing woman.

PEDIATRIC USE

Safety and effectiveness of Alteplase, Recombinant in children has not been established.

ADVERSE REACTIONS
BLEEDING

The most frequent adverse reaction associated with Alteplase, Recombinant is bleeding. The type of bleeding associated with thrombolytic therapy can be divided into two broad categories:

Internal bleeding, involving the gastrointestinal tract, genitourinary tract, retroperitoneal or intracranial sites.
Superficial or surface bleeding, observed mainly at invaded or disturbed sites (e.g., venous cutdowns, arterial punctures, sites of recent surgical intervention).

The following incidence of significant internal bleeding (estimated as > 250 cc blood loss) has been reported in studies in over 800 patients treated at all doses:

	Total Dose ≤ 100 mg	Total Dose > 100 mg
gastrointestinal	5%	5%
genitourinary	4%	4%
ecchymosis	1%	< 1%
retroperitoneal	< 1%	< 1%
epistaxis	< 1%	< 1%
gingival	< 1%	< 1%

The incidence of intracranial bleeding (ICB) in patients treated with Alteplase, Recombinant is as follows:

Dose	Number of Patients	%
100 mg	3272	0.4
150 mg	1779	1.3
1-1.4 mg/kg	237	0.4

These data indicate that a dose of 150 mg of Alteplase, Recombinant should not be used because it has been associated with an increase in intracranial bleeding.

Recent data indicate that the incidence of stroke in 6 randomized double-blind placebo controlled trials[2,5-9,11] is not significantly different in the Alteplase, Recombinant treated patients compared to those treated with placebo (37/3161, 1.2% versus 27/3092, 0.9%, respectively) (p = 0.26).

Should serious bleeding in a critical location (intracranial, gastrointestinal, retroperitoneal, pericardial) occur, Alteplase, Recombinant therapy should be discontinued immediately, along with any concomitant therapy with heparin.

Fibrin which is part of the hemostatic plug formed at needle puncture sites will be lysed during Alteplase, Recombinant therapy.

Therefore, Alteplase, Recombinant therapy requires careful attention to potential bleeding sites, e.g., catheter insertion sites, arterial puncture sites.

ALLERGIC REACTIONS

Allergic type reactions, e.g., anaphylactoid reaction, laryngeal edema, rash, and urticaria have been reported very rarely (less than 0.02%). A cause and effect relationship to Alteplase, Recombinant therapy has not been established. When such reactions occur, they usually respond to conventional therapy.

OTHER ADVERSE REACTIONS

Other adverse reactions have been reported, principally nausea and/or vomiting, hypotension, and fever. These reactions are frequent sequelae of myocardial infarction and may or may not be attributable to Alteplase, Recombinant therapy.

DOSAGE AND ADMINISTRATION

Alteplase, Recombinant is for intravenous administration only. Extravasation of Alteplase, Recombinant infusion can cause ecchymosis and/or inflammation. Management consists of terminating the infusion at that IV site and application of local therapy.

ACUTE MYOCARDIAL INFARCTION

Administer Alteplase, Recombinant as soon as possible after the onset of symptoms.

The recommended dose is 100 mg administered as 60 mg (34.8 million IU) in the first hour (of which 6 to 10 mg is administered as a bolus over the first 1-2 minutes), 20 mg (11.6 million IU) over the second hour, and 20 mg (11.6 million IU) over the third hour. For smaller patients (less than 65 kg), a dose of 1.25 mg/kg administered over 3 hours, as described above, may be used.[12]

a. The bolus dose may be prepared in one of the following ways:

1. By removing 6 to 10 mL from the vial of reconstituted (1 mg/mL) Alteplase, Recombinant using a syringe and needle. If this method is used with the 20 mg or 50 mg vials, the syringe should not be primed with air and the needle should be inserted into the Alteplase, Recombinant vial stopper. If the 100 mg vial is used, the needle should be inserted away from the puncture mark made by the transfer device.
2. By removing 6 to 10 mL from a port (second injection site) on the infusion line after the infusion set is primed.
3. By programming an infusion pump to deliver a 6 to 10 mL (1 mg/mL) bolus at the initiation of the infusion.

b. The remainder of the Alteplase, Recombinant dose may be administered as follows:

20 mg, 50 mg vials, administer using either a polyvinyl chloride bag or glass vial and infusion set
100 mg vials, insert the spike end of an infusion set through the same puncture site created by the transfer device in the stopper of the vial of reconstituted Alteplase, Recombinant. Hang the Alteplase, Recombinant vial from the plastic molded capping attached to the bottom of the vial.

Although the use of anticoagulants and antiplatelet drugs during and following administration of Alteplase, Recombinant has not been shown to be of unequivocal benefit, heparin has been administered concomitantly for 24 hours or longer in more than 90% of patients. Aspirin and/or dipyridamole have been given either during and/or following heparin treatment.

PULMONARY EMBOLISM

The recommended dose is 100 mg administered by intravenous infusion over two hours. Heparin therapy should be instituted or reinstituted near the end of or immediately following the Alteplase, Recombinant infusion when the partial thromboplastin time or thrombin time returns to twice normal or less.

The dose may be administered using the instructions described above in Acute Myocardial Infarction (b).

A DOSE OF 150 MG OF ALTEPLASE, RECOMBINANT, SHOULD NOT BE USED BECAUSE IT HAS BEEN ASSOCIATED WITH AN INCREASE IN INTRACRANIAL BLEEDING.

RECONSTITUTION AND DILUTION

Alteplase, Recombinant should be reconstituted by aseptically adding the appropriate volume of the accompanying Sterile Water for Injection, USP to the vial. It is important that Alteplase, Recombinant be reconstituted only with Sterile Water for Injection, USP, without preservatives. Do not use Bacteriostatic Water for Injection, USP. The reconstituted preparation results in a colorless to pale yellow transparent solution containing Alteplase, Recombinant 1 mg/mL at approximately pH 7.3. The osmolality of this solution is approximately 215 mOsm/kg.

Because Alteplase, Recombinant contains no antibacterial preservatives, it should be reconstituted immediately before use. The solution may be used for intravenous administration within 8 hours following reconstitution when stored between 2-30°C (36-86°F). Before further dilution or administration, the product should be visually inspected for particulate matter and discoloration prior to administration whenever solution and container permit.

Alteplase, Recombinant may be administered as reconstituted at 1 mg/mL. As an alternative, the reconstituted solution may be diluted further immediately before administration in an equal volume of 0.9% Sodium Chloride Injection, USP or 5% Dextrose Injection, USP to yield a concentration of 0.5 mg/mL. Either polyvinyl chloride bags or glass vials are acceptable. Alteplase, Recombinant is stable for up to 8 hours in these solutions at room temperature. Exposure to light has no effect on the stability of these solutions. Excessive agitation during dilution should be avoided; mixing should be accomplished with gentle swirling and/or slow inversion. Do not use other infusion solutions, e.g., Sterile Water for Injection, USP or preservative-containing solutions for further dilution.

20 MG AND 50 MG VIALS

Reconstitution should be carried out using a large bore needle (e.g., 18 gauge) and a syringe, directing the stream of Sterile Water for Injection, USP into the lyophilized cake. **DO NOT USE IF VACUUM IS NOT PRESENT.** Slight foaming upon reconstitution is not unusual; standing undisturbed for several minutes is usually sufficient to allow dissipation of any large bubbles.

No other medication should be added to infusion solutions containing Alteplase, Recombinant. Any unused infusion solution should be discarded.

100 MG VIALS

Reconstitution should be carried out using the transfer device provided, adding the contents of the accompanying 100 mL vial of Sterile Water for Injection, USP to the contents of the 100 mg vial of Alteplase, Recombinant powder. Slight foaming upon reconstitution is not unusual; standing undisturbed for several minutes is usually sufficient to allow dissipation of any large bubbles. Please refer to the accompanying Instructions for Reconstitution and Administration. **100 MG VIALS DO NOT CONTAIN VACUUM.**

100 MG VIAL RECONSTITUTION

1. Use aseptic technique throughout.
2. Remove the protective flip-caps from one vial of Alteplase, Recombinant and one vial of Sterile Water for Injection, USP (SWFI).
3. Open the package containing the transfer device by peeling the paper label off the package.
4. Remove the protective cap from one end of the transfer device and keeping the vial of SWFI upright, insert the piercing pin vertically into the center of the stopper of the vial of SWFI.
5. Remove the protective cap from the other end of the transfer device. **DO NOT INVERT THE VIAL OF SWFI.**
6. Holding the vial of Alteplase, Recombinant upside-down, position it so that the center of the stopper is directly over the exposed piercing pin of the transfer device.
7. Push the vial of Alteplase, Recombinant down so that the piercing pin is inserted through the center of the Alteplase, Recombinant vial stopper.
8. Invert the two vials so that the vial of Alteplase, Recombinant is on the bottom (upright) and the vial of SWFI is upside-down, allowing the SWFI to flow down through the transfer device. Allow the entire contents of the vial of SWFI to flow into the Alteplase, Recombinant vial (approximately 0.5 cc of SWFI will remain in the diluent vial). Approximately two minutes are required for this procedure.
9. Remove the transfer device and the empty SWFI vial from the Alteplase, Recombinant vial. Safely discard both the transfer device and the empty diluent vial according to institutional procedures.
10. Swirl gently to dissolve the Alteplase, Recombinant powder. **DO NOT SHAKE.**

No other medication should be added to infusion solutions containing Alteplase, Recombinant. Any unused infusion solution should be discarded.

STORAGE

Store lyophilized Alteplase, Recombinant at controlled room temperature not to exceed 30°C (86°F), or under refrigeration (2-8°C/36-46°F). Protect the lyophilized material during extended storage from excessive exposure to light.

Do not use beyond the expiration date stamped on the vial.

REFERENCES

1. Mueller H, Rao AK, Forman SA, et al, Thrombolysis in Myocardial Infarction (TIMI): Comparative studies of coronary reperfusion and systemic fibrinogenolysis with two forms of recombinant tissue-type plasminogen activator. J Am Coll Card 1987; 10:479-490. 2. Topol EJ, Morriss DC, Smalling RW, et al, A multicenter, randomized, placebo-controlled trial of a new form of intravenous recombinant tissue-type plasminogen activator (Alteplase, Recombinant) in acute myocardial infarction. J Am Coll Card 1987; 9:1205-1213. 3. De Wood MA, Spores J, Notske R, et al, Prevalence of total coronary occlusion during the early hours of transmural myocardial infarction. New Engl J Med 1980: 303:897-902. 4. Chesebro JH, Knatterud G, Roberts R, et al, Thrombolysis in Myocardial Infarction (TIMI) Trial, Phase I: A comparison between intravenous tissue plasminogen activator and intravenous streptokinase. Circulation July, 1987; 76(1):142-154. 5. Guerci AD, Gerstenblith G, Brinker JA, et al, A randomized trial of intravenous tissue plasminogen activator for acute myocardial infarction with subsequent randomization to elective coronary angioplasty. New Engl J Med 1987; 317:1613-1618. 6. O'Rourke M, Baron D, Keogh A, et al, Limitation of myocardial infarction by early infusion of recombinant tissue-plasminogen activator. Circulation 1988; 77:1311-1315. 7. Wilcox RG, von der Lippe G, Olsson CG, et al, Trial of tissue plasminogen activator for mortality reduction in acute myocardial infarction: ASSET. Lancet 1988; 2:525-530. 8. Hampton JR, The University of Nottingham, Personal Communication. 9. Van de Werf F, Arnold AER, et al, Effect of intravenous tissue-plasminogen activator on infarct size, left ventricular function and survival in patients with acute myocardial infarction. Br Med J 1988; 297:1374-1379. 10. Goldhaber SZ, Kessler CM, Heit J, et al, A randomized controlled trial of recombinant tissue plasminogen activator in the treatment of acute pulmonary embolism. Lancet 1988; 2:293-298. 11. National Heart Foundation of Australia Coronary Thrombolysis Group: Coronary thrombolysis and myocardial infarction salvage by tissue plasminogen activator given up to 4 hours after onset of myocardial infarction. Lancet 1988; 1:203-207. 12. Califf RM, Stump D, Thornton D, et al, Hemorrhagic complications after tissue plasminogen activator (t-PA) therapy for acute myocardial infarction. Circulation 1987; 76:IV-1.

J CODES

Per 10 mg IV—J2996

HOW SUPPLIED

POWDER FOR INJECTION: 20 MG

BRAND/MANUFACTURER	NDC	SIZE	AWP
○ BRAND ACTIVASE: Genentech	50242-0044-12	1s	$550.00

POWDER FOR INJECTION: 50 MG

BRAND/MANUFACTURER	NDC	SIZE	AWP
○ BRAND ACTIVASE: Genentech	50242-0044-13	1s	$1375.00

POWDER FOR INJECTION: 100 MG

BRAND/MANUFACTURER	NDC	SIZE	AWP
○ BRAND ACTIVASE: Genentech	50242-0085-27	1s	$2750.00

Altretamine

WARNINGS

1. ALTRETAMINE SHOULD ONLY BE GIVEN UNDER THE SUPERVISION OF A PHYSICIAN EXPERIENCED IN THE USE OF ANTINEOPLASTIC AGENTS.

2. PERIPHERAL BLOOD COUNTS SHOULD BE MONITORED AT LEAST MONTHLY, PRIOR TO THE INITIATION OF EACH COURSE OF ALTRETAMINE, AND AS CLINICALLY INDICATED (SEE "*ADVERSE REACTIONS*").

3. BECAUSE OF THE POSSIBILITY OF ALTRETAMINE-RELATED NEUROTOXICITY, NEUROLOGIC EXAMINATION SHOULD BE PERFORMED REGULARLY DURING ALTRETAMINE ADMINISTRATION (SEE "*ADVERSE REACTIONS*").

DESCRIPTION

Altretamine is a synthetic cytotoxic antineoplastic s-triazine derivative. Altretamine capsules contain 50 mg of Altretamine for oral administration. Altretamine, known chemically as N,N,N',N'',N''-hexamethyl-1,3,5-triazine-2,4,6-triamine.

Its empirical formula is $C_9H_{18}N_6$ with a molecular weight of 210.28. Altretamine is a white crystalline powder, melting at 172° ± 1°C. Altretamine is practically insoluble in water but increasingly soluble at pH 3 and below.

Following is its chemical structure:

CLINICAL PHARMACOLOGY

The precise mechanism by which Altretamine exerts its cytotoxic effect is unknown, although a number of theoretical possibilities have been studied. Structurally, Altretamine resembles the alkylating agent triethylenemelamine, yet *in vitro* tests for alkylating activity of Altretamine and its metabolites have been negative. Altretamine has been demonstrated to be efficacious for certain ovarian tumors resistant to classical alkylating agents. Metabolism of Altretamine is a requirement for cytotoxicity. Synthetic monohydroxymethylmelamines, and products of Altretamine metabolism, *in vitro* and *in vivo*, can form covalent adducts with tissue macromolecules including DNA, but the relevance of these reactions to antitumor activity is unknown.

Altretamine is well-absorbed following oral administration in humans, but undergoes rapid and extensive demethylation in the liver, producing variation in altretamine plasma levels. The principal metabolites are pentamethylmelamine and tetramethylmelamine.

Pharmacokinetic studies were performed in a limited number of patients and should be considered preliminary. After oral administration of Altretamine to 11 patients with advanced ovarian cancer in doses of 120-300 mg/m^2, peak plasma levels (as measured by gas-chromatographic assay) were reached between 0.5 and 3 hours, varying from 0.2 to 20.8 mg/l. Half-life of the β-phase of elimination ranged from 4.7 to 10.2 hours. Altretamine and metabolites show binding to plasma proteins. The free fractions of altretamine, pentamethylmelamine and tetramethylmelamine are 6%, 25% and 50%, respectively.

Following oral administration of ^{14}C-ring-labeled altretamine (4 mg/kg), urinary recovery of radioactivity was 61% at 24 hours and 90% at 72 hours. Human urinary metabolites were N-demethylated homologues of altretamine with < 1% unmetabolized altretamine excreted at 24 hours.

After intraperitoneal administration of ^{14}C-ring-labeled Altretamine to mice, tissue distribution was rapid in all organs, reaching a maximum at 30 minutes. The excretory organs (liver and kidney) and the small intestine showed high concentrations of radioactivity, whereas relatively low concentrations were found in other organs, including the brain.

There have been no formal pharmacokinetic studies in patients with compromised hepatic and/or renal function, though Altretamine has been administered both concurrently and following nephrotoxic drugs such as cisplatin.

Altretamine has been administered in 4 divided doses, with meals and at bedtime, though there is no pharmacokinetic data on this schedule nor information from formal interaction studies about the effect of food on its bioavailability or pharmacokinetics.

In two studies in patients with persistent or recurrent ovarian cancer following first-line treatment with cisplatin and/or alkylating agent-based combinations, Altretamine was administered as a single agent for 14 or 21 days of a 28 day cycle. In the 51 patients with measurable or evaluable disease, there were 6 clinical complete responses, 1 pathologic complete response, and 2 partial responses for an overall response rate of 18%. The duration of these responses ranged from 2 months in a patient with a palpable pelvic mass to 36 months in a patient who achieved a pathologic complete response. In some patients, tumor regression was associated with improvement in symptoms and performance status.

INDICATIONS AND USAGE
Altretamine is indicated for use as a single agent in the palliative treatment of patients with persistent or recurrent ovarian cancer following first-line therapy with a cisplatin and/or alkylating agent-based combination.

UNLABELED USES
Altretamine has been used alone or as an adjunct in the treatment of breast and small cell lung carcinoma.

CONTRAINDICATIONS
Altretamine is contraindicated in patients who have shown hypersensitivity to it. Altretamine should not be employed in patients with preexisting severe bone marrow depression or severe neurologic toxicity. Altretamine has been administered safely, however, to patients heavily pretreated with cisplatin and/or alkylating agents, including patients with preexisting cisplatin neuropathies. Careful monitoring of neurologic function in these patients is essential.

WARNINGS
See boxed *"Warnings"*.

Concurrent administration of Altretamine and antidepressants of the monoamine oxidase (MAO) inhibitor class may cause severe orthostatic hypotension. Four patients, all over 60 years of age, were reported to have experienced symptomatic hypotension after 4 to 7 days of concomitant therapy with Altretamine and MAO inhibitors.

Altretamine causes mild to moderate myelosuppression and neurotoxicity. Blood counts and a neurologic examination should be performed prior to the initiation of each course of therapy and the dose of Altretamine adjusted as clinically indicated (see *"Dosage and Administration"*).

PREGNANCY: CATEGORY D
Altretamine has been shown to be embryotoxic and teratogenic in rats and rabbits when given at doses 2 and 10 times the human dose. Altretamine may cause fetal damage when administered to a pregnant woman. If Altretamine is used during pregnancy, or if the patient becomes pregnant while taking the drug, the patient should be appraised of the potential hazard to the fetus. Women of childbearing potential should be advised to avoid becoming pregnant.

PRECAUTIONS
GENERAL
Neurologic examination should be performed regularly (see *"Adverse Reactions"*).

LABORATORY TESTS
Peripheral blood counts should be monitored at least monthly, prior to the initiation of each course of Altretamine, and as clinically indicated (see *"Adverse Reactions"*).

DRUG INTERACTIONS
Concurrent administration of Altretamine and antidepressants of the MAO inhibitor class may cause severe orthostatic hypotension (see *"Warnings"* section). Cimetidine, an inhibitor of microsomal drug metabolism, increased Altretamine's half-life and toxicity in a rat model.

Data from a randomized trial of Altretamine and cisplatin plus or minus pyridoxine in ovarian cancer indicated that pyridoxine significantly reduced neurotoxicity; however, it adversely affected response duration suggesting that pyridoxine should not be administered with Altretamine and/or cisplatin (1).

CARCINOGENESIS, MUTAGENESIS AND IMPAIRMENT OF FERTILITY
The carcinogenic potential of Altretamine has not been studied in animals, but drugs with similar mechanisms of action have been shown to be carcinogenic. Altretamine was weakly mutagenic when tested in strain TA100 of *Salmonella typhimurium*. Altretamine administered to female rats 14 days prior to breeding through the gestation period had no adverse effect on fertility, but decreased postnatal survival at 120 mg/m^2/day and was embryocidal at 240 mg/m^2/day. Administration of 120 mg/m^2/day Altretamine to male rats for 60 days prior to mating resulted in testicular atrophy, reduced fertility and a possible dominant lethal mutagenic effect. Male rats treated with Altretamine at 450 mg/m^2/day for 10 days had decreased spermatogenesis, atrophy of testes, seminal vesicles and ventral prostate.

PREGNANCY
Pregnancy Category D: see *"Warnings"* section.

NURSING MOTHERS
It is not known whether Altretamine is excreted in human milk. Because there is a possibility of toxicity in nursing infants secondary to Altretamine treatment of the mother, it is recommended that breast feeding be discontinued if the mother is treated with Altretamine.

PEDIATRIC USE
The safety and effectiveness of Altretamine in children have not been established.

ADVERSE REACTIONS
GASTROINTESTINAL
With continuous high-dose daily Altretamine, nausea and vomiting of gradual onset occur frequently. Although in most instances these symptoms are controllable with antiemetics, at times the severity requires Altretamine dose reduction or, rarely, discontinuation of Altretamine therapy. In some instances, a tolerance of these symptoms develops after several weeks of therapy. The incidence and severity of nausea and vomiting are reduced with moderate-dose administration of Altretamine. In 2 clinical studies of single-agent Altretamine utilizing a moderate, intermittent dose and schedule, only 1 patient (1%) discontinued Altretamine due to severe nausea and vomiting.

NEUROTOXICITY
Peripheral neuropathy and central nervous system symptoms (mood disorders, disorders of consciousness, ataxia, dizziness, vertigo) have been reported. They are more likely to occur in patients receiving continuous high-dose daily Altretamine than moderate-dose Altretamine administered on an intermittent schedule. Neurologic toxicity has been reported to be reversible when therapy is discontinued. Data from a randomized trial of Altretamine and cisplatin plus or minus pyridoxine in ovarian cancer indicated that pyridoxine significantly reduced neurotoxicity; however, it adversely affected response duration suggesting that pyridoxine should not be administered with Altretamine and/or cisplatin (1).

HEMATOLOGIC
Altretamine causes mild to moderate dose-related myelosuppression. Leukopenia below 3000 WBC/mm^3 occurred in < 15% of patients on a variety of intermittent or continuous dose regimens. Less than 1% had leukopenia below 1000 WBC/mm^3. Thrombocytopenia below 50,000 platelets/mm^3 was seen in < 10% of patients. When given in doses of 8-12 mg/kg/day over a 21 day course, nadirs of leukocyte and platelet counts were reached by 3-4 weeks, and normal counts were regained by 6 weeks. With continuous administration at doses of 6-8 mg/kg/day, nadirs are reached in 6-8 weeks (median).

Data in the following table are based on the experience of 76 patients with ovarian cancer previously treated with a cisplatin-based combination regimen who received single-agent Altretamine. In one study, Altretamine, 260 mg/m^2/day, was administered for 14 days of a 28 day cycle. In another study, Altretamine, 6-8 mg/kg/day, was administered for 21 days of a 28 day cycle.

ADVERSE EXPERIENCES IN 76 PREVIOUSLY TREATED OVARIAN CANCER PATIENTS RECEIVING SINGLE-AGENT ALTRETAMINE

	%	%
Gastrointestinal		
Nausea and Vomiting	33	
Mild to Moderate		32
Severe		1
Increased Alkaline Phosphatase	9	
Neurologic		
Peripheral Sensory Neuropathy	31	
Mild		22
Moderate to Severe		9
Anorexia and Fatigue	1	
Seizures	1	

ADVERSE EXPERIENCES IN 76 PREVIOUSLY TREATED OVARIAN CANCER PATIENTS RECEIVING SINGLE-AGENT ALTRETAMINE

	%	%
Hematologic		
Leukopenia	5	
WBC 2000-2999/mm^3		4
WBC < 2000/mm^3		1
Thrombocytopenia	9	
Platelets 75,000-99,000/mm^3		6
Platelets < 75,000/mm^3		3
Anemia	33	
Mild		20
Moderate to Severe		13
Renal		
Serum Creatinine 1.6-3.75 mg/dl	7	
BUN	9	
25-40 mg%		5
41-60 mg%		3
> 60 mg%		1

Additional adverse reaction information is available from 13 single-agent Altretamine studies (total of 1014 patients) conducted under the auspices of the National Cancer Institute. The treated patients had a variety of tumors and many were heavily pretreated with other chemotherapies; most of these trials utilized high, continuous daily doses of Altretamine (6-12 mg/kg/day). In general, adverse reaction experiences were similar in the two trials described above. Additional toxicities, not reported in the above table, included hepatic toxicity, skin rash, pruritus and alopecia, each occurring in < 1% of patients.

OVERDOSAGE
No case of acute overdosage in humans has been described. The oral LD50 dose in rats was 1050 mg/kg and 437 mg/kg in mice.

DOSAGE AND ADMINISTRATION
Altretamine is administered orally. Doses are calculated on the basis of body surface area.

Altretamine may be administered either for 14 or 21 consecutive days in a 28 day cycle at a dose of 260 mg/m^2/day. The total daily dose should be given as 4 divided oral doses after meals and at bedtime. There is no pharmacokinetic information supporting this dosing regimen and the effect of food on Altretamine bioavailability or pharmacokinetics has not been evaluated.

Altretamine should be temporarily discontinued (for 14 days or longer) and subsequently restarted at 200 mg/m^2/day for any of the following situations:

1) Gastrointestinal intolerance unresponsive to symptomatic measures;
2) White blood count < 2000/mm^3 or granulocyte count < 1000/mm^3;
3) Platelet count < 75,000/mm^3;
4) Progressive neurotoxicity.

If neurologic symptoms fail to stabilize on the reduced dose schedule, Altretamine should be discontinued indefinitely. Procedures for proper handling and disposal of anticancer drugs should be considered. Several guidelines on this subject have been published (2-8). There is no general agreement that all of the procedures recommended in the guidelines are necessary or appropriate.

Store at controlled room temperature 15°-30°C (59°-86°F).

REFERENCES
1. Wiernik PH, et al. Hexamethylmelamine and Low or Moderate Dose Cisplatin With or Without Pyridoxine for Treatment of Advanced Ovarian Carcinoma: A Study of the Eastern Cooperative Oncology Group. *Cancer Investigation* 10(1): 1-9, 1992. 2. Recommendations for the Safe Handling of Parenteral Antineoplastic Drugs. NIH Publication No. 83-2621. For sale by the Superintendent of Documents, U.S. Government Printing Office, Washington, D.C. 20402. 3. AMA Council Report. Guidelines for Handling Parenteral Antineoplastics. *Journal of the American Medical Association* March 15, 1985. 4. National Study Commission on Cytotoxic Exposure—Recommendation for Handling Cytotoxic Agents. Available from Louis P. Jeffrey, Sc.D., Director of Pharmacy Services, Rhode Island Hospital, 593 Eddy Street, Providence, Rhode Island 02902. 5. Clinical Oncological Society of Australia: Guidelines and Recommendations for Safe Handling of Antineoplastic Agents. *Medical Journal of Australia* 1:426-428, 1983. 6. Jones, RB, et al. Safe Handling of Chemotherapeutic Agents: A Report from the Mount Sinai Medical Center. *CA—A Cancer Journal for Clinicians* Sept/Oct, 258-263, 1983. 7. American Society of Hospital Pharmacists Technical Assistance Bulletin on Handling Cytotoxic Drugs in Hospitals. *American Journal of Hospital Pharmacy* 42:131-137, 1985. 8. OSHA Work Practice Guidelines for Personnel Dealing with Cytotoxic (Antineoplastic) Drugs. *American Journal of Hospital Pharmacy* 43:1193-1204, 1986.

HOW SUPPLIED
CAPSULE: 50 MG

BRAND/MANUFACTURER	NDC	SIZE	AWP
○ **BRAND**			
HEXALEN: U.S. Bioscience	58178-0001-70	100s	$348.92

Aluminum Chloride (Hexahydrate)

ALUMINUM CHLORIDE 20% W/V SOLUTION
A solution of Aluminum Chloride (Hexahydrate) 20% w/v in Anhydrous Ethyl Alcohol (S.D. Alcohol 40%) 93% v/v.

ALUMINUM CHLORIDE 6.25% W/V SOLUTION
A solution of Aluminum Chloride (Hexahydrate) 6.25% w/v in Anhydrous Ethyl Alcohol (S.D. Alcohol 40%) 96% v/v.

INDICATION
ALUMINUM CHLORIDE 20% W/V SOLUTION
An aid in the management of hyperhidrosis.

ALUMINUM CHLORIDE 6.25% W/V SOLUTION
For topical application as an antiperspirant (anhidrotic).

DIRECTIONS
Apply Aluminum Chloride to the affected area once a day, *only at bedtime*. To help prevent irritation, the area should be completely dry prior to application. Do not apply Aluminum Chloride to broken, irritated or recently shaved skin.

Apply Aluminum Chloride Hexahydrate in Anhydrous Ethyl Alcohol to the axillae at bedtime or as directed by physician. To help prevent irritation, the area should be completely dry prior to application. Do not apply Aluminum Chloride Hexahydrate in Anhydrous Ethyl Alcohol to broken or irritated skin. Keep container tightly closed.

FOR MAXIMUM EFFECT
Your doctor may instruct you to cover the treated area with saran wrap held in place by a snug fitting "T" or body shirt, mitten or sock. (Never hold saran in place with tape.) Wash the treated area the following morning. Excessive sweating may be stopped after two or more treatments. Thereafter, apply Aluminum Chloride once or twice weekly or as needed.

NOTICE
Aluminum Chloride may produce a burning or prickling sensation. Keep cap tightly closed when not in use to prevent evaporation.

ADVERSE REACTIONS
Transient stinging or itching may occur. It is not evidence of contact sensitivity and may be prevented or reduced by applying Aluminum Chloride Hexahydrate in Anhydrous Ethyl Alcohol only to skin which is completely dry or by removing the solution with soap and water.

WARNING
For external use only. Keep out of the reach of children. Avoid contact with the eyes. If irritation or sensitization occurs, discontinue use or consult with a physician. Aluminum Chloride may be harmful to certain metals and fabrics. Keep away from open flame.

HOW SUPPLIED
SOLUTION: 6.25%

BRAND/MANUFACTURER	NDC	SIZE	AWP
○ **BRAND**			
XERAC AC: Person & Covey	00096-0709-35	35 ml	$5.78
	00096-0709-60	60 ml	$7.72

SOLUTION: 20%

BRAND/MANUFACTURER	NDC	SIZE	AWP
○ **BRAND**			
DRYSOL: Person & Covey	00096-0707-35	35 ml	$6.63
	00096-0707-37	37.5 ml	$6.06

Alupent *SEE* METAPROTERENOL SULFATE

Amantadine Hydrochloride

DESCRIPTION
Amantadine Hydrochloride is designated chemically as 1-adamantanamine hydrochloride.

Amantadine Hydrochloride is a stable white or nearly white crystalline powder, freely soluble in water and soluble in alcohol and in chloroform.

Amantadine Hydrochloride has pharmacological actions as both an antiParkinson and an antiviral drug.

Amantadine Hydrochloride is available in capsules and syrup.

Following is its chemical structure:

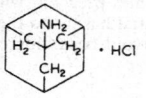

CLINICAL PHARMACOLOGY
Amantadine Hydrochloride is readily absorbed, is not metabolized, and is excreted unchanged in the urine by glomerular filtration and tubular secretion.

After oral administration of a single dose of 100 mg, maximum blood levels are reached, based on the mean time of the peak urinary excretion rate, in approximately 4 hours; the peak excretion rate is approximately 5 mg/hr; the mean half-life of the excretion rate approximates 15 hours.

Compared with otherwise healthy adult individuals, the clearance of Amantadine Hydrochloride is significantly reduced in adult patients with renal insufficiency. The elimination half-life increases two to three fold when creatinine clearance is less than 40 mL/min./1.73m², and averages eight days in patients on chronic maintenance hemodialysis.

The renal clearance of Amantadine Hydrochloride is reduced and plasma levels are increased in otherwise healthy elderly patients age 65 years and older. The drug plasma levels in elderly patients receiving 100 mg daily have been reported to approximate those determined in younger adults taking 200 mg daily. Whether these changes are due to the normal decline in renal function or other age related factors is not known.

The mechanism of action of Amantadine Hydrochloride in the treatment of Parkinson's disease and drug-induced extrapyramidal reactions is not known. It has been shown to cause an increase in dopamine release in the animal brain. The drug does not possess anticholinergic activity in animal tests at doses similar to those used clinically. The antiviral activity of Amantadine Hydrochloride against influenza A virus is not completely understood. The mode of action of Amantadine Hydrochloride appears to be the prevention of the release of infectious viral nucleic acid into the host cell. Amantadine Hydrochloride does not appear to interfere with the immunogenicity of inactivated influenza A virus vaccine.

INDICATIONS AND USAGE
PARKINSON'S DISEASE/SYNDROME
Amantadine Hydrochloride is indicated in the treatment of idiopathic Parkinson's disease (Paralysis Agitans), postencephalitic parkinsonism, and symptomatic parkinsonism which may follow injury to the nervous system by carbon monoxide intoxication. It is indicated in those elderly patients believed to develop parkinsonism in association with cerebral arteriosclerosis. In the treatment of Parkinson's disease, Amantadine Hydrochloride is less effective than levodopa, (−)-3-(3,4-dihydroxyphenyl)-L-alanine, and its efficacy in comparison with the anticholinergic antiparkinson drugs has not yet been established.

DRUG-INDUCED EXTRAPYRAMIDAL REACTIONS
Amantadine Hydrochloride is indicated in the treatment of drug-induced extrapyramidal reactions. Although anticholinergic-type side effects have been noted with Amantadine Hydrochloride when used in patients with drug-induced extrapyramidal reactions, there is a lower incidence of these side effects than that observed with the anticholinergic antiparkinson drugs.

INFLUENZA A VIRUS RESPIRATORY TRACT ILLNESS
Prophylaxis: Amantadine Hydrochloride is indicated in the prevention or chemoprophylaxis of influenza A virus illness. Amantadine Hydrochloride should be considered especially for high risk individuals, close household or hospital ward contacts of index cases, immunocompromised patients, health care and community services personnel. In the prophylaxis of influenza early vaccination as periodically recommended by the Centers for Disease Control's Immunization Practices Advisory Committee is the method of choice. When early vaccination is not feasible, or when the vaccine is contraindicated or not available, Amantadine Hydrochloride can be used for chemoprophylaxis against influenza A virus illness. Because Amantadine Hydrochloride does not appear to suppress antibody response, it can be used chemoprophylactically in conjunction with inactivated influenza A virus vaccine until protective antibody responses develop.

Treatment: Amantadine Hydrochloride is also indicated in the treatment of uncomplicated respiratory tract illness caused by influenza A virus strains. There are as yet no well-controlled clinical studies demonstrating treatment with Amantadine Hydrochloride will avoid the development of influenza A virus pneumonitis or other complications in high risk patients.

There is no clinical evidence indicating that Amantadine Hydrochloride is effective in the prophylaxis or treatment of viral respiratory tract illnesses other than those caused by influenza A virus strains.

UNLABELED USES
Amantadine Hydrochloride is used alone or as an adjunct in the treatment of multiple sclerosis and postherpetic neuralgia.

CONTRAINDICATIONS
Amantadine Hydrochloride is contraindicated in patients with known hypersensitivity to the drug.

WARNINGS
A small number of suicidal attempts, some of which have been fatal, have been reported in patients treated with Amantadine Hydrochloride. The incidence of suicidal attempts is not known and the pathophysiologic mechanism is not understood. Suicidal attempts and suicidal ideation have been reported in patients with and without prior history of psychiatric illness. Amantadine Hydrochloride can exacerbate mental problems in patients with a history of psychiatric disorders or substance abuse. Patients who attempt suicide may exhibit abnormal mental states which include disorientation, confusion, depression, personality changes, agitation, aggressive behavior hallucinations, paranoia, other psychotic reactions, and somnolence or insomnia. Because of the possibility of serious adverse effects, caution should be observed when prescribing Amantadine Hydrochloride to patients being treated with drugs having CNS effects, or for whom the potential risks outweigh the benefit of treatment. Because some patients have attempted suicide by overdosing with amantadine, prescriptions

should be written for the smallest quantity consistent with good patient management.

Patients with a history of epilepsy or other "seizures" should be observed closely for possible increased seizure activity. Patients with a history of congestive heart failure or peripheral edema should be followed closely as there are patients who developed congestive heart failure while receiving Amantadine Hydrochloride.

Patients with Parkinson's disease improving on Amantadine Hydrochloride should resume normal activities gradually and cautiously, consistent with other medical considerations, such as the presence of osteoporosis or phlebothrombosis.

Patients receiving Amantadine Hydrochloride who note central nervous system effects or blurring of vision should be cautioned against driving or working in situations where alertness and adequate motor coordination are important.

PRECAUTIONS
Amantadine Hydrochloride should not be discontinued abruptly since a few patients with Parkinson's disease experienced a parkinsonian crisis, i.e., a sudden marked clinical deterioration when this medication was suddenly stopped. The dose of anticholinergic drugs or of Amantadine Hydrochloride should be reduced if atropine-like effects appear when these drugs are used concurrently.

Neuroleptic Malignant Syndrome (NMS): Sporadic cases of possible Neuroleptic Malignant Syndrome (NMS) have been reported in association with dose reduction or withdrawal of Amantadine Hydrochloride therapy.

NMS is an uncommon but life-threatening syndrome characterized by fever or hyperthermia; neurologic findings including muscle rigidity, involuntary movements, altered consciousness; other disturbances such as autonomic dysfunction, tachycardia, tachypnea, hyper- or hypotension; laboratory findings such as creatine phosphokinase elevation, leukocytosis, and increased serum myoglobin.

The diagnostic evaluation of patients with this syndrome is complicated. In arriving at a diagnosis, it is important to identify cases where the clinical presentation includes both serious medical illness (e.g., pneumonia, systemic infection, etc.) and untreated or inadequately treated extrapyramidal signs and symptoms (EPS). Other important considerations in the differential diagnosis include central anticholinergic toxicity, heat stroke, drug fever and primary central nervous system (CNS) pathology.

The management of NMS should include: 1) intensive symptomatic treatment and medical monitoring, and 2) treatment of any concomitant serious medical problems for which specific treatments are available. There is no general agreement about specific pharmacological treatment regimens for uncomplicated NMS.

Other: Because Amantadine Hydrochloride is not metabolized and is mainly excreted in the urine, it accumulates in the plasma and in the body when renal function declines. Thus, the dose of Amantadine Hydrochloride should be reduced in patients with renal impairment and in individuals who are 65 years of age or older. The dose of Amantadine Hydrochloride may need careful adjustment in patients with congestive heart failure, peripheral edema, or orthostatic hypotension.

Care should be exercised when administering Amantadine Hydrochloride to patients with liver disease, a history of recurrent eczematoid rash, or to patients with psychosis or severe psychoneurosis not controlled by chemotherapeutic agents. Rare instances of reversible elevation of liver enzymes have been reported in patients receiving Amantadine Hydrochloride, though a specific relationship between the drug and such changes has not been established. Careful observation is required when Amantadine Hydrochloride is administered concurrently with central nervous system stimulants.

No long-term studies in animals have been performed to evaluate the carcinogenic potential of Amantadine Hydrochloride. The mutagenic potential of the drug has not yet been determined in experimental systems.

Pregnancy Category C: Amantadine Hydrochloride has been shown to be embryotoxic and teratogenic in rats at 50 mg/kg/day, about 12 times the recommended human dose, but not at 37 mg/kg/day. Embryotoxic and teratogenic drug effects were not seen in rabbits which received up to 25 times the recommended human dose. There are no adequate and well-controlled studies in pregnant women.

Amantadine Hydrochloride should be used during pregnancy only if the potential benefit justifies the potential risk to the embryo or the fetus.

Nursing Mothers: Amantadine Hydrochloride is excreted in human milk. Use is not recommended in nursing mothers.

Pediatric Use: The safety and efficacy of Amantadine Hydrochloride in newborn infants, and infants below the age of 1 year have not been established.

ADVERSE REACTIONS
The adverse reactions reported most frequently (5-10%) are: nausea, dizziness (lightheadedness), and insomnia.

Less frequently (1-5%) reported adverse reactions are: depression, anxiety, irritability, hallucinations, confusion, anorexia, dry mouth, constipation, ataxia, livedo reticularis, peripheral edema, orthostatic hypotension, headache, somnolence, nervousness, dream abnormality, agitation, dry nose, diarrhea and fatigue.

Infrequently (0.1-1%) occurring adverse reactions are: congestive heart failure, psychosis, urinary retention, dyspnea, fatigue, skin rash, vomiting, weakness, slurred speech, euphoria, confusion, thinking abnormality, amnesia, hyperkinesia, hypertension, decreased libido, and visual disturbance, including punctuate subepithelial or other corneal opacity, corneal edema, decreased visual acuity, sensitivity to light, and optic nerve palsy.

Rare (less than 0.1%) occurring adverse reactions are instances of convulsion, leukopenia, neutropenia, eczematoid dermatitis, oculogyric episodes, suicidal attempt, suicide, and suicidal ideation (see *"Warnings")*.

Rare (less than 0.1%) occurring adverse reactions are instances of convulsion, leukopenia, neutropenia, eczematoid dermatitis, oculogyric episodes, suicidal attempt, suicide, and suicidal ideation (see *"Warnings")*.

OVERDOSAGE

There is no specific antidote. Deaths have been reported from overdose with Amantadine Hydrochloride. The lowest reported acute lethal dose was 2 grams. However, slowly administered intravenous physostigmine in 1 and 2 mg doses in an adult[1] at 1 to 2 hour intervals and 0.5 mg doses in a child[2] at 5 to 10 minute intervals up to a maximum of 2 mg/hour have been reported to be effective in the control of central nervous system toxicity caused by Amantadine Hydrochloride. For acute overdosing, general supportive measures should be employed along with immediate gastric lavage or induction of emesis. Fluids should be forced, and if necessary, given intravenously. Hemodialysis does not remove significant amounts of Amantadine Hydrochloride; in patients with renal failure, a four hour hemodialysis removed 7 to 15 mg after a single 300 mg oral dose.[3] The pH of the urine has been reported to influence the excretion rate of Amantadine Hydrochloride. Since the excretion rate of Amantadine Hydrochloride increases rapidly when the urine is acidic, the administration of urine acidifying drugs may increase the elimination of the drug from the body. The blood pressure, pulse, respiration and temperature should be monitored. The patient should be observed for hyperactivity and convulsions: if required, sedation, and anticonvulsant therapy should be administered. The patient should be observed for the possible development of arrhythmias and hypotension; if required, appropriate antiarrhythmic and antihypotensive therapy should be given. The blood electrolytes, urine pH and urinary output should be monitored. If there is no record of recent voiding, catheterization should be done. The possibility of multiple drug ingestion by the patient should be considered.

DOSAGE AND ADMINISTRATION
DOSAGE FOR PARKINSONISM
Adult: The usual dose of Amantadine Hydrochloride is 100 mg twice a day when used alone. Amantadine Hydrochloride has an onset of action usually within 48 hours.

The initial dose of Amantadine Hydrochloride is 100 mg daily for patients with serious associated medical illnesses or who are receiving high doses of other antiparkinson drugs. After one to several weeks at 100 mg once daily, the dose may be increased to 100 mg twice daily, if necessary.

Occasionally, patients whose responses are not optimal with Amantadine Hydrochloride at 200 mg daily may benefit from an increase up to 400 mg daily in divided doses. However, such patients should be supervised closely by their physicians.

Patients initially deriving benefit from Amantadine Hydrochloride not uncommonly experience a fall-off of effectiveness after a few months. Benefit may be regained by increasing the dose to 300 mg daily. Alternatively, temporary discontinuation of Amantadine Hydrochloride for several weeks, followed by reinitiation of the drug, may result in regaining benefit in some patients. A decision to use other antiparkinson drugs may be necessary.

DOSAGE FOR CONCOMITANT THERAPY
Some patients who do not respond to anticholinergic antiparkinson drugs may respond to Amantadine Hydrochloride. When Amantadine Hydrochloride or anticholinergic antiparkinson drugs are each used with marginal benefit, concomitant use may produce additional benefit.

When Amantadine Hydrochloride and levodopa are initiated concurrently, the patient can exhibit rapid therapeutic benefits. Amantadine Hydrochloride should be held constant at 100 mg daily or twice daily while the daily dose of levodopa is gradually increased to optimal benefit.

When Amantadine Hydrochloride is added to optimal well-tolerated doses of levodopa, additional benefit may result, including smoothing out the fluctuations in improvement which sometimes occur in patients on levodopa alone. Patients who require a reduction in their usual dose of levodopa because of development of side effects may possibly regain lost benefit with the addition of Amantadine Hydrochloride.

DOSAGE FOR DRUG-INDUCED EXTRAPYRAMIDAL REACTIONS
Adult: The usual dose of Amantadine Hydrochloride is 100 mg twice a day. Occasionally, patients whose responses are not optimal with Amantadine Hydrochloride at 200 mg daily may benefit from an increase up to 300 mg daily in divided doses.

DOSAGE FOR PROPHYLAXIS OF INFLUENZA A VIRUS ILLNESS AND TREATMENT OF UNCOMPLICATED INFLUENZA A VIRUS ILLNESS
Normal Renal Function:
Adult: The adult daily dosage of Amantadine Hydrochloride is 200 mg: two 100 mg capsules (or four teaspoonfuls of syrup) as a single daily dose, or the daily dosage may be split into one capsule of 100 mg (or two teaspoonfuls of syrup) twice a day. If central nervous system effects develop on once-a-day dosage, a split dosage schedule may reduce such complaints. In persons 65 years of age or older, the daily dosage of Amantadine Hydrochloride is 100 mg.

---

1 D.F. Casey, N. Engl. J. Med. 298:516, 1978.
2 C.D. Berkowitz, J. Pediatr. 95:144, 1979.
3 V.W. Horadam, et al., Ann. Intern. Med. 94:454, 1981.

Children: 1 yr.-9 yrs. of age: The total daily dose should be calculated on the basis of 2 to 4 mg/lb/day (4.4 to 8.8 mg/kg/day), but not to exceed 150 mg per day.
9 yrs.-12 yrs. of age: The total daily dose is 200 mg given as one capsule of 100 mg (or two teaspoonfuls of syrup) twice a day.

Impaired Renal Function: Depending upon creatinine clearance, the following dosage adjustments are recommended:

Creatinine Clearance (mL/min./1.73m²)	Amantadine Hydrochloride Dosage
30-50	200 mg 1st day and 100 mg each day thereafter
15-29	200 mg 1st day followed by 100 mg on alternate days
< 15	200 mg every 7 days

The recommended dosage for patients on hemodialysis is 200 mg every 7 days.

Prophylactic dosing should be started in anticipation of an influenza A outbreak and before or after contact with individuals with influenza A virus respiratory tract illness.

Amantadine Hydrochloride should be continued daily for at least 10 days following a known exposure. If Amantadine Hydrochloride is used chemoprophylactically in conjunction with inactivated influenza A virus vaccine until protective antibody responses develop, then it should be administered for 2 to 3 weeks after the vaccine has been given. When inactivated influenza A virus vaccine is unavailable or contraindicated, Amantadine Hydrochloride should be administered for up to 90 days in case of possible repeated and unknown exposures. Treatment of influenza A virus illness should be started as soon as possible, preferably within 24 to 48 hours, after onset of signs and symptoms, and should be continued for 24 to 48 hours after the disappearance of signs and symptoms.

Store at controlled room temperature (59°-86°F, 15°-30°C).

HOW SUPPLIED
CAPSULE: 100 MG

AVERAGE UNIT PRICE (AVAILABLE SIZES)

BRAND	$0.84	GENERIC A-RATED AVERAGE PRICE (GAAP)	
GENERIC	$0.33	100s	$33.70
HCFA FUL (100s ea)	$0.19	500s	$135.32

BRAND/MANUFACTURER	NDC	SIZE	AWP
◆ BRAND			
➤ SYMMETREL: Du Pont Multi	00056-0105-70	100s	$84.72
	00056-0105-85	500s	$411.84
◆ GENERICS			
Medirex	57480-0300-06	30s	$14.85
Rugby	00536-3090-01	100s	$25.55
SYMADINE: Solvay	00032-4140-01	100s	$27.75
Caremark	00339-5779-12	100s	$27.75
Chase	54429-3185-01	100s	$30.00
Warner Chilcott	00047-0853-24	100s	$30.18
Qualitest	00603-2163-21	100s	$30.59
Qualitest	00603-2164-21	100s	$30.59
Moore,H.L.	00839-7250-06	100s	$31.05
Major	00904-3430-60	100s	$31.50
Major	00904-3431-60	100s	$31.50
Parmed	00349-8613-01	100s	$31.50
Geneva	00781-2105-01	100s	$31.50
Goldline	00182-1258-01	100s	$31.50
Rosemont	00832-1015-00	100s	$31.50
URL	00677-1128-01	100s	$32.40
Schein	00364-2146-01	100s	$32.42
URL	00677-1452-01	100s	$32.90
Lemmon	00093-0548-01	100s	$32.93
Martec	52555-0122-01	100s	$33.00
Purepac	00228-2291-10	100s	$34.24
Intl Labs	00665-4140-06	100s	$34.75
Moore,H.L.	00839-7471-06	100s	$35.71
Aligen	00405-4042-01	100s	$36.20
Mason Dist	11845-0354-01	100s	$36.26
Duramed	51285-0803-02	100s	$36.58
Invamed	52189-0211-24	100s	$36.58
U.S. Trading	56126-0364-11	100s ud	$20.46
Raway	00686-0481-20	100s ud	$29.50
Major	00904-3430-61	100s ud	$49.05
Medirex	57480-0300-01	100s ud	$49.50
UDL	51079-0481-20	100s ud	$59.78
Major	00904-3430-40	500s	$119.65
Major	00904-3431-40	500s	$119.65
Chase	54429-3185-05	500s	$122.30
Parmed	00349-8613-05	500s	$122.30
Rosemont	00832-1015-50	500s	$122.30
Moore,H.L.	00839-7250-12	500s	$129.53
Qualitest	00603-2163-28	500s	$130.78
Qualitest	00603-2164-28	500s	$130.78
Duramed	51285-0803-04	500s	$177.95
Invamed	52189-0211-29	500s	$177.95

◆ RATED THERAPEUTICALLY EQUIVALENT; ◇ THERAPEUTIC EQUIVALENCE UNCONFIRMED; ○ UNRATED

SYRUP: 50 MG/5 ML

AVERAGE UNIT PRICE (AVAILABLE SIZES)		GENERIC A-RATED AVERAGE PRICE (GAAP)	
BRAND	$0.17	480 ml	$63.25
GENERIC	$0.13		
HCFA FUL (480 ml)	$0.11		

BRAND/MANUFACTURER	NDC	SIZE	AWP
◆ **BRAND**			
SYMMETREL: Du Pont Multi	00056-0205-16	480 ml	$80.22
◆ **GENERICS**			
Rugby	00536-2665-85	480 ml	$57.50
Copley	38245-0180-07	480 ml	$59.95
Qualitest	00603-1010-58	480 ml	$59.95
Barre	00472-0833-16	480 ml	$61.51
Endo	60951-0656-16	480 ml	$62.15
Goldline	00182-6016-40	480 ml	$63.00
Aligen	00405-2140-16	480 ml	$63.11
King Pharm	60793-0113-12	480 ml	$68.04
Major	00904-3432-16	480 ml	$70.70

TABLETS: 100 MG

BRAND/MANUFACTURER	NDC	SIZE	AWP
◆ **GENERICS**			
URL	00677-1346-01	100s	$32.00

Ambenonium Chloride

DESCRIPTION

Ambenonium Chloride, is [Oxalylbis (iminoethylene)] bis[(o-chlorobenzyl) diethylammonium] dichloride, a white crystalline powder, soluble in water to 20 percent (w/v).

Following is its chemical structure:

CLINICAL PHARMACOLOGY

The compound is a cholinesterase inhibitor with all the pharmacologic actions of acetylcholine, both the muscarinic and nicotinic types. Cholinesterase inactivates acetylcholine. Like neostigmine, Ambenonium Chloride suppresses cholinesterase but has the advantage of longer duration of action and fewer side effects on the gastrointestinal tract. The longer duration of action also results in more even strength, better endurance, and greater residual effect during the night and on awakening than is produced by shorter-acting anti-cholinesterase compounds.

INDICATION AND USAGE

This drug is indicated for the treatment of myasthenia gravis.

CONTRAINDICATIONS

Routine administration of atropine with Ambenonium Chloride is contraindicated since belladonna derivatives may suppress the parasym-pathomimetic (muscarinic) symptoms of excessive gastrointestinal stimulation, leaving only the more serious symptoms of fasciculation and paralysis of voluntary muscles as signs of overdosage.

Ambenonium Chloride should not be administered to patients receiving mecamylamine, a ganglionic blocking agent.

WARNINGS

Because this drug has a more prolonged action than other antimyasthenic drugs, simultaneous administration with other cholinergics is contraindicated except under strict medical supervision. The overlap in duration of action of several drugs complicates dosage schedules. Therefore, when a patient is to be given the drug, the administration of all other cholinergics should be suspended until the patient has been stabilized. In most instances the myasthenic symptoms are effectively controlled by its use alone.

PRECAUTIONS

Great care and supervision are required, since the warning of overdosage is minimal and the requirements of patients vary tremendously. It must be borne in mind constantly that a narrow margin exists between the first appearance of side effects and serious toxic effects. Caution in increasing the dosage is essential.

The drug should be used with caution in patients with asthma or in patients with mechanical intestinal or urinary obstruction.

Usage in Pregnancy: Safe use of this drug during pregnancy has not been established. Therefore, before use of Ambenonium Chloride in pregnant women or women of childbearing potential, the potential benefits should be weighed against possible risks to mother and fetus.

ADVERSE REACTIONS

Adverse effects of anticholinesterase agents such as Ambenonium Chloride usually result from overdosage and include excessive salivation, abdominal cramps, diarrhea, miosis, urinary urgency, sweating, and vomiting. (See *"Overdosage"*.)

DOSAGE AND ADMINISTRATION

The oral dose must be individualized according to the patient's response because the disease varies widely in its severity in different patients and because patients vary in their sensitivity to cholinergic drugs. Since the point of maximum therapeutic effectiveness with optimal muscle strength and no gastrointestinal disturbances is a highly critical one, the close supervision of a physician familiar with the disease is necessary.

Because its action is longer, administration of Ambenonium Chloride is necessary only every three or four hours, depending on the clinical response. Usually medication is not required throughout the night, so that the patient can sleep uninterruptedly.

For the patient with moderately severe myasthenia, from 5 mg to 25 mg of Ambenonium Chloride three or four times daily is an effective dose. In some patients a 5 mg dose is effective, whereas other patients require as much as from 50 mg to 75 mg per dose. The physician should start with a 5 mg dose, carefully observing the effect of the drug on the patient. The dosage may then be increased gradually to determine the effective and safe dose. The longer duration of action of Ambenium Chloride makes it desirable to adjust dosage at intervals of one to two days to avoid drug accumulation and overdosage. (See *"Overdosage"*.)

In addition to individual variations in dosage requirements, the amount of cholinergic medication necessary to control symptoms may fluctuate in each patient, depending on his activity and the current status of the disease, including spontaneous remission. A few patients have required greater doses for adequate control of myasthenic symptoms, but increasing the dosage above 200 mg daily requires exacting supervision of a physician well aware of the signs and treatment of overdosage with cholinergic medication.

Edrophonium may be used to evaluate the adequacy of the maintenance dose of anticholinesterase medication. Two mg (0.2 mL) edrophonium are administered intravenously one hour after the last anticholinesterase dose. A transient increase in strength occurring about 30 seconds later and lasting 3 to 5 minutes indicates insufficient maintenance dose. If the dose is adequate or excessive, no change or a transient decrease in strength will occur, sometimes accompanied by muscarinic symptoms.

OVERDOSAGE

When the drug produces overstimulation, the clinical picture is one of increasing parasympathomimetic action that is more or less characteristic when not masked by the use of atropine.

Signs and symptoms of overdosage, including cholinergic crises, vary considerably. They are usually manifested by increasing gastrointestinal stimulation with epigastric distress, abdominal cramps, diarrhea and vomiting, excessive salivation, pallor, cold sweating, urinary urgency, blurring of vision, and eventually fasciculation and paralysis of voluntary muscles, including those of the tongue (thick tongue and difficulty in swallowing), shoulder, neck, and arms. Miosis, increase in blood pressure with or without bradycardia, and finally, subjective sensations of internal trembling, and often severe anxiety and panic may complete the picture. A cholinergic crisis is usually differentiated from the weakness and paralysis of myasthenia gravis insufficiently treated by cholinergic drugs by the fact that myasthenic weakness is not accompanied by any of the above signs and symptoms, except the last two subjective ones (anxiety and panic).

Since the warning of overdosage is minimal, the existence of a narrow margin between the first appearance of side effects and serious toxic effects must be borne in mind constantly. If signs of overdosage occur (excessive gastrointestinal stimulation, excessive salivation, miosis, and more serious fasciculations of voluntary muscles) discontinue temporarily all cholinergic medication and administer from 0.5 mg to 1 mg (1/120 to 1/60 grain) of atropine intravenously. Give other supportive treatment as indicated (artificial respiration, tracheotomy, oxygen, etc).

HOW SUPPLIED
TABLETS: 10 MG

BRAND/MANUFACTURER	NDC	SIZE	AWP
○ **BRAND**			
MYTELASE CHLORIDE: Sanofi Winthrop	00024-1287-04	100s	$79.19

Ambenyl SEE BROMODIPHENHYDRAMINE HYDROCHLORIDE AND CODEINE PHOSPHATE

Amcinonide

DESCRIPTION

The topical corticosteroids constitute a class of primarily synthetic steroids used as anti-inflammatory and antipruritic agents.

TOPICAL LOTION 0.1%
Each gram of Amcinonide topical Lotion contains 1 mg of the active steroid amcinonide.

► SHOWN IN PRODUCT IDENTIFICATION GUIDE

TOPICAL CREAM 0.1%

Each gram of Amcinonide topical Cream contains 1 mg of the active steroid amcinonide.

Certain brands of Amcinonide contain Aquatain®, which is non-staining, water-washable, paraben-free, spermaceti-free, and has a light texture and consistency.

TOPICAL OINTMENT 0.1%

Each gram of Amcinonide topical Ointment contains 1 mg of the active steroid amcinonide in a specially formulated base.

Pregna-1,4-diene-3,20-dione, 21-(acetyloxy)-16,17-[cyclopentylidenebis(oxy)]-9-fluoro-11-hydroxy-, (11β, 16α).

Following is its chemical structure:

CLINICAL PHARMACOLOGY

Topical corticosteroids have anti-inflammatory, antipruritic, and vasoconstrictive actions.

The mechanism of anti-inflammatory activity of the topical corticosteroids is unclear. Various laboratory methods, including vasoconstrictor assays, are used to compare and predict potencies and/or clinical efficacies of the topical corticosteroids. There is some evidence to suggest that a recognizable correlation exists between vasoconstrictor potency and therapeutic efficacy in man.

PHARMACOKINETICS

The extent of percutaneous absorption of topical corticosteroids is determined by many factors, including the vehicle, the integrity of the epidermal barrier, and the use of occlusive dressings.

Topical corticosteroids can be absorbed from normal intact skin. Inflammation and/or other disease processes in the skin increase percutaneous absorption. Occlusive dressings substantially increase the percutaneous absorption of topical corticosteroids (see "Dosage and Administration"). Once absorbed through the skin, topical corticosteroids are handled through pharmacokinetic pathways similar to systemically-administered corticosteroids. Corticosteroids are bound to plasma proteins in varying degrees.

Corticosteroids are metabolized primarily in the liver and are then excreted by the kidneys. Some of the topical corticosteroids and their metabolites are also excreted into the bile.

INDICATIONS AND USAGE

Topical corticosteroids are indicated for the relief of the inflammatory and pruritic manifestations of corticosteroid-responsive dermatoses.

CONTRAINDICATIONS

Topical corticosteroids are contraindicated in those patients with a history of hypersensitivity to any of the components of the preparation.

PRECAUTIONS

GENERAL

Systemic absorption of topical corticosteroids has produced reversible hypothalamic-pituitary-adrenal (HPA) axis suppression, manifestations of Cushing's syndrome, hyperglycemia, and glucosuria in some patients.

Conditions that augment systemic absorption include the application of the more potent steroids, use over large surface areas, prolonged use, and the addition of occlusive dressings. Therefore, patients receiving a large dose of a potent topical steroid applied to a large surface area or under an occlusive dressing should be evaluated periodically for evidence of HPA-axis suppression by using the urinary free-cortisol and ACTH stimulation tests. If HPA-axis suppression is noted, an attempt should be made to withdraw the drug, to reduce the frequency of application, or to substitute with a less potent steroid.

Recovery of HPA-axis function is generally prompt and complete upon discontinuation of the drug.

Infrequently, signs and symptoms of steroid withdrawal may occur, requiring supplemental systemic corticosteroids.

Children may absorb proportionally larger amounts of topical corticosteroids and thus be more susceptible to systemic toxicity (see "Precautions, Pediatric Use").

If irritation develops, topical corticosteroids should be discontinued and appropriate therapy instituted.

In the presence of dermatological infections, the use of an appropriate antifungal or antibacterial agent should be instituted. If a favorable response does not occur promptly, the corticosteroid should be discontinued until the infection has been adequately controlled.

The products are not for ophthalmic use.

INFORMATION FOR THE PATIENT

Patients using topical corticosteroids should receive the following information and instructions.

1. This medication is to be used as directed by the physician. It is for external use only. Avoid contact with the eyes.
2. Patients should be advised not to use this medication for any disorder other than for which it was prescribed.
3. The treated skin area should not be bandaged or otherwise covered or wrapped, as to be occlusive, unless directed by the physician.
4. Patients should report any signs of local adverse reactions, especially those that occur under occlusive dressings.
5. Parents of pediatric patients should be advised not to use tight-fitting diapers or plastic pants on a child being treated in the diaper area, as those garments may constitute occlusive dressings.

LABORATORY TESTS

The following tests may be helpful in evaluating the HPA-axis suppression.
    Urinary free-cortisol test
    ACTH stimulation test

CARCINOGENESIS, MUTAGENESIS, AND IMPAIRMENT OF FERTILITY

Long-term animal studies have not been performed to evaluate the carcinogenic potential of topical corticosteroids or their effect on fertility.

Studies to determine mutagenicity with prednisolone and hydrocortisone have revealed negative results.

PREGNANCY CATEGORY C

Corticosteroids are generally teratogenic in laboratory animals when administered systemically at relatively low dosage levels. The more potent corticosteroids have been shown to be teratogenic after dermal application in laboratory animals. There are no adequate and well-controlled studies in pregnant women on teratogenic effects from topically-applied corticosteroids. Therefore, topical corticosteroids should be used during pregnancy only if the potential benefit justifies the potential risk to the fetus. Drugs of this class should not be used extensively on pregnant patients, in large amounts, or for prolonged periods of time.

NURSING MOTHERS

It is not known whether topical administration of corticosteroids could result in sufficient systemic absorption to produce detectable quantities in breast milk. Systemically-administered corticosteroids are secreted into breast milk in quantities not likely to have a deleterious effect on the infant. Nevertheless, a decision should be made whether to discontinue nursing or to discontinue the drug, taking into account the importance of the drug to the mother.

PEDIATRIC USE

Pediatric patients may demonstrate greater susceptibility to topical corticosteroid-induced HPA-axis suppression and Cushing's syndrome than mature patients because of a higher ratio of skin surface area to body weight.

Hypothalamic-pituitary-adrenal (HPA) axis suppression, Cushing's syndrome, and intracranial hypertension have been reported in children receiving topical corticosteroids. Manifestations of adrenal suppression in children include linear growth retardation, delayed weight gain, low plasma cortisol levels, and absence of response to ACTH stimulation. Manifestations of intracranial hypertension include bulging fontanelles, headaches, and bilateral papilledema.

Administration of topical corticosteroids to children should be limited to the least amount compatible with an effective therapeutic regimen. Chronic corticosteroid therapy may interfere with the growth and development of children.

ADVERSE REACTIONS

In the clinical trials with Amcinonide Lotion, the investigators reported a 4.7% incidence of side effects. In a weekly acceptability evaluation, approximately 20% of the patients treated with Amcinonide Lotion or placebo reported itching, stinging, soreness, or burning at one or more of the visits.

The following local adverse reactions are reported infrequently with topical corticosteroids, but may occur more frequently with the use of occlusive dressings. These reactions are listed in an approximate decreasing order of occurrence.

Burning
Itching
Irritation
Dryness
Folliculitis
Hypertrichosis
Acneiform eruptions
Hypopigmentation
Perioral dermatitis
Allergic contact dermatitis
Maceration of the skin
Secondary infection
Skin atrophy
Striae
Miliaria

OVERDOSAGE

Topically-applied corticosteroids can be absorbed in sufficient amounts to produce systemic effects (see "Precautions").

DOSAGE AND ADMINISTRATION

Topical corticosteroids are generally applied to the affected area as a thin film from two to three times daily depending on the severity of the condition.

The lotion may be applied topically to the specified lesions, particularly to those in hairy areas, two times per day. The lotion should be rubbed into the affected area completely, and the area should be protected from washing, clothing, rubbing, etc. until the lotion has dried.

Occlusive dressings may be a valuable therapeutic adjunct for the management of psoriasis or recalcitrant conditions.

If an infection develops, the use of occlusive dressings should be discontinued and appropriate antimicrobial therapy instituted.

Store at controlled room temperature 15°-30°C (59°-86°F). DO NOT FREEZE.

HOW SUPPLIED
CREAM: 0.1%

BRAND/MANUFACTURER	NDC	SIZE	AWP
○ BRAND			
CYCLOCORT: Fujisawa	57317-0054-15	15 gm	$15.34
	57317-0054-30	30 gm	$22.84
	57317-0054-60	60 gm	$38.38

OINTMENT: 0.1%

BRAND/MANUFACTURER	NDC	SIZE	AWP
○ BRAND			
CYCLOCORT: Fujisawa	57317-0115-15	15 gm	$15.34
	57317-0115-60	60 gm	$38.38

Amen SEE MEDROXYPROGESTERONE ACETATE, ORAL

Americaine SEE BENZOCAINE

A-Methapred SEE METHYLPREDNISOLONE

Amicar SEE AMINOCAPROIC ACID

Amidate SEE ETOMIDATE

Amikacin Sulfate

WARNINGS

PATIENTS TREATED WITH PARENTERAL AMINOGLYCOSIDES SHOULD BE UNDER CLOSE CLINICAL OBSERVATION BECAUSE OF THE POTENTIAL OTOTOXICITY AND NEPHROTOXICITY ASSOCIATED WITH THEIR USE. SAFETY FOR TREATMENT PERIODS WHICH ARE LONGER THAN 14 DAYS HAS NOT BEEN ESTABLISHED.

NEUROTOXICITY, MANIFESTED AS VESTIBULAR AND PERMANENT BILATERAL AUDITORY OTOTOXICITY, CAN OCCUR IN PATIENTS WITH PREEXISTING RENAL DAMAGE AND IN PATIENTS WITH NORMAL RENAL FUNCTION TREATED AT HIGHER DOSES AND/OR FOR PERIODS LONGER THAN THOSE RECOMMENDED. THE RISK OF AMINOGLYCOSIDE-INDUCED OTOTOXICITY IS GREATER IN PATIENTS WITH RENAL DAMAGE. HIGH FREQUENCY DEAFNESS USUALLY OCCURS FIRST AND CAN BE DETECTED ONLY BY AUDIOMETRIC TESTING. VERTIGO MAY OCCUR AND MAY BE EVIDENCE OF VESTIBULAR INJURY. OTHER MANIFESTATIONS OF NEUROTOXICITY MAY INCLUDE NUMBNESS, SKIN TINGLING, MUSCLE TWITCHING AND CONVULSIONS. THE RISK OF HEARING LOSS DUE TO AMINOGLYCOSIDES INCREASES WITH THE DEGREE OF EXPOSURE TO EITHER HIGH PEAK OR HIGH TROUGH SERUM CONCENTRATIONS.

PATIENTS DEVELOPING COCHLEAR DAMAGE MAY NOT HAVE SYMPTOMS DURING THERAPY TO WARN THEM OF DEVELOPING EIGHTH-NERVE TOXICITY, AND TOTAL OR PARTIAL IRREVERSIBLE BILATERAL DEAFNESS MAY OCCUR AFTER THE DRUG HAS BEEN DISCONTINUED. AMINOGLYCOSIDE-INDUCED OTOTOXICITY IS USUALLY IRREVERSIBLE.

AMINOGLYCOSIDES ARE POTENTIALLY NEPHROTOXIC. THE RISK OF NEPHROTOXICITY IS GREATER IN PATIENTS WITH IMPAIRED RENAL FUNCTION AND IN THOSE WHO RECEIVE HIGH DOSES OR PROLONGED THERAPY.

NEUROMUSCULAR BLOCKADE AND RESPIRATORY PARALYSIS HAVE BEEN REPORTED FOLLOWING PARENTERAL INJECTION, TOPICAL INSTILLATION (AS IN ORTHOPEDIC AND ABDOMINAL IRRIGATION OR IN LOCAL TREATMENT OF EMPYEMA), AND FOLLOWING ORAL USE OF AMINOGLYCOSIDES. THE POSSIBILITY OF THESE PHENOMENA SHOULD BE CONSIDERED IF AMINOGLYCOSIDES ARE ADMINISTERED BY ANY ROUTE, ESPECIALLY IN PATIENTS RECEIVING ANESTHETICS, NEUROMUSCULAR BLOCKING AGENTS SUCH AS TUBOCURARINE, SUCCINYLCHOLINE, DECAMETHONIUM, OR IN PATIENTS RECEIVING MASSIVE TRANSFUSIONS OF CITRATE-ANTICOAGULATED BLOOD. IF BLOCKAGE OCCURS, CALCIUM SALTS MAY REVERSE THESE PHENOMENA, BUT MECHANICAL RESPIRATORY ASSISTANCE MAY BE NECESSARY.

RENAL AND EIGHTH-NERVE FUNCTION SHOULD BE CLOSELY MONITORED ESPECIALLY IN PATIENTS WITH KNOWN OR SUSPECTED RENAL IMPAIRMENT AT THE ONSET OF THERAPY AND ALSO IN THOSE WHOSE RENAL FUNCTION IS INITIALLY NORMAL BUT WHO DEVELOP SIGNS OF RENAL DYSFUNCTION DURING THERAPY.

SERUM CONCENTRATIONS OF AMIKACIN SHOULD BE MONITORED WHEN FEASIBLE TO ASSURE ADEQUATE LEVELS AND TO AVOID POTENTIALLY TOXIC LEVELS AND PROLONGED PEAK CONCENTRATIONS ABOVE 35 µG PER ML. URINE SHOULD BE EXAMINED FOR DECREASED SPECIFIC GRAVITY, INCREASED EXCRETION OF PROTEINS, AND THE PRESENCE OF CELLS OR CASTS. BLOOD UREA NITROGEN, SERUM CREATININE, OR CREATININE CLEARANCE SHOULD BE MEASURED PERIODICALLY. SERIAL AUDIOGRAMS SHOULD BE OBTAINED WHERE FEASIBLE IN PATIENTS OLD ENOUGH TO BE TESTED, PARTICULARLY HIGH RISK PATIENTS. EVIDENCE OF OTOTOXICITY (DIZZINESS, VERTIGO, TINNITUS, ROARING IN THE EARS, AND HEARING LOSS) OR NEPHROTOXICITY REQUIRES DISCONTINUATION OF THE DRUG OR DOSAGE ADJUSTMENT.

CONCURRENT AND/OR SEQUENTIAL SYSTEMIC, ORAL OR TOPICAL USE OF OTHER NEUROTOXIC OR NEPHROTOXIC PRODUCTS, PARTICULARLY BACITRACIN, CISPLATIN, AMPHOTERICIN B, CEPHALORIDINE, PAROMOMYCIN, VIOMYCIN, POLYMYXIN B, COLISTIN, VANCOMYCIN, OR OTHER AMINOGLYCOSIDES SHOULD BE AVOIDED. OTHER FACTORS THAT MAY INCREASE RISK OF TOXICITY ARE ADVANCED AGE AND DEHYDRATION.

THE CONCURRENT USE OF AMIKACIN SULFATE WITH POTENT DIURETICS (ETHACRYNIC ACID, OR FUROSEMIDE) SHOULD BE AVOIDED SINCE DIURETICS BY THEMSELVES MAY CAUSE OTOTOXICITY. IN ADDITION, WHEN ADMINISTERED INTRAVENOUSLY, DIURETICS MAY ENHANCE AMINOGLYCOSIDE TOXICITY BY ALTERING ANTIBIOTIC CONCENTRATIONS IN SERUM AND TISSUE.

DESCRIPTION

Amikacin Sulfate is a semisynthetic aminoglycoside antibiotic derived from kanamycin. It is D-Streptamine, 0-3-amino-3-deoxy-α-D-glucopyranosyl-(1→6)-0-[6-amino-6-deoxy-α-D-glucopyranosyl-(1→4)]-N^1-(4-amino-2-hydroxy-1-oxobutyl) 2-deoxy-, (S)-, sulfate (1:2) (salt). Its empirical formula is $C_{22}H_{43}N_5O_{13} \cdot 2H_2SO_4$. Its molecular weight is 781.75.

The dosage form is supplied as a sterile, colorless to light straw-colored solution for IM or IV use.

Amikacin Sulfate is available as 100mg/2 mL vial; 250mg/mL; 500 mg/2 mL; and 1 gram/4 mL with either sodium sulfite or sodium metabisulfite. Vial headspace contains nitrogen.

Following is its chemical structure:

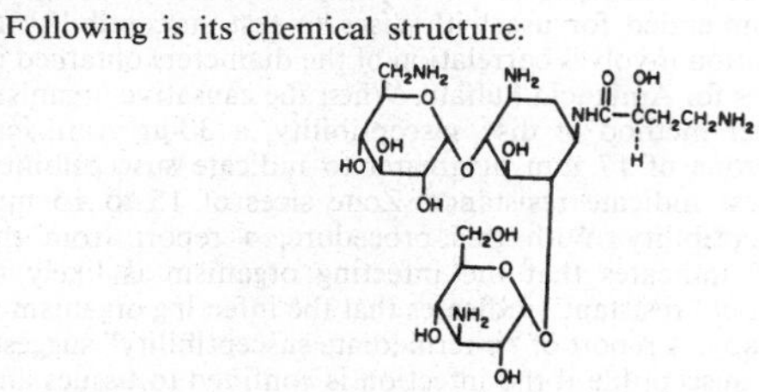

CLINICAL PHARMACOLOGY

Intramuscular Administration: Amikacin Sulfate is rapidly absorbed after intramuscular administration. In normal adult volunteers, average peak serum concentrations of about 12, 16, and 21 µg/mL are obtained 1 hour after intramuscular administration of 250-mg (3.7 mg/kg), 375-mg (5 mg/kg), 500-mg (7.5 mg/kg), single doses, respectively. At 10 hours, serum levels are about 0.3 µg/mL, 1.2 µg/mL, and 2.1 µg/mL, respectively.

Tolerance studies in normal volunteers reveal that Amikacin Sulfate is well tolerated locally following repeated intramuscular dosing, and when given at maximally recommended doses, no ototoxicity or nephrotoxicity has been reported. There is no evidence of drug accumulation with repeated dosing for 10 days when administered according to recommended doses.

With normal renal function, about 91.9% of an intramuscular dose is excreted unchanged in the urine in the first 8 hours, and 98.2% within 24 hours. Mean urine concentrations for 6 hours are 563 μg/mL following a 250-mg dose, 697 μg/mL following a 375-mg dose, and 832 μg/mL following a 500-mg dose.

Preliminary intramuscular studies in newborns of different weights (less than 1.5 kg, 1.5 to 2.0 kg, over 2.0 kg) at a dose of 7.5 mg/kg revealed that, like other aminoglycosides, serum half-life values were correlated inversely with post-natal age and renal clearances of Amikacin Sulfate. The volume of distribution indicates that Amikacin Sulfate, like other aminoglycosides, remains primarily in the extracellular fluid space of neonates. Repeated dosing every 12 hours in all the above groups did not demonstrate accumulation after 5 days.

Intravenous Administration: Single doses of 500 mg (7.5 mg/kg) administered to normal adults as an infusion over a period of 30 minutes produced a mean peak serum concentration of 38 μg/mL at the end of the infusion, and levels of 24 μg/mL, 18 μg/mL, and 0.75 μg/mL at 30 minutes, 1 hour and 10 hours postinfusion, respectively. Eighty-four percent of the administered dose was excreted in the urine in 9 hours and about 94% within 24 hours.

Repeat infusions of 7.5 mg/kg every 12 hours in normal adults were well tolerated and caused no drug accumulation.

General: Pharmacokinetic studies in normal adult subjects reveal the mean serum half-life to be slightly over 2 hours with a mean total apparent volume of distribution of 24 liters (28% of the body weight). By the ultrafiltration technique, reports of serum protein binding range from 0% to 11%. The mean serum clearance rate is about 100 mL/min and the renal clearance rate is 94 mL/min in subjects with normal renal function.

Amikacin is excreted primarily by glomerular filtration. Patients with impaired renal function or diminished glomerular filtration pressure excrete the drug much more slowly (effectively prolonging the serum half-life). Therefore, renal function should be monitored carefully and dosage adjusted accordingly (see suggested dosage schedule under *"Dosage and Administration"*).

Following administration at the recommended dose, therapeutic levels are found in bone, heart, gallbladder, and lung tissue in addition to significant concentrations in urine, bile, sputum, bronchial secretions, interstitial, pleural and synovial fluids.

Spinal fluid levels in normal infants are approximately 10% to 20% of the serum concentrations and may reach 50% when the meninges are inflamed. Amikacin Sulfate has been demonstrated to cross the placental barrier and yield significant concentrations in amniotic fluid. The peak fetal serum concentration is about 16% of the peak maternal serum concentration and maternal and fetal serum half-life values are about 2 and 3.7 hours, respectively.

MICROBIOLOGY
Gram-negative: Amikacin is active *in vitro* against *Pseudomonas* species, *Escherichia coli*, *Proteus* species (indole-positive and indole-negative), *Providencia* species, *Klebsiella-Enterobacter-Serratia* species, *Acinetobacter* (formerly *Mima-Herellea*) species, and *Citrobacter freundii*.

When strains of the above organisms are found to be resistant to other aminoglycosides, including gentamicin, tobramycin and kanamycin, many are susceptible to Amikacin Sulfate *in vitro*.

Gram-positive: Amikacin is active *in vitro* against penicillinase and nonpenicillinase-producing *Staphylococcus* species including methicillin-resistant strains. However, aminoglycosides in general have a low order of activity against other Gram-positive organisms; viz., *Streptococcus pyogenes*, enterococci, and *Streptococcus pneumoniae* (formerly *Diplococcus pneumoniae*).

Amikacin resists degradation by most aminoglycoside inactivating enzymes known to affect gentamicin, tobramycin, and kanamycin.

In vitro studies have shown that Amikacin Sulfate combined with a beta-lactam antibiotic acts synergistically against many clinically significant gram-negative organisms.

Disc Susceptibility Tests: Quantitative methods that require measurement of zone diameters give the most precise estimates of antibiotic susceptibility. One such procedure* has been recommended for use with discs to test susceptibility to Amikacin Sulfate. Interpretation involves correlation of the diameters obtained in the disc test with MIC values for Amikacin Sulfate. When the causative organism is tested by the Kirby-Bauer method of disc susceptibility, a 30-μg Amikacin Sulfate disc should give a zone of 17 mm or greater to indicate susceptibility. Zone sizes of 14 mm or less indicate resistance. Zone sizes of 15 to 16 mm indicate intermediate susceptibility. With this procedure, a report from the laboratory of "susceptible" indicates that the infecting organism is likely to respond to therapy. A report of "resistant" indicates that the infecting organism is not likely to respond to therapy. A report of "intermediate susceptibility" suggests that the organism would be susceptible if the infection is confined to tissues and fluids (eg, urine) in which high antibiotic levels are attained.

INDICATIONS AND USAGE
Amikacin Sulfate is indicated in the short-term treatment of serious infections due to susceptible strains of Gram-negative bacteria, including *Pseudomonas* species, *Escherichia coli*, species of indole-positive and indole-negative *Proteus*, *Providencia* species, *Klebsiella-Enterobacter-Serratia* species, and *Acinetobacter (Mima-Herellea)* species.

Clinical studies have shown Amikacin Sulfate to be effective in bacterial septicemia (including neonatal sepsis); in serious infections of the respiratory tract, bones and joints, central nervous system (including meningitis) and skin

*Bauer, A. W., Kirby, W. M. M., Sherris, J. C., and Turck, M.: Antibiotic Testing by a Standardized Single Disc Method, Am. J. Clin. Pathol. 45:493, 1966; Standardized Disc Susceptibility Test, FEDERAL REGISTER, 37:20527-29, 1972.

and soft tissue; intra-abdominal infections (including peritonitis); and in burns and postoperative infections (including postvascular surgery). Clinical studies have shown Amikacin Sulfate also to be effective in serious complicated and recurrent urinary tract infections due to these organisms. Aminoglycosides, including Amikacin Sulfate injectable, are not indicated in uncomplicated initial episodes of urinary tract infections unless the causative organisms are not susceptible to antibiotics having less potential toxicity.

Bacteriologic studies should be performed to identify causative organisms and their susceptibilities to Amikacin Sulfate. Amikacin Sulfate may be considered as initial therapy in suspected Gram-negative infections and therapy may be instituted before obtaining the results of susceptibility testing. Clinical trials demonstrated that Amikacin Sulfate was effective in infections caused by gentamicin and/or tobramycin-resistant strains of Gram-negative organisms, particularly *Proteus rettgeri*, *Providencia stuartii*, *Serratia marcescens*, and *Pseudomonas aeruginosa*. The decision to continue therapy with the drug should be based on results of the susceptibility tests, the severity of the infection, the response of the patient and the important additional considerations contained in the *"Warnings"* box above.

Amikacin Sulfate has also been shown to be effective in staphylococcal infections and may be considered as initial therapy under certain conditions in the treatment of known or suspected staphylococcal disease such as, severe infections where the causative organism may be either a Gram-negative bacterium or a staphylococcus, infections due to susceptible strains of staphylococci in patients allergic to other antibiotics, and in mixed staphylococcal/Gram-negative infections.

In certain severe infections such as neonatal sepsis, concomitant therapy with a penicillin-type drug may be indicated because of the possibility of infections due to Gram-positive organisms such as streptococci or pneumococci.

UNLABELED USES
Amikacin Sulfate is used alone or as an adjunct in the treatment of mycobacterium avium infection and nocardia infection.

CONTRAINDICATIONS
A history of hypersensitivity to Amikacin Sulfate is a contraindication for its use. A history of hypersensitivity or serious toxic reactions to aminoglycosides may contraindicate the use of any other aminoglycoside because of the known cross-sensitivities of patients to drugs in this class.

WARNINGS
See *"Warnings"* box above.

Aminoglycosides can cause fetal harm when administered to a pregnant woman. Aminoglycosides cross the placenta and there have been several reports of total irreversible, bilateral congenital deafness in children whose mothers received streptomycin during pregnancy. Although serious side effects to the fetus or newborns have not been reported in the treatment of pregnant women with other aminoglycosides, the potential for harm exists. Reproduction studies of Amikacin Sulfate have been performed in rats and mice and revealed no evidence of impaired fertility or harm to the fetus due to Amikacin Sulfate. There are no well controlled studies in pregnant women, but investigational experience does not include any positive evidence of adverse effects to the fetus. If this drug is used during pregnancy, or if the patient becomes pregnant while taking this drug, the patient should be apprised of the potential hazard to the fetus.

Contains sodium bisulfite or metabisulfite, a sulfite that may cause allergic-type reactions including anaphylactic symptoms and life-threatening or less severe asthmatic episodes in certain susceptible people. The overall prevalence of sulfite sensitivity in the general population is unknown and probably low. Sulfite sensitivity is seen more frequently in asthmatic than nonasthmatic people.

PRECAUTIONS
Aminoglycosides are quickly and almost totally absorbed when they are applied topically, except to the urinary bladder, in association with surgical procedures. Irreversible deafness, renal failure, and death due to neuromuscular blockade have been reported following irrigation of both small and large surgical fields with an aminoglycoside preparation.

Amikacin Sulfate is potentially nephrotoxic, ototoxic and neurotoxic. The concurrent or serial use of other ototoxic or nephrotoxic agents should be avoided either systemically or topically because of the potential for additive effects. Increased nephrotoxicity has been reported following concomitant parenteral administration of aminoglycoside antibiotics and cephalosporins. Concomitant cephalosporins may spuriously elevate creatinine determinations.

Since Amikacin Sulfate is present in high concentrations in the renal excretory system, patients should be well hydrated to minimize chemical irritation of the renal tubules. Kidney function should be assessed by the usual methods prior to starting therapy and daily during the course of treatment.

If signs of renal irritation appear (casts, white or red cells, or albumin), hydration should be increased. A reduction in dosage (see *"Dosage and Administration"*) may be desirable if other evidence of renal dysfunction occurs such as decreased creatinine clearance; decreased urine specific gravity; increased BUN, creatinine, or oliguria. If azotemia increases or if a progressive decrease in urinary output occurs, treatment should be stopped.

Note: When patients are well hydrated and kidney function is normal the risk of nephrotoxic reactions with Amikacin Sulfate is low if the dosage recommendations (see *"Dosage and Administration"*) are not exceeded.

Elderly patients may have reduced renal function which may not be evident in routine screening tests such as BUN or serum creatinine. A creatinine clearance determination may be more useful. Monitoring of renal function during treatment with aminoglycosides is particularly important.

Aminoglycosides should be used with caution in patients with muscular disorders such as myasthenia gravis or parkinsonism since these drugs may aggravate muscle weakness because of their potential curare-like effect on the neuromuscular junction.

In vitro mixing of aminoglycosides with beta-lactam antibiotics (penicillin or cephalosporins) may result in a significant mutual inactivation. A reduction in serum half-life or serum level may occur when an aminoglycoside or penicillin-type drug is administered by separate routes. Inactivation of the aminoglycoside is clinically significant only in patients with severely impaired renal function. Inactivation may continue in specimens of body fluids collected for assay, resulting in inaccurate aminoglycoside readings. Such specimens should be properly handled (assayed promptly, frozen, or treated with beta-lactamase).

Cross-allergenicity among aminoglycosides has been demonstrated.

As with other antibiotics, the use of Amikacin Sulfate may result in overgrowth of nonsusceptible organisms. If this occurs, appropriate therapy should be instituted.

Aminoglycosides should not be given concurrently with potent diuretics (See "Warnings" box).

Carcinogenesis, Mutagenesis, Impairment of Fertility: Long term studies in animals to evaluate carcinogenic potential have not been performed, and mutagenicity has not been studied. Amikacin Sulfate administered subcutaneously to rats at doses up to 4 times the human daily dose did not impair male or female fertility.

Pregnancy: Teratogenic Effects Category D (See "Warnings" section).

Nursing Mothers: It is not known whether Amikacin Sulfate is excreted in human milk. Because many drugs are excreted in human milk and because of the potential for serious adverse reactions in nursing infants from Amikacin Sulfate, a decision should be made whether to discontinue nursing or to discontinue the drug, taking into account the importance of the drug to the mother.

Pediatric Use: Aminoglycosides should be used with caution in premature and neonatal infants because of the renal immaturity of these patients and the resulting prolongation of serum half-life of these drugs.

ADVERSE REACTIONS

All aminoglycosides have the potential to induce auditory, vestibular, and renal toxicity and neuromuscular blockade (see "Warnings" box). They occur more frequently in patients with present or past history of renal impairment, of treatment with other ototoxic or nephrotoxic drugs, and in patients treated for longer periods and/or with higher doses than recommended.

Neurotoxicity-Ototoxicity: Toxic effects on the eighth cranial nerve can result in hearing loss, loss of balance, or both. Amikacin Sulfate primarily affects auditory function. Cochlear damage includes high frequency deafness and usually occurs before clinical hearing loss can be detected.

Neurotoxicity-Neuromuscular Blockage: Acute muscular paralysis and apnea can occur following treatment with aminoglycoside drugs.

Nephrotoxicity: Elevation of serum creatinine, albuminuria, presence of red and white cells, casts, azotemia, and oliguria have been reported. Renal function changes are usually reversible when the drug is discontinued.

Other: In addition to those described above, other adverse reactions which have been reported on rare occasions are skin rash, drug fever, headache, paresthesia, tremor, nausea and vomiting, eosinophilia, arthralgia, anemia, and hypotension.

Overdosage: In the event of overdosage or toxic reaction, peritoneal dialysis or hemodialysis will aid in the removal of Amikacin Sulfate from the blood. In the newborn infant, exchange transfusion may also be considered.

DOSAGE AND ADMINISTRATION

The patient's pretreatment body weight should be obtained for calculation of correct dosage. Amikacin Sulfate may be given intramuscularly or intravenously.

The status of renal function should be estimated by measurement of the serum creatinine concentration or calculation of the endogenous creatinine clearance rate. The blood urea nitrogen (BUN) is much less reliable for this purpose. Reassessment of renal function should be made periodically during therapy.

Whenever possible, Amikacin Sulfate concentrations in serum should be measured to assure adequate but not excessive levels. It is desirable to measure both peak and trough serum concentrations intermittently during therapy. Peak concentrations (30 to 90 minutes after injection) above 35 µg per mL and trough concentrations (just prior to the next dose) above 10 µg per mL should be avoided. Dosage should be adjusted as indicated.

Intramuscular Administration for Patients with Normal Renal Function: The recommended dosage for adults, children and older infants (see "Warnings" box) with normal renal function is 15 mg/kg/day divided into 2 or 3 equal doses administered at equally-divided intervals, i.e., 7.5 mg/kg q12h or 5 mg/kg q8h. Treatment of patients in the heavier weight classes should not exceed 1.5 g/day.

When Amikacin Sulfate is indicated in newborns (see "Warnings" box), it is recommended that a loading dose of 10 mg/kg be administered initially to be followed with 7.5 mg/kg every 12 hours.

The usual duration of treatment is 7 to 10 days. It is desirable to limit the duration of treatment to short term whenever feasible. The total daily dose by all routes of administration should not exceed 15 mg/kg/day. In difficult and complicated infections where treatment beyond 10 days is considered, the use of Amikacin Sulfate should be reevaluated. If continued, Amikacin Sulfate serum

levels, and renal, auditory, and vestibular functions should be monitored. At the recommended dosage level, uncomplicated infections due to Amikacin Sulfate-sensitive organisms should respond in 24 to 48 hours. If definite clinical response does not occur within 3 to 5 days, therapy should be stopped and the antibiotic susceptibility pattern of the invading organism should be rechecked. Failure of the infection to respond may be due to resistance of the organism or to the presence of septic foci requiring surgical drainage.

When Amikacin Sulfate is indicated in uncomplicated urinary tract infections, a dose of 250 mg twice daily may be used.

DOSAGE GUIDELINES
ADULTS AND CHILDREN WITH NORMAL RENAL FUNCTION

Patient Weight		Dosage		
		7.5 mg/kg		5mg/kg
lbs.	kg	q12h	OR	q8h
99	45	337.5 mg		225 mg
110	50	375 mg		250 mg
121	55	412.5 mg		275 mg
132	60	450 mg		300 mg
143	65	487.5 mg		325 mg
154	70	525 mg		350 mg
165	75	562.6 mg		375 mg
176	80	600 mg		400 mg
187	85	637.5 mg		425 mg
198	90	675 mg		450 mg
209	95	712.5 mg		475 mg
220	100	750 mg		500 mg

Intramuscular Administration for Patients with Impaired Renal Function: Whenever possible, serum Amikacin Sulfate concentrations should be monitored by appropriate assay procedures. Doses may be adjusted in patients with impaired renal function either by administering normal doses at prolonged intervals or by administering reduced doses at a fixed interval.

Both methods are based on the patient's creatinine clearance or serum creatinine values since these have been found to correlate with aminoglycoside half-lives in patients with diminished renal function. These dosage schedules must be used in conjunction with careful clinical and laboratory observations of the patient and should be modified as necessary. Neither method should be used when dialysis is being performed.

Normal Dosage at Prolonged Intervals: If the creatinine clearance rate is not available and the patient's condition is stable, a dosage interval in hours for the normal dose can be calculated by multiplying the patient's serum creatinine by 9; eg, if the serum creatinine concentration is 2 mg/100 mL, the recommended single dose (7.5 mg/kg) should be administered every 18 hours.

Reduced Dosage at Fixed Time Intervals: When renal function is impaired and it is desirable to administer Amikacin Sulfate at a fixed time interval, dosage must be reduced. In these patients, serum Amikacin Sulfate concentrations should be measured to assure accurate administration of Amikacin Sulfate and to avoid concentrations above 35 µg/mL. If serum assay determinations are not available and the patient's condition is stable, serum creatinine and creatinine clearance values are the most readily available indicators of the degree of renal impairment to use as a guide for dosage.

First, initiate therapy by administering a normal dose, 7.5 mg/kg, as a loading dose. This loading dose is the same as the normally recommended dose which would be calculated for a patient with a normal renal function as described above.

To determine the size of maintenance doses administered every 12 hours, the loading dose should be reduced in proportion to the reduction in the patient's creatinine clearance rate:

$$\frac{\text{Maintenance Dose Every 12 hours}}{} = \frac{\text{observed CC in mL/min}}{\text{normal CC in mL/min}} \times \frac{\text{calculated loading dose in mg}}{}$$

(CC—creatinine clearance rate)

An alternate rough guide for determining reduced dosage at 12-hour intervals (for patients whose steady state serum creatinine values are known) is to divide the normally recommended dose by the patient's serum creatinine.

The above dosage schedules are not intended to be rigid recommendations but are provided as guides to dosage when the measurement of Amikacin serum levels is not feasible.

Intravenous Administration: The individual dose, the total daily dose, and the total cumulative dose of Amikacin Sulfate are identical to the dose recommended for intramuscular administration. The solution for intravenous use is prepared by adding the contents of a 500 mg vial to 100 to 200 mL of sterile diluent such as 0.9% Sodium Chloride or 5% Dextrose in Water or any other compatible solutions listed below.

The solution is administered to adults over a 30 to 60 minute period. The total daily dose should not exceed 15 mg/kg/day and may be divided into either 2 or 3 equally-divided doses at equally-divided intervals.

In pediatric patients the amount of fluid used will depend on the amount of Amikacin Sulfate ordered for the patient. It should be a sufficient amount to infuse the Amikacin Sulfate over a 30 to 60 minute period. Infants should receive a 1- to 2-hour infusion.

▶ SHOWN IN PRODUCT IDENTIFICATION GUIDE

Stability in IV Fluids: Amikacin Sulfate is stable for 24 hours at room temperature at concentrations of 0.25 and 5.0 mg/mL in the following solutions:

5% Dextrose Injection, USP
5% Dextrose and 0.2% Sodium Chloride Injection, USP
5% Dextrose and 0.45% Sodium Chloride Injection, USP
0.9% Sodium Chloride Injection, USP
Lactated Ringer's Injection, USP
Normosol®M in 5% Dextrose Injection, USP (or Plasma-Lyte 56 Injection in 5% Dextrose in Water)
Normosol®R in 5% Dextrose Injection, USP (or Plasma-Lyte 148 Injection in 5% Dextrose in Water)

In the above solutions with Amikacin Sulfate concentrations of 0.25 and 5.0 mg/mL, solutions aged for 60 days at 4°C and then stored at 25°C had utility times of 24 hours.

At the same concentrations, solutions frozen and aged for 30 days at −15°C, thawed, and stored at 25°C had utility times of 24 hours.

Parenteral drug products should be inspected visually for particulate matter and discoloration prior to administration whenever the solution and container permit.

Aminoglycosides administered by any of the above routes should not be physically premixed with other drugs but should be administered separately.

Because of the potential toxicity of aminoglycosides, "fixed dosage" recommendations which are not based upon body weight are not advised. Rather, it is essential to calculate the dosage to fit the needs of each patient.

Amikacin Sulfate is stable at room temperature for 2 years. At times the solution may become a very pale yellow; this does not indicate a decrease in potency.

STORAGE
Store at controlled room temperature 15°-30°C (59°-86°F)

HOW SUPPLIED
INJECTION: 50 MG/ML

BRAND/MANUFACTURER		NDC	SIZE	AWP
◆ **BRAND**				
AMIKIN PEDIATRIC: Apothecon		00015-3015-20	2 ml	$35.24
◆ **GENERICS**				
Gensia		00703-9022-03	2 ml 10s	$385.38

INJECTION: 250 MG/ML

AVERAGE UNIT PRICE (AVAILABLE SIZES)		GENERIC A-RATED AVERAGE PRICE (GAAP)	
BRAND	$30.89	2 ml 10s	$645.25
GENERIC	$31.90	4 ml 10s	$1261.07

BRAND/MANUFACTURER	NDC	SIZE	AWP
◆ **BRAND**			
AMIKIN: Apothecon	00015-3020-20	2 ml	$58.74
	00015-3020-21	2 ml	$68.54
	00015-3023-20	4 ml	$116.08
◆ **GENERICS**			
Elkins-Sinn	00641-0123-23	2 ml 10s	$637.50
Gensia	00703-9032-03	2 ml 10s	$653.00
Elkins-Sinn	00641-2357-43	4 ml 10s	$1200.00
Gensia	00703-9040-03	4 ml 10s	$1322.13

Amikin *SEE* AMIKACIN SULFATE

Amiloride Hydrochloride

DESCRIPTION
Amiloride Hydrochloride, an antikaliuretic-diuretic agent, is a pyrazine-carbonyl-guanidine that is unrelated chemically to other known antikaliuretic or diuretic agents. It is the salt of a moderately strong base (pKa 8.7). It is designated chemically as 3,5-diamino-6-chloro-N-(diaminomethylene) pyrazinecarboxamide monohydrochloride, dihydrate and has a molecular weight of 302.14. Its empirical formula is $C_6H_8ClN_7O \cdot HCl \cdot 2H_2O$ and its structural formula is:

Following is its chemical structure:

$$ \cdot HCl \cdot 2H_2O $$

CLINICAL PHARMACOLOGY
Amiloride Hydrochloride is a potassium-conserving (antikaliuretic) drug that possesses weak (compared with thiazide diuretics) natriuretic, diuretic, and antihypertensive activity. These effects have been partially additive to the effects of thiazide diuretics in some clinical studies. When administered with a thiazide or loop diuretic, Amiloride Hydrochloride has been shown to decrease the enhanced urinary excretion of magnesium which occurs when a thiazide or loop diuretic is used alone. Amiloride Hydrochloride has potassium-conserving activity in patients receiving kaliuretic diuretic agents.

Amiloride Hydrochloride is not an aldosterone antagonist and its effects are seen even in the absence of aldosterone.

Amiloride Hydrochloride exerts its potassium sparing effect through the inhibition of sodium reabsorption at the distal convoluted tubule, cortical collecting tubule and collecting duct; this decreases the net negative potential of the tubular lumen and reduces both potassium and hydrogen secretion and their subsequent excretion. This mechanism accounts in large part for the potassium sparing action of amiloride.

Amiloride Hydrochloride usually begins to act within 2 hours after an oral dose. Its effect on electrolyte excretion reaches a peak between 6 and 10 hours and lasts about 24 hours. Peak plasma levels are obtained in 3 to 4 hours and the plasma half-life varies from 6 to 9 hours. Effects on electrolytes increase with single doses of amiloride HCl up to approximately 15 mg.

Amiloride Hydrochloride is not metabolized by the liver but is excreted unchanged by the kidneys. About 50 percent of a 20 mg dose of Amiloride Hydrochloride is excreted in the urine and 40 percent in the stool within 72 hours. Amiloride Hydrochloride has little effect on glomerular filtration rate or renal blood flow. Because Amiloride Hydrochloride is not metabolized by the liver, drug accumulation is not anticipated in patients with hepatic dysfunction, but accumulation can occur if the hepatorenal syndrome develops.

INDICATIONS AND USAGE
Amiloride Hydrochloride is indicated as adjunctive treatment with thiazide diuretics or other kaliuretic-diuretic agents in congestive heart failure or hypertension to:

a. help restore normal serum potassium levels in patients who develop hypokalemia on the kaliuretic diuretic;
b. prevent development of hypokalemia in patients who would be exposed to particular risk if hypokalemia were to develop, e.g., digitalized patients or patients with significant cardiac arrhythmias.

The use of potassium-conserving agents is often unnecessary in patients receiving diuretics for uncomplicated essential hypertension when such patients have a normal diet. Amiloride Hydrochloride has little additive diuretic or antihypertensive effect when added to a thiazide diuretic.

Amiloride Hydrochloride should rarely be used alone. It has weak (compared with thiazides) diuretic and antihypertensive effects. Used as single agents, potassium sparing diuretics, including Amiloride Hydrochloride, result in an increased risk of hyperkalemia (approximately 10% with Amiloride Hydrochloride. Amiloride Hydrochloride should be used alone only when persistent hypokalemia has been documented and only with careful titration of the dose and close monitoring of serum electrolytes.

CONTRAINDICATIONS
HYPERKALEMIA
Amiloride Hydrochloride should not be used in the presence of elevated serum potassium levels (greater than 5.5 mEq per liter).

ANTIKALIURETIC THERAPY OR POTASSIUM SUPPLEMENTATION
Amiloride Hydrochloride should not be given to patients receiving other potassium-conserving agents, such as spironolactone or triamterene. Potassium supplementation in the form of medication, potassium-containing salt substitutes, or a potassium-rich diet should not be used with Amiloride Hydrochloride except in severe and/or refractory cases of hypokalemia. Such concomitant therapy can be associated with rapid increases in serum potassium levels. If potassium supplementation is used, careful monitoring of the serum potassium level is necessary.

IMPAIRED RENAL FUNCTION
Anuria, acute or chronic renal insufficiency, and evidence of diabetic nephropathy are contraindications to the use of Amiloride Hydrochloride. Patients with evidence of renal functional impairment (blood urea nitrogen [BUN] levels over 30 mg per 100 mL or serum creatinine levels over 1.5 mg per 100 mL) or diabetes mellitus should not receive the drug without careful, frequent and continuing monitoring of serum electrolytes, creatinine, and BUN levels. Potassium retention associated with the use of an antikaliuretic agent is accentuated in the presence of renal impairment and may result in the rapid development of hyperkalemia.

HYPERSENSITIVITY
Amiloride Hydrochloride is contraindicated in patients who are hypersensitive to this product.

WARNINGS
HYPERKALEMIA

LIKE OTHER POTASSIUM-CONSERVING AGENTS, AMILORIDE HYDROCHLORIDE MAY CAUSE HYPERKALEMIA (SERUM POTASSIUM LEVELS GREATER THAN 5.5 MEQ PER LITER) WHICH, IF UNCORRECTED, IS POTENTIALLY FATAL. HYPERKALEMIA OCCURS COMMONLY (ABOUT 10%) WHEN AMILORIDE HYDROCHLORIDE IS USED WITHOUT A KALIURETIC DIURETIC. THIS INCIDENCE IS GREATER IN PATIENTS WITH RENAL IMPAIRMENT, DIABETES MELLITUS (WITH OR WITHOUT RECOGNIZED RENAL INSUFFICIENCY), AND IN THE ELDERLY. WHEN AMILORIDE HYDROCHLORIDE IS USED CONCOMITANTLY WITH A THIAZIDE DIURETIC IN PATIENTS WITHOUT THESE COMPLICATIONS,

THE RISK OF HYPERKALEMIA IS REDUCED TO ABOUT 1-2 PERCENT. IT IS THUS ESSENTIAL TO MONITOR SERUM POTASSIUM LEVELS CAREFULLY IN ANY PATIENT RECEIVING AMILORIDE HYDROCHLORIDE, PARTICULARLY WHEN IT IS FIRST INTRODUCED, AT THE TIME OF DIURETIC DOSAGE ADJUSTMENTS, AND DURING ANY ILLNESS THAT COULD AFFECT RENAL FUNCTION.

The risk of hyperkalemia may be increased when potassium-conserving agents, including Amiloride Hydrochloride, are administered concomitantly with an angiotensin-converting enzyme inhibitor. (See *"Precautions, Drug Interactions."*) Warning signs or symptoms of hyperkalemia include paresthesias, muscular weakness, fatigue, flaccid paralysis of the extremities, bradycardia, shock, and ECG abnormalities. Monitoring of the serum potassium level is essential because mild hyperkalemia is not usually associated with an abnormal ECG.

When abnormal, the ECG in hyperkalemia is characterized primarily by tall, peaked T waves or elevations from previous tracings. There may also be lowering of the R wave and increased depth of the S wave, widening and even disappearance of the P wave, progressive widening of the QRS complex, prolongation of the PR interval, and ST depression.

Treatment of Hyperkalemia: If hyperkalemia occurs in patients taking Amiloride Hydrochloride, the drug should be discontinued immediately. If the serum potassium level exceeds 6.5 mEq per liter, active measures should be taken to reduce it. Such measures include the intravenous administration of sodium bicarbonate solution or oral or parenteral glucose with a rapid-acting insulin preparation. If needed, a cation exchange resin such as sodium polystyrene sulfonate may be given orally or by enema. Patients with persistent hyperkalemia may require dialysis.

DIABETES MELLITUS
In diabetic patients, hyperkalemia has been reported with the use of all potassium-conserving diuretics, including Amiloride Hydrochloride, even in patients without evidence of diabetic nephropathy. Therefore, Amiloride Hydrochloride should be avoided, if possible, in diabetic patients and, if it is used, serum electrolytes and renal function must be monitored frequently.

Amiloride Hydrochloride should be discontinued at least three days before glucose tolerance testing.

METABOLIC OR RESPIRATORY ACIDOSIS
Antikaliuretic therapy should be instituted only with caution in severely ill patients in whom respiratory or metabolic acidosis may occur, such as patients with cardiopulmonary disease or poorly controlled diabetes. If Amiloride Hydrochloride is given to these patients, frequent monitoring of acid-base balance is necessary. Shifts in acid-base balance alter the ratio of extracellular/intracellular potassium, and the development of acidosis may be associated with rapid increases in serum potassium levels.

PRECAUTIONS
GENERAL
Electrolyte Imbalance and Bun Increases: Hyponatremia and hypochloremia may occur when Amiloride Hydrochloride is used with other diuretics and increases in BUN levels have been reported. These increases usually have accompanied vigorous fluid elimination, especially when diuretic therapy was used in seriously ill patients, such as those who had hepatic cirrhosis with ascites and metabolic alkalosis, or those with resistant edema. Therefore, when Amiloride Hydrochloride is given with other diuretics to such patients, careful monitoring of serum electrolytes and BUN levels is important. In patients with pre-existing severe liver disease, hepatic encephalopathy, manifested by tremors, confusion, and coma, and increased jaundice, have been reported in association with diuretics, including Amiloride Hydrochloride.

DRUG INTERACTIONS
When Amiloride Hydrochloride is administered concomitantly with an angiotensin-converting enzyme inhibitor, the risk of hyperkalemia may be increased. Therefore, if concomitant use of these agents is indicated because of demonstrated hypokalemia, they should be used with caution and with frequent monitoring of serum potassium. (See *"Warnings".*)

Lithium generally should not be given with diuretics because they reduce its renal clearance and add a high risk of lithium toxicity. Read circulars for lithium preparations before use of such concomitant therapy.

In some patients, the administration of a non-steroidal anti-inflammatory agent can reduce the diuretic, natriuretic, and antihypertensive effects of loop, potassium-sparing and thiazide diuretics. Therefore, when Amiloride Hydrochloride and non-steroidal anti-inflammatory agents are used concomitantly, the patient should be observed closely to determine if the desired effect of the diuretic is obtained. Since indomethacin and potassium-sparing diuretics, including Amiloride Hydrochloride, each may be associated with increased serum potassium levels, the potential effects on potassium kinetics and renal function should be considered when these agents are administered concurrently.

CARCINOGENICITY, MUTAGENICITY, IMPAIRMENT OF FERTILITY
There was no evidence of a tumorigenic effect when Amiloride Hydrochloride was administered for 92 weeks to mice at doses up to 10 mg/kg/day (25 times the maximum daily human dose). Amiloride Hydrochloride has also been administered for 104 weeks to male and female rats at doses up to 6 and 8 mg/kg/day (15

and 20 times the maximum daily dose for humans, respectively) and showed no evidence of carcinogenicity.

Amiloride Hydrochloride was devoid of mutagenic activity in various strains of *Salmonella typhimurium* with or without a mammalian liver microsomal activation system (Ames test).

PREGNANCY
Pregnancy Category B. Teratogenicity studies with Amiloride Hydrochloride in rabbits and mice given 20 and 25 times the maximum human dose, respectively, revealed no evidence of harm to the fetus, although studies showed that the drug crossed the placenta in modest amounts. Reproduction studies in rats at 20 times the expected maximum daily dose for humans showed no evidence of impaired fertility. At approximately 5 or more times the expected maximum daily dose for humans, some toxicity was seen in adult rats and rabbits and a decrease in rat pup growth and survival occurred.

There are, however, no adequate and well-controlled studies in pregnant women. Because animal reproduction studies are not always predictive of human response, this drug should be used during pregnancy only if clearly needed.

NURSING MOTHERS
Studies in rats have shown that Amiloride Hydrochloride is excreted in milk in concentrations higher than that found in blood, but it is not known whether Amiloride Hydrochloride is excreted in human milk. Because many drugs are excreted in human milk and because of the potential for serious adverse reactions in nursing infants from Amiloride Hydrochloride, a decision should be made whether to discontinue nursing or to discontinue the drug, taking into account the importance of the drug to the mother.

PEDIATRIC USE
Safety and effectiveness in children have not been established.

ADVERSE REACTIONS
Amiloride Hydrochloride is usually well tolerated and, except for hyperkalemia (serum potassium levels greater than 5.5 mEq per liter— see *"Warnings"*), significant adverse effects have been reported infrequently. Minor adverse reactions were reported relatively frequently (about 20%) but the relationship of many of the reports to Amiloride Hydrochloride is uncertain and the overall frequency was similar in hydrochlorothiazide treated groups. Nausea/anorexia, abdominal pain, flatulence, and mild skin rash have been reported and probably are related to Amiloride Hydrochloride. Other adverse experiences that have been reported with Amiloride Hydrochloride are generally those known to be associated with diuresis, or with the underlying disease being treated.

The adverse reactions for Amiloride Hydrochloride listed in the following table have been arranged into two groups: (1) incidence greater than one percent; and (2) incidence one percent or less. The incidence for group (1) was determined from clinical studies conducted in the United States (837 patients treated with Amiloride Hydrochloride). The adverse effects listed in group (2) include reports from the same clinical studies and voluntary reports since marketing. The probability of a causal relationship exists between Amiloride Hydrochloride and these adverse reactions, some of which have been reported only rarely.

Incidence > 1%	Incidence ≤ 1%
Body as a Whole	
Headache*	Back pain
Weakness	Chest pain
Fatigability	Neck/shoulder ache
	Pain, extremities
Cardiovascular	
None	Angina pectoris
	Orthostatic hypotension
	Arrhythmia
	Palpitation
Digestive	
Nausea/anorexia*	Jaundice
Diarrhea*	GI bleeding
Vomiting*	Abdominal fullness
Abdominal pain	GI disturbance
Gas pain	Thirst
Appetite changes	Heartburn
Constipation	Flatulence
	Dyspepsia
Metabolic	
Elevated serum potassium levels (> 5.5 mEq per liter)†	None
Skin	
None	Skin rash
	Itching
	Dryness of mouth
	Pruritus
	Alopecia
Musculoskeletal	
Muscle cramps	Joint pain
	Leg ache
Nervous	
Dizziness	Paresthesia
Encephalopathy	Tremors
	Vertigo

Incidence > 1%	Incidence ≤ 1%
Psychiatric	
None	Nervousness
	Mental confusion
	Insomnia
	Decreased libido
	Depression
	Somnolence
Respiratory	
Cough	Shortness of breath
Dyspnea	
Special Senses	
None	Visual disturbances
	Nasal congestion
	Tinnitus
	Increased intraocular pressure
Urogenital	
Impotence	Polyuria
	Dysuria
	Urinary frequency
	Bladder spasms
	Gynecomastia

* *Reactions occurring in 3% to 8% of patients treated with Amiloride Hydrochloride. (Those reactions occurring in less than 3% of the patients are unmarked.)*
† *See "Warnings".*

CAUSAL RELATIONSHIP UNKNOWN
Other reactions have been reported but occurred under circumstances where a causal relationship could not be established. However, in these rarely reported events, that possibility cannot be excluded. Therefore, these observations are listed to serve as alerting information to physicians.

Activation of probable pre-existing peptic ulcer
Aplastic anemia
Neutropenia
Abnormal liver function

OVERDOSAGE
No data are available in regard to overdosage in humans. The oral LD_{50} of Amiloride Hydrochloride (calculated as the base) is 56 mg/kg in mice and 36 to 85 mg/kg in rats, depending on the strain.

It is not known whether the drug is dialyzable.

The most likely signs and symptoms to be expected with overdosage are dehydration and electrolyte imbalance. These can be treated by established procedures. Therapy with Amiloride Hydrochloride should be discontinued and the patient observed closely. There is no specific antidote. Emesis should be induced or gastric lavage performed. Treatment is symptomatic and supportive. If hyperkalemia occurs, active measures should be taken to reduce the serum potassium levels.

DOSAGE AND ADMINISTRATION
Amiloride Hydrochloride should be administered with food.

Amiloride Hydrochloride, one 5 mg tablet daily, should be added to the usual antihypertensive or diuretic dosage of a kaliuretic diuretic. The dosage may be increased to 10 mg per day, if necessary. More than two 5 mg tablets of Amiloride Hydrochloride daily usually are not needed, and there is little controlled experience with such doses. If persistent hypokalemia is documented with 10 mg, the dose can be increased to 15 mg, then 20 mg, with careful monitoring of electrolytes.

In treating patients with congestive heart failure after an initial diuresis has been achieved, potassium loss may also decrease and the need for Amiloride Hydrochloride should be reevaluated. Dosage adjustment may be necessary. Maintenance therapy may be on an intermittent basis.

If it is necessary to use Amiloride Hydrochloride alone (see *"Indications"*), the starting dosage should be one 5 mg tablet daily. This dosage may be increased to 10 mg per day, if necessary. More than two 5 mg tablets usually are not needed, and there is little controlled experience with such doses. If persistent hypokalemia is documented with 10 mg, the dose can be increased to 15 mg, then 20 mg, with careful monitoring of electrolytes.

STORAGE
Protect from moisture, freezing and excessive heat.

HOW SUPPLIED
TABLETS: 5 MG

BRAND/MANUFACTURER	NDC	SIZE	AWP
◆ **BRAND**			
MIDAMOR: Merck	00006-0092-68	100s	$44.65
◆ **GENERICS**			
Goldline	00182-1828-01	100s	$27.75

Amiloride Hydrochloride with Hydrochlorothiazide

DESCRIPTION
Amiloride Hydrochloride/Hydrochlorothiazide combines the potassium-conserving action of Amiloride Hydrochloride with the natriuretic action of Hydrochlorothiazide.

Amiloride Hydrochloride is designated chemically as 3,5-diamino-6-chloro-N-(diaminomethylene) pyrazinecarboxamide monohydrochloride, dihydrate and has a molecular weight of 302.14. Its empirical formula is $C_6H_8ClN_7O$•Hydrochloride•$2H_2O$.

Hydrochlorothiazide is designated chemically as 6-chloro-3,4-dihydro-2H-1,2,4-benzothiadiazine-7-sulfonamide 1,1-dioxide. Its empirical formula is $C_7H_8ClN_3O_4S_2$.

It is a white, or practically white, crystalline powder with a molecular weight of 297.72, which is slightly soluble in water, but freely soluble in sodium hydroxide solution. Amiloride/HCTZ is available for oral use as tablets containing 5 mg of anhydrous Amiloride Hydrochloride and 50 mg of Hydrochlorothiazide.

CLINICAL PHARMACOLOGY
Amiloride/HCTZ provides diuretic and antihypertensive activity (principally due to the Hydrochlorothiazide component), while acting through the Amiloride component to prevent the excessive potassium loss that may occur in patients receiving a thiazide diuretic. Due to its Amiloride component, the urinary excretion of magnesium is less with Amiloride/HCTZ than with a thiazide or loop diuretic used alone (see *"Precautions"*). The onset of the diuretic action of Amiloride/HCTZ is within 1 to 2 hours and this action appears to be sustained for approximately 24 hours.

AMILORIDE HYDROCHLORIDE
Amiloride Hydrochloride is a potassium-conserving (antikaliuretic) drug that possesses weak (compared with thiazide diuretics) natriuretic, diuretic, and antihypertensive activity. These effects have been partially additive to the effects of thiazide diuretics in some clinical studies. Amiloride Hydrochloride has potassium-conserving activity in patients receiving kaliuretic-diuretic agents.

Amiloride Hydrochloride is not an aldosterone antagonist and its effects are seen even in the absence of aldosterone.

Amiloride Hydrochloride exerts its postassium sparing effect through the inhibition of sodium reabsorption at the distal convoluted tubule, cortical collecting tubule and collecting duct; this decreases the net negative potential of the tubular lumen and reduces both potassium and hydrogen secretion and their subsequent excretion. This mechanism accounts in large part for the potassium sparing action of Amiloride.

Amiloride Hydrochloride usually begins to act within 2 hours after an oral dose. Its effect on electrolyte excretion reaches a peak between 6 and 10 hours and lasts about 24 hours. Peak plasma levels are obtained in 3 to 4 hours and the plasma half-life varies from 6 to 9 hours. Effects on electrolytes increase with single doses of Amiloride Hydrochloride up to approximately 15 mg.

Amiloride Hydrochloride is not metabolized by the liver but is excreted unchanged by the kidneys. About 50 percent of a 20 mg dose of Amiloride Hydrochloride is excreted in the urine and 40 percent in the stool within 72 hours. Amiloride Hydrochloride has little effect on glomerular filtration rate or renal blood flow. Because Amiloride Hydrochloride is not metabolized by the liver, drug accumulation is not anticipated in patients with hepatic dysfunction, but accumulation can occur if the hepatorenal syndrome develops.

HYDROCHLOROTHIAZIDE
The mechanism of the antihypertensive effect of thiazides is unknown. Thiazides do not usually affect normal blood pressure.

Hydrochlorothiazide is a diuretic and antihypertensive. It affects the distal renal tubular mechanism of electrolyte reabsorption. Hydrochlorothiazide increases excretion of sodium and chloride in approximately equivalent amounts. Natriuresis may be accompanied by some loss of potassium and bicarbonate.

After oral use diuresis begins within two hours, peaks in about four hours and lasts about 6 to 12 hours.

Hydrochlorothiazide is not metabolized but is eliminated rapidly by the kidney. When plasma levels have been followed for at least 24 hours, the plasma half-life has been observed to vary between 5.6 and 14.8 hours. At least 61 percent of the oral dose is eliminated unchanged within 24 hours. Hydrochlorothiazide crosses the placental but not the blood-brain barrier and is excreted in breast milk.

INDICATIONS AND USAGE
Amiloride/HCTZ is indicated in those patients with hypertension or with congestive heart failure who develop hypokalemia when thiazides or other kaliuretic diuretics are used alone, or in whom maintenance of normal serum potassium levels is considered to be clinically important, e.g., digitalized patients, or patients with significant cardiac arrhythmias.

The use of potassium-conserving agents is often unnecessary in patients receiving diuretics for uncomplicated essential hypertension when such patients have a normal diet.

◆ RATED THERAPEUTICALLY EQUIVALENT; ◇ THERAPEUTIC EQUIVALENCE UNCONFIRMED; ○ UNRATED

Amilovicle/HCTZ may be used alone or as an adjunct to other antihypertensive drugs, such as methyldopa or beta blockers. Since Amilovicle/HTCZ enhances the action of these agents, dosage adjustments may be necessary to avoid an excessive fall in blood pressure and other unwanted side effects.

This fixed combination drug is not indicated for the initial therapy of edema or hypertension except in individuals in whom the development of hypokalemia cannot be risked.

CONTRAINDICATIONS

HYPERKALEMIA
Amiloride/HCTZ should not be used in the presence of elevated serum potassium levels (greater than 5.5 mEq per liter).

ANTIKALIURETIC THERAPY OR POTASSIUM SUPPLEMENTATION
Amiloride/HCTZ should not be given to patients receiving other potassium-conserving agents, such as spironolactone or triamterene. Potassium supplementation in the form of medication, potassium-containing salt substitutes or a potassium-rich diet should not be used with Amiloride/HCTZ except in severe and/or refractory cases of hypokalemia. Such concomitant therapy can be associated with rapid increases in serum potassium levels. If potassium supplementation is used, careful monitoring of the serum potassium level is necessary.

IMPAIRED RENAL FUNCTION
Anuria, acute or chronic renal insufficiency, and evidence of diabetic nephropathy are contraindications to the use of Amiloride/HCTZ. Patients with evidence of renal functional impairment (blood urea nitrogen [BUN] levels over 30 mg per 100 mL or serum creatinine levels over 1.5 mg per 100 mL) or diabetes mellitus should not receive the drug without careful, frequent and continuing monitoring of serum electrolytes, creatinine, and BUN levels. Potassium retention associated with the use of an antikaliuretic agent is accentuated in the presence of renal impairment and may result in the rapid development of hyperkaiemia.

HYPERSENSITIVITY
Amiloride/HCTZ is contraindicated in patients who are hypersensitive to this product, or to other sulfonamide-derived drugs.

WARNINGS

HYPERKALEMIA
LIKE OTHER POTASSIUM-CONSERVING DIURETIC COMBINATIONS, AMILORIDE/HCTZ MAY CAUSE HYPERKALEMIA (SERUM POTASSIUM LEVELS GREATER THAN 5.5 MEQ PER LITER). IN PATIENTS WITHOUT RENAL IMPAIRMENT OR DIABETES MELLITUS, THE RISK OF HYPERKALEMIA WITH AMILORIDE/HCTZ IS ABOUT 1-2 PERCENT. THIS RISK IS HIGHER IN PATIENTS WITH RENAL IMPAIRMENT OR DIABETES MELLITUS (EVEN WITHOUT RECOGNIZED DIABETIC NEPHROPATHY). SINCE HYPERKALEMIA, IF UNCORRECTED, IS POTENTIALLY FATAL, IT IS ESSENTIAL TO MONITOR SERUM POTASSIUM LEVELS CAREFULLY IN ANY PATIENT RECEIVING AMILORIDE/HCTZ PARTICULARLY WHEN IT IS FIRST INTRODUCED, AT THE TIME OF DOSAGE ADJUSTMENTS, AND DURING ANY ILLNESS THAT COULD AFFECT RENAL FUNCTION.

The risk of hyperkalemia may be increased when potassium-conserving agents, including Amiloride/HCTZ are administered concomitantly with an angiotensin converting enzyme inhibitor: (See *"Precautions, Drug Interactions."*) Warning signs or symptoms of hyperkalemia include paresthesias, muscular weakness, fatigue, flaccid paralysis of the extremities, bradycardia, shock, and ECG abnormalities. Monitoring of the serum potassium level is essential because mild hyperkalemia is not usually associated with an abnormal ECG.

When abnormal, the ECG in hyperkalemia is characterized primarily by tall, peaked T waves or elevations from previous tracings. There may also be lowering of the R wave and increased depth of the S wave, widening and even disappearance of the P wave, progressive widening of the QRS complex, prolongation of the PR interval, and ST depression.

Treatment of Hyperkalemia: If hyperkalemia occurs in patients taking Amiloride/HCTZ the drug should be discontinued immediately. If the serum potassium level exceeds 6.5 mEq per liter, active measures should be taken to reduce it. Such measures include the intravenous administration of sodium bicarbonate solution or oral or parenteral glucose with a rapid-acting insulin preparation. If needed, a cation exchange resin such as sodium polystyrene sulfonate may be given orally or by enema. Patients with persistent hyperkalemia may require dialysis.

DIABETES MELLITUS
In diabetic patients, hyperkalemia has been reported with the use of all potassium-conserving diuretics, including Amiloride Hydrocloride, even in patients without evidence of diabetic nephropathy. Therefore, Amiloride/HCTZ should be avoided, if possible, in diabetic patients and, if it is used, serum electrolytes and renal function must be monitored frequently. Amiloride/HCTZ should be discontinued at least three days before glucose tolerance testing.

METABOLIC OR RESPIRATORY ACIDOSIS
Antikaliuretic therapy should be instituted only with caution in severely ill patients in whom respiratory or metabolic acidosis may occur, such as patients with cardiopulmonary disease or poorly controlled diabetes. If Amiloride/HCTZ is given to these patients, frequent monitoring of acid-base balance is necessary. Shifts in acid-base balance alter the ratio of extracellular/intracellular potassium, and the development of acidosis may be associated with rapid increases in serum potassium levels.

PRECAUTIONS

GENERAL

ELECTROLYTE IMBALANCE AND BUN INCREASES
Determination of serum electrolytes to detect possible electrolyte imbalance should be performed at appropriate intervals.

Patients should be observed for clinical signs of fluid or electrolyte imbalance: i.e., hyponatremia, hypochloremic alkalosis, and hypokalemia. Serum and urine electrolyte determinations are particularly important when the patient is vomiting excessively or receiving parenteral fluids. Warning signs or symptoms of fluid and electrolyte imbalance, irresponsive of cause, include dryness of mouth, thirst, weakness, lethargy, drowsiness, restlessness, confusion, seizures, muscle pains or cramps, muscular fatigue, hypotension, oliguria, tachycardia, and gastrointestinal disturbances such as nausea and vomiting.

Hyponatremia and hypochloremia may occur during the use of thiazides and other diuretics. Any chloride deficit during thiazide therapy is generally mild and may be lessened by the Amiloride Hydrochloride component of Amiloride/HCTZ. Hypochloremia usually does not require specific treatment except under extraordinary circumstances (as in liver disease or renal disease). Dilutional hyponatremia may occur in edematous patients in hot weather; appropriate therapy is water restriction, rather than administration of salt, except in rare instances when the hyponatremia is life-threatening. In actual salt depletion, appropriate replacement is the therapy of choice.

Hypokalemia may develop during thiazide therapy, especially with brisk diuresis, when severe cirrhosis is present, during concomitant use of corticosteroids or ACTH, or after prolonged therapy. However, this usually is prevented by the Amiloride Hydrochloride component of Amiloride/HCTZ.

Interference with adequate oral electrolyte intake will also contribute to hypokalemia. Hypokalemia may cause cardiac arrhythmia and may also sensitize or exaggerate the response of the heart to the toxic effects of digitalis (e.g., increased ventricular irritability).

Thiazides have been shown to increase the urinary excretion of magnesium; this may result in hypomagnesemia. Amiloride Hydrochloride, a component of Amiloride/HCTZ has been shown to decrease the enhanced urinary excretion of magnesium which occurs when a thiazide or loop diuretic is used alone.

Increase in BUN levels have been reported with Amiloride Hydrochloride and with Hydrochlorothiazide. These increases usually have accompanied vigorous fluid elimination, especially when diuretic therapy was used in seriously ill patients, such as those who had hepatic cirrhosis with ascites and metabolic alkalosis, or those with resistant edema. Therefore, when Amiloride/HCTZ is given to such patients, careful monitoring of serum electrolyte and BUN levels is important. In patients with pre-existing severe liver disease, hepatic encephalopathy, manifested by tremors, confusion, and coma, and increased jaundice, have been reported in association with diuretic therapy including Amiloride Hydrochloride and Hydrochlorothiazide.

In patients with renal disease, diuretics may precipitate azotemia. Cumulative effects of the components of Amiloride/HCTZ may develop in patients with impaired renal function. If renal impairment becomes evident, Amiloride/HCTZ should be discontinued (see *"Contraindications"* and *"Warnings"*).

DRUG INTERACTIONS
In some patients, the administration of a nonsteroidal anti-inflammatory agent can reduce the diuretic, natriuretic, and antihypertensive effects of loop, potassium-sparing and thiazide diuretics. Therefore, when Amiloride/HCTZ and nonsteroidal anti-inflammatory agents are used concomitantly, the patient should be observed closely to determine if the desired effect of the diuretic is obtained. Since indomethacin and potassium-sparing diuretics, including Amiloride/HCTZ, each may be associated with increased serum potassium levels, the potential effects on potassium kinetics and renal function should be considered when these agents are administered concurrently.

AMILORIDE HYDROCHLORIDE
When Amiloride Hydrochloride is administered concomitantly with an angiotensin-converting enzyme inhibitor, the risk of hyperkalemia may be increased. Therefore, if concomitant use of these agents is indicated because of demonstrated hypokalemia, they should be used with caution and with frequent monitoring of serum potassium. (See *"Warnings."*)

HYDROCHLOROTHIAZIDE
When given concurrently the following drugs may interact with thiazide diuretics.

Alcohol, Barbiturates, or Narcotics: potentiation of orthostatic hypotension may occur.

Antidiabetic Drugs (Oral Agents and Insulin): dosage adjustment of the antidiabetic drug may be required.

Other Antihypertensive Drugs: additive effect of potentiation.

Cholestyramine and Colestipol Resins: absorption of Hydrochlorothiazide is impaired in the presence of anionic exchange resins. Single doses of either cholestyramine or colestipol resins bind the Hydrochlorothiazide and reduce its absorption from the gastrointestinal tract by up to 85 and 43 percent, respectively.

Corticosteroids, ACTH: intensified electrolyte depletion, particularly hypokalema.

Pressor Amines (e.g., Norepinephrine): possible decreased response to pressor amines but not sufficient to preclude their use.

Skeletal Muscle Relaxants, Nondepolarizing (e.g., Tubocurarine): possible increased responsiveness to the muscle relaxant.

Lithium: generally should not be given with diuretics. Diuretic agents reduce the renal clearance of lithium and add a high risk of lithium toxicity. Refer to the package insert for lithium preparations before use of such preparations with Amiloride/HCTZ.

METABOLIC AND ENDOCRINE EFFECTS
In diabetic patients, insulin requirements may be increased, decreased, or unchanged due to the Hydrochlorothiazide component. Diabetes mellitus that has been latent may become manifest during administration of thiazide diuretics. Because calcium excretion is decreased by thiazides, Amiloride/HCTZ should be discontinued before carrying out tests for parathyroid function. Pathologic changes in the parathyroid glands, with hypercalcemia and hypophosphatemia have been observed in a few patients on prolonged thiazide therapy; however, the common complications of hyperparathyroidism such as renal lithiasis, bone resorption, and peptic ulceration have not been seen.

Hyperuricemia may occur or acute gout may be precipitated in certain patients receiving thiazide therapy.

OTHER PRECAUTIONS
In patients receiving thiazides, sensitivity reactions may occur with or without a history of allergy or bronchial asthma. The possibility of exacerbation or activation of systemic lupus erythematosus has been reported with the use of thiazides.

Increases in cholesterol and triglyceride levels may be associated with thiazide diuretic therapy.

CARCINOGENICITY, MUTAGENICITY, IMPAIRMENT OF FERTILITY
Long-term studies in animals have not been performed to evaluate the effects upon fertility, mutagenicity or carcinogenic potential of Amiloride/HCTZ.

AMILORIDE HYDROCHLORIDE
There was no evidence of a tumorigenic effect when Amiloride Hydrochloride was administered for 92 weeks to mice at doses up to 10 mg/kg/day (25 times the maximum daily human dose). Amiloride Hydrochloride has also been administered for 104 weeks to male and female rats at doses up to 6 and 8 mg/kg/day (15 and 20 times the maximum daily dose for humans, respectively) and showed no evidence of carcinogenicity.

Amiloride Hydrochloride was devoid of mutagenic activity in various strains of *Salmonella typhimurium* with or without a mammalian liver microsomal activation system (Ames test).

HYDROCHLOROTHIAZIDE
Two-year feeding studies in mice and rats conducted under the auspices of the National Toxicology Program (NTP) uncovered no evidence of a carcinogenic potential of Hydrochlorothiazide in female mice (at doses of up to approximately 600 mg/kg/day) or in male and female rats (at doses of up to approximately 100 mg/kg/day). The NTP, however, found equivocal evidence for hepatocarcinogenicity in male mice. Hydrochlorothiazide was not genotoxic *in vitro* in the Ames mutagenicity assay of *Salmonella typhimurium* strains TA 98, TA 100, TA 1535, TA 1537, and TA 1538 and in the Chinese Hamster Ovary (CHO) test for chromosomal aberrations, or *in vivo* in assays using mouse germinal cell chromosomes, Chinese hamster bone marrow chromosomes, and the *Drosophila* sex-linked recessive lethal trait gene. Positive test results were obtained only in the *in vitro* CHO Sister Chromatid Exchange (clastogenicity) and in the Mouse Lymphoma Cell (mutagenicity) assays, using concentrations of Hydrochlorothiazide from 43 to 1300 μg/mL, and in the *Aspergillus nidulans* non-disjunction assay at an unspecified concentration.

Hydrochlorothiazide had no adverse effects on the fertility of mice and rats of either sex in studies wherein these species were exposed, via their diet, to doses of up to 100 and 4 mg/kg, respectively, prior to conception and throughout gestation.

PREGNANCY
Pregnancy Category B. Teratogenicity studies have been performed with combinations of Amiloride Hydrochloride and Hydrochlorothiazide in rabbits and mice at doses up to 25 times the expected maximum daily dose for humans and have revealed no evidence of harm to the fetus. No evidence of impaired fertility in rats was apparent at dosage levels up to 25 times the expected maximum human daily dose. A perinatal and postnatal study in rats showed a reduction in maternal body weight gain during and after gestation at a daily dose of 25 times the expected maximum daily dose for humans. The body weights of alive pups at birth and at weaning were also reduced at this dose level. There are no adequate and well-controlled studies in pregnant women. Because animal reproduction studies are not always predictive of human responses, and because of the data listed below with the individual components, this drug should be used during pregnancy only if clearly needed.

AMILORIDE HYDROCHLORIDE
Teratogenicity studies with Amiloride Hydrochloride in rabbits and mice given 20 and 25 times the maximum human dose, respectively, revealed no evidence of

harm to the fetus, although studies showed that the drug crossed the placenta in modest amounts. Reproduction studies in rats at 20 times the expected maximum daily dose for humans showed no evidence of impaired fertility. At approximately 5 or more times the expected maximum daily dose for humans, some toxicity was seen in adult rats and rabbits and a decrease in rat pup growth and survival occurred.

HYDROCHLOROTHIAZIDE
Teratogenic Effects: Studies in which Hydrochlorothiazide was orally administered to pregnant mice and rats during their respective periods of major organogenesis at doses up to 3000 and 1000 mg Hydrochlorothiazide/kg, respectively, provided no evidence of harm to the fetus. There are, however, no adequate and well-controlled studies in pregnant women.

Nonteratogenic Effects: Thiazides cross the placental barrier and appear in cord blood. There is a risk of fetal or neonatal jaundice, thrombocytopenia, and possibly other adverse reactions that have occurred in adults.

NURSING MOTHERS
Studies in rats have shown that Amiloride is excreted in milk in concentrations higher than that found in blood, but it is not known whether Amiloride Hydrochloride is excreted in human milk. However, thiazides appear in brest milk. Because of the potential for serious adverse reactions in nursing infants, a decision should be made whether to discontinue nursing or to discontinue the drug, taking into account the importance of the drug to the mother.

PEDIATRIC USE
Safety and effectiveness in children have not been established.

ADVERSE REACTIONS
Amiloride/HCTZ is usually well tolerated and significant clinical adverse effects have been reported infrequently. The risk of hyperkalemia (serum potassium levels greater than 5.5 m Eq per liter) with Amiloride/HCTZ is about 1-2 percent in patients without renal impairment or diabetes mellitus (see *"Warnings"*). Minor adverse reactions to Amiloride Hydrochloride have been reported relatively frequently (about 20%) but the relationship of many of the reports to Amiloride Hydrochloride is uncertain and the overall frequency was similar in Hydrochlorothiazide treated groups. Nausea/anorexia, abdominal pain, flatulence, and mild skin rash have been reported and probably are related to Amiloride. Other adverse experiences that have been reported with Amiloride/HCTZ are generally those known to be associated with diuresis, thiazide therapy, or with the underlying disease being treated. Clinical trials have not demonstrated that combining Amiloride and Hydrochlorothiazide increases the risk of adverse reactions over those seen with the individual components.

The adverse reactions for Amiloride/HCTZ listed in the following table have been arranged into two groups: (1) incidence greater than one percent; and (2) incidence one percent or less. The incidence for group (1) was determined from clinical studies conducted in the United States (607 patients treated with Amiloride/HCTZ). The adverse effects listed in group (2) include reports from the same clinical studies and voluntary reports since marketing. The probability of a causal relationship exists between Amiloride/HCTZ and these adverse reactions, some of which have been reported only rarely.

Incidence > 1%	Incidence ≤ 1%
Body as a Whole	
Headache*	Malaise
Weakness*	Chest pain
Fatigue/tiredness	Back pain
	Syncope
Cardiovascular	
Arrhythmia	Tachycardia
	Digitalis toxicity
	Orthostatic hypotension
	Angina pectoris
Digestive	
Nausea/anorexia*	Constipation
Diarrhea	GI bleeding
Gastrointestinal	GI disturbance
pain	Appetite changes
Abdominal pain	Abdominal fullness
	Hiccups
	Thirst
	Vomiting
	Anorexia
	Flatulence
Metabolic	
Elevated serum	Gout
potassium levels	Dehydration
(> 5.5 mEq	Symptomatic
per liter)†	hyponatremia**
Musculoskeletal	
Leg ache	Muscle cramps/spasm
	Joint pain
Nervous	
Dizziness*	Paresthesia/numbness
	Stupor
	Vertigo

Incidence > 1%	Incidence ≤ 1%
Psychiatric	
None	Insomnia
	Nervousness
	Depression
	Sleepiness
	Mental confusion
Respiratory	
Dyspnea	None
Skin	
Rash*	Flushing
Pruritus	Diaphoresis
	Erythema multiforme including
	Stevens-Johnson syndrome
	Exfoliative dermatitis including toxic
	epidermal necrolysis
	Alopecia
Special Senses	
None	Bad taste
	Visual disturbance
	Nasal congestion
Urogenital	
None	Impotence
	Nocturia
	Dysuria
	Incontinence
	Renal dysfunction including renal
	failure
	Gynecomastia

Reactions occurring in 3% to 8% of patients treated with Amiloride/HCTZ (Those reactions occurring in less than 3% of the patients are unmarked.)
† (see "Warnings").
** (see "Precautions").

Other adverse reactions that have been reported with the individual components and within each category are listed in order of decreasing severity:

AMILORIDE:
Body as a Whole: Painful extremities, neck/ shoulder ache, fatigability;

Cardiovascular: Palpitation;

Digestive: Activation of probable pre-existing peptic ulcer, abnormal liver function, jaundice, dyspepsia, heartburn;

Hematologic: Aplastic anemia, neutropenia;

Integumentary: Alopecia, itching, dry mouth;

Nervous System/Psychiatric: Encephalopathy, tremors, decreased libido;

Respiratory: Shortness of breath, cough;

Special Senses: Increased intraocular pressure, tinnitus;

Urogenital: Bladder spasms, polyuria, urinary frequency.

HYDROCHLOROTHIAZIDE:
Digestive: Pancreatitis, jaundice (intrahepatic cholestatic jaundice), sialadenitis, cramping, gastric irritation;

Hematologic: Aplastic anemia, agranulocytosis, leukopenia, hemolytic anemia, thrombocytopenia;

Hypersensitivity: Anaphylactic reactions, necrotizing angiitis (vasculitis, cutaneous vasculitis), respiratory distress including pneumonitis and pulmonary edema, photosensitivity, fever, urticaria, purpura;

Metabolic: Electrolyte imbalance (see "Precautions") hyperglycemia, glycosuria, hyperuricemia;

Nervous System/Psychiatric: Restlessness;

Special Senses: Transient blurred vision, xanthopsia;

Urogenital: Interstitial nephritis (see "Warnings").

OVERDOSAGE
No data are available in regard to overdosage in humans. The oral LD_{50} of the combination drug is 189 and 422 mg/kg for female mice and female rats, respectively.

It is not known whether the drug is dialyzable.

No specific information is available on the treatment of overdosage with Amiloride/HCTZ, and no specific antidote is available. Treatment is symptomatic and supportive. Therapy with Amiloride/HCTZ should be discontinued and the patient observed closely. Suggested measures include induction of emesis and/or gastric lavage.

Amiloride Hydrochloride: No data are available in regard to overdosage in humans.

The oral LD_{50} of Amiloride Hydrochloride (calculated as the base) is 56 mg/kg in mice and 36 to 85 mg/kg in rats, depending on the strain.

The most common signs and symptoms to be expected with overdosage are dehydration and electrolyte imbalance. If hyperkalemia occurs, active measures should be taken to reduce the serum potassium levels.

Hydrochlorothiazide: The oral LD_{50} of Hydrochlorothiazide is greater than 10.0 g/kg in both mice and rats.

The most common signs and symptoms observed are those caused by electrolyte depletion (hypokalemia, hypochloremia, hyponatremia) and dehydration resulting from excessive diuresis. If digitalis has also been administered, hypokalemia may accentuate cardiac arrhythmias.

DOSAGE AND ADMINISTRATION
Amiloride/HCTZ should be administered with food.

The usual starting dosage is 1 tablet a day. The dosage may be increased to 2 tablets a day, if necessary. More than 2 tablets of Amiloride/HCTZ daily usually are not needed and there is no controlled experience with such doses. The daily dose is usually given as a single dose but may be given in divided doses. Once an initial diuresis has been achieved, dosage adjustment may be necessary. Maintenance therapy may be on an intermittent basis.

Keep container tightly closed. Protect from light, moisture, freezing, −20°C (−4°F) and store at room temperature, 15-30 °C (59-86°F).

HOW SUPPLIED
TABLETS: 5 MG-50 MG

AVERAGE UNIT PRICE (AVAILABLE SIZES)		GENERIC A-RATED AVERAGE PRICE (GAAP)	
BRAND	$0.52	100s	$32.54
GENERIC	$0.31	500s	$152.96
HCFA FUL (100s ea)	$0.10	1000s	$272.31

BRAND/MANUFACTURER	NDC	SIZE	AWP
◆ **BRAND**			
➤ MODURETIC 5-50: Merck	00006-0917-68	100s	$49.89
	00006-0917-28	100s ud	$54.00
◆ **GENERICS**			
Biocraft	00332-2205-09	100s	$28.90
Schein	00364-2260-01	100s	$29.55
Mason Dist	11845-0462-01	100s	$29.56
Warner Chilcott	00047-0832-24	100s	$30.41
Moore,H.L.	00839-7446-06	100s	$30.44
Rugby	00536-3044-01	100s	$31.12
Rugby	00536-5699-01	100s	$31.12
Major	00904-2113-60	100s	$32.55
➤ West Point	59591-0162-68	100s	$32.75
Barr	00555-0483-02	100s	$32.86
URL	00677-1223-01	100s	$32.95
Mylan	00378-0577-01	100s	$32.95
Geneva	00781-1119-01	100s	$32.95
Qualitest	00603-2188-21	100s	$33.34
Aligen	00405-4053-01	100s	$33.90
Martec	52555-0338-01	100s	$37.95
Royce	51875-0358-01	100s	$38.00
Goldline	00182-1877-01	100s	$38.00
Raway	00686-0421-20	100s ud	$20.00
Vangard	00615-3516-13	100s ud	$34.97
UDL	51079-0421-20	100s ud	$35.56
Major	00904-2113-61	100s ud	$36.30
Rugby	00536-3044-05	500s	$149.40
Mylan	00378-0577-05	500s	$156.51
Mason Dist	11845-0462-04	1000s	$141.93
Moore,H.L.	00839-7446-16	1000s	$242.33
Biocraft	00332-2205-15	1000s	$255.00
Martec	52555-0338-10	1000s	$255.60
Major	00904-2113-80	1000s	$272.10
Rugby	00536-5699-10	1000s	$280.08
Qualitest	00603-2188-32	1000s	$313.58
Barr	00555-0483-05	1000s	$330.16
Royce	51875-0358-04	1000s	$360.00

Aminess *SEE* AMINO ACIDS, INJECTABLE *AND* AMINO ACIDS/CALCIUM CHLORIDE/DEXTROSE/ELECTROLYTES

Amino Acid and Urea Cream

DESCRIPTION
This cream contains Urea 8.34%, Sodium Propionate 0.50%, Methionine 0.83%, Cystine 0.35%, Inositol 0.83%, Benzalkonium Chloride 0.000004%. Buffered to pH of 5.5.

Amino Acid/Urea Cream is specifically formulated for cervical treatment: Cervicitis (mild), postpartum cervicitis, postpartum cervical tears, postcauterization, postcryosurgery and postconization.

Methionine and Cystine are Amino Acids necessary for wound healing and forming of epithelial tissue. Inositol acts as an essential growth factor and promotes epithelialization.

Urea aids in debridement, dissolves the coagulum and promotes epithelialization. Its solvent action on fibroblasts prevents the formation of excessive tissue—thus preventing stenosis when used as directed.

Benzalkonium Chloride serves to lower surface tension and thus aids in spreading the medication. Along with Sodium Propionate it also exerts a bacteriostatic effect.

Amino Acid/Urea Cream is geared to the higher pH of the healthy cervix in contrast with pH 4 vaginal preparations. With its pH factor of 5.5, Amino Acid/

➤ SHOWN IN PRODUCT IDENTIFICATION GUIDE

Urea Cream promotes faster healing of the cervix, yet will not adversely affect a healthy vagina.

DIRECTIONS

When immediate postpartum bleeding has subsided (usually from 24 to 48 hours after delivery), one applicatorful of Amino Acid/Urea Cream should be applied nightly for four weeks. In mild cervicitis (not requiring cautery or cryosurgery) one applicatorful of Amino Acid/Urea Cream should be injected in the vagina nightly upon retiring for 2 weeks.

A small amount of Amino Acid/Urea Cream should be applied immediately after hot cauterization, hot conization and cryosurgery. One applicatorful should be injected nightly upon retiring for 2 to 4 weeks (the duration of treatment depends on extent of cauterization or hot conization or cryosurgery). During the weekly office visit for (2 to 4 visits) the physician should again apply a small amount of Amino Acid/Urea Cream with a probe or applicator. The canal is to be completely probed on the last visit.

After cold coning, one applicatorful should be injected upon retiring about 24 hours after surgery and nightly thereafter for four weeks. During the four weekly office visits following cold coning, a small amount of Amino Acid/Urea Cream should be applied with a probe or applicator into the canal by the physician. The canal is to be completely probed on the last visit.

REASONS FOR VARIATION OF DIRECTIONS

(1) After hot conization, cauterization and cryosurgery, immediate use of Amino Acid/Urea Cream is indicated to aid in dissolving dead or burned tissue.

(2) After cold coning, there is no dead tissue to slough off. Therefore, a wait of 24 hours or longer is desirable for normal healing to take place and for some fibroblasts to be laid down before applying the Amino Acid/Urea Cream (which has a solvent action on both the fibroblasts and the absorbable sutures). When *nonabsorbable* sutures are used, Amino Acid/Urea Cream can be used immediately.

CONTRAINDICATIONS

Deleterious side effects have not been a problem at the doses recommended. The usual precautions against allergic reactions should be observed.

STORAGE

Store at room temperature.

HOW SUPPLIED
CREAM:

BRAND/MANUFACTURER	NDC	SIZE	AWP
○ BRAND			
AMINO-CERV: Milex	00396-6010-00	82.5 gm doz	$158.40
	00396-6010-10	82.5 gm 12s	$144.00

Amino Acids with Electrolytes, Injectable

DESCRIPTION

Amino Acids/Electrolytes is a sterile, nonpyrogenic solution containing crystalline Amino Acids and Electrolytes. (See related tables).

CLINICAL PHARMACOLOGY

Amino Acids/Electrolytes provides a physiological ratio of biologically utilizable Amino Acids in concentrated form for protein synthesis and wound healing along with maintenance Electrolytes. Given by central venous infusion with concentrated calorie sources such as hypertonic dextrose or fat emulsion, and vitamins and minerals, it provides total parenteral nutrition. The amino acids provide a substrate for protein synthesis as well as sparing body protein and muscle mass. Peripheral intravenous infusions of Amino Acids administered for short periods in selected patients with dextrose and maintenance Electrolytes promote protein anabolism and prevent protein breakdown to meet caloric requirements in stress conditions where oral intake is inadequate. Intravenous fat emulsion may be substituted for part of the carbohydrate calories.

Sodium, the major cation of the extracellular fluid, functions primarily in the control of water distribution, fluid balance, and osmotic pressure of body fluids. Sodium is also associated with chloride and bicarbonate in the regulation of the acid-base equilibrium of body fluid. Potassium, the principal cation of intracellular fluid, participates in carbohydrate utilization and protein synthesis, and is critical in the regulation of nerve conduction and muscle contraction, particularly in the heart.

Chloride, the major extracellular anion, closely follows the metabolism of sodium, and changes in the acid-base balance of the body are reflected by changes in the chloride concentration. Magnesium, a principal cation of soft tissue, is primarily involved in enzyme activity associated with the metabolism of carbohydrates and protein. Magnesium is also involved in neuromuscular irritability.

Phosphate is a major intracellular anion which participates in providing energy for metabolism of substrates and contributes to significant metabolic and enzymatic reactions in almost all organs and tissues. It exerts a modifying influence on calcium levels, a buffering effect on acid-base equilibrium and has a primary role in the renal excretion of hydrogen ions.

Inorganic acetate salts serve as bicarbonate precursors. It is thought that the acetate from lysine acetate and acetic acid, under the condition of parenteral nutrition, does not impact net acid-base balance when renal and respiratory functions are normal. Clinical evidence seems to support this thinking; however, confirmatory experimental evidence is not available.

INDICATIONS AND USAGE

Parenteral nutrition with Amino Acids/Electrolytes is indicated to prevent nitrogen loss or treat negative nitrogen balance in adults and children where (1) the alimentary tract, by the oral, gastrostomy, or jejunostomy route, cannot or should not be used, or adequate protein intake is not feasible by these routes; (2) gastrointestinal absorption of protein is impaired; or (3) protein requirements are substantially increased as with extensive burns; and (4) morbidity and mortality may be reduced by replacing Amino Acids lost from tissue breakdown, thereby preserving tissue reserves, as in acute renal failure. Dosage, route of administration, and concomitant infusion of non-protein calories are dependent on various factors, such as nutritional metabolic status of the patient, anticipated duration of parenteral nutritional support, and vein tolerance. See "Dosage and Administration" for additional information.

Central Venous Nutrition: Central venous infusion should be considered when amino acid solutions are to be admixed with hypertonic dextrose to promote protein synthesis in hypercatabolic or severely depleted patients, or those requiring long-term parenteral nutrition.

AMINO ACID CONTENT (MG/100 ML)

Essential	3%	3.5%			7%		8.5%			10%
Isoleucine $C_6H_{13}NO_2$	210	168	252	231	510	462	590	620	561	660
Leucine $C_6H_{13}NO_2$	270	217	329	350	660	700	770	810	850	1000
Lysine $C_6H_{14}N_2O_2$	220	203	252	368	510	735	620	624	893	1050
Methionine $C_5H_{11}NO_2S$	160	203	140	60	280	120	450	340	146	172
Phenylalanine $C_9H_{11}NO_2$	170	217	154	104	310	209	480	380	253	298
Tyrosine		14	31	95	44	189		44	230	270
Threonine $C_4H_9NO_3$	120	147	182	140	370	280	340	460	340	400
Tryptophan $C_{11}H_2N_2O_2$	46	63	56	70	120	140	130	150	170	200
Valine $C_5H_{11}NO_2$	200	161	280	175	560	350	560	680	425	500
Histidine	85	154	105	105	210	210	240	260	255	300
Cysteine	< 14					< 14				
Nonessential										
Alanine	210	728	448	348	900	695	600	1100	844	993
Arginine	290	364	343	356	690	713	810	850	865	1018
L-Aspartic Acid				245			490		595	700
L-Glutamic Acid				258			517		627	738
Proline	340	147	300	253	610	505	950	750	614	722
Serine	180		147	186	300	371	500	370	450	530
Glycine	420	728	448	175	900	350	1190	1100	450	100
Protein gm/L	29	35	35	35	70	70	82	85	85	100
Nitrogen gm/L	4.6	5.9	5.5	5.4	11.0	10.7	13.0	13.4	13.0	15.3
mOsm/L	405	450	477	425	1013	869	1045	1160	999	1130
pH range	6.8	6.0	5.4	5.4	5.3	5.8	6.5	5.3	5.8	5.8
	6.0-7.0	5.0-7.0	4.5-6.0	5.0-6.5	4.5-6.0	5.0-6.5	6.0-7.0	4.5-6.0	5.0-6.5	5.0-6.5

◆ RATED THERAPEUTICALLY EQUIVALENT; ◇ THERAPEUTIC EQUIVALENCE UNCONFIRMED; ○ UNRATED

ELECTROLYTE CONCENTRATION (MEQ/L)

	3%		3.5%		7%		8.5%			10%
Sodium	35	25	47	36	70	76	60	70	80	87
Potassium	24.5	15	13	13	66	66	60	66	66	66
Magnesium	5	5	3	3	10	10	10	10	10	10
Chloride	41	25	40	37	96	86	60	98	86	86
Phosphate	7	15					40			
Acetate	44	52	58	25	124	50	125	142	61	72
Phosphorus			3.5	3.5	30	30	30			30

ELECTROLYTE CONTENT (MG/100 ML)

	3%		3.5%		7%		8.5%			10%
Sodium Acetate	200	218					690			
Magnesium Acetate	54			21			110			
Potassium Acetate				128			10			
Potassium Chloride	150			97		45	440		45	45
Phosphoric Acid	40			40			230			
Sodium Chloride	120	35	234	120	410	410	410		410	410
Potassium Phosphate		131			522	522	522		522	522
Magnesium Chloride		51	30		102	102	102		102	102
Sodium Phosphate				49						

Peripheral Parenteral Nutrition: For moderately catabolic or depleted patients in whom the central venous route is not indicated, diluted amino acid solutions mixed with 5% dextrose solutions may be infused by peripheral vein, supplemented, if desired, with fat emulsion as a source of nutritional support.

Protein Sparing: In well-nourished, mildly catabolic patients such as routine postsurgical patients who require only short-term parenteral nutrition, protein sparing can be achieved by peripheral infusion of diluted amino acid solutions with or without dextrose or other non-protein calories.

The injection is indicated as a source of nitrogen for patients with adequate stores of body fat, in whom oral nutrition cannot be tolerated, is undesirable or is inadequate.

Some brands are indicated only for short term peripheral administration.

CONTRAINDICATIONS

Amino Acids/Electrolytes is contraindicated in patients with untreated anuria, severe liver disease, renal failure, hepatic coma or encephalopathy, inborn errors of Amino Acid metabolism, or hypersensitivity to one or more Amino Acids present in the solution.

This solution is also contraindicated where the administration of sodium, potassium, magnesium, chloride, phosphate or acetate could be clinically detrimental. Such conditions include hyperkalemia, heart block or myocardial damage, edema due to cardiovascular, renal or hepatic failure, or acid-base imbalance.

WARNINGS

Some brands contain sodium bisulfite, potassium metabisulfite, or sodium hydrosulfite, sulfites that may cause allergic-type reactions including anaphylactic symptoms and life-threatening or less severe asthmatic episodes in certain susceptible people. The overall prevalence of sulfite sensitivity in the general population is unknown and probably low. Sulfite sensitivity is seen more frequently in asthmatic than in nonasthmatic people.

Safe and effective use of Amino Acids/Electrolytes requires a knowledge of nutrition and protein sparing and of fluid and Electrolyte balance as well as clinical expertise in recognition and treatment of the complications which can occur and an appreciation of the role of protein-sparing therapy in relation to other forms of nutritional support. **Frequent clinical evaluation and laboratory determinations are necessary for proper monitoring of parenteral nutrition.** Studies should include blood sugar, serum proteins, kidney and liver function tests, Electrolytes, hemogram, carbon dioxide content, serum osmolarities, blood cultures, and blood ammonia levels.

The intravenous administration of these solutions can cause fluid and/or solute overload resulting in dilution of serum Electrolyte concentrations, overhydration, congested states or pulmonary edema. The risk of dilutional states is inversely proportional to the solute concentration of the solution infused. The risk of solute overload causing congested states with peripheral and pulmonary edema is directly proportional to the concentration of the solution.

Peripheral intravenous infusion of Amino Acids may cause a modest rise in blood urea nitrogen (BUN) as a result of increased protein intake. The BUN may become elevated in patients with impaired renal or hepatic function. Appropriate laboratory tests should be performed periodically and the infusion should be discontinued if the BUN levels exceed postprandial limits and continue to rise. It should be noted that a modest rise in BUN normally occurs as a result of increased protein intake.

Administration of Amino Acids in the presence of impaired renal function or gastrointestinal bleeding may augment an already elevated blood urea nitrogen. Patients with azotemia from any cause should not be infused with Amino Acids without regard to total nitrogen intake.

Administration of Amino Acid solutions to a patient with hepatic insufficiency may result in plasma Amino Acid imbalances, metabolic alkalosis, hyperammonemia, prerenal azotemia, stupor and coma. The use of this injection in such

patients should be considered very carefully by the physicians and the benefits of protein-sparing therapy should outweigh the risk of adverse results.

Some formulations may not be suitable for use in infants who require individualized Electrolyte therapy.

Hyperammonemia is of *special significance in infants* as its occurrence in the syndrome caused by genetic metabolic defects is sometimes associated, although not necessarily in a causal relationship, with mental retardation. This reaction appears to be dose related and is more likely to develop during prolonged therapy. It is essential that blood ammonia be measured frequently in infants. The mechanisms of this reaction are not clearly defined but may involve genetic defects and immature or subclinically impaired liver function.

Conservative doses of Amino Acids should be given, dictated by the nutritional status of the patient. Should symptoms of hyperammonemia develop, Amino Acid administration should be discontinued and the patient's clinical status reevaluated.

Instances of asymptomatic hyperammonemia have been reported in patients without overt liver dysfunction. The mechanisms of this reaction are not clearly defined, but may involve genetic defects and immature or subclinically impaired liver function.

Solutions containing sodium ions should be used with great care, if at all, in patients with congestive heart failure, severe renal insufficiency, and in clinical states in which there is sodium retention with edema. In patients with diminished renal function, administration of solutions containing sodium or potassium ions may result in sodium or potassium retention.

Solutions containing potassium ions should be used with great care, if at all, in patients with hyperkalemia, severe renal failure, and in conditions in which potassium retention is present.

Solutions containing acetate should be used with great care in patients with metabolic or respiratory alkalosis, or in conditions where there is an increased level or an impaired utilization of acetate, such as severe hepatic insufficiency.

Care must be taken to avoid incompatible Electrolyte mixtures. Calcium and additional phosphate may be added to alternate bottles. If additions are made, the admixture must be inspected for solution clarity when mixed, before dispensing from the pharmacy, and immediately before and periodically during administration.

This solution should not be given simultaneously with blood through the same infusion set because of the possibility of pseudoagglutination.

PRECAUTIONS

GENERAL

The electrolyte pattern in some brands is designed for maintenance only during protein-sparing therapy in adults. Losses greater than normal should be monitored and replaced in the usual fashion.

Clinical evaluation and periodic laboratory determinations are necessary to monitor changes in fluid balance, Electrolyte concentrations, and acid-base balance during prolonged parenteral therapy or whenever the condition of the patient warrants such evaluation. Significant deviations from normal concentrations may require the use of additional Electrolyte supplements.

Strongly hypertonic nutrient solutions should be administered through an indwelling intravenous catheter with the tip located in the superior vena cava.

Protein-sparing therapy is intended for short-term usage only (up to 10 to 12 days). If a patient requires an extended period of nutritional support, oral or parenteral regimens should include adequate nonprotein calorie components.

Care should be taken to avoid circulatory overload, particularly in patients with cardiac insufficiency.

Care should be taken to avoid excess fluid accumulation, particularly in patients with renal disease, pulmonary insufficiency and heart disease.

In patients with myocardial infarct, infusion of amino acids should always be accompanied by dextrose, since in anoxia, free fatty acids cannot be utilized by the myocardium, and energy must be produced anaerobically from glycogen or glucose.

Blood sugar levels should be monitored frequently in diabetic patients.

Special care must be taken when giving hypertonic dextrose to a diabetic or prediabetic patient. To prevent severe hyperglycemia in such patients, insulin may be required.

Administration of glucose at a rate exceeding the patient's utilization may lead to hyperglycemia, coma, and death.

Administration of Amino Acids without carbohydrates may result in the accumulation of ketone bodies in the blood. Correction of this ketonemia may be achieved by the administration of carbohydrate. The effect of infusion of Amino Acids, without dextrose, upon carbohydrate metabolism of children is not known at this time.

After appropriate dilution, if Amino Acids/Electrolytes is to be administered by peripheral vein, care should be taken to assure proper placement of the needle within the lumen of the vein. The venipuncture site should be inspected frequently for signs of infiltration or inflammation. If venous thrombosis or phlebitis occurs, discontinue infusions or change infusion site and initiate appropriate treatment.

Extraordinary Electrolyte losses such as may occur during protracted nasogastric suction, vomiting, diarrhea or gastrointestinal fistula drainage may necessitate additional Electrolyte supplementation.

Sodium-containing solutions should be administered with caution to patients receiving corticosteroids or corticotropin, or to other salt-retaining patients. Care should be exercised in administering solutions containing sodium or potassium to patients with renal or cardiovascular insufficiency, with or without congestive heart failure, particularly if they are postoperative or elderly.

Potassium therapy should be guided primarily by serial electrocardiograms, especially in patients receiving digitalis. Serum potassium levels are not necessarily indicative of tissue potassium levels. Solutions containing potassium or magnesium should be used with caution in the presence of cardiac disease, particularly in the presence of renal disease.

Use only if solution is clear and vacuum is present.

Nitrogen intake should be carefully monitored in patients with impaired renal function.

For long-term total nutrition, or if a patient has inadequate fat stores, it is essential to provide adequate exogenous calories concurrently with the amino acids. Concentrated dextrose solutions are an effective source of such calories. Such strongly hypertonic nutrient solutions should be administered through an indwelling intravenous catheter with the tip located in the superior vena cava.

DRUG INTERACTIONS

Administration of barbiturates, narcotics, hypnotics or systemic anesthetics should be adjusted with caution in patients also receiving magnesium-containing solutions because of an additive central depressive effect.

Because of its antianabolic activity, concurrent administration of tetracycline may reduce the protein-sparing effect of infused amino acids.

To minimize the risk of possible incompatibilities arising from mixing this solution with other additives that may be prescribed, the final infusate should be inspected for cloudiness or precipitation immediately after mixing, prior to administration, and periodically during administration.

USAGE IN PREGNANCY

Pregnancy Category C. Animal reproduction studies have not been conducted with Amino Acids/Electrolytes. It is also not known whether Amino Acids/Electrolytes can cause fetal harm when administered to a pregnant woman or can affect reproduction capacity. The safety of the use of Amino Acid solutions has not been demonstrated in pregnant women. In such patients protein-sparing therapy would seem unlikely to have an application that would supervene unknown risks. Amino Acids/Electrolytes should be given to a pregnant woman only if clearly needed.

SPECIAL PRECAUTIONS FOR CENTRAL VENOUS NUTRITION

Administration by central venous catheter should be used only by those familiar with this technique and its complications.

Central venous nutrition may be associated with complications which can be prevented or minimized by careful attention to all aspects of the procedure including solution preparation, administration, and patient monitoring. *It is essential that a carefully prepared protocol, based on current medical practices, be followed, preferably by an experienced team.*

Although a detailed discussion of the complications of central venous nutrition is beyond the scope of this insert, the following summary lists those based on current literature:

Technical: The placement of a central venous catheter should be regarded as a surgical procedure. One should be fully acquainted with various techniques of catheter insertion as well as recognition and treatment of complications. For details of techniques and placement sites, consult the medical literature. X-ray is the best means of verifying catheter placement. Complications known to occur from the placement of central venous catheters are pneumothorax, hemothorax, hydrothorax, artery puncture and transection, injury to the brachial plexus, malposition of the catheter, formation of arterio-venous fistula, phlebitis, thrombosis, and air and catheter embolus.

Septic: The constant risk of sepsis is present during central venous nutrition. Since contaminated solutions and infusion catheters are potential sources of infection, it is imperative that the preparation of parenteral nutrition solutions and the placement and care of catheters be accomplished under controlled aseptic conditions.

Solutions should ideally be prepared in the hospital pharmacy under a laminar flow hood. The key factor in their preparation is careful aseptic technique to avoid inadvertent touch contamination during mixing of solutions and subsequent admixtures.

Parenteral nutrition solutions should be used promptly after mixing. Any storage should be for as brief as possible—preferably less than 24 hours—under refrigeration, and protected from light. Administration time for a single bottle and set should never exceed 24 hours.

Consult the medical literature for a discussion of the management of sepsis during central venous nutrition. In brief, typical management includes replacing the solution being administered with a fresh container and set, and the remaining contents are cultured for bacterial or fungal contamination. If sepsis persists and another source of infection is not identified, the catheter is removed, the proximal tip cultured, and a new catheter reinserted when the fever has subsided. Nonspecific prophylactic antibiotic treatment is not recommended. Clinical experience indicates that the catheter is likely to be the prime source of infection as opposed to aseptically prepared and properly stored solutions.

Metabolic: The following metabolic complications have been reported: metabolic acidosis, hypophosphatemia, alkalosis, hypocalcemia, osteoporosis, hyperosmolar nonketotic states and dehydration, hyperglycemia and glycosuria, osmotic diuresis and dehydration, rebound hypoglycemia, elevated liver enzymes, hypo- and hypervitaminosis, Electrolyte imbalances, and hyperammonemia in children. Frequent clinical evaluation and laboratory determinations are necessary, especially during the first few days of central venous nutrition, to prevent or minimize these complications.

Clinical Evaluation and Laboratory Determinations, at the Discretion of the Attending Physician, are Necessary for Proper Monitoring during Administration: Do not withdraw venous blood for blood chemistries through the peripheral infusion site, as interference with estimations of nitrogen containing substances may occur. Blood studies should include glucose, urea nitrogen, serum electrolytes, ammonia, cholesterol, acid-base balance, serum proteins, kidney and liver function tests, osmolarity and hemogram. White blood count and blood cultures are to be determined if indicated. Urinary osmolality and glucose should be determined as necessary.

ADVERSE REACTIONS

See *"Warnings"* and *"Special Precautions for Central Venous Nutrition."*

Reactions which may occur because of the solution or the technique of administration include febrile response, infection at the site of injection, venous thrombosis or phlebitis extending from the site of injection, extravasation and hypervolemia.

Local reactions of the infusion site, consisting of a warm sensation, erythema, phlebitis and thrombosis, have been reported with peripheral amino acid infusions, especially if other substances, such as antibiotics, are also administered through the same site. In such cases the infusion site should be changed promptly to another vein. Use of large peripheral veins, inline filters, and slowing the rate of infusion may reduce the incidence of local venous irritation. Irritating additive medications may need to be injected at another venous site.

Generalized flushing, fever and nausea have been reported during peripheral administration of Amino Acids.

Symptoms may result from an excess or deficit of one or more of the ions present in the solution; therefore, frequent monitoring of Electrolyte levels is essential.

Hypernatremia may be associated with edema and exacerbation of congestive heart failure due to the retention of water, resulting in an expanded extracellular fluid volume.

Reactions reported with the use of potassium-containing solutions include nausea, vomiting, abdominal pain and diarrhea. The signs and symptoms of potassium intoxication include paresthesias of the extremities, areflexia, muscular or respiratory paralysis, mental confusion, weakness, hypotension, cardiac arrhythmias, heart block, electrocardiographic abnormalities and cardiac arrest. Potassium deficits result in disruption of neuromuscular function, and intestinal ileus and dilatation.

If infused in large amounts, chloride ions may cause a loss of bicarbonate ions, resulting in an acidifying effect.

Abnormally high plasma levels of magnesium can result in flushing, sweating, hypotension, circulatory collapse, and depression of cardiac and central nervous system function. Respiratory depression is the most immediate threat to life. Magnesium deficits can result in tachycardia, hypertension, hyperirritability and psychotic behavior.

Phosphorus deficiency may lead to impaired tissue oxygenation and acute hemolytic anemia. Relative to calcium, excessive phosphorus intake can precipitate hypocalcemia with cramps, tetany and muscular hyperexcitability.

If an adverse reaction does occur, discontinue the infusion, evaluate the patient, institute appropriate therapeutic countermeasures and save the remainder of the fluid for examination if deemed necessary.

OVERDOSAGE

In the event of a fluid or solute overload during parenteral therapy, reevaluate the patient's condition, and institute appropriate corrective treatment.

In the event of overdosage with potassium-containing solutions, discontinue the infusion immediately and institute corrective therapy to reduce serum potassium levels.

Treatment of hyperkalemia includes the following:

1. Dextrose Injection USP, 10% or 25%, containing 10 units of crystalline insulin per 20 grams of dextrose administered intravenously, 300 to 500 mL per hour.
2. Absorption and exchange of potassium using sodium or ammonium cycle cation exchange resin, orally and as retention enema.
3. Hemodialysis and peritoneal dialysis. The use of potassium-containing foods or medications must be eliminated. However, in cases of digitalization, too rapid a lowering of plasma potassium concentration can cause digitalis toxicity.

DOSAGE AND ADMINISTRATION

The total daily dose of Amino Acids/Electrolytes depends on daily protein requirements and on the patient's metabolic and clinical response. The determination of nitrogen balance and accurate daily body weights, corrected for fluid balance, are probably the best means of assessing individual protein requirements.

Recommended Dietary Allowances of protein are approximately 0.9 g/kg of body weight for a healthy adult and 1.4 to 2.2 g/kg for healthy growing infants and children. It must be recognized, however, that protein as well as caloric requirements in traumatized or malnourished patients may be substantially increased. For peripheral intravenous infusion, daily Amino Acid doses of approximately 1.0 to 1.5 g/kg of body weight for adults and 2 to 3 g/kg of body weight for infants with adequate calories are generally sufficient to satisfy protein needs and promote positive nitrogen balance in such patients, although higher doses may be required in severely catabolic states. Such higher doses, especially in infants, must be accompanied by frequent laboratory evaluation. Infusion or ingestion of carbohydrate or lipid will not reduce the nitrogen sparing effect of intravenous Amino Acid infusions at this dose.

For protein sparing in well-nourished patients not receiving significant additional calories, Amino Acid dosages of 1.0 to 1.7 g/kg/day significantly reduce nitrogen losses and spare body protein. If rises in BUN exceed 20 mg% in 48 hours, Amino Acid infusion should be discontinued or rate of administration reduced.

For an Amino Acid solution of specified total concentration, the volume required to meet Amino Acid requirements per 24 hours can be calculated. After making an estimate of the total daily fluid (water) requirement, the balance of fluid needed beyond the volume of Amino Acid solution required can be provided either as a noncarbohydrate or a carbohydrate-containing Electrolyte solution. I.V. lipid emulsion may be substituted for part of the carbohydrate-containing solution.

Fat emulsion coadministration should be considered when prolonged (more than 5 days) parenteral nutrition is required in order to prevent essential fatty acid deficiency (E.F.A.D.). Serum lipids should be monitored for evidence of E.F.A.D. in patients maintained on fat free TPN.

When Amino Acids/Electrolytes is diluted the resulting diluted Electrolyte concentrations must be considered when estimating the patient's daily Electrolyte requirement. Additional Electrolyte supplementation may be needed.

The Electrolyte content of Amino Acids/Electrolytes must be considered when calculating daily Electrolyte intake. Serum Electrolytes, including magnesium and phosphate, should be monitored frequently.

If a patient's nutritional intake is primarily parenteral, vitamins, especially the water soluble vitamins, should also be provided.

As with all intravenous fluid therapy, the goal is to provide adequate water to cover insensible, urinary and other (nasogastric suction, fistula drainage, diarrhea) losses, and electrolytes for replacement and maintenance. Total fluid requirements, as well as Electrolyte and acid-base needs, should be determined frequently and administered appropriately.

Additional Electrolytes should be administered evenly throughout the day, and irritating medications should be injected at an alternate infusion site.

Venous irritation at an infusion site can be minimized by the selection of a large peripheral vein as well as by slowing the rate of infusion.

Parenteral drug products should be inspected visually for particulate matter and discoloration prior to administration, whenever solution and container permit.

Additives may be incompatbile. Complete information is not available. Those additives known to be incompatible should not be used. Consult with pharmacist, if available. If, in the informed judgment of the physician, it is deemed advisable to introduce additives, use aseptic technique. Mix thoroughly when additives have been introduced. Do not store solutions containing additives.

Solutions should be used promptly after mixing. Any storage should be under refrigeration and limited to a brief period of time, preferably less than 24 hours.

Central Venous Nutrition: For severely catabolic, depleted patients or those requiring long-term total parenteral nutrition, central venous nutrition with adequate amounts of exogenous calories should be considered. Calorie-to-nitrogen ratios of at least 100 to 150 nonprotein calories per gram of nitrogen have been recommended to achieve positive nitrogen balance in such patients. These ratios are easily and conveniently attained with the use of concentrated dextrose solutions, supplemented if desired with parenteral fat emulsion.

Admixtures of 3.5 to 4.25% amino acids with 5 to 10% glucose or dextrose may be coinfused with a fat emulsion by peripheral vein to provide approximately 1400 to 2000 kcal/day. Fat emulsion coadministration should be considered when prolonged parenteral nutrition is required in order to prevent essential fatty acid deficiency (EFAD). Serum lipids should be monitored for evidence of EFAD in patients maintained on fat-free total parenteral nutrition.

Amino Acids/Electrolytes 7%, 8.5%, or 10% should only be infused via a central vein when admixed with sufficient dextrose to provide full caloric requirements in patients who require prolonged total parenteral nutrition. I.V. lipid may be administered separately to provide part of the calories, if desired.

Total parenteral nutrition may be started with infusates containing lower concentrations of dextrose; dextrose content may be gradually increased to estimated caloric needs as the patient's glucose tolerance increases. Each gram of dextrose provides approximately 3.4 kcal. Each gram of fat provides 9 kcal.

The average depleted major surgical patient with complications requires between 2500 and 4000 kcal and between 12 and 24 grams of nitrogen per day. An adult patient in an acceptable weight range with restricted activity who is not hypermetabolic, requires about 30 kcal/kg of body weight/day. Average daily adult fluid requirements are between 2500 and 3000 mL and may be much higher with losses from fistula drainage or in severe burns. Typically, a hospitalized patient may lose 12 to 18 grams of nitrogen a day, and in severe trauma the daily loss may be 20 to 25 grams or more.

Some solutions do not contain calcium, and this should be added as indicated.

Serum Electrolytes should be Monitored as Indicated: Electrolytes may be added to the nutrient solution as indicated by the patient's clinical condition and laboratory determinations of plasma values. Major Electrolytes are sodium, chloride, potassium, phosphorus or phosphate, magnesium and calcium. Vitamins, including folic acid and vitamin K are required additives. The trace element supplements should be given when long-term parenteral nutrition is undertaken.

Calcium and phosphorus are added to the solution as indicated. The usual dose of phosphorus added to a liter of TPN solution (containing 25% dextrose) is 12 mM. This requirement is related to the carbohydrate calories delivered. Iron is added to the solution or given intramuscularly in depot form as indicated. Vitamin B_{12}, vitamin K and folic acid are given intramuscularly or added to the solution as desired.

Calcium and phosphorus additives are potentially incompatible when added to the TPN admixture. However, if one additive is added to the amino acid container, and the other to the container of concentrated dextrose, and if the contents of both containers are swirled before they are combined, then the likelihood of physical incompatibility is reduced.

In patients with hyperchloremic or other metabolic acidosis, sodium and potassium may be added as the acetate or lactate salts to provide bicarbonate alternates.

In adults, strongly hypertonic mixtures of amino acids and dextrose may be safely administered only by continuous infusion through a central venous catheter with the tip located in the vena cava. For optimal nitrogen utilization, Amino Acids/Electrolytes appropriately mixed with concentrated dextrose, and vitamins are typically administered over an 8-hour period. Typically, the 7%, 8.5%, or 10% solution is used in equal volume with 50% or 70% dextrose to provide an admixture containing 3.5%, 4.25%, or 5% amino acids and 25% or 35% dextrose.

The rate of intravenous infusion initially should be 2 mL/min and may be increased gradually. If administration rate should fall behind schedule, no attempt to "catch up" to planned intake should be made. In addition to meeting protein needs, the administration rate is also governed, especially during the first few days of therapy by the patient's glucose tolerance estimated by glucose levels in blood and urine. Daily intake of Amino Acids and dextrose should be increased gradually to the maximum required dose as indicated by frequent determination of urine and blood sugar levels. In many patients, provision of adequate calories in the form of hypertonic dextrose may require the administration of exogenous insulin to prevent hyperglycemia and glycosuria. To prevent rebound hypoglycemia, a solution containing 5% dextrose should be administered when hypertonic dextrose infusions are abruptly discontinued.

Peripheral Parenteral Nutrition: For moderately catabolic, depleted patients requiring parenteral nutrition in whom the central venous route is not indicated, Amino Acids/Electrolytes can be mixed with 5% dextrose solutions and administered by peripheral vein.

For example, to prepare a solution of 4.25% Amino Acids/Electrolytes in 2.5% dextrose, aseptically transfer 500 mL of 8.5% Amino Acids/Electrolytes to a one liter intravenous bottle containing 500 mL of 5% dextrose.

Fat provides approximately 9 kcal per gram and parenteral fat emulsion may be administered along with Amino Acid-dextrose solutions through a Y-type administration set to supplement caloric intake. Fat, however, should not be the sole caloric intake since some studies have suggested that glucose is more nitrogen sparing in the stressed patient.

Protein-Sparing: For well-nourished, mildly catabolic patients who require short-term parenteral nutritional support, Amino Acids/Electrolytes can be administered peripherally with or without parenteral carbohydrate calories. Approximately 3 liters per day of 3% Amino Acids/Electrolytes will provide a total of 90 g of Amino Acids and the recommended adult daily intake of principal intra- and extracellular Electrolytes for the stable patient. Therapy should begin with one liter of 3% Amino Acids/Electrolytes on the first day (with supplemental fluids), gradually increasing the dosage until full Amino Acid and fluid requirements are met, to approximately 3 liters of 3% Amino Acids/Electrolytes per day. Such infusates can be prepared by dilution of 8.5% Amino Acids/Electrolytes with Sterile Water for Injection or 5% dextrose solutions to prepare isotonic or slightly hypertonic solutions which may be administered by peripheral vein. When administering diluted amino acid injections, serum electrolyte concentrations should be monitored to ensure that appropriate electrolyte levels are provided. For example, a 4.25% Amino Acids/Electrolytes solution can be prepared by the aseptic transfer of 500 mL of 8.5% Amino Acids/Electrolytes to a half-filled intravenous one liter bottle of Sterile Water for Injection. The resultant solution contains 41 grams of Amino Acids with an osmolarity of approximately 525 mOsmol/liter. An approximately isotonic solution of 3% Amino Acids/Electrolytes can be prepared by aseptic transfer of 350 mL of 8.5% Amino Acids/Electrolytes to a partially filled intravenous one liter bottle containing 650 mL of

Sterile Water for Injection. The resultant solution will provide 29 grams of Amino Acids per liter with an osmolarity of approximately 365 mOsmol/liter.

Pediatric Dosage and Administration: Some forms of Amino Acids/Electrolytes may not be suitable for use in infants whose electrolyte requirements must be "custom tailored" based on serial blood chemistry determinations.

Pediatric requirements for parenteral nutrition are constrained by the greater relative fluid requirements of the infant and greater caloric requirements per kilogram. Amino Acids are probably best administered in a 2.5% concentration. For most pediatric patients on intravenous nutrition, 2.5 grams Amino Acids/kg/day with dextrose alone or with I.V. lipid calories of 100 to 130 kcal/kg/day is recommended. In cases of malnutrition or stress, these requirements may be increased. It is acceptable in pediatrics to start with a nutritional solution of half strength at a rate of about 60 to 70 mL/kg/day. Within 24 to 48 hours the volume and concentration of the solution can be increased until the full strength pediatric solution (Amino Acids and dextrose) is given at a rate of 125 to 150 mL/kg/day.

Supplemental electrolytes and vitamin additives should be administered as deemed necessary by careful monitoring of blood chemistries and nutritional status. Addition of iron is more critical in the infant than the adult because of the increasing red cell mass required for the growing infant. Serum lipids should be monitored for evidence of essential fatty acid deficiency in patients maintained on fat-free TPN. Bicarbonate should not be administered during infusion of the nutritional solution unless deemed absolutely necessary.

To ensure the precise delivery of the small volumes of fluid necessary for total parenteral nutrition in infants, accurately calibrated and reliable infusion systems should be used.

A basic solution for pediatric use should contain 25 grams of Amino Acids and 200 to 250 grams of glucose per 1000 mL, administered from containers containing 250 or 500 mL. Such a solution given at the rate of 145 mL/kg/day provides 130 kcal/kg/day.

When administering diluted amino acid injections, serum Electrolyte concentrations should be monitored to ensure that appropriate Electrolyte levels are provided. Fat emulsion may be given concurrently by central or peripheral vein through a Y-type administration set to provide essential fatty acids and increase caloric intake. Since physiological changes occur rapidly in infants, the daily dose of nutrients/Electrolytes should initially be increased slowly with frequent monitoring of pertinent clinical and metabolic parameters (see *"Warnings"*). Children over 10 kilograms require fewer calories and slightly less protein: generally 50 to 80 calories and 2 grams of protein per kilogram per day is sufficient.

Storage: Exposure of pharmaceutical products to heat should be minimized. Avoid excessive heat. Protect from freezing. It is recommended that the product be stored at room temperature (25°C); however, brief exposure up to 40°C does not adversely affect the product.

Protect from light until use.

HOW SUPPLIED
INJECTION:

BRAND/MANUFACTURER	NDC	SIZE	AWP
○ **BRAND**			
NEPHRAMINE: McGaw	00264-1909-20	250 ml	$62.40
TROPHAMINE: McGaw	00264-1936-10	500 ml	$71.03
FREAMINE III W/ELECTROLYTES: McGaw	00264-1931-10	500 ml	$75.76
TROPHAMINE: McGaw	00264-1934-10	500 ml	$99.31
FREAMINE HBC: McGaw	00264-1935-00	750 ml	$82.15
PROCALAMINE: McGaw	00264-1915-07	1000 ml	$43.45
	00264-1915-00	1000 ml	$47.30
FREAMINE III W/ELECTROLYTES: McGaw	00264-1904-00	1000 ml	$57.82
	00264-1931-00	1000 ml	$133.94
AMINOSYN W/ELECTROLYTES: Abbott Hosp	00074-4343-01	500 ml 3s	$307.19
	00074-4183-01	500 ml 3s	$329.67
TRAVASOL: Clintec	00338-0627-04	1000 ml 6s	$335.30
	00338-0457-04	1000 ml 6s	$581.52
	00338-0459-04	1000 ml 6s	$928.63
AMINOSYN W/ELECTROLYTES: Abbott Hosp	00074-5856-05	1000 ml 6s	$938.72
TRAVASOL: Clintec	00338-0457-06	2000 ml 6s	$711.54
	00338-0459-06	2000 ml 6s	$939.06
	00338-0627-03	500 ml 12s	$401.66
	00338-0457-03	500 ml 12s	$581.49
AMINOSYN II W/ELECTROLYTES: Abbott Hosp	00074-1089-03	500 ml 12s	$885.50
AMINOSYN W/ELECTROLYTES: Abbott Hosp	00074-5852-03	500 ml 12s	$888.06
TRAVASOL: Clintec	00338-0459-03	500 ml 12s	$921.26
AMINOSYN W/ELECTROLYTES: Abbott Hosp	00074-5856-03	500 ml 12s	$938.79
○ **GENERICS**			
HEPATAMINE: McGaw	00264-1937-10	500 ml	$101.90

KIT:

BRAND/MANUFACTURER	NDC	SIZE	AWP
○ **BRAND**			
TRAVASOL: Clintec	00338-0651-98	3s	$143.07

Amino Acids, Injectable

DESCRIPTION
Amino Acids, Injectable, is a sterile, nonpyrogenic, hypertonic solution containing crystalline Amino Acids for intravenous infusion. Some brands of Amino

Acids, Injectable, are supplied in a Pharmacy Bulk Package and are not for direct infusion. (See related table).

CLINICAL PHARMACOLOGY
Amino Acids, Injectable, provides a physiological ratio of biologically utilizable Amino Acids in concentrated form for protein synthesis, wound healing, and reduction of the rate of endogenous protein catabolism. Used with concentrated calorie sources such as hypertonic dextrose or fat emulsion, and with electrolytes, vitamins and minerals, it provides total parenteral nutrition. Administered peripherally as an isotonic solution (3%) without nonprotein calories or with minimal caloric supplementation such as 5% dextrose and sometimes maintenance electrolytes, it provides nutritional support, conserves lean body mass, reduces protein catabolism, and spares body protein. Intravenous fat emulsion may be substituted for part of the carbohydrate calories during either TPN or peripheral vein administration.

Phosphate is a major intracellular anion which participates in providing energy for metabolism of substrates and contributes to significant metabolic and enzymatic reactions in all organs and tissues. It exerts a modifying influence on calcium levels, a buffering effect on acid-base equilibrium and has a primary role in the renal excretion of hydrogen ions.

Some brands contain a high concentration of the branched chain Amino Acids (isoleucine, leucine, and valine) because these Amino Acids have been reported to be metabolically active in the compromised patient.

It is thought that the acetate from lysine acetate and acetic acid, under the condition of parenteral nutrition, does not impact net acid-base balance when renal and respiratory functions are normal. Clinical evidence seems to support this thinking; however, confirmatory experimental evidence is not available.

The amounts of sodium and chloride present are not of clinical significance.

Amino Acids, Injectable, 5.2%—renal formula—is a mixture of Amino Acids specifically designed for patients with acute renal failure who are unable to eat. The use of these essential Amino Acids in the management of the uremic patient is based on the minimal requirements for each of the eight Amino Acids essential in adult nutrition. In renal failure nonspecific nitrogens such as urea, glycine, or ammonium chloride, are broken down in the intestine. The ammonia formed is absorbed into the portal system and incorporated by the liver into nonessential Amino Acids, provided requirements for essential Amino Acids are being met. By this metabolic route, urea nitrogen contributes to protein synthesis when the proper combination of essential Amino Acids, sufficient calories and other required nutrients are administered.

Thus, the administration of essential Amino Acids to uremic patients, particularly those who are protein-deficient, results in the utilization of retained urea in protein synthesis, and may be followed by a drop in BUN and resolution of many of the symptoms associated with azotemia.

Amino Acids, Injectable, 5.2% contains histidine, an Amino Acid considered essential for infant growth, and identified as an essential Amino Acid for uremic patients.

In patients with potentially reversible acute renal failure who cannot eat, maintenance of adequate nutrition may assist in reducing morbidity.

INDICATIONS AND USAGE
Parenteral nutrition with Amino Acids, Injectable, is indicated to prevent nitrogen loss or treat negative nitrogen balance in adults and children where (1) the alimentary tract, by the oral, gastrostomy, or jejunostomy route, cannot or should not be used, or adequate protein intake is not feasible by these routes; (2) gastrointestinal absorption of protein is impaired; or (3) protein requirements are substantially increased or nitrogen homeostasis is substantially impaired as with extensive burns, severe trauma or sepsis; or (4) morbidity and mortality may be reduced by replacing amino acids lost from tissue breakdown, thereby preserving tissue reserves, as in acute renal failure. Dosage, route of administration, and concomitant infusion of nonprotein calories are dependent on various factors, such as nutritional and metabolic status of the patient, anticipated duration of parenteral nutritional support, and vein tolerance. See *"Dosage and Administration"* for additional information.

Supplemental electrolytes, in accordance with the prescription of the attending physician, must be added.

CENTRAL VENOUS NUTRITION
Central venous infusion should be considered when Amino Acid solutions are to be admixed with hypertonic dextrose to promote protein synthesis in hypercatabolic or severely depleted patients, or those requiring long-term parenteral nutrition.

PERIPHERAL PARENTERAL NUTRITION
For moderately catabolic or depleted patients in whom the central venous route is not indicated, diluted Amino Acid solutions mixed with minimal caloric or low dextrose supplementation may be infused by peripheral vein, supplemented, if desired, with fat emulsion.

PROTEIN SPARING
In well-nourished, mildly catabolic patients such as routine postsurgical patients who require only short-term parenteral nutrition, protein sparing can be achieved by peripheral infusion of Amino Acid solutions with or without dextrose.

Amino Acids, Injectable, 5.2%—renal formula—is indicated only as an adjunct to management of patients with potentially reversible acute renal failure who are unable to eat. When infused with hypertonic dextrose as a source of calories and with added appropriate electrolytes and vitamins, Amino Acids,

---

Injectable, 5.2% is suitable as an intravenous source of protein in a parenteral nutritional regimen for such patients.

CONTRAINDICATIONS

Amino Acids, Injectable, is contraindicated in patients with anuria, hepatic coma or encephalopathy, inborn errors of Amino Acid metabolism, severe uncorrected electrolyte or acid-base balance, hyperammonemia or other disorders involving impaired nitrogen utilization, decreased circulating blood volume, severe liver disease, or hypersensitivity to one or more Amino Acids present in the solution.

WARNINGS

Some brands contain sodium bisulfite, potassium metabisulfate or sodium hydrosulfite, sulfites that may cause allergic-type reactions including anaphylactic symptoms and life-threatening or less severe asthmatic episodes in certain susceptible people. The overall prevalence of sulfite sensitivity in the general population is unknown and probably low. Sulfite sensitivity is seen more frequently in asthmatic than in nonasthmatic people.

Safe and effective use of parenteral nutrition requires a knowledge of nutrition as well as clinical expertise in recognition and treatment of the complications which can occur. **Frequent clinical evaluation and laboratory determinations are necessary for proper monitoring of parenteral nutrition.** Studies should include blood sugar, serum proteins, kidney and liver function tests, electrolytes, hemogram, carbon dioxide content, serum osmolarities, blood cultures, and blood ammonia levels.

The intravenous administration of these solutions can cause fluid and/or solute overload resulting in dilution of serum electrolyte concentrations, overhydration, congested states or pulmonary edema. The risk of dilutional states is inversely proportional to the solute or electrolyte concentration of the solution infused. The risk of solute overload causing congested states with peripheral and pulmonary edema is directly proportional to the concentration of the solution.

Administration of Amino Acid solutions in the presence of impaired renal function presents special issues associated with retention of electrolytes.

Administration of Amino Acids in the presence of impaired renal function or gastrointestinal bleeding may augment an already elevated blood urea nitrogen. Appropriate laboratory tests should be performed periodically and infusion discontinued or nitrogen content reduced if BUN levels continue to rise inappropriately. It should be noted that a modest rise in BUN normally occurs as a result of increased protein intake. Patients with azotemia from any cause should not be infused with Amino Acids without regard to total nitrogen intake.

Solutions containing sodium ion should be used with great care, if at all, in patients with congestive heart failure, severe renal insuffiency and in clinical states in which there exists edema with sodium retention.

Solutions which contain potassium ion should be used with great care, if at all, in patients with hyperkalemia, severe renal failure and in conditions in which potassium retention is present.

Solutions containing acetate ion should be used with great care in patients with metabolic or respiratory alkalosis. Acetate should be administered with great care in those conditions in which there is an increased level or an impaired utilization of this ion, such as severe hepatic insufficiency.

Administration of Amino Acid solutions to a patient with hepatic insufficiency may result in plasma Amino Acid imbalances, hyperammonemia, prerenal azotemia, stupor and coma.

Hyperammonemia is of **special significance in infants** as its occurrence in the syndrome caused by genetic metabolic defects is sometimes associated, although not necessarily in a causal relationship, with mental retardation. This reaction appears to be dose related and is more likely to develop during prolonged therapy. It is essential that blood ammonia be measured frequently in infants. Also, instances of asymptomatic hyperammonemia have been reported in patients without overt liver dysfunction. The mechanisms of these reactions are not clearly defined but may involve genetic defects and immature or subclinically impaired liver function.

Conservative doses of Amino Acids should be given, dictated by the nutritional status of the patient. Should symptoms of hyperammonemia develop, Amino Acid administration should be discontinued and the patient's clinical status reevaluated.

Amino Acids, Injectable, 5.2%—renal formula—does not replace dialysis and conventional supportive therapy in patients with renal failure.

Pharmacy Bulk Package injections are for compounding only, not for direct infusion.

Caution should be exercised when admixing Pharmacy Bulk Package Injections. Studies have shown that admixtures of Pharmacy Bulk Package Amino Acids, Fat Emulsion Injection, and high concentration dextrose injection (10 to 70%) are stable over short periods of time. These solutions should be used promptly after admixing. Any storage should be under refrigeration and limited to a brief period of time, preferably less than 24 hours.

These injections should not be administered simultaneously with blood through the same infusion set because of the possibility of pseudoagglutination.

Care must be taken to avoid incompatible electrolyte mixtures. Infusate levels of 10-15 mEq/liter of phosphate, 5 mEq/liter of calcium, and 5-10 mEq/liter of magnesium are rarely incompatible when properly mixed. Higher levels must be added cautiously with adequate mixing (avoid layering) and inspection. Additional calcium and phosphate may be added to alternate bottles. Whatever the electrolyte formula, the infusion must be inspected for solution clarity at the time of mixing, before dispensing from the pharmacy, and immediately before and periodically during administration.

PRECAUTIONS

GENERAL

Clinical evaluation and periodic laboratory determinations are necessary to monitor changes in fluid balance, electrolyte concentrations, and acid-base

COMPOSITION (MG/100 ML)

Essential Amino Acids	3.5%	5%	5.2%	5.5%	7%		8.5%			10%		
Isoleucine	231	330	462	263	462	789	590	561	406	690	660	600
Leucine	350	500	726	340	700	1576	770	850	526	910	1000	730
Lysine	368	525	535	318	735	265	620	893	492	730	1050	580
Methionine	60	86	726	318	120	206	450	146	492	530	172	400
Phenylalanine	104	149	726	340	209	228	480	253	526	560	298	560
Threonine	140	200	330	230	280	272	340	340	356	400	400	420
Tryptophan	70	100	165	99	140	88	130	170	152	150	200	180
Valine	175	250	528	252	350	789	560	425	390	660	500	580
Histidine	105	150	429	241	210	154	240	255	372	280	480	480
Cysteine							< 14			< 16		
Tyrosine	95	135		22	189	33		230	34		270	40
Nonessential Amino Acids												
Alanine	348	497		1140	695	660	600	844	1760	710	993	2070
Arginine	356	509	600	570	713	507	810	865	880	950	1018	1150
Proline	253	361		230	505	448	950	614	356	1120	722	680
Serine	186	265			371	221	500	450		590	530	500
Glycine	175	250		1140	350	660	1190	425	1760	1400	500	1030
L-Aspartic Acid	245	350			490			595			700	
L-Glutamic Acid	258	369			517			627			738	
pH	5.4 (5.0-6.5)	5.4 (5.0-6.5)	5.5 (4.5-6.0)	6.0 (5.0-7.0)	5.8 (5.0-6.5)	5.2 (4.5-6.0)	6.5 (6.0-7.0)	5.8 (5.0-6.5)	6.0 (5.0-7.0)	6.5 (6.0-7.0)	5.8 (5.0-6.5)	6.0 (5.0-7.0)
Osmolarity (mOsmol/L)	308	438	475	575	612	665	810	742	890	950	873	998
Protein equivalent (gm/L)	35	50	52.3	55	70	70	82	85	85	95.6	100	100
Nitrogen (gm/L)	5.4	7.7	7.9	9.3	10.7	11.2	13.0	13.0	14.3	15.3	15.3	16.5

balance during prolonged parenteral therapy or whenever the condition of the patient warrants such evaluation. Significant deviations from normal concentrations may require the use of additional electrolyte supplements. Blood studies should include glucose, urea nitrogen, serum electrolytes, acid-base balance, blood ammonia levels, serum proteins, kidney and liver function tests, serum osmolality and hemogram. Circulating blood volume should be determined if indicated. If sepsis is suspected, blood cultures should be taken.

Strongly hypertonic nutrient solutions should be administered through an indwelling intravenous catheter with the tip located in the superior vena cava.

Care should be taken to avoid circulatory overload, particularly in patients with cardiac insufficiency.

Care should be taken to avoid excess fluid accumulation, particularly in patients with renal disease, pulmonary insufficiency and heart disease.

During protein-sparing therapy in the absence of supporting carbohydrate metabolism, an accumulation of ketone bodies in the blood often occurs. Correction of ketonemia usually can be accomplished by administering some carbohydrates.

Protein-sparing therapy is useful for periods up to 10 to 12 days. Patients requiring nutritional support thereafter should be placed on oral or parenteral regimens that employ adequate nonprotein calorie components.

In patients with myocardial infarct, infusion of Amino Acids should always be accompanied by dextrose, since in anoxia, free fatty acids cannot be utilized by the myocardium, and energy must be produced anaerobically from glycogen or glucose.

It is essential to provide adequate calories concurrently if parenterally administered Amino Acids are to be retained by the body and utilized for protein synthesis. Concentrated dextrose solutions are an effective source of such calories.

With the administration of Amino Acids, Injectable, in combination with highly concentrated dextrose solutions, hyperglycemia, glycosuria and hyperosmolar syndrome may result. Blood and urine glucose should be monitored on a routine basis in patients receiving this therapy.

Sudden cessation in administration of a concentrated dextrose solution may result in insulin reaction due to continued endogenous insulin production. Parenteral nutrition mixtures should be withdrawn slowly.

Special care must be taken when giving hypertonic dextrose to a diabetic or prediabetic patient. To prevent severe hyperglycemia in such patients, insulin may be required.

Administration of glucose at a rate exceeding the patient's utilization may lead to hyperglycemia, coma, and death.

Administration of Amino Acids without carbohydrates may result in the accumulation of ketone bodies in the blood. Correction of this ketonemia may be achieved by the administration of carbohydrate.

After appropriate dilution, if Amino Acids, Injectable, is to be administered by peripheral vein, care should be taken to assure proper placement of the needle or infusion device within the lumen of the vein. The venipuncture site should be inspected frequently for signs of infiltration. If venous thrombosis or phlebitis occurs, discontinue infusions or change infusion site and initiate appropriate treatment.

Because of its antianabolic activity, concurrent administration of tetracycline may reduce the protein sparing effects of infused Amino Acids.

Do not withdraw venous blood for blood chemistries through the peripheral infusion site, as interference with estimations of nitrogen-containing substances may occur.

Intravenously administered Amino Acids should be used with caution in patients with history of renal disease, pulmonary disease, or with cardiac insufficiency so as to avoid excessive fluid accumulation.

Extraordinary electrolyte losses such as may occur during protracted nasogastric suction, vomiting, diarrhea or gastrointestinal fistula drainage may necessitate additional electrolyte supplementation.

Metabolic acidosis can be prevented or readily controlled by adding a portion of the cations in the electrolyte mixture as acetate salts and in the case of hyperchloremic acidosis, by keeping the total chloride content of the infusate to a minimum.

Some solutions contain added phosphorus and some do not. Patients, especially those with hypophosphatemia, may require additional phosphate. To prevent hypocalcemia, calcium supplementation should always accompany phosphate administration. To assure adequate intake, serum levels should be monitored frequently.

Clinically significant hypocalcemia, hypophosphatemia or hypomagnesemia may occur as a result of therapy with Amino Acids, Injectable, 5.2%—renal formula—and hypertonic dextrose; electrolyte replacement may become necessary.

In order to promote urea nitrogen reutilization in patients with renal failure, it is essential to provide adequate calories with minimal amounts of the essential Amino Acids and to restrict the intake of nonessential nitrogen. Hypertonic dextrose solutions are a convenient and metabolically effective source of concentrated calories. Hypertonic solutions should be administered through an indwelling catheter with the tip located in the superior vena cava. When abrupt cessation of hypertonic dextrose is required, monitoring for rebound hypoglycemia should be instituted. Essential fatty acid deficiency (EFAD) is becoming increasingly recognized in patients on long term TPN (more than 5 days). The use of fat emulsion to provide 4—10% of total caloric intake as linoleic acid may prevent EFAD.

Fluid balance should be carefully monitored in patients with renal failure to avoid excessive fluid overload, especially in relation to cardiac insufficiency.

To minimize the risk of possible incompatibilites arising from mixing this solution with other additives that may be prescribed, the final infusate should be inspected for cloudiness or precipitation immediately after mixing, prior to administration, and periodically during administration.

Use only if solution is clear and vacuum is present.

USAGE IN PREGNANCY
Pregnancy Category C. Animal reproduction studies have not been conducted with Amino Acids, Injectable. It is also not known whether Amino Acids, Injectable can cause fetal harm when administered to a pregnant woman or can affect reproduction capacity. Amino Acids, Injectable should be given to a pregnant woman only if clearly needed.

Nitrogen intake should be carefully monitored in patients with impaired renal function.

SPECIAL PRECAUTIONS IN PATIENTS WITH RENAL INSUFFICIENCY
Frequent laboratory studies are necessary in patients with renal insufficiency. In renal failure hyperglycemia may not be reflected by glycosuria. Blood glucose must be determined frequently, often every six hours to guide dosage of dextrose, and insulin should be given, if required.

SPECIAL PRECAUTIONS IN PEDIATRIC PATIENTS
Amino Acids, Injectable, should be used with special caution in pediatric patients with acute renal failure, especially low birth weight infants. Laboratory and clinical monitoring of pediatric patients, especially those who are nutritionally depleted, must be extensive and frequent. See "Dosage and Administration" for additional information.

Frequent monitoring of blood glucose is required in low birth weight or septic infants as hypertonic dextrose infusion involves a greater risk of hyperglycemia in such patients.

The effect of infusion of Amino Acids, without dextrose, upon carbohydrate metabolism of children is not known at this time. Safety and effectiveness have not been established in children for some formulations.

SPECIAL PRECAUTIONS FOR CENTRAL VENOUS NUTRITION
Administration by central venous catheter should be used only by those familiar with this technique and its complications.

Central venous nutrition may be associated with complications which can be prevented or minimized by careful attention to all aspects of the procedure including solution preparation, administration, and patient monitoring. **It is essential that a carefully prepared protocol, based on current medical practices, be followed, preferably by an experienced team.**

Although a detailed discussion of the complications of central venous nutrition is beyond the scope of this insert, the following summary lists those based on current literature:

TECHNICAL
The placement of a central venous catheter should be regarded as a surgical procedure. One should be fully acquainted with various techniques of catheter insertion as well as recognition and treatment of complications. For details of techniques and placement sites, consult the medical literature. X-ray is the best means of verifying catheter placement. Complications known to occur from the placement of central venous catheters are pneumothorax, hemothorax, hydrothorax, artery puncture and transection, injury to the brachial plexus, malposition of the catheter, formation of arteriovenous fistula, phlebitis, thrombosis, and air and catheter embolus.

SEPTIC
The constant risk of sepsis is present during central venous nutrition. Since contaminated solutions and infusion catheters are potential sources of infection, it is imperative that the preparation of parenteral nutrition solutions and the placement and care of catheters be accomplished under controlled aseptic conditions.

Solutions should ideally be prepared in the hospital pharmacy in a laminar flow hood. The key factor in their preparation is careful aseptic technique to avoid inadvertent touch contamination during mixing of solutions and subsequent admixtures.

Parenteral nutrition solutions should be used promptly after mixing. Any storage should be under refrigeration for as brief a time as possible. Administration time for a single bottle and set should never exceed 24 hours.

Consult the medical literature for a discussion of the management of sepsis during central venous nutrition. In brief, typical management includes replacing the solution being administered with a fresh container and set, and the remaining contents are cultured for bacterial or fungal contamination. If sepsis persists and another source of infection is not identified, the catheter is removed, the proximal tip cultured, and a new catheter reinserted when the fever has subsided. Nonspecific, prophylactic antibiotic treatment is not recommended. Clinical experience indicates that the catheter is likely to be the prime source of infection as opposed to aseptically prepared and properly stored solutions.

METABOLIC
The following metabolic complications have been reported: metabolic acidosis, hypophosphatemia, alkalosis, hyperglycemia and glycosuria, osmotic diuresis and dehydration, rebound hypoglycemia, elevated liver enzymes, hypo- and hypervitaminosis, electrolyte imbalances, and hyperammonemia in children. Frequent clinical evaluation and laboratory determinations are necessary, especially during the first few days of central venous nutrition, to prevent or minimize these complications.

ADVERSE REACTIONS

See "Warnings" and "Special Precautions for Central Venous Nutrition."

Reactions which may occur because of the solution or the technique of administration include febrile response, infection at the site of injection, venous thrombosis or phlebitis extending from the site of injection, extravasation and hypervolemia.

Local reactions of the infusion site, consisting of a warm sensation, erythema, phlebitis and thrombosis, have been reported with peripheral Amino Acid infusions, especially if other substances, such as antibiotics, are also administered through the same site. In such cases the infusion site should be changed promptly to another vein. Use of large peripheral veins, inline filters, and slowing the rate of infusion may reduce the incidence of local venous irritation.

Generalized flushing, fever and nausea have been reported during peripheral administration of Amino Acids.

Metabolic, fluid, electrolyte and acid-base imbalances can occur unless appropriate monitoring and corrective management are accomplished during therapy.

Symptoms may result from an excess or deficit of one or more of the ions present in the solution; therefore, frequent monitoring of electrolyte levels is essential.

If electrolyte supplementation is required during peripheral infusion, it is recommended that additives be administered throughout the day in order to avoid possible venous irritation. Irritating additive medications may require injection at another site and should not be added directly to the Amino Acid infusate.

Phosphorous deficiency may lead to impaired tissue oxygenation and acute hemolytic anemia. Relative to calcium, excessive phosphorus intake can precipitate hypocalcemia with cramps, tetany and muscular hyperexcitability.

If an adverse reaction does occur, discontinue the infusion, evaluate the patient, institute appropriate therapeutic countermeasures and save the remainder of the fluid for examination if deemed necessary.

OVERDOSAGE

In the event of a fluid or solute overload during parenteral therapy, reevaluate the patient's condition, and institute appropriate corrective treatment.

DOSAGE AND ADMINISTRATION

The total daily dose of Amino Acids, Injectable, depends on daily protein requirements and on the patient's metabolic and clinical response. The determination of nitrogen balance and accurate daily body weights, corrected for fluid balance, are probably the best means of assessing individual protein requirements.

While Recommended Dietary Allowances of protein are approximately 0.8 to 0.9 g/kg of body weight for a healthy adult and 1.4 to 2.2 g/kg for healthy growing infants and children. It must be recognized that protein as well as caloric requirements in traumatized or malnourished patients may be substantially increased. Daily Amino Acid doses of approximately 1.0 to 1.5 g/kg of body weight for adults and 2 to 3 g/kg of body weight for infants with adequate calories are generally sufficient to satisfy protein needs and promote positive nitrogen balance. Infusion or ingestion of carbohydrate or lipid will not reduce the nitrogen sparing effect of intravenous Amino Acid infusions at this dose.

For the initial treatment of trauma or protein calorie malnutrition, higher doses of protein with corresponding quantities of carbohydrate will be necessary to promote adequate patient response to therapy. The severity of the illness being treated is the primary consideration in determining proper dose level. Higher doses may be required in severely catabolic states. Such higher doses, especially in infants, must be accompanied by frequent laboratory evaluation. Fat emulsion may be supplied to help meet energy requirements.

Fat emulsion coadministration should be considered when prolonged (more than 5 days) parenteral nutrition is required in order to prevent essential fatty acid deficiency (E.F.A.D.). Serum lipids should be monitored for evidence of E.F.A.D. in patients maintained on fat free TPN.

For protein sparing in well-nourished patients not receiving significant additional calories, Amino Acid dosages of 1.0 to 1.7 g/kg/day significantly reduce nitrogen losses and spare body protein. If daily increases in BUN in the range of 10 to 15 mg% for more than three days should occur or if rises in BUN exceed 20 mg% in 48 hours, Amino Acid infusion should be discontinued or rate of administration reduced; if it is discontinued, a regimen with full nonprotein calorie substrates should be adopted.

The provision of sufficient intracellular electrolytes, principally potassium, magnesium, and phosphate, is also required for optimum utilization of Amino Acids. Approximately 60-180 mEq of potassium, 10-30 mEq of magnesium, and 20-80 mEq or 10 to 40 mM of phosphate per day appear necessary to achieve optimum metabolic response. In addition, sufficient quantities of the major extracellular electrolytes (sodium, calcium, and chloride) must be given. In patients with hyperchloremic or other metabolic acidoses, sodium and potassium may be added as the acetate or lactate salts to provide bicarbonate precursor. The electrolyte content of Amino Acids, Injectable must be considered when calculating daily electrolyte intake. Serum electrolytes, including magnesium and phosphorus, should be monitored frequently.

Acceptable total daily administration volumes are dependent upon the fluid balance requirements of the patient. Extreme care should be given to prevent fluctuations of blood osmolarity and serum electrolyte concentrations. Frequent and careful monitoring is mandatory when fluid restricted patients are receiving intravenous nutrition.

If a patient's nutritional intake is primarily parenteral, vitamins, especially the water soluble vitamins, and trace elements should also be provided.

Calcium and phosphorus are added to the solution as indicated. The usual dose of phosphorus added to a liter of TPN solution (containing 25% dextrose) is 12 mM. This requirement is related to the carbohydrate calories delivered. Iron is added to the solution or given intramuscularly in depot form as indicated. Vitamin B_{12}, vitamin K and folic acid are given intramuscularly or added to the solution as desired.

Calcium and phosphorus additives are potentially incompatible when added to the TPN admixture. However, if one additive is added to the Amino Acid container and the other to the container of concentrated dextrose, and if the contents of both containers are swirled before they are combined, and then the likelihood of physical incompatibility is reduced.

In patients with hyperchloremic or other metabolic acidosis, sodium and potassium may be added as the acetate or lactate salts to provide bicarbonate alternates.

Solutions from Pharmacy Bulk Packages should be used promptly after mixing. Any storage should be under refrigeration and limited to a brief period of time, preferably less than 24 hours.

CENTRAL VENOUS NUTRITION

For severely catabolic, depleted patients, those unable to take oral or enteral nourishment for a prolonged period of time, or those requiring long-term total parenteral nutrition, central venous nutrition should be considered. Calorie-to-nitrogen ratios of at least 100 to 150 nonprotein calories per gram of nitrogen have been recommended to achieve positive nitrogen balance in such patients. These ratios are easily and conveniently attained with the use of concentrated dextrose solutions, supplemented if desired with parenteral fat emulsion.

Total parenteral nutrition may be started with infusates containing lower concentrations of dextrose; dextrose content may be gradually increased to estimated caloric needs as the patient's glucose tolerance increases.

Each gram of dextrose provides approximately 3.4 kcal. Each gram of fat provides 9 kcal.

The average depleted major surgical patient with complications requires between 2500 and 4000 kcal and between 12 and 24 grams of nitrogen per day. An adult patient in an acceptable weight range with restricted activity who is not hypermetabolic, requires about 30 kcal/kg of body weight/day. Average daily adult fluid requirements are between 2500 and 3000 mL and may be much higher with losses from fistula drainage or severe burns. Typically, a hospitalized patient may lose 12 to 18 grams of nitrogen a day, and in severe trauma the daily loss may be 20 to 25 grams or more.

In adults, strongly hypertonic mixtures of Amino Acids and dextrose may be safely administered only by continuous infusion through a central venous catheter with the tip located in the vena cava. For optimal nitrogen utilization, 500 mL of Amino Acids, Injectable, appropriately mixed with concentrated dextrose, electrolytes, and vitamins are typically administered over an 8-hour period. If administration rate should fall behind schedule, no attempt to "catch up" to planned intake should be made. In addition to meeting protein needs, the administration rate is also governed, especially during the first few days of therapy by the patient's glucose tolerance. Daily intake of Amino Acids and dextrose should be increased gradually to the maximum required dose as indicated by frequent determination of urine and blood sugar levels. In many patients, provision of adequate calories in the form of hypertonic dextrose may require the administration of exogenous insulin to prevent hyperglycemia and glycosuria. To prevent rebound hypoglycemia, a solution containing 5% dextrose should be administered when hypertonic dextrose infusions are abruptly discontinued.

PERIPHERAL PARENTERAL NUTRITION

For moderately catabolic, depleted patients requiring parenteral nutrition in whom the central venous route is not indicated, Amino Acids, Injectable, can be mixed with hypocaloric energy supplements by peripheral vein. Dextrose in a final concentration of up to 10% and/or lipid emulsion may be administered.

For example, to prepare a solution of 4.25% Amino Acids, Injectable, in 2.5% dextrose, aseptically transfer 500 mL of 8.5% Amino Acids, Injectable, to a one liter intravenous bottle containing 500 mL of 5% dextrose. Each liter of the resultant solution provides 41 grams of protein equivalent and 85 carbohydrate calories with an osmolarity of approximately 530 mOsmol/liter.

As with all intravenous fluid therapy, the primary aim is to provide sufficient water to compensate for insensible, urinary and other (nasogastric suction, fistula drainage, diarrhea) fluid losses. Total fluid requirements, as well as electrolyte and acid-base needs, should be estimated and appropriately administered.

For an Amino Acid solution of specified total concentration, the volume required to meet Amino Acid requirements per 24 hours can be calculated. After making an estimate of the total daily fluid (water) requirement, the balance of fluid needed beyond the volume of Amino Acid solution required can be provided either as a noncarbohydrate or a carbohydrate-containing electrolyte solution.

If desired, only one-half of an estimated daily amino acid requirement of 1.5 g/kg can be given on the first day. Amino Acids together with dextrose in concentrations of 5% to 10% infused into a peripheral vein can be continued while oral nutrition is impaired.

Parenteral fat emulsion may be administered along with Amino Acid-dextrose solution through a Y-type administration set to supplement caloric intake. Fat, however, should not be the sole caloric intake—should not provide more than 60% of the total caloric intake—since some studies have suggested that glucose is more nitrogen sparing in the stressed patient.

PROTEIN SPARING

For well-nourished, mildly catabolic patients who require short-term parenteral nutritional support, both 10% and 8.5% Amino Acid Injections can be administered peripherally with or without parenteral carbohydrate calories. Such infusates can be prepared by dilution of 10% Amino Acid Injection with Sterile Water for Injection USP or 5% Dextrose Injection USP solutions to prepare isotonic or slightly hypertonic solutions which may be administered by peripheral vein.

Depending upon the clinical condition of the patient, approximately 3 liters of solution may be administered per 24 hour period. When used postoperatively, the therapy should begin with 1000 mL on the first postoperative day. Thereafter, the dose may be increased to 3000 mL per day. For example, a 4.25% Amino Acid Injection Solution can be prepared by the aseptic transfer of 500 mL of 8.5% Amino Acid Injection to a half-filled intravenous one liter bottle of Sterile Water for Injection. The resultant solution contains 41 grams of Amino Acids with an osmolarity of approximately 405 mOsmol/liter. An approximately isotonic solution of 3% Amino Acid Injection can be prepared by aseptic transfer of 350mL of 8.5% Amino Acid Injection to a partially filled intravenous one liter bottle containing 650 mL of Sterile Water for Injection. The resultant solution will provide 29 grams of Amino Acids per liter with an osmolarity of approximately 285 mOsmol/liter.

PEDIATRIC DOSAGE AND ADMINISTRATION

Pediatric requirements for parenteral nutrition are constrained by the greater relative fluid requirements of the infant and greater caloric requirements per kilogram. Amino Acids are probably best administered in a 2.5% concentration.

Infants (up to 10 kg) on total parenteral nutrition generally receive 2 to 3 grams of protein, 100 to 150 calories, and 120 to 150 mL of fluid per kilogram of body weight per day. This can be provided in a solution containing approximately 2-1/8% Amino Acids, Injectable, (diluted from 10% Amino Acids, Injectable, and 20% dextrose. Less hypertonic mixtures may be administered by peripheral vein. In cases of malnutrition or stress, these requirements may be increased. Fat emulsion may be given concurrently by central or peripheral vein through a Y-type administration set to provide essential fatty acids and increase caloric intake. Since physiological changes occur rapidly in small infants, it is acceptable in pediatrics to start with a nutritional solution of half strength at a rate of about 60 to 70 mL/kg/day. Within 24 to 48 hours the volume and concentration of the solution can be increased until the full strength pediatric solution (Amino Acids and dextrose) is given at a rate of 125 to 150 mL/kg/day.

Supplemental electrolytes and vitamin additives should be administered as deemed necessary by careful monitoring of blood chemistries and nutritional status. Addition of iron is more critical in the infant than the adult because of the increasing red cell mass required for the growing infant. Serum lipids should be monitored for evidence of essential fatty acid deficiency in patients maintained on fat-free TPN. Bicarbonate should not be administered during infusion of the nutritional solution unless deemed absolutely necessary.

To ensure the precise delivery of the small volumes of fluid necessary for total parenteral nutrition in infants, accurately calibrated and reliable infusion systems should be used.

A basic solution for pediatric use should contain 25 grams of Amino Acids and 200 to 250 grams of glucose per 1000 mL, administered from containers containing 250 or 500 mL. Such a solution given at the rate of 145 mL/kg/day provides 130 kcal/kg/day.

Children over 10 kilograms require fewer calories and slightly less protein; generally 50 to 80 calories and 2 grams of protein per kilogram per day is sufficient.

Parenteral drug products should be inspected visually for particulate matter and discoloration prior to administration, whenever solution and container permit.

Care must be taken to avoid incompatible admixtures. Consult with pharmacist.

Amino Acids, Injectable—Renal Formula: The objective of nutritional management of renal decompensation is to provide sufficient Amino Acid and caloric support for protein synthesis without exceeding the renal capacity to excrete metabolic wastes.

A dosage of 2.4 to 4.7 grams of nitrogen per day (from essential Amino Acids) with adequate calories will maintain nitrogen equilibrium in patients with uremia. If more nitrogen and calories are required in severely stressed patients in acute renal failure who cannot eat, higher dosages may be administered provided great care is taken to avoid exceeding limits of fluid intake or glucose tolerance.

In general, dosage should be guided by fluid, glucose and nitrogen tolerances, as well as the metabolic and clinical response. The rate of rise in BUN generally diminishes with infusion of essential Amino Acids. However, excessive intake of protein or increased protein catabolism may alter this response.

The usual daily dose ranges from 300 to 600 mL of Amino Acids, Injectable, 5.2% — renal formula — equivalent to 2.4 to 4.7 grams of nitrogen in 15.7 to 31 grams of essential Amino Acids. Adequate calories should be administered simultaneously. Each 300 mL of Amino Acids, Injectable — renal formula — mixed under sterile conditions with 500 mL of 70% dextrose will provide a solution of 1.96% of Amino Acids, Injectable — renal formula — in 44% dextrose. This mixture provides a calorie-to-nitrogen ratio of 504:1.

Electrolyte supplementation may be required. Amino Acids, Injectable—renal formula—contains approximately 0.54 mEq/100 mL of potassium.

Elevated phosphorus, potassium and magnesium levels generally decrease during treatment with Amino Acids, Injectable—renal formula. Particular care

should be taken in the presence of cardiac arrhythmias or digitalis toxicity to assure that sufficient quantities of these electrolytes are provided when necessary.

Compatibility of electrolyte additives to the mixtures of Amino Acids, Injectable—renal formula—and hypertonic dextrose must be considered and potentially incompatible ions (calcium, phosphate) may be added to alternate infusion bottles to avoid precipitation.

Children: Pediatric requirements for Amino Acids, Injectable—renal formula—vary greatly depending upon growth, nutritional state and degree of renal insufficiency. A dosage of 0.5 to 1 gram of essential Amino Acids per kilogram of body weight per day will meet the requirements of the majority of pediatric patients. Initial daily dosage of Amino Acids, Injectable—renal formula—should be low and increased slowly; more than one gram of essential Amino Acids per kilogram of body weight per day is not recommended. The total volume of nutritional solution and the rate at which it is administered will vary with the child's age, nutritional and growth state, as well as the degree of renal failure.

Administration: Amino Acids, Injectable 5.2%—renal formula—admixed with sufficient dextrose to provide caloric energy requirements may be safely administered via a central venous catheter with the tip located in the vena cava.

Initial infusion rates should be slow, generally 20 to 30 mL/hour for the first 6 to 8 hours. Increments of 10 mL/hour for each hour are suggested up to a maximum rate of 60 to 100 mL/hour. If administration rates fall behind the scheduled 24 hour dosage, no attempt should be made to catch up to the planned intake. The patient's fluid, nitrogen and glucose tolerance should be the governing factor of the rate of administration. Uremic patients are frequently glucose intolerant especially in association with peritoneal dialysis; insulin may be required to prevent hyperglycemia. When hypertonic dextrose infusion is abruptly discontinued, rebound hypoglycemia may be prevented by administering 5% dextrose.

Storage: Exposure of pharmaceutical products to heat should be minimized. Avoid excessive heat. Protect from freezing. It is recommended that the product be stored at room temperature (25°C); however, brief exposure up to 40°C does not adversely affect the product.

Protect from light until use.

HOW SUPPLIED

INJECTION: 3.5%

BRAND/MANUFACTURER	NDC	SIZE	AWP
○ **BRAND**			
AMINOSYN: Abbott Hosp	00074-2989-05	1000 ml 6s	$341.79
	00074-4154-05	1000 ml 6s	$357.68
AMINOSYN II W/5% DEXTROSE: Abbott Hosp	00074-7701-29	1000 ml 6s	$525.04
	00074-7740-29	1000 ml 6s	$551.33
AMINOSYN II W/25% DEXTROSE: Abbott Hosp	00074-7700-29	1000 ml 6s	$585.53
AMINOSYN II: Abbott Hosp	00074-1083-05	1000 ml 6s	$610.47

INJECTION: 4%

BRAND/MANUFACTURER	NDC	SIZE	AWP
○ **BRAND**			
BRANCHAMIN: Clintec	00338-0477-03	500 ml 18s	$1684.80

INJECTION: 4.25%

BRAND/MANUFACTURER	NDC	SIZE	AWP
○ **BRAND**			
AMINOSYN II W/10% DEXTROSE: Abbott Hosp	00074-7751-29	1000 ml 6s	$597.65
AMINOSYN II W/20% DEXTROSE: Abbott Hosp	00074-7752-29	1000 ml 6s	$603.06
AMINOSYN II W/5% DEXTROSE: Abbott Hosp	00074-7702-29	1000 ml 6s	$607.41
AMINOSYN II W/10% DEXTROSE: Abbott Hosp	00074-7742-29	1000 ml 6s	$626.29

INJECTION: 5%

BRAND/MANUFACTURER	NDC	SIZE	AWP
○ **BRAND**			
AMINOSYN: Abbott Hosp	00074-2990-05	1000 ml 6s	$610.47
AMINOSYN II W/25% DEXTROSE: Abbott Hosp	00074-7744-29	1000 ml 6s	$693.19
AMINOSYN: Abbott Hosp	00074-2990-03	500 ml 12s	$624.01

INJECTION: 5.2%

BRAND/MANUFACTURER	NDC	SIZE	AWP
○ **BRAND**			
AMINESS: Clintec	00338-0488-17	400 ml 10s	$1073.52
AMINOSYN-RF: Abbott Hosp	00074-4072-02	300 ml 12s	$1094.26

INJECTION: 5.5%

BRAND/MANUFACTURER	NDC	SIZE	AWP
○ **BRAND**			
TRAVASOL 5.5%: Clintec	00338-0623-04	1000 ml 6s	$549.24
	00338-0623-06	2000 ml 6s	$672.06
	00338-0623-03	500 ml 12s	$549.23

INJECTION: 6.5%

BRAND/MANUFACTURER	NDC	SIZE	AWP
○ **BRAND**			
RENAMIN: Clintec	00338-0471-03	500 ml 6s	$1800.00
	00338-0471-02	250 ml 12s	$900.00

◆ RATED THERAPEUTICALLY EQUIVALENT; ◇ THERAPEUTIC EQUIVALENCE UNCONFIRMED; ○ UNRATED

INJECTION: 7%

BRAND/MANUFACTURER	NDC	SIZE	AWP
○ BRAND			
AMINOSYN: Abbott Hosp	00074-2996-01	500 ml 3s	$293.84
AMINOSYN HBC 7%: Abbott Hosp	00074-1108-05	1000 ml 6s	$885.92
AMINOSYN-PF 7%: Abbott Hosp	00074-1616-02	250 ml 12s	$641.54
AMINOSYN: Abbott Hosp	00074-2992-03	500 ml 12s	$843.46
AMINOSYN II: Abbott Hosp	00074-1086-03	500 ml 12s	$843.46
AMINOSYN-PF 7%: Abbott Hosp	00074-1616-03	500 ml 12s	$855.86
AMINOSYN HBC 7%: Abbott Hosp	00074-1108-03	500 ml 12s	$885.64

INJECTION: 8.5%

BRAND/MANUFACTURER	NDC	SIZE	AWP
○ BRAND			
FREAMINE III: McGaw	00264-1903-10	500 ml	$72.20
	00264-1903-00	1000 ml	$144.55
AMINOSYN: Abbott Hosp	00074-4041-01	500 ml 3s	$308.73
TRAVASOL 8.5%: Clintec	00338-0625-04	1000 ml 6s	$877.32
AMINOSYN: Abbott Hosp	00074-5855-05	1000 ml 6s	$894.26
AMINOSYN II: Abbott Hosp	00074-1088-05	1000 ml 6s	$894.26
TRAVASOL 8.5%: Clintec	00338-0625-06	2000 ml 6s	$889.56
	00338-0625-03	500 ml 12s	$877.10
AMINOSYN: Abbott Hosp	00074-5855-03	500 ml 12s	$894.05
AMINOSYN II: Abbott Hosp	00074-1088-03	500 ml 12s	$894.05

INJECTION: 10%

BRAND/MANUFACTURER	NDC	SIZE	AWP
○ BRAND			
FREAMINE III: McGaw	00264-1901-10	500 ml	$82.34
	00264-1901-00	1000 ml	$158.23
AMINOSYN: Abbott Hosp	00074-4360-05	1000 ml	$607.92
TRAVASOL 10%: Clintec	00338-0629-04	1000 ml 6s	$1000.80
AMINOSYN-PF 10%: Abbott Hosp	00074-1617-05	1000 ml 6s	$1012.25
AMINOSYN: Abbott Hosp	00074-2991-05	1000 ml 6s	$1020.09
AMINOSYN II: Abbott Hosp	00074-1090-05	1000 ml 6s	$1020.09
TRAVASOL 10%: Clintec	00338-0629-06	2000 ml 6s	$2001.67
AMINOSYN II: Abbott Hosp	00074-7121-07	2000 ml 6s	$2040.24
TRAVASOL 10%: Clintec	00338-0629-02	250 ml 12s	$347.88
	00338-0629-03	500 ml 12s	$1001.23
AMINOSYN: Abbott Hosp	00074-2991-03	500 ml 12s	$1020.59
AMINOSYN II: Abbott Hosp	00074-1090-03	500 ml 12s	$1020.59

INJECTION: 11.4%

BRAND/MANUFACTURER	NDC	SIZE	AWP
○ BRAND			
NOVAMINE: Clintec	00338-0489-04	1000 ml 6s	$1095.94
	00338-0489-03	500 ml 10s	$951.35

INJECTION: 15%

BRAND/MANUFACTURER	NDC	SIZE	AWP
○ BRAND			
NOVAMINE: Clintec	00338-0498-06	2000 ml 4s	$1980.00
	00338-0494-04	1000 ml 6s	$1405.02
AMINOSYN II: Abbott Hosp	00074-7122-07	2000 ml 6s	$3060.33
NOVAMINE: Clintec	00338-0494-03	500 ml 10s	$1123.20

KIT: 8.5%

BRAND/MANUFACTURER	NDC	SIZE	AWP
○ BRAND			
TRAVASOL 8.5%: Clintec	00338-0653-98	3s	$134.07

Amino Acids/Calcium Chloride/Dextrose/Electrolytes

DESCRIPTION

Amino Acids/Calcium Chloride/Dextrose/Electrolytes contains 1000 mL of amino acid injection with electrolytes—a sterile, nonpyrogenic solution for intravenous infusion—and 1000 mL of Dextrose injection with 10 mEq Calcium—a sterile, nonpyrogenic, hyertonic solution of Dextrose, USP in water for injection with added Calcium Chloride, USP dihydrate.

In brands with two chambers, the container must be used only after removing the clamp and thoroughly mixing the contents of the two chambers. Mixing the contents of the upper and lower chambers yields a concentrated source of Amino Acids and carbohydrate calories for intravenous infusion. The composition of this admixture is described in the table below.

SOLUTION COMPOSITION AMINO ACIDS WITH ELECTROLYTES
ESSENTIAL AMINO ACIDS (mg/100 mL)

	7% w/Electrolytes	8.5% w/Electrolytes	10% w/Electrolytes
Isoleucine	462	561	660
Leucine	700	850	1000
Lysine (acetate)*	735	893	1050
Methionine	120	146	172
Phenylalanine	209	253	298
Threonine	280	340	400
Tryptophan	140	170	200
Valine	350	425	500

* *Amount cited is for lysine alone and does not include the acetate salt.*

NONESSENTIAL AMINO ACIDS (mg/100 mL)

	7% w/Electrolytes	8.5% w/Electrolytes	10% w/Electrolytes
Alanine	695	844	993
Arginine	713	865	1018
Aspartic Acid	490	595	700
Glutamic Acid	517	627	738
Glycine	350	425	500
Histidine	210	255	300
Proline	505	614	722
Serine	371	450	530
N-Acetyl-L-Tyrosine	189	230	270

ELECTROLYTES (mEq/L)

	7% w/Electrolytes	8.5% w/Electrolytes	10% w/Electrolytes
Sodium[a] (Na^+)	80	84	94
Potassium (K^+)	66	66	66
Chloride (Cl^-)	86	86	86
Magnesium (Mg^{++})	10	10	10
Phosphorus (P)	30 mM	30 mM	30 mM
Acetate[b] ($C_2H_3O_2^-$)	50.3	61.1	71.8
Sodium Hydrosulfite ($Na_2S_2O_4$) added (mg/100 mL)	60	60	60
Other Characteristics			
Osmolarity (actual mOsm/L)	806	896	1081
pH	5.8	5.8	5.8
range	5.0-6.5	5.0-6.5	5.0-6.5

a   *Includes sodium from the pH adjustor, sodium hydroxide, and from the antioxidant, sodium hydrosulfite, where applicable.*
b   *From lysine acetate.*

LOWER CHAMBER COMPOSITION

Dextrose Injection w/Added Calcium	D50-W w/Ca^{++}	D40-W w/Ca^{++}
Dextrose, hydrous (g/100 mL)	50	40
Energy (kcal/100 mL)	170	136
Osmolarity (actual mOsm/L)	1916	1720
pH	4.3	4.3
range	3.5-6.5	3.5-6.5
Electrolytes (in mEq/L)		
Calcium (Ca^{++})	10	10
Chloride (Cl^-)	10	10

TOTAL COMPOSITION (2000 mL)
Essential Amino Acids (mg/100 mL)

	3.5% w/E in D25-W w/Ca^{++}	4.25% w/E in D20-W w/Ca^{++}	4.25% w/E in D25-W w/Ca^{++}	5% w/E in D25-W w/Ca^{++}
Isoleucine	231	280	280	330
Leucine	350	425	425	500
Lysine (acetate)*	368	446	446	525
Methionine	60	73	73	86
Phenylalanine	104	126	126	149
Threonine	140	170	170	200
Tryptophan	70	85	85	100
Valine	175	212	212	250

* *Amount cited is for lysine alone and does not include the acetate salt.*

Nonessential Amino Acids (mg/100 mL)

	3.5% w/E in D25-W w/ Ca^{++}	4.25% w/E in D20-W w/ Ca^{++}	4.25% w/E in D25-W w/ Ca^{++}	5% w/E in D25-W w/ Ca^{++}
Alanine	348	422	422	496
Arginine	356	432	432	509
Aspartic Acid	245	298	298	350
Glutamic Acid	258	314	314	369
Glycine	175	212	212	250
Histidine	105	128	128	150
Proline	252	307	307	361
Serine	186	225	225	265
N-Acetyl-L-Tyrosine	94	115	115	135

Electrolytes (mEq/L)

	3.5% w/E in D25-W w/Ca^{++}	4.25% w/E in D20-W w/Ca^{++}	4.25% w/E in D25-W w/Ca^{++}	5% w/E in D25-W w/Ca^{++}
Sodium[a] (Na$^+$)	40	42	42	47
Potassium (K$^+$)	33	33	33	33
Chloride (Cl$^-$)	48	48	48	48
Magnesium (Mg^{++})	5	5	5	5
Calcium (Ca^{++})	5	5	5	5
Phosphorus (P)	15 mM	15 mM	15 mM	15 mM
Acetate[b] (C$_2$H$_3$O$_2^-$)	25.2	30.6	30.6	35.9
Sodium Hydrosulfite (Na$_2$S$_2$O$_4$) added (mg/100 mL)	30	30	30	30
Other Characteristics				
Dextrose, hydrous (g/100 mL)	25	20	25	25
Osmolarity (actual mOsm/L)	1556	1353	1563	1645
pH	5.8	5.8	5.8	5.8
range	5.0-6.5	5.0-6.5	5.0-6.5	5.0-6.5
Total Amino Acids (g/L)	35	42.5	42.5	50
Protein Equivalent (g/L)	35	42.5	42.5	50
Total Nitrogen (g/L)	5.35	6.5	6.5	7.65

a Includes sodium from the pH adjustor, sodium hydroxide, and from the antioxidant, sodium hydrosulfite, where applicable.
b From lysine acetate.

The formulations contain the following added ingredients per 100 mL:
Sodium chloride, 205 mg; potassium chloride, 22.4 mg; calcium chloride, dihydrate, 36.8 mg; magnesium chloride, hexahydrate, 51 mg; potassium phosphate, dibasic, 261 mg; and sodium hydrosulfite added, 30 mg.
Sodium Chloride, USP is chemically designated NaCl, a white crystalline powder freely soluble in water.
Potassium Chloride, USP is chemically designated KCl, a white granular powder freely soluble in water.
Calcium Chloride, USP (dihydrate) is chemically designated CaCl$_2$ • 2H$_2$O, deliquescent white granules freely soluble in water.
Magnesium Chloride, USP (hexahydrate) is chemically designated MgCl$_2$ • 6H$_2$O, deliquescent crystals very soluble in water.
Dibasic Potassium Phosphate, USP (anhydrous) is chemically designated K$_2$HPO$_4$, white granules very soluble in water.
Dextrose, USP is chemically designated D-glucose, monohydrate (C$_6$H$_{12}$O$_6$ • H$_2$O), a hexose sugar freely soluble in water.
The formulas for the individual amino acids are as follows:

Essential Amino Acids

Isoleucine, USP	C$_6$H$_{13}$NO$_2$
Leucine, USP	C$_6$H$_{13}$NO$_2$
Lysine Acetate, USP	C$_6$H$_{14}$N$_2$O$_2$ • CH$_3$COOH
Methionine, USP	C$_5$H$_{11}$NO$_2$S
Phenylalanine, USP	C$_9$H$_{11}$NO$_2$
Threonine, USP	C$_4$H$_9$NO$_3$
Tryptophan, USP	C$_{11}$H$_{12}$N$_2$O$_2$
Valine, USP	C$_5$H$_{11}$NO$_2$

Nonessential Amino Acids

Alanine, USP	C$_3$H$_7$NO$_2$
Arginine, USP	C$_6$H$_{14}$N$_4$O$_2$
Aspartic Acid	C$_4$H$_7$NO$_4$
	HO$_2$CCH$_2$CH(NH$_2$)CO$_2$H
Glutamic Acid	C$_5$H$_9$NO$_4$
	HO$_2$CCH$_2$CH$_2$CH(NH$_2$)CO$_2$H
Glycine, USP	C$_2$H$_5$NO$_2$
Histidine, USP	C$_6$H$_9$N$_3$O$_2$
Proline, USP	C$_5$H$_9$NO$_2$
Serine, USP	C$_3$H$_7$NO$_3$
N-Acetyl-L-Tyrosine	C$_{11}$H$_{13}$NO$_4$

CLINICAL PHARMACOLOGY

Amino Acids/Calcium Chloride/Dextrose/Electrolytes provides carbohydrate calories and crystalline amino acids to stimulate protein synthesis, to limit protein catabolism, to minimize liver glycogen depletion and to promote wound healing. The infusion of this mixture through a central venous line should be considered to meet the protein and calorie requirements for patients receiving prolonged total parenteral nutrition. I.V. lipids may be infused simultaneously to provide adequate calories, if desired.

INDICATIONS AND USAGE

Amino Acids/Calcium Chloride/Dextrose/Electrolytes is indicated for central vein infusion in the prevention of nitrogen loss and negative nitrogen balance in cases where (a) the gastrointestinal tract by the oral, gastrostomy or jejunostomy route cannot or should not be used, (b) gastrointestinal absorption of nutrients is impaired or (c) metabolic requirements for protein and calories are substantially increased as with extensive burns and (d) morbidity and mortality may be reduced by replacing amino acids lost from tissue breakdown, thereby preserving tissue reserves, as in acute renal failure. In such patients intravenous feeding for more than a few days would be expected.

Supplemental Electrolytes, multivitamins and trace metals will be required in accordance with the prescription of the attending physician.

CONTRAINDICATIONS

This preparation should not be used in patients with hepatic coma or metabolic disorders involving impaired nitrogen utilization. These solutions are too concentrated for use in infants.

WARNINGS

Solutions of Amino Acids/Calcium Chloride/Dextrose/Electrolytes in Dextrose with a final concentration of 20% or 25% are hypertonic and may not be administered by peripheral vein.

Concentrated Dextrose solutions, if administered too rapidly, may result in significant hyperglycemia and possible hyperosmolar syndrome, characterized by mental confusion and loss of consciousness.

Intravenous infusion of Amino Acids may induce a rise in blood urea nitrogen (BUN), especially in patients with impaired hepatic or renal function. Appropriate laboratory tests should be performed periodically and infusion discontinued if BUN levels exceed normal postprandial limits and continue to rise. It should be noted that a modest rise in BUN normally occurs as a result of increased protein intake.

Administration of Amino Acid solutions to a patient with hepatic insufficiency may result in serum amino acid imbalances, metabolic alkalosis, prerenal azotemia, hyperammonemia, stupor and coma.

Administration of Amino Acid solutions in the presence of impaired renal function may augment an increasing BUN, as does any protein dietary component.

Solutions containing sodium ion should be used with great care, if at all, in patients with congestive heart failure, severe renal insufficiency and in clinical states in which there exists edema with sodium retention.

Solutions containing potassium ions should be used with great care, if at all, in patients with hyperkalemia, severe renal failure and in conditions in which potassium retention is present.

Solutions containing acetate ion should be used with great care in patients with metabolic or respiratory alkalosis. Acetate should be administered with great care in those conditions in which there is an increased level or an impaired utilization of this ion, such as severe hepatic insufficiency.

Some brands of Amino Acids/Calcium Chloride/Dextrose/Electrolytes contain sodium hydrosulfite, a sulfite that may cause allergic-type reactions including anaphylactic symptoms and life-threatening or less severe asthmatic episodes in certain susceptible people. The overall prevalence of sulfite sensitivity in the general population is unknown and probably low. Sulfite sensitivity is seen more frequently in asthmatic than in nonasthmatic people.

Amino Acids/Calcium Chloride/Dextrose/Electrolytes with an Amino Acid concentration greater than 2.5% are too concentrated for administration to infants.

Instances of asymptomatic hyperammonemia have been reported in patients without overt liver dysfunction. The mechanisms of this reaction are not clearly defined, but may involve genetic defects and immature or subclinically impaired liver function.

PRECAUTIONS

Special care must be taken when administering concentrated glucose to diabetic or prediabetic patients. To control and minimize hyperglycemia and consequent glycosuria, it is desirable to monitor blood and urine glucose and, if necessary, add insulin.

Because of its antianabolic activity, concurrent administration of tetracycline may reduce the nitrogen sparing effects of infused amino acids.

Intravenously administered amino acids should be used with caution in patients with history of renal disease, pulmonary disease, or with cardiac insufficiency so as to avoid excessive fluid accumulation.

Nitrogen intake should be carefully monitored in patients with impaired renal function.

Amino Acids/Calcium Chloride/Dextrose/Electrolytes in 20% or 25% Dextrose are indicated for long-term total parenteral nutrition and whenever it is essential

---

◆ RATED THERAPEUTICALLY EQUIVALENT; ◇ THERAPEUTIC EQUIVALENCE UNCONFIRMED; ○ UNRATED

to provide, together with amino acids, adequate amounts of exogenous calories. Concentrated Dextrose is an effective source of such calories. Such strongly hypertonic nutrient solutions should be administered only through an indwelling catheter with the tip located in a large vein; i.e., the superior vena cava.

SPECIAL PRECAUTIONS FOR CENTRAL INFUSIONS
ADMINISTRATION BY CENTRAL VENOUS CATHETER SHOULD BE USED ONLY BY THOSE FAMILIAR WITH THIS TECHNIQUE AND ITS COMPLICATIONS.

Central vein infusion of nutrient solutions requires a knowledge of nutrition as well as clinical expertise in recognition and treatment of complications. Attention must be given to solution preparation, administration and patient monitoring. *It is essential that a carefully prepared protocol based on current medical practices be followed, preferably by an experienced team.*

SUMMARY HIGHLIGHTS OF COMPLICATIONS
(See also Current Medical Literature).

1. Technical: The placement of a central venous catheter should be regarded as a surgical procedure. One should be fully acquainted with various techniques of catheter insertion. For details of technique and placement sites, consult the medical literature. X-ray is the best means of verifying catheter placement. Complications known to occur from the placement of central venous catheters are pneumothorax, hemothorax, hydrothorax, artery puncture and transection, injury to the brachial plexus, malposition of the catheter, formation of arteriovenous fistula, phlebitis, thrombosis and air and catheter emboli.

2. Septic: The constant risk of sepsis is present during administration of total parenteral nutrition. It is imperative that the preparation of the solution and the placement and care of catheters be accomplished under strict aseptic conditions.

Solutions should be used promptly after mixing. Storage should be under refrigeration and limited to a brief period of time, preferably less than 24 hours.

Administration time for a single container and set should never exceed 24 hours.

3. Metabolic: The following metabolic complications have been reported: metabolic acidosis and alkalosis, hypophosphatemia, hypocalcemia, osteoporosis, hyperglycemia, hyperosmolar nonketotic states and dehydration, glycosuria, rebound hypoglycemia, osmotic diuresis and dehydration, elevated liver enzymes, hypo- and hypervitaminosis, electrolyte imbalances and hyperammonemia in children. Frequent evaluations are necessary especially during the first few days of therapy to prevent or minimize these complications.

Administration of glucose at a rate exceeding the patient's utilization rate may lead to hyperglycemia, coma and death.

Pregnancy Category C. Animal reproduction studies have not been conducted with Amino Acids/Calcium Chloride/Dextrose/Electrolytes. It is not known whether this admixture can cause fetal harm when administered to a pregnant woman or can affect reproductive capacity. Amino Acids/Calcium/Dextrose/Electrolytes should be given to pregnant women only if clearly needed. Not for use in infants. See *"Warnings"* and *"Dosage and Administration"*.

Clinical evaluation and laboratory determinations, at the discretion of the attending physician, are necessary for proper monitoring during administration. Do not withdraw venous blood for blood chemistries through the infusion site, as interference with estimations of nitrogen-containing substances may occur. Blood studies should include glucose, urea nitrogen, serum electrolytes, ammonia, triglycerides, acid-base balance, serum proteins, kidney and liver function tests, osmolarity and hemogram. White blood count and blood cultures are to be determined if indicated. Urinary osmolality and glucose should be determined as necessary.

Do not use unless the solutions are clear and container is undamaged. Discard unused portion.

ADVERSE REACTIONS
Hyperosmolar syndrome, resulting from excessively rapid administration of concentrated dextrose may cause mental confusion and/or loss of consciousness.

Reactions which may occur because of the solution or the technique of administration include febrile response, infection at the site of injection, venous thrombosis or phlebitis extending from the site of injection, extravasation and hypervolemia.

Generalized flushing, fever and nausea also have been reported during peripheral infusions of amino acid solutions. Also see *"Warnings"* and *"Precautions"*.

If an adverse reaction does occur, discontinue the infusion, evaluate the patient, institute appropriate therapeutic countermeasures and save the remainder of the fluid for examination if deemed necessary.

OVERDOSAGE
In the event of overhydration or solute overload, re-evaluate the patient and institute appropriate corrective measures. See *"Warnings"* and *"Precautions"*.

DOSAGE AND ADMINISTRATION
The total daily dose of Amino Acids/Calcium Chloride/Dextrose/Electrolytes to be infused depends on daily protein and caloric requirements and on the patient's metabolic and clinical response. In many patients, provision of adequate calories in the form of hypertonic dextrose may require the administration of exogenous insulin to prevent hyperglycemia and glycosuria. To prevent rebound hyperglyce-

mia, a solution containing 5% Dextrose should be administered when hypertonic Dextrose infusions are abruptly discontinued.

As with all intravenous fluid therapy, the parenteral administration of a solution of Amino Acids and Dextrose requires an accurate estimate of the total fluid and Electrolytes needed to compensate for the patient's measurable urinary and other (i.e., nasogastric suction, fistula drainage, diarrhea) daily losses. After estimating the total daily fluid (water) requirements, the appropriate volume to be infused to meet the daily protein requirement of the patient, can be determined. The daily determination of nitrogen balance and accurate body weights, corrected for fluid balance, are probably the best means of assessing individual protein requirements. The balance of fluid needed beyond the volume of the Amino Acid/Dextrose solution can be provided by other solutions suitable for intravenous infusion. I.V. lipid emulsions may also be infused to deliver additional calories if required. Lipid emulsion can be administered to provide up to 3 g fat/kg/day, infused simultaneously with Amino Acids/Calcium Chloride/Dextrose/Electrolytes by means of a Y-connector located near the infusion site, using separate flow controls for each solution. Amino/Acids/Calcium Chloride/Dextrose/Electrolytes may also be premixed in the same container with lipid emulsion. See *"Instructions for Use"*. Vitamins and trace minerals may be prescribed as needed.

Parenteral drug products should be inspected visually for particulate matter and discoloration prior to administration, whenever solution and container permit.

ADULT PATIENTS
The daily nutrient requirements of an average adult patient, not hypermetabolic, in an acceptable weight range and with restricted physical activity, are about 30 kcal/kg of body weight, 12 to 18 grams of nitrogen (or 1.0 to 1.5 g amino acids/kg/day) and between 2500 and 3000 mL of fluids. In depleted and severely traumatized patients such as burned patients or patients who have received major surgery with complications, the requirements for nutrients and fluids may be significantly higher. In such cases, 4000 calories and 25 grams of nitrogen or more may be required daily to achieve nitrogen balance. The fluid losses through drainages and wound surface must be taken into account in calculating the fluid requirements of these patients.

Fat emulsion administration should be considered when prolonged parenteral nutrition is required in order to prevent essential fatty acid deficiency (EFAD). Serum lipids should be monitored for evidence of EFAD in patients maintained on fat-free TPN.

The infusion rate for central vein admixtures of Amino Acids/Calcium/Dextrose/Electrolytes should be 2 mL/min initially and may be gradually increased to deliver the required amounts of Amino Acids and calories. If nutrient administration falls behind schedule, under no circumstances should an attempt to "catch up" to planned intake be made. The rate of nutrient infusion is governed by the protein requirements and by the patient's glucose tolerance estimated by glucose levels in plasma and urine. The maximum rate at which dextrose can be infused without producing glycosuria is 0.5 g/kg/hour; at a rate of 0.8 g/kg/hour, about 95% of the infused Dextrose is retained. Administration of exogenous insulin may be required in order to control hyperglycemia and glycosuria which may occur upon infusion of concentrated glucose solutions. When concentrated Dextrose infusion is abruptly interrupted rebound hypoglycemia may occur, which can be prevented by the administration of 5% or 10% Dextrose solutions. Part of the caloric requirements may be met by the infusion of IV fat emulsions.

Serum Electrolytes Should Be Monitored as Indicated: Electrolytes should be added to the nutrient solution as indicated by the patient's clinical condition and laboratory determinations of plasma values. Major electrolytes are sodium, chloride, potassium, phosphate, magnesium and calcium. All of the aforementioned electrolytes are contained in the Amino Acids/Calcium Chloride/Dextrose/Electrolytes. Supplemental electrolyte additives may be used at the clinician's discretion.

Vitamins, including folic acid and vitamin K, are required. Vitamin K_1 (Phytonadione Injection, USP) is given intramuscularly or intravenously. The trace element supplements should be given when long-term parenteral nutrition is undertaken. Iron is given intramuscularly in depot form or intravenously as indicated.

In patients with hyperchloremic or other metabolic acidosis, supplemental sodium and potassium may be added as the acetate or lactate salts to provide bicarbonate alternates.

In adults, hypertonic mixtures of Amino Acids and Dextrose may be safely administered by continuous infusion through a central venous catheter with the tip located in the vena cava.

PEDIATRIC PATIENTS
Pediatric requirements for parenteral nutrition are constrained by the greater relative fluid requirements of the child and greater caloric requirements per kilogram. These solutions are too concentrated for use in infants, but older pediatric patients can tolerate Amino Acids in concentrations of up to 5%. Dosage is usually prescribed on a g/kg body weight/day basis and patient age as follows: ages 1 to 3 years, 2 to 2.5 g/kg/day; ages 4 to 12 years, 2 g/kg/day; ages 13 to 15 years, 1.7 g/kg/day; ages 16 and above, 1.5 g/kg/day. Energy requirements for children between 1 and 7 years of age are approximately 75 to 90 kcal/kg/day; for children 7 to 12 years of age, 60 to 75 kcal/kg/day; and for ages 12 to 18 years, 30 to 60 kcal/kg/day. Energy intake may be supplemented with intravenous fat emulsion. In cases of malnutrition or stress, these requirements may be increased.

Supplemental Electrolytes and vitamins should be administered as deemed necessary by careful monitoring of blood chemistries and nutritional status. Iron supplementation is more critical in the child than the adult because of the increasing red cell mass required by the growing child. Serum lipids should be monitored for evidence of essential fatty acid deficiency in patients maintained on fat-free TPN. Bicarbonate should not be administered during infusion of the nutritional solution unless deemed absolutely necessary.

To ensure the precise delivery of the small volumes of fluid necessary for total parenteral nutrition in children, accurately calibrated and reliable infusion systems should be used.

Following admixture and/or storage, the contents should be administered within 24 hours.

DRUG INTERACTIONS

Additives may be incompatible. Consult with pharmacist, if available. When introducing additives use aseptic technique, mix thoroughly and do not store.

STORAGE

Exposure of pharmaceutical products to heat should be minimized. Avoid excessive heat. Protect from freezing. It is recommended that the product be stored at room temperature (25° C); however, brief exposure up to 40° C does not adversely affect the product.

Avoid exposure to light.

HOW SUPPLIED

AMINO ACIDS
INJECTION: 3.5%

BRAND/MANUFACTURER	NDC	SIZE	AWP
○ **BRAND**			
AMINOSYN: Abbott Hosp	00074-2989-05	1000 ml 6s	$341.79
	00074-4154-05	1000 ml 6s	$357.68
AMINOSYN II W/5% DEXTROSE: Abbott Hosp	00074-7701-29	1000 ml 6s	$525.04
	00074-7740-29	1000 ml 6s	$551.33
AMINOSYN II W/25% DEXTROSE: Abbott Hosp	00074-7700-29	1000 ml 6s	$585.53
AMINOSYN II: Abbott Hosp	00074-1083-05	1000 ml 6s	$610.47

INJECTION: 4%

BRAND/MANUFACTURER	NDC	SIZE	AWP
○ **BRAND**			
BRANCHAMIN: Clintec	00338-0477-03	500 ml 18s	$1684.80

INJECTION: 4.25%

BRAND/MANUFACTURER	NDC	SIZE	AWP
○ **BRAND**			
AMINOSYN II W/10% DEXTROSE: Abbott Hosp	00074-7751-29	1000 ml 6s	$597.65
AMINOSYN II W/20% DEXTROSE: Abbott Hosp	00074-7752-29	1000 ml 6s	$603.06
AMINOSYN II W/5% DEXTROSE: Abbott Hosp	00074-7702-29	1000 ml 6s	$607.41
AMINOSYN II W/10% DEXTROSE: Abbott Hosp	00074-7742-29	1000 ml 6s	$626.29

INJECTION: 5%

BRAND/MANUFACTURER	NDC	SIZE	AWP
○ **BRAND**			
AMINOSYN II: Abbott Hosp	00074-2990-05	1000 ml 6s	$610.47
AMINOSYN II W/25% DEXTROSE: Abbott Hosp	00074-7744-29	1000 ml 6s	$693.19
AMINOSYN: Abbott Hosp	00074-2990-03	500 ml 12s	$624.01

INJECTION: 5.2%

BRAND/MANUFACTURER	NDC	SIZE	AWP
○ **BRAND**			
AMINESS: Clintec	00338-0488-17	400 ml 10s	$1073.52
AMINOSYN-RF: Abbott Hosp	00074-4072-02	300 ml 12s	$1094.26

INJECTION: 5.5%

BRAND/MANUFACTURER	NDC	SIZE	AWP
○ **BRAND**			
TRAVASOL 5.5%: Clintec	00338-0623-04	1000 ml 6s	$549.24
	00338-0623-06	2000 ml 6s	$672.06
	00338-0623-03	500 ml 12s	$549.23

INJECTION: 6.5%

BRAND/MANUFACTURER	NDC	SIZE	AWP
○ **BRAND**			
RENAMIN: Clintec	00338-0471-03	500 ml 6s	$1800.00
	00338-0471-02	250 ml 12s	$900.00

INJECTION: 7%

BRAND/MANUFACTURER	NDC	SIZE	AWP
○ **BRAND**			
AMINOSYN: Abbott Hosp	00074-2996-01	500 ml 3s	$293.84
AMINOSYN HBC 7%: Abbott Hosp	00074-1108-05	1000 ml 6s	$885.92
AMINOSYN-PF 7%: Abbott Hosp	00074-1616-02	250 ml 12s	$641.54
AMINOSYN: Abbott Hosp	00074-2992-03	500 ml 12s	$843.46
AMINOSYN II: Abbott Hosp	00074-1086-03	500 ml 12s	$843.46
AMINOSYN-PF 7%: Abbott Hosp	00074-1616-03	500 ml 12s	$855.86
AMINOSYN HBC 7%: Abbott Hosp	00074-1108-03	500 ml 12s	$885.64

INJECTION: 8.5%

BRAND/MANUFACTURER	NDC	SIZE	AWP
○ **BRAND**			
FREAMINE III: McGaw	00264-1903-10	500 ml	$72.20
	00264-1903-00	1000 ml	$144.55
AMINOSYN: Abbott Hosp	00074-4041-01	500 ml 3s	$308.73
TRAVASOL 8.5%: Clintec	00338-0625-04	1000 ml 6s	$877.32
AMINOSYN II: Abbott Hosp	00074-5855-05	1000 ml 6s	$894.26
TRAVASOL 8.5%: Clintec	00338-0625-06	2000 ml 6s	$889.56
	00338-0625-03	500 ml 12s	$877.10
AMINOSYN: Abbott Hosp	00074-5855-03	500 ml 12s	$894.05
AMINOSYN II: Abbott Hosp	00074-1088-03	500 ml 12s	$894.05

INJECTION: 10%

BRAND/MANUFACTURER	NDC	SIZE	AWP
○ **BRAND**			
FREAMINE III: McGaw	00264-1901-10	500 ml	$82.34
	00264-1901-00	1000 ml	$158.23
AMINOSYN: Abbott Hosp	00074-4360-05	1000 ml	$607.92
TRAVASOL 10%: Clintec	00338-0629-04	1000 ml 6s	$1000.80
AMINOSYN-PF 10%: Abbott Hosp	00074-1617-05	1000 ml 6s	$1012.25
AMINOSYN: Abbott Hosp	00074-2991-05	1000 ml 6s	$1020.09
AMINOSYN II: Abbott Hosp	00074-1090-05	1000 ml 6s	$1020.09
TRAVASOL 10%: Clintec	00338-0629-06	2000 ml 6s	$2001.67
AMINOSYN: Abbott Hosp	00074-7121-07	2000 ml 6s	$2040.24
TRAVASOL 10%: Clintec	00338-0629-02	250 ml 12s	$347.88
	00338-0629-03	500 ml 12s	$1001.23
AMINOSYN: Abbott Hosp	00074-2991-03	500 ml 12s	$1020.59
AMINOSYN II: Abbott Hosp	00074-1090-03	500 ml 12s	$1020.59

INJECTION: 11.4%

BRAND/MANUFACTURER	NDC	SIZE	AWP
○ **BRAND**			
NOVAMINE: Clintec	00338-0489-04	1000 ml 6s	$1095.94
	00338-0489-03	500 ml 10s	$951.35

INJECTION: 15%

BRAND/MANUFACTURER	NDC	SIZE	AWP
○ **BRAND**			
NOVAMINE: Clintec	00338-0498-06	2000 ml 4s	$1980.00
	00338-0494-04	1000 ml 6s	$1405.02
AMINOSYN II: Abbott Hosp	00074-7122-07	2000 ml 6s	$3060.33
NOVAMINE: Clintec	00338-0494-03	500 ml 10s	$1123.20

KIT: 8.5%

BRAND/MANUFACTURER	NDC	SIZE	AWP
○ **BRAND**			
TRAVASOL 8.5%: Clintec	00338-0653-98	3s	$134.07

AMINO ACIDS/DEXTROSE/ELECTROLYTES
INJECTION:

BRAND/MANUFACTURER	NDC	SIZE	AWP
○ **BRAND**			
AMINOSYN II 3.5% W/ELEC, 25% DEX W/CALC: Abbott Hosp	00074-7756-29	1000 ml 6s	$636.19
AMINOSYN II 4.25% W/ELEC, 20% DEX W/CALC: Abbott Hosp	00074-7753-29	1000 ml 6s	$639.83
AMINOSYN II 4.25% W/ELEC, 25% DEX W/CALC: Abbott Hosp	00074-7757-29	1000 ml 6s	$659.42

KIT:

BRAND/MANUFACTURER	NDC	SIZE	AWP
○ **BRAND**			
TRAVASOL: Clintec	00338-0783-98	3s	$232.99
	00338-0785-98	3s	$253.68
	00338-0787-98	3s	$302.61
	00338-0789-98	3s	$323.42
	00338-0626-03	500 gm 6s	$478.32
	00338-0644-03	500 gm 6s	$503.93
TRAVASOL 10%: Clintec	00338-0644-06	2000 gm 6s	$2001.67

◆ RATED THERAPEUTICALLY EQUIVALENT; ◇ THERAPEUTIC EQUIVALENCE UNCONFIRMED; ○ UNRATED

9-Aminoacridine Hydrochloride/ Polyoxyethylene Nonyl Phenol/ Sodium Dioctyl Sulfosuccinate/ Sodium Edetate

DESCRIPTION

9-Aminoacridine/Polyoxyethylene Nonyl Phenol/Sodium Dioctyl Sulfosuccinate/ Sodium Edetate suppositories contain a combination of trichomonacidal and bactericidal agents and provide continued medication by gradual liquefaction.

Each vaginal suppository contains:

9-Aminoacridine Hydrochloride	6.00 mg
Polyoxyethylene Nonyl Phenol	5.25 mg
Sodium Edetate	0.66 mg
Sodium Dioctyl Sulfosuccinate	0.07 mg

in a polyethylene glycol base containing glycerin and citric acid.

Medicated Douche Liquid Concentrate contains a combination of Polyoxyethylene Nonyl Phenol, Sodium Edetate and Sodium Dioctyl Sulfosuccinate, a complex proven to be an effective trichomonacide when used as a vaginal douche.

CLINICAL PHARMACOLOGY

9-Aminoacridine is a broad-spectrum anti-infective of extensive medical acceptance for the topical treatment of bacterial infections. The combination of Polyoxyethylene Nonyl Phenol, Sodium Edetate, and Sodium Dioctyl Sulfosuccinate is a trichomonacide which when in solution and diluted disintegrates the flagellates through marked changes in surface tension.

INDICATIONS AND USAGE

The liquid/suppository regimen is indicated for the specific treatment, in adults, of vaginitis, as evidenced by pruritus, malodorous leukorrhea, erythema of the vaginal mucosa, dyspareunia, caused by Trichomonas vaginalis and mixed vaginal infections complicated by bacterial moiety.

The presence of trichomonads can be established by a hanging drop mount preparation of the discharge from the posterior fornix and confirmed by cultures grown on STS medium; the atypical bacterial moiety can be identified by examination of gram-stained preparations of smeared vaginal secretions.

CONTRAINDICATIONS

Douching is not recommended during pregnancy. The medicated douche and suppositories are spermicidal and should not be used when the patient is trying to conceive.

PRECAUTIONS

General: The full course of therapy must be completed to eliminate the infecting micro-organisms from the vagina. It is generally desirable to continue treatment through the menses in order to guard against potential flare-ups since the presence of blood favors the rapid growth of Trichomonas. Recurrence of vaginitis often indicates extravaginal foci or infection in cervical, vestibular and urethral glands, etc. or reinfection by the sexual partner.

Information for Patients: During treatment, patient should refrain from intercourse, or the partner should wear a prophylactic. To prevent flare-ups after completion of therapy and for continued vaginal cleanliness, the patient is advised to continue with the liquid as a regular douche, but no more than twice weekly unless otherwise directed by physician.

Laboratory Tests: No patient should be considered cured until cultures on STS medium and gram-stained preparations of smeared vaginal secretions, taken at monthly intervals for 3 months following treatment, show absence of trichomonads and a return to the normal vaginal bacterial flora.

ADVERSE REACTIONS

No significant reactions have been reported to date for the suppositories or liquid. Any minor irritation is generally relieved by discontinuance of douche for 24 hours.

OVERDOSAGE

Antidote: Copious use of water. The dilute solution is nontoxic.

DOSAGE & ADMINISTRATION

Office Treatment (Adult): For the treatment of vaginal trichomoniasis and mixed vaginal infections, best results are obtained by scrubbing the vagina with the liquid, diluted 1:100 by the physician in the office; 3 scrubs the first week, 2 the second. A suppository is inserted after each office scrub in the liquid/suppository regimen. Patient should be instructed to continue treatment at home.

Home Treatment: The combination douche and suppositories (liquid/suppository regimen) is recommended for home use. The usual daily home treatment is medicated douche in the morning, followed by a suppository inserted deep in the vagina, using the tip of finger, and a second suppository inserted in like manner at bedtime for a period of 14 days. Treatment should be omitted the night and morning preceding an office visit. In chronic or stubborn cases, therapy may be repeated with no interval between courses. The liquid/suppository regimen may be continued throughout the menstrual cycle. It is advisable to continue treatment through two menstrual periods. Patients should be reexamined 3 days after home treatment has been discontinued.

The full course of therapy must be completed to eliminate the infecting micro-organisms from the vagina. No patient should be considered cured until vaginal smears or cultures, taken at monthly intervals for 3 months following treatment, show absence of trichomonads and a return to the normal vaginal flora.

HOW SUPPLIED
SUPPOSITORY:

BRAND/MANUFACTURER	NDC	SIZE	AWP
○ BRAND			
VAGISEC PLUS: Schmid	00234-0810-00	28s doz	$179.55

Amino-Cerv *SEE* **AMINO ACID AND UREA CREAM**

Aminobenzoate Potassium

DESCRIPTION

This member of the vitamin B complex is chemically Aminobenzoate Potassium, U.S.P.

> ## INDICATIONS
>
> BASED ON A REVIEW OF THIS DRUG BY THE NATIONAL ACADEMY OF SCIENCES-NATIONAL RESEARCH COUNCIL AND/OR OTHER INFORMATION, FDA HAS CLASSIFIED THE INDICATIONS AS FOLLOWS:
> "POSSIBLY" EFFECTIVE: AMINOBENZOATE POTASSIUM IS POSSIBLY EFFECTIVE IN THE TREATMENT OF SCLERODERMA, DERMATOMYOSITIS, MORPHEA, LINEAR SCLERODERMA, PEMPHIGUS, AND PEYRONIE'S DISEASE.
> FINAL CLASSIFICATION OF THE LESS-THAN-EFFECTIVE INDICATIONS REQUIRES FURTHER INVESTIGATION.

Aminobenzoate Potassium offers a means of treatment of serious and often chronic entities involving fibrosis and nonsuppurative inflammation.

PHARMACOLOGY

P-Aminobenzoate is considered a member of the vitamin B complex. Small amounts are found in cereal, eggs, milk and meats. Detectable amounts are normally present in human blood, spinal fluid, urine, and sweat. PABA is a component of several biologically important systems, and it participates in a number of fundamental biological processes. It has been suggested that the antifibrosis action of Aminobenzoate Potassium is due to its mediation of increased oxygen uptake at the tissue level. Fibrosis is believed to occur from either too much serotonin or too little monoamine oxidase activity over a period of time. Monoamine oxidase requires an adequate supply of oxygen to function properly. By increasing oxygen supply at the tissue level Aminobenzoate Potassium may enhance MAO activity and prevent or bring about regression of fibrosis.

CLINICAL USES

Peyronies Disease: 21 patients with Peyronie's disease were placed on Aminobenzoate Potassium therapy for periods ranging from 3 months to 2 years. Pain disappeared from 16 of 16 cases in which it had been present. There was objective improvement in penile deformity in 10 of 17 patients, and decrease in plaque size in 16 of 21. The authors suggest that this medication offers no hazard of further local injury as may result from other therapy. There were no significant untoward effects encountered on long term Aminobenzoate Potassium therapy.

Scleroderma: Of 135 patients with diffuse systemic sclerosis treated with Aminobenzoate Potassium every patient but one has shown softening of the involved skin if treatment has been continued for 3 months or longer. The responses have been reported in a number of publications. The treatment program consists of systemic antifibrosis therapy with Aminobenzoate Potassium, physical therapy, including deep breathing exercises and dynamic traction splints where indicated, and bethanechol chloride for relief of dysphagia as well as small doses of reserpine for amelioration of Raynaud's phenomena.

Dermatomyositis: Five patients with scleroderma and 2 with dermatomyositis were treated with Aminobenzoate Potassium. There was striking clinical improvement in each patient. Doses of 15-20 grams per day were well tolerated, and patients were easily able to take these doses.

Morphea and Linear Scleroderma: All 14 patients with localized forms of scleroderma placed on longterm Aminobenzoate Potassium treatment showed

➤ SHOWN IN PRODUCT IDENTIFICATION GUIDE

softening of the sclerotic component of their disorder. Treatment is particularly indicated in patients where persistent compressive sclerosis may contribute even greater disfigurement or functional embarrassment from secondary pressure atrophy.

CONTRAINDICATIONS

Aminobenzoate Potassium should not be administered to patients taking sulfonamides.

PRECAUTIONS

Should anorexia or nausea occur, therapy is interrupted until the patient is eating normally again. This permits prompt subsidence of symptoms and also avoids the possible development of hypoglycemia. Give cautiously to patients with renal disease. If a hypersensitivity reaction should occur, Aminobenzoate Potassium should be stopped.

USAGE IN PREGNANCY
Safety for use in pregnancy or during lactation has not been established.

SIDE EFFECTS

Anorexia, nausea, fever and rash have occurred infrequently and subside with omission of the drug. Often, desensitization can be accomplished and treatment resumed.

DOSAGE AND ADMINISTRATION

The average adult daily dose of Aminobenzoate Potassium is 12 grams, usually given in four to six divided doses. Tablets and capsules 0.5 gram are given at the rate of 4 tablets or capsules 6 times daily, or 6 given four times daily, usually with meals, and at bed-time with a snack. Tablets must be dissolved in an adequate amount of liquid to prevent gastrointestinal upset.

Aminobenzoate Potassium Packets contain 2 grams pure drug each, and 6 Packets are given for a total of 12 grams Aminobenzoate Potassium daily.

Aminobenzoate Potassium Powder is used to prepare solutions, which are kept refrigerated, but for no longer than one week. 100 grams Aminobenzoate Potassium powder make 1 quart of 10% solution when dissolved in potable tap water. Children are given 1 gram Aminobenzoate Potassium daily in divided doses for each 10 lbs. of body weight.

HOW SUPPLIED
CAPSULE: 0.5 GM

BRAND/MANUFACTURER	NDC	SIZE	AWP
○ BRAND			
POTABA: Glenwood	00516-0051-25	250s	$55.27
	00516-0051-10	1000s	$204.96

CAPSULE: 2 GM

BRAND/MANUFACTURER	NDC	SIZE	AWP
○ BRAND			
POTABA: Glenwood	00516-0052-50	50s	$41.41

POWDER:

BRAND/MANUFACTURER	NDC	SIZE	AWP
○ BRAND			
POTABA: Glenwood	00516-0053-01	100 gm	$43.34
	00516-0053-16	454 gm	$146.00

TABLETS: 0.5 GM

BRAND/MANUFACTURER	NDC	SIZE	AWP
○ BRAND			
POTABA: Glenwood	00516-0054-01	100s	$23.38
	00516-0054-10	1000s	$196.40

Aminocaproic Acid

DESCRIPTION

Aminocaproic Acid is 6-aminohexanoic acid, which acts as an inhibitor of fibrinolysis.

Its chemical formula is $C_6H_{13}NO_2$. Its molecular weight is 131.7

Aminocaproic Acid is soluble in water, acids, and alkalies: it is sparingly soluble in methanol and practically insoluble in chloroform.

Aminocaproic Acid injection for intravenous administration, is a sterile pyrogen free solution containing 250 mg/mL of Aminocaproic Acid with Benzyl Alcohol 0.9% as preservative and Water for Injection qs 100%. Hydrochloric acid may be added to adjust pH to approximately 6.8 during manufacture.

Aminocaproic Acid syrup 25%, for oral administration, contains 250 mg/mL of Aminocaproic Acid with potassium sorbate 0.2% and sodium benzoate 0.1% as preservatives.

Each Aminocaproic Acid Tablet, for oral administration, contains 500 mg of Aminocaproic Acid.

Following is its chemical structure:

$$H_2C(CH_2)_3CH_2COOH$$
$$NH_2$$

CLINICAL PHARMACOLOGY

The fibrinolysis-inhibitory effects of Aminocaproic Acid appear to be exerted principally via inhibition of plasminogen activators and to a lesser degree through antiplasmin activity.

In adults, oral absorption appears to be a zero-order process with an absorption rate of 5.2 g/hr. The mean lag time in absorption is 10 minutes. After a single oral dose of 5 g, absorption was complete (F=1). Mean ± SD peak plasma concentrations (164 ± 28 mcg/mL) were reached within 1.2 ± 0.45 hours.

After oral administration, the apparent volume of distribution was estimated to be 23.1 ± 6.6 L (mean ± SD). Correspondingly, the volume of distribution after intravenous administration has been reported to be 30.0 ± 8.2 L. After prolonged administration, Amicocaproic Acid has been found to distribute throughout extravascular and intravascular compartments of the body, penetrating human red blood cells as well as other tissue cells.

Renal excretion is the primary route of elimination, whether Aminocaproic Acid is administered orally or intravenously. Sixty-five percent of the dose is recovered in the urine as unchanged drug and 11% of the dose appears as the metabolite adipic acid. Renal clearance (116 mL/min) approximates endogenous creatinine clearance. The total body clearance is 169 mL/min. The terminal elimination half-life for Aminocaproic Acid is approximately 2 hours.

INDICATIONS AND USAGE

Aminocaproic Acid iss useful in enhancing hemostasis when fibrinolysis contributes to bleeding. In life-threatening situations, fresh whole blood transfusions, fibrinogen infusions, and other emergency measures may be required.

Fibrinolytic bleeding may frequently be associated with surgical complications following heart surgery (with or without cardiac bypass procedures) and portacaval shunt; hematological disorders such as aplastic anemia, abruptio placentae, hepatic cirrhosis, neoplastic disease such as carcinoma of the prostate, lung, stomach, and cervix.

Urinary fibrinolysis, usually a normal physiological phenomenon, may frequently be associated with life-threatening complications following severe trauma, anoxia, and shock. Symptomatic of such complications is surgical hematuria (following prostatectomy and nephrectomy) or nonsurgical hematuria (accompanying polycystic or neoplastic diseases of the genitourinary system). (See "Warnings".)

UNLABELED USES
Aminocaproic Acid is used alone or as an adjunct in the treatment of hereditary angioedema, Kasabach Merritt syndrome, menorrhagia, hematuria induced by sickle cell hemoglobinopathy. It is also used in streptokinase overdose, amegakarycytic thrombocytopenia, and prophylaxis against the occurrence of secondary hemorrhage following traumatic hyphema. Aminocaproic Acid is also prescribed to prevent rebleeding from ruptured aneurysms in subarachnoid hemorrhage.

CONTRAINDICATIONS

Aminocaproic Acid should not be used when there is evidence of an active intravascular clotting process.

When there is uncertainty as to whether the cause of bleeding is primary fibrinolysis or disseminated intravascular coagulation (DIC), this distinction must be made before administering Aminocaproic Acid.

The following tests can be applied to differentiate the two conditions:

■ Platelet count is usually decreased in DIC but normal in primary fibrinolysis.
■ Protamine paracoagulation test is positive in DIC; a precipitate forms when protamine sulphate is dropped into citrated plasma. The test is negative in the presence of primary fibrinolysis.
■ The euglobulin clot lysis test is abnormal in primary fibrinolysis but normal in DIC.

Aminocaproic Acid must not be used in the presence of DIC without concomitant heparin.

WARNINGS

In patients with upper urinary tract bleeding, Aminocaproic Acid administration has been known to cause intrarenal obstruction in the form of glomerular capillary thrombosis, or clots in the renal pelvis and ureters. For this reason, Aminocaproic Acid should not be used in hematuria of upper urinary tract origin, unless the possible benefits outweigh the risk.

Subendocardial hemorrhages have been observed in dogs given intravenous infusions of 0.2 times the maximum human therapeutic dose of Aminocaproic Acid and in monkeys given eight times the maximum human therapeutic dose of Aminocaproic Acid.

Fatty degeneration of the myocardium has been reported in dogs given intravenous doses of Aminocaproic Acid at 0.8 to 3.3 times the maximum human therapeutic dose and in monkeys given intravenous doses of Aminocaproic Acid at six times the maximum human therapeutic dose.

Rarely, skeletal muscle weakness with necrosis of muscle fibers has been reported following prolonged administration. Clinical presentation may range from mild myalgias with weakness and fatigue to a severe proximal myopathy with rhabdomyolysis, myoglobinuria, and acute renal failure. Muscle enzymes, especially creatine phosphokinase (CPK) are elevated. CPK levels should be monitored in patients on long-term therapy. Aminocaproic Acid administration should be stopped if a rise in CPK is noted. Resolution follows discontinuation of Aminocaproic Acid; however, the syndrome may recur if Aminocaproic Acid is restarted.

The possibility of cardiac muscle damage should also be considered when skeletal myopathy occurs. One case of *cardiac* and *hepatic lesions* observed in man has been reported. The patient received 2 g of Aminocaproic Acid every 6 hours for a total dose of 26 g. Death was due to continued cerebrovascular hemorrhage. Necrotic changes in the heart and liver were noted at autopsy.

PRECAUTIONS

General: Aminocaproic Acid inhibits both the action of plasminogen activators and, to a lesser degree, plasmin activity. The drug should NOT be administered without a definite diagnosis, and/or laboratory finding indicative of hyperfibrinolysis (hyperplasminemia).*

Rapid intravenous administration of the drug should be avoided since this may induce hypotension, bradycardia, and/or arrhythmia.

Inhibition of fibrinolysis by Aminocaproic Acid may theoretically result in clotting or thrombosis. However, there is no definite evidence that administration of Aminocaproic Acid has been responsible for the few reported cases of intravascular clotting which followed this treatment. Rather, it appears that such *intravascular clotting* was most likely due to the patient's preexisting clinical condition, eg, the presence of DIC. It has been postulated that *extravascular clots* formed *in vivo* may not undergo spontaneous lysis as do normal clots.

Reports have appeared in the literature of an increased incidence of certain neurological deficits such as hydrocephalus, cerebral ischemia, or cerebral vasospasm associated with the use of antifibrinolytic agents in the treatment of subarachnoid hemorrhage (SAH). All of these events have also been described as part of the natural course of SAH, or as a consequence of diagnostic procedures such as angiography. Drug relatedness remains unclear.

Thrombophlebitis, a possibility with all intravenous therapy, should be guarded against by strict attention to the proper insertion of the needle and the fixing of its position.

Laboratory Tests: The use of Aminocaproic Acid should be accompanied by tests designed to determine the amount of fibrinolysis present. There are presently available (a) general tests such as those for the determination of the lysis of a clot of blood or plasma and (b) more specific tests for the study of various phases of fibrinolytic mechanisms. These latter tests include both semiquantitative and quantitative techniques for the determination of profibrinolysin, fibrinolysin, and antifibrinolysin.

Drug/Laboratory Test Interactions: Prolongation of the template bleeding time has been reported during continous intravenous infusion of Aminocaproic Acid at dosages exceeding 24 g/day. Platelet function studies in these patients have not demonstrated any significant platelet dysfunction. However, *in vitro* studies have shown that at high concentrations (7.4 mMol/L or 0.97 mg/mL and greater) EACA inhibits ADP and collagen-induced platelet aggregation, the release of ATP and serotonin, and the binding of fibrinogen to the platelets in a concentration-response manner. Following a 10 g bolus of Aminocaproic Acid, transient peak plasma concentrations of 4.6 mMol/L or 0.60 mg/mL have been obtained. The concentration of Aminocaproic Acid necessary to maintain inhibition of fibrinolysis is 0.99 mMol/L or 0.13 mg/mL. Administration of a 5 g bolus followed by 1 to 1.25 g/hr should achieve and sustain plasma levels of 0.13 mg/mL. Thus, concentrations which have been obtained *in vivo* clinically in patients with normal renal function are considerably lower than the *in vitro* concentrations found to induce abnormalities in platelet function tests. However, higher plasma concentrations of Aminocaproic Acid may occur in patients with severe renal failure.

Carcinogenesis, Mutagenesis, Impairment of Fertility: Long-term studies in animals to evaluate the carcinogenic potential of Aminocaproic Acid and studies to evaluate its mutagenic potential have not been conducted. Dietary administration of an equivalent of the maximum human therapeutic dose of Aminocaproic Acid to rats of both sexes impaired fertility as evidenced by decreased implantations, litter sizes and number of pups born.

Pregnancy: Pregnancy Category C. Animal teratological studies have not been conducted with Aminocaproic Acid. It is also not known whether Aminocaproic Acid can cause fetal harm when administered to a pregnant woman or can affect reproduction capacity. Aminocaproic Acid should be given to a pregnant woman only if clearly needed.

Nursing Mothers: It is not known whether this drug is excreted in human milk. Because many drugs are exereted in human milk, caution should be exercised when Aminocaproic Acid is administered to a nursing woman.

Pediatric Use: Safety and effectiveness in children have not been established.

ADVERSE REACTIONS

Occasionally nausea, cramps, diarrhea, hypotension, dizziness, tinnitus, malaise, conjunctival suffusion, nasal stuffiness, headache, and skin rash have been reported as results of the administration of Aminocaproic Acid. Only rarely has it been necessary to discontinue or reduce medication because of one or more of these effects. Myopathy (see *"Warnings"*) may be accompanied by general weakness, fatigue, and elevated serum enzymes. Rarely, rhabdomyolysis with myoglobinuria and renal failure may occur.

There have also been some reports of dry ejaculation during the period of Aminocaproic Acid treatment. These have been reported to date only in hemophilia patients who received the drug after undergoing dental surgical procedures. However, this symptom resolved in all patients within 24 to 48 hours of completion of therapy.

Two cases of convulsions have been reported to occur following intravenous administration of Aminocaproic Acid.

OVERDOSAGE

Signs, symptoms, laboratory findings, and complications have not been reported in association with acute overdosage of Aminocaproic Acid. Concentrations of Aminocaproic Acid in biologic fluids related to toxicity and/or death in humans are not known. Further, the single dose of Aminocaproic Acid causing symptoms of overdosage or considered to be life-threatening is unknown. The intravenous and oral LD$_{50}$ of Aminocaproic Acid were 3.0 and 12.0 g/kg, respectively in the mouse and 3.2 and 16.4 g/kg, respectively, in the rat. An intravenous infusion dose of 2.3 g/kg was lethal in the dog. On intravenous administration, tonic-clonic convulsions were observed in dogs and mice.

No treatment for overdosage is known, although evidence exists that Aminocaproic Acid removed by hemodialysis and may be removed by peritoneal dialysis.

DOSAGE AND ADMINISTRATION

Intravenous: Aminocaproic Acid Injection is administered by infusion, utilizing the usual compatible intravenous vehicles (eg, Sterile Water for Injection, Sodium Chloride for Injection, 5% Dextrose or Ringer's Injection). Although Sterile Water for Injection is compatible for intravenous injection the resultant solution is hypo-osmolar, RAPID INJECTION OF AMINOCAPROIC ACID INJECTION UNDILUTED INTO A VEIN IS NOT RECOMMENDED.

For the treatment of *acute* bleeding syndromes due to elevated fibrinolytic activity, it is suggested that 16 to 20 mL (4 to 5 g) of Aminocaproic Acid injection in 250 mL of diluent be administered by infusion during the first hour of treatment, followed by a continuing infusion at the rate of 4 mL (1 g) per hour in 50 mL of diluent. This method of treatment would ordinarily be continued for about 8 hours or until the bleeding situation has been controlled.

Parenteral drug products should be inspected visually for particulate matter and discoloration prior to administration, whenever solution and container permit.

Oral Therapy: If the patient is able to take medication by mouth, an identical dosage regimen may be followed by administering Aminocaproic Acid Tablets or Aminocaproic Acid Syrup 25% as follows: For the treatment of acute bleeding syndromes due to elevated fibrinolytic activity, it is suggested that 10 tablets (5 g) or 4 teaspoonfuls of syrup (5 g) of Aminocaproic Acid be administered during the first hour of treatment, followed by a continuing rate of 2 tablets (1 g) or 1 teaspoonful of syrup (1.25 g) per hour. This method of treatment would ordinarily be continued for about 8 hours or until the bleeding situation has been controlled.

Injection: Store at controlled room temperature, 15°-30°C (59°-86°F). DO NOT FREEZE.

Syrup: Store at controlled room temperature, 15°-30°C (59°-86°F). Dispense in tight containers. DO NOT FREEZE.

Tablets: Store at controlled room temperature, 15°-30°C (59°-86°F). Dispense in tight containers.

REFERENCES

*Stefanini, M, Dameshek, W: The Hemorrhagic Disorders, Ed. 2, New York, Grune and Stratton, 1962; pp. 510-514.

HOW SUPPLIED
INJECTION: 250 MG/ML

AVERAGE UNIT PRICE (AVAILABLE SIZES)			
BRAND	$0.81		
GENERIC	$0.32		

BRAND/MANUFACTURER	NDC	SIZE	AWP
◆ BRAND			
AMICAR: Immunex	00205-4668-37	20 ml	$16.24
◆ GENERICS			
Amer Regent	00517-9120-05	20 ml 5s	$13.44
Elkins-Sinn	00641-2235-43	20 ml 10s	$100.25
Abbott Hosp	00074-4346-73	20 ml 25s	$168.33

SYRUP: 1.25 GM/5 ML

BRAND/MANUFACTURER	NDC	SIZE	AWP
○ BRAND			
AMICAR: Immunex	00005-4667-65	480 ml	$391.28

TABLETS: 500 MG

BRAND/MANUFACTURER	NDC	SIZE	AWP
○ BRAND			
AMICAR: Immunex	00005-4665-23	100s	$156.75

Aminoglutethimide

DESCRIPTION

Aminoglutethimide is an inhibitor of adrenocortical steroid synthesis, available as 250-mg tablets for oral administration. Its chemical name is 3-(4-aminophenyl)-3-ethyl-2, 6-piperidinedione.

Aminoglutethimide is a fine, white or creamy white, crystalline powder. It is very slightly soluble in water, and readily soluble in most organic solvents. It forms water-soluble salts with strong acids. Its molecular weight is 232.28.

Following is its chemical structure:

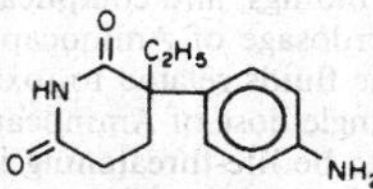

CLINICAL PHARMACOLOGY

Aminoglutethimide inhibits the enzymatic conversion of cholesterol to Δ^5-pregnenolone, resulting in a decrease in the production of adrenal glucocorticoids, mineralocorticoids, estrogens, and androgens.

Aminoglutethimide blocks several other steps in steroid synthesis, including the C-11, C-18, and C-21 hydroxylations and the hydroxylations required for the aromatization of androgens to estrogens, mediated through the binding of Aminoglutethimide to cytochrome P-450 complexes.

A decrease in adrenal secretion of cortisol is followed by an increased secretion of pituitary adrenocorticotropic hormone (ACTH), which will overcome the blockade of adrenocortical steroid synthesis by Aminoglutethimide. The compensatory increase in ACTH secretion can be suppressed by the simultaneous administration of hydrocortisone. Since Aminoglutethimide increases the rate of metabolism of dexamethasone but not that of hydrocortisone, the latter is preferred as the adrenal glucocorticoid replacement.

Although Aminoglutethimide inhibits the synthesis of thyroxine by the thyroid gland, the compensatory increase in thyroid-stimulating hormone (TSH) is frequently of sufficient magnitude to overcome the inhibition of thyroid synthesis due to Aminoglutethimide. In spite of an increase in TSH, Aminoglutethimide has not been associated with increased prolactin secretion.

Note: Aminoglutethimide was marketed previously as an anticonvulsant but was withdrawn from marketing for that indication in 1966 because of the effects on the adrenal gland.

PHARMACOKINETICS

Aminoglutethimide is rapidly and completely absorbed after oral administration. In 6 healthy male volunteers, maximum plasma levels of Aminoglutethimide averaged 5.9 µg/ml at a median of 1.5 hours after ingestion of two 250-mg tablets. The bioavailability of tablets is equivalent to equal doses given as a solution. After ingestion of a single oral dose, 34-54% is excreted in the urine as unchanged drug during the first 48 hours, and an additional fraction as the N-acetyl derivative.

The half-life of Aminoglutethimide in normal volunteers given single oral doses averaged 12.5 ± 1.6 hours.

Upon withdrawal of therapy with Aminoglutethimide the ability of the adrenal glands to synthesize steroid returns, usually within 72 hours.

INDICATIONS AND USAGE

Aminoglutethimide is indicated for the suppression of adrenal function in selected patients with Cushing's syndrome. Morning levels of plasma cortisol in patients with adrenal carcinoma and ectopic ACTH-producing tumors were reduced on the average to about one half of the pretreatment levels, and in patients with adrenal hyperplasia to about two thirds of the pretreatment levels, during 1-3 months of therapy with Aminoglutethimide. Data available from the few patients with adrenal adenoma suggest similar reductions in plasma cortisol levels. Measurements of plasma cortisol showed reductions to at least 50% of baseline or to normal levels in one third or more of the patients studied, depending on diagnostic groups and time of measurement.

Because Aminoglutethimide does not affect the underlying disease process, it is used primarily as an interim measure until more definitive therapy such as surgery can be undertaken or in cases where such therapy is not appropriate. Only small numbers of patients have been treated for longer than 3 months. A decreased effect or "escape phenomenon" seems to occur more frequently in patients with pituitary-dependent Cushing's syndrome, probably because of increasing ACTH levels in response to decreasing glucocorticoid levels. Aminoglutethimide should be used only in those patients who are responsive to treatment.

UNLABELED USES

Aminoglutethimide is used as an adjunct in the treatment of adrenal, breast, and prostate carcinoma and in the treatment of hypertension.

CONTRAINDICATIONS

Aminoglutethimide is contraindicated in those patients with serious forms, and/or severe manifestations, of hypersensitivity to glutethimide or Aminoglutethimide.

WARNINGS

Aminoglutethimide may cause adrenocortical hypofunction, especially under conditions of stress, such as surgery, trauma, or acute illness. Patients should be carefully monitored and given hydrocortisone and mineralocorticoid supplements as indicated. Dexamethasone should not be used. (See *"Precautions, Drug Interactions"*.)

Aminoglutethimide also may suppress aldosterone production by the adrenal cortex and may cause orthostatic or persistent hypotension. The blood pressure should be monitored in all patients at appropriate intervals. Patients should be advised of the possible occurrence of weakness and dizziness as symptoms of hypotension, and of measures to be taken should they occur.

The effects of Aminoglutethimide may be potentiated if it is taken in combination with alcohol.

Aminoglutethimide can cause fetal harm when administered to a pregnant woman. In the earlier experience with the drug in about 5000 patients, two cases

of pseudohermaphroditism were reported in female infants whose mothers were treated with Aminoglutethimide and concomitant anticonvulsants. Normal pregnancies have also occurred in patients treated with Aminoglutethimide.

When administered to rats at doses ½ and 1¼ times the maximum daily human dose, Aminoglutethimide caused a decrease in fetal implantation, an increase in fetal deaths, and a variety of teratogenic effects. The compound also caused pseudohermaphroditism in rats treated with approximately 3 times the maximum daily human dose. If this drug must be used during pregnancy, or if the patient becomes pregnant while taking the drug, the patient should be apprised of the potential hazard to the fetus.

PRECAUTIONS

GENERAL

This drug should be administered only by physicians familiar with its use and hazards. Therapy should be initiated in a hospital. (See *"Dosage and Administration."*)

INFORMATION FOR PATIENTS

Patients should be warned that drowsiness may occur and that they should not drive, operate potentially dangerous machinery, or engage in other activities that may become hazardous because of decreased alertness.

Patients should also be warned of the possibility of hypotension and its symptoms (see *"Warnings"*).

LABORATORY TESTS

Hypothyroidism may occur in association with Aminoglutethimide; hence, appropriate clinical observations should be made and laboratory studies of thyroid function performed as indicated. Supplementary thyroid hormone may be required. Hematologic abnormalities in patients receiving Aminoglutethimide have been reported (see *"Adverse Reactions"*). Therefore, baseline hematologic studies should be performed, followed by periodic hematologic evaluation.

Since elevations in SGOT, alkaline phosphatase, and bilirubin have been reported, appropriate clinical observations and regular laboratory studies should be performed before and during therapy.

Serum electrolyte levels should be determined periodically.

DRUG INTERACTIONS

Aminoglutethimide accelerates the metabolism of dexamethasone; therefore, if glucocorticoid replacement is needed, hydrocortisone should be prescribed.

Aminoglutethimide diminishes the effect of coumarin and warfarin.

CARCINOGENESIS, MUTAGENESIS, IMPAIRMENT OF FERTILITY

A 2-year carcinogenicity study of Aminoglutethimide conducted in rats at doses of 10-60 mg/kg/day (approximately 0.04 to 0.2 times the maximum daily therapeutic dose based on surface area, mg/m²) revealed a highly statistically dose-related trend in the incidence of benign and malignant neoplasms of the adrenal cortex and thyroid follicular cells in both sexes. A borderline statistically significant increase (0.05 level) in ovarian tubular adenomas was observed at 60 mg/kg/day. Urinary bladder papillomas also showed a statistically significant dose-related trend in males.

Aminoglutethimide affects fertility in female rats (see *"Warnings"*). The relevance of these findings to humans is not known.

PREGNANCY CATEGORY D

See *"Warnings"*.

NURSING MOTHERS

It is not known whether this drug is excreted in human milk. Because many drugs are excreted in human milk and because of the potential for serious adverse reactions in nursing infants from Aminoglutethimide, a decision should be made whether to discontinue nursing or to discontinue the drug, taking into account the importance of the drug to the mother.

PEDIATRIC USE

Safety and effectiveness in children have not been established (see *"Clinical Studies in Children"*).

ADVERSE REACTIONS

Untoward effects have been reported in about 2 out of 3 patients with Cushing's syndrome who were treated for 4 or more weeks with Aminoglutethimide as the only adrenocortical suppressant.

The most frequent and reversible side effects were drowsiness (approximately 1 in 3 patients), morbilliform skin rash (1 in 6 patients), nausea and anorexia (each approximately 1 in 8 patients), and dizziness (about 1 in 20 patients). The dizziness was possibly caused by lowered vascular resistance or orthostasis. These reactions often disappear spontaneously with continued therapy.

OTHER EFFECTS OBSERVED

Hematologic: Single instances of neutropenia, leukopenia (patient received concomitant *o,p'*-DDD), pancytopenia (patient received concomitant 5-fluorouracil), and agranulocytosis occurred in 4 of 27 patients with Cushing's syndrome caused by adrenal carcinoma who were treated for at least 4 weeks. In 1 patient with adrenal hyperplasia, hemoglobin levels and hematocrit decreased during the course of treatment with Aminoglutethimide. From the earlier experience with the drug used as an anticonvulsant in 1,214 patients, transient leukopenia was the only hematologic effect and was reported once; Coombs'-negative hemolytic anemia also occurred once. In approximately 300 patients with nonadrenal malignancy, 1 in 25 showed some degree of anemia, and 1 in 150 developed pancytopenia during treatment with Aminoglutethimide.

Endocrine: Adrenal insufficiency occurred in about 1 in 30 patients with Cushing's syndrome who were treated with Aminoglutethimide for 4 or more weeks. This insufficiency tended to involve glucocorticoids as well as mineralocorticoids. Hypothyroidism is occasionally associated with thyroid enlargement and may be detected or confirmed by measuring plasma levels of the thyroid hormone. Masculinization and hirsutism have occasionally occurred in females, as has precocious sexual development in males.

Central Nervous System: Headache was reported in about 1 in 20 patients.

Cardiovascular: Hypotension, occasionally orthostatic occurred in 1 in 30 patients receiving Aminoglutethimide. Tachycardia occurred in 1 in 40 patients.

Gastrointestinal and Liver: Vomiting occurred in 1 in 30 patients. Isolated instances of abnormal findings on liver function tests were reported. Suspected hepatotoxicity occurred in less than 1 in 1000 patients.

Skin: In addition to rash (1 in 6 patients, and often reversible with continued therapy), pruritus was reported in 1 in 20 patients. These may be allergic or hypersensitive reactions. Urticaria has occurred rarely.

Miscellaneous: Fever was reported in several patients who were treated with Aminoglutethimide for less than 4 weeks; some of these patients also received other drugs. Myalgia occurred in 1 in 30 patients.

Pulmonary hypersensitivity, including allergic alveolitis and interstitial alveolar infiltrates, has occurred rarely.

OVERDOSAGE

ACUTE TOXICITY
No deaths due to overdosage with Aminoglutethimide have been reported.

The highest known doses that have been survived are 7 g (33-year-old woman) and 7.5-10.0 g (16-year-old girl).

Oral LD_{50}'s (mg/kg): rats, 1800; dogs > 100. Intravenous LD_{50}'s (mg/kg): rats, 156; dogs > 100.

SIGNS AND SYMPTOMS
An acute overdose with Aminoglutethimide may reduce the production of steroids in the adrenal cortex to a degree that is clinically relevant. The following manifestations may be expected:

Respiratory Function: Respiratory depression, hyperventilation.

Cardiovascular System: Hypotension, hypovolemic shock due to dehydration.

Central Nervous System Muscles: Somnolence, lethargy, coma, ataxia, dizziness, fatigue. (Extreme weakness has been reported with divided doses of 3 g daily.)

Gastrointestinal System: Nausea, vomiting.

Renal Function: Loss of sodium and water.

Laboratory Findings: Hyponatremia, hypochloremia, hyperkalemia, hypoglycemia.

The signs and symptoms of acute overdosage with Aminoglutethimide may be aggravated or modified if alcohol, hypnotics, tranquilizers, or tricyclic antidepressants have been taken at the same time.

TREATMENT
Symptomatic treatment of overdosage is recommended. Since Aminoglutethimide and glutethimide are chemically related, measures that have been used in successfully removing glutethimide from the body might be useful in removing Aminoglutethimide.

Gastric lavage and unspecified supportive treatment have been employed. Full consciousness following deep coma was regained 40 hours or less after ingestion of 3 or 4 g without lavage. No evidence of hematologic, renal, or hepatic effects was subsequently found.

Close monitoring should be provided, and appropriate measures taken to support vital functions, if necessary.

If deficiency of circulating glucocorticoid develops, an intravenous infusion of a soluble hydrocortisone preparation (100 mg of hydrocortisone sodium succinate in 500 mL of isotonic sodium chloride solution) and 50 mL of 40% glucose solution should be given within 3 hours. After the initial infusion is completed, an intravenous administration of hydrocortisone, 10 mg per hour, should be continued until the patient is able to take oral cortisone.

If hypovolemia or hypotension occurs, an intravenous administration of norepinephrine, 10 mg, in 500 mL of isotonic sodium chloride should be administered according to the patient's needs and response. After rehydration, 500 mL of plasma or blood should be given for maintenance of sufficient circulatory volume.

Dialysis may be considered in severe intoxication.

DOSAGE AND ADMINISTRATION

ADULTS
Treatment should be instituted in a hospital until a stable dosage regimen is achieved. Therapy should be initiated with 250 mg orally four times daily, preferably at 6-hour intervals. Adrenocortical response should be followed by careful monitoring of plasma cortisol levels until the desired level of suppression is achieved. If the level of cortisol suppression is inadequate, the dosage may be increased in increments of 250 mg daily at intervals of 1-2 weeks to a total daily dose of 2 g. Dose reduction or temporary discontinuation of therapy may be required in the event of adverse effects, including extreme drowsiness, severe skin rash, or excessively low cortisol levels. If a skin rash persists for longer than 5-8 days or becomes severe, the drug should be discontinued. It may be possible to reinstate therapy at a lower dosage following the disappearance of a mild or

moderate rash. Mineralocorticoid replacement (e.g., fludrocortisone) may be necessary. If glucocorticoid replacement therapy is needed, 20-30 mg of hydrocortisone orally in the morning will replace endogenous secretion.

Protect from light.

Dispense in tight, light-resistant container.

Do not store above 86° F(30° C).

CLINICAL STUDIES IN CHILDREN
Clinical investigations included 9 patients aged 2½ to 16 years; 4 of these were aged 10 or less. Seven of the patients received other therapies (drugs or irradiation) either with Aminoglutethimide or within a short period before initiation of therapy with Aminoglutethimide Diagnoses included 5 patients with adrenal carcinoma, 3 with adrenal hyperplasia, and 1 with ectopic ACTH-producing tumor. Duration of treatment ranged from 3 days to 6½ months. Dosages ranged from 0.375 g to 1.5 g daily. In general, smaller doses were used for younger patients; for example, a 2½-year-old received 0.5-0.75 g daily, a 3½-year-old received 0.5 g daily, and all others over 10 years of age received 0.75-1.5 g daily. Results are difficult to evaluate because of the concomitant therapy, duration of therapy, or inadequate laboratory documentation. Most patients did show decreases in plasma or urinary steroids at some time during treatment, but these may have been due to other therapeutic modalities or their combinations.

HOW SUPPLIED
TABLETS: 250 MG

BRAND/MANUFACTURER	NDC	SIZE	AWP
○ **BRAND**			
CYTADREN: Ciba Pharm	00083-0024-30	100s	$100.34

Aminohippurate Sodium

DESCRIPTION
Aminohippurate Sodium* is an agent to measure effective renal plasma flow (ERPF). It is the Sodium salt of para-aminohippuric acid. It is water soluble, lipid-insoluble, and has a pKa of 3.83. The empirical formula of the anhydrous salt is $C_9H_9N_2NaO_3$.

It is provided as a sterile, nonpreserved 20 percent aqueous solution for injection, with a pH of 6.7 to 7.6. Each 10 mL contains: Aminohippurate Sodium 2 g.

Following is its chemical structure:

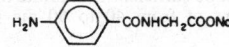

CLINICAL PHARMACOLOGY
Aminohippurate Sodium is filtered by the glomeruli and is actively secreted by the proximal tubules. At low plasma concentrations (1.0 to 2.0 mg/100 mL), an average of 90 percent of Aminohippurate Sodium is cleared by the kidneys from the renal blood stream in a single circulation. It is ideally suited for measurement of ERPF since it has a high clearance, is essentially nontoxic at the plasma concentrations reached with recommended doses and its analytical determination is relatively simple and accurate. Aminohippurate Sodium is also used to measure the functional capacity of the renal tubular secretory mechanism or transport maximum (Tm_{PAH}). This is accomplished by elevating the plasma concentration to levels (40-60 mg/100 mL) sufficient to saturate the maximal capacity of the tubular cells to secrete Aminohippurate Sodium. Inulin clearance is generally measured during Tm_{PAH} determinations since glomerular filtration rate (GFR) must be known before calculations of secretory Tm measurements can be done (see *"Calculations"*).

INDICATIONS AND USAGE
Estimation of effective renal plasma flow.

Measurement of the functional capacity of the renal tubular secretary mechanism.

CONTRAINDICTIONS
Hypersensitivity to this product or to its components.

PRECAUTIONS
GENERAL
Intravenous solutions must be given with caution to patients with low cardiac reserve, since a rapid increase in plasma volume can precipitate congestive heart failure.

For measurement of ERPF, small doses of Aminohippurate Sodium are used. However, in research procedures to measure Tm_{PAH}, high plasma levels are required to saturate the capacity of the tubular cells. During these procedures the intravenous administration of Aminohippurate Sodium solutions should be carried out slowly and with caution. The patient should be continuously observed for any adverse reactions.

DRUG INTERACTIONS
Renal clearance measurements of Aminohippurate Sodium cannot be made with any significant accuracy in patients receiving sulfonamides, procaine, or thiazole-sulfone. These compounds interfere with chemical color development essential to the analytical procedures.

* Formerly referred to as Sodium para-Aminohippurate.

Probenecid depresses tubular secretion of certain weak acids such as Aminohippurate Sodium. Therefore, patients receiving probenecid will have erroneously low ERPF and Tm_{PAH} values.

CARCINOGENESIS, MUTAGENESIS, IMPAIRMENT OF FERTILITY
Long-term studies in animals have not been done to evaluate any effects upon fertility or carcinogenic potential of Aminohippurate Sodium.

PREGNANCY
Pregnancy Category C: Animal reproduction studies have not been done with Aminohippurate Sodium. It is also not known whether Aminohippurate Sodium can cause fetal harm when given to a pregnant woman or can affect reproduction capacity. Aminohippurate Sodium should be given to a pregnant woman only if clearly needed.

NURSING MOTHERS
It is not known whether this drug is excreted in human milk. Because many drugs are excreted in human milk, caution should be exercised when Aminohippurate Sodium is administered to a nursing woman.

PREDIATRIC USE
Safety and effectiveness in children have not been established.

ADVERSE REACTIONS
Vasomotor disturbances, flushing, tingling, nausea, vomiting, and cramps may occur.

Patients may have a sensation of warmth or the desire to defecate or urinate during or shortly following initiation of infusion.

OVERDOSAGE
The intravenous LD_{50} in female mice is 7.22 g/kg.

DOSAGE AND ADMINISTRATION
FOR INTRAVENOUS USE ONLY
Clearance measurements using single injection technics are generally inaccurate, particularly in the measurement of ERPF. For this reason, intravenous infusions at fixed rates are used to sustain the plasma Aminohippurate Sodium concentration at the desired level.

To measure ERPF, the concentration of Aminohippurate Sodium in the plasma should be maintained at 2 mg per 100 mL, which can be achieved with a priming dose of 6 to 10 mg/kg and an infusion dose of 10 to 24 mg/min.

As a research procedure for the measurement of Tm_{PAH}, the plasma level of Aminohippurate Sodium must be sufficient to saturate the capacity of the tubular secretory cells. Concentrations of from 40 to 60 mg per 100 mL are usually necessary.

Technical details of these tests may be found in Smith[1]; Wesson[2]; Bauer[3]; Pitts[4]; and Schnurr.[5]

Parenteral drug products should be inspected visually for particulate matter and discoloration prior to use, whenever solution and container permit. *Note:* The normal color range for this product is a colorless to yellow/brown solution. The efficacy is not affected by color changes within this range.

CALCULATIONS
Effective Renal Plasma Flow (ERPF): The clearance of Aminohippurate Sodium (PAH), which is extracted almost completely from the plasma during its passage through the renal circulation, constitutes a measure of ERPF. Hence:

ERPF	=	$\dfrac{U_{PAH}V}{P_{PAH}}$
Where U_{PAH}	=	concentration of PAH (mg/mL) in the urine
V	=	rate of urine excretion (mL/min), and
P_{PAH}	=	plasma concentration of PAH (mg/mL).
Example: U_{PAH}	=	8.0 mg/mL
V	=	1.5 mL/min
P_{PAH}	=	0.02 mg/mL
ERPF	=	$\dfrac{8.0 \times 1.5}{0.02}$ = 600 mL/min.

Based on PAH clearance studies, the normal values for ERPF are:

men 675 ± 150 mL/min
women 595 ± 125 mL/min.

MAXIMUM TUBULAR SECRETORY MECHANISM (Tm_{PAH})
The quantity of PAH, secreted by the tubules (Tm_{PAH}) is given by the difference between the total rate of excretion ($U_{PAH}V$) and the quantity filtered by the glomeruli (GFR × P_{PAH}). Hence:
$$Tm_{PAH}V = U_{PAH}V - (GFR \times P_{PAH} \times 0.83)$$
The factor, 0.83, corrects for that portion of PAH which is bound to plasma protein and hence is unfilterable.

Example:	U_{PAH}	=	9.55 mg/mL
	V	=	16.68 mL/min
	GFR	=	120 mL/min
	P_{PAH}	=	0.60 mg/mL

Then Tm_{PAH} = 9.55 × 16.68 − (120 × 0.60 × 0.83) = 100 mg/min.
Average normal values of Tm_{PAH} are 80-90 mg/min. The value of the expression $U_{PAH}V$, used in calculations of ERPF and Tm_{PAH}, may be found by determining the amount of PAH in a measured volume of urine excreted within a specific period of time.

These calculations are based on a body surface area of 1.73 m^2. Corrections for variations in surface area are made by multiplying the values obtained for ERPF and Tm_{PAH} by 1.73/A, where A is the subject surface area.

STORAGE
Avoid storage at temperatures below −20°C (−4°F) and above 40°C (104°F)

REFERENCES
1. Smith, H.W.: Lectures on the kidney, University Extension Division, University of Kansas, Lawrence, Kansas, 1943. 2. Wesson, L. G., Jr.: "Physiology of the Human Kidney," New York, Grune & Stratton, 1969, pp. 632-655. 3. Bauer, J. D.; Ackermann, P. G.; Toro, G.: "Brays Clinical Laboratory Methods," ed. 7, St. Louis, Mosby, 1968. 4. Pitts, R. F.: "Physiology of the Kidney and Body Fluids," ed. 2, Chicago, Year Book Medical Publishers, 1968. 5. Schnurr, E., Lahme, W., Kuppers, H.: Measurement of renal clearance of inulin and PAH in the steady state without urine collection; Clinical Nephrology, *13*(1): (26-29), 1980.

HOW SUPPLIED
INJECTION: 20%

BRAND/MANUFACTURER	NDC	SIZE	AWP
◆ **GENERICS**			
Merck	00006-3395-11	10 ml	$5.51

Aminophylline

DESCRIPTION
Aminophylline, a xanthine bronchodilator, is a 2:1 complex of theophylline and ethylenediamine and has the chemical name 1H-Purine-2,6,-dione,3,7-dihydro-1,3-dimethyl-, compounded with 1,2-ethanediamine (2:1). It occurs as white or slightly yellowish granules or powder with slight ammoniacal odor and bitter taste.

Aminophylline is available as tablets, and controlled-release tablets for oral administration and as a solution for injection.

Each tablet contains:
Aminophylline (as dihydrate) ....100 or 200 mg
(equivalent to 79 or 158 mg anhydrous theophylline)

Each controlled-release tablet contains:
Aminophylline (as dihydrate) ....225 mg
(equivalent to 178 mg anhydrous theophylline)

Each mL of solution for injection contains:
Aminophylline (as dihydrate) ....25 mg
(equivalent to 19.7 mg anhydrous theophylline)

Aminophylline (dihydrate) is approximately 79% of anhydrous theophylline by weight and contains between 157 mg and 175 mg of ethylenediamine for every gram of anhydrous theophylline.

Aminophylline for injection is a sterile, nonpyrogenic solution; it is administered by slow intravenous injection or diluted and administered by intravenous infusion.

The solution is intended for use only as a single-dose injection. When smaller doses are required the unused portion should be discarded.

Following is its chemical structure:

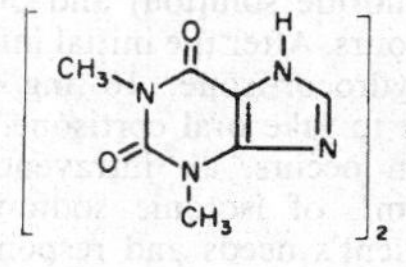

CLINICAL PHARMACOLOGY
AMINOPHYLLINE SHOULD BE CONSIDERED A MIXTURE OF THEOPHYLLINE AND BASE. THE ACTIVITY IS THAT OF THEOPHYLLINE ALONE.

Theophylline directly relaxes the smooth muscle of the bronchial airways and pulmonary blood vessels, thus acting mainly as a bronchodilator and smooth muscle relaxant. It has also been demonstrated that Aminophylline has a potent effect on diaphragmatic contractility in normal persons and may then be capable of reducing fatigability and thereby improve contractility in patients with chronic obstructive airways disease. The exact mode of action remains unsettled. Although theophylline does cause inhibition of phosphodiesterase with a resultant increase in intracellular cyclic AMP, other agents similarly inhibit the enzyme producing a rise of cyclic AMP but are unassociated with any demonstrable bronchodilation. Other mechanisms proposed include an effect on translocation of intracellular calcium; prostaglandin antagonism; stimulation of catecholamines endogenously; inhibition of cyclic guanosine monophosphate metabolism and adenosine receptor antagonism. None of these mechanisms has been proved, however.

In vitro, theophylline, the active moiety of Aminophylline has been shown to act synergistically with beta agonists and there are now available data which do demonstrate an additive effect *in vivo* with combined use.

PHARMACOKINETICS

The half-life of theophylline is influenced by a number of known variables. It may be prolonged in chronic alcoholics, particularly those with liver disease (cirrhosis or alcoholic liver disease), in patients with impaired renal function or congestive heart failure, and in those patients taking certain other drugs (see *"Precautions, Drug Interactions"*).

Older adults (over age 55) and patients with chronic obstructive pulmonary disease, with or without cor pulmonale, may also have much slower clearance rates; in these individuals the theophylline half-life may exceed 24 hours. High fever for prolonged periods may reduce the rate of theophylline elimination.

Newborns and neonates have extremely slow clearance rates compared to older infants and children, i.e., those over 1 year. Older children have rapid clearance rates while most non-smoking adults have clearance rates between these two extremes. In premature neonates the decreased clearance is related to oxidative pathways that have yet to be established.

THEOPHYLLINE ELIMINATION CHARACTERISTICS

	Half-Life (in hours)	
	Range	Mean
Children	1- 9	3.7
Adults	3-15	7.7

In cigarette smokers (1-2 packs/day) the mean half-life is 4-5 hours, much shorter than in non-smokers. The increase in clearance associated with smoking is presumably due to stimulation of the hepatic metabolic pathway by components of cigarette smoke. The duration of this effect after cessation of smoking is unknown but may require 6 months to 2 years before the rate approaches that of the nonsmoker.

In single dose studies with 12 normal male volunteers (while fasting), Aminophylline 225 mg tablets produced a mean peak theophylline level of 2.8 mcg/mL at 5 hours following administration and having an average elimination half-life of 9.1 hours.

A multiple-dose bioavailability study in normal adult males comparing an equal total daily dosage of Aminophylline tablets administered every 6 hours to Aminophylline controlled-release tablets administered every 12 hours showed that subjects given Aminophylline controlled-release tablets had a serum theophylline level of 8-20 mcg/mL for a longer time period than those receiving the immediate-release product.

INDICATIONS AND USAGE

For the relief and/or prevention of symptoms of asthma (tablets) or relief of acute bronchial asthma (injection) and for reversible bronchospasm associated with chronic bronchitis and emphysema.

UNLABELED USES

Aminophylline is used alone or as an adjunct in the treatment of Cheyne-Stokes respiration, cystic fibrosis, essential tremor, and severe headache. It is also used to improve exercise-induced myocardial ischemia in patients with stable angina pectoris, in bronchopulmonary dysplasia, and cerebral vasospasm.

CONTRAINDICATIONS

This product is contraindicated in individuals who have shown hypersensitivity to its components, including ethylenediamine.

It is also contraindicated in patients with active peptic ulcer disease, and in individuals with underlying seizure disorders (unless receiving appropriate anticonvulsant medications).

WARNINGS

Serum levels above 20 mcg/mL are rarely found after appropriate administration of the recommended doses. However, in individuals in whom theophylline plasma clearance is reduced *for any reason,* even conventional doses may result in increased serum levels and potential toxicity. Reduced theophylline clearance has been documented in the following readily identifiable groups: 1) patients with impaired renal or liver function; 2) patients over 55 years of age, particularly males and those with chronic lung disease; 3) those with cardiac failure from any cause; 4) patients with sustained high fever; 5) neonates and infants under 1 year of age; and 6) those patients taking certain drugs (see *"Precautions, Drug Interactions"*). Frequently, such patients have markedly prolonged theophylline serum levels following discontinuation of the drug. Decreased theophylline clearance may occur following immunization for influenza, with active influenza, or other viral illnesses and also with high fever for prolonged periods. This may be specially true in infants and the elderly.

Reduction of dosage and laboratory monitoring is especially appropriate in the above individuals.

Serious side effects such as ventricular arrhythmias, convulsions or even death may appear as the first sign of toxicity without any previous warning. Elderly patients with serum concentrations above 20 µg/mL are more likely to experience serious side effects such as ventricular arrhythmias or convulsions than are younger patients. Less serious signs of theophylline toxicity (i.e., nausea and restlessness) may occur frequently when initiating therapy, but are usually transient; when such signs are persistent during maintenance therapy, they are often associated with serum concentrations above 20 mcg/mL. Stated differently, *serious toxicity is not reliably preceded by less severe side effects.* A serum concentration measurement is the only reliable method of predicting potentially life-threatening toxicity.

Many patients who require theophylline exhibit tachycardia due to their underlying disease process so that the cause/effect relationship to elevated serum theophylline concentrations may not be appreciated.

Theophylline products may cause or worsen arrhythmias and any significant change in rate and/or rhythm warrants monitoring and further investigation.

Studies in laboratory animals (minipigs, rodents, and dogs) recorded the occurrence of cardiac arrhythmias and sudden death (with histologic evidence of myocardial necrosis) when beta-agonists and methylxanthines were administered concurrently. The significance of these findings when applied to humans is currently unknown.

PRECAUTIONS

GENERAL

On the average, theophylline half-life is shorter in cigarette and marijuana smokers than in non-smokers, but smokers can have half-lives as long as non-smokers. Theophylline should not be administered concurrently with other xanthines. Use with caution in patients with hypoxemia, hypertension, or those with a history of peptic ulcer. Theophylline may occasionally act as a local irritant to the G.I. tract when administered orally, although gastrointestinal symptoms are more commonly centrally mediated and associated with serum drug concentrations over 20 mcg/mL.

INFORMATION FOR PATIENTS

The physician should reinforce the importance of taking only the prescribed dose at the recommended time interval between doses. The patient should alert the physician if symptoms occur repeatedly, especially near the end of the dosing interval.

For such measurements, the serum sample should be obtained at the time of peak concentration—1 to 2 hours after administration of immediate-release products and 4 to 6 hours after administration of controlled-release tablets. It is important that the patient will not have missed or taken additional doses during the previous 48 hours and that dosing intervals will have been reasonably equally spaced. DOSAGE ADJUSTMENT BASED ON SERUM THEOPHYLLINE MEASUREMENTS WHEN THESE INSTRUCTIONS HAVE NOT BEEN FOLLOWED MAY RESULT IN RECOMMENDATIONS THAT PRESENT RISK OF TOXICITY TO THE PATIENT.

DRUG INTERACTIONS

Toxic synergism with ephedrine has been documented and may occur with other sympathomimetic bronchodilators. In addition, the following drug interactions have been demonstrated:

Theophylline with:

Allopurinol (high-dose)	Increased serum theophylline levels
Cimetidine	Increased serum theophylline levels
Ciprofloxacin	Increased serum theophylline levels
Erythromycin, Troleandomycin	Increased serum theophylline levels
Lithium carbonate	Increased renal excretion of lithium
Norfloxacin	Increased serum theophylline levels
Oral Contraceptives	Increased serum theophylline levels
Phenytoin	Decreased theophylline and phenytoin serum levels
Propranolol	Increased serum theophylline levels
Rifampin	Decreased serum theophylline levels

DRUG-LABORATORY TEST INTERACTIONS

Currently available analytical methods, including high pressure liquid chromatography and immunoassay techniques, for measuring serum theophylline levels are specific. Metabolites and other drugs generally do not affect the results. Other new analytic methods are also now in use. The physician should be aware of the laboratory method used and whether other drugs will interfere with the assay for theophylline.

DRUG-FOOD INTERACTIONS

Available data suggest that drug administration at the time of food ingestion may influence the absorption characteristics of some or all xanthine controlled-release products resulting in serum values different from those found after administration in the fasting state.

A drug-food effect, if any, would likely have its greatest clinical significance when high xanthine serum levels are being maintained and/or when large scale single doses (greater than 13 mg/kg or 900 mg of theophylline or 16 mg/kg or 1100 mg for Aminophylline) of a controlled-release xanthine product are given. The influence of the type and amount of food on performance of controlled-release xanthine products is under study at this time.

CARCINOGENESIS, MUTAGENESIS, AND IMPAIRMENT OF FERTILITY

Long-term carcinogencity studies have not been performed with theophylline.

Chromosome-breaking activity was detected in human cell cultures at concentrations of theophylline up to 50 times the therapeutic serum concentration in humans. Theophylline was not mutagenic in the dominant lethal assay in male mice given theophylline intraperitoneally in doses up to 30 times the maximum daily human oral dose.

Studies to determine the effect on fertility have not been performed with theophylline.

Pregnancy Category C: Animal reproduction studies have not been conducted with theophylline or Aminophylline. It is not known whether theophylline can cause fetal harm when administered to a pregnant woman or can affect reproduction capacity. Xanthines should be given to a pregnant woman only if clearly needed.

NURSING MOTHERS

Theophylline is distributed into breast milk and may cause irritability or other signs of toxicity in nursing infants. Because of the potential for serious adverse reactions in nursing infants from theophylline, a decision should be made whether to discontinue nursing or to discontinue the drug, taking into account the importance of the drug to the mother.

PEDIATRIC USE

Immediate-release tablets and injection: Sufficient numbers of infants under the age of 1 year have not been studied in clinical trials to support use in this age group; however, there is evidence recorded that the use of dosage recommendations for older infants and young children (16 mg/kg/24 hours) may result in the development of toxic serum levels. Such findings very probably reflect differences in the metabolic handling of the drug related to absent or undeveloped enzyme systems. Consequently, the use of the drug in this age group should carefully consider the associated benefits and risks. If used, the maintenance dose must be conservative and in accord with the following guidelines:

Initial Maintenance Dosage of Theophylline: 1.0 mg theophylline (anhydrous) = 1.3 mg Aminophylline (dihydrate)

Premature Infants: Up to 24 days postnatal age - - 1.0 mg/kg q12h
    Beyond 24 days postnatal age - - 1.5 mg/kg q12h

Infants 6 to 52 Weeks: $[(0.2 \times \text{age in weeks}) + 5.0] \times$ kg body wt = 24 hour dose in mg.

Up to 26 Weeks: divide into q8h dosing intervals.

From 26-52 Weeks: divide into q6h dosing intervals.

Final Dosage: should be guided by serum concentration after a steady state (no further accumulation of drug) has been achieved.

Safety and effectiveness in children under 6 years of age have not been established with controlled-release Aminophylline tablets.

ADVERSE REACTIONS

The following adverse reactions have been observed, but there has not been enough systematic collection of data to support an estimate of their frequency. The most consistent adverse reactions are usually due to overdosage.
1. *Gastrointestinal:* Nausea, vomiting, epigastric pain, hematemesis, diarrhea.
2. *Central Nervous System:* Headaches, irritability, restlessness, insomnia, reflex hyperexcitability, muscle twitching, clonic and tonic generalized convulsions.
3. *Cardiovascular:* Palpitation, tachycardia, extrasystoles, flushing, hypotension, circulatory failure, ventricular arrhythmias.
4. *Respiratory:* Tachypnea.
5. *Renal:* Potentiation of diuresis.
6. *Others:* Alopecia, hyperglycemia and inappropriate ADH syndrome, rash (consider ethylenediamine), Stevens-Johnson syndrome.

OVERDOSAGE

Tablets: Management: It is suggested that the management principles (consistent with the clinical status of the patient when first seen) outlined below be instituted and that simultaneous contact with a Regional Poison Control Center be established. In this way, both updated information and individualization regarding required therapy may be provided.

When potential oral overdose is established and seizure has not occurred:
a) If patient is alert and seen within the early hours after ingestion, induction of emesis may be of value. Gastric lavage has been demonstrated to be of no value in influencing outcome in patients who present more than 1 hour after ingestion.
b) Administer a cathartic. Sorbitol solution is reported to be of value.
c) Administer repeated doses of activated charcoal and monitor theophylline serum levels.
d) Prophylactic administration of phenobarbital has been shown to increase the seizure threshold in laboratory animals and administration of this drug can be considered.
2. If patient presents with a seizure:
a) Establish an airway.
b) Administer oxygen.
c) Treat the seizure with intravenous diazepam, 0.1 to 0.3 mg/kg up to 10 mg. If seizures cannot be controlled, the use of general anesthesia should be considered.
d) Monitor vital signs, maintain blood pressure and provide adequate hydration.
3. Post-Seizure Coma:
a) Maintain airway and oxygenation.
b) If overdose is a result of oral medication, follow above recommendations to prevent absorption of the drug, but intubation and lavage will have to be

performed instead of inducing emesis, and the cathartic and charcoal will need to be introduced via a large-bore gastric lavage tube.
c) Continue to provide full supportive care and adequate hydration while waiting for the drug to be metabolized. In general, the drug is metabolized sufficiently rapidly so as not to warrant consideration of dialysis. If repeated oral activated charcoal is ineffective (as noted by stable or rising serum levels) charcoal hemoperfusion may be indicated.

Injection: Management of Toxic Symptoms:
1. Discontinue drug immediately.
2. There is no known specific antidote.
3. Treatment is supportive and symptomatic.
4. Avoid administration of sympathomimetic drugs.
5. Administer intravenous fluids, oxygen and other supportive measures to prevent hypotension; correct dehydration and acid-base imbalance.
6. For hyperthermia, use a cooling blanket or give sponge baths as necessary.
7. Maintain patient airway and use artificial respiration in case of respiratory depression.
8. Control convulsions with intravenous diazepam (0.1 to 0.3 mg/kg up to 10 mg). If seizures cannot be controlled, the use of general anesthesia should be considered.
9. Monitor serum theophylline levels until below 20 mcg/mL.

DOSAGE AND ADMINISTRATION

Effective use of theophylline (i.e., the concentration of drug in the serum associated with optimal benefit and minimal risk of toxicity) is considered to occur when the theophylline concentration is maintained from 10 to 20 mcg/mL. The early studies from which these levels were derived were carried out in patients immediately or shortly after recovery from acute exacerbations of their disease (some hospitalized with status asthmaticus).

Although the 20 mcg/mL level remains appropriate as a critical value (above which toxicity is more likely to occur) for safety purposes, additional data are now available which indicate that the serum theophylline concentrations required to produce maximum physiologic benefit may, in fact, fluctuate with the degree of bronchospasm present and are variable. Therefore, the physician should individualize the range appropriate to the patient's requirements, based on both symptomatic response and improvement in pulmonary function. It should be stressed that serum theophylline concentrations maintained at the upper level of the 10 to 20 mcg/mL range may be associated with potential toxicity when factors known to reduce theophylline clearance are operative. (See *"Warnings"*).

If it is not possible to obtain serum level determinations, restriction of the daily dose (in otherwise healthy adults) to not greater than 13 mg/kg/day, to a maximum of 900 mg of theophylline in divided doses or not greater than 16 mg/kg/day of Aminophylline will result in relatively few patients exceeding serum levels of 20 mcg/mL and the resultant greater risk of toxicity.

Theophylline does not distribute into fatty tissue. Dosage should be calculated on the basis of lean (ideal) body weight where mg/kg doses are presented.

Caution should be exercised for younger children who cannot complain or minor side effects. Older adults, those with cor pulmonale, congestive heart failure, and/or liver disease may have unusually low dosage requirements and thus may experience toxicity at the maximal dosage recommended below.

FREQUENCY OF DOSING

When immediate-release products with rapid absorption (such as immediate-release tablets or liquids) are used, dosing to maintain serum levels generally requires administration every 6 hours. This is particularly true in children, but dosing intervals up to 8 hours may be satisfactory in adults since they eliminate the drug at a slower rate. Some children, and adults requiring higher than average doses (those having rapid rates of clearance; e.g., half-lives of under 6 hours) may benefit and be more effectively controlled during chronic therapy when given products with sustained-release characteristics since these provide longer dosing intervals and/or less fluctuation in serum concentration between dosing. Rapid metabolizers (such as smokers and children) may require larger doses and more frequent administration.

Dosage guidelines are approximations only and the wide range of theophylline clearance between individuals (particularly those with concomitant disease) makes indiscriminate usage hazardous. Each patient should be titrated with an immediate release product to establish the appropriate dosage and serum theophylline levels used for any dosage adjustment after transfer to controlled-release tablets.

DOSAGE GUIDELINES

I. Acute symptoms of bronchospasm requiring rapid attainment of Theophylline serum levels for bronchodilation:

Note: Status asthmaticus should be considered a medical emergency and is defined as that degree of bronchospasm which is not rapidly responsive to usual doses of conventional bronchodilators. Optimal therapy for such patients frequently requires both *additional medication,* parenterally administered, and *close monitoring,* preferably in an intensive care setting.

Controlled-release Aminophylline tablets are not intended for patients experiencing an acute episode of bronchospasm (associated with asthma, chronic bronchitis, or emphysema). Such patients require *rapid* relief of symptoms and should be treated with an immediate release or intravenous theophylline preparation (or other bronchodilators) and not with controlled release products.

A. Patients not currently receiving theophylline products. (* = equivalent dosage of theophylline)

AMINOPHYLLINE DOSAGE

	Oral Loading	Maintenance	Oral
Children age: 1 to under 9 years	6.3 mg/kg *(5.0)	1.0 mg/kg/hr *(0.79)	5.1 mg/kg g 6 hours (4.0)
Children age: 9 to under 16 years and smokers	6.3 mg/kg *(5.0)	0.8 mg/kg/hr *(0.63)	3.8 mg/kg g 6 hours (3.0)
Otherwise healthy nonsmoking adults adults	6.3 mg/kg *(5.0)	0.5 mg/kg/hr *(0.40)	3.8 mg/kg g 8 hours (3.0)
Older patients and patients with cor pulmonale	6.3 mg/kg *(5.0)	0.3 mg/kg/hr *(0.24)	2.5 mg/kg g 8 (2.0)
Patients with congestive heart failure	6.3 mg/kg *(5.0)	0.1-0.2 mg/kg/ *(0.08-0.16)	1.3-2.5 mg/kg g 12 hours (1.0-2.0)

B. Patients currently receiving theophylline products:

Determine, where possible, the time, amount, dosage form, and route of administration of the last dose the patient received.

The loading dose for theophylline is based on the principle that each 0.5 mg/kg of theophylline administered as a loading dose will result in a 1 mcg/mL increase in serum theophylline concentration. Ideally, the loading dose should be deferred if a serum theophylline concentration can be obtained rapidly.

If this is not possible, the clinician must exercise his judgment in selecting a dose based on the potential for benefit and risk. When there is sufficient respiratory distress to warrant a small risk, then 2.5 mg/kg of theophylline administered in rapidly absorbed form is likely to increase the serum concentration by approximately 5 mcg/mL. If the patient is not experiencing theophylline toxicity, this is unlikely to result in dangerous adverse effects.

Subsequent to the decision regarding modification of the loading dose for this group of patients, the maintenance dosage recommendations are the same as those described above.

Principles of I.V. Therapy: The loading dose of Aminophylline can be given by very slow I.V. push or, more conveniently, may be infused in a small quantity (usually 100 to 200 mL) of 5% Dextrose Injection, USP or 0.9% Sodium Chloride Injection, USP. Do not exceed the rate of 25 mg/min.

Thereafter, maintenance therapy can be administered by a large volume infusion to deliver the desired amount of drug each hour. Aminophylline is compatible with most commonly used I.V. solutions.

Oral therapy should be substituted for intravenous Aminophylline as soon as adequate improvement is achieved.

Intravenous Admixture Incompatibility: Although there have been reports of Aminophylline precipitating in acidic media, these reports do not apply to the dilute solutions found in intravenous infusions. Aminophylline injection should not be mixed in a syringe with other drugs but should be added separately to the intravenous solution.

When an intravenous solution containing an Aminophylline is given "piggyback", the intravenous system already in place should be turned off while the Aminophylline is infused if there is a potential problem with admixture incompatibility.

Because of the alkalinity of Aminophylline containing solutions, drugs known to be alkali labile should be avoided in admixtures. These include epinephrine HCl, norepinephrine bitartrate, isoproterenol HCl and penicillin G potassium. It is suggested that specialized literature be consulted before preparing admixtures with Aminophylline and other drugs.

Parenteral drug products should be inspected visually for particulate matter and discoloration prior to administration, whenever solution and container permit. Do not administer unless solution is clear and container is undamaged. Discard unused portion. Do not use if crystals have separated from solution.

II. Chronic Therapy: Theophylline is a treatment for the management of reversible bronchospasm (asthma, chronic bronchitis and emphysema) to prevent symptoms and maintain patent airways. A dosage form which allows small incremental doses is desirable for initiating therapy. A liquid preparation should be considered for children to permit both greater ease of and more accurate dosage adjustment. It is recommended that the appropriate dosage be established using an immediate-release preparation. Slow clinical titration is generally preferred to assure acceptance and safety of the medication, and to allow the patient to develop tolerance to transient caffeine-like side effects.

Initial Dose: 16 mg/kg/24 hours of 400 mg/24 hours (whichever is less) of theophylline in divided doses at 6 or 8 hour intervals.

Increasing Dose: The above dosage may be increased in approximately 25 percent increments at 3 day intervals so long as the drug is tolerated; until clinical response is satisfactory or the maximum dose as indicated in Section III (below) is reached. The serum concentration may be checked at these intervals, but at a minimum, should be determined at the end of this adjustment period.

It is important that no patient be maintained on any dosage that is not tolerated. When instructing patients to increase dosage according to the schedule above, they should be told not to take a subsequent dose if apparent side effects occur and to resume therapy at a lower dose once adverse effects have disappeared.

If the total 24-hour dose can be given by use of the available strength of this product, the patient can usually be switched to controlled-release Aminophylline tablets giving one-half of the daily dose at 12-hour intervals. However, certain patients such as the young, smokers, and some non-smoking adults are likely to metabolize theophylline rapidly and require dosing at 8-hour intervals. Such patients can generally be identified as having trough serum concentrations lower than desired or repeatedly exhibiting symptoms near the end of the dosing interval.

III. Maximum Dose of Theophylline Where the Serum Concentration is not Measured:

WARNING: DO NOT ATTEMPT TO MAINTAIN ANY DOSE THAT IS NOT TOLERATED.

Not to exceed the following or 900 mg (*1100-1140 mg) whichever is less (* = aminophylline dihydrate):

Age 6 - under 9 years	24 mg/kg/day *(30.4 mg/kg/day)
Age 9 - under 12 years	20 mg/kg/day *(25.3 mg/kg/day)
Age 12 - under 16 years	18 mg/kg/day *(22.8 mg/kg/day)
Age 16 years and older	13 mg/kg/day *(16.5 mg/kg/day)

IV. Measurement of Serum Theophylline Concentrations During Chronic Therapy: **If If the above maximum doses are to be maintained or exceeded, serum theophylline measurement is essential.** (See *"Precautions, Laboratory Tests,"* for guidance.)

V. Final Adjustment of Dosage: Dosage adjustment, using the following table, may be necessary after serum theophylline measurement. If the patient is taking controlled-release Aminophylline, he or she may need to be transferred to an immediate-release product for titration. Then, if the final 24 hour dose can be given using controlled-release Aminophylline mg 225, the patient may be transferred back to controlled-release Aminophylline.

If serum theophylline is:		Directions:
Within desired range		Maintain dosage if tolerated.
Too high	20 to 25 mcg/mL	Decrease doses by about 10% and recheck serum level after 3 days.
	25 to 30 mcg/mL	Skip the next dose and decrease subsequent doses by about 25%. Recheck serum level after 3 days.
	Over 30 mcg/mL	Skip next 2 doses and decrease subsequent doses by 50%. Recheck serum level after 3 days.
Too low		Increase dosage by 25% at 3 day intervals until either the desired serum concentration and/or clinical response is achieved. The total daily dose may need to be administered at more frequent intervals if symptoms occur repeatedly at the end of a dosing interval.

The serum concentration may be rechecked at appropriate intervals, but at least at the end of any adjustment period. When the patient's condition is otherwise clinically stable and none of the recognized factors which alter elimination are present, measurement of serum levels need be repeated only every 6 to 12 months.

STORAGE

Store at controlled room temperature, 15° to 30°C (59° to 86°F).

Protect injection from light. Keep syringes in carton until time of use.

Use single-dose container. Discard unused portion.

Protect tablets from moisture. Dispense in a tight, light-resistant container.

J CODES

Up to 250 mg IV—J0280

HOW SUPPLIED
INJECTION: 25 MG/ML

AVERAGE UNIT PRICE (AVAILABLE SIZES)		GENERIC A-RATED AVERAGE PRICE (GAAP)	
GENERIC	$0.36	10 ml 25s	$42.88
		20 ml 25s	$55.49

BRAND/MANUFACTURER	NDC	SIZE	AWP
◆ GENERICS			
Moore,H.L.	00839-5673-30	10 ml	$1.20
Abbott Hosp	00074-4909-03	10 ml 10s	$149.51
Abbott Hosp	00074-4906-03	20 ml 10s	$158.65
Amer Regent	00517-3810-25	10 ml 25s	$19.69
Abbott Hosp	00074-7385-01	10 ml 25s	$51.36
Abbott Hosp	00074-5921-01	10 ml 25s	$57.59

➤ SHOWN IN PRODUCT IDENTIFICATION GUIDE

BRAND/MANUFACTURER	NDC	SIZE	AWP
Amer Regent	00517-3820-25	20 ml 25s	$22.19
Abbott Hosp	00074-7386-01	20 ml 25s	$64.42
Abbott Hosp	00074-5922-01	20 ml 25s	$79.86

SOLUTION: 105 MG/5 ML

AVERAGE UNIT PRICE (AVAILABLE SIZES)		GENERIC A-RATED AVERAGE PRICE (GAAP)	
GENERIC	$0.05	240 ml	$11.88

BRAND/MANUFACTURER	NDC	SIZE	AWP
◆ GENERICS			
Schein	00364-7342-76	240 ml	$11.00
URL	00677-0789-42	240 ml	$11.15
Major	00904-2616-09	240 ml	$11.90
Rugby	00536-0202-59	240 ml	$12.13
Barre	00472-0873-08	240 ml	$12.32
Roxane	00054-3045-63	500 ml	$18.01
Roxane	00054-8049-16	10 ml 40s ud	$23.04
Roxane	00054-8050-16	15 ml 40s ud	$24.05

SUPPOSITORY: 250 MG

BRAND/MANUFACTURER	NDC	SIZE	AWP
◆ GENERICS			
Qualitest	00603-8020-10	10s	$13.12

SUPPOSITORY: 500 MG

BRAND/MANUFACTURER	NDC	SIZE	AWP
◆ GENERICS			
Qualitest	00603-8022-10	10s	$14.48

TABLET, EXTENDED RELEASE: 225 MG

BRAND/MANUFACTURER	NDC	SIZE	AWP
○ BRAND			
PHYLLOCONTIN: Purdue Frederick	00034-0225-80	100s	$33.22

TABLETS: 100 MG

AVERAGE UNIT PRICE (AVAILABLE SIZES)		GENERIC A-RATED AVERAGE PRICE (GAAP)	
GENERIC	$0.03	100s	$3.77
HCFA FUL (100s ea)	$0.03	1000s	$17.50

BRAND/MANUFACTURER	NDC	SIZE	AWP
◆ GENERICS			
Richlyn	00115-2150-01	100s	$2.07
West-Ward	00143-1020-01	100s	$2.47
Rugby	00536-3046-01	100s	$2.92
Geneva	00781-1214-01	100s	$3.45
Schein	00364-0004-01	100s	$3.45
Goldline	00182-0109-01	100s	$3.45
Roxane	00054-4025-25	100s	$3.50
Aligen	00405-4060-01	100s	$3.90
Major	00904-2273-60	100s	$4.20
Roxane	00054-8025-25	100s ud	$8.26
West-Ward	00143-1020-10	1000s	$11.32
Richlyn	00115-2150-03	1000s	$15.90
Goldline	00182-0109-10	1000s	$16.50
Roxane	00054-4025-31	1000s	$18.00
Major	00904-2273-80	1000s	$19.95
Rugby	00536-3046-10	1000s	$20.33
Moore,H.L.	00839-5053-16	1000s	$20.51

TABLETS: 100 MG

BRAND/MANUFACTURER	NDC	SIZE	AWP
◇ GENERICS			
URL	00677-0003-01	100s	$3.45
URL	00677-0003-10	1000s	$20.30

TABLETS: 200 MG

AVERAGE UNIT PRICE (AVAILABLE SIZES)		GENERIC A-RATED AVERAGE PRICE (GAAP)	
GENERIC	$0.04	100s	$5.23
HCFA FUL (100s ea)	$0.04	1000s	$27.93

BRAND/MANUFACTURER	NDC	SIZE	AWP
◆ GENERICS			
Richlyn	00115-2158-01	100s	$3.30
West-Ward	00143-1025-01	100s	$3.68
Roxane	00054-4026-25	100s	$4.03
Geneva	00781-1318-01	100s	$4.35
Moore,H.L.	00839-1011-06	100s	$4.90
Rugby	00536-3060-01	100s	$5.28
Major	00904-2283-60	100s	$5.30
Goldline	00182-0110-01	100s	$5.40
Aligen	00405-4061-01	100s	$5.64

BRAND/MANUFACTURER	NDC	SIZE	AWP
Schein	00364-0005-01	100s	$5.99
Roxane	00054-8026-25	100s ud	$9.66
West-Ward	00143-1025-10	1000s	$16.99
Parmed	00349-2009-10	1000s	$19.75
Richlyn	00115-2158-03	1000s	$25.35
Geneva	00781-1318-10	1000s	$25.85
Roxane	00054-4026-31	1000s	$26.42
Goldline	00182-0110-10	1000s	$33.00
Rugby	00536-3060-10	1000s	$33.33
Major	00904-2283-80	1000s	$33.40
Moore,H.L.	00839-1011-16	1000s	$37.26

Aminophylline/Ephedrine Hydrochloride/Guaifenesin/ Phenobarbital

DESCRIPTION

Each tablet contains:

Aminophylline (anhydrous) .... 130 mg
Ephedrine Hydrochloride .... 16 mg
Phenobarbital .... 8 mg (Warning: may be habit-forming)
Guaifenesin .... 100 mg

INDICATIONS

Aminophylline/Ephedrine Hydrochloride/Guaifenesin/Phenobarbital gives prompt symptomatic relief in bronchial asthma, emphysema and asthmatic bronchitis. This combination dilates the bronchi and liquefies the mucus plugs. The Phenobarbital minimizes the side-effect (nervousness) of Ephedrine. The product is buffered for gastric tolerance.

This combination should be prescribed when acne or tuberculosis co-exist, during pregnancy, or when iodide intolerance is present.

CONTRAINDICATIONS

Aminophylline/theophylline is contraindicated in the presence of severe cardiac arrhythmias and in patients with massive myocardial damage. Ephedrine is contraindicated in the presence of severe heart disease, severe hypertension and in hyperthyroidism.

Phenobarbital is contraindicated in porphyria and in patients with known Phenobarbital sensitivity.

PRECAUTIONS

Aminophylline/theophylline should be avoided in patients with massive myocardial damage and/or severe cardiac arrhythmias, and severe agitation.

Ephedrine should be used with caution in the presence of severe cardiac disease, particularly arrhythmias and angina pectoris, it should be avoided in hyperthyroidism and severe hypertension.

Phenobarbital may be habit-forming. Avoid overdosage.

ADVERSE REACTIONS

Aminophylline/theophylline may cause cardiac arrhythmias and aggravate severe myocardial disease; may cause headaches and tachycardia; vomiting and dizziness are not uncommon. Ephedrine may cause nervousness, tachycardia, extrasystole and ventricular arrhythmias in patients hypersensitive to CNS stimulation. Also, Ephedrine may cause urinary retention, especially in the presence of partial prostatic obstruction. Psychoneurosis may be aggravated. Pre-existing anginal pain will be aggravated. Phenobarbital may produce severe skin rash; avoid overdosage; may be habit-forming.

DOSAGE

One tablet with full glass of water, 3 or 4 times daily, as required. Divide tablet for child's dose.

HOW SUPPLIED
TABLETS:

BRAND/MANUFACTURER	NDC	SIZE	AWP
○ BRAND			
MUDRANE GG-2: Poythress	00095-0033-01	100s	$21.00

Aminosalicylic Acid

DESCRIPTION

Aminosalicylic Acid granules are a delayed release granule preparation of Aminosalicylic Acid (p-aminosalicylic acid; (4-aminosalicylic acid) for use with other anti-tuberculosis drugs for the treatment of all forms of active tuberculosis due to susceptible strains of tubercle bacilli. The granules are designed for gradual release to avoid high peak levels not useful (and perhaps toxic) with bacteriostatic drugs. Aminosalicylic Acid is rapidly degraded in acid media; the protective acid-resistant outer coating is rapidly dissolved in neutral media so a mildly acidic food such as orange, apple or tomato juice, yogurt or apple sauce should be used.

◆ RATED THERAPEUTICALLY EQUIVALENT; ◇ THERAPEUTIC EQUIVALENCE UNCONFIRMED; ○ UNRATED

Aminosalicylic Acid (p-aminosalicylic acid) is 4-Amino-2-hydroxybenzoic acid. Aminosalicylic Acid granules are the free base of Aminosalicylic Acid and do NOT contain sodium or a sugar. The molecular formula is $C_7H_7NO_3$ with a molecular weight of 153.14. With heat p-aminosalicylic acid is decarboxylated to produce CO_2 and m-aminophenol. If the airtight packets are swollen, storage has been improper. DO NOT USE if packets are swollen or the granules have lost their tan color and are dark brown or purple.

The packets contain 4 grams of Aminosalicylic Acid for oral administration three times a day by sprinkling on apple sauce or yogurt to be eaten without chewing. Suspension in an acidic fruit drink such as orange juice or tomato juice will protect the coating for at least 2 hours. Swirling the juice in the glass will help resuspend the granules if they sink.

Following is its chemical structure:

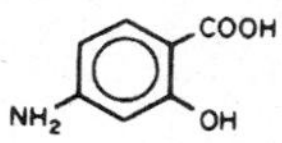

CLINICAL PHARMACOLOGY

Mechanism of Action: Aminosalicylic Acid is bacteriostatic against Mycobacterium tuberculosis. It inhibits the onset of bacterial resistance to streptomycin and isoniazid. The mechanism of action has been postulated to be inhibition of folic acid synthesis (but without potentiation with antifolic compounds) and/or inhibition of synthesis of the cell wall component, mycobactin, thus reducing iron uptake by M. tuberculosis.

Characteristics: The two major considerations in the clinical pharmacology of Aminosalicylic Acid are the prompt production of a toxic inactive metabolite under acid conditions and the short serum half life of one hour for the free drug. Both are discussed below.

After two hours in simulated gastric fluid, 10% of unprotected Aminosalicylic Acid is decarboxylated to form meta-aminophenol, a known hepatotoxin. The acid-resistant coating of the Aminosalicylic Acid granules protects against degradation in the stomach. The small granules are designed to escape the usual restriction on gastric emptying of large particles. Under neutral conditions such as are found in the small intestine or in neutral foods, the acid-resistant coating is dissolved within one minute. Care must be taken in the administration of these granules to protect the acid-resistant coating by maintaining the granules in an acidic food during dosage administration. Patients who have neutralized gastric acid with antacids will not need to protect the acid resistant coating with an acidic food since no acid is present to spoil the drug. Antacids may influence the absorption of other medications and are not necessary for Aminosalicylic Acid consumed with an acidic food.

Because Aminosalicylic Acid granules are protected by an enteric coating, absorption does not commence until they leave the stomach; the soft skeletons of the granules remain and may be seen in the stool.

Absorption and Excretion: In a single 4 gram pharmacokinetic study with food in normal volunteers the initial time to a 2 µg/mL serum level of Aminosalicylic Acid was 2 hours with a range of 45 minutes to 24 hours; the median time to peak was 6 hours with a range of 1.5 to 24 hours; the mean peak level was 20 µg/mL with a range of 9 to 35 µg/mL; a level of 2 µg/mL was maintained for an average of 7.9 hours with a range of 5 to 9; a level of 1 µg/mL was maintained for an average of 8.8 hours with a range of 6 to 11.5 hours. The recommended schedule is 4 grams every 8 hours.

80% of Aminosalicylic Acid is excreted in the urine, with 50% or more of the dosage excreted in acetylated form. The acetylation process is not genetically determined as is the case for isoniazid. Aminosalicylic Acid is excreted by glomerular filtration; although previously reported otherwise, probenecid, a tubular blocking agent, does not enhance plasma concentration. In a 1954 study thyroxine synthesis but not iodide uptake was reported reduced about 40% when the sodium salt (not Aminosalicylic Acid granules) of Aminosalicylic Acid was administered one hour before radio-iodine; the sodium salt typically produces a serum level over 120 µg/mL at one hour lasting one hour. Occasional goiter development can be prevented by the administration of thyroxine but not iodide.

Penetration into the cerebrospinal fluid occurs only if the meninges are inflamed.

Approximately 50-60% of Aminosalicylic Acid is protein bound; binding is reported to be reduced 50% in kwashiorkor.

Microbiology: The Aminosalicylic Acid MIC for M. tuberculosis in 7H11 agar was less than 1.0 µg/mL for nine strains including three multidrug resistant strains, but 4 and 8 µg/mL for two other multidrug resistant strains. The 90% inhibition in 7H12 broth (Bactec) showed little dose response but was interpreted as being less than or equal to 0.12-0.25 µg/mL for eight strains of which three were multi-resistant, 0.50 µg/mL for one resistant strain, questionable for four non-resistant strains and greater than 1 µg/mL for one non-resistant and three resistant strains. Aminosalicylic Acid is not active *in vitro* against M. avium.

INDICATIONS AND USAGE

Aminosalicylic Acid is indicated for the treatment of tuberculosis in combination with other active agents. It is most commonly used in patients with Multi-drug Resistant TB (MDR-TB) or in situations when therapy with isoniazid and rifampin is not possible due to a combination of resistance and/or intolerance. When Aminosalicylic Acid is added to the treatment regimen in patients with proven or suspected drug resistance, it should be accompanied by at least one and preferably two other new agents to which the patient's organism is known or expected to be susceptible.

UNLABELED USES

Aminosalicylic Acid is used alone or as an adjunct in the treatment of Crohn's disease.

CONTRAINDICATIONS

Hypersensitivity to any component of this medication.

Severe renal disease.

Patients with severe renal disease will accumulate Aminosalicylic Acid and its acetyl metabolite but will continue to acetylate thus leading exclusively to the inactive acetylated form; deacetylation, if any, is not significant.

The half life of free Aminosalicylic Acid in renal disease is 30.8 minutes in comparison to 26.4 minutes in normal volunteers, but the half life of the inactive metabolite is 309 minutes in uremic patients in comparison to 51 minutes in normal volunteers. Although Aminosalicylic Acid passes dialysis membranes, the frequency of dialysis usually is not comparable to the half-life of 50 minutes for the free acid. Patients with end stage renal disease should not receive Aminosalicylic Acid.

WARNINGS

Liver Function

In one retrospective study of 7492 patients on rapidly absorbed Aminosalicylic Acid preparations, drug-induced hepatitis occurred in 38 patients (0.5%); in these 38 the first symptom usually appeared within three months of the start of therapy with a rash as the most common event followed by fever and much less frequently by GI disturbances of anorexia, nausea or diarrhea. Only one patient was diagnosed on routine biochemistry.

Premonitory symptoms in 90% of the patients preceded jaundice by a few days to several weeks. The mean time of onset was 33 days with a range of 7-90 days. Half of the adverse reactions occurred during the third, fourth or fifth weeks. When Aminosalicylic Acid-induced hepatitis was diagnosed, hepatomegaly was invariably present with lymphadenopathy in 46%, leucocytosis in 79%, and eosinophilia in 55%. Prompt recognition with discontinuation led to the recovery of all 38 patients. If recognized in the premonitory stage, the reaction is reported to "settle" in 24 hours and no jaundice ensues. From other reported studies the failure to recognize the reaction can result in a mortality of up to 21%. The patient must be monitored carefully during the first three months of therapy and treatment must be discontinued immediately at the first sign of a rash, fever or other premonitory signs of intolerance.

PRECAUTIONS

(1) General: All drugs should be stopped at the first sign suggesting a hypersensitivity reaction. They may be restarted one at a time in very small but gradually increasing doses to determine whether the manifestations are drug-induced and, if so, which drug is responsible.

Desensitization has been accomplished successfully in 15 of 17 patients starting with 10 mg Aminosalicylic Acid given as a single dose. The dosage is doubled every 2 days until reaching a total of 1 gram after which the dosage is divided to follow the regular schedule of administration. If a mild temperature rise or skin reaction develops, the increment is to be dropped back one level or the progression held for one cycle. Reactions are rare after a total dosage of 1.5 grams.

Patients with hepatic disease may not tolerate Aminosalicylic Acid as well as normal patients, even though the metabolism in patients with hepatic disease has been reported to be comparable to that in normal volunteers.

(2) Information for Patients: The patient should be advised that the first signs of hypersensitivity include a rash, often followed by fever, and much less frequently, GI disturbances of anorexia, nausea or diarrhea. If such symptoms develop, the patient should immediately cease taking the medication and arrange for a prompt clinical visit.

Patients should be advised that poor compliance in taking anti-TB medication often leads to treatment failure, and, not infrequently, to the development of resistance of the organisms in the individual patient.

Patients should be advised that the skeleton of the granules may be seen in the stool.

The coating to protect the Aminosalicylic Acid granules dissolves promptly under neutral conditions; the granules therefore should be administered by sprinkling on acidic foods such as apple sauce or yogurt or by suspension in a fruit drink which will protect the coating, but the granules sink and will have to be swirled. The coating will last at least 2 hours in either system. All juices tested to date have been satisfactory; tested are: tomato, orange, grapefruit, grape, cranberry, apple, "fruit punch".

Patients should be advised NOT to use if the packets are swollen or the granules have lost their tan color and are dark brown or purple. The patient should inform the pharmacist or physician immediately and return the medication.

(3) Laboratory Tests: Aminosalicylic Acid has been reported to interfere technically with the serum determinations of albumin by dye-binding, SGOT by the azoene dye method and with qualitative urine tests for ketones, bilirubin, urobilinogen or porphobilinogen.

(4) Drug Interactions: Aminosalicylic Acid at a dosage of 12 grams in a rapidly available form has been reported to produce a 20 percent reduction in the acetylation of isoniazid, especially in patients who are rapid acetylators; INH serum levels, half lives and excretions in fast acetylators still remain half of the levels seen in slow acetylators with or without p-aminosalicylic acid. The effect is

dose related and, while it has not been studied with the current delayed release preparation, the lower serum levels with this preparation will result in a reduced effect on the acetylation of INH.

Aminosalicylic Acid has previously been reported to block the absorption of rifampin. A subsequent report has shown that this blockade was due to an excipient not included in Aminosalicylic Acid granules. Oral administration of a solution containing both Aminosalicylic Acid and rifampin showed full absorption of each product.

As a result of competition, Vitamin B_{12} absorption has been reduced 55% by 5 grams of Aminosalicylic Acid with clinically significant erythrocyte abnormalities developing after depletion; patients on therapy of more than one month should be considered for maintenance B_{12}.

A malabsorption syndrome can develop in patients on Aminosalicylic Acid but is usually not complete. The complete syndrome includes steatorrhea, an abnormal small bowel pattern on x-ray, villus atrophy, depressed cholesterol, reduced D-xylose and iron absorption. Triglyceride absorption always is normal.

In one literature report 8 hours after the last dosage of Aminosalicylic Acid at 2 gm qid serum digoxin levels were reduced 40% in two of ten patients but not changed in the remaining eight.

(5) Carcinogenesis, Mutagenesis, Impairment of Fertility: Sodium aminosalicylate produced an occipital bone defect, probably with a dose response, when administered to ten pregnant Wistar rats at five doses from 3.85 to 385 mg/kg from days 6 to 14. There were no significant changes from controls in any group in corpora lutea, early resorptions, total resorptions, fetal death, litter size, or hematomas. For all except the 77 mg/kg group, fetal weights were significantly greater than controls. Chinchilla rabbits on 5 mg/kg from days 7 to 14 did not show any significant differences as compared to controls for the same parameters studied.

Sodium Aminosalicylic Acid was not mutagenic in Ames tester strain TA 100. In human lymphocyte cultures *in vitro* clastogenic effects of achromatic, chromatid, isochromatic breaks or chromatid translocations were not seen at 153 or 600 µg/mL. At 1500 and 3000 µg/mL there was a dose related increase in chromatid aberrations.

Patients on isoniazid and Aminosalicylic Acid have been reported to have an increased number of chromosomal aberrations as compared to controls.

(6) Pregnancy: Pregnancy Category C: Aminosalicylic Acid has been reported to produce occipital malformations in rats when given at doses within the human dose range. Although there probably is a dose response, the frequency of abnormalities was comparable to controls at the highest level tested (two times the human dosage). When administered to rabbits at 5 mg/kg, throughout all three trimesters, no teratogenic or embryocidal effects were seen. Literature reports on Aminosalicylic Acid in pregnant women always report coadministration of other medications. Because there are no adequate and well controlled studies of Aminosalicylic Acid in humans, Aminosalicylic Acid granules should be given to a pregnant woman only if clearly needed.

(7) Nursing Mothers: After administration of a different preparation of Aminosalicylic Acid to one patient, the maximum concentration in the milk was 1 µg/mL at 3 hours with a half-life of 2.5 hours; the maximum maternal plasma concentration was 70 µg/mL at two hours.

ADVERSE EFFECTS
The most common side effect is gastrointestinal intolerance manifested by nausea, vomiting, diarrhea, and abdominal pain.

Hypersensitivity Reactions: Fever, skin eruptions of various types, including exfoliative dermatitis, infectious mononucleosis-like, or lymphoma-like syndrome, leucopenia, agranulocytosis, thrombocytopenia, Coombs' positive hemolytic anemia, jaundice, hepatitis, pericarditis, hypoglycemia, optic neuritis, encephalopathy, Leoffler's syndrome, and vasculitis and a reduction in prothrombin.

Crystalluria may be prevented by the maintenance of urine at a neutral or an alkaline pH.

OVERDOSAGE
Overdosage has not been reported.

DOSAGE AND ADMINISTRATION
Aminosalicylic Acid granules should be administered with other drugs to which the organism is known or expected to be susceptible. It is most commonly administered to patients with Multi-drug Resistant TB (MDR-TB) or in other situations in which therapy with isoniazid or rifampin is not possible due to a combination of resistance and/or intolerance. The adult dosage of four grams (one packet) three times per day or correspondingly smaller doses in children should be given by sprinkling on apple sauce or yogurt or by swirling in the glass to suspend the granules in an acidic drink such as tomato or orange juice.

DO NOT USE if the packet is swollen or the granules have lost their tan color, turning dark brown or purple.

Store below 77°F (25°C). AVOID EXCESSIVE HEAT.

HOW SUPPLIED
For Paser Granules availability contact Jacobus Pharmaceuticals.

Aminosyn *SEE* AMINO ACIDS, INJECTABLE *AND* AMINO ACIDS/CALCIUM CHLORIDE/DEXTROSE/ELECTROLYTES

Aminosyn with Electrolytes *SEE* AMINO ACIDS WITH ELECTROLYTES, INJECTABLE

Amiodarone Hydrochloride

DESCRIPTION
Amiodarone Hydrochloride is a member of a new class of antiarrhythmic drugs with predominantly Class III (Vaughan Williams' classification) effects, available for oral administration as white, scored tablets containing 200 mg of Amiodarone Hydrochloride. Amiodarone HCl is a benzofuran derivative: 2-butyl-3-benzofuranyl 4-[2-(diethylamino)-ethoxy]-3-5-diiodophenyl ketone, hydrochloride. It is not chemically related to any other available antiarrhythmic drug.

Amiodarone HCl is a white to cream-colored crystalline powder. It is slightly soluble in water, soluble in alcohol, and freely soluble in chloroform. It contains 37.3% iodine by weight.

Following is its chemical structure:

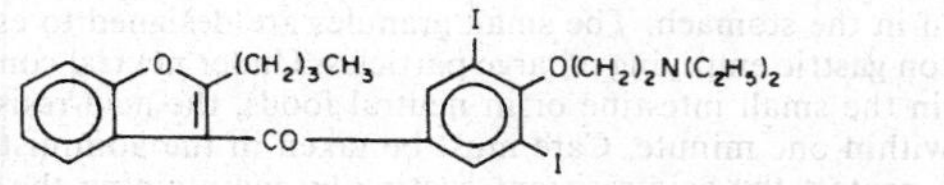

CLINICAL PHARMACOLOGY
ELECTROPHYSIOLOGY/MECHANISMS OF ACTION
In animals. Amiodarone HCl is effective in the prevention or suppression of experimentally induced arrhythmias. The antiarrhythmic effect of Amiodarone HCl may be due to at least two major properties: 1) a prolongation of the myocardial cell-action potential duration and refractory period and 2) noncompetitive alpha- and beta-adrenergic inhibition.

Amiodarone HCl prolongs the duration of the action potential of all cardiac fibers while causing minimal reduction of dV/dt (maximal upstroke velocity of the action potential). The refractory period is prolonged in all cardiac tissues. Amiodarone HCl increases the cardiac refractory period without influencing resting membrane potential, except in automatic cells where the slope of the prepotential is reduced, generally reducing automaticity. These electrophysiologic effects are reflected in a decreased sinus rate of 15 to 20%, increased PR and QT intervals of about 10%, the development of U-waves, and changes in T-wave contour. These changes should not require discontinuation of Amiodarone HCl, as they are evidence of its pharmacological action, although Amiodarone HCl can cause marked sinus bradycardia or sinus arrest and heart block. On rare occasions, QT prolongation has been associated with worsening of arrhythmia (see *"Warnings"*).

HEMODYNAMICS
In animal studies and after intravenous administration in man, Amiodarone HCl relaxes vascular smooth muscle, reduces peripheral vascular resistance (afterload), and slightly increases cardiac index. After oral dosing, however Amiodarone HCl produces no significant change in left ventricular ejection fraction (LVEF), even in patients with depressed LVEF. After acute intravenous dosing in man, Amiodarone HCl may have a mild negative inotropic effect.

PHARMACOKINETICS
Following oral administration in man, Amiodarone HCl is slowly and variably absorbed. The bioavailability of Amiodarone HCl is approximately 50%, but has varied between 35 and 65% in various studies. Maximum plasma concentrations are attained 3 to 7 hours after a single dose. Despite this, the onset of action may occur in 2 to 3 days, but more commonly takes 1 to 3 weeks, even with loading doses. Plasma concentrations with chronic dosing at 100 to 600 mg/day are approximately dose proportional, with a mean 0.5 mg/L increase for each 100 mg/day. These means, however, include considerable individual variability.

Amiodarone HCl has a very large but variable volume of distribution, averaging about 60 L/kg because of extensive accumulation in various sites, especially adipose tissue and highly perfused organs, such as the liver, lung, and spleen. One major metabolite of Amiodarone HCl, desethylamiodarone, has been identified in man; it accumulates to an even greater extent in almost all tissues. The pharmacological activity of this metabolite, however, is not known. During chronic treatment, the plasma ratio of metabolite to parent compound is approximately one.

The main route of elimination is via hepatic excretion into bile, and some enterohepatic recirculation may occur. However, its kinetics in patients with hepatic insufficiency have not been elucidated. Amiodarone HCl has a very low plasma clearance with negligible renal excretion, so that it does not appear necessary to modify the dose in patients with renal failure. In patients with renal impairment, the plasma concentration of Amiodarone HCl is not elevated. Neither Amiodarone HCl nor its metabolite is dailyzable.

In patients following discontinuation of chronic oral therapy, Amiodarone HCl has been shown to have a biphasic elimination with an initial one-half reduction of plasma levels after 2.5 to 10 days. A much slower terminal plasma-elimination phase shows a half-life of the parent compound ranging from 26 to 107 days, with a mean of approximately 53 days and most patients in the 40- to 55-day range. In the absence of a loading-dose period, steady-state plasma concentrations, at constant oral dosing, would therefore be reached between 130 and 535 days, with an average of 265 days. For the metabolite, the mean plasma-elimination half-life was approximately 61 days. These data probably reflect an initial elimination of the drug from well-perfused tissue (the 2.5- to 10-day half-life phase), followed by a terminal phase representing extremely slow elimination from poorly perfused tissue compartments such as fat.

The considerable intersubject variation both phases of elimination, as well as uncertainty as to what compartment is critical to drug effect, requires attention to individual responses once arrhythmia control is achieved with loading doses because the correct maintenance dose is determined, in part, by the elimination rates. Daily maintenance doses of Amiodarone HCl should be based on individual patient requirements (see *"Dosage and Administration"*).

Amiodarone HCl and its metabolite have a limited transplacental transfer of approximately 10 to 50%. The parent drug and its metabolite have been detected in breast milk. Amiodarone HCl is highly protein-bound (approximately 96%). Although electrophysiologic effects, such as prolongation of QTc, can be seen within hours after a parenteral dose of Amiodarone HCl, effects on abnormal rhythms are not seen before 2 to 3 days and usually require 1 to 3 weeks, even when a loading dose is used. There may be a continued increase in effect for longer periods still. There is evidence that the time to effect is shorter when a loading-dose regimen is used.

Consistent with the slow rate of elimination, antiarrhythmic effects persist for weeks or months after Amiodarone HCl is discontinued, but the time of recurrence is variable and unpredictable. In general, when the drug is resumed after recurrence of the arrhythmia, control is established relatively rapidly compared to the initial response, presumably because tissue stores were not wholly depleted at the time of recurrence.

PHARMACODYNAMICS
There is no well-established relationship of plasma concentration to effectiveness, but it does appear that concentrations much below 1 mg/L are often ineffective and that levels above 2.5 mg/L are generally not needed. Within individuals dose reductions and ensuing decreased plasma concentrations can result in loss of arrhythmia control. Plasma-concentrations measurements can be used to identify patients whose levels are unusually low, and who might benefit from a dose increase, or unusually high, and who might have dosage reduction in the hope of minimizing side effects. Some observations have suggested a plasma concentration, dose, or dose/duration relationship for side effects such as pulmonary fibrosis, liver-enzyme elevations, corneal deposits and facial pigmentation, peripheral neuropathy, gastrointestinal and central nervous system effects.

MONITORING EFFECTIVENESS
Predicting the effectiveness of any antiarrhythmic agent in long-term prevention of recurrent ventricular tachycardia and ventricular fibrillation is difficult and controversial, with highly qualified investigators recommending use of ambulatory monitoring, programmed electrical stimulation with various stimulation regimens, or a combination of these, to assess response. There is no present consensus on many aspects of how best to assess effectiveness, but there is a reasonable consensus on some aspects:

1. If a patient with a history of cardiac arrest does not manifest a hemodynamically unstable arrhythmia during electocardiographic monitoring prior to treatment, assessment of the effectiveness of Amiodarone HCl requires some provocative approach, either exercise or programmed electrical stimulation (PES).
2. Whether provocation is also needed in patients who do manifest their life-threatening arrhythmia spontaneously is not settled, but there are reasons to consider PES or other provocation in such patients. In the fraction of patients whose PES-inducible arrhythmia can be made noninducible by Amiodarone HCl (a fraction that has varied widely in various series from less than 10% to almost 40%, perhaps due to different stimulation criteria), the prognosis has been almost uniformly excellent, with very low recurrence (ventricular tachycardia or sudden death) rates. More controversial is the meaning of continued inducibility. There has been an impression that continued inducibility in Amiodarone HCl patients may not foretell a poor prognosis but, in fact, many observers have found greater recurrence rates in patients who remain inducible than in those who do not. A number of criteria have been proposed, however, for identifying patients who remain inducible but who seem likely nonetheless to do well on Amiodarone HCl. These criteria include increased difficulty of induction (more stimuli or more rapid stimuli), which has been reported to predict a lower rate of recurrence, and ability to tolerate the induced ventricular tachycardia without severe symptoms, a

finding that has been reported to correlate with better survival but not with lower recurrence rates. While these criteria require confirmation and further study in general, *easier* inducibility or *poorer* tolerance of the induced arrhythmia should suggest consideration of a need to revise treatment.

Several predictors of success not based on PES have also been suggested, including complete elimination of all nonsustained ventricular tachycardia on ambulatory monitoring and very low premature ventricular-beat rates (less than 1 VPB/1,000 normal beats).

While these issues remain unsettled for Amiodarone HCl, as for other agents, the prescriber of Amiodarone HCl should have access to (direct or through referral), and familiarity with, the full range of evaluatory procedures used in the care of patients with life-threatening arrhythmias.

It is difficult to describe the effectiveness rates of Amiodarone HCl, as these depend on the specific arrhythmia treated, the success criteria used, the underlying cardiac disease of the patient, the number of drugs tried before resorting to Amiodarone HCl, the duration of follow-up, the dose of Amiodarone HCl, the use of additional antiarrhythmic agents, and many other factors. As Amiodarone HCl has been studied principally in patients with refractory life-threatening ventricular arrhythmias, in whom drug therapy must be selected on the basis of response and cannot be assigned arbitrarily, randomized comparisons with other agents or placebo have not been possible. Reports of series of treated patients with a history of cardiac arrest and mean follow-up of one year or more have given mortality (due to arrhythmia) rates that were highly variable, ranging from less than 5% to over 30%, with most series in the range of 10 to 15%. Overall arrhythmia-recurrence rates (fatal and nonfatal) also were highly variable (and, as noted above, depended on response to PES and other measures), and depend on whether patients who do not seem to respond initially are included. In most cases, considering only patients who seemed to respond well enough to be placed on long-term treatment, recurrence rates have ranged from 20 to 40% in series with a mean follow-up of a year or more.

INDICATIONS AND USAGE
Because of its life-threatening side effects and the substantial management difficulties associated with its use (see *"Warnings"* below), Amiodarone HCl is indicated only for the treatment of the following documented, life-threatening recurrent ventricular arrhythmias when these have not responded to documented adequate doses of other available antiarrhythmics or when alternative agents could not be tolerated.
   1. Recurrent ventricular fibrillation.
   2. Recurrent hemodynamically unstable ventricular tachycardia.

As is the case for other antiarrhythmic agents, there is no evidence from controlled trials that the use of Amiodarone HCl favorably affects survival.

Amiodarone HCl should be used only by physicians familiar with and with access to (directly or through referral) the use of all available modalities for treating recurrent life-threatening ventricular arrhythmias, and who have access to appropriate monitoring facilities, including in-hospital and ambulatory continuous electrocardiographic monitoring and electrophysiologic techniques. Because of the life-threatening nature of the arrhythmias treated, potential interactions with prior therapy, and potential exacerbation of the arrhythmia, initiation of therapy with Amiodarone HCl should be carried out in the hospital.

UNLABELED USES
Amiodarone HCl is used alone or as an adjunct in the treatment of angina, arrhythmias secondary to hypertrophic cardiomyopathy, and ventricular arrhythmias in patients with Chagasic myocarditis. It is also used in the treatment of paroxysmal atrial fibrillation, supraventricular tachycardia, and tachycardia in Wolff-Parkinson White syndrome.

CONTRAINDICATIONS
Amiodarone HCl is contraindicated in severe sinus-node dysfunction, causing marked sinus bradycardia; second- and third-degree atrioventricular block; and when episodes of bradycardia have caused syncope (except when used in conjunction with a pacemaker).

Amiodarone HCl is contraindicated in patients with a known hypersensitivity to the drug.

WARNINGS
AMIODARONE HCL IS INTENDED FOR USE ONLY IN PATIENTS WITH THE INDICATED LIFE-THREATENING ARRHYTHMIAS BECAUSE ITS USE IS ACCOMPANIED BY SUBSTANTIAL TOXICITY.

AMIODARONE HCL HAS SEVERAL POTENTIALLY FATAL TOXICITIES, THE MOST IMPORTANT OF WHICH IS PULMONARY TOXICITY (HYPERSENSITIVITY PNEUMONITIS OR INTERSTITIAL/ALVEOLAR PNEUMONITIS) THAT HAS RESULTED IN CLINICALLY MANIFEST DISEASE AT RATES AS HIGH AS 10 TO 17% IN SOME SERIES OF PATIENTS WITH VENTRICULAR ARRHYTHMIAS GIVEN DOSES AROUND 400 MG/DAY, AND AS ABNORMAL DIFFUSION CAPACITY WITHOUT SYMPTOMS IN A MUCH HIGHER PERCENTAGE OF PATIENTS. PULMONARY TOXICITY HAS BEEN FATAL ABOUT 10% OF THE TIME. LIVER INJURY IS COMMON WITH AMIODARONE HCL BUT IS USUALLY MILD AND EVIDENCED ONLY BY ABNORMAL LIVER ENZYMES. OVERT LIVER DISEASE CAN OCCUR, HOWEVER, AND HAS BEEN FATAL IN A FEW CASES. LIKE OTHER ANTIARRHYTHMICS, AMIODARONE HCL CAN EXACERBATE THE ARRHYTHMIA, E.G., BY MAKING THE ARRHYTHMIA LESS WELL TOLERATED OR MORE DIFFICULT TO

REVERSE. THIS HAS OCCURRED IN 2 TO 5% OF PATIENTS IN VARIOUS SERIES, AND SIGNIFICANT HEART BLOCK OR SINUS BRADYCARDIA HAS BEEN SEEN IN 2 TO 5%. ALL OF THESE EVENTS SHOULD BE MANAGEABLE IN THE PROPER CLINICAL SETTING IN MOST CASES. ALTHOUGH THE FREQUENCY OF SUCH PROARRHYTHMIC EVENTS DOES NOT APPEAR GREATER WITH AMIODARONE HCL THAN WITH MANY OTHER AGENTS USED IN THIS POPULATION, THE EFFECTS ARE PROLONGED WHEN THEY OCCUR.

EVEN IN PATIENTS AT HIGH RISK OF ARRHYTHMIC DEATH, IN WHOM THE TOXICITY OF AMIODARONE HCL IS AN ACCEPTABLE RISK, AMIODARONE HCL POSES MAJOR MANAGEMENT PROBLEMS THAT COULD BE LIFE-THREATENING IN A POPULATION AT RISK OF SUDDEN DEATH, SO THAT EVERY EFFORT SHOULD BE MADE TO UTILIZE ALTERNATIVE AGENTS FIRST.

THE DIFFICULTY OF USING AMIODARONE HCL EFFECTIVELY AND SAFELY ITSELF POSES A SIGNIFICANT RISK TO PATIENTS. PATIENTS WITH THE INDICATED ARRHYTHMIAS MUST BE HOSPITALIZED WHILE THE LOADING DOSE OF AMIODARONE HCL IS GIVEN, AND A RESPONSE GENERALLY REQUIRES AT LEAST ONE WEEK, USUALLY TWO OR MORE. BECAUSE ABSORPTION AND ELIMINATION ARE VARIABLE, MAINTENANCE-DOSE SELECTION IS DIFFICULT, AND IT IS NOT UNUSUAL TO REQUIRE DOSAGE DECREASE OR DISCONTINUATION OF TREATMENT. IN A RETROSPECTIVE SURVEY OF 192 PATIENTS WITH VENTRICULAR TACHYARRHYTHMIAS, 84 REQUIRED DOSE REDUCTION AND 18 REQUIRED AT LEAST TEMPORARY DISCONTINUATION BECAUSE OF ADVERSE EFFECTS, AND SEVERAL SERIES HAVE REPORTED 15 TO 20% OVERALL FREQUENCIES OF DISCONTINUATION DUE TO ADVERSE REACTIONS. THE TIME AT WHICH A PREVIOUSLY CONTROLLED LIFE-THREATENING ARRHYTHMIA WILL RECUR AFTER DISCONTINUATION OR DOSE ADJUSTMENT IS UNPREDICTABLE, RANGING FROM WEEKS TO MONTHS. THE PATIENT IS OBVIOUSLY AT GREAT RISK DURING THIS TIME AND MAY NEED PROLONGED HOSPITALIZATION. ATTEMPTS TO SUBSTITUTE OTHER ANTIARRHYTHMIC AGENTS WHEN AMIODARONE HCL MUST BE STOPPED WILL BE MADE DIFFICULT BY THE GRADUALLY, BUT UNPREDICTABLY, CHANGING AMIODARONE BODY BURDEN. A SIMILAR PROBLEM EXISTS WHEN AMIODARONE HCL IS NOT EFFECTIVE; IT STILL POSES THE RISK OF AN INTERACTION WITH WHATEVER SUBSEQUENT TREATMENT IS TRIED.

PULMONARY TOXICITY

Amiodarone HCl may cause a clinical syndrome of cough and progressive dyspnea accompanied by functional, radiographic, gallium-scan, and pathological data consistent with pulmonary toxicity, the frequency of which varies from 2 to 7% in most reports, but is as high as 10 to 17% in some reports. Therefore, when Amiodarone HCl therapy is initiated, a baseline chest x-ray and pulmonary-function tests, including diffusion capacity, should be performed. The patient should return for a history, physical exam, and chest x-ray every 3 to 6 months.

Preexisting pulmonary disease does not appear to increase the risk of developing pulmonary toxicity; however, these patients have a poorer prognosis if pulmonary toxicity does develop.

Pulmonary toxicity secondary to Amiodarone HCl seems to result from either indirect or direct toxicity as represented by hypersensitivity pneumonitis or interstitial/alveolar pneumonitis, respectively.

Hypersensitivity pneumonitis usually appears earlier in the course of therapy, and rechallenging these patients with Amiodarone HCl results in a more rapid recurrence of greater severity. Bronchoalveolar lavage is the procedure of choice to confirm this diagnosis, which can be made when a T suppressor/cytotoxic (CD8-positive) lymphocytosis is noted. Steroid therapy should be instituted and Amiodarone HCl therapy discontinued in these patients.

Interstitial/alveolar pneumonitis may result from the release of oxygen radicals and/or phospholipidosis and is characterized by findings of diffuse alveolar damage, interstitial pneumonitis or fibrosis in lung biopsy specimens. Phospholipidosis (foamy cells, foamy macrophages), due to inhibition of phospholipase, will be present in most cases of Amiodarone HCl induced pulmonary toxicity; however, these changes also are present in approximately 50% of all patients on Amiodarone HCl therapy. These cells should be used as markers of therapy, but not as evidence of toxicity. A diagnosis of Amiodarone-HCl induced interstitial/alveolar pneumonitis should lead, at a minimum, to dose reduction or preferably, to withdrawal of the Amiodarone HCl to establish reversibility, especially if other acceptable antiarrhythmic therapies are available. Where these measures have been instituted, a reduction in symptoms of amiodarone-induced pulmonary toxicity was usually noted within the first week, and a clinical improvement was greatest in the first two to three weeks. Chest X-ray changes usually resolve within two to four months. According to some experts, steroids may prove beneficial. Prednisone in doses of 40 to 60 mg/day or equivalent doses of other steroids have been given and tapered over the course of several weeks depending upon the condition of the patient. In some cases re-challenge with Amiodarone HCl at a lower dose has not resulted in return of toxicity. Recent reports suggest that the use of lower loading and maintenance doses of Amiodarone-HCl are associated with a decreased incidence of Amiodarone HCl induced pulmonary toxicity.

In a patient receiving Amiodarone HCl, any new respiratory symptoms should suggest the possibility of pulmonary toxicity, and the history, physical exam, chest X-ray, and pulmonary-function tests (with diffusion capacity) should be repeated and evaluated. A 15% decrease in diffusion capacity has a high sensitivity but only a moderate specificity for pulmonary toxicity; as the decrease in diffusion capacity approaches 30%, the sensitivity decreases but the specificity increases. A gallium scan also may be performed as part of the diagnostic workup.

Fatalities, secondary to pulmonary toxicity, have occurred in approximately 10% of cases. However, in patients with life threatening arrhythmias, discontinuation of Amiodarone HCl therapy due to suspected drug-induced pulmonary toxicity should be undertaken with caution, as the most common cause of death in these patients is sudden cardiac death. Therefore, every effort should be made to rule out other causes of respiratory impairment (i.e., congestive heart failure with Swan-Ganz catheterization if necessary, respiratory infection, pulmonary embolism, malignancy, etc.) before discontinuing Amiodarone HCl in these patients. In addition, bronchoalveolar lavage, transbronchial lung biopsy, and/or open lung biopsy may be necessary to confirm the diagnosis, especially in those cases where no acceptable alternative therapy is available.

If a diagnosis of Amiodarone HCl-induced hypersensitivity pneumonitis is made, Amiodarone HCl should be discontinued, and treatment with steroids should be instituted. If a diagnosis of Amiodarone HCl interstitial/alveolar pneumonitis is made, steroid therapy should be instituted and, preferably Amiodarone HCl discontinued or at a minimum, reduced in dosage. Some cases of Amiodarone HCl induced interstitial/alveolar pneumonitis may resolve following a reduction in Amiodarone HCl dosage in conjunction with the administration of steroids. In some patients, rechallenge at a lower dose has not resulted in return of interstitial/alveolar pneumonitis; however, in some patients (perhaps because of severe alveolar damage) the pulmonary lesions have not been reversible.

WORSENED ARRHYTHMIA

Amiodarone HCl like other antiarrhythmics, can cause serious exacerbation of the presenting arrhythmia, a risk that may be enhanced by the presence of concomitant antiarrhythmics. Exacerbation has been reported in about 2 to 5% in most series, and has included new ventricular fibrillation, incessant ventricular tachycardia, increased resistance to cardioversion, and polymorphic ventricular tachycardia associated with QT prolongation (Torsade de Pointes).

In addition, Amiodarone HCl has caused symptomatic bradycardia or sinus arrest with suppression of escape foci in 2 to 4% of patients.

LIVER INJURY

Elevations of hepatic enzyme levels are seen frequently in patients exposed to Amiodarone HCl and in most cases are asymptomatic. If the increase exceeds three times normal, or doubles in a patient with an elevated baseline, discontinuation of Amiodarone HCl or dosage reduction should be considered. In a few cases in which biopsy has been done, the histology has resembled that of alcoholic hepatitis or cirrhosis. Hepatic failure has been a rare cause of death in patients treated with Amiodarone HCl.

PREGNANCY: PREGNANCY CATEGORY D

Amiodarone HCl has been shown to be embryotoxic (increased fetal resorption and growth retardation) in the rat when given orally at a dose of 200 mg/kg/day (18 times the maximum recommended maintenance dose). Similar findings have been noted in one strain of mice at a dose of 5 mg/kg/day (approximately 1/2 the maximum recommended maintenance dose) and higher, but not in a second strain nor in the rabbit at doses up to 100 mg/kg/day (9 times the maximum recommended maintenance dose).

Neonatal hypo or hyperthyroidism: Amiodarone HCl can cause fetal harm when administered to a pregnant woman. Although Amiodarone HCl use during pregnancy is uncommon, there have been a small number of published reports of congenital goiter/hypothyroidism and hyperthyroidism. If Amiodarone HCl is used during pregnancy, or if the patient becomes pregnant while taking Amiodarone HCL the patient should be apprised of the potential hazard to the fetus.

In general, Amiodarone HCl should be used during pregnancy only if the potential benefit to the mother justifies the unknown risk to the fetus.

PRECAUTIONS

CORNEAL MICRODEPOSITS: IMPAIRMENT OF VISION

Corneal microdeposits appear in the majority of adults treated with Amiodarone HCl. They are usually discernible only by slit-lamp examination, but give rise to symptoms such as visual halos or blurred vision in as many as 10% of patients. Corneal microdeposits are reversible upon reduction of dose or termination of treatment. Asymptomatic microdeposits are not a reason to reduce dose or discontinue treatment.

PHOTOSENSITIVITY

Amiodarone HCl has induced photosensitization in about 10% of patients; some protection may be afforded by the use of sun-barrier creams or protective clothing. During long-term treatment, a blue-gray discoloration of the exposed skin may occur. The risk may be increased in patients of fair complexion or those with excessive sun exposure, and may be related to cumulative dose and duration of therapy.

◆ RATED THERAPEUTICALLY EQUIVALENT; ◇ THERAPEUTIC EQUIVALENCE UNCONFIRMED; ○ UNRATED

THYROID ABNORMALITIES

Amiodarone HCl inhibits peripheral conversion of thyroxine (T_4) to triiodothyronine (T_3) and may cause increased thyroxine levels, decreased T_3 levels, and increased levels of inactive reverse T_3 (rT_3) in clinically euthyroid patients. It is also a potential source of large amounts of inorganic iodine. Because of its release of inorganic iodine, or perhaps for other reasons. Amiodarone HCl can cause either hypothyroidism or hyperthyroidism. Thyroid function should be monitored prior to treatment and periodically therafter, particularly in elderly patients, and in any patient with a history of thyroid nodules, goiter, or other thyroid dysfunction. Because of the slow elimination of Amiodarone HCl and its metabolites, high plasma iodide levels, altered thyroid function, and abnormal thyroid function tests may persist for several weeks or even months following Amiodarone HCl withdrawal.

Hypothyroidism has been reported in 2 to 4% of patients in most series, but in 8 to 10% in some series. This condition may be identified by relevant clinical symptoms and particularly by elevated serum TSH levels. In some clinically hypothyroid Amiodarone-treated patients, free thyroxine index values may be normal. Hypothyroidism is best managed by Amiodarone HCl dose reduction and/or thyroid hormone supplement. However, therapy must be individualized, and it may be necessary to discontinue Amiodarone HCl in some patients. Hyperthyroidism occurs in about 2% of patients receiving Amiodarone HCl but the incidence may be higher among patients with prior inadequate dietary iodine intake. Amiodarone HCl-induced hyperthyroidism usually poses a greater hazard to the patient than hypothyroidism because of the possibility of arrhythmia breakthrough or aggravation. In fact, IF ANY NEW SIGNS OF ARRHYTHMIA APPEAR, THE POSSIBILITY OF HYPERTHYROIDISM SHOULD BE CONSIDERED. Hyperthyroidism is best identified by relevant clinical symptoms and signs, accompanied usually by abnormally elevated levels of serum T_3 RIA, and further elevations of serum T_4, and a subnormal serum TSH level (using a sufficiently sensitive TSH assay). The finding of a flat TSH response to TRH is confirmatory of hyperthyroidism and may be sought in equivocal cases. Since arrhythmia break-throughs may accompany Amiodarone HCl-induced hyperthyroidism, aggressive medical treatment is indicated including, if possible, dose reduction or withdrawal of Amiodarone HCl. The institution of antithyroid drugs, beta-adrenergic blockers and/or temporary corticosteroid therapy may be necessary. The action of antithyroid drugs may be especially delayed in Amiodarone-induced, thyrotoxicosis because of substantial quantities of preformed thyroid hormones stored in the gland. Radioactive iodine therapy is contraindicated because of the low radioiodine uptake associated with Amiodarone-induced hyperthyroidism. Experience with thyroid surgery in this setting is extremely limited, and this form of therapy runs the theoretical risk of inducing thyroid storm. Amiodarone HCl-induced hyperthyroidism may be followed by a transient period of hypothyroidism.

SURGERY

HYPOTENSION POSTBYPASS

Rare occurrences of hypotension upon discontinuation of cardiopulmonary bypass during open-heart surgery in patients receiving Amiodarone HCl have been reported. The relationship of this event to Amiodarone HCl therapy is unknown.

Adult Respiratory Distress Syndrome (ARDS): Postoperatively, rare occurrences of ARDS have been reported in patients receiving Amiodarone HCl therapy who have undergone either cardiac or noncardiac surgery. Although patients usually respond well to vigorous respiratory therapy, in rare instances the outcome has been fatal. One possible mechanism of this deleterious effect may be the generation of superoxide radicals during oxygenation; therefore, the operative FiO_2 should be kept as close to room air as possible.

LABORATORY TESTS

Elevations in liver enzymes (SGOT and SGPT) can occur. Liver enzymes in patients on relatively high maintenance doses should be monitored on a regular basis. Persistent significant elevations in the liver enzymes or hepatomegaly should alert the physician to consider reducing the maintenance dose of Amiodarone HCl or discontinuing therapy.

Amiodarone HCl alters the results of thyroid-function tests, causing an increase in serum T_4 and serum reverse T_3, and a decline in serum T_3 levels. Despite these biochemical changes, most patients remain clinically euthyroid.

DRUG INTERACTIONS

Although only a small number of drug-drug interactions with Amiodarone HCl have been explored formally, most of these have shown such an interaction. The potential for other interactions should be anticipated, particularly for drugs with potentially serious toxicity, such as other antiarrhythmics. If such drugs are needed, their dose should be reassessed and, where appropriate, plasma concentration measured.

In view of the long and variable half-life of Amiodarone HCl, potential for drug interactions exists not only with concomitant medication but also with drugs administered after discontinuation of Amiodarone HCl.

Digitalis: Administration of Amiodarone HCl to patients receiving digoxin therapy regularly results in an increase in the serum digoxin concentration that may reach toxic levels with resultant clinical toxicity. *On initiation of Amiodarone HCl, the need for digitalis therapy should be reviewed and the dose reduced by approximately 50% or discontinued .* If digitalis treatment is continued, serum levels should be closely monitored and patients observed for clinical evidence of toxicity. These precautions probably should apply to digitoxin administration as well.

Anticoagulants: Potentiation of warfarin-type anticoagulant response is almost always seen in patients receiving Amiodarone HCl and can result in serious or fatal bleeding. *The dose of the anticoagulant should be reduced by one-third to one-half, and prothrombin times should be monitored closely .*

Antiarrhythmic Agents: Other antiarrhythmic drugs, such as quinidine, procainamide, disopyramide, and phenytoin, have been used concurrently with Amiodarone HCl.

There have been case reports of increased steady-state levels of quinidine, procainamide and phenytoin during concomitant therapy with Amiodarone HCl. In general, any added antiarrhythmic drug should be initiated at a lower than usual dose with careful monitoring.

In general, combination of Amiodarone HCl with other antiarrhythmic therapy should be reserved for patients with life-threatening threatening ventricular arrhythmias who are incompletely responsive to a single agent or incompletely responsive to Amiodarone HCl. During transfer to Amiodarone HCl the dose levels of previously administered agents should be reduced by 30 to 50% several days after the addition of Amiodarone HCl when arrhythmia suppression should be beginning. The continued need for the other antiarrhythmic agent should be reviewed after the effects of Amiodarone HCl have been established, and discontinuation ordinarily should be attempted. If the treatment is continued, these patients should be particularly carefully monitored for adverse effects, especially conduction disturbances and exacerbation of tachyarrhythmias, as Amiodarone HCl is continued. In Amiodarone HCl-treated patients who require additional antiarrhythmic therapy, the initial dose of such agents should be approximately half of the usual recommended dose.

Amiodarone HCl should be used with caution in patients receiving beta-blocking agents or calcium antagonists because of the possible potentiation of bradycardia, sinus arrest, and AV block; if necessary, Amiodarone HCl can continue to be used after insertion of a pacemaker in patients with severe bradycardia or sinus arrest. (See related table).

ELECTROLYTE DISTURBANCES

Since antiarrhythmic drugs may be ineffective or may be arrhythmogenic in patients with hypokalemia, any potassium or magnesium deficiency should be corrected before instituting Amiodarone HCl therapy.

CARCINOGENESIS, MUTAGENESIS, IMPAIRMENT OF FERTILITY

Amiodarone HCl reduced fertility of male and female rats at a dose level of 90 mg/kg/day (8 $\times$ highest recommended human maintenance dose). Amiodarone HCl caused a statistically significant, dose-related increase in the incidence of thyroid tumors (follicular adenoma and/or carcinoma) in rats. The incidence of thyroid tumors was greater than control even at the lowest dose level of Amiodarone HCl tested, i.e., 5 mg/kg/day or approximately equal to ½ the highest recommended human maintenance dose. Mutagenicity studies (Ames, micronucleus, and lysogenic tests) with Amiodarone HCl were negative.

PREGNANCY: PREGNANCY CATEGORY D
See *"Warnings"*.

LABOR AND DELIVERY

It is not known whether the use of Amiodarone HCl during labor or delivery has any immediate or delayed adverse effects. Preclinical studies in rodents have not shown any effect of Amiodarone HCl on the duration of gestation or on parturition.

NURSING MOTHERS

Amiodarone HCl is excreted in human milk, suggesting that breast-feeding could expose the nursing infant to a significant dose of the drug. Nursing offspring of lactating rats administered Amiodarone HCl have been shown to be less viable and have reduced body-weight gains. Therefore, when Amiodarone HCl therapy is indicated, the mother should be advised to discontinue nursing.

PEDIATRIC USE

The safety and effectiveness of Amiodarone HCl in children have not been established.

ADVERSE REACTIONS

Adverse reactions have been very common in virtually all series of patients treated with Amiodarone HCl for ventricular arrhythmias, with relatively large doses of drug (400 mg/day and above) occurring in about three-fourths of all patients and causing discontinuation in 7 to 18%. The most serious reactions are pulmonary toxicity, exacerbation of arrhythmia, and rare serious liver injury (see *"Warnings"*), but other adverse effects constitute important problems. They are often reversible with dose reduction and virtually always reversible with cessation of Amiodarone HCl treatment. Most of the adverse effects appear to become more frequent with continued treatment beyond six months, although rates appear to remain relatively constant beyond one year. The time and dose relationships of adverse effects are under continued study.

Neurologic problems are extremely common, occurring in 20 to 40% of patients and including malaise and fatigue, tremor and involuntary movements, poor coordination and gait, and peripheral neuropathy; they are rarely a reason to stop therapy and may respond to dose reductions.

Gastrointestinal complaints, most commonly nausea, vomiting, constipation, and anorexia, occur in about 25% of patients but rarely require discontinuation of drug. These commonly occur during high-dose administration (i.e., loading dose) and usually respond to dose reduction or divided doses. Asymptomatic corneal microdeposits are present in virtually all adult patients who have been on drug for

SUMMARY OF DRUG INTERACTIONS WITH AMIODARONE HCL

Concomitant Drug	Onset (days)	Interaction Magnitude	Recommended Dose Reduction of Concomitant Drug
Warfarin	3 to 4	Increases prothrombin time by 100%	⅓ to ½
Digoxin	1	Increases serum concentration by 70%	½
Quinidine	2	Increases serum concentration by 33%	⅓ to ½ (or discontinue)
Procainamide	< 7	Increases plasma concentration by 55%, NAPA* concentration by 33%	⅓ (or discontinue)

* NAPA = n-acetyl procainamide.

more than 6 months. Some patients develop eye symptoms of halos, photophobia, and dry eyes. Vision is rarely affected and drug discontinuation is rarely needed.

Dermatological adverse reactions occur in about 15% of patients, with photosensitivity being most common (about 10%). Sunscreen and protection from sun exposure may be helpful, and drug discontinuation is not usually necessary. Prolonged exposure to Amiodarone HCl occasionally results in a blue-gray pigmentation. This is slowly and occasionally incompletely reversible on discontinuation of drug but is of cosmetic importance only.

Cardiovascular adverse reactions, other than exacerbation of the arrhythmias, include the uncommon occurrence of congestive heart failure (3%) and bradycardia. Bradycardia usually responds to dosage reduction but may require a pacemaker for control. CHF rarely requires drug discontinuation. Cardiac conduction abnormalities occur infrequently and are reversible on discontinuation of drug.

The following side-effect rates are based on a retrospective study of 241 patients treated for 2 to 1.515 days (mean 441.3 days).

THE FOLLOWING SIDE EFFECTS WERE REPORTED IN 10 TO 33% OF PATIENTS:
Gastrointestinal: Nausea and vomiting.

THE FOLLOWING SIDE EFFECTS WERE EACH REPORTED IN 4 TO 9% OF PATIENTS:
Dermatologic: Solar dermatitis/photosensitivity.

Neurologic: Malaise and fatigue, tremor/abnormal involuntary movements, lack of coordination, abnormal gait/ataxia, dizziness, paresthesias.

Gastrointestinal: Constipation, anorexia.

Ophthalmologic: Visual disturbances.

Hepatic: Abnormal liver-function tests.

Respiratory: Pulmonary inflammation or fibrosis.

THE FOLLOWING SIDE EFFECTS WERE EACH REPORTED IN 1 TO 3% OF PATIENTS:
Thyroid: Hypothyroidism, hyperthyroidism.

Neurologic: Decreased libido, insomnia, headache, sleep disturbances.

Cardiovascular: Congestive heart failure, cardiac arrhythmias, SA node dysfunction.

Gastrointestinal: Abdominal pain.

Hepatic: Nonspecific hepatic disorders.

Other: Flushing, abnormal taste and smell, edema, abnormal salivation, coagulation abnormalities.

THE FOLLOWING SIDE EFFECTS WERE EACH REPORTED IN LESS THAN 1% OF PATIENTS:
Blue skin discoloration, rash, spontaneous ecchymosis, alopecia, hypotension, and cardiac conduction abnormalities. Rare occurrences of hepatitis, cholestatic hepatitis, cirrhosis, optic neuritis, epididymitis, vasculitis, pseudotumor cerebri, and thrombocytopenia have been reported in patients receiving Amiodarone HCl.

In surveys of almost 5,000 patients treated in open U.S. studies and in published reports of treatment with Amiodarone HCl, the adverse reactions most frequently requiring discontinuation of Amiodarone HCl included pulmonary infiltrates or fibrosis, paroxysmal ventricular tachycardia, congestive heart failure, and elevation of liver enzymes. Other symptoms causing discontinuations less often included visual disturbances, solar dermatitis, blue skin discoloration, hyperthyroidism and hypothyrodism.

OVERDOSAGE
There have been a few reported cases of Amiodarone HCl overdose in which 3 to 8 grams were taken. There were no deaths or permanent sequelae. Animal studies indicate that Amiodarone HCl has a high oral LD$_{50}$ (> 3,000 mg/kg).

In addition to general supportive measures, the patient's cardiac rhythm and blood pressure should be monitored, and if bradycardia ensues, a β-adrenergic agonist or a pacemarker may be used. Hypotension with inadequate tissue perfusion should be treated with positive inotropic and/or vasopressor agents. Neither Amiodarone HCl nor its metabolite is dialyzable.

DOSAGE AND ADMINISTRATION
BECAUSE OF THE UNIQUE PHARMACOKINETIC PROPERTIES, DIFFICULT DOSING SCHEDULE, AND SEVERITY OF THE SIDE EFFECTS IF PATIENTS ARE IMPROPERLY MONITORED, AMIODARONE HCL

SHOULD BE ADMINISTERED ONLY BY PHYSICIANS WHO ARE EXPERIENCED IN THE TREATMENT OF LIFE-THREATENING ARRHYTHMIAS, WHO ARE THOROUGHLY FAMILIAR WITH THE RISKS AND BENEFITS OF AMIODARONE HCL THERAPY, AND WHO HAVE ACCESS TO LABORATORY FACILITIES CAPABLE OF ADEQUATELY MONITORING THE EFFECTIVENESS AND SIDE EFFECTS OF TREATMENT.

In order to insure that an antiarrhythmic effect will be observed without waiting several months, loading doses are required. A uniform, optimal dosage schedule for administration of Amiodarone HCl has not been determined. Individual patient titration is suggested according to the following guidelines.

For Life-Threatening Ventricular Arrhythmias, such as Ventricular Fibrillation or Hemodynamically Unstable Ventricular Tachycardia: Close monitoring of the patients is indicated during the loading phase, particularly until risk of recurrent ventricular tachycardia or fibrillation has abated. Because of the serious nature of the arrhythmia and the lack of predictable time course of effect, loading should be performed in a hospital setting. Loading doses of 800 to 1,600 mg/day are required for 1 to 3 weeks (occasionally longer) until initial therapeutic response occurs. (Administration of Amiodarone HCl in divided doses with meals is suggested for total daily doses of 1,000 mg or higher, or when gastrointestinal intolerance occurs.) If side effects become excessive, the dose should be reduced. Elimination of recurrence of ventricular fibrillation and tachycardia usually occurs within 1 to 3 weeks, along with reduction in complex and total ventricular ectopic beats.

Upon starting Amiodarone HCl therapy, an attempt should be made to gradually discontinue prior antiarrhythmic drugs (see section on "Drug Interactions"). When adequate arrhythmia control is achieved, or if side effects become prominent, Amiodarone HCl dose should be reduced to 600 to 800 mg/day for one month and then to the maintenance dose, usually 400 mg/day (see "Clinical Pharmacology—Monitoring Effectiveness"). Some patients may require larger maintenance doses, up to 600 mg/day, and some can be controlled on lower doses. Amiodarone HCl may be administered as a single daily dose, or in patients with severe gastrointestinal intolerance, as a b.i.d. dose. In each patient, the chronic maintenance dose should be determined according to antiarrhythmic effect as assessed by symptoms, Holter recordings, and/or programmed electrical stimulation and by patient tolerance. Plasma concentrations may be helpful in evaluating nonresponsiveness or unexpectedly severe toxicity (see "Clinical Pharmacology").

The lowest effective dose should be used to prevent the occurrence of side effects. In all instances, the physician must be guided by the severity of the individual patient's arrhythmia and response to therapy. When dosage adjustments are necessary, the patient should be closely monitored for an extended period of time because of the long and variable half-life of Amiodarone HCl and the difficulty in predicting the time required to attain a new steady-state level of drug. Dosage suggestions are summarized below:

	Loading Dose (Daily)	Adjustment and Maintenance Dose (Daily)		
Ventricular Arrhythmias	1 to 3 weeks	~ 1 month	usual maintenance	
	800 to 1,600 mg	600 to 800 mg	400 mg	

Keep tightly closed.
Store at Room Temperature, Approx. 25 °C (77 °F).
Protect from light.

HOW SUPPLIED
TABLETS: 200 MG

BRAND/MANUFACTURER	NDC	SIZE	AWP
◇ BRAND			
CORDARONE: Wyeth-Ayerst	00008-4188-04	60s	$163.71
	00008-4188-06	100s	$250.01

Amipaque SEE METRIZAMIDE

Amitriptyline Hydrochloride

DESCRIPTION
Amitriptyline Hydrochloride is 3-(10,11-dihydro-5H-dibenzo [a,d] cycloheptene-5-ylidene)-N,N-dimethyl-1-propanamine hydrochloride. Its empirical formula is $C_{20}H_{23}N \cdot HCl$

Amitriptyline Hydrochloride a dibenzocycloheptadiene derivative, has a molecular weight of 313.87. It is a white, odorless, crystalline compound which is freely soluble in water.

Amitriptyline Hydrochloride is supplied as 10 mg, 25 mg, 50 mg, 75 mg, 100 mg, and 150 mg tablets and as a sterile solution for intramuscular use.

Following is its chemical structure:

CHCH$_2$CH$_2$N(CH$_3$)$_2$ • HCl

ACTIONS

Amitriptyline HCl is an antidepressant with sedative effects. Its mechanism of action in man is not known. It is not a monoamine oxidase inhibitor and it does not act primarily by stimulation of the central nervous system.

Amitriptyline inhibits the membrane pump mechanism responsible for uptake of norepinephrine and serotonin in adrenergic and serotonergic neurons. Pharmacologically this action may potentiate or prolong neuronal activity since reuptake of these biogenic amines is important physiologically in terminating transmitting activity. This interference with the reuptake of norepinephrine and/or serotonin is believed by some to underlie the antidepressant activity of Amitriptyline.

INDICATIONS

For the relief of symptoms of depression. Endogenous depression is more likely to be alleviated than are other depressive states.

UNLABELED USES

Amitriptyline is used alone or as an adjunct in the treatment of bulimia nervosa and diabetic neuropathy, and in prophylaxis of migraine headache. It is also used in combination with lithium to stabilize hypertension, and in the treatment of neurogenic pain, postherpetic neuralgia, panic attacks, and posttraumatic stress disorder. Amitriptyline is also used in trichotillomania and vulvodynia (chronic vulvar burning).

CONTRAINDICATIONS

Amitriptyline HCl is contraindicated in patients who have shown prior hypersensitivity to it.

It should not be given concomitantly with monoamine oxidase inhibitors. Hyperpyretic crises, severe convulsions, and deaths have occurred in patients receiving tricyclic antidepressant and monoamine oxidase inhibiting drugs simultaneously. When it is desired to replace a monoamine oxidase inhibitor with Amitriptyline HCl, a minimum of 14 days should be allowed to elapse after the former is discontinued. Amitriptyline HCl should then be initiated cautiously with gradual increase in dosage until optimum response is achieved.

This drug is not recommended for use during the acute recovery phase following myocardial infarction.

WARNINGS

Amitriptyline HCl may block the antihypertensive action of guanethidine or similarly acting compounds.

It should be used with caution in patients with a history of seizures and, because of its atropine-like action, in patients with a history of urinary retention, angle-closure glaucoma or increased intraocular pressure. In patients with angle-closure glaucoma, even average doses may precipitate an attack.

Patients with cardiovascular disorders should be watched closely. Tricyclic antidepressant drugs, including Amitriptyline HCl, particularly when given in high doses, have been reported to produce arrhythmias, sinus tachycardia, and prolongation of the conduction time. Myocardial infarction and stroke have been reported with drugs of this class.

Close supervision is required when Amitriptyline HCl is given to hyperthyroid patients or those receiving thyroid medication.

Amitriptyline HCl may enhance the response to alcohol and the effects of barbiturates and other CNS depressants. In patients who may use alcohol excessively, it should be borne in mind that the potentiation may increase the danger inherent in any suicide attempt or overdosage. Delirium has been reported with concurrent administration of Amitriptyline and disulfiram.

Usage in Pregnancy: Teratogenic effects were not observed in mice, rats, or rabbits when Amitriptyline was given orally at doses of 2 to 40 mg/kg/day (up to 13 times the maximum recommended human dose*). Studies in the literature have shown Amitriptyline to be teratogenic in mice and hamsters when given by various routes of administration at doses of 28 to 100 mg/kg/day (9 to 33 times the maximum recommended human dose), producing multiple malformations. Another study in the rat reported that an oral dose of 25 mg/kg/day (8 times the maximum recommended human dose) produced delays in ossification of fetal vertebral bodies without other signs of embryotoxicity. In rabbits, an oral dose of 60 mg/kg/day (20 times the maximum recommended human dose) was reported to cause incomplete ossification of the cranial bones.

Amitriptyline has been shown to cross the placenta. Although a causal relationship has not been established, there have been a few reports of adverse events, including CNS effects, limb deformities, or developmental delay, in infants whose mothers had taken Amitriptyline during pregnancy.

---

* Based on a maximum recommended Amitriptyline dose of 150 mg/day or 3 mg/kg/day for a 50 kg patient.

There are no adequate or well-controlled studies in pregnant women. Amitriptyline HCl should be used during pregnancy only if the potential benefit to the mother justifies the potential risk to the fetus.

Nursing Mothers: Amitriptyline is excreted into breast milk. In one report in which a patient received Amitriptyline 100 mg/day while nursing her infant, levels of 83-141 ng/mL were detected in the mother's serum. Levels of 135-151 ng/mL were found in the breast milk, but no trace of the drug could be detected in the infant's serum.

Because of the potential for serious adverse reactions in nursing infants from Amitriptyline, a decision should be made whether to discontinue nursing or to discontinue the drug, taking into account the importance of the drug to the mother.

Usage in Children: In view of the lack of experience with the use of this drug in children, it is not recommended at the present time for patients under 12 years of age.

PRECAUTIONS

Schizophrenic patients may develop increased symptoms of psychosis; patients with paranoid symptomatology may have an exaggeration of such symptoms. Depressed patients, particularly those with known manic-depressive illness, may experience a shift to mania or hypomania. In these circumstances the dose of Amitriptyline may be reduced or a major tranquilizer such as perphenazine may be administered concurrently.

When Amitriptyline HCl is given with anticholinergic agents or sympathomimetic drugs, including epinephrine combined with local anesthetics, close supervision and careful adjustment of dosages are required.

Hyperpyrexia has been reported when Amitriptyline HCl is administered with anticholinergic agents or with neuroleptic drugs, particularly during hot weather.

Paralytic ileus may occur in patients taking tricyclic antidepressants in combination with anticholinergic-type drugs.

Cimetidine is reported to reduce hepatic metabolism of certain tricyclic antidepressants, thereby delaying elimination and increasing steady-state concentrations of these drugs. Clinically significant effects have been reported with the tricyclic antidepressants when used concomitantly with cimetidine. Increases in plasma levels of tricyclic antidepressants, and in the frequency and severity of side effects, particularly anticholinergic, have been reported when cimetidine was added to the drug regimen. Discontinuation of cimetidine in well-controlled patients receiving tricyclic antidepressants and cimetidine may decrease the plasma levels and efficacy of the antidepressants.

Caution is advised if patients receive large doses of ethchlorvynol concurrently. Transient delirium has been reported in patients who were treated with one gram of ethchlorvynol and 75-150 mg of Amitriptyline HCl.

The possibility of suicide in depressed patients remains until significant remission occurs. Potentially suicidal patients should not have access to large quantities of this drug. Prescriptions should be written for the smallest amount feasible.

Concurrent administration of Amitriptyline HCl and electroshock therapy may increase the hazards associated with such therapy. Such treatment should be limited to patients for whom it is essential.

When possible, the drug should be discontinued several days before elective surgery.

Both elevation and lowering of blood sugar levels have been reported.

Amitriptyline HCl should be used with caution in patients with impaired liver function.

Information for Patients: While on therapy with Amitriptyline HCl, patients should be advised as to the possible impairment of mental and/or physical abilities required for performance of hazardous tasks, such as operating machinery or driving a motor vehicle.

ADVERSE REACTIONS

Within each category the following adverse reactions are listed in order of decreasing severity. Included in the listing are a few adverse reactions which have not been reported with this specific drug. However, pharmacological similarities among the tricyclic antidepressant drugs require that each of the reactions be considered when Amitriptyline is administered.

Cardiovascular: Myocardial infarction; stroke; nonspecific ECG changes and changes in AV conductor; heart block; arrhythmias; hypotension, particularly orthostatic hypotension; syncope; hypertension; tachycardia; palpitation.

CNS and Neuromuscular: Coma; seizures; hallucinations; delusions; confusional states; disorientation; incoordination; ataxia; tremors; peripheral neuropathy; numbness, tingling, and paresthesias of the extremities; extrapyramidal symptoms including abnormal involuntary movements and tardive dyskinesia; dysarthria; disturbed concentration; excitement; anxiety; insomnia; restlessness; nightmares; drowsiness; dizziness; weakness; fatigue; headache; syndrome of inappropriate ADH (antidiuretic hormone) secretion; tinnitus; alteration in EEG patterns.

Anticholinergic: Paralytic ileus; hyperpyrexia; urinary retention, dilatation of the urinary tract; constipation; blurred vision, disturbance of accommodation, increased intraocular pressure, mydriasis; dry mouth.

Allergic: Skin rash; urticaria; photosensitization; edema of face and tongue.

Hematologic: Bone marrow depression including agranulocytosis, leukopenia, thrombocytopenia; purpura; eosinophilia.

Gastrointestinal: Rarely hepatitis (including altered liver function and jaundice); nausea; epigastric distress; vomiting; anorexia; stomatitis; peculiar taste; diarrhea; parotid swelling; black tongue.

Endocrine: Testicular swelling and gynecomastia in the male; breast enlargement and galactorrhea in the female; increased or decreased libido; impotence; elevation and lowering of blood sugar levels.

Other: Alopecia; edema; weight gain or loss; urinary frequency; increased perspiration.

Withdrawal Symptoms: After prolonged administration, abrupt cessation of treatment may produce nausea, headache, and malaise. Gradual dosage reduction has been reported to produce, within two weeks, transient symptoms including irritability, restlessness, and dream and sleep disturbance. These symptoms are not indicative of addiction. Rare instances have been reported of mania or hypomania occurring within 2-7 days following cessation of chronic therapy with tricyclic antidepressants.

Causal Relationship Unknown: Other reactions, reported under circumstances where a causal relationship could not be established, are listed to serve as alerting information to physicians.

Body as a Whole: Lupus-like syndrome (migratory arthritis, positive ANA and rheumatoid factor).

Digestive: Hepatic failure, ageusia.

DOSAGE AND ADMINISTRATION

ORAL DOSAGE
Dosage should be initiated at a low level and increased gradually, noting carefully the clinical response and any evidence of intolerance.

Initial Dosage for Adults: For outpatients 75 mg of Amitriptyline HCl a day in divided doses is usually satisfactory. If necessary, this may be increased to a total of 150 mg per day. Increases are made preferably in the late afternoon and/or bedtime doses. A sedative effect may be apparent before the antidepressant effect is noted, but an adequate therapeutic effect may take as long as 30 days to develop.

An alternate method of initiating therapy in outpatients is to begin with 50 to 100 mg Amitriptyline HCl at bedtime. This may be increased by 25 or 50 mg as necessary in the bedtime dose to a total of 150 mg per day.

Hospitalized patients may require 100 mg a day initially. This can be increased gradually to 200 mg a day if necessary. A small number of hospitalized patients may need as much as 300 mg a day.

Adolescent and Elderly Patients: In general, lower dosages are recommended for these patients. Ten mg 3 times a day with 20 mg at bedtime may be satisfactory in adolescent and elderly patients who do not tolerate higher dosages.

Maintenance: The usual maintenance dosage of Amitriptyline HCl is 50 to 100 mg per day. In some patients 40 mg per day is sufficient. For maintenance therapy the total daily dosage may be given in a single dose preferably at bedtime. When satisfactory improvement has been reached, dosage should be reduced to the lowest amount that will maintain relief of symptoms. It is appropriate to continue maintenance therapy 3 months or longer to lessen the possibility of relapse.

INTRAMUSCULAR DOSAGE
Initially, 20 to 30 mg (2 to 3 mL) four times a day.

When Amitriptyline HCl Injection is administered intramuscularly, the effects may appear more rapidly than with oral administration.

When Amitriptyline HCl Injection is used for initial therapy in patients unable or unwilling to take Amitriptyline HCl tablets, the tablets should replace the injection as soon as possible.

USAGE IN CHILDREN
In view of the lack of experience with the use of this drug in children, it is not recommended at the present time for patients under 12 years of age.

PLASMA LEVELS
Because of the wide variation in the absorption and distribution of tricyclic antidepressants in body fluids, it is difficult to directly correlate plasma levels and therapeutic effect. However, determination of plasma levels may be useful in identifying patients who appear to have toxic effects and may have excessively high levels, or those in whom lack of absorption or noncompliance is suspected. Adjustments in dosage should be made according to the patient's clinical response and not on the basis of plasma levels.**

OVERDOSAGE
Manifestations: High doses may cause temporary confusion, disturbed concentration, or transient visual hallucinations. Overdosage may cause drowsiness; hypothermia; tachycardia and other arrhythmic abnormalities, such as bundle branch block; ECG evidence of impaired conduction; congestive heart failure; dilated pupils; disorders of ocular motility; convulsions; severe hypotension; stupor; coma; and polyradiculoneuropathy. Other symptoms may be agitation, hyperactive reflexes, muscle rigidity, vomiting, hyperpyrexia, or any of those listed under *"Adverse Reactions"*. There has been a report of fatal dysrhythmia occuring as late as 56 hours after Amitriptyline overdose.

All patients suspected of having taken an overdosage should be admitted to a hospital as soon as possible. *Treatment* is symptomatic and supportive. Empty the

** Hollister LE: JAMA 1979;241:2350-2533.

stomach as quickly as possible by emesis followed by gastric lavage upon arrival at the hospital. Following gastric lavage, activated charcoal may be administered. Twenty to 30 g of activated charcoal may be given every four to six hours during the first 24 to 48 hours after ingestion. An ECG should be taken and close monitoring of cardiac function instituted if there is any sign of abnormality. Maintain an open airway and adequate fluid intake; regulate body temperature.

The intravenous administration of 1-3 mg of physostigmine salicylate is reported to reverse the symptoms of tricyclic antidepressant poisoning. Because physostigmine is rapidly metabolized, the dosage of physostigmine should be repeated as required particularly if life threatening signs such as arrhythmias, convulsions, and deep coma recur or persist after the initial dosage of physostigmine. Because physostigmine itself may be toxic, it is not recommended for routine use.

Standard measures should be used to manage circulatory shock and metabolic acidosis. Cardiac arrhythmias may be treated with neostigmine, pyridostigmine, or propranolol. Should cardiac failure occur, the use of digitalis should be considered. Close monitoring of cardiac function for not less than five days is advisable.

Anticonvulsants may be given to control convulsions. Amitriptyline increases the CNS depressant action but not the anticonvulsant action of barbiturates; therefore, an inhalation anesthetic, diazepam, or paraldehyde is recommended for control of convulsions.

Dialysis is of no value because of low plasma concentrations of the drug.

Since overdosage is often deliberate, patients may attempt suicide by other means during the recovery phase.

Deaths by deliberate or accidental overdosage have occurred with this class of drugs.

Storage: Store tablets in a well-closed container. Avoid storage at temperatures above 30°C (86°F). In addition, certain brands of 10 mg Amitriptyline tablets must be protected from light and stored in a well-closed, light-resistant container.

Protect injection from freezing and avoid storage above 30°C (86°F).

METABOLISM
Studies in man following oral administration of ^{14}C-labeled drug indicated that Amitriptyline is rapidly absorbed and metabolized. Radioactivity of the plasma was practically negligible, although significant amounts of radioactivity appeared in the urine by 4 to 6 hours and one-half to one-third of the drug was excreted within 24 hours.

Amitriptyline is metabolized by N-demethylation and bridge hydroxylation in man, rabbit, and rat. Virtually the entire dose is excreted as glucuronide or sulfate conjugate of metabolites, with little unchanged drug appearing in the urine. Other metabolic pathways may be involved.

REFERENCES
Ayd FJ Jr: Amitriptyline (ELAVIL) therapy for depressive reactions. Psychosomatics 1960:1:320-325. Diamond S: Human metabolization of amitriptyline tagged with carbon 14. Curr Ther Res, Mar 1965, pp 170-175. Dorfman W: Clinical experiences with amitriptyline (ELAVIL): A preliminary report. Psychosomatics 1960:1:153-155. Fallette JM, Stasney CR, Mintz AA: Amitriptyline poisoning treated with physostigmine. South Med J 1970; 63:1492-1493. Hollister LE, Overall JE, Johnson M, et al: Controlled comparison of amitriptyline, imipramine and placebo in hospitalized depressed patients. J Nerv Ment Dis 1964: 139:370-375. Hordern A, Burt CG, Holt NF: Depressive states: A pharmacotherapeutic study, Springfield study. Springfield, Ill, Charles C. Thomas, 1965. Klerman GL, Cole JO: Clinical pharmacology of imipramine and related antidepressant compounds. Int J Psychiatry 1976:3:267-304. McConaghy N, Joffe AD, Kingston WR, et al: Correlation of clinical features of depressed outpatients with response to amitriptyline and protriptyline. Br J Psychiatry 1968: 114:103-106. McDonald IM, Perkins M, Marjerrison G, et al: A controlled comparison of amitriptyline and electroconvulsive therapy in the treatment of depression. Am J Psychiatry 1966:122: 1427-1431. Slovis T, Ott J, Teitelbaum, et al: Physostigmine therapy in acute tricyclic antidepressant poisoning. Clin Toxicol 1971;4: 451-459. Symposium on depression with special studies of a new antidepressant, amitriptyline. Dis Nerv Syst, (Sect 2) May 1961, pp 5-56.

J CODES
Up to 20 mg IM—J1320

HOW SUPPLIED
INJECTION: 10 MG/ML

BRAND/MANUFACTURER	NDC	SIZE	AWP
◆ **BRAND**			
ELAVIL: Stuart	00038-0049-10	10 ml	$8.54

TABLET: 10 MG

AVERAGE UNIT PRICE (AVAILABLE SIZES)		GENERIC A-RATED AVERAGE PRICE (GAAP)	
BRAND	$0.18	100s	$6.07
GENERIC	$0.05	1000s	$31.96
HCFA FUL (100s ea)	$0.02		

BRAND/MANUFACTURER	NDC	SIZE	AWP
◆ **BRAND**			
▶ ELAVIL: Stuart	00038-0040-10	100s	$17.87
	00038-0040-34	1000s	$170.32
◆ **GENERICS**			
Medirex	57480-0301-06	30s	$4.45
▶ Rugby	00536-3071-01	100s	$2.55
Major	00904-0200-60	100s	$3.55

◆ **RATED THERAPEUTICALLY EQUIVALENT;** ◇ **THERAPEUTIC EQUIVALENCE UNCONFIRMED;** ○ **UNRATED**

BRAND/MANUFACTURER	NDC	SIZE	AWP
➤ Geneva	00781-1486-01	100s	$3.60
Biocraft	00332-2120-09	100s	$3.74
Qualitest	00603-2212-21	100s	$3.90
Sidmak	50111-0366-01	100s	$4.00
Martec	52555-0975-01	100s	$4.00
Mutual	53489-0104-01	100s	$4.00
Goldline	00182-1018-01	100s	$4.00
Roxane	00054-4041-25	100s	$4.21
URL	00677-0475-01	100s	$4.28
Schein	00364-0573-01	100s	$4.30
Parmed	00349-1040-01	100s	$4.40
Moore,H.L.	00839-6191-06	100s	$4.52
Purepac	00228-2131-10	100s	$4.53
Mylan	00378-2610-01	100s	$4.60
Aligen	00405-4066-01	100s	$4.68
ENDEP: Roche Prod	00140-0106-01	100s	$15.56
U.S. Trading	56126-0133-11	100s ud	$3.21
Raway	00686-0131-20	100s ud	$4.00
➤ Geneva	00781-1486-13	100s ud	$7.75
Vangard	00615-0828-13	100s ud	$8.31
Major	00904-0200-61	100s ud	$8.96
Roxane	00054-8041-25	100s ud	$9.20
UDL	51079-0131-20	100s ud	$12.62
Medirex	57480-0301-01	100s ud	$12.65
Goldline	00182-1018-89	100s ud	$12.80
➤ Rugby	00536-3071-10	1000s	$16.35
Major	00904-0200-80	1000s	$26.50
➤ Geneva	00781-1486-10	1000s	$26.70
Qualitest	00603-2212-32	1000s	$28.90
Mutual	53489-0104-10	1000s	$29.75
Moore,H.L.	00839-6191-16	1000s	$31.39
URL	00677-0475-10	1000s	$31.70
Purepac	00228-2131-96	1000s	$31.72
Aligen	00405-4066-03	1000s	$33.85
Schein	00364-0573-02	1000s	$33.95
Biocraft	00332-2120-15	1000s	$35.66
Sidmak	50111-0366-03	1000s	$36.00
Goldline	00182-1018-10	1000s	$36.00
Parmed	00349-1040-10	1000s	$39.60
Mylan	00378-2610-10	1000s	$41.40

TABLET: 10 MG

BRAND/MANUFACTURER	NDC	SIZE	AWP
◇ GENERICS			
Copley	38245-0206-10	100s	$2.40
Copley	38245-0206-20	1000s	$15.65

TABLET: 25 MG

AVERAGE UNIT PRICE (AVAILABLE SIZES)		GENERIC A-RATED AVERAGE PRICE (GAAP)	
BRAND	$0.36	100s	$8.76
GENERIC	$0.07	1000s	$44.74
HCFA FUL (100s ea)	$0.02		

BRAND/MANUFACTURER	NDC	SIZE	AWP
◆ BRAND			
➤ ELAVIL: Stuart	00038-0045-10	100s	$35.83
	00038-0045-39	100s ud	$39.31
	00038-0045-34	1000s	$340.01
	00038-0045-50	5000s	$1660.30
◆ GENERICS			
Medirex	57480-0302-06	30s	$7.29
Major	00904-0201-52	60s	$2.30
➤ Rugby	00536-3072-01	100s	$3.07
➤ Geneva	00781-1487-01	100s	$3.90
Aligen	00405-4067-01	100s	$4.94
Schein	00364-0574-01	100s	$5.20
Major	00904-0201-60	100s	$5.25
Qualitest	00603-2213-21	100s	$5.25
URL	00677-0476-01	100s	$5.70
Mutual	53489-0105-01	100s	$5.70
Biocraft	00332-2122-09	100s	$6.00
Sidmak	50111-0367-01	100s	$6.75
Goldline	00182-1019-01	100s	$6.75
Martec	52555-0976-01	100s	$6.80
Purepac	00228-2132-10	100s	$7.11
Parmed	00349-1041-01	100s	$7.45
Roxane	00054-4042-25	100s	$8.44
Moore,H.L.	00839-6192-06	100s	$8.71
➤ Mylan	00378-2625-01	100s	$8.75
ENDEP: Roche Prod	00140-0107-01	100s	$30.74
Raway	00686-0107-20	100s ud	$4.55
➤ Geneva	00781-1487-13	100s ud	$8.95
Vangard	00615-0829-13	100s ud	$9.42
Major	00904-0201-61	100s ud	$9.51
Roxane	00054-8042-25	100s ud	$14.18
UDL	51079-0107-20	100s ud	$14.80
Medirex	57480-0302-01	100s ud	$14.85
Goldline	00182-1019-89	100s ud	$15.00
➤ Rugby	00536-3072-10	1000s	$18.90
Major	00904-0201-80	1000s	$29.50
➤ Geneva	00781-1487-10	1000s	$32.25
Qualitest	00603-2213-32	1000s	$32.55
Schein	00364-0574-02	1000s	$35.08
URL	00677-0476-10	1000s	$35.30
Mutual	53489-0105-10	1000s	$35.30
Aligen	00405-4067-03	1000s	$36.62
Martec	52555-0976-10	1000s	$37.00
Moore,H.L.	00839-6192-16	1000s	$39.22
Purepac	00228-2132-96	1000s	$46.49
Biocraft	00332-2122-15	1000s	$57.04
Sidmak	50111-0367-03	1000s	$58.10
Goldline	00182-1019-10	1000s	$58.10
Parmed	00349-1041-10	1000s	$59.00
Roxane	00054-4042-31	1000s	$71.46
➤ Mylan	00378-2625-10	1000s	$78.75

TABLET: 25 MG

BRAND/MANUFACTURER	NDC	SIZE	AWP
◇ GENERICS			
Copley	38245-0207-10	100s	$2.85
Copley	38245-0207-20	1000s	$20.35

For additional alternatives, turn to the section beginning on page 2859.

Amitriptyline Hydrochloride with Chlordiazepoxide

DESCRIPTION

Amitriptyline Hydrochloride/Chlordiazepoxide combines for oral administration, Chlordiazepoxide, an agent for the relief of anxiety and tension, and Amitriptyline, an antidepressant. It is available in double strength tablets, each containing 10 mg Chlordiazepoxide and 25 mg Amitriptyline (as the Hydrochloride salt); and in tablets each containing 5 mg Chlordiazepoxide and 12.5 mg Amitriptyline (as the Hydrochloride salt). Chlordiazepoxide is a benzodiazepine with the formula 7-chloro-2-(methylamino),-5-phenyl-3H-1,4-benzodiazepine 4-oxide. It is a slightly yellow crystalline material and is insoluble in water. The molecular weight is 299.76.

Amitriptyline is a dibenzocycloheptadiene derivative. The formula is 10,11-dihydro-N,N-dimethyl-5H-dibenzo[a,d] cycloheptene-$\Delta^{5,\gamma}$-propylamine Hydrochloride. It is a white or practically white crystalline compound that is freely soluble in water. The molecular weight is 313.87.

ACTIONS

Both components of Amitriptyline Hydrochloride/Chlordiazepoxide exert their action in the central nervous system. Extensive studies with Chlordiazepoxide in many animal species suggest action in the limbic system. Recent evidence indicates that the limbic system is involved in emotional response. Taming action was observed in some species. The mechanism of action of Amitriptyline in man is not known, but the drug appears to interfere with the reuptake of norepinephrine into adrenergic nerve endings. This action may prolong the sympathetic activity of biogenic amines.

INDICATIONS

Amitriptyline Hydrochloride/Chlordiazepoxide is indicated for the treatment of patients with moderate to severe depression associated with moderate to severe anxiety.

The therapeutic response to Amitriptyline Hydrochloride/Chlordiazepoxide occurs earlier and with fewer treatment failures than when either Amitriptyline or Chlordiazepoxide is used alone.

Symptoms likely to respond in the first week of treatment include: insomnia, feelings of guilt or worthlessness, agitation, psychic and somatic anxiety, suicidal ideation and anorexia.

CONTRAINDICATIONS

Amitriptyline Hydrochloride/Chlordiazepoxide is contraindicated in patients with hypersensitivity to either benzodiazepines or tricyclic antidepressants. It should not be given concomitantly with a monoamine oxidase inhibitor. Hyperpyretic crises, severe convulsions and deaths have occurred in patients receiving a tricyclic antidepressant and a monoamine oxidase inhibitor simultaneously. When it is desired to replace a monoamine oxidase inhibitor with Amitriptyline Hydrochloride/Chlordiazepoxide a minimum of 14 days should be allowed to elapse after the former is discontinued. Limbitrol should then be initiated cautiously with gradual increase in dosage until optimum response is achieved.

This drug is contraindicated during the acute recovery phase following myocardial infarction.

➤ SHOWN IN PRODUCT IDENTIFICATION GUIDE

WARNINGS

Because of the atropine-like action of the Amitriptyline component, great care should be used in treating patients with a history of urinary retention or angle-closure glaucoma. In patients with glaucoma, even average doses may precipitate an attack. Severe constipation may occur in patients taking tricyclic antidepressants in combination with anticholinergic-type drugs.

Patients with cardiovascular disorders should be watched closely. Tricyclic antidepressant drugs, particularly when given in high doses, have been reported to produce arrhythmias, sinus tachycardia and prolongation of conduction time. Myocardial infarction and stroke have been reported in patients receiving drugs of this class.

Because of the sedative effects of Amitriptyline Hydrochloride/Chlordiazepoxide patients should be cautioned about combined effects with alcohol or other CNS depressants. The additive effects may produce a harmful level of sedation and CNS depression.

Patients receiving Amitriptyline Hydrochloride/Chlordiazepoxide should be cautioned against engaging in hazardous occupations requiring complete mental alertness, such as operating machinery or driving a motor vehicle.

Usage in Pregnancy: Safe use of Amitriptyline Hydrochloride/Chlordiazepoxide during pregnancy and lactation has not been established. Because of the Chlordiazepoxide component, please note the following:

An increased risk of congenital malformations associated with the use of minor tranquilizers (Chlordiazepoxide, diazepam and meprobamate) during the first trimester of pregnancy has been suggested in several studies. Because use of these drugs is rarely a matter of urgency, their use during this period should almost always be avoided. The possibility that a woman of childbearing potential may be pregnant at the time of institution of therapy should be considered. Patients should be advised that if they become pregnant during therapy or intend to become pregnant they should communicate with their physicians about the desirability of discontinuing the drug.

Withdrawal symptoms of the barbiturate type have occurred after the discontinuation of benzodiazepines. (See *"Drug Abuse and Dependence"* section.)

PRECAUTIONS

General: Use with caution in patients with a history of seizures.

Close supervision is required when Amitriptyline Hydrochloride/Chlordiazepoxide is given to hyperthyroid patients or those on thyroid medication.

The usual precautions should be observed when treating patients with impaired renal or hepatic function.

Patients with suicidal ideation should not have easy access to large quantities of the drug. The possibility of suicide in depressed patients remains until significant remission occurs.

Essential Laboratory Tests: Patients on prolonged treatment should have periodic liver function tests and blood counts.

Drug and Treatment Interactions: Because of its Amitriptyline component, Amitriptyline Hydrochloride/Chlordiazepoxide may block the antihypertensive action of guanethidine or compounds with a similar mechanism of action.

The effects of concomitant administration of Amitriptyline Hydrochloride/Chlordiazepoxide and other psychotropic drugs have not been evaluated. Sedative effects may be additive.

Cimetidine is reported to reduce hepatic metabolism of certain tricyclic antidepressants and benzodiazepines, thereby delaying elimination and increasing steady state concentrations of these drugs. Clinically significant effects have been reported with the tricyclic antidepressants when used concomitantly with cimetidine (Tagamet).

The drug should be discontinued several days before elective surgery.

Concurrent administration of ECT and Amitriptyline Hydrochloride/Chlordiazepoxide should be limited to those patients for whom it is essential.

Pregnancy: See *"Warnings"* section.

Nursing Mothers: It is not known whether this drug is excreted in human milk. As a general rule, nursing should not be undertaken while a patient is on a drug, since many drugs are excreted in human milk.

Pediatric Use: Safety and effectiveness in children below the age of 12 years have not been established.

Elderly Patients: In elderly and debilitated patients it is recommended that dosage be limited to the smallest effective amount to preclude the development of ataxia oversedation, confusion or anticholinergic effects.

Information for Patients: To assure the safe and effective use of benzodiazepines, patients should be informed that, since benzodiazepines may produce psychological and physical dependence, it is advisable that they consult with their physician before either increasing the dose or abruptly discontinuing this drug.

ADVERSE REACTIONS

Adverse reactions to Amitriptyline Hydrochloride/Chlordiazepoxide are those associated with the use of either component alone. Most frequently reported were drowsiness, dry mouth, constipation, blurred vision, dizziness and bloating. Other side effects occurring less commonly included vivid dreams, impotence, tremor, confusion and nasal congestion. Many symptoms common to the depressive state, such as anorexia, fatigue, weakness, restlessness and lethargy, have been reported as side effects of treatment with both Amitriptyline Hydrochloride/Chlordiazepoxide and Amitriptyline.

Granulocytopenia, jaundice and hepatic dysfunction of uncertain etiology have also been observed rarely with Amitriptyline Hydrochloride/Chlordiazepoxide.

When treatment with Amitriptyline Hydrochloride/Chlordiazepoxide is prolonged, periodic blood counts and liver function tests are advisable.

Note: Included in the listing which follows are adverse reactions which have not been reported with Amitriptyline Hydrochloride/Chlordiazepoxide. However, they are included because they have been reported during therapy with one or both of the components or closely related drugs.

Cardiovascular: Hypotension, hypertension, tachycardia, palpitations, myocardial infarction, arrhythmias, heart block, stroke.

Psychiatric: Euphoria, apprehension, poor concentration, delusions, hallucinations, hypomania and increased or decreased libido.

Neurologic: Incoordination, ataxia, numbness, tingling and paresthesias of the extremities, extrapyramidal symptoms, syncope, changes in EEG patterns.

Anticholinergic: Disturbance of accommodation, paralytic ileus, urinary retention, dilatation of urinary tract.

Allergic: Skin rash, urticaria, photosensitization, edema of face and tongue, pruritus.

Hematologic: Bone marrow depression including agranulocytosis, eosinophilia, purpura, thrombocytopenia.

Gastrointestinal: Nausea, epigastric distress, vomiting, anorexia, stomatitis, peculiar taste, diarrhea, black tongue.

Endocrine: Testicular swelling and gynecomastia in the male, breast enlargement, galactorrhea and minor menstrual irregularities in the female, elevation and lowering of blood sugar levels, and syndrome of inappropriate ADH (antidiuretic hormone) secretion.

Other: Headache, weight gain or loss, increased perspiration, urinary frequency, mydriasis, jaundice, alopecia, parotid swelling.

DRUG ABUSE AND DEPENDENCE

Withdrawal symptoms, similar in character to those noted with barbiturates and alcohol (convulsions, tremor, abdominal and muscle cramps, vomiting and sweating), have occurred following abrupt discontinuance of Chlordiazepoxide.

The more severe withdrawal symptoms have usually been limited to those patients who had received excessive doses over an extended period of time. Generally milder withdrawal symptoms (*e.g.*, dysphoria and insomnia) have been reported following abrupt discontinuance of benzodiazepines taken continuously at therapeutic levels for several months. Withdrawal symptoms (*e.g.*, nausea, headache and malaise) have also been reported in association with abrupt Amitriptyline discontinuation. Consequently, after extended therapy, abrupt discontinuation should generally be avoided and a gradual dosage tapering schedule followed. Addiction-prone individuals (such as drug addicts or alcoholics) should be under careful surveillance when receiving Chlordiazepoxide or other psychotropic agents because of the predisposition of such patients to habituation and dependence.

OVERDOSAGE

There has been limited experience with Amitriptyline Hydrochloride/Chlordiazepoxide overdosage *per se*; the manifestations of overdosage and recommendations for treatment are based on clinical experience with its components. Primary concern should be with the dangers associated with Amitriptyline overdosage. Deaths by deliberate or accidental overdosage have occurred with this class of drugs.

All patients suspected of having an overdosage of Amitriptyline Hydrochloride/Chlordiazepoxide should be admitted to a hospital as soon as possible.

Manifestations: High doses may cause drowsiness, temporary confusion, disturbed concentration or transient visual hallucinations. Overdosage may cause hypothermia, tachycardia and other arrhythmias, ECG evidence of impaired conduction (such as bundle branch block), congestive heart failure, dilated pupils, convulsions, severe hypotension, stupor and coma. Other symptoms may be agitation, hyperactive reflexes, muscle rigidity, vomiting, hyperpyrexia or any of those listed under *"Adverse Reactions."*

Treatment: Empty the stomach as quickly as possible by emesis or lavage. In the comatose patient a cuff endotracheal tube should be placed in position prior to either of these measures. The instillation of activated charcoal into the stomach also should be considered. If the patient is stuporous but responds to stimuli, only close observation and nursing care may be required. It is essential to maintain an adequate airway and fluid intake. Body temperature should be watched closely and appropriate measures taken should deviations occur.

The intramuscular or slow intravenous administration of 1 to 3 mg in adults (or 0.5 mg in children) of physostigmine salicylate[1-3] has been reported to reverse the manifestations of Amitriptyline overdosage. Because of its relatively short half-life, additional doses may be needed at intervals of 30 minutes to 2 hours.

Convulsions may be treated by the use of an inhalation anesthetic rather than the use of barbiturates. Cardiac monitoring is advisable, and the cautious use of digitalis or other antiarrhythmic agents should be considered if serious cardiovascular abnormalities occur. Serum potassium levels should be monitored and kept within normal limits by the use of appropriate I.V. fluids. Standard measures including oxygen, I.V. fluids, plasma expanders and corticosteroids may be used to control circulatory shock.

Dialysis is unlikely to be of value, as it has not proven useful in overdosages of either Amitriptyline or Chlordiazepoxide.

◆ RATED THERAPEUTICALLY EQUIVALENT; ◇ THERAPEUTIC EQUIVALENCE UNCONFIRMED; ○ UNRATED

Since many suicidal attempts involve multiple drugs including barbiturates, the possibility of dialysis being beneficial for removal of other drugs should not be overlooked.

Treatment should be continued for at least 48 hours, along with cardiac monitoring in patients who do not respond to therapy promptly. Since relapses are frequent, patients should be hospitalized until their conditions remain stable without physostigmine for at least 24 hours.

Since overdosage is often deliberate, patients may attempt suicide by other means during the recovery phase.

REFERENCES:
1. Granacher RP, Baldessarini RJ: Physostigmine: Its use in acute anticholinergic syndrome with antidepressant and antiparkinson drugs. *Arch Gen Psychiatry* 32:375-380, March 1975. 2. Burks JS, Walker JE, Rumack BH, Ott JE: Tricyclic antidepressant poisoning: Reversal of coma, choreoathetosis, and myoclonus by physostigmine. *JAMA* 230:1405-1407, Dec. 9, 1974. 3. Snyder BD, Blonde L, McWhirter WR: Reversal of Amitriptyline intoxication by physostigmine. *JAMA* 230:1433-1434, Dec. 9, 1974.

DOSAGE AND ADMINISTRATION
Optimum dosage varies with the severity of the symptoms and the response of the individual patient. When a satisfactory response is obtained, dosage should be reduced to the smallest amount needed to maintain the remission. The larger portion of the total daily dose may be taken at bedtime. In some patients, a single dose at bedtime may be sufficient. In general, lower dosages are recommended for elderly patients.

Amitriptyline Hydrochloride/Chlordiazepoxide (double strength) Tablets are recommended in an initial dosage of three or four tablets daily in divided doses; this may be increased to six tablets daily as required. Some patients respond to smaller doses and can be maintained on two tablets daily.

Amitriptyline Hydrochloride/Chlordiazepoxide Tablets in an initial dosage of three or four tablets daily in divided doses may be satisfactory in patients who do not tolerate higher doses.

HOW SUPPLIED
TABLETS (C-IV): 12.5 MG-5 MG

AVERAGE UNIT PRICE (AVAILABLE SIZES)		GENERIC A-RATED AVERAGE PRICE (GAAP)	
BRAND	$0.65	100s	$32.49
GENERIC	$0.32	500s	$155.20
HCFA FUL (100s ea)	$0.18		

BRAND/MANUFACTURER	NDC	SIZE	AWP
◆ **BRAND**			
LIMBITROL: Roche Prod	00140-0070-01	100s	$64.55
	00140-0070-49	100s ud	$66.58
	00140-0070-14	500s	$321.66
◆ **GENERICS**			
Schein	00364-2157-01	100s	$26.50
URL	00677-1142-01	100s	$30.00
Qualitest	00603-2690-21	100s	$30.10
Mylan	00378-0211-01	100s	$31.95
Aligen	00405-0037-01	100s	$32.44
Parmed	00349-8657-01	100s	$36.95
Moore,H.L.	00839-7279-06	100s	$39.49
Qualitest	00603-2690-28	500s	$136.94
Mylan	00378-0211-05	500s	$151.80
Moore,H.L.	00839-7279-12	500s	$176.85

TABLETS (C-IV): 25 MG-10 MG

AVERAGE UNIT PRICE (AVAILABLE SIZES)		GENERIC A-RATED AVERAGE PRICE (GAAP)	
BRAND	$0.92	100s	$44.52
GENERIC	$0.45	500s	$224.94
HCFA FUL (100s ea)	$0.24		

BRAND/MANUFACTURER	NDC	SIZE	AWP
◆ **BRAND**			
LIMBITROL DS: Roche Prod	00140-0071-01	100s	$91.13
	00140-0071-49	100s ud	$93.18
	00140-0071-14	500s	$454.61
◆ **GENERICS**			
Schein	00364-2158-01	100s	$34.75
URL	00677-1143-01	100s	$40.20
Qualitest	00603-2691-01	100s	$41.08
Aligen	00405-0038-01	100s	$41.80
Mylan	00378-0277-01	100s	$44.50
Parmed	00349-8658-01	100s	$49.95
Moore,H.L.	00839-7280-06	100s	$59.33
Qualitest	00603-2691-28	500s	$197.75
Mylan	00378-0277-05	500s	$211.40
Moore,H.L.	00839-7280-12	500s	$265.68

Amitriptyline Hydrochloride with Perphenazine

DESCRIPTION
Amitriptyline Hydrochloride/Perphenazine, a broad-spectrum psychotherapeutic agent for the management of outpatients and hospitalized patients with psychoses or neuroses characterized by mixtures of anxiety or agitation with symptoms of depression, is a combination of Amitriptyline Hydrochloride and Perphenazine (Amtriptyline HCl/Perphenazine). Since such syndromes can occur in patients with various degrees of intensity of mental illness, Amitriptyline HCl/Perphenazine tablets are provided in multiple combinations to afford dosage flexibility for optimum management.

Amitriptyline HCl/Perphenazine is a combination of Perphenazine, a piperazine phenothiazine, and Amitriptyline HCl, a dibenzo- cycloheptadiene.

PERPHENAZINE
Perphenazine is 4-[3-(2-chloro-10 *H*-phenothiazin-10-yl)-propyl] -1-piperazineethanol. Its empirical formula is $C_{21}H_{26}ClN_3OS$.

Perphenazine has a molecular weight of 403.97. It is a white, odorless, bitter-tasting powder that is insoluble in water.

AMITRIPTYLINE HYDROCHLORIDE
Amitriptyline Hydrochloride is 3-(10,11-dihydro-5 *H*-dibenzo [*a,d*]cyclohepten-5-ylidene)-*N,N*-dimethyl-1-propanamine hydrochloride. Its empirical formula is $C_{20}H_{23}N \cdot HCl$.

Amitriptyline HCl, a dibenzocycloheptadiene derivative, has a molecular weight of 313.87. It is a white, odorless, crystal line compound which is freely soluble in water.

Each tablet contains:

Amitriptyline HCl/Perphenazine 2-10	
Perphenazine	2 mg
Amitriptyline HCl	10mg
Amitriptyline HCl/Perphenazine 2-25	
Perphenazine	2 mg
Amitriptyline HCl	25 mg
Amitriptyline HCl/Perphenazine 4-10	
Perphenazine	4 mg
Amitriptyline HCl	10 mg
Amitriptyline HCl/Perphenazine 4-25	
Perphenazine	4 mg
Amitriptyline HCl	25 mg
Amitriptyline HCl/Perphenazine 4-50	
Perphenazine	4 mg
Amitriptyline HCl	50 mg

ACTIONS
Perphenazine: In common with all members of the piperazine group of phenothiazine derivatives, Perphenazine has greater behavioral potency than phenothiazine derivatives of other groups without a corresponding increase in autonomic, hematologic, or hepatic side effects.

Extrapyramidal effects, however, may occur more frequently. These effects are interpreted as neuropharmacologic. They usually regress after discontinuation of the drug. Perphenazine is a potent tranquilizer and also a potent antiemetic. Orally, its milligram potency is about five or six times that of chlorpromazine with respect to behavorial effects. It is capable of alleviating symptoms of anxiety, tension, psychomotor excitement, and other manifestations of emotional stress without apparent dulling of mental acuity.

Amitriptyline HCl is an antidepressant with sedative effects. Its mechanism of action in man is not known. It is not a monoamine oxidase inhibitor and it does not act primarily by stimulation of the central nervous system.

INDICATIONS
Amitriptyline HCl/Perphenazine is recommended for treatment of (1) patients with *moderate to severe anxiety and/or agitation and depressed mood*, (2) patients with *depression in whom anxiety and/or agitation are severe*, and (3) patients with *depression and anxiety in association with chronic physical disease*. In many of these patients anxiety masks the depressive state so that, although therapy with a tranquilizer appears to be indicated, the administration of a tranquilizer alone will not be adequate.

Schizophrenic patients who have associated depressive symptoms should be considered for therapy with Amitriptyline HCl/Perphenazine.

Many patients presenting symptoms such as agitation, anxiety, insomnia, psychomotor retardation, functional somatic complaints, a feeling of tiredness, loss of interest, and anorexia have responded well to therapy with Amitriptyline HCl/Perphenazine.

CONTRAINDICATIONS
Amitriptyline HCl/Perphenazine is contraindicated in depression of the central nervous system from drugs (barbiturates, alcohol, narcotics, analgesics, antihistamines); in the presence of evidence of bone marrow depression; and in patients known to be hypersensitive to Phenothiazines or Amitriptyline.

It should not be given concomitantly with monoamine oxidase inhibitors. Hyperpyretic crises, severe convulsions, and deaths have occurred in patients receiving tricyclic antidepressants and monoamine oxidase inhibitors simultaneously. When it is desired to replace a monoamine oxidase inhibitor with Amitriptyline HCl/Perphenazine, a minimum of 14 days should be allowed to elapse after the former is discontinued. Amitriptyline HCl/Perphenazine should then be initiated cautiously with gradual increase in dosage until optimum response is achieved.

Amitriptyline HCl is not recommended for use during the acute recovery phase following myocardial infarction.

➤ SHOWN IN PRODUCT IDENTIFICATION GUIDE

WARNINGS

TARDIVE DYSKINESIA

Tardive dyskinesia, a syndrome consisting of potentially irreversible, involuntary dyskinetic movements may develop in patients treated with neuroleptic (antipsychotic) drugs. Although the prevalence of the syndrome appears to be highest among the elderly, especially elderly women, it is impossible to rely upon prevalence estimates to predict, at the inception of neuroleptic treatment, which patients are likely to develop the syndrome. Whether neuroleptic drug products differ in their potential to cause tardive dyskinesia is unknown.

Both the risk of developing the syndrome and the likelihood that it will become irreversible are believed to increase as the duration of treatment and the total cumulative dose of neuroleptic drugs administered to the patient increase. However, the syndrome can develop, although much less commonly, after relatively brief treatment periods at low doses. There is no known treatment for established cases of tardive dyskinesia, although the syndrome may remit, partially or completely, if neuroleptic treatment is withdrawn. Neuroleptic treatment, itself, however, may suppress (or partially suppress) the signs and symptoms of the syndrome and thereby may possibly mask the underlying disease process. The effect that symptomatic suppression has upon the long-term course of the syndrome is unknown.

Given these considerations, neuroleptics should be prescribed in a manner that is most likely to minimize the occurrence of tardive dyskinesia. Chronic neuroleptic treatment should generally be reserved for patients who suffer from a chronic mental illness that, 1) is known to respond to neuroleptic drugs, and, 2) for whom alternative, equally effective, but potentially less harmful treatments are *not* available or appropriate. In patients who do require chronic treatment, the smallest dose and the shortest duration of treatment producing a satisfactory clinical response should be sought. The need for continued treatment should be reassessed periodically.

If signs and symptoms of tardive dyskinesia appear in a patient on neuroleptics, drug discontinuation should be considered. However, some patients may require treatment despite the presence of the syndrome.

(For further information about the description of tardive dyskinesia and its clinical detection, please refer to the section on *"Adverse Reactions".*)

NEUROLEPTIC MALIGNANT SYNDROME (NMS)

A potentially fatal symptom complex sometimes referred to as Neuroleptic Malignant Syndrome (NMS) has been reported in association with antipsychotic drugs. Clinical manifestations of NMS are hyperpyrexia, muscle rigidity, altered mental status and evidence of autonomic instability (irregular pulse or blood pressure, tachycardia, diaphoresis, and cardiac dysrhythmias).

The diagnostic evaluation of patients with this syndrome is complicated. In arriving at a diagnosis, it is important to identify cases where the clinical presentation includes both serious medical illness (e.g., pneumonia, systemic infection, etc.) and untreated or inadequately treated extrapyramidal signs and symptoms (EPS). Other important considerations in the differential diagnosis include central anticholinergic toxicity, heat stroke, drug fever and primary central nervous system (CNS) pathology.

The management of NMS should include 1) immediate discontinuation of antipsychotic drugs and other drugs not essential to concurrent therapy, 2) intensive symptomatic treatment and medical monitoring, and 3) treatment of any concomitant serious medical problems for which specific treatments are available. There is no general agreement about specific pharmacological treatment regimens for uncomplicated NMS.

If a patient requires antipsychotic drug treatment after recovery from NMS, the potential reintroduction of drug therapy should be carefully considered. The patient should be carefully monitored, since recurrences of NMS have been reported.

GENERAL

Amitriptyline HCl/Perphenazine should not be given concomitantly with guanethidine or similarly acting compounds, since Amitriptyline, like other tricyclic antidepressants, may block the antihypertensive effect of these compounds.

Because of the atropine-like activity of Amitriptyline, Amitriptyline HCl/Perphenazine should be used with caution in patients with a history of urinary retention, or with angle-closure glaucoma or increased intraocular pressure. In patients with angle-closure glaucoma, even average doses may precipitate an attack. It should be used with caution also in patients with convulsive disorders. Dosage of anticonvulsive agents may have to be increased.

Patients with cardiovascular disorders should be watched closely. Tricyclic antidepressants, including Amitriptyline HCl, particularly when given in high doses, have been reported to produce arrhythmias, sinus tachycardia, and prolongation of the conduction time. Myocardial infarction and stroke have been reported with drugs of this class.

Close supervision is required when Amitriptyline HCl is given to hyperthyroid patients or those receiving thyroid medication.

Amitriptyline HCl/Perphenazine may enhance the response to alcohol and the effects of barbiturates and other CNS depressants. In patients who may use alcohol excessively, it should be borne in mind that the potentiation may increase the danger inherent in any suicide attempt or overdosage. Delirium has been reported with concurrent administration of Amitriptyline and disulfiram.

Usage in Pregnancy: Amitriptyline HCl/Perphenazine is not recommended for use in pregnant patients or in nursing mothers at this time. Reproduction studies in rats have shown no fetal abnormalities; however, clinical experience and follow-up in pregnancy have been limited, and the possibility of adverse effects on fetal development must be considered.

Usage in Children: Since dosage for children has not been established. Amitriptyline HCl/Perphenazine is not recommended for use in children.

PRECAUTIONS

GENERAL

The possibility of suicide in depressed patients remains during treatment and until significant remission occurs. Such patients should not have access to large quantities of this drug.

Perphenazine: As with all phenothiazine compounds, Perphenazine should not be used indiscriminately. Caution should be observed in giving it to patients who have previously exhibited severe adverse reactions to other phenothiazines.

Some of the untoward actions of Perphenazine tend to appear more frequently when high doses are used. However, as with other phenothiazine compounds, patients receiving Perphenazine in any dosage should be kept under close supervision.

The antiemetic effect of Perphenazine may obscure signs of toxicity due to overdosage of other drugs, or render more difficult the diagnosis of disorders such as brain tumors or intestinal obstruction.

A significant, not otherwise explained, rise in body temperature may suggest individual intolerance to Perphenazine, in which case Amitriptyline HCl/Perphenazine should be discontinued.

Neuroleptic drugs elevate prolactin levels; the elevation persists during chronic administration. Tissue culture experiments indicate that approximately one third of human breast cancers are prolactin dependent *in vitro,* a factor of potential importance if the prescription of these drugs is contemplated in a patient with a previously detected breast cancer. Although disturbances such as galactorrhea, amenorrhea, gynecomastia, and impotence have been reported, the clinical significance of elevated serum prolactin levels is unknown for most patients. An increase in mammary neoplasms has been found in rodents after chronic administration of neuroleptic drugs. Neither clinical studies nor epidemiologic studies conducted to date, however, have shown an association between chronic administration of these drugs and mammary tumorigenesis; the available evidence is considered too limited to be conclusive at this time.

Amitriptyline Hydrochloride: Depressed patients, particularly those with known manic depressive illness, may experience a shift to mania or hypomania. Patients with paranoid symptomatology may have an exaggeration of such symptoms. The tranquilizing effect of Amitriptyline HCl/Perphenazine seems to reduce the likelihood of these effects.

Concurrent administration of Amitriptyline HCl and electro-shock therapy may increase the hazards associated with such therapy. Such treatment should be limited to patients for whom it is essential.

Discontinue the drug several days before elective surgery if possible.

Both elevation and lowering of blood sugar levels have been reported.

Amitriptyline HCl should be used with caution in patients with impaired liver function.

INFORMATION FOR PATIENTS

While on therapy with Amitriptyline HCl/Perphenazine, patients should be advised as to the possible impairment of mental and/or physical abilities required for performance of hazardous tasks, such as operating machinery or driving a motor vehicle.

DRUG INTERACTIONS

Perphenazine: If hypotension develops, epinephrine should not be employed, as its action is blocked and partially reversed by Perphenazine.

Phenothiazines may potentiate the action of central nervous system depressants (opiates, analgesics, antihistamines, barbiturates, alcohol) and atropine. In concurrent therapy with any of these, Amitriptyline HCl/Perphenazine should be given in reduced dosage. Phenothiazines also may potentiate the action of heat and phosphorous insecticides.

Amitriptyline Hydrochloride: When Amitriptyline HCl is given with anticholinergic agents or sympathomimetic drugs, including epinephrine combined with local anesthetics, close supervision and careful adjustment of dosages are required.

Hyperpyrexia has been reported when Amitriptyline HCl is administered with anticholinergic agents or with neuroleptic drugs, particularly during hot weather.

Paralytic ileus may occur in patients taking tricyclic antidepressants in combination with anticholinergic-type drugs.

Cimetidine is reported to reduce hepatic metabolism of certain tricyclic antidepressants, thereby delaying elimination and increasing steady-state concentrations of these drugs. Clinically significant effects have been reported with the tricyclic antidepressants when used concomitantly with cimetidine. Increases in plasma levels of tricyclic antidepressants, and in the frequency and severity of side effects, particularly anticholinergic, have been reported when cimetidine was added to the drug regimen. Discontinuation of cimetidine in well-controlled patients receiving tricyclic antidepressants and cimetidine may decrease the plasma levels and efficacy of the antidepressants.

Caution is advised if patients receive large doses of ethchlorvynol concurrently. Transient delirium has been reported in patients who were treated with 1 g of ethchlorvynol and 75-150 mg of Amitriptyline HCl.

ADVERSE REACTIONS

To date, clinical evaluation of Amitriptyline HCl/Perphenazine has not revealed any adverse reactions peculiar to the combination. The adverse reactions that occurred were limited to those that have been reported previously for Perphenazine and Amitriptyline. Treatment with Amitriptyline HCl/Perphenazine is commonly associated with sedation, hypotension, neurological impairments, and dry mouth.

PERPHENAZINE

The common acute neurological effects of neuroleptic drugs, including Perphenazine, consist of dystonia, akathisia or motor restlessness, and pseudoparkinsonism.

More chronic use of neuroleptics may be associated with the development of tardive dyskinesia. The salient features of this syndrome are described in the *"Warnings"* section and below.

The following adverse reactions have been reported and, within each category, are listed in order of decreasing severity.

Neurological: Tardive dyskinesia: The syndrome is characterized by involuntary choreoathetoid movements which variously involve the tongue, face, mouth, lips, or jaw (e.g., protrusion of the tongue, puffing of cheeks, puckering of the mouth, chewing movements), trunk and extremities. The severity of the syndrome and the degree of impairment produced vary widely.

The syndrome may become clinically recognizable either during treatment, upon dosage reduction, or upon withdrawal of treatment. Movements may decrease in intensity and may disappear altogether if further treatment with neuroleptics is withheld. It is generally believed that reversibility is more likely after short rather than long term neuroleptic exposure. Consequently, early detection of tardive dyskinesia is important. To increase the likelihood of detecting the syndrome at the earliest possible time, the dosage of neuroleptic drug should be reduced periodically (if clinically possible) and the patient observed for signs of the disorder. It has been suggested that fine vermicular movements of the tongue may be an early sign of the syndrome, and that the full-blown syndrome may not develop if medication is stopped when lingual vermiculation appears.

1. Dystonia

This may present as acute, reversible torticollis, opisthotonos, carpopedal spasm, trismus, dysphagia, respiratory difficulty, oculogyric crisis, and protrusion of the tongue. Treatment consists of the parenteral administration of either an anticholinergic antiparkinsonian agent or diphenhydramine.

2. Akathisia

Akathisia presents as constant motor restlessness. The patient with akathisia often complains, *when asked,* about his/her inability to stop moving. Akathisia should *not* be treated with an increased dose of neuroleptic; rather, the dose of antipsychotic may be lowered until the motor restlessness has subsided. The efficacy of anticholinergic treatment of this side effect is unestablished.

3. Pseudoparkinsonism

Pseudoparkinsonism refers to a drug-induced state similar to the classic syndrome. Generally, anticholinergic antiparkinsonian agents (i.e., benztropine, biperiden, procylidine, or trihexphenidyl) and amantadine are helpful in alleviating symptoms that cannot be managed by neuroleptic dose reduction. The value of prophylactic antiparkinsonian drug therapy has not been established. The need for continued use of antiparkinsonian medication should be re-evaluated periodically.

Cardiovascular: Hypotension, hypertension, tachycardia, peripheral edema, occasional change in pulse rate, ECG abnormalities (quinidine-like effect), reversed epinephrine effect.

CNS and Neuromuscular: Neuroleptic malignant syndrome (see *"Warnings"*); extrapyramidal symptoms, including acute dyskinesia (see *Neurological*); reactivation of psychoses and production of catatonic-like states; paradoxical excitement; ataxia; muscle weakness; hypnotic effects; mild insomnia; lassitude; headache; hyperflexia; altered cerebrospinal fluid proteins.

Autonomic: Urinary frequency or incontinence, dry mouth or salivation, nasal congestion.

Allergic: Anaphylactoid reactions, laryngeal edema, asthma, angioneurotic edema.

Hematologic: Blood dyscrasias including pancytopenia, agranulocytosis, leukopenia, thrombocytopenic purpura, eosinophilia.

Gastrointestinal: Liver damage (jaundice, biliary stasis), obstipation, vomiting, nausea, constipation, anorexia.

Dermatologic: Eczema up to exfoliative dermatitis, urticaria, erythema, itching, photosensitivity.

Ophthalmic: Pigmentation of the cornea and lens, blurred vision.

Endocrine: Lactation, galactorrhea, hyperglycemia, gynecomastia, disturbances in menstrual cycle.

Other: False-positive pregnancy tests, including immunologic.

Other adverse reactions that should be considered because they have been reported with various phenothiazine compounds, but not with perphenazine, include:

CNS and Neuromuscular: Grand mal convulsions, cerebral edema.

Gastrointestinal: Polyphagia.

Dermatologic: Photophobia, pigmentation.

Ophthalmic: Pigmentary retinopathy.

Endocrine: Failure of ejaculation.

AMITRIPTYLINE HYDROCHLORIDE

Within each category the following adverse reactions are listed in order of decreasing severity. Included in the listing are a few adverse reactions which have not been reported with this specific drug. However, pharmacological similarities among the tricyclic antidepressant drugs require that each of the reactions be considered when amitriptyline is administered.

Cardiovascular: Myocardial infarction; stroke; heart block; arrhythmias; hypotension, particularly orthostatic hypotension; hypertension; tachycardia; palpitation.

CNS and Neuromuscular: Coma; seizures; hallucinations; delusions; confusional states; disorientation; incoordination; ataxia; tremors; peripheral neuropathy; numbness, tingling, and paresthesias of the extremities; extrapyramidal symptoms; dysarthria; disturbed concentration; excitement; anxiety; insomnia; restlessness; nightmares; drowsiness; dizziness; weakness; fatigue; headache; syndrome of inappropriate ADH (antidiuretic hormone) secretion; tinnitus; alteration in EEG patterns.

Anticholinergic: Paralytic ileus; hyperpyrexia; urinary retention, dilation of the urinary tract; constipation; blurred vision, disturbance of accommodation, increased intraocular pressure, mydriasis; dry mouth.

Allergic: Skin rash; urticaria; photosensitization; edema of face and tongue.

Hematologic: Bone marrow depression including agranulocytosis, leukopenia, thrombocytopenia; purpura; eosinophilia.

Gastrointestinal: Rarely hepatitis (including altered liver function and jaundice); nausea; epigastric distress; vomiting; anorexia; stomatitis; peculiar taste; diarrhea; parotid swelling; black tongue.

Endocrine: Testicular swelling and gynecomastia in the male; breast enlargement and galactorrhea in the female; increased or decreased libido; elevation and lowering of blood sugar levels.

Other: Alopecia; edema; weight gain or loss; urinary frequency; increased perspiration.

Withdrawal Symptoms: After prolonged administration, abrupt cessation of treatment may produce nausea, headache, and malaise. Gradual dosage reduction has been reported to produce within two weeks, transient symptoms including irritability, restlessness, and dream and sleep disturbance. These symptoms are not indicative of addition. Rare instances have been reported of mania or hypomania occurring within 2-7 days following cessation of chronic therapy with tricyclic antidepressants.

OVERDOSAGE

Manifestations: High doses may cause temporary confusion, disturbed concentration, or transient visual hallucinations. Overdosage may cause drowsiness; hypothermia; tachycardia and other arrhythmic abnormalities, such as bundle branch block; ECG evidence of impaired conduction; congestive heart failure; dilated pupils; disorders of ocular motility; convulsions; severe hypotension; stupor; and coma. Other symptoms may be agitation, hyperactive reflexes, muscle rigidity, vomiting, hyperpyrexia, or any of the adverse reactions listed for perphenazine or amitriptyline.

Levarterenol (norepinephrine) may be used to treat hypotension, but not epinephrine.

All patients suspected of having taken an overdosage should be admitted to a hospital as soon as possible. *Treatment* is symptomatic and supportive. Empty the stomach as quickly as possible by emesis followed by gastric lavage upon arrival at the hospital. Saline emetics should not be used as the antiemetic effect of perphenazine may cause retention of the saline load and subsequent hypernatremia. Following gastric lavage, activated charcoal may be administered. Twenty to 30 g of activated charcoal may be given every four to six hours during the first 24 to 48 hours after ingestion. An ECG should be taken and close monitoring of cardiac function instituted if there is any sign of abnormality. Maintain an open airway and adequate fluid intake; regulate body temperature.

The intravenous administration of 1-3 mg of physostigmine salicylate is reported to reverse the symptoms of tricyclic antidepressant poisoning. Because physostigmine is rapidly metabolized, the dosage of physostigmine should be repeated as required particularly if life threatening signs such as arrhythmias, convulsions, and deep coma recur or persist after the initial dosage of physostigmine. On this basis, in severe overdosage with perphenazine-amitriptyline combinations, symptomatic treatment of central anticholinergic effects with physostigmine salicylate should be considered. Because physostigmine itself may be toxic, it is not recommended for routine use.

Standard measures should be used to manage circulatory shock and metabolic acidosis. Cardiac arrhythmias may be treated with neostigmine, pyridostigmine, or propranolol. Should cardiac failure occur, the use of digitalis should be considered. Close monitoring of cardiac function for not less than five days is advisable.

Anticonvulsants may be given to control convulsions. Amitriptyline and perphenazine increase the CNS depressant action but not the anticonvulsant action of barbiturates; therefore, an inhalation anesthetic, diazepam, or paraldehyde is recommended for control of convulsions. The management of acute symptoms of parkinsonism resulting from Perphenazine intoxication may be treated with appropriate doses of benztropine mesylate or diphenhydramine hydrochloride.

Dialysis is of no value because of low plasma concentrations of the drug.

Since overdosage is often deliberate, patients may attempt suicide by other means during the recovery phase.

Deaths by deliberate or accidental overdosage have occurred with this class of drugs.

DOSAGE AND ADMINISTRATION

Since dosage for children has not been established, Amitriptyline HCl/Perphenazine is not recommended for use in children.

The total daily dose of Amitriptyline HCl/Perphenazine should not exceed four tablets of the 4-50 or eight tablets of any other dosage strength.

INITIAL DOSAGE

In psychoneurotic patients when anxiety and depression are of such a degree as to warrant combined therapy, one tablet of Amitriptyline HCl/Perphenazine 2-25 or Amitriptyline HCl/Perphenazine 4-25 three or four times a day or one tablet of Amitriptyline HCl/Perphenazine 4-50 twice a day is recommended. *In more severely ill patients with schizophrenia,* Amitriptyline HCl/Perphenazine 4-25 is recommended in an initial dose of two tablets three times a day. If necessary, a fourth dose may be given at bedtime.

In elderly patients and adolescents, and some other patients in whom anxiety tends to predominate, Amitriptyline HCl/Perphenazine 4-10 may be administered three or four times a day initially, then adjusted as required for subsequent adequate therapy.

MAINTENANCE DOSAGE

Depending on the condition being treated, therapeutic response may take from a few days to a few weeks or even longer. After a satisfactory response is noted, dosage should be reduced to the smallest amount necessary to obtain relief from the symptoms for which Amitriptyline HCl/Perphenazine is being administered. A useful maintenance dosage is one tablet of Amitriptyline HCl/Perphenazine 2-25 or 4-25 two to four times a day or one tablet of Amitriptyline HCl/Perphenazine 4-50 twice a day. Amitriptyline HCl/Perphenazine 2-10 and 4-10 can be used to increase flexibility in adjusting maintenance dosage to the lowest amount consistent with relief of symptoms. In some patients, maintenance dosage is required for many months.

STORAGE

Store Amitriptyline HCl/Perphenazine Tablets in a well-closed container. Avoid storage at temperatures above 40°C (104°F). In addition, Amitriptyline HCl/Perphenazine Tablets 2-10 must be protected from light and stored in a well-closed, light-resistant container.

HOW SUPPLIED
TABLETS: 2 MG-10 MG

BRAND/MANUFACTURER	NDC	SIZE	AWP
◆ GENERICS			
Caraco	57664-0133-08	100s	$11.70

TABLETS: 2 MG-25 MG

AVERAGE UNIT PRICE (AVAILABLE SIZES)			
GENERIC	$0.15		

BRAND/MANUFACTURER	NDC	SIZE	AWP
◆ GENERICS			
Caraco	57664-0135-08	100s	$15.90
Caraco	57664-0135-13	500s	$69.80

TABLETS: 4 MG-10 MG

BRAND/MANUFACTURER	NDC	SIZE	AWP
◆ GENERICS			
Caraco	57664-0138-08	100s	$13.50

TABLETS: 4 MG-25 MG

AVERAGE UNIT PRICE (AVAILABLE SIZES)			
GENERIC	$0.16		

BRAND/MANUFACTURER	NDC	SIZE	AWP
◆ GENERICS			
Caraco	57664-0139-08	100s	$17.25
Caraco	57664-0139-13	500s	$78.00

TABLETS: 10 MG-2 MG

AVERAGE UNIT PRICE (AVAILABLE SIZES)		GENERIC A-RATED AVERAGE PRICE (GAAP)	
BRAND	$0.57	100s	$19.99
GENERIC	$0.18	500s	$80.45
HCFA FUL (100s ea)	$0.06		

BRAND/MANUFACTURER	NDC	SIZE	AWP
◆ BRAND			
▶ TRIAVIL 2-10: Merck	00006-0914-68	100s	$55.83
	00006-0914-28	100s ud	$60.40
	00006-0914-74	500s	$267.86
◆ GENERICS			
Aligen	00405-4787-01	100s	$15.00
Goldline	00182-1235-01	100s	$17.00
Rugby	00536-3077-01	100s	$17.31

BRAND/MANUFACTURER	NDC	SIZE	AWP
Qualitest	00603-5115-21	100s	$17.68
Major	00904-1820-60	100s	$18.40
Geneva	00781-1265-01	100s	$18.45
Royce	51875-0247-01	100s	$18.95
Moore,H.L.	00839-6225-06	100s	$19.24
Martec	52555-0460-01	100s	$19.30
Mylan	00378-0330-01	100s	$19.95
Parmed	00349-8882-01	100s	$20.85
U.S. Trading	56126-0182-11	100s ud	$13.56
Major	00904-7636-61	100s ud	$29.13
Geneva	00781-1265-13	100s ud	$35.00
Mason Dist	11845-0163-03	500s	$51.64
Rugby	00536-3077-05	500s	$51.90
Qualitest	00603-5115-25	500s	$75.51
Goldline	00182-1235-05	500s	$80.00
Major	00904-1820-40	500s	$86.40
Geneva	00781-1265-05	500s	$87.64
Mylan	00378-0330-05	500s	$88.50
Royce	51875-0247-02	500s	$89.10
Martec	52555-0460-05	500s	$90.80
Moore,H.L.	00839-6225-12	500s	$91.13
Parmed	00349-8882-05	500s	$92.29

TABLETS: 10 MG-2 MG

BRAND/MANUFACTURER	NDC	SIZE	AWP
◇ BRAND			
▶ ETRAFON 2-10: Schering	00085-0287-04	100s	$59.60
	00085-0287-08	100s ud	$62.86

TABLETS: 10 MG-4 MG

AVERAGE UNIT PRICE (AVAILABLE SIZES)		GENERIC A-RATED AVERAGE PRICE (GAAP)	
BRAND	$0.61	100s	$21.88
GENERIC	$0.21	500s	$90.36
HCFA FUL (100s ea)	$0.08		

BRAND/MANUFACTURER	NDC	SIZE	AWP
◆ BRAND			
▶ TRIAVIL 4-10: Merck	00006-0934-68	100s	$62.46
	00006-0934-74	500s	$298.48
◆ GENERICS			
Aligen	00405-4789-01	100s	$19.00
Goldline	00182-1237-01	100s	$19.00
Mason Dist	11845-0165-01	100s	$19.09
Rugby	00536-3078-01	100s	$19.19
Qualitest	00603-5117-21	100s	$19.54
Major	00904-1840-60	100s	$20.30
Schein	00364-2128-01	100s	$20.30
Geneva	00781-1266-01	100s	$20.35
Royce	51875-0249-01	100s	$21.20
Martec	52555-0462-01	100s	$21.60
Mylan	00378-0042-01	100s	$23.50
Moore,H.L.	00839-6226-06	100s	$24.30
Major	00904-7638-61	100s ud	$37.02
Qualitest	00603-5117-28	500s	$83.87
Royce	51875-0249-02	500s	$96.85

TABLETS: 10 MG-4 MG

BRAND/MANUFACTURER	NDC	SIZE	AWP
◇ BRAND			
ETRAFON-A: Schering	00085-0119-04	100s	$62.68
	00085-0119-08	100s ud	$66.18

TABLETS: 25 MG-2 MG

AVERAGE UNIT PRICE (AVAILABLE SIZES)		GENERIC A-RATED AVERAGE PRICE (GAAP)	
BRAND	$0.72	100s	$25.52
GENERIC	$0.23	500s	$101.95
HCFA FUL (100s ea)	$0.08		

BRAND/MANUFACTURER	NDC	SIZE	AWP
◆ BRAND			
▶ TRIAVIL 2-25: Merck	00006-0921-68	100s	$71.08
	00006-0921-28	100s ud	$75.65
	00006-0921-74	500s	$339.19
◆ GENERICS			
Aligen	00405-4788-01	100s	$19.50
Rugby	00536-3082-01	100s	$21.94
Goldline	00182-1236-01	100s	$22.00
Qualitest	00603-5116-21	100s	$22.61
Major	00904-1825-60	100s	$23.40
Geneva	00781-1273-01	100s	$23.40
Parmed	00349-8883-01	100s	$24.08
Royce	51875-0248-01	100s	$24.15
Moore,H.L.	00839-6217-06	100s	$24.50
Martec	52555-0461-01	100s	$24.65
▶ Mylan	00378-0442-01	100s	$24.95
Major	00904-7637-61	100s	$33.64

◆ RATED THERAPEUTICALLY EQUIVALENT; ◇ THERAPEUTIC EQUIVALENCE UNCONFIRMED; ○ UNRATED

BRAND/MANUFACTURER	NDC	SIZE	AWP
Geneva	00781-1273-13	100s ud	$43.00
Mason Dist	11845-0164-03	500s	$66.50
Rugby	00536-3082-05	500s	$66.83
Qualitest	00603-5116-28	500s	$92.40
Goldline	00182-1236-05	500s	$105.00
Major	00904-1825-40	500s	$109.75
Geneva	00781-1273-05	500s	$111.15
Royce	51875-0248-02	500s	$112.60
▶ Mylan	00378-0442-05	500s	$112.95
Parmed	00349-8883-05	500s	$113.37
Martec	52555-0461-05	500s	$114.85
Moore,H.L.	00839-6217-12	500s	$116.10

TABLETS: 25 MG-2 MG

BRAND/MANUFACTURER	NDC	SIZE	AWP
◇ BRAND			
▶ ETRAFON 2-25: Schering	00085-0598-04	100s	$75.79
	00085-0598-08	100s ud	$78.98

TABLETS: 25 MG-4 MG

AVERAGE UNIT PRICE (AVAILABLE SIZES)		GENERIC A-RATED AVERAGE PRICE (GAAP)	
BRAND	$0.78	100s	$25.32
GENERIC	$0.24	500s	$113.59
HCFA FUL (100s ea)	$0.10		

BRAND/MANUFACTURER	NDC	SIZE	AWP
◆ BRAND			
▶ TRIAVIL 4-25: Merck	00006-0946-68	100s	$77.41
	00006-0946-28	100s ud	$81.96
	00006-0946-74	500s	$370.04
◆ GENERICS			
Aligen	00405-4790-01	100s	$21.00
Goldline	00182-1238-01	100s	$24.00
Rugby	00536-3083-01	100s	$24.25
Qualitest	00603-5118-21	100s	$25.11
Major	00904-1845-60	100s	$25.80
Geneva	00781-1267-01	100s	$25.83
Royce	51875-0250-01	100s	$26.25
Martec	52555-0464-01	100s	$26.78
Moore,H.L.	00839-6227-06	100s	$26.99
Mylan	00378-0574-01	100s	$27.50
Parmed	00349-8885-01	100s	$28.00
U.S. Trading	56126-0183-11	100s ud	$10.20
U.S. Trading	56126-0184-11	100s ud	$14.70
Geneva	00781-1267-13	100s ud	$48.00
Mason Dist	11845-0166-03	500s	$73.58
Rugby	00536-3083-05	500s	$73.95
Qualitest	00603-5118-28	500s	$104.86
Goldline	00182-1238-05	500s	$115.00
Major	00904-1845-40	500s	$120.95
Mylan	00378-0574-05	500s	$122.50
Geneva	00781-1267-05	500s	$122.69
Royce	51875-0250-02	500s	$124.30
Martec	52555-0464-05	500s	$126.78
Moore,H.L.	00839-6227-12	500s	$127.56
Parmed	00349-8885-05	500s	$137.30
Parmed	00349-8885-10	1000s	$91.75

TABLETS: 25 MG-4 MG

BRAND/MANUFACTURER	NDC	SIZE	AWP
◇ BRAND			
▶ ETRAFON FORTE: Schering	00085-0720-04	100s	$82.32
	00085-0720-08	100s ud	$85.56

TABLETS: 50 MG-4 MG

AVERAGE UNIT PRICE (AVAILABLE SIZES)		GENERIC A-RATED AVERAGE PRICE (GAAP)	
BRAND	$1.29	100s	$38.06
GENERIC	$0.38		
HCFA FUL (100s ea)	$0.18		

BRAND/MANUFACTURER	NDC	SIZE	AWP
◆ BRAND			
▶ TRIAVIL 4-50: Merck	00006-0517-60	60s	$78.01
	00006-0517-68	100s	$127.83
◆ GENERICS			
Qualitest	00603-5119-21	100s	$37.78
Mylan	00378-0073-01	100s	$41.50
Moore,H.L.	00839-7233-06	100s	$43.27
Geneva	00781-1268-01	100s	$53.97
U.S. Trading	56126-0185-11	100s ud	$13.80

Amlodipine Besylate

DESCRIPTION

Amlodipine is the besylate salt of Amlodipine, a long-acting calcium channel blocker.

Amlodipine is chemically described as (R.S.) 3-ethyl-5-methyl-2-(2-aminoe-thoxymethyl)-4-(2-chlorophenyl)-1,4-dihydro-6-methyl-3,5-pyridinedicarboxylate benzenesulphonate. Its empirical formula is $C_{20}H_{25}ClN_2O_5 \cdot C_6H_6O_3S$.

Amlodipine besylate is a white crystalline powder with a molecular weight of 567.1. It is slightly soluble in water and sparingly soluble in ethanol. Amlodipine is available as a 2.5 mg, 5 mg and 10 mg tablet for oral administration.

Following is its chemical structure:

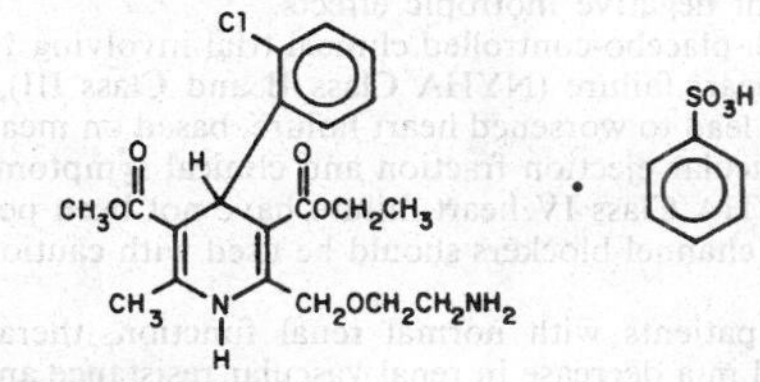

CLINICAL PHARMACOLOGY

Mechanism of Action: Amlodipine is a dihydropyridine calcium antagonist (calcium ion antagonist or slow channel blocker) that inhibits the transmembrane influx of calcium ions into vascular smooth muscle and cardiac muscle. Experimental data suggest that Amlodipine binds to both dihydropyridine and nondihydropyridine binding sites. The contractile processes of cardiac muscle and vascular smooth muscle are dependent upon the movement of extracellular calcium ions into these cells through specific ion channels. Amlodipine inhibits calcium ion influx across cell membranes selectively, with a greater effect on vascular smooth muscle cells than on cardiac muscle cells. Negative inotropic effects can be detected *in vitro* but such effects have not been seen in intact animals at therapeutic doses. Serum calcium concentration is not affected by Amlodipine. Within the physiologic pH range, Amlodipine is an ionized compound (pKa = 8.6), and its kinetic interaction with the calcium channel receptor is characterized by a gradual rate of association and dissociation with the receptor binding site, resulting in a gradual onset of effect.

Amlodipine is a peripheral arterial vasodilator that acts directly on vascular smooth muscle to cause a reduction in peripheral vascular resistance and reduction in blood pressure.

The precise mechanisms by which Amlodipine relieves angina have not been fully delineated, but are thought to include the following:

Exertional Angina: In patients with exertional angina, Amlodipine reduces the total peripheral resistance (afterload) against which the heart works and reduces the rate pressure product, and thus myocardial oxygen demand, at any given level of exercise.

Vasospastic Angina: Amlodipine has been demonstrated to block constriction and restore blood flow in coronary arteries and arterioles in response to calcium, potassium epinephrine, serotonin, and thromboxane A_2 analog in experimental animal models and in human coronary vessels *in vitro*. This inhibition of coronary spasm is responsible for the effectiveness of Amlodipine in vasospastic (Prinzmetal's or variant) angina.

Pharmacokinetics and Metabolism: After oral administration of therapeutic doses of Amlodipine, absorption produces peak plasma concentrations between 6 and 12 hours. Absolute bioavailability has been estimated to be between 64 and 90%. The bioavailability of Amlodipine is not altered by the presence of food.

Amlodipine is extensively (about 90%) converted to inactive metabolites via hepatic metabolism with 10% of the parent compound and 60% of the metabolites excreted in the urine. *Ex vivo* studies have shown that approximately 93% of the circulating drug is bound to plasma proteins in hypertensive patients. Elimination from the plasma is biphasic with a terminal elimination half-life of about 30-50 hours. Steady state plasma levels of Amlodipine are reached after 7 to 8 days of consecutive daily dosing.

The pharmacokinetics of Amlodipine are not significantly influenced by renal impairment. Patients with renal failure may therefore receive the usual initial dose.

Elderly patients and patients with hepatic insufficiency have decreased clearance of Amlodipine with a resulting increase in AUC of approximately 40-60%, and a lower initial dose may be required.

Pharmacodynamics: Hemodynamics—Following administration of therapeutic doses to patients with hypertension, Amlodipine produces vasodilation resulting in a reduction of supine and standing blood pressures. These decreases in blood pressure are not accompanied by a significant change in heart rate or plasma catecholamine levels with chronic dosing. Although the acute intravenous administration of Amlodipine decreases arterial blood pressure and increases heart rate in hemodynamic studies of patients with chronic stable angina, chronic administration of oral Amlodipine in clinical trials did not lead to clinically significant changes in heart rate or blood pressures in normotensive patients with angina.

With chronic once daily oral administration, antihypertensive effectiveness is maintained for at least 24 hours. Plasma concentrations correlate with effect in both young and elderly patients. The magnitude of reduction in blood pressure with Amlodipine is also correlated with the height of pretreatment elevation; thus, individuals with moderate hypertension (diastolic pressure 105-114 mmHg) had about a 50% greater response than patients with mild hypertension (diastolic pressure 90-104 mmHg). Normotensive subjects experienced no clinically significant change in blood pressures (−1/−2 mmHg).

As with other calcium channel blockers, hemodynamic measurements of cardiac function at rest and during exercise (or pacing) in patients with normal ventricular function treated with Amlodipine have generally demonstrated a small increase in cardiac index without significant influence on dP/dt or on left ventricular end diastolic pressure or volume. In hemodynamic studies, Amlodipine has not been associated with a negative inotropic effect when administered in the therapeutic dose range to intact animals and man, even when co-administered with beta-blockers to man. Similar findings, however, have been observed in normals or well-compensated patients with heart failure with agents possessing significant negative inotropic effects.

In a double-blind, placebo-controlled clinical trial involving 118 patients with well compensated heart failure (NYHA Class II and Class III), treatment with Amlodipine did not lead to worsened heart failure, based on measures of exercise tolerance, left ventricular ejection fraction and clinical symptomatology. Studies in patients with NYHA Class IV heart failure have not been performed and, in general, all calcium channel blockers should be used with caution in any patient with heart failure.

In hypertensive patients with normal renal function, therapeutic doses of Amlodipine resulted in a decrease in renal vascular resistance and an increase in glomerular filtration rate and effective renal plasma flow without change in filtration fraction or proteinuria.

Electrophysiologic Effects: Amlodipine does not change sinoatrial nodal function or atrioventricular conduction in intact animals or man. In patients with chronic stable angina, intravenous administration of 10 mg did not significantly alter A-H and H-V conduction and sinus node recovery time after pacing. Similar results were obtained in patients receiving Amlodipine and concomitant beta blockers. In clinical studies in which Amlodipine was administered in combination with beta-blockers to patients with either hypertension or angina, no adverse effects on electrocardiographic parameters were observed. In clinical trials with angina patients alone. Amlodipine therapy did not alter electrocardiographic intervals or produce higher degrees of AV blocks.

Effects in Hypertension: The antihypertensive efficacy of Amlodipine has been demonstrated in a total of 15 double-blind, placebo-controlled, randomized studies involving 800 patients on Amlodipine and 538 on placebo. Once daily administration produced statistically significant placebo-corrected reductions in supine and standing blood pressures at 24 hours postdose, averaging about 12/6 mmHg in the standing position and 13/7 mmHg in the supine position in patients with mild to moderate hypertension. Maintenance of the blood pressure effect over the 24 hour dosing interval was observed, with little difference in peak and trough effect. Tolerance was not demonstrated in patients studied for up to 1 year. The 3 parallel, fixed dose, dose response studies showed that the reduction in supine and standing blood pressures was dose-related within the recommended dosing range. Effects on diastolic pressure were similar in young and older patients. The effect on systolic pressure was greater in older patients, perhaps because of greater baseline systolic pressure. Effects were similar in black and white patients.

Effects in Chronic Stable Angina: The effectiveness of 5-10 mg/day of Amlodipine in exercise-induced angina has been evaluated in 8 placebo-controlled, double-blind clinical trials of up to 6 weeks duration involving 1038 patients (684 Amlodipine, 354 placebo) with chronic stable angina. In 5 of the 8 studies significant increases in exercise time (bicycle or treadmill) were seen with the 10 mg dose. Increases in symptom-limited exercise time averaged 12.8% (63 sec) for Amlodipine 10 mg, and averaged 7.9% (38 sec) for Amlodipine 5 mg, Amlodipine 10 mg also increased time to 1 mm ST segment deviation in several studies and decreased angina attack rate. The sustained efficacy of Amlodipine in angina patients has been demonstrated over long-term dosing. In patients with angina there were no clinically significant reductions in blood pressures (4/1 mmHg) or changes in heart rate (+ 0.3 bpm).

Effects in Vasospastic Angina: In a double-blind, placebo-controlled clinical trial of 4 weeks duration in 50 patients, Amlodipine therapy decreased attacks by approximately 4/week compared with a placebo decrease of approximately 1/week (p < 0.01). Two of 23 Amlodipine and 7 of 27 placebo patients discontinued from the study due to lack of clinical improvement.

INDICATIONS AND USAGE

1. HYPERTENSION

Amlodipine is indicated for the treatment of hypertension. It may be used alone or in combination with other antihypertensive agents.

2. CHRONIC STABLE ANGINA

Amlodipine is indicated for the treatment of chronic stable angina. Amlodipine may be used alone or in combination with other antianginal agents.

3. VASOSPASTIC ANGINA (PRINZMETAL'S OR VARIANT ANGINA)

Amlodipine is indicated for the treatment of confirmed or suspected vasospastic angina. Amlodipine may be used as monotherapy or in combination with other antianginal drugs.

CONTRAINDICATIONS

Amlodipine is contraindicated in patients with known sensitivity to Amlodipine.

WARNINGS

Increased Angina and/or Myocardial Infarction: Rarely, patients, particularly those with severe obstructive coronary artery disease, have developed documented increased frequency, duration and/or severity of angina or acute myocardial infarction on starting calcium channel blocker therapy or at the time of dosage increase. The mechanism of this effect has not been elucidated.

PRECAUTIONS

General: Since the vasodilation induced by Amlodipine is gradual in onset, acute hypotension has rarely been reported after oral administration of Amlodipine. Nonetheless, caution should be exercised when administering Amlodipine as with any other peripheral vasodilator particularly in patients with severe aortic stenosis.

Use in Patients with Congestive Heart Failure: Although hemodynamic studies and a controlled trial in NYHA Class II-III heart failure patients have shown that Amlodipine did not lead to clinical deterioration as measured by exercise tolerance, left ventricular ejection fraction and clinical symptomatology, studies have not been performed in patients with NYHA Class IV heart failure. In general, all calcium channel blockers should be used with caution in patients with heart failure.

Beta-Blocker Withdrawal: Amlodipine is not a beta-blocker and therefore gives no protection against the dangers of abrupt beta-blocker withdrawal; any such withdrawal should be by gradual reduction of the dose of beta-blocker.

Patients with Hepatic Failure: Since Amlodipine is extensively metabolized by the liver and the plasma elimination half-life (t ½) is 56 hours in patients with impaired hepatic function caution should be exercised when administering Amlodipine to patients with severe hepatic impairment.

Drug Interactions: In vitro data in human plasma indicate that Amlodipine has no effect on the protein binding of drugs tested (digoxin, phenytoin, warfarin, and indomethacin). Special studies have indicated that the co-administration of Amlodipine with digoxin did not change serum digoxin levels or digoxin renal clearance in normal volunteers; that co-administration with cimetidine did not alter the pharmacokinetics of Amlodipine; and that co-administration with warfarin did not change the warfarin prothrombin response time.

In clinical trials, Amlodipine has been safely administered with thiazide diuretics, beta-blockers, angiotensin converting enzyme inhibitors, long-acting nitrates, sublingual nitroglycerin, digoxin, warfarin, non-steroidal anti-inflammatory drugs, antibiotics, and oral hypoglycemic drugs.

Drug/Laboratory Test Interactions: None known.

Carcinogenesis, Mutagenesis, Impairment of Fertility: Rats and mice treated with Amlodipine in the diet for two years, at concentrations calculated to provide daily dosage levels of 0.5, 1.25, and 2.5 mg/kg/day showed no evidence of carcinogenicity. The highest dose (for mice, similar to, and for rats twice* the maximum recommended clinical dose of 10 mg on a mg/m² basis), was close to the maximum tolerated dose for mice but not for rats.

Mutagenicity studies revealed no drug related effects at either the gene or chromosome levels.

There was no effect on the fertility of rats treated with Amlodipine (males for 64 days and females 14 days prior to mating) at doses up to 10 mg/kg/day (8 times the maximum recommended human dose of 10 mg on a mg/m² basis).

Pregnancy Category C: No evidence of teratogenicity or other embryo/fetal toxicity was found when pregnant rats or rabbits were treated orally with up to 10 mg/kg Amlodipine (respectively 8 times* and 23 times* the maximum recommended human dose of 10 mg on a mg/m² basis) during their respective periods of major organogenesis. However, litter size was significantly decreased (by about 50%) and the number of intrauterine deaths was significantly increased (about 5-fold) in rats administered 10 mg/kg Amlodipine for 14 days before mating and throughout mating and gestation. Amlodipine has been shown to prolong both the gestation period and the duration of labor in rats at this dose. There are no adequate and well-controlled studies in pregnant women. Amlodipine should be used during pregnancy only if the potential benefit justifies the potential risk to the fetus.

Nursing Mothers: It is not known whether Amlodipine is excreted in human milk. In the absence of this information, it is recommended that nursing be discontinued while Amlodipine is administered.

Pediatric Use: Safety and effectiveness of Amlodipine in children have not been established.

ADVERSE REACTIONS

Amlodipine has been evaluated for safety in more than 11,000 patients in U.S. and foreign clinical trials. In general, treatment with Amlodipine was well-tolerated at doses up to 10 mg daily. Most adverse reactions reported during therapy with Amlodipine were of mild or moderate severity. In controlled clinical trials directly comparing Amlodipine (N = 1730) in doses up to 10 mg to placebo (N = 1250), discontinuation of Amlodipine due to adverse reactions was required in only about 1.5% of patients and was not significantly different from placebo (about 1%). The most common side effects are headache and edema. The incidence (%) of side effects which occurred in a dose related manner are as follows:

Adverse Event	2.5 mg N = 275	5.0 mg N = 296	10.0 mg N = 268	Placebo N = 520
Edema	1.8	3.0	10.8	0.6
Dizziness	1.1	3.4	3.4	1.5
Flushing	0.7	1.4	2.6	0.0
Palpitation	0.7	1.4	4.5	0.6

* Based on patient weight of 50 kg.

Other adverse experiences which were not clearly dose related but which were reported with an incidence greater than 1.0% in placebo-controlled clinical trials include the following:

PLACEBO CONTROLLED STUDIES

	Amlodipine (%) (N = 1730)	Placebo (%) (N = 1250)
Headache	7.3	7.8
Fatigue	4.5	2.8
Nausea	2.9	1.9
Abdominal Pain	1.6	0.3
Somnolence	1.4	0.6

For several adverse experiences that appear to be drug and dose related, there was a greater incidence in women than men associated with Amlodipine treatment as shown in the following table:

	Amlodipine		Placebo	
ADR	M = % (N = 1218)	F = % (N = 512)	M = % (N = 914)	F = % (N = 336)
Edema	5.6	14.6	1.4	5.1
Flushing	1.5	4.5	0.3	0.9
Palpitations	1.4	3.3	0.9	0.9
Somnolence	1.3	1.6	0.8	0.3

The following events occurred in ≤ 1% but > 0.1% of patients in controlled clinical trials or under conditions of open trials or marketing experience where a causal relationship is uncertain; they are listed to alert the physician to a possible relationship:

Cardiovascular: arrhythmia (including ventricular tachycardia and atrial fibrillation), bradycardia, chest pain, hypotension, peripheral ischemia, syncope, tachycardia, postural dizziness, postural hypotension.

Central and Peripheral Nervous System: hypoesthesia, paresthesia, tremor, vertigo.

Gastrointestinal: anorexia, constipation, dyspepsia,** dysphagia, diarrhea, flatulence, vomiting, gingival hyperplasia.

General: asthenia,** back pain, hot flushes, malaise, pain, rigors, weight gain.

Musculo-skeletal System: arthralgia, arthrosis, muscle cramps,** myalgia.

Psychiatric: sexual dysfunction (male** and female), insomnia, nervousness, depression, abnormal dreams, anxiety, depersonalization.

Respiratory System: dyspnea,** epistaxis.

Skin and Appendages: pruritus,** rash,** rash erythematous, rash maculopapular.

Special Senses: abnormal vision, conjunctivitis, diplopia, eye pain, tinnitus.

Urinary System: micturition frequency, micturition disorder, nocturia.

Autonomic Nervous System: dry mouth, sweating increased.

Metabolic and Nutritional: thirst.

Hemopoietic: purpura.

The following events occurred in ≤ 0.1% of patients: cardiac failure, pulse irregularity, extrasystoles, skin discoloration, urticaria, skin dryness, alopecia, dermatitis, muscle weakness, twitching, ataxia, hypertonia, migraine, cold and clammy skin, apathy, agitation, amnesia, gastritis, increased appetite, loose stools, coughing, rhinitis, dysuria, polyuria, parosmia, taste perversion, abnormal visual accommodation, and xerophthalmia.

Other reactions occurred sporadically and cannot be distinguished from medications or concurrent disease states, such as myocardial infarction and angina.

Amlodipine therapy has not been associated with clinically significant changes in routine laboratory tests. No clinically relevant changes were noted in serum potassium, serum glucose, total triglycerides, total cholesterol, HDL cholesterol, uric acid, blood urea nitrogen, creatinine or liver function tests.

Amlodipine has been used safely in patients with chronic obstructive pulmonary disease, well compensated congestive heart failure, peripheral vascular disease, diabetes mellitus, and abnormal lipid profiles.

OVERDOSAGE
Single oral doses of 40 mg/kg and 100 mg/kg in mice and rats, respectively, caused deaths. A single oral dose of 4 mg/ kg or higher in dogs caused a marked peripheral vasodilation and hypotension.

Overdosage might be expected to cause excessive peripheral vasodilation with marked hypotension and possibly a reflex tachycardia. In humans, experience with intentional overdosage of Amlodipine is limited. Reports of intentional overdosage include a patient who ingested 250 mg and was asymptomatic and was

** These events occurred in less than 1% in placebo controlled trials, but the incidence of these side effects was between 1% and 2% in all multiple dose studies.

not hospitalized; another (120 mg) was hospitalized, underwent gastric lavage and remained normotensive; the third (105 mg) was hospitalized and had hypotension (90/50 mmHg) which normalized following plasma expansion. A patient who took 70 mg Amlodipine and an unknown quantity of benzodiazepine in a suicide attempt, developed shock which was refractory to treatment and died the following day with abnormally high benzodiazepine plasma concentration. A case of accidental drug overdose has been documented in a 19 month old male who ingested 30 mg Amlodipine (about 2 mg/kg). During the emergency room presentation, vital signs were stable with no evidence of hypotension, but a heart rate of 180 bpm. Ipecac was administered 3.5 hours after ingestion and on subsequent observation (overnight) no sequelae were noted.

If massive overdose should occur, active cardiac and respiratory monitoring should be instituted. Frequent blood pressure measurements are essential. Should hypotension occur, cardiovascular support including elevation of the extremities and the judicious administration of fluids should be initiated. If hypotension remains unresponsive to these conservative measures, administration of vasopressors (such as phenylephrine), should be considered with attention to circulating volume and urine output. Intravenous calcium gluconate may help to reverse the effects of calcium entry blockade. As Amlodipine is highly protein bound, hemodialysis is not likely to be of benefit.

DOSAGE AND ADMINISTRATION
The usual initial antihypertensive oral dose of Amlodipine is 5 mg once daily with a maximum dose of 10 mg once daily. Small, fragile, or elderly individuals, or patients with hepatic insufficiency may be started on 2.5 mg once daily and this dose may be used when adding Amlodipine to other antihypertensive therapy.

Dosage should be adjusted according to each patient's need. In general, titration should proceed over 7 to 14 days so that the physician can fully assess the patient's response to each dose level. Titration may proceed more rapidly, however, if clinically warranted, provided the patient is assessed frequently.

The recommended dose for chronic stable or vasospastic angina is 5-10 mg, with the lower dose suggested in the elderly and in patients with hepatic insufficiency. Most patients will require 10 mg for adequate effect. See Adverse Reactions section for information related to dosage and side effects.

Co-administration with Other Antihypertensive and/or Antianginal Drugs. Amlodipine has been safely administered with thiazides, ACE inhibitors, beta-blockers, long-acting nitrates, and/or sublingual nitroglycerin.

Tablets: Store bottles at controlled room temperature, 59° to 86°F (15° to 30°C) and dispense in tight, light-resistant containers (USP).

HOW SUPPLIED
TABLETS: 2.5 MG

BRAND/MANUFACTURER	NDC	SIZE	AWP
○ BRAND ➤ NORVASC: Pfizer Labs	00069-1520-66	100s	$113.35

TABLETS: 5 MG

BRAND/MANUFACTURER	NDC	SIZE	AWP
○ BRAND ➤ NORVASC: Pfizer Labs	00069-1530-66 00069-1530-72	100s 300s	$113.35 $333.24

TABLETS: 10 MG

BRAND/MANUFACTURER	NDC	SIZE	AWP
○ BRAND ➤ NORVASC: Pfizer Labs	00069-1540-66	100s	$196.14

Ammonium Chloride

DESCRIPTION
Ammonium Chloride Injection, USP, 100 mEq, is a sterile, nonpyrogenic concentrated solution of Ammonium Chloride (NH_4Cl) in water for injection administered (after dilution) by the intravenous route. Each mL contains 267.5 mg of Ammonium Chloride 5 mEq of Ammonium and 5 mEq of Chloride) and edetate disodium (anhydrous) 2 mg added as a stabilizer. pH 4.4 (4.0 to 6.0). May contain hydrochloric acid for pH adjustment. 10 mOsmol/mL (calc.). It is intended to be used only after dilution in a larger volume of isotonic (0.9%) sodium chloride injection.

The solution contains no bacteriostat, antimicrobial agent or added buffer (except for pH adjustment) and is intended only for dilution as a single-dose additive. When smaller doses are required the unused portion should be discarded with the entire additive unit.

Ammonium Chloride Injection, USP is an electrolyte replenisher and systemic acidifier.

Ammonium Chloride, USP is chemically designated NH_4Cl, colorless crystals or white granular powder freely soluble in water.

CLINICAL PHARMACOLOGY
The Ammonium ion (NH_4^+) in the body plays an important role in the maintenance of acid-base balance. The kidney uses ammonium (NH_4^+) in place of sodium (Na^+) to combine with fixed anions in maintaining acid-base balance, especially as a homeostatic compensatory mechanism in metabolic acidosis.

➤ SHOWN IN PRODUCT IDENTIFICATION GUIDE

When a loss of hydrogen ions (H^+) occurs and serum chloride (Cl^-) decreases, sodium is made available for combination with bicarbonate (HCO_3^-). This creates an excess of sodium bicarbonate ($NaHCO_3$) which leads to a rise in blood pH and a state of metabolic alkalosis.

The therapeutic effects of ammonium chloride depend upon the ability of the kidney to utilize ammonia in the excretion of an excess of fixed anions and the conversion of ammonia to urea by the liver, thereby liberating hydrogen (H^+) and Chloride (Cl^-) ions into the extracellular fluid.

INDICATIONS AND USAGE

Ammonium Chloride Injection, USP, after dilution in isotonic sodium chloride injection, may be indicated in the treatment of patients with (1) hypochloremic states and (2) metabolic alkalosis.

UNLABELED USES

Ammonium Chloride is used alone or as an adjunct in the treatment of Ménière's disease, phencyclidine intoxication, and premenstrual syndrome.

CONTRAINDICATIONS

Ammonium Chloride is contraindicated in patients with severe impairment of renal or hepatic function.

Ammonium Chloride should not be administered when metabolic alkalosis due to vomiting of hydrochloric acid is accompanied by loss of sodium (excretion of sodium bicarbonate in the urine).

PRECAUTIONS

Patients receiving Ammonium Chloride should be constantly observed for symptoms of ammonia toxicity (pallor, sweating, retching, irregular breathing, bradycardia, cardiac arrhythmias, local and general twitching, tonic convulsions and coma).

It should be used with caution in patients with high total CO_2 and buffer base secondary to primary respiratory acidosis.

Intravenous administration should be slow to avoid local irritation and toxic effects.

When exposed to low temperatures, concentrated solutions of Ammonium Chloride may crystallize. If crystals are observed, the vial should be warmed to room temperature in a water bath prior to use.

Do not administer unless the solution is clear and seal is intact. Discard unused portion.

Pregnancy Category C: Animal reproduction studies have not been conducted with Ammonium Chloride. It is also not known whether Ammonium Chloride can cause fetal harm when administered to a pregnant woman or can affect reproduction capacity. Ammonium Chloride should be given to a pregnant woman only if clearly needed.

ADVERSE REACTIONS

Rapid intravenous administration of Ammonium Chloride may be accompanied by pain or irritation at the site of injection or along the venous route.

Reactions which may occur because of the solution or the technique of administration include febrile response, infection at the site of injection, venous thrombosis or phlebitis extending from the site of injection, extravasation and hypervolemia (from large volume diluent).

If an adverse reaction does occur, discontinue the infusion, evaluate the patient, institute appropriate therapeutic countermeasures and save the remainder of the fluid for examination if deemed necessary.

OVERDOSAGE

Overdosage of Ammonium Chloride has resulted in a serious degree of metabolic acidosis, disorientation, confusion and coma. Should metabolic acidosis occur following overdosage, the administration of an alkalinizing solution such as sodium bicarbonate or sodium lactate will serve to correct the acidosis.

DOSAGE AND ADMINISTRATION

Ammonium Chloride Injection, USP is administered intravenously and must be diluted before use. Solutions for intravenous infusion should not exceed a concentration of 1% to 2% of ammonium chloride.

Dosage is dependent upon the condition and tolerance of the patient. It is recommended that the contents of one to two vials (100 to 200 mEq) be added to 500 or 1000 mL of isotonic (0.9%) sodium chloride injection. The rate of intravenous infusion should not exceed 5 mL per minute in adults (approximately 3 hours for infusion of 1000 mL).

Dosage should be monitored by repeated serum bicarbonate determinations.

Parenteral drug products should be inspected visually for particulate matter and discoloration prior to administration, whenever solution and container permit. See "Precautions".

Store at controlled room temperature, 15° to 30°C (59° to 86°F).

HOW SUPPLIED
INJECTION: 5 MEQ/ML

BRAND/MANUFACTURER	NDC	SIZE	AWP
◆ GENERICS			
Abbott Hosp	00074-6043-01	20 ml 25s	$116.97

Ammonium Lactate

DESCRIPTION

Ammonium Lactate specially formulates 12% lactic acid neutralized with ammonium hydroxide as Ammonium Lactate to provide a lotion pH of 4.5-5.5. Lactic acid is a racemic mixture of 2-hydroxypropanoic acid.

CLINICAL PHARMACOLOGY

It is generally accepted that the water content of the stratum corneum is a controlling factor in maintaining skin flexibility. When the stratum corneum contains more than 10% water, it remains soft and pliable; however, when the water content drops below 10%, the stratum corneum becomes less flexible and rough, and may exhibit scaling and cracking and the underlying skin may become irritated.

Symptomatic relief of dry skin is provided by skin protectants containing hygroscopic substances (humectants) which increase skin moisture. Lactic acid, an α-hydroxy acid, is reported to be one of the most effective naturally occurring humectants in the skin. The α-hydroxy acids (and their salts), in addition to having beneficial effects on dry skin, have also been shown to reduce excessive epidermal keratinization in patients with hyperkeratotic conditions (e.g., ichthyosis).

Pharmacokinetics: The mechanism of action of topically applied neutralized lactic acid is not yet known.

INDICATIONS AND USAGE

Ammonium Lactate is indicated for the treatment of dry, scaly skin (xerosis) and ichthyosis vulgaris and for temporary relief of itching associated with these conditions.

CONTRAINDICATIONS

Known hypersensitivity to any of the label ingredients.

PRECAUTIONS

General: For external use only. Avoid contact with eyes, lips or mucous membranes. Caution is advised when used on the face of fair-skinned individuals since irritation may occur. A mild, transient stinging may occur on application to abraded or inflamed areas or in individuals with sensitive skin.

Carcinogenesis, Mutagenesis, Impairment of Fertility: Ammonium Lactate was nonmutagenic in the Ames/Salmonella/ Microsome Plate Assay. Reproductive studies in rats given lactic acid orally showed no effect on the sex ratio of the offspring.

Pregnancy (Category C): Animal reproduction studies have not been conducted with Ammonium Lactate. It is also not known whether Ammonium Lactate can cause fetal harm when administered to a pregnant woman or can affect reproduction capacity. Ammonium Lactate should be given to a pregnant woman only if clearly needed.

Nursing Mothers: Although lactic acid is a normal constituent of blood and tissues, it is not known to what extent this drug affects normal lactic acid levels in human milk. Because many drugs are excreted in human milk, caution should be exercised when Ammonium Lactate is administered to a nursing woman.

Pediatric Use: Safety and effectiveness of Ammonium Lactate have been demonstrated in infants and children. No unusual toxic effects were reported.

ADVERSE REACTIONS

The most frequent adverse experiences in patients with xerosis are transient stinging (1 in 30 patients), burning (1 in 30 patients), erythema (1 in 50 patients) and peeling (1 in 60 patients). Other adverse reactions which occur less frequently are irritation, eczema, petechiae, dryness and hyperpigmentation.

Due to the more severe initial skin conditions associated with ichthyosis, there was a higher incidence of transient stinging, burning and erythema (each occurring in 1 in 10 patients).

OVERDOSAGE

The oral administration of Ammonium Lactate to rats and mice showed this drug to be practically nontoxic ($LD_{50} > 15$ ml/kg).

DOSAGE AND ADMINISTRATION

Shake well. Apply to the affected areas and rub in thoroughly. Use twice daily or as directed by a physician.

Store at controlled room temperature, (15°-30°C; 59°-86°F).

HOW SUPPLIED
LOTION: 12%

BRAND/MANUFACTURER	NDC	SIZE	AWP
○ BRAND			
LAC-HYDRIN: Westwood-Squibb	00072-5712-08	225 gm	$22.19
	00072-5712-14	400 gm	$34.95

◆ RATED THERAPEUTICALLY EQUIVALENT; ◇ THERAPEUTIC EQUIVALENCE UNCONFIRMED; ○ UNRATED

Ammonium Molybdate

DESCRIPTION

Ammonium Molybdate is a sterile, nonpyrogenic solution for use as molybdenum additive to solutions for total parenteral nutrition (TPN).

Each mL contains:

Ammonium Molybdate tetrahydrate [$(NH_4)_6MO_7O_{24} \cdot 4H_2O$]
(equivalent to Molybdenum 25 mcg) ....46 mcg
Water for Injection ....q.s.

Hydrochloric acid and/or ammonium hydroxide for pH adjustment.

CLINICAL PHARMACOLOGY

Molybdenum is a constituent of the enzymes xanthine oxidase, sulfite oxidase, and aldehyde oxidase. Among other reactions, xanthine oxidase catalyzes conversion of xanthine and hypoxanthine to uric acid; sulfite oxidase converts sulfite to sulfate, and aldehyde oxidase detoxifies a variety of harmful organic molecules (such as aldehydes into acids).

In humans, molybdenum deficiency resulting from prolonged TPN support has been reported in literature. The deficiency syndrome included tachycardia, tachypnea, headache, night blindness, nausea, vomiting, central scotomas, culminating in generalized edema, lethargy, disorientation, and coma. The biochemical changes associated with the syndrome were: hypermethioninemia, hypouricemia, hypouricuria, low urinary excretion of inorganic sulfate and elevated urinary excretion of thiosulfate. Supplementation of TPN solutions with Molybdenum has been reported to alleviate the symptoms and normalize the biochemical abnormalities.

In animals, diet induced molybdenum deficiency has been produced experimentally with tungstate. The deficiency symptoms are characterized by decreased weight gain, food consumption, and life expectancy and deranged microbiological processes in the rumen. Renal xanthine calculi have been reported in sheep grazing on low-Molybdenum pasture.

Tissue storage of molybdenum varies with the intake levels and are affected by the amount of copper and sulfate in the diet. Consistent levels are observed in liver, kidney, and adrenal cortex.

Molybdenum is primarily excreted via kidneys. Some excretion through bile also occurs.

INDICATIONS AND USAGE

Ammonium Molybdate is indicated for use as a supplement to TPN solutions. Administration of Ammonium Molybdate in TPN solutions helps prevent depletion of endogenous stores and subsequent deficiency symptoms.

CONTRAINDICATIONS

■ Ammonium Molybdate should not be given undiluted by direct injection into a peripheral vein because of the potential of infusion phlebitis.

■ Ammonium Molybdate without copper supplementation should not be given to copper-deficient patients.

WARNINGS

■ Molybdenum has been reported to promote the mobilization of tissue copper, and increase urinary excretion of copper both in humans and animals. Excessive amounts of Molybdenum can therefore produce copper deficiency. The metabolism of copper in patients receiving Molybdenum supplements in TPN solution should be frequently checked.

■ Purine and sulfur metabolic profiles should be frequently carried out in patients receiving Molybdenum supplements in TPN solutions.

■ Ammonium Molybdate is a hypotonic solution and should be administered in admixtures only.

PRECAUTIONS

As molybdenum is excreted in urine and bile, molybdenum supplements may need to be adjusted, reduced or omitted in renal dysfunction and bile duct obstruction.

Molybdenum metabolism has been reported to be inversely related to copper, sulfate ions, tungsten, methionine, and cysteine.

PREGNANCY CATEGORY C
Animal reproduction studies have not been conducted with Ammonium Molybdate. It is also not known whether Ammonium Molybdate can cause fetal harm when administered to a pregnant woman or can affect reproduction capacity. Ammonium Molybdate should be given to a pregnant woman only if clearly needed.

Molybdenum has been reported to cross placenta. Molybdenum has also been detected in cow and sheep milk.

ADVERSE REACTIONS

Toxic symptoms are unlikely to occur at the recommended dosage level.

OVERDOSAGE

In humans, consumption of food grown in molybdeniferous soils, estimated to provide 10 to 15 mg Molybdenum/day, has been associated with goutlike syndrome with increased blood levels of Molybdenum uric acid, and xanthine oxidase.

In animals, cattle grazing on molybdeniferous pastures have been reported to develop molybdenosis known as "teart" or "peat scours." The condition is characterized by diarrhea, bone deformities, growth failure, alopecia, and anemia. Similar conditions except diarrhea, have been experimentally induced in rats, chickens, and sheep maintained on high dietary Molybdenum intakes.

No information on the treatment of molybdenosis in humans is available. Among animals, treatment with copper, sulfate ions, and tungsten has been reported to enhance excretion of Molybdenum thus imparting protection against molybdenosis. The sulfur-containing amino acids, methionine and cysteine, have also been reported to afford limited protection against molybdenosis in sheep.

DOSAGE AND ADMINISTRATION

Ammonium Molybdate provides 25 mcg molybdenum/mL. For metabolically stable adults receiving TPN, the suggested additive dosage level is 20 to 120 mcg molybdenum/day. For pediatric patients, the additive dosage level should be calculated by extrapolation.

In an adult, molybdenum deficiency state resulting from prolonged TPN support, intravenous administration of molybdenum as ammonium molybdate at 163 mcg/day for 21 days has been reported to reverse deficiency symptoms without toxicity.

Aseptic addition of Ammonium Molybdate to TPN solutions under a laminar flow hood is recommended. Molybdenum is physically compatible with the electrolytes and other trace elements usually present in amino acid/dextrose solutions used for TPN. Monitoring of sulfur and purine metabolism is suggested as a guideline. Since copper and molybdenum are antagonistic to each other, frequent monitoring of blood copper levels should be carried out during TPN supplementation with Ammonium Molybdate.

Parenteral drug products should be inspected visually for particulate matter and discoloration prior to administration, whenever solution and container permit.

Store injection at controlled room temperature, 15°-30°C (59°-86°F). Do not permit to freeze.

HOW SUPPLIED
INJECTION: 25 MCG/ML

BRAND/MANUFACTURER	NDC	SIZE	AWP
◆ BRAND			
MOLYPEN: Fujisawa	00469-4900-30	10 ml	$8.65

Amobarbital Sodium

Caution: These products are to be used under the direction of a physician.

The intravenous administration of Amobarbital Sodium carries with it the potential dangers inherent in the intravenous use of any potent hypnotic.

DESCRIPTION

The barbiturates are nonselective central nervous system (CNS) depressants that are primarily used as sedative hypnotics. In subhypnotic doses, they are also used as anticonvulsants. The barbiturates and their sodium salts are subject to control under the Federal Controlled Substances Act.

Amobarbital Sodium is a white, friable, granular powder that is odorless, has a bitter taste, and is hygroscopic. It is very soluble in water, soluble in alcohol, and practically insoluble in ether and chloroform. Amobarbital Sodium is sodium 5-ethyl-5-isopentylbarbiturate and has the empirical formula $C_{11}H_{17}N_2NaO_3$. Its molecular weight is 248.26.

Amobarbital Sodium is a substituted pyrimidine derivative in which the basic structure is barbituric acid, a substance that has no CNS activity.

Vials Amobarbital Sodium are for parenteral administration. The vials contain 250 mg (1 mmol) or 500 mg (2 mmol) sterile Amobarbital Sodium.

Following is its chemical structure:

$$CH_3CH_2$$
$$(CH_3)_2CHCH_2CH_2$$

CLINICAL PHARMACOLOGY

Barbiturates are capable of producing all levels of CNS mood alteration, from excitation to mild sedation, hypnosis, and deep coma. Overdosage can produce death. In high enough therapeutic doses, barbiturates induce anesthesia.

Barbiturates depress the sensory cortex, decrease motor activity, alter cerebellar function, and produce drowsiness, sedation, and hypnosis.

Barbiturate-induced sleep differs from physiologic sleep. Sleep laboratory studies have demonstrated that barbiturates reduce the amount of time spent in the rapid eye movement (REM) phase of sleep or the dreaming stage. Also, Stages III and IV sleep are decreased. Following abrupt cessation of barbiturates used regularly, patients may experience markedly increased dreaming, nightmares and/or insomnia. Therefore, withdrawal of a single therapeutic dose over 5 or 6 days has been recommended to lessen the REM rebound and disturbed sleep that contribute to the drug withdrawal syndrome (for example, the dose should be decreased from 3 to 2 doses/day for 1 week).

In studies, secobarbital sodium and pentobarbital sodium have been found to lose most of their effectiveness for both inducing and maintaining sleep by the end of 2 weeks of continued drug administration, even with the use of multiple doses. As with secobarbital sodium and pentobarbital sodium, other barbiturates (including Amobarbital) might be expected to lose their effectiveness for inducing and maintaining sleep after about 2 weeks. The short- intermediate-, and to a lesser degree, long-acting barbiturates have been widely prescribed for treating insomnia. Although the clinical literature abounds with claims that the short-acting barbiturates are superior for producing sleep whereas the intermediate-acting compounds are more effective in maintaining sleep, controlled studies have failed to demonstrate these differential effects. Therefore, as sleep medications, the barbiturates are of limited value beyond short-term use.

Barbiturates have little analgesic action at subanesthetic doses. Rather, in subanesthetic doses, these drugs may increase the reaction to painful stimuli. All barbiturates exhibit anticonvulsant activity in anesthetic doses. However, of the drugs in this class, only phenobarbital, mephobarbital, and metharbital are effective as oral anticonvulsants in subhypnotic doses.

Barbiturates are respiratory depressants, and the degree of respiratory depression is dependent upon the dose. With hypnotic doses, respiratory depression produced by barbiturates is similar to that which occurs during physiologic sleep and is accompanied by a slight decrease in blood pressure and heart rate.

Studies in laboratory animals have shown that barbiturates cause reduction in the tone and contractility of the uterus, ureters, and urinary bladder. However, concentrations of the drugs required to produce this effect in humans are not reached with sedative-hypnotic doses.

Barbiturates do not impair normal hepatic function but have been shown to induce liver microsomal enzymes, thus increasing and/or altering the metabolism of barbiturates and other drugs (see *"Drug Interactions"* under *"Precautions"*).

Pharmacokinetics: Barbiturates are absorbed in varying degrees following oral or parenteral administration. The salts are more rapidly absorbed than are the acids. The rate of absorption is increased if the sodium salt is ingested as a dilute solution or taken on an empty stomach.

The onset of action for oral administration of barbiturates varies from 20 to 60 minutes. For intramuscular (IM) administration, the onset of action is slightly faster. Following intravenous (IV) administration, the onset of action ranges from almost immediately for pentobarbital sodium to 5 minutes for phenobarbital sodium. Maximal CNS depression may not occur until 15 minutes or more after IV administration for phenobarbital sodium. Duration of action, which is related to the rate at which the barbiturates are redistributed throughout the body, varies among persons and in the same person from time to time. Amobarbital Sodium, an intermediate-acting barbiturate, is a CNS depressant. For the oral form, the onset of sedative and hypnotic action is 3/4 to 1 hour, with a duration of action ranging from 6 to 8 hours. These values should serve as a guide but not be used to predict exact duration of effect. No studies have demonstrated that the different routes of administration are equivalent with respect to bioavailability.

Barbiturates are weak acids that are absorbed and rapidly distributed to all tissues and fluids, with high concentrations in the brain, liver, and kidneys. Lipid solubility of the barbiturates is the dominant factor in their distribution within the body. The more lipid soluble the barbiturate, the more rapidly it penetrates all tissues of the body. Barbiturates are bound to plasma and tissue proteins to a varying degree, with the degree of binding increasing directly as a function of lipid solubility.

Phenobarbital has the lowest lipid solubility, lowest plasma binding, lowest brain protein binding, the longest delay in onset of activity, and the longest duration of action. At the opposite extreme is secobarbital, which has the highest lipid solubility, highest plasma protein binding, highest brain protein binding, the shortest delay in onset of activity, and the shortest duration of action. Amobarbital Sodium is classified as an intermediate barbiturate. The plasma half-life for Amobarbital Sodium in adults ranges between 16 and 40 hours, with a mean of 25 hours.

Barbiturates are metabolized primarily by the hepatic microsomal enzyme system, and the metabolic products are excreted in the urine and, less commonly, in the feces. Only a negligible amount of Amobarbital Sodium is eliminated unchanged in the urine.

INDICATIONS AND USAGE
A. Sedative
B. Hypnotic, for the short-term treatment of insomnia, since it appears to lose its effectiveness for sleep induction and sleep maintenance after 2 weeks (see *"Clinical Pharmacology"*).
C. Preanesthetic

UNLABELED USES
Amobarbital Sodium is used alone or as an adjunct in the treatment of catatonic and negativistic reactions, conversion reactions, and tinnitus. It is also used in surgical epilepsy programs for diagnostic and prognostic purposes.

CONTRAINDICATIONS
Amobarbital Sodium is contraindicated in patients who are hypersensitive to barbiturates, in patients with a history of manifest or latent prophyria, and in patients with marked impairment of liver function or respiratory disease in which dyspnea or obstruction is evident.

WARNINGS
1. Habit Forming: Amobarbital Sodium may be habit forming. Tolerance, psychological and physical dependence may occur with continued use (see *"Drug Abuse and Dependence"* and *"Pharmacokinetics"* under *"Clinical Pharmacology"*). Patients who have psychological dependence on barbiturates may increase the dosage or decrease the dosage interval without consulting a physician and may subsequently develop a physical dependence on barbiturates. In order to minimize the possibility of overdosage or the development of dependence, the prescribing and dispensing of sedative-hypnotic barbiturates should be limited to the amount required for the interval until the next appointment. Abrupt cessation after prolonged use in a person who is dependent on the drug may result in withdrawal symptoms, including delirium, convulsions, and possibly death. Barbiturates should be withdrawn gradually from any patient known to be taking excessive doses over long periods of time (see *"Drug Abuse and Dependence"*).

2. Intravenous Administration: Too rapid administration may cause respiratory depression, apnea, laryngospasm, or vasodilation with fall in blood pressure.

3. Acute or Chronic Pain: Caution should be exercised when barbiturates are administered to patients with acute or chronic pain, because paradoxical excitement could be induced or important symptoms could be masked. However, the use of barbiturates as sedatives in the postoperative surgical period and as adjuncts to cancer chemotherapy is well established.

4. Usage in Pregnancy: Barbiturates can cause fetal damage when administered to a pregnant woman. Retrospective, case-controlled studies have suggested a connection between the maternal consumption of barbiturates and a higher than expected incidence of fetal abnormalities. Barbiturates readily cross the placental barrier and are distributed throughout fetal tissues; the highest concentrations are found in the placenta, fetal liver, and brain. Fetal blood levels approach maternal blood levels following parenteral administration.

Withdrawal symptoms occur in infants born to women who receive barbiturates throughout the last trimester of pregnancy (see *"Drug Abuse and Dependence"*).

If Amobarbital Sodium is used during pregnancy or if the patient becomes pregnant while taking this drug, the patient should be apprised of the potential hazard to the fetus.

5. Synergistic Effects: The concomitant use of alcohol or other CNS depressants may produce additive CNS-depressant effects.

PRECAUTIONS
General: Barbiturates may be habit forming. Tolerance and psychological and physical dependence may occur with continuing use (see *"Drug Abuse and Dependence"*).

Barbiturates should be administered with caution, if at all, to patients who are mentally depressed, have suicidal tendencies, or have a history of drug abuse. Particular caution is also indicated before administering barbiturates to patients who have abused other classes of drugs (see *"Warnings"*).

Elderly or debilitated patients may react to barbiturates with marked excitement, depression, or confusion. In some persons, especially children, barbiturates repeatedly produce excitement rather than depression.

In patients with hepatic damage, barbiturates should be administered with caution and initially in reduced doses. Barbiturates should not be administered to patients showing the premonitory signs of hepatic coma.

Parenteral solutions of barbiturates are highly alkaline. Therefore, extreme care should be taken to avoid perivascular extravasation or intra-arterial injection. Extravascular injection may cause local tissue damage with subsequent necrosis; consequences of intra-arterial injection may vary from transient pain to gangrene of the limb. Any complaint of pain in the limb warrants stopping the injection.

The systemic effects of exogenous and endogenous corticosteroids may be diminished by amobarbital sodium. Thus, this product should be administered with caution to patients with borderline hypoadrenal function, regardless of whether it is of pituitary or of primary adrenal origin.

Information for Patients: The following information should be given to patients receiving barbiturates.

1. The use of barbiturates carries with it an associated risk of psychological and/or physical dependence.
2. Barbiturates may impair the mental and/or physical abilities required for the performance of potentially hazardous tasks, such as driving a car or operating machinery. The patient should be cautioned accordingly.
3. Alcohol should not be consumed while taking barbiturates. The concurrent use of the barbiturates with other CNS depressants (eg, alcohol, narcotics, tranquilizers, and antihistamines) may result in additional CNS-depressant effects.

Laboratory Tests: Prolonged therapy with barbiturates should be accompanied by periodic evaluation of organ systems, including hematopoietic, renal, and hepatic systems (see *"General"* under *"Precautions"* and *"Adverse Reactions"*).

Drug Interactions: Most reports of clinically significant drug interactions occurring with the barbiturates have involved phenobarbital. However, the application of these data to other barbiturates appears valid and warrants serial blood level determinations of the relevant drugs when there are multiple therapies.

1. Anticoagulants: Phenobarbital lowers the plasma levels of dicumarol and causes a decrease in anticoagulant activity as measured by the prothrombin time. Barbiturates can induce hepatic microsomal enzymes, resulting in increased metabolism and decreased anticoagulant response of oral anticoagulants (eg, warfarin, acenocoumarol, dicumarol, and phenprocoumon). Patients stabilized on anticoagulant therapy may require dosage adjustments if barbiturates are added to or withdrawn from their dosage regimen.

2. Corticosteroids: Barbiturates appear to enhance the metabolism of exogenous corticosteroids, probably through the induction of hepatic microsomal enzymes. Patients stabilized on corticosteroid therapy may require dosage adjustments if barbiturates are added to or withdrawn from their dosage regimen.

3. Griseofulvin: Phenobarbital appears to interfere with the absorption of orally administered griseofulvin, thus decreasing its blood level. The effect of the resultant decreased blood levels of griseofulvin on therapeutic response has not been established. However, it would be preferable to avoid concomitant administration of these drugs.

4. Doxycycline: Phenobarbital has been shown to shorten the half-life of doxycycline for as long as 2 weeks after barbiturate therapy is discontinued.

This mechanism is probably through the induction of hepatic microsomal enzymes that metabolize the antibiotic. If Amobarbital Sodium and doxycycline are administered concurrently, the clinical response to doxycycline should be monitored closely.

5. Phenytoin, Sodium Valproate, Valproic Acid: The effect of barbiturates on the metabolism of phenytoin appears to be variable. Some investigators report an accelerating effect, whereas others report no effect. Because the effect of barbiturates on the metabolism of phenytoin is not predictable, phenytoin and barbiturate blood levels should be monitored more frequently if these drugs are given concurrently. Sodium valproate and valproic acid appear to increase the Amobarbital Sodium serum levels; therefore, Amobarbital Sodium blood levels should be closely monitored and appropriate dosage adjustments made as clinically indicated.

6. CNS Depressants: The concomitant use of other CNS depressants, including other sedatives or hypnotics, antihistamines, tranquilizers, or alcohol, may produce additive depressant effects.

7. Monoamine Oxidase Inhibitors (MAOIs): MAOIs prolong the effects of barbiturates, probably because metabolism of the barbiturate is inhibited.

8. Estradiol, Estrone, Progesterone, and Other Steroidal Hormones: Pretreatment with or concurrent administration of phenobarbital may decrease the effect of estradiol by increasing its metabolism. There have been reports of patients treated with antiepileptic drugs (eg, phenobarbital) who become pregnant while taking oral contraceptives. An alternate contraceptive method might be suggested to women taking barbiturates.

Carcinogenesis:
1. Animal Data: Phenobarbital sodium is carcinogenic in mice and rats after lifetime administration. In mice, it produced benign and malignant liver cell tumors. In rats, benign liver cell tumors were observed very late in life.

2. Human Data: In a 29-year epidemiologic study of 9,136 patients who were treated on an anticonvulsant protocol that included phenobarbital, results indicated a higher than normal incidence of hepatic carcinoma. Previously, some of these patients had been treated with thorotrast, a drug that is known to produce hepatic carcinomas. Thus, this study did not provide sufficient evidence that phenobarbital sodium is carcinogenic in humans.

A retrospective study of 84 children with brain tumors matched to 73 normal controls and 78 cancer controls (malignant disease other than brain tumors) suggested an association between exposure to barbiturates prenatally and an increased incidence of brain tumors.

Usage in Pregnancy:
1. *Teratogenic Effects. Pregnancy Category D:* See *"Usage in Pregnancy"* under *"Warnings"*.

2. *Nonteratogenic Effects:* Reports of infants suffering from long-term barbiturate exposure in utero included the acute withdrawal syndrome of seizures and hyperirritability from birth to a delayed onset of up to 14 days (see *"Drug Abuse and Dependence"*).

Labor and Delivery: Hypnotic doses of barbiturates do not appear to impair uterine activity significantly during labor. Full anesthetic doses of barbiturates decrease the force and frequency of uterine contractions. Administration of sedative-hypnotic barbiturates to the mother during labor may result in respiratory depression in the newborn. Premature infants are particularly susceptible to the depressant effects of barbiturates. If barbiturates are used during labor and delivery, resuscitation equipment should be available.

Data are not available to evaluate the effect of barbiturates when forceps delivery or other intervention is necessary or to determine the effect of barbiturates on the later growth, development, and functional maturation of the child.

Nursing Mothers: Caution should be exercised when Amobarbital Sodium is administered to a nursing woman because small amounts of barbiturates are excreted in the milk.

Usage in Children: Safety and effectiveness have not been established in children below the age of 6 years.

ADVERSE REACTIONS
The following adverse reactions and their incidence were compiled from surveillance of thousands of hospitalized patients who received barbiturates. Because such patients may be less aware of certain of the milder adverse effects of barbiturates, the incidence of these reactions may be somewhat higher in fully ambulatory patients.

MORE THAN 1 IN 100 PATIENTS
The most common adverse reaction, estimated to occur at a rate of 1 to 3 patients per 100, is the following:

Nervous System: Somnolence

LESS THAN 1 IN 100 PATIENTS
Adverse reactions estimated to occur at a rate of less than 1 in 100 patients are listed below, grouped by organ system and by decreasing order of occurrence:

Nervous System: Agitation, confusion, hyperkinesia, ataxia, CNS depression, nightmares, nervousness, psychiatric disturbance, hallucinations, insomnia, anxiety, dizziness, abnormality in thinking.

Respiratory System: Hypoventilation, apnea, postoperative atelectasis.

Cardiovascular System: Bradycardia, hypotension, syncope.

Digestive System: Nausea, vomiting, constipation.

Other Reported Reactions: Headache, injection site reactions, hypersensitivity reactions (angioedema, skin rashes, exfoliative dermatitis), fever, liver damage, megaloblastic anemia following chronic phenobarbital use.

DRUG ABUSE AND DEPENDENCE
Controlled Substance: Amorbarbital Sodium is a Schedule II drug.

Dependence: Barbiturates may be habit-forming. Tolerance, psychological dependence, and physical dependence may occur, especially following prolonged use of high doses of barbiturates. Daily administration in excess of 400 mg of pentobarbital or secobarbital for approximately 90 days is likely to produce some degree of physical dependence. A dosage of 600 to 800 mg for at least 35 days is sufficient to produce withdrawal seizures. The average daily dose for the barbiturate addict is usually about 1.5 g. As tolerance to barbiturates develops, the amount needed to maintain the same level of intoxication increases; tolerance to a fatal dosage, however, does not increase more than twofold. As this occurs, the margin between intoxicating dosage and fatal dosage becomes smaller.

Symptoms of acute intoxication with barbiturates include unsteady gait, slurred speech, and sustained nystagmus. Mental signs of chronic intoxication include confusion, poor judgment, irritability, insomnia, and somatic complaints.

Symptoms of barbiturate dependence are similar to those of chronic alcoholism. If an individual appears to be intoxicated with alcohol to a degree that is radically disproportionate to the amount of alcohol in his or her blood, the use of barbiturates should be suspected. The lethal dose of a barbiturate is far less if alcohol is also ingested.

The symptoms of barbiturate withdrawal can be severe and may cause death. Minor withdrawal symptoms may appear 8 to 12 hours after the last dose of a barbiturate. These symptoms usually appear in the following order: anxiety, muscle twitching, tremor of hands and fingers, progressive weakness, dizziness, distortion in visual perception, nausea, vomiting, insomnia, and orthostatic hypotension. Major withdrawal symptoms (convulsions and delirium) may occur within 16 hours and last up to 5 days after abrupt cessation of barbiturates. The intensity of withdrawal symptoms gradually declines over a period of approximately 15 days. Individuals susceptible to barbiturate abuse and dependence include alcoholics and opiate abusers, as well as other sedative-hypnotic and amphetamine abusers.

Drug dependence on barbiturates arises from repeated administration on a continuous basis, generally in amounts exceeding therapeutic dose levels. The characteristics of drug dependence on barbiturates include: (a) a strong desire or need to continue taking the drug; (b) a tendency to increase the dose; (c) a psychic dependence on the effects of the drug related to subjective and individual appreciation of those effects; and (d) a physical dependence on the effects of the drug, requiring its presence for maintenance of homeostasis and resulting in a definite, characteristic, and self-limited abstinence syndrome when the drug is withdrawn.

Treatment of barbiturate dependence consists of cautious and gradual withdrawal of the drug. Barbiturate-dependent patients can be withdrawn by using a number of different withdrawal regimens. In all cases, withdrawal requires an extended period of time. One method involves substituting a 30-mg dose of phenobarbital for each 100- to 200-mg dose of barbiturate that the patient has been taking. The total daily amount of phenobarbital is then administered in 3 or 4 divided doses, not to exceed 600 mg daily. If signs of withdrawal occur on the first day of treatment, a loading dose of 100 to 200 mg of phenobarbital may be administered IM in addition to the oral dose. After stabilization on phenobarbital the total daily dose is decreased by 30 mg/day as long as withdrawal is proceeding smoothly. A modification of this regimen involves initiating treatment at the patient's regular dosage level and decreasing the daily dosage by 10% if tolerated by the patient.

Infants that are physically dependent on barbiturates may be given phenobarbital, 3 to 10 mg/kg/day. After withdrawal symptoms (hyperactivity, disturbed sleep, tremors, and hyperreflexia) are relieved, the dosage of phenobarbital should be gradually decreased and completely withdrawn over a 2-week period.

OVERDOSAGE
The toxic dose of barbiturates varies considerably. In general, an oral dose of 1 g of most barbiturates produces serious poisoning in an adult. Toxic effects and fatalities have occurred following overdoses of Amobarbital Sodium alone and in combination with other CNS depressants. Death commonly occurs after 2 to 10 g of ingested barbiturate. The sedated, therapeutic blood levels of Amobarbital range between 2 to 10 μg/mL; the usual lethal blood level ranges from 40 to 80 μg/mL. Barbiturate intoxication may be confused with alcoholism, bromide

QUANTITY OF STERILE WATER FOR INJECTION REQUIRED TO DILUTE THE CONTENTS OF A GIVEN VIAL OF AMOBARBITAL SODIUM TO OBTAIN THE PERCENTAGES LISTED. SOLUTIONS DERIVED WILL BE IN WEIGHT/VOLUME.

Amobarbital Sodium

Vial Number	Content in Weight	1%	2.5%	5%	10%	20%
386	250 mg	25 mL	10 mL	5 mL	2.5 mL	1.25mL
387	0.5 g	50 mL	20 mL	10 mL	5 mL	2.5 mL

intoxication, and various neurologic disorders. Potential tolerance must be considered when evaluating significance of dose and plasma concentration.

Signs and Symptoms: Symptoms of oral overdose may occur within 15 minutes beginning with CNS depression, absent or sluggish reflexes, underventilation, hypotension, and hypothermia and may progress to pulmonary edema and death. Hemorrhagic blisters may develop, especially at pressure points.

In extreme overdose, all electrical activity in the brain may cease, in which case a "flat" EEG normally equated with clinical death cannot be accepted. This effect is fully reversible unless hypoxic damage occurs. Consideration should be given to the possibility of barbiturate intoxication even in situations that appear to involve trauma.

Complications such as pneumonia, pulmonary edema, cardiac arrhythmias, congestive heart failure, and renal failure may occur. Uremia may increase CNS sensitivity to barbiturates if renal function is impaired. Differential diagnosis should include hypoglycemia, head trauma, cerebrovascular accidents, convulsive states, and diabetic coma.

Treatment: To obtain up-to-date information about the treatment of overdose, a good resource is your certified Regional Poison Control Center. Telephone numbers of certified poison control centers are listed in the *Physicians' Desk Reference (PDR).* In managing overdosage, consider the possibility of multiple drug overdoses, interaction among drugs, and unusual drug kinetics in your patient.

Protect the patient's airway and support ventilation and perfusion. Meticulously monitor and maintain, within acceptable limits, the patient's vital signs, blood gases, serum electrolytes, etc. Absorption of drugs from the gastrointestinal tract may be decreased by giving activated charcoal, which, in many cases, is more effective than emesis or lavage; consider charcoal instead of or in addition to gastric emptying. Repeated doses of charcoal over time may hasten elimination of some drugs that have been absorbed. Safeguard the patient's airway when employing gastric emptying or charcoal.

Diuresis and peritoneal dialysis are of little value; hemodialysis and hemoperfusion enhance drug clearance and should be considered in serious poisoning. If the patient has chronically abused sedatives, withdrawal reactions may be manifest following acute overdose.

PREPARATION OF SOLUTION
Solutions of Amobarbital Sodium should be made up aseptically with Sterile Water for Injection. The accompanying table will aid in preparing solutions of various concentrations. Ordinarily, a 10% solution is used. After Sterile Water for Injection is added, the vial should be rotated to facilitate solution of the powder. **Do not shake the vial.**

Several minutes may be required for the drug to dissolve completely, but under no circumstances should a solution be injected if it has not become absolutely clear within 5 minutes. Also, a solution that forms a precipitate after clearing should not be used. Amobarbital Sodium hydrolyzes in solution or on exposure to air. Not more than 30 minutes should elapse from the time the vial is opened until its contents are injected. Prior to administration, parenteral drug products should be inspected visually for particulate matter and discoloration whenever solution containers permit. (See related table).

DOSAGE AND ADMINISTRATION
The dose of Amobarbital Sodium must be individualized with full knowledge of its particular characteristics and recommended rate of administration. Factors of consideration are the patient's age, weight, and condition. The maximum single dose for an adult is 1 g.

Intramuscular Use: Intramuscular injection of the sodium salts of barbiturates should be made deeply into a large muscle. The average intramuscular dose ranges from 65 mg to 0.5 g. A volume of 5 mL (irrespective of concentration) should not be exceeded at any one site because of possible tissue irritation. Twenty percent solutions may be used so that a small volume can contain a large dose. After IM injection of a hypnotic dose, the patient's vital signs should be monitored. Superficial intramuscular or subcutaneous injections may be painful and may produce sterile abscesses or sloughs.

Intravenous Use: Intravenous injection is restricted to conditions in which other routes are not feasible, either because the patient is unconscious (as in cerebral hemorrhage, eclampsia, or status epilepticus), because the patient resists (as in delirium), or because prompt action is imperative. Slow IV injection is essential, and patients should be carefully observed during administration. This requires that blood pressure, respiration, and cardiac function be maintained, vital signs be recorded and equipment for resuscitation and artificial ventilation be available. The rate of IV injection for adults should not exceed 50 mg/min to prevent sleep or sudden respiratory depression. The final dosage is determined to a great extent by the patient's reaction to the slow administration of the drug.

Adults:
a. Sedative: 30 to 50 mg given 2 or 3 times daily.
b. Hypnotic: 65 to 200 mg at bedtime.

Special Patient Population: Dosage should be reduced in the elderly or debilitated because these patients may be more sensitive to barbiturates. Dosage should be reduced for patients with impaired renal function or hepatic disease. Ordinarily, an intravenous dose of 65 mg to 0.5 g may be given to a child 6 to 12 years of age.

J CODES
Up to 125 mg IM,IV—J0300

HOW SUPPLIED
POWDER FOR INJECTION (C-II): 0.5 GM

BRAND/MANUFACTURER	NDC	SIZE	AWP
○ **BRAND**			
AMYTAL SODIUM: Lilly	00002-7215-10	10s	$82.49
	00002-7215-25	25s	$189.01

Amobarbital Sodium and Secobarbital Sodium

DESCRIPTION
The barbiturates are nonselective central nervous system (CNS) depressants that are primarily used as sedative hypnotics. In subhypnotic doses, they are also used as anticonvulsants. The barbiturates and their sodium salts are subject to control under the Federal Controlled Substances Act.

Amobarbital Sodium/Secobarbital Sodium is a combination of equal parts of Secobarbital Sodium, USP, and Amobarbital Sodium, USP, barbituric acid derivatives that occur as white, odorless, bitter powders. They are very soluble in water, soluble in alcohol, and practically insoluble in ether and in chloroform.

Amobarbital Sodium and Secobarbital Sodium is a combination of 2 substituted pyrimidine derivatives in which the basic structure of each is barbituric acid, a substance which has no CNS activity.

Each Capsule contains 50 mg (0.19 mmol) Secobarbital Sodium and 50 mg (0.2 mmol) Amobarbital Sodium.

Each Capsule contains 100 mg (0.38 mmol) Secobarbital Sodium and 100 mg (0.4 mmol) Amobarbital Sodium.

Chemically, Secobarbital Sodium is sodium 5-allyl-5-(1-methylbutyl) barbiturate, with the empirical formula $C_{12}H_{17}N_2NaO_3$. Its molecular weight is 260.27.

Amobarbital Sodium is sodium 5-ethyl-5-isopentylbarbiturate, with the empirical formula $C_{11}H_{17}N_2NaO_3$. Its molecular weight is 248.26.

CLINICAL PHARMACOLOGY
Barbiturates are capable of producing all levels of CNS mood alteration, from excitation to mild sedation, to hypnosis, and deep coma. Overdosage can produce death. In high enough therapeutic doses, barbiturates induce anesthesia. Barbiturates depress the sensory cortex, decrease motor activity, alter cerebellar function and produce drowsiness, sedation, and hypnosis.

Barbiturate-induced sleep differs from physiologic sleep. Sleep laboratory studies have demonstrated that barbiturates reduce the amount of time spent in the rapid eye movement (REM) phase of sleep or the dreaming stage. Also, Stages III and IV sleep are decreased. Following abrupt cessation of barbiturates used regularly, patients may experience markedly increased dreaming nightmares, and/or insomnia. Therefore, withdrawal of a single therapeutic dose over 5 or 6 days has been recommended to lessen the REM rebound and disturbed sleep that contribute to the drug withdrawal syndrome (for example, the dose should be decreased from 3 to 2 doses/day for 1 week).

In studies, Secobarbital Sodium and pentobarbital sodium have been found to lose most of their effectiveness for both inducing and maintaining sleep by the end of 2 weeks of continued drug administration even with the use of multiple doses. As with Secobarbital Sodium and pentobarbital sodium, other barbiturates (including Amobarbital) might be expected to lose their effectiveness for inducing and maintaining sleep after about 2 weeks. The short-, intermediate-, and to a lesser degree, long-acting barbiturates have been widely prescribed for treating insomnia. Although the clinical literature abounds with claims that the short-acting barbiturates are superior for producing sleep whereas the intermediate-acting compounds are more effective in maintaining sleep, controlled studies have failed to demonstrate these differential effects. Therefore, as sleep medications, the barbiturates are of limited value beyond short-term use.

Barbiturates have little analgesic action at subanesthetic doses. Rather, in subanesthetic doses these drugs may increase the reaction to painful stimuli. All barbiturates exhibit anticonvulsant activity in anesthetic doses. However, of the

---

◆ RATED THERAPEUTICALLY EQUIVALENT; ◇ THERAPEUTIC EQUIVALENCE UNCONFIRMED; ○ UNRATED

drugs in this class, only phenobarbital, mephobarbital, and metharbital are effective as oral anticonvulsants in subhypnotic doses.

Barbiturates are respiratory depressants, and the degree of respiratory depression is dependent upon the dose. With hypnotic doses, respiratory depression produced by barbiturates is similar to that which occurs during physiologic sleep and is accompanied by a slight decrease in blood pressure and heart rate.

Studies in laboratory animals have shown that barbiturates cause reduction in the tone and contractility of the uterus, ureters, and urinary bladder. However, concentrations of the drugs required to produce this effect in humans are not reached with sedative-hypnotic doses.

Barbiturates do not impair normal hepatic function but have been shown to induce liver microsomal enzymes, thus increasing and/or altering the metabolism of barbiturates and other drugs. (See *"Drug Interactions"* under *"Precautions"*.)

Pharmacokinetics: Barbiturates are absorbed in varying degrees following oral or parenteral administration. The salts are more rapidly absorbed than are the acids. The rate of absorption is increased if the sodium salt is ingested as a dilute solution or taken on an empty stomach.

The onset of action for oral administration of barbiturates varies from 20 to 60 minutes. Duration of action, which is related to the rate at which the barbiturates are redistributed throughout the body, varies among persons and in the same person from time to time.

Secobarbital Sodium is classified as a short-acting barbiturate. When administered orally, its onset of action is 10 to 15 minutes and its duration of action ranges from 3 to 4 hours. Amobarbital Sodium is classified as an intermediate-acting barbiturate. When administered orally, the onset of sedative and hypnotic action is ¾ to 1 hour with a duration of action ranging from 6 to 8 hours.

No studies have demonstrated that the different routes of administration are equivalent with respect to bioavailability.

Barbiturates are weak acids that are absorbed and rapidly distributed to all tissues and fluids, with high concentrations in the brain, liver, and kidneys. Lipid solubility of the barbiturates is the dominant factor in their distribution within the body. The more lipid soluble the barbiturate, the more rapidly it penetrates all tissues of the body. Barbiturates are bound to plasma and tissue proteins to a varying degree with the degree of binding increasing directly as a function of lipid solubility.

Phenobarbital has the lowest lipid solubility, lowest plasma binding, lowest brain protein binding, the longest delay in onset of activity, and the longest duration of action. At the opposite extreme is Secobarbital, which has the highest lipid solubility, highest plasma protein binding, highest brain protein binding, the shortest delay in onset of activity, and the shortest duration of action. The plasma half-life for Secobarbital Sodium in adults ranges between 15 to 40 hours with a mean of 28 hours; and for Amobarbital Sodium, between 16 to 40 hours with a mean of 25 hours.

Barbiturates are metabolized primarily by the hepatic microsomal enzyme system, and the metabolic products are excreted in the urine and, less commonly, in the feces. The excretion of unmetabolized barbiturates is one feature that distinguishes the long-acting category from those belonging to other categories, which are almost entirely metabolized. The inactive metabolites of the barbiturates are excreted as conjugates of glucuronic acid.

INDICATIONS AND USAGE

A. Hypnotic, for the short-term treatment of insomnia, since it appears to lose its effectiveness for sleep induction and sleep maintenance after 2 weeks. (See *"Clinical Pharmacology"*.)

B. Preanesthetic

CONTRAINDICATIONS

Amobarbital Sodium/Secobarbital Sodium is contraindicated in patients who are hypersensitive to barbiturates. It is also contraindicated in patients with a history of manifest or latent porphyria, marked impairment of liver function, or respiratory disease in which dyspnea or obstruction is evident.

WARNINGS

1. Habit-Forming: Amobarbital Sodium/Secobarbital Sodium may be habit-forming. Tolerance, psychologic and physical dependence may occur with continued use (see *"Drug Abuse and Dependence"* and *"Pharmacokinetics"* under *"Clinical Pharmacology"*). Patients who have psychologic dependence on barbiturates may increase the dosage or decrease the dosage interval without consulting a physician and may subsequently develop a physical dependence on barbiturates. In order to minimize the possibility of overdosage or the development of dependence, the prescribing and dispensing of sedative-hypnotic barbiturates should be limited to the amount required for the interval until the next appointment. The abrupt cessation after prolonged use in a person who is dependent on the drug may result in withdrawal symptoms, including delirium, convulsions, and possibly death. Barbiturates should be withdrawn gradually from any patient known to be taking excessive doses over long periods of time (see *"Drug Abuse and Dependence"*).

2. Acute or Chronic Pain: Caution should be exercised when barbiturates are administered to patients with acute or chronic pain, because paradoxical excitement could be induced or important symptoms could be masked.

3. Usage in Pregnancy: Barbiturates can cause fetal damage when administered to a pregnant woman. Retrospective, case-controlled studies have suggested a connection between the material consumption of barbiturates and a higher than expected incidence of fetal abnormalities. Barbiturates readily cross the placental barrier and are distributed throughout fetal tissues; the highest concentrations are found in the placenta, fetal liver, and brain.

Withdrawal symptoms occur in infants born to women who receive barbiturates throughout the last trimester of pregnancy (see *"Drug Abuse and Dependence"*). If Amobarbital Sodium/Secobarbital Sodium is used during pregnancy or if the patient becomes pregnant while taking this drug, the patient should be apprised of the potential hazard to the fetus.

4. Synergistic Effects: The concomitant use of alcohol or other CNS depressants may produce additive CNS depressant effects.

PRECAUTIONS

General: Barbiturates may be habit-forming. Tolerance and psychologic and physical dependence may occur with continuing use (see *"Drug Abuse and Dependence"*).

Barbiturates should be administered with caution, if at all, to patients who are mentally depressed or who have suidical tendencies. Particular caution is also indicated before administering barbiturates to patients who have abused other classes of drugs.

Elderly or debilitated patients may react to barbiturates with marked excitement, depression, or confusion. In some persons, barbiturates repeatedly produce excitement rather than depression.

In patients with hepatic damage, barbiturates should be administered with caution and initially in reduced doses. Barbiturates should not be administered to patients showing the premonitory signs of hepatic coma.

Information for Patients: The following information should be given to patients receiving barbiturates.

1. The use of barbiturates carries with it an associated risk of psychologic and/or physical dependence. The patient should be warned against increasing the dose of the drug without consulting a physician.

2. Barbiturates may impair the mental and/or physical abilities required for the performance of potentially hazardous tasks, such as driving a car or operating machinery. The patient should be cautioned accordingly.

3. Alcohol should not be consumed while taking barbiturates. The concurrent use of the barbiturates with other CNS depressants (e.g., alcohol, narcotics, tranquilizers, and antihistamines) may result in additional CNS depressant effects.

Laboratory Tests: Prolonged therapy with barbiturates should be accompanied by periodic evaluation of organ systems, including hematopoietic, renal, and hepatic systems (see *"General"* under *"Precautions"* and *"Adverse Reactions"*).

Drug Interactions: Most reports of clinically significant drug interactions occurring with the barbiturates have involved phenobarbital. However, the application of these data to other barbiturates appears valid and warrants serial blood level determinations of the relevant drugs when there are multiple therapies.

1. Anticoagulants: Phenobarbital lowers the plasma levels of dicumarol and causes a decrease in anticoagulant activity as measured by the prothrombin time. Barbiturates can induce hepatic microsomal enzymes resulting in increased metabolism and decreased anticoagulant response of oral anticoagulants (eg, warfarin, acenocoumarol, dicumarol, and phenprocoumon). Patients stabilized on anticoagulant therapy may require dosage adjustments if barbiturates are added to or withdrawn from their dosage regimen.

2. Corticosteroids: Barbiturates appear to enhance the metabolism of exogenous corticosteroids, probably through the induction of hepatic microsomal enzymes. Patients stabilized on corticosteroid therapy may require dosage adjustments if barbiturates are added to or withdrawn from their dosage regimen.

3. Griseofulvin: Phenobarbital appears to interfere with the absorption of orally administered griseofulvin, thus decreasing its blood level. The effect of the resultant decreased blood levels of griseofulvin on therapeutic response has not been established. However, it would be preferable to avoid concomitant administration of these drugs.

4. Doxycycline: Phenobarbital has been shown to shorten the half-life of doxycycline for as long as 2 weeks after barbiturate therapy is discontinued.

This mechanism is probably through the induction of hepatic microsomal enzymes that metabolize the antibiotic. If barbiturates and doxycycline are administered concurrently, the clinical response to doxycycline should be monitored closely.

5. Phenytoin, Sodium Valproate, Valproic Acid: The effect of barbiturates on the metabolism of phenytoin appears to be variable. Some investigators report on accelerating effect, whereas others report no effect. Because the effect of barbiturates on the metabolism of phenytoin is not predictable, phenytoin and barbiturate blood levels should be monitored more frequently if these drugs are given concurrently. Sodium valproate and valproic acid appear to decrease barbiturate metabolism; therefore, barbiturate blood levels should be monitored and appropriate dosage adjustments made as indicated.

6. CNS Depressants: The concomitant use of other CNS depressants, including other sedatives or hypnotics, antihistamines, tranquilizers, or alcohol, may produce additive depressant effects.

7. Monoamine Oxidase Inhibitors (MAOI): MAOI prolong the effects of barbiturates, probably because metabolism of the barbiturate is inhibited.

8. Estradiol, Estrone, Progesterone, and Other Steroidal Hormones: Pretreatment with or concurrent administration of phenobarbital may decrease the effect of estradiol by increasing its metabolism. There have been reports of patients treated with antiepileptic drugs (eg, phenobarbital) who become pregnant while taking oral contraceptives. An alternate contraceptive method might be suggested to women taking barbiturates.

Carcinogenesis:
1. Animal Data. Phenobarbital sodium is carcinogenic in mice and rats after lifetime administration. In mice, it produced benign and malignant liver cell tumors. In rats, benign liver cell tumors were observed very late in life.

2. Human Data: In a 29-year epidemiologic study of 9,136 patients who were treated on an anticonvulsant protocol that included phenobarbital, results indicated a higher than normal incidence of hepatic carcinoma. Previously, some of these patients had been treated with thorotrast, a drug that is known to produce hepatic carcinomas. Thus, this study did not provide sufficient evidence that phenobarbital sodium is carcinogenic in humans.

A retrospective study of 84 children with brain tumors matched to 73 normal controls and 78 cancer controls (malignant disease other than brain tumors) suggested an association between exposure to barbiturates prenatally and an increased incidence of brain tumors.

Pregnancy:
1. Teratogenic Effects. Pregnancy Category D: See *"Usage in Pregnancy"* under *"Warnings".*

2. Nonteratogenic Effects: Reports of infants suffering from long-term barbiturate exposure *in utero* included the acute withdrawal syndrome of seizures and hyperirritability from bith to a delayed onset of up to 14 days (see *"Drug Abuse and Dependence"*).

Labor and Delivery: Hypnotic doses of barbiturates do not appear to impair uterine activity significantly during labor. Full anesthetic doses of barbiturates decrease the force and frequency of uterine contractions. Administration of sedative-hypnotic barbiturates to the mother during labor may result in respiratory depression in the newborn. Premature infants are particularly susceptible to the depressant effects of barbiturates. If barbiturates are used during labor and delivery, resuscitation equipment should be available.

Data are not available to evaluate the effect of barbiturates when forceps delivery or other intervention is necessary, or to determine the effect of barbiturates on the later growth, development, and functional maturation of the child.

Nursing Mothers: Caution should be exercised when Amobarbital Sodium/Secobarbital Sodium is administered to a nursing woman because small amounts of barbiturates are excreted in the milk.

ADVERSE REACTIONS

The following adverse reactions and their incidence were compiled from surveillance of thousands of hospitalized patients who received barbiturates. Because such patients may be less aware of certain of the milder adverse effects of barbiturates, the incidence of these reactions may be somewhat higher in fully ambulatory patients.

MORE THAN 1 IN 100 PATIENTS
The most common adverse reaction, estimated to occur at a rate of 1 to 3 patients per 100, is the following:

Nervous System: Somnolence

LESS THAN 1 IN 100 PATIENTS
Adverse reactions estimated to occur at a rate of less than 1 in 100 patients are listed below, grouped by organ system and by decreasing order of occurrence:

Nervous System: Agitation, confusion, hyperkinesia, ataxia, CNS depression, nightmares, nervousness, psychiatric disturbance, hallucinations, insomnia, anxiety, dizziness, abnormality in thinking.

Respiratory System: Hypoventilation, apnea

Cardiovascular System: Bradycardia, hypotension, syncope

Digestive System: Nausea, vomiting, constipation

Other Reported Reactions: Headache, injection site reactions, hypersensitivity reactions (angioedema, skin rashes, exfoliative dermatitis), fever, liver damage, megaloblastic anemia following chronic phenobarbital use

DRUG ABUSE AND DEPENDENCE

Controlled Substance: Amobarbital Sodium/Secobarbital Sodium is a Schedule II drug.

Dependence: Barbiturates may be habit-forming. Tolerance, psychologic dependence, and physical dependence may occur especially following prolonged use of high doses of barbiturates. Daily administration in excess of 400 mg of pentobarbital or Secobarbital for approximately 90 days is likely to produce some degree of physical dependence. A dosage of 600 to 800 mg for at least 35 days is sufficient to produce withdrawal seizures. The average daily dose for the barbiturate addict is usually about 1.5 g. As tolerance to barbiturates develops, the amount needed to maintain the same level of intoxication increases; tolerance to a fatal dosage, however, does not increase more than twofold. As this occurs, the margin between intoxicating dosage and fatal dosage becomes smaller.

Symptoms of acute intoxication with barbiturates include unsteady gait, slurred speech, and sustained nystagmus. Mental signs of chronic intoxication include confusion, poor judgment, irritability, insomnia, and somatic complaints.

Symptoms of barbiturate dependence are similar to those of chronic alcoholism. If an individual appears to be intoxicated with alcohol to a degree that is radically disproportionate to the amount of alcohol in his or her blood, the use of barbiturates should be suspected. The lethal dose of a barbiturate is far less if alcohol is also ingested.

The symptoms of barbiturate withdrawal can be severe and may cause death. Minor withdrawal symptoms may appear 8 to 12 hours after the last dose of a barbiturate. These symptoms usually appear in the following order: anxiety, muscle twitching, tremor of hands and fingers, progressive weakness, dizziness, distortion in visual perception, nausea, vomiting, insomnia, and orthostatic hypotension. Major withdrawal symptoms (convulsions and delirium) may occur within 16 hours and last up to 5 days after abrupt cessation of barbiturates. The intensity of withdrawal symptoms gradually declines over a period of approximately 15 days. Individuals susceptible to barbiturate abuse and dependence include alcoholics and opiate abusers, as well as other sedative-hypnotic and amphetamine abusers.

Drug dependence on barbiturates arises from repeated administration on a continuous basis, generally in amounts exceeding therapeutic dose levels. The characteristics of drug dependence on barbiturates include: (a) a strong desire or need to continue taking the drug; (b) a tendency to increase the dose; (c) a psychic dependence on the effects of the drug related to subjective and individual appreciation of those effects; and (d) a physical dependence on the effects of the drug, requiring its presence for maintenance of homeostasis and resulting in a definite, characteristic, and self-limited abstinence syndrome when the drug is withdrawn.

Treatment of barbiturate dependence consists of cautious and gradual withdrawal of the drug. Barbiturate-dependent patients can be withdrawn by using a number of different withdrawal regimens. In all cases, withdrawal requires an extended period of time. One method involves substituting a 30-mg dose of phenobarbital for each 100- to 200-mg dose of barbiturate that the patient has been taking. The total daily amount of phenobarbital is then administered in 3 or 4 divided doses, not to exceed 600 mg daily. If signs of withdrawal occur on the first day of treatment, a loading dose of 100 to 200 mg of phenobarbital may be administered IM in addition to the oral dose. After stabilization on phenobarbital, the total daily dose is decreased by 30 mg/day as long as withdrawal is proceeding smoothly. A modification of this regimen involves initiating treatment at the patient's regular dosage level and decreasing the daily dosage by 10% if tolerated by the patient.

Infants that are physically dependent on barbiturates may be given phenobarbital, 3 to 10 mg/kg/day. After withdrawal symptoms (hyperactivity, disturbed sleep, tremors, and hyperreflexia) are relieved, the dosage of phenobarbital should be gradually decreased and completely withdrawn over a 2-week period.

OVERDOSAGE

The toxic dose of barbiturates varies considerably. In general, an oral dose of 1 g of most barbiturates produces serious poisoning in an adult. Death commonly occurs after 2 to 10 g of ingested barbiturate. The sedated, therapeutic blood levels of Secobarbital range between 0.5 to 5 µg/mL; the usual lethal blood level ranges from 15 to 40 µg/mL. Barbiturate intoxication may be confused with alcoholism, bromide intoxication, and various neurologic disorders. Potential tolerance must be considered when evaluating significance of dose and plasma concentration.

Signs and Symptoms: Symptoms of oral overdose may occur within 15 minutes beginning with CNS depression, underventilation, hypotension, and hypothermia and may progress to pulmonary edema and death. Hemorrhagic blisters may develop, especially at pressure points.

In extreme overdose, all electrical activity in the brain may cease, in which case a "flat" EEG normally equated with clinical death cannot be accepted. This effect is fully reversible unless hypoxic damage occurs. Consideration should be given to the possibility of barbiturate intoxication even in situations that appear to involve trauma.

Complications such as pneumonia, pulmonary edema, cardiac arrhythmias, congestive heart failure, and renal failure may occur. Uremia may increase CNS sensitivity to barbiturates if renal function is impaired.

Treatment: To obtain up-to-date information about the treatment of overdose, a good resource is your certified Regional Poison Control Center. Telephone numbers of certified poison control centers are listed in the *Physicians' Desk Reference (PDR).* In managing overdosage, consider the possibility of multiple drug overdoses, interaction among drugs, and unusual drug kinetics in your patient.

Protect the patient's airway and support ventilation and perfusion. Meticulously monitor and maintain, within acceptable limits, the patient's vital signs, blood gases, serum electrolytes, etc. Absorption of drugs from the gastrointestinal tract may be decreased by giving activated charcoal, which, in many cases, is more effective than emesis or lavage; consider charcoal instead of, or in addition to gastric emptying. Repeated doses of charcoal over time may hasten elimination of some drugs that have been absorbed. Safeguard the patient's airway when employing gastric emptying or charcoal.

Diuresis and peritoneal dialysis are of little value; hemodialysis and hemoperfusion enhance drug clearance and should be considered in serious poisoning. If the patient has chronically abused sedatives, withdrawal reactions may be manifest following acute overdose.

DOSAGE AND ADMINISTRATION

The dose of Amobarbital Sodium/Secobarbital Sodium must be individualized with full knowledge of its particular characteristics and recommended rate of administration. Factors of consideration are the patient's age, weight, and condition.

◆ RATED THERAPEUTICALLY EQUIVALENT; ◇ THERAPEUTIC EQUIVALENCE UNCONFIRMED; ○ UNRATED

Adults: 100 mg (50 mg each of Secobarbital Sodium and Amobarbital Sodium) to 200 mg (100 mg each of Secobarbital Sodium and Amobarbital Sodium) at bedtime or 1 hour preoperatively.

Special Patient Population: Dosage should be reduced in the elderly or debilitated because these patients may be more sensitive to barbiturates. Dosage should be reduced for patients with impaired renal function or hepatic disease.

Storage: Store at controlled room temperature, 59° to 86°F (15° to 30°C). Dispense in a tight container.

HOW SUPPLIED
CAPSULE (C-II): 100 MG-100 MG

BRAND/MANUFACTURER	NDC	SIZE	AWP
○ **BRAND**			
TUINAL: Lilly	00002-0665-02	100s	$22.87

CAPSULE (C-II): 200 MG-200 MG

BRAND/MANUFACTURER	NDC	SIZE	AWP
○ **BRAND**			
TUINAL: Lilly	00002-0666-02	100s	$30.52

Amoxapine

DESCRIPTION
Amoxapine is an antidepressant of the dibenzoxazepine class, chemically distinct from the dibenzazepines, dibenzocycloheptenes, and dibenzoxepines.

It is designated chemically as 2-chloro-11-(1-piperazinyl) dibenz-[b,f][1,4] oxazepine. The molecular weight is 313.8. The empirical formula is $C_{17}H_{16}ClN_3O$.

Amoxapine is supplied for oral administration as 25 mg, 50 mg, 100 mg, and 150 mg tablets.

Following is its chemical structure:

CLINICAL PHARMACOLOGY
Amoxapine is an antidepressant with a mild sedative component to its action. The mechanism of its clinical action in man is not well understood. In animals, Amoxapine reduced the uptake of norepinephrine and serotonin and blocked the response of dopamine receptors to dopamine. Amoxapine is not a monoamine oxidase inhibitor.

Amoxapine is absorbed rapidly and reaches peak blood levels approximately 90 minutes after ingestion. It is almost completely metabolized. The main route of excretion is the kidney. *In vitro* tests show that Amoxapine binding to human serum is approximately 90%.

In man, Amoxapine serum concentration declines with a half-life of 8 hours. However, the major metabolite, 8-hydroxyAmoxapine, has a biologic half-life of 30 hours. Metabolites are excreted in the urine in conjugated form as glucuronides.

Clinical studies have demonstrated that Amoxapine has a more rapid onset of action than either amitriptyline or imipramine. The initial clinical effect may occur within 4 to 7 days and occurs within 2 weeks in over 80% of responders.

INDICATIONS AND USAGE
Amoxapine is indicated for the relief of symptoms of depression in patients with neurotic or reactive depressive disorders as well as endogenous and psychotic depressions. It is indicated for depression accompanied by anxiety or agitation.

CONTRAINDICATIONS
Amoxapine is contraindicated in patients who have shown prior hypersensitivity to dibenzoxazepine compounds. It should not be given concomitantly with monoamine oxidase inhibitors. Hyperpyretic crises, severe convulsions, and deaths have occurred in patients receiving tricyclic antidepressants and monoamine oxidase inhibitors simultaneously. When it is desired to replace a monoamine oxidase inhibitor with Amoxapine, a minimum of 14 days should be allowed to elapse after the former is discontinued. Amoxapine should then be initiated cautiously with gradual increase in dosage until optimum response is achieved. The drug is not recommended for use during the acute recovery phase following myocardial infarction.

WARNINGS
Tardive Dyskinesia: Tardive dyskinesia, a syndrome consisting of potentially irreversible, involuntary, dyskinetic movements may develop in patients treated with neuroleptic (ie, antipsychotic) drugs. (Amoxapine is not an antipsychotic, but it has substantive neuroleptic activity.) Although the prevalence of the syndrome appears to be highest among the elderly, especially elderly women, it is impossible to rely upon prevalence estimates to predict, at the inception of neuroleptic treatment, which patients are likely to develop the syndrome. Whether neuroleptic drug products differ in their potential to cause tardive dyskinesia is unknown.

Both the risk of developing the syndrome and the likelihood that it will become irreversible are believed to increase as the duration of treatment and the total cumulative dose of neuroleptic drugs administered to the patient increase. However, the syndrome can develop, although much less commonly, after relatively brief treatment periods at low doses. There is no known treatment for established cases of tardive dyskinesia, although the syndrome may remit, partially or completely, if neuroleptic treatment is withdrawn. Neuroleptic treatment itself, however, may suppress (or partially suppress) the signs and symptoms of the syndrome and thereby may possibly mask the underlying disease process. The effect that symptomatic suppression has upon the long-term course of the syndrome is unknown.

Given these considerations, neuroleptics should be prescribed in a manner that is most likely to minimize the occurrence of tardive dyskinesia. Chronic neuroleptic treatment should generally be reserved for patients who suffer from a chronic illness that 1) is known to respond to neuroleptic drugs, and 2) for whom alternative, equally effective, but potentially less harmful treatments are not available or appropriate. In patients who do require chronic treatment, the smallest dose and the shortest duration of treatment producing a satisfactory clinical response should be sought. The need for continued treatment should be reassessed periodically.

If signs and symptoms of tardive dyskinesia appear in a patient on neuroleptics, drug discontinuation should be considered. However, some patients may require treatment despite the presence of the syndrome.

(For further information about the description of tardive dyskinesia and its clinical detection, please refer to the sections on *"Information for the Patient"* and *"Adverse Reactions".*)

Neuroleptic Malignant Syndrome (NMS): A potentially fatal symptom complex sometimes referred to as Neuroleptic Malignant Syndrome (NMS) has been reported in association with antipsychotic drugs and with Amoxapine. Clinical manifestations of NMS are hyperpyrexia, muscle rigidity, altered mental status and evidence of autonomic instability (irregular pulse or blood pressure, tachycardia, diaphoresis, and cardiac dysrhythmias).

The diagnostic evaluation of patients with this syndrome is complicated. In arriving at a diagnosis, it is important to identify cases where the clinical presentation includes both serious medical illness (eg, pneumonia, systemic infection, etc) and untreated or inadequately treated extrapyramidal signs and symptoms (EPS). Other important considerations in the differential diagnosis include central anticholinergic toxicity, heat stroke, drug fever, and primary central nervous system (CNS) pathology.

The management of NMS should include 1) immediate discontinuation of antipsychotic drugs and other drugs not essential to concurrent therapy, 2) intensive symptomatic treatment and medical monitoring, and 3) treatment of any concomitant serious medical problems for which specific treatments are available. There is no general agreement about specific pharmacological treatment regimens for uncomplicated NMS.

If a patient requires antipsychotic drug treatment after recovery from NMS, the potential reintroduction of drug therapy should be carefully considered. The patient should be carefully monitored since recurrences of NMS have been reported.

Amoxapine should be used with caution in patients with a history of urinary retention, angle-closure glaucoma, or increased intraocular pressure. Patients with cardiovascular disorders should be watched closely. Tricyclic antidepressant drugs, particularly when given in high doses, can induce sinus tachycardia, changes in conduction time, and arrhythmias. Myocardial infarction and stroke have been reported with drugs of this class.

Extreme caution should be used in treating patients with a history of convulsive disorder or those with overt or latent seizure disorders.

PRECAUTIONS
General: In prescribing the drug it should be borne in mind that the possibility of suicide is inherent in any severe depression, and persists until a significant remission occurs; the drug should be dispensed in the smallest suitable amount. Manic depressive patients may experience a shift to the manic phase. Schizophrenic patients may develop increased symptoms of psychosis; patients with paranoid symptomatology may have an exaggeration of such symptoms. This may require reduction of dosage or the addition of a major tranquilizer to the therapeutic regimen. Antidepressant drugs can cause skin rashes and/or "drug fever" in susceptible individuals. These allergic reactions may, in rare cases, be severe. They are more likely to occur during the first few days of treatment, but may also occur later. Amoxapine should be discontinued if rash and/or fever develop. Amoxapine possesses a degree of dopamine-blocking activity which may cause extrapyramidal symptoms in <1% of patients. Rarely, symptoms indicative of tardive dyskinesia have been reported.

Information for the Patient: Given the likelihood that some patients exposed chronically to neuroleptics will develop tardive dyskinesia, it is advised that all patients in whom chronic use is contemplated be given, if possible, full information about this risk. The decision to inform patients and/or their guardians must obviously take into account the clinical circumstances and the competency of the patient to understand the information provided.

Patients should be warned of the possibility of drowsiness that may impair performance of potentially hazardous tasks such as driving an automobile or operating machinery.

Drug Interactions: See *"Contraindications"* about concurrent usage of tricyclic antidepressants and monoamine oxidase inhibitors. Paralytic ileus may occur in patients taking tricyclic antidepressants in combination with anticholinergic drugs. Amoxapine may enhance the response to alcohol and the effects of barbiturates and other CNS depressants. Serum levels of several tricyclic antidepressants have been reported to be significantly increased when cimetidine is administered concurrently. Although such an interaction has not been reported to date with Amoxapine, specific interaction studies have not been done, and the possibility should be considered.

Therapeutic Interactions: Concurrent administration with electroshock therapy may increase the hazards associated with such therapy.

Carcinogenesis, Impairment of Fertility: In a 21-month toxicity study at three dose levels in rats, pancreatic islet cell hyperplasia occurred with slightly increased incidence at doses 5 to 10 times the human dose. Pancreatic adenocarcinoma was detected in low incidence in the mid-dose group only, and may possibly have resulted from endocrine-mediated organ hyperfunction. The significance of these findings to man is not known.

Treatment of male rats with 5 to 10 times the human dose resulted in a slight decrease in the number of fertile matings. Female rats receiving oral doses within the therapeutic range displayed a reversible increase in estrous cycle length.

Pregnancy: Pregnancy Category C: Studies performed in mice, rats, and rabbits have demonstrated no evidence of teratogenic effect due to Amoxapine. Embryotoxicity was seen in rats and rabbits given oral doses approximating the human dose. Fetotoxic effects (intrauterine death, stillbirth, decreased birth weight) were seen in animals studied at oral doses 3 to 10 times the human dose. Decreased postnatal survival (between days 0 to 4) was demonstrated in the offspring of rats at 5 to 10 times the human dose. There are no adequate and well-controlled studies in pregnant women. Amoxapine should be used during pregnancy only if the potential benefit justifies the potential risk to the fetus.

Nursing Mothers: Amoxapine, like many other systemic drugs, is excreted in human milk. Because effects of the drug on infants are unknown, caution should be exercised when Amoxapine is administered to nursing women.

Pediatric Use: Safety and effectiveness in children below the age of 16 have not been established.

ADVERSE REACTIONS
Adverse reactions reported in controlled studies in the United States are categorized with respect to incidence below. Following this is a listing of reactions known to occur with other antidepressant drugs of this class but not reported to date with Amoxapine.

INCIDENCE GREATER THAN 1%
The most frequent types of adverse reactions occurring with Amoxapine in controlled clinical trials were sedative and anticholinergic: these included drowsiness (14%), dry mouth (14%), constipation (12%), and blurred vision (7%). Less frequently reported reactions are:

CNS and Neuromuscular: anxiety, insomnia, restlessness, nervousness, palpitations, tremors, confusion, excitement, nightmares, ataxia, alterations in EEG patterns.

Allergic: edema, skin rash.

Endocrine: elevation of prolactin levels.

Gastrointestinal: nausea.

Other: dizziness, headache, fatigue, weakness, excessive appetite, increased perspiration.

INCIDENCE LESS THAN 1%
Anticholinergic: disturbances of accommodation, mydriasis, delayed micturition, urinary retention, nasal stuffiness.

Cardiovascular: hypotension, hypertension, syncope, tachycardia.

Allergic: drug fever, urticaria, photosensitivity, pruritus, rarely vasculitis, hepatitis.

CNS and Neuromuscular: tingling, paresthesias of the extremities, tinnitus, disorientation, seizures, hypomania, numbness, incoordination, disturbed concentration, hyperthermia, extrapyramidal symptoms, including, rarely, tardive dyskinesia. Neuroleptic malignant syndrome has been reported. (See "Warnings".)

Hematologic: leukopenia, agranulocytosis.

Gastrointestinal: epigastric distress, vomiting, flatulence, abdominal pain, peculiar taste, diarrhea.

Endocrine: increased or decreased libido, impotence, menstrual irregularity, breast enlargement and galactorrhea in the female, syndrome of inappropriate antidiuretic hormone secretion.

Other: lacrimation, weight gain or loss, altered liver function, painful ejaculation.

DRUG RELATIONSHIP UNKNOWN
The following reactions have been reported very rarely, and occurred under uncontrolled circumstances where a drug relationship was difficult to assess. These observations are listed to serve as alerting information to physicians.

Anticholinergic: paralytic ileus.

Cardiovascular: atrial arrhythmias (including atrial fibrillation), myocardial infarction, stroke, heart block.

CNS and Neuromuscular: hallucinations.

Hematologic: thrombocytopenia, eosinophilia, purpura, petechiae.

Gastrointestinal: parotid swelling.

Endocrine: change in blood glucose levels.

Other: pancreatitis, hepatitis, jaundice, urinary frequency, testicular swelling, anorexia, alopecia.

ADDITIONAL ADVERSE REACTIONS
The following reactions have been reported with other antidepressant drugs, but not with Amoxapine

Anticholinergic: sublingual adenitis, dilation of the urinary tract.

CNS and Neuromuscular: delusions.

Gastrointestinal: stomatitis, black tongue.

Endocrine: gynecomastia.

OVERDOSAGE
Signs and Symptoms: Toxic manifestations of Amoxapine overdosage differ significantly from those of other tricyclic antidepressants. Serious cardiovascular effects are seldom if ever observed. However, CNS effects—particularly grand mal convulsions—occur frequently, and treatment should be directed primarily toward prevention or control of seizures. Status epilepticus may develop and constitutes a neurologic emergency. Coma and acidosis are other serious complications of substantial Amoxapine overdosage in some cases. Renal failure may develop 2 to 5 days after toxic overdosage in patients who may appear otherwise recovered. Acute tubular necrosis with rhabdomyolysis and myoglobinuria is the most common renal complication in such cases. This reaction probably occurs in less than 5% of overdose cases, and typically in those who have experienced multiple seizures.

Treatment: Treatment of Amoxapine overdosage should be symptomatic and supportive, but with special attention to prevention or control of seizures. If the patient is conscious, induced emesis followed by gastric lavage with appropriate precautions to prevent pulmonary aspiration should be accomplished as soon as possible. Following lavage, activated charcoal may be administered to reduce absorption, and repeated administrations may facilitate drug elimination. An adequate airway should be established in comatose patients and assisted ventilation instituted if necessary. Seizures may respond to standard anticonvulsant therapy such as intravenous diazepam and/or phenytoin. The value of physostigmine appears less certain. Status epilepticus, should it develop, requires vigorous treatment such as that described by Delgado-Escueta et al (*N Engl J Med* 1982; 306:1337-1340).

Convulsions, when they occur, typically begin within 12 hours after ingestion. Because seizures may occur precipitously in some overdosage patients who appear otherwise relatively asymptomatic, the treating physician may wish to consider prophylactic administration of anticonvulsant medication during this period.

Treatment of renal impairment, should it occur, is the same as that for nondrug-induced renal dysfunction.

Serious cardiovascular effects are remarkably rare following Amoxapine overdosage, and the ECG typically remains within normal limits except for sinus tachycardia. Hence, prolongation of the QRS interval beyond 100 milliseconds within the first 24 hours is *not* a useful guide to the severity of overdosage with this drug.

Fatalities and, rarely, neurologic sequelae have resulted from prolonged status epilepticus in Amoxapine overdosage patients. While the lethal dose appears higher than that of other tricyclic antidepressants (80% of lethal Amoxapine overdosages have involved ingestion of 3 grams or more), many factors other than amount ingested are important in assessing probability of survival. These include age and physical condition of the patient, concomitant ingestion of other drugs, and especially the interval between drug ingestion and initiation of emergency treatment.

DOSAGE AND ADMINISTRATION
Effective dosage of Amoxapine may vary from one patient to another. Usual effective dosage is 200 to 300 mg daily. Three weeks constitutes an adequate period of trial providing dosage has reached 300 mg daily (or lower level of tolerance) for at least 2 weeks. If no response is seen at 300 mg, dosage may be increased, depending upon tolerance, up to 400 mg daily. Hospitalized patients who have been refractory to antidepressant therapy and who have no history of convulsive seizures may have dosage raised cautiously up to 600 mg daily in divided doses.

Amoxapine may be given in a single daily dose, not to exceed 300 mg, preferably at bedtime. If the total daily dosage exceeds 300 mg, it should be given in divided doses.

Initial Dosage for Adults: Usual starting dosage is 50 mg two or three times daily. Depending upon tolerance, dosage may be increased to 100 mg two or three times daily by the end of the first week. (Initial dosage of 300 mg daily may be given, but notable sedation may occur in some patients during the first few days of therapy at this level). Increases above 300 mg daily should be made only if 300 mg daily has been ineffective during a trial period of at least 2 weeks. When effective dosage is established, the drug may be given in a single dose (not to exceed 300 mg) at bedtime.

Elderly Patients: In general, lower dosages are recommended for these patients. Recommended starting dosage of Amoxapine is 25 mg two or three times daily. If no intolerance is observed, dosage may be increased by the end of the first week to 50 mg two or three times daily. Although 100 to 150 mg daily may be adequate for many elderly patients, some may require higher dosage. Careful increases up to 300 mg daily are indicated in such cases.

Once an effective dosage is established, Amoxapine may conveniently be given in a single bedtime dose, not to exceed 300 mg.

Maintenance: Recommended maintenance dosage of Amoxapine is the lowest dose that will maintain remission. If symptoms reappear, dosage should be increased to the earlier level until they are controlled.

For maintenance therapy at dosages of 300 mg or less, a single dose at bedtime is recommended.

Tablets: Store at Controlled Room Temperature 15°-30° C (59°-86° F).

HOW SUPPLIED
TABLETS: 25 MG

AVERAGE UNIT PRICE (AVAILABLE SIZES)		GENERIC A-RATED AVERAGE PRICE (GAAP)	
BRAND	$0.75	100s	$51.81
GENERIC	$0.52		
HCFA FUL (100s ea)	$0.43		

BRAND/MANUFACTURER	NDC	SIZE	AWP
◆ **BRAND**			
ASENDIN: Lederle Labs	00005-5389-23	100s	$74.56
◆ **GENERICS**			
Schein	00364-2432-01	100s	$41.50
Warner Chilcott	00047-0314-24	100s	$43.85
Mason Dist	11845-0394-01	100s	$46.58
Moore,H.L.	00839-7604-06	100s	$46.70
Qualitest	00603-2240-21	100s	$49.20
Parmed	00349-8702-01	100s	$51.95
Martec	52555-0539-01	100s	$52.87
URL	00677-1432-01	100s	$52.90
Geneva	00781-1844-01	100s	$52.90
Major	00904-3994-60	100s	$52.95
Rugby	00536-3003-01	100s	$52.97
Watson	52544-0379-01	100s	$61.48
Goldline	00182-1043-01	100s	$61.48
Aligen	00405-4076-01	100s	$64.72
Major	00904-3994-61	100s ud	$45.10

TABLETS: 50 MG

AVERAGE UNIT PRICE (AVAILABLE SIZES)		GENERIC A-RATED AVERAGE PRICE (GAAP)	
BRAND	$1.23	100s	$83.67
GENERIC	$0.84		
HCFA FUL (100s ea)	$0.70		

BRAND/MANUFACTURER	NDC	SIZE	AWP
◆ **BRAND**			
ASENDIN: Lederle Labs	00005-5390-23	100s	$121.29
	00005-5390-60	100s ud	$133.53
	00005-5390-31	500s	$576.14
◆ **GENERICS**			
Schein	00364-2433-01	100s	$67.75
Mason Dist	11845-0395-01	100s	$73.25
Warner Chilcott	00047-0315-24	100s	$74.40
Moore,H.L.	00839-7605-06	100s	$76.48
Parmed	00349-8703-01	100s	$82.95
Rugby	00536-3004-01	100s	$83.85
Geneva	00781-1845-01	100s	$83.93
Major	00904-3995-60	100s	$84.20
URL	00677-1378-01	100s	$85.38
Qualitest	00603-2241-21	100s	$85.41
Martec	52555-0540-01	100s	$86.85
Aligen	00405-4077-01	100s	$99.95
Watson	52544-0380-01	100s	$99.95
Goldline	00182-1044-01	100s	$99.95
Major	00904-3995-61	100s ud	$70.69
Watson	52544-0380-05	500s	$474.34

TABLETS: 100 MG

AVERAGE UNIT PRICE (AVAILABLE SIZES)		GENERIC A-RATED AVERAGE PRICE (GAAP)	
BRAND	$2.09	100s	$139.42
GENERIC	$1.39		
HCFA FUL (100s ea)	$1.17		

BRAND/MANUFACTURER	NDC	SIZE	AWP
◆ **BRAND**			
ASENDIN: Lederle Labs	00005-5391-23	100s	$202.34
	00005-5391-60	100s ud	$214.83
◆ **GENERICS**			
Schein	00364-2434-01	100s	$112.50
Warner Chilcott	00047-0316-24	100s	$118.74
Mason Dist	11845-0396-01	100s	$124.92
Moore,H.L.	00839-7606-06	100s	$128.99
Qualitest	00603-2242-21	100s	$134.80
Geneva	00781-1846-01	100s	$134.87
Major	00904-3996-60	100s	$135.70
URL	00677-1379-01	100s	$138.72
Rugby	00536-3005-01	100s	$138.77

BRAND/MANUFACTURER	NDC	SIZE	AWP
Parmed	00349-8709-01	100s	$139.95
Martec	52555-0541-01	100s	$143.47
Aligen	00405-4078-01	100s	$166.83
Watson	52544-0381-01	100s	$166.83
Goldline	00182-1045-01	100s	$166.83

TABLETS: 150 MG

AVERAGE UNIT PRICE (AVAILABLE SIZES)		GENERIC A-RATED AVERAGE PRICE (GAAP)	
BRAND	$3.19	30s	$65.57
GENERIC	$2.21		

BRAND/MANUFACTURER	NDC	SIZE	AWP
◆ **BRAND**			
ASENDIN: Lederle Labs	00005-5392-38	30s	$95.69
◆ **GENERICS**			
Schein	00364-2435-30	30s	$53.50
Geneva	00781-1847-31	30s	$56.00
Warner Chilcott	00047-0317-15	30s	$57.70
Mason Dist	11845-0397-08	30s	$59.92
Moore,H.L.	00839-7607-19	30s	$60.95
Major	00904-3997-46	30s	$62.95
Qualitest	00603-2243-16	30s	$63.15
URL	00677-1380-07	30s	$66.83
Rugby	00536-3006-07	30s	$66.86
Martec	52555-0542-30	30s	$67.85
Aligen	00405-4079-30	30s	$78.90
Watson	52544-0382-30	30s	$78.90
Goldline	00182-1046-17	30s	$78.90
Watson	52544-0382-01	100s	$249.85

Amoxicillin

DESCRIPTION

Amoxicillin is a semisynthetic antibiotic, an analog of ampicillin, with a broad spectrum of bactericidal activity against many gram-positive and gram-negative microorganisms. Chemically it is D-(−)-α-amino-p-hydroxybenzyl penicillin trihydrate.

Following is its chemical structure:

$$HO \longleftarrow \left\langle \text{—} \right\rangle \text{—} \underset{\underset{NH_2}{|}}{\overset{\overset{H}{|}}{C}} \text{—} CONH \text{—} \cdots \quad CH_3 \cdot 3H_2O$$

ACTIONS

PHARMACOLOGY

Amoxicillin is stable in the presence of gastric acid and may be given without regard to meals. It is rapidly absorbed after oral administration. It diffuses readily into most body tissues and fluids, with the exception of brain and spinal fluid, except when meninges are inflamed. The half-life of Amoxicillin is 61.3 minutes. Most of the Amoxicillin is excreted unchanged in the urine; its excretion can be delayed by concurrent administration of probenecid. Amoxicillin is not highly protein-bound. In blood serum Amoxicillin is approximately 20% protein-bound as compared to 60% for penicillin G.

Orally administered doses of 250 mg and 500 mg Amoxicillin capsules result in average peak blood levels 1 to 2 hours after administration in the range of 3.5 mcg/mL to 5.0 mcg/mL and 5.5 mcg/mL to 7.5 mcg/mL, respectively.

Orally administered doses of Amoxicillin suspension 125 mg/5 mL and 250 mg/5 mL result in average peak blood levels 1 to 2 hours after administration in the range of 1.5 mcg/mL to 3.0 mcg/mL and 3.5 mcg/mL to 5.0 mcg/mL, respectively. Amoxicillin chewable tablets, 125 mg and 250 mg, produced blood levels similar to those achieved with the corresponding doses of Amoxicillin oral suspensions.

Detectable serum levels are observed up to 8 hours after an orally administered dose of Amoxicillin. Following a 1 gram dose and utilizing a special skin window technique to determine levels of the antibiotic, it was noted that therapeutic levels were found in the interstitial fluid. Approximately 60% of an orally administered dose of Amoxicillin is excreted in the urine within 6 to 8 hours.

MICROBIOLOGY

Amoxicillin is similar to ampicillin in its bactericidal action against susceptible organisms during the stage of active multiplication. It acts through the inhibition of biosynthesis of cell wall mucopeptide. *In vitro* studies have demonstrated the susceptibility of most strains of the following gram-positive bacteria: alpha- and beta-hemolytic streptococci, *Diplococcus pneumoniae*, nonpenicillinase-producing staphylococci, and *Streptococcus faecalis*. It is active *in vitro* against many strains of *Haemophilus influenzae*, *Neisseria gonorrhoeae*, *Escherichia coli* and *Proteus mirabilis*. Because it does not resist destruction by penicillinase, it is not effective against penicillinase-producing bacteria, particularly resistant staphylococci. All strains of *Pseudomonas* and most strains of *Klebsiella* and *Enterobacter* are resistant.

Disk Susceptibility Tests: Quantitative methods that require measurement of zone diameters give the most precise estimates of antibiotic susceptibility. One such procedure* has been recommended for use with disks for testing susceptibility to ampicillin-class antibiotics. Interpretations correlate diameters of the disk test with MIC values for Amoxicillin. With this procedure, a report from the laboratory of "susceptible" indicates that the infecting organism is likely to respond to therapy. A report of "resistant" indicates that the infecting organism is not likely to respond to therapy. A report of "intermediate susceptibility" suggests that the organism would be susceptible if high dosage is used, or if the infection is confined to tissues and fluids (e.g., urine), in which high antibiotic levels are attained.

INDICATIONS
Amoxicillin is indicated in the treatment of infections due to susceptible strains of the following:

Gram-negative organisms: H. influenzae, E. coli, P. mirabilis and *N. gonorrhoeae.*

Gram-positive organisms Streptococci (including *Streptococcus faecalis*), D. *pneumoniae* and nonpenicillinase-producing staphylococci.

Therapy may be instituted prior to obtaining results from bacteriological and susceptibility studies to determine the causative organisms and their susceptibility to Amoxicillin. Indicated surgical procedures should be performed.

UNLABELED USES
Amoxicillin is used alone or as an adjunct in the treatment of Lyme Disease (caused by infection with the spirochete, Borrelia burgdorferi infection) and for prophylaxis against bacterial endocarditis.

CONTRAINDICATIONS
A history of allergic reaction to any of the penicillins is a contraindication.

WARNINGS
SERIOUS AND OCCASIONALLY FATAL HYPERSENSITIVITY (ANAPHYLACTOID) REACTIONS HAVE BEEN REPORTED IN PATIENTS ON PENICILLIN THERAPY. ALTHOUGH ANAPHYLAXIS IS MORE FREQUENT FOLLOWING PARENTERAL THERAPY, IT HAS OCCURRED IN PATIENTS ON ORAL PENICILLINS. THESE REACTIONS ARE MORE LIKELY TO OCCUR IN INDIVIDUALS WITH A HISTORY OF SENSITIVITY TO MULTIPLE ALLERGENS. THERE HAVE BEEN REPORTS OF INDIVIDUALS WITH A HISTORY OF PENICILLIN HYPERSENSITIVITY WHO HAVE EXPERIENCED SEVERE REACTIONS WHEN TREATED WITH CEPHALOSPORINS. BEFORE THERAPY WITH ANY PENICILLIN, CAREFUL INQUIRY SHOULD BE MADE CONCERNING PREVIOUS HYPERSENSITIVITY REACTIONS TO PENICILLINS, CEPHALOSPORINS OR OTHER ALLERGENS. IF AN ALLERGIC REACTION OCCURS, APPROPRIATE THERAPY SHOULD BE INSTITUTED AND DISCONTINUANCE OF AMOXICILLIN THERAPY CONSIDERED. SERIOUS ANAPHYLACTOID REACTIONS REQUIRE IMMEDIATE EMERGENCY TREATMENT WITH EPINEPHRINE. OXYGEN, INTRAVENOUS STEROIDS AND AIRWAY MANAGEMENT, INCLUDING INTUBATION, SHOULD ALSO BE ADMINISTERED AS INDICATED.

Pseudomembranous colitis has been reported with nearly all antibacterial agents, including Amoxicillin and may range in severity from mild to life-threatening. Therefore, it is important to consider this diagnosis in patients who present with diarrhea subsequent to the administration of antibacterial agents.

Treatment with antibacterial agents alters the normal flora of the colon and may permit overgrowth of clostridia. Studies indicate that a toxin produced by *Clostridium difficile* is a primary cause of 'antibiotic-associated colitis.'

Mild cases of pseudomembranous colitis usually respond to drug discontinuation alone. In moderate to severe cases, consideration should be given to management with fluids and electrolytes, protein supplementation and treatment with an antibacterial drug clinically effective against *C. difficile* colitis.

USAGE IN PREGNANCY
Safety for use in pregnancy has not been established.

PRECAUTIONS
As with any potent drug, periodic assessment of renal, hepatic and hematopoietic function should be made during prolonged therapy. The possibility of superinfections with mycotic or bacterial pathogens should be kept in mind during therapy. If superinfections occur (usually involving *Enterobacter, Pseudomonas* or *Candida*), the drug should be discontinued and/or appropriate therapy instituted.

ADVERSE REACTIONS
As with other penicillins, it may be expected that untoward reactions will be essentially limited to sensitivity phenomena. They are more likely to occur in individuals who have previously demonstrated hypersensitivity to penicillins and in those with a history of allergy, asthma, hay fever or urticaria. The following adverse reactions have been reported as associated with the use of penicillins:

Gastrointestinal: Nausea, vomiting and diarrhea.

Hypersensitivity Reactions: Erythematous maculopapular rashes and urticaria have been reported.

Note: Urticaria, other skin rashes and serum-sickness-like reactions may be controlled with antihistamines and, if necessary, systemic corticosteroids. When-

ever such reactions occur, Amoxicillin should be discontinued unless, in the opinion of the physician, the condition being treated is life-threatening and amendable only to Amoxicillin therapy.

Liver: A moderate rise in serum glutamic oxaloacetic transaminase (SGOT) has been noted, but the significance of this finding is unknown.

Hemic and Lymphatic Systems: Anemia, thrombocytopenia, thrombocytopenic purpura, eosinophilia, leukopenia and agranulocytosis have been reported during therapy with penicillins. These reactions are usually reversible on discontinuation of therapy and are believed to be hypersensitivity phenomena.

Central Nervous System: Reversible hyperactivity, agitation, anxiety, insomnia, confusion, behavioral changes, and/or dizziness have been reported rarely.

DOSAGE AND ADMINISTRATION
Infections of the ear, nose and throat due to streptococci, pneumococci, nonpenicillinase-producing staphylococci and *H. influenzae;*

Infections of the genitourinary tract due to *E. coli, Proteus mirabilis* and *Streptococcus facealis;*

Infections of the skin and soft-tissues due to streptococci, susceptible staphylococci and *E. coli:*

USUAL DOSAGE
Adults: 250 mg every 8 hours.
   Children: 20 mg/kg/day in divided doses every 8 hours.
   Children weighing 20 kg or more should be dosed according to the adult recommendations.
   In severe infections or those caused by less susceptible organisms:
   500 mg every 8 hours for adults and 40 mg/kg/day in divided doses every 8 hours for children may be needed.

Infections of the lower respiratory tract due to streptococci, pneumococci, nonpenicillinase-producing staphylococci and *H. influenzae:*

USUAL DOSAGE:
Adults: 500 mg every 8 hours.
   Children: 40 mg/kg/day in divided doses every 8 hours.
   Children weighing 20 kg or more should be dosed according to the adult recommendations.

Gonorrhea, acute uncomplicated ano-genital and urethral infections due to *N. gonorrhoeae* (males and females):
USUAL DOSAGE:
Adults: 3 grams as a single oral dose.
   Prepubertal children: 50 mg/kg Amoxicillin combined with 25 mg/kg probenecid as a single dose.
   Note: SINCE PROBENECID IS CONTRAINDICATED IN CHILDREN UNDER 2 YEARS, THIS REGIMEN SHOULD NOT BE USED IN THESE CASES.
   Cases of gonorrhea with a suspected lesion of syphilis should have dark-field examinations before receiving Amoxicillin, and monthly serological tests for a minimum of 4 months. Larger doses may be required for stubborn or severe infections.
   The children's dosage is intended for individuals whose weight will not cause a dosage to be calculated greater than that recommended for adults.
   It should be recognized that in the treatment of chronic urinary tract infections, frequent bacteriological and clinical appraisals are necessary. Smaller doses than those recommended above should not be used. Even higher doses may be needed at times. In stubborn infections, therapy may be required for several weeks. It may be necessary to continue clinical and/or bacteriological follow-up for several months after cessation of therapy. Except for gonorrhea, treatment should be continued for a minimum of 48 to 72 hours beyond the time that the patient becomes asymptomatic or evidence of bacterial eradication has been obtained. It is recommended that there be at least 10 days' treatment for any infection caused by hemolytic streptococci to prevent the occurrence of acute rheumatic fever or glomerulonephritis.

DOSAGE AND ADMINISTRATION OF PEDIATRIC DROPS
Usual dosage for all indications except infections of the lower respiratory tract:
   Under 6 kg (13 lbs): 0.75 mL every 8 hours.
   6 to 7 kg (13 to 15 lbs): 1.0 mL every 8 hours.
   8 kg (16 to 18 lbs): 1.25 mL every 8 hours.
Infections of the lower respiratory tract:
   Under 6 kg (13 lbs): 1.25 mL every 8 hours.
   6 to 7 kg (13 to 15 lbs): 1.75 mL every 8 hours.
   8 kg (16 to 18 lbs): 2.25 mL every 8 hours.

Children weighing more than 8 kg (18 lbs) should receive the appropriate dose of the Oral Suspension 125 mg or 250 mg/5 mL.

After reconstitution, the required amount of suspension should be placed directly on the child's tongue for swallowing. Alternate means of administration are to add the required amount of suspension to formula, milk, fruit juice, water, ginger ale or cold drinks. These preparations should then be taken immediately. To be certain the child is receiving full dosage, such preparations should be consumed in entirety.

DIRECTIONS FOR MIXING ORAL SUSPENSION
Prepare suspension at time of dispensing as follows: Tap bottle until all powder flows freely. Add approximately ⅓ of the total amount of water for reconstitution (see table below) and shake vigorously to wet powder. Add remainder of the water and again shake vigorously.

---

* Bauer, A. W., Kirby, W. M. M., Sherris J. C., and Turck, M.: Antibiotic Testing by a Standardized Single Disc Method, Am. J. Clin. Pathol., 45:493, 1966. Standardized Disc Susceptibility Test, Federal Register 37:20527-29, 192.

◆ RATED THERAPEUTICALLY EQUIVALENT; ◇ THERAPEUTIC EQUIVALENCE UNCONFIRMED; ○ UNRATED

125 MG PER 5 ML

Bottle Size	Amount of Water Required for Reconstitution
80 mL	62 mL
100 mL	78 mL
150 mL	116 mL
Each teaspoonful (5 mL) will contain 125 mg Amoxicillin.	
125 mg unit dose	5 mL

250 MG PER 5 ML

Bottle Size	Amount of Water Required for Reconstitution
80 mL	59 mL
100 mL	74 mL
150 mL	111 mL
Each teaspoonful (5 mL) will contain 250 mg Amoxicillin.	
250 mg unit dose	5 mL

DIRECTIONS FOR MIXING PEDIATRIC DROPS

Prepare pediatric drops at time of dispensing as follows: Add the required amount of water (see table below) to the bottle and shake vigorously. Each mL of suspension will then contain Amoxicillin trihydrate equivalent to 50 mg Amoxicillin.

Bottle Size	Amount of Water Required for Reconstitution
15 mL	12 mL
30 mL	23 mL

NOTE: SHAKE BOTH ORAL SUSPENSION AND PEDIATRIC DROPS WELL BEFORE USING. Keep bottle tightly closed. Any unused portion of the reconstituted suspension must be discarded after 14 days. Refrigeration preferable, but not required.

HOW SUPPLIED
CAPSULE: 250 MG

AVERAGE UNIT PRICE (AVAILABLE SIZES)		GENERIC A-RATED AVERAGE PRICE (GAAP)	
BRAND	$0.21	100s	$20.81
GENERIC	$0.22	500s	$88.99
HCFA FUL (100s ea)	$0.08	1000s	$120.89

BRAND/MANUFACTURER	NDC	SIZE	AWP
◆ BRAND			
➤ AMOXIL: SK Beecham Pharm	00029-6006-30	100s	$21.60
	00029-6006-32	500s	$102.90
◆ GENERICS			
Novopharm	55953-0724-27	30s	$5.87
UDL	51079-0600-97	45s	$60.00
Raway	00686-3107-09	100s	$9.95
Novopharm	55953-0724-40	100s	$12.40
Rugby	00536-0070-01	100s	$12.53
Schein	00364-2040-01	100s	$15.00
Major	00904-2617-60	100s	$15.95
Mylan	00378-0204-01	100s	$16.33
Moore,H.L.	00839-6037-06	100s	$16.73
Martec	52555-0148-01	100s	$17.30
Geneva	00781-2020-01	100s	$19.80
SENOX: Seneca	47028-0053-01	100s	$19.95
Goldline	00182-1070-01	100s	$20.95
Biocraft	00332-3107-09	100s	$20.95
➤ WYMOX: Wyeth-Ayerst	00008-0559-01	100s	$21.05
URL	00677-0660-01	100s	$21.67
Du Pont Multi	00056-0153-70	100s	$21.79
Aligen	00405-4083-01	100s	$22.05
Lederle Std Prod	00005-3144-23	100s	$22.39
TRIMOX: Apothecon	00003-0101-50	100s	$23.89
TRIMOX: Apothecon	00003-0101-51	100s	$23.89
Warner Chilcott	00047-0730-24	100s	$24.76
Qualitest	00603-2266-21	100s	$24.97
Medirex	57480-0455-01	100s	$26.10
VHA Supply	00015-7278-73	100s	$33.25
Raway	00686-0600-20	100s ud	$12.25
Novopharm	55953-0724-01	100s ud	$15.29
Major	00904-2617-61	100s ud	$23.95
UDL	51079-0600-20	100s ud	$26.10
Goldline	00182-1070-89	100s ud	$26.50
VHA Supply	00015-7278-62	100s ud	$35.71
Novopharm	55953-0724-70	500s	$56.83
Schein	00364-2040-05	500s	$60.75
Rugby	00536-0070-04	500s	$61.12
Major	00904-2617-40	500s	$61.25
Geneva	00781-2020-05	500s	$73.62
Moore,H.L.	00839-6037-12	500s	$75.45
URL	00677-0660-05	500s	$75.50
Mylan	00378-0204-05	500s	$76.11
Martec	52555-0148-05	500s	$78.00
➤ WYMOX: Wyeth-Ayerst	00008-0559-02	500s	$94.50
Goldline	00182-1070-05	500s	$99.85
Biocraft	00332-3107-13	500s	$99.85
Du Pont Multi	00056-0153-85	500s	$101.95
Lederle Std Prod	00005-3144-31	500s	$106.64
Parmed	00349-0190-05	500s	$107.75
Aligen	00405-4083-02	500s	$110.12
TRIMOX: Apothecon	00003-0101-60	500s	$113.78

BRAND/MANUFACTURER	NDC	SIZE	AWP
Warner Chilcott	00047-0730-30	500s	$118.82
Qualitest	00603-2266-28	500s	$118.95
Novopharm	55953-0724-80	1000s	$107.98
Parmed	00349-0190-10	1000s	$133.80

CAPSULE: 500 MG

AVERAGE UNIT PRICE (AVAILABLE SIZES)		GENERIC A-RATED AVERAGE PRICE (GAAP)	
BRAND	$0.39	50s	$18.51
GENERIC	$0.36	100s	$36.29
HCFA FUL (100s ea)	$0.23	500s	$164.09
		1000s	$219.73

BRAND/MANUFACTURER	NDC	SIZE	AWP
◆ BRAND			
➤ AMOXIL: SK Beecham Pharm	00029-6007-30	100s	$40.40
	00029-6007-32	500s	$189.90
◆ GENERICS			
Novopharm	55953-0716-27	30s	$8.85
UDL	51079-0601-97	45s	$60.00
Raway	00686-3109-07	50s	$9.50
Novopharm	55953-0716-33	50s	$12.40
Schein	00364-2041-50	50s	$15.00
➤ Mylan	00378-0205-89	50s	$15.76
Moore,H.L.	00839-6038-04	50s	$16.19
Martec	52555-0149-00	50s	$16.70
Major	00904-2618-51	50s	$16.95
Rugby	00536-0080-06	50s	$17.10
➤ WYMOX: Wyeth-Ayerst	00008-0560-01	50s	$19.70
URL	00677-0661-02	50s	$20.25
Lederle Std Prod	00005-3145-18	50s	$20.94
➤ TRIMOX: Apothecon	00003-0109-45	50s	$22.33
Aligen	00405-4084-50	50s	$23.35
Goldline	00182-1071-19	50s	$23.35
➤ Biocraft	00332-3109-07	50s	$23.35
Qualitest	00603-2267-19	50s	$23.35
Novopharm	55953-0716-40	100s	$23.27
➤ Warner Chilcott	00047-0731-24	100s	$24.95
Aligen	00405-4084-01	100s	$30.67
URL	00677-0661-01	100s	$39.00
Geneva	00781-2613-01	100s	$39.00
Du Pont Multi	00056-0154-70	100s	$39.95
➤ TRIMOX: Apothecon	00003-0109-55	100s	$41.68
➤ TRIMOX: Apothecon	00003-0109-51	100s	$44.66
Medirex	57480-0456-01	100s	$49.00
Raway	00686-0601-20	100s ud	$19.00
Novopharm	55953-0716-01	100s ud	$26.15
Goldline	00182-1071-89	100s ud	$45.50
UDL	51079-0601-20	100s ud	$49.00
Rugby	00536-0080-02	250s	$85.46
Novopharm	55953-0716-70	500s	$110.77
Aligen	00405-4084-02	500s	$117.50
Schein	00364-2041-05	500s	$135.00
Major	00904-2618-40	500s	$145.10
➤ Mylan	00378-0205-05	500s	$145.88
Martec	52555-0149-05	500s	$146.90
Moore,H.L.	00839-6038-12	500s	$148.49
➤ Warner Chilcott	00047-0731-30	500s	$166.79
Rugby	00536-0080-05	500s	$170.91
Qualitest	00603-2267-28	500s	$172.88
URL	00677-0661-05	500s	$174.98
Geneva	00781-2613-05	500s	$175.00
➤ WYMOX: Wyeth-Ayerst	00008-0560-02	500s	$175.50
➤ TRIMOX: Apothecon	00003-0109-60	500s	$182.70
Goldline	00182-1071-05	500s	$184.48
➤ Biocraft	00332-3109-13	500s	$184.48
Du Pont Multi	00056-0154-85	500s	$194.50
Lederle Std Prod	00005-3145-31	500s	$196.85
Parmed	00349-0999-05	500s ud	$189.00
Novopharm	55953-0716-80	1000s	$210.46
Parmed	00349-0999-10	1000s	$229.00

For additional alternatives, turn to the section beginning on page 2859.

Amoxicillin with Clavulanate Potassium

DESCRIPTION

Amoxicillin/Clavulanate Potassium is an oral Antibacterial combination consisting of the semisynthetic antibiotic Amoxicillin and the β-lactamase inhibitor, clavulanate potassium (the potassium salt of clavulanic acid). Amoxicillin is an analog of ampicillin, derived from the basic penicillin nucleus, 6-aminopenicillanic acid. Chemically, Amoxicillin is D-(-)-α-amino-p-hydroxybenzyl-penicillin trihydrate.

Clavulanic acid is produced by the fermentation of *Streptomyces clavuligerus*. It is a β-lactam structurally related to the penicillins and possesses the ability to inactivate a wide variety of β-lactamases by blocking the active sites of these enzymes. Clavulanic acid is particularly active against the clinically important plasmid mediated β-lactamases frequently responsible for transferred drug resistance to penicillins and cephalosporins. Chemically clavulanate potassium is potassium Z-(3R, 5R)-2-(β-hydroxyethylidene) clavam-3-carboxylate.

Amoxicillin/Clavulanate Potassium 250 mg and 500 mg tablet contains 250 mg and 500 mg amoxicillin as the trihydrate, respectively, together with 125 mg clavulanic acid as the potassium salt. Each 125 mg chewable tablet and each teaspoonful (5 mL) of reconstituted Amoxicillin/Clavulanate Potassium 125 mg/5 mL oral suspension contain 125 mg amoxicillin and 31.25 mg clavulanic acid as the potassium salt while each 250 mg chewable tablet and each 5 mL of reconstituted Amoxicillin/Clavulanate Potassium 250 mg/5 mL oral suspension contain 250 mg amoxicillin and 62.5 mg clavulanic acid as the potassium salt.

Each Amoxicillin/Clavulanate Potassium tablet contains 0.63 mEq potassium. Each 125 mg chewable tablet and each 5 mL of reconstituted Amoxicillin/Clavulanate Potassium 125 mg/5 mL oral suspension contain 0.16 mEq Potassium. Each 250 mg chewable tablet and each 5 mL of reconstituted Amoxicillin/Clavulanate Potassium 250 mg/5 mL oral suspension contain 0.32 mEq Potassium.

CLINICAL PHARMACOLOGY

Amoxicillin and Clavulanate Potassium are well absorbed from the gastrointestinal tract after oral administration of Amoxicillin/Clavulanate Potassium. Amoxicillin/Clavulanate Potassium is stable in the presence of gastric acid and may be given without regard to meals.

Oral administration of 1 Amoxicillin/Clavulanate Potassium 250 mg or Amoxicillin/Clavulanate Potassium 500 mg tablet provides average peak serum concentrations 1 to 2 hours after dosing of 4.4 mcg/mL and 7.6 mcg/mL, respectively, for amoxicillin and 2.3 mcg/mL for clavulanic acid. The areas under the serum concentration curves obtained during the first 6 hours after dosing were 11.4 mcg/mL.hr. and 20.2 mcg/mL.hr. for amoxicillin, respectively, when 1 Amoxicillin/Clavulanate Potassium 250 mg or 500 mg tablet was administered to adult volunteers. The corresponding area under the serum concentration curve for clavulanic acid was 5 mcg/mL.hr. Oral administration of 5 mL of Amoxicillin/Clavulanate Potassium 250 mg/5 mL suspension or the equivalent dose of 10 mL Amoxicillin/Clavulanate Potassium 125 mg/5 mL suspension provides average peak serum concentrations approximately 1 hour after dosing of 6.9 mcg/mL for amoxicillin and 1.6 mcg/mL for clavulanic acid. The areas under the serum concentration curves obtained during the first 6 hours after dosing were 12.6 mcg/mL.hr. for amoxicillin and 2.9 mcg/mL.hr. for clavulanic acid when 5 mL of Amoxicillin/Clavulanate Potassium 250 mg/5 mL suspension or equivalent dose of 10 mL of Amoxicillin/Clavulanate Potassium 125 mg/5 mL suspension was administered to adult volunteers. One Amoxicillin/Clavulanate Potassium 250 mg chewable tablet or 2 Amoxicillin/Clavulanate Potassium 125 mg chewable tablets are equivalent to 5 mL of Amoxicillin/Clavulanate Potassium 250 mg/5 mL suspension and provide similar serum levels of amoxicillin and clavulanic acid.

Amoxicillin serum concentrations achieved with Amoxicillin/Clavulanate Potassium are similar to those produced by the oral administration of equivalent doses of amoxicillin alone. The half-life of amoxicillin after the oral administration of Amoxicillin/Clavulanate Potassium is 1.3 hours and that of clavulanic acid is 1.0 hour.

Approximately 50% to 70% of the amoxicillin and approximately 25% to 40% of the clavulanic acid are excreted unchanged in urine during the first 6 hours after administration of a single Amoxicillin/Clavulanate Potassium 250 mg or 500 mg tablet or 10 mL of Amoxicillin/Clavulanate Potassium 250 mg/5 mL suspension.

Concurrent administration of probenecid delays amoxicillin excretion but does not delay renal excretion of clavulanic acid.

Neither component in Amoxicillin/Clavulanate Potassium is highly protein-bound; clavulanic acid has been found to be approximately 30% bound to human serum and amoxicillin approximately 20% bound.

Amoxicillin diffuses readily into most body tissues and fluids with the exception of the brain and spinal fluids. The results of experiments involving the administration of clavulanic acid to animals suggest that this compound, like amoxicillin, is well distributed in body tissues.

Two hours after oral administration of a single 35 mg/kg dose of Amoxicillin/Clavulanate Potassium suspension to fasting children, average concentrations of 3.0 mcg/mL of amoxicillin and 0.5 mcg/mL of clavulanic acid were detected in middle ear effusions.

Microbiology: Amoxicillin is a semisynthetic antibiotic with a broad spectrum of bactericidal activity against many gram-positive and gram-negative microorganisms. Amoxicillin is, however, susceptible to degradation by β-lactamases and therefore the spectrum of activity does not include organisms which produce these enzymes. Clavulanic acid is a β-lactam, structurally related to the penicillins, which possesses the ability to inactivate a wide range of β-lactamase enzymes commonly found in microorganisms resistant to penicillins and cephalosporins. In particular, it has good activity against the clinically important plasmid mediated β-lactamases frequently responsible for transferred drug resistance.

The formulation of amoxicillin with clavulanic acid in Amoxicillin/Clavulanate Potassium protects amoxicillin from degradation by β-lactamase enzymes and effectively extends the antibiotic spectrum of amoxicillin to include many bacteria normally resistant to amoxicillin and other β-lactam antibiotics. Thus Amoxicillin/Clavulanate Potassium possesses the distinctive properties of a broad-spectrum antibiotic and a β-lactamase inhibitor.

While *in vitro* studies have demonstrated the susceptibility of most strains of the following organisms, clinical efficacy for infections other than those included in the *"Indications and Usage"* section has not been documented:

Gram-Positive Bacteria: Staphylococcus aureus (β-lactamase and non-β-lactamase producing), *Staphylococcus epidermidis* (β-lactamase and non-β-lactamase producing), *Staphylococcus saprophyticus* (β-lactamase and non-β-lactamase producing), *Streptococcus faecalis** (*Enterococcus*), *Streptococcus pneumoniae** (D. *pneumoniae*), *Streptococcus pyogenes**, *Streptococcus viridans**
  * These are non-β-lactamase-producing strains and therefore are susceptible to Amoxicillin alone.

Anaerobes: Clostridium species*, *Peptococcus* species*, *Peptostreptococcus* species*

Gram-Negative Bacteria: Hemophilus influenzae (β-lactamase and non-β-lactamase producing), *Moraxella (Branhamella) catarrhalis* (β-lactamase and non-β-lactamase producing); *Escherichia coli* (β-lactamase and non-β-lactamase producing), *Klebsiella* species (All known strains are β-lactamase producing), *Enterobacter* species (Although most strains of *Enterobacter* species are resistant *in vitro*, clinical efficacy has been demonstrated with Amoxicillin/Clavulanate Potassium in urinary tract infections caused by these organisms.), *Proteus mirabilis* (β-lactamase and non-β-lactamase producing), *Proteus vulgaris* (β-lactamase and non-β-lactamase producing), *Neisseria gonorrhoeae* (β-lactamase and non-β-lactamase producing), *Legionella* species (β-lactamase and non-β-lactamase producing).

Anaerobes: Bacteroides species, including *B. fragilis* (β-lactamase and non-β-lactamase producing).

SUSCEPTIBILITY TESTING

Diffusion Technique: For Kirby-Bauer method of susceptibility testing, a 30 mcg Amoxicillin/Clavulanate Potassium (20 mcg Amoxicillin + 10 mcg clavulanic acid) diffusion disk should be used. With this procedure, a report from the laboratory of "Susceptible" indicates that the infecting organism is likely to respond to Amoxicillin/Clavulanate Potassium therapy and a report of "Resistant" indicates that the infecting organism is not likely to respond to therapy. An "intermediate susceptibility" report suggests that the infecting organism would be susceptible to Amoxicillin/Clavulanate Potassium if the higher dosage is used or if the infection is confined to tissues or fluids (e.g., urine) in which high antibiotic levels are attained.

Dilution Techniques: Broth or agar dilution methods may be used to determine the minimal inhibitory concentration (MIC) value for susceptibility of bacterial isolates to Amoxicillin/Clavulanate Potassium. Tubes should be inoculated to contain 10^4 to 10^5 organisms/mL or plates "spotted" with 10^3 to 10^4 organisms. The recommended dilution method employs a constant Amoxicillin/clavulanic acid ratio of 2 to 1 in all tubes with increasing concentrations of Amoxicillin. MICs are reported in terms of Amoxicillin concentration in the presence of clavulanic acid at a constant 2 parts Amoxicillin to 1 part clavulanic acid. (See related table).

INDICATIONS AND USAGE

Amoxicillin/Clavulanate Potassium is indicated in the treatment of infections caused by susceptible strains of the designated organisms in the conditions listed below:

Lower Respiratory Tract Infections—caused by β-lactamase-producing strains of *Hemophilus influenzae* and *Moraxella (Branhamella) catarrhalis.*

Otitis Media—caused by β-lactamase-producing strains of *Hemophilus influenzae* and *Moraxella (Branhamella) catarrhalis.*

Sinusitis—caused by β-lactamase-producing strains of *Hemophilus influenzae* and *Moraxella (Branhamella) catarrhalis.*

Skin and Skin Structure Infections—caused by β-lactamase-producing strains of *Staphylococcus aureus, Escherichia coli* and *Klebsiella* spp.

Urinary Tract Infections—caused by β-lactamase-producing strains of *Escherichia coli, Klebsiella* spp. and *Enterobacter* spp.

While Amoxicillin/Clavulanate Potassium is indicated only for the conditions listed above, infections caused by ampicillin-susceptible organisms are also amenable to Amoxicillin/Clavulanate Potassium treatment due to its Amoxicillin content. Therefore, mixed infections caused by ampicillin-susceptible organisms and β-lactamase-producing organisms susceptible to Amoxicillin/Clavulanate Potassium should not require the addition of another antibiotic.

Bacteriological studies, to determine the causative organisms and their susceptibility to Amoxicillin/Clavulanate Potassium should be performed together with any indicated surgical procedures. Therapy may be instituted prior to obtaining the results from bacteriological and susceptibility studies to determine the causative organisms and their susceptibility to Amoxicillin/Clavulanate Potassium when there is reason to believe the infection may involve any of the β-lactamase-producing organisms listed above. Once the results are known, therapy should be adjusted, if appropriate.

UNLABELED USES

Amoxicillin/Clavulanate Potassium is used in the treatment of chancroid secondary to beta-lactamase-producing *H. Ducreyi*, Gonorrhea, and otorhinolaryngological infections.

CONTRAINDICATIONS

A history of allergic reactions to any penicillin is a contraindication.

WARNINGS

SERIOUS AND OCCASIONALLY FATAL HYPERSENSITIVITY (ANAPHYLACTOID) REACTIONS HAVE BEEN REPORTED IN PATIENTS ON PENICILLIN THERAPY. ALTHOUGH ANAPHYLAXIS IS MORE FRE-

QUENT FOLLOWING PARENTERAL THERAPY, IT HAS OCCURRED IN PATIENTS ON ORAL PENICILLINS. THESE REACTIONS ARE MORE LIKELY TO OCCUR IN INDIVIDUALS WITH A HISTORY OF PENICILLIN HYPERSENSITIVITY AND/OR A HISTORY OF SENSITIVITY TO MULTIPLE ALLERGENS. THERE HAVE BEEN REPORTS OF INDIVIDUALS WITH A HISTORY OF PENICILLIN HYPERSENSITIVITY WHO HAVE EXPERIENCED SEVERE REACTIONS WHEN TREATED WITH CEPHALOSPORINS. BEFORE INITIATING THERAPY WITH ANY PENICILLIN, CAREFUL INQUIRY SHOULD BE MADE CONCERNING PREVIOUS HYPERSENSITIVITY REACTIONS TO PENICILLINS, CEPHALOSPORINS OR OTHER ALLERGENS. IF AN ALLERGIC REACTION OCCURS, AMOXICILLIN/CLAVULANATE POTASSIUM SHOULD BE DISCONTINUED AND THE APPROPRIATE THERAPY INSTITUTED. SERIOUS ANAPHYLACTOID REACTIONS REQUIRE IMMEDIATE EMERGENCY TREATMENT WITH EPINEPHRINE. OXYGEN, INTRAVENOUS STEROIDS AND AIRWAY MANAGEMENT, INCLUDING INTUBATION, SHOULD ALSO BE ADMINISTERED AS INDICATED.

Pseudomembranous colitis has been reported with nearly all antibacterial agents, including Amoxicillin/Clavulanate Potassium and has ranged in severity from mild to life-threatening. Therefore, it is important to consider this diagnosis in patients who present with diarrhea subsequent to the administration of antibacterial agents.

Treatment with antibacterial agents alters the normal flora of the colon and may permit overgrowth of clostridia. Studies indicate that a toxin produced by Clostridium difficile is 1 primary cause of "antibiotic associated colitis."

Mild cases of pseudomembranous colitis usually respond to drug discontinuation alone. In moderate to severe cases, consideration should be given to management with fluids and electrolytes, protein supplementation and treatment with an antibacterial drug clinically effective against C. difficile colitis.

PRECAUTIONS

General: While Amoxicillin/Clavulanate Potassium possesses the characteristic low toxicity of the penicillin group of antibiotics, periodic assesment of organ system functions, including renal, hepatic and hematopoietic function, is advisable during prolonged therapy.

A high percentage of patients with mononucleosis who receive ampicillin develop a skin rash. Thus, ampicillin class antibiotics should not be administered to patients with mononucleosis.

The possibility of superinfections with mycotic or bacterial pathogens should be kept in mind during therapy. If superinfections occur (usually involving Pseudomonas or Candida), the drug should be discontinued and/or appropriate therapy instituted.

Drug Interactions: Probenecid decreases the renal tubular secretion of Amoxicillin. Concurrent use with Amoxicillin/Clavulanate Potassium may result in increased and prolonged blood levels of Amoxicillin.

The concurrent administration of allopurinol and ampicillin increases substantially the incidence of rashes in patients receiving both drugs as compared to patients receiving ampicillin alone. It is not known whether this potentiation of ampicillin rashes is due to allopurinol or the hyperuricemia present in these patients. There are no data with Amoxicillin/Clavulanate Potassium and allopurinol administered concurrently.

Amoxicillin/Clavulanate Potassium should not be co-administered with disulfiram.

Drug/Laboratory Test Interactions: Oral administration of Amoxicillin/Clavulanate Potassium will result in high urine concentrations of Amoxicillin. High urine concentrations of ampicillin may result in false-positive reactions when testing for the presence of glucose in urine using Clinitest®, Benedict's Solution or Fehling's Solution. Since this effect may also occur with Amoxicillin and therefore Amoxicillin/Clavulanate Potassium, it is recommended that glucose tests based on enzymatic glucose oxidase reactions (such as Clinistix® or Tes-Tape®) be used.

Following administration of ampicillin to pregnant women a transient decrease in plasma concentration of total conjugated estriol, estriol-glucuronide, conjugated estrone and estradiol has been noted. This effect may also occur with Amoxicillin and therefore Amoxicillin/Clavulanate Potassium.

Carcinogenesis, Mutagenesis, Impairment of Fertility: Long-term studies in animals have not been performed to evaluate carcinogenic or mutagenic potential.

Pregnancy (Category B): Reproduction studies have been performed in mice and rats at doses up to ten (10) times the human dose and have revealed no evidence of impaired fertility or harm to the fetus due to Amoxicillin/Clavulanate Potassium. There are, however, no adequate and well-controlled studies in pregnant women. Because animal reproduction studies are not always predictive of human response, this drug should be used during pregnancy only if clearly needed.

Labor and Delivery: Oral ampicillin class antibiotics are generally poorly absorbed during labor. Studies in guinea pigs have shown that intravenous administration of ampicillin decreased the uterine tone, frequency of contractions, height of contractions and duration of contractions. However, it is not known whether the use of Amoxicillin/Clavulanate Potassium in humans during labor or delivery has immediate or delayed adverse effects on the fetus, prolongs the duration of labor, or increases the likelihood that forceps delivery or other obstetrical intervention or resuscitation of the newborn will be necessary.

Nursing Mothers: Ampicillin class antibiotics are excreted in the milk; therefore, caution should be exercised when Amoxicillin/Clavulanate Potassium is administered to a nursing woman.

ADVERSE REACTIONS

Amoxicillin/Clavulanate Potassium is generally well tolerated. The majority of side effects observed in clinical trials were of a mild and transient nature and less than 3% of patients discontinued therapy because of drug-related side effects. The most frequently reported adverse effects were diarrhea/loose stools (9%), nausea (3%), skin rashes and urticaria (3%), vomiting (1%) and vaginitis (1%). The overall incidence of side effects, and in particular diarrhea, increased with the higher recommended dose. Other less frequently reported reactions include: abdominal discomfort, flatulence and headache.

The following adverse reactions have been reported for ampicillin class antibiotics:

Gastrointestinal: Diarrhea, nausea, vomiting, indigestion, gastritis, stomatitis, glossitis, black "hairy" tongue, enterocolitis and pseudomembranous colitis. Onset of pseudomembranous colitis symptoms may occur during or after antibiotic treatment (see "Warnings").

Hypersensitivity Reactions: Skin rashes, urticaria, angioedema, serum sickness-like reactions (urticaria or skin rash accompanied by arthritis, arthralgia, myalgia and frequently fever), erythema multiforme (rarely Stevens-Johnson Syndrome) and an occasional case of exfoliative dermatitis have been reported. These reactions may be controlled with antihistamines and, if necessary, systemic corticosteroids. Whenever such reactions occur, the drug should be discontinued, unless the opinion of the physician dictates otherwise. Serious and occasional fatal hypersensitivity (anaphylactic) reactions can occur with oral penicillin (see "Warnings").

Liver: A moderate rise in AST (SGOT) and/or ALT (SGPT) has been noted in patients treated with ampicillin class antibiotics but the significance of these findings is unknown. Hepatic dysfunction, including increases in serum transaminases (AST and/or ALT), serum bilirubin and/or alkaline phosphatase, has been infrequently reported with Amoxicillin/Clavulanate Potassium. The histologic findings on liver biopsy have consisted of predominantly cholestatic, hepatocellular or mixed cholestatic-hepatocellular changes. The onset of signs/symptoms of hepatic dysfunction may occur during or after therapy. Complete resolution has occurred with time.

Hemic and Lymphatic Systems: Anemia, thrombocytopenia, thrombocytopenic purpura, eosinophilia, leukopenia and agranulocytosis have been reported during therapy with penicillins. These reactions are usually reversible on discontinuation of therapy and are believed to be hypersensitivity phenomena. A slight thrombocytosis was noted in less than 1% of the patients treated with Amoxicillin/Clavulanate Potassium.

Central Nervous System: Reversible hyperactivity, agitation, anxiety, insomnia, confusion, behavioral changes, and/or dizziness have been reported rarely.

OVERDOSAGE

Amoxicillin may be removed from circulation by hemodialysis.

RECOMMENDED AMOXICILLIN/CLAVULANATE POTASSIUM SUSCEPTIBILITY RANGES[1,2]

ORGANISMS	RESISTANT	INTERMEDIATE	SUSCEPTIBLE	MIC[3] CORRELATES mcg/mL R	S
Gram-Negative Enteric Bacteria	≤ 13 mm	14 to 17 mm	≥ 18 mm	≥ 32/16	≤ 8/4
Staphylococcus[4] and	≤ 19mm	—	≥ 20 mm		≤ 4/2
Hemophilus spp.					≤ 4/2

[1] The non-β-lactamase-producing organisms which are normally susceptible to ampicillin, such as streptococci, will have similar zone sizes as for ampicillin disks.
[2] The quality control cultures should have the following assigned daily ranges for Amoxicillin/Clavulanate Potassium:

		Disks	MIC Range (mcg/mL)
E. coli	(ATCC 25922)	19 to 25 mm	2/1 to 8/4
S. aureus	(ATCC 25923)	28 to 36 mm	0.25/0.12 to 0.5/0.25
E. coli	(ATCC 35218)	18 to 22 mm	4/2 to 16/8

[3] Expressed as concentration of Amoxicillin/clavulanic acid.
[4] Organisms which show susceptibility to Amoxicillin/Clavulanate Potassium but are resistant to methicillin/oxacillin should be considered resistant.

The molecular weight, degree of protein binding and pharmacokinetic profile of clavulanic acid together with information from a single patient with renal insufficiency all suggest that this compound may also be removed by hemodialysis.

DOSAGE AND ADMINISTRATION

The Amoxicillin/Clavulanate Potassium 250 mg tablet and the 250 mg chewable tablet do *not* contain the same amount of clavulanic acid (as the potassium salt). The Amoxicillin/Clavulanate Potassium 250 mg tablet contains 125 mg of clavulanic acid, whereas the 250 mg chewable tablet contains 62.5 mg of clavulanic acid. Therefore, the Amoxicillin/Clavulanate Potassium 250 mg tablet and the 250 mg chewable tablet should *not* be substituted for each other, as they are not interchangeable.

Since both the Amoxicillin/Clavulanate Potassium 250 mg and 500 mg tablets contain the same amount of clavulanic acid (125 mg, as the potassium salt), 2 Amoxicillin/Clavulanate Potassium 250 mg tablets are not equivalent to 1 Amoxicillin/Clavulanate Potassium 500 mg tablet. Therefore, 2 Amoxicillin/Clavulanate Potassium 250 mg tablets should not be substituted for 1 Amoxicillin/Clavulanate Potassium 500 mg tablet for treatment of more severe infections.

DOSAGE:

Adults: The usual adult dose is 1 Amoxicillin/Clavulanate Potassium 250 mg tablet every 8 hours. For more severe infections and infections of the respiratory tract, the dose should be 1 Amoxicillin/Clavulanate Potassium 500 mg tablet every 8 hours.

Children: The usual dose is 20 mg/kg/day, based on Amoxicillin component, in divided doses every 8 hours. For otitis media, sinusitis and lower respiratory tract infections, the dose should be 40 mg/kg/day, based on the Amoxicillin component, in divided doses every 8 eight hours. Severe infections should be treated with the higher recommended dose. Children weighing 40 kg and more should be dosed according to the adult recommendations.

Due to the different Amoxicillin to clavulanic acid ratios in the Amoxicillin/Clavulanate Potassium 250 mg tablet (250/125) versus the Amoxicillin/Clavulanate Potassium 250 mg chewable tablet (250/62.5), the Amoxicillin/Clavulanate Potassium 250 mg tablet should not be used until the child weighs at least 40 kg and more.

DIRECTIONS FOR MIXING ORAL SUSPENSION

Prepare a suspension at time of dispensing as follows: Tap bottle until all the powder flows freely. Add approximately ⅔ of the total amount of water for reconstitution (see table below) and shake vigorously to suspend powder. Add remainder of the water and again shake vigorously.

AMOXICILLIN/CLAVULANATE POTASSIUM 125 MG/5 ML SUSPENSION

Bottle Size	Amount of Water Required for Reconstitution
75 mL	67 mL
150 mL	134 mL

Each teaspoonful (5 mL) will contain 125 mg Amoxicillin and 31.25 mg of clavulanic acid as the potassium salt.

AMOXICILLIN/CLAVULANATE POTASSIUM 250 MG/5 ML SUSPENSION

Bottle Size	Amount of Water Required for Reconstitution
75 mL	65 mL
150 mL	130 mL

Each teaspoonful (5 mL) will contain 250 mg Amoxicillin and 62.5 mg of clavulanic acid as the potassium salt.

NOTE: SHAKE ORAL SUSPENSION WELL BEFORE USING.

Reconstituted suspension must be stored under refrigeration and discarded after 10 days.

Administration: The absorption of Amoxicillin/Clavulanate Potassium is unaffected by food. Therefore, Amoxicillin/Clavulanate Potassium may be administered without regard to meals.

HOW SUPPLIED
CHEW TABLET: 125 MG-31.25 MG

BRAND/MANUFACTURER	NDC	SIZE	AWP
○ BRAND			
▶ AUGMENTIN: SK Beecham Pharm	00029-6073-47	30s	$26.25

CHEW TABLET: 250 MG-62.5 MG

BRAND/MANUFACTURER	NDC	SIZE	AWP
○ BRAND			
▶ AUGMENTIN: SK Beecham Pharm	00029-6074-47	30s	$50.00

POWDER FOR RECONSTITUTION: 125 MG-31.25 MG/5ML

BRAND/MANUFACTURER	NDC	SIZE	AWP
○ BRAND			
AUGMENTIN: SK Beecham Pharm	00029-6085-39	75 ml	$13.40
	00029-6085-22	150 ml	$26.25

POWDER FOR RECONSTITUTION: 250 MG-62.5 MG/5 ML

BRAND/MANUFACTURER	NDC	SIZE	AWP
○ BRAND			
AUGMENTIN: SK Beecham Pharm	00029-6090-39	75 ml	$25.55
	00029-6090-22	150 ml	$50.00

TABLETS: 250 MG-125 MG

BRAND/MANUFACTURER	NDC	SIZE	AWP
○ BRAND			
▶ AUGMENTIN: SK Beecham Pharm	00029-6075-27	30s	$55.95
	00029-6075-31	100s ud	$191.30

TABLETS: 500 MG-125 MG

BRAND/MANUFACTURER	NDC	SIZE	AWP
○ BRAND			
▶ AUGMENTIN: SK Beecham Pharm	00029-6080-27	30s	$78.00
	00029-6080-31	100s ud	$266.40

Amoxil SEE AMOXICILLIN

Amphetamine

> AMPHETAMINES HAVE A HIGH POTENTIAL FOR ABUSE. THEY SHOULD THUS BE TRIED ONLY IN WEIGHT REDUCTION PROGRAMS FOR PATIENTS IN WHOM ALTERNATIVE THERAPY HAS BEEN INEFFECTIVE. ADMINISTRATION OF AMPHETAMINES FOR PROLONGED PERIODS OF TIME IN OBESITY MAY LEAD TO DRUG DEPENDENCE AND MUST BE AVOIDED. PARTICULAR ATTENTION SHOULD BE PAID TO THE POSSIBILITY OF SUBJECTS OBTAINING AMPHETAMINES FOR NON-THERAPEUTIC USE OR DISTRIBUTION TO OTHERS, AND THE DRUGS SHOULD BE PRESCRIBED OR DISPENSED SPARINGLY.

DESCRIPTION

A single entity amphetamine product combining the neutral sulfate salts of dextroamphetamine and amphetamine, with the dextro isomer of Amphetamine saccharate and d, 1 Amphetamine aspartate.

Each Tablet Contains:	10 mg.	20 mg.
Dextroamphetamine Saccharate	2.5 mg.	5 mg.
Amphetamine Aspartate	2.5 mg.	5 mg.
Dextroamphetamine Sulfate	2.5 mg.	5 mg.
Amphetamine Sulfate	2.5 mg.	5 mg.

Following is its chemical structure:

$$\left[\bigcirc \begin{array}{c} CH_2\ CHNH_2 \\ | \\ CH_3 \end{array} \right]_2$$

ACTIONS

Amphetamines are non-catecholamine sympathomimetic amines with CNS stimulant activity. Peripheral actions include elevation of systolic and diastolic blood pressures and weak bronchodilator and respiratory stimulant action. Drugs of this class used in obesity are commonly known as "anorectics" or "anorexigenics". It has not been established, however, that the action of such drugs in treating obesity is primarily one of appetite suppression. Other central nervous system actions, or metabolic effect, may be involved, for example.

Adult obese subjects instructed in dietary management and treated with "anorectic" drugs, lose more weight on the average than those treated with placebo and diet, as determined in relatively short-term clinical trials.

The magnitude of increased weight loss of drug-treated patients over placebo-treated patients is only a fraction of a pound a week. The rate of weight loss is greater in the first weeks of therapy for both drug and placebo subjects and tends to decrease in succeeding weeks. The origins of the increased weight loss due to the various possible drug effects are not established. The amount of weight loss associated with the use of an "anorectic" drug varies from trial to trial, and the increased weight loss appears to be related in part to variables other than the drug prescribed, such as the physician-investigator, the population treated, and the diet prescribed. Studies do not permit conclusions as to the relative importance of the drug and non-drug factors on weight loss. The natural history of obesity is measured in years, whereas the studies cited are restricted to a few weeks duration, thus, the total impact of drug-induced weight loss over that of diet alone must be considered clinically limited.

There is neither specific evidence which clearly establishes the mechanism whereby Amphetamine produces mental and behavioral effects in children, nor conclusive evidence regarding how these effects relate to the condition of the central nervous system.

◆ RATED THERAPEUTICALLY EQUIVALENT; ◇ THERAPEUTIC EQUIVALENCE UNCONFIRMED; ○ UNRATED

INDICATIONS

In Attention Deficit Disorder with Hyperactivity: Amphetamine is indicated as an integral part of a total treatment program which typically includes other remedial measures (psychological, educational, social) for a stabilizing effect in children with behavioral syndrome characterized by the following group of developmentally inappropriate symptoms: moderate to severe distractibility, short attention span, hyperactivity, emotional lability, and impulsivity. The diagnosis of the syndrome should not be made with finality when these symptoms are only of comparatively recent origin. Nonlocalizing (soft) neurological signs, learning disability and abnormal EEG may or may not be present, and a diagnosis of central nervous system dysfunction may or may not be warranted.

Exogenous Obesity: as a short-term (a few weeks) adjunct in a regimen of weight reduction based on caloric restriction, for patients refractory to alternative therapy, e.g., repeated diets, group programs, and other drugs. The limited usefulness of Amphetamines (see *"Actions"*) should be weighed against possible risks inherent in use of the drug, such as those described below.

Narcolepsy

UNLABELED USES

Amphetamines are used as an adjunct in the treatment of psychiatric disorders, including Obsessive-Compulsive Disorder and Resistant Depression.

CONTRAINDICATIONS

Advanced arteriosclerosis, symptomatic cardiovascular disease, moderate to severe hypertension, hyperthyroidism, known hypersensitivity or idiosyncrasy to the sympathomimetic amines, glaucoma.

Agitated states.

Patients with a history of drug abuse.

During or within 14 days following the administration of monoamine oxidase inhibitors (hypertensive crises may result).

WARNINGS

When tolerance to the "anorectic" effect develops, the recommended dose should not be exceeded in an attempt to increase the effect; rather, the drug should be discontinued. Clinical experience suggests that in psychotic children, administration of Amphetamine may exacerbate symptoms of behavior disturbance and thought disorder. Data are inadequate to determine whether chronic administration of Amphetamine may be associated with growth inhibition: therefore, growth should be monitored during treatment.

Usage in Nursing Mothers: Amphetamines are excreted in human milk. Mothers taking Amphetamines should be advised to refrain from nursing.

PRECAUTION

General: Caution is to be exercised in prescribing Amphetamines for patients with even mild hypertension.

The least amount feasible should be prescribed or dispensed at one time in order to minimize the possibility of overdosage.

Certain brands of Amphetamines contain FD&C Yellow #6, which may cause allergic-type reactions (including bronchial asthma) in certain susceptible individuals. Although the overall incidence of FD&C Yellow #6 sensitivity in the general population is low, it is frequently seen in patients who also have aspirin hypersensitivity.

Information for Patients: Amphetamines may impair the ability of the patient to engage in potentially hazardous activities such as operating machinery or vehicles; the patient should therefore be cautioned accordingly.

Drug Interactions: Acidifying agents—Gastrointestinal acidifying agents (guanethidine, reserpine, glutamic acid HCl, ascorbic acid, fruit juices, etc.) lower absorption of Amphetamines.

Urinary acidifying agents (ammonium chloride, sodium acid phosphate, etc.) increase the concentration of the ionized species of the Amphetamine molecule, thereby increasing urinary excretion. Both groups of agents lower blood levels and efficacy of Amphetamines.

Adrenergic blockers—Adrenergic blockers are inhibited by Amphetamines.

Alkalinizing agents—Gastrointestinal alkalinizing agents (sodium bicarbonate, etc.) increase absorption of Amphetamines. Urinary alkalinizing agents (acetazolamide, some thiazides) increase the concentration of the non-ionized species of the Amphetamine molecule, thereby decreasing urinary excretion. Both groups of agents increase blood levels and therefore potentiate the actions of Amphetamines.

Antidepressants, tricyclic—Amphetamines may enhance the activity of tricyclic or sympathomimetic agents; d-amphetamine with desipramine or protriptyline and possibly other tricyclics cause striking and sustained increases in the concentration of d-amphetamine in the brain; cardiovascular effects can be potentiated.

MAO inhibitors—MAOI antidepressants, as well as a metabolite of furazolidone, slow Amphetamine metabolism. This slowing potentiates, Amphetamines increasing their effect on the release of norepinephrine and other monoamines from adrenergic nerve endings; this can cause headaches and other signs of hypertensive crisis. A variety of neurological toxic effects and malignant hyperpyrexia can occur, sometimes with fatal results.

Antihistamines—Amphetamines—Amphetamines may counteract the sedative effect of antihistamines.

Antihypertensives—Amphetamines may antagonize the hypotensive effects of antihypertensives. Chlorpromazine—Chlorpromazine blocks dopamine and norepinephrine reuptake, thus inhibiting the central stimulant effects of Amphetamines, and can be used to treat Amphetamine poisoning.

Ethosuximide—Amphetamines may delay intestinal absorption of ethosuximide.

Haloperidol—Haloperidol blocks dopamine and norepinephrine reuptake, thus inhibiting the central stimulant effects of Amphetamines.

Lithium carbonate—The antiobesity and stimulatory effects of Amphetamines may be inhibited by lithium carbonate.

Meperidine—Amphetamines potentiate the analgesic effect of meperidine.

Methenamine therapy—Urinary excretion of Amphetamines is increased, and efficacy is reduced, by acidifying agents used in methenamine therapy.

Norepinephrine—Amphetamines enhance the adrenergic effect of norepinephrine.

Phenobarbital—Amphetamines may delay intestinal absorption of phenobarbital; co-administration of phenobarbital may produce a synergistic anticonvulsant action.

Phenytoin—Amphetamines may delay intestinal absorption of phenytoin; co-administration of phenytoin may produce a synergistic anticonvulsant action.

Propoxyphene—In cases of propoxyphene overdosage, amphetamine CNS stimulation is potentiated and fatal convulsions can occur.

Veratrum alkaloids—Amphetamines inhibit the hypotensive effect of veratrum alkaloids.

DRUG/LABORATORY TEST INTERACTIONS:

■ Amphetamines can cause a significant elevation in plasma corticosteroid levels. This increase is greatest in the evening.

■ Amphetamines may interfere with urinary steroid determinations.

Carcinogenesis/Mutagenesis: Mutagenicity studies and long-term studies in animals to determine the carcinogenic potential of Amphetamine, have not been performed.

Pregnancy—Teratogenic Effects: Pregnancy Category C. Amphetamine has been shown to have embryotoxic and teratogenic effects when administered to A/Jax mice and C57BL mice in doses approximately 41 times the maximum human dose. Embryotoxic effects were not seen in New Zealand white rabbits given the drug in doses 7 times the human dose nor in rats given 12.5 times the maximum human dose. There are no adequate and well-controlled studies in pregnant women. Amphetamine should be used during pregnancy only if the potential benefit justifies the potential risk to the fetus.

Nonteratogenic Effects: Infants born to mothers dependent on Amphetamines have an increased risk of premature delivery and low birth weight. Also, these infants may experience symptoms of withdrawal as demonstrated by dysphoria, including agitation, and significant lassitude.

Pediatric Use: Long-term effects of Amphetamines in children have not been well established. Amphetamines are not recommended for use as anorectic agents in children under 12 years of age, or in children under 3 years of age with Attention Deficit Disorder with Hyperactivity described under *"Indications and Usage"*.

Clinical experience suggests that in psychotic children, administration of Amphetamines may exacerbate symptoms of behavior disturbance and thought disorder.

Amphetamines have been reported to exacerbate motor and phonic tics and Tourette's syndrome.

Therefore, clinical evaluation for tics and Tourette's syndrome in children and their families should precede use of stimulant medications.

Data are inadequate to determine whether chronic administration of Amphetamines may be associated with growth inhibition; therefore, growth should be monitored during treatment.

Drug treatment is not indicated in all cases of Attention Deficit Disorder with Hyperactivity and should be considered only in light of the complete history and evaluation of the child. The decision to prescribe Amphetamines should depend on the physician's assessment of the chronicity and severity of the child's symptoms and their appropriateness for his/her age. Prescription should not depend solely on the presence of one or more of the behavioral characteristics.

When these symptoms are associated with acute stress reactions, treatment with Amphetamines is usually not indicated.

ADVERSE REACTIONS

Cardiovascular: Palpitations, tachycardia, elevation of blood pressure.

Central Nervous System: Psychotic episodes at recommended doses (rare), overstimulation, restlessness, dizziness, insomnia, euphoria, dyskinesia, dysphoria, tremor, headache, exacerbation of motor and phonic tics and Tourette's syndrome.

Gastrointestinal: Dryness of the mouth, unpleasant taste, diarrhea, constipation, other gastrointestinal disturbances. Anorexia and weight loss may occur as undesirable effects when Amphetamines are used for other than the anorectic effect.

Allergic: Urticaria.

Endocrine: Impotence, changes in libido.

DRUG ABUSE AND DEPENDENCE

Dextroamphetamine sulfate is a Schedule II controlled substance.

Amphetamines have been extensively abused. Tolerance, extreme psychological dependence, and severe social disability have occurred. There are reports of patients who have increased the dosage to many times that recommended. Abrupt cessation following prolonged high dosage administration results in extreme fatigue and mental depression; changes are also noted on the sleep EEG. Manifestations of chronic intoxication with Amphetamines include severe dermatoses, marked insomnia, irritability, hyperactivity, and personality changes. The most severe manifestation of chronic intoxication is psychosis, often clinically indistinguishable from schizophrenia. This is rare with oral Amphetamines.

OVERDOSAGE

Individual patient response to Amphetamines varies widely. While toxic symptoms occasionally occur as an idiosyncrasy at doses as low as 2 mg., they are rare with doses of less than 15 mg; 30 mg. can produce severe reactions, yet doses of 400 to 500 mg. are not necessarily fatal.

In rats, the oral LD_{50} of dextroamphetamine sulfate is 96.8 mg./kg.

SYMPTOMS—Manifestations of acute overdosage with Amphetamines include restlessness, tremor, hyperreflexia rapid respiration, confusion, assaultiveness, hallucinations, panic states, hyperpyrexia and rhabdomolysis.

Fatigue and depression usually follow the central stimulation.

Cardiovascular effects include arrhythmias, hypertension or hypotension and circulatory collapse.

Gastrointestinal symptoms include nausea, vomiting, diarrhea, and abdominal cramps. Fatal poisoning is usually preceded by convulsions and coma.

TREATMENT

Management of acute Amphetamine intoxication is largely symptomatic and includes gastric lavage and sedation with a barbiturate. Experience with hemodialysis or peritoneal dialysis is inadequate to permit recommendation in this regard. Acidification of the urine increases Amphetamine excretion. If acute, severe hypertension complicates Amphetamine overdosage, administration of intravenous phentolamine has been suggested. However, a gradual drop in blood pressure will usually result when sufficient sedation has been achieved. Chlorpromazine antagonizes the central stimulant effects of Amphetamines and can be used to treat Amphetamine intoxication.

Saline cathartics are useful for hastening the evacuation of pellets that have not already released medication.

DOSAGE AND ADMINISTRATION

Regardless of indication, Amphetamines should be administered at the lowest effective dosage and should be individually adjusted. Late evening doses should be avoided because of the resulting insomnia.

Narcolepsy: Usual dose 5 to 60 milligrams per day in divided doses, depending on the individual patient response. Narcolepsy seldom occurs in children under 12 years of age; however, when it does, dextroamphetamine sulfate, may be used. The suggested initial dose for patients aged 6–12 is 5 mg. daily; daily dose may be raised in increments of 5 mg. at weekly intervals until optimal response is obtained. In patients 12 years of age and older, start with 10 mg. daily; daily dosage may be raised in increments of 10 mg. at weekly intervals until optimal response is obtained. If bothersome adverse reactions appear (e.g., insomnia or anorexia), dosage should be reduced. Give first dose on awakening; additional doses (1 or 2) at intervals of 4 to 6 hours.

Attention Deficit Disorder with Hyperactivity: Not recommended for children under 3 years of age.

In children from 3 to 5 years of age, start with 2.5 mg. daily, daily dosage may be raised in increments of 2.5 mg. at weekly intervals until optimal response is obtained.

In children 6 years of age and older, start with 5 mg. once or twice daily; daily dosage may be raised in increments of 5 mg. at weekly intervals until optimal response is obtained. Only in rare cases will it be necessary to exceed a total of 40 milligrams per day. Give first dose on awakening; additional doses (1 or 2) at intervals of 4 to 6 hours.

Where possible, drug administration should be interrupted occasionally to determine if there is a recurrence of behavioral symptoms sufficient to require continued therapy.

Exogenous Obesity: Usual adult dose is 5 to 30 mg. per day in divided doses, taken 30 to 60 minutes before meals. Not recommended for use in children under 12 years of age.

Dispense in tight containers as defined in the USP.

HOW SUPPLIED
TABLETS (C-II): 10 MG

BRAND/MANUFACTURER	NDC	SIZE	AWP
○ **BRAND**			
OBETROL: Rexar	00477-5432-01	100s	$46.06
	00477-5432-05	500s	$258.92
	00477-5432-10	1000s	$502.50
○ **GENERICS**			
ADDERALL: Richwood	58521-0032-01	100s	$46.06

TABLETS (C-II): 20 MG

BRAND/MANUFACTURER	NDC	SIZE	AWP
○ **BRAND**			
OBETROL: Rexar	00477-5433-01	100s	$67.03
	00477-5433-05	500s	$380.83
	00477-5433-10	1000s	$731.00

BRAND/MANUFACTURER	NDC	SIZE	AWP
○ **GENERICS**			
ADDERALL: Richwood	58521-0033-01	100s	$67.03

Amphotericin B, Injectable

> **WARNING**
>
> THIS DRUG SHOULD BE USED *PRIMARILY* FOR TREATMENT OF PATIENTS WITH PROGRESSIVE AND POTENTIALLY LIFE-THREATENING FUNGAL INFECTIONS; IT SHOULD NOT BE USED TO TREAT NONINVASIVE FORMS OF FUNGAL DISEASE SUCH AS ORAL THRUSH, VAGINAL CANDIDASIS AND ESOPHAGEAL CANDIDIASIS IN PATIENTS WITH NORMAL NEUTROPHIL COUNTS.

DESCRIPTION

Amphotericin B is an antifungal polyene antibiotic obtained from a strain of *Streptomyces nodosus*. Amphotericin B is designated chemically as [1R-(1R*,3S*,5R*,6R*,9R*,11R*,15S*,16R*,17R*,18S*,19E,21E, 23E,25E,27E,29E,31E,33R*,35S*,36R*,37S*)]-33[(3-Amino-3,6-dideoxy-β-D-man-nopyranosyl)oxy]-1,3,5,6,9,11,17,37-octahydroxy-15,16, 18-trimethyl-13-oxo-14,39-dioxabicyclo[33.3.1]nonatriaconta-19,21,23, 25, 27, 29, 31-heptaene-36-carboxylic acid. Its molecular formula is $C_{47}H_{73}NO_{17}$ and molecular weight is 924.09.

Each vial contains a sterile, nonpyrogenic, lyophilized cake (which may partially reduce to powder following manufacture) providing 50 mg Amphotericin B and 41 mg sodium desoxycholate with 20.2 mg sodium phosphates as a buffer. Crystalline Amphotericin B is insoluble in water; therefore, the antibiotic is solubilized by the addition of sodium desoxycholate to form a mixture which provides a colloidal dispersion for intravenous infusion following reconstitution.

At the time of manufacture the air in the vial is replaced by nitrogen.

Following is its chemical structure:

CLINICAL PHARMACOLOGY
MICROBIOLOGY

Amphotericin B shows a high order of *in vitro* activity against many species of fungi. *Histoplasma capsulatum, Coccidioides immitis, Candida* species, *Blastomyces dermatitidis, Rhondotorula, Cryptococcus neoformans, Sporothrix schenckii, Mucor mucedo,* and *Aspergillus fumigatus* are all inhibited by concentrations of Amphotericin B ranging from 0.03 to 1.0 mcg/mL *in vitro*. While *Candida albicans* is generally quite susceptible to Amphotericin B, non-*albicans* species may be less susceptible. *Pseudallescheria boydii* and *Fusarium* sp. are often resistant to Amphotericin B. The antibiotic is without effect on bacteria, rickettsiae, and viruses.

SUSCEPTIBILITY TESTING

Standarized techniques for susceptibility testing for antifungal agents have not been established and results of susceptibility studies have not been correlated with clinical outcomes.

PHARMACOKINETICS

Amphotericin B is fungistatic or fungicidal depending on the concentration obtained in body fluids and the susceptibility of the fungus. The drug acts by binding to steroids in the cell membrane of susceptible fungi with a resultant change in membrane permeability allowing leakage of intracellular components. Mammalian cell membranes also contain sterols and it has been suggested that the damage to human cells and fungal cells may share common mechanisms.

An initial intravenous infusion of 1 to 5 mg of Amphotericin B per day, gradually increased to 0.4 to 0.6 mg/kg daily, produces peak plasma concentrations ranging from approximately 0.5 to 2 mcg/mL. Following a rapid initial fall, plasma concentrations plateau at about 0.5 mcg/mL. An elimination half-life of approximately 15 days follows an initial plasma half-life of about 24 hours. Amphotericin B circulating in plasma is highly bound (> 90%) to plasma proteins and is poorly dialyzable. Approximately two thirds of concurrent plasma concentrations have been detected in fluids from inflamed pleura, peritoneum, synovium, and aqueous humor. Concentrations in the cerebrospinal fluid seldom exceed 2.5 percent of those in the plasma. Little Amphotericin B penetrates into vitreous humor or normal amniotic fluid. Complete details of tissue distribution are not known.

Amphotericin B is excreted very slowly (over weeks to months) by the kidneys with two to five percent of a given dose being excreted in the biologically active form. Details of possible metabolic pathways are not known. After treatment is

---

◆ RATED THERAPEUTICALLY EQUIVALENT; ◇ THERAPEUTIC EQUIVALENCE UNCONFIRMED; ○ UNRATED

discontinued, the drug can be detected in the urine for at least seven weeks due to the slow disappearance of the drug. The cumulative urinary output over a seven day period amounts to approximately 40 percent of the amount of drug infused.

INDICATIONS AND USAGE
Amphotericin B should be administered primarily to patients with progressive, potentially life-threatening fungal infections. This potent drug should not be used to treat noninvasive fungal infections, such as oral thrush, vaginal candidiasis and esophageal candidiasis in patients with normal neutrophil counts.

Amphotericin B is specifically intended to treat potentially life-threatening fungal infections: aspergillosis, cryptococcosis (torulosis), North American blastomycosis, systemic candidiasis, coccidioidomycosis, histoplasmosis, zygomycosis including mucromycosis due to susceptible species of the genera *Absidia, Mucor* and *Rhizopus,* and infections due to related susceptible species of *Conidiobolus* and *Basidiobolus,* and sporotrichosis.

Amphotericin B may be useful in the treatment of American mucocutaneous leishmaniasis, but it is not the drug of choice as primary therapy.

CONTRAINDICATIONS
This product is contraindicated in those patients who have shown hypersensitivity to Amphotericin B or any other component in the formulation unless, in the opinion of the physician, the condition requiring treatment is life-threatening and amenable only to Amphotericin B therapy.

WARNINGS
Amphotericin B is frequently the only effective treatment available for potentially life-threatening fungal disease. In each case, its possible life-saving benefit must be balanced against its untoward and dangerous side effects.

PRECAUTIONS
GENERAL
Amphotericin B should be administered intravenously under close-clinical observation by medically trained personnel. It should be reserved for treatment of patients with progressive, potentially life-threatening fungal infections due to susceptible organisms (see *"Indications and Usage"*).

Acute reactions including fever, shaking chills, hypotension, anorexia, nausea, vomiting, headache, and tachypnea are common 1 to 3 hours after starting an intravenous infusion. These reactions are usually more severe with the first few doses of Amphotericin B and usually diminish with subsequent doses.

Rapid intravenous infusion has been associated with hypotension, hypokalemia, arrhythmias, and shock and should, therefore, be avoided (see *"Dosage and Administration"*).

Amphotericin B should be used with care in patients with reduced renal function; frequent monitoring of renal function is recommended (see *"Precautions, Laboratory Tests"* and *"Adverse Reactions"*). In some patients hydration and sodium repletion prior to Amphotericin B administration may reduce the risk of developing nephrotoxicity. Supplemental alkali medication may decrease renal tubular acidosis complications.

Since acute pulmonary reactions have been reported in patients given Amphotericin B during or shortly after leukocyte transfusions, it is advisable to temporally separate these infusions as far as possible and to monitor pulmonary function (see *"Precautions, Drug Interactions"*).

Whenever medication is interrupted for a period longer than seven days, therapy should be resumed by starting with the lowest dosage level, e.g., 0.25 mg/kg of body weight, and increased gradually as outlined under *"Dosage and Administration."*

LABORATORY TESTS
Renal function should be monitored frequently during Amphotericin B therapy (see *"Adverse Reactions"*). It is also advisable to monitor on a regular basis liver function, serum electrolytes (particularly magnesium and potassium), blood counts, and hemoglobin concentrations. Laboratory test results should be used as a guide to subsequent dosage adjustments.

DRUG INTERACTIONS
When administered concurrently, the following drugs may interact with Amphotericin B:

Antineoplastic Agents: may enhance the potential for renal toxicity, bronchospasm and hypotension. Antineoplastic agents (e.g., nitrogen mustard, etc.) should be given concomitantly only with great caution.

Corticosteroids and Corticotropin (ACTH): may potentiate Amphotericin B-induced hypokalemia which may predispose the patient to cardiac dysfunction. Avoid concomitant use unless necessary to control side effects of Amphotericin B. If used concomitantly, closely monitor serum electrolytes and cardiac function (see *"Adverse Reactions"*).

Digitalis Glycosides: Amphotericin B-induced hypokalemia may potentiate digitalis toxicity. Serum potassium levels and cardiac function should be closely monitored and any deficit promptly corrected.

Flucytosine: while a synergistic relationship with Amphotericin B has been reported, concomitant use may increase the toxicity of flucytosine by possibly increasing its cellular uptake and/or impairing its renal excretion.

Imidazoles (e.g., ketoconazole, miconazole, clotrimazole, fluconazole, etc.): In vitro and animal studies with the combination of Amphotericin B and imidazoles may induce fungal resistance to Amphotericin B. Combination therapy should be administered with caution, especially in immunocompromised patients.

Other Nephrotoxic Medications: agents such as aminoglycosides, cyclosporine, and pentamidine may enhance the potential for drug-induced renal toxicity, and should be used concomitantly only with great caution. Intensive monitoring of renal function is recommended in patients requiring any combination of nephrotoxic medications (see *"Precautions, Laboratory Tests"*).

Skeletal Muscle Relaxants: Amphotericin B-induced hypokalemia may enhance the curariform effect of skeletal muscle relaxants (e.g., tubocurarine). Serum potassium levels should be monitored and deficiencies corrected.

Leukocyte Transfusions: acute pulmonary toxicity has been reported in patients receiving intravenous Amphotericin B and leukocyte transfusions (see *"Precautions, General"*).

CARCINOGENESIS, MUTAGENESIS, IMPAIRMENT OF FERTILITY
No long-term studies in animals have been performed to evaluate carcinogenic potential. There also have been no studies to determine mutagenicity or whether this medication affects fertility in males or females.

PREGNANCY: TERATOGENIC EFFECTS, PREGNANCY CATEGORY B
Reproduction studies in animals have revealed no evidence of harm to the fetus due to Amphotericin B for injection. Systemic fungal infections have been successfully treated in pregnant women and Amphotericin B for injection without obvious effects to the fetus, but the number of cases reported has been small. Because animal reproduction studies are not always predictive of human response, and adequate and well-controlled studies have not been conducted in pregnant women, this drug should be used during pregnancy only if clearly indicated.

NURSING MOTHERS
It is not known whether Amphotericin B is excreted in human milk. Because many drugs are excreted in human milk and considering the potential toxicity of Amphotericin B, it is prudent to advise a nursing mother to discontinue nursing.

PEDIATRIC USE
Safety and effectiveness in pediatric patients have not been established through adequate and well-controlled studies. Systemic fungal infections have been successfully treated in pediatric patients without reports of unusual side effects. Amphotericin B for Injection when administered to pediatric patients should be limited to the smallest dose compatible with an effective therapeutic regimen.

ADVERSE REACTIONS
Although some patients may tolerate full intravenous doses of Amphotericin B without difficulty, most will exhibit some intolerance, often at less than the full therapeutic dose.

Tolerance may be improved by treatment with aspirin, anti-pyretics (e.g., acetaminophen), antihistamines, or antiemetics. Meperidine (25 to 50 mg IV) has been shown in some patients to decrease the duration of shaking chills and fever that may accompany the infusion of Amphotericin B.

Administration of Amphotericin B on alternate days may decrease anorexia and phlebitis.

Intravenous administration of small doses of adrenal corticosteroids just prior to or during the Amphotericin B infusion may help decrease febrile reactions. Dosage and duration of such corticosteroid therapy should be kept to a minimum (see *"Precautions, Drug Interactions"*).

Addition of heparin (1000 units per infusion), and the use of a pediatric scalp-vein needle may lessen the incidence of thrombophlebitis. Extravasation may cause chemical irritation.

The adverse reactions most commonly observed are:

General (body as a whole): fever (sometimes accompanied by shaking chills usually occurring within 15 to 20 minutes after initiation of treatment); malaise; weight loss.

Cardiopulmonary: hypotension; tachypnea.

Gastrointestinal: anorexia; nausea; vomiting; diarrhea; dyspepsia; cramping epigastric pain.

Hematologic: normochromic, normocytic anemia.

Local: pain at the injection site with or without phlebitis or thrombophlebitis.

Musculoskeletal: generalized pain, including muscle and joint pains.

Neurologic: headache.

Renal: decreased renal function and renal function abnormalities including: azotemia, hypokalemia, hyposthenuria, renal tubular acidosis; and nephrocalcinosis. These usually improve with interruption of therapy. However, some permanent impairment often occurs, especially in those patients receiving large amounts (over 5 g) of Amphotericin B or receiving other nephrotoxic agents. In some patients hydration and sodium repletion prior to Amphotericin B administration may reduce the risk of developing nephrotoxicity. Supplemental alkali medication may decrease renal tubular acidosis.

The following adverse reactions have also been reported:

General (body as a whole): flushing.

Allergic: anaphylactoid and other allergic reactions; bronchospasm; wheezing.

Cardiopulmonary: cardiac arrest; shock; cardiac failure; pulmonary edema; hypersensitivity pneumonitis; arrhythmias, including ventricular fibrillation; dyspnea; hypertension.

Dermatologic: rash, in particular maculopapular; pruritis.

➤ SHOWN IN PRODUCT IDENTIFICATION GUIDE

Gastrointestinal: acute liver failure; hepatitis; jaundice; hemorrhagic gastroenteritis; melena.

Hematologic: agranulocytosis; coagulation defects; thrombocytopenia; leukopenia; eosinophilia; leukocytosis.

Neurologic: convulsions; hearing loss; tinnitus; transient vertigo; visual impairment; diplopia; peripheral neuropathy; other neurologic symptoms.

Renal: acute renal failure; anuria; oliguria.

ALTERED LABORATORY FINDINGS
Serum Electrolytes: Hypomagnesemia; hypo- and hyperkalemia; hypocalcemia.

Liver Function Tests: Elevations of AST, ALT, GGT, bilirubin, and alkaline phosphatase.

Renal Function Tests: Elevations of BUN and serum creatinine.

OVERDOSAGE
Amphotericin B overdoses can result in cardio-respiratory arrest. If an overdose is suspected, discontinue therapy and monitor the patient's clinical status (e.g., cardio-respiratory, renal, and liver function, hematologic status, serum electrolytes) and administer supportive therapy, as required. Amphotericin B is not hemodialyzable.

Prior to reinstituting therapy, the patient's condition should be stabilized (including correction of electrolyte deficiencies, etc.).

DOSAGE AND ADMINISTRATION
Caution: **Under no circumstances should a total daily dose of 1.5 mg/kg be exceeded. Amphotericin B overdoses can result in cardio-respiratory arrest** (*see* "*Overdosage*").

Amphotericin B should be administered by *slow* intravenous infusion. Intravenous infusion should be given over a period of approximately 2 to 6 hours (depending on the dose) observing the usual precautions for intravenous therapy (see "*Precautions, General*"). The recommended concentration for intravenous infusion is 0.1 mg/mL (1 mg/10 mL).

Since patient tolerance varies greatly, the dosage of Amphotericin B must be individualized and adjusted according to the patient's clinical status (e.g., site and severity of infection, etiologic agent, cardio-renal function, etc.).

A single intravenous *test dose* (1 mg in 20 mL of 5% dextrose solution) administered over 20–30 minutes may be preferred. The patient's temperature, pulse, respiration, and blood pressure should be recorded every 30 minutes for 2 to 4 hours.

In patients with *good cardio-renal function* and a *well tolerated test dose,* therapy is usually initiated with a daily dose of 0.25 mg/kg of body weight. However, in those patients having *severe and rapidly progressive fungal infection,* therapy may be initiated with a daily dose of 0.3 mg/kg of body weight. In patients with *impaired cardio-renal function* or a *severe reaction to the test dose,* therapy should be initiated with smaller daily doses (i.e., 5 to 10 mg).

Depending on the patient's cardio-renal status (see "*Precautions, Laboratory Tests*"), doses may gradually be increased by 5 to 10 mg per day to final daily dosage of 0.5 to 0.7 mg/kg.

There are insufficient data presently available to define total dosage requirements and duration of treatment necessary for eradication of specific mycoses. The optimal dose is unknown. Total daily dosage may range up to 1.0 mg/kg per day or up to 1.5 mg/kg when given on alternate days.

Sporotrichosis: Therapy with intravenous Amphotericin B for sporotrichosis has ranged up to nine months with a total dose up to 2.5 g.

Aspergillosis: Aspergillosis has been treated with Amphotericin B intravenously for a period up to 11 months with a total dose up to 3.6 g.

Rhinocerebral phycomycosis: This fulminating disease generally occurs in association with diabetic ketoacidosis. It is, therefore, imperative that diabetic control be restored in order for treatment with Amphotericin B to be successful. In contradistinction, pulmonary phycomycosis, which is more common in association with hematologic malignancies, is often an incidental finding at autopsy. A cumulative dose of at least 3 g of Amphotericin B is recommended to treat rhinocerebral phycomycosis. Although a total dose of 3 to 4 g will infrequently cause lasting renal impairment, this would seem a reasonable minimum where there is clinical evidence of invasion of deep tissue. Since rhinocerebral phycomycosis usually follows a rapidly fatal course, the therapeutic approach must necessarily be more aggressive than that used in more indolent mycoses.

PREPARATION OF SOLUTIONS
Reconstitute as follows: An initial concentrate of 5 mg Amphotericin B per mL is first prepared by rapidly expressing 10 mL Sterile Water for Injection USP *without a bacteriostatic agent* directly into the lyophillized cake, using a sterile needle (minimum diameter: 20 gauge) and syringe. Shake the vial immediately until the colloidal solution is clear. The infusion solution, providing 0.1 mg Amphotericin B per mL, is then obtained by further dilution (1:50) with 5% Dextrose Injection USP *of pH above 4.2.* The pH of each container of Dextrose Injection should be ascertained before use. Commercial Dextrose Injection usually has a pH above 4.2; however, if it is below 4.2, then 1 or 2 mL of buffer should be added to the Dextrose Injection before it is used to dilute the concentrated solution of Amphotericin B. The recommended buffer has the following composition:

Dibasic sodium phosphate (anhydrous)	1.59 g
Monobasic sodium phosphate (anhydrous)	0.96 g
Water for Injection USP	qs 100.0 mL

The buffer should be sterilized before it is added to the Dextrose Injection, either by filtration through a bacterial retentive stone, mat, or membrane, or by autoclaving for 30 minutes at 15 lb pressure (121°C).

CAUTION: Aseptic technique must be strictly observed in all handling, since no preservative or bacteriostatic agent is present in the antibiotic or in the materials used to prepare it for administration. *All entries into the vial or into the diluents must be made with a sterile needle. Do not reconstitute with saline solutions. The use of any diluent other than the ones recommended or the presence of a bacteriostatic agent* (e.g., benzyl alcohol) *in the diluent may cause precipitation of the antibiotic. Do not use the initial concentrate or the infusion solution if there is any evidence of precipitation or foreign matter in either one.*

An in-line membrane filter may be used for intravenous infusion of Amphotericin B; *however, the mean pore diameter of the filter should not be less than 1.0 micron in order to assure passage of the antibiotic dispersion.*

Prior to reconstitution, Amphotericin B should be stored in the refrigerator, protected against exposure to light. The concentrate (5 mg Amphotericin B per mL after reconstitution with 10 mL Sterile Water for Injection USP) may be stored in the dark, at room temperature for 24 hours, or at refrigerator temperatures for one week with minimal loss of potency and clarity. Any unused material should then be discarded. Solutions prepared for intravenous infusion (0.1 mg or less Amphotericin B per mL) should be used promptly after preparation and should be protected from light during administration.

HOW SUPPLIED
POWDER FOR INJECTION: 50 MG

AVERAGE UNIT PRICE (AVAILABLE SIZES)

BRAND	$35.13	GENERIC A-RATED AVERAGE PRICE (GAAP)	
GENERIC	$34.90	1s	$34.90

BRAND/MANUFACTURER	NDC	SIZE	AWP
◆ **BRAND**			
FUNGIZONE INTRAVENOUS: Apothecon	00003-0437-30	1s	$29.64
FUNGIZONE FOR TISSUE CULTURE: Apothecon	00003-0437-60	1s	$40.61
◆ **GENERICS**			
AMPHOCIN: Pharmacia	00013-1405-44	1s	$34.54
Pharma-Tek	39822-1055-05	1s	$35.25

Amphotericin B, Topical

DESCRIPTION
Amphotericin B cream and lotion for dermatologic use contain the antifungal antibiotic Amphotericin B at a concentration of 3% (30 mg/g for the cream, 30 mg/ml for the lotion).

CLINICAL PHARMACOLOGY
Amphotericin B is an antibiotic with antifungal activity produced by a strain of *Streptomyces nodosus.* It has been shown to exhibit greater *in vitro* activity than nystatin against *Candida* (Monilia) *albicans.* In clinical studies involving cutaneous and mucocutaneous candidal infections, results with topical preparations of Amphotericin B were comparable to those obtained with nystatin in similar formulations.

Although Amphotericin B exhibits some *in vitro* activity against the superficial dermatophytes (ringworm organisms), it has not demonstrated an effectiveness *in vivo* on topical application. Amphotericin B has no significant effect either *in vitro* or clinically against gram-positive or gram-negative bacteria, or viruses.

INDICATIONS AND USAGE
Amphotericin B cream and lotion are indicated in the treatment of cutaneous and mucocutaneous mycotic infections caused by Candida (Monilia) species.

CONTRAINDICATIONS
Amphotericin B cream and lotion are contraindicated in patients with a history of hypersensitivity to any of their components.

PRECAUTIONS
Should a reaction of hypersensitivity occur the drug should be immediately withdrawn and appropriate measures taken. These preparations are not for ophthalmic use.

ADVERSE REACTIONS
No evidence of any systemic toxicity or side effects has been observed during or following the use of Amphotericin B cream or during or following even prolonged, intensive and extensive application of Amphotericin B lotion.

The cream is usually well tolerated by all age groups. The lotion is extremely well tolerated by all age groups, including infants, even when therapy must be continued for many months. Neither is a primary irritant and both apparently have only a slight sensitizing potential. The cream may have a "drying" effect on some skin, and local irritation characterized by erythema, pruritus, or a burning sensation sometimes occurs, particularly in intertriginous areas. Local intolerance to the lotion, which seldom occurs, has included increased pruritus with or without other subjective or objective evidence of local irritation, or exacerbation of preexisting candidal lesions; allergic contact dermatitis is rare.

DOSAGE AND ADMINISTRATION
Amphotericin B cream and lotion should be applied liberally to the candidal lesions two to four times daily. Duration of therapy depends on individual patient

---

◆ RATED THERAPEUTICALLY EQUIVALENT; ◇ THERAPEUTIC EQUIVALENCE UNCONFIRMED; ○ UNRATED

response. Intertriginous lesions usually respond within a few days, and treatment may be completed in one to three weeks. Similarly, candidiasis of the diaper area, perleche, and glabrous skin lesions usually clear in one to two weeks. Interdigital (erosio) lesions may require two to four weeks of intensive therapy, paronychias also require relatively prolonged therapy, and those onychomycoses which respond may require several months or more of treatment. (Relapses are frequently encountered in the last three clinical conditions).

Note: When rubbed into the lesion, the cream discolors the skin minimally; the lotion does not stain the skin, although nail lesions may be stained. The patient should be informed that any discoloration of fabrics may be removed by handwashing the fabric with soap and warm water.

Store the lotion at room temperature; avoid freezing.

HOW SUPPLIED
CREAM: 3%

BRAND/MANUFACTURER	NDC	SIZE	AWP
○ BRAND FUNGIZONE CREAM: Apothecon	00003-0411-20	20 gm	$29.21

LOTION: 3%

BRAND/MANUFACTURER	NDC	SIZE	AWP
○ BRAND FUNGIZONE LOTION: Apothecon	00003-0412-30	30 ml	$40.07

Ampicillin

DESCRIPTION
Ampicillin is a semisynthetic penicillin derived from the basic penicillin nucleus, 6-amino-penicillanic acid. It is available as capsules, a powder for oral suspension, and an injection for intramuscular (IM) or intravenous (IV) use.

Each capsule contains:
Ampicillin (anhydrous) ....250 or 500 mg

Each 5 ml of reconstituted suspension contains:
Ampicillin ....125 or 250 mg

Each unit of injection contains:
Ampicillin Sodium ....125, 250, or 500 mg; 1 or 2 gm
(3.1 mEq sodium/gm Ampicillin)

Ampicillin is designated chemically as (2S,5R,6R)-6-[(R)-2-Amino-2- phenylace-tamido]-3,3-dimethyl-7-oxo-4-thia-1-aza-bicyclo [3.2.0] heptane-2-carboxylic acid. The molecular formula for Ampicillin is $C_{16}H_{19}N_3O_4S$ with a molecular weight of 349.40.

Note: Ampicillin contains 3.1 milliequivalents of sodium per gram of Ampicillin as the sodium salt.

Following is its chemical structure:

CLINICAL PHARMACOLOGY
Ampicillin is bactericidal at low concentrations and is clinically effective not only against the gram-positive organisms usually susceptible to penicillin G, but also against a variety of gram-negative organisms. It is stable in the presence of gastric acid and is well absorbed from the gastrointestinal tract. It diffuses readily into most body tissues and fluids; however, penetration into the cerebrospinal fluid and brain occurs only with meningeal inflammation. Ampicillin is excreted largely unchanged in the urine; its excretion can be delayed by concurrent administration of probenecid which inhibits the renal tubular secretion of Ampicillin. In blood serum, Ampicillin is the least bound of all the penicillins; an average of about 20% of the drug is bound to the plasma proteins as compared to 60 to 90% for the other penicillins. Blood serum levels of approximately 2mcg/ml are attained within 1 to 2 hours following a 250 mg oral dose given to fasting adults. Detectable amounts persist for about 6 hours.

Blood-level determinations were made in 60 normal male volunteers receiving a total of 116 separate dosages with anhydrous Ampicillin. Of these volunteers 57 also received Ampicillin trihydrate in crossover studies. Results show statistically significant higher blood levels at the ½-, 1-, and 2-hour periods with the anhydrous form. After the first two hours, the same high and persistent blood levels were observed with both forms. The studies utilized oral suspensions given as a single 250 mg dose of each drug. Assay was performed against sarcina lutea. MIC of the test organism was 0.005 mcg per ml.

Blood serum levels obtained on IM injection are proportionate to the dose administered. Levels of approximately 40 mcg/ml per 1-gram IM dose are attained at one-half hour. Higher levels are attainable with IV injection, depending on the dose and rate of administration.

MICROBIOLOGY
While *in vitro* studies have demonstrated the susceptibility of most strains of the following microorganisms, clinical efficacy for infections other than those included in the *"Indications and Usage"* section has not been documented.

GRAM-POSITIVE
Alpha- and beta-hemolytic streptococci, *Streptococcus pneumoniae,* staphylococci (non-penicillinase-producing strains), *Bacillus anthracis, Clostridium* spp., *Corynebacterium xerosis,* and most strains of enterococci.

GRAM-NEGATIVE
Hemophilus influenzae, Neisseria gonorrhoeae, Neisseria meningitidis, Proteus mirabilis, and many strains of Salmonella (including *S. typhosa*), Shigella, and *Escherichia coli.*

Note: Ampicillin is inactivated by penicillinase and therefore is ineffective against penicillinase-producing organisms including certain strains (penicillin G-resistant) of staphylococci, *Pseudomonas aeruginosa, P. vulgaris, Klebsiella pneumoniae, Enterobacter aerogenes,* and some strains of *E. coli;* Ampicillin is not active against Rickettsia, Mycoplasma, and "large viruses" (Miyagawanella).

Testing for Susceptibility: The invading organism should be cultured and its susceptibility demonstrated as a guide to therapy. If the Kirby-Bauer method of disc susceptibility is used, a 10 mcg Ampicillin disc should be used to determine the relative *in vitro* susceptibility.

INDICATIONS AND USAGE
Ampicillin is indicated in the treatment of infections caused by susceptible strains of the following microorganisms:

Infections of the genitourinary tract including gonorrhea: E. coli, P. mirabilis, enterococci, *Shigella, S. typhosa* and other *Salmonella,* and non-penicillinase-producing *N. gonorrhoeae. Infections of the respiratory tract:* Non-penicillinase-producing *H. influenzae* and staphylococci, streptococci including *streptococcus pneumoniae,* and pneumococci.

Infections of the gastrointestinal tract: Shigella, S. typhosa and other *Salmonella, E. coli, P. mirabilis,* and enterococci.

Meningitis: N. meningitidis. Since it is effective against the commonest pathogens causing meningitis, it may be used intravenously as initial therapy before the results of bacteriology are available.

Bacteriology studies to determine the causative organisms and their sensitivity to ampicillin should be performed. Therapy may be instituted prior to the results of susceptibility testing.

It is advisable to reserve the parenteral form of this drug for moderately severe and severe infections and for patients who are unable to take the oral forms (capsules or oral suspension). A change to oral Ampicillin may be made as soon as appropriate.

In patients at particularly high risk for bacterial endocarditis (e.g., those with prosthetic heart valves), the American Heart Association recommends the use of parenteral prophylactic antibiotics prior to dental procedures and surgery of the upper respiratory tract and before genitourinary- or gastrointestinal-tract surgery and instrumentation.[1] (See *"Dosage"*.)

UNLABELED USES
Ampicillin is used alone or as an adjunct in the treatment of *Bordetella Pertussis* infections (whooping cough) and *Helicobacter Pylori* infections, and to protect patients with preterm premature rupture of the membranes in preterm labor.

CONTRAINDICATIONS
The use of this drug is contraindicated in individuals with a history of a previous hypersensitivity reaction to any of the penicillins. Ampicillin is also contraindicated in infections caused by penicillinase-producing organisms.

WARNINGS
Serious and occasionally fatal hypersensitivity (anaphylactic) reactions have been reported in patients on penicillin therapy. Although anaphylaxis is more frequent following parenteral administration, it has occurred in patients on oral penicillins. These reactions are more apt to occur in individuals with a history of penicillin hypersensitivity and/or a history of sensitivity to multiple allergens.

There have been well-documented reports of individuals with a history of penicillin hypersensitivity who experienced severe hypersensitivity reactions when treated with cephalosporins. Before initiating therapy with any penicillin, careful inquiry should be made concerning previous hypersensitivity reactions to penicillins, cephalosporins, or other allergens. If an allergic reaction occurs, the drug should be discontinued and appropriate therapy should be instituted.

Serious anaphylactoid reactions require immediate emergency treatment with epinephrine. Oxygen, antihistamines, intravenous steroids, and airway management, including intubation, should also be administered as indicated.

PRECAUTIONS
GENERAL
Prolonged use of antibiotics may promote the overgrowth of nonsusceptible organisms, including fungi. Should superinfection occur, appropriate measures should be taken. Patients with gonorrhea who also have syphilis should be given additional appropriate parenteral penicillin treatment.

Treatment with Ampicillin does not preclude the need for surgical procedures, particularly in staphylococcal infections.

INFORMATION FOR THE PATIENT

1. The patient should inform the physician of any history of sensitivity to allergens, including previous hypersensitivity reactions to penicillins and cephalosporins (see *"Warnings"*).
2. The patient should discontinue Ampicillin and contact the physician immediately if any side effect occurs (see *"Warnings"*).
3. Ampicillin should be taken with a full glass (8 oz) of water, one-half hour before or two hours after meals.
4. Diabetic patients should consult with the physician before changing diet or dosage of diabetes medication (see *"Precautions—Drug/Laboratory Test Interaction"*).

LABORATORY TESTS

In prolonged therapy, and particularly with high dosage regimens, periodic evaluation of the renal, hepatic, and hematopoietic systems is recommended.

In streptococcal infections, therapy must be sufficient to eliminate the organism (10 days minimum); otherwise, the sequelae of streptococcal disease may occur. Cultures should be taken following completion of treatment to determine whether streptococci have been eradicated.

Cases of gonococcal infection with a suspected lesion of syphilis should have dark-field examinations ruling out syphilis before receiving Ampicillin. Patients who do not have suspected lesions of syphilis and are treated with Ampicillin should have a follow-up serologic test for syphilis each month for four months to detect syphilis that may have been masked by treatment for gonorrhea.

DRUG INTERACTIONS

When administered concurrently, the following drugs may interact with Ampicillin:

Allopurinol: Increased possibility of skin rash, particularly in hyperuricemic patients, may occur.

Bacteriostatic Antibiotics: Chloramphenicol, erythromycins, sulfonamides, or tetracyclines may interfere with the bactericidal effect of penicillins. This has been demonstrated *in vitro;* however, the clinical significance of this interaction is not well-documented.

Oral Contraceptives: May be less effective and increased breakthrough bleeding may occur.

Probenecid: May decrease renal tubular secretion of Ampicillin resulting in increased blood levels and/or Ampicillin toxicity.

DRUG/LABORATORY TEST INTERACTION

After treatment with Ampicillin, a false-positive reaction for glucose in the urine may occur with copper sulfate tests (Benedict's solution, Fehling's solution) but not with enzyme based tests.

CARCINOGENESIS, MUTAGENESIS, IMPAIRMENT OF FERTILITY

Long-term studies in animals have not been performed to evaluate carcinogenesis, mutagenesis, or impairment of fertility in males or females.

PREGNANCY

Teratogenic Effects: Category B. Reproduction studies in animals have revealed no evidence of impaired fertility or harm to the fetus due to penicillin. There are, however, no adequate and well-controlled studies in pregnant women. Because animal reproduction studies are not always predictive of human response, penicillin should be used during pregnancy only if clearly needed.

LABOR AND DELIVERY

Oral Ampicillin-class antibiotics are poorly absorbed during labor. Studies in guinea pigs showed that intravenous administration of Ampicillin slightly decreased the uterine tone and frequency of contractions, but moderately increased the height and duration of contractions. However, it is not known whether use of these drugs in humans during labor or delivery has immediate or delayed adverse effects on the fetus, prolongs the duration of labor, or increases the likelihood that forceps delivery or other obstetrical intervention or resuscitation of the newborn will be necessary.

NURSING MOTHERS

Ampicillin-class antibiotics are excreted in milk. Ampicillin use by nursing mothers may lead to sensitization of infants; therefore, a decision should be made whether to discontinue nursing or to discontinue Ampicillin, taking into account the importance of the drug to the mother.

PEDIATRIC USE

Penicillins are excreted primarily unchanged by the kidney; therefore, the incompletely developed renal function in neonates and young infants will delay the excretion of penicillin. Administration to neonates and young infants should be limited to the lowest dosage compatible with an effective therapeutic regimen (see *"Dosage and Administration"*).

ADVERSE REACTIONS

As with other penicillins, it may be expected that untoward reactions will be essentially limited to sensitivity phenomena. They are more likely to occur in individuals who have previously demonstrated hypersensitivity to penicillins and in those with a history of allergy, asthma, hay fever, or urticaria.

The following adverse reactions have been reported as associated with the use of Ampicillin:

Gastrointestinal: glossitis, stomatitis, nausea, vomiting, enterocolitis, pseudo-membranous colitis, and diarrhea. These reactions are usually associated with oral dosage forms of the drug.

Hypersensitivity Reactions: an erythematous, mildly pruritic, maculopapular skin rash has been reported fairly frequently. The rash, which usually does not develop within the first week of therapy, may cover the entire body including the soles, palms, and oral mucosa. The eruption usually disappears in three to seven days. Other hypersensitivity reactions that have been reported are: skin rash, pruritus, urticaria, erythema multiforme, and an occasional case of exfoliative dermatitis. Anaphylaxis is the most serious reaction experienced and has usually been associated with the parenteral dosage form of the drug.

Note: Urticaria, other skin rashes, and serum sickness-like reactions may be controlled with antihistamines and, if necessary, systemic corticosteroids. Whenever such reactions occur, Ampicillin should be discontinued, unless, in the opinion of the physician, the condition being treated is life-threatening and amenable only to Ampicillin therapy. Serious anaphylactic reactions require emergency measures (see *"Warnings"*).

Liver: A moderate elevation in the serum glutamic-oxalo-acetic transaminase (SGOT) has been noted, particularly in infants, but the significance of this finding is unknown.

Hemic and Lymphatic Systems: Anemia, thrombocytopenia, thrombocytopenic purpura, eosinophilia, leukopenia, and agranulocytosis have been reported during therapy with penicillins. These reactions are usually reversible on discontinuation of therapy and are believed to be hypersensitivity phenomena.

Other adverse reactions that have been reported with the use of Ampicillin are laryngeal stridor and high fever. An occasional patient may complain of sore mouth or tongue as with any oral penicillin preparation.

OVERDOSAGE

In case of overdosage, discontinue medication, treat symptomatically and institute supportive measures as required. In patients with renal function impairment, Ampicillin-class antibiotics can be removed by hemodialysis but not by peritoneal dialysis.

DOSAGE AND ADMINISTRATION

CAPSULES AND ORAL SUSPENSION

Adults and Children weighing over 20 kg:

For Genitourinary- or Gastrointestinal-tract Infections Other than Gonorrhea in Men and Women: The usual dose is 500 mg q.i.d. in equally spaced doses (i.e., 500 mg every 6 hours); larger doses may be required for severe or chronic infections.

For the Treatment of Gonorrhea in both Men and Women: A single oral dose of 3.5 grams of Ampicillin with 1 gram of probenecid administered simultaneously is recommended. Physicians are cautioned to use no less than the above recommended dosage for the treatment of gonorrhea. Follow-up cultures should be obtained from the original site(s) of infection in males within 4 to 7 days and in females 7 to 14 days after therapy. In women, it is also desirable to obtain culture test-of-cure from both the endocervical and anal canals. Prolonged intensive therapy is needed for complications such as prostatitis and epididymitis.

All gonorrhea patients should have a serologic test for syphilis at the time of diagnosis. Patients with negative serology and no suspected lesions of syphilis should have a follow-up test for syphilis monthly for 4 months to detect possible syphilis masked by gonorrhea therapy.

Patients with gonorrhea who also have syphilis should be given additional treatment appropriate to the stage of syphilis.

For Respiratory-tract Infections: The usual dose is 250 mg q.i.d. in equally spaced doses (i.e., 250 mg every 6 hours).

Children weighing 20 kg or less:

For genitourinary- or gastrointestinal-tract infections: The usual dose is 100 mg/kg/day total, administered q.i.d. in equally divided and spaced doses (i.e., every 6-8 hours).

For respiratory infections: The usual dose is 50 mg/kg/day total, administered in equally divided and spaced doses three to four times daily (i.e., every 8 to every 6 hours).

Doses for children should not exceed doses recommended for adults.

INJECTION (SEE RELATED TABLE).

A change to oral Ampicillin may be made as soon as appropriate.

ALL DOSAGE FORMS

In all patients, irrespective of age and weight: Larger doses may be required for severe or chronic infections. Although Ampicillin is resistant to degradation by gastric acid, it should be administered at least one-half hour before or two hours after meals for maximal absorption. Except for the single-dose regimen for gonorrhea referred to above, therapy should be continued for a minimum of 48 to 72 hours after the patient becomes asymptomatic or evidence of bacterial eradication has been obtained. In infections caused by hemolytic strains of streptococci, a minimum of 10 days' treatment is recommended to guard against the risk of rheumatic fever or glomerulonephritis (see *"Precautions—Laboratory Tests"*).

In the treatment of chronic urinary or gastrointestinal infections, frequent bacteriologic and clinical appraisal is necessary during therapy and may be necessary for several months afterwards. Stubborn infections may require

DOSAGE (IM OR IV)

Infection	Organisms	Adults	Children*
Respiratory tract	streptococci, pneumococci, nonpenicillianse-producing staphylococci, H. influenzae	250-500 mg q. 6 h.	25-50 mg/kg/day In equal doses q. 6h.
Gastrointestinal tract	susceptible pathogens	500 mg q. 6 h.	50 mg/kg/day in equal doses q. 6 h.
Genitourinary tract	susceptible gram-negative or gram-positive pathogens	500 mg q. 6 h.	50 mg/kg/day in equal doses q. 6 h.
Urethritis (acute) in adult males	N. gonorrhoeae	500 mg b.i.d. for 1 day (IM)	
Bacterial meningitis	N. meningitidis, H. influenzae (Initial treatment is usually by IV drip, followed by frequent [q. 3-4 h.] IM Injections.)	8-14 gm/day	100-200 mg/kg/day
Bacterial endocarditis prophylaxis (See "Indications.") Dental procedures and oral/ respiratory tract surgery	S. viridans	Ampicillin 1-2 gm PLUS gentamicin 1.5 mg/kg (Both IM or IV 30 minutes before procedure)	Ampicillin 50 mg/kg PLUS gentamicin 2 mg/kg
	(Initial treatment is followed by either: One full parenteral dose 8 hours later; or oral penicillin V, 1 gm, 6 hours later.)		
Genitourinary/gastrointestinal tract procedures		Ampicillin 2.0 gm PLUS gentamicin 1.5 mg/kg (Both IM or IV 30 minutes before procedure)	Ampicillin 50 mg/kg PLUS gentamicin 2.0 mg/kg
	(Initial treatment may be followed by one full parenteral dose 8 hours later.)		

*   *Children's dosage recommendations are intended for those whose weight will not result in a dosage higher than for the adult.*

treatment for several weeks. Smaller doses than those indicated above should not be used.

ADMINISTRATION (IV OR IM)
Parenteral drug products should be inspected visually for particulate matter and discoloration prior to administration, whenever solution and container permit.

Conventional Vials: 125 mg, 250 mg, 500 mg, 1 gm, and 2 gm.

Intramuscular Use:
125-mg vial: Add 1 ml sterile water for injection, or bacteriostatic water for injection to give a final concentration of 125 mg/ml. For fractional doses, withdraw the Ampicillin sodium solution as follows:

Dose	Withdraw
25 mg	0.2 ml
50 mg	0.4 ml
75 mg	0.6 ml
100 mg	0.8 ml
125 mg	1.0 ml

250-mg vial: Add 0.9 ml sterile water for injection, or bacteriostatic water for injection to give a final concentration of 250 mg/ml. For fractional doses, withdraw the Ampicillin sodium solution as follows:

Dose	Withdraw
125 mg	0.5 ml
150 mg	0.6 ml
175 mg	0.7 ml
200 mg	0.8 ml
225 mg	0.9 ml
250 mg	1.0 ml

For dilution of 500-mg, 1-g, and 2-g vials, dissolve contents of a vial with the amount of sterile water for injection or bacteriostatic water for injection listed in the table below:

Label Claim	Recommended Amount of Diluent	Withdrawable Volume	Concentration in mg/ml
500 mg	1.8 ml	2.0 ml	250 mg
1.0 gm	3.4 ml	4.0 ml	250 mg
2.0 gm	6.8 ml	8.0 ml	250 mg

While the 1-gm and 2-gm vials are primarily for intravenous use, they may be administered intramuscularly when the 250-mg or 500-mg vials are unavailable. In such instances, dissolve in 3.4 or 6.8 ml sterile water for injection, or bacteriostatic water for injection to give a final concentration of 250mg/ml.
The above solutions must be used within one hour after reconstitution.

DIRECT INTRAVENOUS USE
125-mg, 250-mg, and 500-mg vials: Add 5 ml sterile water for injection or bacteriostatic water for injection and withdraw the entire contents; the dose should be injected over a period of 3 to 5 minutes.
1-gm and 2-gm vials: Add 10 ml sterile water for injection or bacteriostatic water for injection and withdraw the entire contents; administer slowly over a period of at least 10 to 15 minutes. Caution: More rapid administration may

result in convulsive seizures. The above solutions should be used within one hour after reconstitution.

To reconstitute for continuous intravenous infusion, dissolve the contents of 125-mg, 250-mg, 500-mg vials in 5 ml and the 1-g and 2-gm vials in 10 ml sterile water for injection, or bacteriostatic water for injection and transfer directly to acceptable large-volume IV fluids. Stability of the resulting solution at room temperature or under refrigeration will vary with the bulk fluid. (See tables.)

For Administration by Intravenous Drip Stability studies on Ampicillin Sodium in various intravenous solutions indicate the drug will lose less than 10% activity at room temperature (70°F) for the time periods and concentrations stated:

IV Solution	Concentrations	Stability Periods
Sterile water for injection	Up to 30 mg/ml	8 hours
Isotonic sodium chloride	Up to 30 mg/ml	8 hours
M/6 Sodium lactate solution	Up to 30 mg/ml	8 hours
5% Dextrose in water	Up to 20 mg/ml	2 hours
5% Dextrose in 0.45% sodium chloride	Up to 2 mg/ml	4 hours
10% Invert sugar	Up to 2 mg/ml	4 hours
Lactated Ringer's solution	Up to 30 mg/ml	8 hours

If the solutions below are stored under refrigeration, they will remain stable for the time periods indicated:

IV Solution	Concentrations	Stability Periods
Sterile water for injection	30 mg/ml	48 hours
Sterile water for injection	Up to 20 mg/ml	72 hours
Isotonic sodium chloride	30 mg/ml	48 hours
Isotonic sodium chloride	Up to 20 mg/ml	72 hours
Lactated Ringer's solution	Up to 30 mg/ml	24 hours
M/6 sodium lactate solution	Up to 30 mg/ml	8 hours
5% dextrose in water	Up to 20 mg/ml	4 hours
5% dextrose in 0.4% sodium chloride	Up to 10 mg/ml	4 hours
10% invert sugar	Up to 20 mg/ml	3 hours

PIGGYBACK UNITS (for Intravenous Drip Use)—Use sterile water for injection or isotonic sodium chloride.

500-mg Bottle: Add a minimum of 50 ml water or saline, and shake well. If lower concentrations are desired, the solution could be further diluted with up to a total of 100 ml of diluent.

Diluent Amount	Solution Concentration
50 ml	10 mg/ml
100 ml	5 mg/ml

One-Gram Bottle: Add a minimum of 49 ml water or saline, and shake well. If lower concentrations are desired, the solution could be further diluted with up to a total of 99 ml of diluent.

Diluent Amount	Solution Concentration
49 ml	20 mg/ml
99 ml	10 mg/ml

➤ SHOWN IN PRODUCT IDENTIFICATION GUIDE

Two-Gram Bottle: Add 99 ml water or saline, and shake well. The resulting solution will contain 20 mg/ml.

Caution: Administer slowly by intravenous route over a period of at least 10 to 15 minutes. More rapid administration may result in convulsive seizures.

The reconstituted solution must be used within 8 hours if stored at room temperature or within 72 hours if stored under refrigeration.

To reconstitute for continuous intravenous infusion, dissolve the contents of the 500-mg, 1-g, or 2-g piggyback unit in 10 ml sterile water for injection or bacteriostatic water for injection and transfer directly to acceptable large-volume IV fluids. Stability of the resulting solution at room temperature or under refrigeration will vary with bulk fluid used. (See tables.)

STORAGE
Keep tightly closed.
Dispense in a tight container.
Store at room temperature, approximately 25° C (77°F).
Shake suspension well before using.
When suspension is stored in refrigerator discard unused portion after 14 days, or when stored at room temperature discard unused portion after 7 days (250 mg per 5 ml). When stored in refrigerator discard unused portion after 14 days (125 mg per 5 ml).

REFERENCES
1. American Heart Association. Prevention of bacterial endocarditis. Circulation 1984; 70:1123A-1127A.

J CODES
Up to 500 mg IM,IV—J0290

HOW SUPPLIED

AMPICILLIN
CAPSULE: 250 MG

AVERAGE UNIT PRICE (AVAILABLE SIZES)		GENERIC A-RATED AVERAGE PRICE (GAAP)	
GENERIC	$0.11	100s	$12.46
HCFA FUL (100s ea)	$0.07	500s	$50.59
		1000s	$91.26

BRAND/MANUFACTURER	NDC	SIZE	AWP
◆ GENERICS			
Raway	00686-3111-09	100s	$5.95
Schein	00364-2001-01	100s	$8.50
Lederle Std Prod	00005-3586-23	100s	$8.55
Rugby	00536-0010-01	100s	$10.43
Moore,H.L.	00839-5087-06	100s	$11.00
PRINCIPEN: Apothecon	00003-0122-50	100s	$11.26
URL	00677-0010-01	100s	$11.65
Major	00904-2017-60	100s	$11.75
Mylan	00378-0115-01	100s	$11.76
Geneva	00781-2555-01	100s	$11.76
Biocraft	00332-3111-09	100s	$11.93
Goldline	00182-0163-01	100s	$11.93
Qualitest	00603-2290-21	100s	$11.93
Parmed	00349-1003-01	100s	$11.95
Aligen	00405-4089-01	100s	$12.11
Warner Chilcott	00047-0402-24	100s	$14.86
VHA Supply	00015-7992-65	100s	$18.57
Raway	00686-0602-20	100s ud	$10.00
PRINCIPEN: Apothecon	00003-0122-51	100s ud	$11.26
UDL	51079-0602-20	100s ud	$17.20
Goldline	00182-0163-89	100s ud	$18.85
VHA Supply	00015-7992-68	100s ud	$20.98
Schein	00364-2001-05	500s	$37.75
PRINCIPEN: Apothecon	00003-0122-60	500s	$39.88
Lederle Std Prod	00005-3586-31	500s	$40.76
Geneva	00781-2555-05	500s	$41.55
Parmed	00349-1003-05	500s	$43.13
Moore,H.L.	00839-5087-12	500s	$44.67
Rugby	00536-0010-05	500s	$46.35
Major	00904-2017-40	500s	$46.40
URL	00677-0010-05	500s	$50.57
Mylan	00378-0115-05	500s	$50.62
TOTACILLIN: SK Beecham Pharm	00029-6615-32	500s	$52.25
Biocraft	00332-3111-13	500s	$57.51
Goldline	00182-0163-05	500s	$57.51
Qualitest	00603-2290-28	500s	$57.51
Aligen	00405-4089-02	500s	$59.32
➤ OMNIPEN: Wyeth-Ayerst	00008-0053-05	500s	$62.71
Warner Chilcott	00047-0402-30	500s	$71.62
Schein	00364-2001-02	1000s	$72.50
Rugby	00536-0010-10	1000s	$88.05
Biocraft	00332-3111-15	1000s	$113.22

CAPSULE: 500 MG

AVERAGE UNIT PRICE (AVAILABLE SIZES)		GENERIC A-RATED AVERAGE PRICE (GAAP)	
GENERIC	$0.21	100s	$22.02
HCFA FUL (100s ea)	$0.13	500s	$97.64

BRAND/MANUFACTURER	NDC	SIZE	AWP
◆ GENERICS			
Raway	00686-3313-09	100s	$10.95
Lederle Std Prod	00005-3587-23	100s	$15.85
➤ PRINCIPEN: Apothecon	00003-0134-50	100s	$16.99
Schein	00364-2002-01	100s	$17.75
Moore,H.L.	00839-5130-06	100s	$18.87
Rugby	00536-0016-01	100s	$19.35
Major	00904-2073-60	100s	$19.95
Geneva	00781-2999-01	100s	$20.80
Goldline	00182-0641-01	100s	$21.00
URL	00677-0011-01	100s	$21.25
Biocraft	00332-3113-09	100s	$21.29
Qualitest	00603-2291-21	100s	$21.29
MARCILLIN: Marnel	00682-9113-01	100s	$21.60
➤ Mylan	00378-0116-01	100s	$22.00
Aligen	00405-4090-01	100s	$24.19
➤ OMNIPEN: Wyeth-Ayerst	00008-0309-03	100s	$25.70
Parmed	00349-1006-01	100s	$25.95
Warner Chilcott	00047-0404-24	100s	$26.51
➤ PRINCIPEN: Apothecon	00003-0134-51	100s ud	$16.99
Raway	00686-0603-20	100s ud	$17.55
Goldline	00182-0641-89	100s ud	$32.00
UDL	51079-0603-20	100s ud	$33.00
VHA Supply	00015-7993-68	100s ud	$35.55
➤ PRINCIPEN: Apothecon	00003-0134-60	500s	$72.78
Lederle Std Prod	00005-3587-31	500s	$75.83
Schein	00364-2002-05	500s	$80.60
Geneva	00781-2999-05	500s	$83.50
Major	00904-2073-40	500s	$86.50
Moore,H.L.	00839-5130-12	500s	$88.68
Rugby	00536-0016-05	500s	$89.55
URL	00677-0011-05	500s	$101.00
➤ Mylan	00378-0116-05	500s	$101.38
Parmed	00349-1006-05	500s	$101.38
Biocraft	00332-3113-13	500s	$102.70
Goldline	00182-0641-05	500s	$102.70
Qualitest	00603-2291-28	500s	$102.70
TOTACILLIN: SK Beecham Pharm	00029-6620-32	500s	$104.55
Aligen	00405-4090-02	500s	$117.20
➤ OMNIPEN: Wyeth-Ayerst	00008-0309-06	500s	$120.94
Warner Chilcott	00047-0404-30	500s	$127.90

For additional alternatives, turn to the section beginning on page 2859.

Ampicillin Sodium and Sulbactam Sodium

DESCRIPTION
Ampicillin Sodium/Sulbactam Sodium an injectable antibacterial combination consisting of the semisynthetic antibiotic ampicillin sodium and the beta-lactamase inhibitor sulbactam sodium for intravenous and intramuscular administration.

Ampicillin Sodium is derived from the penicillin nucleus, 6-aminopenicillanic acid. Chemically, it is monosodium (2S,5R,6R)-6 [(R)-2-amino-2-phenylacetamido]-3,3-dimethyl-7-oxo-4-thia-1-azabicy- clo[3.2.0]heptane-2-carboxylate and has a molecular weight of 371.39. Its chemical formula is $C_{16}H_{18}N_3NaO_4S$.

Sulbactam Sodium is a derivative of the basic penicillin nucleus. Chemically, Sulbactam Sodium is sodium penicillinate sulfone: sodium (2S, 5R)-3,3-dimethyl-7-oxo-4-thia-1-azabicyclo[3.2.0] heptane-2-carboxylate 4,4-dioxide. Its chemical formula is $C_8H_{10}NNaO_5S$ with a molecular weight of 255.22.

CLINICAL PHARMACOLOGY
General: Immediately after completion of a 15-minute intravenous infusion of Ampicillin Sodium/Sulbactam Sodium peak serum concentrations of ampicillin and sulbactam are attained. Ampicillin serum levels are similar to those produced by the administration of equivalent amounts of ampicillin alone. Peak Ampicillin serum levels ranging from 109 to 150 mcg/mL are attained after administration of 2000 mg of Ampicillin plus 1000 mg Sulbactam and 40 to 71 mcg/mL after administration of 1000 mg Ampicillin plus 500 mg Sulbactam. The corresponding mean peak serum levels for sulbactam range from 48 to 88 mcg/mL and 21 to 40 mcg/mL, respectively. After an intramuscular injection of 1000 mg Ampicillin plus 500 mg Sulbactam, peak Ampicillin serum levels ranging from 8 to 37 mcg/mL and peak Sulbactam serum levels ranging from 6 to 24 mcg/mL are attained.

◆ RATED THERAPEUTICALLY EQUIVALENT; ◇ THERAPEUTIC EQUIVALENCE UNCONFIRMED; ○ UNRATED

The mean serum half-life of both drugs is approximately 1 hour in healthy volunteers.

Approximately 75 to 85% of both Ampicillin and Sulbactam are excreted unchanged in the urine during the first 8 hours after administration of Ampicillin Sodium/Sulbactam Sodium to individuals with normal renal function. Somewhat higher and more prolonged serum levels of Ampicillin and Sulbactam can be achieved with the concurrent administration of probenecid.

In patients with impaired renal function the elimination kinetics of Ampicillin and Sulbactam are similarly affected, hence the ratio of one to the other will remain constant whatever the renal function. The dose Ampicillin Sodium/Sulbactam Sodium in such patients should be administered less frequently in accordance with the usual practice for Ampicillin (see "Dosage and Administration").

Ampicillin has been found to be approximately 28% reversibly bound to human serum protein and Sulbactam approximately 38% reversibly bound.

The following average levels of Ampicillin and Sulbactam were measured in the tissues and fluids listed:

CONCENTRATION OF AMPICILLIN SODIUM/SULBACTAM SODIUM IN VARIOUS BODY TISSUES AND FLUIDS

Fluid or Tissue	Dose (grams) Ampicillin/Sulbactam	Concentration (mcg/mL or mcg/g) Ampicillin/Sulbactam
Peritoneal Fluid	0.5/0.5 IV	7/14
Blister Fluid (Cantharides)	0.5/0.5 IV	8/20
Tissue Fluid	1/0.5 IV	8/4
Intestinal Mucosa	0.5/0.5 IV	11/18
Appendix	2/1 IV	3/40

Penetration of both Ampicillin and Sulbactam into cerebrospinal fluid in the presence of inflamed meninges has been demonstrated after IV administration of Ampicillin Sodium/Sulbactam Sodium.

MICROBIOLOGY

Ampicillin is similar to benzyl penicillin in its bactericidal action against susceptible organisms during the stage of active multiplication. It acts through the inhibition of cell wall mucopeptide biosynthesis. Ampicillin has a broad spectrum of bactericidal activity against many gram-positive and gram-negative aerobic and anaerobic bacteria. (Ampicillin is, however, degraded by beta-lactamases and therefore the spectrum of activity does not normally include organisms which produce these enzymes.)

A wide range of beta-lactamases found in microorganisms resistant to penicillins and cephalosporins have been shown in biochemical studies with cell free bacterial systems to be irreversibly inhibited by Sulbactam. Although Sulbactam alone possesses little useful antibacterial activity except against the *Neisseriaciae*, whole organism studies have shown that Sulbactam restores ampicillin activity against beta-lactamase producing strains. In particular, Sulbactam has good inhibitory activity against the clinically important plasmid mediated beta-lactamases most frequently responsible for transferred drug resistance. Sulbactam has no effect on the activity of ampicillin against ampicillin susceptible strains.

The presence of Sulbactam in the Ampicillin Sodium/Sulbactam Sodium formulation effectively extends the antibiotic spectrum of Ampicillin to include many bacteria normally resistant to it and to other beta-lactam antibiotics. Thus, Ampicillin Sodium/Sulbactam Sodium possesses the properties of a broad-spectrum antibiotic and a beta-lactamase inhibitor.

While *in vitro* studies have demonstrated the susceptibility of most strains of the following organisms, clinical efficacy for infections other than those included in the indications section has not been documented.

Gram-Positive Bacteria: Staphylococcus aureus (beta-lactamase and non-beta-lactamase producing), *Staphylococcus epidermidis* (beta-lactamase and non-beta-lactamase producing), *Staphylococcus saprophyticus* (beta-lactamase and non-beta-lactamase producing), *Streptococcus faecalis*[†] (Enterococcus), *Streptococcus pneumoniae*[†] (formerly *D. pneumoniae*), *Streptococcus pyogenes*[†] *Streptococcus viridans*[†]

Gram-Negative Bacteria: Hemophilus influenzae (beta-lactamase and non-beta-lactamase producing). *Moraxella (Branhamella) catarrhalis* (beta-lactamase and non-beta-lactamase producing). *Escherichia coli* (beta-lactamase and non-beta-lactamase producing). *Klebsiella* species (all known strains are beta-lactamase producing). *Proteus mirabilis* (beta-lactamase and non-beta-lactamase producing). *Proteus vulgaris, Providencia rettgeri, Providencia stuartii, Morganella morganii,* and *Neisseria gonorrhoeae* (beta-lactamase and non-beta-lactamase producing).

Anaerobes: Clostridium species[†], *Peptococcus* species[†], *Peptostreptococcus* species, *Bacteroides* species, including *B. fragilis.*

SUSCEPTIBILITY TESTING

Diffusion Technique: For the Kirby-Bauer method of susceptibility testing, a 20 mcg (10 mcg Ampicillin + 10 mcg sulbactam) diffusion disk should be used. The method is one outlined in the NCCLS publication M2-A4.[1] With this procedure, a report from the laboratory of "Susceptible" indicates that the infecting organism is likely to respond to Ampicillin Sodium/Sulbactam Sodium therapy and a report of "Resistant" indicates that the infecting organism is not likely to respond to therapy. An "Intermediate" susceptibility report suggests that the infecting organism would be susceptible to Ampicillin Sodium/Sulbactam Sodium if a higher dosage is used or if the infection is confined to tissues or fluids (e.g., urine) in which high antibiotic levels are attained.

Dilution Techniques: Broth or agar dilution methods may be used to determine the minimal inhibitory concentration (MIC) value for susceptibility of bacterial isolates to Ampicillin/Sulbactam. The method used is one outlined in the NCCLS publication M7-A2.[2] Tubes should be inoculated to contain 10^5 to 10^6 organisms/mL or plates "spotted" with 10^4 organisms.

The recommended dilution method employs a constant Ampicillin/Sulbactam ratio of 2:1 in all tubes with increasing concentrations of Ampicillin. MIC's are reported in terms of Ampicillin concentration in the presence of Sulbactam at a constant 2 parts Ampicillin to 1 part Sulbactam.

RECOMMENDED AMPICILLIN/SULBACTAM SUSCEPTIBILITY RANGES[1,2,3]

	Resistant	Intermediate	Susceptible
Gram(-) and *Staphylococcus* Bauer/Kirby Zone Sizes	≤ 11 mm	12-13 mm	≥ 14 mm
MIC (mcg of ampicillin/mL)	≥ 32	16	≤ 8
Hemophilus influenzae Bauer/Kirby Zone Sizes	≤ 19	-	≥ 20
MIC (mcg of ampicillin/mL)	≥ 4	-	≥ 2

[1] The non-beta-lactamase producing organisms which are normally susceptible to ampicillin, such as Streptococci, will have similar zone sizes as for ampicillin disks.

[2] Staphylococci resistant to methicillin, oxacillin, or nafcillin must be considered resistant to Ampicillin Sodium/Sulbactam Sodium.

[3] The quality control cultures should have the following assigned daily ranges for ampicillin/sulbactam.

		Disks	Mode MIC (mcg/mL Ampicillin/mcg/mL Sulbactam)
E. coli	(ATCC 25922)	20-24 mm	2/1
S. aureus	(ATCC 25923)	29-37 mm	0.12/0.06
E. coli	(ATCC 35218)	13-19 mm	8/4

INDICATIONS AND USAGE

Ampicillin Sodium/Sulbactam Sodium is indicated for the treatment of infections due to susceptible strains of the designated microorganisms in the conditions listed below.

Skin and Skin Structure Infections: caused by beta-lactamase producing strains of *Staphylococcus aureus,*[*] *Escherichia coli,*[*] *Klebsiella* spp.[*] (including *K. pneumoniae*), *Proteus mirabilis,*[*] *Bacteroides fragilis.*[*] *Enterobacter* spp.,[*] and *Acinetobacter calcoaceticus.*[*]

Intra-Abdominal Infections: caused by beta-lactamase producing strains of *Escherichia coli, Klebsiella* spp. (including *K. pneumoniae*[*]), *Bacteroides* spp. (including *B. fragilis*), and *Enterobacter* spp.[*]

Gynecological Infections: caused by beta-lactamase producing strains of *Escherichia coli,*[*] and *Bacteroides* spp.[*] (including *B. fragilis*).[*]

While Ampicillin Sodium/Sulbactam Sodium is indicated only for the conditions listed above, infections caused by Ampicillin-susceptible organisms are also amenable to treatment with Ampicillin Sodium/Sulbactam Sodium due to its Ampicillin content. Therefore, mixed infections caused by Ampicillin-susceptible organisms and beta-lactamase producing organisms susceptible to Ampicillin Sodium/Sulbactam Sodium should not require the addition of another antibiotic.

[†] These are not beta-lactamase producing strains and, therefore, are susceptible to ampicillin alone.

[*] Efficacy for this organism in this organ system was studied in fewer than 10 infections.

Appropriate culture and susceptibility tests should be performed before treatment in order to isolate and identify the organisms causing infection and to determine their susceptibility to Ampicillin Sodium/Sulbadam Sodium.

Therapy may be instituted prior to obtaining the results from bacteriological and susceptibility studies, when there is reason to believe the infection may involve any of the betalactamase producing organisms listed above in the indicated organ systems. Once the results are known, therapy should be adjusted if appropriate.

CONTRAINDICATIONS

The use of Ampicillin Sodium/Sulbactam Sodium is contraindicated in individuals with a history of hypersensitivity reactions to any of the penicillins.

WARNINGS

SERIOUS AND OCCASIONALLY FATAL HYPERSNSITIVITY (ANAPHYLACTIC) REACTIONS HAVE BEEN REPORTED IN PATIENTS ON PENICILLIN THERAPY. THESE REACTIONS ARE MORE APT TO OCCUR IN INDIVIDUALS WITH A HISTORY OF PENICILLIN HYPERSENSITIVITY AND/OR HYPERSENSITIVITY REACTIONS TO MULTIPLE ALLERGENS. THERE HAVE BEEN REPORTS OF INDIVIDUALS WITH A HISTORY OF PENICILLIN HYPERSENSITIVITY WHO HAVE EXPERIENCED SEVERE REACTIONS WHEN TREATED WITH CEPHALOSPORINS. BEFORE THERAPY WITH A PENICILLIN, CAREFUL INQUIRY SHOULD BE MADE CONCERNING PREVIOUS HYPERSENSITIVITY REACTIONS TO PENICILLINS, CEPHALOSPORINS, AND OTHER ALLERGENS. IF AN ALLERGIC REACTION OCCURS, AMPICILLIN SODIUM/SULBACTAM SODIUM SHOULD BE DISCONTINUED AND THE APPROPRIATE THERAPY INSTITUTED.

SERIOUS ANAPHYLACTOID REACTIONS REQUIRE IMMEDIATE EMERGENCY TREATMENT WITH EPINEPHRINE, OXYGEN, INTRAVENOUS STEROIDS, AND AIRWAY MANAGEMENT, INCLUDING INTUBATION, SHOULD ALSO BE ADMINISTERED AS INDICATED.

Pseudomembranous colitis has been reported with nearly all antibacterial agents, including Ampicillin Sodium/Sulbadam Sodium, and has ranged in severity from mild to life-threatening. Therefore, it is important to consider this diagnosis in patients who present with diarrhea subsequent to the administration of antibacterial agents.

Treatment with antibacterial agents alters the normal flora of the colon and may permit overgrowth of clostridia. Studies indicate that toxin produced by *Clostridium difficile* is one primary cause of "antibiotic-associated colitis."

Mild cases of pseudomembranous colitis usually respond to drug discontinuation alone. In moderate to severe cases, consideration should be given to management with fluids and electrolytes, protein supplementation and treatment with an antibacterial drug clinically effective against *C. difficile* colitis.

PRECAUTIONS

General: A high percentage of patients with mononucleosis who receive ampicillin develop a skin rash. Thus, Ampicillin class antibiotics should not be administered to patients with mononucleosis. In patients treated with Ampicillin Sodium/Sulbactam Sodium the possibility of superinfections with mycotic or bacterial pathogens should be kept in mind during therapy. If superinfections occur (usually involving *Pseudomonas* or *Candida*), the drug should be discontinued and/or appropriate therapy instituted.

Drug Interactions: Probenecid decreases the renal tubular secretion of Ampicillin and Sulbactam. Concurrent use of probenecid with Ampicillin Sodium/Sulbactam Sodium may result in increased and prolonged blood levels of Ampicillin and Sulbactam. The concurrent administration of allopurinol and Ampicillin increases substantially the incidence of rashes in patients receiving both drugs as compared to patients receiving Ampicillin alone. It is not known whether this potentiation of Ampicillin rashes is due to allopurinol or the hyperuricemia present in these patients. There are no data with Ampicillin Sodium/Sulbactam Sodium and allopurinol administered concurrently Ampicillin Sodium/Sulbactam Sodium and aminoglycosides should not be reconstituted together due to the *in vitro* inactivation of aminoglycosides by the Ampicillin component of Ampicillin Sodium/Sulbactam Sodium.

Drug/Laboratory Test Interactions: Administration of Ampicillin Sodium/Sulbactam Sodium will result in high urine concentration of Ampicillin. High urine concentrations of Ampicillin may result in false positive reactions when testing for the presence of glucose in urine using Clinitest®, Benedict's Solution or Fehling's Solution. It is recommended that glucose tests based on enzymatic glucose oxidase reactions (such as Clinistix® or Testape®) be used. Following administration of Ampicillin to pregnant women, a transient decrease in plasma concentration of total conjugated estriol, estriol-glucuronide, conjugated estrone and estradiol has been noted. This effect may also occur with Ampicillin Sodium/Sulbactam Sodium.

Carcinogenesis, Mutagenesis, Impairment of Fertility: Long-term studies in animals have not been performed to evaluate carcinogenic or mutagenic potential.

Pregnancy Category B: Reproduction studies have been performed in mice, rats, and rabbits at doses up to ten (10) times the human dose and have revealed no evidence of impaired fertility or harm to the fetus due to Ampicillin Sodium/Sulbactam Sodium. There are, however, no adequate and well controlled studies in pregnant women. Because animal reproduction studies are not always predictive of human response, this drug should be used during pregnancy only if clearly needed. (See *"Drug/Laboratory Test Interactions"*.)

Labor and Delivery: Studies in guinea pigs have shown that intravenous administration of Ampicillin decreased the uterine tone, frequency of contractions, height of contractions, and duration of contractions. However, it is not known whether the use of Ampicillin Sodium/Sulbactam Sodium in humans during labor or delivery has immediate or delayed adverse effects on the fetus, prolongs the duration of labor, or increases the likelihood that forceps delivery or other obstetrical intervention or resuscitation of the newborn will be necessary.

Nursing Mothers: Low concentrations of Ampicillin and sulbactam are excreted in the milk: therefore, caution should be exercised when Ampicillin Sodium/Sulbactam Sodium is administered to a nursing woman.

Pediatric Use: The efficacy and safety of Ampicillin Sodium/Sulbactam Sodium have not been established in infants and children under the age of 12.

ADVERSE REACTIONS

Ampicillin Sodium/Sulbactam Sodium is generally well tolerated. The following adverse reactions have been reported.

LOCAL ADVERSE REACTIONS
Pain at IM injection site—16%
Pain at IV injection site—3%
Thrombophlebitis—3%

SYSTEMIC ADVERSE REACTIONS
The most frequently reported adverse reactions were diarrhea in 3% of the patients and rash in less than 2% of the patients.

Additional systemic reactions reported in less than 1% of the patients were: itching, nausea, vomiting, candidiasis, fatigue, malaise, headache, chest pain, flatulence, abdominal distension, glossitis, urine retention, dysuria, edema, facial swelling, erythema, chills, tightness in throat, substernal pain, epistaxis and mucosal bleeding.

ADVERSE LABORATORY CHANGES
Adverse laboratory changes without regard to drug relationship that were reported during clinical trials were:

Hepatic: Increased AST (SGOT), ALT (SGPT), alkaline phosphatase, and LDH.

Hematologic: Decreased hemoglobin, hematocrit, RBC, WBC, neurophils, lymphocytes, platelets and increased lymphocytes, monocytes, basophils, eosinophils, and platelets.

Blood Chemistry: Decreased serum albumin and total proteins.

Renal: Increased BUN and creatinine.

Urinalysis: Presence of RBC's and hyaline casts in urine. The following adverse reactions have been reported with ampicillin-class antibiotics and can also occur with Ampicillin Sodium/Sulbactam Sodium.

Gastrointestinal: Gastritis, stomatitis, black "hairy" tongue, and enterocolitis. Onset of pseudomembranous colitis symptoms may occur during or after antibiotic treatment. (See *"Warnings"*.)

Hypersensitivity Reactions: Urticaria, erythema multiforme, and an occasional case of exfoliative dermatitis have been reported. These reactions may be controlled with antihistamines and, if necessary, systemic corticosteroids. Whenever such reactions occur, the drug should be discontinued, unless the opinion of the physician dictates otherwise. Serious and occasional fatal hypersensitivity (anaphylactic) reactions can occur with a penicillin. (See *"Warnings"*.)

Hematologic: In addition to the adverse laboratory changes listed above for Ampicillin Sodium/Sulbactam Sodium, agranulocytosis has been reported during therapy with penicillins. All of these reactions are usually reversible on discontinuation of therapy and are believed to be hypersensitivity phenomena. Some individuals have developed positive direct Coombs Tests during treatment with Ampicillin Sodium/Sulbactam Sodium, as with other beta-lactam antibiotics.

OVERDOSAGE

Neurological adverse reactions, including convulsions, may occur with the attainment of high CSF levels of beta-lactams. Ampicillin may be removed from circulation by hemodialysis. The molecular weight, degree of protein binding and pharmacokinetics profile of Sulbactam suggest that this compound may also be removed by hemodialysis.

DOSAGE AND ADMINISTRATION

Ampicillin Sodium/Sulbactam Sodium may be administered by either the IV or the IM routes.

For IV administration, the dose can be given by slow intravenous injection over at least 10-15 minutes or can also be delivered, in greater dilutions with 50-100 mL of a compatible diluent as an intravenous infusion over 15-30 minutes.

Ampicillin Sodium/Sulbactam Sodium may be administered by deep intramuscular injection. (See *"Preparation for Intramuscular Injection"*.) The recommended adult dosage of Ampicillin Sodium/Sulbactam Sodium is 1.5 g (1 g Ampicillin as the sodium salt plus 0.5 g Sulbactam as the sodium salt) to 3 g (2 g Ampicillin as the sodium salt plus 1 g Sulbactam as the sodium salt) every six hours. This 1.5 to 3 g range represents the total of Ampicillin content plus the Sulbactam content of Ampicillin Sodium/Sulbactam Sodium and corresponds to a range of 1 g Ampicillin/0.5 g Sulbactam to 2 g Ampicillin/1 g Sulbactam. The total dose of Sulbactam should not exceed 4 grams per day.

IMPAIRED RENAL FUNCTION
In patients with impairment of renal function the elimination kinetics of ampicillin and sulbactam are similarly affected, hence the ratio of one to the other will remain constant whatever the renal function. The dose of Ampicillin Sodium/Sulbactam Sodium in such patients should be administered less frequently in accordance with the usual practice for Ampicillin and according to the following recommendations:

AMPICILLIN SODIUM/SULBACTAM SODIUM DOSAGE GUIDE FOR PATIENTS WITH RENAL IMPAIRMENT

Creatinine Clearance (mL/min/1.73m²)	Ampicillin/Sulbactam Half-Life (Hours)	Recommended Ampicillin Sodium/ Sulbactam Sodium Dosage
≥ 30	1	1.5-3.0 g q 6h-q 8h
15-29	5	1.5-3.0 g q 12h
5-14	9	1.5-3.0 g q 24h

When only serum creatinine is available, the following formula (based on sex, weight, and age of the patient) may be used to convert this value into creatinine clearance. The serum creatinine should represent a steady state of renal function.

Males $\quad \dfrac{\text{weight (kg)} \times (140\text{—age})}{72 \times \text{serum creatinine}}$

Females $\quad 0.85 \times$ above value

COMPATABILITY, RECONSTITUTION AND STABILITY

Ampicillin Sodium/Sulbactam Sodium sterile powder is to be stored at or below 30°C (86°F) prior to reconstitution.

When concomitant therapy with aminoglycosides is indicated, Ampicillin Sodium/Sulbactam Sodium and aminoglycosides should be reconstituted and administered separately, due to the *in vitro* inactivation of aminoglycosides by any of the aminopenicillins.

General Dissolution Procedures: Ampicillin Sodium/Sulbactam Sodium sterile powder for intravenous and intramuscular use may be reconstituted with any of the compatible diluents described in this insert. Solutions should be allowed to stand after dissolution to allow any foaming to dissipate in order to permit visual inspection for complete solubilization.

PREPARATION FOR INTRAVENOUS USE

1.5 g and 3.0 g Bottles: Ampicillin Sodium/Sulbactam Sodium sterile powder in piggy-back units may be reconstituted directly to the desired concentrations using any of the following parenteral diluents. Reconstitution of Ampicillin Sodium/Sulbactam Sodium at the specified concentrations, with these diluents provide stable solutions for the time periods indicated in the following table; (After the indicated time periods any unused portions of solutions should be discarded.)

Diluent	Maximum Concentration (mg/mL) Ampicillin/Sulbactam	Use Periods
Sterile Water for Injection	45 (30/15)	8 hrs @ 25°C
	45 (30/15)	48 hrs @ 4°C
	30 (20/10)	72 hrs @ 4°C
0.9% Sodium Chloride Injection	45 (30/15)	8 hrs @ 25°C
	45 (30/15)	48 hrs @ 4°C
	30 (20/10)	72 hrs @ 4°C
5% Dextrose Injection	30 (20/10)	2 hrs @ 25°C
	30 (20/10)	4 hrs @ 4°C
	3 (2/1)	4 hrs @ 25°C
Lactated Ringer's Injection	45 (30/15)	8 hrs @ 25°C
	45 (30/15)	24 hrs @ 4°C
M/6 Sodium Lactate Injection	45 (30/15)	8 hrs @ 25°C
	45 (30/15)	8 hrs @ 4°C
5% Dextrose in 0.45% Saline	3 (2/1)	4 hrs @ 25°C
	15 (10/5)	4 hrs @ 4°C
10% Invert Sugar	3 (2/1)	4 hrs @ 25°C
	30 (20/10)	3 hrs @ 4°C

If piggyback bottles are unavailable, standard vials of Ampicillin Sodium/ Sulbactam Sodium sterile powder may be used. Initially, the vials may be reconstituted with Sterile Water for Injection to yield solutions containing 375 mg Ampicillin Sodium/Sulbactam Sodium per mL (250 mg Ampicillin/125 mg Sulbactam per mL). An appropriate volume should then be immediately diluted with a suitable parenteral diluent to yield solutions containing 3 to 45 mg Ampicillin Sodium/Sulbactam Sodium per mL (2 to 30 mg Ampicillin/1 to 15 mg sulbactam per mL).

1.5 g Vials: Ampicillin Sodium/Sulbactam Sodium in the ADD-Vantage® system is intended as a single dose for intravenous administration after dilution with the ADD-Vantage® Flexible Diluent Container containing 50 mL, 100 mL or 250 mL of 0.9% Sodium Chloride Injection, USP.

3 g ADD-Vantage® Vials: Ampicillin Sodium/Sulbactam Sodium in the ADD-Vantage® system is intended as a single dose for intravenous administration after dilution with the ADD-Vantage® Flexible Diluent Container containing 100 mL or 250 mL of 0.9% Sodium Chloride Injection, USP.

Ampicillin Sodium/Sulbactam Sodium in the ADD-Vantage® system is to be reconstituted with 0.9% Sodium Chloride Injection, USP only. See *"Instructions for use of the ADD-Vantage® Vial"*. Reconstitution of Ampicillin Sodium/ Sulbactam Sodium at the specified concentration, with 0.9% Sodium Chloride Injection, USP provides stable solutions for the time period indicated below.

Diluent	Maximum Concentration (mg/mL) (Ampicillin/Sulbactam)	Use Period
0.9% Sodium Chloride Injection	30 (20/10)	8 hrs @ 25°C

IN 0.9% SODIUM CHLORIDE INJECTION, USP

The final diluted solution of Ampicillin Sodium/Sulbactam sodium should be completely administered *within 8 hours* in order to assure proper potency.

PREPARATION FOR INTRAMUSCULAR INJECTION

1.5 g and 3.0 g Standard Vials: Vials for intramuscular use may be reconstituted with Sterile Water for Injection USP, 0.5% Lidocaine Hydrochloride Injection USP or 2% Lidocaine Hydrochloride Injection USP. Consult the following table for recommended volumes to be added to obtain solutions containing 375 mg Ampicillin Sodium/Sulbactam Sodium per mL (250 mg ampicillin/125 mg sulbactam per mL). *Note:* Use only freshly prepared solutions and administer within one hour after preparation.

Ampicillin Sodium/ Sulbactam Sodium Vial Size	Volume of Diluent to be Added	Withdrawal Volume*
1.5 g	3.2 mL	4.0 mL
3.0 g	6.4 mL	8.0 mL

* *There is sufficient excess present to allow withdrawal and administration of the stated volumes.*

Animal Pharmacology: While reversible glycogenosis was observed in laboratory animals, this phenomenon was dose-and time-dependent and is not expected to develop at the therapeutic doses and corresponding plasma levels attained during the relatively short periods of combined ampicillin/sulbactam therapy in man.

REFERENCES
1. National Committee for Clinical Laboratory Standards, *Performance Standards for Antimicrobial Disk Susceptibility Tests*—Fourth Edition. Approved Standard NCCLS Document M2-A4, Vol. 10, No. 7 NCCLS. Villanova, PA. April 1990. 2. National Committee for Clinical Laboratory Standards, *Methods for Dilution Antimicrobial Susceptibility Tests for Bacteria that Grow Aerobically*. Second Edition. Approved Standard NCCLS Document M7-A2. Vol. 10, No 8 NCCLS. Villanova, PA. April 1990.

HOW SUPPLIED
POWDER FOR INJECTION: 1 GM-0.5 GM

BRAND/MANUFACTURER	NDC	SIZE	AWP
○ **BRAND**			
UNASYN: Roerig,J.B.	00049-0013-83	10s	$63.54
	00049-0031-83	10s	$67.41
	00049-0022-83	10s	$73.63

POWDER FOR INJECTION: 2 GM-1 GM

BRAND/MANUFACTURER	NDC	SIZE	AWP
○ **BRAND**			
UNASYN: Roerig,J.B.	00049-0014-83	10s	$119.93
	00049-0032-83	10s	$123.80
	00049-0023-83	10s	$130.63

Amrinone Lactate

DESCRIPTION

Amrinone Lactate injection represents a new class of cardiac inotropic agents distinct from digitalis glycosides or catecholamines. Amrinone Lactate is designated chemically as 5-Amino[3,4'-bipyridin]-6(1H)-one 2-hydroxypropanate.

Amrinone is a pale yellow crystalline compound with a molecular weight of 187.2 and an empirical formula of $C_{10}H_9N_3O$. Each mole of lactic acid has a molecular weight of 90.08 and an empirical formula of $C_3H_6O_3$. The solubilities of Amrinone Lactate at pH's 4.1, 6.0, and 8.0 are 25, 0.9, and 0.7 mg/mL, respectively.

Amrinone Lactate injection is available as a sterile solution in 20 mL ampuls for intravenous administration. Each mL contains Amrinone Lactate equivalent to 5 mg of base and 0.25 mg of sodium metabisulfite added as a preservative in Water for Injection. All dosages expressed in the package insert are expressed in terms of the base, Amrinone. The pH is adjusted to between 3.2 to 4.0 with lactic acid or sodium hydroxide. The total concentration of lactic acid can vary between 5.0 mg/mL and 7.5 mg/mL.

➤ SHOWN IN PRODUCT IDENTIFICATION GUIDE

Following is its chemical structure:

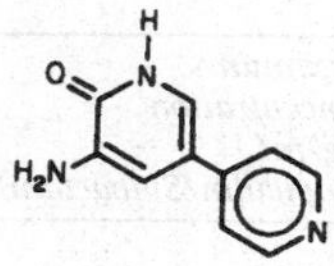

CLINICAL PHARMACOLOGY

Amrinone Lactate injection is a positive inotropic agent with vasodilator activity, different in structure and mode of action from either digitalis glycosides or catecholamines.

The mechanism of its inotropic and vasodilator effects has not been fully elucidated.

With respect to its inotropic effect, experimental evidence indicates that it is not a beta-adrenergic agonist. It inhibits myocardial cyclic adenosine monophosphate (c-AMP) phosphodiesterase activity and increases cellular levels of c-AMP. Unlike digitalis, it does not inhibit sodium-potassium adenosine triphosphatase activity.

With respect to its vasodilatory activity, Amrinone Lactate reduces afterload and preload by its direct relaxant effect on vascular smooth muscle.

PHARMACOKINETICS

Following intravenous bolus (1 to 2 minutes) injection of 0.68 mg/kg to 1.2 mg/kg to normal volunteers, Amrinone Lactate had a volume of distribution of 1.2 liters/kg, and following a distributive phase half-life of about 4.6 minutes in plasma, had a mean apparent first-order terminal elimination half-life of about 3.6 hours. In patients with congestive heart failure receiving infusions of Amrinone Lactate the mean apparent first-order terminal elimination half-life was about 5.8 hours.

Amrinone has been shown in one study to be 10% to 22% bound to human plasma protein by ultrafiltration in vitro, and in another study 35% to 49% bound by either ultrafiltration or equilibrium dialysis.

The primary route of excretion in man is *via* the urine as both Amrinone Lactate and several metabolites (N-glycolyl, N-acetate, O-glucuronide and N-glucuronide). In normal volunteers, approximately 63% of an oral dose of ^{14}C-labelled amrinone was excreted in the urine over a 96-hour period. In the first 8 hours, 51% of the radioactivity in the urine was Amrinone with 5% as the N-acetate, 8% as the N-glycolate, and less than 5% for each glucuronide. Approximately 18% of the administered dose was excreted in the feces in 72 hours. In a 24-hour nonradioactive intravenous study, 10% to 40% of the dose was excreted in urine as unchanged Amrinone Lactate with the N-acetyl metabolite representing less than 2% of the dose.

In congestive heart failure patients, after a loading bolus dose, steady-state plasma levels of about 2.4 μg/mL were able to be maintained by an infusion of 5 μg/kg/min to 10 μg/kg/min. In some congestive heart failure patients, with associated compromised renal and hepatic perfusion, it is possible that plasma levels of Amrinone Lactate may rise during the infusion period; therefore, in these patients, it may be necessary to monitor the hemodynamic response and/or drug level. The principal measures of patient response include cardiac index, pulmonary capillary wedge pressure, central venous pressure, and their relationship to plasma concentrations. Additionally, measurements of blood pressure, urine output, and body weight may prove useful, as may such clinical symptoms as orthopnea, dyspnea, and fatigue.

PHARMACODYNAMICS

In patients with depressed myocardial function, Amrinone Lactate injection produces a prompt increase in cardiac output due to its inotropic and vasodilator actions.

Following a single intravenous bolus dose of Amrinone Lactate of 0.75 mg/kg to 3 mg/kg in patients with congestive heart failure, dose-related maximum increases in cardiac output occur (of about 28% at 0.75 mg/kg to about 61% at 3 mg/kg). The peak effect occurs within 10 minutes at all doses. The duration of effect depends upon dose, lasting about ½ hour at 0.75 mg/kg and approximately 2 hours at 3 mg/kg.

Over the same range of doses, pulmonary capillary wedge pressure and total peripheral resistance show dose-related decreases (mean maximum decreases of 29% in pulmonary capillary wedge pressure and 29% in systemic vascular resistance). At doses up to 3.0 mg/kg dose-related decreases in diastolic pressure (up to 13%) have been observed. Mean arterial pressure decreases (9.7%) at a dose of 3.0 mg/kg. The heart rate is generally unchanged.

The changes in hemodynamic parameters are maintained during continuous intravenous infusion and for several hours thereafter.

Amrinone Lactate injection is effective in fully digitalized patients without causing signs of cardiac glycoside toxicity. Its inotropic effects are additive to those of digitalis. In cases of atrial flutter/fibrillation, it is possible that Amrinone Lactate may increase ventricular response because of its slight enhancement of A/V conduction. In these cases, prior treatment with digitalis is recommended.

Improvement in left ventricular function and relief of congestive heart failure in patients with ischemic heart disease have been observed. The improvement has occurred without inducing symptoms or electrocardiographic signs of myocardial ischemia.

At constant heart rate and blood pressure, increases in cardiac output occur without measurable increases in myocardial oxygen consumption or changes in arteriovenous oxygen difference.

Inotropic activity is maintained following repeated intravenous doses of Amrinone Lactate. Administration of Amrinone Lactate produces hemodynamic and symptomatic benefits to patients not satisfactorily controlled by conventional therapy with diuretics and cardiac glycosides.

INDICATIONS AND USAGE

Amrinone Lactate injection is indicated for the short-term management of congestive heart failure. Because of limited experience and potential for serious adverse effects (see *"Adverse Reactions"*), Amrinone Lactate should be used only in patients who can be closely monitored and who have not responded adequately to digitalis, diuretics, and/or vasodilators. Although most patients have been studied hemodynamically for periods only up to 24 hours, some patients were studied for longer periods and demonstrated consistent hemodynamic and clinical effects. The duration of therapy should depend on patient responsiveness.

UNLABELED USES

Amrinone Lactate is used alone or as an adjunct in the treatment of low cardiac output after open heart surgery.

CONTRAINDICATIONS

Amrinone Lactate injection is contraindicated in patients who are hypersensitive to it.

It is also contraindicated in those patients known to be hypersensitive to bisulfites.

WARNING

Contains sodium metabisulfite, a sulfite that may cause allergic-type reactions including anaphylactic symptoms and life-threatening or less severe asthmatic episodes in certain susceptible people. The overall prevalence of sulfite sensitivity in the general population is unknown and probably low. Sulfite sensitivity is seen more frequently in asthmatic than in nonasthmatic people.

PRECAUTIONS

GENERAL

Amrinone Lactate injection should not be used in patients with severe aortic or pulmonic valvular disease in lieu of surgical relief of the obstruction. Like other inotropic agents, it may aggravate outflow tract obstruction in hypertrophic subaortic stenosis.

During intravenous therapy with Amrinone Lactate injection, blood pressure and heart rate should be monitored and the rate of infusion slowed or stopped in patients showing excessive decreases in blood pressure.

Patients who have received vigorous diuretic therapy may have insufficient cardiac filling pressure to respond adequately to Amrinone Lactate injection, in which case cautious liberalization of fluid and electrolyte intake may be indicated.

Supraventricular and ventricular arrhythmias have been observed in the very high-risk population treated. While Amrinone Lactate per se has not been shown to be arrhythmogenic, the potential for arrhythmia, present in congestive heart failure itself, may be increased by any drug or combination of drugs.

Thrombocytopenia and hepatotoxicity have been noted (see *"Adverse Reactions"*).

USE IN ACUTE MYOCARDIAL INFARCTION

No clinical trials have been carried out in patients in the acute phase of postmyocardial infarction. Therefore, Amrinone Lactate injection is not recommended in these cases.

LABORATORY TESTS

Fluid and Electrolytes: Fluid and electrolyte changes and renal function should be carefully monitored during Amrinone Lactate therapy. Improvement in cardiac output with resultant diuresis may necessitate a reduction in the dose of diuretic. Potassium loss due to excessive diuresis may predispose digitalized patients to arrhythmias. Therefore, hypokalemia should be corrected by potassium supplementation in advance of or during Amrinone Lactate use.

DRUG INTERACTIONS

In a relatively limited experience, no untoward clinical manifestations have been observed in patients in which Amrinone Lactate injection was used concurrently with the following drugs: digitalis glycosides; lidocaine, quinidine; metoprolol, propranolol; hydralazine, prazosin; isosorbide dinitrate, nitroglycerine; chlorthalidone, ethacrynic acid, furosemide, hydrochlorothiazide, spironolactone; captopril; heparin, warfarin; potassium supplements; insulin, diazepam.

One case report of excessive hypotension has been reported when Amrinone Lactate was used concurrently with disopyramide. Until additional experience is available, concurrent administration with disopyramides should be undertaken with caution.

CHEMICAL INTERACTIONS

A chemical interaction occurs slowly over a 24-hour period when the intravenous solution of Amrinone Lactate injection is mixed *directly* with dextrose(glucose)-containing solutions. **THEREFORE, AMRINONE LACTATE INJECTION SHOULD NOT BE DILUTED WITH SOLUTIONS THAT CONTAIN DEXTROSE (GLUCOSE) PRIOR TO INJECTION.**

A chemical interaction occurs immediately, which is evidenced by the formation of a precipitate when furosemide is injected into an intravenous line of an infusion of Amrinone Lactate. Therefore, furosemide should not be administered in intravenous lines containing Amrinone Lactate.

◆ RATED THERAPEUTICALLY EQUIVALENT; ◇ THERAPEUTIC EQUIVALENCE UNCONFIRMED; ○ UNRATED

CARCINOGENESIS, MUTAGENESIS, IMPAIRMENT OF FERTILITY

There was no suggestion of a carcinogenic potential with Amrinone Lactate when administered orally for up to two years to rats and mice at dose levels up to the maximally tolerated dose of 80 mg/kg/day.

The mouse micronucleus test (at 7.5 to 10 times the maximum human dose) and the Chinese hamster ovary chromosome aberration assay were positive indicating both clastogenic potential and suppression of the number of polychromatic erythrocytes. However, the Ames Salmonella assay, mouse lymphoma study, and cultured human lymphocyte metaphase analysis were all negative. The clastogenic effects are in contrast to negative results obtained in the rat male and female fertility studies, and a three-generation study in rats, both with oral dosing.

Slight prolongation of the rat gestation period was seen in these studies at dose levels of 50 mg/kg/day and 100 mg/kg/day. Dystocia occurred in dams receiving 100 mg/kg/day resulting in increased numbers of stillbirths, decreased litter size, and poor pup survival.

PREGNANCY CATEGORY C

In New Zealand white rabbits, Amrinone Lactate has been shown to produce fetal skeletal and gross external malformations at oral doses of 16 mg/kg and 50 mg/kg which were toxic for the rabbit. Studies in French Hy/Cr rabbits using oral doses up to 32 mg/kg/day did not confirm this finding. No malformations were seen in rats receiving Amrinone Lactate intravenously at the maximum dose used, 15 mg/kg/day (approximately the recommended daily intravenous dose for patients with congestive heart failure). There are no adequate and well-controlled studies in pregnant women. Amrinone Lactate should be used during pregnancy only if the potential benefit justifies the potential risk to the fetus.

NURSING MOTHERS

Caution should be exercised when Amrinone Lactate is administered to nursing women, since it is not known whether it is excreted in human milk.

PEDIATRIC USE

Safety and effectiveness in children have not been established.

ADVERSE REACTIONS

Thrombocytopenia: Intravenous Amrinone Lactate injection resulted in platelet count reductions to below 100,000/mm^3 or normal limits in 2.4 percent of the patients.

It is more common in patients receiving prolonged therapy. To date, in closely-monitored clinical trials, in patients whose platelet counts were not allowed to remain depressed, no bleeding phenomena have been observed.

Platelet reduction is dose dependent and appears due to a decrease in platelet survival time. Several patients who developed thrombocytopenia while receiving Amrinone Lactate had bone marrow examinations which were normal. There is no evidence relating platelet reduction to immune response or to a platelet activating factor.

Gastrointestinal Effects: Gastrointestinal adverse reactions reported with Amrinone Lactate injection during clinical use included nausea (1.7%), vomiting (0.9%), abdominal pain (0.4%), and anorexia (0.4%).

Cardiovascular Effects: Cardiovascular adverse reactions reported with Amrinone Lactate injection include arrhythmia (3%) and hypotension (1.3%).

Hepatic Toxicity: In dogs, at IV doses between 9 mg/kg/day and 32 mg/kg/day, Amrinone Lactate showed dose-related hepatotoxicity manifested either as enzyme elevation or hepatic cell necrosis or both. Hepatotoxicity has been observed in man following long-term oral dosing and has been observed, in a limited experience (0.2%), following intravenous administration of Amrinone Lactate. There have also been rare reports of enzyme and bilirubin elevation and jaundice.

Hypersensitivity: There have been reports of several apparent hypersensitivity reactions in patients treated with oral Amrinone Lactate for about two weeks. Signs and symptoms were variable but included pericarditis, pleuritis and ascites (1 case), myositis with interstitial shadowing on chest x-ray and elevated sedimentation rate (1 case) and vasculitis with nodular pulmonary densities, hypoxemia, and jaundice (1 case). The first patient died, not necessarily of the possible reaction, while the last two resolved with discontinuation of therapy. None of the cases were rechallenged so that attribution to Amrinone Lactate is not certain, but possible hypersensitivity reactions should be considered in any patient maintained for a prolonged period on Amrinone Lactate.

General: Additional adverse reactions observed in intravenous Amrinone Lactate clinical studies include fever (0.9%), chest pain (0.2%), and burning at the site of injection (0.2%).

MANAGEMENT OF ADVERSE REACTIONS

Platelet Count Reductions: Asymptomatic platelet count reduction (to < 150,000/mm^3) may be reversed within one week of a decrease in drug dosage. Further, with no change in drug dosage, the count may stabilize at lower than pre-drug levels without any clinical sequelae. Pre-drug platelet counts and frequent platelet counts during therapy are recommended to assist in decisions regarding dosage modifications.

Should a platelet count less than 150,000/mm^3 occur, the following actions may be considered:

■ Maintain total daily dose unchanged, since in some cases counts have either stabilized or returned to pretreatment levels.
■ Decrease total daily doses.

■ Discontinue Amrinone Lactate if, in the clinical judgment of the physician, risk exceeds the potential benefit.

Gastrointestinal Side Effects: While gastrointestinal side effects were seen infrequently with intravenous therapy, should severe or debilitating ones occur, the physician may wish to reduce dosage or discontinue the drug based on the usual benefit-to-risk considerations.

Hepatic Toxicity: In clinical experience to date with intravenous administration, hepatotoxicity has been observed rarely. If acute marked alterations in liver enzymes occur together with clinical symptoms suggesting an idiosyncratic hypersensitivity reaction, Amrinone Lactate therapy should be promptly discontinued.

If less than marked enzyme alterations occur without clinical symptoms, these nonspecific changes should be evaluated on an individual basis. The clinician may wish to continue Amrinone Lactate, reduce dosage, or discontinue the drug based on the usual benefit/risk considerations.

OVERDOSAGE

A death has been reported with a massive accidental overdose (840 mg over three hours by initial bolus and infusion) of Amrinone Lactate, although causal relation is uncertain. Diligence should be exercised during product preparation and administration.

Doses of Amrinone Lactate injection may produce hypotension because of its vasodilator effect. If this occurs, Amrinone Lactate administration should be reduced or discontinued. No specific antidote is known, but general measures for circulatory support should be taken.

In rats, the LD$_{50}$ of Amrinone Lactate was 102 mg/kg or 130 mg/kg intravenously in two different studies and 132 mg/kg orally (intragastrically); as a suspension in aqueous gum tragacanth the oral LD$_{50}$ was 239 mg/kg.

DOSAGE AND ADMINISTRATION

Loading doses of Amrinone Lactate injection should be administered as supplied (undiluted). Infusions of Amrinone Lactate injection may be administered in normal, or half normal saline solution to a concentration of 1 mg/mL to 3 mg/mL. Diluted solutions should be used within 24 hours.

Amrinone Lactate injection may be injected into running dextrose (glucose) infusions through a Y-Connector or directly into the tubing where preferable.

CHEMICAL INTERACTIONS

A chemical interaction occurs slowly over a 24-hour period when the intravenous solution of Amrinone Lactate injection is mixed *directly* with dextrose (glucose)-containing solutions. **THEREFORE, AMRINONE LACTATE INJECTION SHOULD NOT BE DILUTED WITH SOLUTIONS THAT CONTAIN DEXTROSE (GLUCOSE) PRIOR TO INJECTION.**

A chemical interaction occurs immediately, which is evidenced by the formation of a precipitate when furosemide is injected into an intravenous line of an infusion of Amrinone Lactate. Therefore, furosemide should not be administered in intravenous lines containing Amrinone Lactate.

The following procedure is recommended for the administration of Amrinone Lactate injection:

1. Initiate therapy with a 0.75 mg/kg loading dose given slowly over 2 to 3 minutes. (See related table).

2. Continue therapy with a maintenance infusion between 5 µg/kg/min and 10 µg/kg/min.

3. Based on clinical response, an additional loading dose of 0.75 mg/kg may be given 30 minutes after the initiation of therapy.

4. The rate of infusion usually ranges from 5 µg/kg/min to 10 µg/kg/min such that the recommended total daily dose (including loading doses) does not exceed 10 mg/kg. A limited number of patients studied at higher doses support a dosage regimen up to 18 mg/kg/day for shortened durations of therapy.

The following infusion rate chart may be used to assure that the calculations are made correctly.

To utilize the chart, the concentration of Amrinone Lactate infusion solution used must be 2.5 mg/mL (2500 µg/mL). This concentration is prepared by mixing the Amrinone Lactate solution with an equal volume of diluent (normal or half normal saline). (See related table).

5. The rate of administration and the duration of therapy should be adjusted according to the response of the patient. The physician may wish to reduce or titrate the infusion downward based on clinical responsiveness or untoward effects.

The above dosing regimens can be expected to place most patients' plasma concentration of Amrinone Lactate at approximately 3 µg/mL. Increases in cardiac index show a linear relationship to plasma concentration of a range of 0.5 µg/mL to 7 µg/mL. No observations have been made at greater plasma concentrations.

Patient improvement may be reflected by increases in cardiac output, reduction in pulmonary capillary wedge pressure, and such clinical responses as a lessening of dyspnea and an improvement in other symptoms of heart failure, such as orthopnea and fatigue.

Monitoring central venous pressure (CVP) may be valuable in the assessment of hypotension and fluid balance management. Prior correction or adjustment of fluid/electrolytes is essential to obtain satisfactory response with Amrinone Lactate.

Parenteral drug products should be inspected visually and should not be used if particulate matter or discoloration is observed.

➤ SHOWN IN PRODUCT IDENTIFICATION GUIDE

LOADING DOSE DETERMINATION

Patient Weight in kg	30	40	50	60	0.75 Mg/Kg (Undiluted)					
					70	80	90	100	110	120
mL of undiluted Amrinone Lactate Inj	4.5	6.0	7.5	9.0	10.5	12.0	13.5	15.0	16.5	18.0

AMRINONE LACTATE I.V. INFUSION RATE (ML/HR) CHART

Patient Weight in kg	30	40	50	60	Using 2.5 mg/mL Infusion Concentration*					
					70	80	90	100	110	120
Dosage: 5.0 µg/kg/min	4	5	6	7	8	10	11	12	13	14
7.5 µg/kg/min	5	7	9	11	13	14	16	18	20	22
10.0 µg/kg/min	7	10	12	14	17	19	22	24	26	29

Example: A 70 kg patient would require a loading dose of 10.5 mL of undiluted Amrinone Lactate. If the physician selects a dose of 7.5 µg/kg/min for the infusion, the flow rate would be 13 mL/hr at the 2.5 mg/mL concentration of Amrinone Lactate.

* *Dilution:* To prepare the 2.5 mg/mL concentration recommended for infusion mix Amrinone Lactate with an equal volume of diluent. For example, mix three 20 mL ampuls of Amrinone Lactate (3 × 20 mL = 60 mL) with 60 mL of diluent for a total volume of 120 mL of the final 2.5 mg/mL solution of Amrinone Lactate.

Protect Amrinone Lactate ampuls from light. Ampul packaging is light resistant for protection during storage. Store at room temperature.

HOW SUPPLIED
INJECTION: 5 MG/ML

BRAND/MANUFACTURER	NDC	SIZE	AWP
○ BRAND			
INOCOR I.V.: Sanofi Winthrop	00024-0888-20	20 ml 25s	$1448.66

Amyl Nitrite

DESCRIPTION
Amyl Nitrite is a rapidly acting vasodilator administered by inhalation. 0.3 ml is supplied in a covered thin glass capsule which is easily crushed between the fingers. Amyl Nitrite is a clear, yellowish liquid having a peculiar ethereal, fruity odor. It is volatile, even at low temperatures, and is flammable.

Following is its chemical structure:

$$CH_3CH(CH_3)CH_2CH_2-O-N=O$$

CLINICAL PHARMACOLOGY
Amyl Nitrite causes a non specific relaxation of smooth muscle with the most prominent actions occurring in vascular smooth muscle. This effect on vascular smooth muscle results in coronary vasodilation and decreased systemic vascular resistance and left ventricular preload and afterload. Myocardial ischemia is relieved in patients with angina pectoris, with an abatement of chest pain and possibly other related symptoms. Amyl Nitrite vapors are absorbed rapidly through the pulmonary alveoli, manifesting therapeutic effects within one minute after inhalation. The drug is metabolized rapidly, probably by hydrolytic denitration; approximately one-third of the inhaled Amyl Nitrite is excreted in the urine.

INDICATIONS AND USAGE
Amyl Nitrite is indicated for the rapid relief of angina pectoris. Its effect appears within 30 seconds and lasts for approximately 3 to 5 minutes.

UNLABELED USES
Amyl Nitrite is used alone or as an adjunct in the treatment to prevent postoperative erections.

CONTRAINDICATIONS
Since it may increase intraocular and intracranial pressures, Amyl Nitrite is contraindicated or should be used with great caution in patients with glaucoma, recent head trauma or cerebral hemorrhage.

Amyl Nitrite can cause harm to the fetus when it is administered to a pregnant woman because it significantly reduces systemic blood pressure and blood flow on the maternal side of the placenta.

WARNINGS
Transient episodes of dizziness, weakness, or syncope or other signs of cerebral ischemia due to postural hypotension may develop following inhalation of Amyl Nitrite, particularly if the patient is standing immobile. To hasten recovery, measures which facilitate venous return such as head-low posture, deep breathing and movement of extremities may be used.

CAUTION
Amyl Nitrite is very flammable. Do not use where it might become ignited.

PRECAUTIONS
General: Tolerance to Amyl Nitrite may develop with repeated use of the drug for prolonged periods of time. Tolerance may be minimized by beginning with the smallest effective dose and alternating the drug with another coronary vasodilator.

High doses of Nitrites may produce methemoglobinemia, especially in individuals with methemoglobin reductase deficiency or other metabolic abnormality that interferes with the normal conversion of methemoglobin back to hemoglobin.

Patient Information: Amyl Nitrite should be taken by the patient when seated or lying down.

Drug Interactions: Taking Amyl Nitrite after drinking alcohol may worsen side effects and may cause severe hypotension and cardiovascular collapse.

Carcinogenesis, Mutagenesis, Fertility Impairment: Adequate long term studies to establish adverse carcinogenic potential of this drug have not been reported.

Pregnancy: Teratogenic effects: Category C. Animal studies have not been conducted with Amyl Nitrite. It is also not known whether Amyl Nitrite can cause fetal harm when administered to a pregnant woman or can affect reproduction capacity. Amyl Nitrite should be given to a pregnant woman only if clearly needed.

Nursing Mothers: It is not known whether this drug is excreted in human milk. Because many drugs care excreted in human milk, caution should be exercised when Amyl Nitrite is administered to a nursing woman.

Pediatric Use: Safety and effectiveness in children have not been established.

ADVERSE REACTIONS
Mild transitory headache, dizziness and flushing of the face are common with the use of Amyl Nitrite. The following adverse reactions may occur in susceptible patients: syncope, involuntary passing of urine and feces, hypotension, pallor, cold sweat, tachycardia, restlessness, weakness, vomiting and nausea. Excessively high doses of Amyl Nitrite administered chronically may cause methemoglobinemia.

DRUG ABUSE AND DEPENDENCE
Abuse: Volatile Nitrites are abused for sexual stimulation, with headache as a common side effect.

Dependence: Tolerance to Nitrites can develop; conditions and duration have not been established.

OVERDOSAGE
Symptoms: Inhaled doses of 5 to 10 drops of Amyl Nitrite may cause violent flushing of the face, accompanied by a feeling of imminent bursting of the head and very excessive heart action. The inhalation of larger amounts may produce a feeling of suffocation and muscular weakness. Symptoms comparable to shock may be produced (such as weakness, restlessness, sweating, pallor, nausea, vomiting, syncope and incontinence) attributable to pooling of blood in the postarteriolar vessels and failure of the venous blood to return to the heart.

Treatment: Measures which facilitate venous return such as head-low posture, deep breathing and movement of extremities may be used. The use of epinephrine aggravates the shock-like reaction. Methylene blue should be injected for treatment of severe methemoglobinemia with dyspnea. For treating cyanide poisoning, methylene blue is contraindicated where nitrites cause iatrogenic methemoglobinemia.

DOSAGE AND ADMINISTRATION
With the patient in recumbent or seated position a capsule of Amyl Nitrite is held away from the face, crushed between the fingers, and held under the patient's

---

◆ RATED THERAPEUTICALLY EQUIVALENT; ◇ THERAPEUTIC EQUIVALENCE UNCONFIRMED; ○ UNRATED

nose. Two to six inhalations of the vapors from the capsule are usually sufficient to promptly produce therapeutic effects. Caution is recommended to avoid inhalation of excessive amounts of the drug when it is administered by someone other than the patient. If necessary, the dose may be repeated in 3 to 5 minutes.

The capsule contents are **FLAMMABLE** and should be protected from light. Storage should be in a cool place, 8°-15°C (46°-59°F).

HOW SUPPLIED
SOLUTION:

BRAND/MANUFACTURER	NDC	SIZE	AWP
○ GENERICS			
Moore,H.L.	00839-6462-03	12s	$3.85
Newton	17113-0001-12	12s	$4.55
Alexander, James	46414-2222-01	12s	$4.75
Pharma-Tek	39822-9950-02	12s	$5.95
Allscrips	54569-3157-00	0.3 ml 12s	$4.75
CMC-Cons	00223-7002-12	0.3 ml 12s	$6.00

Amyl Nitrite/Sodium Nitrite/
Sodium Thiosulfate

DESCRIPTION
Each cyanide antidote package contains:
12 ampoules Amyl Nitrite Inhalants, USP, 5 min (0.3 mL).
2 ampoules Sodium Nitrite Injection, USP, 300 mg in 10 mL of sterile water.
2 vials or ampoules of Sodium Thiosulfate Injection, USP, 12.5 g in 50 mL of sterile water.

The package also contains 1 sterile 10 mL plastic, disposable syringe with 22-gauge needle, 1 sterile 60 mL plastic disposable syringe, 1 sterile disposable 20-gauge needle, 1 stomach tube, 1 nonsterile 60 mL syringe, 1 tourniquet, and 1 set of instructions for the treatment of cyanide poisoning.

ACTIONS
Sodium Nitrite reacts with hemoglobin to form methemoglobin. The latter removes cyanide ions from various tissues and couples with them to become cyanmethemoglobin, which has a relatively low toxicity. The function of Sodium Thiosulfate is to convert cyanide to thiocyanate, probably by an enzyme known as rhodanese. The combined mechanism may thus be expressed in a chemical manner.

$NaNO_2$ + Hemoglobin = Methemoglobin
HCN + Methemoglobin = Cyanmethemoglobin
$Na_2S_2O_3$ + HCN + O = HSCN

The combination of Sodium Nitrite and Sodium Thiosulfate is the best therapy against cyanide and hydrocyanic acid poisoning. The 2 substances intravenously injected, one after the other (nitrite followed by the thiosulfate) are capable of detoxifying approximately 20 lethal doses of sodium cyanide in dogs and are effective even after respiration has stopped. As long as the heart is still beating, the chances of recovery by utilizing this method are very good.

There is not only a summation but also a definite potentiation of action when the nitrite and the thiosulfate are administered together.

INDICATION
Indicated for the treatment of cyanide poisoning.

WARNING
Both Sodium Nitrite and Amyl Nitrite in excessive doses induce dangerous methemoglobinemia and can cause death. The amounts found in a single cyanide antidote package are not excessive for an adult. The doses for children should be calculated on a surface area or on a weight basis with the dosage adjusted so that excessive methemoglobin is not formed.

If signs of excessive methemoglobinemia develop (i.e., blue skin and mucous membranes, vomiting, shock, and coma), 1% methylene blue solution should be given intravenously. A total dose of 1 to 2 mg/kg of body weight should be administered over a period of 5 to 10 minutes and should be repeated in 1 hour if necessary.

In addition, oxygen inhalation and transfusion of whole fresh blood should be considered.

DOSAGE AND ADMINISTRATION
Personnel should acquire some skill in the proper method of administering the contents of this package prior to an emergency. Cyanide poisoning is rapidly fatal. The patient seldom survives many hours. The prevention of death demands a quick diagnosis and the prompt use of specific antidotes. No valuable time should be lost. Even though the diagnosis is doubtful, the therapy recommended should be instituted immediately. For best results, the physician should be acquainted beforehand with the following steps:

1. Instruct an assistant how to break an ampoule of Amyl Nitrite, one at a time, in a handkerchief and hold it in front of the patient's mouth for 15 seconds—followed by a rest for 15 seconds. Then reapply until Sodium Nitrite can be administered. This interrupted schedule is important because continuous use of Amyl Nitrite may prevent adequate oxygenation.

2. Discontinue administration of Amyl Nitrite and inject intravenously 300 mg (10 mL of a 3% solution) of Sodium Nitrite at the rate of 2.5 to 5 mL/minute. The recommended dose of Sodium Nitrite for children is 6 to 8 mL/square meter (approximately 0.2 mL/kg of body weight) but is not to exceed 10 mL.
3. Immediately thereafter, inject 12.5 g (50 mL of a 25% solution) of Sodium Thiosulfate for adults. The dosage for children is 7 g/square meter of body surface area, but dosage should not exceed 12.5 g. The same needle and vein may be used.
4. If the poison was taken by mouth, gastric lavage should be performed as soon as possible, but this should not delay the treatments outlined above. Lavage may be done concurrently by a third person—a physician or a nurse, if one is available. One should take quick action without waiting for positive diagnostic tests.

The patient should be watched closely for at least 24 to 48 hours. If signs of poisoning reappear, injection of both Sodium Nitrite and Sodium Thiosulfate should be repeated, but each in one-half of the original dose. Even it the patient seems perfectly well, the medication may be given for prophylactic purposes 2 hours after the first injections.

If respiration has ceased but the pulse is palpable, artificial respiration should be applied at once. The purpose is not to revive, per se, but to keep the heart beating. The gauze sponge or handkerchief containing Amyl Nitrite should be laid over the patient's nose, for it may hasten the resumption of respiratory movements. When signs of breathing appear, injection of the above solutions should be made promptly.

SOURCE OF CYANIDE POISONING
Certain plants produce free hydrocyanic acid or cyanogenetic glycosides which may become a source of poisoning to human beings or animals. It is said that the formation of hydrocyanic acid in these plants is due to their inability to convert all the available amino acids into proteins. Thus, it is a side reaction in protein metabolism. Bitter almonds, cherry, plum, peach, apricot, apple, and pear seeds, cassava, and certain bamboo sprouts are all capable of inducing symptoms of cyanide poisoning in human subjects when taken in sufficient quantities. Chokecherry, arrow grass, Sudan grass, and sorghum, owing to their hydrocyanic acid content, have been responsible for death of livestock. Poisoning by chokecherry seeds in man also has been reported.

Sodium or potassium cyanide is extensively used in metallurgy for extraction of gold and silver from their ores, in electroplating, for cleaning of metal by both the dip and the electrolytic processes, for organic synthesis, for dehairing hides, and for partial sterilization of soil.

Hydrocyanic acid is a most effective agent for the fumigation of ships, army posts, navy stations, large buildings, flour mills, and private dwellings which have been infested with mice, rats, moths, bedbugs, cockroaches, or carpet beetles. It is also used for the control of scale insects on citrus trees. Various commodities, such as nutmeats, beans, peas, seeds of different kinds, and baled cotton, are fumigated with hydrocyanic acid in vacuum chambers.

DIAGNOSIS
To establish a diagnosis of cyanide poisoning before death, positive proof of the presence of cyanide by chemical tests of body fluids is necessary; but to make an immediate, tentative diagnosis, circumstantial evidence usually is sufficient. If a person works with cyanide or is in proximity to fumigation activities and is suddenly taken ill, to suspect cyanide poisoning is justifiable; or, if an individual is discovered unconscious and a cyanide container is found nearby, suicidal intent may be considered probable. Clinically, the odor of bitter almond oil on the breath is highly suggestive of cyanide poisoning, but its absence does not rule out that possibility. Other signs, although not specific or pathognomonic, consist of rapid respiration (later slow and gasping), accelerated pulse, vomiting, and convulsions which are followed by coma and cyanosis. The toxic effect of cyanide is due to the suppression of cellular respiration by inhibition of the action of catalysts which promote the utilization of oxygen. The latter remains unabsorbed from the capillaries, and the venous blood appears bright red. Cyanosis is therefore a late manifestation, occurring when circulatory failure is approaching. If a person is suspected of having taken the poison by mouth, his stomach should be emptied and the contents analyzed. If he is poisoned by gaseous hydrocyanic acid, a 20 mL sample of venous blood should be drawn and similarly examined.

PREPARATION FOR EMERGENCIES
Personnel should be instructed in the proper method of administering the contents of this package prior to an emergency.

For the successful treatment of cyanide poisoning, a kit composed of the following articles may be installed in emergency cabinets, ambulances, and chemical laboratories or carried at all times with fumigation equipment.

12 pearls of Amyl Nitrite; 2 ampoules of Sodium Nitrite, 300 mg in 10 mL of sterile water; 2 ampoules of Sodium Thiosulfate injection, 12.5 g in 50 mL of sterile water; 1 sterile 10-mL syringe with a 22-gauge needle; 1 sterile 60-mL plastic disposable syringe; 1 sterile disposable 20-gauge needle; 1 stomach tube (not necessary with fumigation equipment); 1 nonsterile 60-mL syringe; and 1 tourniquet.

With the addition of certain preservatives, these solutions remain stable in ampoules for several years. It is, however, possible to make ampoules of dry crystals of each product which can be dissolved in sterile distilled water at the time of injection. If the ampoules are not available, the Nitrite and the Thiosulfate may be weighed separately and dissolved in sterile water or, if the latter is not available, in tap water. These solutions may then be injected promptly. The urgency required in the treatment of cyanide poisoning justifies the omission of sterilization. Animal experimentation has shown that infection very rarely occurs following intravenous injection, even though the drug solutions are not sterilized. If injection is made intramuscularly or subcutaneously, the nonsterilized solutions more frequently cause abscess formation.

The same combination of Sodium Nitrite and Sodium Thiosulfate has been advocated in treating sheep and cattle poisoned by eating cyanogenetic plants.

HOW SUPPLIED
KIT:

BRAND/MANUFACTURER	NDC	SIZE	AWP
○ GENERICS			
Pasadena	00418-0821-00	1s	$99.00
Lilly	00002-2385-01	1s	$140.29

Amylase/Cellulase/Lipase/Protease

DESCRIPTION
Amylase/Cellulase/Lipase/Protease Capsules are derived from fungal, plant and animal sources and are designed for oral digestive enzyme supplement therapy.

Each capsule contains:

Lipase	75 mg
Amylase	30 mg
Protease	6 mg
Cellulase	2 mg

CLINICAL PHARMACOLOGY
Diminution of secretions from exocrine glands is often a result of the normal aging process. Amylase/Cellulase/Lipase/Protease capsules provide a balanced combination of natural proteolytic, amylolytic, cellulolytic and lipolytic enzymes to enhance digestion of proteins, starch and fat in the gastrointestinal tract. These enzymes do not exert any systemic pharmacologic effects. Amylase/Cellulase/Lipase/Protease capsules should be considered an enzyme supplement and not an enzyme replacement therapy. Enzymes in Amylase/Cellulase/Lipase/Protease capsules are basically derived from fungal and plant sources and possess a broad spectrum of pH activity. Enzymes are promptly released from the capsule and are bioavailable for digestion of food in the stomach and intestines.

INDICATIONS AND USAGE
For the relief of functional indigestion when due to enzyme deficiency or imbalance. Amylase/Cellulase/Lipase/Protease capsules relieve symptoms due to faulty digestion including the sensation of fullness after meals, dyspepsia, flatulence, abdominal distention and intolerance to certain foods.

CONTRAINDICATIONS
There are no known contraindications to the administration of digestive enzymes. These enzymes do not attack living tissues and do not present any danger to the patient with ulceration or inflammation in the digestive tract.

WARNINGS
Do not administer to patients who are allergic to pork products.

PRECAUTIONS
INFORMATION FOR PATIENTS
If capsules are opened, avoid inhalation of the powder. Sensitive individuals may experience allergic reactions.

CARCINOGENESIS, MUTAGENESIS, IMPAIRMENT OF FERTILITY
Long-term studies in animals have not been performed to evaluate carcinogenic, mutagenic or impairment of fertility potential of Amylase/Cellulase/Lipase/Protease capsules.

PREGNANCY: PREGNANCY CATEGORY C
Animal reproduction studies have not been conducted with Amylase/Cellulase/Lipase/Protease capsules. It is also not known whether Amylase/Cellulase/Lipase/Protease capsules can cause fetal harm when administered to a pregnant woman or can affect reproduction capacity. Amylase/Cellulase/Lipase/Protease capsules should be given to a pregnant woman only if clearly needed.

NURSING MOTHERS
It is not known whether Amylase/Cellulase/Lipase/Protease capsules are excreted in human milk. Because many drugs are excreted in human milk, caution should be exercised when Amylase/Cellulase/Lipase/Protease capsules are administered to a nursing woman.

ADVERSE REACTIONS
Virtually unknown. Occasionally, a slight looseness of the stool may be noticed. If so, dosage should be reduced. Finely powdered pancreatic enzyme may be irritating to the mucous membranes and respiratory tract. Inhalation of the airborne powder may precipitate an asthma attack in sensitive individuals.

OVERDOSAGE
No systemic toxicity occurs. Excessive dosage may, however, produce a laxative effect.

DOSAGE AND ADMINISTRATION
1 or 2 capsules taken with each meal or snack. Dosage may be adjusted depending on individual requirements for relief of symptoms due to digestive enzyme deficiency. In patients who experience difficulty in swallowing the capsule, it may be opened and the contents sprinkled on the food. When opening the capsules, avoid inhalation of the powder (see "Precautions" and "Adverse Reactions").

Store at controlled room temperature 15°–30°C (59°–86°F).

HOW SUPPLIED
CAPSULE:

BRAND/MANUFACTURER	NDC	SIZE	AWP
○ BRAND			
KU-ZYME: Schwarz	00091-3522-01	100s	$35.19

Amytal Sodium SEE AMOBARBITAL SODIUM

Ana-Guard SEE EPINEPHRINE, SYSTEMIC

Ana-Kit SEE CHLORPHENIRAMINE MALEATE AND EPINEPHRINE HYDROCHLORIDE

Anafranil SEE CLOMIPRAMINE HYDROCHLORIDE

Anaprox SEE NAPROXEN

Anaspaz SEE HYOSCYAMINE SULFATE

Anatuss LA SEE GUAIFENESIN AND PSEUDOEPHEDRINE HYDROCHLORIDE

Ancef SEE CEFAZOLIN SODIUM

Ancobon SEE FLUCYTOSINE

Android SEE METHYLTESTOSTERONE

Anectine SEE SUCCINYLCHOLINE CHLORIDE

Anestacon SEE LIDOCAINE HYDROCHLORIDE, LOCAL ANESTHESIA AND LIDOCAINE, TOPICAL

Anexsia SEE ACETAMINOPHEN WITH HYDROCODONE BITARTRATE

Anisindione

DESCRIPTION
Anisindione Tablets contain a synthetic anticoagulant, Anisindione, an indanedione derivative. Each tablet contains 50 mg Anisindione.

Following is its chemical structure:

ACTIONS

Like phenindione, to which it is related chemically, anisindione exercises its therapeutic action by reducing the prothrombin activity of the blood.

INDICATIONS

Anisindione is indicated for the prophylaxis and treatment of venous thrombosis and its extension, the treatment of atrial fibrillation with embolization, the prophylaxis and treatment of pulmonary embolism, and as an adjunct in the treatment of coronary occlusion.

CONTRAINDICATIONS

All contraindications to oral anticoagulant therapy are relative rather than absolute. Contraindications should be evaluated for each patient, giving consideration to the need for and the benefits to be achieved by anticoagulant therapy, the potential dangers of hemorrhage, the expected duration of therapy, and the quality of patient monitoring and compliance.

Hemorrhagic Tendencies or Blood Dyscrasias: In general, oral anticoagulants are contraindicated in patients who are bleeding or who have hemorrhagic blood dyscrasias or hemorrhagic tendencies (eg, hemophilia, polycythemia vera, purpura, leukemia) or a history of bleeding diathesis. They are contraindicated in patients with recent cerebral hemorrhage, active ulceration of the gastrointestinal tract, including ulcerative colitis, or open ulcerative, traumatic, or surgical wounds. Oral anticoagulants may be contraindicated in patients with recent or contemplated brain, eye, or spinal cord surgery or prostatectomy, and in those undergoing regional or lumbar block anesthesia or continuous tube drainage of the small intestine. Oral anticoagulants may be contraindicated in patients who have severe renal or hepatic disease, subacute bacterial endocarditis, pericarditis, polyarthritis, diverticulitis, visceral carcinoma, or aneurysm. Other conditions in which the oral anticoagulants may be contraindicated include severe or malignant hypertension, eclampsia or preeclampsia, threatened abortion, emaciation, malnutrition, and vitamin C or K deficiencies. Since a high degree of patient cooperation is required for the outpatient use of oral anticoagulants, a lack of such cooperation is a relative contraindication to their use.

Pregnancy: Anisindione is contraindicated in pregnancy because the drug crosses the placental barrier. Oral anticoagulants may cause fetal damage when administered to pregnant women. Fetal or neonatal hemorrhage and intrauterine fetal death have occurred even when maternal prothrombin times were within the therapeutically accepted range. Maternal use of warfarin and anisindione during the first trimester of pregnancy has been reported to cause hypoplastic nasal structures, or other signs of the Conradi-Hunermann syndrome in the offspring. These patients received other drugs in addition to anticoagulants and a positive causal relationship has not been established. If oral anticoagulants must be used during pregnancy, or if the patient becomes pregnant while taking one of these drugs, the patient should be apprised of the potential hazard to the fetus. The possibility of termination of the pregnancy should be considered in light of these risks.

As an alternative to the use of oral anticoagulants in pregnant patients, the use of heparin, which does not cross the placenta, should be considered.

WARNINGS

Anisindione should be reserved for patients who cannot tolerate the coumarins.

Oral anticoagulants are potent drugs with prolonged and cumulative effects. Treatment must be individualized according to patient response, and the benefit expected from anticoagulant therapy should be weighed against the possible hazards associated with the use of these drugs.

Oral anticoagulants should not be used in the treatment of acute completed strokes due to the risk of fatal cerebral hemorrhage (see *"Indications"*).

Because agranulocytosis and hepatitis have been associated with the use of Anisindione, liver function and blood studies should be performed periodically. Patients should be instructed to report to the physician symptoms such as marked fatigue, chills, fever, or sore throat; the drug should be discontinued promptly since these symptoms may signal the onset of severe toxicity. If leukopenia or evidence of hypersensitivity occurs, the drug should be discontinued. Because of the possibility of renal damage associated with the use of phenindione, the urine should be tested periodically for albumin whenever phenindione or any indanedione anticoagulant is used.

Relatively minor bleeding episodes and hemorrhage occur in 2% to 10% of patients treated with oral anticoagulants. Bleeding will vary in intensity, and may be related to the quality of patient monitoring, compliance on the part of the patient, the incidence of potentially hemorrhagic lesions, or the extent of anticoagulation induced. Severe and moderate hypertension, severe to moderate hepatic and renal insufficiency, and infectious diseases or disturbances of intestinal flora as in sprue, or with antibiotic therapy may increase the risks associated with anticoagulant therapy.

Occasionally, fatal hemorrhages can occur. Massive hemorrhage from organ systems may involve cerebral, pericardial, pulmonary, adrenal, hepatic, spinal, gastrointestinal, or genito-urinary sites. Gastrointestinal hemorrhage may be secondary to peptic ulceration or silent neoplasm and is responsible for 25% of all deaths due to oral anticoagulant therapy. Bleeding complications in the genitourinary tract may range in severity from microscopic hematuria to gross hematuria to extensive uterine hemorrhage.

Hemorrhagic necrosis and/or gangrene of the skin and subcutaneous tissue, petechial and purpuric hemorrhage, ecchymosis, epistaxis, hematemesis, or hemoptysis, may also occur. Hemorrhage and necrosis have in some cases been reported to result in death or permanent disability. Necrosis appears to be associated with local thrombosis and usually appears within a few days of the start of anticoagulant therapy. In severe cases of necrosis, treatment through debridement or amputation of the affected tissue, limb, breast, or penis has been reported. Careful diagnosis is required to determine whether necrosis is caused by an underlying disease. Anisindione therapy should be discontinued when Anisindione is suspected to be the cause of developing necrosis and heparin therapy may be considered for anticoagulation. Although various treatments have been attempted, no treatment for necrosis has been considered uniformly effective. (See below for information on predisposing conditions.) The risks of anticoagulant therapy may be increased in patients with known or suspected hereditary, familial, or clinical deficiency in protein C. This condition, which should be suspected if there is a history of recurrent episodes of thromboembolic disorders in the patient or in the family, has been associated with an increased risk of developing necrosis following warfarin administration, and may be expected following Anisindione therapy. Skin necrosis may occur in the absence of protein C deficiency. It has been reported that initiation of anticoagulation therapy with heparin for 4 to 5 days before initiation of therapy with Anisindione may minimize the incidence of this reaction. Anisindione therapy should be discontinued when it is suspected to be the cause of developing necrosis and heparin therapy may be considered for anticoagulation.

Concurrent use of anticoagulants with streptokinase, urokinase, or alteplase (recombinant) is not recommended and may be hazardous. (Consult the product information accompanying those preparations.)

Abrupt cessation of anticoagulant therapy is not generally recommended; if possible, taper the dose gradually over 3 to 4 weeks.

PRECAUTIONS

General: Periodic determination of prothrombin time or other suitable coagulation test is essential. The availability of suitable laboratory facilities to monitor therapy accurately with oral anticoagulants is mandatory, both to assure adequate anticoagulation and to avoid toxicity due to overdosage. The dosage of oral anticoagulants depends on the clinical response as monitored by prothrombin time determinations (see *"Dosage and Administration"*). Since heparin prolongs the one-stage prothrombin time, a period of at least 5 hours should elapse after the last intravenous dose and after the last subcutaneous dose of heparin before drawing blood to determine the prothrombin time when heparin and Anisindione have been given together. In addition to adequate laboratory facilities, a supply of oral or parenteral phytonadione (vitamin K_1) and a source of whole blood or plasma should be available when emergency treatment of acute overdosage is required (see *"Overdosage"*).

A number of factors including environmental, mental, medical, and nutritional states may affect an individual's response to anticoagulant therapy. Factors which increase sensitivity to the drug and lengthen prothrombin time include: initial hypoprothrombinemia, increased age, poor nutritional status, vitamin K deficiency or malabsorption, congestive heart failure or vascular damage, hepatic disorders including hepatitis or obstructive jaundice, biliary fistula, febrile states, hyperthyroidism, preparatory bowel sterilization, recent surgery, and x-ray therapy.

Factors which may decrease the response to oral anticoagulants and shorten the prothrombin time include: pregnancy, diabetes mellitus, hyperlipidemia, hypothyroidism, hypercholesterolemia, and hereditary or acquired resistance.

Information for Patients: The physician should instruct patients:
■ To follow carefully the physician's directions for taking this drug and not to alter these directions without authorization.
■ To follow carefully the physician's directions for the periodic blood test (prothrombin time) required to assure that the correct dose of the drug is being used.
■ To discuss with the physician any other medication (prescription or nonprescription) to be used.
■ To report to the physician any abnormal bleeding, such as blood in the urine, blood in the stool (a black, tarry appearance), bleeding from the gums or nose, patches of discoloration or bruises on the arms, legs, or toes, or excessive bleeding following minor cuts (eg, while shaving).
■ To discuss with the physician any plan to become pregnant or to report any pregnancy promptly.

Laboratory Tests: The need for careful control of the degree of anticoagulation, as determined by changes in prothrombin activity, cannot be over-emphasized. It should be noted, however, that bleeding during anticoagulant therapy may not always correlate with prothrombin activity.

In long-term therapy with anticoagulants, periodic laboratory evaluation of organ systems, including hematopoietic, renal, and hepatic studies, should be performed (see *"Warnings"*).

Drug Interactions: Addition or deletion of any drug from the therapeutic regimen of patients receiving oral anticoagulants may affect patient response to the anticoagulant. Frequent determination of prothrombin time and close monitoring of the patient is essential to ascertain when adjustment of dosage of anticoagulant may be needed.

Because of the variability of individual patient response, multiple interacting mechanisms with some drugs, the dependency of the extent of the interaction on the dosage and duration of therapy, and the possible administration of several interacting drugs simultaneously, it is difficult to predict the direction and degree of the ultimate effect of concomitant medications on anticoagulant response. For example, since cholestyramine may reduce the gastrointestinal absorption of both the oral anticoagulants and vitamin K, the net effects are unpredictable. Chloral hydrate may cause an increased prothrombin response by displacing the anticoagulant from protein binding sites or a diminished prothrombin response through increased metabolism of the unbound drug by hepatic enzyme induction, thus leading to inter-patient variation in ultimate prothrombin effect. An interacting drug which leads to a decrease in prothrombin time necessitating an increased dose of oral anticoagulant to maintain an adequate degree of anticoagulation may, if abruptly discontinued, increase the risk of subsequent bleeding.

Drugs that have been reported to diminish oral anticoagulant response, ie, decreased prothrombin time response, in man significantly include: adrenocortical steroids; alcohol*; antacids; antihistamines; barbiturates; carbamazepine; chloral hydrate*; chlordiazepoxide; cholestyramine; diet high in vitamin K; diuretics*; ethchlorvynol; gluthetimide; griseofulvin; haloperidol; meprobamate; oral contraceptives; paraldehyde; primidone; ranitidine*; rifampin; unreliable prothrombin time determinations; vitamin C; warfarin sodium underdosage.

Drugs that reportedly may increase oral anticoagulant response, ie, increased prothrombin response, in man include: alcohol*; allopurinol; aminosalicyclic acid; amiodarone; anabolic steroids; antibiotics; bromelains; chloral hydrate*; chlorpropamide; chymotrypsin; cimetidine; cinchophen; clofibrate; dextran; dextrothyroxine; diazoxide; dietary deficiencies; diflunisal; diuretics*; disulfiram; drugs affecting blood elements; ethacrynic acid; fenoprofen; glucagon; hepatotoxic drugs; ibuprofen; indomethacin; influenza virus vaccine; inhalation anesthetics; mefenamic acid; methyldopa; methylphenidate; metronidazole; miconazole; monoamine oxidase inhibitors; nalidixic acid; naproxen; oxolinic acid; oxyphenbutazone; pentoxifylline; phenylbutazone; phenyramidol; phenytoin; prolonged hot weather; prolonged narcotics; pyrazolones; quinidine; quinine; ranitidine*; salicylates; sulfinpyrazone; sulfonamides, long acting; sulindac; thyroid drugs; tolbutamide; triclofos sodium; trimethoprim/sulfamethoxazole; unreliable prothrombin time determinations; warfarin sodium overdosage.

Oral anticoagulants may potentiate the hypoglycemic action of hypoglycemic agents, eg, tolbutamide and chlorpropamide, by inhibiting their metabolism in the liver. Because oral anticoagulants may interfere with the hepatic metabolism of phenytoin, toxic levels of the anticonvulsant may occur when an oral anticoagulant and phenytoin are administered concurrently.

Drugs that reduce the number of blood platelets by causing bone marrow depression (such as antineoplastic agents) or drugs which inhibit platelet function (eg, aspirin and other non-steroidal anti-inflammatory drugs, dipyridamole, hydrochloroquine, clofibrate, dextran) may increase the bleeding tendency produced by anticoagulants without altering prothrombin time determinations. The beneficial effects on arterial thrombus formation from combined therapy with anti-platelet and anticoagulant medication must be weighed against an increased risk of inducing hemorrhage.

Drug/Laboratory Test Interferences: Dicumarol and indanedione anticoagulants, including Anisindione, or their metabolites may color alkaline urine red-orange, which may interfere with spectrophotometrically determined urinary laboratory tests. The color reverses when the test sample is acidified *in vitro* to a pH below 4.

Carcinogenesis, Mutagenesis, Impairment of Fertility: Long-term dosing studies to determine the carcinogenic potential of oral anticoagulants, including Anisindione, have not been done. Information on mutagenesis is unknown.

Pregnancy: Teratogenic and other effects—Pregnancy Category X: (See *"Contraindications".*)

Labor and Delivery: Anisindione is contraindicated in pregnancy. If oral anticoagulants are used in pregnant women, they should not be administered during the first trimester, and should be discontinued prior to labor and delivery.

Some clinicians suggest the replacement of oral anticoagulants with heparin therapy before term. Heparin is withheld during early labor and reinstituted 6 hours postpartum. After 5 to 7 days, therapy with oral anticoagulants may be resumed if indicated.

See *"Contraindications"* for the use of oral anticoagulants in pregnancy.

Nursing Mothers: Oral anticoagulants or their metabolites are excreted in the milk of nursing mothers, possibly in amounts sufficient to cause a prothrombopenic state and bleeding in the newborn. As a general rule, nursing should not be undertaken while a patient is receiving an oral anticoagulant.

Pediatric Use: The use of oral anticoagulants in children is not well documented. However, they may be beneficial in children with rare thromboembolic disorder secondary to other disease states such as the nephrotic syndrome or congenital heart lesions. Heparin is probably the initial anticoagulant of choice because of its immediate onset of action.

ADVERSE REACTIONS
Multisystem adverse reactions have been reported, and some may be serious enough to warrant hospital admission. In general, they may be divided into 2 categories: those which involve abnormal bleeding and other effects which do not. Hemorrhage and/or necrosis are among the hazards of treatment with any anticoagulant and are the main serious complications of therapy. For additional discussion of possible hemorrhagic complications following oral anticoagulant therapy see *"Warnings"*. Although most of the adverse reactions for oral

---

* Increased and decreased prothrombin time responses have been reported.

anticoagulant drugs have been reported for warfarin, dicumarol, and phenindione, all the drugs within this class have similar pharmacologic and clinical properties, and require the same degree of caution in monitoring adverse reactions regardless of the drug administered.

Some indanediones (phenindione) have been associated with undesirable reactions which have not been reported with the coumarins and are not counterbalanced by advantages, thus perhaps favoring the use of the coumarin-type anticoagulants. Changing from one chemical type of oral anticoagulant to the other may eliminate an adverse reaction, such as rash or diarrhea. Dermatitis is the only untoward reaction consistently associated with Anisindione therapy.

Adverse reactions reported following therapy with either coumarin or indanedione anticoagulants include: nausea, diarrhea, pyrexia, dermatitis or exfoliative dermatitis, urticaria, alopecia, and sore mouth or mouth ulcers.

Side effects which have additionally been reported for coumarin derivatives include: vomiting, abdominal cramps, anorexia, priapism, erythemia, and necrosis of the skin and other tissues, manifesting as purple toes and cutaneous gangrene. There is no reason to expect that some or all of these adverse reactions might not occur in patients receiving Anisindione.

Additional side effects attributed to the indanedione anticoagulants include: headache, sore throat, blurred vision, paralysis of accommodation, steatorrhea, hepatitis, jaundice, liver damage, renal tubular necrosis, albuminuria, anuria, myeloid immaturity, agranulocytosis, leukocyte agglutinins, red cell aplasia, atypical mononuclear cells, leukopenia, leukocytosis, anemia, thrombocytopenia, and eosinophilia.

Phenprocoumon-induced delayed callus formation following bone fracture has been reported.

OVERDOSAGE
Vitamin K_1 is a specific antidote for anticoagulants, such as Anisindione, which reduce prothrombin activity in the blood. Vitamin K_1 may be administered orally or by injection, if the patient is not bleeding or if bleeding is slight. A few hours after administration of vitamin K_1 preparations, such as phytonadione, prothrombin activity increases and clotting time decreases. In the presence of more active hemorrhage, however, transfusions of whole blood or plasma are required until the desired level of prothrombin activity is achieved. Treatment with vitamin K_1 preparations is only adjunctive in such cases.

DOSAGE AND ADMINISTRATION
Initial dosage of Anisindione Tablets is 300 mg the first day, 200 mg the second day, and 100 mg the third day. With initiation of treatment, prothrombin activity decreases rapidly to 50 percent of baseline values within six hours; thereafter, it decreases slowly until it reaches 15 to 30 percent of baseline values in 48 to 72 hours.

Maintenance dosage is established from daily prothrombin-time determinations for each patient, although with Anisindione Tablets, the uniform, predictable action of the drug makes it possible to reduce the frequency of prothrombin-time determinations in some cases. Maintenance dosage will vary between 25 to 250 mg a day and should be set to keep the prothrombin time two to two and one-half times the normal value. The dose may be repeated for many days; Anisindione does not accumulate in the body.

Prothrombin activity returns to normal within 24 to 72 hours after treatment with the drug is discontinued. Some studies suggest that gradual reduction of dosage over a two-week period may decrease the frequency of recurrence of thromboembolic disease by preventing a rapid rise in prothrombin activity.

HOW SUPPLIED
TABLETS: 50 MG

BRAND/MANUFACTURER	NDC	SIZE	AWP
○ BRAND			
MIRADON: Schering	00085-0795-05	100s	$35.82

Anistreplase

DESCRIPTION
Anistreplase is the p-anisoylated derivative of the lys-plasminogen-streptokinase activator complex prepared *in vitro* by acylating human plasma-derived, purified, heat-treated, lys-plasminogen and purified streptokinase from group C β-hemolytic streptococci. Anistreplase has a molecular weight of about 131,000. Each vial of Anistreplase is supplied as a sterile, lyophilized, white to off-white powder containing 30 units of Anistreplase, < 3 mg dimethylsulfoxide, < 0.2 mg sodium hydroxide and the following buffers and stabilizers: 150 μg p-amidinophenyl-p′-anisate (acylating agent), 100 mg mannitol, 46 mg L-lysine, 30 mg albumin (human), < 2 mg glycerol, and 1.3 mg E-aminocaproic acid. Anistreplase is intended only for intravenous (I.V.) injection after reconstitution with Sterile Water for Injection, USP. The preparation contains no preservatives and is intended to be used as a single dose. Potency is expressed in units of Anistreplase by using a reference standard which is specific for Anistreplase and is not comparable with units used for other fibrinolytics.

CLINICAL PHARMACOLOGY
Anistreplase is an inactive derivative of a fibrinolytic enzyme with the catalytic center of the activator complex temporarily blocked by an anisoyl group. The anisoyl group does not decrease the high fibrin-binding ability of the complex. Anistreplase is made *in vitro* from lys-plasminogen and streptokinase. Anistre-

---

◆ RATED THERAPEUTICALLY EQUIVALENT; ◇ THERAPEUTIC EQUIVALENCE UNCONFIRMED; ○ UNRATED

plase differs from the complex initially formed *in vivo* upon administration of streptokinase, the latter complex contains predominately glu-plasminogen. Activation of Anistreplase occurs with release of the anisoyl group by deacylation, a non-enzymatic first-order process with a half-life *in vitro* in human blood of about 2 hours. In solution, deacylation of Anistreplase starts immediately and the enzymatically active lys-plasminogen-streptokinase activator complex is progressively formed. The production of plasmin from plasminogen by deacylated Anistreplase can take place in the bloodstream or within the thrombus; the latter process is catalytically more efficient but both may contribute to thrombolysis. The half-life of fibrinolytic activity of the circulating Anistreplase is 70 to 120 minutes (mean 94 minutes).

A number of controlled clinical studies have been performed with Anistreplase to demonstrate benefit. Heparin anticoagulation was administered to all patients routinely following (about 4 to 6 hours) dosing with Anistreplase.

Randomized, controlled studies have demonstrated that Anistreplase reduces mortality when administered within 6 hours of the onset of the symptoms of acute myocardial infarction (AMI). The benefit of mortality reduction occurs acutely and is maintained for at least one year.

In a study of 1258 patients (AIMS trial), mortality at 30 days postinfarction was decreased (47.2%, p = 0.0001) in patients receiving Anistreplase as compared with placebo. At one year, the reduction in mortality was maintained (38%, p = 0.001). The incidence of heart failure was less in patients treated with Anistreplase (17.9%) compared with patients who received placebo (23.3%).[1,2] Similar mortality results were obtained from a smaller, randomized, controlled trial.[1,3]

In a double-blind, randomized trial of Anistreplase compared with heparin bolus, left ventricular function was improved and infarction size reduced. There was significantly (p < 0.01, two sample t-test) higher left ventricular ejection fraction (LVEF) for the Anistreplase treatment group (53%) compared with the heparin treatment group (47.5%) when measured 4 days after treatment (intent-to-treat analysis). This difference was maintained when patients were reexamined by radionuclide ventriculography at day 19, even when patients who experienced successful angioplasty were excluded from the analysis (p = 0.04). About 3 weeks after treatment, mean infarct size was 24% lower in the patients treated with Anistreplase compared with those treated with heparin (n = 188, p = 0.02).[1,4] Similarly, if those patients who experienced successful angioplasty were excluded from the analysis, the mean infarct size in patients treated with Anistreplase was significantly less than that of heparin-treated patients (p < 0.01).

In randomized, comparative studies reperfusion rates of between 50% and 68% have been reported in patients receiving Anistreplase within 6 hours of symptom onset. However, for maximum rates of reperfusion, treatment should be initiated as soon as possible after onset of symptoms.

In two studies,[1,5,6] Anistreplase and intracoronary (IC) streptokinase were compared in patients with angiographically proven coronary artery occlusion. Reperfusion occurred about 45 minutes after the start of therapy for both treatment groups. When therapy was initiated within 4 hours of onset of AMI symptoms reperfusion rates of 59% (n = 87) and 68% (n = 41) were observed for Anistreplase compared with 59% (n = 85) and 70% (n = 43) for IC streptokinase. Of those patients who had coronary artery reperfusion, angiographically demonstrated reocclusion occurred within 24 hours in 3% to 4% of those treated with Anistreplase and in 7% to 12% of those treated with streptokinase.[1,5,6]

In a well-controlled, randomized study, a patency rate of 72% was obtained with Anistreplase compared with 53% for I.V. streptokinase. Patency for the 107 patients was determined by posttreatment angiography.[1,7]

Anistreplase was also found to have a favorable risk/benefit profile in elderly patients (> 65 years, n = 940) who participated in clinical trials. Use of Anistreplase in patients over 75 years old has not been adequately studied.

INDICATIONS AND USAGE

Anistreplase is indicated for use in the management of acute myocardial infarction (AMI) in adults, for the lysis of thrombi obstructing coronary arteries, the reduction of infarct size, the improvement of ventricular function following AMI, and the reduction of mortality associated with AMI. Treatment should be initiated as soon as possible after the onset of AMI symptoms (see *"Clinical Pharmacology"*).

UNLABELED USES

Anistreplase is used alone or as an adjunct in the treatment of pulmonary embolism.

CONTRAINDICATIONS

Because thrombolytic therapy increases the risk of bleeding, Anistreplase is contraindicated in the following situations:

- active internal bleeding
- history of cerebrovascular accident
- recent (within 2 months) intracranial or intraspinal surgery or trauma (see *"Warnings"*)
- intracranial neoplasm, arteriovenous malformation, or aneurysm
- known bleeding diathesis
- severe, uncontrolled hypertension

Anistreplase should not be administered to patients having experienced severe allergic reactions to either this product or streptokinase.

WARNINGS

Bleeding: (See *"Adverse Reactions."*) The most common complication associated with Anistreplase therapy is bleeding. The types of bleeding associated with thrombolytic therapy can be divided into two broad categories:

1. Internal bleeding involving the gastrointestinal tract, genitourinary tract, retroperitoneal, ocular, or intracranial sites.
2. Superficial or surface bleeding, observed mainly at invaded or disturbed sites (e.g., venous cutdowns, arterial punctures, sites of recent surgical intervention).

The concomitant use of heparin anticoagulation may contribute to the bleeding. Some of the hemorrhagic episodes occurred one or more days after the effects of Anistreplase had dissipated, but while heparin therapy was continuing.

As fibrin is lysed during Anistreplase therapy, bleeding from recent puncture sites may occur. Therefore, thrombolytic therapy requires careful attention to all potential bleeding sites (including catheter insertion sites, arterial and venous puncture sites, cutdown sites, and needle puncture sites).

Intramuscular injections and nonessential handling of the patient should be avoided during treatment with Anistreplase. Venipunctures should be performed carefully and only as required.

Should an arterial puncture be necessary following administration of Anistreplase, it is preferable to use an upper-extremity vessel that is accessible to manual compression. A pressure dressing should be applied, and the puncture site should be checked frequently for evidence of bleeding.

Each patient being considered for therapy with Anistreplase should be carefully evaluated and anticipated benefits should be weighed against potential risks associated with therapy.

In the following conditions, the risks of Anistreplase therapy may be increased and should be weighed against the anticipated benefits:

- recent (within 10 days) major surgery (e.g., coronary artery bypass graft, obstetrical delivery, organ biopsy previous puncture of noncompressible vessels)
- cerebrovascular disease
- recent gastrointestinal or genitourinary bleeding (within 10 days)
- recent trauma (within 10 days) including cardiopulmonary resuscitation
- hypertension: systolic BP ≥ 180 mmHg and/or diastolic BP ≥ 110 mmHg
- high likelihood of left heart thrombus (e.g., mitral stenosis with atrial fibrillation)
- subacute bacterial endocarditis
- acute pericarditis
- hemostatic defects including those secondary to severe hepatic or renal disease
- pregnancy
- age > 75 years (Use of Anistreplase in patients over 75 years old has not been adequately studied.)
- diabetic hemorrhagic retinopathy or other hemorrhagic ophthalmic conditions
- septic thrombophlebitis or occluded AV cannula at seriously infected site
- patients currently receiving oral anticoagulants (e.g., warfarin sodium)
- any other condition in which bleeding constitutes a significant hazard or would be particularly difficult to manage because of its location

Arrhythmias: Coronary thrombolysis may result in arrhythmias associated with reperfusion. These arrhythmias (such as sinus bradycardia, accelerated idioventricular rhythm, ventricular premature depolarizations, ventricular tachycardia) are not different from those often seen in the ordinary course of acute myocardial infarction and may be managed with standard antiarrhythmic measures. It is recommended that antiarrhythmic therapy for bradycardia and/or ventricular irritability be available when injections of Anistreplase are administered.

Hypotension: Hypotension, sometimes severe, not secondary to bleeding or anaphylaxis, has occasionally been observed soon after intravenous Anistreplase administration. Patients should be monitored closely and, should symptomatic or alarming hypotension occur, appropriate symptomatic treatment should be administered.

PRECAUTIONS

General: Standard management of myocardial infarction should be implemented concomitantly with Anistreplase treatment. Invasive procedures should be minimized (see *"Warnings"*). Anaphylactoid reactions have rarely been reported in patients who received Anistreplase. Accordingly, adequate treatment provisions such as epinephrine should be available for immediate use.

Readministration: Because of the increased likelihood of resistance due to antistreptokinase antibody, Anistreplase may not be as effective if administered more than 5 days after prior Anistreplase or streptokinase therapy, particularly between 5 days and 12 months. Increased antistreptokinase antibody levels after Anistreplase or streptokinase may also increase the risk of allergic reactions following readministration.

Repeated administration of Anistreplase within one week of the initial dose has occurred in a small number of patients treated for AMI and non-AMI conditions. The incidence of hematomas/bruising was somewhat greater in those patients who received repeat doses of Anistreplase but otherwise the adverse event profile was similar to those who received one dose.

Laboratory Tests: Intravenous administration of Anistreplase will cause marked decreases in plasminogen and fibrinogen and increases in thrombin time (TT), activated partial thromboplastin time (APTT), and prothrombin time (PT).

Results of coagulation tests and/or measures of fibrinolytic activity performed during Anistreplase therapy may be unreliable unless specific precautions are taken to prevent *in vitro* artifacts. Anistreplase, when present in blood in pharmacologic concentrations, remains active under *in vitro* conditions. This can lead to degradation of fibrinogen in blood samples removed for analysis. Collection of blood samples in the presence of aprotinin (2000 to 3000 KIU/mL) can, to some extent, mitigate this phenomenon.

Drug Interactions: The interaction of Anistreplase with other cardioactive drugs has not been studied. In addition to bleeding associated with heparin and vitamin K antagonists, drugs that alter platelet function (such as aspirin and dipyridamole) may increase the risk of bleeding if administered prior to Anistreplase therapy.

Use of Anticoagulants: Anistreplase alone or in combination with antiplatelet agents and anticoagulants may cause bleeding complications. Therefore, careful monitoring is advised, especially at arterial puncture sites. In clinical studies, a majority of patients treated received anticoagulant therapy postdosing with Anistreplase during their hospital stay and a minority received heparin pretreatment with Anistreplase. The use of antiplatelet agents increased the incidence of bleeding events similarly in patients treated with Anistreplase or non-thrombolytic therapy. There was no evidence of a synergistic effect of combined Anistreplase and antiplatelet agents on bleeding events. In addition, there was no difference in the incidence of hemorrhagic CVAs in Anistreplase-treated patients who did or did not receive aspirin.

Carcinogenesis, Mutagenesis, Impairment of Fertility: Long-term studies in animals have not been performed to evaluate the carcinogenic potential or the effect on fertility. Studies to determine mutagenicity and chromosomal aberration assays in human lymphocytes were negative at all concentrations tested.

Pregnancy (Category C): Animal reproduction studies have not been conducted with Anistreplase. It is also not known whether Anistreplase can cause fetal harm when administered to a pregnant woman or can affect reproduction capacity. Anistreplase should be given to a pregnant woman only if clearly needed.

Nursing Mothers: It is not known whether Anistreplase is excreted in human milk. Because many drugs are excreted in human milk, the physician should decide whether the patient should discontinue nursing or not receive Anistreplase.

Pediatric Use: Safety and effectiveness of Anistreplase in children have not been established.

ADVERSE REACTIONS

Bleeding: The incidence of bleeding (major or minor) varied widely from study to study and may depend on the use of arterial catheterization and other invasive procedures, patient population, and/or concomitant therapy. The overall incidence of bleeding in patients treated with Anistreplase in clinical trials (n = 5275) was 14.6%, with nonpuncture-site bleeding occurring in 10.2%, and puncture-site bleeding occurring in 5.7%, of these patients. Bleeding at the puncture site occurred more frequently in clinical trials in which the patients underwent immediate coronary catheterization (13.3%, n = 637) compared with those who did not (3.0%, n = 2023). The incidence of presumed intracranial bleeding within 7 days postdosing with Anistreplase was 0.57% (n = 5275; 0.34% etiology confirmed hemorrhagic; 0.23% etiology not confirmed) compared to 0.16% (n = 1249) after nonthrombolytic therapy.

In the AIMS trial the overall incidence of bleeding in patients treated with Anistreplase was 14.8% compared with 3.8% for placebo. The incidence of specific bleeding events was:

Type of Bleeding	ANISTREPLASE (n = 500)	Placebo (n = 501)
Puncture site	4.6%	< 1%
Nonpuncture site hematoma	2.8%	< 1%
Hematuria/ Genitourinary	2.4%	< 1%
Hemoptysis	2.2%	< 1%
Gastrointestinal hemorrhage	2.0%	1.4%
Intracranial	1.0%	< 1%
Gum/Mouth hemorrhage	1.0%	0
Epistaxis	< 1%	< 1%
Anemia	< 1%	< 1%
Eye hemorrhage	< 1%	< 1%
Hemorrhage (unspecified)	< 1%	0

In this study there was no difference between Anistreplase and placebo in the incidence of major bleeding events.

Should serious bleeding (not controlled by local pressure) occur in a critical location (intracranial, gastrointestinal, retroperitoneal, pericardial), any concomitant heparin should be terminated immediately and the administration of protamine to reverse heparinization should be considered. If necessary, the bleeding tendency can be reversed with appropriate replacement therapy.

Minor bleeding can be anticipated mainly at invaded or disturbed sites. If such bleeding occurs, local measures should be taken to control the bleeding (see *"Warnings"*).

Cardiovascular: The most frequently reported adverse experiences in Anistreplase clinical trials (n = 5275) were arrhythmia/conduction disorders which were reported in 38% of patients treated with Anistreplase and 46% of nonthrombolytic control patients. Hypotension occurred in 10.4% of patients treated with Anistreplase compared to 7.9% for patients who received nonthrombolytic treatment (see *"Warnings"*).

Allergic-type Reactions: Anaphylactic and anaphylactoid reactions have been observed rarely (0.2%) in patients treated with Anistreplase and are similar in incidence to streptokinase (0.1% anaphylactic shock in one study). These included symptoms such as bronchospasm or angioedema. Other milder or delayed effects such as urticaria, itching, flushing, rashes and eosinophilia have been occasionally observed. A delayed purpuric rash appearing one to two weeks after treatment has been reported in 0.3% of patients. The rash may also be associated with arthralgia, ankle edema, gastrointestinal symptoms, mild hematuria and mild proteinuria. This syndrome was self-limiting and without long-term sequelae.

Risk of Viral Transmission: Six batches of Anistreplase (five different batches of lys-plasminogen) were used in clinical trials designed specifically to monitor possible hepatitis non-A, non-B transmission. No case of hepatitis was diagnosed in patients receiving Anistreplase. Lys-plasminogen is derived from human plasma obtained from FDA approved sources and tested for absence of viral contamination, including human immunodeficiency virus type-1 (HIV-1) and hepatitis B surface antigen. The manufacturing process includes a vapor-heat treatment step for inactivation of viruses. The entire manufacturing process has also been validated to yield a cumulative reduction of $\geq 10^{21}$ fold HIV-1 infectious particles, i.e., $\geq 10^6$ infectious particles removed by vapor-heat treatment and a cumulative total of $\geq 10^{15}$ infectious particles removed by the various steps in the purification process.

Causal Relationship Unknown: Since the following experiences may also be associated with AMI or other therapy, the causal relationship to Anistreplase administration is unknown. The following adverse experiences were infrequently (< 10%) reported in clinical trials:

Body as a Whole—chills, fever, headache, shock;

Cardiovascular—cardiac rupture, chest pain, emboli;

Dermatology—purpura, sweating;

Gastrointestinal—nausea and/or vomiting;

Hemic and Lymphatic—thrombocytopenia;

Metabolic and Nutritional—elevated transaminase levels;

Musculoskeletal—arthralgia;

Nervous—agitation, dizziness, paresthesia, tremor, vertigo;

Respiratory—dyspnea, lung edema.

DOSAGE AND ADMINISTRATION

Administer Anistreplase as soon as possible after the onset of symptoms. The recommended dose is 30 units of Anistreplase administered only by intravenous injection over 2 to 5 minutes into an intravenous line or vein.

RECONSTITUTION:
1. Slowly add 5 mL of *Sterile Water for Injection, USP,* by directing the stream of fluid against the side of the vial.
2. Gently roll the vial, mixing the dry powder and fluid. **Do not shake.** Try to minimize foaming.
3. The reconstituted preparation is a colorless to pale yellow transparent solution. Before administration, the product should be visually inspected for particulate matter and discoloration.
4. Withdraw the entire contents of the vial.
5. The reconstituted solution should not be further diluted before administration or added to any infusion fluids. No other medications should be added to the vial or syringe containing Anistreplase.
6. If Anistreplase is not administered within 30 minutes of reconstitution, it should be discarded.

Storage: Store lyophilized Anistreplase between 2° and 8°C (36° to 46°F).
Do not use beyond the expiration date printed on the vial.

REFERENCES
1. Data on File. SmithKline Beecham Pharmaceuticals, Philadelphia. 2. AIMS Trial Study Group. Effect of intravenous APSAC on mortality after acute myocardial infarction: preliminary report of a placebo-controlled clinical trial. Lancet 1988; 1:545–9. 3. Meinertz T, Kasper W, Schumacher M, Just H for the APSAC multicenter trial group. The German multicenter trial of anisoylated plasminogen streptokinase activator complex versus heparin for acute myocardial infarction. Am J Cardiol 1988; 62:347–51. 4. Bassand JP, Machecourt J, Cassagnes J, et al. Multicenter trial of intravenous anisoylated plasminogen streptokinase activator complex (APSAC) in acute myocardial infarction: effects on infarct size and left ventricular function. J Am Coll Cardiol 1989; 13:988–97. 5. Anderson JL, Rothbard RL, Hackworthy RA, et al. Multicenter reperfusion trial of intravenous anisoylated plasminogen streptokinase activator complex (APSAC) in acute myocardial infarction: controlled comparison with intracoronary streptokinase. J Am Coll Cardiol 1988; 11:1153–63. 6. Bonnier HJRM, Visser RF, Klomps HC, Hoffmann HJML and the Dutch Invasive Reperfusion Study Group. Comparison of intravenous anisoylated plasminogen streptokinase activator complex and intracoronary streptokinase in acute myocardial infarction. Am J Cardiol 1988; 62:25–30. 7. Brochier ML, Quilliet L, Kulbertus H, et al. Intravenous anisoylated plasminogen streptokinase activator complex versus intravenous streptokinase in evolving myocardial infarction: preliminary data from a randomized multicentre study. Drugs 1987; 33(Suppl 3):140–5.

HOW SUPPLIED
POWDER FOR INJECTION: 30 U

BRAND/MANUFACTURER	NDC	SIZE	AWP
○ **BRAND**			
EMINASE: SK Beecham Pharm	57294-0030-20	1s	$2233.70

◆ RATED THERAPEUTICALLY EQUIVALENT; ◇ THERAPEUTIC EQUIVALENCE UNCONFIRMED; ○ UNRATED

Ansaid SEE FLURBIPROFEN, ORAL

Antabuse SEE DISULFIRAM

Antazoline Phosphate and Naphazoline Hydrochloride

DESCRIPTION

Antazoline Phosphate/Naphazoline Hydrochloride is a combination of an antihistamine and a vasoconstrictor prepared as a sterile solution for ophthalmic administration having the following composition:

Antazoline Phosphate ....5 mg/mL
Naphazoline Hydrochloride ....0.5 mg/mL

The chemical name for Naphazoline Hydrochloride is 1 H-imidazole,4,5-dihydro-2-(1-naphthalenyl-methyl)-,monohydrochloride.

The chemical name for Anatozoline Phosphate is 1 H-imidazole-2-methanamine,4,5-dihydro-N-phenyl-N-(phenylmethyl)-, phosphate (1:1).

CLINICAL PHARMACOLOGY

Naphazoline Hydrochloride is an alpha-sympathetic receptor agonist (sympathomimetic) producing vasoconstriction. Antazoline Phosphate is an H_1-receptor antagonist producing antihistaminic effects.

INDICATIONS AND USAGE

Antazoline Phosphate/Naphazoline Hydrochloride Ophthalmic Solution is indicated for relief of signs and symptoms of allergic conjunctivitis.

CONTRAINDICATIONS

Contraindicated in the presence of an anatomically narrow angle or in narrow angle glaucoma or in persons hypersensitive to one or more of the components of this preparation. Antazoline Phosphate/Naphazoline Hydrochloride is contraindicated while soft contact lenses are being worn.

WARNINGS

Patients under therapy with monoamine oxidase (MAO) inhibitors may experience a severe hypertensive crisis if given a sympathomimetic drug. (See "Precautions"). Use of drugs in this pharmacologic class may cause CNS depression leading to unconsciousness and/or coma. Marked reduction in body temperature may occur in children, especially infants. Patients are advised not to wear contact lenses during treatment with Antazoline Phosphate/Naphazoline Hydrochloride.

PRECAUTIONS

General: Use with caution in the presence of hypertension, cardiovascular abnormalities, hyperglycemia (diabetes), hyperthyroidism, ocular infection or injury and when other medications are being used.

Information to the Patient: For topical use only. To prevent contaminating the dropper tip and solution, care should be taken not to touch the eyelids or surrounding areas with the dropper tip of the bottle. Keep bottle tightly closed when not in use. Protect from light. Do not use if the solution has darkened. Patients should be advised to discontinue the drug and consult a physician if relief is not obtained within 48 hours of therapy; if irritation, blurring or redness persists or increases; or if symptoms of systemic absorption occur, i.e., dizziness, headache, nausea, decrease in body temperature or drowsiness.

Overuse of this product may produce increased redness/irritation of the eyes.

Drug Interactions: Concurrent use of maprotiline or tricyclic antidepressants and Naphazoline may potentiate the pressor effect of Naphazoline. Patients under therapy with MAO inhibitors may experience a severe hypertensive crisis if given a sympathomimetic drug. (See "Warnings".)

Carcinogenesis, Mutagenesis, Impairment of Fertility: There have been no long-term studies done using Naphazoline and/or Antazoline in animals to evaluate carcinogenic or mutagenic potential.

Pregnancy: Pregnancy Category C. Animal reproduction studies have not been conducted with Naphazoline and/or Antazoline. It is also not known whether Naphazoline and/or Antazoline can cause fetal harm when administered to a pregnant woman or can affect reproduction capacity. Antazoline Phosphate/Naphazoline Hydrochloride Ophthalmic Solution should be given to a pregnant woman only if clearly needed. There are no available data on the effect of the drug on later growth, development, and functional maturation of the child.

Nursing Mothers: It is not known whether Naphazoline and/or Antazoline are excreted in human milk. Because many drugs are excreted in human milk, caution should be exercised when these drugs are administered to a nursing woman.

Pediatric Use: Safety and effectiveness in children have not been established. (See "Warnings".)

ADVERSE REACTIONS

Ocular: The most frequent complaint with the use of Antazoline Phosphate/Naphazoline Hydrochloride Ophthalmic Solution is that of mild transient stinging/burning. Other adverse experiences that have been reported with Naphazoline and/or Antazoline include mydriasis, increased redness, irritation, blurring, punctate keratitis, lacrimation, increased intraocular pressure.

Systemic: Dizziness, headache, nausea, sweating, nervousness, drowsiness, weakness, hypertension, cardiac irregularities and hyperglycemia.

DOSAGE AND ADMINISTRATION

Instill one to two drops in the conjunctival sac(s) every two hours as needed, but not to exceed four times per day.

Keep tightly closed when not in use. Protect from light.
Do not store above 25°C (79°F).

HOW SUPPLIED
DROP: 0.5%-0.05%

BRAND/MANUFACTURER	NDC	SIZE	AWP
◆ BRAND			
VASOCON-A: Iolab	00058-2880-15	15 ml	$13.32

Anthra-Derm SEE ANTHRALIN

Anthralin

DESCRIPTION

Anthralin is a pale yellow topical cream containing 0.1%, 0.25%, 0.5% or 1.0% (HP) Anthralin USP in a base of white petrolatum, sodium lauryl sulfate, catostearyl alcohol, ascorbic acid, salicylic acid, chlorocreasol and purified water.

Following is its chemical structure:

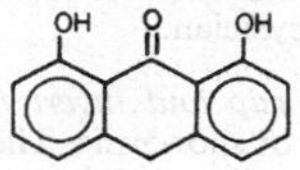

CLINICAL PHARMACOLOGY

Although the precise mechanism of Anthralin's antipsoriatic action is not fully understood, *in vitro* evidence suggests that its antimitotic effect results from inhibition of DNA synthesis. Additionally, the chemically reducing properties of Anthralin may upset oxidative metabolic processes, providing a further slowing down of epidermal mitosis.

Absorption in man has not been finally determined, but in a limited clinical study of Anthralin, no traces of anthraquinone metabolites were detected in the urine of subjects treated; however, caution is advised in patients with renal disease.

INDICATIONS AND USAGE

An aid in the topical treatment of quiescent or chronic psoriasis. Treatment should be coninued until the skin is entirely clear, *i.e.,* when there is nothing to feel with the fingers and the texture is normal.

CONTRAINDICATIONS

Do not use Anthralin on the face, or for acute or actively inflamed psoriatic eruptions. Do not use if sensitive to any of the ingredients.

WARNINGS

Avoid contact with the eyes or mucous membranes. Anthralin should not normally be applied to intertriginous skin areas and high strengths should not be used on these sites. Remove any unintended residue which may be deposited behind the ears. Avoid applying to the folds and creases of the skin. Discontinue use if a sensitivity reaction occurs or if excessive irritation develops on uninvolved skin areas. Keep out of the reach of children.

PRECAUTIONS

For external use only. To prevent the possibility of staining clothing or bed linen while gaining experience in using Anthralin, it may be advisable to use protective dressings. To prevent the possibility of discoloration, particularly where Anthralin HP (1.0%) has been used, always rinse the bath/shower with hot water immediately after washing/showering and then use a suitable cleanser to remove any deposit on the surface of the bath or shower. Contact with fabrics, plastics and other materials may cause staining and should be avoided. Always wash hands thoroughly after use.

Long-term studies in animals have not been performed to evaluate the carcinogenic potential of the drug. Although Anthralin has been found to have tumor-promoting properties on mouse skin, there have been no reports to suggest carcinogenic effects in humans after many years of clinical use.

As long-term use of topical corticosteroids may destabilize psoriasis, and withdrawal may also give rise to a "rebound" phenomenon, an interval of at least one week should be allowed between the discontinuance of such steroids and the commencement of Anthralin therapy. Petrolatum or a suitably bland emollient may usefully be applied during the intervening period.

PREGNANCY

Pregnancy Category C. Animal reproduction studies have not been conducted with Anthralin. It is also not known whether Anthralin can cause fetal harm when administered to a pregnant woman or can affect reproduction capacity. Anthralin should be given to a pregnant woman only if clearly needed.

NURSING MOTHERS

It is not known whether this drug is excreted in human milk. Because many drugs are excreted in milk and because of the potential for tumorigenicity shown for anthralin in animal studies, a decision should be made whether to discontinue nursing or to discontinue the drug, taking into account the importance of the drug to the mother.

PEDIATRIC USE

Safety and effectiveness in children have not been specifically established.

ADVERSE REACTIONS

Very few instances of contact allergic reactions to Anthralin have been reported. However, transient primary irritation of normal skin or uninvolved skin surrounding the treated lesions is more frequently seen and may occasionally be severe. Application of Anthralin must be restricted to the psoriatic lesions. If the initial treatment produces excessive soreness or if the lesions spread, reduce frequency of application and, in extreme cases, discontinue use and consult physician. Some temporary discoloration of hair and fingernails may arise during the period of treatment but should be minimized by careful application. Anthralin may stain skin, hair or fabrics. Staining of fabrics may be permanent, so contact should be avoided.

DOSAGE AND ADMINISTRATION

Generally, it is recommended that Anthralin be applied once a day or as directed by a physician. Anthralin is known to be a potential skin irritant. The irritant potential of Anthralin is directly related to the strength being used and each patient's individual tolerance. Therefore, where the response to Anthralin treatment has not previously been established, always commence treatment for at least one week using 0.1% Anthralin. Increase to the 0.25%, 0.5% and 1.0% (HP) strengths when directed by a physician.

To open the tube, unscrew the cap and invert to pierce membrane. Apply as directed and remove by washing or showering. The optimal period of contact will vary according to the strength used and the patient's response to treatment.

FOR THE SKIN

Apply sparingly only to the psoriatic lesions and rub gently and carefully into the skin until absorbed. It is most important to avoid applying an excessive quantity which may cause unnecessary soiling and staining of the clothing and/or bed linen. At the end of each period of treatment, a bath or shower should be taken to remove any surplus cream (which may have become red/brown in color). The margins of the lesions may gradually become stained purple/brown as treatment progresses, but this will disappear after cessation of treatment.

FOR THE SCALP

Comb the hair to remove scalar debris and, after suitably parting, rub the cream well into the lesions. Keep Anthralin away from the eyes. Care should be taken to avoid application of the cream to uninvolved scalp margins. Remove any unintended residue which may be deposited behind the ears. At the end of each period of contact, wash the hair and scalp to remove any surplus cream (which may have become red/brown in color). Keep tightly capped when not in use.

Store at controlled room temperature, 15°–30°C (59°–88°F).

HOW SUPPLIED
CREAM: 0.1%

BRAND/MANUFACTURER	NDC	SIZE	AWP
○ BRAND			
DRITHOCREME: Dermik	00066-7200-50	50 gm	$19.01
○ GENERICS			
ANTHRA-TEX: Syosset	47854-0604-05	30 gm	$5.25

CREAM: 0.25%

BRAND/MANUFACTURER	NDC	SIZE	AWP
○ BRAND			
DRITHOCREME: Dermik	00066-7201-50	50 gm	$20.47
DRITHO-SCALP: Dermik	00066-7204-50	50 gm	$21.20
○ GENERICS			
ANTHRA-TEX: Syosset	47854-0642-05	30 gm	$5.40

CREAM: 0.5%

BRAND/MANUFACTURER	NDC	SIZE	AWP
○ BRAND			
DRITHOCREME: Dermik	00066-7202-50	50 gm	$22.87
DRITHO-SCALP: Dermik	00066-7205-50	50 gm	$23.50
○ GENERICS			
ANTHRA-TEX: Syosset	47854-0689-05	30 gm	$5.55

CREAM: 1%

BRAND/MANUFACTURER	NDC	SIZE	AWP
○ BRAND			
DRITHOCREME: Dermik	00066-7203-50	50 gm	$26.84
○ GENERICS			
ANTHRA-TEX: Syosset	47854-0690-05	30 gm	$5.90

OINTMENT: 0.1%

BRAND/MANUFACTURER	NDC	SIZE	AWP
○ BRAND			
ANTHRA-DERM: Dermik	00066-0010-15	45 gm	$21.14

OINTMENT: 0.25%

BRAND/MANUFACTURER	NDC	SIZE	AWP
○ BRAND			
ANTHRA-DERM: Dermik	00066-0025-15	45 gm	$21.14

OINTMENT: 0.5%

BRAND/MANUFACTURER	NDC	SIZE	AWP
○ BRAND			
ANTHRA-DERM: Dermik	00066-0050-15	45 gm	$22.43

OINTMENT: 1%

BRAND/MANUFACTURER	NDC	SIZE	AWP
○ BRAND			
ANTHRA-DERM: Dermik	00066-0100-15	45 gm	$22.81

POWDER:

BRAND/MANUFACTURER	NDC	SIZE	AWP
○ GENERICS			
	53118-0700-25	25 gm	$41.25
	17137-0208-02	25 gm	$58.80
	53118-0700-01	100 gm	$131.45
	17137-0208-04	100 gm	$196.00

Anti-Inhibitor Coagulant Complex

Caution: This product is to be used only in patients with inhibitors to Factor VIII.

Warning: This is a potent drug with potential hazards. For maximal safety and efficacy, carefully read and follow directions below.

DESCRIPTION

Anti-Inhibitor Coagulant Complex is a sterile product prepared from pooled human plasma with subsequent alcohol fractionation to Cohn Fraction IV. It contains, in concentrated form, variable amounts of activated and precursor vitamin K-dependent clotting factors. Factors of the kinin generating system are also present. The product is standardized by its ability to correct the clotting time of Factor VIII deficient plasma or Factor VIII deficient plasma which contains inhibitors to Factor VIII.

Laboratory testing of several lots of Anti-Inhibitor Coagulant Complex, Heat Treated, has shown the presence of Factor VIII coagulant antigen (VIII:CAg). Although anamnestic response to this antigen following administration of the product was not observed during the clinical trials, the possibility of such a response does exist.

Each lot of Anti-Inhibitor Coagulant Complex is assayed and labeled for units of Hyland Factor VIII correctional activity. Factor VIII correctional activity may not be exclusively related to the efficacious component(s). (See *"Clinical Pharmacology."*)

During the manufacturing process, this product was heated for 6 days at 60°C. This heating step is designed to reduce the risk of transmission of hepatitis and other viral diseases. However, no procedure has been shown to be totally effective in removing hepatitis infectivity from Anti-Inhibitor Coagulant Complex.

Anti-Inhibitor Coagulant Complex must be administered intravenously.

CLINICAL PHARMACOLOGY

The Factor VIII correctional activity of Anti-Inhibitor Coagulant Complex is thought to be, in part, related to the Factor Xa content of the product. It is additionally hypothesized that the elevated Factor VII-VIIa content of this product is also a contributing factor in the *in vivo* reestablishment of normal hemostasis by way of Factor X activation in conjunction with tissue factor, phospholipid and ionic calcium.

Control of thrombin formation is regulated by (1) the presence of antithrombin III and other serine protease inhibitors which neutralize Factors IXa and Xa, (2) the short biological half-lifes of Factors VII and VIIa and (3) the presence of the circulating Factor VIII inhibitor which additionally controls overactivation of the intrinsic coagulation system.

In work with human immunodeficiency virus (HIV), substantial reduction in viral content has been reported in a recent study of the effects of ethanol fractionation, the process by which Anti-Inhibitor Coagulant Complex is manufactured. Wells, *et al.* report 1 to 4 log reduction in each fractionation step they examined.[1]

◆ RATED THERAPEUTICALLY EQUIVALENT; ◇ THERAPEUTIC EQUIVALENCE UNCONFIRMED; ○ UNRATED

The effectiveness of the 6-day heating step in reducing viral infectivity was assessed by *in vitro* viral inactivation studies, using, as markers, viruses not commonly found in plasma. When known quantities of these viruses were added to the product, the heat treatment employed inactivated the following quantities of virus:

Sindbis	10.0 Log$_{10}$	(1.68 Log$_{10}$/day)
Vesicular stomatitis	5.0 Log$_{10}$	(0.84 Log$_{10}$/day)
Herpes simplex	1.6 Log$_{10}$	(0.26 Log$_{10}$/day)
HIV	4.5 Log$_{10}$	(2 Log$_{10}$/day)

In separate experiments, HIV was also studied and these data are reported in the table above.

A retrospective study conducted with patients receiving unheated Anti-Inhibitor Coagulant Complex supports the effectiveness of the purification process in reducing viral burden in the product. In the study, none of the patients who received that product exclusively seroconverted for HIV antibodies, while 56% of those patients who received other treatment modalities seroconverted during the three year study.[2]

INDICATIONS AND USAGE
Anti-Inhibitor Coagulant Complex is indicated for use in patients with Factor VIII inhibitors who are bleeding or are to undergo surgery.[3-6] The intravenous administration of this preparation is intended to control bleeding episodes in such patients.

Approximately 10% of individuals with hemophilia A (classical hemophilia) have laboratory-measurable inhibitors to Factor VIII.[7] For these patients, the treatment of choice depends upon the following factors: the severity of the bleeding episode, the existing level of inhibitor and whether the patient responds to infusion of Factor VIII with increasing antibody titers (anamnestic rise of Factor VIII antibody).

The following table is presented as a guide in determining the preferred therapy with respect to the use of Anti-Inhibitor Coagulant Complex or Antihemophilic Factor (Human) in patients with Factor VIII inhibitors. Inhibitor level categories are given in the shaded areas of the table and the corresponding recommended product or products are given in the unshaded areas. Other regimens have been proposed.[8]

PRESENT LEVEL OF FACTOR VIII INHIBITOR

Historical Maximum Level of Factor VIII Inhibitor	<2 B.U.[a]	2-10 B.U.	>10 B.U.
<2 B.U.	AHF[b]	AICC[c] or AHF	AICC
2-10 B.U.	AICC or AHF	AICC or AHF	AICC
>10 B.U.	AICC	AICC	AICC

[a] B.U. designates Bethesda Units.
[b] AHF designates Antihemophilic Factor (Human).
[c] AICC designates Anti-Inhibitor Coagulant Complex.

Patients whose present Factor VIII inhibitor levels are greater than 10 Bethesda Units, as well as patients whose inhibitor levels are historically known to rise to greater than 10 Bethesda Units following treatment with Antihemophilic Factor (Human), should be treated with Anti-Inhibitor Coagulant Complex.

Patients whose present Factor VIII inhibitor levels are between 2 and 10 Bethesda Units and whose inhibitor levels are historically known to remain in this range following treatment with Antihemophilic Factor (Human) may be treated with either Antihemophilic Factor (Human) or Anti-Inhibitor Coagulant Complex, depending on the patient's clinical history and the severity of the bleeding episode.

Patients with Factor VIII inhibitor levels of less than 2 Bethesda Units whose inhibitor levels are historically known to remain at 2 Bethesda Units or less following treatment with Antihemophilic Factor (Human) may be treated with appropriate doses of Antihemophilic Factor (Human).

For patients who have low levels of Factor VIII inhibitor and whose history does not include adequate laboratory indications of an anamnestic response to Antihemophilic Factor (Human), the treatment of choice should be based on clinical judgment. In such patients who are having non-critical or minor bleeding episodes, the use of Anti-Inhibitor Coagulant Complex will maintain the inhibitor at a low level and allow the use of other coagulant therapeutic agents in subsequent major emergencies.

CONTRAINDICATIONS
The use of Anti-Inhibitor Coagulant Complex contraindicated in patients with signs of fibrinolysis and in patients with disseminated intravascular coagulation (DIC).

WARNINGS
This product is prepared from pooled human plasma which may contain the causative agents of hepatitis and other viral diseases. Prescribed manufacturing procedures utilized at the plasma collection centers, plasma testing laboratories, and the fractionation facilities are designed to reduce the risk of transmitting viral infection. However, the risk of viral infectivity from this product cannot be totally eliminated.

Individuals who receive infusions of blood or plasma products may develop signs and/or symptoms of some viral infections, particularly non A, non B hepatitis.

If the infusion of the concentrate occurs more than 1 hour following reconstitution, there may be increased prekallikrein activator (PKA) with consequent hypotension.

PRECAUTIONS
GENERAL
Identification of the clotting deficiency as that caused by the presence of Factor VIII inhibitors is essential before the administration of Anti-Inhibitor Coagulant Complex is initiated.

Signs and/or symptoms of hypotension may occur with this product. In these cases, stopping the infusion allows the symptoms to disappear. With all but the most reactive individuals, the infusion may be resumed at a slower rate.

If signs of intravascular coagulation occur, the infusion should be stopped and the patient monitored for DIC by the appropriate laboratory tests. Symptoms of DIC include changes in blood pressure and pulse rate, respiratory distress, chest pain and cough. Laboratory indications of DIC include prolonged thrombin time, prothrombin time and partial thromboplastin time tests. Other indications of DIC are decreased fibrinogen concentration, decreased platelet count and/or the presence of fibrin split products.

Special caution should be taken in the use of this concentrate in newborns, where a high morbidity and mortality may be associated with hepatitis, and in individuals with preexisting liver disease.

LABORATORY TESTS
In some cases, laboratory tests such as the activated partial thromboplastin time test may not correlate with clinical response, in that the appearance of hemostatic improvement may occur without a reduction of partial thromboplastin time. However, the prothrombin time would be expected to be shortened.

In children, fibrinogen levels should be determined prior to the initial infusion and monitored during the course of the treatment.

DRUG INTERACTIONS
Since only limited data are available on the administration of highly activated prothrombin complex products together with antifibrinolytic agents such as epsilonaminocaproic acid (EACA) or tranexamic acid,[6] the concomitant use of Anti-Inhibitor Coagulant Complex with such agents is not recommended.

PREGNANCY
Pregnancy Category C. Animal reproduction studies have not been conducted with Anti-Inhibitor Coagulant Complex. It is also not known whether Anti-Inhibitor Coagulant Complex can cause fetal harm when administered to a pregnant woman or can affect reproduction capacity. Anti-Inhibitor Coagulant Complex, should be given to a pregnant woman only if clearly needed.

ADVERSE REACTIONS
As with other plasma preparations, reactions manifested by fever, chills or indications of protein sensitivity may be observed with the administration of Anti-Inhibitor Coagulant Complex. Signs and/or symptoms of high prekallikrein activity, such as changes in blood pressure or pulse rate, may also be observed. It is advisable that appropriate medications be available for the treatment of acute allergic reactions or acute vasoactive reactions should they occur.

A rate of infusion that is too rapid may cause headache, flushing, and changes in pulse rate and blood pressure. In such instances, stopping the infusion allows the symptoms to disappear promptly. With all but the most reactive individuals, infusion may be resumed at a slower rate.

DOSAGE AND ADMINISTRATION
Each bottle of Anti-Inhibitor Coagulant Complex is labeled with the number of Hyland Factor VIII Correctional Units that it contains. One Hyland Factor VIII Correctional Unit is that quantity of activated prothrombin complex which, upon addition to an equal volume of Factor VIII deficient or inhibitor plasma, will correct the clotting time (ellagic acid-activated partial thromboplastin time) to 35 seconds (normal).

The recommended dosage range is 25 to 100 Hyland Factor VIII Correctional Units per kg of body weight, depending upon the severity of hemorrhage. If no hemostatic improvements is observed approximately 6 hours following the initial administration, the dosage should be repeated.

Subsequent dosage and administration intervals should be adjusted according to the patient's clinical response. (See *"Laboratory Tests."*)

RECONSTITUTION: USE ASEPTIC TECHNIC
1. Bring Anti-Inhibitor Coagulant Complex (dry concentrate) and Sterile Water for Injection, USP, (diluent) to room temperature.
2. Remove caps from concentrate and diluent bottles to expose central portions of rubber stoppers.
3. Cleanse stoppers with germicidal solution.
4. Remove protective covering from one end of the double-ended needle and insert exposed needle through diluent stopper.
5. Remove protective covering from other end of the double-ended needle. Invert diluent bottle over the upright concentrate bottle, then rapidly insert free end of the needle through the concentrate bottle stopper at its center. Vacuum in the concentrate bottle will draw in diluent.
6. Disconnect the two bottles by removing needle from the diluent bottle, then remove needle from concentrate bottle stopper. Swirl or rotate the concentrate bottle until all material is dissolved.

Parenteral drug products should be inspected visually for particulate matter and discoloration prior to administration, whenever solution and container permit.

Note: Do not refrigerate after reconstitution.

RATE OF ADMINISTRATION

It is recommended that Anti-Inhibitor Coagulant Complex be infused initially at a rate of 2 mL/min. If infusion at this rate is well tolerated, the administration rate may be gradually increased to 10 mL/min.

ADMINISTRATION: USE ASEPTIC TECHNIQUE

When reconstitution of Anti-Inhibitor Coagulant Complex is complete, its infusion should commence as soon as practical; however, it must be completed within 1 hour. The reconstituted solution should be at room temperature during infusion.

A. Intravenous Drip Infusion

When a Hyland administration set is used, follow directions for use printed on the administration set container. When an administration set from another source is used, follow directions accompanying that set where necessary. The use of a Hyland administration set is recommended as it contains a suitable filter.

B. Intravenous Syringe Injection

1. Attach filter needle to syringe and draw back plunger to admit air into the syringe.
2. Insert needle into the reconstituted Anti-Inhibitor Coagulant Complex.
3. Inject air into bottle and then withdraw the reconstituted material into the syringe.
4. Remove and discard the filter needle from the syringe: attach a suitable needle and inject intravenously as instructed under *"Rate of Administration."*
5. If patient is to receive more than one bottle of concentrate, the contents of two bottles may be drawn into the same syringe by drawing up each bottle through a separate unused filter needle. This practice lessens the loss of concentrate. Please note, filter needles are intended to filter the contents of a single bottle of Anti-Inhibitor Coagulant Complex only.

Storage

Anti-Inhibitor Coagulant Complex should be stored under ordinary refrigeration (2 to 8°C, 36 to 46°F). Avoid freezing to prevent damage to the diluent bottle.

REFERENCES

1. Wells MA, Wittek AE, Epstein JS, *et al:* Inactivation and partition of human T-cell lymphotropic virus, type III, during ethanol fractionation. *Transfusion* 26:210-213, 1986 2. Gazengel C, Larrieu MJ: Lack of seroconversion for LAV/HTLV-III in patients exclusively given unheated activated prothrombin complex prepared with ethanol step. *Lancet* 2:1189, 1985 3. Kurczynski EM, Penner JA: Activated prothrombin concentrate for patients with factor VIII inhibitors. *New Eng J Med* 291:164-167, 1974 4. Penner JA, Kelley PE: Management of patients with factor VIII or IX inhibitors. *Semin Thromb Hemostas* 1:386-399, 1975 5. Buchanan GR, Kevy SV: Use of prothrombin complex concentrates in hemophiliacs with inhibitors: Clinical and laboratory studies. *Pediatrics* 62:767-774, 1978 6. Mannucci PM, Federici F, Vigano S, *et al:* Multiple dental extractions with a new prothrombin complex concentrate in two patients with factor VIII inhibitors. *Thromb Res* 15:359:364, 1979 7. Shapiro SS: Antibodies to blood coagulation factors. *Clinics in Haematology* 8:207-214, 1979 8. Roberts HR: Hemophiliacs with inhibitors: Therapeutic options: *New Eng J Med* 305:757-758, 1981

BIBLIOGRAPHY

Fekete LF, Holst SL, Peetoom F, *et al:* 'Auto' Factor IX Concentrate: A new therapeutic approach to treatment of hemophilia A patients with inhibitors. *Proceedings, 14th International Congress of Hematology.* Sao Paulo, Brazil, 1972
Kelly P, Penner JA: Antihemophilic factor inhibitors: Management with prothrombin complex concentrates. *JAMA* 236:2061, 1976
Seligsohn U, Kasper CK, Østerud B, *et al:* Activated factor VII. Presence in factor IX concentrates and persistence in the circulation after infusion. *Blood* 53:828, 1979
Abildgaard CF, Penner JA, Watson-Williams EJ: Anti-Inhibitor Coagulant Complex (Autoplex) for treatment of factor VIII inhibitors in hemophilia. *Blood* 56:978, 1980

HOW SUPPLIED
POWDER FOR INJECTION:

BRAND/MANUFACTURER	NDC	SIZE	AWP
◇ **BRAND**			
AUTOPLEX T: Baxter Biotech	00944-0650-01	1s	$1.30
◇ **GENERICS**			
FEIBA-VH: Immuno-U.S.	54129-0222-04	1s	$1.30

Anticoagulant Citrate Phosphate Dex *SEE ANTICOAGULANT CITRATE PHOSPHATE DEXTROSE*

Anticoagulant Citrate Phosphate Dextrose

DESCRIPTION

Anticoagulant Citrate Phosphate Dextrose is a sterile, nonpyrogenic solution of citric acid, sodium citrate, monobasic sodium phosphate and dextrose in water for injection intended only for use with Receptal Autologous Transfusion Systems for emergency hemothorax procedures or other autologous blood transfusion procedures.

Each 100 mL of Anticoagulant Citrate Phosphate Dextrose Solution (CPD Solution) contains citric acid (anhydrous) 299 mg, sodium citrate (dihydrate) 2.63 g, monobasic sodium phosphate (monohydrate) 222 mg, dextrose, hydrous 2.55 g in water for injection. The solution is hypertonic, 566 mOsmol/liter (calc.); pH 5.6 (5.0 - 6.0).

It contains no bacteriostat, antimicrobial agent or added buffer and is intended for use only in a single procedure. When smaller volumes are required, the unused portion should be discarded.

Anticoagulant Citrate Phosphate Dextrose Solution is an anticoagulant for use in autologous blood transfusion procedures.

Citric Acid, USP is chemically designated citric acid, anhydrous $CH_2(COOH)C(OH)(COOH)CH_2COOH$, a colorless, translucent crystal or white, granular to fine, crystalline powder very soluble in water.

Sodium Citrate, USP is chemically designated sodium citrate, dihydrate $CH_2(COONa)C(OH)(COONa)CH_2COONa \cdot 2H_2O$, a colorless crystal or white, crystalline powder hydrous form freely soluble in water.

Monobasic Sodium Phosphate, USP (monohydrate) is chemically designated $NaH_2PO_4 \cdot H_2O$, a colorless transparent crystal or white, crystalline powder freely soluble in water.

Dextrose, USP is chemically designated $C_6H_{12}O_6 \cdot H_2O$ (D-glucose monohydrate), a hexose sugar freely soluble in water.

Water for Injection, USP is chemically designated H_2O.

CLINICAL PHARMACOLOGY

Anticoagulant Citrate Phosphate Dextrose Solution, USP acts as an anticoagulant by the action of the citrate ion chelating calcium, thus making calcium unavailable to the coagulation system. When mixed with autologous blood collected for reinfusion in a ratio of 1 part CPD Solution to 7 parts blood (14 mL solution per 100 mL of whole blood), it prevents coagulation in the Receptal Autologous Transfusion System by inhibiting the several calcium dependent steps of the coagulation cascade.

Citric acid, sodium citrate and monobasic sodium phosphate are in the proper proportions to buffer the solution at the optimal pH for blood. Dextrose provides a substrate for glycolysis.

INDICATIONS AND USAGE

Add appropriate amounts of Anticoagulant Citrate Phosphate Dextrose Solution, USP (14 mL per 100 mL autologous blood collected) via a volume control I.V. set to the Receptal Autologous Transfusion System used to collect blood for reinfusion.

CONTRAINDICATIONS

Not for direct intravenous infusion. Do not store collected blood in sterile collection reservoir.

PRECAUTIONS

Aseptic technique must be maintained.

If a citrate anticoagulant blood is administered by rapid autotransfusion, citrate toxicity and circulatory depression may be seen. To monitor toxicity, frequent blood gas samples to check pH and serum calcium levels are required.

Do not use unless solution is clear, seal is intact and vacuum present. Discard unused portion.

Pregnancy Category C: Animal reproduction studies have not been conducted with this solution. It is also not known whether it can cause fetal harm when used to anticoagulate autologous blood administered to a pregnant woman or if it can affect reproduction capacity. It should be given to a pregnant woman only if clearly needed.

ADVERSE REACTIONS

Too rapid administration of CPD Solution–treated autologous blood may result in citrate toxicity. One gram of calcium chloride may be administered prophylactically for each 1000 mL autologous blood reinfused.

OVERDOSAGE

In event of overinfusion or solute overload following reinfusion of autologous blood anticoagulated with CPD Solution, re-evaluate the patient and institute appropriate corrective measures. See *"Precautions"* and *"Adverse Reactions".*

DOSAGE AND ADMINISTRATION

The amount of CPD Solution added to the Receptal Autologous Transfusion System is dependent on the amount of autologous blood collected. The ratio is 1 part CPD Solution to 7 parts blood (14 mL CPD to 100 mL blood).

CPD Solution should be inspected visually for particulate matter and discoloration prior to use, whenever solution container permits. See *"Precautions."*

DRUG INTERACTIONS

Additives may be incompatible. Consult with pharmacist, if available. When introducing additives, use aseptic technique, mix thoroughly and do not store.

Exposure of pharmaceutical products to heat should be minimized. Protect from freezing. It is recommended that the product be stored at room temperature (25° C); however, brief exposure up to 40°C does not adversely affect the product.

◆ RATED THERAPEUTICALLY EQUIVALENT; ◇ THERAPEUTIC EQUIVALENCE UNCONFIRMED; ○ UNRATED

HOW SUPPLIED
SOLUTION:

BRAND/MANUFACTURER	NDC	SIZE	AWP
○ **BRAND**			
ANTICOAGULANT CITRATE PHOSPHATE DEX:	00074-1967-04	500 ml 6s	$143.78
Abbott Hosp			

Antihemophilic Factor

DESCRIPTION
Antihemophilic Factor (Recombinant) is a sterile, stable, purified, dried concentrate which has been manufactured by recombinant DNA technology. Antihemophilic Factor is intended for use in therapy of classical hemophilia (hemophilia A). Antihemophilic Factor is produced by Baby Hamster Kidney (BHK) cells or Chinese Hamster Ovary (CHO) into which the human factor VIII (FVIII) gene has been introduced. Antihemophilic Factor is a highly purified glycoprotein consisting of multiple peptides including an 80 kD and various extensions of the 90 kD subunit. It has the same biological activity as FVIII derived from human plasma. In addition to the use of the classical purification methods of ion exchange chromatography and size exclusion chromatography, monoclonal antibody immunoaffinity chromatography is utilized along with other steps designed to purify recombinant factor VIII (rAHF) and remove contaminating substances. The final preparation is stabilized with Albumin (Human) and lyophilized. The concentration of Antihemophilic Factor is approximately 100 IU/mL. The product contains no preservatives.

Each vial of Antihemophilic Factor contains the labeled amount of rAHF in international units (IU). One IU, as defined by the World Health Organization standard for blood coagulation factor VIII, human, is approximately equal to the level of factor VIII activity found in 1.0 mL of fresh pooled human plasma. Antihemophilic Factor must be administered by the intravenous route.

CLINICAL PHARMACOLOGY
The clinical trial of one brand of Antihemophilic Factor has included 168 patients, enrolled over a 55-month period. A total of 16,186 infusions have been utilized in this trial. The study was conducted in several stages.

Initial pharmacokinetic studies were conducted in 17 asymptomatic hemophilic patients, comparing pharmacokinetics of plasma-derived Antihemophilic Factor (Human) (pdAHF) and Antihemophilic Factor. The mean biologic half-life of rAHF was 15.8 hours. The mean biologic half-life of pdAHF in the same individuals was 13.9 hours. A similar degree of shortening of the activated partial thromboplastin time was seen with both rAHF and pdAHF. The mean *in vivo* recovery of rAHF was similar to pdAHF, with a linear dose-response relationship. The recovery and half-life of rAHF was consistent with initial results following 13 weeks of exclusive treatment with one brand of Antihemophilic Factor. Subsequently, 826 recovery studies were conducted in 58 hemophilic patients participating in later clinical studies. Mean recovery from this group was 2.48% per IU/kg infused.

Fourteen (14) subjects from initial pharmacokinetic studies commenced home treatment with rAHF. Forty-four (44) additional subjects were then enrolled who treated themselves at home exclusively with rAHF. A total of 12,730 infusions have been administered under this portion of the study, of which 1,021 were given in clinic for recovery studies, 7,339 were given for treatment of bleeds, 4,361 were given as prophylaxis, 5 for minor surgery not requiring hospitalization, and 4 for unspecified reason.

Forty-eight (48) patients have received rAHF on 63 occasions for surgical procedures or in-hospital treatment of serious hemorrhage. Eleven (11) received rAHF for the first time in this study, while 37 were already on study or study participants under an investigation of previously untreated patients. Hemostatis has been satisfactory in all cases, with no adverse reactions.

In a study of previously untreated patients, a total of 3,254 infusions have been administered to 96 patients over a 48-month enrollment period. Hemostasis was successfully achieved in all cases.

During the analytical characterization of Antihemophilic Factor, analyses for carbohydrate structure revealed the presence of terminal galactose α1 3 galactose residues. Since naturally occurring antibody to this structure has been reported in humans, a trial in 18 patients was performed in which the half-life and recovery of rAHF with high levels on this carbohydrate residue was compared to that with one brand of Antihemophilic Factor, which contains low levels of this structure. As in the normal population, all patients had preexisting endogenous antibody to galactose α1 3 galactose in titers ranging from 1:320 to 1:5120 and no significant change in antibody level was noted during the study. While the mean recovery for one brand of Antihemophilic Factor in the study, 2.76-%/IU/kg (N = 43), was significantly different from that of rAHF with high levels of residues, 2.43%/IU/kg (N = 155; p = 0.0001), the recovery for rAHF with high levels of galactose α1 → 3 galactose is not significantly different from the 2.48%/IU/kg recovery obtained in the larger study from the 58 patients treated with one brand of Antihemophilic Factor mentioned above. Based on these results, the galactose α1→3 galactose residue appears to have no clinical significance.

INDICATIONS AND USAGE
Antihemophilic Factor is indicated for the treatment of classical hemophilia (hemophilia A) in which there is a demonstrated deficiency of activity of the plasma clotting factor, factor VIII. Antihemophilic Factor provides a means of temporarily replacing the missing clotting factor in order to correct or prevent bleeding episodes, or in order to perform emergency and elective surgery in hemophiliacs.

Antihemophilic Factor can also be used for treatment of hemophilia A in certain patients with inhibitors to factor VIII. In clinical studies of Antihemophilic Factor, patients who developed inhibitors on study continued to manifest a clinical response when inhibitor titers were less than 10 Bethesda Units (B.U.) per mL. When an inhibitor is present, the dosage requirement for factor VIII is variable. The dosage can be determined only by clinical response, and by monitoring of circulating factor VIII levels after treatment (see *"Dosage and Administration"*).

Antihemophilic Factor does not contain von Willebrand's factor and therefore is not indicated for the treatment of von Willebrand's disease.

UNLABELED USES
Antihemophilic Factor is used alone or as an adjunct in the treatment of Von Willebrand's Disease.

CONTRAINDICATIONS
Due to the fact that Antihemophilic Factor (Recombinant) contains trace amounts of mouse protein (maximum 0.03 ng/IU rAHF) and hamster protein (maximum 0.04 ng/IU rAHF), it should be administered with caution to individuals with previous hypersensitivity to pdAHF or known hypersensitivity to biologic preparations with trace amounts of murine or hamster or bovine proteins.

Assays to detect seroconversion to mouse and hamster protein were conducted on all patients on study. No patient has developed specific antibody titers against these proteins after commencing study, and no allergic reactions have been associated with rAHF infusions. Although no reactions were observed, patients should be warned of the theoretical possibility of a hypersensitivity reaction, and altered to the early signs of such a reaction (e.g., hives, generalized uticaria, wheezing and hypotension). Patients should be advised to discontinue use of the product and contact their physician if such symptoms occur.

WARNINGS
None.

PRECAUTIONS
GENERAL
Antihemophilic Factor is intended for the treatment of bleeding disorders arising from a deficiency in factor VIII. This deficiency should be proven prior to administrating Antihemophilic Factor.

The development of circulating neutralizing antibodies to factor VIII may occur during the treatment of patients with hemophilia A. In a study of previously untreated patients, conducted with one brand of Antihemophilic Factor, inhibitor antibodies have developed in 17 of the 92 patients (18.5%) who have had at least one follow-up titer. The incidence of antibodies is 15/56 (26.7%) in patients with severe disease (< 2% factor VIII), 2/18 (11%) in patients with moderate disease (2-5% factor VIII) and 0/18 in patients with mild disease (> 5% factor VIII). Ten of the antibodies were higher titer (> 10 Bethesda Units), three were low titer, and four were low titer and transient. Studies most closely resembling the design of the study of inhibitor development with Antihemophilic Factor have reported incidences of inhibitor formation ranging between 18.4 and 52% for patients treated with pdAHF.[3-6] The incidence of inhibitor formation in previously untreated patients treated with Antihemophilic Factor Recombinant, appears to be consistent with that reported in the literature, however, the true immunogenicity of Antihemophilic Factor is not known at present. Patients treated with rAHF should be carefully monitored for the development of antibodies to rAHF by appropriate clinical observation and laboratory tests.

CARCINOGENESIS, MUTAGENESIS, IMPAIRMENT OF FERTILITY
In vitro evaluation of the mutagenic potential of Antihemophilic Factor failed to demonstrate reverse mutation or chromosomal aberrations at doses substantially greater than the maximum expected clinical dose. *In vivo* evaluation of rAHF using doses ranging between 10 and 40 times the expected clinical maximum also indicated that Antihemophilic Factor does not possess a mutagenic potential. Long-term investigations of carcinogenic potential in animals have not been performed.

PEDIATRIC USE
Antihemophilic Factor has been proven to be safe and efficacious in newborns and children while under investigation as previously treated and previously untreated patients (see *"Clinical Pharmacology"* and *"Precautions"*).

PREGNANCY CATEGORY C
Animal reproduction studies have not been conducted with Antihemophilic Factor. It is also not known whether Antihemophilic Factor can cause fetal harm when administered to a pregnant woman or can affect reproduction capacity. Antihemophilic Factor should be given to a pregnant woman only if clearly needed.

ADVERSE REACTIONS
During the clinical studies conducted with one brand of Antihemophilic Factor in previously treated patients, 47 out of 12,932 infusions (0.36%) were associated with 58 reported minor adverse reactions. Of these, 19 reactions were local to the injection site (e.g., burning, pruritus, erythema); and 39 were systemic complaints (dizziness, nausea, chest discomfort, sore throat, cold feet, unusual taste in mouth, and slight decrease in blood pressure). In the study with previously untreated patients, 3,254 infusions have been associated with 11 minor adverse reactions

(0.34%): two reports of erythema at the injection site, one of facial flushing related to the infusion, one report of diarrhea, two reports of nonspecific rash, two reports of fever, and three reports of emesis. Side effects reported with another brand were flushing, nausea, mild fatigue, and nosebleeds. No serious reactions have been reported, and all reactions have been self-limited.

DOSAGE AND ADMINISTRATION
Each bottle of Antihemophilic Factor has the rAHF content in international units per bottle stated on the label of the bottle. The reconstituted product must be administered intravenously by either direct syringe injection or drip infusion. The product must be administered within 3 hours after reconstitution.

GENERAL APPROACH TO TREATMENT AND ASSESSMENT OF TREATMENT EFFICACY
The dosages described below are presented as general guidance. It should be emphasized that the dosage of Antihemophilic Factor required for (hemostasis) must be individualized according to the needs of the patient, the severity of the deficiency, the severity of the hemorrhage, the presence of inhibitors, and the factor VIII level desired. It is often critical to follow the course of therapy with factor VIII level assays.

The clinical effect of Antihemophilic Factor is the most important element in evaluating the effectiveness of treatment. It may be necessary to administer more Antihemophilic Factor than would be estimated in order to attain satisfactory clinical results. If the calculated dose fails to attain the expected factor VIII levels, or if bleeding is not controlled after administration of the calculated dosage, the presence of a circulating inhibitor in the patient should be suspected. Its presence should be substantiated and the inhibitor level quantitated by appropriate laboratory tests. When an inhibitor is present, the dosage requirement for rAHF is extremely variable and the dosage can be determined only by the clinical response.

Some patients with low titer inhibitors (< 10 B.U.) can be successfully treated with factor VIII without a resultant anamnestic rise in inhibitor titer.[7] Factor VIII levels and clinical response to treatment must be assessed to insure adequate response. Use of alternative treatment products, such as Factor IX Complex concentrates, Antihemophilic Factor (Porcine) or Anti-Inhibitor Coagulant Complex, may be necessary for patients with anamnestic responses to factor VIII treatment and/or high titer inhibitors.

CALCULATION OF DOSAGE
The in vivo percent elevation in factor VIII level can be estimated by multiplying the dose of rAHF per kilogram of body weight (IU/kg) by 2%. This method of calculation is based on clinical findings by Abildgaard et al.,[8] and is illustrated in the following examples.

$$\text{Expected \% factor VIII increase} = \frac{\text{\# units administered} \times 2\%/\text{IU/kg}}{\text{body weight (kg)}}$$

Example for a 70 kg adult:

$$\frac{1400 \text{ IU} \times 2\%/\text{IU}}{70 \text{ kg}} = 40\%$$

or

$$\text{Dosage required (IU)} = \frac{\text{body weight (kg)} \times \text{desired \% factor VIII increase}}{2\%/\text{IU/kg}}$$

Example for a 15 kg child:

$$\frac{15 \text{ kg} \times 100\%}{2\%/\text{IU/kg}} = 750 \text{ IU required}$$

The dosage necessary to achieve hemostasis depends upon the type and severity of the bleeding episode, according to the following general guidelines:

MILD HEMORRHAGE
Mild superficial or early hemorrhages may respond to a single dose of 10 IU per kg,[9] leading to an in vivo rise of approximately 20% in the factor VIII level. Therapy need not be repeated unless there is evidence of further bleeding.

MODERATE HEMORRHAGE
For more serious bleeding episodes (e.g., definite hemarthroses, known trauma), the factor VIII level should be raised to 30-50% by administering approximately 15-25 IU per kg. If further therapy is required, a repeat infusion can be given at 12-24 hours.[10]

SEVERE HEMORRHAGE
In patients with life-threatening bleeding or possible hemorrhage involving vital structures (e.g., central nervous system, retropharyngeal and retroperitoneal spaces, iliopsoas sheath), the factor VIII level should be raised to 80-100% of normal in order to achieve hemostasis. This may be achieved with an initial rAHF (Antihemophilic Factor) dose of 40-50 IU per kg and a maintenance dose of 20-25 IU per kg every 8-12 hours.[11,12]

SURGERY
For major surgical procedures, the factor VIII level should be raised to approximately 100% by giving a preoperative dose of 50 IU/kg. The factor VIII level should be checked to assure that the expected level is achieved before the patient goes to surgery. In order to maintain hemostatic levels, repeat infusions may be necessary every 6 to 12 hours initially, and for a total of 10 to 14 days until healing is complete. The intensity of factor VIII replacement therapy

required depends on the type of surgery and postoperative regimen employed. For minor surgical procedures, less intensive treatment schedules may provide adequate hemostasis.[11,12]

PROPHYLAXIS
Factor VIII concentrates may also be administered on a regular schedule for prophylaxis of bleeding, as reported by Nilsson, et al.[13]

RECONSTITUTION
Vacuum Transfer

1. Warm the unopened diluent and the concentrate to room temperature (NMT 37°C, 99°F).
2. After removing the caps, aseptically cleanse the rubber stoppers of both bottles.
3. Remove the protective cover from the plastic transfer-needle cartridge and penetrate the stopper of the diluent bottle.
4. Remove the remaining portion of the plastic cartridge, invert the diluent bottle and penetrate the rubber seal on the concentrate bottle with the needle at an angle. Alternate method of transferring sterile water: With a sterile needle and syringe, withdraw the appropriate volume of diluent and transfer to the bottle of lyophilized concentrate.
5. The vacuum will draw the diluent into the concentrate bottle. Hold the diluent bottle at an angle to the concentrate bottle in order to direct the jet of diluent against the wall of the concentrate bottle. Avoid excessive foaming.
6. After removing the diluent bottle and transfer needle, swirl continuously until completely dissolved.
7. After the concentrate powder is completely dissolved, withdraw solution into the syringe through the filter needle. Replace the filter needle with the administration set provided and inject intravenously.
8. If the same patient is to receive more than one bottle, the contents of two bottles may be drawn into the same syringe through a separate unused filter needle before attaching the vein needle.

RATE OF ADMINISTRATION
The rate of administration should be adapted to the response of the individual patient, but administration of the entire dose in 5 to 10 minutes or less is well-tolerated.

Parenteral drug products should be inspected visually for particulate matter and discoloration prior to administration, whenever solution and container permit.

STORAGE
Antihemophilic Factor should be stored under refrigeration (2-8°C; 35-46°F). Storage of lyophilized powder at room temperature (up to 25°C or 77°F) for 3 months, such as in home treatment situations, may be done without loss of factor VIII activity. Freezing should be avoided, as breakage of the diluent bottle might occur. Do not use beyond the expiration date indicated on the bottle.

REFERENCES
1. Lawn RM, Vehar GA: The molecular genetics of hemophilia. Sci Am 254(3):48-54, 1986. 2. Schwartz RS, Abildgaard CF, Aledort LM, et al: Human recombinant DNA-derived antihemophilic factor (factor VIII) in the treatment of hemophilia A. N Engl J Med 323(26):1800-5, 1990. 3. Lusher JM: Viral safety and inhibitor development associated with monoclonal antibody-purified FVIIIc. Ann Hematol 63(3):138-41, 1991. 4. Addiego JE Jr, Gomperts E, Liu S-L, et al: Treatment of hemophilia A with a highly purified factor VIII concentrate prepared by anti-FVIIIc immunoaffinity chromatography. Thromb Haemost 67(1):19-27, 1992. 5. Schwarzinger I, Pabinger I, Korninger C, et al: Incidence of inhibitors in patients with severe and moderate hemophilia A treated with factor VIII concentrates. Am J Hematol 24(3):241-5, 1987. 6. Ehrenforth S, Kreuz W. Scharrer I, et al: Incidence of development of factor VIII and factor IX inhibitors in hemophiliacs. Lancet 339(8793):594-8, 1992. 7. Kasper CK: Complications of hemophilia A treatment: factor VIII inhibitors, Ann NY Acad Sci 614:97-105, 1991. 8. Abildgaard CF, Simone JV, Corrigan JJ, et al: Treatment of hemophilia with glycine-precipitated Factor VIII, N Engl J Med 275(9):471-5, 1966. 9. Britton M, Harrison J, Abildgaard CF: Early treatment of hemophilic hemarthroses with minimal dose of new factor VIII concentrate, J Pediatr 85(2):245-7, 1974. 10. Abildgaard CF: Current concepts in the management of hemophilia. Semin Hematol 12(3):223-32, 1975. 11. Hilgartner MW: Factor replacement therapy. In: Hilgartner MW, Pochedly C, eds.: Hemophilia in the child and adult. New York, Raven Press, 1989, pp 1-26. 12. Kasper CK, Dietrich SL: Comprehensive management of haemophilia. Clin Haematol 14(2):489-512, 1985. 13. Nilsson IM, Berntorp E, Lofqvist T, et al: Twenty-five years' experience of prophylactic treatment in severe haemophilia A and B. J Intern Med 232(1):25-32, 1992.

HOW SUPPLIED
POWDER FOR INJECTION:

BRAND/MANUFACTURER	NDC	SIZE	AWP
○ **BRAND**			
BIOCLATE: Armour	00053-8110-01	1s	$1.18
	00053-8110-02	1s	$1.18
	00053-8110-04	1s	$1.18
HELIXATE: Armour	00053-8120-01	1s	$1.18
	00053-8120-02	1s	$1.18
	00053-8120-04	1s	$1.18
RECOMBINATE: Baxter Biotech	00944-2938-01	1s	$1.18
	00944-2938-02	1s	$1.18
	00944-2938-03	1s	$1.18

◆ RATED THERAPEUTICALLY EQUIVALENT; ◇ THERAPEUTIC EQUIVALENCE UNCONFIRMED; ○ UNRATED

POWDER FOR INJECTION: 1 I.U.

BRAND/MANUFACTURER	NDC	SIZE	AWP
○ **BRAND**			
KOGENATE: Miles Biol	00161-0670-20	1s	$1.18
	00161-0670-30	1s	$1.18
	00161-0670-50	1s	$1.18

Antihemophilic Factor, Human

DESCRIPTION

Antihemophilic Factor (Human), Factor VIII:C Pasteurized, Monoclonal Antibody Purified is a sterile, stable, lyophilized concentrate of Factor VIII:C with reduced amounts of vWf:Ag and purified of extraneous plasma-derived protein by use of affinity chromatography. A murine monoclonal antibody to Wf:Ag is used as an affinity ligand to first isolate the Factor VIII Complex. Factor VIII:C is then dissociated from vWf:Ag, recovered, formulated and provided as a sterile lyophilized powder.[1,2,3] The concentrate as formulated contains Albumin (Human) as a stabilizer, resulting in a concentrate with a specific activity between 5 and 10 units/mg of total protein. In the absence of this added Albumin (Human) stabilizer, specific activity has been determined to exceed 3000 units/mg of protein.[4] Antihemophilic Factor, Human has been prepared from pooled human plasma and is intended for use in therapy of classical hemophilia (Hemophilia A).

The concentrate has been pasteurized by heating at 60°C for 10 hours in aqueous solution form during its manufacture in order to further reduce the risk of viral transmission.[5] However, no procedure has been shown to be totally effective in removing viral infectivity from coagulant factor concentrates. (See *"Clinical Pharmacology"* and *"Warnings."*)

Antihemophilic Factor, Human is a highly purified preparation of Factor VIII:C. When stored as directed, it will maintain its labeled potency for the period indicated on the container and package labels.[8,9]

Upon reconstitution, a clear, colorless solution is obtained, containing 50 to 150 times as much Factor VIII:C as does an equal volume of plasma.

Each vial contains the labeled amount of antihemophilic factor (AHF) activity as expressed in terms of International Units of antihemophilic activity. One unit of antihemophilic activity is equivalent to that quantity of AHF present in one mL of normal human plasma. When reconstituted as recommended, the resulting solution contains approximately 300 to 450 millimoles of sodium ions per liter and has 2 to 3 times the tonicity of saline. It contains approximately 2-5 millimoles of calcium ions per liter, contributed as calcium chloride, approximately 1 to 2% Albumin (Human), 0.8% mannitol, and 1.2 mM histidine. The pH is adjusted with hydrochloric acid and/or sodium hydroxide. Certain brands of Antihemophilic Factor, Human also contain trace amounts ($\leq$ 50 ng per 100 I.U of AHF) of the murine monoclonal antibody used in its purification (see *"Clinical Pharmacology"*).

Antihemophilic Factor, Human is to be administered only intravenously.

CLINICAL PHARMACOLOGY

Factor VIII:C is the coagulant portion of the Factor VIII complex circulating in plasma. It is noncovalently associated with the von Willebrand protein responsible for von Willebrand factor activity. These two proteins have distinct biochemical and immunological properties and are under separate genetic control. Factor VIII:C acts as a cofactor for Factor IX to activate Factor X in the intrinsic pathway of blood coagulation.[6] Hemophilia A, an hereditary disorder of blood coagulation due to decreased levels of Factor VIII:C, results in profuse bleeding into joints, muscles or internal organs as a result of a trauma. Antihemophilic Factor (Human), Factor VIII:C Pasteurized, Monoclonal Antibody Purified provides an increase in plasma levels of AHF, thereby enabling temporary correction of Hemophilia A bleeding.

Clinical evaluation of Antihemophilic Factor, Human Factor VIII:C Pasteurized, Monoclonal Antibody Purified concentrate for its half-life characteristics in hemophilic patients showed it to be comparable to other commercially available Antihemophilic Factor (Human) concentrates. The mean half-life obtained from six patients was 17.5 hours with a mean recovery of 1.9 Units/dl rise/U/kg.

The pasteurization process used in the manufacture of this concentrate has demonstrated *in vitro* inactivation of human immunodeficiency virus (HIV) and several model viruses. In two separate studies, HIV was reduced by $\geq$ 7.0 $\log_{10}$ to an undetectable level and by 10.5 $\log_{10}$, respectively. In addition to HIV, studies were also performed using three lipid containing model viruses and one non-lipid, encapsulated model virus. Vesicular stomatitis (VSV) was reduced by $\geq$ 6.79 $\log_{10}$ to undetectable, Sindbis was reduced by $\geq$ 6.48 $\log_{10}$ to undetectable and Vaccinia was reduced by $\geq$ 5.36 $\log_{10}$ to detectable. Murine encephalomyocarditis (EMC), a non-lipid, encapsulated model virus, was reduced by $\geq$ 7.1 $\log_{10}$ to undetectable.

Evidence of the capability of the purification and preparative steps used in the production of Antihemophilic Factor (Human), Factor VIII:C Pasteurized, Monoclonal Antibody Purified, to reduce viral bioburden was obtained in studies involving the addition of known quantities of virus to cryoprecipitate. These studies were conducted using an earlier form of the concentrate which had not undergone liquid pasteurization (Antihemophilic Factor (Human), Monoclonal Antibody Purified, Factor VIII:C, Heat-Treated). These studies provide evidence of the viral removal potential of the purification and preparative steps of the manufacturing process (exclusive of heat treatment) which are common to both concentrates. In one study, the viruses used were human immunodeficiency virus

(HIV), sindbis virus, vesicular stomatitis virus (VSV) and pseudorabies virus (PsRV). A comparison of the cumulative mean reductions for all viruses tested with the individual values obtained in each experiment indicates that the combined effects of the manufacturing steps, which purify the Factor VIII:C and prepare the concentrate in a final sterile container as a lyophilized powder, contribute viral reduction capabilities of approximately 5 to 6 logs. In a separate study, aluminum hydroxide treatment followed by antibody affinity chromatography reduced vaccinia virus infectivity by 4.81 logs. These studies indicate that the purification and preparative steps of the manufacturing process are capable of providing a nonspecific, viral reduction of approximately 5 to 6 logs, independent of the pasteurization process.

Certain brands of Antihemophilic Factor, Human, contain trace amounts of mouse protein[7] ($\leq$ 50 ng per 100 I.U. of AHF). In a study using an earlier form of the concentrate which had not undergone pasteurization Antihemophilic Factor, Human, a number of patients sero-negative for anti-HIV-1 were monitored to determine whether they would develop antibody or experience adverse reactions as a result of repeated exposure. These patients were treated on multiple occasions. Prestudy serum measurements of 27 patients for human anti-mouse IgG showed that, prior to treatment, 6 of them had either detectable antibody to mouse proteins or cross-reactive proteins. These patients continued to demonstrate similar or lower antibody levels during the study. Of the remaining 21 patients, 6 were shown to have low antibody levels on one or more occasions. In no case was observance of low antibody level associated with an anamnestic response or with any clinical adverse reaction. Patients were observed for time periods ranging from 2 to 30 months.

INDICATIONS AND USAGE

Antihemophilic Factor (Human), Factor VIII:C Pasteurized, Monoclonal Antibody Purified is indicated for treatment of classical hemophilia (Hemophilia A). Affected individuals frequently require therapy following minor accidents. Surgery, when required in such individuals, must be preceded by temporary corrections of the clotting abnormality. Presurgical correction of severe AHF deficiency can be accomplished with a small volume of Antihemophilic Factor, Human.

Antihemophilic Factor, Human is not effective in controlling the bleeding of patients with von Willebrand's disease.

CONTRAINDICATIONS

Known hypersensitivity to mouse protein is a contraindication to Antihemophilic Factor (Human), Factor VIII:C Pasteurized, Monoclonal Antibody Purified.

WARNINGS

This product is prepared from pooled human plasma which may contain the causative agents of hepatitis and other viral diseases. Prescribed manufacturing procedures utilized at the plasma collection centers, plasma testing laboratories, and the fractionation facilities are designed to reduce the risk of transmitting viral infection. However, the risk of viral infectivity from this product cannot be totally eliminated. Accordingly, the benefits and risks of treatment with this concentrate should be carefully assessed prior to use. Individuals who receive infusions of blood or plasma products may develop signs and/or symptoms of some viral infections, particularly nonA, nonB hepatitis.

PRECAUTIONS

General: Most brands of Antihemophilic Factor (Human) concentrates contain naturally occurring blood group specific antibodies. When large or frequently repeated doses of product are needed, patients should be monitored by means of hematocrit and direct Coombs tests for signs of progressive anemia.

FORMATION OF ANTIBODIES TO MOUSE PROTEIN

Although no hypersensitivity reactions have been observed, because certain brands of Antihemophilic Factor, Human contain trace amounts of mouse protein ($\leq$ 50 ng per 100 I.U. of AHF), the possibility exists that patients treated with Antihemophilic Factor, Human may develop hypersensitivity to the mouse proteins.

INFORMATION FOR PATIENTS

Patients should be informed of the early signs of hypersensitivity reactions including hives, generalized urticaria, tightness of the chest, wheezing, hypotension, and anaphylaxis, and should be advised to discontinue use of the concentrate and contact their physician if these symptoms occur.

PREGNANCY CATEGORY C

Animal reproduction studies have not been conducted with Antihemophilic Factor (Human), Factor VIII:C Pasteurized, Monoclonal Antibody Purified. It is also not known whether Antihemophilic Factor, Human can cause fetal harm when administered to a pregnant woman or can affect reproduction capacity. Antihemophilic Factor, Human should be given to a pregnant woman only if clearly needed.

ADVERSE REACTIONS

Products of this type are known to cause allergic reactions, mild chills, nausea or stinging at the infusion site.

DOSAGE AND ADMINISTRATION

Antihemophilic Factor (Human), Factor VIII:C Pasteurized, Monoclonal Antibody Purified is for intravenous administration only. As a general rule 1 unit of AHF activity per kg will increase the circulating AHF level by 2%.[10] The following formula provides a guide for dosage calculations:

Number of AHF I.U. Required	=	Body weight (in kg)	X	desired Factor VIII increase (% normal)	X	0.5[10]

Although dosage must be individualized according to the needs of the patient (weight, severity of hemorrhage, presence of inhibitors), the following general dosages are suggested.[11]

1. Mild Hemorrhages: Minor hemorrhagic episodes will generally subside with a single infusion if a level of 30% or more is attained.

2. Moderate Hemorrhage and Minor Surgery: For more serious hemorrhages and minor surgical procedures, the patient's Factor VIII level should be raised to 30–50% of normal, which usually requires an initial dose of 15–25 I.U. per kg. If further therapy is required a maintenance dose is 10–15 I.U. per kg every 8–12 hours.

3. Severe Hemorrhage: In hemorrhages near vital organs (neck, throat, subperitoneal) it may be desirable to raise the Factor VIII level to 80–100% of normal which can be achieved with an initial dose of 40–50 I.U. per kg and a maintenance dose of 20–25 I.U. per kg every 8–12 hours.

4. Major Surgery: For surgical procedures a dose of AHF sufficient to achieve a level 80–100% of normal should be given an hour prior to surgery. A second dose, half the size of the priming dose, should be given five hours after the first dose. Factor VIII levels should be maintained at a daily minimum of at least 30% for a period of 10–14 days postoperatively. Close laboratory control to maintain AHF plasma levels deemed appropriate to maintain hemostasis is recommended.

RECONSTITUTION

1. Warm both the diluent and Antihemophilic Factor (Human), Factor VIII:C Pasteurized, Monoclonal Antibody Purified in unopened vials to room temperature [not above 37°C (98°F)].
2. Remove the caps from both vials to expose the central portions of the rubber stoppers.
3. Treat the surface of the rubber stoppers with antiseptic solution and allow them to dry.
4. Using aseptic technique, insert one end of the double-end needle into the rubber stopper of the diluent vial. Invert the diluent vial and insert the other end of the double-end needle into the rubber stopper of the vial. Direct the diluent, which will be drawn in by vacuum, over the entire surface of the Antihemophilic Factor, Human cake. (In order to assure transfer of all the diluent, adjust the position of the tip of the needle in the diluent vial to the inside edge of the diluent stopper.) Rotate the vial to ensure complete wetting of the cake during the transfer process.
5. Remove the diluent vial to release the vacuum, *then remove the double-end needle,* from the Antihemophilic Factor, Human vial.
6. Gently swirl the vial until the powder is dissolved and the solution is ready for administration. The concentrate routinely and easily reconstitutes within one minute. To assure sterility, Antihemophilic Factor, Human should be administered within three hours after reconstitution.
7. Parenteral drug preparations should be inspected visually for particulate matter and discoloration prior to administration, whenever solution and container permit.

ADMINISTRATION

Caution: This kit contains *two* devices, a stainless steel 5 micron filter needle, individually labeled as a 5 micron filter needle and contained in a separate blister pack, and an all plastic 5 micron vented filter spike which is supplied with the four-item administration components blister pack, either of which may be used to withdraw the reconstituted product for administration. The withdrawal directions specific for each of these alternate devices must be followed *exactly* for whichever device is chosen for use as described below. Product loss or inability to withdraw product will result if the improper instructions are followed.

A. Administration using the Stainless Steel *Filter Needle* for Withdrawal (This item is individually packaged in a separate, labeled blister pack.)

Intravenous Injection: Plastic disposable syringes are recommended with Antihemophilic Factor (Human), Factor VIII:C Pasteurized, Monoclonal Antibody Purified solution. The ground glass surface of all-glass syringes tend to stick with solutions of this type.

1. Using aseptic technique, attach the *filter needle* to a sterile disposable syringe.
2. *Draw air into the syringe* equal to or greater than the contents of the vial.
3. Insert the filter needle into the stopper of the Antihemophilic Factor, Human vial, invert the vial, position the filter needle above the level of the liquid and inject all of the air into the vial.
4. Pull the filter needle back down below the level of the liquid until the *tip is at the inside edge of the stopper.*
5. Withdraw the reconstituted solution into the syringe *being careful to always keep the tip of the needle below the level of the liquid.*

Caution: Failure to inject air into the vial, or allowing air to pass through the filter needle while filling the syringe with reconstituted solution, may cause the needle to clog.
6. Discard the filter needle. Perform venipuncture using the enclosed winged needle with microbore tubing. Attach the syringe to the luer end of the tubing.
Caution: Use of other winged needles without microbore tubing, although compatible with the concentrate, will result in a larger retention of solution within the winged infusion set.
7. Administer solution intravenously at a rate (approximately 2 mL/minute) comfortable to the patient.

B. Administration using the all plastic *Vented Filter Spike* for Withdrawal (This spike is supplied in the four-item Administration Components pack.)

Intravenous Injection: Plastic disposal syringes are recommended with Antihemophilic Factor (Human), Factor VIII:C Pasteurized, Monoclonal Antibody Purified solution. The ground glass surface of all-glass syringes tend to stick with solutions of this type.

1. Using aseptic technique, attach the *vented filter spike* to a sterile disposable syringe.
CAUTION: DO NOT INJECT AIR INTO THE ANTIHEMOPHILIC FACTOR, HUMAN VIAL. The self-venting feature of the vented filter spike precludes the need to inject air in order to facilitate withdrawal of the reconstituted solution. The injection of air could cause partial product loss through the vent filter.
Caution: The use of other, non-vented filter needles or spikes without the proper procedure may result in an air lock and prevent the complete transfer of the concentrate.
2. Insert the vented filter spike into the stopper of the Antihemophilic Factor, Human vial, invert the vial, and position the filter spike so that the orifice is at the inside edge of the stopper.
3. Withdraw the reconstituted solution into the syringe.
4. Discard the filter spike. Perform venipuncture using the enclosed winged needle with microbore tubing. Attach the syringe to the luer end of the tubing.
Caution: Use of other winged needles without microbore tubing, although compatible with the concentrate, will result in a larger retention of solution within the winged infusion set.
5. Administer solution intravenously at a rate (approximately 2 mL/minute) comfortable to the patient.

STORAGE

When stored at refrigerator temperature, 2°–8°C (36°–46°F), Antihemophilic Factor (Human), Factor VIII:C Pasteurized, Monoclonal Antibody Purified is stable for the period indicated by the expiration date on its label. Within this period, Antihemophilic Factor, Human may be stored at room temperature not to exceed 30°C (86°F), for up to 6 months.

Avoid freezing which may damage container for the diluent.

REFERENCES

1. W. Terry, A. Schreiber, C. Tarr, M. Hrinda, W. Curry, and F. Feldman, "Human Factor VIII:C Produced Using Monoclonal Antibodies," in *Research in Clinic and Laboratory,* Vol. XVI, (#1), 202 (1986) from the XVIIth International Congress of the World Federation of Hemophilia. 2. A.B. Schreiber, "The Preclinical Characterization of Monoclate Factor VIII C Antihemophilic Factor Human," *Semin Hematol* 25 (2 Suppl. 1), 1988, pp. 27–32. 3. E. Berntorp and I.M. Nilsson, "Biochemical Properties of Human Factor VIII C Monoclate Purified Using Monoclonal Antibody to VWF," *Thromb Res* O (Suppl. 7), 1987, p. 60, from the Satellite Symposia of the XIth International Congress on Thrombosis and Haemostasis, Brussels, Belguim, July 11, 1987. 4. S. Chandra, C.C. Huang, R.L. Weeks, K. Beatty and F. Feldman, "Purity of a Factor VIII:C Preparation (Monoclate) Manufactured by Monoclonal Immunoaffinity Chromatography Technique," from the XVIII International Congress of the World Federation of Hemophilia, May 1988. 5. B. Spire, D. Dormont, F. Barre-Sinousii, L. Montagnier, and J.C. Chermann, "Inactivation of Lumphadenopathy Associated Virus by Heat, Gamma Rays, and Ultraviolet Light," *Lancet,* Jan. 26, 1985, p.188. 6. L.W. Hoyer, "The Factor VIII Complex: Structure and Function," *Blood* 58 (1981), p.1. 7. F. Feldman, S. Chandra, R. Kleszynski, C.C. Huang and R.L. Weeks, "Measurement of Murine Protein Levels in Monoclonal Antibody Purified Coagulation Factor," from the XVIII International Congress of the World Federation of Hemophilia, May 1988. 8. F. Feldman, R. Kleszynski, L. Ho, R. Kling, S. Chandra and C.C. Huang, "Validation of Coagulation Test Methods for Evaluation of Monoclate (Factor VIII:C) Potencies," from the XVIII International Congress of the World Federation of Hemophilia, May 1988. 9. S. Chandra, C.C. Huang, L. Ho, R. Kling, R.L. Weeks and F. Feldman, "Studies on the Stability of Factor VIII:C (Monoclate) in Lyophilized and Solution Form," from the XVIII International Congress of the World Federation of Hemophilia, May 1988. 10. C.F. Abilgaard, J.V. Simone, J.J. Corrigan, et al., "Treatment of Hemophilia with Glycine—Precipitated Factor VIII," *New Eng J Med,* 275 (1966), p.471. 11. C.K. Kasper, "Hematologic Care," *Comprehensive Management of Hemophilia,* ed. Boone, D.C., Philadelphia, F.A. Davis Co., (1976) pp. 2–20.

BIBLIOGRAPHY

1. Hershman, R.J., Naconti, S.B., and Shulman, N.R., "Prophylactic Treatment of Factor VIII Deficiency." *Blood* 35 (1970), p. 189. 2. Kasper, C.K., Dietrich, S.I. and Rapaport, S.K. "Hemophilia Prophylaxis in Factor VIII Concentrate." *Arch. Int. Med.* 125 (1970), p. 1004. 3. Biggs, R., ed. "The Treatment of Hemophilia A and B and von Willebrands Disease." Oxford: Blackwell, 1978. 4. Fulcher, C.A., Zimmerman, T.S., "Characterization of the Human Factor VIII Procoagulant Protein With a Heterologous Precipitating Antibody." *Proc. Natl. Acad. Sci.* 79 (1982), pp. 1648–1652. 5. Levine, P.H., "Factor VIII C Purified from Plasma Via Monoclonal Antibodies Human Studies." *Semin Hematol* 25 (2 Suppl. 1), 1988, pp. 38–41.

◆ RATED THERAPEUTICALLY EQUIVALENT; ◇ THERAPEUTIC EQUIVALENCE UNCONFIRMED; ○ UNRATED

HOW SUPPLIED
POWDER FOR INJECTION:

BRAND/MANUFACTURER	NDC	SIZE	AWP
BRAND			
PROFILATE OSD: Alpha Therapeutic	49669-4300-01	1s	$0.90
	49669-4300-02	1s	$0.90
HUMATE-P: Armour	00053-7605-01	1s	$1.30
	00053-7605-02	1s	$1.30
	00053-7605-04	1s	$1.30
GENERICS			
Amer Red Cross	52769-0460-01	1s	$0.83
MELATE: Melville	13143-0321-54	1s	$0.90
MELATE: Melville	13143-0321-55	1s	$0.90
MELATE: Melville	13143-0321-56	1s	$0.90
MONOCLATE-P: Armour	00053-7656-01	1s	$0.90
MONOCLATE-P: Armour	00053-7656-02	1s	$0.90
MONOCLATE-P: Armour	00053-7656-04	1s	$0.90

POWDER FOR INJECTION: 1 I.U.

BRAND/MANUFACTURER	NDC	SIZE	AWP
GENERICS			
ALPHANATE: Alpha Therapeutic	49669-4500-01	1s	$0.70
KOATE-HP: Miles Biol	00192-0664-20	1s	$0.90
KOATE-HP: Miles Biol	00192-0664-30	1s	$0.90
KOATE-HP: Miles Biol	00192-0664-50	1s	$0.90
KOATE-HP: Miles Biol	00192-0664-60	1s	$0.90

Antihemophilic Factor, Porcine

WARNING

THIS IS A POTENT DRUG WITH POTENTIAL HAZARDS. FOR MAXIMAL SAFETY AND EFFICACY CAREFULLY READ AND FOLLOW DIRECTIONS BELOW.

DESCRIPTION
Antihemophilic Factor, Porcine is a highly purified, sterile, freeze-dried concentrate of Porcine Antihemophilic Factor (Factor VIII:C) in the form of a white lyophilized powder for reconstitution with 20 mL Sterile Water for Injection, U.S.P. Each vial contains between 400 and 700 Porcine units of Factor VII:C. The assayed amount of activity is stated on the label, but may vary depending on the type of assay and hemophilic substrate plasma used. The Factor VIII specific activity for each vial is greater than 15 Porcine units/mg of protein. The level of platelet aggregating factor (Porcine von Willebrand factor) is 1 unit to 5 or more Porcine units of Factor VIII:C. The sodium ion concentration is not more than 200 millimoles per liter and the citrate ion concentration not more than 55 millimoles per liter. Each batch of Antihemophilic Factor, Porcine is screened for porcine viruses. Antihemophilic Factor, Porcine is administered intravenously. The preparation contains no preservative.

CLINICAL PHARMACOLOGY
Porcine Factor VIII:C can replace human Factor VIII:C in the human blood coagulation cascade, and has been shown to be effective in controlling bleeding in patients with congenital Factor VIII:C deficiency (Hemophilia A).[1,2] Circulating antibodies to Factor VIII:C occur in 10-15% of severe hemophiliacs,[3] and may also arise in nonhemophiliacs who consequently develop a state of acquired hemophilia. These antibodies generally show a weaker neutralizing activity against Porcine Factor VIII:C than against human Factor VIII:C and Antihemophilic Factor, Porcine can thus be used to produce a hemostatic level of Factor VIII:C in patients whose antibody level precludes treatment with human Factor VIII concentrates.[4,5]

The activity of a patient's antibody against Antihemophilic Factor, Porcine can be determined in the laboratory using a modification of the Bethesda assay[6] and this value used as a guide to the likely effectiveness of Antihemophilic Factor, Porcine in the individual patient. (See "Indications and Usage".)

After infusion of Antihemophilic Factor, Porcine the level in the circulation can be monitored by measurement of Factor VIII:C in the patient's plasma. Recovery and half-life of Antihemophilic Factor, Porcine will vary, being dependent on both the level and the kinetics of the patient's antibody, and it is thus desirable to monitor pre- and post-infusion Factor VIII:C levels for each dose of Antihemophilic Factor, Porcine. This information will assist in determination of dose size and frequency. (See "Dosage and Administration".)

Recovery of Factor VIII:C has been reported to improve with successive doses of Antihemophilic Factor, Porcine possibly as a result of saturation of circulating antibody.[5]

No evidence of human viral infection has been reported with the use of Antihemophilic Factor, Porcine.

INDICATIONS AND USAGE
Antihemophilic Factor, Porcine is intended for the treatment of congenital hemophiliacs with antibodies to Factor VIII:C and also for previously nonhemophilic patients with spontaneously acquired inhibitors to human Factor VIII:C.

Use of Antihemophilic Factor, Porcine is indicated for patients with inhibitors who are bleeding or *who are to undergo surgery.*

Antihemophilic Factor, Porcine has not been known to transmit hepatitis or human immunodeficiency virus (HIV).[7] It may therefore be justified to consider Antihemophilic Factor, Porcine as a primary treatment option in acquired inhibitor patients.

Antihemophilic Factor, Porcine treatment is not normally indicated in patients with an antibody titer of less than 5 Bethesda units/mL (BU/mL) against human Factor VIII:C and is likely to be ineffective in patients with an antibody titer of greater than 50 BU/mL against human Factor VIII. If a patient has an antibody titer of greater than 50 BU/mL against human Factor VIII:C the activity of the antibody against Porcine Factor VIII should be determined. An antibody titer of less than 15-20 BU/mL against Porcine Factor VIII:C indicates suitability for treatment with Antihemophilic Factor, Porcine.

UNLABELED USES
Antihemophilic Factor, Porcine is used alone or as an adjunct in the treatment of von Willebrand's Disease.

CONTRAINDICATIONS
Antihemophilic Factor, Porcine should not be used to treat patients who have previously suffered acute allergic reaction to Antihemophilic Factor, Porcine.

WARNINGS
ACUTE INFUSION REACTIONS
On rare occasions Antihemophilic Factor, Porcine administration has been associated with anaphylaxis. Adrenaline, hydrocortisone and facilities for cardiopulmonary resuscitation should be available in case such a reaction occurs.

PRECAUTIONS
IMMUNE RESPONSE TO ANTIHEMOPHILIC FACTOR, PORCINE
Infusion of Antihemophilic Factor, Porcine may be followed by a rise in plasma levels of antibody to both human and Porcine Factor VIII:C[8,9] Inhibitor levels should therefore be monitored both during and after treatment.

GENERAL
Hydrocortisone and/or antihistamine may help to prevent or alleviate side effects to Antihemophilic Factor, Porcine and may thus be prescribed as a precautionary measure.

Following reconstitution Antihemophilic Factor, Porcine must not be frozen. Any dose not used within 3 hours of reconstitution should be discarded.

Antihemophilic Factor, Porcine is for administration by intravenous route only.

Antihemophilic Factor, Porcine is not recommended for use in home treatment programs.

LABORATORY TESTS
The activity of the patient's antibody against Antihemophilic Factor, Porcine can be determined using a modification of the Bethesda assay[6] in which Antihemophilic Factor, Porcine is diluted to 1 Porcine U/mL in hemophilic plasma and used as substrate for the assay.

CARCINOGENESIS, MUTAGENESIS, IMPAIRMENT OF FERTILITY
Long term studies have not been conducted with Antihemophilic Factor, Porcine.

PREGNANCY CATEGORY C
Antihemophilic Factor, Porcine. Animal reproduction studies have not been conducted with Antihemophilic Factor, Porcine. It is also not known whether Antihemophilic Factor, Porcine can cause fetal harm when administered to a pregnant woman or can affect reproduction capacity. Antihemophilic Factor, Porcine should be given to a pregnant woman only if clearly needed.

ADVERSE REACTIONS
MILD INFUSION REACTIONS
Antihemophilic Factor, Porcine may give rise to reactions such as fever, chills, headache, nausea, vomiting and skin rashes. Such reactions have been reported to occur after approximately 10% of infusions[4] and are more common after the first infusion in a course of treatment. Reactions tend to lessen in frequency and severity as further infusions are given.

THROMBOCYTOPENIA
Acute thrombocytopenia has been reported to occur on rare occasions.[5] Monitoring of the platelet count during the treatment period is thus recommended.

DOSAGE AND ADMINISTRATION
The dosage of Antihemophilic Factor, Porcine required for control of bleeding varies for individual patients, but is dependent upon the patient's weight, the level of circulating antibody and the type of hemorrhage and desired plasma Factor VIII level.

It is commonly observed that recovery of Factor VIII:C increases during a course of treatment, possibly as a result of saturation of circulating antibody. It is therefore desirable to monitor pre- and postinfusion levels of Factor VIII:C for each dose. This is of particular importance during long courses of treatment when variation in the patient's antibody level may give rise to considerable variation in the recovery of Factor VIII:C in the plasma.

INITIAL DOSE
Because of the variation in patient response and the possible variation in the assayed unitage (see "Description") each patient should be monitored closely.

Rather than relying upon a particular laboratory value for recovery of Factor VIII:C, clinical response should be used to assess efficacy. In view of the difficulty in managing hemophiliacs with inhibitors close consultation with a regional comprehensive hemophilia center is advised.

1. If the patient's antihuman Factor VIII:C antibody level is less than 50 BU/mL an initial dose of 100 to 150 Porcine Units per Kg body weight is recommended.

2. If the patient's antibody titer to human Factor VIII:C is greater than 50 BU/mL the activity of the antibody against Antihemophilic Factor, Porcine should be determined. An antiporcine Factor VIII:C antibody level of more than 20 Bethesda units indicates that the patient is unlikely to benefit from treatment with Antihemophilic Factor, Porcine. For lower titers, a dose of 100 to 150 Porcine Units per Kg is recommended.

3. If a patient has previously been treated with Antihemophilic Factor, Porcine this may provide a guide as to his likely response and therefore assist in estimation of the preliminary dose.

SUBSEQUENT DOSES

Following administration of the initial dose, if the recovery of Factor VIII:C in the patient's plasma is not sufficient, a further higher dose should be administered. If recovery after the second dose is still insufficient, a third and higher dose may prove effective. As previously noted, the recovery of Factor VIII:C tends to improve with successive doses.

DETERMINATION OF THE ACTIVITY OF THE INHIBITOR AGAINST ANTIHEMOPHILIC FACTOR, PORCINE

A modification of the Bethesda assay[6] is recommended. Antihemophilic Factor, Porcine should be diluted to 1 Porcine unit per mL in hemophilic plasma and used as a substrate in the Bethesda assay.

RECONSTITUTION AND ADMINISTRATION

1. Warm the unopened vials of Antihemophilic Factor, Porcine to between 20°C and 37°C.

2. Clean the exposed central portion of the rubber stopper with antiseptic immediately prior to piercing.

3. Using a sterile needle and a syringe slowly inject 20 mL of Sterile Water for Injection, U.S.P. into the vial.

4. Withdraw the needle and shake the vial gently avoiding frothing, until the powder is completely dissolved. This usually takes less than 5 minutes.

5. Parenteral drug products should be inspected visually for particulate matter and discoloration prior to administration, whenever solution and container permit.

6. Withdraw the solution into a syringe using a filter needle.

7. Replace the filter needle with a sterile injection needle and administer intravenously at a rate of not more than 2-5 mL per minute.

8. Following reconstitution, Antihemophilic Factor, Porcine must not be stored. Any dose not used within 3 hours of reconstitution should be discarded.

STORAGE

Antihemophilic Factor, Porcine should be stored at a temperature of minus 15°C to minus 20°C and should be used before the expiration date stated on the package. Reconstituted Antihemophilic Factor, Porcine must not be stored, and should be used within 3 hours.

REFERENCES

1. Macfarlane RG, Mallam PC, Witts LJ, Bidwell E, Biggs R, Fraenkel GJ, Honey GE, Taylor KB. Surgery in haemophilia. The use of animal antihaemophilic globulin and human plasma in thirteen cases. Lancet 1957;2:251. 2. Biggs R, Macfarlane RG. (eds): Treatment of haemophilia and other coagulation disorders. Oxford, Blackwell Scientific 1966. 3. Shapiro SS, Hultin M. Acquired inhibitors to the blood coagulation factors. Semin. Thromb. Hemostas. 1975;1:336. 4. Kernoff PBA, Thomas ND, Lilley PA, Matthews KB, Goldman E, Tuddenham EGD. Clinical experience with polyelectrolyte-fractionated porcine factor VIII concentrate in the treatment of haemophiliacs with antibodies to factor VIII. Blood 1984;63:31. 5. Gatti L, Mannucci PM. Use of porcine factor VIII in the management of seventeen patients with factor VIII antibodies. Thromb. Haemostas. 1984;51:379. 6. Kasper CK, Aledort LM, Counts RB, Edson JR, Frantantoni J, Green D, Hampton JW, Hilgartner MW, Lazerson J, Levine PH, McMillan CW, Pool JG, Shapiro SS, Shulman NR, Van Eys J. A more uniform measurement of factor VIII inhibitors. Thrombos. Diathes. Haemorrh. 1975;34:869. 7. Lusher JM. Factor VIII inhibitors-etiology, characterization, natural history and management. Annals of the New York Academy of Sciences 1987;509:96. 8. Hewitt P, Mackie IJ, Machin SJ. Highly Purified Factor VIII in Haemophilia A. Lancet 1982;1:741. 9. Verroust F, Allain JP. Immune response induced by porcine factor VIII in severe hemophiliacs with antibody to factor VIII. Thromb. Haemostas. 1982;48:238.

HOW SUPPLIED
POWDER FOR INJECTION:

BRAND/MANUFACTURER	NDC	SIZE	AWP
○ BRAND			
HYATE: C: Porton	55688-0106-02	1s	$1.56

Antilirium *SEE* PHYSOSTIGMINE SALICYLATE

Antipyrine and Benzocaine

DESCRIPTION

Each mL contains:

Antipyrine	54.0 mg
Benzocaine	54.0 mg
Glycerin dehydrated q.s. to	1.0 mL

(contains not more than 0.6% moisture)
(also contains oxyquinoline sulfate)

TOPICAL DECONGESTANT AND ANALGESIC

Antipyrine/Benzocaine is an otic solution. The solution congeals at 0°C (32°F), but returns to normal consistency, unchanged, at room temperature.

CLINICAL PHARMACOLOGY

Antipyrine/Benzocaine combines the hygroscopic property of dehydrated glycerin with the analgesic action of Antipyrine and Benzocaine to relieve pressure, reduce inflammation and congestion, and alleviate pain and discomfort in acute otitis media. Antipyrine/Benzocaine does not blanch the tympanic membrane or mask the landmarks and, therefore, does not distort the otoscopic picture.

INDICATIONS AND USAGE

ACUTE OTITIS MEDIA OF VARIOUS ETIOLOGIES

—prompt relief of pain and reduction of inflammation in the congestive and serous stages

—adjuvant therapy during systemic antibiotic administration for resolution of the infection

Because of the close anatomical relationship of the eustachian tube to the nasal cavity, otitis media is a frequent problem, especially in children in whom the tube is shorter, wider, and more horizontal than in adults.

REMOVAL OF CERUMEN

—facilitates the removal of excessive or impacted cerumen

CONTRAINDICATIONS

Hypersensitivity to any of the components or substances related to them.

Perforated tympanic membrane is considered a contraindication to the use of any medication in the external ear canal.

WARNINGS

Discontinue promptly if sensitization or irritation occurs.

PRECAUTIONS

CARCINOGENESIS, MUTAGENESIS, IMPAIRMENT OF FERTILITY

No long-term studies in animals or humans have been conducted

PREGNANCY CATEGORY C

Animal reproduction studies have not been conducted with Antipyrine/Benzocaine. It is also not known whether Antipyrine/Benzocaine can cause fetal harm when administered to a pregnant woman, or can affect reproduction capacity. Antipyrine/Benzocaine should be given to a pregnant woman only if clearly needed.

NURSING MOTHERS

It is not known whether this drug is excreted in human milk. Because many drugs are excreted in human milk, caution should be exercised when Antipyrine/Benzocaine is administered to a nursing woman.

DOSAGE AND ADMINISTRATION

ACUTE OTITIS MEDIA

Instill Antipyrine/Benzocaine permitting the solution to run along the wall of the canal until it is filled. Avoid touching the ear with dropper. Then moisten a cotton pledget with Antipyrine/Benzocaine and insert into meatus. Repeat every one to two hours until pain and congestion are relieved.

REMOVAL OF CERUMEN

Before: Instill Antipyrine/Benzocaine three times daily for two or three days to help detach cerumen from wall of canal and facilitate removal.

After: Antipyrine/Benzocaine is useful for drying out the canal or relieving discomfort.

Before and after removal of cerumen, a cotton pledget moistened with Antipyrine/Benzocaine should be inserted into the meatus following instillation.

Note: Do not rinse dropper after use.

Replace dropper in bottle after each use. Hold dropper assembly by screw cap and, without compressing the rubber bulb, insert into drug container and screw down tightly.

Protect the solution from light and heat, and do not use if it is brown or contains a precipitate.

Discard this product six months after dropper is first placed in the drug solution.

Storage: Store at room temperature (approximately 25° C).

◆ RATED THERAPEUTICALLY EQUIVALENT; ◇ THERAPEUTIC EQUIVALENCE UNCONFIRMED; ○ UNRATED

BRAND/MANUFACTURER	NDC	SIZE	AWP
○ **BRAND**			
AURALGAN: Wyeth-Ayerst	00046-1000-10	10 ml	$12.73

For additional alternatives, turn to the section beginning on page 2859.

Antipyrine/Benzocaine/ Phenylephrine Hydrochloride

DESCRIPTION

Antipyrine/Benzocaine/Phenylephrine Hydrochloride Otic Solution, analgesic-decongestant ear drops, contains:

Antipyrine USP	5%
Benzocaine USP	5%
Phenylephrine Hydrochloride USP	0.25%

Sodium metabisulfite and edetate disodium USP in propylene glycol USP.

Antipyrine is an analgesic with local anesthetic action.
  Benzocaine is a local anesthetic.
  Phenylephrine Hydrochloride is a sympathomimetic amine with local vasoconstriction or decongestant action.

CLINICAL PHARMACOLOGY

Topical application of Phenylephrine produces vasoconstriction mainly by a direct effect on α-adrenergic receptors. The effects of Phenylephrine are similar to those of epinephrine. However, Phenylephrine is considered less CNS and cardio-stimulatory than epinephrine Phenylephrine, after its absorption, is metabolized in the liver and the intestine by the enzyme monoamine oxidase (MAO). The type, route and rate of excretion of metabolites have not been defined.

Antipyrine is believed to have analgesic and local anesthetic effects on the nerve endings. After absorption, it is slowly metabolized in the liver by oxidation and conjugated with glucuronic acid and is excreted in the urine mainly in the conjugated form.

Like other local anesthetics, Benzocaine acts by blocking nerve conduction first in autonomic, then in sensory and finally in motor nerve fibers. Its effect appears to be due to decreased nerve cell membrane permeability to sodium ions or competition with calcium ions for membrane binding sites. A vasoconstrictor, such as Phenylephrine, is added to decrease the rate of absorption and prolong the duration of action of the anesthetic. Ester-type anesthetics, which include Benzocaine, after absorption are comparatively rapidly degraded by esterases mainly in the liver and excreted in the urine as metabolites and in small amounts as the unchanged drug.

INDICATIONS AND USAGE

Antipyrine/Benzocaine/Phenylephrine Otic Solution may be used as a topical anesthetic in the external auditory canal to relieve ear pain.

It may be used concomitantly with systemic antibiotics as in the treatment of acute otitis media.

CONTRAINDICATIONS

Antipyrine/Benzocaine/Phenylephrine Otic Solution or any medication for use in the external ear canal is contraindicated in the presence of perforated tympanic membrane or ear discharge and in individuals with a history of hypersensitivity to any of its ingredients.

WARNINGS

As with all drugs containing a sympathomimetic or an anesthetic, systemic reactions may occur after local application. Phenylephrine may cause blanching and a feeling of coolness in the skin. Allergic and idiosyncratic reactions to local anesthetics have been observed infrequently. Such reactions are unlikely because absorption from the skin of the ear drum or the external ear canal is minimal.

Discontinue promptly if sensitization or irritation occurs. Cross-sensitivity reactions between the members of the *caine* group or local anesthetics have been reported. Contains *sodium metabisulfite*, a sulfite that may cause allergic-type reactions including anaphylactic symptoms and life-threatening or less severe asthmatic episodes in certain susceptible people. The overall prevalence of sulfite sensitivity in the general population is unknown and probably low. Sulfite sensitivity is seen more frequently in asthmatic than in nonasthmatic people.

PRECAUTIONS

General: Drugs containing a sympathomimetic should be used with caution in the elderly and in patients with hypertension, increased intraocular pressure, diabetes mellitus, ischemic heart disease, hyperthyroidism and prostatic hypertrophy.

High plasma levels of Benzocaine and Antipyrine may cause CNS stimulation with nausea and vomiting. Such levels, however, are unlikely to be attained following local application in the external ear.

Drug Interactions: MAO inhibitors and β-adrenergic blockers enhance the effects of sympathomimetics. Benzocaine is hydrolyzed in the body to p-aminobenzoic acid which competes with the antibacterial action of sulfonamides. However, these are unlikely to occur because of the limited absorption from the external ear canal.

Carcinogenesis, Mutagenesis, Impairment of Fertility: There have been no studies in animals or humans to evaluate the carcinogenesis, mutagenesis or impairment of fertility for Antipyrine/Benzocaine/Phenylephrine Otic Solution.

Pregnancy: Category C. Animal reproduction studies have not been conducted with Antipyrine/Benzocaine/Phenylephrine Otic Solution. It is also not known whether Antipyrine/Benzocaine/Phenylephrine Otic Solution can cause fetal harm when a administered to a pregnant woman or can effect reproduction capacity. Antipyrine/Benzocaine/Phenylephrine Otic Solution should be given to a pregnant woman only if clearly needed.

Nursing Mothers: It is not known whether this drug is excreted in human milk. Because many drugs are excreted in human milk, caution should be exercised when Antipyrine/Benzocaine/Phenylephrine Otic Solution is administered to a nursing woman.

Pediatric Use: Safety and effectiveness in children below the age of 12 has not been established.

ADVERSE REACTIONS

Following its absorption, Phenylephrine may produce a pressor response or cause restlessness, anxiety, nervousness, weakness, pallor, headache and dizziness. Absorption of Benzocaine and Antipyrine in the plasma may cause chills, nausea, vomiting, tinnitus and agranulocytosis. Such reactions are unlikely following application of Antipyrine/Benzocaine/Phenylephrine Otic Solution on the external ear canal.

Benzocaine can cause a hypersensitivity reaction consisting of rash, urticaria and edema. Individuals frequently exposed to ester-type local anesthetics can develop contact dermatitis characterized by erythema and pruritus which may progress to vesiculation and oozing.

OVERDOSAGE

It is more likely to be associated with accidental or deliberate ingestion rather than cutaneous absorption. Phenylephrine present in Antipyrine/Benzocaine/Phenylephrine Otic Solution, if absorbed, may cause hypertension, headache, vomiting and palpitations. Effects of Benzocaine overdosage may include yawning, restlessness, excitement, nausea and vomiting. Antipyrine overdosage may cause giddiness, tremor, sweating and skin eruptions.

Treatment is symptomatic. If ingestion of the contents of a bottle or more of Antipyrine/Benzocaine/Phenylephrine Otic Solution is recent or food is present in the stomach, induction of emesis with ipecac syrup, gastric emptying and lavage and introduction of activated charcoal may be recommended.

DOSAGE AND ADMINISTRATION

Using the dropper, instill Antipyrine/Benzocaine/Phenylephrine Otic Solution in the external ear canal allowing the solution to run into the canal unit filled. Insert a cotton pledget into the meatus after moistening with the otic solution. Repeat every 2 to 4 hours, if necessary, until pain is relieved.
  Replace dropper in bottle without rinsing.
  Store at 15°-30°C (59°-86°F).

HOW SUPPLIED
DROP: 5%-5%-0.25%

BRAND/MANUFACTURER	NDC	SIZE	AWP
○ **BRAND**			
TYMPAGESIC: Savage	00281-7363-39	13 ml	$11.28

Antithrombin III (Human)

DESCRIPTION

Antithrombin III (Human) is a sterile, stable, lyophilized preparation of purified Human Antithrombin III.

Antithrombin III is prepared from pooled units of human plasma from normal donors by modifications and refinements of the cold ethanol method of Cohn.[1] When reconstituted, Antithrombin III has a pH of 6.0–7.5, a sodium content of 110–210 mEq/L, a chloride content of 110–210 mEq/L, an alanine content of 0.075–0.125 M and a heparin content of not more than 0.004 unit/IU AT-III. Antithrombin III contains no preservative and must be administered by the intravenous route. In addition, Antithrombin III has been heat-treated in solution at 60°C ± 0.5°C for not less than 10 hours.

Each vial of Antithrombin III contains the labeled amount of antithrombin III in international units (IU) per vial. The potency assignment has been determined with a standard calibrated against a World Health Organization (WHO) Antithrombin III reference preparation.

CLINICAL PHARMACOLOGY

Antithrombin III (AT-III), an alpha$_2$-glycoprotein of molecular weight 58,000, is normally present in human plasma at a concentration of approximately 12.5 mg/dL[2,3] and is the major plasma inhibitor of thrombin.[4] Inactivation of thrombin by AT-III occurs by formation of a covalent bond resulting in an inactive 1:1 stoichiometric complex between the two, involving an interaction of the active serine of thrombin and an arginine reactive site on AT-III.[4] AT-III is also capable of inactivating other components of the coagulation cascade including factors IXa, Xa, XIa, and XIIa, as well as plasmin.[4]

The neutralization rate of serine proteases by AT-III proceeds slowly in the absence of heparin, but is greatly accelerated in the presence of heparin.[4] As the therapeutic antithrombotic effect in vivo of heparin is mediated by AT-III, heparin is ineffective in the absence or near absence of AT-III.[4-8]

The prevalence of the hereditary deficiency of AT-III is estimated to be one per 2000 to 5000 in the general population.[4,7] The pattern of inheritance is autosomal dominant. In affected individuals, spontaneous episodes of thrombosis and pulmonary embolism may be associated with AT-III levels of 40%–60% of normal.[7] These episodes usually appear after the age of 20, the risk increasing with age and in association with surgery, pregnancy and delivery. The frequency of thromboembolic events in hereditary antithrombin III (AT-III) deficiency during pregnancy has been reported to be 70%, and several studies of the beneficial use of Antithrombin III (Human) concentrates during pregnancy in women with hereditary deficiency have been reported.[9-11] In many cases, however, no precipitating factor can be identified for venous thrombosis or pulmonary embolism.[7] Greater than 85% of individuals with hereditary AT-III deficiency have had at least one thrombotic episode by the age of 50 years.[7] In about 60% of patients thrombosis is recurrent. Clinical signs of pulmonary embolism occur in 40% of affected individuals.[7] In some individuals, treatment with oral anticoagulants leads to an increase of the endogenous levels of AT-III, and treatment with oral anticoagulants may be effective in the prevention of thrombosis in such individuals.[6,7]

In clinical studies of Antithrombin III (Human) conducted in 10 asymptomatic subjects with hereditary deficiency of AT-III, the mean in vivo recovery of AT-III was 1.6% per unit per kg administered based on immunologic AT-III assays, and 1.4% per unit per kg administered based on functional AT-III assays.[12] The mean 50% disappearance time (the time to fall to 50% of the peak plasma level following an initial administration) was approximately 22 hours and the biologic half-life was 2.5 days based on immunologic assays and 3.8 days based on functional assays of AT-III.[12] These values are similar to the half-life for radiolabeled Antithrombin III (Human) reported in the literature of 2.8–4.8 days.[13-15]

In clinical studies of Antithrombin III none of the 13 patients with hereditary AT-III deficiency and histories of thromboembolism treated prophylactically on 16 separate occasions with Antithrombin III or high thrombotic risk situations (11 surgical procedures, 5 deliveries) developed a thrombotic complication. Heparin was also administered in 3 of the 11 surgical procedures and all 5 deliveries. Eight patients with hereditary AT-III deficiency were treated therapeutically with Antithrombin III as well as heparin for major thrombotic or thromboembolic complications, with seven patients recovering. Treatment with Antithrombin III reversed heparin resistance in two patients with hereditary AT-III deficiency being treated for thrombosis or thromboembolism.

During clinical investigation of Antithrombin III, none of 12 subjects monitored for a median of 8 months (range 2–19 months) after receiving Antithrombin III, became antibody positive to human immunodeficiency virus (HIV-1). None of 14 subjects monitored for $\geq$ 3 months demonstrated any evidence of hepatitis, either non-A, non-B hepatitis or hepatitis B.

INDICATIONS AND USAGE

Antithrombin III is indicated for the treatment of patients with hereditary Antithrombin III deficiency in connection with surgical or obstetrical procedures or when they suffer from thromboembolism.

Subjects with AT-III deficiency should be informed about the risk of thrombosis in connection with pregnancy and surgery and about the inheritance of the disease.

The diagnosis of hereditary Antithrombin III (AT-III) deficiency should be based on a clear family history of venous thrombosis as well as decreased plasma AT-III levels, and the exclusion of acquired deficiency.

AT-III in plasma may be measured by amidolytic assays using synthetic chromogenic substrates, by clotting assays, or by immunoassays. The latter does not detect all hereditary AT-III deficiencies.[16]

The AT-III level in neonates of parents with hereditary AT-III deficiency should be measured immediately after birth. (Fatal neonatal thromboembolism, such as aortic thrombi in children of women with hereditary Antithrombin III deficiency, has been reported.)[17]

Plasma levels of AT-III are lower in neonates than adults, averaging approximately 60% in normal term infants.[18,19] AT-III levels in premature infants may be much lower.[18,19] Low plasma AT-III levels, especially in a premature infant, therefore, do not necessarily indicate hereditary deficiency. It is recommended that testing and treatment with Antithrombin III (Human) of neonates be discussed with an expert on coagulation.[11]

UNLABELED USES

Antithrombin III (Human) is also used alone or as an adjunct in the treatment of acquired Antithrombin deficiency, including disseminated intravascular coagulation.

CONTRAINDICATIONS

None known.

WARNINGS

This product is prepared from pooled human plasma which may contain the causative agents of hepatitis and other viral diseases. Prescribed manufacturing procedures utilized at the plasma collection centers, plasma testing laboratories, and the fractionation facilities are designed to reduce the risk of transmitting viral infection. However, the risk of viral infectivity from this product cannot be totally eliminated.

Individuals who receive multiple infusions of blood or plasma products may develop signs and/or symptoms of some viral infections, particularly non-A, non-B hepatitis. The anticoagulant effect of heparin is enhanced by concurrent treatment with Antithrombin III in patients with hereditary AT-III deficiency. Thus, in order to avoid bleeding, reduced dosage of heparin is recommended during treatment with Antithrombin III.

PRECAUTIONS

GENERAL

1. Administer within 3 hours after reconstitution. Do not refrigerate after reconstitution.
2. Administer only by the intravenous route.
3. Antithrombin III should be given alone, without mixing with other agents or diluting solutions.
4. Administration equipment and any reconstituted Antithrombin III not used should be appropriately discarded.

The diagnosis of hereditary Antithrombin III (AT-III) deficiency should be based on a clear family history of venous thrombosis as well as decreased plasma AT-III levels, and the exclusion of acquired deficiency.

LABORATORY TESTS

It is recommended that AT-III plasma levels be monitored during the treatment period. Functional levels of AT-III in plasma may be measured by amidolytic assays using chromogenic substrates or by clotting assays.

DRUG INTERACTIONS

The anticoagulant effect of heparin is enhanced by concurrent treatment with Antithrombin III in patients with hereditary AT-III deficiency. Thus, in order to avoid bleeding, reduced dosage of heparin is recommended during treatment with Antithrombin III.

PREGNANCY CATEGORY C

Animal reproduction studies have not been conducted with Antithrombin III. It is also not known whether Antithrombin III can cause fetal harm when administered to a pregnant woman or can affect reproduction capacity. Antithrombin III should be given to a pregnant woman only if clearly needed.

PEDIATRIC USE

Safety and effectiveness in children have not been established. The AT-III level in neonates of parents with hereditary AT-III deficiency should be measured immediately after birth. (Fatal neonatal thromboembolism, such as aortic thrombi in children of women with hereditary Antithrombin III deficiency, has been reported.)[17]

Plasma levels of AT-III are lower in neonates than adults, averaging approximately 60% in normal term infants.[18,19] AT-III levels in premature infants may be much lower.[18,19] Low plasma AT-III levels, especially in a premature infant, therefore, do not necessarily indicate hereditary deficiency. It is recommended that testing and treatment with Antithrombin III (Human) of neonates be discussed with an expert on coagulation.[11]

ADVERSE REACTIONS

In clinical studies involving Antithrombin III, adverse reactions were reported in association with 17 of the 340 infusions during the clinical studies. Included were dizziness (7), chest tightness (3), nausea (3), foul taste in mouth (3), chills (2), cramps (2), shortness of breath (1), chest pain (1), film over eye (1), lightheadedness (1), bowel fullness (1), hives (1), fever (1), and oozing and hematoma formation (1). If adverse reactions are experienced, the infusion rate should be decreased, or if indicated, the infusion should be interrupted until symptoms abate.

DOSAGE AND ADMINISTRATION

Each bottle of Antithrombin III has the functional activity, in international units (IU), stated on the label of the bottle. The potency assignment has been determined with a standard calibrated against a World Health Organization Antithrombin III reference preparation.

Dosage should be determined on an individual basis based on the pre-therapy plasma Antithrombin III (AT-III) level, in order to increase plasma AT-III levels to the level found in normal human plasma (100%). Dosage of Antithrombin III can be calculated from the following formula:

$$\text{Units required (IU)} = \frac{[\text{desired - baseline AT-III level*}] \times \text{weight (kg)}}{1.4}$$

expressed as % normal level based on functional AT-III assay

The above formula is based on an expected incremental in vivo recovery above baseline levels for Antithrombin III of 1.4% per IU per kg administered.[12] Thus, if a 70 kg individual has a baseline AT-III level of 57%, in order to increase plasma AT-III to 120%, the initial Antithrombin III dose would be [(120 − 57) × 70] / 1.4 = 3150 IU total.

However, recovery may vary, and initially levels should be drawn at baseline and 20 minutes postinfusion. Subsequent doses can be calculated based on the recovery of the first dose. These recommendations are intended only as a guide for therapy. The exact loading dose and maintenance intervals should be individualized for each patient.

It is recommended that following an initial dose of Antithrombin III, plasma levels of AT-III be initially monitored at least every 12 hours and before the next infusion of Antithrombin III to maintain plasma AT-III levels greater than 80%. In some situations, e.g., following surgery,[20] hemorrhage or acute thrombosis, and during intravenous heparin administration,[13,21-23] the half-life of Antithrombin III (Human) has been reported to be shortened. In such conditions, plasma AT-III levels should be monitored more frequently, and Antithrombin III (Human) administered as necessary.

When an infusion of Antithrombin III is indicated for a patient with hereditary deficiency to control an acute thrombotic episode or prevent thrombosis following surgical or obstetrical procedures, it is desirable to raise the AT-III level to normal and maintain this level for 2 to 8 days, depending on the indication for treatment, type and extent of surgery, patient's medical condition, past history and physician's judgment. Concomitant administration of heparin in each of these situations should be based on the medical judgment of the physician.

As a general recommendation, the following therapeutic program may be utilized as a starting program for treatment, modifying the program based on the actual plasma AT-III levels achieved:

a) An initial loading dose of Antithrombin III calculated to elevate the plasma AT-III level to 120%, assuming an expected rise over the baseline plasma AT-III level of 1.4% (functional activity) per IU per kg of Antithrombin III administered. Thus, if an individual has a baseline AT-III level of 57%, the initial Antithrombin III dose would be (120 − 57)/1.4 = 45 IU/kg.

b) Measure preinfusion and 20 minutes postinfusion (peak) plasma Antithrombin III levels following the initial dose, plasma Antithrombin III level after 12 hours, then preceding the next infusion (trough level). Subsequently measure Antithrombin III levels preceding and 20 minutes after each infusion until predictable peak and trough levels have been achieved, generally between 80%-120%. Plasma levels between 80%-120% may be maintained by administration of maintenance doses of 60% of the initial loading dose, administered every 24 hours. Adjustments in the maintenance dose and/or interval between doses should be made based on actual plasma AT-III levels achieved.

The above recommendations for dosing are provided as a general guideline for therapy only. The exact loading and maintenance dosages and dosing intervals should be individualized for each subject, based on the individual clinical conditions, response to therapy, and actual plasma AT-III levels achieved. In some situations, e.g., following surgery,[20] with hemorrhage or acute thrombosis and during intravenous heparin administration,[13,21-23] in vivo survival of infused Antithrombin III has been reported to be shortened, resulting in the need to administer Antithrombin III more frequently.

Antithrombin III should be reconstituted with Sterile Water for Injection, USP and brought to room temperature prior to administration. Antithrombin III should be filtered through a sterile filter needle as supplied in the package prior to use, and should be administered within 3 hours following reconstitution. Antithrombin III may be infused over 10-20 minutes. Antithrombin III must be administered intravenously.

Parenteral drug products should be inspected visually for particulate matter and discoloration prior to administration, whenever solution and container permit.

RECONSTITUTION
Vacuum Transfer

1. Warm the unopened diluent and the concentrate to room temperature (NMT 37°C, 99°F).
2. After removing the plastic flip-top caps, aseptically cleanse the rubber stoppers of both bottles.
3. Remove the protective cover from the plastic transfer needle cartridge with tamper-proof seal and penetrate the stopper of the diluent bottle.
4. Remove the remaining portion of the plastic cartridge, invert the diluent bottle and penetrate the rubber seal on the concentrate bottle with the needle at an angle. Alternate method of transferring sterile water: With a sterile needle and syringe, withdraw the appropriate volume of diluent and transfer to the bottle of lyophilized concentrate.
5. The vacuum will draw the diluent into the concentrate bottle. Hold the diluent bottle at an angle to the concentrate bottle in order to direct the jet of diluent against the wall of the concentrate bottle. Avoid excessive foaming.
6. After removing the diluent bottle and transfer needle swirl continuously until completely dissolved.
7. After the concentrate powder is completely dissolved, withdraw solution into the syringe through the filter needle which is supplied in the package. Replace the filter needle with an administration set (not provided) and inject intravenously.
8. If the same patient is to receive more than one bottle, the contents of two bottles may be drawn into the same syringe through a separate unused filter needle before attaching the vein needle.

RATE OF ADMINISTRATION
The rate of administration should be adapted to the response of the individual patient, but administration of the entire dose in 10 to 20 minutes is generally well-tolerated.

Antithrombin III (Human) should be stored under refrigeration (2°-8°C; 35°-46°F). Freezing should be avoided as breakage of the diluent bottle might occur.

REFERENCES
1. Cohn EJ, Strong LE, Hughes WL Jr, et al: Preparation and properties of serum and plasma proteins. IV. A system for the separation into fractions of the protein and lipoprotein components of biological tissues and fluids. *J Am Chem Soc* 68(3):459-75, 1946. 2. Rosenberg RD, Bauer KA, Marcum JA: Antithrombin III "the heparin-Antithrombin system." *Rev Hematol* 2:351-416, 1986. 3. Murano G, Williams L, Miller-Andersson M: Some properties of Antithrombin-III and its concentration in human plasma. *Thromb Res* 18(1-2):259-62, 1980. 4. Rosenberg RD: Action and interactions of Antithrombin and heparin. *N Engl J Med* 292(3):146-51, 1975. 5. Winter JH, Fenech A, Ridley W, et al: Familial Antithrombin III deficiency. *Q J Med* 51(204):373-95, 1982. 6. Marciniak E, Farley CH, DeSimone PA: Familial thrombosis due to Antithrombin III deficiency. *Blood* 43(2):219-31, 1974. 7. Thaler E, Lechner K: Antithrombin III deficiency and thromboembolism. *Clin Haematol* 10(2):369-90, 1981. 8. Blauhut B, Necek S, Kramar H, et al: Activity of Antithrombin III and effect of heparin on coagulation in shock. *Thromb Res* 19(6):775-82, 1980. 9. Samson D, Stirling Y, Woolf L, et al: Management of planned pregnancy in a patient with cogenital Antithrombin III deficiency. *Br J Haematol* 56(2):243-9, 1984. 10. Brandt P: Observations during the treatment of Antithrombin-III deficient women with heparin and Antithrombin concentrate during pregnancy, parturition, and abortion. *Thromb Res* 22(1-2):15-24, 1981. 11. Hellgren M, Tengborn L, Abildgaard U: Pregnancy in women with congenital Antithrombin III deficiency; experience of treatment with heparin and Antithrombin. *Gynecol Obstet Invest* 14(2):127-41, 1982. 12. Schwartz RS, Bauer KA, Rosenberg RD, et al: Clinical experience with Antithrombin III concentrate in treatment of congenital and acquired deficiency of Antithrombin. *Am J Med* 87 (Suppl 3B): 53S-60S, 1989. 13. Collen D, Schetz J, de Cock F, et al: Metabolism of Antithrombin III (heparin cofactor) in man; effects of venous thrombosis and of heparin administration. *Eur J Clin Invest* 7(1):27-35, 1977. 14. Knot EAR, de Jong E, ten Cate JW, et al. Purified radiolabeled Antithrombin III metabolism in three families with hereditary AT III deficiency: application of a three-compartment model. *Blood* 67(1):93-8, 1986. 15. Tengborn L, Frohm B, Nilsson LE, et al: Antithrombin III concentrate; its catabolism in health and in Antithrombin III deficiency. *Scand J Clin Lab Invest* 41(5):469-77, 1981. 16. Sas G, Blasko G, Banhegyi D, et al: Abnormal Antithrombin III (antithronbin II "Budapest") as a cause of familial thrombophilia. *Thromb Diath Haemorrh* 32(1):105-15, 1974. 17. Bjarke B, Herin P, Blomback M: Neonatal aortic thrombosis. A possible clinical manifestation of congenital Antithrombin III deficiency. *Acta Paediatr Scand* 63:297-301, 1974. 18. Hathaway WE, Bonnar J: Perinatal coagulation, New York, Grune & Stratton, 1978, p. 68. 19. Peters M, Jansen E, ten Cate JW, et al: Neonatal Antithrombin III. *Br J Haematol* 58(4):579-87, 1984. 20. Mannucci PM, Boyer C, Wolf M, et al: Treatment of cogenital Antithrombin III deficiency with concentrates. *Br J Haematol* 50(3):531-5, 1982. 21. Marciniak E, Gockerman JP: Heparin-induced decrease in circulating Antithrombin-III. *Lancet* 2(8038):581-4, 1977. 22. O'Brien JR, Etherington MD: Effect of heparin and warfarin on Antithrombin III. *Lancet* 2(8050):1232, 1977. 23. Kakkar VV, Bentley PG, Scully MF, et al: Antithrombin III and heparin. *Lancet* 1(8159):103-4, 1980.

J CODES
Per IU IV—J7197

HOW SUPPLIED
POWDER FOR INJECTION:

BRAND/MANUFACTURER	NDC	SIZE	AWP
GENERICS			
ATNATIV: Baxter Biotech	00944-0996-01	1s	$625.00

POWDER FOR INJECTION: 1 I.U.

BRAND/MANUFACTURER	NDC	SIZE	AWP
BRAND			
THROMBATE III: Miles Biol	00192-0603-20	1s	$0.86
	00192-0603-30	1s	$0.86

Antivenin *SEE* MICRURUS FULVIUS

Antivenin (Crotalidae) Polyvalent

IMPORTANT
Pit viper bites may cause severe tissue damage or fatal envenomation, or both. The physician responsible for treatment of an envenomated patient should be familiar with this prescribing information and the pertinent medical literature concerning current concepts of first-aid and general supportive therapy as presented in the references listed at the end of this prescribing information.

COMPOSITION
Antivenin (Crotalidae) Polyvalent is a refined and concentrated preparation of serum globulins obtained by fractionating blood from healthy horses immunized with the following venoms: *Crotalus adamanteus* (Eastern diamod rattlesnake), *C. atrox* (Western diamond rattlesnake), *C. durissus terrificus* (tropical rattlesnake, Cascabel), and *Bothrops atrox* ("Fer-de-lance"). The product is standardized by its ability to neutralize the lethal action of standard venoms by intravenous injection in mice.[1] Dried from the frozen state, the lyophilized serum has a moisture content of less than 1% and is soluble on addition of the diluent contained in each package (Bacteriostatic Water for Injection, USP, with preservative: 0.001% phenylmercuric nitrate).

Antivenin (Crotalidae) Polyvalent (hereinafter referred to as Antivenin) contains protective substances capable of neutralizing the toxic effects of venoms of crotalids (pit vipers) native to North, Central, and South America, including rattlesnakes *(Crotalus, Sistrurus);* copperhead and cottonmouth moccasins *(A gkistrodon)* including *A. halys* of Korea and Japan; the Fer-de-lance and other species of *Bothrops;* the tropical rattler *(Crotalus durissus* and similar species); the Cantil *(A. bilineatus);* and bushmaster *(Lachesis mutus)* of South and Central America.

INDICATION
Antivenin is indicated only for the treatment of envenomation caused by bites of those crotalids (pit vipers) specified in the immediately preceding paragraph.

PIT VIPER BITES AND ENVENOMATION
The symptoms, signs, and severity of snake-venom poisoning resulting from pit viper bites depend on many factors, including, but not limited to, the following variables: species, age, and size of the biting snake; the number and location of bite(s); the depth of venom deposit by the snake's fangs; the condition of the snake's fangs and venom glands; the length of time the snake "hangs on"; the age, general health, and size of the victim; the type and efficacy of any first-aid treatment rendered in an attempt to remove venom and how soon such treatment was applied. In any venomous snake bite, the actual amount of venom introduced into the victim is always an unknown. Even the type of clothing or leg-footwear through which the snake's fangs pass may affect the amount of venom delivered by the bite. Although most North American pit vipers tend to bite and introduce venom superficially, their fangs may get hung-up in the subcutaneous tissues during the biting act and can penetrate deeper tissues during the attempt to release the bitten part. In some bites the fangs may penetrate into muscle. In such cases, the usual local superficial manifestations of envenomation may not appear early in the course of poisoning. In bites by some species, systemic evidence of envenomation may be present in the absence of significant local manifestations. It may be difficult to determine the severity of envenomation during the first several hours after a pit viper bite and estimates of severity may need to be revised as poisoning progresses. It must be remembered, too, that not all pit viper bites result in envenomation. In approximately 20% of rattlesnake bites, the snake may not inject any venom. The local and systemic symptoms and signs of envenomation include the following:

LOCAL
Fang puncture(s).

Swelling: edema is usually seen around the site of bite within five minutes. It may progress rapidly and involve the entire extremity within an hour. More than 95% of all snakebites are inflicted on extremities.[2] Generally, however, edema spreads more slowly, usually over a period of 8 or more hours. Swelling is usually most severe following envenomation by the Eastern diamondback; less severe after bites by the Western diamondback, prairie, timber, red, Pacific, Mojave, and blacktailed rattlers, the sidewinder and cottonmouth moccasins; least severe after bites by copperheads, massasaugas, and pygmy rattlers.

Ecchymosis and discoloration of the skin: often appear in the area of the bite within a few hours. Vesicles may form within a few hours and are usually present at 24 hours. Hemorrhagic blebs and petechiae are common. Necrosis may develop, necessitating amputation of an extremity or a portion thereof.

Pain: frequently a complaint of the victim beginning shortly after the bite by most pit vipers. Pain may be absent after bites by Mojave rattlers.

SYSTEMIC
Weakness; faintness; nausea; sweating; numbness or tingling around the mouth, tongue, scalp, fingers, toes, site of bite; muscle fasciculations; hypotension; prolongation of bleeding and clotting times; hemoconcentration, early followed by a decrease in erythrocytes; thrombocytopenia; hematuria; proteinuria; vomiting, including hematemesis; melena; hemoptysis; epistaxis. In fatal poisoning, a frequent cause of death is associated with destruction of erythrocytes and changes in capillary permeability, especially of the pulmonary vascular system, leading to pulmonary edema; hemoconcentration usually occurs early, probably as a result of plasma loss secondary to vascular permeability; the hemoglobin may fall, and bleeding may occur throughout the body as early as 6 hours after the bite. Renal involvement is not uncommon. Mojave rattler venom may cause neuromuscular changes leading to respiratory failure.

An estimate of the severity of envenomation should be made as soon as possible and before any Antivenin is administered. The amount (volume) of the first dose of Antivenin is determined on this estimate of severity. Every symptom, sign, laboratory-test result, and any other pertinent information should be considered in estimating severity—local manifestations; systemic manifestations, including abnormal laboratory findings; species and size of the biting snake, if known; number and location of bite(s); size and health of the patient; type of first-aid treatment rendered; and interval between bite and arrival for treatment. Russell et al.[3] and Wingert and Wainschel[4] grade severity as follows:

No envenomention: no local or systemic manifestations.

Minimal envenomation: local swelling and other local changes; no systemic manifestations; normal laboratory findings.

Moderate envenomation: swelling progressing beyond the site of bite and one or more systemic manifestations; abnormal laboratory findings, for example, a fall in hematocrit or platelets.

Severe envenomation: marked local response, severe systemic manifestations and significant alteration in laboratory findings.

Parrish and Hayes,[5] McCollough and Gennaro[6] and Watt and Gennaro[7] have used a Grade 0 (no envenomation) through Grade IV (very severe) classification of severity which was developed for the most part in treatment of envenomation by the Eastern diamondback and timber rattlers. This classification is more dependent on local manifestations, or the absence thereof, as the venoms of these species seem to be more consistent in inducing local tissue damage.

Any suspected envenomation should be treated as a medical emergency, and until careful observation provides clear evidence that envenomation has not occurred or is minimal, the following procedures are recommended:

Monitor vital signs at frequent intervals: Blood pressure, pulse, respiration.

Draw sufficient blood as soon as possible for baseline laboratory studies, including type and cross-match, CBC, hematocrit, platelet count, prothrombin time, clot retraction, bleeding and coagulation times, BUN, electrolytes, bilirubin. Some of these studies may need to be repeated at daily intervals, or less, depending on the severity of envenomation and the response to treatment. During the first 4 or 5 days of severe envenomations, hemoglobin, hematocrit, and platelet counts should be carried out several times a day.

Obtain urine samples at frequent intervals for analysis, with special attention to microscopic examination for presence of erythrocytes.

Chart fluid intake and urine output.

Measure and record the circumference of the bitten extremity just proximal to the bite and at one or more additional points each several inches closer to the trunk. Repeat measurements every 15-30 minutes to obtain information about progression of edema.

Have available and ready for immediate use: oxygen, resuscitation equipment including airway, tourniquet, epinephrine, injectable antihistaminic agents and corticosteroids.

Start an intravenous infusion in one or two extremities: one line to be used for supportive therapy, if needed, such as whole blood, plasma, packed red cells, specific clotting factors, platelet transfusion, plasma expanders; the other line to be used for administration of Antivenin and electrolytes. Carry out and interpret a skin test for horse-serum sensitivity. (See "Precautions" section below.)

DOSAGE AND ADMINISTRATION
Before administration, read "Precautions" and "Systemic Reactions" sections below. Since the possibility of a severe immediate reaction (anaphylaxis) exists whenever a horse-serum-containing product is administered, appropriate therapeutic agents, including a tourniquet, airway, oxygen, epinephrine, an injectable pressor amine, and corticosteroid, must be available and ready for immediate use. Constant attendance and observation of the patient for untoward reactions are mandatory when Antivenin is administered. Should any systemic reaction occur, administration should be discontinued immediately and appropriate treatment initiated.

The intravenous route of administration is preferred, and probably should always be used for moderate or severe envenomation. Intravenous administration is mandatory if venom-induced shock is present. To be most effective, Antivenin should be administered within 4 hours of the bite; it is less effective when given after 8 hours and may be of questionable value after 12 hours. However, it is recommended that Antivenin therapy be given in severe poisonings, even if 24 hours have elapsed since the time of the bite. It should be kept in mind that maximum blood levels of Antivenin may not be obtained for 8 or more hours after intramuscular administration.

For intravenous-drip use, prepare a 1:1 to 1:10 dilution of reconstituted Antivenin in Sodium Chloride Injection, USP, or 5% Dextrose Injection, USP. To avoid foaming, mix by gently swirling rather than shaking. Allow the initial 5 to 10 mL to infuse over a 3- to 5-minute period, with careful observation of the patient for evidence of untoward reaction. If no symptoms or signs of an immediate systemic reaction appear, continue the infusion with delivery at the maximum safe rate for intravenous fluid administration. The dilution of Antivenin to be used, the type of electrolyte solution used for dilution, and the rate of intravenous delivery of the diluted Antivenin must take into consideration the age, weight, and cardiac status of the patient; the severity of envenomation; the total amount and type of parenteral fluids it is anticipated will be given or are needed; and the interval between bite and initiation of specific therapy.

It is important to give as soon as possible the entire initial dose of Antivenin as based on the best estimate of the severity of envenomation at the time treatment is begun. The following initial doses are recommended:[3,4,8]

No envenomation: none

Minimal envenomation: 20-40 mL (contents of 2 to 4 vials)

Moderate envenomation: 50-90 mL (contents of 5 to 9 vials)

Severe envenomation: 100-150 mL or more (contents of 10 to 15 or more vials)
These recommended initial-dosage volumes are in general accord with those of others.[5-7,9]

The need for additional Antivenin must be based on the clinical response to the initial dose and continuing assessment of the severity of poisoning. If swelling continues to progress or if systemic symptoms or signs of envenomation increase in severity or if new manifestations appear, for example, fall in hematocrit or hypotension, administer an additional 10 to 50 mL (contents of 1 to 5 vials) intravenously.

Envenomation by large snakes in children or small adults requires larger doses of Antivenin. The amount administered to a child is not based on weight.

If Antivenin is given intramuscularly, it should be given into a large muscle mass, preferably the gluteal area, with care to avoid nerve trunks. Antivenin should never be injected into a finger or toe.

The effectiveness of corticosteroids in treatment of envenomation per se or venom shock is not resolved. Russell[3] and others[9,10] believe corticosteroids may mask the seriousness of hypovolemia in moderate or severe poisoning and have little, if any, effect on the local-tissue response to rattler venoms. Corticosteroids should not be given simultaneously with Antivenin on a routine basis or during the acute state of envenomation; however, their use may be necessary to treat immediate allergic reactions to Antivenin, and corticosteroids are the agents of choice for treating serious delayed reactions to Antivenin.

Snakes' mouths do not harbor *Clostridium tetani*. However, appropriate tetanus prophylaxis is indicated, since tetanus spores may be carried into the fang puncture wounds by dirt present on skin at time of bite or by nonsterile first-aid procedures.

A broad-spectrum antibiotic in adequate dosage is indicated if local tissue damage is evident.

Shock following envenomation is treated like shock resulting from hypovolemia from any cause, including administration of whole blood, plasma, albumin, or other plasma expanders, as indicated.

Aspirin or codeine is usually adequate for relieving pain. Sedation with phenobarbital or mild tranquilizers may be used if indicated, but not in the presence of respiratory failure.

The bitten extremity should not be packed in ice, and socalled "cryotherapy" is contraindicated.

Compartment syndromes may complicate pit viper envenomations, especially those caused by bites on the lower extremities. Prompt surgical consultation is indicated whenever a closed-compartment syndrome is suspected.[3,12]

Defibrination and disseminated intravascular coagulation (DIC) syndromes have been associated with envenomation caused by some pit vipers native to the United States, and appropriate therapy may be indicated.[3,9,10,13-17]

TECHNIC FOR RECONSTITUTING THE DRIED ANTIVENIN
Pry off the small metal disc in the cap over the diaphragms of the vials of Antivenin and diluent. Swab the exposed surface of the rubber diaphragms of both vials with an appropriate germicide. With a sterile 10 mL syringe and needle, withdraw the diluent (Bacteriostatic Water for Injection, USP, containig phenylmercuric nitrate 1:100,000) from the vial of diluent and inject it into the vial of Antivenin. Gentle agitation will hasten complete dissolution of the lyophilized Antivenin.

PRECAUTIONS
Before administration of any product prepared from horse serum, appropriate measures must be taken in an effort to detect the presence of dangerous sensitivity: (1) A careful review of the patient's history, including any report of (a) asthma, hay fever, urticaria, or other allergic manifestations; (b) allergic reactions upon exposure to horses; and (c) prior injections of horse serum. (2) A suitable test for detection of sensitivity. A skin test should be performed in every patient prior to administration, regardless of clinical history.

Skin test: Inject intracutaneously 0.02 to 0.03 mL of a 1:10 dilution of Normal Horse Serum or Antivenin. A control test on the opposite extremity, using Sodium Chloride Injection, USP, facilitates interpretation. Use of larger amounts for the skin-test dose increases the likelihood of false-positive reactions, and in the exquisitely sensitive patient, increases the risk of a systemic reaction from the skin-test dose. A 1:100 or greater dilution should be used for preliminary skin testing if the history suggests sensitivity. A positive reaction to a skin test occurs within five to thirty minutes and is manifested by a wheal with or without pseudopodia and surrounding erythema. In general, the shorter the interval between injection and the beginning of the skin reaction, the greater the sensitivity.

If the history is negative for allergy and the result of a skin test is negative, proceed with administration of Antivenin as outlined above. If the history is positive and a skin test is strongly positive, administration may be dangerous, especially if the positive sensitivity test is accompanied by systemic allergic manifestations. In such instances, the risk of administering Antivenin must be weighed against the risk of withholding it, keeping in mind that severe envenomation can be fatal. (See last paragraph of this section.)

A negative allergic history and absence of reaction to a properly applied skin test do not rule out the possibility of an immediate reaction. Also, a negative skin test has no bearing on whether or not delayed serum reactions (serum sickness) will occur after administration of the full dose.

If the history is negative, and the skin test is mildly or questionably positive, administer as follows to reduce the risk of a severe immediate systemic reaction: (a) Prepare, in separate sterile vials or syringes, 1:100 and 1:10 dilutions of Antivenin. (b) Allow at least 15 minutes between injections and proceed with the next dose if no reaction follows the previous dose. (c) Inject subcutaneously, using a tuberculin-type syringe, 0.1, 0.2, and 0.5 mL of the 1:100 dilution at 15-minute intervals; repeat with the 1:10 dilution, and finally undiluted Antivenin. (d) If a systemic reaction occurs after any injection, place a tourniquet proximal to the site of injections and administer an appropriate dose of epinephrine, 1:1000, proximal to the tourniquet or into another extremity. Wait at least 30 minutes before injecting another dose. The amount of the next dose should be the same as the last that did not evoke a reaction. (e) If no reaction occurs after 0.5 mL of undiluted Antivenin has been administered, switch to the intramuscular route and continue doubling the dose at 15-minute intervals until the entire dose has been

injected intramuscularly or proceed to the intravenous route as described above under *"Dosage and Administration."*

Obviously, if the just-described schedule is used, 3 to 5 or more hours would be required to administer the initial dose suggested for a moderate or severe envenomation, and time is an important factor in neutralization of venom in a critically ill patient. Wingert and Wainschel[4] have described a procedure based on the experience of their group which they have used in some severely envenomated patients who have positive sensitivity tests: 50 to 100 mg of diphenhydramine hydrochloride is given intravenously, followed by slow intravenous infusion of diluted Antivenin for 15 to 20 minutes while carefully observing the patient for symptoms and signs of anaphylaxis; if anaphylaxis does not occur, Antivenin is continued, maintaining close observation of the patient. Patients who require Antivenin but develop signs of impending anaphylaxis in spite of this or the procedure described earlier present a difficult problem, and consultation should be sought.

SYSTEMIC REACTIONS
A. The immediate reaction (shock, anaphylaxis) usually occurs within 30 minutes. Symptoms and signs may develop before the needle is withdrawn and may include apprehension, flushing, itching, urticaria; edema of the face, tongue, and throat; cough, dyspnea, cyanosis, vomiting, and collapse.

B. Serum sickness usually occurs 5 to 24 days after administration. The incubation period may be less than 5 days, especially in those who have received horse-serum-containing preparations in the past. The usual symptoms and signs are malaise, fever, urticaria, lymphadenopathy, edema, arthralgia, nausea, and vomiting. Occasionally, neurological manifestations develop, such as meningismus or peripheral neuritis. Peripheral neuritis usually involves the shoulders and arms. Pain and muscle weakness are frequently present, and permanent atrophy may develop.

REFERENCES
1. Gingrich, W. & Hohenadel, J.: Standardization of polyvalent antivenin. "Venoms", edited by E. Buckley and N. Porges. Publication No. 44, Amer. Assoc. for the Advancement of Science, Washington, D.C., 1956, Pages 337-80. 2. Parrish, H.: Incidence of treated snakebite in the United States. Pub. Hlth. Rep. *81*:269, 1966. 3. Russell, F., et al.: Snake venom poisoning in the United States. Experiences with 550 cases. JAMA *233*:341, 1975. Russell, F.: Venomous bites and stings: Poisonous snakes. In The Merck Manual of Diagnosis and Therapy, pp. 2450-2456, 14th Ed., 1982. 4. Wingert, W. and Wainschel, J.: Diagnosis and management of envenomation by poisonous snakes. South. Med. J. *68*:1015, 1975. 5. Parrish, H. & Hayes, R.: Hospital management of pit viper venenations. Clinical Toxicol. *3*:501, 1970. 6. McCollough, N. & Gennaro, J.: Diagnosis, symptoms, treatment and sequelae of envenomation by *Crotalus adamanteus* and Genus *Agkistrodon*. J. Florida Med. Assoc. *55*:327, 1968. 7. Watt, C. & Gennaro, J.: Pit viper bites in South Georgia and North Florida. Tr. South. Surg. Assoc. *77*:378, 1966. 8. Minton, S.: Venom Diseases: Snakebite. In Textbook of Medicine, P. Beeson and W. McDermott (Eds.), pp. 88-92; Saunders, Philadelphia, 1975. 9. Van Mierop, L.: Snakebite symposium. J. Florida Med. Assoc. *63*:101, 1976. 10. Arnold, R.: Treatment of snakebite. JAMA *236*:1843, 1976; Controversies and hazards in the treatment of pit viper bites. South Med. J. *72*:902, 1979. 11. Poisonous Snakes of the World. U.S. Government Printing Office, Washington, D.C., NAVMED, 1965. 12. Garfin, S. et al.: Rattlesnake bites: Current concepts. Clin. Orthop. *140*:50, 1979; Role of surgical decompression in treatment of rattlesnake bites. Surg. Forum *30*:502, 1979. 13. Van Mierop, L. & Kitchen, C.: Defibrination syndrome following bites by the Eastern diamondback rattlesnake. J. Florida Med. Assoc. *67*:21, 1980. 14. Hasiba, U. et al.: DIC-like syndrome after envenomation by the snake, *Crotalus horvidis horridus*. New Eng. J. Med. *292*:505, 1975. 15. Weiss, H. et al.: Afibrinogenemia in man following the bite of a rattlesnake (*Crotalus adamanteus*). Am. J. Med. *47*:625, 1969. 16. Sivaprasad, R. & Cantini, E.: Western diamondback rattlesnake (*Crotalus atrox*) poisoning. Postgrad. Med. *71*:223, 1982. 17. Sabback, M. et al.: A study of the treatment of pit viper envenomization in 45 patients. J. Trauma. *17*:569, 1977.

HOW SUPPLIED
KIT:

BRAND/MANUFACTURER	NDC	SIZE	AWP
○ **BRAND**			
ANTIVENIN POLYVALENT: Wyeth-Ayerst	00008-0332-04	1s	$188.30

Antivenin (Latrodectus Mactans)

DESCRIPTION
Antivenin (Latrodectus Mactans) is a sterile, nonpyrogenic preparation derived by drying a frozen solution of specific venom-neutralizing globulins obtained from the blood serum of healthy horses immunized against venom of black widow spiders (Latrodectus Mactans). It is standardized by biological assay on mice, in terms of one dose of antivenin neutralizing the venom in not less than 6000 mouse LD_{50} of Latrodectus Mactans. Thimerosal (mercury derivative) 1:10,000 is added as a preservative. When constituted as specified, it is opalescent, ranging in color from light (straw) to very dark (iced tea), and contains not more than 20.0 percent of solids.

Each vial contains not less than 6000 Antivenin units. One unit of Antivenin will neutralize one average mouse lethal dose of black widow spider venom when the Antivenin and the venom are injected simultaneously in mice under suitable conditions.

CLINICAL PHARMACOLOGY
The pharmacological mode of action is unknown and metabolic and pharmacokinetic data in humans are unavailable.

INDICATIONS AND USAGE

Antivenin (Latrodectus mactans) is used to treat patients with symptoms due to bites by the black widow spider (Latrodectus mactans). Early use of the Antivenin is emphasized for prompt relief.

Local muscular cramps begin from 15 minutes to several hours after the bite which usually produces a sharp pain similar to that caused by puncture with a needle. The exact sequence of symptoms depends somewhat on the location of the bite. The venom acts on the myoneural junctions or on the nerve endings, causing an ascending motor paralysis or destruction of the peripheral nerve endings. The groups of muscles most frequently affected at first are those of the thigh, shoulder, and back. After a varying length of time, the pain becomes more severe, spreading to the abdomen, and weakness and tremor usually develop. The abdominal muscles assume a boardlike rigidity, but tenderness is slight.

Respiration is thoracic. The patient is restless and anxious. Feeble pulse, cold, clammy skin, labored breathing and speech, light stupor, and delirium may occur. Convulsions also may occur, particularly in small children. The temperature may be normal or slightly elevated. Urinary retention, shock, cyanosis, nausea and vomiting, insomnia, and cold sweats also have been reported. The syndrome following the bite of the black widow spider may be confused easily with any medical or surgical condition with acute abdominal symptoms.

The symptoms of black widow spider bite increase in severity for several hours, perhaps a day, and then very slowly become less severe, gradually passing off in the course of two or three days except in fatal cases. Residual symptoms such as general weakness, tingling, nervousness, and transient muscle spasm may persist for weeks or months after recovery from the acute stage.

If possible, the patient should be hospitalized. Other additional measures giving greatest relief are prolonged warm baths and intravenous injection of 10 mL of 10 percent solution of calcium gluconate repeated as necessary to control muscle pain. Morphine also may be required to control pain. Barbiturates may be used for extreme restlessness. However, as the venom is a neurotoxin, it can cause respiratory paralysis. This must be borne in mind when considering use of morphine or a barbiturate. Adrenocorticosteroids have been used with varying degrees of success. Supportive therapy is indicated by the condition of the patient. Local treatment of the site of the bite is of no value. Nothing is gained by applying a tourniquet or by attempting to remove venom from the site of the bite by incision and suction.

In otherwise healthy individuals between the ages of 16 and 60, the use of Antivenin may be deferred and treatment with muscle relaxants may be considered.

WARNINGS

Prior to treatment with any product prepared from horse serum, a careful review of the patient's history should be taken emphasizing prior exposure to horse serum or any allergies. Serious sickness and even death could result from the use of horse serum in a sensitive patient. A skin or conjunctival test should be performed prior to administration of Antivenin.

Skin test: Inject into (not under) the skin not more than 0.02 mL of the test material (1:10 dilution of normal horse serum in physiologic saline). Evaluate result in 10 minutes. A positive reaction is an urticarial wheal surrounded by a zone of erythema. A control test using Sodium Chloride Injection facilitates interpretation of the results.

Conjunctival Test: For adults instill into the conjunctival sac one drop of a 1:10 dilution of horse serum and for children one drop of 1:100 dilution. Itching of the eye and reddening of the conjunctiva indicate a positive reaction, usually within 10 minutes.

Patients should be observed for serum sickness for an average of 8 to 12 days following administration of Antivenin. *Desensitization should be attempted only when the administration of Antivenin is considered necessary to save life.* Epinephrine must be available in case of untoward reaction.

Desensitization: If the history is positive or the results of the sensitivity tests are mildly or questionably positive, Antivenin should be administered as follows to reduce the risk of an immediate severe allergic reaction:

1. In separate sterile vials or syringes prepare 1:10 or 1:100 dilutions of Antivenin in Sodium Chloride for Injection.
2. Allow at least 15 but preferably 30 minutes between injections and only proceed with the next dose if no reactions occurred following the previous dose.
3. Using a tuberculin syringe, inject subcutaneously 0.1, 0.2 and 0.5 mL of the 1:100 dilution at 15 or 30 minute intervals; repeat with the 1:10 dilution, and finally the undiluted Antivenin.
4. If there is a reaction after any of the injections, place a tourniquet proximal to the sites of injection and administer epinephrine, 1:1000 (0.3 to 1.0 mL subcutaneously, 0.05 to 0.1 mL intravenously), proximal to the tourniquet or into another extremity. Wait at least 30 minutes before giving another injection of Antivenin, the amount of which should be the same as the last one not evoking a reaction.
5. If no reaction has occurred after 0.5 mL of undiluted Antivenin has been given, it is probably safe to continue the dose at 15 minute intervals until the entire dose has been injected.

PRECAUTIONS

CARCINOGENESIS, MUTAGENESIS, IMPAIRMENT OF FERTILITY
No long term studies in animals have been performed to evaluate the potential for carcinogenesis, mutagenesis, or impairment of fertility.

PREGNANCY
Pregnancy Category C. Animal reproduction studies have not been conducted with Black Widow Spider Antivenin. It is also not known whether Black Widow Spider Antivenin can cause fetal harm when administered to a pregnant woman or can affect reproduction capacity. Black Widow Spider Antivenin should be given to a pregnant woman only if clearly needed.

NURSING MOTHERS
It is not known whether this drug is excreted in human milk. Because many drugs are excreted in human milk, caution should be exercised when Black Widow Spider Antivenin is administered to a nursing woman.

PEDIATRIC USE
Controlled clinical studies for safety and effectiveness in children have not been conducted; however, there have been virtually no adverse effects reported in those children who have received the product.

ADVERSE REACTIONS

Anaphylaxis and serum sickness have been reported following use of Antivenin.

DOSAGE AND ADMINISTRATION

Using a sterile syringe, remove from the accompanying vial 2.5 mL of Sterile Diluent for Antivenin and inject into the vial of Antivenin. With the needle still in the rubber stopper, shake the vial to dissolve the contents completely.

Parenteral drug products should be inspected visually for particulate matter prior to administration, whenever solution and container permit (see *"Description"*).

The dose for adults and children is the entire contents of a restored vial (2.5 mL) of Antivenin. It may be given intramuscularly, preferably in the region of the anterolateral thigh so that a tourniquet may be applied in the event of a systemic reaction. Symptoms usually subside in 1 to 3 hours. Although one dose of Antivenin usually is adequate, a second dose may be necessary in some cases.

Antivenin also may be given intravenously in 10 to 50 mL of saline solution over a 15 minute period. It is the preferred route in severe cases, or when the patient is under 12, or in shock. One restored vial usually is enough.

Antivenin must be stored and shipped at 2–8°C (36–46°F). When reconstituted as directed, the color of Antivenin ranges from light (straw) to very dark (iced tea), but the color has no effect on potency. *Do not freeze.*

HOW SUPPLIED
POWDER FOR INJECTION:

BRAND/MANUFACTURER	NDC	SIZE	AWP
○ GENERICS			
Merck	00006-4084-00	1s	$24.80

Antivenin Polyvalent *SEE* ANTIVENIN
(CROTALIDAE) POLYVALENT

Antivert *SEE* MECLIZINE HYDROCHLORIDE

Antrocol *SEE* ATROPINE SULFATE AND PHENOBARBITAL

Anturane *SEE* SULFINPYRAZONE

Anusol-HC *SEE* HYDROCORTISONE, RECTAL

A.P.L. *SEE* GONADOTROPIN, CHORIONIC

Aplisol *SEE* TUBERCULIN

Aplitest *SEE* TUBERCULIN

Appecon *SEE* PHENDIMETRAZINE TARTRATE

◆ RATED THERAPEUTICALLY EQUIVALENT; ◇ THERAPEUTIC EQUIVALENCE UNCONFIRMED; ○ UNRATED

Apraclonidine Hydrochloride

DESCRIPTION

Apraclonidine Hydrochloride is an alpha adrenergic agonist in a sterile isotonic solution for topical application to the eye. Apraclonidine Hydrochloride is a white to off-white powder and is highly soluble in water. Its chemical name is 2-[(4-amino-2,6 dichlorophenyl) imino]imidazolidine monohydrochloride with an empirical formula of $C_9H_{11}Cl_3N_4$ and a molecular weight of 281.6.

Each mL of Apraclonidine ophthalmic solution contains: Apraclonidine 11.5 mg equivalent to Apraclonidine base 10 mg.

Following is its chemical structure:

CLINICAL PHARMACOLOGY

Apraclonidine is a relatively selective, alpha adrenergic agonist and does not have significant membrane stabilizing (local anesthetic) activity. When instilled into the eye, Apraclonidine HCl ophthalmic solution has the action of reducing intraocular pressure. Ophthalmic Apraclonidine has minimal effect on cardiovascular parameters.

Optic nerve head damage and visual field loss may result from an acute elevation in intraocular pressure that can occur after argon or Nd:YAG laser surgical procedures. Elevated intraocular pressure, whether acute or chronic in duration, is a major risk factor in the pathogenesis of visual field loss. The higher the peak or spike of intraocular pressure, the greater the likelihood of visual field loss and optic nerve damage especially in patients with previously compromised optic nerves. The onset of action with Apraclonidine HCl ophthalmic solution can usually be noted within one hour and the maximum intraocular pressure reduction usually occurs three to five hours after application of a single dose. The precise mechanism of the ocular hypotensive action of Apraclonidine HCl ophthalmic solution is not completely established at this time. Aqueous fluorophotometry studies in man suggest that its predominant action may be related to a reduction of aqueous formation. Controlled clinical studies of patients requiring argon laser trabeculoplasty, argon laser iridotomy or Nd:YAG posterior capsulotomy showed that Apraclonidine HCl ophthalmic solution controlled or prevented the postsurgical intraocular pressure rise typically observed in patients after undergoing those procedures. After surgery, the mean intraocular pressure was 1.2 to 4.0 mmHg below the corresponding presurgical baseline pressure before Apraclonidine HCl ophthalmic solution treatment. With placebo treatment, postsurgical pressures were 2.5 to 8.4 mmHg higher than their corresponding presurgical baselines. Overall, only 2% of patients treated with Apraclonidine HCl ophthalmic solution had severe intraocular pressure elevations (spike $\geq$ 10 mmHg) during the first three hours after laser surgery, whereas 22% of placebo-treated patients responded with severe pressure spikes (Table 1). Of the patients that experienced a pressure spike after surgery, the peak intraocular pressure was above 30 mmHg in most patients (Table 2) and was above 50 mmHg in seven placebo-treated patients and one Apraclonidine HCl ophthalmic solution-treated patient. (See related tables).

INDICATIONS AND USAGE

Apraclonidine HCl ophthalmic solution is indicated to control or prevent postsurgical elevations in intraocular pressure that occur in patients after argon laser trabeculoplasty, argon laser iridotomy or Nd:YAG posterior capsulotomy.

CONTRAINDICATION

Apraclonidine HCl ophthalmic solution is contraindicated for patients receiving monoamine oxidase inhibitor therapy and for patients with hypersensitivity to any component of this medication or to clonidine.

General: Since Apraclonidine HCl ophthalmic solution is a potent depressor of intraocular pressure, patients who develop exaggerated reductions in intraocular pressure should be closely monitored.

Although the acute administration of two drops of Apraclonidine HCl ophthalmic solution has minimal effect on heart rate or blood pressure in clinical studies evaluating patients undergoing anterior segment laser surgery, the preclinical pharmacologic profile of this drug suggests that caution should be observed in treating patients with severe cardiovascular disease including hypertension.

The possibility of a vasovagal attack occurring during laser surgery should be considered and caution used in patients with history of such episodes.

Topical ocular administration of two drops of 0.5%, 1.0% and 1.5% Apraclonidine HCl ophthalmic solution to New Zealand albino rabbits three times daily for one month resulted in sporadic and transient instances of minimal corneal cloudiness in the 1.5% group only. No histopathological changes were noted in those eyes. No adverse ocular effects were observed in cynomolgus monkeys treated with two drops of 1.5% Apraclonidine HCl ophthalmic solution applied three times daily for three months. No corneal changes were observed in 320 humans given at least one dose of 1.0% Apraclonidine HCl ophthalmic solution.

Drug Interactions: Interactions with other agents have not been investigated.

Carcinogenesis, Mutagenesis, Impairment of Fertility: In a variety of *in vitro* cell assays, Apraclonidine was nonmutagenic. Studies addressing carcinogenesis and the impairment of fertility have not been conducted.

Pregnancy: Pregnancy Category C: There are no adequate and well controlled studies of Apraclonidine HCl ophthalmic solution in pregnant women. Animal reproduction studies have not been conducted with Apraclonidine HCl. This medication should be used in pregnancy only if the potential benefit to the mother justifies the potential risk to the fetus.

Nursing Mothers: It is not known if topically applied Apraclonidine HCl ophthalmic solution is excreted in human milk. A decision should be considered to discontinue nursing temporarily for the one day on which Apraclonidine HCl ophthalmic solution is used.

Pediatric Use: Safety and effectiveness in children have not been established.

ADVERSE REACTIONS

The following adverse events were reported in association with the use of Apraclonidine HCl ophthalmic solution in laser surgery: ocular injection (1.8%), upper lid elevation (1.3%), irregular heart rate (0.7%), ocular inflammation (0.45%), nasal decongestion (0.45%), conjunctival blanching (0.4%) and mydriasis (0.4%).

The following adverse events were observed in investigational studies dosing Apraclonidine HCl ophthalmic solution once or twice daily for up to 28 days in nonlaser studies.

Ocular: Conjunctival blanching, upper lid elevation, mydriasis, burning, discomfort, foreign body sensation, dryness, itching, hypotony, blurred or dimmed vision, allergic response, conjunctival microhemorrhage.

Table 1
INCIDENCE OF INTRAOCULAR PRESSURE SPIKES $\geq$ 10 MMHG

| | | | Treatment | | | |
| | | | Apraclonidine | | Placebo | |
Study	Laser Procedure	P-Value	[a]N	(%)	[a]N	(%)
1	Trabeculoplasty	< 0.05	0/40	(0%)	6/35	(17%)
2	Trabeculoplasty	= 0.06	2/41	(5%)	8/42	(19%)
1	Iridotomy	< 0.05	0/11	(0%)	4/10	(40%)
2	Iridotomy	= 0.05	0/17	(0%)	4/19	(21%)
1	Nd:YAG Capsulotomy	< 0.05	3/80	(4%)	19/83	(23%)
2	Nd:YAG Capsulotomy	< 0.05	0/83	(0%)	22/81	(27%)

[a]N = Number Spikes/Number Eyes.

Table 2
MAGNITUDE OF POSTSURGICAL INTRAOCULAR PRESSURE IN TRABECULOPLASTY, IRIDOTOMY AND ND:YAG CAPSULOTOMY PATIENTS WITH SEVERE PRESSURE SPIKES $\geq$ 10 MMHG

| | | Maximum Postsurgical Intraocular Pressure (mmHg) | | | |
Treatment	Total Spikes	20-29 mmHg	30-39 mmHg	40-49 mmHg	> 50 mmHg
Apraclonidine HCl	8	1	4	2	1
Placebo	78	16	47	8	7

➤ SHOWN IN PRODUCT IDENTIFICATION GUIDE

Gastrointestinal: Abdominal pain, diarrhea, stomach discomfort, emesis.

Cardiovascular: Bradycardia, vasovagal attack, palpitations, orthostatic episode.

Central Nervous System: Insomnia, dream disturbances, irritability, decreased libido.

Other: Taste abnormalities, dry mouth, nasal burning or dryness, headache, head cold sensation, chest heaviness or burning, clammy or sweaty palms, body heat sensation, shortness of breath, increased pharyngeal secretion, extremity pain or numbness, fatigue, paresthesia, pruritus not associated with rash.

OVERDOSAGE

No information is available on overdosage in humans. The oral LD_{50} of the drug ranged from 3-8 mg/kg in mice and 38-107 mg/kg in rats. The intravenous LD_{50} of the drug ranged from 6-9 mg/kg in mice and 9-21 mg/kg in rats. LD_{50} values in these ranges are indicative of a drug with a high degree of toxicity.

DOSAGE AND ADMINISTRATION

One drop of Apraclonidine HCl ophthalmic solution should be instilled in the scheduled operative eye one hour before initiating anterior segment laser surgery and a second drop should be instilled to the same eye immediately upon completion of the laser surgical procedure. Use a separate container for each single-drop dose and discard each container after use.

Store at room temperature: Protect from light.

HOW SUPPLIED
DROP: 0.5%

BRAND/MANUFACTURER	NDC	SIZE	AWP
○ **BRAND** IOPIDINE: Alcon Labs	00065-0665-05	5 ml	$33.75

DROP: 1%

BRAND/MANUFACTURER	NDC	SIZE	AWP
○ **BRAND** IOPIDINE: Alcon Labs	00065-0660-10	0.1 ml 24s	$142.50

Apresazide *SEE* HYDRALAZINE HYDROCHLORIDE WITH HYDROCHLOROTHIAZIDE

Apresoline *SEE* HYDRALAZINE HYDROCHLORIDE

Aprotinin

DESCRIPTION

Aprotinin, $C_{284}H_{432}N_{84}O_{79}S_7$, is a natural proteinase inhibitor obtained from bovine lung. Aprotinin (molecular weight of 6512 daltons) consists of 58 amino acid residues that are arranged in a single polypeptide chain, cross-linked by three disulfide bridges. It is supplied as a clear, colorless, sterile isotonic solution for intravenous administration. Each milliliter contains 10,000 KIU (Kallikrein Inhibitor Units (1.4 mg/mL) and 9 mg sodium chloride in water for injection.

Following is its chemical structure:

```
        55
        |
Arg-Pro-Asp-Phe-Cys-Leu-Glu-Pro-Pro-Tyr-Thr-Gly-Pro-Cys-Lys-Ala
 1               5                          14  16     18
                                                    38
                                                    |
Arg-Ile-Ile-Arg-Tyr-Phe-Tyr-Asn-Ala-Lys-Ala-Gly-Leu-Cys-Gln-Thr
 17                23                            30     32
                   14
                    |
Phe-Val-Tyr-Gly-Gly-Cys-Arg-Ala-Lys-Arg-Asn-Asn-Phe-Lys-Ser-Ala
 33                36                               48
       30        5
        |         |
Glu-Asp-Cys-Met-Arg-Thr-Cys-Gly-Gly-Ala
 49                55          58
```

CLINICAL PHARMACOLOGY

Mechanism of Action: Aprotinin is a protease inhibitor with a variety of effects on the coagulation system. It inhibits plasmin and kallikrein, thus directly affecting fibrinolysis. It also inhibits the contact phase activation of coagulation which both initiates coagulation and promotes fibrinolysis. In addition to these effects on the clotting and lysis cascades in blood, Aprotinin preserves the adhesive glycoproteins in the platelet membrane making them resistant to damage from the increased plasmin levels and mechanical injury that occur during cardiopulmonary bypass (CPB). The net effect is to inhibit both fibrinolysis and turnover of coagulation factors, and to decrease bleeding, although the precise mechanism of this effect is unclear.

Patients undergoing cardiac surgery with extracorporeal circulation by a heart-lung machine (cardiopulmonary bypass; CPB) develop adverse changes of their blood components, blood cells and specific coagulation proteins. These changes cause a transient hemostatic defect during the intraoperative and immediate postoperative period which may result in diffuse bleeding despite correct surgical technique. At times, this blood loss is severe enough to require multiple blood transfusions and even surgical re-exploration.

Pharmacokinetics: The studies comparing the pharmacokinetics of Aprotinin in healthy volunteers, cardiac patients undergoing surgery with cardiopulmonary bypass, and women undergoing hysterectomy suggest linear pharmacokinetics over the dose range of 50,000 KIU to 2 million KIU. After intravenous (i.v.) injection, rapid distribution of Aprotinin occurs into the total extracellular space, leading to a rapid initial decrease in plasma Aprotinin concentration. Following this distribution phase, a plasma half-life of about 150 minutes is observed. At later time points, (i.e., beyond 5 hours after dosing) there is a terminal elimination phase with a half-life of about 10 hours.

Average steady state intraoperative plasma concentrations were 250 KIU/mL in patients (n = 20) treated with Aprotinin during cardiac surgery by administration of the following dosage regimen: 2 million KIU i.v. loading dose, 2 million KIU into the pump prime volume, 500,000 KIU per hour of operation as continuous intravenous infusion (Regimen A). Average steady state intraoperative plasma concentrations were 137 KIU/mL (n = 10) after administration of exactly half of Regimen A: 1 million KIU i.v. loading dose, 1 million KIU into the pump prime volume, 250,000 KIU per hour of operation as continuous intravenous infusion (Regimen B).

Following a single i.v. dose of radiolabeled Aprotinin, approximately 25-40% of the radioactivity is excreted in the urine over 48 hours. After a 30 minute infusion of 1 million KIU, about 2% is excreted as unchanged drug. After a larger dose of 2 million KIU infused over 30 minutes, urinary excretion of unchanged Aprotinin accounts for approximately 9% of the dose. Animal studies have shown that Aprotinin is accumulated primarily in the kidney. Aprotinin, after being filtered by the glomeruli, is actively reabsorbed by the proximal tubules in which it is stored in phagolysosomes. Aprotinin is slowly degraded by lysosomal enzymes. The physiological renal handling of Aprotinin is similar to that of other small proteins, e.g. insulin.

CLINICAL TRIALS

Two placebo-controlled, double-blind studies of Aprotinin were conducted in the United States involving 236 patients undergoing repeat coronary artery bypass graft (CABG) surgery, of whom 209 were valid for efficacy analysis. The following treatments were used in the studies: Aprotinin Regimen A (2 million KIU i.v. loading dose, 2 million KIU into the pump prime volume, 500,000 KIU per hour of surgery as a continuous intravenous infusion); Aprotinin Regimen B, exactly one half of Regimen A (1 million KIU i.v. loading dose, 1 million KIU into the pump prime volume, 250,000 KIU per hour of surgery as a continuous intravenous infusion); and placebo (normal saline). In the two studies fewer patients receiving either regimen of Aprotinin required any donor blood:

REPEAT CABG PATIENTS WHO REQUIRED DONOR BLOOD

	Aprotinin Regimen A	Aprotinin Regimen B	Placebo
Study 1	22/53 (42%)*	23/49 (47%)*	40/52 (77%)
Study 2	7/23 (30%)*	Not Studied	23/32 (72%)

$p \leq 0.002$ compared to placebo

The number of units of donor blood required by patients was also reduced by both regimens:

UNITS OF DONOR BLOOD REQUIRED BY REPEAT CABG PATIENTS

Study 1

	Aprotinin Regimen A	Aprotinin Regimen B	Placebo
Mean ± SE	1.8 ± 0.6*	2.0 ± 0.6**	3.5 ± 0.6
Range	0-24	0-18	0-34
Median	0	0	2

$p \leq 0.001$ compared to placebo, ANOVA on ranks
**$p = 0.005$ compared to placebo, ANOVA on ranks*

Study 2

	Aprotinin Regimen A	Placebo
Mean ± SE	0.4 ± 0.8*	3.3 ± 0.7
Range	0-5	0-20
Median	0	4

$p = 0.0001$ compared to placebo, ANOVA on ranks

Study 2 also included 151 patients undergoing primary CABG surgery; 74 of the patients receiving Aprotinin and 67 of the patients receiving placebo were valid for efficacy analysis. Fewer patients receiving Aprotinin required any donor blood:

PRIMARY CABG PATIENTS WHO REQUIRED DONOR BLOOD

	Aprotinin Regimen A	Placebo
Study 2	28/74 (38%)*	35/67 (52%)

$p = 0.052$ compared to placebo

◆ RATED THERAPEUTICALLY EQUIVALENT; ◇ THERAPEUTIC EQUIVALENCE UNCONFIRMED; ○ UNRATED

UNITS OF DONOR BLOOD REQUIRED BY PRIMARY CABG PATIENTS

Study 2

	Aprotinin Regimen A	Placebo
Mean ± SE	1.1 ± 0.3*	2.1 ± 0.3
Range	0-10	0-15
Median	0	1

p = 0.0246 compared to placebo, ANOVA on ranks

In these studies there was no diminution of benefit with age. Male and female patients received benefits from Aprotinin in terms of a reduction in the average number of units of donor blood transfused. Male patients did better than female patients in terms of the percentage of patients who required any donor blood transfusions. However, the number of female patients studied was small.

A double-blind, randomized, Canadian study compared Aprotinin (n = 28) and placebo (n = 23) in primary cardiac surgery patients (mainly CABG) requiring cardiopulmonary bypass who were treated with aspirin within 48 hours of surgery. The mean total blood loss (1209.7 mL vs. 2532.3 mL) and the mean number of units of packed red blood cells transfused (1.6 units vs. 4.3 units) were significantly less (p < 0.008) in the Aprotinin group compared to the placebo group.

In a U.S. randomized placebo controlled study of Aprotinin Regimen A versus placebo in 212 patients undergoing primary aortic and/or mitral valve replacement or repair, no benefit was found for Aprotinin in terms of the need for transfusion or the number of units of blood required.

INDICATIONS AND USAGE

Aprotinin is indicated for prophylactic use to reduce perioperative blood loss and the need for blood transfusion in patients undergoing cardiopulmonary bypass in the course of repeat coronary artery bypass graft surgery. Aprotinin is also indicated in selected cases of primary coronary artery bypass graft surgery where the risk of bleeding is especially high (impaired hemostasis, e.g., presence of aspirin or other coagulopathy) or where transfusion is unavailable or unacceptable. This selected use of Aprotinin in primary CABG patients is based on the risk of renal dysfunction and on the risk of anaphylaxis (should a second procedure be needed).

CONTRAINDICATIONS

Hypersensitivity to Aprotinin.

WARNINGS

None

PRECAUTIONS

General: Test Dose and Use of H_1 Antihistamine: All patients treated with Aprotinin should first receive a test dose to assess the potential for allergic reactions. The test dose of 1 mL Trasylol® should be administered intravenously at least 10 minutes prior to the loading dose. Particular caution is necessary when administering Aprotinin (even test doses) to patients who have received Aprotinin in the past because of the risk of anaphylaxis. In re-exposure cases, intravenous administration of an H_1-histamine antagonist (antihistamine) is recommended shortly before the loading dose of Aprotinin.

Loading Dose: The loading dose of Aprotinin should be given intravenously to patients in the supine position over a 20-30 minute period. Rapid intravenous administration of Aprotinin can cause a transient fall in blood pressure. (See "Dosage and Administration.")

Allergic Reactions: Patients who experience any allergic reaction to the test dose of Aprotinin should not receive further administration of the drug. Even after the uneventful administration of the 1 mL test dose, or without previous exposure to Aprotinin, the full therapeutic dose may cause anaphylaxis. If this happens, the infusion should be stopped immediately and emergency treatment for anaphylaxis should be applied. Patients with a history of allergic reactions to drugs or other agents may be at greater risk of developing an allergic reaction.

Use of Aprotinin in patients undergoing deep hypothermic circulatory arrest: An increase in both renal failure and mortality compared to age matched historical controls has been reported in patients receiving Aprotinin while undergoing deep hypothermic circulatory arrest in connection with surgery of the aortic arch. The strength of this association is uncertain because there are no data from randomized studies to confirm or refute these findings.

Drug Interactions: Aprotinin is known to have antifibrinolytic activity and, therefore, may inhibit the effects of fibrinolytic agents.

In a study of nine patients with untreated hypertension, Aprotinin intravenously infused in a dose of 2 million KIU over two hours blocked the acute hypotensive effect of 100mg of captopril. Aprotinin, in the presence of heparin, has been found to prolong the activated clotting time (ACT) as measured by the Hemochron® method or similar surface activation methods. However, Aprotinin should not be viewed as a heparin sparing agent (see "Laboratory Monitoring of Anticoagulation During Cardiopulmonary Bypass").

Carcinogenesis, Mutagenesis, Impairment of Fertility: Long-term animal studies to evaluate the carcinogenic potential of Aprotinin or studies to determine the effect of Aprotinin on fertility have not been performed.

Results of microbial *in vitro* testing using *Salmonella typyhimurlum* and *Bacillus subtilis* indicate that Aprotinin is not a mutagen.

Pregnancy: Teratogenic Effects: Pregnancy Category B: Reproduction studies have been performed in rats at intravenous doses up to 200,000 KIU/kg/day for 11 days, and in rabbits at intravenous doses up to 100,000 KIU/kg/day for 13 days, 2.4 and 1.2 times the human dose on a mg/kg basis and 0.37 and 0.36 times the human mg/m² dose. They have revealed no evidence of impaired fertility or harm to the fetus due to Aprotinin. There are, however, no adequate and well-controlled studies in pregnant women. Because animal reproduction studies are not always predictive of human response, this drug should be used during pregnancy only if clearly needed.

Nursing Mother: Not applicable.

Pediatric Use: Safety and effectiveness in children have not been established.

Laboratory Monitoring of Anticoagulation During Cardiopulmonary Bypass: Aprotinin prolongs whole blood clotting time of heparinized blood as determined by the Hemochron® method or similar surface activation methods. In the event of prolonged extracorporeal circulation, patients may require additional heparin, even in the presence of activated clotting time (ACT) levels that appear to represent adequate anticoagulation. Therefore, in patients on cardiopulmonary bypass (CPB) who are receiving Aprotinin, the standard system of monitoring heparinization during CPB, by keeping the ACT above 400-450 seconds, may lead to inadequate anticoagulation. In patients undergoing cardiopulmonary bypass with Aprotinin therapy, standard loading doses of heparin should be employed. However, additional heparin should be administered either in a fixed-dose regimen based on patient weight and duration of CPB, or on the basis of heparin levels measured by a method, such as protamine titration, that is not affected by Aprotinin.

ADVERSE REACTIONS

Studies analyzed to date indicate that Aprotinin is generally well-tolerated. The adverse events reported are frequent sequelae of open-heart surgery and are not necessarily attributable to Aprotinin therapy. Adverse events reported up to the time of discharge from three double-blind, placebo-controlled studies conducted in the United States involving 599 patients undergoing cardiac surgery with cardiopulmonary bypass (Study 1 - repeat CABG; Study 2 - repeat and primary CABG; Study 3 - primary cardiac valve replacement or repair) are listed in the following tables. The table lists only those events which occurred in 2% or more of the Aprotinin treated patients without regard to causal relationship.

	Aprotinin Treated Patients (N = 384) % of Patients	Placebo-Treated Patients (N = 235) % of Patients
Any Event	70	70
Atrial fibrillation	25	22
Myocardial Infarction	10	7
Heart failure	8	6
Atrial flutter	7	4
Ventricular tachycardia	5	4
Fever	5	3
Hypotension	4	3
Pneumonia	4	3
Respiratory disorder	4	3
Heart arrest	3	1
Congestive heart failure	3	1
Supraventricular tachycardia	3	2
Kidney failure	3	1
Sepsis	3	1
Apnea	3	1
Confusion	3	2
Heart block	2	1
Shock	2	1
Asthma	2	0
Dyspnea	2	0
Surgery*	2	1

*   These surgical procedures included: rethoracotomy, pacemaker implantation, mitral valve repair, vena cava filter placement, femoral thrombectomy and chest drainage in the Aprotinin group and balloon placement, pacemaker placement and tracheostomy in the placebo group.

Certain other significant events (pericarditis, ventricular fibrillation, pleural effusion, and pneumothorax) were observed in patients given Aprotinin but were more common in the placebo group.

In a pooled analysis of the three U.S. placebo-controlled studies, in patients undergoing cardiopulmonary bypass there was a trend toward an increased incidence of myocardial infarction in patients given Aprotinin. Further, in the study of patients undergoing primary or repeat CABG (Study 2), in which graft patency was evaluated by ultrafast computerized tomography (CT), a trend was seen toward an increased incidence of saphenous vein graft closure in patients who received Aprotinin Regimen A versus placebo. Neither of these trends reached statistical significance and whether there is an effect of Aprotinin on reinfarction or vein graft closure is uncertain. No increase in mortality in the Aprotinin group was observed.

Less frequent adverse events of concern, without regard to drug relationship, in open-heart surgery patients treated with Aprotinin in clinical trials in the United

States were: phlebitis (1.4%), kidney tubular necrosis (1.4%), convulsion (0.8%), cerebral embolism (0.8%), liver damage (0.5%), acute kidney failure (0.5%), cerebrovascular accident (0.5%), lung edema (0.5%), hemolysis (0.5%), allergic reaction (0.5%).

LABORATORY FINDINGS

Serum Creatinine: Pooled data from the three U.S. placebo-controlled studies showed a statistically significant increase in the incidence of post-operative renal dysfunction in the Aprotinin-treated group. The incidence of serum creatinine elevations $\geq$ 0.5 mg/dL above baseline was 23 percent in Aprotinin-treated (Regimen A) patients compared to 12 percent in the placebo group (p = 0.002). In patients undergoing coronary artery bypass graft procedures only (Studies 1, 2), the rates were 20 percent in the Aprotinin group and 13 percent in the placebo group (p = 0.115). Postoperative renal dysfunction was observed somewhat more frequently in association with primary cardiac valve procedures (30% for Aprotinin Regimen A, and 14% for Regimen B versus 8% for placebo). In the majority of instances the renal dysfunction was not severe and was reversible. A total of 4 percent of Aprotinin-treated (Regimen A) patients and 1 percent of the placebo group had a serum creatinine increase of $\geq$ 2 mg/dL above the preoperative value.

Patients with baseline elevations in serum creatinine were not at increased risk of developing postoperative renal dysfunction following Aprotinin treatment. In Aprotinin treated patients, there was a mean increase in creatinine of 0.16 mg/dL after the high dose regimen (A) which was statistically significant compared to placebo and a mean increase of 0.05 mg/dL after the low dose regimen (B) which was not significant.

Serum Glucose: In the hours after cardiopulmonary bypass surgery, the serum glucose was increased; however, the average serum glucose increase in patients treated with the high dose regimen (61 mg/dL) was less than in the placebo treated group (78 mg/dL).

Serum Transaminases: In U.S. controlled studies, there was a significantly greater incidence of treatment emergent abnormal liver function tests in all Aprotinin treated (Regimen A and Regimen B) patients (6%) compared to placebo treated patients (2%). The percent of primary CABG patients developing an elevation of ALT (alanine amino transferase; formerly SGPT, serum glutamic pyruvic transaminase) greater than 1.8 times the upper limit of normal was not higher in the Aprotinin treated group compared to the placebo group. Among the repeat CABG patients, the percent of subjects developing an elevation of ALT of this magnitude was significantly higher in the Aprotinin treated group. This suggests an indirect effect possibly related to the risk of repeated surgery and attendant myocardial dysfunction rather than a primary drug effect. There were no differences between drug treated and placebo groups in the incidence of elevated ALT greater than 3.0 times the upper limit of normal.

Serum Creatine Kinase (CK): There was a trend toward an increased incidence of elevated serum creatine kinase (CK) with increased MB fractions in Aprotinin treated patients.

Partial Thromboplastin Time (PTT) and Activated Clotting Time (ACT): Significant elevations in the partial thromboplastin time (PTT) and activated clotting time (ACT) in Aprotinin treated patients are expected in the hours after surgery due to circulating concentrations of Aprotinin which are known to inhibit activation of the intrinsic clotting system by contact with a foreign surface, a method used in these tests (see *"Laboratory Monitoring of Anticoagulation During Cardiopulmonary Bypass"*).

Hypersensitivity and Anaphylaxia: Anaphylactic reactions in patients receiving Aprotinin have been reported in less than 0.5% of cases in post-marketing experience outside the U.S. Such reactions are more likely to occur with repeated administration. The following table describes the reported incidence of anaphylactic reactions with Aprotinin treatment.

REPORTED INCIDENCE OF ANAPHYLAXIS WITH APROTININ TREATMENT

	No prior Aprotinin exposure		Prior Aprotinin exposure	
	total	fatal	total	fatal
U.S. controlled studies	0/398	0/398	0/0	0/0
Foreign controlled studies	7/1996	1/1996	0/0	0/0
U.S. open studies	0/299	0/299	1/6	1/6
Foreign open studies	3/1873	1/1873	1*	0/0
Foreign marketing	5/140,000	1/140,000	13/7000	4/7000

* *patient was treated a second time in violation of study protocol*

The symptoms of hypersensitivity-type reactions can range from skin eruptions, itching, dyspnea, nausea and tachycardia to fatal anaphylactic shock with circulatory failure. If hypersensitivity reactions occur during injection or infusion, administration should be stopped immediately. Emergency treatment should be initiated.

OVERDOSAGE

The maximum amount of Aprotinin that can be safely administered in single or multiple doses has not been determined. Doses up to 17.5 million KIU have been administered within a 24 hour period without any apparent toxicity. There is one poorly documented case, however, of a patient who received a large, but not well determined, amount of Aprotinin (in excess of 15 million KIU) in 24 hours. The patient, who had pre-existing liver dysfunction, developed hepatic and renal failure postoperatively and died. Autopsy showed hepatic necrosis and extensive renal tubular and glomerular necrosis. The relationship of these findings to Aprotinin therapy is unclear.

DOSAGE AND ADMINISTRATION

Aprotinin given prophylactically in both dose regimens A and B to high-risk patients undergoing repeat CABG surgery significantly reduced the donor blood transfusion requirement relative to placebo treatment. The experience with the lower dose of Aprotinin Regimen B (see *"Clinical Trials"*) is, however, limited. Regimen A appeared more effective than Regimen B in patients given aspirin preoperatively.

Aprotinin is supplied as a solution containing 10,000 KIU/mL, which is equal to 1.4 mg/mL. All intravenous doses of Aprotinin should be administered through a central line. **DO NOT ADMINISTER ANY OTHER DRUG USING THE SAME LINE.** Both regimens include a 1 mL test dose, a loading dose, a dose to be added to the priming fluid of the cardiopulmonary bypass circuit ("pump prime" dose), and a constant infusion dose. Regimen A is described in the table below:

Test Dose	Loading Dose	*"Pump Prime" Dose*	Constant Infusion Dose
1 mL (1.4mg, or 10,000 KIU)	200 mL (280mg, or 2.0 million KIU)	200 mL (280mg, or 2.0 million KIU)	50 mL/hr (70mg/hr or 500,000 KIU/ hr)

The 1 mL test dose should be administered intravenously at least 10 minutes before the loading dose. With the patient in a supine position, the loading dose is given slowly over 20-30 minutes, after induction of anesthesia but prior to sternotomy. When the loading dose is complete, it is followed by the constant infusion dose, which is continued until surgery is complete and the patient leaves the operating room. The "pump prime" dose is added to the priming fluid of the cardiopulmonary bypass circuit, by replacement of an aliquot of the priming fluid, prior to the institution of cardiopulmonary bypass. Total doses of more than 7 million KIU have not been studied in controlled trials.

Renal and Hepatic Impairment: No formal studies of the pharmacokinetics of Aprotinin in patients with pre-existing renal insufficiency have been conducted. However, in the placebo-controlled clinical trials conducted in the United States, patients with mildly elevated pretreatment serum creatinine levels did not have a notably higher incidence of clinically significant post-treatment elevations in serum creatinine following Aprotinin Regimen A compared to administration of placebo. Changes in Aprotinin pharmacokinetics with age or impaired renal function are not great enough to require any dose adjustment. No pharmacokinetic data from patients with pre-existing hepatic disease treated with Aprotinin are available.

Parenteral drug products should be inspected visually for particulate matter and discoloration prior to administration whenever solution and container permit. Discard any unused portion.

COMPATIBILITY

Aprotinin is incompatible *in vitro* with corticosteroids, heparin, tetracyclines, and nutrient solutions containing amino acids or fat emulsion. If Aprotinin is to be given concomitantly with another drug, each drug should be administered separately through different venous lines or catheters.

STORAGE

Aprotinin should be stored between 2° and 25°C (36°-77°F).
Protect from freezing.

HOW SUPPLIED
INJECTION: 10,000 KIU/ML

BRAND/MANUFACTURER	NDC	SIZE	AWP
○ **BRAND**			
TRASYLOL: Miles Pharm	00026-8196-36	100 ml	$180.00
	00026-8197-63	200 ml	$360.00

Aquachloral Supprettes *SEE* CHLORAL HYDRATE

Aquamephyton *SEE* PHYTONADIONE

Aquasol A *SEE* VITAMIN A

Aquatensen *SEE* METHYCLOTHIAZIDE

◆ RATED THERAPEUTICALLY EQUIVALENT; ◇ THERAPEUTIC EQUIVALENCE UNCONFIRMED; ○ UNRATED

Aralen *SEE* CHLOROQUINE

Aramine *SEE* METARAMINOL BITARTRATE

Arco-Lase Plus *SEE* ATROPINE SULFATE/
HYOSCYAMINE SULFATE/PANCREATIC ENZYMES/PHENOBARBITAL

Arduan *SEE* PIPECURONIUM BROMIDE

Aredia *SEE* PAMIDRONATE DISODIUM

Arfonad *SEE* TRIMETHAPHAN CAMSYLATE

Arginine Hydrochloride

DESCRIPTION
Each 100 mL of Arginine Hydrochloride for intravenous use contains 10 g of L-Arginine Hydrochloride, USP in Water for Injection, USP. L-arginine is a naturally occurring amino acid.

Arginine Hydrochloride is hypertonic (950 mOsmol/liter) and contains 47.5 mEq of chloride ion per 100 mL of solution. The pH is adjusted to 5.6 (5.0-6.5) with Arginine base or Hydrochloric acid.

Following is its chemical structure:

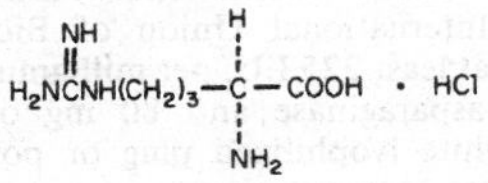

$$H_2NCNH(CH_2)_3 - C - COOH \cdot HCl$$

CLINICAL PHARMACOLOGY
Intravenous infusion of Arginine Hydrochloride often induces a pronounced rise in the plasma level of human growth hormone (HGH) in subjects with intact pituitary function. This rise is usually diminished or absent in patients with impairment of this function.

EXPECTED PLASMA LEVELS OF HGH IN NG/ML

Patient	Control Range	Range of Peak Response to Arginine
Normal	0-6	10-30
Pituitary deficient	0-4	0-10

These ranges are based on the mean values of plasma HGH levels calculated from the data of several clinical investigators and reflect their experiences with various methods of radioimmunoassay. Upon gaining experience with this diagnostic test, each clinician will establish his/her own ranges for control and peak levels of HGH.

L-arginine is a normal metabolite in animals and man and has a low order of toxicity.

INDICATIONS AND USAGE
Arginine Hydrochloride is indicated as an intravenous stimulant to the pituitary for the release of human growth hormone in patients where the measurement of pituitary reserve for HGH can be of diagnostic usefulness. It can be used as a diagnostic aid in such conditions as panhypopituitarism, pituitary dwarfism, chromophobe adenoma, postsurgical craniopharyngioma, hypophysectomy, pituitary trauma, acromegaly, gigantism and problems of growth and stature.

If the insulin hypoglycemia test has indicated a deficiency of pituitary reserve for HGH, a test with Arginine Hydrochloride is advisable to confirm the negative response. This can be done after a waiting period of one day. As patients may not respond to Arginine Hydrochloride during the first test, the unresponsive patient should be tested again to confirm the negative result. A second test can be performed after a waiting period of one day. Some patients who respond to Arginine Hydrochloride do not respond to insulin and vice versa. The rate of false positive responses for Arginine Hydrochloride is approximately 32%, and the rate of false negatives is approximately 27%.

UNLABELED USES
Arginine Hydrochloride is used alone or as an adjunct in the treatment of liver disease associated with elevated blood ammonia levels in patients with hepatic encephalopathy. It is also used as a diagnostic test in diabetes mellitus and in identification of distal renal tubular acidosis.

CONTRAINDICATIONS
The administration of Arginine Hydrochloride is contraindicated in persons having highly allergic tendencies.

WARNINGS
Arginine Hydrochloride should always be administered by intravenous injection because of its hypertonicity.

A suitable antihistaminic drug should be available in the event that an allergic reaction occurs.

Arginine Hydrochloride is a diagnostic aid and is not intended for therapeutic use.

PRECAUTIONS
GENERAL
Arginine Hydrochloride is a hypertonic (950 mOsmol/liter) and acidic (average pH of 5.6) solution that can irritate tissues. Care should be used to insure administration of Arginine Hydrochloride through a patent catheter within a patent vein. Excessive rates of infusion may result in local irritation and in flushing, nausea, or vomiting. Inadequate dosing or prolongation of the infusion period may diminish the stimulus to the pituitary and nullify the test.

The Arginine in Arginine Hydrochloride can be metabolized resulting in nitrogen-containing products for excretion. The effect of an acute amino acid or nitrogen burden upon patients with impairment of renal function should be considered when Arginine Hydrochloride is to be administered.

The chloride content of Arginine Hydrochloride is 47.5 mEq per 100 mL of solution, and the effect of infusing this amount of chloride into patients with electrolyte imbalance should be evaluated before the test is undertaken.

It should be noted that the basal and post-stimulation levels of growth hormone are elevated in patients who are pregnant or are taking oral contraceptives.

CARCINOGENESIS, MUTAGENESIS, AND IMPAIRMENT OF FERTILITY
Long term animal studies have not been performed to evaluate the carcinogenic potential, the mutagenic potential or the effect on fertility of intravenously administered Arginine Hydrochloride.

PREGNANCY CATEGORY B
Reproduction studies have been performed in rabbits and mice at doses 12 times the human dose and have revealed no evidence of impaired fertility or harm to the fetus due to Arginine Hydrochloride. There have been no adequate or well controlled studies for the use of Arginine Hydrochloride in pregnant women. Because animal reproduction studies are not always predictive of human response, this drug should not be used during pregnancy.

Nursing Mothers: It is not known whether intravenous adminstration of Arginine Hydrochloride could result in significant quantities of Arginine in breast milk. Systematically administered amino acids are secreted into breast milk in quantities not likely to have a deleterious effect on the infant. Nevertheless, caution should be exercised when Arginine Hydrochloride is to be administered to nursing women.

ADVERSE REACTIONS
Adverse reactions associated with 1670 infusions in premarketing studies were as follows:

Nonspecific side effects consisting of nausea, vomiting, headache, flushing, numbness and local venous irritation were reported in approximately 3% of the patients.

One patient had an allergic reaction which was manifested as a confluent macular rash with reddening and swelling of the hands and face. The rash subsided rapidly after the infusion was terminated and 50 mg of diphenhydramine were administered. One patient had an apparent decrease in platelet count from 150,000 to 60,000. One patient with a history of acrocyanosis had an exacerbation of this condition following infusion of Arginine Hydrochloride.

OVERDOSAGE
An overdosage may cause a transient metabolic acidosis with hyperventilation. The acidosis will be compensated and the base deficit will return to normal following completion of the infusion. If the condition persists, the deficit should be determined and corrected by a calculated dose of an alkalizing agent.

DOSAGE AND ADMINISTRATION
The intravenous dose for adults is 300 mL (30 g Arginine Hydrochloride). The intravenous dose for children is 5 mL (0.5 g Arginine Hydrochloride) per kilogram of body weight.

The intravenous infusion of Arginine Hydrochloride is a part of the test for measurement of pituitary reserve of human growth hormone and, for successful administration of the test, clinical conditions and procedures should be as follows:

1. The test should be scheduled in the morning following a normal night's sleep, and an overnight fast should continue through the test period.
2. Patients must be placed at bed rest for at least 30 minutes before the infusion begins. Care should be taken to minimize apprehension and distress. This is particularly important in children.
3. Arginine Hydrochloride should be infused through an indwelling needle or soft catheter placed in an antecubital vein or other suitable vein. Blood samples should be taken by venipuncture from the contra-lateral arm.
4. A desirable schedule for drawing blood samples is at −30, 0, 30, 60, 90, 120 and 150 minutes.

5. Arginine Hydrochloride should be infused beginning at zero time at a uniform rate which will permit the recommended dose to be administered in 30 minutes.

6. Blood samples should be promptly centrifuged and the plasma stored at −20°C until assayed by one of the published radioimmunoassay procedures.

7. Diagnostic test results showing a deficiency of pituitary reserve for HGH should be confirmed by a second test with Arginine Hydrochloride or one may elect to confirm with the insulin hypoglycemia test. A waiting period of one day is advised between tests.

Parenteral drug products should be inspected visually for particulate matter and discoloration prior to administration whenever solution and container permit.

Exposure of pharmaceutical products to heat should be minimized. Avoid excessive heat. It is recommended that the product be stored at room temperature (25°C); however, brief exposure up to 40°C does not adversely affect the product. Solution that has been frozen must not be used.

DIRECTIONS FOR USE OF I.V. CONTAINER

The important feature of this container is that **it is a closed system**. That is, **no** unfiltered air comes in contact with the solution. The spike is thrust through a solid stopper, the air enters through a bacterial air filter, and only filtered air enters the bottle then or during the infusion. The rubber stopper surface beneath the metal seal is sterile.

A special air-inletting, air-filtering set with a bacterial air filter is required. **No airway needle is needed.**

1. Use only if solution is clear and seal is intact: Carefully examine bottle for evidence of damage, e.g., dents or other evidence of damage to metal cap, small cracks, dents in seal, or areas of dried powder on exterior. **Do not administer contents if such damage is found.** Also check for safe assembly of bail and band.

2. Remove tamperproof metal seal and metal disc from bottle to expose rubber stopper, taking care that you do not contaminate the target site of the stopper with fingers, hair, clothing, etc. **Immediately perform step #3.**

3. With shut-off clamp closed, remove sterility protector from spike of administration set and immediately insert set with a quick thrust into center of stopper with bottle upright on table. (Push straight in—don't twist—twisting may cause stopper coring.)

4. Promptly invert bottle to automatically establish fluid level in drip chamber and to check for vacuum by observing rising filtered air bubbles. *Discard bottle if there is no vacuum or if the solution is not clear.*

5. Clear tubing of air. Proceed with infusion.

Caution: While the top of the rubber stopper is sterile, as soon as the seal and disc are removed the stopper is exposed. The longer the time between removal of the seal and disc and the piercing of the stopper, the greater the chance of contamination of the stopper.

Note: When medication is to be added to the bottle:

A. See #1 and #2 above.

B. Add medications before attaching administration set. Vacuum should be observed at this point, by sucking in of additive container content, since vacuum may be lost during this procedure and not observable during administration set insertion.

C. If medications have been placed in bottle through stopper, it is recommended that the face of the stopper be swabbed immediately before piercing with administration set.

CONTINUED USE OF SOLUTIONS AND SETS

Procedure differs with every hospital for the length of time solutions and administration sets may be used continuously. Some recommend change of both every 8 hours, others recommend change of both every 24 hours, and others recommend change of solutions every 8 hours and change of sets every 24 hours. The shorter the period of use the less the possibility of multiplication of organisms inadvertently introduced.

HOW SUPPLIED
INJECTION: 10%

BRAND/MANUFACTURER	NDC	SIZE	AWP
○ BRAND			
R-GENE 10: Pharmacia	00601-0436-24	300 ml 10s	$1062.50

Aristocort *SEE* TRIAMCINOLONE, TRIAMCINOLONE ACETONIDE, TOPICAL *AND* TRIAMCINOLONE DIACETATE

Aristospan Injection *SEE* TRIAMCINOLONE HEXACETONIDE

Armour Thyroid *SEE* THYROID

Artane *SEE* TRIHEXYPHENIDYL HYDROCHLORIDE

Asacol *SEE* MESALAMINE

Asbron G *SEE* GUAIFENESIN AND THEOPHYLLINE

Asendin *SEE* AMOXAPINE

Asparaginase

> **WARNING**
>
> IT IS RECOMMENDED THAT ASPARGINASE BE ADMINISTERED TO PATIENTS ONLY IN A HOSPITAL SETTING UNDER THE SUPERVISION OF A PHYSICIAN WHO IS QUALIFIED BY TRAINING AND EXPERIENCE TO ADMINISTER CANCER CHEMOTHERAPEUTIC AGENTS, BECAUSE OF THE POSSIBILITY OF SEVERE REACTIONS, INCLUDING ANAPHYLAXIS AND SUDDEN DEATH. THE PHYSICIAN MUST BE PREPARED TO TREAT ANAPHYLAXIS AT EACH ADMINISTRATION OF THE DRUG.
>
> IN THE TREATMENT OF EACH PATIENT THE PHYSICIAN MUST WEIGH CAREFULLY THE POSSIBILITY OF ACHIEVING THERAPEUTIC BENEFIT VERSUS THE RISK OF TOXICITY. THE FOLLOWING DATA SHOULD BE THOROUGHLY REVIEWED BEFORE ADMINISTERING THE COMPOUND.

DESCRIPTION

Asparaginase contains the enzyme L-asparagine amidohydrolase, type EC-2, derived from *Escherichia coli.* It is a white crystalline powder that is freely soluble in water and practically insoluble in methanol, acetone and chloroform. Its activity is expressed in terms of International Units (I.U.) according to the recommendation of the International Union of Biochemistry. The specific activity of Asparaginase is at least 225 I.U. per milligram of protein and each vial contains 10,000 I.U. of asparaginase and 80 mg of mannitol, an inactive ingredient, as a sterile, white lyophilized plug or powder for intravenous or intramuscular injection after reconstitution.

CLINICAL PHARMACOLOGY
ACTION

In a significant number of patients with acute leukemia, particularly lymphocytic, the malignant cells are dependent on an exogenous source of asparagine for survival. Normal cells, however, are able to synthesize asparagine and thus are affected less by the rapid depletion produced by treatment with the enzyme asparaginase. This is a unique approach to therapy based on a metabolic defect in asparagine synthesis of some malignant cells. Asparaginase, derived from *Escherichia coli,* is effective in inducing remissions in some patients with acute lymphocytic leukemia.

ASPARAGINE DEPENDENCE TEST

An asparagine dependence test has been utilized during the investigational studies. In this test leukemic cells obtained from some marrow cultures could be shown to require asparagine *in vitro,* suggesting sensitivity to asparaginase therapy *in vivo.* However, present data indicate that the correlation between asparagine dependence in such tests and the final response to therapy is sufficiently poor that the test is not recommended as a basis for selection of patients for treatment.

PHARMACOKINETICS AND METABOLISM

In a study in patients with metastatic cancer and leukemia, initial plasma levels of L-asparaginase following intravenous administration were correlated to dose. Daily administration resulted in a cumulative increase in plasma levels.

Plasma half-life varied from 8 to 30 hours; it did not appear to be influenced by dosage, either single or repetitive, and could not be correlated with age, sex, surface area, renal or hepatic function, diagnosis or extent of disease. Apparent volume of distribution was approximately 70–80% of estimated plasma volume. There was some slow movement of asparaginase from vascular to extravascular, extracellular space. L-asparaginase was detected in the lymph. Cerebrospinal fluid levels were less than 1% of concurrent plasma levels. Only trace amounts appeared in the urine.

In a study in which patients with leukemia and metastatic cancer received intramuscular L-asparaginase, peak plasma levels of asparaginase were reached 14 to 24 hours after dosing. Plasma half-life was 39 to 49 hours. No asparaginase was detected in the urine.

INDICATIONS AND USAGE

Asparaginase is indicated in the therapy of patients with acute lymphocytic leukemia. This agent is useful primarily in combination with other chemotherapeutic agents in the induction of remissions of the disease in children. Asparaginase should not be used as the sole induction agent unless combination therapy is deemed inappropriate. Asparaginase is not recommended for maintenance therapy.

◆ RATED THERAPEUTICALLY EQUIVALENT; ◇ THERAPEUTIC EQUIVALENCE UNCONFIRMED; ○ UNRATED

UNLABELED USES
Asparaginase is used as an adjunct in the treatment of acute nonlymphocytic leukemia (ANLL).

CONTRAINDICATIONS
Asparaginase is contraindicated in patients with pancreatitis or a history of pancreatitis. Acute hemorrhagic pancreatitis, in some instances fatal, has been reported following Asparaginase administration. Asparaginase is also contraindicated in patients who have had previous anaphylactic reactions to it.

WARNINGS
Allergic reactions to Asparaginase are frequent and may occur during the primary course of therapy. They are not completely predictable on the basis of the intradermal skin test. Anaphylaxis and death have occurred even in a hospital setting with experienced observers.

Once a patient has received Asparaginase as part of a treatment regimen, retreatment with this agent at a later time is associated with increased risk of hypersensitivity reactions. In patients found by skin testing to be hypersensitive to asparaginase, and in any patient who has received a previous course of therapy with Asparaginase, therapy with this agent should be instituted or reinstituted only after successful desensitization, and then only if in the judgement of the physician the possible benefit is greater than the increased risk. Desensitization itself may be hazardous. (See "Dosage and Administration, Intradermal Skin Test.")

In view of the unpredictability of the adverse reactions to Asparaginase, it is recommended that this product be used in a hospital setting. Asparaginase has an adverse effect on liver function in the majority of patients. Therapy with Asparaginase may increase pre-existing liver impairment caused by prior therapy or the underlying disease. Because of this there is a possibility that asparaginase may increase the toxicity of other medications.

The administration of Asparaginase *intravenously concurrently with or immediately before* a course of vincristine and prednisone may be associated with increased toxicity. (See "Dosage and Administration, Recommended Induction Regimens.")

PRECAUTIONS
GENERAL
This drug may be a contact irritant and both powder and solution must be handled and administered with care. Inhalation of dust or vapors and contact with skin or mucous membranes, especially those of the eyes, must be avoided. In case of contact, wash with copious amounts of water for at least 15 minutes.

Asparaginase has been reported to have immunosuppressive activity in animal experiments. Accordingly, the possibility that use of the drug in man may predispose to infection should be considered.

Asparaginase toxicity is reported to be greater in adults than in children.

LABORATORY TESTS
The fall in circulating lymphoblasts often is quite marked; normal or below normal leukocyte counts are noted frequently within the first several days after initiating therapy. This may be accompanied by a marked rise in serum uric acid. The possible development of uric acid nephropathy should be borne in mind. Appropriate preventive measures should be taken, e.g., allopurinol, increased fluid intake, alkalization of urine. As a guide to the effects of therapy, the patient's peripheral blood count and bone marrow should be monitored frequently.

Frequent serum amylase determinations should be obtained to detect early evidence of pancreatitis. If pancreatitis occurs, therapy should be stopped and not reinstituted.

Blood sugar should be monitored during therapy with Asparaginase because hyperglycemia may occur.

DRUG INTERACTIONS
Tissue culture and animal studies indicate that Asparaginase can diminish or abolish the effect of methotrexate on malignant cells. This effect on methotrexate activity persists as long as plasma asparagine levels are suppressed. These results would seem to dictate against the clinical use of methotroxate with Asparaginase or during the period following Asparaginase therapy when plasma asparagine levels are below normal.

DRUG/LABORATORY TEST INTERACTIONS
L-asparaginase has been reported to interfere with the interpretation of thyroid function tests by producing a rapid and marked reduction in serum concentrations of thyroxine-binding globulin within two days after the first dose. Serum concentrations of thyroxine-binding globulin returned to pretreatment values within four weeks of the last dose of L-asparaginase.

ANIMAL TOXICOLOGY
A one-month intravenous toxicity study of Asparaginase in dogs at doses of 250, 1000, and 2000 I.U./kg/day revealed reduced serum total protein and albumin with loss of body weight at the highest dose level and anorexia, emesis, and diarrhea at all dosage levels. A similar study in monkeys at doses of 100, 300, and 1000 I.U./kg/day also revealed reduction of serum total protein and albumin and body weight loss at all dosage levels. Bromsulfalein retention and fatty changes in the liver were noted in monkeys that were given 300 and 1000 I.U./kg/day. The rabbit was unusually sensitive to Asparaginase since a single intravenous dose of 1000 I.U./kg caused hypocalcemia associated with necrosis of the parathyroid cells, convulsions, and death in about one third of the animals. Some rabbits that died showed small thymic and lymph node hemorrhages and necrosis of the germinal centers in the lymph nodes and spleen. The intravenous administration of calcium gluconate alleviated or prevented the adverse effects.

Changes in the pancreatic islets (not pancreatitis) ranging from edema to necrosis were observed in the rabbits in the acute intravenous toxicity studies (doses of 12,500 to 50,000 I.U./kg) but not in rabbits that received 1000 I.U./kg. The anatomical changes and the hypocalcemia found in the rabbits were not observed in the subacute intravenous studies in the dogs and monkeys.

CARCINOGENESIS, MUTAGENESIS, IMPAIRMENT OF FERTILITY
The intraperitoneal injection of 2500 I.U./kg/day for 4 days in newborn Swiss mice resulted in a small increase in pulmonary adenomas; lymphatic leukemia was not increased.

L-asparaginase at concentrations of 152-909 I.U./plate was not mutagenic in the Ames microbial mutagen test with or without metabolic activation.

There are no adequate studies on the effects of Asparaginase on fertility.

PREGNANCY
Pregnancy Category C. In mice and rats Asparaginase has been shown to retard the weight gain of mothers and fetuses when given in doses of more than 1000 I.U./kg (the recommended human dose). Resorptions, gross abnormalities and skeletal abnormalities were observed. The intravenous administration of 50 or 100 I.U./kg (one-twentieth or one-tenth of the human dose) to pregnant rabbits on Day 8 and 9 of gestation resulted in dose dependent embryotoxicity and gross abnormalities. There are no adequate and well-controlled studies in pregnant women. Asparaginase should be used during pregnancy only if the potential benefit justifies the potential risk to the fetus.

NURSING MOTHERS
It is not known whether this drug is secreted in human milk. Because many drugs are secreted in human milk and because of the potential for serious adverse reactions in nursing infants from Asparaginase, a decision should be made whether to discontinue nursing or to discontinue the drug, taking into account the importance of the drug to the mother.

ADVERSE REACTIONS
Allergic reactions, including skin rashes, urticaria, arthralgia, respiratory distress, and acute anaphylaxis have been reported. (See "Warnings.") Acute reactions have occurred in the absence of a positive skin test and during continued maintenance of therapeutic serum levels of Asparaginase. In children with advanced leukemia, a lower incidence of anaphylaxis has been reported with intramuscular administration, although there was a higher incidence of milder hypersensitivity reactions than with intravenous administration.

Fatal hyperthermia has been reported.

Pancreatitis, sometimes fulminant and fatal, has occurred during or following therapy with Asparaginase.

Hyperglycemia with glucosuria and polyuria has been reported in low incidence. Serum and urine acetone usually have been absent or negligible in these patients; this syndrome thus resembles hyperosmolar, nonketotic, hyperglycemia induced by a variety of other agents. This complication usually responds to discontinuance of Asparaginase, judicious use of intravenous fluid, and insulin, but may be fatal on occasion.

In addition to hypofibrinogenemia, depression of various other clotting factors has been reported. Most marked has been a decrease in plasma levels of factors V and VIII with a variable decrease in factors VII and IX. A decrease in circulating platelets has occurred in low incidence which, together with the increased levels of fibrin degradation products in the serum, may indicate development of a consumption coagulopathy. Bleeding has been a problem in only a minority of patients with demonstrable coagulopathy. However, intracranial hemorrhage and fatal bleeding associated with low fibrinogen levels have been reported. Increased fibrinolytic activity, apparently compensatory in nature, also has occurred.

Some patients have shown central nervous system effects consisting of depression, somnolence, fatigue, coma, confusion, agitation, and hallucinations varying from mild to severe. Rarely, a Parkinson-like syndrome has occurred, with tremor and a progressive increase in muscular tone. These side effects usually have reversed spontaneously after treatment was stopped. Therapy with Asparaginase is associated with an increase in blood ammonia during the conversion of asparagine to aspartic acid by the enzyme. No clear correlation exists between the degree of elevation of blood ammonia levels and the appearance of CNS changes. Chills, fever, nausea, vomiting, anorexia, abdominal cramps, weight loss, headache, and irritability may occur and usually are mild.

Azotemia, usually pre-renal, occurs frequently. Acute renal shut down and fatal renal insufficiency have been reported during treatment: Proteinuria has occurred infrequently.

A variety of liver function abnormalities have been reported, including elevations of SGOT, SGPT, alkaline phosphatase, bilirubin (direct and indirect), and depression of serum albumin, cholesterol (total and esters), and plasma fibrinogen.

Increases and decreases of total lipids have occurred. Marked hypoalbuminemia associated with peripheral edema has been reported. However, these abnormalities usually are reversible on discontinuance of therapy and some reversal may occur during the course of therapy. Fatty changes in the liver have been documented by biopsy. Malabsorption syndrome has been reported.

Rarely, transient bone marrow depression has been observed, as evidenced by a delay in return of hemoglobin or hematocrit levels to normal in patients undergoing hematologic remission of leukemia. Marked leukopenia has been reported.

OVERDOSAGE

The acute intravenous LD$_{50}$ of Asparaginase for mice was about 500,000 I.U./kg and for rabbits about 22,000 I.U./kg.

DOSAGE AND ADMINISTRATION

As a component of selected multiple agent induction regimens, Asparaginase may be administered by either the intravenous or the intramuscular route. When administered intravenously this enzyme should be given over a period of not less than thirty minutes through the side arm of an already running infusion of Sodium Chloride Injection or Dextrose Injection 5% (D$_5$W). Asparaginase has little tendency to cause phlebitis when given intravenously. Anaphylactic reactions require the immediate use of epinephrine, oxygen, and intravenous steroids.

When administering Asparaginase intramuscularly, the volume at a single injection site should be limited to 2 ml. If a volume greater than 2 ml is to be administered, two injection sites should be used.

Unfavorable interactions of Asparaginase with some antitumor agents have been demonstrated. It is recommended therefore, that Asparaginase be used in combination regimens only by physicians familiar with the benefits and risks of a given regimen. During the period of its inhibition of protein synthesis and cell replication Asparaginase may interfere with the action of drugs such as methotrexate which require cell replication for their lethal effect. Asparaginase may interfere with the enzymatic detoxification of other drugs, particularly in the liver.

RECOMMENDED INDUCTION REGIMENS

When using chemotherapeutic agents in combination for the induction of remissions in patients with acute lymphocytic leukemia, regimens are sought which provide maximum chance of success while avoiding excessive cumulative toxicity or negative drug interactions.

One of the following combination regimens incorporating Asparaginase is recommended for acute lymphocytic leukemia in children:

In the regimens below, Day 1 is considered to be the first day of therapy.

REGIMEN I

Prednisone: 40 mg/square meter of body surface area per day orally in three divided doses for 15 days, followed by tapering of the dosage as follows:
20 mg/square meter for 2 days, 10 mg/square meter for 2 days, 5 mg/square meter for 2 days, 2.5 mg/square meter for 2 days and then discontinue.

Vincristine Sulfate: 2 mg/square meter of body surface area intravenously once weekly on Days 1, 8, and 15 of the treatment period. The maximum single dose should not exceed 2.0 mg.

Asparaginase: 1,000 I.U./kg/day intravenously for ten successive days beginning on Day 22 of the treatment period.

REGIMEN II

Prednisone: 40 mg/square meter of body surface area per day orally in three divided doses for 28 days (the total daily dose should be to the nearest 2.5 mg), following which the dosage of prednisone should be discontinued gradually over a 14 day period.

Vincristine Sulfate: 1.5 mg/square meter of body surface area intravenously weekly for four doses, on Days 1, 8, 15, and 22 of the treatment period. The maximum single dose should not exceed 2.0 mg.

Asparaginase: 6,000 I.U./square meter of body surface area intramuscularly on Days 4, 7, 10, 13, 16, 19, 22, 25, and 28 of the treatment period. When a remission is obtained with either of the above regimens, appropriate maintenance therapy must be instituted. Asparaginase should not be used as part of a maintenance regimen. The above regimens do not preclude a need for special therapy directed toward the prevention of central nervous system leukemia.

It should be noted that Asparaginase has been used in combination regimens other than those recommended above. It is important to keep in mind that Asparaginase administered intravenously concurrently with or immediately before a course of vincristine and prednisone may be associated with increased toxicity. Physicians using a given regimen should be thoroughly familiar with its benefits and risks. Clinical data are insufficient for a recommendation concerning the use of combination regimens in adults. Asparaginase toxicity is reported to be greater in adults than in children.

Use of Asparaginase as the sole induction agent should be undertaken only in an unusual situation when a combined regimen is inappropriate because of toxicity or other specific patient-related factors, or in cases refractory to other therapy. When Asparaginase is to be used as the sole induction agent for children or adults the recommended dosage regimen is 200 I.U./kg/day intravenously for 28 days. When complete remissions were obtained with this regimen, they were of short duration, 1 to 3 months. Asparaginase has been used as the sole induction agent in other regimens. Physicians using a given regimen should be thoroughly familiar with its benefits and risks.

Patients undergoing induction therapy must be carefully monitored and the therapeutic regimen adjusted according to response and toxicity.

Such adjustments should always involve decreasing dosages of one or more agents or discontinuation depending on the degree of toxicity. Patients who have received a course of Asparaginase, if retreated, have an increased risk of hypersensitivity reactions. Therefore, retreatment should be undertaken only when the benefit of such therapy is weighed against the increased risk.

INTRADERMAL SKIN TEST

Because of the occurrence of allergic reactions, an intradermal skin test should be performed prior to the initial administration of Asparaginase and when Asparaginase is given after an interval of a week or more has elapsed between doses. The skin test solution may be prepared as follows: Reconstitute the contents of a 10,000 I.U. vial with 5.0 ml of diluent. From this solution (2,000 I.U./ml) withdraw 0.1 ml and inject it into another vial containing 9.9 ml of diluent, yielding a skin test solution of approximately 20.0 I.U./ml. Use 0.1 ml of this solution (about 2.0 I.U.) for the intradermal skin test. The skin test site should be observed for at least one hour for the appearance of a wheal or erythema either of which indicates a positive reaction. An allergic reaction even to the skin test dose in certain sensitized individuals may rarely occur. A negative skin test reaction does not preclude the possibility of the development of an allergic reaction.

DESENSITIZATION:

DESENSITIZATION SHOULD BE PERFORMED BEFORE ADMINISTERING THE FIRST DOSE OF ASPARAGINASE IN INITIATION OF THERAPY IN POSITIVE REACTORS, AND ON RETREATMENT OF ANY PATIENT IN WHOM SUCH THERAPY IS DEEMED NECESSARY AFTER CAREFULLY WEIGHING THE INCREASED RISK OF HYPERSENSITIVITY REACTIONS. RAPID DESENSITIZATION OF THE PATIENT MAY BE ATTEMPTED WITH PROGRESSIVELY INCREASING AMOUNTS OF INTRAVENOUSLY ADMINISTERED ASPARAGINASE PROVIDED ADEQUATE PRECAUTIONS ARE TAKEN TO TREAT AN ACUTE ALLERGIC REACTION SHOULD IT OCCUR. ONE REPORTED SCHEDULE BEGINS WITH A TOTAL OF 1 I.U. GIVEN INTRAVENOUSLY AND DOUBLES THE DOSE EVERY 10 MINUTES, PROVIDED NO REACTION HAS OCCURRED, UNTIL THE ACCUMULATED TOTAL AMOUNT GIVEN EQUALS THE PLANNED DOSES FOR THAT DAY.

FOR CONVENIENCE THE FOLLOWING TABLE IS INCLUDED TO CALCULATE THE NUMBER OF DOSES NECESSARY TO REACH THE PATIENT'S TOTAL DOSE FOR THAT DAY.

Injection Number	Asparaginase Dose in I.U.	Accumulated Total Dose
1	1	1
2	2	3
3	4	7
4	8	15
5	16	31
6	32	63
7	64	127
8	128	255
9	256	511
10	512	1023
11	1024	2047
12	2048	4095
13	4096	8191
14	8192	16383
15	16384	32767
16	32768	65535
17	65536	131071
18	131072	262143

FOR EXAMPLE: A PATIENT WEIGHING 20 KG WHO IS TO RECEIVE 200 I.U./KG (TOTAL DOSE 4000 I.U.) WOULD RECEIVE INJECTIONS 1 THROUGH 12 DURING DESENSITIZATION.

DIRECTIONS FOR RECONSTITUTION

Parenteral drug products should be inspected visually for particulate matter and discoloration prior to administration whenever solution and container permit. When reconstituted Asparaginase should be a clear, colorless solution. If the solution becomes cloudy, discard.

FOR INTRAVENOUS USE

Reconstitute with Sterile Water for Injection or with Sodium Chloride Injection. The volume recommended for reconstitution is 5 ml for the 10,000 unit vials. Ordinary shaking during reconstitution does not inactivate the enzyme. This solution may be used for direct intravenous administration within an eight hour period following restoration. For administration by infusion, solutions should be diluted with the isotonic solutions, Sodium Chloride Injection or Dextrose Injection 5%. These solutions should be infused within eight hours and only if clear.

Occasionally, a very small number of gelatinous fiber-like particles may develop on standing. Filtration through a 5.0 micron filter during administration will remove the particles with no resultant loss in potency. Some loss of potency has been observed with the use of a 0.2 micron filter.

FOR INTRAVASCULAR USE

When Asparaginase is administered intramuscularly according to the schedule cited in the induction regimen, reconstitution is carried out by adding 2 ml Sodium Chloride Injection to the 10,000 unit vial. The resulting solution should be used within eight hours and only if clear.

Personnel preparing Asparaginase should avoid drug contact with skin, mucous membranes, or eyes and avoid inhaling the dust or vapor.

Store at 2–8°C (36-46°F). Asparaginase does not contain a preservative. Unused, reconstituted solution should be stored at 2 to 8°C (36 to 46°F) and discarded after eight hours, or sooner if it becomes cloudy.

J CODES
10,000 units IV,IM—J9020

HOW SUPPLIED
POWDER FOR INJECTION: 10,000 IU

BRAND/MANUFACTURER	NDC	SIZE	AWP
○ **BRAND**			
ELSPAR: Merck	00006-4612-00	1s	$52.38

Aspirin

DESCRIPTION
Aspirin Delayed-release Tablets, USP enteric coated tablets contain 15 grains (975 mg) aspirin for oral administration. The enteric coating is designed to prevent the release of aspirin in the stomach and thereby reduce gastric irritation and total occult blood loss. The pharmacologic effects of aspirin include analgesia, antipyresis, antiinflammatory activity, and antirheumatic activity.

Following is its chemical structure:

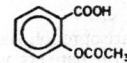

CLINICAL PHARMACOLOGY
Aspirin is a salicylate that has demonstrated antiinflammatory, analgesic, antipyretic, and antirheumatic activity.

Aspirin's mode of action as an antiinflammatory and antirheumatic agent may be due to inhibition of synthesis and release of prostaglandins.

Aspirin appears to produce analgesia by virtue of both a peripheral and CNS effect. Peripherally, Aspirin acts by inhibiting the synthesis and release of prostaglandins. Acting centrally, it would appear to produce analgesia at a hypothalamic site in the brain, although the mode of action is not known.

Aspirin also acts on the hypothalamus to produce antipyresis; heat dissipation is increased as a result of vasodilation and increased peripheral blood flow. Aspirin's antipyretic activity may also be related to inhibition of synthesis and release of prostaglandins.

In a crossover study, Aspirin at a dose of one tablet (15 grains) three times a day produced an average fecal blood loss of 1.54 ml per day. Uncoated Aspirin at a dosage of three 5 grain tablets given three times a day caused an average fecal blood loss of 4.33 ml per day.

Aspirin Tablets are enteric coated. This coating acts to prevent the release of Aspirin in the stomach but permits the tablet to dissolve with resultant absorption in the upper portion of the small intestine. This reduces any gastric irritation that may occur with uncoated aspirin but does delay the onset of action. Aspirin is rapidly hydrolyzed primarily in the liver to salicylic acid, which is conjugated with glycine (forming salicyluric acid) and glucuronic acid and excreted largely in the urine. As a result of the rapid hydrolysis, plasma concentrations of Aspirin are always low and rarely exceed 20 mcg/ml at ordinary therapeutic doses. The peak salicylate level for uncoated Aspirin occurs in about 2 hours; however with enteric coated Aspirin tablets this is delayed. A direct correlation between salicylate plasma levels and clinical analgesic effectiveness has not been definitely established, but effective analgesia is usually achieved at plasma levels of 15 to 30 mg per 100 ml. Effective antiinflammatory activity is usually achieved at salicylate plasma levels of 20 to 30 mg per 100 ml. There is also poor correlation between toxic symptoms and plasma salicylate concentrations, but most patients exhibit symptoms of salicylism at plasma salicylate levels of 35 mg per 100 ml. The plasma half-life for Aspirin is approximately 15 minutes; that for salicylate lengthens as the dose increases: Doses of 300 to 650 mg have a half-life of 3.1 to 3.2 hours; with doses of 1 gram, the half-life is increased to 5 hours and with 2 grams it is increased to about 9 hours.

Salicylates are excreted mainly by the kidney. Studies in man indicate that salicylate is excreted in the urine as free salicylic acid (10%), salicyluric acid (75%), salicylic phenolic (10%), and acyl (5%) glucuronides and gentisic acid.

INDICATIONS AND USAGE
Aspirin is indicated in the long-term palliative treatment of mild to moderate pain and inflammation of arthritic and other inflammatory conditions.

UNLABELED USES
Aspirin is used alone or as an adjunct in the treatment of Kawasaki syndrome, thromboembolism after surgery, and unstable angina.

CONTRAINDICATIONS
Aspirin should not be used in patients who have previously exhibited hypersensitivity to Aspirin and/or nonsteroidal anti-inflammatory agents.

Aspirin should not be given to patients with a recent history of gastrointestinal bleeding or in patients with bleeding disorders (eg, hemophilia).

WARNINGS
Aspirin tablets should be used with caution when anticoagulants are prescribed concurrently, for Aspirin may depress the concentration of prothrombin in plasma and thereby increase bleeding time. Large doses of salicylates have a hypoglycemic action and may enhance the effect of the oral hypoglycemics. Consequently, they should not be given concomitantly; if however, this is necessary, the dosage of the hypoglycemic agent must be reduced while the salicylate is given. This hypoglycemic action may also affect the insulin requirements of diabetics.

Although salicylates in large doses are uricosuric agents, smaller amounts may decrease the uricosuric effects of probenecid, sulfinpyrazone, and phenylbutazone.

PRECAUTIONS
General: Aspirin tablets should be administered with caution to patients with asthma, nasal polyps, or nasal allergies.

In patients receiving large doses of Aspirin and/or prolonged therapy, mild salicylate intoxication (salicylism) may develop that may be reversed by reduction in dosage.

Although the fecal blood loss with coated Aspirin is less than that with uncoated Aspirin tablets, the coated tablets should be administered with caution to patients with a history of gastric distress, ulcer, or bleeding problems. Occult gastrointestinal bleeding occurs in many patients but is not correlated with gastric distress. The amount of blood lost is usually insignificant clinically, but with prolonged administration, it may result in iron deficiency anemia.

Sodium excretion produced by spironolactone may be decreased in the presence of salicylates.

Salicylates can produce changes in thyroid function tests.

Salicylates should be used with caution in patients with severe hepatic damage, preexisting hypoprothrombinemia, or Vitamin K deficiency, and in those undergoing surgery.

DRUG INTERACTIONS
Anticoagulants: See "Warnings".

Hypoglycemic Agents: See "Warnings".

Uricosuric Agents: Aspirin may decrease the effects of probenecid, sulfinpyrazone, and phenylbutazone.

Spironolactone: See *"General Precautions"* above.

Alcohol: Has a synergistic effect with Aspirin in causing gastrointestinal bleeding.

Corticosteroids: Concomitant administration with Aspirin may increase the risk of gastrointestinal ulceration and may reduce serum salicylate levels.

Pyrazolone Derivatives (phenylbutazone, oxyphenbutazone, and possibly dipyrone): Concomitant administration with Aspirin may increase the risk of gastrointestinal ulceration.

Nonsteroidal Anti-inflammatory Agents: Aspirin is contraindicated in patients who are hypersensitive to nonsteroidal anti-inflammatory agents.

Urinary Alkalinizers: Decrease Aspirin effectiveness by increasing the rate of salicylate renal excretion.

Phenobarbital: Decreases Aspirin effectiveness by enzyme induction.

Phenytoin: Serum phenytoin levels may be increased by Aspirin.

Propranolol: May decrease Aspirin's anti-inflammatory action by competing for the same receptors.

Antacids: Aspirin should not be given concurrently with antacids, since an increase in the pH of the stomach may affect the enteric coating of the tablets.

Usage in Pregnancy: It has been reported that adverse effects were increased in the mother and fetus following chronic ingestion of Aspirin. Prolonged pregnancy and labor with increased bleeding before and after delivery, as well as decreased birth weight and increased rate of stillbirth were correlated with high blood salicylate levels. Because of possible adverse effects on the neonate and the potential for increased maternal blood loss, Aspirin should be avoided during the last three months of pregnancy.

ADVERSE REACTIONS
Gastrointestinal: Dyspepsia, thirst, nausea, vomiting, diarrhea, acute reversible hepatotoxicity, gastrointestinal bleeding, and/or ulceration.

Special Senses: Tinnitus, vertigo, reversible hearing loss and dimness of vision.

Hematologic: Prolongation of bleeding time, leukopenia, thrombocytopenia, purpura, decreased plasma iron concentration and shortened erythrocyte survival time.

Dermatologic and Hypersensitivity: Urticaria, angioedema, pruritus, sweating, various skin eruptions, asthma, and anaphylaxis.

Neurologic: Mental confusion, drowsiness and dizziness.

Body as a Whole: Headache and fever.

OVERDOSAGE
Overdosage of 200 to 500 mg/kg is in the fatal range. Early symptoms are CNS stimulation with vomiting, hyperpnea, hyperactivity, and possibly convulsions. This progresses quickly to depression, coma, respiratory failure, and collapse. These symptoms are accompanied by severe electrolyte disturbances.

➤ SHOWN IN PRODUCT IDENTIFICATION GUIDE

In the treatment of salicylate overdosage, intensive supportive therapy should be instituted immediately. Plasma salicylate levels should be measured in order to determine the severity of the poisoning and to provide a guide for therapy.

Emptying of the stomach should be accomplished as soon as possible with ipecac syrup unless the patient is depressed. In depressed patients use airway protected gastric lavage. Delay absorption with activated charcoal and give a saline cathartic. Proceed according to Standard Reference Procedures for Salicylate Intoxication.

Storage: Store at controlled room temperature 15° to 30°C (59° to 86°F).

DOSAGE AND ADMINISTRATION

Usual Adult Dosage: Two to three tablets 3 to 4 times daily.

If necessary, dosage may be increased until relief is obtained, but dosage should be maintained slightly below that which produces tinnitus. Plasma salicylate levels may also be helpful in determining proper dosage (see *"Clinical Pharmacology"* section).

HOW SUPPLIED
ENTERIC COATED TABLETS: 975 MG

BRAND/MANUFACTURER	NDC	SIZE	AWP
○ **BRAND**			
EASPRIN: Parke-Davis	00071-0490-24	100s	$34.89
○ **GENERICS**			
Rugby	00536-3321-01	100s	$11.55
URL	00677-1347-01	100s	$12.50
Goldline	00182-1065-01	100s	$13.20
DASPRIN: Diane	52938-0975-10	100s	$15.00

TABLET, EXTENDED RELEASE: 800 MG

BRAND/MANUFACTURER	NDC	SIZE	AWP
○ **BRAND**			
ZORPRIN: Boots Pharm	00048-0057-01	100s	$30.30
○ **GENERICS**			
Moore,H.L.	00839-7269-06	100s	$8.03
Aligen	00405-4100-01	100s	$9.00
SLOPRIN: Econolab	55053-0514-01	100s	$9.00
Parmed	00349-8784-01	100s	$9.79
Rugby	00536-3320-01	100s	$11.12
URL	00677-1172-01	100s	$11.25
Major	00904-0585-60	100s	$12.85
Cheshire	55175-1693-00	100s	$13.49
Duramed	51285-0824-02	100s	$14.35
Able	53265-0156-10	100s	$14.50

TABLET, EXTENDED RELEASE: 975 MG

BRAND/MANUFACTURER	NDC	SIZE	AWP
○ **GENERICS**			
Moore,H.L.	00839-7404-06	100s	$11.48
Duramed	51285-0806-02	100s	$13.31
Invamed	52189-0220-24	100s	$13.31
Major	00904-0582-60	100s	$14.50
Invamed	52189-0220-29	500s	$65.30

Aspirin and Carisoprodol

DESCRIPTION

Aspirin/Carisoprodol is a combination product containing Carisoprodol, a centrally-acting muscle relaxant, plus Aspirin, an analgesic with antipyretic and anti-inflammatory properties. Each tablet contains Carisoprodol 200 mg and Aspirin 325 mg. Chemically, Carisoprodol is N-isopropyl-2-methyl-2-propyl-1,3-propanediol dicarbamate. Its empirical formula is $C_{12}H_{24}N_2O_4$, with a molecular weight of 260.33.

CLINICAL PHARMACOLOGY

Aspirin: Aspirin is a non-narcotic analgesic with anti-inflammatory and antipyretic activity. Inhibition of prostaglandin biosynthesis appears to account for most of its anti-inflammatory and for at least part of its analgesic and anti-pyretic properties.

Aspirin is rapidly absorbed and almost totally hydrolyzed to salicylic acid following oral administration. Although Aspirin has a half-life of only about 15 minutes, the apparent biologic half-life of salicylic acid in the therapeutic plasma concentration range is between 6 and 12 hours. Salicylic acid is eliminated by renal excretion and by biotransformation to inactive metabolites. Clearance of salicylic acid in the high-dose range is sensitive to urinary pH (see *"Drug Interactions"*) and is reduced by renal dysfunction.

Carisoprodol: Carisoprodol is a centrally-acting muscle relaxant that does not directly relax tense skeletal muscles in man. The mode of action of Carisoprodol in relieving acute muscle spasm of local origin has not been clearly identified, but may be related to its sedative properties. In animals, Carisoprodol has been shown to produce muscle relaxation by blocking interneuronal activity and depressing transmission of polysynaptic neurons in the spinal cord and in the descending reticular formation of the brain. The onset of action is rapid and lasts four to six hours.

Carisoprodol is metabolized in the liver and is excreted by the kidneys. It is dialyzable by peritoneal and hemodialysis.

INDICATIONS AND USAGE

Aspirin/Carisoprodol is indicated as an adjunct to rest, physical therapy, and other measures for the relief of pain, muscle spasm, and limited mobility associated with acute, painful musculoskeletal conditions.

CONTRAINDICATIONS

Acute intermittent porphyria; bleeding disorders; allergic or idiosyncratic reactions to Carisoprodol, Aspirin or related compounds.

WARNINGS

On very rare occasions, the first dose of Carisoprodol has been followed by an idiosyncratic reaction with symptoms appearing within minutes or hours. These may include extreme weakness, transient quadriplegia, dizziness, ataxia, temporary loss of vision, diplopia, mydriasis, dysarthia, agitation, euphoria, confusion, and disorientation. Although symptoms usually subside over the course of the next several hours, discontinue Aspirin/Carisoprodol and initiate appropriate supportive and symptomatic therapy, which may include epinephrine and/or antihistamines. In severe cases, corticosteroids may be necessary. Severe reactions have been manifested by asthmatic episodes, fever, weakness, dizziness, angioneurotic edema, smarting eyes, hypotension, and anaphylactoid shock.

The effects of Carisoprodol with agents such as alcohol, other CNS depressants, or psychotropic drugs may be additive. Appropriate caution should be exercised with patients who may take one or more of these agents simultaneously with Aspirin/Carisoprodol.

PRECAUTIONS

GENERAL

To avoid excessive accumulation of Carisoprodol, Aspirin, or their metabolites, use Aspirin/Carisoprodol with caution in patients with compromised liver or kidney function, or in elderly or debilitated patients (see *"Clinical Pharmacology"*).

Use with caution in patients with history of gastritis or peptic ulcer, in patients on anticoagulant therapy, and in addiction-prone individuals.

INFORMATION FOR PATIENTS

Caution patients that this drug may impair the mental and/or physical abilities required for the performance of potentially hazardous tasks such as driving a motor vehicle or operating machinery.

Caution patients with a predisposition for gastrointestinal bleeding that concomitant use of Aspirin and alcohol may have an additive effect in this regard.

Caution patients that dosage of medications used for gout, arthritis, or diabetes may have to be adjusted when Aspirin is administered or discontinued (see *"Drug Interactions"*).

DRUG INTERACTIONS

Clinically important interactions may occur when certain drugs are administered concomitantly with Aspirin or Aspirin-containing drugs.

1. Oral Anticoagulants: By interfering with platelet function or decreasing plasma prothrombin concentration, Aspirin enhances the potential for bleeding in patients on anticoagulants.

2. Methotrexate: Aspirin enhances the toxic effects of this drug.

3. Probenecid and Sulfinpyrazone: large doses of Aspirin reduce the uricosuric effect of both drugs. Renal excretion of salicylate may also be reduced.

4. Oral Antidiabetic Drugs: enhancement of hypoglycemia may occur.

5. Antacids: to the extent that they raise urinary pH, antacids may substantially decrease plasma salicylate concentrations: conversely, their withdrawal can result in a substantial increase.

6. Ammonium Chloride: this and other drugs that acidify a relatively alkaline urine can elevate plasma salicylate concentrations.

7. Ethyl Alcohol: enhanced Aspirin-induced fecal blood loss has been reported.

8. Corticosteroids: salicylate plasma levels may be decreased when adrenal corticosteroids are given, and may be increased substantially when they are discontinued.

CARCINOGENESIS, MUTAGENESIS, IMPAIRMENT OF FERTILITY

No long-term studies have been done with Aspirin/Carisoprodol.

PREGNANCY—TERATOGENIC EFFECTS

Pregnancy Category C. Adequate animal reproduction studies have not been conducted with Aspirin/Carisoprodol. It is also not known whether Aspirin/Carisoprodol can cause fetal harm when administered to a pregnant woman or can affect reproduction capacity. Aspirin/Carisoprodol should be given to a pregnant woman only if clearly needed.

Studies in rodents have shown salicylates to be teratogenic when given in early gestation, and embryocidal when given in later gestation in doses considerably greater than usual therapeutic doses in humans. Studies in women who took Aspirin during pregnancy have not demonstrated an increased incidence of congenital abnormalities in the offspring.

LABOR AND DELIVERY

Ingestion of Aspirin near term or prior to delivery may prolong delivery or lead to bleeding in mother, fetus, or neonate.

◆ RATED THERAPEUTICALLY EQUIVALENT; ◇ THERAPEUTIC EQUIVALENCE UNCONFIRMED; ○ UNRATED

NURSING MOTHERS
Carisoprodol is excreted in human milk in concentrations two-to-four times that in maternal plasma. Aspirin is excreted in human milk in moderate amounts and can produce a bleeding tendency in nursing infants. Because of the potential for serious adverse reactions in nursing infants, a decision should be made whether to discontinue nursing or the drug, taking into account the importance of the drug to the mother.

PEDIATRIC USE
Safety and effectiveness in children below the age of twelve have not been established.

ADVERSE REACTIONS
If severe reactions occur, discontinue Aspirin/Carisoprodol and initiate appropriate symptomatic and supportive therapy.

The following side effects which have occurred with the administration of the individual ingredients alone may also occur with the combination.

Carisoprodol: Central Nervous System: Drowsiness is the most frequent complaint and along with other CNS effects may require dosage reduction. Observed less frequently are dizziness, vertigo and ataxia. Tremor, agitation, irritability, headache, depressive reactions, syncope, and insomnia have been infrequent or rare.

Idiosyncratic: Idiosyncratic reactions are very rare. They are usually seen within the period of the first to fourth dose in patients having had no previous contact with the drug (see *"Warnings"*).

Allergic: Skin rash, erythema multiforme, pruritus, eosinophilia, and fixed drug eruptions with cross-reaction to meprobamate have been reported. If allergic reactions occur, discontinue Aspirin/Carisoprodol and treat symptomatically. In evaluating possible allergic reactions, also consider allergy to excipients (information on excipients is available to physicians on request).

Cardiovascular: Tachycardia, postural hypotension, and facial flushing.

Gastrointestinal: Nausea, vomiting, epigastric distress and hiccup.

Hematologic: No serious blood dyscrasias have been attributed to Carisoprodol alone. Leukopenia and pancytopenia have been reported, very rarely, in situations in which other drugs or viral infections may have been responsible.

Aspirin: The most common adverse reactions associated with the use of Aspirin have been gastrointestinal, including nausea, vomiting, gastritis, occult bleeding, constipation and diarrhea. Gastric erosion, angioedema, asthma, rash, pruritus and urticaria have been reported less commonly. Tinnitus is a sign of high serum salicylate levels (see *"Overdosage"*).

Aspirin Intolerance: Allergic type reactions in Aspirin-sensitive individuals may involve the respiratory tract or the skin. Symptoms of the former range from rhinorrhea and shortness of breath to severe asthma, and the latter may consist of urticaria, edema, rash, or angioedema (giant hives). These may occur independently or in combination.

DRUG ABUSE AND DEPENDENCE
Abuse: In clinical use, abuse has been rare.

Dependence: In clinical use, dependence with Aspirin/Carisoprodol has been rare and there have been no reports of significant abstinence signs. Nevertheless, the following information on the individual ingredients should be kept in mind.

Carisoprodol: In dogs, no withdrawal symptoms occurred after abrupt cessation of Carisoprodol from dosages as high as 1 gm/kg/day. In a study in man, abrupt cessation of 100 mg/kg/day (about five times the recommended daily adult dosage) was followed in some subjects by mild withdrawal symptoms such as abdominal cramps, insomnia, chills, headache, and nausea. Delirium and convulsions did not occur (see *"Precautions"*).

OVERDOSAGE
Signs and Symptoms: Any of the following which have been reported with the individual ingredients may occur and may be modified to a varying degree by the effects of the other ingredients present in Aspirin/Carisoprodol.

Aspirin: Headache, tinnitus, hearing difficulty, dim vision, dizziness, lassitude, hyperpnea, rapid breathing, thirst, nausea, vomiting, sweating and occasionally diarrhea are characteristic of mild to moderate salicylate poisoning. Salicylate poisoning should be considered in children with symptoms of vomiting, hyperpnea, and hyperthermia.

Hyperpnea is an early sign of salicylate poisoning, but dyspnea supervenes at plasma levels above 50 mg/dl. These respiratory changes eventually lead to serious acid-base disturbances. Metabolic acidosis is a constant finding in infants but occurs in older children only with severe poisoning; adults usually exhibit respiratory alkalosis initially and acidosis terminally.

Other symptoms of severe salicylate poisoning include hyperthermia, dehydration, delirium, and mental disturbances. Skin eruptions, GI hemorrhage, or pulmonary edema are less common. Early CNS stimulation is replaced by increasing depression, stupor, and coma. Death is usually due to respiratory failure or cardiovascular collapse.

Carisoprodol: Stupor, coma, shock, respiratory depression and, very rarely, death. Overdosage with Carisoprodol in combination with alcohol, other CNS depressants, or psychotropic agents can have additive effects, even when one of the agents has been taken in the usually recommended dosage.

Treatment: General: Provide symptomatic and supportive treatment, as indicated. Any drug remaining in the stomach should be removed using appropriate procedures and caution to protect the airway and prevent aspiration, especially in the stuporous or comatose patient. Incomplete gastric emptying with delayed absorption of Carisoprodol has been reported as a cause for relapse. Should respiration or blood pressure become compromised, respiratory assistance, central nervous system stimulants, and pressor agents should be administered cautiously, as indicated.

Aspirin: Since there are no specific antidotes for salicylate poisoning, the aim of treatment is to enhance elimination of salicylate and prevent or reduce further absorption; to correct any fluid, electrolyte or metabolic imbalance; and to provide general and cardiorespiratory support. If acidosis is present, intravenous sodium bicarbonate must be given, along with adequate hydration, until salicylate levels decrease to within the therapeutic range. To enhance elimination, forced diuresis and alkalinization of the urine may be beneficial. The need for hemoperfusion or hemodialysis is rare and should be used only when other measures have failed.

Carisoprodol: The following have been used successfully in overdosage with the related drug meprobamate: diuretics, osmotic (mannitol) diuresis, peritoneal dialysis, and hemodialysis (see *"Clinical Pharmacology"*). Careful monitoring of urinary output is necessary and caution should be taken to avoid overhydration. Carisoprodol can be measured in biological fluid by gas chromatography (Douglas, J. F., et al: *J Pharm Sci* 58: 145, 1969).

DOSAGE AND ADMINISTRATION
Usual Adult Dosage: 1 or 2 tablets, four times daily.

Not recommended for use in children under age twelve (see *"Precautions"*).

Store at controlled room temperature 15°-30°C (59°-86°F). Protect from moisture.

Dispense in a tight container.

HOW SUPPLIED
TABLETS: 325 MG-200 MG

AVERAGE UNIT PRICE (AVAILABLE SIZES)		GENERIC A-RATED AVERAGE PRICE (GAAP)	
BRAND	$1.52	100s	$82.30
GENERIC	$0.82	500s	$405.27
HCFA FUL (100s ea)	$0.58		

BRAND/MANUFACTURER	NDC	SIZE	AWP
◆ BRAND			
➤ SOMA COMPOUND: Wallace	00037-2103-01	100s	$152.80
	00037-2103-85	100s ud	$153.83
	00037-2103-03	500s	$746.58
◆ GENERICS			
Qualitest	00603-2583-21	100s	$72.50
Rugby	00536-3429-01	100s	$72.53
Major	00904-0356-60	100s	$73.20
URL	00677-1068-01	100s	$74.35
Par	49884-0246-01	100s	$88.48
Goldline	00182-1821-01	100s	$88.48
Moore,H.L.	00839-7162-06	100s	$92.88
Parmed	00349-8475-01	100s	$95.95
Rugby	00536-3429-05	500s	$336.52
Major	00904-0356-40	500s	$338.80
Par	49884-0246-05	500s	$429.13
Goldline	00182-1821-05	500s	$429.13
Moore,H.L.	00839-7162-12	500s	$433.15
Parmed	00349-8475-05	500s	$464.89

Aspirin and Methocarbamol

DESCRIPTION
Each tablet contains:

Methocarbamol .... 400 mg
Aspirin, USP .... 325 mg

The chemical name of Methocarbamol is 3-(2-Methoxyphenoxy)-1,2-propanediol 1-Carbamate.

ACTIONS
Aspirin and Methocarbamol provides a double approach to the management of discomforts associated with musculoskeletal disorders.

Methocarbamol: The mechanism of action of Methocarbamol in humans has not been established, but may be due to general central nervous system depression. It has no direct action on the contractile mechanism of striated muscle, the motor end plate or the nerve fiber.

Aspirin: Aspirin is a mild analgesic with anti-inflammatory and antipyretic activity.

INDICATIONS
Aspirin and Methocarbamol is indicated as an adjunct to rest, physical therapy, and other measures for the relief of discomfort associated with acute, painful musculoskeletal conditions. The mode of action of Methocarbamol has not been

clearly identified but may be related to its sedative properties. Methocarbamol does not directly relax tense skeletal muscles in man.

CONTRAINDICATIONS

Hypersensitivity to Methocarbamol or Aspirin.

WARNINGS

Since Methocarbamol may possess a general central nervous system depressant effect, patients receiving Aspirin and Methocarbamol should be cautioned about combined effects with alcohol and other CNS depressants.

PRECAUTIONS

Products containing Aspirin should be administered with caution to patients with gastritis or peptic ulceration, or those receiving hypoprothrombinemic anticoagulants.

Methocarbamol may cause a color interference in certain screening tests for 5-hydroxyindoleacetic acid (5-HIAA) and vanillymandelic acid (VMA).

Pregnancy: Safe use of Aspirin and Methocarbamol has not been established with regard to possible adverse effects upon fetal development. Therefore, Aspirin and Methocarbamol should not be used in women who are or may become pregnant and particularly during early pregnancy unless in the judgment of the physician the potential benefits outweigh the possible hazards.

Nursing Mothers: It is not known whether Methocarbamol is secreted in human milk; however, Aspirin does appear in human milk in moderate amounts. It can produce a bleeding tendency either by interfering with the function of the infant's platelets or by decreasing the amount of prothrombin in the blood. The risk is minimal if the mother takes the aspirin just after nursing and if the infant has an adequate store of vitamin K. As a general rule, nursing should not be undertaken while a patient is on a drug.

Pediatric Use: Safety and effectiveness in children 12 years of age and below have not been established.

Use in Activities Requiring Mental Alertness: Aspirin and Methocarbamol may rarely cause drowsiness. Until the patient's response has been determined, he should be cautioned against the operation of motor vehicles or dangerous machinery.

ADVERSE REACTIONS

The most frequent adverse reaction to Methocarbamol is dizziness or light-headedness and nausea. This occurs in about one in 20-25 patients. Less frequent reactions are drowsiness, blurred vision, headache, fever, allergic manifestations such as urticaria, pruritus, and rash.

Adverse reactions that have been associated with the use of Aspirin include: nausea and other gastrointestinal discomfort, gastritis, gastric erosion, vomiting, constipation, diarrhea, angio-edema, asthma, rash, pruritus, urticaria.

Gastrointestinal discomfort may be minimized by taking Aspirin and Methocarbamol with food.

OVERDOSAGE

Toxicity due to overdosage of Methocarbamol is unlikely; however, acute overdosage of Aspirin may cause symptoms of salicylate intoxication.

Treatment of Overdosage: Supportive therapy for 24 hours, as Methocarbamol is excreted within that time. If salicylate intoxication occurs, especially in children, the hyperpnea may be controlled with sodium bicarbonate. Judicious use of 5% CO_2 with 95% O_2 may be of benefit. Abnormal electrolyte patterns should be corrected with appropriate fluid therapy.

DOSAGE AND ADMINISTRATION

Adults and children over 12 years of age: Two tablets four times daily. Three tablets four times daily may be used in severe conditions for one to three days in patients who are able to tolerate salicylates. These dosage recommendations provide respectively 3.2 and 4.8 grams of Methocarbamol per day.

Store at controlled room temperature, between 15°C and 30°C (59°F and 86°F).
Dispense in well-closed container.

HOW SUPPLIED
TABLETS: 325 MG-400 MG

AVERAGE UNIT PRICE (AVAILABLE SIZES)		GENERIC A-RATED AVERAGE PRICE (GAAP)	
BRAND	$0.46	100s	$23.44
GENERIC	$0.23	500s	$111.85
HCFA FUL (100s ea)	$0.19		

BRAND/MANUFACTURER	NDC	SIZE	AWP
◆ BRAND			
ROBAXISAL: Robins Pharm	00031-7469-63	100s	$47.30
	00031-7469-70	500s	$220.19
◆ GENERICS			
Moore,H.L.	00839-6284-06	100s	$19.24
Rugby	00536-4028-01	100s	$22.29
Major	00904-0227-60	100s	$23.25
Aligen	00405-4641-01	100s	$23.94
URL	00677-0579-01	100s	$23.95
Goldline	00182-1911-01	100s	$24.00
Zenith	00172-2813-60	100s	$24.30
Par	49884-0249-01	100s	$24.85
Qualitest	00603-4489-21	100s	$25.11

BRAND/MANUFACTURER	NDC	SIZE	AWP
Major	00904-0227-40	500s	$105.50
Zenith	00172-2813-70	500s	$114.55
Par	49884-0249-05	500s	$115.50

Aspirin and Pentazocine Hydrochloride

DESCRIPTION

Each tablet contains Aspirin, USP, 325 mg and Pentazocine Hydrochloride, USP, equivalent to 12.5 mg base.

Pentazocine is a member of the benzazocine series (also known as the benzomorphan series). Chemically, pentazocine is 1,2,3,4,5,6-hexahydro-6, 11-dimethyl-3-(3-methyl-2-butenyl)-2, 6-methano-3-benzazocin-8-ol, a white, crystal-line substance soluble in acidic aqueous solutions.

Chemically, Aspirin is benzoic acid, 2-(acetyloxy)-,.

CLINICAL PHARMACOLOGY

Pentazocine is a potent analgesic which when administered orally is approximately equivalent, on a mg for mg basis in analgesic effect to codeine. Two tablets of Aspirin/Pentazocine HCl when administered orally have the additive analgesic effect equivalent to 25 mg of Pentazocine HCl plus 650 mg of Aspirin. Aspirin/Pentazocine HCl provides the analgesic effects of Pentazocine and the analgesic, anti-inflammatory, and antipyretic actions of Aspirin.

Onset of significant analgesia usually occurs between 15 and 30 minutes after oral administration, and duration of action is usually three hours or longer. Onset and duration of action and the degree of pain relief are related both to dose and the severity of pretreatment pain. Pentazocine weakly antagonizes the analgesic effects of morphine, meperidine, and phenazocine; in addition, it produces incomplete reversal of cardiovascular, respiratory, and behavioral depression induced by morphine and meperidine. Pentazocine has about 1/50 the antagonistic activity of nalorphine. It also has sedative activity.

INDICATION AND USAGE

For the relief of moderate pain.

CONTRAINDICATIONS

Aspirin/Pentazocine HCl should not be administered to patients who are hypersensitive to either Pentazocine or salicylates, or in any situation where Aspirin is contraindicated.

WARNINGS

Drug Dependence: There have been instances of psychological and physical dependence on parenteral Pentazocine in patients with a history of drug abuse, and rarely, in patients without such a history. Abrupt discontinuance following the extended use of parenteral Pentazocine has resulted in withdrawal symptoms. There have been a few reports of dependence and of withdrawal symptoms with orally administered Pentazocine. Patients with a history of drug dependence should be under close supervision while receiving Aspirin/Pentazocine HCl orally. There have been rare reports of possible abstinence syndromes in newborns after prolonged use of Pentazocine during pregnancy.

In prescribing Aspirin/Pentazocine HCl for chronic use, the physician should take precautions to avoid increases in dose by the patient and to prevent the use of the drug in anticipation of pain rather than for the relief of pain.

Head Injury and Increased Intracranial Pressure: The respiratory depressant effects of Pentazocine and its potential for elevating cerebrospinal fluid pressure may be markedly exaggerated in the presence of head injury, other intracranial lesions, or a preexisting increase in intracranial pressure. Furthermore, Pentazocine can produce effects which may obscure the clinical course of patients with head injuries. In such patients, Aspirin/Pentazocine HCl must be used with extreme caution and only if its use is deemed essential.

Usage in Pregnancy: Safe use of Pentazocine during pregnancy (other than labor) has not been established. Animal reproduction studies have not demonstrated teratogenic or embryotoxic effects. However, Aspirin/Pentazocine HCl should be administered to pregnant patients (other than labor) only when, in the judgment of the physician, the potential benefits outweigh the possible hazards. Patients receiving Pentazocine during labor have experienced no adverse effects other than those that occur with commonly used analgesics. Aspirin/Pentazocine HCl tablets should be used with caution in women delivering premature infants.

Acute CNS Manifestations: Patients receiving therapeutic doses of Pentazocine have experienced hallucinations (usually visual), disorientation, and confusion which have cleared spontaneously within a period of hours. The mechanism of this reaction is not known. Such patients should be closely observed and vital signs checked. If the drug is reinstituted it should be done with caution since these acute CNS manifestations may recur.

Due to the potential for increased CNS depressant effects, alcohol should be used with caution in patients who are currently receiving Pentazocine.

Usage in Children: Because clinical experience in children under 12 years of age is limited, administration of Aspirin/Pentazocine HCl in this age group is not recommended.

◆ RATED THERAPEUTICALLY EQUIVALENT; ◇ THERAPEUTIC EQUIVALENCE UNCONFIRMED; ○ UNRATED

Ambulatory Patients: Since sedation, dizziness, and occasional euphoria have been noted, ambulatory patients should be warned not to operate machinery, drive cars, or unnecessarily expose themselves to hazards.

Other: Because of its Aspirin content, Aspirin/Pentazocine HCl should be used with caution in the presence of peptic ulcer, in conjunction with anticoagulant therapy, or in any situation where the effects of Aspirin may be deleterious.

PRECAUTIONS
Certain Respiratory Conditions: Although respiratory depression has rarely been reported after oral administration of Pentazocine, Aspirin/Pentazocine HCl should be administered with caution to patients with respiratory depression from any cause, severely limited respiratory reserve, severe bronchial asthma and other obstructive respiratory conditions, or cyanosis.

Impaired Renal or Hepatic Function: Decreased metabolism of the drug by the liver in extensive liver disease may predispose to accentuation of side effects. Although laboratory tests have not indicated that Pentazocine causes or increases renal or hepatic impairment, Aspirin/Pentazocine HCl should be administered with caution to patients with such impairment.

Myocardial Infarction: As with all drugs, Aspirin/Pentazocine HCl should be used with caution in patients with myocardial infarction who have nausea or vomiting.

Biliary Surgery: Narcotic drug products are generally considered to elevate biliary tract pressure for varying periods following administration. Some evidence suggests that Pentazocine may differ in this respect (ie, it causes little or no elevation in biliary tract pressures). The clinical significance of these findings, however, is not yet known.

Patients Receiving Narcotics: Pentazocine is a mild narcotic antagonist. Some patients previously given narcotics, including methadone for the daily treatment of narcotic dependence, have experienced withdrawal symptoms after receiving Pentazocine.

CNS Effect: Caution should be used when Pentazocine is administered to patients prone to seizures. Seizures have occurred in a few such patients in association with the use of Pentazocine although no cause and effect relationship has been established.

ADVERSE REACTIONS
Reactions reported after oral administration of Pentazocine or Aspirin/Pentazocine HCl include:

Gastrointestinal: nausea, vomiting; infrequently constipation; and rarely abdominal distress, anorexia, diarrhea.

CNS Effects: dizziness, light-headedness, hallucinations, sedation, euphoria, headache, confusion, disorientation; infrequently weakness, disturbed dreams, insomnia, syncope, visual blurring and focusing difficulty, depression; and rarely tremor, irritability, excitement, tinnitus.

Autonomic: sweating; infrequently flushing; and rarely chills.

Allergic: infrequently rash; and rarely urticaria, edema of the face, and angioneurotic edema.

Cardiovascular: infrequently decrease in blood pressure, tachycardia.

Hematologic: rarely depression of white blood cells (especially granulocytes), which is usually reversible, moderate transient eosinophilia.

Other: rarely respiratory depression, urinary retention, paresthesia, toxic epidermal necrolysis, and angioneurotic edema.

OVERDOSAGE
Manifestations: Clinical experience with Pentazocine overdosage has been insufficient to define the signs of this condition. Signs of salicylate overdosage include headache, dizziness, confusion, tinnitus, diaphoresis, thirst, nausea, vomiting, diarrhea, tachycardia, tachypnea, Kussmaul breathing, convulsions, and coma. Death is usually from respiratory failure.

Treatment: Treatment for overdosage of Aspirin/Pentazocine HCl should include treatment for salicylate poisoning as outlined in standard references.

Oxygen, intravenous fluids, vasopressors, and other supportive measures should be employed as indicated. Assisted or controlled ventilation should also be considered. For respiratory depression due to overdosage or unusual sensitivity to Pentazocine, parenteral naloxone is a specific and effective antagonist.

DOSAGE AND ADMINISTRATION
Adults: The usual adult dose is tablets three or four times a day.

Children Under 12 Years of Age: Since clinical experience in children under 12 years of age is limited, administration of Aspirin/Pentazocine HCl in this age group is not recommended.

Duration of Therapy: Patients with chronic pain who receive Pentazocine orally for prolonged periods have only rarely been reported to experience withdrawal symptoms when administration was abruptly discontinued (see *"Warnings"*). Tolerance to the analgesic effect of Pentazocine has also been reported only rarely. Significant abnormalities of liver and kidney function tests have not been reported, even after prolonged administration of Pentazocine.

Aspirin with Butalbital

DESCRIPTION
Each Aspirin/Butalbital tablet for oral administration contains:

Butalbital, (Warning: May be habit forming) ....50 mg
Aspirin ....650 mg

Butalbital, 5-allyl-5-isobutylbarbituric acid, a white odorless crystalline powder having a slightly bitter taste, is a short to intermediate-acting barbiturate.

Aspirin, salicylic acid acetate, is a non-opiate analgesic, anti-inflammatory and antipyretic agent. It occurs as a white, crystalline tabular or needle-like powder and is odorless or has a faint odor.

CLINICAL PHARMACOLOGY
Pharmacologically, Aspirin/Butalbital combines the analgesic properties of Aspirin with the anxiolytic and muscle relaxant properties of Butalbital.

INDICATIONS AND USAGE
Aspirin/Butalbital is indicated for the relief of the symptom complex of tension (or muscle contraction) headache.

CONTRAINDICATIONS
Hypersensitivity to Aspirin or barbiturates. Patients with porphyria.

PRECAUTIONS
1. General: Aspirin/Butalbital should be used with caution in patients with certain medical problems, including those with a history of asthma, allergies and nasal polyps. Also, the drug must be prescribed carefully for patients with hemophilia or other bleeding problems, peptic ulcer, renal impairment, or a history of drug abuse or dependence.

2. Information for Patients: Aspirin/Butalbital may impair mental and/or physical abilities required for the performance of potentially hazardous tasks, such as driving a car or operating machinery. The patient should be cautioned accordingly.

3. Drug Interactions: Patients receiving narcotic analgesics, antipsychotics, antianxiety agents, or other CNS depressants (including alcohol) concomitantly with Aspirin/Butalbital may exhibit additive CNS depressant effects. When combined therapy is contemplated, the dose of one or both agents should be reduced.

Drugs	Effect
Aspirin w/anti-inflammatory agents	Increased ulcerogenic effects
Butalbital w/coumarin anticoagulants	Decreased effect of anti-coagulant because of increased metabolism resulting from enzyme induction.
Butalbital w/tricyclic anti-depressants	Decreased blood levels of the anti-depressant

4. Usage in Pregnancy: Adequate studies have not been performed in animals to determine whether this drug affects fertility in males or females, has teratogenic potential or has other adverse effects on the fetus. While there are no well-controlled studies in pregnant women, over twenty years of marketing and clinical experience does not include any positive evidence of adverse effects on the fetus. Although there is no clearly defined risk, such experience cannot exclude the possibility of infrequent or subtle damage to the human fetus. Aspirin/Butalbital should be used in pregnant women only when clearly needed.

5. Nursing Mothers: The effects of Aspirin/Butalbital on infants of nursing mothers are not known. Salicylates and barbiturates are excreted in the breast milk of nursing mothers. The serum levels in infants are believed to be insignificant with therapeutic doses.

6. Pediatric Use: Safety and effectiveness in children below the age of 12 have not been established.

ADVERSE REACTIONS
The most frequent adverse reactions are drowsiness and dizziness. Less frequent reactions are lightheadedness and gastrointestinal disturbances including nausea, vomiting and flatulence. Mental confusion or depression can occur due to intolerance or overdosage of Butalbital.

Several cases of dermatological reactions including toxic epidermal necrolysis and erythema multiforme have been reported.

DRUG ABUSE AND DEPENDENCE
Prolonged use of barbiturates can produce drug dependence, characterized by psychic dependence, and less frequently, physical dependence and tolerance. The abuse liability of Aspirin/Butalbital is similar to that of other barbiturate-containing drug combinations. Caution should be exercised when prescribing

medication for patients with a known propensity for taking excessive quantities of drugs, which is not uncommon in patients with chronic tension headache.

OVERDOSAGE

Symptoms: The toxic effects of acute overdosage of Aspirin/Butalbital are attributable mainly to its barbiturate component, and, to a lesser extent, Aspirin. Symptoms attributable to *acute Aspirin poisoning* include hyperpnea; acid-base disturbances with development of metabolic acidosis; vomiting and abdominal pain; tinnitus; hyperthermia; hypoprothrombinemia; restlessness; delirium; convulsions. Symptoms attributable to *acute barbiturate poisoning* include drowsiness, confusion, and coma; respiratory depression; hypotension; shock.

Treatment: Treatment consists primarily of management of barbiturate intoxication and the correction of the acid-base imbalance due to salicylism. Vomiting should be induced mechanically or with emetics in the conscious patient. Gastric lavage may be used if the pharyngeal and laryngeal reflexes are present and if less than four hours have elapsed since ingestion. A cuffed endotracheal tube should be inserted before gastric lavage of the unconscious patient and when necessary to provide assisted respiration. Diuresis, alkalinization of the urine, and correction of electrolyte disturbances should be accomplished through administration of intravenous fluids such as 1% sodium bicarbonate in 5% dextrose injection. Meticulous attention should be given to maintaining adequate pulmonary ventilation. Correction of hypotension may require the administration of norepinephrine bitartrate or phenylephrine hydrochloride by intravenous infusion. In severe cases of intoxication, peritoneal dialysis, hemodialysis, or exchange transfusion may be lifesaving. Hypoprothrombinemia should be treated with Vitamin K, intravenously.

DOSAGE AND ADMINISTRATION

Oral: One tablet every four hours as needed. Do not exceed 6 tablets per day.
   Medication should be taken with food or a full glass of water or milk to lessen gastric irritation caused by Aspirin.

Storage: Store in a tight container, below 30°C (86°F). Protect from moisture.

HOW SUPPLIED
TABLETS: 650 MG-50 MG

BRAND/MANUFACTURER	NDC	SIZE	AWP
○ BRAND			
AXOTAL: Savage	00281-1301-17	100s	$45.05

Aspirin with Codeine Phosphate

DESCRIPTION
Aspirin/Codeine is supplied in tablet form for oral administration. Each tablet contains Aspirin (acetylsalicylic acid) 325 mg, Codeine Phosphate in one of the following strengths: No. 3, 30 mg and No. 4, 60 mg (Warning—may be habit-forming).
   Aspirin/Codeine has analgesic, antipyretic and anti-inflammatory effects.
   The components of Aspirin/Codeine have the following chemical names:
   a. Aspirin (acetylsalicylic acid): 2-(acetyloxy)benzoic acid
   b. Codeine Phosphate U.S.P.: 7,8-didehydro-4, 5α-epoxy-3-methoxy-17-methylmorphinan-6α-ol phoshate (1:1) (salt) hemihydrate

CLINICAL PHARMACOLOGY
Aspirin: The analgesic, anti-inflammatory and antipyretic effects of Aspirin are believed to result from inhibition of the synthesis of certain prostaglandins. Aspirin interferes with clotting mechanisms primarily by diminishing platelet aggregation; at high doses prothrombin synthesis can be inhibited.
   Aspirin in solution is rapidly absorbed from the stomach and from the upper small intestine. About 50 percent of an oral dose is absorbed in 30 minutes and peak plasma concentrations are reached in about 40 minutes. Higher than normal stomach pH or the presence of food slightly delays absorption.
   Once absorbed, Aspirin is mainly hydrolyzed to salicylic acid and distributed to all body tissues and fluids, including fetal tissue, breast milk and the central nervous system (CNS). Highest concentrations are found in plasma, liver, renal cortex, heart and lung.
   From 50 to 80 percent of the salicylic acid and its metabolites in plasma are loosely bound to proteins. The plasma half-life of total salicylate is about 3.0 hours, with a 650 mg dose. Higher doses of Aspirin cause increases in plasma salicylate half-life. Metabolism occurs primarily in the hepatocytes. The major metabolites are salicyluric acid (75%), the phenolic and acyl glucuronides of salicylate (15%), and gentisic and gentisuric acid (< 1%).
   Almost all of a therapeutic dose of Aspirin is excreted through the kidneys, either as salicylic acid or the above-mentioned metabolic products. Renal clearance of salicylates is greatly augmented by an alkaline urine, as is proproduced by concurrent administration of sodium bicarbonate or potassium citrate.
   Toxic salicylate blood levels are usually above 30 mg/100 mL. The single lethal dose of Aspirin in normal adults is approximately 25 to 30 g, but patients have recovered from much larger doses with appropriate treatment.

Codeine: Codeine probably exerts its analgesic effect through actions on opiate receptors in the CNS.
   Codeine is readily absorbed from the gastrointestinal tract, and a therapeutic dose reaches peak analgesic effectiveness in about 2 hours and persists for 4 to 6

hours. Oral Codeine (60 mg) given to healthy males has been shown to achieve peak blood levels of 0.016 mg/100 mL at approximately one hour post-dose. The Codeine plasma half-life for a 60 mg oral dose is about 2.9 hours. Blood levels causing CNS depression begin at 0.05 to 0.19 mg/100 mL. The single lethal dose of Codeine in adults is estimated to be approximately 0.5 to 1.0 g.
   Codeine is rapidly distributed from blood to body tissues and taken up preferentially by parenchymatous organs such as liver, spleen and kidney. It passes the blood-brain barrier and is found in fetal tissue and breast milk.
   The drug is not bound by plasma proteins nor is it accumulated in body tissues. Codeine is metabolized in liver to morphine and norcodeine, each representing about 10 percent of the administered dose of Codeine. About 90 percent of the dose is excreted within 24 hours, primarily through the kidneys. Urinary excretion products are free and glucuronide-conjugated Codeine (about 70%), free and conjugated norcodeine (about 10%), free and conjugated morphine (about 10%), normorphine (under 4%) and hydrocodone (< 1%). The remainder of the dose appears in the feces.

INDICATIONS AND USAGE
Aspirin/Codeine is indicated for the relief of mild, moderate, and moderate to severe pain.

CONTRAINDICATIONS
Aspirin/Codeine is contraindicated under the following conditions:
   (1) hypersensitivity or intolerance to Aspirin or Codeine,
   (2) severe bleeding, disorders of coagulation or primary hemostasis, including hemophilia, hypoprothrombinemia, von Willebrand's disease, the thrombocytopenias, thrombasthenia and other ill-defined hereditary platelet dysfunctions, as well as such associated conditions as severe vitamin K deficiency and severe liver damage,
   (3) anticoagulant therapy, and
   (4) peptic ulcer, or other serious gastrointestinal lesions
   (5) children or teenagers with the symptoms of chicken pox or influenza. Reye's Syndrome has been reported to be associated with Aspirin use in this population.

WARNINGS
Therapeutic doses of Aspirin can cause anaphylactic shock and other severe allergic reactions. A history of allergy is often lacking.
   Significant bleeding can result from Aspirin therapy in patients with peptic ulcer or other gastrointestinal lesions, and in patients with bleeding disorders. Aspirin administered preoperatively may prolong the bleeding time.
   In the presence of head injury or other intracranial lesions, the respiratory depressant effects of Codeine and other narcotics may be markedly enhanced, as well as their capacity for elevating cerebrospinal fluid pressure. Narcotics also produce other CNS depressant effects, such as drowsiness, that may further obscure the clinical course of patients with head injuries.
   Codeine or other narcotics may obscure signs on which to judge the diagnosis or clinical course of patients with acute abdominal conditions.

PRECAUTIONS
General: Aspirin/Codeine should be prescribed with caution for certain special-risk patients such as the elderly or debilitated, and those with severe impairment of renal or hepatic function, gallbladder disease or gallstones, respiratory impairment, cardiac arrhythmias, inflammatory disorders of the gastrointestinal tract, hypothyroidism, Addison's disease, prostatic hypertrophy or urethral stricture, coagulation disorders, head injuries, or acute abdominal conditions. Aspirin/Codeine should not be prescribed for long-term therapy unless specifically indicated.
   Precautions should be taken when administering salicylates to persons with known allergies. Hypersensitivity to Aspirin is particularly likely in patients with nasal polyps, and relatively common in those with asthma.

Information for Patients: Aspirin/Codeine may impair the mental and/or physical abilities required for the performance of potentially hazardous tasks such as driving a car or operating machinery. Such tasks should be avoided while taking Aspirin/Codeine.
   Alcohol and other CNS depressants may produce an additive CNS depression when taken with Aspirin Codeine and should be avoided.
   Codeine may be habit-forming when used over long periods or in high doses. Patients should take the drug only for as long as it is prescribed, in the amounts prescribed, and no more frequently than prescribed.

Laboratory Tests: Hypersensitivity to Aspirin cannot be detected by skin testing or radioimmunoassay procedures. The primary screening tests for detecting a bleeding tendency are platelet count, bleeding time, activated partial thromboplastin time and prothrombin time.
   In patients with severe hepatic or renal disease, effects of therapy should be monitored with serial liver and/or renal function tests.

Drug Interactions: Aspirin/Codeine may *enhance* the effects of:
   (1) monoamine oxidase (MAO) inhibitors,
   (2) oral anticoagulants, causing bleeding by inhibiting prothrombin formation in the liver and displacing anticoagulants from plasma protein binding sites,
   (3) oral antidiabetic agents and insulin, causing hypoglycemia by contributing an additive effect, and by displacing the oral antidiabetic agents from secondary binding sites,
   (4) 6-mercaptopurine and methotrexate, causing bone marrow toxicity and blood dyscrasias by displacing these drugs from secondary binding sites,
   (5) penicillins and sulfonamides, increasing their blood levels by displacing these drugs from protein binding sites,

(6) nonsteroidal anti-inflammatory agents, increasing the risk of peptic ulceration and bleeding by contributing additive effects,

(7) other narcotic analgesics, alcohol, general anesthetics, tranquilizers such as chlordiazepoxide, sedative-hypnotics, or other CNS depressants, causing increased CNS depression,

(8) corticosteroids, potentiating steroid anti-inflammatory effects by displacing steroids from protein binding sites. Aspirin intoxication may occur with corticosteroid withdrawal because steroids promote renal clearance of salicylates.

Aspirin/Codeine may *diminish* the effects of:

(1) uricosuric agents such as probenecid and sulfinpyrazone, reducing their effectiveness in the treatment of gout. Aspirin competes with these agents for protein binding sites.

Aspirin and its metabolites may be caused to accumulate in the body, perhaps to toxic levels, by para-aminosalicylic acid, furosemide, and vitamin C.

DRUG/LABORATORY TEST INTERACTIONS

Aspirin: Aspirin may interfere with the following laboratory determinations in blood: serum amylase, fasting blood glucose, carbon dioxide, cholesterol, protein, protein bound iodine, uric acid, prothrombin time, bleeding time, and spectrophotometric detection of barbiturates. Aspirin may interfere with the following laboratory determinations in urine: glucose, 5-hydroxyindoleacetic acid, Gerhardt ketone, vanillymandelic acid (VMA), protein, uric acid, and diacetic acid.

Codeine: Codeine may increase serum amylase levels.

Carcinogenesis, Mutagenesis, Impairment of Fertility: No adequate long-term studies have been conducted in animals to determine whether Codeine has a potential for carcinogenesis, mutagenesis, or impairment of fertility.

Adequate long-term studies have been conducted in mice and rats with Aspirin, alone or in combination with other drugs, in which no evidence of carcinogenesis was seen. No adequate studies have been conducted in animals to determine whether Aspirin has a potential for mutagenesis or impairment of fertility.

Pregnancy: Teratogenic Effects: Pregnancy Category C. Animal reproduction studies have not been conducted with Aspirin with Codeine. It is also not known whether Aspirin with Codeine can cause fetal harm when administered to a pregnant woman or can affect reproduction capacity. Aspirin/Codeine should be given to a pregnant woman only if clearly needed.

Reproductive studies in rats and mice have shown Aspirin to be teratogenic and embryocidal at four to six times the human therapeutic dose. Studies in pregnant women, however, have not shown that Aspirin increases the risk of abnormalities when administered during the first trimester of pregnancy. In controlled studies involving 41,337 pregnant women and their offspring, there was no evidence that Aspirin taken during pregnancy caused stillbirth, neonatal death or reduced birthweight. In controlled studies of 50,282 pregnant women and their offspring, Aspirin administration in moderate and heavy doses during the first four lunar months of pregnancy showed no teratogenic effect.

Reproduction studies have been performed in rabbits and rats at doses up to 150 times the human dose and have revealed no evidence of impaired fertility or harm to the fetus due to Codeine.

Nonteratogenic Effects: Therapeutic doses of Aspirin in pregnant women close to term may cause bleeding in mother, fetus, or neonate. During the last 3 months of pregnancy regular use of Aspirin may cause problems in the unborn child or complications during delivery.

Labor and Delivery: Ingestion of Aspirin prior to delivery may prolong delivery or lead to bleeding in the mother or neonate. Use of Codeine during labor may lead to respiratory depression in the neonate.

Nursing Mothers: Aspirin and Codeine are excreted in breast milk in small amounts, but the significance of their effects on nursing infants is not known. Because of the potential for serious adverse reactions in nursing infants from Aspirin/Codeine a decision should be made whether to discontinue nursing or to discontinue the drug, taking into account the importance of the drug to the mother.

ADVERSE REACTIONS

Codeine: The most frequently observed adverse reactions to Codeine include light-headedness, dizziness, drowsiness, nausea, vomiting, constipation and depression of respiration. Less common reactions to Codeine include euphoria, dysphoria, pruritus and skin rashes.

Aspirin: Mild Aspirin intoxication (salicylism) can occur in response to chronic use of large doses. Manifestations include nausea, vomiting, hearing impairment, tinnitus, diminished vision, headache, dizziness, drowsiness, mental confusion, hyperpnea, hyperventilation, tachycardia, sweating and thirst.

Therapeutic doses of Aspirin can induce mild or severe allergic reactions manifested by skin rashes, urticaria, angioedema, rhinorrhea, asthma, abdominal pain, nausea, vomiting, or anaphylactic shock. A history of allergy is often lacking, and allergic reactions may occur even in patients who have previously taken Aspirin without any ill effects. Allergic reactions to Aspirin are most likely to occur in patients with a history of allergic disease, especially in patients with nasal polyps or asthma.

Some patients are unable to take Aspirin or other salicylates without developing nausea or vomiting. Occasional patients respond to Aspirin (usually in large doses) with dyspepsia or heartburn, which may be accompanied by occult bleeding.

Excessive bruising or bleeding is sometimes seen in patients with mild disorders of primary hemostasis who regularly use low doses of Aspirin.

Prolonged use of Aspirin can cause painless erosion of gastric mucosa, occult bleeding and, infrequently, iron-deficiency anemia. High doses of Aspirin can exacerbate symptoms of peptic ulcer and, occasionally, cause extensive bleeding.

Excessive bleeding can follow injury or surgery in patients with or without known bleeding disorders who have taken therapeutic doses of Aspirin within the preceding 10 days. Hepatotoxicity has been reported in association with prolonged use of large doses of Aspirin in patients with lupus erythematosus, rheumatoid Arthritis and rheumatic disease. Bone marrow depression, manifested by weakness, fatigue, or abnormal bruising or bleeding, has occasionally been reported.

In patients with glucose-6-Phosphate dehydrogenase deficiency, Aspirin can cause a mild degree of hemolytic anemia. In hyperuricemic persons, low doses of Aspirin may reduce the effectiveness of uricosuric therapy or precipitate an attack of gout.

DRUG ABUSE AND DEPENDENCE

Like other medications containing a narcotic analgesic, Aspirin/Codeine is controlled by the Drug Enforcement Administration and is classified under Schedule III.

Aspirin/Codeine can produce drug dependence of the morphine type, therefore, it has a potential for being abused. Psychic dependence, physical dependence and tolerance may develop on repeated administration.

The dependence liability of Codeine has been found to be too small to permit a full definition of its characteristics. Studies indicate that addiction to Codeine is extremely uncommon and requires very high parenteral doses.

When dependence on Codeine occurs at therapeutic doses, it appears to require from one to two months to develop, and withdrawal symptoms are mild. Most patients on long-term oral Codeine therapy show no signs of physical dependence upon abrupt withdrawal.

OVERDOSAGE

Severe intoxication, caused by overdose of Aspirin with Codeine may produce: skin eruptions, dyspnea, vertigo, double vision, delusions, hallucinations, garbled speech, excitability, restlessness, delirium, constricted pupils, a positive Babinski sign, respiratory depression (slow and shallow breathing; Cheyne-Stokes respiration), cyanosis, clammy skin, muscle flaccidity, circulatory collapse, stupor and coma. In children, difficulty in hearing, tinnitus, dim vision, headache, dizziness, drowsiness, confusion, rapid breathing, sweating, thirst, nausea, vomiting, hyperpyrexia, dehydration and convulsions are prominent signs. The most severe manifestations from Aspirin result from cardiovascular and respiratory insufficiency secondary to acid-base and electrolyte disturbances, complicated by hyperthermia and dehydration. The most severe manifestations from Codeine are associated with respiratory depression.

Respiratory alkalosis is characteristic of the early phase of intoxication with Aspirin while hyperventilation is occurring, but is quickly followed by metabolic acidosis in most people with severe intoxication. This occurs more readily in children. Hypoglycemia may occur in children who have taken large overdoses. Other laboratory findings associated with Aspirin intoxication include ketonuria, hyponatremia, hypokalemia, and occasionally proteinuria. A slight rise in lactic dehydrogenase and hydroxybutyric dehydrogenase may occur.

Concentrations of Aspirin in plasma above 30 mg/100 mL are associated with toxicity. (See *"Clinical Pharmacology"* section for information on factors influencing Aspirin blood levels.) The single lethal dose of Aspirin in adults is probably about 25 to 30 g, but is not known with certainty.

The toxic plasma concentration of Codeine is not known with certainty. Experimental production of mild to moderate CNS depression in healthy, nontolerant subjects occurred at plasma concentrations of 0.05 to 0.19 mg/100 mL when Codeine was given by intravenous infusion. The single lethal dose of Codeine in adults is estimated to be from 0.5 to 1.0 g. It is also estimated that 5 mg/kg could be fatal in children. Hemodialysis and peritoneal dialysis can be performed to reduce the body Aspirin content. Codeine is theoretically dialyzable but the procedure has not been clinically established.

Treatment of overdosage consists primarily of support of vital functions, management of Codeine-induced respiratory depression, increasing salicylate elimination, and correcting the acid-base imbalance due primarily to salicylism.

In a comatose patient, primary attention should be given to establishment of adequate respiratory exchange through provisions of a patent airway and the institution of assisted or controlled ventilation. The narcotic antagonist naloxone is a specific antidote for respiratory depression which may result from overdose or unusual sensitivity to narcotics. Therefore, an appropriate dose of an antagonist should be administered, preferably by the intravenous route, simultaneously with efforts at respiratory resuscitation. Since the duration of action of Aspirin with Codeine may exceed that of the antagonist, the patient should be kept under continued surveillance and repeated doses of the antagonist should be administered as needed to maintain adequate respiration. A narcotic antagonist should not be administered in the absence of clinically significant respiratory or cardiovascular depression.

Gastric emptying (Syrup of Ipecac) and/or lavage is recommended as soon as possible after ingestion, even if the patient has vomited spontaneously. (Apomorphine should not be used as an emetic for Aspirin/Codeine, since it may potentiate hypotension and respiratory depression.) Administration of activated charcoal as a slurry is beneficial after lavage and/or emesis, if less than three hours have passed since ingestion. Charcoal adsorption should *not* be employed prior to emesis or lavage.

Severity of Aspirin intoxication is determined by measuring the blood salicylate level. Acid-base status should be closely followed with serial blood gas and serum pH measurements. Fluid and electrolyte balance should also be regularly monitored.

A serum salicylate level of 30 mg/100 mL or higher indicates a need for enhanced salicylate excretion that can be achieved through body-fluid supplementation and urine alkalinization if renal function is normal. In mild intoxication, urine flow can be increased by forcing oral fluids and giving potassium citrate capsules.

(DO NOT GIVE BICARBONATE BY MOUTH SINCE IT INCREASES THE RATE OF SALICYLATE ABSORPTION.)

In severe cases, hyperthermia and hypovolemia, as well as respiratory depression are the major immediate threats to life. Children should be sponged with tepid water. Replacement fluid should be administered intravenously and augmented with sufficient bicarbonate to correct acidosis, with monitoring of plasma electrolytes and pH, to promote alkaline diuresis of salicylate if renal function is normal. Complete control may also require infusion of glucose to control hypoglycemia.

Potassium deficiency may also be corrected through the infusion, once adequate urinary output is assured. Plasma or plasma expanders may be needed if fluid replacement is insufficient to maintain normal blood pressure or adequate urinary output.

In patients with renal insufficiency or in cases of life-threatening intoxication, dialysis is usually required. Peritoneal dialysis or exchange transfusion is indicated in infants and young children, and hemodialysis in older patients.

Oxygen, intravenous fluids, vasopressors and other supportive measures should be employed as needed.

DOSAGE AND ADMINISTRATION

Dosage is adjusted according to the severity of pain and the response of the patient. It may occasionally be necessary to exceed the usual dosage recommended below when pain is severe or the patient has become tolerant to the analgesic effect of Codeine. Aspirin/Codeine is given orally. The usual adult dose for Aspirin/Codeine 30mg is one or two tablets every four hours as required. The usual adult dose for Aspirin/Codeine 60mg is one tablet every four hours as required.

Aspirin/Codeine should be taken with food or a full glass of milk or water to lessen gastric irritation.

Store at 15° to 30°C (59° to 86°F) in a dry place and protect from light.

HOW SUPPLIED
TABLETS (C-III): 325 MG-15 MG

BRAND/MANUFACTURER	NDC	SIZE	AWP
○ GENERICS			
Halsey Pharm	00879-0441-01	100s	$7.48
Parmed	00349-8655-01	100s	$8.95
Halsey Pharm	00879-0441-10	1000s	$52.10
Parmed	00349-8655-10	1000s	$58.38

TABLETS (C-III): 325 MG-30 MG

BRAND/MANUFACTURER	NDC	SIZE	AWP
○ BRAND			
▶ EMPIRIN W/CODEINE: Burr Wellcome	00081-0220-55	100s	$33.67
	00081-0220-70	500s	$165.10
○ GENERICS			
Southwood	58016-0226-10	10s	$4.37
Allscrips	54569-0300-01	12s	$1.20
Quality Care	60346-0560-12	12s	$2.52
Pharm Corp/America	51655-0817-54	15s	$2.70
Quality Care	60346-0560-15	15s	$2.86
Southwood	58016-0226-15	15s	$5.83
Allscrips	54569-0300-01	20s	$2.00
Quality Care	60346-0560-20	20s	$3.30
Southwood	58016-0226-20	20s	$6.36
Southwood	58016-0226-24	24s	$6.73
Quality Care	60346-0560-25	25s	$4.24
Allscrips	54569-0300-02	30s	$3.01
Pharm Corp/America	51655-0817-24	30s	$4.55
Quality Care	60346-0560-30	30s	$4.57
Southwood	58016-0226-30	30s	$7.78
Rugby	00536-3328-01	100s	$8.93
Moore,H.L.	00839-7857-06	100s	$9.30
Major	00904-3900-60	100s	$9.40
Moore,H.L.	00839-6435-06	100s	$9.71
Qualitest	00603-2361-21	100s	$10.55
Geneva	00781-1660-01	100s	$10.80
Goldline	00182-1225-01	100s	$10.85
Zenith	00172-3984-60	100s	$10.85
Martec	52555-0333-01	100s	$10.95
Halsey Pharm	00879-0442-01	100s	$10.95
▶ URL	00677-0647-01	100s	$11.23
Schein	00364-0540-01	100s	$11.97
Parmed	00349-4082-01	100s	$12.95
Aligen	00405-0021-01	100s	$13.44
Southwood	58016-0226-00	100s	$15.91
Halsey Pharm	00879-0442-05	500s	$36.50
Rugby	00536-3328-05	500s	$41.63
Geneva	00781-1660-05	500s	$51.30
Major	00904-3900-80	1000s	$70.45
Halsey Pharm	00879-0442-10	1000s	$74.80
Moore,H.L.	00839-6435-16	1000s	$81.66

BRAND/MANUFACTURER	NDC	SIZE	AWP
Qualitest	00603-2361-32	1000s	$93.50
Zenith	00172-3984-80	1000s	$93.55
Martec	52555-0333-10	1000s	$93.80
Parmed	00349-4082-10	1000s	$109.95

TABLETS (C-III): 325 MG-60 MG

BRAND/MANUFACTURER	NDC	SIZE	AWP
○ BRAND			
EMPIRIN W/CODEINE: Burr Wellcome	00081-0225-55	100s	$78.65
	00081-0225-70	500s	$392.20
○ GENERICS			
Pharm Corp/America	51655-0818-54	15s	$3.80
Allscrips	54569-0280-02	15s	$6.50
Pharm Corp/America	51655-0818-24	30s	$5.40
Allscrips	54569-0280-03	30s	$7.85
Allscrips	54569-0280-00	50s	$10.55
Moore,H.L.	00839-6776-06	100s	$12.00
Major	00904-3907-60	100s	$14.65
Allscrips	54569-0280-01	100s	$15.35
Rugby	00536-3329-01	100s	$15.75
Moore,H.L.	00839-7858-06	100s	$15.92
Quality Care	60346-0936-00	100s	$16.66
Halsey Pharm	00879-0443-01	100s	$17.75
Geneva	00781-1875-01	100s	$18.25
▶ URL	00677-0676-01	100s	$18.35
Goldline	00182-1226-01	100s	$18.40
Qualitest	00603-2362-21	100s	$18.40
Zenith	00172-3985-60	100s	$18.40
Martec	52555-0334-01	100s	$18.97
Southwood	58016-0227-00	100s	$19.03
Parmed	00349-8337-01	100s	$19.53
Schein	00364-0541-01	100s	$20.29
Aligen	00405-0022-01	100s	$20.67
Major	00904-3907-40	500s	$56.95
Halsey Pharm	00879-0443-05	500s	$83.75
Zenith	00172-3985-70	500s	$86.25
Halsey Pharm	00879-0443-10	1000s	$129.95
Parmed	00349-8337-10	1000s	$171.15

Aspirin with Hydrocodone Bitartrate

DESCRIPTION
Each tablet contains:

Hydrocodone Bitartrate* .... 5 mg
Aspirin .... 500 mg
WARNING: May be habit forming.

Hydrocodone Bitartrate is an opioid analgesic and antitussive and occurs as fine, white crystals or as a crystalline powder. It is affected by light. The chemical name is: 4,5α-epoxy-3-methoxy-17-methylmorphinan-6-one tartrate (1:1) hydrate (2:5). The molecular formula is $C_{18}H_{21}NO_3 \cdot C_4H_6O_6 \cdot 2\frac{1}{2}H_2O$.

Aspirin, salicylic acid acetate, is a non-opiate, salicylate analgesic, anti-inflammatory, and antipyretic which occurs as a white, crystalline tabular or needle-like powder and is odorless or has a faint odor. The molecular formula is $C_9H_8O_4$.

CLINICAL PHARMACOLOGY
Hydrocodone: Hydrocodone is a semisynthetic narcotic analgesic and antitussive with multiple actions qualitatively similar to those of codeine. Most of these involve the central nervous system and smooth muscle. The precise mechanism of action of Hydrocodone and other opiates is not known, although it is believed to relate to the existence of opiate receptors in the central nervous system. In addition to analgesia, narcotics may produce drowsiness, changes in mood and mental clouding.

Radioimmunoassay techniques have recently been developed for the analysis of Hydrocodone in human plasma. After a 10 mg oral dose of Hydrocodone Bitartrate, a mean peak serum drug level of 23.6 ng/mL and an elimination half-life of 3.8 hours were found.

Aspirin: The analgesic, anti-inflammatory and antipyretic effects of Aspirin are believed to result from inhibition of the synthesis of certain prostaglandins. Aspirin interferes with clotting mechanisms primarily by diminishing platelet aggregation; at high doses prothrombin synthesis can be inhibited.

Aspirin in solution is rapidly absorbed from the stomach and from the upper small intestine. About 50 percent of an oral dose is absorbed in 30 minutes and peak plasma concentrations are reached in about 40 minutes. Higher than normal stomach pH or the presence of food slightly delays absorption.

Once absorbed, Aspirin is mainly hydrolyzed to salicylic acid and distributed to all body tissues and fluids, including fetal tissue, breast milk and the central nervous system (CNS). Highest concentrations are found in plasma, liver, renal cortex, heart and lung.

From 50 to 80 percent of salicylic acid and its metabolites in plasma are loosely bound to protein. The plasma half-life of total salicylate is about 3.0 hours, with a

---

◆ RATED THERAPEUTICALLY EQUIVALENT; ◇ THERAPEUTIC EQUIVALENCE UNCONFIRMED; ○ UNRATED

650 mg dose. Higher doses of Aspirin cause increases in plasma salicylate half-life. Almost all of a therapeutic dose of Aspirin is excreted through the kidneys, either as salicyclic acid or its metabolites. Renal clearance of salicylate is greatly augmented by an alkaline urine, as is produced by concurrent administration of sodium bicarbonate or potassium citrate.

Toxic salicylate blood levels are usually above 30 mg/100 mL. The single lethal dose of Aspirin in normal adults is approximately 25-30 g, but patients have recovered from much larger doses with appropriate treatment.

INDICATIONS AND USAGE
For the relief of moderate to moderately severe pain.

CONTRAINDICATIONS
Hydrocodone Bitartrate and Aspirin Tablets are contraindicated under the following conditions:

(1) hypersensitivity or intolerance to Hydrocodone or Aspirin.

(2) severe bleeding, disorders of coagulation or primary hemostasis, including hemophilia, hypoprothrombinemia, von Willebrand's disease, thrombocytopenias, thrombasthenia and other ill-defined hereditary platelet dysfunctions, severe vitamin K deficiency and severe liver damage.

(3) anticoagulant therapy.

(4) peptic ulcer, or other serious gastrointestinal lesions.

WARNINGS
Drugs of this class, salicylates, have been reported to be associated with the development of Reyes Syndrome in children or teenagers with chicken pox, influenza, and influenza-like infections.

Hydrocodone: Respiratory Depression: At high doses or in sensitive patients, Hydrocodone may produce dose-related respiratory depression by acting directly on the brain stem respiratory center. Hydrocodone also affects the center that controls respiratory rhythm, and may produce irregular and periodic breathing.

Head Injury and Increased Intracranial Pressure: The respiratory depressant effects of narcotics and their capacity to elevate cerebrospinal fluid pressure may be markedly exaggerated in the presence of head injury, other intracranial lesions or a pre-existing increase in intracranial pressure. Furthermore, narcotics produce adverse reactions which may obscure the clinical course of patients with head injuries.

Acute Abdominal Conditions: The administration of narcotics may obscure the diagnosis or clinical course of patients with acute abdominal conditions.

Aspirin: Allergic Reactions: Therapeutic doses of Aspirin can cause anaphylactic shock and other severe allergic reactions. A history of allergy is often lacking.

Bleeding: Significant bleeding can result from Aspirin therapy in patients with peptic ulcer or other gastrointestinal lesions, and in patients with bleeding disorders. Aspirin administered preoperatively may prolong bleeding time.

PRECAUTIONS
Special Risk Patients: As with any narcotic analgesic agent. Aspirin and Hydrocodone Bitartrate Tablets should be used with caution in elderly or debilitated patients and those with severe impairment of hepatic or renal function, gallbladder disease or gallstones, respiratory impairment, cardiac arrhythmias, inflammatory disorders of the gastrointestinal tract, hypothyroidism, Addison's disease, prostatic hypertrophy or urethral stricture, coagulation disorders, head injuries or acute abdominal conditions. The usual precautions should be observed and the possibility of respiratory depression should not be overlooked.

Precautions should be taken when administering salicylates to persons with known allergies. Hypersensitivity to Aspirin is particularly likely in patients with nasal polyps, and relatively common with asthma.

Information for Patients: Aspirin and Hydrocodone Bitartrate Tablets, like all narcotics, may impair the mental and/or physical abilities required for the performance of potentially hazardous tasks such as driving a car or operating machinery; patients should be cautioned accordingly.

Cough Reflex: Hydrocodone suppresses the cough reflex; as with all narcotics, caution should be exercised when Aspirin and Hydrocodone Bitartrate Tablets are used postoperatively and in patients with pulmonary disease.

Laboratory Tests: Hypersensitivity to Aspirin cannot be detected by skin testing or radioimmunoassay procedures.

DRUG INTERACTIONS
Aspirin: Aspirin may *enhance* the effects of:

(1) oral anticoagulants, causing bleeding by inhibiting prothrombin formation in the liver and displacing anticoagulants from plasma protein binding sites.

(2) oral antidiabetic agents and insulin, causing hypoglycemia by contributing an additive effect, and by displacing the oral antidiabetic agents from secondary binding sites.

(3) 6-mercaptopurine and methotrexate, causing bone marrow toxicity and blood dyscrasias by displacing these drugs from secondary binding sites.

(4) non-steroidal anti-inflammatory agents, increasing the risk of peptic ulceration and bleeding by contributing additive effects.

(5) corticosteroids, potentiating anti-inflammatory effects by displacing steroids from protein binding sites. Aspirin intoxication may occur with corticosteroid withdrawal because steroids promote renal clearance of salicylates.

Aspirin may *diminish* the effects of uricosuric agents, such as probenecid and sulfinpyrazone, in the treatment of gout by competing for protein binding sites.

Hydrocodone: Patients receiving other narcotic analgesics, antipsychotics, anti-anxiety agents, or other CNS depressants (including alcohol) concomitantly with Aspirin/Hydrocodone Bitartrate Tablets may exhibit additive CNS depression. When combined therapy is contemplated, the dose of one or both agents should be reduced.

The use of MAO inhibitors or tricyclic antidepressants with Hydrocodone preparations may increase the effect of either the antidepressant or Hydrocodone.

The concurrent use of anticholinergics with Hydrocodone, as with all narcotics, may produce paralytic ileus.

DRUG/LABORATORY TEST INTERACTIONS
Aspirin: Aspirin may interfere with the following laboratory determinations.

In Blood: serum amylase, fasting blood glucose, carbon dioxide, cholesterol, protein, protein bound iodine, uric acid, prothrombin time, bleeding time and spectrophotometric detection of barbiturates.

In Urine: glucose, 5-hydroxyindoleacetic acid, Gerhardt ketone, vanillylmandelic acid (VMA), protein, uric acid, and diacetic acid.

PREGNANCY
Teratogenic Effects: Pregnancy Category C.

Aspirin: Reproductive studies in rats and mice have shown Aspirin to be teratogenic and embryocidal at four to six times the human therapeutic dose. Studies in pregnant women, however, have not shown that Aspirin increases the risk of abnormalities when administered during the first trimester of pregnancy. In controlled studies involving 41,337 pregnant women and their offspring, there was no evidence that Aspirin taken during pregnancy caused stillbirth, neonatal death or reduced birthweight. In controlled studies of 50,282 pregnant women and their offspring, Aspirin administration in moderate and heavy doses during the first four months of pregnancy showed no teratogenic effect.

Hydrocodone: Hydrocodone has been shown to be teratogenic in hamsters when given in doses 700 times the human dose. There are no adequate and well-controlled studies in pregnant women. Aspirin/Hydrocodone Bitartrate Tablets should be used during pregnancy only if the potential benefit justifies the potential risk to the fetus.

NONTERATOGENIC EFFECTS
Aspirin: Therapeutic doses of Aspirin in pregnant women close to term may cause bleeding in the mother, fetus, or neonate. During the last six months of pregnancy, regular use of Aspirin in high doses may prolong pregnancy and delivery.

Hydrocodone: Babies born to mothers who have been taking opioids regularly prior to delivery will be physically dependent. The withdrawal signs include irritability and excessive crying, tremors, hyperactive reflexes, increased respiratory rate, increased stools, sneezing, yawning, vomiting, and fever. The intensity of the syndrome does not always correlate with the duration of maternal opioid use or dose. There is no consensus on the best method of managing withdrawal. Chloropromazine 0.7 to 1 mg/kg q6h, and paregoric 2 to 4 drops/kg q4h, have been used to treat withdrawal symptoms in infants. The duration of therapy is 4 to 28 days, with the dosage decreased as tolerated.

Labor and Delivery: As with all narcotics, administration of Aspirin/Hydrocodone Bitartrate Tablets to the mother shortly before delivery may result in some degree of respiratory depression in the newborn, especially if higher doses are used. Ingestion of Aspirin prior to delivery may prolong delivery or lead to bleeding in the mother or neonate.

Nursing Mothers: Aspirin is excreted in human milk in a small amount; the significance of its effect on nursing infants is not known. It is not known whether Hydrocodone is excreted in human milk. Because many drugs are excreted in human milk and because of the potential for serious adverse reactions in nursing infants, a decision should be made whether to discontinue nursing or to discontinue the drug, taking into account the importance of the drug to the mother.

Pediatric Use: Safety and effectiveness in children have not been established.

ADVERSE REACTIONS
The most frequently observed adverse reactions include light-headedness, dizziness, sedation, nausea and vomiting. These effects seem to be more prominent in ambulatory than in nonambulatory patients and some of these adverse reactions may be alleviated if the patient lies down.

Other adverse reactions include:

CENTRAL NERVOUS SYSTEM
Aspirin: Headache, drowsiness and mental confusion can occur in response to chronic use of large doses.

Hydrocodone: Drowsiness, mental clouding, lethargy, impairment of mental and physical performance, anxiety, fear, dysphoria, psychic dependence, mood changes.

GASTROINTESTINAL SYSTEM
Aspirin: Some patients are unable to take Aspirin or other salicylates without developing nausea or vomiting. Occasional patients respond to Aspirin (usually large doses) with dyspepsia or heartburn, which may be accompanied by occult bleeding. Excessive bruising or bleeding is sometimes seen in patients with mild disorders or primary hemostasis who regularly use low doses of Aspirin.

Prolonged use of Aspirin can cause painless erosion of gastric mucosa, occult bleeding and infrequently, iron-deficiency anemia. High doses of Aspirin can exacerbate symptoms of peptic ulcer and, occasionally, cause extensive bleeding. Excessive bleeding can follow injury or surgery in patients with or without known bleeding disorders who have taken therapeutic doses of Aspirin within the preceding 10 days. Hepatotoxicity has been reported in association with prolonged use of large doses of Aspirin in patients with lupus erythematosus, rheumatoid arthritis and rheumatic disease.

Hydrocodone: The antiemetic phenothiazines are useful in suppressing the nausea and vomiting which may occur (see above); however, some phenothiazine derivatives seem to be antianalgesic and to increase the amount of narcotic required to produce pain relief, while other phenothiazines reduce the amount of narcotic required to produce a given level of analgesia. Prolonged administration of Aspirin and Hydrocodone Bitartrate Tablets may produce constipation.

HEMATOLOGIC
Aspirin: Bone marrow depression, manifested by weakness, fatigue or abnormal bruising or bleeding, has occasionally been reported with Aspirin.

In patients with glucose-6-phosphate dehydrogenase deficiency, Aspirin can cause a mild degree of hemolytic anemia.

RESPIRATORY
Hydrocodone: Hydrocodone Bitartrate may produce dose related respiratory depression by acting directly on the brain stem respiratory center. Hydrocodone also affects the center that controls respiratory rhythm, and may produce irregular and periodic breathing.

If significant respiratory depression occurs, it may be antagonized by the use of naloxone hydrochloride. Apply other supportive measures when indicated.

Aspirin: Hyperpnea and hyperventilation can occur in response to chronic use of large doses.

CARDIOVASCULAR
Aspirin: Tachycardia can occur in response to chronic use of large doses of Aspirin.

GENITOURINARY
Hydrocodone: Ureteral spasm, spasm of vesical sphincters and urinary retention have been reported.

METABOLIC
Aspirin: In hyperuricemic persons, low doses of Aspirin may reduce the effectiveness of uricosuric therapy or precipitate an attack of gout.

ALLERGIC
Aspirin: Therapeutic doses of Aspirin can induce mild or severe allergic reactions manifested by skin rashes, urticaria, angioedema, rhinorrhea, asthma, abdominal pain, nausea, vomiting, or anaphylactic shock. A history of allergy is often lacking, and allergic reactions may occur even in patients who have previously taken Aspirin without any ill effects. Allergic reactions to Aspirin are most likely to occur in patients with a history of allergic disease, especially in patients with nasal polyps or asthma.

OTHER
Aspirin: Sweating and thirst can occur in response to chronic use of large doses of Aspirin.

DRUG ABUSE AND DEPENDENCE
Aspirin and Hydrocodone Bitartrate Tablets are subject to the Federal Controlled Substance Act [Schedule CIII].

Psychic dependence, physical dependence, and tolerance may develop upon repeated administration of narcotics; therefore, Aspirin and Hydrocodone Bitartrate Tablets should be prescribed and administered with caution. However, psychic dependence is unlikely to develop when Aspirin and Hydrocodone Bitartrate Tablets are used for a short time for the treatment of pain.

Physical dependence, the condition in which continued administration of the drug is required to prevent the appearance of a withdrawal syndrome, assumes clinically significant proportions only after several weeks of continued narcotic use, although some mild degree of physical dependence may develop after a few days of narcotic therapy. Tolerance, in which increasingly large doses are required in order to produce the same degree of analgesia, is manifested initially by shortened duration of analgesic effect, and subsequently by decreases in the intensity of analgesia. The rate of development of tolerance varies among patients.

OVERDOSAGE
ASPIRIN
Signs and Symptoms: The most severe manifestations from Aspirin results from cardiovascular and respiratory insufficiency secondary to acid-base and electrolyte disturbances, complicated by hyperthermia and dehydration.

Respiratory alkalosis is characteristic of the early phase of intoxication with Aspirin while hyperventilation is occurring, but is quickly followed by metabolic acidosis in most people with severe intoxication.

Concentrations of Aspirin in plasma above 30 mg/100 ml are associated with toxicity (see "Clinical Pharmacology" section) for information on factors influencing aspirin blood levels. The single lethal dose of aspirin in adults is probably about 25-30 g, but is not known with certainty.

Hemodialysis and peritoneal dialysis can be performed to reduce the body Aspirin content.

Treatment: Treatment consists primarily of supporting vital functions, increasing salicylate elimination, and correcting the acid-base imbalance due primarily to salicylism.

Gastric emptying (Syrup of Ipecac) and/or lavage is recommended as soon as possible after ingestion, even if the patient has vomited spontaneously. Administration of activated charcoal as a slurry is beneficial after lavage and/or emesis, if less than three hours have passed since ingestion. Charcoal adsorption should *not* be employed prior to emesis of lavage.

Severity of Aspirin intoxication is determined by measuring the blood salicylate level. Acid-base status should be closely followed with serial blood gas and serum pH measurements. Fluid and electrolyte balance should also be regularly monitored.

In severe cases, hyperthermia and hypovolemia are the major immediate threats to life. Children should be sponged with tepid water. Replacement fluid should be administered intravenously and augmented with sufficient bicarbonate to correct acidosis, with monitoring of plasma electrolytes and pH, to promote alkaline diuresis of salicylate if renal function is normal. Complete control may also require infusion of glucose to control hypoglycemia.

In patients with renal insufficiency or in cases of life-threatening intoxication, dialysis is usually required. Peritoneal dialysis or exchange transfusion is indicated in infants and young children and hemodialysis in older patients.

HYDROCODONE
Signs and Symptoms: Serious overdose with Hydrocodone is characterized by respiratory depression (a decrease in respiratory rate and/or tidal volume, Cheyne-Stokes respiration, cyanosis), extreme somnolence progressing to stupor or coma, skeletal muscle flaccidity, cold and clammy skin, and sometimes bradycardia and hypotension. In severe overdosage, apnea, circulatory collapse, cardiac arrest and death may occur.

Treatment: Primary attention should be given to the reestablishment of adequate respiratory exchange through provision of a patent airway and institution of assisted or controlled ventilation. If significant respiratory depression occurs, it may be antagonized by the use of naloxone hydrochloride intravenously (see package insert for dosage and full information). Naloxone promptly reverses the effects of morphine-like opioid antagonists such as Hydrocodone. In patients who are physically dependent, small doses of naloxone may be sufficient not only to antagonize respiratory depression, but also to precipitate withdrawal phenomena. The dose of naloxone should therefore be adjusted accordingly in such patients. Since the duration of action of Hydrocodone may exceed that of the antagonist, the patient should be kept under continued surveillance and repeated doses of the antagonist should be administered as needed to maintain adequate respiration.

A narcotic antagonist should not be administered in the absence of clinically significant respiratory or cardiovascular depression. Oxygen, intravenous fluids, vasopressors and other supportive measures should be employed as indicated.

Gastric emptying may be useful in removing unabsorbed drug.

DOSAGE AND ADMINISTRATION
Dosage should be adjusted according to the severity of the pain and the response of the patient. However, tolerance to Hydrocodone can develop with continued use and the incidence of untoward effects is dose related.

The usual adult dosage is one or two tablets every four to six hours as needed for pain. The total 24 hour dose should not exceed 8 tablets.

Aspirin and Hydrocodone Bitartrate Tablets should be taken with food or a full glass of milk or water to lessen gastric irritation.

Store at controlled room temperature, 15°-30°C (59°-86°F).

Protect from moisture.

Dispense in a tight, light-resistant container as defined in the USP/NF with a child-resistant closure.

HOW SUPPLIED
TABLETS (C-III): 500 MG-5 MG

BRAND/MANUFACTURER	NDC	SIZE	AWP
◆ **BRAND**			
PANASAL 5/500: ECR	00095-0131-01	100s	$27.00

TABLETS (C-III): 500 MG-5 MG

BRAND/MANUFACTURER	NDC	SIZE	AWP
○ **BRAND**			
AZDONE: Central	00131-2821-37	100s	$29.30
DAMASON-P: Mason Pharm	12758-0057-01	100s	$37.68
LORTAB ASA: Whitby	50474-0500-01	100s	$47.94
DAMASON-P: Mason Pharm	12758-0057-05	500s	$162.18
AZDONE: Central	00131-2821-43	1000s	$253.40
DAMASON-P: Mason Pharm	12758-0057-10	1000s	$316.81

Aspirin with Meprobamate

DESCRIPTION
Each tablet contains 200 mg Meprobamate and 325 mg Aspirin.

ACTIONS
Meprobamate is a carbamate derivative which has been shown (in animal and/or human studies) to have effects at multiple sites in the central nervous system, including the thalamus and limbic system.

Aspirin, acetylsalicylic acid, is a nonnarcotic analgesic with antipyretic and anti-inflammatory properties.

INDICATIONS
As an adjunct in the short-term treatment of pain accompanied by tension and/or anxiety in patients with musculo-skeletal disease. Clinical trials have demonstrated that in these situations relief of pain is somewhat greater than with aspirin alone.

The effectiveness of Aspirin/Meprobamate in long-term use, that is, more than 4 months, has not been assessed by systematic clinical studies. The physician should periodically reassess the usefulness of the drug for the individual patient.

CONTRAINDICATIONS
ASPIRIN
Allergic or idiosyncratic reactions to Aspirin or related compounds.

MEPROBAMATE
Acute intermittent porphyria and allergic or idiosyncratic reactions to Meprobamate or related compounds, such as carisoprodol, mebutamate, or carbromal.

WARNINGS
ASPIRIN
Salicylates should be used with extreme caution in patients with peptic ulcer, asthma, coagulation abnormalities, hypoprothrombinemia, vitamin K deficiency, or in those on anticoagulant therapy.

In rare instances, the use of Aspirin in persons allergic to salicylates may result in life-threatening allergic episodes.

MEPROBAMATE
DRUG DEPENDENCE
Physical dependence, psychological dependence, and abuse have occurred. Chronic intoxication from prolonged ingestion of, usually, greater-than-recommended doses is manifested by ataxia, slurred speech, and vertigo. Therefore, careful supervision of dose and amounts prescribed is advised, as well as avoidance of prolonged administration, especially for alcoholics and other patients with a known propensity for taking excessive quantities of drugs.

Sudden withdrawal of the drug after prolonged and excessive use may precipitate recurrence of preexisting symptoms such as anxiety, anorexia, or insomnia, or withdrawal reactions such as vomiting, ataxia, tremors, muscle twitching, confusional states, hallucinosis, and, rarely, convulsive seizures. Such seizures are more likely to occur in persons with central-nervous-system damage or preexistent or latent convulsive disorders. Onset of withdrawal symptoms occurs usually within 12 to 48 hours after discontinuation of Meprobamate; symptoms usually cease within the next 12- to 48-hour period.

When excessive dosage has continued for weeks or months, dosage should be reduced gradually over a period of 1 to 2 weeks rather than abruptly stopped. Alternatively, a short-acting barbiturate may be subsituted, then gradually withdrawn.

POTENTIALLY HAZARDOUS TASKS
Patients should be warned that Meprobamate may impair the mental or physical abilities required for performance of potentially hazardous tasks, such as driving or operating machinery.

ADDITIVE EFFECTS
Since CNS-suppressant effects of Meprobamate and alcohol or Meprobamate and other psychotropic drugs may be additive, appropriate caution should be exercised with patients who take more than one of these agents simultanteously.

USAGE IN PREGNANCY AND LACTATION
An increased risk of congenital malformations associated with the use of minor tranquilizers (Meprobamate, chlordiaz-epoxide, and diazepam) during the first trimester of pregnancy has been suggested in several studies. Because use of these drugs is rarely a matter of urgency, their use during this period should almost always be avoided. The possibility that a woman of childbearing potential may be pregnant at the time of institution of therapy should be considered. Patients should be advised that if they become pregnant during therapy or intend to become pregnant they should communicate with their physicians about the desirability of discontinuing the drug.

Meprobamate passes the placental barrier. It is present both in umbilical-cord blood at or near maternal plasma levels and in breast milk of lactating mothers at concentrations two to four times that of maternal plasma. When use of Meprobamate is contemplated in breast-feeding patients, the drug's higher concentrations in breast milk as compared to maternal plasma levels should be considered.

USAGE IN CHILDREN
Preparations containing Aspirin should be kept out of the reach of children Aspirin/Meprobamate is not recommended for patients 12 years of age and under.

PRECAUTIONS
ASPIRIN
Salicylates antagonize the uricosuric activity of probenecid and sulfinpyrazone. Salicylates are reported to enhance the hypoglycemic effect of the sulfonylurea antidiabetic drugs.

MEPROBAMATE
The lowest effective dose should be administered, particularly to elderly and/or debilitated patients, in order to preclude oversedation.

Meprobamate is metabolized in the liver and excreted by the kidney; to avoid its excess accumulation, caution should be exercised in the administration to patients with compromised liver or kidney function. Meprobamate occasionally may precipitate seizures in epileptic patients.

The drug should be prescribed cautiously and in small quantities to patients with suicidal tendencies.

ADVERSE REACTIONS
ASPIRIN
Aspirin may cause epigastric discomfort, nausea, and vomiting. Hypersensitivity reactions, including urticaria, angioneurotic edema, purpura, asthma, and anaphylaxis, may rarely occur.

Patients receiving large doses of salicylates may develop tinnitus.

MEPROBAMATE
Central Nervous System: Drowsiness, ataxia, dizziness, slurred speech, headache, vertigo, weakness, paresthesias, impairment of visual accommodation, euphoria, overstimulation, paradoxical excitement, fast EEG activity.

Gastrointestinal: Nausea, vomiting, diarrhea.

Cardiovascular: Palpitation, tachycardia, various forms of arrhythmia, transient ECG changes, syncope, hypotensive crisis.

Allergic or Idiosyncratic: Milder reactions are characterized by an itchy, urticarial, or erythematous maculopapular rash which may be generalized or confined to the groin.

Other reactions have included leukopenia, acute nonthrombocytopenic purpura, petechiae, ecchymoses, eosinophilia, peripheral edema, adenopathy, fever, fixed-drug eruption with cross-reaction to carisoprodol, and cross-sensitivity between Meprobamate/mebutamate and Meprobamate/carbromal.

More severe hypersensitivity reactions, rarely reported, include hyperpyrexia, chills, angioneurotic edema, bronchospasm, oliguria, and anuria. Also, anaphylaxis, exfoliative dermatitis, stomatitis, and proctitis. Stevens-Johnson syndrome and bullous dermatitis have occurred.

Hematologic (See also "Allergic or Idiosyncratic"): Agranulocytosis, aplastic anemia have been reported, although no causal relationship has been established, and thrombocytopenic purpura.

Other: Exacerbation of porphyric symptoms.

DOSAGE AND ADMINISTRATION
The usual dosage of Aspirin/Meprobamate is one or two tablets, each tablet containing Meprobamate, 200 mg, and Aspirin, 325 mg, orally 3 to 4 times daily as needed for the relief of pain when tension or anxiety is present.

Aspirin/Meprobamate is not recommended for patients 12 years of age and under.

OVERDOSAGE
Treatment of overdose with Aspirin/Meprobamate is essentially symptomatic and supportive. Any drug remaining in the stomach should be removed. Induction of vomiting or gastric lavage may be indicated. Activated charcoal may reduce absorption of both Aspirin and Meprobamate.

Overdosage with Aspirin produces the usual symptoms and signs of salicylate intoxication. Observation and treatment should include management of hyperthermia, specific parenteral electrolyte therapy for ketoacidosis and dehydration, watching for evidence of hemorrhagic manifestations due to hypoprothrombinemia which, if it occurs, usually requires whole-blood transfusions.

Suicidal attempts with Meprobamate have resulted in drowsiness, lethargy, stupor, ataxia, coma, shock, vasomotor and respiratory collapse. Some suicidal attempts have been fatal. The following data have been reported in the literature and from other sources. These data are not expected to correlate with each case (considering factors such as individual susceptibility and length of time from ingestion to treatment) but represent the usual ranges reported.

Acute simple overdose (Meprobamate alone): Death has been reported with ingestion of as little as 12 grams Meprobamate and survival with as much as 40 grams.

BLOOD LEVELS
0.5 to 2.0 mg percent represents the usual blood-level range of Meprobamate after therapeutic doses. The level may occasionally be as high as 3.0 mg percent.

3 to 10 mg percent usually corresponds to findings of mild-to-moderate symptoms of overdosage, such as stupor or light coma.

10 to 20 mg percent usually corresponds to deeper coma, requiring more intensive treatment. Some fatalities occur.

At levels greater than 20 mg percent, more fatalities than survivals can be expected.

Acute combined overdose (Meprobamate with other psychotropic drugs or alcohol): Since effects can be additive, a history of ingestion of a low dose of Meprobamate plus any of these compounds (or of a relatively low blood or tissue level) cannot be used as a prognostic indicator.

In cases where excessive doses have been taken, sleep ensues rapidly and blood pressure, pulse, and respiratory rates are reduced to basal levels. Any drug remaining in the stomach should be removed and symptomatic treatment given. Should respiration or blood pressure become compromised, respiratory assistance, central-nervous-system stimulants, and pressor agents should be administered cautiously as indicated. Diuresis, osmotic (mannitol) diuresis, peritoneal dialysis, and hemodialysis have been used successfully in removing both Aspirin and Meprobamate. Alkalinization of the urine increases the excretion of salicylates. Careful monitoring of urinary output is necessary, and caution should be taken to avoid overhydration. Relapse and death, after initial recovery, have been attributed to incomplete gastric emptying and delayed absorption.

Store at room temperature, approx. 25°C (77°F).
Keep tightly closed.
Protect from light.
Dispense in light-resistant, tight container.

HOW SUPPLIED
TABLETS (C-IV): 325 MG-200 MG

AVERAGE UNIT PRICE (AVAILABLE SIZES)	
BRAND	$0.91
GENERIC	$0.20

BRAND/MANUFACTURER	NDC	SIZE	AWP
◆ BRAND			
EQUAGESIC: Wyeth-Ayerst	00008-0091-02	100s	$67.14
MICRAININ: Wallace	00037-0120-01	100s	$114.41
◆ GENERICS			
EPROMATE-M: Major	00904-0671-60	100s	$20.90
EPROMATE-M: Major	00904-0671-40	500s	$98.05

Aspirin/Butalbital/Caffeine

DESCRIPTION
Each Aspirin/Butalbital/Caffeine Tablet or Capsule for oral administration contains: Aspirin, USP, 325 mg; Butalbital, USP, 50 mg (Warning: May be habit forming); Caffeine, USP, 40 mg.

Butalbital, 5-allyl-5-isobutyl-barbituric acid, a white odorless crystalline powder; is a short- to intermediate-acting barbiturate.

TABLETS
Active Ingredients: Aspirin, USP, Butalbital, USP, and Caffeine, USP.

CAPSULES
Active Ingredients: Aspirin, USP, Butalbital, USP, and Caffeine, USP.

Certain brands of Aspirin/Butalbital/Caffeine may also include: benzyl alcohol, butylparaben, color additives including FD&C Blue #1, FD&C Green #3, FD&C Yellow #6, edetate calcium disodium, methylparaben, propylparaben, silicon dioxide, sodium propionate.

ACTIONS
Pharmacologically, Aspirin/Butalbital/Caffeine combines the analgesic properties of Aspirin with the anxiolytic and muscle relaxant properties of Butalbital.

The clinical effectiveness of Aspirin/Butalbital/Caffeine in tension headache has been established in double-blind, placebo-controlled, multi-clinic trials. A factorial design study compared Aspirin/Butalbital/Caffeine with each of its major components. This study demonstrated that each component contributes to the efficacy of Aspirin/Butalbital/Caffeine in the treatment of the target symptoms of tension headache (headache pain, psychic tension, and muscle contraction in the head, neck, and shoulder region). For each symptom and the symptom complex as a whole Aspirin/Butalbital/Caffeine was shown to have significantly superior clinical effects to either component alone.

INDICATIONS
Aspirin/Butalbital/Caffeine is indicated for the relief of the symptom complex of tension (or muscle contraction) headache.

CONTRAINDICATIONS
Hypersensitivity to Aspirin, Barbiturates, or Caffeine. Patients with porphyria.

WARNINGS
DRUG DEPENDENCY
Prolonged use of barbiturates can produce drug dependence, characterized by psychic dependence, and less frequently, physical dependence and tolerance. The abuse liability of Aspirin/Butalbital/Caffeine is similar to that of other barbiturate-containing drug combinations. Caution should be exercised when prescribing medication for patients with a known propensity for taking excessive quantities of drugs, which is not uncommon in patients with chronic tension headache.

USE IN AMBULATORY PATIENTS
Aspirin/Butalbital/Caffeine may impair the mental and/or physical abilities required for the performance of potentially hazardous tasks, such as driving a car or operating machinery. The patient should be cautioned accordingly. Central Nervous System depressant effects of Butalbital may be additive with those of other CNS depressants. Concurrent use with other sedative-hypnotics or alcohol should be avoided. When such combined therapy is necessary, the dose of one or more agents may need to be reduced.

USE IN PREGNANCY
Adequate studies have not been performed in animals to determine whether this drug affects fertility in males or females, has teratogenic potential, or has other adverse effects on the fetus. While there are no well-controlled studies in pregnant women, over twenty years of marketing and clinical experience does not include any positive evidence of adverse effects on the fetus. Although there is no clearly defined risk, such experience cannot exclude the possibility of infrequent or subtle damage to the human fetus. Aspirin/Butalbital/Caffeine should be used in pregnant women only when clearly needed.

NURSING MOTHERS
The effects of Aspirin/Butalbital/Caffeine on infants of nursing mothers are not known. Salicylates and barbiturates are excreted in the breast milk of nursing mothers. The serum levels in infants are believed to be insignificant with therapeutic doses.

PRECAUTIONS
Salicylates should be used with extreme caution in the presence of peptic ulcer or coagulation abnormalities.

PEDIATRIC USE
Safety and effectiveness in children below the age of 12 have not been established.

ADVERSE REACTIONS
The most frequent adverse reactions are drowsiness and dizziness. Less frequent adverse reactions are light-headedness and gastrointestinal disturbances including nausea, vomiting, and flatulence. A single incidence of bone marrow suppression has been reported with the use of Aspirin/Butalbital/Caffeine. Several cases of dermatological reactions including toxic epidermal necrolysis and erythema multiforme have been reported.

OVERDOSAGE
The toxic effects of acute overdosage of Aspirin/Butalbital/Caffeine are attributable mainly to its barbiturate component, and, to a lesser extent, Aspirin. Because toxic effects of Caffeine occur in very high dosages only, the possibility of significant Caffeine toxicity from Aspirin/Butalbital/Caffeine overdosage is unlikely. Symptoms attributable to *acute barbiturate poisoning* include drowsiness, confusion, and coma; respiratory depression; hypotension; shock. Symptoms attributable to *acute Aspirin poisoning* include hyperpnea; acid-base disturbances with development of metabolic acidosis; vomiting and abdominal pain; tinnitus; hyperthermia; hypoprothrombinemia; restlessness; delirium; convulsions. *Acute Caffeine poisoning* may cause insomnia, restlessness, tremor, and delirium; tachycardia and extrasystoles. *Treatment* consists primarily of management of barbiturate intoxication and the correction of the acid-base imbalance due to salicylism. Vomiting should be induced mechanically or with emetics in the conscious patient. Gastric lavage may be used if the pharyngeal and laryngeal reflexes are present and if less than 4 hours have elapsed since ingestion. A cuffed endotracheal tube should be inserted before gastric lavage of the unconscious patient and when necessary to provide assisted respiration. Diuresis, alkalinization of the urine, and correction of electrolyte disturbances should be accomplished through administration of intravenous fluids such as 1% sodium bicarbonate in 5% dextrose in water. Meticulous attention should be given to maintaining adequate pulmonary ventilation. Correction of hypotension may require the administration of levarterenol bitartrate or phenylephrine hydrochloride by intravenous infusion. In severe cases of intoxication, peritoneal dialysis, hemodialysis, or exchange transfusion may be lifesaving. Hypoprothrombinemia should be treated with Vitamin K, intravenously.

DOSAGE AND ADMINISTRATION
One or 2 tablets or capsules every 4 hours. Total daily dose should not exceed 6 tablets or capsules.

STORE AND DISPENSE
Below 77°F (25°C), tight container.

HOW SUPPLIED
CAPSULE (C-III): 325 MG-50 MG-40 MG

AVERAGE UNIT PRICE (AVAILABLE SIZES)		GENERIC A-RATED AVERAGE PRICE (GAAP)	
BRAND	$0.51	100s	$36.93
GENERIC	$0.32		

BRAND/MANUFACTURER	NDC	SIZE	AWP
◆ BRAND			
FIORINAL: Sandoz Pharm	00078-0103-13	25s ud	$16.26
	00078-0103-05	100s	$45.06
	00078-0103-08	500s	$215.52
◆ GENERICS			
Lannett	00527-1552-01	100s	$33.75
Qualitest	00603-2550-21	100s	$36.70
Goldline	00182-0140-01	100s	$37.00
ISOLLYL: Rugby	00536-3933-01	100s	$37.10
Major	00904-3934-60	100s	$37.35
Aligen	00405-0029-01	100s	$39.70
Lannett	00527-1552-10	1000s	$38.90

TABLETS (C-III): 325 MG-50 MG-40 MG

AVERAGE UNIT PRICE (AVAILABLE SIZES)		GENERIC A-RATED AVERAGE PRICE (GAAP)	
BRAND	$0.46	100s	$8.39
GENERIC	$0.06	1000s	$33.98
HCFA FUL (100s ea)	$0.04		

BRAND/MANUFACTURER	NDC	SIZE	AWP
◆ BRAND			
▶ FIORINAL: Sandoz Pharm	00078-0104-05	100s	$45.06
	00078-0104-06	100s ud	$49.26
	00078-0104-09	1000s	$421.44

◆ RATED THERAPEUTICALLY EQUIVALENT; ◇ THERAPEUTIC EQUIVALENCE UNCONFIRMED; ○ UNRATED

BRAND/MANUFACTURER	NDC	SIZE	AWP
◆ GENERICS			
Mason Dist	11845-0239-01	100s	$3.44
West-Ward	00143-1785-01	100s	$4.35
Geneva	00781-1435-01	100s	$4.45
Schein	00364-0677-01	100s	$4.50
Major	00904-3892-60	100s	$4.50
Qualitest	00603-2548-21	100s	$4.60
FORTABS: URL	00677-0827-01	100s	$4.85
Caremark	00339-4083-12	100s	$4.95
FIORMOR: Moore,H.L.	00839-6733-06	100s	$5.60
Parmed	00349-8299-01	100s	$5.95
➤ ISOLLYL: Rugby	00536-3937-01	100s	$6.44
Goldline	00182-1631-01	100s	$7.27
Purepac	00228-2023-10	100s	$7.49
Aligen	00405-0026-01	100s	$13.75
URL	00677-1439-01	100s	$37.05
West-Ward	00143-1785-25	100s ud	$15.00
Lannett	00527-1043-10	1000s	$16.00
Major	00904-3892-80	1000s	$25.00
West-Ward	00143-1785-10	1000s	$26.15
Qualitest	00603-2548-32	1000s	$26.71
Schein	00364-0677-02	1000s	$28.02
Parmed	00349-8299-10	1000s	$30.98
Geneva	00781-1435-10	1000s	$33.25
FIORMOR: Moore,H.L.	00839-6733-16	1000s	$34.29
FORTABS: URL	00677-0827-10	1000s	$34.50
➤ ISOLLYL: Rugby	00536-3937-10	1000s	$35.55
Goldline	00182-1631-10	1000s	$56.67
Purepac	00228-2023-96	1000s	$60.66

Aspirin/Butalbital/Caffeine/Codeine Phosphate

DESCRIPTION

Aspirin/Butalbital/Caffeine/Codeine Phosphate is supplied in capsule form for oral administration.

Each capsule contains:

Codeine Phosphate, USP	30 mg (½ g)

Warning: May be habit forming.

Butalbital, USP	50 mg

Warning: May be habit forming.

Caffeine, USP	40 mg
Aspirin, USP	325 mg

Codeine Phosphate occurs as fine, white, needle-shaped crystals, or white, crystalline powder. It is affected by light. Its chemical name is 7,8-didehydro-4,5α-epoxy-3-methoxy-17-methylmorphinan-6α-ol phosphate (1:1)(salt) hemihydrate.
Butalbital, 5-allyl-5-isobutyl-barbituric acid, a white odorless crystalline powder, is a short- to intermediate-acting barbiturate. Its molecular weight is 224.26 and its empirical formula is $C_{11}H_{16}N_2O_3$.

Caffeine, 1,3,7-trimethylxanthine, is a central nervous stimulant which occurs as a white powder or white glistening needles.

Aspirin is benzoic acid, 2-(acetyloxy)-, with an empirical formula of $C_9H_8O_4$.

CLINICAL PHARMACOLOGY

Aspirin/Butalbital/Caffeine/Codeine Phosphate (ASA/Butalbital/Caff/Cod) is a combination drug product intended as a treatment for tension headache.

ASA/Butalbital/Caff consists of a fixed combination of Caffeine 40 mg, Butalbital 50 mg, and Aspirin 325 mg. The role each component plays in the relief of the complex of symptoms known as tension headache is incompletely understood.

PHARMACOKINETICS

Bioavailability: The bioavailability of the components of the fixed combination of ASA/Butalbital/Caff/Cod is identical to their bioavailability when ASA/Butalbital/Caff/Cod is administered separately in equivalent molar doses.

The behavior of the individual components is described below.

ASPIRIN

The systemic availability of Aspirin after an oral dose is highly dependent on the dosage form, the presence of food, the gastric emptying time, gastric pH, antacids, buffering agents, and particle size. These factors affect not necessarily the extent of absorption of total salicylates but more the stability of Aspirin prior to absorption.

During the absorption process and after absorption, Aspirin is mainly hydrolyzed to salicylic acid and distributed to all body tissues and fluids, including fetal tissues, breast milk, and the central nervous system (CNS). Highest concentrations are found in plasma, liver, renal cortex, heart, and lung. In plasma, about 50%-80% of the salicylic acid and its metabolites are loosely bound to plasma proteins.

The clearance of total salicylates is subject to saturable kinetics; however, first-order elimination kinetics are still a good approximation for doses up to 650 mg. The plasma half-life for Aspirin is about 12 minutes and for salicylic acid and/or total salicylates is about 3.0 hours.

The elimination of therapeutic doses is through the kidneys either as salicylic acid or other biotransformation products. The renal clearance is greatly augmented by an alkaline urine as is produced by concurrent administration of sodium bicarbonate or potassium citrate.

The biotransformation of Aspirin occurs primarily in the hepatocytes. The major metabolites are salicyluric acid (75%), the phenolic and acyl glucuronides of salicylate (15%), and gentisic and gentisuric acid (1%). The bioavailability of the Aspirin component of ASA/Butalbital/Caff/Cod capsules is equivalent to that of a solution except for a slower rate of absorption. A peak concentration of 8.80 μg/mL was obtained at 40 minutes after a 650 mg dose.

See *"Overdosage"* for toxicity information.

CODEINE

Codeine is readily absorbed from the gastrointestinal tract. It is rapidly distributed from the intravascular spaces to the various body tissues, with preferential uptake by parenchymatous organs such as the liver, spleen, and kidney. Codeine crosses the blood-brain barrier, and is found in fetal tissue and breast milk. Codeine is not bound to plasma proteins and does not accumulate in body tissues.

The plasma half-life is about 2.9 hours. The elimination of codeine is primarily via the kidneys, and about 90% of an oral dose is excreted by the kidneys within 24 hours of dosing. The urinary secretion products consist of free and glucuronide-conjugated codeine (about 70%), free and conjugated norcodeine (about 10%), free and conjugated morphine (about 10%), normorphine (4%), and hydrocodone (1%). The remainder of the dose is excreted in the feces.

At therapeutic doses, the analgesic effect reaches a peak within 2 hours and persists between 4 and 6 hours.

The bioavailability of the Codeine component of ASA/Butalbital/Caff/Cod capsules is equivalent to that of a solution. Peak concentrations of 198 ng/mL were obtained at 1 hour after a 60 mg dose.

See *"Overdosage"* for toxicity information.

BUTALBITAL

Butalbital is well absorbed from the gastrointestinal tract and is expected to distribute to most of the tissues in the body. Barbiturates, in general, may appear in milk and readily cross the placental barrier. They are bound to plasma and tissue proteins to a varying degree and binding increases directly as a function of lipid solubility.

Elimination of Butalbital is primarily via the kidney (59%-88% of the dose) as unchanged drug or metabolites. The plasma half-life is about 35 hours. Urinary excretion products included parent drug (about 3.6% of the dose), 5-isobutyl-5-(2,3-dihydroxypropyl) barbituric acid (about 24% of the dose), 5-allyl-5(3-hydroxy-2-methyl-1-propyl) barbituric acid (about 4.8% of the dose), products with the barbituric acid ring hydrolyzed with excretion of urea (about 14% of the dose), as well as unidentified materials. Of the material excreted in the urine, 32% was conjugated.

The bioavailability of the Butalbital component of ASA/Butalbital/Caff/Cod capsules is equivalent to that of a solution except for a decrease in the rate of absorption. A peak concentration of 2020 ng/mL is obtained at about 1.5 hours after a 100 mg dose.

See *"Overdosage"* for toxicity information.

CAFFEINE

Like most xanthines, Caffeine is rapidly absorbed and distributed in all body tissues and fluids, including the CNS, fetal tissues, and breast milk.

Caffeine is cleared rapidly through metabolism and excretion in the urine. The plasma half-life is about 3 hours. Hepatic biotransformation prior to excretion results in about equal amounts of 1-methyl-xanthine and 1-methyluric acid. Of the 70% of the dose that has been recovered in the urine, only 3% was unchanged drug.

The bioavailability of the Caffeine component for ASA/Butalbital/Caff/Cod capsules is equivalent to that of a solution except for a slightly longer time to peak. A peak concentration of 1660 ng/mL was obtained in less than an hour for an 80 mg dose.

See *"Overdosage"* for toxicity information.

INDICATIONS

ASA/Butalbital/Caff/Cod is indicated for the relief of the symptom complex of tension (or muscle contraction) headache.

Evidence supporting the efficacy of ASA/Butalbital/Caff/Cod is derived from 2 multi-clinic trials that compared patients with tension headache randomly assigned to 4 parallel treatments: ASA/Butalbital/Caff/Cod Codeine, ASA/Butalbital/Caff and placebo. Response was assessed over the course of the first 4 hours of each of 2 distinct headaches, separated by at least 24 hours. ASA/Butalbital/Caff/Cod proved statistically significantly superior to each of its components (ASA/Butalbital/Caff, Codeine) and to placebo on measures of pain relief.

Evidence supporting the efficacy and safety of ASA/Butalbital/Caff/Cod in the treatment of multiple recurrent headaches is unavailable. Caution in this regard is required because Codeine and Butalbital are habit-forming and potentially abusable.

CONTRAINDICATIONS

ASA/Butalbital/Caff/Cod is contraindicated under the following conditions:

1. Hypersensitivity or intolerance to Aspirin, Caffeine, Butalbital or Codeine.

2. Patients with a hemorrhagic diathesis (e.g., hemophilia, hypoprothrombinemia, von Willebrand's disease, the thrombocytopenias, thrombasthenia and other

ill-defined hereditary platelet dysfunctions, severe vitamin K deficiency and severe liver damage.)

3. Patients with the syndrome of nasal polyps, angioedema and bronchospastic reactivity to Aspirin or other nonsteroidal anti-inflammatory drugs. Anaphylactoid reactions have occurred in such patients.

4. Peptic ulcer or other serious gastrointestinal lesions.

5. Patients with porphyria.

WARNINGS

Therapeutic doses of Aspirin can cause anaphylactic shock and other severe allergic reactions. It should be ascertained if the patient is allergic to Aspirin, although a specific history of allergy may be lacking.

Significant bleeding can result from Aspirin therapy in patients with peptic ulcer or other gastrointestinal lesions, and in patients with bleeding disorders.

Aspirin administered pre-operatively may prolong the bleeding time.

In the presence of head injury or other intracranial lesions, the respiratory depressant effects of Codeine and other narcotics may be markedly enhanced, as well as their capacity for elevating cerebrospinal fluid pressure. Narcotics also produce other CNS depressant effects, such as drowsiness, that may further obscure the clinical course of patients with head injuries.

Codeine or other narcotics may obscure signs on which to judge the diagnosis or clinical course of patients with acute abdominal conditions.

Butalbital and Codeine are both habit-forming and potentially abusable. Consequently, the extended use of ASA/Butalbital/Caff/Cod is not recommended.

Results from epidemiologic studies indicate an association between Aspirin and Reye Syndrome. Caution should be used in administering this product to children, including teenagers, with chicken pox or flu.

PRECAUTIONS
GENERAL

ASA/Butalbital/Caff/Cod should be prescribed with caution for certain special-risk patients such as the elderly or debilitated, and those with severe impairment of renal or hepatic function, coagulation disorders, or head injuries.

Aspirin should be used with caution in patients on anticoagulant therapy and in patients with underlying hemostatic defects.

Precautions should be taken when administering salicylates to persons with known allergies. Hypersensitivity to Aspirin is particularly likely in patients with nasal polyps, and relatively common in those with asthma.

INFORMATION FOR PATIENTS

Patients should be informed that ASA/Butalbital/Caff/Cod contains Aspirin and should not be taken by patients with an Aspirin allergy.

ASA/Butalbital/Caff/Cod may impair the mental and/or physical abilities required for performance of potentially hazardous tasks such as driving a car or operating machinery. Such tasks should be avoided while taking ASA/Butalbital/Caff/Cod.

Alcohol and other CNS depressants may produce an additive CNS depression when taken with ASA/Butalbital/Caff/Cod, and should be avoided.

Codeine and Butalbital may be habit-forming. Patients should take the drug only for as long as it is prescribed, in the amounts prescribed, and no more frequently than prescribed.

LABORATORY TESTS

In patients with severe hepatic or renal disease, effects of therapy should be monitored with serial liver and/or renal function tests.

DRUG INTERACTIONS

The CNS effects of Butalbital may be enhanced by monoamine oxidase (MAO) inhibitors.

In patients receiving concomitant corticosteroids and chronic use of Aspirin, withdrawal of corticosteroids may result in salicylism because corticosteroids enhance renal clearance of salicylates and their withdrawal is followed by return to normal rates of renal clearance.

ASA/Butalbital/Caff/Cod may enhance the effects of:

1. Oral anticoagulants, causing bleeding by inhibiting prothrombin formation in the liver and displacing anticoagulants from plasma protein binding sites.

2. Oral antidiabetic agents and insulin, causing hypoglycemia by contributing an additive effect, if dosage of ASA/Butalbital/Caff/Cod exceeds maximum recommended daily dosage.

3. 6-mercaptopurine and methotrexate, causing bone marrow toxicity and blood dyscrasias by displacing these drugs from secondary binding sites, and, in the case of methotrexate, also reducing its excretion.

4. Non-steroidal anti-inflammatory agents, increasing the risk of peptic ulceration and bleeding by contributing additive effects.

5. Other narcotic analgesics, alcohol, general anesthetics, tranquilizers such as chlordiazepoxide, sedative-hypnotics, or other CNS depressants, causing increased CNS depression.

ASA/Butalbital/Caff/Cod may diminish the effects of:

Uricosuric agents such as probenecid and sulfinpyrazone, reducing their effectiveness in the treatment of gout. Aspirin competes with these agents for protein binding sites.

DRUG/LABORATORY TEST INTERACTIONS

Aspirin: Aspirin may interfere with the following laboratory determinations in blood: serum amylase, fasting blood glucose, cholesterol, protein, serum glutamic-oxalacetic transaminase (SGOT), uric acid, prothrombin time and bleeding time. Aspirin may interfere with the following laboratory determinations in urine:

glucose, 5-hydroxyindoleacetic acid, Gerhardt ketone, vanillylmandelic acid (VMA), uric acid, diacetic acid, and spectrophotometric detection of barbiturates.

Codeine: Codeine may increase serum amylase levels.

CARCINOGENESIS, MUTAGENESIS, IMPAIRMENT OF FERTILITY

Adequate long-term studies have been conducted in mice and rats with Aspirin, alone or in combination with other drugs, in which no evidence of carcinogenesis was seen. No adequate studies have been conducted in animals to determine whether Aspirin has a potential for mutagenesis or impairment of fertility. No adequate studies have been conducted in animals to determine whether Butalbital has a potential for carcinogenesis, mutagenesis, or impairment of fertility.

USAGE IN PREGNANCY
TERATOGENIC EFFECTS:

Pregnancy Category C: Animal reproduction studies have not been conducted with ASA/Butalbital/Caff/Cod. It is also not known whether ASA/Butalbital/Caff/Cod can cause fetal harm when administered to a pregnant woman or can affect reproduction capacity. ASA/Butalbital/Caff/Cod should be given to a pregnant woman only when clearly needed.

NONTERATOGENIC EFFECTS:

Although ASA/Butalbital/Caff/Cod was not implicated in the birth defect, a female infant was born with lissencephaly, pachygyria and heterotopic gray matter. The infant was born 8 weeks prematurely to a woman who had taken an average of 90 ASA/Butalbital/Caff/Cod capsules each month from the first few days of pregnancy. The child's development was mildly delayed and from one year of age she had partial simple motor seizures.

Withdrawal seizures were reported in a two-day-old male infant whose mother had taken a Butalbital-containing drug during the last 2 months of pregnancy. Butalbital was found in the infant's serum. The infant was given phenobarbital 5 mg/kg, which was tapered without further seizure or other withdrawal symptoms.

Studies of Aspirin use in pregnant women have not shown that Aspirin increases the risk of abnormalities when administered during the first trimester of pregnancy. In controlled studies involving 41,337 pregnant women and their offspring, there was no evidence that Aspirin taken during pregnancy caused stillbirth, neonatal death or reduced birth weight. In controlled studies of 50,282 pregnant women and their offspring, Aspirin administration in moderate and heavy doses during the first four lunar months of pregnancy showed no teratogenic effect.

Reproduction studies have been performed in rabbits and rats at doses up to 150 times the human dose and have revealed no evidence of impaired fertility or harm to the fetus due to Codeine.

Therapeutic doses of Aspirin in pregnant women close to term may cause bleeding in mother, fetus, or neonate. During the last 6 months of pregnancy, regular use of Aspirin in high doses may prolong pregnancy and delivery.

LABOR AND DELIVERY

Ingestion of Aspirin prior to delivery may prolong delivery or lead to bleeding in the mother or neonate. Use of codeine during labor may lead to respiratory depression in the neonate.

NURSING MOTHERS

Aspirin, Caffeine, barbiturates and Codeine are excreted in breast milk in small amounts, but the significance of their effects on nursing infants is not known. Because of potential for serious adverse reactions in nursing infants from ASA/Butalbital/Caff/Cod a decision should be made whether to discontinue nursing or to discontinue the drug, taking into account the importance of the drug to the mother.

PEDIATRIC USE

Safety and effectiveness in children below the age of 12 have not been established.

ADVERSE REACTIONS
COMMONLY OBSERVED

The most commonly reported adverse events associated with the use of ASA/Butalbital/Caff/Cod and not reported at an equivalent incidence by placebo-treated patients were nausea and/or abdominal pain, drowsiness, and dizziness.

ASSOCIATED WITH TREATMENT DISCONTINUATION

Of the 382 patients treated with ASA/Butalbital/Caff/Cod in controlled clinical trials, three (0.8%) discontinued treatment with ASA/Butalbital/Caff/Cod because of adverse events. One patient each discontinued treatment for the following reasons: gastrointestinal upset; light-headedness and heavy eyelids; and drowsiness and generalized tingling.

INCIDENCE IN CONTROLLED CLINICAL TRIALS

The following table summarizes the incidence rates of the adverse events reported by at least 1% of the ASA/Butalbital/Caff/Cod treated patients in controlled clinical trials comparing ASA/Butalbital/Caff/Cod to placebo, and provides a comparison to the incidence rates reported by the placebo-treated patients.

The prescriber should be aware that these figures cannot be used to predict the incidence of side effects in the course of usual medical practice where patient characteristics and other factors differ from those that prevailed in the clinical trials. Similarly, the cited frequencies cannot be compared with figures obtained from other clinical investigations involving different treatments, uses, and investigators.

◆ RATED THERAPEUTICALLY EQUIVALENT; ◇ THERAPEUTIC EQUIVALENCE UNCONFIRMED; ○ UNRATED

ADVERSE EVENTS REPORTED BY AT LEAST 1% OF ASA/ BUTALBITAL/CAFF/COD TREATED PATIENTS DURING PLACEBO CONTROLLED CLINICAL TRIALS

	Incidence Rate of Adverse Events	
Body System/ Adverse Event	ASA/Butalbital/Caff/Cod (N = 382)	Placebo (N = 377)
Central Nervous		
Drowsiness	2.4%	0.5%
Dizziness/ Light-headedness	2.6%	0.5%
Intoxicated Feeling	1.0%	0%
Gastrointestinal		
Nausea/ Abdominal Pain	3.7%	0.8%

OTHER ADVERSE EVENTS REPORTED DURING CONTROLLED CLINICAL TRIALS
The listing that follows represents the proportion of the 382 patients exposed to ASA/Butalbital/Caff/Cod while participating in the controlled clinical trials who reported, on at least one occasion, an adverse event of the type cited. All reported adverse events, except those already presented in the previous table, are included. It is important to emphasize that, although the adverse events reported did occur while the patient was receiving ASA/Butalbital/Caff/Cod, the adverse events were not necessarily caused by ASA/Butalbital/Caff/Cod.

Adverse events are classified by body system and frequency. "Frequent" is defined as an adverse event which occurred in at least 1/100 (1%) of the patients; all adverse events listed in the previous table are frequent. "Infrequent" is defined as an adverse event that occurred in less than 1/100 patients but at least 1/1000 patients. All adverse events tabulated below are classified as infrequent.

Central Nervous: headache, shaky feeling, tingling, agitation, fainting, fatigue, heavy eyelids, high energy, hot spells, numbness, and sluggishness.

Autonomic Nervous: dry mouth and hyperhidrosis.

Gastrointestinal: vomiting, difficulty swallowing, and heartburn.

Cardiovascular: tachycardia.

Musculoskeletal: leg pain and muscle fatigue.

Genitourinary: diuresis.

Miscellaneous: pruritus, fever, earache, nasal congestion, and tinnitus.

Voluntary reports of adverse drug events, temporally associated with ASA/ Butalbital/Caff/Cod that have been received since market introduction and that were not reported in clinical trials by the patients treated with ASA/Butalbital/ Caff/Cod, are listed below. Many or most of these events may have no causal relationship with the drug and are listed according to body system.

Central Nervous: Abuse, addiction, anxiety, depression, disorientation, hallucination, hyperactivity, insomnia, libido decrease, nervousness, neuropathy, psychosis, sedation, sexual activity increase, slurred speech, twitching, unconsciousness, vertigo.

Autonomic Nervous: epistaxis, flushing, miosis, salivation.

Gastrointestinal: anorexia, appetite increased, constipation, diarrhea, esophagitis, gastroenteritis, gastrointestinal spasm, hiccup, mouth burning, pyloric ulcer.

Cardiovascular: chest pain, hypotensive reaction, palpitations, syncope.

Skin: erythema, erythema multiforme, exfoliative dermatitis, hives, rash, toxic epidermal necrolysis.

Urinary: kidney impairment, urinary difficulty.

Miscellaneous: allergic reaction, anaphylactic shock, cholangiocarcinoma, drug interaction with erythromycin (stomach upset), edema.

The following adverse drug event may be borne in mind as potential effects of the components of ASA/Butalbital/Caff/Cod. Potential effects of high dosage are listed in the *"Overdosage"* section of this monograph.

Aspirin: occult blood loss, hemolytic anemia, iron deficiency anemia, gastric distress, heartburn, nausea, peptic ulcer, prolonged bleeding time, acute airway obstruction, renal toxicity when taken in high doses for prolonged periods, impaired urate excretion, hepatitis.

Caffeine: cardiac stimulation, irritability, tremor, dependence, nephrotoxicity, hyperglycemia.

Codeine: nausea, vomiting, drowsiness, light-headedness, constipation, pruritus.

DRUG ABUSE AND DEPENDENCE
ASA/Butalbital/Caff/Cod is controlled by the Drug Enforcement Administration and is classified under Schedule III.

CODEINE
Codeine can produce drug dependence of the morphine type and, therefore, has the potential for being abused. Psychological dependence, physical dependence, and tolerance may develop upon repeated administration and it should be prescribed and administered with the same degree of caution appropriate to the use of other oral narcotic medications.

BUTALBITAL
Barbiturates may be habit forming: Tolerance, psychological dependence, and physical dependence may occur especially following prolonged use of high doses of barbiturates. The average daily dose for the barbiturate addict is usually about 1,500 mg. As tolerance to barbiturates develops, the amount needed to maintain the same level of intoxication increases; tolerance to a fatal dosage, however, does not increase more than two-fold. As this occurs, the margin between an intoxication dosage and fatal dosage becomes smaller. The lethal dose of a barbiturate is far less if alcohol is also ingested. Major withdrawal symptoms (convulsions and delirium) may occur within 16 hours and last up to 5 days after abrupt cessation of these drugs. Intensity of withdrawal symptoms gradually declines over a period of approximately 15 days. Treatment of barbiturate dependence consists of cautious and gradual withdrawal of the drug. Barbiturate-dependent patients can be withdrawn by using a number of different withdrawal regimens. One method involves initiating treatment at the patient's regular dosage level and gradually decreasing the daily dosage as tolerated by the patient.

OVERDOSAGE
The toxic effects of acute overdosage of ASA/Butalbital/Caff/Cod capsules are attributable mainly to the barbiturate and Codeine components, and, to a lesser extent, Aspirin. Because toxic effects of Caffeine occur in very high dosages only, the possibility of significant Caffeine toxicity from ASA/Butalbital/Caff/Cod overdosage is unlikely.

SIGNS AND SYMPTOMS
Symptoms attributable to *acute barbiturate poisoning* include drowsiness, confusion, and coma; respiratory depression; hypotension; shock. Symptoms attributable to *acute Aspirin poisoning* include hyperpnea; acid-base disturbances with development of metabolic acidosis; vomiting and abdominal pain; tinnitus, hyperthermia; hypoprothrombinemia; restlessness; delirium; convulsions. *Acute Caffeine poisoning* may cause insomnia, restlessness, tremor, and delirium; tachycardia and extrasystoles. Symptoms of *acute Codeine poisoning* include the triad of: pinpoint pupils, marked depression of respiration, and loss of consciousness. Convulsions may occur.

TREATMENT
The following paragraphs describe one approach to the treatment of overdose with ASA/Butalbital/Caff/Cod. However, because strategies for the management of an overdose continually evolve, consultation with a regional poison control center is strongly encouraged.

Treatment consists primarily of management of barbiturate intoxication, reversal of the effects of Codeine, and the correction of the acid-base imbalance due to salicylism. Vomiting should be induced mechanically or with emetics in the conscious patient. Gastric lavage may be used if the pharyngeal and laryngeal reflexes are present and if less than 4 hours have elapsed since ingestion. A cuffed endotracheal tube should be inserted before gastric lavage of the unconscious patient and when necessary to provide assisted respiration. Diuresis, alkalinization of the urine, and correction of electrolyte disturbances should be accomplished through administration of intravenous fluids such as 1% sodium bicarbonate and 5% dextrose in water.

Meticulous attention should be given to maintaining adequate pulmonary ventilation. Correction of hypotension may require the administration of levarterenol bitartrate or phenylephrine hydrochloride by intravenous infusion. In severe cases of intoxication, peritoneal dialysis, hemodialysis, or exchange transfusion may be lifesaving. Hypoprothrombinemia should be treated with vitamin K, intravenously.

Methemoglobinemia over 30% should be treated with methylene blue by slow intravenous administration.

Naloxone, a narcotic antagonist, can reverse respiratory depression and coma associated with opioid overdose. Typically, a dose of 0.4 mg to 2 mg is given parenterally and may be repeated if an adequate response is not achieved. Since the duration of action of Codeine may exceed that of the antagonist, the patient should be kept under continued surveillance and repeated doses of the antagonist should be administered as needed to maintain adequate respiration. A narcotic antagonist should not be administered in the absence of clinically significant respiratory or cardiovascular depression.

TOXIC AND LETHAL DOSES
Butalbital: toxic dose 1.0 g (adult); lethal dose 2.0-5.0 g

Aspirin: toxic blood level greater than 30 mg/100 mL; lethal dose 10-30 g (adult)

Caffeine: toxic dose greater than 1.0 g; lethal dose unknown

Codeine: lethal dose 0.5-1.0 g (adult)

DOSAGE AND ADMINISTRATION
One or 2 capsules every 4 hours. Total daily dosage should not exceed 6 capsules.

Extended and repeated use of this product is not recommended because of the potential for physical dependence.

HOW SUPPLIED
CAPSULE (C-III): 325 MG-50 MG-40 MG-30 MG

BRAND/MANUFACTURER	NDC	SIZE	AWP
○ **BRAND**			
➤ FIORINAL W/CODEINE: Sandoz Pharm	00078-0107-13	25s ud	$29.64
	00078-0107-05	100s	$94.56

➤ SHOWN IN PRODUCT IDENTIFICATION GUIDE

TABLETS (C-III): 325 MG-50 MG-40 MG-30 MG

BRAND/MANUFACTURER	NDC	SIZE	AWP
○ **GENERICS**			
Major	00904-3932-60	100s	$28.45

Aspirin/Caffeine/Dihydrocodeine Bitartrate

DESCRIPTION
Each Aspirin/Caffeine/Dihydrocodeine Bitartrate capsule contains 356. 4 mg Aspirin, 30 mg Caffeine, and 16 mg Dihydrocodeine Bitartrate. (Warning—may be habit-forming)

ACTIONS
Aspirin/Caffeine/Dihydrocodeine Bitartrate contains the nonnarcotic antipyretic-analgesic, Aspirin.

Dihydrocodeine Bitartrate is a semisynthetic narcotic analgesic, related to codeine, with multiple actions qualitatively similar to those of codeine; the most prominent of these involve the central nervous system and organs with smooth-muscle components. The principal action of therapeutic value is analgesia.

INDICATIONS
For the relief of moderate to moderately severe pain.

CONTRAINDICATIONS
Hypersensitivity to Dihydrocodeine, codeine, or Aspirin.

WARNINGS
Salicylates should be used with extreme caution in the presence of peptic ulcer or coagulation abnormalities.

DRUG DEPENDENCE
Dihydrocodeine can produce drug dependence of the codeine type and therefore has the potential of being abused. Psychic dependence, physical dependence, and tolerance may develop upon repeated administration of Dihydrocodeine, and it should be prescribed and administered with the same degree of caution appropriate to the use of other oral narcotic-containing medications.

Like other narcotic-containing medications, Dihydrocodeine is subject to the provisions of the Federal Controlled Substances Act.

USAGE IN AMBULATORY PATIENTS
Dihydrocodeine may impair the mental and/or physical abilities required for the performance of potentially hazardous tasks, such as driving a car or operating machinery. The patient using Aspirin/Caffeine/Dihydrocodeine Bitartrate should be cautioned accordingly.

INTERACTIONS WITH OTHER CENTRAL NERVOUS SYSTEM DEPRESSANTS
Patients receiving other narcotic analgesics, general anesthetics, tranquilizers, sedative-hypnotics, or other CNS depressants (including alcohol) concomitantly with Aspirin/Caffeine/Dihydrocodeine Bitartrate may exhibit an additive CNS depression. When such combined therapy is contemplated, the dose of one or both agents should be reduced.

USAGE IN PREGNANCY
Reproduction studies have not been performed in animals. There is no adequate information on whether this drug may affect fertility in human males and females or has a teratogenic potential or other adverse effect on the fetus.

USAGE IN CHILDREN
Preparations containing Aspirin should be kept out of the reach of children. Aspirin/Caffeine/Dihydrocodeine Bitartrate is not recommended for patients 12 years of age and under. Since there is no experience in children who have received this drug, safety and efficacy in children have not been established.

PRECAUTIONS
Aspirin/Caffeine/Dihydrocodeine Bitartrate should be given with caution to certain patients, such as the elderly or debilitated.

ADVERSE REACTIONS
The most frequently observed reactions include light-headedness, dizziness, drowsiness, sedation, nausea, vomiting, constipation, pruritus, and skin reactions.

DOSAGE AND ADMINISTRATION
Dosage should be adjusted according to the severity of the pain and the response of the patient Aspirin/Caffeine/Dihydrocodeine Bitartrate is given orally. The usual adult dose is two capsules every 4 hours as needed for pain.

DRUG INTERACTIONS
The CNS-depressant effects of Aspirin/Caffeine/Dihydrocodeine Bitartrate may be additive with that of other CNS depressants. See *"Warnings"*.

Aspirin may enhance the effects of anticoagulants and inhibit the uricosuric effects of uricosuric agents.

Store at room temperature (approximately 25°C).
Keep tightly closed.
Dispense in tight container.

**HOW SUPPLIED
CAPSULE (C-III): 356.4 MG-30 MG-16 MG**

AVERAGE UNIT PRICE (AVAILABLE SIZES)

BRAND	$0.70

BRAND/MANUFACTURER	NDC	SIZE	AWP
◆ **BRAND**			
SYNALGOS-DC: Wyeth-Ayerst	00008-4191-01	100s	$72.03
	00008-4191-02	500s	$342.50

Aspirin/Caffeine/Orphenadrine Citrate

ACTIONS
Aspirin/Caffeine/Orphenadrine Citrate is a centrally acting (brain stem) compound which in animals selectively blocks facilitatory functions of the reticular formation. Orphenadrine does not produce myoneural block, nor does it affect crossed extensor reflexes. Orphenadrine prevents nicotine-induced convulsions but not those produced by strychnine.

Chronic administration of Aspirin/Caffeine/Orphenadrine Citrate (ASA/Caff/Orphenadrine) to dogs and rats has revealed no drug-related toxicity. No blood or urine changes were observed, nor were there any macroscopic or microscopic pathological changes detected. Extensive experience with combinations containing Aspirin and Caffeine has established them as safe agents. The addition of Orphenadrine Citrate does not alter the toxicity of Aspirin and Caffeine. The mode of therapeutic action of Orphenadrine has not been clearly identified, but may be related to its analgesic properties. Orphenadrine Citrate also possesses anticholinergic actions.

INDICATIONS
1. Symptomatic relief of mild to moderate pain of acute musculoskeletal disorders.

2. The Orphenadrine component is indicated as an adjunct to rest, physical therapy, and other measures for the relief of discomfort associated with acute painful musculoskeletal conditions.

The mode of action of Orphenadrine has not been clearly identified, but may be related to its analgesic properties. ASA/Caff/Orphenadrine does not directly relax tense skeletal muscles in man.

CONTRAINDICATIONS
Because of the mild anticholinergic effect of Orphenadrine, ASA/Caff/Orphenadrine should not be used in patients with glaucoma, pyloric or duodenal obstruction, achalasia, prostatic hypertrophy or obstructions at the bladder neck. ASA/Caff/Orphenadrine is also contraindicated in patients with myasthenia gravis and in patients known to be sensitive to Aspirin or Caffeine.

The drug is contraindicated in patients who have demonstrated a previous hypersensitivity to the drug.

WARNINGS
Reye Syndrome may develop in individuals who have chicken pox, influenza, or flu symptoms. Some studies suggest possible association between the development of Reye Syndrome and the use of medicines containing salicylate or Aspirin. ASA/Caff/Orphenadrine contains aspirin and therefore are not recommended for use in patients with chicken pox, influenza, or flu symptoms.

ASA/Caff/Orphenadrine may impair the ability of the patient to engage in potentially hazardous activities such as operating machinery or driving a motor vehicle; ambulatory patients should therefore be cautioned accordingly.

Aspirin should be used with extreme caution in the presence of peptic ulcers and coagulation abnormalities.

USAGE IN PREGNANCY
Since safety of the use of this preparation in pregnancy, during lactation, or in the childbearing age has not been established, use of the drug in such patients requires that the potential benefits of the drug be weighed against its possible hazard to the mother and child.

USAGE IN CHILDREN
The safe and effective use of this drug in children has not been established. Usage of this drug in children under 12 years of age is not recommended.

PRECAUTIONS
Confusion, anxiety and tremors have been reported in a few patients receiving propoxyphene and Orphenadrine concomitantly. As these symptoms may be simply due to an additive effect, reduction of dosage and/or discontinuation of one or both agents is recommended in such cases.

Safety of continuous long term therapy with ASA/Caff/Orphenadrine has not been established; therefore, if ASA/Caff/Orphenadrine is prescribed for prolonged use, periodic monitoring of blood, urine and liver function values is recommended.

◆ RATED THERAPEUTICALLY EQUIVALENT; ◇ THERAPEUTIC EQUIVALENCE UNCONFIRMED; ○ UNRATED

ADVERSE REACTIONS

Side effects of ASA/Caff/Orphenadrine are those seen with Aspirin and Caffeine or those usually associated with mild anticholinergic agents. These may include tachycardia, palpitation, urinary hesitancy or retention, dry mouth, blurred vision, dilatation of the pupil, increased intraocular tension, weakness, nausea, vomiting, headache, dizziness, constipation, drowsiness, and rarely, urticaria and other dermatoses. Infrequently, an elderly patient may experience some degree of confusion. Mild central excitation and occasional hallucinations may be observed. These mild side effects can usually be eliminated by reduction in dosage. One case of aplastic anemia associated with the use of ASA/Caff/Orphenadrine has been reported. No causal relationship has been established. Rare G.I. hemorrhage due to Aspirin content may be associated with the administration of ASA/Caff/Orphenadrine. Some patients may experience transient episodes of light-headedness, dizziness or syncope.

DOSAGE AND ADMINISTRATION

ASA/Caff/Orphenadrine: Adults 1 to 2 tablets 3 to 4 times daily.

ASA/Caff/Orphenadrine double strength: Adults ½ to 1 tablet 3 to 4 times daily.

ASA/CAFF/Orphenadrine contains Orphenadrine Citrate (2-dimethylamino-ethyl 2-methylbenzhydryl ether citrate) 25 mg, Aspirin 385 mg, and Caffeine 30 mg.

ASA/Caff/Orphenadrine double strength contains Orphenadrine Citrate 50 mg, Aspirin 770 mg, and Caffeine 60 mg.

Store below 30°C (86°F).

HOW SUPPLIED
TABLETS: 385 MG-30 MG-25 MG

BRAND/MANUFACTURER	NDC	SIZE	AWP
○ **BRAND**			
NORGESIC: 3M Pharm	00089-0231-10	100s	$80.16
	00089-0231-50	500s	$380.34

TABLETS: 770 MG-60 MG-50 MG

BRAND/MANUFACTURER	NDC	SIZE	AWP
○ **BRAND**			
NORGESIC FORTE: 3M Pharm	00089-0233-10	100s	$116.34
	00089-0233-50	500s	$552.06
○ **GENERICS**			
Allscrips	54569-1613-01	20s	$13.25
Allscrips	54569-1613-00	30s	$16.90
Allscrips	54569-1613-02	100s	$43.55

Aspirin/Caffeine/Propoxyphene Hydrochloride

DESCRIPTION

Propoxyphene Hydrochloride, USP is an odorless, white crystalline powder with a bitter taste. It is freely soluble in water. Chemically, it is $(2S, 3R)\text{-}(^+)\text{-}4\text{-}$ (Dimethylamino)-3-methyl- 1,2-diphenyl-2-butanol propionate (ester) hydrochloride. Its molecular weight is 375.94.

Each capsule of Aspirin/Caffeine/Propoxyphene Hydrochloride contains 65 mg (172.9 µmol) Propoxyphene Hydrochloride, 389 mg (2,159 µmol) Aspirin, and 32.4 mg (166.8 µmol) Caffeine.

CLINICAL PHARMACOLOGY

Propoxyphene is a centrally acting narcotic analgesic agent. Equimolar doses of Propoxyphene Hydrochloride or napsylate provide similar plasma concentrations. Following administration of 65, 130, or 195 mg of Propoxyphene Hydrochloride, the bioavailability of Propoxyphene is equivalent to that of 100, 200, or 300 mg respectively of Propoxyphene napsylate. Peak plasma concentrations of Propoxyphene are reached in 2 to 2 ½ hours. After a 65-mg oral dose of Propoxyphene Hydrochloride, peak plasma levels of 0.05 to 0.1 µg/mL are achieved.

Repeated doses of Propoxyphene at 6-hour intervals lead to increasing plasma concentrations, with a plateau after the ninth dose at 48 hours.

Propoxyphene is metabolized in the liver to yield norpropoxyphene. Propoxyphene has a half-life of 6 to 12 hours, whereas that of norpropoxyphene is 30 to 36 hours.

Norpropoxyphene has substantially less central-nervous-system-depressant effect than Propoxyphene, but a greater local anesthetic effect, which is similar to that of amitriptyline antiarrhythmic agents, such as lidocaine and quinidine.

In animal studies in which Propoxyphene and norpropoxyphene were continuously infused in large amounts, intracardiac conduction time (PR and QRS intervals) was prolonged. Any intracardiac conduction delay attributable to high concentrations of norpropoxyphene may be of relatively long duration.

ACTIONS

Propoxyphene is a mild narcotic analgesic structurally related to methadone. The potency of Propoxyphene Hydrochloride is from two-thirds to equal that of Codeine.

The combination of Propoxyphene with a mixture of Aspirin and Caffeine produces greater analgesia than that produced by either Propoxyphene or Aspirin and Caffeine administered alone.

INDICATIONS

Aspirin/Caffeine/Propoxyphene Hydrochloride is indicated for the relief of mild to moderate pain, either when pain is present alone or when it is accompanied by fever.

CONTRAINDICATION

Hypersensitivity to Propoxyphene, Aspirin, or Caffeine.

WARNINGS

- DO NOT PRESCRIBE PROPOXYPHENE FOR PATIENTS WHO ARE SUICIDAL OR ADDICTION-PRONE.
- PRESCRIBE PROPOXYPHENE WITH CAUTION FOR PATIENTS TAKING TRANQUILIZERS OR ANTIDEPRESSANT DRUGS AND PATIENTS WHO USE ALCOHOL IN EXCESS.
- TELL YOUR PATIENTS NOT TO EXCEED THE RECOMMENDED DOSE AND TO LIMIT THEIR INTAKE OF ALCOHOL.

PROPOXYPHENE PRODUCTS IN EXCESSIVE DOSES, EITHER ALONE OR IN COMBINATION WITH OTHER CNS DEPRESSANTS, INCLUDING ALCOHOL, ARE A MAJOR CAUSE OF DRUG-RELATED DEATHS. FATALITIES WITHIN THE FIRST HOUR OF OVERDOSAGE ARE NOT UNCOMMON. IN A SURVEY OF DEATHS DUE TO OVERDOSAGE CONDUCTED IN 1975, IN APPROXIMATELY 20% OF THE FATAL CASES, DEATH OCCURRED WITHIN THE FIRST HOUR (5% OCCURRED WITHIN 15 MINUTES). PROPOXYPHENE SHOULD NOT BE TAKEN IN DOSES HIGHER THAN THOSE RECOMMENDED BY THE PHYSICIAN. THE JUDICIOUS PRESCRIBING OF PROPOXYPHENE IS ESSENTIAL TO THE SAFE USE OF THIS DRUG. WITH PATIENTS WHO ARE DEPRESSED OR SUICIDAL, CONSIDERATION SHOULD BE GIVEN TO THE USE OF NON-NARCOTIC ANALGESICS. PATIENTS SHOULD BE CAUTIONED ABOUT THE CONCOMITANT USE OF PROPOXYPHENE PRODUCTS AND ALCOHOL BECAUSE OF POTENTIALLY SERIOUS CNS-ADDITIVE EFFECTS OF THESE AGENTS. BECAUSE OF ITS ADDED DEPRESSANT EFFECTS, PROPOXYPHENE SHOULD BE PRESCRIBED WITH CAUTION FOR THOSE PATIENTS WHOSE MEDICAL CONDITION REQUIRES THE CONCOMITANT ADMINISTRATION OF SEDATIVES, TRANQUILIZERS, MUSCLE RELAXANTS, ANTIDEPRESSANTS, OR OTHER CNS-DEPRESSANT DRUGS. PATIENTS SHOULD BE ADVISED OF THE ADDITIVE DEPRESSANT EFFECTS OF THESE COMBINATIONS.

MANY OF THE PROPOXYPHENE-RELATED DEATHS HAVE OCCURRED IN PATIENTS WITH PREVIOUS HISTORIES OF EMOTIONAL DISTURBANCES OR SUICIDAL IDEATION OR ATTEMPTS AS WELL AS HISTORIES OF MISUSE OF TRANQUILIZERS, ALCOHOL, AND OTHER CNS-ACTIVE DRUGS. SOME DEATHS HAVE OCCURRED AS A CONSEQUENCE OF THE ACCIDENTAL INGESTION OF EXCESSIVE QUANTITIES OF PROPOXYPHENE ALONE OR IN COMBINATION WITH OTHER DRUGS. PATIENTS TAKING PROPOXYPHENE SHOULD BE WARNED NOT TO EXCEED THE DOSAGE RECOMMENDED BY THE PHYSICIAN.

Drug Dependence: Propoxyphene, when taken in higher-than-recommended doses over long periods of time, can produce drug dependence characterized by psychic dependence and, less frequently, physical dependence and tolerance. Propoxyphene will only partially suppress the withdrawal syndrome in individuals physically dependent on morphine or other narcotics. The abuse liability of Propoxyphene is qualitatively similar to that of codeine although quantitatively less, and Propoxyphene should be prescribed with the same degree of caution appropriate to the use of codeine.

Usage in Ambulatory Patients: Propoxyphene may impair the mental and/or physical abilities required for the performance of potentially hazardous tasks, such as driving a car or operating machinery. The patient should be cautioned accordingly.

Warning: Reye syndrome is a rare but serious disease which can follow flu or chickenpox in children and teenagers. Although the cause of Reye syndrome is unknown, some reports claim aspirin (or salicylates) may increase the risk of developing this disease.

PRECAUTIONS

General: Salicylates should be used with extreme caution in the presence of peptic ulcer or coagulation abnormalities. Propoxyphene should be administered with caution to patients with hepatic or renal impairment since higher serum concentrations or delayed elimination may occur.

Drug Interactions: The CNS-depressant effect of Propoxyphene is additive with that of other CNS depressants, including alcohol.

Salicylates may enhance the effect of anticoagulants and inhibit the uricosuric effect of uricosuric agents.

As is the case with medicinal agents, Propoxyphene may slow the metabolism of a concomitantly administered drug. Should this occur, the higher serum concentrations of that drug may result in increased pharmacologic or adverse effects of that drug. Such occurrences have been reported when Propoxyphene was administered to patients on antidepressants, anticonvulsants, or warfarin-like

➤ SHOWN IN PRODUCT IDENTIFICATION GUIDE

drugs. Severe neurologic signs, including coma, have occurred with concurrent use of carbamazepine.

Usage in Pregnancy: Safe use in pregnancy has not been established relative to possible adverse effects on fetal development. Instances of withdrawal symptoms in the neonate have been reported following usage during pregnancy. Therefore, Propoxyphene should not be used in pregnant women unless, in the judgment of the physician, the potential benefits outweigh the possible hazards. Aspirin does not appear to have teratogenic effects. However, prolonged pregnancy and labor with increased bleeding before and after delivery, decreased birth weight, and increased rate of stillbirth were reported with high blood salicylate levels. Because of possible adverse effects on the neonate and the potential for increased maternal blood loss, aspirin should be avoided during the last 3 months of pregnancy.

Usage in Nursing Mothers: Low levels of Propoxyphene have been detected in human milk. In postpartum studies involving nursing mothers who were given Propoxyphene, no adverse effects were noted in infants receiving mother's milk.

Usage in Children: Propoxyphene is not recommended for use in children, because documented clinical experience has been insufficient to establish safety and a suitable dosage regimen in the pediatric age group.

Usage in the Elderly: The rate of Propoxyphene metabolism may be reduced in some patients. Increased dosing interval should be considered.

A Patient Information Sheet is available for this product.

ADVERSE REACTIONS
In a survey conducted in hospitalized patients, less than 1% of patients taking Propoxyphene Hydrochloride at recommended doses experienced side effects. The most frequently reported have been dizziness, sedation, nausea, and vomiting. Some of these adverse reactions may be alleviated if the patient lies down.

Other adverse reactions include constipation, abdominal pain, skin rashes, light-headedness, headache, weakness, euphoria, dysphoria, hallucinations, and minor visual disturbances.

Propoxyphene therapy has been associated with abnormal liver function tests and, more rarely, with instances of reversible jaundice (including cholestatic jaundice).

Renal papillary necrosis may result from chronic aspirin use, particularly when the dosage is greater than recommended and when combined with acetaminophen.

Subacute painful myopathy has occurred following chronic Propoxyphene overdosage.

MANAGEMENT OF OVERDOSAGE
In all cases of suspected overdosage, call your regional poison control center to obtain the most up-to-date information about the treatment of overdosage. This recommendation is made because, in general, information regarding the treatment of overdosage may change more rapidly than do package inserts.

Initial consideration should be given to the management of the CNS effects of Propoxyphene overdosage. Resuscitative measures should be initiated promptly.

Symptoms of Propoxyphene Overdosage: The manifestations of acute overdosage with Propoxyphene are those of narcotic overdosage. The patient is usually somnolent, but may be stuporous or comatose and convulsing. Respiratory depression is characteristic. The ventilatory rate and/or tidal volume is decreased, which results in cyanosis and hypoxia. Pupils, initially pinpoint, may become dilated as hypoxia increases. Cheyne-Stokes respiration and apnea may occur. Blood pressure and heart rate are usually normal initially, but blood pressure falls and cardiac performance deteriorates, which ultimately results in pulmonary edema and circulatory collapse, unless the respiratory depression is corrected and adequate ventilation is restored promptly. Cardiac arrhythmias and conduction delay may be present. A combined respiratory-metabolic acidosis occurs, owing to retained CO_2 (hypercapnia) and to lactic acid formed during anaerobic glycolysis. Acidosis may be severe if large amounts of salicylates have also been ingested. Death may occur.

Treatment of Propoxyphene Overdosage: Attention should be directed first to establishing a patent airway and to restoring ventilation. Mechanically assisted ventilation, with or without oxygen, may be required, and positive-pressure respiration may be desirable if pulmonary edema is present. The narcotic antagonist naloxone will markedly reduce the degree of respiratory depression, and 0.4 to 2 mg should be administered promptly, preferably intravenously. If the desired degree of counteraction with improvement in respiratory function is not obtained, naloxone should be repeated at 2- to 3-minute intervals. The duration of action of the antagonist may be brief. If no response is observed after 10 mg of naloxone have been administered, the diagnosis of propoxyphene toxicity should be questioned. Naloxone may also be administered by continuous intravenous infusion.

Treatment of Propoxyphene Overdosage in Children: The usual initial dose of naloxone in children is 0.01 mg/kg body weight given intravenously. If this dose does not result in the desired degree of clinical improvement, a subsequent increased dose of 0.1 mg/kg body weight may be administered. If an IV route of administration is not available, naloxone may be administered IM or subcutaneously in divided doses. If necessary, naloxone can be diluted with sterile water for injection.

Blood gases, pH, and electrolytes should be monitored in order that acidosis and any electrolyte disturbance present may be corrected promptly. Acidosis, hypoxia, and generalized CNS depression predispose to the development of cardiac arrhythmias. Ventricular fibrillation or cardiac arrest may occur and

necessitate the full complement of cardiopulmonary resuscitation (CPR) measures. Respiratory acidosis rapidly subsides as ventilation is restored and hypercapnia eliminated, but lactic acidosis may require intravenous bicarbonate for prompt correction.

Electrocardiographic monitoring is essential. Prompt correction of hypoxia, acidosis, and electrolyte disturbance (when present) will help prevent these cardiac complications and will increase the effectiveness of agents administered to restore normal cardiac function.

In addition to the use of a narcotic antagonist, the patient may require careful titration with an anticonvulsant to control convulsions. Analeptic drugs (for example, caffeine or amphetamine) should not be used because of their tendency to precipitate convulsions.

General supportive measures, in addition to oxygen, include, when necessary, intravenous fluids, vasopressor-inotropic compounds, and, when infection is likely, anti-infective agents. Gastric lavage may be useful, and activated charcoal can adsorb a significant amount of ingested Propoxyphene. Dialysis is of little value in poisoning due to Propoxyphene. Efforts should be made to determine whether other agents, such as alcohol, barbiturates, tranquilizers, or other CNS depressants, were also ingested, since these increase CNS depression as well as cause specific toxic effects.

Symptoms of Salicylate Overdosage: Such symptoms include central nausea and vomiting, tinnitus and deafness, vertigo and headaches, mental dullness and confusion, diaphoresis, rapid pulse, and increased respiration and respiratory alkalosis.

Treatment of Salicylate Overdosage: When Aspirin/Caffeine/ Propoxyphene Hydrochloride has been ingested, the clinical picture may be complicated by salicylism.

The treatment of acute salicylate intoxication includes minimizing drug absorption, promoting elimination through the kidneys, and correcting metabolic derangements affecting body temperature, hydration, acid-base balance, and electrolyte balance. The technique to be employed for eliminating salicylate from the bloodstream depends on the degree of drug intoxication.

If the patient is seen within 4 hours of ingestion, the stomach should be emptied by inducing vomiting or by gastric lavage as soon as possible.

The nomogram of Done is a useful prognostic guide in which the expected severity of salicylate intoxication is based on serum salicylate levels and the time interval between ingestion and taking the blood sample.

Exchange transfusion is most feasible for a small infant. Intermittent peritoneal dialysis is useful for cases of moderate severity in adults. Intravenous fluids alkalinized by the addition of sodium bicarbonate or potassium citrate are helpful. Hemodialysis with the artificial kidney is the most effective means of removing salicylate and is indicated for the very severe cases of salicylate intoxication.

DOSAGE AND ADMINISTRATION
These products are given orally. The usual dosage of Propoxyphene Hydrochloride is 65 mg every 4 hours as needed for pain.

The usual dosage of Aspirin/Caffeine/Propoxyphene Hydrochloride is 65 mg Propoxyphene Hydrochloride, 389 mg Aspirin, and 32.4 mg Caffeine every 4 hours as needed for pain.

The maximum recommended dose of Propoxyphene Hydrochloride is 390 mg/day.

Consideration should be given to a reduced total daily dosage in patients with hepatic or renal impairment.

Store at controlled room temperature, 59° to 86°F (15° to 30°C).

HOW SUPPLIED
CAPSULE (C-IV): 389 MG-32.4 MG-65 MG

AVERAGE UNIT PRICE (AVAILABLE SIZES)		GENERIC A-RATED AVERAGE PRICE (GAAP)	
BRAND	$0.33	100s	$23.00
GENERIC	$0.19	500s	$91.34
HCFA FUL (100s ea)	$0.08	1000s	$90.59

BRAND/MANUFACTURER	NDC	SIZE	AWP
◆ **BRAND**			
DARVON COMPOUND-65: Lilly	00002-3111-02	100s	$34.29
	00002-3111-03	500s	$163.02
◆ **GENERICS**			
PC-CAP: Alra	51641-0323-01	100s	$13.50
Geneva	00781-2367-01	100s	$20.30
Goldline	00182-1673-01	100s	$21.45
URL	00677-0828-01	100s	$23.05
Qualitest	00603-5460-21	100s	$23.10
Major	00904-7701-60	100s	$23.20
Moore,H.L.	00839-1561-06	100s	$23.27
Lemmon	00093-0686-01	100s	$24.50
Rugby	00536-4374-01	100s	$24.95
Schein	00364-0668-01	100s	$25.00
Aligen	00405-0173-01	100s	$25.79
Mylan	00378-0131-01	100s	$25.95
PC-CAP: Alra	51641-0323-11	100s ud	$25.00
DOXAPHENE COMPOUND: Major	00904-2170-40	500s	$41.25
PC-CAP: Alra	51641-0323-05	500s	$58.50
Major	00904-7701-40	500s	$79.15
Aligen	00405-0173-02	500s	$90.78
Goldline	00182-1673-05	500s	$99.00

◆ RATED THERAPEUTICALLY EQUIVALENT; ◇ THERAPEUTIC EQUIVALENCE UNCONFIRMED; ○ UNRATED

BRAND/MANUFACTURER	NDC	SIZE	AWP
Rugby	00536-4374-05	500s	$109.85
Qualitest	00603-5460-28	500s	$110.10
Lemmon	00093-0686-05	500s	$116.45
Mylan	00378-0131-05	500s	$116.95
Moore,H.L.	00839-1561-16	1000s	$79.64
Goldline	00182-1673-10	1000s	$91.80
PC-CAP: Alra	51641-0323-10	1000s	$92.50
Major	00904-7701-80	1000s	$94.50
Geneva	00781-2367-10	1000s	$94.50

Aspirin/Carisoprodol/Codeine Phosphate

DESCRIPTION

Aspirin/Carisoprodol/Codeine Phosphate is a combination product containing Carisoprodol, a centrally-acting muscle relaxant, plus Aspirin, an analgesic with antipyretic and anti-inflammatory properties and Codeine Phosphate, a centrally-acting narcotic analgesic. Each tablet contains Carisoprodol 200 mg, Aspirin 325 mg, and Codeine Phosphate 16 mg. Chemically, Carisoprodol is N-isopropyl-2-methyl-2-propyl-1,3-propanediol dicarbamate. Its empirical formula is $C_{12}H_{24}N_2O_4$, with a molecular weight of 260.33.

Certain brands of Aspirin/Carisoprodol/Codeine Phosphate contain sodium metabisulfite (see *"Warnings"*).

CLINICAL PHARMACOLOGY

Carisoprodol: Carisoprodol is a centrally-acting muscle relaxant that does not directly relax tense skeletal muscles in man. The mode of action of Carisoprodol in relieving acute muscle spasm of local origin has not been clearly identified, but may be related to its sedative properties. In animals, Carisoprodol has been shown to produce muscle relaxation by blocking interneuronal activity and depressing transmission of polysynaptic neurons in the spinal cord and in the descending reticular formation of the brain. The onset of action is rapid and lasts four to six hours.

Carisoprodol is metabolized in the liver and is excreted by the kidneys. It is dialyzable by peritoneal and hemodialysis.

Aspirin: Aspirin is a non-narcotic analgesic with anti-inflammatory and antipyretic activity. Inhibition of prostaglandin biosynthesis appears to account for most of its anti-inflammatory and for at least part of its analgesic and antipyretic properties.

Aspirin is rapidly absorbed and almost totally hydrolyzed to salicyclic acid following oral administration. Although Aspirin has a half-life of only about 15 minutes, the apparent biologic half-life of salicyclic acid in the therapeutic plasma concentration range is between 6 and 12 hours. Salicyclic acid is eliminated by renal excretion and by biotransformation to inactive metabolites. Clearance of salicyclic acid in the high-dose range is sensitive to urinary pH (see *"Drug Interactions"*) and is reduced by renal dysfunction.

Codeine Phosphate: Codeine Phosphate is a centrally-acting narcotic-analgesic. Its actions are qualitatively similar to morphine, but its potency is substantially less.

Clinical studies have shown that combining Aspirin and Codeine produces a significant additive effect in analgesic efficacy.

INDICATIONS AND USAGE

Aspirin/Carisoprodol/Codeine Phosphate (Aspirin/Carisoprodol/Codeine) is indicated as an adjunct to rest, physical therapy, and other measures for the relief of pain, muscle spasm, and limited mobility associated with acute, painful musculoskeletal conditions when the additional action of Codeine is desired.

CONTRAINDICATIONS

Acute intermittent porphyria; bleeding disorders; allergic or idiosyncratic reactions to Carisoprodol, Aspirin, Codeine, or related compounds.

WARNINGS

On very rare occasions, the first dose of Carisoprodol has been followed by idiosyncratic reactions, with symptoms appearing within minutes or hours. These may include extreme weakness, transient quadriplegia, dizziness, ataxia, temporary loss of vision, diplopia, mydriasis, dysarthria, agitation, euphoria, confusion, and disorientation. Although symptoms usually subside over the course of the next several hours, discontinue Aspirin/Carisoprodol/Codeine and initiate appropriate supportive and symptomatic therapy, which may include epinephrine and/or antihistamines. In severe cases, corticosteroids may be necessary. Severe reactions have been manifested by asthmatic episodes, fever, weakness, dizziness, angioneurotic edema, smarting eyes, hypotension, and anaphylactoid shock.

The effects of Carisoprodol with agents such as alcohol, other CNS depressants, or psychotropic drugs may be additive. Appropriate caution should be exercised with patients who take one or more of these agents simultaneously with Aspirin/Carisoprodol/Codeine.

Contains sodium metabisulfite, a sulfite that may cause allergic-type reactions including anaphylactic symptoms and life-threatening or less severe asthmatic episodes in certain susceptible people. The overall prevalence of sulfite sensitivity in the general population is unknown and probably low. Sulfite sensitivity is seen more frequently in asthmatic then in nonasthmatic people.

PRECAUTIONS

General: To avoid excessive accumulation of Carisoprodol, Aspirin, or their metabolites, use Aspirin/Carisoprodol/Codeine with caution in patients with compromised liver or kidney function, or in elderly or debilitated patients (see *"Clinical Pharmacology"*).

Use with caution in patients with history of gastritis or peptic ulcer, in patients on anticoagulant therapy, and in addiction-prone individuals.

Information for Patients: Caution patients that this drug may impair the mental and/or physical abilities required for the performance of potentially hazardous tasks such as driving a motor vehicle or operating machinery.

Caution patients with a predisposition for gastrointestinal bleeding that concomitant use of Aspirin and alcohol may have an additive effect in this regard.

Caution patients that dosage of medications used for gout, arthritis, or diabetes may have to be adjusted when Aspirin is administered or discontinued (see *"Drug Interactions"*).

Drug Interactions: Clinically important interactions may occur when certain drugs are administered concomitantly with Aspirin or Aspirin-containing drugs.

1. *Oral Anticoagulants:* By interfering with platelet function or decreasing plasma prothrombin concentration, Aspirin enhances the potential for bleeding in patients on anticoagulants.
2. *Methotrexate:* Aspirin enhances the toxic effects of this drug.
3. *Probenecid and Sulfinpyrazone:* large doses of Aspirin reduce the uricosuric effect of both drugs. Renal excretion of salicylate may also be reduced.
4. *Oral Antidiabetic Drugs:* enhancement of hypoglycemia may occur.
5. *Antacids:* to the extent that they raise urinary pH, antacids may substantially decrease plasma salicylate concentrations; conversely, their withdrawal can result in a substantial increase.
6. *Ammonium Chloride:* this and other drugs that acidify a relatively alkaline urine can elevate plasma salicylate concentrations.
7. *Ethyl Alcohol:* enhanced Aspirin-induced fecal blood loss has been reported.
8. *Corticosteroids:* salicylate plasma levels may be decreased when adrenal corticosteroids are given, and may be increased substantially when they are discontinued.

Carcinogenesis, Mutagenesis, Impairment of Fertility: No long-term studies have been done with Aspirin/Carisoprodol/Codeine.

Pregnancy—Teratogenic Effects: Pregnancy Category C: Adequate animal reproduction studies have not been conducted with Aspirin/Carisoprodol/Codeine. It is also not known whether Aspirin/Carisoprodol/Codeine can cause fetal harm when administered to a pregnant woman or can affect reproduction capacity. Aspirin/Carisoprodol/Codeine should be given to a pregnant woman only if clearly needed. Studies in rodents have shown salicylates to be teratogenic when given in early gestation, and embryocidal when given in later gestation in doses considerably greater than usual therapeutic doses in humans. Studies in women who took Aspirin during pregnancy have not demonstrated an increased incidence of congenital abnormalities in the offspring.

Labor and Delivery: Ingestion of Aspirin near term or prior to delivery may prolong delivery or lead to bleeding in mother, fetus, or neonate.

Nursing Mothers: Carisoprodol is excreted in human milk in concentrations two-to-four times that in maternal plasma. Aspirin is excreted in human milk in moderate amounts and can produce a bleeding tendency in nursing infants. Because of the potential for serious adverse reactions in nursing infants, a decision should be made whether to discontinue nursing or the drug, taking into account the importance of the drug to the mother.

Pediatric Use: Safety and effectiveness in children below the age of twelve have not been established.

ADVERSE REACTIONS

If severe reactions occur, discontinue Aspirin/Carisoprodol/Codeine and initiate appropriate symptomatic and supportive therapy.

The following side effects which have occurred with the administration of the individual ingredients alone may also occur with the combination.

Carisoprodol: Central Nervous System: Drowsiness is the most frequent complaint and along with other CNS effects may require dosage reduction. Observed less frequently are dizziness, vertigo and ataxia. Tremor, agitation, irritability, headache, depressive reactions, syncope, and insomnia have been infrequent or rare.

Idiosyncratic: Idiosyncratic reactions are very rare. They are usually seen within the period of the first to fourth dose in patients having had no previous contact with the drug (see *"Warnings"*).

Allergic: Skin rash, erythema multiforme, pruritus, eosinophilia, and fixed drug eruptions with cross-reaction to meprobamate have been reported. If allergic reactions occur, discontinue Aspirin/Carisoprodol/Codeine and treat symptomatically. In evaluating possible allergic reactions, also consider allergy to excipients (information on excipients is available to physicians on request).

Cardiovascular: Tachycardia, postural hypotension, and facial flushing.

Gastrointestinal: Nausea, vomiting, epigastric distress and hiccup.

Hematologic: No serious blood dyscrasias have been attributed to Carisoprodol alone. Leukopenia and pancytopenia have been reported, very rarely, in situations in which other drugs or viral infections may have been responsible.

▶ **SHOWN IN PRODUCT IDENTIFICATION GUIDE**

Aspirin: The most common adverse reactions associated with the use of Aspirin have been gastrointestinal, including nausea, vomiting, gastritis, occult bleeding, constipation and diarrhea. Gastric erosion, angioedema, asthma, rash, pruritus and urticaria have been reported less commonly. Tinnitus is a sign of high serum salicylate levels (see *"Overdosage"*).

Aspirin Intolerance: Allergic type reactions in Aspirin-sensitive individuals may involve the respiratory tract or the skin. Symptoms of the former range from rhinorrhea and shortness of breath to severe asthma, and the latter may consist of urticaria, edema, rash, or angioedema (giant hives). These may occur independently or in combination.

Codeine Phosphate: Nausea, vomiting, constipation, miosis, sedation, and dizziness have been reported.

DRUG ABUSE AND DEPENDENCE
Controlled Substance: Schedule C-III (see *"Precautions"*).

Abuse: In clinical use, abuse has been rare.

Dependence: In clinical use, dependence with Aspirin/Carisoprodol/Codeine has been rare and there have been no reports of significant abstinence signs. Nevertheless, the following information on the individual ingredients should be kept in mind.

Carisoprodol: In dogs, no withdrawal symptoms occurred after abrupt cessation of Carisoprodol from dosages as high as 1 gm/kg/day. In a study in man, abrupt cessation of 100 mg/kg/day (about five times the recommended daily adult dosage) was followed in some subjects by mild withdrawal symptoms such as abdominal cramps, insomnia, chills, headache, and nausea. Delirium and convulsions did not occur (see *"Precautions"*).

Codeine Phosphate: Drug dependence of the morphine type may result.

OVERDOSAGE
Signs and Symptoms: Any of the following which have been reported with the individual ingredients may occur and may be modified to a varying degree by the effects of the other ingredients present in Aspirin/Carisoprodol/Codeine.

Carisoprodol: Stupor, coma, shock, respiratory depression and, very rarely, death. Overdosage with Carisoprodol in combination with alcohol, other CNS depressants, or psychotropic agents can have additive effects, even when one of the agents has been taken in the usually recommended dosage.

Aspirin: Headache, tinnitus, hearing difficulty, dim vision, dizziness, lassitude, hyperpnea, rapid breathing, thirst, nausea, vomiting, sweating and occasionally diarrhea are characteristic of mild to moderate salicylate poisoning. Salicylate poisoning should be considered in children with symptoms of vomiting, hyperpnea, and hyperthermia.

Hyperpnea is an early sign of salicylate poisoning, but dyspnea supervenes at plasma levels above 50 mg/dl. These respiratory changes eventually lead to serious acid-base disturbances. Metabolic acidosis is a constant finding in infants but occurs in older children only with severe poisoning: adults usually exhibit respiratory alkalosis initially and acidosis terminally.

Other symtoms of severe salicylate poisoning include hyperthermia, dehydration, delirium, and mental disturbances. Skin eruptions, GI hemorrhage, or pulmonary edema are less common. Early CNS stimulation is replaced by increasing depression, stupor, and coma. Death is usually due to respiratory failure or cardiovascular collapse.

Codeine Phosphate: pinpoint pupils, CNS depression, coma, respiratory depression, and shock.

Treatment: General: Provide symptomatic and supportive treatment, as indicated. Any drug remaining in the stomach should be removed using appropriate procedures and caution to protect the airway and prevent aspiration, especially in the stuporous or comatose patient. Incomplete gastric emptying with delayed absorption of Carisoprodol has been reported as a cause for relapse. Should respiration or blood pressure become compromised, respiratory assistance, central nervous system stimulants, and pressor agents should be administered cautiously, as indicated.

Carisoprodol: The following have been successfully in overdosage with the related drug meprobamate: diuretics, osmotic (mannitol) diuresis, peritoneal dialysis, and hemodialysis (see *"Clinical Pharmacology"*). Careful monitoring of urinary output is necessary and caution should be taken to avoid overhydration. Carisoprodol can be measured in biological fluid by gas chromatography (Douglas, J.F., et al: *J Pharm Sci* 58: 145, 1969).

Aspirin: Since there are no specific antidotes for salicylate poisoning, the aim of treatment is to enhance elimination of salicylate and prevent or reduce further absorption; to correct any fluid, electrolyte or metabolic imbalance; and to provide general and cardiorespiratory support. If acidosis is present, intravenous sodium bicarbonate must be given, along with adequate hydration, until salicylate levels decrease to within the therapeutic range. To enhance elimination, forced diuresis and alkalinization of the urine may be beneficial. The need for hemoperfusion or hemodialysis is rare and should be used when other measures have failed.

Codeine Phosphate: Narcotic antagonists, such as nalorphine and levallorphan, may be indicated.

DOSAGE AND ADMINISTRATION
Usual Adult Dosage: 1 or 2 tablets, four times daily. Not recommended for use in children under age twelve.

Store at controlled room temperature 15°-30°C (59°-86°F). Protect from moisture.

Dispense in a tight container.

HOW SUPPLIED
TABLETS (C-III): 325 MG-200 MG-16 MG

BRAND/MANUFACTURER	NDC	SIZE	AWP
○ BRAND			
➤ SOMA COMPOUND W/CODEINE: Wallace	00037-2403-01	100s	$158.16

Aspirin/Oxycodone Hydrochloride/Oxycodone Terephthalate

DESCRIPTION
Each tablet of Aspirin/Oxycodone contains:

Aspirin, U.S.P.	325 mg
Oxycodone Hydrochloride	4.50 mg*
WARNING: May be habit forming	
Oxycodone Terephthalate	0.38 mg**
WARNING: May be habit forming	

* 4.50 mg Oxycodone Hydrochloride is equivalent to 4.0338 mg of Oxycodone.
** 0.38 mg Oxycodone Terephthalate is equivalent to 0.3008 mg of Oxycodone.

Each tablet of Aspirin/Oxycodone(half-strength) contains:

Aspirin, U.S.P.	325 mg
Oxycodone Hydrochloride	2.25 mg*
WARNING: May be habit forming	
Oxycodone Terephthalate	0.19 mg**
WARNING: May be habit forming	

* 2.25 mg Oxycodone Hydrochloride is equivalent to 2.0169 mg of Oxycodone.
** 0.19 mg Oxycodone Terephthalate is equivalent to 0.1504 mg of Oxycodone.

The Oxycodone component is 14-hydroxydihydrocodeinone, a white odorless crystalline powder which is derived from the opium alkaloid, thebaine.

ACTIONS
The principal ingredient, Oxycodone, is a semisynthetic narcotic analgesic with multiple actions qualitatively similar to those of morphine; the most prominent of these involve the central nervous system and organs composed of smooth muscle. The principal actions of therapeutic value of Oxycodone are analgesia and sedation.

Oxycodone is similar to codeine and methadone in that it retains at least one-half of its analgesic activity when administered orally.

Tablets also contain the non-narcotic antipyretic-analgesic, Aspirin.

INDICATIONS
For the relief of moderate to moderately severe pain.

CONTRAINDICATIONS
Hypersensitivity to Oxycodone or Aspirin.

WARNINGS
Drug Dependence: Oxycodone can produce drug dependence of the morphine type and, therefore, has the potential for being abused. Psychic dependence, physical dependence and tolerance may develop upon repeated administration of Aspirin/Oxycodone and it should be prescribed and administered with the same degree of caution appropriate to the use of other oral narcotic-containing medications. Like other narcotic containing medications, Aspirin/Oxycodone are subject to the Federal Controlled Substances Act.

Usage in Ambulatory Patients: Oxycodone may impair the mental and/or physical abilities required for the performance of potentially hazardous tasks such as driving a car or operating machinery. The patient using Aspirin/Oxycodone should be cautioned accordingly.

Interaction with Other Central Nervous System Depressants: Patients receiving other narcotic analgesics, general anesthetics, phenothiazines, other tranquilizers, sedative-hypnotics or other CNS depressants (including alcohol) concomitantly with Aspirin/Oxycodone may exhibit an additive CNS depression. When such combined therapy is contemplated, the dose of one or both agents should be reduced.

Usage in Pregnancy: Safe use in pregnancy has not been established relative to possible adverse effects on fetal development. Therefore, Aspirin/Oxycodone should not be used in pregnant women unless, in the judgment of the physician, the potential benefits outweigh the possible hazards.

Usage in Children: Aspirin/Oxycodone should not be administered to children. Aspirin/Oxycodone (half strength) containing half the amount of Oxycodone, can be considered. (See *"Dosage and Administration"*).

Reye Syndrome is a rare but serious disease which can follow flu or chicken pox in children and teenagers. While the cause of Reye Syndrome is unknown, some

---

◆ RATED THERAPEUTICALLY EQUIVALENT; ◇ THERAPEUTIC EQUIVALENCE UNCONFIRMED; ○ UNRATED

reports claim Aspirin (or salicylates) may increase the risk of developing this disease.

Salicylates should be used with caution in the presence of peptic ulcer or coagulation abnormalities.

PRECAUTIONS

Head Injury and Increased Intracranial Pressure: The respiratory depressant effects of narcotics and their capacity to elevate cerebrospinal fluid pressure may be markedly exaggerated in the presence of head injury, other intracranial lesions or a pre-existing increase in intracranial pressure. Furthermore, narcotics produce adverse reactions which may obscure the clinical course of patients with head injuries.

Acute Abdominal Conditions: The administration of Aspirin/Oxycodone or other narcotics may obscure the diagnosis or clinical course in patients with acute abdominal conditions.

Special Risk Patients: Aspirin/Oxycodone should be given with caution to certain patients such as the elderly or debilitated, and those with severe impairment of hepatic or renal function, hypothyroidism, Addison's disease, and prostatic hypertrophy or urethral stricture.

ADVERSE REACTIONS

The most frequently observed adverse reactions include lightheadedness, dizziness, sedation, nausea and vomiting. These effects seem to be more prominent in ambulatory than in nonambulatory patients, and some of these adverse reactions may be alleviated if the patient lies down.

Other adverse reactions include euphoria, dysphoria, constipation and pruritus.

DRUG ABUSE AND DEPENDENCE

Aspirin/Oxycodone tablets are a Schedule II controlled substance. Oxycodone can produce drug dependence and has the potential for being abused. (See *"Warnings".*)

DOSAGE AND ADMINISTRATION

Dosage should be adjusted according to the severity of the pain and the response of the patient. It may occasionally be necessary to exceed the usual dosage recommended below in cases of more severe pain or in those patients who have become tolerant to the analgesic effect of narcotics. Aspirin/Oxycodone is given orally. Aspirin/Oxycodone: The usual adult dose is one tablet every 6 hours as needed for pain.

Aspirin/Oxycodone (half-strength): Adults—One or two tablets every six hours. Children 12 years and older—One-half tablet every six hours. Children 6 to 12 years—One-quarter tablet every six hours. Aspirin/Oxycodone (half-strength) is not indicated for children under 6 years of age.

Store at controlled room temperature (59°-86°F, 15°-30°C).

DRUG INTERACTIONS

The CNS depressant effects of Aspirin/Oxycodone may be additive with that of other CNS depressants. (See *"Warnings".*)

Aspirin may enhance the effect of anticoagulants and inhibit the uricosuric effects of uricosuric agents.

MANAGEMENT OF OVERDOSAGE

Signs and Symptoms: Serious overdose with Aspirin/Oxycodone is characterized by respiratory depression (a decrease in respiratory rate and/or tidal volume, Cheyne-Stokes respiration, cyanosis), extreme somnolence progressing to stupor or coma, skeletal muscle flaccidity, cold and clammy skin, and sometimes bradycardia and hypotension. In severe overdosage, apnea, circulatory collapse, cardiac arrest and death may occur. The ingestion of very large amounts of Aspirin/Oxycodone may, in addition, result in acute salicylate intoxication.

Treatment: Primary attention should be given to the reestablishment of adequate respiratory exchange through provision of a patent airway and the institution of assisted or controlled ventilation. The narcotic antagonist naloxone Hydrochloride is a specific antidote against respiratory depression which may result from overdosage or unusual sensitivity to narcotics, including Oxycodone. Therefore, an appropriate dose of naloxone Hydrochloride should be administered (usual initial adult dose: 0.4 mg-2 mg) preferably by the intravenous route, simultaneously with efforts at respiratory resuscitation. Since the duration of action of Oxycodone may exceed that of the antagonist, the patient should be kept under continued surveillance and repeated doses of the antagonist should be administered as needed to maintain adequate respiration.

Oxygen, intravenous fluids, vasopressors and other supportive measures should be employed as indicated.

Gastric emptying may be useful in removing unabsorbed drug.

HOW SUPPLIED
TABLETS (C-II): 325 MG-4.5 MG-0.38 MG

AVERAGE UNIT PRICE (AVAILABLE SIZES)		GENERIC A-RATED AVERAGE PRICE (GAAP)	
BRAND	$0.60	100s	$23.01
GENERIC	$0.22	500s	$101.72
HCFA FUL (100s ea)	$0.20		

BRAND/MANUFACTURER	NDC	SIZE	AWP
◆ BRAND			
PERCODAN-DEMI: Du Pont Pharma	00590-0166-70	100s	$49.80
▶ PERCODAN: Du Pont Pharma	00590-0135-70	100s	$65.22
	00590-0135-85	500s	$316.56
	00590-0135-90	1000s	$617.16

BRAND/MANUFACTURER	NDC	SIZE	AWP
◆ GENERICS			
Parmed	00349-8831-01	100s	$18.95
▶ ROXIPRIN: Roxane	00054-4653-25	100s	$20.84
Rugby	00536-5671-01	100s	$21.35
Goldline	00182-1508-01	100s	$22.95
ENDODAN: Endo	60951-0610-70	100s	$23.00
▶ ROXIPRIN: Roxane	00054-8653-24	100s ud	$30.94
Parmed	00349-8831-05	500s	$93.95
Rugby	00536-5671-05	500s	$101.41
ENDODAN: Endo	60951-0610-85	500s	$103.50
Goldline	00182-1508-05	500s	$108.00
▶ ROXIPRIN: Roxane	00054-4653-31	1000s	$202.16

Astemizole

DESCRIPTION

Astemizole is a histamine H_1-receptor antagonist available in scored white tablets for oral use. Astemizole is chemically designated as 1-[(4-fluorophenyl)-methyl]-*N*-[1-[2-(4-methoxyphenyl)ethyl]-4-   piperidinyl]-1*H*-benzimidazol-2-amine, with a molecular weight of 458.58.

The empirical formula is $C_{28}H_{31}FN_4O$.

Astemizole is a white to slightly off-white powder; it is insoluble in water, slightly soluble in ethanol and soluble in chloroform and methanol.

Following is its chemical structure:

CLINICAL PHARMACOLOGY

Astemizole is a long-acting, selective histamine H_1-receptor antagonist. Receptor binding studies in animals demonstrated that at pharmacological doses Astemizole occupies peripheral H_1-receptors but does not reach H_1-receptors in the brain. Whole body autoradiographic studies in rats, radiolabel tissue distribution studies in dogs and radioligand binding studies of guinea pig brain H_1-receptors have shown that Astemizole does not readily cross the blood-brain barrier. Screening studies in rats at effective antihistaminic doses showed no anticholinergic effects. Studies in humans using the recommended dosage regimens have not been performed to determine whether Astemizole is associated with a different frequency of anticholinergic effects than therapeutic doses of other antihistamines.

The absorption of Astemizole is reduced by 60% when taken with meals. In single oral dose studies Astemizole was rapidly absorbed from the gastrointestinal tract; peak plasma concentrations of unchanged Astemizole were reached within one hour. Due to extensive first pass metabolism and significant tissue distribution, plasma concentrations of unchanged drug were low. Elimination of unchanged Astemizole occurred with a half-life of approximately one day. Elimination of Astemizole plus hydroxylated metabolites, considered together to represent the pharmacologically active fraction in plasma, was biphasic with half-lives of 20 hours for the distribution phase and 7-11 days for the elimination phase. The pharmacokinetics of Astemizole plus hydroxylated metabolites are dose proportional following single doses of 10 to 30 mg.

Following chronic administration, steady state plasma concentrations of Astemizole plus hydroxylated metabolites (mainly desmethylastemizole) were reached within four to eight weeks; concentrations of the metabolites are substantially higher than those of unchanged Astemizole plus hydroxylated metabolites decayed biphasically with an initial half-life of 7–9 days, with plasma concentrations being reduced by 75% within this phase, and with a terminal half-life of about 19 days. The initial phase ($t_{1/2} = 7–9$ days) appears to determine the time to reach steady state plasma concentrations of Astemizole plus hydroxylated metabolites. Steady state plasma concentrations of unchanged Astemizole were reached by 6 days (with a range of 6–9 days); unchanged Astemizole was eliminated from plasma with a half-life of approximately 2 days (with a range of 1–2.5 days).

Excretion and metabolism studies with ^{14}C-labeled Astemizole on volunteers demonstrated that the drug is almost completely metabolized in the liver and primarily excreted in the feces.

Interpatient variability in pharmacokinetic parameters may be greater in patients with liver disease as compared to normal subjects. Systematic evaluation of the pharmacokinetics in patients with hepatic or renal dysfunction has not been performed.

The *in-vitro* plasma protein binding of unchanged Astemizole (100 ng/mL) was 96.7% with 2.3% being found as free drug in the plasma water. In human blood with an astemizole concentration of 100 ng/mL, 61.5% of astemizole was bound to the plasma proteins, with 36.2% being distributed to the blood cell fraction. The concentration of astemizole found in the blood was the same as that found in the plasma fraction of the blood. Binding studies for the astemizole metabolite(s) which achieve much higher concentrations than astemizole under chronic dosing conditions have not been conducted.

INDICATIONS AND USAGE

Astemizole tablets are indicated for the relief of symptoms associated with seasonal allergic rhinitis and chronic idiopathic urticaria. Astemizole should not be used as a p r n product for immediate relief of symptoms. Patients should be advised not to increase the dose in an attempt to accelerate the onset of action.

Clinical studies have not been conducted to evaluate the effectiveness of Astemizole in the common cold.

UNLABELED USES.
Astemizole is used alone or as an adjunct in the treatment of asthma.

CONTRAINDICATIONS

CONCOMITANT ADMINISTRATION OF ASTEMIZOLE WITH ERYTHROMYCIN IS CONTRAINDICATED BECAUSE ERYTHROMYCIN IS KNOWN TO IMPAIR THE CYTOCHROME P450 ENZYME SYSTEM WHICH ALSO INFLUENCES ASTEMIZOLE METABOLISM. THERE HAVE BEEN TWO REPORTS TO DATE OF SYNCOPE WITH TORSADES DE POINTES, REQUIRING HOSPITALIZATION, IN PATIENTS TAKING COMBINATIONS OF ASTEMIZOLE 10 MG DAILY WITH ERYTHROMYCIN. IN EACH CASE THE QT INTERVALS WERE PROLONGED BEYOND 650 MILLISECONDS AT THE TIME OF THE EVENT: ONE PATIENT ALSO RECEIVED KETOCONAZOLE AND THE OTHER PATIENT ALSO HAD HYPOKALEMIA.

CONCOMITANT ADMINISTRATION OF ASTEMIZOLE WITH KETOCONAZOLE TABLETS IS CONTRAINDICATED BECAUSE AVAILABLE HUMAN PHARMACOKINETIC DATA INDICATE THAT ORAL KETOCONAZOLE SIGNIFICANTLY INHIBITS THE METABOLISM OF ASTEMIZOLE, RESULTING IN ELEVATED PLASMA LEVELS OF ASTEMIZOLE AND DESMETHYLASTEMIZOLE. DATA SUGGEST THAT CARDIOVASCULAR EVENTS ARE ASSOCIATED WITH ELEVATION OF ASTEMIZOLE AND/OR ASTEMIZOLE METABOLITE LEVELS, RESULTING IN ELECTROCARDIOGRAPHIC QT PROLONGATION.

CONCOMITANT ADMINISTRATION OF ASTEMIZOLE WITH ITRACONAZOLE IS ALSO CONTRAINDICATED BASED ON THE CHEMICAL RESEMBLANCE OF ITRACONAZOLE AND KETOCONAZOLE. IN-VITRO DATA SUGGEST THAT ITRACONAZOLE HAS A LESS PRONOUNCED EFFECT ON THE BIOTRANSFORMATION SYSTEM RESPONSIBLE FOR THE METABOLISM OF ASTEMIZOLE COMPARED TO KETOCONAZOLE.

(See *"Warnings"* and *"Precautions: Drug Interactions"*).

Astemizole is contraindicated in patients with known hypersensitivity to astemizole or any of the inactive ingredients.

WARNINGS

QT PROLONGATION/VENTRICULAR ARRHYTHMIAS

RARE CASES OF SERIOUS CARDIOVASCULAR ADVERSE EVENTS INCLUDING DEATH, CARDIAC ARREST, QT PROLONGATION, TORSADES DE POINTES, AND OTHER VENTRICULAR ARRHYTHMIAS HAVE BEEN OBSERVED IN PATIENTS EXCEEDING RECOMMENDED DOSES OF ASTEMIZOLE. WHILE THE MAJORITY OF SUCH EVENTS HAVE OCCURRED FOLLOWING SUBSTANTIAL OVERDOSES OF ASTEMIZOLE, TORSADES DE POINTES (ARRHYTHMIAS) HAVE VERY RARELY OCCURRED AT REPORTED DOSES AS LOW AS 20–30 MG DAILY (2–3 TIMES THE RECOMMENDED DAILY DOSE). DATA SUGGEST THAT THESE EVENTS ARE ASSOCIATED WITH ELEVATION OF ASTEMIZOLE AND/OR ASTEMIZOLE METABOLITE LEVELS, RESULTING IN ELECTROCARDIOGRAPHIC QT PROLONGATION.

THESE EVENTS HAVE ALSO OCCURRED AT 10 MG DAILY IN A FEW PATIENTS WITH POSSIBLE AUGMENTING CIRCUMSTANCES (SEE *"CONTRAINDICATIONS,"* AND *"WARNING PARAGRAPHS"* BELOW *"WARNINGS BOX")*. IN VIEW OF THE POTENTIAL FOR CARDIAC ARRHYTHMIAS, ADHERENCE TO THE RECOMMENDED DOSE SHOULD BE EMPHASIZED.

DO NOT EXCEED THE RECOMMENDED DOSE OF 10 MG (ONE TABLET) DAILY.

SOME PATIENTS APPEAR TO INCREASE THE DOSE OF ASTEMIZOLE IN AN ATTEMPT TO ACCELERATE THE ONSET OF ACTION. PATIENTS SHOULD BE ADVISED NOT TO DO THIS AND NOT TO USE ASTEMIZOLE AS A P R N PRODUCT FOR IMMEDIATE RELIEF OF SYMPTOMS.

CONCOMITANT ADMINISTRATION OF ASTEMIZOLE WITH KETOCONAZOLE TABLETS, ITRACONAZOLE, OR ERYTHROMYCIN IS CONTRAINDICATED. (SEE *"CONTRAINDICATIONS"* AND *"PRECAUTIONS: DRUG INTERACTIONS")*.

SINCE ASTEMIZOLE IS EXTENSIVELY METABOLIZED BY THE LIVER, THE USE OF ASTEMIZOLE IN PATIENTS WITH SIGNIFICANT HEPATIC DYSFUNCTION SHOULD GENERALLY BE AVOIDED.

IN SOME CASES, SEVERE ARRHYTHMIAS HAVE BEEN PRECEDED BY EPISODES OF SYNCOPE. SYNCOPE IN PATIENTS RECEIVING ASTEMIZOLE SHOULD LEAD TO IMMEDIATE DISCONTINUATION OF TREATMENT AND APPROPRIATE CLINICAL EVALUATION, INCLUDING ELECTROCARDIOGRAPHIC TESTING (LOOKING FOR QT PROLONGATION AND VENTRICULAR ARRHYTHMIA).

(SEE *"CLINICAL PHARMACOLOGY," "CONTRAINDICATIONS," "WARNINGS," "PRECAUTIONS,"* AND *"DOSAGE AND ADMINISTRATION.")*

Patients known to have conditions leading to QT prolongation may experience QT prolongation and/or ventricular arrhythmia with Astemizole at recommended doses. The effect of Astemizole in patients who are receiving agents which alter the QT interval is unknown. However, in view of Astemizole's known potential for QT prolongation, it is advisable to avoid its use in patients with QT prolongation syndrome or who are taking medications which are reported to prolong QT intervals (including probucol, certain antiarrhythmics, certain tricyclic antidepressants, certain phenothiazines, certain calcium channel blockers such as bepridil, and terfenadine), patients with electrolyte abnormalities such as hypokalemia or hypomagnesemia, or those taking diuretics with potential for inducing electrolyte abnormalities.

Rare cases of cardiovascular events have been observed in patients with hepatic dysfunction. Systematic evaluation of the pharmacokinetics of Astemizole in patients with hepatic dysfunction has not been performed. Since Astemizole is extensively metabolized by the liver, the use of Astemizole in patients with significant hepatic dysfunction should generally be avoided.

PRECAUTIONS

GENERAL

Caution should be given to potential anticholinergic (drying effects) in patients with lower airway diseases.

Caution should be used in patients with cirrhosis or other liver diseases. (See *"Clinical Pharmacology"* section.) Astemizole does not appear to be dialyzable.

Caution should also be used when treating patients with renal impairment.

DRUG INTERACTIONS:

See *"Contraindications"* and *"Warnings"* sections for discussion of information regarding potential drug interactions.

KETOCONAZOLE/ITRACONAZOLE

Concomitant administration of ketoconazole tablets or itraconazole with Astemizole is contraindicated. (See *"Contraindications"* and *"Warnings Box.")*

Due to the chemical similarity of fluconazole, metronidazole, and miconazole i.v. to ketoconazole, concomitant use of these products with Astemizole is not recommended.

MACROLIDES (INCLUDING ERYTHROMYCIN)

Concomitant administration of erythromycin with Astemizole is contraindicated. (See *"Contraindications"* and *"Warnings"* box.) Concomitant administration of Astemizole with other macrolide antibiotics, including troleandomycin, azithromycin, and clarithromycin, is not recommended.

INFORMATION FOR PATIENTS

Patients taking Astemizole should receive the following information and instructions. Antihistamines are prescribed to reduce allergic symptoms. Patients taking Astemizole should be advised 1) to adhere to the recommended dose, and 2) that the use of excessive doses may lead to serious cardiovascular events. Some patients appear to increase the dose of Astemizole in an attempt to accelerate the onset of action. *PATIENTS SHOULD BE ADVISED NOT TO DO THIS* and not to use Astemizole as a p r n product for immediate relief of symptoms. Patients should be questioned about use of any other prescription or over-the-counter medication, and should be cautioned regarding the potential for life-threatening arrhythmias with concurrent use of ketoconazole, itraconazole, or erythromycin. Patients should be advised to consult the physician before concurrent use of other medications with Astemizole. Patients should be questioned about pregnancy or lactation before starting Astemizole therapy, since the drug should be used in pregnancy or lactation only if the potential benefit justifies the potential risk to fetus or baby. (See *"Pregnancy"* subsection.) In addition, patients should be instructed to take Astemizole on an empty stomach, e.g., at least 2 hours after a meal. No additional food should be taken for at least 1 hour after-dosing. Patients should also be instructed to store this medication in a tightly closed container in a cool, dry place, away from heat or direct sunlight, and away from children.

CARCINOGENESIS, MUTAGENESIS, IMPAIRMENT OF FERTILITY

Carcinogenic potential has not been revealed in rats given 260× the recommended human dose of Astemizole for 24 months, or in mice given 400× the recommended human dose for 18 months. Micronucleus, dominant lethal, sister chromatid exchange and Ames tests of Astemizole have not revealed mutagenic activity.

Impairment of fertility was not observed in male or female rats given 200× the recommended human dose.

PREGNANCY: PREGNANCY CATEGORY C

Teratogenic effects were not observed in rats administered 200× the recommended human dose or in rabbits given 200× the recommended human dose. Maternal toxicity was seen in rabbits administered 200× the recommended human dose. Embryocidal effects accompanied by maternal toxicity were observed at 100× the recommended human dose in rats. Embryotoxicity or maternal toxicity was not observed in rats or rabbits administered 50× the recommended human dose. There are no adequate and well controlled studies in pregnant women. Astemizole should be used during pregnancy only if the potential benefit justifies the potential risk to the fetus. Metabolites may remain in the body for as long as 4 months after the end of dosing, calculated on the basis of 6 times the terminal half-life. (See *"Clinical Pharmacology"* section.)

NURSING MOTHERS

It is not known whether this drug is excreted in human milk. Because certain drugs are known to be excreted in human milk, caution should be exercised when Astemizole is administered to a nursing woman. Astemizole is excreted in the milk of dogs.

PEDIATRIC USE

Safety and efficacy in children under 12 years of age has not been demonstrated.

ADVERSE REACTIONS

For information regarding cardiovascular adverse events (e.g. cardiac arrest, ventricular arrhythmias), please see *"Contraindications"* and *"Warnings"* box. In some cases, recognition of severe arrhythmias has been preceded by episodes of syncope. Similarly, rare cases of hypotension, palpitations, and dizziness have also been reported with Astemizole use, which may reflect undetected ventricular arrhythmia.

The reported incidences of adverse reactions listed in the following table are derived from controlled clinical studies in adults. In these studies the usual maintenance dose of Astemizole was 10 mg once daily.

PERCENT OF PATIENTS REPORTING

	Controlled Studies*		
Adverse Event	*Astemizole (N = 1630) %*	*Placebo (N = 1109) %*	*Classical** (N = 304) %*
Central Nervous System			
Drowsiness	7.1	6.4	22.0
Headache	6.7	9.2	3.3
Fatigue	4.2	1.6	11.8
Appetite increase	3.9	1.4	0.0
Weight increase	3.6	0.7	1.0
Nervousness	2.1	1.2	0.3
Dizzy	2.0	1.8	1.0
Gastrointestinal System			
Nausea	2.5	2.9	1.3
Diarrhea	1.8	2.0	0.7
Abdominal pain	1.4	1.2	0.7
Eye, Ear, Nose, and Throat			
Mouth dry	5.2	3.8	7.9
Pharyngitis	1.7	2.3	0.3
Conjunctivitis	1.2	1.2	0.7
Other			
Arthralgia	1.2	1.6	0.0

* *Duration of treatment in Controlled Studies ranged from 7 to 182 Days*
** *Classical Drugs: Clemastine (N = 137); Chlorpheniramine (N = 100); Pheniramine Maleate (N = 47); d-Chlorpheniramine (N = 20)*

Adverse reaction information has been obtained from more than 7500 patients in all clinical trials. Weight gain has been reported in 3.6% of Astemizole treated patients involved in controlled studies, with an average treatment duration of 53 days. In 46 of the 59 patients for whom actual weight gain data was available, the average weight gain was 3.2 kg.

Less frequently occurring adverse experiences reported in clinical trials or spontaneously from marketing experience with Astemizole include: angioedema, asymptomatic liver enzyme elevations, bronchospasm, depression, edema, epistaxis, hepatitis, myalgia, palpitation, paresthesia, photosensitivity, pruritus, and rash.

Marketing experiences include isolated cases of convulsions. A causal relationship with Astemizole has not been established.

OVERDOSAGE

In the event of overdosage, supportive measures including gastric lavage and emesis should be employed. Substantial overdoses of Astemizole can cause death, cardiac arrest, QT prolongation, torsades de pointes, and other ventricular arrhythmias. These events can also occur, although rarely, at doses (20–30 mg) close to the recommended dose (10 mg/daily). (See *"Warnings"* box and *"Dosage and Administration."*)

Seizures and syncope have also been reported with overdose and may be associated with a cardiac event.

Overdose patients should be carefully monitored as long as the QT interval is prolonged or arrhythmias are present. In some cases, this has been up to six days. In overdose cases in which ventricular arrhythmias are associated with significant QT prolongation, treatment with antiarrhythmics known to prolong QT intervals is not recommended Astemizole does not appear to be dialyzable.

Oral LD_{50} values for Astemizole were 2052 mg/kg in mice and 3154 mg/kg in rats. In neonatal rats, the oral LD_{50} was 905 mg/kg in males and 1235 mg/kg in females.

DOSAGE AND ADMINISTRATION

The recommended dosage for adults and children 12 years of age and older is 10 mg (1 tablet) once daily.

DO NOT EXCEED THE RECOMMENDED DOSE. Patients should be advised not to increase the dose of Astemizole in an attempt to accelerate the onset of action. (See *"Warnings"* box.) USE OF ASTEMIZOLE IN PATIENTS TAKING KETOCONAZOLE, ITRACONAZOLE, OR ERYTHROMYCIN IS CONTRAINDICATED. (See *"Contraindications,"* *"Warnings,"* and *"Precautions: Drug Interactions".*)

Studies evaluating the need for dosage adjustments for patients with hepatic or renal dysfunction have not been performed. Since Astemizole is extensively metabolized by the liver, use of Astemizole in patients with significant hepatic dysfunction should generally be avoided.

Astemizole should be taken on an empty stomach, e.g., at least two hours after a meal. There should be no additional food intake for at least one hour postdosing.

Store tablets at room temperature (59°–86°F) (15°–30°C).

Protect from moisture.

HOW SUPPLIED
TABLETS: 10 MG

BRAND/MANUFACTURER	NDC	SIZE	AWP
○ **BRAND**			
► HISMANAL: Janssen	50458-0510-13	30s	$53.10
	50458-0510-10	100s	$177.02

Atarax *SEE* HYDROXYZINE

Atenolol

DESCRIPTION

Atenolol, a synthetic, beta₁-selective (cardioselective) adrenoreceptor blocking agent, may be chemically described as benzeneacetamide, 4-[2'-hydroxy-3'[(1-methyl-ethyl)amino]propoxyl]-. Its molecular formula is $C_{14}H_{22}N_2O_3$.

Atenolol (free base) has a molecular weight of 266. It is a relatively polar hydrophilic compound with a water solubility of 26.5 mg/mL at 37°C and a log partition coefficient (octanol/water) of 0.23. It is freely soluble in 1N HCl (300 mg/mL at 25°C) and less soluble in chloroform (3 mg/mL at 25°C).

Atenolol is available as 25, 50 and 100 mg tablets for oral administration. Atenolol for parenteral administration is available as Atenolol I.V. Injection containing 5 mg atenolol in 10 mL sterile, isotonic, citrate-buffered, aqueous solution. The pH of the solution is 5.5-6.5.

Following is its chemical structure:

$$OCH_2CHCH_2NHCH(CH_3)_2$$
$$|$$
$$OH$$

$$CH_2CONH_2$$

CLINICAL PHARMACOLOGY

Atenolol is a beta₁-selective (cardioselective) beta-adrenergic receptor blocking agent without membrane stabilizing or intrinsic sympathomimetic (partial agonist) activities. This preferential effect is not absolute, however, and at higher doses, Atenolol inhibits beta₂-adrenoreceptors, chiefly located in the bronchial and vascular musculature.

Pharmacokinetics and Metabolism: In man, absorption of an oral dose is rapid and consistent but incomplete. Approximately 50% of an oral dose is absorbed from the gastrointestinal tract, the remainder being excreted unchanged in the feces. Peak blood levels are reached between two (2) and four (4) hours after ingestion. Unlike propranolol or metoprolol, but like nadolol, Atenolol undergoes little or no metabolism by the liver, and the absorbed portion is eliminated primarily by renal excretion. Over 85% of an intravenous dose is excreted in urine within 24 hours compared with approximately 50% for an oral dose. Atenolol also differs from propranolol in that only a small amount (6%–16%) is bound to proteins in the plasma. This kinetic profile results in relatively consistent plasma drug levels with about a fourfold interpatient variation.

The elimination half-life of oral Atenolol is approximately 6 to 7 hours, and there is no alteration of the kinetic profile of the drug by chronic administration. Following intravenous administration, peak plasma levels are reached within 5 minutes. Declines from peak levels are rapid (5- to 10-fold) during the first 7 hours; thereafter, plasma levels decay with a half-life similar to that of orally administered drug. Following oral doses of 50 mg or 100 mg, both beta-blocking and antihypertensive effects persist for at least 24 hours. When renal function is impaired, elimination of Atenolol is closely related to the glomerular filtration rate; significant accumulation occurs when the creatinine clearance falls below 35 mL/min/1.73m². (See *"Dosage and Administration"*).

Pharmacodynamics: In standard animal or human pharmacological tests, beta-adrenoreceptor blocking activity of Atenolol has been demonstrated by: (1) reduction in resting and exercise heart rate and cardiac output, (2) reduction of systolic and diastolic blood pressure at rest and on exercise, (3) inhibition of

	Conventional Therapy Plus Atenolol (n = 244)		Conventional Therapy Alone (n = 233)	
Deaths	7	(2.9%)	16	(6.9%)
Cardiogenic Shock	1	(0.4%)	4	(1.7%)
Development of Ventricular Septal Defect	0	(0%)	2	(0.9%)
Development of Mitral Regurgitation	0	(0%)	2	(0.9%)
Renal Failure	1	(0.4%)	0	(0%)
Pulmonary Emboli	3	(1.2%)	0	(0%)

In the subsequent International Study of Infarct Survival (ISIS-1) including over 16,000 patients of whom 8,037 were randomized to receive Atenolol treatment, the dosage of intravenous and subsequent oral Atenolol was either discontinued or reduced for the following reasons:

REASONS FOR REDUCED DOSAGE

	IV Atenolol Reduced Dose (< 5 mg)*		Oral Partial Dose	
Hypotension/ Bradycardia	105	(1.3%)	1168	(14.5%)
Cardiogenic Shock	4	(.04%)	35	(.44%)
Reinfarction	0	(0%)	5	(.06%)
Cardiac Arrest	5	(.06%)	28	(.34%)
Heart Block (> first degree)	5	(.06%)	143	(1.7%)
Cardiac Failure	1	(.01%)	233	(2.9%)
Arrhythmias	3	(.04%)	22	(.27%)
Bronchospasm	1	(.01%)	50	(.62%)

* Full dosage was 10 mg and some patients received less than 10 mg but more than 5 mg.

During postmarketing experience with Atenolol, the following have been reported in temporal relationship to the use of the drug: elevated liver enzymes and/or bilirubin, headache, impotence, Peyronie's disease, psoriasiform rash or exacerbation of psoriasis, purpura, reversible alopecia, and thrombocytopenia. Atenolol, like other beta blockers, has been associated with the development of antinuclear antibodies (ANA) and lupus syndrome.

POTENTIAL ADVERSE EFFECTS

In addition, a variety of adverse effects have been reported with other beta-adrenergic blocking agents, and may be considered potential adverse effects of Atenolol.

Hematologic: Agranulocytosis.

Allergic: Fever, combined with aching and sore throat, laryngospasm, and respiratory distress.

Central Nervous System: Reversible mental depression progressing to catatonia: visual disturbances; hallucinations; an acute reversible syndrome characterized by disorientation of time and place; short-term memory loss; emotional lability with slightly clouded sensorium; and, decreased performance on neuropsychometrics.

Gastrointestinal: Mesenteric arterial thrombosis, ischemic colitis.

Other: Erythematous rash, Raynaud's phenomenon.

Miscellaneous: There have been reports of skin rashes and/or dry eyes associated with the use of beta-adrenergic blocking drugs. The reported incidence is small, and in most cases, the symptoms have cleared when treatment was withdrawn. Discontinuance of the drug should be considered if any such reaction is not otherwise explicable. Patients should be closely monitored following cessation of therapy. (See "Dosage and Administration".)

The oculomucocutaneous syndrome associated with the beta blocker practolol has not been reported with Atenolol. Furthermore, a number of patients who had previously demonstrated established practolol reactions were transferred to Atenolol therapy with subsequent resolution or quiescence of the reaction.

OVERDOSAGE

Overdosage with Atenolol has been reported with patients surviving acute doses as high as 5 g. One death was reported in a man who may have taken as much as 10 g acutely.

The predominant symptoms reported following Atenolol overdose are lethargy, disorder of respiratory drive, wheezing, sinus pause and bradycardia. Additionally, common effects associated with overdosage of any beta-adrenergic blocking agent and which might also be expected in Atenolol overdose are congestive heart failure, hypotension, bronchospasm and/or hypoglycemia.

Treatment of overdose should be directed to the removal of any unabsorbed drug by induced emesis, gastric lavage, or administration of activated charcoal. Atenolol can be removed from the general circulation by hemodialysis. Other treatment modalities should be employed at the physician's discretion and may include:

Bradycardia: Atropine intravenously. If there is no response to vagal blockade, give isoproterenol cautiously. In refractory cases, a transvenous cardiac pacemaker may be indicated.

Heart Block (Second or Third Degree): Isoproterenol or transvenous cardiac pacemaker.

Cardiac Failure: Digitalize the patient and administer a diuretic. Glucagon has been reported to be useful.

Hypotension: Vasopressors such as dopamine or norepinephrine (levarterenol). Monitor blood pressure continuously.

Bronchospasm: A beta$_2$ stimulant such as isoproterenol or terbutaline and/or aminophylline.

Hypoglycemia: Intravenous glucose.

Based on the severity of symptoms, management may require intensive support care and facilities for applying cardiac and respiratory support.

DOSAGE AND ADMINISTRATION

Hypertension: The initial dose of Atenolol is 50 mg given as one tablet a day either alone or added to diuretic therapy. The full effect of this dose will usually be seen within one to two weeks. If an optimal response is not achieved, the dosage should be increased to Atenolol 100 mg given as one tablet a day. Increasing the dosage beyond 100 mg a day is unlikely to produce any further benefit.

Atenolol may be used alone or concomitantly with other antihypertensive agents including thiazide-type diuretics, hydralazine, prazosin, and alpha-methyldopa.

Angina Pectoris: The initial dose of Atenolol is 50 mg given as one tablet a day. If an optimal response is not achieved within one week, the dosage should be increased to Atenolol 100 mg given as one tablet a day. Some patients may require a dosage of 200 mg once a day for optimal effect. Twenty-four hour control with once daily dosing is achieved by giving doses larger than necessary to achieve an immediate maximum effect. The maximum early effect on exercise tolerance occurs with doses of 50 to 100 mg, but at these doses the effect at 24 hours is attenuated, averaging about 50% to 75% of that observed with once a day oral doses of 200 mg.

Acute Myocardial Infarction: In patients with definite or suspected acute myocardial infarction, treatment with Atenolol I.V. Injection should be initiated as soon as possible after the patient's arrival in the hospital and after eligibility is established. Such treatment should be initiated in a coronary care or similar unit immediately after the patient's hemodynamic condition has stabilized. Treatment should begin with the intravenous administration of 5 mg Atenolol over 5 minutes followed by another 5 mg intravenous injection 10 minutes later. Atenolol I.V. Injection should be administered under carefully controlled conditions including monitoring of blood pressure, heart rate, and electrocardiogram. Dilutions of Atenolol I.V. Injection in Dextrose Injection USP, Sodium Chloride Injection USP, or Sodium Chloride and Dextrose Injection may be used. These admixtures are stable for 48 hours if they are not used immediately.

In patients who tolerate the full intravenous dose (10 mg), Atenolol Tablets 50 mg should be initiated 10 minutes after the last intravenous dose followed by another 50 mg oral dose 12 hours later. Thereafter Atenolol can be given orally either 100 mg once daily or 50 mg twice a day for a further 6-9 days or until discharge from the hospital. If bradycardia or hypotension requiring treatment or any other untoward effects occur Atenolol should be discontinued.

Data from other beta blocker trials suggest that if there is any question concerning the use of IV beta blocker or clinical estimate that there is a contraindication, the IV beta blocker may be eliminated and patients fulfilling the safety criteria may be given Atenolol Tablets 50 mg twice daily or 100 mg once a day for at least seven days (if the IV dosing is excluded).

Although the demonstration of efficacy of Atenolol is based entirely on data from the first seven postinfarction days, data from other beta blocker trials suggest that treatment with beta blockers that are effective in the postinfarction setting may be continued for one to three years if there are no contraindications. Atenolol is an additional treatment to standard coronary care unit therapy.

Elderly Patients or Patients with Renal Impairment: Atenolol is excreted by the kidneys; consequently dosage should be adjusted in cases of severe impairment of renal function. Some reduction in dosage may also be appropriate for the elderly, since decreased kidney function is a physiologic consequence of aging. Atenolol excretion would be expected to decrease with advancing age.

No significant accumulation of Atenolol occurs until creatinine clearance falls below 35 mL/min/1.73 m^2. Accumulation of atenolol and prolongation of its half-life were studied in subjects with creatinine clearance between 5 and 105 mL/min. Peak plasma levels were significantly increased in subjects with creatinine clearances below 30 mL/min.

The following maximum oral dosages are recommended for elderly, renally-impaired patients and for patients with renal impairment due to other causes:

Creatinine Clearance (mL/min/1.73m^2)	Atenolol Elimination Half-Life (h)	Maximum Dosage
15–35	16–27	50 mg daily
<15	>27	25 mg daily

Some renally-impaired or elderly patients being treated for hypertension may require a lower starting dose of Atenolol, 25 mg given as one tablet a day. If this 25 mg dose is used, assessment of efficacy must be made carefully. This should include measurement of blood pressure just prior to the next dose ("trough" blood pressure) to ensure that the treatment effect is present for a full 24 hours. Although a similar dosage reduction may be considered for elderly and/or renally-impaired patients being treated for indications other than hypertension, data are not available for these patient populations.

Patients on hemodialysis should be given 25 mg or 50 mg after each dialysis; this should be done under hospital supervision as marked falls in blood pressure can occur.

Cessation of Therapy in Patients with Angina Pectoris: If withdrawal of Atenolol therapy is planned, it should be achieved gradually and patients should be carefully observed and advised to limit physical activity to a minimum. Parenteral drug products should be inspected visually for particulate matter and discoloration prior to administration, whenever solution and container permit.

Injection: Protect from light. Keep ampules in outer packaging until time of use. Store at room temperature.

Tablets: Store at controlled room temperature, 15°–30°C (59°–86°F). Dispense in well-closed, light resistant containers.

Injection: Protect from light. Keep ampules in outer packaging until time of use. Store at room temperature.

HOW SUPPLIED
INJECTION: 0.5 MG/ML

BRAND/MANUFACTURER	NDC	SIZE	AWP
○ **BRAND**			
TENORMIN: Zeneca	00310-0108-10	10 ml 6s	$17.70

TABLETS: 25 MG

AVERAGE UNIT PRICE (AVAILABLE SIZES)		GENERIC A-RATED AVERAGE PRICE (GAAP)	
GENERIC	$0.67	100s	$67.28
HCFA FUL (100s ea)	$0.16		

BRAND/MANUFACTURER	NDC	SIZE	AWP
◆ **BRAND**			
▶ TENORMIN: Zeneca	00310-0107-10	100s	$85.01
◆ **GENERICS**			
IPR	54921-0107-10	100s	$63.85
Goldline	00182-1001-01	100s	$67.00
Lederle Std Prod	00005-3218-43	100s	$67.00
West Point	59591-0007-68	100s	$70.25
Geneva	00781-1078-01	100s	$70.30
Rugby	00536-3325-01	100s	$70.74
UDL	51079-0759-20	100s ud	$61.80
Rugby	00536-3325-05	500s	$335.90
Lederle Std Prod	00005-3218-34	1000s	$619.75

TABLETS: 50 MG

AVERAGE UNIT PRICE (AVAILABLE SIZES)		GENERIC A-RATED AVERAGE PRICE (GAAP)	
BRAND	$0.86	90s	$64.55
GENERIC	$0.65	100s	$66.50
HCFA FUL (100s ea)	$0.12	750s	$475.69
		1000s	$608.79

BRAND/MANUFACTURER	NDC	SIZE	AWP
◆ **BRAND**			
▶ TENORMIN: Zeneca	00310-0105-10	100s	$86.74
	00310-0105-39	100s ud	$86.74
	00310-0105-34	1000s	$857.08
◆ **GENERICS**			
Allscrips	54569-3432-02	3s	$2.15
Allscrips	54569-3432-03	6s	$4.30
Medirex	57480-0446-06	30s	$19.28
Allscrips	54569-8008-00	90s	$64.55
Allscrips	54569-8507-00	90s	$64.55
Qualitest	00603-2371-01	100s	$61.25
Novopharm	55953-0039-40	100s	$61.25
Aligen	00405-4107-01	100s	$61.50
▶ Schein	00364-2513-01	100s	$61.50
Major	00904-7634-60	100s	$65.00
▶ IPR	54921-0105-10	100s	$65.02
Martec	52555-0531-01	100s	$65.40
Rugby	00536-3330-01	100s	$65.55
Mason Dist	11845-0489-01	100s	$66.12
URL	00677-1478-01	100s	$66.16
▶ Apothecon	00003-5040-50	100s	$66.90
Moore,H.L.	00839-7723-06	100s	$67.49
Moore,H.L.	00839-7741-06	100s	$67.49
Goldline	00182-1004-01	100s	$68.26
▶ Lederle Std Prod	00005-3219-43	100s	$68.26
Mutual	53489-0529-01	100s	$70.00
▶ Geneva	00781-1506-01	100s	$71.72
Allscrips	54569-8008-01	100s	$71.72
▶ Mylan	00378-0231-01	100s	$71.75

BRAND/MANUFACTURER	NDC	SIZE	AWP
West Point	59591-0263-68	100s	$71.75
UDL	51079-0684-20	100s ud	$62.91
Vangard	00615-3532-13	100s ud	$63.43
▶ Schein	00364-2513-90	100s ud	$64.16
Medirex	57480-0446-01	100s ud	$64.25
▶ IPR	54921-0105-39	100s ud	$65.02
Goldline	00182-1004-89	100s ud	$69.00
▶ Geneva	00781-1506-13	100s ud	$72.56
Allscrips	54569-8507-01	180s	$129.10
Glasgow	60809-0102-55	750s ud	$475.69
Glasgow	60809-0102-72	750s ud	$475.69
Qualitest	00603-2371-32	1000s	$567.38
Novopharm	55953-0039-80	1000s	$567.38
▶ Schein	00364-2513-02	1000s	$582.95
▶ IPR	54921-0105-34	1000s	$588.00
Major	00904-7634-80	1000s	$590.00
Moore,H.L.	00839-7741-16	1000s	$593.99
Martec	52555-0531-10	1000s	$595.50
Mason Dist	11845-0489-04	1000s	$599.42
▶ Apothecon	00003-5040-75	1000s	$600.00
URL	00677-1478-10	1000s	$623.00
Mutual	53489-0529-10	1000s	$623.00
Rugby	00536-3330-10	1000s	$623.68
Goldline	00182-1004-10	1000s	$631.42
▶ Lederle Std Prod	00005-3219-50	1000s	$631.43
SCS Pharm	00905-5711-52	1000s	$633.94
▶ Geneva	00781-1506-10	1000s	$634.56
Moore,H.L.	00839-7723-16	1000s	$635.99
▶ Mylan	00378-0231-10	1000s	$636.50

TABLETS: 100 MG

AVERAGE UNIT PRICE (AVAILABLE SIZES)		GENERIC A-RATED AVERAGE PRICE (GAAP)	
BRAND	$$ 1.30	30s	$29.97
GENERIC	$0.96	100s	$96.66
HCFA FUL (100s ea)	$0.18	1000s	$905.51

BRAND/MANUFACTURER	NDC	SIZE	AWP
◆ **BRAND**			
▶ TENORMIN: Zeneca	00310-0101-10	100s	$130.10
	00310-0101-39	100s ud	$130.10
◆ **GENERICS**			
Allscrips	54569-3654-01	3s	$2.93
Allscrips	54569-3654-02	6s	$5.94
Allscrips	54569-3654-00	30s	$29.27
Medirex	57480-0447-06	30s	$30.67
Allscrips	54569-8590-00	90s	$87.82
Schein	00364-2514-01	100s	$89.75
Rugby	00536-3331-01	100s	$89.85
Qualitest	00603-2372-21	100s	$91.85
Novopharm	55953-0401-40	100s	$91.85
Major	00904-7635-60	100s	$94.50
Martec	52555-0534-01	100s	$94.50
IPR	54921-0101-10	100s	$94.94
Mason Dist	11845-0490-01	100s	$94.96
SCS Pharm	00905-5721-31	100s	$96.23
Apothecon	00003-5240-50	100s	$96.24
Mutual	53489-0530-01	100s	$96.50
Aligen	00405-4108-01	100s	$96.80
URL	00677-1479-01	100s	$96.90
West Point	59591-0265-68	100s	$97.65
Geneva	00781-1507-01	100s	$98.90
Goldline	00182-1005-01	100s	$99.95
Lederle Std Prod	00005-3220-43	100s	$99.95
Moore,H.L.	00839-7724-06	100s	$101.24
Moore,H.L.	00839-7742-06	100s	$101.24
Mylan	00378-0757-01	100s	$101.50
Schein	00364-2514-90	100s ud	$93.25
UDL	51079-0685-20	100s ud	$94.35
IPR	54921-0101-39	100s ud	$94.94
Vangard	00615-3533-13	100s ud	$99.78
Geneva	00781-1507-13	100s ud	$99.95
Goldline	00182-1005-89	100s ud	$99.95
Medirex	57480-0447-01	100s ud	$102.25
URL	00677-1479-10	1000s	$896.00
Mutual	53489-0530-10	1000s	$896.00
Lederle Std Prod	00005-3220-34	1000s	$924.54

Atenolol with Chlorthalidone

DESCRIPTION
Atenolol/Chlorthalidone is for the treatment of hypertension. It combines the antihypertensive activity of two agents: a beta$_1$-selective (cardioselective) hydrophilic blocking agent (Atenolol) and a monosulfonamyl diuretic (Chlorthalidone). Atenolol is Benzeneacetamide, 4-[2'-hydroxy-3'-[(1-methylethyl) amino] propoxy]. Its molecular formula is $C_{14}H_{22}N_2O_3$.

Atenolol (free base) is a relatively polar hydrophilic compound with a water solubility of 26.5 mg/mL at 37°C. It is freely soluble in 1N HCl (300 mg/mL at 25°C) and less soluble in chloroform (3 mg/mL at 25°C).

Chlorthalidone is 2-Chloro-5-(1-hydroxy-3-oxo-1 isoindolinyl) benzene sulfonamide. Its molecular formula is $C_{14}H_{11}ClN_2O_4S$.

Chlorthalidone has a water solubility of 12 mg/100 mL at 20°C.

CLINICAL PHARMACOLOGY

ATENOLOL/CHLORTHALIDONE

Atenolol and Chlorthalidone have been used singly and concomitantly for the treatment of hypertension. The antihypertensive effects of these agents are additive, and studies have shown that there is no interference with bioavailability when these agents are given together in the single combination tablet. Therefore, this combination provides a convenient formulation for the concomitant administration of these two entities. In patients with more severe hypertension, Atenolol/Chlorthalidone may be administered with other antihypertensives such as vasodilators.

ATENOLOL

Atenolol is a beta$_1$-selective (cardioselective) beta-adrenergic receptor blocking agent without membrane stabilizing or intrinsic sympathomimetic (partial agonist) activities. This preferential effect is not absolute, however, and at higher doses, Atenolol inhibits beta$_2$-adrenoreceptors, chiefly located in the bronchial and vascular musculature.

Pharmacodynamics: In standard animal or human pharmacological tests, beta-adrenoreceptor blocking activity of Atenolol has been demonstrated by: (1) reduction in resting and exercise heart rates and cardiac output, (2) reduction of systolic and diastolic blood pressure at rest and on exercise, (3) inhibition of isoproterenol induced tachycardia and (4) reduction in reflex orthostatic tachycardia.

A significant beta-blocking effect of Atenolol, as measured by reduction of exercise tachycardia, is apparent within one hour following oral administration of a single dose. This effect is maximal at about 2 to 4 hours and persists for at least 24 hours. The effect at 24 hours is dose related and also bears a linear relationship to the logarithm of plasma Atenolol concentration. However, as has been shown for all beta-blocking agents, the antihypertensive effect does not appear to be related to plasma level.

In normal subjects, the beta$_1$-selectivity of Atenolol has been shown by its reduced ability to reverse the beta$_2$-mediated vasodilating effect of isoproterenol as compared to equivalent beta-blocking doses of propranolol. In asthmatic patients, a dose of Atenolol producing a greater effect on resting heart rate than propranolol resulted in much less increase in airway resistance. In a placebo controlled comparison of approximately equipotent oral doses of several beta blockers, Atenolol produced a significantly smaller decrease of FEV_1 than nonselective beta blockers, such as propranolol and unlike those agents did not inhibit bronchodilation in response to isoproterenol.

Consistent with its negative chronotropic effect due to beta blockade of the SA node, Atenolol increases sinus cycle length and sinus node recovery time. Conduction in the AV node is also prolonged. Atenolol is devoid of membrane stabilizing activity, and increasing the dose well beyond that producing beta blockade does not further depress myocardial contractility. Several studies have demonstrated a moderate (approximately 10%) increase in stroke volume at rest and exercise.

In controlled clinical trials, Atenolol given as a single daily dose, was an effective antihypertensive agent providing 24-hour reduction of blood pressure. Atenolol has been studied in combination with thiazide-type diuretics and the blood pressure effects of the combination are approximately additive. Atenolol is also compatible with methyldopa, hydralazine and prazosin, the combination resulting in a larger fall in blood pressure than with the single agents. The dose range of Atenolol is narrow, and increasing the dose beyond 100 mg once daily is not associated with increased antihypertensive effect. The mechanisms of the antihypertensive effects of beta-blocking agents have not been established. Several mechanisms have been proposed and include: (1) competitive antagonism of catecholamines at peripheral (especially cardiac) adrenergic neuron sites, leading to decreased cardiac output, (2) a central effect leading to reduced sympathetic outflow to the periphery and (3) suppression of renin activity.

The results from long-term studies have not shown any diminution of the antihypertensive efficacy of Atenolol with prolonged use.

Pharmacokinetics and Metabolism: In man, absorption of an oral dose is rapid and consistent but incomplete. Approximately 50% of an oral dose is absorbed from the gastrointestinal tract, the remainder being excreted unchanged in the feces. Peak blood levels are reached between 2 and 4 hours after ingestion. Unlike propranolol or metoprolol, but like nadolol, hydrophilic Atenolol undergoes little or no metabolism by the liver, and the absorbed portion is eliminated primarily by renal excretion. Atenolol also differs from propranolol in that only a small amount (6-16%) is bound to proteins in the plasma. This kinetic profile results in relatively consistent plasma drug levels with about a fourfold interpatient variation. There is no information as to the pharmacokinetic effect of Atenolol on Chlorthalidone.

The elimination half-life of Atenolol is approximately 6 to 7 hours and there is no alteration of the kinetic profile of the drug by chronic administration. Following doses of 50 mg or 100 mg, both beta-blocking and antihypertensive effects persist for at least 24 hours. When renal function is impaired, elimination of Atenolol is closely related to the glomerular filtration rate; but significant accumulation does not occur until the creatinine clearance falls below 35 mL/min/1.73m^2.

CHLORTHALIDONE

Chlorthalidone is a monosulfonamyl diuretic which differs chemically from thiazide diuretics in that a double ring system is incorporated in its structure. It is an oral diuretic with prolonged action and low toxicity. The diuretic effect of the drug occurs within 2 hours of an oral dose. It produces diuresis with greatly increased secretion of sodium and chloride. At maximal therapeutic dosage, Chlorthalidone is approximately equal in its diuretic effect to comparable maximal therapeutic doses of benzothiadiazine diuretics. The site of action appears to be the cortical diluting segment of the ascending limb of Henle's loop of the nephron.

INDICATIONS AND USAGE

Atenolol/Chlorthalidone is indicated in the treatment of hypertension. This fixed dose combination drug is not indicated for initial therapy of hypertension. If the fixed dose combination represents the dose appropriate to the individual patient's needs, it may be more convenient than the separate components.

CONTRAINDICATIONS

Atenolol/Chlorthalidone is contraindicated in patients with: sinus bradycardia; heart block greater than first degree; cardiogenic shock; overt cardiac failure (see "*Warnings*"); anuria; hypersensitivity to this product or to sulfonamide-derived drugs.

WARNINGS

Cardiac Failure: Sympathetic stimulation is necessary in supporting circulatory function in congestive heart failure, and beta blockade carries the potential hazard of further depressing myocardial contractility and precipitating more severe failure. In patients who have congestive heart failure controlled by digitalis and/or diuretics, Atenolol/Chlorthalidone should be administered cautiously. Both digitalis and Atenolol slow AV conduction.

IN PATIENTS WITHOUT A HISTORY OF CARDIAC FAILURE, continued depression of the myocardium with beta-blocking agents over a period of time can, in some cases, lead to cardiac failure. At the first sign or symptom of impending cardiac failure, patients receiving Atenolol/Chlorthalidone should be digitalized and/or given additional diuretic therapy. Observe the patient closely. If cardiac failure continues despite adequate digitalization and diuretic therapy, Atenolol/Chlorthalidone therapy should be withdrawn.

Renal and Hepatic Disease and Electrolyte Disturbances: Since Atenolol is excreted via the kidneys Atenolol/Chlorthalidone should be used with caution in patients with impaired renal function.

In patients with renal disease, thiazides may precipitate azotemia. Since cumulative effects may develop in the presence of impaired renal function, if progressive renal impairment becomes evident, Atenolol/Chlorthalidone should be discontinued. In patients with impaired hepatic function or progressive liver disease, minor alterations in fluid and electrolyte balance may precipitate hepatic coma. Atenolol/Chlorthalidone should be used with caution in these patients.

Ischemic Heart Disease: Following abrupt cessation of therapy with certain beta-blocking agents in patients with coronary artery disease, exacerbations of angina pectoris and, in some cases, myocardial infarction have been reported. Therefore, such patients should be cautioned against interruption of therapy without the physician's advice. Even in the absence of overt angina pectoris, when discontinuation of Atenolol/Chlorthalidone is planned, the patient should be carefully observed and should be advised to limit physical activity to a minimum Atenolol/Chlorthalidone should be reinstated if withdrawal symptoms occur. Because coronary artery disease is common and may be unrecognized, it may be prudent not to discontinue Atenolol/Chlorthalidone therapy abruptly even in patients treated only for hypertension.

Bronchospastic Diseases: **PATIENTS WITH BRONCHOSPASTIC DISEASE SHOULD, IN GENERAL, NOT RECEIVE BETA BLOCKERS. Because of its relative beta$_1$-selectivity, however, Atenolol/Chlorthalidone may be used with caution in patients with bronchospastic disease who do not respond to or cannot tolerate, other antihypertensive treatment. Since beta$_1$-selectivity is not absolute, the lowest possible dose of Atenolol/Chlorthalidone should be used and a beta$_2$-stimulating agent (bronchodilator) should be made available. If dosage must be increased, dividing the dose should be considered in order to achieve lower peak blood levels.**

Anesthesia and Major Surgery: It is not advisable to withdraw beta-adrenoreceptor blocking drugs prior to surgery in the majority of patients. However, care should be taken when using anesthetic agents such as those which may depress the myocardium. Vagal dominance, if it occurs, may be corrected with atropine (1-2 mg IV).

Beta blockers are competitive inhibitors of beta-receptor agonists and their effects on the heart can be reversed by administration of such agents; eg, dobutamine or isoproterenol with caution (see section on "*Overdosage*").

Metabolic and Endocrine Effects: Atenolol/Chlorthalidone may be used with caution in diabetic patients. Beta blockers may mask tachycardia occurring with hypoglycemia, but other manifestations such as dizziness and sweating may not be significantly affected. At recommended doses Atenolol does not potentiate insulin-induced hypoglycemia and, unlike nonselective beta blockers, does not delay recovery of blood glucose to normal levels.

Insulin requirements in diabetic patients may be increased, decreased or unchanged; latent diabetes mellitus may become manifest during Chlorthalidone administration.

Beta-adrenergic blockade may mask certain clinical signs (eg, tachycardia) of hyperthyroidism. Abrupt withdrawal of beta blockade might precipitate a thyroid

---

storm; therefore, patients suspected of developing thyrotoxicosis from whom Atenolol/Chlorthalidone therapy is to be withdrawn should be monitored closely.

Because calcium excretion is decreased by thiazides, Atenolol/Chlorthalidone should be discontinued before carrying out tests for parathyroid function. Pathologic changes in the parathyroid glands, with hypercalcemia and hypophosphatemia, have been observed in a few patients on prolonged thiazide therapy; however, the common complications of hyperparathyroidism such as renal lithiasis, bone resorption, and peptic ulceration have not been seen.

Hyperuricemia may occur, or acute gout may be precipitated in certain patients receiving thiazide therapy.

WARNINGS

Pregnancy and Fetal Injury: Atenolol/Chlorthalidone can cause fetal harm when administered to a pregnant woman. Atenolol and thiazides cross the placental barrier and appear in cord blood. No studies have been performed on the use of Atenolol/Chlorthalidone in the first trimester and the possibility of fetal injury cannot be excluded. Atenolol has been used under close supervision for the treatment of hypertension in the third trimester. Administration of Atenolol for longer periods to pregnant women in the management of mild to moderate hypertension has been associated with intrauterine growth retardation. If Atenolol/Chlorthalidone is used during pregnancy, or if the patient becomes pregnant while taking this drug, the patient should be apprised of the potential hazard to the fetus.

Atenolol/Chlorthalidone was studied for teratogenic potential in the rat and rabbit. Doses of Atenolol/Chlorthalidone of 8/2, 80/20, and 240/60 mg/kg/day were administered orally to pregnant rats with no evidence of embryofetotoxicity observed. Two studies were conducted in rabbits. In the first study, pregnant rabbits were dosed with 8/2, 80/20, and 160/40 mg/kg/day of Atenolol/Chlorthalidone. No teratogenic effects were noted, but embryonic resorptions were observed at all dose levels (ranging from approximately 5 times to 100 times the maximum recommended human dose*). In the second rabbit study, doses of Atenolol/Chlorthalidone were 4/1, 8/2, and 20/5 mg/kg/day. No teratogenic or embryotoxic effects were demonstrated.

Atenolol: Atenolol has been shown to produce a dose-related increase in embryo/fetal resorptions in rats at doses equal to or greater than 50 mg/kg/day or 25 or more times the maximum recommended human antihypertensive dose. Although similar effects were not seen in rabbits, the compound was not evaluated in rabbits at doses above 25 mg/kg/day or 12.5 times the maximum recommended human antihypertensive dose.*

Chlorthalidone: Thiazides cross the placental barrier and appear in cord blood. The use of Chlorthalidone and related drugs in pregnant women requires that the anticipated benefits of the drug be weighed against possible hazards to the fetus. These hazards include fetal or neonatal jaundice, thrombocytopenia and possibly other adverse reactions which have occurred in the adult.

PRECAUTIONS

General: Atenolol/Chlorthalidone may aggravate peripheral arterial circulatory disorders.

Electrolyte and Fluid Balance Status: Periodic determination of serum electrolytes to detect possible electrolyte imbalance should be performed at appropriate intervals.

Patients should be observed for clinical signs of fluid or electrolyte imbalance; ie, hyponatremia, hypochloremic alkalosis, and hypokalemia. Serum and urine electrolyte determinations are particularly important when the patient is vomiting excessively or receiving parenteral fluids. Warning signs or symptoms of fluid and electrolyte imbalance include dryness of the mouth, thirst, weakness, lethargy, drowsiness, restlessness, muscle pains or cramps, muscular fatigue, hypotension, oliguria, tachycardia, and gastrointestinal disturbances such as nausea and vomiting.

Measurement of potassium levels is appropriate especially in elderly patients, those receiving digitalis preparations for cardiac failure, patients whose dietary intake of potassium is abnormally low, or those suffering from gastrointestinal complaints.

Hypokalemia may develop especially with brisk diuresis, when severe cirrhosis is present, or during concomitant use of corticosteroids or ACTH.

Interference with adequate oral electrolyte intake will also contribute to hypokalemia. Hypokalemia can sensitize or exaggerate the response of the heart to the toxic effects of digitalis (eg, increased ventricular irritability). Hypokalemia may be avoided or treated by use of potassium supplements or foods with a high potassium content.

Any chloride deficit during thiazide therapy is generally mild and usually does not require specific treatment except under extraordinary circumstances (as in liver disease or renal disease). Dilutional hyponatremia may occur in edematous patients in hot weather: appropriate therapy is water restriction rather than administration of salt except in rare instances when the hyponatremia is life-threatening. In actual salt depletion, appropriate replacement is the therapy of choice.

Drug Interactions: Atenolol/Chlorthalidone may potentiate the action of other antihypertensive agents used concomitantly. Patients treated with Atenolol/Chlorthalidone plus a catecholamine depletor (eg, reserpine) should be closely observed for evidence of hypotension and/or marked bradycardia which may produce vertigo, syncope or postural hypotension.

Thiazides may decrease arterial responsiveness to norepinephrine. This diminution is not sufficient to preclude the therapeutic effectiveness of norepinephrine. Thiazides may increase the responsiveness to tubocurarine.

Lithium generally should not be given with diuretics because they reduce its renal clearance and add a high risk of lithium toxicity. Read circulars for lithium preparations before use of such preparations with Atenolol/Chlorthalidone.

Beta blockers may exacerbate the rebound hypertension which can follow the withdrawal of cloridine. If the two drugs are coadministered, the beta blocker should be withdrawn several days before the gradual withdrawal of clonidine. If replacing clonidine by beta-blocker therapy, the introduction of beta blockers should be delayed for several days after clonidine administration has stopped.

While taking beta blockers, patients with a history of anaphylactic reaction to a variety of allergens may have a more severe reaction on repeated challenge, either accidental, diagnostic or therapeutic. Such patients may be unresponsive to the usual doses of epinephrine used to treat the allergic reaction.

Other Precautions: In patients receiving thiazides, sensitivity reactions may occur with or without a history of allergy or bronchial asthma. The possible exacerbation or activation of systemic lupus erythematosus has been reported. The antihypertensive effects of thiazides may be enhanced in the postsympathectomy patient.

Carcinogenesis, Mutagenesis, Impairment of Fertility: Two long-term (maximum dosing duration of 18 or 24 months) rat studies and one long-term (maximum dosing duration of 18 months) mouse study, each employing dose levels as high as 300 mg/kg/day or 150 times the maximum recommended human antihypertensive dose,* did not indicate a carcinogenic potential of Atenolol. A third (24 month) rat study, employing doses of 500 and 1,500 mg/kg/day (250 and 750 times the maximum recommended human antihypertensive dose*) resulted in increased incidences of benign adrenal medullary tumors in males and females, mammary fibroadenomas in females, and anterior pituitary adenomas and thyroid parafollicular cell carcinomas in males. No evidence of a mutagenic potential of Atenolol was uncovered in the dominant lethal test (mouse), in vivo cytogenetics test (Chinese hamster) or Ames test (*S typhimurium*).

Fertility of male or female rats (evaluated at dose levels as high as 200 mg/kg/day or 100 times the maximum recommended human dose*) was unaffected by Atenolol administration.

Animal Toxicology: Six month oral studies were conducted in rats and dogs using Atenolol/Chlorthalidone doses up to 12.5 mg/kg/day (Atenolol/Chlorthalidone 10/2.5 mg/kg/day—approximately five times the maximum recommended human antihypertensive dose*). There were no functional or morphological abnormalities resulting from dosing either compound alone or together other than minor changes in heart rate, blood pressure and urine chemistry which were attributed to the known pharmacologic properties of Atenolol and/or Chlorthalidone.

Chronic studies of Atenolol performed in animals have revealed the occurrence of vacuolation of epithelial cells of Brunner's glands in the duodenum of both male and female dogs at all tested dose levels (starting at 15 mg/kg/day or 7.5 times the maximum recommended human antihypertensive dose*) and increased incidence of atrial degeneration of hearts of male rats at 300 but not 150 mg Atenolol/kg/day (150 and 75 times the maximum recommended human antihypertensive dose*, respectively).

Use in Pregnancy: Pregnancy Category D. See *"Warnings—Pregnancy and Fetal Injury"*.

Nursing Mothers: Atenolol is excreted in human breast milk at a ratio of 1.5 to 6.8 when compared to the concentration in plasma. Caution should be exercised when Atenolol is administered to a nursing woman. Clinically significant bradycardia has been reported in breast fed infants. Premature infants, or infants with impaired renal function, may be more likely to develop adverse effects.

Pediatric Use: Safety and effectiveness in children have not been established.

ADVERSE REACTIONS

Atenolol/Chlorthalidone is usually well tolerated in properly selected patients. Most adverse effects have been mild and transient. The adverse effects observed for Atenolol/Chlorthalidone are essentially the same as those seen with the individual components.

Atenolol: The frequency estimates in the following table were derived from controlled studies in which adverse reactions were either volunteered by the patient (US studies) or elicited, eg, by checklist (foreign studies). The reported frequency of elicited adverse effects was higher for both Atenolol and placebo-treated patients than when these reactions were volunteered. Where frequency of adverse effects for Atenolol and placebo is similar, causal relationship to Atenolol is uncertain. (See related table).

During postmarketing experience, the following have been reported in temporal relationship to the use of the drug: elevated liver enzymes and/or bilirubin, headache, impotence, Peyronie's disease, psoriasiform rash or exacerbation of psoriasis, purpura, reversible alopecia, and thrombocytopenia. Atenolol/Chlorthalidone, like other beta blockers, has been associated with the development of antinuclear antibodies (ANA) and lupus syndrome.

Chlorthalidone: Cardiovascular: orthostatic hypotension: Gastrointestinal: anorexia, gastric irritation, vomiting, cramping, constipation, jaundice (intrahepatic cholestatic jaundice), pancreatitis; CNS: vertigo, paresthesias, xanthopsia; Hematologic: leukopenia, agranulocytosis, thrombocytopenia, aplastic anemia; Hyper-

---

* Based on the maximum dose of 100 mg/day in a 50 kg patient

sensitivity: purpura, photosensitivity, rash, urticaria, necrotizing angiitis (vasculitis) (cutaneous vasculitis), Lyell's syndrome (toxic epidermal necrolysis); Miscellaneous: hyperglycemia, glycosuria, hyperuricemia, muscle spasm, weakness, restlessness. Clinical trials of Atenolol/Chlorthalidone conducted in the United States (89 patients treated with Atenolol/Chlorthalidone) revealed no new or unexpected adverse effects.

Potential Adverse Effects: In addition, a variety of adverse effects not observed in clinical trials with Atenolol but reported with other beta-adrenergic blocking agents should be considered potential adverse effects of Atenolol. Nervous System: Reversible mental depression progressing to catatonia: hallucinations; an acute reversible syndrome characterized by disorientation for time and place, short-term memory loss, emotional lability, slightly clouded sensorium, and decreased performance on neuropsychometrics; visual disturbance; Cardiovascular: Intensification of AV block (see *"Contraindications"*): Gastrointestinal: Mesenteric arterial thrombosis, ischemic colitis; Hematologic: Agranulocytosis; Allergic: Erythematous rash, fever combined with aching and sore throat, laryngospasm and respiratory distress.

Other: Raynaud's phenomenon.

Miscellaneous: There have been reports of skin rashes and/or dry eyes associated with the use of beta-adrenergic blocking drugs. The reported incidence is small, and, in most cases, the symptoms have cleared when treatment was withdrawn. Discontinuance of the drug should be considered if any such reaction is not otherwise explicable. Patients should be closely monitored following cessation of therapy.

The oculomucocutaneous syndrome associated with the beta blocker practolol has not been reported with Atenolol. Furthermore, a number of patients who had previously demonstrated established practolol reactions were transferred to Atenolol therapy with subsequent resolution or quiescence of the reaction.

Clinical Laboratory Test Findings: Clinically important changes in standard laboratory parameters were rarely associated with the administration of Atenolol/Chlorthalidone. The changes in laboratory parameters were not progressive and usually were not associated with clinical manifestations. The most common changes were increases in uric acid and decreases in serum potassium.

OVERDOSAGE

No specific information is available with regard to overdosage and Atenolol/Chlorthalidone in humans. Treatment should be symptomatic and supportive and directed to the removal of any unabsorbed drug by induced emesis or administration or activated charcoal. Atenolol can be removed from the general circulation by hemodialysis. Further consideration should be given to dehydration, electrolyte imbalance and hypotension by established procedures.

Atenolol: Overdosage with Atenolol has been reported with patients surviving acute doses as high as 5 g. One death was reported in a man who may have taken as much as 10 g acutely.

The predominant symptoms reported following Atenolol overdose are lethargy, disorder of respiratory drive, wheezing, sinus pause, and bradycardia. Additionally, common effects associated with overdosage of any beta-adrenergic blocking agent are congestive heart failure, hypotension, bronchospasm, and/or hypoglycemia. Other treatment modalities should be employed at the physician's discretion and may include.

Bradycardia: Atropine 1-2 mg intravenously. If there is no response to vagal blockade, give isoproterenol cautiously. In refractory cases, a transvenous cardiac pacemaker may be indicated. Glucagon in a 10 mg intravenous bolus has been reported to be useful. If required, this may be repeated or followed by an intravenous infusion of glucagon 1-10 mg/h depending on response.

Heart Block (Second or Third Degree): Isoproterenol or transvenous pacemaker.
Congestive Heart Failure: Digitalize the patient and administer a diuretic. Glucagon has been reported to be useful.
Hypotension: Vasopressors such as dopamine or norepinephrine (levarterenol). Monitor blood pressure continuously.
Bronchospasm: A beta$_2$-stimulant such as isoproterenol or terbutaline and/or aminophylline.
Hypoglycemia: Intravenous glucose.
Electrolyte Disturbance: Monitor electrolyte levels and renal function. Institute measures to maintain hydration and electrolytes.

Based on the severity of symptoms, management may require intensive support care and facilities for applying cardiac and respiratory support.

Chlorthalidone: Symptoms of Chlorthalidone overdose include nausea, weakness, dizziness and disturbances of electrolyte balance.

DOSAGE AND ADMINISTRATION

DOSAGE MUST BE INDIVIDUALIZED (see *"Indications"*).

Chlorthalidone is usually given at a dose of 25 mg daily: the usual initial dose of Atenolol is 50 mg daily. Therefore, the initial dose should be one Atenolol/Chlorthalidone 50 tablet given once a day. If an optimal response is not achieved, the dosage should be increased to one Atenolol/Chlorthalidone 100 tablet given once a day. When necessary, another antihypertensive agent may be added gradually beginning with 50 percent of the usual recommended starting dose to avoid an excessive fall in blood pressure.

Since Atenolol is excreted via the kidneys, dosage should be adjusted in cases of severe impairment of renal function. No significant accumulation of Atenolol occurs until creatinine clearance falls below 35 mL/min/1.73m^2 (normal range is 100-150 mL/min/1.73m^2); therefore, the following maximum dosages are recommended for patients with renal impairment.

Creatinine Clearance (mL/min/1.73m^2)	Atenolol Elimination Half-life (hrs)	Maximum Dosage
15-35	16-27	50 mg daily
< 15	> 27	50 mg every other day

Store at controlled room temperature, 15°-30°C (59°-86°F). Dispense in well-closed, light-resistant containers.

HOW SUPPLIED
TABLETS: 50 MG-25 MG

AVERAGE UNIT PRICE (AVAILABLE SIZES)			GENERIC A-RATED AVERAGE PRICE (GAAP)	
BRAND		$0.99		
GENERIC		$0.83	100s	$82.97

BRAND/MANUFACTURER	NDC	SIZE	AWP
◆ BRAND			
➤ TENORETIC 50: Zeneca	00310-0115-10	100s	$99.02

	Volunteered (US Studies)			Total—Volunteered and Elicited (Foreign + US Studies)	
	Atenolol n = 164 %	Placebo n = 206 %		Atenolol n = 399 %	Placebo n = 407 %
Cardiovascular					
Bradycardia	3	0		3	0
Cold Extremities	0	0.5		12	5
Postural Hypotension	2	1		4	5
Leg Pain	0	0.5		3	1
Central Nervous System/ Neuromuscular					
Dizziness	4	1		13	6
Vertigo	2	0.5		2	0.2
Light-Headedness	1	0		3	0.7
Tiredness	0.6	0.5		26	13
Fatigue	3	1		6	5
Lethargy	1	0		3	0.7
Drowsiness	0.6	0		2	0.5
Depression	0.6	0.5		12	9
Dreaming	0	0		3	1
Gastrointestinal					
Diarrhea	2	0		2	3
Nausea	4	1		3	1
Respiratory (see *"Warnings"*)					
Wheeziness	0	0		3	3
Dyspnea	0.6	1		6	4

◆ RATED THERAPEUTICALLY EQUIVALENT; ◇ THERAPEUTIC EQUIVALENCE UNCONFIRMED; ○ UNRATED

BRAND/MANUFACTURER	NDC	SIZE	AWP
◆ GENERICS			
Qualitest	00603-2374-21	100s	$79.80
Goldline	00182-1942-01	100s	$80.00
IPR	54921-0115-10	100s	$80.12
Schein	00364-2527-01	100s	$80.12
Moore,H.L.	00839-7807-06	100s	$80.57
Martec	52555-0547-01	100s	$80.80
Rugby	00536-3332-01	100s	$82.40
Major	00904-7881-60	100s	$85.65
Geneva	00781-1315-01	100s	$88.13
Aligen	00405-4103-01	100s	$92.14

TABLETS: 100 MG-25 MG

AVERAGE UNIT PRICE (AVAILABLE SIZES)		GENERIC A-RATED AVERAGE PRICE (GAAP)	
BRAND	$1.39	100s	$116.32
GENERIC	$1.16		

BRAND/MANUFACTURER	NDC	SIZE	AWP
◆ BRAND			
► TENORETIC 100: Zeneca	00310-0117-10	100s	$138.98
◆ GENERICS			
Qualitest	00603-2375-21	100s	$111.45
Goldline	00182-1943-01	100s	$112.00
IPR	54921-0117-10	100s	$112.45
Schein	00364-2528-01	100s	$112.45
Moore,H.L.	00839-7808-06	100s	$113.09
Martec	52555-0548-01	100s	$113.10
Rugby	00536-3333-01	100s	$115.65
Major	00904-7882-60	100s	$120.25
Geneva	00781-1316-01	100s	$123.69
Aligen	00405-4104-01	100s	$129.03

Atgam SEE LYMPHOCYTE IMMUNE GLOBULIN

Ativan SEE LORAZEPAM

Atovaquone

DESCRIPTION

Atovaquone is an antiprotozoal agent. The chemical name of Atovaquone is *trans*-2-[4-(4-chlorophenyl)cyclohexyl]-3-hydroxy-1,4-naphthalenedione. Atovaquone is a yellow crystalline solid that is practically insoluble in water. It has a molecular weight of 366.84 and the molecular formula $C_{22}H_{19}ClO_3$.

Atovaquone tablets are for oral administration. Each film-coated tablet contains 250 mg.

Following is its chemical structure:

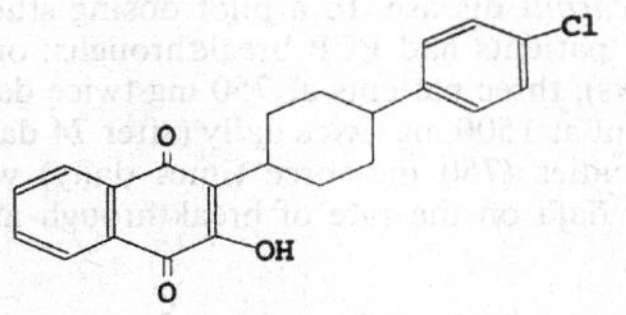

CLINICAL PHARMACOLOGY

Mechanism of Action: Atovaquone is a hydroxy-1,4-naphthoquinone, an analog of ubiquinone, with antipneumocystis activity. The mechanism of action against *P. carinii* has not been fully elucidated. In *Plasmodium* species, the site of action appears to be the cytochrome bc_1 complex (Complex III). Several metabolic enzymes are linked to the mitochondrial electron transport chain via ubiquinone. Inhibition of electron transport by atovaquone will result in indirect inhibition of these enzymes. The ultimate metabolic effects of such blockade may include inhibition of nucleic acid and ATP synthesis.

MICROBIOLOGY

Pneumocystis carinii: Several laboratories, using different *in vitro* methodologies, have shown the IC_{50} (50% Inhibitory Concentration) of Atovaquone against rat *P. carinii* to be in the range of 0.1 to 3.0 µg/mL.

Pharmacokinetics: Atovaquone is a highly lipophilic compound with a low aqueous solubility. Pharmacokinetic and bioavailability studies indicate that the bioavailability of the drug is low, variable, and decreases significantly with single doses above 750 mg. Following single-dose administration of Atovaquone to fasted normal volunteers, the Atovaquone plasma concentration-time profile displayed a distinct double-peak, with the first peak occurring between 1 and 8 hours after dosing and the second peak occurring 24 to 96 hours post-dose. This

double-peak profile is suggestive of enterohepatic cycling, whereby drug in the systemic circulation is excreted into the bile and is subsequently reabsorbed.

The bioavailability of Atovaquone is increased approximately 3-fold when administered with meals. In particular, fat has been shown to enhance absorption significantly. In one study, 18 volunteers received a single dose of 500 mg Atovaquone after an overnight fast and following a breakfast (23 g fat: 642 kCal). The mean (± SD) AUC values were 93.8 ± 45.7 and 288 ± 77 hr. µg/mL, under fasting and fed conditions, respectively. In another volunteer study where Atovaquone was administered under fasting conditions, with 28 g butter (23 g fat) and 56 g butter (46 g fat) on toast, mean AUC values increased 2.7- and 4.0-fold, respectively, compared to the fasting state. Significant differences in the bioavailability of Atovaquone have been observed between normal volunteers or HIV-seropositive asymptomatic volunteers and AIDS patients. Steady-state Atovaquone plasma concentrations in the AIDS patients are about one-third to one-half the levels achieved in the asymptomatic HIV-infected volunteers. The reasons for this difference are not clear.

Atovaquone has a long half-life in normal volunteers (2.9 ± 0.8 days: n = 27) and in AIDS patients (2.2 ± 0.6 days; n = 14), due to presumed enterohepatic cycling and eventual fecal elimination. In a study where ^{14}C-labelled Atovaquone was administered to healthy volunteers, greater than 94% of the dose was recovered in the feces over 21 days. There was little or no excretion of Atovaquone in the urine (less than 0.6%). There is no evidence that the drug is metabolized in man. Atovaquone is extensively bound to plasma proteins (> 99.9%). *In vitro* binding interaction studies with phenytoin (15 µg/mL) did not show mutual displacement from binding proteins.

During a multiple-dose study of Atovaquone administered with food in cohorts of 4 HIV-seropositive asymptomatic volunteers, dose-proportionality was demonstrated for dosage regimens of 100 to 750 mg once daily. However, at doses above 750 mg once daily with food, the relative oral bioavailability decreased. The maximum dose tested, 3000 mg once daily, produced a mean ± SD steady-state average plasma concentration of 40.0 ± 19.0 µg/mL compared to 26.9 ± 10.0 µg/mL in volunteers receiving 750 mg once daily. In a multiple-dose escalation study (Table 1) conducted in volunteers with AIDS, where a single cohort of 15 individuals received 15- to 17-day consecutive courses of Atovaquone administered with food at regimens of 750, 1500, 3000 mg once daily, 750 mg twice daily, and 1500 mg twice daily, the lack of dose proportionality was also demonstrated; however, there was a modest increase in concentrations with increasing total daily dose. Altering dose intervals without changing total daily dose did not affect concentrations. In this study, the C_{max}/C_{min} concentration ratio values were low; approximately 1.5, and independent of the dosage regimen.

Table 1
ATOVAQUONE AUC VALUES AND PLASMA CONCENTRATIONS IN VOLUNTEERS WITH AIDS*

	Once Daily with Food		
	750 mg (n = 15)	1500 mg (n = 15)	3000 mg (n = 14)
Steady-State AUC (hr·µg/mL)	181 ± 84	253 ± 126	322 ± 135
Steady-State Average Concentrations (µg/mL)	7.5 ± 3.5	10.6 ± 5.3	13.4 ± 5.6
	Twice Daily with Food		
	750 mg (n = 12)	1500 mg (n = 13)	
Steady-State AUC (hr·µg/mL)	231 ± 59	314 ± 109	
Steady-State Average Concentrations (µg/mL)	9.6 ± 2.5	13.1 ± 4.5	

* Mean ± SD

In the controlled efficacy trials for the treatment of PCP where AIDS patients received 750 mg Atovaquone three times daily, the mean steady-state Atovaquone concentration was 13.9 ± 6.8 µg/mL (n = 191).

In a human study where volunteers receive Atovaquone at a dose of 750 mg four times daily for two weeks, the cerebrospinal fluid levels in three volunteers were 0.04 µg/mL, 0.14 µg/mL and 0.26 µg/mL. The corresponding CSF/plasma ratios were less than 1%.

The pharmacokinetics of Atovaquone have been evaluated in 10 immunocompromised children (age; 5 months to 13 years; weight: 3.5 to 85.5 kg). The mean half-life was 2.7 ± 1.6 days. A dosage regimen of 10 mg/kg once daily achieved a steady-state average concentration of 7.5 ± 4.6 µg/mL (range 2.5 to 15.2 µg/mL). For 3 of these children who also received a dosage regimen of 40 mg/kg once daily, a steady-state average concentration of 14.0 ± 2.2 µg/mL (range 10.9 to 15.6 µg/mL) was achieved.

The pharmacokinetics of Atovaquone has not been studied in patients with hepatic or renal impairment.

INDICATIONS AND USAGE

Atovaquone is indicated for the acute oral treatment of mild to moderate *Pneumocystis carinii* pneumonia in patients who are intolerant to trimethoprim-sulfamethoxazole (TMP-SMX).

This indication is based on the results of a randomized, double-blind trial comparing Atovaquone to TMP-SMX in AIDS patients with mild to moderate PCP (defined in the study protocol as an alveolar-arterial oxygen diffusion gradient $[(A\text{-}a)DO_2]^1 \leq 45$ mmHg and $PaO_2 \geq 60$ mmHg on room air) and a randomized trial comparing Atovaquone to intravenous pentamidine isethionate in patients with mild to moderate PCP intolerant to trimethoprim or sulfa-antimicrobials. These studies are summarized below:

TMP-SMX Comparative Study: This double-blind, randomized trial initiated in 1990 was designed to compare the safety and efficacy of Atovaquone to that of TMP-SMX for the treatment of AIDS patients with histologically confirmed PCP. Only patients with mild to moderate PCP were eligible for enrollment.

A total of 408 patients were enrolled into the trial at 37 study centers. Eight-six patients without histologic confirmation of PCP were excluded from the efficacy analyses. Of the 322 patients with histologically confirmed PCP, 160 were randomized to receive Atovaquone and 162 to TMP-SMX.

Study participants randomized to Atovaquone treatment were to receive 750 mg Atovaquone (three 250 mg tablets) three times daily for 21 days and those randomized to TMP-SMX were to receive 320 mg TMP plus 1600 mg SMX three times daily for 21 days.

Therapy success was defined as improvement in clinical and respiratory measures persisting at least four weeks after cessation of therapy. Therapy failures included lack of response, treatment discontinuation due to an adverse experience, and unevaluable.

There was a significant difference ($P = 0.03$) in mortality rates between the treatment groups. Among the 322 patients with confirmed PCP, 13 of 160 (8%) patients treated with Atovaquone and four of 162 (2.5%) patients receiving TMP-SMX died during the 21-day treatment course or 8-week follow-up period. In the intent-to-treat analysis for all 408 randomized patients, there were 16 (8%) deaths in the Atovaquone arm and seven (3.4%) deaths in the TMP-SMX arm ($P = 0.051$). Of the 13 patients treated with Atovaquone who died, 4 died of PCP and 5 died with a combination of bacterial infections and PCP; bacterial infections did not appear to be a factor in any of the 4 deaths among TMP-SMX-treated patients.

A correlation between plasma Atovaquone concentrations and death was demonstrated; in general, patients with lower plasma concentrations were more likely to die. For those patients for whom day 4 Atovaquone plasma concentration data are available, 5 (63%) of the 8 patients with concentrations $< \mu g/mL$ died during participation in the study. However, only 1 (2.0%) of the 49 patients with day 4 plasma concentrations ≥ 5 µg/mL died.

Sixty-two percent of patients on Atovaquone and 64% of patients on TMP-SMX were classified as protocol-defined therapy successes (Table 2).

Table 2

OUTCOME OF TREATMENT FOR PCP-POSITIVE PATIENTS ENROLLED IN THE TMP-SMX COMPARATIVE STUDY

Outcome of Therapy*	Number of patients (% of Total)		
	Atovaquone (n = 160)	TMP-SMX (n = 162)	P Value
Therapy Success	99 (62%)	103 (64%)	0.75
Therapy Failure			
-Lack of Response	28 (17%)	10 (6%)	< 0.01
-Adverse Experience	11 (7%)	33 (20%)	< 0.01
-Unevaluable	22 (14%)	16 (0%)	0.28
Required Alternate PCP Therapy During Study	55 (34%)	55 (34%)	0.95

* *As defined by the protocol and described in study description above.*

The failure rate due to lack of response was significantly larger for Atovaquone patients while the failure rate due to adverse experiences was significantly larger for TMP-SMX patients.

There were no significant differences in the effect of either treatment on additional indicators of response (i.e., arterial blood gas measurements, vital signs, serum LDH levels, clinical symptoms, and chest radiographs).

Pentamidine Comparative Study: This unblinded, randomized trial initiated in 1991 was designed to compare the safety and efficacy of Atovaquone to that of pentamidine for the treatment of histologically confirmed mild or moderate PCP in AIDS patients. Approximately 80% of the patients had a history of intolerance to trimethoprim or sulfa-antimicrobials (the primary therapy group) or were experiencing intolerance to TMP-SMX with treatment of an episode of PCP at the time of enrollment in the study (the salvage treatment group).

Patients randomized to Atovaquone were to receive 750 mg Atovaquone (three 250 mg tablets) three times daily for 21 days and those randomized to pentamidine isethionate were to receive a 3 to 4 mg/kg single intravenous infusion daily for 21 days.

A total of 174 patients were enrolled into the trial at 22 study centers. Thirty-nine patients without histologic confirmation of PCP were excluded from the efficacy analyses. Of the 135 patients with histologically confirmed PCP, 70 were randomized to receive Atovaquone and 65 to pentamidine. One hundred and ten

(110) of these were in the primary therapy group and 25 were in the salvage therapy group. One patient in the primary therapy group randomized to receive pentamidine did not receive study medication.

There was no difference in mortality rates between the treatment groups. Among the 135 patients with confirmed PCP, 10 of 70 (14%) patients randomized to Atovaquone and nine of 65 (14%) patients randomized to pentamidine died during the 21-day treatment course or 8-week follow-up period. In the intent-to-treat analysis for all randomized patients, there were 11 (12.5%) deaths in the Atovaquone arm and 12 (14%) deaths in the pentamidine arm. For those patients for whom day 4 Atovaquone plasma concentration are available, 3 of 5 (60%) patients with concentrations < 5 µg/mL died during participation in the study. However, only 2 of 21 (9%) patients with day 4 plasma concentrations ≥ 5 µg/mL died.

The therapeutic outcomes for the 134 patients who received study medication in this trial are presented in Table 3.

Table 3

OUTCOME OF TREATMENT FOR PCP-POSITIVE PATIENTS ENROLLED IN THE PENTAMIDINE COMPARATIVE STUDY

Outcome of Therapy	Primary Treatment		
	Atovaquone (n = 56)	Pentamidine (n = 53)	P Value
Therapy Success	32 (57%)	21 (40%)	0.09
Therapy Failure			
-Lack of Response	16 (29%)	9 (17%)	0.18
-Adverse Experience	2 (3.6%)	19 (36%)	< 0.01
-Unevaluable	6 (11%)	4 (8%)	0.75
Required Alternate PCP Therapy During Study	19 (34%)	29 (55%)	0.04

Outcome of Therapy	Salvage Treatment		
	Atovaquone (n = 14)	Pentamidine (n = 11)	P Value
Therapy Success	13 (93%)	7 (64%)	0.14
Therapy Failure			
-Lack of Response	0	0	—
-Adverse Experience	0	3 (27%)	0.07
-Unevaluable	1 (7%)	1 (9%)	1.00
Required Alternate PCP Therapy During Study	0	4 (36%)	0.03

Data on Chronic Use: Atovaquone has not been systematically evaluated as a chronic suppressive agent to prevent the development of PCP in patients at high risk for *Pneumocystis carinii* disease. In a pilot dosing study of Atovaquone in AIDS patients, 5 of 31 patients had PCP breakthroughs: one patient at 750 mg once daily (after 20 days), three patients at 750 mg twice daily (after 14, 70, and 97 days), and one patient at 1500 mg twice daily (after 74 days). The dose used in the acute treatment studies (750 mg three times daily) was not studied and, therefore, there are no data on the rate of breakthrough at this dose.

UNLABELED USES

Atovaquone is used alone or as an adjunct in the treatment of toxoplasmosis in patients with acquired immunodeficiency syndrome.

CONTRAINDICATIONS

Atovaquone tablets are contraindicated for patients who develop or have a history of potentially life-threatening allergic reactions to any of the components of the formulation.

WARNINGS

Clinical experience with Atovaquone has been limited to patients with mild to moderate PCP [$(A\text{-}a)DO_2 \geq 45$ mmHg]. Treatment of more severe episodes of PCP has not been systematically studied with this agent. Also, the efficacy of Atovaquone in patients who are failing therapy with TMP-SMX has not been systematically studied Atovaquone has not been evaluated as an agent for PCP prophylaxis.

PRECAUTIONS

General: Absorption of orally administered Atovaquone is limited but can be significantly increased when the drug is taken with food Atovaquone plasma concentrations have been shown to correlate with the likelihood of successful treatment and survival. Therefore, parenteral therapy with other agents should be considered for patients who have difficulty taking Atovaquone with food (see *Clinical Pharmacology*). Gastrointestinal disorders may limit absorption of orally administered drugs. Patients with these disorders also may not achieve plasma concentrations of Atovaquone associated with response to therapy in controlled trials.

Based upon the spectrum of *in vitro* antimicrobial activity, Atovaquone is not effective therapy for concurrent pulmonary conditions such as bacterial, viral or fungal pneumonia or mycobacterial diseases. Clinical deterioration in patients may be due to infections with other pathogens, as well as progressive PCP. All patients with acute PCP should be carefully evaluated for other possible causes of pulmonary disease and treated with additional agents as appropriate.

Information for Patients: The importance of taking the prescribed dose of Atovaquone should be stressed. Patients should be instructed to take their daily doses of Atovaquone with meals as the presence of food will significantly improve the absorption of the drug.

Drug Interactions: Atovaquone is highly bound to plasma protein (> 99.9%). Therefore, caution should be used when administering Atovaquone concurrently with other highly plasma protein bound drugs with narrow therapeutic indices as competition for binding sites may occur. The extent of plasma protein binding of Atovaquone in human plasma is not affected by the presence of therapeutic concentrations of phenytoin (15 µg/mL), nor is the binding of phenytoin affected by the presence of Atovaquone.

Drug/Laboratory Test Interactions: It is not known if Atovaquone interferes with clinical laboratory test or assay results.

Carcinogenesis, Mutagenesis, Impairment of Fertility: Carcinogenicity studies in rats and mice have not been completed. Atovaquone was negative with or without metabolic activation in the Ames *Salmonella* mutagenicity assay, the Mouse Lymphoma mutagenesis assay, and the Cultured Human Lymphocyte cytogenetic assay. No evidence of genotoxicity was observed in the *in vivo* Mouse Micronucleus assay.

Pregnancy: Pregnancy Category C. Atovaquone was not teratogenic and did not cause reproductive toxicity in rats at plasma concentrations up to 5 times the estimated human exposure. Atovaquone caused maternal toxicity in rabbits at plasma concentrations that were approximately equal to the estimated human exposure. Mean fetal body lengths and weights were decreased and there were higher numbers of early resorption and post-implantation loss per dam. It is not clear whether these effects were caused by Atovaquone or were secondary to maternal toxicity. Concentrations of Atovaquone in rabbit fetuses averaged 30% of the concurrent maternal plasma concentrations. In a separate study in rats given a single ^{14}C-radiolabelled dose, concentrations of radiocarbon in rat fetuses were 18% (middle gestation) and 60% (late gestation) of concurrent maternal plasma concentrations. There are no adequate and well-controlled studies in pregnant women. Atovaquone should be used during pregnancy only if the potential benefit justifies the potential risk to the fetus.

Nursing Mothers: It is not known whether Atovaquone is excreted into human milk. Because many drugs are excreted into human milk, caution should be exercised when Atovaquone is administered to a nursing woman. In a rat study, Atovaquone concentrations in the milk were 30% of the concurrent Atovaquone concentrations in the maternal plasma.

Pediatric Use: There are no efficacy studies in children. Clinical experience with Atovaquone in the pediatric population is limited to a pharmacokinetic and safety study. No children under 4 months of age participated in the phase I trial.

Geriatric Use: Atovaquone has not been systematically evaluated in patients greater than 65 years of age. Caution should be exercised when treating elderly patients reflecting the greater frequency of decreased hepatic, renal and cardiac function in this population.

ADVERSE REACTIONS

Because many patients who participated in clinical trials with Atovaquone had complications of advanced HIV disease, it was often difficult to distinguish adverse events caused by Atovaquone from those caused by underlying medical conditions. There were no life-threatening or fatal adverse experiences caused by Atovaquone.

Table 4 summarizes all the clinical adverse experiences reported by ≥ 5% of the study population during the TMP-SMX comparative study of Atovaquone (n = 408), regardless of attribution.

Table 4

TREATMENT-EMERGENT ADVERSE EXPERIENCES IN THE TMP-SMX COMPARATIVE PCP TREATMENT STUDY

Treatment-Emergent Adverse Experience	Number of Patients with Treatment-Emergent Adverse Experience (% of Total)	
	Atovaquone (n = 203)	TMP-SMX (n = 205)
Rash (including maculopapular)	47 (23%)	69 (34%)*
Nausea	43 (21%)	90 (44%)*
Diarrhea	39 (19%)*	15 (7%)
Headache	33 (16%)	44 (22%)
Vomiting	29 (14%)	72 (35%)*
Fever	28 (14%)	52 (25%)*
Insomnia	20 (10%)	18 (9%)

Treatment-Emergent Adverse Experience	Number of Patients with Treatment-Emergent Adverse Experience (% of Total)	
	Atovaquone (n = 203)	TMP-SMX (n = 205)
Asthenia	17 (8%)	16 (8%)
Pruritus	11 (5%)	18 (9%)
Monilia, Oral	11 (5%)	21 (10%)
Abdominal Pain	9 (4%)	15 (7%)
Constipation	7 (3%)	35 (17%)*
Dizziness	7 (3%)	17 (8%)*
No. Patients Discontinuing Therapy due to an Adverse Experience	19 (9%)	50 (24%)*
No. Patients Reporting at least one Adverse Experience	127 (63%)	134 (65%)

* P = < 0.05

Although an equal percentage of patients receiving Atovaquone and TMP-SMX reported at least one adverse experience, more patients receiving TMP-SMX required discontinuation of therapy due to an adverse event. Nine percent of patients receiving Atovaquone were prematurely discontinued from therapy due to an adverse event versus 24% of patients receiving TMP-SMX. Four percent of patients receiving Atovaquone had therapy discontinued due to development of rash. The majority of cases of rash among patients receiving Atovaquone were mild and did not require the discontinuation of dosing. The only other clinical adverse experience that led to premature discontinuation of Atovaquone dosing by more than one patient was the development of vomiting (< 1%). Twenty-four percent of patients receiving TMP-SMX were prematurely discontinued from therapy due to an adverse experience versus 9% of patients receiving Atovaquone. The most common adverse experience requiring discontinuation of dosing in the TMP-SMX group was rash (8%).

Laboratory test abnormalities reported for ≥ 5% of the study population during the treatment period are summarized in Table 5. Two percent of patients treated with Atovaquone and 7% of patients treated with TMP-SMX had therapy prematurely discontinued due to elevations in ALT/AST. In general, patients treated with Atovaquone developed fewer abnormalities in measures of hepatocellular function (ALT, AST, alkaline phosphatase) or amylase values than patients treated with TMP-SMX.

Table 5

TREATMENT-EMERGENT LABORATORY TEST ABNORMALITIES IN THE TMP-SMX COMPARATIVE PCP TREATMENT STUDY

Laboratory Test Abnormality	Patients Developing a Laboratory Test Abnormality (% of Total)	
	Atovaquone	TMP-SMX
Anemia (Hgb < 8.0 gm/dL)	6%	7%
Neutropenia (ANC < 750 c/mm^3)	3%	9%
Elevated ALT (> 5 × ULN)	6%	16%
Elevated AST (> 5 × ULN)	4%	14%
Elevated Alkaline Phosphatase (> 2.5 × ULN)	8%	6%
Elevated Amylase (> 1.5 × ULN)	7%	12%
Hyponatremia (< 0.96 × LLN)	7%	26%

ULN = upper limit of normal range
LLN = lower limit of normal range

Table 6 summarizes the clinical adverse experiences reported by ≥ 5% of the primary therapy study population (n = 144) during the comparative trial of Atovaquone and intravenous pentamidine, regardless of attribution. A slightly lower percentage of patients who received Atovaquone reported occurrence of adverse events than did those who received pentamidine (63% vs 72%). However, only 7% of patients discontinued treatment with Atovaquone due to adverse events while 41% of patients who received pentamidine discontinued treatment for this reason (P < 0.001). Of the five patients who discontinued therapy with Atovaquone, three reported rash (4%). Rash was not severe in any patient. No other reason for discontinuation of Atovaquone was cited more than once. The most frequently cited reasons for discontinuation of pentamidine therapy were hypoglycemia (11%) and vomiting (9%).

Table 6
TREATMENT-EMERGENT ADVERSE EXPERIENCES IN THE PENTAMIDINE COMPARATIVE PCP TREATMENT STUDY (PRIMARY THERAPY GROUP)

| Treatment-Emergent Adverse Experience | Number of Patients with Treatment-Emergent Adverse Experience (% of Total) | |
	Atovaquone (n = 73)	Pentamidine (n = 71)
Fever	29 (40%)	18 (25%)
Nausea	16 (22%)	26 (37%)
Rash	16 (22%)	9 (13%)
Diarrhea	15 (21%)	22 (31%)
Insomnia	14 (19%)	10 (14%)
Headache	13 (18%)	20 (28%)
Vomiting	10 (14%)	12 (17%)
Cough	10 (14%)*	1 (1%)
Abdominal Pain	7 (10%)	8 (11%)
Pain	7 (10%)	7 (10%)
Sweat	7 (10%)	2 (3%)
Monilia, Oral	7 (10%)	2 (3%)
Asthenia	6 (8%)	10 (14%)
Dizziness	6 (8%)	10 (14%)
Anxiety	5 (7%)	7 (10%)
Anorexia	5 (7%)	7 (10%)
Sinusitis	5 (7%)	4 (6%)
Dyspepsia	4 (5%)	7 (10%)
Rhinitis	4 (5%)	5 (7%)
Taste Perversion	2 (3%)	9 (13%)*
Hypoglycemia	1 (1%)	11 (15%)*
Hypotension	1 (1%)	7 (10%)*
No. Patients Discontinuing Therapy due to an Adverse Expereince	5 (7%)	29 (41%)†
No. Patients Reporting at least one Adverse Experience	46 (63%)	51 (72%)

* P = < 0.05
† P = < 0.001

Laboratory test abnormalities reported in ≥ 5% of patients in the pentamidine comparative study are presented in Table 7. Laboratory abnormality was reported as the reason for discontinuation of treatment in two of 73 patients who received Atovaquone. One patient (1%) had elevated creatinine and BUN levels and one patient (1%) had elevated amylase levels. Laboratory abnormalities were the sole or contributing factor in 14 patients who prematurely discontinued pentamidine therapy. In the 71 patients who received pentamidine, laboratory parameters most frequently reported as reasons for discontinuation were hypoglycemia (11%), elevated creatinine levels (6%), and leukopenia (4%).

Table 7
TREATMENT-EMERGENT LABORATORY TEST ABNORMALITIES IN THE PENTAMIDINE COMPARATIVE PCP TREATMENT STUDY

| Laboratory Test Abnormality | Patients Developing a Laboratory Test Abnormality (% of Total) | |
	Atovaquone	Pentamidine
Anemia (Hgb < 8.0 gm/dL)	4%	9%
Neutropenia (ANC < 750 cells/mm^3)	5%	9%
Hyponatremia (< 0.96 × LLN)	10%	10%
Hyperkalemia (> 1.18 × ULN)	0%	5%
Alkaline Phosphatase (> 2.5 × ULN)	5%	2%
Hyperglycemia (> 1.8 × ULN)	9%	13%
Elevated AST (> 5 × ULN)	0%	5%
Elevated Amylase (< 1.5 +11 ULN)	8%	4%
Elevated Creatinine (> 1.5 × ULN)	0%	7%

ULN = upper limit of normal range
LLN = lower limit of normal range

OVERDOSAGE
There have been no reports of overdosage from the oral administration of Atovaquone.

DOSAGE AND ADMINISTRATION
Adults: The recommended oral dose is 750 mg (three 250 mg tablets) administered with food three times a day for 21 days (total daily dose 2250 mg). Failure to administer Atovaquone with food may result in lower Atovaquone plasma concentrations and may limit response to therapy (see "Clinical Pharmacology" and "Precautions").

Dispense in well-closed container as defined in U.S.P., if product package is subdivided.

HOW SUPPLIED
TABLETS: 250 MG

BRAND/MANUFACTURER	NDC	SIZE	AWP
○ BRAND MEPRON: Burr Wellcome	00081-0126-62	200s	$532.67

Atracurium Besylate

This drug should be used only by adequately trained individuals familiar with its actions, characteristics, and hazards.

DESCRIPTION
Atracurium Besylate is an intermediate-duration, nondepolarizing, skeletal muscle relaxant for intravenous administration. Atracurium Besylate is designated as 2,2′-[pentamethylenebis(oxycarbonylethyl-ene)]bis(1,2,3,4-tetrahydro-6, 7-dimethoxy-2-methyl-1-veratrylisoquinolinium) dibenzenesulfonate. It has a molecular weight of 1243.49, and its molecular formula is $C_{65}H_{82}N_2O_{18}S_2$.

Atracurium Besylate is a complex molecule containing four sites at which different stereochemical configurations can occur. The symmetry of the molecule, however, results in only ten, instead of sixteen, possible different isomers. The manufacture of Atracurium Besylate results in these isomers being produced in unequal amounts but with a consistent ratio. Those molecules in which the methyl group attached to the quaternary nitrogen projects on the opposite side to the adjacent substituted-benzyl moiety predominate by approximately 3:1.

Atracurium Besylate Injection is a sterile, non-pyrogenic aqueous solution. Each mL contains 10 mg Atracurium Besylate. The pH is adjusted to 3.25-3.65 with benzenesulfonic acid. The multiple dose vial contains 0.9% benzyl alcohol added as a preservative. Atracurium Besylate slowly loses potency with time at the rate of approximately 6% per *year* under refrigeration (5°C). Atracurium Besylate Injection should be refrigerated at 2° to 8°C (36° to 46°F) to preserve potency. Rate of loss in potency increases to approximately 5% per *month* at 25°C (77°F). Upon removal from refrigeration to room temperature storage conditions (25°C/77°F), use Atracurium Besylate Injection within 14 days even if rerefrigerated.

Following is its chemical structure:

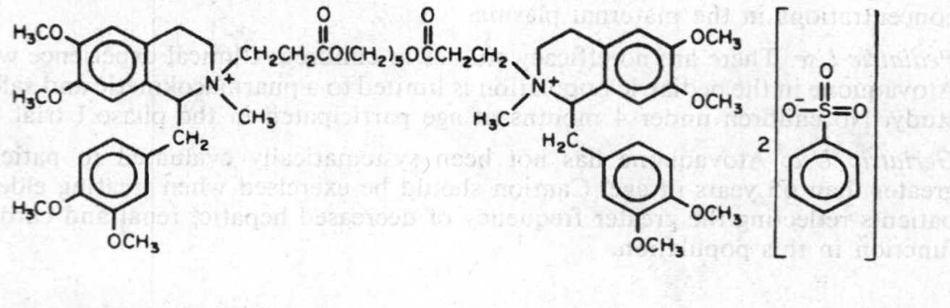

CLINICAL PHARMACOLOGY
Atracurium Besylate is a nondepolarizing skeletal muscle relaxant. Nondepolarizing agents antagonize the neurotransmitter action of acetylcholine by binding competitively with cholinergic receptor sites on the motor end-plate. This antagonism is inhibited, and neuromuscular block reversed, by acetylcholinesterase inhibitors such as neostigmine, edrophonium, and pyridostigmine.

Atracurium Besylate can be used most advantageously if muscle twitch response to peripheral nerve stimulation is monitored to assess degree of muscle relaxation.

The duration of neuromuscular blockade produced by Atracurium Besylate is approximately one-third to one-half the duration of blockade by d-tubocurarine, metocurine, and pancuronium at initially equipotent doses. As with other nondepolarizing neuromuscular blockers, the time to onset of paralysis decreases and the duration of maximum effect increases with increasing Atracurium Besylate doses.

The ED$_{95}$ (dose required to produce 95% suppression of the muscle twitch response with balanced anesthesia) has averaged 0.23 mg/kg (0.11 to 0.26 mg/kg in various studies). An initial Atracurium Besylate dose of 0.4 to 0.5 mg/kg generally produces maximum neuromuscular blockade within 3 to 5 minutes of injection, with good or excellent intubation conditions within 2 to 2.5 minutes in most patients. Recovery from neuromuscular blockade (under balanced anesthesia) can be expected to begin approximately 20 to 35 minutes after injection. Under balanced anesthesia, recovery to 25% of control is achieved approximately 35 to 45 minutes after injection, and recovery is usually 95% complete approximately 60-70 minutes after injection. The neuromuscular blocking action of Atracurium Besylate is enhanced in the presence of potent inhalation anesthetics. Isoflurane and enflurane increase the potency of Atracurium Besylate and prolong neuromuscular blockade by approximately 35%; however, halo-

◆ RATED THERAPEUTICALLY EQUIVALENT; ◇ THERAPEUTIC EQUIVALENCE UNCONFIRMED; ○ UNRATED

thane's potentiating effect (approximately 20%) is marginal (see *"Dosage and Administration"*).

Repeated administration of maintenance doses of Atracurium Besylate has no cumulative effect on the duration of neuromuscular blockade if recovery is allowed to begin prior to repeat dosing. Moreover, the time needed to recover from repeat doses does not change with additional doses. Repeat doses can therefore be administered at relatively regular intervals with predictable results. After an initial dose of 0.4 to 0.5 mg/kg under balanced anesthesia, the first maintenance dose (suggested maintenance dose is 0.08 to 0.10 mg/kg) is generally required within 20 to 45 minutes, and subsequent maintenance doses are usually required at approximately 15 to 25 minute intervals.

Once recovery from Atracurium Besylate's neuromuscular blocking effects begins, it proceeds more rapidly than recovery from d-tubocurarine, metocurine, and pancuronium. Regardless of Atracurium Besylate dose, the time from start of recovery (from complete block) to complete (95%) recovery is approximately 30 minutes under balanced anesthesia, and approximately 40 minutes under halothane, enflurane or isoflurane. Repeated doses have no cumulative effect on recovery rate.

Reversal of neuromuscular blockade produced by Atracurium Besylate can be achieved with an anticholinesterase agent such as neostigmine, edrophonium, or pyridostigmine, in conjunction with an anticholinergic agent such as atropine or glycopyrrolate. Under balanced anesthesia, reversal can usually be attempted approximately 20 to 35 minutes after an initial Atracurium Besylate dose of 0.4 to 0.5 mg/kg, or approximately 10 to 30 minutes after a 0.08 to 0.10 mg/kg maintenance dose, when recovery of muscle twitch has started. Complete reversal is usually attained within 8-10 minutes of the administration of reversing agents. Rare instances of breathing difficulties, possibly related to incomplete reversal, have been reported following attempted pharmacologic antagonism of Atracurium Besylate induced neuromuscular blockade. As with other agents in this class, the tendency for residual neuromuscular block is increased if reversal is attempted at deep levels of blockade or if inadequate doses of reversal agents are employed.

The pharmacokinetics of Atracurium Besylate in man are essentially linear within the 0.3 to 0.6 mg/kg dose range. The elimination half-life is approximately 20 minutes. THE DURATION OF NEUROMUSCULAR BLOCKADE PRODUCED BY ATRACURIUM BESYLATE DOES NOT CORRELATE WITH PLASMA PSEUDOCHOLINESTERASE LEVELS AND IS NOT ALTERED BY THE ABSENCE OF RENAL FUNCTION. This is consistent with the results of *in vitro* studies which have shown that Atracurium Besylate is inactivated in plasma via two nonoxidative pathways: ester hydrolysis, catalyzed by nonspecific esterases; and Hofmann elimination, a nonenzymatic chemical process which occurs at physiological pH. Some placental transfer occurs in humans.

Radiolabel studies demonstrated that Atracurium Besylate undergoes extensive degradation in cats, and that neither kidney nor liver plays a major role in its elimination. Biliary and urinary excretion were the major routes of excretion of radioactivity (totaling > 90% of the labeled dose within 7 hours of dosing), of which Atracurium Besylate represented only a minor fraction. The metabolites in bile and urine were similar, including products of Hofmann elimination and ester hydrolysis. Atracurium Besylate is a less potent histamine releaser than d-tubocurarine or metocurine. Histamine release is minimal with initial Atracurium Besylate doses up to 0.5 mg/kg, and hemodynamic changes are minimal within the recommended dose range. A moderate histamine release and significant falls in blood pressure have been seen following 0.6 mg/kg of Atracurium Besylate. The histamine and hemodynamic responses were poorly correlated. The effects were generally short-lived and manageable, but the possibility of substantial histamine release in sensitive individuals or in patients in whom substantial histamine release would be especially hazardous (e.g., patients with significant cardiovascular disease) must be considered.

It is not known whether the prior use of other nondepolarizing neuromuscular blocking agents has any effect on the activity of Atracurium Besylate. The prior use of succinylcholine decreases by approximately 2 to 3 minutes the time to maximum blockade induced by Atracurium Besylate, and may increase the depth of blockade. Atracurium Besylate should be administered only after a patient recovers from succinylcholine-induced neuromuscular blockade.

INDICATIONS AND USAGE
Atracurium Besylate is indicated, as an adjunct to general anesthesia, to facilitate endotracheal intubation and to provide skeletal muscle relaxation during surgery or mechanical ventilation.

CONTRAINDICATIONS
Atracurium Besylate is contraindicated in patients known to have a hypersensitivity to it.

WARNINGS
ATRACURIUM BESYLATE SHOULD BE USED ONLY BY THOSE SKILLED IN AIRWAY MANAGEMENT AND RESPIRATORY SUPPORT. EQUIPMENT AND PERSONNEL MUST BE IMMEDIATELY AVAILABLE FOR ENDOTRACHEAL INTUBATION AND SUPPORT OF VENTILATION, INCLUDING ADMINISTRATION OF POSITIVE PRESSURE OXYGEN. ADEQUACY OF RESPIRATION MUST BE ASSURED THROUGH ASSISTED OR CONTROLLED VENTILATION. ANTICHOLINESTERASE REVERSAL AGENTS SHOULD BE IMMEDIATELY AVAILABLE.

DO NOT GIVE ATRACURIUM BESYLATE BY INTRAMUSCULAR ADMINISTRATION.

Atracurium Besylate has no known effect on consciousness, pain threshold, or cerebration. It should be used only with adequate anesthesia.

Atracurium Besylate Injection, which has an acid pH, should not be mixed with alkaline solutions (e.g., barbiturate solutions) in the same syringe or administered simultaneously during intravenous infusion through the same needle. Depending on the resultant pH of such mixtures, Atracurium Besylate may be inactivated and a free acid may be precipitated.

Atracurium Besylate Injection 10 mL multiple dose vials contain benzyl alcohol. Benzyl alcohol has been associated with an increased incidence of neurological and other complications in newborn infants which are sometimes fatal. Atracurium Besylate Injection 5 mL single use vials do not contain benzyl alcohol.

PRECAUTIONS
General: Although Atracurium Besylate is a less potent histamine releaser than d-tubocurarine or metocurine, the possibility of substantial histamine release in sensitive individuals must be considered. Special caution should be exercised in administering Atracurium Besylate to patients in whom substantial histamine release would be especially hazardous (e.g., patients with clinically significant cardiovascular disease) and in patients with any history (e.g., severe anaphylactoid reactions or asthma) suggesting a greater risk of histamine release. In these patients, the recommended initial Atracurium Besylate dose is lower (0.3 to 0.4 mg/kg) than for other patients and should be administered slowly or in divided doses over one minute.

Since Atracurium Besylate has no clinically significant effects on heart rate in the recommended dosage range, it will not counteract the bradycardia produced by many anesthetic agents or vagal stimulation. As a result, bradycardia during anesthesia may be more common with Atracurium Besylate than with other muscle relaxants.

Atracurium Besylate may have profound effects in patients with myasthenia gravis, Eaton-Lambert syndrome, or other neuromuscular diseases in which potentiation of nondepolarizing agents has been noted. The use of a peripheral nerve stimulator is especially important for assessing neuromuscular blockade in these patients. Similar precautions should be taken in patients with severe electrolyte disorders or carcinomatosis.

Multiple factors in anesthesia practice are suspected of triggering malignant hyperthermia (MH), a potentially fatal hypermetabolic state of skeletal muscle. Halogenated anesthetic agents and succinylcholine are recognized as the principal pharmacologic triggering agents in MH-susceptible patients; however, since MH can develop in the absence of established triggering agents, the clinician should be prepared to recognize and treat MH in any patient scheduled for general anesthesia. Reports of MH have been rare in cases in which Atracurium Besylate has been used. In studies of MH-susceptible animals (swine) and in a clinical study of MH susceptible patients, Atracurium Besylate did not trigger this syndrome.

Resistance to nondepolarizing neuromuscular blocking agents may develop in burn patients. Increased doses of non-depolarizing muscle relaxants may be required in burn patients and are dependent on the time elapsed since the burn injury and the size of the burn.

The safety of Atracurium Besylate has not been established in patients with bronchial asthma.

Long-Term Use in Intensive Care Unit (ICU): When there is a need for long-term mechanical ventilation, the benefits to risk ratio of neuromuscular blockade must be considered. There is only limited information available on the efficacy and safety of long-term (days to weeks) intravenous Atracurium infusion to facilitate mechanical ventilation in the ICU. These data suggest that there is wide interpatient variability in dosage requirements and that these requirements may decrease or increase with time.

Little information is available on the plasma levels or clinical consequences of Atracurium metabolites that may accumulate during days to weeks of Atracurium administration in ICU patients. Laudanosine, a major biologically active metabolite of Atracurium without neuromuscular blocking activity, produces transient hypotension and, in higher doses, cerebral excitatory effects (generalized muscle twitching and seizures) when administered to several species of animals. There have been rare reports of seizures in ICU patients who have received Atracurium or other agents. These patients usually had predisposing causes (such as head trauma, cerebral edema, hypoxic encephalopathy, viral encephalitis, uremia). There are insufficient data to determine whether or not laudanosine contributes to seizures in ICU patients.

WHENEVER THE USE OF ATRACURIUM BESYLATE OR ANY NEUROMUSCULAR BLOCKING AGENT IS CONTEMPLATED IN THE ICU, IT IS RECOMMENDED THAT NEUROMUSCULAR TRANSMISSION BE MONITORED CONTINUOUSLY DURING ADMINISTRATION WITH THE HELP OF A NERVE STIMULATOR. ADDITIONAL DOSES OF ATRACURIUM BESYLATE OR ANY OTHER NEUROMUSCULAR BLOCKING AGENT SHOULD NOT BE GIVEN BEFORE THERE IS A DEFINITE RESPONSE TO T_1 OR TO THE FIRST TWITCH. IF NO RESPONSE IS ELICITED, INFUSION ADMINISTRATION SHOULD BE DISCONTINUED UNTIL A RESPONSE RETURNS.

The effects of hemodialysis, hemoperfusion and hemofiltration on plasma levels of Atracurium and its metabolites are unknown.

Drug Interactions: Drugs which may enhance the neuromuscular blocking action of Atracurium Besylate include: enflurane; isoflurane; halothane; certain antibiotics, especially the aminoglycosides and polymyxins; lithium; magnesium salts; procainamide; and quinidine.

If other muscle relaxants are used during the same procedure, the possibility of a synergistic or antagonist effect should be considered.

The prior administration of succinylcholine does not enhance the duration, but quickens the onset and may increase the depth, of neuromuscular blockade induced by Atracurium Besylate. Atracurium Besylate should not be administered until a patient has recovered from succinylcholine-induced neuromuscular blockade.

Carcinogenesis, Mutagenesis, Impairment of Fertility: Carcinogenesis and fertility studies have not been performed. Atracurium was evaluated in a battery of three short-term mutagenicity tests. It was non-mutagenic in both the Ames Salmonella assay at concentrations up to 1000 µg/plate, and in a rat bone marrow cytogenicity assay at up to paralyzing doses. A positive response was observed in the mouse lymphoma assay under conditions (80 and 100 µg/mL, in the absence of metabolic activation) which killed over 80% of the treated cells; there was no mutagenicity at 60 µg/mL and lower, concentrations which killed up to half of the treated cells. A far weaker response was observed in the presence of metabolic activation at concentrations (1200 µg/mL and higher) which also killed over 80% of the treated cells.

Mutagenicity testing is intended to simulate chronic (years to lifetime) exposure in an effort to determine potential carcinogenicity. Thus, a single positive mutagenicity response for a drug used infrequently and/or briefly is of questionable clinical relevance.

Pregnancy: Teratogenic Effects: Pregnancy Category C. Atracurium Besylate has been shown to be potentially teratogenic in rabbits when given in doses up to approximately one-half the human dose. There are no adequate and well-controlled studies in pregnant women. Atracurium Besylate should be used during pregnancy only if the potential benefit justifies the potential risk to the fetus.

Atracurium Besylate was administered subcutaneously on days 6 through 18 of gestation to non-ventilated Dutch rabbits. Treatment groups were given either 0.15 mg/kg once daily or 0.10 mg/kg twice daily. Lethal respiratory distress occurred in two 0.15 mg/kg animals and in one 0.10 mg/kg animal, with transient respiratory distress or other evidence of neuromuscular blockade occurring in 10 of 19 and in 4 of 20 of the 0.15 mg/kg and 0.10 mg/kg animals, respectively. There was an increased incidence of certain spontaneously occurring visceral and skeletal anomalies or variations in one or both treated groups when compared to nontreated controls. The percentage of male fetuses was lower (41% vs. 51%) and the postimplantation losses were increased (15% vs. 8%) in the group given 0.15 mg/kg once daily when compared to the controls; the mean numbers of implants (6.5 vs. 4.4) and normal live fetuses (5.4 vs. 3.8) were greater in this group when compared to the control group.

Labor and Delivery: It is not known whether muscle relaxants administered during vaginal delivery have immediate or delayed adverse effects on the fetus or increase the likelihood that resuscitation of the newborn will be necessary. The possibility that forceps delivery will be necessary may increase.

Atracurium Besylate (0.3 mg/kg) has been administered to 26 pregnant women during delivery by cesarean section. No harmful effects were attributable to Atracurium Besylate in any of the newborn infants, although small amounts of Atracurium Besylate were shown to cross the placental barrier. The possibility of respiratory depression in the newborn infant should always be considered following cesarean section during which a neuromuscular blocking agent has been administered. In patients receiving magnesium sulfate, the reversal of neuromuscular blockade may be unsatisfactory and Atracurium Besylate dose should be lowered as indicated.

Nursing Mothers: It is not known whether this drug is excreted in human milk. Because many drugs are excreted in human milk, caution should be exercised when Atracurium Besylate is administered to a nursing woman.

Pediatric Use: Safety and effectiveness in children below the age of 1 month have not been established.

ADVERSE REACTIONS

Observed in Controlled Clinical Studies: Atracurium Besylate was well tolerated and produced few adverse reactions during extensive clinical trials. Most adverse reactions were suggestive of histamine release. In studies including 875 patients, Atracurium Besylate was discontinued in only one patient (who required treatment for bronchial secretions), and six other patients required treatment for adverse reactions attributable to Atracurium Besylate (wheezing in one, hypotension in five). Of the five patients who required treatment for hypotension, three had a history of significant cardiovascular disease. The overall incidence rate for clinically important adverse reactions, therefore, was 7/875 or 0.8%. The table below includes all adverse reactions reported attributable to Atracurium Besylate during clinical trials with 875 patients. (See related table).

Most adverse reactions were of little clinical significance unless they were associated with significant hemodynamic changes. The table below summarizes the incidences of substantial vital sign changes noted during Atracurium Besylate clinical trials with 530 patients, without cardiovascular disease, in whom these parameters were assessed. (See related table).

Observed in Clinical Practice: Based on initial clinical practice experience in approximately 3 million patients who received Atracurium Besylate in the U.S. and in the United Kingdom, spontaneously reported adverse reactions were uncommon (approximately 0.01-0.02%). The following adverse reactions are among the most frequently reported, but there are insufficient data to support an estimate of their incidence.

General: Allergic reactions (anaphylatic or anaphylactoid responses) which, in rare instances, were severe (e.g., cardiac arrest)

Musculoskeletal: Inadequate block, prolonged block

Cardiovascular: Hypotension, vasodilatation (flushing), tachycardia, bradycardia

Respiratory: Dyspnea, bronchospasm, laryngospasm

Integumentary: Rash, urticaria, reaction at injection site.

There have been rare reports of seizures in ICU patients following long-term infusion of atracurium to support mechanical ventilation. There are insufficient data to define the contribution, if any, of atracurium and/or its metabolite laudanosine. (See "Precautions, Long-Term Use in Intensive Care Unit [ICU]").

OVERDOSAGE

There has been limited experience with Atracurium Besylate overdosage. The possibility of iatrogenic overdosage can be minimized by carefully monitoring muscle twitch response to peripheral nerve stimulation. Excessive doses of Atracurium Besylate can be expected to produce enhanced pharmacological effects. Overdosage may increase the risk of histamine release and cardiovascular effects, especially hypotension. If cardiovascular support is necessary, this should include proper positioning, fluid administration, and the use of vasopressor agents if necessary. The patient's airway should be assured, with manual or mechanical ventilation maintained as necessary. A longer duration of neuromuscular blockade may result from overdosage and a peripheral nerve stimulator should be used to monitor recovery. Recovery may be facilitated by administration of an anticholinesterase reversing agent such as neostigmine, edrophonium, or pyridostigmine, in conjunction with an anticholinergic agent such as atropine or glycopyrrolate. The appropriate package inserts should be consulted for prescribing information.

Three pediatric patients (3 weeks, 4 and 5 months of age) unintentionally received doses of 0.8 mg/kg to 1.0 mg/kg of Atracurium Besylate. The time to 25% recovery (50 to 55 minutes) following these doses, which were 5 to 6 times the ED$_{95}$ dose, was moderately longer than the corresponding time observed following doses 2.0 to 2.5 times the Atracurium Besylate ED$_{95}$ dose in infants (22 to 36 minutes). Cardiovascular changes were minimal. Nonetheless the possibility of cardiovascular changes must be considered in the case of overdose.

An adult patient (17 years of age) unintentionally received an initial dose of 1.3 mg/kg of Atracurium Besylate. The time from injection to 25% recovery (83 minutes) was approximately twice that observed following maximum recommended doses in adults (35-45 minutes). The patient experienced moderate hemodynamic changes (13% increase in mean arterial pressure and 27% increase in heart rate) which persisted for 40 minutes and did not require treatment.

The intravenous LD$_{50}$'s determined in non-ventilated male and female albino mice and male Wistar rats were 1.9, 2.01 and 1.31 mg/kg, respectively. Deaths occurred within 2 minutes and were caused by respiratory paralysis. The subcutaneous LD$_{50}$ determined in non-ventilated male Wistar rats was 282.8 mg/kg. Tremors, ptosis, loss of reflexes and respiratory failure preceded death which occurred 45-120 minutes after injection.

DOSAGE AND ADMINISTRATION

To avoid distress to the patient Atracurium Besylate should not be administered before unconsciousness has been induced. Atracurium Besylate should not be mixed in the same syringe, or administered simultaneously through the same needle, with alkaline solutions (e.g., barbiturate solutions).

Atracurium Besylate should be administered intravenously. *Do not give Atracurium Besylate by intramuscular administration.* Intramuscular administration of Atracurium Besylate may result in tissue irritation and there are no clinical data to support this route of administration.

The use of a peripheral nerve stimulator to monitor muscle twitch suppression and recovery will permit the most advantageous use of Atracurium Besylate and minimize the possibility of overdosage.

PERCENT OF PATIENTS REPORTING ADVERSE REACTIONS

	Initial Atracurium Besylate Dose (mg/kg)			
Adverse Reaction	0.00-0.30 (n = 485)	0.31-0.50* (n = 366)	≥ 0.60 (n = 24)	Total (n = 875)
Skin Flush	1.0%	8.7%	29.2%	5.0%
Erythema	0.6%	0.5%	0%	0.6%
Itching	0.4%	0%	0%	0.2%
Wheezing/Bronchial Secretions	0.2%	0.3%	0%	0.2%
Hives	0.2%	0%	0%	0.1%

* Includes the recommended initial dosage range for most patients.

◆ RATED THERAPEUTICALLY EQUIVALENT; ◇ THERAPEUTIC EQUIVALENCE UNCONFIRMED; ○ UNRATED

PERCENT OF PATIENTS SHOWING ≥ 30% VITAL SIGN CHANGES FOLLOWING ADMINISTRATION OF ATRACURIUM BESYLATE

| Vital Sign Change | Initial Atracurium Besylate Dose (mg/kg) | | | |
	0.00-0.30 (n = 365)	0.31-0.50* (n = 144)	≥ 0.60 (n = 21)	Total (n = 530)
Mean Arterial Pressure				
Increase	1.9%	2.8%	0%	2.1%
Decrease	1.1%	2.1%	14.3%	1.9%
Heart Rate				
Increase	1.6%	2.8%	4.8%	2.1%
Decrease	0.8%	0%	0%	0.6%

* Includes the recommended initial dosage range for most patients.

Parenteral drug products should be inspected visually for particulate matter and discoloration prior to administration, whenever solution and container permit.

BOLUS DOSES FOR INTUBATION AND MAINTENANCE OF NEUROMUSCULAR BLOCKADE

Adults: An Atracurium Besylate dose of 0.4 to 0.5 mg/kg (1.7 to 2.2 times the ED$_{95}$) given as an intravenous bolus injection, is the recommended initial dose for most patients. With this dose, good or excellent conditions for nonemergency intubation can be expected in 2 to 2.5 minutes in most patients, with maximum neuromuscular blockade achieved approximately 3 to 5 minutes after injection. Clinically required neuromuscular blockade generally lasts 20 to 35 minutes under balanced anesthesia. Under balanced anesthesia, recovery to 25% of control is achieved approximately 35 to 45 minutes after injection, and recovery is usually 95% complete approximately 60 minutes after injection.

Atracurium Besylate is potentiated by isoflurane or enflurane anesthesia. The same initial Atracurium Besylate dose of 0.4 to 0.5 mg/kg may be used for intubation prior to administration of these inhalation agents; however, if Atracurium Besylate is first administered under steady state of isoflurane or enflurane, the initial Atracurium Besylate dose should be reduced by approximately one-third, i.e., to 0.25 to 0.35 mg/kg, to adjust for the potentiating effects of these anesthetic agents. With halothane, which has only a marginal (approximately 20%) potentiating effect on Atracurium Besylate, smaller dosage reductions may be considered.

Atracurium Besylate doses of 0.08 to 0.10 mg/kg are recommended for maintenance of neuromuscular blockade during prolonged surgical procedures. The first maintenance dose will generally be required 20 to 45 minutes after the initial Atracurium Besylate injection, but the need for maintenance doses should be determined by clinical criteria. Because Atracurium Besylate lacks cumulative effects, maintenance doses may be administered at relatively regular intervals for each patient, ranging approximately from 15 to 25 minutes under balanced anesthesia, slightly longer under isoflurane or enflurane. Higher Atracurium Besylate doses (up to 0.2 mg/kg) permit maintenance dosing at longer intervals.

Children and Infants: No Atracurium Besylate dosage adjustments are required for pediatric patients two years of age or older. An Atracurium Besylate dose of 0.3 to 0.4 mg/kg is recommended as the initial dose for infants (1 month to 2 years of age) under halothane anesthesia. Maintenance doses may be required with slightly greater frequency in infants and children than in adults.

Special Considerations: An initial Atracurium Besylate dose of 0.3 to 0.4 mg/kg, given slowly or in divided doses over one minute, is recommended for adults, children, or infants with significant cardiovascular disease and for adults, children, or infants with any history (e.g., severe anaphylactoid reactions or asthma) suggesting a greater risk of histamine release. Dosage reductions must be considered also in patients with neuromuscular disease, severe electrolyte disorders, or carcinomatosis in which potentiation of neuromuscular blockade or difficulties with reversal have been demonstrated. There has been no clinical experience with Atracurium Besylate in these patients, and no specific dosage adjustments can be recommended. No Atracurium Besylate dosage adjustments are required for patients with renal disease.

An initial Atracurium Besylate dose of 0.3 to 0.4 mg/kg is recommended for adults following the use of succinylcholine for intubation under balanced anesthesia. Further reductions may be desirable with the use of potent inhalation anesthetics. The patient should be permitted to recover from the effects of succinylcholine prior to Atracurium Besylate administration. Insufficient data are available for recommendation of a specific initial Atracurium Besylate dose for administration following the use of succinylcholine in children and infants.

Use by Infusion: After administration of a recommended initial bolus dose of Atracurium Besylate (0.3 to 0.5 mg/kg), a diluted solution of Atracurium Besylate can be administered by continuous infusion to adults and children aged 2 or more years for maintenance of neuromuscular blockade during extended surgical procedures. Long-term intravenous infusion to support mechanical ventilation in the intensive care unit has not been studied sufficiently to support dosage recommendations (see *"Precautions: Long-Term Use in Intensive Care Unit"*).

Infusion of Atracurium Besylate should be individualized for each patient. The rate of administration should be adjusted according to the patient's response as determined by peripheral nerve stimulation. Accurate dosing is best achieved using a precision infusion device.

Infusion of Atracurium Besylate should be initiated only after early evidence of spontaneous recovery from the bolus dose. An initial infusion rate of 9 to 10 µg/kg/min may be required to rapidly counteract the spontaneous recovery of

neuromuscular function. Thereafter, a rate of 5 to 9 µg/kg/min should be adequate to maintain continuous neuromuscular blockade in the range of 89 to 99% in most pediatric and adult patients under balanced anesthesia. Occasional patients may require infusion rates as low as 2 µg/kg/min or as high as 15 µg/kg/min.

The neuromuscular blocking effect of Atracurium Besylate administered by infusion is potentiated by enflurane or isoflurane and, to a lesser extent, by halothane. Reduction in the infusion rate of Atracurium Besylate should, therefore, be considered for patients receiving inhalation anesthesia. The rate of Atracurium Besylate infusion should be reduced by approximately one-third in the presence of steady-state enflurane or isoflurane anesthesia; smaller reductions should be considered in the presence of halothane.

In patients undergoing cardiopulmonary bypass with induced hypothermia, the rate of infusion of Atracurium Besylate required to maintain adequate surgical relaxation during hypothermia (25° to 28°C) has been shown to be approximately half the rate required during normothermia.

Spontaneous recovery from neuromuscular blockade following discontinuation of Atracurium Besylate infusion may be expected to proceed at a rate comparable to that following administration of a single bolus dose.

Atracurium Besylate infusion solutions may be prepared by admixing Atracurium Besylate Injection with an appropriate diluent such as 5% Dextrose Injection USP, 0.9% Sodium Chloride Injection USP, or 5% Dextrose and 0.9% Sodium Chloride Injection USP. Infusion solutions should be used within 24 hours of preparation. Unused solutions should be discarded. Solutions containing 0.2 mg/mL or 0.5 mg/mL Atracurium Besylate in the above diluents may be stored either under refrigeration or at room temperature for 24 hours without significant loss of potency. Care should be taken during admixture to prevent inadvertent contamination. Visually inspect prior to administration.

Spontaneous degradation of Atracurium Besylate has been demonstrated to occur more rapidly in lactated Ringer's solution than in 0.9% sodium chloride solution. Therefore, it is recommended that Lactated Ringer's Injection USP not be used as a diluent in preparing solutions of Atracurium Besylate for infusion.

The amount of infusion solution required per minute will depend upon the concentration of Atracurium Besylate in the infusion solution, the desired dose of Atracurium Besylate, and the patient's weight. The following tables provide guidelines for delivery, in mL/hr (equivalent to microdrops/min when 60 micro drops = 1 mL), of Atracurium Besylate solutions in concentrations of 0.2 mg/mL (20 mg in 100 mL) or 0.5 mg/mL (50 mg in 100 mL) with an infusion pump or a gravity flow device.

ATRACURIUM BESYLATE INFUSION RATES FOR A CONCENTRATION OF 0.2 MG/ML

| Patient Weight (Kg) | Drug Delivery Rate (µg/kg/min) | | | | | |
| | 5 | 6 | 7 | 8 | 9 | 10 |
	Infusion Delivery Rate (mL/hr)					
30	45	54	63	72	81	90
35	53	63	74	84	95	105
40	60	72	84	96	108	120
45	68	81	95	108	122	135
50	75	90	105	120	135	150
55	83	99	116	132	149	165
60	90	108	126	144	162	180
65	98	117	137	156	176	195
70	105	126	147	168	189	210
75	113	135	158	180	203	225
80	120	144	168	192	216	240
90	135	162	189	216	243	270
100	150	180	210	240	270	300

ATRACURIUM BESYLATE INFUSION RATES FOR A CONCENTRATION OF 0.5 MG/ML

| Patient Weight (Kg) | Drug Delivery Rate (µg/kg/min) | | | | | |
| | 5 | 6 | 7 | 8 | 9 | 10 |
	Infusion Delivery Rate (mL/hr)					
30	18	22	25	29	32	36
35	21	25	29	34	38	42
40	24	29	34	38	43	48

Patient Weight	Drug Delivery Rate (µg/kg/min)					
	5	6	7	8	9	10
(Kg)	Infusion Delivery Rate (mL/hr)					
45	27	32	38	43	49	54
50	30	36	42	48	54	60
55	33	40	46	53	59	66
60	36	43	50	58	65	72
65	39	47	55	62	70	78
70	42	50	59	67	76	84
75	45	54	63	72	81	90
80	48	58	67	77	86	96
90	54	65	76	86	97	108
100	60	72	84	96	108	120

Atracurium Besylate Injection should be refrigerated at 2° to 8°C (36° to 46°F) to preserve potency. DO NOT FREEZE. Upon removal from refrigeration to room temperature storage conditions (25°C/77°F), use Atracurium Besylate Injection within 14 days even if rerefrigerated.

HOW SUPPLIED
INJECTION: 10 MG/ML

BRAND/MANUFACTURER	NDC	SIZE	AWP
○ BRAND			
TRACRIUM: Burr Wellcome	00081-0940-44	5 ml 10s	$259.74
	00081-0940-95	10 ml 10s	$483.53

Atrohist Sprinkle *SEE* CHLORPHENIRAMINE MALEATE AND PSEUDOEPHEDRINE HYDROCHLORIDE

Atromid-S *SEE* CLOFIBRATE

Atropine Sulfate and Difenoxin Hydrochloride

DESCRIPTION
Each tablet contains:

Difenoxin (as the Hydrochloride) ....1.0 mg
  Warning—May be habit forming.
Atropine Sulfate ....0.025 mg

Difenoxin Hydrochloride, 1-(3-cyano-3,3-diphenylpropyl)-4-phenyl-4-piperidine-carboxylic acid monohydrochloride, is an orally administered antidiarrheal agent which is chemically related to the narcotic meperidine.
  Atropine Sulfate is present to discourage deliberate overdosage.
  Atropine Sulfate, an anticholinergic, is endo (±)-α-(hydroxymethyl) benzeneacetic acid 8-methyl-8-azabicyclo[3.2.1] oct-3-yl ester sulfate (2:1) (salt) monohydrate.

CLINICAL PHARMACOLOGY
Animal studies have shown that Difenoxin Hydrochloride manifests its antidiarrheal effect by slowing intestinal motility. The mechanism of action is by a local effect on the gastrointestinal wall.
  Difenoxin is the principal active metabolite of diphenoxylate.
  Following oral administration of Atropine Sulfate/Difenoxin Hydrochloride (Atropine/Difenoxin), Difenoxin is rapidly and extensively absorbed. Mean peak plasma levels of approximately 160 ng/mL occurred within 40 to 60 minutes in most patients following an oral dose of 2mg. Plasma levels decline to less than 10% of their peak values within 24 hours and to less than 1% of their peak values within 72 hours. This decline parallels the appearance of Difenoxin and its metabolites in the urine. Difenoxin is metabolized to an inactive hydroxylated metabolite. Both the drug and its metabolites are excreted, mainly as conjugates, in urine and feces.

INDICATIONS AND USAGE
Atropine/Difenoxin is indicated as adjunctive therapy in the management of acute nonspecific diarrhea and acute exacerbations of chronic functional diarrhea.

CONTRAINDICATIONS
Atropine/Difenoxin is contraindicated in patients with diarrhea associated with organisms that penetrate the intestinal mucosa (toxigenic *E. coli, Salmonella* species, *Shigella*) and pseudomembranous colitis associated with broad spectrum antibiotics. Antiperistaltic agents should not be used in these conditions because they may prolong and/or worsen diarrhea.
  Atropine/Difenoxin is *contraindicated in children under 2 years of age* because of the decreased margin of safety of drugs in this class in younger age groups.

Atropine/Difenoxin is contraindicated in patients with a known hypersensitivity to difenoxin, atropine, or any of the inactive ingredients, and in patients who are jaundiced.

WARNINGS
ATROPINE/DIFENOXIN IS *NOT* AN INNOCUOUS DRUG AND DOSAGE RECOMMENDATIONS SHOULD BE STRICTLY ADHERED TO. ATROPINE/DIFENOXIN IS NOT RECOMMENDED FOR CHILDREN UNDER 2 YEARS OF AGE. OVERDOSAGE MAY RESULT IN SEVERE RESPIRATORY DEPRESSION AND COMA, POSSIBLY LEADING TO PERMANENT BRAIN DAMAGE OR DEATH (SEE "OVERDOSAGE"). THEREFORE, KEEP THIS MEDICATION OUT OF THE REACH OF CHILDREN.
  FLUID AND ELECTROLYTE BALANCE—THE USE OF ATROPINE/DIFENOXIN DOES NOT PRECLUDE THE ADMINISTRATION OF APPROPRIATE FLUID AND ELECTROLYTE THERAPY. DEHYDRATION, PARTICULARLY IN CHILDREN, MAY FURTHER INFLUENCE THE VARIABILITY OF RESPONSE TO ATROPINE/DIFENOXIN AND MAY PREDISPOSE TO DELAYED DIFENOXIN INTOXICATION. DRUG-INDUCED INHIBITION OF PERISTALSIS MAY RESULT IN FLUID RETENTION IN THE COLON, AND THIS MAY FURTHER AGGRAVATE DEHYDRATION AND ELECTROLYTE IMBALANCE.
  IF SEVERE DEHYDRATION OR ELECTROLYTE IMBALANCE IS MANIFESTED, ATROPINE/DIFENOXIN SHOULD BE WITHHELD UNTIL APPROPRIATE CORRECTIVE THERAPY HAS BEEN INITIATED.

Ulcerative Colitis: In some patients with acute ulcerative colitis, agents which inhibit intestinal motility or delay intestinal transit time have been reported to induce toxic megacolon. Consequently, patients with acute ulcerative colitis should be carefully observed and Atropine/Difenoxin therapy should be discontinued promptly if abdominal distention occurs or if other untoward symptoms develop.

Liver and Kidney Disease: Atropine/Difenoxin should be used with extreme caution in patients with advanced hepatorenal disease and in all patients with abnormal liver function tests since hepatic coma may be precipitated.

Atropine: A subtherapeutic dose of Atropine has been added to Difenoxin Hydrochloride to discourage deliberate overdosage. Usage of Atropine/Difenoxin in recommended doses is not likely to cause prominent anticholinergic side effects, but Atropine/Difenoxin should be avoided in patients in whom anticholinergic drugs are contraindicated. The warnings and precautions for use of anticholinergic agents should be observed.
  In children, signs of atropinism may occur even with recommended doses of Atropine/Difenoxin, particularly in patients with Down's Syndrome.

PRECAUTIONS
INFORMATION FOR PATIENTS
CAUTION PATIENTS TO ADHERE STRICTLY TO RECOMMENDED DOSAGE SCHEDULES. THE MEDICATION SHOULD BE KEPT OUT OF REACH OF CHILDREN SINCE ACCIDENTAL OVERDOSAGE MAY RESULT IN SEVERE, EVEN FATAL, RESPIRATORY DEPRESSION. Atropine/Difenoxin may produce drowsiness or dizziness. The patient should be cautioned regarding activities requiring mental alertness, such as driving or operating dangerous machinery.

DRUG INTERACTIONS
Since the chemical structure of Difenoxin Hydrochloride is similar to meperidine hydrochloride, the concurrent use of Atropine/Difenoxin with monoamine oxidase inhibitors may, in theory, precipitate a hypertensive crisis.
  Atropine/Difenoxin may potentiate the action of barbiturates, tranquilizers, narcotics, and alcohol. When these medications are used concomitantly with Atropine/Difenoxin the patient should be closely monitored.
  Diphenoxylate Hydrochloride, from which the principal active metabolite difenoxin is derived, was found to inhibit the hepatic microsomal enzyme system at a dose of 2 mg/kg/day in studies conducted with male rats. Therefore, difenoxin has the potential to prolong the biological half-lives of drugs for which the rate of elimination is dependent on the microsomal drug metabolizing enzyme system.

CARCINOGENESIS, MUTAGENESIS, IMPAIRMENT OF FERTILITY
No evidence of carcinogenesis was found in a long-term study of Difenoxin Hydrochloride/Atropine in the rat. In this 104 week study, rats received dietary doses of 0, 1.25, 2.5, or 5 mg/kg/day Difenoxin/Atropine (20:1 ratio).
  No experiments have been conducted to determine the mutagenic potential of Atropine/Difenoxin. Atropine/Difenoxin did not significantly impair fertility in rats.

PREGNANCY/TERATOGENIC EFFECTS
Pregnancy Category C. Reproduction studies in rats and rabbits with doses at 31 and 61 times the human therapeutic dose respectively, on a mg/kg basis, demonstrated no evidence of teratogenesis due to Atropine/Difenoxin.
  Pregnant rats receiving oral doses of Difenoxin Hydrochloride/Atropine 20 times the maximum human dose had an increase in delivery time as well as a significant increase in the percent of stillbirths.
  Neonatal survival in rats was also reduced with most deaths occurring within four days of delivery.
  There are no well controlled studies in pregnant women. Atropine/Difenoxin should be used during pregnancy only if the potential benefit justifies the potential risk to the fetus.

◆ RATED THERAPEUTICALLY EQUIVALENT; ◇ THERAPEUTIC EQUIVALENCE UNCONFIRMED; ○ UNRATED

NURSING MOTHERS

Because of the potential for serious adverse reactions in nursing infants from Atropine/Difenoxin, a decision should be made whether to discontinue nursing or to discontinue the drug, taking into account the importance of the drug to the mother.

PEDIATRIC USE

SAFETY AND EFFECTIVENESS IN CHILDREN BELOW THE AGE OF 12 HAVE NOT BEEN ESTABLISHED. ATROPINE/DIFENOXIN IS CONTRAINDICATED IN CHILDREN UNDER 2 YEARS OF AGE. See *"Overdosage"* section for information on hazards from accidental poisoning in children.

ADVERSE REACTIONS

In view of the small amount of Atropine present (0.025 mg/tablet), effects such as dryness of the skin and mucous membranes, flushing, hyperthermia, tachycardia and urinary retention are very unlikely to occur, except perhaps in children.

Many of the adverse effects reported during clinical investigation of Atropine/ Difenoxin are difficult to distinguish from symptoms associated with the diarrheal syndrome. However, the following events were reported at the stated frequencies:

Gastrointestinal: Nausea, 1 in 15 patients; vomiting, 1 in 30 patients; dry mouth, 1 in 30 patients; epigastric distress, 1 in 100 patients; and constipation, 1 in 300 patients.

Central Nervous System: Dizziness and light-headedness, 1 in 20 patients; drowsiness, 1 in 25 patients; and headache, 1 in 40 patients; tiredness, nervousness, insomnia and confusion ranged from 1 in 200 to 1 in 600 patients.

Other Less Frequent Reactions: Burning eyes and blurred vision occurred in a few cases.

The following adverse reactions have been reported in patients receiving chemically-related drugs: numbness of extremities, euphoria, depression, sedation, anaphylaxis, angioneurotic edema, urticaria, swelling of the gums, pruritus, toxic megacolon, paralytic ileus, pancreatitis, and anorexia.

THIS MEDICATION SHOULD BE KEPT IN A CHILD-RESISTANT CONTAINER AND OUT OF THE REACH OF CHILDREN SINCE AN OVERDOSAGE MAY RESULT IN SEVERE RESPIRATORY DEPRESSION AND COMA, POSSIBLY LEADING TO PERMANENT BRAIN DAMAGE OR DEATH.

DRUG ABUSE AND DEPENDENCE

Atropine/Difenoxin tablets are a Schedule IV controlled substance.

Addiction to (dependence on) Difenoxin Hydrochloride is theoretically possible at high dosage. Therefore, the recommended dosage should not be exceeded. Because of the structural and pharmacological similarities of Difenoxin Hydrochloride to drugs with a definite addiction potential, Atropine/Difenoxin should be administered with considerable caution to patients who are receiving addicting drugs, to individuals known to be addiction prone, or to those in whom histories suggest may increase the dosage on their own initiative.

OVERDOSAGE

DIAGNOSIS AND TREATMENT

In the event of overdosage (initial signs may include dryness of the skin and mucous membranes, flushing, hyperthermia and tachycardia followed by lethargy or coma, hypotonic reflexes, nystagmus, pinpoint pupils and respiratory depression) gastric lavage, establishment of a patent airway and possibly mechanically assisted respiration are advised.

The narcotic antagonist naloxone may be used in the treatment of respiratory depression caused by narcotic analgesics or pharmacologically related compounds such as Atropine/Difenoxin tablets. When naloxone is administered intravenously, the onset of action is generally apparent within two minutes. Naloxone may also be administered subcutaneously or intramuscularly providing a slightly less rapid onset of action but a more prolonged effect.

To counteract respiratory depression caused by Atropine/Difenoxin overdosage, the following dosage schedule for naloxone should be followed:

Adult Dosage: The usual initial adult dose of naloxone is 0.4 mg (one mL) administered intravenously. If respiratory function does not adequately improve after the initial dose, the same IV dose may be repeated at two-to-three minute intervals.

Children: The usual adult dose of naloxone for children is 0.01 mg/kg of body weight administered intravenously and repeated at two-to-three minute intervals if necessary.

Since the duration of action of Difenoxin Hydrochloride is longer than that of naloxone, improvement of respiration following administration may be followed by recurrent respiratory depression. Consequently, continuous observation is necessary until the effect of Difenoxin Hydrochloride on respiration (which effect may persist for many hours) has passed. Supplemental intramuscular doses of naloxone may be utilized to produce a longer lasting effect. TREAT ALL POSSIBLE ATROPINE/DIFENOXIN OVERDOSAGES AS SERIOUS AND MAINTAIN MEDICAL OBSERVATION FOR AT LEAST 48 HOURS, PREFERABLY UNDER CONTINUOUS HOSPITAL CARE.

Although signs of overdosage and respiratory depression may not be evident soon after ingestion of Difenoxin Hydrochloride, respiratory depression may occur from 12 to 30 hours later.

DOSAGE AND ADMINISTRATION

The recommended starting dose of Atropine/Difenoxin tablets in adults is 2 tablets (2 mg), then 1 tablet (1 mg) after each loose stool or 1 tablet (1 mg) every 3

to 4 hours as needed, but the total dosage during any 24-hour treatment period should not exceed 8 tablets (8 mg). In the treatment of diarrhea, if clinical improvement is not observed in 48 hours, continued administration of this type medication is not recommended.

For acute diarrheas and acute exacerbations of functional diarrhea, treatment beyond 48 hours is usually not necessary.

Studies in children below the age of 12 have been inadequate to evaluate the safety and effectiveness of Atropine/Difenoxin in this age group. Atropine/ Difenoxin is contraindicated in children under 2 years of age.

Store at controlled room temperature, 15°–30°C (59°–86°F).

HOW SUPPLIED
TABLETS (C-IV): 0.025 MG-1 MG

BRAND/MANUFACTURER	NDC	SIZE	AWP
BRAND			
MOTOFEN: Carnrick	00086-0074-05	50s	$22.80
	00086-0074-10	100s	$40.80

Atropine Sulfate and Diphenoxylate Hydrochloride

DESCRIPTION

Each Atropine Sulfate/Diphenoxylate Hydrochloride tablet and each 5 ml of Atropine Sulfate/Diphenoxylate Hydrochloride liquid for oral use contains:

Diphenoxylate Hydrochloride ....2.5 mg
(Warning—May be habit forming.)
Atropine Sulfate ....0.025 mg

Diphenoxylate Hydrochloride, an antidiarrheal, is ethyl 1-(3-cyano-3,3-diphenyl-propyl)-4-phenylisonipecotate monohydrochloride.
Atropine Sulfate, an anticholinergic, is endo-(±)-α-(hydroxymethyl) benzeneacetic acid 8-methyl-8-azabicyclo[3.2.1] oct-3-yl ester Sulfate (2:1) (salt) monohydrate.

IMPORTANT INFORMATION
Atropine/Diphenoxylate is classified as a Schedule V controlled substance by federal law. Diphenoxylate Hydrochloride is chemically related to the narcotic meperidine. Therefore, in case of overdosage, treatment is similar to that for meperidine or morphine intoxication, in which prolonged and careful monitoring is essential. Respiratory depression may be evidenced as late as 30 hours after ingestion and may recur in spite of an initial response to narcotic antagonists. A subtherapeutic amount of Atropine Sulfate is present to discourage deliberate overdosage. ATROPINE/DIPHENOXYLATE IS *NOT* AN INNOCUOUS DRUG AND DOSAGE RECOMMENDATIONS SHOULD BE STRICTLY ADHERED TO, ESPECIALLY IN CHILDREN. KEEP THIS AND ALL MEDICATIONS OUT OF REACH OF CHILDREN.

CLINICAL PHARMACOLOGY

Diphenoxylate is rapidly and extensively metabolized in man by ester hydrolysis to diphenoxylic acid (difenoxine), which is biologically active and the major metabolite in the blood. After a 5-mg oral dose of carbon-14 labeled Diphenoxylate Hydrochloride in ethanolic solution was given to three healthy volunteers, an average of 14% of the drug plus its metabolites was excreted in the urine and 49% in the feces over a four-day period. Urinary excretion of the unmetabolized drug constituted less than 1% of the dose, and Diphenoxylic acid plus its glucuronide conjugate constituted about 6% of the dose. In a 16-subject crossover bioavailability study, a linear relationship in the dose range of 2.5 to 10 mg was found between the dose of Diphenoxylate Hydrochloride (given as Atropine/Diphenoxylate liquid) and the peak plasma concentration, the area under the plasma concentration-time curve, and the amount of Diphenoxylic acid excreted in the urine. In the same study the bioavailability of the tablet compared with an equal dose of the liquid was approximately 90%. The average peak plasma concentration of Diphenoxylic acid following ingestion of four 2.5-mg tablets was 163 ng/ml at about 2 hours, and the elimination half-life of Diphenoxylic acid was approximately 12 to 14 hours.

In dogs, Diphenoxylate Hydrochloride has a direct effect on circular smooth muscle of the bowel that conceivably results in segmentation and prolongation of gastrointestinal transit time. The clinical antidiarrheal action of Diphenoxylate Hydrochloride may thus be a consequence of enhanced segmentation that allows increased contact of the intraluminal contents with the intestinal mucosa.

INDICATIONS AND USAGE

Atropine/Diphenoxylate is effective as adjunctive therapy in the management of diarrhea.

CONTRAINDICATIONS

Atropine/Diphenoxylate is contraindicated in patients with

1. Known hypersensitivity to Diphenoxylate or Atropine.
2. Obstructive jaundice.
3. Diarrhea associated with pseudomembranous enterocolitis or enterotoxin-producing bacteria.

➤ SHOWN IN PRODUCT IDENTIFICATION GUIDE

WARNINGS

ATROPINE/DIPHENOXYLATE IS NOT AN INNOCUOUS DRUG AND DOSAGE RECOMMENDATIONS SHOULD BE STRICTLY ADHERED TO, ESPECIALLY IN CHILDREN. ATROPINE/DIPHENOXYLATE IS NOT RECOMMENDED FOR CHILDREN UNDER 2 YEARS OF AGE. OVERDOSAGE MAY RESULT IN SEVERE RESPIRATORY DEPRESSION AND COMA, POSSIBLY LEADING TO PERMANENT BRAIN DAMAGE OR DEATH (See "Overdosage"). THEREFORE, KEEP THIS MEDICATION OUT OF THE REACH OF CHILDREN.

THE USE OF ATROPINE/DIPHENOXYLATE SHOULD BE ACCOMPANIED BY APPROPRIATE FLUID AND ELECTROLYTE THERAPY, WHEN INDICATED. IF SEVERE DEHYDRATION OR ELECTROLYTE IMBALANCE IS PRESENT, ATROPINE/DIPHENOXYLATE SHOULD BE WITHHELD UNTIL APPROPRIATE CORRECTIVE THERAPY HAS BEEN INITIATED. DRUG-INDUCED INHIBITION OF PERISTALSIS MAY RESULT IN FLUID RETENTION IN THE INTESTINE, WHICH MAY FURTHER AGGRAVATE DEHYDRATION AND ELECTROLYTE IMBALANCE.

ATROPINE/DIPHENOXYLATE SHOULD BE USED WITH SPECIAL CAUTION IN YOUNG CHILDREN BECAUSE THIS AGE GROUP MAY BE PREDISPOSED TO DELAYED DIPHENOXYLATE TOXICITY AND BECAUSE OF THE GREATER VARIABILITY OF RESPONSE IN THIS AGE GROUP.

Antiperistaltic agents may prolong and/or worsen diarrhea associated with organisms that penetrate the intestinal mucosa (toxigenic *E. coli, Salmonella, Shigella*), and pseudomembranous enterocolitis associated with broad-spectrum antibiotics. Antiperistaltic agents should not be used in these conditions.

In some patients with acute ulcerative colitis, agents that inhibit intestinal motility or prolong intestinal transit time have been reported to induce toxic megacolon. Consequently, patients with acute ulcerative colitis should be carefully observed and Atropine/Diphenoxylate therapy should be discontinued promptly if abdominal distention occurs or if other untoward symptoms develop.

Since the chemical structure of Diphenoxylate Hydrochloride is similar to that of meperidine Hydrochloride, the concurrent use of Atropine/Diphenoxylate with monoamine oxidase (MAO) inhibitors may, in theory, precipitate hypertensive crisis.

Atropine/Diphenoxylate should be used with extreme caution in patients with advanced hepatorenal disease and in all patients with abnormal liver function since hepatic coma may be precipitated.

Diphenoxylate Hydrochloride may potentiate the action of barbiturates, tranquilizers, and alcohol. Therefore, the patient should be closely observed when any of these are used concomitantly.

PRECAUTIONS

General: Since a subtherapeutic dose of Atropine has been added to the Diphenoxylate Hydrochloride, consideration should be given to the precautions relating to the use of Atropine. In children, Atropine/Diphenoxylate should be used with caution since signs of atropinism may occur even with recommended doses, particularly in patients with Down's syndrome.

Information for Patients: INFORM THE PATIENT (PARENT OR GUARDIAN) NOT TO EXCEED THE RECOMMENDED DOSAGE AND TO KEEP ATROPINE/DIPHENOXYLATE OUT OF THE REACH OF CHILDREN AND IN A CHILD-RESISTANT CONTAINER. INFORM THE PATIENT OF THE CONSEQUENCES OF OVERDOSAGE, INCLUDING SEVERE RESPIRATORY DEPRESSION AND COMA, POSSIBLY LEADING TO PERMANENT BRAIN DAMAGE OR DEATH. Atropine/Diphenoxylate may produce drowsiness or dizziness. The patient should be cautioned regarding activities requiring mental alertness, such as driving or operating dangerous machinery. Potentiation of the action of alcohol, barbiturates, and tranquilizers with concomitant use of Atropine/Diphenoxylate should be explained to the patient. The physician should also provide the patient with other information in this labeling, as appropriate.

Drug interactions: Known drug interactions include barbiturates, tranquilizers, and alcohol Atropine/Diphenoxylate may interact with MAO inhibitors (see *"Warnings"*).

In studies with male rats, Diphenoxylate Hydrochloride was found to inhibit the hepatic microsomal enzyme system at a dose of 2 mg/kg/day. Therefore, Diphenoxylate has the potential to prolong the biological half-lives of drugs for which the rate of elimination is dependent on the microsomal drug metabolizing enzyme system.

Carcinogenesis, Mutagenesis, Impairment of Fertility: No long-term study in animals has been performed to evaluate carcinogenic potential. Diphenoxylate Hydrochloride was administered to male and female rats in their diets to provide dose levels of 4 and 20 mg/kg/day throughout a three-litter reproduction study. At 50 times the human dose (20 mg/kg/day), female weight gain was reduced and there was a marked effect on fertility as only 4 of 27 females became pregnant in three test breedings. The relevance of this finding to usage of Atropine/Diphenoxylate in humans is unknown.

Pregnancy: Pregnancy Category C. Diphenoxylate Hydrochloride has been shown to have an effect on fertility in rats when given in doses 50 times the human dose (see above discussion). Other findings in this study include a decrease in maternal weight gain of 30% at 20 mg/kg/day and of 10% at 4 mg/kg/day. At 10 times the human dose (4 mg/kg/day), average litter size was slightly reduced.

Teratology studies were conducted in rats, rabbits, and mice with Diphenoxylate Hydrochloride at oral doses of 0.4 to 20 mg/kg/day. Due to experimental design and small numbers of litters, embryotoxic, fetotoxic, or teratogenic effects

cannot be adequately assessed. However, examination of the available fetuses did not reveal any indication of teratogenicity.

There are no adequate and well-controlled studies in pregnant women. Atropine/Diphenoxylate should be used during pregnancy only if the anticipated benefit justifies the potential risk to the fetus.

Nursing Mothers: Caution should be exercised when Atropine/Diphenoxylate is administered to a nursing woman, since the physicochemical characteristics of the major metabolite, Diphenoxylic acid, are such that it may be excreted in breast milk and since it is known that Atropine is excreted in breast milk.

Pediatric Use: Atropine/Diphenoxylate may be used as an adjunct to the treatment of diarrhea but should be accompanied by appropriate fluid and electrolyte therapy, if needed. Atropine/Diphenoxylate *is not recommended for children under 2 years of age.* Atropine/Diphenoxylate should be used with special caution in young children because of the greater variability of response in this age group. See *"Warnings"* and *"Dosage and Administration."* In case of accidental ingestion by children, see *"Overdosage"* for recommended treatment.

ADVERSE REACTIONS

At *therapeutic* doses, the following have been reported; they are listed in decreasing order of severity, but not of frequency:

Nervous system: numbness of extremities, euphoria, depression, malaise/lethargy, confusion, sedation/drowsiness, dizziness, restlessness, headache.

Allergic: anaphylaxis, angioneurotic edema, urticaria, swelling of the gums, pruritus.

Gastrointestinal system: toxic megacolon, paralytic ileus, pancreatitis, vomiting, nausea, anorexia, abdominal discomfort.

The following Atropine Sulfate effects are listed in decreasing order of severity, but not of frequency: hyperthermia, tachycardia, urinary retention, flushing, dryness of the skin and mucous membranes. These effects may occur, especially in children.

THIS MEDICATION SHOULD BE KEPT IN A CHILD-RESISTANT CONTAINER AND OUT OF THE REACH OF CHILDREN SINCE AN OVERDOSAGE MAY RESULT IN SEVERE RESPIRATORY DEPRESSION AND COMA, POSSIBLY LEADING TO PERMANENT BRAIN DAMAGE OR DEATH.

DRUG ABUSE AND DEPENDENCE

Controlled Substance: Atropine/Diphenoxylate is classified as a Schedule V controlled substance by federal regulation. Diphenoxylate Hydrochloride is chemically related to the narcotic analgesic meperidine.

Drug Abuse and Dependence: In doses used for the treatment of diarrhea, whether acute or chronic, Diphenoxylate has not produced addiction.

Diphenoxylate Hydrochloride is devoid of morphine-like subjective effects at therapeutic doses. At high doses it exhibits codeine-like subjective effects. The dose which produces anti-diarrheal action is widely separated from the dose which causes central nervous system effects. The insolubility of Diphenoxylate Hydrochloride in commonly available aqueous media precludes intravenous self-administration. A dose of 100 to 300 mg/day, which is equivalent to 40 to 120 tablets, administered to humans for 40 to 70 days, produced opiate withdrawal symptoms. Since addiction to Diphenoxylate Hydrochloride is possible at high doses, the recommended dosage should not be exceeded.

OVERDOSAGE

RECOMMENDED DOSAGE SCHEDULES SHOULD BE STRICTLY FOLLOWED. THIS MEDICATION SHOULD BE KEPT IN A CHILD-RESISTANT CONTAINER AND OUT OF THE REACH OF CHILDREN, SINCE AN OVERDOSAGE MAY RESULT IN SEVERE, EVEN FATAL, RESPIRATORY DEPRESSION.

Diagnosis: Initial signs of overdosage may include dryness of the skin and mucous membranes, mydriasis, restlessness, flushing, hyperthermia, and tachycardia followed by lethargy or coma, hypotonic reflexes, nystagmus, pinpoint pupils, and respiratory depression. Respiratory depression may be evidenced as late as 30 hours after ingestion and may recur despite an initial response to narcotic antagonists. TREAT ALL POSSIBLE ATROPINE/DIPHENOXYLATE OVERDOSAGES AS SERIOUS AND MAINTAIN MEDICAL OBSERVATION FOR AT LEAST 48 HOURS, PREFERABLY UNDER CONTINUOUS HOSPITAL CARE.

Treatment: In the event of overdose, induction of vomiting, gastric lavage, establishment of a patient airway, and possibly mechanically assisted respiration are advised. *In vitro* and animal studies indicate that activated charcoal may significantly decrease the bioavailability of Diphenoxylate. In noncomatose patients, a slurry of 100 g of activated charcoal can be administered immediately after the induction of vomiting or gastric lavage.

A pure narcotic antagonist (eg, naloxone) should be used in the treatment of respiratory depression caused by Atropine/Diphenoxylate. When a narcotic antagonist is administered intravenously, the onset of action is generally apparent within two minutes. It may also be administered subcutaneously or intramuscularly, providing a slightly less rapid onset of action but a more prolonged effect.

To counteract respiratory depression caused by Atropine/Diphenoxylate overdosage, the following dosage schedule for the narcotic antagonist naloxone Hydrochloride should be followed:

Adult dosage: An initial dose of 0.4 mg to 2 mg of naloxone Hydrochloride may be administered intravenously. If the desired degree of counteraction and improvement in respiratory function is not obtained, it may be repeated at 2- to 3-minute intervals. If no response is observed after 10 mg of naloxone Hydrochloride has been administered, the diagnosis of narcotic-induced or partial narcotic-induced toxicity should be questioned. Intramuscular or subcutaneous administration may be necessary if the intravenous route is not available.

Children: The usual initial dose in children is 0.01 mg/kg body weight given I.V. If this dose does not result in the desired degree of clinical improvement, a subsequent dose of 0.1 mg/kg body weight may be administered. If an I.V. route of administration is not available, naloxone Hydrochloride may be administered I.M. or S.C. in divided doses. If necessary, naloxone Hydrochloride can be diluted with sterile water for injection.

Following initial improvement of respiratory function, repeated doses of naloxone Hydrochloride may be required to counteract recurrent respiratory depression. Supplemental intramuscular doses of naloxone Hydrochloride may be utilized to produce a longer-lasting effect.

Since the duration of action of Diphenoxylate Hydrochloride is longer than that of naloxone Hydrochloride, improvement of respiration following administration may be followed by recurrent respiratory depression. Consequently, continuous observation is necessary until the effect of Diphenoxylate Hydrochloride on respiration has passed. This effect may persist for many hours. The period of observation should extend over at least 48 hours, preferably under continuous hospital care. Although signs of overdosage and respiratory depression may not be evident soon after ingestion of Diphenoxylate Hydrochloride, respiratory depression may occur from 12 to 30 hours later.

DOSAGE AND ADMINISTRATION
DO NOT EXCEED RECOMMENDED DOSAGE.
Adults: The recommended initial dosage is two Atropine/Diphenoxylate tablets four times daily or 10 ml (two regular teaspoonfuls) of Atropine/Diphenoxylate liquid four times daily (20 mg per day). Most patients will require this dosage until initial control has been achieved, after which the dosage may be reduced to meet individual requirements. Control may often be maintained with as little as 5 mg (two tablets or 10 ml of liquid) daily.

Clinical improvement of acute diarrhea is usually observed within 48 hours. If clinical improvement of chronic diarrhea after treatment with a maximum daily dose of 20 mg of Diphenoxylate Hydrochloride is not observed within 10 days, symptoms are unlikely to be controlled by further administration.

Children: Atropine/Diphenoxylate is not recommended in children under 2 years of age and should be used with special caution in young children (See "Warnings" and "Precautions"). The nutritional status and degree of dehydration must be considered. In children under 13 years of age, use Atropine/Diphenoxylate liquid. Do not use Atropine/Diphenoxylate tablets for this age group.

Only the plastic dropper should be used when measuring Atropine/Diphenoxylate liquid for administration to children.

Dosage Schedule for Children: The recommended initial total daily dosage of Atropine/Diphenoxylate liquid for children is 0.3 to 0.4 mg/kg, administered in four divided doses. The following table provides an *approximate* initial daily dosage recommendation for children.

| Age (years) | Approximate weight | | Dosage in ml (four times daily) |
	(kg)	(lb)	
2	11-14	24-31	1.5-3.0
3	12-16	26-35	2.0-3.0
4	14-20	31-44	2.0-4.0
5	16-23	35-51	2.5-4.5
6-8	17-32	38-71	2.5-5.0
9-12	23-55	51-121	3.5-5.0

These pediatric schedules are the best approximation of an average dose recommendation which may be adjusted downward according to the overall nutritional status and degree of dehydration encountered in the sick child. Reduction of dosage may be made as soon as initial control of symptoms has been achieved. Maintenance dosage may be as low as one-fourth of the initial daily dosage. If no response occurs within 48 hours, Atropine/Diphenoxylate is unlikely to be effective.

KEEP THIS AND ALL MEDICATIONS OUT OF THE REACH OF CHILDREN.

A plastic dropper calibrated in increments of ½ ml (¼ mg) with a capacity of 2 ml (1 mg) accompanies each 2-oz bottle of Atropine/Diphenoxylate liquid. Only this plastic dropper should be used when measuring Atropine/Diphenoxylate liquid for administration to children.

HOW SUPPLIED
SOLUTION (C-V): 0.025 MG-2.5 MG/5 ML

AVERAGE UNIT PRICE (AVAILABLE SIZES)	
BRAND	$0.21
GENERIC	$0.13

BRAND/MANUFACTURER	NDC	SIZE	AWP
◆ BRAND			
LOMOTIL: Searle	00025-0066-02	60 ml	$12.50

BRAND/MANUFACTURER	NDC	SIZE	AWP
◆ GENERICS			
Roxane	00054-3194-46	60 ml	$6.28
Roxane	00054-8191-16	5 ml 40s ud	$32.49
Roxane	00054-8171-16	10 ml 40s ud	$53.54

TABLETS (C-V): 0.025 MG-2.5 MG

AVERAGE UNIT PRICE (AVAILABLE SIZES)		GENERIC A-RATED AVERAGE PRICE (GAAP)	
BRAND	$0.40	100s	$6.58
GENERIC	$0.06	500s	$15.23
HCFA FUL (100s ea)	$0.02	1000s	$27.81

BRAND/MANUFACTURER	NDC	SIZE	AWP
◆ BRAND			
LOMOTIL: Searle	00025-0061-31	100s	$42.30
	00025-0061-34	100s ud	$44.80
	00025-0061-51	500s	$200.78
	00025-0061-52	1000s	$374.22
	00025-0061-55	2500s	$912.14
◆ GENERICS			
Major	00904-0032-60	100s	$2.80
Rugby	00536-3763-01	100s	$3.14
Goldline	00182-1006-01	100s	$3.30
Qualitest	00603-3360-21	100s	$3.80
Caremark	00339-4037-12	100s	$4.16
Moore,H.L.	00839-6120-06	100s	$4.46
URL	00677-1531-01	100s	$4.75
LONOX: Geneva	00781-1262-01	100s	$4.80
DI-ATRO: MD Pharm	43567-0535-07	100s	$6.35
Roxane	00054-4200-25	100s	$7.30
UDL	51079-0067-20	100s ud	$6.87
UDL	51079-0067-21	100s ud	$6.87
Vangard	00615-0429-13	100s ud	$7.03
Vangard	00615-0429-47	100s ud	$7.03
Goldline	00182-8180-89	100s ud	$7.50
LONOX: Geneva	00781-1262-13	100s ud	$8.95
Roxane	00054-8200-25	100s ud	$11.80
Roxane	00054-8200-24	100s ud	$17.55
UDL	51079-0067-91	120s ud	$60.00
Rugby	00536-3763-05	500s	$9.38
Goldline	00182-1006-05	500s	$12.30
LONOX: Geneva	00781-1262-05	500s	$13.25
Schein	00364-0449-05	500s	$17.79
DI-ATRO: MD Pharm	43567-0535-11	500s	$23.45
Rugby	00536-3763-10	1000s	$13.06
Qualitest	00603-3360-32	1000s	$18.10
Goldline	00182-1006-10	1000s	$19.20
Major	00904-0032-80	1000s	$19.70
Moore,H.L.	00839-6120-16	1000s	$20.86
Aligen	00405-0080-03	1000s	$22.61
URL	00677-1531-10	1000s	$24.85
LONOX: Geneva	00781-1262-10	1000s	$24.90
Schein	00364-0449-02	1000s	$25.89
Parmed	00349-8019-10	1000s	$27.95
DI-ATRO: MD Pharm	43567-0535-12	1000s	$30.00
Purepac	00228-2049-96	1000s	$34.28
Mylan	00378-0415-10	1000s	$37.42
Roxane	00054-4200-31	1000s	$70.49

Atropine Sulfate and Edrophonium Chloride

DESCRIPTION
Atropine Sulfate/Edrophonium Chloride Injection, for intravenous use, is a sterile, nonpyrogenic, nondepolarizing neuromuscular relaxant antagonist. Atropine Sulfate/Edrophonium Chloride is a combination drug containing a rapid acting acetylcholinesterase inhibitor, Edrophonium Chloride, and an anticholinergic, atropine sulfate. Chemically, Edrophonium Chloride is ethyl (m-hydroxyphenyl) dimethylammonium chloride. Its molecular formula is $C_{10}H_{16}ClNO$ and molecular weight is 201.70.

Chemically, Atropine Sulfate is endo-(±)-alpha-(hydroxymethyl)-8-methyl- 8-azabicyclo [3.2.1]oct-3-yl benzeneacetate sulfate (2:1) monohydrate.

Its molecular formula is $(C_{17}H_{23}NO_3)_2 \cdot H_2SO_4 \cdot H_2O$ and molecular weight is 694.84.

5 mL Ampuls: 10 mg Edrophonium Chloride and 0.14 mg Atropine Sulfate.

15 mL Multidose Vials: 10 mg Edrophonium Chloride and 0.14 mg Atropine Sulfate.

CLINICAL PHARMACOLOGY
PHARMACODYNAMICS
Atropine Sulfate/Edrophonium Chloride Injection is a combination of an anticholinesterase agent, which antagonizes the action of nondepolarizing neuromuscular blocking drugs, and a parasympatholytic (anticholinergic) drug, which prevents the muscarinic effects caused by inhibition of acetylcholine breakdown by the anticholinesterase. Edrophonium Chloride antagonizes the effect of nondepolarizing neuromuscular blocking agents primarily by inhibiting or

inactivating acetylcholinesterase. By inactivating the acetylcholinesterase enzyme, acetylcholine is not hydrolyzed as rapidly by acetylcholinesterase and is thereby allowed to accumulate. The greater quantity of acetylcholine reaching the sites of nicotinic cholinergic postjunctional receptors improves transmission of impulses across the myoneural junction. The concomitant, unavoidable accumulation of acetylcholine at the sites of muscarinic cholinergic transmission occurring at the parasympathetic, postganglionic receptors of the autonomic nervous system may cause *bradycardia, bronchoconstriction, increased secretions,* and other parasym-pathomimetic side effects. The magnitude of these muscarinic side effects can be expected to vary from patient to patient depending upon the amount of vagal nerve activity present. Atropine Sulfate counteracts these side effects.

Intravenous Edrophonium Chloride in doses of 0.5 to 1.0 mg/kg promptly antagonizes the effects of nondepolarizing muscle relaxants reaching the maxi-mum antagonism within 1.2 minutes. A plateau of maximal antagonism is sustained for 70 minutes[1]. Intravenous Atropine Sulfate has an immediate effect on heart rate which reaches a peak in 2 to 16 minutes and lasts 170 minutes after an average 0.02 mg/kg dose.

PHARMACOKINETICS
Edrophonium Chloride: Edrophonium Chloride given intravenously shows first order elimination in a two compartment open pharmacokinetic model[3]. Onset of reversal of muscle relaxant induced depression in twitch tension occurs within three minutes. Edrophonium is primarily renally excreted with 67% of the dose appearing in the urine[4]. Hepatic metabolism and biliary excretion have also been demonstrated in animals[4,8]. While infants and children have been shown to have a reduced plasma half-life and an increased clearance of Edrophonium, doses in children are not significantly different from adults on a mg/kg basis although they are more variable in effect. Conversely, elderly subjects (> 75 years old) have a prolonged plasma half-life and a reduced clearance. Studies have shown that in spite of these changes the onset and duration of action is unchanged in these patients. (See related table).

Atropine Sulfate: Atropine Sulfate given intravenously shows first order elimina-tion in a two compartment open model[7]. Approximately 57% of a dose of atropine appears in the urine as unchanged drug. Tropine is the primary hepatic metabolite of atropine and it accounts for approximately 30% of the dose[2]. Atropine is only 14 ± 9% bound to plasma proteins[7]. Atropine clearance in children under 2 years old and in the elderly is decreased in relation to normal healthy adults. (See related table).

INDICATIONS AND USAGE
Atropine Sulfate/Edrophonium Chloride Injection is recommended as a reversal agent or antagonist of nondepolarizing neuromuscular blocking agents. It is not effective against depolarizing neuromuscular blocking agents. It is also useful if used adjunctively in the treatment of respiratory depression caused by curare overdosage.

The appropriateness of the specific fixed ratio of Edrophonium and Atropine contained in Atropine Sulfate/Edrophonium Chloride has not been evaluated in myasthenia agravis. Therefore, Atropine Sulfate/Edrophonium Chloride is not recommended for use in the differential diagnosis of this condition.

CONTRAINDICATIONS
Atropine Sulfate/Edrophonium Chloride Injection is not to be used in patients with known hypersensitivity to either of the components, or in patients with intestinal or urinary obstruction of mechanical type. Atropine sulfate is contrain-dicated in the presence of acute glaucoma, adhesions (synechiae) between the iris and lens of the eye, and pyloric stenosis.

WARNINGS
Atropine Sulfate/Edrophonium Chloride Injection should be used with caution in patients with bronchial asthma or cardiac arrhythmias. Cardiac arrest has been reported to occur in digitalized patients as well as in jaundiced subjects receiving cholinesterase inhibitors. In patients with cardiovascular disease, given anesthesia with narcotic and nitrous oxide without a potent inhalational agent, there is increased risk for clinically significant bradycardia. In patients receiving beta-adrenergic blocking agents there is increased risk for excessive bradycardia from unopposed parasympathetic vagal tone. Such patients should receive Atropine Sulfate alone prior to Atropine Sulfate/Edrophonium Chloride. Isolated instances of respiratory arrest have also been reported following the administration of edrophonium chloride. Additional Atropine Sulfate (1 mg) should be available for immediate use to counteract severe cholinergic reaction which may occur in hypersensitive individuals when Atropine Sulfate/Edrophonium Chloride is used.

Atropine Sulfate/Edrophonium Chloride contains sodium sulfite, a sulfite that may cause allergic-type reactions including anaphylactic symptoms and life-threatening or less severe asthmatic episodes in certain susceptible people. The overall prevalence of sulfite sensitivity in the general population is unknown and probably low. Sulfite sensitivity is seen more frequently in asthmatic than in nonasthmatic people.

There is a potential for tissue irritation by extravascular injection.

PRECAUTIONS
General: As with any antagonist of nondepolarizing muscle relaxants, adequate recovery of voluntary respiration and neuromuscular transmission must be obtained prior to the discontinuation of respiratory assistance. Should a patient develop 'anticholinesterase insensitivity" for brief or prolonged periods. The patient should be carefully monitored and the dosage of anticholinesterase drugs reduced or withheld until the patient again becomes sensitive to them. Use with caution in patients with prostatic hypertrophy and in debilitated patients with chronic lung disease.

When used in therapeutic doses, Atropine can cause dryness of the mouth. This effect is additive when the product is administered with other drugs that can cause dryness of the mouth.

Since Atropine Sulfate slows gastric emptying and gastrointestinal motility, it may interfere with the absorption of other medications. The effect of Atropine on dryness of the mouth may be increased if it is given with other drugs that have anticholinergic action (tricyclic antidepressants, antipsychotics, some antihista-mines, and antiparkinsonism drugs).

Drug Interactions: Atropine Sulfate/Edrophonium Chloride, Injection should not be administered prior to the administration of any nondepolarizing muscle relaxants. It should be administered with caution to patients with symptoms of myasthenic weakness who are also on anticholinesterase drugs. Anticholinesterase overdosage (cholinergic crisis) symptoms may mimic underdosage (myasthenic weakness), so the use of this drug may worsen the condition of these patients (see "Overdosage" section for treatment).

Narcotic analgesics, except when combined with potent inhaled anesthetics, appear to potentiate the effect of edrophonium on the sinus node and conduction system, increasing both the frequency and duration of bradycardia. In patients with cardiovascular disease, given anesthesia with narcotic and nitrous oxide without a potent inhalational agent, there is increased risk for clinically significant bradycardia. In patients receiving beta-adrenergic blocking agents there is increased risk for excessive bradycardia from unopposed parasympathetic vagal tone. Such patients should receive Atropine Sulfate alone prior to Atropine Sulfate/Edrophonium Chloride.

TABLE OF PHARMACEKINETIC VALUES FOR EDROPHONIUM CHLORIDE

Population	hr ± S.D.	L/kg ± S.D.	± S.D.	N	Cl mL/kg/min	Ref.
Adults	1.8 ± 0.6	1.1 ± 0.2	9.6 ± 2.7	10		3
Anephric Patients* †	3.4 ± 1.0	0.68 ± 0.13	2.7 ± 1.4	6		4
Infants (3 wks-11 mos)	1.2 ± 0.5	1.2 ± 0.2	17.8± 1.2	4		5
Children (1-6 yr)	1.6 ± 0.5	1.2 ± 0.7	14.2 ± 7.3	5		6
Elderly* (over 75 yr)	‡1.4 ± 0.3	0.6 ± 0.1	5.1 ± 1	5		6

T1/2β = Elimination half-life
VD = Volume of distribution
Cl = Clearance

* *No adjustments of edrophonium dosage are required because elimination of non-depolarizing muscle relaxants is similarly decreased.*
† *Values for anephric patients were calculated using a non-compartmental model.*
‡ *From a study using a different, less sensitive HPLC method and fitting C vs T data to a biexponential curve.*

TABLE OF PHARMACOKINETIC VALUES FOR ATROPINE SULFATE

Population	T1/2b hr ± S.D.	VD L/kg ± S.D.	S.D.	N	Cl mL/kg/min	Ref.
Adults	3.0 ± 0.9	1.6 ± 0.4	6.8 ± 2.9	8		7
Children (0.08-10 yrs)	4.8 ± 3.5	2.2 ± 1.5	6.4 ± 3.9	13		7
Elderly* (65-75 yrs)	10.0 ± 7.3	1.8 ± 1.2	2.9 ± 1.9	10		7

T1/2β = Elimination half-life
VD = Volume of distribution
Cl = Clearance

* *No dose adjustment required because the cardiovascular effect of atropine is diminished in the elderly.*

♦ RATED THERAPEUTICALLY EQUIVALENT; ◇ THERAPEUTIC EQUIVALENCE UNCONFIRMED; ○ UNRATED

Compared to muscle relaxants with some vagolytic activity, muscle relaxants with no vagolytic effects, i.e., vecuronium, may be associated with a slightly higher incidence of vagotonic effects such as bradycardia and first-degree heart block when reversed with Atropine Sulfate/Edrophonium Chloride.

Pregnancy Category C: Animal reproduction studies have not been conducted with Atropine Sulfate/Edrophonium Chloride. It is also not known whether Atropine Sulfate/Edrophonium Chloride can cause fetal harm when administered to a pregnant woman or can affect reproduction capacity. Atropine Sulfate/Edrophonium Chloride should be used during pregnancy only if the potential benefit justifies the potential risk to the fetus.

Labor and Delivery: The effect of Atropine Sulfate/Edrophonium Chloride on the mother and fetus, on the duration of labor or delivery, in the possibility that a forceps delivery or other intervention or resuscitation of the newborn will be necessary, is not known. The effect of the combination drug on the later growth, development and functional maturation of the child is also unknown.

Nursing Mothers: The safety of Atropine Sulfate/Edrophonium Chloride during lactation in humans has not been established.

Pediatric Use: Safety and effectiveness in children have not been established. Pediatric patients may have increased vagal tone. The effect of fixed ratios of edrophonium and atropine on heart rate in such patients has not been evaluated.

ADVERSE REACTIONS

Cardiovascular: Arrhythmias Frequency > 10%: junctional rhythm, bradycardia, tachycardia;

Frequency 3-10%: first and second degree A-V block, P Wave changes, atrial premature contractions;

Frequency 1-3%: third degree A-V block, ventricular premature contractions;

Frequency less than 1%: 3 second R-R interval.

Of the patients who experienced any arrhythmias, 85% had the onset within two minutes, 74% no longer had any arrhythmias after 10 minutes. Arrhythmias related to increased vagal tone, bradycardia, second and third degree heart block respond to treatment with 0.2 - 0.4 mg of Atropine IV (Bigeminy or ventricular ectopy may be treated with lidocaine 50 mg IV).

Adverse experiences reported for anticholinesterase agents such as edrophonium chloride, but not observed in the 235 patients studied with Atropine Sulfate/Edrophonium Chloride Injection:

Cardiovascular: Nonspecific EKG changes, fall in cardiac output leading to hypotension;

Respiratory: Increased tracheobronchial secretions, laryngospasm, bronchiolar constriction and respiratory muscle paralysis;

Neurologic: Convulsions, dysarthria, dysphonia, and dysphagia;

Gastrointestinal: Nausea, vomiting, increased peristalsis, increased gastric and intestinal secretions, diarrhea, abdominal cramps;

Musculoskeletal: Weakness and fasciculations;

Miscellaneous: Increased urinary frequency, diaphoresis, increased lacrimation, pupillary constriction, diplopia, and conjunctival hyperemia.

Untoward reactions to atropine sulfate generally are dose-related. Individual tolerance varies greatly but systemic doses of 0.5 to 10 mg are likely to produce the following effects, which were not observed in the 235 patients treated with Atropine Sulfate/Edrophonium Chloride.

Neurologic: Speech disturbances and restlessness with asthenia;

Dermatologic: Flushed, dry skin, formation of a scartatiniform rash;

Miscellaneous: Dryness of the nose and mouth, thirst, blurred vision, photophobia, slight mydriasis. Atropine may produce fever through inhibition of heat loss by evaporation.

OVERDOSAGE

Muscarinic symptoms (nausea, vomiting, diarrhea, sweating, increased bronchial and salivary secretions and bradycardia) may appear with overdosage (cholinergic crisis) of Atropine Sulfate/Edrophonium Chloride Injection, but may be managed by the use of additional atropine sulfate. Obstruction of the airway by bronchial secretions can arise and may be managed with suction (especially if tracheostomy has been performed).

Should Edrophonium Chloride overdosage occur:
1. Maintain respiratory exchange.
2. Monitor cardiac function.

Appropriate measures should be taken if convulsions occur or shock is present.

Principal manifestations of overdosage (poisoning) with Atropine Sulfate are delirium, tachycardia and fever. In the treatment of Atropine poisoning, respiratory assistance and symptomatic support are indicated. Death is usually due to paralysis of the medullary centers.

In the clinical studies performed with Atropine Sulfate/Edrophonium Chloride, there were no reported overdoses and therefore no clinical information is available regarding overdosing with Atropine Sulfate/Edrophonium Chloride.

DOSAGE AND ADMINISTRATION

Dosages of Atropine Sulfate/Edrophonium Chloride Injection range from 0.05-0.1 mL/kg given slowly over 45 seconds to 1 minute at a point of at least 5% recovery of twitch response to neuromuscular stimulation (95% block). The dosage delivered is 0.5-1.0 mg/kg of edrophonium chloride and 0.007-0.014 mg/kg of atropine sulfate. A total dosage of 1.0 mg/kg of edrophonium chloride should

rarely be exceeded. Response should be monitored carefully and assisted or controlled ventilation secured. Satisfactory reversal permits adequate voluntary respiration and neuromuscular transmission (as tested with a peripheral nerve stimulator). Recurarization has not been reported after satisfactory reversal has been attained.

Parenteral drug products should be inspected visually for particulate matter and discoloration prior to administration.

REFERENCES

1. Cronnelly R, Morris RB, Miller RD: Edrophonium: Duration of action and atropine requirement in humans during halothane anesthesia. Anesthesiology 1982;57:261-266. 2. Hinderling PH, Gundert-Remy U, Schmidlin O, Heinzel G: Integrated pharmacokinetics and pharmacodynamics of atropine in healthy humans. I: Pharmacokinetics: II: Pharmacodynamics. J Pharmaceutical Sci 1985; 74:I-703-710; II-711-717. 3. Morris RB, Cronnelly R, Miller RD, Stanski DR, Fahey MR: Pharmacokinetics of edrophonium and neostigmine when antagonizing d-tubocurarine neuromuscular blockade in man. Anesthesiology 1981; 54:399-402. 4. Morris RB, Cronnelly R, Miller RD, Stanski DR, Fahey MR: Pharmacokinetics of edrophonium in anephric and renal transplant patients. Br J Anaesth 1981;53:1311-1313. 5. Fisher DM, Cronnelly R, Sharma M, Miller RD: Clinical pharmacology of edrophonium in infants and children. Anesthesiology 1984; 61:428-433. 6. Silverberg PA, Mattee RS, Ornstein E, Young WL, Diaz J: Pharmacokinetics and pharmacodynamics of edrophonium in the elderly. Anesth Analg 1986;65PS,142. 7. Virtanen R, Kanto J, Lisalo E, Lisalo EU, Salo M, Sjovall S: Pharmacokinetic studies on atropine with special reference to age. Acta Anaesthesiol Scand 1982;26:297-300. 8. Back DJ, Calvey TN: Excretion of ^{14}C-edrophonium and its metabolites in bile: role of the liver cell and the peribiliary vascular plexus. Br J Pharmacol., 1972;44:534 Rev. 2 - 94

HOW SUPPLIED
INJECTION: 0.14 MG/ML-10 MG/ML

BRAND/MANUFACTURER	NDC	SIZE	AWP
BRAND			
ENLON-PLUS: Ohmeda	10019-0180-05	5 ml ud	$4.95
	10019-0195-15	15 ml	$10.29

Atropine Sulfate and Meperidine Hydrochloride

DESCRIPTION
Each mL contains 0.4 mg/mL Atropine Sulfate and 50 mg/mL Meperidine Hydrochloride. Warning: May be habit forming. The solution may contain sodium acetate buffer, not more than 1.5 mg sodium metabisulfite, and 5 mg phenol. The pH is adjusted with sodium hydroxide or acetic acid.

CLINICAL PHARMACOLOGY
Meperidine is a synthetic narcotic analgesic structurally unlike the opium alkaloids but with multiple actions qualitatively similar to those of morphine. The most prominent of these involve the central nervous system and organs composed of smooth muscle. Analgesia and sedation are the principal actions of therapeutic value. Some evidence suggests that Meperidine may produce less smooth-muscle spasm, constipation, and depression of the cough reflex than morphine in equianalgesic doses. Meperidine in parenteral doses of 60 mg to 80 mg has the analgesic effect of approximately 10 mg of morphine. Maximum analgesia occurs 30 to 50 minutes after an intramuscular injection of Meperidine; the duration of action is 2 to 4 hours.

Atropine, a belladonna alkaloid, blocks the actions of acetylcholine at postganglionic parasympathetic neuroeffector junctions. There is considerable variation in endorgan sensitivity to this antimuscarinic activity. The small doses of Atropine used as preoperative medication inhibit primarily salivary, tracheobronchial, and sweat secretion. Atropine also exhibits central nervous system activity, usually confined to mild vagal stimulation in clinical dosage. Conventional doses of atropine injected for preanesthetic medication normally have little ocular effect except in a few patients predisposed to narrow-angle glaucoma.

INDICATIONS AND USAGE
For preoperative sedation and antisecretory effect.

CONTRAINDICATIONS
Hypersensitivity to Atropine or Meperidine.

Atropine and other drugs with anticholinergic properties are contraindicated in the presence of narrow-angle glaucoma. Routine screening for a shallow anterior chamber may help to avoid precipitating a first attack of acute angle-closure glaucoma. Atropine should not be used in patients with organic pyloric stenosis.

Meperidine is contraindicated in patients who are receiving monoamine oxidase inhibitors (MAOI) or those who have received such agents within 14 days. Therapeutic doses of Meperidine have inconsistently precipitated unpredictable, severe, and occasionally fatal reactions in patients who have received such agents within 14 days. The mechanism of these reactions is unclear. Some have been characterized by coma, severe respiratory depression, cyanosis, and hypotension, and have resembled the syndrome of acute narcotic overdose. In other reactions the predominant manifestations have been hyperexcitability, convulsions, tachycardia, hyperpyrexia, and hypertension.

Although it is not known that other narcotics are free of the risk of such reactions virtually all of the reported reactions have occurred with Meperidine. If a narcotic is needed in such patients, a sensitivity test should be performed in which repeated, small, incremental doses of morphine are administered over the course of several hours while the patient's condition and vital signs are under careful observation. (Intravenous hydrocortisone or prednisolone has been used to treat severe reactions, with the addition of intravenous chlorpromazine in those cases exhibiting hypertension and hyperpyrexia. The usefulness and safety of narcotic antagonists in the treatment of these reactions are unknown.)

WARNINGS

Drug Dependence: Meperidine can produce drug dependence of the morphine type and, therefore, has the potential for being abused. Psychic dependence, physical dependence, and tolerance may develop upon repeated administration of Meperidine, and it should be prescribed and administered with the same degree of caution appropriate to the use of morphine. The combination of Atropine and Meperidine is subject to provisions of the Drug Enforcement Administration (Schedule II).

Interaction with Other Central Nervous System Depressants: Atropine in therapeutic doses acts to stimulate medulla and higher cerebral centers. Toxic doses of Atropine produce central excitation, hallucinations, or delirium, while still larger doses produce central depression.

Meperidine should be used with caution and reduced dosage in patients concurrently receiving other narcotic analgesics, general anesthetics, phenothiazines, sedative-hypnotics, tranquilizers, tricyclic antidepressants and other CNS depressants including alcohol. Respiratory depression, hypotension, and profound sedation or coma may result from additive CNS depression.

Cardiac Conditions: Atropine and Meperidine Hydrochloride Injection must be used with caution in patients with cardiac disease and decompensation, since alterations in cardiac rate and conduction may result. A possible vagolytic action may produce dangerous increases in ventricular rate in patients with supraventricular tachycardias.

Hypotensive Effect: The administration of Meperidine may result in severe hypotension in an individual whose ability to maintain his blood pressure has already been compromised by a depleted blood volume or concurrent administration of drugs such as certain andrenolytic phenothiazines or certain anesthetics.

Head Injury and Increased Intracranial Pressure: The respiratory depressant effects of Meperidine and its capacity to elevate cerebrospinal fluid pressure may be markedly exaggerated in the presence of head injury, intracranial lesions, or preexisting increase in intracranial pressure. Furthermore, narcotics produce adverse reactions which may obscure the clinical course of patients with head injuries. In such patients, Meperidine must be used with extreme caution and only if deemed essential.

Obstetrical Use: When used as an obstetrical analgesic, meperidine crosses the placental barrier and can produce respiratory depression in the newborn. Resuscitation may be required (see *"Overdosage"*).

Obstructive Gastrointestinal Conditions: Caution must be used in the administration of Atropine and Meperidine Hydrochloride Injection to patients with obstructive gastrointestinal conditions, since marked decreases in motility and tone may occur, resulting in obstruction and gastric retention.

Obstructive Urinary Tract Condition: Patients with prostatic hypertrophy, urethral stricture, or other conditions of the urinary tract predisposing to urinary retention should be administered Atropine and Meperidine Hydrochloride Injection with caution. Elderly males should receive this agent with caution.

Asthma and Other Respiratory Conditions: Meperidine should be used with extreme caution in patients having an acute asthmatic attack, patients with chronic obstructive pulmonary disease or cor pulmonale, patients having a substantially decreased respiratory reserve, and patients with preexisting respiratory depression, hypoxia, or hypercapnia. In such patients, even usual therapeutic doses of narcotics may decrease respiratory drive while simultaneously increasing airway resistance to the point of apnea.

Glaucoma: While Atropine is contraindicated in patients predisposed to narrow-angle glaucoma, parenteral Atropine may generally be administered to patients with open-angle glaucoma without significant increases in intraocular pressure occurring. Caution should be exercised and an ophthalmologist informed if a shallow anterior chamber is detected, so that an undesirable rise in intraocular pressure may be prevented or treated appropriately.

Acute glaucoma may be precipitated by Atropine in susceptible individuals. The parenteral administration of Atropine to persons over 40 should be preceded by careful ophthalmological screening. If eye pain occurs in a patient receiving Atropine, the drug should be discontinued as this may be an indication of undiagnosed glaucoma.

Intravenous Use: If necessary, Meperidine may be given intravenously, but the injection should be given very slowly, preferably in the form of a diluted solution. Rapid intravenous injection of narcotic analgesics, including Meperidine, increases the incidence of adverse reactions; severe respiratory depression, apnea, hypotension, peripheral circulatory collapse, and cardiac arrest have occurred. Meperidine should not be administered intravenously unless a narcotic antagonist and the facilities for assisted or controlled respiration are immediately available. When Meperidine is given parenterally, especially intravenously, the patient should be lying down.

May contain sodium metabisulfite, a sulfite that may cause allergic-type reactions including anaphylactic symptoms and life-threatening or less severe asthmatic episodes in certain susceptible people. The overall prevalence of sulfite sensitivity in the general population is unknown and probably low. Sulfite sensitivity is seen more frequently in asthmatic than in nonasthmatic people.

PRECAUTIONS

Usage in Ambulatory Patients: Meperidine may impair the mental and/or physical abilities required for the performance of potentially hazardous tasks such as driving a car or operating machinery. The patient should be cautioned accordingly. Meperidine, like other narcotics, may produce orthostatic hypotension in ambulatory patients.

Acute Abdominal Conditions: The administration of Meperidine or other narcotics may obscure the diagnosis or clinical course in patients with acute abdominal conditions.

Convulsions: Meperidine may worsen seizure control in patients with convulsive disorders. If dosage is escalated substantially above recommended levels because of tolerance development, convulsions may occur in individuals without a history of convulsive disorders.

Usage in Pregnancy and Lactation: Atropine and Meperidine should not be used in pregnant women prior to the labor period, unless in the judgment of the physician the potential benefits outweigh the possible hazards, because safe use in pregnancy prior to labor has not been established relative to possible adverse effects on fetal development.

Atropine and Meperidine appear in trace amounts in the milk of nursing mothers. To avoid possible unwanted sedative or anticholinergic effects in the infant, Atropine and Meperidine should not be administered to a nursing mother.

Pulmonary Disease: Although the belladonna alkaloids can induce bronchodilation, they are less effective than other agents. Because Atropine exerts a drying effect on bronchial secretions, it must be used with caution in patients with chronic lung disease. Repeated administration of this agent can produce viscid bronchial secretions that may dangerously obstruct airflow and predispose to infection.

Body Temperature: Atropine and other anticholinergics must be used with caution in patients with fever because loss of body heat through sweating is inhibited by these agents. In infants and small children, even moderate doses may produce "Atropine fever". In persons of normal body temperature, increased temperature will occur only when room temperature and humidity are elevated.

Additive Anticholinergic Effects: Numerous drugs such as phenothiazines, tricyclic antidepressants, antihistamines, and antiparkinsonian agents, possess anticholinergic activity. When Atropine is administered concomitantly with such agents, the incidence and degree of undesirable anticholinergic effects may be increased.

Special Risk Patients: Infants and young children are especially sensitive to the effects of belladonna alkaloids. Special caution must be used if it is felt desirable to administer Atropine to children under six years of age.

Atropine and Meperidine should be given with caution and the initial dose reduced in elderly or debilitated patients, and those with significant renal or hepatic impairment, hypothyroidism, or Addison's disease.

ADVERSE REACTIONS

The major side effects of Atropine can be attributed to its antimuscarinic action. These include dryness of the mouth, blurred vision, photophobia, confusion, headache, dizziness, tachycardia, palpitations, flushing, urinary hesitancy or retention, constipation, abdominal distention, nausea, vomiting, loss of libido and impotency. Anhidrosis may produce heat intolerance and impairment of temperature regulation in a hot environment. Larger or toxic doses may produce such central effects as restlessness, tremor, fatigue, locomotor difficulties, delirium, followed by hallucinations, depression, and ultimately, medullary paralysis and death.

Hypersensitivity reactions will occasionally occur with the belladonna alkaloids; these are usually seen as skin rashes, on occasion progressing to exfoliation.

The major hazards of Meperidine, as with other narcotic analgesics, are respiratory depression and, to a lesser degree, circulatory depression; respiratory arrest, shock, and cardiac arrest have occurred.

The most frequently observed reactions include light-headedness, dizziness, sedation, nausea, vomiting, and sweating. These effects seem to be more prominent in ambulatory patients and in those who are not experiencing severe pain. In such individuals, lower doses are advisable. Some adverse reactions in ambulatory patients may be alleviated if the patient lies down.

Other adverse reactions to Meperidine include:

Central Nervous System: Euphoria, dysphoria, weakness, headache, agitation, tremor, uncoordinated muscle movements, transient hallucinations and disorientation, visual disturbances.

Gastrointestinal: Dry mouth, constipation, biliary tract spasm.

Cardiovascular: Flushing of the face, tachycardia, bradycardia, palpitations, faintness, syncope.

Genitourinary: Urinary retention.

Allergic: Pruritus, urticaria, other skin rashes, wheal and flare over the vein with IV injection.

Other: Pain at the injection site; local tissue irritation and induration following subcutaneous injection, particularly when repeated; antidiuretic effect.

DOSAGE AND ADMINISTRATION

Do not use Atropine and Meperidine in children under 10 years of age (see *"Precautions"*).

◆ RATED THERAPEUTICALLY EQUIVALENT; ◇ THERAPEUTIC EQUIVALENCE UNCONFIRMED; ○ UNRATED

For preoperative medication, the average dosage recommendations are:

Children: Ages 10 to 12 years (average, well-developed patients): Atropine, 0.4 mg and Meperidine Hydrochloride, 50 mg.

Adults: Atropine, 0.4 mg and Meperidine Hydrochloride, 50 mg, 75 mg, and 100 mg.

The appropriate dose of Atropine and Meperidine Hydrochloride Injection should be administered intramuscularly 30 to 90 minutes prior to the beginning of anesthesia for maximum effectiveness.

Warning: Barbiturates are not chemically compatible in solution with Meperidine and should not be mixed in the same syringe. Since numerous other chemical incompatibilities have been reported with Meperidine Injection, the appropriate literature on Atropine and Meperidine should be consulted before any drug is mixed with this combination in the same syringe.

OVERDOSAGE

ATROPINE

Symptoms: Serious overdosage with Atropine is characterized by widespread paralysis of parasympathetically innervated organs. Dry mucous membranes, widely dilated and nonresponsive pupils, tachycardia, fever and cutaneous flush are especially prominent, as are mental and neurological symptoms. Disorientation, mania, hallucinations, gait disturbances and incoordination may suggest an acute toxic psychosis. Such symptoms may last 48 hours or longer; in instances of severe intoxication, respiratory depression, coma, circulatory collapse, and death may occur.

Doses of 10 mg or less have been fatal in children, but the fatal dose of Atropine in adults is not known. Doses of 200 mg of Atropine have been used therapeutically in mental illness; survival has been reported after doses of 1,000 mg.

Treatment: Supportive treatment should be administered as indicated. If respiration is depressed, artifical respiration with oxygen is necessary. Alcohol sponges or a hypothermia blanket may be required to reduce fever, especially in children. Catheterization may be necessary if urinary retention occurs. Since Atropine elimination takes place through the kidney, urinary output must be maintained and increased if possible; intravenous fluids may be indicated. Because of the patient's photophobia, the room should be darkened.

Physostigmine is the rational physiological antidote to the belladonna alkaloids, because it will reverse the dangerous central nervous system effects as well as the peripheral effects. Physostigmine has a short duration of action, and repeated doses are likely to be required. Neostigmine, pilocarpine, and methacholine are of little real benefit, since they do not penetrate the blood-brain barrier.

MEPERIDINE

Symptoms: Serious overdose with Meperidine is characterized by respiratory depression (a decrease in respiratory rate and/or tidal volume, Cheyne-Stokes respiration, cyanosis), extreme somnolence progressing to stupor or coma, skeletal muscle flaccidity, cold and clammy skin, and sometimes bradycardia and hypotension. In severe overdosage, particularly by the intravenous route, apnea, circulatory collapse, cardiac arrest, and death may occur.

Treatment: Primary attention should be given to the reestablishment of adequate respiratory exchange through provision of a patent airway and institution of assisted or controlled ventilation. The narcotic antagonists, naloxone hydrochloride, nalorphine hydrochloride, and levallorphan tartrate, are specific antidotes against respiratory depression which may result from overdosage or unusual sensitivity to narcotics, including Meperidine. Therefore, an appropriate dose of one of these antagonists should be administered, preferably by the intravenous route, simultaneously with efforts at respiratory resuscitation.

An antagonist should only be administered in the presence of clinically significant respiratory or cardiovascular depression induced by a narcotic. Oxygen, intravenous fluids, vasopressors, and other supportive measures should be employed as indicated.

Note: In an individual physically dependent on narcotics, the administration of the usual dose of a narcotic antagonist will precipitate an acute withdrawal syndrome. The severity of this syndrome will depend on the degree of physical dependence and the dose of antagonist administered. The use of narcotic antagonists in such individuals should be avoided if possible. If a narcotic antagonist must be used to treat serious respiratory depression in the physically dependent patient, the antagonist should be administered with extreme care and only one-fifth to one-tenth the usual initial dose administered.

Note: Do not use if solution is discolored or contains a precipitate.

HOW SUPPLIED

INJECTION (C-II): 0.4 MG/ML-50 MG/ML

BRAND/MANUFACTURER	NDC	SIZE	AWP
◆ **BRAND**			
ATROPINE AND DEMEROL: Sanofi Winthrop	00024-0021-02	1 ml 10s	$7.45

INJECTION (C-II): 0.4 MG/ML-75 MG/ML

BRAND/MANUFACTURER	NDC	SIZE	AWP
◆ **BRAND**			
ATROPINE AND DEMEROL: Sanofi Winthrop	00024-0022-02	1 ml 10s	$8.15

Atropine Sulfate and Phenobarbital

DESCRIPTION

Each tablet or 5 ml (teaspoonful) of elixir contains:

Phenobarbital (¼ gr) ....16 mg.
(Warning: May Be Habit-Forming)
Atropine Sulfate ....0.195 mg.

ACTIONS

This drug combination provides the natural belladonna alkaloid Atropine Sulfate in a specific, fixed ratio combined with Phenobarbital to provide peripheral anticholinergic/antispasmodic action and mild sedation.

INDICATIONS

BASED ON A REVIEW OF THIS DRUG BY THE NATIONAL ACADEMY OF SCIENCES-NATIONAL RESEARCH COUNCIL AND/OR OTHER INFORMATION, FDA HAS CLASSIFIED THE INDICATIONS AS "POSSIBLY" EFFECTIVE.

FOR USE AS ADJUNCTIVE THERAPY IN THE TREATMENT OF PEPTIC ULCER.

IT SHOULD BE NOTED AT THIS POINT IN TIME THAT THERE IS A LACK OF CONCURRENCE AS TO THE VALUE OF ANTICHOLINERGICS/ANTISPASMODICS IN THE TREATMENT OF GASTRIC ULCER. IT HAS NOT BEEN SHOWN CONCLUSIVELY WHETHER ANTICHOLINERGIC/ANTISPASMODIC DRUGS AID IN THE HEALING OF A PEPTIC ULCER, DECREASE THE RATE OF RECURRENCES, OR PREVENT COMPLICATION.

MAY ALSO BE USEFUL IN THE IRRITABLE BOWEL SYNDROME (IRRITABLE COLON, SPASTIC COLON, MUCOUS COLITIS), AND ACUTE ENTEROCOLITIS.

FINAL CLASSIFICATION OF THE LESS-THAN-EFFECTIVE INDICATIONS REQUIRES FURTHER INVESTIGATION.

CONTRAINDICATIONS

Glaucoma, obstructive uropathy (for example, bladder neck obstruction due to prostatic hypertrophy); obstructive disease of the gastrointestinal tract (as in achalasia, pyloroduodental stenosis, etc.); paralytic ileus, intestinal atony of the elderly or debilitated patient; unstable cardiovascular status in acute hemorrhage; severe ulcerative colitis especially if complicated by toxic megacolon; myasthenia gravis; hiatal hernia associated with reflux esophagitis.

Phenobarbital is contraindicated in acute intermittent porphyria. A sensitivity to Phenobarbital contraindicates the use of belladonna alkaloids with Phenobarbital and in those patients in whom Phenobarbital produces restlessness and/or excitement.

WARNINGS

Belladonna alkaloids with Phenobarbital should be used in pregnancy, lactation, or in women of childbearing age only, when in the judgment of the physician, the expected benefits outweigh the potential hazards to the mother and child.

In the presence of a high environmental temperature, heat prostration can occur with the drug use (fever and heatstroke due to decreased sweating). Diarrhea may be an early symptom of incomplete intestinal obstruction, especially in patients with ileostomy or colostomy. In this instance treatment with this drug would be inappropriate and possibly harmful.

Belladonna alkaloids with Phenobarbital may produce drowsiness or blurred vision. In this event, the patient should be warned not to engage in activities requiring mental alertness such as operating a motor vehicle or other machinery, or perform hazardous work while taking this drug.

Phenobarbital in patients taking anticoagulants may decrease the effect of the anticoagulant and thus require larger doses of the anticoagulant for optimal effect. When the Phenobarbital is discontinued, the dose of the anticoagulant may have to be decreased. Barbiturates may thus decrease the action of anticoagulant drugs.

Phenobarbital may be habit-forming and should not be administered to individuals known to be addiction prone or to those with a history of physical and/or psychological dependence upon habit-forming drugs.

Since barbiturates are metabolized in the liver, use with initial small doses and caution in patients with hepatic dysfunction.

PRECAUTIONS

Use with caution in patients with:
Autonomic neuropathy.
Hepatic or renal disease.
Hyperthyroidism, coronary heart disease, congestive heart failure, cardiac arrhythmias, and hypertension.
It should be noted that the use of anticholinergic/antispasmodic drugs in the treatment of gastric ulcer may produce a delay in gastric emptying time and may

complicate such therapy (antral stasis). Do not rely on the use of the drug in the presence of complication of biliary tract disease.

Investigate any tachycardia before giving anticholinergic (Atropine-like) drugs since they may increase the heart rate.

With overdosage, a curare-like action may occur.

ADVERSE REACTIONS

Adverse reactions may include xerostomia; urinary hesitancy and retention; blurred vision and tachycardia; palpitations; mydriasis; cycloplegia; increased ocular tension; loss of taste sense; headache; nervousness; drowsiness; weakness; dizziness; insomnia; nausea; vomiting; impotence; suppression of lactation; constipation; bloated feeling; severe allergic reaction or drug idiosyncrasies including anaphylaxis; urticaria and other dermal manifestations; and decreased sweating. Elderly patients may react with symptoms of excitement, agitation, drowsiness, and other untoward manifestations to even small doses of the drug.

Phenobarbital may produce excitement in some patients rather than a sedative effect. An occasional patient may experience musculoskeletal pain. Some patients may acquire a sensitivity to barbiturates and experience allergic phenomena and/or dermatologic response.

In patients habituated to barbiturates, abrupt withdrawal may produce delirium or convulsions.

MANAGEMENT OF OVERDOSAGE

The signs and symptoms of overdose are headache, nausea, vomiting, blurred vision, dilated pupils, hot, dry skin, dizziness, dryness of the mouth, difficulty in swallowing, CNS stimulation. Treatment should consist of gastric lavage, emetics, and activated charcoal. If indicated, parenteral cholinergic agents such as bethanechol chloride USP should be used.

DOSAGE AND ADMINISTRATION

The dosage should be adjusted to the needs of the individual patient to assure symptomatic control with a minimum of adverse effects.

ATROPINE SULFATE AND PHENOBARBITAL TABLETS
Adults: One or two tablets three or four times a day according to condition and severity of symptoms.

ATROPINE SULFATE AND PHENOBARBITAL ELIXIR
Adults: One or two teaspoonsful of elixir three or four times a day according to condition and severity of symptoms.

Children (elixir):

Body weight	Starting Dosage
15 lbs.	0.5 cc
30 lbs.	1 cc
45 lbs.	1.5 cc
60 lbs.	2 cc
90 lbs.	3 cc

Dosage may be repeated every 4 to 6 hours as needed; dosage adjustments may be necessary.

HOW SUPPLIED
ELIXIR: 0.195 MG-16 MG/ML

BRAND/MANUFACTURER	NDC	SIZE	AWP
○ BRAND			
ANTROCOL: Poythress	00095-0042-16	480 ml	$21.00

Atropine Sulfate, Injectable

DESCRIPTION

Atropine Sulfate, Injectable, is a sterile, nonpyrogenic isotonic solution of Atropine Sulfate monohydrate in water for injection with sodium chloride sufficient to render the solution isotonic. It is administered parenterally by subcutaneous, intramuscular or intravenous injection.

Each milliliter (mL) contains Atropine Sulfate, monohydrate 0.1 mg (adult strength) or 0.05 mg (pediatric strength), and sodium chloride, 9 mg. May contain sodium hydroxide and/or sulfuric acid for pH adjustment 0.308 mOsmol/mL (calc.). pH 4.2 (3.0 to 6.5).

The solution contains no bacteriostat, antimicrobial agent or added buffer (except for pH adjustment) and is intended for use only as a single-dose injection. When smaller doses are required the unused portion should be discarded.

Atropine Sulfate Injectable is a parenteral anticholinergic agent and muscarinic antagonist.

Atropine Sulfate Injectable is chemically designated 1α H, 5α H-Tropan-3-α ol (±)-tropate (ester), sulfate (2:1) (salt) monohydrate, $(C_{17}H_{23}NO_3)_2 \cdot H_2SO_4 \cdot H_2O$, colorless crystals or white crystalline powder very soluble in water.

Atropine, a naturally occurring belladonna alkaloid, is a racemic mixture of equal parts of d- and l-hyocyamine, whose activity is due almost entirely to the levo isomer of the drug.

Sodium Chloride is chemically designated NaCl, a white crystalline powder freely soluble in water.

Following is its chemical structure:

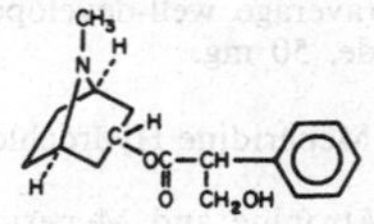

CLINICAL PHARMACOLOGY

Atropine Sulfate Injectable is commonly classified as an anticholinergic or antiparasympathetic (parasympatholytic) drug. More precisely, however, it is termed an antimuscarinic agent since it antagonizes the muscarine-like actions of acetylcholine and other choline esters.

Atropine inhibits the muscarinic actions of acetylcholine on structures innervated by postganglionic cholinergic nerves, and on smooth muscles which respond to endogenous acetylcholine but are not so innervated. As with other antimuscarinic agents, the major action of atropine is a competitive or surmountable antagonism which can be overcome by increasing the concentration of acetylcholine at receptor sites of the effector organ (e.g., by using anticholinesterase agents which inhibit the enzymatic destruction of acetylcholine). The receptors antagonized by atropine are the peripheral structures that are stimulated or inhibited by muscarine (i.e., exocrine glands and smooth and cardiac muscle). Responses to postganglionic cholinergic nerve stimulation also may be inhibited by atropine but this occurs less readily than with responses to injected (exogenous) choline esters.

Atropine-induced parasympathetic inhibition may be preceded by a transient phase of stimulation, especially on the heart where small doses first slow the rate before characteristic tachycardia develops due to paralysis of vagal control. Atropine exerts a more potent and prolonged effect on heart, intestine and bronchial muscle than scopolamine, but its action on the iris, ciliary body and certain secretory glands is weaker than that of scopolamine. Unlike the latter, atropine in clinical doses does not depress the central nervous system but may stimulate the medulla and higher cerebral centers. Although mild vagal excitation occurs, the increased respiratory rate and (sometimes) increased depth of respiration produced by atropine are more probably the result of bronchiolar dilatation. Accordingly, atropine is an unreliable respiratory stimulant and large or repeated doses may depress respiration.

Adequate doses of atropine abolish various types of reflex vagal cardiac slowing or asystole. The drug also prevents or abolishes bradycardia or asystole produced by injection of choline esters, anticholinesterase agents or other parasympathomimetic drugs, and cardiac arrest produced by stimulation of the vagus. Atropine also may lessen the degree of partial heart block when vagal activity is an etiologic factor. In some patients with complete heart block, the idioventricular rate may be accelerated by Atropine; in others, the rate is stabilized. Occasionally a large dose may cause atrioventricular (A-V) block and nodal rhythm.

Atropine Sulfate Injectable in clinical doses counteracts the peripheral dilatation and abrupt decrease in blood pressure produced by choline esters. However, when given by itself, atropine does not exert a striking or uniform effect on blood vessels or blood pressure. Systemic doses slightly raise systolic and lower diastolic pressures and can produce significant postural hypotension. Such doses also slightly increase cardiac output and decrease central venous pressure. Occasionally, therapeutic doses dilate cutaneous blood vessels, particularly in the "blush" area (atropine flush), and may cause atropine "fever" due to suppression of sweat gland activity in infants and small children.

Atropine disappears rapidly from the blood following injection and is distributed throughout the body. Much of the drug is destroyed by enzymatic hydrolysis, particularly in the liver; from 13 to 50% is excreted unchanged in the urine. Traces are found in various secretions, including milk. Atropine readily crosses the placental barrier and enters the fetal circulation.

Sodium chloride added to render the solution isotonic for injection of the active ingredient is present in amounts insufficient to affect serum electrolyte balance of sodium (Na^+) and chloride (Cl^-) ions.

INDICATIONS AND USAGE

Atropine Sulfate Injectable is indicated (1) as an antisialogogue for preanesthetic medication to prevent or reduce secretions of the respiratory tract, (2) to restore cardiac rate and arterial pressure during anesthesia when vagal stimulation produced by intra-abdominal surgical traction causes a sudden decrease in pulse rate and cardiac action, (3) to lessen the degree of atrioventricular (A-V) heart block when increased vagal tone is a major factor in the conduction defect as in some cases due to digitalis, (4) to overcome severe bradycardia and syncope due to a hyperactive carotid sinus reflex, (5) as an antidote (with external cardiac massage) for cardiovascular collapse from the injudicious use of a choline ester (cholinergic) drug, (6) in the treatment of anticholinesterase poisoning from organophosphorus insecticides, and (7) as an antidote for the "rapid" type of mushroom poisoning due to the presence of the alkaloid, muscarine, in certain species of fungus such as *Amanita muscaria*.

UNLABELED USES
Atropine Sulfate is used alone or as an adjunct in the treatment of bronchial asthma and anoxic seizures.

CONTRAINDICATIONS

Atropine generally is contraindicated in patients with glaucoma, pyloric stenosis or prostatic hypertrophy, except in doses ordinarily used for preanesthetic medication.

◆ RATED THERAPEUTICALLY EQUIVALENT; ◇ THERAPEUTIC EQUIVALENCE UNCONFIRMED; ○ UNRATED

WARNINGS

Atropine is a highly potent drug and due care is essential to avoid overdosage, especially with intravenous administration. Children are more susceptible than adults to the toxic effects of anticholinergic agents.

PRECAUTIONS

Do not administer unless solution is clear and seal is intact.
Discard unused portion.

Atropine Sulfate Injectable should be used with caution in all individuals over 40 years of age. Conventional systemic doses may precipitate acute glaucoma in susceptible patients, convert partial organic pyloric stenosis into complete obstruction, lead to complete urinary retention in patients with prostatic hypertrophy or cause inspissation of bronchial secretions and formation of dangerous viscid plugs in patients with chronic lung disease.

Pregnancy Category C: Animal reproduction studies have not been conducted with atropine. It also is not known whether atropine can cause fetal harm when given to a pregnant woman or can affect reproduction capacity. Atropine should be given to a pregnant woman only if clearly needed.

ADVERSE REACTIONS

Most of the side effects of atropine are directly related to its antimuscarinic action. Dryness of the mouth, blurred vision, photophobia and tachycardia commonly occur with chronic administration of therapeutic doses. Anhidrosis also may occur and produce heat intolerance or impair temperature regulation in persons living in a hot environment. Constipation and difficulty in micturition may occur in elderly patients. Occasional hypersensitivity reactions have been observed, especially skin rashes which in some instances progressed to exfoliation.

Adverse effects following single or repeated injections of atropine are most often the result of excessive dosage. These include palpitation, dilated pupils, difficulty in swallowing, hot dry skin, thirst, dizziness, restlessness, tremor, fatigue and ataxia. Toxic doses lead to marked palpitation, restlessness and excitement, hallucinations, delirium and coma. Depression and circulatory collapse occur only with severe intoxication. In such cases, blood pressure declines and death due to respiratory failure may ensue following paralysis and coma.

OVERDOSAGE

In the event of toxic overdosage (see *"Adverse Reactions"*), a short acting barbiturate or diazepam may be given as needed to control marked excitement and convulsions. Large doses for sedation should be avoided because central depressant action may coincide with the depression occurring late in atropine poisoning. Central stimulants are not recommended. Physostigmine, given as an atropine antidote by slow intravenous injection of 1 to 4 mg (0.5 to 1.0 mg in children), rapidly abolishes delirium and coma caused by large doses of atropine. Since physostigmine is rapidly destroyed, the patient may again lapse into coma after one to two hours, and repeated doses may be required. Artificial respiration with oxygen may be necessary. Ice bags and alcohol sponges help to reduce fever, especially in children.

The fatal adult dose of atropine is not known; 200 mg doses have been used and doses as high as 1000 mg have been given.

In children, 10 mg or less may be fatal. With a dose as low as 0.5 mg, undesirable minimal symptoms or responses of overdosage may occur. These increase in severity and extent with larger doses of the drug (excitement, hallucinations, delirium and coma with a dose of 10 mg or more).

DOSAGE AND ADMINISTRATION

Atropine Sulfate Injectable may be administered subcutaneously, intramuscularly or intravenously. The average adult dose is 0.5 mg (5 mL of a 0.1 mg/mL solution), range 0.4 to 0.6 mg (4 to 6 mL). As an antisialogogue it is usually injected intramuscularly prior to induction of anesthesia. This produces only minimal blocking of vagal activity. In children, the dosage ranges from 0.1 mg (2 mL of a a 0.05 mg solution) in the newborn to 0.06 mg (6 mL of a 0.1 mg/mL solution) in a child age 12 years, injected subcutaneously 30 minutes before surgery. During surgery, the drug is given intravenously when reduction in pulse rate and cessation of cardiac action are due to increased vagal activity; however, if the anesthetic is cyclopropane, doses less than 0.4 mg should be used and should be given slowly to avoid the possible production of ventricular arrhythmia. Usual doses are used to reduce severe bradycardia and syncope associated with hyperactive carotid sinus reflex. For bradyarrhythmias the usual intravenous adult dosage ranges from 0.4 to 1 mg (4 to 10 mL of a 0.1 mg/mL solution) every one to two hours as needed; larger doses up to a maximum of 2 mg may be required. In children, intravenous dosage ranges from 0.01 to 0.03 mg (0.2 to 0.6 mL of a 0.05 mg/mL solution) per kg of body weight. Atropine is also a specific antidote for cardiovascular collapse resulting from injudicious administration of choline ester. When cardiac arrest has occurred, external cardiac massage or other method of resuscitation is required to distribute the drug after intravenous injection.

In anticholinesterase poisoning from exposure to insecticides, large doses of at least 2 to 3 mg (20 to 30 mL of a 0.1 mg/mL solution) should be administered parenterally and repeated until signs of atropine intoxication appear. In the "rapid" type of mushroom poisoning, atropine should be given in doses sufficient to control parasympathomimetic signs before coma and cardiovascular collapse supervene.

Parenteral drug products should be inspected visually for particulate matter and discoloration prior to administration, whenever solution and container permit. See *"Precautions"*.

Store at controlled room temperature, 15° to 30°C (59° to 86°F).

J CODES
Up to 0.3 mg IV,IM,SC—J0460

HOW SUPPLIED
INJECTION: 0.05 MG/ML

BRAND/MANUFACTURER	NDC	SIZE	AWP
◆ GENERICS			
Abbott Hosp	00074-7897-01	5 ml 10s	$92.86

INJECTION: 0.1 MG/ML

AVERAGE UNIT PRICE (AVAILABLE SIZES)			
GENERIC	$1.78		

BRAND/MANUFACTURER	NDC	SIZE	AWP
◆ GENERICS			
Abbott Hosp	00074-4910-01	5 ml 10s	$117.44
Abbott Hosp	00074-4911-01	10 ml 10s	$121.24

INJECTION: 0.4 MG/ML

AVERAGE UNIT PRICE (AVAILABLE SIZES)			
GENERIC	$0.59		

BRAND/MANUFACTURER	NDC	SIZE	AWP
◆ GENERICS			
Fujisawa	00469-1234-25	1 ml	$1.12
Fujisawa	00469-0234-25	20 ml	$1.33

INJECTION: 0.5 MG/ML

BRAND/MANUFACTURER	NDC	SIZE	AWP
◆ GENERICS			
Fujisawa	00469-0243-25	1 ml	$1.33

INJECTION: 1 MG/ML

BRAND/MANUFACTURER	NDC	SIZE	AWP
◆ GENERICS			
Fujisawa	00469-0246-25	1 ml	$1.12

Atropine Sulfate, Ophthalmic

DESCRIPTION

Atropine Sulfate Ophthalmic Solution, 1% USP, and Atropine Sulfate Ophthalmic Ointment, 1% USP, are sterile topical anticholinergics for ophthalmic use.

Its molecular formula is $(C_{17}H_{23}NO_3)_2.H_2SO_4.H_2O$ and its molecular weight is 694.84.

Chemical name: Benzeneacetic acid, α-(hydroxymethyl)-,8-methyl-8- azabicyclo-(3,2.1)oct-3-yl ester, *endo-*(±)-, sulfate (2:1) (salt), mono- hydrate.

Each mL Contains: Atropine Sulfate Ophthalmic Solution, 1%, USP, contains in each mL of solution: Atropine Sulfate, USP, 1% (10mg).

Each Gram Contains: Atropine Sulfate Ophthalmic Ointment, 1%, USP, contains in each gram of ointment Atropine Sulfate, USP, 1% (10mg).

CHEMICAL PHARMACOLOGY

The anticholinergic effect of this product blocks the responses of the sphincter muscle of the iris and the accommodative muscle of the ciliary body to cholinergic stimulation, producing pupiliary dilation (mydriasis) and paralysis of accommodation (cycloplegia).

INDICATIONS AND USAGE

For mydriasis and/or cycloplegia. For cycloplegic refraction, for pupillary dilation desired in inflammatory conditions of the iris and uveal tract.

CONTRAINDICATIONS

This product should not be used in patients with primary glaucoma or a predisposition to narrow anterior chamber angle glaucoma. This product should not be used in children who have previously had a severe systemic reaction to Atropine. This product should not be used in those persons showing hypersensitivity to any component of this preparation.

WARNINGS

For topical use only — not for injection. Do not touch dropper tip to any surface, as this may contaminate the solution. In infants and small children, use with extreme caution. Excessive use in children or in certain individuals with a previous history of susceptibility to belladonna alkaloids may produce systemic symptoms of Atropine poisoning. If this occurs, discontinue medication, and use appropriate therapy as outlined in *"Overdosage"* section.

PRECAUTIONS

To avoid excessive systemic absorption, the lacrimal sac should be compressed by digital pressure for two to three minutes after installation. To avoid inducing angle closure glaucoma, an estimation of the depth of the angle of the anterior chamber should be made. Administration of Atropine in infants requires great caution.

Patient Warning: Patients should be advised not to drive or engage in other hazardous activities while pupils are dilated. Patients may experience sensitivity to light and should protect eyes in bright illumination during dilation.

Parents should be warned not to get this preparation in their children's mouth and to wash their own hands and the child's hands following administration.

Carcinogenesis, Mutagenesis, Impairment of Fertility: No studies have been conducted in animals or in humans to evaluate the potential of these effects.

Pregnancy Category C: Animal reproduction studies have not been performed with Atropine. It is also not known whether Atropine can cause fetal harm when administered to a pregnant woman or can affect reproduction capacity. Atropine should be given to pregnant women only if clearly needed.

Pediatric Use: (See *"Contraindications"* and *"Warnings"* sections.)

ADVERSE REACTIONS

Prolonged use may produce local irritation characterized by follicular conjunctivitis, vascular congestion, adema, exudate, and an aczematoid dermatitis. Severe reactions are manifested by hypotension with progressive respiratory depression. Coma and death have been reported in the very young.

OVERDOSAGE

Systemic atropine toxicity is manifested by flushing and dryness of the skin (a rash may be present in children), blurred vision, a rapid and irregular pulse, fever, abdominal distinsion in infants, mental aberration (hallucinosis) and loss of neuromuscular coordination.

Atropine poisoning, although distressing, is rarely fatal, even with large doses of Atropine, and is self-limited if the cause is recognized and the Atropine medication is discontinued. In severe intoxication, physostigmine salicylate may be administered parenterally to provide more prompt relief of the intoxication. Give physostigmine salicylate as 1-5 mL IV of dilution containing 1 mg in 5 mL of saline. The smaller dose is for children, and injection should take not less than two minutes. EKG control is advisable. Dosage can be repeated every five minutes up to a total dose of 2 mg in children and 6 mg in adults every 30 minutes. Physostigmine is contraindicated in hypotensive reactions. Atropine (1 mg) should be available for immediate injection if physostigmine causes bradycardia, convulsions or bronchconstriction. In infants and small children, the body surface must be kept moist.

Use extreme caution when employing short-acting barbiturates to control excitement.

DOSAGE AND ADMINISTRATION

Atropine Sulfate Solution: 1 or 2 drops in the eye(s) three times or as directed by a physician.

Atropine Sulfate Ointment: A small amount in the conjunctival sac once or twice a day or as directed by a physician.

FOR OPHTHALMIC USE ONLY

Storage: Store at controlled room temperature, 15° - 30°C (59° - 86°F).

KEEP OUT OF REACH OF CHILDREN.

HOW SUPPLIED

DROP: 0.5%

BRAND/MANUFACTURER	NDC	SIZE	AWP
○ **BRAND**			
ISOPTO ATROPINE: Alcon Ophthalmic	00998-0302-05	5 ml	$9.38

For additional alternatives, turn to the section beginning on page 2859.

Atropine Sulfate, Oral

DESCRIPTION

Atropine is a white, crystalline alkaloid that may be extracted from belladonna root and hyoscyamine or may be produced synthetically. It is used in the form of Atropine Sulfate because this compound has much greater solubility in water.

Atropine Sulfate is an anticholinergic drug. The empirical formula of Atropine Sulfate is $(C_{17}H_{23}NO_3)_2 \cdot H_2SO_4 \cdot H_2O$, and the molecular weight is 694.84.

Atropine Sulfate, Oral, is intended for oral use only. Each tablet contains Atropine Sulfate 0.4 mg (0.58 μmol).

CLINICAL PHARMACOLOGY

Atropine has 2 main actions. The most important therapeutic action is the inhibition of smooth muscle and glands innervated by postganglionic cholinergic nerves. Atropine also has central-nervous-system activity, which may be either stimulating or depressing depending on the dose.

Following the administration of usual clinical doses (0.5 to 1 mg), Atropine produces stimulation of the medulla and higher cerebral centers. This effect is manifested by mild central vagal excitation and moderate respiratory stimulation.

In addition to its effect on the central nervous system, Atropine Sulfate acts peripherally as a competitive antagonist of the muscarinic actions of acetylcholine. It does not prevent the release of acetylcholine but antagonizes the effect of acetylcholine on the effector cells. These actions include vasodilation; drying of the mouth; increase in pulse rate; inhibition of contractions of the gastrointestinal tract, ureter, and bladder; and reduction of salivary, bronchial, gastric, and sweat gland secretions. Following clinical and larger doses, Atropine Sulfate causes dilation of the pupils (mydriasis) and paralysis of accommodation (cycloplegia) and, in narrow-angle glaucoma, can increase intraocular pressure.

INDICATIONS AND USAGE

Atropine Sulfate, Oral, is used to reduce salivation and bronchial secretions.

The antispasmodic action of Atropine Sulfate, Oral, is useful in pylorospasm and other spastic conditions of the gastrointestinal tract. For ureteral and biliary colic, concomitant use of Atropine and morphine may be indicated.

CONTRAINDICATIONS

Glaucoma; adhesions (synechiae) between the iris and lens of the eye; asthma.

PRECAUTIONS

General: Doses of 0.5 to 1 mg of Atropine are mildly stimulating to the central nervous system. Larger doses may produce mental disturbances; still larger doses are depressing. Death from Atropine poisoning, though rare, is usually due to paralysis of the medullary centers.

Information for Patients: When used in therapeutic doses, Atropine can cause dryness of the mouth. This effect is additive when the product is administered with other drugs that can cause dryness of the mouth.

Patients with prostatism can have difficulty urinating and may require catheterization.

Patients receiving chronic treatment can develop blurred vision and should not be involved in activities that require clear vision.

Drug Interactions: Since Atropine Sulfate slows gastric emptying and gastrointestinal motility, it may interfere with the absorption of other medications. The potential of Atropine to cause mouth dryness may be increased if it is given with other drugs that have anticholinergic action (tricyclic antidepressants, antipsychotics, some antihistamines, and antiparkinsonism drugs).

Usage in Pregnancy. Pregnancy Category C: Animal reproduction studies have not been conducted with Atropine Sulfate. It is also not known whether Atropine Sulfate can cause fetal harm when administered to a pregnant woman or can affect reproduction capacity. Atropine Sulfate should be given to a pregnant woman only if clearly needed.

Nursing Mothers: Caution should be exercised when Atropine Sulfate is administered to a nursing woman.

ADVERSE REACTIONS

Individual tolerance varies greatly, but these systemic doses are likely to produce the following effects:

0.5 mg: Slight dryness of nose and mouth; bradycardia.

1 mg: Greater dryness of nose and mouth with thirst; slowing, then acceleration of heart; slight mydriasis.

2 mg: Very dry mouth; tachycardia with palpitations; mydriasis, slight blurring of near vision; flushed dry skin.

5 mg: Increase in above symptoms plus disturbance of speech; difficulty in swallowing; headache; hot, dry skin; restlessness with asthenia.

10 mg and over: Above symptoms to extreme degree plus ataxia, excitement, disorientation, hallucinations, delirium, and coma.

A scarlatiniform rash may occur. Atropine may produce fever, particularly in children, through inhibition of heat loss by evaporation. Although large doses of Atropine may cause an alarming condition, recovery is usual.

OVERDOSAGE

Signs and Symptoms: Symptoms of Atropine overdose include mydriasis, tachycardia, decreased salivation and sweating, diminished bowel sounds, urinary retention, hypertension, and vasodilation. CNS symptoms include anxiety, disorientation, hallucinations, hyperactivity, and convulsions or coma. Hyperthermia may occur.

Treatment: To obtain up-to-date information about the treatment of overdose, a good resource is your certified regional poison control center. Telephone numbers of certified poison control centers are listed in the *Physicians' Desk Reference (PDR)*. In managing overdosage consider the possibility of multiple drug overdoses, interaction among drugs, and unusual drug kinetics in your patient.

The fatal dose of Atropine in children may be as low as 10 mg. In an adult, a dose of 10 mg usually produces severe distress, but recovery after 1,000 mg has

---

◆ RATED THERAPEUTICALLY EQUIVALENT; ◇ THERAPEUTIC EQUIVALENCE UNCONFIRMED; ○ UNRATED

been reported. Information is scant on serum concentrations that may be toxic or lethal. The oral median lethal dose in rats is 622 mg/kg.

Protect the patient's airway and support ventilation and perfusion. Meticulously monitor and maintain, within acceptable limits, the patient's vital signs, blood gases, serum electrolytes, etc. Absorption of drugs from the gastrointestinal tract may be decreased by giving activated charcoal, which, in many cases, is more effective than emesis or lavage; consider charcoal instead of or in addition to gastric emptying. Repeated doses of charcoal over time may hasten elimination of some drugs that have been absorbed. Safeguard the patient's airway when employing gastric emptying or charcoal.

Physostigmine may reverse some of the effects of Atropine overdose in some patients, but it should be used cautiously while closely monitoring and supporting the patient's airway, ventilation, and cardiac rhythm. Cholinergic toxicity from physostigmine may include bronchospasm, bronchorrhea, bradycardia, asystole, diaphoresis, incontinence, and seizures. If used, give physostigmine slowly because rapid injection may cause seizures. The effects of physostigmine may be short-lived and repeated doses may be necessary for continued improvement.

Forced diuresis, peritoneal dialysis, hemodialysis, or charcoal hemoperfusion have not been established as beneficial for an overdose of Atropine.

DOSAGE AND ADMINISTRATION
The usual oral adult dose of Atropine is 0.4 mg.

Suggested doses for children are as follows:

7-16 lb.—0.1 mg
17-24 lb.—0.15 mg
24-40 lb.—0.2 mg
40-65 lb.—0.3 mg
65-90 lb.—0.4 mg
Over 90 lb.—0.4 mg

These doses may be exceeded in certain cases.

HOW SUPPLIED
TABLETS: 0.4 MG

BRAND/MANUFACTURER	NDC	SIZE	AWP
○ **GENERICS**			
SAL-TROPINE: Hope	60267-0742-30	100s	$26.95

Atropine Sulfate/Benzoic Acid/ Hyoscyamine/Methenamine/ Methylene Blue/Phenyl Salicylate

DESCRIPTION
This product is a combination of antiseptics (Methenamine, Methylene Blue, Phenyl Salicylate, Benzoic Acid) and parasympatholytics (Atropine Sulfate, Hyoscyamine).

Each tablet contains: Methenamine 40.8 mg. Phenyl Salicylate 18.1 mg, Methylene Blue 5.4 mg, Benzoic Acid 4.5 mg, Atropine Sulfate 0.03 mg and Hyoscyamine 0.03 mg.

CLINICAL PHARMACOLOGY
Methenamine itself does not have antiseptic, irritant, or toxic properties in the urine. Methenamine, in an acid urine (pH 6 or below), hydrolyzes into formaldehyde within the urinary tract providing mild antiseptic activity.[1] When given as directed and the daily urine volume is 1000 to 1500 mL, a daily dose of 2 grams will yield a urinary concentration of 18-60 mcg/mL of free formaldehyde in the urine. This is more than the minimal inhibitory dose of formaldehyde which must be available for most urinary tract pathogens. Methenamine is readily absorbed from the gastrointestinal tract and is rapidly excreted almost entirely in the urine. Methylene Blue and Benzoic Acid are mild but effective antiseptics which contribute to the antiseptic properties of Methenamine. Phenyl Salicylate is a mild analgesic and antipyretic with weak antiseptic activity. All of these compounds are readily absorbed from the gastrointestinal tract and excreted in the urine. Through parasympatholytic action, Atropine and Hyoscyamine relax smooth muscle spasms resulting from parasympathetic stimulation.[2]

INDICATIONS AND USAGE
This combination is indicated for the relief of discomfort of the lower urinary tract caused by hypermotility resulting from inflammation or diagnostic procedures and in the treatment of cystitis, urethritis, and trigonitis when caused by organisms which maintain or produce an acid urine and are susceptible to formaldehyde.

CONTRAINDICATIONS
Glaucoma, urinary bladder neck obstruction, pyloric or duodenal obstruction, or cardiospasm. Hypersensitivity to any of the ingredients.

WARNINGS
Do not exceed recommended dose. Methenamine may combine with sulfonamides in the urine to give mutual antagonism and should not be used with sulfonamides.

PRECAUTIONS
Administer with caution to persons with known idiosyncrasy to Atropine-like compounds and to patients suffering from cardiac disease. Bacteriological studies of the urine may be helpful in following the patient response. Methylene Blue interferes with the analysis for some urinary components such as free formaldehyde. Drugs and/or foods which produce an alkaline urine should be restricted.[3]

Patient should be advised that the urine may become blue to blue-green and the feces may be discolored as a result of excretion of Methylene Blue. Methenamine preparations should not be given to patients taking sulfonamides since insoluble precipitates may form with formaldehyde in the urine. No known long-term animal studies have been performed to evaluate carcinogenic potential. The precautions related to drug interaction, diagnostic interference, medical problems and side effects to use of belladonna alkaloids, should be observed.

Pregnancy Category C: Animal reproduction studies have not been conducted with this combination. It is also not known whether this combination can cause fetal harm when administered to a pregnant woman or can affect reproduction capacity. This combination should be given to a pregnant woman only if clearly needed.

Nursing Mothers: It is not known whether this drug is excreted in human milk. Because many drugs are excreted in human milk, caution should be exercised when these combination tablets are administered to a nursing woman.

Prolonged Use: There have been no studies to establish the safety of prolonged use in humans.

ADVERSE REACTIONS
Prolonged use may result in a generalized skin rash, pronounced dryness of the mouth, flushing, difficulty in initiating micturition, rapid pulse, dizziness or blurring of vision. If any of these reactions occurs, discontinue use immediately. Acute urinary retention may be precipitated in prostatic hypertrophy. See *"Overdosage"*.

DRUG ABUSE AND DEPENDENCE
A dependence on the use of this combination has not been reported and due to the nature of its ingredients, abuse of this combination is not expected.

OVERDOSAGE
By exceeding the recommended dosage of this combination, symptomology related to the overdose of its individual active ingredients may be expected as follows:

Atropine Sulfate, Hyoscyamine: Symptoms associated with an overdose of this combination will most probably be manifested in the symptoms related to overdosage of the alkaloids Atropine Sulfate and Hyoscyamine. Such symptoms as dryness of mucous membranes; dilation of pupils; hot, dry, flushed skin; hyperpyrexia; tachycardia; palpitations; elevated blood pressure; coma; circulatory collapse and death from respiratory failure can occur due to overdosage of these alkaloids.

Methenamine: If large amounts of the drug (2-8 gm daily) are used over extended periods (3-4 weeks), bladder and gastrointestinal irritation, painful and frequent micturition, albuminuria and gross hematuria may be expected.

Methylene Blue: Symptoms of Methylene Blue overdose associated with the overdosage of this combination are not expected to be discernible from those associated with the other active ingredients in this combination.

Benzoic Acid: Symptoms of Benzoic Acid overdosage associated with the overdosage of this combination are not expected to be discernible from those associated with the other active ingredients in this combination.

Phenyl Salicylate: Symptoms of Phenyl Salicylate overdosage include burning pain in throat and mouth, white necrotic lesions in the mouth, abdominal pain, vomiting, bloody diarrhea, pallor, sweating, weakness, headache, dizziness and tinnitus. The symptoms, however, are not expected to be discernible from those associated with the other active ingredients in this combination.

DOSAGE AND ADMINISTRATION
Adults: Two tablets four times daily. See *"Precautions"*.

Usual pediatric dosage: Children up to 6 years of age—Use is not recommended. Children 6 years of age and older—Dosage must be individualized by physician.

Storage: Store in a dry place at room temperature.

HOW SUPPLIED
TABLET:

BRAND/MANUFACTURER	NDC	SIZE	AWP
○ **BRAND**			
TRAC TABS 2X: Hyrex	00314-0408-01	100s	$15.90
URISED: Polymedica	00998-2183-10	100s	$40.94
	00998-2183-20	500s	$191.94
TRAC TABS 2X: Hyrex	00314-0408-10	1000s	$134.00
○ **GENERICS**			
URL	00677-1393-01	100s	$8.95
U-SEPT: Pharmacist's Choice	54979-0145-01	100s	$8.95
Eon	00185-0230-01	100s	$8.95

➤ SHOWN IN PRODUCT IDENTIFICATION GUIDE

BRAND/MANUFACTURER	NDC	SIZE	AWP
UAA: EconoMed	38130-0046-01	100s	$8.98
ATROSEPT: Geneva	00781-1341-01	100s	$8.99
Alphagen	59743-0016-01	100s	$9.05
URITIN: Goldline	00182-0850-01	100s	$9.75
Qualitest	00603-6311-21	100s	$9.78
URIDON MODIFIED: Rugby	00536-4757-01	100s	$9.89
URAPINE: Major	00904-3286-60	100s	$10.60
URI-SEP SC: Moore,H.L.	00839-7796-06	100s	$12.08
URETRON: Marin	12539-0110-01	100s	$18.00
URIMAR T: Marnel	00682-0333-01	100s	$24.50
URETRON DS: Marin	12539-0144-01	100s	$26.65
URO BLUE: McNeil,R.A.	12830-0301-01	100s	$27.40
DOLSED: Amer Urological	00539-0708-01	100s	$29.69
PROSED/DS: Star	00076-0108-03	100s	$36.96
Parmed	00349-2345-10	1000s	$55.89
CYSTEMMS-V: Truxton	00463-6259-10	1000s	$56.00
URIDON MODIFIED: Rugby	00536-4757-10	1000s	$60.94
Qualitest	00603-6311-32	1000s	$65.11
URAPINE: Major	00904-3286-80	1000s	$71.95
ATROSEPT: Geneva	00781-1341-10	1000s	$80.91
U-SEPT: Pharmacist's Choice	54979-0145-10	1000s	$84.50
UAA: EconoMed	38130-0046-10	1000s	$84.75
Eon	00185-0230-10	1000s	$84.95
Alphagen	59743-0016-10	1000s	$86.40
URI-SEP SC: Moore,H.L.	00839-7796-16	1000s	$107.99
DOLSED: Amer Urological	00539-0708-10	1000s	$202.50

Atropine Sulfate/Hyoscyamine Sulfate/Pancreatic Enzymes/ Phenobarbital

COMPOSITION
Same as Pancreatic Enzymes plus the addition of Hyoscyamine Sulfate 0.10 mg., Atropine Sulfate 0.02 mg. and Phenobarbital ⅛ gr. (Warning: may be habit forming).

ACTION AND USES
Gastrointestinal disturbances, such as cramps, bloating, spasms, diarrhea, nausea, vomiting and peptic ulcer. The enzymes correct the digestive insufficiencies.

The antispasmodic and phenobarbital contribute to the symptomatic relief of hypermotility and nervous tension, which usually accompanies functional disturbances of the bowel.

ADMINISTRATION AND DOSAGE
One tablet following meals.

SIDE EFFECTS
May cause rapid pulse, dryness of mouth and blurred vision.

CONTRAINDICATIONS
This product is contraindicated in the presence of glaucoma or prostatic hypertrophy.

HOW SUPPLIED
TABLETS:

BRAND/MANUFACTURER	NDC	SIZE	AWP
○ BRAND			
ARCO-LASE PLUS: Arco	00275-0045-02	50s	$5.00

Atropine and Demerol SEE ATROPINE SULFATE AND MEPERIDINE HYDROCHLORIDE

Atropisol SEE ATROPINE SULFATE, OPHTHALMIC

Atrovent SEE IPRATROPIUM BROMIDE

A/T/S SEE ERYTHROMYCIN, TOPICAL

Attenuvax SEE MEASLES VIRUS VACCINE

Augmentin SEE AMOXICILLIN WITH CLAVULANATE POTASSIUM

Auralgan SEE ANTIPYRINE AND BENZOCAINE

Auranofin

AURANOFIN CONTAINS GOLD AND, LIKE OTHER GOLD-CONTAINING DRUGS, CAN CAUSE GOLD TOXICITY, SIGNS OF WHICH INCLUDE: FALL IN HEMOGLOBIN, LEUKOPENIA BELOW 4,000 WBC/CU MM, GRANULOCYTES BELOW 1,500/CU MM, DECREASE IN PLATELETS BELOW 150,000/CU MM, PROTEINURIA, HEMATURIA, PRURITUS, RASH, STOMATITIS OR PERSISTENT DIARRHEA. THEREFORE, THE RESULTS OF

RECOMMENDED LABORATORY WORK (SEE "PRECAUTIONS") SHOULD BE REVIEWED BEFORE WRITING EACH AURANOFIN PRESCRIPTION. LIKE OTHER GOLD PREPARATIONS, AURANOFIN IS ONLY INDICATED FOR USE IN SELECTED PATIENTS WITH ACTIVE RHEUMATOID ARTHRITIS. PHYSICIANS PLANNING TO USE AURANOFIN SHOULD BE EXPERIENCED WITH CHRYSOTHERAPY AND SHOULD THOROUGHLY FAMILIARIZE THEMSELVES WITH THE TOXICITY AND BENEFITS OF AURANOFIN.

IN ADDITION, THE FOLLOWING PRECAUTIONS SHOULD BE ROUTINELY EMPLOYED:

1. THE POSSIBILITY OF ADVERSE REACTIONS SHOULD BE EXPLAINED TO PATIENTS BEFORE STARTING THERAPY.

2. PATIENTS SHOULD BE ADVISED TO REPORT PROMPTLY ANY SYMPTOMS SUGGESTING TOXICITY. (SEE "PRECAUTIONS— INFORMATION FOR PATIENTS.").

DESCRIPTION
Auranofin is available in oral form as capsules containing 3 mg Auranofin.

Auranofin is (2,3,4,6-tetra-O-acetyl-1-thio-β-D-glycopyranosato-S-) (triethylphosphine) gold.

Auranofin contains 29% gold.

Following is its chemical structure:

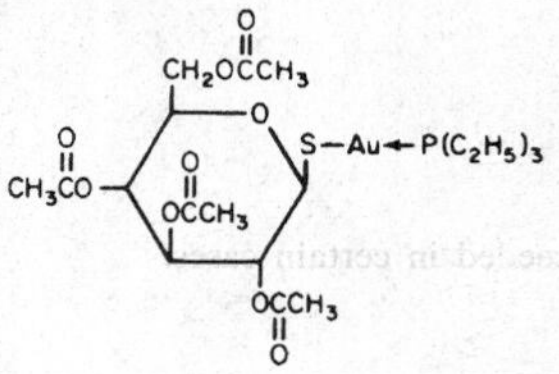

CLINICAL PHARMACOLOGY
The mechanism of action of Auranofin is not understood. In patients with adult rheumatoid arthritis, Auranofin may modify disease activity as manifested by synovitis and associated symptoms, and reflected by laboratory parameters such as ESR. There is no substantial evidence, however, that gold-containing compounds induce remission or rheumatoid arthritis.

Pharmacokinetics: Pharmacokinetic studies were performed in rheumatoid arthritis patients, not in normal volunteers. Auranofin is rapidly metabolized and intact Auranofin has never been detected in the blood. Thus, studies of the pharmacokinetics of Auranofin have involved measurement of gold concentrations. Approximately 25% of the gold in Auranofin is absorbed.

The mean terminal plasma half-life of Auranofin gold at steady state was 26 days (range 21 to 31 days; n = 5). The mean terminal body half-life was 80 days (range 42 to 128; n = 5). Approximately 60% of the absorbed gold (15% of the administered dose) from a single dose of Auranofin is excreted in urine; the remainder is excreted in the feces.

In clinical studies, steady state blood-gold concentrations are achieved in about three months. In patients on 6 mg Auranofin/day, mean steady state blood-gold concentrations were 0.68 ± 0.45 mcg/mL (n = 63 patients). In blood, approximately 40% of Auranofin gold is associated with red cells, and 60% associated with serum proteins. In contrast, 99% of injectable gold is associated with serum proteins.

Mean blood-gold concentrations are proportional to dose; however, no correlation between blood-gold concentrations and safety or efficacy has been established.

INDICATIONS AND USAGE
Auranofin is indicated in the management of adults with active classical or definite rheumatoid arthritis (ARA criteria) who have had an insufficient therapeutic response to, or are intolerant of, an adequate trial of full doses of one or more nonsteroidal anti-inflammatory drugs. Auranofin should be added to a comprehensive baseline program, including nondrug therapies.

Unlike anti-inflammatory drugs, Auranofin does not produce an immediate response. Therapeutic effects may be seen after three to four months of treatment, although improvement has not been seen in some patients before six months. When cartilage and bone damage has already occurred, gold cannot reverse structural damage to joints caused by previous disease. The greatest potential benefit occurs in patients with active synovitis, particularly in its early stage.

In controlled clinical trials comparing Auranofin with injectable gold, Auranofin was associated with fewer dropouts due to adverse reactions, while injectable gold was associated with fewer dropouts for inadequate or poor therapeutic effect. Physicians should consider these findings when deciding on the use of Auranofin in patients who are candidates for chrysotherapy.

UNLABELED USES:
Auranofin is used alone or as an adjunct in the treatment of asthma and psoriatic arthritis.

CONTRAINDICATIONS
Auranofin is contraindicated in patients with a history of any of the following gold-induced disorders anaphylactic reactions, necrotizing enterocolitis, pulmo-

nary fibrosis, exfoliative dermatitis, bone marrow aplasia or other severe hematologic disorders.

WARNINGS

Danger signs of possible gold toxicity include fall in hemoglobin, leukopenia below 4,000 WBC/cu mm, granulocytes below 1,500/cu mm, decrease in platelets below 150,000/cu mm, proteinuria, hematuria, pruritus, rash, stomatitis or persistent diarrhea.

Thrombocytopenia has occurred in 1-3% of patients (See "Adverse Reactions"), treated with Auranofin some of whom developed bleeding. The thrombocytopenia usually appears to be peripheral in origin and is usually reversible upon withdrawal of Auranofin. Its onset bears no relationship to the duration of Auranofin therapy and its course may be rapid. While patients' platelet counts should normally be monitored at least monthly (see "Precautions—Laboratory Tests"), the occurrence of a precipitous decline in platelets or a platelet count less than 100,000/cu mm or signs and symptoms (e.g., purpura, ecchymoses or petechiae) suggestive of thrombocytopenia indicates a need to immediately withdraw Auranofin and other therapies with the potential to cause thrombocytopenia, and to obtain additional platelet counts. No additional Auranofin should be given unless the thrombocytopenia resolves and further studies show it was not due to gold therapy.

Proteinuria has developed in 3-9% of patients (see "Adverse Reactions") treated with Auranofin. If clinically significant proteinuria or microscopic hematuria is found (See "Precautions—Laboratory Tests"), Auranofin and other therapies with the potential to cause proteinuria or microscopic hematuria should be stopped immediately.

PRECAUTIONS

General: The safety of concomitant use of Auranofin with injectable gold, hydroxychloroquine, penicillamine, immunosuppressive agents (e.g., cyclophosphamide, azathioprine, or methotrexate) or high doses of corticosteroids has not been established.

Medical problems that might affect the signs or symptoms used to detect Auranofin toxicity should be under control before starting Auranofin.

The potential benefits of using Auranofin in patients with progressive renal disease, significant hepatocellular disease, inflammatory bowel disease, skin rash or history of bone marrow depression should be weighed against 1) the potential risks of gold toxicity on organ systems previously compromised or with decreased reserve, and 2) the difficulty in quickly detecting and correctly attributing the toxic effect. The following adverse reactions have been reported with the use of gold preparations and require modification of Auranofin treatment or additional monitoring. See "Adverse Reactions" for the approximate incidence of those reactions specifically reported with Auranofin.

Gastrointestinal Reactions: Gastrointestinal reactions reported with gold therapy include diarrhea/loose stools, nausea, vomiting, anorexia and abdominal cramps. The most common reaction to Auranofin is diarrhea/loose stools reported in approximately 50% of the patients. This is generally manageable by reducing the dosage (e.g., from 6 mg daily to 3 mg) and in only 6% of the patients is it necessary to discontinue Auranofin permanently.

Ulcerative enterocolitis is a rare serious gold reaction. Therefore, patients with gastrointestinal symptoms should be monitored for the appearance of gastrointestinal bleeding.

Cutaneous Reactions: Dermatitis is the most common reaction to injectable gold therapy and the second most common reaction to Auranofin. Any eruption, especially if pruritic, that develops during treatment should be considered a gold reaction until proven otherwise. Pruritis often exists before dermatitis becomes apparent, and therefore should be considered to be a warning signal of a cutaneous reaction. Gold dermatitis may be aggravated by exposure to sunlight or an actinic rash may develop. The most serious form of cutaneous reaction reported with injectable gold is generalized exfoliative dermatitis.

Mucous Membrane Reactions: Stomatitis, another common gold reaction, may be manifested by shallow ulcers on the buccal membranes, on the borders of the tongue, and on the palate or in the pharynx. Stomatitis may occur as the only adverse reaction or with a dermatitis. Sometimes diffuse glossitis or gingivitis develops. A metallic taste may precede these oral mucous membrane reactions and should be considered a warning signal.

Renal Reactions: Gold can produce a nephrotic syndrome or glomerulitis with proteinuria and hematuria. These renal reactions are usually relatively mild and subside completely if recognized early and treatment is discontinued. They may become severe and chronic if treatment is continued after the onset of the reaction. Therefore it is important to perform urinalyses regularly and to discontinue treatment promptly if proteinuria or hematuria develops.

Hematologic Reactions: Blood dyscrasias including leukopenia, granulocytopenia, thrombocytopenia and aplastic anemia have all been reported as reactions to injectable gold and Auranofin. These reactions may occur separately or in combination at anytime during treatment. Because they have potentially serious consequences, blood dyscrasias should be constantly watched for through regular monitoring (at least monthly) of the formed elements of the blood throughout treatment.

Miscellaneous Reactions: Rare reactions attributed to gold include cholestatic jaundice; gold bronchitis and interstitial pneumonitis and fibrosis; peripheral neuropathy; partial or complete hair loss; fever.

Information for Patients: Patients should be advised of the possibility of toxicity from Auranofin and of the signs and symptoms that they should report promptly. (Patient information sheets are available.)

Women of childbearing potential should be warned of the potential risks of Auranofin therapy during pregnancy (See "Precautions—Pregnancy").

Laboratory Tests: CBC with differential, platelet count, urinalysis, and renal and liver function tests should be performed prior to Auranotin therapy to establish a baseline and to identify any preexisting conditions.

CBC with differential, platelet count and urinalysis should then be monitored at least monthly; other parameters should be monitored as appropriate.

Drug Interactions: In a single patient-report, there is the suggestion that concurrent administration of Auranofin and phenytoin may have increased phenytoin blood levels.

Carcinogenesis/Mutagenesis: In a 24-month study in rats, animals treated with Auranofin at 0.4, 1.0 or 2.5 mg/kg/day orally (3, 8 or 21 times the human dose) or gold sodium thiomalate at 2 or 6 mg/kg injected twice weekly (4 or 12 times the human dose) were compared to untreated control animals.

There was a significant increase in the frequency of renal tubular cell karyomegaly and cytomegaly and renal adenoma in the animals treated with 1.0 or 2.5 mg/kg/day of Auranofin and 2 or 6 mg/kg twice weekly of gold sodium thiomalate. Malignant renal epithelial tumors were seen in the 1.0 mg/kg/day and the 2.5 mg/kg/day Auranofin and in the 6 mg/kg twice weekly gold sodium thiomalate-treated animals.

In a 12-month study, rats treated with Auranofin at 23 mg/kg/day (192 times the human dose) developed tumors of the renal tubular epithelium, whereas those treated with 3.6 mg/kg/day (30 times the human dose) did not.

In an 18-month study in mice given oral Auranofin at doses of 1, 3 and 9 mg/kg/day (8, 24 and 72 times the human dose), there was no statistically significant increase above controls in the instances of tumors.

In the mouse lymphoma forward mutation assay, Auranofin at high concentrations (313 to 700 ng/mL) induced increases in the mutation frequencies in the presence of a rat liver microsomal preparation. Auranofin produced no mutation effects in the Ames test (Salmonella), in the in vitro assay (Forward and Reverse Mutation Inducement Assay with Saccharomyces), in the in vitro transformation of BALB/T3 cell mouse assay or in the Dominant Lethal Assay.

Pregnancy: Teratogenic Effects—Pregnancy Category C. Use of Auranofin by pregnant women is not recommended. Furthermore, women of childbearing potential should be warned of the potential risks of Auranofin therapy during pregnancy. (See below.)

Pregnant rabbits given Auranofin at doses of 0.5, 3 or 6 mg/kg/day (4.2 to 50 times the human dose) had impaired food intake, decreased maternal weights, decreased fetal weights and an increase above controls in the incidence of resorptions, abortions and congenital abnormalities, mainly abdominal defects such as gastroschisis and umbilical hernia.

Pregnant rats given Auranofin at a dose of 5 mg/kg/day (42 times the human dose) had an increase above controls in the incidence of resorptions and a decrease in litter size and weight linked to maternal toxicity. No such effects were found in rats given 2.5 mg/kg/day (21 times the human dose).

Pregnant mice given Auranofin at a dose of 5 mg/kg/day (42 times the human dose) had no teratogenic effects.

There are no adequate and well-controlled Auranofin studies in pregnant women.

Nursing Mothers: Nursing during Auranofin therapy is not recommended. Following Auranofin administration to rats and mice, gold is excreted in milk. Following the administration of injectable gold, gold appears in the milk of nursing women; human data on Auranofin are not available.

Pediatric Use: Auranofin is not recommended for use in children because its safety and effectiveness have not been established.

ADVERSE REACTIONS

The adverse reactions incidences listed below are based on observations of 1) 4,784 Auranofin-treated patients in clinical trials (2,474 U.S., 2,310 foreign), of whom 2,729 were treated more than one year and 573 for more than three years; and 2) postmarketing experience. The highest incidence is during the first six months of treatment; however, reactions can occur after many months of therapy. With rare exceptions, all patients were on concomitant nonsteroidal anti-inflammatory therapy; some of them were also taking low dosages of corticosteroids.

REACTIONS OCCURRING IN MORE THAN 1% OF AURANOFIN-TREATED PATIENTS

Gastrointestinal: loose stools or diarrhea (47%); abdominal pain (14%); nausea with or without vomiting (10%); constipation; anorexia*, flatulence*; dyspepsia*; dyegeusia.

Dermatological: rash (24%); pruritus (17%); hair loss; urticaria.

Mucous Membrane: stomatitis (13%); conjunctivitis*; glossitis.

Hematological: anemia; leukopenia; thrombocytopenia; eosinophilia.

Renal: proteinuria*; hematuria.

Hepatic: elevated liver enzymes.

---

* Reactions marked with an asterisk occurred in 3-9% of the patients. The other reactions listed occurred in 1-3%

REACTIONS OCCURRING IN LESS THAN 1% OF AURANOFIN-TREATED PATIENTS

Gastrointestinal: dysphagia; gastrointestinal bleeding[†], melena[†]; positive stool for occult blood[†]; ulcerative enterocolitis.

Dermatological: angioedema.

Mucous Membrane: gingivitis[†].

Hematological: aplastic anemia; neutropenia[†]; agranulocytosis; pure red cell aplasia; pancytopenia.

Hepatic: jaundice.

Respiratory: interstitial pneumonitis.

Neurological: peripheral neuropathy.

Ocular: gold deposits in the lens or cornea unassociated clinically with eye disorders or visual impairment.

REACTIONS REPORTED WITH INJECTABLE GOLD PREPARATIONS, BUT NOT WITH AURANOTIN (BASED ON CLINICAL TRIALS AND ON POSTMARKETING EXPERIENCE)
Cutaneous Reactions: generalized exfoliative dermatitis.

INCIDENCE OF ADVERSE REACTIONS FOR SPECIFIC CATEGORIES— 18 COMPARATIVE TRIALS

	Auranofin (445 patients)	Injectable Gold (445 patients)
Proteinuria	0.9%	5.4%
Rash	26 %	39 %
Diarrhea	42.5%	13 %
Stomatitis	13 %	18 %
Anemia	3.1%	2.7%
Leukopenia	1.3%	2.2%
Thrombocytopenia	0.9%	2.2%
Elevated liver function tests	1.9%	1.7%
Pulmonary	0.2%	0.2%

OVERDOSAGE
The acute oral LD$_{50}$ for Auranofin is 310 mg/kg in adult mice and 265 mg/kg in adult rats. The minimum lethal dose in rats is 30 mg/kg.

In case of acute overdosage, immediate induction of emesis or gastric lavage and appropriate supportive therapy are recommended.

Auranofin overdosage experience is limited. A 50-year-old female, previously on 6 mg Auranofin daily, took 27 mg (9 capsules) daily for 10 days and developed an encephalopathy and peripheral neuropathy. Auranofin was discontinued and she eventually recovered.

There has been no experience with treating Auranofin overdosage with modalities such as chelating agents. However, they have been used with injectable gold and may be considered for Auranofin overdosage.

DOSAGE AND ADMINISTRATION
Usual Adult Dosage: The usual adult dosage of Auranofin is 6 mg daily, given either as 3 mg twice daily or 6 mg once daily. Initiation of therapy at dosages exceeding 6 mg daily is not recommended because it is associated with an increased incidence of diarrhea. If response is inadequate after six months, an increase to 9 mg (3 mg three times daily) may be tolerated. If response remains inadequate after a three-month trial of 9 mg daily, Auranofin therapy should be discontinued. Safety at dosages exceeding 9 mg daily has not been studied.

Transferring from Injectable Gold: In controlled clinical studies, patients on injectable gold have been transferred to Auranofin by discontinuing the injectable agent and starting oral therapy with Auranofin, 6 mg daily. When patients are transferred to Auranofin they should be informed of its adverse reaction profile, in particular the gastrointestinal reactions. (See *"Precautions—Information for Patients."*) At six months, control of disease activity of patients transferred to Auranofin and those maintained on the injectable agent was not different. Data beyond six months are not available.

Storage: Store at controlled room temperature (59°-86°F). Dispense in a tight, light-resistant container.

HOW SUPPLIED
CAPSULE: 3 MG

BRAND/MANUFACTURER	NDC	SIZE	AWP
○ BRAND			
RIDAURA: SK Beecham Pharm	00007-4879-18	60s	$65.80

Aureomycin *SEE* CHLORTETRACYCLINE
HYDROCHLORIDE

[†] Reactions marked with a dagger occurred in 0.1-1% of the patients. The other reactions listed occurred in less than 0.1%.

Aurolate *SEE* GOLD SODIUM THIOMALATE

Aurothioglucose

> **WARNINGS**
> PHYSICIANS PLANNING TO USE AUROTHIOGLUCOSE SUSPENSION SHOULD THOROUGHLY FAMILIARIZE THEMSELVES WITH ITS TOXICITY AND ITS BENEFITS. THE POSSIBILITY OF TOXIC REACTIONS SHOULD ALWAYS BE EXPLAINED TO THE PATIENT BEFORE STARTING THERAPY. PATIENTS SHOULD BE WARNED TO REPORT PROMPTLY ANY SYMPTOM SUGGESTING TOXICITY. BEFORE *EACH* INJECTION OF AURO-THIOGLUCOSE SUSPENSION, THE PHYSICIAN SHOULD REVIEW THE RESULTS OF LABORATORY WORK AND SEE THE PATIENT TO DETERMINE THE PRESENCE OR ABSENCE OF ADVERSE REACTIONS, SINCE SOME OF THESE CAN BE SEVERE OR EVEN FATAL.

DESCRIPTION
Aurothioglucose is a sterile suspension, for **intramuscular injection only**. Aurothioglucose Suspension is an antiarthritic agent which is absorbed gradually following intramuscular injection, producing a therapeutically desired prolonged effect.

The empirical formula for Aurothioglucose is $C_6H_{11}AuO_5S$; the molecular weight is 392.18. Chemically it is (1-Thio-D-glucopyranosato) gold.

Aurothioglucose is a nearly odorless, yellow powder which is stable in air. An aqueous solution is unstable on long standing. Aurothioglucose is freely soluble in water but practically insoluble in acetone, in alcohol, in chloroform, and in ether.

Following is its chemical structure:

CLINICAL PHARMACOLOGY
Although the mechanism of action is not well understood, gold compounds have been reported to decrease synovial inflammation and retard cartilage and bone destruction. Gold is absorbed from injection sites, reaching peak concentration in blood in four to six hours. Following a single intramuscular injection of 50 mg Aurothioglucose Suspension in each of two patients, peak serum levels were about 235 mcg/dl in one patient and 450 mcg/dl in the other. In plasma, 95% is bound to the albumin fraction. Approximately 70% of the gold is eliminated in the urine and approximately 30% in the feces. When a standard weekly treatment schedule is followed, approximately 40% of the administered dose is excreted each week, and the remainder is excreted over a longer period. The biological half-life of gold salts following a single 50 mg dose has been reported to range from 3 to 27 days. Following successive weekly doses, the half-life increases and may be 14 to 40 days after the third dose and up to 168 days after the eleventh weekly dose.

After the initial injection, the serum level of gold rises sharply and declines over the next week. Peak levels with aqueous preparations are higher and decline faster than those with oily preparations. Weekly administration produces a continuous rise in the basal value for several months, after which the serum level becomes relatively stable. After a standard weekly dose, considerable individual variation in the levels of gold has been found. A steady decline in gold levels occurs when the interval between injections is lengthened, and small amounts may be found in the serum for months after discontinuance of therapy. The incidence of toxic reactions is apparently unrelated to the plasma level of gold, but it may be related to the cumulative body content of gold.

Storage of gold in human tissues is dependent upon organ mass as well as upon the concentration of gold. Therefore, tissues having the highest gold levels (weight/weight) do not necessarily contain the greatest total amounts of gold. The major depots, in decreasing order of total gold content, are the bone marrow, liver, skin, and bone, accounting for approximately 85% of body gold. The highest concentrations of gold are found in the lymph nodes, adrenal glands, liver, kidneys, bone marrow, and spleen. Relatively small concentrations are found in articular structures.

Gold passes the blood-brain barrier in hamsters.

Transfer of gold across the human placenta at the twentieth week of pregnancy has been documented. The placenta showed numerous gold deposits and smaller amounts were detected in the fetal liver and kidneys; other tissues provided no evidence of gold deposition.

Gold is excreted into human milk in significant amounts and trace amounts can be demonstrated in the blood of nursing infants. (See *"Precautions, Nursing Mothers."*)

INDICATIONS AND USAGE
Aurothioglucose Suspension is indicated for the adjunctive treatment of early active rheumatoid arthritis (both of the adult and juvenile types) not adequately controlled by other anti-inflammatory agents and conservative measures. In chronic, advanced cases of rheumatoid arthritis, gold therapy is less valuable.

◆ RATED THERAPEUTICALLY EQUIVALENT; ◇ THERAPEUTIC EQUIVALENCE UNCONFIRMED; ○ UNRATED

Antirheumatic measures such as salicylates and other anti-inflammatory drugs (both steroidal and nonsteroidal) may be continued after initiation of gold therapy. After improvement commences, these measures may be discontinued slowly as symptoms permit.

See *"Precautions, Laboratory Tests"* and *"Dosage and Administration."*

UNLABELED USES:
Aurothioglucose is used alone or as an adjunct in the treatment of pemphigus and asthma.

CONTRAINDICATIONS
A history of known hypersensitivity to any component of Aurothioglucose Suspension contraindicates its use. Gold therapy is contraindicated in patients with uncontrolled diabetes mellitus, severe debilitation, systemic lupus erythematosus, renal disease, hepatic dysfunction, uncontrolled congestive heart failure, marked hypertension, agranulocytosis, other blood dyscrasias, or hemorrhagic diathesis; or if there is a history of infectious hepatitis. Patients who recently have had radiation, and those who have developed severe toxicity from previous exposure to gold or other heavy metals should not receive Aurothioglucose Suspension.

Urticaria, eczema, and colitis are also contraindications. Gold therapy is usually contraindicated in pregnancy. (See *"Precautions, Usage in Pregnancy."*)

Gold salts should not be used with penicillamine (See *"Management of Adverse Reactions"*) or antimalarials. The safety of coadministration with immunosuppressive agents other than corticosteroids has not been established.

WARNINGS
The following signs should be considered danger signals of gold toxicity, and no additional injection should be given unless further studies reveal some other cause for their presence: rapid reduction of hemoglobin, leukopenia (WBC below 4000/cu mm), eosinophilia above 5%, platelet count below 100,000/cu mm, albuminuria, hematuria, pruritus, dermatitis, stomatitis, jaundice, and petechiae.

Effects that may occur immediately following an injection, or at any time during gold therapy, include: anaphylactic shock, syncope, bradycardia, thickening of the tongue, difficulty in swallowing and breathing, and angioneurotic edema. If such effects are observed, treatment with Aurothioglucose Suspension should be discontinued.

Tolerance to gold usually decreases with advancing age. Diabetes mellitus or congestive heart failure should be under control before gold therapy is instituted.

Aurothioglucose Suspension should be used with extreme caution in patients with: skin rash, hypersensitivity to other medications, or a history of renal or liver disease.

PRECAUTIONS
General: Before **each** injection, the physician should personally check the patient for adverse reactions and inquiry should be made regarding pruritus, rash, sore mouth, indigestion, and metallic taste. The patient should be observed for at least 15 minutes following each injection. (See also *"Laboratory Tests."*)

Patients with HLA-D locus histocompatibility antigens DRw2 and DRw3 may have a genetic predisposition to develop certain toxic reactions, such as proteinuria, during treatment with gold or D-penicillamine.

Aurothioglucose Suspension should be used with caution in patients with compromised cardiovascular or cerebral circulation.

Information for Patients:
1. Promptly report to the physician any unusual symptoms such as pruritus (itching), rash, sore mouth, indigestion, or metallic taste.
2. Increased joint pain may occur for one or two days after an injection and usually subsides after the first few injections.
3. Exposure to sunlight or artificial ultraviolet light should be minimized.
4. Careful oral hygiene is recommended in conjunction with therapy.
5. Patients should be aware of potential hazards if they become pregnant while receiving gold therapy. (See *"Usage in Pregnancy."*)

Laboratory Tests: Before treatment is started, a complete blood count, platelet count, and urinalysis should be done to serve as reference points. Since gold therapy is usually contraindicated in pregnant patients, pregnancy should be ruled out before treatment is started. Throughout the treatment period, urinalysis should be repeated prior to each injection, and complete blood cell and platelet counts should be performed every two weeks. A platelet count is indicated any time that purpura or ecchymosis occurs.

Drug Interactions: Drug interactions have not been reported. (See *"Contraindications."*)

Carcinogenesis, Mutagenesis, and Impairment of Fertility: Renal adenomas developed in rats receiving an injectable gold product similar to Aurothioglucose Suspension at doses of 2 mg/kg weekly for 46 weeks, followed by 6 mg/kg daily for 47 weeks. These doses were higher and administered more frequently than the recommended human doses. The adenomas were similar histologically to those produced by chronic administration of other gold compounds and heavy metals, such as lead or nickel.

Renal tubular cell neoplasia consisting of renal adenoma and adenocarcinoma were noted in a dose-response relationship in another study in rats using daily intramuscular doses of 3 mg/kg and 6 mg/kg for up to 2 years. These doses were higher and were administered more frequently than the recommended human doses. In this same study, sarcomas at the injection site occurred in some rats but their numbers were not sufficient to demonstrate a dose-response relationship.

No report of renal adenoma or sarcoma at the injection site in man in association with the use of Aurothioglucose Suspension has been received.

Gold compounds have not been studied for evaluation of mutagenesis.

Gold sodium thiomalate given subcutaneously did not adversely affect fertility or reproductive performance.

Usage in Pregnancy: Gold therapy is usually contraindicated in pregnant patients. The patient should be warned about the hazards of becoming pregnant while on gold therapy. Rheumatoid arthritis frequently improves when the patient becomes pregnant, thereby eliminating the need for gold therapy. The potential nephrotoxicity of gold should not be superimposed on the increased renal burden which normally occurs in pregnancy and hence, gold therapy should be discontinued upon recognition of pregnancy unless continued use is required in an individual case. The slow excretion of gold and its persistence in body tissues after discontinuation of treatment should be kept in mind when a woman of childbearing potential being treated with gold plans to become pregnant.

Pregnancy Category C: Gold sodium thiomalate administered subcutaneously, a route not used clinically, has been shown to be teratogenic during the organogenic period in rats and rabbits when given in doses 140 and 175 times, respectively, the usual human dose. Hydrocephalus and microphthalmia were the malformations observed in rats when gold sodium thiomalate was administered at a dose of 25 mg/kg/day from day 6 through day 15 of gestation. In rabbits, limb defects and gastroschisis were the malformations observed when gold sodium thiomalate was administered at doses of 20 to 45 mg/kg/day from day 6 through day 18 of gestation.

Gold compounds administered orally to rabbits from days 6 through 18 of pregnancy resulted in the occurrence of abdominal defects, such as gastroschisis and umbilical hernia; anomalies of the brain, heart, lung, and skeleton: and microphthalmia.

The administration of excessive doses of gold-containing compounds during pregnancy in the above studies was toxic to the mothers and their embryos; the embryotoxic effects probably were secondary to maternal toxicity. Therefore, the significance of these findings in relation to human use is unknown.

There are no adequate and well-controlled studies with Aurothioglucose Suspension in pregnant women. Extensive clinical experience with Aurothioglucose Suspension has not demonstrated human teratogenicity.

Nursing Mothers: Gold has been demonstrated in the milk of lactating mothers. In one patient, a total dose of 135 mg of gold thioglucose was given during the postpartum period. Samples of the maternal milk and urine, and samples of red blood cells and serum of the mother and child were evaluated by atomic absorption spectrophotometry. Trace amounts of gold appeared in the serum and red blood cells of the nursing offspring. It has been postulated that this may be the cause of unexplained rashes, nephritis, hepatitis, and hematologic aberrations in the nursing infants of mothers treated with gold. Because of the potential for serious adverse reactions in nursing infants, a decision should be made whether to discontinue nursing or to discontinue the gold therapy, taking into account the importance of the drug to the mother. The slow excretion of gold and its persistence in the mother after discontinuation of treatment should be kept in mind.

Pediatric Use: Safety and effectiveness in children below the age of six years have not been established.

ADVERSE REACTIONS
Adverse reactions to gold therapy may occur at any time during treatment or many months after therapy has been discontinued. The incidence of toxic reactions is apparently unrelated to the plasma level of gold, but it may be related to the cumulative body content of gold. Higher than conventional dosage schedules may increase the occurrence and severity of toxicity. Severe effects are most common after 300 to 500 mg have been administered.

Cutaneous Reactions: Dermatitis is the most common reaction. Pruritus should be considered a warning signal of an impending cutaneous reaction. Erythema and occasionally the more severe reactions such as papular, vesicular, and exfoliative dermatitis leading to alopecia and shedding of the nails may occur. Chrysiasis (gray-to-blue pigmentation) has been reported, especially on photoexposed areas. Gold dermatitis may be aggravated by exposure to sunlight, or an actinic rash may develop.

Mucous Membrane Reactions: Stomatitis is the second most common adverse reaction. Shallow ulcers on the buccal membranes, on the borders of the tongue and on the palate, diffuse glossitis, or gingivitis may be preceded by the sensation of metallic taste. Careful oral hygiene is recommended. Inflammation of the upper respiratory tract, pharyngitis, gastritis, colitis, tracheitis, and vaginitis have also been reported. Conjunctivitis is rare.

Renal Reactions: Nephrotic syndrome or glomerulitis with hematuria, which is usually relatively mild, subsides completely if recognized early and treatment is discontinued. These reactions become severe and chronic if gold therapy is continued after their onset. Therefore, it is important to perform a urinalysis before each injection and to discontinue treatment promptly if proteinuria or hematuria develops.

Hematologic Reactions: Although rare, blood dyscrasias, including granulocytopenia, agranulocytosis, thrombocytopenia with or without purpura, leukopenia, eosinophilia, panmyelopathy, hemorrhagic diathesis, and hypoplastic and aplastic anemia, have been reported. These reactions may occur separately or in combination.

Nitritoid and Allergic Reactions: These reactions, which may rarely occur with Aurothioglucose Suspension and which resemble anaphylactoid effects, include flushing, fainting, dizziness, sweating, malaise, weakness, nausea, and vomiting.

Miscellaneous Reactions: On rare occasions, gastrointestinal symptoms, i.e., nausea, vomiting, colic, anorexia, abdominal cramps, diarrhea, ulcerative enterocolitis, and headache have been reported.

There have been rare reports of iritis and corneal ulcers. Transient, asymptomatic gold deposits in the cornea or conjunctiva may occur.

Other reported reactions include encephalitis, immunological destruction of the synovia, EEG abnormalities, intrahepatic cholestasis, hepatitis with jaundice, toxic hepatitis, acute yellow atrophy, peripheral neuritis, gold bronchitis, pulmonary injury manifested by interstitial pneumonitis or fibrosis, fever, and partial or complete hair loss.

Less common but more severe effects that may occur shortly after an injection or at any time during gold therapy include: anaphylactic shock, syncope, bradycardia, thickening of the tongue, difficulty in swallowing and breathing, and angioneurotic edema. If they are observed, treatment with Aurothioglucose Suspension should be discontinued.

Arthralgia may occur for one or two days after an injection and usually subsides after the first few injections. The mechanism of the transient increase in rheumatic symptoms after injection of gold (the so-called nonvasomotor postinjection reaction) is unknown. These reactions are usually mild but occasionally may be so severe that treatment is stopped prematurely.

MANAGEMENT OF ADVERSE REACTIONS
In the event of toxic reactions, gold therapy should be discontinued immediately.

In the presence of mild reactions, it may be sufficient to discontinue the administration of Aurothioglucose Suspension for a short period and then to resume treatment with smaller doses.

Dermatitis and pruritus may respond to soothing lotions, other appropriate antipruritic treatment, or topical glucocorticoids.

If dermatitis or stomatitis becomes severe or spreads, systemic glucocorticoid treatment may be indicated. For renal, hematologic, and most other adverse reactions, glucocorticoids may be required in larger doses and for a longer time than for dermatologic reactions. Often this treatment may be required for many months because of the slow elimination of gold from the body.

If severe adverse reactions do not improve with steroid treatment in patients who receive large doses of gold, a chelating agent, such as dimercaprol (BAL), may be used. In one case, it was reported that penicillamine was beneficial in the treatment of gold-induced thrombocytopenia. Adjunctive use of an anabolic steroid with other drugs (i.e., BAL, penicillamine, and corticosteroids) may contribute to recovery of bone marrow deficiency.

In the presence of severe or idiosyncratic reactions, treatment with Aurothioglucose Suspension should not be reinstituted.

OVERDOSAGE
Overdosage resulting from too rapid increases in dosing with Aurothioglucose Suspension will be manifested by rapid appearance of toxic reactions, particularly those relating to renal damage, such as hematuria, proteinuria, and to hematologic effects, such as thrombocytopenia and granulocytopenia. Other toxic effects, including fever, nausea, vomiting, diarrhea, and various skin disorders such as papulovesicular lesions, urticaria, and exfoliative dermatitis, all attended with severe pruritus, may develop. Treatment consists of prompt discontinuation of the medication, and early administration of dimercaprol. Specific supportive therapy should be given for the renal and hematologic complications. (See also *"Management of Adverse Reactions"* above).

DOSAGE AND ADMINISTRATION
Adults: The usual dosage schedule for the intramuscular administration of Aurothioglucose is as follows: first dose, 10 mg; second and third doses, 25 mg; fourth and subsequent doses, 50 mg. The interval between doses is one week. The 50 mg dose is continued at weekly intervals until 0.8 to 1.0 g Aurothioglucose has been given. If the patient has improved and has exhibited no sign of toxicity, the 50 mg dose may be continued many months longer, at three- to four-week intervals. A weekly dose above 50 mg is usually unnecessary and contraindicated; the tendency in gold therapy is toward lower dosage. With this in mind, it may eventually be established that a 25 mg dose is the one of choice. If no improvement has been demonstrated after a total administration of 1.0 g of Aurothioglucose reevaluated.

Children 6 to 12 years: one-fourth of the adult dose, governed chiefly by body weight, not to exceed 25 mg per dose. Aurothioglucose Suspension should be injected **intramuscularly**, (preferably intragluteally), **never intravenously**. The patient should be lying down and should remain recumbent for approximately 10 minutes after the injection. The vial should be thoroughly shaken in order to suspend all of the active material. Heating the vial to body temperature (by immersion in warm water) will facilitate drawing the suspension into the syringe. An 18-gauge, 1½-inch needle is recommended for depositing the preparation deep into the muscular tissue. For obese patients, an 18-gauge, 2-inch needle may be used. The site usually selected for injection is the upper outer quadrant of the gluteal region.

Note: Shake the vial in horizontal position before the dose is withdrawn. Needle and syringe must be dry. The patient should be observed for at least 15 minutes following each injection.

Shake well before using. Store between 0° and 30°C (32° and 86°F). Protect from light. Store in carton until contents are used.

J CODES
Up to 50 mg IM—J2910

HOW SUPPLIED
INJECTION: 50 MG/ML

BRAND/MANUFACTURER	NDC	SIZE	AWP
○ BRAND			
SOLGANAL: Schering	00085-0460-03	10 ml	$107.30

Autoplex T *SEE ANTI-INHIBITOR COAGULANT COMPLEX*

AVC *SEE SULFANILAMIDE*

Aventyl HCl *SEE NORTRIPTYLINE HYDROCHLORIDE*

Axid Pulvules *SEE NIZATIDINE*

Axotal *SEE ASPIRIN WITH BUTALBITAL*

Azactam *SEE AZTREONAM*

Azatadine Maleate

DESCRIPTION
Azatadine Maleate is an antihistamine having the empirical formula, $C_{20}H_{22}N_2 \cdot 2C_4H_4O_4$ and the chemical name, 6,11-Dihydro-11-(1-methyl-4-piperidylidene-5H-benzo [5,6] cyclohepta [1,2-b] pyridine maleate (1:2).

The molecular weight of Azatadine Maleate is 522.55. It is a white to off-white powder and is very soluble in water and soluble in alcohol.

It is available as tablets, each containing 1 mg Azatadine Maleate.

Following is its chemical structure:

CLINICAL PHARMACOLOGY
Azatadine Maleate is an antihistamine, related to cyproheptadine, with antiserotonin, anticholinergic (drying), and sedative effects.

Antihistamines competitively antagonize those pharmacological effects of histamine which are mediated through activation of histamine H_1-receptor sites on effector cells. Histamine-related allergic reactions and tissue injury are blocked or diminished in intensity. Antihistamines antagonize the vasodilator effect of endogenously released histamine, especially in small vessels, and mitigate the effect of histamine which results in increased capillary permeability and edema formation. As consequences of these actions, antihistamines antagonize the physiological manifestations of histamine release in the nose following antigen-antibody interactions, such as congestion related to vascular engorgement, mucosal edema, and profuse, watery secretion, and irritation and sneezing resulting from histamine action on afferent nerve terminals.

Pharmacokinetic studies in normal volunteers dosed orally with radio-labeled Azatadine Maleate show that the drug is readily absorbed with peak plasma levels at about four hours after dosing. Approximately 50% of the drug is excreted in the urine within five days after administration of a single dose, and no evidence of drug accumulation was seen after daily dosing for 30 days. The elimination half-life of Azatadine Maleate, based on plasma radioactivity, was approximately 9 hours. Approximately 20% of the drug is excreted unchanged and extensive conjugation of the drug and its metabolites occurs. Azatadine Maleate is minimally bound to plasma protein.

While the antihistamines have not been studied for passage through the blood-brain and placental barriers, the occurrence of pharmacologic effects in the central nervous system and in the newborn indicate presence of the drug.

INDICATIONS AND USAGE
Azatadine Maleate tablets are indicated for the treatment of perennial and seasonal allergic rhinitis and chronic urticaria.

◆ RATED THERAPEUTICALLY EQUIVALENT; ◇ THERAPEUTIC EQUIVALENCE UNCONFIRMED; ○ UNRATED

CONTRAINDICATIONS

Antihistamines *should NOT* be used to treat lower respiratory tract symptoms, including asthma.

Antihistamines, including Azatadine Maleate, are also contraindicated in patients hypersensitive to this medication and to other antihistamines of similar chemical structure, and in patients receiving monoamine oxidase inhibitor therapy. (See *"Drug Interactions."*)

WARNINGS

Antihistamines should be used with caution in patients with narrow angle glaucoma; stenosing peptic ulcer; pyloroduodenal obstruction; and urinary bladder obstruction due to symptomatic prostatic hypertrophy and narrowing of the bladder neck.

Use with CNS Depressants: Antihistamines have additive effects with alcohol and other CNS depressants (hypnotics, sedatives, tranquilizers, etc.).

Use in Activities Requiring Mental Alertness: Patients should be warned about engaging in activities requiring mental alertness, such as driving a car or operating certain appliances, machinery, etc., until their response to this medication has been determined.

Use in Patients Approximately 60 Years or Older: Antihistamines are more likely to cause dizziness, sedation, and hypotension in patients over 60 years of age.

PRECAUTIONS

General: Azatadine Maleate has an atropine-like action and therefore should be used with caution in patients with: a history of bronchial asthma; increased intraocular pressure; hyperthyroidism; cardiovascular disease; hypertension.

Information for Patients: This information is intended to aid in the safe and effective use of this medication. It is not a disclosure of all possible adverse or intended effects.

1. Antihistamines may cause drowsiness.
2. Patients taking antihistamines should not engage in activities requiring mental alertness, such as driving a car or operating machinery, certain appliances, etc., until their response to this medication has been determined.
3. Alcohol or other sedative drugs may enhance the drowsiness caused by antihistamines.
4. Patients should not take this medication if they are receiving a monoamine oxidase (MAO) inhibitor, or if they are receiving oral anticoagulants.
5. This medication should not be given to children less than 12 years of age.

Drug Interactions: MAO inhibitors prolong and intensify the anticholinergic and sedative effects of antihistamines. Additive effects may occur from the concomitant use of antihistamines with tricyclic antidepressants. (See also *"Warnings"*.)

Drug/Laboratory Test Interaction: Antihistamines should be discontinued about four days prior to skin testing procedures since these drugs may prevent or diminish otherwise positive reactions to dermal reactivity indicators.

Carcinogenesis, Mutagenesis, and Impairment of Fertility: Long-term oral dosing studies with Azatadine Maleate in rats and mice showed no evidence of carcinogenesis. No mutagenic effect was seen in a dominant lethal assay study in mice dosed with Azatadine Maleate orally and intraperitoneally. There was no impairment of fertility in rats fed Azatadine Maleate at doses greater than 150 times the recommended human daily dose.

Pregnancy Category B: Reproduction studies have been performed in rats and rabbits at doses up to 188 times and 38 times, respectively, the human dose and have revealed no evidence of impaired fertility or harm to the fetus due to Azatadine Maleate. There are, however, no adequate and well-controlled studies in pregnant women. Because animal reproduction studies are not always predictive of human response, this drug should be used during pregnancy only if clearly needed. (See *"Non-Teratogenic Effects"*.)

Non-Teratogenic Effects: Antihistamines should not be used in the third trimester of pregnancy because newborns and premature infants may have severe reactions, such as convulsions, to them.

Nursing Mothers: It is not known whether this drug is excreted in human milk. However, certain antihistamines are known to be excreted in human milk in low concentration.

Because of the higher risk of antihistamines for infants generally and for newborns and prematures in particular, a decision should be made whether to discontinue nursing or to discontinue the drug, taking into account the importance of the drug to the mother.

Pediatric Use: Safety and effectiveness in children below the age of 12 years have not been established.

ADVERSE REACTIONS

Slight to moderate drowsiness may occur with Azatadine Maleate. Other possible side effects common to antihistamines in general include (the most frequent are italicized):

General: urticaria, drug rash, anaphylactic shock, photosensitivity, excessive perspiration, chills, dryness of mouth, nose, and throat.

Cardiovascular: hypotension, headache, palpitations, tachycardia, extrasystoles.

Hematologic: hemolytic anemia, hypoplastic anemia, thrombocytopenia, agranulocytosis.

Nervous: sedation, sleepiness, dizziness, vertigo, tinnitus, acute labyrinthitis, *disturbed coordination*, fatigue, confusion, restlessness, excitation, nervousness,

tremor, irritability, insomnia, euphoria, paresthesias, blurred vision, diplopia, hysteria, neuritis, convulsions.

Gastrointestinal: epigastric distress, anorexia, nausea, vomiting, diarrhea, constipation.

Genitourinary: urinary frequency, difficult urination, urinary retention, early menses.

Respiratory: thickening of bronchial secretions, tightness of chest and wheezing, nasal stuffiness.

DRUG ABUSE AND DEPENDENCE

There is no information to indicate that abuse or dependency occurs with Azatadine Maleate.

OVERDOSAGE

In the event of overdosage, emergency treatment should be started immediately.

Manifestations: Antihistamine overdosage effects may vary from central nervous system depression (sedation, apnea, diminished mental alertness, cardiovascular collapse) to stimulation (insomnia, hallucinations, tremors or convulsions) to death. Other signs and symptoms may be dizziness, tinnitus, ataxia, blurred vision, and hypotension. Stimulation is particularly likely in children, as are atropine-like signs and symptoms (dry mouth; fixed, dilated pupils; flushing; hyperthermia; and gastrointestinal symptoms).

Treatment: The patient should be induced to vomit, even if emesis has occurred spontaneously. Pharmacologic vomiting by the administration of ipecac syrup is a preferred method. However, vomiting should not be induced in patients with impaired consciousness. The action of ipecac is facilitated by physical activity and by the administration of 8 to 12 fluid ounces of water. If emesis does not occur within fifteen minutes, the dose of ipecac should be repeated. Precautions against aspiration must be taken, especially in infants and children. Following emesis, any drug remaining in the stomach may be adsorbed by activated charcoal administered as a slurry with water. If vomiting is unsuccessful or contraindicated, gastric lavage should be performed. Physiologic saline solution is the lavage solution of choice, particularly in children. In adults, tap water can be used; however, as much as possible of the amount administered should be removed before the next instillation. Saline cathartics, such as milk of magnesia, draw water into the bowel by osmosis and, therefore, may be valuable for their action in rapid dilution of bowel content. Dialysis is of little value in antihistamine poisoning. After emergency treatment, the patient should continue to be medically monitored.

Treatment of the signs and symptoms of overdosage is symptomatic and supportive. *Stimulants* (analeptic agents) should *not* be used. Vasopressors may be used to treat hypotension. Short acting barbiturates, diazepam, or paraldehyde may be administered to control seizures. Hyperpyrexia, especially in children, may require treatment with tepid water sponge baths or a hypothermic blanket. Apnea is treated with ventilatory support.

DOSAGE AND ADMINISTRATION

DOSAGE SHOULD BE INDIVIDUALIZED ACCORDING TO THE NEEDS AND THE RESPONSE OF THE PATIENT.

Azatadine Maleate tablets are not recommended for use in children under 12 years of age.

The usual adult dosage is 1 or 2 mg, twice a day.

Store between 2° and 30°C (36° and 86°F).

HOW SUPPLIED
TABLETS: 1 MG

BRAND/MANUFACTURER	NDC	SIZE	AWP
BRAND OPTIMINE: Schering	00085-0282-03	100s	$81.94

Azatadine Maleate with Pseudoephedrine Sulfate

DESCRIPTION

Azatadine Maleate/Pseudoephedrine Sulfate (Azatadine/Pseudoephedrine) Long-Acting Antihistamine/Decongestant Tablets contain 1 mg Azatadine Maleate, USP in the tablet coating and 120 mg Pseudoephedrine Sulfate, USP, equally distributed between the tablet coating and the barrier-coated core. Following ingestion, the two active components in the coating are quickly liberated; release of the decongestant in the core is delayed for several hours.

Azatadine Maleate is an antihistamine having the empirical formula, $C_{20}H_{22}N_2 \cdot 2C_4H_4O_4$, the chemical name, 6,11-Dihydro-11-(1-methyl-4-piperidylidene)-5H-benzo [5,6] cyclohepta [1,2-b] pyridine Maleate (1:2).

The molecular weight of Azatadine Maleate is 522.54. Azatadine Maleate is a white to off-white powder and is very soluble in water and soluble in alcohol.

Pseudoephedrine Sulfate, a sympathomimetic amine, is a salt of Pseudoephedrine, one of the naturally occurring alkaloids obtained from various species of the plant *Ephedra*. The empirical formula for Pseudoephedrine Sulfate is $(C_{10}H_{15}NO)_2 \cdot H_2SO_4$: the chemical name is Benzenemethanol, α-[1-(methylamino)ethyl]-, [S-(R*, R*)]-, Sulfate (2:1) (salt).

The molecular weight of Pseudoephedrine Sulfate is 428.56. It is a white to off-white crystal or powder, very soluble in water, freely soluble in alcohol, and sparingly soluble in chloroform.

CLINICAL PHARMACOLOGY

Azatadine Maleate is an antihistamine, related to cyproheptadine, with antiserotonin, anticholinergic (drying), and sedative effects. Antihistamines appear to compete with histamine for histamine H_1-receptor sites on effector cells. The antihistamines antagonize those pharmacological effects of histamine which are mediated through activation of H_1-receptor sites and thereby reduce the intensity of allergic reactions and tissue injury response involving histamine release. Antihistamines antagonize the vasodilator effect of endogenously released histamine, especially in small vessels, and mitigate the effect of histamine which results in increased capillary permeability and edema formation. As consequences of these actions, antihistamines antagonize the physiological manifestations of histamine release in the nose following antigen-antibody interaction, such as congestion related to vascular engorgement, mucosal edema, and profuse, watery secretion, and irritation and sneezing resulting from histamine action on afferent nerve terminals.

Pseudoephedrine Sulfate (d-isoephedrine Sulfate) is an orally effective nasal decongestant which appears to exert its sympathomimetic effect indirectly, predominantly through release of adrenergic mediators from post-ganglionic nerve terminals. In effective recommended oral dosage, Pseudoephedrine Sulfate produces minimal other sympathomimetic effects, such as pressor activity and CNS stimulation. Use of an orally administered vasoconstrictor for shrinkage of congested nasal mucosa has several advantages: a) it produces a gradual but sustained decongestant effect, causing little, if any, "rebound" congestion; b) it facilitates shrinkage of swollen mucosa in upper respiratory areas that are relatively inaccessible to topically applied sprays or drops; c) it relieves nasal obstruction without the additional irritation that may result from local medication.

Pseudoephedrine passes through the blood-brain and placental barriers. While the antihistamines have not been studied systematically for passage through these barriers, the occurrence of pharmacologic effects in the central nervous system and in newborns indicate presence of the drug.

Following administration of the two drugs to normal volunteers in either a single Azatadine/Pseudoephedrine long-acting tablet or similar doses in two conventional Pseudoephedrine Sulfate tablets and a conventional tablet of Azatadine Maleate, the blood levels of Pseudoephedrine and the urinary excretion of Azatadine showed that the Azatadine/Pseudoephedrine long-acting tablet is bioequivalent to the conventional dosage forms. The apparent elimination half-life of Pseudoephedrine in Azatadine/Pseudoephedrine long-acting tablet was approximately 6 1/2 hours. The apparent elimination of half-life of Azatadine Maleate (available from the outer layer of the Azatadine/Pseudoephedrine long-acting tablet or from the conventional Azatadine Maleate tablet) was approximately 12 hours.

INDICATIONS AND USAGE

Azatadine/Pseudoephedrine Long-Acting Antihistamine/Decongestant Tablets are indicated for the relief of the symptoms of upper respiratory mucosal congestion in perennial and allergic rhinitis, and for the relief of nasal congestion and eustachian tube congestion. Analgesics, antibiotics, or both may be administered concurrently, when indicated.

CONTRAINDICATIONS

Antihistamines *should not* be used to treat lower respiratory tract symptoms, including asthma.

This product is contraindicated in patients with narrow-angle glaucoma or urinary retention, and in patients receiving monoamine oxidase (MAO) inhibitor therapy or within ten days of stopping such treatment. (See *"Drug Interactions"* section.) It is also contraindicated in patients with severe hypertension, severe coronary artery disease, hyperthyroidism, and in those who have shown hypersensitivity or idiosyncrasy to its components, to adrenergic agents, or to other drugs of similar chemical structures. Manifestations of patient idiosyncrasy to adrenergic agents include: insomnia, dizziness, weakness, tremor, or arrhythmias.

WARNINGS

Azatadine/Pseudoephedrine long-acting tablets should be used with considerable caution in patients with: stenosing peptic ulcer, pyloroduodenal obstruction, urinary bladder obstruction due to symptomatic prostatic hypertrophy, or narrowing of the bladder neck. It should also be administered with caution to patients with cardiovascular disease, including hypertension or ischemic heart disease; increased intraocular pressure (see *"Contraindications"*); diabetes mellitus, or in patients receiving digitalis or oral anticoagulants.

Central nervous system stimulation and convulsions or cardiovascular collapse with accompanying hypotension may be produced by sympathomimetics.

Do not exceed recommended dosage.

Use in Activities Requiring Mental Alertness: Patients should be warned about engaging in activities requiring mental alertness, such as driving a car or operating appliances, machinery, etc.

Use in Patients Approximately 60 Years and Older: Antihistamines are more likely to cause dizziness, sedation, and hypotension in patients over 60 years of age. In these patients, sympathomimetics are also more likely to cause adverse reactions, such as confusion, hallucinations, convulsions, CNS depression, and death. For this reason, before considering the use of a repeat-action formulation, the safe use of a short-acting sympathomimetic in that particular patient should be demonstrated.

PRECAUTIONS

General: Because of the atropine-like action of antihistamines, this product should be used with caution in patients with a history of bronchial asthma.

Information for Patients:
1. Products containing antihistamines may cause drowsiness.
2. Patients should not engage in activities requiring mental alertness, such as driving or operating machinery or appliances.
3. Alcohol or other sedative drugs may enhance the drowsiness caused by antihistamines.
4. Patients should not take Azatadine/Pseudoephedrine long-acting tablets if they are receiving a monoamine oxidase inhibitor or within 10 days of stopping such treatment, or if they are receiving oral anticoagulants.
5. This medication should not be given to children less than 12 years of age.

Drug Interactions: MAO inhibitors prolong and intensify the effects of antihistamines. Concomitant use of antihistamines with alcohol, tricyclic antidepressants, barbiturates, or other central nervous system depressants may have an additive effect.

When sympathomimetic drugs are given to patients receiving monoamine oxidase inhibitors, hypertensive reactions, including hypertensive crises, may occur. The antihypertensive effects of methyldopa, mecamylamine, reserpine, and veratrum alkaloids may be reduced by sympathomimetics. Beta-adrenergic blocking agents may also interact with sympathomimetics. Increased ectopic pacemaker activity can occur when Pseudoephedrine is used concomitantly with digitalis. Antacids increase the rate of absorption of Pseudoephedrine, while kaolin decreases it.

Drug/Laboratory Test Interactions: The *in vitro* addition of Pseudoephedrine to sera containing the cardiac isoenzyme MB of serum creatine phosphokinase progressively inhibits the activity of the enzyme. The inhibition becomes complete over six hours.

Carcinogenesis, Mutagenesis, and Impairment of Fertility: There is no animal or laboratory study of the mixture of Azatadine Maleate and Pseudoephedrine Sulfate to evaluate carcinogenesis or mutagenesis. Reproduction studies of this mixture in rats showed no evidence of impaired fertility.

Pregnancy Category C: Retarded fetal development and the presence of angulated hyoid wings were seen in the offspring of pregnant rabbits administered Azatadine/Pseudoephedrine long-acting tablets at about 12.5 times and 5 times the recommended human dosage, respectively; increased resorption was noted at about 25 times the human dosage. A decreased survival rate at day 21 was seen in rat pups born of mothers given Azatadine/Pseudoephedrine long-acting tablets during pregnancy at a dose about 12.5 times the human dosage. There are no adequate and well-controlled studies in pregnant women. Azatadine/Pseudoephedrine long-acting tablets should be used during pregnancy only if the potential benefits to the mother justify the potential risks to the infant. (See *"Nonteratogenic Effects"*.)

Nonteratogenic Effects: Antihistamines should not be used in the third trimester of pregnancy, because newborns and premature infants may have severe reactions to them such as convulsions.

Nursing Mothers: It is not known whether these drugs are excreted in human milk. However, certain antihistamines and sympathomimetics are known to be excreted in human milk. Because of the higher risks of antihistamines for infants generally and for newborns and prematures in particular, a decision should be made whether to discontinue nursing or to discontinue the drug, taking into account the importance of the drug to the mother.

There is a report of irritability, excessive crying and disturbed sleeping patterns in a nursing infant whose mother had taken a product containing an antihistamine and Pseudoephedrine.

Pediatric use: Safety and effectiveness in children below the age of 12 years have not been established.

ADVERSE REACTIONS

The following adverse reactions are associated with antihistamine and sympathomimetic drugs. (Those adverse reactions which occur most frequently with the antihistamines appear in italics.)

General: Urticaria, drug rash, anaphylactic shock, photosensitivity, excessive perspiration, chills, dryness of mouth, nose, and throat.

Cardiovascular: Hypertension (see *"Contraindications"* and *"Warnings"*), hypotension, arrhythmias and cardiovascular collapse, headache, palpitations, extrasystoles, tachycardia, angina.

Hematologic: Hemolytic anemia, hypoplastic anemia, thrombocytopenia, agranulocytosis.

Central Nervous System: Sedation, sleepiness, dizziness, vertigo, tinnitus, acute labyrinthitis, *disturbed coordination,* fatigue, mydriasis, confusion, restlessness, excitation, nervousness, tension, tremor, irritability, insomnia, euphoria, paresthesias, blurred vision, hysteria, neuritis, convulsions, fear, anxiety, hallucinations, CNS depression, weakness, pallor.

Gastrointestinal: Epigastric distress, anorexia, nausea, vomiting, diarrhea, constipation, abdominal cramps.

Genitourinary: Urinary frequency, urinary retention, dysuria, early menses.

◆ RATED THERAPEUTICALLY EQUIVALENT; ◇ THERAPEUTIC EQUIVALENCE UNCONFIRMED; ○ UNRATED

Respiratory: Thickening of bronchial secretions, tightness of chest and wheezing, nasal stuffiness, respiratory difficulty.

DRUG ABUSE AND DEPENDENCE

There is no information to indicate that abuse or dependency occurs with Azatadine Maleate.

Pseudoephedrine, like other central nervous system stimulants, has been abused. At high doses, subjects commonly experience an elevation of mood, a sense of increased energy and alertness, and decreased appetite. Some individuals become anxious, irritable, and loquacious. In addition to the marked euphoria, the user experiences a sense of markedly enhanced physical strength and mental capacity. With continued use, tolerance develops, the user increases the dose, and toxic signs and symptoms appear. Depression may follow rapid withdrawal.

OVERDOSAGE

In the event of overdosage, emergency treatment should be started immediately.

Manifestations of overdosage may vary from central nervous system depression (sedation, apnea, diminished mental alertness, cyanosis, coma, cardiovascular collapse) to stimulation (insomnia, hallucinations, tremors, or convulsions) to death. Other signs and symptoms may be euphoria, excitement, tachycardia, palpitations, thirst, perspiration, nausea, dizziness, tinnitus, ataxia, blurred vision, and hypertension or hypotension. Stimulation is particularly likely in children, as are atropine-like signs and symptoms (dry mouth; fixed, dilated pupils, flushing; hyperthermia; and gastrointestinal symptoms).

In large doses sympathomimetics may give rise to giddiness, headache, nausea, vomiting, sweating, thirst, tachycardia, precordial pain, palpitations, difficulty in micturition, muscular weakness and tenseness, anxiety, restlessness, and insomnia. Many patients can present a toxic psychosis with delusions and hallucinations. Some may develop cardiac arrhythmias, circulatory collapse, convulsions, coma, and respiratory failure.

The oral LD_{50} of the mixture of the two drugs in mature rats and mice was greater than 1700 mg/kg and 600 mg/kg, respectively.

Treatment: The patient should be induced to vomit, even if emesis has occurred spontaneously. Pharmacologically induced vomiting by the administration of ipecac syrup is a preferred method. However, vomiting should not be induced in patients with impaired consciousness. The action of ipecac is facilitated by physical activity and by the administration of eight to twelve fluid ounces of water. If emesis does not occur within fifteen minutes, the dose of ipecac should be repeated. Precautions against aspiration must be taken, especially in infants and children. Following emesis, any drug remaining in the stomach may be adsorbed by activated charcoal administered as a slurry with water. If vomiting is unsuccessful or contraindicated, gastric lavage should be performed. Isotonic and one-half isotonic saline are the lavage solutions of choice. Saline cathartics, such as milk of magnesia, draw water into the bowel by osmosis and therefore may be valuable for their action in rapid dilution of bowel content. Dialysis is of little value in antihistamine poisoning. After emergency treatment the patient should continue to be medically monitored.

Treatment of the signs and symptoms of overdosage is symptomatic and supportive. Stimulants (analeptic agents) should *not* be used. Vasopressors may be used to treat hypotension. Short-acting barbiturates, diazepam, or paraldehyde may be administered to control seizures. Hyperpyrexia, especially in children, may require treatment with tepid water sponge baths or a hypothermic blanket. Apnea is treated with ventilatory support.

DOSAGE AND ADMINISTRATION

Azatadine/Pseudoephedrine long-acting tablets *Are Not Intended For Use in Children Under 12 Years of Age.* The usual adult dosage is one tablet twice a day.

Store between 2° and 30°C (36° and 86°F).

HOW SUPPLIED
TABLETS: 1 MG-120 MG

BRAND/MANUFACTURER	NDC	SIZE	AWP
○ BRAND			
▶ TRINALIN REPETABS: Schering	00085-0703-04	100s	$83.20

Azathioprine

> **WARNING**
> CHRONIC IMMUNOSUPPRESSION WITH THIS PURINE ANTIMETABOLITE INCREASES *RISK OF NEOPLASIA* IN HUMANS. PHYSICIANS USING THIS DRUG SHOULD BE VERY FAMILIAR WITH THIS RISK AS WELL AS WITH THE MUTAGENIC POTENTIAL TO BOTH MEN AND WOMEN AND WITH POSSIBLE HEMATOLOGIC TOXICITIES. SEE *"WARNINGS"*.

DESCRIPTION

Azathioprine an immunosuppressive antimetabolite, is available in tablet form for oral administration and 100 mg vials for intravenous injection. Each scored tablet contains 50 mg Azathioprine.

Each 100 mg vial contains Azathioprine, as the sodium salt, equivalent to 100 mg Azathioprine sterile lyophilized material and sodium hydroxide to adjust pH.

Azathioprine is insoluble in water, but may dissolved with addition of one molar equivalent of alkalie. The sodium salt of Azthioprine is sufficiently soluble to make a 10 mg/mL water solution which is stable for 24 hours at 59° to 77°F (15° to 25°C). Azathioprine is stable in solution at neutral or acid pH but hydrolysis to mercaptopurine occurs in excess sodium hydroxide (0.1N), especially on warming. Conversion to mercaptopurine also occurs in the presence of sulfhydryl compounds such as cysteine, glutathione and hydrogen sulfide.

Azathioprine is chemically 6-[1-methyl-4-nitroimidazol-5-yl)thio] purine. It is an imidazoyl derivative of 6-mercaptopurine and many of its biological effects are similar to those of the parent compound.

Following is its chemical structure:

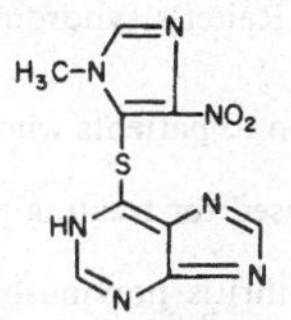

CLINICAL PHARMACOLOGY

Metabolism[1]: Azathioprine is well absorbed following oral administration. Maximum serum radioactivity occurs at one to two hours after oral ^{35}S-Azathioprine and decays with a half-life of five hours. This is not an estimate of the half-life of Azathioprine itself but is the decay rate for all ^{35}S-containing metabolites of the drug. Because of extensive metabolism, only a fraction of the radioactivity is present as Azathioprine. Usual doses produce blood levels of Azathioprine, and of mercaptopurine derived from it, which are low (< 1 µg/mL). Blood levels are of little predictive value for therapy since the magnitude and duration of clinical effects correlate with thiopurine nucleotide levels in tissues rather than with plasma drug levels. Azathioprine and mercaptopurine are moderately bound to serum proteins (30%) and are partially dialyzable.

Azathioprine is cleaved *in vivo* to mercaptopurine. Both compounds are rapidly eliminated from blood and are oxidized or methylated in erythrocytes and liver; no Azathioprine or mercaptopurine is detectable in urine after eight hours. Conversion to inactive 6-thiouric acid by xanthine oxidase is an important degradative pathway, and the inhibition of this pathway in patients receiving allopurinol is the basis for the Azathioprine dosage reduction required in these patients (see *"Drug Interactions"* under *"Precautions"*). Proportions of metabolites are different in individual patients, and this presumably accounts for variable magnitude and duration of drug effects. Renal clearance is probably not important in predicting biological effectiveness or toxicities, although dose reduction is practiced in patients with poor renal function.

Homograft Survival[1,2]: Summary information from transplant centers and registries indicates relatively universal use of Azathioprine with or without other immunosuppressive agents.[3,4,5] Although the use of Azathioprine for inhibition of renal homograft rejection is well established, the mechanism(s) for this action are somewhat obscure. The drug suppresses hypersensitivities of the cell-mediated type and causes variable alterations in antibody production. Suppression of T-cell effects, including ablation of T-cell suppression, is dependent on the temporal relationship to antigenic stimulus or engraftment. This agent has little effect on established graft rejections or secondary responses.

Alterations in specific immune responses or immunologic functions in transplant recipients are difficult to relate specifically to immunosuppression by Azathioprine. These patients have subnormal responses to vaccines, low numbers of T-cells, and abnormal phagocytosis by peripheral blood cells, but their mitogenic responses, serum immunoglobulins and secondary antibody responses are usually normal.

Immunoinflammatory Response: Azathioprine suppresses disease manifestations as well as underlying pathology in animal models of autoimmune disease. For example, the severity of adjuvant arthritis is reduced by Azathioprine. The mechanisms whereby Azathioprine affects Autoimmune diseases are not known. Azathioprine is immunosuppressive, delayed hypersensitivity and cellular cytotoxicity tests being suppressed to a greater degree than are antibody responses. In the rat model of adjuvant arthritis, Azathioprine has been shown to inhibit the lymph node hyperplasia which precedes the onset of the signs of the disease. Both the immunosuppressive and therapeutic effects in animal models are dose-related. Azathioprine is considered a slow-acting drug and effects may persist after the drug has been discontinued.

INDICATIONS AND USAGE

Azathioprine is indicated as an adjunct for the prevention of rejection in renal homotransplantation. It is also indicated for the management of severe, active rheumatoid arthritis unresponsive to rest, aspirin or other nonsteroidal anti-inflammatory drugs, or to agents in the class of which gold is an example.

Renal Homotransplantation: Azathioprine is indicated as an adjunct for the prevention of rejection in renal homotransplantation. Experience with over 16,000 transplants shows a five-year patient survival of 35% to 55%, but this is dependent on donor, match for HLA antigens, and antidonor or anti B-cell alloantigen antibody and other variables. The effect of Azathioprine on these variables has not been tested in controlled trials.

Rheumatoid Arthritis[6,7]: Azathioprine is indicated only in adult patients meeting criteria for classic or definite rheumatoid arthritis as specified by the American Rheumatism Association.[8] Azathioprine should be restricted to patients with severe, active and erosive disease not responsive to conventional management including rest, aspirin, or other nonsteroidal drugs or to agents in the class of which gold is an example. Rest, physiotherapy, and salicylates should be continued while Azathioprine is given, but it may be possible to reduce the dose of corticosteroids in patients on Azathioprine. The combined use of Azathioprine with gold, antimalarials, or penicillamine has not been studied for either added benefit or unexpected adverse effects. The use of Azathioprine with these agents cannot be recommended.

UNLABELED USES
Azathioprine is used alone or as an adjunct in the treatment of Crohn's disease, actinic dermatitis, and Duchenne's dystrophy. It is also used in the treatment of myasthenia gravis, pemphigus, Reiter's syndrome, and ulcerative colitis.

CONTRAINDICATIONS
Azathioprine should not be given to patients who have shown hypersensitivity to the drug.

Azathioprine should not be used for treating rheumatoid arthritis in pregnant women.

Patients with rheumatoid arthritis previously treated with alkylating agents (cyclophosphamide, chlorambucil, melphalan, or others) may have a prohibitive risk of neoplasia if treated with Azathioprine.[9]

WARNINGS
Severe *leukopenia and/or thrombocytopenia* may occur in patients on Azathioprine Macrocytic anemia and severe bone marrow depression may also occur. Hematologic toxicities are dose related and may be more severe in renal transplant patients whose homograft is undergoing rejection. It is suggested that patients on Azathioprine have complete blood counts, including platelet counts, weekly during the first month, twice monthly for the second and third months of treatment, then monthly or more frequently if dosage alterations or other therapy changes are necessary. Delayed hematologic suppression may occur. Prompt reduction in dosage or temporary withdrawal of the drug may be necessary if there is a rapid fall in, or persistently low leukocyte count or other evidence of bone marrow depression. Leukopenia does not correlate with therapeutic effect; therefore the dose should not be increased intentionally to lower the white blood cell count.

Serious infections are a constant hazard for patients receiving chronic immunosuppression, especially for homograft recipients. Fungal, viral, bacterial and protozoal infections may be fatal and should be treated vigorously. Reduction of Azathioprine dosage and/or use of other drugs should be considered.

Azathioprine is mutagenic in animals and humans, carcinogenic in animals, and may increase the patient's *risk of neoplasia*. Renal transplant patients are known to have an increased risk of malignancy, predominantly skin cancer and reticulum cell or lymphomatous tumors.[10] The risk of post-transplant lymphomas may be increased in patients who receive aggressive treatment with immonosuppressive drugs.[11] The degree of immunosuppression is determined not only by the immunosuppressive regimen but also by a number of other patient factors. The number of immunosuppressive agents may not necessarily increase the risk of post-transplant lymphomas. However, transplant patients who receive multiple immunosuppressive agents may be at risk for over-immunosuppression, therefore, immunosuppressive drug therapy should be maintained at the lowest effective levels. Information is available on the spontaneous neoplasia risk in rheumatoid arthritis,[12,13] and on neoplasia following immunosuppressive therapy of other autoimmune diseases.[14,15] It has not been possible to define the precise risk of neoplasia due to Azathioprine.[16] The data suggest the risk may be elevated in patients with rheumatoid arthritis, though lower than for renal transplant patients.[11,13] However, acute myelogenous leukemia as well as solid tumors have been reported in patients with rheumatoid arthritis who have received Azathioprine. Data on neoplasia in patients receiving Azathioprine can be found under "Adverse Reactions".

Azathioprine has been reported to cause temporary depression in spermatogenesis and reduction in sperm viability and sperm count in mice at doses 10 times the human therapeutic dose[17]; a reduced percentage of fertile matings occurred when animals received 5 mg/kg.[18]

Pregnancy: "Pregnancy Category D": Azathioprine can cause fetal harm when administered to a pregnant woman. Azathioprine should not be given during pregnancy without careful weighing of risk versus benefit. Whenever possible, use of Azathioprine in pregnant patients should be avoided. This drug should not be used for treating rheumatoid arthritis in pregnant women.[19]

Azathioprine is teratogenic in rabbits and mice when given in doses equivalent to the human dose (5 mg/kg daily). Abnormalities included skeletal malformations and visceral anomalies.[18]

Limited immunologic and other abnormalities have occurred in a few infants born of renal allograft recipients on Azathioprine. In a detailed case report,[20] documented lymphopenia, diminished IgG and IgM levels, CMV infection, and a decreased thymic shadow were noted in an infant born to a mother receiving 150 mg Azathioprine and 30 mg prednisone daily throughout pregnancy. At ten weeks most features were normalized. DeWitte et al[21] reported pancytopenia and severe immune deficiency in a preterm infant whose mother received 125 mg Azathioprine and 12.5 mg prednisone daily. There have been two published reports of abnormal physical findings. Williamson and Karp[22] described an infant born with preaxial polydactyly whose mother received Azathioprine 200 mg daily and prednisone 20 mg every other day during pregnancy. Tallent et al[23] described an infant with a large myelomeningocele in the upper lumbar region, bilateral dislocated hips, and bilateral talipes equinovarus. The father was on long-term Azathioprine therapy.

Benefit versus risk must be weighed carefully before use of Azathioprine in patients of reproductive potential. There are no adequate and well-controlled studies in pregnant women. If this drug is used during pregnancy or if the patient becomes pregnant while taking this drug, the patient should be apprised of the potential hazard to the fetus. Women of childbearing age should be advised to avoid becoming pregnant.

PRECAUTIONS
General: A gastrointestinal hypersensitivity reaction characterized by severe nausea and vomiting has been reported.[24,25,26] These symptoms may also be accompanied by diarrhea, rash, fever, malaise, myalgias, elevations in liver enzymes, and occasionally, hypotension. Symptoms of gastrointestinal toxicity most often develop within the first several weeks of Azathioprine therapy and are reversible upon discontinuation of the drug. The reaction can recur within hours after rechallenge with a single dose of Azathioprine.

INFORMATION FOR PATIENTS
Patients being started on Azathioprine should be informed of the necessity of periodic blood counts while they are receiving the drug and should be asked to report any unusual bleeding or bruising to their physician. They should be informed of the danger of infection while receiving Azathioprine and asked to report signs and symptoms of infection to their physician. Careful dosage instructions should be given to the patient, especially when Azathioprine is being administered in the presence of impaired renal function or concomitantly with allopurinol (see "Dosage and Administration" and "Drug Interactions" under "Precautions"). Patients should be advised of the potential risks of the use of Azathioprine during pregnancy and during the nursing period. The increased risk of neoplasia following Azathioprine therapy should be explained to the patient.

Laboratory Tests: See "Warnings" and "Adverse Reactions".

DRUG INTERACTIONS:
Use with Allopurinol: The principal pathway for detoxification of Azathioprine is inhibited by allopurinol. Patients receiving Azathioprine and allopurinol concomitantly should have a dose reduction of Azathioprine, to approximately 1/3 to 1/4 the usual dose.

Use with Other Agents Affecting Myelopoesis: Drugs which may affect leukocyte production, including co-trimoxazole, may lead to exaggerated leukopenia, especially in renal transplant recipients.[27]

Use with Angiotensin Converting Enzyme Inhibitors: The use of angiotensin converting enzyme inhibitors to control hypertension in patients on azathioprine has been reported to induce severe leukopenia.[28]

Carcinogenesis, Mutagenesis, Impairment of Fertility: See "Warnings" section.

Pregnancy: Teratogenic Effect. Pregnancy Category D. See "Warnings" section.

Nursing Mother: The use of Azathioprine in nursing mothers is not recommend. Azathioprine or its metabolites are transferred at low levels, both transplacentally and in breast milk.[29,30,31] Because of the potential for tumorigenicity shown for Azathioprine, a decision should be made whether to discontinue nursing or discontinue the drug, taking into account the importance of the drug to the mother.

Pediatric Use: Safety and efficacy of Azathioprine in children have not been established.

ADVERSE REACTIONS
The principal and potentially serious toxic effects of Azathioprine are hematologic and gastrointestinal. The risks of secondary infection and neoplasia are also significant (see "Warnings"). The frequency and severity of adverse reactions depend on the dose and duration of Azathioprine as well as on the patient's underlying disease or concomitant therapies. The incidence of hematologic toxicities and neoplasia encountered in groups of renal homograft recipients is significantly higher than that in studies employing Azathioprine for rheumatoid arthritis. The relative incidences in clinical studies are summarized below:

Toxicity	Renal Homograft	Rheumatoid Arthritis
Leukopenia Any Degree	> 50%	28%
< 2500/mm³	16%	5.3%
Infections	20%	> 1%
Neoplasia Lymphoma	0.5%	*
Others	2.8%	

* Data on the rate and risk of neoplasia among persons with rheumatoid arthritis treated with Azathioprine are limited. The incidence of lymphoproliferative disease in patients with RA appears to be significantly higher than that in the general population.[12] In one completed study, the rate of lymphoproliferative disease in RA patients receiving more than recommended doses of Azathioprine (5 mg/kg/day) was 1.8 cases per 1000 patient years of follow-up, compared with 0.8 cases per 1000 patient years of follow-up in those not receiving Azathioprine.[13] However, the proportion of the increased risk attributable to the Azathioprine dosage or to other therapies (i.e., alkylating agents) received by patients treated with Azathioprine cannot be determined.

Hematologic: Leukopenia and/or thrombocytopenia are dose dependent and may occur late in the course of Azathioprine therapy. Dose reduction or temporary withdrawal allows reversal of these toxicities. Infection may occur as a secondary manifestation of bone marrow suppression or leukopenia, but the incidence of infection in renal homotransplantation is 30 to 60 times that in rheumatoid arthritis. Macrocytic anemia and/or bleeding have been reported in two patients on Azathioprine.

Gastrointestinal: Nausea and vomiting may occur within the first few months of Azathioprine therapy, and occurred in approximately 12% of 676 rheumatoid arthritis patients. The frequency of gastric disturbance often can be reduced by administration of the drug in divided doses and/or after meals. However, in some patients, nausea and vomiting may be severe and may be accompanied by symptoms such as diarrhea, fever, malaise, and myalgias (see *"Precautions"*). Vomiting with abdominal pain may occur rarely with a hypersensitivity pancreatitis. Hepatotoxicity manifest by elevation of serum alkaline phosphatase, bilirubin, and/or serum transaminases is known to occur following Azathioprine use, primarily in allograft recipients. Hepatotoxicity has been uncommon (less than 1%) in rheumatoid arthritis patients. Hepatotoxicity following transplantation most often occurs within 6 months of transplantation and is generally reversible after interruption of Azathioprine. A rare, but life-threatening hepatic veno-occlusive disease associated with chronic administration of Azathioprine has been described in transplant patients and in one patient receiving Azathioprine for panuveitis.[32,33,34] Periodic measurement of serum transaminases, alkaline phosphatase and bilirubin is indicated for early detection of hepatotoxicity. If hepatic veno-occlusive disease is clinically suspected, Azathioprine should be permanently withdrawn.

Others: Additional side effects of low frequency have been reported. These include skin rashes (approximately 2%), alopecia, fever, arthralgias, diarrhea, steatorrhea, and negative nitrogen balance (all less than 1%).

OVERDOSAGE

The oral LD_{50}s for single doses of Azathioprine in mice and rats are 2500 mg/kg and 400 mg/kg, respectively. Very large doses of this antimetabolite may lead to marrow hypoplasia, bleeding, infection, and death. About 30% of Azathioprine is bound to serum proteins, but approximately 45% is removed during an 8-hour hemodialysis.[35] A single case has been reported of a renal transplant patient who ingested a single dose of 7500 mg Azathioprine. The immediate toxic reactions were nausea, vomiting, and diarrhea, followed by mild leukopenia and mild abnormalities in liver function. The white blood cell count, SGOT, and bilirubin returned to normal six days after the overdose.

DOSAGE AND ADMINISTRATION

Renal Homotransplantation: The dose of Azathioprine required to prevent rejection and minimize toxicity will vary with individual patients; this necessitates careful management. The initial dose is usually 3 to 5 mg/kg daily, beginning at the time of transplant. Azathioprine is usually given as a single daily dose on the day of, and in a minority of cases one to three days before, transplantation. Azathioprine is often initiated with the intravenous administration of the sodium salt, with subsequent use of tablets (at the same dose level) after the post-operative period. Intravenous administration of the sodium salt is indicated only in patients unable to tolerate oral medications. Dose reduction to maintenance levels of 1 to 3 mg/kg daily is usually possible. The dose of Azathioprine should not be increased to toxic levels because of threatened rejection. Discontinuation may be necessary for severe hematologic or other toxicity, even if rejection of the homograft may be a consequence of drug withdrawal.

Rheumatoid Arthritis: Azathioprine is usually given on a daily basis. The initial dose should be approximately 1.0 mg/kg (50 to 100 mg) given as a single dose or on a twice daily schedule. The dose may be increased, beginning at six to eight weeks and thereafter by steps at four-week intervals, if there are no serious toxicities and if initial response is unsatisfactory. Dose increments should be 0.5 mg/kg daily, up to a maximum dose of 2.5 mg/kg/day. Therapeutic response occurs after several weeks of treatment, usually six to eight; an adequate trial should be a minimum of 12 weeks. Patients not improved after twelve weeks can be considered refractory. Azathioprine may be continued long-term in patients with clinical response, but patients should be monitored carefully, and gradual dosage reduction should be attempted to reduce risk of toxicities.

Maintenance therapy should be at the lowest effective dose, and the dose given can be lowered decrementally with changes of 0.5 mg/kg or approximately 25 mg daily every four weeks while other therapy is kept constant. The optimum duration of maintenance Azathioprine has not been determined. Azathioprine can be discontinued abruptly, but delayed effects are possible.

Use in Renal Dysfunction: Relatively oliguric patients, especially those with tubular necrosis in the immediate post-cadaveric transplant period, may have delayed clearance of Azathioprine or its metabolites, may be particularly sensitive to this drug and are usually given lower doses.

Parenteral Administration: Add 10 mL of Sterile Water for Injection, and swirl until a clear solution results. This solution, equivalent to 100 mg Azathioprine, is for intravenous use only; it has a pH of approximately 9.6, and it should be used within twenty-four hours. Further dilution into sterile saline or dextrose is usually made for infusion; the final volume depends on time for the infusion, usually 30 to 60 minutes but as short as 5 minutes and as long as 8 hours for the daily dose.

Parenteral drug products should be inspected visually for particulate matter and discoloration prior to administration, whenever solution and container permit.

Procedures for proper handling and disposal of this immunosuppressive antimetabolite drug should be considered. Several guidelines on this subject have been published.[36-42]

There is no general agreement that all of the procedures recommended in the guidelines are necessary or appropriate.

Tablets: Store at 15° to 25°C (59° to 77°F) in a dry place and protect from light.

Injection: Store at 15° to 25°C (59° to 77°F) and protect from light. Dissolve in Sterile Water for Injection (see *"Parenteral Administration"* under *"Dosage and Administration"*).

REFERENCES

1. Elion GB, Hitchings GH. Azathioprine. In: Sartorelli AC, Johns DG, eds. *Antineoplastic and Immunosuppressive Agents Pt II*. New York, NY: Springer Verlag; 1975: chap 48. 2. McIntosh J. Hansen P, Ziegler J, et al. Defective immune and phagocytic functions in uraemia and renal transplantation. *Int Arch Allergy Appl Immunol.* 1976;15:544-549. 3. Renal Transplant Registry Advisory Committee. The 12th report of the Human Renal Transplant Registry. *JAMA.* 1975;233:787-796. 4. McGeown M. Immunosuppression for kidney transplantation. *Lancet.* 1973;2:310-312. 5. Simmons RL, Thompson EJ, Yunis EJ, et al. 115 patients with first cadaver kidney transplants followed two to seven and a half years: a multifactorial analysis. *Am J Med.* 1977;62:234-242. 6. Fye K, Talal N. Cytotoxic drugs in the treatment of rheumatoid arthritis. *Ration Drug Ther.* 1975;9:1-5. 7. Davis JD, Muss HB, Turner RA. Cytotoxic agents in the treatment of rheumatoid arthritis. *South Med. J.* 1978;71:58-64. 8. McEwen C. The diagnosis and differential diagnosis of rheumatoid arthritis. In: Hollander JL, ed. *Arthritis and Allied Conditions: A Textbook of Rheumatology.* 8th ed. Philadelphia, PA: Lea and Febiger; 1972:403-418. 9. Hoover R, Fraumeni, JF. Drug-induced cancer. *Cancer.* 1981;47:1071-1080. 10. Hoover R, Fraumeni JF Jr. Risk of cancer in renal transplant recipients. *Lancet.* 1973;2:55-57. 11. Wilkinson AH, Smith JL, Hunsicker LG, et al. Increased frequency of post-transplant lymphomas in patients treated with cyclosporine, azathioprine, and prednisone. *Transplantation.* 1989;47:293-296. 12. Prior P, Symmons DPM, Hawkins CF, et al. Cancer morbidity in rheumatoid arthritis. *Ann Rheum Dis* 1984; 43:128-131. 13. Silman, AJ, Petrie J, Hazelman B, et al. Lymphoproliferative cancer and other malignancy in patients with rheumatoid arthritis treated with azathioprine: a 20 year follow up study. *Ann Rheum Dis.* 1988; 47:988-992. 14. Louie S, Schwartz RS. Immunodeficiency and pathogenesis of lymphoma and leukemia. *Semin Hematol.* 1978;15:117-138. 15. Wang KK, Czaja AJ, Beaver SJ, et al. Extra hepatic malignancy following long-term immunosuppressive therapy of severe hepatitis B surface antigen-negative chronic active hepatitis. *Hepatology.* 1989; 10:39-43. 16. Sieber SM, Adamson RH. Toxicity of antineoplastic agents in man: chromosomal aberrations, antifertility effects, congenital malformations, and carcinogenic potential. In: Klein G, Weinhouse S, eds. *Advances in Cancer Research.* New York, NY: Academic Press; 1975;22:57-155. 17. Clark JM. The mutagenicity of azathioprine in mice, *Drosophila Melanogaster and Neurospora Crassa. Mut Res.* 1975; 28:87-99. 18. Data on file, Burroughs Wellcome Co. 19. Tagatz GE, Simmons RL. Pregnancy after renal transplantation. *Ann Intern Med.* 1975:82:113-114. Editorial Notes. 20. Cote CJ, Meuwissen HJ, Pickering RJ. Effects on the neonate of prednisone and azathioprine administered to the mother during pregnancy. *J Pediatr.* 1974; 85:324-328. 21. DeWitte DB, Buick MK, Stephen EC, et al. Neonatal pancytopenia and severe combined immunodeficiency associated with antenatal administration of azathioprine and prednisone. *J Pediatr.* 1984;105:625-628. 22. Williamson RA, Karp LE. Azathioprine teratogenicity: review of the literature and case report. *Obstet Gynecol.* 1981;58:247-250. 23. Tallent MB, Simmons RL, Najarian JS. Birth defects in child of male recipient of kidney transplant. *JAMA.* 1970;211:1854-1855. 24. Assini JF, Hamilton R, Strosberg JM. Adverse reactions to azathioprine mimicking gastroenteritis. *J Rheumatol.* 1986;13:1117-1118. 25. Cochrane D, Adamson AR, Halsey JP. Adverse reactions to azathioprine mimicking gastroenteritis. *J Rheumatol.* 1987;14:1075. 26. Cox J, Daneshmend JK, Hawkey CJ, et al. Devastating diarrhoea caused by azathioprine: management difficulty in inflammatory bowel disease. *Gut.* 1988;29:686-688. 27. Bradley PP, Warden GD, Maxwell JG, et al. Neutropenia and thrombocytopenia in renal allograft recipients treated with trimethoprim-sulfamethoxazole. *Ann Int Med.* 1980;93:560-562. 28. Kirchertz EJ, Grone HJ, Rieger J, et al. Successful low dose captopril rechallenge following drug-induced leucopenia. *Lancet.* 1981;1234:1362-1363. 29. Nelson D, Bugge C. Data on file, Burroughs Wellcome Co. 30. Saarikoski S, Seppala M. Immunosuppression during pregnancy: transmission of azathioprine and its metabolites from the mother to the fetus. *Am J Obstet Gynecol.* 1973:115:1100-1106. 31. Coulam CB, Moyer TP, Jiang NS, et al. Breast-feeding after renal transplantation. *Transplant Proc.* 1982;14:605-609. 32. Read AE, Wiesner RH, LaBrecque DR, et al. Hepatic veno-occlusive disease associated with renal transplantation and azathioprine therapy. *Ann Intern Med.* 1986;104:651-655. 33. Katzka DA, Saul SH, Jorkasky D, et al. Azathioprine and hepatic venocclusive disease in renal transplant patients. *Gastroenterology.* 1986:90:446-454. 34. Weitz H. Gokel JM, Loeschke K, et al. Veno-occlusive disease of the liver in patients receiving immunosuppressive therapy. *Virchows Arch A.* 1982:395:245-256. 35. Schusziarra V, Ziekursch V, Schlamp R, et al. Pharmacokinetics of azathioprine under haemodialysis. *Int J Clin Pharmacol Biopharm.* 1976;14:298-302. 36. Recommendations for the safe handling of parenteral antineoplastic drugs. Washington, DC: Division of Safety, National Institutes of Health; 1983. US Dept of Health and Human Services, Public Health Service publication NIH 83-2621. 37. AMA Council on Scientific Affairs. Guidelines for handling parenteral antineoplastics. *JAMA.* 1985;253:1590-1591. 38. National Study Commission on Cytotoxic Exposure. Recommendations for handling cytotoxic agents. 1984. Available from Louis P. Jeffrey, ScD, Director of Pharmacy Services, Rhode Island Hospital, 593 Eddy Street, Providence, RI 02902. 39. Clinical Oncological Society of Australia. Guidelines and recommendations for safe handling of antineoplastic agents. *Med J Australia.* 1983;1:426-428. 40. Jones RB, Frank R, Mass T. Safe handling of chemotherapeutic agents: a report from the Mount Sinai Medical Center. *CA-A Cancer J for Clin.* 1983;33:258-263. 41. American Society of Hospital Pharmacists. ASHP technical assistance bulletin on handling cytotoxic and hazardous drugs. *Am J Hosp Pharm.* 1990;47:1033-1049. 42. Yodaiken RE, Bennett D. OSHA work-practice guidelines for personnel dealing with cytotoxic (antineoplastic) drugs. *Am J Hosp Pharm.* 1986;43:1193-1204.

J CODES

Tab, 50 mg ORAL K0119
Vial, 100 mg IV K0120
Tab, 50 mg, 100s ea ORAL—J7500
Vial,100 mg, 20 ml ea IV—J7501

HOW SUPPLIED
POWDER FOR INJECTION: 100 MG

BRAND/MANUFACTURER	NDC	SIZE	AWP
◆ BRAND			
IMURAN: Burr Wellcome	00081-0598-71	1s	$88.42

TABLETS: 50 MG

BRAND/MANUFACTURER	NDC	SIZE	AWP
○ BRAND			
▶ IMURAN: Burr Wellcome	00081-0597-55	100s	$113.35
	00081-0597-56	100s ud	$113.35

Azdone SEE ASPIRIN WITH HYDROCODONE BITARTRATE

Azithromycin

DESCRIPTION

Azithromycin is an azalide, a subclass of macrolide antibiotics, for oral administration. Azithromycin has the chemical name (2R,3S,4R,5R,8R,10R,11R,12S,13S,14R)-13-[(2,6-dideoxy-3-C-methyl-3-O-methyl-a-L-ribo-hexopyranosyl) oxy] -2-ethyl-3,4,10-trihydroxy-3,5,6,8,10,12,14-heptamethyl -11- [[3,4,6-trideoxy-3-(dimethylamino) -β-D-xylo-hexopyranosyl[oxy[-1-oxa-6-azacyclopentadecan-15-one. Azithromycin is derived from erythromycin; however, it differs chemically from erythromycin in that a methyl-substituted nitrogen atom is incorporated into the lactone ring.

Azithromycin, as the dihydrate, is a white crystalline powder with a chemical formula of $C_{38}H_{72}N_2O_{12}2H_2O$ and a molecular weight of 785.0.

Following is its chemical structure:

CLINICAL PHARMACOLOGY

Following oral administration Azithromycin is rapidly absorbed and widely distributed throughout the body. Rapid distribution of Azithromycin into tissues and high concentration within cells result in significantly higher Azithromycin concentrations in tissues than in plasma or serum.

The pharmacokinetic parameters of Azithromycin in plasma after dosing as per labeled recommendations (i.e., 500 mg loading dose on day 1 followed by 250 mg q.d. on days 2 through 5) in healthy young adults (age 18-40 years old) are portrayed in the following chart:

PK Parameter (Mean)	Total n = 12 Day 1	Day 5
C_{max}(µg/mL)	0.41	0.24
T_{max}(h)	2.5	3.2
AUC 0-24 (µg•h/mL)	2.6	2.1
C_{min}(µg/mL)	0.05	0.05
Urinary Excret.		
(% dose)	4.5	6.5

In this study, there was no significant difference in the disposition of Azithromycin between male and female subjects. Plasma concentrations of Azithromycin declined in a poly-phasic pattern resulting in an average terminal half-life of 68 hours. On the recommended dosing regimen, C_{min} and C_{max} remained essentially unchanged from day 2 through day 5 of therapy. However, without a loading dose Azithromycin C_{min} levels required 5 to 7 days to reach steady-state. When studied in healthy elderly subjects from age 65 to 85 years, the pharmacokinetic parameters of Azithromycin in elderly men were similar to those in young adults; however, in elderly women, although higher peak concentrations (increased by 30 to 50%) were observed, no significant accumulation occurred.

The high values for apparent steady-state volume of distribution (31.1 L/kg) and plasma clearance (630 mL/min) suggest that the prolonged half-life is due to extensive uptake and subsequent release of drug from tissues. Selected tissue (or fluid) to plasma/serum concentration ratios are shown in the following table:

AZITHROMYCIN CONCENTRATIONS FOLLOWING RECOMMENDED CLINICAL DOSAGE REGIMEN

Tissue or Fluid	Time After Dose (h)	Tissue or Fluid Concentration (µg/g or µg/mL)[1]	Corresponding Plasma or Serum Level (µg/mL)	Tissue (Fluid) Plasma (Serum) Ratio[1]
Skin	72-96	0.4	0.012	35
Lung	72-96	4.0	0.012	>100
Sputum*	2-4	1.0	0.64	2
Sputum**	10-12	2.9	0.1	30
Tonsil***	9-18	4.5	0.03	>100
Tonsil***	180	0.9	0.006	>100
Cervix****	19	2.8	0.04	70

[1] High tissue concentrations should not be interpreted to be quantitatively related to clinical efficacy. The antimicrobial activity of Azithromycin is pH related. Azithromycin is concentrated in cell lysosomes which have a low intraorganelle pH, at which the drug's activity is reduced. However, the extensive distribution of drug to tissues may be relevant to clinical activity.
* Sample obtained 2-4 hours after the first dose.
** Sample was obtained 10-12 hours after the first dose.
*** Dosing regimen of 2 doses of 250 mg each, separated by 12 hours.
**** Sample was obtained 19 hours after a single 500 mg dose.

The extensive tissue distribution was confirmed by examination of additional tissues and fluids (bone, ejaculum, prostate, ovary, uterus, salpinx, stomach, liver, and gallbladder). As there are no data from adequate and well-controlled studies of Azithromycin treatment of infections in these additional body sites, the clinical significance of these tissue concentration data is unknown.

Only very low concentrations were noted in cerebrospinal fluid (less than 0.01 µg/mL) in the presence of non-inflamed meninges.

The serum protein binding of Azithromycin is variable in the concentration range approximating human exposure, decreasing from 51% at 0.02 µg/mL to 7% at 2 µg/mL. Biliary excretion of Azithromycin, predominantly as unchanged drug, is a major route of elimination. Over the course of a week, approximately 6% of the administered dose appears as unchanged drug in urine.

There are no pharmacokinetic data available from studies in hepatically- or renally-impaired individuals. Food decreases the absorption of Azithromycin, reducing the C_{max} by 52% and the AUC by 43%.

The AUC of Azithromycin was unaffected by co-administration of an aluminum and magnesium hydroxide antacid on Azithromycin; however, the C_{max} was reduced by 24%. Administration of cimetidine (800 mg) two hours prior to Azithromycin had no effect on Azithromycin absorption.

The effect of Azithromycin on the plasma levels or pharmacokinetics of theophylline administered in multiple doses adequate to reach therapeutic steady-state plasma levels is not known. (See "Precautions".)

MICROBIOLOGY

Azithromycin acts by binding to the 50S ribosomal subunit of susceptible organisms and thus interfering with microbial protein synthesis. Nucleic acid synthesis is not affected. Azithromycin concentrates in phagocytes and fibroblasts as demonstrated by in vitro incubation techniques. Using such methodology, the ratio of intracellular to extracellular concentration was > 30 after one hour incubation. In In vivo studies suggest that concentration in phagocytes may contribute to drug distribution to inflamed tissues.

Azithromycin has been shown to be active against most strains of the following organisms—both in vitro and in clinical infections. (See "Indications and Usage.")

GRAM-POSITIVE AEROBES
Staphylococcus aureus
Streptococcus agalactiae
Streptococcus pneumoniae
Streptococcus pyogenes

Note: Azithromycin demonstrates cross-resistance with erythromycin-resistant gram-positive strains. Most strains of Enterococcus faecalis and methicillin-resistant staphylococci are resistant to Azithromycin.

GRAM-NEGATIVE AEROBES
Haemophilus influenzae
Moraxella catarrhalis

OTHER ORGANISMS
Chlamydia trachomatis

Beta-lactamase production should have no effect on Azithromycin activity.

Azithromycin exhibits in vitro minimum inhibitory concentrations of 2.0 µg/mL or less against most strains of the following organisms. The safety and efficacy of Azithromycin in treating infections due to these organisms have not been established in adequate and well-controlled trials. The following in vitro data are available; however, their clinical significance is unknown.

GRAM-POSITIVE AEROBES
Streptococci (Groups C, F, G)
Viridans group streptococci

ANAEROBIC BACTERIA
Bacteroides bivius
Clostridium perfringens

GRAM-NEGATIVE AEROBES
Bordetella pertussis
Campylobacter jejuni
Haemophilus ducreyi
Legionella pneumophila
Peptostreptococcus species

OTHER ORGANISMS
Borrelia burgdorferi
Mycoplasma pneumoniae
Treponema pallidum

Ureaplasma urealyticum

SUSCEPTIBILITY TESTS

Diffusion Techniques: Quantitative methods that require measurement of zone diameters give the most precise estimate of the susceptibility of bacteria to antimicrobial agents. One such standard procedure[1] which has been recommended for use with disks to test susceptibility of organisms to Azithromycin uses the 15-μg Azithromycin disk. Interpretation involves the correlation of the diameter obtained in the disk test with the minimum inhibitory concentration (MIC) for Azithromycin.

Reports from the laboratory giving results of the standard single-disk susceptibility test with a 15-μg Azithromycin disk should be interpreted according to the following criteria:

Zone Diameter (mm)	Interpretation
≥ 18	(S) Susceptible
14-17	(I) Intermediate
≥ 13	(R) Resistant

A report of "Susceptible" indicates that the pathogen is likely to respond to monotherapy with Azithromycin. A report of "Intermediate" indicates that the result be considered equivocal, and, if the organism is not fully susceptible to alternative clinically feasible drugs, the test should be repeated. This category provides a buffer zone which prevents small uncontrolled technical factors from causing major discrepancies in interpretations. A report of 'Resistant' indicates that achievable drug concentrations are unlikely to be inhibitory and other therapy should be selected.

Standardized procedures require the use of laboratory control organisms. The 15-μg Azithromycin disk should give the following zone diameter:

Organism	Zone diameter (mm)
S. aureus ATCC 25923	21-26

Dilution Techniques: Use a standardized dilution method[2] (broth, agar, microdilution) or equivalent with Azithromycin powder. The MIC values obtained should be interpreted according to the following criteria:

MIC (μg/mL)	Interpretation
≤ 2	(S) Susceptible
4	(I) Intermediate
≤ 8	(R) Resistant

The *in vitro* potency of Azithromycin is markedly affected by the pH of the microbiological growth medium during incubation. Incubation in CO_2 atmosphere will result in lowering of media pH (7.2 to 6.6, 18 hours in 10% CO_2) and an apparent reduction in *in vitro* potency of Azithromycin. Thus, the initial pH of the growth medium should be 7.2-7.4, and the CO_2 content of the incubation atmosphere should be as low as practical.

Azithromycin can be solubilized for *in vitro* testing by dissolving in a minimum amount of 95% ethanol and diluting to working concentration with water.

As with standard diffusion methods, dilution methods require the use of laboratory control organisms. Standard Azithromycin powder should provide the following MIC values:

Organism	MIC (μg/mL)
E. coli ATCC 25922	2.0-8.0
E. faecalis ATCC 29212	1.0-4.0
S. aureus ATCC 29213	0.25-1.0

INDICATIONS AND USAGE

Azithromycin is indicated for the treatment of individuals 16 years of age and older with mild to moderate infections (pneumonia: *see "Warnings"*) caused by susceptible strains of the designated microorganisms in the specific conditions listed below:

LOWER RESPIRATORY TRACT
Acute bacterial exacerbations of chronic obstructive pulmonary disease due to *Haemophilus influenzae, Moraxella catarrhalis*, or *Streptococcus pneumoniae.*

Community-acquired pneumonia of mild severity due to *Streptococcus pneumoniae* or *Haemophilus influenzae* in patients appropriate for outpatient oral therapy.

Note: Azithromycin should not be used in patients with pneumonia who are judged to be inappropriate for outpatient oral therapy because of moderate to severe illness or risk factors such as any of the following:

patients with nosocomially acquired infections,
patients with known or suspected bacteremia,
patients requiring hospitalization,
elderly or debilitated patients, or
patients with significant underlying health problems that may compromise their ability to respond to their illness (including immunodeficiency or functional asplenia).

UPPER RESPIRATORY TRACT
Streptococcal pharyngitis/tonsillitis—As an alternative to first line therapy of acute pharyngitis/tonsillitis due to *Streptococcus pyogenes* occurring in individuals who cannot use first line therapy.

Note: Penicillin is the usual drug of choice in the treatment of *Streptococcus pyogenes* infections and the prophylaxis of rheumatic fever Azithromycin is often effective in the eradication of susceptible strains of *Streptococcus pyogenes* from the nasopharynx. Because some strains are resistant to Azithromycin susceptibility tests should be performed when patients are treated with Azithromycin Data establishing efficacy of Azithromycin in subsequent prevention of rheumatic fever are not available.

SKIN AND SKIN STRUCTURE
Uncomplicated skin and skin structure infections due to *Staphylococcus aureus, Streptococcus pyogenes*, or *Streptococcus agalactiae.* Abscesses usually require surgical drainage.

SEXUALLY TRANSMITTED DISEASES
Non-gonococcal urethritis and cervicitis due to *Chlamydia trachomatis.*

Azithromycin, at the recommended dose, should not be relied upon to treat gonorrhea or syphilis. Antimicrobial agents used in high doses for short periods of time to treat non-gonococcal urethritis may mask or delay the symptoms of incubating gonorrhea or syphilis. All patients with sexually-transmitted urethritis or cervicitis should have a serologic test for syphilis and appropriate cultures for gonorrhea performed at the time of diagnosis. Appropriate antimicrobial therapy and follow-up tests for these diseases should be initiated if infection is confirmed.

Appropriate culture and susceptibility tests should be performed before treatment to determine the causative organism and its susceptibility to azithromycin. Therapy with Azithromycin may be initiated before results of these tests are known; once the results become available, antimicrobial therapy should be adjusted accordingly.

UNLABELED USES
Azithromycin is used alone or as an adjunct in the treatment of disseminated mycobacterium avium-intracellulare complex infections in male patients with AIDS.

CONTRAINDICATIONS
Azithromycin is contraindicated in patients with known hypersensitivity to Azithromycin, erythromycin, or any macrolide antibiotic.

WARNINGS
Rare serious allergic reactions, including angioedema and anaphylaxis, have been reported in patients on Azithromycin therapy. (See *"Contraindications".*) Despite initially successful symptomatic treatment of the allergic symptoms when symptomatic therapy was discontinued, the allergic symptoms recurred soon thereafter in some patients without further Azithromycin exposure. These patients required prolonged periods of observation and symptomatic treatment. The relationship of these episodes to the long tissue half-life of Azithromycin and subsequent prolonged exposure to antigen is unknown at present.

If an allergic reaction occurs, the drug should be discontinued and appropriate therapy should be instituted. Physicians should be aware that reappearance of the allergic symptoms may occur when symptomatic therapy is discontinued.

In the treatment of pneumonia, Azithromycin has only been shown to be safe and effective in the treatment of community-acquired pneumonia of mild severity due to *Streptococcus pneumoniae* or *Haemophilus influenzae* in patients appropriate for outpatient oral therapy. Azithromycin should not be used in patients with pneumonia who are judged to be inappropriate for outpatient oral therapy because moderate to severe illness or risk factors such as any of the following: patients with nosocomially acquired infections, patients with known or suspected bacteremia, patients, or patients with significant underlying health problems that may compromise their ability to respond to their illness (including immunodeficiency or functional asplenia). Pseudomembranous colitis has been reported with nearly all antibacterial agents and may range in severity from mild to life-threatening. Therefore, it is important to consider this diagnosis in patients who present with diarrhea subsequent to the administration of antibacterial agents.

Treatment with antibacterial agents alters the normal flora of the colon and may permit overgrowth of clostridia. Studies indicate that a toxin produced by *Clostridium difficile* is a primary cause of "antibiotic-associated colitis."

After the diagnosis of pseudomembranous colitis has been established, therapeutic measures should be initiated. Mild cases of pseudomembranous colitis usually respond to discontinuation of the drug alone. In moderate to severe cases, consideration should be given to management with fluids and electrolytes, protein supplementation, and treatment with an antibacterial drug clinically effective against *Clostridium difficile* colitis.

PRECAUTIONS

General: Because Azithromycin is principally eliminated via the liver, caution should be exercised when Azithromycin is administered to patients with impaired hepatic function. There are no data regarding Azithromycin usage in patients with renal impairment; thus, caution should be exercised when prescribing Azithromycin in these patients.

The following adverse event has not been reported in clinical trials with Azithromycin, an azalide. However, it has been reported with macrolide products: ventricular arrhythmias, including ventricular tachycardia and *torsades de pointes*, in individuals with prolonged QT intervals.

Information for Patients: Patients should be cautioned to take this medication at least one hour prior to a meal or at least two hours after a meal. This medication should not be taken with food.

Patients should also be cautioned not to take aluminum- and magnesium-containing antacids and Azithromycin simultaneously.

The patient should be directed to discontinue Azithromycin immediately and contact a physician if any signs of an allergic reaction occur.

Drug Interactions: Aluminum- and magnesium-containing antacids reduce the peak serum levels (rate) but not the A.U.C. (extent) of Azithromycin absorption.

Administration of cimetidine (800 mg) two hours prior to Azithromycin had no effect on Azithromycin absorption.

Azithromycin did not affect the plasma levels or pharmacokinetics of theophylline administered as a single intravenous dose. The effect of Azithromycin on the plasma levels of pharmacokinetics of theophylline administered in multiple doses resulting in therapeutic steady state levels of theophylline is not known. However, concurrent use of macrolides and theophylline has been associated with increases in the serum concentrations of theophylline. Therefore, until further data are available, prudent medical practice dictates careful monitoring of plasma theophylline levels in patients receiving Azithromycin and theophylline concomitantly.

Azithromycin did not affect the prothrombin time response to a single dose of warfarin. However, prudent medical practice dictates careful monitoring of prothrombin time in all patients treated with Azithromycin and warfarin concomitantly. Concurrent use of macrolides and warfarin in clinical practice has been associated with increased anticoagulant effects.

The following drug interactions have not been reported in clinical trials with Azithromycin, however, no specific drug interaction studies have been performed to evaluate potential drug-drug interaction. Nonetheless, they have been observed with macrolide products. Until further data are developed regarding drug interactions when Azithromycin and these drugs are used concomitantly, careful monitoring of patients is advised:

Digoxin—elevated digoxin levels.

Ergotamine or dihydroergotamine—acute ergot toxicity characterized by severe peripheral vasospasm and dysesthesia.

Triazolam—decrease the clearance of triazolam and thus may increase the pharmacologic effect of triazolam.

Drugs metabolized by the cytochrome P450 system—elevations of serum carbamazepine, cyclosporine, hexobarbital, and phenytoin levels.

Laboratory Test Interactions: There are no reported laboratory test interactions.

Carcinogenesis, Mutagenesis, Impairment of Fertility: Long-term studies in animals have not been performed to evaluate carcinogenic potential. Azithromycin has shown no mutagenic potential in standard laboratory tests: mouse lymphoma assay, human lymphocyte clastogenic assay, and mouse bone marrow clastogenic assay.

Pregnancy: Teratogenic Effects. Pregnancy Category B: Reproduction studies have been performed in rats and mice at doses up to moderately maternally toxic dose levels (i.e., 200 mg/kg/day). These doses, based on a mg/m² basis, are estimated to be 4 and 2 times, respectively, the human daily dose of 500 mg. No evidence of impaired fertility or harm to the fetus due to Azithromycin was found. There are, however, no adequate and well-controlled studies in pregnant women. Because animal reproduction studies are not always predictive of human response, Azithromycin should be used during pregnancy only if clearly needed.

Nursing Mothers: It is not known whether Azithromycin is excreted in human milk. Because many drugs are excreted in human milk, caution should be exercised when Azithromycin is administered to a nursing woman.

Pediatric Use: Safety and effectiveness in children or adolescents under 16 years of age have not been established.

Geriatric Use: Pharmacokinetic parameters in older volunteers (65-85 years old) were similar to those in younger volunteers (18-40 years old) for the 5-day therapeutic regimen. Dosage adjustment does not appear to be necessary for older patients with normal renal and hepatic function receiving treatment with this dosage regimen. (See *"Clinical Pharmacology".*)

ADVERSE REACTIONS

In clinical trials most of the reported side effects were mild to moderate in severity and were reversible upon discontinuation of the drug. Approximately 0.7% of the patients from the multiple-dose clinical trials discontinued Azithromycin therapy because of treatment-related side effects. Most of the side effects leading to discontinuation were related to the gastrointestinal tract, e.g., nausea, vomiting, diarrhea, or abdominal pain. Rare, but potentially serious side effects, were angioedema and cholestatic jaundice.

CLINICAL:

Multiple-dose Regimen: Overall, the most common side effects in patients receiving the multiple-dose regimen of Azithromycin were related to the gastrointestinal system with diarrhea/loose stools (5%), nausea (3%), and abdominal pain (3%) being the most frequently reported.

No other side effects occurred in patients on the multiple-dose regimen of Azithromycin with a frequency greater than 1%. Side effects that occurred with a frequency of 1% or less included the following:

Cardiovascular: Palpitations, chest pain.

Gastrointestinal: Dyspepsia, flatulence, vomiting, melena, and cholestatic jaundice.

Cenitourinary: Monilia, vaginitis, and nephritis.

Nervous System: Dizziness, headache, vertigo, and somnolence.

General: Fatigue.

Allergic: Rash, photosensitivity, and angioedema.

Single 1-gram Dose Regimen: Overall, the most common side effects in patients receiving a single-dose regimen of 1 gram of Azithromycin were related to the gastrointestinal system and were more frequently reported than in patients receiving the multiple-dose regimen.

Side effects that occurred in patients on the single one-gram dosing regimen of Azithromycin with a frequency of 1% or greater included diarrhea/loose stools (7%), nausea (5%), vomiting (2%), and vaginitis (2%).

Laboratory Abnormalities: Significant abnormalities (irrespective of drug relationship) occurring during the clinical trials were reported as follows:

With an incidence of 1-2%, elevated serum creatinine phosphokinase, potassium, ALT (SGPT), GGT, and AST (SGOT). With an incidence of less than 1%, leukopenia, neutropenia, decreased platelet count, elevated serum alkaline phosphatase, bilirubin, BUN, creatinine, blood glucose, LDH, and phosphate.

When follow-up was provided, changes in laboratory tests appeared to be reversible.

In multiple-dose clinical trials involving more than 3000 patients, 3 patients discontinued therapy because of treatment-related liver enzyme abnormalities and 1 because of a renal function abnormality.

DOSAGE AND ADMINISTRATION

(See *"Indications and Usage"*)

Azithromycin should be given at least 1 hour before or 2 hours after a meal.

The recommended dose of Azithromycin for the treatment of individuals 16 years of age and older with mild to moderate acute bacterial exacerbations of chronic obstructive pulmonary disease, pneumonia, pharyngitis/tonsillitis (as second-line therapy), and uncomplicated skin and skin structure infections due to the indicated organisms is: 500 mg as a single dose on the first day followed by 250 mg once daily on days 2 through 5 for a total dose of 1.5 grams of Azithromycin.

The recommended dose of Azithromycin for the treatment of non-gonococcal urethritis and cervicitis due to *C. trachomatis* is: a single 1 gram (1000 mg) dose of Azithromycin.

ANIMAL TOXICOLOGY

Phospholipidosis (intracellular phospholipid binding) has been observed in some tissues of mice, rats, and dogs given multiple doses of Azithromycin. It has been demonstrated in numerous organ systems (e.g., eye, dorsal root ganglia, liver, gallbladder, kidney, spleen, and pancreas) in dogs administered doses which, based on pharmacokinetics, are as low as 2 times greater than the recommended human dose and in rats at doses comparable to the recommended human dose. This effect has been reversible after cessation of Azithromycin treatment. The significance of these findings for humans is unknown.

REFERENCES
1. National Committee for Clinical Laboratory Standards, Performance Standards for Antimicrobial Disk Susceptibility Tests—Fourth Edition. Approved Standard NCCLS Document M2-A4, Vol. 10, No. 7, NCCLS, Villanova, PA, 1990. 2. National Committee for Clinical Laboratory Standards, Methods for Dilution Antimicrobial Susceptibility Tests for Bacteria that Grow Aerobically—Second Edition. Approved Standard NCCLS Document M7-A2, Vol. 10, No. 8, NCCLS, Villanova, PA, 1990.

HOW SUPPLIED
CAPSULE: 250 MG

BRAND/MANUFACTURER	NDC	SIZE	AWP
○ BRAND			
➤ ZITHROMAX Z-PAK: Pfizer Labs	00069-3050-34	18s	$146.25
➤ ZITHROMAX: Pfizer Labs	00069-3050-50	50s	$406.25
	00069-3050-86	50s ud	$390.00

Azmacort *SEE* **TRIAMCINOLONE ACETONIDE, INHALATION**

AzoGantanol *SEE* **PHENAZOPYRIDINE HYDROCHLORIDE AND SULFAMETHOXAZOLE**

◆ RATED THERAPEUTICALLY EQUIVALENT; ◇ THERAPEUTIC EQUIVALENCE UNCONFIRMED; ○ UNRATED

Azo Gantrisin *SEE* PHENAZOPYRIDINE
HYDROCHLORIDE AND SULFISOXAZOLE

Aztreonam

DESCRIPTION

Aztreonam is the first member of a new class of antibiotics classified as monobactams. These agents were originally isolated from *Chromobacterium violaceum*. Aztreonam is a totally synthetic bactericidal antibiotic with activity against a wide spectrum of gram-negative aerobic pathogens.

The monobactams, having a unique monocyclic beta-lactam nucleus, are structurally different from other beta-lactam antibiotics (e.g., penicillins, cephalosporins, cephamycins). The sulfonic acid substituent in the 1-position of the ring activates the beta-lactam moiety; an aminothiazolyl oxime side chain in the 3-position and a methyl group in the 4-position confer the specific antibacterial spectrum and beta-lactamase stability.

Aztreonam is designated chemically as (Z)-2-[[[(2-amino-4-thiazolyl) [[(2S, 3S)-2-methyl-4-oxo-1-sulfo-3-azetidinyl]carbamoyl] methylene] amino]oxy]-2-methylpropionic acid.

Aztreonam for Injection is a sterile, nonpyrogenic, sodium-free, white to yellowish-white lyophilized cake containing approximately 780 mg arginine per gram of aztreonam. Following constitution, the product is for intramuscular or intravenous use. Aqueous solutions of the product have a pH in the range of 4.5 to 7.5.

Following is its chemical structure:

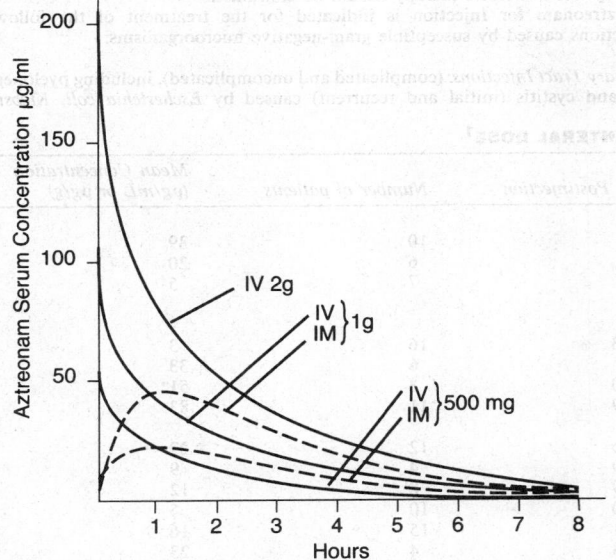

CLINICAL PHARMACOLOGY

Single 30-minute intravenous infusions of 500 mg, 1 g and 2 g doses of Aztreonam in healthy subjects produced peak serum levels of 54, 90 and 204 μg/mL, respectively, immediately after administration; at eight hours, serum levels were 1, 3 and 6 μg/mL, respectively (Figure 1). Single 3-minute intravenous injections of the same doses resulted in serum levels of 58, 125 and 242 μg/mL at five minutes following completion of injection.

Serum concentrations of Aztreonam in healthy subjects following completion of single intramuscular injections of 500 mg and 1 g doses are depicted in Figure 1; maximum serum concentrations occur at about one hour. After identical single intravenous or intramuscular doses of Aztreonam, the serum concentrations of Aztreonam are comparable at one hour (1.5 hours from start of intravenous infusion) with similar slopes of serum concentrations thereafter.

The serum levels of Aztreonam following single 500 mg or 1 g (intramuscular or intravenous) or 2 g (intravenous) doses of Aztreonam exceed the MIC90 for *Neisseria* sp., *H. influenzae* and most genera of the *Enterobacteriaceae* for eight hours (for *Enterobacter* sp., the eight hour serum levels exceed the MIC for 80 percent of strains). For *Ps. aeruginosa*, a single 2 g intravenous dose produces

serum levels that exceed the MIC90 for approximately four to six hours. All of the above doses of Aztreonam result in average urine levels of Aztreonam that exceed the MIC90 for the same pathogens for up to 12 hours.

The serum half-life of Aztreonam averaged 1.7 hours (1.5 to 2.0) in subjects with normal renal function, independent of the dose and route of administration. In healthy subjects, based on a 70 kg person, the serum clearance was 91 mL/min and renal clearance was 56 mL/min; the apparent mean volume of distribution at steady-state averaged 12.6 liters, approximately equivalent to extracellular fluid volume.

In a study of healthy elderly male subjects (65 to 75 years of age), the average elimination half-life of Aztreonam was slightly longer than in young healthy males.

In patients with impaired renal function, the serum half-life of Aztreonam is prolonged (see *"Dosage and Administration, Renal Impairment"*). The serum half-life of Aztreonam is only slightly prolonged in patients with hepatic impairment since the liver is a minor pathway of excretion. Average urine concentrations of Aztreonam were approximately 1100, 3500 and 6600 μg/mL within the first two hours following single 500 mg, 1 g and 2 g intravenous doses of Aztreonam (30-minute infusions), respectively. The range of average concentrations for Aztreonam in the 8 to 12 hour urine specimens in these studies was 25 to 120 μg/mL. After intramuscular injection of single 500 mg and 1 g doses of Aztreonam, urinary levels were approximately 500 and 1200 μg/mL, respectively, within the first two hours, declining to 180 and 470 μg/mL in the six to eight hour specimens. In healthy subjects, Aztreonam is excreted in the urine about equally by active tubular secretion and glomerular filtration. Approximately 60 to 70 percent of an intravenous or intramuscular dose was recovered in the urine by eight hours. Urinary excretion of a single parenteral dose was essentially complete by 12 hours after injection. About 12 percent of a single intravenous radiolabeled dose was recovered in the feces. Unchanged Aztreonam and the inactive beta-lactam ring hydrolysis product of Aztreonam were present in feces and urine.

Intravenous or intramuscular administration of a single 500 mg or 1 g dose of Aztreonam every eight hours for seven days to healthy subjects produced no apparent accumulation of Aztreonam or modification of its disposition characteristics; serum protein binding averaged 56 percent and was independent of dose. An average of about 6 percent of a 1 g intramuscular dose was excreted as a microbiologically inactive open beta-lactam ring hydrolysis product (serum half-life approximately 26 hours) of Aztreonam in the zero to eight hour urine collection on the last day of multiple dosing.

Renal function was monitored in healthy subjects given Aztreonam: standard tests (serum creatinine, creatinine clearance, BUN, urinalysis and total urinary protein excretion) as well as special tests (excretion of N-acetyl-β-glucosaminidase, alanine aminopeptidase and β2-microglobulin) were used. No abnormal results were obtained. Aztreonam achieves measurable concentrations in the following body fluids and tissues: (See related table).

The concentration of Aztreonam in saliva at 30 minutes after a single 1 g intravenous dose (9 patients) was 0.2 μg/mL; in breast milk at two hours after a single 1 g intravenous dose (6 patients), 0.2 μg/mL, and at six hours after a single 1 g intramuscular dose (6 patients), 0.3 μg/mL; in amniotic fluid at six to eight hours after a single 1 g intravenous dose (5 patients), 2 μg/mL. The concentration of Aztreonam in peritoneal fluid obtained one to six hours after multiple 2 g intravenous doses ranged between 12 and 90 μg/mL in 7 of 8 patients studied.

Aztreonam given intravenously rapidly reaches therapeutic concentrations in peritoneal dialysis fluid; conversely, Aztreonam given intraperitoneally in dialysis fluid rapidly produces therapeutic serum levels.

Concomitant administration of probenecid or furosemide and Aztreonam causes clinically insignificant increases in the serum levels of Aztreonam. Single-dose intravenous pharmacokinetic studies have not shown any significant interaction between Aztreonam and concomitantly administered gentamicin, nafcillin sodium, cephradine, clindamycin or metronidazole. No reports of disulfiram-like reactions with alcohol ingestion have been noted; this is not unexpected since Aztreonam does not contain a methyl-tetrazole side chain.

The implications of the following information for predicting the occurrence of hypersensitivity reactions to Aztreonam have not been established. The number of patients included in immunologic studies is too small to draw firm conclusions with regard to clinical practice:

A study in rabbits suggests that antibodies produced in response to benzylpenicillin and to cephalothin show little cross-reactivity with Aztreonam, and antibodies produced in response to Aztreonam show little cross-reactivity with benzylpenicillin and cephalothin.

In a group of 22 subjects with positive skin tests to penicillin reagents, three also had positive skin tests to Aztreonam. One was negative on retesting, one was confirmed as positive, and the third subject refused further evaluation. The 20 subjects with negative Aztreonam skin tests were given one injection of Aztreonam 1 g IM. There were no immediate hypersensitivity reactions, but one subject later developed a localized rash that was compatible with a fixed drug eruption.

In 36 subjects receiving multiple doses of Aztreonam over a seven-day period, no IgE antibody response was detectable and only one subject demonstrated an IgG response.

MICROBIOLOGY

Aztreonam exhibits potent and specific activity *in vitro* against a wide spectrum of gram-negative aerobic pathogens including *Pseudomonas aeruginosa*. The bactericidal action of Aztreonam results from the inhibition of bacterial cell wall synthesis due to a high affinity of Aztreonam for penicillin binding protein 3

➤ SHOWN IN PRODUCT IDENTIFICATION GUIDE

(PBP3). Aztreonam, unlike the majority of beta-lactam antibiotics, does not induce beta-lactamase activity and its molecular structure confers a high degree of resistance to hydrolysis by beta-lactamases (i.e., penicillinases and cephalosporinases) produced by most gram-negative and gram-positive pathogens; it is therefore usually active against gram-negative aerobic organisms that are resistant to antibiotics hydrolyzed by beta-lactamases. Aztreonam maintains its antimicrobial activity over a pH range of 6 to 8 *in vitro*, as well as in the presence of human serum and under anaerobic conditions. Aztreonam is active *in vitro* and is effective in laboratory animal models and clinical infections against most strains of the following organisms, including many that are multiply-resistant to other antibiotics (i.e., certain cephalosporins, penicillins, and aminoglycosides):

Escherichia coli
Enterobacter species
Klebsiella pneumoniae and *K. oxytoca*
Proteus mirabilis
Pseudomonas aeruginosa
Serratia marcescens
Haemophilus influenzae (including ampicillin-resistant and other penicillinase-producing strains)
Citrobacter species

While *in vitro* studies have demonstrated the susceptibility to Aztreonam of most strains of the following organisms, clinical efficacy for infections other than those included in the *"Indications and Usage"* section has not been documented:

Neisseria gonorrhoeae (including penicillinase-producing strain)
Proteus vulgaris
Morganella morganii (formerly *Proteus morganii*)
Providencia species, including *P. stuartii* and *P. retti* (formerly *Proteus rettgeri*)
Pseudomonas species
Shigella species
Pasteurella multocida
Yersinia enterocolitica
Aeromonas hydrophila
Neisseria meningitidis

Aztreonam and aminoglycosides have been shown to be synergistic *in vitro* against most strains of *Ps. aeruginosa*, many strains of *Enterobacteriaceae*, and other gram-negative aerobic bacilli.

Alterations of the anaerobic intestinal flora by broad spectrum antibiotics may decrease colonization resistance, thus permitting overgrowth of potential pathogens, e.g., *Candida* and *Clostridia* species. Aztreonam has little effect on the anaerobic intestinal microflora in *in vitro* studies. *Clostridium difficile* and its cytotoxin were not found in animal models following administration of Aztreonam (see *"Adverse Reactions, Gastrointestinal"*).

SUSCEPTIBILITY TESTING
Diffusion Technique: Quantitative procedures that require measurement of zone diameters give precise estimates of microbial susceptibility to antibiotics. One such method, recommended for use with the Aztreonam 30 µg disk, is the National Committee of Clinical Laboratory Standards (NCCLS) approved procedure. Only a 30 µg Aztreonam disk should be used: there are no suitable surrogate disks.

Results of laboratory tests using 30 µg Aztreonam disks should be interpreted using the following criteria:

Zone Diameter (mm)	Interpretation
≥ 22	(S) Susceptible
16-21	(I) Intermediate (Moderate Susceptibility)
≤ 15	(R) Resistant

Dilution Technique: Broth or agar dilution methods may be used to determine the minimal inhibitory concentration (MIC) of Aztreonam

MIC test results should be interpreted according to the concentrations of Aztreonam that can be attained in serum, tissues and body fluids.

MIC (µg/mL)	Interpretation
≤ 8	(S) Susceptible
16	(I) Intermediate (Moderate Susceptibility)
≥ 32	(R) Resistant

For any susceptibility test, a report of "susceptible" indicates that the pathogen is likely to respond to Aztreonam therapy: a report of "resistant" indicates that the pathogen is not likely to respond. A report of "intermediate" (moderate susceptibility) indicates that the pathogen is expected to be susceptible to Aztreonam if high dosages are used, or if the infection is confined to tissues and fluids (e.g., urine, bile) in which high Aztreonam levels are attained.

The quality control cultures should have the following assigned daily ranges for Aztreonam:

	Disks	Mode MIC (µg/mL)
E. coli (ATCC 25922)	28-36 mm	0.06-0.25
Ps. aeruginosa (ATCC 27853)	23-29 mm	2.0-8.0

INDICATIONS AND USAGE
Before initiating treatment with Aztreonam, appropriate specimens should be obtained for isolation of the causative organism(s) and for determination of susceptibility to Aztreonam. Treatment with Aztreonam may be started empirically before results of the susceptibility testing are available; subsequently, appropriate antibiotic therapy should be continued.

Aztreonam for Injection is indicated for the treatment of the following infections caused by susceptible gram-negative microorganisms:

Urinary Tract Infections: (complicated and uncomplicated), including pyelonephritis and cystitis (initial and recurrent) caused by *Escherichia coli*, *Klebsiella*

EXTRAVASCULAR CONCENTRATIONS OF AZTREONAM AFTER A SINGLE PARENTERAL DOSE[1]

Fluid or Tissue	Dose (g)	Route	Hours Postinjection	Number of patients	Mean Concentration (µg/mL or µg/g)
Fluids					
bile	1	IV	2	10	39
blister fluid	1	IV	1	6	20
bronchial secretion	2	IV	4	7	5
cerebrospinal fluid (inflamed meninges)	2	IV	0.9-4.3	16	3
pericardial fluid	2	IV	1	6	33
pleural fluid	2	IV	1.1-3.0	3	51
synoval fluid	2	IV	0.8-1.9	11	83
Tissues					
atrial appendage	2	IV	0.9-1.6	12	22
endometrium	2	IV	0.7-1.9	4	9
fallopian tube	2	IV	0.7-1.9	8	12
fat	2	IV	1.3-2.0	10	5
femur	2	IV	1.0-2.1	15	16
gallbladder	2	IV	0.8-1.3	4	23
kidney	2	IV	2.4-5.6	5	67
large intestine	2	IV	0.8-1.9	9	12
liver	2	IV	0.9-2.0	6	47
lung	2	IV	1.2-2.1	6	22
myometrium	2	IV	0.7-1.9	9	11
ovary	2	IV	0.7-1.9	7	13
prostate	1	IM	0.8-3.0	8	8
skeletal muscle	2	IV	0.3-0.7	6	16
skin	2	IV	0.0-1.0	8	25
sternum	2	IV	1	6	6

[1] *Tissue penetration is regarded as essential to therapeutic efficacy, but specific tissue levels have not been correlated with specific therapeutic effects.*

pneumoniae, Proteus mirabilis, Pseudomonas aeruginosa, Enterobacter cloacae, Klebsiella oxyteca*, *Citrobacter* species* and *Serratia marcescens**.

Lower Respiratory Tract Infections, including pneumonia and bronchitis caused by *Escherichia coli, Klebsiella pneumoniae, Pseudomonas aeruginosa, Haemophilus influenzae, Proteus mirabilis, Enterobacter* species and *Serratia marcescens**.

Septicemia caused by *Escherichia coli, Klebsiella pneumoniae, Pseudomonas aeruginosa, Proteus mirabilis**, *Serratia marcescens** and *Enterobacter* species.

Skin and Skin-Structure Infections, including those associated with post-operative wounds, ulcers and burns caused by *Escherichia coli, Proteus mirabilis, Serratia marcescens, Enterobacter* species*, *Pseudomonas aeruginosa, Klebsiella pneumoniae* and *Citrobacter* species*.

Intra-abdominal Infections, including peritonitis caused by *Escherichia coli, Klebsiella* species including *K. pneumoniae, Enterobacter* species including *E. cloacae**, *Pseudomonas aeruginosa, Citrobacter* species* including *C. freundii* and *Serratia* species* including *S. marcescens**.

Gynecologic Infections, including endometritis and pelvic cellulitis caused by *Escherichia coli, Klebsiella pneumoniae**, *Enterobacter* species* including *E. cloacae** and *Proteus mirabilis**.

Aztreonam is indicated for adjunctive therapy to surgery in the management of infections caused by susceptible organisms, including abscesses, infections complicating hollow viscus perforations, cutaneous infections and infections of serous surfaces. Aztreonam is effective against most of the commonly encountered gram-negative aerobic pathogens seen in general surgery.

CONCURRENT THERAPY
Concurrent initial therapy with other antimicrobial agents and Aztreonam is recommended before the causative organism(s) is known in seriously ill patients who are also at risk of having an infection due to gram-positive aerobic pathogens. If anaerobic organisms are also suspected as etiologic agents, therapy should be initiated using an anti-anaerobic agent concurrently with Aztreonam (see *"Dosage and Administration"*). Certain antibiotics (e.g., cefoxitin, imipenem) may induce high levels of beta-lactamase *in vitro* in some gram-negative aerobes such as *Enterobacter* and *Pseudomonas* species, resulting in antagonism to many beta-lactam antibiotics including Aztreonam. These *in vitro* findings suggest that such beta-lactamase inducing antibiotics not be used concurrently with Aztreonam. Following identification and susceptibility testing of the causative organism(s), appropriate antibiotic therapy should be continued.

UNLABELED USES
Aztreonam is used alone or as an adjunct in the treatment of bone and joint infections.

CONTRAINDICATIONS
Aztreonam is contraindicated in patients with known allergy to this antibiotic.

WARNINGS
Careful inquiry should be made for a history of hypersensitivity reaction to any antibiotic or other drugs. Antibiotics should be given with caution to any patient who has had some form of allergy, particularly to drugs. It is recommended that patients who have had immediate hypersensitivity reactions (e.g., anaphylactic or urticarial) to penicillins and/or cephalosporins should be followed with special care. If an allergic reaction to Aztreonam occurs, discontinue the drug and institute supportive treatment as appropriate (e.g., maintenance of ventilation, pressor amines, antihistamines, corticosteroids). Serious hypersensitivity reactions may require epinephrine and other emergency measures.

Pseudomembranous colitis has been reported with nearly all antibacterial agents, including Aztreonam and may range in severity from mild to life-threatening. Therefore, it is important to consider this diagnosis in patients who present with diarrhea subsequent to the administration of antibacterial agents.

Treatment with antibacterial agents alters the normal flora of the colon and may permit overgrowth of clostridia. Studies indicate that a toxin produced by *Clostridium difficile* is one primary cause of "antibiotic-associated colitis."

After the diagnosis of pseudomembranous colitis has been established, therapeutic measures should be initiated. Mild cases of pseudomembranous colitis usually respond to drug discontinuation alone. In moderate to severe cases, consideration should be given to management with fluids and electrolytes, protein supplementation, and treatment with an antibacterial drug effective against *C. difficile*.

PRECAUTIONS
GENERAL
In patients with impaired hepatic or renal function, appropriate monitoring is recommended during therapy.

If an aminoglycoside is used concurrently with Aztreonam especially if high dosages of the former are used or if therapy is prolonged, renal function should be monitored because of the potential nephrotoxicity and ototoxicity of aminoglycoside antibiotics.

The use of antibiotics may promote the overgrowth of nonsusceptible organisms, including gram-positive organisms (*Staphylococcus aureus* and *Streptococcus faecalis*) and fungi. Should superinfection occur during therapy, appropriate measures should be taken.

---

* Efficacy for this organism in this organ system was studied in fewer than ten infections.

CARCINOGENESIS, MUTAGENESIS, IMPAIRMENT OF FERTILITY
Carcinogenicity studies in animals have not been performed. Genetic toxicology studies performed *in vivo* and *in vitro* with Aztreonam in several standard laboratory models revealed no evidence of mutagenic potential at the chromosomal or gene level.

Two-generation reproduction studies in rats at daily doses up to 20 times the maximum recommended human dose, prior to and during gestation and lactation, revealed no evidence of impaired fertility. There was a slightly reduced survival rate during the lactation period in the offspring of rats that received the highest dosage, but not in offspring of rats that received five times the maximum recommended human dose.

PREGNANCY PREGNANCY CATEGORY B
Aztreonam crosses the placenta and enters the fetal circulation.

Studies in pregnant rats and rabbits, with daily doses up to 15 and 5 times, respectively, the maximum recommended human dose, revealed no evidence of embryo- or fetotoxicity or teratogenicity. No drug induced changes were seen in any of the maternal, fetal, or neonatal parameters that were monitored in rats receiving 15 times the maximum recommended human dose of Aztreonam during late gestation and lactation.

There are no adequate and well-controlled studies in pregnant women. Because animal reproduction studies are not always predictive of human response, Aztreonam should be used during pregnancy only if clearly needed.

NURSING MOTHERS
Aztreonam is excreted in breast milk in concentrations that are less than 1 percent of concentrations determined in simultaneously obtained maternal serum; consideration should be given to temporary discontinuation of nursing and use of formula feedings.

PEDIATRIC USE
Safety and effectiveness have not been established in infants and children.

ADVERSE REACTIONS
Local reactions such as phlebitis/thrombophlebitis following IV administration, and discomfort/swelling at the injection site following IM administration occurred at rates of approximately 1.9 percent and 2.4 percent, respectively.

Systemic reactions (considered to be related to therapy or of uncertain etiology) occurring at an incidence of 1 to 1.3 percent include diarrhea, nausea and/or vomiting, and rash. Reactions occurring at an incidence of less than 1 percent are listed within each body system in order of decreasing severity:

Hypersensitivity: anaphylaxis, anigioedema, bronchospasm.

Hematologic: panctopenia, neutropenia, thrombocytopenia, anemia, leukocytosis, thrombocytosis.

Gastrointestinal: abdominal cramps; rare cases of *C. difficile*-associated diarrhea, including pseudomembranous colitis, or gastrointestinal bleeding have been reported. Onset of pseudomembranous colitis symptoms may occur during or after antibiotic treatment (see *"Warnings"*).

Dermatologic: toxic epidermal necrolysis, purpura, erythema multiforme, exfoliative dermatitis, urticaria, petechiae, pruritus.

Cardiovascular: hypotension, transient ECG changes (ventricular bigeminy and PVC).

Respiratory: one patient experienced flushing, chest pain, and dyspnea.

Hepatobiliary: hepatitis, jaundice.

Nervous System: seizure, confusion, vertigo, paresthesia, insomnia, dizziness.

Musculoskeletal: muscular aches.

Special Senses: tinnitus, diplopia, mouth ulcer, altered taste, numb tongue, sneezing and nasal congestion, halitosis.

Other: vaginal candidiasis, vaginitis, breast tenderness.

Body as a Whole: weakness, headache, fever, malaise, diaphoresis.

ADVERSE LABORATORY CHANGES
Adverse laboratory changes without regard to drug relationship that were reported during clinical trials were:

Hepatic: elevations of AST (SGOT), ALT (SGPT), and alkaline phosphatase; signs or symptoms of hepatobiliary dysfunction occurred in less than 1 percent of recipients (see above).

Hematologic: increases in prothrombin and partial thromboplastin times, eosinophilia, positive Coombs test.

Renal: increases in serum creatinine.

OVERDOSAGE
If necessary, Aztreonam may be cleared from the serum by hemodialysis and/or peritoneal dialysis.

DOSAGE AND ADMINISTRATION
Aztreonam for Injection may be administered intravenously or by intramuscular injection. Dosage and route of administration should be determined by susceptibility of the causative organisms, severity and site of infection, and the condition of the patient.

AZTREONAM DOSAGE GUIDELINES: ADULTS

Type of Infection	Dose*	Frequency (hours)
Urinary tract infections	500 mg or 1 g	8 or 12
Moderately severe systemic infections	1 g or 2 g	8 or 12
Severe systemic or life-threatening infections	2 g	6 or 8

* Maximum recommended dose is 8 g per day.

The intravenous route is recommended for patients requiring single doses greater than 1 g or those with bacterial septicemia, localized parenchymal abscess (e.g., intra-abdominal abscess), peritonitis or other severe systemic or life-threatening infections. Because of the serious nature of infections due to *Pseudomonas aeruginosa*, dosage of 2 g every six or eight hours is recommended, at least upon initiation of therapy, in systemic infections caused by this organism.

The duration of therapy depends on the severity of infection. Generally, Aztreonam should be continued for at least 48 hours after the patient becomes asymptomatic or evidence of bacterial eradication has been obtained. Persistent infections may require treatment for several weeks. Doses smaller than those indicated should not be used.

RENAL IMPAIRMENT

Prolonged serum levels of Aztreonam may occur in patients with transient or persistent renal insufficiency. Therefore, the dosage of Aztreonam should be halved in patients with estimated creatinine clearances between 10 and 30 mL/min/1.73 m² after an initial loading dose of 1 g or 2 g.

When only the serum creatinine concentration is available, the following formula (based on sex, weight, and age of the patient) may be used to approximate the creatinine clearance (Clcr). The serum creatinine should represent a steady state of renal function.

$$\text{Males:} \quad \text{Clcr} = \frac{\text{weight (kg)} \times (140 - \text{age})}{72 \times \text{serum creatinine (mg/dL)}}$$

Females: $0.85 \times$ above value

In patients with severe renal failure (creatinine clearance less than 10 mL/min/1.73 m²), such as those supported by hemodialysis, the usual dose of 500 mg, 1 g or 2 g should be given initially. The maintenance dose should be one-fourth of the usual initial dose given at the usual fixed interval of 6, 8 or 12 hours. For serious or life-threatening infections, in addition to the maintenance doses, one-eight of the initial dose should be given after each hemodialysis session.

DOSAGE IN THE ELDERLY

Renal status is a major determinant of dosage in the elderly; these patients in particular may have diminished renal function. Serum creatinine may not be an accurate determinant of renal status. Therefore, as with all antibiotics eliminated by the kidneys, estimates of creatinine clearance should be obtained, and appropriate dosage modifications made if necessary.

PREPARATION OF PARENTERAL SOLUTIONS
GENERAL

Upon the addition of the diluent to the container, contents should be shaken **immediately** and **vigorously**. Constituted solutions are not for multiple-dose use; should the entire volume in the container not be used for a single-dose, the unused solution must be discarded.

Depending upon the concentration of Aztreonam and diluent used, reconstituted Aztreonam for Injection yields a colorless to light straw yellow solution which may develop a slight pink tint on standing (potency is not affected). Parenteral drug products should be inspected visually for particulate matter and discoloration whenever solution and container permit.

ADMIXTURES WITH OTHER ANTIBIOTICS

Intravenous infusion solutions of Aztreonam for Injection not exceeding 2% w/v prepared with Sodium Chloride Injection USP 0.9% or Dextrose Injection USP 5%, to which clindamycin phosphate, gentamicin sulfate, tobramycin sulfate, or cefazolin sodium have been added at concentrations usually use clinically, are stable for up to 48 hours at room temperature or seven days under refrigeration. Ampicillin sodium admixtures with Aztreonam in Sodium Chloride Injection USP 0.9% are stable for 24 hours at room temperature and 48 hours under refrigeration; stability in Dextrose Injection USP 5% is two hours at room temperature and eight hours under refrigeration.

Aztreonam-cloxacillin sodium and aztreonam-vancomycin hydrochloride admixtures are stable in Dianeal® 137 (Peritoneal Dialysis Solution) with 4.25% Dextrose for up to 24 hours at room temperature.

Aztreonam is incompatible with nafcillin sodium, cephradine, and metronidazole.

Other admixtures are not recommended since compatibility data are not available.

INTRAVENOUS (IV) SOLUTIONS

For Bolus Injection: The contents of an Aztreonam for Injection 15 mL or 30mL capacity vial should be constituted with 6 to 10 mL Sterile Water for Injection USP.

For Infusion: Contents of the 100 mL capacity bottle should be constituted to a final concentration not exceeding 2 percent w/v (at least 50 mL of any appropriate infusion solution listed below per gram Aztreonam. These solutions may be frozen immediately after constitution in the original container (see Stability below).

If the contents of a 15 mL or 30 mL capacity vial are to be transferred to an appropriate infusion solution, each gram of Aztreonam should be initially constituted with at least 3 mLd Sterile Water for Injection USP. Further dilution may be obtained with one of the following intravenous infusion solutions:

Sodium Chloride Injection USP, 0.9%
Ringer's Injection USP
Lactated Ringer's Injection USP
Dextrose Injection USP, 5% or 10%
Dextrose and Sodium Chloride Injection USP, 5%:0.9%, 5%:0.45% or 5%:0.2%
Sodium Lactate Injection USP (M/6 Sodium Lactate)
Ionosol® B and 5% Dextrose
Isolyte® E
Isolyte® E with 5% Dextrose
Isolyte® M with 5% Dextrose
Normosol®-R
Normosol®-R and 5% Dextrose
Normosol®-M and 5% Dextrose
Mannitol Injection USP, 5% or 10%
Lactated Ringer's and 5% Dextrose Injection
Plasma-Lyte® M and 5% Dextrose
10% Travert® Injection
10% Travert® and Electrolyte No. 1 Injection
10% Travert® and Electrolyte No. 2 Injection
10% Travert® and Electrolyte No. 3 Injection

INTRAMUSCULAR (IM) SOLUTIONS

The contents of an Aztreonam for Injection 15 mL or 30 mL capacity vial should be constituted with at least 3 mL of an appropriate diluent per gram Aztreonam. The following diluents may be used:

Sterile Water for Injection USP
Bacteriostatic Water for Injection USP (with benzyl alcohol or with methyl- and propylparabens)
Sodium Chloride Injection USP, 0.9%
Bacteriostatic Sodium Chloride Injection USP (with benzyl alcohol)

STABILITY OF IV AND IM SOLUTIONS

Aztreonam solutions for IV infusions at concentration not exceeding 2% w/v must be used within 48 hours following constitution if kept at controlled room temperature (59°-86°F/15°-30°C) or within seven days if refrigerated (36°-46° F/2°-8°C).

Frozen Aztreonam infusion solutions may be stored for up to three months at −4°F/−20°C; frozen solutions may be thawed at controlled room temperature or by overnight refrigeration. Solutions that have been thawed and maintained at controlled room temperature or under refrigeration should be used within 24 or 72 hours after removal from the freezer, respectively. Solutions should not be refrozen.

Aztreonam solutions at concentrations exceeding 2% w/v, except those prepared with Sterile Water for Injection USP or Sodium Chloride Injection USP, should be used promptly after preparation: the two excepted solutions must be used within 48 hours if stored at controlled room temperature or within seven days if refrigerated.

INTRAVENOUS ADMINISTRATION

Bolus Injection: A bolus injection may be used to initiate therapy. The dose should be **slowly** injected directly into a vein, or the tubing of a suitable administration set, over a period of three to five minutes (see next paragraph regarding flushing of tubing).

Infusion: With any intermittent infusion of Aztreonam and another drug with which it is not pharmaceutically compatible, the common delivery tube should be flushed before and after delivery of Aztreonam with any appropriate infusion solution compatible with both drug solutions; the drugs should not be delivered simultaneously. Any Aztreonam infusion should be completed within a 20 to 60 minute period. With use of a *Y-type administrated set,* careful attention should be given to the calculated volume of Aztreonam solution required so that the entire dose will be infused. A *volume control administration set* may be used to deliver an initial dilution of Aztreonam For Injection (see Preparation Of Parenteral Solutions, For Infusion) into a compatible infusion solution during administration: in this case, the final dilution of Aztreonam should provide a concentration not exceeding 2% w/v.

INTRAMUSCULAR ADMINISTRATION

The dose should be given by deep injection into a large muscle mass (such as the upper outer quadrant of the gluteus maximus or lateral part of the thigh). Aztreonam is well tolerated and should not be admixed with any local anesthetic agent.

Store original packages at room temperature; avoid excessive heat.

◆ RATED THERAPEUTICALLY EQUIVALENT; ◇ THERAPEUTIC EQUIVALENCE UNCONFIRMED; ○ UNRATED

HOW SUPPLIED

POWDER FOR INJECTION: 20 MG/ML

BRAND/MANUFACTURER	NDC	SIZE	AWP
○ **BRAND**			
AZACTAM: Squibb, E.R.	00003-2230-51	24s	$401.79

POWDER FOR INJECTION: 40 MG/ML

BRAND/MANUFACTURER	NDC	SIZE	AWP
○ **BRAND**			
AZACTAM: Squibb, E.R.	00003-2240-51	24s	$745.28

POWDER FOR INJECTION: 500 MG

BRAND/MANUFACTURER	NDC	SIZE	AWP
○ **BRAND**			
AZACTAM: Squibb, E.R.	00003-2550-10	1s	$7.51

POWDER FOR INJECTION: 1 GM

BRAND/MANUFACTURER	NDC	SIZE	AWP
○ **BRAND**			
AZACTAM: Squibb, E.R.	00003-2560-10	1s	$14.35
	00003-2560-20	1s	$15.10

POWDER FOR INJECTION: 2 GM

BRAND/MANUFACTURER	NDC	SIZE	AWP
○ **BRAND**			
AZACTAM: Squibb, E.R.	00003-2570-10	1s	$28.66
	00003-2570-20	1s	$30.21

Azulfidine *SEE* SULFASALAZINE

B. & O. Suprettes *SEE* BELLADONNA ALKALOIDS AND OPIUM

Bacampicillin Hydrochloride

DESCRIPTION
Bacampicillin is a member of the ampicillin class of semi-synthetic penicillins derived from the basic penicillin nucleus: 6-aminopenicillanic acid. Bacampicillin, as well as ampicillin and other ampicillin analogues, is acid resistant and suitable for oral administration.

Bacampicillin is the Hydrochloride salt of 1-ethoxycarbonyloxyethyl ester of ampicillin and is available as a tablet. During the process of absorption from the gastrointestinal tract Bacampicillin is hydrolyzed rapidly to ampicillin, a well characterized and effective antibacterial agent. Each 400 mg tablet of Bacampicillin is chemically equivalent to 280 mg of ampicillin.

Chemically Bacampicillin is 1'-ethoxycarbonyloxyethyl-6-(D-α aminophenylacetamide) - penicillinate Hydrochloride. It has a molecular weight of 501.96.

Following is its chemical structure:

ACTIONS
CLINICAL PHARMACOLOGY
Bacampicillin is characterized by its more complete and more rapid absorption from the GI tract than ampicillin. Bacampicillin tablets of 400 mg, 800 mg, and 1600 mg have provided ampicillin peak serum concentrations of 7.9, 12.9, and 20.1 mcg/mL. These peak levels are approximately three times the levels obtained with administration of equivalent amounts of ampicillin. The areas-under-the-serum-concentration curves obtained during the first 6 hours were 24.8 and 12.9 mcg/mL/hr., when Bacampicillin Hydrochloride 800 mg and ampicillin 500 mg were administered to adults. (See graph.)

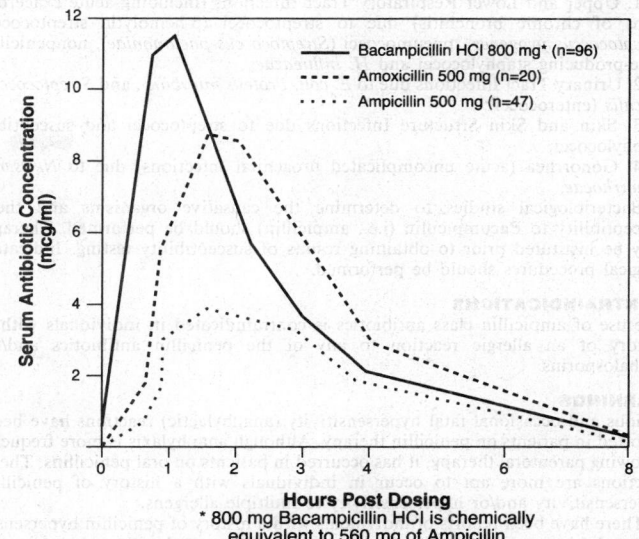

Hours Post Dosing
* 800 mg Bacampicillin HCl is chemically equivalent to 560 mg of Ampicillin

In fasting adult volunteers, a 400 mg dose of the tablet gave a peak serum ampicillin concentration of 7.2 mcg/mL. In fasting pediatric patients a 12.5 mg/kg dose provided a peak of 8.4 mcg/mL.

After oral administration of Bacampicillin tablet, ampicillin activity in serum peaks at 0.7-0.9 hours (compared to 1.5-2.0 hours after administration of ampicillin). Serum ampicillin half-life is 1.1 hours after either Bacampicillin or ampicillin administration.

Peak tissue and body fluid ampicillin concentrations also are higher after administration of Bacampicillin. Utilizing a special skin window technique to determine ampicillin levels, therapeutic levels in the interstitial fluid were higher and more prolonged after Bacampicillin than after ampicillin administration. Bacampicillin is stable in the presence of gastric acid. Food does not retard absorption of Bacampicillin tablets which may be given without regard to meals. Bacampicillin has been shown to be rapidly and well absorbed after oral administration, with about 75% of a given dose being recoverable in the urine as active ampicillin within 8 hours of administration. Urinary excretion can be delayed by concurrent administration of probenecid. The active moiety of Bacampicillin (i.e., ampicillin) diffuses readily into most body tissues and fluids. In serum, ampicillin is only 20% protein-bound, compared to 60-90% for other penicillins.

MICROBIOLOGY
Bacampicillin per se has no *in vitro* antibacterial activity and owes its *in vitro* bactericidal activity to the parent compound, ampicillin. The ampicillin class of penicillins (including Bacampicillin) has a broad spectrum of activity against many gram-negative and gram-positive bacteria. Like other penicillins, the ampicillin class of penicillins inhibits the synthesis of cell wall mucopeptide.

Ampicillin class antibiotics are inactivated by β-lactamases produced by certain strains of *Enterobacter, Citrobacter, Haemophilus influenzae,* and *Escherichia coli,* and by most strains of staphylococci and indole-positive *Proteus* spp. Ampicillin class antibiotics are not active against *Pseudomonas, Klebsiella,* or *Serratia* spp.

SUSCEPTIBILITY TESTING
Elution Technique: For the automated method of susceptibility testing (i.e., Autobac®), gram-negative organisms should be tested with the 4.5 mcg ampicillin elution disk, while gram-positive organisms should be tested with the 0.22 mcg disk.

Diffusion Technique: For the Kirby-Bauer method of susceptibility testing, a 10 mcg ampicillin diffusion disk should be used. With this procedure, a laboratory report of "susceptible" indicates that the infecting organism is likely to respond to Bacampicillin therapy, and a report of "resistant" indicates that the infecting organism is not likely to respond to therapy. An "intermediate susceptibility" report suggests that the infecting organism would be susceptible to Bacampicillin if a high dosage is used or if the infection is confined to tissues and fluids (e.g., urine) in which high antibiotic levels are attained.

Dilution Techniques. Broth or agar dilution methods may be used to determine the minimal inhibitory concentration (MIC) value for susceptibility of bacterial isolates to Bacampicillin. Since Bacampicillin per se has no *in vitro* activity, ampicillin powder should be used in a twofold concentration series of the antibiotic prepared in either broth (in tubes) or agar (in petri plates). Tubes should be inoculated to contain 10^4 to 10^5 organisms/mL or plates "spotted" with 10^3 to 10^4 organisms.

INDICATIONS AND USAGE
Bacampicillin is indicated for the treatment of the following infections when caused by ampicillin-susceptible organisms:

1. Upper and Lower Respiratory Tract Infections (including acute exacerbations of chronic bronchitis) due to streptococci (β-hemolytic streptococci, *Streptococcus pyogenes*), pneumococci (*Streptococcus pneumoniae*), nonpenicillinase-producing staphylococci and *H. influenzae*;

2. Urinary Tract Infections due to *E. coli, Proteus mirabilis* , and *Streptococcus faecalis* (enterococci);

3. Skin and Skin Structure Infections due to streptococci and susceptible staphylococci;

4. Gonorrhea (acute uncomplicated urogenital infections) due to *Neisseria gonorrhoeae*.

Bacteriological studies to determine the causative organisms and their susceptibility to Bacumpicillin (i.e., ampicillin) should be performed. Therapy may be instituted prior to obtaining results of susceptibility testing. Indicated surgical procedures should be performed.

CONTRAINDICATIONS

The use of ampicillin class antibiotics is contraindicated in individuals with a history of an allergic reaction to any of the penicillin antibiotics and/or cephalosporins.

WARNINGS

Serious and occasional fatal hypersensitivity (anaphylactic) reactions have been reported in patients on penicillin therapy. Although anaphylaxis is more frequent following parenteral therapy, it has occurred in patients on oral penicillins. These reactions are more apt to occur in individuals with a history of penicillin hypersensitivity and/or hypersensitivity to multiple allergens.

There have been reports of individuals with a history of penicillin hypersensitivity who have experienced severe reactions when treated with cephalosporins. Before therapy with a penicillin, careful inquiry should be made concerning previous hypersensitivity reactions to penicillins, cephalosporins, and other allergens.

IF AN ALLERGIC REACTION OCCURS, THE DRUG SHOULD BE DISCONTINUED AND THE APPROPRIATE THERAPY INSTITUTED. SERIOUS ANAPHYLACTOID REACTIONS REQUIRE IMMEDIATE EMERGENCY TREATMENT WITH EPINEPHRINE. OXYGEN, INTRAVENOUS STEROIDS, AND AIRWAY MANAGEMENT, INCLUDING INTUBATION, SHOULD ALSO BE ADMINISTERED AS INDICATED.

PRECAUTIONS

1. General: The possibility of superinfections with mycotic or bacterial pathogens should be kept in mind during therapy. If superinfections occur (usually involving *Aerobacter, Pseudomonas,* or *Candida*), the drug should be discontinued and appropriate therapy instituted.

As with any potent agent, it is advisable to check periodically for organ system dysfunction during prolonged therapy. This includes renal, hepatic, and hematopoietic systems and is particularly important in prematures, neonates, and patients with liver or renal impairments.

A high percentage of patients with mononucleosis who receive ampicillin develop a skin rash. Thus, ampicillin class antibiotics should not be administered to patients with mononucleosis.

2. Clinically Significant Drug Interactions: The concurrent administration of allopurinol and ampicillin increases substantially the incidence of rashes in patients receiving both drugs as compared to patients receiving ampicillin alone. It is not known whether this potentiation of ampicillin rashes is due to allopurinol or the hyperuricemia present in these patients. There are no data available on the incidence of rash in patients treated concurrently with Bacampicillin and allopurinol. Bacampicillin should not be co-administered with Antabuse (disulfiram).

3. Drug and Laboratory Test Interactions: When testing for the presence of glucose in urine using Clinitest®, Benedict's Solution, or Fehling's Solution, high urine concentrations of ampicillin may result in false-positive reactions. Therefore, it is recommended that glucose tests based on enzymatic glucose oxidase reactions (such as Clinistix® or Testape®) be used.

Following administration of ampicillin to pregnant women a transient decrease in plasma concentration of total conjugated estriol, estriol-glucuronide, conjugated estrone and estradiol, has been noted.

4. Pregnancy Category B: Reproduction studies have been performed in mice and rats a Bacampicillin doses of up to 750 mg/kg (more than 25 times the human dose) and have revealed no evidence of impaired fertility or harm to the fetus due to Bacampicillin.

There are, however, no adequate and well controlled studies in pregnant women. Because animal reproduction studies are not always predictive of human response, this drug should be used during pregnancy only if clearly needed.

5. Carcinogenesis, Mutagenesis, Impairment of Fertility: No carcinogenicity or mutagenicity studies were conducted. No impairment of fertility and no significant effect on general reproductive performance was observed in rats administered oral doses of up to 750 mg/kg of Bacampicillin per day prior to and during mating and gestation. In addition Bacampicillin caused no drug-related effects on the reproductive organs of rats or dogs receiving daily oral doses of up to 800 and 650 mg/kg respectively for 6 months.

6. Labor and Delivery: Oral ampicillin class antibiotics are generally poorly absorbed during labor. Studies in guinea pigs showed that intravenous administration of ampicillin decreased the uterine tone, frequency of contractions, height of contractions, and duration of contractions. However, it is not known whether use of Bacampicillin in humans during labor or delivery has immediate or delayed adverse effects on the fetus, prolongs the duration of labor, or increases the likelihood that forceps delivery or other obstetrical intervention or resuscitation of the newborn will be necessary.

7. Nursing Mothers: Ampicillin class antibiotics are excreted in milk; therefore, caution should be exercised when ampicillin class antibiotics are administered to a nursing woman.

8. Pediatric Use: Bacampicillin tablets are indicated for children weighing 25 kg or more.

ADVERSE REACTIONS

As with other penicillins, it may be expected that untoward reactions will be essentially limited to sensitivity phenomena. They are more likely to occur in individuals who have previously demonstrated hypersensitivity to penicillins and in those with a history of allergy, asthma, hay fever, or urticaria.

In well controlled clinical trials conducted in the U.S. the most frequent adverse reactions to Bacampicillin were epigastric upset (2%) and diarrhea (2%). Increased dosage may result in an increased incidence of diarrhea. In the same clinical trials the most frequent adverse effects for amoxicillin were diarrhea (4%) and nausea (2%).

The following adverse reactions have been reported for ampicillin.

Gastrointestinal: diarrhea, gastritis, stomatitis, nausea, vomiting, glossitis, black "hairy" tongue, enterocolitis, and pseudomembranous colitis.

Hypersensitivity Reactions: skin rashes, urticaria, erythema multiforme, and an occasional case of exfoliative dermatitis. These reactions may be controlled with antihistamines and, if necessary, systemic corticosteroids. Whenever such reactions occur, the drug should be discontinued, unless the opinion of the physician dictates otherwise.

Serious and occasional fatal hypersensitivity (anaphylactic) reactions can occur with oral penicillins. (See *"Warnings."*)

Liver: A moderate rise in serum glutamic oxaloacetic transaminase (SGOT) has been noted in some ampicillin treated patients, but the significance of this finding is unknown. In well controlled clinical trials no difference was noted between ampicillin and Bacampicillin with regard to the incidence of liver function test abnormalities.

Hemic and Lymphatic Systems: Anemia, thrombocytopenia, thrombocytopenic purpura, eosinophilia, leukopenia, and agranulocytosis have been reported during therapy with penicillins. These reactions are usually reversible on discontinuation of therapy and are believed to be hypersensitivity phenomena.

DOSAGE AND ADMINISTRATION

Bacampicillin tablets may be given without regard to meals.

UPPER RESPIRATORY TRACT INFECTIONS (including otitis media) due to streptococci, pneumococci, nonpenicillinase-producing straphylococci and *H. influenzae*;
URINARY TRACT INFECTIONS due to *E. coli, Proteus mirabilis*, and *Streptococcus faecalis*;
SKIN AND SKIN STRUCTURES INFECTIONS due to streptococci and susceptible staphylococci:

USUAL DOSAGE
Adults: 1 × 400 mg tablet every 12 hours (for patients weighing 25 kg or more).
Children: (≥ 25kg) 25 mg/kg per day in 2 equally divided doses at 12 hour intervals.

IN SEVERE INFECTIONS OR THOSE CAUSED BY LESS SUSCEPTIBLE ORGANISMS:

USUAL DOSAGE
Adults: 2 × 400 mg tablets every 12 hours (for patients weighing 25 kg or more).
Children: (≥ 25 kg) 50 mg/kg per day in 2 equally divided doses at 12 hour intervals.

LOWER RESPIRATORY TRACT INFECTIONS due to streptococci, pneumococci, nonpenicillinase-producing staphylococci, and *H. influenzae*:

USUAL DOSAGE
Adults: 2 × 400 mg tablets every 12 hours (for patients weighing 25 kg or more).
Children: (≥ 25 kg) 50 mg/kg per day in 2 equally divided doses at 12 hour intervals.

GONORRHEA—acute uncomplicated urogenital infections due to *N. gonorrhoeae* (males and females):
1.6 grams (4 × 400 mg tablet plus 1 gram probenecid) as a single oral dose.

No pediatric dosage has been established.

Cases of gonorrhea with a suspected lesion of syphilis should have dark field examination before receiving Bacampicillin and monthly serological tests for a minimum of four months. Larger doses may be required for stubborn or severe infections.

It should be recognized that in the treatment of chronic urinary tract infections, frequent bacteriological and clinical appraisals are necessary. Smaller doses than those recommended above should not be used. In stubborn infections, therapy may be required for several weeks. It may be necessary to continue clinical and/or bacteriological follow-up for several months after cessation of therapy. Except for gonorrhea, treatment should be continued for a minimum of

48 to 72 hours beyond the time that the patient becomes asymptomatic or evidence of bacterial eradication has been obtained.

IT IS RECOMMENDED THAT THERE BE AT LEAST 10 DAYS' TREATMENT FOR ANY INFECTION CAUSED BY HEMOLYTIC STREPTOCOCCI TO PREVENT THE OCCURRENCE OF ACUTE RHEUMATIC FEVER OR GLOMERULONEPHRITIS.

HOW SUPPLIED
TABLETS: 400 MG

BRAND/MANUFACTURER	NDC	SIZE	AWP
○ BRAND			
SPECTROBID: Roerig,J.B.	00049-0350-66	100s	$209.75

Bacitracin and Polymyxin, Ophthalmic

DESCRIPTION
Each gram contains Polymyxin 10,000 units, Bacitracin Zinc 500 units, special white petrolatum qs.

ACTIONS
Polymyxin B attacks gram-negative bacilli, including virtually all strains of *Pseudomonas aeruginosa* and *H influenzae* species.

Bacitracin is active against most gram-positive bacilli and cocci, including hemolytic streptococci.

INDICATIONS
For the treatment of superficial ocular infections involving the conjunctiva and/or cornea caused by organisms susceptible to Polymyxin B Sulfate and Bacitracin Zinc.

CONTRAINDICATIONS
This product is contraindicated in those individuals who have shown hypersensitivity to any of its components.

WARNINGS
Ophthalmic ointments may retard corneal healing.

PRECAUTIONS
As with other antibiotic preparations, prolonged use may result in overgrowth of nonsusceptible organisms, including fungi. Appropriate measures should be taken if this occurs.

DOSAGE AND ADMINISTRATION
Apply the ointment every 3 or 4 hours, depending on the severity of the infection.

HOW SUPPLIED
OINTMENT: 500 U/GM-10,000 U/GM

AVERAGE UNIT PRICE (AVAILABLE SIZES)		GENERIC A-RATED AVERAGE PRICE (GAAP)	
BRAND	$4.13	3.5 gm	$4.19
GENERIC	$1.42	3.75 gm	$5.82
HCFA FUL (3.5 gm)	$0.64		

BRAND/MANUFACTURER	NDC	SIZE	AWP
◆ BRAND			
POLYSPORIN: Burr Wellcome	00081-0797-86	3.75 gm	$15.50
◆ GENERICS			
OCUMYCIN: Bausch&Lomb Pharm	24208-0555-55	3.5 gm	$3.43
AK-POLY-BAC: Akorn	17478-0238-35	3.5 gm	$4.94
POLYCIN-B: Ocusoft	54799-0515-35	3.5 gm	$5.65
Schein	00364-2552-70	3.75 gm	$4.15
OCUMYCIN: Parmed	00349-8725-38	3.75 gm	$7.49

Bacitracin Zinc/Neomycin Sulfate/ Polymyxin B Sulfate, Ophthalmic

DESCRIPTION
Bacitracin Zinc/Neomycin Sulfate/Polymyxin B Sulfate, Ophthalmic is a sterile antimicrobial ointment for ophthalmic use. Each gram contains: Polymyxin B Sulfate 10,000 units, Bacitracin Zinc 400 units, Neomycin Sulfate equivalent to 3.5 mg Neomycin base, and special white petrolatum, q.s.

Polymyxin B Sulfate is the Sulfate salt of Polymyxin B_1 and B_2 which are produced by the growth of *Bacillus polymyxa* (Prazmowski) Migula (Fam. Bacillaceae). It has a potency of not less than 6,000 Polymyxin B units per mg, calculated on an anhydrous basis.

Bacitracin Zinc is the Zinc salt of Bacitracin, a mixture of related cyclic polypeptides (mainly Bacitracin A) produced by the growth of an organism of the *licheniformis* group of *Bacillus subtilis* (Fam. Bacillaceae). It has a potency of not less than 40 Bacitracin units per mg.

Neomycin Sulfate is the Sulfate salt of Neomycin B and C, which are produced by the growth of *Streptomyces fradiae* Waksman (Fam. Streptomycetaceae). It has

a potency equivalent of not less than 600 µg of Neomycin standard per mg, calculated on an anhydrous basis.

CLINICAL PHARMACOLOGY
A wide range of antibacterial action is provided by the overlapping spectra of Polymyxin B Sulfate, Bacitracin and Neomycin. The spectrum of action encompasses most bacterial pathogens capable of causing external infections of the eye and its adnexa.

Polymyxin B is bactericidal for a variety of gram-negative organisms. It increases the permeabilty of the bacterial cell membrane by interacting with the phospholipid components of the membrane.

Bacitracin is bactericidal for a variety of gram-positive and gram-negative organisms. It interferes with bacterial cell wall synthesis by inhibition of the regeneration of phospholipid receptors involved in peptidoglycan synthesis.

Neomycin is bactericidal for many gram-positive and gram-negative organisms. It is an aminoglycoside antibiotic which inhibits protein synthesis by binding with ribosomal RNA and causing misreading of the bacterial genetic code.

When used topically, Polymyxin B, Bacitracin and Neomycin are rarely irritating, and absorption from the intact skin or mucous membrane is insignificant. The incidence of skin sensitization to this combination has been shown to be low on normal skin.[1,2] Since these antibiotics are seldom used systemically, the patient is spared sensitization to those antibiotics which might later be required systemically.

Microbiology: Polymyxin B Sulfate, Bacitracin Zinc and Neomycin Sulfate together are considered active against the following microorganisms: *Staphylococcus aureus*, streptococci, including *Streptococcus pneumoniae*, *Escherichia coli*, *Haemophilus influenzae*, *Klebsiella-Enterobacter* species, *Neisseria* species and *Pseudomonas aeruginosa*. The product does not provide adequate coverage against *Serratia marcescens*.

INDICATIONS AND USAGE
Bacitracin/Neomycin/Polymyxin is indicated in the short-term treatment of superficial external ocular infections caused by organisms susceptible to one or more of the antibiotics contained therein.

CONTRAINDICATIONS
This product is contraindicated in those individuals who have shown hypersensitivity to any of its components.

WARNINGS
The manifestations of sensitization to Neomycin are usually itching, reddening and edema of the conjunctiva and eyelid. It may be manifest simply as a failure to heal. During long-term use of Neomycin-containing products, periodic examination for such signs is advisable, and the patient should be told to discontinue the product if they are observed. These symptoms subside quickly on withdrawing the medication. Neomycin-containing applications should be avoided for the patient thereafter.

PRECAUTIONS
General: As with other antibiotic preparations, prolonged use may result in overgrowth of nonsusceptible organisms including fungi. Appropriate measures should be taken if this occurs.

Allergic cross-reactions may occur which could prevent the use of any or all of the following antibiotics for the treatment of future infections: kanamycin, paromomycin, streptomycin, and possibly gentamicin.

Information for Patients: If redness, irritation, swelling or pain persists or increases, discontinue use and contact your physician.

Avoid contaminating the applicator tip with material from the eye, fingers, or other source. This caution is necessary if the sterility of the ointment is to be preserved.

ADVERSE REACTIONS
Neomycin Sulfate may cause cutaneous and conjunctival sensitization. A precise incidence of hypersensivity reactions (primarily skin rash) due to topical Neomycin is not known.

DOSAGE AND ADMINISTRATION
Apply the ointment every 3 or 4 hours for 7 to 10 days, depending on the severity of the infection.

Store at 15° to 25°C (59° to 77°F).

REFERENCES
1. Leyden JJ; Kligman AM. Contact dermatitis to Neomycin Sulfate, *JAMA*. 1979; 242(12): 1276-1278. 2. Prystowsky SD, Allen AM, Smith RW, Nonomura JH, Odom RB, Akers WA. Allergic contact hypersensitivity to nickel, neomycin, ethylenediamine, and benzocaine: Relationships between age, sex, history of exposure, and reactivity to standard patch tests and use tests in a general population. *Arch Dermatol.* 1979; 115: 959-962.

HOW SUPPLIED
OINTMENT: 400 U-3.5 MG-10,000 U/GM

AVERAGE UNIT PRICE (AVAILABLE SIZES)		GENERIC A-RATED AVERAGE PRICE (GAAP)	
BRAND	$4.43	3.5 gm	$3.94
GENERIC	$1.13		
HCFA FUL (3.5 gm)	$1.17		

BRAND/MANUFACTURER	NDC	SIZE	AWP
◆ BRAND			
NEOSPORIN: Burr Wellcome	00081-0732-86	3.5 gm	$15.50

BRAND/MANUFACTURER	NDC	SIZE	AWP
◆ **GENERICS**			
OCUTRICIN: Bausch&Lomb Pharm	24208-0780-55	3.5 gm	$2.39
OCUTRICIN: Bausch&Lomb Pharm	24208-0782-35	3.5 gm	$2.73
Fougera	00168-0027-38	3.5 gm	$3.96
AK-SPORE OINTMENT: Akorn	17478-0235-35	3.5 gm	$5.10
NEOCIDIN: Major	00904-3012-38	3.5 gm	$5.50

Bacitracin Zinc/Hydrocortisone/ Neomycin Sulfate/Polymyxin B Sulfate

DESCRIPTION

Each gram of Ointment contains:

Bacitracin Zinc ....400 units
Hydrocortisone ....10 mg (1%)
Neomycin Sulfate
equivalent to 3.5 mg Neomycin base
Polymyxin B Sulfate ....5,000 units

Each gram of Ophthalmic Ointment contains:

Bacitracin Zinc ....400 units
Hydrocortisone ....10 mg (1%)
Neomycin Sulfate equivalent to 3.5 mg Neomycin base
Polymyxin B Sulfate ....10,000 units

Polymyxin B Sulfate/Bacitracin Zinc/Neomycin Sulfate/Hydrocortisone ointment is a topical antibacterial ointment. Polymyxin B Sulfate-Bacitracin Zinc-Neomycin Sulfate-Hydrocortisone is a sterile antimicrobial and anti-inflammatory ointment for ophthalmic use.

Polymyxin B Sulfate is the sulfate salt of Polymyxin B_1 and B_2, which are produced by the growth of *Bacillus polymyxa* (Prazmowski) Migula (Fam. Bacillaceae). It has a potency of not less than 6,000 Polymyxin B units per mg, calculated on an anhydrous basis.

Bacitracin zinc is the zinc salt of Bacitracin, a mixture of related cyclic polypeptides (mainly Bacitracin A) produced by the growth of an organism of the *licheniformis* group of *Bacillus subtilis* (Fam. Bacillaceae). It has a potency of not less than 40 Bacitracin units per mg.

Neomycin Sulfate is the sulfate salt of Neomycin B and C, which are produced by the growth of *Streptomyces fradiae* Waksman (Fam. Streptomycetaceae). It has a potency equivalent of not less than 600 μg of Neomycin standard per mg, calculated on an anhydrous basis.

Hydrocortisone, 11β, 17, 21-trihydroxypregn-4-ene-3, 20-dione, is an anti-inflammatory hormone.

CLINICAL PHARMACOLOGY

Corticoids suppress the inflammatory response to a variety of agents and they may delay healing. Since corticoids may inhibit the body's defense mechanism against infection, a concomitant antimicrobial drug may be used when this inhibition is considered to be clinically significant in a particular case.

The anti-infective components in the combination are included to provide action against specific organisms susceptible to them. Polymyxin B Sulfate, Bacitracin Zinc and Neomycin Sulfate together are considered active against the following microorganisms: *Staphylococcus aureus*, streptococci, including *Streptococcus pneumoniae*, *Escherichia coli*, *Haemophilus influenzae*, *Klebsiella-Enterobacter* species, *Neisseria* species and *Pseudomonas aeruginosa*.

The product does not provide adequate coverage against *Seratia marcescens*.

When used topically, Polymyxin B, Bacitracin and Neomycin are rarely irritating, and absorption from the intact skin or mucous membrane is insignificant. The incidence of skin sensitization to this combination has been shown to be low on normal skin.[1,2] Since these antibiotics are seldom used systemically, the patient is spared sensitization to those antibiotics which might later be required systemically.

When a decision to administer both a corticoid and antimicrobials is made, the administration of such drugs in combination has the advantage of greater patient compliance and convenience, with the added assurance that the intended dosage of both drugs is administered, plus assured compatibility of ingredients when both types of drug are in the same formulation and particularly that the intended volume of each drug is delivered simultaneously, thereby avoiding dilution of either medication by successive applications.

The relative potency of corticosteroids depends on the molecular structure, concentration and release from the vehicle.

INDICATIONS AND USAGE

Ointment: For the treatment of corticosteroid-responsive dermatoses with secondary infection. It has not been demonstrated that this steroid-antibiotic combination provides greater benefit than the steroid component alone after 7 days of treatment (see "Warnings" section).

Ophthalmic Ointment: For steroid-responsive inflammatory ocular conditions for which a corticosteroid is indicated and where bacterial infection or a risk of bacterial ocular infection exists.

Ocular steroids are indicated in inflammatory conditions of the palpebral and bulbar conjunctiva, cornea and anterior segment of the globe where the inherent risk of steroid use in certain infective conjunctivitides is accepted to obtain a diminution in edema and inflammation. They are also indicated in chronic anterior uveitis and corneal injury from chemical, radiation, or thermal burns, or penetration of foreign bodies. The use of a combination drug with an anti-infective component is indicated where the risk of infection is high or where there is an expectation that potentially dangerous numbers of bacteria will be present in the eye.

The particular anti-infective drugs in this product are active against the following common bacterial eye pathogens: *Staphylococcus aureus*, streptococci, including *Streptococcus pneumoniae*, *Escherichia coli*, *Haemophilus influenzae*, *Klebsiella Enterobacter* species, *Neisseria* species, and *Pseudomonas aeruginosa*.

CONTRAINDICATIONS

Ointment: Not for use in the eyes or in the external ear canal if the eardrum is perforated. This product is contraindicated in tuberculous, fungal or viral lesions of the skin (herpes simplex, vaccinia and varicella). This product is contraindicated in those individuals who have shown hypersensitivity to any of its components.

Ophthalmic Ointment: Epithelial herpes simplex keratitis (dendritic keratitis), vaccinia, varicella, and many other viral diseases of the cornea and conjunctiva. Mycobacterial infection of the eye. Fungal diseases of ocular structures. Hypersensitivity to a component of the medication. (Hypersensitivity to the antibiotic component occurs at a higher rate than for other components.)

The use of these combinations is always contraindicated after uncomplicated removal of a corneal foreign body.

WARNINGS

Ointment: Because of the concern of nephrotoxicity and ototoxicity associated with Neomycin, this combination should not be used over a wide area or for extended periods of time.

Ophthalmic Ointment: Prolonged use may result in glaucoma, with damage to the optic nerve, defects in visual acuity and fields of vision, and posterior subcapsular cataract formation. Prolonged use may suppress the host response and thus increase the hazard of secondary ocular infections. In those diseases causing thinning of the cornea or sclera, perforations have been known to occur with the use of topical steroids. In acute purulent conditions of the eye, steroids may mask infection or enhance existing infection. If these products are used for 10 days or longer, intraocular pressure should be routinely monitored even though it may be difficult in children and uncooperative patients.

Employment of steroid medication in the treatment of herpes simplex requires great caution.

Neomycin Sulfate may cause cutaneous sensitization. A precise incidence of hypersensitivity reactions (primarily skin rash) due to topical Neomycin is not known.

The manifestations of sensitization to Neomycin are usually itching, reddening and edema of the conjunctiva and eyelid. It may be manifest simply as a failure to heal. During long-term use of Neomycin-containing products, periodic examination for such signs is advisable, and the patient should be told to discontinue the product if they are observed. These symptoms subside quickly on withdrawing the medication. Neomycin-containing applications should be avoided for the patient thereafter.

PRECAUTIONS

GENERAL

Ointment: As with any antibiotic preparation, prolonged use may result in the overgrowth of nonsusceptible organisms, including fungi. Appropriate measures should be taken if this occurs. Use of steroids on infected areas should be supervised with care as anti-inflammatory steroids may encourage spread of infection. If this occurs, steroid therapy should be stopped and appropriate antibacterial drugs used. Generalized dermatological conditions may require systemic corticosteroid therapy.

Signs and symptoms of exogenous hyperadrenocorticism can occur with the use of topical corticosteroids, including adrenal suppression. Systemic absorption of topically applied steroids will be increased if extensive body surface areas are treated or if occlusive dressings are used. Under these circumstances, suitable precautions should be taken when long-term use is anticipated.

Ophthalmic Ointment: The initial prescription and renewal of the medication order beyond 8 grams should be made by a physician only after examination of the patient with the aid of magnification, such as slit lamp biomicroscopy and, where appropriate, fluorescein staining.

The possibility of persistent fungal infections of the cornea should be considered after prolonged steroid dosing.

Allergic cross-reactions may occur which could prevent the use of any or all of the following antibiotics for the treatment of future infections: kanamycin, paromomycin, streptomycin, and possibly gentamicin.

Information for Patients: If redness, irritation, swelling or pain persists or increases, discontinue use and notify physician. Do not use in the eyes.

Laboratory Tests: Systemic effects of excessive levels of hydrocortisone may include a reduction in the number of circulating eosinophils and a decrease in urinary excretion of 17-hydroxycorticosteroids.

Carcinogenesis, Mutagenesis, Impairment of Fertility: Long-term studies in animals (rats, rabbits, mice) showed no evidence of carcinogenicity attributable to oral administration of corticosteroids.

◆ RATED THERAPEUTICALLY EQUIVALENT; ◇ THERAPEUTIC EQUIVALENCE UNCONFIRMED; ○ UNRATED

Pregnancy: Teratogenic Effects: Pregnancy Category C. Corticosteroids have been shown to be teratogenic in rabbits when applied topically at concentrations of 0.5% on days 6-18 of gestation and in mice when applied topically at a concentration of 15% on days 10-13 of gestation. There are no adequate and well-controlled studies in pregnant women. Corticosteroids should be used during pregnancy only if the potential benefit justifies the potential risk to the fetus.

Nursing Mothers: Hydrocortisone appears in human milk following oral administration of the drug. Since systemic absorption of Hydrocortisone may occur when applied topically, caution should be exercised when this combination is used by a nursing woman.

Pediatric Use: Sufficient percutaneous absorption of Hydrocortisone can occur in infants and children during prolonged use to cause cessation of growth, as well as other systemic signs and symptoms of hyperadrenocorticism.

ADVERSE REACTIONS

Ointment: Neomycin occasionally causes skin sensitization. Ototoxicity and nephrotoxicity have also been reported (see *"Warnings"* section). Adverse reactions have occurred with topical use of antibiotic combinations including Neomycin, Bacitracin and Polymyxin B. Exact incidence figures are not available since no denominator of treated patients is available. The reaction occurring most often is allergic sensitization. In one clinical study, using a 20% Neomycin patch, Neomycin-induced allergic skin reactions occurred in two of 2,175 (0.09%) individuals in the general population.[1] In another study, the incidence was found to be approximately 1%.[2] The following local adverse reactions have been reported with topical corticosteroids, especially under occlusive dressings: burning, itching, irritation, dryness, folliculitis, hypertrichosis, acneiform eruptions, hypopigmentation, perioral dermatitis, allergic contact dermatitis, maceration of the skin, secondary infection, skin atrophy, striae and miliaria. When steroid preparations are used for long periods of time in intertriginous areas or over extensive body areas, with or without occlusive non-permeable dressings, striae may occur; also there exists the possibility of systemic side effects when steroid preparations are used over larger areas or for a long period of time.

Ophthalmic Ointment: Adverse reactions have occurred with steroid/anti-infective combination drugs which can be attributed to the steroid component, the anti-infective component, or the combination. Reactions occurring most often from the presence of the anti-infective ingredient are localized hypersensitivity, including itching, swelling and conjunctival erythema. Local irritation on instillation has also been reported. Exact incidence figures are not available since no denominator of treated patients is available.

The reactions due to the steroid component in decreasing order of frequency are: elevation of intraocular pressure (IOP) with possible development of glaucoma, and infrequent optic nerve damage; posterior subcapsular cataract formation; and delayed wound healing.

Secondary Infection: The development of secondary infection has occurred after use of combinations containing steroids and antimicrobials. Fungal infections of the cornea are particularly prone to develop coincidentally with long-term applications of steroid. The possibility of fungal invasion must be considered in any persistent corneal ulceration where steroid treatment has been used.

Secondary bacterial ocular infection following suppression of host responses also occurs.

DOSAGE AND ADMINISTRATION

Ointment: A thin film is applied 2 to 4 times daily to the affected area.

Ophthalmic Ointment: Apply the ointment in the affected eye every 3 or 4 hours, depending on the severity of the condition.

Not more than 8 g should be prescribed initially and the prescription should not be refilled without further evaluation as outlined in *"Precautions"* above.

Store at 15° to 25°C (59° to 77°F).

REFERENCES

1. Leyden JJ, Kligman AM: Contact dermatitis to neomycin sulfate. *JAMA* 1979;242:1276-1278. 2. Prystowsky SD, Allen AM, Smith RW, et al: Allergic contact hypersensivity to nickel, neomycin, ethylenediamine, and benzocaine. *Arch Dermatol* 1979;115:959-962.

HOW SUPPLIED
OINTMENT: 400 U-1%-3.5 MG-10,000 U

AVERAGE UNIT PRICE (AVAILABLE SIZES)		GENERIC A-RATED AVERAGE PRICE (GAAP)	
BRAND	$2.84	3.5 gm	$4.52
GENERIC	$1.25		

BRAND/MANUFACTURER	NDC	SIZE	AWP
◆ BRAND			
CORTISPORIN: Burr Wellcome	00081-0197-86	3.75 gm	$15.72
	00081-0196-88	15 gm	$22.36
◆ GENERICS			
AK-SPORE HC: Akorn	17478-0232-35	3.5 gm	$4.50
NEOTRICIN HC: Bausch&Lomb Pharm	24208-0786-35	3.5 gm	$4.52
Fougera	00168-0029-38	3.5 gm	$4.53
Moore,H.L.	00839-6658-43	3.75 gm	$4.25

Bacitracin, Ophthalmic

DESCRIPTION
Bacitracin Ophthalmic Ointment, USP (Sterile) is a sterile antimicrobial ointment formulated for ophthalmic use to contain Bacitracin.

The antibiotic consists of 3 separate compounds, Bacitracin A, B and C; Bacitracin A is the chief constituent. Bacitracin occurs as a white to pale buff, hygroscopic powder and is freely soluble in water and soluble in alcohol.

Each gram contains: Bacitracin, USP, 500 units

Following is its chemical structure:

CLINICAL PHARMACOLOGY
Bacitracin is a polypeptide produced by an organism of the licheniformis group of *Bacillus subtilisi.* It has a range of anti-bacterial activity similar to that of penicillin; however, there are some penicillin-resistant organisms which are Bacitracin-sensitive. *In vitro* tests indicate that the drug is strongly inhibitory for hemolytic streptococci, pneumococci, gonococci, meningococci, and *Clostridia.* In addition, some strains of coagulase-positive *Staphylococcus aureus* obtained from clinical infections were found to be completely inhibited *in vitro.* Bacitracin is not inhibited by products of bacterial growth, and it exhibits activity against organisms that acquire resistance to penicillin.

Bacitracin inhibits bacterial cell wall synthesis preventing the incorporation of amino acids and nucleotides into the cell wall. It is ineffective against fungi.

INDICATIONS AND USAGE
For the treatment of superficial ocular infections involving the conjunctiva and/or cornea caused by Bacitracin susceptible organisms.

CONTRAINDICATIONS
This product is contraindicated in those individuals who have shown hypersensitivity to any of its components.

WARNINGS
Ophthalmic ointments may retard corneal healing.

PRECAUTIONS
Bacitracin Ophthalmic Ointment should not be used in deep-seated ocular infections or in those that are likely to become systemic. In such cases appropriate systemic antibiotic therapy should also be employed. As with other antibiotic preparations, prolonged use may result in overgrowth of non-susceptible organisms, including fungi. Appropriate measures should be taken if this occurs.

INFORMATION TO PATIENTS
If redness, irritation, swelling or pain persists or increases, discontinue use and contact your physician.

Avoid contaminating the applicator tip with material from the eye, fingers, or other source. This caution is necessary if the sterility of the ointment is to be preserved.

ADVERSE REACTIONS
Bacitracin has such a low incidence of allergenicity that for all practical purposes side reactions are essentially nonexistent. However, if such reaction should occur, therapy should be discontinued.

DOSAGE AND ADMINISTRATION
Pull down lower eyelid and apply a small amount (approximately ¼ inch) of ointment directly into the conjunctival sac 1-3 times daily. In blepharitis all scales and crusts should be carefully removed and the ointment then spread uniformly over the lid margins. Patients should take care to avoid gross contamination of the ointment when applying the ointment directly to the infected eye. (See *"Information to Patients."*)

Duration of therapy should be determined by the judgment of the physician and the response of the patient to therapy.

Store at controlled room temperature, 15° - 30° C (59° - 86° F).

KEEP OUT OF REACH OF CHILDREN.

HOW SUPPLIED
OINTMENT: 500 U/GM

AVERAGE UNIT PRICE (AVAILABLE SIZES)		GENERIC A-RATED AVERAGE PRICE (GAAP)	
GENERIC	$0.95	3.5 gm	$3.31
HCFA FUL (3.5 gm)	$0.77		

BRAND/MANUFACTURER	NDC	SIZE	AWP
◆ GENERICS			
Parmed	00349-8726-38	3.5 gm	$2.36
Schein	00364-7174-70	3.5 gm	$2.60
Moore,H.L.	00839-5493-43	3.5 gm	$2.82
Bausch&Lomb Pharm	24208-0565-55	3.5 gm	$2.85
AK-TRACIN: Akorn	17478-0233-35	3.5 gm	$3.13
Fougera	00168-0026-38	3.5 gm	$3.37

► SHOWN IN PRODUCT IDENTIFICATION GUIDE

BRAND/MANUFACTURER	NDC	SIZE	AWP
Major	00904-2625-38	3.5 gm	$3.40
Goldline	00182-1698-31	3.5 gm	$3.60
Ocusoft	54799-0514-35	3.5 gm	$5.65

Baclofen

DESCRIPTION

Baclofen, is a muscle relaxant and antispastic, available as 10-mg and 20-mg tablets for oral administration and solution for injection. Its chemical name is 4-amino-3-(4-chlorophenyl)-butanoic acid.

Baclofen USP is a white to off-white, odorless or practically odorless crystalline powder, with a molecular weight of 213.66. It is slightly soluble in water, very slightly soluble in methanol, and insoluble in chloroform.

Baclofen Injection is a sterile, pyrogen-free, isotonic solution free of antioxidents, preservatives or other potentially neurotoxic additives indicated only for intrathecal administration. The drug is stable in solution at 37° C and compatible with CSF. Each mL of Baclofen Injection contains Baclofen U.S.P. 500 mcg or 2000 mcg and sodium chloride 9 mg in Water for Injection; pH range is 5-7. Each ampule is intended for SINGLE USE ONLY. Discard any unused portion. *DO NOT AUTOCLAVE.*

Following is its chemical structure:

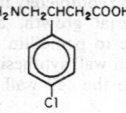

ACTIONS

The precise mechanism of action of Baclofen is not fully known. Baclofen is capable of inhibiting both monosynaptic and polysynaptic reflexes at the spinal level, possibly by decreasing excitatory neurotransmitter release from primary afferent terminals, although actions at supraspinal sites may also occur and contribute to its clinical effect. Although Baclofen is an analog of the putative inhibitory neurotransmitter gamma-aminobutyric acid (GABA), and may exert its effects by stimulation of the GABA$_B$ receptor subtype, there is no conclusive evidence that actions on GABA systems are involved in the production of its clinical effects. In studies with animals, and in people, Baclofen has been shown to have general CNS depressant properties as indicated by the production of sedation with tolerance, somnolence, ataxia, and respiratory and cardiovascular depression. Baclofen is rapidly and extensively absorbed and eliminated. Absorption may be dose-dependent, being reduced with increasing doses. Baclofen is excreted primarily by the kidney in unchanged form and there is relatively large intersubject variation in absorption and/or elimination.

Baclofen Injection when introduced directly into the intrathecal space permits effective CSF concentrations to be achieved with resultant plasma concentrations 100 times less than those occurring with oral administration.

PHARMACODYNAMICS OF BACLOFEN INJECTION

Intrathecal Bolus: The onset of action is generally one-half hour to one hour after an intrathecal bolus. Peak spasmolytic effect is seen at approximately four hours after dosing and effects may last four to eight hours. Onset, peak response, and duration of action may vary with individual patients depending on the dose and severity of symptoms.

Continuous Infusion: Baclofen Injection's antispastic action is first seen at 6 to 8 hours after initiation of continuous infusion. Maximum activity is observed in 24 to 48 hours.

PHARMACOKINETICS OF BACLOFEN INJECTION

The pharmacokinetics of CSF clearance of Baclofen Injection calculated from intrathecal bolus or continuous infusion studies approximates CSF turnover, suggesting elimination is by bulk-flow removal of CSF.

Intrathecal Bolus: After a bolus lumbar injection of 50 or 100 mcg Baclofen Injection in seven patients, the average CSF elimination half-life was 1.51 hours over the first four hours and the average CSF clearance was approximately 30 ml/hour.

Continuous Infusion: The mean CSF clearance for Baclofen Injection was approximately 30 ml/hour in a study involving ten patients on continuous intrathecal infusion.

Concurrent plasma concentrations of Baclofen during intrathecal administration are expected to be low (0.5 ng/ml).

Limited pharmacokinetic data suggest that a lumbar-cisternal concentration gradient of about 4:1 is established along the neuroaxis during Baclofen infusion. This is based upon simultaneous CSF sampling via cisternal and lumbar tap in 5 patients receiving continuous Baclofen infusion at the lumbar level at doses associated with therapeutic efficacy; the inter-patient variability was great. The gradient was not altered by position.

INDICATIONS

Baclofen is useful for the alleviation of signs and symptoms of spasticity resulting from multiple sclerosis, particularly for the relief of flexor spasms and concomitant pain, clonus, and muscular rigidity.

Patients should have reversible spasticity so that Baclofen treatment will aid in restoring residual function.

Baclofen may also be of some value in patients with spinal cord injuries and other spinal cord diseases.

Baclofen is not indicated in the treatment of skeletal muscle spasm resulting from rheumatic disorders.

The efficacy of Baclofen in spasticity of cerebral origins, e.g., stroke, cerebral palsy, and Parkinson's disease, has not been established and, therefore, it is not recommended for these conditions.

Baclofen Injection is indicated for use in the management of severe spasticity of spinal cord origin in patients who are unresponsive to oral baclofen therapy or experience intolerable CNS side effects at effective doses. Baclofen Injection is intended for use by the intrathecal route in single bolus test doses (via spinal catheter or lumbar puncture) and, for chronic use, only in implantable pumps approved by the FDA specifically for the administration of baclofen intrathecal into the intrathecal space.

Evidence supporting the efficacy of Baclofen Injection was obtained in randomized, controlled investigations that compared the effects of either a single intrathecal dose or a three day intrathecal infusion of Baclofen Injection to placebo in patients with severe spasticity and spasms due to either spinal cord trauma or multiple sclerosis. Baclofen Injection was superior to placebo on both principal outcome measures employed: change from baseline in the Ashworth rating of spasticity and the frequency of spasms.

Baclofen Injection therapy may be considered an alternative to destructive neurosurgical procedures. Prior to implantation of a device for chronic intrathecal infusion of Baclofen Injection, patients must show a response to Baclofen Injection in a screening trial (see *"Dosage and Administration"*).

UNLABELED USES

Baclofen is used alone or as an adjunct in the treatment of tardive dyskinesia, tardive dystonia, nocturnal myoclonus, and trigeminal neuralgia.

CONTRAINDICATIONS

Hypersensitivity to Baclofen.

Baclofen Injection is not recommended for intravenous, intramuscular, subcutaneous or epidural administration.

WARNINGS

Abrupt Drug Withdrawal: Hallucination and seizures have occurred on abrupt withdrawal of Baclofen. Therefore, except for serious adverse reactions, the dose should be reduced slowly when the drug is discontinued.

Impaired Renal Function: Because Baclofen is primarily excreted unchanged through the kidneys, it should be given with caution, and it may be necessary to reduce the dosage.

Stroke: Baclofen has not significantly benefited patients with stroke. These patients have also shown poor tolerability to the drug.

Pregnancy: Pregnancy Category C: Baclofen has been shown to increase the incidence of omphaloceles (ventral hernias) in fetuses of rats given approximately 13 times on a mg/kg basis, or 3 times on a mg/m^2 basis, the maximum dose recommended for human use, at a dose which caused significant reductions in food intake and weight gain in dams. This abnormality was not seen in mice or rabbits. There was also an increased incidence of incomplete sternebral ossification in fetuses of rats given approximately 13 times the maximum recommended human dose, and an increased incidence of unossified phalangeal nuclei of forelimbs and hindlimbs in fetuses of rabbits given approximately 7 times the maximum recommended human dose. In mice, no teratogenic effects were observed, although reductions in mean fetal weight with consequent delays in skeletal ossification were present when dams were given 17 or 34 times the human daily dose. There are no adequate and well-controlled studies in pregnant women. Baclofen should be used during pregnancy only if the benefit clearly justifies the potential risk to the fetus.

Baclofen Injection is for use in single bolus intrathecal injections (via a catheter placed in the lumbar intrathecal space or injection by lumbar puncture) and in implantable pumps approved by the FDA specifically for the intrathecal administration of Baclofen. Because of the possibility of potentially life-threatening CNS depression, cardiovascular collapse, and/or respiratory failure, physicians must be adequately trained and educated in chronic intrathecal infusion therapy.

The pump system should not be implanted until the patient's response to bolus Baclofen Injection is adequately evaluated. Evaluation (consisting of a screening procedure: see *"Dosage and Administration"*) requires that Baclofen Injection be administered into the intrathecal space via a catheter or lumbar puncture. Because of the risks associated with the screening procedure and the adjustment of dosage following pump implantation, these phases must be conducted in a medically supervised and adequately equipped environment following the instructions outlined in the *"Dosage and Administration"* section.

Resuscitative Equipment Should Be Available.

Following surgical implantation of the pump, particularly during the initial phases of pump use, the patient should be monitored closely until it is certain that the patient's response to the infusion is acceptable and reasonably stable. On each occasion that the dosing rate of the pump and/or the concentration of Baclofen Injection in the reservoir is adjusted, close medical monitoring is required until it is certain that the patient's response to the infusion is acceptable and reasonably stable.

It is mandatory that the patient, all patient care givers, and the physicians responsible for the patient receive adequate information regarding the risks of this mode of treatment. All medical personnel and care givers should be instructed in 1) the signs and symptoms of overdose, 2) procedures to be followed in the event of overdose and 3) proper home care of the pump and insertion site.

Overdose: Signs of overdose may appear suddenly or insidiously. Acute massive overdose may present as coma. Less sudden and/or less severe forms of overdose may present with signs of CNS depression, excessive salivation, dizziness, nausea and/or vomiting, somnolence, and cephalad progression of hypotonia. Should overdose appear likely, the patient should be taken immediately to a hospital for assessment and emptying of the pump reservoir. In the cases reported to date, overdose has generally been related to pump malfunction or dosing error. (See *"Drug Overdose, Symptoms and Treatment"*).

Seizures have been reported during overdose with and withdrawal from Baclofen Injection as well as in patients maintained on therapeutic doses of Baclofen Injection.

Fatalities: There were 13 deaths occurring among the 438 patients treated with Baclofen Injection in pre-marketing studies evaluated as of April 1991. Because these patients were treated under uncontrolled clinical settings, it is impossible to determine definitively what role, if any, Baclofen Injection played in their deaths.

As a group, the patients who died were relatively young (mean age was 47 with a range from 25 to 63), but the majority suffered from severe spasticity of many years duration, were nonambulatory, had various medical complications such as pneumonia, urinary tract infections, and decubiti, and/or had received multiple concomitant medications. A case-by-case review of the clinical course of the 13 patients who died failed to reveal any unique signs, symptoms, or laboratory results that would suggest that treatment with Baclofen Injection caused their deaths. Two patients, however, did suffer sudden and unexpected death within 2 weeks of pump implantation.

One patient, a 44 year-old male with MS, died in hospital on the second day following pump implantation. An autopsy demonstrated severe fibrosis of the coronary conduction system. A second patient, a 52 year-old woman with MS and a history of an inferior wall myocardial infarction, was found dead in bed 12 days after pump implantation, 2 hours after having had documented normal vital signs. An autopsy revealed pulmonary congestion and bilateral pleural effusions. It is impossible to determine whether Baclofen Injection contributed to these deaths.

PRECAUTIONS

Safe use of Baclofen tablets in children under age 12, and of Baclofen Injection in children under age 18, has not been established, and it is, therefore, not recommended for use in children.

Because of the possibility of sedation, patients should be cautioned regarding the operation of automobiles or other dangerous machinery, and activities made hazardous by decreased alertness. Patients should also be cautioned that the central nervous system effects of Baclofen may be additive to those of alcohol and other CNS depressants.

Baclofen should be used with caution where spasticity is utilized to sustain upright posture and balance in locomotion or whenever spasticity is utilized to obtain increased function.

In patients with epilepsy, the clinical state and electroencephalogram should be monitored at regular intervals, since deterioration in seizure control and EEG have been reported occasionally in patients taking Baclofen.

Patients suffering from psychotic disorders, schizophrenia, or confusional states should be treated cautiously with Baclofen Injection and kept under careful surveillance, because exacerbations of these conditions have been observed with oral administration.

Baclofen Injection should be used with caution in patients with a history of autonomic dysreflexia. The presence of nociceptive stimuli or abrupt withdrawal of Baclofen Injection may cause an autonomic dysreflexic episode.

NURSING MOTHERS

In mothers treated with oral Baclofen in therapeutic doses, the active substance passes into the breast milk. It is not known whether detectable levels of drug are present in breast milk of nursing mothers receiving Baclofen Injection. As a general rule, nursing should be undertaken while a patient is receiving Baclofen Injection only if the potential benefit justifies the potential risks to the infant.

A dose-related increase in incidence of ovarian cysts and a less marked increase in enlarged and/or hemorrhagic adrenal glands was observed in female rats treated chronically with Baclofen.

Ovarian cysts have been found by palpation in about 4% of the multiple sclerosis patients that were treated with Baclofen for up to one year. In most cases these cysts disappeared spontaneously while patients continued to receive the drug. Ovarian cysts are estimated to occur spontaneously in approximately 1% to 5% of the normal female population.

SCREENING

Patients should be infection-free prior to the screening trial with Baclofen Injection because the presence of a systemic infection may interfere with an assessment of the patient's response to bolus Baclofen Injection.

PUMP IMPLANTATION

Patients should be infection-free prior to pump implantation because the presence of infection may increase the risk of surgical complications. Moreover, a systemic infection may complicate attempts to adjust the pump's dosing rate.

PUMP DOSE ADJUSTMENT AND TITRATION

In most patients, it will be necessary to increase the dose gradually over time to maintain effectiveness; a sudden requirement for substantial dose escalation typically indicates a catheter complication (i.e., catheter kink or dislodgement).

Reservoir refilling must be performed by fully trained and qualified personnel following the directions provided by the pump manufacturer. Refill intervals should be carefully calculated to prevent depletion of the reservoir, as this would result in the return of severe spasticity.

Strict aseptic technique in filling is required to avoid bacterial contamination and serious infection. A period of observation appropriate to the clinical situation should follow each refill or manipulation of the drug reservoir.

Extreme caution must be used when filling an FDA approved implantable pump equipped with an injection port that allows direct access to the intrathecal catheter. Direct injection into the catheter through the access port may cause a life-threatening overdose.

ADDITIONAL CONSIDERATIONS PERTAINING TO DOSAGE ADJUSTMENT

It may be important to maintain some degree of muscle tone and allow occasional spasms to help support circulatory function and possibly prevent the formation of deep vein thrombosis.

An attempt should be made to discontinue concomitant oral antispasticity medication to avoid possible overdose or adverse drug interactions, preferably prior to initiation of Baclofen Injection infusion, with careful monitoring by the physician. Abrupt reduction or discontinuation of concomitant antispastics, however, during chronic Baclofen Injection therapy should be avoided.

LABORATORY TESTS

No specific laboratory tests are deemed essential for the management of patients on Baclofen Injection.

DRUG INTERACTIONS

There is inadequate systematic experience with the use of Baclofen Injection in combination with other medications to predict specific drug-drug interactions. Interactions attributed to the combined use of Baclofen Injection and epidural morphine include hypotension and dyspnea.

CARCINOGENESIS, MUTAGENESIS AND IMPAIRMENT OF FERTILITY

No increase in tumors was seen in rats receiving Baclofen orally for two years at approximately 30-60 times on a mg/kg basis, or 10-20 times on a mg/m2 basis, the maximum oral dose recommended for human use. Mutagenicity assays with Baclofen have not been performed.

ADVERSE REACTIONS

BACLOFEN TABLETS

The most common is transient drowsiness (10-63%). In one controlled study of 175 patients, transient drowsiness was observed in 63% of those receiving Baclofen compared to 36% of those in the placebo group. Other common adverse reactions are dizziness (5-15%), weakness (5-15%) and fatigue (2-4%). Others reported:

Neuropsychiatric: Confusion (1-11%), headache (4-8%), insomnia (2-7%); and, rarely, euphoria, excitement, depression, hallucinations, paresthesia, muscle pain, tinnitus, slurred speech, coordination disorder, tremor, rigidity, dystonia, ataxia, blurred vision, nystagmus, strabismus, miosis, mydriasis, diplopia, dysarthria, epileptic seizure.

Cardiovascular: Hypotension (0-9%). Rare instances of dyspnea, palpitation, chest pain, syncope.

Gastrointestinal: Nausea (4-12%), constipation (2-6%); and, rarely, dry mouth, anorexia, taste disorder, abdominal pain, vomiting, diarrhea, and positive test for occult blood in stool.

Genitourinary: Urinary frequency (2-6%); and rarely, enuresis, urinary retention, dysuria, impotence, inability to ejaculate, nocturia, hematuria.

Other: Instances of rash, pruritus, ankle edema, excessive perspiration, weight gain, nasal congestion.

Some of the CNS and genitourinary symptoms may be related to the underlying disease rather than a drug therapy. The following laboratory tests have been found to be abnormal in a few patients receiving Baclofen: increased SGOT, elevated alkaline phosphatase, and elevation of blood sugar.

BACLOFEN INJECTION

Commonly Observed: In pre-marketing clinical trials, the most commonly observed adverse events associated with use of Baclofen Injection which were not seen at an equivalent incidence among placebo-treated patients were: drowsiness, dizziness, nausea, hypotension, headache, seizures, and weakness.

Associated with Discontinuation of Treatment: 6/244 patients receiving Baclofen Injection in pre-marketing clinical studies in the U.S. discontinued treatment due to adverse events. There were two cases each of unacceptable, posture impairing hypotonicity, pump pocket infection, and meningitis. All seven patients who developed coma secondary to overdose had treatment temporarily suspended, but all were subsequently re-started and were not, therefore, considered to be true discontinuations.

Fatalities: (see *"Warnings"*).

Incidence in Controlled Trials: Experience with Baclofen Injection obtained in parallel, placebo-controlled, randomized studies provides only a limited basis for estimating the incidence of adverse events because the studies were of very brief duration (up to three days of infusion) and involved only a total of 63 patients. The following events occurred among the 31 patients receiving Baclofen Injection in two randomized, placebo-controlled trials: hypotension(2), dizziness/lightheadedness(2), headache(2), dyspnea(1). No adverse events were reported among the 32 patients receiving placebo in these studies.

Events Observed during the Pre-marketing Evaluation of Baclofen Injection: Adverse events associated with the use of Baclofen Injection reflect experience gained with a cohort of 244 patients followed prospectively in the United States. They received Baclofen Injection for periods of one day (screening) (N = 244) to over six years (maintenance) (N = 4). The usual screening bolus dose administered prior to pump implantation in these studies was 50-75 mcg. The maintenance dose ranged from 12 mcg to 1500 mcg per day.

Because of the open, uncontrolled nature of the experience, a causal linkage between events observed and the administration of Baclofen Injection cannot be reliably assessed in many cases and many of the adverse events reported are known to occur in association with the underlying conditions being treated. Nonetheless, many of the more commonly reported reactions—drowsiness, dizziness, headache, nausea, hypotension, hypotonia and coma—appear clearly drug-related.

Adverse experiences reported during all domestic studies (both controlled and uncontrolled) are shown in the following table. None of these adverse experiences led to a discontinuation of treatment:

INCIDENCE OF MOST FREQUENT ADVERSE EVENTS IN PROSPECTIVELY MONITORED CLINICAL TRIALS

Adverse Event	Number of Patients N = 244 Screening[a]	Reporting N = 214 Titration[b]	Events N = 214 Maintenance[c]
Drowsiness	13	11	18
Weakness, Lower Extremities	1	11	15
Dizziness/Lightheadedness	6	5	12
Seizures	1	4	11
Headache	0	3	9
Nausea/Vomiting	3	5	3
Numbness/Itching/Tingling	2	1	8
Hypotension	3	0	5
Blurred Vision	0	2	5
Constipation	0	2	5
Hypotonia	2	3	2
Speech Slurred	0	1	6
Coma (Overdose)	0	4	3
Lethargy	1	0	4
Weakness, Upper Extremities	1	0	4
Hypertension	1	2	2
Dyspnea	1	2	1

[a] *Following administration of test bolus*
[b] *Two month period following implant*
[c] *Beyond two months following implant*
(N = total number of patients entering each period)

In addition to the more common (1% or more) adverse events reported in the prospectively followed 244 domestic patients, experience from an additional 194 patients (total of 438) exposed to Baclofen Injection has been reported. In the total cohort, the following adverse events, not described in the table, and arranged in decreasing order of frequency, and classified by body system, were reported:

Central Nervous System: Respiratory depression, difficulty concentrating, decreased coordination, confusion, memory loss/forgetfulness, insomnia, nystagmus, accommodation disorder, anxiety, hypothermia, burning buttocks/feet, cerebellar dysmetria, cerebrovascular accident, depression, disorientation, unsteady gait/balance alteration, hallucinations, moodiness, paranoia, head/neck pressure, responsiveness delayed, somnolence, difficulty swallowing, and vertigo.

Gastrointestinal: Dry mouth, diarrhea/bowel incontinence, decreased appetite, dehydration, ileus, and decreased taste.

Cardiovascular: Hypertension, bradycardia, deep vein thrombosis, skin flushing, diaphoresis, orthostatic hypotension, paleness, and swelling of lower extremities.

Special Senses: Double vision.

Respiratory: Dyspnea, chest tightness, aspiration pneumonia.

Genitourinary: Urinary incontinence, sluggish bladder, bladder spasms, sexual dysfunction.

Skin and Appendages: Urticaria of face and hands, alopecia, and face edema.

Miscellaneous: Fatigue, septicemia, weight loss, accidental injury, subdural hemorrhage, suicide attempt, and suicide ideation.

OVERDOSAGE
BACLOFEN TABLETS
Signs and Symptoms: Vomiting, muscular hypotonia, drowsiness, accommodation disorders, coma, respiratory depression, and seizures.

Treatment: In the alert patient, empty the stomach promptly by induced emesis followed by lavage. In the obtunded patient, secure the airway with a cuffed endotracheal tube before beginning lavage (do not induce emesis). Maintain adequate respiratory exchange, do not use respiratory stimulants.

BACLOFEN INJECTION
Special attention must be given to recognizing the signs and symptoms of overdosage, especially during the initial screening and dose-titration phase of treatment, but also during re-introduction of Baclofen Injection after a period of interruption in therapy.

Symptoms of Baclofen Injection Overdose: drowsiness, light-headedness, dizziness, somnolence, respiratory depression, seizures, rostral progression of hypotonia and loss of consciousness progressing to coma of up to 24-hr duration. In all seven cases reported, coma was reversible without sequelae after infusion was stopped.

Symptoms of Baclofen Injection overdose were reported in a sensitive adult patient after receiving a 25 mcg intrathecal bolus.

TREATMENT SUGGESTIONS FOR OVERDOSE
There is no specific antidote for treating overdoses of Baclofen Injection; however, the following steps should ordinarily be undertaken:

1) Residual Baclofen Injection solution should be removed from the pump as soon as possible.
2) Patients with respiratory depression should be intubated if necessary, until the drug is eliminated.

Anecdotal reports suggest that intravenous physostigmine may reverse central side effects, notably drowsiness and respiratory depression. Caution in administering physostigmine intravenously is advised, however, because its use has been associated with the induction of seizures, bradycardia, cardiac conduction disturbances. A total dose of 1-2 mg physostigmine may be tried intravenously over 5-10 minutes. Patients should be monitored closely during this time. Repeat doses of 1 mg may be administered at 30-60 minute intervals in an attempt to maintain adequate respiration and alertness if the patient shows a positive response. Physostigmine may not be effective in reversing large overdoses and patients may need to be maintained with respiratory support.

If lumbar puncture is not contraindicated, consideration should be given to withdrawing 30-40 ml of CSF to reduce CSF Baclofen concentration.

DOSAGE AND ADMINISTRATION
BACLOFEN TABLETS
The determination of optimal dosage requires individual titration. Start therapy at a low dosage and increase gradually until optimum effect is achieved (usually between 40-80 mg daily).
   The following dosage titration schedule is suggested:
   5 mg t.i.d. for 3 days
   10 mg t.i.d. for 3 days
   15 mg t.i.d. for 3 days
   20 mg t.i.d. for 3 days

   Thereafter additional increases may be necessary but the total daily dose should not exceed a maximum of 80 mg daily (20 mg q.i.d.).
   The lowest dose compatible with an optimal response is recommended. If benefits are not evident after a reasonable trial period, patients should be slowly withdrawn from the drug (see *"Warnings, Abrupt Drug Withdrawal"*).

BACLOFEN INJECTION
Refer to the manufacturer's manual for the implantable intrathecal infusion pump for specific instructions and precautions for programming the pump and/or refilling the reservoir.

Screening Phase: Prior to pump implantation and initiation of chronic infusion of Baclofen Injection, patients must demonstrate a positive clinical response to a Baclofen Injection bolus dose administered intrathecally in a screening trial. The screening trial employs Baclofen Injection which must be diluted to a concentration of 50 mcg per mL. The screening procedure is as follows. An initial bolus containing 50 mcg in a volume of 1 mL is administered into the intrathecal space by barbotage over a period of not less than one minute. The patient is observed over the ensuring 4 to 8 hours. A positive response consists of a significant decrease in muscle tone and/or frequency and/or severity of spasms. If the initial response is less than desired, a second bolus injection may be administered 24 hours after the first. This second screening bolus dose consists of 75 mcg in 1.5 mL. Again, the patient should be observed for an interval of 4 to 8 hours. If the response is still inadequate, a final bolus screening dose of 100 mcg in 2 mL may be administered 24 hours later.

Patients who do not respond to a 100 mcg intrathecal bolus should not be considered candidates for an implanted pump for chronic infusion.

Post-Implant Dose Titration Period: To determine the initial total daily dose of Baclofen Injection following implant, the screening dose that gave a positive effect should be doubled and administered over a 24-hour period, unless the efficacy of the bolus dose was maintained for more than 12 hours, in which case the starting daily dose should be the screening dose delivered over a 24-hour period. No dose increases should be given in the first 24 hours (i.e., until the steady state is achieved).
   After the first 24 hours, the daily dosage should be increased slowly by 10%-30% increments and only once every 24 hours, until the desired clinical effect is

achieved. If there is not a substantive clinical response to increases in the daily dose, check for proper pump function and catheter patency. Patients must be monitored closely in a fully equipped and staffed environment during the screening phase and dose-titration period immediately following implant. Resuscitative equipment should be immediately available for use in case of life-threatening or intolerable side effects.

Maintenance Therapy: The clinical goal is to maintain muscle tone as close to normal as possible, and to minimize the frequency and severity of spasms to the extent possible, without inducing intolerable side effects. Very often the maintenance dose needs to be adjusted during the first few months of therapy while patients adjust to changes in life style due to the alleviation of spasticity. During periodic refills of the pump, the daily dose may be increased by 10-40%, but no more than 40%, to maintain adequate symptom control. The daily dose may be reduced by 10-20% if patients experience side effects. Most patients require gradual increases in dose over time to maintain optimal response during chronic therapy. A sudden large requirement for dose escalation suggests a catheter complication (i.e., catheter kink or dislodgement).

Maintenance dosage for long term continuous infusion of Baclofen Injection has ranged from 12 mcg/day to 1500 mcg/day, with most patients adequately maintained on 300 mcg to 800 mcg per day. There is limited experience with daily doses greater than 1000 mcg/day. Determination of the optimal Baclofen Injection dose requires individual titration. The lowest dose with an optimal response should be used.

POTENTIAL NEED FOR DOSE ADJUSTMENTS IN CHRONIC USE
During long term treatment approximately 10% of patients become refractory to increasing doses. There is not sufficient experience to make firm recommendations for tolerance treatment; however, this "tolerance" has been treated on occasion, in hospital, by a "drug holiday" consisting of the gradual reduction of Baclofen Injection over a two week period and switching to alternative methods of spasticity management: After a few days, sensitivity to Baclofen may return, and Baclofen Injection may be restarted at the initial continuous infusion dose.

STABILITY
Parenteral drug products should be inspected for particulate matter and discoloration prior to administration, whenever solution and container permit.

DELIVERY SPECIFICATIONS
The specific concentration that should be used depends upon the total daily dose required as well as the delivery rate of the pump. Baclofen Injection may require dilution when used with certain implantable pumps. Please consult manufacturer's manual for specific recommendations.

DILUTION INSTRUCTION
Screening: Both strengths of Baclofen Injection (10 mg/5 mL and 10mg/20 mL) must be diluted to a 50 mcg/mL concentration for bolus injection into the subarachnoid space.

Maintenance: For patients who require concentrations other than 500 mcg/mL or 2000 mcg/mL, Baclofen Injection *must be diluted.*

Baclofen Injection *must be diluted* with sterile preservative free Sodium Chloride for Injection, U.S.P.

DELIVERY REGIMEN
Baclofen Injection is most often administered in a continuous infusion mode immediately following implant. For those patients implanted with programmable pumps who have achieved relatively satisfactory control on continuous infusion, further benefit may be attained using more complex schedules of Baclofen Injection delivery. For example, patients who have increased spasms at night may require a 20% increase in their hourly infusion rate. Changes in flow rate should be programmed to start two hours before the time of desired clinical effect.

Do not store above 86°F (30°C).

Dispense in tight container (USP).

Do not freeze or heat sterilize solution for injection; does not require refrigeration.

J CODES
10 mg—J0475

HOW SUPPLIED
KIT:

BRAND/MANUFACTURER	NDC	SIZE	AWP
○ **BRAND**			
LIORESAL INTRATHECAL: Medtronic	58281-0560-01	1s	$187.00
	58281-0561-02	1s	$394.00
	58281-0561-04	1s	$732.00

TABLETS: 10 MG

AVERAGE UNIT PRICE (AVAILABLE SIZES)		GENERIC A-RATED AVERAGE PRICE (GAAP)	
BRAND	$0.49	100s	$33.18
GENERIC	$0.33	500s	$158.08
HCFA FUL (100s ea)	$0.13	750s	$230.25
		1000s	$310.49

BRAND/MANUFACTURER	NDC	SIZE	AWP
◆ **BRAND**			
► LIORESAL: Geigy	00028-0023-01	100s	$47.08
	00028-0023-61	100s ud	$49.84

BRAND/MANUFACTURER	NDC	SIZE	AWP
◆ **GENERICS**			
Warner Chilcott	00047-0611-24	100s	$28.30
Qualitest	00603-2408-21	100s	$28.71
Mason Dist	11845-0159-01	100s	$28.86
Rugby	00536-4959-01	100s	$30.88
Major	00904-3365-60	100s	$31.75
Moore,H.L.	00839-7472-06	100s	$32.39
Schein	00364-2312-01	100s	$32.75
URL	00677-1259-01	100s	$32.95
Biocraft	00332-2234-09	100s	$34.50
Caraco	57664-0120-08	100s	$35.15
Zenith	00172-4096-60	100s	$36.10
Goldline	00182-1295-01	100s	$36.10
Aligen	00405-4110-01	100s	$36.20
Martec	52555-0513-01	100s	$36.20
Royce	51875-0255-01	100s	$36.25
Geneva	00781-1641-01	100s	$36.25
Parmed	00349-8925-01	100s	$36.50
U.S. Trading	56126-0402-11	100s ud	$15.23
Vangard	00615-3541-13	100s ud	$23.17
Raway	00686-0668-20	100s ud	$31.00
Major	00904-3365-61	100s ud	$35.76
UDL	51079-0668-20	100s ud	$37.46
Goldline	00182-1295-89	100s ud	$37.50
Schein	00364-2312-90	100s ud	$39.36
Auro	55829-0158-10	100s ud	$40.11
Zenith	00172-4096-65	250s	$88.25
Rugby	00536-4959-05	500s	$136.32
Major	00904-3365-40	500s	$142.85
Qualitest	00603-2408-28	500s	$142.88
Royce	51875-0255-02	500s	$172.19
Martec	52555-0513-05	500s	$173.00
Aligen	00405-4110-02	500s	$181.25
Glasgow	60809-0103-55	750s	$230.25
Glasgow	60809-0103-72	750s ud	$230.25
Moore,H.L.	00839-7472-16	1000s	$289.97
Zenith	00172-4096-80	1000s	$331.00

TABLETS: 20 MG

AVERAGE UNIT PRICE (AVAILABLE SIZES)		GENERIC A-RATED AVERAGE PRICE (GAAP)	
BRAND	$0.88	100s	$57.67
GENERIC	$0.58	500s	$283.66
HCFA FUL (100s ea)	$0.24	1000s	$554.24

BRAND/MANUFACTURER	NDC	SIZE	AWP
◆ **BRAND**			
► LIORESAL: Geigy	00028-0033-01	100s	$86.23
	00028-0033-61	100s ud	$89.27
◆ **GENERICS**			
Warner Chilcott	00047-0612-24	100s	$49.26
Qualitest	00603-2409-21	100s	$51.11
Mason Dist	11845-0160-01	100s	$53.01
Rugby	00536-4960-01	100s	$55.80
Schein	00364-2313-01	100s	$56.00
Moore,H.L.	00839-7473-06	100s	$56.69
URL	00677-1260-01	100s	$56.75
Major	00904-3366-60	100s	$56.90
Caraco	57664-0121-08	100s	$59.95
Biocraft	00332-2236-09	100s	$60.00
Zenith	00172-4097-60	100s	$63.90
Aligen	00405-4111-01	100s	$63.90
Goldline	00182-1296-01	100s	$63.90
Royce	51875-0256-01	100s	$64.08
Martec	52555-0514-01	100s	$64.30
Geneva	00781-1642-01	100s	$64.67
Parmed	00349-8926-01	100s	$65.06
U.S. Trading	56126-0403-11	100s ud	$24.03
Vangard	00615-3542-13	100s ud	$41.16
Raway	00686-0669-20	100s ud	$43.00
Auro	55829-0159-10	100s ud	$65.84
UDL	51079-0669-20	100s ud	$65.85
Goldline	00182-1296-89	100s ud	$69.00
Schein	00364-2313-90	100s ud	$70.02
Zenith	00172-4097-65	250s	$157.75
Qualitest	00603-2409-28	500s	$253.80
Major	00904-3366-40	500s	$256.05
Royce	51875-0256-02	500s	$304.38
Aligen	00405-4111-02	500s	$320.40
Moore,H.L.	00839-7473-16	1000s	$499.48
Zenith	00172-4097-80	1000s	$609.00

Bactrim SEE SULFAMETHOXAZOLE AND TRIMETHOPRIM

Bactroban SEE MUPIROCIN

BAL In Oil SEE DIMERCAPROL

Balanced Salt Solution

DESCRIPTION
Balanced Salt Solution is a sterile intraocular irrigating solution containing essential ions for use during all intraocular surgical procedures, even those requiring a relatively long intraocular perfusion time (e.g., pars plana vitrectomy, phacoemulsification, extracapsular cataract extraction/lens aspiration, anterior segment reconstruction, etc.).

CLINICAL PHARMACOLOGY
None of the components of Balanced Salt Solution are foreign to the eye, and Balanced Salt Solution has no pharmacological action. Human perfused cornea studies[1-3] have shown Balanced Salt Solution to be an effective irrigation solution for providing corneal detumescence and maintaining corneal endothelial integrity during intraocular perfusion. An *in vivo* study[4] in rabbits has shown that Balanced Salt Solution is more suitable than normal saline for intravitreal irrigation. Human *in vivo* studies have demonstrated Balanced Salt Solution to be safe and effective when used during surgical procedures such as pars plana vitrectomy, phacoemulsification, cataract extraction/lens aspiration and anterior segment reconstruction.

INDICATIONS AND USAGE
Balanced Salt Solution is indicated for use as an intraocular irrigating solution during intraocular surgical procedures involving perfusion of the eye and surgical procedures of ears, nose or throat requiring a physiological irrigant.

CONTRAINDICATIONS
There are no specific contraindications to the use of Balanced Salt Solution, however, contraindications for the surgical procedure during which Balanced Salt Solution is to be used should be strictly adhered to.

WARNINGS
For *irrigation* during ophthalmic surgery only. Not for injection or intravenous infusion. Do not use unless product is clear, seal is intact, vacuum is present and container is undamaged. Do not use if product is discolored or contains a precipitate.

PRECAUTIONS
For products that require reconstitution, *do not use Balanced Salt Solution until reconstituted and discard any unused portion six hours after preparation.* DISCARD UNUSED CONTENTS. IF THE PRODUCT DOES NOT CONTAIN A PRESERVATIVE, DO NOT USE THE CONTAINER FOR MORE THAN ONE PATIENT. Do not use additives (products that require reconstitution may be supplied with their own concentrate for mixing). Tissue damage could result if other drugs are added to product. Studies suggest that intraocular irrigating solutions which are isoosmotic with normal aqueous fluids should be used with caution in diabetic patients undergoing vitrectomy since intraoperative lens changes have been observed.[5,6]

There have been reports of corneal clouding or edema following ocular surgery in which Balanced Salt Solution was used as an irrigating solution. As in all surgical procedures appropriate measures should be taken to minimize trauma to the cornea and other ocular tissues.

Carcinogenesis, Mutagenesis, Impairment of Fertility: No long term studies in animals have been performed to evaluate the carcinogenic potential.

Pregnancy: Teratogenic effects. Pregnancy Category C. Animal reproduction studies have not been conducted with Balanced Salt Solution. It is also not known whether Balanced Salt Solution can cause fetal harm when administered to a pregnant woman or can affect reproductive capacity. Balanced Salt Solution should be given to pregnant women only if clearly needed.

Nursing Mothers: Caution should be exercised when Balanced Salt Solution is administered to a nursing mother.

Pediatric Use: Safety and effectiveness in children have not been established.

ADVERSE REACTIONS
Postoperative inflammatory reactions as well as incidents of corneal edema and corneal decompensation have been reported. Their relationship to the use of Balanced Salt Solution has not been established.

When used for intraocular surgery in cases where the corneal endothelium is abnormal, excessive intraocular irrigation (as well as other intraocular manipulations) may contribute to endothelial damage and result in bullous keratopathy.

OVERDOSAGE
The solution has no pharmacological action and thus has no potential for overdosage. However, as with any intraocular surgical procedure, the duration of intraocular manipulation should be kept to a minimum.

DOSAGE AND ADMINISTRATION
The solution should be used according to the technique standardly employed by the operating surgeon. If the bottle does not contain a separate airway tube, use an administration set with an air inlet in the plastic spike. Follow the directions for the particular administration set to be used. Insert the spike aseptically into the bottle through the target area of the rubber stopper. Invert the bottle and allow the fluid to flow the entire length of the tubing to remove air from the tubing before intraocular irrigation begins. If a second bottle is necessary to complete the surgical procedure, insure that the vacuum is vented from the second bottle *before* attachment to the administration set.

For products requiring reconstitution:

Preparation: RECONSTITUTE BALANCED SALT SOLUTION JUST PRIOR TO USE IN SURGERY. FOLLOW THE SAME STRICT ASEPTIC PROCEDURES IN THE RECONSTITUTION OF BALANCED SALT SOLUTION AS IS USED FOR INTRAVENOUS ADDITIVES. CLEAN AND DISINFECT THE RUBBER STOPPERS ON BOTH CONTAINERS BY USING STERILE ALCOHOL WIPES. TRANSFER THE CONCENTRATE FOR MIXING TO THE SOLUTION. Gently agitate the contents to mix the solution. Place a sterile cap on the bottle. Record the time and date of reconstitution and the patient's name on the bottle label.

Storage: Store at 46°-80°F (8°-27°C). Avoid excessive heat; protect from freezing. Discard prepared solution after six hours.

REFERENCES
1. Edelhauser, H. F., Van Horn, D. L., Hyndiuk, R. A., Schultz, R. O., Intraocular Irrigation Solutions: Their Effect on the Corneal Endothelium. *Arch. Ophthalmol.,* 93, 648, 1975. 2. Edelhauser, H. F., Van Horn, D. L., Schultz, R. O., Hyndiuk, R. A., Comparative Toxicity of Intraocular Irrigating Solutions on the Corneal Endothelium, *Am. J. Ophthalmol.,* 81, 473, 1976. 3. Edelhauser, H.F., Gonnering, R., Van Horn, D. L., Intraocular Irrigating Solutions: A Comparative Study of BSS PLUS and Lactated Ringer's Solution, *Arch. Ophthalmol.,* 96, 516, 1978. 4. Moorhead, L. C., Redburn, D. A., Merritt, J., Garcia, C. A., The Effects of Intravitreal Irrigation During Vitrectomy on the Electroretinogram, *Am. J. Ophthalmol.,* 88, 239, 1979. 5. Faulborn, J., Conway, B. P., Machemer, R., Surgical Complications of Pars Plana Vitreous Surgery. *Ophthalmology* 85: 116-125, 1978. 6. Haimann, M. H., and Abrams, G. W., Prevention of Lens Opacification During Diabetic Vitrectomy. *Ophthalmology,* 91:116-121, 1984.

HOW SUPPLIED
SOLUTION:

BRAND/MANUFACTURER	NDC	SIZE	AWP
○ **BRAND**			
BASOL-S: Ocumed	51944-4355-42	15 ml	$4.50
	51944-4355-67	250 ml	$14.50
	51944-4355-83	500 ml	$17.50
BSS: Alcon Surg	00065-0795-25	250 ml 6s	$88.20
	00065-0795-50	500 ml 6s	$109.20
BSS PLUS: Alcon Surg	00065-0800-50	500 ml 6s	$297.60
BSS: Alcon Surg	00065-0795-30	30 ml 20s	$150.00
	00065-0795-15	15 ml 36s	$167.40

Balsa-Derm *SEE* CASTOR OIL/PERU BALSAM/TRYPSIN

Barium Sulfate

DESCRIPTION
Barium Sulfate esophageal cream is a radiopaque contrast medium containing 560 mg per g (100% w/v). Barium Sulfate esophageal cream provides prolonged adherence and residual coating of the esophageal mucosa.

Use of a Half-inch Barium Tablet to Detect Minimal Esophageal Strictures: In addition to demonstrating the presence of a significant narrowing by failure to pass, a tablet of known diameter furnishes a simple method of measuring the true size of the residual lumen at the site of a ring or a stricture. The tablet is flattened from side to side in order that patients may swallow it without difficulty. When held up proximal to a stricture, the patient complains of no special discomfort and fluid easily passes around the tablet. Within half an hour, the tablet will disintegrate and the fragments pass without difficulty. The diameter of half an inch was selected because it corresponds to the external diameter of a 36 French esophagoscope, the size which has been in routine use for esophagoscopy for many years. Transient delay particularly in older individuals at the level of the arch of the aorta or above the hiatus is often seen but a swallow or two of fluid carries the tablet distally without difficulty. The simultaneous visualization of the tablet and the constricted site makes calculation of the diameter of the constriction simple since the magnification factor is directly determined from the known size of the tablet. In inches, the true diameter of the narrowed site is one-half of the ratio of its measured value on the film to the measured value of the tablet.

This tablet has been of greatest use in patients who complain of dysphagia but in whom questionable or no definite findings are discovered by conventional methods. In patients who refuse to drink sufficient amounts of barium, obstruction to the passage of the tablet may nevertheless indicate the presence of important esophageal disease as the cause of symptoms. The difficulties of securing satisfactory films showing complete filling of the pharynx and cricopharyngeal area often make roentgen diagnosis in this region difficult. In such instances failure of the tablet to pass this site freely may be sufficient evidence to warrant further studies, for example, by motion picture techniques. The original assumption that, if a tablet of this diameter passes through the esophagus without delay dysphagia is not likely to be on an obstructive basis, has not been contradicted by further experience.

Barium Sulfate for suspension is a radiopaque contrast medium containing 92% barium sulfate.

Barium Sulfate for suspension is designed to aid in the detailed mucosal examination of the gastrointestinal tract. The high radio-density, low viscosity and suspension stability provides for optimum visualization of mucosal patterns.

It provides a prolonged, uniform, smooth and flexible coating of the gastric and intestinal mucosa.

CLINICAL PHARMACOLOGY
Not applicable. Barium Sulfate is insoluble and is not absorbed.

INDICATIONS AND USAGE
Barium Sulfate esophageal cream is a radiopaque contrast medium for x-ray diagnosis of esophageal disorders. Prolonged retention of residual coat allows adequate time for fluoroscopy and radiography of the esophagus, and for chest studies of heart size and configuration.

Barium Sulfate tablets are indicated for use as an intact-shaped Roentgen contrast medium in esophagoscopy.

Barium Sulfate for suspension is a radiopaque contrast medium for use in gastrointestinal x-ray diagnosis, especially upper G.I. and small bowel examinations.

UNLABELED USES
Barium Sulfate is used alone or as an adjunct in the treatment of intussusception and in the diagnosis of intussusception and appendicitis. Barium Sulfate is also used as a negative oral contrast medium for magnetic resonance imaging.

CONTRAINDICATIONS
None known.

ADVERSE REACTIONS
Constipation may occur with Barium Sulfate preparations taken orally; it can be relieved using a suitable laxative.

DOSAGE AND ADMINISTRATION
Barium Sulfate esophageal cream: One tablespoonful "chewed" thoroughly before swallowing. To enhance palatability use a plastic spoon. Repeat with a second tablespoonful to assure prolonged adherence and coating of the esophageal mucosa.

Store Barium Sulfate esophageal cream at room temperature Avoid excessive heat (104°F).

Barium Sulfate tablets: The patient should be instructed to swallow one tablet, intact, with the aid of one or two swallows of water, just prior to fluoroscopic examination by esophagoscope.

Barium Sulfate for suspension: Administer 60 to 450 grams orally. 150 g Barium Sulfate for suspension added to 250 mL (8.5 fl oz) water will yield 300 mL (10 fl oz) of 35% w/w Barium Sulfate suspension. *Always* add the powder to the water. Density can be increased or decreased according to individual preference.

Store Barium Sulfate for suspension at controlled room temperature, 15°-30°C (59°-86°F).

HOW SUPPLIED
POWDER:

BRAND/MANUFACTURER	NDC	SIZE	AWP
○ **BRAND**			
ESOPHOTRAST: RPR	00075-0824-01	454 gm	$27.31
ORATRAST: RPR	00075-0812-01	11350 gm	$198.12
BAROTRAST: RPR	00075-0821-01	11350 gm	$198.12
○ **GENERICS**			
	00395-0200-01	454 gm	$11.26
	53118-0513-10	480 gm	$10.00
	00395-0200-05	2270 gm	$54.57

TABLETS:

BRAND/MANUFACTURER	NDC	SIZE	AWP
○ **GENERICS**			
BAR-TEST: Glenwood	00516-0130-01	100s	$61.85

Barotrast SEE BARIUM SULFATE

Basol-S SEE BALANCED SALT SOLUTION

BCG

DESCRIPTION
BCG Vaccine for intravesical or percutaneous use, is an attenuated, live culture preparation of the Bacillus of Calmette and Guerin (BCG) strain *Mycobacterium bovis.*[1]

CLINICAL PHARMACOLOGY
INTRAVESICAL USE FOR CARCINOMA IN SITU OF THE BLADDER
BCG induces a granulomatous or inflammatory reaction with histiocytic and leukocytic infiltration at the local site of administration.[2] Intravesical BCG has been used as a therapy for and prophylaxis against recurrent tumors in patients with carcinoma *in situ* (CIS) of the bladder. The precise mechanism of action is unknown. A variety of different treatment regimens have been used with the BCG[3-6] and other BCG substrains.[7-12]

An evaluation of intravesical administration of BCG in patients with carcinoma *in situ* of the urinary bladder was recently completed. Bladder cancer patients were identified who had been treated with BCG under six different Investigational New Drug (IND) applications in which the most important shared aspect was the use of an induction plus maintenance schedule. Comparison of demographic data between the six INDs revealed uniformity. Among these six studies were 119 evaluable patients who received intravesical treatment of CIS of the bladder. Patients with biopsy-proven CIS received BCG (50 mg; $1\text{-}8 \times 10^8$ CFU) intravesically, once weekly for at least 6 weeks and once monthly thereafter for up to 12 months. A longer maintenance was given in some cases. Follow-up cystoscopies were performed at 3 month intervals, as were urine cytologies for most patients (71 of 119). Urine cytology was obtained at the time of the 1989 follow-up for all patients who responded to BCG treatment, (CR and CRNC, see below). The median time post treatment for these follow-up cytologies was 47 months.

The study population consisted of 153 patients; 132 males, 19 females and 2 unidentified as to gender. Thirty patients lacking baseline documentation of CIS and 4 patients lost to follow-up were not evaluable for treatment response. Therefore, 119 patients with biopsy or cystoscopy proven CIS prior to BCG administration were available for efficacy evaluation. Some of these patients had undergone transurethral resection (TUR) one or more weeks prior to BCG, primarily for the treatment of papillomatous disease. The mean age for the CIS population was 68.8 ± 9.7 years s.d. (range: 38-97 years). Sixty-three evaluable patients had received intravesical chemotherapy treatment for their bladder malignancy prior to BCG treatment and had been diagnosed as treatment failures. The treatment had been as follows: thiotepa (30), mitomycin C (10), doxorubicin (1), mitomycin C and thiotepa (14), doxorubicin and thiotepa (1), doxorubicin and mitomycin C (1), thiotepa, mitomycin C and doxorubicin (2), interferon (1), interferon and thiotepa (1), cyclophosphamide IV (1), and cisplatin and thiotepa (1).

For the 119 patients with biopsy or cystoscopy proven CIS the BCG induction dosage consisted of a mean of 6.6 instillations (± 1.5 standard error of the mean). These patients also received a mean of 10.0 maintenance instillations after completing the induction phase. Twenty patients (16.8%) required BCG reinduction at some point in the study. Nine patients in one of the six studies received a percutaneous dose along with intravesical instillation. Data from a recent study show that a percutaneous dose with CIS is unnecessary.[13]

Clinical response criteria were defined as follows:

Complete Histological Response (CR): Complete resolution of carcinoma in situ documented by biopsy or, if a biopsy was not obtained, then by negative cystoscopy. All patients in this category were required to have urine cytology tests that were negative upon examination.

Complete Clinical Response Without Cytology (CRNC): Patients in this category had an apparent complete disappearance of tumor that was not confirmed by urine cytology tests. Complete resolution of carcinoma *in situ* documented by a biopsy or, if a biopsy was not obtained, then by negative cystoscopy.

Failure/Progression: Patients in this category had urine cytology tests that were found to be positive, although biopsy or cystoscopy was negative. This category also includes patients who continued to have evidence of malignant lesions, or a progression to a higher stage or grade; the appearance of new lesions; reappearance of old lesions.

A 75.6 percent response rate was reported for 119 evaluable patients (Table 1).

Table 1
RESPONSE OF PATIENTS TO BCG IN CIS BLADDER CANCER

	Entered	Evaluable	CR	CRNC	Overall Response
No. of Patients	153	119	54	36	90
% Response	—		45.4%	30.2%	75.6%

The median duration of follow-up for the 1989 update, presented in Table 2, is 47 months. Of the 54 patients classified as CR in 1987, 30 remained without evidence of disease (CR) in 1989, whereas 6 patients died of unrelated disease and 18 relapsed. The 15 of 36 patients classified as CRNC in 1987 who remained without evidence of disease in 1989 were all found to meet the criteria of CR status on the basis of negative cytologies. In the interim, 4 CRNC patients died of unrelated diseases, 2 died of unknown causes, and 15 relapsed. Therefore, of the 90 overall responders (75.6%), 36.7 percent of patients relapsed, 13.3 percent died of other diseases, and 50 percent remained in CR. In addition, two patients who relapsed were reinduced in complete response by a second course of BCG.

Table 2
THERAPEUTIC EFFICACY OF BCG IN CIS BLADDER CANCER 1989 STATUS OF 90 RESPONDERS (CR OR CRNC)

Response	1987/CR n = 54	1987/CRNC n = 36	1987 Response n = 90	Percent
CR	30	15	45	50.0
CRNC	0	0	0	0.0
Unrelated Deaths	6	6	12	13.3
Failure	18	15	33	36.7

Among the 119 evaluable patients there was no significant difference in response rates between patients with or without prior intravesical chemotherapy: 45 of 63 (71%) versus 45 of 56 (80%), p > .05. Similarly, for the patients remaining in CR at the time of the 1989 evaluation, there was no significant difference between those with or without prior chemotherapy.

The median duration of response, calculated from the Kaplan-Meier curve as median time to recurrence, is estimated at 4 years or greater. The median duration of follow-up was 47 months. Of the total 90 responders, 45 patients (50%) remained without evidence of disease.

At a median follow-up of 47 months, 85 (71.4%) of the 119 evaluable patients remain alive. Thirteen patients (10.9%) died from causes unrelated to bladder cancer: cardiovascular disease (6 patients), second primary cancer (3 patients), and other (4 patients). Three patients died from unknown causes and bladder cancer cannot be ruled out. The bladder cancer related deaths were 18 (15%) of the 119. Historical data prior to the use of BCG, in a series of CIS patients treated usually with electrofulguration, indicate 82% of the patients recurred, 60% of the patients developed invasive cancer, and 34% of the patients died of their disease within 5 years.[14]

The incidence of cystectomy for 90 patients who achieved a complete response (CR or CRNC) with BCG was 11%. For 29 patients who did not achieve CR or CRNC, the incidence of cystectomy was 55%, which is consistent with cystectomy rates reported in the literature for CIS patients who were not treated with intravesical therapies.[15]

The median time to cystectomy in patients who achieved a complete response (CR or CRNC) exceeded 74 months, whereas the median time to cystectomy for non-responders was 31 months.

In a randomized, actively controlled multicenter study BCG was compared to doxorubicin hydrochloride in the treatment of carcinoma *in situ* of the urinary bladder. The response of 114 eligible patients for evaluation is given in Table 3 below. Among the 54 patients receiving BCG, 74% had a complete response (negative by cystoscopic examination and by urine cytology). The estimated median time to treatment failure (recurrence, progression or death) was 48.2 months (Table 4).

Table 3
RESPONSE OF PATIENTS WITH CARCINOMA *IN SITU* TO TREATMENT WITH BCG OR DOXORUBICIN

	BCG (n = 54)	doxorubicin (n = 60)
Complete Response†	74%	42%
No Response‡	11%	10%
Progressive Disease§	13%	42%
No Evaluation	2%	7%
Total	100%	100%

* Difference is statistically significant (P < 0.01).
† Confirmed by cytology and cystoscopic examination.
‡ Less than a CR or stable disease.
§ Increase of stage or grade.

Table 4
TIME TO RECURRENCE, PROGRESSION OR DEATH: TIME TO TREATMENT FAILURE (TTF)

Treatment	Number Studied	Number Failures	Median TTF
BCG	54	27	48.2 months*
Doxorubicin	60	46	5.9 months*

* Difference is statistically significant (P < 0.01 by stratified logrank test).

The effect of chemotherapy (other than BCG or doxorubicin prior into the controlled study was analysed. Patients in the BCG treated arm who had received prior chemotherapy had a complete response rate of 81% (11/26) as compared to 68% (16/28) in the group who had not received prior chemotherapy (Table 5). This difference was not statistically significant.

Table 5
PRIOR VERSUS NO PRIOR TREATMENT

Prior Treatment*	Study Arm	Response Rate	Median TTF (# Events/N)
Yes	BCG	81%	Not reached (11/26)
Yes	doxorubicin	53%	7.0 months (22/30)
No	BCG	68%	32.8 months (16/28)
No	doxorubicin	30%	3.7 months (24/30)

* Other than BCG and doxorubicin.

No survival advantage of BCG therapy over that for doxorubicin was demonstrated after a 40-72 month follow-up. The median time to death for each group was 23 months and 21 months for BCG and doxorubicin respectively.

The clinical trials carried out with BCG included percutaneous administration of 0.5 mL of BCG Live (Intravesical) solution, which was reconstituted in the diluent provided and further diluted in 50 mL sterile preservative-free saline, with each intravesical dose. Some studies have suggested that this may not be necessary and if severe reactions, such as ulceration, occurred the percutaneous treatment was discontinued.

PERCUTANEOUS USE FOR IMMUNIZATION AGAINST TUBERCULOSIS
Immunization with BCG vaccine lowers the risk of serious complications of primary tuberculosis in children.[16-19] Estimates of efficacy from observational studies in areas where vaccination is performed at birth show that the incidence of tuberculous meningitis and miliary tuberculosis is 50%-100% lower and that the incidence of pulmonary tuberculosis 2%-80% lower in vaccinated children less than 15 years of age than in unvaccinated controls.[16-21] However, estimates of vaccine efficacy may be distorted because of the following: vaccination was not allocated randomly in observational studies; there were differences in BCG strains, methods, and routes of administration; and there were differences in the characteristics of the populations and environments in which the vaccines have been studied.[22]

Some brands are NOT indicated as immunizing agents for the prevention of tuberculosis.

INDICATIONS AND USAGE
INTRAVESICAL USE FOR CARCINOMA *IN SITU* OF THE BLADDER
Intravesical instillation of BCG is indicated for the treatment of carcinoma *in situ* of the bladder in the following situations: (1) primary treatment in the absence of an associated invasive cancer without papillary tumors or with papillary tumors after TUR, (2) secondary treatment in the absence of an associated invasive cancer, in patients failing to respond or relapsing after intravesical chemotherapy with other agents, (3) primary or secondary treatment in the absence of invasive cancer for patients with medical contraindications to radical surgery. BCG is not indicated for the treatment of papillary tumors occurring alone.

PERCUTANEOUS USE FOR IMMUNIZATION AGAINST TUBERCULOSIS.
Exposed tuberculin skin test-negative infants and children: BCG vaccination is recommended for infants and children with negative tuberculin skin test who are (1) at high risk to intimate and prolonged exposure to persistently untreated or ineffectively treated patients with infectious pulmonary tuberculosis and who cannot be removed from the source of exposure and cannot be placed on long-term preventive therapy, or (2) continuously exposed to persons with tuberculosis who have bacilli resistant to isoniazid and rifampin.[22]

Groups with an excessive rate of new infections: BCG vaccination is also recommended for tuberculin-negative infants and children in groups in which the rate of new infections exceeds 1% per year and for whom the usual surveillance and treatment programs have been attempted but are not operationally feasible. These groups include persons without regular access to health care, those for whom usual health care is culturally or socially unacceptable, or groups who have demonstrated an inability to effectively use existing accessible care.

The US Immunization Practices Advisory Committee (ACIP) no longer recommends the use of BCG vaccination of health care workers at risk of repeated exposure to tuberculosis but recommends that these individuals be under tuberculin skin testing surveillance and receive isoniazid prophylaxis in case of tuberculin skin test conversion.[22]

For international travelers, the Centers for Disease Control (CDC) recommends that BCG vaccination be considered only for travelers with insignificant reaction to tuberculin skin test who will be in a high-risk environment for prolonged periods of time without access to tuberculin skin test surveillance.[22]

Some brands are NOT indicated as immunizing agents for the prevention of tuberculosis.

BCG is NOT a vaccine for the prevention of cancer.

CONTRAINDICATIONS
INTRAVESICAL USE FOR CARCINOMA *IN SITU* OF THE BLADDER
BCG should not be used in immunosuppressed patients or persons with congenital or acquired immune deficiencies, whether due to concurrent disease (e.g., AIDS, leukemia, lymphoma) or cancer therapy (e.g., cytotoxic drugs, radiation) BCG should be avoided in asymptomatic carriers with a positive HIV serology and in patients receiving steroids at immunosuppressive doses or other immunosuppressive therapies because of the possibility of the vaccine establishing a systemic infection.

Treatment should be postponed until resolution of a concurrent febrile illness, urinary tract infection, or gross hematuria. Seven to fourteen days should elapse before BCG is administered following biopsy, TUR, or traumatic catheterization.

A positive Mantoux test is a contraindication only if there is evidence of an active tuberculosis infection.

In the absence of safety data, intravesical BCG should not be given to pregnant or lactating women.

PERCUTANEOUS USE FOR IMMUNIZATION AGAINST TUBERCULOSIS
BCG Vaccine for the prevention of tuberculosis should not be given to persons with impaired immune responses, whether they be congenital, disease produced, drug or therapy induced (i.e., cytotoxic drugs and radiation used in cancer therapy). The concurrent use of steroids requires caution because of the possibility of the vaccine establishing a systemic infection. If necessary, the infection can be

treated with anti-tuberculous drugs. Some brands should not be administered as immunizing agents for the prevention of tuberculosis.

WARNINGS

INTRAVESICAL USE FOR CARCINOMA *IN SITU* OF THE BLADDER

BCG IS NOT A VACCINE FOR THE PREVENTION OF CANCER.
There are currently no data on the effectiveness of intravesical installation of BCG in the treatment of invasive bladder cancer.

Since administration of intravesical BCG causes an inflammatory response in the bladder and has been associated with hematuria, urinary frequency, dysuria and bacterial urinary tract infection, careful monitoring of urinary status is required. If there is an increase in the patient's existing symptoms, or if their symptoms persist or if any of these symptoms develop, the patient should be evaluated and managed for urinary tract infection or BCG toxicity.

The use of BCG may cause tuberculin sensitivity. Since this is a valuable aid in the diagnosis of tuberculosis, it may therefore be useful to determine the tuberculin reactivity by PPD skin testing before treatment.

Intravesical instillations should be postponed in the presence of fever, suspected infection, or during treatment with antibiotics, since antimicrobial therapy may interfere with the effectiveness of BCG.

Instillation of BCG onto a bleeding mucosa may promote systemic BCG infection.[23] Death has been reported as a result of systemic BCG infection and sepsis. Patients should be monitored for the presence of symptoms and signs of toxicity after each intravesical treatment. Febrile episodes with flu-like symptoms lasting more than 48 hours, fever $\geq$ 103°F, systemic manifestations increasing in intensity with repeated instillations, or persistent abnormalities of liver function tests suggest systemic BCG infection and require antituberculous therapy (see *"Adverse Reactions"* section). Small bladder capacity has been associated with increased risk of severe local reactions and should be considered in deciding to use BCG therapy.

PERCUTANEOUS USE FOR IMMUNIZATION AGAINST TUBERCULOSIS

Administration should be percutaneous with the multiple puncture disc as described below. DO NOT INJECT INTRAVENOUSLY, SUBCUTANEOUSLY, OR INTRADERMALLY. BCG Vaccine should not be used in infants, children, or adults with severe immune deficiency syndromes. Children with family history of immune deficiency disease should not be vaccinated. If they are, an infectious disease specialist should be consulted and anti-tuberculous therapy[24] administered if clinically indicated.

Some brands should not be administered as immunizing agents for the prevention of tuberculosis.

PRECAUTIONS

General: BCG contains live bacteria and should be used with aseptic technique. All equipment, supplies, and receptacles in contact with BCG should be handled and disposed of as biohazardous.

The possibility of allergic reactions should be assessed. BCG administration should not be attempted in individuals with severe immune deficiency disease. BCG Vaccine should be administered with caution to persons in groups at high risk for HIV infection.

INTRAVESICAL USE FOR CARCINOMA *IN SITU* OF THE BLADDER.

General: Care should be taken not to traumatize the urinary tract or to introduce contaminants into the urinary system. Seven to fourteen days should elapse before BCG is administered following TUR, biopsy, or traumatic catheterization.

If the physician believes that the bladder catheterization has been traumatic (e.g., associated with bleeding or possible false passage), then BCG should not be administered and there must be a treatment delay of at least one week. Subsequent treatment should be resumed as if no interruption in the schedule had occurred. That is, all doses of BCG should be administered even after a temporary halt in administration.

If systemic BCG infection is suspected (i.e., if patients have fever over 39°C (103°F) or persistent fever above 38°C (101°F) over two days or severe malaise), an infectious disease specialist should be consulted and fast acting antituberculosis therapy should be initiated. It should be noted that BCG systemic infections are rarely evidenced by positive cultures.

Information for Patients: Patients should be advised to check with their doctor as soon as possible if there is an increase in their existing symptoms, or if their symptoms persist even after receiving a number of treatment.

BCG is retained in the bladder 2 hours and then voided. Patients should void while seated for safety reasons following instillation of suspension. Within 6 hours after treatment, urine voided should be disinfected for 15 minutes with an equal volume of household bleach before flushing. Patients should be instructed to increase fluid intake to "flush" the bladder in the hours following BCG treatment. Patients may experience burning with the first void after treatment. Patients should be attentive to side effects, such as fever, chills, malaise, flu-like symptoms, or increased fatigue. If patient experiences severe urinary side effects, such as burning or pain on urination, urgency, frequency of urination, blood in urine, joint pain, nausea and vomiting, cough, or skin rash, the physician should be notified.

A cough that develops after administration of BCG could indicate a BCG systemic infection which is life-threatening. If systemic infection occurs it should be treated immediately with antituberculous antibiotics.

Drug Interaction: Drug combinations containing immunosuppressants and/or bone marrow depressants and/or radiation interfere with the development of the immune response or increase the risk of osteomyelitis or disseminated BCG infection, and should not be used in combination with BCG. Antimicrobial therapy for other infections may interfere with the effectiveness of BCG therapy.

Pregnancy Category C: Animal reproduction studies have not been conducted with BCG. It is also not known whether BCG can cause fetal harm when administered to a pregnant woman or can affect reproductive capacity. BCG should be given to a pregnant woman only if clearly needed. Women should be advised not to become pregnant while on therapy.

Nursing Mothers: It is not known whether BCG is excreted in human milk. Because many drugs are excreted in human milk and because of the potential for serious adverse reactions from BCG in nursing infants, a decision should be made whether to discontinue nursing or to discontinue the drug, taking into account the importance of the drug to the mother.

Pediatric Use: Safety and effectiveness of carcinoma *in situ* of the urinary bladder in children have not been established.

PERCUTANEOUS USE FOR IMMUNIZATION AGAINST TUBERCULOSIS.

Normal Reaction: The intensity and duration of the local reaction depends on the depth of penetration of the multiple-puncture disc and individual variations in patients' tissue reactions. The initial skin lesions usually appear within 10-14 days and consist of small red papules at the site. The papules reach maximum diameter (about 3 mm) after 4 to 6 weeks, after which they may scale and then slowly subside. Six months afterward there is usually no visible sign of the vaccination, but on occasion a faintly discernible pattern of the disc points may be visible. On people whose skin tends to keloid formation, there may be slightly more visible evidence of the vaccination.

Vaccination is recommended only for those who are tuberculin negative to a recent skin test with 5 tuberculin units (5TU). Otherwise, vaccination of persons highly sensitive to mycobacterial antigens can result in hypersensitivity reactions including fever, anorexia, myalgia, and neuralgia, which last a few days.

After BCG vaccination, it is usually not possible to clearly distinguish between a tuberculin reaction caused by persistent postvaccination sensitivity and one caused by a virulent suprainfection. Caution is advised in attributing a positive skin test to BCG vaccination. A sharp rise in the tuberculin reaction since the latest test should be further investigated (except in the immediate post vaccination period).

Information For Patients: Keep the vaccination site clean until the local reaction has disappeared.

Drug Interaction: Antimicrobial or immunosuppressive agents may interfere with the development of the immune response and should be used only under medical supervision.

Pregnancy Category C: Animal reproduction studies have not been conducted with BCG. It is also not known whether BCG can cause fetal harm when administered to a pregnant woman or can affect reproduction capacity. BCG should be given to a pregnant woman only if clearly needed.

Nursing Mothers: It is not known whether BCG is excreted in human milk. Because many drugs are excreted in human milk and because of the potential for serious adverse reactions in nursing infants from BCG, a decision should be made whether to discontinue nursing or not to vaccinate, taking into account the importance of tuberculosis vaccination to the mother.

Pediatric Use: See *"Treatment and Schedule"* under *"Dosage and Administration"* section. Precautions should be taken with respect to infants vaccinated with BCG and exposed to persons with active tuberculosis.[25]

Some brands should not be administered as immunizing agents for the prevention of tuberculosis.

ADVERSE REACTIONS

INTRAVESICAL USE FOR CARCINOMA *IN SITU* OF THE BLADDER.

Adverse reactions are often localized to the bladder but may be accompanied by systemic manifestations. Symptoms of bladder irritability, related to the inflammatory response induced by intravesical BCG, are reported in 60 percent of cases. They begin 3-4 hours after instillation and last 24-72 hours. The urinary side effects are usually seen after the third treatment and tend to increase in severity after each administration. There were, however, no long-term urinary complications in this group of patients.

A summary of adverse reactions seen with 674 patients with superficial bladder cancer, including 153 CIS patients treated intravesically with BCG is shown in Table 6.[26] Irritative bladder adverse effects associated with BCG administration can be managed symptomatically with pyridium, propantheline bromide or oxybutynin chloride, and acetaminophen or ibuprofen.[27] Systemic adverse effects such as malaise, fever, and chills may reflect hypersensitivity reactions and can be treated with antihistamines.[27] The "flu-like" syndrome of 1-2 days' duration that frequently accompanies intravesical BCG administration should be managed by standard symptomatic treatment. Symptoms persisting longer than 2 days suggest continued infection, and consideration should be given to therapy with isoniazid. Localized (e.g., prostatitis, epididymitis) as well as systemic infection can occur with intravesical BCG administration. For systemic infection, an infectious diseases specialist should be consulted and the patient promptly treated with antituberculous therapy as advised.[28] At least two deaths have been reported as a result of systemic BCG infection and sepsis.[27] There have been two cases of nephrogenic adenoma, a benign lesion of bladder epithelium, associated with

Table 6
SUMMARY OF ADVERSE EFFECTS SEEN IN 674 PATIENTS WITH SUPERFICIAL BLADDER CANCER, INCLUDING 153 WITH CARCINOMA *IN SITU*

Local Adverse Effects	Number of Patients	Percent (%)	Toxicity by Grade (%)*			
			Mild	Moderate	Severe	Not Stated
Dysuria	401	59.9	28.2	18.1	10.7	2.5
Urinary Frequency	272	40.4	17.2	15.7	7.4	—
Hematuria	175	26.0	8.2	9.6	7.4	0.8
Cystitis	40	5.9	1.6	2.4	1.9	—
Urgency	39	5.8	1.2	1.8	1.3	1.5
Nocturia	30	4.5	1.3	1.8	0.6	0.7
Cramps/Pain	27	4.0	0.9	1.3	0.9	0.9
Urinary Incontinence	16	2.4	0.4	0.9	—	1.2
Urinary Debris	15	2.2	0.2	1.0	0.4	0.6
Genital Inflammation/Abscess	12	1.8	0.3	0.4	0.4	0.6
Urinary Tract Infection	10	1.5	0.2	0.3	0.9	0.2
Urethritis	8	1.2	0.3	0.6	—	0.3
Pyuria	5	0.7	0.2	0.1	0.1	0.3
Epididymitis/Prostatitis	2	0.3	—	—	—	0.3
Urinary Obstruction	2	0.3	—	—	—	0.3
Contracted Bladder	1	0.2	—	—	—	0.2
Orchitis	1	0.2	—	—	—	0.2

Systemic Adverse Effects	Number of Patients	Percent (%)	Toxicity by Grade (%)			
			Mild	Moderate	Severe	Not Stated
Flu-like Syndrome**	224	33.2	9.3	10.9	9.0	4.0
Fever	134	19.9	6.1	5.3	7.6	0.9
Malaise/Fatigue	50	7.4	2.7	3.1	—	1.6
Shaking Chills	22	3.3	0.2	1.5	1.0	0.6
Nausea/Vomiting	20	3.0	1.0	1.6	0.3	—
Arthritis/Myalgia	18	2.7	0.3	1.0	0.4	0.9
Headache/Dizziness	16	2.4	0.3	0.9	—	1.2
Anorexia/Weight Loss	15	2.2	0.4	1.3	0.1	0.5
Allergic	14	2.1	0.6	0.7	0.4	0.3
Cardiac	13	1.9	—	0.3	1.3	0.3
Respiratory (Unclassified)	11	1.6	0.4	0.4	0.2	0.6
Abdominal Pain	10	1.5	—	0.6	0.6	0.3
Anemia	9	1.3	0.2	0.6	0.4	0.1
Diarrhea	8	1.2	0.2	0.6	0.1	0.3
Pneumonitis	8	1.2	0.2	—	0.6	0.4
Gastrointestinal (Unclassified)	7	1.0	0.2	0.1	—	0.7
Neurologic	6	0.9	0.1	—	0.3	0.4
Rash	4	0.6	—	0.4	0.2	—
BCG Sepsis	3	0.4	—	—	0.4	—
Coagulopathy	2	0.3	—	—	0.3	—
Leukopenia	2	0.3	0.2	0.1	—	—
Thrombocytopenia	2	0.3	0.2	0.1	—	—
Hepatic Granuloma	1	0.2	—	—	0.2	—
Hepatitis	1	0.2	—	—	0.2	—

* Grade was determined using ECOG scale of toxicity criteria, Mild = Grade 1, Moderate = Grade 2, Severe = Grade 3 or 4.
** Flu-like syndrome includes fever, shaking chills, malaise and myalgia.

intravesical BCG therapy.[29] In general, the adverse effects of BCG therapy in bladder carcinoma have been of short duration and moderate morbidity.

PERCUTANEOUS USE FOR IMMUNIZATION AGAINST TUBERCULOSIS.
Occasionally, lymphadenopathy of the regional lymph node, which spontaneously resolves itself, is seen in young children. Only rarely does the node create a fistula followed by a short period of drainage. The usual treatment is to maintain cleanliness of the site of drainage and allow the lesion to heal spontaneously without medical intervention.

Other rare events are osteomyelitis, lupoid reactions, disseminated BCG infection, and death. Osteomyelitis has been reported to occur at a rate of about 1 per 1,000,000 vaccinees.[22] Disseminated BCG infection and death are very rare (about 1 per 5,000,000 vaccinees)[30] and occur almost exclusively in children with impaired immune responses. (See related table).

In a controlled multi-center clinical trial comparing BCG therapy and doxorubicin hydrochloride for the intravesical treatment of superficial transitional cell carcinoma with and without carcinoma *in situ* of the bladder, 112 patients received BCG.

In another controlled study using BCG for the treatment of superficial transitional cell carcinoma, with or without carcinoma *in situ*, of the blader, similar adverse reactions were observed. However, two deaths were noted in this study which may have been associated with traumatic catheterization.

The incidence of adverse reactions associated with intravesical BCG therapy is given below. Most local adverse reactions occur following the third intravesical instillation. Symptoms usually begin two to four hours after instillation and persist for 24 to 72 hours. Systemic reactions usually last for 1-3 days after each intravesical instillation.

Table 7
LOCAL REACTIONS (% OF 112 PATIENTS)

Reaction	Total	Severe*
Dysuria	51.8	3.6
Frequency	40.2	1.8
Hematuria	39.3	17.0
Cystitis	29.5	0.0
Urgency	17.9	0.0
Urinary Tract Infection	17.9	1.0
Urinary Incontinence	6.3	0.0
Cramps/Pain	6.3	0.0
Decreased Bladder Capacity	5.4	0.0
Tissue in Urine	0.9	0.0
Local Infection	0.9	0.0

* Severe is defined as grade 3 (severe) or grade 4 (life threatening).

◆ RATED THERAPEUTICALLY EQUIVALENT; ◇ THERAPEUTIC EQUIVALENCE UNCONFIRMED; ○ UNRATED

Table 8:
SYSTEMATIC REACTIONS (% OF 112 PATIENTS)

Reaction	Total	Severe*
Malaise	40.2	2.0
Fever (> 38°C)	38.4	2.6
Chills	33.9	2.6
Anemia	20.5	0.0
Nausea/Vomiting	16.1	0.0
Anorexia	10.7	0.0
Myalgia/Arthralgia/Arthritis	7.1	1.0
Diarrhea	6.3	0.0
Mild Liver Involvement	2.7	0.0
Mild Abdominal Pain	2.7	0.0
Systemic Infection**	2.7	2.0
Pulmonary Infection**	2.7	0.0
Cardiac	2.7	0.0
Headache	1.8	0.0
Hypersensitivity Skin Rash	1.8	0.0
Constipation	0.9	0.0
Dizziness	0.9	0.0
Fatigue	0.9	0.0
Leukopenia	5.4	0.0
Disseminated Intravascular Coagulation	2.7	0.0
Thrombocytopenia	0.9	0.0
Renal Toxicity	9.8	2.0
Genital Pain	9.8	0.0
Flank Pain	0.9	0.0

* Severe is defined as grade 3 (severe) or grade 4 (life threatening).
** Includes both BCG and other infections.

No fatalities associated with the use of BCG were reported in this study. Two fatalities have been reported with the use of BCG in another study after traumatic catheterization or in the presence of urinary infection.

An increased risk of additional primary malignancies has been reported following radiotherapy and chemotherapy for many types of malignancies. No increase in second primary malignancies after treatment with BCG was reported in these studies.

OVERDOSAGE
INTRAVESICAL USE FOR CARCINOMA IN SITU OF THE BLADDER
Overdosage occurs if more than one ampule of BCG is administered per instillation. The patient should be closely monitored for signs of systemic BCG infection and treated with antituberculous medication (see "Adverse Reactions" section).

PERCUTANEOUS USE OF IMMUNIZATION AGAINST TUBERCULOSIS.
Accidental overdosages if treated immediately with anti-tuberculous drugs have not led to complications.[31] If the vaccination response is allowed to progress it can still be treated successfully with anti-tuberculous drugs but complications can include regional adenitis, lupus vulgaris, subcutaneous cold abscesses, ocular lesions, and others.[32]

DOSAGE AND ADMINISTRATION
INTRAVESICAL USE FOR CARCINOMA IN SITU OF THE BLADDER
The intravesical dose consists of one ampule or three vials of BCG suspended in 50 mL preservative-free saline.

Preparation of Agent: The preparation of the BCG suspension should be done using sterile technique. The pharmacist or individual responsible for mixing the agent should wear gloves, mask, and gown to avoid inadvertent exposure of open sores or inhalation of BCG organisms. Draw 1 mL of sterile, preservative-free saline (0.9% Sodium Chloride Injection USP) at 4°-25°C, into a small (e.g., 3 mL) syringe and add to one ampule of BCG to resuspend. Draw the mixture into the syringe and gently expel back into the ampule three times to ensure thorough mixing. This mixing minimizes the clumping of the mycobacteria. Dispense the cloudy BCG suspension into the top end of a catheter-tip syringe which contains 49 mL saline diluent bringing the total volume to 50 mL. Gently rotate the syringe. The suspended BCG should be used immediately after preparation. Discard after 2 hours.

Note: DO NOT filter the contents of the BCG ampule. Precautions should be taken to avoid exposing the BCG to light. Bacteriostatic solutions must be avoided. In addition, use only sterile preservative-free saline, 0.9% Sodium Chloride Injection USP, as diluent and perform all mixing operations in sterile glass or thermosetting plastic containers and syringes.

Apply a sterile pledget of cotton moistened with a suitable antiseptic to the surface of the rubber stoppers of the vials of diluent and BCG product. Allow the antiseptic to act for at least 5 minutes. Draw into a sterile syringe a volume of air equal to the volume of the diluent in the vial. Pierce the centre of the rubber stopper in the vial containing diluent with the sterile needle of the syringe, invert the vial, slowly inject into it the air contained in the syringe and, keeping the point of the needle immersed, withdraw into the syringe 1.0 mL of diluent. Then holding the syringe-plunger steady, withdraw the needle from the vial. Inject this volume of diluent into the vial of freeze-dried material. Shake the vial gently until a fine, even suspension results. Withdraw the entire contents of the reconstituted material into the syringe.

The reconstituted material from three vials (1 dose) is further diluted in an additional 50 mL sterile, preservative-free saline to a final volume of 53 mL for intravesical instillation (and percutaneous injection if it is given, see "Clinical Pharmacology").

Treatment and Schedule: Allow 7-14 days to elapse after bladder biopsy or TUR before BCG is administered. Patients should not drink fluids for 4 hours before treatment and should empty their bladder prior to BCG administration. The reconstituted BCG is instilled into the bladder by gravity flow via the catheter. DO NOT depress plunger and force the flow of the BCG. The BCG is retained in the bladder 2 hours and then voided. Patients unable to retain the suspension for 2 hours should be allowed to void sooner, if necessary. While the BCG is retained in the bladder, the patient may be repositioned from left side to right side and also may alternately lie upon the back and the abdomen, changing these positions every 15 minutes to maximize bladder surface exposure to the agent.

A standard treatment schedule consists of one intravesical instillation per week for 6 weeks. This schedule may be repeated once if tumor remission has not been achieved and if the clinical circumstances warrant. Thereafter, intravesical BCG administration should continue at approximately monthly intervals for at least 6-12 months.

If the physician believes that the bladder catheterization has been traumatic (e.g., associated with bleeding or possible false passage), then BCG should not be administered and there must be a treatment delay of at least one week. Subsequent treatment should be resumed as if no interruption in the schedule had occurred. That is, all doses of BCG should be administered even after a temporary halt in administration.

PERCUTANEOUS USE OF IMMUNIZATION AGAINST TUBERCULOSIS
Preparation of Agent: Using sterile methods, 1 mL of Sterile Water for Injection. USP at 4°-25°C, is added to one ampule of vaccine (see "Pediatric Dose" below for pediatric use). Draw the mixture into a syringe and expel it back into the ampule three times to ensure thorough mixing.

Parenteral drug products should be inspected visually for particulate matter and discoloration prior to administration, whenever solution and container permit. Reconstitution should result in a uniform suspension of the bacilli.

Treatment and Schedule: The vaccine is to be administered after fully explaining the risks and benefits to the vacinee, parent, or guardian. After the vaccine is prepared, the immunizing dose of 0.2-0.3 mL is dropped on the cleansed surface of the skin, and the vaccine is administered percutaneously utilizing a sterile multiple-puncture disc. The multiple-puncture disc is a thin wafer-like stainless steel plate 7/8″ × 1 1/8″, from which 36 points protrude. The disc is held by a magnet type holder. In this method a drop of vaccine is placed on the arm and spread with the wide edge of disc. The disc is placed gently over the vaccine and the magnet is centered. The arm is grasped firmly from underneath, tensing the skin appreciably. Downward pressure is applied on the magnet so the points of the disc are well buried in skin. With pressure still exerted, the disc is rocked forward and backward and from side to side several times. Pressure underneath the arm is then released and the magnet is slid off the disc. In a successful procedure, the points remain in the skin. If the points are on top of the skin, the procedure must be repeated. Remove the disc after successful puncture and spread vaccine evenly over the puncture area with the wide edge of the disc. Discs should only be used once and discarded after autoclaving. Between individual vaccinations the magnet should be sterilized (see instructions for use provided with the device).

After vaccination the vaccine should flow into the wounds and dry. No dressing is required; however, it is recommended that the site be kept dry for 24 hours. The patient should be advised that the vaccine contains live organisms. Although the vaccine will not survive in a dry state, infection of others is possible.

Reconstituted vaccine should be kept refrigerated, protected from exposure to light, and used within 2 hours. Vaccination should be repeated for those who remain tuberculin negative to 5TU of tuberculin after 2-3 months.

Pediatric Dose: In infants less than 1 month old the dosage of vaccine should be reduced by one half, by using 2 mL of sterile water when reconstituting. If a vaccinated infant remains tuberculin negative to 5TU on skin testing, and if indications for vaccination persist, the infant should receive a full dose after 1 year of age.

STORAGE
Storage of the intact ampules of BCG should be at refrigerated temperatures of 2-8°C (36-46°F). This agent contains live bacteria and should be protected from light. The product should not be used after expiration date printed on the label.

BCG vials and the accompanying diluent should be kept in a refrigerator at a temperature between 2° and 8°C (35° and 46°F). It should not be used after the expiration date marked on the vial, otherwise it may be inactive. The product should be used immediately after reconstitution: however, it must not be used after 2 hours. Any reconstituted product which exhibits flocculation or clumping that cannot be dispersed with gentle shaking should not be used.

At no time should the freeze-dried or reconstituted BCG be exposed to sunlight, direct or indirect. Exposure to artificial light should be kept to a minimum.

REFERENCES

1. Guerin C: The history of BCG. *In*: Rosenthal SR (ed): BCG Vaccine: Tuberculosis-Cancer. Littleton, MA, PSG Publishing Co., Inc. 1980, pp. 35-43. 2. Kelley DR, Haaff E, Becich M, et al.: Prognostic value of purified protein derivative skin test and granuloma formation in patients treated with intravesical bacillus Calmette-Guerin, J Urol 1986: 135:268-271. 3. Brosman SA: The use of bacillus Calmette-Guerin in the therapy of bladder carcinoma *in situ*. J Urol 1985; 134:36-39. 4. DeKernion JB, Huang M. Linder A, et al: The management of superficial bladder tumors and carcinoma *in situ* with intravesical bacillus Calmette-Guerin. J Urol 1985; 133:598-601. 5. Guinan P, Batenhorst R: BCG in the treatment of superficial bladder cancer (Abstract). J Urol 1987; 137:180A. 6. Soloway M, Perry A: Bacillus Calmette-Guerin for treatment of superficial transitional cell carcinoma of the bladder in patients who have failed thiotepa and/or mitomycin C. J Urol 1987; 137:871-873. 7. Morales A: Long-term results and complications of intra-cavitary bacillus Calmette-Guerin therapy for bladder cancer. J Urol 1984; 132:457-459. 8. Haaff E, Dresner SM, Ratliff TL, Catalona WJ: Two courses of intravesical bacillus Calmette-Guerin for transitional cell carcinoma of the bladder, J Urol 1986; 136:820-824. 9. Herr HW, Pinsky CM, Whitmore WF, et al.: Effect of intravesical bacillus Calmette-Guerin (BCG) on carcinoma *in situ*. Cancer 1983; 51:1323-1326. 10. Kelley DR, Ratliff T, Catalona WJ, et al.: Intravesical bacillus Calmette-Guerin therapy for superficial bladder cancer. Effect of bacillus Calmette-Guerin viability on treatment results. J Urol 1985; 134:48-53. 11. Schellhammer PF, Ladaga LE, Fillion MB: Bacillus Calmette-Guerin for therapy of superficial transitional cell carcinoma of the bladder. J Urol 1986; 135:261-264. 12. Lamm DL: BCG immunotherapy in bladder cancer. *In* Urology Annual 1987. Vol. 1, Appleton & Lange, Norwalk, CT, 1987; pp. 67-86. 13. Lamm DL, Sarosdy MS, DeHaven JI: Percutaneous, oral, or intravesical BCG administration: What is the optimal route? EORTC Genitourinary Group Monograph 6. BCG in Superficial Bladder Cancer. Alan R. Liss, Inc., New York, NY, 1989: pp. 301-310. 14. Utz DC, Hanash KA, Farrow GM: The plight of the patient with carcinoma *in situ* of the bladder, J Urol 1970; 103: 160-164. 15. Herr HW, Pinsky CM, Whitmore WF Jr., et al.: Longterm effect of intravesical bacillus Calmette-Guerin on flat carcinoma *in situ* of the bladder. J Urol 1986; 135:265-267. 16. Romanus V: Tuberculosis in bacillus Calmette-Guerin immunized and unimmunized children in Sweden: a ten-year evaluation following the cessation of general bacillus Calmette-Guerin immunization of the newborn in 1975. Pediatr Infect Dis 1987; 6:272-280. 17. Smith PG: Case-control studies of the efficacy of BCG against tuberculosis. *In*: International Union Against Tuberculosis, Proceedings of the XXXVIth IUAT World Conference on Tuberculosis and Respiratory Diseases, Singapore. Professional Postgraduate Services, International, Japan, 1987; 73-79. 18. Padunchan S, Konjanart S, Kasiratta S, et al.: The effectiveness of BCG vaccination of the newborn against childhood tuberculosis in Bangkok. Bull WHO 1986; 64:247-258. 19. Tidjani O, Amedone A, ten Dam HG: The protective effect of BCG vaccination of the newborn against childhood tuberculosis in an African community. Tubercle 1986; 67:269-281. 20. Young TK, Hershfield ES: A case-control study to evaluate the effectiveness of BCG vaccination among Canadian Indians. Am J Public Health 1986; 76:783-786. 21. Shapiro C, Cook N, Evans D, et al.: A case-control study of BCG and childhood tuberculosis in Cali, Columbia. Int H Epidemiol 1985; 14:441-446. 22. Morbidity and Mortality Weekly Report 37, No. 43 1988; pp. 663-675. 23. Rawls WH, Lamm DL, Eyollfson MF: Septic complications in the use of bacillus Calmette-Guerin (BCG) for noninvasive transitional cell carcinoma. Presented at: 1988 Annual Meeting, American Urological Association, Boston, MA. 24. Lorin MI, Hsu KHK, Jacob SC: Treatment of tuberculosis in children. *In*: Symposium on anti-infective therapy. Pediatric Clinics of North America, 1983; 30:333-348. 25. Report of the Committee on the Control of Infectious Diseases. American Academy of Pediatrics 1988; 21st Edition. 26. Data on file. Organon Teknika Corporation/Biotechnology Research Institute, Rockville, MD. 27. Lamm DL, Steg A, Boccon-Gibod L, et al.: Complications of bacillus Calmette-Guerin immunotherapy: Review of 2602 patients and comparison of chemotherapy complications. EORTC Genitourinary Group Monograph 6: BCG in Superficial Bladder Cancer. Alan R. Liss, Inc., New York, NY, 1989; pp. 335-355. 28. Standard Therapy for Tuberculosis, 1985. Presented at: National Consensus Conference on Tuberculosis. Chest, 1985; 87 (Suppl):117S-124S. 29. Oates R, Siroky M: Nephrogenic adenoma of urinary bladder due to intravesical BCG therapy. J Urol 1986; 135:186. 30. Mande R: BCG Vaccination. Dawsons, London, 1968. 31. Griffith AH: Ten cases of BCG overdose treated with isoniazid. Tubercle 1963; 44:247-250. 32. Watkins SM: Unusual complications of BCG vaccination. Brit Med J 1971; 1:442.

J CODES

Per vial IV—J9031

HOW SUPPLIED
POWDER FOR INJECTION:

BRAND/MANUFACTURER	NDC	SIZE	AWP
○ **BRAND**			
TICE BCG VACCINE: Organon	00052-0601-01	1s	$147.50

POWDER FOR INJECTION: 27 MG

BRAND/MANUFACTURER	NDC	SIZE	AWP
○ **BRAND**			
THERACYS: Connaught	11793-8802-01	1s	$158.13
○ **GENERICS**			
Pasadena	00418-8802-10	3s	$247.50

Beclomethasone Dipropionate

DESCRIPTION

Beclomethasone Dipropionate Nasal and Oral Inhalation Aerosol: Beclomethasone Dipropionate, USP, is an anti-inflammatory steroid having the chemical name 9-chloro-11β,17,21-trihydroxy-16β-methylpregna-1, 4-diene-3, 20-dione 17,21-dipropionate.

Beclomethasone Dipropionate is a white to creamy-white, odorless powder with a molecular weight of 521.25. It is very slightly soluble in water, very soluble in chloroform, and freely soluble in acetone and in alcohol.

Beclomethasone Dipropionate Nasal Spray: Beclomethasone Dipropionate, monohydrate, is an anti-inflammatory steroid having the chemical name 9-chloro-11β-17,21-trihydroxy-16β-methylpregna-1,4-diene-3,20-dione 17,21-dipropionate, monohydrate.

Beclomethasone Dipropionate, monohydrate is a white to creamy-white, odorless powder with a molecular weight of 539.06. It is very slightly soluble in water, very soluble in chloroform, and freely soluble in acetone and in alcohol.

Beclomethasone Dipropionate Nasal Spray is a metered-dose, manual pump spray unit containing a microcrystalline suspension of Beclomethasone Dipropionate, monohydrate equivalent to 0.042% w/w Beclomethasone Dipropionate, calculated on the dried basis, in an aqueous medium.

Each activation of the Nasal Inhalation Aerosol delivers:
Beclomethasone Dipropionate equivalent ....42 mcg

Each activation of the Nasal Spray pump delivers:
Beclomethasone Dipropionate equivalent ....42 mcg

Each activation of the Oral Inhalation Aerosol delivers:
Beclomethasone Dipropionate equivalent ....42 mcg

Following is its chemical structure:

CLINICAL PHARMACOLOGY

Beclomethasone 17,21-Dipropionate is a diester of Beclomethasone, a synthetic halogenated corticosteroid. Animal studies show that Beclomethasone Dipropionate has potent glucocorticoid and weak mineralocorticoid activity. When Beclomethasone Dipropionate was administered systematically to mice, the anti-inflammatory activity was accompanied by other features typical of glucocorticoid action, including thymic involution, liver glycogen deposition, and pituitary-adrenal suppression. However, after systemic administration of Beclomethasone Dipropionate to rats, the anti-inflammatory action was associated with little or no effect on other tests of glucocorticoid activity.

The mechanisms responsible for the anti-inflammatory action of Beclomethasone Dipropionate are unknown. The precise mechanism of the aerosolized drug's action in the nose or lung is also unknown. Biopsies of nasal mucosa obtained during clinical studies showed no histopathologic changes when Beclomethasone Dipropionate was administered intranasally.

The effects of Beclomethasone Dipropionate on hypothalamic-pituitary-adrenal (HPA) function have been evaluated in adult volunteers by other routes of administration. Studies with Beclomethasone Dipropionate by the intranasal route may demonstrate that there is more or that there is less absorption by this route of administration. There was no suppression of early morning plasma cortisol concentrations when Beclomethasone Dipropionate was administered in a dose of 1,000 mcg per day for 1 month as an oral aerosol or for 3 days by intramuscular injection. However, partial suppression of plasma cortisol concentrations was observed when Beclomethasone Dipropionate was administered in doses of 2,000 mcg per day either by oral aerosol or intramuscular injection. Immediate suppression of plasma cortisol concentrations was observed after single doses of 4,000 mcg of Beclomethasone Dipropionate. Suppression of HPA function (reduction of early morning plasma cortisol levels) has been reported in adult patients who received 1,600-mcg daily doses of oral Beclomethasone Dipropionate for 1 month. In clinical studies using Beclomethasone Dipropionate aerosol intranasally, there was no evidence of adrenal insufficiency. The effect of Beclomethasone Dipropionate Nasal Spray on HPA function was not evaluated but would not be expected to differ from intranasal Beclomethasone Dipropionate aerosol.

In one study in asthmatic children, the administration of inhaled Beclomethasone at recommended daily doses for at least 1 year was associated with a reduction in nocturnal cortisol secretion. The clinical significance of this finding is not clear. It reinforces other evidence, however, that topical Beclomethasone may be absorbed in amounts that can have systemic effects and that physicians should be alert for evidence of systemic effects, especially in chronically treated patients (see *"Precautions"*).

Beclomethasone Dipropionate is sparingly soluble and is poorly mobilized from subcutaneous or intramuscular injection sites. However, systemic absorption occurs after all routes of administration. When given by nasal inhalation in the form of an aqueous or aerosolized suspension, the drug is deposited primarily in the nasal passages; when given to animals by oral inhalation, the drug is deposited in the mouth and nasal passages, the trachea and principal bronchi, and the lung. A portion of the drug is swallowed. Absorption occurs rapidly from all respiratory and gastrointestinal tissues, as indicated by the rapid clearance of radioactively labeled drug from local tissues and appearance of tracer in the circulation. There is no evidence of tissue storage of Beclomethasone Dipropionate or its metabolites. *In vitro* studies have shown that tissue other than the liver (lung slices) can rapidly metabolize Beclomethasone Dipropionate to Beclomethasone 17-monopropionate and more slowly to free Beclomethasone (which has very weak anti-inflammatory activity). However, irrespective of the route of entry (injection, oral, or aerosol), the principal route of excretion of the drug and its metabolites is the feces. Less than 10% of the drug and its metabolites is excreted in the urine. In humans, 12%-15% of an orally administered dose of Beclomethasone Dipropionate is excreted in the urine as both conjugated and free metabolites of the drug.

Studies have shown that the degree of binding to plasma proteins is 87%.

INDICATIONS AND USAGE

Beclomethasone Dipropionate Nasal Inhalation Aerosol is indicated for the relief of the symptoms of seasonal or perennial rhinitis in those cases poorly responsive to conventional treatment.

Beclomethasone Dipropionate, monohydrate, Nasal Spray is indicated for the relief of the symptoms of seasonal or perennial allergic and nonallergic (vasomotor) rhinitis.

Both preparations are also indicated for the prevention of recurrence of nasal polyps following surgical removal.

Clinical studies with Beclomethasone Dipropionate Nasal Inhalation Aerosol in patients with seasonal or peerennial rhinitis have shown that improvement is usually apparent within a few days. Results from two clinical trials have shown that significant symptomatic relief was obtained with Beclomethasone Dipropionate. Nasal Spray within 3 days. With either preparation, however, symptomatic relief may not occur in some patients for as long as 2 weeks. Although systemic effects are minimal at recommended doses, Beclomethasone Dipropionate Nasal. Inhalation Aerosol and Beclomethasone Dipropionate Nasal Spray should not be continued beyond 3 weeks in the absence of significant symptomatic improvement. Both preparations should not be used in the presence of untreated localized infection involving the nasal mucosa.

Clinical studies have shown that treatment of the symptoms associated with nasal polyps may have to be continued for several weeks or more before a therapeutic result can be fully assessed. Recurrence of symptoms due to polyps can occur after stopping treatment, depending on the severity of the disease.

Beclomethasone Dipropionate Oral Inhalation Aerosol is indicated only for patients who require chronic treatment with corticosteroids for control of the symptoms of bronchial asthma. Such patients would include those already receiving systemic corticosteroids, and selected patients who are inadequately controlled on a nonsteroid regimen and in whom steroid therapy has been withheld because of concern over potential adverse effects.

Beclomethasone Dipropionate Oral Inhalation Aerosol is NOT indicated:

1. For relief of asthma that can be controlled by bronchodilators and other nonsteroid medications.

2. In patients who require systemic corticosteroid treatment infrequently.

3. In the treatment of nonasthmatic bronchitis.

CONTRAINDICATIONS

Hypersensitivity to any of the ingredients of any of the preparations contraindicates its use.

Beclomethasone Dipropionate Oral Inhalation Aerosol is contraindicated in the primary treatment of status asthmaticus or other acute episodes of asthma where intensive measures are required.

WARNINGS

The replacement of a systemic corticosteroid with Beclomethasone Dipropionate Nasal Inhalation Aerosol or Beclomethasone Dipropionate, monohydrate Nasal Spray can be accompanied by signs of adrenal insufficiency.

Careful attention must be given when patients previously treated for prolonged periods with systemic corticosteroids are transferred to Beclomethasone Dipropionate Nasal Inhalation Aerosol or Beclomethasone Dipropionate Nasal Spray. This is particularly important in those patients who have associated asthma or other clinical conditions where too rapid a decrease in systemic corticosteroids may cause a severe exacerbation of their symptoms.

Studies have shown that the combined administration of alternate-day prednisone systemic treatment and orally inhaled Beclomethasone increases the likelihood of HPA suppression compared to a therapeutic dose of either one alone. Therefore, Beclomethasone Dipropionate Nasal Inhalation Aerosol and Beclomethasone Dipropionate Nasal Spray treatment should be used with caution in patients already on alternate-day prednisone regimens for any disease.

If recommended doses of intranasal Beclomethasone are exceeded or if individuals are particularly sensitive or predisposed by virtue of recent systemic steroid therapy, symptoms of hypercorticism may occur, including very rare cases of menstrual irregularities, acneiform lesions, and cushingoid features. Because of the possibility of systemic absorption of orally inhaled corticosteroids, including Beclomethasone, patients should be monitored for symptoms of systemic effects such as mental disturbances, increased bruising, weight gain, cushingoid features, and, in children, reduction in growth velocity. If such changes occur, Beclomethasone Dipropionate Nasal or Oral Inhalation Aerosol and Beclomethasone Dipropionate Nasal Spray should be discontinued slowly consistent with accepted procedures for discontinuing oral steroid therapy.

PARTICULAR CARE IS NEEDED IN PATIENTS WHO ARE TRANSFERRED FROM SYSTEMICALLY ACTIVE CORTICOSTEROIDS TO BECLOMETHASONE DIPROPIONATE ORAL INHALATION AEROSOL BECAUSE *DEATHS DUE TO ADRENAL INSUFFICIENCY HAVE OCCURRED IN ASTHMATIC PATIENTS DURING AND AFTER TRANSFER FROM SYSTEMIC CORTICOSTEROIDS TO AEROSOL BECLOMETHASONE DIPROPIONATE.* AFTER WITHDRAWAL FROM SYSTEMIC CORTICOSTEROIDS, A NUMBER OF MONTHS ARE REQUIRED FOR RECOVERY OF HYPOTHALAMIC-PITUITARY-ADRENAL (HPA) FUNCTION. DURING THIS PERIOD OF HPA SUPPRESSION, PATIENTS MAY EXHIBIT SIGNS AND SYMPTOMS OF ADRENAL INSUFFICIENCY WHEN EXPOSED TO TRAUMA, SURGERY, OR INFECTIONS, PARTICULARLY GASTROENTERITIS. ALTHOUGH BECLOMETHASONE DIPROPIONATE ORAL INHALATION AEROSOL MAY PROVIDE CONTROL OF ASTHMATIC SYMPTOMS DURING THESE EPISODES, IT DOES *NOT* PROVIDE THE SYSTEMIC STEROID THAT IS NECESSARY FOR COPING WITH THESE EMERGENCIES.

DURING PERIODS OF STRESS OR A SEVERE ASTHMATIC ATTACK, PATIENTS WHO HAVE BEEN WITHDRAWN FROM SYSTEMIC CORTICOSTEROIDS SHOULD BE INSTRUCTED TO RESUME SYSTEMIC STEROIDS (IN LARGE DOSES) IMMEDIATELY AND TO CONTACT THEIR PHYSICIAN FOR FURTHER INSTRUCTION. THESE PATIENTS SHOULD ALSO BE INSTRUCTED TO CARRY A WARNING CARD INDICATING THAT THEY MAY NEED SUPPLEMENTARY SYSTEMIC STEROIDS DURING PERIODS OF STRESS OR A SEVERE ASTHMA ATTACK. TO ASSESS THE RISK OF ADRENAL INSUFFICIENCY IN EMERGENCY SITUATIONS, ROUTINE TESTS OF ADRENAL CORTICAL FUNCTION, INCLUDING MEASUREMENT OF EARLY MORNING RESTING CORTISOL LEVELS, SHOULD BE PERFORMED PERIODICALLY IN ALL PATIENTS. AN EARLY MORNING RESTING CORTISOL LEVEL MAY BE ACCEPTED AS NORMAL ONLY IF IT FALLS AT OR NEAR THE NORMAL MEAN LEVEL.

Children who are on immunosuppressant drugs are more susceptible to infections than healthy children. Chickenpox and measles, for example, can have a more serious or even fatal course in children on immunosuppresant corticosteroids. In such children, or in adults who have not had these diseases, particular care should be taken to avoid exposure. If exposed, therapy with varicella zoster immune globulin (VZIG) or pooled intravenous immunoglobulin (IVIG), as appropriate, may be indicated. If chickenpox develops, treatment with antiviral agents may be considered.

Beclomethasone Dipropionate Oral Inhalation Aerosol not to be regarded as a bronchodilator and is not indicated for rapid relief of bronchospasm.

Patients should be instructed to contact their physician immediately when episodes of asthma that are not responsive to bronchodilators occur during the course of treatment with Beclomethasone Dipropionate Oral Inhalation Aerosol. During such episodes, patients may require therapy with systemic corticosteroids.

There is no evidence that control of asthma can be achieved by the administration of Beclomethasone Dipropionate Oral Inhalation Aerosol in amounts greater than the recommended doses.

Transfer of patients from systemic steroid therapy to Beclomethasone Dipropionate Oral Inhalation Aerosol may unmask allergic conditions previously suppressed by the systemic steroid therapy, e.g., rhinitis, conjunctivitis, and eczema.

PRECAUTIONS

General: During withdrawal from oral steroids, some patients may experience symptoms of withdrawal, e.g., joint and/or muscular pain, lassitude, and depression, despite maintenance or even improvement of respiratory function (see "*Dosage and Administration*"). Rare instances of nasal septum perforation have been spontaneously reported.

In clinical studies with Beclomethasone Dipropionate administered intranasally, the development of localized infections of the nose and pharynx with *Candida albicans* has occurred only rarely. When such an infection develops, it may require treatment with appropriate local therapy or discontinuation of treatment with Beclomethasone Dipropionate Nasal Inhalation Aerosol or Beclomethasone Dipropionate, Monohydrate Nasal Spray. With Beclomethasone Dipropionate Oral Inhalation Aerosol, localized infections with *Candida albicans or Aspergillus niger* have occurred frequently in the mouth and pharynx and occasionally in the larynx. Positive cultures for oral *Candida* may be present in up to 75% of patients. Although the frequency of clinically apparent infection is considerably lower, these infections may require treatment with appropriate antifungal therapy or discontinuation of treatment with Beclomethasone Dipropionate Oral Inhalation Aerosol.

Beclomethasone Dipropionate is absorbed into the circulation. Use of excessive doses of Beclomethasone Dipropionate Nasal Inhalation Aerosol or Beclomethasone Dipropionate Nasal Spray may suppress HPA function.

In responsive patients, Beclomethasone Dipropionate may permit control of asthmatic symptoms without suppression of HPA function, as discussed below (see "*Clinical Studies*"). Since Beclomethasone Dipropionate is absorbed into the circulation and can be systemically active, the beneficial effects of Beclomethasone Dipropionate Oral Inhalation Aerosol in minimizing or preventing HPA dysfunction may be expected only when recommended dosages are not exceeded.

Beclomethasone Dipropionate Nasal or Oral Inhalation Aerosol and Beclomethasone Dipropionate Nasal Spray should be used with caution, it at all, in patients with active or quiescent tuberculous infections of the respiratory tract; untreated fungal, bacterial, or systemic viral infections; or ocular herpes simplex.

For either preparation to be effective in the treatment of nasal polyps, the aerosol or spray must be able to enter the nose. Therefore, treatment of nasal polyps with these preparations should be considered adjunctive therapy to surgical removal and/or the use of other medications that will permit effective penetration of Beclomethasone Dipropionate Nasal Inhalation Aerosol or Beclomethasone Dipropionate Nasal Spray into the nose. Nasal polyps may recur after any form of treatment.

As with any long-term treatment, patients using Beclomethasone Dipropionate Nasal or Oral Inhalation Aerosol or Beclomethasone Dipropionate Nasal Spray over several months or longer should be examined periodically for possible changes in the nasal mucosa.

The long-term effects of Beclomethasone Dipropionate in human subjects are still unknown. In particular, the local effects of the agent on developmental or immunologic processes in the mouth, pharynx, trachea, and lung are unknown. There is also no information about the possible long-term systemic effects of the agent.

Because of the inhibitory effect of corticosteroids on wound healing, patients who have experienced recent nasal septum ulcers, nasal surgery, or trauma should not use a nasal corticosteroid until healing has occurred.

Although systemic effects have been minimal with recomended doses, this potential increases with excessive doses. Therefore, larger than recommended doses of Beclomethasone Dipropionate Nasal Inhalation Aerosol and Beclomethasone Dipropionate Nasal Spray should be avoided.

Beclomethasone Dipropionate Nasal Inhalation Aerosol: Rare instances of increased intraocular pressure have been reported following the intranasal application of aerosolized corticosteroids.

Beclomethasone Dipropionate Oral Inhalation Aerosol: Pulmonary infiltrates with eosinophilia may occur in patients on Beclomethasone Dipropionate Oral Inhalation Aerosol therapy. Although it is possible that in some patients this state may become manifest because of systemic steroid withdrawal when inhalational steroids are administered, a causative role for Beclomethasone Dipropionate and/or its vehicle cannot be ruled out.

Beclomethasone Dipropionate Nasal Spray: Rarely, immediate hypersensitivity reactions may occur after the intranasal administration of Beclomethasone.

Rare instances of wheezing and increased intraocular pressure have been reported following the intranasal application of aerosolized corticosteroids. Although these have not been observed in clinical trials with Beclomethasone Dipropionate Nasal Spray, vigilance should be maintained.

If persistent nasopharyngeal irritation occurs, it may be an indication for stopping Beclomethasone Dipropionate Nasal Spray.

Information for Patients: Patients being treated with Beclomethasone Dipropionate Nasal or Oral Inhalation Aerosol or Beclomethasone Dipropionate Nasal Spray should receive the following information and instructions. This information is intended to aid in the safe and effective use of this medication. It is not a disclosure of all possible adverse or intended effects. Patients should use these preparations at regular intervals since their effectiveness depends on their regular use. The patient should take the medication as directed. It is not acutely effective, and the prescribed dosage should not be increased. Instead, nasal vasoconstrictors or oral antihistamines may be needed until the effects of Beclomethasone Dipropionate Nasal Inhalation Aerosol or Beclomethasone Dipropionate Nasal Spray are fully manifested. One to 2 weeks may pass before full relief is obtained. The patient should contact the physician if symptoms do not improve, or if the condition worsens, or if sneezing or nasal irritation occurs. For the proper use of either unit and to attain maximum improvement, the patient should read and follow carefully the patient's instructions section of the package insert.

Patients who are on immunosuppressant doses of corticosteroids should be warned to avoid exposure to chickenpox or measles and, if exposed, to obtain medical advice.

Carcinogenesis, Mutagenesis, Impairment of Fertility: Treatment of rats for a total of 95 weeks, 13 weeks by inhalation and 82 weeks by the oral route, resulted in no evidence of carcinogenic activity. Mutagenic studies have not been performed.

Impairment of fertility, as evidenced by inhibition of the estrous cycle in dogs, was observed following treatment by the oral route. No inhibition of the estrous cycle in dogs was seen following treatment with Beclomethasone Dipropionate by the inhalation route.

Pregnancy: Teratogenic Effects: Pregnancy Category C: Like other corticoids, parenteral (subcutaneous) Beclomethasone Dipropionate has been shown to be teratogenic and embryocidal in the mouse and rabbit when given in doses approximately 10 times the human dose. In these studies, Beclomethasone was found to produce fetal resorption, cleft palate, agnathia, microstomia, absence of tongue, delayed ossification, and agenesis of the thymus. No teratogenic or embryocidal effects have been seen in the rat when Beclomethasone Dipropionate was administered by inhalation at 10 times the human dose or orally at 1,000 times the human dose. There are no adequate and well-controlled studies in pregnant women or relating to fetal risk in humans. Beclomethasone Dipropionate should be used during pregnancy only if the potential benefit justifies the potential risk to the fetus.

Nonteratogenic Effects: Hypoadrenalism may occur in infants born of mothers receiving corticosteroids during pregnancy. Such infants should be carefully observed.

Nursing Mothers: It is not known whether Beclomethasone Dipropionate is excreted in human milk. Because other corticosteroids are excreted in human milk, caution should be exercised when Beclomethasone Dipropionate Nasal or Oral Inhalation Aerosol or Beclomethasone Dipropionate, Nasal Spray is administered to a nursing woman.

Pediatric Use: Safety and effectiveness in children below 6 years of age have not been established.

ADVERSE REACTIONS

In general, side effects in clinical studies with both nasal preparations have been primarily associated with irritation of the nasal mucous membranes.

Beclomethasone Dipropionate Nasal Inhalation Aerosol: Adverse reactions reported in controlled clinical trials and long-term open studies in patients treated with Beclomethasone Dipropionate Nasal Inhalation Aerosol are described below.

Sensations of irritation and burning in the nose (11 per 100 patients) following the use of Beclomethasone Dipropionate Nasal Inhalation Aerosol have been reported. Also, occasional sneezing attacks (10 per 100 adult patients) have occurred immediately following the use of the intranasal inhaler. This symptom may be more common in children. Rhinorrhea may occur occasionally (1 per 100 patients).

Localized infections of the nose and pharynx with *Candida albicans* have occurred rarely (see "Precautions").

Transient episodes of epistaxis have been reported in 2 per 100 patients.

Rare cases of ulceration of the nasal mucosa and instances of nasal septum perforation have been spontaneously reported (See "Precautions"). Rare reports of loss of taste and smell have been reported.

Rare instances of increased intraocular pressure have been reported following the intranasal application of aerosolized corticosteroids (see "Precautions").

Rare cases of immediate and delayed hypersensitivity reactions, including urticaria, angioedema, rash, and bronchospasm, have been reported following the oral and intranasal inhalation and administration of Beclomethasone.

Systemic corticosteroid side effects were not reported during controlled clinical trials. If recommended doses are exceeded, however, or if individuals are particularly sensitive, symptoms of hypercorticism, i.e., Cushing's syndrome, could occur.

Beclomethasone Dipropionate Oral Inhalation Aerosol: **Deaths due to adrenal insufficiency have occurred in asthmatic patients during and after transfer from systemic corticosteroids to aerosol Beclomethasone Dipropionate (see "Warnings").**

Suppression of HPA function (reduction of early morning plasma cortisol levels) has been reported in adult patients who received 1,600-mcg daily doses of Beclomethasone Dipropionate Oral Inhalation Aerosol for 1 month. A few patients on Beclomethasone Dipropionate Oral Inhalation Aerosol have complained of hoarseness or dry mouth.

Rare cases of immediate and delayed hypersensitivity reactions, including urticaria, angioedema, rash, and bronchospasm, have been reported after the use of Beclomethasone oral or intranasal inhalers.

Beclomethasone Dipropionate, Monohydrate Nasal Spray: Rarely, immediate hypersensitivity reactions may occur after the intranasal administration of Beclomethasone.

Adverse reactions reported in controlled clinical trials and open studies in patients treated with Beclomethasone Dipropionate Nasal Spray are described below.

Mild nasopharyngeal irritation following the use of Beclomethasone aqueous nasal spray has been reported in up to 24% of patients treated, including occasional sneezing attacks (about 4%) occurring immediately following use of the spray. In patients experiencing these symptoms, none had to discontinue treatment. The incidence of transient irritation and sneezing was approximately the same in the group of patients who received placebo in these studies, implying that these complaints may be related to vehicle components of the formulation.

Fewer than 5 per 100 patients reported headache, nausea, or lightheadedness following the use of Beclomethasone Dipropionate Nasal Spray. Fewer than 3 per 100 patients reported nasal stuffiness nosebleeds, rhinorrhea, or tearing eyes.

Rare cases of ulceration of the nasal mucosa and instances of nasal septum perforation have been spontaneously reported (see "Precautions"). Rare reports of loss of taste and smell have been received.

Rare instances of wheezing and increased intraocular pressure have been reported following the intranasal administration of aerosolized corticosteroids (see "Precautions").

OVERDOSAGE

When used at excessive doses, systemic corticosteroid effects such as hypercorticism and adrenal suppression may appear. If such changes occur, Beclomethasone Dipropionate Nasal or Oral Inhalation Aerosol and Beclomethasone Dipropionate, Monohydrate Nasal Spray should be discontinued slowly consistent with accepted procedures for discontinuing oral steroid therapy. The oral LD_{50} of Beclomethasone Dipropionate is greater than 1 g/kg in rodents. One canister of Beclomethasone Dipropionate Nasal Inhalation Aerosol contains 8.4 mg of Beclomethasone Dipropionate, and one bottle of Beclomethasone Dipropionate Nasal Spray contains Beclomethasone Dipropionate, Monohydrate equivalent to 10.5 mg of Beclomethasone Dipropionate; therefore, acute overdosage is unlikely.

DOSAGE AND ADMINISTRATION

Beclomethasone Dipropionate Nasal Inhalation Aerosol:

Adults and Children 12 Years of Age and Older: The usual dosage is one inhalation (42 mcg) in each nostril two to four times a day (total dose, 168-336 mcg per day). Patients can often be maintained on a maximum dose of one inhalation in each nostril three times a day (252 mcg per day).

Children 6-12 Years of Age: The usual dosage is one inhalation in each nostril three times a day (252 mcg per day). Beclomethasone Dipropionate Nasal

---

Inhalation Aerosol is *not* recommended for children below 6 years of age since safety and efficacy studies have not been conducted in this age-group.

Contents Under Pressure: Do not puncture. Do not use or store near heat or open flame. Exposure to temperatures above 120°F may cause bursting. Never throw container into fire or incinerator. Keep out of reach of children.

Beclomethasone Dipropionate Oral Inhalation Aerosol:

Adults and Children 12 Years of Age and Older: The usual recommended dosage is two inhalations (84 mcg) given three or four times a day. Alternatively, four inhalations (168 mcg) given twice daily have been shown to be effective in some patients. In patients with severe asthma, it is advisable to start with 12-16 inhalations a day and adjust the dosage downward according to the response of the patient. *The maximal daily intake should not exceed 20 inhalations, 840 mcg (0.84 mg), in adults.*

Children 6-12 Years of Age: The usual recommended dosage is one or two inhalations (42-84 mcg) given three or four times a day according to the response of the patient. Alternatively, four inhalations (168 mcg) given twice daily have been shown to be effective in some patients. *The maximal daily intake should not exceed 10 inhalations, 420 mcg (0.42 mg), in children 6-12 years of age.* Insufficient clinical data exist with respect to the administration of Beclomethasone Dipropionate Oral Inhalation Aerosol in children below the age of 6.

Rinsing the mouth after inhalation is advised.

Patients receiving bronchodilators by inhalation should be advised to use the bronchodilator before Beclomethasone Dipropionate Oral Inhalation Aerosol in order to enhance penetration of Beclomethasone Dipropionate into the bronchial tree. After use of an aerosol bronchodilator, several minutes should elapse before use of the Beclomethasone Dipropionate Oral Inhalation Aerosol to reduce the potential toxicity from the inhaled fluorocarbon propellants in the two aerosols.

Different considerations must be given to the following groups of patients in order to obtain the full therapeutic benefit of Beclomethasone Dipropionate Oral Inhalation Aerosol.

Patients Not Receiving Systemic Steroids: The use of Beclomethasone Dipropionate Oral Inhalation Aerosol is straightforward in patients who are inadequately controlled with nonsteroid medications but in whom systemic steroid therapy has been withheld because of concern over potential adverse reactions. In patients who respond to Beclomethasone Dipropionate Oral Inhalation Aerosol, an improvement in pulmonary function is usually apparent within 1-4 weeks after the start of Beclomethasone Dipropionate Oral Inhalation Aerosol.

Patients Receiving Systemic Steroids: In those patients dependent on systemic steroids, transfer to Beclomethasone Dipropionate Oral Inhalation Aerosol and subsequent management may be more difficult because recovery from impaired adrenal function is usually slow. Such suppression has been known to last for up to 12 months. Clinical studies, however, have demonstrated that Beclomethasone Dipropionate Oral Inhalation Aerosol may be effective in the management of these asthmatic patients and may permit replacement or significant reduction in the dosage of systemic corticosteroids.

The patient's asthma should be reasonably stable before treatment with Beclomethasone Dipropionate Oral Inhalation Aerosol is started. Initially, the aerosol should be used concurrently with the patient's usual maintenance dose of systemic steroid. After approximately 1 week, gradual withdrawal of the systemic steroid is started by reducing the daily or alternate-daily dose. The next reduction is made after an interval of 1 or 2 weeks, depending on the response of the patient. Generally, these decrements should not exceed 2.5 mg of prednisone or its equivalent. A slow rate of withdrawal cannot be overemphasized. During withdrawal some patients may experience symptoms of systemically active steroid withdrawal, e.g., joint and/or muscular pain, lassitude, and depression, despite maintenance or even improvement of respiratory function. Such patients should be encouraged to continue with the inhaler but should be watched carefully for objective signs of adrenal insufficiency such as hypotension and weight loss. If evidence of adrenal insufficiency occurs, the systemic steroid dose should be boosted temporarily and thereafter further withdrawal should continue more slowly. *During periods of stress or a severe asthma attack, transfer patients will require supplementary treatment with systemic steroids.* Exacerbations of asthma that occur during the course of treatment with Beclomethasone Dipropionate Oral Inhalation Aerosol should be treated with a short course of systemic steroid that is gradually tapered as these symptoms subside. There is no evidence that control of asthma can be achieved by administration of Beclomethasone Dipropionate Oral Inhalation Aerosol in amounts greater than the recommended doses.

Contents Under Pressure: Do not puncture. Do not use or store near heat or open flame. Exposure to temperatures above 120° F may cause bursting. Never throw container into fire or incinerator. Keep out of reach of children.

Beclomethasone Dipropionate Nasal Spray:

Adults and Children 6 Years of Age and Older: The usual dosage is one or two inhalations (42-84 mcg) in each nostril twice a day (total dose, 168-336 mcg per day).

Beclomethasone Dipropionate Nasal Spray is *not* recommended for children below 6 years of age.

In patients who respond to Beclomethasone Dipropionate Nasal Inhalation Aerosol and to Beclomethasone Dipropionate Nasal Spray, an improvement of the symptoms of seasonal or perennial rhinitis usually becomes apparent within a few days after the start of therapy. However, symptomatic relief may not occur in some patients for as long as 2 weeks. Beclomethasone Dipropionate Nasal Inhalation Aerosol and Beclomethasone Dipropionate Nasal Spray should not be continued beyond 3 weeks in the absence of significant symptomatic improvement.

The therapeutic effects of corticosteroids, unlike those of decongestants, are not immediate. This should be explained to the patient in advance in order to ensure cooperation and continuation of treatment with the prescribed dosage regimen.

In the presence of excessive nasal mucous secretion or edema of the nasal mucosa, the drug may fail to reach the site of intended action. In such cases it is advisable to use a nasal vasoconstrictor during the first 2-3 days of Beclomethasone Dipropionate Nasal Inhalation Aerosol or Beclomethasone Dipropionate Nasal Spray therapy.

Directions for Use: Illustrated Patient's Instructions for Use accompany each package of Beclomethasone Dipropionate Nasal Inhalation Aerosol and Beclomethasone Dipropionate Nasal Spray.

Storage: Store Beclomethasone Dipropionate Nasal and Oral Inhalation Aerosol between 2° and 30°C (36° and 86° F). As with most inhaled medications in aerosol canisters, the therapeutic effect of this medication may decrease when the canister is cold. Shake well before using.

Store Beclomethasone Dipropionate Nasal Spray between 15° and 30° C (59° and 86° F).

ANIMAL PHARMACOLOGY AND TOXICOLOGY
Studies in a number of animal species, including rats, rabbits, and dogs, have shown no unusual toxicity during acute experiments. However, the effects of Beclomethasone Dipropionate in producing signs of glucocorticoid excess during chronic administration by various routes were dose related.

CLINICAL STUDIES
The effects of Beclomethasone Dipropionate on HPA function have been evaluated in adult volunteers. There was no suppression of early morning plasma cortisol concentrations when Beclomethasone Dipropionate was administered in a dose of 1,000 mcg per day for 1 month as an aerosol or for 3 days by intramuscular injection. However, partial suppression of plasma cortisol concentration was observed when Beclomethasone Dipropionate was administered in doses of 2,000 mcg per day either intramuscularly or by aerosol. Immediate suppression of plasma cortisol concentrations was observed after single doses of 4,000 mcg of Beclomethasone Dipropionate.

In one study the effects of Beclomethasone Dipropionate on HPA function were examined in patients with asthma. There was no change in basal early morning plasma cortisol concentrations or in the cortisol responses to tetracosactrin (ACTH 1:24) stimulation after daily administration of 400, 800, or 1,200 mcg of Beclomethasone Dipropionate for 28 days. After daily administration of 1,600 mcg each day for 28 days, there was slight reduction in basal cortisol concentrations and a statistically significant ($p < .01$) reduction in plasma cortisol responses to tetracosactrin stimulation. The effects of a more prolonged period of Beclomethasone Dipropionate administration on HPA function have not been evaluated. However, a number of investigators have noted that when systemic corticosteroid therapy in asthmatic subjects can be replaced with recommended doses of Beclomethasone Dipropionate, there is gradual recovery of endogenous cortisol concentrations to the normal range. There is still no documented evidence of recovery from other adverse systemic corticosteroid-induced reactions during prolonged therapy of patients with Beclomethasone Dipropionate.

Clinical experience has shown that some patients with bronchial asthma who require corticosteroid therapy for control of symptoms can be partially or completely withdrawn from systemic corticosteroids if therapy with Beclomethasone Dipropionate aerosol is substituted. Beclomethasone Dipropionate aerosol is not effective for all patients with bronchial asthma or at all stages of the disease in a given patient.

The early clinical experience has revealed several new problems that may be associated with the use of Beclomethasone Dipropionate by inhalation for treatment of patients with bronchial asthma.

1. There is a risk of adrenal insufficiency when patients are transferred from systemic corticosteroids to aerosol Beclomethasone Dipropionate. Although the aerosol may provide adequate control of asthma during the transfer period, it does not provide the systemic steroid that is needed during acute stress situations. *Deaths due to adrenal insufficiency have occurred in asthmatic patients during and after transfer from systemic corticosteroids to aerosol Beclomethasone Dipropionate* (see '*Warnings*').

2. Transfer of patients from systemic steroid therapy to Beclomethasone Dipropionate aerosol may unmask allergic conditions that were previously controlled by the systemic steroid therapy, e.g., rhinitis, conjunctivitis, and eczema.

3. Localized infections with *Candida albicans* or *Aspergillus niger* have occurred frequently in the mouth and pharynx and occasionally in the larynx. It has been reported that up to 75% of the patients who receive prolonged treatment with Beclomethasone Dipropionate have positive oral cultures for *Candida albicans*. The incidence of clinically apparent infection is considerably lower but may require therapy with appropriate antifungal agents or discontinuation of treatment with Beclomethasone Dipropionate aerosol.

The long-term effects of beclomethasone dipropionate in human subjects are still unknown. In particular, the local effects of the agent on developmental or immunologic processes in the mouth, pharynx, trachea, and lung are unknown. There is also no information about the possible long-term systemic effects of the agent. The possible relevance of the data in animal studies to results in human subjects cannot be evaluated.

HOW SUPPLIED
AEROSOL SOLID INGREDIENTS: 0.042 MG/INH

BRAND/MANUFACTURER	NDC	SIZE	AWP
◇ **BRAND**			
BECLOVENT: Allen & Hanburys	00173-0360-98	16.8 gm	$24.47

AEROSOL SOLID W/ADAPTER: 0.042 MG/INH

BRAND/MANUFACTURER	NDC	SIZE	AWP
◇ **BRAND**			
BECONASE: Allen & Hanburys	00173-0468-00	6.7 gm	$17.23
BECLOVENT: Allen & Hanburys	00173-0469-00	6.7 gm	$17.23
VANCENASE INHALER: Schering	00085-0649-02	7 gm	$30.01
VANCERIL: Key	00085-0736-04	17 gm	$30.01
BECONASE: Allen & Hanburys	00173-0336-02	17 gm	$30.01
BECLOVENT: Allen & Hanburys	00173-0312-88	17 gm	$30.01

SPRAY: 0.042 MG/INH

BRAND/MANUFACTURER	NDC	SIZE	AWP
◇ **BRAND**			
VANCENASE AQ: Schering	00085-0259-02	25 ml	$32.40
BECONASE AQ: Allen & Hanburys	00173-0388-79	25 ml	$32.40

Beclovent SEE BECLOMETHASONE DIPROPIONATE

Becomject-100 SEE VITAMIN B COMPLEX

Beconase SEE BECLOMETHASONE DIPROPIONATE

Belladonna Alkaloids and Butabarbital Sodium

DESCRIPTION
Each Belladonna Alkaloide/Butabarbital Sodium Tablet contains:

Butabarbital Sodium ....15 mg
(Warning: May be habit-forming.)
Belladonna Extract ....15 mg*

Each 5 mL (one teaspoonful) of Belladonna/Butabarbital elixir contains:

Butabarbital Sodium ....15 mg
(Warning: May be habit-forming.)
Belladonna Extract ....15 mg*
Alcohol (by volume) 7%

CLINICAL PHARMACOLOGY
Belladonna/Butabarbital provides natural Belladonna Alkaloids in a specific, fixed ratio combined with Butabarbital Sodium to provide peripheral anticholinergic/antispasmodic action and mild sedation.

INDICATIONS AND USAGE

BASED ON A REVIEW BY THE NATIONAL ACADEMY OF SCIENCES—NATIONAL RESEARCH COUNCIL AND/OR OTHER INFORMATION, FDA HAS CLASSIFIED THE INDICATIONS AS 'POSSIBLY" EFFECTIVE:

FOR USE AS ADJUNCTIVE THERAPY IN THE TREATMENT OF PEPTIC ULCER.

IT SHOULD BE NOTED AT THIS POINT IN TIME THAT THERE IS A LACK OF CONCURRENCE AS TO THE VALUE OF ANTICHOLINERGICS/ANTISPASMODICS IN THE TREATMENT OF GASTRIC ULCER. IT HAS NOT BEEN SHOWN CONCLUSIVEY WHETHER ANTICHOLINERGIC/ANTISPASMODIC DRUGS AID IN THE HEALING OF A PEPTIC ULCER, DECREASE THE RATE OF RECURRENCES, OR PREVENT COMPLICATION.

MAY ALSO BE USEFUL IN THE IRRITABLE BOWEL SYNDROME (IRRITABLE COLON, SPASTIC COLON, MUCOUS COLITIS), AND ACUTE ENTEROCOLITIS.

FINAL CLASSIFICATION OF THE LESS-THAN-EFFECTIVE INDICATION REQUIRES FURTHER INVESTIGATION.

* Total alkaloids (as bases) 0.187 mg, equivalent to 10 minims of tincture of Belladonna.

CONTRAINDICATIONS
Belladonna/Butabarbital tablets and elixir are contraindicated in patients with glaucoma, obstructive uropathy (for example, bladder neck obstruction due to prostatic hypertrophy); obstructive disease of the gastrointestinal tract (as in achalasia, pyloroduodenal stenosis, etc.); paralytic ileus, intestinal atony of the elderly or debilitated patient; unstable cardiovascular status in acute hemorrhage; severe ulcerative colitis especially if complicated by toxic megacolon; myasthenia gravis; hiatal hernia associated with reflex esophagitis.

Belladonna/Butabarbital is contraindicated in patients with acute intermittent porphyria. It is also contraindicated in those with a known sensitivity to either component or barbiturates in general, or in those in whom barbiturates produce restlessness and/or excitement.

WARNINGS
Diarrhea may be an early symptom of incomplete intestinal obstruction, especially in patients with ileostomy or colostomy. In this instance, treatment with Belladonna/Butabarbital would be inappropriate and possibly harmful.

Belladonna/Butabarbital contains butabarbital sodium, a barbiturate, which may be habit-forming. Tolerance, psychological and physical dependence may occur with continued use of barbiturates (see *"Drug Abuse and Dependence"* below).

Use in Pregnancy: Barbiturates can cause fetal damage when administered to a pregnant woman. Retrospective, case-controlled studies have suggested a connection between the maternal consumption of barbiturates and a higher than expected incidence of fetal abnormalities. Following oral administration, barbiturates readily cross the placental barrier and are distributed throughout fetal tissues with highest concentrations found in the placenta, fetal liver, and brain.

Withdrawal symptoms have occurred in infants born to mothers who received barbiturates throughout the last trimester of pregnancy (see *"Drug Abuse and Dependence"* below). If this drug is to be used during pregnancy or if the patient becomes pregnant while taking this drug, the patient should be apprised of the potential hazard to the fetus.

PRECAUTIONS
General: Use of Belladonna/Butabarbital in the treatment of gastric ulcer may produce a delay in gastric emptying time and may complicate such therapy (antral stasis). Do not rely on the use of Belladonna/Butabarbital in the presence of complication of biliary tract disease.

Use with caution in patients with autonomic neuropathy, hyperthyroidism, coronary heart disease, congestive heart failure, cardiac arrhythmias, and hypertension.

Employ caution while administering Belladonna/Butabarbital to those with renal or hepatic disease. Since barbiturates are metabolized in the liver, use with initial small doses and caution in patients with hepatic dysfunction.

Certain brands of Belladonna/Butabarbital elixir contain FD&C Yellow No. 5 (tartrazine) may cause allergic-type reactions (including bronchial asthma) in certain susceptible individuals. Although the overall incidence of FD&C Yellow No. 5 (tartrazine) sensitivity in the general population is low, it is frequently seen in patients who also have aspirin hypersensitivity.

Information for Patients: Belladonna/Butabarbital may produce drowsiness or blurred vision. In this event, the patient should be warned not to engage in activities requiring mental alertness, such as operating a motor vehicle or other machinery, or perform hazardous work while taking this drug.

In the presence of a high environmental temperature, heat prostration can occur (fever and heatstroke due to decreased sweating).

Drug Interactions: Barbiturates stimulate hepatic microsomal enzymes, and may therefore increase the rate of metabolism of some drugs, including the coumarin anticoagulants. Caution is therefore advised in the administration of Belladonna/Butabarbital to patients receiving anticoagulant drugs. Similarly, the systemic effects of exogenous or endogenous corticosteroids may be diminished by concomitant Belladonna/Butabarbital administration.

The concomitant use of other central nervous system depressants, including other sedatives or hypnotics, antihistamines, tranquilizers, or alcohol, may produce additive depressant effects.

Carcinogenesis, Mutagenesis, Impairment of Fertility: Adequate long-term studies in animals to determine the carcinogenic potential of Belladonna/Butabarbital or its components have not been performed. Also, adequate studies of mutagenicity or effects on fertility are not available on Belladonna/Butabarbital or its components.

Pregnancy: Teratogenic Effects - Pregnancy Category C: There are no adequate and well-controlled studies in pregnant women. Belladonna/Butabarbital should be used during pregnancy only if the potential benefits outweigh the potential risk to the fetus (see *"Warnings"*.)

Nursing Mothers: Since small amounts of some barbiturates are excreted in human milk, caution should be exercised when Belladonna/Butabarbital is administered to a nursing woman.

ADVERSE REACTIONS
The following adverse reactions may occur with anticholinergic/sedative combinations, such as Belladonna/Butabarbital.

Gastrointestinal: nausea, vomiting, constipation, bloated feeling.

Cardiovascular: tachycardia and palpitation.

◆ RATED THERAPEUTICALLY EQUIVALENT; ◇ THERAPEUTIC EQUIVALENCE UNCONFIRMED; ○ UNRATED

Ocular: blurred vision, increased intraocular pressure, mydriasis, and cycloplegia.

Musculoskeletal: pain.

Genitourinary: urinary hesitancy and retention.

Central Nervous System: headache, nervousness, drowsiness, weakness, dizziness, insomnia, impotence.

Nasopharyngeal: xerostomia, loss of taste.

Other: decreased sweating, suppression of lactation.

Butabarbital Sodium may paradoxically produce excitement in some patients. In the elderly, excitement, agitation, drowsiness, and other untoward manifestations may occur with even small doses of the drug.

Severe allergic reactions or drug idiosyncrasies, including anaphylaxis, urticaria, or other dermal manifestations may occur after taking Belladonna/Butabarbital or its components.

DRUG ABUSE AND DEPENDENCE

Abuse and Dependence: Because barbiturates may be habit-forming, Belladonna/Butabarbital should not be administered to individuals known to be addiction prone or to those with a history of physical and/or psychological dependence upon habit-forming drugs.

In patients habituated to barbiturates, abrupt withdrawal may produce delirium, convulsions, and possibly death.

OVERDOSAGE

Signs and Symptoms: The manifestations of Belladonna/Butabarbital overdose are extensions of the pharmacologic actions of the individual components. A curare-like action may occur. The signs and symptoms of overdosage include headache, nausea, vomiting, blurred vision, dilated pupils, hot and dry skin, dizziness, dryness of the mouth, difficulty in swallowing, CNS stimulation.

Treatment: When an overdosage of Belladonna/Butabarbital has been taken, measures to reduce intestinal absorption (gastric lavage, administration of emetics or activated charcoal) should be initiated immediately. A patent airway should be maintained and specific therapy instituted based upon signs and symptoms. If indicated, parenteral cholinergic agents such as bethanechol chloride USP should be administered to counteract the effects of the belladonna alkaloids.

DOSAGE AND ADMINISTRATION

Usual Dosage: (usually given one-half hour before meals and at bedtime):

ADULTS
Tablets: One to two tablets four times daily.

Elixir: One to two teaspoonfuls four times daily.

CHILDREN
Elixir: Six years or older: One-half teaspoonful four times daily.

Less than six years of age: One-quarter to one-half teaspoonful four times daily (according to age and weight).

Tablets and Elixir: - Store at controlled room temperature, 15°-30°C (59°-86°F).
Dispense in a tight, light-resistant container.
Keep bottle tightly closed.

HOW SUPPLIED

ELIXIR:

BRAND/MANUFACTURER	NDC	SIZE	AWP
○ BRAND			
BUTIBEL: Wallace	00037-0044-16	480 ml	$65.81

TABLETS:

BRAND/MANUFACTURER	NDC	SIZE	AWP
○ BRAND			
BUTIBEL: Wallace	00037-0046-60	100s	$39.59

Belladonna Alkaloids and Opium

DESCRIPTION

Each suppository contains:

B & O No. 15A
Powdered Opium* 30mg
Powdered Belladonna Extract 16.2mg
B & O No. 16A
Powdered Opium* 60mg
Powdered Belladonna Extract 16.2mg
* *Warning - may be habit forming*

This drug falls into the pharmacologic/therapeutic class of narcotic analgesic/antispasmotic agents.

The pharmacologically active principles present in Belladonna Alkaloids extract component are atropine and scopolamine.

Opium contains more than a score of Alkaloids, the principal ones being morphine (10%), narcotine (6%), papaverine (1%) and codeine (0.5%).

CLINICAL PHARMACOLOGY

Through its parasympatholytic action, atropine relaxes smooth muscle resulting from parasympathetic stimulation. It is the dl isomer of l-hyoscyamine and therefore exhibits the same clinical effects. It is, however, approximately one-half as active peripherally as l-hyoscyamine, the latter being the major active plant alkaloid. The dl isomer atropine is formed during the process of isolation of the Belladonna extract.[1]

Morphine, the major active principle of powdered Opium, is responsible for the action of powdered Opium although the other alkaloids present also contribute to it. The sedative and analgesic action of morphine, the effect desired by inclusion of powdered Opium, are thought to be due to its depressant effect on the cerebral cortex, hypothalamus and medullary centers. In large doses, the opiates and their analogs also inhibit synaptic conduction in the spinothalamic tracts, depress the function of the reticular formation, the lemniscus and the thalamic relays, and inhibit spinal synaptic reflexes; but these inhibitor actions are not elicited with therapeutic doses of the drug. Moderate doses of powdered Opium should not alter the electroencephalogram.

The action of morphine consists mainly of a descending depression of the central nervous system. It exerts its analgesic action by increasing the pain threshold or the magnitude of stimulus required to evoke pain and by dulling the sensibility or reaction to pain. In addition to its action in abolishing pain, morphine induces a sense of well-being (euphoria) facilitating certain mental processes while retarding others. Upon absorption of morphine, oxidative dealkylation to produce nor-compounds appears to be the first step in the reaction sequence which imparts analgesia. Morphine is conjugated in the liver to form the 3-glucuronide which passes into the bile and is reabsorbed and excreted in the urine. The atropine effect of the belladonna extract serves to eliminate morphine induced smooth muscle spasm without affecting the sedative analgesic action of powdered Opium.[2]

INDICATIONS AND USAGE

Belladonna Alkaloids and Opium Suppositories are used for relief of moderate to severe pain associated with ureteral spasm not responsive to non-narcotic analgesics and to space intervals between injections of opiates.

CONTRAINDICATIONS

Do not use Belladonna Alkaloids and Opium Suppositories in patients suffering from glaucoma, severe hepatic or renal disease, bronchial asthma, narcotic idiosyncrasies, respiratory depression, convulsive disorders, acute alcoholism, delirium tremens and premature labor.

WARNINGS

True addiction may result from Opium usage. These preparations are not recommended for use in children.

PRECAUTIONS

Administer with caution to persons with a known idiosyncrasy to atropine or atropine-like compounds; to persons known to be sensitive to or addicted to morphine or morphine-like drugs; to persons with cardiac disease, incipient glaucoma or prostatic hypertrophy. Caution should be used in the administration of this drug to old and debilitated patients and patients with increased intracranial pressure, toxic psychosis and myxedema.

Pregnancy Category C: Animal studies have not been conducted with Belladonna Alkaloids and Opium Suppositories. It is also not known whether Belladonna Alkaloids and Opium Suppositories can affect reproduction capacity. The active principles of Belladonna Alkaloids and Opium Suppositories, atropine and morphine, are known to enter the fetal circulation. Regular use of Opium Alkaloids during pregnancy has resulted in addiction of the fetus leading to withdrawal symptoms in the neonate. Belladonna Alkaloids and Opium Suppositories therefore should be used by a pregnant woman with caution and only when clearly indicated.

Nursing Mothers: It is not known whether this drug is excreted in human milk. Because many drugs are excreted in human milk, caution should be exercised when Belladonna Alkaloids and Opium Suppositories are administered to a nursing woman.

ADVERSE REACTIONS

Belladonna may cause drowsiness, dry mouth, urinary retention, photophobia, rapid pulse, dizziness and blurred vision. Opium usage may result in constipation, nausea or vomiting. Pruritis and urticaria may occasionally occur.

DRUG ABUSE AND DEPENDENCE

Because of their content of opium, Belladonna Alkaloids and Opium Suppositories are considered as Schedule II drugs by the Drug Enforcement Administration. No data exists on chronic abuse effects or dependence characteristics of Belladonna Alkaloids and Opium Suppositories.

OVERDOSAGE

As with morphine and related narcotics, overdosage is characterized by respiratory depression, pinpoint pupils and coma. Respiratory depression may be reversed by intravenous administration of naloxone hydrochloride. In addition, supportive measures such as oxygenation, intravenous fluids and vasopressors should be used as indicated. As with atropine derivatives, hot, dry, flushed skin; dry mouth and hyperpyrexia may occur.

► SHOWN IN PRODUCT IDENTIFICATION GUIDE

DOSAGE AND ADMINISTRATION

Adults: One Belladonna Alkaloids and Opium Suppository rectally once or twice daily, not to exceed four doses daily or as recommended by the physician. Moisten finger and Suppository with water before inserting. Not recommended for use in children 12 and under. Absorption is dependent on body hydration and not on body temperature. Store at room temperature. DO NOT refrigerate.

REFERENCES

1. Gilman, A. G., Goodman, L.S. & Gilman, A. 6th Edition, *The Pharmacological Basis of Therapeutics*, MacMillan Pub. Co., N.Y. 1980, pp. 121-127. 2. Ibid, pp. 494-513.

HOW SUPPLIED
SUPPOSITORY (C-II): 15 MG-60 MG

BRAND/MANUFACTURER	NDC	SIZE	AWP
○ GENERICS			
Wyeth-Ayerst	00008-0330-01	20s	$43.91

SUPPOSITORY (C-II): 16.2 MG-30 MG

BRAND/MANUFACTURER	NDC	SIZE	AWP
○ BRAND			
B. & O. SUPPRETTES 15-A: Polymedica	00998-5015-75	12s	$29.88

SUPPOSITORY (C-II): 16.2 MG-60 MG

BRAND/MANUFACTURER	NDC	SIZE	AWP
○ BRAND			
B. & O. SUPPRETTES 16-A: Polymedica	00998-5016-75	12s	$34.00
○ GENERICS			
	00574-7040-12	12s ud	$16.50
	00574-7040-20	20s ud	$27.50

Belladonna Alkaloids/ Chlorpheniramine Maleate/ Phenylephrine Hydrochloride/ Phenylpropanolamine Hydrochloride

DESCRIPTION

Each prolonged action tablet contains:

Chlorpheniramine Maleate (CPM) ....8 mg
Phenylephrine Hydrochloride ....25 mg
Phenylpropanolamine Hydrochloride (PPA) ....50 mg
Hyoscyamine Sulfate ....0.19 mg
Atropine Sulfate ....0.04 mg
Scopolamine Hydrobromide ....0.01 mg

This product acts continuously for 10 to 12 hours. It is an oral antihistaminic, nasal decongestant and anti-secretory preparation.

INDICATIONS AND USAGE

These tablets provide relief of the symptoms resulting from irritation of sinus, nasal and upper respiratory tract tissues. Phenylephrine and phenylpropanolamine combine to exert a vasconstructive and decongestive action while chlorpheramine maleate decreases the symptoms of watering eyes, post nasal drip and sneezing which may be associated with an allergic-like response. The belladonna alkaloids, hyoscyamine, atropine and scopolamine further augment the anti-secretory activity of the tablets.

CONTRAINDICATIONS

Hypersensitivity to antihistamines or sympathomimetics.

This product is contraindicated in children under 12 years of age and in patients with glaucoma, bronchial asthma and women who are pregnant. Concomitant use of MAO inhibitors is contraindicated.

WARNINGS

These tablets may cause drowsiness. Patients should be warned of possible additive effects caused by taking antihistamines with alcohol, hypnotics or tranquilizers.

PRECAUTIONS

These tablets contain Belladonna Alkaloids, and must be administered with care to those patients with urinary bladder neck obstruction. Caution should be exercised when the tablets are given to patients with hypertension, cardiac or peripheral vascular disease or hyperthyroidism. Patients should avoid driving a motor vehicle or operating dangerous machinery. (See *"Warnings."*)

ADVERSE REACTIONS

Hypersensitivity reactions such as rash, urticaria, leukopenia, agranulocytosis, and thrombocytopenia may occur. Large overdoses may cause tachypnea, delirium, fever, stupor, coma and respiratory failure.

Gastrointestinal: nausea, vomiting, diarrhea, constipation, epigastric distress.

Genitourinary System: urinary frequency and dysuria.

Cardiovascular: tightness of the chest, palpitation, tachycardia, hypotension/hypertension.

Central Nervous System: drowsiness, giddiness, faintness, dizziness, headache, incoordination, mydriasis, hyperirritability, nervousness, and insomnia.

Metabolic/Endocrine: lassitude, anorexia.

Miscellaneous: dryness of mucous membranes, xerostomia.

Respiratory: thickening of bronchial secretions.

Special Senses: tinnitus, visual disturbances, blurred vision.

OVERDOSAGE

Since the action of sustained release products may continue for as long as 12 hours, treatment of overdoses directed at reversing the effects of the drug and supporting the patient should be maintained for at least that length of time. In children and infants, antihistamine overdosage may produce convulsions and death.

DOSAGE AND ADMINISTRATION

Adults and children 12 years of age and older, one tablet every 12 hours, morning and evening, not to exceed 2 tablets in 24 hours. Not recommended for children under 12 years of age. Tablets are to be swallowed whole.

Store at controlled room temperature 15°-30°C (59°-86°F). Dispense in tight, light-resistant containers.

HOW SUPPLIED
TABLET, EXTENDED RELEASE:

BRAND/MANUFACTURER	NDC	SIZE	AWP
○ GENERICS			
ROLATUSS SR: Major	00904-1198-60	100s	$11.95
DECONHIST: Goldline	00182-1317-01	100s	$12.15
Q-TUSS: Qualitest	00603-5549-21	100s	$15.40
TUSS DELAY: Norton,HN	50732-0609-01	100s	$17.28
PRO-TUSS: Econolab	55053-0073-01	100s	$19.80
RU-TAB: Moore,H.L.	00839-7440-06	100s	$20.79
PHENCHLOR S.H.A.: Rugby	00536-4410-01	100s	$23.76
STAHIST: Huckaby	58407-0370-01	100s	$25.24
PHENAHIST-TR: Williams,T.E.	51189-0084-01	100s	$28.95
PANNAZ: Pan Amer	00525-0777-01	100s	$34.80
RU-TUSS: Boots Pharm	00048-0058-01	100s	$54.80
ATROHIST PLUS: Adams	53014-0024-10	100s	$68.86
PRO-TUSS: URL	00677-1418-01	300s	$13.00
ROLATUSS SR: Major	00904-1198-40	500s	$53.95
TUSS DELAY: Norton,HN	50732-0609-05	500s	$79.19
PHENCHLOR S.H.A.: Rugby	00536-4410-05	500s	$90.92
RU-TUSS: Boots Pharm	00048-0058-05	500s	$254.70
ROLATUSS SR: Major	00904-1198-80	1000s	$100.45
TUSS DELAY: Norton,HN	50732-0609-10	1000s	$150.23
PRO-TUSS: Econolab	55053-0073-10	1000s	$188.00

Belladonna Alkaloids/Ergotamine Tartrate/Phenobarbital

DESCRIPTION

Each Belladonna Alkaloids/Ergotamine Tartrate/Phenobarbital tablet contains: Phenobarbital, USP, (Warning: may be habit forming), 40 mg; Ergotamine Tartrate, USP, 0.6 mg; Bellafoline® (levorotatory alkaloids of Belladonna) 0.2 mg.

CLINICAL PHARMACOLOGY

Based on the concept that functional disorders frequently involve hyperactivity of both the sympathetic and parasympathetic nervous systems, the ingredients in Belladonna Alkaloids/Ergotamine Tartrate/Phenobarbital (Belladonna/Ergotamine/Phenobarbital) are combined to provide a balanced preparation designed to correct imbalance of the autonomic nervous system. The intergrated action of Belladonna/Ergotamine/Phenobarbital is effected through the combined administration of Ergotamine and the levorotatory alkaloids of Belladonna, specific inhibitors of the sympathetic and parasympathetic respectively, reinforced by the synergistic action of Phenobarbital in dampening the cortical centers. It should be noted that on a weight basis the levorotatory alkaloids of Belladonna have approximately twice the pharmacological effects as do the usual racemic mixtures.

INDICATIONS AND USAGE

Belladonna/Ergotamine/Phenobarbital is employed in the management of disorders characterized by nervous tension and exaggerated autonomic response: *Menopausal disorders* with hot flushes, sweats, restlessness and insomnia; *cardiovascular disorders* with palpitation, tachycardia, chest oppression and vasomotor disturbances; *gastrointestinal disorders* with hypermotility, hypersecretion, "nervous stomach," and alternately diarrhea and constipation; interval treatment of *recurrent, throbbing headache.*

CONTRAINDICATIONS

Peripheral vascular disease, coronary heart disease, hypertension, impaired hepatic or renal function, sepsis, pregnancy, nursing mothers and glaucoma. The

---

◆ RATED THERAPEUTICALLY EQUIVALENT; ◇ THERAPEUTIC EQUIVALENCE UNCONFIRMED; ○ UNRATED

concomitant administration of Ergotamine and dopamine should be avoided, due to the increased potential for ischemic vasoconstriction. Phenobarbital is contraindicated in patients with a history of manifest or latent porphyria. Phenobarbital is contraindicated in those patients in whom the drug produces restlessness and/or excitement. Belladonna/Ergotamine/Phenobarbital is contraindicated in patients with a demonstrated hypersensitivity to any of the components.

WARNINGS
Total weekly dosage of Ergotamine Tartrate should not exceed 10 mg. (This dosage corresponds to 16 Belladonna/Ergotamine/Phenobarbital tablets.) Due to the presence of a barbiturate, may be habit forming.

PRECAUTIONS
Even though the Ergotamine Tartrate content of this product is low and untoward effects have been rare and of minor significance, caution should be exercised if large or prolonged dosage is contemplated, and physicians should be alert to possible peripheral vascular complications in patients sensitive to ergot. Due to the presence of the anticholinergic agent, special caution should be exercised in the use of this drug in patients with bronchial asthma or obstructive uropathy.

Belladonna/Ergotamine/Phenobarbital contains FD&C Yellow #5 (tartrazine) which may cause allergic-type reactions (including bronchial asthma) in certain susceptible individuals. Although the overall incidence of FD&C Yellow #5 (tartrazine) sensitivity in the general population is low, it is frequently seen in patients who also have aspirin hypersensitivity.

INFORMATION FOR PATIENTS
Patients on large or prolonged dosage should be asked to report numbness or tingling of extremities, claudication or other symptoms of peripheral vasoconstriction.

DRUG INTERACTION
Oral Anticoagulants: Phenobarbital may lower the plasma levels of dicumarol (name previously used: bishydroxycoumarin) and may cause a decrease in anticoagulant activity as measured by the prothrombin time. More frequent monitoring of prothrombin time responses is indicated whenever Phenobarbital is initiated or discontinued, and the dosage of anticoagulants should be adjusted accordingly.

CNS Depressants: Combined administration of Phenobarbital and CNS depressants such as alcohol, tricyclic antidepressants, phenothiazines and narcotic analgesics may result in a potentiation of the depressant action.

Beta Adrenergic Blocking Agents: Although proof is lacking, several reports in the literature suggest a possible interaction between ergot alkaloids and beta adrenergic blocking agents. This interaction may result in excessive vasoconstriction. Although many patients can apparently take propranolol and ergot alkaloids without ill effects, there is enough evidence of an interaction to dictate closer surveillance of patients so treated.

Hepatic Metabolism: Through the mechanism of enzyme induction caused by Phenobarbital, a number of substances have been shown to be metabolized at an increased rate. In these cases, clinical responses should be closely monitored and appropriate dosage adjustments made. Included are such substances as griseofulvin, quinidine, doxycycline and estrogen. Although the meaning of published reports regarding the effects of Phenobarbital on estrogen metabolism are unclear at this time, if avoidance of pregnancy is critical, consideration should be given to alternative methods of contraception.

Phenytoin, Sodium Valproate, Valproic Acid: The effect of barbiturates on the metabolism of phenytoin appears to be variable. Some investigators report an accelerating effect, while others report no effect. Because the effect of barbiturates on the metabolism of phenytoin is not predictable, phenytoin and barbiturate blood levels should be monitored more frequently if these drugs are given concurrently. Sodium valproate and valproic acid appear to decrease barbiturate metabolism; therefore, barbiturate blood levels should be monitored and appropriate dosage adjustments made as indicated.

Tricyclic Antidepressants: Due to the presence of levorotatory alkaloids of Belladonna, concomitant administration of tricyclic antidepressants may result in additive anticholinergic effects.

CARCINOGENESIS
No data are available on the long-term potential for carcinogenicity in animals or humans.

PREGNANCY
Pregnancy Category X—due to the potential uterotonic effects of the ergot alkaloids, the use of Belladonna/Ergotamine/Phenobarbitol during pregnancy is contraindicated. See *"Contraindications"* section.

NURSING MOTHERS
A number of ergot alkaloids inhibit the secretion of prolactin. Therefore, Belladonna/Ergotamine/Phenobarbital is contraindicated in nursing mothers. See *"Contraindications"* section.

PEDIATRIC USE
Safety and effectiveness in children have not been established.

ADVERSE REACTIONS
Tingling and other paresthesias of the extremities, blurred vision, palpitations, dry mouth, decreased sweating, decreased gastrointestinal motility, urinary retention, tachycardia, flushing, and drowsiness occur rarely.

DRUG ABUSE AND DEPENDENCE
Barbiturates may be habit-forming. Tolerance, psychological dependence, and physical dependence may occur especially following prolonged use of high doses. Daily administration in excess of 400 mg of Pentobarbital or secobarbital for approximately 90 days is likely to produce some degree of physical dependence. By way of comparison, the Phenobarbital component of Belladonna/Ergotamine/Phenobarbital at the highest recommended daily dosage amounts to 80 mg.

OVERDOSAGE
Management of Overdosage: While severe symptoms of overdosage with Belladonna/Ergotamine/Phenobarbital have not been reported, theoretically they could occur. It is imperative to note that overdosage symptoms with Belladonna/Ergotamine/Phenobarbital may be attributable to any one or more of the three active ingredients. Which toxic manifestation might predominate in any individual case would be impossible to predict but one should be alert to the various possibilities. When anticholinergic/antispasmodic drugs are taken in sufficient overdose to produce such severe symptoms, prompt treatment should be instituted. Gastric lavage and other measures to limit intestinal absorption should be initiated without delay.

Cholinesterase inhibitors administered parenterally may be necessary for treatment of the serious manifestations of anticholinergic overdosage. Additionally, symptomatic therapy, including oxygen, sedatives and control of hyperthermia may be necessary.

Acute barbiturate overdosage symptoms with Belladonna/Ergotamine/Phenobarbital, while possible, have not been reported. While the usual procedures for handling barbiturate poisoning should be employed, keep in mind the possibility of anticholinergic overdosing effects.

Acute ergot overdosage symptoms with Belladonna/Ergotamine/Phenobarbital, while possible, have not been reported. The usual procedures for handling ergot overdosage include the administration of a peripheral vasodilator to counteract the vasopasm.

DOSAGE AND ADMINISTRATION
One tablet in the morning and one tablet in the evening.

HOW SUPPLIED
TABLET, EXTENDED RELEASE:

BRAND/MANUFACTURER	NDC	SIZE	AWP
GENERICS			
BEL-PHEN-ERGOT: Goldline	00182-1990-01	100s	$45.45

TABLETS:

BRAND/MANUFACTURER	NDC	SIZE	AWP
GENERICS			
BELLAMOR: Moore,H.L.	00839-7370-06	100s	$31.85
BELLAMINE: Major	00904-2548-60	100s	$37.45
SPASTRIN: Horizon Prod	54580-0124-01	100s	$37.95
Geneva	00781-1701-01	100s	$37.98
SPASTRIN: Econolab	55053-0124-01	100s	$41.75
BEL-TABS: URL	00677-1171-01	100s	$45.40
BEL-PHEN-ERGOT: Goldline	00182-1847-01	100s	$45.45
PHENERBEL-S: Rugby	00536-4234-01	100s	$53.62
BELLASPAS: Qualitest	00603-2424-21	100s	$56.31
BELLAPHEN-S: Pecos	59879-0121-01	100s	$70.00

Belladonna and Phenobarbital

DESCRIPTION
Each Belladonna/Phenobarbital tablet, capsule or 5 mL (teaspoonful) of elixir contains:

Phenobarbital (¼ gr) ....16.2 mg (Warning: May be habit forming)
Hyoscyamine Sulfate ....0.1037 mg
Atropine Sulfate ....0.0194 mg
Scopolamine Hydrobromide ....0.0065 mg

Each Belladonna/Phenobarbital extended-release tablet contains:
Phenobarbital (¾ gr) ....48.6 mg (Warning: May be habit forming)
Hyoscyamine Sulfate ....0.3111 mg
Atropine Sulfate ....0.0582 mg
Scopolamine Hydrobromide ....0.0195 mg

Each extended-release tablet contains the equivalent of three regular tablets. Extended-release tablets are designed to release the ingredients gradually to provide effects for up to twelve (12) hours.

ACTIONS
This drug combination provides natural Belladonna alkaloids in a specific, fixed ratio combined with Phenobarbital to provide peripheral anticholinergic/antispasmodic action and mild sedation.

➤ SHOWN IN PRODUCT IDENTIFICATION GUIDE

INDICATIONS

> BASED ON A REVIEW OF THIS DRUG BY THE NATIONAL ACADEMY OF SCIENCES—NATIONAL RESEARCH COUNCIL AND/OR OTHER INFORMATION, FDA HAS CLASSIFIED THE FOLLOWING INDICATIONS AS "POSSIBLY" EFFECTIVE:
>
> FOR USE AS ADJUNCTIVE THERAPY IN THE TREATMENT OF IRRITABLE BOWEL SYNDROME (IRRITABLE COLON, SPASTIC COLON, MUCOUS COLITIS) AND ACUTE ENTEROCOLITIS.
>
> MAY ALSO BE USEFUL AS ADJUNCTIVE THERAPY IN THE TREATMENT OF DUODENAL ULCER. IT HAS NOT BEEN SHOWN CONCLUSIVELY WHETHER ANTICHOLINERGIC/ANTISPASMODIC DRUGS AID IN THE HEALING OF A DUODENAL ULCER, DECREASE THE RATE OF RECURRENCES OR PREVENT COMPLICATIONS.

CONTRAINDICATIONS

Glaucoma, obstructive uropathy (for example, bladder neck obstruction due to prostatic hypertrophy); obstructive disease of the gastrointestinal tract (as in achalasia, pyloroduodenal stenosis, etc.); paralytic ileus, intestinal atony of the elderly or debilitated patient; unstable cardiovascular status in acute hemorrhage; severe ulcerative colitis especially if complicated by toxic megacolon; myasthenia gravis; hiatal hernia associated with reflux esophagitis.

Belladonna/Phenobarbital is contraindicated in patients with known hypersensitivity to any of the ingredients. Phenobarbital is contraindicated in acute intermittent porphyria and in those patients in whom Phenobarbital produces restlessness and/or excitement.

WARNINGS

In the presence of a high environmental temperature, heat prostration can occur with Belladonna alkaloids (fever and heatstroke due to decreased sweating).

Diarrhea may be an early symptom of incomplete intestinal obstruction, especially in patients with ileostomy or colostomy. In this instance treatment with this drug would be inappropriate and possibly harmful.

Belladonna/Phenobarbital may produce drowsiness or blurred vision. The patient should be warned, should these occur, not to engage in activities requiring mental alertness, such as operating a motor vehicle or other machinery, and not to perform hazardous work.

Phenobarbital may decrease the effect of anticoagulants, and necessitate larger doses of the anticoagulant for optimal effect. When the Phenobarbital is discontinued, the dose of the anticoagulant may have to be decreased.

Phenobarbital may be habit forming and should not be administered to individuals known to be addiction prone or to those with a history of physical and/or psychological dependence upon drugs.

Since barbiturates are metabolized in the liver, they should be used with caution and initial doses should be small in patients with hepatic dysfunction.

PRECAUTIONS

Use with caution in patients with: autonomic neuropathy, hepatic or renal disease, hyperthyroidism, coronary heart disease, congestive heart failure, cardiac arrhythmias, tachycardia, and hypertension.

Belladonna alkaloids may produce a delay in gastric emptying (antral stasis) which would complicate the management of gastric ulcer.

Theoretically, with overdosage, a curare-like action may occur.

Carcinogenesis, Mutagenesis. Long-term studies in animals have not been performed to evaluate carcinogenic potential.

Pregnancy Category C: Animal reproduction studies have not been conducted with Belladonna/Phenobarbital. It is not known whether Belladonna/Phenobarbital can cause fetal harm when administered to a pregnant woman or can affect reproduction capacity. Belladonna/Phenobarbital should be given to a pregnant woman only if clearly needed.

Nursing Mothers: It is not known whether this drug is excreted in human milk. Because many drugs are excreted in human milk, caution should be exercised when Belladonna/Phenobarbital is administered to a nursing mother.

ADVERSE REACTIONS

Adverse reactions may include xerostomia; urinary hesitancy and retention; blurred vision; tachycardia; palpitation; mydriasis; cycloplegia; increased ocular tension; loss of taste sense; headache; nervousness; drowsiness; weakness; dizziness; insomnia; nausea; vomiting; impotence; suppression of lactation; constipation; bloated feeling; musculoskeletal pain; severe allergic reaction or drug idiosyncrasies, including anaphylaxis, urticaria and other dermal manifestations; and decreased sweating. Elderly patients may react with symptoms of excitement, agitation, drowsiness, and other untoward manifestations to even small doses of the drug.

Phenobarbital may produce excitement in some patients, rather than a sedative effect. In patients habituated to barbiturates, abrupt withdrawal may produce delirium or convulsions.

OVERDOSAGE

The signs and symptoms of overdose are headache, nausea, vomiting, blurred vision, dilated pupils, hot and dry skin, dizziness, dryness of the mouth, difficulty in swallowing, CNS stimulation. Treatment should consist of gastric lavage, emetics, and activated charcoal. If indicated, parenteral cholinergic agents such as physostigmine or bethanechol chloride should be added.

DOSAGE AND ADMINISTRATION

The dosage of Belladonna/Phenobarbital should be adjusted to the needs of the individual patient to assure symptomatic control with a minimum of adverse effects.

Belladonna/Phenobarbital Tablets or Capsules: Adults: One or two Belladonna/Phenobarbital tablets or capsules three of four times a day according to condition and severity of symptoms.

Belladonna and Phenobarbital extended-release tablets: One tablet every 12 hours. If indicated, one tablet every 8 hours may be given.

Elixir: Adults: One or two teaspoonfuls of elixir three or four times a day according to conditions and severity of symptoms.

Children (Elixir)—may be dosed every 4 or 6 hours:

	Starting Dosage	
Body Weight	q4h	q6h
10 lb (4.5 kg)	0.5 mL	0.75 mL
20 lb (9.1 kg)	1.0 mL	1.5 mL
30 lb (13.6 kg)	1.5 ml	2.0 mL
50 lb (22.7 kg)	½ tsp	¾ tsp
75 lb (34.0 kg)	¾	1 tsp
100 lb (45.4 kg)	1 tsp	1 ½ tsp

Store at controlled room temperature, between 15°C and 30°C (59°F and 86°F). Dispense in tight, light-resistant container.

HOW SUPPLIED
CAPSULE:

BRAND/MANUFACTURER	NDC	SIZE	AWP
○ BRAND			
▶ DONNATAL: Robins Pharm	00031-4207-63	100s	$13.74

CHEW TABLET:

BRAND/MANUFACTURER	NDC	SIZE	AWP
○ BRAND			
KINESED: Stuart	00038-0220-10	100s	$16.32

ELIXIR:

AVERAGE UNIT PRICE (AVAILABLE SIZES)	
GENERIC	$0.01

BRAND/MANUFACTURER	NDC	SIZE	AWP
◆ GENERICS			
Cenci,H.R.	00556-0053-04	120 ml	$2.50
Cenci,H.R.	00556-0053-16	480 ml	$4.50
Cenci,H.R.	00556-0053-28	3840 ml	$23.00

ELIXIR:

BRAND/MANUFACTURER	NDC	SIZE	AWP
○ BRAND			
DONNATAL: Robins Pharm	00031-4221-12	120 ml	$5.74
	00031-4221-25	480 ml	$20.33
	00031-4221-29	3840 ml	$143.65
	00031-4221-13	5 ml 100s ud	$91.29
○ GENERICS			
Allscrips	54569-3251-00	120 ml	$0.97
Moore,H.L.	00839-5018-65	120 ml	$2.01
Veratex	17022-1446-03	120 ml	$2.25
Pennex	00426-8009-04	120 ml	$3.36
Pennex	00832-8009-04	120 ml	$3.40
Cheshire	55175-1672-00	120 ml	$5.10
Southwood	58016-0700-24	120 ml	$5.17
SPACOL: Dayton	52041-0043-33	120 ml	$6.50
Southwood	58016-0700-40	200 ml	$8.60
Moore,H.L.	00839-5018-69	480 ml	$4.31
Qualitest	00603-1030-58	480 ml	$4.55
DONNAPINE: Major	00904-0981-16	480 ml	$4.80
Pennex	00832-8009-16	480 ml	$4.90
Moore,H.L.	00839-7850-69	480 ml	$6.21
Halsey Pharm	00879-0059-16	480 ml	$6.70
Aligen	00405-2350-16	480 ml	$7.78
HYOSOPHEN: Rugby	00536-0100-85	480 ml	$9.57
Goldline	00182-0686-40	480 ml	$9.60
Pennex	00426-8009-16	480 ml	$9.90
R.I.D.	54807-0125-16	480 ml	$16.62
Veratex	17022-1446-09	3840 ml	$15.95
Moore,H.L.	00839-5018-70	3840 ml	$17.54
DONNAPINE: Major	00904-0981-28	3840 ml	$22.45
DONNAPINE: Major	00904-1981-28	3840 ml	$22.45
SPASTEMMS: Truxton	00463-9023-28	3840 ml	$24.00
Pennex	00832-8009-28	3840 ml	$24.00
Moore,H.L.	00839-7850-70	3840 ml	$42.24
Halsey Pharm	00879-0059-28	3840 ml	$44.75
Goldline	00182-0686-41	3840 ml	$61.65
Pennex	00426-8009-28	3840 ml	$67.70
HYOSOPHEN: Rugby	00536-0100-90	3840 ml	$68.91
UDL	51079-0318-10	5 ml 50s ud	$15.60

◆ RATED THERAPEUTICALLY EQUIVALENT; ◇ THERAPEUTIC EQUIVALENCE UNCONFIRMED; ○ UNRATED

TABLET, EXTENDED RELEASE:

BRAND/MANUFACTURER	NDC	SIZE	AWP
○ **BRAND**			
▶ DONNATAL EXTENTABS: Robins Pharm	00031-4235-63	100s	$39.25
	00031-4235-70	500s	$181.7

TABLETS:

BRAND/MANUFACTURER	NDC	SIZE	AWP
○ **BRAND**			
▶ DONNATAL: Robins Pharm	00031-4250-63	100s	$12.33
DONNATAL NO. 2: Robins Pharm	00031-4264-63	100s	$15.01
CHARDONNA-2: Schwarz	00091-0202-01	100s	$17.61
▶ DONNATAL: Robins Pharm	00031-4250-64	100s ud	$13.60
	00031-4250-74	1000s	$110.08
○ **GENERICS**			
Allscrips	54569-0427-06	6s	$0.08
Allscrips	54569-0427-00	10s	$0.13
Cheshire	55175-0229-01	12s	$3.00
Allscrips	54569-0427-05	15s	$0.19
Allscrips	54569-0427-04	20s	$0.25
Pharm Corp/America	51655-0119-52	20s	$1.70
Cheshire	55175-0229-02	20s	$3.00
Southwood	58016-0709-20	20s	$4.15
Allscrips	54569-0427-01	30s	$0.38
Phys Total Care	54868-0031-04	30s	$1.39
Cheshire	55175-0229-03	30s	$3.50
Southwood	58016-0709-30	30s	$4.29
Allscrips	54569-0427-09	40s	$0.51
Southwood	58016-0709-40	40s	$4.58
Southwood	58016-0709-42	42s	$4.62
Allscrips	54569-0427-07	50s	$0.63
Southwood	58016-0709-50	50s	$4.86
Allscrips	54569-0427-02	60s	$0.76
Allscrips	54569-0427-08	100s	$1.26
SPASMOLIN: Richlyn	00115-4652-01	100s	$1.29
DONNAPINE: Major	00904-3741-60	100s	$1.90
Southwood	58016-0709-00	100s	$5.83
BELLATAL: Richwood	58521-0162-01	100s	$8.25
ANTISPAS: R.I.D.	54807-0126-01	100s	$11.91
BARBIDONNA: Wallace	00037-0301-92	100s	$44.58
BARBIDONNA: Wallace	00037-0311-92	100s	$49.98
DONNAPINE: Major	00904-3741-61	100s ud	$5.83
BELLATAL: Richwood	58521-0162-05	500s	$16.40
BARBIDONNA: Wallace	00037-0301-96	500s	$207.37
Veratex	17022-0679-06	1000s	$5.95
SEDAPAR: Parmed	00349-2355-10	1000s	$9.60
SPASMOLIN: Richlyn	00115-4652-03	1000s	$9.90
SPASTEMMS: Truxton	00463-6181-10	1000s	$9.90
HAPONAL: URL	00677-0074-10	1000s	$14.28
Major	00904-3741-80	1000s	$17.25
Moore, H.L.	00839-5055-16	1000s	$17.54
HYOSOPHEN: Rugby	00536-3920-10	1000s	$17.99
Goldline	00182-1048-10	1000s	$18.00
HYPERSED: EconoMed	38130-0048-10	1000s	$29.80
Rexar	00478-5477-10	1000s	$31.00
HYONATAL: Jones-Western	52604-6790-08	1008s	$19.44
HYOSOPHEN: Rugby	00536-3920-50	5000s	$57.50
Moore, H.L.	00839-5055-20	5000s	$82.89
Rexar	00478-5477-50	5000s	$148.33

Bellergal-S SEE BELLADONNA ALKALOIDS/ERGOTAMINE TARTRATE/PHENOBARBITAL

Benadryl SEE DIPHENHYDRAMINE HYDROCHLORIDE

Benazepril Hydrochloride

USE IN PREGNANCY

WHEN USED IN PREGNANCY DURING THE SECOND AND THIRD TRIMESTERS, ACE INHIBITORS CAN CAUSE INJURY AND EVEN DEATH TO THE DEVELOPING FETUS. WHEN PREGNANCY IS DETECTED, BENAZEPRIL HYDROCHLORIDE SHOULD BE DISCONTINUED AS SOON AS POSSIBLE. SEE "WARNINGS, FETAL/NEONATAL MORBIDITY AND MORTALITY."

DESCRIPTION

Benazepril Hydrochloride is a white to off-white crystalline powder, soluble (> 100 mg/mL) in water, in ethanol, and in methanol. Benzepril's chemical name is 3-[[1-(ethoxy-carbonyl)-3-phenyl-(1S)-propyl]amino]-2,3,4,5-tetrahydro-2-oxo-1H-1-(3S)-benzazepine-1-acetic acid monohydrochloride. Its empirical formula is $C_{24}H_{28}N_2O_5 \cdot HCl$, and its molecular weight is 460.96.

Benazeprilat, the active metabolite of Benazepril, is a non-sulfhydryl angiotensin-converting enzyme inhibitor. Benazepril is converted to benazeprilat by hepatic cleavage of the ester group.

Benazepril Hydrochloride is supplied as tablets containing 5 mg, 10 mg, 20 mg, and 40 mg of Benazepril for oral administration.

Following is its chemical structure:

CLINICAL PHARMACOLOGY

MECHANISM OF ACTION

Benazepril and benazeprilat inhibit angiotensin-converting enzyme (ACE) in human subjects and animals. ACE is a peptidyl dipeptidase that catalyzes the conversion of angiotensin 1 to the vasoconstrictor substance, angiotensin II. Angiotensin II also stimulates aldosterone secretion by the adrenal cortex.

Inhibition of ACE results in a decreased plasma angiotensin II, which leads to decreased vasopressor activity and to decreased aldosterone secretion. The latter decrease may result in a small increase in serum potassium. Hypertensive patients treated with Benazepril Hydrochloride alone for up to 52 weeks had elevations of serum potassium of up to 0.2 mEq/L. Similar patients treated with Benazepril Hydrochloride and hydrochlorothiazide for up to 24 weeks had no consistent changes in their serum potassium (see "Precautions").

Removal of angiotensin II negative feedback on renin secretion leads to increased plasma renin activity. In animal studies, Benazepril had no inhibitory effect on the vasopressor response to angiotensin II and did not interfere with the hemodynamic effects of the autonomic neurotransmitters acetylcholine, epinephrine, and norepinephrine.

ACE is identical to kininase, an enzyme that degrades bradykinin. Whether increased levels of bradykinin, a potent vasodepressor peptide, play a role in the therapeutic effects of Benazepril Hydrochloride remains to be elucidated.

While the mechanism through which Benazepril lowers blood pressure is believed to be primarily suppression of the renin-angiotensin-aldosterone system, Benazepril has an antihypertensive effect even in patients with low-renin hypertension. In particular Benazepril Hydrochloride was antihypertensive in all races studied, although it was somewhat less effective in blacks than in nonblacks.

PHARMACOKINETICS AND METABOLISM

Following oral administration of Benazepril Hydrochloride, peak plasma concentrations of Benazepril are reached within 0.5-1.0 hours. The extent of absorption is at least 37% as determined by urinary recovery and is not significantly influenced by the presence of food in the GI tract.

Cleavage of the ester group (primarily in the liver) converts Benazepril to its active metabolite, benazeprilat. Peak plasma concentrations of Benazeprilat are reached 1-2 hours after drug intake in the fasting state and 2-4 hours after drug intake in the nonfasting state. The serum protein binding of Benazepril is about 96.7% and that of Benazeprilat about 95.3%, as measured by equilibrium dialysis; on the basis of in vitro studies, the degree of protein binding should be unaffected by age, hepatic dysfunction, or concentration (over the concentration range of 0.24-23.6 μmol/L).

Benazepril is almost completely metabolized to benazeprilat, which has much greater ACE inhibitory activity than Benazepril, and to the glucuronide conjugates of Benazepril and benazeprilat. Only trace amounts of an administered dose of Benazepril Hydrochloride can be recovered in the urine as unchanged Benazepril, while about 20% of the dose is excreted as Benazeprilat, 4% as Benazepril glucuronide, and 8% as benazeprilat glucuronide.

The kinetics of Benazepril are approximately dose-proportional within the dosage range of 10-80 mg.

The effective half-life of accumulation of benazeprilat following multiple dosing of Benazepril Hydrochloride is 10-11 hours. Thus, steady-state concentrations of benazeprilat should be reached after 2 or 3 doses of Benazepril Hydrochloride given once daily.

The kinetics did not change, and there was no significant accumulation during chronic administration (28 days) of once-daily doses between 5 mg and 20 mg. Accumulation ratios based on AUC and urinary recovery of Benazeprilat were 1.19 and 1.27, respectively.

When dialysis was started two hours after ingestion of 10 mg of Benazepril, approximately 6% of benazeprilat was removed in 4 hours of dialysis. The parent compound Benazepril, was not detected in the dialysate.

The disposition of Benazepril and benazeprilat in patients with mild-to-moderate renal insufficiency (creatinine clearance > 30 mL/min) is similar to that in patients with normal renal function. In patients with creatinine clearance ≤ 30 mL/min, peak benazeprilat levels and the initial (alpha phase) half-life increase, and time to steady-state may be delayed (see "Dosage and Administration").

Benazepril and benazeprilat are cleared predominantly by renal excretion in healthy subjects with normal renal function. Nonrenal (i.e., biliary) excretion accounts for approximately 11-12% of Benazeprilat excretion in healthy subjects. In patients with renal failure, biliary clearance may compensate to an extent for deficient renal clearance.

In patients with hepatic dysfunction due to cirrhosis, levels of Benazeprilat are essentially unaltered. The pharamcokinetics of Benazepril and benazeprilat do not appear to be influenced by age.

▶ SHOWN IN PRODUCT IDENTIFICATION GUIDE

In studies in rats given ¹⁴C-Benazepril, Benazepril and its metabolites crossed the blood-brain barrier only to an extremely low extent. Multiple doses of Benazepril did not result in accumulation in any tissue except the lung, where, as with other ACE inhibitors in similar studies, there was a slight increase in concentration due to slow elimination in that organ.

Some placental passage occurred when the drug was administered to pregnant rats.

PHARMACODYNAMICS

Single and multiple doses of 10 mg or more of Benazepril Hydrochloride cause inhibition of plasma ACE activity by at least 80-90% for at least 24 hours after dosing. Pressor responses to exogenous angiotensin I were inhibited by 60-90% (up to 4 hours postdose) at the 10 mg dose.

Administration of Benazepril Hydrochloride to patients with mild-to-moderate hypertension results in reduction of both supine and standing blood pressure to about the same extent with no compensatory tachycardia. Symptomatic postural hypotension is infrequent, although it can occur in patients who are salt- and/or volume-depleted (see *"Warnings"*).

In single-dose studies, Benazepril Hydrochloride lowered blood pressure within 1 hour, with peak reductions achieved 2-4 hours after dosing. The antihypertensive effect of a single dose persisted for 24 hours. In multiple dose studies, once-daily doses of 20-80 mg decreased seated pressure (systolic/diastolic) 24 hours after dosing by about 6-12/4-7 mmHg. The trough values represent reductions of about 50% of that seen at peak.

Four dose-response studies using once-daily dosing were conducted in 470 mild-to-moderate hypertensive patients not using diuretics. The minimal effective once-daily dose of Benazepril Hydrochloride was 10 mg; but further falls in blood pressure, especially at morning trough, were seen with higher doses in the studied dosing range (10-80 mg). In studies comparing the same daily dose of Benazepril Hydrochloride given as a single morning dose or as a twice-daily dose, blood pressure reductions at the time of morning trough blood levels were greater with the divided regimen.

During chronic therapy, the maximum reduction in blood pressure with any dose is generally achieved after 1-2 weeks. The antihypertensive effects of Benazepril Hydrochloride have continued during therapy for at least two years. Abrupt withdrawal of Benazepril Hydrochloride has not been associated with a rapid increase in blood pressure.

In patients with mild-to-moderate hypertension, Benazepril Hydrochloride 10-20 mg was similar in effectiveness to captopril, hydrochlorothiazide, nifedipine SR, and propranolol.

The antihypertensive effects of Benazepril Hydrochloride were not appreciably different in patients receiving high- or low-sodium diets.

In hemodynamic studies in dogs, blood pressure reduction was accompanied by a reduction in peripheral arterial resistance, with an increase in cardiac output and renal blood flow and little or no change in heart rate. In normal human volunteers, single doses of Benazepril caused an increase in renal blood flow but had no effect on glomerular filtration rate.

Use of Benazepril Hydrochloride in combination with thiazide diuretics gives a blood-pressure-lowering effect greater than that seen with either agent alone. By blocking the renin-angiotensin-aldosterone axis, administration of Benazepril Hydrochloride tends to reduce the potassium loss associated with the diuretic.

INDICATIONS AND USAGE

Benazepril Hydrochloride is indicated for the treatment of hypertension. It may be used alone or in combination with thiazide diuretics. In using Benazepril Hydrochloride, consideration should be given to the fact that another angiotensin-converting enzyme inhibitor, captopril, has caused agranulocytosis, particularly in patients with renal impairment or collagen-vascular disease. Available data are insufficient to show that Benazepril Hydrochloride does not have a similar risk (see *"Warnings"*).

UNLABELED USES

Benazepril is used alone or as an adjunct in the treatment of congestive heart failure.

CONTRAINDICATIONS

Benazepril Hydrochloride is contraindicated in patients who are hypersensitive to this product or to any other ACE inhibitor.

WARNINGS

ANAPHYLACTOID AND POSSIBLY RELATED REACTIONS

Presumably because angiotensin-converting enzyme inhibitors affect the metabolism of eicosanoids and polypeptides, including endogenous bradykinin, patients receiving ACE inhibitors (including Benazepril Hydrochloride) may be subject to a variety of adverse reactions, some of them serious.

Angioedema: Angioedema of the face, extremities, lips, tongue, glottis, and larynx has been reported in patients treated with angiotensin-converting enzyme inhibitors. In U.S. clinical trials, symptoms consistent with angioedema were seen in none of the subjects who received placebo and in about 0.5% of the subjects who received Benazepril Hydrochloride. Angioedema associated with laryngeal edema can be fatal. If laryngeal stridor or angioedema of the face, tongue, or glottis occurs, treatment with Benazepril Hydrochloride should be discontinued and appropriate therapy instituted immediately. **Where there is involvement of the tongue, glottis, or larynx, likely to cause airway obstruction, appropriate therapy, e.g., subcutaneous epinephrine injection 1:1000 (0.3 mL to 0.5 mL) should be promptly administered (see "Adverse Reactions").**

HYPOTENSION

Anaphylactoid Reactions During Desensitization: Two patients undergoing desensitizing treatment with hymenoptera venom while receiving ACE inhibitors sustained life-threatening anaphylactoid reactions. In the same patients, these reactions were avoided when ACE inhibitors were temporarily withheld, but they reappeared upon inadvertent rechallenge.

Anaphylactoid Reactions During Membrane Exposure: Anaphylactoid reactions have been reported in patients dialyzed with high-flux membranes and treated concomitantly with an ACE inhibitor. Anaphylactoid reactions have also been reported in patients undergoing low-density lipoprotein apheresis with dextran sulfate absorption (a procedure dependent upon devices not approved in the United States). Benazepril Hydrochloride can cause symptomatic hypotension. Like other ACE inhibitors, Benazepril has been only rarely associated with hypotension in uncomplicated hypertensive patients. Symptomatic hypotension is most likely to occur in patients who have been volume- and/or salt-depleted as a result of prolonged diuretic therapy, dietary salt restriction, dialysis, diarrhea, or vomiting. Volume- and/or salt-depletion should be corrected before initiating therapy with Benazepril Hydrochloride.

In patients with congestive heart failure, with or without associated renal insufficiency, ACE inhibitor therapy may cause excessive hypotension, which may be associated with oliguria or azotemia and, rarely, with acute renal failure and death. In such patients, Benazepril Hydrochloride therapy should be started under close medical supervision; they should be followed closely for the first 2 weeks of treatment and whenever the dose of Benazepril or diuretic is increased.

If hypotension occurs, the patient should be placed in a supine position, and, if necessary, treated with intravenous infusion of physiological saline. Benazepril Hydrochloride treatment usually can be continued following restoration of blood pressure and volume.

NEUTROPENIA/AGRANULOCYTOSIS

Another angiotensin-converting enzyme inhibitor, captopril, has been shown to cause agranulocytosis and bone marrow depression, rarely in uncomplicated patients, but more frequently in patients with renal impairment, especially if they also have a collagen-vascular disease such as systemic lupus erythematosus or scleroderma. Available data from clinical trials of Benazepril are insufficient to show that Benazepril does not cause agranulocytosis at similar rates. Monitoring of white blood cell counts should be considered in patients with collagen-vascular disease, especially if the disease is associated with impaired renal function.

FETAL/NEONATAL MORBIDITY AND MORTALITY

ACE inhibitors can cause fetal and neonatal morbidity and death when administered to pregnant women.

Several dozen cases have been reported in the world literature. When pregnancy is detected, ACE inhibitors should be discontinued as soon as possible.

The use of ACE inhibitors during the second and third trimesters of pregnancy has been associated with fetal and neonatal injury, including hypotension, neonatal skull hypoplasia, anuria, reversible or irreversible renal failure, and death. Oligohydramnios has also been reported, presumably resulting from decreased fetal renal function; oligohydramnios in this setting has been associated with fetal limb contractures, craniofacial deformation, and hypoplastic lung development. Prematurity, intrauterine growth retardation, and patent ductus arteriosus have also been reported, although it is not clear whether these occurrences were due to the ACE inhibitor exposure.

These adverse effects do not appear to have resulted from intrauterine ACE inhibitor exposure that has been limited to the first trimester. Mothers whose embryos and fetuses are exposed to ACE inhibitors only during the first trimester should be so informed. Nonetheless, when patients become pregnant, physicians should make every effort to discontinue the use of Benazepril as soon as possible.

Rarely (probably less often than once in every thousand pregnancies), no alternative to ACE inhibitors will be found. In these rare cases, the mothers should be apprised of the potential hazards to their fetuses, and serial ultrasound examinations should be performed to assess the intraamniotic environment.

If oligohydramnios is observed, Benazepril should be discontinued unless it is considered life-saving for the mother. Contraction stress testing (CST), a nonstress test (NST), or biophysical profiling (BPP) may be appropriate, depending upon the week of pregnancy. Patients and physicians should be aware, however, that oligohydramnios may not appear until after the fetus has sustained irreversible injury.

Infants with histories of *in utero* exposure to ACE inhibitors should be closely observed for hypotension, oliguria, and hyperkalemia. If oliguria occurs, attention should be directed toward support of blood pressure and renal perfusion. Exchange transfusion or dialysis may be required as means of reversing hypotension and/or substituting for disordered renal function. Benazepril, which crosses the placenta, can theoretically be removed from the neonatal circulation by these means; there are occasional reports of benefit from these maneuvers with another ACE inhibitor, but experience is limited.

No teratogenic effects of Benazepril Hydrochloride were seen in studies of pregnant rats, mice, and rabbits. On a mg/m² basis, the doses used in these studies were 60 times (in rats), 9 times (in mice), and more than 0.8 times (in rabbits) the maximum recommended human dose (assuming a 50 kg woman). On a mg/kg basis these multiples are 300 times (in rats), 90 times (in mice) and more than 3 times (in rabbits) the maximum recommended human dose.

HEPATIC FAILURE

Rarely, ACE inhibitors have been associated with a syndrome that starts with cholestatic jaundice and progresses to fulminant hepatic necrosis and (sometimes) death. The mechanism of this syndrome is not understood. Patients receiving ACE inhibitors who develop jaundice or marked elevations of hepatic enzymes should discontinue the ACE inhibitor and receive appropriate medical follow-up.

PRECAUTIONS
GENERAL
Impaired Renal Function: As a consequence of inhibiting the renin-angiotensin-aldosterone system, changes in renal function may be anticipated in susceptible individuals. In patients with severe congestive heart failure whose renal function may depend on the activity of the renin-angiotensin-aldosterone system, treatment with angiotensin-converting enzyme inhibitors, including Benazepril Hydrochloride, may be associated with oliguria and/or progressive azotemia and (rarely) with acute renal failure and/or death. In a small study of hypertensive patients with renal artery stenosis in a solitary kidney or bilateral renal artery stenosis, treatment with Benazepril Hydrochloride was associated with increases in blood urea nitrogen and serum creatinine; these increases were reversible upon discontinuation of Benazepril Hydrochloride or diuretic therapy, or both. When such patients are treated with ACE inhibitors, renal function should be monitored during the first few weeks of therapy. Some hypertensive patients with no apparent preexisting renal vascular disease have developed increases in blood urea nitrogen and serum creatinine, usually minor and transient, especially when Benazepril Hydrochloride has been given concomitantly with a diuretic. This is more likely to occur in patients with preexisting renal impairment. Dosage reduction of Benazepril Hydrochloride and/or discontinuation of the diuretic may be required. **Evaluation of the hypertensive patient should always include assessment of renal function (see** *"Dosage and Administration"*).

Hyperkalemia: In clinical trials, hyperkalemia (serum potassium at least 0.5 mEq/L greater than the upper limit of normal) occurred in approximately 1% of hypertensive patients receiving Benazepril Hydrochloride. In most cases, these were isolated values which resolved despite continued therapy. Risk factors for the development of hyperkalemia include renal insufficiency, diabetes mellitus, and the concomitant use of potassium-sparing diuretics, potassium supplements, and/or potassium-containing salt substitutes, which should be used cautiously, if at all, with Benazepril Hydrochloride (see *"Drug Interactions"*).

Cough: Presumably due to the inhibition of the degradation of endogenous bradykinin, persistent nonproductive cough has been reported with all ACE inhibitors, always resolving after discontinuation of therapy. ACE inhibitor-induced cough should be considered in the differential diagnosis of cough.

Impaired Liver Function: In patients with hepatic dysfunction due to cirrhosis, levels of Benazeprilat are essentially unaltered (see *"Warnings, Hepatic Failure"*.)

Surgery/Anesthesia: In patients undergoing surgery or during anesthesia with agents that produce hypotension, Benazepril will block the angiotensin II formation that could otherwise occur secondary to compensatory renin release. Hypotension that occurs as a result of this mechanism can be corrected by volume expansion.

INFORMATION FOR PATIENTS
Pregnancy: Female patients of childbearing age should be told about the consequences of second- and third-trimester exposure to ACE inhibitors, and they should also be told that these consequences do not appear to have resulted from intrauterine ACE inhibitor exposure that has been limited to the first trimester. These patients should be asked to report pregnancies to their physicians as soon as possible.

Angioedema: Angioedema, including laryngeal edema, can occur with treatment with ACE inhibitors, especially following the first dose. Patients should be so advised and told to report immediately any signs or symptoms suggesting angioedema (swelling of face, eyes, lips, or tongue, or difficulty in breathing) and to take no more drug until they have consulted with the prescribing physician.

Symptomatic Hypotension: Patients should be cautioned that lightheadedness can occur, especially during the first days of therapy, and it should be reported to the prescribing physician. Patients should be told that if syncope occurs, Benazepril Hydrochloride should be discontinued until the prescribing physician has been consulted.

All patients should be cautioned that inadequate fluid intake or excessive perspiration, diarrhea, or vomiting can lead to an excessive fall in blood pressure, with the same consequences of lightheadedness and possible syncope.

Hyperkalemia: Patients should be told not to use potassium supplements or salt substitutes containing potassium without consulting the prescribing physician.

Neutropenia: Patients should be told to promptly report any indication of infection (e.g., sore throat, fever), which could be a sign of neutropenia.

DRUG INTERACTIONS
Diuretics: Patients on diuretics, especially those in whom diuretic therapy was recently instituted, may occasionally experience an excessive reduction of blood pressure after initiation of therapy with Benazepril Hydrochloride. The possibility of hypotensive effects with Benazepril Hydrochloride can be minimized by either discontinuing the diuretic or increasing the salt intake prior to initiation of treatment with Benazepril Hydrochloride. If this is not possible, the starting dose should be reduced (see *"Dosage and Administration"*).

Potassium Supplements and Potassium-Sparing Diuretics: Benazepril Hydrochloride can attenuate potassium loss caused by thiazide diuretics. Potassium-sparing diuretics (spironolactone, amiloride, triamterene, and others) or potassium supplements can increase the risk of hyperkalemia. Therefore, if concomitant use

of such agents is indicated, they should be given with caution, and the patient's serum potassium should be monitored frequently.

Oral Anticoagulants: Interaction studies with warfarin and acenocoumarol failed to identify any clinically important effects on the serum concentrations or clinical effects of these anticoagulants.

Lithium: Increased serum lithium levels and symptoms of lithium toxicity have been reported in patients receiving ACE inhibitors during therapy with lithium. These drugs should be coadministered with caution, and frequent monitoring of serum lithium levels is recommended. If a diuretic is also used, the risk of lithium toxicity may be increased.

Other: No clinically important pharmacokinetic interactions occurred when Benazepril Hydrochloride was administered concomitantly with hydrochlorothiazide, chlorthalidone, furosemide, digoxin, propranolol, atenolol, naproxen, or cimetidine.

Benazepril Hydrochloride has been used concomitantly with beta-adrenergic-blocking agents, calcium-channel-blocking agents, diuretics digoxin, and hydralazine, without evidence of clinically important adverse interactions. Benazepril, like other ACE inhibitors, has had less than additive effects with beta-adrenergic blockers, presumably because both drugs lower blood pressure by inhibiting parts of the renin-angiotensin system.

CARCINOGENSIS, MUTAGENESIS, IMPAIRMENT OF FERTILITY
No evidence of carcinogenicity was found when Benazepril was administered to rats and mice for up to two years at doses of up to 150 mg/kg/day. When compared on the basis of body weights, this dose is 110 times the maximum recommended human dose. When compared on the basis of body surface areas, this dose is 18 and 9 times (rats and mice, respectively) the maximum recommended human dose (calculations assume a patient weight of 60 kg). No mutagenic activity was detected in the Ames test in bacteria (with or without metabolic activation), in an in vitro test for forward mutations in cultured mammalian cells, or in a nucleus anomaly test. In doses of 50-500 mg/kg/day (6-60 times the maximum recommended human dose based on mg/m^2 comparison and 37-375 times the maximum recommended human dose based on a mg/kg comparison), Benazepril Hydrochloride had no adverse effect on the reproductive performance of male and female rats.

PREGNANCY CATEGORIES C (FIRST TRIMESTER) AND D (SECOND AND THIRD TRIMESTERS)
See *"Warnings, Fetal/Neonatal Morbidity and Mortality"*.

NURSING MOTHERS
Minimal amounts of unchanged Benazepril and of Benazeprilat are excreted into the breast milk of lactating women treated with Benazepril. A newborn child ingesting entirely breast milk would receive less than 0.1% of the mg/kg maternal dose of Benazepril and benazeprilat.

GERIATRIC USE
Of the total number of patients who received Benazepril in U.S. clinical studies of Benazepril Hydrochloride, 18% were 65 or older while 2% were 75 or older. No overall differences in effectiveness or safety were observed between these patients and younger patients, and other reported clinical experience has not identified differences in responses between the elderly and younger patients, but greater sensitivity of some older individuals cannot be ruled out.

PEDIATRIC USE
Safety and effectiveness in children have not been established.

ADVERSE REACTIONS
Benazepril Hydrochloride has been evaluated for safety in over 6000 patients with hypertension; over 700 of these patients were treated for at least one year. The overall incidence of reported adverse events was comparable in Benazepril Hydrochloride and placebo patients.

The reported side effects were generally mild and transient, and there was no relation between side effects and age, duration of therapy, or total dosage within the range of 2 to 80 mg. Discontinuation of therapy because of a side effect was required in approximately 5% of U.S. patients treated with Benazepril Hydrochloride and in 3% of patients treated with placebo.

The most common reasons for discontinuation were headache (0.6%) and cough (0.5%). (See *"Precautions, Cough"*). The side effects considered possibly or probably related to study drug that occurred in U.S. placebo-controlled trials in more than 1% of patients treated with Benazepril Hydrochloride are shown below.

PATIENTS IN U.S. PLACEBO-CONTROLLED STUDIES

	Benazepril Hydrochloride (N = 964)		PLACEBO (N = 496)	
	N	%	N	%
Headache	60	6.2	21	4.2
Dizziness	35	3.6	12	2.4
Fatigue	23	2.4	11	2.2
Somnolence	15	1.6	2	0.4
Postural Dizziness	14	1.5	1	0.2
Nausea	13	1.3	5	1.0
Cough	12	1.2	5	1.0

Other adverse experiences reported in controlled clinical trials (in less than 1% of Benazepril patients), and rarer events seen in postmarketing experience, include the following (in some, a causal relationship to drug use is uncertain):

Cardiovascular: Symptomatic hypotension was seen in 0.3% of patients, postural hypotension in 0.4%, and syncope in 0.1%; these reactions led to discontinuation of therapy in 4 patients who had received Benazepril monotherapy and in 9 patients who had received Benazepril with hydrochlorothiazide (see *"Precautions"* and *"Warnings"*). Other reports include angina pectoris, palpitations, and peripheral edema.

Renal: Of hypertensive patients with no apparent preexisting renal disease, about 2% have sustained increases in serum creatinine to at least 150% of their baseline values while receiving Benazepril Hydrochloride, but most of these increases have disappeared despite continuing treatment. A much smaller fraction of these patients (less than 0.1%) developed simultaneous (usually transient) increases in blood urea nitrogen and serum creatinine.

Fetal/Neonatal Morbidity and Mortality: (see *"Warnings, Fetal/Neonatal Morbidity and Mortality"*.)

Angioedema: Angioedema has been reported in patients receiving ACE inhibitors. During clinical trials in hypertensive patients with Benazepril, 0.5% of patients experienced edema of the lips or face without other manifestations of angioedema. Angioedema associated with laryngeal edema and/or shock may be fatal. If angioedema of the face, extremities, lips, tongue, or glottis and/or larynx occurs, treatment with Benazepril Hydrochloride should be discontinued and appropriate therapy instituted immediately (see *"Warnings"*).

Gastrointestinal: Constipation, gastritis, vomiting, and melena.

Dermatologic: Apparent hypersensitivity reactions (manifested by dermatitis, pruritus, or rash), photosensitivity and flushing.

Neurologic and Psychiatric: Anxiety, decreased libido, hypertonia, insomnia, nervousness, and paresthesia.

Other: Arthralgia, arthritis, asthenia, asthma, bronchitis, dyspnea, impotence, infection, myalgia, sinusitis, sweating, and urinary tract infection.

CLINICAL LABORATORY TEST FINDINGS

Creatinine and Blood Urea Nitrogen: Of hypertensive patients with no apparent preexisting renal disease, about 2% have sustained increases in serum creatinine to at least 150% of their baseline values while receiving Benazepril Hydrochloride, but most of these increases have disappeared despite continuing treatment. A much smaller fraction of these patients (less than 0.1%) developed simultaneous (usually transient) increases in blood urea nitrogen and serum creatinine. None of these increases required discontinuation of treatment. Increases in these laboratory values are more likely to occur in patients with renal insufficiency or those pretreated with a diuretic and, based on experience with other ACE inhibitors, would be expected to be especially likely in patients with renal artery stenosis (see *"Precautions, General"*).

Potassium: Since Benazepril decreases aldosterone secretion, elevation of serum potassium can occur. Potassium supplements and potassium-sparing diuretics should be given with caution, and the patient's serum potassium should be monitored frequently (see *"Precautions"*).

Hemoglobin: Decreases in hemoglobin (a low value and a decrease of 5 g/dL) were rare, occurring in only 1 of 2014 patients receiving Benazepril Hydrochloride alone and in 1 of 1357 patients receiving Benazepril Hydrochloride plus a diuretic. No U.S. patients discontinued treatment because of decreases in hemoglobin.

Other (causal relationships unknown): Clinically important changes in standard laboratory tests were rarely associated with Benazepril Hydrochloride administration. Elevations of uric acid, blood glucose, serum bilirubin, and liver enzymes (see *"Warnings"*) have been reported, as have scattered incidents of hyponatremia, electrocardiographic changes, leukopenia, eosinophilia, and proteinuria. In U.S. trials, less than 0.5% of patients discontinued treatment because of laboratory abnormalities.

OVERDOSAGE

Single oral doses of 3 g/kg Benazepril were associated with significant lethality in mice. Rats however, tolerated single oral doses of up to 6 g/kg. Reduced activity was seen at 1 g/kg in mice and at 5 g/kg in rats. Human overdoses of Benazepril have not been reported, but the most common manifestation of human Benazepril overdosages is likely to be hypotension. Laboratory determinations of serum levels of Benazepril and its metabolites are not widely available, and such determinations have, in any event, no established role in the management of Benazepril overdose.

No data are available to suggest physiological maneuvers (e.g., maneuvers to change the pH of the urine) that might accelerate elimination of Benazepril and its metabolities. Benazepril is only slightly dialyzable, but dialysis might be considered in overdosed patients with severely impaired renal function (see *"Warnings"*).

Angiotensin II could presumably serve as a specific antagonist-antidote in the setting of Benazepril overdose, but angiotensin II is essentially unavailable outside of scattered research facilities. Because the hypotensive effect of Benazepril is achieved through vasodilation and effective hypovolemia, it is reasonable to treat Benazepril overdose by infusion of normal saline solution.

DOSAGE AND ADMINISTRATION

The recommended initial dose for patients not receiving a diuretic is 10 mg once-a-day. The usual maintenance dosage range is 20-40 mg per day administered as a single dose or in two equally divided doses. A dose of 80 mg gives an increased response, but experience with this dose is limited. The divided regimen was more effective in controlling trough (predosing) blood pressure than the same dose given as a once-daily regimen. Dosage adjustment should be based on measurement of peak (2-6 hours after dosing) and trough responses. If a once-daily regimen does not give adequate trough response an increase in dosage or divided administration should be considered. If blood pressure is not controlled with Benazepril Hydrochloride alone, a diuretic can be added.

Total daily doses above 80 mg have not been evaluated.

Concomitant administration of Benazepril Hydrochloride with potassium supplements, potassium salt substitutes, or potassium-sparing diuretics can lead to increases of serum potassium (see *"Precautions"*).

In patients who are currently being treated with a diuretic, symptomatic hypotension occasionally can occur following the initial dose of Benazepril Hydrochloride. To reduce the likelihood of hypotension, the diuretic should, if possible, be discontinued two to three days prior to beginning therapy with Benazepril Hydrochloride (see *"Warnings"*). Then, if blood pressure is not controlled with Benazepril Hydrochloride alone, diuretic therapy should be resumed.

If the diuretic cannot be discontinued, an initial dose of 5 mg Benazepril Hydrochloride should be used to avoid excessive hypotension.

DOSAGE ADJUSTMENT IN RENAL IMPAIRMENT

For patients with a creatinine clearance < 30 mL/min/1.73 m² (serum creatinine > 3 mg/dL), the recommended initial dose is 5 mg Benazepril Hydrochloride once daily. Dosage may be titrated upward until blood pressure is controlled or to a maximum total daily dose of 40 mg (see *"Warnings"*).

Storage: Do not store above 86 ° F (30 ° C). Protect from moisture.
Dispense in tight container (USP).

HOW SUPPLIED
TABLETS: 5 MG

BRAND/MANUFACTURER	NDC	SIZE	AWP
○ **BRAND**			
▶ LOTENSIN: Ciba Pharm	00083-0059-30	100s	$63.63
	00083-0059-32	100s ud	$63.63

TABLETS: 10 MG

BRAND/MANUFACTURER	NDC	SIZE	AWP
○ **BRAND**			
▶ LOTENSIN: Ciba Pharm	00083-0063-30	100s	$63.63
	00083-0063-32	100s ud	$63.63

TABLETS: 20 MG

BRAND/MANUFACTURER	NDC	SIZE	AWP
○ **BRAND**			
▶ LOTENSIN: Ciba Pharm	00083-0079-30	100s	$63.63
	00083-0079-32	100s ud	$63.63

TABLETS: 40 MG

BRAND/MANUFACTURER	NDC	SIZE	AWP
○ **BRAND**			
▶ LOTENSIN: Ciba Pharm	00083-0094-30	100s	$63.63
	00083-0094-32	100s ud	$63.63

Benazepril Hydrochloride with Hydrochlorothiazide

> **USE IN PREGNANCY**
> WHEN USED IN PREGNANCY DURING THE SECOND AND THIRD TRIMESTERS, ACE INHIBITORS CAN CAUSE INJURY AND EVEN DEATH TO THE DEVELOPING FETUS. WHEN PREGNANCY IS DETECTED, BENAZEPRIL HYDROCHLORIDE/HYDROCHLOROTHIAZIDE SHOULD BE DISCONTINUED AS SOON AS POSSIBLE. SEE *"WARNINGS, FETAL/NEONATAL MORBIDITY AND MORTALITY."*

DESCRIPTION

Benazepril Hydrochloride is a white to off-white crystalline powder, soluble (> 100 mg/mL) in water, in ethanol, and in methanol. Benazepril Hydrochloride's chemical name is 3-[[1-(ethoxycarbonyl)-3-phenyl-(1S)-propyl]amino]- 2,3,4,5-tetrahydro-2-oxo-1-*H*-1-(3S)-benzazepine-1-acetic acid monohydrochloride.

Its empirical formula is $C_{24}H_{28}N_2O_5$.HCl, and its molecular weight is 460.96.

Benazeprilat, the active metabolite of Benazepril, is a nonsulfhydryl angiotensin-converting enzyme inhibitor. Benazepril is converted to benazeprilat by hepatic cleavage of the ester group.

Hydrochlorothiazide (HCTZ) USP is a white, or practically white, practically odorless, crystalline powder. It is slightly soluble in water; freely soluble in sodium hydroxide solution in *n*-butylamine, and in dimethylformamide; sparingly soluble in methanol; and insoluble in ether, in chloroform, and in dilute mineral acids. Hydrochlorothiazide's chemical name is 6-chloro-3,4-dihydro-2 *H*-1,2,4-benzothi-adiazine-7-sulfonamide 1,1-dioxide.

Its empirical formula is $C_7H_8ClN_8O_4S_2$, and its molecular weight is 297.73. Hydrochlorothiazide is a thiazide diuretic. The combination of Benazepril Hydrochloride and Hydrochlorothiazide is available for oral use in the following strengths:

Each tablet contains:

5/6.25 Benazepril, Hydrochlorothiazide ....5 mg, 6.25 mg
10/12.5 Benazepril, Hydrochlorothiazide ....10 mg, 12.5 mg
20/12.5 Benazepril, Hydrochlorothiazide ....20 mg, 12.5 mg
20/25 Benazepril, Hydrochlorothiazide ....20 mg, 25 mg

CLINICAL PHARMACOLOGY

MECHANISM OF ACTION

Benazepril and benazeprilat inhibit angiotensin-converting enzyme (ACE) in human subjects and in animals. ACE is a peptidyl dipeptidase that catalyzes the conversion of angiotensin I to the vasoconstrictor substance, angiotensin II. Angiotensin II also stimulates aldosterone secretion by the adrenal cortex.

Inhibition of ACE results in decreased plasma angiotensin II, which leads to decreased vasopressor activity and to decreased aldosterone secretion. The latter decrease may result in a small increase of serum potassium. Hypertensive patients treated with Benazepril alone for up to 52 weeks had elevations of serum potassium of up to 0.2 mEq/L. Similar patients treated with Benazepril and Hydrochlorothiazide for up to 24 weeks had no consistent changes in their serum potassium (see *"Precautions"*).

Removal of angiotensin II negative feedback on renin secretion leads to increased plasma renin activity. In animal studies, Benazepril had no inhibitory effect on the vasopressor response to angiotensin II and did not interfere with the hemodynamic effects of the autonomic neutrotransmitters acetylcholine, epinephrine, and norepinephrine.

ACE is identical to kininase, an enzyme that degrades bradykinin. Whether increased levels of bradykinin, a potent vasodepressor peptide, play a role in the therapeutic effects of Benazepril/HCTZ remains to be elucidated.

While the mechanism through which Benazepril lowers blood pressure is believed to be primarily suppression of the renin-angiotensin-aldosterone system, Benazepril has an antihypertensive effect even in patients with low-renin hypertension.

Hydrochlorothiazide is a thiazide diuretic. Thiazides affect the renal tubular mechanisms of electrolyte reabsorption, directly increasing excretion of sodium and chloride in approximately equivalent amounts. Indirectly, the diuretic action of Hydrochlorothiazide reduces plasma volume, with consequent increases in plasma renin activity, increases in aldosterone secretion, increases in urinary potassium loss, and decreases in serum potassium. The renin-aldosterone link is mediated by angiotensin, so coadministration of an ACE inhibitor tends to reverse the potassium loss associated with these diuretics.

The mechanism of the antihypertensive effect of thiazides is unknown.

PHARMACOKINETICS AND METABOLISM

Following oral administration of Benazepril/HCTZ peak plasma concentrations of Benazepril are reached within 0.5-1.0 hours. As determined by urinary recovery, the extent of absorption is at least 37%. The absorption of Hydrochlorothiazide is somewhat slower (1-2.5 hours) and somewhat more complete (50-80%). In fasting subjects, the rate and extent of absorption of Benazepril and Hydrochlorothiazide the combination are not different, respectively, from the rate and extent of absorption of Benazepril and hydrochlorothiazide from immediate-release monotherapy formulations.

The absorption of Benazepril tablets is not influenced by the presence of food in the gastrointestinal tract, but possible effects of food upon absorption of either component Benazepril/HCTZ tablets have not been studied. The reported studies of food effects of Hydrochlorothiazide absorption have been inconclusive. The absorption of Hydrochlorothiazide is increased by agents that reduces gastrointestinal motility, but it is reported to be reduced by 50% in patients with congestive heart failure.

Cleavage of the ester group (primarily in the liver) converts Benazepril to its active metabolite, benazeprilat. Peak plasma concentrations of benazeprilat are reached 1-2 hours after drug intake in the fasting state and 2-4 hours after drug intake in the nonfasting state. The serum protein binding of Benazepril is about 96.7% and that of benazeprilat about 95.3%, as measured by equilibrium dialysis; on the basis of *in vitro* studies, the degree of protein binding should be unaffected by age, hepatic dysfunction, or—over the concentration range of 0.24-23.6 μ mol/L—concentration.

Hydrochlorothiazide is not metabolized. Its apparent volume of distribution is 3.6-7.8 L/kg, and its measured plasma protein binding is 67.9%. The drug also accumulates in red blood cells, so that whole blood levels are 1.6-1.8 times those measured in plasma.

In studies of rats given ^{14}C-Benazepril, Benazepril and its metabolites crossed the blood-brain barrier only to an extremely low extent. Multiple doses of Benazepril did not result in accumulation in any tissue except the lung, where, as with other ACE inhibitors in similar studies, there was a slight increase in concentration due to slow elimination in that organ.

Some placental passage occurred when Benazepril was administered to pregnant rats. In humans, Hydrochlorothiazide crosses the placenta freely, and levels in umbilical-cord blood are similar to those in the maternal circulation.

Benazepril is almost completely metabolized to benazeprilat, which has much greater ACE inhibitory activity than Benazepril, and to the glucuronide conjugates of Benazepril and benazeprilat. Only trace amounts of an administered dose of Benazepril can be recovered unchanged in the urine; about 20% of the dose is excreted as benazeprilat, 4% as benazepril glucuronide, and 8% as benazeprilat glucuronide. In patients with hepatic dysfunction due to cirrhosis, levels of benazeprilat are essentially unaltered. Similarly, the pharmacokinetics of Benazepril and benazeprilat do not appear to be influenced by age.

The kinetics of Benazepril are dose-proportional within the dosage range of 5-20 mg. Small deviations from dose proportionality were observed when the broader range of 2-80 mg was studied, possibly due to the saturable binding of the compound to ACE.

The effective half-life of accumulation of benazeprilat following multiple dosing of Benazepril Hydrochloride is 10-11 hours. Thus, steady-state concentrations of benazeprilat should be reached after 2 or 3 doses of Benazepril Hydrochloride given once daily.

During chronic administration (28 days) of once-daily doses of Benazepril between 5 mg and 20 mg, the kinetics did not change, and there was no significant accumulation. Accumulation ratios based on AUC and urinary recovery of benazeprilat were 1.19 and 1.27, respectively.

When dialysis was started 2 hours after ingestion of 10 mg of Benazepril, approximately 6% of benazeprilat was removed in 4 hours of dialysis. The parent compound, Benazepril, was not detected in the dialysate.

Benazepril and benazeprilat are cleared predominantly by renal excretion in healthy subjects with normal renal function. Nonrenal (i.e., biliary) excretion accounts for approximately 11-12% of benazeprilat excretion in healthy subjects. In patients with renal failure, biliary clearance may compensate to an extent for deficient renal clearance.

The disposition of Benazepril and benazeprilat in patients with mild-to-moderate renal insufficiency (creatinine clearance > 30 mL/min) is similar to that in patients with normal renal function. In patients with creatinine clearance ≤ 30 mL/min, peak benazeprilat levels and the initial (alpha phase) half-life increase, and time to steady state may be delayed (see *"Dosage and Administration"*).

Thiazide diuretics are eliminated by the kidney, with a terminal half-life of 5-15 hours. In a study of patients with impaired renal function (mean creatinine clearance of 19 mL/min), the half-life of Hydrochlorothiazide elimination was lengthened to 21 hours.

PHARMACODYNAMICS

Single and multiple doses of 10 mg or more of *Benazepril* cause inhibition of plasma ACE activity by at least 80-90% for at least 24 hours after dosing. For up to 4 hours after a 10-mg dose, pressor responses to exogenous angiotensin I were inhibited by 60-90%.

Administration of Benazepril to patients with mild-to-moderate hypertension results in a reduction of both supine and standing blood pressure to about the same extent, with no compensatory tachycardia. Symptomatic postural hypotension is infrequent, although it can occur in patients who are salt and/or volume depleted (see *"Warnings, Hypotension"*).

In single-dose studies, Benazepril lowered blood pressure within 1 hour, with peak reductions achieved 2-4 hours after dosing. The antihypertensive effect of a single dose persisted for 24 hours. In multiple-dose studies, once-daily doses of 20-80 mg decreased seated pressure (systolic/diastolic) 24 hours after dosing by about 6-12/4-7 mmHg. The reductions at trough are about 50% of those seen at peak.

Four dose-response studies of Benazepril monotherapy using once-daily dosing were conducted in 470 mild-to-moderate hypertensive patients not using diuretics. The minimal effective once-daily dose of Benazepril was 10 mg; further falls in blood pressure, especially at morning trough, were seen with higher doses in the studied dosing range (10-80 mg). In studies comparing the same daily dose of Benazepril given as a single morning dose or as a twice-daily dose, blood pressure reductions at the time of morning trough blood levels were greater with the divided regimen.

During chronic therapy with Benazepril, the maximum reduction in blood pressure with any given dose is generally achieved after 1-2 weeks. The antihypertensive effects of Benazepril have continued during therapy for at least 2 years. Abrupt withdrawal of Benazepril has not been associated with a rapid increase in blood pressure.

In patients with mild-to-moderate hypertension, total daily doses of Benazepril HCl 20-40 mg were similar in effectiveness to total daily doses of captopril 50-100 mg, Hydrochlorothiazide 25-50 mg, nifedipine SR 40-80 mg, and propranolol 80-160 mg.

The antihypertensive effects of Benazepril were not appreciably different in patients receiving high- or low-sodium diets.

In hemodynamic studies in dogs, blood pressure reduction was accompanied by a reduction in peripheral arterial resistance, with an increase in cardiac output and renal blood flow and little or no change in heart rate. In normal human volunteers, single doses of Benazepril caused an increase in renal blood flow but had no effect on glomerular filtration rate.

In clinical trials of *Benazepril/Hydrochlorothiazide* using Benazepril doses of 5-20 mg and Hydrochlorothiazide doses of 6.25-25 mg, the antihypertensive effects were sustained for at least 24 hours, and they increased with increasing dose of either component. Although Benazepril monotherapy is somewhat less effective in blacks than in nonblacks, the efficacy of combination therapy appears to be independent of race.

By blocking the renin-angiotensin-aldosterone axis, administration of Benazepril tends to reduce the potassium loss associated with the diuretic. In clinical trials of Benazepril/HCTZ, the average change in serum potassium was near zero in subjects who received 5/6.25 mg or 20/12.5 mg, but the average subject who received 10/12.5 mg or 20/25 mg experienced a mild reduction in serum potassium, similar to that experienced by the average subject receiving the same dose of Hydrochlorothiazide monotherapy.

INDICATIONS AND USAGE
Benazepril/HCTZ is indicated for the treatment of hypertension. In using Benazepril/HCTZ consideration should be given to the fact that another angiotensin-converting-enzyme inhibitor, captopril, has caused agranulocytosis, particularly in patients with renal impairment or collagen-vascular disease. Available data are insufficient to show that Benazepril does not have a similar risk (see "Warnings, Neutropenia/Agranulocytosis").

CONTRAINDICATIONS
Benazepril/HCTZ is contraindicated in patients who are anuric. Benazepril/HCTZ is also contraindicated in patients who are hypersensitive to Benazepril, to any other ACE inhibitor, to Hydrochlorothiazide, or to other sulfonamide-derived drugs. Hypersensitivity reactions are more likely to occur in patients with a history of allergy or bronchial asthma.

WARNINGS
ANAPHYLACTOID AND POSSIBLY RELATED REACTIONS
Presumably because angiotensin-converting enzyme inhibitors affect the metabolism of eicosanoids and polypeptides, including endogenous bradykinin, patients receiving ACE inhibitors (including Benazepril/HCTZ may be subject to a variety of adverse reactions, some of them serious.

Angioedema: Angioedema of the face, extremities, lips, tongue, glottis, and larynx has been reported in patients treated with angiotensin-converting-enzyme inhibitors. In U.S. clinical trials, symptoms consistent with angioedema were seen in none of the subjects who received placebo and in about 0.5% of the subjects who received Benazepril. Angioedema associated with laryngeal edema can be fatal. If laryngeal stridor or angioedema of the face, tongue, or glottis occurs, treatment with Benazepril/HCTZ should be discontinued and appropriate therapy instituted immediately. *When involvement of the tongue, glottis, or larynx appears likely to cause airway obstruction, appropriate therapy, e.g., subcutaneous epinephrine injection 1:1000 (0.3-0.5 mL) should be promptly administered* (see "Precautions" and "Adverse Reactions").

Anaphylactoid Reactions During Desensitization: Two patients undergoing desensitizing treatment with hymenoptera venom while receiving ACE inhibitors sustained life-threatening anaphylactoid reactions. In the same patients, these reactions were avoided when ACE inhibitors were temporarily withheld, but they reappeared upon inadvertent rechallenge.

Anaphylactoid Reactions During Membrane Exposure: Anaphylactoid reactions have been reported in patients dialyzed with high-flux membranes and treated concomitantly with an ACE inhibitor. Anaphylactoid reactions have also been reported in patients undergoing low-density lipoprotein apheresis with dextran sulfate absorption (a procedure dependent upon devices not approved in the United States).

HYPOTENSION
Benazepril/HCTZ can cause symptomatic hypotension. Like other ACE inhibitors, Benazepril has been only rarely associated with hypotension in uncomplicated hypertensive patients. Symptomatic hypotension is most likely to occur in patients who have been volume and/or salt depleted as a result of prolonged diuretic therapy, dietary salt restriction, dialysis, diarrhea, or vomiting. Volume and/or salt depletion should be corrected before initiating therapy with Benazepril/HCTZ.

Benazepril/HCTZ should be used cautiously in patients receiving concomitant therapy with other antihypertensives. The thiazide component of Benazepril/HCTZ may potentiate the action of other antihypertensive drugs, especially ganglionic or peripheral adrenergic-blocking drugs. The antihypertensive effects of the thiazide component may also be enhanced in the postsympathectomy patient.

In patients with congestive heart failure, with or without associated renal insufficiency, ACE inhibitor therapy may cause excessive hypotension, which may be associated with oliguria, azotemia, and (rarely) with acute renal failure and death. In such patient, Benazepril/HCTZ therapy should be started under close medical supervision; they should be followed closely for the first 2 weeks of treatment and whenever the dose of Benazepril or diuretic is increased.

If hypotension occurs, the patient should be placed in a supine position, and, if necessary, treated with intravenous infusion of physiological saline Benazepril/HCTZ treatment usually can be continued following restoration of blood pressure and volume.

IMPAIRED RENAL FUNCTION
Benazepril/HCTZ should be used with caution in patients with severe renal disease. Thiazides may precipitate azotemia in such patients, and the effects of repeated dosing may be cumulative.

When the renin-angiotensin-aldosterone system is inhibited by Benazepril, changes in renal function may be anticipated in susceptible individuals. In patients with *severe congestive heart failure,* whose renal function may depend on the activity of the renin-angiotensin-aldosterone system, treatment with angiotensin-converting enzyme inhibitors (including Benazepril) may be associated with oliguria and/or progressive azotemia and (rarely) with acute renal failure and/or death.

In a small study of hypertensive patients with *unilateral or bilateral renal artery stenosis,* treatment with Benazepril was associated with increases in blood urea nitrogen and serum creatinine; these increases were reversible upon discontinuation of Benazepril therapy, concomitant diuretic therapy, or both. When such patients are treated with Benzepril/HCTZ, renal function should be monitored during the first few weeks of therapy.

Some Benazepril-treated hypertensive patients with no *apparent preexisting renal vascular disease* have developed increases in blood urea nitrogen and serum creatinine, usually minor and transient, especially when Benazepril has been given concomitantly with a diuretic. Dosage reduction of Benazepril/HCTZ may be required. *Evaluation of the hypertensive patient should always include assessment of renal function* (see "Dosage and Administration").

NEUTROPENIA/AGRANULOCYTOSIS
Another angiotensin-converting enzyme inhibitor, captopril, has been shown to cause agranulocytosis and bone marrow depression, rarely in uncomplicated patients (incidence probably less than once per 10,000 exposures) but more frequently (incidence possibly as great as once per 1000 exposures) in patients with renal impairment, especially those who also have collagen-vascular diseases such as systemic lupus erythematosus or scleroderma. Available data from clinical trials of Benazepril are insufficient to show that Benazepril does not cause agranulocytosis at similar rates. Monitoring of white blood cell counts should be considered in patients with collagen-vascular disease, especially if the disease is associated with impaired renal function.

FETAL/NEONATAL MORBIDITY AND MORTALITY
ACE inhibitors can cause fetal and neonatal morbidity and death when administered to pregnant women. Several dozen cases have been reported in the world literature. When pregnancy is detected, Benazepril/HCTZ should be discontinued as soon as possible.

The use of ACE inhibitors during the second and third trimesters of pregnancy has been associated with fetal and neonatal injury, including hypotension, neonatal skull hypoplasia, anuria, reversible or irreversible renal failure, and death. Oligohydramnios has also been reported, presumably resulting from decreased fetal renal function, oligohydramnios in this setting has been associated with fetal limb contractures, craniofacial deformation, and hypoplastic lung development. Prematurity, intrauterine growth retardation, and patent ductus arteriosus have also been reported, although it is not clear whether these occurrences were due to the ACE inhibitor exposure.

These adverse effects do not appear to have resulted from intrauterine ACE inhibitor exposure that has been limited to the first trimester. Mothers whose embryos and fetuses are exposed to ACE inhibitors only during the first trimester should be so informed. Nonetheless, when patients become pregnant, physicians should make every effort to discontinue the use of Benazepril as soon as possible.

Rarely (probably less often than once in every thousand pregnancies), no alternative to ACE inhibitors will be found. In these rare cases, the mothers should be apprised of the potential hazards to their fetuses, and serial ultrasound examinations should be performed to assess the intraamniotic environment.

If oligohydramnios is observed, Benazepril should be discontinued unless it is considered life-saving for the mother. Contraction stress testing (CST), a nonstress test (NST), or biophysical profiling (BPP) may be appropriate, depending upon the week of pregnancy. Patients and physicians should be aware, however, that oligohydramnios may not appear until after the fetus has sustained irreversible injury.

Infants with histories of in utero exposure to ACE inhibitors should be closely observed for hypotension, oliguria, and hyperkalemia. If oliguria occurs, attention should be directed toward support of blood pressure and renal perfusion. Exchange transfusion or peritoneal dialysis may be required as means of reversing hypotension and/or substituting for disordered renal function. Benazepril, which crosses the placenta, can theoretically be removed from the neonatal circulation by these means; there are occasional reports of benefit from these maneuvers, but experience is limited.

Intrauterine exposure to thiazide diuretics is associated with fetal or neonatal jaundice, thrombocytopenia, and possibly other adverse reactions that have occurred in adults.

No teratogenic effects were seen when Benazepril and Hydrochlorothiazide were administered to pregnant rats at a dose ratio of 4:5. On a mg/kg basis, the doses used were up to 167 times the maximum recommended human dose. Similarly, no teratogenic effects were seen when Benazepril and Hydrochlorothiazide were administered to pregnant mice at total doses up to 160 mg/kg/day, with Benazepril: Hydrochlorothiazide ratios of 15:1. When Hydrochlorothiazide was orally administered without Benazepril to pregnant mice and rats during their respective periods of major organogenesis, at doses up to 3000 and 1000 mg/kg/day respectively, there was no evidence of harm to the fetus. Similarly, no teratogenic effects of Benazepril were seen in studies of pregnant rats, mice and rabbits; on a mg/kg basis, the doses used in these studies were 300 times (in rats), 90 times (in mice), and more than 3 times (in rabbits) the maximum recommended human dose.

HEPATIC FAILURE
Rarely, ACE inhibitors have been associated with a syndrome that starts with cholestatic jaundice and progresses to fulminant hepatic necrosis and (sometimes) death. The mechanism of this syndrome is not understood. Patients receiving ACE inhibitors who develop jaundice or marked elevations of hepatic enzymes should discontinue the ACE inhibitor and receive appropriate medical follow-up.

IMPAIRED HEPATIC FUNCTION

Benazepril/HCTZ should be used with caution in patients with impaired hepatic function or progressive liver disease, since minor alterations of fluid and electrolyte balance may precipitate hepatic coma (see *"Hepatic Failure"* above). In patients with hepatic dysfunction due to cirrhosis, levels of benazeprilat are essentially unaltered. No formal pharmacokinetic studies have been carried out in hypertensive patients with impaired liver function.

SYSTEMIC LUPUS ERYTHEMATOSUS

Thiazide diuretics have been reported to cause exacerbation or activation of systemic lupus erythematosus.

PRECAUTIONS

GENERAL

Derangements of Serum Electrolytes: In clinical trials of Benazepril monotherapy, hyperkalemia (serum potassium at least 0.5 mEq/L greater than the upper limit of normal) occurred in approximately 1% of hypertensive patients receiving Benazepril. In most cases, these were isolated values which resolved despite continued therapy. Risk factors for the development of hyperkalemia included renal insufficiency, diabetes mellitus, and the concomitant use of potassium-sparing diuretics, potassium supplements, and/or potassium-containing salt substitutes.

Conversely, treatment with thiazide diuretics has been associated with hypokalemia, hyponatremia, and hypochloremic alkalosis. These disturbances have sometimes been manifest as one or more or dryness of mouth, thirst, weakness, lethargy, drowsiness, restlessness, muscle pains or cramps, muscular fatigue, hypotension, oliguria, tachycardia, nausea, and vomiting. Hypokalemia can also sensitize or exaggerate the response of the heart to the toxic effects of digitalis. The risk of hypokalemia is greatest in patients with cirrhosis of the liver, in patients experiencing a brisk diuresis, in patients who are receiving inadequate oral intake of electrolytes, and in patients receiving concomitant therapy with corticosteroids or ACTH.

The opposite effects of Benazepril and Hydrochlorothiazide on serum potassium will approximately balance each other in many patients, so that no net effect upon serum potassium will be seen. In other patients, one or the other effect may be dominant. Initial and periodic determinations of serum electrolytes to detect possible electrolyte imbalance should be performed at appropriate intervals.

Chloride deficits are generally mild and require specific treatment only under extraordinary circumstances (e.g., in liver disease or renal disease). Dilutional hyponatremia may occur in edematous patients; appropriate therapy is water restriction rather than administration of salt, except in rare instances when the hyponatremia is life-threatening. In actual salt depletion, appropriate replacement is the therapy of choice.

Calcium excretion is decreased by thiazides. In a few patients on prolonged thiazide therapy, pathological changes in the parathyroid gland have been observed, with hypercalcemia and hypophosphatemia. More serious complications of hyperparathyroidism (renal lithiasis, bone resorption, and peptic ulceration) have not been seen.

Thiazides increase the urinary excretion of magnesium, and hypomagnesemia may result.

Other Metabolic Disturbances: Thiazide diuretics tend to reduce glucose tolerance and to raise serum levels of cholesterol, triglycerides, and uric acid. These effects are usually minor, but frank gout or overt diabetes may be precipitated in susceptible patients.

Cough: Presumably due to the inhibition of the degradation of endogenous bradykinin, persistent nonproductive cough has been reported with all ACE inhibitors, always resolving after discontinuation of therapy. ACE inhibitor-induced cough should be considered in the differential diagnosis of cough.

Surgery/Anesthesia: In patients undergoing surgery or during anesthesia with agents that produce hypotension, Benazepril will block the angiotensin II formation that could otherwise occur secondary to compensatory renin release. Hypotension that occurs as a result of this mechanism can be corrected by volume expansion.

INFORMATION FOR PATIENTS

Angioedema: Angioedema, including laryngeal edema, can occur with treatment with ACE inhibitors, especially following the first dose. A patient receiving Benazepril/HCTZ should be told to report immediately any signs or symptoms suggesting angioedema (swelling of face, eyes, lips, or tongue, or difficulty in breathing) and to take no more drug until after consulting with the prescribing physician.

Pregnancy: Female patients of childbearing age should be told about the consequences of second- and third-trimester exposure to ACE inhibitors, and they should also be told that these consequences do not appear to have resulted from intrauterine ACE inhibitor exposure that has been limited to the first trimester. These patients should be asked to report pregnancies to their physicians as soon as possible.

Symptomatic Hypotension: A patient receiving Benazepril/HCTZ should be cautioned that light-headedness can occur, especially during the first days of therapy, and that it should be reported to the prescribing physician. The patient should be told that if syncope occurs Benazepril/HCTZ should be discontinued until the physician has been consulted.

All patients should be cautioned that inadequate fluid intake, excessive perspiration, diarrhea, or vomiting can lead to an excessive fall in blood pressure, with the same consequences of light-headedness and possible syncope.

Hyperkalemia: A patient receiving Benazepril/HCTZ should be told not to use potassium supplements or salt substitutes containing potassium without consulting the prescribing physician.

Neutropenia: Patients should be told to promptly report any indication of infection (e.g., sore throat, fever), which could be a sign of neutropenia.

LABORATORY TESTS

The Hydrochlorothiazide component of Benazepril/HCTZ may decrease serum PBI levels without signs of thyroid disturbance.

Therapy with Benazepril/HCTZ should be interrupted for a few days before carrying out tests of parathyroid function.

DRUG INTERACTIONS

Potassium Supplements and Potassium-Sparing Diuretics: As noted above (Derangements of Serum Electrolytes), the net effect of Benazepril/HCTZ may be to elevate a patient's serum potassium, to reduce it, or to leave it unchanged. Potassium-sparing diuretics (spironolactone, amiloride, triamterene, and others) or potassium supplements can increase the risk of hyperkalemia. If concomitant use of such agents is indicated, they should be given with caution, and the patient's serum potassium should be monitored frequently.

Lithium: Increased serum lithium levels and symptoms of lithium toxicity have been reported in patients receiving ACE inhibitors during therapy with lithium. Because renal clearance of lithium is reduced by thiazides, the risk of lithium toxicity is presumably raised further when, as in therapy with Benazepril/HCTZ a thiazide diuretic is coadministered with the ACE inhibitor. Benazepril/HCTZ and lithium should be coadministered with caution, and frequent monitoring of serum lithium levels is recommended.

Other: Benazepril has been used concomitantly with beta-adrenergic-blocking agents, calcium-blocking agents, cimetidine, diuretics, digoxin, hydralazine, and naproxen without evidence of clinically important adverse interactions. Other ACE inhibitors have had less than additive effects with beta-adrenergic blockers, presumably because drugs of both classes lower blood pressure by inhibiting parts of the renin-angiotensin system.

Interaction studies with warfarin and acenocoumarol have failed to identify any clinically important effects of Benazepril on the serum concentrations or clinical effects of these anticoagulants.

Insulin requirements in diabetic patients may be increased, decreased, or unchanged.

Thiazides may decrease arterial responsiveness to norepinephrine, but not enough to preclude effectiveness of the pressor agent for therapeutic use.

Thiazides may increase the responsiveness to tubocurarine. The diuretic, natriuretic, and antihypertensive effects of thiazide diuretics may be reduced by concurrent administration of nonsteroidal anti-inflammatory agents.

Cholestyramine and colestipol resins: Absorption of hydrochlorothiazide is impaired in the presence of anionic exchange resins. Single doses of either cholestyramine or colestipol resins bind the Hydrochlorothiazide and reduce its absorption from the gastrointestinal tract by up to 85% and 43%, respectively.

CARCINOGENESIS, MUTAGENESIS, IMPAIRMENT OF FERTILITY

No evidence of carcinogenicity was found when Benazepril was given to rats and mice for 104 weeks at doses up to 150 mg/kg/day. On a body-weight basis, this dose is over 100 times the maximum recommended human dose; on a body-surface-area basis, this dose is 18 times (rats) and 9 times (mice) the maximum recommended human dose. No mutagenic activity was detected in the Ames test in bacteria (with or without metabolic activation), in an *in vitro* test for forward mutations in cultured mammalian cells, or in a nucleus anomaly test. At doses of 50-500 mg/kg/day (38-375 times the maximum recommended human dose on a body-weight basis; 6-61 times the maximum recommended dose on a body-surface-weight-area basis), Benazepril had no adverse effect on the reproductive performance of male and female rats.

Under the auspices of the National Toxicology Program, rats and mice received Hydrochlorothiazids in their feed for two years, at doses up to 600 mg/kg/day in mice and up to 100 mg/kg/day in rats. These studies uncovered no evidence of a carcinogenic potential of Hydrochlorothiazide in rats or female mice, but there was equivocal evidence of hepatocarcinogenicity in male mice. Hydrochlorothiazide was not genotoxic in *in vitro* assays using strains TA 98, TA 100, TA 1535, TA 1537, and TA 1538 of *Salmonella typhimurium* (the Ames test); in the Chinese Hamster Ovary (CHO) test for chromosomal aberrations; or in *in vivo* assays using mouse germinal cell chromosomes. Chinese hamster bone marrow chromosomes; and the *Drosophila* sex-linked recessive lethal trait gene. Positive test results were obtained in the *in vitro* CHO Sister Chromatid Exchange (clastogenicity) test and in the Mouse Lymphoma Cell (mutagenicity) assays, using concentrations of Hydrochlorothiazide of 43-1300 μg/mL. Positive test results were also obtained in the *Aspergillus nidulans* nondisjunction assay, using an unspecified concentration of Hydrochlorothiazide.

Hydrochlorothiazide had no adverse effects on the fertility of mice and rats of either sex in studies wherein these species were exposed, via their diets, to doses up to 100 and 4 mg/kg/day, respectively, prior to mating and throughout gestation.

PREGNANCY

Pregnancy Categories C first trimester and D second and third trimesters: See *"Warnings, Fatal/National Morbidity and Mortality".*

NURSING MOTHERS

Minimal amounts of unchanged Benazepril and of benazeprilat are excreted into the breast milk of lactating women treated with Benazepril, so that a newborn child ingesting nothing but breast milk would receive less than 0.1% of the maternal doses of Benazepril and benazeprilat. Thiazides, on the other hand, are definitely excreted into breast milk. Because of the potential for serious adverse reactions in nursing infants from Hydrochlorothiazide and the unknown effects of Benazepril in infants, a decision should be made whether to discontinue nursing or to discontinue Benazepril/HCTZ in U.S. clinical studies of Benazepril/HCTZ 19% were 65 or older while about 1.5% were 75 or older. Overall differences in effectiveness or safety were not observed between these patients and younger patients, and other reported clinical experience has not identified differences in responses between the elderly and younger patients, but greater sensitivity of some older individuals cannot be ruled out.

PEDIATRIC USE

Safety and effectiveness in children have not been established.

ADVERSE REACTIONS

Benazepril/HCTZ has been evaluated for safety in over 2500 patients with hypertension; over 500 of these patients were treated for at least 6 months, and over 200 were treated for more than 1 year.

The reported side effects were generally mild and transient, and there was no relationship between side effects and age, sex, race, or duration of therapy. Discontinuation of therapy due to side effects was required in approximately 7% of U.S. patients treated with Benazepril/HCTZ and in 4% of patients treated with placebo.

The most common reasons for discontinuation of therapy with Benazepril/HCTZ in U.S. studies were cough (1.0%, see *"Precautions"*), "dizziness" (1.0%), headache (0.6%), and fatigue (0.6%).

The side effects considered possibly or probably related to study drug that occurred in U.S. placebo-controlled trials in more than 1% of patients treated with Benazepril/HCTz are shown in the table below.

REACTIONS POSSIBLY OR PROBABLY DRUG RELATED

	Patients in U.S. Placebo Controlled Studies Benazepril/HCTZ N= 655		Placebo N= 235	
	N	%	N	%
"Dizziness"	41	6.3	8	3.4
Fatigue	34	5.2	6	2.6
Postural Dizziness	23	3.5	1	0.4
Headache	20	3.1	10	4.3
Cough	14	2.1	3	1.3
Hypertonia	10	1.5	3	1.3
Vertigo	10	1.5	2	0.9
Nausea	9	1.4	2	0.9
Impotence	8	1.2	0	0.0
Somnolence	8	1.2	1	0.4

Other side effects considered possibly or probably related to study drug that occurred in U.S. placebo-controlled trials in 0.3% to 1.0% of patients treated with Benazepril/HCTZ were the following:

Angioedema: Edema of the lips or face without other manifestations of angioedema (0.3%). See *"Warnings, Angioedema."*

Cardiovascular: Hypotension (seen in 0.6% of patients), postural hypotension (0.3%), palpitations, and flushing.

Gastrointestinal: Vomiting, diarrhea, dyspepsia, anorexia, and constipation.

Neurologic and Psychiatric: Insomnia, nervousness, paresthesia, libido decrease, dry mouth, taste perversion, and tinnitus.

Dermatologic: Rash and sweating.

Other: Gout, urinary frequency, arthralgia, myalgia, asthenia, and pain (including chest pain and abdominal pain). Other adverse experiences reported in 0.3% or more of Benazepril/HCTZ patients in U.S. controlled clinical trials were the following; asterisked entries occurred in more than 1% of patients (in some, causal relationship to Benazepril/HCTZ is uncertain).

Angioedema: Edema of the lips or face without other manifestations of angioedema. See *"Warnings, Angioedema."*

Cardiovascular: Syncope, peripheral vascular disorder, and tachycardia.

Body as a Whole: Infection, back pain,* flu syndrome,* fever, chills, and neck pain.

Gastrointestinal: Gastroenteritis, flatulence, and tooth disorder.

Neurologic and Psychiatric: Hypesthesia, abnormal vision, abnormal dreams, and retinal disorder.

Respiratory: Upper respiratory infection,* epistaxis, bronchitis, rhinitis,* sinusitis,* and voice alteration.

Other: Photosensitivity, conjunctivitis, arthritis, pruritus, urinary tract infection, and urinary frequency.

Fetal/Neonatal Morbidity and Mortality: See *"Warnings, Fetal/Neonatal Morbidity and Mortality".*

Monotherapy with Benazepril has been evaluated for safety in over 6000 patients. In clinical trials, the observed adverse reactions to Benazepril were similar to those seen in trials of Benazepril/HCTZ.

Hydrochlorothiazide: has been extensively prescribed for many years, but there has not been enough systematic collection of data to support an estimate of the frequency of the observed adverse reactions. Within organ-system groups, the reported reactions are listed here in decreasing order of severity, without regard to frequency.

Cardiovascular: Orthostatic hypotension (may be potentiated by alcohol, barbiturates, or narcotics).

Digestive: Pancreatitis, jaundice (intrahepatic cholestatic) (see *"Warnings")* sialadenitis, vomiting, diarrhea, cramping, nausea, gastric irritation, constipation, and anorexia.

Neurologic: Vertigo, light-headedness, transient blurred vision, headache, paresthesia, xanthopsia, weakness, and restlessness.

Musculoskeletal: Muscle spasm.

Hematologic: Aplastic anemia, agranulocytosis, leukopenia, and thrombocytopenia.

Metabolic: Hyperglycemia, glycosuria, and hyperuricemia.

Hypersensitivity: Necrotizing angiitis, Stevens-Johnson syndrome, respiratory distress (including pneumonitis and pulmonary edema) purpura, urticaria, rash, and photosensitivity.

CLINICAL LABORATORY TEST FINDINGS

Serum Electrolytes: See *"Precautions".*

Creatinine: Minor reversible increases in serum creatinine were observed in patients with essential hypertension treated with Benazepril/HCTZ. Such increases occurred most frequently in patients with renal artery stenosis (see *"Precautions").*

PBI and Tests of Parathyroid Function: See *"Precautions".*

Other (Causal Relationships Unknown): Other clinically important changes in standard laboratory tests were rarely associated with Benazepril/HCTZ administration. Elevations in blood urea nitrogen, uric acid, glucose, SGOT, and SGPT (see *"Warnings")* have been reported. In the somewhat larger patient population exposed to Benazepril monotherapy in U.S. trials, the same abnormalities were reported, together with scattered accounts of hyponatremia, melena, electrocardiographic changes, leukopenia, eosinophilia, and proteinuria.

OVERDOSAGE

No specific information is available on the treatment of overdosage with Benazepril/HCTZ treatment should be symptomatic and supportive. Therapy with Benazepril/HCTZ should be discontinued, and the patient should be observed. Dehydration electrolyte imbalance, and hypotension should be treated by established procedures.

Single oral doses of 1 g/kg of Benazepril caused reduced activity in mice, and doses of 3 g/kg were associated with significant lethality. Reduction of activity in rats is not seen until they had received doses of 5 g/kg, and doses of 6 g/kg were not lethal. In single-dose studies of Hydrochlorothiazide, most rats survived doses up to 2.75 g/kg.

Data from human overdoses of Benazepril are scanty, but the most common manifestation of human Benazepril overdosage is likely to be hypotension. In human Hydrochlorothiazide overdose, the most common signs and symptoms observed have been those of dehydration and electrolyte depletion (hypokalemia, hypochloremia, hyponatremia). If digitalis has also been administered, hypokalemia may accentuate cardiac arrhythmias.

Laboratory determinations of serum levels of Benazepril and its metabolites are not widely available, and such determinations have, in any event, no established role in the management of Benazepril overdose.

No data are available to suggest physiological maneuvers (e.g., maneuvers to change the pH of the urine) that might accelerate elimination of Benazepril and its metabolites. Benazeprilat is only slightly dialyzable, but dialysis might be considered in overdosed patients with severely impaired renal function (see *"Warnings").*

Angiotensin II could presumably serve as a specific antagonist-antidote in the setting of benazepril overdose, but angiotensin II is essentially unavailable outside of scattered research facilities. Because the hypotensive effect of Benazepril is achieved through vasodilation and effective hypovolemia, it is reasonable to treat Benazepril overdose by infusion of normal saline solution.

DOSAGE AND ADMINISTRATION

Benazepril is an effective treatment of hypertension in once-daily doses of 10-80 mg, while Hydrochlorothiazide is effective in doses of 25-100 mg. In clinical trials of Benazepril/Hydrochlorothiazide combination therapy using Benazepril doses of 5-20 mg and Hydrochlorothiazide doses of 6.25-25 mg, the antihypertensive effects increased with increasing dose of either component.

The side effects (see *"Warnings")* of Benazepril are generally rare and apparently independent of dose; those of Hydrochlorothiazide are a mixture of dose-dependent phenomena (primarily hypokalemia) and dose-independent phenomena (e.g., pancreatitis), the former much more common than the latter. Therapy with any combination of Benazepril and Hydrochlorothiazide will be associated with both sets of dose-independent side effects, but regimens in which Benazepril is combined with low doses of Hydrochlorothiazide produce minimal effects on serum potassium. In clinical trials of Benazepril/HCTZ the average change in serum potassium was near zero in subjects who received 5/6 25 mg or 20/12.5 mg, but the average subject who received 10/12.5 mg or 20/25 mg experienced a mild reduction in serum potassium, similar to that experienced by the average subject receiving the same dose of Hydrochlorothiazide monotherapy.

To minimize dose-independent side effects, it is usually appropriate to begin combination therapy only after a patient has failed to achieve the desired effect with monotherapy.

Therapy Guided by Clinical Effect: A patient whose blood pressure is not adequately controlled with Benazepril monotherapy may be switched to Benazepril/HCTZ 10/12.5 or Benazepril/HCTZ 20/12.5. Further increases of either or both components could depend on clinical response. The Hydrochlorothiazide dose should generally not be increased until 2-3 weeks have elapsed. Patients whose blood pressures are adequately controlled with 25 mg of daily Hydrochlorothiazide, but who experience significant potassium loss with this regimen, may achieve similar blood-pressure control without electrolyte disturbance if they are switched to Benazepril/HCTZ 5/6.25.

Replacement Therapy: The combination may be substituted for the titrated individual components.

Use in Renal Impairment: Regimens of therapy with Benazepril/HCTZ need not take account of renal function as long as the patient's creatinine clearance is > 30 mL/min/1.73m^2 (serum creatinine roughly ≤ 3 mg/dL or 265 μ mol/L). In patients with more severe renal impairment, loop diuretics are preferred to thiazides, so Benazepril/HCTZ is not recommended (see *"Warnings"*).

Storage: Do not store above 86°F (30°C). Protect from moisture and light. Dispense in tight, light-resistant container (USP).

HOW SUPPLIED
TABLETS: 5 MG-6.25 MG

BRAND/MANUFACTURER	NDC	SIZE	AWP
○ **BRAND**			
▶ LOTENSIN HCT: Ciba Pharm	00083-0057-30	100s	$63.63

TABLETS: 10 MG-12.5 MG

BRAND/MANUFACTURER	NDC	SIZE	AWP
○ **BRAND**			
▶ LOTENSIN HCT: Ciba Pharm	00083-0072-30	100s	$63.63

TABLETS: 20 MG-12.5 MG

BRAND/MANUFACTURER	NDC	SIZE	AWP
○ **BRAND**			
▶ LOTENSIN HCT: Ciba Pharm	00083-0074-30	100s	$63.63

TABLETS: 20 MG-25 MG

BRAND/MANUFACTURER	NDC	SIZE	AWP
○ **BRAND**			
▶ LOTENSIN HCT: Ciba Pharm	00083-0075-30	100s	$63.63

Bendroflumethiazide and Nadolol

DESCRIPTION
Bendroflumethiazide/Nadolol for oral administration combines two antihypertensive agents: Nadolol, a nonselective beta-adrenergic blocking agent, and Bendroflumethiazide, a thiazide diuretic-antihypertensive.

NADOLOL
Nadolol is a white crystalline powder. It is freely soluble in ethanol, soluble in hydrochloric acid, slightly soluble in water and in chloroform, and very slightly soluble in sodium hydroxide.

Nadolol is designated chemically as 1-(*tert*-butylamino) -3-[(5,6,7,8-tetrahydro-*cis*-6,7-dihydroxy-1-naphthyl)oxy]-2-propanol.

The molecular formula of Nadolol is $C_{17}H_{27}NO_4$ and its molecular weight is 309.40. The CAS number is 42200-33-9.

BENDROFLUMETHIAZIDE
Bendroflumethiazide is a white crystalline powder. It is soluble in alcohol and in sodium hydroxide, and insoluble in hydrochloric acid, water, and chloroform.

Bendroflumethiazide is designated chemically as 3-benzyl-3,4-dihydro-6-(trifluoromethyl)-2*H*-1,2,4- benzothiadiazine-7-sulfonamide 1,1-dioxide.

The molecular formula of Bendroflumethiazide is $C_{15}H_{14}F_3N_3O_4S_2$ and molecular weight is 421.41. The CAS number is 73-48-3.

CLINICAL PHARMACOLOGY
NADOLOL
Nadolol is a nonselective beta-adrenergic receptor blocking agent. Clinical pharmacology studies have demonstrated beta-blocking activity by showing (1) reduction in heart rate and cardiac output at rest and on exercise, (2) reduction of systolic and diastolic blood pressure at rest and on exercise, (3) inhibition of

isoproterenol-induced tachycardia, and (4) reduction of reflex orthostatic tachycardia.

Nadolol specifically competes with beta-adrenergic receptor agonists for available beta receptor sites; it inhibits both the beta$_1$ receptors located chiefly in cardiac muscle and the beta$_2$ receptors located chiefly in the bronchial and vascular musculature, inhibiting the chronotropic, inotropic, and vasodilator responses to beta-adrenergic stimulation proportionately. Nadolol has no intrinsic sympathomimetic activity and, unlike some other beta-adrenergic blocking agents, Nadolol has little direct myocardial depressant activity and does not have an anesthetic-like membrane-stabilizing action. Animal and human studies show that Nadolol slows the sinus rate and depresses AV conduction. In dogs, only minimal amounts of Nadolol were detected in the brain relative to amounts in blood and other organs and tissues. Nadolol has low lipophilicity as determined by octanol/water partition coefficient, a characteristic of certain beta-blocking agents that has been correlated with the limited extent to which these agents cross the blood-brain barrier, their low concentration in the brain, and low incidence of CNS-related side effects.

In controlled clinical studies, Nadolol at doses of 40 to 320 mg/day has been shown to decrease both standing and supine blood pressure, the effect persisting for approximately 24 hours after dosing.

The mechanism of the antihypertensive effects of beta-adrenergic receptor blocking agents has not been established; however, factors that may be involved include (1) competitive antagonism of catecholamines at peripheral (non-CNS) adrenergic neuron sites (especially cardiac) leading to decreased cardiac output, (2) a central effect leading to reduced tonic-sympathetic nerve outflow to the periphery, and (3) suppression of renin secretion by blockade of the beta-adrenergic receptors responsible for renin release from the kidneys.

While cardiac output and arterial pressure are reduced by Nadolol therapy, renal hemodynamics are stable, with preservation of renal blood flow and glomerular filtration rate.

By blocking catecholamine-induced increases in heart rate, velocity and extent of myocardial contraction, and blood pressure, Nadolol generally reduces the oxygen requirements of the heart at any given level of effort, making it useful for many patients in the long-term management of angina pectoris. On the other hand, Nadolol can increase oxygen requirements by increasing left ventricular fiber length and end diastolic pressure, particularly in patients with heart failure.

Although beta-adrenergic receptor blockade is useful in treatment of angina and hypertension, there are also situations in which sympathetic stimulation is vital. For example, in patients with severely damaged hearts, adequate ventricular function may depend on sympathetic drive. Beta-adrenergic blockade may worsen AV block by preventing the necessary facilitating effects of sympathetic activity on conduction. Beta$_2$-adrenergic blockade results in passive bronchial constriction by interfering with endogenous adrenergic bronchodilator activity in patients subject to bronchospasm and may also interfere with exogenous bronchodilators in such patients.

Absorption of Nadolol after oral dosing is variable, averaging about 30%. Peak serum concentrations of Nadolol usually occur in 3 to 4 hours after oral administration and the presence of food in the gastrointestinal tract does not affect the rate or extent of Nadolol absorption. Approximately 30% of the Nadolol present in serum is reversibly bound to plasma protein.

Unlike many other beta-adrenergic blocking agents, Nadolol is not metabolized by the liver and is excreted unchanged, principally by the kidneys.

The half-life of therapeutic doses of Nadolol is about 20 to 24 hours, permitting once-daily dosage. Because Nadolol is excreted predominantly in the urine, its half-life increases in renal failure (see *"Precautions, General,"* and *"Dosage and Administration"*). Steady state serum concentrations of Nadolol are attained in 6 to 9 days with once-daily dosage in persons with normal renal function. Because of variable absorption and different individual responsiveness, the proper dosage must be determined by titration.

Exacerbation of angina and, in some cases, myocardial infarction and ventricular dysrhythmias have been reported after abrupt discontinuation of therapy with beta-adrenergic blocking agents in patients with coronary artery disease. Abrupt withdrawal of these agents in patients without coronary artery disease has resulted in transient symptoms, including tremulousness, sweating, palpitation, headache, and malaise. Several mechanisms have been proposed to explain these phenomena, among them increased sensitivity to catecholamines because of increased numbers of beta receptors.

BENDROFLUMETHIAZIDE
The mechanism of action of Bendroflumethiazide results in an interference with the renal tubular mechanism of electrolyte reabsorption. At maximal therapeutic dosage all thiazides are approximately equal in their diuretic potency.

Thiazides increase excretion of sodium and chloride in approximately equivalent amounts. Natriuresis causes a secondary loss of potassium and bicarbonate.

The mechanism of the antihypertensive effect of thiazides is unknown. Thiazides do not affect normal blood pressure.

Onset of action of thiazides occurs in 2 hours and the peak effect at about 4 hours. Duration of action persists for approximately 6 to 12 hours. Thiazides are eliminated rapidly by the kidney.

INDICATIONS
Bendroflumethiazide/Nadolol is indicated in the management of hypertension.

This fixed combination drug is not indicated for initial therapy of hypertension. If the fixed combination represents the dose titrated to the individual patient's needs, it may be more convenient than the separate components.

CONTRAINDICATIONS

NADOLOL

Nadolol is contraindicated in bronchial asthma, sinus bradycardia and greater than first degree conduction block, cardiogenic shock, and overt cardiac failure (see *"Warnings"*).

BENDROFLUMETHIAZIDE

Bendroflumethiazide is contraindicated in anuria. It is also contraindicated in patients who have previously demonstrated hypersensitivity to Bendroflumethiazide or other sulfonamide-derived drugs.

WARNINGS

NADOLOL

Cardiac Failure: Sympathetic stimulation may be a vital component supporting circulatory function in patients with congestive heart failure, and its inhibition by beta-blockade may precipitate more severe failure. Although beta-blockers should be avoided in overt congestive heart failure, if necessary, they can be used with caution in patients with a history of failure who are well compensated, usually with digitalis and diuretics. Beta-adrenergic blocking agents do not abolish the inotropic action of digitalis on heart muscle.

In Patients Without a History of Heart Failure, continued use of beta-blockers can, in some cases, lead to cardiac failure. Therefore, at the first sign or symptom of heart failure, the patient should be digitalized and/or treated with diuretics, and the response observed closely, or Nadolol should be discontinued (gradually, if possible).

EXACERBATION OF ISCHEMIC HEART DISEASE FOLLOWING ABRUPT WITHDRAWAL

HYPERSENSITIVITY TO CATECHOLAMINES HAS BEEN OBSERVED IN PATIENTS WITHDRAWN FROM BETA-BLOCKER THERAPY; EXACERBATION OF ANGINA AND, IN SOME CASES, MYOCARDIAL INFARCTION HAVE OCCURRED AFTER *ABRUPT* DISCONTINUATION OF SUCH THERAPY. WHEN DISCONTINUING CHRONICALLY ADMINISTERED NADOLOL, PARTICULARLY IN PATIENTS WITH ISCHEMIC HEART DISEASE, THE DOSAGE SHOULD BE GRADUALLY REDUCED OVER A PERIOD OF 1 TO 2 WEEKS AND THE PATIENT SHOULD BE CAREFULLY MONITORED. IF ANGINA MARKEDLY WORSENS OR ACUTE CORONARY INSUFFICIENCY DEVELOPS, NADOLOL ADMINISTRATION SHOULD BE REINSTITUTED PROMPTLY, AT LEAST TEMPORARILY, AND OTHER MEASURES APPROPRIATE FOR THE MANAGEMENT OF UNSTABLE ANGINA SHOULD BE TAKEN. PATIENTS SHOULD BE WARNED AGAINST INTERRUPTION OR DISCONTINUATION OF THERAPY WITHOUT THE PHYSICIAN'S ADVICE. BECAUSE CORONARY ARTERY DISEASE IS COMMON AND MAY BE UNRECOGNIZED, IT MAY BE PRUDENT NOT TO DISCONTINUE NADOLOL THERAPY ABRUPTLY EVEN IN PATIENTS TREATED ONLY FOR HYPERTENSION.

Nonallergic Bronchospasm (eg, chronic bronchitis, emphysema): PATIENTS WITH BRONCHOSPASTIC DISEASES SHOULD IN GENERAL NOT RECEIVE BETA-BLOCKERS. Nadolol should be administered with caution since it may block bronchodilation produced by endogenous or exogenous catecholamine stimulation of beta$_2$ receptors.

Major Surgery: Because beta blockade impairs the ability of the heart to respond to reflex stimuli and may increase the risks of general anesthesia and surgical procedures, resulting in protracted hypotension or low cardiac output, it has generally been suggested that such therapy should be withdrawn several days prior to surgery. Recognition of the increased sensitivity to catecholamines of patients recently withdrawn from beta-blocker therapy, however, has made this recommendation controversial. If possible, beta-blockers should be withdrawn well before surgery takes place. In the event of emergency surgery, the anesthesiologist should be informed that the patient is on beta-blocker therapy. The effects of Nadolol can be reversed by administration of beta-receptor agonists such as isoproterenol, dopamine, dobutamine, or levarterenol. Difficulty in restarting and maintaining the heart beat has also been reported with beta-adrenergic receptor blocking agents.

Diabetes and Hypoglycemia: Beta-adrenergic blockade may prevent the appearance of premonitory signs and symptoms (eg, tachycardia and blood pressure changes) of acute hypoglycemia. This is especially important with labile diabetics.

Beta-blockade also reduces the release of insulin in response to hyperglycemia; therefore, it may be necessary to adjust the dose of antidiabetic drugs.

Thyrotoxicosis: Beta-adrenergic blockade may mask certain clinical signs (eg, tachycardia) of hyperthyroidism. Patients suspected of developing thyrotoxicosis should be managed carefully to avoid abrupt withdrawal of beta-adrenergic blockade which might precipitate a thyroid storm.

BENDROFLUMETHIAZIDE

Thiazides should be used with caution in severe renal disease. In patients with renal disease, thiazides may precipitate azotemia. Cumulative effects of the drug may develop in patients with impaired renal function.

Thiazides should be used with caution in patients with impaired hepatic function or progressive liver disease, since minor alterations of fluid and electrolyte balance may precipitate hepatic coma.

Sensitivity reactions may occur in patients with or without a history of allergy or bronchial asthma.

The possibility of exacerbation or activation of systemic lupus erythematosus has been reported.

Lithium generally should not be given with diuretics; diuretic agents reduce the renal clearance of lithium and add a high risk of lithium toxicity. Refer to the package insert for lithium preparations before use of such concomitant therapy.

PRECAUTIONS

GENERAL

NADOLOL

Nadolol should be used with caution in patients with impaired renal function (see *"Dosage and Administration"*).

BENDROFLUMETHIAZIDE

Periodic determination of serum electrolytes to detect possible electrolyte imbalance should be performed at appropriate intervals.

All patients receiving thiazide therapy should be observed for clinical signs of fluid or electrolyte imbalance, namely: hyponatremia, hypochloremic alkalosis, and hypokalemia. Serum and urine electrolyte determinations are particularly important when the patient is vomiting excessively or receiving parenteral fluids. Warning signs or symptoms of fluid and electrolyte imbalance may include: dryness of the mouth, thirst, weakness, lethargy, drowsiness, restlessness, muscle pains or cramps, muscular fatigue, hypotension, oliguria, tachycardia, and gastrointestinal disturbances, such as nausea and vomiting.

Hypokalemia may develop especially with brisk diuresis or when severe cirrhosis is present.

Interference with adequate oral electrolyte intake will also contribute to hypokalemia. Hypokalemia can sensitize or exaggerate the response of the heart to the toxic effects of digitalis (eg, increased ventricular irritability). Concurrent administration of a potassium sparing diuretic or potassium supplements may be indicated in these patients.

Any chloride deficit is generally mild and usually does not require specific treatment except under extraordinary circumstances (as in liver disease or renal disease). Dilutional hyponatremia may occur in edematous patients in hot weather; appropriate therapy is water restriction, rather than administration of salt except in rare instances when the hyponatremia is life threatening. In actual salt depletion, appropriate replacement is the therapy of choice.

Hyperuricemia may occur or frank gout may be precipitated in certain patients receiving thiazide therapy.

Latent diabetes mellitus may become manifest during thiazide administration.

The antihypertensive effect of thiazide diuretics may be enhanced in the postsympathectomy patient.

If progressive renal impairment becomes evident, as indicated by a rising nonprotein nitrogen or blood urea nitrogen (BUN), a careful reappraisal of therapy is necessary with consideration given to withholding or discontinuing diuretic therapy.

Thiazides may decrease serum PBI levels without signs of thyroid disturbance.

Calcium excretion is decreased by thiazides. Pathological changes in the parathyroid gland with hypercalcemia and hypophosphatemia have been observed in a few patients on prolonged thiazide therapy. The common complications of hyperparathyroidism such as renal lithiasis, bone resorption, and peptic ulceration have not been seen. Thiazides should be discontinued before carrying out tests for parathyroid function.

Thiazides have been shown to increase the urinary excretion of magnesium; this may result in hypomagnesemia.

INFORMATION FOR PATIENTS

Patients, especially those with evidence of coronary artery insufficiency, should be warned against interruption or discontinuation of therapy without the physician's advice. Although cardiac failure rarely occurs in properly selected patients, patients being treated with beta-adrenergic blocking agents should be advised to consult the physician at the first sign or symptom of impending failure.

The patient should also be advised of a proper course in the event of an inadvertently missed dose.

The patient should be informed of symptoms that would suggest potential adverse effects and told to report them promptly.

LABORATORY TESTS

Serum electrolyte levels should be regularly monitored (see *"Warnings, Bendroflumethiazide,"* also *"Precautions, General, Bendroflumethiazide"*).

DRUG INTERACTIONS

NADOLOL

When administered concurrently the following drugs may interact with beta-adrenergic receptor blocking agents:

Anesthetics, General: exaggeration of the hypotension induced by general anesthetics (see *"Warnings, Nadolol, Major Surgery"*).

Antidiabetic Drugs (Oral Agents and Insulin): hypoglycemia or hyperglycemia; adjust dosage of antidiabetic drug accordingly (see *"Warnings, Nadolol, Diabetes and Hypoglycemia"*).

Catecholamine-depleting Drugs (eg, reserpine): additive effect; monitor closely for evidence of hypotension and/or excessive bradycardia (eg, vertigo, syncope, postural hypotension).

◆ RATED THERAPEUTICALLY EQUIVALENT; ◇ THERAPEUTIC EQUIVALENCE UNCONFIRMED; ○ UNRATED

Response to Treatment for Anaphylactic Reaction: While taking beta-blockers, patients with a history of severe anaphylactic reaction to a variety of allergens may be more reactive to repeated challenge, either accidental, diagnostic, or therapeutic. Such patients may be unresponsive to the unusual doses of epinephrine used to treat allergic reaction.

BENDROFLUMETHIAZIDE

When administered concurrently, the following drugs may interact with Bendroflumethiazide:

Alcohol, Barbiturates, or Narcotics: potentiation of orthostatic hypotension may occur.

Amphotericin B, Corticosteroids, or Corticotropin (ACTH): may intensify electrolyte imbalance, particularly hypokalemia. Monitor potassium levels; use potassium replacements if necessary.

Anticoagulants (Oral): dosage adjustments of anticoagulant medication may be necessary since Bendroflumethiazide may decrease their effects.

Antigout Medications: dosage adjustments of antigout medication may be necessary since Bendroflumethiazide may raise the level of blood uric acid.

Other Antihypertensive Medications (eg, ganglionic or peripheral adrenergic blocking agents): dosage adjustments may be necessary since Bendroflumethiazide may potentiate their effects.

Antidiabetic Drugs (Oral Agents and Insulin): since thiazides may elevate blood glucose levels, dosage adjustments of antidiabetic agents may be necessary.

Calcium Salts: increased serum calcium levels due to decreased excretion may occur. If calcium must be prescribed monitor serum calcium levels and adjust calcium dosage accordingly.

Cardiac Glycosides: enhanced possibility of digitalis toxicity associated with hypokalemia. Monitor potassium levels; use potassium replacement if necessary.

Cholestyramine Resin and Colestipol HCL: may delay or decrease absorption of Bendroflumethiazide. Sulfonamide diuretics should be taken at least 1 hour before or 4 to 6 hours after these medications.

Diazoxide: enhanced hyperglycemic, hyperuricemic, and antihypertensive effects. Be cognizant of possible interaction; monitor blood glucose and serum uric acid levels.

Lithium Salts: may enhance lithium toxicity due to reduced renal clearance. Avoid concurrent use; if lithium must be prescribed monitor serum lithium levels and adjust lithium dosage accordingly (see *"Warnings"*).

MAO Inhibitors: dosage adjustments of one or both agents may be necessary since hypotensive effects are enhanced.

Nondepolarizing Muscle Relaxants, Preanesthetics and Anesthetics Used in Surgery (eg, tubocurarine chloride and gallamine triethiodide): effects of these agents may be potentiated; dosage adjustments may be required. Monitor and correct any fluid and electrolyte imbalances prior to surgery if feasible.

Nonsteroidal Anti-inflammatory Agents: in some patients the administration of a nonsteroidal anti-inflammatory agent can reduce the diuretic, natriuretic, and antihypertensive effect of loop, potassium-sparing or thiazide diuretics. Therefore, when Bendroflumethiazide and nonsteroidal anti-inflammatory agents are used concomitantly, the patient should be observed closely to determine if the desired effect of the diuretic is obtained.

Methenamine: possible decrease effectiveness due to alkalinization of the urine.

Pressor Amines (eg, Norepinephrine): decreased arterial responsiveness, but not sufficient to preclude effectiveness of the pressor agent for therapeutic use. Use caution in patients taking both medications who undergo surgery. Administer preanesthetic and anesthetic agents in reduced dosage and if possible, discontinue Bendroflumethiazide 1 week prior to surgery.

Probenecid or Sulfinpyrazone: increased dosage of these agents may be necessary since Bendroflumethiazide may have hyperuricemic effects.

DRUG/LABORATORY TEST INTERACTIONS

Bendroflumethiazide may produce false-negative results with the phentolamine and tyramine tests; may interfere with the phenosulfonphthalein test due to decreased excretion; and it may cause diagnostic interference of serum electrolyte levels, blood and urine glucose levels, and a decrease in serum PBI levels without signs of thyroid disturbance.

CARCINOGENESIS, MUTAGENESIS, IMPAIRMENT OF FERTILITY
NADOLOL

In chronic oral toxicologic studies (1 to 2 years) in mice, rats, and dogs, Nadolol did not produce any significant toxic effects. In 2-year oral carcinogenicity studies in rats and mice, Nadolol did not produce any neoplastic, preneoplastic, or nonneoplastic pathologic lesions. In fertility and general reproductive performance studies in rats, Nadolol caused no adverse effect.

BENDROFLUMETHIAZIDE

Studies have not been performed to evaluate carcinogenic potential, mutagenesis, or whether this drug adversely affects fertility in males or females.

PREGNANCY—TERATOGENIC EFFECTS
NADOLOL

Category C: In animal reproduction studies with Nadolol, evidence of embryo- and fetotoxicity was found in rabbits, but not in rats or hamsters, at doses 5 to 10

times greater (on a mg/kg basis) than the maximum indicated human dose. No teratogenic potential was observed in any of these species. There are no adequate and well-controlled studies in pregnant women. Nadolol should be used during pregnancy only if the potential benefit justifies the potential risk to the fetus. Neonates whose mothers are receiving Nadolol at parturition have exhibited bradycardia, hypoglycemia, and associated symptoms.

BENDROFLUMETHIAZIDE

Category C: Animal reproduction studies have not been conducted with Bendroflumethiazide. It is also not known whether this drug can cause fetal harm when administered to a pregnant woman or can affect reproduction capacity. Bendroflumethiazide should be given to a pregnant woman only if clearly needed.

PREGNANCY—NONTERATOGENIC EFFECTS

Thiazides cross the placental barrier and appear in cord blood. The use of thiazides in pregnant women requires that the anticipated benefit be weighed against possible hazards to the fetus. These hazards include fetal or neonatal jaundice, thrombocytopenia, and possibly other adverse reactions which have occurred in the adult.

NURSING MOTHERS

Both Nadolol and Bendroflumethiazide are excreted in human milk. Because of the potential for serious adverse reactions in nursing infants from both drugs, a decision should be made whether to discontinue nursing or to discontinue therapy taking into account the importance of Bendroflumethiazide/Nadolol to the mother.

PEDIATRIC USE

Safety and effectiveness in children have not been established.

ADVERSE REACTIONS
NADOLOL

Most adverse effects have been mild and transient and have rarely required withdrawal of therapy.

Cardiovascular: Bradycardia with heart rates of less than 60 beats per minute occurs commonly, and heart rates below 40 beats per minute and/or symptomatic bradycardia were seen in about 2 of 100 patients. Symptoms of peripheral vascular insufficiency, usually of the Raynaud type, have occurred in approximately 2 of 100 patients. Cardiac failure, hypotension, and rhythm/conduction disturbances have each occurred in about 1 of 100 patients. Single instances of first degree and third degree heart block have been reported; intensification of AV block is a known effect of beta-blockers (see also *"Contraindications," "Warnings,"* and *"Precautions"*).

Central Nervous System: Dizziness or fatigue has been reported in approximately 2 of 100 patients; paresthesias, sedation, and change in behavior have each been reported in approximately 6 of 1000 patients.

Respiratory: Bronchospasm has been reported in approximately 1 of 1000 patients (see *"Contraindications"* and *"Warnings"*).

Gastrointestinal: Nausea, diarrhea, abdominal discomfort, constipation, vomiting, indigestion, anorexia, bloating, and flatulence have been reported in 1 to 5 of 1000 patients.

Miscellaneous: Each of the following has been reported in 1 to 5 of 1000 patients: rash; pruritus; headache; dry mouth, eyes, or skin; impotence or decreased libido; facial swelling; weight gain; slurred speech; cough; nasal stuffiness; sweating; tinnitus; blurred vision. Reversible alopecia has been reported infrequently.

The following adverse reactions have been reported in patients taking Nadolol and/or other beta-adrenergic blocking agents, but no causal relationship to Nadolol has been established.

Central Nervous System: Reversible mental depression progressing to catatonia; visual disturbances; hallucinations; an acute reversible syndrome characterized by disorientation for time and place, short-term memory loss, emotional lability with slightly clouded sensorium, and decreased performance on neuropsychometrics.

Gastrointestinal: Mesenteric arterial thrombosis; ischemic colitis; elevated liver enzymes.

Hematologic: Agranulocytosis; thrombocytopenic or nonthrombocytopenic purpura.

Allergic: Fever combined with aching and sore throat; laryngospasm; respiratory distress.

Miscellaneous: Pemphigoid rash; hypertensive reaction in patients with pheochromocytoma; sleep disturbances; Peyronie's disease.

The oculomucocutaneous syndrome associated with the beta-blocker practolol has not been reported with Nadolol.

BENDROFLUMETHIAZIDE

Gastrointestinal System: nausea, vomiting, cramping and anorexia are not uncommon; diarrhea, constipation, gastric irritation, abdominal bloating, jaundice (intrahepatic cholestatic jaundice), hepatitis, and sialadenitis occasionally-occur; and pancreatitis has been reported.

Central Nervous System: dizziness, vertigo, paresthesia, headache, and xanthopsia occasionally occur.

Hematologic: leukopenia, agranulocytosis, thrombocytopenia, hemolytic anemia, and aplastic anemia have been reported.

Dermatologic Hypersensitivity: purpura, exfoliative dermatitis, pruritus, ecchymosis, urticaria, necrotizing, angiitis (vasculitis, cutaneous vasculitis), respiratory distress including pneumonitis, fever, and anaphylactic reactions occasionally occur; photosensitivity and rash have been reported.

Cardiovascular: Orthostatic hypotension may occur and may be potentiated by coadministration with certain other drugs (eg, alcohol, barbiturates, narcotics, other antihypertensive medications, etc.; see *"Precautions, Drug Interactions".*)

Other: muscle spasm, weakness, or restlessness is not uncommon; hyperglycemia, glycosuria, metabolic acidosis in diabetic patients, hyperuricemia, allergic glomerulonephritis, and transient blurred vision occasionally occur.

Whenever adverse reactions are moderate or severe, thiazide dosage should be reduced or therapy withdrawn.

OVERDOSAGE

In the event of overdosage, Nadolol may cause excessive bradycardia, cardiac failure, hypotension, or bronchospasm. In addition to the expected diuresis, overdosage of Bendroflumethiazide may produce varying degrees of lethargy which may progress to coma with minimal depression of respiration and cardiovascular function and without significant serum electrolyte changes or dehydration. The mechanism of thiazide-induced CNS depression is unknown. Gastrointestinal irritation may occur. Transitory increase in BUN has been reported, and serum electrolyte changes may occur, especially in patients with impaired renal function.

TREATMENT

Nadolol can be removed from the general circulation by hemodialysis. In determining the duration of corrective therapy, note must be taken of the long duration of the effect of Nadolol. In addition to gastric lavage, the following measures should be employed, as appropriate.

Excessive Bradycardia: Administer atropine (0.25 to 1.0 mg). If there is no response to vagal blockade, administer isoproterenol cautiously.

Cardiac Failure: Administer a digitalis glycoside and diuretic. It has been reported that glucagon may also be useful in this situation.

Hypotension: Administer vasopressors, eg, epinephrine or levarterenol. (There is evidence that epinephrine may be the drug of choice.)

Bronchospasm: Administer a beta₂-stimulating agent and/or a theophylline derivative.

Stupor or Coma: Supportive therapy as warranted.

Gastrointestinal Effects: Symptomatic treatment as needed.

BUN and/or Serum Electrolyte Abnormalities: Institute supportive measures as required to maintain hydration, electrolyte balance, respiration, and cardiovascular and renal function.

DOSAGE AND ADMINISTRATION

DOSAGE MUST BE INDIVIDUALIZED (SEE *"INDICATIONS"*). BENDROFLUMETHIAZIDE/NADOLOL MAY BE ADMINISTERED WITHOUT REGARD TO MEALS.

Bendroflumethiazide is usually given at a dose of 5 mg daily. The usual initial dose of Nadolol is 40 mg once daily whether used alone or in combination with a diuretic. Bendroflumethiazide in Bendroflumethiazide/Nadolol is 30% more bioavailable than that of 5 mg Bendroflumethiazide tablets. Conversion from 5 mg Bendroflumethiazide to Bendroflumethiazide/Nadolol represents a 30% increase in dose of Bendroflumethiazide.

The initial dose of Bendroflumethiazide/Nadolol may therefore be the 40 mg/5 mg tablet once daily. When the antihypertensive response is not satisfactory, the dose may be increased by administering the 80 mg/5 mg tablet once daily.

When necessary, another antihypertensive agent may be added gradually beginning with 50% of the usual recommended starting dose to avoid an excessive fall in blood pressure.

Dosage Adjustment in Renal Failure: Absorbed Nadolol is excreted principally by the kidneys and, although nonrenal elimination does occur, dosage adjustments are necessary in patients with renal impairment. The following dose intervals are recommended:

Creatinine Clearance (ml/min/1.73m²)	Dosage Interval (hours)
> 50	24
31-50	24-36
10-30	24-48
< 10	40-60

STORAGE

Keep bottle tightly closed. Store at room temperature; avoid excessive heat.

HOW SUPPLIED
TABLETS: 5 MG-40 MG

BRAND/MANUFACTURER	NDC	SIZE	AWP
○ BRAND			
CORZIDE 40/5: Bristol Labs	00003-0283-50	100s	$124.90

TABLETS: 5 MG-80 MG

BRAND/MANUFACTURER	NDC	SIZE	AWP
○ BRAND			
CORZIDE 80/5: Bristol Labs	00003-0284-50	100s	$164.78

Bendroflumethiazide

DESCRIPTION

Bendroflumethiazide is a benzothiadiazine derivative containing a benzyl and a trifluoromethyl group. It is a potent oral diuretic and antihypertensive agent. Bendroflumethiazide is designated chemically as 3-benzyl-3,4-dihydro-6-(trifluoromethyl)-2H-1,2,4-benzothiadia- zine-7-sulfonamide 1,1-dioxide.

It has a chemical formula of $C_{15}H_{14}F_3N_3O_4S_2$ and a molecular weight of 421.41.

It is available as tablets providing 5 or 10 mg Bendroflumethiazide.

Following is its chemical structure:

CLINICAL PHARMACOLOGY

Thiazides affect the renal tubular mechanism of electrolyte reabsorption. At maximal therapeutic dosage all thiazides are approximately equal in their diuretic potency.

Thiazides increase excretion of sodium and chloride in approximately equivalent amounts. Natriuresis causes a secondary loss of potassium and bicarbonate.

The mechanism of the antihypertensive effect of thiazides is unknown. Thiazides do not affect normal blood pressure.

Onset of action of thiazides occurs in two hours and the peak effect at about four hours. Duration of action persists for approximately six to 12 hours. Thiazides are eliminated rapidly by the kidney.

INDICATIONS AND USAGE

Bendroflumethiazide is indicated as adjunctive therapy in edema associated with congestive heart failure, hepatic cirrhosis, and corticosteroid and estrogen therapy.

Bendroflumethiazide has also been found useful in edema due to various forms of renal dysfunction such as: nephrotic syndrome, acute glomerulonephritis, and chronic renal failure.

Bendroflumethiazide tablets are indicated in the management of hypertension either as the sole therapeutic agent or to enhance the effectiveness of other antihypertensive drugs in the more severe forms of hypertension.

Usage in Pregnancy: The routine use of diuretics in an otherwise healthy woman is inappropriate and exposes mother and fetus to unnecessary hazard. Diuretics do not prevent development of toxemia of pregnancy, and there is no satisfactory evidence that they are useful in the treatment of developed toxemia.

Edema during pregnancy may arise from pathological causes or from the physiologic and mechanical consequences of pregnancy. Thiazides are indicated in pregnancy when edema is due to pathologic causes, just as they are in the absence of pregnancy (however, see *"Precautions, Pregnancy: Nonteratogenic Effects"* below). Dependent edema in pregnancy, resulting from restriction of venous return by the expanded uterus, is properly treated through elevation of the lower extremities and use of support hose; use of diuretics to lower intravascular volume in this case is illogical and unnecessary. There is hypervolemia during normal pregnancy which is harmful to neither the fetus nor the mother (in the absence of cardiovascular disease), but which is associated with edema, including generalized edema, in the majority of pregnant women. If this edema produces discomfort, increased recumbency will often provide relief. In rare instances, this edema may cause extreme discomfort which is not relieved by rest. In these cases, a short course of diuretics may provide relief and may be appropriate.

CONTRAINDICATIONS

Bendroflumethiazide is contraindicated in anuria.

It is also contraindicated in patients who have previously demonstrated hypersensitivity to it or other sulfonamide-derived drugs.

WARNINGS

Thiazides should be used with caution in severe renal disease. In patients with renal disease, thiazides may precipitate azotemia. Cumulative effects of the drug may develop in patients with impaired renal function.

Thiazides should be used with caution in patients with impaired hepatic function or progressive liver disease, since minor alterations of fluid and electrolyte balance may precipitate hepatic coma.

Sensitivity reactions may occur in patients with or without a history of allergy or bronchial asthma.

The possibility of exacerbation or activation of systemic lupus erythematosus has been reported.

◆ RATED THERAPEUTICALLY EQUIVALENT; ◇ THERAPEUTIC EQUIVALENCE UNCONFIRMED; ○ UNRATED

Lithium generally should not be given with diuretics; diuretic agents reduce the renal clearance of lithium and add a high risk of lithium toxicity. Refer to the package insert for lithium preparations before use of such concomitant therapy.

PRECAUTIONS

GENERAL
Periodic determination of serum electrolytes to detect possible electrolyte imbalance should be performed at appropriate intervals.

All patients receiving thiazide therapy should be observed for clinical signs of fluid or electrolyte imbalance, namely: hyponatremia, hypochloremic alkalosis, and hypokalemia. Serum and urine electrolyte determinations are particularly important when the patient is vomiting excessively or receiving parenteral fluids. Warning signs or symptoms of fluid and electrolyte imbalance may include: dryness of the mouth, thirst, weakness, lethargy, drowsiness, restlessness, muscle pains or cramps, muscular fatigue, hypotension, oliguria, tachycardia, and gastrointestinal disturbances such as nausea and vomiting.

Hypokalemia may develop, especially with brisk diuresis or when severe cirrhosis is present.

Interference with adequate oral electrolyte intake will also contribute to hypokalemia. Hypokalemia can sensitize or exaggerate the response of the heart to the toxic effects of digitalis (e.g., increased ventricular irritability). Concurrent administration of a potassium-sparing diuretic or potassium supplements may be indicated in these patients.

Any chloride deficit is generally mild and usually does not require specific treatment except under extraordinary circumstances (as in liver disease or renal disease). Dilutional hyponatremia may occur in edematous patients in hot weather; appropriate therapy is water restriction, rather than administration of salt, except in rare instances when the hyponatremia is life threatening. In actual salt depletion, appropriate replacement is the therapy of choice.

Hyperuricemia may occur or frank gout may be precipitated in certain patients receiving thiazide therapy.

Latent diabetes mellitus may become manifest during thiazide administration.

The antihypertensive effect of thiazide diuretics may be enhanced in the postsympathectomy patient.

If progressive renal impairment becomes evident, as indicated by a rising nonprotein nitrogen or blood urea nitrogen (BUN), a careful reappraisal of therapy is necessary with consideration given to withholding or discontinuing diuretic therapy.

Thiazides may decrease serum PBI levels without signs of thyroid disturbance.

Calcium excretion is decreased by thiazides. Pathological changes in the parathyroid gland with hypercalcemia and hypophosphatemia have been observed in a few patients on prolonged thiazide therapy. The common complications of hyperparathyroidism such as renal lithiasis, bone resorption, and peptic ulceration have not been seen. Thiazides should be discontinued before carrying out tests for parathyroid function.

Thiazides have been shown to increase the urinary excretion of magnesium; this may result in hypomagnesemia.

INFORMATION FOR PATIENTS
The patient should be advised to take the medication at the same time each day as prescribed to minimize the inconvenience of diuresis, warned against interruption or discontinuation of medication even though he may feel well, and advised about a proper course in the event of an inadvertent missed dose.

The patient should be informed of symptoms that would suggest potential adverse effects and told to report them promptly.

LABORATORY TESTS
During therapy, the patient's serum electrolyte levels should be regularly monitored. (See "Warnings"; "Precautions: General".)

DRUG INTERACTIONS
When administered concurrently, the following drugs may interact with Bendroflumethiazide:

Alcohol, Barbiturates, or Narcotics: Potentiation of orthostatic hypotension may occur.

Amphotericin B, Corticosteroids, or Corticotropin (ACTH): may intensify electrolyte imbalance, particularly hypokalemia. Monitor potassium levels; use potassium replacements if necessary.

Anticoagulants (Oral): dosage adjustments of anticoagulant medication may be necessary since Bendroflumethiazide may decrease their effects.

Antigout Medications: dosage adjustments of antigout medication may be necessary since Bendroflumethiazide may raise the level of blood uric acid.

Other Antihypertensive Medications (e.g., ganglionic or peripheral adrenergic blocking agents): dosage adjustments may be necessary since Bendroflumethiazide may potentiate their effects.

Antidiabetic Drugs (oral agents and insulin): since thiazides may elevate blood glucose levels, dosage adjustments of antidiabetic agents may be necessary.

Calcium Salts: increased serum calcium levels due to decreased excretion may occur. If calcium must be prescribed monitor serum calcium levels and adjust calcium dosage accordingly.

Cardiac Glycosides: enhanced possibility of digitalis toxicity associated with hypokalemia. Monitor potassium levels; use potassium replacement if necessary.

Cholestyramine Resin and Colestipol HCl: may delay or decrease absorption of Bendroflumethiazide. Sulfonamide diuretics should be taken at least one hour before or four to six hours after these medications.

Diazoxide: enhanced hyperglycemic, hyperuricemic, and antihypertensive effects. Be cognizant of possible interaction; monitor blood glucose and serum uric acid levels.

Lithium Salts: may enhance lithium toxicity due to reduced renal clearance. Avoid concurrent use; if lithium must be prescribed monitor serum lithium levels and adjust lithium dosage accordingly. (See "Warnings".)

MAO Inhibitors: dosage adjustments of one or both agents may be necessary since hypotensive effects are enhanced.

Nondepolarizing Muscle Relaxants, Preanesthetics and Anesthetics Used in Surgery (e.g., tubocurarine chloride and gallamine triethiodide): effects of these agents may be potentiated; dosage adjustments may be required. Monitor and correct any fluid and electrolyte imbalances prior to surgery if feasible.

Nonsteroidal Anti-inflammatory Agents: in some patients, the administration of a nonsteroidal anti-inflammatory agent can reduce the diuretic, natriuretic, and antihypertensive effect of loop, potassium-sparing or thiazide diuretics. Therefore, when Bendroflumethiazide and nonsteroidal anti-inflammatory agents are used concomitantly, the patient should be observed closely to determine if the desired effect of the diuretic is obtained.

Methenamine: possible decreased effectiveness due to alkalinization of the urine.

Pressor Amines (e.g., norepinephrine): decreased arterial responsiveness, but not sufficient to preclude effectiveness of the pressor agent for therapeutic use. Use caution in patients taking both medications who undergo surgery. Administer preanesthetic and anesthetic agents in reduced dosage, and if possible, discontinue Bendroflumethiazide one week prior to surgery.

Probenecid or Sulfinpyrazone: increased dosage of these agents may be necessary since Bendroflumethiazide may have hyperuricemic effects.

DRUG/LABORATORY TEST INTERACTIONS
Bendroflumethiazide may produce false-negative results with the phentolamine and tyramine tests; may interfere with the phenosulfonphthalein test due to decreased excretion; and may cause diagnostic interference of serum electrolyte level blood and urine glucose levels, and a decrease in serum PBI levels without signs of thyroid disturbance.

CARCINOGENESIS, MUTAGENESIS, IMPAIRMENT OF FERTILITY
Studies have not been performed to evaluate carcinogenic potential, mutagenesis, or whether this drug adversely affects fertility in males or females.

PREGNANCY: TERATOGENIC EFFECTS
Category C. Animal reproduction studies have not been conducted with Bendroflumethiazide. It is also not known whether Bendroflumethiazide can cause fetal harm when administered to a pregnant woman or can affect reproduction capacity. Bendroflumethiazide should be given to a pregnant woman only if clearly needed (see "Indications").

PREGNANCY: NONTERATOGENIC EFFECTS
Thiazides cross the placental barrier and appear in cord blood. The use of thiazides in pregnant women requires that the anticipated benefit be weighed against possible hazards to the fetus. These hazards include fetal or neonatal jaundice, thrombocytopenia, and possibly other adverse reactions which have occurred in the adult.

NURSING MOTHERS
Because of the potential for serious adverse reactions in nursing infants from Bendroflumethiazide, a decision should be made whether to discontinue nursing or to discontinue the drug, taking into account the importance of the drug to the mother.

PEDIATRIC USE
Safety and effectiveness in children have not been established.

ADVERSE REACTIONS
Gastrointestinal: nausea, vomiting, cramping and anorexia are not uncommon; diarrhea, constipation, gastric irritation, abdominal bloating, jaundice (intrahepatic cholestatic jaundice), hepatitis, and sialadenitis occasionally occur; and pancreatitis has been reported.

Central Nervous System: dizziness, vertigo, paresthesias, headache, and xanthopsia occasionally occur.

Hematologic: leukopenia, agranulocytosis, thrombocytopenia, hemolytic anemia, and aplastic anemia have been reported.

Dermatologic-Hypersensitivity: purpura, exfoliative dermatitis, pruritus, ecchymosis, urticaria, necrotizing angiitis (vasculitis, cutaneous vasculitis), respiratory distress including pneumonitis, fever, and anaphylactic reactions occasionally occur; photosensitivity and rash have been reported.

Cardiovascular: orthostatic hypotension may occur and may be potentiated by coadministration with certain other drugs (e.g., alcohol, barbiturates, narcotics, other antihypertensive medications, etc., (see "Precautions: Drug Interactions".)

Other: muscle spasm, weakness, or restlessness is not uncommon; hyperglycemia, glycosuria, metabolic acidosis in diabetic patients, hyperuricemia, allergic glomerulonephritis, and transient blurred vision occasionally occur.

Whenever adverse reactions are moderate or severe, thiazide dosage should be reduced or therapy withdrawn.

OVERDOSAGE

Symptoms of overdosage may be manifested in several ways: temporary elevation of BUN; gastrointestinal irritation; and lethargy progressing to coma with minimal depression of respiration and cardiovascular function and without significant serum electrolyte changes or dehydration. Serum electrolyte changes may occur, especially in patients with impaired renal function. The mechanism of thiazide-induced central nervous system depression is unknown.

Treatment is essentially supportive. Evacuation of gastric contents may be useful provided aspiration is avoided in unconscious patients. In conscious patients, induced vomiting using Ipecac Syrup USP is helpful in removing the drug from the stomach. Cathartics should be avoided since they tend to enhance the loss of fluid and electrolytes. Electrolyte levels and renal function should be monitored, and supportive measures instituted to maintain hydration, electrolyte balance, respiration, and cardiovascular-renal function as required. Gastrointestinal irritation is usually of short duration and may be treated symptomatically.

DOSAGE AND ADMINISTRATION

Therapy should be individualized according to patient response and titrated to obtain maximal therapeutic response as well as the lowest dose possible to maintain that therapeutic response and minimize side effects.

Diuretic: The usual dose is 5 mg once daily, preferably given in the morning. To initiate therapy, doses up to 20 mg may be given once daily or divided into two doses. A single daily dose of 2.5 to 5 mg should suffice for maintenance.

Alternatively, intermittent therapy may be advantageous in many patients. By administering the preparation every other day or on a three to five day per week schedule, electrolyte imbalance is less likely to occur; however, the possibility still exists.

In general, the lowest dosage that achieves the therapeutic response should be employed.

Antihypertensive: The suggested initial dosage is 5 to 20 mg daily. Maintenance dosage may range from 2.5 to 15 mg per day depending on the individual response of the patient. When the diuretic is used with other antihypertensive agents, lower maintenance doses for each drug are usually sufficient.

Storage: Dispense in tight containers. Store at room temperature; avoid excessive heat.

HOW SUPPLIED

TABLETS: 5 MG

BRAND/MANUFACTURER	NDC	SIZE	AWP
○ BRAND			
NATURETIN-5: Apothecon	00003-0606-50	100s	$77.28

TABLETS: 10 MG

BRAND/MANUFACTURER	NDC	SIZE	AWP
○ BRAND			
NATURETIN-10: Apothecon	00003-0618-50	100s	$118.93

Bendroflumethiazide and Rauwolfia Serpentina

WARNING

THIS FIXED COMBINATION DRUG IS NOT INDICATED FOR INITIAL THERAPY OF HYPERTENSION. HYPERTENSION REQUIRES THERAPY TITRATED TO THE INDIVIDUAL PATIENT. IF THE FIXED COMBINATION REPRESENTS THE DOSAGE SO DETERMINED, ITS USE MAY BE MORE CONVENIENT IN PATIENT MANAGEMENT. THE TREATMENT OF HYPERTENSION IS NOT STATIC, BUT MUST BE REEVALUATED AS CONDITIONS IN EACH PATIENT WARRANT.

DESCRIPTION

Bendroflumethiazide/Rauwolfia is an antihypertensive agent for oral administration.

Each tablet contains 50 mg powdered Rauwolfia Serpentina composed of not less than 0.15 percent and not more than 0.2 percent of reserpine-rescinnamine group alkaloids calculated as reserpine, combined with 4 mg Bendroflumethiazide.

Reserpine is a white to slightly yellow crystalline powder, insoluble in water, very slightly soluble in ether and alcohol, slightly soluble in benzene, and freely soluble in acetic acid and chloroform. It is designated chemically as methyl 18β-hydroxy-11, 17α-dimethoxy-3β,20α-yohimban-16β-carboxylate 3,4,5-trimethoxybenzoate (ester). Bendroflumethiazide is a white to cream crystalline powder, practically insoluble in water, and freely soluble in acetone and alcohol. It is designated chemically as 3-benzyl-3,4-dihydro-6-(trifluoromethyl)-2H-1,2,4-benzothiadiazine-7-sulfonamide 1,1-dioxide.

CLINICAL PHARMACOLOGY

Either of the components of Bendroflumethiazide/Rauwolfia, when administered alone, may produce a reduction of blood pressure in hypertension. When the two agents are administered simultaneously, the action of the one appears to supplement that of the other so that a hypotensive effect may be produced which is greater than that produced by either agent alone. Thus, hypertension which does not adequately respond to either drug alone may frequently respond to the combination of both drugs.

RAUWOLFIA SERPENTINA

Rauwolfia Serpentina probably exerts its antihypertensive effects through depletion of tissue stores of catecholamines (epinephrine and norepinephrine) from peripheral sites. By contrast, its sedative and tranquilizing properties are thought to be related to depletion of catecholamines and serotonin (5-hydroxytryptamine) from the brain.

Following absorption from the gastrointestinal tract, Rauwolfia alkaloids concentrate in tissues with high lipid content. The drug crosses the blood-brain barrier and the placenta.

The Rauwolfia alkaloids are characterized by slow onset of action and sustained effect. Cardiovascular and central nervous system effects may persist following discontinuation of therapy. The Rauwolfia alkaloids are metabolized in the liver to inactive compounds that are excreted primarily in the urine. Unchanged alkaloids are excreted primarily in the feces.

BENDROFLUMETHIAZIDE

The mechanism of action of Bendroflumethiazide results in an interference with the renal tubular mechanism of electrolyte reabsorption. At maximal therapeutic dosage all thiazides are approximately equal in their diuretic potency.

Thiazides increase excretion of sodium and chloride in approximately equivalent amounts. Natriuresis causes a secondary loss of potassium and bicarbonate.

The mechanism of the antihypertensive effect of thiazides is unknown. Thiazides do not affect normal blood pressure.

Onset of action of thiazides occurs in two hours and the peak effect at about four hours. Duration of action persists for approximately six to 12 hours. Thiazides are eliminated rapidly by the kidney.

INDICATIONS AND USAGE

Bendroflumethiazide/Rauwolfia is indicated for hypertension (see boxed "Warning").

Usage in Pregnancy: The routine use of diuretics in an otherwise healthy woman is inappropriate and exposes mother and fetus to unnecessary hazard. Diuretics do not prevent development of toxemia of pregnancy, and there is no satisfactory evidence that they are useful in the treatment of developed toxemia.

Edema during pregnancy may arise from pathological causes or from the physiologic and mechanical consequences of pregnancy. Thiazides are indicated in pregnancy when edema is due to pathologic causes, just as they are in the absence of pregnancy (however, see "Precautions" below). Dependent edema in pregnancy, resulting from restriction of venous return by the expanded uterus, is properly treated through elevation of the lower extremities and use of support hose; use of diuretics to lower intravascular volume in this case is illogical and unnecessary. There is hypervolemia during normal pregnancy which is harmful to neither the fetus nor the mother (in the absence of cardiovascular disease), but which is associated with edema, including generalized edema, in the majority of pregnant women. If this edema produces discomfort, increased recumbency will often provide relief. In rare instances, this edema may cause extreme discomfort which is not relieved by rest. In these cases, a short course of diuretics may provide relief and may be appropriate.

CONTRAINDICATIONS

RAUWOLFIA SERPENTINA

Rauwolfia Serpentina is contraindicated in patients who have previously demonstrated hypersensitivity to this agent: those with a history of mental depression (especially with suicidal tendencies); active peptic ulcer; ulcerative colitis; and in patients receiving electroconvulsive therapy.

BENDROFLUMETHIAZIDE

Bendroflumethiazide is contraindicated in anuria. It is also contraindicated in patients who have previously demonstrated hypersensitivity to Bendroflumethiazide or other sulfonamide-derived drugs.

WARNINGS

Sensitivity reactions may occur in patients with or without a history of allergy or bronchial asthma.

RAUWOLFIA SERPENTINA

Reserpine may cause mental depression. Recognition of depression may be difficult because this condition may often be disguised by somatic complaints (Masked Depression). The drug should be discontinued at first signs of depression such as despondency, early morning insomnia, loss of appetite, impotence, or self-deprecation. Drug-induced depression may persist for several months after drug withdrawal and may be severe enough to result in suicide.

Rauwolfia Serpentina may impair the mental and physical abilities required for the performance of tasks requiring alertness, such as driving or operating heavy machinery.

◆ RATED THERAPEUTICALLY EQUIVALENT; ◇ THERAPEUTIC EQUIVALENCE UNCONFIRMED; ○ UNRATED

BENDROFLUMETHIAZIDE

Thiazides should be used with caution in severe renal disease. In patients with renal disease, thiazides may precipitate azotemia. Cumulative effects of the drug may develop in patients with impaired renal function.

Thiazides should be used with caution in patients with impaired hepatic function or progressive liver disease, since minor alterations of fluid and electrolyte balance may precipitate hepatic coma.

Sensitivity reactions may occur in patients with or without a history of allergy or bronchial asthma.

The possibility of exacerbation or activation of systemic lupus erythematosus has been reported.

Lithium generally should not be given with diuretics; diuretic agents reduce the renal clearance of lithium and add a high risk of lithium toxicity. Refer to the package insert for lithium preparations before use of such concomitant therapy.

PRECAUTIONS
GENERAL
This product contains FD&C Yellow No. 5 (tartrazine) which may cause allergic-type reactions (including bronchial asthma) in certain susceptible individuals. Although the overall incidence of FD&C Yellow No. 5 (tartrazine) sensitivity in the general population is low, it is frequently seen in patients who also have aspirin hypersensitivity.

RAUWOLFIA SERPENTINA
Because Rauwolfia preparations increase gastrointestinal motility and secretion, this drug should be used cautiously in patients with a history of peptic ulcer, ulcerative colitis, or gallstones where biliary colic may be precipitated. Patients on high dosage should be observed carefully at regular intervals to detect possible reactivation of peptic ulcer.

Chronic administration of Rauwolfia alkaloids may increase serum prolactin levels and decrease urinary catecholamine and vanilmandelic acid (VMA) excretion. Therefore, any diagnostic tests performed for these determinations should be interpreted with caution.

Caution should be exercised when treating hypertensive patients with renal insufficiency since they adjust poorly to lowered blood pressure levels.

Preoperative withdrawal of Rauwolfia Serpentina does not insure that circulatory instability will not occur. It is important that the anesthesiologist be aware of the patient's drug intake and consider this in the overall management since hypotension has occurred in patients receiving rauwolfia preparations. Anticholinergic and/or adrenergic drugs (metaraminol, norepinephrine) have been employed to treat adverse vagocirculatory effects.

BENDROFLUMETHIAZIDE
Periodic determination of serum electrolytes to detect possible electrolyte imbalance should be performed at appropriate intervals.

All patients receiving thiazide therapy should be observed for clinical signs of fluid or electrolyte imbalance, namely: hyponatremia, hypochloremic alkalosis, and hypokalemia. Serum and urine electrolyte determinations are particularly important when the patient is vomiting excessively or receiving parenteral fluids. Warning signs or symptoms of fluid and electrolyte imbalance may include: dryness of the mouth, thirst, weakness, lethargy, drowsiness, restlessness, muscle pains or cramps, muscular fatigue, hypotension, oliguria, tachycardia, and gastrointestinal disturbances such as nausea and vomiting.

Hypokalemia may develop, especially with brisk diuresis or when severe cirrhosis is present.

Interference with adequate oral electrolyte intake will also contribute to hypokalemia. Hypokalemia can sensitize or exaggerate the response of the heart to the toxic effects of digitalis (e.g., increased ventricular irritability). Concurrent administration of a potassium-sparing diuretic or potassium supplements may be indicated in these patients.

Any chloride deficit is generally mild and usually does not require specific treatment except under extraordinary circumstances (as in liver disease or renal disease). Dilutional hyponatremia may occur in edematous patients in hot weather; appropriate therapy is water restriction, rather than administration of salt, except in rare instances when the hyponatremia is life-threatening. In actual salt depletion, appropriate replacement is the therapy of choice.

Hyperuricemia may occur or frank gout may be precipitated in certain patients receiving thiazide therapy.

Latent diabetes mellitus may become manifest during thiazide administration.

The antihypertensive effect of thiazide diuretics may be enhanced in the postsympathectomy patient.

If progressive renal impairment becomes evident, as indicated by a rising nonprotein nitrogen or blood urea nitrogen (BUN), a careful reappraisal of therapy is necessary with consideration given to withholding or discontinuing diuretic therapy.

Calcium excretion is decreased by thiazides. Pathological changes in the parathyroid gland with hypercalcemia and hypophosphatemia have been observed in a few patients on prolonged thiazide therapy. The common complications of hyperparathyroidism such as renal lithiasis, bone resorption, and peptic ulceration have not been seen. Thiazides should be discontinued before carrying out tests for parathyroid function.

Thiazides have been shown to increase the urinary excretion of magnesium; this may result in hypomagnesemia.

INFORMATION FOR THE PATIENT
The patient should be informed of symptoms that would suggest potential adverse effects and told to report them promptly.

Patients should be warned against taking this medication for any disorder other than for which it was prescribed, or discontinuing medication unless instructed by the physician.

The patient should also be advised of a proper course in the event of an inadvertently missed dose.

Caution patients that the drug may impair mental and/or physical abilities required for performance of hazardous tasks, such as operating machinery or driving a motor vehicle.

LABORATORY TESTS
Serum electrolyte levels should be regularly monitored (see *"Warnings, Bendroflumethiazide,"* also *"Precautions, General, Bendroflumethiazide"*).

DRUG INTERACTIONS
RAUWOLFIA SERPENTINA
When administered concurrently the following drugs may interact with Rauwolfia alkaloids:

Alcohol/CNS Depressants: may increase the CNS depressant effects of these drugs or the Rauwolfia alkaloids.

Other Antihypertensives/Diuretics: antihypertensive effects may be potentiated.

Digitalis Glycosides/Quinidine: may result in cardiac arrhythmias.

Levodopa: effects of levodopa may be inhibited.

Methotrimeprazine: may result in increased orthostatic hypotension.

Monoamine Oxidase (MAO) Inhibitors: may result in excessive excitation, hypertension, and sympathetic response.

Sympathomimetics (Direct-acting): Rauwolfia alkaloids may prolong their effects: (Indirect-acting): Rauwolfia alkaloids may inhibit their action.

Tricyclic Antidepressants: the antidepressant effects of these drugs and the antihypertensive effects of Rauwolfia alkaloids may be decreased.

BENDROFLUMETHIAZIDE
When administered concurrently the following drugs may interact with Bendroflumethiazide:

Alcohol, Barbiturates, or Narcotics: potentiation of orthostatic hypotension may occur.

Amphotericin B, Corticosteroids or Corticotropin (ACTH): may intensify electrolyte imbalance, particularly hypokalemia. Monitor potassium levels; use potassium replacements if necessary.

Anticoagulants (Oral): dosage adjustments of anticoagulant medication may be necessary since Bendroflumethiazide may decrease their effects.

Antigout Medications: dosage adjustments of antigout medication may be necessary since Bendroflumethiazide may raise the level of blood uric acid.

Other Antihypertensive Medications (e.g., Ganglionic or Peripheral Adrenergic Blocking Agents): dosage adjustments may be necessary since bendroflumethiazide may potentiate their effects.

Antidiabetic Drugs (Oral Agents and Insulin): since thiazides may elevate blood glucose levels, dosage adjustments of anti-diabetic agents may be necessary.

Calcium Salts: increased serum calcium levels due to decreased excretion may occur. If calcium must be prescribed monitor serum calcium levels and adjust calcium dosage accordingly.

Cardiac Glycosides: enhanced possibility of digitalis toxicity associated with hypokalemia. Monitor potassium levels: use potassium replacement if necessary.

Cholestyramine Resin and Colestipol HCL: may delay or decrease absorption of Bendroflumethiazide. Sulfonamide diuretics should be taken at least one hour before or four to six hours after these medications.

Diazoxide: enhanced hyperglycemic, hyperuricemic, and antihypertensive effects. Be cognizant of possible interaction: monitor blood glucose and serum uric acid levels.

Lithium Salts: may enhance lithium toxicity due to reduced renal clearance. Avoid concurrent use: if lithium must be prescribed monitor serum lithium levels and adjust lithium dosage accordingly. (See *"Warnings, Bendroflumethiazide."*)

MAO Inhibitors: dosage adjustments of one or both agents may be necessary since hypotensive effects are enhanced.

Nondepolarizing Muscle Relaxants, Preanesthetics and Anesthetics Used in Surgery (e.g., Tubocurarine Chloride and Gallamine Triethiodide): effects of these agents may be potentiated; dosage adjustments may be required. Monitor and correct any fluid and electrolyte imbalances prior to surgery if feasible.

Nonsteroidal Anti-Inflammatory Agents: In some patients, the administration of nonsteroidal anti-inflammatory agent can reduce the diuretic, natriuretic, and antihypertensive effect of loop, potassium-sparing or thiazide diuretics. Therefore, when Bendroflumethiazide and nonsteroidal anti-inflammatory agents are used concomitantly, the patient should be observed closely to determine if the desired effect of the diuretic is obtained.

Methenamine: possible decreased effectiveness due to alkalinization of the urine.

Pressor Amines (e.g., Norepinephrine): decreased arterial responsiveness, but not sufficient to preclude effectiveness of the pressor agent for therapeutic use. Use caution in patients taking both medications who undergo surgery. Administer preanesthetic and anesthetic agents in reduced dosage, and if possible, discontinue Bendroflumethiazide one week prior to surgery.

Probenecid or Sulfinpyrazone: increased dosage of these agents may be necessary since Bendroflumethiazide may have hyperuricemic effects.

DRUG/LABORATORY TEST INTERACTIONS
RAUWOLFIA SERPENTINA
Since Rauwolfia alkaloids slightly decrease absorbance readings obtained on urinary steroid colorimetric determinations (e.g., modified Glenn-Nelson technique or Holtorff Koch modification of Zimmerman reaction), false low results may be obtained.

BENDROFLUMETHIAZIDE
Bendroflumethiazide may produce false-negative results with the phentolamine and tyramine tests; may interfere with the phenosulfonphthalein test due to decreased excretion: and it may cause diagnostic interference of serum electrolyte levels, blood and urine glucose levels, and a decrease in serum PBI levels without signs of thyroid disturbance.

CARCINOGENESIS, MUTAGENESIS, IMPAIRMENT OF FERTILITY
RAUWOLFIA SERPENTINA
Studies have not been conducted to evaluate the carcinogenic or mutagenic potential of Rauwolfia Serpentina or its potential to affect male or female fertility adversely. Rodent studies have, however, shown that the rauwolfia alkaloid reserpine is an animal tumorigen, causing an increased incidence of mammary fibroadenomas in female mice, malignant tumors of the seminal vesicles in male mice, and malignant adrenal medullary tumors in male rats. These findings arose in two year studies in which the drug was administered in the feed at concentrations of 5 and 10 ppm-about 100 to 300 times the usual human dose. The breast neoplasms are thought to be related to reserpine's prolactin-elevating effect. Several other prolactin-elevating drugs have also been associated with an increased incidence of mammary neoplasia in rodents.

The extent to which these findings indicate a risk to humans is uncertain. Tissue culture experiments show that about one-third of human breast tumors are prolactin-dependent *in vitro*, a factor of considerable importance if the use of the drug is contemplated in a patient with previously detected breast cancer. The possibility of an increased risk of breast cancer in reserpine users has been studied extensively; however, no firm conclusion has emerged. Although a few epidemiologic studies have suggested a slightly increased risk (less than twofold in all studies except one) in women who have used reserpine, other studies of generally similar design have not confirmed this. Epidemiologic studies conducted using other drugs (neuroleptic agents) that, like reserpine, increase prolactin levels and therefore would be considered rodent mammary carcinogens, have not shown an association between chronic administration of the drug and human mammary tumorigenesis. While long-term clinical observation has not suggested such an association, the available evidence is considered too limited to be conclusive at this time. An association of reserpine intake with pheochromocytoma or tumors of the seminal vesicles has not been explored.

BENDROFLUMETHIAZIDE
Studies have not been conducted to evaluate the carcinogenic or mutagenic potential of Bendroflumethiazide or its potential to affect male or female fertility adversely.

PREGNANCY: TERATOGENIC EFFECTS
Category C. Animal reproduction studies have not been conducted with Rauwolfia alkaloids or Bendroflumethiazide. There are no adequate and well-controlled studies in pregnant women. Since Rauwolfia alkaloids and thiazides cross the placental barrier and appear in cord blood, drugs in these classes should be used during pregnancy only if the potential benefit justifies the potential risk to the fetus.

PREGNANCY: NONTERATOGENIC EFFECTS
RAUWOLFIA SERPENTINA
Increased respiratory secretions, nasal congestion, cyanosis and hypothermia, and anorexia are potential hazards in neonates of Rauwolfia alkaloid-treated mothers.

BENDROFLUMETHIAZIDE
Potential hazards include fetal or neonatal jaundice, thrombocytopenia, and possibly other adverse reactions which have occurred in the adult.

NURSING MOTHERS
Both Rauwolfia Serpentina and Bendroflumethiazide are excreted in human milk. Because of the potential for serious adverse reactions in nursing infants from both drugs, a decision should be made whether to continue nursing or to discontinue therapy taking into account the importance of this preparation to the mother.

PEDIATRIC USE
Safety and effectiveness in children have not been established.

ADVERSE REACTIONS
The following adverse reactions (categorized by organ system in decreasing order of severity) have been observed with Bendroflumethiazide and Rauwolfia Serpentina; there is, however, insufficient data to support an estimate of their frequency.

RAUWOLFIA SERPENTINA
Cardiovascular: Bradycardia: arrhythmias, particularly when used concurrently with digitalis or quinidine (see *"Precautions, Drug Interactions"*); angina-like symptoms.

Central Nervous System: CNS sensitization manifested by optic atrophy, glaucoma, uveitis, deafness, and dull sensorium; extrapyramidal tract symptoms; rare parkinsonian disease; depression; paradoxical anxiety; nightmares; nervousness; drowsiness.

Gastrointestinal: Gastrointestinal bleeding; hypersecretion and increased intestinal motility; dryness of mouth.

Respiratory: Dyspnea; epistaxis; nasal congestion.

Other: Conjunctival injection; dysuria; muscular aches; weight gain; breast engorgement; pseudolactation; impotence or decreased libido; gynecomastia.

These reactions are usually reversible and disappear when the drug is discontinued.

BENDROFLUMETHIAZIDE
Central Nervous System: Vertigo; paresthesia; xanthopsia.

Hematologic: Leukopenia (agranulocytopenia); agranulocytosis; thrombocytopenia; aplastic anemia: hemolytic anemia.

Cardiovascular: Orthostatic hypotension (may be aggravated by alcohol, barbiturates, or narcotics—see *"Precautions, Drug Interactions, Bendroflumethiazide"*).

Gastrointestinal: Gastric irritation: abdominal cramps or bloating; constipation: pancreatitis: sialadenitis.

Hypersensitivity: Ecchymosis; skin photosensitivity; exfoliative dermatitis; urticaria; necrotizing angiitis (vasculitis, cutaneous vasculitis); fever; respiratory distress including pneumonitis; anaphylactic reactions.

Other: Hyperglycemia; glycosuria: occasional metabolic acidosis in diabetic patients: hyperuricemia: muscle spasm or cramps; weakness; restlessness; transient blurred vision.

Whenever adverse reactions are moderate or severe, thiazide dosage should be reduced or therapy withdrawn.

COMMON TO BENDROFLUMETHIAZIDE AND RAUWOLFIA SERPENTINA
Gastrointestinal: Anorexia: nausea: vomiting; diarrhea.

Central Nervous System: Headache: dizziness.

Hypersensitivity: Purpura; pruritus; rash.

OVERDOSAGE
RAUWOLFIA SERPENTINA
In the event of overdosage, Rauwolfia Serpentina may cause CNS depression ranging from drowsiness to coma, flushing of the skin, bradycardia, hypotension, conjunctival congestion, and pupillary constriction. Hypothermia, central respiratory depression, mental depression, diarrhea, vomiting, ptosis, miosis, and extrapyramidal signs such as stiffness, leg pain, and tremors may also occur.

Treatment is symptomatic. Provided the patient is not comatose or convulsing, evacuation of stomach contents by emesis or gastric lavage is recommended: precautions should be taken to preclude aspiration of contents by the patient, and to protect the airway. An activated charcoal slurry may then be administered. Bradycardia and parasympathetic effects may be relieved with appropriate anticholinergic medication. Hypotension and coma usually respond to conservative supportive therapy. In cases of severe hypotension, treatment with a vasopressor having direct action upon vascular smooth muscle or a direct-acting sympathomimetic (see *"Precautions, Drug Interactions"*) is recommended. Rapid infusion of IV solutions intended to raise arterial blood pressure should be avoided, since cardiac status in Rauwolfia poisoning is uncertain. Because the effects of Rauwolfia alkaloids are long acting, patients should be carefully observed for at least 72 hours.

BENDROFLUMETHIAZIDE
In addition to the expected diuresis, overdosage of Bendroflumethiazide may produce varying degrees of lethargy which may progress to coma with minimal depression of respiration and cardiovascular function and without significant serum electrolyte changes or dehydration. The mechanism of thiazide-induced CNS depression is unknown. Gastrointestinal irritation may occur. Transitory increase in BUN has been reported, and serum electrolyte changes may occur, especially in patients with impaired renal function.

In addition to gastric lavage and supportive therapy for stupor or coma, symptomatic treatment of gastrointestinal effects may be needed. Cathartics should be avoided since they tend to enhance the loss of fluid and electrolytes. Measures as required to maintain hydration, electrolyte balance, respiration, and cardiovascular and renal function should be instituted.

DOSAGE AND ADMINISTRATION
As determined by individual titration (see boxed *"Warning"*). Usual dosage may range from one to four tablets daily.

Keep and dispense in tightly closed containers. Store at room temperature; avoid excessive heat.

◆ RATED THERAPEUTICALLY EQUIVALENT; ◇ THERAPEUTIC EQUIVALENCE UNCONFIRMED; ○ UNRATED

HOW SUPPLIED
TABLETS: 4 MG-50 MG

BRAND/MANUFACTURER	NDC	SIZE	AWP
○ **BRAND**			
RAUZIDE: Apothecon	00003-0769-51	100s	$103.32
○ **GENERICS**			
Rugby	00536-4502-01	100s	$43.28
RONDAMETH: Major	00904-2537-60	100s	$44.95
FLUMEZIDE: Econolab	55053-0069-01	100s	$54.89

Benemid SEE PROBENECID

Benoquin SEE MONOBENZONE

Benoxinate Hydrochloride and Fluorescein Sodium

DESCRIPTION
This product is a sterile ophthalmic solution combining the disclosing action of Fluorescein Sodium with the anesthetic action of Benoxinate Hydrochloride.

Each ml contains:

Benoxinate Hydrochloride, U.S.P. 0.4%
Fluorescein Sodium, U.S.P. 0.25%

ACTIONS
Benoxinate HCl/Fluorescein Sodium is a disclosing agent with rapid anesthetic action and short duration. Benoxinate HCl 0.4% produces anesthesia in less than 15 seconds. Using one drop, duration of action averages slightly over 15 minutes. Fluorescein Sodium 0.25% produces reproducible results through reliable and uniform fluorescence.

INDICATIONS
For procedures in which a topical ophthalmic anesthetic agent in conjunction with a disclosing agent are indicated: corneal anesthesia of short duration, e.g., tonometry, gonioscopy, removal of corneal foreign bodies, and for short corneal and conjunctival procedures.

CONTRAINDICATIONS
Known hypersensitivity to the components of this preparation.

WARNING
Prolonged use of a topical ocular anesthetic is not recommended. It may produce permanent corneal opacification with accompanying visual loss.

ADVERSE REACTIONS
Occasional temporary stinging, burning, conjunctival redness.

Rare, severe, immediate-type, apparently hyperallergic corneal reaction, with acute, intense, and diffuse epithelial keratitis, a gray, ground-glass appearance, sloughing or large areas of necrotic epithelium, corneal filaments and sometimes, iritis with descemetitis.

DOSAGE & ADMINISTRATION
Usual dosage (removal of foreign bodies and sutures, and for tonometry):
1 to 2 drops (in single instillations) in each eye before operating.

Deep ophthalmic anesthesia:
Benoxinate HCl 0.4% solution: 2 drops in each eye at 90 second intervals for 3 instillations.

Note: Because the blink reflex is temporarily eliminated, it is suggested that the eye be covered with a patch following this procedure.

HOW SUPPLIED
DROP:

BRAND/MANUFACTURER	NDC	SIZE	AWP
○ **BRAND**			
FLU-OXINATE: Pasadena	00418-9920-05	5 ml	$6.95

SOLUTION: 0.25%-0.4%

BRAND/MANUFACTURER	NDC	SIZE	AWP
○ **BRAND**			
FLURESS: Akorn	00077-0628-55	5 ml	$11.44

Bentiromide

DESCRIPTION
Bentiromide is a peptide for oral administration which carries the marker PABA (para-aminobenzoic acid). Bentiromide is formulated as a 7.5 mL solution containing 500 mg Bentiromide in a 40% propylene glycol solution. Bentiromide is a screening test for the assessment of exocrine pancreatic insufficiency.

Following is its chemical structure:

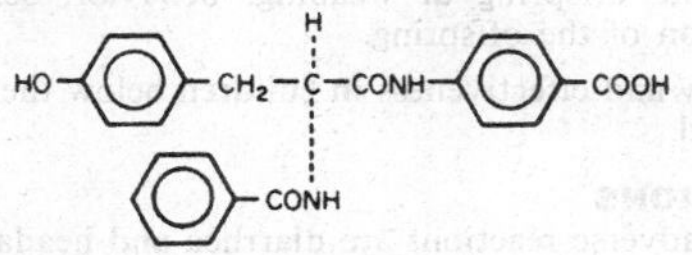

CLINICAL PHARMACOLOGY
Following oral administration of Bentiromide; the agent is selectively cleaved by pancreatic chymotrypsin with the liberation of PABA (para-aminobenzoic acid). PABA is readily absorbed through the intestinal mucosa under normal conditions of absorption, conjugated primarily by the liver and rapidly excreted in the urine. PABA is detected in the urine using the Smith modification of the Bratton-Marshall method of analysis (see References). This method is suitable for detecting both conjugated and unconjugated arylamines. It is not known whether Bentiromide or PABA crosses either the placental barrier or the blood brain barrier.

Under conditions of normal exocrine pancreatic function, normal gastric emptying, normal gut function and normal kidney function, over 50% of the PABA contained in Bentiromide (500 mg of Bentiromide contains 170 mg of PABA) appears in the urine within six hours following administration of this agent.

INDICATIONS AND USAGE
Bentiromide is indicated as a screening test for pancreatic exocrine insufficiency.

Bentiromide may also be used to monitor the adequacy of supplemental pancreatic therapy.

CONTRAINDICATIONS
Bentiromide is contraindicated in individuals who have previously shown hypersensitivity to the product or to PABA.

PRECAUTIONS
General: Proper use of Bentiromide requires (1) close attention to the technical details of drug administration and of urine collection, handling and assay for arylamine levels, (2) awareness that "false positive" and "false negative" results can occur (see *"Interpretation of Results"*).

Repeat dosings of this agent, should be scheduled at intervals of seven days or more to assure complete metabolism and excretion of prior doses of the drug.

In testing of diabetic patients, suitable adjustments in insulin may need to be made in order to accommodate the fasting patient.

Hypersensitivity: A single case of hypersensitivity to bentiromide has been reported (see *"Adverse Reactions"*). It is not possible to determine the frequency of sensitization, but no other cases have been reported in more than 6000 cases reported in the literature, in about 1000 patients studied in clinical trials, or in Japanese postmarketing experience. Following administration of Bentiromide, patients should remain in a medical setting and be observed.

Information for Patients: The full text of patient information is reprinted at the end of the labeling.

Laboratory Tests: Because it has not been established whether concurrent gastrointestinal diagnostic testing interferes with the results of the test, all such testing should be conducted at least 24 hours before or after dosing with Bentiromide.

Drug Interactions: Drugs may compete for binding sites with methotrexate.

Assay Interactions: Drugs that are metabolized to primary arylamines may cause interference in the assay and yield a false elevation of test results. These drugs include the following: acetaminophen, phenacetin, benzocaine, chloramphenicol, lidocaine, procaine, procainamide, sulfonamides and thiazide diuretics. PABA-containing drugs such as sunscreens or certain multiple vitamin preparations may also falsely elevate test results. Drugs such as those listed above should be discontinued three days prior to the administration of Bentiromide. In adults, oral pancreatic enzyme supplements should be discontinued five days prior to the administration of Bentiromide. In cystic fibrotic children the time interval is reduced to one day.

Carcinogenesis, Mutagenesis, Impairment of Fertility: Long-term studies of carcinogenicity have not been performed. No effects on fertility, embryogenesis and delivery were observed in rats dosed at daily levels as high as 1000 mg/kg (100 times the human dose) during pregnancy. In rabbits this dose level was associated with a high frequency of fetal death and resorption, probably due to maternal emaciation. No maternal or embryo-fetal-toxicity occurred in rabbits with 500 mg/kg (50 times the human dose).

Usage in Pregnancy: Pregnancy Category B. Reproduction studies performed in rats and rabbits revealed no evidence of impaired fertility or harm to the fetus due to Bentiromide at doses up to 100 and 50 times the human dose, respectively. There are, however, no adequate and well-controlled studies in pregnant women. Because animal reproduction studies are not always predictive of human response, this drug should be used during pregnancy only if clearly needed.

Nursing Mothers: It is not known whether this drug is excreted in human milk. Because many drugs are excreted in human milk, caution should be exercised when Bentiromide is administered to a nursing woman. In rats dosed with Bentiromide at levels up to 1000 mg/kg during the perinatal period and during lactation, no effect was seen on the functional development, morphological characteristics of the offspring at weaning, behavior, sexual maturation or reproductive function of the offspring.

Pediatric Use: Safety and effectiveness in children below the age of 6 years have not been established.

ADVERSE REACTIONS
The most frequent adverse reactions are diarrhea and headache. These occur in less than one in 50 patients. Flatulence, nausea, vomiting and weakness occur rarely, in approximately 1 out of 160 patients. These side effects are transient in nature and rarely require symptomatic therapy. Acute respiratory distress and stridor, requiring symptomatic therapy, has been reported in one patient following a second dose of Bentiromide; the patient had developed coughing and choking after his first dose (see *"Contraindications"*).

Other adverse reactions reported for which a causal relationship to Bentiromide has not been established include abdominal pain, drowsiness, light-headedness, heartburn and transient elevations of liver function tests.

OVERDOSAGE
This product is packaged in unit dose bottles and overdose is unlikely. If overdosage occurs treatment should be symptomatic.

DOSAGE AND ADMINISTRATION
Administration: Bentiromide is administered following an overnight fast. The urine is to be voided prior to administration of the drug. The drug is administered in a single 500 mg dose, followed immediately by 250 mL of water. In patients less than 12 years of age, the dose should be calculated on the basis of 14 mg/kg body weight. The patient is then given another 250 mL of water at post-dosing hour 2 and should receive up to an additional 500 mL of water during the post-dosing hours 2 through 6. Drinking of water is encouraged in order to promote diuresis. A total collection of urine is obtained during 0-6 hours post-dosing. The volume of the collection is measured and a 10 mL sample is retained for analysis. The fast is broken following completion of urine collection. Should re-testing with Bentiromide become necessary, subsequent administrations should be separated by intervals of at least 7 days to avoid interference of test results by prior Bentiromide dosings. In the testing of diabetic patients, suitable adjustment of insulin may need to be made in order to accommodate the fasting procedure.

Analysis of Urine: Arylamines are assayed in the urine using the Smith modification of the Bratton-Marshall test.

The analysis for urinary arylamines consists of hydrolysis of PABA conjugates to free PABA with hydrochloric acid, formation of the diazonium salt of PABA with sodium nitrite and the condensation of PABA with N-(1-naphthyl) ethylene-diamine dihydrochloride (NEDA) to form a colored compound which is assayed colorimetrically (see References below).

Interpretation of Results: PABA recovery in the urine following administration of 500 mg of Bentiromide is dependent upon the chymotrypsin present in the gut. Total 6 hour post-dosing urinary arylamine recovery levels obtained in a study of healthy subjects and in patients with well-established exocrine pancreatic insufficiency are displayed in the graph below.

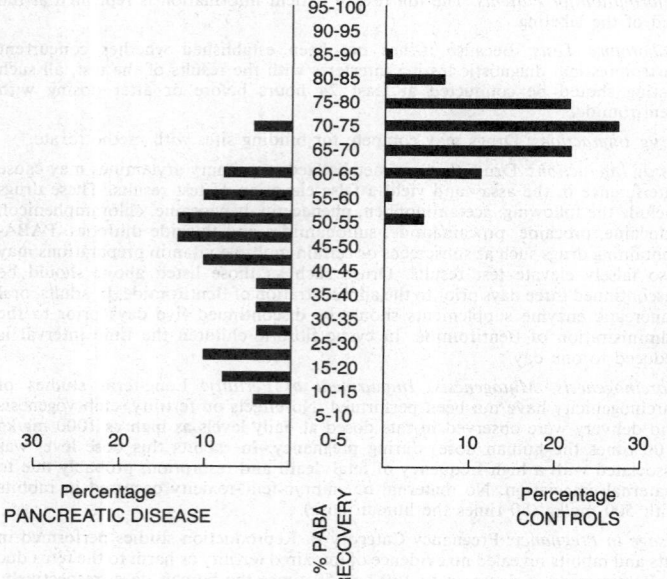

The distribution of PABA recovery shows that all healthy subjects with normal pancreatic function had a recovery of 50% or more; only in patients with pancreatic disease were PABA recoveries below 50%. At the same time, some of the patients with documented pancreatic insufficiency had recoveries indistinguishable from normal subjects.

The overlap of recoveries in normal and abnormal persons precludes designation of any specific value as diagnostic of abnormal pancreatic exocrine function. The smaller the urinary arylamine recovery, the greater the likelihood that the patient has diminished exocrine pancreatic function. The Bentiromide test result can be affected by gastric retention, impaired gut mucosal function, severe hepatic insufficiency, or chronic renal insufficiency. In these instances, an abnormally low recovery of urinary arylamines can be expected.

Concurrent use of drugs that result in the urinary excretion of arylamines or the concurrent use of pancreatic enzyme supplements can result in a false elevation of test value (see *"Assay Interactions"*).

A negative Bentiromide test in the face of a clinical history or other findings suggesting pancreatic exocrine insufficiency should not lead to termination of the search for a pancreatic etiology of maldigestion or other pancreatic disease. A good response to an oral pancreatic enzyme supplement would be confirmatory of a positive Bentiromide test. Store at room temperature.

REFERENCES
INFORMATION FOR PATIENTS
How This Test Works: After Bentiromide is swallowed, it is broken down by the pancreas, similarly to the way the pancreas breaks down food. After Bentiromide is broken down, a part of it goes into the urine.

Bentiromide is used to test how well your pancreas is working. Your doctor will do this by testing your urine after you take the drug. The urine is collected during a six hour period, starting with when you took the drug. Your doctor will need your help to make this an accurate test.

Follow These Instruction Carefully: If you don't follow Instructions exactly, the test might have to be done over again.

INSTRUCTIONS
1. Don't eat any food after midnight before taking this test. If you have eaten since last night, it might change the test results.
2. Urinate before taking the drug. You should have an empty bladder. If you have already urinated this morning, this is O.K.
3. Drink the drug first, then drink a large glass of water (8 oz). You'll also be asked to drink at least one more glass of water during the six hours after dosing. This is to make sure there is plenty of urine to test.
4. Collect ALL the urine you pass for exactly six hours after taking the drug. You will be given a container for collecting the urine.

OTHER DRUGS
If you are taking any of the following drugs they may ruin this test:

1. Acetaminophen (found in aspirin substitutes that you can buy without a prescription).
2. Sulfa drugs
3. "Water pills" (diuretics)
4. Local anesthetics, such as benzocaine and lidocaine.
5. Sunscreen and multiple vitamin preparations containing PABA (para-amino-benzoic acid) or PABA alone.

Let your doctor know which drugs you are taking, or have taken recently. These include drugs prescribed by the doctor or ones purchased without a prescription.

If you take pancreatic supplements you should have discontinued these at least five days ago in order to produce useful results.

SIDE EFFECTS
Some side effects, such as diarrhea, headaches, nausea and vomiting have been reported with this drug. Flatulence (gas) and weakness have been reported but these are rare. If you experience *any* discomfort or unusual change let your physician know about it at once.

HOW SUPPLIED
SOLUTION: 500 MG

BRAND/MANUFACTURER	NDC	SIZE	AWP
○ BRAND			
CHYMEX: Savage	00281-1803-41	7.5 ml	$58.60

Bentyl *SEE* DICYCLOMINE HYDROCHLORIDE

Benzac *SEE* BENZOYL PEROXIDE

Benzagel *SEE* BENZOYL PEROXIDE

Benzamycin *SEE* BENZOYL PEROXIDE AND ERYTHROMYCIN

◆ RATED THERAPEUTICALLY EQUIVALENT; ◇ THERAPEUTIC EQUIVALENCE UNCONFIRMED; ○ UNRATED

Benzocaine

DESCRIPTION

Benzocaine, a local anesthetic, is chemically ethyl p-aminobenzoate, $C_9H_{11}NO_2$, with a molecular weight of 165.19.

CLINICAL PHARMACOLOGY

Benzocaine reversibly stabilizes the neuronal membrane which decreases its permeability to sodium ions. Depolarization of the neuronal membrane is inhibited thereby blocking the initiation and conduction of nerve impulses.

INDICATIONS AND USAGE

Benzocaine Otic is indicated for relief of pain and pruritus in acute congestive and serous otitis media, acute swimmer's ear, and other forms of otitis externa.

Benzocaine Anesthetic Lubricant is indicated for general use as a lubricant and topical anesthetic on intratracheal catheters and pharyngeal and nasal airways to obtund the pharyngeal and tracheal reflexes; on nasogastric and endoscopic tubes; urinary catheters; laryngoscopes; proctoscopes; sigmoidoscopes and vaginal specula.

CONTRAINDICATIONS

In the presence of a perforated tympanic membrane or ear discharge.

Known allergy or hypersensitivity to Benzocaine.

WARNINGS

Indiscriminate use of anesthetic ear drops may mask symptoms of fulminating infection of the middle ear.

PRECAUTIONS

General: Medication should be discontinued if sensitivity or irritation occurs.

Carcinogenesis, Mutagenesis, Impairment of Fertility: Long-term studies in animals or humans to evaluate the carcinogenic and mutagenic potential or the effect on fertility have not been conducted.

Pregnancy Category C: Animal reproduction studies have not been conducted with Benzocaine Otic. It is also not known whether Benzocaine Otic can cause fetal harm when administered to a pregnant woman or can affect reproduction capacity. Benzocaine Otic should be given to a pregnant woman only if clearly needed.

Nursing Mothers: It is not known whether this drug is excreted in human milk. Because many drugs are excreted in human milk, caution should be exercised when Benzocaine Otic is administered to a nursing woman.

Pediatric Use: Do not use infants under 1 year of age.

ADVERSE REACTIONS

Contact dermatitis and/or hypersensitivity to Benzocaine can cause burning, stinging, pruritus, tenderness, erythema, rash, urticaria and edema. Rarely, Benzocaine may induce methemoglobinemia causing respiratory distress and cyanosis. Intravenous methylene blue is the specific therapy for this condition.

DOSAGE AND ADMINISTRATION

Instill 4-5 drops of Benzocaine Otic in the external auditory canal, then insert a cotton pledget into the meatus. Application may be repeated every one to two hours if necessary.

Apply evenly to exterior of tube or instrument prior to use.

Keep tightly closed. Store at 15°-30°C (59°-86°F).

Keep out of the reach of children.

HOW SUPPLIED
DROP:

BRAND/MANUFACTURER	NDC	SIZE	AWP
○ **BRAND**			
AMERICAINE: Fisons Presc	00585-0377-51	15 ml	$12.76

GEL:

BRAND/MANUFACTURER	NDC	SIZE	AWP
○ **BRAND**			
AMERICAINE ANESTHETIC LUBRICANT: Fisons Presc	00585-0376-16	30 gm	$13.09
	00585-0376-62	2.5 gm 144s	$307.87

Benzocaine/Butamben/Tetracaine

ACTIVE INGREDIENTS

Benzocaine	14.0%
Butyl Aminobenzoate	2.0%
Tetracaine Hydrochloride	2.0%

Benzocaine/Butamben/Tetracaine Spray 56 g including propellant.
Benzocaine/Butamben/Tetracaine Liquid 56 g.
Benzocaine/Butamben/Tetracaine Hospital Gel 29 g Tube.
Benzocaine/Butamben/Tetracaine Ointment 37 g Jar.

ACTION

Benzocaine/Butamben/Tetracaine produces anesthesia rapidly in approximately 30 seconds.

INDICATIONS

Benzocaine/Butamben/Tetracaine is a topical anesthetic indicated for the production of anesthesia of accessible mucous membrane.

Benzocaine/Butamben/Tetracaine Spray is indicated for use to control pain or gaging. Benzocaine/Butamben/Tetracaine in all forms is indicated for use to control pain.

DOSAGE AND ADMINISTRATION

Benzocaine/Butamben/Tetracaine Spray should be applied for approximately one second or less for normal anesthesia. Only limited quantity of Benzocaine/Butamben/Tetracaine is required for anesthesia. Spray in excess of two seconds is contraindicated. Average expulsion rate of residue from spray, at normal temperatures, is 200 mg. per second. Tissue need not be dried prior to application of Benzocaine/Butamben/Tetracaine. Benzocaine/Butamben/Tetracaine should be applied directly to the site where pain control is required.

Benzocaine/Butamben/Tetracaine Liquid or Benzocaine/Butamben/Tetracaine Ointment may be applied with a cotton pledget or directly to tissue. Cotton pledget should not be held in position for extended periods of time, since local reactions to benzoate topical anesthetics are related to the length of time of application.

ADVERSE REACTION

Systemic reactions to Benzocaine/Butamben/Tetracaine have not been reported. Localized allergic reactions may occur after prolonged or repeated use. Dehydration of the epithelium or an escharotic effect may result from prolonged contact. Allergic reactions are known to occur in some patients with preparations containing Benzocaine.

Usage in Pregnancy: Safe use of Benzocaine/Butamben/Tetracaine has not been established with respect to possible adverse effects upon fetal development. Therefore Benzocaine/Butamben/Tetracaine should not be used during early pregnancy, unless in the judgment of a physician the potential benefits outweigh the unknown hazards.

Routine precaution for the use of any topical anesthetic should be observed when Benzocaine/Butamben/Tetracaine is used.

CONTRAINDICATIONS

Benzocaine/Butamben/Tetracaine is not for injection.

Do not use on the eyes.

To avoid excessive systemic absorption, Benzocaine/Butamben/Tetracaine should not be applied to large areas of denuded or inflamed tissue.

Benzocaine/Butamben/Tetracaine should not be administered to patients who are hypersensitive to any of its ingredients.

Individual dosage of Tetracaine hydrochloride in excess of 20 mg. is contraindicated. Benzocaine/Butamben/Tetracaine should not be used under dentures or cotton rolls, as retention of the active ingredients under a denture or cotton roll could possibly cause an escharotic effect.

JETCO-SPRAY® CANNULA

The autoclavable, stainless steel Jetco cannula for Benzocaine/Butamben/Tetracaine Spray is specially designed for accessibility and application of Benzocaine/Butamben/Tetracaine at the required site of pain control.

The Jetco cannula is supplied in various lengths and shapes.

The Jetco cannula is inserted firmly onto the protruding plastic tubing on each bottle of Benzocaine/Butamben/Tetracaine Spray.

The Jetco cannula be removed and re-inserted as many times as required for cleansing or sterilization.

HOW SUPPLIED
AEROSOL LIQUID: 14%-2%-2%

BRAND/MANUFACTURER	NDC	SIZE	AWP
○ **BRAND**			
CETACAINE: Cetylite	10223-0201-01	56 ml	$30.00

GEL: 14%-2%-2%

BRAND/MANUFACTURER	NDC	SIZE	AWP
○ **BRAND**			
CETACAINE: Cetylite	10223-0215-01	29 gm	$7.00

KIT:

BRAND/MANUFACTURER	NDC	SIZE	AWP
○ **BRAND**			
CETACAINE: Cetylite	10223-0201-03	56 gm	$41.00

LIQUID: 14%-2%-2%

BRAND/MANUFACTURER	NDC	SIZE	AWP
○ **BRAND**			
CETACAINE: Cetylite	10223-0202-01	56 ml	$8.50

➤ SHOWN IN PRODUCT IDENTIFICATION GUIDE

OINTMENT: 14%-2%-2%

BRAND/MANUFACTURER	NDC	SIZE	AWP
○ **BRAND**			
CETACAINE: Cetylite	10223-0210-01	37 gm	$8.00

Benzonatate

DESCRIPTION

Benzonatate, a nonnarcotic oral antitussive agent, is 2, 5, 8, 11, 14, 17, 20, 23, 26-nonaxaoctacosan-28-yl p-(butylamino) benzoate, with a molecular weight of 603.7.

Each Benzonatate Perle contains:

Benzonatate, USP ....100 mg

Following is its chemical structure:

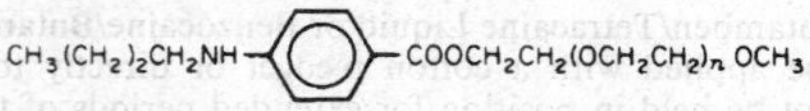

$$CH_3(CH_2)_2CH_2NH \longrightarrow COOCH_2CH_2(OCH_2CH_2)_n \, OCH_3$$

CLINICAL PHARMACOLOGY

Benzonatate acts peripherally by anesthetizing the stretch receptors located in the respiratory passages, lungs, and pleura by dampening their activity and thereby reducing the cough reflex at its source. It begins to act within 15 to 20 minutes and its effect lasts for 3 to 8 hours. Benzonatate has no inhibitory effect on the respiratory center in recommended dosage.

INDICATIONS AND USAGE

Benzonatate is indicated for the symptomatic relief of cough.

CONTRAINDICATIONS

Hypersensitivity to Benzonatate or related compounds.

WARNINGS

Severe hypersensitivity reactions (including bronchospasm, laryngospasm and cardiovascular collapse) have been reported which are possibly related to local anesthesia from sucking or chewing the perle instead of swallowing it. Severe reactions have required intervention with vasopressor agents and supportive measures.

Isolated instances of bizarre behavior, including mental confusion and visual hallucinations, have also been reported in patients taking Benzonatate in combination with other prescribed drugs.

PRECAUTIONS

Benzonatate is chemically related to anesthetic agents of the paramino-benzoic acid class (e.g. procaine; tetracaine) and has been associated with adverse CNS effects possibly related to a prior sensitivity to related agents or interaction with concomitant medication.

Information for Patients: Release of Benzonatate from the perle in the mouth can produce a temporary local anesthesia of the oral mucosa and choking could occur. Therefore, the perles should be swallowed without chewing.

Usage in Pregnancy: Pregnancy Category C. Animal reproduction studies have not been conducted with Benzonatate. It is also not known whether Benzonatate can cause fetal harm when administered to a pregnant woman or can affect reproduction capacity. Benzonatate should be given to a pregnant woman only if clearly needed.

Nursing Mothers: It is not known whether this drug is excreted in human milk. Because many drugs are excreted in human milk caution should be exercised when Benzonatate is administered to a nursing woman.

Carcinogenesis, Mutagenesis, Impairment of Fertility: Carcinogenicity, mutagenicity, and reproduction studies have not been conducted with Benzonatate.

Pediatric Use: Safety and effectiveness in children below the age of 10 has not been established.

ADVERSE REACTIONS

Potential Adverse Reactions to Benzonatate may include:

Hypersensitivity reactions including bronchospasm, laryngospasm, cardiovascular collapse possibly related to local anesthesia from chewing or sucking the perle.

CNS: sedation; headache; dizziness; mental confusion; visual hallucinations.

GI: constipation, nausea, GI upset.

Dermatologic: pruritus; skin eruptions.

Other: nasal congestion; sensation of burning in the eyes; vague "chilly" sensation; numbness of the chest; hypersensitivity. Rare instances of deliberate or accidental overdose have resulted in death.

OVERDOSAGE

Overdose may result in death.

The drug is chemically related to tetracaine and other topical anesthetics and shares various aspects of their pharmacology and toxicology. Drugs of this type are generally well absorbed after ingestion.

SIGNS AND SYMPTOMS

If perles are chewed or dissolved in the mouth, oropharyngeal anesthesia will develop rapidly. CNS stimulation may cause restlessness and tremors which may proceed to clonic convulsions followed by profound CNS depression.

TREATMENT

Evacuate gastric contents and administer copious amounts of activated charcoal slurry. Even in the conscious patient, cough and gag reflexes may be so depressed as to necessitate special attention to protection against aspiration of gastric contents and orally administered materials.

Convulsions should be treated with a short-acting barbiturate given intravenously and carefully titrated for the smallest effective dosage.

Intensive support of respiration and cardiovascular-renal function is an essential feature of the treatment of severe intoxication from overdosage.

Do not use CNS stimulants.

DOSAGE AND ADMINISTRATION

Adults and Children over 10: Usual dose is one 100 mg perle t.i.d. as required. If necessary, up to 6 perles daily may be given.

HOW SUPPLIED
CAPSULE: 100 MG

AVERAGE UNIT PRICE (AVAILABLE SIZES)		GENERIC A-RATED AVERAGE PRICE (GAAP)	
BRAND	$0.74	100s	$54.86
GENERIC	$0.55		

BRAND/MANUFACTURER	NDC	SIZE	AWP
◆ **BRAND**			
➤ TESSALON PERLES: Forest Pharm	00456-0688-01	100s	$75.91
	00456-0688-02	500s	$360.50
◆ **GENERICS**			
Inwood	00258-3654-01	100s	$49.95
Lemmon	00093-0060-01	100s	$51.12
Rugby	00536-5566-01	100s	$54.12
Moore,H.L.	00839-7795-06	100s	$55.15
Moore,H.L.	00839-7797-06	100s	$55.15
Aligen	00405-4115-01	100s	$55.50
Sidmak	50111-0851-01	100s	$55.50
URL	00677-1472-01	100s	$55.58
Qualitest	00603-2426-21	100s	$55.60
Schein	00364-2536-01	100s	$56.39
Major	00904-7737-60	100s	$57.15
Martec	52555-0484-01	100s	$57.15

Benzoyl Peroxide

DESCRIPTION

Benzoyl Peroxide is a topical antibacterial agent, classified as a keratolytic, with the following formula: $C_{14}H_{10}O_4$.

Following is its chemical structure:

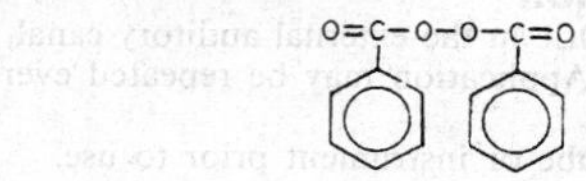

$$O=C-O-O-C=O$$

CLINICAL PHARMACOLOGY

The effectiveness of Benzoyl Peroxide in the treatment of acne vulgaris is primarily attributable to its antibacterial activity, especially with respect to *Propionibacterium acnes*, the predominant organism in sebaceous follicles and comedones. The antibacterial activity of this compound is presumably due to the release of active or free-radical oxygen capable of oxidizing bacterial proteins. This action, combined with its mild keratolytic effect, is believed to be responsible for its usefulness in acne. In acne patients treated topically with Benzoyl Peroxide, resolution of the acne usually coincides with reduction in the level of *P. acnes* and free fatty acids (FFA). Mild desquamation is another observed action of topically applied Benzoyl Peroxide and may also play a role in the drug's effectiveness in acne. Studies also indicate that topical Benzoyl Peroxide may exert a sebostatic effect with a resultant reduction of skin surface lipids.

Benzoyl Peroxide has been shown to be absorbed by the skin, where it is metabolized to benzoic acid and then excreted as benzoate in the urine.

There is no evidence of systemic toxicity caused by Benzoyl Peroxide in humans.

INDICATIONS AND USAGE

Benzoyl Peroxide Emollient Gel is indicated for the topical treatment of mild to moderate acne vulgaris and as an adjunct in therapeutic regimens including antibiotics, retinoic acid products and sulfur or salicylic acid-containing preparations. Benzoyl Peroxide Emollient Gel has been shown effective in the treatment of the following acne lesion types: papules, pustules, open and closed comedones. Clinical studies have demonstrated therapeutic response after two to three weeks.

Benzoyl Peroxide Gel and Cleansing Lotion are indicated for the topical treatment of mild to moderate acne vulgaris and as an adjunct in therapeutic regimens including antibiotics, retinoic acid products and sulfur or salicylic acid-

---

◆ RATED THERAPEUTICALLY EQUIVALENT; ◇ THERAPEUTIC EQUIVALENCE UNCONFIRMED; ○ UNRATED

containing preparations. Benzoyl Peroxide Gel has been shown effective in the treatment of the following acne lesion types: papules, pustules, open and closed comedones. Clinical studies have demonstrated therapeutic response after two to three weeks. Benzoyl Peroxide Gel may also be used as adjunctive treatment for nodulo-cystic acne (acne conglobata), although its effectiveness for this condition has not been proven.

Benzoyl Peroxide Wash is indicated for the topical treatment of mild to moderate acne. In more severe cases, it may be used as an adjunct in therapeutic regimens including Benzoyl Peroxide Gels, antibiotics, retinoic acid products and sulfur/salicylic acid-containing preparations. The improvement of the treated condition is dependent on the degree and type of acne, the frequency of use of Benzoyl Peroxide Wash and the nature of other therapies employed.

Benzoyl Peroxide Bar is indicated for the topical treatment of acne. It may be used as an adjunct in therapeutic regimens including Benzoyl Peroxide Gels, antibiotics, retinoic acid products and sulfur/salicylic acid-containing preparations. The improvement of the treated condition is dependent on the degree and type of acne, the frequency of use of Benzoyl Peroxide Bar and the nature of other therapies employed.

CONTRAINDICATIONS
This product should not be used in patients known to be sensitive to Benzoyl Peroxide or any of the product's other ingredients.

PRECAUTIONS
General: Avoid contact with eyes and other mucous membranes. For external use only. In patients known to be sensitive to the following substances, there is a possibility of cross-sensitization: benzoic acid derivatives (including certain topical anesthetics) and cinnamon.

If severe irritation develops, discontinue use and institute appropriate therapy. After the reaction clears, treatment may often be resumed with less frequent application.

Information for Patients: This product may bleach colored fabric or hair. Concurrent use with PABA-containing sunscreens may result in transient discoloration of the skin.

If excessive irritation develops, discontinue use and consult your physician.

Carcinogenesis, Mutagenesis, Impairment of Fertility: Based upon considerable evidence, Benzoyl Peroxide is not considered to be a carcinogen. However, in several studies, using mice known to be highly susceptible to cancer, there was evidence for Benzoyl Peroxide as a tumor promoter. The clinical significance of these findings to human is unknown. Benzoyl Peroxide has been found to be inactive as a mutagen in the *Ames Salmonella* and other assays, including the mouse dominant lethal assay. This assay is frequently used to assess the effect of substances on spermatogenesis. There are no published data indicating it impairs fertility.

Pregnancy (Category C): Animal reproduction studies have not been conducted with Benzoyl Peroxide. It is also not known whether Benzoyl Peroxide can cause fetal harm when administered to a pregnant woman or can affect reproductive capacity. Benzoyl Peroxide should be given to a pregnant woman only if clearly needed.

There are no available data on the effect of Benzoyl Peroxide on the later growth, development and functional maturation of the unborn child.

Nursing Mothers: It is not known whether this drug is excreted in human milk. Because many drugs are excreted in human milk, caution should be exercised when Benzoyl Peroxide is administered to a nursing woman.

Pediatric Use: Safety and effectiveness in children below the age of 12 have not been established.

ADVERSE REACTIONS
Adverse reactions which may be encountered with topical Benzoyl Peroxide include excessive drying (manifested by marked peeling, erythema and possible edema), and allergic contact sensitization.

Excessive erythema and peeling most frequently appear during the initial phase of drug use and may normally be controlled by reducing frequency of use.

Excessive dryness would appear to occur in approximately 2 patients in 50.

Pertinent literature indicates that allergic sensitization to Benzoyl Peroxide may occur in 10 to 25 patients in 1,000. There is one reference that reports an occurrence of sensitization in 5 of 100 patients.

OVERDOSAGE
In the event that excessive scaling, erythema or edema occur, the use of this preparation should be discontinued. If the reaction is judged to be due to excessive use and not allergenicity, after symptoms and signs subside, a reduced dosage schedule may be cautiously tried.

To hasten resolution of the adverse effects, emollients, cool compresses and/or topical corticosteroid preparations may be used.

DOSAGE AND ADMINISTRATION
Benzoyl Peroxide Emollient Gel should be gently rubbed into all affected areas once or twice daily. Suitable cleansing of the affected areas should precede application. In fair-skinned individuals or under excessively drying conditions, it is suggested that therapy be initiated with one application daily. The degree of drying or peeling may be controlled by modification of dose frequency or drug concentration. The use of Benzoyl Peroxide Emollient Gel (2.5, 5, 10%) may be continued as long as deemed necessary.

Benzoyl Peroxide Gel (2.5, 5, 10%) should be gently rubbed into all affected areas once or twice daily. Suitable cleansing of the affected area should precede application. In fair-skinned individuals or under excessively drying conditions, it is suggested that therapy be initiated with one application daily. The degree of drying or peeling may be controlled by modification of dose frequency or drug concentration. The use of Benzoyl Peroxide Gel may be continued as long as deemed necessary.

Benzoyl Peroxide (5 or 10%) Wash and Cleansing Lotion: Shake well before use. Wash affected areas once or twice daily, (Cleansing Lotion: once daily during the first week and twice a day thereafter as tolerated), avoiding contact with eyes or mucous membranes. Wet skin areas to be treated prior to administration; apply Benzoyl Peroxide Wash to the hands and wash the affected areas, work to a full lather, rinse thoroughly and pat dry. The amount of drying or peeling may be controlled by modification of dose frequency or drug concentration.

Benzoyl Peroxide (10%) Bar: Wash entire area gently with fingertips for 1 to 2 minutes 2 or 3 times daily or as physician directs. Rinse well. The desired degree of dryness and peeling may be obtained by regulating frequency of use.

Store at controlled room temperature (59°-86°F); some brands require storage below 75°F.

HOW SUPPLIED
BAR: 10%

BRAND/MANUFACTURER	NDC	SIZE	AWP
○ **BRAND**			
DESQUAM-X 10: Westwood-Squibb	00072-2000-04	112.5 gm	$7.34

GEL: 2.5%

BRAND/MANUFACTURER	NDC	SIZE	AWP
◆ **GENERICS**			
Qualitest	00603-7713-82	45 gm	$7.62

GEL: 2.5%

BRAND/MANUFACTURER	NDC	SIZE	AWP
◇ **GENERICS**			
Glades	59366-2742-02	45 gm	$7.60

GEL: 2.5%

BRAND/MANUFACTURER	NDC	SIZE	AWP
○ **BRAND**			
DESQUAM-X 2.5: Westwood-Squibb	00072-6300-01	45 gm	$8.72
DESQUAM-E: Westwood-Squibb	00072-6003-45	45 gm	$9.24
PANOXYL AQ 2.5: Stiefel	00145-2375-06	56.7 gm	$9.94
BENZAC W: Galderma	00299-3590-60	60 gm	$12.06
BENZAC AC: Galderma	00299-3620-60	60 gm	$12.38
BENZAC W: Galderma	00299-3590-90	90 gm	$14.56
BENZAC AC: Galderma	00299-3620-90	90 gm	$14.88
PANOXYL AQ 2.5: Stiefel	00145-2375-08	113.4 gm	$13.42
○ **GENERICS**			
BEN-AQUA: Syosset	47854-0657-06	45 gm	$8.00
BEN-AQUA: Syosset	47854-0657-09	120 gm	$15.00

GEL: 4%

BRAND/MANUFACTURER	NDC	SIZE	AWP
○ **BRAND**			
BREVOXYL: Stiefel	00145-2374-06	42.5 gm	$11.33
	00145-2374-08	90 gm	$15.88

GEL: 5%

AVERAGE UNIT PRICE (AVAILABLE SIZES)		GENERIC A-RATED AVERAGE PRICE (GAAP)	
GENERIC	$0.16	45 gm	$7.95

BRAND/MANUFACTURER	NDC	SIZE	AWP
◆ **GENERICS**			
Qualitest	00603-7714-82	45 gm	$7.94
Qualitest	00603-7711-82	45 gm	$7.96
Qualitest	00603-7714-87	93 gm	$11.56

GEL: 5%

BRAND/MANUFACTURER	NDC	SIZE	AWP
◇ **GENERICS**			
Glades	59366-2743-02	45 gm	$7.95
Glades	59366-2745-02	45 gm	$7.95
Glades	59366-2743-03	90 gm	$11.55

GEL: 5%

BRAND/MANUFACTURER	NDC	SIZE	AWP
○ **BRAND**			
DESQUAM-X 5: Westwood-Squibb	00072-6621-01	45 gm	$9.17
DESQUAM-E: Westwood-Squibb	00072-6103-45	45 gm	$9.49
PERSA-GEL: Ortho Pharm	00062-8610-31	45 gm	$10.02
PERSA-GEL W: Ortho Pharm	00062-8630-31	45 gm	$10.02
BENZAGEL-5: Dermik	00066-0430-15	45 gm	$13.75
PANOXYL 5: Stiefel	00145-2372-06	56.7 gm	$10.99
PANOXYL AQ 5: Stiefel	00145-2376-06	56.7 gm	$10.99
BENZAC W: Galderma	00299-3600-01	60 gm	$12.50
BENZAC AC: Galderma	00299-3625-60	60 gm	$12.88
BENZAC: Galderma	00299-3655-01	60 gm	$13.38
DESQUAM-X 5: Westwood-Squibb	00072-6621-03	90 gm	$16.30
BENZAC W: Galderma	00299-3600-09	90 gm	$16.44
BENZAC AC: Galderma	00299-3625-90	90 gm	$16.75
PERSA-GEL: Ortho Pharm	00062-8610-03	90 gm	$17.82
PERSA-GEL W: Ortho Pharm	00062-8630-03	90 gm	$17.82
BENZAGEL-5: Dermik	00066-0430-30	90 gm	$18.95
PANOXYL 5: Stiefel	00145-2372-08	113.4 gm	$15.29
PANOXYL AQ 5: Stiefel	00145-2376-08	113.4 gm	$15.29
○ **GENERICS**			
Moore,H.L.	00839-6186-52	45 gm	$1.61
CMC-Cons	00223-4254-45	45 gm	$2.25
Interstate	00814-1150-73	45 gm	$2.55
SYOXIN: Syosset	47854-0550-06	45 gm	$2.95
PEROXIN A 5: Dermol	50744-0551-06	45 gm	$3.72
CLEARPLEX: Med-Derm	45565-0530-10	45 gm	$3.75
Rugby	00536-4089-56	45 gm	$5.68
ZEROXIN: Syosset	47854-0550-05	45 gm	$8.25
BEN-AQUA: Syosset	47854-0591-06	45 gm	$8.25
ZEROXIN: Syosset	47854-0550-09	120 gm	$5.40
BEN-AQUA: Syosset	47854-0591-09	120 gm	$15.00

GEL: 10%

AVERAGE UNIT PRICE (AVAILABLE SIZES)		GENERIC A-RATED AVERAGE PRICE (GAAP)	
GENERIC	$0.17	**45 gm**	$8.37

BRAND/MANUFACTURER	NDC	SIZE	AWP
◆ **GENERICS**			
Qualitest	00603-7712-82	45 gm	$8.36
Qualitest	00603-7715-82	45 gm	$8.37
Qualitest	00603-7715-87	93 gm	$12.08

GEL: 10%

BRAND/MANUFACTURER	NDC	SIZE	AWP
◇ **GENERICS**			
Glades	59366-2744-02	45 gm	$8.36
Glades	59366-2746-02	45 gm	$8.36
Glades	59366-2744-03	90 gm	$12.10

GEL: 10%

BRAND/MANUFACTURER	NDC	SIZE	AWP
○ **BRAND**			
DESQUAM-X 10: Westwood-Squibb	00072-6721-01	45 gm	$9.35
DESQUAM-E: Westwood-Squibb	00072-6203-45	45 gm	$9.66
PERSA-GEL: Ortho Pharm	00062-8600-31	45 gm	$10.80
PERSA-GEL W: Ortho Pharm	00062-8620-31	45 gm	$10.80
BENZAGEL-10: Dermik	00066-0431-15	45 gm	$14.16
PANOXYL 10: Stiefel	00145-2373-06	56.7 gm	$11.44
PANOXYL AQ 10: Stiefel	00145-2377-06	56.7 gm	$11.44
BENZAC W: Galderma	00299-3610-01	60 gm	$13.06
BENZAC AC: Galderma	00299-3630-60	60 gm	$13.25
BENZAC: Galderma	00299-3665-01	60 gm	$13.88
DESQUAM-X 10: Westwood-Squibb	00072-6721-03	90 gm	$16.59
BENZAC W: Galderma	00299-3610-09	90 gm	$17.19
BENZAC AC: Galderma	00299-3630-90	90 gm	$17.50
PERSA-GEL: Ortho Pharm	00062-8600-03	90 gm	$18.36
PERSA-GEL W: Ortho Pharm	00062-8620-03	90 gm	$18.36
BENZAGEL-10: Dermik	00066-0431-30	90 gm	$19.55
PANOXYL 10: Stiefel	00145-2373-08	113.4 gm	$15.97
PANOXYL AQ 10: Stiefel	00145-2377-08	113.4 gm	$15.97
○ **GENERICS**			
Moore,H.L.	00839-6187-52	45 gm	$1.74
CMC-Cons	00223-4256-45	45 gm	$2.50
Interstate	00814-1151-73	45 gm	$2.63
PEROXIN A 10: Dermol	50744-0592-06	45 gm	$3.84
CLEARPLEX: Med-Derm	45565-0531-10	45 gm	$3.94
SYOXIN: Syosset	47854-0551-06	45 gm	$4.40
Rugby	00536-4092-56	45 gm	$6.91
ZEROXIN: Syosset	47854-0551-05	45 gm	$8.50
BEN-AQUA: Syosset	47854-0592-06	45 gm	$8.50
ACNIGEL: Ampharco	59015-0100-01	85.05 gm	$11.00
ZEROXIN: Syosset	47854-0551-09	120 gm	$6.65
BEN-AQUA: Syosset	47854-0592-09	120 gm	$16.00

LIQUID: 2.5%

BRAND/MANUFACTURER	NDC	SIZE	AWP
○ **BRAND**			
BENZAC AC: Galderma	00299-3635-08	240 ml	$17.44

LIQUID: 5%

AVERAGE UNIT PRICE (AVAILABLE SIZES)	
GENERIC	$0.06

BRAND/MANUFACTURER	NDC	SIZE	AWP
◆ **GENERICS**			
Qualitest	00603-7716-48	150 ml	$9.96
Qualitest	00603-7716-56	240 ml	$12.85

LIQUID: 5%

BRAND/MANUFACTURER	NDC	SIZE	AWP
◇ **GENERICS**			
Glades	59366-2737-04	120 ml	$8.47
Glades	59366-2738-05	150 ml	$9.95
Glades	59366-2739-08	240 ml	$12.85

LIQUID: 5%

BRAND/MANUFACTURER	NDC	SIZE	AWP
○ **BRAND**			
BENZAC W: Galderma	00299-3670-04	120 ml	$11.25
DESQUAM-X WASH: Westwood-Squibb	00072-6905-05	150 ml	$12.04
BENZAC W: Galderma	00299-3670-08	240 ml	$16.88
BENZAC AC: Galderma	00299-3640-08	240 ml	$19.63
○ **GENERICS**			
Rugby	00536-0810-95	30 ml	$2.77

For additional alternatives, turn to the section beginning on page 2859.

Benzoyl Peroxide and Erythromycin

DESCRIPTION

Each gram of Benzoyl Peroxide/Erythromycin topical gel contains, as dispensed, 30 mg (3%) of Erythromycin and 50 mg (5%) of Benzoyl Peroxide.

Benzoyl Peroxide ($C_{14}H_{10}O_4$) is an antibacterial and keratolytic agent.

Erythromycin ($C_{37}H_{67}NO_{13}$) is produced by a strain of *Streptomyces erythraeus* and belongs to the macrolide group of antibiotics.

CLINICAL PHARMACOLOGY

Erythromycin is a bacteriostatic macrolide antibiotic, but may be bactericidal in high concentrations. Although the mechanism by which erythromycin acts in reducing inflammatory lesions of acne vulgaris is unknown, it is presumably due to its antibiotic action. Antagonism has been demonstrated between clindamycin and Erythromycin.

Benzoyl Peroxide is an antibacterial agent which has been shown to be effective against *Propionibacterium acnes,* an anaerobe found in sebaceous follicles and comedones. The antibacterial action of Benzoyl Peroxide is believed to be due to the release of active oxygen. Benzoyl Peroxide has a keratolytic and desquamative effect which may also contribute to its efficacy.

Benzoyl Peroxide has been shown to be absorbed by the skin where it is converted to benzoic acid.

INDICATIONS AND USAGE

Benzoyl Peroxide/Erythromycin is indicated for the topical control of acne vulgaris.

CONTRAINDICATIONS

Benzoyl Peroxide/Erythromycin is contraindicated in those patients with a history of hypersensitivity to Erythromycin, Benzoyl Peroxide or any of the other listed ingredients.

PRECAUTIONS

General: For external use only. Not for ophthalmic use. Avoid contact with eyes and mucous membranes. Concomitant topical acne therapy should be used with caution because a possible cumulative irritancy effect may occur, especially with peeling, desquamating or abrasive agents. If severe irritation develops, discontinue use and institute appropriate therapy.

The use of antibiotic agents may be associated with the overgrowth of antibiotic-resistant organisms. If this occurs, administration of this drug should be discontinued and appropriate measures taken.

Information for Patients: Patients using Benzoyl Peroxide/Erythromycin should receive the following information and instructions:

1. Benzoyl Peroxide/Erythromycin is for external use only. Avoid contact with the eyes and mucous membranes.

2. Patients should not use any other topical acne preparation unless otherwise directed by physician.

3. Benzoyl Peroxide/Erythromycin may bleach hair or colored fabric.

4. If excessive irritation or dryness should occur, patient should discontinue medication and consult physician.

5. Discard product after 3 months and obtain fresh material.

◆ RATED THERAPEUTICALLY EQUIVALENT; ◇ THERAPEUTIC EQUIVALENCE UNCONFIRMED; ○ UNRATED

Carcinogenesis, Mutagenesis and Impairment of Fertility: Long-term studies in animals have not been performed to evaluate carcinogenic potential or the effect on fertility.

Pregnancy Category C: Animal reproduction studies have not been conducted with Benzoyl Peroxide/Erythromycin. It is also not known whether Benzoyl Peroxide/Erythromycin can cause fetal harm when administered to a pregnant woman or can affect reproduction capacity. Benzoyl Peroxide/Erythromycin should be given to a pregnant woman only if clearly needed.

Nursing Mothers: It is not known whether this drug is excreted in human milk. Because many drugs are excreted in human milk, caution should be exercised when Benzoyl Peroxide/Erythromycin is administered to a nursing woman.

Pediatric Use: Safety and effectiveness in children under the age of 12 have not been established.

ADVERSE REACTIONS
Adverse reactions which may occur include dryness, erythema and pruritus. Of a total of 153 patients treated with Benzoyl Peroxide/Erythromycin during clinical trials, 4 patients experienced adverse reactions, of whom three experienced dryness and one an urticarial reaction which responded well to symptomatic treatment.

DOSAGE AND ADMINISTRATION
Benzoyl Peroxide/Erythromycin should be applied twice daily, morning and evening, or as directed by physician, to affected areas after the skin is thoroughly washed, rinsed with warm water and gently patted dry.

DISPENSING INFORMATION
Benzoyl Peroxide/Erythromycin is supplied in a package containing 20 g of Benzoyl Peroxide gel and a plastic vial containing 0.8 g of active Erythromycin powder. Prior to dispensing, tap vial gently until powder flows freely, add 3 mL of ethyl alcohol 70% (to the mark) and shake well to dissolve Erythromycin. Add this solution to gel and stir until homogeneous in appearance (1-1½ minutes). Benzoyl Peroxide/Erythromycin should then be stored under refrigeration. Place a 3-month expiration date on the label.

Note: *Prior* to reconstitution, store at room temperature.

After reconstitution, store in a cold place, preferably in a refrigerator. Do not freeze. Keep tightly closed. Keep out of the reach of children.

HOW SUPPLIED
GEL: 50 MG-30 MG/GM

BRAND/MANUFACTURER	NDC	SIZE	AWP
○ **BRAND** BENZAMYCIN: Dermik	00066-0510-23	23.3 gm	$23.51

Benzoyl Peroxide with Sulfur

DESCRIPTION
Benzoyl Peroxide/Sulfur Lotion Regular and Benzoyl Peroxide/Sulfur Lotion Strong are topical preparations containing Benzoyl Peroxide and Sulfur as the active ingredients.

Benzoyl Peroxide Sulfur Lotion Regular contains: 5% Benzoyl Peroxide and 2% Sulfur.

Benzoyl Peroxide/Sulfur Lotion Strong contains: 10% Benzoyl Peroxide and 5% Sulfur.

CLINICAL PHARMACOLOGY
The exact mode of action of Benzoyl Peroxide and Sulfur in acne vulgaris is unknown. Benzoyl Peroxide and Sulfur are believed to exert a beneficial effect because of their antimicrobial activity and their mild keratolytic action.

INDICATIONS AND USAGE
Benzoyl Peroxide/Sulfur Lotion Regular and Benzoyl Peroxide/Sulfur Lotion Strong are indicated in the treatment of acne vulgaris. See *"Dosage and Administration"* section for information on frequency and duration of drug use.

CONTRAINDICATIONS
Benzoyl Peroxide/Sulfur Lotion Regular and Benzoyl Peroxide/Sulfur Lotion Strong are contraindicated in persons who have shown hypersensitivity to Benzoyl Peroxide, Sulfur, or to any of the other ingredients in the products.

PRECAUTIONS
Benzoyl Peroxide/Sulfur Lotion Regular and Benzoyl Peroxide/Sulfur Lotion Strong are for external use only. They should not be permitted to contact the eyes or mucosal membranes. *Avoid contact with hair, fabrics or carpeting as Benzoyl Peroxide will cause bleaching.*

Long-term studies utilizing rats and mice have been performed to evaluate the carcinogenic potential of Benzoyl Peroxide. Benzoyl Peroxide showed no carcinogenic activity in these studies.

Pregnancy Category C: Animal reproduction studies have not been conducted with Benzoyl Peroxide/Sulfur Lotion Regular or Benzoyl Peroxide/Sulfur Lotion Strong. It is also not known whether Benzoyl Peroxide/Sulfur Lotion Regular or Benzoyl Peroxide/Sulfur Lotion Strong can cause fetal harm when administered to a pregnant woman or can affect reproduction capacity. Benzoyl Peroxide/Sulfur Lotion Regular or Benzoyl Peroxide/Sulfur Lotion Strong should be given

to a pregnant woman only if clearly needed. It is not known whether this drug is excreted in human milk. Because many drugs are excreted in human milk, caution should be exercised when Benzoyl Peroxide/Sulfur Lotion Regular or Benzoyl Peroxide/Sulfur Lotion Strong is administered to a nursing woman.

ADVERSE REACTIONS
Contact sensitization reactions are associated with the use of topical benzoyl peroxide and sulfur products and may be expected to occur in 10 to 25 of 1000 patients. The most frequent adverse reactions associated with Benzoyl Peroxide and Sulfur use are excessive erythema and peeling which may be expected to occur in 5 of 100 patients. Excessive erythema and peeling most frequently appear during the initial phase of drug use and may normally be controlled by reducing frequency of use.

DOSAGE AND ADMINISTRATION
Shake well. It is recommended that therapy be initiated with Benzoyl Peroxide/Sulfur Lotion Regular, applying the medication to the affected areas once a day during the first week, and twice a day thereafter as tolerated. Frequency of use should be adjusted to obtain the desired clinical response. Therapy with Benzoyl Peroxide/Sulfur Lotion Strong may be initiated in patients who demonstrate accommodation to Benzoyl Peroxide/Sulfur Lotion Regular.

Gentle cleansing of the affected areas with a non-medicated soap prior to application of Benzoyl Peroxide/Sulfur Lotion Regular or Benzoyl Peroxide/Sulfur Lotion Strong may be beneficial. Clinically visible improvement will normally occur by the third week of therapy. Maximum lesion reduction may be expected after approximately eight to twelve weeks of drug use. Continuing use of the drug is normally required to maintain a satisfactory clinical response.

Benzoyl Peroxide/Sulfur Lotion Regular and Benzoyl Peroxide/Sulfur Lotion Strong should be stored at controlled room temperature, 15°-30°C (59°-86°F).

HOW SUPPLIED
LOTION: 10%-5%

BRAND/MANUFACTURER	NDC	SIZE	AWP
○ **BRAND** SULFOXYL STRONG: Stiefel	00145-3519-07	60 ml	$11.51

LOTION: 5%-2%

BRAND/MANUFACTURER	NDC	SIZE	AWP
○ **BRAND** SULFOXYL REGULAR: Stiefel	00145-3518-07	60 ml	$10.79

Benzphetamine Hydrochloride

DESCRIPTION
Benzphetamine tablets contain the anorectic agent Benzphetamine Hydrochloride. Benzphetamine Hydrochloride is a white crystalline powder readily soluble in water and 95% ethanol. The chemical name for Benzphetamine Hydrochloride is *d*-N,α-Dimethyl-N-(phenylmethyl)-benzeneethanamine hydrochloride and its molecular weight is 275.82.

Each Benzphetamine Hydrochloride tablet, for oral administration, contains 50 mg of Benzphetamine Hydrochloride.

Following is its chemical structure:

$$\text{C}_6\text{H}_5-\text{CH}_2\text{CH}-\overset{\overset{\displaystyle \text{CH}_3}{|}}{\underset{\underset{\displaystyle \text{CH}_3}{|}}{\text{N}}}-\text{CH}_2-\text{C}_6\text{H}_5 \cdot \text{HCl}$$

CLINICAL PHARMACOLOGY
Benzphetamine Hydrochloride is a sympathomimetic amine with pharmacologic activity similar to the prototype drugs of this class used in obesity, the amphetamines. Actions include central nervous system stimulation and elevation of blood pressure. Tachyphylaxis and tolerance have been demonstrated with all drugs of this class in which these phenomena have been looked for.

Drugs of this class used in obesity are commonly known as "anorectics" or "anorexigenics." It has not been established, however, that the action of such drugs in treating obesity is primarily one of appetite suppression. Other central nervous system actions, or metabolic effects, may be involved.

Adult obese subjects instructed in dietary management and treated with "anorectic" drugs, lose more weight on the average than those treated with placebo and diet, as determined in relatively short term clinical trials.

The magnitude of increased weight loss of drug treated patients over placebo treated patients is only a fraction of a pound a week. The rate of weight loss is greatest in the first weeks of therapy for both drug and placebo subjects and tends to decrease in succeeding weeks. The possible origins of the increased weight loss due to the various drug effects are not established. The amount of weight loss associated with the use of an "anorectic" drug varies from trial to trial, and the increased weight loss appears to be related in part to variables other than the drug prescribed, such as the physician-investigator, the population treated, and the diet prescribed. Studies do not permit conclusions as to the relative importance of the drug and nondrug factors on weight loss.

The natural history of obesity is measured in years, whereas the studies cited are restricted to a few weeks duration; thus, the total impact of drug induced weight loss over that of diet alone must be considered to be clinically limited.

Pharmacokinetic data in humans are not available.

INDICATIONS AND USAGE

Benzphetamine HCl tablets are indicated in the management of exogenous obesity as a short term adjunct (a few weeks) in a regimen of weight reduction based on caloric restriction. The limited usefulness of agents of this class (see "Clinical Pharmacology") should be weighed against possible risks inherent in their use such as those described below.

CONTRAINDICATIONS

Benzphetamine HCl tablets are contraindicated in patients with advanced arteriosclerosis, symptomatic cardiovascular disease, moderate to severe hypertension, hyperthyroidism, known hypersensitivity or idiosyncrasy to sympathomimetic amines, and glaucoma. Benzphetamine should not be given to patients who are in an agitated state or who have a history of drug abuse.

Hypertensive crises have resulted when sympathomimetic amines have been used concomitantly or within 14 days following use of monoamine oxidase inhibitors. Benzphetamine HCl should not be used concomitantly with other CNS stimulants.

Benzphetamine HCl may cause fetal harm when administered to a pregnant woman. Amphetamines have been shown to be teratogenic and embryotoxic in mammals at high multiples of the human dose. Benzphetamine HCl is contraindicated in women who are or may become pregnant. If this drug is used during pregnancy, or if the patient becomes pregnant while taking this drug, the patient should be apprised of the potential hazard to the fetus.

WARNINGS

When tolerance to the anorectic effect develops, the recommended dose should not be exceeded in an attempt to increase the effect; rather, the drug should be discontinued.

PRECAUTIONS

General: Insulin requirements in diabetes mellitus may be altered in association with use of anorexigenic drugs and the concomitant dietary restrictions.

Psychological disturbances have been reported in patients who receive an anorectic agent together with a restrictive dietary regime.

Caution is to be exercised in prescribing amphetamines for patients with even mild hypertension. The least amount feasible should be prescribed or dispensed at one time in order to minimize the possibility of overdosage.

Information for Patients: Amphetamines may impair the ability of the patient to engage in potentially hazardous activities such as operating machinery or driving a motor vehicle; the patient should therefore be cautioned accordingly.

Drug Interactions: Hypertensive crises have resulted when sympathomimetic amines have been used concomitantly or within 14 days following use of monoamine oxidase inhibitors. Benzphetamine HCl should not be used concomitantly with other CNS stimulants.

Amphetamines may decrease the hypotensive effect of antihypertensives. Amphetamines may enhance the effects of tricyclic antidepressants.

Urinary alkalinizing agents increase blood levels and decrease excretion of amphetamines. Urinary acidifying agents decrease blood levels and increase excretion of amphetamines.

Carcinogenesis, Mutagenesis, Impairment of Fertility: Animal studies to evaluate the potential for carcinogenesis, mutagenesis or impairment of fertility have not been performed.

Pregnancy: Pregnancy Category X. (See "Contraindications" section.)

Nursing Mothers: Amphetamines are excreted in human milk. Mothers taking amphetamines should be advised to refrain from nursing.

Pediatric Use: Use of Benzphetamine HCl is not recommended in children under 12 years of age.

ADVERSE REACTIONS

The following have been associated with the use of Benzphetamine HCl:

Cardiovascular: Palpitation, tachycardia, elevation of blood pressure. There have been isolated reports of cardiomyopathy associated with chronic amphetamine use.

CNS: Overstimulation, restlessness, dizziness, insomnia, tremor, sweating, headache; rarely, psychotic episodes at recommended doses; depression following withdrawal of the drug.

Gastrointestinal: Dryness of the mouth, unpleasant taste, nausea, diarrhea, other gastrointestinal disturbances.

Allergic: Urticaria and other allergic reactions involving the skin.

Endocrine: Changes in libido.

DRUG ABUSE AND DEPENDENCE

Benzphetamine is a controlled substance under the Controlled Substance Act by the Drug Enforcement Administration and has been assigned to Schedule III.

Benzphetamine Hydrochloride is related chemically and pharmacologically to the amphetamines. Amphetamines and related stimulant drugs have been extensively abused and the possibility of abuse of Benzphetamine HCl tablets should be kept in mind when evaluating the desirability of including a drug as part of a weight reduction program. Abuse of amphetamines and related drugs may be associated with intense psychological dependence and severe social dysfunction. There are reports of patients who have increased the dosage to many times that recommended. Abrupt cessation following prolonged high dosage administration

results in extreme fatigue and mental depression; changes are also noted on the sleep EEG. Manifestations of chronic intoxication with anorectic drugs include severe dermatoses, marked insomnia, irritability, hyperactivity, and personality changes. The most severe manifestation of chronic intoxication is psychosis, often clinically indistinguishable from schizophrenia.

OVERDOSAGE

Manifestations of Overdosage: Acute overdosage with amphetamines may result in restlessness, tremor, tachypnea, confusion, assaultiveness and panic states. Fatigue and depression usually follow the central stimulation. Cardiovascular effects include arrhythmias, hypertension or hypotension, and circulatory collapse. Gastrointestinal symptoms include nausea, vomiting, diarrhea, and abdominal cramps. Hyperpyrexia and rhabdomyolysis have been reported and can lead to a number of associated complications. Fatal poisoning is usually preceded by convulsions and coma.

TREATMENT OF OVERDOSAGE

(See "Warnings".) Information concerning the effects of overdosage with Benzphetamine HCl tablets is extremely limited. The following is based on experience with other anorectic agents.

Management of acute amphetamine intoxication is largely symptomatic and includes sedation with a barbiturate. If hypertension is marked, the use of a nitrite or rapidly acting alpha receptor blocking agent should be considered. Experience with hemodialysis or peritoneal dialysis is inadequate to permit recommendations in this regard.

Acidification of the urine increases amphetamine excretion. The oral LD_{50} is 174 mg/kg in mice and 104 mg/kg in rats. The intraperitoneal LD_{50} in mice is 153 mg/kg.

DOSAGE AND ADMINISTRATION

Dosage should be individualized according to the response of the patient. The suggested dosage ranges from 25 to 50 mg one to three times daily. Treatment should begin with 25 to 50 mg once daily with subsequent increase in individual dose or frequency according to response. A single daily dose is preferably given in mid-morning or mid-afternoon, according to the patient's eating habits. In an occasional patient it may be desirable to avoid late afternoon administration. Use of Benzphetamine HCl is not recommended in children under 12 years of age.

Store at controlled room temperature, 15°-30° C (59°-86° F).

HOW SUPPLIED
TABLETS (C-III): 50 MG

BRAND/MANUFACTURER	NDC	SIZE	AWP
○ BRAND			
DIDREX: Upjohn	00009-0024-01	100s	$44.48
	00009-0024-02	500s	$219.76

Benzquinamide Hydrochloride

DESCRIPTION

Benzquinamide Hydrochloride is a nonamine-depleting benzoquinolizine derivative, chemically unrelated to the phenothiazines and to other antiemetics.

Chemically, Benzquinamide Hydrochloride is N,N-diethyl-1,3,4,6,7,11b-hexahydro-2-hydroxy-9,10-dimethoxy-2H-benzo-[a]quinolizine-3-carboxamide acetate hydrochloride. The empirical formula is $C_{22}H_{32}N_2O_5 \cdot HCl$ and the molecular weight is 441.

Benzquinamide Hydrochloride for injection contains 50 mg/vial of benzquinamide. When reconstituted with 2.2 ml of proper diluent, each vial yields 2 ml of a solution containing Benzquinamide Hydrochloride equivalent to 25 mg/ml of benzquinamide. When reconstituted this product maintains its potency for 14 days at room temperature.

Following is its chemical structure:

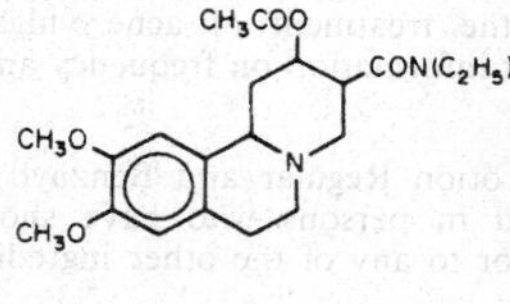

ACTIONS

Benzquinamide Hydrochloride exhibited antiemetic, antihistaminic, mild anticholinergic and sedative action in animals. Studies conducted in dogs and human volunteers have demonstrated suppression of apomorphine-induced vomiting; however, relevance to clinical efficacy has not been established. The mechanism of action in humans is unknown. The onset of antiemetic activity in humans usually occurs within 15 minutes.

Benzquinamide Hydrochloride metabolism has been studied in animals and in man. In both species, 5-10% of an administered dose is excreted unchanged in the urine. The remaining drug undergoes metabolic transformation in the liver by at least three pathways to a spectrum of metabolites which are excreted in the urine and in the bile, from which the more polar metabolites are not reabsorbed but are excreted in the feces. The half-life in plasma of Benzquinamide Hydrochloride is about 40 minutes. More than 95% of an administered dose was excreted within 72 hours in animal studies using C14-labeled Benzquinamide Hydrochloride. In blood, Benzquinamide Hydrochloride is about 58% bound to plasma protein.

INDICATIONS
Benzquinamide Hydrochloride is indicated for the prevention and treatment of nausea and vomiting associated with anesthesia and surgery.

Since the incidence of postoperative and postanesthetic vomiting has decreased with the adoption of modern techniques and agents, the prophylactic use of Benzquinamide Hydrochloride should be restricted to those patients in whom emesis would endanger the results of surgery or result in harm to the patient.

UNLABELED USES
Benzquinamide Hydrochloride is used alone or as an adjunct in the treatment of nausea and vomiting due to chemotherapy.

CONTRAINDICATIONS
Benzquinamide Hydrochloride is contraindicated in individuals who have demonstrated hypersensitivity to the drug.

WARNINGS
USE IN PREGNANCY
No teratogenic effects of Benzquinamide Hydrochloride were demonstrated in reproduction studies in chick embryos, mice, rats and rabbits. The relevance of these data to the human is not known. However, safe use of this drug in pregnancy has not been established and its use in pregnancy is not recommended.

USE IN CHILDREN
As the data available at present are insufficient to establish proper dosage in children, the use of Benzquinamide Hydrochloride in children is not recommended.

INTRAVENOUS USE
Sudden increase in blood pressure and transient arrhythmias (premature ventricular and auricular contractions) have been reported following intravenous administration of Benzquinamide Hydrochloride. Until a more predictable pattern of the effect of intravenous Benzquinamide Hydrochloride has been established, the intramuscular route of administration is considered preferable. The intravenous route of administration should be restricted to patients without cardiovascular disease and receiving no preanesthetic and/or concomitant cardiovascular drugs.

If patients receiving pressor agents or epinephrine-like drugs are also given Benzquinamide Hydrochloride, the latter should be given in fractions of the normal dose. Blood pressure should be monitored. Safeguards against hypertensive reactions are particularly important in hypertensive patients.

PRECAUTIONS
Benzquinamide Hydrochloride, like other antiemetics, may mask signs of overdosage of toxic drugs or may obscure diagnosis of such conditions as intestinal obstruction and brain tumor.

ADVERSE REACTIONS
The following adverse reactions have been reported in subjects who have received Benzquinumide Hydrochloride. However, drowsiness appears to be the most common reaction. One case of pronounced allergic reaction has been encountered, characterized by pyrexia and urticaria.

SYSTEM AFFECTED
Autonomic Nervous System: Dry mouth, shivering, sweating, hiccoughs, flushing, salivation, blurred vision.

Cardiovascular System: Hypertension, hypotension, dizziness, atrial fibrillation, premature auricular and ventricular contractions.

Hypertensive episodes have occurred after IM and IV administration.

Central Nervous System: Drowsiness, insomnia, restlessness, headache, excitement, nervousness.

Gastrointestinal System: Anorexia, nausea.

Musculoskeletal System: Twitching, shaking/tremors, weakness.

Skin: Hives/rash.

Other Systems: Fatigue, shaking chills, increased temperature.

DOSAGE AND ADMINISTRATION
Intramuscular: 50 mg (0.5 mg/kg-1.0 mg/kg)
First dose may be repeated in one hour with subsequent doses every 3-4 hours, as necessary. The precautions applicable to all intramuscular injections should be observed. Benzquinamide Hydrochloride should be injected well within the mass of a larger muscle. The deltoid area should be used only if well developed. Injections should not be made into the lower and mid-thirds of the upper arm. Aspiration of the syringe should be carried out to avoid inadvertent intravascular injection. Therapeutic blood levels and demonstrable antiemetic activity appear within fifteen minutes of intramuscular administration. When the objective of therapy is the prevention of nausea and vomiting, intramuscular adminstration is recommended at least fifteen minutes prior to emergence from anesthesia.

Intravenous: 25 mg (0.2 mg/kg-0.4 mg/kg as a single dose) administered slowly (1 ml per 0.5 to 1 minute). Subsequent doses should be given intramuscularly.

The intravenous route of administration should be restricted to patients without cardiovascular disease (see *"WARNINGS"*). If it is necessary to use Benzquinamide Hydrochloride intravenously in elderly or debilitated patients,

Benzquinamide Hydrochloride should be administered cautiously and the lower dose range is recommended.

This preparation must be initially reconstituted with 2.2 ml of sterile water for injection, bacteriostatic water for injection with benzyl alcohol or with methylparaben and propylparaben. This procedure yields 2 ml of a solution equivalent to 25 mg Benzquinamide Hydrochloride ml, which maintains its potency for 14 days at room temperature.

OVERDOSAGE
Manifestations: On the basis of acute animal toxicology studies, gross Benzquinamide Hydrochloride overdosage in humans might be expected to manifest itself as a combination of Central Nervous System stimulant and depressant effects. This speculation is derived from experimental studies in which intravenous doses of Benzquinamide Hydrochloride, at least 150 times the human therapeutic dose, were administered to dogs.

Treatment: There is no specific antidote for Benzquinamide Hydrochloride overdosage. General supportive measures should be instituted, as indicated. Atropine may be helpful. Although there has been no direct experience with dialysis, it is not likely to be of value, since Benzquinamide Hydrochloride is extensively bound to plasma protein.

J CODES
Up to 50 mg IM,IV—J0510

HOW SUPPLIED
INJECTION: 50 MG

BRAND/MANUFACTURER	NDC	SIZE	AWP
○ **BRAND**			
EMETE-CON: Roerig,J.B.	00049-6690-14	1 ml 10s	$57.62

Benzthiazide

DESCRIPTION
Benzthiazide is a diuretic for oral administration. Each tablet contains 50 mg Benzthiazide.

Benzthiazide is a white, crystalline powder with a characteristic odor, freely soluble in alkaline solution.

The chemical name is 6-chloro-3-[[(phenylmethyl) thio]methyl] -2H-1,2,4-benzothiadiazine-7-sulfonamide 1,1-dioxide.

Following is its chemical structure:

CLINICAL PHARMACOLOGY
Benzthiazide is a diuretic and antihypertensive. It affects the renal tubular mechanism of electrolyte reabsorption. At maximal therapeutic dosage, all thiazides are approximately equal in their diuretic potency. The mechanism whereby thiazides function in the control of hypertension is unknown. Benzthiazide increases excretion of sodium and chloride in approximately equivalent amounts. Natriuresis may be accompanied by some loss of potassium and bicarbonate.

In humans, Benzthiazide is excreted in the urine almost entirely unchanged. Following a single oral dose of Benzthiazide tablets or Benzthiazide solution, 1% and 4.3% of the respective doses were recovered in the urine in 24 hr. The relative bioavailability of Benzthiazide tablets was determined to be about 25% in reference to Benzthiazide solution.

INDICATIONS AND USAGE
Benzthiazide is indicated as adjunctive therapy in edema associated with congestive heart failure, hepatic cirrhosis and corticosteroid and estrogen therapy.

Benzthiazide has also been found useful in edema due to various forms of renal dysfunction as: nephrotic syndrome; acute glomerulonephritis; and chronic renal failure.

Benzthiazide is indicated in the management of hypertension either as the sole therapeutic agent or to enhance the effectiveness of other antihypertensive drugs in the more severe forms of hypertension.

Use in Pregnancy: The routine use of diuretics in an otherwise healthy woman is inappropriate and exposes mother and fetus to unnecessary hazard. Diuretics do not prevent development of toxemia of pregnancy, and there is no satisfactory evidence that they are useful in the treatment of developed toxemia.

Edema during pregnancy may arise from pathological causes or from the physiologic and mechanical consequences of pregnancy. Thiazides are indicated in pregnancy when edema is due to pathologic causes, just as they are in the absence of pregnancy (however, see *"Warnings,"* below). Dependent edema in pregnancy, resulting from restriction of venous return by the expanded uterus, is properly treated through elevation of the lower extremities and use of support hose; use of diuretics to lower intravascular volume in this case is illogical and unnecessary. There is hypervolemia during normal pregnancy which is harmful to neither the fetus nor the mother (in the absence of cardiovascular disease), but which is associated with edema, including generalized edema, in the majority of pregnant women. If this edema produces discomfort, increased recumbency will often provide relief. In rare instances, this edema may cause extreme discomfort which is not relieved by rest. In these cases, a short course of diuretics may provide relief and may be appropriate.

CONTRAINDICATIONS
Anuria. Hypersensitivity to this or other sulfonamide-derived drugs.

WARNINGS
Thiazides should be used with caution in severe renal disease. In patients with renal disease, thiazides may precipitate azotemia. Cumulative effects of the drug may develop in patients with impaired renal function.

Thiazides should be used with caution in patients with impaired hepatic function or progressive liver disease, since minor alterations of fluid and electrolyte balance may precipitate hepatic coma.

Sensitivity reactions may occur inpatients with a history of allergy or bronchial asthma.

The possibility of exacerbation or activation of systemic lupus erythematosus has been reported.

Latent diabetes mellitus may become manifest during thiazide administration: hyperuricemia or frank gout may also be precipitated in certain patients. The antihypertensive effect of the drug may be enhanced in the postsympathectomy patient.

PRECAUTIONS
General: All patients receiving thiazide therapy should be observed for clinical signs of fluid or electrolyte imbalance: namely, hyponatremia, hypochloremic alkalosis, and hypokalemia.

Dilutional hyponatremia may occur in edematous patients in hot weather; appropriate therapy is water restriction, rather than administration of salt except in rare instances when hyponatremia is life threatening.

In actual salt depletion, appropriate replacement is the therapy of choice. Any chloride deficit is generally mild and usually does not require specific treatment except under extraordinary circumstances (as in liver disease or renal disease).

Hypokalemia may develop with thiazides as with any other potent diuretic especially with brisk diuresis. Inadequate oral electrolyte intake will also contribute to hypokalemia. Certain brands of Benzthiazide contain FD&C Yellow No. 5 (tartrazine) which may cause allergic-type reactions (including bronchial asthma) in certain susceptible individuals. Although the overall incidence of FD&C Yellow No. 5 (tartrazine) sensitivity in the general population is low, it is frequently seen in patients who have aspirin hypersensitivity.

Information for Patients: Warning signs of electrolyte imbalance are: dryness of mouth, thirst, weakness, lethargy, drowsiness, restlessness, muscle pains or cramps, muscular fatigue, hypotension, oliguria, tachycardia, and gastrointestinal disturbances such as nausea and vomiting.

Laboratory Tests: Periodic determination of serum electrolytes to detect possible electrolyte imbalance should be performed at appropriate intervals. When the patient is vomiting excessively or receiving parenteral fluids, serum and urine electrolyte determinations are particularly important. In patients with renal impairment, nonprotein nitrogen or blood urea nitrogen level should be tested periodically; rising values would indicate progressive renal impairment and careful reappraisal of therapy is necessary with consideration given to withholding or discontinuing diuretic therapy.

Drug Interaction: Thiazides may add to or potentiate the action of other hypotensive drugs. Potentiation occurs with ganglionic or peripheral adrenergic-blocking drugs.

Thiazides may increase the responsiveness to tubocurarine. Thiazides may decrease arterial responsiveness to norepinephrine. This diminution is not sufficient to preclude effectiveness of the pressor agent for therapeutic use.

Insulin requirement in diabetic patients may be increased, decreased, or unchanged.

Medication such as digitalis may also influence serum electrolytes. Digitalis therapy may exaggerate metabolic effects of hypokalemia especially with reference to myocardial activity.

Drug/Laboratory Test Interactions: Thiazides may decrease serum PBI levels without signs of thyroid disturbance.

Carcinogenesis, Mutagenesis, Impairment of Fertility: No animal carcinogenicity or mutagenesis studies on Benzthiazide are known.

Pregnancy Teratogenic Effects: Pregnancy Category C. Benzthiazide has an embryocidal effect in rats when given in doses several hundred times the human dose. Benzthiazide can cause fetal harm when administered to a pregnant woman. Fetal or neonatal jaundice has been reported. Thrombocytopenia and possibly other adverse reactions have occurred in the adult. If this drug is used during pregnancy, or if patient becomes pregnant while taking this drug, the patient should be apprised of the potential hazard to the fetus.

Thiazides cross the placental barrier and appear in cord blood.

Nursing mothers: It is not known whether this drug is excreted in human milk. Because many drugs are excreted in human milk, caution should be exercised when Benzthiazide is administered to a nursing mother.

Pediatric use: Safety and effectiveness in children have not been established.

ADVERSE REACTIONS
The following adverse reactions have been observed, but there is not enough systematic collection of data to support an estimate of their frequency.

Gastrointestinal System: jaundice (intrahepatic cholestatic jaundice); pancreatitis; gastric irritation; vomiting; cramping; nausea; anorexia; diarrhea; constipation.

Central Nervous System: dizziness; restlessness; paresthesia; headache; xanthopsia.

Hematologic: aplastic anemia; thrombocytopenia; agranulocytosis; leukopenia.

Dermatologic-Hypersensitivity: necrotizing angiitis (vasculitis) (cutaneous vasculitis); purpura; urticaria; rash; photosensitivity.

Cardiovascular: Orthostatic hypotension may occur and may be aggravated by alcohol, barbiturates or narcotics.

Other: hyperglycemia; glycosuria; hyperuricemia; weakness; muscle spasm.

Whenever adverse reactions are moderate or severe, thiazide dosage should be reduced or therapy withdrawn.

OVERDOSAGE
Symptoms of overdosage include electrolyte imbalance and signs of potassium deficiency such as confusion, dizziness, muscular weakness, and gastrointestinal disturbances. General supportive measures including replacement of fluids and electrolytes may be indicated in treatment of overdosage.

DOSAGE AND ADMINISTRATION
Therapy should be individualized according to patient response. This therapy should be titrated to gain maximal therapeutic response as well as the minimal dose possible to maintain that therapeutic response.

	Diuretic	Antihypertensive
Benzthiazide	50 to 200 mg	50 to 200 mg

Edema: Initiation of Diuresis: 50 to 200 mg daily should be used for several days, or until dry weight is attained. With 100 mg or more daily, it is generally preferable to administer Benzthiazide in two doses, following morning and evening meals.

Maintenance of Diuresis: 50 to 150 mg daily depending upon the patient's response. To maintain effectiveness, reduction to minimal effective dosage should be gradual.

Hypertension: Initiation of Antihypertensive Therapy: 50 to 100 mg daily is the average dose. It may be given in two doses of 25 mg or 50 mg each after breakfast and after lunch. This dosage may be continued until a therapeutic drop in blood pressure occurs.

Maintenance of Antihypertensive Therapy: Dosage should be adjusted according to the patient response, either upward to as much as 50 mg q.i.d. or downward to the minimal effective dosage level.

Store: Store at controlled room temperature, between 15°C and 30°C (59°F and 86°F).

Dispense in tight container.

HOW SUPPLIED
TABLETS: 50 MG

BRAND/MANUFACTURER	NDC	SIZE	AWP
◇ **BRAND**			
EXNA: Robins Pharm	00031-5449-63	100s	$18.78

Benztropine Mesylate

DESCRIPTION
Benztropine Mesylate is a synthetic compound containing structural features found in atropine and diphenhydramine. It is designated chemically as 8-azabicyclo[3.2.1] octane, 3-(diphenylmethoxy)-,*endo*, methanesulfonate. Its empirical formula is $C_{21}H_{25}NO \cdot CH_4O_3S$.

Benztropine Mesylate is a crystalline white powder, very soluble in water, and has a molecular weight of 403.54.

Benztropine Mesylate is supplied as tablets in three strengths (0.5 mg, 1 mg, and 2 mg per tablet), and as a sterile injection for intravenous and intramuscular use. Each milliliter of the injection contains 1 mg of Benztropine Mesylate.

Following is its chemical structure:

ACTIONS
Benztropine possesses both anticholinergic and antihistaminic effects, although only the former have been established as therapeutically significant in the management of parkinsonism.

In the isolated guinea pig ileum, the anticholinergic activity of this drug is about equal to that of atropine; however, when administered orally to unanesthetized cats, it is only about half as active as atropine.

◆ RATED THERAPEUTICALLY EQUIVALENT; ◇ THERAPEUTIC EQUIVALENCE UNCONFIRMED; ○ UNRATED

In laboratory animals, its antihistaminic activity and duration of action approach those of pyrilamine maleate.

INDICATIONS
For use as an adjunct in the therapy of all forms of parkinsonism.

Useful also in the control of extrapyramidal disorders (except tardive dyskinesia—see "Precautions") due to neuroleptic drugs (e.g., phenothiazines).

CONTRAINDICATIONS
Hypersensitivity to Benztropine tablets or to any component of Benztropine injection.

Because of its atropine-like side effects, this drug is contraindicated in children under three years of age, and should be used with caution in older children.

WARNINGS
Safe use in pregnancy has not been established. Benztropine may impair mental and/or physical abilities required for performance of hazardous tasks, such as operating machinery or driving a motor vehicle.

When Benztropine is given concomitantly with phenothiazines, haloperidol, or other drugs with anticholinergic or antidopaminergic activity, patients should be advised to report gastrointestinal complaints, fever or heat intolerance promptly. Paralytic ileus, hyperthermia and heat stroke, all of which have sometimes been fatal, have occurred in patients taking anticholinergic-type antiparkinsonism drugs, including Benztropine, in combination with phenothiazines and/or tricyclic antidepressants.

Since Benztropine contains structural features of atropine, it may produce anhidrosis. For this reason, it should be administered with caution during hot weather, especially when given concomitantly with other atropine-like drugs to the chronically ill, the alcoholic, those who have central nervous system disease, and those who do manual labor in a hot environment. Anhidrosis may occur more readily when some disturbance of sweating already exists. If there is evidence of anhidrosis, the possibility of hyperthermia should be considered. Dosage should be decreased at the discretion of the physician so that the ability to maintain body heat equilibrium by perspiration is not impaired. Severe anhidrosis and fatal hyperthermia have occurred.

PRECAUTIONS
General: Since Benztropine has cumulative action, continued supervision is advisable. Patients with a tendency to tachycardia and patients with prostatic hypertrophy should be observed closely during treatment.

Dysuria may occur, but rarely becomes a problem. Urinary retention has been reported with Benztropine.

The drug may cause complaints of weakness and inability to move particular muscle groups, especially in large doses. For example, if the neck has been rigid and suddenly relaxes, it may feel weak, causing some concern. In this event, dosage adjustment is required.

Mental confusion and excitement may occur with large doses, or in susceptible patients. Visual hallucinations have been reported occasionally. Furthermore, in the treatment of extrapyramidal disorders due to neuroleptic drugs (e.g., phenothiazines), in patients with mental disorders, occasionally there may be intensification of mental symptoms. In such cases, antiparkinsonian drugs can precipitate a toxic psychosis. Patients with mental disorders should be kept under careful observation, especially at the beginning of treatment or if dosage is increased.

Tardive dyskinesia may appear in some patiens on long-term therapy with phenothiazines and related agents, or may occur after therapy with these drugs has been discontinued. Antiparkinsonism agents do not alleviate the symptoms of tardive dyskinesia, and in some instances may aggravate them. Benztropine is not recommended for use in patients with tardive dyskinesia.

The physician should be aware of the possible occurrence of glaucoma. Although the drug does not appear to have any adverse effect on simple glaucoma, it probably should not be used in angle-closure glaucoma.

Drug Interactions: Antipsychotic drugs such as phenothiazines or haloperidol; tricyclic antidepressants (see "Warnings").

ADVERSE REACTIONS
The adverse reactions below, most of which are anticholinergic in nature, have been reported and within each category are listed in order of decreasing severity.

Cardiovascular: Tachycardia.

Digestive: Paralytic ileus, constipation, vomiting, nausea, dry mouth. If dry mouth is so severe that there is difficulty in swallowing or speaking, or loss of appetite and weight, reduce dosage, or discontinue the drug temporarily.

Slight reduction in dosage may control nausea and still give sufficient relief of symptoms. Vomiting may be controlled by temporary discontinuation, followed by resumption at a lower dosage.

Nervous System: Toxic psychosis, including confusion, disorientation, memory impairment, visual hallucinations; exacerbation of pre-existing psychotic symptoms; nervousness; depression; list-lessness; numbness of fingers.

Special Senses: Blurred vision, dilated pupils.

Urogenital: Urinary retention, dysuria.

Metabolic/Immune or Skin: Occasionally, an allergic reaction, e.g., skin rash, develops. If this can not be controlled by dosage reduction, the medication should be discontinued.

Other: Heat stroke, hyperthermia, fever.

DOSAGE AND ADMINISTRATION
Benztropine tablets should be used when patients are able to take oral medication.

The injection is especially useful for psychotic patients with acute dystonic reactions or other reactions that make oral medication difficult or impossible. It is recommended also when a more rapid response is desired than can be obtained with the tablets.

Since there is no significant difference in onset of effect after intravenous or intramuscular injection, usually there is no need to use the intravenous route. The drug is quickly effective after either route, with improvement sometimes noticeable a few minutes after injection. In emergency situations, when the condition of the patient is alarming, 1 to 2 mL of the injection normally will provide quick relief. If the parkinsonian effect begins to return, the dose can be repeated. Because of cumulative action, therapy should be initiated with a low dose which is increased gradually at five or six-day intervals to the smallest amount necessary for optimal relief. Increases should be made in increments of 0.5 mg, to a maximum of 6 mg, or until optimal results are obtained without excessive adverse reactions.

Postencephalitic and Idiopathic Parkinsonism: The usual daily dose is 1 to 2 mg, with a range of 0.5 to 6 mg orally or parenterally.

As with any agent used in parkinsonism, dosage must be individualized according to age and weight, and the type of parkinsonism being treated. Generally, older patients and thin patients cannot tolerate large doses. Most patients with postencephalitic parkinsonism need fairly large doses and tolerate them well. Patients with a poor mental outlook are usually poor candidates for therapy.

In idiopathic parkinsonism, therapy may be initiated with a single daily dose of 0.5 to 1 mg at bedtime. In some patients, this will be adequate; in others 4 to 6 mg a day may be required.

In postencephalitic parkinsonism, therapy may be initiated in most patients with 2 mg a day in one or more doses. In highly sensitive patients, therapy may be initiated with 0.5 mg at bedtime, and increased as necessary.

Some patients experience greatest relief by taking the entire dose at bedtime; others react more favorably to divided doses, two to four times a day. Frequently, one dose a day is sufficient, and divided doses may be unnecessary or undesirable.

The long duration of action of this drug makes it particularly suitable for bedtime medication when its effects may last throughout the night, enabling patients to turn in bed during the night more easily, and to rise in the morning.

When Benztropine is started, do not terminate therapy with other antiparkinsonian agents abruptly. If the other agents are to be reduced or discontinued, it must be done gradually. Many patients obtain greatest relief with combination therapy.

Benztropine may be used concomitantly with Carbidopa-Levodopa or with levodopa, in which case periodic dosage adjustment may be required in order to maintain optimum response.

Drug-Induced Extrapyramidal Disorders: In treating extrapyramidal disorders due to neuroleptic drugs (e.g., phenothiazines), the recommended dosage is 1 to 4 mg once or twice a day orally or parenterally. Dosage must be individualized according to the need of the patient. Some patients require more than recommended: others do not need as much.

In acute dystonic reactions, 1 to 2 mL of the injection usually relieves the condition quickly. After that, the tablets, 1 to 2 mg twice a day, usually prevent recurrence.

When extrapyramidal disorders develop soon after initiation of treatment with neuroleptic drugs (e.g., phenothiazines), they are likely to be transient. One to 2 mg of Benztropine tablets two or three times a day usually provides relief within one or two days. After one or two weeks, the drug should be withdrawn to determine the continued need for it. If such disorders recur, Benztropine can be reinstituted.

Certain drug-induced extrapyramidal disorders that develop slowly may not respond to Benztropine.

OVERDOSAGE
Manifestations: May be any of those seen in atropine poisoning or antihistamine overdosage: CNS depression, preceded or followed by stimulation; confusion; nervousness; listlessness; intensification of mental symptoms or toxic psychosis in patients with mental illness being treated with neuroleptic drugs (e.g., phenothiazines); hallucinations (especially visual); dizziness; muscle weakness; ataxia; dry mouth; mydriasis; blurred vision; palpitations; tachycardia; elevated blood pressure; nausea; vomiting; dysuria; numbness of fingers; dysphagia; allergic reactions, e.g., skin rash; headache; hot, dry, flushed skin; delirium; coma; shock; convulsions; respiratory arrest; anhidrosis; hyperthermia; glaucoma; constipation.

Treatment: Physostigmine salicylate, 1 to 2 mg, SC or IV, reportedly will reverse symptoms of anticholinergic intoxication. A second injection may be given after 2 hours if required. Otherwise treatment is symptomatic and supportive. Induce emesis or perform gastric lavage (contraindicated in precomatose, convulsive, or psychotic states). Maintain respiration. A short-acting barbiturate may be used for CNS excitement, but with caution to avoid subsequent depression; supportive care for depression (avoid convulsant stimulants such as picrotoxin, pentylenetetrazol, or bemegride); artificial respiration for severe respiratory depression; a local miotic for mydriasis and cycloplegia; ice bags or other cold applications and alcohol sponges for hyperpyrexia, a vasopressor and fluids for circulatory collapse. Darken room for photophobia.

J CODES
IM,IV—J0515

HOW SUPPLIED

INJECTION: 1 MG/ML

BRAND/MANUFACTURER	NDC	SIZE	AWP
○ BRAND			
COGENTIN: Merck	00006-3275-16	2 ml 6s	$40.46

TABLETS: 0.5 MG

AVERAGE UNIT PRICE (AVAILABLE SIZES)		GENERIC A-RATED AVERAGE PRICE (GAAP)	
BRAND	$0.17	100s	$7.69
GENERIC	$0.08		
HCFA FUL (100s ea)	$0.03		

BRAND/MANUFACTURER	NDC	SIZE	AWP
◆ BRAND			
➤ COGENTIN: Merck	00006-0021-68	100s	$16.93
◆ GENERICS			
Medirex	57480-0305-06	30s	$4.25
Qualitest	00603-2430-21	100s	$5.10
Moore,H.L.	00839-7002-06	100s	$5.25
Rugby	00536-3370-01	100s	$5.38
Goldline	00182-1299-01	100s	$5.65
Invamed	52189-0208-24	100s	$5.70
URL	00677-0994-01	100s	$5.95
Major	00904-1055-60	100s	$5.95
Schein	00364-0834-01	100s	$6.00
Geneva	00781-1347-01	100s	$6.51
Martec	52555-0457-01	100s	$6.90
Par	49884-0164-01	100s	$7.05
Parmed	00349-8941-01	100s	$7.36
Duramed	51285-0827-02	100s	$9.21
Aligen	00405-4116-01	100s	$9.60
U.S. Trading	56126-0164-11	100s ud	$4.89
Goldline	00182-1299-89	100s ud	$6.99
Raway	00686-0220-20	100s ud	$7.85
Auro	55829-0164-10	100s ud	$10.43
Major	00904-1055-61	100s ud	$11.44
UDL	51079-0220-20	100s ud	$14.12
Medirex	57480-0305-01	100s ud	$14.15

TABLETS: 1 MG

AVERAGE UNIT PRICE (AVAILABLE SIZES)		GENERIC A-RATED AVERAGE PRICE (GAAP)	
BRAND	$0.22	100s	$9.61
GENERIC	$0.09	750s	$101.10
HCFA FUL (100s ea)	$0.03	1000s	$60.73

BRAND/MANUFACTURER	NDC	SIZE	AWP
◆ BRAND			
➤ COGENTIN: Merck	00006-0635-68	100s	$19.34
	00006-0635-28	100s ud	$23.56
◆ GENERICS			
Medirex	57480-0306-06	30s	$5.82
Major	00904-1056-52	60s	$3.50
Qualitest	00603-2431-21	100s	$5.40
Invamed	52189-0209-24	100s	$6.40
Goldline	00182-1700-01	100s	$6.40
Schein	00364-0703-01	100s	$6.75
Geneva	00781-1357-01	100s	$6.88
Martec	52555-0458-01	100s	$7.10
Major	00904-1056-60	100s	$7.45
Parmed	00349-8942-01	100s	$7.50
URL	00677-0993-01	100s	$8.10
Mutual	53489-0183-01	100s	$8.10
➤ Par	49884-0165-01	100s	$8.25
Duramed	51285-0828-02	100s	$10.51
Moore,H.L.	00839-6771-06	100s	$10.52
Aligen	00405-4117-01	100s	$10.90
U.S. Trading	56126-0165-11	100s ud	$4.88
Raway	00686-0221-10	100s ud	$7.50
Goldline	00182-1700-89	100s ud	$10.99
Auro	55829-0165-10	100s ud	$11.80
Vangard	00615-2548-13	100s ud	$13.48
Major	00904-1056-61	100s ud	$13.85
UDL	51079-0221-20	100s ud	$19.32
Medirex	57480-0306-01	100s ud	$19.40
Sandocare	58345-0831-65	640s ud	$41.60
Glasgow	60809-0109-55	750s ud	$101.10
Glasgow	60809-0109-72	750s ud	$101.10
Major	00904-1056-80	1000s	$37.20
Qualitest	00603-2431-32	1000s	$43.15
Schein	00364-0703-02	1000s	$49.50
Invamed	52189-0209-30	1000s	$51.00
Goldline	00182-1700-10	1000s	$51.00
Geneva	00781-1357-10	1000s	$53.29
Parmed	00349-8942-10	1000s	$54.45
URL	00677-0993-10	1000s	$54.50
Mutual	53489-0183-10	1000s	$54.50
Martec	52555-0458-10	1000s	$54.90
➤ Par	49884-0165-10	1000s	$80.00
Duramed	51285-0828-05	1000s	$102.97
Moore,H.L.	00839-6771-16	1000s	$102.99

TABLETS: 2 MG

AVERAGE UNIT PRICE (AVAILABLE SIZES)		GENERIC A-RATED AVERAGE PRICE (GAAP)	
BRAND	$0.24	100s	$11.26
GENERIC	$0.11	750s	$119.70
HCFA FUL (100s ea)	$0.04	1000s	$88.94

BRAND/MANUFACTURER	NDC	SIZE	AWP
◆ BRAND			
➤ COGENTIN: Merck	00006-0060-68	100s	$24.38
	00006-0060-28	100s ud	$28.63
	00006-0060-82	1000s	$203.35
◆ GENERICS			
Medirex	57480-0307-06	30s	$5.96
Major	00904-1057-52	60s	$4.10
Rugby	00536-3372-01	100s	$6.88
Qualitest	00603-2432-21	100s	$6.93
Invamed	52189-0210-24	100s	$8.00
Schein	00364-0704-01	100s	$8.50
Goldline	00182-1701-01	100s	$8.50
Geneva	00781-1367-01	100s	$9.38
Martec	52555-0459-01	100s	$9.80
Major	00904-1057-60	100s	$9.95
Par	49884-0166-01	100s	$10.10
Parmed	00349-8943-01	100s	$10.58
URL	00677-0995-01	100s	$10.75
Mutual	53489-0184-01	100s	$10.75
Moore,H.L.	00839-6772-06	100s	$12.54
Duramed	51285-0829-02	100s	$13.25
Aligen	00405-4118-01	100s	$13.75
U.S. Trading	56126-0166-11	100s ud	$5.61
Raway	00686-0222-20	100s ud	$8.00
Auro	55829-0166-10	100s ud	$13.35
Goldline	00182-1701-89	100s ud	$14.99
Major	00904-1057-61	100s ud	$16.48
Medirex	57480-0307-01	100s ud	$19.85
UDL	51079-0222-20	100s ud	$19.86
Rugby	00536-3372-05	500s	$29.75
Sandocare	58345-0832-65	640s ud	$56.50
Glasgow	60809-0110-55	750s ud	$119.70
Glasgow	60809-0110-72	750s ud	$119.70
Major	00904-1057-80	1000s	$62.10
Qualitest	00603-2432-32	1000s	$65.11
Invamed	52189-0210-30	1000s	$66.00
Geneva	00781-1367-10	1000s	$70.39
Schein	00364-0704-02	1000s	$75.00
Goldline	00182-1701-10	1000s	$75.00
URL	00677-0995-10	1000s	$89.00
Mutual	53489-0184-10	1000s	$89.00
Parmed	00349-8943-10	1000s	$89.77

Benzylpenicilloyl Polylysine

DESCRIPTION

Benzylpenicilloyl Polylysine injection USP is a skin test antigen used in assessing a patient's allergy status to penicillin.

Benzylpenicilloyl Polylysine is a sterile solution in a concentration of 6.0×10^{-5} $\underline{M}$ (Benzylpenicilloyl) in 0.01 $\underline{M}$ phosphate buffer and 0.15 $\underline{M}$ sodium chloride and water for injection. The Benzylpenicilloyl polylysine is a derivative of poly-l-lysine, where the epsilon amino groups are substituted with Benzylpenicilloyl groups (50-70%) forming Benzylpenicilloyl alpha amide. Each single dose ampul contains 0.25 mL of Benzylpenicilloy/Polylysine.

Benzylpenicilloyl/Polylysine (Benzylpenicilloyl Polylysine injection USP) is a clear, colorless, sterile solution supplied in ampuls containing 0.25 mL.

CLINICAL PHARMACOLOGY

Benzylpenicilloyl Polylysine reacts specifically with Benzylpenicilloyl skin sensitizing antibodies (reagins: IgE class) to initiate release of chemical mediators which produce an immediate wheal and flare reaction at a skin test site. All individuals exhibiting a positive skin test to Benzylpenicilloyl Polylysine possess reagins against the Benzylpenicilloyl group which is a haptene. A haptene is a low molecular weight chemical which, when conjugated to a carrier, e.g., poly-l-lysine, has the properties under appropriate conditions of an antigen with the haptene's specificity. It is to be noted that individuals who have previously received therapeutic penicillin may have positive skin test reactions to Benzylpenicilloyl Polylysine as well as to a number of other non-Benzylpenicilloyl haptenes. The latter are designated as minor determinants, in that they are present in lesser amounts than the major determinant, Benzylpenicilloyl. The minor determinants may nevertheless be associated with examples of significant clinical hypersensitivity.

Virtually everyone who receives penicillin develops specific antibodies to the drug as measured by hemagglutination studies, but (a) positive skin tests to various penicillin and penicillin-derived reagents become positive in less than 10% of patients who have tolerated penicillin in the past and (b) allergic responses are infrequent (less than 1%).

Many individuals reacting positively to Benzylpenicilloyl Polylysine will not develop a systemic allergic reaction on subsequent exposure to therapeutic penicillin. Thus, the Benzylpenicilloyl Polylysine skin test facilitates assessing the local allergic skin reactivity of a patient to Benzylpenicilloyl.

◆ RATED THERAPEUTICALLY EQUIVALENT; ◇ THERAPEUTIC EQUIVALENCE UNCONFIRMED; ○ UNRATED

INDICATIONS AND USAGE

Benzylpenicilloyl Polylysine is useful as an adjunct in assessing the risk of administering penicillin (benzylpenicillin or penicillin G) when it is the preferred drug of choice in adult patients who have previously received penicillin and have a history of clinical penicillin hypersensitivity. In this situation, a negative skin test to Benzylpenicilloyl Polylysine is associated with an incidence of allergic reactions of less than 5% after the administration of therapeutic penicillin, whereas the incidence may be more than 20% in the presence of a positive skin test to Benzylpenicilloyl Polylysine.

These allergic reactions are predominantly dermatologic. Because of the extremely low incidence of anaphylactic reactions, there are insufficient data at present to document that a decreased incidence of anaphylactic reactions following the administration of penicillin will occur in patients with a negative skin test to Benzylpenicilloyl Polylysine. Similarly, when deciding the risk of proposed penicillin treatment, there are not enough data at present to permit relative weighing in individual cases of a history of clinical penicillin hypersensitivity as compared to positive skin tests to Benzylpenicilloyl Polylysine and/or minor penicillin determinants.

It should be borne in mind that no reagent, test, or combination of tests will completely assure that a reaction to penicillin therapy will not occur.

CONTRAINDICATIONS

Benzylpenicilloyl Polylysine is contraindicated in those patients who have exhibited either a systemic or marked local reaction to its previous administration. Patients known to be extremely hypersensitive to penicillin should not be skin tested.

WARNINGS

There are insufficient data to assess the potential danger of sensitization to repeated skin testing with Benzylpenicilloyl Polylysine.

Rarely, a systemic allergic reaction (see below) may follow a skin test with Benzylpenicilloyl Polylysine. This can be avoided by making the first application by scratch test and very carefully following the instructions below in administering the intradermal test, using the intradermal route only if the scratch test has been entirely negative.

Skin testing with penicillin and/or other penicillin-derived reagents should not be performed simultaneously.

PRECAUTIONS

GENERAL:
There are insufficient data derived from well-controlled studies to determine the value of the Benzylpenicilloyl Polylysine skin test as a means of assessing the risk of administering therapeutic penicillin (when penicillin is the preferred drug of choice) in the following situations:

(1) Adult patients who give no history of clinical penicillin hypersensitivity.

(2) Pediatric patients.

In addition, there are no data at present to assess the clinical value of Benzylpenicilloyl Polylysine where exposure to penicillin is suspected as a cause of a drug reaction and in patients who are undergoing routine allergy evaluation.

Furthermore, there are no data relating the clinical value of Benzylpenicilloyl Polylysine skin tests to the risk of administering semi-synthetic penicillins (phenoxymethyl penicillin, ampicillin, carbenicillin, dicloxacillin, methicillin, nafcillin, oxacillin, phenethicillin) and cephalosporin-derived antibiotics.

Recognition that the following clinical outcomes are possible makes it imperative for the physician to weigh risk to benefit in every instance where the decision to administer or not to administer penicillin is based in part on a Benzylpenicilloyl Polylysine skin test.

(1) An allergic reaction to therapeutic penicillin may occur in a patient with a negative skin test to Benzylpenicilloyl Polylysine.

(2) It is possible for a patient to have an anaphylactic reaction to therapeutic penicillin in the presence of a negative Benzylpenicilloyl Polylysine skin test and a negative history of clinical penicillin hypersensitivity.

(3) If penicillin is the absolute drug of choice in a life-threatening situation, successful desensitization with therapeutic penicillin may be possible irrespective of a positive skin test and/or a positive history of clinical penicillin hypersensitivity.

PREGNANCY-PREGNANCY CATEGORY C:

Animal reproduction studies have not been conducted with Benzylpenicilloyl Polylysine. It is not known whether Benzylpenicilloyl Polylysine can cause fetal harm when administered to a pregnant woman or can affect reproduction capacity. The hazards of skin testing in such patients should be weighed against the hazard of penicillin therapy without skin testing.

ADVERSE REACTIONS

Occasionally, patients may develop an intense local inflammatory response at the skin test site. Rarely, patients will develop a systemic allergic reaction, manifested by generalized erythema, pruritus, angioneurotic edema, urticaria, dyspnea, and/or hypotension. The usual methods of treating a skin test antigen-induced reaction—the application of a venous occlusion tourniquet proximal to the skin test site and administration of epinephrine (and, at times, an injection of an antihistamine)—are recommended and will usually control the reaction. As a rule, systemic allergic reactions following skin test procedures are of short duration and controllable, but the patient should be kept under observation for several hours.

DOSAGE AND ADMINISTRATION

SKIN TESTING DOSAGE AND TECHNIQUE

Scratch Testing: Skin testing is usually performed on the inner volar aspect of the forearm. The skin test material should always be applied first by the scratch technique. After preparing the skin surface, a sterile 20 gauge needle should be used to make a 3-5 mm scratch of the epidermis. Very little pressure is required to break the epidermal continuity. If bleeding occurs, prepare a second site and scratch more lightly with the needle—sufficient to produce a non-bleeding scratched surface. Apply a small drop of Benzylpenicilloyl Polylysine solution to the scratch and rub gently with an applicator, toothpick, or the side of the needle. Observe for the appearance of a wheal, erythema, and the occurrence of itching at the test site during the succeeding 15 minutes at which time the solution over the scratch is wiped off. A positive reaction is unmistakable and consists of the development within 10 minutes of a pale wheal, usually with pseudopods, surrounding the scratch site and varying in diameter from 5 to 15 mm (or more). This wheal may be surrounded by a variable diameter of erythema, and accompanied by a variable degree of itching. The most sensitive individuals develop itching almost instantly, and the wheal and erythema are prompt in their appearance. As soon as a positive response as defined above is clearly evident, the solution over the scratch should be immediately wiped off. If the scratch test is either negative or equivocally positive (less than 5 mm wheal and little or no erythema, and no itching), an intradermal test may be performed.

The Intradermal Test: Using a tuberculin syringe with a ⅜" to ⅝" long, 26 to 30 gauge, short bevel needle, withdraw the contents of the ampul. Prepare a sterile skin test area on the upper, outer arm, sufficiently below the deltoid muscle to permit proximal application of a tourniquet later, if necessary. Be sure to eject all air from the syringe through the needle, then insert the needle, bevel up, immediately below the skin surface.

Inject an amount of Benzylpenicilloyl Polylysine sufficient to raise the smallest possible perceptible bleb. This volume will be between 0.01 and 0.02 mL. Using a separate syringe and needle, inject a like amount of saline as a control at least 1½ inches removed from the test site. Most skin reactions will develop within 5-15 minutes and response to the skin test is read as follows:

(-) Negative response—no increase in size of original bleb and/or no greater reaction than the control site.

(±) Ambiguous response—wheal being only slightly larger than initial injection bleb, with or without accompanying erythematous flare and larger than the control site.

(+) Positive response—itching and marked increase in size of original bleb. Wheal may exceed 20 mm in diameter and exhibit pseudopods.

The control site should be completely reactionless. If it exhibits a wheal greater than 2-3 mm, repeat the test, and if the same reaction is observed, a physician experienced with allergy skin testing should be consulted.

As with all parenteral drug products, Benzylpenicilloyl Polylysine should be inspected visually for particulate matter and discoloration prior to administration, whenever solution and container permit.

Benzylpenicilloyl Polylysine is stable only when kept under refrigeration. It is, therefore, recommended that test materials subjected to ambient temperatures for over a day be discarded.

HOW SUPPLIED

INJECTION:

BRAND/MANUFACTURER	NDC	SIZE	AWP
○ **BRAND** PRE-PEN: Schwarz	00091-1640-05	0.25 ml 5s	$67.33

Bepridil Hydrochloride

DESCRIPTION

Bepridil Hydrochloride is a calcium channel blocker that has well characterized anti-anginal properties and known but poorly characterized type 1 anti-arrhythmic and anti-hypertensive properties. It has inhibitory effects on both the slow calcium and fast sodium inward currents in myocardial and vascular smooth muscle, interferes with calcium binding to calmodulin, and blocks both voltage and receptor operated calcium channels. It is not related chemically to other calcium channel blockers such as diltiazem hydrochloride, nifedipine and verapamil hydrochloride.

Bepridil Hydrochloride monohydrate is a white to off-white, crystalline powder with a bitter taste. It is slightly soluble in water, very soluble in ethanol, methanol and chloroform, and freely soluble in acetone. The molecular weight of Bepridil Hydrochloride monohydrate is 421.02. Its molecular formula is $C_{24}H_{34}N_2O \cdot HCl \cdot H_2O$.

Bepridil Hydrochloride is (±)-β-[(2-Methylpropoxy)methyl]-N-(phenylmethyl)-1 -pyrrolidineethanamine monohydrochloride monohydrate.

Bepridil Hydrochloride is available as film-coated tablets for oral use containing 200, 300, or 400 mg of Bepridil Hydrochloride monohydrate.

► SHOWN IN PRODUCT IDENTIFICATION GUIDE

Following is its chemical structure:

$$(CH_3)_2CHCH_2OCH_2CHCH_2 - N \quad \cdot HCl \cdot H_2O$$

CLINICAL PHARMACOLOGY

Bepridil Hydrochloride inhibits the transmembrane influx of calcium ions into cardiac and vascular smooth muscle. This has been demonstrated in isolated myocardial and vascular smooth muscle preparations in which both the slope of the calcium dose response curve and the maximum calcium-induced inotropic response were significantly reduced by Bepridil Hydrochloride. In cardiac myocytes *in vitro* Bepridil Hydrochloride was shown to be tightly bound to actin. A negative inotropic effect can be seen in the isolated guinea pig atria.

In *in vitro* studies, Bepridil Hydrochloride has also been demonstrated to inhibit the sodium inward current. Reductions in the maximal upstroke velocity and the amplitude of the action potential, as well as increases in the duration of the normal action potential, have been observed. Additionally, Bepridil Hydrochloride has been shown to possess local anesthetic activity in isolated myocardial preparations. It effects electrophysiological changes that are observed with several classes of anti-arrhythmic agents.

CLINICAL STUDIES

In controlled clinical studies with 200-400 mg of Bepridil Hydrochloride, given as a once daily dose, exercise tolerance was improved and angina frequency and daily niitroglycerin use was reduced compared to placebo. Improvement in exercise performance was dose related. In one controlled clinical study, Bepridil Hydrochloride was added to propranolol in daily doses of up to 240 mg. The 200-400 mg dose of Bepridil Hydrochloride was well tolerated (patients entered were not allowed to be in NYHA Class III or IV heart failure) and there was an added effect of Bepridil Hydrochloride on exercise tolerance.

In another controlled clinical study, Bepridil Hydrochloride in doses of up to 400 mg/day, significantly improved exercise tolerance compared to diltiazem hydrochloride in patients refractory to diltiazem hydrochloride therapy.

Mechanism of Action: The precise mechanism of action for Bepridil Hydrochloride as an anti-anginal agent remains to be fully determined, but is believed to include the following mechanisms: Bepridil Hydrochloride regularly reduces heart rate and arterial pressure at rest and at a given level of exercise by dilating peripheral arterioles and reducing total peripheral resistance (after-load) against which the heart works. In exercise tolerance tests in patients with stable angina the heart rate/blood pressure product was reduced with Bepridil Hydrochloride for a given work load.

Hemodynamic Effects: Bepridil Hydrochloride produces dose dependent slowing of the heart, and reflex tachycardia is not seen. The mean decrease in heart rate in US clinical trials was 3 b.p.m. Orally administered Bepridil Hydrochloride also produces modest decreases (less than 5 mm Hg) in systolic and diastolic blood pressure in normotensive patients and somewhat larger decreases in hypertensive patients.

Intravenous administration of Bepridil Hydrochloride is associated with a modest reduction in left ventricular contractility (dP/dt), and increased filling pressure, but radionuclide cineangiography studies in angina patients demonstrated improvement in ejection fraction at rest and during exercise following oral Bepridil Hydrochloride therapy. Patients with impaired cardiac function [overt heart failure] were not included in these studies.

Electrophysiological Effects. Intravenous administration of Bepridil Hydrochloride in man prolongs the effective refractory periods of the atria and ventricles, and the functional refractory period of the AV node. There was a tendency for the AV node effective refractory period and A-H interval to be increased as well. Intravenous and oral administration of Bepridil Hydrochloride slow heart rate, prolong the QT and QTc intervals, and alter the morphology of the T-wave (indentation). In clinical trials with angina patients, the mean percent prolongation of the QTc interval was approximately 8%, and of QT about 10%. The prolongation of QT is dose related, varying from about 0.030 sec at doses of 200 mg once a day to 0.055 sec at 400 mg once a day. Upon cessation of therapy, the ECG gradually normalizes. No instances of greater than first-degree heart block have been observed in US controlled or open clinical studies with Bepridil Hydrochloride, and first-degree heart block occurred in 0.2% of patients in these studies.

Pulmonary Function: In healthy subjects and asthmatic patients, intravenous Bepridil Hydrochloride did not cause bronchoconstriction. Bepridil Hydrochloride has been safely used in asthmatic patients and in patients with chronic obstructive lung disease.

Pharmacokinetics and Metabolism: In studies with healthy volunteers, Bepridil Hydrochloride is rapidly and completely absorbed after oral administration. The time to peak bepridil plasma concentration is about 2 to 3 hours. Over a ten day period, approximately 70% of a single dose of Bepridil Hydrochloride is excreted in the urine and 22% in the feces, as metabolites. Excretion of unmetabolized drug is negligible. In healthy male volunteers, the relationship between dose and steady-state blood levels of Bepridil Hydrochloride was linear over the range of 200 to 400 mg/day. Elimination of Bepridil Hydrochloride is biphasic, with a distribution half-life of about 2 hours. The terminal elimination half-life following the cessation of multiple dosing averaged 42 hours (range 26-64 hours). However,

during a given dosing interval, decay from the peak concentration occurs relatively rapidly indicating a dosing interval half-life shorter than 24 hours. Following once-daily dosing with therapeutic doses, steady-state was reached in about 8 days in healthy volunteers. The clearance of Bepridil Hydrochloride decreases after multiple dosing.

Clearance of Bepridil Hydrochloride in angina patients was lower than that in healthy volunteers, resulting in higher average plasma Bepridil Hydrochloride concentrations. At steady state, maximum Bepridil Hydrochloride concentrations averaged 2332 ng/mL (range 1451 to 3609) and mean minimum concentrations were 1174 ng/mL (range 226 to 2639) in angina patients following 300 mg/day doses of Bepridil Hydrochloride.

Bepridil Hydrochloride is more than 99% bound to plasma proteins. Administration of Bepridil Hydrochloride after a meal resulted in a clinically insignificant delay in time to peak concentration, but neither peak Bepridil Hydrochloride plasma levels nor the extent of absorption was changed.

Bepridil Hydrochloride passes through the placental barrier. Bepridil Hydrochloride may cause uterine hypotonia.

INDICATIONS AND USAGE

CHRONIC STABLE ANGINA
(CLASSIC EFFORT-ASSOCIATED ANGINA)

Bepridil Hydrochloride is indicated for the treatment of chronic stable angina (classic effort-associated angina). Because Bepridil Hydrochloride has caused serious ventricular arrhythmias, including torsades de pointes type ventricular tachycardia, and the occurrence of cases of agranulocytosis associated with its use (see *"Warnings"*), it should be reserved for patients who have failed to respond optimally to, or are intolerant of, other anti-anginal medication.

Bepridil Hydrochloride may be used alone or in combination with beta blockers and/or nitrates. Controlled clinical studies have shown an added effect when Bepridil Hydrochloride is administered to patients already receiving propranolol.

UNLABELED USES

Bepridil Hydrochloride is used alone or as an adjunct in the treatment of supraventricular and ventricular arrhythmias.

CONTRAINDICATIONS

Bepridil Hydrochloride is contraindicated in patients with a known sensitivity to it. Bepridil Hydrochloride is contraindicated in (1) patients with a history of serious ventricular arrhythmias (see *"Warnings—Induction of New Serious Arrhythmias"*), (2) patients with sick sinus syndrome or patients with second- or third-degree AV block, except in the presence of a functioning ventricular pacemaker, (3) patients with hypotension (less than 90 mm Hg systolic), (4) patients with uncompensated cardiac insufficiency, (5) patients with congenital QT interval prolongation (see *"Warnings"*), and (6) patients taking other drugs that prolong QT interval (see *"Precautions—Drug Interactions"*).

WARNINGS

INDUCTION OF NEW SERIOUS ARRHYTHMIAS

BEPRIDIL HYDROCHLORIDE HAS CLASS 1 ANTI-ARRHYTHMIC PROPERTIES AND, LIKE OTHER SUCH DRUGS, CAN INDUCE NEW ARRHYTHMIAS, INCLUDING VT/VF. IN ADDITION, BECAUSE OF ITS ABILITY TO PROLONG THE QT INTERVAL, BEPRIDIL HYDROCHLORIDE CAN CAUSE TORSADES DE POINTES TYPE VENTRICULAR TACHYCARDIA. BECAUSE OF THESE PROPERTIES BEPRIDIL HYDROCHLORIDE SHOULD BE RESERVED FOR PATIENTS IN WHOM OTHER ANTI-ANGINAL AGENTS DO NOT OFFER A SATISFACTORY EFFECT.

IN US CLINICAL TRIALS, THE QT AND QTC INTERVALS WERE COMMONLY PROLONGED BY BEPRIDIL HYDROCHLORIDE IN A DOSE-RELATED FASHION. WHILE THE MEAN PROLONGATION OF QTC WAS 8% AND OF QT WAS 10%. INCREASES OF 25% OR MORE WERE NOT UNCOMMON, OCCURRING IN 5% OF THE STUDIED POPULATION FOR QTC AND 8.7% OF THE STUDIED POPULATION FOR QT. INCREASED QT AND QTC MAY BE ASSOCIATED WITH TORSADES DE POINTES TYPE VT, WHICH WAS SEEN AT LEAST BRIEFLY, IN ABOUT 1.0% OF PATIENTS IN US TRIALS; IN MANY CASES, HOWEVER, PATIENTS WITH MARKED PROLONGATION OF QTC WERE TAKEN OFF BEPRIDIL HYDROCHLORIDE THERAPY. ALL OF THE US PATIENTS WITH TORSADES DE POINTES HAD A PROLONGED QT INTERVAL AND RELATIVELY LOW SERUM POTASSIUM. FRENCH MARKETING EXPERIENCE HAS REPORTED OVER ONE HUNDRED VERIFIED CASES OF TORSADES DE POINTES. WHILE THIS NUMBER, BASED ON TOTAL USE, REPRESENTS A RATE OF ONLY 0.01%, THE TRUE RATE IS UNDOUBTEDLY MUCH HIGHER, AS SPONTANEOUS REPORTING SYSTEMS ALL SUFFER FROM SUBSTANTIAL UNDER REPORTING.

TORSADES DE POINTES IS A POLYMORPHIC VENTRICULAR TACHYCARDIA OFTEN BUT NOT ALWAYS ASSOCIATED WITH A PROLONGED QT INTERVAL, AND OFTEN DRUG INDUCED. THE RELATION BETWEEN THE DEGREE OF QT PROLONGATION AND THE DEVELOPMENT OF TORSADES DE POINTES IS NOT LINEAR AND THE LIKELIHOOD OF TORSADES APPEARS TO BE INCREASED BY HYPOKALEMIA, USE OF POTASSIUM WASTING DIURETICS, AND THE

PRESENCE OF ANTECEDENT BRADYCARDIA. WHILE THE SAFE UPPER LIMIT OF QT IS NOT DEFINED, IT IS SUGGESTED THAT THE INTERVAL NOT BE PERMITTED TO EXCEED 0.52 SECONDS DURING TREATMENT. IF DOSE REDUCTION DOES NOT ELIMINATE THE EXCESSIVE PROLONGATION, BEPRIDIL HYDROCHLORIDE SHOULD BE STOPPED.

BECAUSE MOST DOMESTIC AND FOREIGN CASES OF TORSADES HAVE DEVELOPED IN PATIENTS WITH HYPOKALEMIA, USUALLY RELATED TO DIURETIC USE OR SIGNIFICANT LIVER DISEASE, IF CONCOMITANT DIURETICS ARE NEEDED, LOW DOSES AND ADDITION OR PRIMARY USE OF A POTASSIUM SPARING DIURETIC SHOULD BE CONSIDERED AND SERUM POTASSIUM SHOULD BE MONITORED. BEPRIDIL HYDROCHLORIDE HAS BEEN ASSOCIATED WITH THE USUAL RANGE OF PRO-ARRHYTHMIC EFFECTS CHARACTERISTIC OF CLASS 1 ANTIARRHYTHMICS (INCREASED PREMATURE VENTRICULAR CONTRACTION RATES, NEW SUSTAINED VT, AND VT/VF THAT IS MORE RESISTANT TO SINUS RHYTHM CONVERSION). USE IN PATIENTS WITH SEVERE ARRHYTHMIAS (WHO ARE MOST SUSCEPTIBLE TO CERTAIN PRO-ARRHYTHMIC EFFECTS) HAS BEEN LIMITED, SO THAT RISK IN THESE PATIENTS IS NOT DEFINED.

IN THE NATIONAL HEART, LUNG AND BLOOD INSTITUTE'S CARDIAC ARRHYTHMIA SUPPRESSION TRIAL (CAST), A LONG-TERM, MULTI-CENTERED, RANDOMIZED, DOUBLE-BLIND STUDY IN PATIENTS WITH ASYMPTOMATIC NON-LIFE-THREATENING VENTRICULAR ARRHYTHMIAS WHO HAD MYOCARDIAL INFARCTIONS MORE THAN SIX DAYS BUT LESS THAN TWO YEARS PREVIOUSLY, AN EXCESS MORTALITY/NON-FATAL CARDIAC ARREST RATE WAS SEEN IN PATIENTS TREATED WITH ENCAINIDE OR FLECAINIDE (56/730) COMPARED WITH THAT SEEN IN PATIENTS ASSIGNED TO MATCHED PLACEBO-TREATED GROUPS (22/725). THE APPLICABILITY OF THESE RESULTS TO OTHER POPULATIONS (E.G., THOSE WITHOUT RECENT MYOCARDIAL INFARCTION) OR TO OTHER ANTIARRHYTHMIC DRUGS IS UNCERTAIN, BUT AT PRESENT IT IS PRUDENT TO CONSIDER ANY DRUG DOCUMENTED TO PROVOKE NEW SERIOUS ARRHYTHMIAS OR WORSENING OF PRE-EXISTING ARRHYTHMIAS AS HAVING A SIMILAR RISK AND TO AVOID THEIR USE IN THE POSTINFARCTION PERIOD.

Agranulocytosis: In US clinical trials of over 800 patients treated with Bepridil Hydrochloride for up to five years, two cases of marked leukopenia and neutropenia were reported. Both patients were diabetic and elderly. One died with overwhelming gram-negative sepsis, itself a possible cause of marked leukopenia. The other patient recovered rapidly when Bepridil Hydrochloride was stopped.

Congestive Heart Failure: Congestive heart failure has been observed infrequently (about 1%) during US controlled clinical trials, but experience with the use of Bepridil Hydrochloride in patients with significantly impaired ventricular function is limited. There is little information on the effect of concomitant administration of Bepridil Hydrochloride and digoxin; therefore, caution should be exercised in treating patients with congestive heart failure.

Hepatic Enzyme Elevation: In US clinical studies with Bepridil Hydrochloride in about 1000 patients and subjects, clinically significant (at least 2 times the upper limit of normal) transaminase elevations were observed in approximately 1% of the patients. None of these patients became clinically symptomatic or jaundiced and values returned to normal when the drug was stopped.

Hypokalemia: In clinical trials Bepridil Hydrochloride has not been reported to reduce serum potassium levels. Because hypokalemia has been associated with ventricular arrhythmias, potassium insufficiency should be corrected before Bepridil Hydrochloride therapy is initiated and normal potassium concentrations should be maintained during Bepridil Hydrochloride therapy. Serum potassium should be monitored periodically.

PRECAUTIONS
GENERAL
Caution should be exercised when using Bepridil Hydrochloride in patients with left bundle branch block or sinus bradycardia (less than 50 b.p.m.). Care should also be exercised in patients with serious hepatic or renal disorders because such patients have not been studied and Bepridil Hydrochloride is highly metabolized, with metabolites excreted primarily in the urine.

RECENT MYOCARDIAL INFARCTION
In US clinical trials with Bepridil Hydrochloride patients with myocardial infarctions within three months prior to initiation of drug treatment were excluded. The initiation of Bepridil Hydrochloride therapy in such patients, therefore, cannot be recommended.

PULMONARY INFILTRATION
There have been cases of noninfective, noncardiogenic pulmonary interstitial infiltrates (with or without the presence of eosinophilia), including cases of pulmonary fibrosis in patients taking Bepridil Hydrochloride. These cases may present as dyspnea or cough within a few weeks of commencing Bepridil Hydrochloride: infiltrates may be seen on chest x-ray.

Although the relationship of pulmonary infiltration to Bepridil Hydrochloride is unclear, any patient who develops dyspnea or cough of unspecified etiology should be adequately evaluated. If other causes cannot be identified, discontinuation of Bepridil Hydrochloride therapy should be considered.

INFORMATION FOR PATIENTS
Since QT prolongation is not associated with defined symptomatology, patients should be instructed on the importance of maintaining any potassium supplementation or potassium sparing diuretic, and the need for routine electrocardiograms and periodic monitoring of serum potassium.

The following Patient Information is printed on the carton label of each unit of use bottle:

As with any medication that you take, you should notify your physician of any changes in your overall condition. Be sure to follow your physician's instructions regarding follow-up visits. Please notify any physician who treats you for a medical condition that you are taking Bepridil Hydrochloride as well as any other medications.

DRUG INTERACTIONS
Nitrates: The concomitant use of Bepridil Hydrochloride with long- and short-acting nitrates has been safely tolerated in patients with stable angina pectoris. Sublingual nitroglycerin may be taken if necessary for the control of acute angina attacks during Bepridil Hydrochloride therapy.

Beta-blocking Agents: The concomitant use of Bepridil Hydrochloride and beta-blocking agents has been well tolerated in patients with stable angina. Available data are not sufficient, however, to predict the effects of concomitant medication on patients with impaired ventricular function or cardiac conduction abnormalities (see *"Clinical Pharmacology"* and *"Dosage and Administration"*).

Digoxin: In controlled studies in healthy volunteers, Bepridil Hydrochloride either had no effect (one study) or was associated with modest increases, about 30% (two studies) in steady-state serum digoxin concentrations. Limited clinical data in angina patients receiving concomitant Bepridil Hydrochloride and digoxin therapy indicate no discernible changes in serum digoxin levels. Available data are neither sufficient to rule out possible increases in serum digoxin with concomitant treatment in some patients, nor other possible interactions, particularly in patients with cardiac conduction abnormalities (see also *"Warnings—Congestive Heart Failure"*).

Oral Hypoglycemics: Bepridil Hydrochloride has been safely used in diabetic patients without significantly lowering their blood glucose levels or altering their need for insulin or oral hypoglycemic agents.

General Interactions: Certain drugs could increase the likelihood of potentially serious adverse effects with Bepridil Hydrochloride. In general, these are drugs that have one or more pharmacologic activities similar to Bepridil Hydrochloride, including anti-arrhythmic agents such as quinidine and procainamide, cardiac glycosides and tricyclic anti-depressants. Anti-arrhythmics and tricyclic anti-depressants could exaggerate the prolongation of the QT interval observed with Bepridil Hydrochloride. Cardiac glycosides could exaggerate the depression of AV nodal conduction observed with Bepridil Hydrochloride.

CARCINOGENESIS, MUTAGENESIS, IMPAIRMENT OF FERTILITY
No evidence of carcinogenicity was revealed in one lifetime study in mice at dosages up to 60 times (for a 60 kg subject) the maximum recommended dosage in man. Unilateral follicular adenomas of the thyroid were observed in a study in rats following lifetime administration of high doses of Bepridil Hydrochloride, i.e., ≥ 100 mg/kg/day (20 times the usual recommended dose in man). No mutagenic or other genotoxic potential of Bepridil Hydrochloride was found in the following standard laboratory tests: the Micronucleus Test for Chromosomal Effects, the Liver Microsome Activated Bacterial Assay for Mutagenicity, the Chinese Hamster Ovary Cell Assay for Mutagenicity, and the Sister Chromatid Exchange Assay. No intrinsic effect on fertility by Bepridil Hydrochloride was demonstrated in rats.

In monkeys, at 200 mg/kg/day, there was a decrease in testicular weight and spermatogenesis. There were no systematic studies in man related to this point. In rats, at doses up to 300 mg/kg/day, there was no observed alteration of mating behavior nor of reproductive performance.

USAGE IN PREGNANCY
Pregnancy Category C. Reproductive studies (fertility and peri-postnatal) have been conducted in rats. Reduced litter size at birth and decreased pup survival during lactation was observed at maternal dosages 37 times (on a mg/kg basis) the maximum daily recommended therapeutic dosage. In teratology studies, no effects were observed in rats or rabbits at these same dosages. There are no well-controlled studies in pregnant women. Use Bepridil Hydrochloride in pregnant or nursing women only if the potential benefit justifies the potential risk.

NURSING MOTHERS
Bepridil Hydrochloride is excreted in human milk. Bepridil Hydrochloride concentration in human milk is estimated to reach about one third the concentration in serum. Because of the potential for serious adverse reactions in nursing infants from Bepridil Hydrochloride a decision should be made whether to discontinue nursing or to discontinue the drug, taking into account the importance of the drug to the mother.

PEDIATRIC USE
The safety and effectiveness of Bepridil Hydrochloride in children have not been established.

➤ SHOWN IN PRODUCT IDENTIFICATION GUIDE

ADVERSE REACTIONS

Adverse reactions were assessed in placebo and active-drug controlled trials of 4-12 weeks duration and longer-term uncontrolled studies. The most common side effects occurring more frequently than in control groups were upper gastrointestinal complaints (nausea, dyspepsia or GI distress) in about 22%, diarrhea in about 8%, dizziness in about 15%, asthenia in about 10% and nervousness in about 7%. The adverse reactions seen in at least 2% of Bepridil Hydrochloride patients in controlled trials are shown in the following table. (See related table).

In one twelve week controlled study, daily doses of 200, 300, and 400 mg were compared to placebo. The following table shows the rates of more common reactions (at least 5% in at least one Bepridil Hydrochloride group).

ADVERSE EXPERIENCES BY BODY SYSTEM AND TREATMENT IN GREATER THAN 5% OF BEPRIDIL HYDROCHLORIDE PATIENTS IN CONTROLLED TRIALS

Adverse Reaction	Bepridil HCl 200 mg (N = 43)	Bepridil HCl 300 mg (N = 46)	Bepridil HCl 400 mg (N = 44)	Placebo (N = 44)
Body as a Whole				
Asthenia	13.95	6.52	11.36	2.27
Headache	6.98	8.70	13.64	15.91
Cardiovascular/Respiratory				
Palpitations	0.00	6.52	4.55	0.00
Dyspnea	2.33	8.70	0.00	2.27
Gastrointestinal				
G.I. Distress	6.98	0.00	4.55	4.55
Nausea	6.98	26.09	18.18	2.27
Anorexia	0.00	2.17	6.82	2.27
Diarrhea	0.00	10.87	6.82	2.27
Central Nervous System				
Drowsy	6.98	6.52	0.00	4.55
Dizziness	11.63	15.22	27.27	6.82
Tremor	6.98	0.00	4.55	0.00
Tremor of Hand	9.30	0.00	4.55	0.00
Psychiatric				
Nervous	11.63	8.70	11.36	0.00
Special Senses				
Tinnitus	0.00	6.52	2.27	2.27

Adverse experiences in long-term open studies were generally similar to those seen in controlled trials.

Although adverse experiences were frequent (at least one being reported in 71% of patients participating in controlled clinical trials), most were well-tolerated. About 15% of patients however, discontinued Bepridil Hydrochloride treatment because of adverse experiences. In controlled clinical trials, these were principally gastrointestinal (1.0%), dizziness (1.0%) ventricular arrhythmias (1.0%) and syncope (0.6%). The major reasons for discontinuation, with comparison to control agents, are shown below.

MOST COMMON EVENTS RESULTING IN DISCONTINUATION

Adverse Reaction	Bepridil HCl (N = 515) n (%)	Placebo (N = 288) n (%)	Positive Control (N = 119) n (%)
Dizziness	5 (0.97)	0 (0.0)	2 (1.68)
Gastrointestinal Symptoms	5 (0.97)	0 (0.0)	5 (4.20)
Ventricular Arrhythmia	5 (0.97)	0 (0.0)	0 (0.0)
Syncope	3 (0.58)	0 (0.0)	0 (0.0)

Across all controlled and uncontrolled trials Bepridil Hydrochloride was evaluated in over 800 patients with chronic angina. In addition to the adverse reactions noted above, the following were observed in 0.5 to 2.0% of the Bepridil Hydrochloride patients or are rarer, but potentially important events seen in clinical studies or reported in post marketing experience. In most cases it is not possible to determine whether there is a causal relationship to Bepridil Hydrochloride treatment.

Body as a Whole: Fever, pain, myalgic asthenia, superinfection, flu syndrome.

Cardiovascular/Respiratory: Sinus tachycardia, sinus bradycardia, hypertension vasodilation, edema, ventricular premature contractions, ventricular tachycardia, prolonged QT interval, rhinitis, cough, pharyngitis.

Gastrointestinal: Flatulence, gastritis, appetite increase, dry mouth, constipation.

Musculoskeletal: Arthritis.

Central Nervous System: Fainting, vertigo, akathisia, drowsiness, insomnia, tremor.

Psychiatric: Depression, anxiousness, adverse behavior effect.

Skin: Rash, sweating, skin irritation.

Special Senses: Blurred vision, tinnitus, taste change.

Urogenital: Loss of libido, impotence.

Abnormal Lab Values: Abnormal liver function test, SGPT increase.

Certain cardiovascular events, such as acute myocardial infarction (about 3% of patients) worsened heart failure (1.9%), worsened angina (4.5%), severe arrhythmia (about 2.4% VT/VF) and sudden death (1.6%) have occurred in patients receiving Bepridil Hydrochloride, but have not been included as adverse events because they appear to be, and cannot be distinguished from, manifestations of the patient's underlying cardiac disease. Such events as torsades de pointes arrhythmias, prolonged QT/QTc, bradycardia, first degree heart block, which are probably related to Bepridil Hydrochloride are included in the tables.

OVERDOSAGE

In the event of overdosage, we recommend close observation in a cardiac care facility for a minimum of 48 hours and use of appropriate supportive measures in addition to gastric lavage. Beta-adrenergic stimulation or parenteral administration of calcium solutions may increase transmembrane calcium ion influx.

ADVERSE EXPERIENCES BY BODY SYSTEM AND TREATMENT IN GREATER THAN 2% OF BEPRIDIL HYDROCHLORIDE PATIENTS IN CONTROLLED TRIALS

Adverse Reaction	Bepridil HCl (N = 529)	Nifedipine (N = 50)	Propranolol (N = 88)	Diltiazem (N = 41)	Placebo (N = 190)
Body as a Whole					
Asthenia	9.83	22.00	22.73	12.20	7.37
Headache	11.34	22.00	13.64	7.32	14.21
Flu Syndrome	2.08	8.00	2.27	—α	1.05
Cardiovascular/Respiratory					
Palpitations	2.27	6.00	2.27	0.00	1.58
Dyspnea	3.59	4.00	5.68	4.88	2.11
Respiratory Infection	2.84	4.00	3.41	4.88	3.68
Gastrointestinal					
Dyspepsia	6.81	4.00	5.68	4.88	1.58
G.I. Distress	4.35	10.00	6.82	—α	2.11
Nausea	12.29	14.00	11.36	2.44	3.68
Dry Mouth	3.40	0.00	0.00	2.44	2.63
Anorexia	3.02	0.00	2.27	0.00	1.58
Diarrhea	7.75	2.00	9.09	2.44	2.63
Abdominal Pain	3.02	4.00	1.14	—α	3.16
Constipation	2.84	6.00	1.14	4.88	2.11
Central Nervous System					
Drowsy	3.78	4.00	4.55	—α	3.68
Insomnia	2.65	6.00	3.41	—α	1.05
Dizziness	14.74	30.00	10.23	4.88	9.47
Tremor	4.91	4.00	0.00	—α	1.05
Tremor of Hand	3.02	4.00	0.00	—α	0.53
Paresthesia	2.46	2.00	1.14	4.88	3.16
Psychiatric					
Nervous	7.37	16.00	1.14	2.44	3.68

α No data available.

◆ RATED THERAPEUTICALLY EQUIVALENT; ◇ THERAPEUTIC EQUIVALENCE UNCONFIRMED; ○ UNRATED

Clinically significant hypotensive reactions or high-degree AV block should be treated with vasopressor agents or cardiac pacing, respectively. Ventricular tachycardia should be handled by cardioversion and, if persistent, by overdrive pacing.

There has been one experience with overdosage in which a patient inadvertently took a single dose of 1600 mg of Bepridil Hydrochloride. The patient was observed for 72 hours in intensive care, but no significant adverse experiences were noted.

DOSAGE AND ADMINISTRATION

Therapy with Bepridil Hydrochloride should be individualized according to each patient's response and the physician's clinical judgement. The usual starting dose of Bepridil Hydrochloride is 200 mg once daily. After 10 days, dosage may be adjusted upward depending upon the patient's response (e.g., ability to perform activities of daily living, QT interval, heart rate, and frequency and severity of angina). This long interval for dosage adjustment is needed because steady-state blood levels are not achieved until 8 days of therapy. In clinical trials, most patients were maintained at a dose of Bepridil Hydrochloride of 300 mg once daily. The maximum daily dose of Bepridil Hydrochloride is 400 mg and the established minimum effective dose is 200 mg daily.

The starting dose for elderly patients does not differ from that for young patients. After therapeutic response is demonstrated, however, elderly patients may require more frequent monitoring.

Food does not interfere with the absorption of Bepridil Hydrochloride (see *"Clinical Pharmacology—Pharmacokinetics and Metabolism"*). If nausea is experienced with Bepridil Hydrochloride, the drug may be given at meals or at bedtime.

Bepridil Hydrochloride has not been studied adequately in patients with impaired hepatic or renal function. It is therefore possible that dosage adjustments may be necessary in these patients.

CONCOMITANT USE WITH OTHER AGENTS
The concomitant use of Bepridil Hydrochloride and beta-blocking agents in patients without heart failure is safely tolerated. Physicians wishing to switch patients from beta-blocker therapy to Bepridil Hydrochloride therapy may initiate Bepridil Hydrochloride before terminating the beta blocker in the usual gradual fashion (see *"Clinical Pharmacology"* and *"Precautions"*).

HOW SUPPLIED
TABLETS: 200 MG

AVERAGE UNIT PRICE (AVAILABLE SIZES)			
BRAND		$2.42	

BRAND/MANUFACTURER	NDC	SIZE	AWP
◆ BRAND			
➤ VASCOR: McNeil Pharm	00045-0682-30	30s	$70.10
	00045-0682-33	90s	$210.30
	00045-0682-10	100s ud	$257.08

TABLETS: 300 MG

AVERAGE UNIT PRICE (AVAILABLE SIZES)			
BRAND		$2.95	

BRAND/MANUFACTURER	NDC	SIZE	AWP
◆ BRAND			
➤ VASCOR: McNeil Pharm	00045-0683-30	30s	$85.52
	00045-0683-33	90s	$256.57
	00045-0683-10	100s ud	$313.56

TABLETS: 400 MG

AVERAGE UNIT PRICE (AVAILABLE SIZES)			
BRAND		$3.30	

BRAND/MANUFACTURER	NDC	SIZE	AWP
◆ BRAND			
➤ VASCOR: McNeil Pharm	00045-0684-30	30s	$94.45
	00045-0684-33	90s	$289.36
	00045-0684-10	100s ud	$353.63

Beractant

DESCRIPTION

Beractant Intratracheal Suspension is a sterile, non-pyrogenic pulmonary surfactant intended for intratracheal use only. It is a natural bovine lung extract containing phospholipids, neutral lipids, fatty acids, and surfactant-associated proteins to which colfosceril palmitate (dipalmitoylphosphatidylcholine), palmitic acid, and tripalmitin are added to standardize the composition and to mimic surface-tension lowering properties of natural lung surfactant. The resulting composition provides 25 mg/mL phospholipids (including 11.0-15.5 mg/mL disaturated phosphatidylcholine), 0.5-1.75 mg/mL triglycerides, 1.4-3.5 mg/mL free fatty acids, and less than 1.0 mg/mL protein. It is suspended in 0.9% sodium chloride solution, and heat-sterilized Beractant contains no preservatives. Its protein content consists of two hydrophobic, low molecular weight, surfactant-associated proteins commonly known as SP-B and SP-C. It does not contain the hydrophilic, large molecular weight surfactant-associated protein known as SP-A.

Each mL of Beractant contains 25 mg of phospholipids. It is an off-white to light brown liquid supplied in single-use glass vials containing 8 mL (200 mg phospholipids).

CLINICAL PHARMACOLOGY

Endogenous pulmonary surfactant lowers surface tension on alveolar surfaces during respiration and stabilizes the alveoli against collapse at resting transpulmonary pressures. Deficiency of pulmonary surfactant causes Respiratory Distress Syndrome (RDS) in premature infants Beractant replenishes surfactant and restores surface activity to the lungs of these infants.

ACTIVITY

In vitro Beractant reproducibly lowers minimum surface tension to less than 8 dynes/cm as measured by the pulsating bubble surfactometer and Wilhelmy Surface Balance. *In situ*, Beractant restores pulmonary compliance to excised rat lungs artificially made surfactant-deficient. *In vivo*, single Beractant doses improve lung pressure-volume measurements, lung compliance, and oxygenation in premature rabbits and sheep.

ANIMAL METABOLISM

Beractant is administered directly to the target organ, the lungs, where biophysical effects occur at the alveolar surface. In surfactant-deficient premature rabbits and lambs, alveolar clearance of radio-labelled lipid components of Beractant is rapid. Most of the dose becomes lung-associated within hours of administration, and the lipids enter endogenous surfactant pathways of reutilization and recycling. In surfactant-sufficient adult animals, Beractant clearance is more rapid than in premature and young animals. There is less reutilization and recycling of surfactant in adult animals.

Limited animal experiments have not found effects of Beractant on endogenous surfactant metabolism. Precursor incorporation and subsequent secretion of saturated phosphatidylcholine in premature sheep are not changed by Beractant treatments.

No information is available about the metabolic fate of the surfactant-associated proteins in Beractant. The metabolic disposition in humans has not been studied.

CLINICAL STUDIES

Clinical effects of Beractant were demonstrated in six single-dose and four multiple-dose randomized, multicenter, controlled clinical trials involving approximately 1700 infants. Three open trials, including a Treatment IND, involved more than 4800 infants. Each dose of Beractant in all studies was 100 mg phospholipids/kg birth weight and was based on published experience with Beractant TA, a lyophilized powder dosage form of Beractant having the same composition.

PREVENTION STUDIES

Infants of 600-1250 g birth weight and 23 to 29 weeks estimated gestational age were enrolled in two *multiple-dose* studies. A dose of Beractant was given within 15 minutes of birth to prevent the development of RDS. Up to three additional doses in the first 48 hours, as often as every 6 hours, were given if RDS subsequently developed and infants required mechanical ventilation with an FiO_2 ≥ 0.30. Results of the studies at 28 days of age are shown in Table 1.

Table 1
STUDY 1

	Beractant	Control	P-Value
Number infants studied	119	124	
Incidence of RDS (%)	27.6	63.5	< 0.001
Death due to RDS (%)	2.5	19.5	< 0.001
Death or BPD due to RDS (%)	48.7	52.8	0.536
Death due to any cause (%)	7.6	22.8	0.001
Air Leaks[a] (%)	5.9	21.7	0.001
Pulmonary interstitial emphysema (%)	20.8	40.0	0.001

STUDY 2[b]

	Beractant	Control	P-Value
Number infants studied	91	96	
Incidence of RDS (%)	28.6	48.3	0.007
Death due to RDS (%)	1.1	10.5	0.006
Death or BPD due to RDS (%)	27.5	44.2	0.018
Death due to any cause[c] (%)	16.5	13.7	0.633
Air Leaks[a] (%)	14.5	19.6	0.374
Pulmonary interstitial emphysema (%)	26.5	33.2	0.298

[a] *Pneumothorax or pneumopericardium*
[b] *Study discontinued when Treatment IND initiated*
[c] *No cause of death in the Beractant group was significantly increased; the higher number of deaths in this group was due to the sum of all causes.*

RESCUE STUDIES

Infants of 600-1750 g birth weight with RDS requiring mechanical ventilation and an FiO_2 ≥ 0.40 were enrolled in two *multiple-dose* rescue studies. The initial dose of Beractant was given after RDS developed and before 8 hours of age. Infants could receive up to three additional doses in the first 48 hours, as often as every 6 hours, if they required mechanical ventilation and an $FiO_2 \geq 0.30$. Results of the studies at 28 days of age are shown in Table 2.

Table 2
STUDY 3ᵃ

	Beractant	*Control*	*P-Value*
Number infants studied	198	193	
Death due to RDS (%)	11.6	18.1	0.071
Death or BPD due to RDS (%)	59.1	66.8	0.102
Death due to any cause (%)	21.7	26.4	0.285
Air Leaksᵇ (%)	11.8	29.5	< 0.001
Pulmonary interstitial emphysema (%)	16.3	34.0	< 0.001

STUDY 4

	Beractant	*Control*	*P-Value*
Number infants studied	204	203	
Death due to RDS (%)	6.4	22.3	< 0.001
Death or BPD due to RDS (%)	43.6	63.4	< 0.001
Death due to any cause (%)	15.2	28.2	0.001
Air Leaksᵇ (%)	11.2	22.2	0.005
Pulmonary interstitial emphysema (%)	20.8	44.4	< 0.001

ᵃ Study discontinued when Treatment IND initiated
ᵇ Pneumothorax or pneumopericardium

ACUTE CLINICAL EFFECTS

Marked improvements in oxygenation may occur within minutes of administration of Beractant.

All controlled clinical studies with Beractant provided information regarding the acute effects of Beractant on the arterial-alveolar oxygen ratio (a/APO_2), FiO_2, and mean airway pressure (MAP) during the first 48 to 72 hours of life. Significant improvements in these variables were sustained for 48-72 hours in Beractant-treated infants in four single-dose and two multiple-dose rescue studies and in two multiple-dose prevention studies. In the single-dose prevention studies, FiO_2 improved significantly.

INDICATIONS AND USAGE

Beractant is indicated for prevention and treatment ("rescue") of Respiratory Distress Syndrome (RDS) (hyaline membrane disease) in premature infants. Beractant significantly reduces the incidence of RDS, mortality due to RDS and air leak complications.

PREVENTION

In premature infants less than 1250 g birth weight or with evidence of surfactant deficiency, give Beractant as soon as possible, preferably within 15 minutes of birth.

RESCUE

To treat infants with RDS confirmed by x-ray and requiring mechanical ventilation, give Beractant as soon as possible, preferably by 8 hours of age.

CONTRAINDICATIONS

None known.

WARNINGS

Beractant is intended for intratracheal use only.

BERACTANT CAN RAPIDLY AFFECT OXYGENATION AND LUNG COMPLIANCE. Therefore, its use should be restricted to a highly supervised clinical setting with immediate availability of clinicians experienced with intubation, ventilator management, and general care of premature infants. Infants receiving Beractant should be frequently monitored with arterial or transcutaneous measurement of systemic oxygen and carbon dioxide.

DURING THE DOSING PROCEDURE, TRANSIENT EPISODES OF BRADYCARDIA AND DECREASED OXYGEN SATURATION HAVE BEEN REPORTED. If these occur, stop the dosing procedure and initiate appropriate measures to alleviate the condition. After stabilization, resume the dosing procedure.

PRECAUTIONS

GENERAL

Rales and moist breath sounds can occur transiently after administration. Endotracheal suctioning or other remedial action is not necessary unless clear-cut signs of airway obstruction are present.

Increased probability of post-treatment nosocomial sepsis in Beractant-treated infants was observed in the controlled clinical trials (Table 3). The increased risk for sepsis among Beractant-treated infants was not associated with increased mortality among these infants. The causative organisms were similar in treated and control infants. There was no significant difference between groups in the rate of post-treatment infections other than sepsis.

Use of Beractant in infants less than 600 g birth weight or greater than 1750 g birth weight has not been evaluated in controlled trials. There is no controlled experience with use of Beractant in conjunction with experimental therapies for RDS (eg, high-frequency ventilation or extracorporeal membrane oxygenation).

No information is available on the effects of doses other than 100 mg phospholipids/kg, more than four doses, dosing more frequently than every 6 hours, or administration after 48 hours of age.

CARCINOGENESIS, MUTAGENESIS, IMPAIRMENT OF FERTILITY

Reproduction studies in animals have not been completed. Mutagenicity studies were negative. Carcinogenicity studies have not been performed with Beractant.

ADVERSE REACTIONS

The most commonly reported adverse experiences were associated with the dosing procedure. In the multiple-dose controlled clinical trials, transient bradycardia occurred with 11.9% of *doses*. Oxygen desaturation occurred with 9.8% of *doses*.

Other reactions during the dosing procedure occurred with fewer than 1% of doses and included endotracheal tube reflux, pallor, vasoconstriction, hypotension, endotracheal tube blockage, hypertension, hypocarbia, hypercarbia, and apnea. No deaths occurred during the dosing procedure, and all reactions resolved with symptomatic treatment.

The occurrence of concurrent illnesses common in premature infants was evaluated in the controlled trials. The rates in all controlled studies are in Table 3.

Table 3

Concurrent Event	All Controlled Studies		
	Beractant (%)	*Control (%)*	*P-Valueᵃ*
Patent ductus arteriosus	46.9	47.1	0.814
Intracranial hemorrhage	48.1	45.2	0.241
Severe intracranial hemorrhage	24.1	23.3	0.693
Pulmonary air leaks	10.9	24.7	< 0.001
Pulmonary interstitial emphysema	20.2	38.4	< 0.001
Necrotizing enterocolitis	6.1	5.3	0.427
Apnea	65.4	59.6	0.283
Severe apnea	46.1	42.5	0.114
Post-treatment sepsis	20.7	16.1	0.019
Post-treatment infection	10.2	9.1	0.345
Pulmonary hemorrhage	7.2	5.3	0.166

ᵃ P-value comparing groups in controlled studies

When all controlled studies were pooled, there was no difference in intracranial hemorrhage. However, in one of the single-dose rescue studies and one of the multiple-dose prevention studies, the rate of intracranial hemorrhage was significantly higher in Beractant patients than control patients (63.3% v 30.8%, P = 0.001: and 48.8% v 34.2%, P = 0.047, respectively). The rate in a Treatment IND involving approximately 4400 infants was lower than in the controlled trials.

In the controlled clinical trials, there was no effect of Beractant on results of common laboratory tests: white blood cell count and serum sodium, potassium, bilirubin, creatinine.

More than 3700 pretreatment and post-treatment serum samples were tested by Western Blot immunoassay for antibodies to surfactant-associated proteins SP-B and SP-C. No IgG or IgM antibodies were detected.

Several other complications are known to occur in premature infants. The following conditions were reported in the controlled clinical studies. The rates of the complications were not different in treated and control infants, and none of the complications were attributed to Beractant.

Respiratory: lung consolidation, blood from the endotracheal tube, deterioration after weaning, respiratory decompensation, subglottic stenosis, paralyzed diaphragm, respiratory failure.

Cardiovascular: hypotension, hypertension, tachycardia, ventricular tachycardia, aortic thrombosis, cardiac failure, cardio-respiratory arrest, increased apical pulse, persistent fetal circulation, air embolism, total anomalous pulmonary venous return.

Gastrointestinal: abdominal distention, hemorrhage, intestinal perforations, volvulus, bowel infarct, feeding intolerance, hepatic failure, stress ulcer.

Renal: renal failure, hematuria.

Hematologic: coagulopathy, thrombocytopenia, disseminated intravascular coagulation.

Central Nervous System: seizures.

Endocrine/Metabolic: adrenal hemorrhage, inappropriate ADH secretion, hyperphosphatemia.

Musculoskeletal: inguinal hernia.

Systemic: fever, deterioration.

FOLLOW-UP EVALUATIONS

To date, no long-term complications or sequelae of Beractant therapy have been found.

SINGLE-DOSE STUDIES

Six-month adjusted-age follow-up evaluations of 232 infants (115 treated) demonstrated no clinically important differences between treatment groups in

---

◆ RATED THERAPEUTICALLY EQUIVALENT; ◇ THERAPEUTIC EQUIVALENCE UNCONFIRMED; ○ UNRATED

pulmonary and neurologic sequelae, incidence or severity of retinopathy of prematurity, rehospitalizations, growth, or allergic manifestations.

MULTIPLE-DOSE STUDIES

Six-month adjusted age follow-up evaluations have not been completed. Preliminarily, in 605 (333 treated) of 916 surviving infants, there are trends for decreased cerebral palsy and need for supplemental oxygen in Beractant infants. Wheezing at the time of examination tended to be more frequent among Beractant infants, although there was no difference in bronchodilator therapy.

Twelve-month follow-up data from the multiple-dose studies have been completed in 328 (171 treated) of 909 surviving infants. To date no significant differences between treatments have been found, although there is a trend toward less wheezing in Beractant infants in contrast to the six month results.

OVERDOSAGE

Overdosage with Beractant has not been reported. Based on animal data, overdosage might result in acute airway obstruction. Treatment should be symptomatic and supportive.

Rales and moist breath sounds can transiently occur after Beractant is given, and do not indicate overdosage. Endotracheal suctioning or other remedial action is not required unless clear-cut signs of airway obstruction are present.

DOSAGE AND ADMINISTRATION

For Intratracheal Administration Only. Beractant should be administered by or under the supervision of clinicians experienced in intubation, ventilator management, and general care of premature infants.

Marked improvements in oxygenation may occur within minutes of administration of Beractant. Therefore, frequent and careful clinical observation and monitoring of systemic oxygenation are essential to avoid hyperoxia.

Review of audiovisual instructional materials describing dosage and administration procedures is recommended before using Beractant.

DOSAGE

Each dose of Beractant is 100 mg of phospholipids/kg birth weight (4 mL/kg). The BERACTANT DOSING CHART shows the total dosage for a range of birth weights.

BERACTANT DOSING CHART

Weight (grams)	Total Dose (mL)	Weight (grams)	Total Dose (mL)
600- 650	2.6	1301-1350	5.4
651- 700	2.8	1351-1400	5.6
701- 750	3.0	1401-1450	5.8
751- 800	3.2	1451-1500	6.0
801- 850	3.4	1501-1550	6.2
851- 900	3.6	1551-1600	6.4
901- 950	3.8	1601-1650	6.6
951-1000	4.0	1651-1700	6.8
1001-1050	4.2	1701-1750	7.0
1051-1100	4.4	1751-1800	7.2
1101-1150	4.6	1801-1850	7.4
1151-1200	4.8	1851-1900	7.6
1201-1250	5.0	1901-1950	7.8
1251-1300	5.2	1951-2000	8.0

Four doses of Beractant can be administered in the first 48 hours of life. Doses should be given no more frequently than every 6 hours.

DIRECTIONS FOR USE

Beractant should be inspected visually for discoloration prior to administration. The color of Beractant is off-white to light brown. If settling occurs during storage, swirl the vial gently (DO NOT SHAKE) to redisperse. Some foaming at the surface may occur during handling and is inherent in the nature of the product.

Beractant is stored refrigerated (2-8°C). Before administration, Beractant should be warmed by standing at room temperature for at least 20 minutes or warmed in the hand for at least 8 minutes. *Artificial Warming Methods Should Not Be Used.* If a prevention dose is to be given, preparation of Beractant should begin before the infant's birth.

Unopened, unused vials of Beractant that have been warmed to room temperature may be returned to the refrigerator within 8 hours of warming, and stored for future use. Drug should not be warmed and returned to the refrigerator more than once. Each single-use vial of Beractant should be entered only once. Used vials with residual drug should be discarded.

Beractant does not require reconstitution or sonication before use.

DOSING PROCEDURES
GENERAL

Beractant is administered intratracheally by instillation through a 5 French end-hole catheter inserted into the infant's endotracheal tube with the tip of the catheter protruding just beyond the end of the endotracheal tube above the infant's carina. Before inserting the catheter through the endotracheal tube, the length of the catheter should be shortened. Beractant should not be instilled into a mainstem bronchus.

It is important to ensure homogenous distribution of Beractant throughout the lungs. In the controlled clinical trials, each dose was divided into four quarter-doses. Each quarter-dose was administered with the infant in a different position. The sequence of positions was:

- Head and body inclined slightly down, head turned to the right
- Head and body inclined slightly down, head turned to the left
- Head and body inclined slightly up, head turned to the right
- Head and body inclined slightly up, head turned to the left

The dosing procedure is facilitated if one person administers the dose while another person positions and monitors the infant.

FIRST DOSE

Determine the total dose of Beractant from the BERACTANT DOSING CHART based on the infant's birth weight. Slowly withdraw the entire contents of the vial into a plastic syringe through a large-gauge needle (eg, at least 20 gauge). *Do not filter Beractant and avoid shaking.*

Attach the premeasured 5 French end-hole catheter to the syringe. Fill the catheter with Beractant. Discard excess Beractant, through the catheter so that only the total dose to be given remains in the syringe.

Before administering Beractant, assure proper placement and patency of the endotracheal tube. At the discretion of the clinician, the endotracheal tube may be suctioned before administering Beractant. The infant should be allowed to stabilize before proceeding with dosing.

In the prevention strategy, weigh, intubate and stabilize the infant. Administer the dose as soon as possible after birth, preferably within 15 minutes. Position the infant appropriately and gently inject the first quarter-dose through the catheter over 2-3 seconds.

After administration of the first quarter-dose, remove the catheter from the endotracheal tube. Manually ventilate with a hand-bag with sufficient oxygen to prevent cyanosis, at a rate of 60 breaths/minute, and sufficient positive pressure to provide adequate air exchange and chest wall excursion.

In the rescue strategy, the first dose should be given as soon as possible after the infant is placed on a ventilator for management of RDS. In the clinical trials, immediately before instilling the first quarter-dose, the infant's ventilator settings were changed to rate 60/minute, inspiratory time 0.5 second, and FiO_2 1.0.

Position the infant appropriately and gently inject the first quarter-dose through the catheter over 2-3 seconds. After administration of the first quarter-dose, remove the catheter from the endotracheal tube. Return the infant to the mechanical ventilator.

In both strategies, ventilate the infant for at least 30 seconds or until stable. Reposition the infant for instillation of the next quarter-dose.

Instill the remaining quarter-doses using the same procedures. After instillation of each quarter-dose, remove the catheter and ventilate for at least 30 seconds or until the infant is stabilized. After instillation of the final quarter-dose, remove the catheter without flushing it. Do not suction the infant for 1 hour after dosing unless signs of significant airway obstruction occur.

After completion of the dosing procedure, resume usual ventilator management and clinical care.

REPEAT DOSES

The dosage of Beractant for repeat doses is also 100 mg phospholipids/kg and is based on the infant's birth weight. The infant should not be reweighed for determination of the Beractant dosage. Use the BERACTANT DOSING CHART to determine the total dosage.

The need for additional doses of Beractant is determined by evidence of continuing respiratory distress. Using the following criteria for redosing, significant reductions in mortality due to RDS were observed in the multiple-dose clinical trials with Beractant.

Dose no sooner than 6 hours after the preceding dose if the infant remains intubated and requires at least 30% inspired oxygen to maintain a PaO_2 less than or equal to 80 torr.

Radiographic confirmation of RDS should be obtained before administering additional doses to those who received a prevention dose.

Prepare Beractant and position the infant for administration of each quarter-dose as previously described. After instillation of each quarter-dose, remove the dosing catheter from the endotracheal tube and ventilate the infant for at least 30 seconds or until stable.

In the clinical studies, ventilator settings used to administer repeat doses were different than those used for the first dose. For repeat doses, the FiO_2 was increased by 0.20 or an amount sufficient to prevent cyanosis. The ventilator delivered a rate of 30/minute with an inspiratory time less than 1.0 second. If the infant's pretreatment rate was 30 or greater, it was left unchanged during Beractant instillation.

Manual hand-bag ventilation should not be used to administer repeat doses. *During the dosing procedure, ventilator settings may be adjusted at the discretion of the clinician to maintain appropriate oxygenation and ventilation. After completion of the dosing procedure, resume usual ventilator management and clinical care.*

DOSING PRECAUTIONS

If an infant experiences bradycardia or oxygen desaturation during the dosing procedure, stop the dosing procedure and initiate appropriate measures to alleviate the condition. After the infant has stabilized, resume the dosing procedure. Rales and moist breath sounds can occur transiently after administration of Beractant. Endotracheal suctioning or other remedial action is unnecessary unless clear-cut signs of airway obstruction are present.

Store unopened vials at refrigeration temperature (2-8°C). Protect from light. Store vials in carton until ready for use. Vials are for single use only. Upon opening, discard unused drug.

HOW SUPPLIED
INJECTION: 25 MG/ML

BRAND/MANUFACTURER	NDC	SIZE	AWP
○ BRAND			
SURVANTA INTRATRACHEAL: Ross Pharm	00074-1040-08	8 ml	$688.82

Berocca SEE VITAMIN B COMPLEX WITH VITAMIN C

Berocca Plus SEE VITAMINS, MULTIPLE WITH MINERALS

Beta-carotene

DESCRIPTION

Beta-carotene, precursor of vitamin A, is a carotenoid pigment occurring naturally in green and yellow vegetables. Chemically, Beta-carotene has the empirical formula $C_{40}H_{56}$ and a calculated molecular weight of 536.85. Trans-beta-carotene is a red, crystalline compound which is insoluble in water.

Following is its chemical structure:

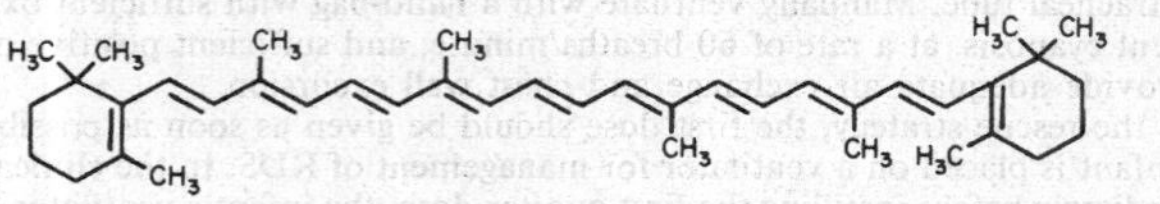

CLINICAL PHARMACOLOGY

Beta-carotene, a provitamin A, belongs to the class of carotenoid pigments. In terms of its vitamin activity, 6 μg of dietary Beta-carotene is considered equivalent to 1 μg of vitamin A (retinol). Bioavailability of Beta-carotene depends on the presence of fat in the diet to act as a carrier, and bile in the intestinal tract for its absorption. Beta-carotene is metabolized, primarily in the intestine, to vitamin A at a rate of approximately 50% to 60% of normal dietary intake and falls off rapidly as intake goes up. In humans, an appreciable amount of unchanged Beta-carotene is absorbed and stored in various tissues, especially the depot fat. Small amounts may be converted to vitamin A in the liver. The vitamin A derived from Beta-carotene follows the same metabolic pathway as that from dietary sources. The major route of elimination is fecal excretion. Excessive ingestion of carotenes is not harmful, but it may cause yellow coloration of the skin, which disappears upon reduction or cessation of intake.

INDICATIONS AND USAGE

Beta-carotene is used to reduce the severity of photosensitivity reactions in patients with erythropoietic protoporphyria (EPP).

UNLABELED USES
Beta-carotene is used as an adjunct in the treatment of polymorphous light eruptions.

CONTRAINDICATIONS

Beta-carotene is contraindicated in patients with known hypersensitivity to the drug.

WARNINGS

Beta-carotene has not been shown to be effective as a sunscreen.

PRECAUTIONS

General: Beta-carotene should be used with caution in patients with impaired renal or hepatic function because safe use in the presence of these conditions has not been established.

Information for Patients: Patients receiving Beta-carotene should be advised against taking supplementary vitamin A since Beta-carotene administration will fulfill normal vitamin A requirements. They should be cautioned to continue sun protection, and forewarned that their skin may appear slightly yellow while receiving Beta-carotene.

Carcinogenesis, Mutagenesis, Impairment of Fertility: Long-term studies in animals to determine carcinogenesis have not been completed. *In vitro* and *in vivo* studies to evaluate mutagenic potential were negative. No effects on fertility in male rats were observed at doses as high as 500 mg/kg/day (100 times the recommended human dose).

Pregnancy: Teratogenic Effects: Pregnancy Category C. Beta-carotene has been shown to be fetotoxic (*i.e.*, cause an increase in resorption rate), but not teratogenic when given to rats at doses 300 to 400 times the maximum recommended human dose. No such fetotoxicity was observed at 75 times the maximum recommended human dose or less. A three-generation reproduction study in rats receiving Beta-carotene at a dietary concentration of 0.1% (1000 ppm) has revealed no evidence of impaired fertility or effect on the fetus. There are no adequate and well-controlled studies in pregnant women. Beta-carotene should be used during pregnancy only if the potential benefit justifies the potential risk to the fetus.

Nursing Mothers: It is not known whether this drug is excreted in human milk. Because many drugs are excreted in human milk, caution should be exercised when Beta-carotene is administered to a nursing mother.

ADVERSE REACTIONS

Some patients may have occasional loose stools while taking Beta-carotene. This reaction is sporadic and may not require discontinuance of medication. Other reactions which have been reported rarely are ecchymoses and arthralgia.

OVERDOSAGE

There are no reported cases of overdosage. The oral LD_{50} of Beta-carotene (suspended in 5% gum acacia solution) in mice and rats is greater than 20,000 mg/kg. No lethality was observed in mice following administration of 30-mg beadlet capsules (ground and suspended in 5% gum acacia) at a dose of 1200 mg/kg Beta-carotene.

DOSAGE AND ADMINISTRATION

Beta-carotene may be administered either as a single daily dose or in divided doses, preferably with meals.

Usage in Children: The usual dosage for children under 14 is 30 to 150 mg (1 to 5 capsules) per day. Capsules may be opened and the contents mixed in orange juice or tomato juice to aid administration.

Usage in Adults: The usual adult dosage is 30 to 300 mg (1 to 10 capsules) per day.

Dosage should be adjusted depending on the severity of the symptoms and the response of the patient. Several weeks of therapy are necessary to accumulate enough Beta-carotene in the skin to exert its effect. Patients should be instructed not to increase exposure to sunlight until they appear carotenemic (first seen as yellowness of palms and soles). This usually occurs after two to six weeks of therapy. Exposure to the sun may then be increased gradually. The protective effect is not total and each patient should establish his or her own limits of exposure.

HOW SUPPLIED
CAPSULE: 30 MG

BRAND/MANUFACTURER	NDC	SIZE	AWP
○ BRAND			
SOLATENE: Roche Labs	00004-0115-01	100s	$55.30

Betadine 5% SEE POVIDONE-IODINE

Betagan SEE LEVOBUNOLOL HYDROCHLORIDE, OPHTHALMIC

Betamethasone Acetate and Betamethasone Sodium Phosphate

DESCRIPTION

Each mL of Betamethasone Acetate/Betamethasone Sodium Phosphate suspension contains: 3.0 mg Betamethasone Acetate and 3.0 mg Betamethasone as Betamethasone Sodium Phosphate. It is a sterile, aqueous suspension with a pH between 6.8 and 7.2.

The formula for Betamethasone Acetate is $C_{24}H_{31}FO_6$ with a molecular weight of 434.50. Chemically it is 9-Fluoro-11β,17,21-trihydroxy-16β-methylpregna-1,4-diene-3,20-dione 21-acetate.

The formula for Betamethasome Sodium Phosphate is $C_{22}H_{28}FNa_2O_8P$ with a molecular weight of 546.41. Chemically it is 9-Fluoro-11β, 17, 21-trihydroxy-16β-methylpregna-1, 4-diene-3, 20-dione 21-(disodium phosphate).

Betamethasone Acetate is a white to creamy white, odorless powder that sinters and resolidifies at about 165°C, and remelts at about 200°C-220°C with decomposition. It is practically insoluble in water, but freely soluble in acetone, and is soluble in alcohol and in chloroform.

Betamethasone Sodium Phosphate is a white to practically white, odorless powder, and is hygroscopic. It is freely soluble in water and in methanol, but is practically insoluble in acetone and in chloroform.

ACTIONS

Naturally occurring glucocorticoids (hydrocortisone), which also have salt-retaining properties, are used as replacement therapy in adrenocortical deficiency states. Their synthetic analogs are primarily used for their potent anti-inflammatory effects in disorders of many organ systems.

Betamethasone Sodium Phosphate, a soluble ester, provides prompt activity, while Betamethasone Acetate is only slightly soluble and affords sustained activity.

Glucocorticoids cause profound and varied metabolic effects. In addition, they modify the body's immune responses to diverse stimuli.

INDICATIONS

When oral therapy is not feasible and the strength, dosage form, and route of administration of the drug reasonably lend the preparation to the treatment of the

---

◆ RATED THERAPEUTICALLY EQUIVALENT; ◇ THERAPEUTIC EQUIVALENCE UNCONFIRMED; ○ UNRATED

condition, Betamethasone Acetate/Betamethasone Sodium Phosphate suspension for intramuscular use is indicated as follows:

Endocrine Disorders: Primary or secondary adrenocortical insufficiency (hydrocortisone or cortisone is the drug of choice: synthetic analogs may be used in conjunction with mineralocorticoids where applicable; in infancy mineralocorticoid supplementation is of particular importance).

Acute adrenocortical insufficiency (hydrocortisone or cortisone is the drug of choice: mineralocorticoid supplementation may be necessary, particularly when synthetic analogs are used); preoperatively and in the event of serious trauma or illness in patients with known adrenal insufficiency or when adrenocortical reserve is doubtful; shock unresponsive to conventional therapy if adrenocortical insufficiency exists or is suspected; congenital adrenal hyperplasia; nonsuppurative thyroiditis; hypercalcemia associated with cancer.

Rheumatic Disorders: As adjunctive therapy for short-term administration (to tide the patient over an acute episode or exacerbation) in: post-traumatic osteoarthritis; synovitis of osteoarthritis; rheumatoid arthritis, including juvenile rheumatoid arthritis (selected cases may require low-dose maintenance therapy); acute and subacute bursitis; epicon dylitis; acute nonspecific tenosynovitis; acute gouty arthritis; psoriatic arthritis; ankylosing spondylitis.

Collagen Disease: During an exacerbation or as maintenance therapy in selected cases of systemic lupus erythematosus, acute rheumatic carditis.

Dermatologic Disease: Pemphigus, severe erythema multiforme (Stevens-Johnson syndrome), exfoliative dermatitis, bullous dermatitis herpetiformis, severe seborrheic dermatitis, severe psoriasis, mycosis fungoides.

Allergic States: Control of severe or incapacitatin allergic conditions intractable to adequate trials of conventional treatment in: bronchial asthma, contact dermatitis, atopic dermatitis, serum sickness, seasonal or perennial allergic rhinitis, drug hypersensitivity reactions, urticarial transfusion reactions, acute noninfectious laryngeal, edema (epinephrine is the drug of first choice.)

Ophthalmic Diseases: Severe acute and chronic allergic and inflammatory processes involving the eye, such as: herpes zoster ophthalmicus, iritis and iridocyclitis, chorioretinitis, diffuse posterior uveitis and choroiditis, optic neuritis, sympathetic ophthalmia, anterior segment inflammation, allergic conjunctivitis, allergic corneal marginal ulcers, keratitis.

Gastrointestinal Diseases: To tide the patient over a critical period of disease in: ulcerative colitis—(systemic therapy), regional enteritis—(systemic therapy).

Respiratory Diseases: Symptomatic sarcoidosis, berylliosis, fulminating or disseminated pulmonary tuberculosis when used concurrently with appropriate antituberculous chemotherapy. Loeffler's syndrome not manageable by other means, aspiration pneumonitis.

Hematologic Disorders: Acquired (autoimmune) hemolytic anemia, secondary thrombocytopenia in adults, erythroblastopenia (RBC anemia), congenital (erythroid) hypoplastic anemia.

Neoplastic Diseases: For palliative management of: leukemias and lymphomas in adults, acute leukemia of childhood.

Edematous States: To induce diuresis or remission of proteinuria in the nephrotic syndrome, without uremia of the idiopathic type or that due to lupus erythematosus.

Miscellaneous: Tuberculous meningitis with subarachnoid block or impending block when used concurrently with appropriate antituberculous chemotherapy, trichinosis with neurologic or myocardial involvement.

When the strength and dosage form of the drug lend the preparation to the treatment of the condition, the *intra-articular or soft tissue administration* of Betamethasone Acetate/Betamethasone Sodium Phosphate suspension is indicated as adjunctive therapy for short-term administration (to tide the patient over an acute episode or exacerbation in: synovitis of osteoarthritis, rheumatoid arthritis, acute and subacute bursitis, acute gouty arthritis, epicondylitis, acute nonspecific, tenosynovitis, post-traumatic osteoarthritis.

When the strength and dosage form of the drug lend the preparation to the treatment of the condition, the *intralesional administration* of Betamethasone Acetate/Betamethasone Sodium Phosphate suspension is indicated for: keloids; localized hypertrophic infiltrated, inflammatory lesions of lichen planus, psoriatic plaques, granuloma annulare, and lichen simplex chronicus (neurodermatitis); discoid lupus erythematosus; necrobiosis lipoidica diabeticorum: alopecia areata.

Betamethasone Acetate/Betamethasone Sodium Phosphate suspension may also be useful in cystic tumors of an aponeurosis or tendon (ganglia).

CONTRAINDICATIONS
Betamethasone Acetate/Betamethasone Sodium Phosphate suspension is contraindicated in systemic fungal infections.

WARNINGS
Betamethasone Acetate/Betamethasone Sodium Phosphate suspension should not be administered intravenously.

In patients on corticosteroid therapy subjected to any unusual stress, increased dosage of rapidly acting corticosteroids before, during, and after the stressful situation is indicated.

Corticosteroids may mask some signs of infection, and new infections may appear during their use. There may be decreased resistance and inability to localize infection when corticosteroids are used.

Prolonged use of corticosteroids may produce posterior sub-capsular cataracts, glaucoma with possible damage to the optic nerves, and may enhance the establishment of secondary ocular infections due to fungi or viruses.

Betamethasone Acetate/Betamethasone Sodium Phosphate suspension contains two Betamethasone esters, one of which, Betamethasone Sodium Phosphate, disappears rapidly from the injection site. The potential for systemic effect produced by the soluble portion of Betamethasone Acetate/Betamethasone Sodium Phosphate suspension should therefore be taken into account by the physician when using the drug. Average and large doses of cortisone or hydrocortisone can cause elevation of blood pressure, salt and water retention, and increased excretion of potassium. These effects are less likely to occur with the synthetic derivatives except when used in large doses. Dietary salt restriction and potassium supplementation may be necessary. All corticosteroids increase calcium excretion.

While on corticosteroid therapy patients should not be vaccinated against smallpox. Other immunization procedures should not be undertaken in patients who are on corticosteroids, especially in high doses, because of possible hazards of neurological complications and lack of antibody response.

Persons who are on drugs which suppress the immune system are more susceptible to infections than healthy individuals. Chickenpox and measles, for example, can have a more serious or even fatal course in non-immune children or adults on corticosteroids. In such children, or adults who have not had these diseases, particular care should be taken to avoid exposure. How the dose, route, and duration of corticosteroid administration affects the risk of developing a disseminated infection is not known. The contribution of the underlying disease and/or prior corticosteroid treatment to the risk is also not known. If exposed to chickenpox, prophylaxis with varicella-zoster immune globulin (VZIG) may be indicated. If exposed to measles, prophylaxis with pooled intramuscular immunoglobulin (IG) may be indicated. (See the respective package inserts for complete VZIG and IG prescribing information.) If chickenpox develops, treatment with antiviral agents may be considered.

The use of Betamethasone Acetate/Betamethasone Sodium Phosphate suspension in active tuberculosis should be restricted to those cases of fulminating or disseminated tuberculosis in which the corticosteroid is used for the management of the disease in conjunction with appropriate antituberculous regimen.

If corticosteroids are indicated in patients with latent tuberculosis or tuberculin reactivity, close observation is necessary as reactivation of the disease may occur. During prolonged corticosteroid therapy, these patients should receive chemoprophylaxis.

Because rare instances of anaphylactoid reactions have occurred in patients receiving parenteral corticosteroid therapy, appropriate precautionary measures should be taken prior to administration, especially when the patient has a history of allergy to any drug.

Usage in Pregnancy: Since adequate human reproduction studies have not been done with corticosteroids, the use of these drugs in pregnancy, nursing mothers, or women of childbearing potential requires that the possible benefits of the drug be weighed against the potential hazards to the mother and embryo or fetus. Infants born of mothers who have received substantial doses of corticosteroids during pregnancy should be carefully observed for signs of hypoadrenalism.

PRECAUTIONS
Information for Patients: Persons who are on immunosuppressent doses of corticosteroids should be warned to avoid exposure to chickenpox or measles. Patients should also be advised that if they are exposed, medical advice should be sought without delay.

General: Drug-induced secondary adrenocortical insufficiency may be minimized by gradual reduction of dosage. This type of relative insufficiency may persist for months after discontinuation of therapy; therefore, in any situation of stress occurring during that period, hormone therapy should be reinstituted. Since mineralocorticoid secretion may be impaired, salt and or a mineralocorticoid should be administered concurrently.

There is an enhanced effect of corticosteroids in patients with hypothyroidism and in those with cirrhosis.

Corticosteroids should be used cautiously in patients with ocular herpes simplex for fear of corneal perforation.

The lowest possible dose of corticosteroid should be used to control the condition under treatment, and when reduction in dosage is possible, the reduction must be gradual.

Psychic derangements may appear when corticosteroids are used, ranging from euphoria, insomnia, mood swings, personality changes, and severe depression to frank psychotic manifestations. Also, existing emotional instability or psychotic tendencies may be aggravated by corticosteroids.

Aspirin should be used cautiously in conjunction with corticosteroids in hypoprothrombinemia.

Steroids should be used with caution in nonspecific ulcerative colitis, if there is a probability of impending perforation, abscess or other pyogenic infection, also in diverticulitis, fresh intestinal anastomoses, active or latent peptic ulcer, renal insufficiency, hypertension, osteoporosis, and myasthenia gravis.

Growth and development of infants and children on prolonged corticosteroid therapy should be carefully followed.

The following additional precautions also apply for parenteral corticosteroids. **Intra-articular injection of a corticosteroid may produce systemic as well as local effects.**

Appropriate examination of any joint fluid present is necessary to exclude a septic process.

A marked increase in pain accompanied by local swelling, further restriction of joint motion, fever, and malaise are suggestive of septic arthritis. If this complication occurs and the diagnosis of sepsis is confirmed, appropriate antimicrobial therapy should be instituted.

Local injection of a steroid into a previously infected joint is to be avoided. Corticosteroids should not be injected into unstable joints. The slower rate of absorption by intramuscular administration should be recognized.

ADVERSE REACTIONS

Fluid and Electrolyte Disturbances: Sodium retention, fluid retention, congestive heart failure in susceptible patients, potassium loss, hypokalemic alkalosis, hypertension.

Musculoskeletal: muscle weakness, steroid myopathy, loss of muscle mass, osteoporosis, vertebral compression fractures, aseptic necrosis of femoral and humeral heads, pathologic fracture of long bones.

Gastrointestinal: peptic ulcer with possible subsequent perforation and hemorrhage, pancreatitis, abdominal distention, ulcerative esophagitis.

Dermatologic: impaired wound healing, thin fragile skin, petechiae and ecchymoses, facial erythema, increased sweating, may suppress reactions to skin tests.

Neurological: convulsions, increased intracranial pressure with papilledema (pseudotumor cerebri) usually after treatment, vertigo, headache.

Endocrine: menstrual irregularities; development of cushingoid state; suppression of growth in children; secondary adrenocortical and pituitary unresponsiveness, particularly in times of stress, as in trauma, surgery, or illness; decreased carbohydrate tolerance; manifestations of latent diabetes mellitus; increased requirements for insulin or oral hypoglycemic agents in diabetics.

Ophthalmic: posterior subcapsular cataracts, increased intraocular pressure, glaucoma, exophthalmos.

Metabolic: negative nitrogen balance due to protein catabolism.

The following *additional* adverse reactions are related to parenteral corticosteroid therapy: rare instances of blindness associated with intralesional therapy around the face and head, hyperpigmentation or hypopigmentation, subcutaneous and cutaneous atrophy, sterile abscess, post-injection flare (following intra-articular use), charcotlike arthropathy.

DOSAGE AND ADMINISTRATION

The initial dosage of Betamethasone Acetate/Betamethasone Sodium Phosphate suspension may vary from 0.5 to 9.0 mg per day depending on the specific disease entity being treated. In situations of less severity, lower doses will generally suffice while in selected patients higher initial doses may be required. Usually the parenteral dosage ranges are one-third to one-half the oral dose given every 12 hours. However, in certain overwhelming, acute, life-threatening situations, administration in dosages exceeding the usual dosages may be justified and may be in multiples of the oral dosages.

The initial dosage should be maintained or adjusted until a satisfactory response is noted. If after a reasonable period of time there is a lack of satisfactory clinical response, Betamethasone Acetate/Betamethasone Sodium Phosphate suspension should be discontinued and the patient transferred to other appropriate therapy. *It should be emphasized that dosage requirements are variable and must be individualized on the basis of the disease under treatment and the response of the patient.* After a favorable response is noted, the proper maintenance dosage should be determined by decreasing the initial drug dosage in small decrements at appropriate time intervals until the lowest dosage which will maintain an adequate clinical response is reached. It should be kept in mind that constant monitoring is needed in regard to drug dosage. Included in the situations which may make dosage adjustments necessary are changes in clinical status secondary to remissions or exacerbations in the disease process, the patient's individual drug responsiveness, and the effect of patient exposure to stressful situations not directly related to the disease entity under treatment; in this latter situation it may be necessary to increase the dosage of Betamethasone Acetate/Betamethasone Sodium Phosphate suspension for a period of time consistent with the patient's condition. If after long-term therapy the drug is to be stopped, it is recommended that it be withdrawn gradually rather than abruptly.

If coadministration of a local anesthetic is desired, Betamethasone Acetate/Betamethasone Sodium Phosphate suspension may be mixed with 1% or 2% lidocaine hydrochloride, using the formuations which do not contain parabens. Similar local anesthetics may also be used. Diluents containing methylparaben, propylparaben, phenol, etc., should be avoided since these compounds may cause flocculation of the steroid. The required dose of Betamethasone Acetate/Betamethasone Sodium Phosphate suspension is first withdrawn from the vial into the syringe. The local anesthetic is then drawn in, and the syringe shaken briefly. *Do not inject local anesthetics into the vial of* Betamethasone Acetate/Betamethasone Sodium Phosphate *suspension.*

Bursitis, Tenosynovitis, Peritendinitis: In acute subdeltoid, subacromial, olecranon, and prepatellar bursitis, one intrabursal injection of 1.0 mL Betamethasone Acetate/Betamethasone Sodium Phosphate suspension can relieve pain and restore full range of movement. Several intrabursal injections of corticosteroids are usually required in recurrent acute bursitis and in acute exacerbations of chronic bursitis. Partial relief of pain and some increase in mobility can be expected in both conditions after one or two injections. Chronic bursitis may be treated with reduced dosage once the acute condition is controlled. In tenosynovitis and tendinitis, three or four local injections at intervals of one to two weeks between injections are given in most cases. Injections should be made into the affected tendon sheaths rather than into the tendons themselves. In ganglions of joint capsules and tendon sheaths, injection of 0.5 mL directly into the ganglion cysts has produced marked reduction in the size of the lesions.

Rheumatoid Arthritis and Osteoarthritis: Following intra-articular administration of 0.5 to 2.0 mL of Betamethasone Acetate/Betamethasone Sodium Phosphate suspension, relief of pain, soreness, and stiffness may be experienced. Duration of relief varies widely in both diseases. Intra-articular injection—Betamethasone Acetate/Betamethasone Sodium Phosphate suspension is well tolerated in joints and periarticular tissues. There is virtually no pain on injection, and the "secondary flare" that sometimes occurs a few hours after intra-articular injection of corticosteroids has not been reported with Betamethasone Acetate/Betamethasone Sodium Phosphate suspension. Using sterile technique, a 20- to 24-gauge needle on an empty syringe is inserted into the synovial cavity, and a few drops of synovial fluid are withdrawn to confirm that the needle is in the joint. The aspirating syringe is replaced by a syringe containing Betamethasone Acetate/Betamethasone Sodium Phosphate suspension and injection is then made into the joint.

RECOMMENDED DOSES FOR INTRA-ARTICULAR INJECTION

| | | Injection | |
Size of joint	Location	Dose (mL)
Very Large	Hip	1.0-2.0
Large	Knee, Ankle, Shoulder	1.0
Medium	Elbow, Wrist	0.5-1.0
Small (Metacarpophalangeal, interphalangeal)	Hand	0.25-0.5
(Sternoclavicular)	Chest	

A portion of the administered dose of Betamethasone Acetate/Betamethasone Sodium Phosphate suspension is absorbed systemically following intra-articular injection. In patients being treated concomitantly with oral or parenteral corticosteroids, especially those receiving large doses, the systemic absorption of the drug should be considered in determining intra-articular dosage.

Dermatologic Conditions: In intralesional treatment, 0.2 mL/sq cm of Betamethasone Acetate/Betamethasone Sodium Phosphate suspension is injected intradermally (not subcutaneously) using a tuberculin syringe with a 25-gauge, ½-inch needle. Care should be taken to deposit a uniform depot of medication intradermally. A total of no more than 1.0 mL at weekly intervals is recommended.

Disorders of the Foot: A tuberculin syringe with a 25-gauge, 3/4-inch needle is suitable for most injections into the foot. The following doses are recommended at intervals of three days to a week.

Diagnosis	Suspension Dose (mL)
Bursitis	
under heloma durum or heloma molle	0.25-0.5
under calcaneal spur	0.5
over hallux rigidus or digiti quinti varus	0.5
Tenosynovitis, periostitis of cuboid	0.5
Acute gouty arthritis	0.5-1.0

Storage: Shake well before using.
Store between 2° and 25°C (36° and 77°F).
Protect from light.

HOW SUPPLIED

BETAMETHASONE ACETATE/BETAMETHASONE SODIUM PHOSPHATE
INJECTION: 3 MG-3 MG/ML

BRAND/MANUFACTURER	NDC	SIZE	AWP
○ BRAND			
CELESTONE SOLUSPAN: Schering	00085-0566-05	5 ml	$18.47

BETAMETHASONE
SYRUP: 0.6 MG/5 ML

BRAND/MANUFACTURER	NDC	SIZE	AWP
○ BRAND			
CELESTONE: Schering	00085-0942-05	120 ml	$31.02

◆ RATED THERAPEUTICALLY EQUIVALENT; ◇ THERAPEUTIC EQUIVALENCE UNCONFIRMED; ○ UNRATED

TABLETS: 0.6 MG

BRAND/MANUFACTURER	NDC	SIZE	AWP
○ **BRAND**			
CELESTONE: Schering	00085-0011-01	21s ud	$27.58
	00085-0011-05	100s	$124.18

Betamethasone Dipropionate with Clotrimazole Cream

DESCRIPTION

Betamethasone Dipropionate/Clotrimazole Cream contains a combination of Betamethasone Dipropionate, USP, a synthetic corticosteroid, and Clotrimazole, USP, a synthetic antifungal agent, for dermatologic use.

Betamethasone Dipropionate has the chemical name 9-Fluoro-11β, 17,21-trihydroxy-16β-methylpregna-1,4-diene-3,20-dione 17,21-Dipropionate, with the empirical formula $C_{28}H_{37}FO_7$ and a molecular weight of 504.6.

Betamethasone Dipropionate is a white to creamy white, odorless crystalline powder, insoluble in water.

Chemically, Clotrimazole is 1-(o-Chloro-α,α-diphenyl benzyl) imidazole, with the empirical formula $C_{22}H_{17}ClN_2$ and a molecular weight of 344.8.

Clotrimazole is an odorless, white crystalline powder, insoluble in water and soluble in ethanol.

Each gram of Betamethasone Dipropionate/Clotrimazole Cream contains 0.64 mg Betamethasone Dipropionate, usp (equivalent to 0.5 mg Betamethasone), and 10.0 mg Clotrimazole, usp, in a hydrophilic emollient cream consisting of purified water, mineral oil, white petrolatum, cetearyl alcohol, ceteareth-30, propylene glycol, sodium phosphate monobasic, and phosphoric acid; benzyl alcohol as preservative.

Betamethasone Dipropionate/Clotrimazole Cream is a smooth, uniform, white to off-white cream.

CLINICAL PHARMACOLOGY

BETAMETHASONE DIPROPIONATE

Betamethasone Dipropionate, a corticosteroid, is effective in the treatment of corticosteroid-responsive dermatoses primarily because of its anti-inflammatory, antipruritic, and vasoconstrictive actions. However, while the physiologic, pharmacologic, and clinical effects of corticosteroids are well-known, the exact mechanisms of their actions in each disease are uncertain. Betamethasone Dipropionate, a corticosteroid, has been shown to have topical (dermatologic) and systemic pharmacologic and metabolic effects characteristic of this class of drugs.

CLOTRIMAZOLE

Clotrimazole is a broad-spectrum, antifungal agent that is used for the treatment of dermal infections caused by various species of pathogenic dermatophytes, yeasts, and *Malasezia furfur*. The primary action of Clotrimazole is against dividing and growing organisms.

In vitro, Clotrimazole exhibits fungistatic and fungicidal activity against isolates of *Trichophyton robrum, Trichophyton mentagrophytes, Epidermophyton floccosum* and *Microsporum canis*. In general, the *in vitro* activity of Clotrimazole corresponds to that of tolnafiate and griseofulxin against the mycelia of dermatophytes (*Trichophyton, Microsporum*, and *Epidermophyton*).

In vivo studies in guinea pigs infected with *Trichophyton mentagrophytes* have shown no measurable loss of Clotrimazole activity due to combination with Betamethasone Dipropionate.

Strains of fungi having a natural resistance to Clotrimazole have not been reported.

No single-step or multiple-step resistance to Clotrimazole has developed during successive passages of *Trichophyton mentagrophytes.*

In studies of the mechanism of action in fungal cultures. The minimum fungicidal concentration of Clotrimazole caused leakage of intracellular phosphorous compounds into the ambient medium with concomitant breakdown of cellular nucleic acids, and accelerated potassium efflux. Both of these events began rapidly and extensively after addition of the drug to the cultures.

Clotrimazole appears to be minimally absorbed following topical application to the skin. Six hours after the application of radioactive Clotrimazole 1% cream and 1% solution onto intact and acutely inflamed skin, the concentration of Clotrimazole varied from 100 mcg/cm^3 in the stratum corneum, to 0.5 to 1 mcg/cm^3 in the stratum reticulare, and 0.1 mcg/cm^3 in the subcutis. No measureable amount of radioactivity (< 0.001 mcg/ml) was found in the serum within 48 hours after application under occlusive dressing of 0.5 ml of the solution or 0.8 g of the cream.

Pharmacokinetics: The extent of percutaneous absorption of topical corticosteroids is determined by many factors including the vehicle, the integrity of the epidermal barrier, and the use of occlusive dressings. (See *"Dosage and Administration"* section.)

Topical corticosteroids can be absorbed from normal intact skin. Inflammation and/or other disease processes in the skin increase percutaneous absorption. Occlusive dressings substantially increase the percutaneous absorption of topical corticosteroids. (See *"Dosage and Administration"* section.)

Once absorbed through the skin, topical corticosteroids are handled through pharmacokinetic pathways similar to systemically administered corticosteroids. Corticosteroids are bound to plasma proteins in varying degrees. Corticosteroids are metabolized primarily in the liver and are then excreted by the kidneys. Some of the topical corticosteroids and their metabolities are also excreted into the bile.

BETAMETHASONE DIPROPIONATE/CLOTRIMAZOLE

In clinical studies of tinea corporis, tinea cruris and tinea pedis, patients treated with Betamethasone Dipropionate/Clotrimazole Cream showed a better clinical response at the first return visit than patients treated with Clotrimazole cream. In tinea corporis and tinea cruris, the patient returned three days after starting treatment, and in tinea pedis, after one week. Mycological cure rates observed in patients treated with Betamethasone Dipropionate/Clotrimazole Cream were as good as or better than in those patients treated with Clotrimazole cream.

In these same clinical studies, patients treated with Betamethasone Dipropionate/Clotrimazole Cream showed statistically significantly better clinical responses and mycological cure rates when compared with patients treated with Betamethasone Dipropionate cream.

INDICATIONS AND USAGE

Betamethasone Dipropionate/Clotrimazole Cream is indicated for the topical treatment of the following dermal infections: tinea pedis, tinea cruris, and tinea corporis due to *Trichophyton rubrum, Trichophyton mentagrophytes. Epidermophyton floccosum*, and *Microsporum canis*.

CONTRAINDICATIONS

Betamethasone Dipropionate/Clotrimazole Cream is contraindicated in patients who are sensitive to Betamethasone Dipropionate, Clotrimazole, other corticosteroids or imidazoles, or to any ingredient in this preparation.

PRECAUTIONS

General: Systemic absorption of topical corticosteroids has produced reversible hypothalamic-pituitary-adrenal (HPA) axis suppression, manifestations of Cushing's syndrome, hyperglycemia, and glucosuria in some patients.

Conditions which augment systemic absorption include the application of the more potent steroids, use over large surface areas, prolonged use, and the addition of occlusive dressings. (See *"Dosage and Administration"* section.)

Therefore, patients receiving a large dose of a potent topical steroid applied to a large surface area should be evaluated periodically for evidence of HPA axis suppression by using the urinary free cortisol and ACTH stimulation tests. If HPA axis suppression is noted, an attempt should be made to withdraw the drug, to reduce the frequency of application, or to substitute a less potent steroid.

Recovery of HPA axis function is generally prompt and complete upon discontinuation of the drug. Infrequently, signs and symptoms of steroid withdrawal may occur, requiring supplemental systemic corticosteroids.

Children may absorb proportionally larger amounts of topical corticosteroids and thus be more susceptible to systemic toxicity. (See *"Precautions-Pediatric Use."*)

If irritation or hypersensitivity develops with the use of Betamethasone Dipropionate/Clotrimazole Cream, treatment should be discontinued and appropriate therapy instituted.

Information for Patients Patients using Betamethasone Dipropionate/Clotrimazole Cream should receive the following information and instructions:

1. This medication is to be used as directed by the physician. It is for external use only. Avoid contact with the eyes.

2. The medication is to be used for the full prescribed treatment time, even though the symptoms may have improved. Notify the physician if there is no improvement after one week of treatment for tinea cruris or tinea corporis, or after two weeks for tinea pedis.

3. Patients should be advised not to use this medication for any disorder other than for which it was prescribed.

4. The treated skin areas should not be bandaged or otherwise covered or wrapped as to be occluded. (See *"Dosage and Administration"* section.)

5. When using this medication in the groin area, patients should be advised to use the medication for two weeks only, and to apply the cream sparingly. The physician should be notified if the condition persists after two weeks. Patients should also be advised to wear loose fitting clothing. (See *"Dosage and Administration"* section.)

6. Patients should report any signs of local adverse reactions.

7. Patients should avoid sources of infection or reinfection.

Laboratory Tests: If there is a lack of response to Betamethasone Dipropionate/Clotrimazole Cream, appropriate microbiological studies should be repeated to confirm the diagnosis and rule out other pathogens before instituting another course of antimycotic therapy.

The following tests may be helpful in evaluating HPA axis suppression due to the corticosteroid component:

Urinary free cortisol test
ACTH stimulation test

Carcinogenesis, Mutagenesis, Impairment of Fertility: There are no animal or laboratory studies with the combination Betamethasone Dipropionate and Clotrimazole to evaluate carcinogenesis, mutagenesis or impairment of fertility.

An 18-month oral dosing study with Clotrimazole in rats has not revealed any carcinogenic effect.

In tests for mutagenesis, chromosomes of the spermatophores of Chinese hamsters which have been exposed to Clotrimazole were examined for structural changes during the metaphase. Prior to testing, the hamsters had received five oral Clotrimazole doses of 100 mg/kg body weight. The resuits of this study showed that Clotrimazole had no mutagenic effect.

Pregnancy Category C: There have been no teratogenic studies performed with the combination Betamethasone Dipropionate and Clotrimazole.

Corticosteroids are generally teratogenic in laboratory animals when administered systemically at relatively low dosage levels. The more potent corticosteroids have been shown to be teratogenic after dermal application in laboratory animals.

Studies in pregnant rats with *intravaginal* doses up to 100 mg/kg have revealed no evidence of harm to the fetus due to Clotrimazole.

High *oral* doses of Clotrimazole in rats and mice ranging from 50 to 120 mg/kg resulted in embryotoxicity (possibly secondary to maternal toxicity), impairment of mating, decreased litter size and number of viable young and decreased pup survival to weaning. However, Clotrimazole was *not* teratogenic in mice, rabbits and rats at oral doses up to 200, 180 and 100 mg/kg, respectively. Oral absorption in the rat amounts to approximately 90% of the administered dose.

There are no adequate and well-controlled studies in pregnant women on teratogenic effects from a topically applied combination of Betamethasone Dipropionate and Clotrimazole. Therefore Betamethasone Dipropionate/Clotrimazole Cream should be used during pregnancy only if the potential benefit justifies the potential risk to the fetus.

Drugs containing corticosteroids should not be used extensively on pregnant patients, in large amounts, or for prolonged periods of time.

Nursing Mothers: It is not known whether this drug is excreted in human milk. Because many drugs are excreted in human milk, caution should be exercised when Betamethasone Dipropionate/ Clotrimazole Cream is used by a nursing woman.

Pediatric Use: Safety and effectiveness in children below the age of 12 have not been established with Betamethasone Dipropionate/ Clotrimazole Cream.

Pediatric patients may demonstrate greater susceptibility to topical corticosteroid-induced HPA axis suppression and Cushing's syndrome than mature patients because of a larger skin surface area to body weight ratio. Hypothalamic-pituitary-adrenal (HPA) axis suppression, Cushing's syndrome, and intracranial hypertension have been reported in children receiving topical corticosteroids. Manifestations of adrenal suppression in children include linear growth retardation, delayed weight gain, low plasma cortisol levels, and absence of response to ACTH stimulation.

Manifestations of intracarnial hypertension include bulging fontanelles, headaches, and bilateral papilledema.

Administration of topical dermatologics containing a corticosteroid to children should be limited to the least amount compatible with an effective therapeutic regimen. Chronic corticosteroid therapy may interfere with the growth and development of children.

The use of Betumethasone Dipropionate/Clotrimazole Cream in diaper dermatitis is not recommended.

ADVERSE REACTIONS
The following adverse reactions have been reported in connection with the use of Betumethasone Dipropionate/Clotrimazole Cream; paresthesia in 5 of 270 patients, maculopapular rash, edema, and secondary infection, each in 1 of 270 patients.

The following local adverse reactions are reported infrequently when topical corticosteroids are used as recommended. These reactions are listed in an approximate decreasing order of occurrence: burning, itching, irritation, dryness, folliculitis, hypertrichosis, acneiform eruptions, hypopigmentation, perioral dermatitis, allergic contact dermatitis, maceration of the skin, secondary infection, skin atrophy, striae, and miliaria.

Adverse reactions reported with the use of Clotrimazole are as follows: erythema, stinging, blistering, peeling, edema, pruritus, urticaria, and general irritation of the skin.

OVERDOSAGE
Acute overdosage with topical application of Betamethasone Dipropionate/Clotrimazole Cream is unlikely and would not be expected to lead to a life-threatening situation.

Topically applied corticosteroids can be absorbed in sufficient amounts to produce systemic effects. (See *"Precautions."*)

DOSAGE AND ADMINISTRATION
Gently massage sufficient Betamethasone Dipropionate/Clotrimazole Cream into the affected and surrounding skin areas twice a day, in the morning and evening for two weeks in tinea cruris and tinea corporis and for four weeks in tinea pedis. The use of Betamethasone Dipropionate/Clotrimazole Cream for longer than four weeks is not recommended.

Clinical improvement, with relief of erythema and pruritus, usually occurs within three to five days of treatment. If a patient with tinea cruris and tinea corporis shows no clinical improvement after one week of treatment with Betamethasone Dipropionate/Clotrimazole Cream, the diagnosis should be reviewed. In tinea pedis, the treatment should be applied for two weeks prior to making that decision.

Treatment with Betamethasone Dipropionate/Clotrimazole Cream should be discontinued if the condition persists after two weeks in tinea cruris and tinea corporis, and after four weeks in tinea pedis. Alternate therapy may then be instituted with Clotrimazole Cream, a product containing an antifungal only.

Betamethasone Dipropionate/Clotrimazole Cream should *not* be used with occlusive dressings.

Store between 2° and 30°C (36° and 86°F).

HOW SUPPLIED
CREAM: 0.5 MG-10 MG/GM

BRAND/MANUFACTURER	NDC	SIZE	AWP
○ **BRAND**			
LOTRISONE: Schering	00085-0924-01	15 gm	$16.13
	00085-0924-02	45 gm	$33.80

Betamethasone Sodium Phosphate

DESCRIPTION
Betamethasone Sodium Phosphate injection is a sterile, aqueous solution containing in each mL: 4.0 mg Betamethasone Sodium Phosphate, USP, equivalent to 3.0 mg Betamethasone alcohol; 10 mg dibasic Sodium Phosphate; 0.1 mg edetate disodium; 3.2 mg sodium bisulfite; and 5.0 mg phenol as preservative. The pH is adjusted to approximately 8.5 with Sodium hydroxide.

The formula for Betamethasone Sodium Phosphate is $C_{22}H_{28}FNa_2O_8P$ and has a molecular weight of 516.41. Chemically, it is 9-Fluoro-11β,17,21-trihydroxy-16β-methylpregna-1,4-diene-3,20 -dione 21-(disodium phosphate).

Betamethasone Sodium Phosphate is a white to practically white, odorless powder, and is hygroscopic. Betamethasone Sodium Phosphate is freely soluble in water and methanol and is practically insoluble in acetone and chloroform.

Following is its chemical structure:

ACTIONS
Naturally occurring glucocorticoids (hydrocortisone), which also have salt-retaining properties, are used as replacement therapy in adrenocortical deficiency states. Their synthetic analogs are primarily used for their potent anti-inflammatory effects in disorders of many organ systems.

Glucocorticoids cause profound and varied metabolic effects. In addition, they modify the body's immune responses to diverse stimuli.

INDICATIONS
When oral therapy is not feasible and the strength, dosage form, and route of administration of the drug reasonably lend the preparation to the treatment of the condition the *"intravenous or intramuscular use"* of Betamethasone Sodium Phosphate Injection is indicated as follows:

Endocrine Disorders: Primary or secondary adrenocortical insufficiency (hydrocortisone or cortisone is the drug of choice; synthetic analogs may be used in conjunction with mineralocorticoids where applicable; in infancy, mineralocorticoid supplementation is of particular importance).

Acute adrenocortical insufficiency (hydrocortisone or cortisone is the drug of choice; mineralocorticoid supplementation may be necessary, particularly when synthetic analogs are used).

Preoperatively and in the event of serious trauma or illness, in patients with known adrenal insufficiency or when adrenocortical reserve is doubtful.

Shock unresponsive to conventional therapy if adrenocortical insufficiency exists or is suspected.

Congenital adrenal hyperplasia. Nonsuppurative thyroiditis. Hypercalcemia associated with cancer.

Rheumatic Disorders: As adjunctive therapy for short-term administration (to tide the patient over an acute episode or exacerbation) in:
Posttraumatic osteoarthritis.
Synovitis of osteoarthritis.
Rheumatoid arthritis, including juvenile rheumatoid arthritis (selected cases may require low-dose maintenance therapy).
Acute and subacute bursitis.
Epicondylitis.
Acute nonspecific tenosynovitis.
Acute gouty arthritis.
Psoriatic arthritis.
Ankylosing spondylitis.

Collagen Diseases: During an exacerbation or as maintenance therapy in selected cases of:
Systemic lupus erythematosus.
Acute rheumatic carditis.

Dermatologic Diseases:
Pemphigus.
Severe erythema multiforme (Stevens-Johnson syndrome).
Exfoliative dermatitis.

◆ RATED THERAPEUTICALLY EQUIVALENT; ◇ THERAPEUTIC EQUIVALENCE UNCONFIRMED; ○ UNRATED

Bullous dermatitis herpetiformis.
Severe seborrheic dermatitis.
Severe psoriasis.
Mycosis fungoides.

Allergic States: Control of severe or incapacitating allergic conditions intractable to adequate trials of conventional treatment in:
Bronchial asthma.
Contact dermatitis.
Atopic dermatitis.
Serum sickness.
Seasonal or perennial allergic rhinitis.
Drug hypersensitivity reactions.
Urticarial transfusion reactions.
Acute noninfectious laryngeal edema (epinephrine is the drug of first choice).

Ophthalmic Diseases: Severe, acute and chronic allergic and inflammatory processes involving the eye, such as:
Herpes zoster ophthalmicus.
Iritis, iridocyclitis.
Chorioretinitis.
Diffuse posterior uveitis and choroiditis.
Optic neuritis.
Sympathetic ophthalmia.
Anterior segment inflammation.
Allergic conjunctivitis.
Allergic corneal marginal ulcers.
Keratitis.

Gastrointestinal Diseases: To tide the patient over a critical period of the disease in:
Ulcerative colitis-(Systemic therapy).
Regional enteritis-(Systemic therapy).

Respiratory Diseases:
Symptomatic sarcoidosis.
Berylliosis.
Fulminating or disseminated pulmonary tuberculosis when used concurrently with appropriate antituberculous chemotherapy.
Loeffler's syndrome not manageable by other means.
Aspiration pneumonitis.

Hematologic Disorders: Acquired (autoimmune) hemolytic anemia. Idopathic thrombocytopenic purpura in adults (I.V. only; I.M. administration is contraindicated).
Secondary thrombocytopenia in adults.
Erythroblastopenia (RBC anemia).
Congenital (erythroid) hypoplastic anemia.

Neoplastic Diseases: For palliative management of:
Leukemias and lymphomas in adults.
Acute leukemia of childhood.

Edematous States: To induce a diuresis or remission of proteinuria in the nephrotic syndrome, without uremia, of the idiopathic type or that due to lupus erythematosus.

Miscellaneous:
Tuberculous meningitis with subarachnoid block or impending block when used concurrently with appropriate antituberculous chemotherapy.
Trichinosis with neurologic or myocardial involvement.
When the strength and dosage form of the drug lend the preparation to the treatment of the condition, *the intra-articular or soft tissue administration* of Betamethasone Sodium Phosphate Injection is indicated as adjunctive therapy for short-term administration (to tide the patient over an acute episode or exacerbation) in:
Synovitis of osteoarthritis.
Rheumatoid arthritis.
Acute and subacute bursitis.
Acute gouty arthritis.
Epicondylitis.
Acute nonspecific tenosynovitis.
Post-traumatic osteoarthritis.
When the strength and dosage form of the drug lend the preparation to the treatment of the condition the *intralesional administration* of Betamethasone Sodium Phosphate Injection is indicated for: Keloids, localized hypertrophic, infiltrated, inflammatory lesions of: lichen planus, psoriatic plaques, granuloma annulare, and lichen simplex chronicus (neurodermatitis); discoid lupus erythematosus; necrobiosis lipoidica diabeticorum; alopecia areata.
Betamethasone Sodium Phosphate injection may also be useful in cystic tumors of an aponeurosis or tendon (ganglia).

CONTRAINDICATIONS
Betamethasone Sodium Phosphate injection is contraindicated in systemic fungal infections.

WARNINGS
In patients on corticosteroid therapy subjected to any unusual stress, increased dosage of rapidly acting corticosteroids before, during, and after the stressful situation is indicated.

Corticosteroids may mask some signs of infection, and new infections may appear during their use. There may be decreased resistance and inability to localize infection when corticosteroids are used.
Prolonged use of corticosteroids may produce posterior subcapsular cataracts, glaucoma with possible damage to the optic nerves, and may enhance the establishment of secondary ocular infections due to fungi or viruses.
Average and large doses of cortisone or hydrocortisone can cause elevation of blood pressure, salt and water retention, and increased excretion of potassium. These effects are less likely to occur with the synthetic derivatives except when used in large doses. Dietary salt restriction and potassium supplementation may be necessary. All corticosteroids increase calcium excretion.
WHILE ON CORTICOSTEROID THERAPY, PATIENTS SHOULD NOT BE VACCINATED AGAINST SMALLPOX. OTHER IMMUNIZATION PROCEDURES SHOULD NOT BE UNDERTAKEN IN PATIENTS WHO ARE ON CORTICOSTEROIDS, ESPECIALLY IN HIGH DOSES, BECAUSE OF POSSIBLE HAZARDS OF NEUROLOGICAL COMPLICATIONS AND LACK OF ANTIBODY RESPONSE.
Children who are on immunosuppressant drugs are more susceptible to infections than healthy children. Chickenpox and measles, for example, can have a more serious or even fatal course in children on immunosuppressant corticosteroids. In such children, or in adults who have not had these diseases, particular care should be taken to avoid exposure. If exposed, therapy with varicella zoster immune globulin (VZIG) or pooled intravenous immunoglobulin (IVIG), as appropriate, may be indicated. If chickenpox develops, treatment with antiviral agents may be considered.
The use of Betamethasone Sodium Phosphate Injection in active tuberculosis should be restricted to those cases of fulminating or disseminated tuberculosis in which the corticosteroid is used for the management of the disease in conjunction with appropriate antituberculous regimen.
If corticosteroids are indicated in patients with latent tuberculosis or tuberculin reactivity, close observation is necessary as reactivation of the disease may occur. During prolonged corticosteroid therapy, these patients should receive chemoprophylaxis.
Because rare instances of anaphylactoid reactions have occurred in patients receiving parenteral corticosteroid therapy, appropriate precautionary measures should be taken prior to administration, especially when the patient has a history of allergy to any drug.

Usage in Pregnancy: Since adequate human reproduction studies have not been done with corticosteroids, the use of these drugs in pregnancy, nursing mothers, or women of childbearing potential requires that the possible benefits of the drug be weighted against the potential hazards to the mother and embryo or fetus. Infants born to mothers who have received substantial doses of corticosteroids during pregnancy should be carefully observed for signs of hypoadrenalism.

PRECAUTIONS
INFORMATION FOR PATIENTS
Patients who are on immunosuppressant doses of corticosteroids should be warned to avoid exposure to chickenpox or measles and, if exposed, to obtain medical advice.
Drug-induced secondary adrenocortical insufficiency may be minimized by gradual reduction of dosage. This type of relative insufficiency may persist for months after discontinuation of therapy; therefore, in any situation of stress occurring during that period, hormone therapy should be reinstituted. Since mineralocorticoid secretion may be impaired, salt and/or a mineralocorticoid should be administered concurrently.
There is an enhanced effect of corticosteroids in patients with hypothyroidism and in those with cirrhosis.
Corticosteroids should be used cautiously in patients with ocular herpes simplex for fear of corneal perforation.
The lowest possible dose of corticosteroid should be used to control the condition under treatment, and when reduction in dosage is possible, the reduction must be gradual.
Psychic derangements may appear when corticosteroids are used, ranging from euphoria, insomnia, mood swings, personality changes, and severe depression to frank psychotic manifestations. Also, existing emotional instability or psychotic tendencies may be aggravated by corticosteroids.
Aspirin should be used cautiously in conjunction with corticosteroids in hypoprothrombinemia.
Steroids should be used with caution in nonspecific ulcerative colitis, if there is a probability of impending perforation, abscess or other pyogenic infection, also in diverticulitis, fresh intestinal anastomoses, active or latent peptic ulcer, renal insufficiency, hypertension, osteoporosis, and myasthenia gravis. Growth and development of infants and children on prolonged corticosteroid therapy should be carefully followed.

The following additional precautions also apply for parenteral corticosteroids: Intra-articular injection of a corticosteroid may produce systemic as well as local effects.
Appropriate examination of any joint fluid present is necessary to exclude a septic process.
A marked increase in pain accompanied by local swelling, further restriction of joint motion, fever, and malaise are suggestive of septic arthritis. If this complication occurs and the diagnosis of sepsis is confirmed, appropriate antimicrobial therapy should be instituted.
Local injection of a steroid into a previously infected joint is to be avoided.
Corticosteroids should not be injected into unstable joints.

The slower rate of absorption by intramuscular administration should be recognized.

ADVERSE REACTIONS

Fluid and electrolyte disturbances: sodium retention; fluid retention; congestive heart failure in susceptible patients; potassium loss; hypokalemic alkalosis; hypertension.

Musculoskeletal: Muscle weakness; steroid myopathy; loss of muscle mass; osteoporosis; vertebral compression fractures; aseptic necrosis of femoral and humoral heads; pathologic fracture of long bones.

Gastrointestinal: Peptic ulcer with possible subsequent perforation and hemorrhage; pancreatitis; abdominal distention; ulcerative esophagitis.

Dermatologic: Impaired wound healing; thin fragile skin; petechiae and ecchymoses; facial erythema; increased sweating; may suppress reactions to skin tests.

Neurological: Convulsions; increased intracranial pressure with papilledema (pseudotumor cerebri) usually after treatment; vertigo; headache.

Endocrine: Menstrual irregularities; development of cushingoid state; suppression of growth in children; secondary adrenocortical and pituitary unresponsiveness, particularly in times of stress, as in trauma, surgery or illness; decreased carbohydrate tolerance; manifestations of latent diabetes mellitus; increased requirements for insulin or oral hypoglycemic agents in diabetics.

Ophthalmic: Posterior subcapsular cataracts; increased intraocular pressure; glaucoma; exophthalmos.

Metabolic: Negative nitrogen balance due to protein catabolism.

The following *additional* adverse reactions are also related to parenteral corticosteroid therapy: rare instances of blindness associated with intralesional therapy around the face and head; hyperpigmentation or hypopigmentation; subcutaneous and cutaneous atrophy; sterile abscess; postinjection flare (following intra-articular use); charcotlike arthropathy.

DOSAGE AND ADMINISTRATION

The initial dosage of parenterally administered Betamethasone may vary up to 9.0 mg per day depending on the specific disease entity being treated. In situations of less severity, lower doses will generally suffice while in selected patients higher initial doses may be required. Usually the parenteral dosage ranges are one-third to one-half the 12-hourly oral dose. However, in certain overwhelming, acute, life-threatening situations, administrations in dosages exceeding the usual dosages may be justified and may be in multiples of the oral dosages.

The initial dosage should be maintained or adjusted until a satisfactory response is noted. If after a reasonable period of time there is a lack of satisfactory clinical response, Betamethasone Sodium Phosphate injection should be discontinued and the patient transferred to other appropriate therapy. *It should be emphasized that dosage requirements are variable and must be individualized on the basis of the disease under treatment and the response of the patient.* After a favorable response is noted, the proper maintenance dosage should be determined by decreasing the initial drug dosage in small decrements at appropriate time intervals until the lowest dosage which will maintain an adequate clinical response is reached. It should be kept in mind that constant monitoring is needed in regard to drug dosage. Included in the situations which may make dosage adjustments necessary are changes in clinical status secondary to remissions or exacerbations in the disease process, the patient's individual drug responsiveness, and the effect of patient exposure to stressful situations not directly related to the disease entity under treatment; in this latter situation it may be necessary to increase dosage of Betamethasone Sodium Phosphate injection for a period of time consistent with the patient's condition. If after long-term therapy the drug is to be stopped, it is recommended that it be withdrawn gradually rather than abruptly.

Protect from freezing.
Protect from light.

J CODES
Up to 6 mg IV,OTH—J0700

HOW SUPPLIED
INJECTION: 3 MG/ML

BRAND/MANUFACTURER	NDC	SIZE	AWP
◆ BRAND			
CELESTONE PHOSPHATE: Schering	00085-0879-05	5 ml	$13.62

INJECTION: 4 MG/ML

AVERAGE UNIT PRICE (AVAILABLE SIZES)		GENERIC A-RATED AVERAGE PRICE (GAAP)	
GENERIC	$2.28	5 ml	$11.38

BRAND/MANUFACTURER	NDC	SIZE	AWP
◆ GENERICS			
Schein	00364-6751-53	5 ml	$8.33
Steris	00402-0217-05	5 ml	$8.33
Insource	58441-1118-05	5 ml	$8.76
Genl Inject	52584-0217-05	5 ml	$8.76
Hyrex	00314-6392-75	5 ml	$11.50
Goldline	00182-3009-62	5 ml	$13.50
SELESTOJECT: Mayrand	00259-0349-05	5 ml	$20.50

Betamethasone, Topical

DESCRIPTION
Betamethasone, Topical, is available as a cream, an ointment, a lotion, and a gel.

Each gm of cream contains:
Betamethasone Benzoate ....0.25 mg
or
Betamethasone Dipropionate ....0.64 mg (equivalent to 0.5 mg Betamethasone)

Each gm of ointment contains:
Betamethasone Dipropionate ....0.64 mg (equivalent to 0.5 mg Betamethasone)

Each gm of lotion contains:
Betamethasone Benzoate ....0.25 mg
or
2 Betamethasone Diproprionate ....0.64 mg (equivalent to 0.5 mg Betamethasone)

Each gm of gel contains:
Bethamethasone Benzoate ....0.25 mg
or
Betamethasone Dipropionate ....0.64 mg (equivalent to 0.5 mg Betamethasone)

Each gram of the 0.1% cream contains:
Betamethasone Valerate ....1.2 mg (equivalent to 1 mg Betamethasone).

Betamethasone, Topical, is a synthetic adrenocorticosteroid for dermatologic use. Betamethasone, an analog of prednisolone, has a high degree of corticosteroid activity and a slight degree of mineralocorticoid activity. Betanethesone benzoate is an active fluorinated corticosteroid, the 17-benzoate ester of Betamethasone, having the chemical formula 9-fluoro-11β, 17, 21-trihydroxy-16β-methylpregna-1, 4-diene-3, 20-dione 17-benzoate. Betamethasone dipropionate is the 17,21 dipropionate ester of Betamethasone. Betamethasone dipropionate is included in a class of compounds consisting primarily of synthetic corticosteroids for use topically as anti-inflammatory and antipruritic agents.

Chemically, Betamethasone dipropionate is 9-fluoro-11β, 17,21-trihydroxy-16β-methylpregna-1,4-diene-3,20- dione 17, 21-dipropionate, with the empirical formula $C_{28}H_{37}FO_7$, and a molecular weight of 504.6. Betamethasone valerate USP (Pregna-1, 4-diene-3, 20-dione, 9-fluoro-11, 21-dihydroxy-16-methyl-17-[(1-oxo-pentyl)oxy]-,(11β, 16β)- has a molecular formula of $C_{27}H_{37}FO_6$ and a molecular weight of 476.58 (CAS Registry Number 2152-44-5).

Betamethasone Dipropionate is a white to creamy white, odorless crystalline powder, insoluble in water.

Following is its chemical structure:

CLINICAL PHARMACOLOGY
The corticosteroids are a class of compounds comprising steroid hormones secreted by the adrenal cortex and their synthetic analogs. In pharmacologic doses, corticosteroids are used primarily for their anti-inflammatory and/or immunosuppressive effects.

Topical corticosterids, such as Betamethastone, are effective in the treatment of corticosteroid-responsive dermatoses primarily because of their anti-inflammatory, anti-pruritic, and vasoconstrictive actions. However, while the physiologic, pharmacologic, and clinical effects of the corticosteroids are well-known, the exact mechanisms of their actions in each disease are uncertain. However corticosteroids are thought to act by the induction of phospholipase A_2 inhibitory proteins, collectively called lipocortins. It is postulated that these proteins control the biosynthesis of potent mediators of inflammation, such as prostaglandins and leukotrienes, by inhibiting the release of their common precursor, arahidonic acid. Arachidonic acid is released from membrane phospholipids by phospholipase A_2. Various laboratory methods including vasoconstrictor assays, are used to compare and predict potencies and/or clinical efficacies of the topical corticosteroids. There is some evidence to suggest that a recognizable correlation exists between vasoconstrictor potency and therapeutic efficacy in man. Betamethasone has been shown to have topical (dermatologic) and systemic pharmacologic and metabolic effects characteristic of this class of drugs.

Pharmacokinetics: The extent of percutaneous absorption of topical corticosteroids is determined by many factors including the vehicle, the integrity of the epidermal barrier, and the use of occlusive dressings. (See *"Dosage and Administration"* section.)

Topical corticosteroids can be absorbed through normal intact skin. Inflammation and/or other disease processes in the skin may increase percutaneous absorption. Occlusive dressings substantially increase the percutaneous absorption of topical corticosteroids. Thus, occlusive dressings may be a valuable therapeutic adjunct for treatment of resistant dermatoses. Occlusive dressings with hydrocortisone for up to 24 hours have not been demonstrated to increase penetration; however, occlusion of hydrocortisone for 96 hours markedly enhances penetration. (See "Dosage and Administration" section.)

Once absorbed through the skin, topical corticosteroids enter pharmacokinetic pathways similar to systemically administered corticosteroids. Corticosteroids are bound to plasma proteins in varying degrees, are metabolized primarily in the liver and excreted by the kidneys. Some of the topical corticosteroids and their metabolites are also excreted into the bile. Betamethasone Dipropionate Cream was applied once daily at 7 grams per day for one week to diseased skin, in patients with psoriasis or atopic dermatitis, to study its effects on the hypothalamic-pituitary-adrenal (HPA) axis. The results suggested that the drug caused a slight lowering of adrenal corticosteroid secretion, although in no case did plasma cortisol levels go below the lower limit of the normal range.

Betamethasone Dipropionate Lotion was applied once daily at 7 mL per day for 21 days to diseased skin (in patients with scalp psoriasis), to study its effects on the hypothalamic-pituitary-adrenal (HPA) axis. In 2 out of 11 patients, the drug lowered plasma cortisol levels below normal limits. Adrenal depression in these patients was transient, and returned to normal within a week. In one of these patients, plasma cortisol levels returned to normal while treatment continued.

At 14 g per day, Betamethasone Dipropionate Ointment was shown to depress the plasma levels of adrenal cortical hormones following repeated application to diseased skin in patients with psoriasis. Adrenal depression in these patients was transient, and rapidly returned to normal upon cessation of treatment. At 7 g per day (3.5 g bid), Betamethasone Dipropionate Ointment was shown to cause inimal inhibition of the hypothalamic-pituitary-adrenal (HPA) axis when applied two times daily for two to three weeks, in normal patients and in patients with psoriasis and eczematous disorders.

With 6 to 7 g of Betamethasone Dipropionate Ointment applied once daily for 3 weeks, no significant inhibition of the HPA axis was observed in patients with psoriasis and atopic dermatitis, as measured by plasma cortisol and 24 hour urinary 17-hydroxycorticosteroid levels.

INDICATIONS AND USAGE

Topical corticosteroids are indicated for relief of the inflammatory and pruritic manifestations of corticosteroid-responsive dermatoses.

Betamethasone Dipropionate lotion or gel is intended for short-term treatment of the inflammatory and pruritic manifestations of moderate to severe corticosteroid-responsive dermatoses.

Treatment beyond two weeks is not recommended for Betamethasone Dipropionate lotion or gel. The total dosage should not exceed 50 mL per week of the lotion or 50 gm per week of the gel because of potential for the drug to suppress the hypothalamic-pituitary-adrenal axis.

UNLABELED USES

Betamethasone Diproprionate, Topical, is used alone or as an adjunct in the treatment of urticaria pigmentosa and skin hypopigmentation (vitiligo).

CONTRAINDICATIONS

Topical corticosteroid products are contraindicated in patients who are hypersensitive to corticosteroids or to any ingredient in the preparations.

Betamethasone Benzoate preparations are not for ophthalmic use.

PRECAUTIONS

General: Systemic absorption of topical corticosteroids can produce reversible hypothalamic-pituitary-adrenal (HPA) axis suppression with the potential for glucocorticosteroid insufficiency after withdrawal of treatment. Manifestations of Cushing's syndrome, hyperglycemia, and glucosuria can also be produced in some patients by systemic absorption of topical corticosteroids while on treatment. Betamethasone Dipropionate lotion has been shown to suppress the HPA axis at 7 mL per day.

Conditions which augment systemic absorption include the application of the more potent corticosteroids, use over large surface areas, prolonged use, and the addition of occlusive dressings. (See "Dosage and Administration" section.)

At 7 g per day (applied once dailyor as 3.5 g twice daily), Betanethasone Dipropionate gel was shown to cause inhibition of the HPA axis following application for one, two or three weeks to diseased skin in some patients with psoriasis or atopic dermatitis. These effects were reversible upon discontinuation of treatment.

Patients receiving a large dose of a potent topical steroid applied to a large surface area should be evaluated periodically for evidence of HPA axis suppression by using the urinary free cortisol and ACTH stimulation tests. Patients should not be treated with Betamethasone Dipropionate gel or lotion for more than 2 weeks at a time, and amounts greater than 50 g per week of the gel or 50 ml per week of the lotion should not be used because of the potential for the drug to suppress the HPA axis. If HPA axis suppression is noted, an attempt should be made to withdraw the drug, to reduce the frequency of application, or to substitute a less potent steroid.

Recovery of HPA axis function is generally prompt and complete upon discontinuation of the drug. Infrequently, signs and symptoms of steroid withdrawal or glucocorticoid insufficiency may occur, requiring supplemental systemic corticosteroids.

Children may absorb proportionally larger amounts of topical corticosteroids due to their larger skin surface to body mass ratio and thus be more susceptible to systemic toxicity. (See "Precautions—Pediatric Use".)

If irritation develops, topical corticosteroids should be discontinued and appropriate therapy instituted. Allergic contact dermatitis with corticosteroids is usually diagnosed by observing failure to heal rather than noting clinical exacerbation as with most topical products not containing corticosteroids. Such an observation should be corroborated with appropriate diagnostic patch testing.

In the presence of dermatological infections, the use of an appropriate antifungal or antibacterial agent should be instituted. If a favorable response does not occur promptly, the corticosteroid should be discontinued until the infection has been adequately controlled.

Betamethasone Dipropionate gel should not be used in the treatment of rosacea or perioral dermatitis, and it should not be used on the face, groin, or in the axillae.

Information for Patients: Patients using topical corticosteroids should receive the following information and instructions. This information is intended to aid in the safe and effective use of this medication. It is not a disclosure of all possible adverse or intended effects.

1. This medication is to be used as directed by the physician and should not be used longer than the prescribed time period. It is for external use only. Avoid contact with the eyes.

2. Patients should be advised not to use this medication for any disorder other than that for which it was prescribed.

3. The treated skin areas should not be bandaged or other wise covered or wrapped so as to be occlusive unless directed by the physician. (See "Dosage and Administration" section.)

4. Patients should report any sign of local adverse reactions.

5. Parents of pediatric patients should be advised not to use tight-fitting diapers or plastic pants on a child being treated in the diaper area, as these garments may constitute occlusive dressings.

Laboratory Tests: The following tests may be helpful in evaluating HPA axis suppression:
Urinary free cortisol test
ACTH stimulation test
Morning plasma-cortisol test

Carcinogenesis, Mutagenesis, and Impairment of Fertility: Long-term animal studies have not been performed to evaluate the carcinogenic potential or the effect on fertility of topically applied corticosteroids. Studies in rabbits, mice and rats using intramuscular doses up to 1.0, 33 and 2.0 mg/kg, respectively, resulted in dose related increases in fetal resorptions in the rabbits and mice.

Studies to determine mutagenicity with prednisolone and hydrocortisone have revealed negative results.

Pregnancy Category C: Corticosteroids are generally teratogenic in laboratory animals when administered systemically at relatively low dosage levels. The more potent corticosteroids have been shown to be teratogenic after dermal application in laboratory animals. Betamethasone Dipropionate has not been tested for teratogenicity by this route, however, it appears to be fairly well-absorbed percutaneously. Betamethasone Dipropionate has been shown to be teratogenic in rabbits when given by the intramuscular route at doses of 0.05 mg/kg. This dose is approximately 26 times the human topical dose of Betamethasone Dipropionate Gel assuming human percutaneous absorption of approximately 3% and the use in a 70 kg person of 7 g per day. The abnormalities observed included umbilical hernias, cephalocele and cleft palate. There are no adequate and well-controlled studies of the teratogenic effects of topically applied corticosteroids in pregnant women. Therefore, topical corticosteroids should be used during pregnancy only if the potential benefit justifies the potential risk to the fetus. Drugs of this class should not be used extensively on pregnant patients, in large amounts, or for prolonged periods of time.

Nursing Mothers: It is not known whether topical administration of corticosteroids can result in sufficient systemic absorption to produce detectable quantities in breast milk. Systemically administered corticosteroids appear in human milk and could suppress growth, interfere with endogenous corticosteroid production, or cause other untoward effects. Because many drugs are excreted in human milk, caution should be exercised when a topical corticosteroid is administered to a nursing woman. A decision should be made whether to discontinue nursing or to discontinue the drug, taking into account the importance of the drug to the mother.

Pediatric Use: Use of Betamethasone Dipropionate cream, ointment, and gel in children under 12 years is not recommended. The safety and efficacy of Betamethasone Dipropionate lotion when used in children under 12 years of age have not been established.

Pediatric patients may demonstrate greater susceptibility to topical corticosteroid-induced HPA axis suppression and Cushing's syndrome than mature patients because of a larger skin surface area to body weight ratio. They are also at greater risk of glucocorticoid insufficiency after withdrawal of treatment.

Hypothalamic-pituitary-adrenal (HPA) axis suppression Cushing's syndrome, and intracranial hypertension have been reported in children receiving topical corticosteroids. Manifestations of adrenal suppression in children include linear growth retardation, delayed weight gain, low plasma cortisol levels, and absence of response to ACTH stimulation. Manifestations of intracranial hypertension include bulging fontanelles, headaches, and bilateral papilledema. Administration of topical corticosteroids to children should be limited to the least amount compatible with an effective therapeutic regimen. Chronic corticosteroid therapy may interfere with the growth and development of children. Adverse effects, including striae, have been reported with inappropriate use of topical corticosteroids in infants and children.

ADVERSE REACTIONS

The only local adverse reaction reported to be possibly or probably related to treatment with Betamethasone Dipropionate cream during controlled clinical studies was stinging. It occurred in 0.4% of the 242 patients or subjects involved in the studies. The overall incidence of drug-related adverse reactions in the Betamethasone Dipropionate lotion clinical studies was 5%. The adverse reactions that were reported to be possibly or probably related to treatment with Betamethasone Dipropionate lotion during controlled clinical studies involving 327 patients or normal volunteers were as follows: folliculitis occurred in 2%, burning and acneiform papules each occurred in 1%, and hyperesthesia and irritation each occurred in less than 1% of patients. The local adverse reactions that were reported with Betamethasone Dipropionate ointment applied either once or twice a day during clinical studies are as follows: erythema, 3 per 767 patients; folliculitis, 2 per 767 patients; pruritus, 2 per 767 patients; vesiculation, 1 per 767 patients.

In controlled clinical trials, the total incidence of adverse events associated with the use of Betamethasone Dipropionate gel was 10%. These included stinging or burning in 6% of patients, dry skin in 4% of patients, and pruritus in 2% of patients. Less frequently reported adverse reactions were irritation, skin atrophy, telangiectasia, erythema, cracking/tightening of the skin, follicular rash, and allergic contact dermatitis.

The following local adverse reactions are reported infrequently when topical corticosteroids are used as recommended but may occur more frequently with the use of occlusive dressings. These reactions are listed in approximate decreasing order of occurrence: burning, itching, irritation, dryness, folliculitis, hypertrichosis, acneiform eruptions, hypopigmentation, perioral dermatitis, allergic contact dermatitis, maceration of the skin, secondary infection, skin atrophy, striae, miliaria. These reactions may occur more frequently with super-high potency corticosteroids, such as Betamethasone Dipropionate Gel: acneiform eruptions, hypopigmentation, perioral dermatitis, secondary infection, striae and miliaria.

Systemic absorption of topical corticosteroids has produced reversible hypothalamicpituitary-adrenal (HPA) axis suppression, manifestation of Cushing's syndrome, hyperglycemia and glucosuria in some patients.

OVERDOSAGE

Topically applied corticosteroids can be absorbed in sufficient amounts to produce systemic effects. (See "Precautions.")

DOSAGE AND ADMINISTRATION

Apply a thin film of Betanethasone Dipropionate cream or ointment to the affected skin areas once or twice daily. Treatment with either Betamethasone Dipropionate cream or ointment should be limited to 45 g per week.

Apply a few drops of Betamethasone Dipropionate lotion to the affected area once or twice daily and massage lightly until the lotion disappears. Treatment must be limited to 14 days, and amounts greater than 50 mL per week should not be used.

Apply a thin layer of Betamethasone Dipropionate gel to the affected skin once or twice daily and rub in gently and completely.

Betamethasone Dipropionate gel is a super-high potency topical corticosteroid; therefore, treatment should be limited to two weeks, and amounts greater than 50 g per week should not be used. *Betamethasone Dipropionate products should not be used with occlusive dressings.* Apply Betamethasone Benzoate cream, lotion, or gel to the affected area as thin film from two to four times daily depending on the severity of the condition.

Store between 15° and 30°C (59° and 86°F).

HOW SUPPLIED

BETAMETHASONE BENZOATE

CREAM: 0.025%

BRAND/MANUFACTURER	NDC	SIZE	AWP
○ **BRAND**			
UTICORT: Parke-Davis	00071-3027-15	60 gm	$36.72

GEL: 0.025%

BRAND/MANUFACTURER	NDC	SIZE	AWP
○ **BRAND**			
UTICORT: Parke-Davis	00071-3025-11	15 gm	$13.81
	00071-3025-15	60 gm	$36.72

BETAMETHASONE DIPROPIONATE

CREAM: 0.05%

AVERAGE UNIT PRICE (AVAILABLE SIZES)		GENERIC A-RATED AVERAGE PRICE (GAAP)	
BRAND	$1.01	15 gm	$6.77
GENERIC	$0.37	45 gm	$12.93
HCFA FUL (15 gm)	$0.23		
HCFA FUL (45 gm)	$0.15		

BRAND/MANUFACTURER	NDC	SIZE	AWP
◆ **BRAND**			
DIPROSONE: Schering	00085-0853-02	15 gm	$18.86
	00085-0853-03	45 gm	$34.61
◆ **GENERICS**			
Thames	49158-0213-20	15 gm	$4.30
Raway	00686-0055-15	15 gm	$4.50
Rugby	00536-5030-20	15 gm	$4.68
Moore,H.L.	00839-7049-47	15 gm	$5.12
Qualitest	00603-7728-74	15 gm	$5.31
BETANATE: Mason Dist	11845-0381-01	15 gm	$5.38
Taro	51672-1274-01	15 gm	$5.40
Schein	00364-7409-72	15 gm	$5.40
NMC	23317-0380-15	15 gm	$5.57
Major	00904-0766-36	15 gm	$5.65
Geneva	00781-7009-27	15 gm	$6.25
Fougera	00168-0055-15	15 gm	$6.25
Goldline	00182-5010-51	15 gm	$6.90
DEL-BETA: Del-Ray	00316-0175-15	15 gm	$9.34
MAXIVATE: Westwood-Squibb	00072-9410-15	15 gm	$13.37
ALPHATREX: Savage	00281-0055-15	15 gm	$14.44
Thames	49158-0213-27	45 gm	$8.60
Raway	00686-0055-46	45 gm	$8.95
Moore,H.L.	00839-7049-52	45 gm	$9.17
BETANATE: Mason Dist	11845-0381-01	45 gm	$9.62
Taro	51672-1274-06	45 gm	$9.90
Qualitest	00603-7728-83	45 gm	$10.08
Schein	00364-7409-80	45 gm	$10.20
NMC	23317-0380-45	45 gm	$10.43
Major	00904-0766-45	45 gm	$10.57
Rugby	00536-5030-26	45 gm	$10.71
Geneva	00781-7009-19	45 gm	$11.50
Fougera	00168-0055-46	45 gm	$12.29
Goldline	00182-5010-60	45 gm	$12.55
DEL-BETA: Del-Ray	00316-0175-45	45 gm	$17.45
ALPHATREX: Savage	00281-0055-46	45 gm	$26.30
MAXIVATE: Westwood-Squibb	00072-9410-45	45 gm	$28.61

CREAM: 0.05%

BRAND/MANUFACTURER	NDC	SIZE	AWP
○ **GENERICS**			
CMC-Cons	00223-4260-15	15 gm	$4.25
Allscrips	54569-1113-00	15 gm	$6.42
TELADAR: Dermol	50744-0108-15	15 gm	$6.72
Cheshire	55175-0365-05	15 gm	$7.00
DEL-BETA: Del-Ray	00316-0176-15	15 gm	$9.34
Southwood	58016-6338-01	15 gm	$10.12
CMC-Cons	00223-4260-45	45 gm	$7.50
TELADAR: Dermol	50744-0108-45	45 gm	$12.60
Allscrips	54569-2556-00	45 gm	$12.61
DEL-BETA: Del-Ray	00316-0176-45	45 gm	$17.45
CMC-Cons	00223-4260-60	60 gm	$17.50
Phys Total Care	54868-0973-01	450 gm	$5.60
Phys Total Care	54868-0973-02	1350 gm	$10.13

LOTION: 0.05%

AVERAGE UNIT PRICE (AVAILABLE SIZES)		GENERIC A-RATED AVERAGE PRICE (GAAP)	
BRAND	$0.96	20 ml	$4.98
GENERIC	$0.25	60 ml	$15.24
HCFA FUL (20 ml)	$0.32		
HCFA FUL (60 ml)	$0.19		

BRAND/MANUFACTURER	NDC	SIZE	AWP
◆ **BRAND**			
DIPROSONE: Schering	00085-0028-04	20 ml	$23.22
DIPROSONE: Schering	00085-0028-06	60 ml	$45.71
◆ **GENERICS**			
Thames	49158-0245-40	20 ml	$4.30
Clay-Park	45802-0021-97	20 ml	$4.32
NMC	23317-0382-20	20 ml	$5.64
Lemmon	00093-0302-60	20 ml	$5.65
Thames	49158-0245-32	60 ml	$9.50
Copley	38245-0611-12	60 ml	$10.00
Moore,H.L.	00839-7202-53	60 ml	$10.52
Clay-Park	45802-0021-46	60 ml	$10.80
Major	00904-0768-03	60 ml	$11.55
Rugby	00536-5038-61	60 ml	$11.56
NMC	23317-0382-60	60 ml	$11.75
Barre	00472-0708-02	60 ml	$11.75
Geneva	00781-7041-61	60 ml	$11.88
Schein	00364-2102-58	60 ml	$13.80
Fougera	00168-0057-60	60 ml	$14.12
Goldline	00182-1787-68	60 ml	$14.25
Lemmon	00093-0302-39	60 ml	$14.35
ALPHATREX: Savage	00281-0057-60	60 ml	$33.43
MAXIVATE: Westwood-Squibb	00072-9490-60	60 ml	$39.34

LOTION: 0.05%

BRAND/MANUFACTURER	NDC	SIZE	AWP
○ **GENERICS**			
Raway	00686-0057-60	60 ml	$10.30

◆ RATED THERAPEUTICALLY EQUIVALENT; ◇ THERAPEUTIC EQUIVALENCE UNCONFIRMED; ○ UNRATED

BRAND/MANUFACTURER	NDC	SIZE	AWP
Cheshire	55175-2796-06	60 ml	$10.73
*DEL-BETA: Del-Ray	00316-0177-02	60 ml	$12.15
Allscrips	54569-1556-00	60 ml	$14.77
Southwood	58016-3246-01	60 ml	$19.11

OINTMENT: 0.05%

AVERAGE UNIT PRICE (AVAILABLE SIZES)		GENERIC A-RATED AVERAGE PRICE (GAAP)	
BRAND	$1.01	15 gm	$7.60
GENERIC	$0.54	45 gm	$14.52
HCFA FUL (15 gm)	$0.38		
HCFA FUL (45 gm)	$0.23		

BRAND/MANUFACTURER	NDC	SIZE	AWP
◆ BRAND			
DIPROSONE: Schering	00085-0510-04	15 gm	$18.86
	00085-0510-06	45 gm	$34.61
◆ GENERICS			
Goldline	00182-5011-60	5 gm	$12.55
Raway	00686-0056-15	15 gm	$4.50
Rugby	00536-5034-20	15 gm	$4.69
NMC	23317-0381-15	15 gm	$5.57
Major	00904-0767-36	15 gm	$5.65
Moore,H.L.	00839-7110-47	15 gm	$5.74
Fougera	00168-0056-15	15 gm	$6.82
MAXIVATE: Westwood-Squibb	00072-9450-15	15 gm	$13.37
ALPHATREX: Savage	00281-0056-15	15 gm	$14.44
Rugby	00536-5034-26	45 gm	$8.56
Raway	00686-0056-46	45 gm	$8.95
Moore,H.L.	00839-7110-52	45 gm	$9.44
NMC	23317-0381-45	45 gm	$10.43
Major	00904-0767-45	45 gm	$10.45
Fougera	00168-0056-46	45 gm	$13.42
ALPHATREX: Savage	00281-0056-46	45 gm	$26.30
MAXIVATE: Westwood-Squibb	00072-9450-45	45 gm	$28.61

OINTMENT: 0.05%

BRAND/MANUFACTURER	NDC	SIZE	AWP
○ GENERICS			
CMC-Cons	00223-4261-15	15 gm	$3.75
Allscrips	54569-1114-00	15 gm	$8.22
CMC-Cons	00223-4261-45	45 gm	$7.50
Allscrips	54569-2613-00	45 gm	$15.26

SPRAY: 0.1%

BRAND/MANUFACTURER	NDC	SIZE	AWP
○ BRAND			
DIPROSONE: Schering	00085-0475-06	85 ml	$18.86

For additional alternatives, turn to the section beginning on page 2859.

Betapace SEE SOTALOL HYDROCHLORIDE

Betaseron SEE INTERFERON BETA-1B

Betaxolol Hydrochloride, Ophthalmic

DESCRIPTION

Betaxolol Hydrochloride a cardioselective beta-adrenergic receptor blocking agent in a sterile isotonic solution or a sterile resin suspension. Betaxolol Hydrochloride is a white, crystalline powder, soluble in water, with a molecular weight of 343.89. The chemical structure is presented below:

Empirical Formula: $C_{18}H_{29}NO_3 \cdot HCl$

Chemical Name:
(±)-1-[p-[2-(Cyclopropylmethoxy)ethyl]phenoxy]-3-(isopropylamino)-2- propanol hydrochloride.

Each mL of Betaxolol Hydrochloride ophthalmic solution contains: Active: 5.6 mg Betaxolol Hydrochloride equivalent to Betaxolol base 5 mg; each mL of Betaxolol Hydrochloride Ophthalmic Suspension contains: Active: Betaxolol Hydrochloride 2.8 mg equivalent to 2.5 mg of Betaxolol base. Preservative: Benzalkonium Chloride 0.01%.

Following is its chemical structure:

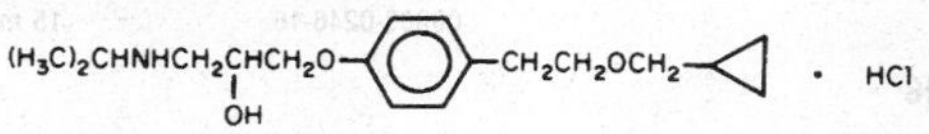

CLINICAL PHARMACOLOGY

Betaxolol Hydrochloride a cardioselective (beta-1-adrenergic) receptor blocking agent, does not have significant membrane-stabilizing (local anesthetic) activity and is devoid of intrinsic sympathomimetic action. Orally administered beta-adrenergic blocking agents reduce cardiac output in healthy subjects and patients with heart disease. In patients with severe impairment of myocardial function, beta-adrenergic receptor antagonists may inhibit the sympathetic stimulatory effect necessary to maintain adequate cardiac function.

When instilled in the eye Betaxolol Hydrochloride has the action of reducing elevated as well as normal intraocular pressure, whether or not accompanied by glaucoma. Ophthalmic Betaxolol Hydrochloride has minimal effect on pulmonary and cardiovascular parameters.

Ophthalmic Betaxolol Hydrochloride (one drop in each eye) was compared to timolol and placebo in a three-way crossover study challenging nine patients with reactive airway disease who were selected on the basis of having at least a 15% reduction in the forced expiratory volume in one second (FEV_1) after administration of ophthalmic timolol. Betaxolol Hydrochloride had no significant effect on pulmonary function as measured by FEV_1, Forced Vital Capacity (FVC) and FEV_1/FVC. Additionally, the action of isoproterenol, a beta stimulant, administered at the end of the study was not inhibited by ophthalmic Betaxolol Hydrochloride. In contrast, ophthalmic timolol significantly decreased these pulmonary functions.

FEV₁—PERCENT CHANGE FROM BASELINE[1]

	Means		
	Betaxolol 1.0%[a]	Timolol 0.5%	Placebo
Baseline	1.6	1.4	1.4
60 Minutes	2.3	-25.7*	5.8
120 Minutes	1.6	-27.4*	7.5
240 Minutes	-6.4	-26.9*	6.9
Isoproterenol[b]	36.1	-12.4*	42.8

[1] Schoene, R.B., et al., Am. J. Ophthal. 97:86, 1984.
[a] Twice the clinical concentration.
[b] Inhaled at 240 minutes; measurement at 270 minutes.
* Timolol statistically different from Betaxolol and placebo ($p < 0.05$).

No evidence of cardiovascular beta-adrenergic blockade during exercise was observed with Betaxolol Hydrochloride in a double-masked, three-way crossover study in 24 normal subjects comparing ophthalmic Betaxolol Hydrochloride, timolol and placebo for effect on blood pressure and heart rate. Mean arterial blood pressure was not affected by any treatment; however, ophthalmic timolol produced a significant decrease in the mean heart rate.

MEAN HEART RATES[1]

	Treatment		
Bruce Stress Exercise Test Minutes	Betaxolol 1%[a]	Timolol 0.5%	Placebo
0	79.2	79.3	81.2
2	130.2	126.0	130.4
4	133.4	128.0*	134.3
6	136.4	129.2*	137.9
8	139.8	131.8*	139.4
10	140.8	131.8*	141.3

[1] Atkins, J. M., et al., Am. J. Oph. 99:173-175, Feb., 1985.
[a] Twice the clinical concentration.
* Mean pulse rate significantly lower for timolol than Betaxolol Hydrochloride or placebo ($p < 0.05$).

Clinical Studies: Optic nerve head damage and visual field loss are the result of a sustained elevated intraocular pressure and poor ocular perfusion Betaxolol Hydrochloride ophthalmic solution and suspension have the action of reducing elevated as well as normal intraocular pressure, and the mechanism of ocular hypotensive action appears to be a reduction of aqueous production as demonstrated by tonography and aqueous fluorophotometry. The onset of action with Betaxolol Hydrochloride can generally be noted within 30 minutes and the maximal effect can usually be detected 2 hours after topical administration. A single dose provides a 12-hour reduction in intraocular pressure. Clinical observation of glaucoma patients treated with Betaxolol Hydrochloride ophthalmic solution for up to three years shows that the intraocular pressure lowering effect is well maintained.

In controlled, double-masked studies, the magnitude and duration of the ocular hypotensive effect of Betaxolol Hydrochloride ophthalmic suspension and Betaxolol Hydrochloride ophthalmic solution were clinically equivalent. Betaxolol Hydrochloride suspension was significantly more comfortable than Betaxolol Hydrochloride solution.

Clinical studies show that topical Betaxolol Hydrochloride ophthalmic solution reduces mean intraocular pressure 25% from baseline. In trials using 22 mmHg as a generally accepted index of intraocular pressure control, Betaxolol Hydrochloride ophthalmic solution was effective in more than 94% of the population studied, of which 73% were treated with the beta blocker alone. In controlled, double-masked studies, the magnitude and duration of the ocular hypotensive effect of Betaxolol Hydrochloride ophthalmic solution and ophthalmic timolol solution were clinically equivalent.

Betaxolol Hydrochloride ophthalmic solution has also been used successfully in glaucoma patients who have undergone a laser trabeculoplasty and have needed additional long-term ocular hypotensive therapy.

➤ SHOWN IN PRODUCT IDENTIFICATION GUIDE

Betaxolol Hydrochloride ophthalmic solution has been well tolerated in glaucoma patients wearing hard or soft contact lenses and in aphakic patients.

Betaxolol Hydrochloride ophthalmic solution does not produce miosis or accommodative spasm which are frequently seen with miotic agents. The blurred vision and night blindness often associated with standard miotic therapy are not associated with Betaxolol Hydrochloride ophthalmic solution. Thus, patients with central lenticular opacities avoid the visual impairment caused by a constricted pupil.

INDICATIONS AND USAGE

Betaxolol Hydrochloride has been shown to be effective in lowering intraocular pressure and is indicated in the treatment of ocular hypertension and chronic open-angle glaucoma. It may be used alone or in combination with other anti-glaucoma drugs.

In clinical studies Betaxolol Hydrochloride ophthalmic solution was safely used to lower intraocular pressure in 47 patients with both glaucoma and reactive airway disease who were followed for a mean period of 15 months. However, caution should be used in treating patients with severe reactive airway disease or a history of asthma.

CONTRAINDICATIONS

Hypersensitivity to any component of this product. Betaxolol Hydrochloride is contraindicated in patients with sinus bradycardia, greater than a first degree atrioventricular block, cardiogenic shock, or patients with overt cardiac failure.

WARNING

Topically applied beta-adrenergic blocking agents may be absorbed systemically. The same adverse reactions found with systemic administration of beta-adrenergic blocking agents may occur with topical administration. For example, severe respiratory reactions and cardiac reactions, including death due to bronchospasm in patients with asthma, and rarely death in association with cardiac failure, have been reported with topical application of beta-adrenergic blocking agents.

Betaxolol Hydrochloride has been shown to have a minor effect on heart rate and blood pressure in clinical studies. Caution should be used in treating patients with a history of cardiac failure or heart block. Treatment with Betaxolol Hydrochloride should be discontinued at the first signs of cardiac failure.

PRECAUTIONS

GENERAL

Information for Patients: Do not touch dropper tip to any surface as this may contaminate the contents. Do not use with contact lenses in eyes.

Diabetes Mellitus: Beta-adrenergic blocking agents should be administered with caution in patients subject to spontaneous hypoglycemia or to diabetic patients (especially those with labile diabetes) who are receiving insulin or oral hypoglycemic agents. Beta-adrenergic receptor blocking agents may mask the signs and symptoms of acute hypoglycemia.

Thyrotoxicosis: Beta-adrenergic blocking agents may mask certain clinical signs (e.g., tachycardia) of hyperthyroidism.

Patients suspected of developing thyrotoxicosis should be managed carefully to avoid abrupt withdrawal of beta-adrenergic blocking agents, which might precipitate a thyroid storm.

Muscle Weakness: Beta-adrenergic blockade has been reported to potentiate muscle weakness consistent with certain myasthenic symptoms (e.g., diplopia, ptosis, and generalized weakness).

Major Surgery: Consideration should be given to the gradual withdrawal of beta-adrenergic blocking agents prior to general anesthesia because of the reduced ability of the heart to respond to beta-adrenergically mediated sympathetic reflex stimuli.

Pulmonary: Caution should be exercised in the treatment of glaucoma patients with excessive restriction of pulmonary function. There have been reports of asthmatic attacks and pulmonary distress during Betaxolol Hydrochloride treatment. Although rechallenges of some such patients with ophthalmic Betaxolol Hydrochloride have not adversely affected pulmonary function test results, the possibility of adverse pulmonary effects in patients sensitive to beta blockers cannot be ruled out.

Risk from Anaphylactic Reaction: While taking beta-blockers, patients with a history of atopy or a history of severe anaphylactic reaction to a variety of allergens may be more reactive to repeated accidental, diagnostic, or therapeutic challenge with such allergens. Such patients may be unresponsive to the usual doses of epinephrine used to treat anaphylactic reactions.

DRUG INTERACTIONS

Patients who are receiving a beta-adrenergic blocking agent orally and Betaxolol Hydrochloride should be observed for a potential additive effect either on the intraocular pressure or on the known systemic effects of beta blockade.

Close observation of the patient is recommended when a beta-blocker is administered to patients receiving catecholamine-depleting drugs such as reserpine, because of possible additive effects and the production of hypotension and/or bradycardia.

Betaxolol Hydrochloride is an adrenergic blocking agent; therefore, caution should be exercised in patients using concomitant adrenergic psychotropic drugs.

Ocular: In patients with angle-closure glaucoma, the immediate treatment objective is to re-open the angle by constriction of the pupil with a miotic agent. Betaxolol Hydrochloride has little or no effect on the pupil. When Betaxolol Hydrochloride is used to reduce elevated intraocular pressure in angle-closure glaucoma, it should be used with a miotic and not alone.

CARCINOGENESIS, MUTAGENESIS, IMPAIRMENT OF FERTILITY

Life-time studies with Betaxolol Hydrochloride have been completed in mice at oral doses of 6, 20 or 60 mg/kg/day and in rats at 3, 12 or 48 mg/kg/day; Betaxolol Hydrochloride demonstrated no carcinogenic effect. Higher dose levels were not tested.

In a variety of *in vitro* and *in vivo* bacterial and mammalian cell assays, Betaxolol Hydrochloride was nonmutagenic.

Pregnancy: Pregnancy Category C: Reproduction, teratology, and peri- and postnatal studies have been conducted with orally administered Betaxolol Hydrochloride in rats and rabbits. There was evidence of drug related postimplantation loss in rabbits and rats at dose levels above 12 mg/kg and 128 mg/kg, respectively. Betaxolol Hydrochloride was not shown to be teratogenic, however, and there were no other adverse effects on reproduction at subtoxic dose levels. There are no adequate and well-controlled studies in pregnant women. Betaxolol Hydrochloride should be used during pregnancy only if the potential benefit justifies the potential risk to the fetus.

Nursing Mothers: It is not known whether Betaxolol Hydrochloride is excreted in human milk. Because many drugs are excreted in human milk, caution should be exercised when Betaxolol Hydrochloride is administered to nursing women.

Pediatric Use: Safety and effectiveness in children have not been established.

ADVERSE REACTIONS

The following adverse reactions have been reported in clinical trials with Betaxolol Hydrochloride ophthalmic solution.

Ocular: Discomfort of short duration was experienced by one in four patients, but none discontinued therapy; occasional tearing has been reported. Rare instances of decreased corneal sensitivity, erythema, itching sensation, corneal punctate staining, keratitis, anisocoria, edema, and photophobia have been reported.

Additional medical events reported with Betaxolol Hydrochloride ophthalmic suspension include blurred vision, foreign body sensation, dryness of the eyes, inflammation, discharge, ocular pain, decreased acuity, and crustly lashes.

Systemic: Systemic reactions following administration of Betaxolol Hydrochloride ophthalmic solution or Betaxolol Hydrochloride ophthalmic suspension have been rarely reported. These include:

Cardiovascular: Bradycardia, heart block and congestive failure.

Pulmonary: Pulmonary distress characterized by dyspnea, bronchospasm, thickened bronchial secretions, asthma and respiratory failure.

Central Nervous System: Insomnia, dizziness, vertigo, headaches, depression, lethargy, and increase in signs and symptoms of myasthenia gravis.

Other: Hives, toxic epidermal necrolysis, hair loss and glossitis.

OVERDOSAGE

No information is available on overdosage of humans. The oral LD_{50} of the drug ranged from 350-920 mg/kg in mice and 860-1050 mg/kg in rats. The symptoms which might be expected with an overdose of a systemically administered beta-1-adrenergic receptor blocker agent are bradycardia, hypotension and acute cardiac failure. A topical overdose of Betaxolol Hydrochloride may be flushed from the eye(s) with warm tap water.

DOSAGE AND ADMINISTRATION

The recommended dose is one to two drops of Betaxolol Hydrochloride in the affected eye(s) twice daily. In some patients, the intraocular pressure lowering responses to Betaxolol Hydrochloride may require a few weeks to stabilize. As with any new medication, careful monitoring of patients is advised.

If the intraocular pressure of the patient is not adequately controlled on this regimen, concomitant therapy with pilocarpine and other miotics, and/or epinephrine and/or carbonic anhydrase inhibitors can be instituted.

Store at room temperature; store suspension upright and shake well before using.

HOW SUPPLIED
DROP: 0.25%

BRAND/MANUFACTURER	NDC	SIZE	AWP
○ **BRAND**			
BETOPTIC S: Alcon Labs	00065-0246-20	2.5 ml	$9.63
	00065-0246-05	5 ml	$18.38
	00065-0246-10	10 ml	$35.00
	00065-0246-15	15 ml	$51.63

DROP: 0.5%

BRAND/MANUFACTURER	NDC	SIZE	AWP
○ **BRAND**			
BETOPTIC: Alcon Labs	00065-0245-20	2.5 ml ud	$9.63
	00065-0245-05	5 ml	$18.38
	00065-0245-10	10 ml	$35.00
	00065-0245-15	15 ml	$51.63

◆ RATED THERAPEUTICALLY EQUIVALENT; ◇ THERAPEUTIC EQUIVALENCE UNCONFIRMED; ○ UNRATED

Betaxolol Hydrochloride, Oral

DESCRIPTION

Betaxolol Hydrochloride is a β_1-selective (cardioselective) adrenergic receptor blocking agent available as 10-mg and 20-mg tablets for oral administration. Betaxolol Hydrochloride is chemically described as 2-propanol, 1-[4-[2-(cyclopropyl-methoxy)ethyl]phenoxy]-3-[(1-methylethyl)amino]-, hydrochloride, ($\pm$).

Betaxolol Hydrochloride is a water-soluble white crystalline powder with a molecular formula of $C_{18}H_{29}NO_3.HCl$ and a molecular weight of 343.9. It is freely soluble in water, ethanol, chloroform, and methanol, and has a pKa of 9.4.

Following is its chemical structure:

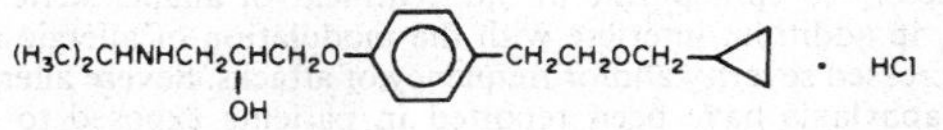

CLINICAL PHARMACOLOGY

Betaxolol Hydrochloride is a β_1-selective (cardioselective) adrenergic receptor blocking agent that has week membrane-stabilizing activity and no intrinsic sympathomimetic (partial agonist) activity. The preferential effect on β_1 receptors is not absolute, however, and some inhibitory effects on β_2 receptors (found chiefly in the bronchial and vascular musculature) can be expected at higher doses.

Pharmacokinetics and metabolism: In man, absorption of an oral dose is complete. There is a small and consistent first-pass effect resulting in an absolute bioavailability of 89% $\pm$ 5% that is unaffected by the concomitant ingestion of food or alcohol. Mean peak blood concentrations of 21.6 ng/mL (range 16.3 to 27.9 ng/mL) are reached between 1.5 and 6 (mean about 3) hours after a single oral dose, in healthy volunteers, of 10 mg of Betaxolol Hydrochloride Peak concentrations for 20-mg and 40-mg doses are 2 and 4 times that of a 10-mg dose and have been shown to be linear over the dose range of 5 to 40 mg. The peak to trough ratio of plasma concentrations over 24 hours is 2.7. The mean elimination half-life in various studies in normal volunteers ranged from about 14 to 22 hours after single oral doses and is similar in chronic dosing. Steady state plasma concentrations are attained after 5 to 7 days with once-daily dosing in persons with normal renal function.

Betaxolol Hydrochloride is approximately 50% bound to plasma proteins. It is eliminated primarily by liver metabolism and secondarily by renal excretion. Following oral administration, greater than 80% of a dose is recovered in the urine as Betaxolol Hydrochloride and its metabolites. Approximately 15% of the dose administered is excreted as unchanged drug, the remainder being metabolites whose contribution to the clinical effect is negligible.

Steady state studies in normal volunteers and hypertensive patients found no important differences in kinetics. In patients with hepatic disease, elimination half-life was prolonged by about 33%, but clearance was unchanged, leading to little change in AUC. Dosage reductions have not routinely been necessary in these patients. In patients with chronic renal failure undergoing dialysis, mean elimination half-life was approximately doubled, as was AUC, indicating the need for a lower initial dosage (5 mg) in these patients. The clearance of Betaxolol Hydrochloride by hemodialysis was 0.015 L/h/kg and by peritoneal dialysis, 0.010 L/h/kg. In one study patients (n = 8) with stable renal failure, not on dialysis, with mean creatinine clearance of 27 ml/min showed slight increases in elimination half-life and AUC, but no change in C_{max}. In a second study of 30 hypertensive patients with mild to severe renal impairment, there was a reduction in clearance of Betaxolol Hydrochloride with increasing degrees of renal insufficiency. Inulin clearance (mL/min/1.73 m^2) ranged from 70 to 107 in 7 patients with mild impairment, 41 to 69 in 14 patients with moderate impairment, and 8 to 37 in 9 patients with severe impairment. Clearance following oral dosing was reduced significantly in patients with moderate and severe renal impairment (26% and 35%, respectively) when compared with those with mildly impaired renal function. In the severely impaired group, the mean C_{max} and the mean elimination half-life tended to increase (28% and 24%, respectively) when compared with the mildly impaired group. A starting dose of 5 mg is recommended in patients with severe renal impairment. (See *"Dosage and Administration."*)

Studies in elderly patients (n = 10) gave inconsistent results but suggest some impairment of elimination, with one small study (n = 4) finding a mean half-life of 30 hours. A starting dose of 5 mg is suggested in older patients.

Pharmacodynamics: Clinical pharmacology studies have demonstrated the beta-adrenergic receptor blocking activity of Betaxolol Hydrochloride by (1) reduction in resting and exercise heart rate, cardiac output, and cardiac work load, (2) reduction of systolic and diastolic blood pressure at rest and during exercise, (3) inhibition of isoproterenol-induced tachycardia, and (4) reduction of reflex orthostatic tachycardia.

The β_1 selectivity of Betaxolol Hydrochloride in man was shown in three ways: (1) In normal subjects, 10- and 40-mg oral doses of Betaxolol Hydrochloride, which reduced resting heart rate at least as much as 40 mg of propranolol, produced less inhibition of isoproterenol-induced increases in forearm blood flow and finger tremor than propranolol. In this study, 10 mg of Betaxolol Hydrochloride was at least comparable to 50 mg of atenolol. Both doses of Betaxolol Hydrochloride, and the one dose of atenolol, however, had more effect on the isoproterenol-induced changes than placebo (indicating some β_2 effect at clinical

doses) and the higher dose of Betaxolol Hydrochloride, was more inhibitory than the lower. (2) In normal subjects, single intravenous doses of Betaxolol Hydrochloride and propranolol, which produced equal effects on exercise-induced tachycardia, had differing effects on insulin-induced hypoglycemia, with propranolol, but not Betaxolol Hydrochloride, prolonging the hypoglycemia compared with placebo. Neither drug affected the maximum extent of the hypoglycemic response. (3) In a single-blind crossover study in asthmatics (n = 10), intravenous infusion over 30 minutes of low doses of Betaxolol Hydrochloride (1.5 mg) and propranolol (2 mg) had similar effects on resting heart rate but had differing effects on FEV_1 and forced vital capacity, with propranolol causing statistically significant (10% to 20%) reductions from baseline in mean values for both parameters while Betaxolol Hydrochloride had no effect on mean values. While blood levels were not measured, the dose of Betaxolol Hydrochloride used in this study would be expected to produce blood concentrations, at the time of the pulmonary function studies, considerably lower than those achieved during antihypertensive therapy with recommended doses of Betaxolol Hydrochloride. In a randomized double-blind, placebo-controlled crossover (4 × 4 Latin Square) study in 10 asthmatics Betaxolol Hydrochloride (about 5 or 10 mg IV) had little effect on isoproterenol-induced increases in FEV_1; in contrast, propranolol (about 7 mg IV) inhibited the response.

Consistent with its negative chronotropic effect, due to betablockade of the SA node, and lack of intrinsic sympathomimetic activity, Betaxolol Hydrochloride increases sinus cycle length and sinus node recovery time. Conduction in the AV node is also prolonged.

Significant reductions in blood pressure and heart rate were observed 24 hours after dosing in double-blind, placebo-controlled trials with doses of 5 to 40 mg administered once daily. The antihypertensive response to Betaxolol Hydrochloride was similar at peak blood levels (3 to 4 hours) and at trough (24 hours). In a large randomized, parallel dose-response study of 5, 10, and 20 mg, the antihypertensive effects of the 5-mg dose were roughly half of the effects of the 20-mg dose (after adjustment for placebo effects) and the 10-mg dose gave more than 80% of the antihypertensive response to the 20-mg dose. The effect of increasing the dose from 10 mg to 20 mg was thus small. In this study, while the antihypertensive response to Betaxolol Hydrochloride showed a dose-response relationship, the heart rate response (reduction in HR) was not dose related. In other trials, there was little evidence of a greater antihypertensive response to 40 mg than to 20 mg. The maximum effect of each dose was achieved within 1 or 2 weeks. In comparative trials against propranolol, atenolol, and chlorthalidone Betaxolol Hydrochloride appeared to be at least as effective as the comparative agent.

Betaxolol Hydrochloride is studied in combination with thiazide-type diuretics and the blood pressure effects of the combination appear additive. Betaxolol Hydrochloride has also been used concurrently with methyldopa, hydralazine, and prazosin.

The mechanism of the antihypertensive effects of beta-adrenergic receptor blocking agents has not been established. Several possible mechanisms have been proposed, however, including: (1) competitive antagonism of catecholamines at peripheral (especially cardiac) adrenergic-neuronal sites, leading to decreased cardiac output, (2) a central effect leading to reduced sympathetic outflow to the periphery, and (3) suppression of renin activity.

The results from long-term studies have not shown any diminution of the antihypertensive effect of Betaxolol Hydrochloride with prolonged use.

INDICATIONS AND USAGE

Betaxolol Hydrochloride is indicated in the management of hypertension. It may be used alone or concomitantly with other antihypertensive agents, particularly thiazide-type diuretics.

UNLABELED USES

Betaxolol Hydrochloride is used alone or as an adjunct in the treatment of angina pectoris.

CONTRAINDICATIONS

Betaxolol Hydrochloride is contraindicated in patients with known hypersensitivity to the drug.

Betaxolol Hydrochloride is contraindicated in patients with sinus bradycardia, heart block greater than first degree, cardiogenic shock, and overt cardiac failure (see *"Warnings"*).

WARNINGS

Cardiac Failure: Sympathetic stimulation may be a vital component supporting circulatory function in congestive heart failure, and beta-adrenergic receptor blockade carries the potential hazard of further depressing myocardial contractility and precipitating more severe heart failure. In hypertensive patients who have congestive heart failure controlled by digitalis and diuretics, beta-blockers should be administered cautiously. Both digitalis and beta-adrenergic receptor blocking agents slow AV conduction.

In Patients without a History of Cardiac Failure: Continued depression of the myocardium with beta-blocking agents over a period of time can, in some cases, lead to cardiac failure. Therefore, at the first sign or symptom of cardiac failure, discontinuation of Betaxolol Hydrochloride should be considered. In some cases beta-blocker therapy can be continued while cardiac failure is treated with cardiac glycosides, diuretics, and other agents, as appropriate.

Exacerbation of Angina Pectoris upon Withdrawal: Abrupt cessation of therapy with certain beta-blocking agents in patients with coronary artery disease has been followed by exacerbations of angina pectoris and, in some cases, myocardial infarction has been reported. Therefore, such patients should be warned against interruption of therapy without the physician's advice. Even in the absence of overt angina pectoris, when discontinuation of Betaxolol Hydrochloride is planned, the patient should be carefully observed and therapy should be reinstituted, at least temporarily, if withdrawal symptoms occur.

Bronchospastic Diseases: **PATIENTS WITH BRONCHOSPASTIC DISEASE SHOULD NOT IN GENERAL RECEIVE BETA-BLOCKERS. Because of its relative β_1 selectivity (cardioselectivity), low doses of Betaxolol Hydrochloride may be used with caution in patients with bronchospastic disease who do not respond to or cannot tolerate alternative treatment. Since β_1 selectivity is not absolute and is inversely related to dose, the lowest possible dose of Betaxolol Hydrochloride should be used (5 to 10 mg once daily) and a bronchodilator should be made available. If dosage must be increased, divided dosage should be considered to avoid the higher peak blood levels associated with once-daily dosing.**

Anesthesia and Major Surgery: The necessity, or desirability, of withdrawal of a beta-blocking therapy prior to major surgery is controversial. Beta-adrenergic receptor blockade impairs the ability of the heart to respond to beta-adrenergically mediated reflex stimuli. While this might be of benefit in preventing arrhythmic response, the risk of excessive myocardial depression during general anesthesia may be increased and difficulty in restarting and maintaining the heart beat has been reported with beta-blockers. If treatment is continued, particular care should be taken when using anesthetic agents which depress the myocardium, such as ether, cyclopropane, and trichloroethylene, and it is prudent to use the lowest possible dose of Betaxolol Hydrochloride. Betaxolol Hydrochloride, like other beta-blockers, is a competitive inhibitor of beta-receptor agonists and its effect on the heart can be reversed by cautious administration of such agents (eg, dobutamine or isoproterenol—see *"Overdosage"*). Manifestations of excessive vagaltone (eg, profound bradycardia, hypotension) may be corrected with atropine 1 to 3 mg IV in divided doses.

Diabetes and Hypoglycemia: Beta-blockers should be used with caution in diabetic patients. Beta-blockers may mask tachycardia occurring with hypoglycemia (patients should be warned of this), although other manifestations such as dizziness and sweating may not be significantly affected. Unlike nonselective beta-blockers, Betaxolol Hydrochloride does not prolong insulin-induced hypoglycemia.

Thyrotoxicosis: Beta-adrenergic blockade may mask certain clinical signs of hyperthyroidism (eg, tachycardia). Abrupt withdrawal of beta-blockade might precipitate a thyroid storm; therefore, patients known or suspected of being thyrotoxic from whom Betaxolol Hydrochloride is to be withdrawn should be monitored closely (see *"Dosage and Administration: Cessation of Therapy"*).

PRECAUTIONS

General. Beta-adrenoceptor blockade can cause reduction of intraocular pressure. Since Betaxolol Hydrochloride is marketed as an ophthalmic solution for treatment of glaucoma, patients should be told that Betaxolol Hydrochloride may interfere with the glaucoma-screening test. Withdrawal may lead to a return of increased intraocular pressure. Patients receiving beta-adrenergic blocking agents orally and beta-blocking ophthalmic solutions should be observed for potential additive effects either on the intraocular pressure or on the known systemic effects of beta-blockade.

Impaired Hepatic or Renal Function. Betaxolol Hydrochloride is primarily metabolized in the liver to metabolites that are inactive and then excreted by the kidneys; clearance is somewhat reduced in patients with renal failure but little changed in patients with hepatic disease. Dosage reductions have not routinely been necessary when hepatic insufficiency is present (see *"Dosage and Administration"*) but patients should be observed. Patients with severe renal impairment and those on dialysis require a reduced dose. (See *"Dosage and Administration."*)

Information for Patients: Patients, especially those with evidence of coronary artery insufficiency, should be warned against interruption or discontinuation of Betaxolol Hydrochloride therapy without the physician's advice.

Although cardiac failure rarely occurs in appropriately selected patients, patients being treated with beta-adrenergic blocking agents should be advised to consult a physician at the first sign or symptom of failure.

Patients should know how they react to this medicine before they operate automobiles and machinery or engage in other tasks requiring alertness. Patients should contact their physician if any difficulty in breathing occurs, and before surgery of any type. Patients should inform their physicians or dentists that they are taking Betaxolol Hydrochloride. Patients with diabetes should be warned that beta-blockers may mask tachycardia occurring with hypoglycemia.

Drug Interactions: The following drugs have been coadministered with Betaxolol Hydrochloride and have not altered its pharmacokinetics: cimetidine, nifedipine, chlorthalidone, and hydrochlorothiazide. Concomitant administration of Betaxolol Hydrochloride with the oral anticoagulant warfarin has been shown not to potentiate the anticoagulant effect of warfarin.

Catecholamine-depleting drugs (eg, reserpine) may have an additive effect when given with beta-blocking agents. Patients treated with a beta-adrenergic receptor blocking agent plus a catecholamine depletor should therefore be closely observed for evidence of hypotension or marked bradycardia, which may produce vertigo, syncope, or postural hypotension.

Should it be decided to discontinue therapy in patients receiving beta-blockers and clonidine concurrently, the beta-blocker should be discontinued slowly over several days before the gradual withdrawal of clonidine.

Literature reports suggest that oral calcium antagonists may be used in combination with beta-adrenergic blocking agents when heart function is normal, but should be avoided in patients with impaired cardiac function. Hypotension, AV conduction disturbances, and left ventricular failure have been reported in some patients receiving beta-adrenergic blocking agents when an oral calcium antagonist was added to the treatment regimen. Hypotension was more likely to occur if the calcium antagonist were a dihydropyridine derivative, eg, nifedipine, while left ventricular failure and AV conduction disturbances, including complete heart block, were more likely to occur with either verapamil or diltiazem.

Risk of Anaphylactic Reaction: Although it is known that patients on beta-blockers may be refractory to epinephrine in the treatment of anaphylactic shock, beta-blockers can, in addition, interfere with the modulation of allergic reaction and lead to an increased severity and/or frequency of attacks. Severe allergic reactions including anaphylaxis have been reported in patients exposed to a variety of allergens either by repeated challenge, or accidental contact, and with diagnostic or therapeutic agents while receiving beta-blockers. Such patients may be unresponsive to the usual doses of epinephrine used to treat allergic reaction.

Carcinogenesis, Mutagenesis, Impairment of Fertility. Lifetime studies with Betaxolol Hydrochloride in mice at oral dosages of 6, 20, and 60 mg/kg/day (up to 90 × the maximum recommended human dose [MRHD] based on 60-kg body weight) and in rats at 3, 12, or 48 mg/kg/day (up to 72 × MRHD) showed no evidence of a carcinogenic effect. In a variety of *in vitro* and *in vivo* bacterial and mammalian cell assays, Betaxolol Hydrochloride was nonmutagenic. Betaxolol Hydrochloride did not adversely affect fertility or mating performance of male or female rats at doses up to 256 mg/kg/day (380 × MRHD).

Pregnancy: Pregnancy Category C. In a study in which pregnant rats received Betaxolol Hydrochloride at doses of 4, 40, or 400 mg/kg/day, the highest dose (600 × MRHD) was associated with increased postimplantation loss, reduced litter size and weight, and an increased incidence of skeletal and visceral abnormalities, which may have been a consequence of drug-related maternal toxicity. Other than a possible increased incidence of incomplete descent of testes and sternebral reductions, Betaxolol Hydrochloride at 4 mg/kg/day and 40 mg/kg/day (6 × MRHD and 60 × MRHD) caused no fetal abnormalities. In a second study with a different strain of rat, 200 mg Betaxolol Hydrochloride/kg/day (300 × MRHD) was associated with maternal toxicity and an increase in resorptions, but no teratogenicity. In a study in which pregnant rabbits received doses of 1, 4, 12, or 36 mg Betaxolol Hydrochloride/kg/day (54 × MRHD), a marked increase in postimplantation loss occurred at the highest dose, but no drug-related teratogenicity was observed. The rabbit is more sensitive to Betaxolol Hydrochloride than other species because of higher bioavailability resulting from saturation of the first-pass effect. In a peri- and postnatal study in rats at doses of 4, 32, and 256 mg Betaxolol Hydrochloride/kg/day (380 × MRHD), the highest dose was associated with a marked increase in total litter loss within 4 days postpartum. In surviving offspring, growth and development were also affected.

There are no adequate and well-controlled studies in pregnant women Betaxolol Hydrochloride should be used during pregnancy only if the potential benefit justifies the potential risk to the fetus.

Nursing Mothers: Since Betaxolol Hydrochloride is excreted in human milk in sufficient amounts to have pharmacological effects in the infant, caution should be exercised when Betaxolol Hydrochloride is administered to a nursing mother.

Pediatric Use: Safety and efficacy in children have not been established.

Elderly Patients: Betaxolol Hydrochloride may produce bradycardia more frequently in elderly patients. In general, patients 65 years of age and older had a higher incidence rate of bradycardia (heart rate < 50 BPM) than younger patients in U.S. clinical trials. In a double-blind study in Europe, 19 elderly patients (mean age = 82) received Betaxolol Hydrochloride 20 mg daily. Dosage reduction to 10 mg or discontinuation was required for 6 patients due to bradycardia (see *"Dosage and Administration"*).

ADVERSE REACTIONS

Most adverse reactions have been mild and transient and are typical of beta-adrenergic blocking agents, eg, bradycardia, fatigue, dyspnea, and lethargy. Withdrawal of therapy in U.S. and European controlled clinical trials has been necessary in about 3.5% of patients, principally because of bradycardia, fatigue, dizziness, headache, and impotence. Frequency estimates of adverse events were derived from controlled studies in which adverse reactions were volunteered and elicited in U.S. studies and volunteered and/or elicited in European studies.

In the U.S. the placebo-controlled hypertension studies lasted for 4 weeks, while the active-controlled hypertension studies had a 22- to 24-week double-blind phase. The following doses were studied: Betaxolol Hydrochloride—5, 10, 20, and 40 mg once daily; atenolol—25, 50, and 100 mg once daily; and propranolol—40, 80, and 160 mg b.i.d.

Betaxolol Hydrochloride like other beta-blockers, has been associated with the development of antinuclear antibodies (ANA). In controlled clinical studies, conversion of ANA from negative to positive occurred in 5.3% of the patients treated with Betaxolol Hydrochloride, 6.3% of the patients treated with atenolol, 4.9% of the patients treated with propranolol, and 3.2% of the patients treated with placebo.

Betaxolol Hydrochloride adverse events reported with a 2% or greater frequency, and selected events with lower frequency, in U.S. controlled studies are: (See related table).

Of the above adverse reactions [listed in Table 1] associated with the use of Betaxolol Hydrochloride, only bradycardia was clearly dose related, but there was a suggestion of dose relatedness for fatigue, lethargy, and dyspepsia.

In Europe, the placebo-controlled study lasted for 4 weeks, while the comparative studies had a 4- to 52-week double-blind phase. The following doses were studied: Betaxolol Hydrochloride 20 and 40 mg once daily and atenolol 100 mg once daily. From European controlled hypertension clinical trials, the following adverse events reported by 2% or more patients and selected events with lower frequency are presented:

Table 2

Dose Range	Betaxolol (N = 155) 20-40 mg q.d.	Atenolol (N = 81) 100 mg q.d.	Placebo (N = 60)
Body System/ Adverse Reaction	(%)	(%)	(%)
Cardiovascular			
Bradycardia (heart rate < 50 BPM)	5.8	5.0	0
Symptomatic bradycardia	1.9	2.5	0
Palpitation	1.9	3.7	1.7
Edema	1.3	1.2	0
Cold extremities	1.9	0	0
Central Nervous System			
Headache	14.8	9.9	23.3
Dizziness	14.8	17.3	15.0
Fatigue	9.7	18.5	0
Asthenia	7.1	0	16.7
Insomnia	5.0	3.7	3.3
Paresthesia	1.9	2.5	0
Gastrointestinal			
Nausea	5.8	1.2	0
Dyspepsia	3.9	7.4	3.3
Diarrhea	1.9	3.7	0
Musculoskeletal			
Chest pain	7.1	6.2	5.0
Joint pain	5.2	4.9	1.7
Myalgia	3.2	3.7	3.3

The only adverse event whose frequency clearly rose with increasing dose was bradycardia. Elderly patients were especially susceptible to bradycardia, which in some cases responded to dose-reduction (see "Precautions").

Table 1

Dose Range Body System/ Adverse Reaction	Betaxolol (N = 509) 5-40 mg q.d.* (%)	Propranolol (N = 73) 40-160 mg b.i.d. (%)	Atenolol (N = 75) 25-100 mg q.d. (%)	Placebo (N = 109) (%)
Cardiovascular				
Bradycardia (heart rate < 50 BPM)	8.1	4.1	12.0	0
Symptomatic bradycardia	0.8	1.4	0	0
Edema	1.8	0	0	1.8
Central Nervous System				
Headache	6.5	4.1	5.3	15.6
Dizziness	4.5	11.0	2.7	5.5
Fatigue	2.9	9.6	4.0	0
Lethargy	2.8	4.1	2.7	0.9
Psychiatric				
Insomnia	1.2	8.2	2.7	0
Nervousness	0.8	1.4	2.7	0
Bizarre dreams	1.0	2.7	1.3	0
Depression	0.8	2.7	4.0	0
Autonomic				
Impotence	1.2†	0	0	0
Respiratory				
Dyspnea	2.4	2.7	1.3	0.9
Pharyngitis	2.0	0	4.0	0.9
Rhinitis	1.4	0	4.0	0.9
Upper respiratory infection	2.6	0	0	5.5
Gastrointestinal				
Dyspepsia	4.7	6.8	2.7	0.9
Nausea	1.6	1.4	0	0
Diarrhea	2.0	6.8	8.0	0.9
Musculoskeletal				
Chest pain	2.4	1.4	2.7	0.9
Arthralgia	3.1	0	4.0	1.8
Skin				
Rash	1.2	0	0	0

*   Five patients received 80 mg q.d.
†   N = 336 males; impotence is a known possible adverse effect of this pharmacological class.

The following selected (potentially important) adverse events have been reported at an incidence of less than 2% in U.S. controlled and open, long-term clinical studies, European controlled clinical trials, or in marketing experience. It is not known whether a causal relationship exists between Betaxolol Hydrochloride and these events; they are listed to alert the physician to a possible relationship:

Autonomic: flushing, salivation, sweating.

Body as a whole: allergy, fever, malaise, pain, rigors.

Cardiovascular: angina pectoris, arrhythmia, atrioventricular block, heart failure, hypertension, hypotension, myocardial infarction, thrombosis, syncope.

Central and Peripheral Nervous System: ataxia, neuralgia, neuropathy, numbness, speech disorder, stupor, tremor, twitching.

Gastrointestinal: anorexia, constipation, dry mouth, increased appetite, mouth ulceration, rectal disorders, vomiting, dysphagia.

Hearing and Vestibular: earache, labyrinth disorders, tinnitus, deafness.

Hematologic: anemia, leucocytosis, lymphadenopathy, purpura, thrombocytopenia.

Liver and Biliary: increased AST, increased ALT.

Metabolic and Nutritional: acidosis, diabetes, hypercholesterolemia, hyperglycemia, hyperkalemia, hyperlipemia, hyperuricemia, hypokalemia, weight gain, weight loss, thirst, increased LDH.

Musculoskeletal: arthropathy, neck pain, muscle cramps, tendonitis.

Psychiatric: abnormal thinking, amnesia, impaired concentration, confusion, emotional lability, hallucinations, decreased libido.

Reproductive Disorders: Female: breast pain, breast fibroadenosis, menstrual disorder; Male: Peyronie's disease, prostatitis.

Respiratory: bronchitis, bronchospasm, cough, epistaxis, flu, pneumonia, sinusitis.

Skin: alopecia, eczema, erythematous rash, hypertrichosis, pruritus, skin disorders.

Special Senses: abnormal taste, taste loss.

Urinary System: cystitis, dysuria, micturition disorder, oliguria, proteinuria, abnormal renal function, renal pain.

Vascular: cerebrovascular disorder, intermittent claudication, leg cramps, peripheral ischemia, thrombophlebitis.

Vision: abnormal lacrimation, abnormal vision, blepharitis, ocular hemorrhage, conjunctivitis, dry eyes, iritis, cataract, scotoma.

► SHOWN IN PRODUCT IDENTIFICATION GUIDE

Potential Adverse Effects: Although not reported in clinical studies with Betaxolol Hydrochloride, a variety of adverse effects have been reported with other beta-adrenergic blocking agents and may be considered potential adverse effects of Betaxolol Hydrochloride:

Central Nervous System: Reversible mental depression progressing to catatonia, an acute reversible syndrome characterized by disorientation for time and place, short-term memory loss, emotional lability with slightly clouded sensorium, and decreased performance on neuropsychometric tests.

Allergic: Fever combined with aching and sore throat, laryngospasm, respiratory distress.

Hematologic: Agranulocytosis, thrombocytopenic purpura, and nonthrombocytopenic purpura.

Gastrointestinal: Mesenteric arterial thrombosis, ischemic colitis.

Miscellaneous: Raynaud's phenomena. There have been reports of skin rashes and/or dry eyes associated with the use of beta-adrenergic blocking drugs. The reported incidence is small, and in most cases, the symptoms have cleared when treatment was withdrawn. Discontinuation of the drug should be considered if any such reaction is not otherwise explicable. Patients should be closely monitored following cessation of therapy.

The oculomucocutaneous syndrome associated with the beta-blocker practolol has not been reported with Betaxolol Hydrochloride during investigational use and extensive foreign experience. However, dry eyes have been reported.

OVERDOSAGE

No specific information on emergency treatment of overdosage with Betaxolol Hydrochloride is available. The most common effects expected are bradycardia, congestive heart failure, hypotension, bronchospasm, and hypoglycemia. In one acute overdosage of Betaxolol Hydrochloride, a 16-year-old female recovered fully after ingesting 460 mg.

Oral LD_{50}s are 350 to 400 mg Betaxolol Hydrochloride kg in mice and 860 to 980 mg/kg in rats.

In the case of overdosage, treatment with Betaxolol Hydrochloride should be stopped and the patient carefully observed. Hemodialysis or peritoneal dialysis does not remove substantial amounts of the drug. In addition to gastric lavage, the following therapeutic measures are suggested if warranted:

Hypotension: Use sympathomimetic pressor drug therapy, such as dopamine, dobutamine, or norepinephrine. In refractory cases of overdosage of other beta-blockers, the use of glucagon hydrochloride has been reported to be useful.

Bradycardia: Atropine should be administered. If there is no response to vagal blockade, isoproterenol should be administered cautiously. In refractory cases the use of a transvenous cardiac pacemaker may be considered.

Acute Cardiac Failure: Conventional therapy including digitalis, diuretics, and oxygen should be instituted immediately.

Bronchospasm: Use a β_2-agonist. Additional therapy with aminophylline may be considered.

Heart Block 2nd- or 3rd-degree. Use isoproterenol or a transvenous cardiac pacemaker.

DOSAGE AND ADMINISTRATION

The initial dose of Betaxolol Hydrochloride in hypertension is ordinarily 10 mg once daily either alone or added to diuretic therapy. The full antihypertensive effect is usually seen within 7 to 14 days. If the desired response is not achieved the dose can be doubled after 7 to 14 days. Increasing the dose beyond 20 mg has not been shown to produce a statistically significant additional antihypertensive effect; but the 40-mg dose has been studied and is well tolerated. An increased effect (reduction) on heart rate should be anticipated with increasing dosage. If monotherapy with Betaxolol Hydrochloride does not produce the desired response, the addition of a diuretic agent or other antihypertensive should be considered (see "Drug Interactions").

DOSAGE ADJUSTMENTS FOR SPECIFIC PATIENTS

Patients with Renal Failure: In patients with renal impairment, clearance of Betaxolol Hydrochloride declines with decreasing renal function.

In patients with severe renal impairment and those undergoing dialysis the initial dose of Betaxolol Hydrochloride is 5 mg once daily. If the desired response is not achieved, dosage may be increased by 5 mg/day increments every 2 weeks to a maximum dose of 20 mg/day.

Patients with Hepatic Disease: Patients with hepatic disease do not have significantly altered clearance. Dosage adjustments are not routinely needed.

Elderly Patients: Consideration should be given to reduction in the starting dose to 5 mg in elderly patients. These patients are especially prone to beta-blocker-induced bradycardia, which appears to be dose related and sometimes responds to reductions in dose.

Cessation of Therapy: If withdrawal of Betaxolol Hydrochloride therapy is planned, it should be achieved gradually over a period of about 2 weeks. Patients should be carefully observed and advised to limit physical activity to a minimum.

Store below 86°F (30°C).

HOW SUPPLIED
TABLETS: 10 MG

BRAND/MANUFACTURER	NDC	SIZE	AWP
○ BRAND			
► KERLONE: Searle	00025-5101-31	100s	$69.37
	00025-5101-34	100s ud	$72.82

TABLETS: 20 MG

BRAND/MANUFACTURER	NDC	SIZE	AWP
○ BRAND			
► KERLONE: Searle	00025-5201-31	100s	$104.04
	00025-5201-34	100s ud	$109.23

Bethanechol Chloride

DESCRIPTION

Bethanechol Chloride, a cholinergic agent, is a synthetic ester which is structurally and pharmacologically related to acetylcholine.

It is designated chemically as 2-[(aminocarbonyl)oxy]-N,N, N-trimethyl-1-propanaminium chloride. Its empirical formula is $C_7H_{17}ClN_2O_2$

It is a white, hygroscopic crystalline compound having a slight amine-like odor, freely soluble in water, and has a molecular weight of 196.68.

Bethanechol Chloride is supplied as 5 mg, 10 mg, 25 mg, and 50 mg tablets for oral use. Inactive ingredients in the tablets are calcium phosphate, lactose, magnesium stearate, and starch.

Bethanechol Chloride is also supplied as a sterile solution *for subcutaneous use only*. The sterile solution is essentially neutral. Each milliliter contains Bethanechol Chloride, 5 mg, and Water for Injection, q.s., 1 mL. It may be autoclaved at 120° C for 20 minutes without discoloration or loss of potency.

Following is its chemical structure:

$$\left[\begin{array}{c} CH_3CHCH_2N^+(CH_3)_3 \\ | \\ OCONH_2 \end{array} \right] Cl^-$$

CLINICAL PHARMACOLOGY

Bethanechol Chloride acts principally by producing the effects of stimulation of the parasympathetic nervous system. It increases the tone of the detrusor urinae muscle, usually producing a contraction sufficiently strong to initiate micturition and empty the bladder. It stimulates gastric motility, increases gastric tone, and often restores impaired rhythmic peristalsis.

Stimulation of the parasympathetic nervous system releases acetylcholine at the nerve endings. When spontaneous stimulation is reduced and therapeutic intervention is required, acetylcholine can be given, but it is rapidly hydrolyzed by cholinesterase, and its effects are transient. Bethanechol Chloride is not destroyed by cholinesterase and its effects are more prolonged than those of acetylcholine.

Effects on the GI and urinary tracts sometimes appear within 30 minutes after oral administration of Bethanechol Chloride, but more often 60-90 minutes are required to reach maximum effectiveness. Following oral administration, the usual duration of action of Bethanechol Chloride is one hour, although large doses (300-400 mg) have been reported to produce effects for up to six hours. Subcutaneous injection produces a more intense action on bladder muscle than does oral administration of the drug.

Because of the selective action of Bethanechol Chloride, nicotinic symptoms of cholinergic stimulation are usually absent or minimal when orally or subcutaneously administered in therapeutic doses, while muscarinic effects are prominent. Muscarinic effects usually occur within 5-15 minutes after subcutaneous injection, reach a maximum in 15-30 minutes, and disappear within two hours. Doses that stimulate micturition and defecation and increase peristalsis do not ordinarily stimulate ganglia or voluntary muscles. Therapeutic test doses in normal human subjects have little effect on heart rate, blood pressure, or peripheral circulation.

Bethanechol Chloride does not cross the blood-brain barrier because of its charged quaternary amine moiety. The metabolic fate and mode of excretion of the drug have not been elucidated.

A clinical study[*] was conducted on the relative effectiveness of oral and subcutaneous doses of Bethanechol Chloride on the stretch response of bladder muscle in patients with urinary retention. Results showed that 5 mg of the drug given subcutaneously stimulated a response that was more rapid in onset and of larger magnitude than an oral dose of 50 mg, 100 mg, or 200 mg. All the oral doses, however, had a longer duration of effect than the subcutaneous dose. Although the 50 mg oral dose caused little change in intravesical pressure in this study, this dose has been found in other studies to be clinically effective in the rehabilitation of patients with decompensated bladders.

INDICATIONS AND USAGE

For the treatment of acute postoperative and postpartum nonobstructive (functional) urinary retention and for neurogenic atony of the urinary bladder with retention.

[*] Diokno, A. C.; Lapides, J., Urol. *10*: 23-24, July 1988.

CONTRAINDICATIONS

Hypersensitivity to Bethanechol Chloride tablets or to any component of Bethanechol Chloride injection, hyperthyroidism, peptic ulcer, latent or active bronchial asthma, pronounced bradycardia or hypotension, vasomotor instability, coronary artery disease, epilepsy, and parkinsonism.

Bethanechol Chloride should not be employed when the strength or integrity of the gastrointestinal or bladder wall is in question, or in the presence of mechanical obstruction: when increased muscular activity of the gastrointestinal tract or urinary bladder might prove harmful, as following recent urinary bladder surgery, gastrointestinal resection and anastomosis, or when there is possible gastrointestinal obstruction: in bladder neck obstruction, spastic gastrointestinal disturbances, acute inflammatory lesions of the gastrointestinal tract, or peritonitis; or in marked vagotonia.

WARNING

The sterile solution is for subcutaneous use only. It should never be given intramuscularly or intravenously: Violent symptoms of cholinergic over-stimulation, such as circulatory collapse, fall in blood pressure, abdominal cramps, bloody diarrhea, shock, or sudden cardiac arrest are likely to occur if the drug is given by either of these routes. Although rare, these same symptoms have occurred after subcutaneous injection, and may occur in cases of hypersensitivity or overdosage.

PRECAUTIONS

GENERAL
In urinary retention, if the sphincter fails to relax as Bethanechol Chloride contracts the bladder, urine may be forced up the ureter into the kidney pelvis. If there is bacteriuria, this may cause reflux infection.

INFORMATION FOR PATIENTS
Bethanechol Chloride tablets should preferably be taken one hour before or two hours after meals to avoid nausea or vomiting. Dizziness, lightheadedness or fainting may occur, especially when getting up from a lying or sitting position.

DRUG INTERACTIONS
Special care is required if this drug is given to patients receiving ganglion blocking compounds because a critical fall in blood pressure may occur. Usually, severe abdominal symptoms appear before there is such a fall in the blood pressure.

CARCINOGENESIS, MUTAGENESIS, IMPARIMENT OF FERTILITY
Long-term studies in animals have not been performed to evaluate the effects upon fertility, mutagenic or carcinogenic potential of Bethanechol Chloride.

PREGNANCY
Pregnancy Category C: Animal reproduction studies have not been conducted with Bethanechol Chloride. It is also not known whether Bethanechol Chloride can cause fetal harm when administered to a pregnant woman or can affect reproduction capacity. Bethanechol Chloride should be given to a pregnant woman only if clearly needed.

NURSING MOTHERS
It is not known whether this drug is secreted in human milk. Because many drugs are secreted in human milk and because of the potential for serious adverse reactions from Bethanechol Chloride in nursing infants, a decision should be made whether to discontinue nursing or to discontinue the drug, taking into account the importance of the drug to the mother.

PEDIATRIC USE
Safety and effectiveness in children have not been established.

ADVERSE REACTIONS

Adverse reactions are rare following oral administration of Bethanechol Chloride, but are more common following subcutaneous injection. Adverse reactions are more likely to occur when dosage is increased.

The following adverse reactions have been observed:

Body as a Whole: malaise;

Digestive: abdominal cramps or discomfort, colicky pain, nausea and belching, diarrhea, borborygmi, salivation;

Renal: urinary urgency;

Nervous System: headache;

Cardiovascular: a fall in blood pressure with reflex tachycardia, vasomotor response;

Skin: flushing producing a feeling of warmth, sensation of heat about the face, sweating;

Respiratory: bronchial constriction, asthmatic attacks;

Special Senses: lacrimation, miosis.

Causal Relationship Unknown: The following adverse reactions have been reported, and a causal relationship to therapy with Bethanechol Chloride has not been established:

Body as a Whole: hypothermia;

Nervous System: seizures.

OVERDOSAGE

Early signs of overdosage are abdominal discomfort, salivation, flushing of the skin ("hot feeling"), sweating, nausea and vomiting.

Atropine is a specific antidote: The recommended dose for adults is 0.6 mg (1/100 grain). Repeat doses can be given every two hours, according to clinical response. The recommended dosage in infants and children up to 12 years of age is 0.01 mg/kg (to a maximum single dose of 0.4 mg) repeated every two hours as needed until the desired effect is obtained, or adverse effects of atropine preclude further usage. Subcutaneous injection of atropine is preferred except in emergencies when the intravenous route may be employed. When Bethanechol Chloride is administered subcutaneously, a syringe containing a dose of atropine sulfate should always be available to treat symptoms of toxicity.

The oral LD_{50} of Bethanechol Chloride is 1510 mg/kg in the mouse.

DOSAGE AND ADMINISTRATION

Dosage and route of administration must be individualized, depending on the type and severity of the condition to be treated.

Preferably give the drug when the stomach is empty. If taken soon after eating, nausea and vomiting may occur.

Oral: The usual adult dosage is 10 to 50 mg three or four times a day. The minimum effective dose is determined by giving 5 or 10 mg initially and repeating the same amount at hourly intervals until satisfactory response occurs or until a maximum of 50 mg has been given. The effects of the drug sometimes appear within 30 minutes and usually within 60 to 90 minutes. They persist for about an hour.

Subcutaneous: The usual dose is 1 mL (5 mg), although some patients respond satisfactorily to as little as 0.5 mL (2.5 mg). The minimum effective dose is determined by injecting 0.5 mL (2.5 mg) initially and repeating the same amount at 15 to 30 minute intervals to a maximum of four doses until satisfactory response is obtained, unless disturbing reactions appear. The minimum effective dose may be repeated thereafter three or four times a day as required.

Rarely, single doses up to 2 mL (10 mg) may be required. Such large doses may cause severe reactions and should be used only after adequate trial of single doses of 0.5 to 1 mL (2.5 to 5 mg) has established that smaller doses are not sufficient.

Bethanechol Chloride is usually effective in 5 to 15 minutes after subcutaneous injection.

If necessary, the effects of the drug can be abolished promptly by atropine (see "*Overdosage*").

Parenteral drug products should be inspected visually for particulate matter and discoloration prior to administration, whenever solution and container permit.

Store Tables Bethanechol Chloride in a tightly-closed container.

Avoid storage at temperatures above 40°C (104°F).

Avoid storage of Injection Bethanechol Chloride at temperatures below -20°C (-4°F) and above 40°C (104°F).

J CODES
Up to 5 mg SC—J0520

HOW SUPPLIED
INJECTION: 5 MG/ML

BRAND/MANUFACTURER	NDC	SIZE	AWP
◆ BRAND			
URECHOLINE: Merck	00006-7786-29	1 ml 6s	$29.89

TABLETS: 5 MG

AVERAGE UNIT PRICE (AVAILABLE SIZES)		GENERIC A-RATED AVERAGE PRICE (GAAP)	
BRAND	$0.34	100s	$7.85
GENERIC	$0.08		
HCFA FUL (100s ea)	$0.02		

BRAND/MANUFACTURER	NDC	SIZE	AWP
◆ BRAND			
URECHOLINE: Merck	00006-0403-68	100s	$34.43
◆ GENERICS			
Major	00904-0590-60	100s	$3.20
Qualitest	00603-2455-21	100s	$3.28
Sidmak	50111-0323-01	100s	$4.01
Goldline	00182-0453-01	100s	$4.01
Aligen	00405-4123-01	100s	$4.22
UDL	51079-0053-40	100s	$5.25
U.S. Trading	56126-0215-11	100s ud	$4.07
Goldline	00182-0453-89	100s ud	$6.00
UDL	51079-0053-20	100s ud	$12.20
Vangard	00615-2556-13	100s ud	$13.02
Major	00904-0590-61	100s ud	$13.47
Auro	55829-0167-10	100s ud	$14.64
Medirex	57480-0426-01	100s ud	$14.65
Sidmak	50111-0323-03	1000s	$37.68

TABLETS: 10 MG

AVERAGE UNIT PRICE (AVAILABLE SIZES)		GENERIC A-RATED AVERAGE PRICE (GAAP)	
BRAND	$0.69	100s	$9.16
GENERIC	$0.08	1000s	$31.88
HCFA FUL (100s ea)	$0.02		

BRAND/MANUFACTURER	NDC	SIZE	AWP
◆ BRAND			
URECHOLINE: Merck	00006-0412-68	100s	$64.55
DUVOID: Roberts Pharm	54092-0101-01	100s	$72.27
URECHOLINE: Merck	00006-0412-28	100s ud	$67.26

BRAND/MANUFACTURER	NDC	SIZE	AWP
DUVOID: Roberts Pharm	54092-0101-52	100s ud	$71.61
◆ GENERICS			
Rugby	00536-3365-01	100s	$3.21
Qualitest	00603-2456-21	100s	$3.56
URL	00677-0506-01	100s	$4.15
Schein	00364-0349-01	100s	$4.25
Martec	52555-0422-01	100s	$4.70
Sidmak	50111-0324-01	100s	$5.01
Goldline	00182-0454-01	100s	$5.01
Geneva	00781-1254-01	100s	$5.05
Aligen	00405-4124-01	100s	$5.27
Parmed	00349-2129-01	100s	$5.50
Moore,H.L.	00839-6209-06	100s	$6.01
MYOTONACHOL: Glenwood	00516-0021-01	100s	$23.75
U.S. Trading	56126-0216-11	100s ud	$4.44
Goldline	00182-0454-89	100s ud	$6.60
Raway	00686-0054-20	100s ud	$9.50
Vangard	00615-2557-13	100s ud	$15.71
Major	00904-0591-61	100s ud	$16.88
UDL	51079-0054-20	100s ud	$17.90
Medirex	57480-0413-01	100s ud	$17.90
Auro	55829-0168-10	100s ud	$18.85
Major	00904-0591-80	1000s	$17.95
Rugby	00536-3365-10	1000s	$21.36
URL	00677-0506-10	1000s	$25.55
Moore,H.L.	00839-6209-16	1000s	$28.15
Qualitest	00603-2456-32	1000s	$34.90
Martec	52555-0422-10	1000s	$40.25
Sidmak	50111-0324-03	1000s	$42.99
Parmed	00349-2129-10	1000s	$43.90

TABLETS: 25 MG

AVERAGE UNIT PRICE (AVAILABLE SIZES)		GENERIC A-RATED AVERAGE PRICE (GAAP)	
BRAND	$1.04	100s	$13.95
GENERIC	$0.11	1000s	$44.16
HCFA FUL (100s ea)	$0.03		

BRAND/MANUFACTURER	NDC	SIZE	AWP
◆ BRAND			
URECHOLINE: Merck	00006-0457-68	100s	$97.83
DUVOID: Roberts Pharm	54092-0102-01	100s	$109.25
URECHOLINE: Merck	00006-0457-28	100s ud	$99.79
DUVOID: Roberts Pharm	54092-0102-52	100s ud	$106.95
◆ GENERICS			
Rugby	00536-3369-01	100s	$4.21
Schein	00364-0410-01	100s	$4.75
URL	00677-0507-01	100s	$5.20
Qualitest	00603-2457-21	100s	$5.50
Parmed	00349-2429-01	100s	$5.90
Martec	52555-0423-01	100s	$6.30
Moore,H.L.	00839-6210-06	100s	$6.41
Sidmak	50111-0325-01	100s	$6.73
Goldline	00182-0455-01	100s	$6.73
Geneva	00781-1250-01	100s	$6.75
Aligen	00405-4125-01	100s	$7.08
UDL	51079-0123-40	100s	$11.09
MYOTONACHOL: Glenwood	00516-0022-01	100s	$50.06
U.S. Trading	56126-0217-11	100s ud	$5.39
Goldline	00182-0455-89	100s ud	$7.05
Raway	00686-0123-20	100s ud	$13.00
Major	00904-0592-61	100s ud	$23.61
Auro	55829-0169-10	100s ud	$26.20
Vangard	00615-2558-13	100s ud	$26.77
UDL	51079-0123-20	100s ud	$32.04
Medirex	57480-0427-01	100s ud	$32.10
Major	00904-0592-70	250s	$8.90
Rugby	00536-3369-10	1000s	$33.57
Major	00904-0592-80	1000s	$34.80
Schein	00364-0410-02	1000s	$37.75
URL	00677-0507-10	1000s	$40.55
Qualitest	00603-2457-32	1000s	$45.30
Martec	52555-0423-10	1000s	$46.00
Moore,H.L.	00839-6210-16	1000s	$47.52
Sidmak	50111-0325-03	1000s	$49.13
Goldline	00182-0455-10	1000s	$49.13
Parmed	00349-2429-10	1000s	$50.25
Aligen	00405-4125-03	1000s	$51.72

TABLETS: 50 MG

AVERAGE UNIT PRICE (AVAILABLE SIZES)		GENERIC A-RATED AVERAGE PRICE (GAAP)	
BRAND	$1.64	100s	$18.23
GENERIC	$0.17	1000s	$102.88
HCFA FUL (100s ea)	$0.06		

BRAND/MANUFACTURER	NDC	SIZE	AWP
◆ BRAND			
URECHOLINE: Merck	00006-0460-68	100s	$137.71
DUVOID: Roberts Pharm	54092-0103-01	100s	$169.00
	54092-0103-52	100s ud	$184.70

BRAND/MANUFACTURER	NDC	SIZE	AWP
◆ GENERICS			
Rugby	00536-3366-01	100s	$8.60
Major	00904-0593-60	100s	$9.00
URL	00677-0940-01	100s	$9.15
Schein	00364-0590-01	100s	$9.28
Qualitest	00603-2458-21	100s	$10.11
Sidmak	50111-0326-01	100s	$11.46
Martec	52555-0424-01	100s	$11.70
Aligen	00405-4126-01	100s	$12.06
Moore,H.L.	00839-6537-06	100s	$12.41
Parmed	00349-8009-01	100s	$13.15
Raway	00686-0056-20	100s ud	$16.00
Goldline	00182-1023-89	100s ud	$18.00

Betoptic SEE BETAXOLOL HYDROCHLORIDE, OPHTHALMIC

Biavax II SEE RUBELLA AND MUMPS VACCINE

Biaxin SEE CLARITHROMYCIN

Bichloracetic Acid Kahlenberg SEE DICHLOROACETIC ACID

Bicillin SEE PENICILLIN G BENZATHINE AND PENICILLIN G BENZATHINE AND PENICILLIN G PROCAINE

Bicitra SEE CITRIC ACID AND SODIUM CITRATE

BiCNU SEE CARMUSTINE

Bidex SEE GUAIFENESIN

Bile Salts/Pancreatin/Pepsin

DESCRIPTION

Each dual coated tablet contains:

Pepsin (N.F. equivalent) ....250 mg
Pancreatin (N.F. equivalent) ....300 mg
Bile Salts ....150 mg

Pepsin, the proteolytic enzyme of the stomach, initiates protein digestion and carries it to the peptone stage. The absence of Pepsin, however, can apparently be compensated for completely by the action of intestinal and pancreatic secretions.

Pancreatin contains proenzymes, chiefly amylase, protease, and lipase, which are activated by the intestinal juice.

Age resulting in metabolic slowdown and consequently diminished enzyme secretion is the most common cause of pancreatic insufficiency.

Exocrine pancreatic insufficiency has several common origins, including cystic fibrosis, alcoholism and surgical resection of portions of the pancreas. The pancreas has a large functional reserve capacity, and malabsorption usually does not occur until pancreatic enzyme output is reduced by more than 90 percent. Malabsorption secondary to pancreatic insufficiency is treated by replacement of the missing pancreatic enzymes by the administration of exogenous pancreatic extracts.

Bile Salts action is favorable for normal digestion and absorption, especially of fats. Bile and pancreatic juice appear to stimulate cell proliferation in intestinal crypts.

ACTIONS

Bile Salts/Pancreatin/Pepsin promotes more complete digestion of carbohydrates, proteins, and fats. Bile Salts/Pancreatin/Pepsin enhances proteolysis by its peptic and tryptic activity; carbohydrate digestion by amylolytic activity; and fat emulsification and transport by lipolytic activity; and enhances the action of bile salts.

Bile Salts/Pancreatin/Pepsin releases the digestive enzymes consecutively from two specially constructed tablet sections. The outer layer of Bile Salts/Pancreatin/Pepsin dissolves in the acid gastric content releasing pepsin; the inner tablet of

Bile Salts/Pancreatin/Pepsin which is protected by an enteric coating, disintegrates in the alkaline medium of the small intestine and releases Pancreatin and Bile Salts.

INDICATIONS AND USAGE
Bile Salts/Pancreatin/Pepsin is indicated for the management of gastrointestinal disturbances associated with a diminished secretion of pancreatic enzymes. Bile Salts/Pancreatin/Pepsin is also recommended for the relief of steatorrhea and symptoms such as flatulence, fermentative or putrefactive dyspepsia, pyrosis, postprandial distress, epigastric fullness, and belching; in some patients, these symptoms are associated with vague digestive complaints with no evidence of specific disease entity.

Digestive enzymes secretion is frequently diminished in older persons; therefore, Bile Salts/Pancreatin/Pepsin is a useful digestive supplement in geriatric patients.

CONTRAINDICATIONS
Biliary tract obstruction.

WARNINGS
Do not take this product if you are allergic to pork. Do not take this product unless directed by a physician. Do not exceed the labeled dose unless directed by a physician. Do not chew tablets. Swallow tablets quickly to lessen potential for mouth irritation.

ADVERSE REACTIONS
Rash may occur in patients who are hypersensitive to any of the ingredients.

DOSAGE AND ADMINISTRATION
Two (2) tablets with each meal, or as directed by the physician. Bile Salts/Pancreatin/Pepsin tablets should be swallowed whole, do not crush or chew.

Store at controlled room temperature, 15° - 30°C (59° - 86°F).

Dispense in a tight and light-resistant container.

HOW SUPPLIED
TABLETS:

BRAND/MANUFACTURER	NDC	SIZE	AWP
○ GENERICS			
DIGEPEPSIN: Kenwood	00482-0020-06	60s	$9.90

Bilopaque Sodium SEE TYROPANOATE SODIUM

Biltricide SEE PRAZIQUANTEL

Bioclate SEE ANTIHEMOPHILIC FACTOR

Biperiden

DESCRIPTION
Each Biperiden Tablet for oral administration contains 2 mg Biperiden Hydrochloride. Other ingredients may include corn syrup, lactose, magnesium stearate, potato starch and tale. Each 1 mL Biperiden Ampule for intramuscular or intravenous administration contains 5 mg Biperiden lactate in an aqueous 1.4 percent sodium lactate solution. No added preservative. Biperiden is an anticholinergic agent. Biperiden is α-5-Norbornen-2-yl-α-phenyl-1-piperidine-propanol. It is a white, crystalline, odorless powder, slightly soluble in water and alcohol. It is stable in air at normal temperatures.

Following is its chemical structure:

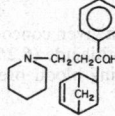

CLINICAL PHARMACOLOGY
Biperiden is a weak peripheral anticholinergic agent. It has, therefore, some antisecretory, antispasmodic and mydriatic effects. In addition, Biperiden possesses nicotinolytic activity. Parkinsonism is thought to result from an imbalance between the excitatory (cholinergic) and inhibitory (dopaminergic) systems in the corpus striatum. The mechanism of action of centrally active anticholinergic drugs such as Biperiden is considered to relate to competitive antagonism of acetylcholine at cholinergic receptors in the corpus striatum, which then restores the balance.

The parenteral form of Biperiden is an effective and reliable agent for the treatment of acute episodes of extrapyramidal disturbances sometimes seen during treatment with neuroleptic agents. Akathisia, akinesia, dyskinetic tremors, rigor, oculogyric crisis, spasmodic torticollis, and profuse sweating are markedly reduced or eliminated. With parenteral Biperiden, these drug-induced disturbances are rapidly brought under control. Subsequently, this can usually be maintained with oral doses which may be given with transquilizer therapy in psychotic and other conditions requiring an uninterrupted therapeutic program.

Pharmacokinetics and Metabolism. Only limited pharmacokinetic studies of Biperiden in humans are available. The serum concentration at 1 to 1.5 hours following a single, 4 mg oral dose was 4-5 ng/mL. Plasma levels (0.1-0.2 ng/mL) could be determined up to 48 hours after dosing. Six hours after an oral dose of 250 mg/kg in rats, 87% of the drug had been absorbed. The metabolism of Biperiden is also incompletely understood, but does involve hydroxylation. In normal volunteers a single 10 mg intravenous dose of Biperiden seemed to cause a transient rise in plasma cortisol and prolactin. No change in GH, LH, FSH, or TSH levels were seen. Biperiden lactate (10 mg/mL) was not irritating to the tissue of rabbits when injected intramuscularly (1.0 mL) into the sacrospinalis muscles and intradermally (0.25 mL) and subcutaneously (0.5 mL) into the shaved abdominal skin.

INDICATIONS AND USAGE
■ As an adjunct in the therapy of all forms of parkinsonism (idiopathic, postencephalitic, arteriosclerotic)
■ Control of extrapyramidal disorders secondary to neuroleptic drug therapy (e.g., phenothiazines).

CONTRAINDICATIONS
1) Hypersensitivity to Biperiden 2) Narrow angle glaucoma 3) Bowel obstruction 4) Megacolon

WARNINGS
Isolated instances of mental confusion, euphoria, agitation and disturbed behavior have been reported in susceptible patients. Also, the central anticholinergic syndrome can occur as an adverse reaction to properly prescribed anticholinergic medication, although it is more frequently due to overdosage. It may also result from concomitant administration of an anticholinergic agent and a drug that has secondary anticholinergic actions (see *"Drug Interactions"* and *"Overdosage"* sections). Caution should be observed in patients with manifest glaucoma, though no prohibitive rise in intraocular pressure has been noted following either oral or parenteral administration. Patients with prostatism, epilepsy or cardiac arrhythmia should be given this drug with caution. Occasionally, drowsiness may occur, and patients who drive a car or operate any other potentially dangerous machinery should be warned of this possibility. As with other drugs acting on the central nervous system, the consumption of alcohol should be avoided during Biperiden therapy.

PRECAUTIONS
Drug Interactions. The central anticholinergic syndrome can occur when anticholinergic agents such as Biperiden are administered concomitantly with drugs that have secondary anticholinergic actions, e.g., certain narcotic analgesics such as meperidine, the phenothiazines and other antipsychotics, tricyclic antidepressants, certain antiarrhythmics such as the quinidine salts, and antihistamines. See *"Overdosage"* section for signs and symptoms of the central anticholinergic syndrome, and for treatment.

Pregnancy: Pregnancy Category C. Animal reproduction studies have not been conducted with Biperiden. It is also not known whether Biperiden can cause fetal harm when administered to a pregnant woman or can affect reproduction capacity. Biperiden should be given to a pregnant woman only if clearly needed.

Nursing Mothers. It is not known whether this drug is excreted in human milk. Because many drugs are excreted in human milk, caution should be exercised when Biperiden is administered to a nursing woman.

Pediatric Use. Safety and effectiveness in children have not been established.

ADVERSE REACTIONS
Atropine-like side effects such as dry mouth; blurred vision: drowsiness; euphoria or disorientation; urinary retention; postural hypotension; constipation; agitation; disturbed behavior may be seen. There usually are no significant changes in blood pressure or heart rate in patients who have been given the parenteral form of Biperiden. Mild transient postural hypotension and bradycardia may occur. These side effects can be minimized or avoided by slow intravenous administration. No local tissue reactions have been reported following intramuscular injection. If gastric irritation occurs following oral administration, it can be avoided by administering the drug during or after meals.

The central anticholinergic syndrome can occur as an adverse reaction to properly prescribed anticholinergic medication, See *"Overdosage"* section for signs and symptoms of the central anticholinergic syndrome, and for treatment.

OVERDOSAGE
Signs and Symptoms: Overdosage with Biperiden produces typical central symptoms of atropine intoxication (the central anticholinergic syndrome). Correct diagnosis depends upon recognition of the peripheral signs of parasympathetic blockade including dilated and sluggish pupils; warm, dry skin: facial flushing; decreased secretions of the mouth, pharynx, nose, and bronchi; foul-smelling breath; elevated temperature, tachycardia, cardiac arrhythmias, decreased bowel sounds, and urinary retention. Neuropsychiatric signs such as delirium, disorientation, anxiety, hallucinations, illusions, confusion, incoherence, agitation, hyperactivity, ataxia, loss of memory, paranoia, combativeness, and seizures may be present. The condition can progress to stupor, coma, paralysis, and cardiac and respiratory arrest and death.

Treatment: Treatment of acute overdose revolves around symptomatic and supportive therapy. If Biperiden was administered orally, gastric lavage or other measures to limit absorption should be instituted. A small dose of diazepam or a short acting barbiturate may be administered if CNS excitation is observed. Phenothiazines are contraindicated because the toxicity may be intensified due to their antimuscarinic action, causing coma. Respiratory support, artificial respiration or vasopressor agents may be necessary. Hyperpyrexia must be reversed, fluid volume replaced and acid-base balance maintained. Urinary catheterization may be necessary.

Routine use of physostigmine for overdose is controversial. Delirium, hallucinations, coma, and supraventricular tachycardia (not ventricular tachycardias or conduction defects) seem to respond. If indicated, 1 mg (half this amount for children or the elderly) may be given intramuscularly or by slow intravenous infusion. If there is no response within 20 minutes, an additional 1 mg dose may be given; this may be repeated until a total of 4 mg has been administered, a reversal of the toxic effects occur or excessive cholinergic signs are seen. Frequent monitoring of clinical signs should be done. Since physostigmine is rapidly destroyed, additional injections may be required every one or two hours to maintain control. The relapse intervals tend to lengthen as the toxic anticholinergic agent is metabolized, so the patient should be carefully observed for 8 to 12 hours following the last relapse.

Toxicity in Animals: The LD_{50} of Biperiden in the white mouse is 545 mg/kg orally, 195 mg/kg subcutaneously, and 56 mg/kg intravenously. The acute oral toxicity (LD_{50}) in rats is 750 mg/kg. The intraperitoneal toxicity (LD_{50}) of Biperiden lactate in rats was 270 mg/kg and the intravenous toxicity (LD_{50}) in dogs is 222 mg/kg. In dogs under general anesthesia, respiratory arrest occurred at 33 mg/kg (intravenous) and circulatory standstill at 45 mg/kg (intravenous). The oral LD_{50} in dogs was 340 mg/kg. Chronic toxicity studies in both rat and dog have been reported.

DOSAGE AND ADMINISTRATION
DRUG INDUCED EXTRAPYRAMIDAL SYMPTOMS
Parenteral: The average adult dose is 2 mg intramuscularly or intravenously. May be repeated every half-hour until there is resolution of symptoms, but not more than four consecutive doses should be given in a 24-hour period.

Note: Parenteral drug products should be inspected visually for particulate matter and discoloration prior to administration, whenever solution and container permit.

Oral: One tablet one to three times daily.

Parkinson's Disease: Oral: The usual beginning dose is one tablet three or four times daily. The dosage should be individualized with the dose titrated upward to a maximum of 8 tablets (16 mg) per 24 hours.

Storage: All dosage forms of Biperiden should be stored at 59°-86°F (15°-30°C). Dispense in tight, light-resistant container as defined in USP.

HOW SUPPLIED
TABLETS: 2 MG

BRAND/MANUFACTURER	NDC	SIZE	AWP
○ BRAND			
AKINETON HCL: Knoll	00044-0120-02	100s	$23.99
	00044-0120-04	1000s	$177.50

Bisoprolol Fumarate

DESCRIPTION
Bisoprolol Fumarate is a synthetic beta$_1$-selective (cardioselective) adrenoceptor blocking agent. The chemical name for Bisoprolol Fumarate is (±)-1-[4-[[2-(1-Methylethoxy) ethoxy]methyl]-phenoxy] -3-[(1-methylethyl)amino]-2-propanol (E) -2- butenedioate (2:1) (salt). It possesses an asymmetric carbon atom in its structure and is provided as a racemic mixture. The S(-)enantiomer is responsible for most of the beta-blocking activity. Its empirical formula is $(C_{18}H_{31}NO_4)_2 \cdot C_4H_4O_4$. Bisoprolol Fumarate has a molecular weight of 766.97. It is a white crystalline powder which is approximately equally hydrophilic and lipophilic, and is readily soluble in water, methanol, ethanol, and chloroform.

Bisoprolol Fumarate is available as 5 and 10 mg tablets for oral administration.

Following is its chemical structure:

CLINICAL PHARMACOLOGY
Bisoprolol Fumarate is a beta$_1$-selective (cardioselective) adrenoceptor blocking agent without significant membrane stabilizing activity or intrinsic sympathomimetic activity in its therapeutic dosage range. Cardioselectivity is not absolute, however, and at higher doses ($\geq$ 20 mg Bisoprolol Fumarate also inhibits beta$_2$-adrenoceptors, chiefly located in the bronchial and vascular musculature; to retain selectivity, it is therefore important to use the lowest effective dose.

Pharmacokinetics and Metabolism: The absolute bioavailability after a 10 mg oral dose of Bisoprolol Fumarate is about 80%. Absorption is not affected by the presence of food. The first pass metabolism of Bisoprolol Fumarate is about 20%. Binding to serum proteins is approximately 30%. Peak plasma concentrations occur within 2-4 hours of dosing with 5 to 20 mg, and mean peak values range from 16 ng/mL at 5 mg to 70 ng/mL at 20 mg. Once daily dosing with Bisoprolol Fumarate results in less than twofold intersubject variation in peak plasma levels. The plasma elimination half-life is 9-12 hours and is slightly longer in elderly patients, in part because of decreased renal function in that population. Steady state is attained within 5 days of once daily dosing. In both young and elderly populations, plasma accumulation is low; the accumulation factor ranges from 1.1 to 1.3, and is what would be expected from the first order kinetics and once daily dosing. Plasma concentrations are proportional to the administered dose in the range of 5 to 20 mg. Pharmacokinetic characteristics of the two enantiomers are similar. Bisoprolol Fumarate is eliminated equally by renal and nonrenal pathways with about 50% of the dose appearing unchanged in the urine and the remainder appearing in the form of inactive metabolites. In humans, the known metabolites are labile or have no known pharmacologic activity. Less than 2% of the dose is excreted in the feces. Bisoprolol Fumarate is not metabolized by cytochrome P450 II D6 (debrisoquin hydroxylase).

In subjects with creatinine clearance less than 40 mL/min, the plasma half-life is increased approximately threefold compared to healthy subjects.

In patients with cirrhosis of the liver, the elimination of Bisoprolol Fumarate is more variable in rate and significantly slower than that in healthy subjects, with plasma half-life ranging from 8.3 to 21.7 hours.

Pharmacodynamics: The most prominent effect of Bisoprolol Fumarate is the negative chronotropic effect, resulting in a reduction in resting and exercise heart rate. There is a fall in resting and exercise cardiac output with little observed change in stroke volume, and only a small increase in right atrial pressure, or pulmonary capillary wedge pressure, at rest or during exercise.

Findings in short-term clinical hemodynamics studies with Bisoprolol Fumarate are similar to those observed with other beta-blocking agents.

The mechanism of action of its antihypertensive effects has not been completely established. Factors which may be involved include:

1. Decreased cardiac output,
2. Inhibition of renin release by the kidneys,
3. Diminution of tonic sympathetic outflow from the vasomotor centers in the brain.

In normal volunteers, Bisoprolol Fumarate therapy resulted in a reduction of exercise- and isoproterenol-induced tachycardia. The maximal effect occurred within 1 to 4 hours post-dosing. Effects persisted for 24 hours at doses equal to or greater than 5 mg.

Electrophysiology studies in man have demonstrated that Bisoprolol Fumarate significantly decreases heart rate, increases sinus node recovery time, prolongs AV node refractory periods, and, with rapid atrial stimulation, prolongs AV nodal conduction.

Beta$_1$-selectivity of Bisoprolol Fumarate has been demonstrated in both animal and human studies. No effects at therapeutic doses on beta$_2$-adrenoreceptor density have been observed. Pulmonary function studies have been conducted in healthy volunteers, asthmatics, and patients with chronic obstructive pulmonary disease (COPD). Doses of Bisoprolol Fumarate ranged from 5 to 60 mg, atenolol from 50 to 200 mg, metoprolol from 100 to 200 mg, and propranolol from 40 to 80 mg. In some studies, slight, asymptomatic increases in airways resistance (AWR) and decreases in forced expiratory volume (FEV_1) were observed with doses of Bisoprolol Fumarate 20 mg and higher, similar to the small increases in AWR also noted with the other cardioselective beta-blockers. The changes induced by beta-blockade with all agents were reversed by bronchodilator therapy.

Bisoprolol Fumarate had minimal effect on serum lipids during antihypertensive studies. In U.S. placebo-controlled trials, changes in total cholesterol averaged +0.8% for Bisoprolol Fumarate-treated patients, and +0.7% for placebo. Changes in triglycerides averaged +19% for Bisoprolol Fumarate-treated patients, and +17% for placebo.

Bisoprolol Fumarate has also been given concomitantly with thiazide diuretics. Even very low doses of hydrochlorothiazide (6.25 mg) were found to be additive with Bisoprolol Fumarate in lowering blood pressure in patients with mild-to-moderate hypertension.

CLINICAL STUDIES
In two randomized double-blind placebo-controlled trials conducted in the U.S., reductions in systolic and diastolic blood pressure and heart rate 24 hours after dosing in patients with mild-to-moderate hypertension are shown below. In both studies, mean systolic/diastolic blood pressures at baseline were approximately 150/100 mm Hg, and mean heart rate was 76 bpm. Drug effect is calculated by subtracting the placebo effect from the overall change in blood pressure and heart rate. (See related table).

Blood pressure responses were seen within one week of treatment and changed little thereafter. They were sustained for 12 weeks and for over a year in studies of longer duration.

Blood pressure returned to baseline when Bisoprolol Fumarate was tapered over two weeks in a long-term study.

◆ RATED THERAPEUTICALLY EQUIVALENT; ◇ THERAPEUTIC EQUIVALENCE UNCONFIRMED; ○ UNRATED

Overall, significantly greater blood pressure reductions were observed on Bisoprolol Fumarate than on placebo, regardless of race, age, or gender. There were no significant differences in response between black and non-black patients.

INDICATIONS AND USAGE

Bisoprolol Fumarate is indicated in the management of hypertension. It may be used alone or in combination with other antihypertensive agents.

UNLABELED USES

Bisoprolol Fumarate is used alone or as an adjunct in the treatment of angina pectoris.

CONTRAINDICATIONS

Bisoprolol Fumarate is contraindicated in patients with cardiogenic shock, overt cardiac failure, second or third degree AV block, and marked sinus bradycardia.

WARNINGS

Cardiac Failure: Sympathetic stimulation is a vital components supporting circulatory function in the setting of congestive heart failure, and beta-blockade may result in further depression of myocardial contractility and precipitate more severe failure. In general, beta-blocking agents should be avoided in patients with overt congestive failure. However, in some patients with compensated cardiac failure it may be necessary to utilize them. In such a situation, they must be used cautiously.

In Patients Without a History of Cardiac Failure: Continued depression of the myocardium with beta-blockers can, in some patients, precipitate cardiac failure. At the first signs or symptoms of heart failure, discontinuation of Bisoprolol Fumarate should be considered. In some cases, beta-blocker therapy can be continued while heart failure is treated with other drugs.

Abrupt Cessation of Therapy: Exacerbation of angina pectoris, and, in some instances, myocardial infarction or ventricular arrhythmia, have been observed in patients with coronary artery disease following abrupt cessation of therapy with beta-blockers. Such patients should, therefore, be cautioned against interruption or discontinuation of therapy without the physician's advice. Even in patients without overt coronary artery disease, it may be advisable to taper therapy with Bisoprolol Fumarate over approximately 1 week with the patient under careful observation. If withdrawal symptoms occur, Bisoprolol Fumarate therapy should be reinstituted, at least temporarily.

Peripheral Vascular Disease: Beta-blockers can precipitate or aggravate symptoms of arterial insufficiency in patients with peripheral vascular disease. Caution should be exercised in such individuals.

Bronchospastic Disease: PATIENTS WITH BRONCHOSPASTIC DISEASE SHOULD, IN GENERAL, NOT RECEIVE BETA-BLOCKERS. Because of its relative beta$_1$-selectivity, however, Bisoprolol Fumarate may be used with caution in patients with bronchospastic disease who do not respond to, or who cannot tolerate other antihypertensive treatment. Since beta$_1$-selectivity is not absolute, the lowest possible dose of Bisoprolol Fumarate should be used, with therapy starting at 2.5 mg. A beta$_2$ agonist (bronchodilator) should be made available.

Anesthesia and Major Surgery: If Bisoprolol Fumarate treatment is to be continued perioperatively, particular care should be taken when anesthetic agents which depress myocardial function such as ether, cyclopropane, and trichloroethylene, are used. (See *"Overdosage"* for information on treatment of bradycardia and hypertension.)

Diabetes and Hypoglycemia: Beta-blockers may mask some of the manifestations of hypoglycemia, particularly tachycardia. Nonselective beta-blockers may potentiate insulin-induced hypoglycemia and delay recovery of serum glucose levels. Because of its beta$_1$-selectivity, this is less likely with Bisoprolol Fumarate. However, patients subject to spontaneous hypoglycemia, or diabetic patients receiving insulin or oral hypoglycemic agents, should be cautioned about these possibilities and Bisoprolol Fumarate should be used with caution.

Thyrotoxicosis: Beta-adrenergic blockade may mask clinical signs of hyperthyroidism, such as tachycardia. Abrupt withdrawal of beta-blockade may be followed by an exacerbation of the symptoms of hyperthyroidism or may precipitate thyroid storm.

PRECAUTIONS

Impaired Renal or Hepatic Function: Use caution in adjusting the dose of Bisoprolol Fumarate in patients with renal or hepatic impairment (see *"Clinical Pharmacology"* and *"Dosage and Administration"*).

Drug Interactions: Bisoprolol Fumarate should not be combined with other beta-blocking agents. Patients receiving catecholamine-depleting drugs, such as reserpine or guanethidine, should be closely monitored, because the added beta-adrenergic blocking action of Bisoprolol Fumarate may produce excessive reduction of sympathetic activity. In patients receiving concurrent therapy with clonidine, if therapy is to be discontinued, it is suggested that Bisoprolol Fumarate be discontinued for several days before the withdrawal of clonidine.

Bisoprolol Fumarate should be used with care when myocardial depressants or inhibitors of AV conduction, such as certain calcium antagonists [particularly of the phenylalkylamine (verapamil) and benzothiazepine (diltiazem) classes], or antiarrhythmic agents, such as disopyramide, are used concurrently.

Concurrent use of rifampin increases the metabolic clearance of Bisoprolol Fumarate, resulting in a shortened elimination half-life of Bisoprolol Fumarate. However, initial dose modification is generally not necessary. Pharmacokinetic studies document no clinically relevant interactions with other agents given concomitantly, including thiazide diuretics, digoxin and cimetidine. There was no effect of Bisoprolol Fumarate on prothrombin time in patients on stable doses of warfarin.

Risk of Anaphylactic Reaction: While taking beta-blockers, patients with a history of severe anaphylactic reaction to a variety of allergens may be more reactive to repeated challenge, either accidental, diagnostic, or therapeutic. Such patients may be unresponsive to the usual doses of epinephrine used to treat allergic reactions.

Information for Patients: Patients, especially those with coronary artery disease, should be warned about discontinuing use of Bisoprolol Fumarate without a physician's supervision. Patients should also be advised to consult a physician if any difficulty in breathing occurs, or if they develop signs or symptoms of congestive heart failure or excessive bradycardia.

Patients subject to spontaneous hypoglycemia, or diabetic patients receiving insulin or oral hypoglycemic agents, should be cautioned that beta-blockers may mask some of the manifestations of hypoglycemia, particularly tachycardia, and Bisoprolol Fumarate should be used with caution.

Patients should know how they react to this medicine before they operate automobiles and machinery or engage in other tasks requiring alertness.

Carcinogenesis, Mutagenesis, Impairment of Fertility: Long-term studies were conducted with oral Bisoprolol Fumarate administered in the feed of mice (20 and 24 months) and rats (26 months). No evidence of carcinogenic potential was seen in mice dosed up to 250 mg/kg/day or rats dosed up to 125 mg/kg/day. On a body-weight basis, these doses are 625 and 312 times, respectively, the maximum recommended human dose (MRHD) of 20 mg, (or 0.4 mg/kg/day based on a 50 kg individual); on a body-surface-area-basis, these doses are 59 times (mice) and 64 times (rats) the MRHD. The mutagenic potential of Bisoprolol Fumarate was evaluated in the microbial mutagenicity (Ames) test, the point mutation and chromosome aberration assays in Chinese hamster V79 cells, the unscheduled DNA synthesis test, the micronucleus test in mice, and the cytogenetics assay in rats. There was no evidence of mutagenic potential in these *in vitro* and *in vivo* assays.

Reproduction studies in rats did not show any impairment of fertility at doses up to 150 mg/kg/day of Bisoprolol Fumarate, or 375 and 77 times the MRHD on the basis of body-weight and body-surface-area respectively.

Pregnancy Category C: In rats, Bisoprolol Fumarate was not teratogenic at doses up to 150 mg/kg/day which is 375 and 77 times the MRHD on the basis of body-weight and body-surface-area, respectively. Bisoprolol Fumarate was fetotoxic (increased late resorptions) at 50 mg/kg/day and maternotoxic (decreased food intake and body-weight gain) at 150 mg/kg/day. The fetotoxicity in rats occurred at 125 times the MRHD on a body-weight-basis and 26 times the MRHD on the

SITTING SYSTOLIC/DIASTOLIC PRESSURE (BP) AND HEART RATE (HR) MEAN DECREASE (Δ) AFTER 3 TO 4 WEEKS

Study A		Bisoprolol Fumarate		
	Placebo	5 mg	10 mg	20 mg
n =	61	61	61	61
Total ΔBP (mm Hg)	5.4/3.2	10.4/8.0	11.2/10.9	12.8/11.9
Drug Effect[a]	—	5.0/4.8	5.8/7.7	7.4/8.7
Total ΔHR (bpm)	0.5	7.2	8.7	11.3
Drug Effect[a]	—	6.7	8.2	10.8

Study B		Bisoprolol Fumarate	
	Placebo	2.5 mg	10 mg
n =	56	59	62
Total ΔBP (mm Hg)	3.0/3.7	7.6/8.1	13.5/11.2
Drug Effect[a]	—	4.6/4.4	10.5/7.5
Total ΔHR (bpm)	1.6	3.8	10.7
Drug Effect[a]	—	2.2	9.1

[a] *Observed total change from baseline minus placebo.*

basis of body-surface-area. The maternotoxicity occurred at 375 times the MRHD on a body-weight basis and 77 times the MRHD on the basis of body-surface-area. In rabbits, Bisoprolol Fumarate was not teratogenic at doses up to 12.5 mg/kg/day, which is 31 and 12 times the MRHD based on body-weight and body-surface-area, respectively, but was embryolethal (increased early resorptions) at 12.5 mg/kg/day.

There are no adequate and well-controlled studies in pregnant women. Bisoprolol Fumarate should be used during pregnancy only if the potential benefit justifies the potential risk to the fetus.

Nursing Mothers: Small amounts of Bisoprolol Fumarate (< 2% of the dose) have been detected in the milk of lactating rats. It is not known whether this drug is excreted in human milk. Because many drugs are excreted in human milk caution should be exercised when Bisoprolol Fumarate is administered to nursing women.

Use in Elderly Patients: Bisoprolol Fumarate has been used in elderly patients with hypertension. Response rates and mean decreases in systolic and diastolic blood pressure were similar to the decreases in younger patients in the U.S. clinical studies. Although no dose response study was conducted in elderly patients, there was a tendency for older patients to be maintained on higher doses of Bisoprolol Fumarate.

Observed reductions in heart rate were slightly greater in the elderly than in the young and tended to increase with increasing dose. In general, no disparity in adverse experience reports or dropouts for safety reasons was observed between older and younger patients. Dose adjustment based on age is not necessary.

Pediatric Use: Safety and effectiveness in children have not been established.

ADVERSE REACTIONS

Safety data are available in more than 30,000 patients or volunteers. Frequency estimates and rates of withdrawal of therapy for adverse events were derived from two U.S. placebo-controlled studies.

In Study A, doses of 5, 10 and 20 mg Bisoprolol Fumarate were administered for 4 weeks. In Study B, doses of 2.5, 10 and 40 mg of Bisoprolol Fumarate were administered for 12 weeks. A total of 273 patients were treated with 5-20 mg of Bisoprolol Fumarate; 132 received placebo.

Withdrawal of therapy for adverse events was 3.3% for patients receiving Bisoprolol Fumarate and 6.8% for patients on placebo. Withdrawals were less than 1% for either bradycardia or fatigue/lack of energy.

The following table presents adverse experiences, whether or not considered drug related, reported in at least 1% of patients in these studies, for all patients studied in placebo controlled clinical trials (2.5-40 mg), as well as for a sub-group that was treated with doses within the recommended dosage range (5-20 mg). Of the adverse events listed in the table, bradycardia, diarrhea, asthenia, fatigue and sinusitis appear to be dose related.

Body System/ Adverse Experience	*All Adverse Experiences (%^{a})*		
		Bisoprolol Fumarate	
	Placebo (n = 132) %	5 to 20 mg (n = 273) %	2.5 to 40 mg (n = 404) %
Skin			
increased sweating	1.5	0.7	1.0
Musculoskeletal			
arthralgia	2.3	2.2	2.7
Central Nervous System			
dizziness	3.8	2.9	3.5
headache	11.4	8.8	10.9
hypoaesthesia	0.8	1.1	1.5
Autonomic Nervous System			
dry mouth	1.5	0.7	1.3
Heart Rate/Rhythm			
bradycardia	0	0.4	0.5
Psychiatric			
vivid dreams	0	0	0
insomnia	2.3	1.5	2.5
depression	0.8	0	0.2
Gastrointestinal			
diarrhea	1.5	2.6	3.5
nausea	1.5	1.5	2.2
vomiting	0	1.1	1.5
Respiratory			
bronchospasm	0	0	0
cough	4.5	2.6	2.5
dyspnea	0.8	1.1	1.5
pharyngitis	2.3	2.2	2.2
rhinitis	3.0	2.9	4.0
sinusitis	1.5	2.2	2.2
URI	3.8	4.8	5.0
Body as a Whole			
asthenia	0	0.4	1.5
chest pain	0.8	1.1	1.5
fatigue	1.5	6.6	8.2
edema (peripheral)	3.8	3.7	3.0

^{a} *Percentage of patients with event.*

The following is a comprehensive list of adverse experiences reported with Bisoprolol Fumarate in worldwide studies, or in post marketing experience (in italics):

Central Nervous System: Dizziness, vertigo, headache, paresthesia, hypoaesthesia, somnolence, anxiety/restlessness, decreased concentration/memory.

Autonomic Nervous System: Dry mouth.

Cardiovascular: Bradycardia, palpitations and other rhythm disturbances, cold extremities, claudication, hypotension, orthostatic hypotension, chest pain, congestive heart failure dyspnea on exertion.

Psychiatric: Vivid dreams, insomnia, depression.

Gastrointestinal: Gastric/epigastric/abdominal pain, gastritis, dyspepsia, nausea, vomiting, diarrhea, constipation.

Musculoskeletal: Muscle/joint pain, back/neck pain, muscle cramps, twitching/tremor.

Skin: Rash, acne, eczema, skin irritation, pruritus, flushing, sweating, alopecia, *angioedema, exfoliative dermatitis.*

Special Senses: Visual disturbances, ocular pain/pressure, abnormal lacrimation, tinnitus, earache, taste abnormalities.

Metabolic: Gout.

Respiratory: Asthma/bronchospasm, bronchitis, coughing, dyspnea, pharyngitis, rhinitis, sinusitis, URI.

Genitourinary: Decreased libido/impotence, *Peyronie's disease,* cystitis, renal colic.

Hematologic: Purpura.

General: Fatigue, asthenia, chest pain, malaise, edema, weight gain.

In addition, a variety of adverse effects have been reported with other beta-adrenergic blocking agents and should be considered potential adverse effects of Bisoprolol Fumarate.

Central Nervous System: Reversible mental depression progressing to catatonia, hallucinations, an acute reversible syndrome characterized by disorientation to time and place, emotional lability, slightly clouded sensorium.

Allergic: Fever, combined with aching and sore throat, laryngospasm, respiratory distress.

Hematologic: Agranulocytosis, thrombocytopenia, thrombocytopenic purpura.

Gastrointestinal: Mesenteric arterial thrombosis, ischemic colitis.

Miscellaneous: The oculomucocutaneous syndrome associated with the beta-blocker practolol has not been reported with Bisoprolol Fumarate during investigational use or extensive foreign marketing experience.

Laboratory Abnormalities: In clinical trials, the most frequently reported laboratory change was an increase in serum triglycerides, but this was not a consistent finding. Sporadic liver test abnormalities have been reported. In the U.S. controlled trials experience with Bisoprolol Fumarate treatment for 4-12 weeks, the incidence of concomitant elevations in SGOT and SGPT of between 1-2 times normal was 3.9%, compared to 2.5% for placebo. No patient had concomitant elevations greater than twice normal.

In the long-term, uncontrolled experience with Bisoprolol Fumarate treatment for 6 to 18 months, the incidence of one or more concomitant elevations in SGOT and SGPT of between one-two times normal was 6.2%. The incidence of multiple occurrences was 1.9%. For concomitant elevations in SGOT and SGPT of greater than twice normal, the incidence was 1.5%. The incidence of multiple occurrences was 0.3%. In many cases these elevations were attributed to underlying disorders, or resolved during continued treatment with Bisoprolol Fumarate.

Other laboratory changes included small increases in uric acid, creatinine, BUN, serum potassium, glucose, and phosphorus, and decreases in WBC and platelets. These were generally not of clinical importance and rarely resulted in discontinuation of Bisoprolol Fumarate.

As with other beta-blockers, ANA conversions have also been reported on Bisoprolol Fumarate. About 15% of patients in long-term studies converted to a positive titer, although about one-third of these patients subsequently reconverted to a negative titer while on continued therapy.

OVERDOSAGE

The most common signs expected with overdosage of a beta-blocker are bradycardia, hypotension, congestive heart failure, bronchospasm, and hypoglycemia. To date, a few cases of overdose (maximum: 2000 mg) with Bisoprolol Fumarate have been reported. Bradycardia and/or hypotension were noted. Sympathomimetic agents were given in some cases, and all patients recovered.

In general, if overdose occurs, Bisoprolol Fumarate therapy should be stopped and supportive and symptomatic treatment should be provided. Limited data suggest that Bisoprolol Fumarate is not dialyzable. Based on the expected pharmacologic actions and recommendations for other beta-blockers, the following general measures should be considered when clinically warranted:

Bradycardia. Administer IV atropine. If the response is inadequate, isoproterenol or another agent with positive chronotropic properties may be given cautiously. Under some circumstances, transvenous pacemaker insertion may be necessary.

Hypotension: IV fluids and vasopressors should be administered. Intravenous glucagon may be useful.

◆ RATED THERAPEUTICALLY EQUIVALENT; ◇ THERAPEUTIC EQUIVALENCE UNCONFIRMED; ○ UNRATED

Heart Block (second or third degree): Patients should be carefully monitored and treated with isoproterenol infusion or transvenous cardiac pacemaker insertion, as appropriate.

Congestive Heart Failure: Initiate conventional therapy (i.e., digitalis, diuretics, inotropic agents, vasodilating agents).

Bronchospasm: Administer bronchodilator therapy such as isoproterenol and/or aminophylline.

Hypoglycemia: Administer IV glucose.

DOSAGE AND ADMINISTRATION

The dose of Bisoprolol Fumarate must be individualized to the needs of the patient. The usual starting dose is 5 mg once daily. In some patients, 2.5 mg may be an appropriate starting dose (see *"Bronchospastic Disease* in *Warnings"*). If the antihypertensive effect of 5 mg is inadequate, the dose may be increased to 10 mg and then, if necessary, to 20 mg once daily.

Patients with Renal or Hepatic Impairment: In patients with hepatic impairment (hepatitis or cirrhosis) or renal dysfunction (creatinine clearance less than 40 mL/min), the initial daily dose should be 2.5 mg and caution should be used in dose-titration. Since limited data suggest that Bisoprolol Fumarate is not dialyzable, drug replacement is not necessary in patients undergoing dialysis.

Elderly Patients: It is not necessary to adjust the dose in the elderly unless there is also significant renal or hepatic dysfunction (see above and *"Use in Elderly Patients"* in *"Precautions"*).

Children: There is no pediatric experience with Bisoprolol Fumarate.

Store at controlled room temperature 15°-30°C (59°-86°F). Dispense in tight containers as defined in the USP.

HOW SUPPLIED
TABLETS: 5 MG

BRAND/MANUFACTURER	NDC	SIZE	AWP
○ **BRAND**			
➤ ZEBETA: Lederle Labs	00005-3816-38	30s	$25.33

TABLETS: 10 MG

BRAND/MANUFACTURER	NDC	SIZE	AWP
○ **BRAND**			
➤ ZEBETA: Lederle Labs	00005-3817-38	30s	$25.33

Bisoprolol Fumarate with Hydrochlorothiazide

DESCRIPTION

Bisoprolol Fumarate/Hydrochlorothiazide is indicated for the treatment of hypertension. It combines two antihypertensive agents in a once-daily dosage: a synthetic beta$_1$-selective (cardioselective) adrenoceptor blocking agent (Bisoprolol Fumarate) and a benzothiadiazine diuretic (Hydrochlorothiazide).

Bisoprolol Fumarate is chemically described as (±)-1-[4-[[2-(1-methylethoxy)ethoxy]methyl]phenoxy]-3- [(1-methylethyl)amino]-2-propanol(*E*)-2-butenedioate (2:1) (salt). It possesses an asymmetric carbon atom in its structure and is provided as a racemic mixture. The S(-) enantiomer is responsible for most of the beta-blocking activity. Its empirical formula is $(C_{18}H_{31}NO_4)_2 \cdot C_4H_4O_4$ and it has a molecular weight of 766.97.

Bisoprolol Fumarate is a white crystalline powder, approximately equally hydrophilic and lipophilic, and readily soluble in water, methanol, ethanol, and chloroform.

Hydrochlorothiazide (HCTZ) is 6-Chloro-3,4-dihydro-2H-1,2,4- benzothiadiazine-7-sulfonamide 1.1-dioxide. It is a white, or practically white, practically odorless crystalline powder. It is slightly soluble in water, sparingly soluble in dilute sodium hydroxide solution, freely soluble in n-butylamine and dimethylformamide, soluble in methanol, and insoluble in ether, chloroform, and dilute mineral acids. Its empirical formula is $C_7H_8ClN_3O_4S_2$ and it has a molecular weight of 297.73.

Each Bisoprolol/HCTZ 2.5 mg/6.25 mg tablet for oral administration contains:	
Bisoprolol Fumarate	2.5 mg
Hydrochlorothiazide	6.25 mg

Each Bisoprolol/HCTZ 5 mg/6.25 mg tablet for oral administration contains:	
Bisoprolol Fumarate	5 mg
Hydrochlorothiazide	6.25 mg

Each Bisoprolol/HCTZ 10 mg/6.25 mg tablet for oral administration contains:	
Bisoprolol Fumarate	10 mg
Hydrochlorothiazide	6.25 mg

CLINICAL PHARMACOLOGY

Bisoprolol Fumarate and HCTZ have been used individually and in combination for the treatment of hypertension. The antihypertensive effects of these agents are additive; HCTZ 6.25 mg significantly increases the antihypertensive effect of Bisoprolol Fumarate. The incidence of hypokalemia with the Bisoprolol Fumarate and HCTZ 6.25 mg combination (B/H) is significantly lower than with HCTZ 25 mg. In clinical trials of Bisoprolol/HCTZ mean changes in serum potassium for patients treated with Bisoprolol/HCTZ 2.5/6.25 mg, 5/6.25 mg or 10/6.25 mg or placebo were less than ± 0.1 mEq/L. Mean changes in serum potassium for patients treated with any dose of Bisoprolol in combination with HCTZ 25 mg ranged from -0.1 to -0.3 mEq/L. Bisoprolol Fumarate is a beta$_1$-selective (cardioselective) adrenoceptor blocking agent without significant membrane stabilizing or intrinsic sympathomimetic activities in its therapeutic dose range. At higher doses (≥ 20 mg) Bisoprolol Fumarate also inhibits beta$_2$-adrenoreceptors located in bronchial and vascular musculature. To retain relative selectivity, it is important to use the lowest effective dose.

Hydrochlorothiazide is a benzothiadiazine diuretic. Thiazides affect renal tubular mechanisms of electrolyte reabsorption and increase excretion of sodium and chloride in approximately equivalent amounts. Natriuresis causes a secondary loss of potassium.

PHARMACOKINETICS AND METABOLISM:

Bisoprolol/HCTZ: In healthy volunteers, both Bisoprolol Fumarate and Hydrochlorothiazide are well absorbed following oral administration of Bisoprolol/HCTZ. No change is observed in the bioavailability of either agent when given together in a single tablet. Absorption is not affected whether Bisoprolol/HCTZ is taken with or without food. Mean peak Bisoprolol Fumarate plasma concentrations of about 9.0 ng/mL, 19 ng/mL and 36 ng/mL occur approximately 3 hours after the administration of the 2.5 mg/6.25 mg, 5 mg/6.25 mg and 10 mg/6.25 mg combination tablets, respectively. Mean peak plasma Hydrochlorothiazide concentrations of 30 ng/mL occur approximately 2.5 hours following the administration of the combination. Dose proportional increase in plasma Bisoprolol concentrations are observed between the 2.5 and 5, as well as between the 5 and 10 mg doses. The elimination of T$_{1/2}$ of Bisoprolol ranges from 7 to 15 hours and of Hydrochlorothiazide ranges from 4 to 10 hours. The percent of dose excreted unchanged in urine is about 55% for Bisoprolol and about 60% for Hydrochlorothiazide.

Bisoprolol Fumarate: The absolute bioavailability after a 10 mg oral dose of Bisoprolol Fumarate is about 80%. The first pass metabolism of Bisoprolol Fumarate is about 20%.

The pharmacokinetic profile of Bisoprolol Fumarate has been examined following single doses and at steady state. Binding to serum proteins is approximately 30%. Peak plasma concentrations occur within 2 to 4 hours of dosing with 2.5 to 20 mg, and mean peak values range from 9.0 ng/mL at 2.5 mg to 70 ng/mL at 20 mg. Once-daily dosing with Bisoprolol Fumarate results in less than twofold intersubject variation in peak plasma concentrations. Plasma concentrations are proportional to the administered dose in the range of 2.5 to 20 mg. The plasma elimination half-life is 9 to 12 hours and is slightly longer in elderly patients, in part because of decreased renal function. Steady state is attained within 5 days with once-daily dosing. In both young and elderly populations, plasma accumulation is low; the accumulation factor ranges from 1.1 to 1.3, and is what would be expected from the half-life and once-daily dosing. Bisoprolol is eliminated equally by renal and nonrenal pathways with about 50% of the dose appearing unchanged in the urine and the remainder in the form of inactive metabolites. In humans, the known metabolites are labile or have no known pharmacologic activity. Less than 2% of the dose is excreted in the feces. The pharmacokinetic characteristics of the two enantiomers are similar. Bisoprolol is not metabolized by cytochrome P450 II D6 (debrisoquin hydroxylase).

In subjects with creatinine clearance less than 40 mL/min, the plasma half-life is increased approximately threefold compared to healthy subjects.

In patients with liver cirrhosis, the rate of elimination of Bisoprolol is more variable and significantly slower than that in healthy subjects, with a plasma half-life ranging from 8 to 22 hours.

In elderly subjects, mean plasma concentrations at steady state are increased, in part attributed to lower creatinine clearance. However, no significant differences in the degree of Bisoprolol accumulation is found between young and elderly populations.

Hydrochlorothiazide: Hydrochlorothiazide is well absorbed (65% to 75%) following oral administration. Absorption of Hydrochlorothiazide is reduced in patients with congestive heart failure.

Peak plasma concentrations are observed within 1 to 5 hours of dosing, and range from 70 to 490 ng/mL following oral doses of 12.5 to 100 mg. Plasma concentrations are linearly related to the administered dose. Concentrations of Hydrochlorothiazide are 1.6 to 1.8 times higher in whole blood than in plasma. Binding to serum proteins has been reported to be approximately 40% to 68%. The plasma elimination half-life has been reported to be 6 to 15 hours. Hydrochlorothiazide is eliminated primarily by renal pathways. Following oral doses of 12.5 to 100 mg, 55% to 77% of the administered dose appears in urine and greater than 95% of the absorbed dose is excreted in urine as unchanged drug. Plasma concentrations of Hydrochlorothiazide are increased and the elimination half-life is prolonged in patients with renal disease.

PHARMACODYNAMICS:

Bisoprolol Fumarate: Findings in clinical hemodynamics studies with Bisoprolol Fumarate are similar to those observed with other beta-blockers. The most prominent effect is the negative chronotropic effect, giving a reduction in resting and exercise heart rate. There is a fall in resting and exercise cardiac output with little observed change in stroke volume, and only a small increase in right atrial pressure, or pulmonary capillary wedge pressure at rest or during exercise.

In normal volunteers, Bisoprolol Fumarate therapy resulted in a reduction of exercise- and isoproterenol-induced tachycardia. The maximal effect occurred within 1 to 4 hours postdosing. Effects generally persisted for 24 hours at doses of 5 mg or greater.

In controlled clinical trials, Bisoprolol Fumarate given as a single daily dose has been shown to be an effective antihypertensive agent when used alone or concomitantly with thiazide diuretics (see *"Clinical Studies"*).

The mechanism of Bisoprolol Fumarate's antihypertensive effect has not been completely established. Factors that may be involved include:
1. Decreased cardiac output
2. Inhibition of renin release by the kidneys
3. Diminution of tonic sympathetic outflow from vasomotor centers in the brain

Beta$_1$-selectivity of Bisoprolol Fumarate has been demonstrated in both animal and human studies. No effects at therapeutic doses on beta$_2$-adrenoreceptor density have been observed. Pulmonary function studies have been conducted in healthy volunteers, asthmatics, and patients with chronic obstructive pulmonary disease (COPD). Doses of Bisoprolol Fumarate ranged from 5 to 60 mg, atenolol from 50 to 200 mg, metoprolol from 100 to 200 mg, and propranolol from 40 to 80 mg. In some studies, slight, asymptomatic increases in airway resistance (AWR) and decreases in forced expiratory volume (FEV$_1$) were observed with doses of Bisoprolol Fumarate 20 mg and higher, similar to the small increases in AWR noted with other cardioselective beta-blocking agents. The changes induced by beta-blockade with all agents were reversed by bronchodilator therapy.

Electrophysiology studies in man have demonstrated that Bisoprolol Fumarate significantly decreases heart rate, increases sinus node recovery time, prolongs AV node refractory periods, and, with rapid atrial stimulation, prolongs AV nodal conduction.

Hydrochlorothiazide: Acute effects of thiazides are thought to result from a reduction in blood volume and cardiac output, secondary to a natriuretic effect, although a direct vasodilatory mechanism has also been proposed. With chronic administration, plasma volume returns toward normal, but peripheral vascular resistance is decreased.

Thiazides do not affect normal blood pressure. Onset of action occurs within 2 hours of dosing, peak effect is observed at about 4 hours, and activity persists for up to 24 hours.

CLINICAL STUDIES

In controlled clinical trials, Bisoprolol Fumarate/Hydrochlorothiazide 6.25 mg has been shown to reduce systolic and diastolic blood pressure throughout a 24-hour period when administered once daily. The effects on systolic and diastolic blood pressure reduction of the combination of Bisoprolol Fumarate and Hydrochlorothiazide were additive. Further, treatment effects were consistent across age groups (< 60, ≥ 60 years), racial groups (black, nonblack), and gender (male, female).

In two randomized, double-blind, placebo-controlled trials conducted in the U.S., reductions in systolic and diastolic blood pressure and heart rate 24 hours after dosing in patients with mild-to-moderate hypertension are shown below.

In both studies mean systolic/diastolic blood pressure and heart rate at baseline were approximately 151/101 mm Hg and 77 bpm. (See related table).

Blood pressure responses were seen within 1 week of treatment but the maximum effect was apparent after 2 to 3 weeks of treatment. Overall, significantly greater blood pressure reductions were observed on Bisoprolol/HCTZ than on placebo. Further, blood pressure reductions were significantly greater for each of the Bisoprolol Fumarate plus Hydrochlorothiazide combinations than for either of the components used alone regardless of race, age, or gender. There were no significant differences in response between black and nonblack patients.

INDICATIONS AND USAGE
Bisoprolol/HCTZ is indicated in the management of hypertension.

CONTRAINDICATIONS
Bisoprolol/HCTZ is contraindicated in patients in cardiogenic shock, overt cardiac failure (see *"Warnings"*), second or third degree AV block, marked sinus bradycardia, anuria, and hypersensitivity to either component of this product or to other sulfonamide-derived drugs.

WARNINGS
Cardiac Failure: In general, beta-blocking agents should be avoided in patients with overt congestive failure. However, in some patients with compensated cardiac failure, it may be necessary to utilize these agents. In such situations, they must be used cautiously.

Patients Without a History of Cardiac Failure: Continued depression of the myocardium with beta-blockers can, in some patients, precipitate cardiac failure. At the first signs or symptoms of heart failure, discontinuation of Bisoprolol/HCTZ should be considered. In some cases Bisoprolol/HCTZ therapy can be continued while heart failure is treated with other drugs.

Abrupt Cessation of Therapy: Exacerbations of angina pectoris and, in some instances, myocardial infarction or ventricular arrhythmia, have been observed in patients with coronary artery disease following abrupt cessation of therapy with beta-blockers. Such patients should, therefore, be cautioned against interruption or discontinuation of therapy without the physician's advice. Even in patients without overt coronary artery disease, it may be advisable to taper therapy with Bisoprolol/HCTZ over approximately 1 week with the patient under careful observation. If withdrawal symptoms occur, beta-blocking agent therapy should be reinstituted, at least temporarily.

Peripheral Vascular Disease: Beta-blockers can precipitate or aggravate symptoms of arterial insufficiency in patients with peripheral vascular disease. Caution should be exercised in such individuals.

Bronchospastic Disease: PATIENTS WITH BRONCHOSPASTIC PULMONARY DISEASE SHOULD, IN GENERAL, NOT RECEIVE BETA-BLOCKERS. Because of the relative beta$_1$-selectivity of Bisoprolol Fumarate, Bisoprolol/HCTZ may be used with caution in patients with bronchospastic disease who do not respond to, or who cannot tolerate other antihypertensive treatment. Since beta$_1$-selectivity is not absolute, the lowest possible dose of Bisoprolol/HCTZ should be used. A beta$_2$ agonist (bronchodilator) should be made available.

Anesthesia and Major Surgery: If Bisoprolol/HCTZ treatment is to be continued perioperatively, particular care should be taken when anesthetic agents that depress myocardial function, such as ether, cyclopropane, and trichloroethylene, are used (see *"Overdosage"*) for information on treatment of bradycardia and hypotension.

Diabetes and Hypoglycemia: Beta-blockers may mask some of the manifestations of hypoglycemia, particularly tachycardia. Nonselective beta-blockers may potentiate insulin-induced hypoglycemia and delay recovery of serum glucose levels. Because of its beta$_1$-selectivity, this is less likely with Bisoprolol Fumarate. However, patients subject to spontaneous hypoglycemia, or diabetic patients receiving insulin or oral hypoglycemic agents, should be cautioned about these possibilities. Also, latent diabetes mellitus may become manifest and diabetic patients given thiazides may require adjustment of their insulin dose. Because of the very low dose of HCTZ employed, this may be less likely with Bisoprolol/HCTZ.

Thyrotoxicosis: Beta-adrenergic blockade may mask clinical signs of hyperthyroidism, such as tachycardia. Abrupt withdrawal of beta-blockade may be followed by an exacerbation of the symptoms of hyperthyroidism or may precipitate thyroid storm.

Renal Disease: Cumulative effects of the thiazides may develop in patients with impaired renal function. In such patients, thiazides may precipitate azotemia. In subjects with creatinine clearance less than 40 mL/min, the plasma half-life of Bisoprolol Fumarate is increased up to threefold, as compared to healthy subjects. If progressive renal impairment becomes apparent, Bisoprolol/HCTZ should be discontinued. (see *"Pharmacokinetics and Metabolism."*)

Hepatic Disease: Bisoprolol/HCTZ should be used with caution in patients with impaired hepatic function or progressive liver disease. Thiazides may alter fluid and electrolyte balance, which may precipitate hepatic coma. Also, elimination of Bisoprolol Fumarate is significantly slower in patients with cirrhosis than in healthy subjects. (see *"Pharmacokinetics and Metabolism."*)

PRECAUTIONS
General: Electrolyte and Fluid Balance Status: Although the probability of developing hypokalemia is reduced with Bisoprolol/HCTZ because of the very low dose of HCTZ employed, periodic determination of serum electrolytes should be performed, and patients should be observed for signs of fluid or electrolyte disturbances, ie, hyponatremia, hypochloremic alkalosis, and hypokalemia and hypomagnesemia. Thiazides have been shown to increase the urinary excretion of magnesium; this may result in hypomagnesemia. Warning signs or symptoms of fluid and electrolyte imbalance include dryness of mouth, thirst, weakness, lethargy, drowsiness, restlessness, muscle pains or cramps, muscular fatigue, hypotension, oliguria, tachycardia, and gastrointestinal disturbances such as nausea and vomiting. Hypokalemia may develop, especially with brisk diuresis when severe cirrhosis is present, during concomitant use of corticosteroids or

SITTING SYSTOLIC/DIASTOLIC PRESSURE (BP) AND HEART RATE (HR) MEAN DECREASE (Δ) AFTER 3-4 WEEKS

	Study 1			Study 2		
n=	Placebo 75	B5/H6.25 mg 150	Placebo 56	H6.25 mg 23	B2.5/H6.25 mg 28	B10/H6.25 mg 25
Total Δ BP (mm Hg)	-2.9/-3.9	-15.8/-12.6	-3.0/-3.7	-6.6/-5.8	-14.1/-10.5	-15.3/-14.3
Drug Effect[a]	—/—	-12.9/-8.7	—/—	-3.6/-2.1	-11.1/-6.8	-12.3/-10.6
Total ΔHR (bpm)	-0.3	-6.9	-1.6	-0.8	-3.7	-9.8
Drug Effect[a]	—	-6.6	—	+0.8	-2.1	-8.2

[a] *Observed mean change from baseline minus placebo.*

adrenocorticotropic hormone (ACTH) or after prolonged therapy. Interference with adequate oral electrolyte intake will also contribute to hypokalemia. Hypokalemia and hypomagnesemia can provoke ventricular arrhythmias or sensitize or exaggerate the response of the heart to the toxic effects of digitalis. Hypokalemia may be avoided or treated by potassium supplementation or increased intake of potassium-rich foods.

Dilutional hyponatremia may occur in edematous patients in hot weather; appropriate therapy is water restriction rather than salt administration, except in rare instances when the hyponatremia is life-threatening. In actual salt depletion, appropriate replacement is the therapy of choice.

Parathyroid Disease: Calcium excretion is decreased by thiazides, and pathologic changes- in the parathyroid glands, with hypercalcemia and hypophosphatemia, have been observed in a few patients on prolonged thiazide therapy.

Hyperuricemia: Hyperuricemia or acute gout may be precipitated in certain patients receiving thiazide diuretics. Bisoprolol Fumarate, alone or in combination with HCTZ, has been associated with increases in uric acid. However, in U.S. clinical trials, the incidence of treatment-related increases in uric acid was higher during therapy with HCTZ 25 mg (25%) than with B/H 6.25 mg (10%). Because of the very low dose of HCTZ employed, hyperuricemia may be less likely with Bisoprolol/HCTZ.

Drug Interactions: Bisoprolol/HCTZ may potentiate the action of other antihypertensive agents used concomitantly. Bisoprolol/HCTZ should not be combined with other beta-blocking agents. Patients receiving catecholamine-depleting drugs, such as reserpine or guanethidine, should be closely monitored because the added beta-adrenergic blocking action of Bisoprolol Fumarate may produce excessive reduction of sympathetic activity. In patients receiving concurrent therapy with clonidine, if therapy is to be discontinued, it is suggested that Bisoprolol/HCTZ be discontinued for several days before the withdrawal of clonidine. Bisoprolol/HCTZ should be used with caution when myocardial depressants or inhibitors of AV conduction, such as certain calcium antagonists (particularly of the phenylalkylamine [verapamil] and benzothiazepine [diltiazem] classes), or antiarrhythmic agents, such as disopyramide, are used concurrently.

Bisoprolol Fumarate: Concurrent use of rifampin increases the metabolic clearance of Bisoprolol Fumarate, shortening its elimination half-life. However, initial dose modification is generally not necessary. Pharmacokinetic studies document no clinically relevant interactions with other agents given concomitantly, including thiazide diuretics, digoxin and cimetidine. There was no effect of Bisoprolol Fumarate on prothrombin times in patients on stable doses of warfarin.

Risk of Anaphylactic Reaction: While taking beta-blockers, patients with a history of severe anaphylactic reaction to a variety of allergens may be more reactive to repeated challenge, either accidental, diagnostic, or therapeutic. Such patients may be unresponsive to the usual doses of epinephrine used to treat allergic reactions.

Hydrochlorothiazide: When given concurrently the following drugs may interact with thiazide diuretics.

Alcohol, barbiturates, or narcotics—potentiation of orthostatic hypotension may occur.

Antidiabetic drugs (oral agents and insulin)—dosage adjustment of the antidiabetic drug may be required.

Other antihypertensive drugs—additive effect or potentiation.

Cholestyramine and colestipol resins—absorption of Hydrochlorothiazide is impaired in the presence of anionic exchange resins. Single doses of cholestyramine and colestipol resins bind the Hydrochlorothiazide and reduce its absorption in the gastrointestinal tract by up to 85 and 43 percent, respectively.

Corticosteroids, ACTH—intensified electrolyte depletion, particularly hypokalemia.

Pressor amines (eg, norepinephrine)—possible decreased response to pressor amines but not sufficient to preclude their use.

Skeletal muscle relaxants, nondepolarizing (eg, tubocurarine)—possible increased responsiveness to the muscle relaxant.

Lithium—generally should not be given with diuretics. Diuretic agents reduce the renal clearance of lithium and add a high risk of lithium toxicity. Refer to the package insert for lithium preparations before use of such preparations with Bisoprolol/HCTZ.

Nonsteroidal anti-inflammatory drugs—in some patients, the administration of a nonsteroidal anti-inflammatory agent can reduce the diuretic natriuretic, and antihypertensive effects of loop, potassium-sparing and thiazide diuretics. Therefore, when Bisoprolol/HCTZ and nonsteroidal anti-inflammatory agents are used concomitantly, the patient should be observed closely to determine if the desired effect of the diuretic is obtained.

In patients receiving thiazides, sensitivity reactions may occur with or without a history of allergy or bronchial asthma. Photosensitivity reactions and possible exacerbation or activation of systemic lupus erythematosus have been reported in patients receiving thiazides. The antihypertensive effects of thiazides may be enhanced in the post-sympathectomy patient.

Laboratory Test Interactions: Based on reports involving thiazides. Bisoprolol/HCTZ may decrease serum levels of protein-bound iodine without signs of thyroid disturbance.

Because it includes a thiazide, Bisoprolol/HCTZ should be discontinued before carrying out tests for parathyroid function (see *"Precautions—Parathyroid Disease"*).

INFORMATION FOR PATIENTS

Patients, especially those with coronary artery disease, should be warned against discontinuing use of Bisoprolol/HCTZ without a physician's supervision. Patients should also be advised to consult a physician if any difficulty in breathing occurs, or if they develop other signs or symptoms of congestive heart failure or excessive bradycardia.

Patients subject to spontaneous hypoglycemia, or diabetic patients receiving insulin or oral hypoglycemic agents, should be cautioned that beta-blockers may mask some of the manifestations of hypoglycemia, particularly tachycardia, and Bisoprolol Fumarate should be used with caution.

Patients should know how they react to this medicine before they operate automobiles and machinery or engage in other tasks requiring alertness. Patients should be advised that photosensitivity reactions have been reported with thiazides.

Carcinogenesis, Mutagenesis, Impairment of Fertility:

Carcinogenesis: Bisoprolol/HCTZ: Long-term studies have not been conducted with the Bisoprolol/HCTZ combination.

Bisoprolol Fumarate: Long-term studies were conducted with oral Bisoprolol Fumarate administered in the feed of mice (20 and 24 months) and rats (26 months). No evidence of carcinogenic potential was seen in mice dosed up to 250 mg/kg/day or rats dosed up to 125 mg/kg/day. On a body-weight basis, these doses are 625 and 312 times, respectively, the maximum recommended human dose (MRHD) of 20 mg, or 0.4 mg/kg/day, based on 50 kg individuals; on a body-surface-area basis, these doses are 59 times (mice) and 64 times (rats) the MRHD.

Hydrochlorothiazide: Two-year feeding studies in mice and rats, conducted under the auspices of the National Toxicology Program (NTP), treated mice and rats with doses of Hydrochlorothiazide up to 600 and 100 mg/kg/day, respectively. On a body-weight basis, these doses are 2400 times (in mice) and 400 times (in rats) the MRHD of Hydrochlorothiazide (12.5 mg/day) in Bisoprolol/HCTZ. On a body-surface-area basis, these doses are 226 times (in mice) and 82 times (in rats) the MRHD. These studies uncovered no evidence of carcinogenic potential of Hydrochlorothiazide in rats or female mice, but there was equivocal evidence of hepatocarcinogenicity in male mice.

Mutagenesis: Bisoprolol/HCTZ: The mutagenic potential of the Bisoprolol/HCTZ combination was evaluated in the microbial mutagenicity (Ames) test, the point mutation and chromosomal aberration assays in Chinese hamster V79 cells, and the micronucleus test in mice. There was no evidence of mutagenic potential in these *in vitro* and *in vivo* assays.

Bisoprolol Fumarate: The mutagenic potential of Bisoprolol Fumarate was evaluated in the microbial mutagenicity (Ames) test, the point mutation and chromosome aberration assays in Chinese hamster V79 cells, the unscheduled DNA synthesis test, the micronucleus test in mice, and the cytogenetics assay in rats. There was no evidence of mutagenic potential in these *in vitro* and *in vivo* assays.

Hydrochlorothiazide: Hydrochlorothiazide was not genotoxic in *in vitro* assays using strains TA 98, TA 100, TA 1535, TA 1537 and TA 1538 of *Salmonella typhimurium* (the Ames test); in the Chinese Hamster Ovary (CHO) test for chromosomal aberrations; or in *in vivo* assays using mouse germinal cell chromosomes, Chinese hamster bone marrow chromosomes, and the *Drosophila* sex-linked recessive lethal trait gene. Positive test results were obtained in the *in vitro* CHO Sister Chromatid Exchange (clastogenicity) test and in the mouse Lymphoma Cell (mutagenicity) assays, using concentrations of Hydrochlorothiazide of 43 to 1300 µg/mL. Positive test results were also obtained in the *Aspergillus nidulans* nondisjunction assay, using an unspecified concentration of Hydrochlorothiazide.

Impairment of Fertility: Bisoprolol/HCTZ: Reproduction studies in rats did not show any impairment of fertility with the Bisoprolol/HCTZ combination doses containing up to 30 mg/kg/day of Bisoprolol Fumarate in combination with 75 mg/kg/day of Hydrochlorothiazide. On a body-weight basis, these doses are 75 and 300 times, respectively, the MRHD of Bisoprolol Fumarate and Hydrochlorothiazide. On a body-surface-area basis, these study doses are 15 and 62 times, respectively, the MRHD.

Bisoprolol Fumarate: Reproduction studies in rats did not show any impairment of fertility at doses up to 150 mg/kg/day of Bisoprolol Fumarate, or 375 and 77 times the MRHD on the basis of body-weight and body-surface-area, respectively.

Hydrochlorothiazide: Hydrochlorothiazide had no adverse effects on the fertility of mice and rats of either sex in studies wherein these species were exposed, via their diet, to doses of up to 100 and 4 mg/kg/day, respectively, prior to mating and throughout gestation. Corresponding multiples of maximum recommended human doses are 400 (mice) and 16 (rats) on the basis of body-weight and 38 (mice) and 3.3 (rats) on the basis of body-surface-area.

Pregnancy: Teratogenic Effects-Pregnancy Category C: Bisoprolol/HCTZ in rats, the Bisoprolol Fumarate/Hydrochlorothiazide (B/H) combination was not teratogenic at doses up to 51.4 mg/kg/day of Bisoprolol Fumarate in combination with 128.6 mg/kg/day of Hydrochlorothiazide. Bisoprolol Fumarate and Hydrochlorothiazide doses used in the rat study are, as multiples of the MRHD in the combination, 129 and 514 times greater, respectively, on a body-weight basis, and 26 and 106 times greater, respectively, on the basis of body-surface-area. The drug combination was maternotoxic (decreased body weight and food consumption) at B5.7/H14.3 (mg/kg/day) and higher, and fetotoxic (increased late resorptions) at B17.1/H42.9 (mg/kg/day) and higher. Maternotoxicity was present at 14/57 times the MRHD of B/H, respectively, on a body-weight basis, and 3/12 times the

MRHD of B/H doses, respectively, on the basis of body-surface-area. Fetotoxicity was present at 43/172 times the MRHD of B/H, respectively, on a body-weight basis, and 9/35 times the MRHD of B/H doses, respectively, on the basis of body-surface-area. In rabbits, the B/H combination was not teratogenic at doses of B10/H25 (mg/kg/day). Bisoprolol Fumarate and Hydrochlorothiazide used in the rabbit study were not teratogenic at 25/100 times the B/H MRHD, respectively, on a body-weight basis, and 10/40 times the B/H MRHD, respectively, on the basis of body-surface-area. The drug combination was maternotoxic (decreased body weight) at B1/H2.5 (mg/kg/day) and higher, and fetotoxic (increased resorptions) at B10/H25 (mg/kg/day). The multiples of the MRHD for the B/H combination that were maternotoxic were, respectively, 2.5/10 (on the basis of body-weight) and 1/4 (on the basis of body-surface-area), and for fetotoxicity were, respectively, 25/100 (on the basis of body-weight) and 10/40 (on the basis of body-surface-area).

There are no adequate and well-controlled studies with Bisoprolol/HCTZ in pregnant women. Bisoprolol/HCTZ should be used during pregnancy only if the potential benefit justifies the risk to the fetus.

Bisoprolol Fumarate: In rats, Bisoprolol Fumarate was not teratogenic at doses up to 150 mg/kg/day, which were 375 and 77 times the MRHD on the basis of body-weight and body-surface-area, respectively. Bisoprolol Fumarate was fetotoxic (increased late resorptions) at 50 mg/kg/day and maternotoxic (decreased food intake and body-weight gain) at 150 mg/kg/day. The fetotoxicity in rats occurred at 125 times the MRHD on a body-weight basis and 26 times the MRHD on the basis of body-surface-area. The maternotoxicity occurred at 375 times the MRHD on a body-weight basis and 77 times the MRHD on the basis of body-surface-area. In rabbits, Bisoprolol Fumarate was not teratogenic at doses up to 12.5 mg/kg/day, which is 31 and 12 times the MRHD based on body-weight and body-surface-area, respectively, but was embryolethal (increased early resorptions) at 12.5 mg/kg/day.

Hydrochlorothiazide: Hydrochlorothiazide was orally administered to pregnant mice and rats during respective periods of major organogenesis at doses up to 3000 and 1000 mg/kg/day, respectively. At these doses, which are multiples of the MRHD equal to 12,000 for mice and 4000 for rats, based on body-weight, and equal to 1129 for mice and 824 for rats, based on body-surface-area, there was no evidence of harm to the fetus. There are, however, no adequate and well-controlled studies in pregnant women. Because animal reproduction studies are not always predictive of human response, this drug should be used during pregnancy only if clearly needed.

Nonteratogenic Effects: Thiazides cross the placental barrier and appear in the cord blood. The use of thiazides in pregnant women requires that the anticipated benefit be weighted against possible hazards to the fetus. These hazards include fetal or neonatal jaundice, pancreatitis, thrombocytopenia, and possibly other adverse reactions which have occurred in the adult.

Nursing Mothers: Bisoprolol Fumarate alone or in combination with HCTZ has not been studied in nursing mothers. Thiazides are excreted in human breast milk. Small amounts of Bisoprolol Fumarate (< 2% of the dose) have been detected in the milk of lactating rats. Because of the potential for serious adverse reactions in nursing infants, a decision should be made whether to discontinue nursing or to discontinue the drug, taking into account the importance of the drug to the mother.

Use in Elderly Patients: In clinical trials, at least 270 patients treated with Bisoprolol Fumurate plus HCTZ were 60 years of age or older. HCTZ added significantly to the antihypertensive effect of Bisoprolol in elderly hypertensive patients. No overall differences in effectiveness or safety were observed between these patients and younger patients. Other reported clinical experience has not identified differences in responses between the elderly and younger patients, but greater sensitivity of some older individuals cannot be ruled out.

Pediatric Use: Safety and effectiveness of Bisoprolol/HCTZ in children have not been established.

ADVERSE REACTIONS

Bisoprolol/HCTZ: Bisoprolol Fumarate/H6.25 mg is well tolerated in most patients. Most adverse effects (AEs) have been mild and transient. In more than 65,000 patients treated worldwide with Bisoprolol Fumarate, occurrences of bronchospasm have been rare. Discontinuation rates for AEs were similar for B/H6.25 mg and placebo-treated patients.

In the United States, 252 patients received Bisoprolol Fumarate (2.5, 5, 10, or 40 mg)/H6.25 mg and 144 patients received placebo in two controlled trials. In Study 1, Bisoprolol Fumarate 5/H6.25 mg was administered for 4 weeks. In Study 2, Bisoprolol Fumarate 2.5, 10 or 40/H6.25 mg was administered for 12 weeks. All adverse experiences, whether drug related or not, and drug related adverse experiences in patients treated with B2.5-10/H6.25 mg, reported during comparable, 4 week treatment periods by at least 2% of Bisoprolol Fumarate/H6.25 mg-treated patients (plus additional selected adverse experiences) are presented in the following table: (See related table).

Other adverse experiences that have been reported with the individual components are listed below.

BISOPROLOL FUMARATE

In clinical trials worldwide, a variety of other AEs, in addition to those listed above, have been reported. While in many cases it is not known whether a causal relationship exists between Bisoprolol and these AEs, they are listed to alert the physician to a possible relationship.

Central Nervous System: Unsteadiness, vertigo, syncope, paresthesia, hyperesthesia, sleep disturbance/vivid dreams, depression, anxiety/restlessness, decreased concentration/memory.

Cardiovascular: Palpitations and other rhythm disturbances, cold extremities, claudication, hypotension, orthostatic hypotension, chest pain, congestive heart failure.

Gastrointestinal: Gastric/epigastric/abdominal pain, peptic ulcer, gastritis, vomiting, constipation, dry mouth.

Musculoskeletal: Arthralgia, muscle/joint pain, back/neck pain, twitching/tremor.

Skin: Rash, acne, eczema, psoriasis, skin irritation, pruritus, purpura, flushing, sweating, alopecia, dermatitis, exfoliative dermatitis (very rarely).

Special Senses: Visual disturbances, ocular pain/pressure, abnormal lacrimation, tinnitus, decreased hearing, earache, taste abnormalities.

Metabolic: Gout.

Respiratory: Asthma, bronchitis, dyspnea, pharyngitis, sinusitis.

Genitourinary: Peyronie's disease (very rarely), cystitis, renal colic, polyuria.

General: Malaise, edema, weight gain, angioedema.

In addition, a variety of adverse effects have been reported with other beta-adrenergic blocking agents and should be considered potential adverse effects:

Central Nervous System: Reversible mental depression progressing to catatonia, hallucinations, an acute reversible syndrome characterized by disorientation to time and place, emotional lability, slightly clouded sensorium.

Allergic: Fever, combined, with aching and sore throat, laryngospasm, and respiratory distress.

Hematologic: Agranulocytosis, thrombocytopenia.

Gastrointestinal: Mesenteric arterial thrombosis and ischemic colitis.

Miscellaneous: The oculomucocutaneous syndrome associated with the beta-blocker practolol has not been reported with Bisoprolol Fumarate during investigational use or extensive foreign marketing experience.

HYDROCHLOROTHIAZIDE:
The following adverse experiences, in addition to those listed in the above table, have been reported with Hydrochlorothiazide (generally with doses of 25 mg or greater).

General: Weakness.

Central Nervous System: Vertigo, paresthesia, restlessness.

Cardiovascular: Orthostatic hypotension (may be potentiated by alcohol, barbiturates, or narcotics).

Gastrointestinal: Anorexia, gastric irritation, cramping, constipation, jaundice (intrahepatic cholestatic jaundice), pancreatitis, cholecystitis, sialadenitis, dry mouth.

Musculoskeletal: Muscle spasm.

Hypersensitive Reactions: Purpura, photosensitivity, rash, urticaria, necrotizing angiitis (vasculitis and cutaneous vasculitis), fever, respiratory distress including pneumonitis and pulmonary edema, anaphylactic reactions.

Special Senses: Transient blurred vision, xanthopsia.

Metabolic: Gout.

Genitourinary: Sexual dysfunction, renal failure, renal dysfunction, interstitial nephritis.

LABORATORY ABNORMALITIES

Bisoprolol/HCTZ: Because of the low dose of Hydrochlorothiazide in Bisoprolol/HCTZ adverse metabolic effects with B/H6.25 mg are less frequent and of smaller magnitude than with HCTZ 25 mg. Laboratory data on serum potassium from the U.S. placebo-controlled trials are shown in the following table: (See related table).

Treatment with both beta blockers and thiazide diuretics is associated with increases in uric acid. However, the magnitude of the change in patients treated with B/H6.25 mg was smaller than in patients treated with HCTZ 25 mg. Mean increases in serum triglycerides were observed in patients treated with Bisoprolol Fumarate and Hydrochlorothiazide 6.25 mg. Total cholesterol was generally unaffected, but small decreases in HDL cholesterol were noted.

Other laboratory abnormalities that have been reported with the individual components are listed below.

Bisoprolol Fumarate: In clinical trials, the most frequently reported laboratory change was an increase in serum triglycerides, but this was not a consistent finding.

Sporadic liver test abnormalities have been reported. In the U.S. controlled trials experience with Bisoprolol Fumarate treatment for 4 to 12 weeks, the incidence of concomitant elevations in SGOT and SGPT of between 1 and 2 times normal was 3.9%, compared to 2.5% for placebo. No patient had concomitant elevations greater than twice normal.

In the long-term, uncontrolled experience with Bisoprolol Fumarate treatment for 6 to 18 months, the incidence of one or more concomitant elevations in SGOT and SGPT of between 1 and 2 times normal was 6.2%. The incidence of multiple occurrence was 1.9%. For concomitant elevations in SGOT and SGPT of greater than twice normal, the incidence was 1.5%. The incidence of multiple occurrences was 0.3%. In many cases these elevations were attributed to underlying disorders, or resolved during continued treatment with Bisoprolol Fumarate.

Other laboratory changes included small increases in uric acid, creatinine, BUN, serum potassium, glucose, and phosphorus and decreases in WBC and platelets. There have been occasional reports of eosinophilia. These were generally not of clinical importance and rarely resulted in discontinuation of Bisoprolol Fumarate.

As with other beta-blockers, ANA conversions have also been reported on Bisoprolol Fumarate. About 15% of patients in long-term studies converted to a positive titer, although about one-third of these patients subsequently reconverted to a negative titer while on continued therapy.

Hydrochlorothiazide: Hyperglycemia, glycosuria, hyperuricemia, hypokalemia and other electrolyte imbalances (see "Precautions"), hyperlipidemia, hypercalcemia, leukopenia, agranulocytosis, thrombo- cytopenia, aplastic anemia, and hemolytic anemia have been associated with HCTZ therapy.

OVERDOSAGE

While there have been no reports of overdose with Bisoprolol/HCTZ several cases of overdose with Bisoprolol Fumarate have been reported (maximum: 2000 mg). Bradycardia and/or hypotension were noted. Sympathomimetic agents were given in some cases, and all patients recovered.

The most frequently observed signs expected with overdosage of a beta-blocker are bradycardia and hypotension. Lethargy is also common, and with severe overdoses, delirium, coma, convulsions, and respiratory arrest have been reported to occur. Congestive heart failure, bronchospasm, and hypoglycemia may occur, particularly in patients with underlying conditions. With thiazide diuretics, acute intoxication is rare. The most prominent feature of overdose is acute loss of fluid and electrolytes. Signs and symptoms include cardiovascular (tachycardia, hypotension, shock), neuromuscular (weakness, confusion, dizziness, cramps of the calf muscles, paresthesia, fatigue, impairment of consciousness), gastrointestinal (nausea, vomiting, thirst), renal (polyuria, oliguria, or anuria [due to hemoconcentration]), and laboratory findings (hypokalemia, hyponatremia, hy-

pochloremia, alkalosis, increased BUN [especially in patients with renal insufficiency]).

If overdosage of Bisoprolol/HCTZ is suspected, therapy with Bisoprolol/HCTZ should be discontinued and the patient observed closely. Treatment is symptomatic and supportive: there is no specific antidote. Limited data suggest Bisoprolol Fumarate is not dialyzable; similarly, there is no indication that Hydrochlorothiazide is dialyzable. Suggested general measures include induction of emesis and/or gastric lavage, administration of activated charcoal, respiratory support, correction of fluid and electrolyte imbalance, and treatment of convulsions. Based on the expected pharmacologic actions and recommendations for other beta-blockers and Hydrochlorothiazide, the following measures should be considered when clinically warranted:

Bradycardia: Administer IV atropine. If the response is inadequate, isoproterenol or another agent with positive chronotropic properties may be given cautiously. Under some circumstances, transvenous pacemaker insertion may be necessary.

Hypotension, Shock: The patient's legs should be elevated. IV fluids should be administered and lost electrolytes (potassium, sodium) replaced. Intravenous glucagon may be useful. Vasopressors should be considered.

Heart Block (second or third degree): Patients should be carefully monitored and treated with isoproterenol infusion or transvenous cardiac pacemaker insertion, as appropriate.

Congestive Heart Failure: Initiate conventional therapy (ie, digitalis, diuretics, vasodilating agents, inotropic agents).

Bronchospasm: Administer a bronchodilator such as isopreterenol and/or aminophylline.

Hypoglycemia: Administer IV glucose.

Surveillance: Fluid and electrolyte balance (especially serum potassium) and renal function should be monitored until normalized.

% OF PATIENTS WITH ADVERSE EXPERIENCES*

Body System/ Adverse Experience	All Adverse Experiences		Drug-related Adverse Experiences	
	Placebo[†] (n = 144) %	B2.5-40/H6.25[†] (n = 252) %	Placebo[†] (n = 144) %	B2.5-10/H6.25[†] (n = 221) %
Cardiovascular				
bradycardia	0.7	1.1	0.7	0.9
arrhythmia	1.4	0.4	0.0	0.0
peripheral ischemia	0.9	0.7	0.9	0.4
chest pain	0.7	1.8	0.0	0.9
Respiratory				
bronchospasm	0.0	0.0	0.0	0.0
cough	1.0	2.2	0.7	1.5
rhinitis	2.0	0.7	0.7	0.9
URI	2.3	2.1	0.0	0.0
Body as a Whole				
asthenia	0.0	0.0	0.0	0.0
fatigue	2.7	4.6	1.7	3.0
peripheral edema	0.7	1.1	0.7	0.9
Central Nervous System				
dizziness	1.8	5.1	1.8	3.2
headache	4.7	4.5	2.7	0.4
Musculoskeletal				
muscle cramps	0.7	1.2	0.7	1.1
myalgia	1.4	2.4	0.0	0.0
Psychiatric				
insomnia	2.4	1.1	2.0	1.2
somnolence	0.7	1.1	0.7	0.9
loss of libido	1.2	0.4	1.2	0.4
impotence	0.7	1.1	0.7	1.1
Gastrointestinal				
diarrhea	1.4	4.3	1.2	1.1
nausea	0.9	1.1	0.9	0.9
dyspepsia	0.7	1.2	0.7	0.9

* *Averages adjusted to combine across studies.*
† *Combined across studies.*

SERUM POTASSIUM DATA FROM U.S. PLACEBO CONTROLLED STUDIES

	Placebo[†] (n = 130*)	B 2.5/H 6.25 mg (n = 28*)	B 5/H 6.25 mg (n = 149*)	B 10/H 6.25 mg (n = 28*)	HCTZ 25 mg[†] (n = 142*)
Potassium					
Mean Change[a] (mEq/L)	+ 0.04	+ 0.11	-0.08	0.00	-0.30
% Hypokalemia[b]	0.0%	0.0%	0.7%	0.0%	5.5%

* *Patients with normal serum potassium at baseline.*
a *Mean change from baseline at Week 4.*
b *Percentage of patients with abnormality at Week 4.*
† *Combined across studies*

DOSAGE AND ADMINISTRATION

Bisoprolol is an effective treatment of hypertension in once-daily doses of 2.5-40 mg, while Hydrochlorothiazide is effective in doses of 15-50 mg. In clinical trials of Bisoprolol/Hydrochlorothiazide combination therapy using Bisoprolol doses of 2.5-20 mg and Hydrochlorothiazide doses of 6.25-25 mg, the antihypertensive effects increased with increasing doses of either component.

The adverse effects (see *"Warnings"*) of Bisoprolol are a mixture of dose-dependent phenomena (primarily bradycardia, diarrhea, asthenia and fatigue) and dose-independent phenomena (eg, occasional rash); those of Hydrochlorothiazide are a mixture of dose-dependent phenomena (primarily hypokalemia) and dose-independent phenomena (eg, possibly pancreatitis); the dose-dependent phenomena for each being much more common than the dose-independent phenomena. The latter consist of those few that are truly idiosyncratic in nature or those that occur with such low frequency that a dose relationship may be difficult to discern.

Therapy with a combination of Bisoprolol and Hydrochlorothiazide will be associated with both sets of dose-independent adverse effects, and to minimize these, it may be appropriate to begin combination therapy only after a patient has failed to achieve the desired effect with monotherapy. On the other hand, regimens that combine low doses of Bisoprolol and Hydrochlorothiazide should produce minimal dose dependent adverse effects, eg, bradycardia, diarrhea, asthenia and fatigue, and minimal dose-dependent adverse metabolic effects, ie, decreases in serum potassium (see *"Clinical Pharmacology"*).

Therapy Guided by Clinical Effect: A patient whose blood pressure is not adequately controlled with 2.5-20 mg Bisoprolol daily may instead be given Bisoprolol/HCTZ. Patients whose blood pressures are adequately controlled with 50 mg of Hydrochlorothiazide daily, but who experience significant potassium loss with this regimen, may achieve similar blood pressure control without electrolyte disturbance if they are switched to Bisoprolol/HCTZ.

Initial Therapy: Antihypertensive therapy may be initiated with the lowest dose of Bisoprolol/HCTZ one 2.5/6.25 mg tablet once daily. Subsequent titration (14 day intervals) may be carried out with Bisoprolol/HCTZ tablets up to the maximum recommended dose 20/12.5 mg (two 10/6.25 mg tablets) once daily, as appropriate.

Replacement Therapy: The combination may be substituted for the titrated individual components.

Cessation of Therapy: If withdrawal of Bisoprolol/HCTZ therapy is planned, it should be achieved gradually over a period of about 2 weeks. Patients should be carefully observed.

Patients with Renal or Hepatic Impairment: As noted in the *"Warnings"* section, caution must be used in dosing/titrating patients with hepatic impairment or renal dysfunction. Since there is no indication that Hydrochlorothiazide is dialyzable, and limited data suggest that Bisoprolol is not dialyzable, drug replacement is not necessary in patients undergoing dialysis.

Elderly Patients: Dosage adjustment on the basis of age is not usually necessary, unless there is also significant renal or hepatic dysfunction (see above and *"Warnings"* section).

Children: There is no pediatric experience with Bisoprolol/HCTZ.

Storage: Store at controlled room temperature, 15-30°C (59-86°F), in a well-closed container.

HOW SUPPLIED
TABLETS: 2.5 MG-6.25 MG

BRAND/MANUFACTURER	NDC	SIZE	AWP
○ **BRAND**			
▶ ZIAC: Lederle Labs	00005-3238-23	100s	$84.41

TABLETS: 5 MG-6.25 MG

BRAND/MANUFACTURER	NDC	SIZE	AWP
○ **BRAND**			
▶ ZIAC: Lederle Labs	00005-3234-23	100s	$84.41

TABLETS: 10 MG-6.25 MG

BRAND/MANUFACTURER	NDC	SIZE	AWP
○ **BRAND**			
▶ ZIAC: Lederle Labs	00005-3235-38	30s	$25.33

Bitolterol Mesylate

DESCRIPTION

Bitolterol Mesylate is the di-*p*-toluate ester of the β-adrenergic bronchodilator *N-t*-butylarterenol (colterol). It has a molecular weight of 557.7. Bitolterol Mesylate is known chemically as 4-[2-[(1,1-dimethylethyl) amino]-1-hydroxyethyl]-1,2-phenylene 4-methylbenzoate (ester) methanesulfonate (salt).

Bitolterol Mesylate, Metered Dose Inhaler, is a complete aerosol unit for oral inhalation. It consists of a plastic-coated bottle of ready-to-use aerosol solution and a detachable plastic mouthpiece with built-in nebulizer.

Each bottle provides at least 300 actuations. Each actuation delivers a measured dose of 0.37 mg of Bitolterol Mesylate as a fine, even mist.

Bitolterol Inhalation Solution contains 0.2% Bitolterol Mesylate.

Each mL of Bitolterol Inhalation Solution, 0.2% contains 2.0 mg of Bitolterol Mesylate.

Following is its chemical structure:

CLINICAL PHARMACOLOGY

Bitolterol Mesylate is administered as a prodrug which is hydrolyzed by esterases in tissue and blood to the active moiety colterol. Bitolterol Mesylate administered as an inhaled aerosol, has a rapid (3 to 4 minutes) onset of bronchodilator activity. The duration of action with Bitolterol Mesylate is at least 5 hours in most patients and 8 or more hours in 25% to 35% of patients, based on 15% or greater increase in forced expiratory volume in one second (FEV$_1$), as demonstrated in 3 month isoproterenol controlled multicenter trials. Based on mean maximal expiratory flow (MMEF) measurements, the duration of action is 6 to 7 hours. The duration of bronchodilator action with Bitolterol Mesylate in these trials is longer than that seen with isoproterenol, especially in steroid-dependent patients. Duration of effect was reduced over time in steroid-dependent asthmatic patients where the duration was 3.5 to 5 hours for FEV$_1$. The mean maximum increase in FEV$_1$ over baseline in the majority of patients was 39% to 42% and occurred by 30 to 60 minutes, similar to that seen in the isoproterenol group.

Bitolterol Mesylate is a beta adrenergic agonist which has been shown by in vitro and in vivo pharmacological studies in animals to exert a preferential effect on beta$_2$ adrenergic receptors, such as those located in bronchial smooth muscle. However, controlled clinical trials in patients who were administered the drug have not revealed a preferential beta$_2$ adrenergic effect. At doses that produced long duration of bronchodilator activity (up to 8 hours in some patients) with a mean maximum bronchodilating effect of approximately 40% increase in FEV$_1$ (forced expiration volume in one second), a less than 10 beat per minute mean maximum increase in heart rate was seen. The effect on the heart rate was transient and similar to the increases seen in the isoproterenol treated patients in these studies.

Although blood levels of colterol formed by gradual release from the pro-drug (Bitolterol) in the lungs are too low to be measured by currently available assay methods, data on disposition are available from oral studies in man. Following oral administration of 5.9 mg tritiated Bitolterol Mesylate to man, radioactivity measurements indicated mean maximum colterol concentration in blood of approximately 2.1 μg/mL one hour after medication. Urinary excretion data indicate that 83 percent of the radioactivity of this oral dose was excreted within the first 24 hours. By 72 hours, 85.6 percent of the tritium had been excreted in the urine and 8.1 percent in the feces. Most of the radioactivity was excreted as conjugated colterol; free colterol accounted for 2.1 to 3.7 percent of the total radioactivity excreted in the urine. No intact Bitolterol was detected in urine.

The pharmacologic effects of β-adrenergic drugs including Bitolterol Mesylate are attributable to stimulation of adenyl cyclase, the enzyme which catalyzes the conversion of adenosine triphosphate (ATP) to cyclic-3', 5'-adenosine monophosphate (c-AMP). Increased c-AMP levels are associated with relaxation of bronchial smooth muscle and with inhibition of release of mediators of immediate hypersensitivity from cells, especially from mast cells.

In a six week clinical trial in which 24 asthmatic patients received Bitolterol Mesylate and theophylline concurrently, improvement in pulmonary function was enhanced over that seen with either drug alone. No potentiation of side effects was observed, and 24-hour ECG recordings (Holter monitoring) indicated no greater degree of cardiac toxicity with Bitolterol Mesylate alone or in combination with theophylline than that which occurred with theophylline alone.

Bitolterol Mesylate did not adversely affect arterial oxygen tension in a blood-gas study in 24 atshmatic patients. However, a decrease in arterial oxygen tension has been reported with other adrenergic bronchodilators and could be anticipated to occur with Bitolterol Mesylate as well.

In repetitive dosing studies, continued effectiveness was demonstrated throughout the 3 month period of treatment in the majority of patients. In steroid-dependent asthmatics, the median duration of bronchodilator activity as measured by FEV$_1$ was greater on the first test day as compared with later test days, but patient response remained constant throughout the balance of the three-month period. Recent studies in laboratory animals (minipigs, rodents, and dogs) recorded the occurence of cardiac arrhythmias and sudden death (with histologic evidence of myocardial necrosis) when beta agonists and methylxanthines were administered concurrently. The significance of these findings when applied to humans is currently unknown.

INDICATIONS AND USAGE

Bitolterol Mesylate is indicated for both prophylactic and therapeutic use as a bronchodilator for bronchial asthma and for reversible bronchospasm. It may be used with or without concurrent theophylline and/or steroid therapy.

CONTRAINDICATIONS

Bitolterol Mesylate is contraindicated in patients who are hypersensitive to any of its ingredients.

WARNINGS

As with other β-adrenergic aerosols, Bitolterol Mesylate should not be used in excess. Use of aerosolized β-adrenergic drugs may have a deleterious cardiac effect. Paradoxical bronchoconstriction has been reported with administration of β-adrenergic agents. Immediate hypersensitivity (allergic) reactions can occur after the administration of Bitolterol Mesylate. In such instances, the drug should be discontinued immediately and alternative therapy instituted.

In controlled clinical studies, clinically significant increases in pulse rate, increases and decreases in systolic and diastolic blood pressure have been demonstrated in individual patients after administration of Bitolterol Mesylate. Therefore, caution should be exercised when administering Bitolterol Mesylate to patients with underlying cardiovascular disease. Even though the changes may be significant in a small number of patients, these changes occur within a short period of time after administration and have not been shown to be persistent.

If an unusual smell or taste is noted with use of this product, the patient should discontinue use in consultation with his/her physician.

PRECAUTIONS

General. As with all β-adrenergic stimulating agents, caution should be used when administering Bitolterol Mesylate to patients with cardiovascular disease such as ischemic heart disease or hypertension. Caution is also advised in patients with hyperthyroidism, diabetes melitus, cardiac arrhythmias, convulsive disorders or unusual responsiveness to β-adrenergic agonists. Significant changes in systolic and diastolic blood pressure have been seen in individual patients and could be expected to occur in some patients after use of any β-adrenergic aerosol bronchodilator.

Information for Patients. The effects of Bitolterol Mesylate may last up to eight hours or longer. It should not be used more often than recommended and the patient should not increase the number of inhalations or frequency of use without first asking the physician. If symptoms of asthma get worse, adverse reactions occur, or the patient does not respond to the usual dose, the patient should be instructed to contact the physician immediately. The patient should be advised to see the Illustrated Directions for Use.

Drug Interactions. Other sympathomimetic aerosol bronchodilators should not be used concomitantly with Bitolterol Mesylate. If additional adrenergic drugs are to be administered by any route, they should be used with caution to avoid deleterious cardiovascular effects.

Bitolterol Mesylate should be administered with caution to patients being treated with monoamine oxidase inhibitors or tricyclic antidepressants, since the action of Bitolterol on the vascular system may be potentiated.

Carcinogenesis, Mutagenesis, and Impairment of Fertility. No tumorigenicity (and specifically no increase in leiomyomas) was observed in a two year oral study in Sprague-Dawley CD rats at doses of Bitolterol Mesylate corresponding to 23 or 114 times the maximal daily human inhalational dose. Bitolterol Mesylate was not tumorigenic in an 18 month oral study in Swiss-Webster mice at doses up to 568 times the maximal daily human inhalational dose.

Ames Salmonella and mouse lymphoma mutation assays in vitro revealed no mutagenesis due to Bitolterol Mesylate. Reproductive studies in male and female rats revealed no significant effects on fertility at doses of Bitolterol Mesylate up to 364 times the maximal daily human inhalational dose.

Teratogenic Effects-Pregnancy Category C. No teratogenic effects were seen in rats and rabbits after oral doses of Bitolterol Mesylate up to 557 times the maximal daily human inhalational dose and in mice after oral doses up to 284 times the maximal daily human inhalational dose.

When Bitolterol Mesylate was injected subcutaneously into mice at doses of 2 mg/kg, 10 mg/kg, 20mg/kg (corresponding to 23, 114, and 227 times the maximal daily human inhalational dose) cleft palate incidences of 5.7 percent, 3.8 percent, and 3.3 percent (compared with 0.9 percent in controls) were found. Cleft palate induction with isoproterenol at 10 mg/kg SC as the positive control was 10.7 percent. Since no well-controlled studies in pregnant women are available. Bitolterol Mesylate should be used during pregnancy only if the potential benefit justifies the potential risk to the fetus.

Nursing Mothers. It is not known whether Bitolterol Mesylate is excreted in human milk. Because many drugs are excreted in human milk, caution should be exercised when Bitolterol Mesylate is administered to a nursing woman.

Pediatric Use. Safety and effectiveness of Bitolterol Mesylate in children 12 years of age or younger has not been established.

ADVERSE REACTIONS

The results of all clinical trials with Bitolterol Mesylate in 492 patients showed the following side effects.

CNS: Tremors (14%), nervousness (5%), headache (4%), dizziness (3%), lightheadedness (3%), insomnia (< 1%), hyperkinesia (< 1%).

Gastrointestinal: Nausea (3%).

Oro-Pharyngeal: Throat irritation (5%).

Cardiovascular: The overall incidence of cardiovascular effects was approximately 5% of patients and these effects included palpitations (approximately 3%), and chest discomfort (approximately 1%). Tachycardia was seen in less than 1%. Premature ventricular contractions and flushing were rarely seen.

Respiratory: Coughing (4%), bronchospasm (< 1%), dyspnea (< 1%), chest tightness (< 1%).

Clinical relevance or relationship to Bitolterol Mesylate administration of rarely reported elevations of SGOT, decrease in platelets, decreases in WBC levels or proteinuria are not known.

In comparing the adverse reactions for Bitolterol Mesylate treated patients to those of isoproterenol treated patients, during three month clinical trials involving approximately 400 patients, the following moderate to severe reactions, as judged by the investigators, were reported for both steroid and non-steroid dependent patients. The table does not include mild reactions or those occurring only with the first dose.

PERCENT INCIDENCE OF MODERATE TO SEVERE ADVERSE REACTIONS

Reaction	Bitolterol N = 197	Isoproterenol N = 194
Central Nervous System		
Tremors	9.1%	1.5%
Nervousness	1.5%	1.0%
Headache	3.5%	6.1%
Dizziness	1.0%	1.5%
Insomnia	0.5%	0%
Cardiovascular		
Palpitations	1.5%	0%
PVC—Transient Increase	0.5%	0%
Chest Discomfort	0.5%	0%
Respiratory		
Cough	4.1%	1.0%
Bronchospasm	1.0%	0%
Dyspnea	1.0%	0%
Oro-Pharyngeal		
Throat Irritation	3.0%	3.1%
Gastrointestinal		
Nausea (Dyspepsia)	0.5%	0.5%

Note: In most patients, the total isoproterenol dosage was divided into three equally dosed inhalations, administered at three minute intervals. This procedure may have reduced the incidence of adverse reactions observed with isoproterenol.

OVERDOSAGE

Overdosage with Bitolterol Mesylate may be expected to result in exaggeration of those drug effects listed in the *"Adverse Reactions"* section. In such cases therapy with Bitolterol Mesylate and all β-adrenergic stimulating drugs should be stopped, supportive therapy provided, and judicious use of a cardioselective β-adrenergic blocking agent should be considered bearing in mind the possibility that such agents can produce profound bronchospasm. As with all sympathomimetic aerosol medications, cardiac arrest and even death may be associated with abuse. The oral LD$_{50}$ of Bitolterol Mesylate in rats was greater than 5000 mg/kg and in mice greater than 6000 mg/kg.

DOSAGE AND ADMINISTRATION

The usual dose to relieve bronchospasm for adults and children over 12 years of age is two inhalations at an interval of at least one to three minutes followed by a third inhalation if needed. For prevention of bronchospasm, the usual dose is two inhalations every 8 hours. The dose of Bitolterol Mesylate should never exceed 3 inhalations every 6 hours or 2 inhalations every 4 hours. Medical consultation should be sought prior to an increase in the frequency of dosing because this may indicate a need for reevaluation of the patient's condition.

Bitolterol Mesylate Inhalation Solution, 0.2% can be administered by nebulization to adults and children over 12 years of age. As with all medications, the physician should begin therapy with the lowest effective dose according to the individual patient's requirements following manufacturer's dosage recommendation. Bitolterol Mesylate should be administered during a ten to fifteen minute period. The treatment period can be adjusted by varying the amount of diluent placed in the nebulizer with the medication. The total volume (medication plus diluent) is usually adjusted to 2.0 mL to 4.0 mL. Safety of the treatment should be monitored by measuring blood pressure and pulse.

Clinical studies were conducted with two types of nebulizer systems.

Intermittent Aerosol Flow (Patient Activated Nebulizer): This nebulizer is operated by a patient activated valve to permit the release of aerosol mist only during inspiration.

Continuous Aerosol Flow Nebulizer: This nebulizer generates a continuous flow of mist while the patient inhales and exhales through an exhaust port. The nebulizer resulting in the loss of some medication through the nebulizer resulting in the loss of some medication through the nebulizer resulting in the loss of some medication through an exhaust port.

When using these types of nebulizer systems the following dosing regimens are recommended:

BITOLTEROL MESYLATE INHALATION SOLUTION, 0.2%

Doses	Intermittent Flow Nebulization		Continuous Flow Nebulization	
	Volume	Bitolterol Mesylate	Volume	Bitolterol Mesylate
Usual Dose	0.5 mL	1.0 mg	1.25 mL	2.5 mg
Decreased Dose	0.25 mL	0.5 mg	0.75 mL	1.5 mg

Doses	Intermittent Flow Nebulization		Continuous Flow Nebulization	
	Volume	Bitolterol Mesylate	Volume	Bitolterol Mesylate
Increased Dose	0.75 mL	1.5 mg	1.75 mL	3.5 mg

Up to 1.0 mL of Bitolterol Mesylate Inhalation Solution, 0.2% (2.0 mg Bitolterol Mesylate), can be administered with the intermittent flow system to severely obstructed patients.

The usual frequency of treatments is three times a day. Treatments may be increased up to four times daily, however the interval between treatments should not be less than four hours. For some patients two treatments a day may be adequate.

The maximum daily dose should not exceed 8.0 mg Bitolterol Mesylate with an intermittent flow nebulization system or 14.0 mg Bitolterol Mesylate with a continuous flow nebulization system. Bitolterol Mesylate Inhalation Solution, 0.2% should be added to the nebulizer just prior to use and should not be left in the nebulizer.

Bitolterol Mesylate Inhalation Solution, 0.2% should not be mixed with other drugs such as cromolyn sodium or acetylcysteine at clinically recommended doses due to chemical and/or physical incompatibilities.

Solution: Do not use the solution if it is discolored or contains a precipitate.
Store at controlled room temperature between 15°C and 30°C (59°F and 86°F).

J CODES
0.2% per 10 ml INH—J7627

HOW SUPPLIED
AEROSOL LIQUID: 0.2%

BRAND/MANUFACTURER	NDC	SIZE	AWP
○ **BRAND** TORNALATE: Dura	51479-0011-03	30 ml	$12.18
	51479-0011-06	60 ml	$23.07

AEROSOL LIQUID W/ADAPTER: 0.8%

BRAND/MANUFACTURER	NDC	SIZE	AWP
○ **BRAND** TORNALATE: Dura	51479-0012-02	15 ml	$32.21
	51479-0012-01	15 ml	$34.28

Blenoxane SEE BLEOMYCIN SULFATE

Bleomycin Sulfate

WARNING
IT IS RECOMMENDED THAT BLEOMYCIN SULFATE BE ADMINISTERED UNDER THE SUPERVISION OF A QUALIFIED PHYSICIAN EXPERIENCED IN THE USE OF CANCER CHEMOTHERAPEUTIC AGENTS.

APPROPRIATE MANAGEMENT OF THERAPY AND COMPLICATIONS IS POSSIBLE ONLY WHEN ADEQUATE DIAGNOSTIC AND TREATMENT FACILITIES ARE READILY AVAILABLE.

PULMONARY FIBROSIS IS THE MOST SEVERE TOXICITY ASSOCIATED WITH BLEOMYCIN SULFATE. THE MOST FREQUENT PRESENTATION IS PNEUMONITIS OCCASIONALLY PROGRESSING TO PULMONARY FIBROSIS. ITS OCCURRENCE IS HIGHER IN ELDERLY PATIENTS AND IN THOSE RECEIVING GREATER THAN 400 UNITS TOTAL DOSE, BUT PULMONARY TOXICITY HAS BEEN OBSERVED IN YOUNG PATIENTS AND THOSE TREATED WITH LOW DOSES.

A SEVERE IDIOSYNCRATIC REACTION CONSISTING OF HYPOTENSION, MENTAL CONFUSION, FEVER, CHILLS, AND WHEEZING HAS BEEN REPORTED IN APPROXIMATELY 1% OF LYMPHOMA PATIENTS TREATED WITH BLEOMYCIN SULFATE.

DESCRIPTION
Bleomycin Sulfate is a mixture of cytotoxic glycopeptide antibiotics isolated from a strain of *Streptomyces verticillus*. It is freely soluble in water.
Note: A unit of Bleomycin Sulfate is equal to the formerly used milligram activity. The term milligram activity is a misnomer and was changed to units to be more precise.

Following is its chemical structure:

(Main component: Bleomycin A₂, in which *R* is $(CH_3)_2S^+CH_2CH_2CH_2—$)

ACTION
Although the exact mechanism of action of Bleomycin Sulfate is unknown, available evidence would seem to indicate that the main mode of action is the inhibition of DNA synthesis with some evidence of lesser inhibition of RNA and protein synthesis.

In mice, high concentrations of Bleomycin Sulfate are found in the skin, lungs, kidneys, peritoneum, and lymphatics. Tumor cells of the skin and lungs have been found to have high concentrations of Bleomycin Sulfate in contrast to the low concentrations found in hematopoietic tissue. The low concentrations of Bleomycin Sulfate found in bone marrow may be related to high levels of Bleomycin Sulfate degradative enzymes found in that tissue.

In patients with a creatinine clearance of > 35 mL per minute, the serum or plasma terminal elimination half-life of Bleomycin Sulfate is approximately 115 minutes. In patients with a creatinine clearance of < 35 mL per minute, the plasma or serum terminal elimination half-life increases exponentially as the creatinine clearance decreases. In humans, 60% to 70% of an administered dose is recovered in the urine as active Bleomycin Sulfate.

INDICATIONS
Bleomycin Sulfate should be considered a palliative treatment. It has been shown to be useful in the management of the following neoplasms either as a single agent or in proven combinations with other approved chemotherapeutic agents:

Squamous Cell Carcinoma: Head and neck (including mouth, tongue, tonsil, nasopharynx, oropharynx, sinus, palate, lip, buccal mucosa, gingiva, epiglottis, larynx), skin, penis, cervix, and vulva. The response to Bleomycin Sulfate is poorer in patients with head and neck cancer previously irradiated.

Lymphomas: Hodgkin's, reticulum cell sarcoma, lymphosarcoma.

Testicular Carcinoma: Embryonal cell, choriocarcinoma, and teratocarcinoma.

UNLABELED USES
Bleomycin Sulfate is used alone or as an adjunct in the treatment of advanced AIDS-related Kaposi's sarcoma.

CONTRAINDICATIONS
Bleomycin Sulfate is contraindicated in patients who have demonstrated a hypersensitive or an idiosyncratic reaction to it.

WARNINGS
Patients receiving Bleomycin Sulfate must be observed carefully and frequently during and after therapy. It should be used with extreme caution in patients with significant impairment of renal function or compromised pulmonary function.

Pulmonary toxicities occur in 10% of treated patients. In approximately 1%, the nonspecific pneumonitis induced by Bleomycin Sulfate progresses to pulmonary fibrosis, and death. Although this is age and dose related, the toxicity is unpredictable. Frequent roentgenograms are recommended.

Idiosyncratic reactions similar to anaphylaxis have been reported in 1% of lymphoma patients treated with Bleomycin Sulfate. Since these usually occur after the first or second dose, careful monitoring is essential after these doses.

Renal or hepatic toxicity, beginning as a deterioration in renal or liver function tests, have been reported infrequently. These toxicities may occur, however, at any time after initiation of therapy.

Usage in Pregnancy: Safe use of Bleomycin Sulfate in pregnant women has not been established.

ADVERSE REACTIONS
Pulmonary: This is potentially the most serious side effect, occurring in approximately 10% of treated patients. The most frequent presentation is pneumonitis occasionally progressing to pulmonary fibrosis. Approximately 1% of patients treated have died of pulmonary fibrosis. Pulmonary toxicity is both dose and age related, being more common in patients over 70 years of age and in those receiving over 400 units total dose. This toxicity, however, is unpredictable and has been seen occasionally in young patients receiving low doses.

Because of lack of specificity of the clinical syndrome, the identification of patients with pulmonary toxicity due to Bleomycin Sulfate has been extremely difficult. The earliest symptom associated with Bleomycin Sulfate pulmonary toxicity is dyspnea. The earliest sign is fine rales.

Radiographically Bleomycin Sulfate-induced pneumonitis produces nonspecific patchy opacities, usually of the lower lung fields.

The most common changes in pulmonary function tests are a decrease in total lung volume and a decrease in vital capacity. However, these changes are not predictive of the development of pulmonary fibrosis.

The microscopic tissue changes due to Bleomycin Sulfate toxicity include bronchiolar squamous metaplasia, reactive macrophages, atypical alveolar epithelial cells, fibrinous edema, and interstitial fibrosis. The acute stage may involve capillary changes and subsequent fibrinous exudation into alveoli producing a change similar to hyaline membrane formation and progressing to a diffuse interstitial fibrosis resembling the Hamman-Rich syndrome. These microscopic findings are nonspecific; eg, similar changes are seen in radiation pneumonitis and pneumocystic pneumonitis.

To monitor the onset of pulmonary toxicity, roentgenograms of the chest should be taken every 1 to 2 weeks. If pulmonary changes are noted, treatment should be discontinued until it can be determined if they are drug related. Recent studies have suggested that sequential measurement of the pulmonary diffusion capacity for carbon monoxide (DL_{co}) during treatment with Bleomycin Sulfate may be an indicator of subclinical pulmonary toxicity. It is recommended that the DL_{co} be monitored monthly if it is to be employed to detect pulmonary toxicities, and thus the drug should be discontinued when the DL_{co} falls below 30% to 35% of the pretreatment value.

Because of Bleomycin Sulfate's sensitization of lung tissue, patients who have received Bleomycin Sulfate are at greater risk of developing pulmonary toxicity when oxygen is administered in surgery. While long exposure to very high oxygen concentrations is a known cause of lung damage, after Bleomycin Sulfate administration, lung damage can occur at lower concentrations that are usually considered safe. Suggestive preventive measures are:

(1) Maintain Fl O_2 at concentrations approximating that of room air (25%) during surgery and the postoperative period.

(2) Monitor carefully fluid replacement, focusing more on colloid administration rather than crystalloid.

Sudden onset of an acute chest pain syndrome suggestive of pleuropericarditis has been rarely reported during Bleomycin Sulfate infusions. Although each patient must be individually evaluated, further courses of Bleomycin Sulfate do not appear to be contraindicated.

Idiosyncratic Reactions: In approximately 1% of the lymphoma patients treated with Bleomycin Sulfate an idiosyncratic reaction, similar to anaphylaxis clinically, has been reported. The reaction may be immediate or delayed for several hours, and usually occurs after the first or second dose.

It consists of hypotension, mental confusion, fever, chills, and wheezing. Treatment is symptomatic including volume expansion, pressor agents, antihistamines, and corticosteroids.

Integument and Mucous Membranes: These are the most frequent side effects being reported in approximately 50% of treated patients. These consist of erythema, rash, striae, vesiculation, hyperpigmentation, and tenderness of the skin.

Hyperkeratosis, nail changes, alopecia, pruritus, and stomatitis have also been reported. It was necessary to discontinue Bleomycin Sulfate therapy in 2% of treated patients because of these toxicities.

Skin toxicity is a relatively late manifestation usually developing in the 2nd and 3rd week of treatment after 150 to 200 units of Bleomycin Sulfate have been administered and appears to be related to the cumulative dose.

Other: Vascular toxicities coincident with the use of Bleomycin Sulfate in combination with other antineoplastic agents have been reported rarely. The events are clinically heterogeneous and may include myocardial infarction, cerebrovascular accident, thrombotic microangiopathy (HUS) or cerebral arteritis. Various mechanisms have been proposed for these vascular complications. There are also reports of Raynaud's phenomenon occurring in patients treated with Bleomycin Sulfate in combination with vinblastine with or without cisplatin or, in a few cases, with Bleomycin Sulfate as a single agent.

It is currently unknown if the cause of Raynaud's phenomenon in these cases is the disease, underlying vascular compromise, Bleomycin Sulfate, vinblastine, hypomagnesemia, or a combination of any of these factors.

Fever, chills, and vomiting were frequently reported side effects. Anorexia and weight loss are common and may persist long after termination of this medication. Pain at tumor site, phlebitis, and other local reactions were reported infrequently.

DOSAGE

Because of the possibility of an anaphylactoid reaction, lymphoma patients should be treated with two units or less for the first two doses. If no acute reaction occurs, then the regular dosage schedule may be followed.

The following dose schedule is recommended: *Squamous cell carcinoma, lymphosarcoma, reticulum cell sarcoma, testicular carcinoma*—0.25 to 0.50 units/kg (10 to 20 units/m^2) given intravenously, intramuscularly, or subcutaneously weekly or twice weekly.

Hodgkin's Disease—0.25 to 0.50 units/kg (10 to 20 units/m^2) given intravenously, intramuscularly, or subcutaneously weekly or twice weekly. After a 50% response, a maintenance dose of one unit daily or five units weekly intravenously or intramuscularly should be given.

Pulmonary toxicity of Bleomycin Sulfate appears to be dose related with a striking increase when the total dose is over 400 units. Total doses over 400 units should be given with great caution.

Note: **When Bleomycin Sulfate is used in combination with other antineoplastic agents, pulmonary toxicities may occur at lower doses.**

Improvement of Hodgkin's Disease and testicular tumors is prompt and noted within 2 weeks. If no improvement is seen by this time, improvement is unlikely. Squamous cell cancers respond more slowly, sometimes requiring as long as 3 weeks before any improvement is noted.

ADMINISTRATION

Bleomycin Sulfate may be given by the intramuscular, intravenous, or subcutaneous routes.

Intramuscular or Subcutaneous: Dissolve the contents of a Bleomycin Sulfate vial in 1 to 5 mL of Sterile Water for Injection, USP, Sodium Chloride for Injection, USP, or Bacteriostatic Water for Injection, USP.

Intravenous: Dissolve the contents of the vial in 5 mL or more of physiologic saline, and administer slowly over a period of 10 minutes.

STABILITY

The sterile powder is stable under refrigeration (2°-8°C) and and should not be used after the expiration date is reached Bleomycin Sulfate is stable for 24 hours at room temperature in Sodium Chloride.

Procedures for proper handling and disposal of anticancer drugs should be considered. Several guidelines on this subject have been published.[1-7] There is no general agreement that all of the procedures recommended in the guidelines are necessary or appropriate.

REFERENCES
1. Recommendations for the Safe Handling of Parenteral Antineoplastic Drugs. NIH Publication No. 83-2621. For sale by the Superintendent of Documents, US Government Printing Office, Washington, D.C. 20402. 2. AMA Council Report. Guidelines for Handling Parenteral Antineoplastics, *JAMA.* 1985: 253 (11):1590-1592. 3. National Study Commission on Cytotoxic Exposure—Recommendations for Handling Cytotoxic Agents. Available from Louis P. Jeffrey, Sc.D., Chairman, National Study Commission on Cytotoxic Exposure, Massachusetts College of Pharmacy and Allied Health Sciences, 179 Longwood Avenue, Boston, Massachusetts 02115. 4. Clinical Oncological Society of Australia. Guidelines and Recommendations for Safe Handling of Antineoplastic Agents. *Med J Australia.*1983; 1:426-428. 5. Jones, RB, et. al. Safe handling of chemotherapeutic agents: A Report from the Mount Sinai Medical Center, *CA—A Cancer J for Clinicians.* 1983; (Sept/Oct) 258-263. 6. American Society of Hospital Pharmacists Technical Assistance Bulletin on Handling Cytotoxic and Hazardous Drugs. *Am J Hosp Pharm.* 1990; 47:1033-1049. 7. OSHA Work-Practice Guidelines for Personnel Dealing with Cytotoxic (Antineoplasic) Drugs, *Am J Hosp Pharm.* 1986; 43:1193-1204.

HOW SUPPLIED
POWDER FOR INJECTION: 15 U

BRAND/MANUFACTURER	NDC	SIZE	AWP
○ **BRAND**			
BLENOXANE: Bristol-Myer Onc/Hiv	00015-3010-20	1s	$276.29

Bleph-10 SEE SULFACETAMIDE SODIUM, OPHTHALMIC

Blephamide SEE PREDNISOLONE AND SULFACETAMIDE SODIUM

Blocadren SEE TIMOLOL MALEATE, ORAL

Bontril SEE PHENDIMETRAZINE TARTRATE

Botox SEE BOTULINUM TOXIN TYPE A

Botulinum Toxin Type A

DESCRIPTION
Sterile, lyophilized Botulinum Toxin Type A is produced from a culture of the Hall strain of *Clostridium botulinum* grown in a medium containing N-Z amine and yeast extract. It is purified from the culture solution by a series of acid precipitations to a crystalline complex consisting of the active high molecular weight toxin protein and an associated hemagglutinin protein. The crystalline complex is re-dissolved in a solution containing saline and albumin and sterile filtered (0.2 microns) prior to lyophilization. Botulinum Toxin Type A is to be reconstituted with sterile non-preserved saline prior to intramuscular injection.

Each vial of Botulinum Toxin Type A contains 100 units (U) of *Clostridium botulinum* toxin type A. One unit (U) corresponds to the calculated median lethal intraperitoneal dose (LD/50) in mice of the reconstituted Botulinum Toxin Type A injected.

CLINICAL PHARMACOLOGY

Botulinum Toxin Type A blocks neuromuscular conduction by binding to receptor sites on motor nerve terminals, entering the nerve terminals, and inhibiting the release of acetylcholine. When injected intramuscularly at therapeutic doses, Botulinum Toxin Type A produces a localized chemical denervation muscle paralysis. When the muscle is chemically denervated, it atrophies and may develop extrajunctional acetylcholine receptors. There is evidence that the nerve can sprout and reinnervate the muscle, with the weakness thus being reversible.

The paralytic effect on muscles injected with Botulinum Toxin Type A is useful in reducing the excessive, abnormal contractions associated with blepharospasm. When used for the treatment of strabismus, it is postulated that the administration of Botulinum Toxin Type A affects muscle pairs by inducing an atrophic lengthening of the injected muscle and a corresponding shortening of the muscle's antagonist. Following periocular injection of Botulinum Toxin Type A, distant muscles show electrophysiologic changes but no clinical weakness or other clinical change for a period of several weeks or months, parallel to the duration of local clinical paralysis.[1]

In one study, Botulinum Toxin was evaluated in 27 patients with essential blepharospasm. Twenty-six of the patients had previously undergone drug treatment utilizing benztropine mesylate, clonazepam and/or baclofen without adequate clinical results. Three of these patients then underwent muscle stripping surgery still without an adequate outcome. One patient of the 27 was previously untreated. Upon using Botulinum Toxin, 25 of the 27 patients reported improvement within 48 hours. One of the other patients was later controlled with a higher dosage. The remaining patient reported only mild improvement but remained functionally impaired.[2]

In another study, twelve patients with blepharospasm were evaluated in a double-blind, placebo-controlled study. All patients receiving Botulinum Toxin (n = 8) were improved compared with no improvements in the placebo group (n = 4). The mean dystonia score improved by 72%, the self-assessment score rating improved by 61%, and a videotape evaluation rating improved by 39%. The effects of the treatment lasted a mean of 12.5 weeks.[3]

One thousand six hundred eighty-four patients with blepharospasm evaluated in an open trial showed clinical improvement lasting an average of 12.5 weeks prior to the need for re-treatment.[4]

Six hundred seventy-seven patients with strabismus treated with one or more injections of Botulinum Toxin Type A were evaluated in an open trial. Fifty-five percent of these patients were improved to an alignment of 10 prism diopters or less when evaluated 6 months or more following injection[5]. These results are consistent with results from additional open label trials which were conducted for this indication.[4]

INDICATIONS AND USAGE

Botulinum Toxin Type A is indicated for the treatment of strabismus and blepharospasm associated with dystonia, including benign essential blepharospasm or VII nerve disorders in patients 12 years of age and above.

The efficacy of Botulinum Toxin Type A in deviations over 50 prism diopters, in restrictive strabismus, in Duane's syndrome with lateral rectus weakness, and in secondary strabismus caused by prior surgical over-recession of the antagonist is doubtful, or multiple injections over time may be required. Botulinum Toxin Type A is ineffective in chronic paralytic strabismus except to reduce antagonist contracture in conjunction with surgical repair.

Presence of antibodies to Botulinum Toxin Type A may reduce the effectiveness of Botulinum Toxin Type A therapy. In clinical studies, reduction in effectiveness due to antibody production has occurred in one patient with blepharospasm receiving 3 doses of Botulinum Toxin Type A over a 6 week period totalling 92 U, and in several patients with torticollis who received multiple doses experimentally, totalling over 300 U in a one-month period. For this reason, the dose of Botulinum Toxin Type A for strabismus and blepharospasm should be kept as low as possible, in any case below 200 U in a one month period.

CONTRAINDICATIONS

Botulinum Toxin Type A is contraindicated in individuals with known hypersensitivity to any ingredient in the formulation.

WARNINGS

The recommended dosages and frequencies of administration for Botulinum Toxin Type A should not be exceeded. There have not been any reported instances of systemic toxicity resulting from accidental injection or oral ingestion of Botulinum Toxin Type A. Should accidental injection or oral ingestion occur, the person should be medically supervised for several days on an office or outpatient basis for signs or symptoms of systemic weakness or muscle paralysis. The entire contents of a vial is below the estimated dose for systemic toxicity in humans weighing 6 kg. or greater.

The effect of Botulinum Toxin may be potentiated by aminoglycoside antibiotics or any other drugs that interfere with neuromuscular transmission. Caution should be exercised when Botulinum Toxin Type A is used in patients taking any of these drugs.[6]

PRECAUTIONS

General: The safe and effective use of Botulinum Toxin Type A depends upon proper storage of the product, selection of the correct dose, and proper reconstitution and administration techniques. Physicians administering Botulinum Toxin Type A must understand the relevant neuromuscular and orbital anatomy and any alterations to the anatomy due to prior surgical procedures, and standard electromyographic techniques.

As with all biologic products, epinephrine and other precautions as necessary should be available should an anaphylactic reaction occur.

During the administration of Botulinum Toxin Type A for the treatment of strabismus, retrobulbar hemorrhages sufficient to compromise retinal circulation have occurred from needle penetrations into the orbit. It is recommended that appropriate instruments to decompress the orbit be accessible. Ocular (globe) penetrations by needles have also occurred. An ophthalmoscope to diagnose this condition should be available. Reduced blinking from Botulinum Toxin Type A injection of the orbicularis muscle can lead to corneal exposure, persistent epithelial defect and corneal ulceration, especially in patients with VII nerve disorders. One case of corneal perforation in an aphakic eye requiring corneal grafting has occurred because of this effect. Careful testing of corneal sensation in eyes previously operated upon, avoidance of injection into the lower lid area to avoid ectropion, and vigorous treatment of any epithelial defect should be employed. This may require protective drops, ointment, therapeutic soft contact lenses, or closure of the eye by patching or other means.

Information for Patients: Patients with blepharospasm may have been extremely sedentary for a long time. Sedentary patients should be cautioned to resume activity slowly and carefully following the administration of Botulinum Toxin Type A.

Drug Interactions: The effect of Botulinum Toxin may be potentiated by aminoglycoside antibiotics or any other drugs that interfere with neuromuscular transmission. Caution should be exercised when Botulinum Toxin Type A is used in patients taking any of these drugs.[6] (See *"Warnings."*)

Pregnancy: Pregnancy Category C: Animal reproduction studies have not been conducted with Botulinum Toxin Type A. It is also not known whether Botulinum Toxin Type A can cause fetal harm when administered to a pregnant woman or can affect reproduction capacity. Botulinum Toxin Type A should be administered to pregnant women only if clearly needed.

Carcinogenesis, Mutagenesis, Impairment of Fertility: Long term studies in animals have not been performed to evaluate carcinogenic potential of Botulinum Toxin Type A.

Nursing Mothers: It is not known whether this drug is excreted in human milk. Because many drugs are excreted in human milk, caution should be exercised when Botulinum Toxin Type A is administered to a nursing woman.

Pediatric Use: Safety and effectiveness in children below the age of 12 have not been established.

ADVERSE REACTIONS[4]

There have been reports of seven cases of diffuse skin rash and two cases of local swelling of the eyelid skin lasting for several days following eyelid injection.

Strabismus: Inducing paralysis in one or more extraocular muscles may produce spatial disorientation, double vision, or past-pointing. Covering the affected eye may alleviate these symptoms. Extraocular muscles adjacent to the injection site are often affected, causing ptosis or vertical deviation, especially with higher doses of Botulinum Toxin Type A. The incidence rates of these side effects in 2058 adults who received 3650 injections for horizontal strabismus are listed below:

Ptosis	15.7%
Vertical deviation	16.9%

The incidence of ptosis was much less after inferior rectus injection (0.9%) and much greater after superior rectus injection (37.7%).

The incidence rates of these side effects persisting for over 6 months in an enlarged series of 5587 injections of horizontal muscles in 3104 patients are listed below:

Ptosis lasting over 180 days	0.3%
Vertical deviation greater than 2 prism diopters lasting over 180 days	2.1%

In these patients, the injection procedure itself caused 9 scleral perforations. A vitreous hemorrhage occurred and later cleared in one case. No retinal detachment or visual loss occurred in any case. Sixteen retrobulbar hemorrhages occurred. Decompression of the orbit after 5 minutes was done to restore retinal circulation in one case. No eye lost vision from retrobulbar hemorrhage. Five eyes had pupillary change consistent with ciliary ganglion damage (Adies pupil).

Blepharospasm: In 1684 patients who received 4258 treatments (involving multiple injections) for blepharospasm, the incidence rates of adverse reactions per treated eye are listed below:

Ptosis	11.0%
Irritation/Tearing	10.0%
(includes dry eye, lagophthalmos, and photophobia)	

Ectropion, keratitis, diplopia and entropion were reported rarely (incidences less than 1%)

Ecchymosis occurs easily in the soft eyelid tissues. This can be prevented by applying pressure at the injection site immediately after the injection.

In two cases of VII nerve disorder (one case of an aphakic eye) reduced blinking from Botulinum Toxin Type A injection of the orbicularis muscle led to serious corneal exposure, persistent epithelial defect and corneal ulceration. Perforation requiring corneal grafting occurred in one case, an aphakic eye. Avoidance of injection into the lower lid area to avoid ectropion may reduce this hazard. Vigorous treatment of any corneal epithelial defect should be employed. This may require protective drops, ointment, therapeutic soft contact lenses, or closure of the eye by patching or other means.

Two patients previously incapacitated by blepharospasm experienced cardiac collapse attributed to over-exertion within three weeks following Botulinum Toxin Type A therapy. Sedentary patients should be cautioned to resume activity slowly and carefully following the administration of Botulinum Toxin Type A.

DOSAGE AND ADMINISTRATION

Strabismus: Botulinum Toxin Type A is intended for injection into extraocular muscles utilizing the electrical activity recorded from the tip of the injection needle as a guide to placement within the target muscle. Injection without surgical exposure or electromyographic guidance should not be attempted. Physicians should be familiar with electromyographic technique.

An injection Botulinum Toxin Type A is prepared by drawing into a sterile 1.0 mL tuberculin syringe an amount of the properly diluted toxin (see Dilution Table) slightly greater than the intended dose. Air bubbles in the syringe barrel are expelled and the syringe is attached to the electromyographic injection needle, preferably a 1½", 27 gauge needle. Injection volume in excess of the intended dose is expelled through the needle into an appropriate waste container to assure patency of the needle and to confirm that there is no syringe-needle leakage. A new, sterile needle and syringe should be used to enter the vial on each occasion for dilution or removal of Botulinum Toxin Type A.

To prepare the eye for Botulinum Toxin Type A injection, it is recommended that several drops of a local anesthetic and an ocular decongestant be given several minutes prior to injection.

Note: The volume of Botulinum Toxin Type A injected for treatment of strabismus should be between 0.05 mL to 0.15 mL per muscle.

Strabismus Dosage: The initial listed doses of the diluted Botulinum Toxin Type A (see Dilution Table below) typically create paralysis of injected muscles beginning one to two days after injection and increasing in intensity during the first week. The paralysis lasts for 2-6 weeks and gradually resolves over a similar time period. Overcorrections lasting over 6 months have been rare. About one half of patients will require subsequent doses because of inadequate paralytic response of the muscle to the initial dose, or because of mechanical factors such as large deviations or restrictions, or because of the lack of binocular motor fusion to stabilize the alignment.

I. Initial doses in units (abbreviated as U). Use the lower listed doses for treatment of small deviations. Use the larger doses only for large deviations.
   A. For vertical muscles, and for horizontal strabismus of less than 20 prism diopters: 1.25 U to 2.5 U in any one muscle.
   B. For horizontal strabismus of 20 prism diopters to 50 prism diopters: 2.5 U to 5.0 U in any one muscle.
   C. For persistent VI nerve palsy of one month or longer duration: 1.25 U to 2.5 U in the medial rectus muscle.

II. Subsequent doses for residual or recurrent strabismus.
   A. It is recommended that patients be re-examined 7-14 days after each injection to assess the effect of that dose.
   B. Patients experiencing adequate paralysis of the target muscle that require subsequent injections should receive a dose comparable to the initial dose.
   C. Subsequent doses for patients experiencing incomplete paralysis of the target muscle may be increased up to twice the size of the previously administered dose.
   D. Subsequent injections should not be administered until the effects of the previous dose have dissipated as evidenced by substantial function in the injected and adjacent muscles.
   E. The maximum recommended dose as a single injection for any one muscle is 25 U.

Blepharospasm: For blepharospasm, diluted Botulinum Toxin Type A (see Dilution Table) is injected using a sterile, 27-30 gauge needle without electromyographic guidance. 1.25 U to 2.5 U (0.05 mL to 0.1 mL volume at each site) injected into the medial and lateral pre-tarsal orbicularis oculi of the upper lid and into the lateral pretarsal orbicularis oculi of the lower lid is the initial recommended dose. In general, the initial effect of the injections is seen within three days and reaches a peak at one to two weeks post-treatment. Each treatment lasts approximately three months, following which the procedure can be repeated indefinitely. At repeat treatment sessions, the dose may be increased up to two-fold if the response from the initial treatment is considered insufficient—usually defined as an effect that does not last longer than two months. However, there appears to be little benefit obtainable from injecting more than 5.0 Units per site. Some tolerance may be found when Botulinum Toxin Type A is used in treating blepharospasm if treatments are given any more frequently than every three months, and it is rare to have the effect be permanent.

The cumulative dose of Botulinum Toxin Type A in a 30-day period should not exceed 200 U.

DILUTION TECHNIQUE

To reconstitute lyophilized Botulinum Toxin Type A, use sterile normal saline without a preservative; 0.9% sodium chloride injection is the recommended diluent. Draw up the proper amount of diluent in the appropriate size syringe. Since Botulinum Toxin Type A is denatured by bubbling or similar violent agitation, inject the diluent into the vial gently. Discard the vial if a vacuum does not pull the diluent into the vial. Record the date and time of reconstitution on the space on the label. Botulinum Toxin Type A should be administered within 4 hours after reconstitution.

During this time period, reconstituted Botulinum Toxin Type A should be stored in a refrigerator (2° to 8°C). Reconstituted Botulinum Toxin Type A should be clear, colorless and free of particulate matter. Parenteral drug products should be inspected visually for particulate matter and discoloration prior to administration and whenever the solution and the container permit. The use of one vial for more than one patient is not recommended because the product and diluent do not contain a preservative.

DILUTION TABLE

Diluent Added (0.9% Sodium Chloride Injection)	Resulting dose in Units per 0.1 mL
1.0 mL	10.0 U
2.0 mL	5.0 U
4.0 mL	2.5 U
8.0 mL	1.25 U

Note: These dilutions are calculated for an injection volume of 0.1 mL. A decrease or increase in the Botulinum Toxin Type A dose is also possible by administering a smaller or larger injection volume—from 0.05 mL (50% decrease in dose) to 0.15 mL (50% increase in dose).

STORAGE

Store the lyophilized product in a freezer at or below -5°C. Administer Botulinum Toxin Type A within 4 hours after the vial is removed from the freezer and reconstituted. During these four hours, reconstituted Botulinum Toxin Type A should be stored in a refrigerator (2° to 8°C). Reconstituted Botulinum Toxin Type A should be clear, colorless and free of particulate matter.

All vials, including expired vials, or equipment used with the drug should be disposed of carefully as is done with all medical waste.

REFERENCES
1. Sanders D. Massey W, Buckley E. Botulinum toxin for blepharospasm: Single-fiber EMG studies. *Neurology*. 1986:36:545-547. 2. Arthurs B, Flanders M, Codere F, Gauthier S, Dresner S, Stone L. Treatment of blepharospasm with medication, surgery and type A botulinum toxin. *Can J Ophthalmol.* 1987;22:24-28. 3. Jankovic J, Orman J. Botulinum A toxin for cranial-cervical dystonia: A double-blind, placebo-controlled study. *Neurology*, 1987;37:616-623. 4. Data on file, Allergan, Inc. 5. Scott AB. Botulinum toxin treatment of strabismus. American Academy of Ophthalmology, Focal Points 1989: Clinical Modules for Ophthalmologists Vol VII Module 12. 6. Wang YC, Burr DH, Korthals GJ, Sugiyama H. Acute toxicity of aminoglycoside antibiotics as an aid in detecting botulism. *Apply Environ Microbiol.* 1984;48:951-955.

J CODES
Per unit IM—J0585

HOW SUPPLIED
POWDER FOR INJECTION: 100 U

BRAND/MANUFACTURER	NDC	SIZE	AWP
○ BRAND			
BOTOX: Allergan Optical	00023-1145-01	1s	$365.63

Branchamin *SEE* AMINO ACIDS, INJECTABLE *AND* AMINO ACIDS/CALCIUM CHLORIDE/DEXTROSE/ELECTROLYTES

Brethaire *SEE* TERBUTALINE SULFATE

Brethancer *SEE* TERBUTALINE SULFATE

Brethine *SEE* TERBUTALINE SULFATE

Bretylium Tosylate

DESCRIPTION

Bretylium Tosylate Injection is an antifibrillatory and antiarrhythmic agent, intended for intravenous or intramuscular use. Bretylium Tosylate is a white, crystalline powder with an extremely bitter taste. It is freely soluble in water and alcohol. Each mL of sterile, non-pyrogenic solution contains 50 mg Bretylium Tosylate in Water for Injection, USP. The pH is adjusted when necessary, with dilute hydrochloric acid or sodium hydroxide. Bretylium Tosylate contains no preservative.

Following is its chemical structure:

$$\left[\begin{array}{c} \text{CH}_3 \\ \text{CH}_2 - \text{N}^+ - \text{C}_2\text{H}_5 \\ \text{CH}_3 \\ \text{Br} \end{array}\right] \quad \text{CH}_3 - \text{SO}_3^-$$

CLINICAL PHARMACOLOGY

Bretylium Tosylate is a bromobenzyl quaternary ammonium compound which selectively accumulates in sympathetic ganglia and their postganglionic adrenergic neurons where it inhibits norepinephrine release by depressing adrenergic nerve terminal excitability.

Bretylium Tosylate also suppresses ventricular fibrillation and ventricular arrhythmias. The mechanisms of the antifibrillatory and antiarrhythmic actions of Bretylium Tosylate are not established. In efforts to define these mechanisms, the following electrophysiologic actions of Bretylium Tosylate have been demonstrated in animal experiments.

1. Increase in ventricular fibrillation threshold.

2. Increase in action potential duration and effective refractory period without changes in heart rate.

3. Little effect on the rate of rise or amplitude of the cardiac action potential (Phase 0) or in resting membrane potential (Phase 4) in normal myocardium. However, when cell injury slows the rate of rise, decreases amplitude, and lowers resting membrane potential, Bretylium Tosylate transiently restores these parameters toward normal.

4. In canine hearts with infarcted areas Bretylium Tosylate decreases the disparity in action potential duration between normal and infarcted regions.

5. Increase in impulse formation and spontaneous firing rate of pacemaker tissue as well as increased ventricular conduction velocity.

The restoration of injured myocardial cell electrophysiology toward normal, as well as the increase of the action potential duration and effective refractory period without changing their ratio to each other, may be important factors in suppressing re-entry of aberrant impulses and decreasing induced dispersion of local excitable states.

Bretylium Tosylate induces a chemical sympathectomy-like state which resembles a surgical sympathectomy. Catecholamine stores are not depleted by Bretylium Tosylate, but catecholamine effects on the myocardium and on peripheral vascular resistance are often seen shortly after administration because Bretylium Tosylate causes an early release of norepinephrine from the adrenergic postganglionic nerve terminals. Subsequently, Bretylium Tosylate blocks the release of norepinephrine in response to neuron stimulation. Peripheral adrenergic blockade regularly causes orthostatic hypotension but has less effect on supine blood pressure. The relationship of adrenergic blockade to the antifibrillatory and antiarrhythmic actions of Bretylium Tosylate is not clear. In a study in patients with frequent ventricular premature beats, peak plasma concentration of Bretylium Tosylate and peak hypotensive effects were seen within one hour of intramuscular administration, presumably reflecting adrenergic neuronal blockade. However, suppression of premature ventricular beats was not maximal until 6-9 hours after dosing, when mean plasma concentration had declined to less than one-half of peak level. This suggests a slower mechanism, other than neuronal blockade, was involved in suppression of the arrhythmia. On the other hand, antifibrillatory effects can be seen within minutes of an intravenous injection, suggesting that the effect on the myocardium may occur quite rapidly.

Bretylium Tosylate has a positive inotropic effect on the myocardium, but it is not yet certain whether this effect is direct or is mediated by catecholamine release.

Bretylium Tosylate is eliminated intact by the kidneys. No metabolites have been identified following administration of Bretylium Tosylate in man and laboratory animals. In man, approximately 70 to 80% of a ^{14}C-labelled intramuscular dose is excreted in the urine during the first 24 hours, with an additional 10% excreted over the next three days.

The terminal half-life in four normal volunteers averaged 7.8 ± 0.6 hrs (range 6.9-8.1). In one patient with a creatinine clearance of 21.0 mL/min $\times 1.73$ m^2, the half-life was 16 hours. In one patient with a creatinine clearance of 1.0 mL/min $\times 1.73$ m^2 the half-life was 31.5 hours. During hemodialysis this patient's arterial and venous Bretylium Tosylate concentrations declined rapidly, resulting in a half-life of 13 hours. During dialysis there was a two-fold increase in total Bretylium Tosylate clearance.

Effect on Heart Rate: There is sometimes an initial small increase in heart rate when Bretylium Tosylate is administered, but this is an inconsistent and transient occurrence.

Hemodynamic Effects: Following intravenous administration of 5 mg/kg of Bretylium Tosylate to patients with acute myocardial infarction, there was a mild increase in arterial pressure, followed by a modest decrease, remaining within normal limits throughout. Pulmonary artery pressure, pulmonary capillary wedge pressure, right atrial pressure, cardiac index, stroke volume index, and stroke work index were not significantly changed. These hemodynamic effects were not correlated with antiarrhythmic activity.

Onset of Action: Suppression of ventricular fibrillation is rapid, usually occurring within minutes following intravenous administration. Suppression of ventricular tachycardia and other ventricular arrhythmias develops more slowly, usually 20 minutes to 2 hours after parenteral administration.

INDICATIONS AND USAGE

Bretylium Tosylate is indicated in the prophylaxis and therapy of ventricular fibrillation.

Bretylium Tosylate is also indicated in the treatment of life-threatening ventricular arrhythmias, such as ventricular tachycardia, that have failed to respond to adequate doses of a first-line antiarrhythmic agent, such as lidocaine.

Use of Bretylium Tosylate should be limited to intensive care units, coronary care units or other facilities where equipment and personnel for constant monitoring of cardiac arrhythmias and blood pressure are available.

Following injection of Bretylium Tosylate there may be a delay of 20 minutes to 2 hours in the onset of antiarrhythmic action, although it appears to act within minutes in ventricular fibrillation. The delay in effect appears to be longer after intramuscular than after intravenous injection.

CONTRAINDICATIONS

There are no contraindications to use in treatment of ventricular fibrillation or life-threatening refractory ventricular arrhythmias.

WARNINGS

1. HYPOTENSION

Administration of Bretylium Tosylate regularly results in postural hypotension, subjectively recognized by dizziness, light-headedness, vertigo or faintness. Some degree of hypotension is present in about 50% of patients while they are supine. Hypotension may occur at doses lower than those needed to suppress arrhythmias.

> PATIENTS SHOULD BE KEPT IN THE SUPINE POSITION UNTIL TOLERANCE TO THE HYPOTENSIVE EFFECT OF BRETYLIUM TOSYLATE DEVELOPS. TOLERANCE OCCURS UNPREDICTABLY BUT MAY BE PRESENT AFTER SEVERAL DAYS.

Hypotension with supine systolic pressure greater than 75 mm Hg need not be treated unless there are associated symptoms. If supine systolic pressure falls below 75 mm Hg, an infusion of dopamine or norepinephrine may be used to raise blood pressure. When catecholamines are administered, a dilute solution should be employed and blood pressure monitored closely because the pressor effects of the catecholamines are enhanced by Bretylium Tosylate. Volume expansion with blood or plasma and correction of dehydration should be carried out where appropriate.

2. TRANSIENT HYPERTENSION AND INCREASED FREQUENCY OF ARRHYTHMIAS

Due to the initial release of norepinephrine from adrenergic postganglionic nerve terminals by Bretylium Tosylate, transient hypertension or increased frequency of premature ventricular contractions and other arrhythmias may occur in some patients.

3. CAUTION DURING USE WITH DIGITALIS GLYCOSIDES

The initial release of norepinephrine caused by Bretylium Tosylate may aggravate digitalis toxicity. When a life-threatening cardiac arrhythmia occurs in a digitalized patient, Bretylium Tosylate should be used only if the etiology of the arrhythmia does not appear to be digitalis toxicity and other antiarrhythmic drugs are not effective. Simultaneous initiation of therapy with digitalis glycosides and Bretylium Tosylate should be avoided.

4. PATIENTS WITH FIXED CARDIAC OUTPUT

In patients with fixed cardiac output (i.e., severe aortic stenosis or severe pulmonary hypertension), Bretylium Tosylate should be avoided since severe hypotension may result from a fall in peripheral resistance without a compensatory increase in cardiac output. If survival is threatened by the arrhythmia, Bretylium Tosylate may be used but vasoconstrictive catecholamines should be given promptly if severe hypotension occurs.

PRECAUTIONS

GENERAL

1. DILUTION FOR INTRAVENOUS USE

Bretylium Tosylate should be diluted (one part Bretylium Tosylate with at least four parts of Dextrose Injection, USP or Sodium Chloride Injection, USP) prior to intravenous use. Rapid intravenous administration may cause severe nausea and vomiting. Therefore, the diluted solution should be infused over a period greater than 8 minutes. However, in treating existing ventricular fibrillation Bretylium Tosylate should be given as rapidly as possible and may be given without dilution.

2. USE VARIOUS SITES FOR INTRAMUSCULAR INJECTION

When injected intramuscularly, not more than 5 mL should be given in a site, and injection sites should be varied since repeated intramuscular injection into the same site may cause atrophy and necrosis of muscle tissue, fibrosis, vascular degeneration and inflammatory changes.

3. REDUCE DOSAGE IN IMPAIRED RENAL FUNCTION

Since Bretylium Tosylate is excreted principally via the kidney, the dosage interval should be increased in patients with impaired renal function. See 'Clinical Pharmacology' section for information on the effect of reduced renal function on half-life.

DRUG INTERACTIONS

1. Digitalis toxicity may be aggravated by the initial release of norepinephrine caused by Bretylium Tosylate.

2. The pressor effects of catecholamines such as dopamine or norepinephrine are enhanced by Bretylium Tosylate. When catecholamines are administered, dilute solutions should be used and blood pressure should be monitored closely. (See "Warnings".)

3. Although there is little published information on concomitant administration of lidocaine and Bretylium Tosylate, these drugs are often administered concurrently without any evidence of interactions resulting in adverse effects or diminished efficacy.

CARCINOGENESIS, MUTAGENESIS, IMPAIRMENT OF FERTILITY
No data are available on potential for carcinogenicity, mutagenicity or impairment of fertility in animals or humans.

PREGNANCY CATEGORY C
Animal reproduction studies have not been conducted with Bretylium Tosylate. It is also not known whether Bretylium Tosylate can cause harm when administered to a pregnant woman or can affect reproduction capacity. Bretylium Tosylate should be given to pregnant women only if clearly needed.

PEDIATRIC USE
The safety and efficacy of this drug in children has not been established. Bretylium Tosylate has been administered to a limited number of pediatric patients, but such use has been inadequate to define fully proper dosage and limitations for use.

ADVERSE REACTIONS
Hypotension and postural hypotension have been the most frequently reported adverse reactions (see "Warnings" section). Nausea and vomiting occurred in about three percent of patients, primarily when Bretylium Tosylate was administered rapidly by the intravenous route (see "Precautions" section). Vertigo, dizziness, light-headedness and syncope, which sometimes accompanied postural hypotension, were reported in about 7 patients in 1000.

Bradycardia, increased frequency of premature ventricular contractions, transitory hypertension initial increase in arrhythmias (see "Warnings" section), precipitation of anginal attacks, and sensation of substernal pressure have also been reported in a small number of patients, i.e., approximately 1-2 patients in 1000.

Renal dysfunction, diarrhea, abdominal pain, hiccups, erythematous macular rash, flushing, hyperthermia, confusion, paranoid psychosis, emotional lability, lethargy, generalized tenderness, anxiety, shortness of breath, diaphoresis, nasal stuffiness and mild conjunctivitis, have been reported in about 1 patient in 1000. The relationship of Bretylium Tosylate administration to these reactions has not been clearly established.

OVERDOSAGE
In the presence of life threatening arrhythmias, underdosing with Bretylium Tosylate probably presents a greater risk to the patient than potential overdosage. However, one case of accidental overdose has been reported in which a rapidly injected intravenous bolus of 30 mg/kg was given instead of an intended 10 mg/kg dose during an episode of ventricular tachycardia. Marked hypertension resulted, followed by protracted refractory hypotension. The patient expired 18 hours later in asystole, complicated by renal failure and aspiration pneumonitis. Bretylium Tosylate serum levels were 8,000 ng/mL.

The exaggerated hemodynamic response was attributed to the rapid injection of a very large dose while some effective circulation was still present. Neither the total dose nor the serum levels observed in this patient are in themselves associated with toxicity. Total doses of 30 mg/kg are not unusual and do not cause toxicity when given incrementally during cardio-pulmonary resuscitation procedures. Similarly, patients maintained on chronic Bretylium Tosylate therapy have had documented serum levels of 12,000 ng/mL. These levels were achieved after sequential dosage increases over time with no apparent ill effects.

If Bretylium Tosylate is overdosed and symptoms of toxicity develop, administration of nitroprusside or another short acting intravenous antihypertensive agent should be considered for the treatment of the hypertensive response.

Long acting drugs that might potentiate the subsequent hypotensive effects of Bretylium Tosylate should not be used. Hypotension should be treated with appropriate fluid therapy and pressor agents such as dopamine or norepinephrine. Dialysis is probably not useful in the treatment of Bretylium Tosylate overdose.

DOSAGE AND ADMINISTRATION
Bretylium Tosylate is to be used clinically only for treatment of life-threatening ventricular arrhythmias under constant electrocardiographic monitoring. The clinical use of Bretylium Tosylate is for short-term use only. Patients should either be kept supine during the course of Bretylium Tosylate therapy or be closely observed for postural hypotension. The optimal dose schedule for parenteral administration of Bretylium Tosylate has not been determined. There is comparatively little experience with dosages greater than 40 mg/kg/day, although such doses have been used without apparent adverse effects. The following schedule is suggested.

A. FOR IMMEDIATELY LIFE-THREATENING VENTRICULAR ARRHYTHMIAS SUCH AS VENTRICULAR FIBRILLATION OR HEMODYNAMICALLY UNSTABLE VENTRICULAR TACHYCARDIA:
Administer undiluted Bretylium Tosylate at a dosage of 5 mg/kg of body weight by rapid intravenous in injection. Other usual cardiopulmonary resuscitative procedures, including electrical cardioversion, should be employed prior to and following the injection in accordance with good medical practice. If ventricular fibrillation persists, the dosage may be increased to 10 mg/kg and repeated as necessary.

For continuous suppression, dilute Bretylium Tosylate with Dextrose Injection, USP or Sodium Chloride Injection, USP using the table below and administer the diluted solution as a constant infusion of 1 to 2 mg Bretylium Tosylate per minute. When administering Bretylium Tosylate (or any potent medication) by continuous intravenous infusion, it is advisable to use a precision volume control device. An alternative maintenance schedule is to infuse the diluted solution at a dosage of 5 to 10 mg Bretylium Tosylate per kg body weight, over a period greater than 8 minutes, every 6 hours. More rapid infusion may cause nausea and vomiting.

B. OTHER VENTRICULAR ARRHYTHMIAS:
1. Intravenous Use: Bretylium Tosylate must be diluted as described above before intravenous use.

Administer the diluted solution at a dosage of 5 to 10 mg Bretylium Tosylate per kg of body weight by intravenous infusion over a period greater than 8 minutes. More rapid infusion may cause nausea and vomiting. Subsequent doses may be given at 1 to 2 hour intervals if the arrhythmia persists.

For maintenance therapy, the same dosage may be administered every 6 hours, or a constant infusion of 1 to 2 mg Bretylium Tosylate per minute may be given. (See related table.)

2. For intramuscular Injection: Do not dilute Bretylium Tosylate prior to intramuscular injection. Inject 5 to 10 mg Bretylium Tosylate per kg of body weight. Subsequent doses may be given at 1 to 2 hour intervals if the arrhythmia persists. Thereafter maintain the same dosage every 6 to 8 hours.

Intramuscular injection should not be made directly into or near a major nerve, and the site of injection should be varied on repeated injection. No more than 5 mL should be injected intramuscularly in one site. (See "Precautions").

As soon as possible, and when indicated, patients should be changed to an oral antiarrhythmic agent for maintenance therapy.

Store at controlled room temperature 15°-30°C (59°-86°F).

HOW SUPPLIED
INJECTION: 1 GM/ML

AVERAGE UNIT PRICE (AVAILABLE SIZES)				
BRAND	$2.38			
BRAND/MANUFACTURER		NDC	SIZE	AWP
◆ BRAND				
BRETYLOL: Du Pont Multi		00590-0012-71	10 ml 20s	$475.00
		00590-0012-79	20 ml 20s	$950.00

SUGGESTED BRETYLIUM TOSYLATE ADMIXTURE DILUTIONS AND ADMINISTRATION RATES FOR CONTINUOUS INFUSION MAINTENANCE THERAPY ARRANGED IN DESCENDING ORDER OF CONCENTRATION

Preparation				Administration		
Amount of Bretylium Tosylate	Volume of IV Fluid*	Final Volume	Final Conc. (mg/mL)	Dose mg/min.	Microdrops per min.	mL/hr
FOR FLUID RESTRICTED PATIENTS:						
500 mg (10 mL)	50 mL	60 mL	8.3	1.0	7	7
				1.5	11	11
				2.0	14	14
2 g (40 mL)	500 mL	540 mL	3.7	1.0	16	16
1 g (20 mL)	250 mL	270 mL	3.7	1.5	24	24
				2.0	32	32
1 g (20 mL)	500 mL	520 mL	1.9	1.0	32	32
500 mg (10 mL)	250 mL	260 mL	1.9	1.5	47	47
				2.0	63	63

* IV fluid may be either Dextrose Injection, USP or Sodium Chloride Injection, USP.

➤ SHOWN IN PRODUCT IDENTIFICATION GUIDE

INJECTION: 50 MG/ML

AVERAGE UNIT PRICE (AVAILABLE SIZES)		GENERIC A-RATED AVERAGE PRICE (GAAP)	
BRAND	$2.38	10 ml 5s	$144.69
GENERIC	$2.43	10 ml 25s	$349.25

BRAND/MANUFACTURER	NDC	SIZE	AWP
◆ **BRAND**			
BRETYLOL: Du Pont Multi	00590-0012-37	10 ml 5s	$118.75
	00590-0012-10	10 ml 20s	$475.00
◆ **GENERICS**			
Elkins-Sinn	00641-2211-41	10 ml	$23.13
Amer Regent	00517-8810-01	10 ml	$22.44
Elkins-Sinn	00641-1381-34	10 ml 5s	$112.50
Abbott Hosp	00074-9263-01	10 ml 5s	$160.79
Abbott Hosp	00074-9268-01	10 ml 5s	$160.79
Abbott Hosp	00074-9267-01	10 ml 10s	$341.17
Raway	00686-8810-01	10 ml 25s	$100.00
Intl Med Sys	00548-1118-00	10 ml 25s	$598.50

Bretylol SEE BRETYLIUM TOSYLATE

Brevibloc SEE ESMOLOL HYDROCHLORIDE

Brevicon SEE ETHINYL ESTRADIOL AND NORETHINDRONE

Brevital Sodium SEE METHOHEXITAL SODIUM

Brevoxyl SEE BENZOYL PEROXIDE

Bromfed SEE BROMPHENIRAMINE MALEATE AND PSEUDOEPHEDRINE HYDROCHLORIDE

Bromfed-DM SEE BROMPHENIRAMINE/ DEXTROMETHORPHAN/PSEUDOEPHEDRINE

Bromocriptine Mesylate

DESCRIPTION

Bromocriptine Mesylate is an ergot derivative with potent dopamine receptor agonist activity. Each Bromocriptine Mesylate tablet for oral administration contains 2½ mg and each capsule contains 5 mg Bromocriptine Mesylate. Bromocriptine Mesylate is chemically designated as (1) Ergotaman-3', 6', 18-trione, 2-bromo-12'-hydroxy-2'-(1-methyl-ethyl)-5'-(2-methylpropyl)-, (5'α) monomethanesulfonate (salt); (2) 2-bromoergocryptine monomethanesulfonate (salt).

Following is its chemical structure:

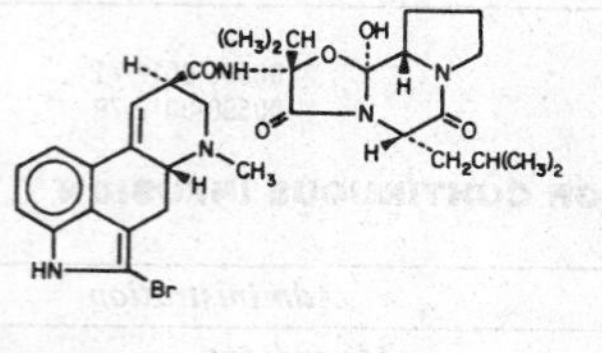

CLINICAL PHARMACOLOGY

Bromocriptine Mesylate is a dopamine receptor agonist, which activates post-synaptic dopamine receptors. The dopaminergic neurons in the tuberoinfundibular process modulate the secretion of prolactin from the anterior pituitary by secreting a prolactin inhibitory factor (thought to be dopamine); in the corpus striatum the dopaminergic neurons are involved in the control of motor function. Clinically, Bromocriptine Mesylate significantly reduces plasma levels of prolactin in patients with physiologically elevated prolactin as well as in patients with hyperprolactinemia. The inhibition of physiological lactation as well as galactorrhea in pathological hyperprolactinemic states is obtained at dose levels that do not affect secretion of other tropic hormones from the anterior pituitary. Experiments have demonstrated that Bromocriptine Mesylate induces long lasting stereotyped behavior in rodents and turning behavior in rats having unilateral lesions in the substantia nigra. These actions, characteristic of those produced by dopamine, are inhibited by dopamine antagonists and suggest a direct action of Bromocriptine Mesylate on striatal dopamine receptors.

Bromocriptine Mesylate is a nonhormonal, nonestrogenic agent that inhibits the secretion of prolactin in humans, with little or no effect on other pituitary hormones, except in patients with acromegaly, where it lowers elevated blood levels of growth hormone in the majority of patients.

In about 75% of cases of amenorrhea and galactorrhea. Bromocriptine Mesylate therapy suppresses the galactorrhea completely, or almost completely, and reinitiates normal ovulatory menstrual cycles.

Menses are usually reinitiated prior to complete suppression of galactorrhea; the time for this on average is 6-8 weeks. However, some patients respond within a few days, and others may take up to 8 months.

Galactorrhea may take longer to control depending on the degree of stimulation of the mammary tissue prior to therapy. At least a 75% reduction in secretion is usually observed after 8-12 weeks. Some patients may fail to respond even after 12 months of therapy.

Bromocriptine Mesylate, by virtue of its ability to inhibit prolactin secretion, acts to prevent physiological lactation in women when therapy is started after delivery and continued for two to three weeks. There is no evidence that Bromocriptine Mesylate acts on the mammary tissues to prevent lactation, as is the case with estrogen-containing preparations.

In many acromegalic patients, Bromocriptine Mesylate produces a prompt and sustained reduction in circulating levels of serum growth hormone.

Bromocriptine Mesylate produces its therapeutic effect in the treatment of Parkinson's disease, a clinical condition characterized by a progressive deficiency in dopamine synthesis in the substantia nigra, by directly stimulating the dopamine receptors in the corpus striatum. In contrast, levodopa exerts its therapeutic effect only after conversion to dopamine by the neurons of the substantia nigra, which are known to be numerically diminished in this patient population.

PHARMACOKINETICS

The pharmacokinetics and metabolism of Bromocriptine Mesylate in human subjects were studied with the help of radioactively labeled drug. Twenty-eight percent of an oral dose was absorbed from the gastrointestinal tract. The blood levels following a 2½ mg dose were in the range of 2-3 ng equivalents/ml. Plasma levels were in the range of 4-6 ng equivalents/ml indicating that the red blood cells did not contain appreciable amounts of drug and/or metabolites. *In vitro* experiments showed that the drug was 90-96% bound to serum albumin.

Bromocriptine Mesylate was completely metabolized prior to excretion. The major route of excretion of absorbed drug was via the bile. Only 2.5-5.5% of the dose was excreted in the urine. Almost all (84.6%) of the administered dose was excreted in the feces in 120 hours.

INDICATIONS AND USAGE

HYPERPROLACTINEMIA-ASSOCIATED DYSFUNCTIONS

Bromocriptine Mesylate is indicated for the treatment of dysfunctions associated with *hyperprolactinemia* including *amenorrhea* with or without *galactorrhea, infertility* or *hypogonadism*. Bromocriptine Mesylate treatment is indicated in patients with *prolactin-secreting adenomas*, which may be the basic underlying endocrinopathy contributing to the above clinical presentations. *Reduction* in tumor size has been demonstrated in both male and female patients with macroadenomas. In cases where adenectomy is elected, a course of Bromocriptine Mesylate therapy may be used to reduce the tumor mass prior to surgery.

ACROMEGALY

Bromocriptine Mesylate therapy is indicated in the treatment of acromegaly. Bromocriptine Mesylate therapy, alone or as adjunctive therapy with pituitary irradiation or surgery, reduces serum growth hormone by 50% or more in approximately one-half of patients treated, although not usually to normal levels.

Since the effects of external pituitary radiation may not become maximal for several years, adjunctive therapy with Bromocriptine Mesylate tablets or capsules offers potential benefit before the effects of irradiation are manifested.

PARKINSON'S DISEASE

Bromocriptine Mesylate tablets or capsules are indicated in the treatment of the signs and symptoms of idiopathic or postencephalitic Parkinson's disease. As adjunctive treatment to levodopa (alone or with a peripheral decarboxylase inhibitor), Bromocriptine Mesylate therapy may provide additional therapeutic benefits in those patients who are currently maintained on optimal dosages of levodopa, those who are beginning to deteriorate (develop tolerance) to levodopa therapy, and those who are experiencing "end of dose failure" on levodopa therapy.

Bromocriptine Mesylate therapy may permit a reduction of the maintenance dose of levodopa and, thus may ameliorate the occurrence and/or severity of adverse reactions associated with long-term levodopa therapy such as abnormal involuntary movements (e.g., dyskinesias) and the marked swings in motor function ("on-off" phenomenon). Continued efficacy of Bromocriptine Mesylate therapy during treatment of more than two years has not been established.

Data are insufficient to evaluate potential benefit from treating newly diagnosed Parkinson's disease with Bromocriptine Mesylate. Studies have shown, however, significantly more adverse reactions (notably nausea, hallucinations, confusion and hypotension) in Bromocriptine Mesylate treated patients than in levodopa/carbidopa treated patients. Patients unresponsive to levodopa are poor candidates for Bromocriptine Mesylate therapy.

◆ RATED THERAPEUTICALLY EQUIVALENT; ◇ THERAPEUTIC EQUIVALENCE UNCONFIRMED; ○ UNRATED

UNLABELED USES
UNLABELED USES
Bromocriptine Mesylate is used alone or as an adjunct in the treatment of benign prostatic hyperplasia, cocaine addiction, dystonia, hypertension, neuroleptic malignant syndrome, and restless leg syndrome.

Prevention of Physiological Lactation (no longer an approved indication); Bromocriptine Mesylate tablets are used for the prevention of physiological lactation (secretion, congestion, and engorgement) occurring:
1. After parturition when the mother elects not to breast feed the infant, or when breast feeding is contraindicated.
2. After stillbirth or abortion.

The physician should keep in mind that the incidence of significant painful engorgement is low and usually responsive to appropriate supportive therapy. In contrast with supportive therapy, Bromocriptine Mesylate prevents the secretion of prolactin, thus inhibiting lactogenesis and the subsequent development of secretion, congestion and engorgement.

Once Bromocriptine Mesylate therapy is stopped, 18% to 40% of patients experience rebound of breast secretion, congestion or engorgement, which is usually mild to moderate in severity.

CONTRAINDICATIONS
Uncontrolled hypertension, toxemia of pregnancy, sensitivity to any ergot alkaloids.

WARNINGS
Since hyperprolactinemia with amenorrhea/galactorrhea and infertility has been found in patients with pituitary tumors, a complete evaluation of the pituitary is indicated before treatment with Bromocriptine Mesylate. If pregnancy occurs during Bromocriptine Mesylate administration, careful observation of these patients is mandatory. Prolactin-secreting adenomas may expand and compression of the optic or other cranial nerves may occur, emergency pituitary surgery becoming necessary. In most cases, the compression resolves following delivery. Reinitiation of Bromocriptine Mesylate treatment has been reported to produce improvement in the visual fields of patients in whom nerve compression has occurred during pregnancy. The safety of Bromocriptine Mesylate treatment during pregnancy to the mother and fetus has not been established.

Symptomatic hypotension can occur in patients treated with Bromocriptine Mesylate for any indication.

In postpartum studies with Bromocriptine Mesylate, decreases in supine systolic and diastolic pressures of greater than 20 mm and 10 mm Hg, respectively, have been observed in almost 30% of patients receiving Bromocriptine Mesylate. On occasion, the drop in supine systolic pressure was as much as 50-59 mm of Hg. Since decreases in blood pressure are frequently noted during the puerperium independent of drug therapy, it is likely that many of these decreases in blood pressure observed with Bromocriptine Mesylate therapy were not drug induced. **While hypotension during the start of therapy with Bromocriptine Mesylate occurs in some patients, 50 cases of hypertension have been reported, sometimes at the initiation of therapy, but often developing in the second week of therapy. Seizures have been reported in 38 cases (including 4 cases of status epilepticus), both with and without the prior development of hypertension occurring mostly in postpartum patients up to 14 days after initiation of treatment. Fifteen cases of stroke during Bromocriptine Mesylate therapy have been reported mostly in postpartum patients whose prenatal and obstetric courses had been uncomplicated. Many of these patients experiencing seizures and/or strokes reported developing a constant and often progressively severe headache hours to days prior to the acute event. Some cases of strokes and seizures during therapy with Bromocriptine Mesylate were also preceded by visual disturbances (blurred vision, and transient cortical blindness). Four cases of acute myocardial infarction have been reported, including 3 cases receiving Bromocriptine Mesylate for the prevention of physiological lactation. The relationship of these adverse reactions to Bromocriptine Mesylate administration is not certain. The use of Bromocriptine Mesylate is not recommended for patients with uncontrolled hypertension or toxemia of pregnancy. Although there is no conclusive evidence which demonstrates the interaction between Bromocriptine Mesylate and other ergot alkaloids, the concomitant use of these medications is not recommended. Particular attention should be paid to patients who have recently received other drugs that can alter the blood pressure. Bromocriptine Mesylate therapy for the prevention of postpartum lactation should not be initiated until the vital signs have been stabilized and no sooner than four hours after delivery.** Periodic monitoring of the blood pressure, particularly during the first weeks of therapy and especially during the postpartum period, is prudent. If hypertension, severe, progressive, or unremitting headache (with or without visual disturbance), or evidence of CNS toxicity develops, drug therapy should be discontinued and the patient should be evaluated promptly.

Long-term treatment (6-36 months) with Bromocriptine Mesylate in doses ranging from 20-100 mg/day has been associated with pulmonary infiltrates, pleural effusion and thickening of the pleura in a few patients. In those instances in which Bromocriptine Mesylate treatment was terminated, the changes slowly reverted towards normal.

PRECAUTIONS
GENERAL
Safety and efficacy of Bromocriptine Mesylate have not been established in patients with renal or hepatic disease. Care should be exercised when administering Bromocriptine Mesylate therapy concomitantly with other medications known to lower blood pressure.

HYPERPROLACTINEMIC STATES
The relative efficacy of Bromocriptine Mesylate versus surgery in preserving visual fields is not known. Patients with rapidly progressive visual field loss should be evaluated by a neurosurgeon to help decide on the most appropriate therapy. Since pregnancy is often the therapeutic objective in many hyperprolactinemic patients presenting with amenorrhea/galactorrhea and hypogonadism (infertility), a careful assessment of the pituitary is essential to detect the presence of a prolactin-secreting adenoma. Patients not seeking pregnancy, or those harboring large adenomas, should be advised to use contraceptive measures, other than oral contraceptives, during treatment with Bromocriptine Mesylate. Since pregnancy may occur prior to reinitiation of menses, a pregnancy test is recommended at least every four weeks during the amenorrheic period, and, once menses are reinitiated, every time a patient misses a menstrual period. Treatment with Bromocriptine Mesylate tablets or capsules should be discontinued as soon as pregnancy has been established. Patients must be monitored closely throughout pregnancy for signs and symptoms that may signal the enlargement of a previously undetected or existing prolactin-secreting tumor. Discontinuation of Bromocriptine Mesylate treatment in patients with known macroadenomas has been associated with rapid regrowth of tumor and increase in serum prolactin in most cases.

USE IN PREGNANCY
In human studies with Bromocriptine Mesylate there have been 1276 reported pregnancies, which have yielded 1109 live and 4 stillborn infants from women who took Bromocriptine Mesylate during pregnancy. The majority of these patients received Bromocriptine Mesylate during the first two to three weeks of pregnancy and several received the drug for up to three months and five were treated for the entire period of gestation. Several studies in the literature reported on the use of Bromocriptine Mesylate during the final weeks of pregnancy to reduce plasma levels of prolactin in cases where possible pituitary tumor expansion occurred. Among the 1113 infants, 37 cases of congenital anomalies have been reported. There were 9 major malformations which included 3 limb reduction defects and 28 minor malformations which include 8 hip dislocations. The total incidence of malformations (3.3%) and the incidence of spontaneous abortions (11%) in this group of pregnancies does not exceed that generally reported for the population at large. There were three hydatidiform moles, two of which occurred in the same patient.

PHYSIOLOGICAL LACTATION
Decreases in the blood pressure are common during the puerperium and, since Bromocriptine Mesylate therapy is known to produce hypotension and, rarely, hypertension in some patients, the drug should not be administered until the vital signs have been stabilized. Because the development of hypertension may be delayed, it is prudent to monitor the blood pressure periodically during the first weeks of therapy. If hypertension, severe, progressive, or unremitting headache (with or without visual disturbance), or evidence of CNS toxicity develops, drug therapy should be discontinued and the patient should be evaluated promptly.

ACROMEGALY
Cold sensitive digital vasospasm has been observed in some acromegalic patients treated with Bromocriptine Mesylate. The response, should it occur, can be reversed by reducing the dose of Bromocriptine Mesylate and may be prevented by keeping the fingers warm. Cases of severe gastrointestinal bleeding from peptic ulcers have been reported, some fatal. Although there is no evidence that Bromocriptine Mesylate increases the incidence of peptic ulcers in acromegalic patients, symptoms suggestive of peptic ulcer should be investigated thoroughly and treated appropriately.

Possible tumor expansion while receiving Bromocriptine Mesylate therapy has been reported in a few patients. Since the natural history of growth hormone secreting tumors is unknown, all patients should be carefully monitored and, if evidence of tumor expansion develops, discontinuation of treatment and alternative procedures considered.

PARKINSON'S DISEASE
Safety during long-term use for more than two years at the doses required for parkinsonism has not been established. As with any chronic therapy, periodic evaluation of hepatic, hematopoietic, cardiovascular, and renal function is recommended. Symptomatic hypotension can occur and, therefore, caution should be exercised when treating patients receiving antihypertensive drugs.

High doses of Bromocriptine Mesylate may be associated with confusion and mental disturbances. Since parkinsonian patients may manifest mild degrees of dementia, caution should be used when treating such patients.

Bromocriptine Mesylate administered alone or concomitantly with levodopa may cause hallucinations (visual or auditory). Hallucinations usually resolve with dosage reduction; occasionally, discontinuation of Bromocriptine Mesylate is required. Rarely, after high doses, hallucinations have persisted for several weeks following discontinuation of Bromocriptine Mesylate.

As with levodopa, caution should be exercised when administering Bromocriptine Mesylate to patients with a history of myocardial infarction who have a residual atrial, nodal, or ventricular arrhythmia.

Retroperitoneal fibrosis has been reported in a few patients receiving long-term therapy (2-10 years) with Bromocriptine Mesylate in doses ranging from 30 to 140 mg daily.

NURSING MOTHERS
Since it prevents lactation, Bromocriptine Mesylate should not be administered to mothers who elect to breast feed infants.

PEDIATRIC USE
Safety and efficacy of Bromocriptine Mesylate have not been established in children under the age of 15.

INFORMATION FOR PATIENTS

When initiating therapy, all patients receiving Bromocriptine Mesylate should be cautioned with regard to engaging in activities requiring rapid and precise responses, such as driving an automobile or operating machinery since dizziness (8-16%), drowsiness (8%), faintness, fainting (8%), and syncope (less than 1%) have been reported early in the course of therapy. Patients receiving Bromocriptine Mesylate for hyperprolactinemic states associated with macroadenoma or those who have had previous transsphenoidal surgery, should be told to report any persistent watery nasal discharge to their physician. Patients receiving Bromocriptine Mesylate for treatment of a macroadenoma should be told that discontinuation of drug may be associated with rapid regrowth of the tumor and recurrence of their original symptoms. Patients receiving Bromocriptine Mesylate for the prevention of physiological lactation should be advised to stop the drug and seek prompt medical attention including blood pressure evaluation should severe, progressive, or unremitting headache develop during therapy.

DRUG INTERACTIONS

Lack or decrease in efficacy may occur in patients receiving Bromocriptine Mesylate when they are treated concurrently with drugs which have dopamine antagonist activity, e.g. phenothiazines, butyrophenones. This may be a problem particularly, for patients treated with Bromocriptine Mesylate for macroadenomas. Although there is no conclusive evidence demonstrating interactions between Bromocriptine Mesylate and other ergot derivatives, the concomitant use of these medications is not recommended.

ADVERSE REACTIONS

HYPERPROLACTINEMIC INDICATIONS

The incidence of adverse effects is quite high (69%) but these are generally mild to moderate in degree. Therapy was discontinued in approximately 5% of patients because of adverse effects. These in decreasing order of frequency are: nausea (49%), headache (19%), dizziness (17%), fatigue (7%), lightheadedness (5%), vomiting (5%), abdominal cramps (4%), nasal congestion (3%), constipation (3%), diarrhea (3%) and drowsiness (3%).

A slight hypotensive effect may accompany Bromocriptine Mesylate treatment. The occurrence of adverse reactions may be lessened by temporarily reducing dosage to one-half tablet two or three times daily. A few cases of cerebrospinal fluid rhinorrhea have been reported in patients receiving Bromocriptine Mesylate for treatment of large prolactinomas. This has occurred rarely, usually only in patients who have received previous transsphenoidal surgery, pituitary radiation, or both, and who were receiving Bromocriptine Mesylate for tumor recurrence. It may also occur in previously untreated patients whose tumor extends into the sphenoid sinus.

PHYSIOLOGICAL LACTATION

Twenty-three percent of patients treated within the recommended dosage range for the prevention of physiological lactation had at least one side effect, but they were generally mild to moderate in degree. Therapy was discontinued in approximately 3% of patients. The most frequently occurring adverse reactions were: headache (10%), dizziness (8%), nausea (7%), vomiting (3%), fatigue (1.0%), syncope (0.7%), diarrhea (0.4%) and cramps (0.4%). Decreases in blood pressure ($\geq$ 20 mm Hg systolic and $\geq$ 10 mm Hg diastolic) occurred in 28% of patients at least once during the first three postpartum days; these were usually of a transient nature. Reports of fainting in the puerperium may possibly be related to this effect. Serious adverse reactions reported include 38 cases of seizures (including 4 cases of status epilepticus), 15 cases of stroke, and 3 cases of myocardial infarction among postpartum patients. Seizure cases were not necessarily accompanied by the development of hypertension. An unremitting and often progressively severe headache, sometimes accompanied by visual disturbance, often preceded by hours to days many cases of seizure and/or stroke. Most patients had shown no evidence of toxemia during the pregnancy. One stroke case was associated with sagittal sinus thrombosis, and another was associated with cerebral and cerebellar vasculitis. One case of myocardial infarction was associated with unexplained disseminated intravascular coagulation and a second occurred in conjunction with use of another ergot alkaloid. The relationship of these adverse reactions to Bromocriptine Mesylate administration has not been established.

ACROMEGALY

The most frequent adverse reactions encountered in acromegalic patients treated with Bromocriptine Mesylate were: nausea (18%), constipation (14%), postural/orthostatic hypotension (6%), anorexia (4%), dry mouth/nasal stuffiness (4%), indigestion/dyspepsia (4%), digital vasospasm (3%), drowsiness/tiredness (3%) and vomiting (2%). Less frequent adverse reactions (less than 2%) were: gastrointestinal bleeding, dizziness, exacerbation of Raynaud's Syndrome, headache and syncope. Rarely (less than 1%) hair loss, alcohol potentiation, faintness, light-headedness, arrhythmia, ventricular tachycardia, decreased sleep requirement, visual hallucinations, lassitude, shortness of breath, bradycardia, vertigo, paresthesia, sluggishness, vasovagal attack, delusional psychosis, paranoia, insomnia, heavy headedness, reduced tolerance to cold, tingling of ears, facial pallor and muscle cramps have been reported.

PARKINSON'S DISEASE

In clinical trials in which Bromocriptine was administered with concomitant reduction in the dose of levodopa/carbidopa, the most common newly appearing adverse reactions were: nausea, abnormal involuntary movements, hallucinations, confusion, "on-off" phenomenon, dizziness, drowsiness, faintness/fainting, vomiting, asthenia, abdominal discomfort, visual disturbance, ataxia, insomnia, depression, hypotension, shortness of breath, constipation, and vertigo. Less

common adverse reactions which may be encountered include: anorexia, anxiety, blepharospasm, dry mouth, dysphagia, edema of the feet and ankles, erythromelalgia, epileptiform seizure, fatigue, headache, lethargy, mottling of skin, nasal stuffiness, nervousness, nightmares, paresthesia, skin rash, urinary frequency, urinary incontinence, urinary retention, and rarely, signs and symptoms of ergotism such as tingling of fingers, cold feet, numbness, muscle cramps of feet and legs or exacerbation of Raynaud's Syndrome.

Abnormalities in laboratory tests may include elevations in blood urea nitrogen, SGOT, SGPT, GGPT, CPK, alkaline phosphatase and uric acid, which are usually transient and not of clinical significance.

DOSAGE AND ADMINISTRATION

GENERAL

It is recommended that Bromocriptine Mesylate be taken with food. Patients should be evaluated frequently during dose escalation to determine the lowest dosage that produces a therapeutic response.

HYPERPROLACTINEMIC INDICATIONS

The initial dosage of Bromocriptine Mesylate is ½ to one 2½ mg tablet daily. An additional 2½ mg tablet may be added to the treatment regimen as tolerated every 3-7 days until an optimal therapeutic response is achieved. The therapeutic dosage usually is 5-7.5 mg and ranges from 2.5-15 mg/day.

In order to reduce the likelihood of prolonged exposure to Bromocriptine Mesylate should an unsuspected pregnancy occur, a mechanical contraceptive should be used in conjunction with Bromocriptine Mesylate therapy until normal ovulatory menstrual cycles have been restored. Contraception may then be discontinued in patients desiring pregnancy.

Thereafter, if menstruation does not occur within 3 days of the expected date, Bromocriptine Mesylate therapy should be discontinued and a pregnancy test performed.

PREVENTION OF PHYSIOLOGICAL LACTATION

Therapy should be started only after the patient's vital signs have been stabilized and no sooner than four hours after delivery. The recommended therapeutic dosage is one 2½ mg tablet of Bromocriptine Mesylate twice daily. The usual dosage range is 2.5-7.5 mg daily. Bromocriptine Mesylate therapy should be continued for 14 days; however, therapy may be given up to 21 days if necessary.

ACROMEGALY

Virtually all acromegalic patients receiving therapeutic benefit from Bromocriptine Mesylate also have reductions in circulating levels of growth hormone. Therefore, periodic assessment of circulating levels of growth hormone will, in most cases, serve as a guide in determining the therapeutic potential of Bromocriptine Mesylate. If, after a brief trial with Bromocriptine Mesylate therapy, no significant reduction in growth hormone levels has taken place, careful assessment of the clinical features of the disease should be made, and if no change has occurred, dosage adjustment or discontinuation of therapy should be considered.

The initial recommended dosage is ½ to one 2½ mg Bromocriptine Mesylate tablet on retiring (with food) for 3 days. An additional ½ to 1 tablet should be added to the treatment regimen as tolerated every 3-7 days until the patient obtains optimal therapeutic benefit. Patients should be reevaluated monthly and the dosage adjusted based on reductions of growth hormone or clinical response. The usual optimal therapeutic dosage range of Bromocriptine Mesylate varies from 20 to 30 mg per day in most patients. The maximal dosage should not exceed 100 mg per day.

Patients treated with pituitary irradiation should be withdrawn from Bromocriptine Mesylate therapy on a yearly basis to assess both the clinical effects of radiation on the disease process as well as the effects of Bromocriptine Mesylate therapy. Usually a four to eight week withdrawal period is adequate for this purpose. Recurrence of the signs/symptoms or increases in growth hormone indicate the disease process is still active and further courses of Bromocriptine Mesylate should be considered.

PARKINSON'S DISEASE

The basic principle of Bromocriptine Mesylate therapy is to initiate treatment at a low dosage and, on an individual basis, increase the daily dosage slowly until a maximum therapeutic response is achieved. The dosage of levodopa during this introductory period should be maintained, if possible. The initial dose of Bromocriptine Mesylate is ½ of a 2½ mg tablet twice daily with meals. Assessments are advised at two week intervals during dosage titration to ensure that the lowest dosage producing an optimal therapeutic response is not exceeded. If necessary, the dosage may be increased every 14 to 28 days by 2½ mg per day with meals. Should it be advisable to reduce the dosage of levodopa because of adverse reactions, the daily dosage of Bromocriptine Mesylate, if increased, should be accomplished gradually in small (2½ mg) increments.

The safety of Bromocriptine Mesylate has not been demonstrated in dosages exceeding 100 mg per day.

Storage:
Below 77°F (25°C); tight, light-resistant container.

HOW SUPPLIED
CAPSULE: 5 MG

BRAND/MANUFACTURER	NDC	SIZE	AWP
○ BRAND			
▶ PARLODEL: Sandoz Pharm	00078-0102-15	30s	$69.36
	00078-0102-05	100s	$219.24

◆ RATED THERAPEUTICALLY EQUIVALENT; ◇ THERAPEUTIC EQUIVALENCE UNCONFIRMED; ○ UNRATED

TABLETS: 2.5 MG

BRAND/MANUFACTURER	NDC	SIZE	AWP
○ **BRAND**			
➤ PARLODEL: Sandoz Pharm	00078-0017-15	30s	$43.14
	00078-0017-05	100s	$143.58
➤ PARLODEL: Sandocare	00078-0017-65	640s ud	$918.84

Bromodiphenhydramine Hydrochloride and Codeine Phosphate

DESCRIPTION

Each 5 mL of Bromodiphenhydramine Hydrochloride/Codeine Phosphate cough syrup contains:

Bromodiphenhydramine Hydrochloride ....12.5 mg
Codeine Phosphate
(Warning-May be habit forming) ....10 mg
Alcohol, 5%

Bromodiphenhydramine Hydrochloride/Codeine Phosphate Cough Syrup has a pH between 5.0 and 6.0.

Chemically, Bromodiphenhydramine Hydrochloride is ethanamine, 2-[(4-bromophenyl) phenyl-methoxy]-N, N-dimethyl-, hydrochloride ($C_{17}H_{20}BrNO\cdot HCl$), with a molecular weight of 370.72.

Chemically, Codeine Phosphate is morphinan-6-ol, 7, 8-didehydro-4, 5-epoxy-3-methoxy-17-methyl-, (5α, 6α)-phosphate (1:1) (salt), hemi- hydrate ($C_{18}H_{21}NO_3H_3\cdot PO_4\cdot 1/2H_2O$) with a molecular weight of 406.37.

Bromodiphenhydramine Hydrochloride/Codeine Phosphate Cough Syrup is an antihistamine and narcotic antitussive for oral administration.

CLINICAL PHARMACOLOGY

Codeine: Codeine exerts its antitussive activity by depressing the medullary (brain) cough center, thereby raising its threshold for incoming cough impulses.

Codeine resembles morphine both structurally, and pharmacologically, but its actions at the doses of Codeine used therapeutically are milder, with less sedation, respiratory depression, and gastrointestinal, urinary, and pupillary effects. Codeine produces an increase in biliary tract pressure, but less than morphine or meperidine.

Codeine has good antitussive activity, although less than that of morphine at equal doses. It is used in preference to morphine, because side effects are infrequent at the usual antitussive dose of Codeine.

Codeine may cause nausea and vomiting by stimulating the chemoreceptor trigger zone (CTZ); however, it may also depress the vomiting center, so that subsequent doses are unlikely to produce vomiting. Nausea is minimal after usual oral doses of Codeine.

Codeine causes histamine release, which may also produce dilation of cutaneous blood vessels, with resultant flushing of the face and neck, pruritus, and sweating.

Codeine is readily absorbed from the gastrointestinal tract following oral administration Codeine is metabolized primarily in the liver by enzymes of the endoplasmic reticulum, where it undergoes 0-demethylation, N-demethylation, and partial conjugation with glucuronic acid. The drug is excreted primarily in the urine, largely as inactive metabolites and small amounts of free and conjugated morphine. Negligible amounts of codeine and its metabolites are found in the feces.

The cough-depressing action, in animal studies, was observed to occur 15 minutes after oral administration of Codeine, peak action at 45 to 60 minutes after ingestion. The duration of action, which is dose-dependent, usually did not exceed three hours.

Bromodiphenhydramine: Antihistamines competitively antagonize various physiological effects of histamine including increased capillary permeability and dilatation, the formation of edema, the "flare" and "itch" response, and gastrointestinal and respiratory smooth-muscle constriction. Within the vascular tree, antihistamines inhibit both the vasoconstrictor and vasodilator effects of histamine. Depending on the dose, antihistamines can produce CNS stimulation or depression. Most antihistamines exhibit central and/or peripheral anticholinergic activity.

Antihistamines are well absorbed following oral administration. Many antihistamines achieve peak blood levels within two to five hours following oral administration.

Tissue distribution of the antihistamine in humans has not been established. Diphenhydramine hydrochloride and probably other antihistamines cross the placenta.

Antihistamines appear to be metabolized in the liver chiefly via mono- and didemethylation and glucuronide conjugation. Antihistamine metabolites and small amounts of unchanged drug are excreted in the urine. Small amounts of the drugs may also be excreted in breast milk.

INDICATIONS AND USAGE

Bromodiphenhydramine Hydrochloride/Codeine Phosphate is indicated for temporary relief of upper respiratory symptoms and coughs associated with allergies or other common cold.

CONTRAINDICATIONS

Use in Newborn or Premature Infants: This drug should not be used in newborn or premature infants. Bromodiphenhydramine Hydrochloride/Codeine Phosphate Cough Syrup is contraindicated in patients with known hypersensitivity to Bromodiphenhydramine Hydrochloride, Codeine Phosphate and any other drugs of similar chemical structures.

WARNINGS

Antihistamines should be used with considerable caution in patients with:
　　Narrow angle glucoma
　　Stenosing peptic ulcer
　　Pyloroduodenal obstruction
　　Bladder neck obstruction
Overdoses of antihistamines may cause hallucinations, convulsions or death, especially in infants and children (see *"Overdosage"*). Therapeutic doses of antihistamines can produce excitation or drowsiness.

Bromodiphenhydramine Hydrochloride/Codeine Phosphate Cough Syrup may have additive effects with alcohol and other CNS depressants (see *"Precautions: Drug Interactions"*).

Patients should be warned about engaging in activities requiring mental alertness such as driving a car or operating appliances, machinery, etc.

Antihistamines are more likely to cause dizziness, sedation, and hypotension in elderly patients.

Dosage of Codeine *should not be increased* if cough fails to respond; an unresponsive cough should be reevaluated in five days or sooner for possible underlying pathology, such as foreign body or lower respiratory tract disease.

Respiratory depression leading to arrest, coma, and death has occurred with the use of Codeine antitussives in young children, particularly in the under-one-year infants whose ability to deactivate the drug is not fully developed.

Administration of Codeine may be accompanied by histamine release resulting in flushing of the face and neck, pruritus, and sweating. It should be used with caution in atopic children.

Narcotics, including Codeine, may produce adverse reactions which may obscure the clinical course of patients with head injuries.

Asthma and Other Respiratory Conditions: Cough suppressants, including codeine, should not be used in asthmatic patients (see *"Contraindications"*). Nor should they be used in acute febrile illness associated with productive cough or in chronic respiratory disease where interference with ability to clear the tracheo-bronchial tree of secretions would have a deleterious effect on the patient's respiratory function.

Hypotensive Effect: Codeine may produce orthostatic hypotension in ambulatory patients.

PRECAUTIONS

General: Bromodiphenhydramine has an atropine-like action and, therefore, should be used with caution in patients with:
　　History of bronchial asthma
　　Increased intraocular pressure
　　Hyperthyroidism
　　Cardiovascular disease
　　Hypertension
At near toxic doses antihistamines can cause hallucinations. They have been abused by some patients to produce intoxication.

The drug abuse and dependence potential of antihistamines remains to be determined.

Codeine should be administered with caution and the initial dose reduced in patients with acute abdominal pathology, convulsive disorders, significant renal or hepatic impairment, fever, hypothyroidism, ulcerative colitis, prostatic hypertrophy, and in the very young or elderly or debilitated individual.

Information for Patients: Bromodiphenhydramine Hydrochloride/Codeine Phosphate Cough Syrup may cause marked drowsiness or may impair the mental and/or physical abilities required for the performance of potentially hazardous tasks, such as driving a vehicle or operating machinery Ambulatory patients should be told to avoid engaging in such activities until it is known that they do not become drowsy or dizzy from the use of this product.

Codeine, like other narcotic analgesics, may produce orthostatic hypotension in some ambulatory patients.

Patients should report any involuntary muscle movements or unusual sensitivity to light.

Patients should be questioned regarding a history of glaucoma, peptic ulcer, urinary retention, or pregnancy before starting therapy with Bromodiphenhydramine Hydrochloride/Codeine Phosphate Cough Syrup.

Patients should be told the sedative effects may be additive if alcohol, sleeping pills, sedatives, or tranquilizers are taken with Bromodiphenhydramine Hydrochloride/Codeine Phosphate Cough Syrup.

Bromodiphenhydramine Hydrochloride/Codeine Phosphate Cough Syrup may cause drowsiness, dizziness, dry mouth, blurred vision, weakness, nausea, headache, or nervousness in some patients.

Patients should be told to store this medicine in a tightly closed container in a dry, cool place away from heat or direct sunlight and out of the reach of children.

Drug Interactions: Bromodiphenhydramine Hydrochloride/Codeine Phosphate Cough Syrup may potentiate the effects of other narcotics, general anesthetics, tranquilizers, sedatives and hypnotics, tricyclic antidepressants, MAO inhibitors, alcohol, and other CNS depressants.

Also, the prominent anticholinergic effects of the tricyclic antidepressants and monoamine oxidase (MAO) inhibitors are additive with those produced by other drugs having a similar action, including antihistamines, and may prolong and intensify the anticholinergic effects of antihistamines. This could result in a toxic confusional and delirious state in the elderly. Bromodiphenhydramine should be used with caution in patients receiving tricyclic antidepressants or MAO inhibitors such as isocarboxazid, pargyline hydrochloride, phenelzine sulfate, tranylcypromine sulfate and other drugs which do not achieve their therapeutic effect by MAO inhibition, but which, nevertheless are powerful MAO inhibitors, eg, Furazolidone procarbazine hydrochloride.

Carcinogenesis, Mutagenesis, Impairment of Fertility: No long-term studies in animals were performed to evaluate the carcinogenic potential of Bromodiphenhydramine Hydrochloride/Codeine Phosphate Cough Syrup.

Pregnancy: Pregnancy Category C. Animal reproduction studies have not been conducted with Bromodiphenhydramine Hydrochloride/Codeine Phosphate cough syrup. It is also not known whether Bromodiphenhydramine Hydrochloride/Codeine Phosphate cough syrup can cause fetal harm when administered to a pregnant woman or can affect reproduction capacity. Bromodiphenhydramine Hydrochloride/Codeine Phosphate cough syrup should be given to a pregnant woman only if clearly needed.

Nursing Mothers: Because of the potential for serious adverse reactions in nursing infants from maternal ingestion of Bromodiphenhydramine Hydrochloride/Codeine Phosphate cough syrup, a decision should be made whether to discontinue nursing or to discontinue the drug, taking into account the importance of the drug to the mother.

Pediatric Use: Safety and effectiveness in children below the age of six have not been established.

ADVERSE REACTIONS
The most frequent adverse reactions are italicized:

General: Urticaria, drug rash, anaphylactic shock, photosensitivity, excessive perspiration, chills, dryness of mouth nose, and throat.

Cardiovascular System: Hypotension, headache, palpitations, tachycardia, extrasystoles.

Hematologic System: Hemolytic anemia, thrombocytopenia, agranulocytosis.

Nervous System: Sedation, sleepiness, dizziness, disturbed coordination, fatigue, confusion, restlessness, excitation nervousness, tremor, irritability, insomnia, euphoria, paresthesia, blurred vision, diplopia, vertigo, tinnitus, acute labyrinthitis, hysteria, neuritis, convulsions.

Gastrointestinal System: Epigastric distress, constipation, anorexia, nausea, vomiting, diarrhea.

Genitourinary System: Urinary frequency, difficult urination, urinary retention.

Respiratory System: Thickening of bronchial secretions, tightness of chest and wheezing, nasal stuffiness.

DRUG ABUSE AND DEPENDENCE
Bromodiphenhydramine Hydrochloride/Codeine Phosphate is a schedule V controlled substance. Codeine can produce drug dependence of the morphine type and, therefore, has the potential for being abused. Psychic dependence, physical depencence, and tolerance may develop upon repeated administration of this drug, and it should be prescribed and administered with the same degree of caution appropriate to the user of other oral narcotic-containing medications. Like other narcotic-containing medications, the drug is subject to the Federal Controlled Substances Act.

OVERDOSAGE
Serious overdosage with Codeine is characterized by respiratory depression (a decrease in respiratory rate and/or tidal volume, Cheyne-Stokes respiration, cyanosis), extreme somnolence progressing to stupor or coma, skeletal muscle flaccidity, cold and clammy skin, and sometimes bradycardia and hypotension. The triad of coma, pinpoint pupils, and respiratory depression is strongly suggestive of opiate poisoning. In severe overdosage, particularly by the intravenous route, apnea, circulatory collapse, cardiac arrest, and death may occur. Bromodiphenhydramine is additive to the depressant effects of Codeine.

It is difficult to determine what constitutes a standard toxic or lethal dose. However, the lethal oral dose of codeine in an adult is reported to be in the range of 0.5 to 1.0 gram. Infants and children are believed to be relatively more sensitive to opiates on a body weight basis. It is estimated that 5 mg/kg could be fatal in children. Elderly patients are also comparatively intolerant to opiates.

Antihistamine overdosage reactions may vary from CNS depression to stimulation. In children, stimulation predominates initially in a syndrome which may include excitement, hallucinations, ataxia, incoordination, muscle twitching, athetosis, hyperthermia, cyanosis, convulsions, tremors, and hyperreflexia followed by postictal depression and cardio-respiratory arrest. Convulsions in children may be preceded by mild depression. Dry mouth, fixed dilated pupils, flushing of the face, and fever are common. In adults, CNS depression, ranging from drowsiness to coma, is more common. The convulsant dose of antihistamines lies near the lethal dose. Convulsions indicate a poor prognosis.

In both children and adults, coma and cardiovascular collapse may occur. Deaths are reported especially in infants and children.

There is no specific therapy for acute overdosage with antihistamines. The latent period from ingestion to appearance of toxic effects is characteristically short (one-half to two hours). General symptomatic and supportive measures should be instituted promptly and maintained for as long as necessary.

Since overdoses of other classes of drugs (ie, tricyclic antidepressants) may also present anticholinergic symptomatology, appropriate toxicological analysis should be performed as soon as possible to identify the causative agent.

In the conscious patient, vomiting should be induced even though it may have occurred spontaneously. If vomiting cannot be induced, gastric lavage is indicated. Adequate precautions must be taken to protect against aspiration, especially in infants and children. Charcoal slurry or other suitable agents should be instilled into the stomach after vomiting or lavage. Saline cathartics or milk of magnesia may be of additional benefit.

In the unconscious patient, the airway should be secured with a cuffed endotracheal tube before attempting to evacuate the gastric contents. Intensive supportive and nursing care is indicated, as for any comatose patient.

If breathing is significantly impaired, maintenance of an adequate airway and mechanical support of respiration is the most effective means of providing adequate oxygenation.

Hypotension is an early sign of impending cardiovascular collapse and should be treated vigorously. Although general supportive measures are important, specific treatment with intravenous infusion of vasopressor titrated to maintain adequate blood pressure may be necessary.

Do not use CNS stimulants.

Convulsions should be controlled by careful administration of diazepam or a short-acting barbiturate, repeated as necessary. Physostigmine may also be considered for use in controlling centrally mediated convulsions.

Ice packs and cooling sponge baths, not alcohol, can aid in reducing the fever commonly seen in children.

The LD_{50} (single oral dose) of Bromodiphenhydramine is 366 mg/kg in the mouse and 602 mg/kg in the rat.

DOSAGE AND ADMINISTRATION
Dosage should be individualized according to the needs and the response of the patient.

Adults—one or two teaspoonfuls every four to six hours, not to exceed 12 teaspoonfuls in 24 hours. Children (total intake of codeine phosphate should not exceed 1 mg/kg/24 hours)—Six to under 12 years of age—one-half to one teaspoonful every six hours.

Not recommended for use in children under 6 years of age.

Store at controlled room temperature 15°-30°C(59°-86°F).

HOW SUPPLIED
SYRUP (C-V): 12.5 MG/5 ML-10 MG/5 ML

AVERAGE UNIT PRICE (AVAILABLE SIZES)		GENERIC A-RATED AVERAGE PRICE (GAAP)	
BRAND	$0.17	120 ml	$3.53
GENERIC	$0.02	480 ml	$11.38
HCFA FUL (480 ml)	$0.02	3840 ml	$81.65

BRAND/MANUFACTURER	NDC	SIZE	AWP
◆ **BRAND**			
AMBENYL: Forest Pharm	00456-0681-04	120 ml	$21.24
	00456-0681-16	480 ml	$76.63
◆ **GENERICS**			
BROMANYL: Aligen	00405-2387-76	120 ml	$3.09
BROMOTUSS W/CODEINE: Rugby	00536-0272-97	120 ml	$3.51
BROMANYL: Barre	00472-1634-04	120 ml	$3.99
BROMANYL: Schein	00364-7405-16	480 ml	$9.25
BROMANYL: Aligen	00405-2387-16	480 ml	$9.93
BROMOTUSS W/CODEINE: Rugby	00536-0272-85	480 ml	$10.43
Pennex	00426-8590-16	480 ml	$10.67
Pennex	00832-8590-16	480 ml	$10.67
AMBOPHEN: Major	00904-0067-16	480 ml	$11.35
BROMANYL: Moore,H.L.	00839-6796-69	480 ml	$11.60
BROMANYL: Qualitest	00603-1040-58	480 ml	$11.75
BROMANYL: Barre	00472-1634-16	480 ml	$11.76
Goldline	00182-1680-40	480 ml	$14.25
AMBOPHEN: Major	00904-0067-28	3840 ml	$75.25
BROMOTUSS W/CODEINE: Rugby	00536-0272-90	3840 ml	$81.39
BROMANYL: Barre	00472-1634-28	3840 ml	$88.32

Brompheniramine Maleate and Pseudoephedrine Hydrochloride

DESCRIPTION

Each capsule contains:

Brompheniramine Maleate	12 mg or 6 mg
Pseudoephedrine Hydrochloride	120 mg or 60 mg

in a specially prepared base to provide prolonged action.

◆ RATED THERAPEUTICALLY EQUIVALENT; ◇ THERAPEUTIC EQUIVALENCE UNCONFIRMED; ○ UNRATED

Each tablet contains:

Brompheniramine Maleate ....4 mg
Pseudoephedrine Hydrochloride ....60 mg

Brompheniramine Maleate/Pseudoephedrine Hydrochloride contains ingredients of the following therapeutic classes: antihistamine and nasal decongestant.

CLINICAL PHARMACOLOGY

Brompheniramine Maleate is an alkylamine type antihistamine. This group of antihistamines are among the most active histamine antagonists and are generally effective in relatively low doses. The drugs are not so prone to produce drowsiness and are among the most suitable agents for day time use; but again, a significant proportion of patients do experience this effect. Pseudoephedrine Hydrochloride is a sympathomimetic which acts predominently on alpha receptors and has little action on beta receptors. It therefore functions as an oral nasal decongestant with minimal CNS stimulation.

INDICATIONS

For the temporary relief of symptoms of seasonal and perenial allergic rhinitis, and vasomotor rhinitis, including nasal obstruction (congestion).

CONTRAINDICATIONS

Hypersensitivity to any of the ingredients. Also contraindicated in patients with severe hypertension, severe coronary artery disease, patients on MAO inhibitor therapy, patients with narrow-angle glaucoma, urinary retention, peptic ulcer and during an asthmatic attack.

WARNINGS

Considerable caution should be exercised in patients with hypertension, diabetes mellitus, ischemic heart disease, hyperthyroidism, increased intraocular pressure and prostatic hypertrophy. The elderly (60 years or older) are more likely to exhibit adverse reactions.

Anthistamines may cause excitability, especially in children. At dosages higher than the recommended dose, nervousness, dizziness or sleeplessness may occur.

PRECAUTIONS

General: Caution should be exercised in patients with high blood pressure, heart disease, diabetes or thyroid disease. The antihistamine in this product may exhibit additive effects with other CNS depressants, including alcohol.

Information for Patients: Antihistamine may cause drowsiness and ambulatory patients who operate machinery or motor vehicles should be cautioned accordingly.

Drug Interactions: MAO inhibitors and beta adrenergic blockers increase the effects of sympathomimetics. Sympathomimetics may reduce the antihypertensive effects of methyldopa, mecamylamine, reserpine and veratrum alkaloids. Concomitant use of antihistamines with alcohol and other CNS depressants may have an additive effect.

Pregnancy: The safety of use of this product in pregnancy has not been established.

ADVERSE REACTIONS

Adverse reactions include drowsiness, lassitude, nausea, giddiness, dryness of mouth, blurred vision, cardiac palpitations, flushing, increased irritability or excitement (especially in children).

DOSAGE AND ADMINISTRATION

Brompheniramine Maleate 12 mg and Pseudoephedrine Hydrochloride 120 mg: Adults and children over 12 years of age—1 capsule every 12 hours.

Brompheniramine Maleate 6 mg and Pseudoephedrine Hydrochloride 60 mg Adults and children over 12 years of age—1 or 2 capsules every 12 hours. Children 6 to 12 years of age—1 capsule every 12 hours.

Brompheniramine Maleate/Pseudoephedrine Hydrochloride Tablets: Adults and children 12 and over: One tablet every 4 hours not to exceed 6 doses in 24 hours. Children 6 to 12 years: One-half tablet every 4 hours not to exceed 6 doses in 24 hours. Do not give to children under 6 years except under the advice and supervision of a physician.

Dispense in tight child-resistant containers as defined in USP. Store between 15°-30°C (59°-86°F).

HOW SUPPLIED
CAPSULE, EXTENDED RELEASE: 6 MG-60 MG

BRAND/MANUFACTURER	NDC	SIZE	AWP
○ **BRAND**			
SHELLCAP PD: HTD	60354-0002-04	100s	$12.80
LODRANE LD: ECR	00095-6006-01	100s	$25.20
TOURO A&H: Dartmouth	58869-0301-01	100s	$39.96
BROMFED-PD: Muro	00451-4001-50	100s	$59.14
	00451-4001-60	500s	$267.93

BRAND/MANUFACTURER	NDC	SIZE	AWP
○ **GENERICS**			
DALLERGY-JR.: Laser	00277-0176-01	100s	$29.96
Goldline	00182-1054-01	100s	$30.00
Qualitest	00603-2506-21	100s	$32.22
BROMADRINE PD: Rugby	00536-4449-01	100s	$35.62
NALFED-PD: Econolab	55053-0222-01	100s	$39.95
ULTRABROM PD: WE Pharm	59196-0004-01	100s	$41.25
RESPAHIST: Respa Pharm	60575-0825-19	100s	$44.00
Jerome Stevens	50564-0526-01	100s	$66.98

For additional alternatives, turn to the section beginning on page 2859.

Brompheniramine Maleate, Injectable

DESCRIPTION

Brompheniramine Maleate, Injectable (an antihistaminic compound), is a sterile solution of Brompheniramine Maleate in water for injection.

Brompheniramine Maleate, Injectable, 10 mg/mL may be administered by intramuscular, subcutaneous, or intravenous injection.

Each mL contains: Brompheniramine Maleate 10 mg with methylparaben 0.18% and propylparaben 0.02% as preservatives, in Water for Injection q.s.

Sodium hydroxide and/or hydrochloric acid may have been used to adjust pH. pH range is 6.7 to 7.1.

At the time of manufacture, the air in the containers is replaced by nitrogen.

Following is its chemical structure:

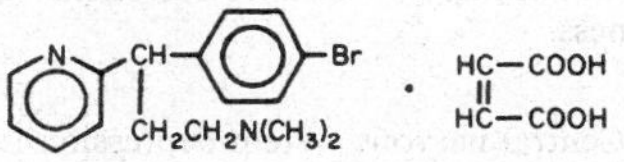

CLINICAL PHARMACOLOGY

Brompheniramine is a histamine antagonist, specifically an H_1-receptor blocking agent belonging to the alkylamine class of antihistamines. Antihistamines appear to compete with histamine for receptor sites on effector cells antagonizing the allergic response which consists of vasodilation, increased vascular permeability, and increased mucus secretion. Brompheniramine also has anticholinergic (drying) and sedative effects. Brompheniramine is well absorbed from the gastrointestinal tract, with peak plasma concentration reached in 5 hours after a single oral dose of 4 mg, and having an excretory half-life on the order of 24 hours. Urinary excretion is the major route of elimination; most as products of bio-degradation. The liver is assumed to be the main site of metabolic transformation.

INDICATIONS AND USAGE

For use in the following conditions when administration of the oral form of the drug is impractical: Amelioration of allergic reactions to blood or plasma.

In anaphylaxis as an adjunct to epinephrine and other standard measures after the acute symptoms have been controlled.

For other uncomplicated allergic conditions of the immediate type when oral therapy is impossible or contraindicated.

CONTRAINDICATIONS

Do not use in newborn or premature infants; in patients known to be hypersensitive to Brompheniramine Maleate; or in patients receiving monoamine oxidase inhibitor therapy.

Antihistamines should not be used to treat lower respiratory tract conditions including acute bronchial asthma. Contraindicated in those persons who have shown hypersensitivity to any component of this preparation.

WARNINGS

In the young child, antihistamines may produce excitation. In the elderly (approximately 60 years or older), antihistamines are more likely to cause dizziness, sedation, and hypotension.

PRECAUTIONS

General: Because Brompheniramine Maleate, Injectable, is an antihistamine, it should be administered with caution to patients with a history of bronchial asthma, narrow angle glaucoma, gastrointestinal obstruction, or prostatic hypertrophy.

Information for Patients: Patients should be warned about engaging in activities requiring mental alertness such as driving a car or operating dangerous machinery until the extent of individual toleration has been established.

Drug Interactions: Antihistamines have an additive effect with alcohol and other CNS depressants (hypnotics, sedatives, tranquilizers, anti-anxiety agents, etc.). MAO inhibitors prolong and intensify the anti-cholinergic (drying) effects of antihistamines.

Carcinogenesis, Mutagenesis: Long-term studies in animals to evaluate carcinogenic or mutagenic potential have not been performed.

Pregnancy: Pregnancy Category B. Reproduction studies have been performed in rats and mice at doses up to 16 times the maximum human dose and have revealed no evidence of impaired fertility or harm to the fetus due to Brompheniramine Maleate. There are, however, no adequate and well-controlled studies in pregnant women. Because animal reproduction studies are not always predictive of human response, this drug should be used during pregnancy only if clearly needed.

Nursing Mothers: It is not known whether this drug is excreted in human milk. Because many drugs are excreted in human milk, caution should be exercised when Brompheniramine Maleate, Injectable is administered to a nursing mother.

Pediatric Use: Brompheniramine Maleate, Injectable, should not be used in newborn or premature infants. In infants and children, especially, antihistamines in overdosage may cause hallucinations, convulsions, or death.

ADVERSE REACTIONS
The most frequent adverse reactions are italicized:

General: Urticaria, drug rash, anaphylactic shock, photosensitivity, excessive perspiration, chills, dryness of mouth, nose and throat.

Cardiovascular System: Hypotension, headache, palpitations, tachycardia, extrasystoles.

Hematologic System: Hemolytic anemia, thrombocytopenia, agranulocytosis.

Nervous System: Sedation, sleepiness, dizziness, disturbed coordination, fatigue, confusion, restlessness, excitation, nervousness, tremor, irritability, insomnia, euphoria, paresthesias, blurred vision, diplopia, vertigo, tinnitus, acute labyrinthitis, hysteria, neuritis, convulsions.

G.I. System: Epigastric distress, anorexia, nausea, vomiting, diarrhea, constipation.

G.U. System: Urinary frequency, difficult urination, urinary retention, early menses.

Respiratory System: Thickening of bronchial secretions, tightness of chest and wheezing, nasal stuffiness.

OVERDOSAGE
Signs and Symptoms: Central nervous system depression is usually the dominant action in adults; it is evidenced by drowsiness, lethargy, fatigue, hypnosis, and coma. Related symptoms include vertigo, ataxia, tinnitus, and blurred vision.

Central nervous hyperexcitability often follows initial sedation; in children excitement is often the first evidence of overdosage. The stimulant phase may include tremors, anxiety, insomnia, excitement, hallucinations, delirium, toxic psychosis, and convulsions. Hyperpyrexia may occur in children.

The terminal phase is one of severe central nervous depression with death from respiratory arrest or cardiovascular collapse.

LD$_{50}$

Species	Route	LD$_{50}$ mg/kg	Range mg/kg
Rat	PO	372	324-428
Rat	PO	207	179-239
Mice	IP	110	100-121
Mice	PO	195	167-228
Dogs	IV	97	85-126

Toxic dosage in humans: There are no absolute figures relative to the toxic dosage of brompheniramine in humans. There have been no reports of Brompheniramine Maleate, Injectable, overdosage in adults.

Removal: There is no information regarding the usefulness of forced diuresis or dialysis in the management of overdosage. Brompheniramine is 80-85% bound to protein in plasma and tissues.

Treatment: There is no specific therapy or known antidote, and treatment is along general symptomatic and supportive lines. Mechanical ventilation and oxygen therapy may be used if indicated. Care should be taken to avoid or carefully control medications which are likely to potentiate the effects of the antihistamine. If convulsions develop, they are best countered by a short-acting depressant such as thiopental, to provide a rapid, transient, and controllable effect. Diazepam is also worthy of a trial. Stimulants should not be used. Vasopressors may be used to treat hypotension.

In view of the anticholinergic manifestation of antihistamines, especially in overdosage, physostigmine may be useful in reversing such symptoms as severe agitation, delirium, and tachycardia.

DOSAGE AND ADMINISTRATION
DOSAGE SHOULD BE INDIVIDUALIZED ACCORDING TO THE NEEDS AND THE RESPONSE OF THE PATIENTS.

Adults: The usual dose is 10 mg. The dosage range is 5 mg to 20 mg. The period of protection is 3 to 12 hours, and twice daily administration is usually all that is necessary. The maximum recommended dose for 24 hours is 40 mg.

Children under 12 years: 0.5 mg per kg per 24 hours, or 15 mg per M^2 per 24 hours, divided into 3-4 doses.

Note: Brompheniramine Maleate, Injectable, 10 mg/mL, may be administered without further dilution intramuscularly or subcutaneously. It may also be administered intravenously either undiluted or diluted 1 to 10 with sterile saline for injection. If given intravenously, the drug should be given slowly, preferably with the patient in a recumbent position. If desired, Brompheniramine Maleate, Injectable may be added to normal saline or 5% glucose or whole blood for intravenous administration.

Parenteral drug products should be inspected visually for particulate matter and discoloration prior to administration, whenever solution and container permit.

Store at controlled room temperature 15°-30° C (59°-86° F). Protect from light to prevent discoloration. Temperatures below 0°C (32°F) may produce crystal formation. If present, dissolve by warming to 30°C (86°F) before using.

J CODES
IM,SC,IV—J0945

HOW SUPPLIED
INJECTION: 10 MG/ML

BRAND/MANUFACTURER	NDC	SIZE	AWP
◆ GENERICS			
ND-STAT: Hyrex	00314-2236-70	10 ml	$7.50

For additional alternatives, turn to the section beginning on page 2859.

Brompheniramine Maleate/ Codeine Phosphate/ Phenylpropanolamine Hydrochloride

DESCRIPTION
Each 5 mL (1 teaspoonful) contains:

Brompheniramine Maleate, USP	2.0 mg
Phenylpropanolamine Hydrochloride, USP	12.5 mg
Codeine Phosphate, USP	10.0 mg

(Warning: May be habit forming)

Alcohol 0.95 percent
Antihistamine/Nasal Decongestant Antitussive syrup for oral administration.

CLINICAL PHARMACOLOGY
Brompheniramine Maleate is a histamine antagonist, specifically an H$_1$-receptor-blocking agent belonging to the alkylamine class of antihistamines. Antihistamines appear to compete with histamine for receptor sites on effector cells. Brompheniramine also has anticholinergic (drying) and sedative effects. Among the antihistaminic effects, it antagonizes the allergic response (vasodilatation, increased vascular permeability, increased mucus secretion) of nasal tissue. Brompheniramine is well absorbed from the gastrointestinal tract, with peak plasma concentration after a single oral dose of 4 mg reached in 5 hours; urinary excretion is the major route of elimination, mostly as products of biodegradation; the liver is assumed to be the main site of metabolic transformation.

Phenylpropanolamine Hydrochloride is a sympathomimetic drug which is readily absorbed from the gastrointestinal tract and produces nasal vasoconstriction (decongestion). Phenylpropanolamine stimulates both α and β-adrenergic receptors, similar to ephedrine. Part of its peripheral action is indirect and is due to the displacement of norepinephrine from storage sites, but it also has direct effect on the adrenergic receptors.

Codeine is an opiate analgesic and antitussive. Codeine calms the cough control center.

INDICATIONS AND USAGE
For relief of coughs and upper respiratory symptoms, including nasal congestion, associated with allergy or the common cold.

CONTRAINDICATIONS
Hypersensitivity to any of the ingredients. Do not use in the newborn, in premature infants, in nursing mothers, in patients with severe hypertension or severe coronary artery disease, or in those receiving monoamine oxidase (MAO) inhibitors.

Antihistamines should not be used to treat lower respiratory tract conditions including asthma.

WARNINGS
Especially in infants and small children, antihistamines in overdosage may cause hallucinations, convulsions, death. Codeine may cause or aggravate constipation.

Antihistamines may diminish mental alertness. In the young child, they may produce excitation.

PRECAUTIONS

General: Because of its antihistamine component Brompheniramine Maleate/Codeine Phosphate/Phenylpropanolamine Hydrochloride (Bromphen/Codeine/PPA) Cough Syrup should be used with caution in patients with a history of bronchial asthma, narrow angle glaucoma, gastrointestinal obstruction, or urinary bladder neck obstruction. Because of its sympathomimetic component, Bromphen/Codeine/PPA Cough Syrup should be used with caution in patients with diabetes, hypertension, heart disease, or thyroid disease.

Information for Patients: Patients should be warned about engaging in activities requiring mental alertness, such as driving a car or operating dangerous machinery.

Drug Interactions: Antihistamines have additive effects with alcohol and other CNS depressants (hypnotics, sedatives, tranquilizers, antianxiety agents, etc.) MAO inhibitors prolong and intensify the anticholinergic (drying) effects of antihistamines. MAO inhibitors may enhance the effect of Phenylpropanolamine. Sympathomimetics may reduce the effects of antihypertensive drugs.

Carcinogenesis, Mutagenesis: Long-term studies in animals to evaluate carcinogenic and mutagenic potential have not been performed.

Pregnancy Category C: Animal reproduction studies have not been conducted with Bromphen/Codeine/PPA Cough Syrup. It is also not known whether Bromphen/Codeine/PPA Cough Syrup can cause fetal harm when administered to a pregnant woman or can affect reproduction capacity. Bromphen/Codeine/PPA Cough Syrup should be given to a pregnant woman only if clearly needed. Reproduction studies of Brompheniramine Maleate (one of the components of the Dimetane formulations) in rats and mice at doses up to 16 times the maximum human dose have revealed no evidence of impaired fertility or harm to the fetus.

Nursing Mothers: Because of the higher risk of intolerance of antihistamines in small infants generally, and in new borns and prematures in particular, and the fact that Codeine appears in human milk, Bromphen/Codeine/PPA Cough Syrup is contraindicated in nursing mothers.

ADVERSE REACTIONS

The most frequent adverse reactions to Bromphen/Codeine/PPA Cough Syrup are: sedation; dryness of mouth, nose and throat; thickening of bronchial secretions; dizziness. Other adverse reactions may include:

Dermatologic: Urticaria, drug rash, photosensitivity, pruritus.

Cardiovascular System: Hypotension, hypertension, cardiac arrhythmias.

CNS: Disturbed coordination, tremor, irritability, insomnia, visual disturbances, weakness, nervousness, convulsions, headache, euphoria, and dysphoria.

G. U. System: Urinary frequency, difficult urination.

G. I. System: Epigastric discomfort, anorexia, nausea, vomiting, diarrhea, constipation.

Respiratory System: Tightness of chest and wheezing, shortness of breath. At higher doses, Codeine has most of the disadvantages of morphine including respiratory depression.

Hematologic System: Hemolytic anemia, thrombocytopenia, agranulocytosis.

DRUG ABUSE AND DEPENDENCE

Codeine can produce drug dependence of the morphine type, and therefore has the potential for being abused. Psychic dependence, physical dependence and tolerance may develop upon repeated administration of this drug, and it should be prescribed and administered with the same degree of caution appropriate to the use of other oral narcotic medications. Bromphen/Codeine/PPA Cough Syrup is subject to the Federal Controlled Substances Act (Schedule V).

OVERDOSAGE

Signs and Symptoms: Serious overdose with codeine is characterized by respiratory depression, extreme somnolence progressing to stupor or coma. In severe overdosage, apnea, circulatory collapse, cardiac arrest and death may occur. The central nervous system effects from overdosage of Brompheniramine may vary from depression to stimulation. Anticholinergic effects may also occur. Overdosage of Phenylpropanolamine may be associated with tachycardia, hypertension and cardiac arrhythmias.

Toxic Doses: Doses of 800 mg or more of Codeine have caused partial loss of consciousness, delirium, restlessness, excitement, tremors, convulsions and collapse; or respiratory paralysis with such sequelae as mydriasis, marked vasodilatation, and finally death. A 2½-year-old child survived a dose of 300-900 mg of Brompheniramine; the lethal dose of Phenylpropanolamine is in the range of 50 mg/kg.

Treatment: Respiratory depression should be treated promptly. Oxygen, intravenous fluids, vasopressors and other supportive measures should be employed as indicated. If necessary, reestablishment of adequate respiratory exchange through provision of a patent airway and the institution of assisted or controlled ventilation must be provided. The narcotic antagonist, naloxone, is a specific antidote to Codeine-induced respiratory depression, and should be administered by the intravenous route if appropriate (see package insert for naloxone). Since the duration of action of Codeine may exceed that of the antagonist, the patient should be kept under constant surveillance.

Gastric emptying may be useful in removing unabsorbed drug, either by inducing emesis or lavage; precautions against aspiration must be taken. Stimulants or depressants should be used cautiously and only when specifically indicated. If marked excitement is present, one of the short-acting barbiturates or chloral hydrate may be used.

DOSAGE AND ADMINISTRATION

Adults and children 12 years of age and over: 2 teaspoonfuls every 4 hours. Children 6 to under 12 years: 1 teaspoonful every 4 hours. Children 2 to under 6 years: ½ teaspoonful every 4 hours. Children 6 months to under 2 years: Dosage to be established by physician.

Do not exceed 6 doses during a 24-hour period.

Store at controlled room temperature, between 15°C and 30°C (59°F and 86°F). Dispense in tight, light-resistant container.

HOW SUPPLIED
SYRUP (C-V): 2 MG-10 MG-12.5 MG/5 ML

AVERAGE UNIT PRICE (AVAILABLE SIZES)		GENERIC A-RATED AVERAGE PRICE (GAAP)	
BRAND	$0.06	480 ml	$44.05
GENERIC	$0.03	3840 ml	$44.05
HCFA FUL (480 ml)	$0.03	120 ml	$3.46
		3840 ml	$69.31

BRAND/MANUFACTURER	NDC	SIZE	AWP
◆ **BRAND**			
DIMETANE-DC: Robins Pharm	00031-1833-25	480 ml	$31.54
	00031-1833-29	3840 ml	$226.26
◆ **GENERICS**			
MYPHETANE DC: Pennex	00832-8461-04	120 ml	$2.86
BROMANATE DC: Moore,H.L.	00839-7070-65	120 ml	$3.09
BROMPHEN DC W/CODEINE: Rugby	00536-0262-97	120 ml	$3.15
BROMPHEN DC: Schein	00364-7387-77	120 ml	$3.60
MYPHETANE DC: Pennex	00426-8461-04	120 ml	$3.60
Geneva	00781-6805-04	120 ml	$3.68
BROMANATE DC COUGH: Major	00904-7819-00	120 ml	$3.85
Major	00904-0716-20	120 ml	$3.85
BROMANATE DC COUGH: Barre	00472-1645-04	120 ml	$4.05
BROMANATE DC COUGH: Barre	00472-1645-16	480 ml	$14.05
BROMANATE DC COUGH: Major	00904-7819-16	480 ml	$14.65
BROMPHEN DC W/CODEINE: Rugby	00536-0262-85	480 ml	$15.25
BROMANATE DC: Moore,H.L.	00839-7070-70	3840 ml	$58.98
MYPHETANE DC: Pennex	00832-8461-28	3840 ml	$64.13
BROMPHEN DC W/CODEINE: Rugby	00536-0262-90	3840 ml	$64.35
MYPHETANE DC: Pennex	00426-8461-28	3840 ml	$69.50
BROMANATE DC COUGH: Barre	00472-1645-28	3840 ml	$74.05
BROMANATE DC COUGH: Major	00904-7819-28	3840 ml	$79.45
Major	00904-0716-28	3840 ml	$79.45

Brompheniramine/ Dextromethorphan/ Pseudoephedrine

DESCRIPTION

Brompheniramine/Dextromethorphan/Pseudoephedrine (Bromphen/DM/Pseudoeph) is a cough syrup.

Each 5 mL (1 teaspoonful) contains:

Brompheniramine Maleate, USP	2 mg
Pseudoephedrine Hydrochloride, USP	30 mg
Dextromethorphan Hydrobromide, USP	10 mg

Alcohol 0.95 percent

In a palatable, aromatic vehicle.

Antihistamine/Antitussive/Nasal Decongestant syrup for oral administration.

CLINICAL PHARMACOLOGY

Brompheniramine Maleate is a histamine antagonist, specifically an H_1-receptor-blocking agent belonging to the alkylamine class of antihistamines. Antihistamines appear to compete with histamine for receptor sites on effector cells. Brompheniramine also has anticholinergic (drying) and sedative effects. Among the antihistaminic effects, it antagonizes the allergic response (vasodilatation, increased vascular permeability, increased mucus secretion) of nasal tissue. Brompheniramine is well absorbed from the gastrointestinal tract, with peak plasma concentration after single, oral dose of 4 mg reached in 5 hours; urinary excretion is the major route of elimination, mostly as products of biodegradation; the liver is assumed to be the main site of metabolic transformation.

Pseudoephedrine acts on sympathetic nerve endings and also on smooth muscle, making it useful as a nasal decongestant. The nasal decongestant effect is mediated by the action of pseudoephedrine on α-sympathetic receptors, producing vasoconstriction of the dilated nasal arterioles. Following oral administration, effects are noted within 30 minutes with peak activity occurring at approximately one hour.

Dextromethorphan acts centrally to elevate the threshold for coughing. It has no analgesic or addictive properties. The onset of antitussive action occurs in 15 to 30 minutes after administration and is of long duration.

INDICATIONS AND USAGE

For relief of coughs and upper respiratory symptoms, including nasal congestion, associated with allergy or the common cold.

CONTRAINDICATIONS

Hypersensitivity to any of the ingredients. Do not use in the newborn, in premature infants, in nursing mothers, in patients with severe hypertension or severe coronary artery disease, or in those receiving monoamine oxidase (MAO) inhibitors.

Antihistamines should not be used to treat lower respiratory tract conditions including asthma.

WARNINGS

Especially in infants and small children, antihistamines in overdosage may cause hallucinations, convulsions, and death.

Antihistamines may diminish mental alertness. In the young child, they may produce excitation.

PRECAUTIONS

General: Because of its antihistamine component, Bromphen/DM/Pseudoeph Cough Syrup should be used with caution in patients with a history of bronchial asthma, narrow angle glaucoma, gastrointestinal obstruction, or urinary bladder neck obstruction. Because of its sympathomimetic component, Bromphen/DM/Pseudoeph Cough Syrup should be used with caution in patients with diabetes, hypertension, heart disease, or thyroid disease.

Information for Patients: Patients should be warned about engaging in activities requiring mental alertness, such as driving a car or operating dangerous machinery.

Drug Interactions: Antihistamines have additive effects with alcohol and other CNS depressants (hypnotics, sedatives, tranquilizers, antianxiety agents, etc.). MAO inhibitors prolong and intensify the anticholinergic (drying) effects of antihistamines. MAO inhibitors may enhance the effect of Pseudoephedrine. Sympathomimetics may reduce the effects of antihypertensive drugs.

Carcinogenesis, Mutagenesis, Impairment Of Fertility: Animal studies of Bromphen/DM/Pseudoeph Cough Syrup to assess the carcinogenic and mutagenic potential or the effect on fertility have not been performed.

PREGNANCY

Teratogenic Effects—Pregnancy Category C: Animal reproduction studies have not been conducted with Bromphen/DM/Pseudoeph Cough Syrup. It is also not known whether Bromphen/DM/Pseudoeph Cough Syrup can cause fetal harm when administered to a pregnant woman or can affect reproduction capacity. Bromphen/DM/Pseudoeph Cough Syrup should be given to a pregnant woman only if clearly needed.

Reproduction studies of Brompheniramine Maleate (a component of Bromphen/DM/Pseudoeph Cough Syrup) in rats and mice at doses up to 16 times the maximum human dose have revealed no evidence of impaired fertility or harm to the fetus.

Nursing Mothers: Because of the higher risk of intolerance of antihistamines in small infants generally, and in newborns and prematures in particular, Bromphen/DM/Pseudoeph Cough Syrup is contraindicated in nursing mothers.

ADVERSE REACTIONS

The most frequent adverse reactions to Bromphen/DM/Pseudoeph Cough Syrup are: sedation; dryness of mouth, nose and throat; thickening of bronchial secretions; dizziness. Other adverse reactions may include:

Dermatologic: Urticaria, drug rash, photosensitivity, pruritus.

Cardiovascular System: Hypotension, hypertension, cardiac arrhythmias palpitation.

CNS: Disturbed coordination, tremor, irritability, insomnia, visual disturbances, weakness, nervousness, convulsions, headache, euphoria, and dysphoria.

G. U. Systems: Urinary frequency, difficult urination.

G. I. System: Epigastric discomfort, anorexia, nausea, vomiting, diarrhea, constipation.

Respiratory System: Tightness of chest and wheezing, shortness of breath.

Hematologic System: Hemolytic anemia, thrombocytopenia, agranulocytosis.

OVERDOSAGE

Signs and Symptoms: Central nervous system effects from overdosage of Brompheniramine may vary from depression to stimulation, especially in children. Anticholinergic effects may be noted. Toxic doses of Pseudoephedrine may result in CNS stimulation, tachycardia, hypertension, and cardiac arrhythmias: signs of CNS depression may occasionally be seen. Dextromethorphan in toxic doses will cause drowsiness, ataxia, nystagmus, opisthotonos, and convulsive seizures.

Toxic Doses: Data suggest that individuals may respond in an unexpected manner to apparently small amounts of a particular drug. A 2½-year-old child survived the ingestion of 21 mg/kg of Dextromethorphan exhibiting only ataxia, drowsiness, and fever, but seizures have been reported in 2 children following the ingestion of 13-17 mg/kg. Another 2½-year-old child survived a dose of 300-900 mg of Brompheniramine. The toxic dose of Pseudoephedrine should be less than that of ephedrine, which is estimated to be 50 mg/kg.

Treatment: Induce emesis if patient is alert and is seen prior to 6 hours following ingestion. Precautions against aspiration must be taken, especially in infants and small children. Gastric lavage may be carried out, although in some instances tracheostomy may be necessary prior to lavage. Naloxone hydrochloride 0.005 mg/kg intravenously may be of value in reversing the CNS depression that may occur from an overdose of Dextromethorphan. CNS stimulants may counter CNS depression. Should CNS hyperactivity or convulsive seizures occur, intravenous short-acting barbiturates may be indicated. Hypertensive responses and/or tachycardia should be treated appropriately. Oxygen, intravenous fluids, and other supportive measures should be employed as indicated.

DOSAGE AND ADMINISTRATION

Adults and children 12 years of age and over: 2 teaspoonfuls every 4 hours. Children 6 to under 12 years: 1 teaspoonful every 4 hours. Children 2 to under 6 years: ½ teaspoonful every 4 hours. Children 6 months to under 2 years: Dosage to be established by physician.

Do not exceed 6 doses during a 24-hour period.

Store at controlled room temperature, between 15°C and 30°C (59°F and 86°F). Dispense in tight, light-resistant container.

HOW SUPPLIED
SYRUP: 2 MG-10 MG-30 MG/5 ML

AVERAGE UNIT PRICE (AVAILABLE SIZES)		GENERIC A-RATED AVERAGE PRICE (GAAP)	
BRAND	$0.06	120 ml	$3.75
GENERIC	$0.02	480 ml	$10.39
HCFA FUL (480 ml)	$0.01	3840 ml	$49.08

BRAND/MANUFACTURER	NDC	SIZE	AWP
◆ **BRAND**			
BROMFED-DM: Muro	00451-4101-16	480 ml	$28.36
DIMETANE-DX: Robins Pharm	00031-1836-25	480 ml	$32.00
	00031-1836-29	3840 ml	$231.36
◆ **GENERICS**			
MYPHETANE DX COUGH: Pennex	00832-8482-04	120 ml	$3.30
MYPHETANE DX COUGH: Pennex	00426-8482-04	120 ml	$4.20
Aligen	00405-3660-76	120 ml	$4.42
MYPHETANE DX COUGH: Pennex	00832-8482-16	480 ml	$5.85
BROMATANE DX: Goldline	00182-6022-40	480 ml	$7.95
MYPHETANE DX COUGH: Pennex	00426-8482-16	480 ml	$8.00
BROMANATE DX COUGH: Major	00904-0717-16	480 ml	$8.25
BROMPHEN DX: Rugby	00536-0285-85	480 ml	$13.44
BROMAREST DX: Warner Chilcott	00047-2909-23	480 ml	$18.84
MYPHETANE DX COUGH: Pennex	00832-8482-28	3840 ml	$39.80
BROMANATE DX COUGH: Major	00904-0717-28	3840 ml	$49.45
MYPHETANE DX COUGH: Pennex	00426-8482-28	3840 ml	$58.00

Bronkodyl *SEE* THEOPHYLLINE

Bronkometer *SEE* ISOETHARINE MESYLATE

Bronkosol *SEE* ISOETHARINE HYDROCHLORIDE

Bronkotuss *SEE* CHLORPHENIRAMINE MALEATE/ EPHEDRINE SULFATE/GUAIFENESIN/HYDRIODIC ACID

Brontex *SEE* CODEINE PHOSPHATE WITH GUAIFENESIN

BSS *SEE* BALANCED SALT SOLUTION

Bucladin-S *SEE* BUCLIZINE HYDROCHLORIDE

Buclizine Hydrochloride

Each Tablet Contains:

Buclizine Hydrochloride . . . . .50 mg

DESCRIPTION
Buclizine Hydrochloride is 1-(p-tert-Butylbenzyl) -4- (p-chloro- α -phenylbenzyl) piperazine dihydrochloride. Each tablet contains 50 mg Buclizine Hydrochloride.

◆ RATED THERAPEUTICALLY EQUIVALENT; ◇ THERAPEUTIC EQUIVALENCE UNCONFIRMED; ○ UNRATED

Following is its chemical structure:

ACTIONS

Buclizine Hydrochloride acts centrally to suppress nausea and vomiting.

INDICATIONS

Buclizine Hydrochloride is effective in the management of nausea, vomiting, and dizziness associated with motion sickness.

CONTRAINDICATIONS

Buclizine Hydrochloride, when administered to the pregnant rat, induced fetal abnormalities at doses above the human therapeutic range. Clinical data are not adequate to establish nonteratogenicity in early pregnancy. Until such data are available Buclizine Hydrochloride is contraindicated for use in early pregnancy.

Buclizine Hydrochloride is contraindicated in individuals who have shown a previous hypersensitivity to it.

WARNINGS

Since drowsiness may occur with use of this drug, patients should be warned of this possibility and cautioned against engaging in activities requiring mental alertness, such as driving a car, or operating heavy machinery or appliances. Safe and effective dosage in children has not been established.

PRECAUTION

Certain brands of Buclizine Hydrochloride contain Yellow 5 (tartrazine) which may cause allergic-type reactions (including bronchial asthma) in certain susceptible individuals. Although the overall incidence of Yellow 5 (tartrazine) sensitivity in the general population is low, it is frequently seen in patients who also have aspirin hypersensitivity.

ADVERSE REACTIONS

Occasionally drowsiness, dryness of mouth, headache, and jitteriness are encountered.

DOSAGE AND ADMINISTRATION

Buclizine Hydrochloride Tablets can be taken without swallowing water. Place the Tablet in the mouth and allow it to dissolve, or the tablet may be chewed.

Adults: One tablet usually serves to alleviate nausea. In severe cases, three tablets a day may be taken. The usual maintenance dosage is one tablet twice daily.

In the prevention of motion sickness, one tablet taken at least ½ hour before beginning travel usually suffices. For extended travel, a second tablet may be taken after 4 to 6 hours.

Store at room temperature; avoid excess heat (over 104°F/40°C). Dispense in well-closed light-resistant container.

HOW SUPPLIED
TABLETS: 50 MG

BRAND/MANUFACTURER	NDC	SIZE	AWP
○ **BRAND**			
BUCLADIN-S: Stuart	00038-0864-10	100s	$47.20

Budesonide

DESCRIPTION

Budesonide is an anti-inflammatory glucocorticosteroid. It is designated chemically as 16α, 17α-butylidene-dioxypregna-1,4-diene-11β, 21-diol-3, 20-dione. Budesonide possesses an asymmetric carbon atom in its structure and is provided as the mixture of the two epimers, 22R and 22S. The empirical formula of Budesonide is $C_{25}H_{34}O_6$ and its molecular weight is 430.5.

Budesonide is a white to off-white odorless powder that is practically insoluble in water and in heptane, sparingly soluble in ethanol, and freely soluble in chloroform. Its partition coefficient between octanol and water at pH 7.4 is 1.6×10^3. Budesonide nasal inhaler is a metered-dose pressurized aerosol unit containing a suspension of micronized Budesonide in propellants.

Each actuation releases 50 µg Budesonide from the valve and delivers approximately 32 µg Budesonide from the nasal adapter (dose to patient).

Following is its chemical structure:

CLINICAL PHARMACOLOGY

Budesonide is a glucocorticosteroid having a potent glucocorticoid and weak mineralocorticoid activity. In standard *in vitro* and animal models, Budesonide has an approximately 200 fold higher affinity for the glucocorticoid receptor and a 1000 fold higher topical anti-inflammatory potency than cortisol (rat croton oil ear edema assay). As a measure of systemic activity, Budesonide is 40 times more potent than cortisol when administered subcutaneously and 25 times more potent when administered orally in the rat thymus involution assay.

The precise mechanism of glucocorticosteroid actions on allergic and nonallergic rhinitis is not known. Glucocorticosteroids have been shown to have a wide range of inhibitory activities against multiple cell types (e.g., mast cells, eosinophils, neutrophils, macrophages and lymphocytes) and mediators (e.g., histamine, eicosanoids, leukotrienes and cytokines) involved in allergic and nonallergic/irritant-mediated inflammation.

Corticoids affect the delayed (6 hour) response to an allergen challenge more than the histamine-associated immediate response (20 minute). The clinical significance of these findings is unknown.

Pharmacokinetics: The pharmacokinetics of Budesonide have been studied following nasal, oral and intravenous administration. Pharmacokinetic studies were performed with doses higher than those used clinically because at clinical doses the resulting plasma levels are below the limits of detection.

The results are as follows: (See related table).

Only about 20% of an intranasal dose from the Budesonide nasal inhaler reaches the systemic circulation.

While Budesonide is well absorbed from the G1 tract, the oral bioavailability of Budesonide is low (~ 10%) primarily due to extensive first pass metabolism in the liver. After reaching the systemic circulation plasma levels decline in a log linear manner with an apparent elimination half-life of approximately 2 hours.

Budesonide has a volume of distribution of approximately 200 L and is 88% protein bound in the plasma. Budesonide is a mixture of two epimers, 22R and 22S. In glucocorticoid receptor affinity studies, the 22R form is two times as active as the 22S epimer. It is also preferentially cleared by the liver with an apparent systemic clearance of 1.4 ± 0.3 L/min vs. 1.0 ± 0.2 L/min for the 22S form. *In vitro* studies indicate that the two forms of Budesonide do not interconvert. Budesonide is rapidly and extensively metabolized in man by the liver. *In vitro* studies looking at sites of metabolism showed negligible metabolism in skin, lung, and serum. After intranasal administration of a radiolabeled dose 2/3 of the radioactivity was found in the urine and the remainder in the feces by 96 hours. The primary metabolites of Budesonide in the urine following IV administration are 16α-hydroxyprednisolone (24%) and 6β-hydroxybudesonide (5%). An additional 34% of the radioactivity recovered in the urine were conjugates. No unchanged Budesonide was found in the urine. These results regarding the metabolic fate of Budesonide parallel results obtained in *in vitro* metabolic studies using human liver homogenates.

In vitro studies of the binding of the two primary metabolites to the glucocorticoid receptor indicate that they have less than 1% of the affinity for the receptor as the parent compound Budesonide.

Pharmacodynamics: The effect of intranasal Budesonide at a dosage of two sprays in each nostril morning and evening (total daily dose of 256 µg) on hypothalamic-pituitary-adrenal (HPA) axis function has been evaluated in 275 adults and 61 children following short-term use (< 2 months) and in 113 adults and 116 children following longer use (6—48 months). Early morning plasma cortisol and the short cosyntropin stimulation test (30-60 minutes) were the most commonly performed assessments of HPA function.

Twenty-four hour urinary cortisol levels were determined in 50 adults (short term) and 96 children (long term). There were no statistically significant changes from baseline measurements in early morning plasma cortisol or 24-hour urinary cortisol excretion or in response to cosyntropin.

In a crossover trial using single doses of 200, 400 and 800 µg of an aqueous formulation of Budesonide administered intransally at 10 P.M., a dose-dependent decrease in urinary cortisol excretion was found between 10 P.M. and 8 A.M. the following morning. In another study using intranasal Budesonide administered at 10 P.M., doses four (1024 µg) and eight (2048 µg) times higher than the recommended daily dose (256 µg) were followed by a significant decrease in plasma cortisol levels at 8 A.M. the following morning (17% and 22%, respectively).

A 3 week clinical study in seasonal rhinitis, comparing intranasal Budesonide and orally ingested Budesonide with placebo in 98 patients with allergic rhinitis due to birch pollen, demonstrated that the therapeutic effect of Budesonide can be attributed to the topical effects of Budesonide. Intranasally, 128 µg of Budesonide applied twice daily (55 µg systemically absorbed/day) provided clinically and statistically significant evidence of efficacy, whereas 250 µg of Budesonide ingested twice a day as a capsule (65 µg systemically absorbed/day) was no different from placebo in reducing nasal symptoms.

Clinical Trials: The prophylactic and therapeutic efficacy of intranasal Budesonide has been evaluated in 20 controlled clinical trials of seasonal or perennial rhinitis. The number of patients treated with Budesonide in these studies was 50 male and 33 female patients ages 6 to 12 years old, 77 males and 62 females ages 13 to 18 years old, 185 males and 246 females ages 19 to 64 and 1 male and 2 females over 64. The patients were predominantly caucasian.

Double-blind clinical trials of two to four weeks duration have shown that, compared with placebo, intranasal Budesonide 128 µg b.i.d. (two sprays in each nostril morning and evening) or 256 mg q.d. (four sprays in each nostril in the morning) provides statistically significant relief of nasal symptoms such as blockage, rhinorrhea, itching, and sneezing in adults and children with seasonal allergic rhinitis or perennial allergic rhinitis. Similar improvement has also been demonstrated in adults with nonallergic perennial rhinitis.

The therapeutic effect of intranasal Budesonide compared with placebo has been demonstrated by rhinoscopic examinations, in children and adults with seasonal or perennial allergic rhinitis and adults with nonallergic perennial rhinitis. Biopsies of the nasal mucosa of 50 adult patients after 12 months of treatment and of 10 patients after 3–5 years of therapy showed no histopathological evidence of adverse effects. The clinical significance of either of these findings is unknown.

Individualization of Dosage: It is recommended that the starting dose for all adults be 256 µg daily, as either two sprays in each nostril twice per day, morning and evening, or as four sprays in each nostril once a day in the morning. The effect should be assessed 3–7 days after initiating treatment and then periodically until the patient's symptoms are stable. If adequate relief of symptoms is not achieved after 3 weeks of treatment, then intranasal Budesonide should be discontinued.

In patients who do achieve a good result it is desirable, once the maximum benefit seems to have been achieved, to titrate an individual patient to the minimum effective dose. Because of the generally short duration of therapy for seasonal allergic rhinitis, it is usually not necessary to do this.

In patients with perennial allergic rhinitis, once adequate relief has been obtained the dose should be gradually decreased every 2—4 weeks as long as the desired clinical effect is maintained. If symptoms return, the dose may briefly be increased to the patient's starting dose and then returned to the dose the patient was on before symptoms reoccurred.

As with other aerosolized nasal glucocorticosteroids, the vehicle used to deliver the glucocorticosteroid may cause symptoms that are difficult to distinguish from the patient's rhinitis symptoms. The corticoid may suppress symptoms caused by the vehicle at higher doses but as the dose is decreased symptoms from the vehicle may emerge. If a patient needs chronic treatment and the daily dose cannot be decreased from the starting dose, it may be advisable to try alternative therapy.

INDICATIONS AND USAGE

Intranasal Budesonide is indicated for the management of symptoms of seasonal or perennial allergic rhinitis in adults and children and nonallergic perennial rhinitis in adults.

Intranasal Budesonide is not recommended for treatment of nonallergic rhinitis in children because adequate numbers of such children have not been studied.

CONTRAINDICATIONS

Hypersensitivity to any of the ingredients of this preparation contraindicates its use.

WARNINGS

The replacement of a systemic glucocorticosteroid with a topical glucocorticosteroid can be accompanied by signs of adrenal insufficiency, and in addition some patients may experience symptoms of withdrawal, e.g., joint and/or muscular pain, lassitude and depression. Patients previously treated for prolonged periods with systemic glucocorticosteroids and transferred to topical glucocorticosteroids should be carefully monitored for acute adrenal insufficiency in response to stress. In those patients who have asthma or other clinical conditions requiring long-term systemic glucocorticosteroid treatment, too rapid a decrease in systemic glucocorticosteroids may cause a severe exacerbation of their symptoms.

The use of intranasal Budesonide with alternate-day systemic prednisone could increase the likelihood of hypothalamic-pituitary-adrenal (HPA) suppression compared with a therapeutic dose of either one alone. Therefore, intranasal Budesonide should be used with caution in patients already receiving alternate-day prednisone treatment for any disease. In addition, the concomitant use of intranasal Budesonide with other inhaled glucocorticosteroids could increase the risk of signs or symptoms of hypercorticism and/or suppression of the HPA-axis.

Patients who are on drugs which suppress the immune system are more susceptible to infections than healthy individuals. Chickenpox and measles, for example, can have a more serious or even fatal course in non-immune children or adults on immunosuppressant doses of corticosteroids. In such children or adults who have not had these diseases, particular care should be taken to avoid exposure. How the dose, route and duration of corticosteroid administration affects the risk of developing a disseminated infection is not known. The contribution of the underlying disease and/or prior corticosteroid treatment to the risk is also not known. If exposed to chickenpox, prophylaxis with varicella zoster immune globulin (VZIG) may be indicated. If exposed to measles, prophylaxis with pooled intramuscular immunoglobulin (IG) may be indicated. (See the

respective package insert for complete VZIG and IG prescribing information). If chickenpox develops, treatment with antiviral agents may be considered.

PRECAUTIONS

General: Rarely, immediate hypersensitivity reactions or contact dermatitis may occur after the intranasal administration of Budesonide. Rare instances of wheezing, nasal septum perforation and increased intraocular pressure have been reported following the intranasal application of aerosolized glucocorticosteroids.

Like other glucocorticosteroids, Budesonide is absorbed into the circulation. Use of excessive doses of glucocorticosteroids may lead to signs or symptoms of hypercorticism, suppression of HPA function and/or suppression of growth in children or teenagers. In short term studies of the acute effect of inhaled Budesonide 256 µg/day on lower leg growth (knemometry), it like other inhaled and intramuscular corticoids which have been studied showed a decrease in the rate of lower leg growth. The clinical significance of this finding is not known. In two one-year studies in 92 children taking recommended doses of intranasal Budesonide, height and skeletal stature were consistent with chronological age. Physicians should closely follow the growth of children taking corticoids, by any route, and weigh the benefits of corticoid therapy against the possibility of growth suppression if a child's growth appears slowed.

Although systemic effects have been minimal with recommended doses of intranasal Budesonide, this potential risk increases with larger doses. Therefore, larger than recommended doses of intranasal Budesonide should be avoided. When used at larger doses, systemic glucocorticosteroid effects such as hypercorticism and adrenal suppression may appear. If such changes occur, the dosage of intranasal Budesonide should be discontinued slowly consistent with accepted procedures for discontinuing oral glucocorticosteroid therapy.

In clinical studies with Budesonide administered intranasally, the development of localized infections of the nose and pharynx with Candida albicans has occurred only rarely. When such an infection develops, it may require treatment with appropriate local therapy and discontinuation of treatment with intranasal Budesonide. Patients using intranasal Budesonide over several months or longer should be examined periodically for evidence of Candida infection or other signs of adverse effects on the nasal mucosa.

Intranasal Budesonide should be used with caution, if at all, in patients with active or quiescent tuberculous infections, untreated fungal, bacterial, or systemic viral infections, or ocular herpes simplex.

Because of the inhibitory effect of glucocorticosteroids on wound healing, patients who have experienced recent nasal septal ulcers, nasal surgery, or nasal trauma should not use a nasal glucocorticosteroid until healing has occurred.

Information for Patients: Patients being treated with intranasal Budesonide should receive the following information and instructions.

Patients should use intranasal Budesonide as prescribed. A decrease in symptoms may occur as soon as 24 hours after starting glucocorticosteroid therapy and generally can be expected to occur within a few days of initiating therapy in allergic rhinitis. The patient should contact the physician if symptoms do not improve by three weeks, or if the condition worsens. Nasal irritation and/or burning after use of the spray occur only rarely with this product. The patient should contact the physician if they occur repeatedly.

Patients who are on corticosteroids should be warned to avoid exposure to chickenpox or measles. Patients should also be advised that if they are exposed they should consult their physician without delay.

Carcinogenesis, Mutagenesis, Impairment of Fertility: Longterm studies were conducted in mice and rats using oral administration to evaluate the carcinogenic potential of Budesonide.

There was no evidence of a carcinogenic effect when Budesonide was administered orally for 91 weeks to mice at doses up to 200 µg/kg/day (600 µg/m^2/day).

In a 104-week carcinogenicity study in Sprague-Dawley rats (41), a statistically significant increase in the incidence of gliomas was observed in male rats receiving 50 µg/kg/day (300 µg/m^2/day) orally; no such changes were seen in male rats receiving doses of 10 and 25 µg/kg/day (60 and 150 µg/m^2/day) or in female rats at any dose. Two additional 104-week carcinogenicity studies have been performed with oral Budesonide at doses of 50 µg/kg/day (300 µg/m^2/day) in male Sprague-Dawley and Fischer rats. These studies did not demonstrate an increased glioma incidence in Budesonide treated animals as compared with concurrent controls or reference glucocorticosteroid treated groups (prednisolone and triamcinolone acetonide).

Compared with concurrent control male Sprague-Dawley rats there was a statistically significant increase in the incidence of hepatocellular tumors. This

| Route of Administration | T_{max} (hr) | C_{max}** (nmol/L) | Mean* [range] | | |
			Systemic Availability***	V_D (L)	Clearance (L/min)
Nasal Inhaler (N = 9)	0.6 [0.3-2]	0.52 [0.24-0.88]	21 [16-27]	–	–
Oral Capsule (N = 11)	1.0 [0.5-2]	0.33 [0.19-0.50]	12 [8-20]	–	–
I.V. (N = 11)	-	-	100	201 [102-275]	1.2 [0.8-1.5]

* mean of the two epimers
** dose normalized to a 256 µg dose
*** % of delivered dose

◆ RATED THERAPEUTICALLY EQUIVALENT; ◇ THERAPEUTIC EQUIVALENCE UNCONFIRMED; ○ UNRATED

finding was confirmed in all three steroid groups (Budesonide, prednisolone, triamcinolone acetonide) in the second study in male Sprague-Dawley rats.

The mutagenic potential of Budesonide was evaluated in six different test systems: Ames Salmonella/microsome plate test, mouse micronucleus test, mouse lymphoma test, chromosome aberration test in human lymphocytes, sex-linked recessive lethal test in Drosophila melanogaster, and DNA repair analysis in rat hepatocyte culture. No mutagenic or clastogenic properties of Budesonide were found in any of the tests.

The effect upon fertility and general reproductive performance was studied in rats given Budesonide subcutaneously. At 20 μg/kg/day (120 μg/m^2/day) and higher dose levels, a decrease in maternal body-weight gain was observed along with a decrease in prenatal viability and viability of the young at birth and during lactation. No such effects were noted at the dose level 5 μg/kg/day (30 μg/m^2/day).

Pregnancy: Teratogenic Effects: Pregnancy Category C: As with other glucocorticoids Budesonide has been shown to be teratogenic and embryocidal in rabbits and rats when given subcutaneously in doses exceeding 5 and 100 μg/kg/day (59 and 600 μg/m^2/day), respectively. In these studies Budesonide at 25 μg/kg/day (295 μg/m^2/day) given to rabbits and 500 μg/kg/day (3000 μg/m^2/day) given to rats was found to produce fetal loss, decreased pup weights and skeletal abnormalities. No teratogenic or embryocidal effects have been seen in rats when Budesonide was administered by inhalation at doses of 100—250 μg/kg/day (600—1500 μg/m^2/day, approximately 27—68 times the human recommended starting dose based on μg/kg/day or 4—10 times the human dose based on μg/m^2/day).

There are no adequate and well-controlled studies in pregnant women. Budesonide should be used during pregnancy only if the potential benefit justifies the potential risk to the fetus. Experience with oral glucocorticosteroids since their introduction in pharmacologic, as opposed to physiologic, doses suggests that rodents are more prone to teratogenic effects from glucocorticosteroids than humans. In addition, because there is a natural increase in glucocorticosteroid production during pregnancy, most women will require a lower exogenous glucocorticosteroid dose and many will not need glucocorticosteroid treatment during pregnancy.

Nonteratogenic Effects: Hypoadrenalism may occur in infants born of mothers receiving glucocorticosteroids during pregnancy. Such infants should be carefully observed.

Nursing Mothers: It is not known whether Budesonide is excreted in human milk. Because other glucocorticosteroids are excreted in human milk, caution should be exercised when intranasal Budesonide is administered to nursing women.

Pediatric Use: Safety and effectiveness in children below 6 years of age have not been established. Oral glucocorticosteroids have been shown to cause growth suppression in children and teenagers with extended use. If a child or teenager on any glucocorticosteroid appears to have growth suppression, the possibility that they are particularly sensitive to this effect of glucocorticosteroids should be considered (see *"Precautions"*).

ADVERSE REACTIONS

Adverse reaction information is derived from blinded-controlled clinical trials (see *"Clinical Trials"*), open label studies and marketing experience. In the description below, rates of rare events are derived principally from marketing experience and publications, and accurate estimates of incidence are not possible.

The incidence of common adverse reactions is based upon controlled clinical trials in 606 patients [101 girls and 145 boys (< 19 years of age) and 203 female and 157 male adults] treated with intranasal Budesonide 128 μg twice daily over 2—4 weeks. The most common adverse reactions were symptoms of irritation of the nasal mucous membranes. All common adverse reactions were reported with approximately the same frequency by placebo patients suggesting the possibility that the vehicle or the rhinitis itself was responsible for the symptoms. Sneezing after use of the inhaler occurred in 2% of Budesonide treated patients and in 11% of patients using the placebo.

Systemic glucocorticosteroid side-effects were not reported during controlled clinical studies with intranasal Budesonide. If recommended doses are exceeded, however, or if individuals are particularly sensitive, symptoms of hypercorticism, i.e., Cushing's syndrome, could occur.

INCIDENCE GREATER THAN 1%
(Based on controlled clinical trials).

Respiratory: nasal irritation*, pharyngitis*, cough increased*, epistaxis.

Digestive: dry mouth, dyspepsia.

INCIDENCE LESS THAN 1%
Causal Relationship Probable (Adverse reactions reported only in the literature or from marketing experience, and presumably rarer are *italicized*):

Respiratory: moniliasis, hoarseness, wheezing, nasal pain, *nasal septum mucosal atrophy/necrosis, nasal septum perforation.*

Special Senses: reduced sense of smell, bad taste.

Digestive: nausea.

Skin and Appendages: facial edema, rash, pruritus, *contact dermatitis,* herpes simplex.

---

* Incidence 3 to 9%; incidence of unmarked reactions 1 to 3%.

INCIDENCE LESS THAN 1%
Causal Relationship Unknown (Adverse reactions reported only in the literature or from marketing experience, and presumably rarer are *italicized*):

Respiratory: dyspnea.

Nervous System: nervousness.

Skin and Appendages: alopecia.

Musculoskeletal: myalgia, arthralgia.

OVERDOSAGE
Acute overdosage with this dosage form is unlikely since one canister of Budesonide nasal inhaler only contains approximately 12.7 mg of Budesonide. Chronic overdosage may result in signs/symptoms of hyerpcorticism (see *"Warnings"* and *"Precautions"*).

DOSAGE AND ADMINISTRATION
Adults and children 6 years of age and older: The recommended starting dose is 256 μg daily, given as either two sprays in each nostril morning and evening or as four sprays in each nostril in the morning.

A decrease in symptoms may occur as soon as 24 hours after onset of treatment with intranasal Budesonide but generally it takes 3—7 days to reach maximum benefit.

If no improvement has been obtained by the third week of treatment with intranasal Budesonide, treatment should be discontinued.

After the desired clinical effect has been obtained, the maintenance dose should be reduced to the smallest amount necessary for control of symptoms (see *"Individualization of Dosage, Clinical Pharmacology"* section).

If glucocorticosteroids are discontinued when they still are needed, symptoms may not recur for several days.

At recommended doses, intranasal Budesonide's therapeutic effects are localized to the nose; therefore, concomitant treatment may be necessary to counteract allergic eye symptoms. Doses exceeding 256 μg daily (4 sprays/nostril) are not recommended. Intranasal Budesonide is not recommended for children below 6 years of age or for children with nonallergic perennial rhinitis because adequate numbers of these children have not been studied.

Budesonide nasal inhaler should be stored between 15°C (59°F) and 30°C (86°F) with the valve downwards. Shake well before use.

Contents under pressure: Do not puncture. Do not use or store near heat or open flame. Exposure to temperatures above 50°C (120°F) may cause the canister to explode.

Never throw the container into fire or an incinerator. Keep out of reach of children.

Note: The indented statement below is required by the Federal government's Clean Air Act for all products containing or manufactured with chlorofluorocarbons (CFCs).

WARNING: Contains trichloromonofluoromethane, dichlorotetrafluoroethane, and dichlorodifluoromethane, substances which harm public health and environment by destroying ozone in the upper atmosphere.

A notice similar to the above *"Warning"* has been placed in the patient information leaflet of this product pursuant to EPA regulations.

HOW SUPPLIED
AEROSOL SOLID W/ADAPTER: 0.032 MG/INH

BRAND/MANUFACTURER	NDC	SIZE	AWP
○ **BRAND**			
RHINOCORT: Astra	00186-1075-09	7 gm	$27.00

Bumetanide

> **WARNING**
> BUMETANIDE IS A POTENT DIURETIC WHICH, IF GIVEN IN EXCESSIVE AMOUNTS, CAN LEAD TO A PROFOUND DIURESIS WITH WATER AND ELECTROLYTE DEPLETION. THEREFORE, CAREFUL MEDICAL SUPERVISION IS REQUIRED, AND DOSE AND DOSAGE SCHEDULE HAVE TO BE ADJUSTED TO THE INDIVIDUAL PATIENT'S NEEDS. (SEE *"DOSAGE AND ADMINISTRATION"*.)

DESCRIPTION
Chemically, Bumetanide is 3-(butylamino)-4-phenoxy-5-sulfamoylbenzoic acid. It is a practically white powder having a calculated molecular weight of 364.41.

Following is its chemical structure:

CLINICAL PHARMACOLOGY

Bumetanide is a loop diuretic with a rapid onset and short duration of action. Pharmacological and clinical studies have shown that 1 mg Bumetanide has a diuretic potency equivalent to approximately 40 mg furosemide. The major site of Bumetanide action is the ascending limb of the loop of Henle.

The mode of action has been determined through various clearance studies in both humans and experimental animals. Bumetanide inhibits sodium reabsorption in the ascending limb of the loop of Henle, as shown by marked reduction of free-water clearance (C_{H_2O}) during hydration and tubular free-water reabsorption ($T^C_{H_2O}$) during hydropenia. Reabsorption of chloride in the ascending limb is also blocked by Bumetanide, and Bumetanide is somewhat more chloruretic than natriuretic.

Potassium excretion is also increased by Bumetanide in a dose-related fashion.

Bumetanide may have an additional action in the proximal tubule. Since phosphate reabsorption takes place largely in the proximal tubule, phosphaturia during Bumetanide-induced diuresis is indicative of this additional action. This is further supported by the reduction in the renal clearance of Bumetanide by probenecid, associated with diminution in the natriuretic response. This proximal tubular activity does not seem to be related to an inhibition of carbonic anhydrase. Bumetanide does not appear to have a noticeable action on the distal tubule.

Bumetanide decreases uric acid excretion and increases serum uric acid. Following oral administration of Bumetanide the onset of diuresis occurs in 30 to 60 minutes. Peak activity is reached between 1 and 2 hours. At usual doses (1 to 2 mg) diuresis is larely complete within 4 hours: with higher doses, the diuretic action lasts for 4 to 6 hours. Diuresis starts within minutes following an intravenous injection and reaches maximum levels within 15 to 30 minutes.

Several pharmacokinetic studies have shown that Bumetanide administered orally or parenterally, is eliminated rapidly in humans, with a half-life of between 1 and 1 ½ hours. Plasma protein-binding is in the range of 94% to 96%.

Oral administration of carbon-14 labeled Bumetanide to human volunteers revealed that 81% of the administered radioactivity was excreted in the urine, 45% of it as unchanged drug. Urinary and biliary metabolites identified in this study were formed by oxidation of the N-butyl side chain. Biliary excretion of Bumetanide amounted to only 2% of the administered dose.

INDICATIONS AND USAGE

Bumetanide is indicated for the treatment of edema associated with congestive heart failure, hepatic and renal disease, including the nephrotic syndrome.

Almost equal diuretic response occurs after oral and parenteral administration of Bumetanide. Therefore, if impaired gastrointestinal absorption is suspected or oral administration is not practical Bumetanide should be given by the intramuscular or intravenous route.

Successful treatment with Bumetanide following instances of allergic reactions to furosemide suggests a lack of cross-sensitivity.

UNLABELED USES

Bumetanide is used alone or as an adjunct in the treatment of hypertension nocturia in the elderly, and acute pulmonary edema.

CONTRAINDICATIONS

Bumetanide is contraindicated in anuria. Although Bumetanide can be used to induce diuresis in renal insufficiency, any marked increase in blood urea nitrogen or creatinine, or the development of oliguria during therapy of patients with progressive renal disease, is an indication for discontinuation of treatment with Bumetanide. Bumetanide is also contraindicated in patients in hepatic coma or in states of severe electrolyte depletion until the condition is improved or corrected. Bumetanide is contraindicated in patients hypersensitive to this drug.

WARNINGS

1. Volume and electrolyte depletion: The dose of Bumetanide should be adjusted to the patient's need. Excessive doses or too frequent administration can lead to profound water loss, electrolyte depletion, dehydration, reduction in blood volume and circulatory collapse with the possibility of vascular thrombosis and embolism, particularly in elderly patients.

2. Hypokalemia: Hypokalemia can occur as a consequence of Bumetanide administration. Prevention of hypokalemia requires particular attention in the following conditions: patients receiving digitalis and diuretics for congestive heart failure, hepatic cirrhosis and ascites, states of aldosterone excess with normal renal function, potassium-losing nephropathy, certain diarrheal states, or other states where hypokalemia is thought to represent particular added risks to the patient, *i.e.*, history of ventricular arrhythmias.

In patients with hepatic cirrhosis and ascites, sudden alterations of electrolyte balance may precipitate hepatic encephalopathy and coma. Treatment in such patients is best initiated in the hospital with small doses and careful monitoring of the patient's clinical status and electrolyte balance. Supplemental potassium and/ or spironolactone may prevent hypokalemia and metabolic alkalosis in these patients.

3. Ototoxicity: In cats, dogs and guinea pigs, Bumetanide has been shown to produce ototoxicity. In these test animals Bumetanide was 5 to 6 times more potent than furosemide and, since the diuretic potency of Bumetanide is about 40 to 60 times furosemide, it is anticipated that blood levels necessary to produce ototoxicity will rarely be achieved. The potential exists, however, and must be considered a risk of intravenous therapy, especially at high doses, repeated frequently in the face of renal excretory function impairment. Potentiation of

aminoglycoside ototoxicity has not been tested for Bumetanide. Like other members of this class of diuretics, Bumetanide probably shares this risk.

4. Allergy to sulfonamides. Patients allergic to sulfonamides may show hypersensitivity to Bumetanide.

5. Thrombocytopenia: Since there have been rare spontaneous reports of thrombocytopenia from postmarketing experience, patients should be observed regularly for possible occurrence of thrombocytopenia.

PRECAUTIONS

General: Serum potassium should be measured periodically and potassium supplements or potassium-sparing diuretics added if necessary. Periodic determinations of other electrolytes are advised in patients treated with high doses or for prolonged periods, particularly in those on low salt diets.

Hyperuricemia may occur; it has been asymptomatic in cases reported to date. Reversible elevations of the BUN and creatinine may also occur, especially in association with dehydration and particularly in patients with renal insufficiency. Bumetanide may increase urinary calcium excretion with resultant hypocalcemia.

Diuretics have been shown to increase the urinary excretion of magnesium; this may result in hypomagnesemia.

Laboratory Tests: Studies in normal subjects receiving Bumetanide revealed no adverse effects on glucose tolerance, plasma insulin, glucagon and growth hormone levels, but the possibility of an effect on glucose metabolism exists. Periodic determinations of blood sugar should be done, particularly in patients with diabetes or suspected latent diabetes.

Patients under treatment should be observed regularly for possible occurrence of blood dyscrasias, liver damage or idiosyncratic reactions, which have been reported occasionally in foreign marketing experience. The relationship of these occurrences to Bumetanide use is not certain.

Drug Interactions:

1. Drugs with Ototoxic Potential (see *"Warnings"*): Especially in the presence of impaired renal function, the use of parenterally administered Bumetanide in patients to whom aminoglycoside antibiotics are also being given should be avoided, except in life-threatening conditions.

2. Drugs with Nephrotoxic Potential: There has been no experience on the concurrent use of Bumetanide with drugs known to have a nephrotoxic potential. Therefore, the simultaneous administration of these drugs should be avoided.

3. Lithium: Lithium should generally not be given with diuretics (such as Bumetanide) because they reduce its renal clearance and add a high risk of lithium toxicity.

4. Probenecid: Pretreatment with probenecid reduces both the natriuresis and hyperreninemia produced by Bumetanide. This antagonistic effect of probenecid Bumetanide natriuresis is not due to a direct action on sodium excretion but is probably secondary to its inhibitory effect on renal tubular secretion of bumetanide. Thus probenecid should not be administered concurrently with Bumetanide.

5. Indomethacin: Indomethacin blunts the increases in urine volume and sodium excretion seen during Bumetanide treatment and inhibits the bumetanide-induced increase in plasma renin activity. Concurrent therapy with Bumetanide is thus not recommended.

6. Antihypertensives: Bumetanide may potentiate the effect of various antihypertensive drugs, necessitating a reduction in the dosage of these drugs.

7. Digoxin: Interaction studies in humans have shown no effect on digoxin blood levels.

8. Anticoagulants: Interaction studies in humans have shown Bumetanide to have no effect on warfarin metabolism or on plasma prothrombin activity.

Carcinogenesis, Mutagenesis, Impairment of Fertility: Bumetanide was devoid of mutagenic activity in various strains of *Salmonella typhimurium* when tested in the presence or absence of an *in vitro* metabolic activation system. An 18-month study showed an increase in mammary adenomas of questionable significance in female rats receiving oral doses of 60 mg/kg/day (2000 times a 2-mg human dose). A repeat study at the same doses failed to duplicate this finding.

Reproduction studies were performed to evaluate general reproductive performance and fertility in rats at oral dose levels of 10, 30, 60 or 100 mg/kg/day. The pregnancy rate was slightly decreased in the treated animals; however, the differences were small and not statistically significant.

Pregnancy: Teratogenic Effects: Pregnancy Category C. Bumetanide is neither teratogenic nor embryocidal in mice when given in doses up to 3400 times the maximum human therapeutic dose.

Bumetanide has been shown to be nonteratogenic, but it has a slight embryocidal effect in rats when given in doses of 3400 times the maximum human therapeutic dose and in rabbits at doses of 3.4 times the maximum human therapeutic dose. In one study, moderate growth retardation and increased incidence of delayed ossification of sternebrae were observed in rats at oral doses of 100 mg/kg/day, 3400 times the maximum human therapeutic dose. These effects were associated with maternal weight reductions noted during dosing. No such adverse effects were observed at 30 mg/kg/day (1000 times the maximum human therapeutic dose). No fetotoxicity was observed at 1000 to 2000 times the human therapeutic dose.

In rabbits, a dose-related decrease in litter size and an increase in resorption rate were noted at oral doses of 0.1 and 0.3 mg/kg/day (3.4 and 10 times the maximum human therapeutic dose). A slightly increased incidence of delayed

---

◆ RATED THERAPEUTICALLY EQUIVALENT; ◇ THERAPEUTIC EQUIVALENCE UNCONFIRMED; ○ UNRATED

ossification of sternebrae occurred at 0.3 mg/kg/day; however, no such adverse effects were observed at the dose of 0.03 mg/kg/day. The sensitivity of the rabbit to Bumetanide parallels the marked pharmacologic and toxicologic effects of the drug in this species.

Bumetanide was not teratogenic in the hamster at an oral dose of 0.5 mg/kg/day (17 times the maximum human therapeutic dose). Bumetanide was not teratogenic when given intravenously to mice and rats at doses up to 140 times the maximum human therapeutic dose.

There are no adequate and well-controlled studies in pregnant women. A small investigational experience in the United States and marketing experience in other countries to date have not indicated any evidence of adverse effects on the fetus, but these data do not rule out the possibility of harmful effects. Bumetanide should be given to a pregnant woman only if the potential benefit justifies the potential risk to the fetus.

Nursing Mothers: It is not known whether this drug is excreted in human milk. As a general rule, nursing should not be undertaken while the patient is on Bumetanide since it may be excreted in human milk.

Pediatric Use: Safety and effectiveness in children below the age of 18 have not been established.

ADVERSE REACTIONS
The most frequent clinical adverse reactions considered probably or possibly related to Bumetanide are muscle cramps (seen in 1.1% of treated patients), dizziness (1.1%), hypotension (0.8%), headache (0.6%), nausea (0.6%), and encephalopathy (in patients with preexisting liver disease) (0.6%). One or more of these adverse reactions have been reported in approximately 4.1% of Bumetanide-treated patients.

Less frequent clinical adverse reactions to Bumetanide are impaired hearing (0.5%), pruritus (0.4%), electrocardiogram changes (0.4%), weakness (0.2%), hives (0.2%), abdominal pain (0.2%), arthritic pain (0.2%), musculoskeletal pain (0.2%), rash (0.2%) and vomiting (0.2%). One or more of these adverse reactions have been reported in approximately 2.9% of Bumetanide patients.

Other clinical adverse reactions, which have each occurred in approximately 0.1% of patients, are vertigo, chest pain, ear discomfort, fatigue, dehydration, sweating, hyperventilation, dry mouth, upset stomach, renal failure, asterixis, itching, nipple tenderness, diarrhea, premature ejaculation and difficulty maintaining an erection.

Laboratory abnormalities reported have included hyperuricemia (in 18.4% of patients tested), hypochloremia (14.9%), hypokalemia (14.7%), azotemia (10.6%), hyponatremia (9.2%), increased serum creatinine (7.4%), hyperglycemia (6.6%), and variations in phosphorus (4.5%), CO_2 content (4.3%), bicarbonate (3.1%) and calcium (2.4%). Although manifestations of the pharmacologic action of Bumetanide, these conditions may become more pronounced by intensive therapy.

Also reported have been thrombocytopenia (0.2%) and deviations in hemoglobin (0.8%), prothrombin time (0.8%), hematocrit (0.6%), WBC (0.3%) and differential counts (0.1%). There have been rare spontaneous reports of thrombocytopenia from postmarketing experience.

Diuresis induced by Bumetanide may also rarely be accompanied by changes in LDH (1.0%), total serum bilirubin (0.8%), serum proteins (0.7%), SGOT (0.6%), SGPT (0.5%), alkaline phosphatase (0.4%), cholesterol (0.4%) and creatinine clearance (0.3%). Increases in urinary glucose (0.7%) and urinary protein (0.3%) have also been seen.

OVERDOSAGE
Overdosage can lead to acute profound water loss, volume and electrolyte depletion, dehydration, reduction of blood volume and circulatory collapse with a possibility of vascular thrombosis and embolism. Electrolyte depletion may be manifested by weakness, dizziness, mental confusion, anorexia, lethargy, vomiting and cramps. Treatment consists of replacement of fluid and electrolyte losses by careful monitoring of the urine and electrolyte output and serum electrolyte levels.

DOSAGE AND ADMINISTRATION
Dosage should be individualized with careful monitoring of patient response.

Oral Administration: The usual total daily dosage of Bumetanide is 0.5 to 2 mg and in most patients is given as a single dose.

If the diuretic response to an initial dose of Bumetanide is not adequate, in view of its rapid onset and short duration of action, a second or third dose may be given at 4- to 5-hour intervals up to a maximum daily dose of 10 mg. An intermittent dose schedule, whereby Bumetanide is given on alternate days or for 3 to 4 days with rest periods of 1 to 2 days in between, is recommended as the safest and most effective method for the continued control of edema. In patients with hepatic failure, the dosage should be kept to a minimum, and if necessary, dosage increased very carefully.

Because cross-sensitivity with furosemide has rarely been observed, Bumetanide can be substituted at approximately a 1:40 ratio of Bumetanide to furosemide in patients allergic to furosemide.

Parenteral Administration: Bumetanide may be administered parenterally (IV or IM) to patients in whom gastrointestinal absorption may be impaired or in whom oral administration is not practical.

Parenteral treatment should be terminated and oral treatment instituted as soon as possible.

The usual initial dose is 0.5 to 1 mg intravenously or intramuscularly. Intravenous administration should be given over a period of 1 to 2 minutes. If the response to an initial dose is deemed insufficient, a second or third dose may be given at intervals of 2 to 3 hours, but should not exceed a daily dosage of 10 mg.

Miscibility and Parenteral Solutions: The compatibility tests of Bumetanide injection (0.25 mg/mL, 2-mL ampuls) with 5% dextrose in water, 0.9% sodium chloride, and lactated Ringer's solution in both glass and plasticized PVC (Viaflex) containers have shown no significant absorption effect with either containers, nor a measurable loss of potency due to degradation of the drug. However, solutions should be freshly prepared and used within 24 hours.

Parenteral drug products should be inspected visually for particulate matter and discoloration prior to administration whenever solution and container permit.

Storage: Store all tablets, vials and ampules at 59°-86°F.

HOW SUPPLIED
INJECTION: 0.25 MG/ML

BRAND/MANUFACTURER	NDC	SIZE	AWP
○ **BRAND**			
BUMEX: Roche Labs	00004-1944-06	2 ml 10s	$16.53
	00004-1968-01	2 ml 10s	$16.53
	00004-1969-01	4 ml 10s	$27.75
	00004-1970-01	10 ml 10s	$78.40

TABLETS: 0.5 MG

BRAND/MANUFACTURER	NDC	SIZE	AWP
○ **BRAND**			
➤ BUMEX: Roche Labs	00004-0125-01	100s	$28.14
	00004-0125-49	100s ud	$30.21
	00004-0125-14	500s	$130.02

TABLETS: 1 MG

BRAND/MANUFACTURER	NDC	SIZE	AWP
○ **BRAND**			
➤ BUMEX: Roche Labs	00004-0121-01	100s	$39.52
	00004-0121-49	100s ud	$41.61
	00004-0121-14	500s	$183.11

TABLETS: 2 MG

BRAND/MANUFACTURER	NDC	SIZE	AWP
○ **BRAND**			
➤ BUMEX: Roche Labs	00004-0162-01	100s	$66.83
	00004-0162-07	100s ud	$68.91

Bumex *SEE* BUMETANIDE

Bupivacaine, Bupivacaine with Epinephrine, and Bupivacaine Spinal in Dextrose

DESCRIPTION
Bupivacaine Hydrochloride injections are sterile isotonic solutions that contain a local anesthetic agent with and without Epinephrine (as bitartrate) 1:200,000 and are administered parenterally by injection. See *"Indications and Usage"* for specific uses. Solutions of Bupivacaine Hydrochloride may be autoclaved if they do not contain Epinephrine.

Bupivacaine Hydrochloride injection is chemically designated as 2-piperidine-carboxamide, 1-butyl-N-(2,6-dimethylphenyl)-monohydrochloride, monohydrate.

Epinephrine is (-)-3,4-Dihydroxy-α-[(methylamino)methyl]benzyl alcohol.

Dextrose is D-glucopyranose monohydrate.

The pKa of Bupivacaine Hydrochloride (8.1) is similar to that of lidocaine (7.86). However, Bupivacaine Hydrochloride possesses a greater degree of lipid solubility and is protein bound to a greater extent than lidocaine.

Bupivacaine is related chemically and pharmacologically to the aminoacyl local anesthetics. It is a homologue of mepivacaine and is chemically related to lidocaine. All three of these anesthetics contain an amide linkage between the aromatic nucleus and the amino or piperidine group. They differ in this respect from the procaine-type local anesthetics, which have an ester linkage.

Dosage forms listed as Bupivacaine Hydrochloride-MPF indicate single dose solutions that are Methyl Paraben Free (MPF).

Bupivacaine Hydrochloride-MPF is a sterile isotonic solution containing sodium chloride. Bupivacaine Hydrochloride in multiple dose vials, each mL also contains 1 mg methylparaben as antiseptic preservative. The pH of these solutions is adjusted to between 4.0 and 6.5 with sodium hydroxide and/or hydrochloric acid.

Bupivacaine Hydrochloride-MPF with Epinephrine 1:200,000 (as bitartrate) is a sterile isotonic solution containing sodium chloride.

Each mL contains Bupivacaine Hydrochloride and 0.005 or 0.0091 mg Epinephrine.

Note: The user should have an appreciation and awareness of the formulations and their intended uses. (See *"Dosage and Administration"*.)

CLINICAL PHARMACOLOGY

Local anesthetics block the generation and the conduction of nerve impulses, presumably by increasing the threshold for electrical excitation in the nerve, by slowing the propagation of the nerve impulse, and by reducing the rate of rise of the action potential. In general, the progression of anesthesia is related to the diameter, myelination and conduction velocity of affected nerve fibers. Clinically, the order of loss of nerve function is as follows: (1) pain, (2) temperature, (3) touch, (4) proprioception, and (5) skeletal muscle tone.

Systemic absorption of local anesthetics produces effects on the cardiovascular and central nervous systems. At blood concentrations achieved with therapeutic doses, changes in cardiac conduction, excitability, refractoriness, contractility, and peripheral vascular resistance are minimal. However, toxic blood concentrations depress cardiac conduction and excitability, which may lead to atrioventricular block, ventricular arrhythmias and to cardiac arrest, sometimes resulting in fatalities. In addition, myocardial contractility is depressed and peripheral vasodilation occurs, leading to decreased cardiac output and arterial blood pressure.

Recent clinical reports and animal research suggest that these cardiovascular changes are more likely to occur after unintended intravascular injection of Bupivacaine. Therefore, incremental dosing is necessary.

Following systemic absorption, local anesthetics can produce central nervous system stimulation, depression or both. Apparent central stimulation is usually manifested as restlessness, tremors and shivering, progressing to convulsions, followed, by depression and coma, progressing ultimately to respiratory arrest. However, the local anesthetics have a primary depressant effect on the medulla and on higher centers. The depressed stage may occur without a prior excited stage.

Pharmacokinetics: The rate of systemic absorption of local anesthetics is dependent upon the total dose and concentration of drug administered, the route of administration, the vascularity of the administration site, and the presence or absence of Epinephrine in the anesthetic solution. A dilute concentration of Epinephrine (1:200,000 or 5 µg/mL) usually reduces the rate of absorption and peak plasma concentration of Bupivacaine, permitting the use of moderately larger total doses and sometimes prolonging the duration of action. The onset of action with Bupivacaine is rapid and anesthesia is long-lasting. The duration of anesthesia is significantly longer with Bupivacaine than with any other commonly used local anesthetic. It has also been noted that there is a period of analgesia that persists after the return of sensation, during which time the need for potent analgesics is reduced.

The onset of action following dental injections is usually 2 to 10 minutes and anesthesia may last two or three times longer than lidocaine and mepivacaine for dental use, in many patients up to 7 hours. The duration of anesthetic effect is prolonged by the addition of Epinephrine 1:200,000.

Local anesthetics are bound to plasma proteins in varying degrees. Generally, the lower the plasma concentration of drug, the higher the percentage of drug bound to plasma proteins.

The onset of sensory blockade following spinal block with Bupivacaine Spinal is very rapid (within one minute); maximum motor blockade and maximum dermatome level are achieved within 15 minutes in most cases. Duration of sensory blockade (time to return of complete sensation in the operative site or regression of two dermatomes) following a 12 mg dose averages 2 hours with or without 0.2 mg Epinephrine. The time to return of complete motor ability with 12 mg Bupivacaine Spinal averages 3½ hours without the addition of Epinephrine and 4½ hours if 0.2 mg Epinephrine is added. When compared to equal milligram doses of hyperbaric tetracaine, the duration of sensory blockade was the same but the time to complete motor recovery was significantly longer for tetracaine. Addition of 0.2 mg Epinephrine significantly prolongs the motor blockade and time to first postoperative narcotic with Bupivacaine Spinal.

Local anesthetics appear to cross the placenta by passive diffusion. The rate and degree of diffusion is governed by: (1) the degree of plasma protein binding, (2) the degree of ionization, and (3) the degree of lipid solubility. Fetal/maternal ratios of local anesthetics appear to be inversely related to the degree of plasma protein binding, because only the free, unbound drug is available for placental transfer. Bupivacaine with a high protein binding capacity (95%), has a low fetal/maternal ratio (0.2-0.4). The extent of placental transfer is also determined by the degree of ionization and lipid solubility of the drug. Lipid soluble, nonionized drugs readily enter the fetal blood from the maternal circulation.

Depending upon the route of administration, local anesthetics are distributed to some extent to all body tissues, with high concentrations found in highly perfused organs such as the liver, lungs, heart and brain.

Pharmacokinetic studies on the plasma profile of Bupivacaine after direct intravenous injection suggest a three-compartment open model. The first compartment is represented by the rapid intravascular distribution of the drug. The second compartment represents the equilibration of the drug throughout the highly perfused organs such as the brain, myocardium, lungs, kidneys and liver. The third compartment represents an equilibration of the drug with poorly perfused tissues, such as muscle and fat. The elimination of drug from tissue depends largely upon the ability of binding sites in the circulation to carry it to the liver where it is metabolized.

After injection of Bupivacaine Hydrochloride injection for caudal, epidural or peripheral nerve block in man, peak levels of Bupivacaine in the blood are reached in 30 to 45 minutes, followed by a decline to insignificant levels during the next 3 to 6 hours.

Various pharmacokinetic parameters of the local anesthetics can be significantly altered by the presence of hepatic or renal disease, addition of Epinephrine, factors affecting urinary pH, renal blood flow, the route of drug administration, and the age of the patient. The half-life of Bupivacaine in adults is 2.7 hours and in neonates 8.1 hours.

Amide-type local anesthetics such as Bupivacaine are metabolized primarily in the liver via conjugation with glucuronic acid.

Patients with hepatic disease, especially those with severe hepatic disease, may be more susceptible to the potential toxicities of the amide-type local anesthetics. The major metabolite of Bupivacaine is 2,6-pipecoloxylidide.

The kidney is the main excretory organ for most local anesthetics and their metabolites. Urinary excretion is affected by renal perfusion and factors affecting urinary pH. Only 5% to 6% of Bupivacaine is excreted unchanged in the urine.

When administered in recommended doses and concentrations, Bupivacaine Hydrochloride injection does not ordinarily produce irritation or tissue damage and does not cause methemoglobinemia.

INDICATIONS AND USAGE

Bupivacaine Hydrochloride injection is indicated for the production of local or regional anesthesia or analgesia for surgery, for dental and oral surgery procedures, for diagnostic and therapeutic procedures and for obstetrical procedures. Only the 0.25% and 0.5% concentrations are indicated for obstetrical anesthesia. (See *"Warnings"*.) Bupivacaine Spinal in Dextrose injection is indicated for the production of subarachnoid block (spinal anesthesia).

Experience with nonobstetrical surgical procedures in pregnant patients is not sufficient to recommend use of the 0.75% concentration in these patients. Bupivacaine Hydrochloride injection is not recommended for intravenous regional anesthesia (Bier Block). See *"Warnings"*.

The routes of administration and indicated Bupivacaine Hydrochloride concentrations are:

local infiltration	0.25%
peripheral nerve block	0.25%, 0.5%
retrobulbar block	0.75%
sympathetic block	0.25%
lumbar epidural	0.25%, 0.5% and 0.75% (nonobstetrical)
caudal	0.25%, 0.5%
epidural test dose (see *"Precautions"*)	0.5% with Epinephrine 1:200,000
dental blocks	0.5% with Epinephrine 1:200,000

(See *"Dosage and Administration"* for additional information.) Standard textbooks should be consulted to determine the accepted procedures and techniques for the administration of Bupivacaine Hydrochloride and/or of spinal anesthesia.

Use only the single-dose ampules and single-dose vials for caudal or epidural anesthesia, the multiple-dose vials contain a preservative and, therefore, should not be used for these procedures.

CONTRAINDICATIONS

Bupivacaine Hydrochloride injection is contraindicated in obstetrical paracervical block anesthesia. Its use by this technique has resulted in fetal bradycardia and death.

Bupivacaine Hydrochloride is contraindicated in patients with a known hypersensitivity to it or to any local anesthetic agent of the amide type or to other components of Bupivacaine Hydrochloride solutions.

The following conditions preclude the use of spinal anesthesia:

1. Severe hemorrhage, severe hypotension or shock and arrhythmias, such as complete heart block, which severely restrict cardiac output.
2. Local infection at the site of proposed lumbar puncture.
3. Septicemia.

WARNINGS

THE 0.75% CONCENTRATION OF BUPIVACAINE HYDROCHLORIDE INJECTION IS NOT RECOMMENDED FOR OBSTETRICAL ANESTHESIA. THERE HAVE BEEN REPORTS OF CARDIAC ARREST WITH DIFFICULT RESUSCITATION OR DEATH DURING USE OF BUPIVACAINE FOR EPIDURAL ANESTHESIA IN OBSTETRICAL PATIENTS. IN MOST CASES, THIS HAS FOLLOWED USE OF THE 0.75% CONCENTRATION. RESUSCITATION HAS BEEN DIFFICULT OR IMPOSSIBLE DESPITE APPARENTLY ADEQUATE PREPARATION AND APPROPRIATE MANAGEMENT. CARDIAC ARREST HAS OCCURRED AFTER CONVULSIONS RESULTING FROM SYSTEMIC TOXICITY. PRESUMABLY FOLLOWING UNINTENTIONAL INTRAVASCULAR INJECTION. THE 0.75% CONCENTRATION SHOULD BE RESERVED FOR SURGICAL PROCEDURES WHERE A HIGH DEGREE OF MUSCLE RELAXATION AND PROLONGED EFFECT ARE NECESSARY.

LOCAL ANESTHETICS SHOULD ONLY BE EMPLOYED BY CLINICIANS WHO ARE WELL VERSED IN DIAGNOSIS AND MANAGEMENT OF DOSE-RELATED TOXICITY AND OTHER ACUTE EMERGENCIES WHICH MIGHT ARISE FROM THE BLOCK TO BE EMPLOYED, AND

THEN ONLY AFTER INSURING THE *IMMEDIATE* AVAILABILITY OF OXYGEN, OTHER RESUSCITATIVE DRUGS, CARDIOPULMONARY RESUSCITATIVE EQUIPMENT, AND THE PERSONNEL RESOURCES NEEDED FOR PROPER MANAGEMENT OF TOXIC REACTIONS AND RELATED EMERGENCIES. (SEE ALSO *"ADVERSE REACTIONS," "PRECAUTIONS,"* AND *"OVERDOSAGE.")* DELAY IN PROPER MANAGEMENT OF DOSE-RELATED TOXICITY, UNDERVENTILATION FROM ANY CAUSE AND/OR ALTERED SENSITIVITY MAY LEAD TO THE DEVELOPMENT OF ACIDOSIS, CARDIAC ARREST AND, POSSIBLY, DEATH.

Local anesthetic solutions containing antimicrobial preservatives, i.e. those supplied in multiple dose vials, should not be used for epidural or caudal anesthesia because safety has not been established with regard to intrathecal injection, either intentional or unintentional, of such preservatives. It is essential that aspiration for blood or cerebrospinal fluid (where applicable) be done prior to injecting any local anesthetic, both the original dose and all subsequent doses, to avoid intravascular or subarachnoid injection. However, a negative aspiration does *not* ensure against an intravascular or subarachnoid injection.

Spinal anesthetics should not be injected during uterine contractions, because spinal fluid current may carry the drug further cephalad than desired.

A free flow of cerebrospinal fluid during the performance of spinal anesthesia is indicative of entry into the subarachnoid space. However, aspiration should be performed before the anesthetic solution is injected to confirm entry into the subarachnoid space and to avoid intravascular injection.

Bupivacaine and Epinephrine Injection or other vasopressors should not be used concomitantly with ergot-type oxytocic drugs, because a severe persistent hypertension may occur. Likewise, solutions of Bupivacaine containing a vasoconstrictor, such as Epinephrine, should be used with extreme caution in patients receiving monoamine oxidase (MAO) inhibitors or antidepressants of the triptyline or imipramine types, because severe prolonged hypertension may result. Until further experience is gained in children younger than 12 years (18 years for Bupivacaine Spinal), administration of Bupivacaine in this age group is not recommended.

Mixing or the prior or intercurrent use of any other local anesthetic with Bupivacaine cannot be recommended because of insufficient data on the clinical use of such mixtures.

Reports of cardiac arrest and death have occurred with the use of Bupivacaine for intravenous regional anesthesia (Bier Block). Information on safe dosages or techniques of administration of this product in this procedure are lacking; therefore, Bupivacaine is not recommended for use by this technique.

Prior use of chloroprocaine may interfere with subsequent use of Bupivacaine. Because of this, and because safety of intercurrent use of Bupivacaine and chloroprocaine has not been established, such use is not recommended.

Certain brands of Bupivacaine Hydrochloride with Epinephrine solutions contain sodium metabisulfite, a sulfite that may cause allergic-type reactions including anaphylactic symptoms and life-threatening or less severe asthmatic episodes in certain susceptible people. The overall prevalence of sulfite sensitivity in the general population is unknown and probably low. Sulfite sensitivity is seen more frequently in asthmatic than in nonasthmatic people. Single-dose ampuls and vials of some brands do not contain sodium metabisulfite.

PRECAUTIONS

General: The safety and effectiveness of local and spinal anesthetics depend on proper dosage, correct technique, adequate precautions and readiness for emergencies. Resuscitative equipment, oxygen and other resuscitative drugs should be available for immediate use. (See *"Warnings," "Adverse Reactions,"* and *"Overdosage".)* During major regional nerve blocks, the patient should have I.V. fluids running via an indwelling catheter to assure a functioning intravenous pathway. The lowest dosage of local anesthetic that results in effective anesthesia should be used to avoid high plasma levels and serious adverse effects. The rapid injection of a large volume of local anesthetic solution should be avoided and fractional (incremental) doses should be used when feasible.

Epidural Anesthesia: During epidural administration of Bupivacaine Hydrochloride, concentrated solutions (0.5-0.75%) should be administered in incremental doses of 3 to 5 mL with sufficient time between doses to detect toxic manifestations of unintentional intravascular or intrathecal injection. Injections should be made slowly, with frequent aspirations before and during the injection to avoid intravascular injection. Syringe aspirations should also be performed before and during each supplemental injection in continuous (intermittent) catheter techniques. An intravascular injection is still possible even if aspirations for blood are negative.

During the administration of epidural anesthesia, it is recommended that a test dose be administered initially and the effects monitored before the full dose is given. When using a "continuous" catheter technique, test doses should be given prior to both the original and all reinforcing doses, because plastic tubing in the epidural space can migrate into a blood vessel or through the dura. When clinical conditions permit, the test dose should contain Epinephrine (10 to 15 μg have been suggested) to serve as a warning of unintentional intravascular injection. If injected into a blood vessel, this amount of Epinephrine is likely to produce a transient "Epinephrine response" within 45 seconds, consisting of an increase in heart rate and/or systolic blood pressure, circumoral pallor, palpitations and nervousness in the unsedated patient. The sedated patient may exhibit only a pulse rate increase of 20 or more beats per minute for 15 or more seconds. Therefore, following the test dose, the heart rate should be monitored for a heart rate increase. Patients on beta-blockers may not manifest changes in heart rate, but blood pressure monitoring can detect an evanescent rise in systolic blood pressure. The test dose should also contain 10 to 15 mg of Bupivacaine

Hydrochloride injection or an equivalent dose of a short-acting amide anesthetic such as 30 to 40 mg of lidocaine, to detect an unintentional intrathecal administration. This will be manifested within a few minutes by signs of spinal block (e.g. decreased sensation of the buttocks, paresis of the legs, or, in the sedated patient, absent knee jerk). An intravascular or subarachnoid injection is still possible even if results of the test dose are negative. The test dose itself may produce a systemic toxic reaction, high spinal or Epinephrine-induced cardiovascular effects.

Injection of repeated doses of local anesthetics may cause significant increases in plasma levels with each repeated dose due to slow accumulation of the drug or its metabolites or to slow metabolic degradation. Tolerance to elevated blood levels varies with the physical condition of the patient. Debilitated, elderly patients, acutely ill patients and children should be given reduced doses commensurate with their age and physical condition. Reduced doses may also be indicated in patients with increased intra-abdominal pressure (including obstetrical patients), if otherwise suitable for spinal anesthesia. Local anesthetics should also be used with caution in patients with hypotension or heart block.

Careful and constant monitoring of cardiovascular and respiratory vital signs (adequacy of ventilation) and the patient's state of consciousness should be performed after each local anesthetic injection. It should be kept in mind at such times that restlessness, anxiety, incoherent speech, light-headedness, numbness and tingling of the mouth and lips, metallic taste, tinnitus, dizziness, blurred vision, tremors, twitching, depression, or drowsiness may be early warning signs of central nervous system toxicity.

Local anesthetic solutions containing a vasoconstrictor should be used cautiously and in carefully restricted quantities in areas of the body supplied by end arteries or having otherwise compromised blood supply such as digits, nose, external ear, penis, etc. Patients with hypertensive vascular disease may exhibit exaggerated vasoconstrictor response. Ischemic injury or necrosis may result.

Spinal anesthetics should be used with caution in patients with severe disturbances of cardiac rhythm, shock, or heart block.

Sympathetic blockade occurring during spinal anesthesia may result in peripheral vasodilation and hypotension, the extent depending on the number of dermatomes blocked. Blood pressure should, therefore, be carefully monitored especially in the early phases of anesthesia. Hypotension may be controlled by vasoconstrictors in dosages depending on the severity of hypotension and response of treatment.

The level of anesthesia should be carefully monitored because it is not always controllable in spinal techniques.

Because amide-type local anesthetics such as Bupivacaine are metabolized by the liver, these drugs, especially repeat doses, should be used cautiously in patients with hepatic disease. Patients with severe hepatic disease, because of their inability to metabolize local anesthetics normally, are at a greater risk of developing toxic plasma concentrations. Local anesthetics should also be used with caution in patients with impaired cardiovascular function because they may be less able to compensate for functional changes associated with the prolongation of A-V conduction produced by these drugs. However, dosage recommendations for spinal anesthesia are much lower than dosage recommendations for other major blocks and most experience regarding hepatic and cardiovascular disease dose-related toxicity is derived from these other major blocks.

Serious dose-related cardiac arrhythmias may occur if preparations containing a vasoconstrictor such as Epinephrine are employed in patients during or following the administration of potent inhalation anesthetics. In deciding whether to use these products concurrently in the same patient, the combined action of both agents upon the myocardium, the concentration and volume of vasoconstrictor used, and the time since injection, when applicable, should be taken into account.

Many drugs used during the conduct of anesthesia are considered potential triggering agents for familial malignant hyperthermia. Because it is not known whether amide-type local anesthetics may trigger this reaction and because the need for supplemental general anesthesia cannot be predicted in advance, it is suggested that a standard protocol for management should be available. Early unexplained signs of tachycardia, tachypnea, labile blood pressure and metabolic acidosis may precede temperature elevation. Successful outcome is dependent on early diagnosis, prompt discontinuance of the suspect triggering agent(s) and prompt treatment, including oxygen therapy, dantrolene (consult dantrolene sodium intravenous package insert before using) and other supportive measures.

Use in Head and Neck Area: Small doses of local anesthetics injected into the head and neck area, including retrobulbar, dental and stellate ganglion blocks, may produce adverse reactions similar to systemic toxicity seen with unintentional intravascular injections of larger doses. The injection procedures require the utmost care. Confusion, convulsions, respiratory depression and/or respiratory arrest, and cardiovascular stimulation or depression have been reported. These reactions may be due to intraarterial injection of the local anesthetic with retrograde flow to the cerebral circulation. They also may be due to puncture of the dural sheath of the optic nerve during retrobulbar block with diffusion of any local anesthetic along the subdural space to the mid-brain. Patients receiving these blocks should have their circulation and respiration monitored and be constantly observed. Resuscitative equipment and personnel for treating adverse reactions should be immediately available. Dosage recommendations should not be exceeded. (See *"Dosage and Administration".)*

Use in Opthalmic Surgery: Clinicians who perform retrobulbar blocks should be aware that there have been reports of respiratory arrest following local anesthetic injection. Prior to retrobulbar block, as with all other regional procedures the immediate availability of equipment, drugs, and personnel to manage respiratory

➤ SHOWN IN PRODUCT IDENTIFICATION GUIDE

arrest or depression, convulsions, and cardiac stimulation or depression should be assured (see also *"Warnings"* and *"Use in Head and Neck Area"* above). As with other anesthetic procedures, patients should be constantly monitored following ophthalmic blocks for signs of these adverse reactions, which may occur following relatively low total doses. A concentration of 0.75% Bupivacaine is indicated for retrobulbar block; however this concentration is not indicated for any other peripheral nerve block, including the facial nerve and not indicated for local infiltration, including the conjunctiva (see *"Indications"* and *"Precautions, General"*). Mixing Bupivacaine Hydrochloride with other local anesthetics is not recommended because of insufficient data on the clinical use of such mixtures.

When Bupivacaine Hydrochloride 0.75% is used for retrobulbar block, complete corneal anesthesia usually precedes onset of clinically acceptable external ocular muscle akinesia. Therefore, presence of akinesia rather than anesthesia alone should determine readiness of the patient for surgery.

Use in Dentistry: Because of the long duration of anesthesia, when Bupivacaine 0.5% with Epinephrine is used for dental injections, patients should be cautioned about the possibility of inadvertent trauma to tongue, lips, and buccal mucosa and advised not to chew solid foods or test the anesthetized area by biting or probing.

The following conditions may preclude the use of spinal anesthesia, depending upon the physician's evaluation of the situation and ability to deal with the complications or complaints which may occur:

- Preexisting diseases of the central nervous system, such as those attributable to pernicious anemia, poliomyelitis, syphilis, or tumor.
- Hematological disorders predisposing to coagulopathies or patients on anticoagulant therapy. Trauma to a blood vessel during the conduct of spinal anesthesia may, in some instances, result in uncontrollable central nervous system hemorrhage or soft tissue hemorrhage.
- Chronic backache and preoperative headache.
- Hypotension and hypertension.
- Technical problems (persistent paresthesias, persistent bloody tap).
- Arthritis or spinal deformity.
- Extremes of age.
- Psychosis or other causes of poor cooperation by the patient.

Information for Patients: When appropriate, patients should be informed in advance that they may experience temporary loss of sensation and motor activity, usually in the lower half of the body, following proper administration of caudal, lumbar epidural, or spinal anesthesia. Also, when appropriate, the physician should discuss other information including adverse reactions in the Bupivacaine Hydrochloride package insert.

Patients receiving dental injections of Bupivacaine should be cautioned not to chew solid foods or test the anesthetized area by biting or probing until anesthesia has worn off (up to 7 hours).

Clinically Significant Drug Interactions: The administration of local anesthetic solutions containing Epinephrine or norepinephrine to patients receiving monoamine oxidase inhibitors or tricyclic antidepressants may produce severe, prolonged hypertension. Concurrent use of these agents should generally be avoided. In situations in which concurrent therapy is necessary, careful patient monitoring is essential.

Concurrent administration of vasopressor drugs and or ergot-type oxytocic drugs may cause severe, persistent hypertension or cerebrovascular accidents.

Phenothiazines and butyrophenones may reduce or reverse the pressor effect of Epinephrine.

Carcinogenesis, Mutagenesis, and Impairment of Fertility: Long-term studies in animals of most local anesthetics, including Bupivacaine, to evaluate the carcinogenic potential have not been conducted. Mutagenic potential or the effect on fertility have not been determined. There is no evidence from human data that Bupivacaine may be carcinogenic or mutagenic or that it impairs fertility.

Pregnancy Category C: Decreased pup survival in rats and an embryocidal effect in rabbits have been observed when Bupivacaine Hydrochloride was administered to these species in doses comparable to nine and five times, respectively, the maximum recommended daily human dose (400 mg) or in doses comparable to 230 and 130 times, respectively, the maximum recommended human spinal dose. There are no adequate and well-controlled studies in pregnant women of the effect of Bupivacaine on the developing fetus. Bupivacaine injection should be used during pregnancy only if the potential benefit justifies the potential risk to the fetus. This does not exclude the use of Bupivacaine Hydrochloride injection (0.25% and 0.5% concentrations) at term for obstetrical, anesthesia or analgesia or of Bupivacaine Spinal at term for obstetrical anesthesia. (See *"Labor and Delivery"*.)

Labor and Delivery: See *"Box Warning"* regarding obstetrical use in 0.75% concentration.

Bupivacaine Hydrochloride injection is contraindicated in obstetrical paracervical block anesthesia.

Local anesthetics rapidly cross the placenta, and when used for epidural, caudal or pudendal block anesthesia, can cause varying degrees of maternal fetal and neonatal toxicity. (See *"Pharmacokinetics"* in *"Clinical Pharmacology"*). The incidence and degree of toxicity depend upon the procedure performed, the type and amount of drug used, and the technique of drug administration. Adverse reactions in the parturient, fetus and neonate involve alterations of the central nervous system, peripheral vascular tone and cardiac function.

Spinal anesthesia has a recognized use during labor and delivery. Bupivacaine Hydrochloride, when administered properly, via the epidural route in doses 10 to 12 times the amount used in spinal anesthesia has been used for obstetrical analgesia and anesthesia without evidence of adverse effects on the fetus.

Maternal hypotension has resulted from regional anesthesia. Local anesthetics produce vasodilation by blocking sympathetic nerves. Elevating the patient's legs and positioning her on her left side will help prevent decreases in blood pressure. The fetal heart rate also should be monitored continuously, and electronic fetal monitoring is highly advisable.

Epidural, caudal, pudendal, or spinal anesthesia may alter the forces of parturition through changes in uterine contractility or maternal expulsive efforts. Epidural and spinal anesthesia have been reported to prolong the second stage of labor by removing the parturient's reflex urge to bear down or by interfering with motor function. The use of obstetrical anesthesia may increase the need for forceps assistance.

The use of some local anesthetic drug products during labor and delivery may be followed by diminished muscle strength and tone for the first day or two of life. This has not been reported with Bupivacaine Hydrochloride injection.

It is extremely important to avoid aortocaval compression by the gravid uterus during administration of regional block to parturients. To do this, the patient must be maintained in the left lateral decubitus position or a blanket roll or sandbag may be placed beneath the right hip and the gravid uterus displaced to the left.

Nursing Mothers: It is not known whether local anesthetic drugs are excreted in human milk. Because many drugs are excreted in human milk, caution should be exercised when local anesthetics are administered to a nursing mother.

Pediatric Use: Until further experience is gained in children younger than 12 years, (18 years for Bupivacaine Spinal), administration of Bupivacaine Hydrochloride injection in this age group is not recommended.

ADVERSE REACTIONS

Reactions Bupivacaine Hydrochloride are characteristic of those associated with other amide-type local anesthetics. A major cause of adverse reactions to this group of drugs may be associated with its excessive plasma levels, which may be due to overdosage, unintentional intravascular injection or slow metabolic degradation.

Systemic: The most commonly encountered acute adverse experiences that demand immediate countermeasures are related to the central nervous system and the cardiovascular system. These adverse experiences, such as convulsions and cardiovascular collapse, are generally dose related and due to high plasma levels which may result from overdosage, rapid absorption from the injection site, diminished tolerance or from unintentional intravascular injection of the local anesthetic solution. In addition to systemic dose-related toxicity, unintentional subarachnoid injection of drug during the intended performance of caudal or lumbar epidural block or nerve blocks near the vertebral column (especially in the head and neck region) may result in underventilation or apnea ("Total or High Spinal"). Also, hypotension due to loss of sympathetic tone and respiratory paralysis or underventilation due to cephalad extension of the motor level of anesthesia may occur; these are the adverse experiences most commonly encountered with Bupivacaine Spinal and may lead to secondary cardiac arrest if untreated. Factors influencing plasma protein binding, such as acidosis, systemic diseases that alter protein production or competition with other drugs for protein binding sites, may diminish individual tolerance.

Central Nervous System Reactions: These are characterized by excitation and/or depression. Restlessness, anxiety, dizziness, tinnitus, blurred vision or tremors may occur, possibly proceeding to convulsions. However, excitement may be transient or absent, with depression being the first manifestation of an adverse reaction. This may quickly be followed by drowsiness merging into unconsciousness and respiratory arrest. Other central nervous system effects may be nausea, vomiting, chills, and constriction of the pupils.

The incidence of convulsions associated with the use of local anesthetics varies with the procedure used and the total dose administered. In a survey of studies of epidural anesthesia, overt toxicity progressing to convulsions occurred in approximately 0.1 percent of local anesthetic administrations.

Respiratory paralysis or underventilation secondary to cephalad spread of the level of spinal anesthesia (see *Respiratory System*) and hypotension for the same reason (see *Cardiovascular System*) are the two most commonly encountered central nervous system-related adverse observations with Bupivacaine Spinal which demand immediate countermeasures.

Cardiovascular System Reactions: High doses or unintentional intravascular injection may lead to high plasma levels and related depression of the myocardium, decreased cardiac output, heart block, hypotension, bradycardia, ventricular arrhythmias, including ventricular tachycardia and ventricular fibrillation, and cardiac arrest. (See *"Warnings," "Precautions,"* and *"Overdosage"* sections.)

Hypotension due to loss of sympathetic tone is a commonly encountered extension of the clinical pharmacology of spinal anesthesia. This is more commonly observed in patients with shrunken blood volume, shrunken interstitial fluid volume, cephalad spread of the local anesthetic, and/or mechanical obstruction of venous return. Nausea and vomiting are frequently associated with hypotensive episodes following the administration of spinal anesthesia.

Respiratory System: Respiratory paralysis or underventilation may be noted as a result of upward extension of the level of spinal anesthesia and may lead to secondary hypoxic cardiac arrest if untreated. Preanesthetic medication, intraoperative analgesics and sedatives, as well as surgical manipulation, may contribute to underventilation. This will usually be noted within minutes of the injection of spinal anesthetic solution, but because of differing maximal onset times, differing intercurrent drug usage and differing surgical manipulation, it may occur at any time during surgery or the immediate recovery period.

Allergic: Allergic type reactions are rare and may occur as a result of sensitivity to the local anesthetic or to other formulation ingredients, such as the antimicrobial preservative methylparaben contained in some multiple dose vials or sulfites in some Epinephrine-containing solutions (see *"Warnings"*). These reactions are characterized by signs such as urticaria, pruritus, erythema, angioneurotic edema (including laryngeal edema), tachycardia, sneezing, nausea, vomiting, dizziness, syncope, excessive sweating, elevated temperature, and possibly, anaphylactoid symptomatology (including severe hypotension). Cross sensitivity among members of the amide-type local anesthetic group has been reported. The usefulness of screening for sensitivity has not been definitely established.

Neurologic: The incidence of adverse neurologic reactions associated with the use of local anesthetics may be related to the total dose of local anesthetic administered and are also dependent upon the particular drug used, the route of administration and the physical status of the patient. Many of these effects may be related to local anesthetic techniques, with or without a contribution from the drug.

In the practice of caudal or lumbar epidural block, occasional unintentional penetration of the subarachnoid space by the catheter or needle may occur. Subsequent adverse effects may depend partially on the amount of drug administered intrathecally and the physiological and physical effects of a dural puncture. A high spinal is characterized by paralysis of the legs, loss of consciousness, respiratory paralysis and bradycardia.

Neurologic effects following unintentional subarachnoid administration during epidural or caudal anesthesia may include spinal block by varying magnitude (including high or total spinal block); hypotension secondary to spinal block; urinary retention; fecal and urinary incontinence; loss of perineal sensation and sexual function; persistent anesthesia, paresthesia, weakness, paralysis of the lower extremities and loss of sphincter control, all of which may have slow, incomplete or no recovery; headache; backache; septic meningitis; meningismus; slowing of labor; increased incidence of forceps delivery; or cranial nerve palsies due to traction on nerves from loss of cerebrospinal fluid.

Neurologic effects following spinal anesthesia may include loss of perineal sensation and sexual function: persistent anesthesia, paresthesia, weakness and paralysis of the lower extremities, and loss of sphincter control all of which may have slow, incomplete, or no recovery; hypotension; high or total spinal block; urinary retention; headache; backache; septic meningitis; meningismus; arachnoiditis; slowing of labor; increased incidence of forceps delivery; shivering; cranial nerve palsies due to traction on nerves from loss of cerebrospinal fluid; and fecal and urinary incontinence.

Other: Nausea and vomiting may occur during spinal anesthesia.

Neurologic effects following other procedures or routes of administration may include persistent anesthesia, paresthesia, weakness, paralysis, all of which may have slow, incomplete, or no recovery.

OVERDOSAGE

Acute emergencies from local anesthetics are generally related to high plasma levels encountered during therapeutic use of local anesthetics, to unintended subarachnoid injection of local anesthetic solution, or to underventilation (and perhaps apnea) secondary to upward extension of spinal anesthesia. Hypotension is commonly encountered during the conduct of spinal anesthesia due to relaxation of sympathetic tone, and sometimes, contributory mechanical obstruction of venous return. (See *"Adverse Reactions," "Warnings,"* and *"Precautions".*)

Management of Local Anesthetic Emergencies: The first consideration is prevention, best accomplished by careful and constant monitoring of cardiovascular and respiratory vital signs and the patient's state of consciousness after each local anesthetic injection. At the first sign of change, oxygen should be administered.

The first step in the management of systemic toxic reactions, as well as underventilation or apnea due to unintentional subarachnoid injection of drug solution or to a high or total spinal, consists of **immediate** attention to the establishment and maintenance of a patent airway and effective assisted or controlled ventilation with 100% oxygen with a delivery system capable of permitting immediate positive airway pressure by mask. This may prevent convulsions if they have not already occurred.

If necessary, use drugs to control the convulsions. A 50 to 100 mg bolus I.V. injection of succinylcholine will paralyze the patient without depressing the central nervous or cardiovascular systems and facilitate ventilation. A bolus I.V. dose of 5 to 10 mg of diazepam or 50 to 100 mg of thiopental will permit ventilation and counteract central nervous system stimulation, but these drugs also depress the central nervous system, respiratory and cardiac function, add to postictal depression, and may result in apnea. Intravenous barbiturates, anticonvulsant agents, or muscle relaxants should only be administered by those familiar with their use. Immediately after the institution of these ventilatory measures, the adequacy of the circulation should be evaluated. Supportive treatment of circulatory depression may require administration of intravenous fluids, and, when appropriate, a vasopressor dictated by the clinical situation (such as ephedrine or Epinephrine to enhance myocardial contractile force).

Hypotension due to sympathetic relaxation may be managed by giving intravenous fluids (such as isotonic saline or lactated Ringer's solution), in an attempt to relieve mechanical obstruction of venous return, or by using vasopressors (such as ephedrine which increases the force of myocardial contractions) and, if indicated, by giving plasma expanders or whole blood.

If difficulty is encountered in the maintenance of a patent airway or if prolonged ventilatory support (assisted or controlled) is indicated, endotracheal

intubation, employing drugs and techniques familiar to the clinician, may be indicated after initial administration of oxygen by mask.

Recent clinical data from patients experiencing local anesthetic induced convulsions demonstrated rapid development of hypoxia, hypercarbia and acidosis with Bupivacaine within a minute of the onset of convulsions. These observations suggest that oxygen consumption and carbon dioxide production are greatly increased during local anesthetic convulsions and emphasize the importance of immediate and effective ventilation with oxygen which may avoid cardiac arrest.

If not treated immediately, convulsions with simultaneous hypoxia, hypercarbia and acidosis, plus myocardial depression from the direct effects of the local anesthetic may result in cardiac arrhythmias, bradycardia, asystole, ventricular fibrillation, or cardiac arrest. Respiratory abnormalities, including apnea, may occur. Underventilation or apnea due to unintentional subarachnoid injection of local anesthetic solution or to a high or total spinal may produce these same signs and also lead to cardiac arrest if ventilatory support is not instituted. *If cardiac arrest should occur,* standard cardiopulmonary resuscitative measures should be instituted and maintained for a prolonged period if necessary.

The supine position is dangerous in pregnant women at term because of aortocaval compression by the gravid uterus.

Therefore, during treatment of systemic toxicity, maternal hypotension or fetal bradycardia following regional block, the parturient should be maintained in the left lateral decubitus position if possible, or manual displacement of the uterus off the great vessels be accomplished.

The mean seizure dosage of Bupivacaine in rhesus monkeys was found to be 4.4 mg/kg with mean arterial plasma concentration of 4.5 mcg/mL. The intravenous and subcutaneous LD_{50} in mice is 6 to 8 mg/kg and 38 to 54 mg/kg respectively.

DOSAGE AND ADMINISTRATION

The dose of any local anesthetic administered varies with the anesthetic procedure, the area to be anesthetized, the vascularity of the tissues, the number of neuronal segments to be blocked, the depth of anesthesia and degree of muscle relaxation required, the duration of anesthesia desired, individual tolerance, and the physical condition of the patient. The smallest dose and concentration required to produce the desired result should be administered. Dosages of Bupivacaine Hydrochloride should be reduced for young, elderly and debilitated patients and patients with cardiac and/or liver disease. The rapid injection of a large volume of local anesthetic solution should be avoided and fractional (incremental) doses should be used when feasible.

For specific techniques and procedures, refer to standard textbooks.

In recommended doses, Bupivacaine Hydrochloride produces complete sensory block, but the effect on motor function differs among the three concentrations.

0.25%— when used for caudal, epidural, or peripheral nerve block, produces incomplete motor block. Should be used for operations in which muscle relaxation is not important, or when another means of providing muscle relaxation is used concurrently. Onset of action may be slower than with the 0.5% or 0.75% solutions.

0.5%— provides motor blockade for caudal, epidural, or nerve block, but muscle relaxation may be inadequate for operations in which complete muscle relaxation is essential.

0.75%— produces complete motor block. Most useful for epidural block in abdominal operations requiring complete muscle relaxation, and for retrobulbar anesthesia. Not for obstetrical anesthesia.

The duration of anesthesia with Bupivacaine Hydrochloride is such that for most indications, a single dose is sufficient.

Maximum dosage limit must be individualized in each case after evaluating the size and physical status of the patient, as well as the usual rate of systemic absorption from a particular injection site. Most experience to date is with single doses of Bupivacaine Hydrochloride up to 225 mg with Epinephrine 1:200,000 and 175 mg without Epinephrine, more or less drug may be used depending on individualization of each case.

These doses may be repeated up to once every three hours. In clinical studies to date, total daily doses up to 400 mg have been reported. Until further experience is gained, this dose should not be exceeded in 24 hours. The duration of anesthetic effect may be prolonged by the addition of Epinephrine.

The dosages in Table 1 have generally proved satisfactory and are recommended as a guide for use in the average adult.

These dosages should be reduced for young, elderly or debilitated patients. Until further experience is gained. Bupivacaine Hydrochloride is not recommended for children younger than 12 years. Bupivacaine Hydrochloride is contraindicated for obstetrical paracervical blocks and is not recommended for intravenous regional anesthesia (Bier Block).

Use in Epidural Anesthesia: During epidural administration of Bupivacaine Hydrochloride, 0.5% and 0.75% solutions should be administered in incremental doses of 3 mL to 5 mL, with sufficient time between doses to detect toxic manifestations of unintentional intravascular or intrathecal injection. In obstetrics, only the 0.5% and 0.25% concentrations should be used; incremental doses of 3 mL to 5 mL of the 0.5% solution, not exceeding 50 mg to 100 mg at any dosing interval are recommended. Repeat doses should be preceded by a test dose containing Epinephrine if not contraindicated. Use only the single-dose ampules and single-dose vials for caudal or epidural anesthesia; the multiple-dose vials contain a preservative and therefore should not be used for these procedures.

The extent and degree of spinal anesthesia depend upon several factors including dosage, specific gravity of the anestheic solution, volume of solution used, force of injection, level of puncture, and position of the patient during and immediately after injection.

Seven and one-half mg (7.5 mg or 1.0 mL) Bupivacaine Spinal has generally proven satisfactory for spinal anesthesia for lower extremity and perineal procedures including TURP and vaginal hysterectomy. Twelve mg (12.0 mg or 1.6 mL) has been used for lower abdominal procedures such as abdominal hysterectomy, tubal ligation, and appendectomy. These doses are recommended as a guide for use in the average adult and may be reduced for the elderly or debilitated patients. Because experience with Bupivacaine Spinal is limited in patients below the age of 18 years, dosage recommendations in this age group cannot be made.

Obstetrical Use: Doses as low as 6 mg Bupivacaine Hydrochloride have been used for vaginal delivery under spinal anesthesia. The dose range of 7.5 mg to 10.5 mg (1 mL to 1.4 mL) Bupivacaine Hydrochloride has been used for Cesarean section under spinal anesthesia.

In recommended doses, Bupivacaine Spinal produces complete motor and sensory block.

Test dose for Caudal and Lumbar Epidural Blocks: See "Precautions."

The pulse rate and other signs should be monitored carefully immediately following each test dose administration to detect possible intravascular injection, and adequate time for onset of spinal block should be allotted to detect possible intrathecal injection. An intravascular or subarachnoid injection is still possible even if results of the test dose are negative. The test dose itself may produce a systemic toxic reaction, high spinal or cardiovascular effects from the Epinephrine. (See "Warnings" and "Overdosage".)

Use in Dentistry: The 0.5% concentration with Epinephrine is recommended for infiltration and block injection in the maxillary and mandibular area when a longer duration of local anesthetic action is desired, such as for oral surgical procedures generally associated with significant postoperative pain. The average dose of 1.8 mL (9 mg) per injection site will usually suffice; an occasional second dose of 1.8 mL (9 mg) may be used if necessary to produce adequate anesthesia after making allowance for 2 to 10 minutes onset time. (See "Clinical Pharmacology".) The lowest effective dose should be employed and time should be allowed between injections; it is recommended that the total dose for all injection sites, *spread out* over a single dental sitting, should not ordinarily exceed 90 mg for a healthy adult patient (ten 1.8 mL injections of 0.5% Bupivacaine with Epinephrine, Bupivacaine and Epinephrine). Injections should be made slowly and with frequent aspirations. Until further experience is gained. Bupivacaine in dentistry is not recommended for children younger than 12 years.

Unused portions of solutions in single dose containers, including, Bupivacaine Spinal, should be discarded, since this product form contains no preservatives.

(SEE RELATED TABLE).

Note: Parenteral drug products should be inspected visually for particulate matter and discoloration prior to administration whenever the solution and container permit. The Injection is not to be used if its color is pinkish or darker than slightly yellow or if it contains a precipitate.

SOLUTIONS OF BUPIVACAINE HYDROCHLORIDE SHOULD NOT BE USED FOR THE PRODUCTION OF SPINAL ANESTHESIA (SUBARACHNOID BLOCK) BECAUSE OF INSUFFICIENT DATA TO SUPPORT SUCH USE.

Disinfecting agents containing heavy metals, which cause release of respective ions (mercury, zinc, copper, etc.), should not be used for skin or mucous membrane disinfection since they have been related to incidents of swelling and edema.

When chemical disinfection of the container surface is desired, either isopropyl alcohol (91%) of ethyl alcohol (70%) is recommended. It is recommended that chemical disinfection be accomplished by wiping the ampule or vial stopper

thoroughly with cotton or gauze that has been moistened with the recommended alcohol just prior to use.

Solutions should be stored at controlled room temperature 15° to 30°C (59°-86°F).

Solutions containing Epinephrine should be protected from light.

Bupivacaine Spinal solution may be autoclaved once at 15 pound pressure, 121° C (250° F) for 15 minutes. Do not administer any solution which is discolored or contains particulate matter.

HOW SUPPLIED
INJECTION: 0.25%

AVERAGE UNIT PRICE (AVAILABLE SIZES)

		GENERIC A-RATED AVERAGE PRICE (GAAP)	
BRAND	$0.20		
GENERIC	$0.53	50 ml 25s	$281.73

BRAND/MANUFACTURER	NDC	SIZE	AWP
◆ BRAND			
SENSORCAINE-MPF: Astra	00186-1030-01	30 ml	$4.43
MARCAINE HCL: Sanofi Winthrop	00024-1217-01	50 ml	$6.66
SENSORCAINE: Astra	00186-1031-01	50 ml	$7.30
SENSORCAINE-MPF: Astra	00186-1030-12	10 ml 5s	$15.76
	00186-1030-02	30 ml 5s	$23.21
	00186-1030-91	30 ml 5s	$30.98
	00186-1030-92	30 ml 5s	$32.55
MARCAINE HCL: Sanofi Winthrop	00024-1212-02	50 ml 5s	$42.75
	00024-1212-10	10 ml 10s	$28.96
	00024-1212-30	30 ml 10s	$49.64
◆ GENERICS			
Abbott Hosp	00074-4272-01	20 ml 5s	$46.55
Abbott Hosp	00074-1158-01	30 ml 5s	$31.71
Abbott Hosp	00074-3613-01	2 ml 10s	$45.84
Abbott Hosp	00074-1159-01	10 ml 25s	$101.53
Abbott Hosp	00074-1159-02	30 ml 25s	$154.38
Abbott Hosp	00074-1160-01	50 ml 25s	$241.06
Abbott Hosp	00074-1158-02	50 ml 25s	$263.92
Abbott Hosp	00074-5749-01	50 ml 25s	$340.22

INJECTION: 0.5%

AVERAGE UNIT PRICE (AVAILABLE SIZES)

		GENERIC A-RATED AVERAGE PRICE (GAAP)	
BRAND	$0.22	30 ml 25s	$236.46
GENERIC	$0.33		

BRAND/MANUFACTURER	NDC	SIZE	AWP
◆ BRAND			
SENSORCAINE-MPF: Astra	00186-1033-01	30 ml	$4.79
MARCAINE HCL: Sanofi Winthrop	00024-1218-01	50 ml	$7.29
SENSORCAINE: Astra	00186-1035-01	50 ml	$8.13
SENSORCAINE-MPF: Astra	00186-1033-12	10 ml 5s	$17.20
	00186-1033-02	30 ml 5s	$23.59
	00186-1033-91	30 ml 5s	$33.29
	00186-1033-92	30 ml 5s	$33.29
MARCAINE HCL: Sanofi Winthrop	00024-1213-02	30 ml 5s	$35.98
	00024-1213-10	10 ml 10s	$31.68
	00024-1213-30	30 ml 10s	$54.20
◆ GENERICS			
Abbott Hosp	00074-4273-01	20 ml 5s	$49.99
Abbott Hosp	00074-1161-01	30 ml 5s	$32.42
Abbott Hosp	00074-1162-01	10 ml 25s	$108.36
Abbott Hosp	00074-1162-02	30 ml 25s	$156.16
Abbott Hosp	00074-5748-01	30 ml 25s	$316.77
Abbott Hosp	00074-1163-01	50 ml 25s	$251.16

Table 1.
DOSAGE RECOMMENDATIONS—BUPIVACAINE HYDROCHLORIDE INJECTIONS

		Each Dose		
Type of Block	conc.(%)	(mL)	(mg)	Motor Block[1]
Local Infiltration	0.25[4]	up to max.	up to max.	—
Epidural	0.75[2,4]	10-20	75-150	Complete
	0.5[4]	10-20	50-100	Moderate to complete
	0.25[4]	10-20	25-50	Partial to moderate
Caudal	0.5[4]	15-30	75-150	Moderate to complete
	0.25[4]	15-30	37.5-75	Moderate
Peripheral Nerves	0.5[4]	5 to max.	25 to max.	Moderate to complete
	0.25[4]	5 to max.	12.5 to max.	Moderate to complete
Retrobulbar[3]	0.75[4]	2-4	15-30	Complete
Sympathetic	0.25	20-50	50-125	—
Dental[3]	0.5 w/epi	1.8-3.6 per site	9-18	—
Epidural[3] Test Dose	0.5 w/epi	2-3	10-15 (10-15 mcg Epinephrine)	—

[1] With continuous (intermittent) techniques, repeat doses increase the degree of motor block. The first repeat dose of 0.5% may produce complete motor block. Intercostal nerve block with 0.25% may also produce complete motor block for intra-abdominal surgery.
[2] For single-dose use; not for intermittent (catheter) epidural technique. Not for obstetrical anesthesia.
[3] See PRECAUTIONS.
[4] Solutions with or without Epinephrine.

◆ RATED THERAPEUTICALLY EQUIVALENT; ◇ THERAPEUTIC EQUIVALENCE UNCONFIRMED; ○ UNRATED

INJECTION: 0.75%

AVERAGE UNIT PRICE (AVAILABLE SIZES)

BRAND	$0.42
GENERIC	$0.37

BRAND/MANUFACTURER	NDC	SIZE	AWP
◆ **BRAND**			
SENSORCAINE-MPF: Astra	00186-1037-01	30 ml	$5.00
	00186-1037-12	10 ml 5s	$17.93
	00186-1037-02	30 ml 5s	$27.65
MARCAINE HCL: Sanofi Winthrop	00024-1214-02	30 ml 5s	$36.84
SENSORCAINE-MPF: Astra	00186-1037-92	30 ml 5s	$38.50
SENSORCAINE: Astra	00186-1026-03	2 ml 5s	$33.00
MARCAINE HCL: Sanofi Winthrop	00024-1214-10	10 ml 10s	$32.92
	00024-1214-30	30 ml 10s	$55.93
◆ **GENERICS**			
Abbott Hosp	00074-4274-01	20 ml 5s	$53.44
Abbott Hosp	00074-1164-01	30 ml 5s	$33.31
Abbott Hosp	00074-1165-01	10 ml 25s	$124.09
Abbott Hosp	00074-1165-02	30 ml 25s	$179.31

Buprenex *SEE* BUPRENORPHINE HYDROCHLORIDE

Buprenorphine Hydrochloride

DESCRIPTION

Buprenorphine Hydrochloride is a narcotic under the Controlled Substances Act due to its chemical derivation from thebaine. Chemically, it is 17-(cyclopropylmethyl)-α-(1,1-dimethylethyl)-4, 5-epoxy-18, 19-dihydro-3-hydroxy-6-methoxy-α-methyl-6, 14-ethenomorphinan-7-methanol, hydrochloride [5α, 7α(S)]. Buprenorphine Hydrochloride is a white powder, weakly acidic and with limited solubility in water. Buprenorphine Hydrochloride is a clear, sterile, injectable agonist-antagonist analgesic intended for intravenous or intramuscular administration. Each ml contains 0.324 mg Buprenorphine Hydrochloride (equivalent to 0.3 mg buprenorphine), 50 mg anhydrous dextrose, water for injection and HCl to adjust pH. Buprenorphine Hydrochloride has the molecular formula, $C_{29}H_{41}NO_4 \cdot HCl$, and the molecular weight is 504.09.

Following is its chemical structure:

CLINICAL PHARMACOLOGY

Buprenorphine Hydrochloride is a parenteral opioid analgesic with 0.3 mg Buprenorphine Hydrochloride being approximately equivalent to 10 mg morphine sulfate in analgesic and respiratory depressant effects in adults. Pharmacological effects occur as soon as 15 minutes after intramuscular injection and persist for 6 hours or longer. Peak pharmacologic effects usually are observed at 1 hour. When used intravenously, the times to onset and peak effect are shortened.

The limits of sensitivity of available analytical methodology precluded demonstration of bioequivalence between intramuscular and intravenous routes of administration. In postoperative adults, pharmacokinetic studies have shown elimination half-lives ranging from 1.2-7.2 hours (mean 2.2 hours) after intravenous administration of 0.3 mg of Buprenorphine Hydrochloride. A single, ten-patient, pharmacokinetic study of doses of 3μg/kg in children (age 5-7 years) showed a high inter-patient variability, but suggests that the clearance of the drug may be higher in children than in adults. This is supported by at least one repeat-dose study in postoperative pain that showed an optimal inter-dose interval of 4-5 hours in pediatric patients as opposed to the recommended 6-8 hours in adults.

Buprenorphine Hydrochloride, in common with morphine and other phenolic opioid analgesics, is metabolized by the liver and its clearance is related to hepatic blood flow. Studies in patients anesthetized with 0.5% halothane have shown that this anesthetic decreases hepatic blood flow by about 30%.

Mechanism of Analgesic Action: Buprenorphine Hydrochloride exerts its analgesic effect via high affinity binding to μ subclass opiate receptors in the central nervous system. Although Buprenorphine Hydrochloride may be classified as a partial agonist, under the conditions of recommended use it behaves very much like classical μ agonists such as morphine. One unusual property of Buprenorphine Hydrochloride observed in *in vitro* studies is its very slow rate of dissociation from its receptor. This could account for its longer duration of action than morphine, the unpredictability of its reversal by opioid antagonists, and its low level of manifest physical dependence.

Narcotic Antagonist Activity: Buprenorphine Hydrochloride demonstrates narcotic antagonist activity and has been shown to be equipotent with naloxone as an antagonist of morphine in the mouse tail flick test.

Cardiovascular Effects: Buprenorphine Hydrochloride may cause a decrease or, rarely, an increase in pulse rate and blood pressure in some patients.

Effects on Respiration: Under usual conditions of use in adults, both Buprenorphine Hydrochloride and morphine show similar dose-related respiratory depressant effects. At adult therapeutic doses, 0.3 mg Buprenorphine Hydrochloride can decrease respiratory rate in an equivalent manner to an equianalgesic dose of morphine (10 mg). (See *"Warnings"*.)

INDICATIONS AND USAGE

Buprenorphine Hydrochloride is indicated for the relief of moderate to severe pain.

CONTRAINDICATIONS

Buprenorphine Hydrochloride should not be administered to patients who have been shown to be hypersensitive to the drug.

WARNINGS

Impaired Respiration: As with other potent opioids, clinically significant respiratory depression may occur within the recommended dose range in patients receiving therapeutic doses of Buprenorphine Hydrochloride. Buprenorphine Hydrochloride should be used with caution in patients with compromised respiratory function (e.g., chronic obstructive pulmonary disease, cor pulmonale, decreased respiratory reserve, hypoxia, hypercapnia, or preexisting respiratory depression). Particular caution is advised if Buprenorphine Hydrochloride is administered to patients taking or recently receiving drugs with CNS/respiratory depressant effects. In patients with the physical and/or pharmacological risk factors above, the dose should be reduced by approximately one-half.

NALOXONE MAY NOT BE EFFECTIVE IN REVERSING THE RESPIRATORY DEPRESSION PRODUCED BY BUPRENORPHINE HYDROCHLORIDE. THEREFORE, AS WITH OTHER POTENT OPIOIDS, THE PRIMARY MANAGEMENT OF OVERDOSE SHOULD BE THE REESTABLISHMENT OF ADEQUATE VENTILATION WITH MECHANICAL ASSISTANCE OF RESPIRATION, IF REQUIRED.

Interaction with Other Central Nervous System Depressants: Patients receiving Buprenorphine Hydrochloride in the presence of other narcotic analgesics, general anesthetics, antihistamines, benzodiazepines, phenothiazines, other tranquilizers, sedative/hypnotics or other CNS depressants (including alcohol) may exhibit increased CNS depression. When such combined therapy is contemplated, it is particularly important that the dose of one or both agents be reduced.

Head Injury and Increased Intracranial Pressure: Buprenorphine Hydrochloride, like other potent analgesics, may itself elevate cerebrospinal fluid pressure and should be used with caution in head injury, intracranial lesions and other circumstances where cerebrospinal pressure may be increased. Buprenorphine Hydrochloride can produce miosis and changes in the level of consciousness which may interfere with patient evaluation.

Use in Ambulatory Patients: Buprenorphine Hydrochloride may impair the mental or physical abilities required for the performance of potentially dangerous tasks such as driving a car or operating machinery. Therefore, Buprenorphine Hydrochloride should be administered with caution to ambulatory patients who should be warned to avoid such hazards.

Use in Narcotic-Dependent Patients: Because of the narcotic antagonist activity of Buprenorphine Hydrochloride, use in the physically dependent individual may result in withdrawal effects.

PRECAUTIONS

General: Buprenorphine Hydrochloride should be administered with caution in the elderly, debilitated patients, in children and those with severe impairment of hepatic, pulmonary, or renal function; myxedema or hypothyroidism; adrenal cortical insufficiency (e.g., Addison's disease); CNS depression or coma; toxic psychoses; prostatic hypertrophy or urethral stricture; acute alcoholism, delirium tremens; or kyphoscoliosis.

Because Buprenorphine Hydrochloride is metabolized by the liver, the activity of Buprenorphine Hydrochloride may be increased and/or extended in those individuals with impaired hepatic function or those receiving other agents known to decrease hepatic clearance.

Buprenorphine Hydrochloride has been shown to increase intracholedochal pressure to a similar degree as other opioid analgesics, and thus should be administered with caution to patients with dysfunction of the biliary tract.

Information for Patients: The effects of Buprenorphine Hydrochloride, particularly drowsiness, may be potentiated by other centrally acting agents such as alcohol or benzodiazepines. It is particularly important that in these circumstances patients must not drive or operate machinery. Buprenorphine Hydrochloride has some pharmacologic effects similar to morphine which in susceptible patients may lead to self-administration of the drug when pain no longer exists. Patients must not exceed the dosage of Buprenorphine Hydrochloride prescribed by their physician. Patients should be urged to consult their physician if other prescription medications are currently being used or are prescribed for future use.

Drug Interactions: Drug interactions common to other potent opioid analgesics also may occur with Buprenorphine Hydrochloride. Particular care should be taken when Buprenorphine Hydrochloride is used in combination with central nervous system depressant drugs (see *"Warnings"*). Although specific information is not presently available, caution should be exercised when Buprenorphine

➤ SHOWN IN PRODUCT IDENTIFICATION GUIDE

Hydrochloride is used in combination with MAO inhibitors. There have been reports of respiratory and cardiovascular collapse in patients who received therapeutic doses of diazepam and Buprenorphine Hydrochloride. A suspected interaction between Buprenorphine Hydrochloride and phenprocoumon resulting in purpura has been reported.

Carcinogenesis, Mutagenesis, Impairment of Fertility: The effects of Buprenorphine Hydrochloride on fertility and gestation indices were investigated in rats by the subcutaneous and intramuscular routes at doses 10 to 1,000 times the proposed human doses. Dystocia was noted in dams treated with 1,000 times the human dose. No effects on fertility or gestation were noted in these Segment 1 studies.

Pregnancy: Pregnancy Category C. Reproduction studies have been performed in the rat at doses which ranged from 10 to 1,000 times the proposed human dose by the subcutaneous and intramuscular routes and 160 times the proposed human dose by the intravenous route. By the intramuscular route, Buprenorphine Hydrochloride produced mild but statistically significant ($p < 0.05$) post-implantation losses and early fetal deaths at 10 and 100 but not 1,000 times the proposed human dose. No fetal malformations were noted in rats at any dose when Buprenorphine Hydrochloride was administered by subcutaneous, intramuscular, or intravenous routes. In rabbits, intramuscularly administered Buprenorphine Hydrochloride produced a dose-related trend for extra rib formation which attained statistical significance ($p < 0.01$) at 1,000 times the proposed human dose. By the intravenous route, doses in rats of 40 and 160 times the proposed human dose of Buprenorphine Hydrochloride caused a slight increase in post-implantation losses that may have been treatment-related. No major fetal malformations were noted in drug treated groups when administered by intramuscular or intravenous routes.

There are no adequate and well-controlled studies in pregnant women. Buprenorphine Hydrochloride should be used during pregnancy only if the potential benefit justifies the potential risk to the fetus.

Labor and Delivery: The safety of Buprenorphine Hydrochloride given during labor and delivery has not been established.

Nursing Mothers: An apparent lack of milk production during general reproduction studies with Buprenorphine Hydrochloride in rats caused decreased viability and lactation indices. It is unknown at this time whether or not Buprenorphine Hydrochloride is excreted in human milk. Despite the lack of specific knowledge on this issue, it is reasonable to assume that Buprenorphine Hydrochloride will enter human milk and caution should be exercised in the use of Buprenorphine Hydrochloride when it is administered to nursing mothers.

Pediatric Use: The safety and effectiveness of Buprenorphine Hydrochloride have been established for children between 2 and 12 years of age. Use of Buprenorphine Hydrochloride in children is supported by evidence from adequate and well controlled trials of Buprenorphine Hydrochloride in adults, with additional data from studies of 960 children ranging in age from 9 months to 18 years of age. Data is available from a pharmacokinetic study, several controlled clinical trials, and several large post-marketing studies and case series. The available information provides reasonable evidence that Buprenorphine Hydrochloride may be used safely in children ranging from 2-12 years of age, and that it is of similar effectiveness in children as in adults.

ADVERSE REACTIONS

The most frequent side effect in clinical studies involving 1,133 patients was sedation which occurred in approximately two-thirds of the patients. Although sedated, these patients could easily be aroused to an alert state.

OTHER LESS FREQUENT ADVERSE REACTIONS OCCURRING IN 5-10% OF THE PATIENTS WERE:
Nausea
Dizziness/Vertigo

OCCURRING IN 1-5% OF THE PATIENTS:
Sweating
Hypotension
Vomiting
Moisis
Headache
Nausea/Vomiting
Hypoventilation

THE FOLLOWING ADVERSE REACTIONS WERE REPORTED TO HAVE OCCURRED IN LESS THAN 1% OF THE PATIENTS:
CNS Effect: confusion, blurred vision, euphoria, weakness/fatigue, dry mouth, nervousness, depression, slurred speech, paresthesia.

Cardiovascular: hypertension, tachycardia, bradycardia.

Gastrointestinal: constipation.

Respiratory: dyspnea, cyanosis.

Dermatological: pruritus.

Ophthalmological: diplopia, visual abnormalities.

Miscellaneous: injection site reaction, urinary retention, dreaming, flushing/warmth, chills/cold, tinnitus, conjunctivitis, Wenckebach block, and psychosis.

Other effects observed infrequently include malaise, hallucinations, depersonalization, coma, dyspepsia, flatulence, apnea, rash, amblyopia, tremor, and pallor.

The following reactions have been reported to occur rarely: loss of appetite, dysphoria/agitation, diarrhea, urticaria, and convulsions/lack of muscle coordination.

In the United Kingdom, Buprenorphine Hydrochloride was made available under monitored release regulation during the first year of sale, and yielded data from 1,736 physicians on 9,123 patients (17,120 administrations). Data on 240 children under the age of 18 years were included in this monitored release program. No important new adverse effects attributable to Buprenorphine Hydrochloride were observed.

DRUG ABUSE AND DEPENDENCE

Buprenorphine Hydrochloride is a partial agonist of the morphine type: *i.e.,* it has certain opioid properties which may lead to psychic dependence of the morphine type due to an opiate-like euphoric component of the drug. Direct dependence studies have shown little physical dependence upon withdrawal of the drug. However, caution should be used in prescribing to individuals who are known to be drug abusers or ex-narcotic addicts. The drug may not substitute in acutely dependent narcotic addicts due to its antagonist component and may induce withdrawal symptoms.

OVERDOSAGE

Manifestations: Clinical experience with Buprenorphine Hydrochloride overdosage has been insufficient to define the signs of this condition at this time. Although the antagonist activity of Buprenorphine Hydrochloride may become manifest at doses somewhat above the recommended therapeutic range, doses in the recommended therapeutic range may produce clinically significant respiratory depression in certain circumstances. (see *"Warnings".*)

Treatment: The respiratory and cardiac status of the patients should be monitored carefully. Primary attention should be given to the reestablishment of adequate respiratory exchange through provision of a patent airway and institution of assisted or controlled ventilation. Oxygen, intravenous fluids, vasopressors, and other supportive measures should be employed as indicated. Doxapram, a respiratory stimulant, may be used. **NALOXONE MAY NOT BE EFFECTIVE IN REVERSING THE RESPIRATORY DEPRESSION PRODUCED BY BUPRENORPHINE HYDROCHLORIDE. THEREFORE, AS WITH OTHER POTENT OPIOIDS, THE PRIMARY MANAGEMENT OF OVERDOSE SHOULD BE THE REESTABLISHMENT OF ADEQUATE VENTILATION WITH MECHANICAL ASSISTANCE OF RESPIRATION, IF REQUIRED.**

DOSAGE AND ADMINISTRATION

Adults: The usual dosage for persons 13 years of age and over is 1 ml Buprenorphine Hydrochloride (0.3 mg) given by deep intramuscular or slow (over at least 2 minutes) intravenous injection at up to 6-hour intervals, as needed. Repeat once (up to 0.3 mg) if required, 30 to 60 minutes after initial dosage, giving consideration to previous dose pharmacokinetics, and thereafter only as needed. In high-risk patients (e.g., elderly, debilitated, presence of respiratory disease, etc.) and/or in patients where other CNS depressants are present, such as in the immediate postoperative period, the dose should be reduced by approximately one-half. Extra caution should be exercised with the intravenous route of administration, particularly with the initial dose.

Occasionally, it may be necessary to administer single doses of up to 0.6 mg to adults depending on the severity of the pain and the response of the patient. This dose should only be given I.M. and only to adult patients who are not in a high risk category (see *"Warnings"* and *"Precautions"*). At this time, there are insufficient data to recommend single doses greater than 0.6 mg for long-term use.

Children: Buprenorphine Hydrochloride has been used in children 2-12 years of age at doses between 2-6 micrograms/kg of body weight given every 4-6 hours. There is insufficient experience to recommend a dose in infants below the age of two years, single doses greater than 6 micrograms/kg of body weight, or the use of a repeat or second dose at 30-60 minutes (such as is used in adults). Since there is some evidence that not all children clear Buprenorphine Hydrochloride faster than adults, fixed interval or "round-the-clock" dosing should not be undertaken until the proper inter-dose interval has been established by clinical observation of the child. Physicians should recognize that, as with adults, some pediatric patients may not need to be remedicated for 6-8 hours.

Safety and Handling: Buprenorphine Hydrochloride is supplied in sealed ampuls and poses no known environmental risk to health care providers. Accidental dermal exposure should be treated by removal of any contaminated clothing and rinsing the affected area with water.

Buprenorphine Hydrochloride is a potent narcotic, and like all drugs of this class has been, associated with abuse and dependence among health care providers. To control the risk of diversion, it is recommended that measures appropriate to the health care setting be taken to provide rigid accounting, control of wastage, and restriction of access.

Parenteral drug products should be inspected visually for particulate matter and discoloration prior to administration, whenever solution and container permit.

Avoid excessive heat (over 104°F or 40°C). Protect from prolonged exposure to light.

◆ RATED THERAPEUTICALLY EQUIVALENT; ◇ THERAPEUTIC EQUIVALENCE UNCONFIRMED; ○ UNRATED

HOW SUPPLIED
INJECTION (C-V): 0.3 MG/ML

BRAND/MANUFACTURER	NDC	SIZE	AWP
○ **BRAND**			
BUPRENEX: Reckitt & Colman	12496-0757-01	1 ml 10s	$23.10

Bupropion Hydrochloride

DESCRIPTION

Bupropion Hydrochloride, an antidepressant of the aminoketone class, is chemically unrelated to tricyclic, tetracyclic, or other known antidepressant agents. Its structure closely resembles that of diethylpropion; it is related to phenylethylamines. It is designated as *2-tert-* butylamino-3'-chloropropiophenone hydrochloride. The molecular weight is 276.2. The empirical formula is $C_{13}H_{18}ClNO \cdot HCl$. Bupropion Hydrochloride powder is white, crystalline, and highly soluble in water. It has a bitter taste and produces the sensation of local anesthesia on the oral mucosa.

Bupropion Hydrochloride is supplied for oral administration as 75 mg and 100 mg film-coated tablets.

Following is its chemical structure:

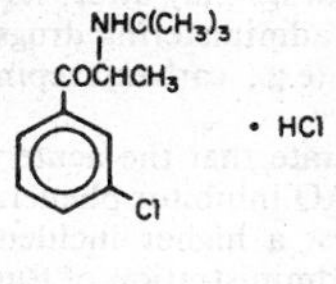

CLINICAL PHARMACOLOGY

PHARMACODYNAMICS AND PHARMACOLOGICAL ACTIONS

The neurochemical mechanism of the antidepressant effect of Bupropion Hydrochloride is not known. Bupropion Hydrochloride does not inhibit monoamine oxidase. Compared to classical tricyclic antidepressants, it is a weak blocker of the neuronal uptake of serotonin and norepinephrine; it also inhibits the neuronal re-uptake of dopamine to some extent.

Bupropion Hydrochloride produces dose-related CNS stimulant effects in animals, as evidenced by increased locomotor activity, increased rates of responding in various schedule-controlled operant behavior tasks, and, at high doses, induction of mild stereotyped behavior.

Bupropion Hydrochloride causes convulsions in rodents and dogs at doses approximately tenfold the dose recommended as the human antidepressant dose.

ABSORPTION, DISTRIBUTION, PHARMACOKINETICS, METABOLISM, AND ELIMINATION

Oral Bioavailability and Single Dose Pharmacokinetics: In man, following oral administration of Bupropion Hydrochloride, peak plasma Bupropion Hydrochloride concentrations are usually achieved within 2 hours, followed by a biphasic decline. The average half-life of the second (post-distributional) phase is approximately 14 hours, with a range of 8 to 24 hours. Six hours after a single dose, plasma Bupropion Hydrochloride concentrations are approximately 30% of peak concentrations. Plasma Bupropion Hydrochloride concentrations are dose-proportional following single doses of 100 to 250 mg; however, it is not known if the proportionality between dose and plasma level is maintained in chronic use.

The absolute bioavailability of Bupropion Hydrochloride tablets in man has not been determined because an intravenous formulation for human use is not available.

However, it appears likely that only a small proportion of any orally administered dose reaches the systemic circulation intact. For example, the absolute bioavailability of Bupropion Hydrochloride in animals (rats and dogs) ranges from 5-20%.

Metabolism: Following oral administration of 200 mg of ^{14}C-bupropion, 87% and 10% of the radioactive dose were recovered in the urine and feces, respectively. However, the fraction of the oral dose of Bupropion Hydrochloride excreted unchanged was only 0.5%, a finding documenting the extensive metabolism of Bupropion Hydrochloride.

Several of the known metabolites of Bupropion Hydrochloride are pharmacologically active, but their potency and toxicity relative to Bupropion Hydrochloride have not been fully characterized. However, because of their longer elimination half-lives, the plasma concentrations of at least two of the known metabolites can be expected, especially in chronic use, to be very much higher than the plasma concentration of Bupropion Hydrochloride. This is of potential clinical importance because factors or conditions altering metabolic capacity (e.g., liver disease, congestive heart failure, age, concomitant medications, etc.) or elimination may be expected to influence the degree and extent of accumulation of these active metabolites.

Furthermore, Bupropion Hydrochloride has been shown to induce its own metabolism in three animal species (mice, rats, and dogs) following subchronic administration. If induction also occurs in humans, the relative contribution of Bupropion Hydrochloride and its metabolites to the clinical effects of Bupropion Hydrochloride may be changed in chronic use.

Plasma and urinary metabolites so far identified include biotransformation products formed via reduction of the carbonyl group and/or hydroxylation of the *tert*-butyl group of Bupropion Hydrochloride. Four basic metabolites have been identified. They are the *erythro-* and *threo-* amino alcohols of Bupropion Hydrochloride, the *erythro-* amino diol of Bupropion Hydrochloride, and a morpholmol metabolite (formed from hydroxylation of the *tert*-butyl group of Bupropion Hydrochloride).

The morpholinol metabolite appears in the systemic circulation almost as rapidly as the parent drug following a single oral dose. Its peak level is three times the peak level of the parent drug; it has a half-life on the order of 24 hours; and its AUC 0-60 hrs is about 15 times that of Bupropion Hydrochloride.

The *threo-* amino alcohol metabolite has a plasma concentration-time profile similar to that of the morpholinol metabolite. The *erythro*-amino alcohol and the *erythro-* amino diol metabolites generally cannot be detected in the systemic circulation following a single oral dose of the parent drug. The morpholinol and the *threo-* amino alcohol metabolites have been found to be half as potent as Bupropion Hydrochloride in animal screening tests for antidepressant drugs.

During a chronic dosing study in 14 depressed patients with left ventricular dysfunction, it was found that there was substantial interpatient variability (two- to fivefold) in the trough steady-state concentrations of Bupropion Hydrochloride and the morpholinol and *threo-* amino alcohol metabolites. In addition, the steady-state plasma concentrations of these metabolites were 10-100 times the steady-state plasma concentrations of the parent drug.

The effect of other disease states and altered organ function on the metabolism and/or elimination of Bupropion Hydrochloride has not been studied in detail. However, the elimination of the major metabolites of Bupropion Hydrochloride may be affected by reduced renal or hepatic function because they are moderately polar compounds and are likely to undergo conjugation in the liver prior to urinary excretion. The preliminary results of a comparative single-dose pharmacokinetic study in normal versus cirrhotic patients indicated that half-lives of the metabolites were prolonged by cirrhosis and that the metabolites accumulated to levels two to three times those in normals. The effect of age on plasma concentrations of Bupropion Hydrochloride and its metabolites has not been characterized.

In vitro tests show that Bupropion Hydrochloride is 80% or more bound to human albumin at plasma concentrations up to 800 micromolar (200 µg/mL).

INDICATIONS AND USAGE

Bupropion Hydrochloride is indicated for the treatment of depression. A physician considering Bupropion Hydrochloride for the management of a patient's first episode of depression should be aware that the drug may cause generalized seizures with an approximate incidence of 0.4% (4/1000). This incidence of seizures may exceed that of other marketed antidepressants by as much as fourfold. This relative risk is only an approximate estimate because no direct comparative studies have been conducted. The efficacy of Bupropion Hydrochloride has been established in three placebo-controlled trials, including two of approximately three weeks duration in depressed inpatients, and one of approximately six weeks duration in depressed outpatients. The depressive disorder of the patients studied corresponds most closely to the Major Depression category of the APA Diagnostic and Statistical Manual III.

Major Depression implies a prominent and relatively persistent depressed or dysphoric mood that usually interferes with daily functioning (nearly every day for at least two weeks); it should include at least four of the following eight symptoms: change in appetite, change in sleep, psychomotor agitation or retardation, loss of interest in usual activities or decrease in sexual drive, increased fatigability, feelings of guilt or worthlessness, slowed thinking or impaired concentration, and suicidal ideation or attempts.

Effectiveness of Bupropion Hydrochloride in long-term use, that is, for more than 6 weeks, has not been systematically evaluated in controlled trials. Therefore, the physician who elects to use Bupropion Hydrochloride for extended periods should periodically reevaluate the long-term usefulness of the drug for the individual patient.

UNLABELED USES

Bupropion Hydrochloride is used alone or as an adjunct in the treatment of attention deficit hyperactivity disorder.

CONTRAINDICATIONS

Bupropion Hydrochloride is contraindicated in patients with a seizure disorder. Bupropion Hydrochloride is also contraindicated in patients with a current or prior diagnosis of bulimia or anorexia nervosa because of a higher incidence of seizures noted in such patients treated with Bupropion Hydrochloride. The concurrent administration of Bupropion Hydrochloride and a monoamine oxidase (MAO) inhibitor is contraindicated. At least 14 days should elapse between discontinuation of an MAO inhibitor and initiation of treatment with Bupropion Hydrochloride. Bupropion Hydrochloride is contraindicated in patients who have shown an allergic response to it.

WARNINGS

Seizures: Bupropion Hydrochloride is associated with seizures in approximately 0.4% (4/1000) of patients treated at doses up to 450 mg/day. This incidence of seizures may exceed that of other marketed antidepressants by as much as fourfold. This relative risk is only an approximate estimate because no direct comparative studies have been conducted. The estimated seizure incidence for Bupropion Hydrochloride increases almost tenfold between 450 and 600 mg/day, which is twice the usually required daily dose (300 mg) and one and one-third the maximum recommended daily dose (450 mg). Given the wide variability among individuals and their capacity to metabolize and eliminate drugs, this disproportionate increase in seizure incidence with dose incrementation calls for caution in dosing.

During the initial development, 25 among approximately 2400 patients treated with Bupropion Hydrochloride experienced seizures. At the time of seizure, 7 patients were receiving daily doses of 450 mg or below, for an incidence of 0.33% (3/1000) within the recommended dose range. Twelve (12) patients experienced seizures at 600 mg per day (2.3% incidence); 6 additional patients had seizures at daily doses between 600 and 900 mg (2.8% incidence).

A separate, prospective study was conducted to determine the incidence of seizure during an 8-week treatment exposure in approximately 3200 additional patients who received daily doses of up to 450 mg. Patients were permitted to continue treatment beyond 8 weeks if clinically indicated. Eight (8) seizures occurred during the initial 8-week treatment period and 5 seizures were reported in patients continuing treatment beyond 8 weeks, resulting in a total seizure incidence of 0.4%.

The risk of seizure appears to be strongly associated with dose and the presence of predisposing factors. A significant predisposing factor (e.g., history of head trauma or prior seizure, CNS tumor, concomitant medications that lower seizure threshold, etc.) was present in approximately one-half of the patients experiencing a seizure. Sudden and large increments in dose may contribute to increased risk. While many seizures occurred early in the course of treatment, some seizures did occur after several weeks at fixed dose.

Recommendations for reducing the risk of seizure: Retrospective analysis of clinical experience gained during the development of Bupropion Hydrochloride suggests that the risk of seizure may be minimized if (1) the total daily dose of Bupropion Hydrochloride does *not* exceed 450 mg, (2) the daily dose is administered t.i.d., with each single dose *not* to exceed 150 mg to avoid high peak concentrations of Bupropion Hydrochloride and/or its metabolites, and (3) the rate of incrementation of dose is very gradual. Extreme caution should be used when Bupropion Hydrochloride is (1) administered to patients with a history of seizure, cranial trauma, or other predisposition(s) toward seizure, or (2) prescribed with other agents (e.g., antipsychotics, other antidepressants, etc.) or treatment regimens (e.g., abrupt discontinuation of a benzodiazepine) that lower seizure threshold.

Potential for Hepatotoxicity: In rats receiving large doses of Bupropion Hydrochloride chronically, there was an increase in incidence of hepatic hyperplastic nodules and hepatocellular hypertrophy. In dogs receiving large doses of Bupropion Hydrochloride chronically, various histologic changes were seen in the liver, and laboratory tests suggesting mild hepatocellular injury were noted. Although scattered abnormalities in liver function tests were detected in patients participating in clinical trials, there is no clinical evidence that Bupropion Hydrochloride acts as a hepatotoxin in humans.

PRECAUTIONS
GENERAL
Agitation and Insomnia: A substantial proportion of patients treated with Bupropion Hydrochloride experience some degree of increased restlessness, agitation, anxiety, and insomnia, especially shortly after initiation of treatment. In clinical studies, these symptoms were sometimes of sufficient magnitude to require treatment with sedative/hypnotic drugs. In approximately 2% of patients, symptoms were sufficiently severe to require discontinuation of Bupropion Hydrochloride treatment.

Psychosis, Confusion, and Other Neuropsychiatric Phenomena: Patients treated with Bupropion Hydrochloride have been reported to show a variety of neuropsychiatric signs and symptoms including delusions, hallucinations, psychotic episodes, confusion, and paranoia. Because of the uncontrolled nature of many studies, it is impossible to provide a precise estimate of the extent of risk imposed by treatment with Bupropion Hydrochloride. In several cases, neuropsychiatric phenomena abated upon dose reduction and/or withdrawal of treatment.

Activation of Psychosis and/or Mania: Antidepressants can precipitate manic episodes in Bipolar Manic Depressive patients during the depressed phase of their illness and may activate latent psychosis in other susceptible patients. Bupropion Hydrochloride is expected to pose similar risks.

Altered Appetite and Weight: A weight loss of greater than 5 pounds occurred in 28% of Bupropion Hydrochloride patients. This incidence is approximately double that seen in comparable patients treated with tricyclics or placebo. Furthermore, while 34.5% of patients receiving tricyclic antidepressants gained weight, only 9.4% of patients treated with Bupropion Hydrochloride did. Consequently, if weight loss is a major presenting sign of a patient's depressive illness, the anorectic and/or weight reducing potential of Bupropion Hydrochloride should be considered.

Suicide: The possibility of a suicide attempt is inherent in depression and may persist until significant remission occurs. Accordingly, prescriptions for Bupropion Hydrochloride should be written for the smallest number of tablets consistent with good patient management.

Use in Patients with Systemic Illness: There is no clinical experience establishing the safety of Bupropion Hydrochloride in patients with a recent history of myocardial infarction or unstable heart disease. Therefore, care should be exercised if it is used in these groups. Bupropion Hydrochloride was well tolerated in patients who had previously developed orthostatic hypotension while receiving tricyclic antidepressants.

Because Bupropion Hydrochloride and its metabolites are almost completely excreted through the kidney and metabolites are likely to undergo conjugation in the liver prior to urinary excretion, treatment of patients with renal or hepatic impairment should be initiated at reduced dosage as Bupropion and its metabolites may accummulate in such patients beyond concentrations expected in patients without renal or hepatic impairment. The patient should be closely monitored for possible toxic effects of elevated blood and tissue levels of drug and metabolites.

INFORMATION FOR PATIENTS
Physicians are advised to discuss the following issues with patients:

Patients should be instructed to take Bupropion Hydrochloride in equally divided doses three or four times a day to minimize the risk of seizure.

Patients should be told that any CNS-active drug like Bupropion Hydrochloride may impair their ability to perform tasks requiring judgment or motor and cognitive skills. Consequently, until they are reasonably certain that Bupropion Hydrochloride does not adversely affect their performance they should refrain from driving an automobile or operating complex, hazardous machinery.

Patients should be told that the use and cessation of use of alcohol may alter the seizure threshold, and, therefore, that the consumption of alcohol should be minimized, and, if possible, avoided completely.

Patients should be advised to inform their physician if they are taking or plan to take any prescription or over-the-counter drugs. Concern is warranted because Bupropion Hydrochloride and other drugs may affect each other's metabolism.

Patients should be advised to notify their physician if they become pregnant or intend to become pregnant during therapy.

DRUG INTERACTIONS
No systematic data have been collected on the consequences of the concomitant administration of Bupropion Hydrochloride and other drugs.

However, animal data suggest that Bupropion Hydrochloride may be an inducer of drug metabolizing enzymes. This may be of potential clinical importance because the blood levels of co-administered drugs may be altered.

Alternatively, because Bupropion Hydrochloride is extensively metabolized, the co-administration of other drugs may affect its clinical activity. In particular, care should be exercised when administering drugs known to affect hepatic drug metabolizing enzyme systems (e.g., carbamazepine, cimetidine, phenobarbital, phenytoin).

Studies in animals demonstrate that the acute toxicity of Bupropion Hydrochloride is enhanced by the MAO inhibitor phenelzine (see *"Contraindications"*).

Limited clinical data suggest a higher incidence of adverse experiences in patients receiving concurrent administration of Bupropion Hydrochloride and L-dopa. Administration of Bupropion Hydrochloride to patients receiving L-dopa concurrently should be undertaken with caution, using small initial doses and small gradual dose increases.

Concurrent administration of Bupropion Hydrochloride and agents which lower seizure threshold should be undertaken only with extreme caution (see *"Warnings"*). Low initial dosing and small gradual dose increases should be employed.

CARCINOGENESIS, MUTAGENESIS, IMPAIRMENT OF FERTILITY
Life-time carcinogenicity studies were performed in rats and mice at doses up to 300 and 150 mg/kg/day, respectively. In the rat study there was an increase in nodular proliferative lesions of the liver at doses of 100 to 300 mg/kg/day; lower doses were not tested. The question of whether or not such lesions may be precursors of neoplasms of the liver is currently unresolved. Similar liver lesions were not seen in the mouse study, and no increase in malignant tumors of the liver and other organs was seen in either study.

Bupropion Hydrochloride produced a borderline positive response (2-3 times control mutation rate) in some strains in the Ames bacterial mutagenicity test, and a high oral dose (300, but not 100 or 200 mg/kg) produced a low incidence of chromosomal aberrations in rats. The relevance of these results in estimating the risk of human exposure to therapeutic doses is unknown.

A fertility study was performed in rats; no evidence of impairment of fertility was encountered at oral doses up to 300 mg/kg/day.

PREGNANCY
Teratogenic Effects: Pregnancy Category B: Reproduction studies have been performed in rabbits and rats at doses up to 15-45 times the human daily dose and have revealed no definitive evidence of impaired fertility or harm to the fetus due to Bupropion Hydrochloride. (In rabbits, a slightly increased incidence of fetal abnormalities was seen in two studies, but there was no increase in any specific abnormality). There are no adequate and well-controlled studies in pregnant women. Because animal reproduction studies are not always predictive of human response, this drug should be used during pregnancy only if clearly needed.

LABOR AND DELIVERY
The effect of Bupropion Hydrochloride on labor and delivery in humans is unknown.

NURSING MOTHERS
Because of the potential for serious adverse reactions in nursing infants from Bupropion Hydrochloride, a decision should be made whether to discontinue nursing or to discontinue the drug, taking into account the importance of the drug to the mother.

PEDIATRIC USE
The safety and effectiveness of Bupropion Hydrochloride in individuals under 18 years old have not been established.

USE IN THE ELDERLY
Bupropion Hydrochloride has not been systematically evaluated in older patients.

ADVERSE REACTIONS
See also *"Warnings"* and *"Precautions"*. Adverse events commonly encountered in patients treated with Bupropion Hydrochloride are agitation, dry mouth, insomnia, headache/migraine, nausea/vomiting, constipation, and tremor.

Adverse events were sufficiently troublesome to cause discontinuation of Bupropion Hydrochloride treatment in approximately ten percent of the 2400 patients and volunteers who participated in clinical trials during the product's initial development. The more common events causing discontinuation include neuropsychiatric disturbances (3.0%), primarily agitation and abnormalities in mental status; gastrointestinal disturbances (2.1%), primarily nausea and vomiting; neurological disturbances (1.7%), primarily seizures, headaches, and sleep disturbances; and dermatologic problems (1.4%), primarily rashes. It is important to note, however, that many of these events occurred at doses that exceed the recommended daily dose.

Accurate estimates of the incidence of adverse events associated with the use of any drug are difficult to obtain. Estimates are influenced by drug dose, detection technique, setting, physician judgments, etc. Consequently, the table below is presented solely to indicate the relative frequency of adverse events reported in representative controlled clinical studies conducted to evaluate the safety and efficacy of Bupropion Hydrochloride under relatively similar conditions of daily dosage (300-600 mg), setting, and duration (3-4 weeks). The figures cited cannot be used to predict precisely the incidence of untoward events in the course of usual medical practice where patient characteristics and other factors must differ from those which prevailed in the clinical trials. These incidence figures also cannot be compared with those obtained from other clinical studies involving related drug products as each group of drug trials is conducted under a different set of conditions.

Finally, it is important to emphasize that the tabulation does not reflect the relative severity and/or clinical importance of the events. A better perspective on the serious adverse events associated with the use of Bupropion Hydrochloride is provided in the *"Warnings"* and *"Precautions"* sections.

TREATMENT EMERGENT ADVERSE EXPERIENCE INCIDENCE IN PLACEBO-CONTROLLED CLINICAL TRIALS* (PERCENT OF PATIENTS REPORTING)

Adverse Experience	*Bupropion Hydrochloride Patients (n = 323)*	*Placebo Patients (n = 185)*
Cardiovascular		
Cardiac Arrhythmias	5.3	4.3
Dizziness	22.3	16.2
Hypertension	4.3	1.6
Hypotension	2.5	2.2
Palpitations	3.7	2.2
Syncope	1.2	0.5
Tachycardia	10.8	8.6
Dermatologic		
Pruritus	2.2	0.0
Rash	8.0	6.5
Gastrointestinal		
Anorexia	18.3	18.4
Appetite Increase	3.7	2.2
Constipation	26.0	17.3
Diarrhea	6.8	8.6
Dyspepsia	3.1	2.2
Nausea/Vomiting	22.9	18.9
Weight Gain	13.6	22.7
Weight Loss	23.2	23.2
Genitourinary		
Impotence	3.4	3.1
Menstrual Complaints	4.7	1.1
Urinary Frequency	2.5	2.2
Urinary Retention	1.9	2.2
Musculoskeletal		
Arthritis	3.1	2.7
Neurological		
Akathisia	1.5	1.1
Akinesia/Bradykinesia	8.0	8.6
Cutaneous Temperature Disturbance	1.9	1.6
Dry Mouth	27.6	18.4
Excessive Sweating	22.3	14.6
Headache/Migraine	25.7	22.2
Impaired Sleep Quality	4.0	1.6
Increased Salivary Flow	3.4	3.8
Insomnia	18.6	15.7
Muscle Spasms	1.9	3.2
Pseudoparkinsonism	1.5	1.6
Sedation	19.8	19.5
Sensory Disturbance	4.0	3.2
Tremor	21.1	7.6
Neuropsychiatric		
Agitation	31.9	22.2
Anxiety	3.1	1.1
Confusion	8.4	4.9
Decreased Libido	3.1	1.6
Delusions	1.2	1.1
Disturbed Concentration	3.1	3.8
Euphoria	1.2	0.5
Hostility	5.6	3.8

Adverse Experience	*Bupropion Hydrochloride Patients (n = 323)*	*Placebo Patients (n = 185)*
Nonspecific		
Fatigue	5.0	8.6
Fever/Chills	1.2	0.5
Respiratory		
Upper Respiratory Complaints	5.0	11.4
Special Senses		
Auditory Disturbance	5.3	3.2
Blurred Vision	14.6	10.3
Gustatory Disturbance	3.1	1.1

* *Events reported by at least 1% Bupropion Hydrochloride patients are included.*

OTHER EVENTS OBSERVED DURING THE DEVELOPMENT OF BUPROPION HYDROCHLORIDE

The conditions and duration of exposure to Bupropion Hydrochloride varied greatly and a substantial proportion of the experience was gained in open and uncontrolled clinical settings. During this experience, numerous adverse events were reported; however, without appropriate controls, it is impossible to determine with certainty which events were or were not caused by Bupropion Hydrochloride. The following enumeration is organized by organ system and describes events in terms of their relative frequency of reporting in the data base. Events of major clinical importance are also described in the *"Warnings"* and *"Precautions"* sections of the labeling. The following definitions of frequency are used: Frequent adverse events are defined as those occurring in at least 1/100 patients. Infrequent adverse events are those occurring in 1/100 to 1/1000 patients, while rare events are those occurring in less than 1/1000 patients.

Cardiovascular: Frequent was edema; infrequent were chest pain, EKG abnormalities (premature beats and non-specific ST-T changes), and shortness of breath/ dyspnea; rare were flushing, pallor, phlebitis and myocardial infarction.

Dermatologic: Frequent were nonspecific rashes; infrequent were alopecia and dry skin; rare were change in hair color, hirsutism and acne.

Endocrine: Infrequent was gynecomastia; rare were glycosuria and hormone level change.

Gastrointestinal: Infrequent were dysphagia, thirst disturbance, and liver damage/ jaundice; rare were rectal complaints, colitis G.I. bleeding, intestinal perforation and stomach ulcer.

Genitourinary: Frequent was nocturia; infrequent were vaginal irritation, testicular swelling, urinary tract infection, painful erection, and retarded ejaculation; rare were dysuria, enuresis, urinary incontinence, menopause, ovarian disorder, pelvic infection, cystitis, dyspareunia, and painful ejaculation.

Hematologic/Oncologic: Rare were lymphadenopathy, anemia and pancytopenia.

Musculoskeletal: Rare was musculoskeletal chest pain.

Neurological: (see *"Warnings"*) Frequent were ataxia/incoordination, seizure, myoclonus, dyskinesia, and dystonia; infrequent were mydriasis, vertigo, and dysarthria; rare were EEG abnormality, abnormal neurological exam, impaired attention, sciatica and aphasia.

Neuropsychiatric: (see *"Precautions"*). Frequent were mania/hypomania, increased libido, hallucinations, decrease in sexual function, and depression; infrequent were memory impairment, depersonalization, psychosis, dysphoria, mood instability, paranoia, formal thought disorder, and frigidity; rare was suicidal ideation.

Oral Complaints: Frequent was stomatitis; infrequent were toothache, bruxism, gum irritation, and oral edema; rare was glossitis.

Respiratory: Infrequent were bronchitis and shortness of breath/dyspnea; rare were epistaxis, rate or rhythm disorder, pneumonia and pulmonary embolism.

Special Senses: Infrequent was visual disturbance; rare was diplopia.

Nonspecific: Frequent were flu-like symptoms; infrequent was nonspecific pain; rare were body odor, surgically related pain, infection, medication reaction and overdose.

POSTINTRODUCTION REPORTS

Voluntary reports of adverse events temporally associated with Bupropion Hydrochloride that have been received since market introduction and which may have no causal relationship with the drug include the following:

Cardiovascular: orthostatic hypotension, third degree heart block

Endocrine: syndrome of inappropriate antidiuretic hormone secretion

Gastrointestinal: esophagitis, hepatitis

Hemic and Lymphatic: ecchymosis, leukocytosis, leukopenia

Musculoskeletal: arthralgia, myalgia, muscle rigidity/fever/rhabdomyolysis

Nervous: coma, delirium, dream abnormalities, paresthesia, unmasking of tardive dyskinesia.

Skin and Appendages: Stevens-Johnson syndrome, angioedema, exfoliative dermatitis, urticaria

Special Senses: tinnitus

DRUG ABUSE AND DEPENDENCE

Humans: Controlled clinical studies conducted in normal volunteers, in subjects with a history of multiple drug abuse, and in depressed patients showed some increase in motor activity and agitation/excitement.

In a population of individuals experienced with drugs of abuse, a single dose of 400 mg Bupropion Hydrochloride produced mild amphetamine-like activity as compared to placebo on the morphine-benzedrine subscale of the Addiction Research Center Index (ARCI) and a score intermediate between placebo and amphetamine on the Liking Scale of the ARCI. These scales measure general feelings of euphoria and drug desirability. Findings in clinical trials, however, are not known to predict the abuse potential of drugs reliably. Nonetheless, evidence from single dose studies does suggest that the recommended daily dosage of Bupropion Hydrochloride when administered in divided doses is not likely to be especially reinforcing to amphetamine or stimulant abusers. However, higher doses, which could not be tested because of the risk of seizure, might be modestly attractive to those who abuse stimulant drugs.

Animals: Studies in rodents have shown that Bupropion Hydrochloride exhibits some pharmacologic actions common to psychostimulants, including increases in locomotor activity and the production of a mild stereotyped behavior and increases in rates of responding in several schedule-controlled behavior paradigms. Drug discrimination studies in rats showed stimulus generalization between Bupropion Hydrochloride and amphetamine and other psychostimulants. Rhesus monkeys have been shown to self-administer Bupropion Hydrochloride intravenously.

OVERDOSAGE

Lethal Doses in Animals: In rats, the acute oral LD_{50} values were 607 mg/kg (males) and 482 mg/kg (females). Respective values for mice were 544 mg/kg and 636 mg/kg. Signs of acute toxicity included labored breathing, salivation, arched back, ptosis, ataxia, and convulsions.

Human Overdose Experience: There has been limited clinical experience with overdosage of Bupropion Hydrochloride. Thirteen over-doses occurred during clinical trials. Twelve patients ingested 850 to 4200 mg and recovered without significant sequelae. Another patient who ingested 9000 mg of Bupropion Hydrochloride and 300 mg of tranylcypromine experienced a grand mal seizure and recovered without further sequelae. Since introduction, Bupropion Hydrochloride overdoses up to 17,500 mg have been reported. Seizure was reported in approximately one-third of all cases. Other serious reactions reported with overdoses of Bupropion Hydrochloride alone included hallucinations, loss of consciousness, and tachycardia. Fever, muscle rigidity, rhabdomyolysis, hypotension, stupor, coma, and respiratory failure have been reported when Bupropion Hydrochloride was part of multiple drug overdoses.

Although most patients recovered without sequelae, deaths associated with overdoses of Bupropion Hydrochloride alone have been reported rarely in patients ingesting massive doses of Bupropion Hydrochloride. Multiple uncontrolled seizures, bradycardia, cardiac failure, and cardiac arrest prior to death were reported in these patients.

Management of Overdose: Following suspected overdose, hospitalization is advised. If the patient is conscious, vomiting should be induced by syrup of ipecac. Activated charcoal also may be administered every 6 hours during the first 12 hours after ingestion. Baseline laboratory values should be obtained. Electrocardiogram and EEG monitoring also are recommended for the next 48 hours. Adequate fluid intake should be provided.

If the patient is stuporous, comatose, or convulsing, airway intubation is recommended prior to undertaking gastric lavage. Although there is little clinical experience with lavage following an overdose of Bupropion Hydrochloride it is likely to be of benefit within the first 12 hours after ingestion since absorption of the drug may not yet be complete.

While diuresis, dialysis, or hemoperfusion are sometimes used to treat drug overdosage, there is no experience with their use in the management of Bupropion Hydrochloride overdose. Because diffusion of Bupropion Hydrochloride from tissue to plasma may be slow, dialysis may be of minimal benefit several hours after overdose.

Based on studies in animals, it is recommended that seizures be treated with an intravenous benzodiazepine preparation and other supportive measures, as appropriate.

Further information about the treatment of overdoses may be available from a poison control center.

DOSAGE AND ADMINISTRATION

General Dosing Considerations: It is particularly important to administer Bupropion Hydrochloride in a manner most likely to minimize the risk of seizure (see "Warnings"). Increases in dose should not exceed 100 mg/day in a 3 day period. Gradual escalation in dosage is also important if agitation, motor restlessness, and insomnia, often seen during the initial days of treatment, are to be minimized. If necessary, these effects may be managed by temporary reduction of dose or the short-term administration of an intermediate to long-acting sedative hypnotic. A sedative hypnotic usually is not required beyond the first week of treatment. Insomnia may also be minimized by avoiding bedtime doses. If distressing, untoward effects supervene, dose escalation should be stopped.

No single dose of Bupropion Hydrochloride should exceed 150 mg. Bupropion Hydrochloride should be administered t.i.d., preferably with at least 6 hours between successive doses.

Usual Dosage for Adults: The usual adult dose is 300 mg/day, given t.i.d. Dosing should begin at 200 mg/day, given as 100 mg b.i.d. Based on clinical response, this dose may be increased to 300 mg/day, given as 100 mg t.i.d., no sooner than 3 days after beginning therapy (see table below).

DOSING REGIMEN

Treatment	Total Daily Dose	Tablet Strength	Number of Tablets		
			Morning	Midday	Evening
1	200 mg	100 mg	1	0	1
4	300 mg	100 mg	1	1	1

Increasing the Dosage Above 300 mg/Day: As with other antidepressants, the full antidepressant effect of Bupropion Hydrochloride may not be evident until 4 weeks of treatment or longer. An increase in dosage, up to a maximum of 450 mg/day, given in divided doses of not more than 150 mg each, may be considered for patients in whom no clinical improvement is noted after several weeks of treatment at 300 mg/day. Dosing above 300 mg/day may be accomplished using the 75 or 100 mg tablets. The 100 mg tablet must be administered q.i.d. with at least 4 hours between successive doses, in order not to exceed the limit of 150 mg in a single dose. Bupropion Hydrochloride should be discontinued in patients who do not demonstrate an adequate response after an appropriate period of treatment at 450 mg/day.

Elderly Patients: In general, older patients are known to metabolize drugs more slowly and to be more sensitive to the anticholinergic, sedative, and cardiovascular side effects of antidepressant drugs. Clinical trials enrolled several hundred patients 60 years of age and older. The experience with these patients and younger ones was similar.

Maintenance: The lowest dose that maintains remission is recommended. Although it is not known how long the patient should remain on Bupropion Hydrochloride, it is generally recognized that acute episodes of depression require several months or longer of antidepressant drug treatment.

Store at 15° to 25°C (59° to 77°F).

HOW SUPPLIED
TABLETS: 75 MG

BRAND/MANUFACTURER	NDC	SIZE	AWP
○ BRAND			
▸ WELLBUTRIN: Burr Wellcome	00081-0177-55	100s	$54.13

TABLETS: 100 MG

BRAND/MANUFACTURER	NDC	SIZE	AWP
○ BRAND			
▸ WELLBUTRIN: Burr Wellcome	00081-0178-55	100s	$72.22

BuSpar *SEE* BUSPIRONE HYDROCHLORIDE

Buspirone Hydrochloride

DESCRIPTION

Buspirone Hydrochloride is an antianxiety agent that is not chemically or pharmacologically related to the benzodiazepines, barbiturates, or other sedative/anxiolytic drugs.

Buspirone Hydrochloride is a white crystalline, water soluble compound with a molecular weight of 422.0. Chemically, Buspirone Hydrochloride is 8-[4-[4-(2-pyrimidinyl)-1-piperazinyl]butyl]-8-azaspiro[4,5]decane- 7,9-dione monohydrochloride. The empirical formula is $C_{21}H_{31}N_5O_2 \cdot HCl$.

Following is its chemical structure:

CLINICAL PHARMACOLOGY

The mechanism of action of buspirone is unknown. Buspirone differs from typical benzodiazepine anxiolytics in that it does not exert anticonvulsant or muscle relaxant effects. It also lacks the prominent sedative effect that is associated with more typical anxiolytics. *In vitro* preclinical studies have shown that buspirone has a high affinity for serotonin ($5\text{-}HT_{1A}$) receptors. Busipirone has no significant affinity for benzodiazepine receptors and does not affect GABA binding *in vitro* or *in vivo* when tested in preclinical models.

Buspirone has moderate affinity for brain D_2-dopamine receptors. Some studies do suggest that buspirone may have indirect effects on other neurotransmitter systems.

◆ RATED THERAPEUTICALLY EQUIVALENT; ◇ THERAPEUTIC EQUIVALENCE UNCONFIRMED; ○ UNRATED

Buspirone HCl is rapidly absorbed in man and undergoes extensive first pass metabolism. In a radiolabeled study, unchanged buspirone in the plasma accounted for only about 1% of the radioactivity in the plasma. Following oral administration, plasma concentrations of unchanged buspirone are very low and variable between subjects. Peak plasma levels of 1 to 6 ng/mL have been observed 40 to 90 minutes after single oral doses of 20 mg. The single-dose bioavailability of unchanged buspirone when taken as a tablet is on the average about 90% of an equivalent dose of solution, but there is large variability.

The effects of food upon the bioavailability of Buspirone HCl have been studied in eight subjects. They were given a 20-mg dose with and without food; the area under the plasma concentration-time curve (AUC) and peak plasma concentration (Cmax) of unchanged buspirone increased by 84% and 116% respectively, but the total amount of buspirone immunoreactive material did not change. This suggests that food may decrease the extent of presystemic clearance of buspirone, but the clinical significance of these findings is unknown. A multiple-dose study conducted in 15 subjects suggests that buspirone has nonlinear pharmacokinetics. Thus, dose increases and repeated dosing may lead to somewhat higher blood levels of unchanged buspirone than would be predicted from results of single-dose studies.

In man, approximately 95% of buspirone is plasma protein bound, but other highly bound drugs, eg, phenytoin, propranolol, and warfarin are not displaced by buspirone from plasma protein *in vitro*. However, *in vitro* binding studies show that buspirone does displace digoxin.

Buspirone is metabolized primarily by oxidation producing several hydroxylated derivatives and a pharmacologically active metabolite, 1-pyrimidinylpiperazine (1-PP). In animal models predictive of anxiolytic potential, 1-PP has about one quarter of the activity of buspirone, but is present in up to 20-fold greater amounts. However, this is probably not important in humans; blood samples from humans chronically exposed to Buspirone HCl do not exhibit high levels of 1-PP; mean values are approximately 3 ng/mL and the highest human blood level recorded among 108 chronically dosed patients was 17 ng/mL, less than 1/200th of 1-PP levels found in animals given large doses of buspirone without signs of toxicity. In a single-dose study using 14C-labeled buspirone, 29% to 63% of the dose was excreted in the urine within 24 hours, primarily as metabolites; fecal excretion accounted for 18 to 38% of the dose. The average elimination half-life of unchanged buspirone after single doses of 10 to 40 mg is about 2 to 3 hours.

The pharmacokinetics of Buspirone HCl in patients with hepatic or renal dysfunction has not been determined, nor has the effect of age. The effect of Buspirone HCl on drug metabolism or concomitant drug disposition has not been investigated.

INDICATIONS AND USAGE

Buspirone HCl is indicated for the management of anxiety disorders or the short-term relief of the symptoms of anxiety. Anxiety or tension associated with the stress of everyday life usually does not require treatment with an anxiolytic.

The efficacy of Buspirone HCl has been demonstrated in controlled clinical trials of outpatients whose diagnosis roughly corresponds to Generalized Anxiety Disorder (GAD). Many of the patients enrolled in these studies also had coexisting depressive symptoms and Buspirone HCl relieved anxiety in the presence of these coexisting depressive symptoms. The patients evaluated in these studies had experienced symptoms for periods of 1 month to over 1 year prior to the study, with an average symptom duration of 6 months. Generalized Anxiety Disorder (300.02) is described in the American Psychiatric Association's Diagnostic and Statistical Manual, III[1] as follows:

Generalized, persistent anxiety (of at least 1 month continual duration), manifested by symptoms from three of the four following categories.

1. Motor tension: shakiness, jitteriness, jumpiness, trembling, tension, muscle aches, fatigability, inability to relax, eyelid twitch, furrowed brow, strained face, fidgeting, restlessness, easy startle.
2. Autonomic hyperactivity: sweating, heart pounding or racing, cold, clammy hands, dry mouth, dizziness, lightheadedness, paresthesias (tingling in hands or feet), upset stomach, hot or cold spells, frequent urination, diarrhea, discomfort in the pit of the stomach, lump in the throat, flushing, pallor, high resting pulse, and respiration rate.
3. Apprehensive expectation: anxiety, worry, fear, rumination, and anticipation of misfortune to self or others.
4. Vigilance and scanning: hyperattentiveness resulting in distractibility, difficulty in concentrating, insomnia, feeling "on edge," irritability, impatience.

The above symptoms would not be due to another mental disorder, such as a depressive disorder or schizophrenia. However, mild depressive symptoms are common in GAD. The effectiveness of Buspirone HCl in long-term use, that is, for more than 3 to 4 weeks, has not been demonstrated in controlled trials. There is no body of evidence available that systematically addresses the appropriate duration of treatment for GAD. However, in a study of long-term use, 264 patients were treated with Buspirone HCl for 1 year without ill effect. Therefore, the physician who elects to use Buspirone HCl for extended periods should periodically reassess the usefulness of the drug for the individual patient.

UNLABELED USES
Buspirone is used alone or as an adjunct in the treatment of chronic alcohol abuse, autism, depression, and obsessive-compulsive disorder. It is also used in panic disorders and agoraphobia with panic attacks, premenstrual syndrome, sexual dysfunction, and alcohol withdrawal.

CONTRAINDICATIONS
Buspirone HCl is contraindicated in patients hypersensitive to buspirone hydrochloride.

WARNINGS
The administration of Buspirone HCl to a patient taking a monoamine oxidase inhibitor (MAOI) may pose a hazard. There have been reports of the occurrence of elevated blood pressure when Buspirone HCl has been added to a regimen including an MAOI. Therefore, it is recommended that Buspirone HCl not be used concomitantly with an MAOI.

Because Buspirone HCl has no established antipsychotic activity, it should not be employed in lieu of appropriate antipsychotic treatment.

PRECAUTIONS
GENERAL
Interference with Cognitive and Motor Performance: Studies indicate that Buspirone HCl is less sedating than other anxiolytics and that it does not produce significant functional impairment. However, its CNS effects in any individual patient may not be predictable. Therefore, patients should be cautioned about operating an automobile or using complex machinery until they are reasonably certain that Buspirone treatment does not affect them adversely.

While formal studies of the interaction of Buspirone HCl with alcohol indicate that buspirone does not increase alcohol-induced impairment in motor and mental performance, it is prudent to avoid concomitant use of alcohol and buspirone.

Potential for Withdrawal Reactions in Sedative/Hypnotic/Anxiolytic Drug Dependent Patients: Because Buspirone HCl does not exhibit cross-tolerance with benzodiazepines and other common sedative/hypnotic drugs, it will not block the withdrawal syndrome often seen with cessation of therapy with these drugs. Therefore, before starting therapy with Buspirone HCl, it is advisable to withdraw patients gradually, especially patients who have been using a CNS-depressant drug chronically, from their prior treatment. Rebound or withdrawal symptoms may occur over varying time periods, depending in part on the type of drug, and its effective half-life of elimination.

The syndrome of withdrawal from sedative/hypnotic/anxiolytic drugs can appear as any combination of irritability, anxiety, agitation, insomnia, tremor, abdominal cramps, muscle cramps, vomiting, sweating, flu-like symptoms without fever, and occasionally, even as seizures.

Possible Concerns Related to Buspirone's Binding to Dopamine Receptors: Because buspirone can bind to central dopamine receptors, a question has been raised about its potential to cause acute and chronic changes in dopamine-mediated neurological function (eg, dystonia, pseudoparkinsonism, akathisia, and tardive dyskinesia). Clinical experience in controlled trials has failed to identify any significant neuroleptic-like activity; however, a syndrome of restlessness, appearing shortly after initiation of treatment, has been reported in some small fraction of buspirone-treated patients. The syndrome may be explained in several ways. For example, buspirone may increase central noradrenergic activity; alternatively, the effect may be attributable to dopaminergic effects (ie, represent akathisia). Obviously, the question cannot be totally resolved at this point in time. Generally, long-term sequelae of any drug's use can be identified only after several years of marketing.

Information for Patients: To assure safe and effective use of Buspirone HCl, the following information and instructions should be given to patients:
1. Inform your physician about any medications, prescription or nonprescription, alcohol, or drugs that you are now taking or plan to take during your treatment with Buspirone HCl.
2. Inform your physician if you are pregnant, or if you are planning to become pregnant, or if you become pregnant while you are taking Buspirone HCl.
3. Inform your physician if you are breastfeeding an infant.
4. Until you experience how this medication affects you, do not drive a car or operate potentially dangerous machinery.

LABORATORY TESTS
There are no specific laboratory tests recommended.

DRUG INTERACTIONS
It is recommended that Buspirone HCl (buspirone hydrochloride) *not* be used concomitantly with MAO inhibitors (see *"Warnings"*). Because the effects of concomitant administration of Buspirone HCl with most other psychotropic drugs have not been studied, the concomitant use of Buspirone HCl with other CNS-active drugs should be approached with caution.

There is one report suggesting that the concomitant use of Desyrel® (trazodone hydrochloride) and Buspirone HCl may have caused 3- to 6-fold elevations on SGPT (ALT) in a few patients. In a similar study, attempting to replicate this finding, no interactive effect on hepatic transaminases was identified.

In a study in normal volunteers, concomitant administration of Buspirone HCl and haloperidol resulted in increased serum haloperidol concentrations. The clinical significance of this finding is not clear.

In vitro, Buspirone does not displace tightly bound drugs like phenytoin, propranolol, and warfarin from serum proteins. However, there has been one report of prolonged prothrombin time when buspirone was added to the regimen of a patient treated with warfarin. The patient was also chronically receiving phenytoin, phenobarbital, digoxin, and Synthroid. *In vitro*, Buspirone may displace less firmly bound drugs like digoxin. The clinical significance of this property is unknown.

► SHOWN IN PRODUCT IDENTIFICATION GUIDE

DRUG/LABORATORY TEST INTERACTIONS

Buspirone is not known to interfere with commonly employed clinical laboratory tests.

CARCINOGENESIS, MUTAGENESIS, IMPAIRMENT OF FERTILITY

No evidence of carcinogenic potential was observed in rats during a 24-month study at approximately 133 times the maximum recommended human oral dose; or in mice, during an 18-month study at approximately 167 times the maximum recommended human oral dose.

With or without metabolic activation, buspirone did not induce point mutations in five strains of *Salmonella typhimurium* (Ames Test) or mouse lymphoma L5178YTK= cell cultures, nor was DNA damage observed with buspirone in Wi-38 human cells. Chromosomal aberrations or abnormalities did not occur in bone marrow cells of mice given one or five daily doses of Buspirone.

PREGNANCY: TERATOGENIC EFFECTS

Pregnancy Category B: No fertility impairment or fetal damage was observed in reproduction studies performed in rats and rabbits at Buspirone doses of approximately 30 times the maximum recommended human dose. In humans, however, adequate and well-controlled studies during pregnancy have *not* been performed. Because animal reproduction studies are not always predictive of human response, this drug should be used during pregnancy only if clearly needed.

LABOR AND DELIVERY

The effect of Buspirone HCl on labor and delivery in women is unknown. No adverse effects were noted in reproduction studies in rats.

NURSING MOTHERS

The extent of the excretion in human milk of buspirone or its metabolites is not known. In rats, however, buspirone and its metabolites are excreted in milk. Buspirone HCl administration to nursing women should be avoided if clinically possible.

PEDIATRIC USE

The safety and effectiveness of Buspirone HCl have not been determined in individuals below 18 years of age.

USE IN THE ELDERLY

Buspirone HCl has not been systematically evaluated in older patients; however, several hundred elderly patients have participated in clinical studies with Buspirone HCl and no unusual adverse age-related phenomena have been identified. In 87 elderly patients for whom dosage data were available, the modal total daily dose of Buspirone HCl was 15 mg per day, the same as that in the total sample of patients treated with Buspirone HCl.

USE IN PATIENTS WITH IMPAIRED HEPATIC OR RENAL FUNCTION

Since Buspirone HCl is metabolized by the liver and excreted by the kidneys, its administration to patients with severe hepatic or renal impairment cannot be recommended.

ADVERSE REACTIONS

(See also "Precautions.")

COMMONLY OBSERVED

The more commonly observed untoward events associated with the use of Buspirone HCl not seen at an equivalent incidence among placebo-treated patients include dizziness, nausea, headache, nervousness, lightheadedness, and excitement.

ASSOCIATED WITH DISCONTINUATION OF TREATMENT

One guide to the relative clinical importance of adverse events associated with Buspirone HCl is provided by the frequency with which they caused drug discontinuation during clinical testing. Approximately 10% of the 2200 anxious patients who participated in the Buspirone HCl premarketing clinical efficacy trials in anxiety disorders lasting 3 to 4 weeks discontinued treatment due to an adverse event. The more common events causing discontinuation included: central nervous system disturbances (3.4%), primarily dizziness, insomnia, nervousness, drowsiness and lightheaded feeling; gastrointestinal disturbances (1.2%), primarily nausea; and miscellaneous disturbances (1.1%), primarily headache and fatigue. In addition, 3.4% of patients had multiple complaints, none of which could be characterized as primary.

INCIDENCE IN CONTROLLED CLINICAL TRIALS

The table that follows enumerates adverse events that occurred at a frequency of 1% or more among Buspirone HCl patients who participated in 4-week, controlled trials comparing Buspirone HCl with placebo. The frequences were obtained from pooled data for 17 trials. The prescriber should be aware that these figures cannot be used to predict the incidence of side effects in the course of usual medical practice where patient characteristics and other factors differ from those which prevailed in the clinical trials. Similarly, the cited frequencies cannot be compared with figures obtained from other clinical investigations involving different treatments, uses, and investigators. Comparison of the cited figures, however, does provide the prescribing physician with some basis for estimating the relative contribution of drug and nondrug factors to the side-effect incidence rate in the population studied.

TREATMENT-EMERGENT ADVERSE EXPERIENCE INCIDENCE IN PLACEBO-CONTROLLED CLINICAL TRIALS*

Adverse Experience	*(Percent of Patients Reporting)* Buspirone HCl (n = 477)	Placebo (n = 464)
Cardiovascular		
Tachycardia/Palpitations	1	1
CNS		
Dizziness	12	3
Drowsiness	10	9
Nervousness	5	1
Insomnia	3	3
Light-headedness	3	—
Decreased Concentration	2	2
Excitement	2	—
Anger/Hostility	2	—
Confusion	2	—
Depression	2	2
EENT		
Blurred Vision	2	—
Gastrointestinal		
Nausea	8	5
Dry Mouth	3	4
Abdominal/Gastric Distress	2	2
Diarrhea	2	—
Constipation	1	2
Vomiting	1	2
Musculoskeletal		
Musculoskeletal Aches/Pains	1	—
Neurological		
Numbness	2	—
Paresthesia	1	—
Incoordination	1	—
Tremor	1	—
Skin		
Skin Rash	1	—
Miscellaneous		
Headache	6	3
Fatigue	4	4
Weakness	2	—
Sweating/Clamminess	1	—

* *Events reported by at least 1% of Buspirone HCl patients are included.*
—*Incidence less than 1%.*

OTHER EVENTS OBSERVED DURING THE ENTIRE PREMARKETING EVALUATION OF BUSPIRONE HCL

During its premarketing assessment, Buspirone HCl was evaluated in over 3500 subjects. This section reports event frequencies for adverse events occurring in approximately 3000 subjects from this group who took multiple doses of Buspirone HCl in the dose range for which Buspirone HCl is being recommended (ie, the modal daily dose of Buspirone HCl fell between 10 and 30 mg for 70% of the patients studied) and for whom safety data were systematically collected. The conditions and duration of exposure to Buspirone HCl varied greatly, involving well-controlled studies as well as experience in open and uncontrolled clinical settings. As part of the total experience gained in clinical studies, various adverse events were reported. In the absence of appropriate controls in some of the studies, a causal relationship to Buspirone HCl treatment cannot be determined. The list includes all undesirable events reasonably associated with the use of the drug.

The following enumeration by organ system describes events in terms of their relative frequency of reporting in this data base. Events of major clinical importance are also described in the "Precautions" section.

The following definitions of frequency are used: Frequent adverse events are defined as those occurring in at least 1/100 patients. Infrequent adverse events are those occurring in 1/100 to 1/1000 patients, while rare events are those occurring in less than 1/1000 patients.

CARDIOVASCULAR

Frequent was nonspecific chest pain; infrequent were syncope, hypotension and hypertension; rare were cerebrovascular accident, congestive heart failure, myocardial infarction, cardiomyopathy and bradycardia.

CENTRAL NERVOUS SYSTEM

Frequent were dream disturbances; infrequent were depersonalization, dysphoria, noise intolerance, euphoria, akathisia, fearfulness, loss of interest, dissociative reaction, hallucinations, suicidal ideation and seizures; rare were feelings of claustrophobia, cold intolerance, stupor, and slurred speech and psychosis.

EENT

Frequent were tinnitus, sore throat, and nasal congestion. Infrequent were redness and itching of the eyes, altered taste, altered smell, and conjunctivitis; rare were inner ear abnormality, eye pain, photophobia, and pressure on eyes.

ENDOCRINE
Rare were galactorrhea and thyroid abnormality.

GASTROINTESTINAL
Infrequent were flatulence, anorexia, increased appetite, salivation, irritable colon and rectal bleeding; rare was burning of the tongue.

GENITOURINARY
Infrequent were urinary frequency, urinary hesitancy, menstrual irregularity and spotting, and dysuria; rare were amenorrhea, pelvic inflammatory disease, enuresis, and nocturia.

MUSCULOSKELETAL
Infrequent were muscle cramps, muscle spasms, rigid/stiff muscles, and arthralgias.

NEUROLOGICAL
Infrequent were involuntary movements and slowed reaction time; rare was muscle weakness.

RESPIRATORY
Infrequent were hyperventilation, shortness of breath, and chest congestion; rare was epistaxis.

SEXUAL FUNCTION
Infrequent were decreased or increased libido; rare were delayed ejaculation and impotence.

SKIN
Infrequent were edema, pruritus, flushing, easy bruising, hair loss, dry skin, facial edema and blisters; rare were acne and thinning of nails.

CLINICAL LABORATORY
Infrequent were increases in hepatic aminotransferases (SGOT, SGPT); rare were eosinophilia, leukopenia, and thrombocytopenia.

MISCELLANEOUS
Infrequent were weight gain, fever, roaring sensation in the head, weight loss, and malaise; rare were alcohol abuse, bleeding disturbance, loss of voice, and hiccoughs.

POSTINTRODUCTION CLINICAL EXPERIENCE
Postmarketing experience has shown an adverse experience profile similar to that given above. Voluntary reports since introduction have included rare occurrences of allergic reactions, cogwheel rigidity, dystonic reactions, ecchymosis, emotional lability, tunnel vision, and urinary retention. Because of the uncontrolled nature of these spontaneous reports, a causal relationship to Buspirone HCl treatment has not been determined.

DRUG ABUSE AND DEPENDENCE
CONTROLLED SUBSTANCE CLASS
Buspirone HCl is not a controlled substance.

PHYSICAL AND PSYCHOLOGICAL DEPENDENCE
In human and animal studies, buspirone has shown no potential for abuse or diversion and there is no evidence that it causes tolerance, or either physical or psychological dependence. Human volunteers with a history of recreational drug or alcohol usage were studied in two double-blind clinical investigations. None of the subjects were able to distinguish between Buspirone HCl and placebo. By contrast, subjects showed a statistically significant preference for methaqualone and diazepam. Studies in monkeys, mice, and rats have indicated that buspirone lacks potential for abuse.

Following chronic administration in the rat, abrupt withdrawal of buspirone did not result in the loss of body weight commonly observed with substances that cause physical dependency.

Although there is no direct evidence that Buspirone HCl causes physical dependence or drug-seeking behavior, it is difficult to predict from experiments the extent to which a CNS-active drug will be misused, diverted, and/or abused once marketed. Consequently, physicians should carefully evaluate patients for a history of drug abuse and follow such patients closely, observing them for signs of Buspirone HCl misuse or abuse (eg, development of tolerance, incrementation of dose, drug-seeking behavior).

OVERDOSAGE
SIGNS AND SYMPTOMS
In clinical pharmacology trials, doses as high as 375 mg/day were administered to healthy male volunteers. As this dose was approached, the following symptoms were observed: nausea, vomiting, dizziness, drowsiness, miosis, and gastric distress. No deaths have been reported in humans either with deliberate or accidental overdosage of Buspirone HCl. Toxicology studies of buspirone yielded the following LD_{50} values: mice, 655 mg/kg; rats, 196 mg/kg; dogs, 586 mg/kg; and monkeys, 356 mg/kg. These dosages are 160-550 times the recommended human daily dose.

RECOMMENDED OVERDOSE TREATMENT
General symptomatic and supportive measures should be used along with immediate gastric lavage. Respiration, pulse, and blood pressure should be monitored as in all cases of drug overdosage. No specific antidote is known to buspirone, and dializability of buspirone has not been determined.

DOSAGE AND ADMINISTRATION
The recommended initial dose is 15 mg daily (5 mg three times a day). To achieve an optimal therapeutic response, at intervals of 2 to 3 days the dosage may be increased 5 mg per day, as needed. The maximum daily dosage should not exceed 60 mg per day. In clinical trials allowing dose titration, divided doses of 20 to 30 mg per day were commonly employed.

Store at room temperature. Protect from temperatures greater than 86° F (30° C). Dispense in a tight, light-resistant container (USP).

REFERENCE
1. American Psychiatric Association, Ed.: Diagnostic and Statistical Manual of Mental Disorders—III, American Psychiatric Association, May 1980.

HOW SUPPLIED
TABLETS: 5 MG

BRAND/MANUFACTURER	NDC	SIZE	AWP
○ **BRAND**			
► BUSPAR: Mead Johnson Pharm	00087-0818-41	100s	$57.82
	00087-0818-43	100s ud	$63.32
	00087-0818-44	500s	$281.11

TABLETS: 10 MG

BRAND/MANUFACTURER	NDC	SIZE	AWP
○ **BRAND**			
► BUSPAR: Mead Johnson Pharm	00087-0819-41	100s	$98.28
	00087-0819-43	100s ud	$107.67
	00087-0819-44	500s	$477.65

Busulfan

> **WARNING**
> BUSULFAN IS A POTENT DRUG. IT SHOULD NOT BE USED UNLESS A DIAGNOSIS OF CHRONIC MYELOGENOUS LEUKEMIA HAS BEEN ADEQUATELY ESTABLISHED AND THE RESPONSIBLE PHYSICIAN IS KNOWLEDGEABLE IN ASSESSING RESPONSE TO CHEMOTHERAPY.
> BUSULFAN CAN INDUCE SEVERE BONE MARROW HYPOPLASIA. REDUCE OR DISCONTINUE THE DOSAGE IMMEDIATELY AT THE FIRST SIGN OF ANY UNUSUAL DEPRESSION OF BONE MARROW FUNCTION AS REFLECTED BY AN ABNORMAL DECREASE IN ANY OF THE FORMED ELEMENTS OF THE BLOOD. A BONE MARROW EXAMINATION SHOULD BE PERFORMED IF THE BONE MARROW STATUS IS UNCERTAIN.
> SEE "WARNINGS" SECTION FOR INFORMATION REGARDING BUSULFAN-INDUCED LEUKEMOGENESIS IN HUMANS.

DESCRIPTION
Busulfan is a bifunctional alkylating agent. Busulfan is known chemically as 1,4-butanediol dimethanesulfonate.

Busulfan is *not* a structural analog of the nitrogen mustards. Busulfan is available in tablet form for oral administration. Each scored tablet contains 2 mg Busulfan.

The activity of Busulfan in chronic myelogenous leukemia was first reported by D.A.G. Galton in 1953.[1]

Following is its chemical structure:

$$CH_3SO_2O(CH_2)_4OSO_2CH_3$$

CLINICAL PHARMACOLOGY
No analytical method has been found which permits the quantitation of nonradiolabeled Busulfan or its metabolites in biological tissues or plasma. All studies of the pharmacokinetics of Busulfan in humans have employed radiolabeled drug using either sulfur-35 (labeling the "carrier" portion of the molecule) or carbon-14 or tritium in the alkane portion of the 4-carbon chain (labels in the "alkylating" portion of the molecule).

Studies with ^{35}*S-Busulfan.* Following the intravenous administration of a single therapeutic dose of ^{35}S-Busulfan, there was rapid disappearance of radioactivity from the blood: 90 to 95% of the ^{35}S-label disappeared within three to five minutes after injection. Thereafter, a constant, low level of radioactivity (1 to 3% of the injected dose) was maintained during the subsequent forty-eight hour period of observation. Following the oral administration of ^{35}S-Busulfan, there was a lag period of one-half to two hours prior to the detection of radioactivity in the blood. However, at four hours the (low) level of circulating radioactivity was comparable to that obtained following intravenous administration. After either oral or intravenous administration of ^{35}S-Busulfan to humans, 45 to 60% of the radioactivity was recovered in the urine in the forty-eight hours after administration; the majority of the total urinary excretion occurred in the first twenty-four hours. In man, over 95% of the urinary sulfur-35 occurs as ^{35}S-methanesulfonic acid.

The fact that urinary recovery of sulfur-35 was equivalent, irrespective of whether the drug was given intravenously or orally, suggests virtually complete absorption by the oral route.

Studies with ^{14}C-Busulfan.[2] Oral and intravenous administration of 1,4-^{14}C-Busulfan showed the same rapid initial disappearance of plasma radioactivity with a subsequent low-level plateau as observed following the administration of ^{35}S-labeled drug. Cumulative radioactivity in the urine after forty-eight hours was 25 to 30% of the administered dose (contrasting with 45 to 60% for ^{35}S-Busulfan) and suggests a slower excretion of the alkylating portion of the molecule and its metabolites than for the sulfonoxymethyl moieties. Regardless of the route of administration, 1,4-^{14}C-Busulfan yielded a complex mixture of at least 12 radiolabeled metabolites in urine; the main metabolite being 3-hydroxy-tetrahydrothiophene-1, 1-dioxide.

Studies with ^{3}H-Busulfan.[3] Human pharmacokinetic studies have been conducted employing Busulfan labeled with tritium on the tetramethylene chain. These experiments confirmed a rapid initial clearance of the radioactivity from plasma, irrespective of whether the drug was given orally or intravenously, and showed a gradual accumulation of radioactivity in the plasma after repeated doses. Urinary excretion of less than 50% of the total dose given suggested a slow elimination of the metabolic products from the body.

There is no experience with the use of dialysis in an attempt to modify the clinical toxicity of Busulfan. One technical difficulty would derive from the extremely poor water solubility of Busulfan. Additionally, all studies of the metabolism of Busulfan employing radiolabeled materials indicate rapid chemical reactivity of the parent compound with prolonged retention of some of the metabolites (particularly the metabolites arising from the "alkylating" portion of the molecule). The effectiveness of dialysis at removing significant quantities of unreacted drug would be expected to be minimal in such a situation.

No information is available regarding the penetration of Busulfan into brain or cerebrospinal fluid.

Biochemical Pharmacology: In aqueous media, Busulfan undergoes a wide range of nucleophilic substitution reactions. While this chemical reactivity is relatively non-specific, alkylation of the DNA is felt to be an important biological mechanism for its cytotoxic effect.[4] Coliphage T7 exposed to Busulfan was found to have the DNA crosslinked by intrastrand crosslinkages, but no interstrand linkages were found.

The metabolic fate of Busulfan has been studied in rats and humans using ^{14}C- and ^{35}S-labeled materials.[2,5,6] In man,[2] as in the rat,[6] almost all of the radioactivity in ^{35}S-labeled Busulfan is excreted in the urine in the form of ^{35}S-methanesulfonic acid. No unchanged drug was found in human urine,[2] although a small amount has been reported in rat urine.[6] Roberts and Warwick demonstrated that the formation of methanesulfonic acid *in vivo* in the rat is not due to a simple hydrolysis of Busulfan to 1,4-butanediol, since only about 4% of 2,3-^{14}C-Busulfan was excreted as carbon dioxide whereas 2,3-^{14}C-1,4-butanediol was converted almost exclusively to carbon dioxide.[5] The predominant reaction of Busulfan in the rat is the alkylation of sulfhydryl groups (particularly cysteine and cysteine-containing compounds) to produce a cyclic sulfonium compound which is the precursor of the major urinary metabolite of the 4-carbon portion of the molecule, 3-hydroxytetrahydrothiophene-1, 1-dioxide.[5] This has been termed a "sulfur-stripping" action of Busulfan and it may modify the function of certain sulfur-containing amino acids, polypeptides, and proteins; whether this action makes an important contribution to the cytotoxicity of Busulfan is unknown.

The biochemical basis for acquired resistance to Busulfan is largely a matter of speculation. Although altered transport of Busulfan into the cell is one possibility, increased intracellular inactivation of the drug before it reaches the DNA is also possible. Experiments with other alkylating agents have shown that resistance to this class of compounds may reflect an acquired ability of the resistant cell to repair alkylation damage more effectively.[4]

INDICATIONS AND USAGE

Busulfan is indicated for the palliative treatment of chronic myelogenous (myeloid, myelocytic, granulocytic) leukemia. Although not curative, Busulfan reduces the total granulocyte mass, relives symptoms of the disease, and improves the clinical state of the patient. Approximately 90% of adults with previously untreated chronic myelogenous leukemia will obtain hematologic remission with regression or stabilization of organomegaly following the use of Busulfan. It has been shown to be superior to splenic irradiation with respect to survival times and maintenance of hemoglobin levels, and to be equivalent to irradiation at controlling splenomegaly.[7]

It is not clear whether Busulfan unequivocally prolongs the survival of responding patients beyond the 31 months experienced by an untreated group of historical controls.[8] Median survival figures of 31-42 months have been reported for several groups of patients treated with Busulfan, but concurrent control groups of patients treated with Busulfan, but concurrent control groups of comparable, untreated patients are not available.[7,9,10,11] The median survival figures reported from different studies will be influenced by the percentage of "poor risk" patients initially entered into the particular study. Patients who are alive two years following the diagnosis of chronic myelogenous leukemia, and who have been treated during that period with Busulfan, are estimated to have a mean annual mortality rate during the second to fifth year which is approximately two-thirds that of patients who received either no treatment, conventional x-ray or ^{32}P-irradiation, or chemotherapy with minimally active drugs.[12]

Busulfan is clearly less effective in patients with chronic myelogenous leukemia who lack the Philadelphia (Ph[1]) chromosome.[13] Also, the so-called "juvenile" type of chronic myelogenous leukemia, typically occurring in young children and associated with the absence of a Philadelphia chromosome, responds poorly to Busulfan.[14] The drug is of no benefit in patients whose chronic myelogenous leukemia has entered a "blastic" phase.

CONTRAINDICATIONS

Busulfan should not be used unless a diagnosis of chronic myelogenous leukemia has been adequately established and the responsible physician is knowledgeable in assessing response to chemotherapy.

Busulfan should not be used in patients whose chronic myelogenous leukemia has demonstrated prior resistance to this drug.

Busulfan is of no value in chronic lymphocytic leukemia, acute leukemia, or in the "blastic crisis" of chronic myelogenous leukemia.

WARNINGS

The most frequent, serious side effect of treatment with Busulfan is the induction of bone marrow failure (which may or may not be anatomically hypoplastic) resulting in severe pancytopenia. The pancytopenia caused by Busulfan may be more prolonged than that induced with other alkylating agents. It is generally felt that the usual cause of Busulfan-induced pancytopenia is the failure to stop administration of the drug soon enough; individual idiosyncrasy to the drug does not seem to be an important factor. *Busulfan should be used with extreme caution and exceptional vigilance in patients whose bone marrow reserve may have been compromised by prior irradiation or chemotherapy, or whose marrow function is recovering from previous cytotoxic therapy.* Although recovery from Busulfan-induced pancytopenia may take from one month to two years, this complication is potentially reversible and the patient should be vigorously supported through any period of severe pancytopenia.[15]

A rare, important complication of Busulfan therapy is the development of bronchopulmonary dysplasia with pulmonary fibrosis.[16] Symptoms have been reported to occur within eight months to ten years after initiation of therapy—the average duration of therapy being four years. The histologic findings associated with "Busulfan lung" mimic those seen following pulmonary irradiation. Clinically, patients have reported the insidious onset of cough, dyspnea, and low-grade fever. Pulmonary function studies have revealed diminished diffusion capacity and decreased pulmonary compliance. It is important to exclude more common conditions (such as opportunistic infections or leukemic infiltration of the lungs) with appropriate diagnostic techniques. If measures such as sputum cultures, virologic studies, and exfoliative cytology fail to establish an etiology for the pulmonary infiltrates, lung biopsy may be necessary to establish the diagnosis. Treatment of established Busulfan-induced pulmonary fibrosis is unsatisfactory; in most cases the patients have died within six months after the diagnosis was established. There is no specific therapy for this complication other than the immediate discontinuation of Busulfan. The administration of corticosteroids has been suggested, but the results have not been impressive or uniformly successful.

Busulfan may cause cellular dysplasia in many organs in addition to the lung. Cytologic abnormalities characterized by giant, hyperchromatic nuclei have been reported in lymph nodes, pancreas, thyroid, adrenal glands, liver, and bone marrow. This cytologic dysplasia may be severe enough to cause difficulty in interpretation of exfoliative cytologic examinations from the lung, bladder, breast, and the uterine cervix.

In addition to the widespread epithelial dysplasia that has been observed during Busulfan therapy, chromosome aberrations have been reported in cells from patients receiving Busulfan.

Busulfan is mutagenic in mice and, possibly, in man.

A number of malignant tumors have been reported in patients on Busulfan therapy and this drug may be a human carcinogen. Four cases of acute leukemia occurred among 243 patients treated with Busulfan as adjuvant chemotherapy following surgical resection of bronchogenic carcinoma. All four cases were from a subgroup of 19 of these 243 patients who developed pancytopenia while taking Busulfan five to eight years before leukemia became clinically apparent. These findings suggest that Busulfan is leukemogenic, although its mode of action is uncertain[17]

Ovarian suppression and amenorrhea with menopausal symptoms commonly occur during Busulfan therapy in premenopausal patients. Busulfan interferes with spermatogenesis in experimental animals, and there have been clinical reports of sterility, azoospermia and testicular atrophy in male patients.

A rare but life-threatening hepatic veno-occlusive disease has been reported following the investigational use of very high doses of Busulfan in combination with cyclophosphamide or other chemotherapeutic agents prior to bone marrow transplantation.[18-24] A clear cause and effect relationship with Busulfan has not been demonstrated. Possible risk factors for the development of hepatic veno-occulusive disease include: total Busulfan dose exceeding 16 mg/kg based on ideal body weight, and concurrent use of multiple alkylating agents. Periodic measurement of serum transaminases, alkaline phosphatase, and bilirubin is indicated for early detection of hepatotoxicity.

Cardiac tamponade has been reported in a small number of patients with thalessemia (2% in one series) who received high doses of Busulfan and cyclophosphamide as the preparatory regimen for bone marrow transplantation. In this series, the cardiac tamponade was often fatal. Abdominal pain and vomiting preceded the tamponade in most patients.

Pregnancy: "Pregnancy Category D": Busulfan may cause fetal harm when administered to a pregnant woman. Although there have been a number of cases reported where apparently normal children have been born after Busulfan treatment during pregnancy,[25] one case has been cited where a malformed baby was delivered by a mother treated with Busulfan. During the pregnancy that resulted in the malformed infant, the mother received x-ray therapy early in the first trimester, mercaptopurine until the third month, then Busulfan until delivery.[26] In pregnant rats, Busulfan produces sterility in both male and female offspring due to the absence of germinal cells in testes and ovaries.[27] Germinal cell aplasia or sterility in offspring of mothers receiving Busulfan during pregnancy has not been reported in humans. There are no adequate and well-controlled studies in pregnant women. If this drug is used during pregnancy, or if the patient becomes pregnant while taking this drug, the patient should be apprised of the potential hazard to the fetus. Women of childbearing potential should be advised to avoid becoming pregnant.

PRECAUTIONS

General: The most consistent, dose-related toxicity is bone marrow suppression. This may be manifest by anemia, leukopenia, thrombocytopenia, or any combination of these. It is imperative that patients be instructed to report promptly the development of fever, sore throat, signs of local infection, bleeding from any site, or symptoms suggestive of anemia. Any one of these findings may indicate Busulfan toxicity; however, they may also indicate transformation of the disease to an acute "blastic" form. Since Busulfan may have a delayed effect, it is important to withdraw the medication temporarily at the first sign of an abnormally large or exceptionally rapid fall in any of the formed elements of the blood. *Patients should never be allowed to take the drug without close medical supervision.*

Seizures have been reported in patients receiving very high, investigational doses of Busulfan.[18,28-32] As with any potentially epileptogenic drug, caution should be exercised when administering very high doses of Busulfan to patients with a history of seizure disorder, head trauma, or receiving other potentially epileptogenic drugs. Some investigators have used prophylactic anticonvulsant therapy in this setting.

Information for Patients: Patients beginning therapy with Busulfan should be informed of the importance of having periodic blood counts and to immediately report any unusual fever or bleeding. Aside from the major toxicity of myelosuppression, patients should be instructed to report any difficulty in breathing, persistent cough or congestion. They should be told that diffuse pulmonary fibrosis is an infrequent but serious and potentially life-threatening complication of long-term Busulfan therapy. Patients should be alerted to report any signs of abrupt weakness, unusual fatigue, anorexia, weight loss, nausea and vomiting, and melanoderma that could be associated with a syndrome resembling adrenal insufficiency. Patients should never be allowed to take the drug without medical supervision and they should be informed that other encountered toxicities to Busulfan include infertility, amenorrhea, skin hyperpigmentation, drug hypersensitivity, dryness of the mucous membranes and rarely cataract formation. Women of childbearing potential should be advised to avoid becoming pregnant. The increased risk of a second malignancy should be explained to the patient.

Laboratory Tests: It is recommended that evaluation of the hemoglobin or hematocrit, total white blood cell count and differential count, and quantitative platelet count be obtained weekly while the patient is on Busulfan therapy. In cases where the cause of fluctuation in the formed elements of the peripheral blood is obscure, bone marrow examination may be useful for evaluation of marrow status. A decision to increase, decrease, continue, or discontinue a given dose of Busulfan must be based not only on the absolute hematologic values, but also on the rapidity with which changes are occurring. The dosage of Busulfan may need to be reduced if this agent is combined with other drugs whose primary toxicity is myelosuppression. Occasional patients may be unusually sensitive to Busulfan administered at standard dosage and suffer neutropenia or thrombocytopenia after a relatively short exposure to the drug. Busulfan should not be used where facilities for complete blood counts, including quantitative platelet counts, are not available at weekly (or more frequent) intervals.

Drug Interactions: Busulfan may cause additive myelosuppression when used with other myelosuppressive drugs.

In one study, 12 of approximately 330 patients receiving continuous Busulfan and thioguanine therapy for treatment of chronic myelogenous leukemia were found to have esophageal varices associated with abnormal liver function tests.[33] Subsequent liver biopsies were performed in four of these patients, all of which showed evidence of nodular regenerative hyperplasia. Duration of combination therapy prior to the appearance of esophageal varices ranged from 6 to 45 months. With the present analysis of the data, no cases of hepatotoxicity have appeared in the Busulfan alone arm of the study. Long-term continuous therapy with thioguanine and Busulfan should be used with caution.

Carcinogenesis, Mutagenesis, Impairment of Fertility: See *"Warnings"* section.

Pregnancy: Teratogenic effects: Pregnancy Category D. See *"Warnings"* sections.

Nonteratogenic effects: There have been reports in the literature of small infants being born after the mothers received Busulfan during pregnancy, in particular, during the third trimester.[34] One case was reported where an infant had mild anemia and neutropenia at birth after Busulfan was administered to the mother from the eighth week of pregnancy to term.[25]

Nursing Mothers: It is not known whether this drug is excreted in human milk. Because of the potential for tumorigenicity shown for Busulfan in animal and human studies, a decision should be made whether to discontinue nursing or to discontinue the drug, taking into account the importance of the drug to the mother.

ADVERSE REACTIONS

Hematological Effects: The most frequent, serious, toxic effect of Busulfan is myelosuppression resulting in leukopenia, thrombocytopenia, and anemia. Myelosuppression is most frequently the result of a failure to discontinue dosage in the face of an undetected decrease in leukocyte or platelet counts.[15]

Pulmonary: Interstitial pulmonary fibrosis has been reported rarely, but it is a clinically significant adverse effect when observed and calls for immediate discontinuation of further administration of the drug. The role of corticosteroids in arresting or reversing the fibrosis has been reported to be beneficial in some cases and without effect in others.[16]

Cardiac: One case of endocardial fibrosis has been reported in a 79-year-old woman who received a total dose of 7,200 mg of Busulfan over a period of nine years for the management of chronic myelogenous leukemia.[35] At autopsy, she was found to have endocardial fibrosis of the left ventricle in addition to interstitial pulmonary fibrosis.

Cardiac tamponade has been reported in a small number of patients with thalassemia who received high doses of Busulfan and cyclophosphamide as the preparatory regimen for bone marrow transplantation (see *"Warnings"*).

Ocular: Busulfan is capable of inducing cataracts in rats and there have been several reports indicating that this is a rare complication in humans. In the few cases reported in humans, cataracts have occurred only after prolonged administration of Busulfan.[36]

Dermatologic: Hyperpigmentation is the most common adverse skin reaction and occurs in 5-10% of patients, particularly those with a dark complexion.

Metabolic: In a few cases, a clinical syndrome closely resembling adrenal insufficiency and characterized by weakness, severe fatigue, anorexia, weight loss, nausea and vomiting, and melanoderma has developed after prolonged Busulfan therapy. The symptoms have sometimes been reversible when Busulfan was withdrawn. Adrenal responsiveness to exogenously administered ACTH has usually been normal. However, pituitary function testing with metyrapone revealed a blunted urinary 17-hydroxycorticosteroid excretion in two patients.[37] Following the discontinuation of Busulfan (which was associated with clinical improvement), rechallenge with metyrapone revealed normal pituitary-adrenal function.

Hyperuricemia and/or hyperuricosuria are not uncommon in patients with chronic myelogenous leukemia. Additional rapid destruction of granulocytes may accompany the initiation of chemotherapy and increase the urate pool. Adverse effects can be minimized by increased hydration, urine alkalinization, and the prophylactic administration of a xanthine oxidase inhibitor such as allopurinol.

Hepatic Effects: Esophageal varices have been reported in patients receiving continuous Busulfan and thioguanine therapy for treatment of chronic myelogenous leukemia (see *"Precautions—Drug Interactions"*). Hepatic veno-occlusive disease has been observed in patients receiving higher than recommended doses of Busulfan (see *"Warnings"*).

Miscellaneous: Other reported adverse reactions include: urticaria, erythema multiforme, erythema nodosum, alopecia, porphyria cutanea tarda, excessive dryness and fragility of the skin with anhidrosis, dryness of the oral mucous membranes and cheilosis, gynecomastia, cholestatic jaundice, and myasthenia gravis. Most of these are single case reports, and in many a clear cause and effect relationship with Busulfan has not been demonstrated.

Seizures (see *"Precautions-General"*) have been observed in patients receiving higher than recommended doses of Busulfan.

OVERDOSAGE

There is no known antidote to Busulfan. The principal toxic effect is on the bone marrow. Survival after a single 140 mg dose has been reported in an 18 kg, 4-year-old child,[38] but hematologic toxicity is likely to be more profound with chronic overdosage. The hematologic status should be closely monitored and vigorous supportive measures instituted if necessary. Induction of vomiting or gastric lavage followed by administration of charcoal would be indicated if ingestion were recent. It is not known whether Busulfan is dialyzable (see *"Clinical Pharmacology"*).

Oral LD_{50} single doses in mice are 120 mg/kg. Two distinct types of toxic response are seen at median lethal doses given intraperitoneally. Within a matter of hours there are signs of stimulation of the central nervous system with convulsions and death on the first day. Mice are more sensitive to this effect than are rats. With doses at the LD_{50} there is also delayed death due to damage to the bone marrow. At three times the LD_{50}, atrophy of the mucosa of the large intestine is found after a week, whereas that of the small intestine is little affected.[39] After doses in the order of 10 times those used therapeutically were added to the diet of rats, irreversible cataracts were produced after several weeks. Small doses had no such effect.[40]

DOSAGE AND ADMINISTRATION

Busulfan is administered orally. The usual adult dose range for *remission induction* is four to eight mg, total dose, daily. Dosing on a weight basis is the same for both children and adults, approximately 60 µg per kg of body weight or 1.8 mg per square meter of body surface, daily. Since the rate of fall of the leukocyte count is dose related, daily doses exceeding four mg per day should be reserved for patients with the most compelling symptoms; the greater the total daily dose, the greater is the possibility of inducing bone marrow aplasia.

A decrease in the leukocyte count is not usually seen during the first ten to fifteen days of treatment; the leukocyte count may actually increase during this period and it should not be interpreted as resistance to the drug, nor should the dose be increased.[41] Since the leukocyte count may continue to fall for more than one month after discontinuing the drug, it is important that Busulfan be discontinued *prior* to the total leukocyte count falling into the normal range. When the total leukocyte count has declined to approximately 15,000/μL the drug should be withheld.

With a constant dose of Busulfan, the total leukocyte count declines exponentially; a weekly plot of the leukocyte count on semi-logarithmic graph paper aids in predicting the time when therapy should be discontinued.[42] With the recommended dose of Busulfan, a normal leukocyte count is usually achieved in twelve to twenty weeks.

During remission, the patient is examined at monthly intervals and treatment resumed with the induction dosage when the total leukocyte count reaches approximately 50,000/μL. When remission is shorter than three months, maintenance therapy of 1 to 3 mg daily may be advisable in order to keep the hematological status under control and prevent rapid relapse.

Procedures for proper handling and disposal of anti-cancer drugs should be considered. Several guidelines on this subject have been published.[43-49]

There is no general agreement that all of the procedures recommended in the guidelines are necessary or appropriate.

REFERENCES

1. Galton DAG. Myleran in chronic myeloid leukemia: results of treatment. *Lancet.* 1953;1:208-213. 2. Nadkarni MV, Trams EG, Smith PK. Preliminary studies on the distribution and fate of TEM, TEPA, and Myleran in the human. *Cancer Res.* 1959;19:713-718. 3. Vodopick H, Hamilton HE, Jackson HL, Peng C-T, Sheets RF. Metabolic fate of tritiated Busulfan in man. *J Lab Clin Med.* 1969;73:266-276. 4. Fox BW. Mechanism of action of methane sulfonates. In: Sartorelli AC, Johns DG, eds. *Antineoplastic and Immunosuppressive Agents,* Part II. Berlin: Springer Verlag; 1975;35-46. 5. Roberts JJ, Warwick GP. The mode of action of alkylating agents, III; the formation of 3-hydroxytetrahydrothiophene-1:1-dioxide from 1:4-dimethanesulphonyloxybutane (Myleran), S-β-L-alanyltetrahydrothiophenium mesylate, tetrahydrothiophene and tetrahydrothiophene-1:1-dioxide in the rat, rabbit and mouse. *Biochem Pharmacol.* 1961;6:217-227. 6. Peng C-T. Distribution and metabolic fate of S[35]-labeled Myleran (Busulfan) in normal and tumor-bearing rats. *J Pharmacol Exp Ther.* 1957;120:229-238. 7. Medical Research Council's Working Party for Therapeutic Trials in Leukemia. Chronic granulocytic leukaemia: comparison of radiotherapy and busulphan therapy. *Br Med J.* 1968;1:201-208. 8. Minot GR, Buckman TE, Isaacs R. Chronic myelogenous leukemia: age incidence, duration, and benefit derived from irradiation. *JAMA.* 1924;82:1489-1494. 9. Haut A, Abbott WS, Wintrobe MM, Cartwright GE. Busulfan in the treatment of chronic myelocytic leukemia; the effect of long term intermittent therapy. *Blood,* 1961;17:1-19. 10. Monfardini S, Gee T, Fried J, Clarkson B. Survival in chronic myelogenous leukemia; influence of treatment and extent of disease at diagnosis. *Cancer.* 1973;31:492-501. 11. Conrad FG. Survival in granulocytic leukemia. *Arch Intern Med.* 1973;131:684-685. 12. Sokal JE. Evaluation of survival data for chronic myelocytic leukemia. *Am J Hematol.* 1976;1:493-500. 13. Ezdinli EZ, Sokal JE, Crosswhite L, Sandberg AA. Philadelphia chromosome-positive and -negative chronic myelocytic leukemia. *Ann Intern Med.* 1970;72:175-182. 14. Smith KL, Johnson W. Classification of chronic myelocytic leukemia in children. *Cancer.* 1974; 34:670-679. 15. Stuart JJ, Crocker DL, Roberts HR. Treatment of Busulfan-induced pancytopenia. *Arch Intern Med.* 1977; 136:1181-1183. 16. Sostman HD, Matthay RA, Putman CE. Cytotoxic drug-induced lung disease. *Am J Med.* 1977;62:608-615. 17. Stott H. Fox W, Girling DJ, Stephens RJ, Galton DAG. Acute leukaemia after busulphan. *Br Med J.* 1977;2:1513-1517. 18. Hartmann O, et al. High-dose Busulfan and cyclophosphamide with autologous bone marrow transplantation support in advanced malignancies in children: A Phase II study. *J Clin Oncol* 1986;4:1804-10. 19. Copelan EA, et al. Marrow transplantation following Busulfan and cyclophosphamide for chronic myelogenous leukemia in accelerated or blastic phase. *Br J Haematol* 1989; 71:487-91. 20. Kirchner H, et al. Allogeneic and autologous bone marrow transplantation (BMT) after high-dose Busulfan and cyclophosphamide treatment. *Blut* 1988;57:198. (abstract) 21. Thompson J, et al. Allogeneic bone marrow transplantation (BMT) following transplant preparation with cyclophosphamide (CTX) and Busulfan (BU). *Proc ASCO* 1989;8:18. (abstract) 22. Geller RB, et al. Allogeneic bone marrow transplatation after high-dose Busulfan and cyclophosphamide in patients with acute non-lymphocytic leukemia. *Blood* 1989; 73-2209-18. 23. Lu C, et al. Preliminary results of high-dose Busulfan and cyclophosphamide with syngeneic or autologous bone marrow rescue. *Cancer Treat Rep* 1984; 68:711-7. 24. Groshow LB, et al. Pharmacokinetics of Busulfan: correlation with veno-occlusive disease in patients undergoing bone marrow transplantation. *Cancer Chemother Pharmacol* 1989; 25:55-61. 25. Dugdal M, Fort AT. Busulfan treatment of leukemia during pregnancy: case report and review of the literature. *JAMA,* 1967:199:131-133. 26. Diamond I, Anderson MM, McCreadie SR. Transplacental transmission of Busulfan (Myleran) in a mother with leukemia: production of fetal malformation and cytomegaly. *Pediatrics* 1960;25:85-90. 27. Bollag W. Cytostatica in der Schwangerschaft. *Schweiz Med Wochenschr,* 1954;84:393-395. 28. Marcus RE, et al. Convulsions due to high-dose Busulfan. *Lancet* 1984;2:1463. (letter) 29. Martell RW, et al. High-dose Busulfan and myoclonic epilepsy. *Ann Intern Med.* 1987;106:173. (letter) 30. Sureda A, et al. High-dose Busulfan and seizures. *Ann Intern Med* 1989; 111:543-4. (letter) 31. Grigg AP, et al. Busulfan and phenytoin. *Ann Intern Med* 1989; 111:1049-50. (letter) 32. Beelen DW, et al. Acute toxicity and first clinical results of intensive post-induction therapy using a modified Busulfan and cyclophosphamide regimen with autologous bone marrow rescue in first remission of acute myeloid leukemia. *Blood* 1989; 74:1507-16. 33. Key NS, Kelly PMA, Emerson PM, Chapman RWG, Allan NC, McGee JO'D: Oesophageal varices associated with Busulfan-thioguanine combination therapy for chronic myeloid leukaemia. *Lancet.* 1987;2:1050-1052. 34. Boros SJ, Reynolds JW. Intrauterine growth retardation following third-trimester exposure to Busulfan. *Am J Obstet Gynecol.* 1977; 129:111-112. 35. Weinberger A. Pinkhas J, Sandbank U, Shaklai M, de Vries A. Endocardial fibrosis following Busulfan treatment. *JAMA.* 1975;231:495. 36. Ravindranathan MP, Paul VJ, Kuriakose ET. Cataract after Busulfan treatment. *Br Med J.* 1972;1:218-219. 37. Vivacqua RJ, Haurani Fl, Erslev AJ. "Selective" pituitary insufficiency secondary to Busulfan. *Ann Intern Med.* 1967;67:380-387. 38. DeOliveira HP, Cruz E. Fonseca A de S, Medeiros M. Accidental ingestion of a toxic dose of Myleran by a child. *Acta Haematol* (Basel) 1963;29:249-255. 39. Sternberg SS, Phillips FS, Scholler J. Pharmacological and pathological effects of alkylating agents. *Ann NY Acad Sci.* 1958;68:811-825. 40. Solomon C, Light AE, deBeer EJ. Cataracts produced in rats by 1,4-dimethanesulfonoxybutane (Myleran). *AMA Arch Ophthal.* 1955;54:850-852. 41. Stryckmans PA: Current concepts in chronic myelogenous leukemia. *Semin Hematol.* 1974;11:101-127. 42. Galton DAG. Chemotherapy of chronic myelocytic leukemia. *Semin Hematol.* 1969;6:323-343. 43. Recommendations for the safe handling of parenteral antineoplastic drugs. Washington, DC: Division of Safety, National Institutes of Health; 1983. US Dept of Health and Human Services, Public Health Service publication NIH 83-2621. 44. AMA Council on Scientific Affairs. Guidelines for handling parenteral antineoplastics. *JAMA.* 1985;253: 1590-1591. 45. National Study Commission on Cytotoxic Exposure. Recommendations for handling cytotoxic agents. 1984. Available from Louis P. Jeffrey, ScD, Director of Pharmacy Services, Rhode Island Hospital, 593 Eddy Street, Providence, Rhode Island 02902. 46. Clinical Oncological Society of Australia. Guidelines and recommendations for safe handling of antineoplastic agents. *Med J Australia.* 1983;1:426-428. 47. Jones RB, Frank R, Mass T. Safe handling of chemotherapeutic agents: a report from the Mount Sinai Medical Center. *CA-A Cancer J for Clin.* 1983;33(Sept/Oct): 258-263. 48. American Society of Hospital Pharmacists. ASHP technical assistance bulletin on handling cytotoxic and hazardous drugs. *AM J Hosp Pharm.* 1990;47:1033-1049. 49. Yodaiken RE, Bennett D. OSHA work-practice guidelines for personnel dealing with cytotoxic (antineoplastic) drugs. *Am J Hosp Pharm.* 1986;43:1193-1204.

HOW SUPPLIED

TABLETS: 2 MG

BRAND/MANUFACTURER	NDC	SIZE	AWP
○ BRAND			
MYLERAN: Burr Wellcome	00081-0713-25	25s	$31.32

Butabarbital Sodium

DESCRIPTION

Butabarbital Sodium is a nonselective central nervous system depressant which is used as a sedative or hypnotic (WARNING: May be habit forming). It is available for oral adminstration as *Tablets* containing 15 mg, 30 mg, 50 mg or 100 mg Butabarbital Sodium; and as *Elixir* containing 30 mg/5 mL.

Butabarbital Sodium occurs as a white, bitter powder which is freely soluble in water and alcohol, but practically insoluble in benzene and ether.

Chemically Butabarbital Sodium is Sodium 5-*sec*-butyl-5-ethylbarbiturate.

Following is its chemical structure:

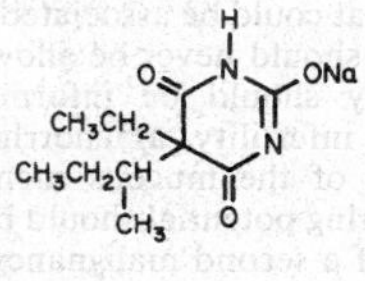

CLINICAL PHARMACOLOGY

Butabarbital Sodium like other barbiturates, is capable of producing all levels of CNS mood alteration from excitation to mild sedation, to hypnosis, and deep coma. Overdosage can produce death. Barbiturates depress the sensory cortex, decrease motor activity, alter cerebellar function, and produce drowsiness, sedation, and hynosis.

Barbiturate-induced sleep differs from physiological sleep. Sleep laboratory studies have demonstrated that barbiturates reduce the amount of time spent in the rapid eye movement (REM) phase of sleep or dreaming stage. Also, Stages III and IV sleep are decreased. Following abrupt cessation of barbiturates used regularly, patients may experience markedly increased dreaming, nightmares, and/or insomnia. Therefore, withdrawal of a single therapeutic dose over 5 or 6 days has been recommended to lessen the REM rebound and disturbed sleep which contribute to drug withdrawal syndrome (for example, decrease the dose from 3 to 2 doses a day for 1 week).

In studies, secobarbital sodium and pentobarbital sodium have been found to lose most of their effectiveness for both inducing and maintaining sleep by the end of 2 weeks of continued drug administration even with the use of multiple doses. As with secobarbital sodium and pentobarbital sodium, other barbiturates might be expected to lose their effectiveness for inducing and maintaining sleep after about 2 weeks. The short-, intermediate-, and, to a lesser degree, long-acting barbiturates have been widely prescribed for treating insomnia. Although the clinical literature abounds with claims that the short-acting barbiturates are superior for producing sleep while the intermediate-acting compounds are more effective in maintaining sleep, controlled studies have failed to demonstrate these differential effects. Therefore, as sleep medications, the barbiturates are of limited value beyond the short-term use.

Barbiturates are respiratory depressants. The degree of respiratory depression is dependent upon dose. With hypnotic doses, respiratory depression produced by barbiturates is similar to that which occurs during physiologic sleep with slight decrease in blood pressure and heart rate.

Barbiturates do not impair normal hepatic function, but have been shown to induce liver microsomal enzymes, thus increasing and/or altering the metabolism of barbiturates and other drugs (see *"Precautions—Drug Interactions"*).

Pharmacokinetics: Butabarbital Sodium is the sodium salt of a weak acid. Barbiturates are weak acids that are absorbed and rapidly distributed to all tissues and fluids with high concentrations in the brain, liver, and kidneys. Barbiturates are bound to plasma and tissue proteins. The rate of absorption is increased if it is ingested as a dilute solution or taken on an empty stomach. Barbiturates are metabolized primarily by the hepatic microsomal enzyme system, and most metabolic products are excreted in the urine. The excretion of unchanged butabarbital in the urine is negligible. Butabarbital Sodium is classified as an intermediate-acting barbiturate. The average plasma half-life for Butabarbital is 100 hours in the adult.

Although variable from patient to patient, Butabarbital has an onset of action of about ¾ to 1 hour, and a duration of action of about 6 to 8 hours.

INDICATIONS AND USAGE

Butabarbital Sodium is indicated for use as a sedative or hypnotic.

Since barbiturates appear to lose their effectiveness for sleep induction and sleep maintenance after 2 weeks, use of Butabarbital Sodium in treating insomnia should be limited to this time (see *"Clinical Pharmacology"* above).

UNLABELED USES
Butabarbital Sodium is also used alone or as an adjunct in the treatment of anxiety disorders.

CONTRAINDICATIONS

Barbiturates are contraindicated in patients with known barbiturate sensivitiy. Barbiturates are also contraindicated in patients with a history of manifest or latent porphyria.

WARNINGS

Habit Forming: Barbiturates may be habit forming. Tolerance, pscyhological and physical dependence may occur with continued use (see *"Drug Abuse and Dependence"* below). Patients who have psychological dependence on barbiturates may increase the dosage or decrease the dosage interval without consulting a physician and may subsequently develop a physical dependence on barbiturates. To minimize the possibility of overdosage or the development of dependence, the prescribing and dispensing of sedative hypnotic barbiturates should be limited to the amount required for the interval until the next appointment. Abrupt cessation after prolonged use in the dependent person may result in withdrawal symptoms, including delirium, convulsions, and possibly death. Barbiturates should be withdrawn gradually from any patient known to be taking excessive dosage over long periods of time. (See *"Drug Abuse and Dependence"* below).

Acute or Chronic Pain: Caution should be exercised when barbiturates are administered to patients with acute or chronic pain, because paradoxical excitement could be induced, or important symptoms could be masked. However, the use of barbiturates as sedatives in the postoperative surgical period, and as adjuncts to cancer chemotherapy, is well established.

Use in Pregnancy: Barbiturates can cause fetal damage when administered to a pregnant woman. Retrospective, case-controlled studies have suggested a connection between the maternal consumption of barbiturates and a higher than expected incidence of fetal abnormalities. Following oral administration, barbiturates readily cross the placental barrier and are distributed throughout fetal tissues with highest concentrations found in the placenta, fetal liver, and brain. Withdrawal symptoms occur in infants born to mothers who receive barbiturates throughout the last trimester of pregnancy (see *"Drug Abuse and Dependence"*). If this drug is used during pregnancy, or if the patient becomes pregnant while taking this drug, the patient should be apprised of the potential hazard to the fetus.

PRECAUTIONS

General: Barbiturates should be administered with caution, if at all, to patients who are mentally depressed, have suicidal tendencies, or a history of drug abuse.

Elderly or debilitated patients may react to barbiturates with marked excitement, depression, and confusion. In some persons, barbiturates repeatedly produce excitement rather than depression.

In patients with hepatic damage, barbiturates should be administered with caution and initially in reduced doses. Barbiturates should not be administered to patients showing the premonitory signs of hepatic coma.

Certain brands of Butabarbital Sodium tablets and elixir contain FD&C Yellow No. 5 (tartrazine) which may cause allergic-type reactions (including bronchial asthma) in certain susceptible individuals. Although the overall incidence of FD&C Yellow No. 5 (tartrazine) sensitivity in the general population is low, it is frequently seen in patients who also have aspirin hypersensitivity.

Information for Patients: Practitioners should give the following information and instructions to patients receiving barbiturates.

The use of barbiturates carries with it an associated risk of psychological and/or physical dependence. The patient should be warned against increasing the dose of the drug without consulting a physician.

Barbiturates may impair mental and/or physical abilities required for the performance of potentially hazardous tasks, such as driving or operating machinery.

Alcohol should not be consumed while taking barbiturates. Concurrent use of the barbiturates with other CNS depressants, including other sedatives or hypnotics, alcohol, narcotics, tranquilizers, and antihistamines, may result in additional CNS depressant effects.

Laboratory Tests: Prolonged therapy with barbiturates should be accompanied by periodic laboratory evaluation of organ systems, including hematopoietic, renal, and hepatic systems (see *"Precautions—General and Adverse Reactions"*).

Drug Interactions: Most reports of clinically significant drug interactions occurring with the barbiturates have involved phenobarbital. However, the application of these data to other barbiturates appears valid and warrants serial blood level determinations of the relevant drugs when there are multiple therapies.

1. *Anticoagulants:* Phenobarbital lowers the plasma levels of dicumarol and causes a decrease in anticoagulant activity as measured by the prothrombin time. Barbiturates can induce hepatic microsomal enzymes resulting in increased metabolism and decreased anticoagulant response of oral anticoagulants (e.g., warfarin, acenocoumarol, dicumarol, and phenprocoumon). Patients stabilized on anticoagulant therapy may require dosage adjustments if barbiturates are added to or withdrawn from their dosage regimen.

2. *Corticosteroids:* Barbiturates appear to enhance the metabolism of exogenous corticosteroids probably through the induction of hepatic microsomal enzymes. Patients stabilized on corticosteroid therapy may require dosage adjustments if barbiturates are added to or withdrawn from their dosage regimen.

3. *Griseofulvin:* Phenobarbital appears to interfere with the absorption of orally administered griseofulvin, thus decreasing its blood level. The effect of the resultant decreased blood levels of griseofulvin on therapeutic response has not been established. However, it would be preferable to avoid concomitant administration of these drugs.

4. *Doxycycline:* Phenobarbital has been shown to shorten the half-life of doxycycline for as long as 2 weeks after barbiturate therapy is discontinued. The mechanism is probably through the induction of hepatic microsomal enzymes that metabolize the antibiotic. If phenobarbital and doxycycline are administered concurrently, the clinical response to doxycycline should be monitored closely.

5. *Phenytoin, Sodium Valproate, Valproic Acid:* The effect of barbiturates on the metabolism of phenytoin appears to be variable. Some investigators report an accelerating effect, while others report no effect. Because the effect of barbiturates on the metabolism of phenytoin is not predictable, phenytoin and barbiturate blood levels should be monitored more frequently if these drugs are given concurrently. Sodium valproate and valproic acid appear to decrease barbiturate metabolism; therefore, barbiturate blood levels should be monitored and appropriate adjustments made as indicated.

6. *Central Nervous System:* The concomitant use of other central nervous system depressants, including other sedatives or hypnotics, antihistamines, tranquilizers, or alcohol, may produce additive depressant effects.

7. *Monoamine Oxidase Inhibitors (MAOI):* MAOI prolong the effects of barbiturates probably because metabolism of the barbiturate is inhibited.

8. *Estradiol, Estrone, Progestrone and Other Steroid Hormones:* Pretreatment with or concurrent administration of phenobarbital may decrease the effect of estradiol by increasing its metabolism. There have been reports of patients treated with antiepileptic drugs (e.g. phenobarbital) who become pregnant while taking oral contraceptives. An alternate contraceptive method might be suggested to women taking phenobarbital.

Carcinogenesis, Mutagenesis, Impairment of Fertility: No long-term studies in animals have been performed with Butabarbital Sodium to determine carcinogenic and mutagenic potential, or effects on fertility.

Pregnancy Teratogenic Effects: Pregnancy Category D (See *"Warnings—Use in pregnancy"* above).

Nonteratogenic Effects: Infants suffering from long-term barbiturate exposure *in utero* may have an acute withdrawal syndrome of seizures and hyperirritability from birth to a delayed onset of up to 14 days (see *"Drugs Abuse and Dependence"*).

Labor and Delivery: Hypnotic doses of barbiturates do not appear to significantly impair uterine activity during labor. Administration of sedative-hypnotic barbiturates to the mother during labor may result in respiratory depression in the newborn. Premature infants are particularly susceptible to the depressant effects of barbiturates. If barbiturates are used during labor and delivery, resuscitation equipment should be available.

Nursing mothers: Caution should be exercised when a barbiturate is administered to a nursing woman since small amounts of some barbiturates are excreted in the milk.

ADVERSE REACTIONS

The following adverse reactions have been observed with the use of barbiturates in hospitalized patients. Because such patients may be less aware of certain of the milder adverse effects of barbiturates, the incidence of these reactions may be somewhat higher in fully ambulatory patients.

More than 1 in 100 Patients: The most common adverse reaction, somnolence, is estimated to occur at a rate of 1 to 3 patients per 100.

Less than 1 in 100 Patients: The most common adverse reactions estimated to occur at a rate of less than 1 in 100 patients listed below, grouped by organ system, and by decreasing order of occurrence are:

Central Nervous System/Psychiatric: Agitation, confusion, hyperkinesia, ataxia, CNS depression, nightmares, nervousness, psychiatric disturbance, hallucinations, insomnia, anxiety, dizziness, thinking abnormality.

Respiratory: Hypoventilation, apnea.

Cardiovascular: Bradycardia, hypotension, syncope.

Gastrointestinal: Nausea, vomiting, constipation.

Other Reported Reactions: Headache, hypersensitivity (angioedema, skin rashes, exfoliative dermatitis), fever, liver damage.

DRUG ABUSE AND DEPENDENCE
Controlled substance: Schedule III.

Abuse and Dependence: Barbiturates may be habit-forming. Tolerance, psychological dependence, and physical dependence may occur especially following prolonged use of high doses of barbiturates. Daily administration in excess of 400 milligrams (mg) of pentobarbital or secobarbital for approximately 90 days is likely to produce some degree of physical dependence. A dosage of from 600 to 800 mg taken for at least 35 days is sufficient to produce withdrawal seizures. The average daily dose for the barbiturate addict is usually about 1.5 grams. As tolerance to barbiturates develops, the amount needed to maintain the same level of intoxication increases; tolerance to a fatal dosage, however, does not increase more than two-fold. As this occurs, the margin between an intoxicating dosage and fatal dosage becomes smaller.

Symptoms of acute intoxication with barbiturates include unsteady gait, slurred speech, and sustained nystagmus. Mental signs of chronic intoxication include confusion, poor judgment, irritability, insomnia, and somatic complaints. Symptoms of barbiturate dependence are similar to those of chronic alcoholism.

If an individual appears to be intoxicated with alcohol to a degree that is radically disproportionate to the amount of alcohol in his or her blood, the use of barbiturates should be suspected. The lethal dose of a barbiturate is far less if alcohol is also ingested.

The symptoms of barbiturate withdrawal can be severe and may cause death. Minor withdrawal symptoms may appear 8 to 12 hours after the last dose of a barbiturate. These symptoms usually appear in the following order: anxiety, muscle twitching, tremor of hands and fingers, progressive weakness, dizziness, distortion in visual perception, nausea, vomiting, insomnia, and orthostatic hypotension. Major withdrawal symptoms (convulsions and delirium) may occur within 16 hours and last up to 5 days after abrupt cessation of these drugs. Intensity of withdrawal symptoms gradually declines over a period of approximately 15 days.

Drug dependence to barbiturates arises from repeated administration of a barbiturate or agent with barbiturate-like effect on a continuous basis, generally in amounts exceeding the therapeutic dose levels. The characteristics of drug dependence to barbiturates include: (a) a strong desire or need to continue taking the drug; (b) a tendency to increase the dose; (c) a psychic dependence on the effects of the drug related to subjective and individual appreciation for those effects; and (d) a physical dependence on the effects of the drug requiring its presence for maintenance of homeostasis and resulting in a definite, characteristic, and self-limited abstinence syndrome when the drug is withdrawn.

Treatment of barbiturate dependence consists of cautious and gradual withdrawal of the drug. Barbiturate-dependent patients can be withdrawn by using a number of different withdrawal regimens. In all cases, withdrawal takes an extended period of time. One method involves initiating treatment at the patient's regular dosage level, in 3 to 4 divided doses, and decreasing the daily dose by 10 percent if tolerated by the patient.

Infants physically dependent on barbiturates may be given phenobarbital 3 to 10 mg/kg/day. After withdrawal symptoms (hyperactivity, disturbed sleep, tremors, hyperreflexia) are relieved, the dosage of phenobarbital should be gradually decreased and completely withdrawn over a 2-week period.

OVERDOSAGE
Signs and Symptoms: The toxic dose of barbiturates varies considerably. In general, an oral dose of 1 gram of most barbiturates produces serious poisoning in an adult. Death commonly occurs after 2 to 10 grams of ingested barbiturates. Symptoms of acute intoxication with barbiturates include unsteady gait, slurred speech, and sustained nystagmus. Mental signs of chronic intoxication include confusion, poor judgment, irritability, insomnia, and somatic complaints. Barbiturate intoxication may be confused with alcoholism, bromide intoxication, and with various neurological disorders.

Acute overdosage with barbiturates is manifested by CNS and respiratory depression which may progress to Cheyne-Stokes respiration, areflexia, construction of the pupils to a slight degree (though in severe poisoning they may show paralytic dilation), oliguria, tachycardia, hypotension, lowered body temperature, and coma. Typical shock syndrome (apnea, circulatory collapse, respiratory arrest, and death) may occur.

In extreme overdose, all electrical activity in the brain may cease, in which case a "flat" EEG normally equated with clinical death cannot be accepted. This effect is fully reversible unless hypoxic damage occurs. Consideration should be given to the possibility of barbiturate intoxication even in situations that appear to involve trauma.

Complications: Pneumonia, pulmonary edema, cardiac arrhythmias, congestive heart failure, and renal failure may occur. Uremia may increase CNS sensitivity to barbiturates if renal function is impaired. Differential diagnosis should include hypoglycemia, head trauma, cerebrovascular accidents, convulsive states, and diabetic coma.

Treatment: Treatment of overdosage is mainly supportive and consists of the following:

1. Maintenance of an adequate airway, with assisted respiration and oxygen administration as necessary.
2. Monitoring of vital signs and fluid balance.
3. If the patient is conscious and has not lost the gag reflex, emesis may be induced with ipecac. Care should be taken to prevent pulmonary aspiration of vomitus. After completion of vomiting, 30 grams activated charcoal in a glass of water may be administered.

4. If emesis is contraindicated, gastric lavage may be performed with a cuffed endotracheal tube in place with the patient in the face down position. Activated charcoal may be left in the emptied stomach and a saline cathartic administered.
5. Fluid therapy and other standard treatment for shock, if needed.
6. If renal function is normal, forced diuresis may aid in the elimination of the barbiturate.
7. Although not recommended as a routine procedure, hemodialysis may be used in severe barbiturate intoxications or if the patient is anuric or in shock.
8. Appropriate nursing care, including rolling patients from side-to-side every 30 minutes, to prevent hypostatic pneumonia, decubiti, aspiration, and other complications of patients with altered states of consciousness.
9. Antibiotics should be given if pneumonia is suspected.

DOSAGE AND ADMINISTRATION
USUAL ADULT DOSAGE
Daytime Sedative: 15 to 30 mg, 3 or 4 times daily.

Bedtime Hypnotic: 50 to 100 mg.

Preoperative Sedative: 50 to 100 mg, 60 to 90 minutes before surgery.

USUAL PEDIATRIC DOSAGE
Preoperative Sedative: 2 to 6 mg/kg maximum 100 mg.

Special Patient Population: Dosage should be reduced in the elderly or debilitated because these patients may be more sensitive to barbiturates. Dosage should be reduced for patients with impaired renal function or hepatic disease (See "*Precautions*").

STORAGE
Store at controlled room temperature 15°-30°C (59°-86°F).
Dispense in a tight container.

HOW SUPPLIED
ELIXIR (C-III): 30 MG/5 ML

AVERAGE UNIT PRICE (AVAILABLE SIZES)		GENERIC A-RATED AVERAGE PRICE (GAAP)	
BRAND	$0.15	480 ml	$6.80
GENERIC	$0.01		
HCFA FUL (480 ml)	$0.01		

BRAND/MANUFACTURER	NDC	SIZE	AWP
◆ BRAND			
BUTISOL SODIUM: Wallace	00037-0110-16	480 ml	$76.37
	00037-0110-28	3840 ml	$567.88
◆ GENERICS			
Rugby	00536-0320-85	480 ml	$5.93
Barre	00472-0933-16	480 ml	$7.67

TABLETS (C-III): 15 MG

AVERAGE UNIT PRICE (AVAILABLE SIZES)	
BRAND	$0.40

BRAND/MANUFACTURER	NDC	SIZE	AWP
◆ BRAND			
BUTISOL SODIUM: Wallace	00037-0112-60	100s	$40.78
	00037-0112-80	1000s	$382.66

TABLETS (C-III): 30 MG

AVERAGE UNIT PRICE (AVAILABLE SIZES)	
BRAND	$0.53

BRAND/MANUFACTURER	NDC	SIZE	AWP
◆ BRAND			
BUTISOL SODIUM: Wallace	00037-0113-60	100s	$54.17
	00037-0113-80	1000s	$512.21
◆ GENERICS			
Parmed	00349-8596-10	1000s	$48.00

TABLETS (C-III): 50 MG

BRAND/MANUFACTURER	NDC	SIZE	AWP
○ BRAND			
BUTISOL SODIUM: Wallace	00037-0114-60	100s	$70.44

TABLETS (C-III): 100 MG

BRAND/MANUFACTURER	NDC	SIZE	AWP
◆ BRAND			
BUTISOL SODIUM: Wallace	00037-0115-60	100s	$83.62

Butibel *SEE BELLADONNA ALKALOIDS AND BUTABARBITAL SODIUM*

Butisol Sodium *SEE BUTABARBITAL SODIUM*

◆ RATED THERAPEUTICALLY EQUIVALENT; ◇ THERAPEUTIC EQUIVALENCE UNCONFIRMED; ○ UNRATED

Butoconazole Nitrate

DESCRIPTION

Butoconazole Nitrate Vaginal Cream 2%, imidazole derivative with antifungal activity. Its chemical name is (±)-1-[4-(p-Chlorophenyl)-2-[(2,6-dichlorophenyl)thio]butyl]- imidazole mononitrate.

Butoconazole Nitrate is a white to off-white crystalline powder with a molecular weight of 474.79. It is sparingly soluble in methanol; slightly soluble in chloroform, methylene chloride, acetone and ethanol; very slightly soluble in ethyl acetate; and practically insoluble in water. It melts at about 159°C with decomposition.

Butoconazole Nitrate Vaginal Cream (20 mg/g) is a water-washable emollient cream.

Following is its chemical structure:

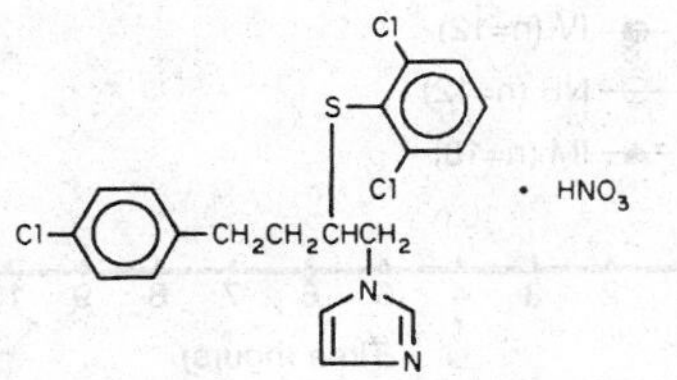

CLINICAL PHARMACOLOGY

Butoconazole Nitrate is an imidazole derivative that has fungicidal activity *in vitro* against *Candida, Trichophyton, Microsporum,* and *Epidermophyton.* It is also active *in vitro* against some gram positive bacteria. Clinically, it is highly effective against vaginal infections induced by strains of *Candida albicans, Candida tropicalis,* and other species of this genus.

The primary site of action of imidazoles appears to be the cell membrane. The permeability of the cell membrane is altered, resulting in a reduced osmotic resistance and viability of the fungus. The exact mechanism of antifungal activity of Butoconazole Nitrate is not known.

Following vaginal administration of Butoconazole Nitrate, 5.5% of the dose is absorbed on average. After vaginal administration peak plasma levels of the drug and its metabolites are attained at 24 hours and the plasma half-life is approximately 21-24 hours.

INDICATIONS AND USAGE

Butoconazole Nitrate Vaginal Cream is indicated for the local treatment of vulvovaginal mycotic infections caused by *Candida* species. The diagnosis should be confirmed by KOH smears and/or cultures.

Butoconazole Nitrate Vaginal Cream can be used in association with oral contraceptive and antibiotic therapy. Butoconazole Nitrate is effective in both nonpregnant and pregnant women, but in pregnant women it should be used only during the second and third trimesters.

CONTRAINDICATIONS

Butoconazole Nitrate Vaginal Cream 2% is contraindicated in patients with a history of hypersensitivity to any of the components of the cream.

PRECAUTIONS

GENERAL

If clinical symptoms persist, microbiological tests should be repeated to rule out other pathogens and to confirm the diagnosis.

If sensitization or irritation is reported during use, the treatment should be discontinued.

INFORMATION FOR THE PATIENT

The patient should be cautioned against premature discontinuation of the medication during menstruation or in response to relief of symptoms.

CARCINOGENESIS

Long-term studies in animals have not been performed to evaluate the carcinogenic potential of this drug.

MUTAGENESIS

Butoconazole Nitrate was not mutagenic when tested on microbial indicator organisms.

IMPAIRMENT OF FERTILITY

No impairment of fertility was seen in rabbits or rats administered Butoconazole Nitrate in oral doses up to 30 mg/kg/day or 100 mg/kg/day respectively.

PREGNANCY

Pregnancy Category C.

In pregnant rats administered 6 mg/kg/day (3-7 times the human dose Butoconazole Nitrate intravaginally during the period of organogenesis, there was an increase in resorption rate and decrease in litter size, but no teratogenicity. Butoconazole Nitrate had no apparent adverse effect when administered orally to pregnant rats throughout organogenesis, at dose levels up to 50 mg/kg/day. Daily oral doses of 100, 300, or 750 mg/kg resulted in fetal malformations (abdominal wall defects, cleft palate), but maternal stress was evident at these higher dose levels. There were no adverse effects on litters of rabbits receiving Butoconazole Nitrate orally, even at maternally stressful dose levels (e.g., 150 mg/kg). There are no adequate and well-controlled studies in pregnant women during the first trimester.

Butoconazole Nitrate, like other azole antimycotic agents, causes dystocia in rats when treatment is extended through parturition. However, this effect was not apparent in rabbits treated with as much as 100 mg/kg/day orally.

In clinical studies, over 200 pregnant patients have used Butoconazole Nitrate cream 2% for 3 or 6 days during the second or third trimester and the drug had no adverse effect on the course of pregnancy. Follow-up reports available on infants born to these women reveal no adverse effects or complications that were attributable to the drug.

NURSING MOTHERS

It is not known whether this drug is excreted in human milk. Because many drugs are excreted in human milk, caution should be exercised when Butoconazole Nitrate is administered to a nursing woman.

PEDIATRIC USE

Safety and effectiveness in children have not been established.

ADVERSE REACTIONS

Of the 561 patients treated with Butoconazole Nitrate cream 2% for 3 or 6 days in controlled clinical trials, 13 (2.3%) reported complaints probably related to therapy. Vulvar/vaginal burning occurred in 2.3%, vulvar itching in 0.9%, and discharge, soreness, swelling, and itching of the fingers each occurred in 0.2%. Nine patients (1.6%) discontinued because of these complaints.

DOSAGE AND ADMINISTRATION

Nonpregnant Patients: The recommended dose is one applicatorful of cream (approximately 5 grams) intravaginally at bedtime for three days. Treatment can be extended for an additional three days if necessary.

Pregnant Patients (2nd and 3rd trimesters only): The recommended dose is one applicatorful of cream (approximately 5 grams) intravaginally at bedtime for six days.

Store at room temperature. Avoid excessive heat, above 40°C (104°F), and avoid freezing.

HOW SUPPLIED
CREAM: 2%

BRAND/MANUFACTURER	NDC	SIZE	AWP
○ BRAND			
FEMSTAT: Syntex	00033-2280-14	28 gm	$19.07
FEMSTAT PREFILL: Syntex	00033-2280-16	5 gm 3s	$20.16

Butorphanol Tartrate

DESCRIPTION

Butorphanol Tartrate is a synthetically derived opioid agonist-antagonist analgesic of the phenanthrene series. The chemical name is (-)- 17-(cyclobutylmethyl) morphinan-3,14-diol [S-(R*,R*)] -2,3-dihydroxybutanedioate (1:1) (salt). The molecular formula is $C_{21}H_{29}NO_2 \cdot C_4H_6O_6$, which corresponds to a molecular weight of 477.55.

Butorphanol Tartrate is a white crystalline substance, soluble in aqueous solution. The dose is expressed as the tartrate salt. One milligram of the salt is equivalent to 0.68 mg of the free base. The n-octanol/aqueous buffer partition coefficient of Butorphanol is 180:1 at pH 7.5.

Butorphanol Tartrate injectable is a sterile, parenteral, aqueous solution of Butorphanol Tartrate for intravenous or intramuscular administration. Each mL of solution contains 1 or 2 mg of Butorphanol Tartrate.

Butorphanol Tartrate nasal spray is an aqueous solution of Butorphanol Tartrate for administration as a metered spray to the nasal mucosa. Each mL of solution contains 10 mg of Butorphanol Tartrate. The pump reservoir must be fully primed prior to initial use. After initial priming each metered spray delivers an average of 1.0 mg of Butorphanol Tartrate. If not used for 48 hours or longer, the unit must be re-primed.

Following is its chemical structure:

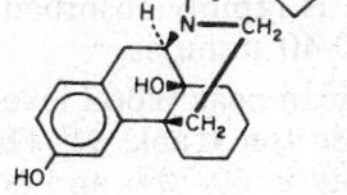

CLINICAL PHARMACOLOGY

GENERAL PHARMACOLOGY AND MECHANISM OF ACTION

Butorphanol Tartrate has narcotic antagonist activity which is approximately equivalent to that of nalorphine, 30 times that of pentazocine and 1/40 that of Butorphanol Tartrate as measured by the antagonism of morphine analgesia in the rat tail flick test.

The exact mechanism of action of Butorphanol Tartrate is unknown. It is felt that the class of narcotic agonist-antagonist analgesics exert their analgesic effect via a central nervous system mechanism. Currently, it is believed the site of action of centrally acting analgesics is subcortical, possibly in the limbic system.

Butorphanol and its major metabolites are agonists at k-opioid receptors and mixed agonist-antagonist at μ-opioid receptors.

Its interactions with these receptors in the central nervous system apparently mediate most of its pharmacologic effects, including analgesia.

In addition to analgesia, CNS effects include depression of spontaneous respiratory activity and cough, stimulation of the emetic center, miosis and sedation. Effects possibly mediated by non-CNS mechanisms include alteration in cardiovascular resistance and capacitance, bronchomotor tone, gastrointestinal secretory and motor activity and bladder sphincter activity.

In an animal model, the dose of the Butorphanol Tartrate required to antagonize morphine analgesia by 50% was similar to that for nalorphine, less than that for pentazocine and more than that for naloxone.

The pharmacological activity of Butorphanol metabolites has not been studied in humans; in animal studies, Butorphanol metabolites have demonstrated some analgesic activity.

In human studies of Butorphanol (see *"Clinical Trials"*), sedation is commonly noted at doses of 0.5 mg or more. Narcosis is produced by 10-12 mg doses of Butorphanol administered over 10-15 minutes intravenously.

Butorphanol, like other mixed agonist-antagonists with a high affinity for the kappa receptor, may produce unpleasant psychotomimetic effects in some individuals.

Nausea and/or vomiting may be produced by doses of 1 mg or more administered by any route.

In human studies involving individuals without significant respiratory dysfunction, 2 mg of Butorphanol IV and 10 mg of morphine sulfate IV depressed respiration to a comparable degree. At higher doses, the magnitude of respiratory depression with Butorphanol is not appreciably increased; however, the duration of respiratory depression is longer. Respiratory depression noted after administration of Butorphanol to humans by any route is reversed by treatment with naloxone, a specific opioid antagonist (see *"Treatment"* in *"Overdosage"*).

Butorphanol Tartrate demonstrates antitussive effects in animals at doses less than those required for analgesia.

Hemodynamic changes noted during cardiac catheterization in patients receiving single 0.025 mg/kg intravenous doses of Butorphanol have included increases in pulmonary artery pressure, wedge pressure and vascular resistance, increases in left ventricular end diastolic pressure and in systemic arterial pressure.

CARDIOVASCULAR EFFECTS
The hemodynamic changes after the intravenous administration of Butorphanol Tartrate are similar to the reported hemodynamic changes after pentazocine. Although smaller than those following pentazocine, these changes are nevertheless in a direction which increases the work of the heart, especially in the pulmonary circuit.

PHARMACODYNAMICS
The analgesic effect of Butorphanol is influenced by the route of administration. Onset of analgesia is within a few minutes for intravenous administration, within 10-15 minutes for intramuscular injection, and within 15 minutes for the nasal spray doses.

Peak analgesic activity occurs within 30-60 minutes following intravenous and intramuscular administration and within 1-2 hours following the nasal spray administration.

The duration of analgesia varies depending on the pain model as well as the route of administration, but is generally 3-4 hours with IM and IV doses as defined by the time 50% of patients required remedication. In postoperative studies, the duration of analgesia with IV or IM Butorphanol was similar to morphine, meperidine and pentazocine when administered in the same fashion at equipotent doses (see *"Clinical Trials"*). Compared to the injectable form and other drugs in this class, Butorphanol Tartrate nasal spray has a longer duration of action (4-5 hours) (see *"Clinical Trials"*).

PHARMACOKINETICS
Butorphanol Tartrate injectable is rapidly absorbed after IM injection and peak plasma levels are reached in 20-40 minutes.

After nasal administration, mean peak blood levels of 0.9-1.04 ng/mL occur at 30-60 minutes after a 1 mg dose (see Table 1). The absolute bioavailability of Butorphanol Tartrate nasal spray is 60-70% and is unchanged in patients with allergic rhinitis. In patients using a nasal vasoconstrictor (oxymetazoline) the fraction of the dose absorbed was unchanged, but the rate of absorption was slowed. The peak plasma concentrations were approximately half those achieved in the absence of the vasoconstrictor.

Following its initial absorption/distribution phase, the single dose pharmacokinetics of Butorphanol by the intravenous, intramuscular, and nasal routes of administration are similar (see Figure 1).

Figure 1

BUTORPHANOL PLASMA LEVELS AFTER IV, IM AND NASAL SPRAY ADMINISTRATION OF 2 MG DOSE

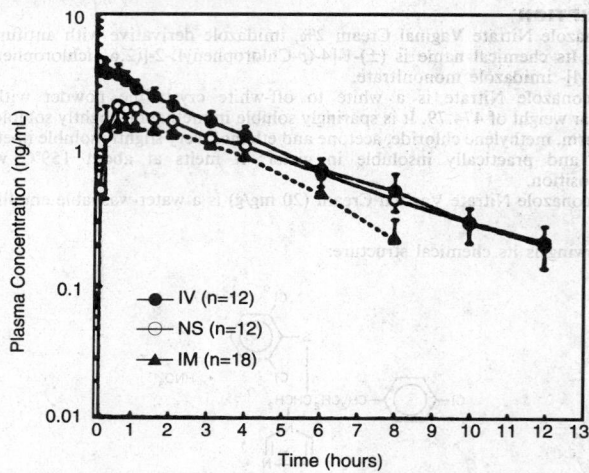

Serum protein binding is independent of concentration over the range achieved in clinical practice (up to 7 ng/mL) with a bound fraction of approximately 80%.

The volume of distribution of Butorphanol varies from 305-901 liters and total body clearance from 52-154 liters/hr (see Table 1). (See related table). Dose proportionality for Butorphanol Tartrate nasal spray has been determined at steady state in doses up to 4 mg at 6 hour intervals. Steady state is achieved within 2 days. The mean peak plasma concentration at steady state was 1.8-fold (maximal 3-fold) following a single dose.

The drug is transported across the blood brain and placental barriers and into human milk (see *"Labor and Delivery"* and *"Nursing Mothers"*).

Butorphanol is extensively metabolized in the liver. Metabolism is qualitatively and quantitatively similar following intravenous, intramuscular, or nasal administration. Oral bioavailability is only 5-17% because of extensive first pass metabolism of Butorphanol.

The major metabolite of Butorphanol is hydroxybutorphanol, while norbutorphanol is produced in small amounts. Both have been detected in plasma following administration of Butorphanol. Preliminary evidence suggests the elimination half-life of hydroxybutorphanol may be greater than that of its parent.

Elimination occurs by urine and fecal excretion. When ^{3}H labelled Butorphanol is administered to normal subjects, most (70-80%) of the dose is recovered in the urine, while approximately 15% is recovered in the feces.

About 5% of the dose is recovered in the urine as Butorphanol. Forty-nine percent is eliminated in the urine as hydroxybutorphanol. Less than 5% is excreted in the urine as norbutorphanol (see also *"Clinical Pharmacology"* above). Butorphanol pharmacokinetics in the elderly differ from younger patients (see *"Table 1"*). The mean absolute bioavailability of Butorphanol Tartrate nasal spray in elderly women (48%) was less than that in elderly men (75%), young men (68%) or young women (70%). Elimination of half-life is increased in the elderly (6.6 hours as opposed to 4.7 hours in younger subjects).

In renally impaired patients with creatinine clearances < 30 mL/min the elimination half-life is approximately doubled and the total body clearance is approximately one half (10.5 hours [clearance 150 L/h] as compared to 5.8 hours [clearance 260 L/h] in normals). No effect was observed on Cmax or Tmax after a single dose.

For further recommendations refer to statements on use in *"Geriatric Patients, Renal Disease, Hepatic Disease"* and statement on *"Drug Interactions"* in the *"Precautions"*, and *"Individualization of Dosage"* sections below.

CLINICAL TRIALS
The effectiveness of opioid analgesics varies in different pain syndromes. Studies with Butorphanol Tartrate injectable have been performed in postoperative (primarily abdominal and orthopedic) pain and pain during labor and delivery, as preoperative and preanesthetic medication, and as a supplement to balanced anesthesia (see below).

Studies with Butorphanol Tartrate nasal spray have been performed in postoperative (general, orthopedic, oral, cesarean section) pain, in post-episiotomy pain, in pain of musculoskeletal origin, and in migraine headache pain (see below).

USE IN THE MANAGEMENT OF PAIN
POSTOPERATIVE ANALGESIA
The analgesic efficacy of Butorphanol Tartrate injectable in postoperative pain was investigated in several double-blind active-controlled studies involving 958 Butorphanol-treated patients. The following doses were found to have approximately equivalent analgesic effect: 2 mg Butorphanol, 10 mg morphine, 40 mg pentazocine and 80 mg meperidine.

After intravenous administration of Butorphanol Tartrate injectable, onset and peak analgesic effect occurred by the time of first observation (30 minutes). After intramuscular administration, pain relief onset occurred at 30 minutes or less, and peak effect occurred between 30 minutes and one hour. The duration of action of

Butorphanol Tartrate injectable was 3-4 hours when defined as the time necessary for pain intensity to return to pretreatment level or the time to retreatment.

The analgesic efficacy of Butorphanol Tartrate nasal spray was evaluated (approximately 35 patients per treatment group) in a general and orthopedic surgery trial. Single doses of Butorphanol Tartrate nasal spray (1 or 2 mg) and IM meperidine (37.5 or 75 mg) were compared. Analgesia provided by 1 and 2 mg doses of Butorphanol Tartrate nasal spray was similar to 37.5 and 75 mg meperidine, respectively, with onset of analgesia within 15 minutes and peak analgesic effect within 1 hour. The median duration of pain relief was 2.5 hours with 1 mg Butorphanol Tartrate nasal spray, 3.5 hours with 2 mg Butorphanol Tartrate nasal spray and 3.3 hours with either dose of meperidine.

In a postcesarean section trial, Butorphanol Tartrate nasal spray administered to 35 patients as two 1 mg doses 60 minutes apart was compared with a single 2 mg dose of Butorphanol Tartrate nasal spray or a single 2 mg IV dose of Butorphanol Tartrate injectable (37 patients each). Onset of analgesia was within 15 minutes for all Butorphanol Tartrate regimens. Peak analgesic effects of 2 mg intravenous Butorphanol Tartrate and Butorphanol Tartrate nasal spray were similar in magnitude. The duration of pain relief provided by both 2 mg Butorphanol Tartrate nasal spray regimens was approximately 4.5 hours and was greater than intravenous Butorphanol Tartrate (2.6 h).

MIGRAINE HEADACHE PAIN

The analgesic efficacy of two 1 mg doses one hour apart of Butorphanol Tartrate nasal spray in migraine headache pain was compared with a single dose of 10 mg IM methadone (31 and 32 patients respectively). Significant onset of analgesia occurred within 15 minutes for both Butorphanol Tartrate nasal spray and IM methadone. Peak analgesic effect occurred at 2 hours for Butorphanol Tartrate nasal spray and 1.5 hours for methadone. The median duration of pain relief was 6 hours with Butorphanol Tartrate nasal spray and 4 hours with methadone as judged by the time when approximately half of the patients remedicated.

In two other trials in patients with migraine headache pain, a 2 mg initial dose of Butorphanol Tartrate nasal spray followed by an additional 1 mg dose 1 hr later (76 patients) was compared with either 75 mg IM meperidine (24 patients) or placebo (72 patients). Onset, peak activity and duration were similar with both active treatments; however, the incidence of adverse experiences (nausea, vomiting, dizziness) was higher in these two trials with the 2 mg initial dose of Butorphanol Tartrate nasal spray than in the trial with the 1 mg initial dose.

PREANESTHETIC MEDICATION

Butorphanol Tartrate injectable (2 mg and 4 mg) and meperidine (80 mg) were studied for use as preanesthetic medication in hospitalized surgical patients. Patients received a single intramuscular dose of either Butorphanol Tartrate injectable or meperidine approximately 90 minutes prior to anesthesia. The anesthesia regimen included barbiturate induction, followed by nitrous oxide and oxygen with halothane or enflurane, with or without a muscle relaxant.

Anesthetic preparation was rated as satisfactory in all 42 Butorphanol Tartrate injectable patients regardless of the type of surgery.

BALANCED ANESTHESIA

Butorphanol Tartrate injectable administered intravenously (mean dose 2 mg) was compared to intravenous morphine sulfate (mean dose 10 mg) as premedication shortly before thiopental induction, followed by balanced anesthesia in 50 ASA Class 1 and 2 patients. Anesthesia was then maintained by repeated intravenous doses, averaging 4.6 mg Butorphanol Tartrate injectable and 22.8 mg morphine per patient.

Anesthetic induction and maintenance were generally rated as satisfactory with both Butorphanol Tartrate injectable (25 patients) and morphine (25 patients) regardless of the type of surgery performed. Emergence from anesthesia was comparable with both agents.

LABOR
(SEE "PRECAUTIONS")

The analgesic efficacy of intravenous Butorphanol Tartrate was studied in pain during labor. In a total of 145 patients Butorphanol Tartrate injectable (1 mg and 2 mg) was as effective as 40 mg and 80 mg of meperidine (144 patients) in the relief of pain in labor with no effect on the duration or progress of labor. Both drugs readily crossed the placenta and entered fetal circulation. The condition of the infants in these studies, determined by Apgar scores at 1 and 5 minutes (8 or above) and time to sustained respiration, showed that Butorphanol Tartrate injectable had the same effects on the infants as meperidine.

In these studies neurobehavioral testing in infants exposed to Butorphanol Tartrate injectable at a mean of 18.6 hours after delivery showed no significant differences between treatment groups.

INDIVIDUALIZATION OF DOSAGE

The usual starting doses of Butorphanol are: 1 mg repeated every 3-4 hours IV; 2 mg repeated every 3-4 hours IM; and 1 mg followed by 1 mg in 60-90 minutes nasally repeated every 3-4 hours (see "Dosage and Administration"). Use of Butorphanol in geriatric patients, patients with renal impairment, patients with hepatic impairment, and during labor requires extra caution (see below and the appropriate sections in "Precautions").

BUTORPHANOL TARTRATE INJECTABLE

For pain relief the recommended initial dosage regimen of Butorphanol Tartrate injectable is 1 mg IV or 2 mg IM with repeated doses every three to four hours, as necessary. This dosage regimen is likely to be effective for the majority of patients. Dosage adjustments of Butorphanol Tartrate injectable should be based on observations of its beneficial and adverse effects. The initial dose in the elderly and in patients with renal or hepatic impairment should generally be half the recommended adult dose (0.5 mg IV and 1.0 mg IM). Repeat doses in these patients should be determined by the patient's response rather than at fixed intervals but will generally be no less than 6 hours (see "Precautions").

The usual preoperative dose is 2 mg IM given 60-90 minutes before surgery or 2 mg IV shortly before induction. This is approximately equivalent in sedative effect to 10 mg morphine or 80 mg of meperidine. This single preoperative dose should be individualized based on age, body weight, physical status, underlying pathological condition, use of other drugs, type of anesthesia to be used and the surgical procedure involved.

During maintenance in balanced anesthesia the usual incremental dose of Butorphanol Tartrate injectable is 0.5 to 1.0 mg IV. The incremental dose may be higher, up to 0.06 mg/kg (4 mg/70 kg), depending on previous sedative, analgesic, and hypnotic drugs administered. The total dose of Butorphanol Tartrate injectable will vary; however, patients seldom require less than 4 mg or more than 12.5 mg (approximately 0.06 to 0.18 mg/kg).

As with other opioids of this class, Butorphanol Tartrate injectable may not provide adequate intraoperative analgesia in every patient or under all conditions. A failure to achieve successful analgesia during balanced anesthesia is commonly reflected by increases in general sympathetic tone. Consequently, if blood pressure or heart rate continue to rise, consideration should be given to adding a potent volatile liquid inhalation anesthetic or another intravenous medication.

Table 1
MEAN PHARMACOKINETIC PARAMETERS OF BUTORPHANOL IN YOUNG AND ELDERLY SUBJECTS[a]

Parameters	Intravenous		Nasal	
	Young	Elderly	Young	Elderly
T_{max}[b] (hr)			0.62 (0.32)[e] (0.15-1.50)[g]	1.03 (0.74) (0.25-3.00)
C_{max}[c] (ng/mL)			1.04 (0.40) (0.35-1.97)	0.90 (0.57) (0.10-2.68)
AUC (inf)[d] (hr.ng/mL)	7.24 (1.57) (4.40-9.77)	8.71 (2.02) (4.76-13.03)	4.93 (1.24) (2.16-7.27)	5.24 (2.27) (0.30-10.34)
Half-life (hr)	4.56 (1.67) (2.06-8.70)	5.61 (1.36) (3.25-8.79)	4.74 (1.57) (2.89-8.79)	6.56 (1.51) (3.75-9.17)
Absolute Bioavailability (%)			69 (16) (44-113)	61 (25) (3-121)
Volume of Distribution[f](L)	487 (155) (305-901)	552 (124) (305-737)		
Total body Clearance (L/hr)	99 (23) (70-154)	82 (21) (52-143)		

a) Young subjects (n=24) are from 20 to 40 years old and elderly (n=24) are greater than 65 years of age.
b) Time to peak plasma concentration, median values.
c) Peak plasma concentration normalized to 1 mg dose.
d) Area under the plasma concentration-time curve after a 1 mg dose.
e) Mean (1 S.D.)
f) Derived from IV data.
g) (range of observed values)

In labor, the recommended initial dose of Butorphanol Tartrate injectable is 1 or 2 mg IM or IV in mothers with fetuses of 37 weeks gestation or beyond and without signs of fetal distress. Dosage adjustments of Butorphanol Tartrate injectable in labor should be based on initial response with consideration given to concomitant analgesic or sedative drugs and the expected time of delivery. A dose should not be repeated in less than four hours nor administered less than four hours prior to the anticipated delivery (see "Precautions").

Since Butorphanol Tartrate nasal spray does not require an injection, it allows the physician to initiate therapy with a low dose and repeat the dose if needed.

The usual recommended dose for initial nasal administration is 1 mg (1 spray in *one* nostril). If adequate pain relief is not achieved within 60-90 minutes, an additional 1 mg dose may be given.

The initial dose sequence outlined above may be repeated in 3-4 hours as required.

For the management of severe pain, an initial dose of 2 mg (1 spray in *each* nostril) may be used in patients who will be able to remain recumbent in the event drowsiness or dizziness occur. In such patients additional doses should not be given for 3-4 hours. The incidence of adverse events is higher with an initial 2 mg dose (see "Clinical Trials").

The initial dose sequence in elderly patients and patients with renal or hepatic impairment should be limited to 1 mg followed by 1 mg in 90-120 minutes. The repeat dose sequence in these patients should be determined by the patient's response rather than at fixed times but will generally be no less than at 6 hour intervals (see "Precautions").

INDICATIONS AND USAGE
Butorphanol Tartrate injection and nasal spray are indicated for the management of moderate to severe pain when the use of an opioid analgesic is appropriate.

Butorphanol Tartrate injectable is also indicated as a preoperative or preanesthetic medication, as a supplement to balanced anesthesia, and for the relief of pain during labor.

UNLABELED USES
Butorphanol Tartrate is used alone or as an adjunct in the treatment of migraine headache and ureteral colic.

CONTRAINDICATIONS
Butorphanol Tartrate injectable and nasal spray are contraindicated in patients hypersensitive to Butorphanol Tartrate or the preservative benzethonium chloride used in some brands.

WARNINGS
PATIENTS DEPENDENT ON NARCOTICS
Because of its opioid antagonist properties, Butorphanol is not recommended for use in patients dependent on narcotics. Such patients should have an adequate period of withdrawal from opioid drugs prior to beginning Butorphanol therapy. In patients taking opioid analgesics chronically, Butorphanol has precipitated withdrawal symptoms such as anxiety, agitation, mood changes, hallucinations, dysphoria, weakness and diarrhea.

Because of the difficulty in assessing opioid tolerance in patients who have recently received repeated doses of narcotic analgesic medication, caution should be used in the administration of Butorphanol to such patients. Detoxification of such patients prior to use should be carefully considered.

USE DURING BALANCED ANESTHESIA
Since the combined respiratory depressant effect of all intravenous medication used during conduct of general anesthesia may lead to under-ventilation or apnea, Butorphanol should be administered during balanced anesthesia only by persons specifically trained in the use of intravenous anesthetics and adjuncts, the maintenance of a patent airway and management of respiratory effects of all intravenous medication administered.

An opioid antagonist, resuscitative and intubation equipment and oxygen should be readily available.

DRUG DEPENDENCE
Special care should be exercised in administering Butorphanol Tartrate to emotionally unstable patients and to those with a history of drug misuse. When long term therapy is contemplated, such patients should be closely supervised. Even though Butorphanol Tartrate has a low physical dependence liability, care should be taken that individuals who may be prone to drug abuse are closely supervised. It is important to avoid increases in dose and frequency of injections by the patient and to prevent the use of the drug in anticipation of pain rather than for the relief of pain.

PRECAUTIONS
GENERAL
Hypotension associated with syncope during the first hour of dosing with Butorphanol Tartrate nasal spray has been reported rarely, particularly in patients with past history of similar reactions to opioid analgesics. Therefore, patients should be advised to avoid activities with potential risks.

HEAD INJURY AND INCREASED INTRACRANIAL PRESSURE
As with other opioids, the use of Butorphanol in patients with head injury may be associated with carbon dioxide retention and secondary elevation of cerebrospinal fluid pressure, drug-induced miosis, and alterations in mental state that would obscure the interpretation of the clinical course of patients with head injuries. In such patients, Butorphanol should be used only if the benefits of use outweigh the potential risks.

DISORDERS OF RESPIRATORY FUNCTION OR CONTROL
Butorphanol may produce respiratory depression, especially in patients receiving other CNS active agents, or patients suffering from CNS diseases or respiratory impairment. It should be administered only with caution and low dosage to patients with respiratory depression (eg, from other medication, uremia, or severe infection), severely limited respiratory reserve, bronchial asthma, obstructive respiratory conditions, or cyanosis.

HEPATIC AND RENAL DISEASE
In patients with severe hepatic or renal disease the initial dosage interval for Butorphanol Tartrate injection and nasal spray should be increased to 6-8 hours until the response has been well characterized. Subsequent doses should be determined by patient response rather than being scheduled at fixed intervals (see "Individualization of Dosage").

Although laboratory tests have not indicated that Butorphanol Tartrate causes or increases renal or hepatic impairment, the drug should be administered with caution to patients with such impairment. Extensive liver disease may predispose to greater side effects and greater activity from the usual clinical dose, possibly the result of decreased metabolism of the drug by the liver.

CARDIOVASCULAR EFFECTS
Because Butorphanol may increase the work of the heart, especially the pulmonary circuit (see "Clinical Pharmacology"), the use of Butorphanol in patients with acute myocardial infarction, ventricular dysfunction, or coronary insufficiency should be limited to those situations where the benefits clearly outweigh the risk, e.g., in patients who are hypersensitive to morphine sulfate or meperidine.

Severe hypertension has been reported rarely during Butorphanol therapy. In such cases, Butorphanol should be discontinued and the hypertension treated with antihypertensive drugs. In patients who are not opioid dependent, naloxone has also been reported to be effective.

BILIARY SURGERY
Clinical studies have not been done to establish the safety of Butorphanol Tartrate administration to patients about to undergo surgery of the biliary tract.

USAGE AS A PREOPERATIVE OR PREANESTHETIC MEDICATION
Slight increases in systolic blood pressure may occur, therefore, caution should be employed when Butorphanol Tartrate is used in the hypertensive patient.

INFORMATION FOR PATIENTS
1. Drowsiness and dizziness related to the use of Butorphanol may impair mental and/or physical abilities required for the performance of potentially hazardous tasks (e.g., driving, operating machinery, etc.).

2. Alcohol should not be consumed while using Butorphanol. Concurrent use of Butorphanol with drugs that affect the central nervous system (e.g., alcohol, barbiturates, tranquilizers, and antihistamines) may result in increased central nervous system depressant effects such as drowsiness, dizziness and impaired mental function.

3. Patients should be instructed on the proper use of Butorphanol Tartrate nasal spray.

DRUG INTERACTIONS
Concurrent use of Butorphanol with central nervous system depressants (e.g., alcohol, barbiturates, tranquilizers, and antihistamines) may result in increased central nervous system depressant effects. When used concurrently with such drugs, the dose of Butorphanol should be the smallest effective dose and the frequency of dosing reduced as much as possible when administered concomitantly with drugs that potentiate the action of opioids.

It is not known if the effects of Butorphanol are altered by concomitant medications that affect hepatic metabolism of drugs (cimetidine, erythromycin, theophylline, etc.), but physicians should be alert to the possibility that a smaller initial dose and longer intervals between doses may be needed.

The fraction of Butorphanol Tartrate nasal spray absorbed is unaffected by the concomitant administration of a nasal vasoconstrictor (oxymetazoline), but the rate of absorption is decreased. Therefore, a slower onset can be anticipated if Butorphanol Tartrate nasal spray is administered concomitantly with, or immediately following, a nasal vasoconstrictor.

No information is available about the use of Butorphanol concurrently with MAO inhibitors.

USE IN AMBULATORY PATIENTS
Drowsiness and dizziness related to the use of Butorphanol may impair mental and/or physical abilities required for the performance of potentially hazardous tasks (e.g., driving, operating machinery, etc.). Patients should be told to use caution in such activities until their individual responses to Butorphanol have been well characterized.

Alcohol should not be consumed while using Butorphanol. Concurrent use of Butorphanol with central nervous system depressants (e.g., alcohol, barbiturates, tranquilizers, and antihistamines) may result in increased central nervous system depressant effects.

Patients should be instructed on the proper use of Butorphanol Tartrate nasal spray.

CARCINOGENESIS, MUTAGENESIS, IMPAIRMENT OF FERTILITY
The carcinogenic potential of Butorphanol has not been adequately evaluated.

◆ RATED THERAPEUTICALLY EQUIVALENT; ◇ THERAPEUTIC EQUIVALENCE UNCONFIRMED; ○ UNRATED

Butorphanol was not genotoxic in *S. typhimurium* or *E. coli* assays or in unscheduled DNA synthesis and repair assays conducted in cultured human fibroblast cells.

Rats treated orally with 160 mg/kg/day (944 mg/sq.m.) had a reduced pregnancy rate. However, a similar effect was not observed with a 2.5 mg/kg/day (14.75 mg/sq.m.) subcutaneous dose.

PREGNANCY

Pregnancy Category C: Reproduction studies in mice, rats and rabbits during organogenesis did not reveal any teratogenic potential to Butorphanol, or evidence of impaired fertility. However, pregnant rats treated subcutaneously with Butorphanol at 1 mg/kg (5.9 mg/sq.m.) had a higher frequency of stillbirths than controls. Butorphanol at 30 mg/kg/oral (5.1 mg/sq.m.) and 60 mg/kg/oral (10.2 mg/sq.m.) also showed higher incidences of post-implantation loss in rabbits.

There are no adequate and well-controlled studies of Butorphanol Tartrate in pregnant women before 37 weeks gestation. Butorphanol Tartrate should be used during pregnancy only if the potential benefit justifies the potential risk to the infant.

LABOR AND DELIVERY

Although there have been rare reports of infant respiratory distress/apnea following the administration of Butorphanol Tartrate injectable during labor, this adverse effect was not attributed to Butorphanol Tartrate injectable as used during controlled clinical trials. The reports of respiratory distress/apnea have been associated with administration of a dose within two hours of delivery, use of multiple doses, use with additional analgesic or sedative drugs, or use in preterm pregnancies.

In a study of 119 patients, the administration of 1 mg of IV Butorphanol Tartrate injectable during labor was associated with transient (10-90 minutes) sinusoidal fetal heart rate patterns, but was not associated with adverse neonatal outcomes. In the presence of an abnormal fetal heart rate pattern, Butorphanol Tartrate injectable should be used with caution.

Butorphanol Tartrate nasal spray is not recommended during labor or delivery because there is no clinical experience with its use in this setting.

Butorphanol Tartrate should be used with caution in women delivering premature infants.

NURSING MOTHERS

Butorphanol has been detected in milk following administration of Butorphanol Tartrate injectable to nursing mothers. The amount an infant would receive is probably clinically insignificant (estimated 4 microgram/liter of milk in a mother receiving 2 mg IM four times a day).

Although there is no clinical experience with the use of Butorphanol Tartrate nasal spray in nursing mothers, it should be assumed that Butorphanol will appear in the milk in similar amounts following the nasal route of administration.

Butorphanol Tartrate has been used safely for labor pain in mothers who subsequently nursed their infants.

PEDIATRIC USE

Butorphanol is not recommended for use in patients below 18 years of age because safety and efficacy have not been established in this population.

GERIATRIC USE

The initial dose of Butorphanol Tartrate injectable recommended for elderly patients is half the usual dose at twice the usual interval. Subsequent doses and intervals should be based on the patient response (see *"Individualization of Dosage"*).

Initially a 1 mg dose of Butorphanol Tartrate nasal spray should generally be used in geriatric patients and 90-120 minutes should elapse before deciding whether a second 1 mg dose is needed (see *"Individualization of Dosage"*).

Due to changes in clearance, the mean half-life of Butorphanol is increased by 25% (to over 6 hours) in patients over the age of 65. Elderly patients may be more sensitive to its side effects. Results from a long-term clinical safety trial suggest that elderly patients may be less tolerant of dizziness due to Butorphanol Tartrate nasal spray than younger patients.

ADVERSE REACTIONS

The most frequent adverse reactions in 1250 patients treated with Butorphanol Tartrate injectable are: sedation (503, 40%), nausea (82.6%), clammy/sweating (76.6%).

Less frequent reactions are: headache (35, 3%), vertigo (33, 3%), floating feeling (33, 3%), dizziness (23, 2%), lethargy (19, 2%), confusion (15, 1%), lightheadedness (12, 1%).

A total of 2446 patients were studied in Butorphanol clinical trials. Approximately half received Butorphanol Tartrate injectable with the remainder receiving Butorphanol Tartrate nasal spray. In nearly all cases the type and incidence of side effects with Butorphanol by any route were those commonly observed with opioid analgesics. The adverse experiences described below are based on data from short- and long-term clinical trials in patients receiving Butorphanol by any route and from post-marketing experience with Butorphanol Tartrate injectable. There has been no attempt to correct for placebo effect or to subtract the frequencies reported by placebo treated patients in controlled trials.

The most frequently reported adverse experiences across all clinical trials with Butorphanol Tartrate injectable and Butorphanol Tartrate nasal spray were somnolence (43%), dizziness (19%), nausea and/or vomiting (13%). In long-term trials with Butorphanol Tartrate nasal spray only, nasal congestion (13%) and insomnia (11%) were frequently reported.

The following adverse experiences were reported at a frequency of 1% or greater, and were considered to be probably related to the use of Butorphanol.

Body as a Whole: asthenia/lethargy*, headache*, sensation of heat

Cardiovascular: VASODILATION*, PALPITATIONS

Digestive: ANOREXIA*, CONSTIPATION*, dry mouth*, nausea and/or vomiting (13%), stomach pain

Nervous: anxiety, confusion*, dizziness (19%), euphoria, floating feeling, INSOMNIA (11%), nervousness, paresthesia, somnolence (43%), TREMOR

Respiratory: BRONCHITIS, COUGH, DYSPNEA*, EPISTAXIS*, NASAL CONGESTIONS (13%), NASAL IRRITATION*, PHARYNGITIS*, RHINITIS*, SINUS CONGESTION*, SINUSITIS, UPPER RESPIRATORY INFECTION*

Skin and Appendages: sweating/clammy*, pruritus

Special Senses: blurred vision, EAR PAIN, TINNITUS*, UNPLEASANT TASTE* (also seen in short-term trials with Butorphanol Tartrate nasal spray).

(Reactions occurring with a frequency of 3-9% are marked with an asterisk.* Reactions reported predominantly from long-term trials with Butorphanol Tartrate nasal spray are CAPITALIZED.)

The following adverse experiences were reported with a frequency of less than 1%, in clinical trials or from post-market experience, and were considered to be probably related to the use of Butorphanol.

Cardiovascular: hypotension, syncope

Nervous: abnormal dreams, agitation, *drug dependence*, dysphoria, hallucinations, hostility

Skin and Appendages: rash/hives

Urogenital: impaired urination

(Reactions reported only from post-marketing experience are *italicized*.)

The following infrequent additional adverse experiences were reported in a frequency of less than 1% of the patients studied in short-term Butorphanol Tartrate nasal spray trials and from post-marketing experiences under circumstances where the association between these events and Butorphanol administration is unknown. They are being listed as alerting information for the physician.

Body as a whole: edema

Cardiovascular: hypertension

Nervous: convulsion, *delusion*, depression

Respiratory: apnea, shallow breathing

(Reactions reported only from postmarketing experience are *italicized*.)

Also possible are: seizures, flushing and warmth, dry mouth, sensitivity to cold, slowing of respiration, and diplopia.

DRUG ABUSE AND DEPENDENCE

Although the mixed agonist-antagonist opioid analgesics, as a class, have lower abuse potential than morphine, all such drugs can be and have been reported to be abused.

Chronic use of Butorphanol Tartrate injectable has been reported to result in mild withdrawal syndromes, and reports of overuse and self-reported addiction have been received.

Among 161 patients who used Butorphanol Tartrate nasal spray for 2 months or longer approximately 3% had behavioral symptoms suggestive of possible abuse. Approximately 1% of these patients reported significant overuse. Symptoms such as anxiety, agitation, and diarrhea were observed. Symptoms suggestive of opioid withdrawal occurred in 2 patients who stopped the drug abruptly after using 16 mg a day or more for longer than 3 months.

Special care should be exercised in administering Butorphanol to emotionally unstable patients and to those with a history of drug misuse. When long-term therapy is necessary, such patients should be closely supervised.

OVERDOSAGE

CLINICAL MANIFESTATIONS

The clinical manifestations of overdose are those of opioid drugs, the most serious of which are hypoventilation, cardiovascular insufficiency and/or coma.

Overdose can occur due to accidental or intentional misuse of Butorphanol, especially in young children who may gain access to the drug in the home.

TREATMENT

The management of suspected Butorphanol overdosage includes maintenance of adequate ventilation, peripheral perfusion, normal body temperature and protection of the airway. Patients should be under continuous observation with adequate serial measures of mental state, responsiveness and vital signs. Oxygen, intravenous fluids, vasopressors, and ventilatory assistance should be available with continual monitoring by pulse oximetry if indicated. In the presence of coma, placement of an artificial airway may be required. An adequate intravenous portal should be maintained to facilitate treatment of hypotension associated with vasodilation.

The use of a specific opioid antagonist such as naloxone should be considered. As the duration of Butorphanol action usually exceeds the duration of action of naloxone, repeated dosing with naloxone may be required.

DOSAGE AND ADMINISTRATION

Factors to be considered in determining the dose are age, body weight, physical status, underlying pathological condition, use of other drugs, type of anesthesia to be used, and surgical procedure involved. Use in the elderly, patients with hepatic or renal disease or in labor requires extra caution (see *"Precautions"* and *"Individualization of Dosage"*). The following doses are for patients who do not have impaired hepatic or renal function and who are not on CNS active agents.

USE FOR PAIN

Intravenous: The usual recommended single dose for IV administration is 1 mg repeated every three to four hours as necessary. The effective dosage range, depending on the severity of pain, is 0.5 to 2 mg repeated every three to four hours.

Intramuscular: The usual recommended single dose for IM administration is 2 mg in patients who will be able to remain recumbent, in the event drowsiness or dizziness occurs. This may be repeated every three to four hours, as necessary. The effective dosage range depending on the severity of pain is 1 to 4 mg repeated every three to four hours. There are insufficient clinical data to recommend single doses above 4 mg.

Children: Since there is no clinical experience in children under 18 years Butorphanol Tartrate is not recommended in this age group.

Concomitant Use with Tranquilizers: According to accepted procedure, the dose of Butorphanol Tartrate should be reduced when administered concomitantly with phenothiazines and other tranquilizers which may potentiate the action of Butorphanol Tartrate.

Nasal Spray: The usual recommended dose for initial nasal administration is 1 mg (1 spray in *one* nostril). Adherence to this dose reduces the incidence of drowsiness and dizziness. If adequate pain relief is not achieved within 60-90 minutes, an additional 1 mg dose may be given.

The initial two dose sequence outlined above may be repeated in 3-4 hours as needed.

Depending on the severity of the pain, an initial dose of 2 mg (1 spray in *each* nostril) may be used in patients who will be able to remain recumbent in the event drowsiness or dizziness occur. In such patients single additional 2 mg doses should not be given for 3-4 hours.

USE AS PREOPERATIVE/PREANESTHETIC MEDICATION

The preoperative medication dosage of Butorphanol Tartrate injectable should be individualized (see *"Individualization of Dosage"*). The usual adult dose is 2 mg IM, administered 60-90 minutes before surgery. This is approximately equivalent in sedative effect to 10 mg morphine or 80 mg meperidine.

USE IN BALANCED ANESTHESIA

For analgesic action during the anesthetic periods, premedication, and maintenance. Some of the factors to be considered in determining the dose are age, body weight, physical status, underlying pathological conditions, use of other drugs, type of anesthesia to be used, and the surgical procedure involved.

The usual dose of Butorphanol Tartrate injectable is 2 mg IV shortly before induction or 2 mg IM 60 to 90 minutes before surgery and/or 0.5 to 1.0 mg IV in increments during anesthesia. Incremental use of intravenous Butorphanol during maintenance in balanced anesthesia must be individualized. The usual incremental dose of Butorphanol is 0.5 to 1 mg intravenously. The increment may be higher, up to 0.06 mg/kg (4 mg/70 kg), depending on previous sedative, analgesic, and hypnotic drugs administered. The total dose of Butorphanol Tartrate injectable will vary; however, patients seldom require less than 4 mg or more than 12.5 mg (approximately 0.06 to 0.18 mg/kg). Butorphanol should not be relied upon as the only intravenous drug to supplement nitrous oxide because it may fail to provide adequate analgesia. A failure to achieve successful analgesia during balanced anesthesia is commonly reflected by increases in general sympathetic tone. Consequently, if blood pressure continues to rise after repeated doses of Butorphanol, consideration should be given to adding a potent volatile liquid inhalational anesthetic or another intravenous medication (such as a thiobarbiturate or benzodiazepine).

The use of Butorphanol Tartrate nasal spray is not recommended, because it has not been studied in induction or maintenance of anesthesia.

LABOR

In patients at full term in early labor a 1-2 mg dose of Butorphanol Tartrate injectable IV or IM may be administered and repeated after 4 hours. Alternative analgesia should be used for pain associated with delivery or if delivery is expected to occur within 4 hours.

If concomitant use of Butorphanol Tartrate with drugs that may potentiate its effects is deemed necessary (see *"Drug Interactions"* in *"Precautions"* section) the lowest effective dose should be employed.

The use of Butorphanol Tartrate nasal spray is not recommended as it has not been studied in labor.

SAFETY AND HANDLING

Butorphanol Tartrate injectable: Ordinary care should be taken to avoid aerosol generation while preparing a syringe for use. Following skin contact, rinsing with cool water is recommended.

Butorphanol Tartrate nasal spray: In the priming process, a certain amount of Butorphanol may be aerosolized; therefore, the pump sprayer should be aimed away from the patient or other people or animals.

The unit should be disposed of by unscrewing the cap, rinsing the bottle, and placing the parts in a waste container.

STORAGE

Store below 86°F (30°C). Parenteral drug products should be inspected visually for particulate matter and discoloration prior to administration, whenever solution and container permit.

HOW SUPPLIED

INJECTION: 1 MG/ML

BRAND/MANUFACTURER	NDC	SIZE	AWP
○ **BRAND**			
STADOL: Apothecon	00015-5645-20	1 ml	$6.92

INJECTION: 2 MG/ML

BRAND/MANUFACTURER	NDC	SIZE	AWP
○ **BRAND**			
STADOL: Apothecon	00015-5646-20	1 ml	$7.22
	00015-5644-20	2 ml	$12.31
	00015-5648-20	10 ml	$62.81

SPRAY: 10 MG/ML

BRAND/MANUFACTURER	NDC	SIZE	AWP
○ **BRAND**			
STADOL NS: Mead Johnson Labs	00087-5650-41	2.5 ml	$57.43

Cafergot *SEE* ERGOTAMINE TARTRATE WITH CAFFEINE

Caffeine with Sodium Benzoate

DESCRIPTION

Caffeine/Sodium Benzoate Injection, USP is a clear sterile solution of Caffeine Alkaloid.

Each mL contains: Caffeine (anhydrous) 125 mg.

The solution is intended for intramuscular or slow intravenous administration only.

CLINICAL PHARMACOLOGY

Caffeine is pharmacologically similar to the other xanthine drugs, such as theobromine and theophylline; however, these three agents differ in the intensity of their actions on various structures. Caffeine's CNS and skeletal muscle effects are greater than those of the other xanthines. In all other areas, theophylline has greater activity than Caffeine, although some studies report that Caffeine has greater diuretic effect than theobromine. The increased levels of intracellular cyclic-AMP mediate most of Caffeine's pharmacologic actions. Caffeine competitively inhibits phosphodiesterase, the enzyme that degrades cyclic 3′ - 5′ adenosine monophosphate. Caffeine stimulates all levels of the CNS. Caffeine's cortical effects are milder and of shorter duration than those of the amphetamines. In slightly larger doses, Caffeine stimulates medullary vagal, vasomotor and respiratory centers, promoting bradycardia, vasoconstriction, and increased respiratory rate.

Caffeine produces a positive inotropic effect on the myocardium and a positive chronotropic effect at the sinoatrial node, causing transient increases in heart rate, force of contraction, cardiac output and heart work. In doses greater than 250 mg, the centrally mediated vagal effects of Caffeine may be masked by increased sinus rates; tachycardia, extrasystoles, or other major ventricular arrhythmias may result.

Caffeine constricts cerebral vasculature. In contrast, the drug directly dilates peripheral blood vessels, decreasing peripheral vascular resistance. The effect of this decrease in peripheral vascular resistance. The effect of this decrease in peripheral vascular resistance (and possibly that of vagal cardiac stimulation) on blood pressure is offset by increased cardiac output (and possibly stimulation of the medullary vasomotor area). The overall effect of Caffeine on heart rate and blood pressure depends on whether CNS or peripheral effects predominate. Therapeutic doses of Caffeine increase blood pressure only slightly.

Caffeine stimulates voluntary skeletal muscle, increasing the force of contraction and decreasing muscular fatigue. The drug also stimulates gastric acid secretion from parietal cells. Caffeine increases renal blood flow and glomerular filtration rate and decreases proximal tubular reabsorption of sodium and water, resulting in mild diuresis.

Caffeine stimulates glycogenolysis and lipolysis, but increases in blood glucose and in plasma lipids are insignificant in normal patients. Tolerance may develop to the diuretic, cardiovascular, and CNS effects of Caffeine.

PHARMACOKINETICS

Caffeine is rapidly distributed throughout the body tissues, readily crossing the placenta and blood-brain barrier. Approximately 17% of the drug is bound to plasma proteins. Caffeine has approximately a half-life (T ½) of 3—4 hours in adults. In adults, the drug is rapidly metabolized in the liver to 1-methyluric acid, 1-methylxanthine and 7-methylxanthine. Caffeine and its metabolites are excreted primarily by the kidneys.

◆ RATED THERAPEUTICALLY EQUIVALENT; ◇ THERAPEUTIC EQUIVALENCE UNCONFIRMED; ○ UNRATED

INDICATIONS AND USAGE

Caffeine/Sodium Benzoate Injection has been used in conjunction with supportive measure to treat respiratory depression associated with overdosage with CNS depressant drugs (e.g., narcotic analgesics, alcohol). However, because of questionable benefit and transient action, most authorities believe Caffeine and other analeptics should not be used in these conditions and recommend other supportive therapy.

CONTRAINDICATIONS

None known.

PRECAUTIONS

Large doses of Caffeine may produce headache, excitement, agitation, a condition resembling anxiety neurosis, scintillating scotoma, hyperesthesia, tinnitus muscle tremors or twitches, diuresis, tachycardia, extrasystoles, and other cardiac arrhythmias. Further CNS depression may occur when already depressed patients are too vigorously treated with Caffeine/Sodium Benzoate Injection.

Caffeine and other xanthines may enhance the cardiac inotropic effects of β-adrenergic stimulating agents. Caffeine has also been reported to increase its own metabolism and that of other drugs, including phenobarbital and aspirin. Caffeine produces false-positive elevations of serum urate as measured by the Bittner method. The drug also produces slight increases in urine levels of vanillylmandelic acid (VMA), catecholamines, and 5-hydroxyindoleacetic acid. Because high urine levels of VMA or catecholamines may result in false-positive diagnosis of pheochromocytoma or neuroblastoma, Caffeine intake should be avoided during tests for these disorders.

Pregnancy: Teratogenic effects: Pregnancy Category C. Animal reproduction studies have not been conducted with Caffeine/Sodium Benzoate Injection. It is also not known whether Caffeine/Sodium Benzoate Injection can cause fetal harm when administered to a pregnant woman or can affect reproduction capacity. Caffeine/Sodium Benzoate Injection should be given to a pregnant woman only if clearly needed.

OVERDOSAGE

Acute toxicity involving Caffeine has been reported rarely. Mild delirium, insomnia, diuresis, dehydration, and fever commonly occur with overdosage. More serious symptoms of overdosage include cardiac arrhythmias and clonic-tonic convulsions. In adults, IV doses of 57 mg/kg of body weight and oral doses of 18.50 grams have been fatal. In one 5-year-old patient, death occurred following oral ingestion of approximately 3 grams of Caffeine. Convulsions may be treated with IV administration of diazepam or a barbiturate such as pentobarbital sodium.

DOSAGE AND ADMINISTRATION

Caffeine/Sodium Benzoate Injection may be administered by intramuscular or slow intravenous injection.

Some clinicians suggest that when used as a mild CNS stimulant to overcome fatigue, oral doses of 100—200 mg of anhydrous Caffeine are required. One manufacturer recommends that citrated caffeine be administered orally in dosages of 65—325 mg (about 32—162 mg of anhydrous Caffeine) 3 times daily. Another manufacturer recommends an oral dosage of 250 mg of anhydrous Caffeine in an extended-release formulation once daily, but warns that the drug should not be administered less than 6 hours before retiring.

Analeptic use of Caffeine is strongly discouraged by most clinicians. However, the manufacturer of Caffeine/Sodium Benzoate Injection recommends intramuscular, or in emergency respiratory failure, intravenous injection of 500 mg of the drug (about 250 mg of anhydrous Caffeine) or a maximum single dose of 1 gram (about 500 mg of anhydrous Caffeine) for the treatment of respiratory depression associated with overdosage of CNS depressants, including narcotic analgesics and alcohol, and with electric shock.

The usual dose is 0.5 g (7 ½ grains) as frequently as directed by the physician. The maximum safe dose is 0.5 g and the total dose in 24 hours should rarely exceed 2.5 g.

Parenteral drug products should be inspected visually for particulate matter prior to administration whenever solution and container permit.

Store at controlled room temperature between 15°—30°C (59°—86°).

HOW SUPPLIED
INJECTION: 250 MG/ML

BRAND/MANUFACTURER	NDC	SIZE	AWP
○ GENERICS			
UDL	51079-0784-11	2 ml	$137.00
Pasadena	00418-1531-10	2 ml 10s	$139.80
Amer Regent	00517-2502-10	2 ml 10s	$187.50
CMC-Cons	00223-7273-10	2 ml 10s	$250.00
CMC-Cons	00223-7273-25	2 ml 25s	$625.00

POWDER:

BRAND/MANUFACTURER	NDC	SIZE	AWP
○ GENERICS			
	17137-0074-04	125 gm	$9.80

Cal-Im *SEE* CALCIUM GLYCEROPHOSPHATE AND CALCIUM LEVULINATE

Calan *SEE* VERAPAMIL HYDROCHLORIDE

Calcibind *SEE* CELLULOSE SODIUM PHOSPHATE

Calcidrine *SEE* CALCIUM IODIDE AND CODEINE

Calcifediol

DESCRIPTION

Calcifediol, USP is the colorless, crystalline monohydrate of 25-hydroxycholecalciferol prepared by chemical synthesis and is identical to the natural vitamin metabolite. Calcifediol has a calculated molecular weight of 418.67 and is soluble in organic solvents but relatively insoluble in water. Chemically, Calcifediol is (5Z, 7E)-9,10-secocholesta-5,7,10(19)-triene-3 β,25-diol monohydrate.

The other names frequently used for 25-hydroxycholecalciferol are 25-hydroxyvitamin D_3, 25-HCC, 25-OHCC, and 25-OHD_3.

Calcifediol for oral administration is available in two strengths: a capsule containing 20 µg Calcifediol and one capsule containing 50 µg Calcifediol.

Following is its chemical structure:

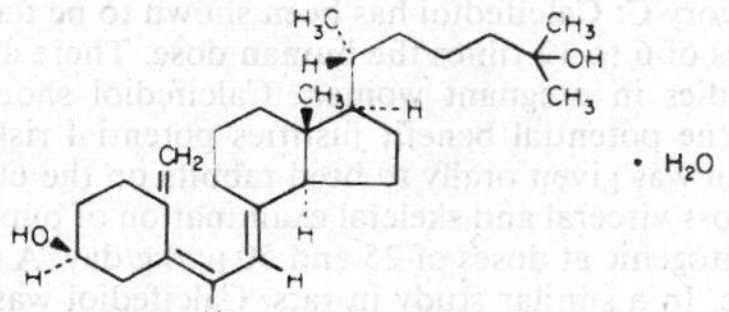

CLINICAL PHARMACOLOGY

The natural supply of vitamin D in man mainly depends on the ultraviolet rays of the sun for conversion of 7-dehydrocholesterol to vitamin D_3 Cholecalciferol). It is now known that vitamin D_3 must be converted to 25-OHD_3 (25-hydroxycholecalciferol) by a vitamin D_3 -hydroxylase enzyme (25-OHase) present in the liver. 25-Hydroxycholecalciferol is the major transport form of vitamin D_3 and can be readily monitored in the serum. It is further converted to 1,25-dihydroxycholecalciferol (1,25-$(OH)_2D_3$) and 24,25-dihydroxycholecalciferol (24,25-$(OH)_2D_3$) in the kidney. 1,25-$(OH)_2D_3$ stimulates resorption of calcium from bone and increases intestinal calcium absorption. The physiologic role of 24,25-$(OH)_2D_3$ has not been clearly established. The metabolic activity of Calcifediol in clinical use appears to be related not only to its conversion to other metabolites but also due to its intrinsic activity.

When administered orally, Calcifediol is rapidly absorbed from the intestine, with peak 25-OHD_3 concentrations in the serum reported after about 4 hours, 25-Hydroxycholecalciferol is known to be transported in blood, bound to a specific plasma protein. The terminal half-life of orally administered calcifediol in the serum is about 16 days.

INDICATIONS AND USAGE

Calcifediol Capsules are indicated in the treatment and management of metabolic bone disease or hypocalcemia associated with chronic renal failure in patients undergoing renal dialysis.

In studies to date it has been shown to increase serum calcium levels, to decrease alkaline phosphatase and parathyroid hormone levels in some patients, to decrease subperiosteal bone resorption in some patients, and to decrease histological signs of hyperparathyroid bone disease and mineralization defects in some patients.

UNLABELED USES

Calcifediol is used alone or as an adjunct in the treatment of osteoporosis and hepatic osteomalacia.

CONTRAINDICATIONS

Calcifediol Capsules should not be given to patients with hypercalcemia or evidence of vitamin D toxicity.

WARNINGS

Since Calcifediol is a metabolite of vitamin D, vitamin D and its derivatives should be withheld during treatment.

Aluminum carbonate or hydroxide gels should be used to control serum phosphorus levels in patients undergoing dialysis.

Overdosage of any form of vitamin D is dangerous (see also *"Overdosage"*). Progressive hypercalcemia may be so severe as to require emergency attention. Chronic hypercalcemia can lead to generalized vascular calcification, nephrocalcinosis, and other soft-tissue calcification. The serum calcium times phosphorus (Ca x P) product should not be allowed to exceed 70. Radiographic and/or slit lamp evaluation of suspect anatomical regions may be useful in the early detection of this condition.

PRECAUTIONS

General: Excessive dosage of Calcifediol capsules induces hypercalcemia and in some instances hypercalciuria; therefore, early in treatment during dosage adjustment, serum calcium should be determined frequently (at least weekly). Should hypercalcemia develop, the drug should be discontinued immediately.

After achieving normocalcemia, the drug may be readministered at a lower dosage. Calcifediol should be given cautiously to patients receiving digitalis, because hypercalcemia in such patients may precipitate cardiac arrhythmias.

Information for the Patient: The patient and his or her parents or spouse should be informed about compliance with dosage instructions, adherence to instructions about diet, calcium supplementation, phosphate binder usage, and avoidance of non-approved prescription drugs. Patients should also be informed about the symptoms of hypercalcemia (see *"Adverse Reactions"*).

Essential Laboratory Tests: Serum calcium, phosphorus and alkaline phosphatase and 24-hour urinary calcium and phosphorus should be determined periodically. During the initial phase of the medication, serum calcium should be determined more frequently (at least weekly).

Drug Interactions: Cholestyramine has been reported to reduce absorption of fat-soluble vitamins; as such, it may impair intestinal absorption of Calcifediol. The administration of anticonvulsants has been shown to affect the Calcifediol requirements in some patients.

Carcinogenesis, Mutagenesis, Impairment of Fertility: Long term studies in animals have not been completed to evaluate the carcinogenic potential of Calcifediol. No significant effects of Calcifediol on fertility and/or general reproductive performances were reported.

Use in Pregnancy: Teratogenic Effects:

Pregnancy Category C: Calcifediol has been shown to be teratogenic in rabbits when given in doses of 6 to 12 times the human dose. There are no adequate and well-controlled studies in pregnant women. Calcifediol should be used during pregnancy only if the potential benefit justifies potential risk to the fetus.

When Calcifediol was given orally to bred rabbits on the 6th through the 18th day of gestation, gross visceral and skeletal examination of pups indicated that the compound was teratogenic at doses of 25 and 50 µg/kg/day. A dose of 5 µg/kg/day was not teratogenic. In a similar study in rats, Calcifediol was not teratogenic at doses up to and including 60 µg/kg/day.

Labor and Delivery: The effect of this drug on the mother and fetus during labor and delivery is not known.

Nursing Mothers: It is not known whether this drug is excreted in human milk. Because many drugs are excreted in human milk, caution should be exercised when Calcifediol is administered to nursing women.

Pediatric Use: The safety and effectiveness of Calcifediol in children have not been established.

ADVERSE REACTIONS

Since Calcifediol is an active metabolite of vitamin D, adverse effects are, in general, similar to those encountered with excessive vitamin D intake. The early and late signs and symptoms of vitamin D intoxication associated with hypercalcemia include:

a. Early: Weakness, headache, somnolence, nausea, vomiting, dry mouth, constipation, muscle pain, bone pain, and metallic taste.

b. Late: Polyuria, polydipsia, anorexia, irritability, weight loss, nocturia, conjunctivitis (calcific), pancreatitis, photophobia, rhinorrhea, pruritus, hyperthermia, decreased libido, elevated BUN, albuminuria, hypercholesterolemia, elevated SGOT and SGPT, ectopic calcification, hypertension, cardiac arrhythmias, and, rarely, overt psychosis.

OVERDOSAGE

Administration of Calcifediol Capsules to patients in excess of their daily requirements can cause hypercalcemia, hypercalciuria, and hyperphosphatemia. High intake of calcium and phosphate concomitant with Calcifediol may lead to similar abnormalities.

TREATMENT OF HYPERCALCEMIA AND OVERDOSAGES

General treatment of hypercalcemia (greater than 1 mg/dL above the upper limit of the normal range) consists of discontinuation of therapy with Calcifediol. Serum calcium measurements should be performed regularly until normocalcemia ensues. Hypercalcemia usually resolves in two to four weeks. When serum calcium levels have returned to within normal limits, therapy with Calcifediol may be re-instituted at a dosage lower than prior therapy. Serum calcium levels should be obtained at least weekly after all dosage changes and subsequent dosage titration. Persistent or markedly elevated calcium levels in dialysis patients may be corrected by dialysis against a calcium-free dialysate.

TREATMENT OF ACCIDENTAL OVERDOSAGE

The treatment of acute accidental overdosage of Calcifediol should consist of general supportive measures. If drug ingestion is discovered within a relatively short time, induction of emesis or gastric lavage may be of benefit in preventing further absorption. If the drug has passed through the stomach, the administration of mineral oil may promote fecal elimination. Serial serum calcium determination, rate of urinary calcium excretion, and an assessment of electrocardiographic abnormalities due to hypercalcemia should be obtained. Such monitoring is critical in patients receiving digitalis. Discontinuation of supplemental calcium and a low calcium diet are also indicated in accidental overdosage. Because the conversion of Calcifediol to 1,25-$(OH)_2D_3$ is tightly regulated by the body's needs, further measures are probably unnecessary. Should persistent and marked hypercalcemia occur, however, there are a variety of therapeutic measures that may be considered, depending on the patient's underlying condition. These include the use of drugs such as phosphates and corticosteroids as well as measures to induce an appropriate forced diuresis. The use of peritoneal dialysis against a calcium-free dialysate may also be considered.

The oral LD_{50} in the rat is > 320 mg/kg.

DOSAGE AND ADMINISTRATION

The optimal daily dose of Calcifediol must be carefully determined for each patient. The recommended initial dosage of Calcifediol is based on the assumption that each patient is receiving an adequate daily intake of calcium from dietary sources or from the addition of calcium supplements. The RDA for calcium in adults is 1000 mg. To ensure that each patient receives an adequate daily intake of calcium, the physician should either prescribe a calcium supplement or instruct the patient in proper dietary measures.

CHRONIC RENAL FAILURE — DIALYSIS PATIENTS

The recommended initial dose of Calcifediol is 300 to 350 µg of Calcifediol weekly, administered on a daily or alternate day schedule. If a satisfactory response in the biochemical parameters and clinical manifestations of the disease state is not observed, dosage may be increased at four-week intervals. During this titration period, serum calcium levels should be obtained at least weekly, and if hypercalcemia is noted the drug should be discontinued until normocalcemia ensues.

Some patients with normal serum calcium levels may respond to doses of 20 µg of Calcifediol every other day. Most patients respond to doses between 50 and 100 µg daily or between 100 and 200 µg on alternate days.

STORAGE

Store at controlled room temperature, 15°-30°C (59°-86°F).

HOW SUPPLIED
CAPSULE: 20 MCG

BRAND/MANUFACTURER	NDC	SIZE	AWP
○ BRAND			
CALDEROL: Organon	00052-0472-60	60s	$48.37

CAPSULE: 50 MCG

BRAND/MANUFACTURER	NDC	SIZE	AWP
○ BRAND			
CALDEROL: Organon	00052-0474-60	60s	$110.32

Calciferol SEE ERGOCALCIFEROL

Calcijex SEE CALCITRIOL

Calcimar SEE CALCITONIN

Calcipotriene

DESCRIPTION

Calcipotriene ointment contains a synthetic vitamin D_3 derivative for topical dermatological use.

Chemically, Calcipotriene is (5Z,7E,22E,24S)-24-cyclopropyl-9,10-secochola-5,7,10(19),22-tetraene-1α, 3β,24-triol-, with the empirical formula $C_{27}H_{40}O_3$, and a molecular weight of 412.6.

Calcipotriene is a white or off-white crystalline substance. Calcipotriene contains 50 µg/g in an ointment base of dibasic sodium phosphate, edetate disodium, mineral oil, petrolatum, propylene glycol, tocopnerol, steareth-2 and water.

Following is its chemical structure:

CLINICAL PHARMACOLOGY

In humans, the natural supply of vitamin D depends mainly on exposure to the ultraviolet rays of the sun for conversion of 7-dehydrocholesterol to vitamin D_3 (cholecalciferol) in the skin. Calcipotriene is a synthetic analog of vitamin D_3.

◆ RATED THERAPEUTICALLY EQUIVALENT; ◇ THERAPEUTIC EQUIVALENCE UNCONFIRMED; ○ UNRATED

Clinical studies with radiolabelled ointment indicate that approximately 6% (± 3%, SD) of the applied dose of Calcipotriene is absorbed systemically when the ointment is applied topically to psoriasis plaques or 5% (± 2.6%, SD) when applied to normal skin, and much of the absorbed active is converted to inactive metabolites within 24 hours of application.

Vitamin D and its metabolites are transported in the blood, bound to specific plasma proteins. The active form of the vitamin, 1.25-dihydroxy vitamin D_3 (calcitriol), is known to be recycled via the liver and excreted in the bile. Calcipotriene metabolism following systemic uptake is rapid, and occurs via a similar pathway to the natural hormone. The primary metabolites are much less potent than the parent compound.

There is evidence that maternal 1.25-dihydroxy vitamin D_3 (calcitriol) may enter the fetal circulation, but it is not known whether it is excreted in human milk. The systemic disposition of Calcipotriene is expected to be similar to that of the naturally occurring vitamin.

CLINICAL STUDIES
Adequate and well-controlled trials of patients treated with Calcipotriene ointment have demonstrated improvement usually beginning after two weeks of therapy. This improvement continued with approximately 70% of patients showing at least marked improvement after 8 weeks of therapy, but only approximately 10% showing complete clearing.

INDICATIONS AND USAGE
Calcipotriene ointment 0.005%, is indicated for the treatment of moderate plaque psoriasis. The safety and effectiveness of topical Calcipotriene ointment in dermatoses other than psoriasis have not been established.

CONTRAINDICATIONS
Calcipotriene ointment is contraindicated in those patients with a history of hypersensitivity to any of the components of the preparation. It should not be used by patients with demonstrated hypercalcemia or evidence of vitamin D toxicity. Calcipotriene ointment should not be used on the face.

PRECAUTIONS
General: Use of Calcipotriene ointment may cause irritation of lesions and surrounding uninvolved skin. If irritation develops, Calcipotriene ointment should be discontinued.

Transient, rapidly reversible elevation of serum calcium has occurred with use of Calcipotriene. If elevation in serum calcium outside the normal range should occur, discontinue treatment until normal calcium levels are restored.

Information for Patients: Patients using Calcipotriene ointment should receive the following information and instructions:

1. This medication is to be used as directed by the physician. It is for external use only. Avoid contact with the face or eyes. As with any topical medication, patients should wash hands after application.
2. This medication should not be used for any disorder other than that for which it was prescribed.
3. Patients should report to their physician any signs of local adverse reactions.

Carcinogenesis, Mutagenesis, Impairment of Fertility: Long-term animal studies have not been conducted to evaluate the carcinogenic potential of Calcipotriene. Studies in rats at doses up to 54 µg/kg/day (318 µg/m²/day) of Calcipotriene indicated no impairment of fertility or general reproductive performance.

Calcipotriene did not elicit any mutagenic effects in the Ames mutagenicity assay, the mouse lymphoma TK locus assay, the human lymphocyte chromosome aberration test or the mouse micronucleus test.

Pregnancy: Teratogenic Effects: Pregnancy Category C: Doses of Calcipotriene up to 36 µg/kg/day (396 µg/m²/day) in the rabbit did not result in teratogenic effects: however, increased maternal and fetal toxicity was observed at 12 µg/kg/day (132 µg/m²/day) and higher. In the rat oral doses of 54 µg/kg/day (318 µg/m²/day) resulted in a significantly higher incidence of skeletal abnormalities consisting primarily of enlarged fontanelles and extra ribs. The enlarged fontanelles are most likely due to Calcipotriene's effect upon calcium metabolism. There are no adequate and well-controlled studies in pregnant women. Therefore, Calcipotriene should be used during pregnancy only if the potential benefit justifies the potential risk to the fetus.

Nursing Mothers: It is not known whether Calcipotriene is excreted in human milk. Because many drugs are excreted in human milk, caution should be exercised when Calcipotriene is administered to a nursing woman.

Pediatric Use: Safety and effectiveness of Calcipotriene in children have not been established. Because of a higher ratio of skin surface area to body mass, children are at greater risk than adults of systemic adverse effects when they are treated with topical medication.

Geriatric Use: Of the total number of patients in clinical studies of Calcipotriene ointment, approximately 12% were 65 or older, while approximately 4% were 75 and over. The results of an analysis of severity of skin-related adverse events showed a statistically significant difference for subjects over 65 years (more severe) compared to those under 65 years (less severe).

ADVERSE REACTIONS
In controlled clinical trials, the most frequent adverse experiences reported for Calcipotriene were burning, itching, and skin irritation, which occurred in approximately 10-15% of patients. Erythema, dry skin, peeling, rash, dermatitis, worsening of psoriasis including development of facial/scalp psoriasis were reported in 1 to 10% of patients. Other experiences reported in less than 1% of

patients included skin atrophy, hyperpigmentation, hypercalcemia, and folliculitis.

OVERDOSAGE
Topically applied Calcipotriene ointment can be absorbed in sufficient amounts to produce systemic effects. Elevated serum calcium has been observed with excessive use of Calcipotriene ointment.

DOSAGE AND ADMINISTRATION
Apply a thin layer of Calcipotriene ointment to the affected skin twice daily and rub in gently and completely. The safety and efficacy of Calcipotriene ointment have been demonstrated in patients treated for eight weeks.

Store at controlled room temperature, 15°-25°C (59°-77°F). Do not freeze.

HOW SUPPLIED
OINTMENT: 0.005%

BRAND/MANUFACTURER	NDC	SIZE	AWP
○ BRAND			
DOVONEX: Westwood-Squibb	00072-2540-03	30 gm	$35.22
	00072-2540-06	60 gm	$70.44
	00072-2540-10	100 gm	$117.40

Calcitonin

DESCRIPTION
Calcitonin is a polypeptide hormone secreted by the parafollicular cells of the thyroid gland in mammals and by the ultimobranchial gland of birds and fish.

Calcitonin Injection, Synthetic is a synthetic polypeptide of 32 amino acids in the same linear sequence that is found in Calcitonin of Salmon or human origin.

It is provided in sterile solution for subcutaneous or intramuscular injection and in vial syringes for subcutaneous administration. Each millimeter contains 200 I.U. (MRC) of Calcitonin-Salmon; each syringe contains Calcitonin-Human for injection 0.5 mg.

The activity of Calcitonin-Salmon is stated in International Units (equal to MRC or Medical Research Council units) based on bio-assay in comparison with the International Reference Preparation of Calcitonin, Salmon for Bioassay, distributed by the National Institute for Biological Standards and Control, Holly Hill, London.

Following is its chemical structure:

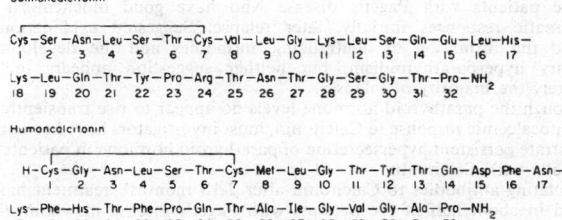

CLINICAL PHARMACOLOGY
Calcitonin acts primarily on bone, but direct renal effects and actions on the gastrointestinal tract are also recognized. Calcitonin-Salmon appears to have actions essentially identical to Calcitonins of mammalian origin, but its potency per mg is greater and it has a longer duration of action. The actions of Calcitonin on bone and its role in normal human bone physiology are still incompletely understood.

Bone: Single injections of Calcitonin cause a marked transient inhibition of the ongoing bone resorptive process. With prolonged use, there is a persistent, smaller decrease in the rate of bone resorption. Histologically this is associated with a decreased number of osteoclasts and an apparent decrease in their resorptive activity. Decreased osteocytic resorption may also be involved. There is some evidence that initially bone formation may be augmented by Calcitonin through increased osteoblastic activity. However, Calcitonin will probably not induce a long-term increase in bone formation. Animal studies indicate that endogenous Calcitonin, primarily through its action on bone, participates with parathyroid hormone in the homeostatic regulation of blood calcium. Thus, high blood calcium levels cause increased secretion of Calcitonin which, in turn, inhibits bone resorption. This reduces the transfer of calcium from bone to blood and tends to return blood calcium to the normal level. The importance of this process in humans has not been determined. In normal adults, who have a relatively low rate of bone resorption, the administration of exogenous Calcitonin results in only a slight decrease in serum calcium. In normal children and in patients with generalized Paget's disease, bone resorption is more rapid and decreases in serum calcium are more pronounced in response to Calcitonin.

Paget's Disease of Bone (osteitis deformans): Paget's disease is a disorder of uncertain etiology characterized by abnormal and accelerated bone formation and resorption in one or more bones. In most patients only small areas of bone are involved and the disease is not symptomatic. In a small fraction of patients, however, the abnormal bone may lead to bone pain and bone deformity, cranial and spinal nerve entrapment, or spinal cord compression. The increased vascularity of the abnormal bone may lead to high output congestive heart failure.

Active Paget's disease involving a large mass of bone may increase the urinary hydroxyproline excretion (reflecting breakdown of collagen-containing bone matrix) and serum alkaline phosphatase (reflecting increased bone formation). Calcitonin, presumably by an initial blocking effect on bone resorption, causes a decreased rate of bone turnover with a resultant fall in the serum alkaline phosphatase and urinary hydroxyproline excretion in approximately 2/3 of patients treated. The metabolic clearance rate of exogenously administered immunoreactive Calcitonin-Human in normal subjects has been determined to be 8.4 ± 1.1 ml/kg per min. The half-life is 1.02 hours after single, subcutaneous doses of 0.5 mg. Evidence to date indicates that the kidney is the principal organ responsible for its degradation, with only small fractions of the parent substance (0.1%) appearing in the urine.

Among 44 patients in clinical studies who had one or more determinations of serum alkaline phosphatase and 29 patients who had one or more determinations of urinary hydroxyproline during the first year of therapy, the following mean percent reductions from baseline were observed:

Time Interval†	Mean % Reduction (n*)	
	Serum Alkaline Phosphatase	Urinary Hydroxyproline
1-3 months	23.4(30)	21.4(20)
4-6 months	41.0(22)	47.4(12)
7-12 months	44.7(25)	56.1(14)

† Duration of treatment at time of observation
* Number of patients evaluated at each time interval

The mean reduction in serum alkaline phosphatase at the final visit compared to baseline for these patients was 36.1% (mean duration of treatment = 18.5 months) and for urinary hydroxyproline was 37.5% (mean duration of treatment = 21.2 months). These biochemical changes appear to correspond to changes toward more normal bone, as evidenced by a small number of documented examples of: 1) radiologic regression of Pagetic lesions, 2) improvement of impaired auditory nerve and other neurologic function, 3) decreases (measured) in abnormally elevated cardiac output. Serial biopsies of Pagetic bone indicate a decrease in the number of osteoclasts per square millimeter of bone during treatment. These improvements occur extremely rarely, if ever, spontaneously (elevated cardiac output may disappear over a period of years when the disease slowly enters a sclerotic phase; in the cases treated with Calcitonin, however, the decreases were seen in less than one year).

Some patients with Paget's disease who have good biochemical and/or symptomatic responses initially, later relapse. Suggested explanations have included the formation of neutralizing antibodies and the development of secondary hyperparathyroidism, but neither suggestion appears to explain adequately the majority of relapses.

Although the parathyroid hormone levels do appear to rise transiently during each hypocalcemic response to Calcitonin, most investigators have been unable to demonstrate persistent hypersecretion of parathyroid hormone in patients treated chronically with Calcitonin.

Circulating antibodies to Calcitonin after 2-18 months' treatment have been reported in about half of the patients with Paget's disease in whom antibody studies were done, but Calcitonin treatment remained effective in many of these cases. Occasionally patients with high antibody titers are found. These patients usually will have suffered a biochemical relapse of Paget's disease and are unresponsive to the acute hypocalcemic effects of Calcitonin.

The risk of diminishing effectiveness as a result of antibody formation or hypersensitivity reactions is less with Calcitonin-Human than with nonhuman forms of the hormone.

Long-term treatment (up to ten or more years in a few patients) with Calcitonin-Human has not been limited by antibody-mediated resistance.

Calcitonin-Human has been shown to be effective in patients who have developed resistance to nonhuman Calcitonins.

Hypercalcemia: In clinical trials, Calcitonin has been shown to lower the elevated serum calcium of patients with carcinoma (with or without demonstrated metastases), multiple myeloma or primary hyperparathyroidism (lesser response). Patients with higher values for serum calcium tend to show greater reduction during Calcitonin therapy. The decrease in calcium occurs about 2 hours after the first injection and lasts for about 6-8 hours. Calcitonin given every 12 hours maintained a calcium lowering effect for about 5-8 days, the time period evaluated for most patients during the clinical studies. The average reduction of 8-hour post-injection serum calcium during this period was about 9 percent.

Kidney: Calcitonin increases the excretion of filtered phosphate, calcium, and sodium by decreasing their tubular reabsorption. In some patients the inhibition of bone resorption by Calcitonin is of such magnitude that the consequent reduction of filtered calcium load more than compensates for the decrease in tubular reabsorption of calcium. The result in these patients is a decrease rather than an increase in urinary calcium.

Transient increases in sodium and water excretion may occur after the initial injection of Calcitonin. In most patients these changes return to pre-treatment levels with continued therapy.

Gastrointestinal Tract: Increasing evidence indicates that Calcitonin has significant actions on the gastrointestinal tract. Short-term administration results in marked transient decreases in the volume and acidity of gastric juice and in the

volume and the trypsin and amylase content of pancreatic juice. Whether these effects continue to be elicited after each injection of Calcitonin during chronic therapy has not been investigated.

Metabolism: The metabolism of Calcitonin-Salmon has not yet been studied clinically. Information from animal studies with Calcitonin-Salmon and from clinical studies with Calcitonins of porcine and human origin suggest that Calcitonin-Salmon is rapidly metabolized by conversion to smaller inactive fragments, primarily in the kidneys, but also in the blood and peripheral tissues. A small amount of unchanged hormone and its inactive metabolites are excreted in the urine.

The metabolic clearance rate of exogenously administered immunoreactive Calcitonin-Human in normal subjects has been determined to be 8.4 ± 1.1 ml/kg per min. The half-life is 1.02 hours after single, subcutaneous doses of 0.5 mg. Evidence to date indicates that the kidney is the principal organ responsible for its degradation, with only small fractions of the parent substance (0.1%) appearing in the urine.

It appears that Calcitonin-Salmon cannot cross the placental barrier and its passage to the cerebrospinal fluid or to breast milk has not been determined.

INDICATIONS AND USAGE

Calcitonin-Salmon and Calcitonin-Human are indicated for the treatment of symptomatic Paget's disease of bone; Calcitonin-Salmon is indicated for the treatment of hypercalcemia, and the treatment of postmenopausal osteoporosis.

Paget's Disease: At the present time effectiveness has been demonstrated principally in patients with moderate to severe disease characterized by polyostotic involvement with elevated serum alkaline phosphatase and urinary hydroxyproline excretion.

Although reduction of serum alkaline phosphatase and urinary hydroxyproline excretion usually occurs within 3 months after initiation of treatment, maximum reductions may not occur until after 6-24 months of continuous treatment.

In these patients, the biochemical abnormalities were substantially improved (more than 30% reduction) in about ⅔ of patients studied, and bone pain was improved in a similar fraction. A small number of documented instances of reversal of neurologic deficits has occurred, including improvement in the basilar compression syndrome, and improvement of spinal cord and spinal nerve lesions. At present there is too little experience to predict the likelihood of improvement of any given neurologic lesion. Hearing loss, the most common neurologic lesion of Paget's disease, is improved infrequently (4 of 29 patients studied audiometrically).

Patients with increased cardiac output due to extensive Paget's disease have had measured decreases in cardiac output while receiving Calcitonin. The number of treated patients in this category is still too small to predict how likely such a result will be.

The large majority of patients with localized, especially monostotic disease do not develop symptoms and most patients with mild symptoms can be managed with analgesics. There is no evidence that the prophylactic use of Calcitonin is beneficial in asymptomatic patients, although treatment may be considered in exceptional circumstances in which there is extensive involvement of the skull or spinal cord with the possibility of irreversible neurologic damage. In these instances treatment would be based on the demonstrated effect of Calcitonin on Pagetic bone, rather than on clinical studies in the patient population in question.

Calcitonin-Human has been reported to cause subjective relief of bone pain and tenderness and a reduction in elevated skin temperature over the affected skeletal areas in some patients.

Hypercalcemia: Calcitonin is indicated for early treatment of hypercalcemic emergencies, along with other appropriate agents, when a rapid decrease in serum calcium is required, until more specific treatment of the underlying disease can be accomplished. It may also be added to existing therapeutic regimens for hypercalcemia such as intravenous fluids and furosemide, oral phosphate or corticosteroids, or other agents.

Postmenopausal Osteoporosis: Calcitonin is indicated for the treatment of postmenopausal osteoporosis in conjunction with adequate calcium and vitamin D intake to prevent the progressive loss of bone mass. No evidence currently exists to indicate whether or not Calcitonin decreases the risk of vertebral crush fractures or spinal deformity. A recent controlled study, which was discontinued prior to completion because of questions regarding its design and implementation, failed to demonstrate any benefit of Calcitonin in fracture rate. No adequate controlled trials have examined the effect of Calcitonin injection on vertebral bone mineral density beyond one year of treatment. Two controlled studies with Calcitonin have shown an increase in total body calcium at one year, followed by a trend to decreasing total body calcium (still above baseline) at two years. The minimum effective dose of Calcitonin for prevention of vertebral bone mineral density loss has not been established. It has been suggested that those postmenopausal patients having increased rates of bone turnover may be more likely to respond to antiresorptive agents such as Calcitonin.

CONTRAINDICATIONS

Clinical allergy to synthetic Calcitonin-Salmon. There are no known contraindications to the use of Calcitonin-Human.

WARNINGS

ALLERGIC REACTIONS

Because Calcitonin is protein in nature, the possibility of a systemic allergic reaction exists. Administration of Calcitonin-Salmon has been reported in a few cases to cause serious allergic-type reactions (e.g. bronchospasms, swelling of the tongue or throat, and anaphylactic shock), and in one case, death due to anaphylaxis. The usual provisions should be made for the emergency treatment of such a reaction should it occur. Allergic reactions should be differentiated from generalized flushing and hypotension.

Skin testing should be considered prior to treatment with Calcitonin-Salmon, particularly for patients with suspected sensitivity to Calcitonin. The following procedure is suggested: Prepare a dilution at 10 I.U. per mL by withdrawing 1/20 mL (0.05 mL) in a tuberculin syringe and filling it to 1.0 mL with sodium chloride injection, USP. Mix well, discard 0.9 mL and inject intracutaneously 0.1 mL (approximately 1 I.U.) on the inner aspect of the forearm. Observe the injection site 15 minutes after injection. The appearance of more than mild erythema or wheal constitutes a positive response.

GENERAL

The incidence of osteogenic sarcoma is known to be increased in Paget's disease. Pagetic lesions, with or without therapy, may appear by X-ray to progress markedly, possibly with some loss of definition of periosteal margins. Such lesions should be evaluated carefully to differentiate these from osteogenic sarcoma.

PRECAUTIONS

1. GENERAL

The administration of Calcitonin possibly could lead to hypocalcemic tetany. Provisions for parenteral calcium administration should be available during the first several administrations of Calcitonin.

2. LABORATORY TESTS

Periodic examinations of urine sediment of patients on chronic therapy are recommended.

Coarse granular casts and casts containing renal tubular epithelial cells were reported in young adult volunteers at bed rest who were given Calcitonin-Salmon to study the effect of immobilization on osteoporosis. There was no other evidence of renal abnormality and the urine sediment became normal after Calcitonin was stopped. Urine sediment abnormalities have not been reported by other investigators.

3. INSTRUCTIONS FOR THE PATIENT

Careful instruction in sterile injection technique should be given to the patient, and to other persons who may administrater Calcitonin.

4. CARCINOGENESIS, MUTAGENESIS, AND IMPAIRMENT OF FERTILITY

An increased incidence of pituitary adenomas has been observed in one-year toxicity studies in Sprague-Dawley rats administered Calcitonin-Salmon at dosages of 20 and 80 I.U./kg/day and in Fisher 344 rats given 80 I.U./kg/day. The relevance of these findings to humans is unknown. Calcitonin-Salmon was not mutagenic in tests using *Salmonella typhimurium*, *Escherichia coli*, and Chinese Hamster V79 cells.

No long-term carcinogenicity studies have been conducted with Calcitonin-Human. Calcitonin-Human was not mutagenic as evaluated by changes in the number of micronuclei in polychromatic bone marrow erythrocytes of male mice. Likewise, in an in vitro human lymphocyte assay for clastogenicity, the compound did not induce any chromosomal aberrations with or without microsomal activation at concentrations as high as 1000 µg/ml. Calcitonin-Human was shown to be mutagenic in various tester strains of *Salmonella typhimurium* and *Escherichia coli* in the Ames assay, but at high concentrations ($\geq$ 1000 µg per plate) and only with microsomal activation. In a Chinese hamster bone marrow study, a marginal increase in the incidence of nuclear anomalies of somatic interphase cells was observed after 2 days at an intraperitoneal dose of 200 mg/kg/day. The clinical significance of these findings is unknown.

5. PREGNANCY: TERATOGENIC EFFECTS. CATEGORY C.

Calcitonin-Salmon has been shown to cause a decrease in fetal birth weights in rabbits when given in doses 14-56 times the dose recommended for human use. Since Calcitonin does not cross the placental barrier, this finding may be due to metabolic effect of Calcitonin on the pregnant animal. Animal reproduction studies have not been conducted with Calcitonin-Human. There are no adequate and well-controlled studies in pregnant women Calcitonin should be used during pregnancy only if the potential benefit justifies the potential risk to the fetus or if it is clearly needed.

6. NURSING MOTHERS

It is not known whether this drug is excreted in human milk. Because Calcitonin is a peptide and subject to digestion in the gastrointestinal tract, it is unlikely that active drug will be absorbed by the nursing infant. However, studies of drug activity after ingestion have not been done in nursing infants. As a general rule, nursing should not be undertaken while a patient is on this drug since many drugs are excreted in human milk. Calcitonin has been shown to inhibit lactation in animals.

7. PEDIATRIC USE

Disorders of bone in children referred to as juvenile Paget's disease have been reported rarely. The relationship of these disorders to adult Paget's disease has not been established and experience with the use of Calcitonin in these disorders is very limited. Safety and effectiveness of Calcitonin in children have not been established. There are no adequate data to support the use of Calcitonin in children.

ADVERSE REACTIONS

CALCITONIN-SALMON:

Gastrointestinal System: Nausea with or without vomiting has been noted in about 10% of patients treated with Calcitonin-Salmon. It is most evident when treatment is first initiated and tends to decrease or disappear with continued administration.

Dermatologic/Hypersensitivity: Local inflammatory reactions at the site of subcutaneous or intramuscular injection have been reported in about 10% of patients. Flushing of face or hands occurred in about 2% to 5% of patients. Skin rashes, nocturia, pruritus of the ear lobes, feverish sensation, pain in the eyes, poor appetite, abdominal pain, edema of feet, and salty taste have been reported in patients treated with Calcitonin-Salmon. Administration of Calcitonin-Salmon has been reported in a few cases to cause serious allergic-type reactions (e.g. bronchospasms, swelling of the tongue or throat, and anaphylactic shock), and in one case, death due to anaphylaxis. (See *"Warnings."*)

CALCITONIN-HUMAN:

The adverse reaction rates listed below are based on studies that included a large proportion of patients with histories of unresponsiveness to nonhuman Calcitonins, a number of whom also had displayed intolerance to those Calcitonins.

Gastrointestinal: Nausea, with or without vomiting, was noted in about 14% to 21% of patients treated with the recommended dose of Calcitonin-Human. Anorexia, diarrhea, epigastric discomfort, or abdominal pain were reported in a few patients. Nausea improved in the majority of patients with continued therapy.

Dermatologic/Hypersensivity: Flushing of face, ears, or hands occurred within minutes of injection in 16% to 21% of patients treated with the recommended dose. Flushing improved in the majority of patients with continued therapy. Skin rashes were reported rarely.

Genitourinary: Increased frequency of urination was noted in about 5% to 10% of patients.

Metabolic: Mild tetanic symptoms were reported rarely during Calcitonin-Human therapy. One patient developed asymptomatic mild hypercalcemia during a study.

Miscellaneous: Rare side effects included chills, chest pressure, weakness, headache, tenderness of palms and soles, dizziness, nasal congestion, shortness of breath, metallic taste, and paresthesia.

OVERDOSAGE

A dose of 1000 I.U. subcutaneously may produce nausea and vomiting as the only adverse effects. Doses of 32 units per kg per day for one or two days demonstrate no other adverse effects. In animals, single doses as high as 1,000 mg/kg produced no mortality or functional or structural organ changes.

Data on chronic high dose administration are insufficient to judge toxicity.

DOSAGE AND ADMINISTRATION

Paget's Disease: The recommended starting dose of Calcitonin-Salmon in Paget's disease is 100 I.U. (0.5 mL) per day administered subcutaneously (preferred for outpatient self-administration) or intramuscularly. The recommended starting dosage of Calcitonin-Human is 0.5 mg daily, given subcutaneously.

Some patients may obtain sufficient clinical and biochemical improvement with a dosage of 0.5 mg two or three times weekly or 0.25 mg daily.

More severe cases (e.g., when there is evidence of mechanically weak bones with osteolytic lesions) may require dosages of up to 1 mg daily (0.5 mg twice daily). Drug effect should be monitored by periodic measurement of serum alkaline phosphatase and 24-hour urinary hydroxyproline (if available) and evaluation of symptoms. A decrease toward normal of the biochemical abnormalities is usually seen, if it is going to occur, within the first few months. Bone pain may also decrease during that time. Improvement of neurologic lesions, when it occurs, requires a longer period of treatment, often more than one year.

Side effects of Calcitonin-Human such as nausea and flushing may be minimized by administration at bedtime. Dose adjustment (e.g. from 0.5 mg to 0.25 mg) may also be helpful in this regard. Treatment with Calcitonin-Human should be continued for 6 months; if symptoms have been relieved, therapy may be discontinued until symptoms or radiologic signs recur. Biochemical parameters will relapse on cessation of therapy and should not be relied on as the basis for a decision to restart therapy.

In many patients doses of 50 I.U. (0.25 mL) per day or every other day are sufficient to maintain biochemical and clinical improvement. At the present time, however, there are insufficient data to determine whether this reduced dose will have the same effect as the higher dose on forming more normal bone structure. It appears preferable, therefore, to maintain the higher dose in any patient with serious deformity or neurological involvement.

In any patient with a good response initially who later relapses, either clinically or biochemically, the possibility of antibody formation should be explored. The patient may be tested for antibodies by an appropriate specialized test or evaluated for the possibility of antibody formation by critical clinical evaluation.

Patient compliance should also be assessed in the event of relapse.

In patients who relapse, because of antibodies or for unexplained reasons, a dosage increase beyond 100 I.U. per day does not usually appear to elicit an improved response.

Hypercalcemia: The recommended starting dose of Calcitonin in hypercalcemia is 4 I.U./kg body weight every 12 hours by subcutaneous or intramuscular injection. If the response to this dose is not satisfactory after one or two days, the dose may be increased to 8 I.U./kg every 12 hours. If the response remains unsatisfactory after two more days, the dose may be further increased to a maximum of 8 I.U./kg every 6 hours.

Postmenopausal Osteoporosis: The recommended dose of Calcitonin Salmon is 100 I.U. per day administered subcutaneously or intramuscularly. Patients should also receive supplemental calcium such as calcium carbonate 1.5 g daily and an adequate vitamin D intake (400 units daily). An adequate diet is also essential.

The minimum effective dose of Calcitonin for the prevention of vertebral bone mineral density loss has not been established. Data from a single one-year placebo-controlled study with Calcitonin-Salmon injection suggested that 100 I.U. every other day might be effective in preserving vertebral bone mineral density. Baseline and interval monitoring of biochemical markers of bone resorption/turnover (*e.g.*, fasting A.M., second-voided urine hydroxyproline to creatinine ratio) and of bone mineral density may be useful in achieving the minimum effective dose.

If the volume of Calcitonin-Salmon to be injected exceeds 2 mL, intramuscular injection is preferable and multiple sites of injection should be used.

Store in refrigerator, 2°-8°C (36°-46°F).

Protect Calcitonin-Human from light and heat. Do not store above 86°F (30° C).

Reconstituted material should be used within 6 hours.

Note: **Parenteral drug products should be inspected visually for particulate matter and discoloration prior to administration, whenever solution and container permit.**

When the dosage is 0.25 mg (one-half of the solution), the remainder of the drug solution is to be discarded.

J CODES
Up to 400 units SC,IM—J0630

HOW SUPPLIED
INJECTION: 200 IU/ML

AVERAGE UNIT PRICE (AVAILABLE SIZES)

BRAND		$16.43		

BRAND/MANUFACTURER	NDC	SIZE	AWP
◆ BRAND			
MIACALCIN: Sandoz Pharm	00078-0149-23	2 ml	$24.90
CALCIMAR: RPR	00075-1306-01	2 ml	$40.81
◆ GENERICS			
OSTEOCALCIN: Arcola	00070-4492-01	2 ml	$28.50

Calcitriol

DESCRIPTION
Calcitriol is synthetically manufactured and is available as a sterile, isotonic, clear, aqueous solution for intravenous injection in 1 mL ampuls and as capsules. Each ampul contains Calcitriol 1 or 2 mcg.

Calcitriol is a colorless, crystalline compound which occurs naturally in humans. It is soluble in organic solvents but relatively insoluble in water. Calcitriol is chemically designated (5Z,7E)-9, 10-secocholesta-5,7,10(19)-triene-1α,3β,25-triol and has the following structural formula:

Molecular Formula: $C_{27}H_{44}O_3$. The other names frequently used for Calcitriol are 1α, 25-dihydroxycholecalciferol, 1α,25-dihydroxyvitamin D3, 1,25-DHCC, 1,25-(OH)2D3 and 1,25-diOHC.

Following is its chemical structure:

CLINICAL PHARMACOLOGY
Calcitriol is the active form of vitamin D3 (cholecalciferol), a synthetic vitamin D analog which is active in the regulation of the absorption of calcium from the gastrointestinal tract and its utilization in the body. The natural or endogenous supply of vitamin D in man mainly depends on ultraviolet light for conversion of 7-dehydrocholesterol to vitamin D3 in the skin. Vitamin D3 must be metabolically activated in the liver and the kidney before it is fully active as a regulator of calcium and phosphorus metabolism at its target tissues. The initial transformation is catalyzed by a vitamin D3-25-hydroxylase enzyme (25-OHase) present in the liver, and the product of this reaction is 25-(OH)D3 (calcifediol). The latter undergoes hydroxylation in the mitochondria of kidney tissue, and this reaction is activated by the renal 25-hydroxyvitamin D3-1-α-hydroxylase to produce 1,25-(OH)2D3 (Calcitriol), the active form of vitamin D3.

The known sites of action of Calcitriol are intestine, bone, kidney and parathyroid gland. A Calcitriol receptor-binding protein appears to exist in the mucosa of human intestine. Calcitriol is the most active known form of vitamin D3 in stimulating intestinal calcium transport. In acutely uremic rats, Calcitriol, has been shown to stimulate intestinal calcium absorption. In bone, Calcitriol, in conjunction with parathyroid hormone, stimulates resorption of calcium; and in

the kidney, Calcitriol increases the tubular reabsorption of calcium. *In-vitro* and *in-vivo* studies have shown that Calcitriol directly suppresses secretion and synthesis of PTH. A vitamin D-resistant state may exist in uremic patients because of the failure of the kidney to adequately convert precursors to the active compound, Calcitriol. Resultant hypocalcemia and secondary hyperparathyroidism are a major cause of the metabolic bone disease of renal failure. However, other bone-toxic substances which accumulate in uremia (e.g., aluminum) may also contribute.

The beneficial effect of Calcitriol in renal osteodystrophy appears to result from correction of hypocalcemia and secondary hyperparathyroidism. It is uncertain whether Calcitriol produces other independent beneficial effects.

Calcitriol when administered by bolus injection is rapidly available in the blood stream. Calcitriol is rapidly absorbed from the intestine. Peak serum concentrations (above basal values) were reached within 3 to 6 hours following oral administration of single doses of 0.25 to 1.0 mcg of Calcitriol. The half-life of Calcitriol elimination from serum was found to range from 3 to 6 hours. Following a single oral dose of 0.5 mcg, mean serum concentrations of Calcitriol rose from a baseline value of 40.0 ± 4.4 (S.D.) pg/ml to 60.0 ± 4.4 pg/ml at 2 hours, and declined to 53.0 ± 6.9 at 4 hours, 50 ± 7.0 at 8 hours, 44 ± 4.6 at 12 hours and 41.5 ± 5.1 at 24 hours. The duration of pharmacologic activity of a single dose of Calcitriol is about 3 to 5 days. Vitamin D metabolites are known to be transported in blood, bound to specific plasma proteins. Enterohepatic recycling and biliary excretion of Calcitriol occurs. Following intravenous administration of radiolabeled Calcitriol in normal subjects, approximately 27% and 7% of the radioactivity appeared in the feces and urine, respectively, within 24 hours. When a 1-mcg oral dose of radiolabeled Calcitriol was administered to normals, approximately 10% of the total radioactivity appeared in urine within 24 hours. Cumulative excretion of radioactivity on the sixth day following intravenous administration of radiolabeled Calcitriol averaged 16% in urine and 49% in feces. The pharmacologic activity of an administered dose of Calcitriol is about 3 to 5 days. Two metabolic pathways for Calcitriol have been identified, conversion to 1,24,25-(OH)3D3 and to calcitroic acid.

INDICATIONS AND USAGE
Calcitriol is indicated in the management of hypocalcemia and the resultant metabolic bone disease in patients undergoing chronic renal dialysis. In these patients, Calcitriol administration enhances calcium absorption and reduces serum alkaline phosphatase levels. It has been shown to significantly reduce elevated parathyroid hormone levels. Reduction of PTH has been shown to result in an improvement in renal osteodystrophy.

Calcitriol is also indicated in the management of hypocalcemia and its clinical manifestations in patients with postsurgical hypoparathyroidism, idiopathic hypoparathyroidism, and pseudohypoparathyroidism.

CONTRAINDICATIONS
Calcitriol should not be given to patients with hypercalcemia or evidence of vitamin D toxicity.

WARNINGS
Since Calcitriol is the most potent metabolite of vitamin D available, vitamin D and its derivatives should be withheld during treatment to avoid possible additive effects and hypercalcemia.

A nonaluminum phosphate-binding compound and a low phosphate diet should be used to control serum phosphorus levels in patients undergoing dialysis.

Overdosage of any form of vitamin D is dangerous (see also *"Overdosage"*). Progressive hypercalcemia due to overdosage of vitamin D and its metabolites may be so severe as to require emergency attention. Chronic hypercalcemia can lead to generalized vascular calcification, nephrocalcinosis and other soft-tissue calcification. The serum calcium times phosphate ($Ca \times P$) product should not be allowed to exceed 70. Radiographic evaluation of suspect anatomical regions may be useful in the early detection of this condition.

Studies in dogs and rats given Calcitriol for up to 26 weeks have shown that small increases of Calcitriol above endogenous levels can lead to abnormalities of calcium metabolism with the potential for calcification of many tissues in the body.

PRECAUTIONS
1. GENERAL
Excessive dosage of Calcitriol induces hypercalcemia and in some instances hypercalciuria; therefore, early in treatment during dosage adjustment, serum calcium and phosphorus should be determined at least twice weekly. In dialysis patients, a fall in serum alkaline phosphatase levels usually antedates the appearance of hypercalcemia and may be an indication of impending hypercalcemia. Should hypercalcemia develop, the drug should be discontinued immediately.

Calcitriol should be given cautiously to patients on digitalis, because hypercalcemia in such patients may precipitate cardiac arrhythmias.

In patients with normal renal function, chronic hypercalcemia may be associated with an increase in serum creatinine. While this is usually reversible, it is important in such patients to pay careful attention to those factors which may lead to hypercalcemia. Calcitriol therapy should always be started at the lowest possible dose and should not be increased without careful monitoring of the serum calcium. An estimate to daily dietary calcium intake should be made and the intake adjusted when indicated.

Patients with normal renal function taking Calcitriol should avoid dehydration. Adequate fluid intake should be maintained.

◆ **RATED THERAPEUTICALLY EQUIVALENT;** ◇ **THERAPEUTIC EQUIVALENCE UNCONFIRMED;** ○ **UNRATED**

2. INFORMATION FOR THE PATIENT

The patient and his or her parents or spouse should be informed about adherence to instructions about diet and calcium supplementation and avoidance of the use of unapproved nonprescription drugs, including magnesium-containing antacids. Patients should also be carefully informed about the symptoms of hypercalcemia (see "Adverse Reactions").

3. ESSENTIAL LABORATORY TESTS

Serum calcium, phosphorus, magnesium and alkaline phosphatase and 24-hour urinary calcium and phosphorus should be determined periodically. During the initial phase of the medication, serum calcium and phosphorus should be determined more frequently (twice weekly).

For dialysis patients, serum calcium, phosphorus, magnesium and alkaline phosphatase should be determined periodically. For hypoparathyroid patients, serum calcium, phosphorus and 24-hour urinary calcium should be determined periodically.

4. DRUG INTERACTIONS

Magnesium-containing antacid and Calcitriol should not be used concomitantly in patients on chronic renal dialysis, because such use may lead to the development of hypermagnesemia.

Cholestyramine has been reported to reduce intestinal absorption of fat-soluble vitamins: as such it may impair intestinal absorption of oral Calcitriol.

5. CARCINOGENESIS, MUTAGENESIS, IMPAIRMENT OF FERTILITY

Long-term studies in animals have not been performed to evaluate the carcinogenic potential of Calcitriol. There was no evidence of mutagenicity as studied by the Ames Method. No significant effects of Calcitriol on fertility and/or general reproductive performance, were reported using oral Calcitriol.

6. USE IN PREGNANCY *PREGNANCY CATEGORY C*:

Teratogenic Effects: Calcitriol given orally has been reported to be teratogenic in rabbits when given in doses 4 and 15 times the dose recommended for human use.

All 15 fetuses in 3 litters at these doses showed external and skeletal abnormalities. However, none of the other 23 litters (156 fetuses) showed significant abnormalities compared with controls.

Teratology studies in rats showed no evidence of teratogenic potential. Although there is evidence that maternal Calcitriol may enter the fetal circulation, there are no adequate and well-controlled studies in pregnant women. Calcitriol should be used during pregnancy only if the potential benefit justifies the potential risk to the fetus.

Nonteratogenic Effects: In the rabbit, dosages of 0.3 mcg/kg/day administered on days 7 to 18 of gestation resulted in 19% maternal mortality, a decrease in mean fetal body weight and a reduced number of newborn surviving to 24 hours. A study of peri- and postnatal development in rats resulted in hypercalcemia in the offspring of dams given Calcitriol at doses of 0.08 or 0.3 mcg/kg/day, hypercalcemia and hypophosphatemia in dams at doses of 0.08 or 0.3 mcg/kg/day, and increased serum urea nitrogen in dams given oral Calcitriol at a dose of 0.3 mcg/kg/day. In another study in rats, maternal weight gain was slightly reduced at a dose of 0.3 mcg/kg/day administered on days 7 to 15 of gestation. The offspring of a woman administered 17 to 36 mcg/day of oral Calcitriol (17 to 144 times the recommended dose) during pregnancy manifested mild hypercalcemia in the first two days of life which returned to normal at day 3.

7. NURSING MOTHERS

It is not known whether this drug is excreted in human milk. Because many drugs are excreted in human milk and because of the potential for serious adverse reactions in nursing infants from Calcitriol, a decision should be made whether to discontinue nursing or to discontinue the drug, taking into account the importance of the drug to the mother.

8. PEDIATRIC USE

Safety and efficacy of Calcitriol in children undergoing dialysis have not been established.

ADVERSE REACTIONS

Adverse effects of Calcitriol are, in general, similar to those encountered with excessive vitamin D intake. The early and late signs and symptoms of vitamin D intoxication associated with hypercalcemia include:

1. EARLY

Weakness, headache, somnolence, nausea, vomiting, dry mouth, constipation, muscle pain, bone pain and metallic taste.

2. LATE

Polyuria, polydipsia, anorexia, weight loss, nocturia, conjunctivitis (calcific), pancreatitis, photophobia, rhinorrhea, pruritus, hyperthermia, decreased libido, elevated BUN, albuminuria, hypercholesterolemia, elevated SGOT and SGPT, ectopic calcification, nephrocalcinosis, hypertension, cardiac arrhythmias and, rarely, overt psychosis.

Occasional mild pain on injection has been observed.

In clinical studies on hypoparathyroidism and pseudohypoparathyroidism, hypercalcemia was noted on at least one occasion in about 1 in 3 patients and hypercalciuria in about 1 in 7. Elevated serum creatinine levels were observed in about 1 in 6 patients (approximately one half of whom had normal levels at baseline).

One case of erythema multiforme was confirmed by rechallenge.

OVERDOSAGE

Administration of Calcitriol to patients in excess of their requirements can cause hypercalcemia, hypercalciuria and hyperphosphatemia. High intake of calcium and phosphate concomitant with Calcitriol may lead to similar abnormalities. High levels of calcium in the dialysate bath may contribute to the hypercalcemia.

1. TREATMENT OF HYPERCALCEMIA AND OVERDOSAGE IN PATIENTS ON HEMODIALYSIS

General treatment of hypercalcemia (greater than 1 mg/dl above the upper limit of normal range) consists of immediate discontinuation of Calcitriol therapy, institution of a low calcium diet and withdrawal of calcium supplements. Serum calcium levels should be determined daily until normocalcemia ensues. Hypercalcemia usually resolves in two to seven days. When serum calcium levels have returned to within normal limits, Calcitriol therapy may be reinstituted at a dose of 0.25 mcg/day or 0.5 mcg less than prior therapy.

Serum calcium levels should be obtained at least twice weekly after all dosage changes and subsequent dosage titration.

Persistent or markedly elevated serum calcium levels may be corrected by dialysis against a calcium-free dialysate.

2. TREATMENT OF ACCIDENTAL OVERDOSAGE OF CALCITRIOL

The treatment of acute accidental overdosage of Calcitriol should consist of general supportive measures. If oral drug ingestion is discovered within a relatively short time, induction of emesis or gastric lavage may be of benefit in preventing further absorption. If the drug has passed through the stomach, the administration of mineral oil may promote its fecal elimination. Serial serum electrolyte determinations (especially calcium), rate of urinary calcium excretion and assessment of electrocardiographic abnormalities due to hypercalcemia should be obtained. Such monitoring is critical in patients receiving digitalis. Discontinuation of supplemental calcium and low calcium diet are also indicated in accidental overdosage. Due to the relatively short duration of the pharmacological action of Calcitriol, further measures are probably unnecessary. Should, however, persistent and markedly elevated serum calcium levels occur, there are a variety of therapeutic alternatives which may be considered, depending on the patients' underlying condition. These include the use of drugs such as phosphates and corticosteroids as well as measures to induce an appropriate forced diuresis. The use of peritoneal dialysis against a calcium-free dialysate has also been reported.

DOSAGE AND ADMINISTRATION

The optimal dose of Calcitriol must be carefully determined for each patient.

The effectiveness of Calcitriol therapy is predicated on the assumption that each patient is receiving an adequate and appropriate daily intake of calcium. The RDA for calcium in adults is 800 to 1200 mg. To ensure that each patient receives an adequate daily intake of calcium, the physician should either prescribe a calcium supplement or instruct the patient in proper dietary measures.

The recommended initial dose of Calcitriol injection is 0.5 mcg (0.01 mcg/kg) administered three times weekly, approximately every other day. Calcitriol injection can be administered as a bolus dose intravenously through the catheter at the end of hemodialysis. If a satisfactory response in the biochemical parameters and clinical manifestations of the disease state is not observed, the dose may be increased by 0.25 to 0.50 mcg at two to four week intervals. During this titration period, serum calcium and phosphorus levels should be obtained at least twice weekly, and if hypercalcemia is noted, the drug should be immediately discontinued until normocalcemia ensues. Most patients undergoing hemodialysis respond to doses between 0.5 and 3.0 mcg (0.01 to 0.05 mcg/kg) three times per week.

Parenteral drug products should be inspected visually for particulate matter and discoloration prior to administration, whenever solution and container permit.

Discard unused portion.

The recommended initial dose of oral Calcitriol is 0.25 mcg/day. If a satisfactory response in the biochemical parameters and clinical manifestations of the disease state is not observed, dosage may be increased by 0.25 mcg/day at four- to eight-week intervals. During this titration period, serum calcium levels should be obtained at least twice weekly, and if hypercalcemia is noted, the drug should be immediately discontinued until normocalcemia ensues.

Patients with normal or only slightly reduced serum calcium levels may respond to oral Calcitriol doses of 0.25 mcg every other day. Most patients undergoing hemodialysis respond to doses between 0.5 and 1 mcg/day.

Oral Calcitriol may normalize plasma ionized calcium in some uremic patients, yet fail to suppress parathyroid hyperfunction. In these individuals with autonomous parathyroid hyperfunction, oral Calcitriol may be useful to maintain normocalcemia, but has not been shown to be adequate treatment for hyperparathyroidism.

Hypoparathyroidism: The recommended initial dose of oral Calcitriol is 0.25 mcg/day given in the morning. If a satisfactory response in the biochemical parameters and clinical manifestations of the disease is not observed, the dose may be increased at two- to four-week intervals. During the dosage titration period, serum calcium levels should be obtained at least twice weekly and, if hypercalcemia is noted oral Calcitriol should be immediately discontinued until normocalcemia ensues. Careful consideration should also be given to lowering the dietary calcium intake.

Most adult patients and pediatric patients age 6 years and older have responded to dosages in the range of 0.5 to 2 mcg daily. Pediatric patients in the 1-5 year age group with hypoparathyroidism have usually been given 0.25 to 0.75

mcg daily. The number of treated patients with pseudohypoparathyroidism less than 6 years of age is too small to make dosage recommendations.

Store at controlled room temperature 15° to 30°C (59° to 86°F).
Protect Oral Calcitriol from heat and light.
Protect Calcitriol Injection from light.

J CODES
1 mcg ampule IM—J0635

HOW SUPPLIED
CAPSULE: 0.25 MCG

BRAND/MANUFACTURER	NDC	SIZE	AWP
○ BRAND			
ROCALTROL: Roche Labs	00004-0143-23	30s	$30.21
	00004-0143-01	100s	$99.23

CAPSULE: 0.5 MCG

BRAND/MANUFACTURER	NDC	SIZE	AWP
○ BRAND			
ROCALTROL: Roche Labs	00004-0144-01	100s	$158.72

INJECTION: 1 MCG/ML

BRAND/MANUFACTURER	NDC	SIZE	AWP
○ BRAND			
CALCIJEX: Abbott Hosp	00074-1200-01	1 ml 50s	$589.00

INJECTION: 2 MCG/ML

BRAND/MANUFACTURER	NDC	SIZE	AWP
○ BRAND			
CALCIJEX: Abbott Hosp	00074-1210-01	1 ml 50s	$1008.00

Calcium Acetate

DESCRIPTION
Each tablet contains 667 mg of Calcium Acetate, USP (anhydrous; $Ca(CH_3COO)_2$; MW = 158.17 grams) equal to 169 mg (8.45 mEq) calcium.

CLINICAL PHARMACOLOGY
Patients with advanced renal insufficiency (creatinine clearance less than 30 ml/min) exhibit phosphate retention and some degree of hyperphosphatemia. The retention of phosphate plays a pivotal role in causing secondary hyperparathyroidism associated with osteodystrophy, and soft tissue calcification. The mechanism by which phosphate retention leads to hyperparathyroidism is not clearly delineated. Therapeutic efforts directed toward the control of hyperphosphatemia include reduction in the dietary intake of phosphate, inhibition of absorption of phosphate in the intestine with phosphate binders, and removal of phosphate from the body by more efficient methods of dialysis. The rate of removal of phosphate by dietary manipulation or by dialysis is insufficient. Dialysis patients absorb 40% to 80% of dietary phosphorous. Therefore, the fraction of dietary phosphate absorbed from the diet needs to be reduced by using phosphate binders in most renal failure patients on maintenance dialysis. Calcium Acetate when taken with meals, combines with dietary phosphate to form insoluble phosphate which is excreted in the feces. Maintenance of serum phosphorus below 6.0 mg/dl is generally considered as a clinically acceptable outcome of treatment with phosphate binders. Calcium Acetate is highly soluble at neutral pH, making the calcium readily available for binding to phosphate in the proximal small intestine.

Orally administered calcium acetate from pharmaceutical dosage forms has been demonstrated to be systemically absorbed up to approximately 40% under fasting conditions and up to approximately 30% under nonfasting conditions. This range represents data from both healthy subjects and renal dialysis patients under various conditions.

INDICATIONS AND USAGE
Calcium Acetate is indicated for the control of hyperphosphatemia in end stage renal failure and does not promote aluminum absorption.

CONTRAINDICATIONS
Patients with hypercalcemia.

WARNINGS
Patients with end stage renal failure may develop hypercalcemia when given calcium with meals. No other calcium supplements should be given concurrently with Calcium Acetate. Progressive hypercalcemia due to overdose of Calcium Acetate, may be severe as to require emergency measures. Chronic hypercalcemia may lead to vascular calcification, and other soft-tissue calcification. The serum calcium level should be monitored twice weekly during the early dose adjustment period. **The serum calcium times phosphate (CaXP) product should not be allowed to exceed 66.** Radiographic evaluation of suspect anatomical region may be helpful in early detection of soft-tissue calcification.

PRECAUTIONS
General: Excessive dosage of Calcium Acetate induces hypercalcemia; therefore, early in the treatment during dosage adjustment serum calcium should be determined twice weekly. Should hypercalcemia develop, the dosage should be reduced or the treatment discontinued immediately depending on the severity of hypercalcemia. Calcium Acetate should not be given to patients on digitalis, because hypercalcemia may precipitate cardiac arrhythmias. Calcium Acetate therapy should always be started at low dose and should not be increased without careful monitoring of serum calcium. An estimate of daily calcium intake should be made initially and the intake adjusted as needed. Serum phosphorus should also be determined periodically.

Information for the Patient: The patient should be informed about compliance with dosage instructions, adherence to instructions about diet and avoidance of the use of nonprescription anatacids. Patients should be informed about the symptoms of hypercalcemia (See "Adverse Reactions" section).

Drug Interactions: Calcium Acetate may decrease the bioavailability of tetracyclines.

Carcinogenesis, Mutagenesis, Impairment of Fertility: Long term animal studies have not been performed to evaluate the carcinogenic potential or effect on fertility of Calcium Acetate.

Pregnancy: Teratogenic Effects: Category C. Animal reproduction studies have not been conducted with Calcium Acetate. It is also not known whether Calcium Acetate can cause fetal harm when administered to a pregnant woman or can affect reproduction capacity. Calcium Acetate should be given to a pregnant woman only if clearly needed.

Pediatric Use: Safety and efficacy of Calcium Acetate have not been established.

ADVERSE REACTIONS
In clinical studies, patients have occasionally experienced nausea during Calcium Acetate therapy. Hypercalcemia may occur during treatment with Calcium Acetate. Mild hypercalcemia (Ca > 10.5 mg/dl) may be asymptomatic or manifest itself as constipation, anorexia, nausea and vomiting. More severe hypercalcemia (Ca > 12 mg/dl) is associated with confusion, delerium, stupor and coma. Mild hypercalcemia is easily controlled by reducing the Calcium Acetate dose or temporarily discontinuing therapy. Severe hypercalcemia can be treated by acute hemodialysis and discontinuing Calcium Acetate therapy.

Decreasing dialysate calcium concentration could reduce the incidence and severity of Calcium Acetate-induced hypercalcemia. The long-term effect of Calcium Acetate on the progression of vascular or soft-tissue calcification has not been determined. Isolated cases of pruritus have been reported which may represent allergic reactions.

OVERDOSAGE
Administration of Calcium Acetate in excess of the appropriate daily dosage can cause severe hypercalcemia (see "Adverse Reactions").

DOSAGE AND ADMINISTRATION
The recommended initial dose of Calcium Acetate for the adult dialysis patient is 2 tablets with each meal. The dosage may be increased gradually to bring serum phosphate value below 6 mg/dl, as long as hypercalcemia does not develop. Most patients require 3-4 tablets with each meal.

Store at controlled room temperature, 15°-30°C.

HOW SUPPLIED
INJECTION: 0.5 MEQ/ML

AVERAGE UNIT PRICE (AVAILABLE SIZES)	
GENERIC	$0.08

BRAND/MANUFACTURER	NDC	SIZE	AWP
◆ GENERICS			
Abbott Hosp	00074-2553-01	10 ml 25s	$24.64
Abbott Hosp	00074-2553-02	50 ml 25s	$83.42
Abbott Hosp	00074-2553-03	100 ml 25s	$187.03

TABLETS: 667 MG

BRAND/MANUFACTURER	NDC	SIZE	AWP
○ BRAND			
PHOSLO: Braintree	52268-0200-01	200s	$17.94

Calcium Disodium Versenate SEE
EDETATE CALCIUM DISODIUM

Calcium Glycerophosphate and Calcium Lactate

COMPOSITION
Calcium Glycerophosphate/Calcium Lactate is a specially processed solution containing Calcium Glycerophosphate and Calcium Lactate. Calcium Glycerophosphate/Calcium Lactate is isotonic, with a pH of about 7 or somewhat above.

◆ RATED THERAPEUTICALLY EQUIVALENT; ◇ THERAPEUTIC EQUIVALENCE UNCONFIRMED; ○ UNRATED

(Other Calcium solutions are usually quite acid, with pH values of 4.5 to 5.5). Each 10 mL Calcium Glycerophosphate/Calcium Lactate solution contains Calcium Glycerophosphate 50 mg, and Calcium Lactate 50 mg, in a physiological solution of sodium chloride, with 0.25% phenol as a preservative.

ADVANTAGES

Intramuscular injections of Calcium Glycerophosphate/Calcium Lactate raise blood serum calcium levels, do not raise the calcium levels above normal. Of conspicuous importance, intramuscular injections of Calcium Glycerophosphate/Calcium Lactate are without pain, inflammatory reactions or sloughing.

INDICATIONS

Wherever Calcium is indicated or in conditions associated with hypocalcemia.

ADMINISTRATION

10 mL 1 to 4 times weekly or as determined by the physician.

USE IN PREGNANCY

Safety for use in pregnancy or during lactation has not been established.

CONTRAINDICATIONS

Hypercalcemia; and in view of the fact that hypercalcemia is associated with sarcoidosis and bone metastasis of neoplastic processes, it should not be used in those conditions. As there is a similarity in the actions of calcium and digitalis on the contractility and excitability of the heart muscle. Calcium Glycerophosphate/Calcium Lactate is contraindicated in fully digitalized patients. **Do not use intramuscularly in infants and young children.**

HOW SUPPLIED
INJECTION:

BRAND/MANUFACTURER	NDC	SIZE	AWP
○ **GENERICS**			
CALPHOSAN: Glenwood	00516-0060-60	60 ml	$14.82
CALPHOSAN: Glenwood	00516-0060-66	60 ml	$14.82
CALPHOSAN: Glenwood	00516-0060-55	125 ml	$24.13

Calcium Glycerophosphate and Calcium Levulinate

DESCRIPTION

Each ml contains: Calcium Glycerophosphate 10mg, Calcium Levulinate 15mg.

ACTIONS

Calcium is the fifth most abundant element in the body and it is essential for many metabolic functions supporting the integrity of the nervous and muscle systems. Hypocalcemia results in tetany and other malfunctions of the neuromuscular system and heart. Prolonged hypocalcemia may be associated with ectodermal defects including the nails, skin and teeth.

INDICATIONS

Acute and chronic hypocalcemia which may result from hypoparathyroidism, simple deficiencies of Vitamin D and conditions associated with intestinal malabsorption.

CONTRAINDICATIONS

Hypercalcemia states. The intraveneous administration of Calcium, injection of parathyroid hormone, or overdosage of Vitamin D may cause hypercalcemia.

WARNING

Do not refrigerate. PROTECT FROM HEAT. Store at controlled room temperature 15°-30° C (59°-86° F). Do not use if precipitate occurs.

PRECAUTIONS

Calcium should be administered with caution in digitalized patients since it may precipitate arrhythmias. Intramuscular Calcium should be infused slowly.

ADVERSE REACTIONS

Hypercalcemia may cause nausea, anorexia, vomiting, constipation, peptic ulcer pain, polydipsia and polyuria.

DOSAGE AND ADMINISTRATION

For subcutaneous, intramuscular or SLOW intravenous injection.

Adults: 5 to 10ml

Children: 6 to 12 years — 3 to 4 mL; 3 to 6 years — 1/2 to 2 mL

Children under 3 years: 1/2 to 1 mL

Give daily for 4 days, then twice weekly for 3 weeks, occasionally as needed for normal blood levels thereafter.

HOW SUPPLIED
INJECTION:

BRAND/MANUFACTURER	NDC	SIZE	AWP
○ **BRAND**			
CAL-IM: Legere	25332-0060-07	100 ml	$9.95

Calcium Iodide and Codeine

DESCRIPTION

Each 5 mL (teaspoonful) contains:

Codeine, USP ....8.4 mg
Warning—May be habit forming
Calcium Iodide, anhydrous ....152 mg

Calcium Iodide/Codeine is an oral antitussive, expectorant syrup.

The chemical formula for Calcium Iodide is CaI_2. Codeine is methylmorphine, a natural alkaloid of opium. The chemical formula for Codeine is $C_{18}H_{21}NO_3 \cdot H_2O$.

CLINICAL PHARMACOLOGY

The major effects of Codeine in man are on the central nervous system. The antitussive effect is produced by depression of the cough reflex. Codeine is rapidly absorbed from the gastrointestinal tract and is metabolized in the liver.

Iodides are readily absorbed from the gastrointestinal tract and are distributed to extracellular fluid as well as gastric and salivary secretions. Iodides are accumulated by the thyroid gland. Excretion occurs mainly through the kidneys.

INDICATIONS AND USAGE

In adults and children as an expectorant, and for symptomatic relief of coughs.

CONTRAINDICATIONS

Calcium Iodide/Codeine should not be used in patients with a history of iodism, or with known hypersensitivity to Iodides or Codeine. Long-term use of Iodide-containing preparations is contraindicated during pregnancy.

WARNINGS

Physiological dependence may develop with the use of Codeine.

Usage During Pregnancy: Calcium Iodide/Codeine syrup can cause fetal harm when administered to a pregnant woman. Maternal ingestion of large amounts of iodides during pregnancy has been associated with development of fetal goiter and resultant acute respiratory distress of the neonate. If this drug is used during pregnancy, or if the patient becomes pregnant while taking this drug, the patient should be apprised of the potential hazard to the fetus.

Severe and occasionally fatal skin eruptions have been reported rarely in patients receiving prolonged administration of iodides.

PRECAUTIONS

Laboratory Tests: Patients who must receive prolonged Iodide therapy should be evaluated periodically for possible depression of thyroid function.

Drug Interactions: The concurrent administration of Calcium Iodide and lithium carbonate may enhance the hypothyroid and goitrogenic effects of either drug.

Laboratory Test Interactions: Elevated values may be obtained on thyroid function tests or protein-bound iodine tests when iodide-containing compounds have been ingested. False positive results may be obtained if iodides have been ingested prior to guaiac or benzidine testing.

Carcinogenesis: No data is available on long-term carcinogenicity in animals or humans.

Pregnancy: Pregnancy Category D. See *"Warnings"* section.

Nursing Mothers: Iodine is excreted in breast milk. Caution should be exercised when Calcium Iodide/Codeine is administered to a nursing woman.

ADVERSE REACTIONS

In decreasing order of severity: severe and sometimes fatal skin eruptions (ioderma) occur rarely after the prolonged use of Iodides. Iodism can occur. Symptoms of iodism include metallic taste, acneform skin lesions, mucous membrane irritation, salivary gland swelling, and gastric distress. These side effects subside quickly upon discontinuance of the Iodide-containing drug.

Codeine may produce vomiting, nausea, and constipation.

OVERDOSAGE

Symptoms of acute Codeine poisoning include respiratory and central nervous system depression, pinpoint pupils and coma. Blood pressure and body temperature may fall.

Acute Iodide poisoning is associated with gastrointestinal irritation. Angioedema with laryngeal swelling may develop. Shock may also occur.

Treatment for overdose of Calcium Iodide/Codeine is:
a. Establish a patient airway and ventilate if needed.
b. Gastric evacuation.
c. Treatment for shock.
d. General supportive measures including replacement of fluids and electrolytes may be indicated.
e. The use of naloxone to antagonize the narcotic depression of the central nervous system should be considered.

➤ SHOWN IN PRODUCT IDENTIFICATION GUIDE

DOSAGE AND ADMINISTRATION

Adults and children over ten years of age, usual dose, 1 to 2 teaspoonfuls every 4 hours. Children 6 to 10 years of age, ½ to 1 teaspoonful every 4 hours. Children 2 to 6 years of age, ½ teaspoonful every 4 hours.

Dispense in a USP tight, light-resistant glass container.

Store below 86°F (30°C).

HOW SUPPLIED

SYRUP (C-V):

BRAND/MANUFACTURER	NDC	SIZE	AWP
○ BRAND CALCIDRINE: Abbott Pharm	00074-5763-16	480 ml	$39.35

Calcium Iodide and Isoproterenol Sulfate

DESCRIPTION

Calcium Iodide/Isoproterenol Sulfate is a bronchodilator, expectorant in a palatable syrup.

Isoproterenol is a sympathomimetic agent which is chemically related to epinephrine. The chemical formula for Isoproterenol Sulfate is 1, 2-Benzenediol, 4-[1-hydroxy-2-[(1-methylethyl) amino] ethyl]-, sulfate (2:1) (salt), dihydrate.

Each teaspoonful of Calcium Iodide/Isoproterenol Sulfate syrup contains 3 mg of Isoproterenol Sulfate and 150 mg of anhydrous Calcium Iodide.

CLINICAL PHARMACOLOGY

Isoproterenol is classified as a catecholamine which acts predominantly on beta receptor sites of peripheral inhibitory and cardiac excitatory sympathetic nerves. Its primary pharmacological actions are to increase both the rate and force of cardiac contractions and to relax the smooth muscle of the bronchi, alimentary tract, and skeletal muscle vasculature. Isoproterenol can prevent or relieve bronchospasm due to drugs as well as that due to disease. The drug lowers peripheral vascular resistance and reduces the diastolic blood pressure. Systolic pressure is unchanged or slightly increased as a consequence of increased cardiac output.

After oral administration, isoproterenol is extensively converted to its sulfate conjugate in the intestinal wall. This presystemic metabolism explains the higher doses and more variable response to isoproterenol by the oral route compared to parenteral administration. The primary excretion product found in urine is the sulfate conjugate (50 to 80% of the dose) with only minor fractions of unchanged drug (5 to 15%) and 3-0 methyl isoproterenol (15% or less).

The coloregenic effects of Isoproterenol are similar to those of epinephrine. However, it causes less hyperglycemia than epinephrine. Isoproterenol can also cause central excitation. Calcium Iodide is an expectorant.

INDICATIONS AND USAGE

Indicated in adults and children for the symptomatic control of bronchospasm in asthma and in allied respiratory disorders such as bronchitis and tracheobronchitis.

CONTRAINDICATIONS

This product should not be used in patients with a history of iodism or with known hypersensitivity to iodides. It is also contraindicated in rare instances in which a patient has demonstrated hypersensitivity to isoproterenol or other sympathomimetic amines.

Use of Isoproterenol is contraindicated in patients with preexisting cardiac arrhythmias because the cardiac stimulant effect may aggravate such disorders.

Long-term use of iodide-containing preparations is contraindicated during pregnancy. (See "Warnings".)

WARNINGS

Bronchial asthma may mask the presence of cardiac asthma (pulmonary edema). A differential diagnosis should be made before instituting therapy.

Usage in Pregnancy: Calcium Iodide/Isoproterenol Sulfate can cause fetal harm when administered to a pregnant woman. Maternal ingestion of large amounts of iodides during pregnancy has been associated with development of fetal goiter and resultant acute respiratory distress of the neonate. If this drug is used during pregnancy, or if the patient becomes pregnant while taking this drug, the patient should be apprised of the potential hazard to the fetus.

PRECAUTIONS

Isoproterenol should be used cautiously in patients with heart disease, hypertension, hyperthyroidism, diabetes, or unstable vasomotor systems.

Patients who must receive prolonged iodide therapy should be evaluated periodically for possible depression of thyroid function.

Drug Interactions: The concurrent administration of Calcium Iodide and lithium carbonate may enhance the hypothyroid and goitrogenic effects of either drug.

Concomitant use of Isoproterenol and MAO inhibitors may induce acute hypertensive crisis.

Propranolol, a beta-adrenergic blocking agent, antagonizes Isoproterenol.

Caution should be exercised when Isoproterenol is used concomitantly with a parenteral or inhalation form of *epinephrine* or other *adrenergic agent* since the effects of these drugs are additive.

Laboratory Test Interactions: Elevated values may be obtained on thyroid function tests, and when testing for protein-bound iodine, when iodine-containing compounds have been ingested.

The use of iodides may cause false positive results when guaiac testing is performed or when testing for benzidine.

Carcinogenesis: No data is available on long-term potential for carcinogenicity in animals or humans.

Pregnancy: Pregnancy Category D. See *"Warnings"* section.

Nursing Mothers: Iodine is excreted in breast milk, therefore, caution should be exercised when Calcium Iodine/Isoproterenol Sulfate is administered to a nursing woman.

ADVERSE REACTIONS

As with other sympathomimetic drugs, isoproterenol may produce undesired side effects. These effects in decreasing order of severity are cardiac arrhythmias, tachycardia, vomiting, dizziness, weakness, nausea, precordial distress and anginal-type pain, headache, palpitation, nervousness, tremor, sweating, and flushing.

Swelling of the parotid glands has been reported with prolonged use of isoproterenol. In such cases the drug should be withdrawn.

Iodism can occur with use of this drug. Symptoms of iodism include metallic taste, acneform skin lesions, mucous membrane irritation, salivary gland swelling, and gastric distress. These side effects subside quickly upon discontinuance of the Iodide-containing drug. Severe and sometimes fatal skin eruptions (ioderma) occur rarely after the prolonged use of iodides.

SYMPTOMS AND TREATMENT OF OVERDOSAGE

Symptoms may include palpitation, tachycardia, restlessness, tremor, sweating, headache, dizziness, weakness, nausea, and vomiting. Blood pressure may at first be elevated slightly. Later, blood pressure may fall and the general picture of "shock" may develop.

Treatment includes general supportive measures. Sedatives may be given for restlessness.

DOSAGE AND ADMINISTRATION

The following suggestions are offered as a general guide to dosage.

Under 3 years: ½ teaspoonful, may be repeated every four to six hours; 3 to 10 years: ½ to 1 teaspoonful, may be repeated every four to six hours; over 10 years and for adults: 1 to 2 teaspoonfuls, may be repeated every four to six hours. Dosage must be adjusted to the response of the patient. Side effects may necessitate dosage reduction.

Store below 77°F (25°C).

HOW SUPPLIED

SYRUP:

BRAND/MANUFACTURER	NDC	SIZE	AWP
○ BRAND NORISODRINE W/CALCIUM IODIDE: Abbott Pharm	00074-6953-01	480 ml	$30.99

Calcium, Injectable

DESCRIPTION

Each ml of Calcium Chloride contains:
Calcium .... 27.3 mg (1.4 mEq)
or 100 mg (13.6 mEq/10 ml)

Each 5 ml of Calcium Gluceptate contains:
Calcium .... 90 mg (4.5 mEq)

Each ml of Calcium Gluconate contains:
Calcium .... 9.3 mg (0.465 mEq)

Calcium, Injectable, Chloride and Gluconate, are for intravenous use only and must not be injected intramuscularly or subcutaneously. Calcium, Injectable, Gluceptate, is suitable for intramuscular or intravenous injection.

CLINICAL PHARMACOLOGY

Calcium is the fifth most abundant element in the body and the major fraction is in the bony structure. Calcium plays important physiological roles, many of which are poorly understood. It is essential for the functional integrity of the nervous and muscular systems. It is necessary for normal cardiac function and is one of the factors that operates in the mechanisms involved in the coagulation of blood. It also functions as an enzyme cofactor and affects the secretory activity of endocrine and exocrine glands. It is essential for maintenance of cell membrane and capillary permeability and is essential to renal function and respiration. Calcium also plays regulatory roles in the release and storage of neurotransmitters and hormones, in the uptake and binding of amino acids, and in cyanocobalamin (vitamin B_{12}) absorption and gastrin secretion.

Calcium Injection in water dissociates to provide calcium (Ca++) and ions. They are normal constituents of the body fluids and are dependent on various physiologic mechanisms for maintenance of balance between intake and output. Approximately 80% of body Calcium is excreted in the feces as insoluble salts; urinary excretion accounts for the remaining 20%.

◆ RATED THERAPEUTICALLY EQUIVALENT; ◇ THERAPEUTIC EQUIVALENCE UNCONFIRMED; ○ UNRATED

INDICATIONS AND USAGE

Calcium, Injectable, is indicated (1) for the treatment of hypocalcemia due to rapid growth or pregnancy and in those conditions requiring a prompt increase in blood plasma Calcium levels, such as neonatal tetany and tetany due to parathyroid deficiency, vitamin D deficiency and alkalosis. Other therapy, such as parathyroid hormone or vitamin D, may be indicated according to the etiology of the tetany. It is also important to institute oral calcium therapy as soon as practicable. (2) in the treatment of magnesium intoxication due to overdosage of magnesium sulfate and (3) to combat the deleterious effects of hyperkalemia as measured by electrocardiographic (ECG), pending correction of the increased potassium level in the extracellular fluid.

Calcium, Injectable, also may be used in cardiac resuscitation when weak or inadequate contractions return following defibrillation or when epinephrine injection has failed to strengthen myocardial contractions.

Calcium salts have been used as adjunctive therapy in a number of conditions, including the following:

Insect bites or stings, such as Black Widow Spider bites.
To decrease capillary permeability in sensitivity reactions, particularly when characterized by urticaria, nonthrombocytopenic purpura and exudative dermatoses such as dermatitis herpetiformis, and for pruritus of eruptions caused by certain drugs.
Rickets and osteomalacia.
As an aid in the management of the acute symptoms in lead colic.

It is also indicated for the prevention of hypocalcemia during exchange transfusions.

Calcium gluconate is also used as an electrolyte supplement in solutions for total parenteral nutrition.

UNLABELED USES

Calcium, Injectable, is used alone or as an adjunct in the treatment of verapamil-induced inotropic effects, postoperative tetany, calcium blocker overdose, and to correct metabolic acidosis in Lowe's syndrome. Oral Calcium is also used for leg cramps in pregnant women and to prevent development of hypertension and osteoporosis.

CONTRAINDICATIONS

Calcium, Injectable, is contraindicated for cardiac resuscitation in the presence of ventricular fibrillation or in patients with the risk of existing digitalis toxicity. Intravenous administration of Calcium is contraindicated when serum Calcium levels are above normal.

WARNINGS

Calcium, Injectable (Chloride and Gluconate), is irritating to veins and *must not be injected into tissues,* since severe necrosis and sloughing may occur. Great care should be taken to avoid extravasation or accidental injection into perivascular tissues.

Calcium, Injectable (Gluceptate), may produce local tissue irritation at the site of intramuscular injection in very small patients. This route of administration should be avoided in such patients except in emergency situations when the intravenous route is not feasible.

Note: If crystallization has occurred, warming may dissolve the precipitate. The Injection must be clear at time of use.

PRECAUTIONS

Do not administer unless solution is clear. Discard unused portion.

Because of its additive effect, Calcium should be administered very cautiously to a patient who is digitalized or who is taking effective doses of digitalis or digitalis-like preparations.

The ionotropic and toxic effects of cardiac glycosides and Calcium are synergistic and arrhythmias may occur if these drugs are given together (particularly when Calcium is given intravenously). Intravenous administration of Calcium should be avoided in patients receiving cardiac glycosides; if necessary, Calcium should be given slowly in small amounts.

Injections should be made slowly through a small needle into a larger vein to minimize venous irritation and avoid undesirable reactions. It is particularly important to prevent a high concentration of Calcium from reaching the heart because of the danger of cardiac syncope. If injected into the ventricular cavity in cardiac resuscitation, it must not be injected into the myocardial tissue.

Rapid injection of Calcium gluconate may cause vasodilation, decreased blood pressure, bradycardia, cardiac arrhythmias, syncope and cardiac arrest.

Calcium complexes tetracycline antibiotics rendering them inactive. The two drugs should not be given at the same time orally nor should they be mixed for parenteral administration.

Calcium, Injectable, has been reported to be incompatible with intravenous solutions containing various drugs. Published data are too varied and/or limited to permit generalizations, and specialized reference should be consulted for specific information.

Transient elevations of plasma 11-hydroxycorticosteroid levels (Glenn-Nelson technique) may occur when intravenous Calcium is administered, but levels return to control values after 1 hour. In addition, intravenous Calcium can produce false-negative values for serum and urinary magnesium.

Pregnancy Category C: Animal reproduction studies have not been conducted with Calcium, Injectable. It also is not known whether Calcium, Injectable, can cause fetal harm when administered to a pregnant woman or can affect reproduction capacity. Calcium, Injectable, should be given to a pregnant woman only if clearly needed.

Nursing Mothers: It is not known whether this drug is excreted in human milk. Because many drugs are excreted in human milk, caution should be exercised when Calcium, Injectable, is administered to a nursing woman.

ADVERSE REACTIONS

Rapid injection may cause the patient to complain of tingling sensations, a Calcium taste, a sense of oppression or "heat wave".

Injections of Calcium are accompanied by peripheral vasodilatation as well as a local "burning" sensation and there may be a moderate fall in blood pressure.

Rapid intravenous injection of Calcium salts may cause vasodilation, decreased blood pressure, bradycardia, cardiac arrhythmias, syncope and cardiac arrest. Use in digitalized patients may precipitate arrhythmias.

Local necrosis and abscess formation may occur with inadvertent intramuscular injection.

Should perivascular infiltration occur, I.V. administration at that site should be discontinued at once. Local infiltration of the affected area with 1% procaine hydrochloride, to which hyaluronidase may be added, will often reduce venospasm and dilute the Calcium remaining in the tissues locally. Local application of heat may also be helpful.

Following intramuscular administration (Gluceptate), mild local reactions may occur; severe inflammatory reactions have not been observed.

DRUG ABUSE AND DEPENDENCE

None known.

OVERDOSAGE

Too rapid injection may produce lowering of blood pressure and cardiac syncope. Persistent hypercalemia from overdosage of Calcium is unlikely because of rapid excretion. Acute hypercalcemic syndrome is characterized by weakness, lethargy, intractable nausea and vomiting, coma, and sudden death, and a markedly elevated plasma Calcium level. In the event of untoward effects from excessive Calcium administration, the drug should be discontinued promptly, the patient reevaluated and appropriate countermeasures instituted, if necessary. See *"Precautions"* and *"Adverse Reactions".*

DOSAGE AND ADMINISTRATION

Calcium Chloride: Calcium, Injectable, is administered only by *slow* intravenous injection (not to exceed 0.7 to 1.5 mEq/min) and/or in cardiac resuscitation, by injection into the ventricular cavity. It must not be injected into the myocardium.

The usual precautions for intravenous therapy should be observed. If time permits, the solution should be warmed to body temperature. The injection should be halted if the patient complains of any discomfort; it may be resumed when symptoms disappear. Following injection, the patient should remain recumbent for a short time.

The usual adult dosage in hypocalcemic disorders ranges from 4.5 to 16 mEq of Calcium (5 to 10 mL) at intervals of 1 to 3 days, depending on the response of the patient and/or results of serum calcium determinations. Repeated injections may be required because of rapid excretion of Calcium.

In magnesium intoxication, an initial adult dose of 4.5 to 9 mEq of Calcium should be administered promptly and the patient observed for signs of recovery before further doses are given.

In hyperkalemic ECG disturbances of cardiac function, the dosage of Calcium Chloride injection should be titrated by constant monitoring of ECG changes during administration.

In cardiac resuscitation, the usual adult dosage ranges from 4.5 to 9 mEq of Calcium intravenously. Care should be taken to avoid injection into the cardiac muscle.

If there has not been sufficient time to establish an intravenous route, intraventricular injection may be administered by personnel who are well trained in the technique and familiar with possible complications. The intravenous needle supplied with the syringe should be broken off and replaced with a suitable intracardiac needle by affixing it firmly to the Luer taper provided on the syringe. After the injection has been completed, the needle/syringe assembly should be removed from the injection site by grasping the needle at the Luer fitting.

The intraventricular dose usually ranges from 200 to 800 mg.

Calcium Gluceptate: Calcium Gluceptate injection, is administered intramuscularly (not to infants or young children except in emergencies when intravenous injection is impossible) or by slow intravenous injection.

The following dosages are based on Calcium Gluceptate injection containing 90 mg of elemental Calcium (4.5 mEq) per 5 mL (equivalent to 10 mL of 10% Calcium Gluconate):

Calcium Gluceptate may be given intramuscularly in 2 to 5 mL doses. When 5 mL are administered, the dose should be injected in the gluteal region or, in infants, in the lateral thigh.

The usual intravenous dose of Calcium Gluceptate is from 5 to 20 mL (90 to 360 mg elemental Calcium). The usual precautions for intravenous therapy should be observed. The solution should be warmed to body temperature and administered slowly (not over 1 to 2 mL per minute). The injection should be halted if the patient complains of any discomfort; it may be resumed when symptoms disappear. Following injection, the patient should remain recumbent for a short time. Repeated injections may be required because of rapid excretion of Calcium.

During exchange transfusions in newborn infants, the usual dose is 0.5 mL after each 100 mL of blood exchanged.

Calcium Gluconate: The dose is dependent on the requirements of the individual patient.

The usual intravenous dose is 5 mL (500 mg) to 20 mL (2 g).

Intravenous Calcium injections must be administered slowly at a rate not to exceed 0.7 to 1.5 mEq/minute (1.5 to 3.2 mL/minute). The injection should be stopped if the patient complains of discomfort. One mEq of Calcium weighs 20 mg.

For producing emergency elevation of serum Calcium, the usual intravenous dose is 7 to 14 mEq (15 to 30.1 mL) in adults, 1 to 7 mEq (2.2 to 15 mL) in children, and less than 1 mEq (2.2 mL) for infants. Depending upon patient response, these doses can be repeated every 1 to 3 days.

For treating hypocalcemic tetany in adults, 4.5 to 16 mEq of Calcium (9.7 to 34.4 mL) may be given intramuscularly until therapeutic response occurs. In children, 0.5 to 0.7 mEq/kg (1.1 to 1.5 mL/kg) may be given intravenously 3 or 4 times daily or until tetany is controlled. Neonatal tetany may be treated with divided doses approximating 2.4 mEq/kg/day (5.2 mL/kg/day).

For treating hyperkalemia with secondary cardiac toxicity, Calcium may be administered intravenously to provide 2.25 to 14 mEq (4.8 to 30.1 mL) while monitoring the ECG. If necessary, doses may be repeated after 1 to 2 minutes.

For treating magnesium intoxication in adults, the initial dose is 4.5 to 9 mEq of Calcium (9.7 to 19.4 mL) given intravenously. Subsequent doses should be adjusted to patient response. If intravenous administration is not possible, 2 to 5 mEq of Calcium (4.3 to 10.8 mL) may be given intramuscularly.

In exchange transfusions in neonates, intravenous Calcium is administered at a dosage of 0.45 mEq Calcium (1 mL)/100mL of citrated blood exchanged.

In adults receiving transfusions of citrated blood, approximately 1.35 mEq of Calcium (2.9 mL) should be given intravenously concurrent with each 100 mL of citrated blood.

In central venous total parenteral nutrition (TPN), Calcium is administered at a concentration of approximately 4.7 mEq (10 mL)/liter of TPN solution. The additive maintenance dose in neonatal TPN is 0.5 mEq Calcium/kg/day (1.1 mL/kg/day).

Parenteral drug products should be inspected visually for particulate matter and discoloration prior to administration whenever solution and container permit. See *"Precautions"*.

The solution should be stored at controlled room temperature 15°-30°C (59°-86°F).

J CODES
Up to 10 ml IV—J0610

HOW SUPPLIED

CALCIUM CHLORIDE
INJECTION: 100 MG/ML

AVERAGE UNIT PRICE (AVAILABLE SIZES)		GENERIC A-RATED AVERAGE PRICE (GAAP)	
GENERIC	$1.005	10 ml 10s	$122.71

BRAND/MANUFACTURER	NDC	SIZE	AWP
◆ GENERICS			
Fujisawa	00469-1140-30	10 ml	$0.78
Abbott Hosp	00074-4928-01	10 ml 10s	$113.64
Abbott Hosp	00074-4928-23	10 ml 10s	$126.47
Abbott Hosp	00074-4908-01	10 ml 10s	$128.01
Abbott Hosp	00074-4928-33	10 ml 25s	$316.17

INJECTION: 100 MG/ML

BRAND/MANUFACTURER	NDC	SIZE	AWP
○ GENERICS			
Moore,H.L.	00839-6673-30	1 ml	$5.33
Allscrips	54569-2237-00	10 ml	$6.56
Astra	00186-0651-01	10 ml 10s	$65.63
VHA Supply	00702-0862-10	10 ml 25s	$11.25
Amer Regent	00517-2710-25	10 ml 25s	$19.69
Astra	00186-1166-04	10 ml 25s	$20.19
CMC-Cons	00223-7277-10	10 ml 25s	$27.50
Intl Med Sys	00548-1004-00	10 ml 25s	$147.75
Intl Med Sys	00548-2004-00	10 ml 25s	$159.00
Intl Med Sys	00548-1006-00	10 ml 25s	$212.63
Intl Med Sys	00548-3004-00	10 ml 25s	$387.75
UDL	51079-0702-45	10 ml 25s ud	$19.89
Raway	00686-2710-25	10 ml 100s	$120.00

CALCIUM GLUCEPTATE
INJECTION: 220 MG/ML

BRAND/MANUFACTURER	NDC	SIZE	AWP
◆ GENERICS			
Abbott Hosp	00074-3894-05	5 ml 25s	$45.72

For additional alternatives, turn to the section beginning on page 2859.

Calderol *SEE* CALCIFEDIOL

Cantil *SEE* MEPENZOLATE BROMIDE

Capastat Sulfate *SEE* CAPREOMYCIN SULFATE

Capitrol *SEE* CHLOROXINE

Capoten *SEE* CAPTOPRIL

Capozide *SEE* CAPTOPRIL WITH HYDROCHLOROTHIAZIDE

Capreomycin Sulfate

> ## WARNINGS
> THIS PREPARATION IS FOR INTRAMUSCULAR USE ONLY.
>
> THE USE OF CAPREOMYCIN SULFATE IN PATIENTS WITH RENAL INSUFFICIENCY OR PREEXISTING AUDITORY IMPAIRMENT MUST BE UNDERTAKEN WITH GREAT CAUTION, AND THE RISK OF ADDITIONAL CRANIAL NERVE VIII IMPAIRMENT OR RENAL INJURY SHOULD BE WEIGHED AGAINST THE BENEFITS TO BE DERIVED FROM THERAPY. *REFER TO* ANIMAL PHARMACOLOGY *FOR ADDITIONAL INFORMATION.*
>
> SINCE OTHER PARENTERAL ANTITUBERCULOSIS AGENTS (STREPTOMYCIN, VIOMYCIN) ALSO HAVE SIMILAR AND SOMETIMES IRREVERSIBLE TOXIC EFFECTS, PARTICULARLY ON CRANIAL NERVE VIII AND RENAL FUNCTION, SIMULTANEOUS ADMINISTRATION OF THESE AGENTS WITH CAPREOMYCIN SULFATE IS NOT RECOMMENDED. USE WITH NONANTITUBERCULOSIS DRUGS (POLYMYXIN A SULFATE, COLISTIN SULFATE, AMIKACIN, GENTAMICIN, TOBRAMYCIN, VANCOMYCIN, KANAMYCIN, AND NEOMYCIN) HAVING OTOTOXIC OR NEPHROTOXIC POTENTIAL SHOULD BE UNDERTAKEN ONLY WITH GREAT CAUTION.
>
> *USAGE IN PREGNANCY*—THE SAFETY OF THE USE OF CAPROMYCIN SULFATE IN PREGNANCY HAS NOT BEEN DETERMINED.
>
> *PEDIATRIC USAGE*—SAFETY OF THE USE OF CAPREOMYCIN SULFATE IN INFANTS AND CHILDREN HAS NOT BEEN ESTABLISHED.

DESCRIPTION
Capreomycin Sulfate is a polypeptide antibiotic isolated from *Streptomyces capreolus*. It is a complex of 4 microbiologically active components, which have been characterized in part: however, complete structural determination of all the components has not been established.

Capreomycin is supplied as the disulfate salt and is soluble in water. In complete solution, it is almost colorless.

Each vial contains the equivalent of 1 g Capreomycin Sulfate activity.

Following is its chemical structure:

$$CH_2-R$$

	R	
Capreomycin IA	OH	$C_{25}H_{44}N_{14}O_8$
Capreomycin IB	H	$C_{25}H_{44}N_{14}O_7$

· 2H₂SO₄ → $\cdot\ 2H_2SO_4$

CLINICAL PHARMACOLOGY
Human Pharamacology: Capreomycin Sulfate is not absorbed in significant quantities from the gastrointestinal tract and must be administered parenterally. In 2 studies of 10 patients each, peak serum concentrations following 1 g of Capreomycin Sulfate given intramuscularly were achieved 1 to 2 hours after administration, and average peak levels reached were 28 and 32 μg/mL respectively (range, 20 to 47 μg/mL). Low serum concentrations were present at 24 hours. However, 1g of Capreomycin Sulfate daily for 30 days or more produced no significant accumulation in subjects with normal renal function. Two patients with marked reduction of renal function had high serum concentrations 24 hours after administration of the drug. When a 1-g dose of Capreomycin

---

◆ RATED THERAPEUTICALLY EQUIVALENT; ◇ THERAPEUTIC EQUIVALENCE UNCONFIRMED; ○ UNRATED

Sulfate was given intramuscularly to normal volunteers, 52% was excreted in the urine within 12 hours.

Paper chromatographic studies indicated that Capreomycin Sulfate is excreted essentially unaltered. Urine concentrations averaged 1.68 µg/mL (average urine volume, 228 mL) during the 6 hours following a 1-g dose.

Microbiology: Capreomycin Sulfate is active against strains of *Mycobacterium tuberculosis* found in humans.

Susceptibility Tests: The in vitro susceptibility of strains of *M. tuberculosis* to Capreomycin Sulfate varies with the media and techniques employed. In general, the minimum inhibitory concentrations for *M. tuberculosis* are lowest in liquid media that are free of egg protein (7H10 or Dubos) and range from 1 to 5 µg/mL when the indirect method is used. Comparable inhibitory concentrations are obtained when 7H10 agar is used for direct susceptibility testing. When indirect susceptibility tests are performed on standard tube slants with 7H10 media, susceptible strains are inhibited by 10 to 25 µg/mL Capreomycin Sulfate. Egg-containing media, such as Lowenstein-Jensen or ATS, require concentrations of 25 to 50 µg/mL to inhibit susceptible strains.

Cross-Resistance: Frequent cross-resistance occurs between Capreomycin Sulfate and viomycin. Varying degrees of cross-resistance between Capreomycin Sulfate and kanamycin and neomycin have been reported. No cross-resistance has been observed between Capreomycin Sulfate and isoniazid, aminosalicylic acid, cycloserine, streptomycin, ethionamide, or ethambutol.

INDICATIONS AND USAGE

Capreomycin Sulfate which is to be used concomitantly with other appropriate antituberculosis agents, is indicated in pulmonary infections caused by Capreomycin Sulfate-susceptible strains of *M. tuberculosis* when the primary agents (isoniazid, rifampin, ethambutol, aminosalicylic acid, and streptomycin) have been ineffective or cannot be used because of toxicity or the presence of resistant tubercle bacilli.

Susceptibility studies should be performed to determine the presence of a Capreomycin Sulfate-susceptible strain of *M. tuberculosis.*

CONTRAINDICATION

Capreomycin Sulfate is contraindicated in patients who are hypersensitive to it.

PRECAUTIONS

General: Audiometric measurements and assessment of vestibular function should be performed prior to initiation of therapy with Capreomycin Sulfate and at regular intervals during treatment.

Renal injury, with tubular necrosis, elevation of the blood urea nitrogen (BUN) or serum creatinine, and abnormal urinary sediment, has been noted. Slight elevation of the BUN and serum creatinine has been observed in a significant number of patients receiving prolonged therapy. The appearance of casts, red cells, and white cells in the urine has been noted in a high percentage of these cases. Elevation of the BUN above 30 mg/100 mL or any other evidence of decreasing renal function with or without a rise in BUN levels calls for careful evaluation of the patient, and the dosage should be reduced or the drug completely withdrawn. The clinical significance of abnormal urine sediment and slight elevation in the BUN (or serum creatinine) observed during long-term therapy with Capreomycin Sulfate has not been established.

The peripheral neuromuscular blocking action that has been attributed to other polypeptide antibiotics (colistin sulfate, polymyxin A sulfate, paromomycin, and viomycin) and to aminoglycoside antibiotics (streptomycin, dihydrostreptomycin, neomycin, and kanamycin) has been studied with Capreomycin Sulfate. A partial neuromuscular blockade was demonstrated after large intravenous doses of Capreomycin Sulfate. This action was enhanced by ether anesthesia (as has been reported for neomycin) and was antagonized by neostigmine.

Caution should be exercised in the administration of antibiotics, including Capreomycin Sulfate, to any patient who has demonstrated some form of allergy, particularly to drugs.

Laboratory Tests: Regular tests of renal function should be made throughout the period of treatment, and reduced dosage should be employed in patients with known or suspected renal impairment.

Renal function studies should be made both before therapy with Capreomycin Sulfate is started and on a weekly basis during treatment.

Since hypokalemia may occur during therapy, serum potassium levels should be determined frequently.

Drug Interactions: For neuromuscular blocking action of this drug, *see* Precautions, General.

Carcinogenesis, Mutagenesis, Impairment of Fertility: Studies have not been performed to determine potential for carcinogenicity, mutagenicity, or impairment of fertility.

Usage in Pregnancy: Pregnancy Category C—Capreomycin Sulfate has been shown to be teratogenic in rats when given in doses 3½ times the human dose. There are no adequate and well-controlled studies in pregnant women. Capreomycin Sulfate should be used during pregnancy only if the potential benefit justifies the potential risk to the fetus (see boxed *"Warnings"* and *"Animal Pharmacology")*.

Nursing Mothers: It is not known whether this drug is excreted in human milk. Because many drugs are excreted in human milk, caution should be exercised when Capreomycin Sulfate is administered to a nursing woman.

Pediatric Use: Safety and effectiveness in children have not been established (see boxed *"Warnings."*).

ADVERSE REACTIONS

Nephrotoxicity: In 36% of 722 patients treated with Capreomycin Sulfate, elevation of the BUN above 20 mg/100 mL has been observed. In many instances, there was also depression of PSP excretion and abnormal urine sediment. In 10% of this series, the BUN elevation exceeded 30 mg/100 mL.

Toxic nephritis was reported in 1 patient with tuberculosis and portal cirrhosis who was treated with Capreomycin Sulfate (1 g) and aminosalicylic acid daily for 1 month. This patient developed renal insufficiency and oliguria and died. Autopsy showed subsiding acute tubular necrosis.

Electrolyte disturbances resembling Bartter's syndrome have been reported in 1 patient.

Ototoxicity: Subclinical auditory loss was noted in approximately 11% of 722 patients undergoing treatment with Capreomycin Sulfate. This was a 5- to 10-decibel loss in the 4,000- to 8,000-CPS range. Clinically apparent hearing loss occurred in 3% of the 722 subjects. Some audiometric changes were reversible. Other cases with permanent loss were not progressive following withdrawal of Capreomycin Sulfate.

Tinnitus and vertigo have occurred.

Liver: Serial tests of liver function have demonstrated a decrease in BSP excretion without change in AST (SGOT) or ALT (SGPT) in the presence of preexisting liver disease. Abnormal results in liver function tests have occurred in many persons receiving Capreomycin Sulfate in combination with other antituberculosis agents that also are known to cause changes in hepatic function. The role of Capreomycin Sulfate in producing these abnormalities is not clear; however, periodic determinations of liver function are recommended.

Blood: Leukocytosis and leukopenia have been observed. The majority of patients treated have had eosinophilia exceeding 5% while receiving daily injections of Capreomycin Sulfate. This has subsided with reduction of the dosage of Capreomycin Sulfate to 2 or 3 g weekly.

Pain and induration at the injection site have been observed. Excessive bleeding at the injection site has been reported. Sterile abscesses have been noted. Rare cases of thrombocytopenia have been reported.

Hypersensitivity: Urticaria and maculopapular skin rashes associated in some cases with febrile reactions have been reported when Capreomycin Sulfate and other antituberculosis drugs were given concomitantly.

OVERDOSAGE

Signs and Symptoms: Nephrotoxicity following the parenteral administration of Capreomycin Sulfate is most closely related to the area under the curve of the serum concentration versus time graph. The elderly patient, patients with abnormal renal function or dehydration, and patients receiving other nephrotoxic drugs are at much greater risk for developing acute tubular necrosis.

Damage to the auditory and vestibular divisions of cranial nerve VIII has been associated with Capreomycin Sulfate given to patients with abnormal renal function or dehydration and in those receiving medications with additive auditory toxicities. These patients often experience dizziness, tinnitus, vertigo, and a loss of high-tone acuity.

Neuromuscular blockage or respiratory paralysis may occur following rapid intravenous administration.

If Capreomycin Sulfate is ingested, toxicity would be unlikely because it is poorly absorbed (less then 1%) from an intact gastrointestinal system.

Hypokalemia, hypocalcemia, hypomagnesemia, and an electrolyte disturbance resembling Bartter's syndrome have been reported to occur in patients with Capreomycin Sulfate toxicity. The subcutaneous median lethal dose in mice was 514 mg/kg.

Treatment: To obtain up-to-date information about the treatment of overdose, a good resource is your certified Regional Poison Control Center. In managing overdosage, consider the possibility of multiple drug overdoses, interaction among drugs, and unusual drug kinetics in your patient.

Protect the patient's airway and support ventilation and perfusion. Meticulously monitor and maintain, within acceptable limits, the patient's vital signs, blood gases, serum electrolytes, etc. Absorption of drugs from the gastrointestinal tract may be decreased by giving activated charcoal, which, in many cases, is more effective than emesis or lavage; consider charcoal instead of or in addition to gastric emptying. Repeated doses of charcoal over time may hasten elimination of some drugs that have been absorbed. Safeguard the patient's airway when employing gastric emptying or charcoal.

Patients who have received an overdose of Capreomycin Sulfate and have normal renal function should be carefully hydrated to maintain a urine output of 3 to 5 mL/kg/h. Fluid balance, electrolytes, and creatinine clearance should be carefully monitored.

Hemodialysis may be effectively used to remove Capreomycin Sulfate in patients with significant renal disease.

DOSAGE AND ADMINISTRATION

Capreomycin Sulfate is for intramuscular use only.

Capreomycin Sulfate should be given by deep intramuscular injection into a large muscle mass, since superficial injection may be associated with increased pain and the development of sterile abscesses.

Capreomycin Sulfate should be dissolved in 2 mL of 0.9% Sodium Chloride Injection or Sterile Water for Injection. Two to 3 minutes should be allowed for complete dissolution. For administration of a 1-g dose, the entire contents of the vial should be given. For dosages lower than 1 g, the accompanying dilution table may be used.

DILUTION TABLE FOR CAPREOMYCIN SULFATE

Diluent Added to 1-g, 10-mL Vial	Volume of Capreomycin Sulfate Solution	Concentration (Approx)
2.15 mL	2.85 mL	350 mg*/mL
2.63 mL	3.33 mL	300 mg*/mL
3.3 mL	4 mL	250 mg*/mL
4.3 mL	5 mL	200 mg*/mL

*   *Equivalent to Capreomycin activity.*

The solution may acquire a pale straw color and darken with time, but this is not associated with loss of potency or the development of toxicity. After reconstitution, solutions of Capreomycin. Sulfate may be stored for 48 hours at room temperature and up to 14 days under refrigeration.

Capreomycin Sulfate is always administered in combination with at least 1 other antituberculosis agent to which the patient's strain of tubercle bacilli is susceptible. The usual dose is 1 g daily (not to exceed 20 mg/kg/day) given intramuscularly for 60 to 120 days, followed by 1 g intramuscularly 2 or 3 times weekly. (*Note*—Therapy for tuberculosis should be maintained for 12 to 24 months. If facilities for administering injectable medication are not available, a change to appropriate oral therapy is indicated on the patient's release from the hospital.)

Patients with reduced renal function should have dosage reduction based on creatinine clearance using the guidelines included in Table 1. These dosages are designed to achieve a mean steady-state Capreomycin level of 10 μg/mL.

Table 1

ESTIMATED DOSAGES TO ATTAIN MEAN STEADY-STATE SERUM CAPREOMYCIN SULFATE CONCENTRATION OF 10 μg/mL (BASED ON CREATININE CLEARANCE)

CrCl (mL/min)	Capreomycin Sulfate Clearance (L/kg/h × 10^{-2})	Half-life (hours)	Dose^a (mg/kg) for the Following Dosing Intervals 24h	48h	72h
0	0.54	55.5	1.29	2.58	3.87
10	1.01	29.4	2.43	4.87	7.30
20	1.49	20.0	3.58	7.16	10.7
30	1.97	15.1	4.72	9.45	14.2
40	2.45	12.2	5.87	11.7	
50	2.92	10.2	7.01	14.0	
60	3.40	8.8	8.16		
80	4.35	6.8	10.4^b		
100	5.31	5.6	12.7^b		
110	5.78	5.2	13.9^b		

^{a} —For patients with renal impairment, initial maintenance dose estimates are given for optional dosing intervals; longer dosing intervals are expected to provide greater peak and lower trough serum Capreomycin Sulfate levels than shorter dosing intervals.

^{b} —The usual dosage for patients with normal renal function is 1,000 mg daily, not to exceed 20 mg/kg/day, for 60 to 120 days, then 1,000 mg 2 to 3 times weekly.

ANIMAL PHARMACOLOGY
In addition to renal and cranial nerve VIII toxicity demonstrated in animal toxicology studies, cataracts developed in 2 dogs on doses of 62 mg/kg and 100 mg/kg for prolonged periods.

In teratology studies, a low incidence of "wavy ribs" was noted in litters of female rats treated with daily doses of 50 mg/kg or more of Capreomycin Sulfate.

HOW SUPPLIED
POWDER FOR INJECTION: 1 GM

BRAND/MANUFACTURER	NDC	SIZE	AWP
○ BRAND			
CAPASTAT SULFATE: Lilly	00002-1485-01	1s	$20.86

Captopril

DESCRIPTION
Captopril is a specific competitive inhibitor of angiotensin I-converting enzyme (ACE), the enzyme responsible for the conversion of angiotensin I to angiotensin II. Captopril is designated chemically as 1-[(2S)-3-mercapto-2-methylpropionyl]-L-proline [MW 217.29].

Captopril is a white to off-white crystalline powder that may have a slight sulfurous odor; it is soluble in water (approx. 160 mg/mL), methanol, and ethanol and sparingly soluble in chloroform and ethyl acetate.

Captopril is available in potencies of 12.5 mg 25 mg, 50 mg, and 100 mg as scored tablets for oral administration.

Following is its chemical structure:

CLINICAL PHARMACOLOGY
MECHANISM OF ACTION
The mechanism of action of Captopril has not yet been fully elucidated. Its beneficial effects in hypertension and heart failure appear to result primarily from suppression of the renin-angiotensin-aldosterone system. However, there is no consistent correlation between renin levels and response to the drug. Renin, an enzyme synthesized by the kidneys, is released into the circulation where it acts on a plasma globulin substrate to produce angiotensin I, a relatively inactive decapeptide. Angiotensin I is then converted by angiotensin converting enzyme (ACE) to angiotensin II, a potent endogenous vasoconstrictor substance. Angiotensin II also stimulates aldosterone secretion from the adrenal cortex, thereby contributing to sodium and fluid retention.

Captopril prevents the conversion of angiotensin I to angiotensin II by inhibition of ACE, a peptidyldipeptide carboxy hydrolase. This inhibition has been demonstrated in both healthy human subjects and in animals by showing that the elevation of blood pressure caused by exogenously administered angiotensin I was attenuated or abolished by Captopril. In animal studies, Captopril did not alter the pressor responses to a number of other agents, including angiotensin II and norepinephrine, indicating specificity of action.

ACE is identical to "bradykininase", and Captopril may also interfere with the degradation of the vasodepressor peptide, bradykinin. Increased concentrations of bradykinin or prostaglandin E_2 may also have a role in the therapeutic effect of Captopril.

Inhibition of ACE results in decreased plasma angiotensin II and increased plasma renin activity (PRA), the latter resulting from loss of negative feedback on renin release caused by reduction in angiotensin II. The reduction of angiotensin II leads to decreased aldosterone secretion, and, as a result, small increases in serum potassium may occur along with sodium and fluid loss.

The antihypertensive effects persist for a longer period of time than does demonstrable inhibition of circulating ACE. It is not known whether the ACE present in vascular endothelium is inhibited longer than the ACE in circulating blood.

PHARMACOKINETICS
After oral administration of therapeutic doses of Captopril, rapid absorption occurs with peak blood levels at about one hour. The presence of food in the gastrointestinal tract reduces absorption by about 30 to 40 percent; Captopril therefore should be given one hour before meals. Based on carbon-14 labeling, average minimal absorption is approximately 75 percent. In a 24-hour period, over 95 percent of the absorbed dose is eliminated in the urine; 40 to 50 percent is unchanged drug; most of the remainder is the disulfide dimer of Captopril and Captopril-cysteine disulfide.

Approximately 25 to 30 percent of the circulating drug is bound to plasma proteins. The apparent elimination half-life for total radioactivity in blood is probably less than 3 hours. An accurate determination of half-life of unchanged Captopril is not, at present, possible, but it is probably less than 2 hours. In patients with renal impairment, however, retention of Captopril occurs (see *"Dosage and Administration"*).

PHARMACODYNAMICS
Administration of Captopril results in a reduction of peripheral arterial resistance in hypertensive patients with either no change, or an increase, in cardiac output. There is an increase in renal blood flow following administration of Captopril and glomerular filtration rate is usually unchanged.

Reductions of blood pressure are usually maximal 60 to 90 minutes after oral administration of an individual dose of Captopril. The duration of effect is dose related. The reduction in blood pressure may be progressive, so to achieve maximal therapeutic effects, several weeks of therapy may be required. The blood pressure lowering effects of Captopril and thiazide-type diuretics are additive. In contrast, Captopril and beta-blockers have a less than additive effect.

Blood pressure is lowered to about the same extent in both standing and supine positions. Orthostatic effects and tachycardia are infrequent but may occur in volume-depleted patients. Abrupt withdrawal of Captopril has not been associated with a rapid increase in blood pressure.

In patients with heart failure, significantly decreased peripheral (systemic vascular) resistance and blood pressure (afterload), reduced pulmonary capillary wedge pressure (preload) and pulmonary vascular resistance, increased cardiac output, and increased exercise tolerance time (ETT) have been demonstrated. These hemodynamic and clinical effects occur after the first dose and appear to persist for the duration of therapy. Placebo controlled studies of 12 weeks duration in patients who did not respond adequately to diuretics and digitalis show no tolerance to beneficial effects on ETT; open studies, with exposure up to 18 months in some cases, also indicate that ETT benefit is maintained. Clinical improvement has been observed in some patients where acute hemodynamic effects were minimal.

The Survival and Ventricular Enlargement (SAVE) study was a multicenter, randomized, double-blind, placebo-controlled trial conducted in 2,231 patients (age 21-79 years) who survived the acute phase of a myocardial infarction and did not have active ischemia. Patients had left ventricular dysfunction (LVD), defined as a resting left ventricular ejection fraction $\leq$ 40%, but at the time of randomization were not sufficiently symptomatic to require ACE inhibitor therapy for heart failure. About half of the patients had had symptoms of heart failure in the past. Patients were given a test dose of 6.25 mg oral Captopril and were randomized within 3-16 days post-infarction to receive either Captopril or placebo in addition to conventional therapy. Captopril was initiated at 6.25 mg or 12.5 mg tid and after two weeks titrated to a target maintenance dose of 50 mg tid. About 80% of patients were receiving the target dose at the end of the study. Patients were followed for a minimum of two years and for up to five years, with an average follow-up of 3.5 years.

Baseline blood pressure was 113/70 mm Hg and 112/70 mm Hg for the placebo and Captopril groups, respectively. Blood pressure increased slightly in both treatment groups during the study and was somewhat lower in the Captopril group (119/74 vs. 125/77 mm Hg at 1 yr).

Therapy with Captopril improved long-term survival and clinical outcomes compared to placebo. The risk reduction for all cause mortality was 19% (P = 0.02) and for cardiovascular death was 21% (P = 0.014). Captopril treated subjects had 22% (P = 0.034) fewer first hospitalizations for heart failure. Compared to placebo, 22% fewer patients receiving Captopril developed symptoms of overt heart failure. There was no significant difference between groups in total hospitalizations for all causes (2056 placebo; 2036 Captopril).

Captopril was well tolerated in the presence of other therapies such as aspirin, beta blockers, nitrates, vasodilators, calcium antagonists and diuretics.

In a multicenter, double-blind, placebo controlled trial, 409 patients, age 18-49 of either gender, with or without hypertension, with type I (juvenile type, onset before age 30) insulin-dependent diabetes mellitus, retinopahy, proteinuria > 500 mg per day and serum creatinine $\leq$ 2.5 mg/dL, were randomized to placebo or Captopril (25 mg tid) and followed for up to 4.8 years (median 3 years). To achieve blood pressure control, additional antihypertensive agents (diuretics, beta blockers, centrally acting agents, or vasodilators) were added as needed for patients in both groups.

The Captopril group had a 51% reduction in risk of doubling of serum creatinine (P < 0.01) and a 51% reduction in risk for the combined endpoint of end-stage renal disease (dialysis or transplantation) or death (P < 0.01). Captopril treatment resulted in a 30% reduction in urine protein excretion within the first 3 months (P < 0.05), which was maintained throughout the trial. The Captopril group had somewhat better blood pressure control than the placebo group, but the effects of Captopril on renal function were greater than would be expected from the group differences in blood pressure reduction alone. Captopril was well-tolerated in this patient population.

In two multicenter, double-blind, placebo controlled studies, a total of 235 normotensive patients with insulin-dependent diabetes mellitus, retinopathy and microalbuminuria (20-200 µg/min) were randomized to placebo or Captopril (50 mg bid) and followed for up to 2 years. Captopril delayed the progression to overt nephropathy (proteinuria $\geq$ 500 mg/day) in both studies (risk reduction 67% to 76%; P < 0.05). Captopril also reduced the albumin excretion rate. However, the long term clinical benefit of reducing the progression from microalbuminuria to proteinuria has not been established.

Studies in rats and cats indicate that Captopril does not cross the blood-brain barrier to any significant extent.

INDICATIONS AND USAGE

Hypertension: Captopril is indicated for the treatment of hypertension.

In using Captopril, consideration should be given to the risk of neutropenia/agranulocytosis (See "Warnings").

Captopril may be used as initial therapy for patients with normal renal function, in whom the risk is relatively low. In patients with impaired renal function, particularly those with collagen vascular disease, Captopril should be reserved for hypertensives who have either developed unacceptable side effects on other drugs, or have failed to respond satisfactorily to drug combinations.

Captopril is effective alone and in combination with other antihypertensive agents, especially thiazide-type diuretics. The blood pressure lowering effects of Captopril and thiazides are approximately additive.

Heart Failure: Captopril is indicated in the treatment of congestive heart failure in combination with diuretics and digitalis. The beneficial effect of Captopril in heart failure does not require the presence of digitalis, however, most controlled clinical trial experience with Captopril has been in patients receiving digitalis, as well as diuretic treatment.

Left Ventricular Dysfunction After Myocardial Infarction: Captopril is indicated to improve survival following myocardial infarction in clinically stable patients with left ventricular dysfunction manifested as an ejection fraction $\leq$ 40% and to reduce the incidence of overt heart failure and subsequent hospitalizations for congestive heart failure in these patients.

Diabetic Nephropathy: Captopril is indicated for the treatment of diabetic nephropathy (proteinuria > 500 mg/day) in patients with type I insulin-dependent diabetes mellitus and retinopathy. Captopril decreases the rate of progression of renal insufficiency and development of serious adverse clinical outcomes (death or need for renal transplantation or dialysis).

UNLABELED USES

Captopril is used alone or as an adjunct in the treatment of angina, idiopathic edema, hypertension associated with scleroderma, renal crisis, and hypertensive crisis. It is also used for the relief of symptoms associated with Raynaud's syndrome, Barter's syndrome, and rheumatoid arthritis.

CONTRAINDICATIONS

Captopril is contraindicated in patients who are hypersensitive to this product or any other angiotensin-converting enzyme inhibitor (e.g., a patient who has experienced angioedema during therapy with any other ACE inhibitor).

WARNINGS

ANGIOEDEMA

Angioedema involving the extremities, face, lips, mucous membranes, tongue, glottis or larynx has been seen in patients treated with ACE inhibitors, including Captopril. If angioedema involves the tongue, glottis or larynx, airway obstruction may occur and be fatal. Emergency therapy, including but not necessarily limited to, subcutaneous administration of a 1:1000 solution of epinephrine should be promptly instituted.

Swelling confined to the face, mucous membranes of the mouth, lips and extremities has usually resolved with discontinuation of Captopril; some cases required medical therapy. (See *"Precautions: Information for Patients"* and *"Adverse Reactions".*)

NEUTROPENIA/AGRANULOCYTOSIS

Neutropenia (<1000/mm³) with myeloid hypoplasia has resulted from use of Captopril. About half of the neutropenic patients developed systemic or oral cavity infections or other features of the syndrome of agranulocytosis.

The risk of neutropenia is dependent on the clinical status of the patient:

- In clinical trials in patients with hypertension who have normal renal function (serum creatinine less than 1.6 mg/dL and no collagen vascular disease), neutropenia has been seen in one patient out of over 8,600 exposed.
- In patients with some degree of renal failure (serum creatinine at least 1.6 mg/dL) but no collagen vascular disease, the risk of neutropenia in clinical trials was about 1 per 500, a frequency over 15 times that for uncomplicated hypertension. Daily doses of Captopril were relatively high in these patients, particularly in view of their diminished renal function. In foreign marketing experience in patients with renal failure, use of allopurinol concomitantly with Captopril has been associated with neutropenia but this association has not appeared in U.S. reports.
- In patients with collagen vascular diseases (e.g., systemic lupus erythematosus, scleroderma) and impaired renal function, neutropenia occurred in 3.7 percent of patients in clinical trials.
- While none of the over 750 patients in formal clinical trials of heart failure developed neutropenia, it has occurred during the subsequent clinical experience. About half of the reported cases had serum creatinine $\geq$ 1.6 mg/dL and more than 75 percent were in patients also receiving procainamide. In heart failure, it appears that the same risk factors for neutropenia are present.

The neutropenia has usually been detected within three months after Captopril was started. Bone marrow examinations in patients with neutropenia consistently showed myeloid hypoplasia, frequently accompanied by erythroid hypoplasia and decreased numbers of megakaryocytes (e.g., hypoplastic bone marrow and pancytopenia); anemia and thrombocytopenia were sometimes seen.

In general, neutrophils returned to normal in about two weeks after Captopril was discontinued, and serious infections were limited to clinically complex patients. About 13 percent of the cases of neutropenia have ended fatally, but almost all fatalities were in patients with serious illness, having collagen vascular disease, renal failure, heart failure or immunosuppressant therapy, or a combination of these complicating factors.

Evaluation of the Hypertensive or Heart Failure Patient Should Always Include Assessment of Renal Function

If Captopril is used in patients with impaired renal function, white blood cell and differential counts should be evaluated prior to starting treatment and at approximately two-week intervals for about three months, then periodically.

In patients with collagen vascular disease or who are exposed to other drugs known to affect the white cells or immune response, particularly when there is impaired renal function, Captopril should be used only after an assessment of benefit and risk, and then with caution.

All patients treated with Captopril should be told to report any signs of infection (e.g., sore throat, fever). If infection is suspected, white cell counts should be performed without delay.

Since discontinuation of Captopril and other drugs has generally led to prompt return of the white count to normal, upon confirmation of neutropenia (neutrophil count < 1000/mm³) the physician should withdraw Captopril and closely follow the patient's course.

PROTEINURIA

Total urinary proteins greater than 1g per day were seen in about 0.7 percent of patients receiving Captopril. About 90 percent of affected patients had evidence of prior renal disease or received relatively high doses of Captopril (in excess of 150 mg/day), or both. The nephrotic syndrome occurred in about one-fifth of proteinuric patients. In most cases, proteinuria subsided or cleared within six months whether or not Captopril was continued. Parameters of renal function, such as BUN and creatinine, were seldom altered in the patients with proteinuria.

HYPOTENSION

Excessive hypotension was rarely seen in hypertensive patients but is a possible consequence of Captopril use in salt/volume depleted persons (such as those treated vigorously with diuretics), patients with heart failure or those patients undergoing renal dialysis. (See *"Precautions: Drug Interactions."*)

In heart failure, where the blood pressure was either normal or low, transient decreases in mean blood pressure greater than 20 percent were recorded in about half of the patients. This transient hypotension is more likely to occur after any of the first several doses and is usually well tolerated, producing either no symptoms or brief mild lightheadedness, although in rare instances it has been associated with arrhythmia or conduction defects. Hypotension was the reason for discontinuation of drug in 3.6 percent of patients with heart failure.

BECAUSE OF THE POTENTIAL FALL IN BLOOD PRESSURE IN THESE PATIENTS, THERAPY SHOULD BE STARTED UNDER VERY CLOSE MEDICAL SUPERVISION.

A starting dose of 6.25 or 12.5 mg tid may minimize the hypotensive effect. Patients should be followed closely for the first two weeks of treatment and whenever the dose of Captopril and/or diuretic is increased. In patients with heart failure, reducing the dose of diuretic, if feasible, may minimize the fall in blood pressure.

Hypotension is not *per se* a reason to discontinue Captopril. Some decrease of systemic blood pressure is a common and desirable observation upon initiation of Captopril treatment in heart failure. The magnitude of the decrease is greatest early in the course of treatment; this effect stabilizes within a week or two, and generally returns to pretreatment levels, without a decrease in therapeutic efficacy, within two months.

FETAL/NEONATAL MORBIDITY AND MORTALITY

ACE inhibitors can cause fetal and neonatal morbidity and death when administered to pregnant women. Several dozen cases have been reported in the world literature. When pregnancy is detected, ACE inhibitors should be discontinued as soon as possible.

The use of ACE inhibitors during the second and third trimesters of pregnancy has been associated with fetal and neonatal injury, including hypotension, neonatal skull hypoplasia, anuria, reversible or irreversible renal failure, and death. Oligohydramnios has also been reported, presumably resulting from decreased fetal renal function; oligohydramnios in this setting has been associated with fetal limb contractures, craniofacial deformation, and hypoplastic lung development. Prematurity, intrauterine growth retardation, and patent ductus arteriosus have also been reported, although it is not clear whether these occurrences were due to the ACE-inhibitor exposure.

These adverse effects do not appear to have resulted from intrauterine ACE-inhibitor exposure that has been limited to the first trimester. Mothers whose embryos and fetuses are exposed to ACE inhibitors only during the first trimester should be so informed. Nonetheless, when patients become pregnant, physicians should make every effort to discontinue the use of Captopril as soon as possible.

Rarely (probably less often than once in every thousand pregnancies), no alternative to ACE inhibitors will be found. In these rare cases, the mothers should be apprised of the potential hazards to their fetuses, and serial ultrasound examinations should be performed to assess the intraamniotic environment.

If oligohydramnios is observed, Captopril should be discontinued unless it is considered life-saving for the mother. Contraction stress testing (CST), a non-stress test (NST), or biophysical profiling (BPP) may be appropriate, depending upon the week of pregnancy. Patients and physicians should be aware, however, that oligohydramnios may not appear until after the fetus has sustained irreversible injury.

Infants with histories of *in utero* exposure to ACE inhibitors should be closely observed for hypotension, oliguria, and hyperkalemia. If oliguria occurs, attention should be directed toward support of blood pressure and renal perfusion. Exchange transfusion or dialysis may be required as a means of reversing hypotension and/or substituting for disordered renal function. While Captopril may be removed from the adult circulatin by hemodialysis, there is inadequate data concerning the effectiveness of hemodialysis for removing it from the circulation of neonates or children. Peritoneal dialysis is not effective for removing Captopril; there is no information concerning exchange transfusion for removing Captopril from the general circulation.

When Captopril was given to rabbits at doses about 0.8 to 70 times (on a mg/kg basis) the maximum recommended human dose, low incidences of craniofacial malformations were seen. No teratogenic effects of Captopril were seen in studies of pregnant rats and hamsters. One a mg/kg basis, the doses used were up to 150 times (in hamsters) and 625 times (in rats) the maximum recommended human dose.

HEPATIC FAILURE

Rarely, ACE inhibitors have been associated with a syndrome that starts with cholestatic jaundice and progresses to fulminant hepatic necrosis and (sometimes) death. The mechanism of this syndrome is not understood. Patients receiving ACE inhibitors who develop jaundice or marked elevations of hepatic enzymes should discontinue the ACE inhibitor and receive appropriate medical follow-up.

PRECAUTIONS

GENERAL

Impaired Renal Function: Hypertension—Some patients with renal disease, particularly those with severe renal artery stenosis, have developed increases in BUN and serum creatinine after reduction of blood pressure with Captopril. Captopril dosage reduction and/or discontinuation of diuretic may be required. For some of these patients, it may not be possible to normalize blood pressure and maintain adequate renal perfusion.

Heart Failure—About 20 percent of patients develop stable elevations of BUN and serum creatinine greater than 20 percent above normal or baseline upon long-term treatment with Captopril. Less than 5 percent of patients, generally those with severe preexisting renal disease, required discontinuation of treatment due to progressively increasing creatinine; subsequent improvement probably depends upon the severity of the underlying renal disease. See *"Clinical Pharmacology," "Dosage and Administration," "Adverse Reactions: Altered Laboratory Findings."*

Hyperkalemia: Elevations in serum potassium have been observed in some patients treated with ACE inhibitors, including Captopril. When treated with ACE inhibitors, patients at risk for the development of hyperkalemia include those with: renal insufficiency; diabetes mellitus; and those using concomitant potassium-sparing diuretics, potassium supplements or potassium-containing salt substitutes; or other drugs associated with increases in serum potassium. In a trial of type I diabetic patients with proteinuria, the incidence of withdrawal of treatment with Captopril for hyperkalemia was 2% (4/207). In two trials of normotensive type I diabetic patients with microalbuminuria, no Captopril group subjects had hyperkalemia (0/116). (See *"Precautions: Information for Patients"* and *"Drug Interactions;" "Adverse Reactions: Altered Laboratory Findings."*)

Cough: Cough has been reported with the use of ACE inhibitors. Characteristically, the cough is nonproductive, persistent and resolves after discontinuation of therapy. ACE inhibitor-induced cough should be considered as part of the differential diagnosis of cough.

Valvular Stenosis: There is concern, on theoretical grounds, that patients with aortic stenosis might be at particular risk of decreased coronary perfusion when treated with vasodilators because they do not develop as much afterload reduction as others.

Surgery/Anesthesia: In patients undergoing major surgery or during anesthesia with agents that produce hypotension, Captopril will block angiotensin II formation secondary to compensatory renin release. If hypotension occurs and is considered to be due to this mechanism, it can be corrected by volume expansion.

HEMODIALYSIS

Recent clinical observations have shown an association of hypersensitivity-like (anaphylactoid) reactions during hemodialysis with high-flux dialysis membranes (e.g., AN69) in patients receiving ACE inhibitors. In these patients, consideration should be given to using a different type of dialysis membrane or a different class of medication.

INFORMATION FOR PATIENTS

Patients should be advised to immediately report to their physician any signs or symptoms suggesting angioedema (e.g., swelling of face, eyes, lips, tongue, larynx and extremities; difficulty in swallowing or breathing; hoarseness) and to discontinue therapy. (See *"Warnings."*)

Patients should be told to report promptly any indication of infection (e.g., sore throat, fever), which may be a sign of neutropenia, or of progressive edema which might be related to proteinuria and nephrotic syndrome.

All patients should be cautioned that excessive perspiration and dehydration may lead to an excessive fall in blood pressure because of reduction in fluid volume. Other causes of volume depletion such as vomiting or diarrhea may also lead to a fall in blood pressure; patients should be advised to consult with the physician.

Patients should be advised not to use potassium-sparing diuretics, potassium supplements or potassium-containing salt substitutes without consulting their physician. (See *"Precautions: General"* and *"Drug Interactions;" "Adverse Reactions."*)

Patients should be warned against interruption or discontinuation of medication unless instructed by the physician. Heart failure patients on Captopril therapy should be cautioned against rapid increases in physical activity.

Patients should be informed that Captopril should be taken one hour before meals (see *"Dosage and Administration"*).

PREGNANCY

Female patients of childbearing age should be told about the consequences of second- and third-trimester exposure to ACE inhibitors, and they should also be told that these consequences do not appear to have resulted from intrauterine ACE-inhibitor exposure that has been limited to the first trimester. These patients should be asked to report pregnancies to their physicians as soon as possible.

DRUG INTERACTIONS

Hypotension—Patients on Diuretic Therapy: Patients on diuretics and especially those in whom diuretic therapy was recently instituted, as well as those on severe dietary salt restriction or dialysis, may occasionally experience a precipitous reduction of blood pressure usually within the first hour after receiving the initial dose of Captopril.

The possibility of hypotensive effects with Captopril can be minimized by either discontinuing the diuretic or increasing the salt intake approximately one week prior to initiation of treatment with Captopril or initiating therapy with small doses (6.25 or 12.5 mg). Alternatively, provide medical supervision for at least one hour after the initial dose. If hypotension occurs, the patient should be placed in a supine position and, if necessary, receive an intravenous infusion of normal saline. This transient hypotensive response is not a contraindication to further doses which can be given without difficulty once the blood pressure has increased after volume expansion.

Agents Having Vasodilator Activity: Data on the effect of concomitant use of other vasodilators in patients receiving Captopril for heart failure are not available; therefore, nitroglycerin or other nitrates (as used for management of angina) or other drugs having vasodilator activity should, if possible, be discontinued before starting Captopril. If resumed during Captopril therapy, such agents should be administered cautiously, and perhaps at lower dosage.

Agents Causing Renin Release: Captopril's effect will be augmented by antihypertensive agents that cause renin release. For example, diuretics (e.g., thiazides) may activate the renin-angiotensin-aldosterone system.

Agents Affecting Sympathetic Activity: The sympathetic nervous system may be especially important in supporting blood pressure in patients receiving Captopril alone or with diuretics. Therefore, agents affecting sympathetic activity (e.g., ganglionic blocking agents or adrenergic neuron blocking agents) should be used with caution. Beta-adrenergic blocking drugs add some further antihypertensive effect to Captopril, but the overall response is less than additive.

Agents Increasing Serum Potassium: Since Captopril decreases aldosterone production, elevation of serum potassium may occur. Potassium-sparing diuretics such as spironolactone, triamterene, or amiloride, or potassium supplements should be given only for documented hypokalemia, and then with caution, since they may lead to a significant increase of serum potassium. Salt substitutes containing potassium should also be used with caution.

Inhibitors Of Endogenous Prostaglandin Synthesis: It has been reported that indomethacin may reduce the antihypertensive effect of Captopril, especially in cases of low renin hypertension. Other nonsteroidal anti-inflammatory agents (e.g., aspirin) may also have this effect.

Lithium: Increased serum lithium levels and symptoms of lithium toxicity have been reported in patients receiving concomitant lithium and ACE inhibitor therapy. These drugs should be coadministered with caution and frequent monitoring of serum lithium levels is recommended. If a diuretic is also used, it may increase the risk of lithium toxicity.

DRUG/LABORATORY TEST INTERACTION
Captopril may cause a false-positive urine test for acetone.

CARCINOGENESIS, MUTAGENESIS AND IMPAIRMENT OF FERTILITY
Two-year studies with doses of 50 to 1350 mg/kg/day in mice and rats failed to show any evidence of carcinogenic potential. The high dose in these studies is 150 times the maximum recommended human dose of 450 mg, assuming a 50-kg subject. On a body-surface-area basis, the high doses for mice and rats are 13 and 26 times the maximum recommended human dose, respectively.

Studies in rats have revealed no impairment of fertility.

ANIMAL TOXICOLOGY
Chronic oral toxicity studies were conducted in rats (2 years), dogs (47 weeks; 1 year), mice (2 years), and monkeys (1 year). Significant drug-related toxicity included effects on hematopoiesis, renal toxicity, erosion/ulceration of the stomach, and variation of retinal blood vessels.

Reductions in hemoglobin and/or hematocrit values were seen in mice, rats, and monkeys at doses 50 to 150 times the maximum recommended human dose (MRHD) of 450 mg, assuming a 50-mg subject. On a body-surface-area, these doses are 5 to 25 times maximum recommended human dose (MRHD). Anemia, leukopenia, thrombocytopenia, and bone marrow suppression occurred in dogs at doses 8 to 30 times MRHD on a body-weight basis (4 to 15 times MRHD on a surface-area basis). The reductions in hemoglobin and hematocrit values in rats and mice were only significant at 1 year and returned to normal with continued dosing by the end of the study. Marked anemia was seen at all dose levels (8 to 30 times MRHD) in dogs, whereas moderate to marked leukopenia was noted only at 15 and 30 times MRHD and thrombocytopenia at 30 times MRHD. The anemia could be reversed upon discontinuation of dosing. Bone marrow suppression occurred to a varying degree, being associated only with dogs that died or were sacrificed in a moribund condition in the 1-year study. However, in the 47-week study at a dose 30 times MRHD, bone marrow suppression was found to be reversible upon continued drug administration.

Captopril caused hyperplasia of the juxtaglomerular apparatus of the kidneys in mice and rats at doses 7 to 200 times MRHD on a body-weight basis (0.6 to 35 times MRHD on a surface-area basis); in monkeys at 20 to 60 times MRHD on a body-weight basis (7 to 20 times MRHD on a surface-area basis); and in dogs at 30 times MRHD on a body-weight basis (15 times MRHD on a surface-area basis).

Gastric erosions/ulcerations were increased in incidence in male rats at 20 to 200 times MRHD on a body-weight basis (3.5 and 35 times MRHD on a surface-area basis); in dogs at 30 times MRHD on a body-weight basis (15 times MRHD on a surface-area basis); and in monkeys at 65 times MRHD on a body-weight basis (20 times MRHD on a surface-area basis). Rabbits developed gastric and intestinal ulcers when given oral doses approximately 30 times MRHD on a body-weight basis (10 times MRHD on a surface-area basis) for only 5 to 7 days.

In the two-year rat study, irreversible and progressive variations in the caliber of retinal vessels (focal sacculations and constrictions) occurred at all dose levels (7 to 200 times MRHD) on a body-weight basis; 1 to 35 times MRHD on a surface-area basis in a dose-related fashion. The effect was first observed in the 88th week of dosing, with a progressively increased incidence thereafter, even after cessation of dosing.

PREGNANCY CATEGORIES C (FIRST TRIMESTER) AND D (SECOND AND THIRD TRIMESTERS)
See *"Warnings: Fetal/Neonatal Morbidity and Mortality."*

NURSING MOTHERS
Concentrations of Captopril in human milk are approximately one percent of those in maternal blood. Because of the potential for serious adverse reactions in nursing infants from Captopril, a decision should be made whether to discontinue nursing or to discontinue the drug, taking into account the importance of Captopril to the mother. (See *"Precautions: Pediatric Use."*)

PEDIATRIC USE
Safety and effectiveness in children have not been established. There is limited experience reported in the literature with the use of Captopril in the pediatric population; dosage, on a weight basis, was generally reported to be comparable to or less than that used in adults.

Infants, especially newborns, may be more susceptible to the adverse hemodynamic effects of Captopril. Excessive, prolonged and unpredictable decreases in blood pressure and associated complications, including oliguria and seizures, have been reported.

Captopril should be used in children only if other measures for controlling blood pressure have not been effective.

ADVERSE REACTIONS
Reported incidences are based on clinical trials involving approximately 7000 patients.

Renal: About one of 100 patients developed proteinuria (see *"Warnings"*).

Each of the following has been reported in approximately 1 to 2 of 1000 patients and are of uncertain relationship to drug use: renal insufficiency, renal failure, nephrotic syndrome, polyuria, oliguria, and urinary frequency.

Hematologic: Neutropenia/agranulocytosis has occurred (see *"Warnings"*). Cases of anemia, thrombocytopenia, and pancytopenia have been reported.

Dermatologic: Rash, often with pruritus, and sometimes with fever, arthralgia, and eosinophilia, occurred in about 4 to 7 (depending on renal status and dose) of 100 patients, usually during the first four weeks of therapy. It is usually maculopapular, and rarely urticarial. The rash is usually mild and disappears within a few days of dosage reduction, short-term treatment with an antihistaminic agent, and/or discontinuing therapy; remission may occur even if Captopril is continued. Pruritus, without rash, occurs in about 2 of 100 patients. Between 7 and 10 percent of patients with skin rash have shown an eosinophilia and/or positive ANA titers. A reversible associated pemphigoid-like lesion, and photosensitivity, have also been reported.

Flushing or pallor has been reported in 2 to 5 of 1000 patients.

Cardiovascular: Hypotension may occur; see *"Warnings and Precautions: Drug Interactions"* for discussion of hypotension with Captopril therapy.

Tachycardia, chest pain, and palpitations have each been observed in approximately 1 of 100 patients.

Angina pectoris, myocardial infarction, Raynaud's syndrome, and congestive heart failure have each occurred in 2 to 3 of 1000 patients.

Dysgeusia: Approximately 2 to 4 (depending on renal status and dose) of 100 patients developed a diminution or loss of taste perception. Taste impairment is reversible and usually self-limited (2 to 3 months) even with continued drug administration. Weight loss may be associated with the loss of taste.

Angioedema: Angioedema involving the extremities, face, lips, mucous membranes, tongue, glottis or larynx has been reported in approximately one in 1000 patients. Angioedema involving the upper airways has caused fatal airway obstruction. (See *"Warnings and Precautions: Information for Patients."*)

Cough: Cough has been reported in 0.5-2% of patients treated with Captopril in clinical trials (see *"Precautions: General, Cough"*).

The following have been reported in about 0.5 to 2 percent of patients but did not appear at increased frequency compared to placebo or other treatments used in controlled trials: gastric irritation, abdominal pain, nausea, vomiting, diarrhea, anorexia, constipation, aphthous ulcers, peptic ulcer, dizziness, headache, malaise, fatigue, insomnia, dry mouth, dyspnea, alopecia, paresthesias.

Other clinical adverse effects reported since the drug was marketed are listed below by body system. In this setting, an incidence or causal relationship cannot be accurately determined.

Body as a Whole: Anaphylactoid reactions (see *"Precautions: Hemodialysis"*).

General: Asthenia, gynecomastia.

Cardiovascular: Cardiac arrest, cerebrovascular accident/insufficiency, rhythm disturbances, orthostatic hypotension, syncope.

Dermatologic: Bullous pemphigus, erythema multiforme (including Stevens-Johnson syndrome), exfoliative dermatitis.

Gastrointestinal: Pancreatitis, glossitis, dyspepsia.

Hematologic: Anemia, including aplastic and hemolytic.

➤ SHOWN IN PRODUCT IDENTIFICATION GUIDE

Hepatobiliary: Jaundice, hepatitis, including rare cases of necrosis, cholestasis.

Metabolic: Symptomatic hyponatremia.

Musculoskeletal: Myalgia, myasthenia.

Nervous/Psychiatric: Ataxia, confusion, depression, nervousness, somnolence.

Respiratory: Bronchospasm, eosinophilic pneumonitis, rhinitis.

Special Senses: Blurred vision.

Urogenital: Impotence.

As with other ACE inhibitors, a syndrome has been reported which may include: fever, myalgia, arthralgia, interstitial nephritis, vasculitis, rash or other dermatologic manifestations, eosinophilia and an elevated ESR.

FETAL/NEONATAL MORBIDITY AND MORTALITY
See *"Warnings: Fetal/Neonatal Morbidity and Mortality."*

ALTERED LABORATORY FINDINGS
Serum Electrolytes: Hyperkalemia: small increases in serum potassium, especially in patients with renal impairment (see *"Precautions"*).

Hyponatremia: particularly in patients receiving a low sodium diet or concomitant diuretics.

BUN/Serum Creatinine: Transient elevations of BUN or serum creatinine especially in volume or salt depleted patients or those with renovascular hypertension may occur. Rapid reduction of longstanding or markedly elevated blood pressure can result in decreases in the glomerular filtration rate and, in turn, lead to increases in BUN or serum creatinine.

Hematologic: A positive ANA has been reported.

Liver Function Tests: Elevations of liver transaminases, alkaline phosphatase, and serum bilirubin have occurred.

OVERDOSAGE
Correction of hypotension would be of primary concern. Volume expansion with an intravenous infusion of normal saline is the treatment of choice for restoration of blood pressure.

While Captopril may be removed from the adult circulation by hemodialysis, there is inadequate data concerning the effectiveness of hemodialysis for removing it from the circulation of neonates or children. Peritoneal dialysis is not effective for removing Captopril; there is no information concerning exchange transfusion for removing Captopril from the general circulation.

DOSAGE AND ADMINISTRATION
Captopril should be taken one hour before meals. Dosage must be individualized.

Hypertension: Initiation of therapy requires consideration of recent antihypertensive drug treatment, the extent of blood pressure elevation, salt restriction, and other clinical circumstances. If possible, discontinue the patient's previous antihypertensive drug regimen for one week before starting Captopril.

The initial dose of Captopril is 25 mg bid or tid. If satisfactory reduction of blood pressure has not been achieved after one or two weeks, the dose may be increased to 50 mg bid or tid. Concomitant sodium restriction may be beneficial when Captopril is used alone.

The dose of Captopril in hypertension usually does not exceed 50 mg tid. Therefore, if the blood pressure has not been satisfactorily controlled after one or two weeks at this dose, (and the patient is not already receiving a diuretic), a modest dose of a thiazide-type diuretic (e.g., hydrochlorothiazide, 25 mg daily), should be added. The diuretic dose may be increased at one- to two-week intervals until its highest usual antihypertensive dose is reached.

If Captopril is being started in a patient already receiving a diuretic, Captopril therapy should be initiated under close medical supervision (see *"Warnings"* and *"Precautions: Drug Interactions"* regarding hypotension), with dosage and titration of Captopril as noted above.

If further blood pressure reduction is required, the dose of Captopril may be increased to 100 mg bid or tid and then, if necessary, to 150 mg bid or tid (while continuing the diuretic). The usual dose range is 25 to 150 mg bid or tid. A maximum daily dose of 450 mg Captopril should not be exceeded.

For patients with severe hypertension (e.g., accelerated or malignant hypertension), when temporary discontinuation of current antihypertensive therapy is not practical or desirable, or when prompt titration to more normotensive blood pressure levels is indicated, diuretic should be continued but other current antihypertensive medication stopped and Captopril dosage promptly initiated at 25 mg bid or tid, under close medical supervision.

When necessitated by the patient's clinical condition, the daily dose of Captopril may be increased every 24 hours or less under continuous medical supervision until a satisfactory blood pressure response is obtained or the maximum dose of Captopril is reached. In this regimen, addition of a more potent diuretic, e.g., furosemide, may also be indicated. Beta-blockers may also; be used in conjuction with Captopril therapy (see *"Precautions: Drug Interactions"*) but the effects of the two drugs are less than additive.

Heart Failure: Initiation of therapy requires consideration of recent diuretic therapy and the possibility of severe salt/volume depletion. In patients with either normal or low blood pressure, who have been vigorously treated with diuretics and who may be hyponatremic and/or hypovolemic, a starting dose of 6.25 or 12.5 mg tid may minimize the magnitude or duration of the hypotensive effect (see *"Warnings: Hypotension"*); for these patients, titration to the usual daily dosage can then occur within the next several days. For most patients the usual initial daily dosage is 25 mg tid. After a dose of 50 mg tid is reached, further

increases in dosage should be delayed, where possible, for at least two weeks to determine if a satisfactory response occurs. Most patients studied have had a satisfactory clinical improvement at 50 or 100 mg tid. A maximum daily dose of 450 mg of Captopril should not be exceeded.

Captopril should generally be used in conjunction with a diuretic and digitalis. Captopril therapy must be initiated under very close medical supervision.

Left Ventricular Dysfunction After Myocardial Infarction: The recommended dose for long-term use in patients following a myocardial infarction is a target maintenance dose of 50 mg tid.

Therapy may be initiated as early as three days following a myocardial infarction. After a single dose of 6.25 mg, Captopril therapy should be initiated at 12.5 mg tid. Captopril should then be increased to 25 mg tid during the next several days and to a target dose of 50 mg tid over the next several weeks as tolerated (See *"Clinical Phamacology"*).

Captopril may be used in patients treated with other postmyocardial infarction therapies, e.g., thrombolytics, aspirin, beta blockers.

Diabetic Nephropathy: The recommended dose of Captopril for long term use to treat diabetic nephropathy is 25 mg tid.

Other antihypertensives such as diuretics, beta blockers, centrally acting agents or vasodilators may be used in conjunction with Captopril if additional therapy is required to further lower blood pressure.

Dosage Adjustment in Renal Impairment: Because Captopril is excreted primarily by the kidneys, excretion rates are reduced in patients with impaired renal function. These patients will take longer to reach steady-state Captopril levels and will reach higher steady-state levels for a given daily dose than patients with normal renal function. Therefore, these patients may respond to smaller or less frequent doses.

Accordingly, for patients with significant renal impairment, initial daily dosage of Captopril should be reduced, and smaller increments utilized for titration, which should be quite slow (one- to two-week intervals). After the desired therapeutic effect has been achieved, the dose should be slowly back-titrated to determine the minimal effective dose. When concomitant diuretic therapy is required, a loop diuretic (e.g., furosemide), rather than a thiazide diuretic, is preferred in patients with severe renal impairment. (See also *"Precautions: Hemodialysis."*)

Storage: Do not store above 86°F. Keep bottles tightly closed (protect from moisture).

HOW SUPPLIED
TABLETS: 12.5 MG

BRAND/MANUFACTURER	NDC	SIZE	AWP
○ **BRAND**			
➤ CAPOTEN: Squibb, E.R.	00003-0450-54	100s	$63.63
	00003-0450-51	100s ud	$65.06
	00003-0450-75	1000s	$629.51
CAPOTEN:	00003-0450-06	5000s	$3304.94

TABLETS: 25 MG

BRAND/MANUFACTURER	NDC	SIZE	AWP
○ **BRAND**			
➤ CAPOTEN: Squibb, E.R.	00003-0452-50	100s	$68.78
	00003-0452-51	100s ud	$70.99
	00003-0452-75	1000s	$680.70
➤ CAPOTEN:	00003-0452-39	5000s	$3573.68

TABLETS: 50 MG

BRAND/MANUFACTURER	NDC	SIZE	AWP
○ **BRAND**			
➤ CAPOTEN: Squibb, E.R.	00003-0482-50	100s	$117.94
	00003-0482-51	100s ud	$120.75
	00003-0482-75	1000s	$1166.90
➤ CAPOTEN:	00003-0482-06	5000s	$6126.23

TABLETS: 100 MG

BRAND/MANUFACTURER	NDC	SIZE	AWP
○ **BRAND**			
➤ CAPOTEN: Squibb, E.R.	00003-0485-50	100s	$160.86
	00003-0485-51	100s ud	$164.74

Captopril with Hydrochlorothiazide

USE IN PREGNANCY
WHEN USED IN PREGNANCY DURING THE SECOND AND THIRD TRIMESTERS, ACE INHIBITORS CAN CAUSE INJURY AND EVEN DEATH TO THE DEVELOPING FETUS. WHEN PREGNANCY IS DETECTED, CAPTOPRIL/ HYDROCHLOROTHIAZIDE SHOULD BE DISCONTINUED AS SOON AS

◆ RATED THERAPEUTICALLY EQUIVALENT; ◇ THERAPEUTIC EQUIVALENCE UNCONFIRMED; ○ UNRATED

POSSIBLE. SEE *"WARNINGS: CAPTOPRIL, FETAL/NEONATAL MORBIDITY AND MORTALITY."*

DESCRIPTION

Captopril/Hydrochlorothiazide Tablets for oral administration combine two antihypertensive agents: Captopril and Hydrochlorothiazide. Captopril, the first of a new class of antihypertensive agents, is a specific competitive inhibitor of angiotensin I-converting enzyme (ACE), the enzyme responsible for the conversion of angiotensin I to angiotensin II. Hydrochlorothiazide is a benzothiadiazide (thiazide) diuretic-antihypertensive. Captopril/Hydrochlorothiazide tablets are available in four combinations of Captopril and Hydrochlorothiazide: 25 mg with 15 mg, 25 mg with 25 mg, 50 mg with 15 mg, and 50 mg with 25 mg.

Captopril is designated chemically as 1-[(2S)-3-mercapto-2-methylpropionyl)]-L-proline; Hydrochlorothiazide is 6-Chloro-3,4-dihydro-2H-1, 2, 4-benzothiadiazine-7-sulfonamide 1,1-dioxide.

Captopril is a white to off-white crystalline powder that may have a slight sulfurous odor; it is soluble in water (approx. 160 mg/mL), methanol, and ethanol and sparingly soluble in chloroform and ethyl acetate.

Hydrochlorothiazide is a white crystalline powder slightly soluble in water but freely soluble in sodium hydroxide solution.

CLINICAL PHARMACOLOGY

CAPTOPRIL

MECHANISM OF ACTION

The mechanism of action of Captopril has not yet been fully elucidated. Its beneficial effects in hypertension and heart failure appear to result primarily from suppression of the renin-angiotensin-aldosterone system. However, there is no consistent correlation between renin levels and response to the drug. Renin, an enzyme synthesized by the kidneys, is released into the circulation where it acts on a plasma globulin substrate to produce angiotensin I, a relatively inactive decapeptide. Angiotensin I is then converted by angiotensin converting enzyme (ACE) to angiotensin II, a potent endogenous vasoconstrictor substance. Angiotensin II also stimulates aldosterone secretion from the adrenal cortex, thereby contributing to sodium and fluid retention.

Captopril prevents the conversion of angiotensin I to angiotensin II by inhibition of ACE, a peptidyldipeptide carboxy hydrolase. This inhibition has been demonstrated in both healthy human subjects and in animals by showing that the elevation of blood pressure caused by exogenously administered angiotensin I was attenuated or abolished by Captopril. In animal studies, Captopril did not alter the pressor responses to a number of other agents, including angiotensin II and norepinephrine, indicating specificity of action.

ACE is identical to "bradykininase", and Captopril may also interfere with the degradation of the vasodepressor peptide, bradykinin. Increased concentrations of bradykinin or prostaglandin E_2 may also have a role in the therapeutic effect of Captopril.

Inhibition of ACE results in decreased plasma angiotensin II and increased plasma renin activity (PRA), the latter resulting from loss of negative feedback on renin release caused by reduction in angiotensin II. The reduction of angiotensin II leads to decreased aldosterone secretion, and as a result, small increases in serum potassium may occur along with sodium and fluid loss.

The antihypertensive effects persist for a longer period of time than does demonstrable inhibition of circulating ACE. It is not known whether the ACE present in vascular endothelium is inhibited longer than the ACE in circulating blood.

PHARMACOKINETICS

After oral administration of therapeutic doses of Captopril, rapid absorption occurs with peak blood levels at about one hour. The presence of food in the gastrointestinal tract reduces absorption by about 30 to 40 percent; Captopril therefore should be given one hour before meals. Based on carbon-14 labeling, average minimal absorption is approximately 75 percent. In a 24-hour period, over 95 percent of the absorbed dose is eliminated in the urine; 40 to 50 percent is unchanged drug; most of the remainder is the disulfide dimer of Captopril and captopril-cysteine disulfide.

Approximately 25 to 30 percent of the circulating drug is bound to plasma proteins. The apparent elimination half-life for total radioactivity in blood is probably less than three hours. An accurate determination of half-life of unchanged Captopril is not, at present, possible, but it is probably less than two hours. In patients with renal impairment, however, retention of Captopril occurs (see *"Dosage and Administration"*).

PHARMACODYNAMICS

Administration of Captopril results in a reduction of peripheral arterial resistance in hypertensive patients with either no change, or an increase, in cardiac output. There is an increase in renal blood flow following administration of Captopril and glomerular filtration rate is usually unchanged. In patients with heart failure, significantly decreased peripheral (systemic vascular) resistance and blood pressure (afterload), reduced pulmonary capillary wedge pressure (preload) and pulmonary vascular resistance, increased cardiac output, and increased exercise tolerance time (ETT) have been demonstrated.

Reductions of blood pressure are usually maximal 60 to 90 minutes after oral administration of an individual dose of Captopril. The duration of effect is dose related and is extended in the presence of a thiazide-type diuretic. The full effect of a given dose may not be attained for 6-8 weeks (see *"Dosage and Administration"*). The blood pressure lowering effects of Captopril and thiazide-type diuretics are additive. In contrast, Captopril and beta-blockers have a less than additive effect.

Blood pressure is lowered to about the same extent in both standing and supine positions. Orthostatic effects and tachycardia are infrequent but may occur in volume-depleted patients. Abrupt withdrawal of Captopril has not been associated with a rapid increase in blood pressure.

Studies in rats and cats indicate that Captopril does not cross the blood-brain barrier to any significant extent.

HYDROCHLOROTHIAZIDE

Thiazides affect the renal tubular mechanism of electrolyte reabsorption. At maximal therapeutic dosage all thiazides are approximately equal in their diuretic potency.

Thiazides increase excretion of sodium and chloride in approximately equivalent amounts. Natriuresis causes a secondary loss of potassium and bicarbonate.

The mechanism of the antihypertensive effect of thiazides is unknown. Thiazides do not affect normal blood pressure. The mean plasma half-life of Hydrochlorothiazide in fasted individuals has been reported to be approximately 2.5 hours. Onset of diuresis occurs in two hours and the peak effect at about four hours. Its action persists for approximately six to twelve hours. Hydrochlorothiazide is eliminated rapidly by the kidney.

INDICATIONS AND USAGE

Captopril/Hydrochlorothiazide Tablets are indicated for the treatment of hypertension. The blood pressure lowering effects of Captopril and thiazides are approximately additive.

This fixed combination drug may be used as initial therapy or substituted for previously titrated doses of the individual components.

When Captopril and Hydrochlorothiazide are given together it may not be necessary to administer Captopril in divided doses to attain blood pressure control at trough (before the next dose). Also, with such a combination, a daily dose of 15 mg of Hydrochlorothiazide may be adequate.

Treatment may, therefore, be initiated with Captopril/Hydrochlorothiazide 25 mg/15 mg once daily. Subsequent titration should be with additional doses of the components (Captopril, Hydrochlorothiazide) as single agents or as Captopril/Hydrochlorothiazide 50 mg/15 mg, 25 mg/25 mg or 50 mg/25 mg (see *"Dosage and Administration"*).

In using Captopril/Hydrochlorothiazide, consideration should be given to the risk of neutropenia/agranulocytosis (see *"Warnings"*).

Captopril/Hydrochlorothiazide may be used for patients with normal renal function, in whom the risk is relatively low. In patients with impaired renal function, particularly those with collagen vascular disease, Captopril/Hydrochlorothiazide should be reserved for hypertensives who have either developed unacceptable side effects on other drugs, or have failed to respond satisfactorily to other drug combinations.

CONTRAINDICATIONS

CAPTOPRIL

This product is contraindicated in patients who are hypersensitive sensitive to Captopril or any other angiotensin-converting enzyme inhibitor (e.g., a patient who has experienced angioedema during therapy with any other ACE inhibitor).

HYDROCHLOROTHIAZIDE

Hydrochlorothiazide is contraindicated in anuria. It is also contraindicated in patients who have previously demonstrated hypersensitivity to Hydrochlorothiazide or other sulfonamide-derived drugs.

WARNINGS

CAPTOPRIL

ANGIOEDEMA

Angioedema involving the extremities, face, lips, mucous membranes, tongue, glottis or larynx has been seen in patients treated with ACE inhibitors, including Captopril. If angioedema involves the tongue, glottis or larynx, airway obstruction may occur and be fatal. Emergency therapy, including but not necessarily limited to, subcutaneous administration of a 1:1000 solution of epinephrine should be promptly instituted.

Swelling confined to the face, mucous membranes of the mouth, lips and extremities has usually resolved with discontinuation of treatment: some cases required medical therapy. (See *"Precautions: Information for Patients"* and *"Adverse Reactions: Captopril."*)

NEUTROPENIA/AGRANULOCYTOSIS

Neutropenia ($< 1000/mm^3$) with myeloid hypoplasia has resulted from use of Captopril. About half of the neutropenic patients developed systemic or oral cavity infections or other features of the syndrome of agranulocytosis.

The risk of neutropenia is dependent on the clinical status of the patient:

In clinical trials in patients with hypertension who have normal renal function (serum creatinine less than 1.6 mg/dL and no collagen vascular disease), neutropenia has been seen in one patient out of over 8,600 exposed.

In patients with some degree of renal failure (serum creatinine at least 1.6 mg/dL) but no collagen vascular disease, the risk of neutropenia in clinical trials was about 1 per 500, a frequency over 15 times that for uncomplicated hypertension. Daily doses of Captopril were relatively high in these patients, particularly in view of their diminished renal function. In foreign marketing experience in patients with renal failure, use of allopurinol concomitantly with Captopril has been associated with neutropenia but this association has not appeared in U.S. reports.

In patients with collagen vascular diseases (e.g., systemic lupus erthematosus, scleroderma) and impaired renal function, neutropenia occurred in 3.7 percent of patients in clinical trials.

While none of the over 750 patients in formal clinical trials of heart failure developed neutropenia, it has occurred during the subsequent clinical experience. About half of the reported cases had serum creatinine ≥ 1.6 mg/dL and more than 75 percent were in patients also receiving procainamide. In heart failure, it appears that the same risk factors for neutropenia are present.

The neutropenia has usually been detected within three months after Captopril was started. Bone marrow examinations in patients with neutropenia consistently showed myeloid hypoplasia, frequently accompanied by erythroid hypoplasia and decreased numbers of megakaryocytes (e.g., hypoplastic bone marrow and pancytopenia); anemia and thrombocytopenia were sometimes seen.

In general, neutrophils returned to normal in about two weeks after Captopril was discontinued, and serious infections were limited to clinically complex patients. About 13 percent of the cases of neutropenia have ended fatally, but almost all fatalities were in patients with serious illness, having collagen vascular disease, renal failure, heart failure or immunosuppressant therapy or a combination of these complicating factors.

EVALUATION OF THE HYPERTENSIVE OR HEART FAILURE PATIENT SHOULD ALWAYS INCLUDE ASSESSMENT OF RENAL FUNCTION.
If Captopril is used in patients with impaired renal function, white blood cell and differential counts should be evaluated prior to starting treatment and at approximately two-week intervals for about three months, then periodically.

In patients with collagen vascular disease or who are exposed to other drugs known to affect the white cells or immune response, particularly when there is impaired renal function, Captopril should be used only after an assessment of benefit and risk, and then with caution.

All patients treated with Captopril should be told to report any signs of infection (e.g., sore throat, fever). If infection is suspected, white cell counts should be performed without delay.

Since discontinuation of Captopril and other drugs has generally led to prompt return of the white count to normal, upon confirmation of neutropenia (neutrophil count < 1000/mm³) the physician should withdraw Captopril and closely follow the patient's course.

PROTEINURIA
Total urinary proteins greater than 1 g per day were seen in about 0.7 percent of patients receiving Captopril. About 90 percent of affected patients had evidence of prior renal disease or received relatively high doses of Captopril (in excess of 150 mg/day), or both. The nephrotic syndrome occurred in about one-fifth of proteinuric patients. In most cases, proteinuria subsided or cleared within six months whether or not Captopril was continued. Parameters of renal function, such as BUN and creatinine, were seldom altered in the patients with proteinuria.

Since most cases of proteinuria occurred by the eighth month of therapy with Captopril, patients with prior renal disease or those receiving Captopril at doses greater than 150 mg per day, should have urinary protein estimations (dipstick on first morning urine) prior to treatment, and periodically thereafter.

HYPOTENSION
Excessive hypotension was rarely seen in hypertensive patients but is a possible consequence of Captopril use in salt/volume depleted persons (such as those treated vigorously with diuretics), patients with heart failure or those patients undergoing renal dialysis. (See "Precautions: Drug Interaction.")

FETAL/NEONATAL MORBIDITY AND MORTALITY
ACE inhibitors can cause fetal and neonatal morbidity and death when administered to pregnant women. Several dozen cases have been reported in the world literature. When pregnancy is detected, ACE inhibitors should be discontinued as soon as possible.

The use of ACE inhibitors during the second and third trimesters of pregnancy has been associated with fetal and neonatal injury, including hypotension, neonatal skull hypoplasia, anuria, reversible or irreversible renal failure, and death. Oligohydramnios has also been reported, presumably resulting from decreased fetal renal function: oligohydramnios in this setting has been associated with fetal limb contractures, craniofacial deformation, and hypoplastic lung development. Prematurity, intrauterine growth retardation, and patent ductus arteriosus have also been reported, although it is not clear whether these occurrences were due to the ACE-inhibitor exposure.

These adverse effects do not appear to have resulted from intrauterine ACE-inhibitor exposure that has been limited to the first trimester. Mothers whose embryos and fetuses are exposed to ACE-inhibitors only during the first trimester should be so informed. Nonetheless, when patients become pregnant, physicians should make every effort to discontinue the use of Captoril as soon as possible.

Rarely (probably less often than once in every thousand pregnancies), no alternative to ACE inhibitors will be found. In these rare cases, the mothers should be apprised of the potential hazards to their fetuses, and serial unltrasound examinations should be performed to assess the intraamniotic environment.

If oligohydramnios is observed, Captopril should be discontinued unless it is considered life-saving for the mother. Contraction stress testing (CST), a non-stress test (NST), or biophysical profiling (BPP) may be appropriate, depending upon the week of pregnancy. Patients and physicians should be aware, however, that oligohydramnios may not appear until after the fetus has sustained irreversible injury.

Infants with histories of *in utero* exposure to ACE inhibitors should be closely observed for hypotension, oliguria, and hyperkalemia. If oliguria occurs, attention should be directed toward support of blood pressure and renal perfusion. Exchange transfusion or dialysis may be required as a means of reversing hypotension and/or substituting for disordered renal function. While Captopril may be removed from the adult circulation by hemodialysis, there is inadequate data concerning the effectiveness of hemodialysis for removing it from the circulation of neonates or children. Peritoneal dialysis is not effective for removing Captopril; there is no information concerning exchange transfusion for removing Captopril from the general circulation.

When Captopril was given to rabbits at doses about 0.8 to 70 times (on a mg/kg basis) the maximum recommended human dose, low incidences of craniofacial malformations were seen. No teratogenic effects of Captopril were seen in studies of pregnant rats and hamsters. On a mg/kg basis, the doses used were up to 150 times (in hamsters) and 625 times (in rats) the maximum recommended human dose.

HYDROCHLOROTHIAZIDE
Thiazides should be used with caution in severe renal disease. In patients with renal disease, thiazides may precipitate azotemia. Cumulative effects of the drug may develop in patients with impaired renal function.

Thiazides should be used with caution in patients with impaired hepatic function or progressive liver disease, since minor alterations of fluid and electrolyte balance may precipitate hepatic coma.

Sensitivity reactions may occur in patients with or without a history of allergy or bronchial asthma.

The possibility of exacerbation or activation of systemic lupus erythematosus has been reported.

In general, lithium should not be given with diuretics (see "Precautions: Drug Interactions, Hydrochlorothiazide").

PRECAUTIONS
GENERAL
CAPTOPRIL
Impaired Renal Function: Some patients with renal disease, particularly those with severe renal artery stenosis, have developed increases in BUN and serum creatinine after reduction of blood pressure with Captopril. Captopril dosage reduction and/or discontinuation of diuretic may be required. For some of these patients, it may not be possible to normalize blood pressure and maintain adequate renal perfusion (see "Clinical Pharmacology," "Dosage and Administration," Adverse Reactions: Altered Laboratory Findings").

Hyperkalemia: Elevations in serum potassium have been observed in some patients treated with ACE inhibitors, including Captopril. When treated with ACE inhibitors, patients at risk for the development of hyperkalemia include those with: renal insufficiency; diabetes mellitus; and those using concomitant potassium-sparing diuretics, potassium supplements or potassium-containing salt substitutes; or other drugs associated with increases in serum potassium. (see "Precautions: Information for Patients" and "Drug Interactions, Captopril;" "Adverse Reactions: Altered Laboratory Findings.")

Cough: Cough has been reported with the use of ACE inhibitors. Characteristically, the cough is nonproductive, persistent and resolves after discontinuation of therapy. ACE inhibitor-induced cough should be considered as part of the differential diagnosis of cough.

Surgery/Anesthesic: In patients undergoing major surgery or during anesthesia with agents that produce hypotension, Captopril will block angiotensin II formation secondary to compensatory renin release. If hypotension occurs and is considered to be due to this mechanism, it can be corrected by volume expansion.

HEMODIALYSIS
Recent clinical observations have shown an association of hypersensitivity-like (anaphylactoid) reactions during hemodialysis with high-flux dialysis membranes (e.g. AN69) in patients receiving ACE inhibitors as medication. In these patients, consideration should be given to using a different type of dialysis membrane or a different class of medication.

HYDROCHLOROTHIAZIDE
Periodic determination of serum electrolytes to detect possible electrolyte imbalance should be performed at appropriate intervals.

All patients receiving thiazide therapy should be observed for clinical signs of fluid or electrolyte imbalance, namely: hyponatremia, hypochloremic alkalosis, and hypokalemia. Serum and urine electrolyte determinations are particularly important when the patient is vomiting excessively or receiving parenteral fluids. Warning signs or symptoms of fluid and electrolyte imbalance may include: dryness of mouth, thirst, weakness, lethargy, drowsiness, restlessness, muscle pains or cramps, muscular fatigue, hypotension, oliguria, tachycardia, and gastrointestinal disturbances such as nausea and vomiting.

Hypokalemia may develop, especially with brisk diuresis, or when severe cirrhosis is present. Interference with adequate oral electrolyte intake will also contribute to hypokalemia. Hypokalemia can sensitize or exaggerate the response of the heart of the toxic effects of digitalis (e.g., increased ventricular irritability). Because Captopril reduces the production of aldolsterone, concomitant therapy with Captopril reduces the diuretic-induced hypokalemia. Fewer patients may require potassium supplements and/or foods with a high potassium content (see "Drug Interactions. Agents Increasing Serum Potassium").

Any chloride deficit is generally mild and usually does not require specific treatment except under extraordinary circumstances (as in liver disease or renal disease). Dilutional hyponatremia may occur in edematous patients in hot weather; appropriate therapy is water restriction, rather than administration of salt except in rare instances when the hyponatremia is life-threatening. In actual salt depletion, appropriate replacement is the therapy of choice.

Hyperuricemia may occur or frank gout may be precipitated in certain patients receiving thiazide therapy.

Latent diabetes mellitus may become manifest during thiazide administration. The antihypertensive effect of thiazide diuretics may be enhanced in the postsympathectomy patients.

If progressive renal impairment becomes evident, as indicated by a rising nonprotein nitrogen or blood urea nitrogen (BUN), a careful reappraisal of therapy is necessary with consideration given to withholding or discontinuing diuretic therapy.

Thiazides may decrease serum PBI levels without signs of thyroid disturbance.

Calcium excretion is decreased by thiazides. Pathological changes in the parathyroid gland with hypercalcemia and hypophosphatemia have been observed in a few patients on prolonged thiazide therapy. The common complications of hyperparathyroidism such as renal lithiasis, bone resorption, and peptic ulceration have not been seen. Thiazides should be discontinued before carrying out tests for parathyroid function.

Thiazides have been shown to increase the urinary excretion of magnesium; this may result in hypomagnesemia.

INFORMATION FOR PATIENTS
Patients should be advised to immediately report to their physician any signs or symptoms suggesting angioedema (e.g., swelling of face, eyes, lips, tongue, larynx and extremities; difficulty in swallowing or breathing; hoarseness) and to discontinue therapy (see *"Warnings: Captopril"*).

Patients should be told to report promptly any indication of infection (e.g., sore throat, fever), which may be a sign of neutropenia, or of progressive edema which might be related to proteinuria and nephrotic syndrome.

All patients should be cautioned that excessive perspiration and dehydration may lead to an excessive fall in blood pressure because of reduction in fluid volume. Other causes of volume depletion such as vomiting or diarrhea may also lead to a fall in blood pressure; patients should be advised to consult with the physician.

Patients should be advised not to use potassium-sparing diuretics, potassium supplements or potassium-containing salt substitutes without consulting their physician (see *"Precautions: General"* and *"Drug Interactions, Captopril;" "Adverse Reactions: Captopril"*).

Patients should be warned against interruption or discontinuation of medication unless instructed by the physician. Heart failure patients on Captopril therapy should be cautioned against rapid increases in physical activity.

Patients should be informed that Captopril/Hydrochlorothiazide Tablets should be taken one hour before meals (see *"Dosage and Administration"*).

Pregnancy: Female patients of childbearing age should be told about the consequences of second- and third-trimester exposure to ACE inhibitors, and they should also be told that these consequences do not appear to have resulted from intrauterine Ace-inhibitor exposure that has been limited to the first trimester. These patients should be asked to report pregnancies to their physicians as soon as possible.

LABORATORY TESTS
Serum electrolyte levels should be regularly monitored (see *"Warnings: Captopril and Hydrochlorothiazide;" "Precautions: General, Hydrochlorothiazide"*).

DRUG INTERACTIONS
CAPTOPRIL
Hypotension—Patients on Diuretic Therapy: Patients on diuretics and especially those in whom diuretic therapy was recently instituted, as well as those on severe dietary salt restrictions or dialysis, may occasionally experience a precipitous reduction of blood pressure usually within the first hour after receiving the initial dose of Captopril.

The possibility of hypotensive effects with Captopril can be minimized by either discontinuing the diuretic or increasing the salt intake approximately one week prior to initiation of treatment with Captopril or initiating therapy with small doses (6.25 or 12.5 mg). Alternatively, provide medical supervision for at least one hour after the initial dose. If hypotension occurs, the patient should be placed in a supine position and, if necessary, receive an intravenous infusion of normal saline. This transient hypotensive response is not a contraindication to further doses which can be given without difficulty once the blood pressure has increased after volume expansion.

Agents Having Vasodilator Activity: Data on the effect of concomitant use of other vasodilators in patients receiving Captopril for heart failure are not available; therefore, nitroglycerin or other nitrates (as used for management of angina) or other drugs having vasodilator activity should, if possible, be discontinued before starting Captopril. If resumed during Captopril therapy, such agents should be administered cautiously, and perhaps at lower dosage.

Agents Causing Renin Release: Captopril's effect will be augmented by antihypertensive agents that cause renin release. For example, diuretics (e.g., thiazides) may activate the renin-angiotensin-aldosterone system.

Agents Affecting Sympathetic Activity: The sympathetic nervous system may be especially important in supporting blood pressure in patients receiving Captopril alone or with diuretics. Therefore, agents affecting sympathetic activity (e.g., ganglionic blocking agents or adrenergic neuron blocking agents) should be used

with caution. Beta-adrenergic blocking drugs add some further antihypertensive effect to Captopril, but the overall response is less than additive.

Agents Increasing Serum Potassium: Since Captopril decreases aldosterone production, elevation of serum potassium may occur. Potassium sparing diuretics such as spironolactone, triamterene, or amiloride, or potassium supplements, should be given only for documented hypokalemia, and then with caution, since they may lead to a significant increase of serum potassium. Salt substitutes containing potassium should also be used with caution.

Inhibitors Of Endogenous Prostaglandin Synthesis: It has been reported that indomethacin may reduce the antihypertensive effect of Captopril, especially in cases of low renin hypertension. Other nonsteroidal anti-inflammatory agents (e.g., aspirin) may also have this effect.

Lithium: Increased serum lithium levels and symptoms of lithium toxicity have been reported in patients receiving concomitant lithium and ACE inhibitor therapy. These drugs should be coadministered with caution and frequent monitoring of serum lithium levels is recommended. If a diuretic is also used, it may increase the risk of lithium toxicity (see *"Precautions: Drug Interactions, Hydrochlorothiazide, Lithium"*).

HYDROCHLOROTHIAZIDE
When administered concurrently the following drugs may interact with thiazide diuretics:

Alcohol, Barbiturates, or Narcotics: potentiation of orthostatic hypotension may occur.

Amphotericin B, Corticosteroids, or Corticotropin (ACTH): may intensify electrolyte imbalance, particularly hypokalemia. Monitor potassium levels; use potassium replacements if necessary.

Anticoagulants (Oral): dosage adjustments of anticoagulant medication may be necessary since Hydrochlorothiazide may decrease their effects.

Antigout Medications: dosage adjustments of antigout medication may be necessary since Hydrochlorothiazide may raise the level of blood uric acid.

Other Antihypertensive Medications (e.g., Ganglionic or Peripheral Adrenergic Blocking Agents): dosage adjustments may be necessary since Hydrochlorothiazide may potentiate their effects.

Antidiabetic Drugs (Oral Agents and Insulin): sine thiazides may elevate blood glucose levels, dosage adjustments of antidiabetic agents may be necessary.

Calcium Salts: Increased serum calcium levels due to decreased excretion may occur. If calcium must be prescribed monitor serum calcium levels and adjust calcium dosage accordingly.

Cardiac Glycosides: enhanced possibility of digitalis toxicity associated with hypokalemia. Monitor potassium levels (see *"Precautions: Drug Interactions, Captopril"*).

Cholestyramine Resin and Colestipol HCL: may delay or decrease absorption of Hydrochlorothiazide. Sulfonamide diuretics should be taken at least one hour before or four to six hours after these medications.

Diazoxide: enhanced hyperglycemic, hyperuricemic, and antihypertensive effects. Be cognizant of possible interaction; monitor blood glucose and serum uric acid levels.

Lithium: diuretic agents reduce the renal clearance of lithium and increase the risk of lithium toxicity. These drugs should be coadministered with caution and frequent monitoring of serum lithium levels is recommended (see *"Precautions: Drug Interactions, Captopril, Lithium"*).

MAO Inhibitors: dosage adjustments of one or both agents may be necessary since hypotensive effects are enhanced.

Nondepolarizing Muscle Relaxants, Preanesthetics and Anesthetics Used in Surgery (e.g., Tubocurarine Chloride and Gallamine Triethiodide): effects of these agents may be potentiated; dosage adjustments may be required. Monitor and correct any fluid and electrolyte imbalances prior to surgery if feasible.

Nonsteroidal anti-inflammatory agents: in some patients, the administration of a nonsteroidal anti-inflammatory agent can reduce the diuretic, natriuretic, and antihypertensive effect of loop, potassium-sparing or thiazide diuretics. Therefore, when Hydrochlorothiazide and nonsteroidal anti-inflammatory agents are used concomitantly, the patient should be observed closely to determine if the desired effect of the diuretic is obtained.

Methenamine: possible decreased effectiveness due to alkalinization of the urine.

Pressor Amines (e.g., Norepinephrine): decreased arterial responsiveness, but not sufficient to preclude effectiveness of the pressor agent for therapeutic use. Use caution in patients taking both medications who undergo surgery. Administer preanesthetic and anesthetic agents in reduced dosage, and if possible, discontinue Hydrochlorothiazide therapy one week prior to surgery.

Probenecid or sulfinpyrazone: increased dosage of these agents may be necessary since Hydrochlorothiazide may have hyperuricemic effect.

DRUG/LABORATORY TEST INTERACTIONS
CAPTOPRIL
Captopril may cause a false-positive urine test for acetone.

HYDROCHLOROTHIAZIDE
Hydrochlorothiazide may cause diagnostic interference of the bentiromide test.

CARCINOGENESIS, MUTAGENESIS, IMPAIRMENT OF FERTILITY
CAPTOPRIL
Two-year studies with doses of 50 to 1350 mg/kg/day in mice and rats failed to show any evidence of carcinogenic potential.

Studies in rats have revealed no impairment of fertility.

ANIMAL TOXICOLOGY
Chronic oral toxicity studies were conducted in rats (2 years), dogs (47 weeks; 1 year), mice (2 years), and monkeys (1 year). Significant drug-related toxicity included effects on hematopoiesis, renal toxicity, erosion/ulceration of the stomach, and variation of retinal blood vessels.

Reductions in hemoglobin and/or hematocrit values were seen in mice, rats, and monkeys at doses 50 to 150 times the maximum recommended human dose (MRHD). Anemia, leukopenia, thrombocytopenia, and bone marrow suppression occurred in dogs at doses 8 to 30 times MRHD. The reductions in hemoglobin and hematocrit values in rats and mice were only significant at 1 year and returned to normal with continued dosing by the end of the study. Marked anemia was seen at all dose levels (8 to 30 times MRHD) in dogs, whereas moderate to marked leukopenia was noted only at 15 and 30 times MRHD and thrombocytopenia at 30 times MRHD. The anemia could be reversed upon discontinuation of dosing. Bone marrow suppression occurred to a varying degree, being associated only with dogs that died or were sacrificed in a moribund condition in the 1 year study. However, in the 47-week study at a dose 30 times MRHD, bone marrow suppression was found to be reversible upon continued drug administration.

Captopril caused hyperplasia of the juxtaglomerular apparatus of the kidneys at doses 7 to 200 times the MRHD in rats and mice, at 20 to 60 times MRHD in monkeys, and at 30 times the MRHD in dogs.

Gastric erosions/ulcerations were increased in incidence at 20 and 200 times MRHD in male rats and at 30 and 65 times MRHD in dogs and monkeys, respectively. Rabbits developed gastric and intestinal ulcers when given oral doses approximately 30 times MRHD for only five to seven days.

In the two-year rat study, irreversible and progressive variations in the caliber of retinal vessels (focal sacculations and constrictions) occurred at all dose levels (7 to 200 times MRHD) in a dose-related fashion. The effect was first observed in the 88th week of dosing, with a progressively increased incidence thereafter, even after cessation of dosing.

HYDROCHLOROTHIAZIDE
Long-term studies in animals have not been performed to evaluate carcinogenic potential, mutagenesis, or whether this drug affects fertility in males or females.

PREGNANCY CATEGORIES C (FIRST TRIMESTER) AND D (SECOND AND THIRD TRIMESTERS)
See *"Warnings: Captopril, Fetal/Neonatal Morbidity and Mortality"*.

PREGNANCY—NONTERATOGENIC EFFECTS
HYDROCHLOROTHIAZIDE
Thiazides cross the placental barrier and appear in cord blood. The use of thiazides in pregnant women requires that the anticipated benefit be weighed against possible hazards to the fetus. These hazards include fetal or neonatal jaundice, thrombocytopenia, and possibly other adverse reactions which have occurred in the adult.

NURSING MOTHERS
Both Captopril and Hydrochlorothiazide are excreted in human milk. Because of the potential for serious adverse reactions in nursing infants from both drugs, a decision should be made whether to discontinue nursing or to discontinue therapy taking into account the importance of Captopril/Hydrochlorothiazide Tablets to the mother. (See *"Precautions: Pediatric Use."*)

PEDIATRIC USE
Safety and effectiveness in children have not been established. There is limited experience reported in the literature with the use of Captopril in the pediatric population; dosage, on a weight basis, was generally reported to be comparable to or less than that used in adults.

Infants, especially newborns, may be more susceptible to the adverse hemodynamic effects of Captopril. Excessive, prolonged and unpredictable decreases in blood pressure and associated complications, including oliguria and seizures, have been reported.

Captopril/Hydrochlorothiazide should be used in children only if other measures for controlling blood pressure have not been effective.

ADVERSE REACTIONS
CAPTOPRIL
Reported incidences are based on clinical trials involving approximately 7000 patients.

Renal: About one of 100 patients developed proteinuria (see *"Warnings"*).

Each of the following has been reported in approximately 1 to 2 of 1000 patients and are of uncertain relationship to drug use: renal insufficiency, renal failure, nephrotic syndrome, polyuria, oliguria, and urinary frequency.

Hematologic: Neutropenia/agranulocytosis has occurred (see *"Warnings"*). Cases of anemia, thrombocytopenia, and pancytopenia have been reported.

Dermatologic: Rash, often with pruritus, and sometimes with fever, arthralgia, and eosinophilia, occurred in about 4 to 7 (depending on renal status and dose) of 100 patients, usually during the first four weeks of therapy. It is usually maculopapular, and rarely urticarial. The rash is usually mild and disappears within a few days of dosage reduction, short-term treatment with an antihistaminic agent, and/or discontinuing therapy; remission may occur even if Captopril is continued. Pruritus, without rash, occurs in about 2 of 100 patients. Between 7 and 10 percent of patients with skin rash have shown eosinophilia and/or positive ANA titers. A reversible associated pemphigoid-like lesion, and photosensitivity, have also been reported.

Flushing or pallor has been reported in 2 to 5 of 1000 patients.

Cardiovascular: Hypotension may occur; see *"Warnings"* and *"Precautions, Drug Interactions"* for discussion of hypotension with Captopril therapy.

Tachycardia, chest pain, and palpitations have each been observed in approximately 1 of 100 patients.

Angina pectoris, myocardial infarction, Raynaud's syndrome, and congestive heart failure have each occurred in 2 to 3 of 1000 patients.

Dysgeusia: Approximately 2 to 4 (depending on renal status and dose) of 100 patients developed a diminution or loss of taste perception. Taste impairment is reversible and usually self-limited (2 to 3 months) even with continued drug administration. Weight loss may be associated with the loss of taste.

Angioedema: Angioedema involving the extremities, face, lips, mucous membranes, tongue, glottis or larynx has been reported in approximately one in 1000 patients. Angioedema involving the upper airways has caused fatal airway obstruction. (see *"Warning: Captopril"* and *"Precautions: Information for Patients."*)

Cough: Cough has been reported in 0.5-2% of patients treated with Captopril in clinical trials (see *"Precautions: General, Captopril, Cough"*).

The following have been reported in about 0.5 to 2 percent of patients but did not appear at increased frequency compared to placebo or other treatments used in controlled trials: gastric irritation, abdominal pain, nausea, vomiting, diarrhea, anorexia, constipation, aphthous ulcers, peptic ulcer, dizziness, headache, malaise, fatigue, insomnia, dry mouth, dyspnea, alopecia, paresthesias.

Other clinical adverse effects reported since the drug was marketed are listed below by body system. In this setting, an incidence or causal relationship cannot be accurately determined.

Body as a Whole: Anaphylactoid reactions (see *"Precautions: Hemodialysis"*).

General: Asthenia, gynecomastia.

Cardiovascular: cardiac arrest, cerebrovascular accident/insufficiency, rhythm disturbances, orthostatic hypotension, syncope.

Dermatologic: bullous pemphigus, erthema multiforme (including Stevens-Johnson syndrome), exfoliative dermatitis.

Gastrointestinal: pancreatitis, glossitis, dyspepsia.

Hematologic: anemia, including aplastic and hemolytic.

Hepatobiliary: jaundice, hepatitis, including rare cases of necrosis, cholestasis.

Metabolic: symptomatic hyponatremia.

Musculoskeletal: myalgia, myasthenia.

Nervous/Psychiatric: ataxia, confusion, depression, nervousness, somnolence.

Respiratory: bronchospasm, eosinophilic pneumonitis, rhinitis.

Special Senses: blurred vision.

Urogenital: impotence.

As with other ACE inhibitors, a syndrome has been reported which may include: fever, myalgia, arthralgia, interstitial nephritis, vasculitis, rash or other dermatologic manifestations, eosinophilia and an elevated ESR.

FETAL/NEONATAL MORBIDITY AND MORTALITY
See *"Warnings: Captopril, Fetal/Neonatal Morbidity and Mortality"*.

HYDROCHLOROTHIAZIDE
Gastrointestinal System: anorexia, gastric irritation, nausea, vomiting, cramping, diarrhea, constipation, jaundice (intrahepatic cholestatic jaundice), pancreatitis, and sialadenitis.

Central Nervous System: dizziness, vertigo, paresthesias, headache, and xanthopsia.

Hematologic: leukopenia, agranulocytosis. thrombocytopenia, aplastic anemia, and hemolytic anemia.

Cardiovascular: orthostatic hypotension.

Hypersensitivity: purpura, photosensitivity, rash, urticaria, necrotizing angiitis (vasculitis; cutaneous vasculitis), fever, respiratory distress including pneumonitis, and anaphylactic reactions.

Other: hyperglycemia, glycosuria, hyperuricemia, muscle spasm, weakness, restlessness, and transient blurred vision. Whenever adverse reactions are moderate or severe, thiazide dosage should be reduced or therapy withdrawn.

ALTERED LABORATORY FINDINGS
Serum Electrolytes: Hyperkalemia: small increase in serum potassium, especially in patients with renal impairment (see *"Precautions: Captopril"*).

Hyponatremia: particularly in patients receiving a low sodium diet or concomitant diuretics.

BUN/Serum Creatinine: Transient elevations of BUN or serum creatinine especially in volume or salt depleted patients or those with renovascular

---

hypertension may occur. Rapid reduction of longstanding or markedly elevated blood pressure can result in decreases in the glomerular filtration rate and, in turn, lead to increases in BUN or serum creatinine.

Hematologic: A positive ANA has been reported.

Liver Function Tests: Elevations of liver transaminases, alkaline phosphatase, and serum bilirubin have occurred.

OVERDOSAGE

CAPTOPRIL

Correction of hypotension would be of primary concern. Volume expansion with an intravenous infusion of normal saline is the treatment of choice for restoration of blood pressure.

While Captopril may be removed from the adult circulation by hemodialysis, there is inadequate data concerning the effectiveness of hemodialysis for removing it from the circulation of neonates or children. Peritoneal dialysis is not effective for removing Captopril: there is no information concerning exchange transfusion for removing Captopril from the general circulation.

HYDROCHLOROTHIAZIDE

In addition to the expected diuresis, overdosage of thiazides may produce varying degrees of lethargy which may progress to coma within a few hours, with minimal depression of respiration and cardiovascular function and without evidence of serum electrolyte changes or dehydration. The mechanism of thiazide-induced CNS depression is unknown. Gastrointestinal irritation and hypermotility may occur. Transitory increase in BUN has been reported, and serum electrolyte changes may occur, especially in patients with impaired renal function.

In addition to gastric lavage and supportive therapy for stupor or coma, symptomatic treatment of gastrointestinal effects may be needed. The degree to which Hydrochlorothiazide is removed by hemodialysis has not been clearly established. Measures as required to maintain hydration, electrolyte balance, respiration, and cardiovascular and renal function should be instituted.

DOSAGE AND ADMINISTRATION

DOSAGE MUST BE INDIVIDUALIZED ACCORDING TO PATIENT'S RESPONSE. Captopril/Hydrochlorothiazide may be substituted for the previously titrated individual components.

Alternatively, therapy may be instituted with a single tablet of Captopril/Hydrochlorothiazide 25 mg/15 mg taken once daily. For patients insufficiently responsive to the initial dose, additional Captopril or Hydrochlorothiazide may be added as individual components or by using Captopril/Hydrochlorothiazide 50 mg/ 15mg, 25 mg/25 mg or 50 mg/25 mg, or divided doses may be used.

Because the full effect of a given dose may not be attained for 6-8 weeks, dosage adjustments should generally be made at 6 week intervals, unless the clinical situation demands more rapid adjustment.

In general, daily doses of Captopril should not exceed 150 mg and of Hydrochlorothiazide should not exceed 50 mg. Captopril/Hydrochlorothiazide Tablets should be taken one hour before meals.

Dosage Adjustment in Renal Impairment: Because Captopril and Hydrochlorothiazide are excreted primarily by the kidneys, excretion rates are reduced in patients with impaired renal function. These patients will take longer to reach steady-state Captopril levels and will reach higher steady-state levels for a given daily dose than patients with normal renal function. Therefore, these patients may respond to smaller or less frequent doses of Captopril/Hydrochlorothiazide.

After the desired therapeutic effect has been achieved, the dose intervals should be increased or the total daily dose reduced until the minimal effective dose is achieved. When concomitant diuretic therapy is required in patients with severe renal impairment, a loop diuretic (e.g., furosemide), rather than a thiazide diuretic is preferred for use with Captopril: therefore, for patients with severe renal dysfunction the Captopril-Hydrochlorothiazide combination tablet is not usually recommended. (See also *"Precautions; Hemodialysis".*)

Keep bottles tightly closed (protect from moisture): do not store above 86°F.

HOW SUPPLIED
TABLETS: 25 MG-15 MG

BRAND/MANUFACTURER	NDC	SIZE	AWP
○ BRAND			
➤ CAPOZIDE 25/15: Squibb, E.R.	00003-0338-50	100s	$70.91

TABLETS: 25 MG-25 MG

BRAND/MANUFACTURER	NDC	SIZE	AWP
○ BRAND			
➤ CAPOZIDE 25/25: Squibb, E.R.	00003-0349-50	100s	$70.91

TABLETS: 50 MG-15 MG

BRAND/MANUFACTURER	NDC	SIZE	AWP
○ BRAND			
➤ CAPOZIDE 50/15: Squibb, E.R.	00003-0384-50	100s	$121.78

TABLETS: 50 MG-25 MG

BRAND/MANUFACTURER	NDC	SIZE	AWP
○ BRAND			
➤ CAPOZIDE 50/25: Squibb, E.R.	00003-0390-50	100s	$121.78

Carafate *SEE* SUCRALFATE

Caramiphen Edisylate with Phenylpropanolamine Hydrochloride

DESCRIPTION

Each 5 mL (one teaspoonful) of liquid contains Caramiphen Edisylate, 6.7 mg; Phenylpropanolamine Hydrochloride, 12.5 mg; and alcohol, 5.0%.

Each sustained release capsule contains Caramiphen Edisylate, 40 mg and Phenylpropanolamine Hydrochloride, 75 mg.

Each sustained release capsule is so prepared that an initial dose is released promptly and the remaining medication is released gradually over a prolonged period.

ACTIONS

Caramiphen Edisylate is a synthetic, non-narcotic cough suppressant, and Phenylpropanolamine Hydrochloride is a vasoconstrictor with decongestant action on nasal and is upper respiratory tract mucosal membranes.

Pharmacokinetics: At steady-state conditions, the following peak levels are reached after the oral administration of a sustained release capsule: 24 ng/mL Caramiphen in 4.6 hours: 200 ng/mL Phenylpropanolamine in 5.5 hours: the half-lives are approximately 11 and 8 hours, respectively.

INDICATIONS

FOR THE SYMPTOMATIC RELIEF OF COUGHS AND NASAL CONGESTION ASSOCIATED WITH COMMON COLDS.

N.B.: A FINAL DETERMINATION HAS NOT BEEN MADE ON THE EFFECTIVENESS OF THIS DRUG COMBINATION IN ACCORDANCE WITH EFFICACY REQUIREMENTS OF THE 1962 AMENDMENTS TO THE FOOD, DRUG AND COSMETIC ACT.

CONTRAINDICATIONS

Hypersensitivity to either of the components; concurrent MAO inhibitor therapy; severe hypertension; bronchial asthma; coronary artery disease.

Do not use Caramiphen Edisylate/Phenylpropanolamine Hydrochloride Liquid in children under 15 pounds or in children less than six months of age.

Do not use Caramiphen Edisylale/Phenylpropanolamine Hydrochloride sustained release capsule in children under 12 years of age.

PRECAUTIONS

Use with caution in patients with cardiovascular disease, glaucoma, prostatic hypertrophy, thyroid disease or diabetes. Use with caution in patients in whom productive cough is desirable to clear excessive secretions from the bronchial tree. Patients taking this medication should be cautioned not to take simultaneously other products containing Phenylpropanolamine Hydrochloride or amphetamines.

Usage in Pregnancy: Safe use in pregnancy has not been established. This drug should not be used in pregnancy, nursing mothers, or women of childbearing potential unless, in the judgment of the physician, the anticipated benefits outweigh the potential risks.

ADVERSE REACTIONS

Adverse effects associated with products containing a centrally acting antitussive or sympathomimetic amine may occur and include: nausea, gastrointestinal upset, diarrhea, constipation, dizziness, drowsiness, nervousness, insomnia, anorexia, weakness, tightness of chest, angina pain, irritability, palpitations, headache, incoordination, tremor, difficulty in urination, dysuria, hypertension, hypotension, visual disturbances.

DOSAGE AND ADMINISTRATION

Adults and children over 12 years—2 teaspoonfuls every 4 hours; do not exceed 12 teaspoonfuls in 24 hours. Children 6 to 12 years—1 teaspoonful every 4 hours; do not exceed 6 teaspoonfuls in 24 hours. Children 2 to 6 years—½ teaspoonful every 4 hours; do not exceed 3 teaspoonfuls in 24 hours. Data are not available on which to base dosage recommendations for children under 2 years of age. **Do not use in children under 15 pounds or less than 6 months old.**

Caramiphen Edisylale/Phenylpropanolamine Hydrochloride sustained release capsule: Adults and children 12 years of age and over—one Caramiphen Edisylate/Phenylpropanolamine Hydrochloride sustained release capsule every 12 hours. **Do not use in children under 12 years of age.**

OVERDOSAGE

Symptoms: May include dryness of mouth, dysphagia, thirst, blurred vision, dilated pupils, photophobia, fever, rapid pulse and respiration, disorientation, dizziness, nausea, fainting, tachycardia, and either excitation or depression of the central nervous system.

Treatment: Immediate evacuation of the stomach should be induced by emesis and gastric lavage, repeated as necessary. Respiratory depression should be treated promptly with oxygen and respiratory stimulants. Do not treat respiratory or CNS depression with analeptics that might precipitate convulsions. If marked excitement occurs, a short-acting barbiturate or chloral hydrate may be used.

Since much of the sustained release capsule medication is coated for gradual release, saline cathartics should be administered to hasten evacuation of pellets that have not already released medication.

HOW SUPPLIED
CAPSULE: 40 MG-75 MG

BRAND/MANUFACTURER	NDC	SIZE	AWP
○ GENERICS			
DE-TUSS: Moore,H.L.	00839-6372-06	100s	$15.92
DE-TUSS: Moore,H.L.	00839-6372-12	500s	$67.89
TUSS VERNADE T.D.:	52765-2152-05	500s	$99.95
TUSS-ADE IMPROVED: Veratex	17022-8922-06	1000s	$88.96

CAPSULE, EXTENDED RELEASE: 40 MG-75 MG

BRAND/MANUFACTURER	NDC	SIZE	AWP
○ GENERICS			
ORDRINE AT: Eon	00185-0345-53	50s	$38.95
TUSS-ALLERGINE: Rugby	00536-4741-01	100s	$11.00
Pioneer	60104-2002-02	100s	$13.75
TUSS GENADE MODIFIED: Goldline	00182-1452-01	100s	$14.40
TUSSOGEST: Major	00904-0322-60	100s	$16.10
RESCAPS-D: Geneva	00781-2847-01	100s	$35.15
ORDRINE AT: Eon	00185-0345-01	100s	$48.75
Parmed	00349-8329-01	100s ud	$11.93
Pioneer	60104-2002-06	500s	$63.25
TUSSOGEST: Major	00904-0322-40	500s	$74.25
ORDRINE AT: Eon	00185-0345-05	500s	$324.95
TUSS-TRUXADE: Truxton	00463-3038-10	1000s	$93.60
Pioneer	60104-2002-08	1000s	$125.40
Parmed	00349-8329-10	1000s ud	$96.38

Carbachol

DESCRIPTION
Carbachol is a cholinergic prepared as a sterile topical ophthalmic solution. The active ingredient is represented by the chemical structure is $[NH_2COOCH_2CH_2N(CH_3)_3]^+Cl^-$.

Chemical name is 2-[(Aminocarbonyl)oxy]- *N,N,N*-trimethylethanaminum chloride.

Each mL contains: Carbachol 0.75%, 1.5%, 2.25%, or 3.0%. Hydroxypropyl Methylcellulose 1.0%.

Following is its chemical structure:

$$NH_2COO(CH_2)_2N^+(CH_3)_3 \quad Cl^-$$

CLINICAL PHARMACOLOGY
A cholinergic (parasympathomimetic) agent. Carbachol has a double action, it not only stimulates the motor endplate of the muscle cell, as do all cholinesters, but it also partially inhibits cholinesterase.

INDICATIONS AND USAGE
For lowering intraocular pressure in the treatment of glaucoma.

CONTRAINDICATIONS
Miotics are contraindicated where constriction is undesirable such as acute iritis. Contraindicated in those persons showing hypersensitivity to any component of this preparation.

WARNINGS
For topical use only. Not for injection. Carbachol should be used with caution in the presence of corneal abrasion to avoid excessive penetration which can produce systemic toxicity; and in patients with acute cardiac failure, bronchial asthma, active peptic ulcer, hyperthyroidism, gastrointestinal spasm, urinary tract obstruction. Parkinson's disease, recent myocardial infarct, systemic hypertension or hypotension. As with all miotics retinal detachment has been reported when used in certain susceptible individuals.

PRECAUTIONS
General: Avoid overdosage.

Information for Patients: The miosis usually causes difficulty in dark adaptation. Patient should be advised to exercise caution in night driving and other hazardous occupations in poor light. Do not touch dropper tip to any surface, as this may contaminate the solution.

Carcinogenesis, Mutagenesis, Impairment of Fertility: There have been no long-term studies done using Carbachol in animals to evaluate carcinogenic potential.

Pregnancy: Pregnancy Category C. Animal reproduction studies have not been conducted with Carbachol. It is also not known whether Carbachol can cause fetal harm when administered to a pregnant women or can affect reproduction capacity. Carbachol should be given to a pregnant woman only if clearly needed.

Nursing Mothers: It is not known whether this drug is excreted in human milk. Because many drugs are excreted in human milk, caution should be exercised when carbachol is administered to a nursing woman.

ADVERSE REACTIONS
Transient symptoms of stinging and burning may occur. This preparation is capable of producing systemic symptoms of a cholinesterase inhibitor even when the epithelium is intact. Transient ciliary and conjunctival injection, headache, and ciliary spasm with resultant temporary decrease of visual acuity may occur. Salivation, syncope, cardiac arrhythmia, gastrointestinal cramping, vomiting, asthma, hypotension, diarrhea, frequent urge to urinate, increased sweating, and irritation of eyes may occur.

OVERDOSAGE
Atropine should be administered parenterally (for dosage refer to Goodman & Gilman or other pharmacology reference).

DOSAGE AND ADMINISTRATION
Instill two drops topically in the eye(s) up to three times daily or as indicated by physician.

Store at 46°-80°F (8°-27°C).

HOW SUPPLIED
DROP: 0.01%

BRAND/MANUFACTURER	NDC	SIZE	AWP
◆ BRAND			
MIOSTAT: Alcon Surg	00065-0023-15	1.5 ml 12s	$264.00

DROP: 0.75%

BRAND/MANUFACTURER	NDC	SIZE	AWP
○ BRAND			
ISOPTO CARBACHOL: Alcon Ophthalmic	00998-0221-15	15 ml	$16.88
	00998-0221-30	30 ml	$19.38

DROP: 1.5%

BRAND/MANUFACTURER	NDC	SIZE	AWP
○ BRAND			
ISOPTO CARBACHOL: Alcon Ophthalmic	00998-0223-15	15 ml	$17.75
	00998-0223-30	30 ml	$24.56

DROP: 2.25%

BRAND/MANUFACTURER	NDC	SIZE	AWP
○ BRAND			
ISOPTO CARBACHOL: Alcon Ophthalmic	00998-0224-15	15 ml	$18.63

DROP: 3%

BRAND/MANUFACTURER	NDC	SIZE	AWP
○ BRAND			
ISOPTO CARBACHOL: Alcon Ophthalmic	00998-0225-15	15 ml	$19.38
	00998-0225-30	30 ml	$25.94

Carbamazepine

> **WARNING**
>
> APLASTIC ANEMIA AND AGRANULOCYTOSIS HAVE BEEN REPORTED IN ASSOCIATION WITH THE USE OF CARBAMAZEPINE DATA FROM A POPULATED-BASED CASE-CONTROL STUDY DEMONSTRATE THAT THE RISK OF DEVELOPING THESE REACTIONS IS 5-8 TIMES GREATER THAN IN THE GENERAL POPULATION.
>
> HOWEVER, THE OVERALL RISK OF THESE REACTIONS IN THE UNTREATED GENERAL POPULATION IS LOW, APPROXIMATELY SIX PATIENTS PER ONE MILLION POPULATION PER YEAR FOR AGRANULOCYTOSIS AND TWO PATIENTS PER ONE MILLION POPULATION PER YEAR FOR APLASTIC ANEMIA.
>
> DUE TO THE SPARSE DATA FROM THIS STUDY, THE RISK ESTIMATE FOR APLASTIC ANEMIA IS UNKNOWN. HOWEVER, THE OVERALL RISK OF THESE REACTIONS IN THE UNTREATED GENERAL POPULATION IS LOW, APPROXIMATELY 4.7 PATIENTS PER 1 MILLION POPULATION PER YEAR FOR AGRANULOCYTOSIS AND 2 PATIENTS PER 1 MILLION POPULATION PER YEAR FOR APLASTIC ANEMIA. ALTHOUGH MOST OF THE CASES OF AGRANULOCYTOSIS (81%) OCCURRED WITHIN 3 MONTHS OF THERAPY, A FEW CASES HAVE BEEN REPORTED AS LATE AS AFTER 5 YEARS OF THERAPY.
>
> ALTHOUGH REPORTS OF TRANSIENT OR PERSISTENT DECREASED PLATELET OR WHITE BLOOD CELL COUNTS ARE NOT UNCOMMON IN ASSOCIATION WITH THE USE OF CARBAMAZEPINE, DATA ARE NOT

AVAILABLE TO ESTIMATE ACCURATELY THEIR INCIDENCE OR OUTCOME. HOWEVER, THE VAST MAJORITY OF THE CASES OF LEUKOPENIA HAVE NOT PROGRESSED TO THE MORE SERIOUS CONDITIONS OF APLASTIC ANEMIA OR AGRANULOCYTOSIS.

BECAUSE OF THE VERY LOW INCIDENCE OF AGRANULOCYTOSIS AND APLASTIC ANEMIA, THE VAST MAJORITY OF MINOR HEMATOLOGIC CHANGES OBSERVED IN MONITORING OF PATIENTS ON CARBAMAZEPINE ARE UNLIKELY TO SIGNAL THE OCCURRENCE OF EITHER ABNORMALITY. NONETHELESS, COMPLETE PRETREATMENT HEMATOLOGICAL TESTING SHOULD BE OBTAINED AS A BASELINE. IF A PATIENT IN THE COURSE OF TREATMENT EXHIBITS LOW OR DECREASED WHITE BLOOD CELL OR PLATELET COUNTS, THE PATIENT SHOULD BE MONITORED CLOSELY. DISCONTINUATION OF THE DRUG SHOULD BE CONSIDERED IF ANY EVIDENCE OF SIGNIFICANT BONE MARROW DEPRESSION DEVELOPS.

Before prescribing Carbamazepine the physician should be thoroughly familiar with the details of this prescribing information, particularly regarding use with other drugs, especially those which accentuate toxicity potential.

DESCRIPTION

Carbamazepine is an anticonvulsant and specific analgesic for trigeminal neuralgia, available for oral administration as chewable tablets of 100 mg, tablets of 200 mg, and as a suspension of 100 mg/5 ml (teaspoon). Its chemical name is 5H-dibenz[b,f]azepine-5-carboxamide.

Carbamazepine USP is a white to off-white powder, practically insoluble in water and soluble in alcohol and in acetone. Its molecular weight is 236.27.

Following is its chemical structure:

CLINICAL PHARMACOLOGY

In controlled clinical trials, Carbamazepine has been shown to be effective in the treatment of psychomotor and grand mal seizures, as well as trigeminal neuralgia.

It has demonstrated anticonvulsant properties in rats and mice with electrically and chemically induced seizures. It appears to act by reducing polysynaptic responses and blocking the post-tetanic potentiation. Carbamazepine greatly reduces or abolishes pain induced by stimulation of the infraorbital nerve in cats and rats. It depresses thalamic potential and bulbar and polysynaptic reflexes, including the linguomandibular reflex in cats. Carbamazepine is chemically unrelated to other anticonvulsants or other drugs used to control the pain of trigeminal neuralgia. The mechanism of action remains unknown.

In clinical studies both suspension and conventional tablet delivered equivalent amounts of drug to the systemic circulation. However, the suspension was absorbed somewhat faster than the tablet. Following a b.i.d. dosage regimen, the suspension has higher peak plasma levels and lower trough levels than those obtained from the tablet formulation for the same dosage regimen. On the other hand, following a t.i.d. dosage regimen, Carbamazepine suspension affords steady-state plasma levels comparable to Carbamazepine tablets given b.i.d. when administered at the same total mg daily dose. Carbamazepine chewable tablets may produce higher peak levels than the same dose given as regular tablets. Carbamazepine in blood is 76% bound to plasma proteins. Plasma levels of Carbamazepine are variable and may range from 0.5-25 µg/ml, with no apparent relationship to the daily intake of the drug. Usual adult therapeutic levels are between 4 and 12 µg/ml. Following chronic oral administration of suspension, plasma levels peak at approximately 1.5 hours compared to 4 to 5 hours after administration of oral tablets. The CSF/serum ratio is 0.22, similar to the 22% unbound Carbamazepine in serum. Because Carbamazepine may induce its own metabolism, the half-life values range from 25-65 hours, with 12-17 hours on repeated doses. Carbamazepine is metabolized in the liver. After oral administration of ^{14}C-carbamazepine, 72% of the administered radioactivity was found in the urine and 28% in the feces. This urinary radioactivity was composed largely of hydroxylated and conjugated metabolites, with only 3% of unchanged Carbamazepine. Transplacental passage of Carbamazepine is rapid (30 to 60 minutes), and the drug is accumulated in fetal tissues, with higher levels found in liver and kidney than in brain and lungs.

INDICATIONS AND USAGE

Epilepsy: Carbamazepine is indicated for use as an anticonvulsant drug. Evidence supporting efficacy of Carbamazepine as an anticonvulsant was derived from active drug-controlled studies that enrolled patients with the following seizure types:

1. Partial seizures with complex symptomatology (psychomotor, temporal lobe). Patients with these seizures appear to show greater improvement than those with other types.

2. Generalized tonic-clonic seizures (grand mal).

3. Mixed seizure patterns which include the above, or other partial or generalized seizures.

Absence seizures (petit mal) do not appear to be controlled by Carbamazepine (see *"Precautions," General*).

Trigeminal Neuralgia: Carbamazepine is indicated in the treatment of the pain associated with true trigeminal neuralgia. Beneficial results have also been reported in glossopharyngeal neuralgia.

This drug is not a simple analgesic and should not be used for the relief of trivial aches or pains.

UNLABELED USES

Carbamazepine is used alone or as an adjunct in the treatment of anxiety, dysphoria, the lightning pains of tabes dorsalis and somatization and other signs of alcohol abstinence syndrome. It is also used in the treatment of tinnitus, benzodiazepine withdrawal, bipolar affective disorder including manic depression, assaultive and aggressive behavior in patients with organic brain syndrome, depression, and chorea. The drug is prescribed to reduce and is used in the treatment of cocaine craving, senile dementia, paroxysmal dysarthria and ataxia associated with multiple sclerosis and depression. It is also used in diabetes insipidus, dystonia, Kluver-Bucy syndrome, postherpetic neuralgia, neurogenic pain, obsessive-compulsive disorder, hemifacial spasm, restless legs (Ekbom's syndrome), psychosis, and panic disorder, and is prescribed as prophylaxis of migraine headache.

CONTRAINDICATIONS

Carbamazepine should not be used in patients with a history of previous bone marrow depression, hypersensitivity to the drug, or known sensitivity to any of the tricyclic compounds, such as amitriptyline, desipramine, imipramine, protriptyline, nortriptyline, etc. Likewise, on theoretical grounds its use with monoamine oxidase inhibitors is not recommended. Before administration of Carbamazepine, MAO inhibitors should be discontinued for a minimum of fourteen days, or longer if the clinical situation permits.

WARNINGS

Patients with a history of adverse hematologic reaction to any drug may be particularly at risk.

Severe dermatologic reactions including toxic epidermal necrolysis (Lyell's syndrome) and Stevens-Johnson syndrome, have been reported with Carbamazepine. These reactions have been extremely rare. However, a few fatalities have been reported.

Carbamazepine has shown mild anticholinergic activity; therefore, patients with increased intraocular pressure should be closely observed during therapy.

Because of the relationship of the drug to other tricyclic compounds, the possibility of activation of a latent psychosis and, in elderly patients, of confusion or agitation should be borne in mind.

PRECAUTIONS

General: Before initiating therapy, a detailed history and physical examination should be made.

Carbamazepine should be used with caution in patients with a mixed seizure disorder that includes atypical absence seizures, since in these patients Carbamazepine has been associated with increased frequency of generalized convulsions (see *"Indications and Usage"*).

Therapy should be prescribed only after critical benefit-to-risk appraisal in patients with a history of cardiac, hepatic or renal damage, adverse hematologic reaction to other drugs, or interrupted courses of therapy with Carbamazepine.

Since a given dose of Carbamazepine suspension will produce higher peak levels than the same dose given as the tablet, it is recommended that patients given the suspension be started on lower doses and increased slowly to avoid unwanted side effects (see *"Dosage and Administration"*).

Information for Patients: Patients should be made aware of the early toxic signs and symptoms of a potential hematologic problem, such as fever, sore throat, ulcers in the mouth, easy bruising, petechial or purpuric hemorrhage, and should be advised to report to the physician immediately if any such signs or symptoms appear.

Since dizziness and drowsiness may occur, patients should be cautioned about the hazards of operating machinery or automobiles or engaging in other potentially dangerous tasks.

Laboratory Tests: Complete pretreatment blood counts, including platelets and possibly reticulocytes and serum iron, should be obtained as a baseline. If a patient in the course of treatment exhibits low or decreased white blood cell or platelet counts, the patient should be monitored closely. Discontinuation of the drug should be considered if any evidence of significant bone marrow depression develops.

Baseline and periodic evaluations of liver function, particularly in patients with a history of liver disease, must be performed during treatment with this drug since liver damage may occur. The drug should be discontinued immediately in cases of aggravated liver dysfunction or active liver disease. Baseline and periodic eye examinations, including slit-lamp, funduscopy and tonometry, are recommended since many phenothiazines and related drugs have been shown to cause eye changes.

Baseline and periodic complete urinalysis and BUN determinations are recommended for patients treated with this agent because of observed renal dysfunction.

Monitoring of blood levels (see *"Clinical Pharmacology"*) has increased the efficacy and safety of anticonvulsants. This monitoring may be particularly useful in cases of dramatic increase in seizure frequency and for verification of compliance. In addition, measurement of drug serum levels may aid in determining the cause of toxicity when more than one medication is being used.

Thyroid function tests have been reported to show decreased values with Carbamazepine administered alone.

Hyponatremia has been reported in association with Carbamazepine use, either alone or in combination with other drugs.

Drug Interactions: The simultaneous administration of phenobarbital, phenytoin, or primidone, or a combination of two, produces a marked lowering of serum levels of Carbamazepine. The effect of valproic acid on Carbamazepine blood levels is not clearly established, although an increase in the ratio of active, 10, 11-epoxide metabolite to parent compound is a consistent finding.

The half-lives of phenytoin, warfarin, doxycycline, and theophylline were significantly shortened when administered concurrently with Carbamazepine. Haloperidol and valproic acid serum levels may be reduced when these drugs are administered with Carbamazepine. The doses of these drugs may therefore have to be increased when Carbamazepine is added to the therapeutic regimen.

Concomitant administration of Carbamazepine with erythromycin, cimetidine, propoxyphene, isoniazid, fluoxetine or calcium channel blockers has been reported to result in elevated plasma levels of carbamazepine resulting in toxicity in some cases. Also, concomitant administration of carbamazepine and lithium may increase the risk of neurotoxic side effects. Alterations of thyroid function have been reported in combination therapy with other anticonvulsant medications.

Breakthrough bleeding has been reported among patients receiving concomitant oral contraceptives and their reliability may be adversely affected.

Carcinogenesis, Mutagenesis, Impairment of Fertility: Carbamazepine, when administered to Sprague-Dawley rats for two years in the diet at doses of 25, 75, and 250 mg/kg/day, resulted in a dose-related increase in the incidence of hepatocellular tumors in females and of benign interstitial cell adenomas in the testes of males.

Carbamazepine must, therefore, be considered to be carcinogenic in Sprague-Dawley rats. Bacterial and mammalian mutagenicity studies using Carbamazepine produced negative results. The significance of these findings relative to the use of Carbamazepine in humans is, at present, unknown.

Pregnancy Category C: Carbamazepine has been shown to have adverse effects in reproduction studies in rats when given orally in dosages 10-25 times the maximum human daily dosage of 1200 mg. In rat teratology studies, 2 of 135 offspring showed kinked ribs at 250 mg/kg and 4 of 119 offspring at 650 mg/kg showed other anomalies (cleft palate, 1; talipes, 1; anophthalmos, 2). In reproduction studies in rats, nursing offspring demonstrated a lack of weight gain and an unkempt appearance at a maternal dosage level of 200 mg/kg.

There are no adequate and well-controlled studies in pregnant women. Epidemiological data suggest that there may be an association between the use of Carbamazepine during pregnancy and congenital malformations, including spina bifida. Carbamazepine should be used during pregnancy only if the potential benefit justifies the potential risk to the fetus.

Retrospective case reviews suggest that, compared with monotherapy, there may be a higher prevalence of teratogenic effects associated with the use of anticonvulsants in combination therapy. Therefore, monotherapy is recommended for pregnant women.

It is important to note that anticonvulsant drugs should not be discontinued in patients in whom the drug is administered to prevent major seizures because of the strong possibility of precipitating status epilepticus with attendant hypoxia and threat to life. In individual cases where the severity and frequency of the seizure disorder are such that removal of medication does not pose a serious threat to the patient, discontinuation of the drug may be considered prior to and during pregnancy, although it cannot be said with any confidence that even minor seizures do not pose some hazard to the developing embryo or fetus.

Labor and Delivery: The effect of Carbamazepine on human labor and delivery is unknown.

Nursing Mothers: During lactation, concentration of Carbamazepine in milk is approximately 60% of the maternal plasma concentration.

Because of the potential for serious adverse reactions in nursing infants from Carbamazepine, a decision should be made whether to discontinue nursing or to discontinue the drug, taking into account the importance of the drug to the mother.

Pediatric Use: Safety and effectiveness in children below the age of 6 years have not been established.

ADVERSE REACTIONS

If adverse reactions are of such severity that the drug must be discontinued, the physician must be aware that abrupt discontinuation of any anticonvulsant drug in a responsive epileptic patient may lead to seizures or even status epilepticus with its life-threatening hazards.

The most severe adverse reactions have been observed in the hemopoietic system (see boxed *"Warning"*), the skin and the cardiovascular system.

The most frequently observed adverse reactions, particularly during the initial phases of therapy, are dizziness, drowsiness, unsteadiness, nausea, and vomiting. To minimize the possibility of such reactions, therapy should be initiated at the low dosage recommended.

The following additional adverse reactions have been reported:

Hemopoietic System: Aplastic anemia, agranulocytosis, pancytopenia, bone marrow depression, thrombocytopenia, leukopenia, leukocytosis, eosinophilia, acute intermittent porphyria.

Skin: Pruritic and erythematous rashes, urticaria, toxic epidermal necrolysis (Lyell's syndrome) (see *"Warnings"*), Stevens-Johnson syndrome (see *"Warnings"*), photosensitivity reactions, alterations in skin pigmentation, exfoliative dermatitis, erythema multiforme and nodosum, purpura, aggravation of disseminated lupus erythematosus, alopecia, and diaphoresis. In certain cases, discontinuation of therapy may be necessary. Isolated cases of hirsutism have been reported, but a causal relationship is not clear.

Cardiovascular System: Congestive heart failure, edema, aggravation of hypertension, hypotension, syncope and collapse, aggravation of coronary artery disease, arrhythmias and AV block, primary thrombophlebitis, recurrence of thrombophlebitis, and adenopathy or lymphadenopathy.

Some of these cardiovascular complications have resulted in fatalities. Myocardial infarction has been associated with other tricyclic compounds.

Liver: Abnormalities in liver function tests, cholestatic and hepatocellular jaundice, hepatitis.

Respiratory System: Pulmonary hypersensitivity characterized by fever, dyspnea, pneumonitis or pneumonia.

Genitourinary System: Urinary frequency, acute urinary retention, oliguria with elevated blood pressure, azotemia, renal failure, and impotence. Albuminuria, glycosuria, elevated BUN and microscopic deposits in the urine have also been reported.

Testicular atrophy occurred in rats receiving Carbamazepine orally from 4 to 52 weeks at dosage levels of 50 to 400 mg/kg/day. Additionally, rats receiving Carbamazepine in the diet for two years at dosage levels of 25, 75, and 250 mg/kg/day had a dose-related incidence of testicular atrophy and aspermatogenesis. In dogs, it produced a brownish discoloration, presumably a metabolite, in the urinary bladder at dosage levels of 50 mg/kg and higher. Relevance of these findings to humans is unknown.

Nervous System: Dizziness, drowsiness, disturbances of coordination, confusion, headache, fatigue, blurred vision, visual hallucinations, transient diplopia, oculomotor disturbances, nystagmus, speech disturbances, abnormal involuntary movements, peripheral neuritis and paresthesias, depression with agitation, talkativeness, tinnitus, and hyperacusis.

There have been reports of associated paralysis and other symptoms of cerebral arterial insufficiency, but the exact relationship of these reactions to the drug has not been established.

Digestive System: Nausea, vomiting, gastric distress and abdominal pain, diarrhea, constipation, anorexia, and dryness of the mouth and pharynx, including glossitis and stomatitis.

Eyes: Scattered, punctate, cortical lens opacities, as well as conjunctivitis have been reported. Although a direct causal relationship has not been established, many phenothiazines and related drugs have been shown to cause eye changes.

Musculoskeletal System: Aching joints and muscles, and leg cramps.

Metabolism: Fever and chills. Inappropriate antidiuretic hormone (ADH) secretion syndrome has been reported. Cases of frank water intoxication, with decreased serum sodium (hyponatremia) and confusion, have been reported in association with Carbamazepine (see *"Precautions, Laboratory Tests"*).

Other: Isolated cases of a lupus erythematosus-like syndrome have been reported. There have been occasional reports of elevated levels of cholesterol, HDL cholesterol and triglycerides in patients taking anticonvulsants.

A case of aseptic meningitis, accompanied by myoclonus and peripheral eosinophilia, has been reported in a patient taking Carbamazepine in combination with other medications. The patient was successfully dechallenged, and the meningitis reappeared upon rechallenge with Carbamazepine.

DRUG ABUSE AND DEPENDENCE

No evidence of abuse potential has been associated with Carbamazepine nor is there evidence of psychological or physical dependence in humans.

OVERDOSAGE

ACUTE TOXICITY

Lowest known lethal dose: adults, > 60 g (39-year-old man). Highest known doses survived: adults, 30 g (31-year-old woman); children, 10 g (6-year-old boy); small children, 5 g (3-year-old girl).

Oral LD_{50} in animals (mg/kg): mice, 1100-3750; rats, 3850-4025; rabbits, 1500-2680; guinea pigs, 920.

SIGNS AND SYMPTOMS

The first signs and symptoms appear after 1-3 hours. Neuromuscular disturbances are the most prominent. Cardiovascular disorders are generally milder, and severe cardiac complications occur only when very high doses (> 60 g) have been ingested.

Respiration: Irregular breathing, respiratory depression.

Cardiovascular System: Tachycardia, hypotension or hypertension, shock, conduction disorders.

Nervous System and Muscles: Impairment of consciousness ranging in severity to deep coma. Convulsions, especially in small children. Motor restlessness, muscular twitching, tremor, athetoid movements, opisthotonos, ataxia, drowsiness, dizziness, mydriasis, nystagmus, adiadochokinesia, ballism, psychomotor disturbances, dysmetria. Initial hyperreflexia, followed by hyporeflexia.

Gastrointestinal Tract: Nausea, vomiting.

Kidneys and Bladder: Anuria or oliguria, urinary retention.

Laboratory Findings: Isolated instances of overdosage have included leukocytosis, reduced leukocyte count, glycosuria and acetonuria. EEG may show dysrhythmias.

Combined Poisoning: When alcohol, tricyclic antidepressants, barbiturates or hydantoins are taken at the same time, the signs and symptoms of acute poisoning with Carbamazepine may be aggravated or modified.

TREATMENT
The prognosis in cases of severe poisoning is critically dependent upon prompt elimination of the drug, which may be achieved by inducing vomiting, irrigating the stomach, and by taking appropriate steps to diminish absorption. If these measures cannot be implemented without risk on the spot, the patient should be transferred at once to a hospital, while ensuring that vital functions are safeguarded. There is no specific antidote.

Elimination of the Drug: Induction of vomiting.
Gastric lavage. Even when more than 4 hours have elapsed following ingestion of the drug, the stomach should be repeatedly irrigated, especially if the patient has also consumed alcohol.

Measures to Reduce Absorption: Activated charcoal, laxatives.

Measures to Accelerate Elimination: Forced diuresis.
Dialysis is indicated only in severe poisoning associated with renal failure. Replacement transfusion is indicated in severe poisoning in small children.

Respiratory Depression: Keep the airways free; resort, if necessary, to endotracheal intubation, artificial respiration, and administration of oxygen.

Hypotension, Shock: Keep the patient's legs raised and administer a plasma expander. If blood pressure fails to rise despite measures taken to increase plasma volume, use of vasoactive substances should be considered.

Convulsions: Diazepam or barbiturates.

Warning: Diazepam or barbiturates may aggravate respiratory depression (especially in children), hypotension, and coma. However, barbiturates should *not* be used if drugs that inhibit monoamine oxidase have also been taken by the patient either in overdosage or in recent therapy (within one week).

Surveillance: Respiration, cardiac function (ECG monitoring), blood pressure, body temperature, pupillary reflexes, and kidney and bladder function should be monitored for several days.

Treatment of Blood Count Abnormalities: If evidence of significant bone marrow depression develops, the following recommendations are suggested: (1) stop the drug, (2) perform daily CBC, platelet and reticulocyte counts, (3) do a bone marrow aspiration and trephine biopsy immediately and repeat with sufficient frequency to monitor recovery.
Special periodic studies might be helpful as follows: (1) white cell and platelet antibodies, (2) ^{59}Fe—ferrokinetic studies, (3) peripheral blood cell typing, (4) cytogenetic studies on marrow and peripheral blood, (5) bone marrow culture studies for colony-forming units, (6) hemoglobin electrophoresis for A_2 and F hemoglobin, and (7) serum folic acid and B_{12} levels.
A fully developed aplastic anemia will require appropriate, intensive monitoring and therapy, for which specialized consultation should be sought.

DOSAGE AND ADMINISTRATION
Monitoring of blood levels has increased the efficacy and safety of anticonvulsants (see *"Precautions, Laboratory Tests"*). Dosage should be adjusted to the needs of the individual patient. A low initial daily dosage with a gradual increase is advised. As soon as adequate control is achieved, the dosage may be reduced very gradually to the minimum effective level. Medications should be taken with meals.
Since a given dose of Carbamazepine suspension will produce higher peak levels than the same dose given as the tablet, it is recommended to start with low doses (children 6-12 years: ½ teaspoon q.i.d.) and to increase slowly to avoid unwanted side effects.
Conversion of patients from oral Carbamazepine tablets to Carbamazepine suspension: Patients should be converted by administering the same number of mg per day in smaller, more frequent doses (i.e., b.i.d. tablets to t.i.d. suspension).

EPILEPSY
(See *"Indications and Usage".*)

Adults and children over 12 years of age—Initial: Either 200 mg b.i.d. for tablets or 1 teaspoon q.i.d. for suspension (400 mg per day). Increase at weekly intervals by adding up to 200 mg per day using a t.i.d. or q.i.d. regimen until the optimal response is obtained. Dosage should generally not exceed 1000 mg daily in children 12 to 15 years of age, and up to 1200 mg daily in patients above 15 years of age. Doses up to 1600 mg daily have been used in adults in rare instances.

Maintenance: Adjust dosage to the minimum effective level, usually 800-1200 mg daily.

Children 6-12 years of age—Initial: Either 100 mg b.i.d. for tablets or ½ teaspoon q.i.d. for suspension (200 mg per day). Increase at weekly intervals by adding up to 100 mg per day using a t.i.d. or q.i.d. regimen until the optimal response is obtained. Dosage generally should not exceed 1000 mg daily.

Maintenance: Adjust dosage to the minimum effective level, usually 400-800 mg daily.

Combination Therapy: Carbamazepine may be used alone or with other anticonvulsants. When added to existing anticonvulsant therapy, the drug should be added gradually while the other anticonvulsants are maintained or gradually decreased, except phenytoin, which may have to be increased (see *"Precautions, Drug Interactions"* and *"Pregnancy, Category C".*).

TRIGEMINAL NEURALGIA
(See *"Indications and Usage".*)

Initial: On the first day, either 100 mg b.i.d. for tablets or ½ teaspoon q.i.d. for suspension for a total daily dose of 200 mg. This daily dose may be increased by up to 200 mg a day using increments of 100 mg every 12 hours for tablets or 50 mg (½ teaspoon) q.i.d. for suspension, only as needed to achieve freedom from pain. Do not exceed 1200 mg daily.

Maintenance: Control of pain can be maintained in most patients with 400 mg to 800 mg daily. However, some patients may be maintained on as little as 200 mg daily, while others may require as much as 1200 mg daily. At least once every 3 months throughout the treatment period, attempts should be made to reduce the dose to the minimum effective level or even to discontinue the drug. (See related table).

STORAGE
Tablets: Do not store above 86°F (30°C).
Protect from moisture. Dispense in tight container (USP).

Suspension: Shake well before using.
Do not store above 86°F (30°C).
Dispense in tight, light-resistant container (USP).

HOW SUPPLIED
CHEW TABLET: 100 MG

AVERAGE UNIT PRICE (AVAILABLE SIZES)		GENERIC A-RATED AVERAGE PRICE (GAAP)	
BRAND	$0.19	100s	$16.71
GENERIC	$0.17		
HCFA FUL (100s ea)	$0.19		

BRAND/MANUFACTURER	NDC	SIZE	AWP
◆ **BRAND**			
▶ TEGRETOL: Basel	58887-0052-30	100s	$18.00
	58887-0052-32	100s ud	$20.26
◆ **GENERICS**			
Rugby	00536-3411-01	100s	$16.00
Goldline	00182-1331-01	100s	$16.20
Warner Chilcott	00047-0242-24	100s	$16.20
Du Pont Multi	00056-0182-70	100s	$16.29
Moore,H.L.	00839-7410-06	100s	$16.86
Schein	00364-2309-01	100s	$17.25
Aligen	00405-4130-01	100s	$18.20

SUSPENSION: 100 MG/5 ML

BRAND/MANUFACTURER	NDC	SIZE	AWP
○ **BRAND**			
TEGRETOL: Basel	58887-0019-76	450 ml	$22.32

TABLETS: 200 MG

AVERAGE UNIT PRICE (AVAILABLE SIZES)		GENERIC A-RATED AVERAGE PRICE (GAAP)	
BRAND	$0.35	100s	$25.13
GENERIC	$0.24	1000s	$198.65
HCFA FUL (100s ea)	$0.16		

BRAND/MANUFACTURER	NDC	SIZE	AWP
◆ **BRAND**			
▶ TEGRETOL: Basel	58887-0027-30	100s	$34.66
	58887-0027-32	100s ud	$37.11
	58887-0027-40	1000s	$343.00
◆ **GENERICS**			
Inwood	00258-3587-01	100s	$17.27
Purepac	00228-2143-10	100s	$23.21
Rugby	00536-3415-01	100s	$23.25
Major	00904-3855-60	100s	$23.25
Schein	00364-2106-01	100s	$23.50
URL	00677-1099-01	100s	$23.95
▶ EPITOL: Lemmon	00093-0090-01	100s	$24.00
Lemmon	00093-0109-01	100s	$24.00
Goldline	00182-1233-01	100s	$24.00
Qualitest	00603-2563-21	100s	$24.00
Moore,H.L.	00839-7177-06	100s	$24.91
ATRETOL: Athena	59075-0554-10	100s	$26.80
Aligen	00405-4131-01	100s	$27.90
Parmed	00349-8924-01	100s	$28.68
Parmed	00349-8977-01	100s	$28.68
Du Pont Multi	00056-0183-70	100s	$29.64
U.S. Trading	56126-0352-11	100s ud	$10.08
Raway	00686-0385-20	100s ud	$19.95
Auro	55829-0173-10	100s ud	$25.31
Vangard	00615-3505-13	100s ud	$31.39
Goldline	00182-1233-89	100s ud	$33.40
UDL	51079-0385-20	100s ud	$35.70
Purepac	00228-2143-50	500s	$116.05
Major	00904-3855-80	1000s	$161.50

DOSAGE INFORMATION: TABLETS AND SUSPENSION

| Indication | Initial Dose | | Subsequent Dose | | Maximum Dose |
	Tablet	Suspension	Tablet	Suspension	Tablet or Suspension
Epilepsy 6-12 years of age	100 mg b.i.d. (200 mg/day)	½ teaspon q.i.d. (200 mg/day)	Add up to 100 mg per day at weekly intervals, t.i.d. or q.i.d.	Add up to 1 teaspoon (100 mg) per day at weekly intervals, t.i.d. or q.i.d.	1000 mg/24 hours
Over 12 years of age	200 mg b.i.d. (400 mg/day)	1 teaspoon q.i.d. (400 mg/day)	Add up to 200 mg per day at weekly intervals, t.i.d. or q.i.d.	Add up to 2 teaspoons (200 mg) per day at weekly intervals, t.i.d. or q.i.d.	1000 mg/24 hours: 12-15 years 1200 mg/24 hours: over 15 years 1600 mg/24 hours: adults, in rare instances
Trigeminal Neuralgia	100 mg b.i.d. on the first day (200 mg/day)	½ teaspoon q.i.d. (200 mg/day)	Add up to 200 mg per day in increments of 100 mg every 12 hours	Add up to 2 teaspoons (200 mg) per day q.i.d.	1200 mg/24 hours

BRAND/MANUFACTURER	NDC	SIZE	AWP
Purepac	00228-2143-96	1000s	$213.65
Lemmon	00093-0109-10	1000s	$220.80

Carbenicillin Indanyl Sodium

DESCRIPTION

Carbenicillin Indanyl Sodium, a semisynthetic penicillin, is the sodium salt of the Indanyl ester of Carbenicillin disodium. The chemical name is:

1-(5-Indanyl)-N-(2-carboxy-3,3-dimethyl-7-oxo-4-thia-1-azabicyclo [3.2.0] hept-6-yl)-2-phenylmalonamate monosodium salt.

The empirical formula is: $C_{26}H_{25}N_2NaO_6S$ and molecular weight is 516.55.

Carbenicillin is freely soluble in water. Each Carbenicillin Indanyl Sodium tablet contains 382 mg of Carbenicillin, 118 mg of Indanyl Sodium ester. Each Carbenicillin Indanyl Sodium tablet contains 23 mg of Sodium.

Following is its chemical structure:

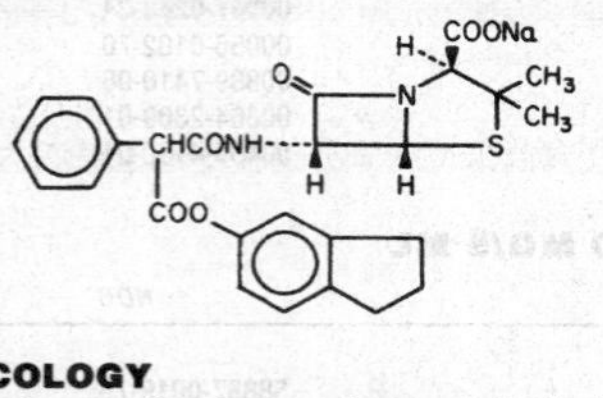

CLINICAL PHARMACOLOGY

Free Carbenicillin is the predominant pharmacologically active fraction of Carbenicillin Indanyl Sodium. Carbenicillin exerts its antibacterial activity by interference with final cell wall synthesis of susceptible bacteria.

Carbenicillin Indanyl Sodium is acid stable, and rapidly absorbed from the small intestine following oral administration. It provides relatively low plasma concentrations of antibiotic and is primarily excreted in the urine. After absorption, Carbenicillin Indanyl Sodium is rapidly converted to Carbenicillin by hydrolysis of the ester linkage. Following ingestion of a single 500 mg tablet of Carbenicillin Indanyl Sodium, a peak Carbenicillin plasma concentration of approximately 6.5 mcg/ml is reached in 1 hour. About 30% of this dose is excreted in the urine unchanged within 12 hours, with another 6% excreted over the next 12 hours.

In a multiple dose study utilizing volunteers with normal renal function, the following mean urine and serum levels of Carbenicillin were achieved:

| Drug | Dose | Mean Urine Concentration of Carbenicillin mcg/ml Hours After Initial Dose | | |
		0-3	3-6	6-24
Carbenicillin Indanyl Sodium	1 tablet q.6 hr	1130	352	292
Carbenicillin Indanyl Sodium	2 tablets q.6 hr	1428	789	809

(See related table).

MICROBIOLOGY

The antibacterial activity of Carbenicillin Indanyl Sodium is due to its rapid conversion to Carbenicillin by hydrolysis after absorption. Though Carbenicillin Indanyl Sodium provides substantial *in vitro* activity against a variety of both gram-positive and gram-negative microorganisms, the most important aspect of its profile is in its antipseudomonal and antiproteal activity. Because of the high urine levels obtained following administration, Carbenicillin Indanyl Sodium has demonstrated clinical efficacy in urinary infections due to susceptible strains of:

Escherichia coli
Proteus mirabilis
Proteus vulgaris
Morganella morganii (formerly *Proteus morganii*)
Pseudomonas species
Providencia rettgeri (formerly *Proteus rettgeri*)
Enterobacter species
Enterococci (*S. faecalis*)

In addition, *in vitro* data, not substantiated by clinical studies, indicate the following pathogens to be usually susceptible to Carbenicillin Indanyl Sodium:
Staphylococcus species (nonpenicillinase producing) *Streptococcus* species

RESISTANCE

Most *Klebsiella* species are usually resistant to the action of Carbenicillin Indanyl Sodium. Some strains of *Pseudomonas* species have developed resistance to Carbenicillin.

SUSCEPTIBILITY TESTING

Carbenicillin disodium Susceptibility Powder or 100 μg. Carbenicillin disodium Susceptibility Discs may be used to determine microbial susceptibility to Carbenicillin Indanyl Sodium using one of the following standard methods recommended by the National Committee for Clinical Laboratory Standards:

M2-A3, "Performance Standards for Antimicrobial Disk Susceptibility Tests"

M7-A, "Methods for Dilution Antimicrobial Susceptibility Tests for Bacteria that Grow Aerobically"

M11-A, "Reference Agar Dilution Procedure for Antimicrobial Susceptibility Testing of Anaerobic Bacteria"

M17-P, "Alternative Methods for Antimicrobial Susceptibility Testing of Anaerobic Bacteria"

Tests should be interpreted by the following criteria:

DISK DIFFUSION
ZONE DIAMETER (MM)

Organisms	Suscept.	Intermed.	Resist.
Enterobacter	≥ 23	18-22	≤ 17
Pseudomonas sp.	≥ 17	14-16	≤ 13

DILUTION MIC (μ/ML)

Organisms	Suscept.	Moderately Suscept.	Resist.
Enterobacter	≤ 16	32	≥ 64
Pseudomonas sp.	≤ 128	—	≥ 156

Interpretations of susceptible, intermediate, and resistant correlate zone size diameters with MIC values. A laboratory report of "susceptible" indicates that the suspected causative microorganism most likely will respond to therapy with Carbenicillin. A laboratory report of "resistant" indicates that the infecting microorganism most likely will not respond to therapy. A laboratory report of "moderately susceptible" indicates that the microorganism is most likely susceptible if a high dosage of Carbenicillin is used, or if the infection is such that high levels of Carbenicillin may be attained as in urine. A report of "intermediate" using the disk diffusion method may be considered an equivocal result, and dilution tests may be indicated.

INDICATIONS AND USAGE

Carbenicillin Indanyl Sodium is indicated in the treatment of acute and chronic infections of the upper and lower urinary tract and in asymptomatic bacteriuria due to susceptible strains of the following organisms:

Escherichia coli
Proteus mirabilis

Mean serum concentrations of Carbenicillin in this study for these dosages are:

Mean Serum Concentration mcg/ml
Hours After Initial Dose

Drug	Dose	½	1	2	4	6	24	25	26	28
Carbenicillin Indanyl Sodium	1 tablet q.6 hr	5.1	6.5	3.2	1.9	0.0	0.4	8.8	5.4	0.4
Carbenicillin Indanyl Sodium	2 tablets q.6 hr	6.1	9.6	7.9	2.6	0.4	0.8	13.2	12.8	3.8

Morganella morganii
   (formerly *Proteus morganii*)
Providencia rettgeri
   (formerly *Proteus rettgeri*)
Proteus vulgaris
Pseudomonas
Enterobacter
Enterococci

Carbenicillin Indanyl Sodium is also indicated in the treatment of prostatitis due to susceptible strains of the following organisms:

Escherichia coli
   Enterococcus (*S. faecalis*)
Proteus mirabilis
Enterobacter sp.

WHEN HIGH AND RAPID BLOOD AND URINE LEVELS OF ANTIBIOTIC ARE INDICATED. THERAPY WITH CARBENICILLIN DISODIUM SHOULD BE INITIATED BY PARENTERAL ADMINISTRATION FOLLOWED, AT THE PHYSICIAN'S DISCRETION, BY ORAL THERAPY.

Note: Susceptibility testing should be performed prior to and during the course of therapy to detect the possible emergence of resistant organisms which may develop.

CONTRAINDICATIONS
Carbenicillin Indanyl Sodium is ordinarily contraindicated in patients who have a known penicillin allergy.

WARNINGS
Serious and occasionally fatal hypersensitivity (anaphylactic) reactions have been reported in patients on oral penicillin therapy. Although anaphylaxis is more frequent following parenteral therapy, it has occurred in patients on oral penicillins. These reactions are more apt to occur in individuals with a history of penicillin hypersensitivity and/or a history of sensitivity to multiple allergens.

There have been reports of individuals with a history of penicillin hypersensitivity who have experienced severe hypersensitivity reactions when treated with a cephalosporin, and vice versa. Before initiating therapy with a penicillin, careful inquiry should be made concerning previous hypersensitivity reactions to penicillins, cephalosporins, or other allergens. If an allergic reaction occurs, the drug should be discontinued and the appropriate therapy instituted.

SERIOUS ANAPHYLACTOID REACTIONS REQUIRE IMMEDIATE EMERGENCY TREATMENT WITH EPINEPHRINE, OXYGEN, INTRAVENOUS STEROIDS AND AIRWAY MANAGEMENT, INCLUDING INTUBATION, SHOULD ALSO BE ADMINISTERED AS INDICATED.

PRECAUTIONS
General: As with any penicillin preparation, an allergic response, including anaphylaxis, may occur particularly in a hypersensitive individual.

Long term use of Carbenicillin Indanyl Sodium may result in the overgrowth of nonsusceptible organisms. If superinfection occurs during therapy, appropriate measures should be taken.

Since Carbenicillin is primarily excreted by the kidney, patients with severe renal impairment (creatinine clearance of less than 10 ml/min) will not achieve therapeutic urine levels of Carbenicillin.

In patients with creatinine clearance of 10-20 ml/min it may be necessary to adjust dosage to prevent accumulation of drug.

Laboratory Tests: As with other penicillins, periodic assessment of organ system function including renal, hepatic, and hematopoietic systems is recommended during prolonged therapy.

Drug Interactions: Carbenicillin Indanyl Sodium blood levels may be increased and prolonged by concurrent administration of probenecid.

Carcinogenesis, Mutagenesis, Impairment of Fertility: There are no long-term animal or human studies to evaluate carcinogenic potential. Rats fed 250-1000 mg/kg/day for 18 months developed mild liver pathology (e.g., bile duct hyperplasia) at all dose levels, but there was no evidence of drug-related neoplasia. Carbenicillin Indanyl Sodium administered at daily doses ranging to 1000 mg/kg had no apparent effect on the fertility or reproductive performance of rats.

Pregnancy Category B: Reproduction studies have been performed at dose levels of 1000 or 500 mg/kg in rats, 200 mg/kg in mice, and at 500 mg/kg in monkeys with no harm to fetus due to Carbenicillin Indanyl Sodium. There are, however, no adequate and well controlled studies in pregnant women. Because animal reproduction studies are not always predictive of human response, this drug should be used during pregnancy only if clearly needed.

Labor and Delivery: It is not known whether the use of Carbenicillin Indanyl Sodium in humans during labor or delivery has immediate or delayed adverse effects on the fetus, prolongs the duration of labor, or increases the likelihood that forceps delivery or other obstetrical intervention or resuscitation of the newborn will be necessary.

Nursing Mothers: Carbenicillin class antibiotics are excreted in milk although the amounts excreted are unknown; therefore, caution should be exercised if administered to a nursing woman.

Pediatric Use: Since only limited clinical data is available to date in children, the safety of Carbenicillin Indanyl Sodium administration in this age group has not yet been established.

ADVERSE REACTIONS
The following adverse reactions have been reported as possibly related to Carbenicillin Indanyl Sodium administration in controlled studies which include 344 patients receiving Carbenicillin Indanyl Sodium.

Gastrointestinal: The most frequent adverse reactions associated with Carbenicillin Indanyl Sodium therapy are related to the gastrointestinal tract. Nausea, bad taste, diarrhea, vomiting, flatulence, and glossitis were reported. Abdominal cramps, dry mouth, furry tongue, rectal bleeding, anorexia, and unspecified epigastric distress were rarely reported.

Dermatologic: Hypersensitivity reactions such as skin rash, urticaria, and less frequently pruritus.

Hematologic: As with other penicillins, anemia, thrombocytopenia, leukopenia, neutropenia, and eosinophilia have infrequently been observed. The clinical significance of these abnormalities is not known.

Miscellaneous: Other reactions rarely reported were hyperthermia, headache, itchy eyes, vaginitis, and loose stools.

Abnormalities of Hepatic Function Tests: Mild SGOT elevations have been observed following Carbenicillin Indanyl Sodium administration.

OVERDOSAGE
Carbenicillin Indanyl Sodium is generally nontoxic. Carbenicillin Indanyl Sodium when taken in excessive amounts may produce mild gastrointestinal irritation. The drug is rapidly excreted in the urine and symptoms are transitory. The usual symptoms of anaphylaxis may occur in hypersensitive individuals.

Carbenicillin blood levels achievable with Carbenicillin Indanyl Sodium are very low, and toxic reactions as a function of overdosage should not occur systematically. The oral LD_{50} in mice is 3,600 mg/kg, in rats 2,000 mg/kg, and in dogs is in excess of 500 mg/kg. The lethal human dose is not known.

Although never reported, the possibility of accumulation of Indanyl should be considered when large amounts of Carbenicillin Indanyl Sodium are ingested. Free indole, which is a phenol derivative, may be potentially toxic. In general 8-15 grams of phenol, and presumably a similar amount of indole, are required orally before toxicity (peripheral vascular collapse) may occur. The metabolic by-products of indole are nontoxic. In patients with hepatic failure it may be possible for unmetabolized indole to accumulate.

The metabolic by products of Carbenicillin Indanyl Sodium, Indanyl sulfate and glucuronide, as well as free Carbenicillin, are dialyzable.

DOSAGE AND ADMINISTRATION
Carbenicillin Indanyl Sodium is available as a coated tablet to be administered orally.

USUAL ADULT DOSE

Urinary Tract Infections

Escherichia coli, Proteus species, and *Enterbacter*	1-2 tablets 4 times daily
Pseudomonas and *Enterococcus*	2 tablets 4 times daily

Prostatitis

Escherichia coli, Proteus mirabilis, Enterobacter and *Enterococcus*	2 tablets 4 times daily

▶ SHOWN IN PRODUCT IDENTIFICATION GUIDE

HOW SUPPLIED
TABLETS: 382 MG

BRAND/MANUFACTURER	NDC	SIZE	AWP
○ **BRAND**			
GEOCILLIN: Roerig,J.B.	00049-1430-66	100s	$173.21
	00049-1430-41	100s ud	$199.10

Carbetapentane/
Chlorpheniramine/Ephedrine/
Phenylephrine

DESCRIPTION

Carbetapentane/Chlorpheniramine/Ephedrine/Phenylephrine is an antitussive/ antihistaminic/ decongestant/bronchodilator combination available for oral administration as *Tablets* and as *Pediatric Suspension*.

Each tablet contains:

Carbetapentane Tannate	.60 mg
Chlorpheniramine Tannate	.5 mg
Ephedrine Tannate	.10 mg
Phenylephrine Tannate	.10 mg

Each 5 ml (one teaspoonful) of the Pediatric Suspension contains:

Carbetapentane Tannate	.30 mg
Chlorpheniramine Tannate	.4 mg
Ephedrine Tannate	.5 mg
Phenylephrine Tannate	.5 mg

CLINICAL PHARMACOLOGY

Carbetapentane/Chlorpheniramine/Ephedrine/Phenylephrine (Carbetapen/Chlorphen/Eph/Phenyleph) combines the antitussive action of Carbetapentane, the antihistaminic action of Chlorpheniramine, the bronchodilator action of Ephedrine, and the sympathomimetic decongestant effect of Phenylephrine.

INDICATIONS AND USAGE

Carbetapen/Chlorphen/Eph/Phenyleph is indicated for the symptomatic relief of cough associated with respiratory tract conditions such as the common cold, bronchial asthma, acute and chronic bronchitis. Appropriate therapy should be provided for the primary disease.

CONTRAINDICATIONS

Carbetapen/Chlorphen/Eph/Phenyleph is contraindicated for newborns, nursing mothers and patients who are sensitive to any of the ingredients or related compounds.

WARNINGS

Use with caution in patients with hypertension, cardiovascular disease, hyperthyroidism, diabetes, narrow angle glaucoma or prostatic hypertrophy. Use with caution or avoid use in patients taking monoamine oxidase (MAO) Inhibitors. This product contains antihistamines which may cause drowsiness and may have additive central nervous system (CNS) effects with alcohol or other CNS depressants (e.g., hypnotics, sedatives, tranquilizers).

PRECAUTIONS

For Carbetapen/Chlorphen/Eph/Phenyleph Pediatric Suspension only: Certain brands of Carbetapen/Clorphen/Eph/Phenyleph contain FD&C Yellow No. 5 (tartrazine) which may cause allergic-type reactions (including bronchial asthma) in certain susceptible individuals. Although the overall incidence of FD&C Yellow No. 5 (tartrazine) sensitivity in the general population is low, it is frequently seen in patients who also have aspirin hypersensitivity.

General: Antihistamines are more likely to cause dizziness, sedation and hypotension in elderly patients. Antihistamines may cause excitation, particularly in children, but their combination with sympathomimetics may cause either mild stimulation or mild sedation.

Information for Patients: Caution patients against drinking alcoholic beverages or engaging in potentially hazardous activities requiring alertness, such as driving a car or operating machinery, while using this product.

Drug Interactions: MAO inhibitors may prolong and intensify the anticholinergic effects of antihistamines and the overall effects of sympathomimetic agents.

Carcinogenesis, Mutagenesis, Impairment of Fertility: No long term animal studies have been performed with Carbetapen/Chlorphen/Eph/Phenyleph.

Pregnancy: Teratogenic Effects: Pregnancy Category C. Animal reproduction studies have not been conducted with Carbetapen/Chlorphen/Eph/Phenyleph. It is also not known whether Carbetapen/ Chlorphen/Eph/Phenyleph can cause fetal harm when administered to a pregnant woman or can affect reproduction capacity. Carbetapen/Chlorphen/Eph/Phenyleph should be given to a pregnant woman only if clearly needed.

Nursing Mothers: Carbetapen/Chlorphen/Eph/Phenyleph should not be administered to a nursing woman.

ADVERSE REACTIONS

Adverse effects associated with Carbetapen/Chlorphen/Eph/Phenyleph at recommended doses have been minimal. The most common have been drowsiness, sedation, dryness of mucous membranes, and gastrointestinal effects. Serious side effects with oral antihistamines or sympathomimetics have been rare.

OVERDOSAGE

Signs and Symptoms: May vary from CNS depression to stimulation (restlessness to convulsions). Antihistamine overdosage in young children may lead to convulsions and death. Atropine-like signs and symptoms may be prominent.

Treatment: Induce vomiting if it has not occurred spontaneously. Precautions must be taken against aspiration especially in infants, children and comatose patients. If gastric lavage is indicated, isotonic or half-isotonic saline solution is preferred. Stimulants should not be used. If hypotension is a problem, vasopressor agents may be considered.

DOSAGE AND ADMINISTRATION

Administer the recommended dose every 12 hours.

Carbetapen/Chlorphen/Eph/Phenyleph Tablets: Adults—1 to 2 tablets.

Carbetapen/Chlorphen/Eph/Phenyleph Pediatric Suspension:

Children over six years of age—5 to 10 mL (1 to 2 teaspoonfuls);

Children two to six years of age—2.5 to 5 mL (1/2 to 1 teaspoonful);

Children under two years of age—Titrate dose individually.
    Store at controlled room temperature 15°-30°C (59°-86°F).
    Dispense in a tight container.

HOW SUPPLIED
SUSPENSION:

BRAND/MANUFACTURER	NDC	SIZE	AWP
○ **BRAND**			
RYNATUSS PEDIATRIC: Wallace	00037-0718-67	240 ml	$94.14
	00037-0718-68	480 ml	$174.44
○ **GENERICS**			
FEN-A-COUGH: TMK	59582-0449-16	473 ml	$41.00
TUSS TAN PEDIATRIC: Econolab	55053-0112-16	473 ml	$43.25
MOORETUSS PEDIATRIC: Moore,H.L.	00839-7432-69	480 ml	$37.11
QUAD-TUSS TANNATE PEDIATRIC: Hi-Tech	50383-0809-16	480 ml	$41.00
TRI-TANNATE PLUS PEDIATRIC: Rugby	00536-2202-85	480 ml	$51.00
RENTAMINE PEDIATRIC: Major	00904-1666-16	480 ml	$52.45
TANORAL-S PEDIATRIC: Econolab	55053-0190-04	120 ml 4s	$52.00

For additional alternatives, turn to the section beginning on page 2859.

Carbidopa and Levodopa

DESCRIPTION

When Carbidopa/Levodopa is to be given to patients who are being treated with Levodopa, Levodopa must be discontinued at least eight hours before therapy with Carbidopa/Levodopa is started. In order to reduce adverse reactions, it is necessary to individualize therapy. See the *"Warnings"* and *"Dosage and Administration"* sections before initiating therapy.

Carbidopa, an inhibitor of aromatic amino acid decarboxylation, is a white, crystalline compound, slightly soluble in water, with a molecular weight of 244.3. It is designated chemically as (--)-L-α-hydrazino-α-methyl-β-(3,4-dihydroxybenzene) propanoic acid, monohydrate.

Its empirical formula is $C_{10}H_{14}N_2O_4 \cdot H_2O$.

Tablet content is expressed in terms of anhydrous Carbidopa which has a molecular weight of 226.3.

Levodopa, an aromatic amino acid, is a white, crystalline compound, slightly soluble in water, with a molecular weight of 197.2. It is designated chemically as (—)-L-α-amino-β-(3,4-dihydroxybenzene) propanoic acid.

Its empirical formula is $C_9H_{11}NO_4$.

Carbidopa/Levodopa is supplied as tablets in three strengths:

Carbidopa/Levodopa 25-100, containing 25 mg of Carbidopa and 100 mg of Levodopa.

Carbidopa/Levodopa 10-100, containing 10 mg of Carbidopa and 100 mg of Levodopa.

Carbidopa/Levodopa 25-250, containing 25 mg of Carbidopa and 250 mg of Levodopa.

Sustained-release Carbidopa/Levodopa tablets contain: 50 mg Carbidopa/200 mg Levodopa or 25 mg Carbidopa/100 mg Levodopa.

ACTIONS

Current evidence indicates that symptoms of Parkinson's disease are related to depletion of dopamine in the corpus striatum. Administration of dopamine is ineffective in the treatment of Parkinson's disease apparently because it does not cross the blood-brain barrier. However, Levodopa, the metabolic precursor of dopamine, does cross the blood-brain barrier, and presumably is converted to dopamine in the basal ganglia. This is thought to be the mechanism whereby Levodopa relieves symptoms of Parkinson's disease.

◆ RATED THERAPEUTICALLY EQUIVALENT; ◇ THERAPEUTIC EQUIVALENCE UNCONFIRMED; ○ UNRATED

When Levodopa is administered orally it is rapidly decarboxylated to dopamine in extracerebral tissues so that only a small portion of a given dose is transported unchanged to the central nervous system. For this reason, large doses of Levodopa are required for adequate therapeutic effect and these may often be attended by nausea and other adverse reactions, some of which are attributable to dopamine formed in extracerebral tissues.

Since Levodopa competes with certain amino acids for transport across the gut wall, the absorption of Levodopa may be impaired in some patients on a high protein diet.

Carbidopa inhibits decarboxylation of peripheral Levodopa. It does not cross the blood-brain barrier and does not affect the metabolism of Levodopa within the central nervous system.

Since its decarboxylase inhibiting activity is limited to extracerebral tissues, administration of Carbidopa with Levodopa makes more Levodopa available for transport to the brain. In dogs, reduced formation of dopamine in extracerebral tissues, such as the heart, provides protection against the development of dopamine-induced cardiac arrhythmias. Clinical studies tend to support the hypothesis of a similar protective effect in humans although controlled data are too limited at the present time to draw firm conclusions.

Patients treated with Levodopa therapy for Parkinson's disease may develop motor fluctuations characterized by end-of-dose failure, peak dose dyskinesia, and akinesia. The advanced form of motor fluctuations ("on-off" phenomenon) is characterized by unpredictable swings from mobility to immobility. Although the causes of the motor fluctuations are not completely understood, *in some patients* they may be attenuated by treatment regimens that produce steady plasma levels of Levodopa.

Sustained-Release Carbidopa/Levodopa contains either 50 mg of Carbidopa and 200 mg of Levodopa, or 25 mg of Carbidopa and 100 mg of Levodopa in a sustained-release dosage form designed to release these ingredients over a 4 to 6 hour period. With Sustained-Release Carbidopa/Levodopa there is less variation in plasma Levodopa levels than with Carbidopa/Levodopa, the conventional formulation. *However, Sustained-Release Carbidopa/Levodopa is less systemically bioavailable than Carbidopa/Levodopa and may require increased daily doses to achieve the same level of symptomatic relief as provided by Carbidopa/Levodopa.*

In clinical trials, patients with moderate to severe motor fluctuations who received Sustained-Release Carbidopa/Levodopa *did not experience quantitatively significant reductions* in "off" time when compared to Sustained-Release Carbidopa/Levodopa. However, global ratings of improvement as assessed by both patient and physician were better during therapy with Sustained-Release Carbidopa/Levodopa than with Carbidopa/Levodopa. In patients without motor fluctuations, Sustained-Release Carbidopa/Levodopa, under controlled conditions, provided the same therapeutic benefit with less frequent dosing when compared to Carbidopa/Levodopa.

Carbidopa reduces the amount of Levodopa required to produce a given response by about 75 percent and, when administered with Levodopa, increases both plasma levels and the plasma half-life of Levodopa, and decreases plasma and urinary dopamine and homovanillic acid.

In clinical pharmacologic studies, simultaneous administration of Carbidopa and Levodopa produced greater urinary excretion of Levodopa in proportion to the excretion of dopamine than administration of the two drugs at separate times.

Pyridoxine hydrochloride (vitamin B$_6$), in oral doses of 10 mg to 25 mg, may reverse the effects of Levodopa by increasing the rate of aromatic amino acid decarboxylation. Carbidopa inhibits this action of pyridoxine.

Elimination half-life of Levodopa in the presence of Carbidopa is about 1.5 hours. Following Sustained-Release Carbidopa/Levodopa, the apparent half-life of Levodopa may be prolonged because of continuous absorption.

In healthy elderly subjects (56-67 years old) the mean time to peak concentration of Levodopa after a single dose of Sustained-Release Carbidopa/Levodopa 50-200 was about 2 hours as compared to 0.5 hours after standard Carbidopa/Levodopa. The maximum concentration of Levodopa after a single dose of Sustained-Release Carbidopa/Levodopa was about 35% of the standard Carbidopa/Levodopa (1151 vs 3256 ng/mL). The extent of availability of Levodopa from Sustained-Release Carbidopa/Levodopa was about 70-75% relative to intravenous Levodopa or standard Carbidopa/Levodopa in the elderly. The absolute bioavailability of Levodopa from Sustained-Release Carbidopa/Levodopa (relative to I.V.) in young subjects was shown to be only about 44%. The extent of availability and the peak concentrations of Levodopa were comparable in the elderly after a single dose and at steady state after t.i.d. administration of Sustained-Release Carbidopa-Levodopa 50-200. In elderly subjects, the average trough levels of Levodopa at steady state after the Sustained-Release tablet were about 2 fold higher than after the standard Carbidopa/Levodopa (163 vs 74 ng/mL).

In these studies, using similar total daily doses of Levodopa, plasma Levodopa concentrations with Sustained-Release Carbidopa/Levodopa fluctuated in a narrower range than with Carbidopa/Levodopa. Because the bioavailability of Levodopa from Sustained-Release Carbidopa/Levodopa relative to Carbidopa/Levodopa is approximately 70-75%, the daily dosage of Levodopa necessary to produce a given clinical response with the sustained-release formulation will usually be higher.

The extent of availability and peak concentrations of Levodopa after a single dose of Sustained-Release Carbidopa/Levodopa 50-200 increased by about 50% and 25%, respectively, when administered with food.

INDICATIONS

Carbidopa/Levodopa is indicated in the treatment of the symptoms of idiopathic Parkinson's disease (paralysis agitans), post-encephalitic parkinsonism, and symptomatic parkinsonism which may follow injury to the nervous system by carbon monoxide intoxication and manganese intoxication. Carbidopa/Levodopa is indicated in these conditions to permit the administration of lower doses of Levodopa with reduced nausea and vomiting, with more rapid dosage titration, with a somewhat smoother response, and with supplemental pyridoxine (vitamin B$_6$).

The incidence of Levodopa-induced nausea and vomiting is less with Carbidopa/Levodopa than with Levodopa. In many patients this reduction in nausea and vomiting will permit more rapid dosage titration.

In some patients a somewhat smoother antiparkinsonian effect results from therapy with Carbidopa/Levodopa than with Levodopa. However, patients with markedly irregular ("on-off") responses to Levodopa have not been shown to benefit from Carbidopa/Levodopa.

Since Carbidopa prevents the reversal of Levodopa effects caused by pyridoxine, Carbidopa/Levodopa can be given to patients receiving supplemental pyridoxine (vitamin B$_6$).

Although the administration of Carbidopa permits control of parkinsonism and Parkinson's disease with much lower doses of Levodopa, there is no conclusive evidence at present that this is beneficial other than in reducing nausea and vomiting, permitting more rapid titration, and providing a somewhat smoother response to Levodopa. *Carbidopa does not decrease adverse reactions due to central effects of Levodopa. By permitting more Levodopa to reach the brain, particularly when nausea and vomiting is not a dose-limiting factor, certain adverse CNS effects, e.g., dyskinesias, may occur at lower dosages and sooner during therapy with Carbidopa/Levodopa than with Levodopa.*

Certain patients who responded poorly to Levodopa have improved when Carbidopa/Levodopa was substituted. This is most likely due to decreased peripheral decarboxylation of Levodopa which results from administration of Carbidopa rather than to a primary effect of Carbidopa on the nervous system. Carbidopa has not been shown to enhance the intrinsic efficacy of Levodopa in parkinsonian syndromes.

In considering whether to give Carbidopa/Levodopa to patients already on Levodopa who have nausea and/or vomiting, the practitioner should be aware that, while many patients may be expected to improve, some do not. Since one cannot predict which patients are likely to improve, this can only be determined by a trial of therapy. It should be further noted that in controlled trials comparing Carbidopa/Levodopa with Levodopa, about half of the patients with nausea and/or vomiting on Levodopa improved spontaneously despite being retained on the same dose of Levodopa during the controlled portion of the trial.

CONTRAINDICATIONS

Monoamine oxidase inhibitors and Carbidopa/Levodopa should not be given concomitantly. These inhibitors must be discontinued at least two weeks prior to initiating therapy with Carbidopa/Levodopa.

Sustained-Release Carbidopa/Levodopa may be administered concomitantly with the manufacturer's recommended dose of an MAO inhibitor with selectivity for MAO type B (e.g., selegiline HCl).

Carbidopa/Levodopa is contraindicated in patients with known hypersensitivity to this drug, and in narrow angle glaucoma.

Because Levodopa may activate a malignant melanoma, it should not be used in patients with suspicious, undiagnosed skin lesions or a history of melanoma.

WARNINGS

When patients are receiving Levodopa, without a decarboxylase inhibitor, Levodopa must be discontinued at least eight hours before Carbidopa/Levodopa is started. Carbidopa/Levodopa should be substituted at a dosage that will provide approximately 25 percent of the previous Levodopa dosage (see *"Dosage and Administration"*). Patients who are taking Carbidopa/Levodopa should be instructed not to take additional Levodopa unless it is prescribed by the physician.

Carbidopa does not decrease adverse reactions due to central effects of Levodopa. By permitting more Levodopa to reach the brain, particularly when nausea and vomiting is not a dose-limiting factor, certain adverse CNS effects, e.g., dyskinesias, will occur at lower dosages and sooner during therapy with Sustained-Release Carbidopa/Levodopa than with Levodopa alone.

As with Levodopa, Carbidopa/Levodopa may cause involuntary movements and mental disturbances. These reactions are thought to be due to increased brain dopamine following administration of Levodopa. All patients should be observed carefully for the development of depression with concomitant suicidal tendencies. Patients with past or current psychoses should be treated with caution. *Because Carbidopa permits more Levodopa to reach the brain and, thus, more dopamine to be formed, dyskinesias may occur at lower dosages and sooner with Carbidopa/Levodopa than with Levodopa.* The occurrence of dyskinesias may require dosage reduction.

Patients receiving Sustained-Release Carbidopa/Levodopa may develop increased dyskinesia compared to Carbidopa/Levodopa.

Carbidopa/Levodopa should be administered cautiously to patients with severe cardiovascular or pulmonary disease, bronchial asthma, renal, hepatic or endocrine disease.

Care should be exercised in administering Carbidopa/Levodopa, as with Levodopa, to patients with a history of myocardial infarction who have residual atrial, nodal, or ventricular arrhythmias. In such patients, cardiac function should be monitored with particular care during the period of initial dosage adjustment, in a facility with provisions for intensive cardiac care.

As with Levodopa there is a possibility of upper gastrointestinal hemorrhage in patients with a history of peptic ulcer. A symptom complex resembling the neuroleptic malignant syndrome including muscular rigidity, elevated body temperature, mental changes, and increased serum creatine phosphokinase has been reported when antiparkinsonian agents were withdrawn abruptly. Therefore, patients should be observed carefully when the dosage of Carbidopa/Levodopa is reduced abruptly or discontinued, especially if the patient is receiving neuroleptics.

CARCINOGENESIS, MUTAGENESIS, IMPAIRMENT OF FERTILITY

In a two-year bioassay of Carbidopa/Levodopa, no evidence of carcinogenicity was found in rats receiving doses of approximately two times the maximum daily human dose of Carbidopa and four times the maximum daily human dose of Levodopa (equivalent to 8 Sustained-Release Carbidopa/Levodopa tablets).

In reproduction studies with Carbidopa/Levodopa, no effects on fertility were found in rats receiving doses of approximately two times the maximum daily human dose of Carbidopa and four times the maximum daily human dose of Levodopa (equivalent to 8 Sustained-Release Carbidopa/Levodopa tablets).

PREGNANCY

Pregnancy Category C.: No teratogenic effects were observed in a study in mice receiving up to 20 times the maximum recommended human dose of Carbidopa/Levodopa There was a decrease in the number of live pups delivered by rats receiving approximately two times the maximum recommended human dose of Carbidopa and approximately five times the maximum recommended human dose of Levodopa during organogenesis. Carbidopa/Levodopa caused both visceral and skeletal malformations in rabbits at all doses and ratios of Carbidopa/Levodopa tested, which ranged from 10 times/5 times the maximum recommended human dose of Carbidopa/Levodopa to 20 times/10 times the maximum recommended human dose of Carbidopa/Levodopa.

There are no adequate or well-controlled studies in pregnant women. Use of Sustained-Release Carbidopa/Levodopa in women of childbearing potential potential requires that the anticipated benefits of the drug be weighed against possible hazards to mother and child.

Carbidopa/Levodopa should not be given to nursing mothers.

Usage in Children: The safety of Carbidopa/Levodopa in patients under 18 years of age has not been established.

PRECAUTIONS

As with Levodopa, periodic evaluations of hepatic, hematopoietic, cardiovascular, and renal function are recommended during extended therapy.

Patients with chronic wide angle glaucoma may be treated cautiously with Carbidopa/Levodopa provided the intraocular pressure is well controlled and the patient is monitored carefully for changes in intraocular pressure during therapy.

INFORMATION FOR PATIENTS

The patient should be informed that the sustained-release formulation of Carbidopa/Levodopa releases these ingredients over a 4 to 6 hour period. It is important that Sustained-Release Carbidopa/Levodopa be taken at regular intervals according to the schedule outlined by the physician. The patient should be cautioned not to change the prescribed dosage regimen and not to add any additional antiparkinson medications, including other Carbidopa/Levodopa preparations, without first consulting the physician.

If abnormal involuntary movements appear or get worse during treatment with Sustained-Release Carbidopa/Levodopa, the physician should be notified, as dosage adjustment may be necessary.

Patients should be advised that sometimes the onset of effect of the first morning dose of Sustained-Release Carbidopa/Levodopa may be delayed for up to 1 hour compared with the response usually obtained from the first morning dose of Carbidopa/Levodopa. The physician should be notified if such delayed responses pose a problem in treatment.

Patients must be advised that the whole or half tablet should be swallowed without chewing or crushing.

NOTE: The suggested advice to patients being treated with Sustained-Release Carbidopa/Levodopa is intended to aid in the safe and effective use of this medication. It is not a disclosure of all possible adverse or intended effects.

LABORATORY TESTS

Abnormalities in laboratory tests may include elevations of liver function tests such as alkaline phosphatase, SGOT (AST), SGPT (ALT), lactic dehydrogenase, and bilirubin. Abnormalities in protein-bound iodine, blood urea nitrogen and positive Coombs test have also been reported. Commonly, levels of blood urea nitrogen, creatinine, and uric acid are lower during administration of Carbidopa/Levodopa than with Levodopa.

Carbidopa/Levodopa may cause a false-positive reaction for urinary ketone bodies when a test tape is used for determination of ketonuria. This reaction will not be altered by boiling the urine specimen. False-negative tests may result with the use of glucose-oxidase methods of testing for glucosuria.

DRUG INTERACTIONS

Caution should be exercised when the following drugs are administered concomitantly with Carbidopa/Levodopa.

Symptomatic postural hypotension can occur when Carbidopa/Levodopa is added to the treatment of a patient receiving antihypertensive drugs. Therefore, when therapy with Carbidopa/Levodopa is started, dosage adjustment of the antihypertensive drug may be required. For patients receiving monoamine oxidase inhibitors, see *"Contraindications"*.

There have been rare reports of adverse reactions, including hypertension and dyskinesia, resulting from the concomitant use of tricyclic antidepressants and Carbidopa/Levodopa. Phenothiazines and butyrophenones may reduce the therapeutic effects of Levodopa. In addition, the beneficial effects of Levodopa in Parkinson's disease have been reported to be reversed by phenytoin and

papaverine. Patients taking these drugs with Carbidopa/Levodopa should be carefully observed for loss of therapeutic response.

ADVERSE REACTIONS

CARBIDOPA/LEVODOPA

The most common serious adverse reactions occurring with Carbidopa/Levodopa are choreiform, dystonic, and other involuntary movements. Other serious adverse reactions are mental changes including paranoid ideation and psychotic episodes, depression with or without development of suicidal tendencies, and dementia. Convulsions also have occurred; however, a causal relationship with Carbidopa/Levodopa has not been established.

A common but less serious effect is nausea.

Less frequent adverse reactions are cardiac irregularities and/or palpitation, orthostatic hypotensive episodes, bradykinetic episodes (the "on-off" phenomenon), anorexia, vomiting, and dizziness.

Rarely, gastrointestinal bleeding, development of duodenal ulcer, hypertension, phlebitis, hemolytic and nonhemolytic anemia, thrombocytopenia, leukopenia, and agranulocytosis have occurred.

Laboratory tests which have been reported to be abnormal are alkaline phosphatase. SGOT (AST), SGPT (ALT), lactic dehydrogenase, bilirubin, blood urea nitrogen, protein-bound iodine, and Coombs test.

Other adverse reactions that have been reported with Levodopa are:

Nervous System: ataxia, numbness, increased hand tremor, muscle twitching, muscle cramps, blepharospasm (which may be taken as an early sign of excess dosage, consideration of dosage reduction may be made at this time), trismus, activation of latent Horner's syndrome.

Psychiatric: confusion, sleepiness, insomnia, nightmares, hallucinations, delusions, agitation, anxiety, euphoria.

Gastrointestinal: dry mouth, bitter taste, sialorrhea, dysphagia, bruxism, hiccups, abdominal pain and distress, constipation, diarrhea, flatulence, burning sensation of tongue.

Metabolic: weight gain or loss, edema.

Integumentary: malignant melanoma (see also *"Contraindications"*), flushing, increased sweating, dark sweat, skin rash, loss of hair.

Genitourinary: urinary retention, urinary incontinence, dark urine, priapism.

Special Senses: diplopia, blurred vision, dilated pupils, oculogyric crises.

Miscellaneous: weakness, faintness, fatigue, headache, hoarseness, malaise, hot flashes, sense of stimulation, bizarre breathing patterns, neuroleptic malignant syndrome.

SUSTAINED-RELEASE CARBIDOPA/LEVODOPA

In controlled clinical trials, patients predominantly with moderate to severe motor fluctuations while on Carbidopa/Levodopa were randomized to therapy with either Carbidopa/Levodopa or Sustained-Release Carbidopa/Levodopa. The adverse experience frequency profile of Sustained-Release Carbidopa/Levodopa did not differ substantially from that of Carbidopa/Levodopa, as shown in Table 1.

Table 1.
CLINICAL ADVERSE EXPERIENCES OCCURRING IN 1% OR GREATER OF PATIENTS

Adverse Experience	Sustained-Release Carbidopa/ Levodopa n=491 %	Carbidopa/ Levodopa n=524 %
Dyskinesia	16.5	12.2
Nausea	5.5	5.7
Hallucinations	3.9	3.2
Confusion	3.7	2.3
Dizziness	2.9	2.3
Depression	2.2	1.3
Urinary tract infection	2.2	2.3
Headache	2.0	1.9
Dream abnormalities	1.8	0.8
Dystonia	1.8	0.8
Vomiting	1.8	1.9
Upper respiratory infection	1.8	1.0
Dyspnea	1.6	0.4
"On-Off" phenomena	1.6	1.6
Back pain	1.6	0.6
Dry mouth	1.4	1.1
Anorexia	1.2	1.1
Diarrhea	1.2	0.6
Insomnia	1.2	1.0
Orthostatic hypotension	1.0	1.1
Shoulder pain	1.0	0.6
Chest pain	1.0	0.8
Muscle cramps	0.8	1.0
Paresthesia	0.8	1.1
Urinary frequency	0.8	1.1
Dyspepsia	0.6	1.1
Constipation	0.2	1.5

Abnormal laboratory findings occurring at a frequency of 1% or greater in approximately 443 patients who received Sustained-Release Carbidopa/Levodopa and 475 who received Carbidopa/Levodopa during controlled clinical trials included: decreased hemoglobin and hematocrit; elevated serum glucose; white blood cells, bacteria and blood in the urine.

The adverse experiences observed in patients in uncontrolled studies were similar to those seen in controlled clinical studies.

Other adverse experiences reported overall in clinical trials in 748 patients treated with Sustained-Release Carbidopa/Levodopa listed by body system in order of decreasing frequency, include:

Nervous System/Psychiatric: Chorea, somnolence, falling, anxiety disorder, disorientation, decreased mental acuity, gait abnormalities, extrapyramidal disorder, agitation, nervousness, sleep disorders, memory impairment.

Body as a Whole: Asthenia, fatigue, abdominal pain, orthostatic effects.

Digestive: Gastrointestinal pain, dysphagia, heartburn.

Cardiovascular: Palpitation, essential hypertension, hypotension, myocardial infarction.

Special Senses: Blurred vision.

Metabolic: Weight loss.

Skin: Rash.

Respiratory: Cough, pharyngeal pain, common cold.

Urogenital: Urinary incontinence.

Musculoskeletal: Leg pain.

Laboratory Tests: Decreased white blood cell count and serum potassium; increased BUN, serum creatinine and serum LDH; protein and glucose in the urine.

Other adverse experiences have been reported with various Carbidopa-Levodopa formulations and may occur with Sustained-Release Carbidopa/Levodopa:

Nervous System/Psychiatric: Mental changes including paranoid ideation, psychotic episodes, depression with suicidal tendencies and dementia; convulsions (however, a causal relationship has not been established); bradykinetic episodes.

Gastrointestinal: Gastrointestinal bleeding, development of duodenal ulcer.

Cardiovascular: Cardiac irregularities, phlebitis.

Hematologic: Hemolytic and nonhemolytic anemia, thrombocytopenia, leukopenia, agranulocytosis.

Laboratory Tests: Abnormalities in alkaline phosphatase, SGOT (AST), SGPT (ALT), lactic dehydrogenase, bilirubin, protein-bound idoine, Coombs test.

Other adverse reactions that have been reported with Levodopa are:

Nervous System: Numbness, increased hand tremor, muscle twitching, blepharospasm (which may be taken as an early sign of excess dosage, consideration of dosage reduction may be made at this time), trismus, activation of latent Horner's syndrome.

Psychiatric: Delusions, euphoria.

Gastrointestinal: Bitter taste, sialorrhea, bruxism, hiccups, flatulence, burning sensation of tongue.

Metabolic: Weight gain, edema.

Integumentary: Malignant melanoma (see also "Contraindications"), flushing, increased sweating, dark sweat, loss of hair.

Genitourinary: Urinary retention, urinary incontinence, dark urine, priapism.

Miscellaneous: Faintness, hoarseness, malaise, hot flashes, sense of stimulation, bizarre breathing patterns, neuroleptic malignant syndrome.

OVERDOSAGE

Management of acute overdosage with Carbidopa/Levodopa is basically the same as management of acute overdosage with Levodopa; however, pyridoxine is not effective in reversing the actions of Carbidopa/Levodopa.

General supportive measures should be employed, along with immediate gastric lavage. Intravenous fluids should be administered judiciously and an adequate airway maintained. Electrocardiographic monitoring should be instituted and the patient carefully observed for the development of arrhythmias; if required, appropriate antiarrhythmic therapy should be given. The possibility that the patient may have taken other drugs as well as Carbidopa/Levodopa should be taken into consideration. To date, no experience has been reported with dialysis; hence, its value in overdosage is not known.

Based on studies in which high doses of Levodopa and/or Carbidopa were administered, a significant proportion of rats and mice given single oral doses of Levodopa of approximately 1500-2000 mg/kg are expected to die. A significant proportion of infant rats of both sexes are expected to die at a dose of 800 mg/kg. A significant proportion of rats are expected to die after treatment with similar doses of Carbidopa. The addition of Carbidopa in a 1:10 ratio with Levodopa increases the dose at which a significant proportion of mice are expected to die to 3360 mg/kg.

DOSAGE AND ADMINISTRATION
CARBIDOPA/LEVODOPA
The optimum daily dosage of Carbidopa/Levodopa must be determined by careful titration in each patient. Carbidopa/Levodopa tablets are available in a 1:4 ratio of Carbidopa to Levodopa (Carbidopa/Levodopa 25-100) as well as 1:10 ratio (Carbidopa/Levodopa 25-250 and Carbidopa/Levodopa MET 10-100). Tablets of the two ratios may be given separately or combined as needed to provide the optimum dosage. Studies show that peripheral dopa decarboxylase is saturated by Carbidopa at approximately 70 to 100 mg a day. Patients receiving less than this amount of Carbidopa are more likely to experience nausea and vomiting.

USUAL INITIAL DOSAGE
Dosage is best initiated with one tablet of Carbidopa/Levodopa 25-100 three times a day. This dosage schedule provides 75 mg of Carbidopa per day. Dosage may be increased by one tablet every day or every other day, as necessary, until a dosage of eight tablets of Carbidopa/Levodopa 25-100 a day is reached.

If Carbidopa/Levodopa 10-100 is used, dosage may be initiated with one tablet three or four times a day. However, this will not provide an adequate amount of Carbidopa for many patients. Dosage may be increased by one tablet every day or every other day until a total of eight tablets (2 tablets q.i.d.) is reached.

HOW TO TRANSFER PATIENTS FROM LEVODOPA
Levodopa must be discontinued at least eight hours before starting Carbidopa/Levodopa. A daily dosage of Carbidopa/Levodopa should be chosen that will provide approximately 25 percent of the previous Levodopa dosage. Patients who are taking less than 1500 mg of Levodopa a day should be started on one tablet of Carbidopa/Levodopa 25-100 three or four times a day. The suggested starting dosage for most patients taking more than 1500 mg of Levodopa is one tablet of Carbidopa/Levodopa 25-250 three or four times a day.

MAINTENANCE
Therapy should be individualized and adjusted according to the desired therapeutic response. At least 70 to 100 mg of Carbidopa per day should be provided. When a greater proportion of Carbidopa is required, one tablet of Carbidopa/Levodopa 25-100 may be substituted for each tablet of Carbidopa/Levodopa 10-100. When more Levodopa is required, Carbidopa/Levodopa 25-250 should be substituted for Carbidopa/Levodopa 25-100 or Carbidopa/Levodopa 10-100. If necessary, the dosage of Carbidopa/Levodopa 25-250 may be increased by one-half or one tablet every day or every other day to a maximum of eight tablets a day. Experience with total daily dosages of Carbidopa greater than 200 mg is limited.

Because both therapeutic and adverse responses occur more rapidly with Carbidopa/Levodopa than with Levodopa alone, patients should be monitored closely during the dose adjustment period. Specifically, involuntary movements will occur more rapidly with Carbidopa/Levodopa than with Levodopa. The occurrence of involuntary movements may require dosage reduction. Blepharospasm may be a useful early sign of excess dosage in some patients.

Current evidence indicates that other standard drugs for Parkinson's disease (except Levodopa) may be continued while Carbidopa/Levodopa is being administered, although their dosage may have to be adjusted.

If general anesthesia is required, Carbidopa/Levodopa may be continued as long as the patient is permitted to take fluids and medication by mouth. If therapy is interrupted temporarily, the usual daily dosage may be administered as soon as the patient is able to take oral medication.

SUSTAINED-RELEASE CARBIDOPA/LEVODOPA
Sustained-Release Carbidopa/Levodopa contains Carbidopa and Levodopa in a 1:4 ration as either the 50-200 tablet or the 25-100 tablet. The daily dosage of Sustained-Release Carbidopa/Levodopa must be determined by careful titration. Patients should be monitored closely during the dose adjustment period, particularly with regard to appearance or worsening of involuntary movements, dyskinesias or nausea. Sustained-Release Carbidopa/Levodopa 50-200 may be administered as whole or as half-tablets which should not be chewed or crushed. Sustained-Release Carbidopa/Levodopa 25-100 may be used in combination with Sustained-Release Carbidopa/Levodopa 50-200 to titrate to the optimum dosage, or as an alternative to the 50-200 half tablet.

Standard drugs for Parkinson's disease, other than Levodopa without a decarboxylase inhibitor, may be used concomitantly while Sustained-Release Carbidopa/Levodopa is being administered, although their dosage may have to be adjusted.

Since Carbidopa prevents the reversal of Levodopa effects caused by pyridoxine, Sustained-Release Carbidopa/Levodopa can be given to patients receiving supplemental pyridoxine (vitamin B_6).

INITIAL DOSAGE
Patients currently treated with conventional Carbidopa/Levodopa preparations: Dosage with Sustained-Release Carbidopa/Levodopa should be substituted at an amount that provides approximately 10% more Levodopa per day, although this may need to be increased to a dosage that provides up to 30% more Levodopa per day depending on clinical response (see "Dosage and Administration, Titration"). The interval between doses of Sustained-Release Carbidopa/Levodopa should be 4-8 hours during the waking day. (See "Clinical Pharmacology, Pharmacodynamics".) A guideline for *initiation* of Sustained-Release Carbidopa/Levodopa is shown in Table 2.

► SHOWN IN PRODUCT IDENTIFICATION GUIDE

Table 2.

GUIDELINES FOR INITIAL CONVERSION FROM CARBIDOPA/ LEVODOPA TO SUSTAINED-RELEASE CARBIDOPA/LEVODOPA

Carbidopa-Levodopa Total Daily Dose* Levodopa (mg)	Suggested Dosage Regimen
300-400	200 mg b.i.d.
500-600	300 mg b.i.d. or 200 mg t.i.d.
700-800	A total of 800 mg in 3 or more divided doses (e.g., 300 mg a.m., 300 mg early p.m. and 200 mg later p.m.)
900-1000	A total of 1000 mg in 3 or more divided doses (e.g., 400 mg a.m., 400 mg early p.m., and 200 mg later p.m.)

*   *For dosing ranges not shown in the table see "Dosage and Administration". Initial Dosage—Patients currently treated with conventional Carbidopa-Levodopa preparations.*

Patients Currently Treated with Levodopa without a Decarboxylase Inhibitor: Levodopa must be discontinued at least eight hours before therapy with Sustained-Release Carbidopa/Levodopa is started. Sustained-Release Carbidopa/ Levodopa should be substituted at a dosage that will provide approximately 25% of the previous Levodopa dosage. In patients with mild to moderate disease, the initial dose is usually 1 tablet of Sustained-Release Carbidopa/Levodopa b.i.d.

Patients not Receiving Levodopa: In patients with mild to moderate disease, the initial recommended dose is 1 tablet of Sustained-Release Carbidopa/Levodopa b.i.d. initial dosage should not be given at intervals of less than 6 hours.

TITRATION WITH SUSTAINED-RELEASE CARBIDOPA/LEVODOPA
Following initiation of therapy, doses and dosing intervals may be increased or decreased depending upon therapeutic response. Most patients have been adequately treated with doses of Sustained-Release Carbidopa/Levodopa that provide 400 to 1600 mg of Levodopa per day, administered as divided doses at intervals ranging from 4 to 8 hours during the waking day. Higher doses (2400 mg or more of Levodopa per day) and shorter intervals (less than 4 hours) have been used, but are not usually recommended.

When doses of Sustained-Release Carbidopa/Levodopa are given at intervals of less than 4 hours, and/or if the divided doses are not equal, it is recommended that the smaller doses be given at the end of the day.

An interval of at least 3 days between dosage adjustments is recommended.

MAINTENANCE
Because Parkinson's disease is progressive, periodic clinical evaluations are recommended; adjustment of the dosage regimen of Sustained-Release Carbidopa/Levodopa may be required.

ADDITION OF OTHER ANTIPARKINSON MEDICATIONS
Anticholinergic agents, dopamine agonists, and amantadine can be given with Sustained-Release Carbidopa/Levodopa. Dosage adjustment of Sustained-Release Carbidopa/Levodopa may be necessary when these agents are added.

A dose of Carbidopa/Levodopa 25-100 or 10-100 (one half or a whole tablet) can be added to the dosage regimen of Sustained-Release Carbidopa/Levodopa in selected patients with advanced disease who need additional Levodopa for a brief time during daytime hours.

INTERRUPTION OF THERAPY
Patients should be observed carefully if abrupt reduction or discontinuation of Sustained-Release Carbidopa/Levodopa is required especially if the patient is receiving neuroleptics. (See "Warnings".)

If general anesthesia is required, Sustained-Release Carbidopa/Levodopa may be continued as long as the patient is permitted to take oral medication. If therapy is interrupted temporarily, the usual dosage should be administered as soon as the patient is able to take oral medication.

STORAGE
CARBIDOPA/LEVODOPA
Carbidopa/Levodopa 10-100 and Carbidopa/Levodopa 25-250 tablets must be protected from light.

SUSTAINED-RELEASE CARBIDOPA/LEVODOPA
Avoid temperatures above 30°C (86°F). Store in a tightly closed container.

HOW SUPPLIED
TABLET, EXTENDED RELEASE: 25 MG-100 MG

BRAND/MANUFACTURER	NDC	SIZE	AWP
○ BRAND			
➤ SINEMET CR: Du Pont Pharma	00056-0601-68	100s	$68.06
	00056-0601-28	100s ud	$72.12

TABLET, EXTENDED RELEASE: 50 MG-200 MG

BRAND/MANUFACTURER	NDC	SIZE	AWP
○ BRAND			
➤ SINEMET CR: Du Pont Pharma	00056-0521-68	100s	$140.88
	00056-0521-28	100s ud	$149.25

TABLETS: 10 MG-100 MG

AVERAGE UNIT PRICE (AVAILABLE SIZES)		GENERIC A-RATED AVERAGE PRICE (GAAP)	
BRAND	$0.63	100s	$56.55
GENERIC	$0.57	500s	$267.50

BRAND/MANUFACTURER	NDC	SIZE	AWP
◆ BRAND			
➤ SINEMET 10-100: Du Pont Pharma	00056-0647-68	100s	$59.88
	00056-0647-28	100s ud	$65.50
◆ GENERICS			
Medirex	57480-0807-06	30s	$19.47
West Point	59591-0247-68	100s	$52.10
Moore,H.L.	00839-7765-06	100s	$52.45
Rugby	00536-5555-01	100s	$52.54
Qualitest	00603-2568-21	100s	$52.60
Schein	00364-2538-01	100s	$53.15
Major	00904-7718-60	100s	$53.95
Lemmon	00093-0292-01	100s	$54.50
Goldline	00182-1948-01	100s	$54.50
Aligen	00405-4134-01	100s	$62.30
Goldline	00182-1948-89	100s ud	$60.65
UDL	51079-0755-20	100s ud	$64.90
Medirex	57480-0807-01	100s ud	$64.90
Goldline	00182-1948-05	500s	$262.50
Lemmon	00093-0292-05	500s	$272.50

TABLETS: 25 MG-100 MG

AVERAGE UNIT PRICE (AVAILABLE SIZES)		GENERIC A-RATED AVERAGE PRICE (GAAP)	
BRAND	$0.69	100s	$61.51
GENERIC	$0.61	500s	$297.03
		750s	$442.50
		1000s	$594.05

BRAND/MANUFACTURER	NDC	SIZE	AWP
◆ BRAND			
➤ SINEMET 25-100: Du Pont Pharma	00056-0650-68	100s	$66.62
	00056-0650-28	100s ud	$70.56
BRAND/MANUFACTURER	NDC	SIZE	AWP
◆ GENERICS			
Medirex	57480-0808-06	30s	$20.85
West Point	59591-0246-68	100s	$58.15
Rugby	00536-5556-01	100s	$58.50
Moore,H.L.	00839-7766-06	100s	$58.50
Qualitest	00603-2569-21	100s	$58.80
Schein	00364-2539-01	100s	$59.21
Lemmon	00093-0293-01	100s	$59.40
Goldline	00182-1949-01	100s	$59.40
Major	00904-7719-60	100s	$59.95
Aligen	00405-4133-01	100s	$62.53
Vangard	00615-3561-13	100s ud	$61.07
Athena	59075-0585-10	100s	$65.25
Goldline	00182-1949-89	100s ud	$65.35
UDL	51079-0756-20	100s ud	$69.30
Medirex	57480-0808-01	100s ud	$69.50
Lemmon	00093-0293-05	500s	$297.00
Goldline	00182-1949-05	500s	$297.05
Glasgow	60809-0113-55	750s	$442.50
Glasgow	60809-0113-72	750s ud	$442.50
Lemmon	00093-0293-10	1000s	$594.00
Goldline	00182-1949-10	1000s	$594.10

TABLETS: 25 MG-250 MG

AVERAGE UNIT PRICE (AVAILABLE SIZES)		GENERIC A-RATED AVERAGE PRICE (GAAP)	
BRAND	$0.88	100s	$78.48
GENERIC	$0.79	500s	$378.75
		1000s	$757.50

BRAND/MANUFACTURER	NDC	SIZE	AWP
◆ BRAND			
➤ SINEMET 25-250: Du Pont Pharma	00056-0654-68	100s	$85.63
	00056-0654-28	100s ud	$90.38
◆ GENERICS			
Medirex	57480-0476-06	30s	$26.99
West Point	59591-0250-68	100s	$71.30
Moore,H.L.	00839-7767-06	100s	$72.09
Schein	00364-2540-01	100s	$73.50
Qualitest	00603-2570-21	100s	$75.14
Rugby	00536-5557-01	100s	$75.20
Major	00904-7720-60	100s	$75.25
Lemmon	00093-0294-01	100s	$76.50
Goldline	00182-1950-01	100s	$76.50
Athena	59075-0587-10	100s	$83.50
Aligen	00405-4132-01	100s	$83.88
Goldline	00182-1950-89	100s ud	$83.70

◆ RATED THERAPEUTICALLY EQUIVALENT; ◇ THERAPEUTIC EQUIVALENCE UNCONFIRMED; ○ UNRATED

BRAND/MANUFACTURER	NDC	SIZE	AWP
UDL	51079-0783-20	100s ud	$88.70
Medirex	57480-0476-01	100s ud	$89.95
Goldline	00182-1950-05	500s	$375.00
Lemmon	00093-0294-05	500s	$382.50
Goldline	00182-1950-10	1000s	$750.00
Lemmon	00093-0294-10	1000s	$765.00

Carbinoxamine Maleate with Pseudoephedrine Hydrochloride

DESCRIPTION

Antihistamine/decongestant for oral use

FOR INFANTS

Carbinoxamine Maleate/Pseudoephedrine Hydrochloride (Carbinoxamine/Pseudoephedrine) Oral Drops

Each dropperful (1 mL) contains Carbinoxamine Maleate, 2 mg; Pseudoephedrine Hydrochloride, 25 mg.

FOR YOUNG CHILDREN

Carbinoxamine/Pseudoephedrine Syrup

Each teaspoonful (5 mL) contains Carbinoxamine Maleate, 4 mg; Pseudoephedrine Hydrochloride, 60 mg.

FOR ADULTS AND CHILDREN 6 YEARS AND OVER

Carbinoxamine/Pseudoephedrine Tablet

Each tablet contains Carbinoxamine Maleate, 4 mg; Pseudoephedrine Hydrochloride, 60 mg.

FOR ADULTS AND CHILDREN 12 YEARS AND OVER

Carbinoxamine/Pseudoephedrine timed-release Tablet

Each timed-release tablet contains Carbinoxamine Maleate, 8 mg; Pseudoephedrine Hydrochloride, 120 mg.

Carbinoxamine Maleate (2-[p-Chloro-α-[2-(dimethylamino) ethoxy]benzyl] pyridine maleate) is one of the ethanolamine class of H_1 antihistamines.

Pseudoephedrine Hydrochloride (Benzenemethanol, α-[1-(methylamino) ethyl]-, [S-(R*, R*)]-, hydrochloride) is the hydrochloride of Pseudoephedrine, a naturally occurring dextrorotatory stereoisomer of ephedrine.

CLINICAL PHARMACOLOGY

Antihistaminic and decongestant actions.

Carbinoxamine Maleate possesses H_1 antihistaminic activity and mild anticholinergic and sedative effects. Serum half-life for Carbinoxamine is estimated to be 10 to 20 hours. Virtually no intact drug is excreted in the urine.

Pseudoephedrine Hydrochloride is an oral sympathomimetic amine that acts as a decongestant to respiratory tract mucous membranes. While its vasoconstrictor action is similar to that of ephedrine, Pseudoephedrine has less pressor effect in normotensive adults. Serum half-life for Pseudoephedrine is 6 to 8 hours. Acidic urine is associated with faster elimination of the drug. About one half of the administered dose is excreted in the urine.

INDICATIONS AND USAGE

For symptomatic relief of seasonal and perennial allergic rhinitis and vasomotor rhinitis.

Carbinoxamine/Pseudoephedrine Oral Drops, Carbinoxamine/Pseudoephedrine Syrup and Carbinoxamine/Pseudoephedrine Tablet are immediate-release dosage forms allowing titration of dose up to four times a day.

Carbinoxamine/Pseudoephedrine timed-release tablets utilizes a gradual-release mechanism providing approximately a 12-hour therapeutic effect, thus allowing twice-daily dosage.

CONTRAINDICATIONS

Patients with hypersensitivity or idiosyncrasy to any ingredients, patients taking monoamine oxidase (MAO) inhibitors, patients with narrow-angle glaucoma, urinary retention, peptic ulcer, severe hypertension or coronary artery disease, or patients undergoing an asthmatic attack.

WARNINGS

Use in Pregnancy: Safety for use during pregnancy has not been established.

Nursing Mothers: Use with caution in nursing mothers.

Special Risk Patients: Use with caution in patients with hypertension or ischemic heart disease, and persons older than 60 years.

PRECAUTIONS

Use with caution in patients with hypertension, heart disease, asthma, hyperthyroidism, increased intraocular pressure, diabetes mellitus and prostatic hypertrophy.

Information for Patients: Avoid alcohol and other CNS depressants while taking these products. Patients sensitive to antihistamines may experience moderate to severe drowsiness. Patients sensitive to sympathomimetic amines may note mild CNS stimulation. While taking these products, exercise care in driving or operating appliances, machinery, etc.

Drug Interactions: Antihistamines may enhance the effects of tricyclic antidepressants, barbiturates, alcohol, and other CNS depressants. MAO inhibitors prolong and intensify the anticholinergic effects of antihistamines. Sympathomimetic amines may reduce the antihypertensive effects of reserpine, veratrum alkaloids, methyldopa and mecamylamine. Effects of sympathomimetics are increased with MAO inhibitors and beta-adrenergic blockers.

Pregnancy Category C.: Animal reproduction studies have not been conducted with these products. It is also not known whether these products can cause fetal harm when administered to a pregnant woman or affect reproduction capacity. Give to pregnant women only if clearly needed.

ADVERSE REACTIONS

Antihistamines: Sedation, dizziness, diplopia, vomiting, diarrhea, dry mouth, headache, nervousness, nausea, anorexia, heartburn, weakness, polyuria and dysuria and, rarely, excitability in children.

Sympathomimetic Amines: Convulsions, CNS stimulation, cardiac arrhythmias, respiratory difficulty, increased heart rate or blood pressure, hallucinations, tremors, nervousness, insomnia, weakness, pallor and dysuria.

OVERDOSAGE

No information is available as to specific results of an overdose of these products. The signs, symptoms and treatment described below are those of H_1 antihistamines and ephedrine overdose.

Symptoms: Should antihistamine effects predominate, central action constitutes the greatest danger. In the small child, symptoms include excitation, hallucination, ataxia, incoordination, tremors, flushed face and fever. Convulsions, fixed and dilated pupils, coma and death may occur in severe cases. In the adult, fever and flushing are uncommon; excitement leading to convulsions and posticial depression is often preceded by drowsiness and coma. Respiration is usually not seriously depressed; blood pressure is usually stable.

Should sympathomimetic symptoms predominate, central effects include restlessness, dizziness, tremor, hyperactive reflexes, talkativeness, irritability and insomnia. Cardiovascular and renal effects include difficulty in micturition, headache, flushing, palpitation, cardiac arrhythmias, hypertension with subsequent hypotension and circulatory collapse. Gastrointestinal effects include dry mouth, metallic taste, anorexia, nausea, vomiting, diarrhea and abdominal cramps.

Treatment: a) Evacuate stomach as condition warrants. Activated charcoal may be useful. *b)* Maintain a non-stimulating environment. *c)* Monitor cardiovascular status. *d)* Do not give stimulants. *e)* Reduce fever with cool sponging. *f)* Support respiration. *g)* Use sedatives or anticonvulsants to control CNS excitation and convulsions. *h)* Physostigmine may reverse anticholinergic symptoms. *i)* Ammonium chloride may acidify the urine to increase excretion of Pseudoephedrine. *j)* Further care is symptomatic and supportive.

DOSAGE AND ADMINISTRATION

Age	Dose*	Frequency*
Carbinoxamine/ Pseudoephedrine Oral Drops for oral use only		
1-3 months	1/4 dropperful (1/4 mL)	q.i.d.
3-6 months	1/2 dropperful (1/2 mL)	q.i.d.
6-9 months	3/4 dropperful (3/4 mL)	q.i.d.
9-18 months	1 dropperful (1 mL)	q.i.d.
Carbinoxamine/ Pseudoephedrine Syrup and Tablet		
18 months- 6 years	1/2 teaspoonful (2.5 mL)	q.i.d.
adults and children 6 years and over	1 teaspoonful (5 mL) or 1 tablet	q.i.d.
Carbinoxamine/ Pseudoephedrine Timed-Release Tablet		
adults and children 12 years and over	1 tablet	b.i.d.

*In mild cases or in particularly sensitive patients, less frequent or reduced doses may be adequate.

Oral Drops and Syrup: Dispense in USP tight glass container.

Tablets: Dispense in USP tight glass container.
Recommended storage: Store below 86°F (30°C).

HOW SUPPLIED

DROP: 2 MG-25 MG/ML

BRAND/MANUFACTURER	NDC	SIZE	AWP
○ BRAND			
RONDEC: Ross Pharm	00074-5783-30	30 ml	$19.49

► SHOWN IN PRODUCT IDENTIFICATION GUIDE

BRAND/MANUFACTURER	NDC	SIZE	AWP
GENERICS			
CHEMDEC: Norton,HN	50732-0887-30	30 ml	$6.50
Aligen	00405-2424-53	30 ml	$14.74
CP ORAL: Pharmacist's Choice	54979-0154-03	30 ml	$14.95

SYRUP: 2 MG-30 MG/5 ML

BRAND/MANUFACTURER	NDC	SIZE	AWP
GENERICS			
PALGIC-DS: Pan Amer	00525-6367-16	480 ml	$25.75

SYRUP: 4 MG-60 MG/5 ML

BRAND/MANUFACTURER	NDC	SIZE	AWP
BRAND			
RONDEC: Ross Pharm	00074-5782-04	120 ml	$8.76
	00074-5782-16	480 ml	$33.34
GENERICS			
CHEMDEC: Norton,HN	50732-0872-04	118 ml	$4.76
CHEMDEC: Norton,HN	50732-0872-16	473 ml	$19.20
CARBODEC: Rugby	00536-0440-85	480 ml	$10.12
RONDAMINE: Major	00904-0705-16	480 ml	$10.30
CARDEC-S: Barre	00472-0727-16	480 ml	$10.60
MALDEC: Cenci,H.R.	00556-0451-16	480 ml	$10.60
CARDEC: Goldline	00182-6034-40	480 ml	$12.00

For additional alternatives, turn to the section beginning on page 2859.

Carbinoxamine Maleate/ Dextromethorphan Hydrobromide/Pseudoephedrine Hydrochloride

DESCRIPTION

Antihistamine/decongestant/antitussive for oral use

FOR ADULTS AND CHILDREN
Carbinoxamine/Dextromethorphan/Pseudoephedrine Syrup

Each teaspoonful (5 mL) contains Carbinoxamine Maleate, 4 mg; Pseudoephedrine Hydrochloride, 60 mg; Dextromethorphan Hydrobromide, 15 mg.

FOR INFANTS
Carbinoxamine/Dextromethorphan/Pseudoephedrine Oral Drops

Each dropperful (1 mL) contains Carbinoxamine Maleate, 2 mg; Pseudoephedrine Hydrochloride, 25 mg; Dextromethorphan Hydrobromide, 4 mg.

Carbinoxamine Maleate (2-[p-Chloro-α-[2-(dimethylamino) ethoxy]benzyl]pyridine maleate) is one of the ethanolamine class of H_1 antihistamines.

Pseudoephedrine Hydrochloride (Benzenemethanol, α-[1-(methylamino) ethyl]-, [S-(R*, R*)]-, hydrochloride) is the Hydrochloride of Pseudoephedrine, a naturally occurring dextrorotatory stereoisomer of ephedrine.

Dextromethorphan Hydrobromide (Morphinan, 3-methoxy-17-methyl-, (9α, 13α, 14α)-, hydrobromide, monohydrate) is the Hydrobromide of d-form racemethorphan.

CLINICAL PHARMACOLOGY

Antihistaminic, decongestant and antitussive actions.

Carbinoxamine Maleate possesses H_1 antihistaminic activity and mild anticholinergic and sedative effects. Serum half-life for Carbinoxamine is estimated to be 10 to 20 hours. Virtually no intact drug is excreted in the urine.

Pseudoephedrine Hydrochloride is an oral sympathomimetic amine that acts as a decongestant to respiratory tract mucous membranes. While its vasoconstrictor action is similar to that of ephedrine, Pseudoephedrine has less pressor effect in normotensive adults. Serum half-life for Pseudoephedrine is 6 to 8 hours. Acidic urine is associated with faster elimination of the drug. About one half of the administered dose is excreted in the urine.

Dextromethorphan Hydrobromide is a nonnarcotic antitussive with effectiveness equal to codeine. It acts in the medulla oblongata to elevate the cough threshold. Dextromethorphan does not produce analgesia or induce tolerance, and has no potential for addition. At usual doses, it will not depress respiration or inhibit ciliary activity. Dextromethorphan is rapidly metabolized, with trace amounts of the parent compound in blood and urine. About one half of the administered dose is excreted in the urine as conjugated metabolites.

INDICATIONS AND USAGE

For relief of coughs and upper respiratory symptoms, including nasal congestion, associated with allergy or the common cold.

CONTRAINDICATIONS

Patients with hypersensitivity or idiosyncrasy to any ingredients, patients taking monoamine oxidase (MAO) inhibitors, patients with narrow-angle glaucoma, urinary retention, peptic ulcer, severe hypertension or coronary artery disease, or patients undergoing an asthmatic attack.

WARNINGS

Use in Pregnancy: Safety for use during pregnancy has not been established.

Nursing Mothers: Use with caution in nursing mothers.

Special Risk Patients: Use with caution in patients with hypertension or ischemic heart disease, and persons older than 60 years.

PRECAUTIONS

Before prescribing medication to suppress or modify cough, identify and provide therapy for the underlying cause of cough.

Use with caution in patients with hypertension, heart disease, asthma, hyperthyroidism, increased intraocular pressure, diabetes mellitus and prostatic hypertrophy.

Information for Patients: Avoid alcohol and other CNS depressants while taking these products. Patients sensitive to antihistamines may experience moderate to severe drowsiness. Patients sensitive to sympathomimetic amines may note mild CNS stimulation. While taking these products, exercise care in driving or operating appliances, machinery, etc.

Drug Interactions: Antihistamines may enhance the effects of tricyclic antidepressants, barbiturates, alcohol, and other CNS depressants. MAO inhibitors prolong and intensify the anticholinergic effects of antihistamines. Sympathomimetic amines may reduce the antihypertensive effects of reserpine, veratrum alkaloids, methyldopa and mecanylamine. Effects of sympathomimetics are increased with MAO inhibitors and beta-adrenergic blockers. The cough-suppressant action of Dextromethorphan and narcotic antitussives are additive.

Pregnancy Category C: Animal reproduction studies have not been conducted with Carbinoxamine/Dextromethorphan/Psuedoephedrine. It is also not known whether these products can cause fetal harm when administered to a pregnant woman or affect reproduction capacity. Give to pregnant women only if clearly needed.

ADVERSE REACTIONS

Antihistamines: Sedation, dizziness, diplopia, vomiting, diarrhea, dry mouth, headache, nervousness, nausea, anorexia, heartburn, weakness, polyuria and dysuria and, rarely, excitability in children.

Sympathomimetic Amines: Convulsions, CNS stimulation, cardiac arrhythmias, respiratory difficulty, increased heart rate or blood pressure, hallucinations, tremors, nervousness, insomnia, weakness, pallor and dysuria.

Dextromethorphan: Drowsiness and GI disturbance.

OVERDOSAGE

No information is available as to specific results of an overdose dose of these products. The signs, symptoms and treatment described below are those of H_1 antihistamine, ephedrine and Dextromethorphan overdose.

Symptoms: Should antihistamine effects predominate, central action constitutes the greatest danger. In the small child, predominant symptoms are excitation, hallucination, ataxia, incoordination, tremors, flushed face and fever. Convulsions, fixed and dilated pupils, coma and death may occur in severe cases. In the adult, fever and flushing are uncommon; excitement leading to convulsions and postictal depression is often preceded by drowsiness and coma. Respiration is usually not seriously depressed; blood pressure is usually stable.

Should sympathomimetic symptoms predominate, central effects include restlessness, dizziness, tremor, hyperactive reflexes, talkativeness, irritability and insomnia. Cardiovascular and renal effects include difficulty in micturition, headache, flushing, palpitation, cardiac arrhythmias, hypertension with subsequent hypotension and circulatory collapse. Gastrointestinal effects include dry mouth, metallic taste, anorexia, nausea, vomiting, diarrhea and abdominal cramps.

Dextromethorphan may cause respiratory depression with a large overdose.

Treatment: a) Evacuate stomach as condition warrants. Activated charcoal may be useful. *b)* Maintain a non-stimulating environment. *c)* Monitor cardiovascular status. *d)* Do not give stimulants. *e)* Reduce fever with cool sponging. *f)* Treat respiratory depression with naloxone if Dextromethorphan toxicity is suspected. *g)* Use sedatives or anti-convulsants to control CNS excitation and convulsions. *h)* Physostigmine may reverse anticholinergic symptoms. *i)* Ammonium chloride may acidify the urine to increase urinary excretion of Pseudoephedrine. *j)* Further care is symptomatic and supportive.

DOSAGE AND ADMINISTRATION

Age	Dose*	Frequency*
Carbinoxamine/Dextromethorphan/Pseudoephedrine Syrup		
18 months-6 years	½ teaspoonful (2.5 mL)	q.i.d.
adults and children 6 years and over	1 teaspoonful (5 mL)	q.i.d.

◆ RATED THERAPEUTICALLY EQUIVALENT; ◇ THERAPEUTIC EQUIVALENCE UNCONFIRMED; ○ UNRATED

Carbinoxamine/Dextromethorphan/Pseudoephedrine Oral Drops

1-3 months	¼ dropperful (¼ mL)	q.i.d.
3-6 months	½ dropperful (½ mL)	q.i.d.
6-9 months	¾ dropperful (¾ mL)	q.i.d.
9-18 months	1 dropperful (1 mL)	q.i.d.

* In mild cases or in particularly sensitive patients, less frequent or reduced doses may be adequate.

Syrup: Dispense in USP tight, light-resistant, glass container. Avoid exposure to excessive heat.

Oral drops: Avoid exposure to excessive heat.

HOW SUPPLIED
DROP: 2 MG-4 MG-25 MG/ML

BRAND/MANUFACTURER	NDC	SIZE	AWP
○ **BRAND**			
RONDEC DM: Ross Pharm	00074-5639-30	30 ml	$23.98
○ **GENERICS**			
Allscrips	54569-3793-00	15 ml	$6.40
BIODEC DM: Bio-Pharm	59741-0134-30	30 ml	$3.10
CARDEC DM: Moore,H.L.	00839-6404-63	30 ml	$4.04
Morton Grove	60432-0951-30	30 ml	$4.34
RONDAMINE DM: Major	00904-0702-30	30 ml	$4.35
CARBOFED-DM: Hi-Tech	50383-0750-01	30 ml	$4.60
CARDEC DM: Qualitest	00603-1060-45	30 ml	$4.66
SILDEC DM: Silarx	54838-0211-30	30 ml	$4.72
CARDEC DM: Goldline	00182-1342-66	30 ml	$4.95
CARDEC DM: Goldline	00182-6171-66	30 ml	$4.95
CARDEC DM: Mason Dist	11845-0457-30	30 ml	$4.95
CHEMDEC DM: Norton,HN	50732-0866-30	30 ml	$5.85
CARBODEC DM: Rugby	00536-0454-75	30 ml	$5.93
CARDEC DM: Barre	00472-0733-31	30 ml	$6.95
CARBODEX DM: Tri-Med	55654-0015-02	30 ml	$6.95
CARDEC-DM: Aligen	00405-2425-53	30 ml	$8.97
TUSSAFED PEDIATRIC: Everett	00642-0797-30	30 ml	$12.35

For additional alternatives, turn to the section beginning on page 2859.

Carbiset *SEE* CARBINOXAMINE MALEATE WITH PSEUDOEPHEDRINE HYDROCHLORIDE

Carbocaine HCl *SEE* MEPIVACAINE HYDROCHLORIDE

Carboplatin

WARNING

CARBOPLATIN SHOULD BE ADMINISTERED UNDER THE SUPERVISION OF A QUALIFIED PHYSICIAN EXPERIENCED IN THE USE OF CANCER CHEMOTHERAPEUTIC AGENTS. APPROPRIATE MANAGEMENT OF THERAPY AND COMPLICATIONS IS POSSIBLE ONLY WHEN ADEQUATE TREATMENT FACILITIES ARE READILY AVAILABLE.

BONE MARROW SUPPRESSION IS DOSE RELATED AND MAY BE SEVERE, RESULTING IN INFECTION AND/OR BLEEDING. ANEMIA MAY BE CUMULATIVE AND MAY REQUIRE TRANSFUSION SUPPORT. VOMITING IS ANOTHER FREQUENT DRUG-RELATED SIDE EFFECT.

ANAPHYLACTIC-LIKE REACTIONS TO CARBOPLATIN HAVE BEEN REPORTED AND MAY OCCUR WITHIN MINUTES OF CARBOPLATIN ADMINISTRATION. EPINEPHRINE, CORTICOSTEROIDS, AND ANTIHISTAMINES HAVE BEEN EMPLOYED TO ALLEVIATE SYMPTOMS.

DESCRIPTION
Carboplatin is a platinum coordination compound that is used as a cancer chemotherapeutic agent. The chemical name for Carboplatin is platinum, diammine [1,1-cyclobutane-dicarboxylato(2)-0,0']-, (SP-4-2).

Carboplatin is a crystalline powder with the molecular formula of $C_6H_{12}N_2O_4Pt$ and a molecular weight of 371.25. It is soluble in water at a rate of approximately 14 mg/mL, and the pH of a 1% solution is 5-7. It is virtually insoluble in ethanol, acetone, and dimethylacetamide.

Following is its chemical structure:

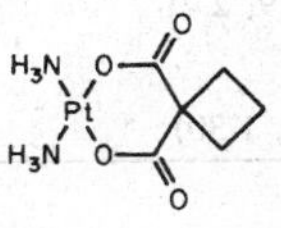

CLINICAL PHARMACOLOGY
Carboplatin, like cisplatin, produces predominantly interstrand DNA cross-links rather than DNA-protein cross-links. This effect is apparently cell-cycle nonspecific. The aquation of carboplatin, which is thought to produce the active species, occurs at a slower rate than in the case of cisplatin. Despite this difference, it appears that both carboplatin and cisplatin induce equal numbers of drug-DNA cross-links, causing equivalent lesions and biological effects. The differences in potencies for Carboplatin and cisplatin appear to be directly related to the difference in aquation rates.

In patients with creatinine clearances of about 60 mL/min or greater, plasma levels of intact Carboplatin decay in a biphasic manner after a 30-minute intravenous infusion of 300 to 500 mg/m² of Carboplatin. The initial plasma half-life (alpha) was found to be 1.1 to 2.0 hours (N = 6), and the postdistribution plasma half-life (beta) was found to be 2.6 to 5.9 hours (N = 6). The total body clearance, apparent volume of distribution, and mean residence time for Carboplatin are 4.4 L/hour, 16 L and 3.5 hours, respectively. The Cmax values and areas under the plasma concentration vs time curves from 0 to infinity (AUC inf) increase linearly with dose, although the increase was slightly more than dose proportional. Carboplatin, therefore, exhibits linear pharmacokinetics over the dosing range studied (300-500 mg/m²).

Carboplatin is not bound to plasma proteins. No significant quantities of protein-free, ultrafilterable platinum-containing species other than Carboplatin are present in plasma. However, platinum from Carboplatin becomes irreversibly bound to plasma proteins and is slowly eliminated with a minimum half-life of 5 days.

The major route of elimination of Carboplatin is renal excretion. Patients with creatinine clearances of approximately 60 mL/min or greater excrete 65% of the dose in the urine within 12 hours and 71% of the dose within 24 hours. All of the platinum in the 24-hour urine is present as Carboplatin. Only 3% to 5% of the administered platinum is excreted in the urine between 24 and 96 hours. There are insufficient data to determine whether biliary excretion occurs.

In patients with creatinine clearances below 60 mL/min the total body and renal clearances of Carboplatin decrease as the creatinine clearance decreases. Carboplatin dosages should therefore be reduced in these patients (see "Dosage and Administration").

CLINICAL STUDIES
USE WITH CYCLOPHOSPHAMIDE FOR INITIAL TREATMENT OF OVARIAN CANCER
In two prospectively randomized, controlled studies conducted by the National Cancer Institute of Canada, Clinical Trials Group (NCIC) and the Southwest Oncology Group (SWOG), 789 chemotherapy naive patients with advanced ovarian cancer were treated with Carboplatin or cisplatin, both in combination with cyclophosphamide every 28 days for six courses before surgical re-evaluation. The following results were obtained from both studies:

COMPARATIVE EFFICACY

(See related tables).

COMPARATIVE TOXICITY
The pattern of toxicity exerted by the Carboplatin-containing regimen was significantly different from that of the cisplatin-containing combinations. Differences between the two studies may be explained by different cisplatin dosages and by different supportive care.

The Carboplatin-containing regimen induced significantly more thrombocytopenia and, in one study, significantly more leukopenia and more need for transfusional support. The cisplatin-containing regimen produced significantly more anemia in one study. However, no significant differences occurred in incidences of infections and hemorrhagic episodes.

Nonhematologic toxicities (emesis, neurotoxicity, ototoxicity, renal toxicity, hypomagnesemia, and alopecia) were significantly more frequent in the cisplatin-containing arms. (See related table).

USE AS A SINGLE AGENT FOR SECONDARY TREATMENT OF ADVANCED OVARIAN CANCER
In two prospective, randomized controlled studies in patients with advanced ovarian cancer previously treated with chemotherapy, Carboplatin achieved six clinical complete responses in 47 patients. The duration of these responses ranged from 45 to 71+ weeks.

INDICATIONS
INITIAL TREATMENT OF ADVANCED OVARIAN CARCINOMA
Carboplatin is indicated for the initial treatment of advanced ovarian carcinoma in established combination with other approved chemotherapeutic agents. One established combination regimen consists of Carboplatin and cyclophosphamide. Two randomized controlled studies conducted by the NCIC and SWOG with Carboplatin vs cisplatin, both in combination with cyclophosphamide, have demonstrated equivalent overall survival between the two groups (see "Clinical Studies" section).

There is limited statistical power to demonstrate equivalence in overall pathologic complete response rates and long-term survival (≥ 3 years) because of the small number of patients with these outcomes; the small number of patients with residual tumor < 2 cm after initial surgery also limits the statistical power to demonstrate equivalence in this subgroup.

SECONDARY TREATMENT OF ADVANCED OVARIAN CARCINOMA
Carboplatin is indicated for the palliative treatment of patients with ovarian carcinoma recurrent after prior chemotherapy, including patients who have been previously treated with cisplatin.

Within the group of patients previously treated with cisplatin, those who have developed progressive disease while receiving cisplatin therapy may have a decreased response rate.

UNLABELED USES
Carboplatin is used alone or as an adjunct in the treatment of metastatic transitional cell carcinoma of the bladder, head and neck cancer, small cell and non-small cell lung cancer, and malignant melanoma.

CONTRAINDICATIONS
Carboplatin is contraindicated in patients with a history of severe allergic reactions to cisplatin or other platinum-containing compounds or mannitol.

Carboplatin should not be employed in patients with severe bone marrow depression or significant bleeding.

WARNINGS
Bone marrow suppression (leukopenia, neutropenia and thrombocytopenia) is dose dependent and is also the dose-limiting toxicity. Peripheral blood counts should be frequently monitored during Carboplatin treatment and, when appropriate, until recovery is achieved. Median nadir occurs at day 21 in patients receiving single-agent Carboplatin. In general, single intermittent courses of

OVERVIEW OF PIVOTAL TRIALS

	NCIC	SWOG
Number of patients randomized	447	342
Median age (years)	60	62
Dose of cisplatin	75 mg/m^2	100 mg/m^2
Dose of Carboplatin	300 mg/m^2	300 mg/m^2
Dose of cyclophosphamid	600 mg/m^2	600 mg/m^2
Residual tumor < 2 cm (number of patients)	39% (174/447)	14% (49/342)

CLINICAL RESPONSE IN MEASURABLE DISEASE PATIENTS

	NCIC	SWOG
Carboplatin (number of patients)	60% (48/80)	58% (48/83)
Cisplatin (number of patients)	58% (49/85)	43% (33/76)
95% C.I. of difference	(=13.9%, 18.6%)	(=2.3%, 31.1%)
(Carboplatin-Cisplatin)		

PATHOLOGIC COMPLETE RESPONSE*

	NCIC	SWOG
Carboplatin (number of patients)	11% (24/224)	10% (17/171)
Cisplatin (number of patients)	15% (33/223)	10% (17/171)
95% C.I. of difference	(=10.7%, 2.5%)	(=6.9%, 6.9%)
(Carboplatin-Cisplatin)		

* 114 Carboplatin and 109 Cisplatin patients did not undergo second-look surgery in NCIC study 90 Carboplatin and 106 Cisplatin patients did not undergo second-look surgery in SWOG study

PROGRESSION-FREE SURVIVAL (PFS)

	NCIC	SWOG
Median		
Carboplatin	59 weeks	49 weeks
Cisplatin	61 weeks	47 weeks
2-year PFS*		
Carboplatin	31%	21%
Cisplatin	31%	21%
95% C.I. of difference (Carboplatin-Cisplatin)	(=9.3, 8.7)	(=9.0, 9.4)
3-year PFS*		
Carboplatin	19%	8%
Cisplatin	23%	14%
95% C.I. of difference (Carboplatin-Cisplatin)	(=11.5, 4.5)	(=14.1, 0.3)
Hazard Ratio**		
95% C.I.	1.10	1.02
(Carboplatin-Cisplatin)	(0.89, 1.35)	(0.81, 1.29)

* Kaplan-Meier Estimates Unrelated deaths occurring in the absence of progression were counted as events (progression) in this analysis.
** Analysis adjusted for factors found to be of prognostic significance were consistent with unadjusted analysis.

SURVIVAL

	NCIC	SWOG
Median		
Carboplatin	110 weeks	86 weeks
Cisplatin	99 weeks	79 weeks
2-year Survival*		
Carboplatin	51.9%	40.2%
Cisplatin	48.4%	39.0%
95% C.I. of difference (Carboplatin-Cisplatin)	(=6.2, 13.2)	(=9.8, 12.2)
3-year Survival*		
Carboplatin	34.6%	18.3%
Cisplatin	33.1%	24.9%
95% C.I. of difference (Carboplatin-Cisplatin)	(=7.7, 10.7)	(=15.9, 2.7)
Hazard Ratio**		
95% C.I.	0.98	1.01
(Carboplatin:Cisplatin)	(0.78, 1.23)	(0.78, 1.30)

* Kaplan-Meier Estimates
** Analysis adjusted for factors found to be of prognostic significance were consistent with unadjusted analysis.

◆ RATED THERAPEUTICALLY EQUIVALENT; ◇ THERAPEUTIC EQUIVALENCE UNCONFIRMED; ○ UNRATED

Carboplatin should not be repeated until leukocyte, neutrophil and platelet counts have recovered.

Since anemia is cumulative, transfusions may be needed during treatment with Carboplatin, particularly in patients receiving prolonged therapy.

Bone marrow suppression is increased in patients who have received prior therapy, especially regimens including cisplatin. Marrow suppression is also increased in patients with impaired kidney function. Initial Carboplatin dosages in these patients should be appropriately reduced (see *"Dosage and Administration"*) and blood counts should be carefully monitored between courses. The use of Carboplatin in combination with other bone marrow suppressing therapies must be carefully managed with respect to dosage and timing in order to minimize additive effects. Carboplatin has limited nephrotoxic potential, but concomitant treatment with aminoglycosides has resulted in increased renal and/or audiologic toxicity, and caution must be exercised when a patient receives both drugs.

Carboplatin can induce emesis, which can be more severe in patients previously receiving emetogenic therapy. The incidence and intensity of emesis have been reduced by using premedication with antiemetics. Although no conclusive efficacy data exist with the following schedules of Carboplatin, lengthening the duration of single intravenous administration to 24 hours or dividing the total dose over five consecutive daily pulse doses has resulted in reduced emesis.

Although peripheral neurotoxicity is infrequent, its incidence is increased in patients older than 65 years and in patients previously treated with cisplatin. Pre-existing cisplatin-induced neurotoxicity does not worsen in about 70% of the patients receiving Carboplatin as secondary treatment.

Loss of vision, which can be complete for light colors, has been reported after the use of Carboplatin with doses higher than those recommended in the package insert. Vision appears to recover totally or to a significant extent within weeks of stopping these high doses.

As in the case of other platinum coordination compounds, allergic reactions to Carboplatin have been reported. These may occur within minutes of administration and should be managed with appropriate supportive therapy.

High dosages of Carboplatin (more than four times the recommended dose) have resulted in severe abnormalities of liver function tests.

Carboplatin may cause fetal harm when administered to a pregnant woman. Carboplatin has been shown to be embryotoxic and teratogenic in rats. There are no adequate and well-controlled studies in pregnant women. If this drug is used during pregnancy, or if the patient becomes pregnant while receiving this drug, the patient should be apprised of the potential hazard to the fetus. Women of childbearing potential should be advised to avoid becoming pregnant.

PRECAUTIONS
General: Needles or intravenous administration sets containing aluminum parts that may come in contact with Carboplatin should not be used for the preparation or administration of the drug. Aluminum can react with carboplatin causing precipitate formation and loss of potency.

Drug Interactions: The renal effects of nephrotoxic compounds may be potentiated by Carboplatin.

Carcinogenesis, Mutagenesis, Impairment of Fertility: The carcinogenic potential of carboplatin has not been studied, but compounds with similar mechanisms of action and mutagenicity profiles have been reported to be carcinogenic. Carboplatin has been shown to be mutagenic both *in vitro* and *in vivo*. It has also been shown to be embryotoxic and teratogenic in rats receiving the drug during organogenesis.

Pregnancy: Pregnancy Category D: (see *"Warnings"*).

Nursing Mothers: It is not known whether Carboplatin is excreted in human milk. Because there is a possibility of toxicity in nursing infants secondary to Carboplatin treatment of the mother, it is recommended that breastfeeding be discontinued if the mother is treated with Carboplatin.

ADVERSE EXPERIENCES IN PATIENTS WITH OVARIAN CANCER NCIC STUDY

		Paraplatin Arm Percent*	Cisplatin Arm Percent*	P-Value**
Bone Marrow				
Thrombocytopenia,	< 100,000/mm^3	70	29	< 0.001
	< 50,000/mm^3	41	6	< 0.001
Neutropenia,	< 2,000 cells/mm^3	97	96	n.s.
	< 1,000 cells/mm^3	81	79	n.s.
Leukopenia,	< 4,000 cells/mm^3	98	97	n.s.
	< 2,000 cells/mm^3	68	52	0.001
Anemia,	< 11 g/dL	91	91	n.s.
	< 8 g/dL	18	12	n.s.
Infections		14	12	n.s.
Bleeding		10	4	n.s.
Transfusions		42	31	0.018
Gastrointestinal				
Nausea and vomiting		93	98	0.010
Vomiting		84	97	< 0.001
Other GI side effects		50	62	0.013
Neurologic				
Peripheral neuropathies		16	42	< 0.001
Ototoxicity		13	33	< 0.001
Other sensory side effects		6	10	n.s.
Central neutrotoxicity		28	40	0.009
Renal				
Serum creatinine elevations		5	13	0.006
Blood urea elevations		17	31	< 0.001
Hepatic				
Bilirubin elevations		5	3	n.s.
SGOT elevations		17	13	n.s.
Alkaline phosphatase elevations		–	–	n.s.
Electrolytes loss				
Sodium		10	20	0.005
Potassium		16	22	n.s.
Calcium		16	19	n.s.
Magnesium		63	88	< 0.001
Other side effects				
Pain		36	37	n.s.
Asthenia		40	33	n.s.
Cardiovascular		15	19	n.s.
Respiratory		8	9	n.s.
Allergic		12	9	n.s.
Genitourinary		10	10	n.s.
Alopecia+		50	62	0.017
Mucositis		10	9	n.s.

* *Values are in percent of evaluable patients*
** *n.s. = not significant, p > 0.05*
+ *May have been affected by cyclophosphamide dosage delivered*

ADVERSE EXPERIENCES IN PATIENTS WITH OVARIAN CANCER SWOG STUDY

	Paraplatin Arm Percent*	Cisplatin Arm Percent*	P-Values**
Bone Marrow			
Thrombocytopenia, $< 100,000/mm^3$	59	35	< 0.001
$< 50,000/mm^3$	22	11	0.006
Neutropenia, $< 2,000\ cells/mm^3$	95	97	n.s.
$< 1,000\ cells/mm^3$	84	78	n.s.
Leukopenia, $< 4,000\ cells/mm^3$	97	97	n.s.
$< 2,000\ cells/mm^3$	76	67	n.s.
Anemia, $< 11\ g/dL$	88	87	n.s.
$< 8\ g/dL$	8	24	< 0.001
Infections	18	21	n.s.
Bleeding	6	4	n.s.
Transfusions	25	33	n.s.
Gastrointestinal			
Nausea and vomiting	94	96	n.s.
Vomiting	82	91	0.007
Other GI side side effects	40	48	n.s.
Neurologic			
Peripheral neuropathies	13	28	0.001
Ototoxicity	12	30	< 0.001
Other sensory side effects	4	6	n.s.
Central neurotoxicity	23	29	n.s.
Renal			
Serum creatinine elevations	7	38	< 0.001
Blood urea elevations	-	-	-
Hepatic			
Bilirubin elevations	5	3	n.s.
SGOT elevations	23	16	n.s.
Alkaline phosphatase elevations	29	20	n.s.
Electrolytes loss			
Sodium	-	29	
Potassium	-	27	
Calcium	-	-	
Magnesium	58	77	< 0.001
Other side effects			
Pain	54	52	n.s.
Asthenia	43	46	n.s.
Cardiovascular	23	30	n.s.
Respiratory	12	11	n.s.
Allergic	10	11	n.s.
Genitourinary	11	13	n.s.
Alopecia+	43	57	0.009
Mucositis	6	11	n.s.

* Values are in percent of evaluable patients
** n.s. = not significant, p > 0.05
+ May have been affected by cyclophosphamide dosage delivered

ADVERSE REACTIONS

For a comparison of toxicities when Carboplatin or cisplatin was given in combination with cyclophosphamide, see the "Comparative Toxicity" subsection of the "Clinical Studies" section.(See related table).

In the narrative section that follows, the incidences of adverse events are based on data from 1,893 patients with various types of tumors who received Carboplatin as single-agent therapy.

Hematologic Toxicity: Bone marrow suppression is the dose-limiting toxicity of Carboplatin. Thrombocytopenia with platelet counts below $50,000/mm^3$ occurs in 25% of the patients (35% of pretreated ovarian cancer patients); neutropenia with granulocyte counts below $1,000/mm^3$ occurs in 16% of the patients (21% of pretreated ovarian cancer patients); leukopenia with WBC counts below $2,000/mm^3$ occurs in 15% of the patients (26% of pretreated ovarian cancer patients). The nadir usually occurs about day 21 in patients receiving single-agent therapy. By day 28, 90% of patients have platelet counts above $100,000/mm^3$; 74% have neutrophil counts above $2,000/mm^3$; 67% have leukocyte counts above $4,000/mm^3$.

Marrow suppression is usually more severe in patients with impaired kidney function. Patients with poor performance status have also experienced a higher incidence of severe leukopenia and thrombocytopenia.

The hematologic effects, although usually reversible, have resulted in infectious or hemorrhagic complications in 5% of the patients treated with Carboplatin, with drug related death occurring in less than 1% of the patients.

Anemia with hemoglobin less than 11 g/dL has been observed in 71% of the patients who started therapy with a baseline above that value. The incidence of anemia increases with increasing exposure to Carboplatin. Transfusions have been administered to 26% of the patients treated with Carboplatin (44% of previously treated ovarian cancer patients).

Bone marrow depression may be more severe when Carboplatin is combined with other bone marrow suppressing drugs or with radiotherapy.

Gastrointestinal Toxicity: Vomiting occurs in 65% of the patients (81% of previously treated ovarian cancer patients) and in about one-third of these patients it is severe. Carboplatin, as a single agent or in combination, is significantly less emetogenic than cisplatin; however, patients previously treated with emetogenic agents, especially cisplatin, appear to be more prone to vomiting. Nausea alone occurs in an additional 10%-15% of patients. Both nausea and vomiting usually cease within 24 hours of treatment and are often responsive to antiemetic measures. Although no conclusive efficacy data exist with the following schedules, prolonged administration of Carboplatin, either by continuous 24-hour infusion or by daily pulse doses given for 5 consecutive days, was associated with less severe vomiting than the single-dose intermittent schedule. Emesis was increased when Carboplatin was used in combination with other emetogenic compounds. Other gastrointestinal effects observed frequently were pain, in 17% of the patients; diarrhea, in 6%; and constipation, also in 6%.

Neurologic Toxicity: Peripheral neuropathies have been observed in 4% of the patients receiving Carboplatin (6% of pretreated ovarian cancer patients) with mild paresthesias occurring most frequently. Carboplatin therapy produces significantly fewer and less severe neurologic side effects than does therapy with cisplatin. However, patients older than 65 years and/or previously treated with cisplatin appear to have an increased risk (10%) for peripheral neuropathies. In 70% of the patients with pre-existing cisplatin-induced peripheral neurotoxicity, there was no worsening of symptoms during therapy with Carboplatin. Clinical ototoxicity and other sensory abnormalities such as visual disturbances and change in taste have been reported in only 1% of the patients. Central nervous system symptoms have been reported in 5% of the patients and appear to be most often related to the use of antiemetics.

Although the overall incidence of peripheral neurologic side effects induced by Carboplatin is low, prolonged treatment, particularly in cisplatin pretreated patients, may result in cumulative neurotoxicity.

Nephrotoxicity: Development of abnormal renal function test results is uncommon, despite the fact that Carboplatin, unlike cisplatin, has usually been administered without high-volume fluid hydration and/or forced diuresis. The incidences of abnormal renal function tests reported are 6% for serum creatinine and 14% for blood urea nitrogen (10% and 22%, respectively, in pretreated ovarian cancer patients). Most of these reported abnormalities have been mild and about one-half of them were reversible.

Creatinine clearance has proven to be the most sensitive measure of kidney function in patients receiving Carboplatin, and it appears to be the most useful test for correlating drug clearance and bone marrow suppression. Twenty-seven percent of the patients who had a baseline value of 60 mL/min or more demonstrated a reduction below this value during Carboplatin therapy.

◆ RATED THERAPEUTICALLY EQUIVALENT; ◇ THERAPEUTIC EQUIVALENCE UNCONFIRMED; ○ UNRATED

Hepatic Toxicity: The incidences of abnormal liver function tests in patients with normal baseline values were reported as follows: total bilirubin, 5%; SGOT, 15%; and alkaline phosphatase, 24%; (5%, 19%, and 37%, respectively, in pretreated ovarian cancer patients). These abnormalities have generally been mild and reversible in about one-half of the cases, although the role of metastatic tumor in the liver may complicate the assessment in many patients. In a limited series of patients receiving very high dosages of Carboplatin and autologous bone marrow transplantation, severe abnormalities of liver function tests were reported.

Electrolyte Changes: The incidences of abnormally decreased serum electrolyte values reported were as follows: sodium, 29%; potassium, 20%; calcium, 22%; and magnesium, 29%; (47%, 28%, 31%, and 43%, respectively, in pretreated ovarian cancer patients). Electrolyte supplementation was not routinely administered concomitantly with Carboplatin, and these electrolyte abnormalities were rarely associated with symptoms.

Allergic reactions: Hypersensitivity to Carboplatin has been reported in 2% of the patients. These allergic reactions have been similar in nature and severity to those reported with other platinum-containing compounds, i.e., rash, urticaria, erythema, pruritus, and rarely bronchospasm and hypotension. These reactions have been successfully managed with standard epinephrine, corticosteriod and antihistamine therapy.

Other Events: Pain and asthenia were the most frequently reported miscellaneous adverse effects; their relationship to the tumor and to anemia was likely. Alopecia was reported (3%). Cardiovascular, respiratory, genitourinary, and mucosal side effects have occurred in 6% or less of the patients. Cardiovascular events (cardiac failure, embolism, cerebrovascular accidents) were fatal in less than 1% of the patients and did not appear to be related to chemotherapy. Cancer-associated hemolytic uremic syndrome has been reported rarely.

OVERDOSAGE
There is no known antidote for Carboplatin overdosage. The anticipated complications of overdosage would be secondary to bone marrow suppression and/or hepatic toxicity.

ADVERSE EXPERIENCES IN PATIENTS WITH OVARIAN CANCER

DOSAGE AND ADMINISTRATION
Note: Aluminum reacts with carboplatin causing precipitate formation and loss of potency, therefore, needles or intravenous sets containing aluminum parts that may come in contact with the drug must not be used for the preparation or administration of Carboplatin.

SINGLE AGENT THERAPY
Carboplatin, as a single agent, has been shown to be effective in patients with recurrent ovarian carcinoma at a dosage of 360 mg/m² I.V. on day 1 every 4 weeks. In general, however, single intermittent courses of Carboplatin should not be repeated until the neutrophil count is at least 2,000 and the platelet count is at least 100,000.

COMBINATION THERAPY WITH CYCLOPHOSPHAMIDE
In the chemotherapy of advanced ovarian cancer, an effective combination for previously untreated patients consists of:
Carboplatin - 300 mg/m² I.V. on day 1 every 4 weeks for six cycles.
Cyclophosphamide - 600 mg/m² I.V. on day 1 every 4 weeks for six cycles. For directions regarding the use and administration of cyclophosphamide please refer to its package insert.
(See "Clinical Studies" section).
Intermittent courses of Carboplatin in combination with cyclophosphamide should not be repeated until the neutrophil count is at least 2,000 and the platelet count is at least 100,000.

DOSE ADJUSTMENT RECOMMENDATIONS
The suggested dose adjustments for single agent or combination therapy shown in the table below are modified from controlled trials in previously treated and untreated patients with ovarian carcinoma. Blood counts were done weekly, and the recommendations are based on the lowest post-treatment platelet or neutrophil value.

	First Line Combination Therapy* Percent	Second Line Single Agent Therapy** Percent
Bone Marrow		
Thrombocytopenia, < 100,000/mm³	66	62
< 50,000/mm³	33	35
Neutropenia, < 2,000 cells/mm³	96	67
< 1,000 cells/mm³	82	21
Leukopenia, < 4,000 cells/mm³	97	85
< 2,000 cells/mm³	71	26
Anemia, < 11 g/dL	90	90
< 8 g/dL	14	21
Infections	16	5
Bleeding	8	5
Transfusions	35	44
Gastrointestinal		
Nausea and vomiting	93	92
Vomiting	83	81
Other GI side effects	46	21
Neurologic		
Peripheral neuropathies	15	6
Ototoxicity	12	1
Other sensory side effects	5	1
Central neurotoxicity	26	5
Renal		
Serum creatinine elevations	6	10
Blood urea elevations	17	22
Hepatic		
Bilirubin elevations	5	5
SGOT elevations	20	19
Alkaline phosphatase elevations	29	37
Electrolytes loss		
Sodium	10	47
Potassium	16	28
Calcium	16	31
Magnesium	61	43
Other side effects		
Pain	44	23
Asthenia	41	11
Cardiovascular	19	6
Respiratory	10	6
Allergic	11	2
Genitourinary	10	2
Alopecia	49	2
Mucositis	8	1

* **Use with cyclophosphamide for initial treatment of ovarian cancer:** *Data are based on the experience of 393 patients with ovarian cancer (regardless of baseline status) who received initial combination therapy with Carboplatin and cyclophosphamide in two randomized controlled studies conducted by SWOG and NCIC (see "Clinical Studies" section). Combination with cyclophosphamide as well as duration of treatment may be responsible for the differences that can be noted in the adverse experience table.*

** **Single agent use for the secondary treatment of ovarian cancer:** *Data are based on the experience of 553 patients with previously treated ovarian carcinoma (regardless of baseline status) who received single-agent Carboplatin.*

Platelets	Neutrophils	Adjusted Dose* (From Prior Course)
> 100,000	> 2,000	125%
50-100,000	500-2,000	No Adjustment
< 50,000	> 500	75%

* *Percentages apply to Carboplatin as a single agent or to both Carboplatin and cyclophosphamide in combination. In the controlled studies, dosages were also adjusted at a lower level (50 to 60%) for severe myelosuppression. Escalations above 125% were not recommended for these studies.*

Carboplatin is usually administered by an infusion lasting 15 minutes or longer. No pre-or post-treatment hydration or forced diuresis is required.

Patients with Impaired Kidney Function: Patients with creatinine clearance values below 60 mL/min are at increased risk of severe bone marrow suppression. In renally-impaired patients who received single-agent Carboplatin therapy, the incidence of severe leukopenia, neutropenia, or thrombocytopenia has been about 25% when the dosage modifications in the table below have been used.

Baseline Creatinine Clearance	Recommended Dose on Day 1
41-59 mL/min	250 mg/m^2
16-40 mL/min	200 mg/m^2

The data available for patients with severely impaired kidney function (creatinine clearance below 15 mL/min) are too limited to permit a recommendation for treatment.[1,2] These dosing recommendations apply to the initial course of treatment. Subsequent dosages should be adjusted according to the patient's tolerance based on the degree of bone marrow suppression.

PREPARATION OF INTRAVENOUS SOLUTIONS
Immediately before use, the content of each vial must be reconstituted with either Sterile Water for Injection, USP, 5% Dextrose in Water (D$_5$W), or 0.9% Sodium Chloride Injection, USP, according to the following schedule:

Vial Strength	Diluent Volume
50 mg	5 mL
150 mg	15 mL
450 mg	45 mL

These dilutions all produce a carboplatin concentration of 10 mg/mL.

Carboplatin can be further diluted to concentrations as low as 0.5 mg/mL with 5% Dextrose in Water (D$_5$W) or 0.9% Sodium Chloride Injection, USP.

STABILITY
Unopened vials of Carboplatin for Injection are stable for the life indicated on the package when stored at controlled room temperature 15°-30°C (59°-86°F), and protected from light.

When prepared as directed, Carboplatin solutions are stable for 8 hours at room temperature (25°C). Since no antibacterial preservative is contained in the formulation, it is recommended that Carboplatin solutions be discarded 8 hours after dilution.

Parenteral drug products should be inspected visually for particulate matter and discoloration prior to administration.

STORAGE
Store the unopened vials at controlled room temperature 15°-30°C (59°-86°F). Protect unopened vials from light. Solutions for infusion should be discarded 8 hours after preparation.

HANDLING AND DISPOSAL
Procedures for proper handling and disposal of anticancer drugs should be considered. Several guidelines on this subject have been published.[3-9] There is no general agreement that all of the procedures recommended in the guidelines are necessary or appropriate.

REFERENCES
1. Egorin, M.J., et al: Phramacokinetics and dosage reduction of cis-diammine (1,1-cyclobutanedicarboxylato) platinum in patients with impaired renal function. *Cancer Res.* 1984; 44:5432-5438. 2. Carboplatin, Etoposide, and Bleomycin for Treatment of Stage IIC Seminoma Complicated by Acute Renal Failure. Cancer Treatment Reports, Vol. 71, No. 11, pp. 1123-1124, November 1987. 3. Recommendations for the Safe Handling of Parenteral Antineoplastic Drugs. NIH Publication No. 83-2621. For sale by the Superintendent of Documents, U.S. Government Printing Office, Washington, DC 20402. 4. AMA Council Report. Guidelines for Handling Parenteral Antineoplastics. *JAMA.* 1985; 253(11): 1590-1592. 5. National Study Commission on Cytotoxic Exposure- Recommendations for Handling Cytotoxic Agents. Available from Louis P. Jeffrey, ScD., Chairman, National Study Commission on Cytotoxic Exposure, Massachusetts College of Pharmacy and Allied Health Sciences, 179 Longwood Avenue, Boston, Massachusetts, 02115. 6. Clinical Oncological Society of Australia: Guidelines and Recommendations for Safe Handling of Antineoplastic Agents. *Med. J. Australia* 1983; 1:426-428. 7. Jones, R.B., et al: Safe Handling of Chemotherapeutic agents: A Report from the Mount Sinai Medical Center. CA-A Cancer Journal for Clinicians, 1983; (Sept/Oct) 258-263. 8. American Society of Hospital Pharmacists Technical Assistance Bulletin on Handling Cytotoxic and Hazardous Drugs. *Am. J. Hosp. Pharm.* 1990;47:1033-1049. 9. OSHA Work-Practice Guidelines for Personnel Dealing with Cytotoxic (Antineoplastic) Drugs. *Am J. Hosp. Pharm.* 1986; 43:1193-1204.

HOW SUPPLIED
POWDER FOR INJECTION: 50 MG

BRAND/MANUFACTURER	NDC	SIZE	AWP
○ BRAND PARAPLATIN: Bristol-Myer Onc/Hiv	00015-3213-30	1s	$78.00

POWDER FOR INJECTION: 150 MG

BRAND/MANUFACTURER	NDC	SIZE	AWP
○ BRAND PARAPLATIN: Bristol-Myer Onc/Hiv	00015-3214-30	1s	$233.96

POWDER FOR INJECTION: 450 MG

BRAND/MANUFACTURER	NDC	SIZE	AWP
○ BRAND PARAPLATIN: Bristol-Myer Onc/Hiv	00015-3215-30	1s	$701.90

Carboprost Tromethamine

DESCRIPTION
Carboprost Tromethamine sterile solution, an oxytocic, contains the Tromethamine salt of the (15S)-15 methyl analogue of naturally occurring prostaglandin F2α in a solution suitable for intramuscular injection.

Four alternate chemical names are:

1. (15S)-15-methyl prostaglandin F2α Tromethamine salt
2. 7-(3α, 5α- dihydroxy-2 β-[(3S)-3-hydroxy-3-methyl-trans-1- octenyl]-1α-cyclopentyl]-*cis*-5-heptenoic acid compound with 2-amino-2-(hydroxymethyl)-1,3-propanediol
3. (15S)-9α, 11α, 15-trihydroxy-15-methyl-prosta-*cis*-5, *trans*-13-*dienoic acid* Tromethamine salt
4. (15S)-15-methyl PGF2α-THAM

The molecular weight of Carboprost Tromethamine is 489.64. It is a white to slightly off-white crystalline powder. It generally melts between 95° and 105° C, depending on the rate of heating.

Carboprost Tromethamine dissolves readily in water at room temperature at a concentration greater than 75 mg/mL.

Each mL contains Carboprost Tromethamine equivalent to 250 mcg of Carboprost, 83 mcg Tromethamine, 9 mg sodium chloride, and 9.45 mg benzyl alcohol added as preservative.

Following is its chemical structure:

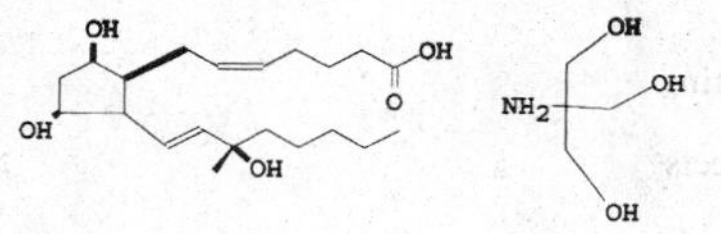

CLINICAL PHARMACOLOGY
Carboprost Tromethamine administered intramuscularly stimulates in the gravid uterus myometrial contractions similar to labor contractions at the end of a full term pregnancy. Whether or not these contractions result from a direct effect of carboprost on the myometrium has not been determined. Nonetheless, they evacuate the products of conception from the uterus in most cases.

Postpartum, the resultant myometrial contractions provide hemostasis at the site of placentation.

Carboprost Tromethamine also stimulates the smooth muscle of the human gastrointestinal tract. This activity may produce the vomiting or diarrhea or both that is common when Carboprost Tromethamine is used to terminate pregnancy and for use postpartum. In laboratory animals and also in humans Carboprost Tromethamine can elevate body temperature. With the clinical doses of Carboprost Tromethamine used for the termination of pregnancy, and for use postpartum, some patients do experience transient temperature increases.

In laboratory animals and in humans large doses of Carboprost Tromethamine can raise blood pressure, probably by contracting the vascular smooth muscle. With the doses of Carboprost Tromethamine used for terminating pregnancy, this effect has not been clinically significant. In laboratory animals and also in humans Carboprost Tromethamine can elevate body temperature. With the clinical doses of Carboprost Tromethamine used for the termination of pregnancy, some patients do experience temperature increases. In some patients, Carboprost Tromethamine may cause transient bronchoconstriction.

Drug plasma concentrations were determined by radioimmunoassay in peripheral blood samples collected by different investigators from 10 patients undergoing abortion. The patients had been injected intramuscularly with 250 micrograms of Carboprost at two hour intervals. Blood levels of drug peaked at an average of 2060 picograms/mL one-half hour after the first injection then declined to an average concentration of 770 picograms/mL two hours after the first injection just before the second injection. The average plasma concentration one-half hour after the second injection was slightly higher (2663 picograms/mL) than that after the first injection and decreased again to an average of 1047 picograms/mL by two hours after the second injection. Plasma samples were collected from 5 of these 10 patients following additional injections of the prostaglandin. The average peak concentrations of drug were slightly higher following each successive injection of the prostaglandin, but always decreased to levels less than the preceding peak values by two hours after each injection.

Five women who had delivery spontaneously at term were treated immediately postpartum with a single injection of 250 micrograms of Carboprost Tromethamine. Peripheral blood samples were collected at several times during the four hours following treatment and Carboprost Tromethamine levels were determined by radioimmunoassay. The highest concentration of Carboprost Tromethamine was observed at 15 minutes in two patients (3009 and 2916 picograms/mL), at 30 minutes in two patients (3097 and 2792 picograms/mL), and at 60 minutes in one patient (2718 picograms/mL).

INDICATIONS AND USAGE

Carboprost Tromethamine is indicated for aborting pregnancy between the 13th and 20th weeks of gestation as calculated from the first day of the last normal menstrual period and in the following conditions related to second trimester abortion:

1. Failure of expulsion of the fetus during the course of treatment by another method;
2. Premature rupture of membranes in intrauterine methods with loss of drug and insufficient or absent uterine activity;
3. Requirement of a repeat intrauterine instillation of drug for expulsion of the fetus;
4. Inadvertent or spontaneous rupture of membranes in the presence of a previable fetus and absence of adequate activity for expulsion.

Carboprost Tromethamine is indicated for the treatment of postpartum hemorrhage due to uterine atony which has not responded to conventional methods of management. Prior treatment should include the use of intravenously administered oxytocin, manipulative techniques such as uterine massage and, unless contraindicated, intramuscular ergot preparations. Studies have shown that in such cases, the use of Carboprost Tromethamine has resulted in satisfactory control of hemorrhage, although it is unclear whether or not ongoing or delayed effects of previously administered ecbolic agents have contributed to the outcome. In a high proportion of cases, Carboprost Tromethamine used in this manner has resulted in the cessation of life threatening bleeding and the avoidance of emergency surgical intervention.

CONTRAINDICATIONS

1. Hypersensitivity to Carboprost Tromethamine
2. Acute pelvic inflammatory disease
3. Patients with active cardiac, pulmonary, renal or hepatic disease

WARNINGS

CARBOPROST TROMETHAMINE LIKE OTHER POTENT OXYTOCIC AGENTS, SHOULD BE USED ONLY WITH STRICT ADHERENCE TO RECOMMENDED DOSAGES. CARBOPROST TROMETHAMINE SHOULD BE USED BY MEDICALLY TRAINED PERSONNEL IN A HOSPITAL WHICH CAN PROVIDE IMMEDIATE INTENSIVE CARE AND ACUTE SURGICAL FACILITIES.

Carboprost Tromethamine does not appear to directly affect the fetoplacental unit. Therefore, the possibility does exist that the previable fetus aborted by Carboprost Tromethamine could exhibit transient life signs. Carboprost Tromethamine is not indicated if the fetus *in utero* has reached the stage of viability. Carboprost Tromethamine should not be considered a feticidal agent.

Evidence from animal studies has suggested that certain other prostaglandins have some teratogenic potential. Although these studies do not indicate that Carboprost Tromethamine is teratogenic, any pregnancy termination with Carboprost Tromethamine that fails should be completed by some other means.

This product contains benzyl alcohol. Benzyl alcohol has been reported to be associated with a fatal "Gasping Syndrome" in premature infants.

PRECAUTIONS

GENERAL

Animal studies lasting several weeks at high doses have shown that prostaglandins of the E and F series can induce proliferation of bone. Such effects have also been noted in newborn infants who have received prostaglandin E1 during prolonged treatment. There is no evidence that short term administration of Carboprost Tromethamine can cause similar bone effects.

As with spontaneous abortion, a process which is sometimes incomplete, abortion induced by Carboprost Tromethamine may be expected to be incomplete in about 20% of cases.

Although the incidence of cervical trauma is extremely small, the cervix should always be carefully examined immediately post-abortion.

Use of Carboprost Tromethamine is associated with transient pyrexia that may be due to its effect on hypothalamic thermoregulation. Temperature elevations exceeding 2°F (1.1°C) were observed in approximately one-eight of the patients who received the recommended dosage regimen. In all cases, temperature returned to normal when therapy ended. Differentiation of postabortion endom-

etritis from drug-induced temperature elevations is difficult, but with increasing clinical experience, the distinctions become more obvious and are summarized below:

ENDOMETRITIS PYREXIA	PYREXIA INDUCED BY CARBOPROST TROMETHAMINE
1. *Time of Onset:* Typical, on third post-abortional day (38° C or higher).	Within 1 to 16 hours after the first injection.
2. *Duration:* Untreated pyrexia and infection continue and may give rise to other pelvic infections.	Temperatures revert to pre-treatment levels after discontinuation of therapy without any other treatment. Temperature elevation occurs whether or not tissue is retained.
3. *Retention:* Products of conception are often retained in the cervical os or uterine cavity.	
4. *Histology:* Endometrium is infiltrated with lymphocytes and some areas are necrotic and hemorrhagic.	Although the endometrial stroma may be edematous and vascular, it is not inflamed.
5. *The Uterus:* Often remains boggy and soft with tenderness over the fundus, and pain on moving the cervix on bimanual examination.	Uterine involution normal and uterus is not tender.
6. *Discharge:* Often associated with foul-smelling lochia and leukorrhea.	Lochia normal.

7. *Cervical Culture:* The culture of pathological organisms from the cervix or uterine cavity after abortion alone does not warrant the diagnosis of septic abortion in the absence of clinical evidence of sepsis. Pathogens have been cultured soon after abortion in patients with no infections. Persistent positive culture with clear clinical signs of infections are significant in the diferential diagnosis.

8. *Blood Count:* Leukocytosis and differential white cell counts do not distinguish between endometritis and Carboprost Tromethamine hyperthermia since total WBC's may increase during infection and transient leukocytosis may also be drug-induced.

Fluids should be forced in patients with drug-induced fever and no clinical or bacteriological evidence of intrauterine infection. Any other simple empirical measures for temperature reduction are unecessary because all fevers induced by Carboprost Tromethamine have been transient or self-limiting.

Increased blood pressure. In the postpartum hemorrhage series, 5/115 (4%) of patients had an increase of blood pressure reported as a side effect. The degree of hypertension was moderate and it is not certain as to whether this was in fact due to a direct effect of Carboprost Tromethamine or a return to a status of pregnancy associated hypertension manifest by the correction of hypovolemic shock. In any event the cases reported did not require specific therapy for the elevated blood pressure.

Use in patients with chorioamnionitis. During the clinical trials with Carboprost Tromethamine, chrioioamnionitis was identified as a complication contributing to postpartum uterine atony and hemorrhage in 8/115 (7%) of cases, 3 of which failed to respond to Carboprost Tromethamine. This complication during labor may have an inhibitory effect on the uterine response to Carboprost Tromethamine similar to what has been reported for other oxytocic agents.[1]

In patients with a history of asthma, hypo- or hypertension, cardiovascular, renal, or hepatic disease, anemia, jaundice, diabetes, or epilepsy, Carboprost Tromethamine should be used cautiously.

As with any oxytocic agent, Carboprost Tromethamine should be used with caution in patients with compromised (scarred) uteri.

DRUG INTERACTIONS

Carboprost Tromethamine may augment the activity of other oxytocic agents. Concomitant use with other oxytocic agents is not recommended.

CARCINOGENESIS, MUTAGENESIS, IMPAIRMENT OF FERTILITY

Carcinogenic bioassay studies have not been conducted in animals with Carboprost Tromethamine due to the limited indications for use and short duration of administration. No evidence of mutagenicity was observed in the Micronucleus Test or Ames Assay.

PREGNANCY: TERATOGENIC EFFECTS: PREGNANCY CATEGORY C

Animal studies do not indicate that Carboprost Tromethamine is teratogenic, however, it has been shown to be embryotoxic in rats and rabbits and any dose which produces increased uterine tone could put the embryo or fetus at risk.

ADVERSE REACTIONS

The adverse effects of Carboprost Tromethamine are generally transient and reversible when therapy ends. The most frequent adverse reactions observed are related to its contractile effect on smooth muscle.

In patients studied, approximately two-thirds experienced vomiting and diarrhea, approximately one-third had nausea, one-eighth had a temperature increase greater than 2°F, and one-fourteenth experienced flushing.

The pretreatment or concurrent administration of antiemetic and antidiarrheal drugs decreases considerably the very high incidence of gastrointestinal effects common with all prostaglandins used for abortion. Their use should be considered

---

1 Duff, Sanders, and Gibbs; The course of labor in term patients with chorioamnionitis; *Am. J. Obstet. Gynecol.*; vol. 147, no. 4, October 15, 1986 pp 391-395.

an integral part of the management of patients undergoing abortion with Carboprost Tromethamine.

Of those patients experiencing a temperature elevation, approximately one-sixteenth had a clinical diagnosis of endometritis. The remaining temperature elevations returned to normal within several hours after the last injection.

Adverse effects observed during the use of Carboprost Tromethamine for abortion and for hemorrhage not all of which are clearly drug related, in decreasing order of frequency include:

Vomiting	Endometritis from IUCD
Diarrhea	Nervousness
Nausea	Nosebleed
Flushing or hot flashes	Sleep disorders
Chills or shivering	Dyspnea
Coughing	Tightness in chest
Headaches	Wheezing
Endometritis	Posterior cervical perforation
Hiccough	Weakness
Dysmenorrhea-like pain	Diaphoresis
Paresthesia	Dizziness
Backache	Blurred vision
Muscular pain	Epigastric pain
Breast tenderness	Excessive thirst
Eye pain	Twitching eyelids
Drowsiness	Gagging, retching
Dystonia	Dry throat
Asthma	Sensation of choking
Injection site pain	Thyroid storm
Tinnitus	Syncope
Vertigo	Palpitations
Vaso-vagal syndrome	Rash
Dryness of mouth	Upper respiratory infection
Hyperventilation	Leg cramps
Respiratory distress	Perforated uterus
Hematemesis	Anxiety
Taste alterations	Chest pain
Urinary tract infection	Retained placental fragment
Septic shock	Shortness of breath
Torticollis	Fullness of throat
Lethargy	Uterine sacculation
Hypertension	Faintness, light-headedness
Tachycardia	Uterine rupture
Pulmonary edema	

The most common complications when Carboprost Tromethamine was utilized for abortion requiring additional treatment after discharge from the hospital were endometritis, retained placental fragments, and excessive uterine bleeding, occurring in about one in every 50 patients.

DOSAGE AND ADMINISTRATION

1. Abortion and Indications 1-4:

An initial dose of 250 micrograms (1 mL) of Carboprost Tromethamine is to be administered deep in the muscle with a tuberculin syringe. Subsequent doses of 250 micrograms should be administered at 1½ to 3½ hour intervals depending on uterine response.

An optional test dose of 100 micrograms (0.4 mL) may be administered initially. The dose may be increased to 500 micrograms (2 mL) if uterine contractility is judged to be inadequate after several doses of 250 micrograms (1 mL).

The total dose administered of Carboprost Tromethamine should not exceed 12 milligrams and continuous administration of the drug for more than two days is not recommended.

2. For Refractory Postpartum Uterine Bleeding:

An initial dose of 250 micrograms (1 mL) of Carboprost Tromethamine is to be given deep, intramuscularly. In clinical trials it was found that the majority of successful cases (73%) responded to single injections.

In some selected cases, however, multiple dosing at intervals of 15 to 90 minutes was carried out with successful outcome. The need for additional injections and the interval at which these should be given can be determined only by the attending physicians as dictated by the course of clinical events. The total dose of Carboprost Tromethamine should not exceed 2 milligrams (8 doses).

Parenteral drug, products should be inspected visually for particulate matter and discoloration prior to administration, whenever solution and container permit.

Carboprost Tromethamine must be refrigerated at 2° to 4°C (36°-39°F).

HOW SUPPLIED
INJECTION: 250 MCG

BRAND/MANUFACTURER	NDC	SIZE	AWP
○ BRAND			
HEMABATE: Upjohn	00009-0856-05	1 ml 10s	$27.36

Cardene *SEE* NICARDIPINE HYDROCHLORIDE

Cardio-Green *SEE* INDOCYANINE GREEN

Cardioplegic Solution

DESCRIPTION

Cardioplegic Solution is a sterile, nonpyrogenic, essentially isotonic, formulation of electrolytes in water for injection. It is a 'core solution' intended for use *only after addition of sodium bicarbonate* to adjust pH prior to administration. After buffering with sodium bicarbonate it is suitable for cardiac instillation (usually with hypothermia) to induce arrest during open heart surgery. Other agents may be added to the solution prior to instillation. (See *"Instructions for Use"*.)

Each 100 mL of solution contains calcium chloride, dihydrate 17.6 mg, magnesium chloride, hexahydrate 325.3 mg, potassium chloride 119.3 mg and sodium chloride 643 mg in water for injection. May contain HCl or NaOH for pH adjustment. Electrolyte content per liter (not including ions for pH adjustment): Calcium (Ca^{++}) 2.4 mEq; magnesium (Mg^{++}) 32 mEq; potassium (K^+) 16 mEq; sodium (Na^+) 110 mEq; chloride (Cl^-) 160 mEq. Osmolar concentration, 304 mOsmol/liter (calc.); pH 3.8 (3.5 — 3.9) prior to sodium bicarbonate addition.

It is required that 10 mL (840 mg) of 8.4% Sodium Bicarbonate Injection, USP (10 mEq each of sodium and bicarbonate) be added aseptically and thoroughly mixed with each 1000 mL of Cardioplegic Solution to adjust pH. Use 10 mL of Abbott List 4900, 8.4% Sodium Bicarbonate Injection, USP, to achieve the approximate pH of 7.8 when measured at room temperature. Use of any other Sodium Bicarbonate Injection may not achieve this pH due to the varying pH's of Sodium Bicarbonate Injections. Due to its inherent instability with other components, sodium bicarbonate must be added just prior to administration. After this addition, the solution must be stored under refrigeration and be used within 24 hours.

The buffered admixture contains the following electrolytes (per liter): Ca^{++} 2.4 mEq, Mg^{++} 32 mEq, K^+ 16 mEq, Na^+ 120 mEq, Cl^- 160 mEq and bicarbonate (HCO_3^-) 10 mEq; osmolar concentration, 324 mOsmol/liter (calc.); pH 7.8 (approx.). If other agents are added, these values may be altered.

The solution contains no bacteriostat, or antimicrobial agent and is intended only for use (after adjusting pH with sodium bicarbonate) in a single operative procedure. When smaller amounts are required, the unused portion should be discarded.

Cardioplegic Solution with added sodium bicarbonate used as a coronary artery infusate induces cardiac arrest, combats ischemic ionic disturbances, buffers ischemic acidosis and protects energy sources for functional recovery after ischemia.

Calcium Chloride, USP is chemically designated calcium chloride, dihydrate $(CaCl_2 • 2 H_2O)$, white fragments or granules freely soluble in water.

Magnesium Chloride, USP is chemically designated magnesium chloride, hexahydrate $(MgCl_2 • 6 H_2O)$, deliquescent flakes or crystals very soluble in water.

Potassium Chloride, USP is chemically designated KCl, a white granular powder freely soluble in water.

Sodium Chloride, USP is chemically designated NaCl, a white crystalline powder freely soluble in water.

Water for Injection, USP is chemically designated H_2O.

CLINICAL PHARMACOLOGY

Cardioplegic Solution with added sodium bicarbonate when cooled and instilled into the coronary artery vasculature, causes prompt arrest of cardiac electromechanical activity, combats intracellular ion losses and buffers ischemic acidosis. When used with hypothermia and ischemia, the action may be characterized as cold ischemic potassium-induced cardioplegia. This is conducive to providing the surgeon with a quiet, relaxed heart and bloodless field of operation.

Calcium (Ca^{++}) ion in low concentration is included in the solution to maintain integrity of cell membrane to ensure that there is no likelihood of calcium paradox during reperfusion.

Magnesium (Mg^{++}) ion may help stabilize the myocardial membrane by inhibiting a myosin phosphorylase, which protects adenosine triphosphate (ATP) reserves for postischemic activity. The protective effects of magnesium and potassium have been shown to be additive.

Potassium (K^+) ion concentration is responsible for prompt cessation of mechanical myocardial contractile activity. The immediacy of the arrest thus preserves energy supplies for postischemic contractile activity in diastole.

The chloride (Cl^-) and sodium (Na^+) ions have no specific role in the production of cardiac arrest. Sodium is essential to maintain ionic integrity of myocardial tissue. The chloride ions are present to maintain the electroneutrality of the solution.

Added bicarbonate (HCO_3^-) anion is included as a buffer to render the solution slightly alkaline and compensate for the metabolic acidosis that accompanies ischemia.

Extemporaneous alternative buffering to the described formulation of this solution is not recommended.

INDICATIONS AND USAGE

Cardioplegic Solution when suitably buffered in combination with ischemia and hypothermia is used to induce cardiac arrest during open heart surgery.

CONTRAINDICATIONS

Cardioplegic Solution must not be administered without the addition of 8.4% Sodium Bicarbonate, Injection, USP, Abbott List 4900.

Not For Intravenous Injection: This solution is only for instillation into cardiac vasculature after buffering with sodium bicarbonate.

WARNINGS

This solution should be used only by those trained to perform open heart surgery. This solution is intended only for use during cardiopulmonary bypass when the coronary circulation is isolated from the systemic circulation. (See *"Indications and Usage".*)

Do not instill the solution into the coronary vasculature unless sodium bicarbonate has been added. If large volumes of Cardioplegic Solution are infused and allowed to return to the heart lung machine without any venting from the right heart, then plasma magnesium and potassium levels may rise. Development of severe hypotension and metabolic acidosis while on bypass has been reported when large volumes (8 to 10 liters) of solution are instilled and allowed to enter the pump and then the systemic circulation. Right heart venting is therefore recommended. The buffered solution with added sodium bicarbonate should be cooled to 4°C prior to administration and used within 24 hours of mixing.

PRECAUTIONS

Myocardial temperature should be monitored during surgery to maintain hypothermia.

Continuous electrocardiogram monitoring is essential to detect changes in myocardial activity during the procedure.

Appropriate equipment to defibrillate the heart following cardioplegia should be readily available.

Inotropic support drugs should be available during postoperative recovery. Do not administer unless solution is clear and container is undamaged. Discard unused portion.

Pregnancy Category C: Animal reproduction studies have not been conducted with Cardioplegic Solution. It is also not known whether this solution can cause fetal harm when administered to a pregnant woman or can affect reproduction capacity. Cardioplegic Solution should be given to a pregnant woman only if clearly needed.

DRUG INTERACTIONS

Additives may be incompatible. Consult with pharmacist, if available. When introducing additives, use aseptic technique, mix thoroughly and do not store. (See *"Instructions For Use"*.)

ADVERSE REACTIONS

Intraoperative and perioperative potential hazards of open heart surgery include myocardial infarction, electrocardiographic abnormalities, and arrhythmias, including ventricular fibrillation. Spontaneous recovery after cardioplegic cardiac arrest may be delayed or absent when circulation is restored. Defibrillation by electric shock may be required to restore normal cardiac function.

OVERDOSAGE

Overzealous instillation of the solution may result in unnecessary dilatation of the myocardial vasculature and leakage into the perivascular myocardium, possibly causing tissue edema. See *"Warnings"*, *"Precautions"*, and *"Adverse Reactions"*.

DOSAGE AND ADMINISTRATION

The following information is suggested as a guide and is subject to variation according to the preference and experience of the surgeon.

It is required that 10 mL (840 mg) of 8.4% Sodium Bicarbonate Injection, USP (10 mEq each of sodium and bicarbonate) be added aseptically and thoroughly mixed with each 1000 mL of cardioplegic solution to adjust pH. Use 10 mL of Abbott 8.4% Sodium Bicarbonate Injection, USP, to achieve the approximate pH of 7.8 when measured at room temperature. Use of any other Sodium Bicarbonate Injection may not achieve this pH due to the varying pH's of Sodium Bicarbonate Injections. Due to its inherent instability with other components, sodium bicarbonate must be added just prior to administration. After this addition, the solution must be used within 24 hours. The solution should be cooled to 4° C prior to use.

Following institution of cardiopulmonary bypass at perfusate temperatures of 28° to 30° C, and after cross-clamping of the ascending aorta, the buffered solution is administered by rapid infusion into the aortic root. The initial rate of infusion may be 300 mL/m²/minute (about 540 mL/min in a 5'8", 70 kg adult with 1.8 square meters of surface area) given for a period of two to four minutes. Concurrent external cooling (regional hypothermia of the pericardium) may be accomplished by instilling a refrigerated (4°C) physiologic solution such as Normosol®-R (balanced electrolyte replacement solution) or Ringer's Injection, USP into the chest cavity.

Should myocardial electromechanical activity persist or recur, the solution may be reinfused at a rate of 300 mL/m²/min for a period of two minutes. Reinfusion of the solution may be repeated every 20 to 30 minutes or sooner if myocardial temperature rises above 15° to 20° C or returning cardiac activity is observed. The regional hypothermia solution around the heart also may be replenished continuously or periodically in order to maintain adequate hypothermia. Suction may be used to remove warmed infusates. An implanted thermistor probe may be used to monitor myocardial temperature.

The volumes of solution instilled into the aortic root may vary depending on the duration or type of open heart surgical procedure.

Parenteral drug products should be inspected visually for particulate matter and discoloration prior to administration, whenever solution and container permit. See *"Precautions."*

INSTRUCTIONS FOR USE

TO OPEN

Tear outer wrap at notch and remove solution container. If supplemental medication is desired, follow directions below before preparing for administration. Some opacity of the plastic due to moisture absorption during the sterilization process may be observed. This is normal and does not affect the solution quality or safety. The opacity will diminish gradually.

To add 10 mL of 8.4% Sodium Bicarbonate Injection, USP, Abbott and other supplemental medication, follow directions below before preparing for administration.

TO ADD MEDICATION
1. Prepare additive port.
2. Using aseptic technique and an additive delivery needle of appropriate length, puncture resealable additive port at target area, inner diaphragm and inject. Withdraw needle after injecting medication.
3. The additive port may be protected by covering with an additive cap.
4. Mix container contents thoroughly.

PREPARATION FOR ADMINISTRATION
(USE ASEPTIC TECHNIQUE)
1. Close flow control clamp of administration set.
2. Remove cover from outlet port at bottom of container.
3. Insert piercing pin of administration set into port with a twisting motion until the set is firmly seated. *Note:* See full directions on administration set carton.
4. Suspend container from hanger.
5. Squeeze and release drip chamber to establish proper fluid level in chamber.
6. Attach aortic infusion device to set.
7. Open flow control clamp to expel air from set and aortic infusion device. Close clamp.
8. Position aortic infusion device to introduce solution into aortic root.
9. Regulate rate of administration with flow control clamp.

Warning: Do not use flexible container in series connections.

Exposure of pharmaceutical products to heat should be minimized. Avoid excessive heat. Protect from freezing. It is recommended that the product be stored at room temperature (25° C); however, brief exposure up to 40°C does not adversely affect the product.

HOW SUPPLIED
SOLUTION:

BRAND/MANUFACTURER	NDC	SIZE	AWP
○ **BRAND**			
PLEGISOL: Abbott Hosp	00074-7969-05	1000 ml 12s	$568.86

Cardioquin SEE QUINIDINE POLYGALACTURONATE

Cardizem SEE DILTIAZEM HYDROCHLORIDE

Cardura SEE DOXAZOSIN MESYLATE

Carisoprodol

DESCRIPTION

Carisoprodol is available as 350 mg round, white tablets. Carisoprodol is N-isopropyl-2-methyl-2-propyl-1,3-propanediol dicarbamate.

Following is its chemical structure:

$$(CH_3)_2CHNHCOOCH_2\overset{\overset{\displaystyle CH_3}{|}}{\underset{\underset{\displaystyle CH_2CH_2CH_3}{|}}{C}}CH_2OOCNH_2$$

ACTIONS

Carisoprodol produces muscle relaxation in animals by blocking interneuronal activity in the descending reticular formation and spinal cord. The onset of action is rapid and the effects last four to six hours.

INDICATIONS

Carisoprodol is indicated as an adjunct to rest, physical therapy, and other measures for the relief of discomfort associated with acute, painful musculoskeletal conditions. The mode of action of this drug has not been clearly identified, but may be related to its sedative properties. Carisoprodol does not directly relax tense skeletal muscles in man.

CONTRAINDICATIONS

Acute intermittent porphyria as well as allergic or idiosyncratic reactions to Carisoprodol or related compounds such as meprobamate, mebutamate, or tybamate.

WARNINGS

Idiosyncratic Reactions: On very rare occasions, the first dose of Carisoprodol has been followed by idiosyncratic symptoms appearing within minutes or hours. Symptoms reported include: extreme weakness, transient quadriplegia, dizziness, ataxia, temporary loss of vision, diplopia, mydriasis, dysarthria, agitation, euphoria, confusion, and disorientation. Symptoms usually subside over the course of the next several hours. Supportive and symptomatic therapy, including hospitalization, may be necessary.

Usage in Pregnancy and Lactation: Safe usage of this drug in pregnancy or lactation has not been established. Therefore, use of this drug in pregnancy, in nursing mothers, or in women of childbearing potential requires that the potential benefits of the drug be weighed against the potential hazards to mother and child. Carisoprodol is present in breast milk of lactating mothers at concentrations two to four times that of maternal plasma. This factor should be taken into account when use of the drug is contemplated in breast-feeding patients.

Usage in Children: Because of limited clinical experience, Carisoprodol is not recommended for use in patients under 12 years of age.

Potentially Hazardous Tasks: Patients should be warned that this drug may impair the mental and/or physical abilities required for the performance of potentially hazardous tasks such as driving a motor vehicle or operating machinery.

Additive Effects: Since the effects of Carisoprodol and alcohol or Carisoprodol and other CNS depressants or psychotropic drugs may be additive, appropriate caution should be exercised with patients who take more than one of these agents simultaneously.

Drug Dependence: In dogs, no withdrawal symptoms occurred after abrupt cessation of Carisoprodol from dosages as high as 1 gm/kg/day. In a study in man, abrupt cessation of 100 mg/kg/day (about five times the recommended daily adult dosage) was followed in some subjects by mild withdrawal symptoms such as abdominal cramps, insomnia, chilliness, headache, and nausea. Delirium and convulsions did not occur. In clinical use, psychological dependence and abuse have been rare, and there have been no reports of significant abstinence signs. Nevertheless, the drug should be used with caution in addiction-prone individuals.

PRECAUTIONS

Carisoprodol is metabolized in the liver and excreted by the kidney; to avoid its excess accumulation, caution should be exercised in administration to patients with compromised liver or kidney function.

ADVERSE REACTIONS

Central Nervous System: Drowsiness and other CNS effects may require dosage reduction. Also observed; dizziness, vertigo, ataxia, tremor, agitation, irritability, headache, depressive reactions, syncope and insomnia (See also *"Idiosyncratic Reactions"* under *"Warnings."*)

Allergic or Idiosyncratic: Allergic or idiosyncratic reactions occasionally develop. They are usually seen within the period of the first to fourth dose in patients having had no previous contact with the drug. Skin rash, erythema multiforme, pruritus, eosinophilia, and fixed drug eruption with cross reaction to meprobamate have been reported with Carisoprodol. Severe reactions have been manifested by asthmatic episodes, fever, weakness, dizziness, angioneurotic edema, smarting eyes, hypotension, and anaphylactoid shock. (See also *"Idiosyncratic Reactions"* under *"Warnings."*) In case of allergic or idiosyncratic reactions to Carisoprodol, discontinue the drug and initiate appropriate symptomatic therapy, which may include epinephrine, antihistamines, and in severe cases corticosteroids. In evaluating possible allergic reactions, also consider allergy to excipients (information on excipients is available to physicians on request).

Cardiovascular: Tachycardia, postural hypotension, and facial flushing.

Gastrointestinal: Nausea, vomiting, hiccup, and epigastric distress.

Hematologic: Leukopenia, in which other drugs or viral infection may have been responsible, and pancytopenia, attributed to phenylbutazone, have been reported. No serious blood dyscrasias have been attributed to Carisoprodol.

OVERDOSAGE

Overdosage of Carisoprodol has produced stupor, coma, shock, respiratory depression, and, very rarely, death. The effects of an overdosage of Carisoprodol and alcohol or other CNS depressants or psychotropic agents can be additive even when one of the drugs has been taken in the usual recommended dosage. Any drug remaining in the stomach should be removed and symptomatic therapy given. Should respiration or blood pressure become compromised, respiratory assistance, central nervous system stimulants, and pressor agents should be administered cautiously as indicated. Carisoprodol is metabolized in the liver and excreted by the kidney. Although Carisoprodol overdosage experience is limited, the following types of treatment have been used successfully with the related drug meprobamate: diuresis, osmotic (mannitol) diuresis, peritoneal dialysis, and hemodialysis (Carisoprodol is dialyzable). Careful monitoring of urinary output is necessary and caution should be taken to avoid overhydration. Observe for possible relapse due to incomplete gastric emptying and delayed absorption. Carisoprodol can be measured in biological fluids by gas chromatography (Douglas, J. F. et al; *J Pharm Sci 58*: 145, 1969).

DOSAGE AND ADMINISTRATION

The usual adult dosage of Carisoprodol is one 350 mg tablet, three times daily and at bedtime. Usage in patients under age 12 is not recommended.

Store at controlled room temperature 15°-30°C (59°-86°F).

Dispense in a tight container.

HOW SUPPLIED
TABLETS: 350 MG

AVERAGE UNIT PRICE (AVAILABLE SIZES)		GENERIC A-RATED AVERAGE PRICE (GAAP)	
BRAND	$1.61	100s	$13.37
GENERIC	$0.11	500s	$57.05
HCFA FUL (100s ea)	$0.07	1000s	$85.90

BRAND/MANUFACTURER	NDC	SIZE	AWP
◆ BRAND			
➤ SOMA: Wallace	00037-2001-01	100s	$162.17
	00037-2001-85	100s ud	$164.02
	00037-2001-03	500s	$787.26
◆ GENERICS			
Pioneer	60104-6018-02	100s	$7.70
Aligen	00405-4141-01	100s	$9.85
➤ Geneva	00781-1050-01	100s	$11.55
Qualitest	00603-2582-21	100s	$12.20
Moore,H.L.	00839-6246-06	100s	$12.22
➤ Schein	00364-0475-01	100s	$12.25
URL	00677-0589-01	100s	$12.35
➤ Rugby	00536-3435-01	100s	$12.35
Mutual	53489-0110-01	100s	$12.35
Major	00904-0355-60	100s	$12.40
Goldline	00182-1079-01	100s	$12.40
Parmed	00349-2120-01	100s	$13.95
Medirex	57480-0345-01	100s ud	$18.90
UDL	51079-0055-20	100s ud	$19.00
Major	00904-0355-61	100s ud	$21.01
Major	00904-0355-70	250s	$14.85
Pioneer	60104-6018-06	500s	$33.00
➤ Geneva	00781-1050-05	500s	$52.85
➤ Schein	00364-0475-05	500s	$59.45
Qualitest	00603-2582-28	500s	$59.55
URL	00677-0589-05	500s	$59.90
Major	00904-0355-40	500s	$59.90
Aligen	00405-4141-02	500s	$59.90
Mutual	53489-0110-05	500s	$59.90
Goldline	00182-1079-05	500s	$59.90
➤ Rugby	00536-3435-05	500s	$60.28
Parmed	00349-2120-05	500s	$62.95
Major	00904-0355-80	1000s	$55.30
Pioneer	60104-6018-08	1000s	$63.14
Moore,H.L.	00839-6246-16	1000s	$66.14
Mutual	53489-0110-10	1000s	$94.60
➤ Schein	00364-0475-02	1000s	$94.64
URL	00677-0589-10	1000s	$99.90
➤ Rugby	00536-3435-10	1000s	$99.98
Goldline	00182-1079-10	1000s	$113.50

Carmustine

WARNINGS

CARMUSTINE SHOULD BE ADMINISTERED UNDER THE SUPERVISION OF A QUALIFIED PHYSICIAN EXPERIENCED IN THE USE OF CANCER CHEMOTHERAPEUTIC AGENTS.

BONE MARROW SUPPRESSION, NOTABLY THROMBOCYTOPENIA AND LEUKOPENIA, WHICH MAY CONTRIBUTE TO BLEEDING AND OVERWHELMING INFECTIONS IN AN ALREADY COMPROMISED PATIENT, IS THE MOST COMMON AND SEVERE OF THE TOXIC EFFECTS OF CARMUSTINE (SEE *"WARNINGS"* AND *"ADVERSE REACTIONS"*).

SINCE THE MAJOR TOXICITY IS DELAYED BONE MARROW SUPPRESSION, BLOOD COUNTS SHOULD BE MONITORED WEEKLY FOR AT LEAST 6 WEEKS AFTER A DOSE (SEE *"ADVERSE REACTIONS"*). AT THE RECOMMENDED DOSAGE, COURSES OF CARMUSTINE SHOULD NOT BE GIVEN MORE FREQUENTLY THAN EVERY 6 WEEKS.

THE BONE MARROW TOXICITY OF CARMUSTINE IS CUMULATIVE AND THEREFORE DOSAGE ADJUSTMENT MUST BE CONSIDERED ON THE BASIS OF NADIR BLOOD COUNTS FROM PRIOR DOSE (SEE *"DOSAGE ADJUSTMENT TABLE"* UNDER *"DOSAGE AND ADMINISTRATION"*).

PULMONARY TOXICITY FROM CARMUSTINE APPEARS TO BE DOSE RELATED. PATIENTS RECEIVING GREATER THAN 1400 MG/M^2 CUMULATIVE DOSE ARE AT SIGNIFICANTLY HIGHER RISK THAN THOSE RECEIVING LESS.

DESCRIPTION

Carmustine is one of the nitrosoureas used in the treatment of certain neoplastic diseases. It is 1,3-bis (2-chloroethyl)-1-nitrosourea. It is lyophilized pale yellow flakes or congealed mass with a molecular weight of 214.06. It is highly soluble in alcohol and lipids, and poorly soluble in water Carmustine is administered by intravenous infusion after reconstitution as recommended. Sterile Carmustine is available in 100 mg single dose vials of lyophilized material.

Following is its chemical structure:

$$ClCH_2CH_2 - \overset{\overset{\displaystyle O}{\|}}{N} - \overset{\underset{\displaystyle N=O}{|}}{C} - NCH_2CH_2Cl$$

CLINICAL PHARMACOLOGY

Although it is generally agreed that Carmustine alkylates DNA and RNA, it is not cross resistant with other alkylators. As with other nitrosoureas, it may also inhibit several key enzymatic processes by carbamoylation of amino acids in proteins.

Intravenously-administered Carmustine is rapidly degraded, with no intact drug detectable after 15 minutes. However, in studies with C-^{14} labeled drug, prolonged levels of the isotope were detected in the plasma and tissue, probably representing radioactive fragments of the parent compound.

It is thought that the antineoplastic and toxic activities of Carmustine may be due to metabolites. Approximately 60% to 70% of a total dose is excreted in the urine in 96 hours and about 10% as respiratory CO_2. The fate of the remainder is undetermined.

Because of the high lipid solubility and the relative lack of ionization at physiological pH, Carmustine crosses the blood-brain barrier quite effectively. Levels of radioactivity in the CSF are $\geq$ 50% of those measured concurrently in plasma.

INDICATIONS AND USAGE

Carmustine is indicated as palliative therapy as a single agent or in established combination therapy with other approved chemotherapeutic agents in the following:

1. Brain tumors—glioblastoma, brainstem glioma, medulloblastoma, astrocytoma, ependymoma, and metastatic brain tumors.

2. Multiple myeloma—in combination with prednisone.

3. Hodgkin's Disease—as secondary therapy in combination with other approved drugs in patients who relapse while being treated with primary therapy, or who fail to respond to primary therapy.

4. Non-Hodgkin's lymphomas—as secondary therapy in combination with other approved drugs for patients who relapse while being treated with primary therapy, or who fail to respond to primary therapy.

UNLABELED USES

Carmustine is used alone or as an adjunct in the treatment of acute lymphoblastic or myeloblastic leukemia.

CONTRAINDICATIONS

Carmustine should not be given to individuals who have demonstrated a previous hypersensitivity to it.

WARNINGS

Since the major toxicity is delayed bone marrow suppression, blood counts should be monitored weekly for at least 6 weeks after a dose (see *"Adverse Reactions"*). At the recommended dosage, courses of Carmustine should not be given more frequently than every 6 weeks.

The bone marrow toxicity of Carmustine is cumulative and therefore dosage adjustment must be considered on the basis of nadir blood counts from prior dose (see *"Dosage Adjustment Table"* under *"Dosage and Administration"*).

Pulmonary toxicity from Carmustine appears to be dose related. Patients receiving greater than 1400 mg/m^2 cumulative dose are at significantly higher risk than those receiving less. Additionally, delayed onset pulmonary fibrosis occurring up to 15 years after treatment has been reported in patients who received Carmustine in childhood and early adolescence (see *"Adverse Reactions"*).

Long term use of nitrosoureas has been reported to be associated with the development of secondary malignancies.

Liver and renal function tests should be monitored periodically (see *"Adverse Reactions"*).

Carmustine may cause fetal harm when administered to a pregnant woman. Carmustine has been shown to be embryotoxic in rats and rabbits and teratogenic in rats when given in doses equivalent to the human dose. There are no adequate and well-controlled studies in pregnant women. If this drug is used during pregnancy, or if the patient becomes pregnant while taking (receiving) this drug, the patient should be apprised of the potential hazard to the fetus. Women of childbearing potential should be advised to avoid becoming pregnant.

Carmustine has been administered through an intra-arterial intracarotid route; this procedure is investigational and has been associated with ocular toxicity.

PRECAUTIONS

General: In all instances where the use of Carmustine is considered for chemotherapy, the physician must evaluate the need and usefulness of the drug against the risks of toxic effects or adverse reactions. Most such adverse reactions are reversible if detected early. When such effects or reactions do occur, the drug should be reduced in dosage or discontinued and appropriate corrective measures should be taken according to the clinical judgment of the physician. Reinstitution of Carmustine therapy should be carried out with caution, and with adequate consideration of the further need for the drug and alertness as to possible recurrence of toxicity.

Laboratory Tests: Due to delayed bone marrow suppression, blood counts should be monitored weekly for at least 6 weeks after a dose.

Baseline pulmonary function studies should be conducted along with frequent pulmonary function tests during treatment. Patients with a baseline below 70% of the predicted Forced Vital Capacity (FVC) or Carbon Monoxide Diffusing Capacity (DL$_{co}$) are particularly at risk.

Since Carmustine may cause liver dysfunction, it is recommended that liver function tests be monitored.

Renal function tests should also be monitored periodically.

Carcinogenesis, Mutagenesis, Impairment of Fertility: Carmustine is carcinogenic in rats and mice, producing a marked increase in tumor incidence in doses approximating those employed clinically. Nitrosourea therapy does have carcinogenic potential in humans (see *"Adverse Reactions"*). Carmustine also affects fertility in male rats at doses somewhat higher than the human dose.

Pregnancy: Pregnancy Category D, see *"Warnings."*

Nursing Mothers: It is not known whether this drug is excreted in human milk. Because many drugs are excreted in human milk and because of the potential for serious adverse reactions in nursing infants from Carmustine, a decision should be made whether to discontinue nursing or to discontinue the drug, taking into account the importance of the drug to the mother.

Pediatric Use: Safety and effectiveness in children have not been established.

ADVERSE REACTIONS

Hematologic Toxicity: The most frequent and most serious toxicity of Carmustine is delayed myelosuppression. It usually occurs 4 to 6 weeks after drug administration and is dose related. Thrombocytopenia occurs at about 4 weeks postadministration and persists for 1 to 2 weeks. Leukopenia occurs at 5 to 6 weeks after a dose of Carmustine and persists for 1 to 2 weeks. Thrombocytopenia is generally more severe than leukopenia. However, both may be dose-limiting toxicities. Carmustine may produce cumulative myelosuppression, manifested by more depressed indices or longer duration of suppression after repeated doses.

The occurrence of acute leukemia and bone marrow dysplasias have been reported in patients following long term nitrosourea therapy.

Anemia also occurs, but is less frequent and less severe than thrombocytopenia or leukopenia.

Pulmonary Toxicity: Pulmonary toxicity characterized by pulmonary infiltrates and/or fibrosis has been reported to occur from 9 days to 43 months after treatment with Carmustine and related nitrosoureas. Most of these patients were receiving prolonged therapy with total doses of Carmustine greater than 1400 mg/m^2. However, there have been reports of pulmonary fibrosis in patients receiving lower total doses. Other risk factors include past history of lung disease and duration of treatment. Cases of fatal pulmonary toxicity with Carmustine have been reported.

Additionally, delayed onset pulmonary fibrosis occurring up to 15 years after treatment has been reported in patients who received Carmustine in childhood and early adolescence in cumulative doses ranging from 770 to 1800 mg/m^2 combined with cranial radiotherapy for intracranial tumors. Chest x-rays have demonstrated pulmonary hypoplasia with upper zone contraction. Gallium scans have been normal in all cases. Thoracic CT scans have demonstrated an unusual pattern of upper zone fibrosis. There appears to be some late reduction of pulmonary function in a substantial percentage of these patients. This form of lung fibrosis may be slowly progressive and has resulted in death in some cases.

Gastrointestinal Toxicity: Nausea and vomiting after IV administration of Carmustine are noted frequently. This toxicity appears within 2 hours of dosing, usually lasting 4 to 6 hours, and is dose related. Prior administration of antiemetics is effective in diminishing and sometimes preventing this side effect.

Hepatotoxicity: A reversible type of hepatic toxicity, manifested by increased transaminase, alkaline phosphatase and bilirubin levels, has been reported in a small percentage of patients receiving Carmustine.

Nephrotoxicity: Renal abnormalities consisting of progressive azotemia, decrease in kidney size and renal failure have been reported in patients who received large cumulative doses after prolonged therapy with Carmustine and related nitrosoureas. Kidney damage has also been reported occasionally in patients receiving lower total doses.

Other Toxicities: Accidental contact of reconstituted Carmustine with skin has caused burning and hyperpigmentation of the affected areas.

Rapid IV infusion of Carmustine may produce intensive flushing of the skin and suffusion of the conjunctiva within 2 hours, lasting about 4 hours. It is also associated with burning at the site of injection although true thrombosis is rare. Neuroretinitis has been reported.

OVERDOSAGE

No proven antidotes have been established for Carmustine overdosage.

DOSAGE AND ADMINISTRATION

The recommended dose of Carmustine as a single agent in previously untreated patients is 150 to 200 mg/m^2 intravenously every 6 weeks. This may be given as a single dose or divided into daily injections such as 75 to 100 mg/m^2 on 2 successive days. When Carmustine is used in combination with other myelosuppressive drugs or in patients in whom bone marrow reserve is depleted, the doses should be adjusted accordingly. Doses subsequent to the initial dose should be adjusted according to the hematologic response of the patient to the preceding dose. The following schedule is suggested as a guide to dosage adjustment:

Nadir After Prior Dose		Percentage of Prior Dose to be Given
Leukocytes/mm³	Platelets/mm³	
> 4000	100,000	100%
3000-3999	75,000-99,999	100%
2000-2999	25,000-74,999	70%
< 2000	< 25,000	50%

A repeat course of Carmustine should not be given until circulating blood elements have returned to acceptable levels (platelets above 100,000/mm³, leukocytes above 4,000/mm³), and this is usually in 6 weeks. An adequate number of neutrophils should be present on a peripheral blood smear. Blood counts should be monitored weekly and repeat courses should not be given before 6 weeks because the hematologic toxicity is delayed and cumulative.

Administration Precautions: As with other potentially toxic compounds, caution should be exercised in handling Carmustine and preparing the solution of Carmustine. Accidental contact of reconstituted Carmustine with the skin has caused transient hyperpigmentation of the affected areas. The use of gloves is recommended. If Carmustine lyophilized material or solution contacts the skin or mucosa, immediately wash the skin or mucosa thoroughly with soap and water.

The reconstituted solution should be used intravenously only and should be administered by IV drip. Injection of Carmustine over shorter periods of time than 1 to 2 hours may produce intense pain and burning at the site of injection.

Preparation of Intravenous Solutions: First, dissolve Carmustine with 3 mL of the supplied sterile diluent (Dehydrated Alcohol Injection, USP). Second, aseptically add 27 mL Sterile Water for Injection, USP. Each mL of resulting solution contains 3.3 mg of Carmustine in 10% ethanol, pH 5.6 to 6.0. Such solutions should be protected from light.

Reconstitution as recommended results in a clear, colorless to yellowish solution which may be further diluted with 5% Dextrose Injection, USP. Parenteral drug products should be inspected visually for particulate matter and discoloration prior to administration, whenever solution and container permit.

Important Note: The lyophilized dosage formulation contains no preservatives and is not intended as a multiple dose vial.

Stability: Unopened vials of the dry drug must be stored in a refrigerator (2°C to 8°C). The recommended storage of unopened vials provides a stable product for 2 years. After reconstitution as recommended, Carmustine is stable for 8 hours at room temperature (25°C), protected from light.

Vials reconstituted as directed and further diluted to a concentration of 0.2 mg/mL in 5% Dextrose Injection, USP should be stored at room temperature, protected from light and utilized within 8 hours.

Glass containers were used for the stability data provided in this section. Only use glass containers for Carmustine administration.

Important Note: Carmustine has a low melting point (30.5° to 32.0°C or 86.9° to 89.6°F). Exposure of the drug to this temperature or above will cause the drug to liquefy and appear as an oil film on the vials. This is a sign of decomposition and vials should be discarded. If there is a question of adequate refrigeration upon receipt of this product, immediately inspect the larger vial in each individual carton. Hold the vial to a bright light for inspection. The Carmustine will appear as a very small amount of dry flakes or dry congealed mass. If this is evident, the Carmustine is suitable for use and should be refrigerated immediately.

Procedures for proper handling and disposal of anticancer drugs should be considered. Several guidelines on this subject have been published.[1-7] There is no general agreement that all of the procedures recommended in the guidelines are necessary or appropriate.

Store dry powder in refrigerator (2° to 8°C).

REFERENCES
1. Recommendations for the Safe Handling of Parenteral Antineoplastic Drugs, NIH Publication No. 83-2621. For sale by the Superintendent of Documents, US Government Printing Office, Washington, DC 20402.   2. AMA Council Report, Guidelines for Handling Parenteral Antineoplastics. *JAMA.* 1985; 253(11); 1590-1592.   3. National Study Commission on Cytotoxic Exposure—Recommendations for Handling Cytotoxic Agents. Available from Louis P. Jeffrey, ScD., Chairman, National Study Commission on Cytotoxic Exposure, Massachusetts College of Pharmacy and Allied Health Sciences, 179 Longwood Avenue, Boston, Massachusetts 02115.   4. Clinical Oncological Society of Australia. Guidelines and Recommendations for Safe Handling of Antineoplastic Agents. *Med J Australia.* 1983; 1:426-428.   5. Jones RB, et al: Safe handling of chemotherapeutic agents; a report from the Mount Sinai Medical Center, *CA—A Cancer J for Clinicians.* 1983; (Sept/Oct) 258-263.   6. American Society of Hospital Pharmacists Technical Assistance Bulletin on Handling Cytotoxic and Hazardous Drugs. *Am J Hosp Pharm.* 1990; 47:1033-1049.   7. OSHA Work-Practice Guidelines for Personnel Dealing with Cytotoxic (Antineoplastic) Drugs. *Am J Hosp Pharm.* 1986; 43:1193-1204.

HOW SUPPLIED
POWDER FOR INJECTION: 100 MG

BRAND/MANUFACTURER	NDC	SIZE	AWP
○ **BRAND**			
BICNU: Bristol-Myer Onc/Hiv	00015-3012-38	1s	$79.53

Carnitor *SEE LEVOCARNITINE*

Carteolol Hydrochloride, Ophthalmic

DESCRIPTION
Carteolol Hydrochloride ophthalmic solution 1% is a nonselective beta-adrenoceptor blocking agent for opthalmic use.

The chemical name for Carteolol Hydrochloride is (±)-5-[3-[(1,1-dimethylethyl)amino]-2-hydroxypropoxy]-3, 4-dihydro-2 (1H)-quinolinone monohydrochloride. Its molecular formula is $C_{16}H_{24}N_2O_3 \cdot HCl$ and its molecular weight is 328.84. Each mL contains 10 mg Carteolol Hydrochloride.

Following is its chemical structure:

CLINICAL PHARMACOLOGY
Carteolol HCl is a nonselective beta-adrenergic blocking agent with associated intrinsic sympathomimetic activity and without significant membrane-stabilizing activity.

Carteolol HCl reduces normal and elevated intraocular pressure (IOP) whether or not accompanied by glaucoma. The exact mechanism of the ocular hypotensive effect of beta-blockers has not been definitely demonstrated.

In general, beta-adrenergic blockers reduce cardiac output in patients in good and poor cardiovascular health. In patients with severe impairment of myocardial function, beta-blockers may inhibit the sympathetic stimulation necessary to maintain adequate cardiac function. Beta-adrenergic blockers may also increase airway resistance in the bronchi and bronchioles due to unopposed parasympathetic activity.

Given topically twice daily in controlled domestic clinical trials ranging from 1.5 to 3 months Carteolol HCl produced a median percent reduction of IOP 22% to 25%. No significant effects were noted on corneal sensitivity, tear secretion, or pupil size.

INDICATIONS AND USAGE
Carteolol HCl ophthalmic solution, 1%, has been shown to be effective in lowering intraocular pressure and may be used in patients with chronic open-angle glaucoma and intraocular hypertension. It may be used alone or in combination with other intraocular pressure lowering medications.

CONTRAINDICATIONS
Carteolol HCl ophthalmic solution is contraindicated in those individuals with bronchial asthma or with a history of bronchial asthma, or severe chronic obstructive pulmonary disease (see *"Warnings"*); sinus bradycardia; second- and third-degree atrioventricular block; overt cardiac failure (see *"Warnings"*); cardiogenic shock; or hypersensitivity to any component of this product.

WARNINGS
Carteolol HCl ophthalmic solution has not been detected in plasma following ocular instillation. However, as with other topically applied ophthalmic preparations, Carteolol HCl may be absorbed systemically. The same adverse reactions found with systemic administration of beta-adrenergic blocking agents may occur with topical administration. For example, severe respiratory reactions and cardiac reactions, including death due to broncho-spasm in patients with asthma, and rarely death in association with cardiac failure, have been reported with topical application of beta-adrenergic blocking agents (see *"Contraindications"*).

Cardiac Failure: Sympathetic stimulation may be essential for support of the circulation in individuals with diminished myocardial contractility, and its inhibition by beta-adrenergic receptor blockade may precipitate more severe failure.

In Patients Without a History of Cardiac Failure: Continued depression of the myocardium with beta-blocking agents over a period of time can, in some cases, lead to cardiac failure. At the first sign or symptom or cardiac failure, Carteolol HCL should be discontinued.

Nonallergic Bronchospasm: In patients with non-allergic bronchospasm or with a history of non-allergic bronchospasm (e.g., chronic bronchitis, emphysema). Carteolol HCl should be administered with caution since it may block bronchodilation produced by endogenous and exogenous catecholamine stimulation of $beta_2$ receptors.

Major Surgery: The necessity or desirability of withdrawal of beta-adrenergic blocking agents prior to major surgery is controversial. Beta-adrenergic receptor blockade impairs the ability of the heart to respond to beta-adrenergically mediated reflex stimuli. This may augment the risk of general anesthesia in surgical procedures. Some patients receiving beta-adrenergic receptor blocking agents have been subject to protracted severe hypotension during anesthesia. For these reasons, in patients undergoing elective surgery, gradual withdrawal of beta-adrenergic receptor blocking agents may be appropriate.

If necessary during surgery, the effects of beta-adrenergic blocking agents may be reversed by sufficient doses of such agonists as isoproterenol, dopamine, dobutamine or levarterenol (See "Overdosage").

Diabetes Mellitus: Beta-adrenergic blocking agents should be administered with caution in patients subject to spontaneous hypoglycemia or to diabetic patients (especially those with labile diabetes) who are receiving insulin or oral hypoglycemic agents. Beta-adrenergic receptor blocking agents may mask the signs and symptoms of acute hypoglycemia.

Thyrotoxicosis: Beta-adrenergic blocking agents may mask certain clinical signs (e.g., tachycardia) of hyperthyroidism. Patients suspected of developing thyrotoxicosis should be managed carefully to avoid abrupt withdrawal of beta-adrenergic blocking agents which might precipitate a thyroid storm.

PRECAUTIONS:
General: Carteolol HCl ophthalmic solution should be used with caution in patients with known hypersensitivity to other beta-adrenoceptor blocking agents.

Use with caution in patients with known diminished pulmonary function.

In patients with angle-closure glaucoma, the immediate objective of treatment is to reopen the angle. This requires constricting the pupil with a miotic. Carteolol HCl has little or no effect on the pupil. When Carteolol HCl is used to reduce elevated intraocular pressure in angle-closure glaucoma, it should be used with a miotic and not alone.

Information to the Patient: For topical use only. To prevent contaminating the dropper tip and solution, care should be taken not to touch the eyelids or surrounding areas with the dropper tip of the bottle. Keep bottle tightly closed when not in use. Protect from light.

Risk from Anaphylactic Reaction: While taking beta-blockers, patients with a history of atopy or a history of severe anaphylactic reaction to a variety of allergens may be more reactive to repeated accidental, diagnostic, or therapeutic challenge with such allergens. Such patients may be unresponsive to the usual doses of epinephrine used to treat anaphylactic reactions.

Muscle Weakness: Beta-adrenergic blockade has been reported to potentiate muscle weakness consistent with certain myasthenic symptoms (e.g., diplopia, ptosis and generalized weakness).

Drug Interactions: Carteolol HCl should be used with caution in patients who are receiving a beta-adrenergic blocking agent orally, because of the potential for additive effects on systemic beta-blockade.

Close observation of the patient is recommended when a beta-blocker is administered to patients receiving catecholamine-depleting drugs such as reserpine, because of possible additive effects and the production of hypotension and/or marked bradycardia, which may produce vertigo, syncope, or postural hypotension.

Carcinogenesis, Mutagenesis, Impairment of Fertility: Carteolol HCl did not produce carcinogenic effects at doses up to 40 mg/kg/day in two-year oral rat and mouse studies. Tests of mutagenicity, including the Ames Test, recombinant (rec)-assay, *in vivo* cytogenetics and dominant lethal assay demonstrated no evidence for mutagenic potential. Fertility of male and female rats and male and female mice was unaffected by administration of carteolol hydrochloride dosages up to 150 mg/kg/day.

Pregnancy: Teratogenic Effects: Pregnancy Category C: Carteolol HCl increased resorptions and decreased fetal weights in rabbits and rats at maternally toxic doses approximately 1052 and 5264 times the maximum recommended human oral dose (10 mg/70 kg/day), respectively. A dose-related increase in wavy ribs was noted in the developing rat fetus when pregnant females received daily doses of approximately 212 times the maximum recommended human oral dose. No such effects were noted in pregnant mice subjected to up to 1052 times the maximum recommended human oral dose. There are no adequate and well-controlled studies in pregnant women. Carteolol HCl should be used during pregnancy only if the potential benefit justifies the potential risk to the fetus.

Nursing Mothers: It is not known whether this drug is excreted in human milk, although in animal studies carteolol has been shown to be excreted in breast milk. Caution should be exercised when Carteolol HCl is administered to nursing mothers.

Pediatric Use: Safety and effectiveness in children have not been established.

ADVERSE REACTIONS:
The following adverse reactions have been reported in clinical trials with Carteolol HCl opthalmic solution.

Ocular: Transient eye irritation, burning, tearing, conjunctival hyperemia and edema occurred in about 1 of 4 patients. Ocular symptoms including blurred and cloudy vision, photophobia, decreased night vision, and ptosis and ocular signs including blepharoconjunctivitis, abnormal corneal staining, and corneal sensitivity occurred occasionally.

Systemic: As is characteristic of nonselective adrenergic blocking agents, Carteolol HCl may cause bradycardia and decreased blood pressure (see "Warnings"). The following systemic events have occasionally been reported with the use of Carteolol HCl cardiac arrhythmia, heart palpitation, dyspnea, asthenia, headache, dizziness, insomnia, sinusitis, and taste perversion.

The following additional adverse reactions have been reported with ophthalmic use of beta₁ and beta₂ (nonselective) adrenergic receptor blocking agents:

Body As a Whole: Headache.

Cardiovascular: Arrhythmia, syncope, heart block, cerebral vascular accident, cerebral ischemia, congestive heart failure, palpitation (see "Warnings").

Digestive: Nausea.

Psychiatric: Depression.

Skin: Hypersensitivity, including localized and generalized rash.

Respiratory: Bronchospasm (predominantly in patients with pre-existing bronchospastic disease), respiratory failure (see "Warnings").

Endocrine: Masked symptoms of hypoglycemia in insulin-dependent diabetics (see "Warnings").

Special Senses: Signs and symptoms of keratitis, blepharoptosis, visual disturbances including refractive changes (due to withdrawal of miotic therapy in some cases), diplopia, ptosis.

Other reactions associated with the oral use of nonselective adrenergic receptor blocking agents should be considered potential effects with ophthalmic use of these agents.

OVERDOSAGE:
No specific information on emergency treatment of overdosage in humans is available. Should accidental ocular overdosage occur, flush eye(s) with water or normal saline. The most common effects expected with overdosage of a beta-adrenergic blocking agent are bradycardia, bronchospasm, congestive heart failure and hypotension.

In case of ingestion, treatment with Carteolol HCl should be discontinued and gastric lavage considered. The patient should be closely observed and vital signs carefully monitored. The prolonged effects of Carteolol HCl must be considered when determining the duration of corrective therapy. On the basis of the pharmacologic profile, the following additional measures should be considered as appropriate:

Symptomatic Sinus Bradycardia or Heart Block: Administer atropine. If there is no response to vagal blockage, administer isoproterenol cautiously.

Bronchospasm: Administer a beta₂-stimulating agent such as isoproterenol and/or a theophylline derivative.

Congestive Heart Failure: Administer diuretics and digitalis glycosides as necessary.

Hypotension: Administer vasopressors such as intravenous dopamine, epinephrine or norepinephrine bitartrate.

DOSAGE AND ADMINISTRATION:
The usual dose is one drop of Carteolol HCl ophthalmic solution, 1%, in the affected eye(s) twice a day.

If the patient's IOP is not at a satisfactory level on this regimen, concomitant therapy with pilocarpine and other miotics, and/or epinephrine or dipivefrin, and/or systemically administered carbonic anhydrase inhibitors, such as acetazolamide, can be instituted.

Store at 15° to 25°C (59° to 77°F) (room temperature) and protect from light.

HOW SUPPLIED
DROP: 1%

BRAND/MANUFACTURER	NDC	SIZE	AWP
○ BRAND			
OCUPRESS: Otsuka	59148-0001-01	5 ml	$15.26
	59148-0001-02	10 ml	$28.78

Carteolol Hydrochloride, Oral

DESCRIPTION
Carteolol Hydrochloride is a synthetic, nonselective, beta-adrenergic receptor blocking agent with intrinsic sympathomimetic activity. It is chemically described as 5-[3-[(1,1-dimethylethyl) amino]-2-hydroxypropoxy]-3,4-dihydro-2(1H)-quinolinone monohydrochloride.

Carteolol Hydrochloride is a stable, white crystalline powder which is soluble in water and slightly soluble in ethanol. The molecular weight is 328.84 and $C_{16}H_{24}N_2O_3 \cdot HCl$ is the empirical formula.

Carteolol Hydrochloride is available as tablets containing either 2.5 mg or 5 mg of Carteolol Hydrochloride for oral administration.

Following is its chemical structure:

CLINICAL PHARMACOLOGY
Carteolol Hydrochloride is a long-acting, nonselective beta-adrenergic receptor blocking agent with intrinsic sympathomimetic activity (ISA) and without significant membrane stabilizing (local anesthetic) activity.

➤ SHOWN IN PRODUCT IDENTIFICATION GUIDE

PHARMACODYNAMICS

Carteolol specifically competes with beta-adrenergic receptor agonists for both beta$_1$-receptors located principally in cardiac muscle and beta$_2$-receptors located in the bronchial and vascular musculature, blocking the chronotropic, inotropic, and vasodilator responses to beta-adrenergic simulation proportionately. Because of its partial agonist activity, however, Carteolol does not reduce resting beta-agonist activity as much as beta-adrenergic blockers lacking this activity. Thus, in clinical trials in man, the decreases in resting pulse rate produced by Carteolol (2-5 beats per minute in various studies) were less than those produced by beta-blockers (nadolol and propranolol) without ISA (10-12 beats per minute). There are also equivocal effects on renin secretion, in contrast to beta-blockers without ISA, which inhibit renin secretion.

In controlled clinical trials Carteolol at doses up to 20 mg as monotherapy or in combination with thiazide type diuretics, produced significantly greater reductions in blood pressure than did placebo, with the full effect seen between two and four weeks. The observed differences from placebo ranged from 3.1 to 6.7 mmHg for supine diastolic blood pressure. The antihypertensive effects of Carteolol are smaller in black populations but do not seem to be affected by age or sex. Doses of Carteolol greater than 10 mg once a day did not produce greater reductions in blood pressure. In fact, doses of 20 mg and above appeared to produce blood pressure reductions less than those produced by 10 mg and below. When Carteolol was compared to nadolol and propanolol, although the differences were not statistically significant in relatively small studies Carteolol at doses up to 20 mg produced supine diastolic blood pressure changes consistently 2 mmHg less than that produced by either nadolol or propranolol.

Although the mechanism of the antihypertensive effect of beta-adrenergic blocking agents has not been established, multiple factors are thought to contribute to the lowering of blood pressure, including diminished response to sympathetic nerve outflow from vasomotor centers in the brain, diminished release of renin from the kidneys, and decreased cardiac output. Carteolol does not have a consistent effect on renin and other agents with ISA have been shown to have less effect than other beta-blockers on resting cardiac output (although they cause the usual decrease in exercise cardiac output so that the difference is of uncertain clinical importance), so that the mechanism of its action is particularly uncertain.

Beta-blockade interferes with endogenous adrenergic bronchodilator activity and diminishes the response to exogenous bronchodilators. This is especially important in patients subject to bronchospasm.

Single intravenous doses of Carteolol (0.5 mg, 1 mg, 2.5 mg and 5 mg) produced statistically, but not clinically, significant increases from baseline in AV node conduction time and RR and PR intervals.

Carteolol Hydrochloride induced no significant alteration in total serum cholesterol and triglycerides.

Following discontinuation of Carteolol treatment in man, pharmacologic activity (evaluated by blockade of the tachycardia induced by isoproterenol or postural changes) is present for 2 to 21 days (median 14 days) after the last dose of Carteolol. Following administration of recommended doses of Carteolol Hydrochloride, both beta-blocking and antihypertensive effects persist for at least 24 hours.

PHARMACOKINETICS AND METABOLISM

Following oral administration in man, peak plasma concentrations of Carteolol usually occur within one to three hours. Carteolol is well absorbed when administered orally as tablets. The presence of food in the gastrointestinal tract somewhat slows the rate of absorption, but the extent of absorption is not appreciably affected. Compared to intravenous administration, the absolute bioavailability of Carteolol tablets is approximately 85%.

The plasma half-life of Carteolol averages approximately six hours. Steady-state serum levels are achieved within one to two days after initiating therapeutic doses of Carteolol in persons with normal renal function. Since approximately 50% to 70% of a Carteolol dose is eliminated unchanged by the kidneys, the half-life is increased in patients with impaired renal function. Significant reductions in the rate of Carteolol elimination (and prolongations of the half-life) occur in patients as creatinine clearance decreases. Therefore, a reduction in maintenance dose and/or prolongation in dosing interval is appropriate (see "Dosage and Administration").

Carteolol is 23-30% bound to plasma proteins in humans. The major metabolites of Carteolol are 8-hydroxycarteolol and the glucuronic acid conjugates of both Carteolol and 8-hydroxycarteolol. In man, 8-hydroxycarteolol is an active metabolite with a half-life of approximately 8 to 12 hours and represents approximately 5% of the administered dose excreted in the urine.

INDICATIONS AND USAGE

Carteolol Hydrochloride is indicated in the management of hypertension. It may be used alone or in combination with other antihypertensive agents, especially thiazide diuretics. Preliminary data indicate that Carteolol does not have a favorable effect on arrhythmias.

UNLABELED USES

Carteolol Hydrochloride is used alone or as an adjunct in the treatment of angina pectoris.

CONTRAINDICATIONS

Carteolol Hydrochloride is contraindicated in patients with: 1) bronchial asthma, 2) severe bradycardia, 3) greater than first degree heart block, 4) cardiogenic shock, and 5) clinically evident congestive heart failure (see "Warnings").

WARNINGS

CONGESTIVE HEART FAILURE

Sympathetic stimulation may be a vital component supporting circulatory function in patients with congestive heart failure, and impairing that support by beta-blockade may precipitate more severe decompensation. Although Carteolol Hydrochloride should be avoided in clinically evident congestive heart failure, it can be used with caution, if necessary, in patients with a history of failure who are well-compensated and are receiving digitalis and diuretics. Beta-adrenergic blocking agents do not abolish the inotropic action of digitalis on heart muscle.

In patients without a history of congestive heart failure, the use of beta-blockers can, in some instances, lead to congestive heart failure. Therefore, at the first sign or symptom of cardiac decompensation, discontinuation of beta-blocker therapy should be considered. The patient should be closely observed and treatment should include a diuretic and/or digitalization as necessary.

EXACERBATION OF ANGINA PECTORIS UPON WITHDRAWAL

In patients with angina pectoris, exacerbation of angina and, in some cases, myocardial infarction, have been reported following abrupt discontinuation of therapy with some beta-blockers. Therefore, such patients should be cautioned against interruption of therapy without a physician's advice. The long persistence of beta-adrenergic blockade following abrupt discontinuation of Carteolol Hydrochloride, however, might be expected to minimize the possibility of this complication. When discontinuation of Carteolol Hydrochloride is planned, dosage should be tapered gradually, as it is with other beta-blockers. If exacerbation of angina occurs when Carteolol Hydrochloride therapy is interrupted, it is advisable to reinstitute Carteolol Hydrochloride or other beta-blocker therapy, at least temporarily, and to take other measures appropriate for the management of unstable angina pectoris.

Patients without clinically recognized angina pectoris should be carefully monitored after withdrawal of Carteolol Hydrochloride therapy, since coronary artery disease may be unrecognized.

NONALLERGIC BRONCHOSPASM (E.G., CHRONIC BRONCHITIS EMPHYSEMA)

Patients with bronchospastic disease generally should not receive beta-blocker therapy and Carteolol is contraindicated in patients with bronchial asthma. If use of Carteolol Hydrochloride is essential, it should be administered with caution since it may block bronchodilation produced by endogenous catecholamine stimulation of beta$_2$-receptors or diminish response to therapy with a beta-receptor agonist.

MAJOR SURGERY

The necessity, or desirability, of withdrawal of beta-blocking therapy prior to major surgery is controversial. Because beta-blockade impairs the ability of the heart to respond to reflex stimuli and may increase risks of general anesthesia and surgical procedures resulting in protracted hypotension or low cardiac output, and difficulty in restarting or maintaining a heartbeat, it has been suggested that beta-blocker therapy should be withdrawn several days prior to surgery. It is also recognized, however, that increased sensitivity to catecholamines of patients recently withdrawn from beta-blocker therapy could increase certain risks. Given the persistence of the beta-blocking activity of Carteolol Hydrochloride, effective withdrawal would take several weeks and would ordinarily be impractical. When beta-blocker therapy is not discontinued, anesthetic agents that depress the myocardium should be avoided. In one study using intravenous Carteolol during surgery, recovery from anesthesia was somewhat delayed in three patients who received Carteolol near the end of anesthesia, and respiratory arrest occurred in one of these patients immediately following administration of intravenous Carteolol.

In the event that Carteolol Hydrochloride treatment is not discontinued before surgery, the anesthesiologist should be informed that the patient is receiving Carteolol Hydrochloride. The effects on the heart of beta-adrenergic blocking agents, such as Carteolol Hydrochloride may be reversed by cautious administration of isoproterenol or dobutamine.

DIABETES MELLITUS AND HYPOGLYCEMIA

Beta-adrenergic blockade may prevent the appearance of premonitory signs and symptoms (e.g., tachycardia and blood pressure changes) of acute hypoglycemia, and it inhibits glycogenolysis, a normal compensatory mechanism for hypoglycemia. This is especially important for patients with labile diabetes mellitus. Beta-blockade also reduces the release of insulin in response to hyperglycemia; therefore, it may be necessary to adjust the dose of antidiabetic agents used to treat hyperglycemia.

THYROTOXICOSIS

Beta-adrenergic blockade may mask certain clinical signs of hyperthyroidism such as tachycardia. Patients suspected of having thyrotoxicosis should be managed carefully to avoid abrupt withdrawal of beta-adrenergic blockade which might precipitate a thyroid storm.

PRECAUTIONS

GENERAL

Impaired Renal Function: Carteolol Hydrochloride should be used with caution in patients with impaired renal function. Patients with impaired renal function clear Carteolol at a reduced rate, and dosage should be reduced accordingly (see "Dosage and Administration").

Beta-adrenoreceptor blockade can cause reduction in intraocular pressure. Therefore, Carteolol Hydrochloride may interfere with glaucoma testing. Withdrawal may lead to a return of increased intraocular pressure.

INFORMATION FOR PATIENTS

Patients, especially those with evidence of coronary artery insufficiency, should be warned against interruption or discontinuation of Carteolol Hydrochloride therapy without the physician's advice. Although cardiac failure rarely occurs in properly selected patients, patients being treated with beta-adrenergic blocking agents should be advised to consult the physician at the first sign or symptom of impending failure (i.e., fatigue with exertion, difficulty breathing, cough or unusually fast heartbeat).

DRUG INTERACTIONS

Catecholamine-depleting drugs (e.g., reserpine) may have an additive effect when given with beta-blocking agents. Therefore, patients treated with Carteolol Hydrochloride plus a catecholamine-depleting agent must be observed carefully for evidence of hypotension and/or excessive bradycardia, which may produce syncope or postural hypotension.

Risk of Anaphylactic Reaction: While taking beta-blockers, patients with a history of severe anaphylactic reaction to a variety of allergens may be more reactive to repeated challenge, either accidental, diagnostic, or therapeutic. Such patients may be unresponsive to the usual doses of epinephrine used to treat allergic reaction.

Concurrent administration of *general anesthetics* and beta-blocking agents may result in exaggeration of the hypotension induced by general anesthetics (see *"Warnings, Major Surgery").*

Blunting of the antihypertensive effect of beta-adrenoreceptor blocking agents by *non-steroidal anti-inflammatory drugs* has been reported. When using these agents concomitantly, patients should be observed carefully to confirm that the desired therapeutic effect has been obtained.

Literature reports suggest that *oral calcium antagonists* may be used in combination with beta-adrenergic blocking agents when heart function is normal, but should be avoided in patients with impaired cardiac function. Hypotension, AV conduction disturbances, and left ventricular failure have been reported in some patients receiving beta-adrenergic blocking agents when an oral calcium antagonist was added to the treatment regimen. Hypotension was more likely to occur if the calcium antagonist were a dihydropyridine derivative, e.g., nifedipine, while left ventricular failure and AV conduction disturbances were more likely to occur with either verapamil or diltiazem.

Intravenous calcium antagonists should be used with caution in patients receiving beta-adrenergic blocking agents. The concomitant use of beta-adrenergic blocking agents with digitalis and either diltiazem or verapamil may have additive effects in prolonging AV conduction time.

Concomitant use of *oral antidiabetic agents* or *insulin* with beta-blocking agents may be associated with hypoglycemia or possibly hyperglycemia. Dosage of the antidiabetic agent should be adjusted accordingly (see *"Warnings, Diabetes Mellitus and Hypoglycemia").*

CARCINOGENESIS, MUTAGENESIS, IMPAIRMENT OF FERTILITY

Carteolol Hydrochloride did not produce carcinogenic effects at doses 280 times the maximum recommended human dose (10 mg/70 kg/day) in two-year oral rat and mouse studies.

Tests of mutagenicity, including the Ames Test, recombinant (rec)-assay, *in vivo* cytogenetics and dominant lethal assay demonstrated no evidence for mutagenic potential. Fertility of male and female rats and male and female mice was unaffected by administration of Carteolol Hydrochloride dosages up to 150 mg/kg/day. This dosage is approximately 1052 times the maximum recommended human dose.

PREGNANCY

Teratogenic Effects: Pregnancy Category C: Carteolol Hydrochloride increased resorptions and decreased fetal weights in rabbits and rats at maternally toxic doses approximately 1052 and 5264 times the maximum recommended human dose (10 mg/70 kg/day), respectively. A dose-related increase in wavy ribs was noted in the developing rat fetus when pregnant females received daily doses of approximately 212 times the maximum recommended human dose. No such effects were noted in pregnant mice subjected to up to 1052 times the maximum recommended human dose. There are no adequate and well-controlled studies in pregnant women. Carteolol Hydrochloride should be used during pregnancy only if the potential benefit justifies the potential risk to the fetus.

NURSING MOTHERS

Studies have not been conducted in lactating humans and, therefore, it is not known whether Carteolol is excreted in human milk. Studies in lactating rats indicate that Carteolol Hydrochloride is excreted in milk. Because many drugs are excreted in human milk, caution should be exercised when Carteolol Hydrochloride is administered to a nursing woman.

PEDIATRIC USE

Safety and effectiveness in children have not been established.

ADVERSE REACTIONS

The prevalence of adverse reactions has been ascertained from clinical studies conducted primarily in the United States. All adverse experiences (events) reported during these studies were recorded as adverse reactions. The prevalence rates presented below are based on combined data from nineteen-placebo-controlled studies of patients with hypertension, angina or dysrhythmias, using once-daily Carteolol at doses up to 60 mg. Table 1 summarizes those adverse experiences reported for patients in these studies where the prevalence in the Carteolol group is 1% or greater and exceeds the prevalence in the placebo group. Asthenia and muscle cramps were the only symptoms that were significantly more common in patients receiving Carteolol than in patients receiving placebo. Patients in clinical trials were carefully selected to exclude those, such as patients with asthma or known bronchospasm, or congestive heart failure, who would be at high risk of experiencing beta-adrenergic blocker adverse effect (see *"Warnings"* and *"Contraindications"*):

Table 1
ADVERSE REACTIONS DURING PLACEBO-CONTROLLED STUDIES

	Placebo (n = 448) %	Carteolol (n = 761) %
Body as a Whole		
†Asthenia	4.0	7.1*
Abdominal Pain	0.4	1.3
Back Pain	1.6	2.1
Chest Pain	1.8	2.2
Digestive System		
Diarrhea	2.0	2.1
Nausea	1.8	2.1
Metabolic/Nutritional Disorders		
Abnormal Lab Test	1.1	1.2
Peripheral Edema	1.1	1.7
Musculoskeletal System		
Arthralgia	1.1	1.2
Muscle Cramps	0.2	2.6*
Lower Extremity Pain	0.2	1.2
Nervous System		
Insomnia	0.7	1.7
Paresthesia	1.1	2.0
Respiratory System		
Nasal Congestion	0.9	1.1
Pharyngitis	0.9	1.1
Skin and Appendages		
Rash	1.1	1.3

† Includes weakness, tiredness, lassitude and fatigue.
* Statistically significant at p=0.05 level.

The adverse experiences were usually mild or moderate in intensity and transient, but sometimes were serious enough to interrupt treatment. The adverse reactions that were most bothersome, as judged by their being reported as reasons for discontinuation of therapy by at least 0.4% of the Carteolol group are shown in Table 2.

Table 2
DISCONTINUATIONS DURING PLACEBO-CONTROLLED STUDIES

	Placebo (n = 448) %	Carteolol (n = 761) %
Body as a Whole		
Asthenia	0.2	0.5
Headache	0.7	0.7
Chest Pain	0.2	0.4
Skin and Appendages		
Rash	0.0	0.4
Sweating	0.2	0.4
Digestive System		
Nausea	0.0	0.4
Overall Adverse Reactions	4.2	3.3

Additional adverse reactions have been reported, but these are, in general, not distinguishable from symptoms that might have occurred in the absence of exposure to Carteolol. The following additional adverse reactions were reported by at least 1% of 1568 patients who received Carteolol in controlled or open, short- or long-term clinical studies, or represent less common, but potentially important, reactions reported in clinical studies or marketing experience (these rarer reactions are shown in italics):

Body as a Whole: fever, infection, injury, malaise, pain, neck pain, shoulder pain

Cardiovascular System: angina pectoris, arrhythmia, *heart failure,* palpitations, *second degree heart block,* vasodilation

Digestive System: acute hepatitis with jaundice, constipation, dyspepsia, flatulence, gastrointestinal disorder

Metabolic/Nutritional Disorder: gout

Musculoskeletal System: pain in extremity, joint disorder, arthritis

Nervous System: abnormal dreams, anxiety, depression, dizziness, nervousness, somnolence

Respiratory System: bronchitis, *bronchospasm,* cold symptoms, cough, dyspnea, flu symptoms, lung disorder, rhinitis, sinusitis, *wheezing*

Skin and Appendages: sweating

Special Senses: blurred vision, conjunctivitis, eye disorder, tinnitus

Urogenital: impotence, urinary frequency, urinary tract infection

In studies of patients with hypertension or angina pectoris where Carteolol and positive reference beta-adrenergic blocking agents [nadolol (n=82) and propranolol (n=50)] have been compared, the differences in prevalence rates between the Carteolol group and the reference agent group were statistically significant (p ≤ 0.05) for the adverse reactions listed in Table 3.

Table 3

ADVERSE REACTIONS DURING POSITIVE-CONTROLLED STUDIES

	Reference Agents (n = 132)	Carteolol (n = 135)
Body as a Whole		
Chest Pain	5.3	0.7
Cardiovascular System		
Bradycardia	4.5	0.0
Digestive System		
Diarrhea	11.4	4.4
Nervous System		
Somnolence	0.8	7.4
Skin and Appendages		
Sweating	5.3	0.7

POTENTIAL ADVERSE REACTIONS

In addition, other adverse reactions not listed above have been reported with other beta-adrenergic blocking agents and should be considered potential adverse reactions of Carteolol Hydrochloride.

Body as a Whole: Fever combined with aching and sore throat.

Cardiovascular System: Intensification of AV block. (See "Contraindications.")

Digestive System: Mesenteric arterial thrombosis, ischemic colitis.

Hemic/Lymphatic System: Agranulocytosis, thrombocytopenic and non-thrombocytopenic purpura.

Nervous System: Reversible mental depression progressing to catatonia; an acute reversible syndrome characterized by disorientation to time and place, short-term memory loss, emotional lability, slightly clouded sensorium, and decreased performance on neuropsychometric testing.

Respiratory System: Laryngospasm, respiratory distress.

Skin and Appendages: Erythematous rash, reversible alopecia.

Urogenital System: Peyronie's disease.

The oculomucocutaneous syndrome associated with the beta-adrenergic blocking agent practolol has not been reported with Carteolol.

OVERDOSAGE

No specific information on emergency treatment of overdosage in humans is available. The most common effects expected with overdosage of a beta-adrenergic blocking agent are bradycardia, bronchospasm, congestive heart failure and hypotension.

In case of overdosage, treatment with Carteolol Hydrochloride should be discontinued and gastric lavage considered. The patient should be closely observed and vital signs carefully monitored. The prolonged effects of Carteolol must be considered when determining the duration of corrective therapy. On the basis of the pharmacologic profile, the following additional measures should be considered as appropriate.

Symptomatic Bradycardia: Administer atropine. If there is no response to vagal blockade, administer isoproterenol cautiously.

Bronchospasm: Administer a beta$_2$-stimulating agent such as isoproterenol and/or a theophylline derivative.

Congestive Heart Failure: Administer diuretics and digitalis glycosides as necessary.

Hypotension: Administer vasopressors such as intravenous dopamine, epinephrine or norepinephrine bitartrate.

DOSAGE AND ADMINISTRATION

Dosage must be individualized. The initial dose of Carteolol Hydrochloride is 2.5 mg given as a single daily oral dose either alone or added to diuretic therapy. If an adequate response is not achieved, the dose can be gradually increased to 5 mg and 10 mg as single daily doses. Increasing the dose above 10 mg per day is unlikely to produce further substantial benefits and, in fact, may decrease the response. The usual maintenance dose of Carteolol is 2.5 or 5 mg once daily.

DOSAGE ADJUSTMENT IN RENAL IMPAIRMENT

Carteolol is excreted principally by the kidneys. When administering Carteolol Hydrochloride to patients with renal impairment, the dosage regimen should be adjusted individually by the physician. Guidelines for dose interval adjustment are shown below:

Creatinine Clearance (mL/min)	Dosage Interval (hours)
>60	24
20-60	48
<20	72

RECOMMENDED STORAGE
Store under controlled room temperature, 59°-86°F (15°-30°C).

HOW SUPPLIED
TABLETS: 2.5 MG

BRAND/MANUFACTURER	NDC	SIZE	AWP
○ **BRAND**			
CARTROL: Abbott Pharm	00074-1664-13	100s	$95.03

TABLETS: 5 MG

BRAND/MANUFACTURER	NDC	SIZE	AWP
○ **BRAND**			
CARTROL: Abbott Pharm	00074-1665-13	100s	$95.03

Cartrol *SEE* CARTEOLOL HYDROCHLORIDE, ORAL

Castor Oil/Peru Balsam/Trypsin

DESCRIPTION
Each 0.82 cc of medication delivered to the wound site contains Trypsin crystallized 0.1 mg, Balsam Peru 72.5 mg, Castor Oil 650.0 mg.

ACTION
Trypsin is intended for debridement of eschar and other necrotic tissue. It appears that in many instances removal of wound debris strengthens humoral defense mechanisms sufficiently to retard proliferation of local pathogens. Balsam Peru is an effective capillary bed stimulant used to increase circulation in the wound site area. Also, Balsam Peru has a mildly bactericidal action. Castor Oil is used to improve epithelialization by reducing premature epithelial desiccation and cornification. Also, it can act as a protective covering and aids in the reduction of pain.

INDICATIONS
For the treatment of decubitus ulcers, varicose ulcers, debridement of eschar, dehiscent wounds and sunburn.

USES
Castor Oil/Peru Balsam/Trypsin is in aerosol form which can be important to healing. It must be remembered, healing starts with a thin sheath of epithelium no more than a cell or two thick. Any rough movement or trauma can quickly destroy the healing tissue. Aerosols have the advantage of eliminating all extraneous physical contact with the wound. Castor Oil/Peru Balsam/Trypsin is easy to apply and quickly reduces odor frequently accompanying a decubitus ulcer. The wound may be left open or a wet bandage may be applied. As a suggestion: keep in mind wounds heal poorly in the presence of hemoglobin or zinc deficiency.

WARNING
Do not spray on fresh arterial clots. Avoid spraying in eyes. Flammable, do not expose to fire or open flame. Contents under pressure. Do not puncture or incinerate. Do not store at temperature above 120°F. Keep out of reach of children. Use only as directed. Intentional misuse by deliberately concentrating and inhaling the contents can be harmful or fatal.

DOSAGE
Apply a minimum of twice daily or as often as necessary. Shake well, press the aerosol valve and coat the wound rapidly but not excessively.

HOW SUPPLIED
AEROSOL LIQUID:

BRAND/MANUFACTURER	NDC	SIZE	AWP
○ **BRAND**			
GRANULEX: Dow Hickam	00514-0001-01	60 ml	$12.75
BALSA-DERM: Major	00904-3678-22	120 ml	$13.45
GRANUMED: Rugby	00536-1371-97	120 ml	$15.27
GRANULEX: Dow Hickam	00514-0001-02	120 ml	$16.95
○ **GENERICS**			
GRANULDERM: Copley	38245-0607-14	120 ml	$14.00
GRANULDERM: Goldline	00182-6056-37	120 ml	$14.00
GRANULDERM: Goldline	00182-6119-37	120 ml	$14.00
GRANUL-DERM: Qualitest	00603-1270-54	120 ml	$14.05
TOPI-CAID: Topi-Cana	59197-0001-01	120 ml	$16.65
DERMUSPRAY: Warner Chilcott	00047-3998-17	120 ml	$16.95

Cataflam *SEE* DICLOFENAC, ORAL

Catapres *SEE* CLONIDINE

◆ RATED THERAPEUTICALLY EQUIVALENT; ◇ THERAPEUTIC EQUIVALENCE UNCONFIRMED; ○ UNRATED

Catarase SEE CHYMOTRYPSIN

Ceclor SEE CEFACLOR

CeeNu SEE LOMUSTINE

Cefaclor

DESCRIPTION
Cefaclor is a semisynthetic cephalosporin antibiotic for oral administration. It is chemically designated as 3-chloro-7-D-(2-phenylglycinamido)-3-cephem-4-carboxylic acid monohydrate. The chemical formula for Cefaclor is $C_{15}H_{14}ClN_3O_4S \cdot H_2O$ and the molecular weight is 385.82.

Each capsule contains Cefaclor monohydrate equivalent to 250 mg (0.68 mmol) or 500 mg (1.36 mmol) anhydrous Cefaclor.

After mixing, each 5 mL of Cefaclor for Oral Suspension will contain Cefaclor monohydrate equivalent to 125 mg (0.34 mmol), 187 mg (0.51 mmol), 250 mg (0.68 mmol), or 375 mg (1.0 mmol) anhydrous Cefaclor.

Following is its chemical structure:

CLINICAL PHARMACOLOGY
Cefaclor is well absorbed after oral administration to fasting subjects. Total absorption is the same whether the drug is given with or without food: however, when it is taken with food, the peak concentration achieved is 50% to 75% of that observed when the drug is administered to fasting subjects and generally appears from three fourths to 1 hour later. Following administration of 250-mg, 500-mg, and 1-g doses to fasting subjects, average peak serum levels of approximately 7, 13, and 23 µg/mL respectively were obtained within 30 to 60 minutes. Approximately 60% to 85% of the drug is excreted unchanged in the urine within 8 hours, the greater portion being excreted within the first 2 hours. During this 8-hour period, peak urine concentrations following the 250-mg, 500-mg, and 1-g doses were approximately 600, 900, and 1,900 µg/mL respectively. The serum half-life in normal subjects is 0.6 to 0.9 hour. In patients with reduced renal function, the serum half-life of Cefaclor is slightly prolonged. In those with complete absence of renal function, the plasma half-life of the intact molecule is 2.3 to 2.8 hours. Excretion pathways in patients with markedly impaired renal function have not been determined. Hemodialysis shortens the half-life by 25% to 30%.

Microbiology: In vitro tests demonstrate that the bactericidal action of the cephalosporins results from inhibition of cell-wall synthesis. Cefaclor is active in vitro against most strains of clinical isolates of the following organisms:

Staphylococci, including coagulase-positive, coagulase-negative, and penicillinase-producing strains (when tested by in vitro methods), exhibit cross-resistance between Cefaclor and methicillin
Streptococcus pyogenes (group A β-hemolytic streptococci)
Streptococcus pneumoniae
Moraxella (Branhamella) catarrhalis
Haemophilus influenzae, including β-lactamase-producing ampicillin-resistant strains
Escherichia coli
Proteus mirabilis
Klebsiella sp
Citrobacter diversus
Neisseria gonorrhoeae
Propionibacterium acnes and *Bacteroides* sp (excluding *Bacteroides fragilis*)
Peptococci
Peptostreptococci

Note: Pseudomonas sp, *Acinetobacter calcoaceticus* (formerly *Mima* sp and *Herellea* sp), and most strains of enterococci (*Enterococcus faecalis* [formerly *Streptococcus faecalis*], group D streptococci), *Enterobacter* sp, indole-positive *Proteus*, and *Serratia* sp are resistant to Cefaclor. When tested by in vitro methods, staphylococci exhibit cross-resistance between Cefaclor and methicillin-type antibiotics.

Disk Susceptibility Tests: Quantitative methods that require measurement of zone diameters give the most precise estimates of antibiotic susceptibility. One such procedure[1] has been recommended for use with disks for testing susceptibility to cephalothin. The currently accepted zone diameter interpretative criteria for the cephalothin disk are appropriate for determining bacterial susceptibility to Cefaclor. With this procedure, a report from the laboratory of "resistant" indicates that the infecting organism is not likely to respond to therapy. A report of "intermediate susceptibility" suggests that the organism would be susceptible if the infection is confined to tissues and fluids (eg, urine) in which high antibiotic levels can be obtained or if high dosage is used.

INDICATIONS AND USAGE
Cefaclor is indicated in the treatment of the following infections when caused by susceptible strains of the designated microorganisms:

Otitis media caused by *S. pneumoniae, H. influenzae*, staphylococci, and *S. pyogenes* (group A β-hemolytic streptococci)

Lower respiratory infections, including pneumonia, caused by *S. pneumoniae, H. influenzae*, and *S. pyogenes* (group A β-hemolytic streptococci)

Upper respiratory infections, including pharyngitis and tonsillitis, caused by *S. pyogenes* (group A β-hemolytic streptococci)

Note: Penicillin is the usual drug of choice in the treatment and prevention of streptococcal infections, including the prophylaxis of rheumatic fever. Cefaclor is generally effective in the eradication of streptococci from the nasopharynx: however, substantial data establishing the efficacy of Cefaclor in the subsequent prevention of rheumatic fever are not available at present.

Urinary tract infections, including pyelonephritis and cystitis, caused by *E. coli, P. mirabilis, Klebsiella* sp, and coagulase-negative staphylococci

Skin and skin structure infections caused by *Staphylococcus aureus* and *S. pyogenes* (group A β-hemolytic streptococci)

Appropriate culture and susceptibility studies should be performed to determine susceptibility of the causative organism to Cefaclor.

UNLABELED USES
Cefaclor is used alone or as an adjunct in the treatment of gonorrhea and respiratory tract infections, including acute bronchitis and acute exacerbation of chronic bronchitis.

CONTRAINDICATION
Cefaclor is contraindicated in patients with known allergy to the cephalosporin group of antibiotics.

WARNINGS
IN PENICILLIN-SENSITIVE PATIENTS, CEPHALOSPORIN ANTIBIOTICS SHOULD BE ADMINISTERED CAUTIOUSLY. THERE IS CLINICAL AND LABORATORY EVIDENCE OF PARTIAL CROSS-ALLERGENICITY OF THE PENICILLINS AND THE CEPHALOSPORINS, AND THERE ARE INSTANCES IN WHICH PATIENTS HAVE HAD REACTIONS, INCLUDING ANAPHYLAXIS, TO BOTH DRUG CLASSSES.

Antibiotics, including Cefaclor should be administered cautiously to any patient who has demonstrated some form of allergy, particularly to drugs.

Pseudomembranous colitis has been reported with virtually all broad-spectrum antibiotics (including macrolides, semisynthetic penicillins, and cephalosporins); therefore, it is important to consider its diagnosis in patients who develop diarrhea in association with the use of antibiotics. Such colitis may range in severity from mild to life threatening.

Treatment with broad-spectrum antibiotics alters the normal flora of the colon and may permit overgrowth of clostrida. Studies indicate that a toxin produced by *Clostridium difficile* is a primary cause of antibiotic-associated colitis.

Mild cases of pseudomembranous colitis usually respond to drug discontinuance alone. In moderate to severe cases, management should include sigmoidoscopy, appropriate bacteriologic studies, and fluid, electrolyte, and protein supplementation. When the colitis does not improve after the drugs has been discontinued, or when it is severe, oral vancomycin is the drug of choice of antibiotic-associated pseudomembranous colitis produced by *C. difficile*. Other causes of colitis should be ruled out.

PRECAUTIONS
General: If an allergic reaction to Cefaclor occurs, the drug should be discontinued, and, if necessary, the patient should be treated with appropriate agents, e.g., pressor amines, antihistamines, or corticosteroids.

Prolonged use of Cefaclor may result in the overgrowth of nonsusceptible organisms. Careful observation of the patient is essential. If superinfection occurs during therapy, appropriate measures should be taken.

Positive direct Coombs' tests have been reported during treatment with the cephalosporin antibiotics. In hematologic studies or in transfusion cross-matching procedures when antiglobulin tests are performed on the minor side or in Coombs' testing of newborns whose mothers have received cephalosporin antibiotics before parturition, it should be recognized that a positive Coombs' test may be due to the drug.

Cefaclor should be administered with caution in the presence of markedly impaired renal function. Since the half-life of Cefaclor in anuria is 2.3 to 2.8 hours, dosage adjustments for patients with moderate or severe renal impairment are usually not required. Clinical experience with Cefaclor under such conditions is limited; therefore, careful clinical observation and laboratory studies should be made.

As with other β-lactam antibiotics, the renal antibiotics, the renal excretion of Cefaclor is inhibited by probenecid.

As a result of administration of Cefaclor a false-positive reaction for glucose in the urine may occur. This has been observed with Benedict's and Fehling's solutions and also with Clinitest® tablets but not with Tes-Tape® (Glucose Enzymatic Test Strip, USP).

► SHOWN IN PRODUCT IDENTIFICATION GUIDE

Broad-spectrum antibiotics should be prescribed with caution in individuals with a history of gastrointestinal disease, particularly colitis.

Pregnancy—Pregnancy Category B: Reproduction studies have been performed in mice and rats at doses up to 12 times the human dose and in ferrets given 3 times the maximum human dose and have revealed no evidence of impaired fertility or harm to the fetus due to Cefaclor. There are, however, no adequate and well-controlled studies in pregnant women. Because animal reproduction studies are not always predictive of human response, this drug should be used during pregnancy only if clearly needed.

Nursing Mothers: Small amounts of Cefaclor have been detected in mother's milk following administration of single 500-mg doses. Average levels were 0.18, 0.20, 0.21, and 0.16 µg/mL at 2, 3, 4, and 5 hours respectively. Trace amounts were detected at 1 hour. The effect on nursing infants is not known. Caution should be exercised when Cefaclor is administered to a nursing woman.

Pediatric Use: Safety and effectiveness of this product for use in infants less than 1 month of age have not been established.

ADVERSE REACTIONS

Adverse effects considered related to therapy with Cefaclor are listed below:

Hypersensitivity reactions have been reported in about 1.5% of patients and include morbilliform eruptions (1 in 100). Pruritus, urticaria, and positive Coombs' tests each occur in less than 1 in 200 patients.

Cases of *serum-sickness-like* reactions have been reported with the use of Cefaclor. These are characterized by findings of erythema multiforme, rashes, and other skin manifestations accompanied by arthritis/arthralgia, with or without fever, and differ from classic serum sickness in that there is infrequently associated lymphaedenopathy and proteinuria, no circulating immune complexes, and no evidence to date of sequelae of the reaction. While further investigation is ongoing, *serum-sickness-like* reactions appear to be due to hypersensitivity and more often occur during or following a second (or subsequent) course of therapy with Cefaclor. Such reactions have been reported more frequently in children than in adults with an overall occurrence ranging from 1 in 200 (0.5% in one focused trial to 2 in 8,346 (0.024%) in overall clinical trials (with an incidence in children in clinical trials of 0.055%) to 1 in 38,000 (0.003%) in spontaneous event reports. Signs and symptoms usually occur a few days after initiation of therapy and subside within a few days after cessation of therapy; occasionally these reactions have resulted in hospitalization, usually of short duration (median hospitalization = two to three days, based on postmarketing surveillance studies). In those requiring hospitalization, the symptoms have ranged from mild to severe at the time of admission with more of the severe reactions occurring in children. Antihistamines and glucocorticoids appear to enhance resolution of the signs and symptoms. No serious sequelae have been reported.

More severe hypersensitivity reactions, including Stevens-Johnson syndrome, toxic epidermal necrolysis, and anaphylaxis, have been reported rarely. Anaphylaxis may be more common in patients with a history of penicillin allergy.

Gastrointestinal symptoms occur in about 2.5% of patients and include diarrhea (1 in 70).

Symptoms of pseudomembranous colitis may appear either during or after antibiotic treatment. Nausea and vomiting have been reported rarely. As with some penicillins and some other cephalosporins, transient hepatitis and cholestatic jaundice have been reported rarely.

Other effects considered related to therapy included eosinophilia (1 in 50 patients), genital pruritus or vaginitis (less than 1 in 100 patients), and, rarely, thrombocytopenia or reversible interstitial nephritis.

Causal Relationship Uncertain: CNS—Rarely, reversible hyperactivity, nervousness, insomnia, confusion, hypertonia, dizziness, and somnolence have been reported.

Transitory abnormalities in clinical laboratory test results have been reported. Although they were of uncertain etiology, they are listed below to serve as alerting information for the physician.

Hepatic: Slight elevations of AST (SGOT), ALT (SGPT), or alkaline phosphatase values (1 in 40).

Hematopoietic: As has also been reported with other β-lactam antibiotics, transient lymphocytosis leukopenia, and, rarely, hemolytic anemia and reversible neutropenia of possible clinical significance.

There have been rare reports of increased prothrombin time with or without clinical bleeding in patients receiving Cefaclor and warfarin concomitantly.

Renal: Slight elevations in BUN or serum creatinine (less than 1 in 500) or abnormal urinalysis (less than 1 in 200).

OVERDOSAGE

Signs and Symptoms: The toxic symptoms following an overdose of Cefaclor may include nausea, vomiting, epigastric distress, and diarrhea. The severity of the epigastric distress and the diarrhea are dose related. If other symptoms are present, it is probable that they are secondary to an underlying disease state, an allergic reaction, or the effects of other intoxication.

Treatment: To obtain up-to-date information about the treatment of overdose, a good resource is your certified Regional Poison Control Center. Telephone numbers of certified poison control centers are listed in the *Physicians' Desk Reference (PDR)*. In managing overdosage, consider the possibility of multiple drug overdoses, interaction among drugs, and unusual drug kinetics in your patient.

Unless 5 times the normal dose of Cefaclor has been ingested, gastrointestinal decontamination will not be necessary.

Protect the patient's airway and support ventilation and perfusion. Meticulously monitor and maintain, within acceptable limits, the patient's vital signs, blood gases, serum electrolytes, etc. Absorption of drugs from the gastrointestinal tract may be decreased by giving activated charcoal, which, in many cases, is more effective than emesis or lavage; consider charcoal instead of, or in addition to, gastric emptying. Repeated doses of charcoal over time may hasten elimination of some drugs that have been absorbed. Safeguard the patient's airway when employing gastric emptying or charcoal.

Forced diuresis, peritoneal dialysis, hemodialysis, or charcoal hemoperfusion have not been established as beneficial for an overdose of Cefaclor.

DOSAGE AND ADMINISTRATION

Cefaclor is administered orally.

Adults: The usual adult dosage is 250 mg every 8 hours. For more severe infections (such as pneumonia) or those caused by less susceptible organisms, doses may be doubled.

Children: The usual recommended daily dosage for children is 20 mg/kg/day in divided doses every 8 hours.

In more serious infections, otitis media, and infections caused by less susceptible organisms, 40 mg/kg/day are recommended, with a maximum dosage of 1 g/day.

CEFACLOR SUSPENSION

Child's Weight	20 mg/kg/day	
	125 mg/5 mL	250 mg/5 mL
9 kg	1/2 tsp t.i.d.	
18 kg	1 tsp t.i.d.	½ tsp t.i.d.
	40 mg/kg/day	
9 kg	1 tsp t.i.d.	½ tsp t.i.d.
18 kg		1 tsp t.i.d.

B.I.D. Treatment Option: For the treatment of otitis media and pharyngitis, the total daily dosage may be divided and administered every 12 hours.

CEFACLOR SUSPENSION

Child's Weight	20 mg/kg/day (Pharyngitis)	
	187 mg/5 mL	375 mg/5 mL
9 kg	½ tsp b.i.d.	
18 kg	1 tsp b.i.d.	½ tsp b.i.d.
	40 mg/kg/day (Otitis Media)	
9 kg	1 tsp b.i.d.	½ tsp b.i.d.
18 kg		1 tsp b.i.d.

Cefaclor may be administered in the presence of impaired renal function. Under such a condition, the dosage usually is unchanged (see *"Precautions"*).

In the treatment of β-hemolytic streptococcal infections, a therapeutic dosage of Cefaclor should be administered for at least 10 days.

Suspension: After mixing, store in a refrigerator. Shake well before using. Keep tightly closed. The mixture may be kept for 14 days without significant loss of potency. Discard unused portion after 14 days.

Capsules: Store at controlled room temperature, 59° to 86°F (15° to 30°C).

HOW SUPPLIED
CAPSULE: 250 MG

BRAND/MANUFACTURER	NDC	SIZE	AWP
◆ GENERICS			
Mylan	00378-7250-01	100s	$185.52

CAPSULE: 250 MG

BRAND/MANUFACTURER	NDC	SIZE	AWP
○ BRAND			
➤ CECLOR: Lilly	00002-3061-15	15s	$32.68
	00002-3061-02	100s	$207.28
	00002-3061-33	100s ud	$211.66

CAPSULE: 500 MG

BRAND/MANUFACTURER	NDC	SIZE	AWP
◆ GENERICS			
Mylan	00378-7500-01	100s	$364.55

CAPSULE: 500 MG

BRAND/MANUFACTURER	NDC	SIZE	AWP
○ BRAND			
➤ CECLOR: Lilly	00002-3062-15	15s	$62.02
	00002-3062-02	100s	$407.32
	00002-3062-33	100s ud	$411.70

◆ RATED THERAPEUTICALLY EQUIVALENT; ◇ THERAPEUTIC EQUIVALENCE UNCONFIRMED; ○ UNRATED

POWDER FOR RECONSTITUTION: 125 MG/5 ML

AVERAGE UNIT PRICE (AVAILABLE SIZES)			
GENERIC	$0.18		

BRAND/MANUFACTURER	NDC	SIZE	AWP
◆ GENERICS			
Mylan	00378-7602-12	75 ml	$13.40
Mylan	00378-7602-06	150 ml	$26.65

POWDER FOR RECONSTITUTION: 125 MG/5 ML

BRAND/MANUFACTURER	NDC	SIZE	AWP
○ BRAND			
CECLOR: Lilly	00002-5057-18	75 ml	$14.97
	00002-5057-68	150 ml	$29.78

POWDER FOR RECONSTITUTION: 187 MG/5 ML

AVERAGE UNIT PRICE (AVAILABLE SIZES)			
GENERIC	$0.27		

BRAND/MANUFACTURER	NDC	SIZE	AWP
◆ GENERICS			
Mylan	00378-7604-09	50 ml	$13.40
Mylan	00378-7604-02	100 ml	$26.65

POWDER FOR RECONSTITUTION: 187 MG/5 ML

BRAND/MANUFACTURER	NDC	SIZE	AWP
○ BRAND			
CECLOR: Lilly	00002-5130-87	50 ml	$14.97
	00002-5130-48	100 ml	$29.78

POWDER FOR RECONSTITUTION: 250 MG/5 ML

AVERAGE UNIT PRICE (AVAILABLE SIZES)			
GENERIC	$0.33		

BRAND/MANUFACTURER	NDC	SIZE	AWP
◆ GENERICS			
Mylan	00378-7610-12	75 ml	$24.86
Mylan	00378-7610-06	150 ml	$48.29

POWDER FOR RECONSTITUTION: 250 MG/5 ML

BRAND/MANUFACTURER	NDC	SIZE	AWP
○ BRAND			
CECLOR: Lilly	00002-5058-18	75 ml	$27.78
	00002-5058-68	150 ml	$53.95

POWDER FOR RECONSTITUTION: 375 MG/5 ML

AVERAGE UNIT PRICE (AVAILABLE SIZES)			
GENERIC	$0.49		

BRAND/MANUFACTURER	NDC	SIZE	AWP
◆ GENERICS			
Mylan	00378-7612-09	50 ml	$24.86
Mylan	00378-7612-02	100 ml	$48.29

POWDER FOR RECONSTITUTION: 375 MG/5 ML

BRAND/MANUFACTURER	NDC	SIZE	AWP
○ BRAND			
CECLOR: Lilly	00002-5132-87	50 ml	$27.78
	00002-5132-48	100 ml	$53.95

Cefadroxil Monohydrate

DESCRIPTION

Cefadroxil Monohydrate is a semisynthetic cephalosporin antibiotic intended for oral administration. It is a white to yellowish-white crystalline powder. It is soluble in water and it is acid-stable. It is chemically designated as 5-Thia-1-azabicyclo[4.2.0]oct-2-ene-2-carboxylic acid, 7-[[amino(4-hydroxyphenyl)acetyl]amino]-3-methyl-8-oxo, monohydrate, [6R-[6α,7β(R*)]]-. It has the formula $C_{16}H_{17}N_3O_5S \cdot H_2O$ and the molecular weight of 381.40.

Cefadroxil Monohydrate is available in 500 mg capsules; 1-g tablets and 125 mg/5ml, 250 mg/5ml, and 500 mg/5ml oral suspension.

Following is its chemical structure:

CLINICAL PHARMACOLOGY

Cefadroxil Monohydrate is rapidly absorbed after oral administration. Following single doses of 500 and 1000 mg, average peak serum concentrations were approximately 16 and 28 µg/mL, respectively. Measurable levels were present 12 hours after administration. Over 90% of the drug is excreted unchanged in the urine within 24 hours. Peak urine concentrations are approximately 1800 µg/mL during the period following a single 500-mg oral dose. Increases in dosage generally produce a proportionate increase in Cefadroxil Monohydrate urinary concentration. The urine antibiotic concentration, following a 1-g dose, was maintained well above the MIC of susceptible urinary pathogens for 20 to 22 hours.

Microbiology: In vitro tests demonstrate that the cephalosporins are bactericidal because of their inhibition of cell-wall synthesis. Cefadroxil has been shown to be active against the following organisms both *in vitro* and in clinical infections (see *"Indications and Usage"*):

Beta- hemolytic streptococci
Staphylococci, including penicillinase-producing strains
Streptococcus (Diplococcus) pneumoniae
Escherichia coli
Proteus mirabilis
Klebsiella species
Moraxella (Branhamella) catarrhalis

Note: Most strains of *Enterococci faecalis* (formerly *Streptococcus faecalis*) and *Enterococcus faecium* (formerly *Streptococcus faecium*) are resistant to Cefadroxil Monohydrate. It is not active against most strains of *Enterobacter* species, *Morganella morganii* (formerly *Proteus morganii*), and *P. vulgaris*. It has no activity against *Pseudomonas* species and *Acinetobacter calcoaceticus* (formerly *Mima* and *Herellea* species.).

Susceptibility Tests: Diffusion Techniques: The use of antibiotic disk susceptibility test methods which measure zone diameter give an accurate estimation of antibiotic susceptibility. One standard procedure[1] which has been recommended for use with disks to test susceptibility of organisms to Cefadroxil uses the cephalosporin class (cephalothin) disk. Interpretation involves the correlation of the diameters obtained in the disk test with the minimum inhibitory concentration (MIC) for Cefadroxil.

Reports from the laboratory giving results of the standard single-disk susceptibility test with a 30 µg cephalothin disk should be interpreted according to the following criteria:

Zone diameter (mm)	Interpretation
≥ 18	(S) Susceptible
15-17	(I) Intermediate
≤ 14	(R) Resistant

A report of "Susceptible" indicates that the pathogen is likely to be inhibited by generally achievable blood levels. A report of "Intermediate susceptibility" suggests that the organism would be susceptible if high dosage is used or if the infection is confined to tissue and fluid (eg, urine) in which high antibiotic levels are attained. A report of "Resistant" indicates that achievable concentrations of the antibiotic are unlikely to be inhibitory and other therapy should be selected.

Standardized procedures require the use of laboratory control organisms. The 30 µg cephalothin disk should give the following zone diameters:

Organism	Zone Diameter (mm)
Staphylococcus aureus	
ATCC 25923	29-37
Escherichia coli ATCC 25922	17-22

Dilution Techniques: When using the NCCLS agar dilution or broth dilution (including microdilution) method[2] or equivalent, a bacterial isolate may be considered susceptible if the MIC (minimum inhibitory concentration) value for cephalothin is 8 µg/mL or less. Organisms are considered resistant if the MIC is 32 µg/mL or greater. Organisms with an MIC value of less than 32 µg/mL but greater than 8 µg/mL are intermediate.

As with standard diffusion methods, dilution procedures require the use of laboratory control organisms. Standard cephalothin powder should give MIC values in the range of 0.12 µg/mL and 0.5 µg/mL for *Staphylococcus aureus* ATCC 29213. For *Escherichia coli* ATCC 25922, the MIC range should be between 4.0 µg/mL and 16.0 µg/mL. For *Streptococcus faecalis* ATCC 29212, the MIC range should be between 8.0 and 32.0 µg/mL.

INDICATIONS AND USAGE

Cefadroxil Monohydrate is indicated for the treatment of patients with infection caused by susceptible strains of the designated organisms in the following diseases:

Urinary tract infections caused by *E. coli, P. mirabilis,* and *Klebsiella* species.
Skin and skin structure infections caused by staphylocci and/or streptococci.
Pharyngitis and tonsillitis caused by group A beta-hemolytic streptococci. (Penicillin is the usual drug of choice in the treatment and prevention of streptococcal infections, including the prophylaxis of rheumatic fever. Cefadroxil Monohydrate is generally effective in the eradication of streptococci from the nasopharynx; however, substantial data establishing the efficacy of Cefadroxil Monohydrate in the subsequent prevention of rheumatic fever are not available at present.)

Note: Culture and susceptibility tests should be initiated prior to and during therapy. Renal function studies should be performed when indicated.

UNLABELED USES
Cefadroxil Monohydrate is used alone or as an adjunct in the treatment of respiratory-tract infections and infections of bone and joints caused by susceptible organisms.

CONTRAINDICATIONS
Cefadroxil Monohydrate is contraindicated in patients with known allergy to the cephalosporin group of antibiotics.

WARNINGS
BEFORE THERAPY WITH CEFADROXIL MONOHYDRATE IS INSTITUTED, CAREFUL INQUIRY SHOULD BE MADE TO DETERMINE WHETHER THE PATIENT HAS HAD PREVIOUS HYPERSENSITIVITY REACTIONS TO CEFADROXIL, CEPHALOSPORINS, PENICILLINS OR OTHER DRUGS. IF THIS PRODUCT IS TO BE GIVEN TO PENICILLIN-SENSITIVE PATIENTS, CAUTION SHOULD BE EXERCISED BECAUSE CROSS-SENSITIVITY AMONG BETALACTAM ANTIBIOTICS HAS BEEN CLEARLY DOCUMENTED AND MAY OCCUR IN UP TO 10% OF PATIENTS WITH A HISTORY OF PENICILLIN ALLERGY. IF AN ALLERGIC REACTION TO CEFADROXIL MONOHYDRATE OCCURS, DISCONTINUE THE DRUG. SERIOUS ACUTE HYPERSENSITIVITY REACTIONS MAY REQUIRE TREATMENT WITH EPINEPHRINE AND OTHER EMERGENCY MEASURES, INCLUDING OXYGEN, INTRAVENOUS FLUIDS, INTRAVENOUS ANTIHISTAMINES, CORTICOSTEROIDS, PRESSOR AMINES, AND AIRWAY MANAGEMENT, AS CLINICALLY INDICATED.

Pseudomembranous colitis has been reported with nearly all antibacterial agents, including Cefadroxil, and may range from mild to life-threatening. Therefore, it is important to consider this diagnosis in patients who present with diarrhea subsequent to the administration of antibacterial agents.

Treatment with antibacterial agents alters the normal flora of the colon and may permit overgrowth of clostridia. Studies indicate that a toxin produced by *Clostridium difficile* is a primary cause of "antibiotic-associated colitis".

After the diagnosis of pseudomembranous colitis has been established, therapeutic measures should be initiated. Mild cases of pseudomembranous colitis usually repond to discontinuation of the drug alone. In moderate to severe cases, consideration should be given to management with fluids and electrolytes, protein supplementation and treatment with an antibacterial drug effective against *Clostridium difficile*.

PRECAUTIONS
General: Cefadroxil Monohydrate should be used with caution in the presence of markedly impaired renal function (creatinine clearance rate of less than 50 mL/min/1.73 M^2). (See *"Dosage and Administration"*.) In patients with known or suspected renal impairment, careful clinical observation and appropriate laboratory studies should be made prior to and during therapy.

Prolonged use of Cefadroxil Monohydrate may result in the overgrowth of nonsusceptible organisms. Careful observation of the patient is essential. If superinfection occurs during therapy, appropriate measures should be taken.

Cefadroxil Monohydrate should be prescribed with caution in individuals with history of gastrointestinal disease, particularly colitis.

Drug/Laboratory Test Interactions: Positive direct Coombs' tests have been reported during treatment with the cephalosporin antibiotics. In hematologic studies or in transfusion cross-matching procedures when antiglobulin tests are performed on the minor side or in Coombs' testing of newborns whose mothers have received cephalosporin antibiotics before parturition, it should be recognized that a positive Coombs' test may be due to the drug.

Carcinogenesis, Mutagenesis, and Impairment of Fertility: No long-term studies have been performed to determine carcinogenic potential. No genetic toxicity tests have been performed.

Pregnancy: Pregnancy Category B: Reproduction studies have been performed in mice and rats at doses up to 11 times the human dose and have revealed no evidence of impaired fertility or harm to the fetus due to Cefadroxil Monohydrate. There are, however, no adequate and well-controlled studies in pregnant women. Because animal reproduction studies are not always predictive of human response, this drug should be used during pregnancy only if clearly needed.

Labor and Delivery: Cefadroxil Monohydrate has not been studied for use during labor and delivery. Treatment should only be given if clearly needed.

Nursing Mothers: Caution should be exercised when Cefadroxil Monohydrate is administered to a nursing mother.

Pediatric Use: See *"Dosage and Administration"*.

ADVERSE REACTIONS
Gastrointestinal: Onset of pseudomembranous colitis symptoms may occur during or after antibiotic treatment (See *"Warnings"*). Nausea and vomiting have been reported rarely. Diarrhea has also occurred.

Hypersensitivity: Allergies (in the form of rash, urticaria, and angioedema) have been observed. These reactions usually subsided upon discontinuation of the drug.

Other adverse reactions have included genital pruritus, genital moniliasis, vaginitis, moderate transient neutropenia, and minor elevations in serum transaminase. Stevens-Johnson syndrome has been rarely reported.

In addition to the adverse reactions listed above which have been observed in patients treated with Cefadroxil, the following adverse reactions and altered laboratory tests have been reported for cephalosporin-class antibiotics:

Anaphylaxis, erythema multiforme, toxic epidermal necrolysis, fever, abdominal pain, superinfection, renal dysfunction, toxic nephropathy, hepatic dysfunction including cholestasis, aplastic anemia, hemolytic anemia, hemorrhage, prolonged prothrombin time, positive Coombs' test, increased BUN, increased creatinine, elevated alkaline phosphatase, elevated aspartate aminotransferase (AST), elevated alanine aminotransferase (ALT), elevated bilirubin, elevated LDH, eosinophilia, pancytopenia, neutropenia, agranlocytosis, thrombocytopenia.

Several cephalosporins have been implicated in triggering seizures, particularly in patients with renal impairment, when the dosage was not reduced (see *"Dosage and Administration"* and *"Overdosage"*). If seizures associated with drug therapy occur, the drug should be discontinued. Anticonvulsant therapy can be given if clinically indicated.

OVERDOSAGE
A study of children under six years of age suggested that ingestion of less than 250 mg/kg of cephalosporins is not associated with significant outcomes. No action is required other than general support and observation. For amounts greater than 250 mg/kg, induce gastric emptying.

In five anuric patients, it was demonstrated that an average of 63% of a 1 g oral dose is extracted from the body during a 6-8 hour hemodialysis session.

DOSAGE AND ADMINISTRATION
Cefadroxil Monohydrate is acid-stable and may be administered orally without regard to meals. Administration with food may be helpful in diminishing potential gastrointestinal complaints occasionally associated with oral cephalosporin therapy.

ADULTS
Urinary Tract Infections: For uncomplicated lower urinary tract infections (ie, cystitis) the usual dosage is 1 or 2 g per day in single (q.d.) or divided doses (b.i.d.).

For all other urinary tract infections the usual dosage is 2 g per day in divided doses (b.i.d.).

Skin and Skin Structure Infections: For skin and skin structure infections the usual dosage is 1 g per day in single (q.d.) or divided doses (b.i.d.).

Pharyngitis and Tonsillitis: Treatment of group A beta-hemolytic streptococcal pharyngitis and tonsillitis—1 g per day in single (q.d.) or divided doses (b.i.d.) for 10 days.

CHILDREN
For urinary tract infections, the recommended daily dosage for children is 30 mg/kg/day in divided doses every 12 hours. For pharyngitis, tonsillitis, and impetigo, the recommended daily dosage for children is 30 mg/kg/day in a single dose or in equally divided doses every 12 hours. For other skin and skin structure infections, the recommended daily dosage is 30 mg/kg/day in equally divided doses every 12 hours. In the treatment of beta-hemolytic streptococcal infections, a therapeutic dosage of Cefadroxil Monohydrate should be administered for at least 10 days. See chart for total daily dosage for children. (See related table).

In patients with renal impairment, the dosage of Cefadroxil Monohydrate should be adjusted according to creatinine clearance rates to prevent drug accumulation. The following schedule is suggested. In adults, the initial dose is 1000 mg of Cefadroxil Monohydrate and the maintenance dose (based on the creatinine clearance rate [mL/min/1.73 M^2]) is 500 mg at the time intervals listed below.

Creatinine Clearances	Dosage Interval
0-10 mL/min	36 hours
10-25 mL/min	24 hours
25-50 mL/min	12 hours

Patients with creatinine clearance rates over 50 mL/min may be treated as if they were patients having normal renal function.

Reconstitution Directions for Oral Suspension

Bottle Size	Reconstitution Directions
100 mL	Suspend in a total of 66 mL water. Method: Tap bottle lightly to loosen powder. Add 66 mL of water in two portions. Shake well after each addition.
75 ml	Suspend in a total of 51 mL water. Method: Tap bottle lightly to loosen powder. Add 51 mL of water in two portions. Shake well after each addition.
50 mL	Suspend in a total of 33 mL water. Method: Tap bottle lightly to loosen powder. Add 33 mL of water in two portions. Shake well after each addition.

After reconstitution, store in refrigerator. Shake well before using. Keep container tightly closed. Discard unused portion after 14 days.

Child's Weight		Daily Dosage of Cefadroxil Monohydrate Suspension		
lbs	kg	125 mg/5 mL	250 mg/5 mL	500 mg/5mL
10	4.5	1 tsp	—	
20	9.1	2 tsp	1 tsp	
30	13.6	3 tsp	1 1/2 tsp	
40	18.2	4 tsp	2 tsp	1 tsp
50	22.7	5 tsp	2 1/2 tsp	1 1/4 tsp
60	27.3	6 tsp	3 tsp	1 1/2 tsp
70 & above	31.8+	—		2 tsp

STORAGE

Capsules: Store at controlled room temperature (15°-30°C).

Suspension: Prior to reconstitution: Store at controlled room temperature (15°-30°C).

REFERENCES

1. National Committee for Clinical Laboratory Standards, Approved Standard, *Performance Standards for Antimicrobial Disk Susceptibility Test*, 4th Edition, Vol. 10(7): M2-A4, Villanova, PA, April, 1990. 2. National Committee for Clinical Laboratory Standards, Approved Standard: *Methods for Dilution Antimicrobial Susceptibility Tests for Bacteria that Grow Aerobically*, 2nd Edition, Vol. 10(8): M7-A2, Villanova, PA, April, 1990.

HOW SUPPLIED
CAPSULE: 500 MG

AVERAGE UNIT PRICE (AVAILABLE SIZES)

BRAND			$3.24	

BRAND/MANUFACTURER		NDC	SIZE	AWP
◆ BRAND				
▶ DURICEF: Princeton		00087-0784-07	20s	$65.85
		00087-0784-46	50s	$161.35
	ULTRACEF: Bristol Labs	00015-7271-50	50s	$171.30
▶ DURICEF: Princeton		00087-0784-42	100s	$306.05
	ULTRACEF: Bristol Labs	00015-7271-60	100s	$324.90
▶ DURICEF: Princeton		00087-0784-44	100s ud	$311.31
	ULTRACEF: Bristol Labs	00015-7271-65	100s ud	$330.53

POWDER FOR RECONSTITUTION: 125 MG/5 ML

AVERAGE UNIT PRICE (AVAILABLE SIZES)

BRAND			$0.17	

BRAND/MANUFACTURER		NDC	SIZE	AWP
◆ BRAND				
DURICEF: Princeton		00087-0786-42	50 ml	$6.65
		00087-0786-41	100 ml	$12.24
	ULTRACEF: Bristol Labs	00015-7283-40	100 ml	$24.98

POWDER FOR RECONSTITUTION: 250 MG/5 ML

AVERAGE UNIT PRICE (AVAILABLE SIZES)

BRAND			$0.23	

BRAND/MANUFACTURER		NDC	SIZE	AWP
◆ BRAND				
DURICEF: Princeton		00087-0782-42	50 ml	$11.72
		00087-0782-41	100 ml	$23.00

POWDER FOR RECONSTITUTION: 500 MG/5 ML

AVERAGE UNIT PRICE (AVAILABLE SIZES)

BRAND			$0.32	

BRAND/MANUFACTURER		NDC	SIZE	AWP
◆ BRAND				
DURICEF: Princeton		00087-0783-42	50 ml	$15.92
		00087-0783-05	75 ml	$23.86
		00087-0783-41	100 ml	$31.85

TABLETS: 1 GM

AVERAGE UNIT PRICE (AVAILABLE SIZES)

BRAND			$5.93	

BRAND/MANUFACTURER		NDC	SIZE	AWP
◆ BRAND				
▶ DURICEF: Princeton		00087-0785-43	50s	$303.62
		00087-0785-42	100s	$581.46
		00087-0785-44	100s ud	$591.58

Cefadyl *SEE* CEPHAPIRIN SODIUM

Cefamandole Nafate

DESCRIPTION

Cefamandole Nafate for Injection, USP is a semisynthetic broad-spectrum cephalosporin antibiotic for parenteral administration. It is 5-Thia-1-azabicyclo[4,2.0]oct-2-ene-2-carboxylic acid, 7-[[(formyloxy) phenylacetyl]amino]-3-[[(1-methyl-1*H*-tetrazol-5-yl)thio]methyl]-8-oxo-, monosodium salt, [6*R*-[6α,7β(*R**)]]. Cefamandole has the empirical formula $C_{19}H_{17}N_6NaO_6S_2$ representing a molecular weight of 512.49. Cefamandole Nafate also contains 63 mg sodium carbonate/g of Cefamandole activity. The total sodium content is approximately 77 mg (3.3 mEq sodium ion) per g of Cefamandole activity. After addition of diluent, Cefamandole Nafate rapidly hydrolyzes to Cefamandole, and both compounds have microbiologic activity in vivo. Solutions of Cefamandole Nafate range from light-yellow to amber, depending on concentration and diluent used. The pH of freshly reconstituted solutions usually ranges from 6.0 to 8.5. Its molecular weight is 512.5.

Following is its chemical structure:

CLINICAL PHARMACOLOGY

After intramuscular administration of a 500-mg dose of Cefamandole to normal volunteers, the mean peak serum concentration was 13 µg/mL. After a 1-g dose, the mean peak concentration was 25 µg/mL. These peaks occurred at 30 to 120 minutes. Following intravenous doses of 1, 2, and 3 g, serum concentrations were 139, 240, and 533 µg/mL respectively at 10 minutes. These concentrations declined to 0.8, 2.2, and 2.9 µg/mL at 4 hours. Intravenous administration of 4-g doses every 6 hours produced no evidence of accumulation in the serum. The half-life after an intravenous dose is 32 minutes; after intramuscular administration, the half-life is 60 minutes.

Sixty-five to 85% of Cefamandole is excreted by the kidneys over an 8-hour period, resulting in high urinary concentrations. Following intramuscular doses of 500 mg and 1 g, urinary concentrations averaged 254 and 1,357 µg/mL respectively. Intravenous doses of 1 and 2 g produced urinary levels averaging 750 and 1,380 µg/mL respectively. Probenecid slows tubular excretion and doubles the peak serum level and the duration of measurable serum concentrations.

The antibiotic reaches therapeutic levels in pleural and joint fluids and in bile and bone.

Microbiology: The bactericidal action of Cefamandole results from inhibition of cell-wall synthesis. Cephalosporins have in vitro activity against a wide range of gram-positive and gram-negative organisms. Cefamandole is usually active against the following organisms in vitro and in clinical infections:

Gram-positive
Staphylococcus aureus, including penicillinase- and nonpenicillinase-producing strains
Staphylococcus epidermidis
β-hemolytic and other streptococci (Most strains of enterococci, eg, *Enterococcus faecalis* [formerly *Streptococcus faecalis*], are resistant.)
Streptococcus pneumoniae
Gram-negative
Escherichia coli
Klebsiella sp
Enterobacter sp (Initially susceptible organisms occasionally may become resistant during therapy.)
Haemophilus influenzae
Proteus mirabilis
Providencia rettgeri (formerly *Proteus rettgeri*)
Morganella morganii (formerly *Proteus morganii*)
Proteus vulgaris (Some strains of *P. vulgaris* have been shown by in vitro tests to be resistant to Cefamandole and other cephalosporins.)
Anaerobic organisms
Gram-positive and gram-negative cocci (including *Peptococcus* and *Peptostreptococcus* sp)
Gram-positive bacilli (including *Clostridium* sp)
Gram-negative bacilli (including *Bacteroides* and *Fusobacterium* sp). Most strains of *Bacteroides fragilis* are resistant.

▶ SHOWN IN PRODUCT IDENTIFICATION GUIDE

Pseudomonas, Acinetobacter calcoaceticus (formerly *Mima* and *Herellea* sp), and most *Serratia* strains are resistant to Cefamandole and certain other cephalosporins. Cefamandole is resistant to degradation by β-lactamases from certain members of the *Enterobacteriaceae*.

Susceptibility Tests: Quantitative methods that require measurement of zone diameters give the most precise estimates of antibiotic susceptibility. One such procedure[1] has been recommended for use with disks to test susceptibility to Cefamandole. Interpretation involves correlation of the diameters obtained in the disk test with minimal inhibitory concentration (MIC) values for Cefamandole.

Reports from the laboratory giving results of the standardized single-disk susceptibility test[1] using a 30-µg Cefamandole disk should be interpreted according to the following criteria:

Susceptible organisms produce zones of 18 mm or greater, indicating that the tested organism is likely to respond to therapy.

Organisms of intermediate susceptibility produce zones of 15 to 17 mm, indicating that the tested organism would be susceptible if high dosage is used or if the infection is confined to tissues and fluids (eg, urine) in which high antibiotic levels are attained.

Resistant organisms produce zones of 14 mm or less, indicating that other therapy should be selected.

For gram-positive isolates, the test may be performed with either the cephalosporin-class disk (30 µg cephalothin) or the Cefamandole disk (30 µg Cefamandole), and a zone of 18 mm is indicative of a Cefamandole-susceptible organism.

Gram-negative organisms should be tested with the Cefamandole disk (using the above criteria), since Cefamandole has been shown by in vitro tests to have activity against certain strains of *Enterobacteriaceae* found resistant when tested with the cephalosporin-class disk. Gram-negative organisms having zones of less than 18 mm around the cephalothin disk are not necessarily of intermediate susceptibility or resistant to Cefamandole.

The Cefamandole disk should not be used for testing susceptibility to other cephalosporins.

A bacterial isolate may be considered susceptible if the MIC value for Cefamandole is not more than 16 µg/mL. Organisms are considered resistant if the MIC is greater than 32 µg/mL.

INDICATIONS AND USAGE

Cefamandole is indicated for the treatment of serious infections caused by susceptible strains of the designated microorganisms in the diseases listed below:

Lower respiratory infections, including pneumonia, caused by *S. pneumoniae, H. influenzae, Klebsiella* sp, *S. aureus* (penicillinase- and non-penicillinase-producing), β-hemolytic streptococci, and *P. mirabilis*

Urinary tract infections caused by *E. coli, Proteus* sp (both indole-negative and indole-positive), *Enterobacter* sp, *Klebsiella* sp, group D streptococci (*Note:* Most enterococci, eg, *E. faecalis*, are resistant), and *S. epidermidis*

Peritonitis caused by *E. coli* and *Enterobacter* sp

Septicemia caused by *E. coli, S aureus* (penicillinase- and non-penicillinase-producing), *S. pneumoniae, S. pyogenes* (group A β-hemolytic streptococci), *H. influenzae*, and *Klebsiella* sp

Skin and skin structure infections caused by *S. aureus* (penicillinase- and non-penicillinase-producing), *S. pyogenes* (group A β-hemolytic streptococci), *H. influenzae, E. coli, Enterobacter* sp, and *P. mirabilis*

Bone and joint infections caused by *S. aureus* (penicillinase- and non-penicillinase-producing)

Clinical microbiologic studies in nongonococcal pelvic inflammatory disease in females, lower respiratory infections, and skin infections frequently reveal the growth of susceptible strains of both aerobic and anaerobic organisms. Cefamandole has been used successfully in those infections in which several organisms have been isolated. Most strains of *B. fragilis* are resistant in vitro; however, infections caused by susceptible strains have been treated successfully.

Specimens for bacteriologic cultures should be obtained in order to isolate and identify causative organisms and to determine their susceptibilities to Cefamandole. Therapy may be instituted before results of susceptibility studies are known; however, once these results become available, the antibiotic treatment should be adjusted accordingly.

In certain cases of confirmed or suspected gram-positive or gram-negative sepsis or in patients with other serious infections in which the causative organism has not been identified Cefamandole may be used concomitantly with an aminoglycoside (see *"Precautions"*). The recommended doses of both antibiotics may be given, depending on the severity of the infection and the patient's condition. The renal function of the patient should be carefully monitored, especially if higher dosages of the antibiotics are to be administered.

Antibiotic therapy of β-hemolytic streptococcal infections should continue for at least 10 days.

Preventive Therapy: The administration of Cefamandole preoperatively, intraoperatively, and postoperatively may reduce the incidence of certain postoperative infections in patients undergoing surgical procedures that are classified as contaminated or potentially contaminated (eg, gastrointestinal surgery, cesarean section, vaginal hysterectomy, or cholecystectomy in high-risk patients such as those with acute cholecystitis, obstructive jaundice, or common-bile-duct stones). In major surgery in which the risk of postoperative infection is low but serious (cardiovascular surgery, neurosurgery, or prosthetic arthroplasty), Cefamandole may be effective in preventing such infections.

The perioperative use of Cefamandole should be discontinued after 48 hours; however, in prosthetic arthroplasty, it is recommended that administration be continued for 72 hours. If signs of infection occur, specimens for culture should be obtained for identification of the causative organism so that appropriate antibiotic therapy may be instituted.

CONTRAINDICATION

Cefamandole is contraindicated in patients with known allergy to the cephalosporin group of antibiotics.

WARNINGS

BEFORE THERAPY WITH CEFAMANDOLE IS INSTITUTED, CAREFUL INQUIRY SHOULD BE MADE TO DETERMINE WHETHER THE PATIENT HAS HAD PREVIOUS HYPERSENSITIVITY REACTIONS TO CEPHALOSPORINS, PENICILLINS, OR OTHER DRUGS. THIS PRODUCT SHOULD BE GIVEN CAUTIOUSLY TO PENICILLIN-SENSITIVE PATIENTS. ANTIBIOTICS SHOULD BE ADMINISTERED WITH CAUTION TO ANY PATIENT WHO HAS DEMONSTRATED SOME FORM OF ALLERGY, PARTICULARLY TO DRUGS. SERIOUS ACUTE HYPERSENSITIVITY REACTIONS MAY REQUIRE EPINEPHRINE AND OTHER EMERGENCY MEASURES.

In newborn infants, accumulation of other cephalosporin class antibiotics (with resulting prolongation of drug half-life) has been reported.

Pseudomembranous colitis has been reported with virtually all broad-spectrum antibiotics (including macrolides, semi-synthetic penicillins, and cephalosporins); therefore, it is important to consider its diagnosis in patients who develop diarrhea in association with the use of antibiotics. Such colitis may range in severity from mild to life threatening.

Treatment with broad-spectrum antibiotics alters the normal flora of the colon and may permit overgrowth of clostridia. Studies indicate that a toxin produced by *Clostridium difficile* is a primary cause of antibiotic-associated colitis.

Mild cases of pseudomembranous colitis usually respond to drug discontinuance alone. In moderate to severe cases, management should include sigmoidoscopy, appropriate bacteriologic studies, and fluid, electrolyte, and protein supplementation. When the colitis does not improve after the drug has been discontinued, or when it is severe, oral vancomycin is the drug of choice for antibiotic-associated pseudomembranous colitis produced by *C. difficile*. Other causes of colitis should be ruled out.

PRECAUTIONS

General: Although Cefamandole rarely produces alteration in kidney function, evaluation of renal status is recommended, especially in seriously ill patients receiving maximum doses.

Prolonged use of Cefamandole may result in the overgrowth of nonsusceptible organisms. Careful observation of the patient is essential. If superinfection occurs during therapy, appropriate measures should be taken.

Nephrotoxicity has been reported following concomitant administration of aminoglycoside antibiotics and cephalosporins.

A false-positive reaction for glucose in the urine may occur with Benedict's or Fehling's solution or with Clinitest® tablets but not with Tes-Tape® (Glucose Enzymatic Test Strip, USP). There may be a false-positive test for proteinuria with acid and denaturization-precipitation tests.

As with other broad-spectrum antibiotics, hypoprothrombinemia, with or without bleeding, has been reported rarely, but it has been promptly reversed by administration of vitamin K. Such episodes usually have occurred in elderly, debilitated, or otherwise compromised patients with deficient stores of vitamin K. Treatment of such individuals with antibiotics possessing significant gram-negative and/or anaerobic activity is thought to alter the number and/or type of intestinal bacterial flora, with consequent reduction in synthesis of vitamin K. Prophylactic administration of vitamin K may be indicated in such patients, especially when intestinal sterilization and surgical procedures are performed.

In a few patients receiving Cefamandole, nausea, vomiting, and vasomotor instability with hypotension and peripheral vasodilatation occurred following the ingestion of ethanol.

Cefamandole inhibits the enzyme acetaldehyde dehydrogenase in laboratory animals. This causes accumulation of acetaldehyde when ethanol is administered concomitantly. Broad-spectrum antibiotics should be prescribed with caution in individuals with a history of gastrointestinal disease, particularly colitis.

Carcinogenesis, Mutagenesis, Impairment of Fertility: Certain β-lactam antibiotics containing the N-methylthiotetrazole side chain have been reported to cause delayed maturity of the testicular germinal epithelium when given to neonatal rats during initial spermatogenic development (6 to 36 days of age). In animals that were treated from 6 to 36 days of age with 1,000 mg/kg/day of Cefamandole (approximately 5 times the maximum clinical dose) the delayed maturity was pronounced and was associated with decreased testicular weights and a reduced number of germinal cells in the leading waves of spermatogenic development. The effect was slight in rats given 50 or 100 mg/kg/day. Some animals that were given 1,000 mg/kg/day during days 6 to 36 were infertile after becoming sexually mature. No adverse effects have been observed in rats exposed in utero, in neonatal rats (4 days of age or younger) treated prior to the initiation of spermatogenesis, or in older rats (more than 36 days of age) after exposure for up to 6 months. The significance to man of these findings in rats is unknown because of differences in the time of initiation of spermatogenesis, rate of spermatogenic development, and duration of puberty.

Usage in Pregnancy—Pregnancy Category B: Reproduction studies have been performed in rats given doses of 500 or 1,000 mg/kg/day and have revealed no evidence of impaired fertility or harm to the fetus due to Cefamandole. There are, however, no adequate and well-controlled studies in pregnant women. Because animal reproduction studies are not always predictive of human response, this drug should be used during pregnancy only if clearly needed.

Nursing Mothers: Caution should be exercised when Cefamandole is administered to a nursing woman.

Usage in Infancy: Cefamandole has been effectively used in this age group, but all laboratory parameters have not been extensively studied in infants between 1 and 6 months of age; safety of this product has not been established in prematures and infants under 1 month of age. Therefore, if Cefamandole is administered to infants, the physician should determine whether the potential benefits outweigh the possible risks involved.

ADVERSE REACTIONS
Gastrointestinal: Symptoms of pseudomembranous colitis may appear either during or after antibiotic treatment. Nausea and vomiting have been reported rarely. As with some penicillins and some other cephalosporins, transient hepatitis and cholestatic jaundice have been reported rarely.

Hypersensitivity: Anaphylaxis, maculopapular rash, urticaria, eosinophilia, and drug fever have been reported. These reactions are more likely to occur in patients with a history of allergy, particularly to penicillin.

Blood: Thrombocytopenia has been reported rarely. Neutropenia has been reported, especially in long courses of treatment. Some individuals have developed positive direct Coombs' tests during treatment with the cephalosporin antibiotics.

Liver: Transient rise in SGOT, SGPT, and alkaline phosphatase levels has been noted.

Kidney: Decreased creatinine clearance has been reported in patients with prior renal impairment. As with some other cephalosporins, transitory elevations of BUN have occasionally been observed with Cefamandole their frequency increases in patients over 50 years of age. In some of these cases, there was also a mild increase in serum creatinine.

Local Reactions: Pain on intramuscular injection is infrequent. Thrombophlebitis occurs rarely.

OVERDOSAGE
The administration of inappropriately large doses of parenteral cephalosporins may cause seizures, particularly in patients with renal impairment. Dosage reduction is necessary when renal function is impaired (see *"Dosage and Administration"*). If seizures occur, the drug should be promptly discontinued; anticonvulsant therapy may be administered if clinically indicated. Hemodialysis may be considered in cases of overwhelming overdosage.

DOSAGE AND ADMINISTRATION
DOSAGE
Adults: The usual dosage range for Cefamandole is 500 mg to 1 g every 4 to 8 hours.

In infections of skin structures and in uncomplicated pneumonia, a dosage of 500 mg every 6 hours is adequate.

In uncomplicated urinary tract infections, a dosage of 500 mg every 8 hours is sufficient. In more serious urinary tract infections, a dosage of 1 g every 8 hours may be needed.

In severe infections, 1-g doses may be given at 4 to 6-hour intervals.

In life-threatening infections or infections due to less susceptible organisms, doses up to 2 g every 4 hours (ie, 12 g/day) may be needed.

Infants and Children: Administration of 50 to 100 mg/kg/day in equally divided doses every 4 to 8 hours has been effective for most infections susceptible to Cefamandole. This may be increased to a total daily dose of 150 mg/kg (not to exceed the maximum adult dose) for severe infections. (See recommendations regarding this age group in *"Warnings"* and *"Precautions."*)

Note: As with antibiotic therapy in general, administration of Cefamandole should be continued for a minimum of 48 to 72 hours after the patient becomes asymptomatic or after evidence of bacterial eradication has been obtained; a minimum of 10 days of treatment is recommended in infections caused by group A β-hemolytic streptococci in order to guard against the risk of rheumatic fever or glomerulonephritis; frequent bacteriologic and clinical appraisal is necessary during therapy of chronic urinary tract infection and may be required for several months after therapy has been completed; persistent infections may require treatment for several weeks; and doses smaller than those indicated above should not be used.

For perioperative use of Cefamandole, the following dosages are recommended:

Adults: 1 or 2 g intravenously or intramuscularly 1/2 to 1 hour prior to the surgical incision followed by 1 or 2 g every 6 hours for 24 to 48 hours.

Children (3 months of age and older): 50 to 100 mg/kg/day in equally divided doses by the routes and schedule designated above.

Note: In patients undergoing prosthetic arthroplasty, administration is recommended for as long as 72 hours.

In patients undergoing cesarean section, the initial dose may be administered just prior to surgery or immediately after the cord has been clamped.

Impaired Renal Function: When renal function is impaired, a reduced dosage must be employed and the serum levels closely monitored. After an initial dose of 1 to 2 g (depending on the severity of infection), a maintenance dosage schedule should be followed (see chart). Continued dosage should be determined by degree of renal impairment, severity of infection, and susceptibility of the causative organism. (See related table).

When only serum creatinine is available, the following formula (based on sex, weight, and age of the patient) may be used to convert this value into creatinine clearance. The serum creatinine should represent a steady state of renal function.

Males:
$$\frac{Weight\ (kg) \times (140 - age)}{72 \times serum\ creatinine}$$

Females: 0.9 × above value

Modes of Administration: Cefamandole may be given intravenously or by deep intramuscular injection into a large muscle mass (such as the gluteus or lateral part of the thigh) to minimize pain.

Intramuscular Administration: Each g of Cefamandole should be diluted with 3 mL of 1 of the following diluents: Sterile Water for Injection, Bacteriostatic Water for Injection, 0.9% Sodium Chloride Injection, or Bacteriostatic Sodium Chloride Injection. Shake well until dissolved.

Intravenous Administration: The intravenous route may be preferable for patients with bacterial septicemia, localized parenchymal abscesses (such as intra-abdominal abscess), peritonitis, or other severe or life-threatening infections when they may be poor risks because of lowered resistance. In those with normal renal function, the intravenous dosage for such infections is 3 to 12 g of Cefamandole daily. In conditions such as bacterial septicemia, 6 to 12 g/day may be given initially by the intravenous route for several days, and dosage may then be gradually reduced according to clinical response and laboratory findings.

If combination therapy with Cefamandole and an aminoglycoside is indicated, each of these antibiotics should be administered in different sites. *Do not mix an aminoglycoside with Cefamandole in the same intravenous fluid container.*

A Solution of 1 g of Cefamandole in 22 mL of Sterile Water for Injection is Isotonic.

The choice of saline, dextrose, or electrolyte solution and the volume to be employed are dicated by fluid and electrolyte management.

For direct intermittent intravenous administration, each g of Cefamandole should be reconstituted with 10 mL of Sterile Water for Injection, 5% Dextrose Injection, or 0.9% Sodium Chloride Injection. Slowly inject the solution into the vein over a period of 3 to 5 minutes, or give it through the tubing of an administration set while the patient is also receiving one of the following intravenous fluids: 0.9% Sodium Chloride Injection; 5% Dextrose Injection; 10% Dextrose Injection; 5% Dextrose and 0.9% Sodium Chloride Injection; 5% Dextrose and 0.45% Sodium Chloride Injection; 5% Dextrose and 0.2% Sodium Chloride Injection; or Sodium Lactate Injection (M/6).

Intermittent intravenous infusion with a Y-type administration set or volume control set can also be accomplished while any of the above-mentioned intravenous fluids are being infused. However, during infusion of the solution containing Cefamandole it is desirable to discontinue the other solution. When this technique is employed, careful attention should be paid to the volume of the solution containing Cefamandole so that the calculated dose will be infused. When a Y-tube hookup is used, 100 mL of the appropriate diluent should be added to the 1- or 2-g piggyback (100-mL) vial. If Sterile Water for Injection is used as the diluent, reconstitute with approximately 20 mL/g to avoid a hypotonic solution.

For continuous intravenous infusion, each g of Cefamandole should be diluted with 10 mL of Sterile Water for Injection. An appropriate quantity of the resulting solution may be added to an IV bottle containing 1 of the following fluids: 0.9% Sodium Chloride Injection; 5% Dextrose Injection; 10% Dextrose Injection; 5% Dextrose and 0.9% Sodium Chloride Injection; 5% Dextrose and 0.45% Sodium Chloride Injection; 5% Dextrose and 0.2% Sodium Chloride Injection; or Sodium Lactate Injection (M/6).

STABILITY
Reconstituted Cefamandole is stable for 24 hours at room temperature (25°C) and for 96 hours if stored under refrigeration (5°C). *During storage at room temperature, carbon dioxide develops inside the vial after reconstitution. This pressure may be dissipated prior to withdrawal of the vial contents, or it may be used to aid withdrawal if the vial is inverted over the syringe needle and the contents are allowed to flow into the syringe.*

Solutions of Cefamandole in Sterile Water for Injection, 5% Dextrose Injection, or 0.9% Sodium Chloride Injection that are frozen immediately after reconstitution in conventional vials in which the drugs are supplied are stable for 6 months when stored at −20°C. **If the product is warmed (to a maximum of 37°C), care should be taken to avoid heating it after the thawing is complete. Once thawed, the solution should not be refrozen.**

REFERENCES
1. Bauer AW, Kirby WMM, et al: Antibiotic susceptibility testing by a standardized single disk method. *Am J Clin Pathol* 1966;45:493. Standardized disk susceptibility test. *Federal Register* 1974;39:19182-19184. National Committee for Clinical Laboratory Standards. Approved Standard: M2-A3 Performance standards for antimicrobial disk susceptibility tests—Fourth Edition, December, 1988. 2. Determined by the ICS agar-dilution method (Ericsson HM, Sherris JC: *Acta Pathol Microbiol Scand* 1971; [suppl 217]: B), or any other method that has been shown to give equivalent results.

CEFAMANDOLE MAINTENANCE DOSAGE GUIDE FOR PATIENTS WITH RENAL IMPAIRMENT

Creatinine Clearance (mL/min/1.73 m²)	Renal Function	Life-Threatening Infections—Maximum Dosage	Less Severe Infections
> 80	Normal	2 g q4h	1-2 g q6h
80-50	Mild Impairment	1.5 g q4h OR 2g q6h	0.75-1.5 g q6h
50-25	Moderate Impairment	1.5 g q6h OR 2 g q8h	0.75-1.5 g q8h
25-10	Severe Impairment	1 g q6h OR 1.25 g q8h	0.5-1 g q8h
10-2	Marked Impairment	0.67 g q8h OR 1 g q12h	0.5-0.75 g q12h
< 2	None	0.5 g q8h OR 0.75 g q12h	0.25-0.5 g q12h

HOW SUPPLIED
POWDER FOR INJECTION: 1 GM

BRAND/MANUFACTURER	NDC	SIZE	AWP
○ BRAND			
MANDOL: Lilly	00002-7068-10	10s	$97.32
	00002-7061-25	25s	$226.62
	00002-7268-25	25s	$239.70
	00002-7208-74	96s	$1019.65

POWDER FOR INJECTION: 2 GM

BRAND/MANUFACTURER	NDC	SIZE	AWP
○ BRAND			
MANDOL: Lilly	00002-7064-10	10s	$181.30
	00002-7269-10	10s	$186.53
	00002-7069-10	10s	$187.97

POWDER FOR INJECTION: 10 GM

BRAND/MANUFACTURER	NDC	SIZE	AWP
○ BRAND			
MANDOL: Lilly	00002-7072-16	6s	$543.89

Cefazolin Sodium

DESCRIPTION
Sterile Cefazolin Sodium is a semi-synthetic cephalosporin for parenteral administration. It is the Sodium salt of 3-[[(5-methyl-1,3,4-thiadiazol-2-yl)thio]-methyl]-8-oxo-7- [2-(1H-tetrazol-1-yl) acetamido]-5-thia-1-azabicyclo [4.2.0] oct-2-ene-2-carboxylic acid.

The Sodium content is 46 mg per gram of Cefazolin.

Cefazolin Sodium in lyophilized form is supplied in vials equivalent to 500 mg or 1 gram of Cefazolin; in "Piggyback" Vials for intravenous admixture equivalent to 1 gram of Cefazolin; and in Pharmacy Bulk Vials equivalent to 5 grams or 10 grams of Cefazolin.

Cefazolin Sodium is also supplied as a frozen, sterile, nonpyrogenic solution of Cefazolin Sodium in an iso-osmotic diluent in plastic containers. After thawing, the solution is intended for intravenous use.

The plastic container is fabricated from specially formulated polyvinyl chloride. Solutions in contact with the plastic container can leach out certain of its chemical components in very small amounts within the expiration period, e.g., di 2-ethylhexyl phthalate (DEHP), up to 5 parts per million. However, the suitability of the plastic has been confirmed in animals according to the USP biological tests for plastic containers as well as by tissue culture toxicity studies.

Its molecular weight is 476.5

Following is its chemical structure:

CLINICAL PHARMACOLOGY
Human Pharmacology: After intramuscular administration of Cefazolin to normal volunteers, the mean serum concentrations were 37 mcg/mL at 1 hour and 3 mcg/mL at 8 hours following a 500 mg dose, and 64 mcg/mL at 1 hour and 7 mcg/mL at 8 hours following a 1 gram dose.

Studies have shown that following intravenous administration of Cefazolin to normal volunteers, mean serum concentrations peaked at approximately 185 mcg/mL and were approximately 4 mcg/mL at 8 hours for a 1 gram dose.

The serum half-life for Cefazolin is approximately 1.8 hours following I.V. administration and approximately 2.0 hours following I.M. administration.

In a study (using normal volunteers) of constant intravenous infusion with dosages of 3.5 mg/kg for 1 hour (approximately 250 mg) and 1.5 mg/kg the next 2 hours (approximately 100 mg) Cefazolin produced a steady serum level at the third hour of approximately 28 mcg/mL.

Studies in patients hospitalized with infections indicate that Cefazolin produces mean peak serum levels approximately equivalent to those seen in normal volunteers.

Bile levels in patients without obstructive biliary disease can reach or exceed serum levels by up to five times; however, in patients with obstructive biliary disease, bile levels of Cefazolin are considerably lower than serum levels (< 1.0 mcg/mL).

In synovial fluid, the Cefazolin level becomes comparable to that reached in serum at about 4 hours after drug administration.

Studies of cord blood show prompt transfer of Cefazolin across the placenta. Cefazolin is present in very low concentrations in the milk of nursing mothers.

Cefazolin is excreted unchanged in the urine. In the first 6 hours approximately 60% of the drug is excreted in the urine and this increases to 70% to 80% within 24 hours. Cefazolin achieves peak urine concentrations of approximately 2400 mcg/mL and 4000 mcg/mL respectively following 500 mg and 1 gram intramuscular doses.

In patients undergoing peritoneal dialysis (2 l/hr.), Cefazolin produced mean serum levels of approximately 10 and 30 mcg/mL after 24 hours' instillation of a dialyzing solution containing 50 mg/l and 150 mg/l, respectively. Mean peak levels were 29 mcg/mL (range 13-44 mcg/mL) with 50 mg/l (three patients), and 72 mcg/mL (range 26-142 mcg/mL) with 150 mg/l (six patients). Intraperitoneal administration of Cefazolin is usually well tolerated.

Controlled studies on adult normal volunteers, receiving 1 gram 4 times a day for 10 days, monitoring CBC, SGOT, SGPT, bilirubin, alkaline phosphatase, BUN, creatinine and urinalysis, indicated no clinically significant changes attributed to Cefazolin.

Microbiology: In vitro tests demonstrate that the bactericidal action of cephalosporins results from inhibition of cell wall synthesis. Cefazolin is active against the following organisms in vitro and in clinical infections:

Staphyloccus aureus (including penicillinase-producing strains)
Staphylococcus epidermidis
Methicillin-resistant staphylococci are uniformly resistant to Cefazolin
Group A beta-hemolytic streptococci and other strains of streptococci (many strains of enterococci are resistant)
Streptococcus pneumoniae
Escherichia coli
Proteus mirabilis
Klebsiella species
Enterobacter aerogenes
Haemophilus influenzae
Most strains of indole positive proteus (*Proteus vulgaris*), *Enterobacter cloacae*, *Morganella morganii* and *Providencia rettgeri* are resistant. *Serratia*, *Pseudomonas*, *Mima*, *Herellea* species are almost uniformly resistant to Cefazolin.

DISK SUSCEPTIBILITY TESTS
Disk Diffusion Technique: Quantitative methods that require measurement of zone diameters give the most precise estimates of antibiotic susceptibility. One such procedure[1] has been recommended for use with disks to test susceptibility to Cefazolin.

Reports from a laboratory using the standardized single-disk susceptibility test[1] with a 30 mcg Cefazolin disk should be interpreted according to the following criteria:

Susceptible organisms produce zones of 18 mm or greater, indicating that the tested organism is likely to respond to therapy.
Organisms of intermediate susceptibility produce zones 15 to 17 mm, indicating that the tested organism would be susceptible if high dosage is used or if the infection is confined to tissues and fluids (e.g., urine), in which high antibiotic levels are attained.
Resistant organisms produce zones of 14 mm or less, indicating that other therapy should be selected.

For gram-positive isolates, a zone of 18 mm is indicative of a Cefazolin-susceptible organism when tested with either the cephalosporin-class disk (30 mcg cephalothin) or the Cefazolin disk (30 mcg Cefazolin).

Gram-negative organisms should be tested with the Cefazolin disk (using the above criteria), since Cefazolin has been shown by in vitro tests to have activity against certain strains of *Enterobacteriaceae* found resistant when tested with the cephalothin disk. Gram-negative organisms having zones of less than 18 mm around the cephalothin disk may be susceptible to Cefazolin.

Standardized procedures require use of control organisms. The 30 mcg Cefazolin disk should give zone diameter between 23 and 29 mm for E coli ATCC 25922 and between 29 and 35 mm for S. aureus ATCC 25923.

The Cefazolin disk should not be used for testing susceptibility to other cephalosporins.

◆ RATED THERAPEUTICALLY EQUIVALENT; ◇ THERAPEUTIC EQUIVALENCE UNCONFIRMED; ○ UNRATED

Dilution techniques: —A bacterial isolate may be considered susceptible if the minimal inhibitory concentration (MIC) for Cefazolin is not more than 16 mcg per mL. Organisms are considered resistant if the MIC is equal to or greater than 64 mcg per mL.

The range of MICs for the control strains are as follows:

S. aureus ATCC 25923, 0.25 to 1.0 mcg/mL
E. coli ATCC 25922, 1.0 to 4.0 mcg/mL

INDICATIONS AND USAGE
Cefazolin is indicated in the treatment of the following serious infections due to susceptible organisms:

Respiratory Tract Infections due to *Streptococcus pneumoniae, Klebsiella* species, *Haemophilus influenzae, Staphylococcus aureus* (penicillin-sensitive and penicillin-resistant) and group A beta-hemolytic streptococci.

Injectable benzathine penicillin is considered to be the drug of choice in treatment and prevention of streptococcal infections, including the prophylaxis of rheumatic fever.

Cefazolin is effective in the eradication of streptococci from the nasopharynx; however, data establishing the efficacy of Cefazolin in the subsequent prevention of rheumatic fever are not available at present.

Urinary Tract Infections due to *Escherichia coli, Proteus mirabilis, Klebsiella* species and some strains of enterobacter and enterococci.

Skin and Skin Structure Infections due to *Staphylococcus cureus* (penicillin-sensitive and penicillin-resistant), group A beta-hemolytic streptococci and other strains of streptococci.

Billiary Tract Infections due to *Escherichia coli*, various strains of streptococci, *Proteus mirabilis, Klebsiella* species and *Staphylococcus aureus.*

Bone and Joint Infections due to *Staphylococcus aureus.*

Genital Infections (i.e., prostatitis, epididymitis) due to *Escherichia coli, Proteus mirabilis, Klebsiella* species and some strains of enterococci.

Septicemia due to *Streptococcus pneumoniae, Staphylococcus aureus* (penicillin-sensitive and penicillin-resistant), *Proteus mirabilis, Escherichia coli* and *Klebsiella* species.

Endocarditis due to *Staphylococcus aureus* (penicillin-sensitive and penicillin-resistant) and group A beta-hemolytic streptococci.

Appropriate culture and susceptibility studies should be performed to determine susceptibility of the causative organism to Cefazolin.

Perioperative Prophylaxis: The prophylactic administration of Cefazolin preoperatively, intraoperatively and postoperatively may reduce the incidence of certain postoperative infections in patients undergoing surgical procedures which are classified as contaminated or potentially contaminated (e.g., vaginal hysterectomy, and cholecystectomy in high-risk patients such as those over 70 years of age, with acute cholecystitis, obstructive jaundice or common duct bile stones).

The perioperative use of Cefazolin may also be effective in surgical patients in whom infection at the operative site would present a serious risk (e.g., during open-heart surgery and prosthetic arthroplasty).

The prophylactic administration of Cefazolin should usually be discontinued within a 24-hour period after the surgical procedure. In surgery where the occurrence of infection may be particularly devastating (e.g., open-heart surgery and prosthetic arthroplasty), the prophylactic administration of Cefazolin may be continued for 3 to 5 days following the completion of surgery.

If there are signs of infection, specimens for cultures should be obtained for the identification of the causative organism so that appropriate therapy may be instituted. (See *"Dosage and Administration."*)

UNLABELED USES
Cefazolin Sodium is used alone or as an adjunct in prophylaxis of peristomal wound infections associated with percutaneous endoscopic gastrostomy and in treatment of pneumococcal pneumonia.

CONTRAINDICATIONS
CEFAZOLIN IS CONTRAINDICATED IN PATIENTS WITH KNOWN ALLERGY TO THE CEPHALOSPORIN GROUP OF ANTIBIOTICS.

WARNINGS
BEFORE CEFAZOLIN THERAPY IS INSTITUTED, CAREFUL INQUIRY SHOULD BE MADE CONCERNING PREVIOUS HYPERSENSITIVITY REACTIONS TO CEPHALOSPORINS AND PENICILLIN. CEPHALOSPORIN C DERIVATIVES SHOULD BE GIVEN CAUTIOUSLY IN PENICILLIN-SENSITIVE PATIENTS.

SERIOUS ACUTE HYPERSENSITIVITY REACTIONS MAY REQUIRE EPINEPHRINE AND OTHER EMERGENCY MEASURES.

There is some clinical and laboratory evidence of partial cross-allergenicity of the penicillins and the cephalosporins. Patients have been reported to have had severe reactions (including anaphylaxis) to both drugs.

Any patient who has demonstrated some form of allergy, particularly to drugs, should receive antibiotics cautiously. No exception should be made with regard to Cefazolin.

---

1 Bauer, A.W.; Kirby, W.M.M.; Sherris, J.C., and Turck, M.: Antibiotic Testing by a Standardized Single Disc Method, Am. J. Clin. Path. 45:493, 1966. Standardized Disc Susceptibility Test, Federal Register 39:19182-19184, 1974.

Pseudomembranous colitis has been reported with nearly all antibacterial agents, including Cefazolin, and has ranged in severity from mild to life-threatening. Therefore, it is important to consider this diagnosis in patients who present with diarrhea subsequent to the administration of antibacterial agents.

Treatment with antibacterial agents alters the normal flora of the colon and may permit overgrowth of clostridia. Studies indicate that a toxin produced by *Clostridium difficile* is one primary cause of "antibiotic-associated colitis."

Mild cases of pseudomembranous colitis usually respond to drug discontinuation alone. In moderate to severe cases, consideration should be given to management with fluids and electrolytes, protein supplementation and treatment with an oral antibiotic drug effective against *C. difficile.*

PRECAUTIONS
GENERAL
Prolonged use of Cefazolin may result in the overgrowth of nonsusceptible organisms. Careful clinical observation of the patient is essential.

When Cefazolin is administered to patients with low urinary output because of impaired renal function, lower daily dosage is required (see *"Dosage and Administration"*). As with other beta-lactam antibiotics, seizures may occur if inappropriately high doses are administered to patients with impaired renal function (see *"Dosage and Administration"*).

Cefazolin, as with all cephalosporins, should be prescribed with caution in individuals with a history of gastrointestinal disease, particularly colitis.

Drug Interactions: Probenecid may decrease renal tubular secretion of cephalosporins when used concurrently, resulting in increased and more prolonged cephalosporin blood levels.

Drug/Laboratory Test Interactions: A false positive reaction for glucose in the urine may occur with Benedict's solution, Fehling's solution or with Clinitest® tablets, but not with enzyme-based tests such as Clinistix® and Tes-Tape®. Positive direct and indirect antiglobulin (Coombs) tests have occurred; these may also occur in neonates whose mothers received cephalosporins before delivery.

Carcinogenesis/Mutagenesis: Mutagenicity studies and long-term studies in animals to determine the carcinogenic potential of Cefazolin have not been performed.

Pregnancy: Teratogenic Effects — Pregnancy Category B. Reproduction studies have been performed in rats, mice and rabbits at doses up to 25 times the human dose and have revealed no evidence of impaired fertility or harm to the fetus due to Cefazolin. There are, however, no adequate and well-controlled studies in pregnant women. Because animal reproduction studies are not always predictive of human response, this drug should be used during pregnancy only if clearly needed.

Labor and Delivery: When Cefazolin has been administered prior to caesarean section, drug levels in cord blood have been approximately one-quarter to one-third of maternal drug levels. The drug appears to have no adverse effect on the fetus.

Nursing Mothers: Cefazolin is present in very low concentrations in the milk of nursing mothers. Caution should be exercised when Cefazolin is administered to a nursing woman.

Pediatric Use: Safety and effectiveness for use in prematures and infants under 1 month of age have not been established. See *"Dosage and Administration"* for recommended dosage in children over 1 month.

The potential for the toxic effect in children from chemicals that may leach from the single-dose I.V. preparation in plastic has not been determined.

ADVERSE REACTIONS
The following reactions have been reported:

Gastrointestinal: Diarrhea, oral candidiasis (oral thrush), vomiting, nausea, stomach cramps, anorexia and pseudomembranous colitis. Onset of pseudomembranous colitis symptoms may occur during or after antibiotic treatment (see *"Warnings"*). Nausea and vomiting have been reported rarely.

Allergic: Anaphylaxis, eosinophilia, itching, drug fever, skin rash, Stevens-Johnson syndrome.

Hematologic: Neutropenia, leukopenia, thrombocytopenia, throm- bocythemia.

Hepatic and Renal: Transient rise in SGOT, SGPT, BUN and alkaline phosphatase levels has been observed without clinical evidence of renal or hepatic impairment.

Local Reactions: Rare instances of phlebitis have been reported at site of injection. Pain at the site of injection after intramuscular administration has occurred infrequently. Some induration has occurred.

Other Reactions: Genital and anal pruritus (including vulvar pruritus, genital moniliasis and vaginitis).

DOSAGE AND ADMINISTRATION
USUAL ADULT DOSAGE

Type of Infection	Dose	Frequency
Moderate to severe infections	500 mg to 1 gram	every 6 to 8 hrs.
Mild infections caused by susceptible gram + cocci	250 mg to 500 mg	every 8 hours

➤ SHOWN IN PRODUCT IDENTIFICATION GUIDE

Type of Infection	Dose	Frequency
Acute, uncomplicated urinary tract infections	1 gram	every 12 hours
Pneumococcal pneumonia	500 mg	every 12 hours
Severe, life-threatening infections (e.g., endocarditis, septicemia)*	1 gram to 1.5 grams	every 6 hours

* In rare instances, doses of up to 12 grams of Cefazolin per day have been used.

PERIOPERATIVE PROPHYLACTIC USE
To prevent postoperative infection in contaminated or potentially contaminated surgery, recommended doses are:

a. 1 gram IV or IM administered 1/2 hour to 1 hour prior to the start of surgery.
b. For lengthy operative procedures (e.g., 2 hours or more), 500 mg to 1 gram IV or IM during surgery (administration modified depending on the duration of the operative procedure).
c. 500 mg to 1 gram IV or IM every 6 to 8 hours for 24 hours postoperatively.

It is important that (1) the preoperative dose be given just (1/2 to 1 hour) prior to the start of surgery so that adequate antibiotic levels are present in the serum and tissues at the time of initial surgical incision; and (2) Cefazolin be administered, if necessary, at appropriate intervals during surgery to provide sufficient levels of the antibiotic at the anticipated moments of greatest exposure to infective organisms.

In surgery where the occurrence of infection may be particularly devastating (e.g., open-heart surgery and prosthetic arthroplasty), the prophylactic administration of Cefazolin may be continued for 3 to 5 days following the completion of surgery.

DOSAGE ADJUSTMENT FOR PATIENTS WITH REDUCED RENAL FUNCTION
Cefazolin may be used in patients with reduced renal function with the following dosage adjustments: Patients with a creatinine clearance of 55 mL/min. or greater or a serum creatinine of 1.5 mg % or less can be given full doses. Patients with creatinine clearance rates of 35 to 54 mL/min. or serum creatinine of 1.6 to 3.0 mg % can also be given full doses but dosage should be restricted to at least 8 hour intervals. Patients with creatinine clearance rates of 11 to 34 mL/min. or serum creatinine of 3.1 to 4.5 mg % should be given 1/2 the usual dose every 12 hours. Patients with creatinine clearance rates of 10 mL/min. or less or serum creatinine of 4.6 mg % or greater should be given 1/2 the usual dose every 18 to 24 hours. All reduced dosage recommendations apply after an initial loading dose appropriate to the severity of the infection. Patients undergoing peritoneal dialysis: See "Human Pharmacology."

PEDIATRIC DOSAGE
In children, a total daily dosage of 25 to 50 mg per kg (approximately 10 to 20 mg per pound) of body weight, divided into three or four equal doses, is effective for most mild to moderately severe infections. Total daily dosage may be increased to 100 mg per kg (45 mg per pound) of body weight for severe infections. Since safety for use in premature infants and in infants under 1 month has not been established, the use of Cefazolin in these patients is not recommended. (See related table).

Weight		50 mg/kg/Day Divided into 3 Doses		50 mg/kg/Day Divided into 4 Doses	
lbs	kg	Approximate Single Dose mg/q8h	Vol. (mL) needed with dilution of 225 mg/mL	Approximate Single Dose mg/q6h	Vol. (mL) needed with dilution of 225 mg/mL
10	4.5	75 mg	0.35 mL	55 mg	0.25 mL
20	9.0	150 mg	0.70 mL	110 mg	0.50 mL
30	13.6	225 mg	1.00 mL	170 mg	0.75 mL
40	18.1	300 mg	1.35 mL	225 mg	1.00 mL
50	22.7	375 mg	1.70 mL	285 mg	1.25 mL

In children with mild to moderate renal impairment (creatinine clearance of 70 to 40 mL/min.), 60 percent of the normal daily dose given in equally divided doses

every 12 hours should be sufficient. In patients with moderate impairment (creatinine clearance of 40 to 20 mL/min.), 25 percent of the normal daily dose given in equally divided doses every 12 hours should be adequate. Children with severe renal impairment (creatinine clearance of 20 to 5 mL/min.) may be given 10 percent of the normal daily dose every 24 hours. All dosage recommendations apply after an initial loading dose.

RECONSTITUTION
PREPARATION OF PARENTERAL SOLUTION
Parenteral drug products should be SHAKEN WELL when reconstituted, and inspected visually for particulate matter prior to administration. If particulate matter is evident in reconstituted fluids, the drug solutions should be discarded. When reconstituted or diluted according to the instructions below, Cefazolin is stable for 24 hours at room temperature or for 10 days if stored under refrigeration (5°C or 41°F). Reconstituted solutions may range in color from pale yellow to yellow without a change in potency.

SINGLE-DOSE VIALS
For I.M. injection, I.V. direct (bolus) injection or I.V. infusion, reconstitute with Sterile Water for Injection according to the following table. SHAKE WELL.

Vial Size	Amount of Diluent	Approximate Concentration	Approximate Available Volume
500 mg	2.0 mL	225 mg/mL	2.2 mL
1 gram	2.5 mL	330 mg/mL	3.0 mL

PHARMACY BULK VIALS
Add Sterile Water for Injection, Bacteriostatic Water for Injection or Sodium Chloride Injection according to the table below. SHAKE WELL.

Vial Size	Amount of Diluent	Approximate Concentration	Approximate Available Volume
5 grams	23 mL	1 gram/5 mL	26 mL
	48 mL	1 gram/10 mL	51 mL
10 grams	45 mL	1 gram/5 mL	51 mL
	96 mL	1 gram/10 mL	102 mL

"PIGGYBACK" VIALS
Reconstitute with 50 to 100 mL of Sodium Chloride Injection or other I.V. solution listed under "Administration". When adding diluent to vial, allow air to escape by using a small vent needle or by pumping the syringe. SHAKE WELL. Administer with primary I.V. fluids, as a single dose.

ADMINISTRATION
Intramuscular Administration: Reconstitute vials with Sterile Water for Injection according to the dilution table above. Shake well until dissolved. Cefazolin should be injected into a large muscle mass. Pain on injection is infrequent with Cefazolin.

Intravenous Administration: Direct (bolus) injection: Following reconstitution according to the above table, further dilute vials with approximately 5 mL Sterile Water for Injection. Inject the solution slowly over 3 to 5 minutes, directly or through tubing for patients receiving parenteral fluids (see list below).

Intermittent or continuous infusion: Dilute reconstituted Cefazolin in 50 to 100 mL of one of the following solutions:

Sodium Chloride Injection, USP
5% or 10% Dextrose Injection, USP
5% Dextrose in Lactated Ringer's Injection, USP
5% Dextrose and 0.9% Sodium Chloride Injection, USP
5% Dextrose and 0.45% Sodium Chloride Injection, USP
5% Dextrose and 0.2% Sodium Chloride Injection, USP
Lactated Ringer's Injection, USP
Inverted Sugar 5% or 10% in Sterile Water for Injection
Ringer's Injection, USP
5% Sodium Bicarbonate Injection, USP

STORAGE
Store in a freezer capable of maintaining a temperature of −20°C (−4°F).

PEDIATRIC DOSAGE GUIDE

Weight		25 mg/kg/Day Divided into 3 Doses		25 mg/kg/Day Divided into 4 Doses	
lbs	kg	Approximate Single Dose mg/q8h	Vol. (mL) needed with dilution of 125 mg/mL	Approximate Single Dose mg/q6h	Vol. (mL) needed with dilution of 125 mg/mL
10	4.5	40 mg	0.35 mL	30 mg	0.25 mL
20	9.0	75 mg	0.60 mL	55 mg	0.45 mL
30	13.6	115 mg	0.90 mL	85 mg	0.70 mL
40	18.1	150 mg	1.20 mL	115 mg	0.90 mL
50	22.7	190 mg	1.50 mL	140 mg	1.10 mL

◆ RATED THERAPEUTICALLY EQUIVALENT; ◇ THERAPEUTIC EQUIVALENCE UNCONFIRMED; ○ UNRATED

THAWING OF PLASTIC CONTAINER

Thaw frozen container at room temperature (25°C or 77°F) or under refrigeration (5°C or 41°F). (DO NOT FORCE THAW BY IMMERSION IN WATER BATHS OR BY MICROWAVE IRRADIATION.)

Containers may be thawed individually after separation from the frozen shingle. A shingle consists of stacked frozen containers. Remove frozen shingle from carton and allow to rest at room temperature until the containers can be easily separated (approximately 5 minutes). Then grasp the body of the container (not the ports, corner, or tail flap) to separate individual units. *Promptly* return unneeded frozen containers to freezer.

Check for minute leaks by squeezing container firmly. If leaks are detected, discard solution as sterility may be impaired.

Do not add supplementary medication.

The container should be visually inspected. Components of the solution may precipitate in the frozen state and will dissolve upon reaching room temperature with little or no agitation. Potency is not affected. Agitate after solution has reached room temperature. If after visual inspection the solution remains cloudy or if an insoluble precipitate is noted or if any seals or outlet ports are not intact, the container should be discarded.

The thawed solution is stable for 10 days under refrigeration (5°C or 41°F) and 48 hours at room temperature (25°C or 77°F). Do not refreeze thawed antibiotics.

Use sterile equipment. It is recommended that the intravenous administration apparatus be replaced at least once every 48 hours.

Caution. Do not use plastic containers in series connections. Such use could result in air embolism due to residual air being drawn from the primary container before administration of the fluid from the secondary container is complete.

PREPARATION FOR ADMINISTRATION
1. Suspend container from eyelet support.
2. Remove plastic protector from outlet port at bottom of container.
3. Attach administration set. Refer to complete directions accompanying set.

J CODES
Up to 500 mg IM,IV—J0690

HOW SUPPLIED
INJECTION: 500 MG

BRAND/MANUFACTURER	NDC	SIZE	AWP
◆ GENERICS			
Fujisawa	00469-2361-30	10 ml 25s	$4.06

INJECTION: 500 MG/50 ML

BRAND/MANUFACTURER	NDC	SIZE	AWP
○ BRAND			
ANCEF: SK Beecham Pharm	00007-3142-04	50 ml 24s	$100.80

INJECTION: 1 GM

BRAND/MANUFACTURER	NDC	SIZE	AWP
○ BRAND			
ANCEF: SK Beecham Pharm	00007-3143-04	50 ml 24s	$136.80

POWDER FOR INJECTION: 500 MG

AVERAGE UNIT PRICE (AVAILABLE SIZES)		GENERIC A-RATED AVERAGE PRICE (GAAP)	
BRAND	$1.62	1s	$3.40
GENERIC	$3.31	10s	$39.28
		25s	$64.98

BRAND/MANUFACTURER	NDC	SIZE	AWP
◆ BRAND			
KEFZOL: Lilly	00002-1497-25	25s	$36.00
ANCEF: Abbott Hosp	00007-3131-16	25s	$37.50
KEFZOL: Lilly	00002-7265-25	25s	$48.00
◆ GENERICS			
Apothecon	00015-7338-12	1s	$1.30
Schein	00364-2464-54	1s	$3.00
Schein	00364-2464-61	1s	$4.50
Fujisawa	00469-2364-00	1s	$4.81
Schein	00364-2464-33	10s	$30.00
Lemmon	00093-0706-03	10s	$37.10
Schein	00364-2464-93	10s	$45.00
Goldline	00182-3047-70	10s	$45.00
VHA	00007-3131-76	25s	$37.50
Geneva	00781-3155-70	25s	$73.68
Lemmon	00093-0704-07	25s	$73.75
Goldline	00182-3046-63	25s	$75.00

POWDER FOR INJECTION: 1 GM

AVERAGE UNIT PRICE (AVAILABLE SIZES)		GENERIC A-RATED AVERAGE PRICE (GAAP)	
BRAND	$3.45	1s	$5.30
GENERIC	$4.75	10s	$47.24
		25s	$113.93

BRAND/MANUFACTURER	NDC	SIZE	AWP
◆ BRAND			
ANCEF: Abbott Hosp	00007-3130-01	1s	$3.00
KEFZOL: Lilly	00002-7011-10	10s	$37.32
ANCEF: Abbott Hosp	00007-3137-05	10s	$38.85

BRAND/MANUFACTURER	NDC	SIZE	AWP
KEFZOL: Lilly	00002-1498-25	25s	$72.00
ANCEF: Abbott Hosp	00007-3130-16	25s	$75.00
KEFZOL: Lilly	00002-7266-25	25s	$84.00
	00002-7202-74	96s	$413.58
◆ GENERICS			
Apothecon	00015-7339-12	1s	$2.48
Fujisawa	00469-2371-30	1s	$8.11
Apothecon	00015-7339-31	10s	$3.06
Fujisawa	00469-2374-00	10s	$8.87
VHA	00007-3137-76	10s	$38.85
Schein	00364-2465-33	10s	$59.00
Schein	00364-2465-93	10s	$65.00
Geneva	00781-3724-46	10s	$66.54
Lemmon	00093-0707-03	10s	$66.60
Goldline	00182-3048-70	10s	$70.00
VHA	00007-3130-76	25s	$75.00
Goldline	00182-3044-63	25s	$78.00
Abbott Hosp	00074-4732-03	25s	$122.31
Geneva	00781-3157-70	25s	$147.10
Lemmon	00093-0705-07	25s	$147.25

POWDER FOR INJECTION: 5 GM

BRAND/MANUFACTURER	NDC	SIZE	AWP
◆ BRAND			
ANCEF: Abbott Hosp	00007-3136-05	10s	$150.00

POWDER FOR INJECTION: 10 GM

AVERAGE UNIT PRICE (AVAILABLE SIZES)		GENERIC A-RATED AVERAGE PRICE (GAAP)	
BRAND	$29.40	1s	$32.47
GENERIC	$36.97	10s	$387.68

BRAND/MANUFACTURER	NDC	SIZE	AWP
◆ BRAND			
KEFZOL: Lilly	00002-7014-16	6s	$172.81
ANCEF: Abbott Hosp	00007-3135-05	10s	$300.00
◆ GENERICS			
Apothecon	00015-7346-39	1s	$18.99
Fujisawa	00469-2382-00	1s	$45.95
VHA	00007-3135-76	10s	$300.00
Lemmon	00093-0709-03	10s	$330.20
Geneva	00781-3726-46	10s	$353.20
Goldline	00182-3045-70	10s	$375.00
Schein	00364-2466-93	10s	$580.00

Cefixime

DESCRIPTION
Cefixime is a semisynthetic, cephalosporin antibiotic for oral administration. Chemically, it is (6R, 7R)-7-[2-(2-Amino-4-thiazolyl) gloxylamido]-8-oxo-3-vinyl-5-thia-1-azabicyclo [4.2.0]oct-2-ene-2-carboxylic acid, 7^2-(Z)-[O-(carboxymethyl) oxime]-trihydrate. Molecular weight = 507.50 as the trihydrate.

Following is its chemical structure:

CLINICAL PHARMACOLOGY
Cefixime, given orally, is about 40% to 50% absorbed whether administered with or without food; however, time to maximal absorption is increased approximately 0.8 hours when administered with food. A single 200 mg tablet of Cefixime produces an average peak serum concentration of approximately 2 mcg/mL (range 1 to 4 mcg/mL); a single 400 mg tablet produces an average peak concentration of approximately 3.7 mcg/mL (range 1.3 to 7.7 mcg/mL). The oral suspension produces average peak concentrations approximately 25% to 50% higher than the tablets, when tested in normal *adult* volunteers. Two hundred milligram and 400 mg doses of oral suspension produce average peak concentrations of 3 mcg/mL (range 1 to 4.5 mcg/mL) and 4.6 mcg/mL (range 1.9 to 7.7 mcg/mL), respectively, when tested in normal *adult* volunteers. The area under the time versus concentration curve is greater by approximately 10% to 25% with the oral suspension than with the tablet after doses of 100 to 400 mg, when tested in normal *adult* volunteers. This increased absorption should be taken into consideration if the oral suspension is to be substituted for the tablet. Because of the lack of bioequivalence, tablets should not be substituted for oral suspension in the treatment of otitis media. (See *"Dosage and Administration."*) Cross-over studies of tablet versus suspension have not been performed in children.

Peak serum concentrations occur between 2 and 6 hours following oral administration of a single 200 mg tablet, a single 400 mg tablet, or 400 mg of suspension of Cefixime. Peak serum concentrations occur between 2 and 5 hours following a single administration of 200 mg of suspension. (See related table).

Pediatric Use: Safety and effectiveness of Cefixime in children aged less than 6 months old have not been established. The incidence of gastrointestinal adverse reactions, including diarrhea and loose stools, in the pediatric patients receiving the suspension, was comparable to the incidence seen in adult patients receiving tablets.

ADVERSE REACTIONS

Most of the adverse reactions observed in clinical trials were of a mild and transient nature. Five percent (5%) of patients in the US trials discontinued therapy because of drug-related adverse reactions. The most commonly seen adverse reactions in US trials of the tablet formulation were gastrointestinal events, which were reported in 30% of adult patients on either the bid or the qd regimen. Clinically mild gastrointestinal side effects occurred in 20% of all patients, moderate events occurred in 9% of all patients, and severe adverse reactions occurred in 2% of all patients. Individual event rates included diarrhea 16%, loose or frequent stools 6%, abdominal pain 3%, nausea 7%, dyspepsia 3%, and flatulence 4%. The incidence of gastrointestinal adverse reactions, including diarrhea and loose stools in pediatric patients receiving the suspension was comparable to the incidence seen in adult patients receiving tablets.

These symptoms usually responded to symptomatic therapy or ceased when Cefixime was discontinued.

Several patients developed severe diarrhea and/or documented pseudomembranous colitis, and a few required hospitalization.

The following adverse reactions have been reported following the use of Cefixime. Incidence rates were less than 1 in 50 (less than 2%), except as noted above for gastrointestinal events.

Gastrointestinal: (See Above): Diarrhea, loose stools, abdominal pain, dyspepsia, nausea, and vomiting. Several cases of documented pseudomembranous colitis were identified during the studies. The onset of pseudomembranous colitis symptoms may occur during or after therapy.

Hypersensitivity Reactions: Skin rashes, urticaria, drug fever, and pruritus. Erythema multiforme, Stevens-Johnson syndrome, and serum sickness-like reactions have been reported.

Hepatic: Transient elevations in SGPT, SGOT, and alkaline phosphatase.

Renal: Transient elevations in BUN or creatinine.

Central Nervous System: Headaches or dizziness.

Hemic and Lymphatic Systems: Transient thrombocytopenia, leukopenia, and eosinophilia. Prolongation in prothrombin time was seen rarely.

Other: Genital pruritus, vaginitis, candidiasis.

In addition to the adverse reactions listed above which have been observed in patients treated with Cefixime, the following adverse reactions and altered laboratory tests have been reported for cephalosporin-class antibiotics:

Adverse Reactions: Allergic reactions including anaphylaxis, toxic epidermal necrolysis, superinfection, renal dysfunction, toxic nephropathy, hepatic dysfunction including cholestasis, aplastic anemia, hemolytic anemia, hemorrhage, and colitis.

Several cephalosporins have been implicated in triggering seizures, particularly in patients with renal impairment when the dosage was not reduced (see *"Dosage and Administration"* and *"Overdosage"*). If seizures associated with drug therapy occur, the drug should be discontinued. Anticonvulsant therapy can be given if clinically indicated.

Abnormal Laboratory Tests: Positive direct Coombs test, elevated bilirubin, elevated LDH, pancytopenia, neutropenia, agranulocytosis.

OVERDOSAGE

Gastric lavage may be indicated; otherwise, no specific antidote exists. Cefixime is not removed in significant quantities from the circulation by hemodialysis or peritoneal dialysis. Adverse reactions in small numbers of healthy adult volunteers receiving single doses up to 2 g of Cefixime did not differ from the profile seen in patients treated at the recommended doses.

DOSAGE AND ADMINISTRATION

Adults: The recommended dose of Cefixime is 400 mg daily. This may be given as a 400 mg tablet daily or as 200 mg tablet every 12 hours. For the treatment of uncomplicated cervical/urethral gonococcal infections, a single oral dose of 400 mg is recommended.

Children: The recommended dose is 8 mg/kg/day of the suspension. This may be administered as a single daily dose or may be given in two divided doses, as 4 mg/kg every 12 hours.

PEDIATRIC DOSAGE CHART

Patient Weight (kg)	Dose/Day mg	Dose/Day mL	Dose/Day tsp of suspension
6.25	50	2.5	0.5
12.5	100	5.0	1.0
18.75	150	7.5	1.5
25.0	200	10.0	2.0
31.25	250	12.5	2.5
37.5	300	15.0	3.0

Children weighing more than 50 kg or older than 12 years should be treated with the recommended adult dose.

Otitis media should be treated with the suspension. Clinical studies of otitis media were conducted with the suspension, and the suspension results in higher peak blood levels than the tablet when administered at the same dose. Therefore, the tablet should not be substituted for the suspension in the treatment of otitis media (see *"Clinical Pharmacology"*).

Efficacy and safety in infants aged less than six months have not been established.

In the treatment of infections due to *S. pyogenes*, a therapeutic dosage of Cefixime should be administered for at least 10 days.

Renal Impairment: Cefixime may be administered in the presence of impaired renal function. Normal dose and schedule may be employed in patients with creatinine clearances of 60 mL/min or greater. Patients whose clearance is between 21 and 60 mL/min or patients who are on renal hemodialysis may be given 75% of the standard dosage at the standard dosing interval (ie, 300 mg daily). Patients whose clearance is < 20 mL/min, or patients who are on continuous ambulatory peritoneal dialysis may be given half the standard dosage at the standard dosing interval (ie, 200 mg daily). Neither hemodialysis nor peritoneal dialysis removes significant amounts of drug from the body.

RECONSTITUTION DIRECTIONS FOR ORAL SUSPENSION

Bottle Size	Reconstitution Directions
100 mL	To reconstitute, suspend with *69 mL water.* Method: Tap the bottle several times to loosen powder contents prior to reconstitution. Add approximately half the total amount of water for reconstitution and shake well. Add the remainder of water and shake well.
75 mL	To reconstitute, suspend with *52 mL water.* Method: Tap the bottle several times to loosen powder contents prior to reconstitution. Add approximately half the total amount of water for reconstitution and shake well. Add the remainder of water and shake well.
50 mL	To reconstitute, suspend with *36 mL water.* Method: Tap the bottle several times to loosen powder contents prior to reconstitution. Add approximately half the total amount of water for reconstitution and shake well. Add the remainder of water and shake well.

After reconstitution, the suspension may be kept for 14 days either at room temperature, or under refrigeration, without significant loss of potency. Keep tightly closed. Shake well before using. Discard unused portion after 14 days.

Prior to Reconstitution: Store at controlled room temperature 15°-30°C (59°-86°F).

REFERENCES

1. Bauer AW, Kirby WMM, Sherris JC, et al: Antibiotic susceptibility testing by a standard single disk method. *Am J Clin Pathol* 1966: 45: 493. 2. National Committee for Clinical Laboratory Standards, Approved Standard: Performance Standards for Antimicrobial Disk Susceptibility Tests (M2-A3), December 1984. 3. Standardized disk susceptibility test. *Federal Register*, 1974; 39 (May 30): 19182-19184.

HOW SUPPLIED
POWDER FOR RECONSTITUTION: 100 MG/5 ML

BRAND/MANUFACTURER	NDC	SIZE	AWP
○ BRAND			
SUPRAX: Lederle Labs	00005-3898-40	50 ml	$29.49
	00005-3898-42	75 ml	$47.08
	00005-3898-46	100 ml	$59.35

TABLETS: 200 MG

BRAND/MANUFACTURER	NDC	SIZE	AWP
○ BRAND			
▶ SUPRAX: Lederle Labs	00005-3899-23	100s	$309.81

TABLETS: 400 MG

BRAND/MANUFACTURER	NDC	SIZE	AWP
○ BRAND			
▶ SUPRAX: Lederle Labs	00005-3897-94	10s	$64.74
	00005-3897-18	50s	$309.81
	00005-3897-23	100s	$607.16
	00005-3897-60	100s ud	$637.50

Cefizox *SEE CEFTIZOXIME SODIUM*

Cefmetazole Sodium

DESCRIPTION

Cefmetazole Sodium is a semisynthetic, cephem antibiotic for intravenous administration. It was originally derived from cephyamycin C, produced by

Streptomyces jumonjinensis. It is now synthetically produced from 7-amino-cephalosporanic acid. It is the sodium salt of (6R-cis)-7-[[[(cyanomethyl)thio]acethyl]amino]-7-methoxy-3- [[(1 - methyl - 1H - tetrazol - 5 - yl)thio]methyl] - 8 - oxo - 5 - thia - 1 - azabicyclo; [4.2.0]oct-2-ene-2-carboxylic acid. The empirical formula is $C_{15}H_{16}N_7O_5S_3Na$.

The molecular weight of Cefmetazole Sodium is 493.51. Cefmetazole Sodium contains 49 mg (2 milliequivalents) of Sodium per gram of Cefmetazole activity. Solutions of Cefmetazole Sodium range from colorless to light amber. The pH of freshly reconstituted solutions ranges from 4.2 to 6.2.

Following is its chemical structure:

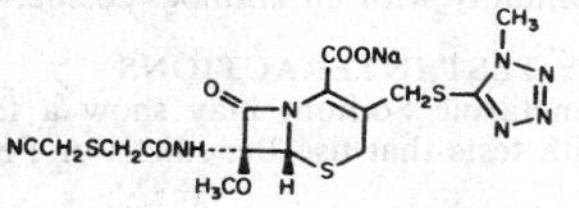

CLINICAL PHARMACOLOGY
Following an intravenous dose of 2 grams administered over 60 minutes to normal volunteers, the mean maximum serum concentration of Cefmetazole was 143 mcg/mL.

SERUM LEVELS (MCG/ML) AFTER INITIAL 60 MINUTE I.V. INFUSIONS

	Time after beginning of infusion					
Dose	*30 min*	*1 hr*	*2 hr*	*4 hr*	*6 hr*	*8 hr*
1 gram	44	73	31	9	3	—
2 gram	92	143	70	20	6	2

Following repeated administration of 2 grams every 6 hours, the mean maximum and trough serum levels of Cefmetazole were 138 and 6 mcg/mL, respectively.

After a 5 minute intravenous infusion of 2 grams to normal volunteers, the mean maximum serum concentration of Cefmetazole was 290 mcg/mL.

SERUM LEVELS (MCG/ML) AFTER 5 MINUTE I.V. INFUSIONS

	Time after beginning of infusion				
Dose	*10 min*	*20 min*	*1hr*	*2 hr*	*4 hr*
1 gram	129	90	43	25	8
2 gram	214	156	91	52	17

The mean plasma or serum elemination half-life after intravenous infusion is approximately 1.2 hours, and the mean plasma clearance is 121 mL/min. Cefmetazole is 65% bound to serum proteins at a concentration of 100 mcg/mL.

Approximately 85% of a dose of Cefmetazole is excreted unchanged in the urine over a 12-hour period resulting in high urinary concentrations. Mean urinary concentrations over collection intervals ranged from 9828 to 52 mcg/mL (mean urine volumes = 104 mL and 645 mL, respectively) in a 12 hour period following a 1 hour I.V. infusion of 2 grams. After a 5 minute I.V. infusion of 2 grams, analogous mean urinary concentrations ranged from 5138 to 46 mcg/mL (mean urine volumes = 183 mL and 575 mL, respectively).

Cefmetazole is excreted by tubular secretion. Probenecid doubles the half-life and increases the duration of measurable plasma concentrations of Cefmetazole; however, the maximum plasma concentrations remain unchanged. In patients with reduced renal function, the plasma clearance is decreased and the half-life of Cefmetazole is prolonged (see *"Dosage and Administration"*).

After a 1 gram I.V. dose, mean concentrations in the gall-bladder wall and the bile at 2.8 hours were 130 mcg/g and 310 mcg/mL, respectively.

After a 1 gram I.V. dose, vaginal, uterine and adnexal tissue concentrations were variable and lower than serum concentrations, ranging from 2.7 to 62.5 mcg/g at 0.1 to 2 hours after the dose.

After a 2 gram dose, the mean maximum concentration in interstitial fluid was 4.5 mcg/mL at one hour after administration and was less than 2 mcg/mL by 4 hours after administration.

Data on CSF levels of Cefmetazole are not available.

MICROBIOLOGY
The bactericidal action of Cefmetazole results from inhibition of cell wall synthesis. Cefmetazole is active *in vitro* against a wide range of aerobic and anaerobic gram-positive and gram-negative organisms. The methoxy group in the 7α position provides Cefmetazole Sodium with a high degree of stability in the presence of beta-lactamases, both penicillinases and cephalosporinases. Cefmetazole is usually active against the following organisms *in vitro* and in clinical infections (see *"Indications and Usage"*).

GRAM-POSITIVE[a]
Staphylococcus aureus[b] (including penicillinase- and non-penicillinase-producing strains)
Staphylococcus epidermidis[b]
Streptococcus pneumoniae
Streptococcus agalactiae
Streptococcus pyogenes

GRAM-NEGATIVE[c]
Escherichia coli
Klebsiella pneumoniae

Klebsiella oxytoca
Haemophilus influenzae (nonpenicillinase-producing strains)
Proteus mirabilis
Proteus vulgaris
Morganella morganii
Providencia stuartii

ANAEROBIC ORGANISMS
Bacteroides fragilis
Bacteroides melaninogenicus
Clostridium perfringens

Note:
   [a] Most strains of enterococci, e.g. *Enterococcus fuecalis* (formerly *Streptococcus faecalis*) are resistant to Cefmetazole.
   [b] Cefmetazole Sodium should not be used for treatment of infections caused by methicillin-resistant staphylocci.
   [c] Cefmetazole is inactive *in vitro* against most strains of *Pseudomonas aeruginosa* and many strains of *Enterobacter* species.

Cefmetazole Sodium has been shown to be active *in vitro* against most strains of the following organisms; however clinical efficacy has not been established.

GRAM-NEGATIVE
Citrobacter diversus
Haemophilus influenzae (penicillinase-producing strains)
Moraxella (Branhamella) catarrhalis
Neisseria gonorrhoeae (penicillinase- and non-penicillinase-producing strains)
Providencia rettgeri
Salmonella species
Shigella species

ANAEROBIC ORGANISMS
Bacteroides bivius
Bacteroides disiens
Bacteroides intermedius
Bacteroides ureolyticus
Peptococcus species
Peptostreptococcus species

SUSCEPTIBILITY TESTING
SUSCEPTIBILITY TESTS: DIFFUSION TECHNIQUES
Quantitative methods that require measurement of zone diameters give an estimate of antibiotic susceptibility. One such procedure[1] has been recommended for use with disks to test susceptibility to Cefmetazole. Interpretation involves correlation of the diameters obtained in the disk test with the minimum inhibitory concentration (MIC) values for Cefmetazole.

Reports from the laboratory giving results of the standardized single disk susceptibility test using a 30 mcg Cefmetazole disk should be interpreted according to the following criteria:

Zone diameter (mm)	*Interpretation*
≥ 16	(S) Susceptible
13-15	(MS) Moderately Susceptible
≤ 12	(R) Resistant

A report of "Susceptible" indicates that the pathogen is likely to be inhibited by generally achievable blood levels. A report of "Moderately Susceptible" indicates that inhibitory concentrations of the antibiotic may well be achieved if high dosage is used or if the infection is confirmed to tissues and fluids (e.g., urine) in which high antibiotic levels are attained. A report of "Resistant" indicates that achievable concentrations of the antibiotic are unlikely to be inhibitory and other therapy should be selected.

Standardized procedures require the use of laboratory control organisms. The 30 mcg disk should give the following zone diameters:

Organism	*Zone diameter (mm)*
E. coli ATCC 25922	26-32
S. aureus ATCC 25923	25-34

Cephalosporin class disks should not be used to test for Cefmetazole susceptibility.

DILUTION TECHNIQUES
In other susceptibility testing procedures, e.g., NCCLS broth microdilution or agar dilution methods[2] or equivalent, a bacterial isolate may be considered susceptible if the MIC value for Cefmetazole is 16 mcg/mL or less. Organisms with an MIC of 32 mcg/mL are considered moderately susceptible. Organisms are considered resistant to Cefmetazole if the MIC is equal to or greater than 64 mcg/mL.

As with standard diffusion methods, dilution procedures require the use of laboratory control organisms. Standard Cefmetazole powder should give MIC values in the range of 0.25-2.0 mcg/mL for *E. coli* ATCC 25922 and in the range of 0.5-2.0 mcg/mL for *S. aureus* ATCC 29213.

INDICATIONS AND USAGE

TREATMENT

Cefmetazole Sodium is indicated for the treatment of serious infections caused by susceptible strains of the designated microorganisms in the following diseases:

Urinary Tract Infections: Complicated or uncomplicated urinary tract infections caused by *Escherichia coli.*

Lower Respiratory Tract Infections: Pneumonia and bronchitis caused by *Streptococcus pneumoniae, Staphylococcus aureus* (penicillinase- and non-penicillinase-producing strains), *Escherichia coli,* and *Haemophilus influenzae* (non-penicillinase producing strains).

Skin and Skin Structure Infections caused by *Staphylococcus aureus* (penicillinase- and non-penicillinase-producing strains), *Staphylococcus epidermidis, Streptococcus pyogenes, Streptococcus agalactiae, Escherichia coli, Proteus mirabilis, Proteus vulgaris**, *Morganella morganii**, *Providencia stuartii**, *Klebsiella pneumoniae, Klebsiella oxytoca**, *Bacteroides fragilis,* and *Bacteroides melaninogenicus**.

Intraabdominal Infections caused by *Escherichia coli, Klebsiella pneumoniae**, *Klebsiella oxytoca**, *Bacteroides fragilis,* and *Clostridium perfringens**.

Appropriate specimens for bacteriological examination should be obtained in order to isolate and identify causative organisms and to determine their susceptibility to Cefmetazole Sodium. Therapy with Cefmetazole Sodium may be instituted before results of susceptibility studies are known; however, once these results become available, antibiotic treatment should be adjusted accordingly.

* Efficacy for the organism in this organ system was studied in fewer than 20 infections.

PROPHYLAXIS

Preoperative administrative of Cefmetazole Sodium may reduce the incidence of certain postoperative infections in patients who undergo cesarean section, abdominal or vaginal hysterectomy, cholecystectomy (high risk patients), and colorectal surgery. These procedures are classified as clean contaminated or potentially contaminated surgery.

If signs and symptoms of an infection develop after surgery, the causative organism should be identified by culture and appropriate therapeutic measures initiated.

CONTRAINDICATIONS

Cefmetazole Sodium is contraindicated in patients with known allergy to Cefmetazole or to the cephalosporin group of antibiotics.

WARNINGS

BEFORE THERAPY WITH CEFMETAZOLE SODIUM IS INSTITUTED, CAREFUL INQUIRY SHOULD BE MADE TO DETERMINE WHETHER THE PATIENT HAS HAD PREVIOUS HYPERSENSITIVITY REACTIONS TO CEFMETAZOLE, CEPHALOSPORINS, PENICILLINS, OR OTHER DRUGS. IF THIS PRODUCT IS TO BE GIVEN TO PENICILLIN-SENSITIVE PATIENTS, CAUTION SHOULD BE EXERCISED BECAUSE CROSS HYPERSENSITIVITY AMONG BETA-LACTAM ANTIBIOTICS HAS BEEN CLEARLY DOCUMENTED AND MAY OCCUR IN UP TO 10% OF PATIENTS WITH A HISTORY OF PENICILLIN ALLERGY. IF AN ALLERGIC REACTION TO CEFMETAZOLE SODIUM OCCURS, DISCONTINUE THE DRUG. SERIOUS ACUTE HYPERSENSITIVITY REACTIONS MAY REQUIRE TREATMENT WITH EPINEPHRINE AND OTHER EMERGENCY MEASURES, INCLUDING OXYGEN, INTRAVENOUS FLUIDS, INTRAVENOUS ANTIHISTAMINES, CORTICOSTEROIDS, PRESSOR AMINES, AND AIRWAY MANAGEMENT, AS CLINICALLY INDICATED.

Pseudomembranous colitis has been reported with nearly all antibacterial agents, including Cefmetazole Sodium, and may range in severity from mild to life-threatening. Therefore, it is important to consider this diagnosis in patients who present with diarrhea subsequent to the administration of antibacterial agents.

Treatment with antibacterial agents alters the normal flora of the colon and may permit overgrowth of clostridia. Studies indicate that a toxin produced by *Clostridium difficile* is the primary cause of "antibiotic-associated colitis".

After the diagnosis of pseudomembranous colitis has been established, therapeutic measures should be initiated. Mild cases of pseudomembranous colitis usually respond to drug discontinuation alone. In moderate to severe cases, consideration should be given to management with fluids and electrolytes, protein supplementation and treatment with an oral antibacterial drug effective against *C. difficile.*

PRECAUTIONS

GENERAL

In patients with transient or persistent reduction in urinary output due to renal insufficiency, the total daily dose of Cefmetazole Sodium should be reduced (see *"Dosage and Administration"*), because high and prolonged serum antibiotic concentrations can occur in such individuals following usual doses.

As with other antibiotics, prolonged use of Cefmetazole Sodium may result in overgrowth of nonsusceptible organisms. Repeated evaluation of the patient's condition is essential. If superinfection occurs during therapy, appropriate measures should be taken.

As with some other cephalosporins, Cefmetazole Sodium may be associated with a fall in prothrombin activity. Those at risk include patients with renal or hepatic impairment, or poor nutritional state, as well as patients receiving a protracted course of antimicrobial therapy. Prothrombin time should be monitored for patients at risk and exogenous Vitamin K administered as indicated.

A disulfiram-like reaction has been reported after ingestion of alcohol (see *"Drug Interactions"*). Therefore, patients should be advised against the ingestion of alcohol-containing beverages during and for 24 hours after the administration of Cefmetazole Sodium.

Antibiotics, including cephalosporins, should be prescribed with caution to individuals with a history of gastrointestinal disease, particularly colitis.

DRUG INTERACTIONS

A disulfiram-like reaction, characterized by flushing, sweating, headache, and tachycardia, has been reported when alcohol was ingested after Cefmetazole Sodium administration. A similar reaction has been reported with other structurally-related cephalosporins.

Although nephrotoxicity has not been noted when Cefmetazole Sodium was given alone, it is possible that nephrotoxicity may be potentiated if Cefmetazole Sodium is used concomitantly with an aminoglycoside.

DRUG/LABORATORY TEST INTERACTIONS

Patients receiving Cefmetazole Sodium may show a false positive result for glucose in the urine with tests that use Benedict's or Fehling's solution.

CARCINOGENESIS, MUTAGENESIS, IMPAIRMENT OF FERTILITY

Long-term carcinogenesis studies of Cefmetazole Sodium have not been performed in animals. Mutagenesis studies of Cefmetazole Sodium, including the Ames test, the unscheduled DNA synthesis test, the mammalian cell foward gene mutation assay, and the dominant lethal test, were all negative. When administered subcutaneously for 35 days to young (6-41 days of age) rats at dosages of 300 mg/kg/day or 1,000 mg/kg/day, Cefmetazole was associated with a reduced number of mature spermatids in the testis and a slight, dose-related reduction of testicular weight. These effects were completely reversible; rats examined 5 and 10 weeks after cessation of the 35 day Cefmetazole treatment regimen at the above doses had normal testicular weights and normal spermatogenesis. In an extension of this study, all aspects of reproductive function were normal in male rats allowed to mate at either 4 to 5 weeks or 7 to 8 weeks after cessation of the 300 or 1,000 mg/kg/day Cefmetazole Sodium treatment regimen. In separate studies, there were no adverse effects on the testicles when Cefmetazole Sodium was given for 30 days to sexually mature male rats at doses up to 2,500 mg/kg/day. The effects of Cefmetazole Sodium on the testes of sexually immature rats are probably due to the methylthiotetrazole side chain which is released from the parent compound by nonenzymatic hydrolysis in the intestine. Rats metabolize the parent compound to release the methylthiotetrazole side chain at a greater rate than humans. There are also species differences in age at onset of spermatogenesis and rate of reproductive maturation. The significance for humans of these testicular changes in sexually immature rats treated with high doses of Cefmetazole Sodium is unknown.

PREGNANCY: PREGNANCY CATEGORY B

Cefmetazole Sodium was not teratogenic or embryocidal when administered to rats or mice at doses up to 2,000 mg/kg/day (approximately 12.5 times the maximum human dose) during the period of organogenesis. There are, however, no adequate and well-controlled studies of Cefmetazole use in pregnant women. Because animal reproduction studies are not always predictive of human response, this drug should be used during pregnancy only if clearly needed.

NURSING MOTHERS

Trace concentrations of Cefmetazole are excreted in human milk; therefore, consideration should be given to temporarily discontinuing nursing during therapy with Cefmetazole Sodium.

PEDIATRIC USE

Safety and effectiveness in children have not been established. For information concerning testicular changes in prepubertal rats, see the *"Carcinogenesis, Mutagenesis, Impairment of Fertility"* subsection.

ADVERSE REACTIONS

Cefmetazole Sodium was generally well-tolerated. Adverse reactions that were reported as possibly or probably related to therapy with Cefmetazole Sodium were:

Gastrointestinal: Diarrhea (3.6%), nausea (1.0%), vomiting, epigastric pain, candidiasis, bleeding. There have been rare reports of pseudomembranous colitis in patients receiving Cefmetazole Sodium. The onset of pseudomembranous colitis symptoms may occur during or after antibiotic treatment (see *"Warnings"*).

Hypersensitivity: Allergic reactions including anaphylaxis and urticaria.

Dermatologic: Rash (1.1%), pruritus, generalized erythema.

Local: Pain and/or swelling at the injection site, phlebitis, thrombophlebitis.

Cardiovascular: Shock, hypotension.

Central Nervous System: Headache, hot flashes.

Respiratory Tract: Pleural effusion, dyspnea, epistaxis, respiratory distress.

Special Senses: Alteration in color perception.

Musculoskeletal: Joint pain and inflammation.

Other: Fever, superinfection, vaginitis.

ADVERSE LABORATORY CHANGES

Adverse laboratory changes that have been reported, without regard to drug relationship, were:

Hepatic: Transient increases in AST (SGOT), ALT (SGPT), alkaline phosphatase, bilirubin, and LDH.

Hematologic: Eosinophillia, leucocytosis, lymphocytosis, granulocytosis, basophilia, monocytosis, thrombocytosis, decreased hemoglobin, decreased hematocrit, decreased RBC, leucopenia, neutropenia, lymphocytopenia, thrombocytopenia, positive Coombs test, prolonged PT and PTT.

Serum Chemistry: Increased glucose, decreased serum albumin, decreased total serum protein.

Renal: Increased BUN, increased creatinine.

In addition to the adverse reactions listed above which have been observed in patients treated with Cefmetazole Sodium, the following adverse reactions and altered laboratory tests have been reported for cephalosporin class antibiotics.

Adverse reactions: Allergic reactions including Stevens-Johnson syndrome, erythema multiforme, toxic epidermal necrolysis, renal dysfunction, toxic nephropathy, hepatic dysfunction including cholestasis, aplastic anemia, hemolytic anemia, hemorrhage.

Several cephalosporins have been implicated in triggering seizures, particularly in patients with renal impairment when the dosage was not reduced (see *"Dosage and Administration"* and *"Overdosage"*). If seizures associated with drug therapy occur, the drug should be discontinued. Anticonvulsant therapy can be given if clinically indicated.

Abnormal Laboratory Tests: Agranulocytosis, pancytopenia.

OVERDOSAGE

Information on overdosage in humans is not available. In the event of serious toxic reactions for overdosage, hemodialysis or peritoneal dialysis may aid in the removal of Cefmetazole from the body, particularly if renal function is compromised. In 7 anuric patients, mean hemodialysis clearance for Cefmetazole was 104 mL/min.

DOSAGE AND ADMINISTRATION
TREATMENT

The usual adult dosage is 2 grams of Cefmetazole Sodium administered intravenously every 6 to 12 hours for 5 to 14 days. Proper dosage should be determined by the condition of the patient, location and severity of the infection, and susceptibility of the causative organisms.

GENERAL GUIDELINES FOR DOSAGE OF CEFMETAZOLE SODIUM

Type of Infection	Daily Dose	Frequency
Urinary Tract	4 grams	2 grams every 12 hours I.V.
Other Sites		
Mild to Moderate	6 grams	2 grams every 8 hours I.V.
Severe to Life-Threatening	8 grams	2 grams every 6 hours I.V.

PROPHYLAXIS

To reduce the incidence of postoperative infection following vaginal hysterectomy, abdominal hysterectomy, cesarean section, colorectal surgery, or cholecystectomy (high risk) in adults, the recommended doses are:

Surgery	Dosing Regimen
Vaginal Hysterectomy	2 grams given as a single dose 30-90 minutes before surgery *or* 1 gram doses given 30-90 minutes before surgery and repeated 8 and 16 hours later
Abdominal Hysterectomy	1 gram doses given 30-90 minutes before surgery and repeated 8 and 16 hours later
Cesarean Section	2 grams given as a single dose after clamping the cord *or* 1 gram doses given after clamping the cord and repeated 8 and 16 hours later
Colorectal[a] Surgery	2 grams given as a single dose 30-90 minutes before surgery *or* 2 gram doses given 30-90 minutes before surgery and repeated 8 and 16 hours later
Cholecystectomy (high risk)	1 gram doses given 30-90 minutes before surgery and repeated 8 and 16 hours later

[a] *All patients studied received preoperative bowel preparation with mechanical cleansing, oral neomycin or kanamycin and oral erythromycin.*

If surgery lasts more than 4 hours, the preoperative dose should be repeated.

IMPAIRED RENAL FUNCTION

For patients with impaired renal function, a reduced dosage schedule should be employed. The following dosage guidelines are derived from clinical pharmacology studies:

DOSAGE GUIDELINES FOR CEFMETAZOLE SODIUM IN ADULTS WITH IMPAIRED RENAL FUNCTION

Renal Function	Creatinine Clearance (mL/min/1.73M^2)	Dose (grams)	Frequency
Mild Impairment	90-50	1-2	Q 12 h
Moderate Impairment	49-30	1-2	Q 16 h
Severe Impairment	29-10	1-2	Q 24 h
Essentially No Function	< 10	1-2	Q 48 h*

* *administered after hemodialysis*

When only the serum creatinine level is available, the following formula (based on sex, weight, and age of the patient) may be used to convert this value into creatinine clearance. The serum creatinine level should represent a steady state of renal function.

Males:
$$\frac{\text{Weight (kg)} \times (140\text{-age})}{72 \times \text{serum creatinine (mg/100 mL)}}$$

Females: $0.85 \times$ above value

PREPARATION OF SOLUTION
GENERAL RECONSTITUTION PROCEDURES

Reconstitute with Sterile Water for Injection, Bacteriostatic Water for Injection, or 0.9 Percent Sodium Chloride Injection. Shake to dissolve and let stand until clear.

Vial Size	Amount of Diluent to be Added (mL)	Approximate Withdrawable Volume (mL)	Approximate Average Concentration (mg/mL)
1 gram	10	10.4	100
1 gram	3.7	4.1	250
2 gram	15	16	125
2 gram	7	8	250

INTRAVENOUS ADMINISTRATION

A solution containing 1 gram or 2 grams of Cefmetazole Sodium Sterile Powder in Sterile Water for Injection, Bacteriostatic Water for Injection, or 0.9 Percent Sodium Chloride Injection can be administered by IV infusion over 10 to 60 minutes. For otherwise healthy patients undergoing elective surgical procedures, a solution containing 1 gram or 2 grams of Cefmetazole Sodium in Sterile Water for Injection, Bacteriostatic Water for Injection, or 0.9 Percent Sodium Chloride Injection can also be injected over three to five minutes. During infusion of the solution containing Cefmetazole Sodium, it is necessary to temporarily discontinue administration of other solutions at the same site.

Solutions of Cefmetazole Sodium, like those of most beta-lactam antibiotics, should not be added to aminoglycoside solutions. If Cefmetazole Sodium and aminoglycosides are to be administered to the same patient, they must be administered separately and not admixed.

COMPATIBILITY AND STABILITY

When reconstituted as described above (Preparation of Solution), Cefmetazole Sodium maintains satisfactory potency for 24 hours at room temperature (25°C, 77°F), for 7 days under refrigeration (8°C, 46°F), and for 6 weeks in the frozen state (at or below -20°C, -4°F).

Primary Cefmetazole solutions (as described in *"Preparation of Solution"*) may be further diluted to concentrations of 1.0 to 20 mg/mL in the following diluents and maintain potency for 24 hours at room temperature (25°C, 77°F), for 7 days under refrigeration (8°C, 46°F), and for 6 weeks in the frozen state (at or below -20°C, -4°F).

0.9 percent Sodium Chloride Injection
5 percent Dextrose Injection
Lactated Ringer's Injection

Reconstituted Cefmetazole Sodium solutions may be stored in glass, Viaflex PL146 or McGaw PAB flexible plastic parenteral solution containers.

Do not refreeze thawed solutions.

At the end of the time periods specified above, any unused solutions or frozen material should be discarded.

The vials should be stored at controlled room temperature 15°-30°C (59°-86°F).

DIRECTIONS FOR USE OF PLASTIC CONTAINERS
STORAGE

Use an appropriate storage module in order to avoid unnecessary handling and to prevent surface contact between bags. Store in a freezer capable of maintaining a temperature of -20°C (-4°F).

THAWING OF PLASTIC CONTAINERS

Thaw frozen bag at room temperature (25°C, 77°F). [DO NOT FORCE THAW BY IMMERSION IN WATER BATHS OR BY MICROWAVE IRRADIATION.]

► SHOWN IN PRODUCT IDENTIFICATION GUIDE

Check for minute leaks by squeezing bag firmly. If leaks are detected, discard solution as sterility may be impaired.

The bag should be visually inspected. Components of the solution may precipitate in the frozen state and will dissolve upon reaching room temperature with little or no agitation. If after visual inspection the solution remains cloudy or if an insoluble precipitate is noted or if any seals or outlet parts are not intact, the bag should be discarded.

The thawed solution is stable for 24 hours under either refrigeration (8°C, 46°F) or at room temperature (25°C, 77°F). Do not refreeze thawed antibiotics.

Caution: Do not use plastic containers in series connections. Such use could result in an embolism due to residual air being drawn from the primary container before administration of the fluid from the secondary container is complete.

PREPARATION FOR ADMINISTRATION:
a. Suspend container(s) from eyelet support.
b. Remove protector from outlet part at bottom of container.
c. Attach administration set. Refer to complete directions accompanying set.

REFERENCES
1. National Committee for Clinical Laboratory Standards Approved Standard: *Performance Standards for Antimicrobial Disk Susceptibility Tests* 3rd Edition, Vol. 4(16): M2-A3, Villanova, PA, December, 1985. 2. National Committee for Clinical Laboratory Standards, Tentative Standard: *Methods for Dilution Antimicrobial Susceptibility Tests for Bacteria That Grow Aerobically*, 2nd Edition, Vol. 8(8): M7-T2, Villanova, PA, December 1988.

HOW SUPPLIED
INJECTION: 1 GM

BRAND/MANUFACTURER	NDC	SIZE	AWP
○ **BRAND**			
ZEFAZONE I.V.: Upjohn	00009-3512-01	50 ml 24s	$240.00

INJECTION: 2 GM

BRAND/MANUFACTURER	NDC	SIZE	AWP
○ **BRAND**			
ZEFAZONE I.V.: Upjohn	00009-3513-01	50 ml 24s	$411.30

POWDER FOR INJECTION: 1 GM

BRAND/MANUFACTURER	NDC	SIZE	AWP
○ **BRAND**			
ZEFAZONE: Upjohn	00009-3471-01	10s	$71.90

POWDER FOR INJECTION: 2 GM

BRAND/MANUFACTURER	NDC	SIZE	AWP
○ **BRAND**			
ZEFAZONE: Upjohn	00009-3477-01	10s	$143.30

Cefobid *SEE* CEFOPERAZONE SODIUM

Cefonicid Sodium

DESCRIPTION
Cefonicid Sodium a sterile, lyophilized, semi-synthetic, bread spectrum cephalosporin antibiotic for intravenous and intramuscular administration, is 5-Thia-1-azabicyclo[4.2.0]oct-2-ene-2-carboxylic acid, 7-[(hydroxyphenyl -acetyl)-amino]-8-oxo-3-[[[1-(sulfomethyl)-1H-tetrazol-5- yl] thio]methyl]-disodium salt, [6R-][6α, 7β(R)]].

Cefonicid Sodium contains 85 mg (3.7 mEq) Sodium per gram of Cefonicid activity.

Following is its chemical structure:

CLINICAL PHARMACOLOGY
HUMAN PHARMACOLOGY
The table below demonstrates the levels and duration of Cefonicid Sodium in serum following intravenous and intramuscular administration of 1 gram to normal volunteers. (See related table).

Serum half-life is approximately 4.5 hours with intravenous and intramuscular administration. Cefonicid Sodium is highly (greater than 90%) and reversibly protein bound.

Cefonicid Sodium is not metabolized; 99% is excreted unchanged in the urine in 24 hours. A 500 mg IM dose provides a high (384 mcg/mL) urinary concentration at 6 to 8 hours. Probenecid, given concurrently with Cefonicid Sodium slows renal excretion, produces higher peak serum levels and significantly increases the serum half-life of the drug (8.2 hours).

Cefonicid Sodium reaches therapeutic levels in the following tissues and fluids: (See related table).

Note: Although Cefonicid Sodium reaches therapeutic levels in bile, those levels are lower than those seen with other cephalosporins, and amounts of Cefonicid Sodium released into the gastrointestinal tract are minute. This small amount of Cefonicid Sodium in the gastrointestinal tract is thought to be the reason for the low incidence of gastrointestinal reactions following therapy with Cefonicid Sodium.

No disulfiram-like reactions were reported in a crossover study conducted in healthy volunteers receiving Cefonicid Sodium and alcohol.

MICROBIOLOGY
The bactericidal action of Cefonicid Sodium results from inhibition of cell-wall synthesis. Cefonicid Sodium is highly resistant to beta-lactamases produced by *Staphylococcus aureus, Haemophilus influenzae, Neisseria gonorrheae* and Richmond type I beta-lactamases. Cefonicid Sodium is resistant to degradation by beta-lactamases from certain members of *Enterobacteriaceae.* Active against a wide range of gram-positive and gram-negative organisms, Cefonicid Sodium is usually active against the following organisms *in vitro* and in clinical situations:

Gram-Positive Aerobes: Staphylococcus aureus (beta-lactamase producing and non-beta-lactamase producing) and *S. epidermidis* (Note: Methicillin-resistant staphylococci are resistant to cephalosporins, including Cefonicid; *Streptococcus pneumoniae, S. pyogenes* (Group A beta-hemolytic *Streptococcus*), and *S. Agalactiae* (Group B *Streptococcus*).

Gram-Negative Aerobes: Escherichia coli; Klebsiella pneumoniae; Providencia rettgeri (formerly *Proteus rettgeri); Proteus vulgaris; Morganella morganii* (formerly *Proteus morganii); Proteus mirabilis;* and *Haemophilus influenzae* (ampicillin-sensitive and -resistant).

The following *in vitro* data are available but their clinical significance is unknown Cefonicid Sodium is usually active against the following organisms *in vitro:*

Gram-Negative Aerobes: Moraxella (formerly *Branhamella) catarrhalis; Klebsiella oxytoca; Enterobacter aerogenes; Neisseria gonorrhoeae* (penicillin-sensitive and -resistant); *Citrobacter freundii* and *C. diversus.*

Gram-Positive Anaerobes: Clostridium perfringens; Peptostreptococcus anaerobius; Peptococcus magnus; P. prevotii; and *Propionibacterium acnes.*

Gram-Negative Anaerobes: Fusobacterium nucleatum.

Cefonicid Sodium is usually inactive *in vitro* against most strains of *Pseudomonas, Serratia, Enterococcus* and *Acinetobacter.* Most strains of *B. fragilis* are resistant.

SUSCEPTIBILITY TESTING
Results from standardized single-disk susceptibility tests using a 30 mcg Cefonicid Sodium disk should be interpreted according to the following criteria:

Zones of 18 mm or greater indicate that the tested organism is susceptible to Cefonicid Sodium and is likely to respond to therapy.
Zones from 15 to 17 mm indicate that the tested organism is of intermediate (moderate) susceptibility, and is likely to respond to therapy if a higher dosage is used or if the infection is confined to tissues and fluids in which high antibiotic levels are attained.
Zones of 14 mm or less indicate that the organism is resistant.

Only the Cefonicid Sodium disk should be used to determine susceptibility, since *in vitro* tests show that Cefonicid Sodium has activity against certain strains not susceptible to other cephalosporins. The Cefonicid Sodium disk should not be used for testing susceptibility to other cephalosporins.

A bacterial isolate may be considered susceptible if the MIC value for Cefonicid Sodium is equal to or less than 8 mcg/mL in accordance with the National Committee for Clinical Laboratory Standards (NCCLS) guidelines. Organisms are considered resistant if the MIC is equal to or greater than 32 mcg/mL. For most organisms the MBC value for Cefonicid Sodium is the same as the MIC value.

The standardized quality control procedure requires use of control organisms. The 30 mcg Cefonicid Sodium disk should give the zone diameters listed below for the quality control strains.

Organism	ATCC	Zone Size Range
E.coli	25922	25 to 29 mm
S. aureus	25923	22 to 28 mm

SERUM CONCENTRATIONS AFTER 1 GRAM ADMINISTRATION (mcg/mL)

Interval	5 min.	15 min.	30 min.	1 hr.	2 hr.	4 hr.	6 hr.	8 hr.	10 hr.	12 hr.	24 hr.
IV	221.3	176.4	147.6	124.2	88.9	61.4	40.0	29.3	20.6	15.2	2.6
IM	13.5	45.9	73.1	98.6	97.1	77.8	54.9	38.5	28.9	20.6	4.5

◆ RATED THERAPEUTICALLY EQUIVALENT; ◇ THERAPEUTIC EQUIVALENCE UNCONFIRMED; ○ UNRATED

INDICATIONS AND USAGE

Due to the long half-life of Cefonicid Sodium a 1 gram dose results in therapeutic serum levels which provide coverage against susceptible organisms (listed below) for 24 hours.

Studies on specimens obtained prior to therapy should be used to determine the susceptibility of the causative organisms to Cefonicid Sodium. Therapy with Cefonicid Sodium may be initiated pending results of the studies; however, treatment should be adjusted according to study findings.

TREATMENT

Cefonicid sodium is indicated in the treatment of infections due to susceptible strains of the microorganisms listed below:

Lower Respiratory Tract Infections: due to *Streptococcus pneumoniae; Klebsiella pneumoniae,** *Escherichia coli*; and *Haemophilus influenzae* (ampicillin-resistant and ampicillin-sensitive).

Urinary Tract Infections: due to *Escherichia coli; Proteus mirabilis* and *Proteus* spp. (which may include the organisms now called *Proteus vulgaris,** *Providencia rettgeri* and *Morganella morganii*); and *Klebsiella pneumoniae.**

Skin and Skin Structure Infections: due to *Staphylococcus aureus* and *S. epidermidis; Streptococcus pyogenes* (Group A *Streptococcus*) and *S. agalactiae* (Group B *Streptococcus*).

Septicemia: due to *Streptococcus pneumoniae* and *Escherichia coli.**

Bone and Joint Infections: due to *Staphylococcus aureus.*

SURGICAL PROPHYLAXIS

Administration of a single 1 gram dose of Cefonicid Sodium before surgery may reduce the incidence of postoperative infections in patients undergoing surgical procedures classified as contaminated or potentially contaminated (e.g., colorectal surgery, vaginal hysterectomy, or cholecystectomy in high-risk patients), or in patients in whom infection at the operative site would present a serious risk (e.g., prosthetic arthroplasty, open heart surgery). Although Cefonicid has been shown to be as effective as cefazolin in prevention of infection following coronary artery bypass surgery, no placebo-controlled trials have been conducted to evaluate any cephalosporin antibiotic in the prevention of infection following coronary artery bypass surgery or prosthetic heart valve replacement.

In cesarean section, the use of Cefonicid Sodium (after the umbilical cord has been clamped) may reduce the incidence of certain postoperative infections.

When administered 1 hour prior to surgical procedures for which it is indicated, a single 1 gram dose of Cefonicid Sodium provides protection from most infections due to susceptible organisms throughout the course of the procedure. Intraoperative and/or postoperative administrations of Cefonicid Sodium are not necessary. Daily doses of Cefonicid Sodium may be administered for 2 additional days in patients undergoing prosthetic arthroplasty or open heart surgery.

If there are signs of infection, the causative organisms should be identified and appropriate therapy determined through susceptibility testing.

Before using Cefonicid Sodium concomitantly with other antibiotics, the prescribing information for those agents should be reviewed for contraindications, warnings, precautions and adverse reactions. Renal function should be carefully monitored.

UNLABELED USES

Cefonocid Sodium is used alone or as an adjunct in the treatment of both complicated and uncomplicated urinary tract infections and uncomplicated gonorrhea.

CONTRAINDICATIONS

Cefonicid Sodium is contraindicated in persons who have shown hypersensitivity to cephalosporin antibiotics.

WARNINGS

BEFORE THERAPY WITH CEFONICID IS INSTITUTED, CAREFUL INQUIRY SHOULD BE MADE TO DETERMINE WHETHER THE PATIENT HAS HAD PREVIOUS HYPERSENSITIVITY REACTIONS TO CEPHALOSPORINS, PENICILLINS OR OTHER DRUGS. THIS PRODUCT SHOULD BE GIVEN CAUTIOUSLY TO PENICILLIN-SENSITIVE PATIENTS. ANTIBIOTICS SHOULD BE ADMINISTERED WITH CAUTION TO ANY PATIENT WHO HAS DEMONSTRATED SOME FORM OF ALLERGY, PARTICULARLY TO DRUGS. SERIOUS ACUTE HYPERSENSITIVITY REACTIONS MAY REQUIRE EPINEPHRINE AND OTHER EMERGENCY MEASURES.

Pseudomembranous colitis has been reported with nearly all antibacterial agents, including Cefonicid Sodium and has ranged in severity from mild to life-threatening. Therefore, it is important to consider this diagnosis in patients who present with diarrhea subsequent to the administration of antibacterial agents.

Treatment with antibacterial agents alters the normal flora of the colon and may permit overgrowth of clostridia. Studies indicate that a toxin produced by *Clostridium difficile* is one primary cause of "antibiotic-associated colitis."

Mild cases of pseudomembranous colitis usually respond to drug discontinuation alone. In moderate to severe cases, consideration should be given to management with fluids and electrolytes, protein supplementation and treatment with an antibacterial drug clinically effective against *C. difficile* colitis.

PRECAUTIONS

General: With any antibiotic, prolonged use may result in overgrowth of nonsusceptible organisms. Careful observation is essential, and appropriate measures should be taken if superinfection occurs.

Drug Interactions: Nephrotoxicity has been reported following concomitant administration of other cephalosporins and aminoglycosides.

Carcinogenesis, Mutagenesis, Impairment of Fertility: Betalactam antibiotics with methyl-thio-tetrazole side chains have been shown to cause testicular atrophy in prepubertal rats, which persisted into adulthood and resulted in decreased spermatogenesis and decreased fertility. Cefonicid, which contains a methylsulfonic-thio-tetrazole moiety, has no adverse effect on the male reproductive system of prepubertal, juvenile or adult rats when given under identical conditions.

Carcinogenicity studies of Cefonicid have not been conducted: however, results of mutagenicity studies (i.e., Ames/Salmonella/microsome plate assay and the micronucleus test in mice) were negative.

Pregnancy: (Category B.) Reproduction studies have been performed in mice, rabbits and rats at doses up to an equivalent of 40 times the usual adult human dose and have revealed no evidence of impaired fertility or harm to the fetus due to Cefonicid Sodium. There are, however, no adequate and well controlled studies in pregnant women. Because animal reproduction studies are not always predictive of human response, this drug should be used in pregnancy only if clearly needed.

Labor and Delivery: In cesarean section, Cetonicid Sodium should be administered only after the umbilical cord has been clamped.

Nursing Mothers: Cefonicid Sodium is excreted in human milk in low concentrations. Caution should be exercised when Cefonicid Sodium is administered to a nursing woman.

Pediatric Use: Safety and effectiveness in children have not been established.

ADVERSE REACTIONS

Cefonicid Sodium is generally well tolerated and adverse reactions have occurred infrequently. The most common adverse reaction has been pain on IM injection. On-therapy conditions occurring in greater than 1% of Cefonicid Sodium treated patients were:

Injection Site Phenomena (5.7%): Pain and/or discomfort on injection: less often, burning, phlebitis at IV site.

Increased Platelets (1.7%).

Increased Eosinophils (2.9%).

Liver Function Test Alterations (1.6%): Increased alkaline phosphatase, increased SGOT, increased SGPT, increased GGTP, increased LDH.

Less frequent on-therapy conditions occurring in less than 1% of Cefonicid Sodium treated patients were:

Hypersensitivity Reactions: Fever, rash, pruritus, erythema, myalgia and anaphylactoid-type reactions have been reported.

Hematology: Decreased WBC, neutropenia, thrombocytopenia, positive Coombs' test.

---

* Efficacy for this organism in this organ system has been demonstrated in fewer than 10 infections.

TISSUE AND BODY FLUID LEVELS

Tissue or Body Fluid	Dosage and Route (No. of Patients Sampled)	Time of Sampling After Dose	Average Tissue or Fluid Levels (mcg/g or mL)
Bone	1 g IM (7)	60 to 90 min.	6.8
	1 g IM (10)	44 to 99 min.	14.0
Gallbladder	1 g IM (10)	60 to 70 min.	15.5
Bile	1 g IM (10)	60 to 70 min.	7.5
Prostate	1 g IM (10)	50 to 115 min.	13.0
Uterine Tissue	1 g IM (6)	60 to 90 min.	17.5
Wound Fluid	1 g IM (10)	60 to 75 min.	37.7
Purulent Wound	1 g IM (9)	60 min.	11.5
Adipose Tissue	1 g IM (5)	60 min.	4.0
Atrial Appendage	1 g IM (7)	77 to 170 min.	7.5
	2 g IM (7)	105 to 170 min.	8.7
	15 mg/kg IV (10)	53 to 160 min.	15.4

► SHOWN IN PRODUCT IDENTIFICATION GUIDE

Renal: Increased BUN and creatinine levels have occasionally been seen. Rare reports of acute renal failure associated with interstitial nephritis, observed with other beta-lactam antibiotics, have also occurred with Cefonicid Sodium.

Gastrointestinal: Diarrhea and pseudomembranous colitis. Onset of pseudomembranous colitis symptoms may occur during or after antibiotic treatment (see "Warnings").

DOSAGE AND ADMINISTRATION

GENERAL

The usual adult dosage is 1 gram of Cefonicid Sodium given once every 24 hours, intravenously of by deep intramuscular injection. Doses in excess of 1 gram daily are rarely necessary; however, in exceptional cases dosage of up to 2 grams given once daily have been well tolerated. When administering 2 gram IM doses once daily, ½ the dose should be administered in different large muscle masses.

OUTPATIENT USE

Cefonicid Sodium has been used (once daily IM or IV) on an outpatient basis. Individuals responsible for outpatient administration of Cefonicid Sodium should be instructed thoroughly in appropriate procedures for storage, reconstitution and administration.

SURGICAL PROPHYLAXIS

When administered 1 hour prior to appropriate surgical procedures (see "Indications and Usage"), a 1 gram dose of Cefonicid Sodium provides protection from most infections due to susceptible organisms throughout the course of the procedure. Intraoperative and/or postoperative administrations of Cefonicid Sodium are not necessary. Daily doses of Cefonicid Sodium may be administered for 2 additional days in patients undergoing prosthetic arthroplasty or open heart surgery.

In cesarean section Cefonicid Sodium should be administered only after the umbilical cord has been clamped.

GENERAL GUIDELINES FOR DOSAGE OF CEFONICID SODIUM, IV OR IM

Type of Infection	Daily Dose (grams)	Frequency
Uncomplicated Urinary Tract	0.5	once every 24 hours
Mild to Moderate	1	once every 24 hours
Severe or Life-Threatening	2*	once every 24 hours
Surgical Prophylaxis	1	1 hour preoperatively

* When administering 2 gram IM doses once daily, 1/2 the dose should be administered in different large muscle masses.

IMPAIRED RENAL FUNCTION

Modification of Cefonicid Sodium dosage is necessary in patients with impaired renal function. Following an initial loading dosage of 7.5 mg/kg IM or IV, the maintenance dosing schedule shown below should be followed. Further dosing should be determined by severity of the infection and susceptibility of the causative organism. (See related table).

Note: It is not necessary to administer additional dosage following dialysis.

PREPARATION OF PARENTERAL SOLUTION

Parenteral drug products should be SHAKEN WELL when reconstituted, and inspected visually for particulate matter prior to administration. If particulate matter is evident in reconstituted fluids, the drug solutions should be discarded.

RECONSTITUTION

Single Dose Vials: For IM injection, IV direct (bolus) injection or IV infusion, reconstitute with Sterile Water for Injection according to the following table. SHAKE WELL.

Vial Size	Diluent to Be Added	Approx. Avail. Volume	Approx. Avg. Concentration
500 mg	2.0 mL	2.2 mL	225 mg/mL
1 gram	2.5 mL	3.1 mL	325 mg/mL

These solutions of Cefonicid Sodium are stable 24 hours at room temperature or 72 hours if refrigerated (5°C). Slight yellowing does not affect potency.

For IV infusion, dilute reconstituted solution in 50 to 100 mL of the parenteral fluids listed under "Administration."

For IM injection, IV direct (bolus) injection or IV infusion, reconstitute with Sterile Water for Injection, Bacteriostatic Water for Injection or Sodium Chloride Injection according to the following table:

Amount of Diluent	Approx. Concentration	Approx. Avail. Volume
25 mL	1 gram/3 mL	31 mL
45 mL	1 gram/5 mL	51 mL

These solutions of Cefonicid Sodium are stable 24 hours at room temperature or 72 hours if refrigerated (5°C). Slight yellowing does not affect potency.

For IV infusion add to parenteral fluids listed under "Administration."

"Piggyback" Vials: Reconstitute with 50 to 100 mL of Sodium Chloride Injection or other IV solution listed under "Administration." Administer with primary IV fluids, as a single dose. These solutions of Cefonicid Sodium are stable 24 hours at room temperature or 72 hours if refrigerated (5°C). Slight yellowing does not affect potency.

A solution of 1 gram of Cefonicid Sodium in 18 mL of Sterile Water for Injection is isotonic.

ADMINISTRATION

IM Injection: Inject well within the body of a relatively large muscle. Aspiration is necessary to avoid inadvertent injection into a blood vessel. When administering 2 gram IM doses once daily, 1/2 the dose should be given in different large muscle masses.

IV Administration: For direct (bolus) injection, administer reconstituted Cefonicid Sodium slowly over 3 to 5 minutes, directly or through tubing for patients receiving parenteral fluids (see list below). For infusion, dilute reconstituted Cefonicid Sodium in 50 to 100 mL of 1 of the following solutions:

0.9% Sodium Chloride Injection, USP
5% Dextrose Injection, USP
5% Dextrose and 0.9% Sodium Chloride Injection, USP
5% Dextrose and 0.45% Sodium Chloride Injection, USP
5% Dextrose and 0.2% Sodium Chloride Injection, USP
10% Dextrose Injection, USP
Ringer's Injection, USP
Lactated Ringer's Injection, USP
5% Dextrose and Lactated Ringer's Injection
10% Invert Sugar in Sterile Water for Injection
5% Dextrose and 0.15% Potassium Chloride Injection
Sodium Lactate Injection, USP

In these fluids Cefonicid Sodium is stable 24 hours at room temperature or 72 hours if refrigerated (5°C). Slight yellowing does not affect potency.

Before reconstitution, Cefonicid sodium should be protected from light and refrigerated (2° to 8°C).

J CODES
1 g IV—J0695

DOSAGE OF CEFONICID SODIUM IN ADULTS WITH REDUCED RENAL FUNCTION

Creatinine Clearance (mL/min per 1.73 M²)	Dosage Regiman *(Monitor renal function and adjust accordingly.)*	
	Mild to Moderate Infections	Severe Infections
79 to 60	10 mg/kg (every 24 hours)	25 mg/kg (every 24 hours)
59 to 40	8 mg/kg (every 24 hours)	20 mg/kg (every 24 hours)
39 to 20	4 mg/kg (every 24 hours)	15 mg/kg (every 24 hours)
19 to 10	4 mg/kg (every 24 hours)	15 mg/kg (every 48 hours)
9 to 5	4 mg/kg (every 3 to 5 days)	15 mg/kg (every 3 to 5 days)
< 5	3 mg/kg (every 3 to 5 days)	4 mg/kg (every 3 to 5 days)

◆ RATED THERAPEUTICALLY EQUIVALENT; ◇ THERAPEUTIC EQUIVALENCE UNCONFIRMED; ○ UNRATED

HOW SUPPLIED
POWDER FOR INJECTION: 1 GM

BRAND/MANUFACTURER	NDC	SIZE	AWP
○ BRAND			
MONOCID: SK Beecham Pharm	00007-4353-01	1s	$26.10
	00007-4354-11	10s	$271.05

Cefoperazone Sodium

DESCRIPTION

Cefoperazone Sodium is a sterile, semisynthetic, broad-spectrum, parenteral cephalosporin antibiotic for intravenous or intramuscular administration. It is the sodium salt of 7-[D(-)-α-(4-ethyl-2,3-dioxo- 1-piperazinecarboxamido)-α-(4-hydroxyphenyl)acetamido]-3-[(l-methyl-1H-tetrazol-5-yl)thiomethyl]-3-cephem-4-carboxylic acid. Its chemical formula is $C_{25}H_{26}N_9NaO_8S_2$ with a molecular weight of 667.65.

Cefoperazone Sodium contains 34 mg sodium (1.5 mEq) per gram. Cefoperazone Sodium is a white powder which is freely soluble in water. The pH of a 25% (w/v) freshly reconstituted solution varies between 4.5-6.5 and the solution ranges from colorless to straw yellow depending on the concentration.

Cefoperazone Sodium in crystalline form is supplied in vials equivalent to 1 g or 2 g of Cefoperazone and in Piggyback Units for intravenous administration equivalent to 1 g or 2 g Cefoperazone. Cefoperazone is also supplied premixed as a frozen, sterile, nonpyrogenic, iso-osmotic solution equivalent to 1 g or 2 g Cefoperazone in plastic containers. After thawing, the solution is intended for intravenous use.

The plastic container is fabricated from specially formulated polyvinyl chloride. Solutions in contact with the plastic container can leach out certain of its chemical components in very small amounts within the expiration period, e.g., di-2-ethylhexyl phthalate (DEHP), up to 5 parts per million. However, the safety of the plastic has been confirmed in tests in animals according to the USP biological tests for plastic containers, as well as by tissue culture toxicity studies.

A pharmacy bulk package is a container of a sterile preparation for parenteral use that contains many single doses.

The pharmacy bulk package is for use in a pharmacy admixture service; it provides many single doses of Cefoperazone for addition to suitable parenteral fluids in the preparation of admixtures for intravenous infusion. (See "Dosage and Administration," and "Directions for Proper Use of Pharmacy Bulk Package".)

Following is its chemical structure:

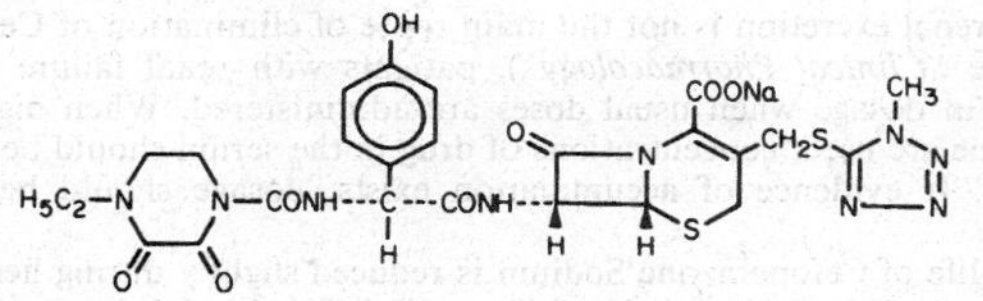

CLINICAL PHARMACOLOGY

High serum and bile levels of Cefoperazone Sodium are attained after a single dose of the drug. Table 1 demonstrates the serum concentrations of Cefoperazone Sodium in normal volunteers following either a single 15-minute constant rate intravenous infusion of 1, 2, 3, or 4 grams of the drug, or a single intramuscular injection of 1 or 2 grams of the drug.

Table 1
CEFOPERAZONE SERUM CONCENTRATIONS

Dose/ Route	Mean Serum Concentrations (mcg/mL)						
	0*	0.5 hr	1 hr	2 hr	4 hr	8 hr	12 hr
1 g IV	153	114	73	38	16	4	0.5
2 g IV	252	153	114	70	32	8	2
3 g IV	340	210	142	89	41	9	2
4 g IV	506	325	251	161	71	19	6
1 g IM	32**	52	65	57	33	7	1
2 g IM	40**	69	93	97	58	14	4

* Hours post-administration, with 0 time being the end of the infusion.
** Values obtained 15 minutes post-injection.

The mean serum half-life of Cefoperazone Sodium is approximately 2.0 hours, independent of the route of administration.

In vitro studies with human serum indicate that the degree of Cefoperazone Sodium reversible protein binding varies with the serum concentration from 93% at 25 mcg/mL of Cefoperazone Sodium to 90% at 250 mcg/mL and 82% at 500 mcg/mL.

Cefoperazone Sodium achieves therapeutic concentrations in the following body tissues and fluids:

Tissue or Fluid	Dose	Concentration
Ascitic Fluid	2 g	64 mcg/mL
Cerebrospinal Fluid (in patients with inflamed meninges)	50 mg/kg	1.8mcg/mL to 8.0 mcg/mL
Urine	2 g	3.286 mcg/mL
Sputum	3 g	6.0 mcg/mL
Endometrium	2 g	74 mcg/g
Myometrium	2 g	54 mcg/g
Palatine Tonsil	1 g	8 mcg/g
Sinus Mucous Membrane	1 g	8 mcg/g
Umbilical Cord Blood	1 g	25 mcg/mL
Amniotic Fluid	1 g	4.8 mcg/mL
Lung	1 g	28 mcg/g
Bone	2 g	40 mcg/g

Cefoperazone Sodium is excreted mainly in the bile. Maximum bile concentrations are generally obtained between one and three hours following drug administration and exceed concurrent serum concentrations by up to 100 times. Reported biliary concentrations of Cefoperazone Sodium range from 66 mcg/mL at 30 minutes to as high as 6000 mcg/mL at 3 hours after an intravenous bolus injection of 2 grams.

Following a single intramuscular or intravenous dose, the urinary recovery of Cefoperazone Sodium over a 12-hour period averages 20-30%. No significant quantity of metabolites has been found in the urine. Urinary concentrations greater than 2200 mcg/mL have been obtained following a 15-minute infusion of a 2 g dose. After an IM injection of 2 g, peak urine concentrations of almost 1000 mcg/mL have been obtained, and therapeutic levels are maintained for 12 hours.

Repeated administration of Cefoperazone Sodium at 12-hour intervals does not result in accumulation of the drug in normal subjects. Peak serum concentrations, areas under the curve (AUC's), and serum half-lives in patients with severe renal insufficiency are not significantly different from those in normal volunteers. In patients with hepatic dysfunction, the serum half-life is prolonged and urinary excretion is increased. In patients with combined renal and hepatic insufficiencies, Cefoperazone Sodium may accumulate in the serum.

Cefoperazone Sodium has been used in pediatrics, but the safety and effectiveness in children have not been established. The half-life of Cefoperazone Sodium in serum is 6-10 hours in low birth-weight neonates.

MICROBIOLOGY

Cefoperazone Sodium is active in vitro against a wide range of aerobic and anaerobic, gram-positive and gram-negative pathogens. The bactericidal action of Cefoperazone Sodium results from the inhibition of bacterial cell wall synthesis. Cefoperazone Sodium has a high degree of stability in the presence of beta-lactamases produced by most gram-negative pathogens. Cefoperazone Sodium is usually active against organisms which are resistant to other beta-lactam antibiotics because of beta-lactamase production. Cefoperazone Sodium is usually active against the following organisms in vitro and in clinical infections:

GRAM-POSITIVE AEROBES
Staphylococcus aureus, penicillinase and non-penicillinase-producing strains
   Staphylococcus epidermidis
   Streptococcus pneumoniae (formerly *Diplococcus pneumoniae*)
   Streptococcus pyogenes (Group A beta-hemolytic streptococci)
   Streptococcus agalactiae (Group B beta-hemolytic streptococci)
   Enterococcus (*Streptococcus faecalis, S. faecium* and *S. durans*)

GRAM-NEGATIVE AEROBES
Escherichia coli
   Klebsiella species (including *K. pneumoniae*)
   Enterobacter species
   Citrobacter species
   Haemophilus influenzae
   Proteus mirabilis
   Proteus vulgaris
   Morganella morganii (formerly *Proteus morganii*)
   Providencia stuartii
   Providencia rettgeri (formerly *Proteus rettgeri*)
   Serratia marcescens
   Pseudomonas aeruginosa
   Pseudomonas species
   Some strains of *Acinetobacter calcoaceticus*
   Neisseria gonorrhoeae

ANAEROBIC ORGANISMS
Gram-positive cocci (including *Peptococcus* and *Peptostreptococcus*)
   Clostridium species
   Bacteroides fragilis
   Other *Bacteroides* species

Cefoperazone Sodium is also active in vitro against a wide variety of other pathogens although the clinical significance is unknown. These organisms include: *Salmonella* and *Shigella* species, *Serratia liquefaciens, N. meningitidis, Bordetella pertussis, Yersinia enterocolitica, Clostridium difficile, Fusobacterium* species, *Eubacterium* species and beta-lactamase producing strains of *H. influenzae* and *N. gonorrhoeae*.

SUSCEPTIBILITY TESTING
Diffusion Technique: For the disk diffusion method of susceptibility testing, a 75 mcg Cefoperazone diffusion disk should be used. Organisms should be tested with the Cefoperazone 75 mcg disk since Cefoperazone has been shown in vitro to be active against organisms which are found to be resistant to other beta-lactam antibiotics.

➤ SHOWN IN PRODUCT IDENTIFICATION GUIDE

Tests should be interpreted by the following criteria:

Zone Diameter	Interpretation
Greater than or equal to 21 mm	Susceptible
16-20 mm	Moderately Susceptible
Less than or equal to 15 mm	Resistant

Quantitative procedures that require measurement of zone diameters give the most precise estimate of susceptibility. One such method which has been recommended for use with the Cefoperazone 75 mcg disk is the NCCLS approved standard. (Performance Standards for Antimicrobic Disk Susceptibility Tests. Second Information Supplement Vol. 2 No. 2 pp. 49-69. Publisher—National Committee for Clinical Laboratory Standards, Villanova, Pennsylvania.)

A report of "susceptible" indicates that the infecting organism is likely to respond to Cefoperazone Sodium therapy and a report of "resistant" indicates that the infecting organism is not likely to respond to therapy. A "moderately susceptible" report suggests that the infecting organism will be susceptible to Cefoperazone Sodium if a higher than usual dosage is used or if the infection is confined to tissues and fluids (e.g., urine or bile) in which high antibiotic levels are attained.

Dilution Techniques: Broth or agar dilution methods may be used to determine the minimal inhibitory concentration (MIC) of Cefoperazone Sodium. Serial twofold dilutions of Cefoperazone should be prepared in either broth or agar. Broth should be inoculated to contain 5×10^5 organisms/mL and agar "spotted" with 10^4 organisms.

MIC test results should be interpreted in light of serum, tissue, and body fluid concentrations of Cefoperazone Sodium. Organisms inhibited by Cefoperazone Sodium at 16 mcg/mL or less are considered susceptible, while organisms with MIC's of 17-63 mcg/mL are moderately susceptible. Organisms inhibited at Cefoperazone Sodium concentrations of greater than or equal to 64 mcg/mL are considered resistant, although clinical cures have been obtained in some patients infected by such organisms.

INDICATIONS AND USAGE

Cefoperazone Sodium is indicated for the treatment of the following infections when caused by susceptible organisms:

Respiratory Tract Infections caused by *S. pneumoniae, H. influenzae, S. aureus* (penicillinase and non-penicillinase producing strains), *S. pyogenes* (Group A beta-hemolytic streptococci), *P. aeruginosa, Klebsiella pneumoniae, E. coli, Proteus mirabilis,* and *Enterobacter* species.

Peritonitis and Other Intra-abdominal Infections caused by *E. coli, P. aeruginosa**, and anaerobic gram-negative bacilli (including *Bacteroides fragilis*).

Bacterial Septicemia caused by *S. pneumoniae, S. agalactiae**, *S. aureus, Pseudomonas aeruginosa**, *E. coli, Klebsiella* spp.*, Klebsiella pneumoniae*, Proteus species* (indole-positive and indole-negative), *Clostridium* spp.* and anaerobic gram-positive cocci.

Infections of the Skin and Skin Structures caused by *S. aureus* (penicillinase and non-penicillinase producing strains), *S. pyogenes**, and *P. aeruginosa.*

Pelvic Inflammatory Disease, Endometritis, and Other Infections of the Female Genital Tract caused by *N. gonorrhoeae, S. epidermidis**, *S. agalactiae, E. coli, Clostridium* spp.*, *Bacteroides* species (including *Bacteroides fragilis*) and anaerobic gram-positive Cocci.

Urinary Tract Infections: caused by *Escherichia coli* and *Pseudomonas aeruginosa.*

Enterococcal Infections: Although Cefoperazone has been shown to be clinically effective in the treatment of infections caused by enterococci in cases of **peritonitis and other intra-abdominal infections, infections of the skin and skin structures, pelvic inflammatory disease, endometritis and other infections of the female genital tract, and urinary tract infection,*** the majority of clinical isolates of enterococci tested are not susceptible to Cefoperazone but fall just at or in the intermediate zone of susceptibility, and are moderately resistant to Cefoperazone. However, *in vitro* susceptibility testing may not correlate directly with *in vivo* results. Despite this, Cefoperazone therapy has resulted in clinical cures of enterococcal infections, chiefly in polymicrobial infections. Cefoperazone should be used in enterococcal infections with care and at doses that achieve satisfactory serum levels of Cefoperazone.

SUSCEPTIBILITY TESTING

Before instituting treatment with Cefoperazone Sodium, appropriate specimens should be obtained for isolation of the causative organism and for determination of its susceptibility to the drug. Treatment may be started before results of susceptibility testing are available.

COMBINATION THERAPY

Synergy between Cefoperazone Sodium and aminoglycosides has been demonstrated with many gram-negative bacilli. However, such enhanced activity of these combinations is not predictable. If such therapy is considered, *in vitro* susceptibility tests should be performed to determine the activity of the drugs in combination, and renal function should be monitored carefully. (See *"Precautions",* and *"Dosage and Administration"* sections.)

---

* Efficacy of this organism in this organ system was studied in fewer than 10 infections.

CONTRAINDICATIONS

Cefoperazone Sodium is contraindicated in patients with known allergy to the cephalosporin-class of antibiotics.

WARNINGS

BEFORE THERAPY WITH CEFOPERAZONE SODIUM IS INSTITUTED, CAREFUL INQUIRY SHOULD BE MADE TO DETERMINE WHETHER THE PATIENT HAS HAD PREVIOUS HYPERSENSITIVITY REACTIONS TO CEPHALOSPORINS, PENICILLINS OR OTHER DRUGS. THIS PRODUCT SHOULD BE GIVEN CAUTIOUSLY TO PENICILLIN-SENSITIVE PATIENTS. ANTIBIOTICS SHOULD BE ADMINISTERED WITH CAUTION TO ANY PATIENT WHO HAS DEMONSTRATED SOME FORM OF ALLERGY, PARTICULARLY TO DRUGS. SERIOUS ACUTE HYPERSENSITIVITY REACTIONS MAY REQUIRE THE USE OF SUBCUTANEOUS EPINEPHRINE AND OTHER EMERGENCY MEASURES.

PSEUDOMEMBRANOUS COLITIS HAS BEEN REPORTED WITH THE USE OF CEPHALOSPORINS (AND OTHER BROAD-SPECTRUM ANTIBIOTICS); THEREFORE, IT IS IMPORTANT TO CONSIDER ITS DIAGNOSIS IN PATIENTS WHO DEVELOP DIARRHEA IN ASSOCIATION WITH ANTIBIOTIC USE.

Treatment with broad-spectrum antibiotics alters normal flora of the colon and may permit overgrowth of clostridia. Studies indicate a toxin produced by *Clostridium difficile* is one primary cause of antibiotic-associated colitis. Cholestyramine and colestipol resins have been shown to bind the toxin *in vitro.*

Mild cases of colitis may respond to drug discontinuance alone.

Moderate to severe cases should be managed with fluid, electrolyte, and protein supplementation as indicated.

When the colitis is not relieved by drug discontinuance or when it is severe, oral vancomycin is the treatment of choice for antibiotic-associated pseudomembranous colitis produced by *C. difficile.* Other causes of colitis should also be considered.

PRECAUTIONS

Although transient elevations of the BUN and serum creatinine have been observed, Cefoperazone Sodium alone does not appear to cause significant nephrotoxicity. However, concomitant administration of aminoglycosides and other cephalosporins has caused nephrotoxicity.

Cefoperazone Sodium is extensively excreted in bile. The serum half-life of Cefoperazone is increased 2-4 fold in patients with hepatic disease and/or biliary obstruction. In general, total daily dosage above 4 g should not be necessary in such patients. If higher dosages are used, serum concentrations should be monitored.

Because renal excretion is not the main route of elimination of Cefoperazone Sodium (see *"Clinical Pharmacology"),* patients with renal failure require no adjustment in dosage when usual doses are administered. When high doses of Cefoperazone are used, concentrations of drug in the serum should be monitored periodically. If evidence of accumulation exists, dosage should be decreased accordingly.

The half-life of Cefoperazone Sodium is reduced slightly during hemodialysis. Thus, dosing should be scheduled to follow a dialysis period. In patients with both hepatic dysfunction and significant renal disease, Cefoperazone Sodium dosage should not exceed 1-2g daily without close monitoring of serum concentrations.

As with other antibiotics, vitamin K deficiency has occurred rarely in patients treated with Cefoperazone Sodium. The mechanism is most probably related to the suppression of gut flora which normally synthesize this vitamin. Those at risk include patients with a poor nutritional status, malabsorption states (e.g., cystic fibrosis), alcoholism, and patients on prolonged hyperalimentation regimens (administered either intravenously or via a naso-gastric tube). Prothrombin time should be monitored in these patients and exogenous vitamin K administered as indicated.

A disulfiram-like reaction characterized by flushing, sweating, headache, and tachycardia has been reported when alcohol (beer, wine) was ingested within 72 hours after Cefoperazone Sodium administration. Patients should be cautioned about the ingestion of alcoholic beverages following the administration of Cefoperazone Sodium. A similar reaction has been reported with other cephalosporins.

Prolonged use of Cefoperazone Sodium may result in the overgrowth of nonsusceptible organisms. Careful observation of the patient is essential. If superinfection occurs during therapy, appropriate measures should be taken.

Cefoperazone Sodium should be prescribed with caution in individuals with a history of gastrointestinal disease, particularly colitis.

DRUG LABORATORY TEST INTERACTIONS

A false-positive reaction for glucose in the urine may occur with Benedict's or Fehling's solution.

CARCINOGENESIS, MUTAGENESIS, IMPAIRMENT OF FERTILITY

Long term studies in animals have not been performed to evaluate carcinogenic potential. The maximum duration of Cefoperazone Sodium animal toxicity studies is six months. In none of the *in vivo* or *in vitro* genetic toxicology studies did Cefoperazone Sodium show any mutagenic potential at either the chromosomal or subchromosomal level. Cefoperazone Sodium produced no impairment of fertility and had no effects on general reproductive performance or fetal development when administered subcutaneously at daily doses up to 500 to 1000 mg/kg prior to and during mating, and to pregnant female rats during gestation. These doses are 10 to 20 times the estimated usual single clinical dose. Cefoperazone Sodium had adverse effects on the testes of prepubertal rats at all

---

◆ RATED THERAPEUTICALLY EQUIVALENT; ◇ THERAPEUTIC EQUIVALENCE UNCONFIRMED; ○ UNRATED

doses tested. Subcutaneous administration of 1000 mg/kg per day (approximately 16 times the average adult human dose) resulted in reduced testicular weight, arrested spermatogenesis, reduced germinal cell population and vacuolation of Sertoli cell cytoplasm. The severity of lesions was dose dependent in the 100 to 1000 mg/kg per day range; the low dose caused a minor decrease in spermatocytes. This effect has not been observed in adult rats. Histologically the lesions were reversible at all but the highest dosage levels. However, these studies did not evaluate subsequent development of reproductive function in the rats. The relationship of these findings to human is unknown.

USAGE IN PREGNANCY

Pregnancy Category B: Reproduction studies have been performed in mice, rats, and monkeys at doses up to 10 times the human dose and have revealed no evidence of impaired fertility or harm to the fetus due to Cefoperazone Sodium. There are, however, no adequate and well controlled studies in pregnant women. Because animal reproduction studies are not always predictive of human response, this drug should be used during pregnancy only if clearly needed.

USAGE IN NURSING MOTHERS

Only low concentrations of Cefoperazone Sodium are excreted in human milk. Although Cefoperazone Sodium passes poorly into breast milk of nursing mothers, caution should be exercised when Cefoperazone Sodium is administered to a nursing woman.

PEDIATRIC USE

Safety and effectiveness in children have not been established. For information concerning testicular changes in prepubertal rats see *"Carcinogenesis, Mutagenesis, Impairment of Fertility"*.

ADVERSE REACTIONS

In clinical studies the following adverse effects were observed and were considered to be related to Cefoperazone Sodium therapy or of uncertain etiology.

Hypersensitivity: As with all cephalosporins, hypersensitivity manifested by skin reactions (1 patient in 45), drug fever (1 in 260), or a change in Coombs' test (1 in 60) has been reported. These reactions are more likely to occur in patients with a history of allergies, particularly to penicillin.

Hematology: As with other beta-lactam antibiotics, reversible neutropenia may occur with prolonged administration. Slight decreases in neutrophil count (1 patient in 50) have been reported. Decreased hemoglobins (1 in 20) or hematocrits (1 in 20) have been reported, which is consistent with published literature on other cephalosporins. Transient eosinophilia has occurred in 1 patient in 10.

Hepatic: Of 1285 patients treated with Cefoperazone in clinical trials, one patient with a history of liver disease developed significantly elevated liver function enzymes during Cefoperazone Sodium therapy. Clinical signs and symptoms of nonspecific hepatitis accompanied these increases. After Cefoperazone Sodium therapy was discontinued, the patient's enzymes returned to pre-treatment levels and the symptomatology resolved. As with other antibiotics that achieve high bile levels, mild transient elevations of liver function enzymes have been observed in 5-10% of the patients receiving Cefoperazone Sodium therapy. The relevance of these findings, which were not accompanied by overt signs or symptoms of hepatic dysfunction, has not been established.

Gastrointestinal: Diarrhea or loose stools has been reported in 1 in 30 patients. Most of these experiences have been mild or moderate in severity and self-limiting in nature. In all cases, these symptoms responded to symptomatic therapy or ceased when Cefoperazone therapy was stopped. Nausea and vomiting have been reported rarely.

Symptoms of pseudomembranous colitis can appear during or for several weeks subsequent to antibiotic therapy (see *"Warnings"*).

Renal Function Tests: Transient elevations of the BUN (1 in 16) and serum creatinine (1 in 48) have been noted.

Local Reactions: Cefoperazone Sodium is well tolerated following intramuscular administration. Occasionally, transient pain (1 in 140) may follow administration by this route. When Cefoperazone Sodium is administered by intravenous infusion some patients may develop phlebitis (1 in 120) at the infusion site.

DOSAGE AND ADMINISTRATION

Sterile Cefoperazone Sodium can be administered by IM or IV injection (following dilution). However, the intent of the pharmacy bulk package is for the preparation of solutions for IV infusion only.

The usual adult daily dose of Cefoperazone Sodium is 2 to 4 grams per day administered in equally divided doses every 12 hours.

In severe infections or infections caused by less sensitive organisms, the total daily dose and/or frequency may be increased. Patients have been successfully treated with a total daily dosage of 6-12 grams divided into 2,3 or 4 administrations ranging from 1.5 to 4 grams per dose.

In a pharmacokinetic study, a total daily dose of 16 grams was administered to severely immunocompromised patients by constant infusion without complications. Steady state serum concentrations were approximately 150 mcg/mL in these patients.

When treating infections caused by *Streptococcus pyogenes*, therapy should be continued for at least 10 days.

Solutions of Cefoperazone Sodium and aminoglycoside should not be directly mixed, since there is a physical incompatibility between them. If combination therapy with Cefoperazone Sodium and an aminoglycoside is comtemplated (see

"Indications") this can be accomplished by sequential intermittent intravenous infusion provided that separate secondary intravenous tubing is used, and that the primary intravenous tubing is adequately irrigated with an approved diluent between doses. It is also suggested that Cefoperazone Sodium be administered prior to the aminoglycoside. *In vitro* testing of the effectiveness of drug combination(s) is recommended.

RECONSTITUTION

The following solutions may be used for the initial reconstitution of Cefoperazone Sodium sterile powder:

Table 2.

SOLUTIONS FOR INITIAL RECONSTITUTION.

5% Dextrose Injection (USP)
5% Dextrose and 0.9% Sodium Chloride Injection (USP)
5% Dextrose and 0.2% Sodium Chloride Injection (USP)
10% Dextrose Injection (USP)
Bacteriostatic Water for Injection [Benzyl Alcohol or Parabens] (USP)*†
0.9% Sodium Chloride Injection (USP)
Normosol® M and 5% Dextrose Injection
Normosol® R
Sterile Water for Injection*

* Not to be used as a vehicle for intravenous infusion
† Preparations containing Benzyl Alcohol should not be used in neonates.

GENERAL RECONSTITUTION PROCEDURES

Cefoperazone Sodium sterile powder for intravenous or intramuscular use may be initially reconstituted with any compatible solution mentioned above in Table 2. Solutions should be allowed to stand after reconstitution to allow any foaming to dissipate to permit visual inspection for complete solubilization. Vigorous and prolonged agitation may be necessary to solubilize Cefoperazone Sodium in higher concentrations (above 333 mg Cefoperazone/mL). The maximum solubility of Cefoperazone Sodium sterile powder is approximately 475 mg Cefoperazone/mL of compatible diluent.

PREPARATION FOR INTRAVENOUS USE

General: Cefoperazone Sodium concentrations between 2 mg/mL and 50 mg/mL are recommended for intravenous administration.

Preparation of Vials: Vials of Cefoperazone Sodium sterile powder may be initially reconstituted with a minimum of 2.8 mL per gram of Cefoperazone Sodium of any compatible reconstituting solution appropriate for intravenous administration listed above in Table 2. For ease of reconstitution the use of 5 mL of compatible solution per gram of Cefoperazone is recommended. The entire quantity of the resulting solution should then be withdrawn for further dilution and administration using any of the following vehicles for intravenous infusion:

Table 3.

VEHICLES FOR INTRAVENOUS INFUSION.

5% Dextrose Injection (USP)
5% Dextrose and Lactated Ringer's Injection
5% Dextrose and 0.9% Sodium Chloride Injection (USP)
5% Dextrose and 0.2% Sodium Chloride Injection (USP)
10% Dextrose Injection (USP)
Lactated Ringer's Injection (USP)
0.9% Sodium Chloride Injection (USP)
Normosol® M and 5% Dextrose Injection
Normosol® R

Preparation of Piggy Back Units: Cefoperazone sterile powder in Piggy Back Units for intravenous use may be prepared by adding between 20 mL and 40 mL of any appropriate diluent listed in Table 2 per gram of Cefoperazone. If 5% Dextrose and Lactated Ringer's Injection or Lactated Ringer's Injection (USP) is the chosen vehicle for administration the Cefoperazone sterile powder should initially be reconstituted using 2.8-5 mL per gram of any compatible reconstituting solution listed in Table 2 prior to the final dilution.

The resulting intravenous solution should be administered in one of the following manners:

Intermittent Infusion: Solutions of Cefoperazone Sodium should be administered over a 15-30 minute time period.

Continuous Infusion: Cefoperazone Sodium can be used for continuous infusion after dilution to a final concentration of between 2 and 25 mg Cefoperazone per mL.

PREPARATION FOR INTRAMUSCULAR INJECTION

Any suitable solution listed above may be used to prepare Cefoperazone Sodium sterile powder for intramuscular injection. When concentrations of 250 mg/mL or more are to be administered, a lidocaine solution should be used. These solutions should be prepared using a combination of Sterile Water for Injection and 2% Lidocaine Hydrochloride Injection (USP) that approximates a 0.5% Lidocaine Hydrochloride Solution. A two-step dilution process as follows is recommended: First, add the required amount of Sterile Water for Injection and agitate until Cefoperazone Sodium powder is completely dissolved. Second, add the required amount of 2% lidocaine and mix.

	Final Cefoperazone Concentration	Step 1 Volume of Sterile Water	Step 2 Volume of 2% Lidocaine	Withdrawable Volume*†
1 g vial	333 mg/mL	2.0 mL	0.6 mL	3 mL
	250 mg/mL	2.8 mL	1.0 mL	4 mL
2 g vial	333 mg/mL	3.8 mL	1.2 mL	6 mL
	250 mg/mL	5.4 mL	1.8 mL	8 mL

When a diluent other than Lidocaine HCl Injection (USP) is used reconstitute as follows:

	Cefoperazone Concentration	Volume of Diluent to be Added	Withdrawable Volume*
1 g vial	333 mg/mL	2.6 mL	3 mL
	250 mg/mL	3.8 mL	4 mL
2 g vial	333 mg/mL	5.0 mL	6 mL
	250 mg/mL	7.2 mL	8 mL

* There is sufficient excess present to allow for withdrawal of the stated volume.
† Final lidocaine concentration will approximate that obtained if a 0.5% Lidocaine Hydrochloride Solution is used as diluent.

DIRECTIONS FOR PROPER USE OF PHARMACY BULK PACKAGE

The 10 gram vial should be reconstituted with 95 mL of sterile water for injection in two separate aliquots in a suitable work area such as a laminar flow hood. Add 45 mL of solution, shake to dissolve and add 50 mL, shake for final solution. The resulting solution will contain 100 mg/mL of Cefoperazone. This closure may be penetrated only one time after reconstitution, if needed, using a suitable sterile transfer device or dispensing set which allows measured dispensing of the contents.

Discard unused solution within 24 hours of initial entry.

> RECONSTITUTED BULK SOLUTIONS SHOULD NOT BE USED FOR DIRECT INFUSION.

Although after reconstitution of the *pharmacy bulk package,* no significant loss of potency occurs for 24 hours at room temperature and for 5 days if refrigerated, transfer individual dose to appropriate intravenous infusion solutions as soon as possible following reconstitution of the bulk package. Discard unused portions of solution held longer than these recommended periods at room temperature or under refrigeration. The stability of the solution which has been transferred into a container varies according to diluent and concentration. (See "Storage and Stability".)

The 10 gram vials may be further diluted with the parenteral diluents listed under Table 3, "Vehicles for Intravenous Infusion". The parenteral diluents and approximate concentrations of Cefoperazone Sodium that provide stable solutions are presented under "Storage and Stability".

Parenteral drug products should be inspected visually for particulate matter and discoloration prior to administration, whenever solution and container permit.

DIRECTIONS FOR USE OF CEFOPERAZONE SODIUM INJECTION IN PLASTIC CONTAINERS

Cefoperazone supplied premixed as a frozen, sterile, iso-osmotic solution in plastic containers is to be administered either as continuous or intermittent infusion.

Thaw container at room temperature. After thawing, check for minute leaks by squeezing bag firmly. If leaks are found, discard solution as sterility may be impaired. Additives should not be introduced into this solution. Do not use if the solution is cloudy or precipitated or if the seal is not intact.

After thawing, the solution is stable for 10 days if stored under refrigeration (5°C) and for 48 hours at room temperature.

DO NOT REFREEZE. Use sterile equipment.

Caution: Do not use plastic container in series connections. Such use could result in air embolism due to residual air being drawn from the primary container before administration of the fluid from the secondary container is complete.

PREPARATION FOR ADMINISTRATION

1. Suspend container from eyelet support.
2. Remove plastic protector from outlet port at bottom of container.
3. Attach administration set. Refer to complete directions accompanying set.

Storage and Stability: Cefoperazone Sodium sterile powder is to be stored at or below 25°C (77°F) and protected from light prior to reconstitution. After reconstitution, protection from light is not necessary.

The following parenteral diluents and approximate concentrations of Cefoperazone provide stable solutions under the following conditions for the indicated time periods. (After the indicated time periods, unused portions of solutions should be discarded.)

Controlled Room Temperature (15°-25°C/59°-77°F) 24 Hours	Approximate Concentrations
Bacteriostatic Water for Injection [Benzyl Alcohol or Parabens] (USP)	300 mg/mL
5% Dextrose Injection (USP)	2 mg to 50 mg/mL
5% Dextrose and Lactated Ringer's Injection	2 mg to 50 mg/mL
5% Dextrose and 0.9% Sodium Chloride Injection (USP)	2 mg to 50 mg/mL
5% Dextrose and 0.2% Sodium Chloride Injection (USP)	2 mg to 50 mg/mL
10% Dextrose Injection (USP)	2 mg to 50 mg/mL
Lactated Ringer's Injection (USP)	2 mg/mL
0.5% Lidocaine Hydrochloride Injection (USP)	300 mg/mL
0.9% Sodium Chloride Injection (USP)	2 mg to 300 mg/mL
Normosol® M and 5% Dextrose Injection	2 mg to 50 mg/mL
Normosol® R	2 mg to 50 mg/mL
Sterile Water for Injection	300 mg/mL

Reconstituted Cefoperazone solutions may be stored in glass or plastic syringes, or in glass or flexible plastic parenteral solution containers.

Refrigerator Temperature (2°-8°C/36°-46°F) 5 Days	Approximate Concentrations
Bacteriostatic Water for Injection [Benzyl Alcohol or Parabens] (USP)	300 mg/mL
5% Dextrose Injection (USP)	2 mg to 50 mg/mL
5% Dextrose and 0.9% Sodium Chloride Injection (USP)	2 mg to 50 mg/mL
5% Dextrose and 0.2% Sodium Chloride Injection (USP)	2 mg to 50 mg/mL
Lactated Ringer's Injection (USP)	2 mg/mL
0.5% Lidocaine Hydrochloride Injection (USP)	300 mg/mL
0.9% Sodium Chloride Injection (USP)	2 mg to 300 mg/mL
Normosol® M and 5% Dextrose Injection	2 mg to 50 mg/mL
Normosol® R	2 mg to 50 mg/mL
Sterile Water for Injection	300 mg/mL

Reconstituted Cefoperazone solutions may be stored in glass or plastic syringes, or in glass or flexible plastic parenteral solution containers.

Freezer Temperature (−20° to −10°C/−4° to 14°F) 3 Weeks	Approximate Concentrations
5% Dextrose Injection (USP)	50 mg/mL
5% Dextrose and 0.9% Sodium Chloride Injection (USP)	2 mg/mL
5% Dextrose and 0.2% Sodium Chloride Injection (USP)	2 mg/mL

5 Weeks	
0.9% Sodium Chloride Injection (USP)	300 mg/mL
Sterile Water for Injection	300 mg/mL

Reconstituted Cefoperazone Sodium solutions may be stored in plastic syringes, or in flexible plastic parenteral solution containers.
Frozen samples should be thawed at room temperature before use. After thawing, unused portions should be discarded. Do not refreeze.

HOW SUPPLIED
POWDER FOR INJECTION: 1 GM

BRAND/MANUFACTURER	NDC	SIZE	AWP
○ **BRAND**			
CEFOBID: Roerig,J.B.	00049-1201-83	10s	$157.89
	00049-1211-83	10s	$168.93

POWDER FOR INJECTION: 2 GM

BRAND/MANUFACTURER	NDC	SIZE	AWP
○ **BRAND**			
CEFOBID: Roerig,J.B.	00049-1202-83	10s	$315.75
	00049-1212-83	10s	$337.88

POWDER FOR INJECTION: 10 GM

BRAND/MANUFACTURER	NDC	SIZE	AWP
○ **BRAND**			
CEFOBID: Roerig,J.B.	00049-1219-28	1s	$151.24

◆ RATED THERAPEUTICALLY EQUIVALENT; ◇ THERAPEUTIC EQUIVALENCE UNCONFIRMED; ○ UNRATED

Cefotan SEE CEFOTETAN DISODIUM

Cefotaxime Sodium

DESCRIPTION

Cefotaxime Sodium is a semisynthetic, broad spectrum cephalosporin antibiotic for parenteral administration. It is the sodium salt of 7-[2- (2-amino-4-thiazolyl) glyoxylamido]-3-(hydroxymethyl)-8-oxo-5-thia-1-azabicycio [4.2.0] oct-2-ene-2-carboxylate 7^2-(Z)-(o-methyloxime), acetate (ester). Cefotaxime Sodium contains approximately 50.5 mg (2.2 mEq) of sodium per gram of cefotaxime activity. Solutions of Cefotaxime Sodium range from very pale yellow to light amber depending on the concentration and the diluent used. The pH of the injectable solutions usually ranges from 5.0 to 7.5.

Cefotaxime Sodium equivalent to 1 gram and 2 grams Cefotaxime, is supplied as frozen, premixed iso-osmotic injections in plastic containers. Solutions range from very pale yellow to light amber. Dextrose Hydrous, USP has been added to adjust osmolality (approximately 1.7 g and 700 mg to the 1 g and 2 g Cefotaxime dosages, respectively). The injections are buffered with sodium citrate hydrous, USP. The pH is adjusted with hydrochloric acid and may be adjusted with sodium hydroxide.

The plastic container is fabricated from a specially designed multilayer plastic (PL 2040). Solutions are in contact with the polyethylene layer of this container and can leach out certain chemical components of the plastic in very small amounts within the expiration period. The suitability of the plastic has been confirmed in tests in animals according to the USP biological tests for plastic containers, as well as by tissue culture toxicity studies.

Following is its chemical structure:

CLINICAL PHARMACOLOGY

Following 1M administration of a single 500 mg or 1 g dose of Cefotaxime Sodium to normal volunteers, mean peak serum concentrations of 11.7 and 20.5 µg/mL respectively were attained within 30 minutes and declined with an elimination half-life of approximately 1 hour. There was a dose-dependent increase in serum levels after the IV administration of 500 mg. 1 g and 2 g of Cefotaxime Sodium (38.9, 101.7, and 214.4 µg/mL respectively) without alteration in the elimination half-life. There is no evidence of accumulation following repetitive IV infusion of 1 g doses every 6 hours for 14 days as there are no alterations of serum or renal clearance. About 60% of the administered dose was recovered from urine during the first 6 hours following the start of the infusion.

Approximately 20-36% of an intravenously administered dose of ^{14}C-cefotaxime is excreted by the kidney as unchanged Cefotaxime and 15-25% as the desacetyl derivative, the major metabolite. The desacetyl metabolite has been shown to contribute to the bactericidal activity. Two other urinary metabolites (M_2 and M_3) account for about 20-25%. They lack bactericidal activity.

A single 50 mg/kg dose of Cefotaxime Sodium was administered as an intravenous infusion over a 10- to 15-minute period to 29 newborn infants grouped according to birth weight and age. The mean half-life of Cefotaxime in infants with lower birth weights ($\leq$ 1500 grams), regardless of age, was longer (4.6 hours) than the mean half-life (3.4 hours) in infants whose birth weight was greater than 1500 grams. Mean serum clearance was also smaller in the lower birth weight infants. Although the differences in mean half-life values are statistically significant for weight, they are not clinically important. Therefore, dosage should be based solely on age. (See "Dosage and Administration" section.)

Additionally, no disulfiram-like reactions were reported in a study conducted in 22 healthy volunteers administered Cefotaxime Sodium and ethanol.

MICROBIOLOGY

The bactericidal activity of Cefotaxime Sodium results from inhibition of cell wall synthesis. Cefotaxime Sodium has in vitro activity against a wide range of gram-positive and gram-negative organisms. Cefotaxime Sodium has a high degree of stability in the presence of beta-lactamases, both penicillinases and cephalosporinases, of gram-negative and gram-positive bacteria. Cefotaxime Sodium has been shown to be a potent inhibitor of β-lactamases produced by certain gram-negative bacteria. Cefotaxime Sodium is usually active against the following microorganisms both in vitro and in clinical infections (see "Indications and Usage").

AEROBES, GRAM-POSITIVE

Staphylococcus aureus, including penicillinase and non-penicillinase producing strains, Staphylococcus epidermidis, Enterococcus species, Streptococcus pyogenes (Group A beta-hemolytic streptococci), Streptococcus agalactiae (Group B streptococci), Streptococcus pneumoniae (formerly Diplococcus pneumoniae).

AEROBES, GRAM-NEGATIVE

Citrobacter species, Enterobacter species, Escherichia coli, Haemophilus influenzae (including ampicillin-resistant H. influenzae), Haemophilus parainfluenzae, Klebsiella species (including K. pneumoniae), Neisseria gonorrhoeae (including penicillinase and nonpenicillinase producing strains), Neisseria meningitidis,

Proteus mirabilis, Proteus vulgaris, Proteus inconstans, Group B, Morganella morganii, Providencia rettgeri, Serratia species, and Acinetobacter species.

Note: Many strains of the above organisms that are multiply resistant to other antibiotics, e.g., penicillins, cephalosporins, and aminoglycosides, are susceptible to Cefotaxime Sodium.

Cefotaxime Sodium is active against some strains of Pseudomonas aeruginosa.

ANAEROBES

Bactervides species, including some strains of B. fragilis, Clostridium species. Note: Most strains of C. difficile are resistant.), Peptococcus species, Peptostreptococcus species, and Fusobacterium species (including F. nucleatum).

Cefotaxime Sodium is highly stable in vitro to four of the five major classes of β-lactamases described by Richmond et al., including type IIIa (TEM) which is produced by many gram-negative bacteria. The drug is also stable to β-lactamase (penicillinase) produced by staphylococci. In addition, Cefotaxime Sodium shows high affinity for penicillin-binding proteins in the cell wall, including PBP, Ib and III.

Cefotaxime Sodium also demonstrates in vitro activity against the following microorganisms although clinical significance is unknown: Salmonella species (including S. typhi), Providencia species, and Shigella species.

Cefotaxime Sodium and aminoglycosides have been shown to be synergistic in vitro against some strains of Pseudomonas aeruginosa.

SUSCEPTIBILITY TESTS

Quantitative methods that require measurement of zone diameters give the most precise estimate of antibiotic susceptibility. One such procedure[1] has been recommended for use with discs to test susceptibility to Cefotaxime Sodium. Interpretation involves correlation of the diameters obtained in the disc test with minimum inhibitory concentration (MIC) values for Cefotaxime Sodium.

Reports from the laboratory giving results of the standardized single-disc susceptibility test using a 30-µg Cefotaxime Sodium disc should be interpreted according to the following criteria:

Susceptible organisms produce zones of 20 mm or greater, indicating that the tested organism is likely to respond to therapy.

Organisms that produce zones of 15 to 19 mm are expected to be susceptible if high dosage is used or if the infection is confined to tissues and fluids (e.g., urine) in which high antibiotic levels are attained.

Resistant organisms produce zones of 14 mm or less, indicating that other therapy should be selected.

Organisms should be tested with the Cefotaxime Sodium disc, since Cefotaxime Sodium has been shown by in vitro tests to be active against certain strains found resistant when other beta lactam discs are used. The Cefotaxime Sodium disc should not be used for testing susceptibility to other cephalosporins. Organisms having zones of less than 18 mm around the cephalothin disc are not necessarily of intermediate susceptibility or resistant to Cefotaxime Sodium.

A bacterial isolate may be considered susceptible if the MIC value for Cefotaxime Sodium is not more than 16 µg/mL. Organisms are considered resistant to Cefotaxime Sodium if the MIC is equal to or greater than 64 µg/mL. Organisms having an MIC value of less than 64 µg/mL but greater than 16µg/mL are expected to be susceptible if high dosage is used or if the infection is confined to tissues and fluids (e.g., urine) in which high antibiotic levels are attained.

INDICATIONS AND USAGE

TREATMENT

Cefotaxime Sodium is indicated for the treatment of patients with serious infections caused by susceptible strains of the designated microorganisms in the diseases listed below.

(1) Lower respiratory tract infections: including pneumonia, caused by Streptococcus pneumoniae (formerly Diplococcus pneumoniae), Streptococcus pyogenes* (Group A streptococci) and other streptococci (excluding enterococci, e.g., Streptococcus faecalis), Staphylococcus aureus (penicillinase and non-penicillinase producing), Escherichia coli, Klebsiella species, Haemohilus influenzae (including ampicillin resistant strains), Haemophilus parainfluenzae, Proteus mirabilis, Serratia marcescens*, Enterobacter species, indole positive Proteus and Pseudomonas species (including P. aeruginosa).

(2) Genitourinary infections: Urinary tract infections caused by Enterococcus species, Staphylococcus epidermidis, Staphylococcus aureus* (penicillinase and non-penicillinase producing), Citrobacter species, Enterobacter species, Escherichia coli, Klebsiella species, Proteus mirabilis, Proteus vulgaris*, Proteus inconstans Group B, Morganella morganii*, Providencia rettgeri*, and Serratia marcescens, and Pseudomonas species (including P. aeruginosa). Also, uncomplicated gonorrhea of single or multiple sites caused by Neisseria gonorrhoeae, including penicillinase producing strains.

(3) Gynecologic infections: including pelvic inflammatory disease, endometritis and pelvic cellulitis caused by Staphylococcus epidermidis, Streptococcus species, Enterococcus species, Enterobacter species*, Klebsiella species*, Escherichia coli, Proteus mirabilis, Bacteroides species (including Bacteroides fragilis*), Clostridium species, and anaerobic cocci (including Peptostreptococcus species and Peptococcus species) and Fusobacterium species (including F. nucleatum*).

(4) Bacteremia/Septicemia: caused by Escherichia coli, Klebsiella species, Serratia marcescens, Staphylococcus aureus, and Streptococcus species (including S. pneumoniae).

(5) Skin and skin structure infections: caused by Staphylococcus aureus (penicillinase and non-penicillinase producing), Staphylococcus epidermidis, Streptococcus

pyogenes (Group A streptococci) and other streptococci, *Enterococcus* species, *Acinetobacter* species*, *Escherichia coli*, *Citrobacter* species (including *C. freundii**). *Enterobacter* species, *Klebsiella* species, *Proteus mirabilis, Proteus vulgaris**, *Morganella morganii, Providencia rettgeri**, *Pseudomonas* species, *Serratia marcescens, Bacteroides* species, and anaerobic cocci (including *Peptostreptococcus** species and *Peptococcus* species).

(6) Intra-abdominal infections: including peritonitis caused by *Streptococcus* species*, *Escherichia coli, Klebsiella* species, *Bacteroides* species, and anaerobic cocci (including *Peptostreptococcus** species and *Peptococcus** species), *Proteus mirabilis**, and *Clostridium* species*.

(7) Bone and/or joint infections: caused by *Staphylococcus aureus* (penicillinase and non-penicillinase producing strains), *Streptococcus* species (including *S. pyogenes**), *Pseudomonas* species (including *P. aeruginosa**), and *Proteus mirabilis**.

(8) Central nervous system infections: e.g., meningitis and ventriculitis, caused by *Neisseria meningitidis, Haemophilus influenzae, Streptococcus pneumoniae, Klebsiella pneumoniae**, and *Escherichia coli**.

(*) Efficacy for this organism, in this organ system, has been studied in fewer than 10 infections.

Although many strains of enterococci (e.g., *S. faecalis*) and *Pseudomonas* species are resistant to Cefotaxime Sodium *in vitro*, Cetotaxime Sodium has been used successfully in treating patients with infections caused by susceptible organisms.

Specimens for bacteriologic culture should be obtained prior to therapy in order to isolate and identify causative organisms and to determine their susceptibilities to Cetotaxime Sodium.

Therapy may be instituted before results of susceptibility studies are known; however, once these results become available, the antibiotic treatment should be adjusted accordingly.

In certain cases of confirmed or suspected gram-positive or gram-negative sepsis or in patients with other serious infections in which the causative organism has not been identified, Cefotaxime Sodium may be used concomitantly with an aminoglycoside. The dosage recommended in the labeling of both antibiotics may be given and depends on the severity of the infection and the patient's condition. Renal function should be carefully monitored, especially if higher dosages of the aminoglycosides are to be administrated or if therapy is prolonged, because of the potential nephrotoxicity and ototoxicity of aminoglycoside antibiotics. Some β-lactam antibiotics also have a certain degree of nephrotoxicity. Although, to date, this has not been noted when Cefotaxime Sodium was given alone, it is possible that nephrotoxicity may be potentiated if Cefotaxime Sodium is used concomitantly with an aminoglycoside.

PREVENTION
The administration of Cefotaxime Sodium preoperatively reduces the incidence of certain infections in patients undergoing surgical procedures (e.g., abdominal or vaginal hysterectomy, gastrointestinal and genitourinary tract surgery) that may be classified as contaminated or potentially contaminated. In patients undergoing cesarean section, intraoperative (after clamping the umbilical cord) and postoperative use of Cefotaxime Sodium may also reduce the incidence of certain postoperative infections. See *"Dosage and Administration"* section.

Effective use for elective surgery depends on the time of administration. To achieve effective tissue levels, Cefotaxime Sodium should be given ½ to 1 ½ hours before surgery. See *"Dosage and Administration"* section.

For patients undergoing gastrointestinal surgery, preoperative bowel preparation by mechanical cleansing as well as with a non-absorbable antibiotic (e.g., neomycin) is recommended.

If there are signs of infection, specimens for culture should be obtained for identification of the causative organism so that appropriate therapy may be instituted.

UNLABELED USES
Cefotaxime is used alone or as an adjunct in the treatment of typhoid fever, Lyme Disease (spirochete species infection due to Borrelia burgdorferi), and ophthalmia neonatorum.

CONTRAINDICATIONS
Cefotaxime Sodium is contraindicated in patients who have shown hypersensitivity to Cefotaxime Sodium or the cephalosporin group of antibiotics.

WARNINGS
BEFORE THERAPY WITH CEFOTAXIME SODIUM IS INSTITUTED, CAREFUL INQUIRY SHOULD BE MADE TO DETERMINE WHETHER THE PATIENT HAS HAD PREVIOUS HYPERSENSITIVITY REACTIONS TO CEFOTAXIME SODIUM, CEPHALOSPORINS, PENICILLINS, OR OTHER DRUGS. THIS PRODUCT SHOULD BE GIVEN WITH CAUTION TO PATIENTS WITH TYPE 1 HYPERSENSITIVITY REACTIONS TO PENICILLIN. ANTIBIOTICS SHOULD BE ADMINISTERED WITH CAUTION TO ANY PATIENT WHO HAS DEMONSTRATED SOME FORM OF ALLERGY, PARTICULARLY TO DRUGS. IF AN ALLERGIC REACTION TO CEFOTAXIME SODIUM OCCURS, DISCONTINUE TREATMENT WITH THE DRUG. SERIOUS HYPERSENSITIVITY REACTIONS MAY REQUIRE EPINEPHRINE AND OTHER EMERGENCY MEASURES.

Pseudomembranous colitis has been reported with the use of cephalosporins (and other broad spectrum antibiotics); therefore, it is important to consider its diagnosis in patients who develop diarrhea in association with antibiotic use.

Treatment with broad spectrum antibiotics alters normal flora of the colon and may permit overgrowth of Clostridia. Studies indicate a toxin produced by *Clostridium difficile* is one primary cause of antibiotic-associated colitis. Cholestyramine and colestipol resins have been shown to bind the toxin *in vitro*.

Mild cases of colitis may respond to drug discontinuance alone.

Moderate to severe cases should be managed with fluid, electrolyte, and protein supplementation as indicated.

When the colitis is not relieved by drug discontinuance or when it is severe, oral vancomycin is the treatment of choice for antibiotic-associated pseudomembranous colitis produced by *C. difficile*. Other causes of colitis should also be considered.

PRECAUTIONS
Cefotaxime Sodium should be prescribed with caution in individuals with a history of gastrointestinal disease, particularly colitis. Cefotaxime Sodium has not been shown to be nephrotoxic; however, because high and prolonged serum antibiotic concentrations can occur from usual doses in patients with transient or persistent reduction of urinary output because of renal insufficiency, the total daily dosage should be reduced when Cefotaxime Sodium is administered to such patients. Continued dosage should be determined by degree of renal impairment, severity of infection, and susceptibility of the causative organism.

Although there is no clinical evidence supporting the necessity of changing the dosage of Cefotaxime Sodium in patients with even profound renal dysfunction, it is suggested that, until further data are obtained, the dose of Cefotaxime Sodium be halved in patients with estimated creatinine clearances of less than 20 mL/min/ 1.73 m^2.

When only serum creatinine is available, the following formula[2] (based on sex, weight, and age of the patient) may be used to convert this value into creatinine clearance. The serum creatinine should represent a steady state of renal function.

Males: $$\frac{\text{Weight (kg)} \times (140 - \text{age})}{72 \times \text{serum creatinine}}$$

Females: $0.85 \times$ above value

As with other antibiotics, prolonged use of Cefotaxime Sodium may result in overgrowth of nonsusceptible organisms. Repeated evaluation of the patient's condition is essential. If superinfection occurs during therapy, appropriate measures should be taken.

As with other beta-lactam antibiotics, granulocytopenia and, more rarely, agranulocytosis may develop during treatment with Cefotaxime Sodium particularly if given over long periods. For courses of treatment lasting longer than 10 days, blood counts should therefore be monitored.

Parenteral antibiotics may be locally irritating to tissues. In rare instances, perivascular extravasation of antibiotics including Cefotaxime Sodium may result in tissue damage requiring surgical intervention. In most cases, perivascular extravasation of Cefotaxime Sodium infusion requires no specific measures beyond changing the infusion site. To minimize the potential for tissue inflammation, infusion sites should be monitored regularly and changed as appropriate.

Drug Interactions: Increased nephrotoxicity has been reported following concomitant administration of cephalosporins and aminoglycoside antibiotics.

Carcinogenesis, Mutagenesis: Long-term studies in animals have not been performed to evaluate carcinogenic potential. Mutagenic tests included a micronucleus and an Ames test. Both tests were negative for mutagenic effects.

Pregnancy (Category B): Reproduction studies have been performed in mice and rats at doses up to 30 times the usual human dose and have revealed no evidence of impaired fertility or harm to the fetus because of Cefotaxime Sodium. However, there are no well-controlled studies in pregnant women. Because animal reproductive studies are not always predictive of human response, this drug should be used during pregnancy only if clearly needed.

Nonteratogenic Effects: Use of the drug in women of childbearing potential requires that the anticipated benefit be weighed against the possible risks.

In perinatal and postnatal studies with rats, the pups in the group given 1200 mg/kg of Cefotaxime Sodium were significantly lighter in weight at birth and remained smaller than pups in the control group during the 21 days of nursing.

Nursing Mothers: Cefotaxime Sodium is excreted in human milk in low concentrations. Caution should be exercised when Cefotaxime Sodium is administered to a nursing woman.

Pediatric Use: The potential for toxic effects in children from chemicals that may leach from the plastic in single dose Galaxy® containers (premixed Cefotaxime Sodium injection) has not been determined.

ADVERSE REACTIONS
Cefotaxime Sodium is generally well tolerated. The most common adverse reactions have been local reactions following IM or IV injection. Other adverse reactions have been encountered infrequently.

THE MOST FREQUENT ADVERSE REACTIONS (GREATER THAN 1%) ARE
Local (4.3%): Injection site inflammation with IV administration. Pain, induration, and tenderness after IM injection.

◆ RATED THERAPEUTICALLY EQUIVALENT; ◇ THERAPEUTIC EQUIVALENCE UNCONFIRMED; ○ UNRATED

Hypersensitivity (2.4%): Rash, pruritus, fever, and eosinophila and less frequently urticaria and anaphylaxis.

Gastrointestinal (1.4%): Colitis, diarrhea, nausea, and vomiting.
Symptoms of pseudomembranous colitis can appear during or after antibiotic treatment.
Nausea and vomiting have been reported rarely.

LESS FREQUENT ADVERSE REACTIONS (LESS THAN 1%) ARE
Hematologic System: Neutropenia, transient leukopenia, eosinophilia, thrombo-cytopenia and agranulocytosis have been reported. Some individuals have developed positive direct Coombs Tests during treatment with Cefotaxime Sodium and other cephalosporin antibiotics. Rare cases of hemolytic anemia have been reported.

Genitourinary System: Moniliasis, vaginitis.

Central Nervous System: Headache.

Liver: Transient elevations in SGOT, SGPT, serum LDH, and serum alkaline phosphatase levels have been reported.

Kidney: As with some other cephalosporins, interstitial nephritis and transient elevations of BUN have been occasionally observed with Cefotaxime Sodium.

DOSAGE AND ADMINISTRATION
ADULTS
Dosage and route of administration should be determined by susceptibility of the causative organisms, severity of the infection, and the condition of the patient (see table for dosage guideline). Cefotaxime Sodium may be administered IM or IV after reconstitution. Premixed Cefotaxime Sodium injection is intended for IV administration after thawing. The maximum daily dosage should not exceed 12 grams.

GUIDELINES FOR DOSAGE OF CEFOTAXIME SODIUM

Type of Infection	Daily Dose (grams)	Frequency and Route
Gonorrhea	1	1 gram IM (single dose)
Uncomplicated infections	2	1 gram every 12 hours IM or IV
Moderate to severe infections	3-6	1-2 grams every 8 hours IM or IV
Infections commonly needing antibiotics in higher dosage (e.g., septicemia)	6-8	2 grams every 6-8 hours IV
Life-threatening infections	up to 12	2 grams every 4 hours IV

To prevent postoperative infection in contaminated or potentially contaminated surgery, the recommended dose is a single 1 gram IM or IV administered 30 to 90 minutes prior to start of surgery.

CESAREAN SECTION PATIENTS
The first dose of 1 gram is administered intravenously as soon as the umbilical cord is clamped. The second and third doses should be given as 1 gram intravenously or intramuscularly at 6 and 12 hours after the first dose.

NEONATES, INFANTS AND CHILDREN
The following dosage schedule is recommended:

Neonates (birth to 1 month):
0-1 week of age . . . . .50 mg/kg IV q 12 h
1-4 weeks of age . . . . .50 mg/kg IV q 8 h

It is not necessary to differentiate between premature and normal-gestational age infants.

Infants and Children (1 month to 12 years): For body weights less than 50 kg, the recommended daily dose is 50 to 180 mg/kg IM or IV of body weight divided into four to six equal doses. The higher dosages should be used for more severe or serious infections, including meningitis. For body weights 50 kg or more, the usual adult dosage should be used: the maximum daily dosage should not exceed 12 grams.

Impaired Renal Function: See "Precautions" section.

Note: As with antibiotic therapy in general, administration of Cefotaxime Sodium should be continued for a minimum of 48 to 72 hours after the patient defervesces or after evidence of bacterial eradication has been obtained; a minimum of 10 days of treatment is recommended for infections caused by Group A beta-hemolytic streptococci in order to guard against the risk of rheumatic fever or glomerulonephritis; frequent bacteriologic and clinical appraisal is necessary during therapy of chronic urinary tract infection and may be required for several months after therapy has been completed; persistent infections may require treatment of several weeks and doses smaller than those indicated above should not be used.

PREPARATION OF CEFOTAXIME SODIUM STERILE

Cefotaxime Sodium for IM or IV administration should be reconstituted as follows:

Strength	Diluent (mL)	Withdrawable Volume (mL)	Approximate Concentration (mg/mL)
500 mg vial* (IM)	2	2.2	230
1g vial* (IM)	3	3.4	300
2g vial* (IM)	5	6.0	330
500 mg vial* (IV)	10	10.2	50
1g vial* (IV)	10	10.4	95
2g vial* (IV)	10	11.0	180
1g infusion	50-100	50-100	20-10
2g infusion	50-100	50-100	40-20
10g bottle	47	52.0	200
10g bottle	97	102.0	100

* *in conventional vials*

Shake to dissolve; inspect for particulate matter and discoloration prior to use. Solutions of Cefotaxime Sodium range from very pale yellow to light amber, depending on concentration, diluent used, and length and condition of storage.

For intramuscular use: Reconstitute VIALS with Sterile Water for Injection or Bacteriostatic Water for Injection as described above.

For intravenous use: Reconstitute VIALS with at least 10 mL of Sterile Water for Injection. Reconstitute INFUSION BOTTLES with 50 or 100 mL of 0.9% Sodium Chloride Injection or 5% Dextrose Injection. For other diluents. see "Compatibility and Stability" section.

Pharmacy Bulk Package: Reconstitute with 47 mL of diluent for an approximate concentration of 200 mg/mL of 97 mL of diluent for an approximate concentration of 100 mg/mL. Stock solutions may be further diluted for IV infusion with diluents as listed in "Compatibility and Stability" section.

Note: Solutions of Cefotaxime Sodium must not be admixed with aminoglycoside solutions. If Cefotaxime Sodium and aminoglycosides are to be administered to the same patient, they must be administered separately and not as mixed injection.
A SOLUTION OF 1 G CEFOTAXIME SODIUM IN 14 ML OF STERILE WATER FOR INJECTION IS ISOTONIC.

IM Administration: As with all IM preparation Cefotaxime Sodium should be injected well within the body of a relatively large muscle such as the upper outer quadrant of the buttock (i.e. gluteus maximus); aspiration is necessary to avoid inadvertent injection into a blood vessel. Individual IM doses of 2 grams may be given if the dose is divided and is administered in different intramuscular sites.

IV Administration: The IV route is preferable for patients with bacteremia, bacterial septicemia, peritonitis, meningitis, or other severe or life-threatening infections, or for patients who may be poor risks because of lowered resistance resulting from such debilitating conditions as malnutrition, trauma, surgery, diabetes, heart failure, or malignancy, particularly if shock is present or impending.
For intermittent IV administration, a solution containing 1 gram or 2 grams in 10 mL of Sterile Water for Injection can be injected over a period of three to five minutes. With an infusion system, it may also be given over a longer period of time through the tubing system by which the patient may be receiving other IV solutions. However, during infusion of the solution containing Cefotaxime Sodium it is advisable to discontinue temporarily the administration of other solutions at the same site.
For the administration of higher doses by continuous IV infusion, a solution of Cefotaxime Sodium may be added to IV bottles containing the solutions discussed below.

Premixed Injection: Store in a freezer capable of maintaining a temperature of 20° C/ −4° F.

THAWING OF PLASTIC CONTAINER
Thaw frozen container at room temperature (22° C/72° F) or under refrigeration (5° C/41° F). [DO NOT FORCE THAW BY IMMERSION IN WATER BATHS OR BY MICROWAVE IRRADIATION.]
Check for minute leaks by squeezing container firmly. If leaks are detected, discard solution as sterility may be impaired.
DO NOT ADD SUPPLEMENTARY MEDICATION.
The container should be visually inspected. Components of the solution may precipitate in the frozen state and will dissolve upon reaching room temperature with little or no agitation. Potency is not affected. Agitate after solution has reached room temperature. If after visual inspection the solution remains cloudy or if an insoluble precipitate is noted or if any seals or outlet ports are not intact, the container should be discarded.
The thawed solution is stable for 10 days under refrigeration (5° C/41° F) or 24 hours at room temperature (25° C/72° F). Do not refreeze thawed antibiotics.

Caution: Do not use plastic containers in series connections. Such use could result in air embolism due to residual air being drawn from the primary container before administration of the fluid from the secondary container is complete.

PREPARATION FOR INTRAVENOUS ADMINISTRATION
1. Suspend container from eyelet support.
2. Remove protector from outlet port at bottom of container.
3. Attach administration set. Refer to complete directions accompanying set.

PREPARATION OF CEFOTAXIME SODIUM STERILE IN ADD-VANTAGE® SYSTEM
Cefotaxime Sodium Sterile 1 g or 2 g may be reconstituted in 50 mL or 100 mL of 5% dextrose or 0.9% sodium chloride in the ADD-Vantage® diluent container. Refer to enclosed, separate INSTRUCTIONS FOR ADD-VANTAGE® SYSTEM.

COMPATIBILITY AND STABILITY
Solutions of Cefotaxime Sodium sterile reconstituted as described above ("*Preparation of Cefotaxime Sodium Sterile*") maintain satisfactory potency for 24 hours at room temperature (at or below 22°C), 10 days under refrigeration (at or below 5°C), and for at least 13 weeks frozen. Solutions may be stored in disposable glass or plastic syringes for 24 hours at room temperature (at or below 22°C), 5 days under refrigeration (at or below 5°C), and 13 weeks frozen.

Reconstituted solutions may be further diluted up to 1000 mL with the following solutions and maintain satisfactory potency for 24 hours at room temperature (at or below 22°C), and at least 5 days under refrigeration (at or below 5°C), 0.9% Sodium Chloride Injection; 5 or 10% Dextrose Injection; 5% Dextrose and 0.9% Sodium Chloride Injection; 5% Dextrose and 0.45% Sodium Chloride Injection; 5% Dextrose and 0.45% Sodium Chloride Injection; 5% Dextrose and 0.2% Sodium Chloride Injection; Lactated Ringers Solution; Sodium Lactate Injection (M/6); 10% Invert Sugar Injection, 8.5% Amino Acid Injection without Electrolytes.

Solutions of Cefotaxime Sodium Sterile reconstituted in 0.9% Sodium Chloride Injection or 5% Dextrose Injection in Viaflex® plastic containers maintain satisfactory potency for 24 hours at room temperature (at or below 22°C), 5 days under refrigeration (at or below 5°C) and 13 weeks frozen. Solutions of Cefotaxime Sodium Sterile reconstituted in 0.9% Sodium Chloride Injection or 5% Dextrose Injection in the ADD-Vantage® flexible containers maintain satisfactory potency for 24 hours at room temperature (at or below 22°C). DO NOT FREEZE.

NOTE: Cefotaxime Sodium solutions exhibit maximum stability in the pH 5-7 range. Solutions of Cefotaxime Sodium should not be prepared with diluents having a pH above 7.5, such as Sodium Bicarbonate Injection.

REFERENCES
1. Bauer, A.W.; Kirby, W.M.M.; Sherris, J.C.; and Turck, M.: Antibiotic Susceptibility Testing by a Standardized Single Disk Method, Am. J. Clin. Pathol., 45:493, 1966; Standardized Disc Susceptibility Test, Federal Register, 39:19182-4, 1974. National Committee for Clinical Laboratory Standards, Approved Standard: ASM-2, Performance Standards for Antimicrobial Disc Susceptibility Tests, July, 1975. 2. Cockcroft, D.W. and Gault, M.H.: Prediction of Creatinine Clearance from Serum Creatinine. Nephron 16:31-41, 1976.

J CODES
Per 1 g IV,IM—J0698

HOW SUPPLIED
INJECTION: 1 GM

BRAND/MANUFACTURER	NDC	SIZE	AWP
○ **BRAND**			
CLAFORAN GALAXY: Hoechst	00039-0037-05	50 ml 24s	$303.85

INJECTION: 2 GM

BRAND/MANUFACTURER	NDC	SIZE	AWP
○ **BRAND**			
CLAFORAN GALAXY: Hoechst	00039-0038-05	50 ml 24s	$510.14

POWDER FOR INJECTION: 500 MG

BRAND/MANUFACTURER	NDC	SIZE	AWP
○ **BRAND**			
CLAFORAN: Hoechst	00039-0017-10	10s	$68.60

POWDER FOR INJECTION: 1 GM

BRAND/MANUFACTURER	NDC	SIZE	AWP
○ **BRAND**			
CLAFORAN: Hoechst	00039-0018-11	10s	$111.80
	00039-0018-10	10s	$114.46
	00039-0018-25	25s	$270.13
	00039-0023-25	25s	$278.95
	00039-0018-50	50s	$510.00
	00039-0023-50	50s	$527.65

POWDER FOR INJECTION: 2 GM

BRAND/MANUFACTURER	NDC	SIZE	AWP
○ **BRAND**			
CLAFORAN: Hoechst	00039-0019-11	10s	$209.95
	00039-0019-10	10s	$211.76
	00039-0019-25	25s	$499.75
	00039-0024-25	25s	$508.58
	00039-0019-50	50s	$944.00
	00039-0024-50	50s	$961.65

POWDER FOR INJECTION: 10 GM

BRAND/MANUFACTURER	NDC	SIZE	AWP
○ **BRAND**			
CLAFORAN: Hoechst	00039-0020-01	1s	$94.40

Cefotetan Disodium

DESCRIPTION
Cefotetan Disodium is a sterile, semisynthetic, broad-spectrum, beta-lactamase resistant, cephalosporin (cephamycin) antibiotic for parenteral administration. It is the disodium salt of [6 R -(6α, 7α)]-7-[[[4- (2-amino-1-carboxy-2-oxoethylidene)-1,3-dithietan-2-yl] carbonyl]amino]-7-methoxy-3-[[(1-methyl-1 H -tetrazol-5-yl)thio]- methyl]-8-oxo-5-thia-1-azabicyclo [4.2.0]oct-2-ene-2-carboxylic acid. Its molecular formula is $C_{17}H_{15}N_7Na_2O_8S_4$ with a molecular weight of 619.57.

Cefotetan Disodium contains approximately 80 mg (3.5 mEq) of sodium per gram of Cefotetan activity. It is a white to pale yellow powder which is very soluble in water. The solution varies from colorless to yellow depending on the concentration. The pH of freshly reconstituted solutions is usually between 4.5 to 6.5

Cefotetan Disodium in the ADD-Vantage Vial is intended for intravenous use only after dilution with the appropriate volume of ADD-Vantage diluent solution.

Cefotetan Disodium is available in two vial strengths containing drug equivalent to 1g and 2g Cefotetan activity respectively.

Following is its chemical structure:

CLINICAL PHARMACOLOGY
High plasma levels of Cefotetan are attained after intravenous and intramuscular administration of single doses to normal volunteers.

PLASMA CONCENTRATIONS AFTER 1.0 GRAM IV[a] OR IM DOSE MEAN PLASMA CONCENTRATION (µg/mL)

	Time After Injection						
Route	15 min	30 min	1h	2h	4h	8h	12h
IV	92	158	103	72	42	18	9
IM	34	56	71	68	47	20	9

[a] *30-minute infusion*

PLASMA CONCENTRATIONS AFTER 2.0 GRAM IV[a] OR IM DOSE MEAN PLASMA CONCENTRATION (µg/mL)

	Time After Injection					
Route	5 min	10 min	1h	3h	5h	9h	12h
IV	237	223	135	74	48	22	12[b]
IM	—	20	75	91	69	33	19

[a] *Injected over 3 minutes*
[b] *Concentrations estimated from regression line*

The plasma elimination half-life of Cefotetan is 3 to 4.6 hours after either intravenous or intramuscular administration. Repeated administration of Cefotetan Disodium does not result in accumulation of the drug in normal subjects.

Cefotetan is 88% plasma protein bound.

No active metabolites of Cefotetan have been detected; however, small amounts (less than 7%) of Cefotetan in plasma and urine may be converted to its tautomer, which has antimicrobial activity similar to the parent drug.

In normal patients, from 51% to 81% of an administered dose of Cefotetan Disodium is excreted unchanged by the kidneys over a 24 hour period, which results in high and prolonged urinary concentrations. Following intravenous doses of 1 gram and 2 grams, urinary concentrations are highest during the first hour and reach concentrations of approximately 1700 and 3500 µg/mL respectively.

In volunteers with reduced renal function, the plasma half-life of Cefotetan is prolonged. The mean terminal half-life of Cefotetan is prolonged. The mean terminal half-life increases with declining renal function, from approximately 4 hours in volunteers with normal renal function to about 10 hours in those with moderate renal impairment. There is a linear correlation between the systemic clearance of Cefotetan and creatinine clearance. When renal function is impaired, a reduced dosing schedule based on creatinine clearance must be used (see "*Dosage and Administration*").[1]

Therapeutic levels of Cefotetan are achieved in many body tissues and fluids including:

skin	ureter
muscle	bladder
fat	maxillary sinus mucosa
myometrium	tonsil
endometrium	bile
cervix	peritoneal fluid

◆ RATED THERAPEUTICALLY EQUIVALENT; ◇ THERAPEUTIC EQUIVALENCE UNCONFIRMED; ○ UNRATED

ovary
kidney

umbilical cord serum
amniotic fluid

MICROBIOLOGY

The bactericidal action of Cefotetan results from inhibition of cell wall synthesis. Cefotetan has *in vitro* activity against a wide range of aerobic and anaerobic gram-positive and gram-negative organisms. The methoxy group in the 7-alpha position provides Cefotetan with a high degree of stability in the presence of beta-lactamases including both penicillinases and cephalosporinases of gram-negative bacteria.

Cefotetan has been shown to be active against most strains of the following organisms **both *in vitro* and in clinical infections** (see *"Indications and Usage"*).

GRAM-NEGATIVE AEROBES

Escherichia coli
Haemophilus influenzae (including ampicillin-resistant strains)
Klebsiella species (including *K pneumoniae*)
Morganella morganii
Neisseria gonorrhoeae (nonpenicillinase-producing strains)
Proteus mirabilis
Proteus vulgaris
Providencia rettgeri
Serratia marcescens

Note: Approximately one-half of the usually clinically significant strains of *Enterobacter* species, (e.g., *E. aerogenes* and *E. cloacae*) are resistant to Cefotetan. Most strains of *Pseudomonas aeruginosa* and *Acinetobacter* species are resistant to Cefotetan.

GRAM-POSITIVE AEROBES

Staphylococcus aureus (including penicillinase- and nonpenicillinase-producing strains)
Staphylococcus epidermidis
Streptococcus agalactiae (group B beta-hemolytic streptococcus)
Streptococcus pneumoniae
Streptococcus pyogenes

Note: Methicillin-resistant staphylococci are resistant to cephalosporins. Some strains of *Staphylococcus epidermidis* and most strains of enterococci, e.g., *Enterococcus faecalis* (formerly *Streptococcus faecalis*) are resistant to Cefotetan.

ANAEROBES

Prevotella bivia (formerly *Bacteroides bivius*)
Prevotella disiens (formerly *Bacteroides disiens*)
Bacteroides fragilis
Prevotella melaninogenica (formerly *Bacteroides melaninogenicus*)
Bacteroides vulgatus
Fusobacterium species
Gram-positive bacilli (including *Clostridium* species)

Note: Many strains of *C. difficile* are resistant (see *"Warnings"*).

Peptococcus niger
Peptostreptococcus species

Note: Many strains of *B. distasonis*, *B. ovatus* and *B. thetaiotaomicron* are resistant to Cefotetan *in vitro*. However, the therapeutic utility of Cefotetan against these organisms cannot be accurately predicted on the basis of *in vitro* susceptibility tests alone.[2]

The following *in vitro* data are available but their clinical significance is unknown. Cefotetan has been shown to be active *in vitro* against most strains of the following organisms:

GRAM-NEGATIVE AEROBES

Citrobacter species (including *C. diversus* and *C. freundii*)
Klebsiella oxytoca
Moraxella (Branhamella) catarrhalis
Neisseria gonorrhoeae (penicillinase-producing strains)
Salmonella species
Serratia species
Shigella species
Yersinia enterocolitica

ANAEROBES

Porphyromonas asaccharolytica (formerly *Bacteroides asaccharolyticus*)
Prevotella oralis (formerly *Bacteroides oralis*)
Bacteroides splanchnicus
Clostridium difficile

Note: Many strains of *C. difficile* are resistant (see *"Warnings"*).

Propionbacterium species
Veillonella species

SUSCEPTIBILITY TESTS

Diffusion Technique: Quantitative methods that require measurement of zone diameters give the most precise estimate of the susceptibility of bacteria to antimicrobial agents. One such procedure[3] that has been recommended for use with disks to test susceptibility of organisms to Cefotetan uses a 30-μg Cefotetan disk. Interpretation involves the correlation of the diameter obtained in the disk test with the minimum inhibitory concentration (MIC) for Cefotetan.

Reports from the laboratory giving results of the standard single-disk susceptibility test with a 30-μg Cefotetan disk should be interpreted according to the following criteria:

Zone Diameter (mm)	Interpretation
≥16	Susceptible
13-15	Moderately Susceptible
≤12	Resistant

A report of "susceptible" indicates that the pathogen is likely to be inhibited by generally achievable blood levels. A report of "moderately susceptible" suggests that the organism would be susceptible if high dosage is used or if the infection is confined to tissues or fluids in which high antimicrobial levels are attained. A report of "resistant" indicates that achievable concentrations are unlikely to be inhibitory, and other therapy should be selected.

Standard procedures require the use of laboratory control organisms. The 30-μg Cefotetan disk should give the following zone diameters:

Zone Diameter (mm)	Organism
28-34	*E. coli* ATCC 25922
17-23	*S. aureus* ATCC 25923

Dilution Techniques: Use a standardized microdilution or agar dilution method[4] (broth, agar, microdilution) or equivalent with Cefotetan powder. The MIC values obtained should be interpreted according to the following criteria:

MIC (μg/mL)	Interpretation
≤16	Susceptible
32	Moderately Susceptible
≥64	Resistant

As with standard diffusion methods, dilution methods require the use of laboratory control organisms. Standard Cefotetan powder should provide the following MIC values:

MIC (μg/mL)	Organism
0.6-0.25	*E. coli* ATCC 25922
4-16	*S. aureus* ATCC 29213

For anaerobic bacteria, the MIC of Cefotetan can be determined by agar or broth dilution (including microdilution) technique.[5]

The MIC values obtained should be interpreted as follows:

MIC (μg/mL)	Interpretation
≤32	Susceptible
≥64	Resistant

As with susceptibility methodology for aerobic bacteria, the dilution methods for anaerobic bacteria must be monitored using laboratory control organisms.

INDICATIONS AND USAGE

TREATMENT

Cefotetan Disodium is indicated for the therapeutic treatment of the following infections when caused by susceptible strains of the designated organisms:

Urinary Tract Infections caused by *E. coli*, *Klebsiella* species (including *K. pneumoniae*), *Proteus mirabilis* and *Proteus* spp (which may include the organisms now called *Proteus vulgaris*, *Providencia rettgeri*, and *Morganella morganii*).

Lower Respiratory Tract Infections caused by *Streptococcus pneumoniae*, *Staphylococcus aureus* (penicillinase- and nonpenicillinase-producing strains), *Haemophilus influenzae* (including ampicillin-resistant strains), *Klebsiella* species (including *K. pneumoniae*), *E. coli*, *Proteus mirabilis*, and *Serratia marcescens**.

Skin and Skin Structure Infections due to *Staphylococcus aureus* (penicillinase- and nonpenicillinase-producing strains), *Staphylococcus epidermidis*, *Streptococcus pyogenes* *Streptococcus* species (excluding enterococci), *Escherichia coli*, *Klebsiella pneumoniae*, *Peptococcus niger**, *Peptostreptococcus* species.

Gynecologic Infections caused by *Staphylococcus aureus*, (including penicillinase- and nonpenicillinase-producing strains), *Staphylococcus epidermidis*, *Streptococcus* species (excluding enterococci), *Streptococcus agalactiae*, *E. coli*, *Proteus mirabilis*, *Neisseria gonorrhoeae*, Bacteroides species (excluding *B. distasonis*, *B. ovatus*, *B. thetaiotaomicron*), *Fusobacterium* species*, and gram-positive anaerobic cocci (including *Peptococcus niger* and *Peptostreptococcus* species.

Cefotetan, like other cephalosporins, has no activity against *Chlamydia trachomatis*. Therefore, when cephalosporins are used in the treatment of pelvic inflammatory disease, and *C. trachomatis* is one of the suspected pathogens, appropriate antichlamydial coverage should be added.

Intra-abdominal Infections caused by *E. coli*, *Klebsiella* species (including *K. pneumoniae*, *Streptococcus* species (excluding enterococci), *Bacteroides* species (excluding *B. distasonis*, *B. ovatus*, *B. thetaiotaomicron*) and *Clostridium* species*.

Bone and Joint Infections caused by *Staphylococcus aureus*.*

---

* Efficacy for this organism in this organ system was studied in fewer than ten infections.

Specimens for bacteriological examination should be obtained in order to isolate and identify causative organisms and to determine their susceptibilities to Cefotetan. Therapy may be instituted before results of susceptibility studies are known; however, once these results become available, the antibiotic treatment should be adjusted accordingly.

In cases of confirmed or suspected gram-positive or gram-negative sepsis or in patients with other serious infections in which the causative organism has not been identified, it is possible to use Cefotetan Disodium concomitantly with an aminoglycoside. Cefotetan combinations with aminoglycosides have been shown to be synergistic *in vitro* against many Enterobacteriaceae and also some other gram-negative bacteria. The dosage recommended in the labeling of both antibiotics may be given and depends on the severity of the infection and the patient's condition.

Note: Increases in serum creatinine have occurred when Cefotetan Disodium was given alone. If Cefotetan Disodium and an aminoglycoside are used concomitantly, renal function should be carefully monitored, because nephrotoxicity may be potentiated.

PROPHYLAXIS
The preoperative administration of Cefotetan Disodium may reduce the incidence of certain postoperative infections in patients undergoing surgical procedures that are classified as clean contaminated or potentially contaminated (e.g., cesarean section, abdominal or vaginal hysterectomy, transurethral surgery, biliary tract surgery, and gastrointestinal surgery).

The prophylactic dose of Cefotetan Disodium should be administered 30-60 minutes prior to surgery. In patients undergoing cesarean section, Cefotetan Disodium should be administered intravenously after the clamping of the umbilical cord.

If there are signs and symptoms of infection, specimens for culture should be obtained for identification of the causative organism so that appropriate therapeutic measures may be initiated.

UNLABELED USES
Cefotetan Disodium is used alone or as an adjunct in the treatment of gonorrhea, acute pelvic inflammatory disease, septicemia, and maxillary sinusitis. It is also prescribed for prophylaxis of endomyometritis.

CONTRAINDICATIONS
Cefotetan Disodium is contraindicated in patients with known allergy to the cephalosporin group of antibiotics.

WARNINGS
BEFORE THERAPY WITH CEFOTETAN DISODIUM IS INSTITUTED, CAREFUL INQUIRY SHOULD BE MADE TO DETERMINE WHETHER THE PATIENT HAS HAD PREVIOUS HYPERSENSITIVITY REACTIONS TO CEFOTETAN DISODIUM, CEPHALOSPORINS, PENICILLINS, OR OTHER DRUGS. IF THIS PRODUCT IS TO BE GIVEN TO PENICILLIN-SENSITIVE PATIENTS, CAUTION SHOULD BE EXERCISED BECAUSE CROSS-HYPERSENSITIVITY AMONG BETA-LACTAM ANTIBIOTICS HAS BEEN CLEARLY DOCUMENTED AND MAY OCCUR IN UP TO 10% OF PATIENTS WITH A HISTORY OF PENICILLIN ALLERGY. IF AN ALLERGIC REACTION TO CEFOTETAN DISODIUM OCCURS, DISCONTINUE THE DRUG. SERIOUS ACUTE HYPERSENSITIVITY REACTIONS MAY REQUIRE TREATMENT WITH EPINEPHRINE AND OTHER EMERGENCY MEASURES, INCLUDING OXYGEN, INTRAVENOUS FLUIDS, INTRAVENOUS ANTIHISTAMINES, CORTICOSTEROIDS, PRESSOR AMINES, AND AIRWAY MANAGEMENT, AS CLINICALLY INDICATED.

Pseudomembranous colitis has been reported with nearly all antibacterial agents, including Cefotetan, and may range from mild to life-threatening. Onset of pseudomembranous colitis symptoms may occur during or after antibiotic treatment or surgical prophylaxis. Therefore, it is important to consider this diagnosis in patients who present with diarrhea subsequent to the administration of antibacterial agents.

Treatment with antibacterial agents alters the normal flora of the colon and may permit overgrowth of clostridia. Studies indicate that a toxin produced by *Clostridium difficile* is a primary cause of "antibiotic-associated colitis".

After the diagnosis of pseudomembranous colitis has been established, therapeutic measures should be initiated. Mild cases of pseudomembranous colitis usually respond to discontinuation of the drug alone. In moderate to severe cases, consideration should be given to management with fluids and electrolytes, protein supplementation, and treatment with an oral antibacterial drug effective against *C. difficile* colitis (see *"Adverse Reactions"*).

In common with many other broad-spectrum antibiotics, Cefotetan Disodium may be associated with a fall in prothrombin activity and, possibly, subsequent bleeding. Those at increased risk include patients with renal or hepatobiliary impairment or poor nutritional state, the elderly, and patients with cancer. Prothrombin time should be monitored and exogenous vitamin K administered as indicated.

Hemolytic anemia has been reported for cephalosporin-class antibiotics. Severe cases of hemolytic anemia, including fatalities, have been reported in association with the administration of Cefotetan Disodium. Such reports are uncommon. If a patient develops a hematologic abnormality subsequent to the administration of Cefotetan, a diagnosis of drug-induced hemolytic anemia should be considered.

PRECAUTIONS
General: As with other broad-spectrum antibiotics, prolonged use of Cefotetan Disodium may result in overgrowth of nonsusceptible organisms. Careful observation of the patient is essential. If superinfection does occur during therapy, appropriate measures should be taken.

Cefotetan Disodium should be used with caution in individuals with a history of gastrointestinal disease, particularly colitis.

Information for Patients: As with some other cephalosporins, a disulfiram-like reaction characterized by flushing, sweating, headache, and tachycardia may occur when alcohol (beer, wine, etc) is ingested within 72 hours after Cefotetan Disodium administration. Patients should be cautioned about the ingestion of alcoholic beverages following the administration of Cefotetan Disodium.

Drug Interactions: Increases in serum creatinine have occurred when Cefotetan Disodium was given alone. If Cefotetan Disodium and an aminoglycoside are used concomitantly, renal function should be carefully monitored, because nephrotoxicity may be potentiated.

Drug/Laboratory Test Interactions: The administration of Cefotetan Disodium may result in a false-positive reaction for glucose in the urine using Clinitest, Benedict's solution, or Fehling's solution. It is recommended that glucose tests based on enzymatic glucose oxidase be used.

As with other cephalosporins, high concentrations of Cefotetan may interfere with measurement of serum and urine creatinine levels by Jaffe reaction and produce false increases in the levels of creatinine reported.

Carcinogenesis, Mutagenesis, Impairment of Fertility: Although long-term studies in animals have not been performed to evaluate carcinogenic potential, no mutagenic potential of Cefotetan was found in standard laboratory tests. Cefotetan has adverse effects on the testes of prepubertal rats. Subcutaneous administration of 500 mg/kg/day (approximately 8-16 times the usual adult human dose) on days 6-35 of life (thought to be developmentally analogous to late childhood and prepuberty in humans) resulted in reduced testicular weight and seminiferous tubule degeneration in 10 of 10 animals. Affected cells included spermatogonia and spermatocytes; Sertoli and Leydig cells were unaffected. Incidence and severity of lesions were dose-dependent; at 120 mg/kg/day (approximately 2-4 times the usual human dose) only 1 of 10 treated animals was affected, and the degree of degeneration was mild.

Similar lesions have been observed in experiments of comparable design with other methylthiotetrazole-containing antibiotics and impaired fertility has been reported, particularly at high dose levels. No testicular effects were observed in 7-week-old rats treated with up to 1000 mg/kg/day SC for 5 weeks, or in infant dogs (3 weeks old) that received up to 300 mg/kg/day IV for 5 weeks. The relevance of these findings to humans is unknown.

Pregnancy: Teratogenic Effects. Pregnancy Category B: Reproduction studies have been performed in rats and monkeys at doses up to 20 times the human dose and have revealed no evidence of impaired fertility or harm to the fetus due to Cefotetan. There are, however, no adequate and well-controlled studies in pregnant women. Because animal reproductive studies are not always predictive of human response, this drug should be used during pregnancy only if clearly needed.

Nursing Mothers: Cefotetan is excreted in human milk in very low concentrations. Caution should be exercised when Cefotetan is administered to a nursing woman.

Pediatric Use: Safety and effectiveness in children have not been established.

ADVERSE REACTIONS
In clinical studies the following adverse effects were considered related to Cefotetan therapy. Those appearing in italics have been reported during postmarketing experience.

Gastrointestinal symptoms occurred in 1.5% of patients, the most frequent were diarrhea (1 in 80) and nausea (1 in 700); *pseudomembranous colitis.* Onset of pseudomembranous colitis symptoms may occur during or after antibiotic treatment or surgical prophylaxis. (See *"Warnings".*)

Hematologic laboratory abnormalities occurred in 1.4% of patients and included eosinophilia (1 in 200), positive direct Coombs' test (1 in 250), and thrombocytosis (1 in 300); *agranulocytosis, hemolytic anemia, leukopenia, thrombocytopenia, and prolonged prothrombin time with or without bleeding.*

Hepatic enzyme elevations occurred in 1.2% of patients and included a rise in ALT (SGPT) (1 in 150), AST (SGOT) (1 in 300), alkaline phosphatase (1 in 700), and LDH (1 in 700).

Hypersensitivity reactions were reported in 1.2% of patients and included rash (1 in 150) and itching (1 in 700); *anaphylactic reactions* and *urticaria.*

Local effects were reported in less than 1.0% of patients and included phlebitis at the site of injection (1 in 300), and discomfort (1 in 500).

Renal: Elevations in BUN and serum creatinine have been reported.

Urogenital: Nephrotoxicity has rarely been reported.

Miscellaneous: Fever

In addition to the adverse reactions listed above which have been observed in patients treated with Cefotetan, the following adverse reactions and altered laboratory tests have been reported for cephalosporin-class antibiotics: pruritus, Stevens-Johnson syndrome, erythema multiforme, toxic epidermal necrolysis, vomiting, abdominal pain, colitis, superinfection, vaginitis including vaginal candidiasis, renal dysfunction, toxic nephropathy, hepatic dysfunction including cholestasis, aplastic anemia, hemorrhage, elevated bilirubin, pancytopenia, and neutropenia.

Several cephalosporins have been implicated in triggering seizures, particularly in patients with renal impairment, when the dosage was not reduced (See *"Dosage and Administration"* and *"Overdosage".*) If seizures associated with drug therapy occur, the drug should be discontinued. Anticonvulsant therapy can be given if clinically indicated.

OVERDOSAGE
Information on overdosage with Cefotetan Disodium in humans is not available. If overdosage should occur, it should be treated symptomatically and hemodialysis considered, particularly if renal function is compromised.

DOSAGE AND ADMINISTRATION
TREATMENT
Cefotetan Disodium in the ADD-Vantage Vial is intended for intravenous infusion only after dilution with the appropriate volume of ADD-Vantage diluent solution.

The usual adult dosage is 1 or 2 grams of Cefotetan Disodium administered intravenously or intramuscularly every 12 hours for 5 to 10 days. Proper dosage and route of administration should be determined by the condition of the patient, severity of the infection, and susceptibility of the causative organism.

GENERAL GUIDELINES FOR DOSAGE OF CEFOTETAN DISODIUM

Type of Infection	Daily Dose	Frequency and Route
Urinary Tract	1-4 grams	500 mg every 12 hours IV or IM 1 or 2 g every 24 hours IV or IM 1 or 2 g every 12 hours IV or IM
Skin & Skin Structure Mild-Moderate[a]	2 grams	2 g every 24 hours IV 1 g every 12 hours IV or IM
Severe	4 grams	2 g every 12 hours IV
Other Sites	2-4 grams	1 or 2 g every 12 hours IV or IM
Severe	4 grams	2 g every 12 hours IV
Life-Threatening	6 grams[b]	3 g every 12 hours IV

[a] *K. pneumoniae* skin and skin structure infections should be treated with 1 or 2 grams every 12 hours IV or IM.
[b] *Maximum daily dosage should not exceed 6 grams.*

If *C. trachomatis* is a suspected pathogen in gynecologic infections, appropriate antichlamydial coverage should be added, since Cefotetan has no activity against this organism.

PROPHYLAXIS
To prevent postoperative infection in clean contaminated or potentially contaminated surgery in adults, the recommended dosage is 1 or 2 g of Cefotetan Disodium administered once, intravenously, 30 to 60 minutes prior to surgery. In patients undergoing cesarean section, the dose should be administered as soon as the umbilical cord is clamped.

IMPAIRED RENAL FUNCTION
When renal function is impaired, a reduced dosage schedule must be employed. The following dosage guidelines may be used.

DOSAGE GUIDELINES FOR PATIENTS WITH IMPAIRED RENAL FUNCTIONS

Creatinine Clearance mL/min	Dose	Frequency
>30	Usual Recommended Dosage*	Every 12 hours
10-30	Usual Recommended Dosage*	Every 24 hours
<10	Usual Recommended Dosage*	Every 48 hours

* *Dose determined by the type and severity of infection, and susceptibility of the causative organism.*

Alternatively, the dosing interval may remain constant at 12 hour intervals, but the dose reduced to one-half the usual recommended dose for patients with a creatinine clearance of 10-30 mL/min, and one-quarter the usual recommended dose for patients with a creatinine clearance of less than 10 mL/min.

When only serum creatinine levels are available, creatinine clearance may be calculated from the following formula. The serum creatinine level should represent a steady state of renal function.

Males:
$$\frac{Weight\ (kg) \times (140 - age)}{72 \times serum\ creatinine\ (mg/100\ mL)}$$

Females: $0.9 \times$ value for males

Cefotetan is dialyzable and it is recommended that for patients undergoing intermittent hemodialysis, one-quarter of the usual recommended dose be given every 24 hours on days between dialysis and one-half the usual recommended dose on the day of dialysis.

PREPARATION OF SOLUTION
For Intravenous Use: Reconstitute with Sterile Water for Injection. Shake to dissolve and let stand until clear.

Vial Size	Amount of Diluent Added (mL)	Approximate Withdrawable Vol (mL)	Approximate Average Concentration (mg/mL)
1 gram	10	10.5	95
2 gram	10-20	11.0-21.0	182-95

Infusion bottles (100 mL) may be reconstituted with 50 to 100 mL of Dextrose Injection 5% or Sodium Chloride Injection 0.9%.

Note: ADD-VANTAGE VIALS ARE NOT TO BE USED IN THIS MANNER.

For ADD-Vantage® Vials: ADD-Vantage Vials of Cefotetan Disodium are to be reconstituted only with Sodium Chloride injection 0.9% or Dextrose Injection 5% in the 50mL, 100mL or 250 mL Flexible Diluent Containers. Cefotetan Disodium supplied in single-use ADD-Vantage Vials should be prepared as directed in the accompanying instruction leaflet.

For Intramuscular Use: Reconstitute with Sterile Water for Injection; Bacteriostatic Water for Injection; Sodium Chloride Injection 0.9%, USP; 0.5% Lidocaine HCl; or 1.0% Lidocaine HCl. Shake to dissolve and let stand until clear.

Vial Size	Amount of Diluent Added (mL)	Approximate Withdrawable Vol (mL)	Approximate Average Concentration (mg/mL)
1 gram	2	2.5	400
2 gram	3	4.0	500

INTRAVENOUS ADMINISTRATION
The intravenous route is preferable for patients with bacteremia, bacterial septicemia, or other severe or life-threatening infections, or for patients who may be poor risks because of lowered resistance resulting from such debilitating conditions as malnutrition, trauma, surgery, diabetes, heart failure, or malignancy, particularly if shock is present or impending.

For intermittent intravenous administration, a solution containing 1 gram or 2 grams of Cefotetan Disodium in Sterile Water for Injection can be injected over a period of three to five minutes. Using an infusion system, the solution may also be given over a longer period of time through the tubing system by which the patient may be receiving other intravenous solutions. Butterfly® or scalp vein-type needles are preferred for this type of infusion. However, during infusion of the solution containing Cefotetan Disodium it is advisable to discontinue temporarily the administration of other solutions at the same site.

Note: Solutions of Cefotetan Disodium must not be admixed with solutions containing aminoglycosides. If Cefotetan Disodium and aminoglycosides are to be administered to the same patient, they must be administered separately and not as a mixed injection.

INTRAMUSCULAR ADMINISTRATION
As with all intramuscular preparations, Cefotetan Disodium should be injected well within the body of a relatively large muscle such as the upper outer quadrant of the buttock (ie, gluteus maximus); aspiration is necessary to avoid inadvertent injection into a blood vessel.

COMPATIBILITY AND STABILITY
Cefotetan Disodium reconstituted as described above (*"Preparation of solution"*) maintains satisfactory potency for 24 hours at room temperature (25°C), for 96 hours under refrigeration (5°C), and for at least 1 week in the frozen state. After reconstitution and subsequent storage in disposable glass or plastic syringes, Cefotetan Disodium is stable for 24 hours at room temperature and 96 hours under refrigeration.

Frozen samples should be thawed at room temperature before use. After the periods mentioned above, any unused solutions or frozen materials should be discarded. Do not refreeze.

ADD-Vantage Vials: Ordinarily, ADD-Vantage vials should be reconstituted only when it is certain that the patient is ready to receive the drug. However, ADD-Vantage vials of Cefotetan Disodium reconstituted as described in Preparation of Solution, for ADD-Vantage Vials, maintains satisfactory potency for 24 hours at room temperature (25° C/77° F). (DO NOT REFRIGERATE OR FREEZE CEFOTETAN DISODIUM IN ADD-VANTAGE VIALS.)

Note: Parenteral drug products should be inspected visually for particulate matter and discoloration prior to administration whenever solution and container permit.

STORAGE
The vials should not be stored at temperatures above 22° C (72° F) and should be protected from light.

REFERENCES
[1] Smith, LeFrock et al. Cefotetan Pharmacokinetics in Volunteers with Various Degrees of Renal Function. Antimicrobial Agents and Chemotherapy. 29(5): 887-893, May 1986.
[2] Sheikh and Bobey. Lack of Predictability of Cefotetan In Vitro Susceptibility Tests Against Cefotetan-Resistant Anaerobic Bacteria in Determining Clinical and Bacterio-

logical Efficacies. Diagn. Microbiol. Infect. Dis. 15:595-600, 1992. [3]National Committee for Clinical Laboratory Standards, Approved Standard: *Performance Standards for Antimicrobial Disk Susceptibility Tests,* 4th Edition, Vol. 10(7): M2-A4, Villanova, PA, April, 1990. [4]National Committee for Clinical Laboratory Standards, Tentative Standard: *Methods for Dilution Antimicrobial Susceptibility Tests for Bacteria That Grow Aerobically,* 2nd Edition, Vol. 10(8): M7-A2, Villanova, PA, April, 1990. [5]National Committee for Clinical Laboratory Standards, Approved Standard: *Methods for Antimicrobial Susceptibility Testing of Anaerobic Bacteria,* 2nd Edition, Vol. 10(15): M11-A2, Villanova, PA, April 1990.

HOW SUPPLIED
POWDER FOR INJECTION: 1 GM

BRAND/MANUFACTURER	NDC	SIZE	AWP
○ **BRAND**			
CEFOTAN: Stuart	00038-0376-10	1s	$11.16
	00038-0376-11	1s	$11.72

POWDER FOR INJECTION: 2 GM

BRAND/MANUFACTURER	NDC	SIZE	AWP
○ **BRAND**			
CEFOTAN: Stuart	00038-0377-20	1s	$21.90
	00038-0377-21	1s	$23.02

POWDER FOR INJECTION: 10 GM

BRAND/MANUFACTURER	NDC	SIZE	AWP
○ **BRAND**			
CEFOTAN: Stuart	00038-0375-10	1s	$118.36

Cefoxitin Sodium

DESCRIPTION
Cefoxitin Sodium is a semi-synthetic, broad-spectrum cepha antibiotic sealed under nitrogen for parenteral administration. It is derived from cephamycin C, which is produced by *Streptomyces lactamdurans.* It is the sodium salt of 3-(hydroxymethyl)-7α-methoxy-8-oxo-7-[2-(2-thienyl) acetamido]-5-thia-1-azabicyclo [4.2.0] oct-2-ene-2-carboxylate carbamate (ester). The empirical formula is $C_{16}H_{16}N_3NaO_7S_2$, and the molecular weight is 449.44.

Cefoxitin Sodium contains approximately 53.8 mg (2.3 milliequivalents) of sodium per gram of Cefoxitin activity. Premixed Intravenous Solution Cefoxitin Sodium is supplied as a sterile, nonpyrogenic, frozen, iso-osmotic solution of Cefoxitin Sodium. Each 50 mL contains Cefoxitin Sodium equivalent to either 1 gram or 2 grams Cefoxitin. Solutions of Cefoxitin Sodium range from colorless to light amber in color. The pH of freshly constituted solutions usually ranges from 4.2 to 7.0.

Following is its chemical structure:

CLINICAL PHARMACOLOGY
CLINICAL PHARMACOLOGY
After intramuscular administration of a 1 gram dose of Cefoxitin Sodium to normal volunteers, the mean peak serum concentration was 24 mcg/mL. The peak occurred at 20 to 30 minutes. Following an intravenous dose of 1 gram, serum concentrations were 110 mcg/mL at 5 minutes, declining to less than 1 mcg/mL at 4 hours. The half-life after an intravenous dose is 41 to 59 minutes; after intramuscular administration, the half-life is 64.8 minutes. Approximately 85 percent of Cefoxitin is excreted unchanged by the kidneys over a 6-hour period, resulting in high urinary concentrations. Following an intramuscular dose of 1 gram, urinary concentrations greater than 3000 mcg/mL were observed. Probenecid slows tubular excretion and produces higher serum levels and increases the duration of measurable serum concentrations.

Cefoxitin passes into pleural and joint fluids and is detectable in antibacterial concentrations in bile.

Clinical experience has demonstrated that Cefoxitin Sodium can be administered to patients who are also receiving carbenicillin, kanamycin, gentamicin, tobramycin, or amikacin (see *"Precautions and Administration").*

MICROBIOLOGY
The bactericidal action of Cefoxitin results from inhibition of cell wall synthesis. Cefoxitin has *in vitro* activity against a wide range of gram-positive and gram-negative organisms. The methoxy group in the 7α position provides Cefoxitin Sodium with a high degree of stability in the presence of beta-lactamases, both penicillinases and cephalosporinases, of gram-negative bacteria. Cefoxitin is usually active against the following organisms *in vitro* and in clinical infections:

Gram-positive:
Staphylococcus aureus, including penicillinase and nonpenicillinase producing strains.
Staphylococcus epidermidis
Beta-hemolytic and other strptococci (most strains of enterococci, e.g., *Streptococcus faecalis,* are resistant)

Streptococcus pneumoniae
Gram-negative:
Escherichia coli
Klebsiella species (including *K. pneumoniae)*
Hemophilus influenzae
Neisseria gonorrhoeae, incuding penicillinase and non-penicillinase producing strains
Proteus mirabilis
Morganella morganii
Proteus vulgaris
Providencia species including *Providencia rettgeri*
Anaerobic organisms:
Peptococcus species
Peptostreptococcus species
Clostridium species
Bacteroides species, including the *B. fragilis* group (includes *B. fragilis, B. distasonis, B. ovatus, B. thetaiotamicron, B. vulgatus)*

Cefoxitin Sodium is inactive *in vitro* against most strains of *Pseudomonas aeruginosa* and enterococci and many strains of *Enterobacter cloacae.*

Methicillin-resistant staphylococci are almost uniformly resistant to Cefoxitin Sodium.

SUSCEPTIBILITY TESTS
For fast-growing aerobic organisms, quantitative methods that require measurements of zone diameters give the most precise estimates of antibiotic susceptibility. One such procedure[*] has been recommended for use with discs to test susceptibility to Cefoxitin. Interpretation involves correlation of the diameters obtained in the disc test with minimal inhibitory concentration (MIC) values for Cefoxitin.

Reports from the laboratory giving results of the standardized single disc susceptibility test[*] using a 30 mcg Cefoxitin disc should be interpreted according to the following criteria: Organisms producing zones of 18 mm or greater are considered susceptible, indicating that the tested organism is likely to respond to therapy.

Organisms of intermediate susceptibility produce zones of 15 to 17 mm, indicating that the tested organism would be susceptible if high dosage is used or if the infection is confined to tissues and fluids (e.g., urine) in which high antibiotic levels are attained.

Resistant organisms produce zones of 14 mm or less, indicating that other therapy should be selected.

The Cefoxitin disc should be used for testing Cefoxitin susceptibility.

Cefoxitin has been shown by *in vitro* tests to have activity against certain strains of *Enterobacteriaceae* found resistant when tested with the cephalosporin class disc. For this reason, the Cefoxitin disc should not be used for testing susceptibility to cephalosporins, and cephalosporin discs should not be used for testing susceptibility to Cefoxitin.

Dilution methods, preferably the agar plate dilution procedure, are most accurate for susceptibility testing of obligate anaerobes.

A bacterial isolate may be considered susceptible if the MIC value for Cefoxitin[†] is not more than 16 mcg/mL. Organisms are considered resistant if the MIC is greater than 32 mcg/mL.

INDICATIONS AND USAGE
Cefoxitin Sodium supplied as a premixed solution in plastic containers is intended for intravenous use only, as dry powder for intramuscular use.

TREATMENT
Cefoxitin Sodium is indicated for the treatment of serious infections caused by susceptible strains of the designated microorganisms in the diseases listed below.

(1) Lower respiratory tract infections, including pneumonia and lung abscess, caused by *Streptococcus pneumoniae,* other streptococci (excluding enterococci, e.g., *Streptococcus faecalis), Staphylococcus aureus* (penicillinase and non-penicillinase producing), *Escherichia coli, Klebsiella* species, *Hemophilus influenzae,* and *Bacteroides* species.

(2) Genitourinary infections. Urinary tract infections caused by *Escherichia coli, Klebsiella* species, *Proteus mirabilis,* indole-positive Proteus (which include the organisms now called *Morganella morganii* and *Proteus vulgaris),* and *Providencia* species (including *Providencia rettgeri).* Uncomplicated gonorrhea due to *Neisseria gonorrhoeae* (penicillinase and nonpenicillinase producing).

(3) Intra-abdominal infections, including peritonitis and intra-abdominal abscess, caused by *Escherichia coli, Klebsiella* species *Bacteroides* species including the *Bacteroides fragilis* group[**], *Clostridium* species.

(4) Gynecological infections, including endometritis, pelvic cellulitis, and pelvic inflammatory disease caused by *Escherichia coli, Neisseria gonorrhoeae* (penicillinase and nonpenicillinase producing), *Bacteroides* species including the *Bacter-*

---

[*] Bauer, A. W.; Kirby, W. M. M.; Sherris, J. C.; Turck, M.: Antibiotic susceptibility testing by a standardized single disc method, Amer. J. Clin. Path. 45: 493-496, Apr. 1966. Standardized disc susceptibility test, Federal Register 37: 20527-20529, 1972. National Committee for Clinical Laboratory Standards: Approved Standard: ASM-2, Performance Standards for Antimicrobial Disc Susceptibility Tests, July 1975.
[†] Determined by the ICS agar dilution method (Ericsson and Sherris, Acta Path. Microbiol. Scand. (B) Suppl. No. 217, 1971) or any other method that has been shown to give equivalent results.
[**] *B. fragilis, B. distasonis, B. ovatus, B. thetaiotaomicron, B. vulgatus.*

oides fragilis group[**], *Clostridium* species, *Peptococcus* species, *Peptostreptococcus* species, and Group B streptococci.

(5) Septicemia caused by *Streptococcus pneumoniae, Staphylococcus aureus* (penicillinase and non-penicillinase producing), *Escherichia coli, Klebsiella* species, and *Bacteroides* species including the *Bacteroides fragilis* group.[**]

(6) Bone and joint infections caused by *Staphylococcus aureus* (penicillinase and non-penicillinase producing).

(7) Skin and skin structure infections caused by *Staphylococcus aureus* (penicillinase and non-penicillinase producing), *Staphylococcus epidermidis,* streptococci (excluding enterococci, e.g., *Streptococcus faecalis), Escherichia coli, Proteus mirabilis, Klebsiella* species, *Bacteroides* species including the *Bacteroides fragilis* group[**], *Clostridium* species, *Peptococcus* species, and *Peptostreptococcus* species.

Appropriate culture and susceptibility studies should be performed to determine the susceptibility of the causative organisms to Cefoxitin Sodium. Therapy may be started while awaiting the results of these studies.

In randomized comparative studies, Cefoxitin Sodium and cephalothin were comparably safe and effective in the management of infections caused by gram-positive cocci and gram-negative rods susceptible to the cephalosporins. Cefoxitin Sodium has a high degree of stability in the presence of bacterial beta-lactamases, both penicillinases and cephalosporinases.

Many infections caused by aerobic and anaerobic gram-negative bacteria resistant to some cephalosporins respond to Cefoxitin Sodium. Similarly, many infections caused by aerobic and anaerobic bacteria resistant to some penicillin antibiotics (ampicillin, carbenicillin, penicillin G) respond to treatment with Cefoxitin Sodium. Many infections caused by mixtures of susceptible aerobic and anaerobic bacteria respond to treatment with Cefoxitin Sodium.

PREVENTION

When compared to placebo in randomized controlled studies in patients undergoing gastrointestinal surgery, vaginal hysterectomy, abdominal hysterectomy and cesarean section, the prophylactic use of Cefoxitin Sodium resulted in a significant reduction in the number of postoperative infections. The prophylactic administration of Cefoxitin Sodium may reduce the incidence of certain postoperative infections in patients undergoing surgical procedures (e.g., hysterectomy, gastrointestinal surgery and transurethral prostatectomy) that are classified as contaminated or potentially contaminated.

The perioperative use of Cefoxitin Sodium may be effective in surgical patients in whom subsequent infection at the operative site would present a serious risk, e.g., prosthetic arthroplasty.

Effective prophylactic use depends on the time of administration. Cefoxitin Sodium usually should be given one-half to one hour before the operation, which is sufficient time to achieve effective levels in the wound during the procedure. Prophylactic administration should usually be stopped within 24 hours since continuing administration of any antibiotic increases the possibility of adverse reactions but, in the majority of surgical procedures, does not reduce the incidence of subsequent infection. However, in patients undergoing prosthetic arthroplasty, it is recommended that Cefoxitin Sodium be continued for 72 hours after the surgical procedure.

If there are signs of infection, specimens for culture should be obtained for identification of the causative organism so that appropriate treatment may be instituted.

CONTRAINDICATIONS

Cefoxitin Sodium is contraindicated in patients who have shown hypersensitivity to Cefoxitin and the cephalosporin group of antibiotics.

WARNINGS

BEFORE THERAPY WITH CEFOXITIN SODIUM IS INSTITUTED, CAREFUL INQUIRY SHOULD BE MADE TO DETERMINE WHETHER THE PATIENT HAS HAD PREVIOUS HYPERSENSITIVITY REACTIONS TO CEFOXITIN, CEPHALOSPORINS, PENICILLINS, OR OTHER DRUGS. THIS PRODUCT SHOULD BE GIVEN WITH CAUTION TO PENICILLIN-SENSITIVE PATIENTS. ANTIBIOTICS SHOULD BE ADMINISTERED WITH CAUTION TO ANY PATIENT WHO HAS DEMONSTRATED SOME FORM OF ALLERGY, PARTICULARLY TO DRUGS. IF AN ALLERGIC REACTION TO 'MEFOXIN' OCCURS, DISCONTINUE THE DRUG, SERIOUS HYPERSENSITIVITY REACTIONS MAY REQUIRE EPINEPHRINE AND OTHER EMERGENCY MEASURES.

Pseudomembranous colitis has been reported with virtually all antibiotics (including cephalosporins); therefore, it is important to consider its diagnosis in patients who develop diarrhea in association with antibiotic use. This colitis may range from mild to life threatening in severity.

Treatment with broad-spectrum antibiotics alters normal flora of the colon and may permit overgrowth of clostridia. Studies indicate a toxin produced by *Clostridium difficile* is one primary cause of antibiotic-associated colitis.

Mild cases of pseudomembranous colitis may respond to drug discontinuance alone. In more severe cases, management may include sigmoidoscopy, appropriate bacteriological studies, fluid, electrolyte and protein supplementation, and the use of a drug such as oral vancomycin as indicated. Isolation of the patient may be advisable. Other causes of colitis should also be considered.

[**] *B. fragilis, B. distasonis, B. ovatus, B. thetaiotaomicron, B. vulgatus.*

PRECAUTIONS

GENERAL

The total daily dose should be reduced when Cefoxitin Sodium is administered to patients with transient or persistent reduction of urinary output due to renal insufficiency (see *"Dosage—Treatment"*), because high and prolonged serum antibiotic concentrations can occur in such individuals from usual doses.

Antibiotics (including cephalosporins) should be prescribed with caution in individuals with a history of gastrointestinal disease, particularly colitis.

As with other antibiotics, prolonged use of Cefoxitin Sodium may result in overgrowth of nonsusceptible organisms. Repeated evaluation of the patient's condition is essential. If superinfection occurs during therapy, appropriate measures should be taken.

Do not use the Premixed Intravenous Solution unless the solution is clear and the seal is intact.

DRUG INTERACTIONS

Increased nephrotoxicity has been reported following concomitant administration of cephalosporins and aminoglycoside antibiotics.

DRUG/LABORATORY TEST INTERACTIONS

As with cephalothin, high concentrations of Cefoxitin (> 100 micrograms/mL) may interfere with measurement of serum and urine creatinine levels by the Jaffe reaction, and produce false increases of modest degree in the levels of creatinine reported. Serum samples from patients treated with Cefoxitin should not be analyzed for creatinine if withdrawn within 2 hours of drug administration.

High concentrations of Cefoxitin in the urine may interfere with measurement of urinary 17-hydroxy-corticosteroids by the Porter-Silber reaction, and produce false increases of modest degree in the levels reported.

A false-positive reaction for glucose in the urine may occur. This has been observed with CLINITEST* reagent tablets.

CARCINOGENESIS, MUTAGENESIS, IMPAIRMENT OF FERTILITY

Long-term studies in animals have not been performed with Cefoxitin to evaluate carcinogenic or mutagenic potential. Studies in rats treated intravenously with 400 mg/kg of Cefoxitin (approximately three times the maximum recommended human dose) revealed no effects on fertility or mating ability.

PREGNANCY

Pregnancy Category B: Reproduction studies performed in rats and mice at parenteral doses of approximately one to seven and one-half times the maximum recommended human dose did not reveal teratogenic or fetal toxic effects, although a slight decrease in fetal weight was observed.

There are, however, no adequate and well-controlled studies in pregnant women. Because animal reproduction studies are not always predictive of human response, this drug should be used during pregnancy only if clearly needed.

In the rabbit, Cefoxitin was associated with a high incidence of abortion and maternal death. This was not considered to be a teratogenic effect but an expected consequence of the rabbit's unusual sensitivity to antibiotic-induced changes in the population of the microflora of the intestine.

NURSING MOTHERS

Cefoxitin Sodium is excreted in human milk in low concentrations. Caution should be exercised when Cefoxitin Sodium is administered to a nursing woman.

PEDIATRIC USE

Safety and efficacy in infants from birth to three months of age have not yet been established in children three months of age and older, higher doses of Cefoxitin Sodium have been associated with an increased incidence of eosinophilia and elevated SGOT.

The potential for toxic effects in children from chemicals that may leach from the single-dose I.V. preparation in plastic has not been determined.

ADVERSE REACTIONS

Cefoxitin Sodium is generally well tolerated. The most common adverse reactions have been local reactions following intravenous or intramuscular injection. Other adverse reactions have been encountered infrequently.

Local Reactions: Thrombophlebitis has occurred with intravenous administration. Pain, duration, and tenderness after intramuscular injections have been reported.

Allergic Reactions: Rash (including exfoliative dermatitis), pruritus, eosinophilia, fever, dyspnea, and other allergic reactions including anaphylaxis and angioedema have been noted.

Cardiovascular: Hypotension

Gastrointestinal: Diarrhea, including documented pseudomembranous colitis which can appear during or after antibiotic treatment. Nausea and vomiting have been reported rarely.

Blood: Eosinophilia, leukopenia, including granulocytopenia, neutropenia, anemia, including hemolytic anemia, thrombocytopenia, and bone marrow depression. A positive direct Coombs test may develop in some individuals, especially those with azotemia.

Liver Function: Transient elevations in SGOT, SGPT, serum LDH, serum alkaline phosphatase; and jaundice have been reported.

Renal Function: Elevations in serum creatinine and/or blood urea nitrogen levels have been observed. As with the cephalosporins, acute renal failure has been reported rarely. The role of Cefoxitin Sodium in changes in renal function tests is

Table 1
GUIDELINES FOR DOSAGE OF CEFOXITIN SODIUM

Type of Infection	Daily Dosage	Frequency and Route
Uncomplicated forms* of infections such as pneumonia, urinary tract infection, cutaneous infection	3-4 grams	1 gram every 6-8 hours IV or IM
Moderately severe or severe infections	6-8 grams	1 grams every 4 hours *or* 2 grams every 6-8 hours IV
Infections commonly needing antibiotics in higher dosage (e.g., gas gangrene)	12 grams	2 grams every 4 hours *or* 3 grams every 6 hours IV

* *Including patients in whom bacteremia is absent or unlikely*

Table 2
MAINTENANCE DOSAGE OF CEFOXITIN SODIUM IN ADULTS WITH REDUCED RENAL FUNCTION

Renal Function	Creatinine Clearance (mL/min)	Dose (grams)	Frequency
Mild impairment	50-30	1-2	every 8-12 hours
Moderate impairment	29-10	1-2	every 12-24 hours
Severe impairment	9-5	0.5-1	every 12-24 hours
Essentially no function	< 5	0.5-1	every 24-48 hours

difficult to assess, since factors predisposing to prerenal azotemia or to impaired renal function usually have been present.

OVERDOSAGE
The acute intravenous LD_{50} in the adult female mouse and rabbit was about 8.0 g/kg and greater than 1.0 g/kg respectively. The acute intraperitoneal LD_{50} in the adult rat was greater than 10.0 g/kg.

DOSAGE
TREATMENT

Adults: The usual adult dosage range is 1 gram to 2 grams every six to eight hours. Dosage and route of administration should be determined by susceptibility of the causative organisms, severity of infection, and the condition of the patient (see Table 1 for dosage guidelines). (See related table).

Cefoxitin Sodium may be used in patients with reduced renal function with the following dosage adjustments:

In Adults with Renal Insufficiency: an initial loading dose of 1 gram to 2 grams may be given. After a loading dose, the recommendations for *maintenance dosage* (Table 2) may be used as a guide. (See related table).

When Only the Serum Creatinine Level is Available: the following formula (based on sex, weight, and age of the patient) may be used to convert this value into creatinine clearance. The serum creatinine should represent a steady state of renal function.

Males:
$$\frac{\text{Weight (kg)} \times (140 - \text{age})}{72 \times \text{serum creatinine (mg/100 mL)}}$$

Females: $0.85 \times$ above value

In Patients Undergoing Hemodialysis: the loading dose of 1 to 2 grams should be given after each hemodialysis, and the maintenance dose should be given as indicated in Table 2. Antibiotic therapy for group A beta-hemolytic streptococcal infections should be maintained for at least 10 days to guard against the risk of rheumatic fever or glomerulonephritis. In staphylococcal and other infections involving a collection of pus, surgical drainage should be carried out where indicated. The recommended dosage of Cefoxitin Sodium *for uncomplicated gonorrhea* is 2 grams intramuscularly, with 1 gram of Probenecid given by mouth at the same time or up to ½ hour before Cefoxitin Sodium.

Infants and Children: The recommended dosage in children three months of age and older is 80 to 160 mg/kg of body weight per day divided into four to six equal doses. The higher dosages should be used for more severe or serious infections. The total daily dosage should not exceed 12 grams.

At this time no recommendation is made for children from birth to three months of age (see "Precautions").

In children with renal insufficiency the dosage and frequency of dosage should be modified consistent with the recommendations for adults (see Table 2).

PREVENTION
General: For prophylactic use in surgery the following doses are recommended:

Adults: 1) 2 grams administered intravenously or intramuscularly just prior to surgery (approximately one-half to one hour before the initial incision).

2) 2 grams every 6 hours after the first dose for no more than 24 hours (continued for 72 hours after prosthetic arthroplasty).

Children (3 months and older): 30 to 40 mg/kg doses may be given at the times designated above.

Obstetric-Gynecologic: For prophylactic use in vaginal hysterectomy, a single 2.0 gram dose administered intramuscularly one-half to one hour prior to surgery is recommended.

For patients undergoing cesarean section, a single 2.0 gram dose should be administered intravenously as soon as the umbilical cord is clamped. A 3-dose regimen may be more effective than a single dose regimen in preventing postoperative infection (esp. endometritis) following cesarean section. Such a regimen would consist of 2.0 grams given intravenously as soon as the umbilical cord is clamped, followed by 2.0 grams 4 and 8 hours after the initial dose.

Transurethral Prostatectomy Patients: One gram administered just prior to surgery; 1 gram every 8 hours for up to five days.

PREPARATION OF SOLUTION
Table 3 is provided for convenience in constituting Cefoxitin Sodium for both intravenous and intramuscular administration. (See related table).

For Intravenous Use: 1 gram should be constituted with at least 10 mL of Sterile Water for Injection, and 2 grams, with 10 or 20 mL. The 10 gram bulk package should be constituted with 43 or 93 mL of Sterile Water for Injection or any of the solutions listed under the *"Intravenous"* portion of the *"Compatibility and Stability"* section. CAUTION: THE 10 GRAM BULK STOCK SOLUTION IS NOT FOR DIRECT INFUSION. One or 2 grams of Cefoxitin Sodium for infusion may be constituted with 50 or 100 mL of 0.9 percent Sodium Chloride Injection, 5 percent or 10 percent Dextrose Injection, or any or the solutions listed under the *"Intravenous"* portion of the *"Compatibility and Stability"* section.

Benzyl alcohol as a preservative has been associated with toxicity in neonates. While toxicity has not been demonstrated in infants greater than three months of age, in whom use of Cefoxitin Sodium may be indicated, small infants in this age range may also be at risk for benzyl alcohol toxicity. Therefore, diluent containing benzyl alcohol should not be used when Cefoxitin Sodium is constituted for administration to infants.

For ADD-Vantage®† *vials,* see separate *"Instructions for Use of Cefoxitin Sodium in ADD-Vantage*® *Vials."* Cefoxitin Sodium in ADD-Vantage®™ vials should be constituted with ADD-Vantage® diluent containers containing 50 mL or 100 mL of either 0.9 percent Sodium Chloride Injection or 5 percent Dextrose Injection. Cefoxitin Sodium in ADD-Vantage® vials is for IV use only.

For Intramuscular Use: each gram of Cefoxitin Sodium may be constituted with 2 mL of Sterile Water for Injection, *or*—

For Intramuscular Use ONLY: each gram of Cefoxitin Sodium may be constituted with 2 mL of 0.5 percent lidocaine hydrochloride solution** (without epinephrine) to minimize the discomfort of intramuscular injection.

ADMINISTRATION
Cefoxitin Sodium may be administered intravenously or intramuscularly after constitution.

Parenteral drug products should be inspected visually for particulate matter and discoloration prior to administration whenever solution and container permit.

INTRAVENOUS ADMINISTRATION
The intravenous route is preferable for patients with bacteremia, bacterial septicemia, or other severe or life-threatening infections, or for patients who may be poor risks because of lowered resistance resulting from such debilitating conditions as malnutrition, trauma, surgery, diabetes, heart failure, or malignancy, particularly if shock is present or impending.

For Intermittent Intravenous Administration: a solution containing 1 gram or 2 grams in 10 mL of Sterile Water for Injection can be injected over a period of

† Registered trademark of Abbott Laboratories.
** See package circular of manufacturer for detailed information concerning contraindications, warnings, precautions, and adverse reactions.

◆ RATED THERAPEUTICALLY EQUIVALENT; ◇ THERAPEUTIC EQUIVALENCE UNCONFIRMED; ○ UNRATED

three to five minutes. Using an infusion system, it may also be given over a longer period of time through the tubing system by which the patient may be receiving other intravenous solutions. However, during infusion of the solution containing Cefoxitin Sodium, it is advisable to temporarily discontinue administration of any other solutions at the same site.

For the Administration of Higher Doses by Continuous Intravenous Infusion: a solution of Cefoxitin Sodium may be added to an intravenous bottle containing 5 percent Dextrose Injection, 0.9 percent Sodium Chloride Injection, 5 percent Dextrose and 0.9 percent Sodium Chloride Injection, or 5 percent Dextrose Injection with 0.02 percent sodium bicarbonate solution. BUTTERFLY† or scalp vein-type needles are preferred for this type of infusion.

The premixed solution is for intravenous use only. Premixed intravenous Solution Cefoxitin Sodium in Galaxy® containers (PL 2040 Plastic) is to be administered either as a continuous or intermittent infusion using sterile equipment. Scalp vein-type needles are preferred for this type of infusion. It is recommended that the intravenous administration apparatus be replaced at least once every 48 hours.

Directions for Use of Galaxy® Containers (PL 2040 Plastic)
Thaw frozen container at room temperature, 25°C (77°F), or under refrigeration, 2-8°C (36-46°F). DO NOT FORCE THAW BY IMMERSION IN WATER BATHS OR BY MICROWAVE IRRADIATION.

After thawing, check for minute leaks by squeezing container firmly. If leaks are detected, discard solution as sterility may be impaired.

The container should be visually inspected for particulate matter and discoloration prior to administration. Components of the solution may precipitate in the frozen state and will dissolve upon reaching room temperature with little or no agitation. Agitate after solution has reached room temperature.

Do not use if the solution is cloudy or a precipitate has formed. If any seals or outlet ports are not intact, the container should be discarded. Solutions of Cefoxitin Sodium tend to darken depending on storage conditions; product potency, however, is not adversely affected.

Additives should not be introduced into this solution.

Caution: Do not use plastic containers in series connections. Such use would result in air embolism due to residual air being drawn from the primary container before administration of the fluid from the secondary container is complete.

PREPARATION FOR INTRAVENOUS ADMINISTRATION:
1. Suspend container from eyelet support.
2. Remove plastic protector from outlet port at bottom of container.
3. Attach administration set. Refer to complete directions accompanying set.

Cefoxitin Sodium may be administered through the tubing system by which the patient may be receiving other intravenous solutions. However, during infusion of the solution containing Cefoxitin Sodium, it is advisable to temporarily discontinue administration of any other solutions at the same site.

Solutions of Cefoxitin Sodium, like those of most beta-lactam antibiotics, should not be added to aminoglycoside solutions (e.g., gentamicin sulfate, tobramycin sulfate, amikacin sulfate) because of potential interaction. However, Cefoxitin Sodium and aminoglycosides may be administered separately to the same patient.

INTRAMUSCULAR ADMINISTRATION
As with all intramuscular preparations, Cefoxitin Sodium should be injected well within the body of a relatively large muscle such as the upper outer quadrant of the buttock (i.e., gluteus maximus); aspiration is necessary to avoid inadvertent injection into a blood vessel.

COMPATIBILITY AND STABILITY
INTRAVENOUS
Cefoxitin Sodium, as supplied in vials or the bulk package and constituted to 1 gram/10 mL with Sterile Water for Injection. Bacteriostatic Water for Injection (see *"Preparation of Solution"*), 0.9 percent Sodium Chloride Injection, or 5 percent Dextrose Injection, maintains satisfactory potency for 24 hours at room temperature, for one week under refrigeration (below 5°C), and for at least 30 weeks in the frozen state.

These primary solutions may be further diluted in 50 to 1000 mL of the following solutions and maintain potency for 24 hours at room temperature and at least 48 hours under refrigeration:

† Registered trademark of Abbott Laboratories.

Sterile Water for Injection†
0.9 percent Sodium Chloride Injection
5 percent or 10 percent Dextrose Injection‡
5 percent Dextrose and 0.9 percent Sodium Chloride Injection
5 percent Dextrose Injection with 0.02 percent sodium bicarbonate solution
5 percent Dextrose Injection with 0.2 percent or 0.45 percent saline solution
Ringer's Injection
Lactated Ringer's Injection‡
5 percent dextrose in Lactated Ringer's Injection‡
5 percent or 10 percent invert sugar in water
10 percent invert sugar in saline solution
5 percent Sodium Bicarbonate Injection
Neut (sodium bicarbonate)*‡
M/6 sodium lactate solution
NORMOSOL-M in D5-W*‡
IONOSOL B w/Dextrose 5 percent*‡
POLYONIC M 56 in 5 percent Dextrose**
Mannitol 5% and 2.5%
Mannitol 10%‡
ISOLYTE*** E
ISOLYTE*** E with 5% dextrose

Cefoxitin Sodium, as supplied in infusion bottles and constituted with 50 to 100 mL of 0.9 percent Sodium Chloride Injection, or 5 percent or 10 percent Dextrose Injection, maintains satisfactory potency for 24 hours at room temperature or for 1 week under refrigeration (below 5°C).

Cefoxitin Sodium supplied in single dose ADD-Vantage® vials should be prepared as directed in the accompanying *"Instructions for Use of Cefoxitin Sodium in Add-Vantage® Vials"* using ADD-Vantage® diluent containers containing 50 mL or 100 mL of either 0.9 percent Sodium Chloride Injection or 5 percent Dextrose Injection. When prepared with either of these diluents, Cefoxitin Sodium maintains satisfactory potency for 24 hours at room temperature.

Limited studies with solutions of Cefoxitin Sodium in 0.9 percent Sodium Chloride Injection, Lactated Ringer's Injection, and 5 percent Dextrose Injection in VIAFLEX† intravenous bags show stability for 24 hours at room temperature, 48 hours under refrigeration or 26 weeks in the frozen state and 24 hours at room temperature thereafter. Also, solutions of Cefoxitin Sodium in 0.9 percent Sodium Chloride Injection show similar stability in plastic tubing, drip chambers, and volume control devices of common intravenous infusion sets. After constitution with Sterile Water for Injection and subsequent storage in disposable plastic syringes, Cefoxitin Sodium is stable for 24 hours at room temperature and 48 hours under refrigeration.

Cefoxitin Sodium, supplied as frozen, premixed, iso-osmotic solution in Galaxy® containers (PL 2040 Plastic), maintains satisfactory potency after thawing for 24 hours at a room temperature of 25°C (77°F) or 21 days under refrigeration, 2-8°C (36-46°F).

After the periods mentioned above, any unused solutions or frozen material should be discarded. Do not refreeze.

INTRAMUSCULAR
Cefoxitin Sodium, as constituted with Sterile Water for Injection, Bacteriostatic Water for Injection, or 0.5 percent or 1 percent lidocaine hydrochloride solution (without epinephrine), maintains satisfactory potency for 24 hours at room temperature, for one week under refrigeration (below 5°C), and for at least 30 weeks in the frozen state.

After the periods mentioned above, any unused solutions or frozen material should be discarded. Do not refreeze.

Cefoxitin Sodium has also been found compatible when admixed in intravenous infusions with the following:

Heparin 0.1 units/mL at room temperature—8 hours
Heparin 100 units/mL at room temperature—24 hours

† In these solutions Cefoxitin Sodium has been found to be stable for a period of one week under refrigeration.
* Registered trademark of Abbott Laboratories.
‡ In these solutions, Cefoxitin Sodium has been found to be stable for a period of one week under refrigeration.
** Registered trademark of Cutter Laboratories, Inc.
***Registered trademark of American Hospital Supply Corporation.
† Registered trademark of Baxter International, Ltd.

Table 3
CEFOXITIN SODIUM: PREPARATION OF SOLUTION

Strength	Amount of Diluent to be Added (mL)*	Approximate Withdrawable Volume (mL)	Approximate Average Concentration (mg/mL)
1 gram Vial	2 (Intramuscular)	2.5	400
2 gram Vial	4 (Intramuscular)	5	400
1 gram Vial	10 (IV)	10.5	95
2 gram Vial	10 or 20 (IV)	11.1 or 21.0	180 or 95
1 gram Infusion Bottle	50 or 100 (IV)	50 or 100	20 or 10
2 gram Infusion Bottle	50 or 100 (IV)	50 or 100	40 or 20
10 gram Bulk	43 or 93 (IV)	49 or 98.5	200 or 100

* Shake to dissolve and let stand until clear.

➤ SHOWN IN PRODUCT IDENTIFICATION GUIDE

M.V.I.[††] concentrate at room temperature 24 hours; under refrigeration 48 hours
BEROCCA[†††] C-500 at room temperature 24 hours; under refrigeration 48 hours
Insulin in Normal Saline at room temperature 24 hours; under refrigeration 48 hours
Insulin in 10% invert sugar at room temperature 24 hours; under refrigeration 48 hours

SPECIAL STORAGE INSTRUCTIONS
Cefoxitin Sodium in the dry state should be stored below 30°C. Avoid exposure to temperatures above 50°C. The dry material as well as solutions tend to darken, depending on storage conditions; product potency, however, is not adversely affected.

J CODES
1 g IV,IM—J0694

HOW SUPPLIED
INJECTION: 1 GM

BRAND/MANUFACTURER	NDC	SIZE	AWP
○ BRAND MEFOXIN: Merck	00006-3545-24	50 ml 24s	$271.23

INJECTION: 2 GM/50 ML

BRAND/MANUFACTURER	NDC	SIZE	AWP
○ BRAND MEFOXIN: Merck	00006-3547-25	50 ml 24s	$482.04

POWDER FOR INJECTION: 1 GM

BRAND/MANUFACTURER	NDC	SIZE	AWP
○ BRAND MEFOXIN: Merck	00006-3368-71	10s	$96.26
	00006-3356-45	25s	$221.21
	00006-3548-45	25s	$230.95

POWDER FOR INJECTION: 2 GM

BRAND/MANUFACTURER	NDC	SIZE	AWP
○ BRAND MEFOXIN: Merck	00006-3369-73	10s	$183.85
	00006-3357-53	25s	$440.83
	00006-3549-53	25s	$450.55

POWDER FOR INJECTION: 10 GM

BRAND/MANUFACTURER	NDC	SIZE	AWP
○ BRAND MEFOXIN: Merck	00006-3388-67	6s	$528.91

Cefpodoxime Proxetil

DESCRIPTION
Cefpodoxime Proxetil is an orally administered, extended spectrum, semi-synthetic antibiotic of the cephalosporin class. The chemical name is (RS)-1-(isopropoxycarbonyloxy)-ethyl (+)-(6R,7R)-7-[2-(2-amino-4-thiazolyl)-2-[(Z)-methoxyimino] acetamido]-3-methoxymethyl-8-oxo-5-thia-1-azabicyclo[4.2.0]oct-2-ene-2-carboxylate.

Its empirical formula is $C_{21}H_{27}N_5O_9S_2$.
The molecular weight of Cefpodoxime Proxetil is 557.6.

Cefpodoxime Proxetil is a prodrug; its active metabolite is Cefpodoxime. All doses of Cefpodoxime Proxetil in this monograph are expressed in terms of the active Cefpodoxime moiety. The drug is supplied both as film-coated tablets and as flavored granules for oral suspension.

Tablets contain Cefpodoxime Proxetil equivalent to 100 mg or 200 mg of Cefpodoxime activity.

Each 5 mL of Cefpodoxime Proxetil Oral Suspension contains Cefpodoxime Proxetil equivalent to 50 mg or 100 mg of Cefpodoxime activity after constitution.

Following is its chemical structure:

[††] Registered trademark of USV Pharmaceutical Corp.
[†††] Registered trademark of Roche Laboratories.

CLINICAL PHARMACOLOGY
ABSORPTION AND EXCRETION
Cefpodoxime Proxetil is a prodrug that is absorbed from the gastrointestinal tract and de-esterified to its active metabolite, Cefpodoxime. Following oral administration of 100 mg of Cefpodoxime Proxetil to fasting subjects, approximately 50% of the administered Cefpodoxime dose was absorbed systemically. Over the recommended dosing range (100 to 400 mg), approximately 29 to 33% of the administered Cefpodoxime dose was excreted unchanged in the urine in 12 hours. There is minimal metabolism of Cefpodoxime in vivo.

EFFECT OF FOOD
The extent of absorption (mean AUC) and the mean peak plasma concentration increased when film-coated tablets were administered with food. Following a 200 mg tablet dose taken with food, the AUC was 21 to 33% higher than under fasting conditions, and the peak plasma concentration averaged 3.1 mcg/mL in fed subjects versus 2.6 mcg/mL in fasted subjects. Time to peak concentration was not significantly different between fed and fasted subjects.

When a 200 mg dose of the suspension was taken with food, the extent of absorption (mean AUC) and mean peak plasma concentration in fed subjects were not significantly different from fasted subjects, but the rate of absorption was slower with food (48% increase in T_{MAX}).

PHARMACOKINETICS OF CEFPODOXIME PROXETIL
FILM-COATED TABLETS
Over the recommended dosing range, (100 to 400 mg), the rate and extent of Cefpodoxime absorption exhibited dose-dependency; dose-normalized C_{max} and AUC decreased by up to 32% with increasing dose. Over the recommended dosing range, the T_{max} was approximately 2 to 3 hours and the $T_{1/2}$ ranged from 2.09 to 2.84 hours. Mean C_{max} was 1.4 mcg/mL for the 100 mg dose, 2.3 mcg/mL for the 200 mg dose, and 3.9 mcg/mL for the 400 mg dose. In patients with normal renal function, neither accumulation nor significant changes in other pharmacokinetic parameters were noted following multiple oral doses of up to 400 mg Q 12 hours.

CEFPODOXIME PLASMA LEVELS (MCG/ML) IN FASTED ADULTS AFTER FILM-COATED TABLET ADMINISTRATION (SINGLE DOSE)

Dose	Time after oral ingestion						
(Cefpodoxime equivalents)	1hr	2hr	3hr	4hr	6hr	8hr	12hr
100 mg	0.98	1.4	1.3	1.0	0.59	0.29	0.08
200 mg	1.5	2.2	2.2	1.8	1.2	0.62	0.18
400 mg	2.2	3.7	3.8	3.3	2.3	1.3	0.38

PHARMACOKINETICS OF CEFPODOXIME PROXETIL SUSPENSION
In adult subjects, a 100 mg dose of oral suspension produced an average peak Cefpodoxime concentration of approximately 1.5 mcg/mL (range: 1.1 to 2.1 mcg/mL), which is equivalent to that reported following administration of the 100 mg tablet. Time to peak plasma concentration and area under the plasma concentration-time curve (AUC) for the oral suspension were also equivalent to those produced with film-coated tablets in adults following a 100 mg oral dose.

The pharmacokinetics of Cefpodoxime were investigated in 18 patients aged 4 to 17 years. Each patient received a single, oral, 5 mg/kg dose of Cefpodoxime oral suspension. Plasma and urine samples were collected for 12 hours after dosing. The plasma levels reported from this study are as follows:

CEFPODOXIME PLASMA LEVELS (MCG/ML) IN FASTED PATIENTS (4 TO 17 YEARS OF AGE) AFTER SUSPENSION ADMINISTRATION

Dose	Time after oral ingestion						
(Cefpodoxime equivalents)	1hr	2hr	3hr	4hr	6hr	8hr	12hr
5 mg/kg[1]	1.6	2.4	2.3	1.9	0.96	0.41	0.091

[1] Dose did not exceed 200 mg.

DISTRIBUTION
Protein binding of Cefpodoxime ranges from 22 to 33% in serum and from 21 to 29% in plasma.

Skin Blister: Following multiple-dose administration every 12 hours for 5 days of 200 mg or 400 mg Cefpodoxime Proxetil, the mean maximum Cefpodoxime concentration in skin blister fluid averaged 1.6 and 2.8 mcg/mL, respectively. Skin blister fluid Cefpodoxime levels at 12 hours after dosing averaged 0.2 and 0.4 mcg/mL for the 200 mg and 400 mg multiple-dose regimens, respectively.

Tonsil Tissue: Following a single, oral 100 mg Cefpodoxime Proxetil film-coated tablet, the mean maximum Cefpodoxime concentration in tonsil tissue averaged 0.24 mcg/g at 4 hours post-dosing and 0.09 mcg/g at 7 hours post-dosing. Equilibrium was achieved between plasma and tonsil tissue within 4 hours of dosing. No detection of Cefpodoxime in tonsillar tissue was reported 12 hours after dosing. These results demonstrated that concentrations of Cefpodoxime exceeded the MIC_{90} of S. pyogenes for at least 7 hours after dosing of 100 mg of Cefpodoxime Proxetil.

Lung Tissue: Following a single, oral 200 mg Cefpodoxime Proxetil film-coated tablet, the mean maximum Cefpodoxime concentration in lung tissue averaged 0.63 mcg/g at 3 hours post-dosing, 0.52 mcg/g at 6 hours post-dosing, and 0.19 mcg/g at 12 hours post-dosing. The results of this study indicated that Cefpodoxime penetrated into lung tissue and produced sustained drug concentra-

---

◆ RATED THERAPEUTICALLY EQUIVALENT; ◇ THERAPEUTIC EQUIVALENCE UNCONFIRMED; ○ UNRATED

tions for at least 12 hours after dosing at levels that exceeded the MIC_{90} for *S. pneumoniae* and *H. influenzae*.

CSF: Adequate data on CSF levels of Cefpodoxime are not available.

EFFECTS OF DECREASED RENAL FUNCTION

Elimination of Cefpodoxime is reduced in patients with moderate to severe renal impairment (< 50 mL/min creatinine clearance). (See *"Precautions"* and *"Dosage and Administration.")* In subjects with mild impairment of renal function (50 to 80 mL/min creatinine clearance), the average plasma half-life of Cefpodoxime was 3.5 hours. In subjects with moderate (30 to 49 mL/min creatinine clearance) or severe renal impairment (5 to 29 mL/min creatinine clearance), the half-life increased to 5.9 to 9.8 hours, respectively. Approximately 23% of the administered dose was cleared from the body during a standard 3-hour hemodialysis procedure.

EFFECT OF HEPATIC IMPAIRMENT (CIRRHOSIS)

Absorption was somewhat diminished and elimination unchanged in patients with cirrhosis. The mean Cefpodoxime $T_{1/2}$ and renal clearance in cirrhotic patients were similar to those derived in studies of healthy subjects. Ascites did not appear to affect values in cirrhotic subjects. No dosage adjustment is recommended in this patient population.

PHARMACOKINETICS IN ELDERLY SUBJECTS

Elderly subjects do not require dosage adjustments unless they have diminished renal function. (See *"Precautions."*) In healthy geriatric subjects, Cefpodoxime half-life in plasma averaged 4.2 hours (vs 3.3 in younger subjects) and urinary recovery averaged 21% after a 400 mg dose was administered every 12 hours. Other pharmacokinetic parameters (C_{max}, AUC, and T_{max}) were unchanged relative to those observed in healthy young subjects.

MICROBIOLOGY

Cefpodoxime is active *in vitro* against a wide range of gram-positive and gram-negative bacteria. Cefpodoxime is highly stable in the presence of beta-lactamase enzymes. As a result, many organisms resistant to penicillins and some cephalosporins, due to the presence of beta-lactamases, may be susceptible to Cefpodoxime.

The bactericidal activity of Cefpodoxime results from its inhibition of cell wall synthesis. Cefpodoxime is usually active against the following organisms *in vitro* and in clinical infections. (See *"Indications and Usage."*)

GRAM-POSITIVE AEROBES

Staphylococcus aureus (including penicillinase-producing strains)
Note: Cefpodoxime is inactive against methicillin-resistant staphylococci.
Staphylococcus saprophyticus
Streptococcus pneumoniae
Streptococcus pyogenes

GRAM-NEGATIVE AEROBES

Escherichia coli
Haemophilus influenzae (including β-lactamase-producing strains)
Klebsiella pneumoniae
Moraxella (Branhamella) catarrhalis
Neisseria gonorrhoeae (including penicillinase-producing strains)
Proteus mirabilis
The following *in vitro* data are available; *however, their clinical significance is unknown.*

Cefpodoxime exhibits *in vitro* minimum inhibitory concentrations of 2.0 mcg/mL or less against most strains of the following organisms. The safety and effectiveness of Cefpodoxime Proxetil in treating infections due to these organisms have not been established in adequate and well-controlled trials.

GRAM-POSITIVE AEROBES

Streptococcus agalactiae
Streptococcus spp. (Groups C, F, G)
Note: Cefpodoxime is inactive against most strains of *Enterococcus*.

GRAM-NEGATIVE AEROBES

Citrobacter diversus
Haemophilus parainfluenzae
Klebsiella oxytoca
Proteus vulgaris
Providencia rettgeri
Note: Cefpodoxime is inactive against most strains of *Pseudomonas* and *Enterobacter*.

ANAEROBES

Peptostreptococcus magnus

SUSCEPTIBILITY TESTING

Diffusion Techniques: Quantitative methods that require measurement of zone diameters give the most precise estimate of the susceptibility of bacteria to antimicrobial agents. One such standardized procedure[1] recommended for use with the 10 mcg Cefpodoxime disk is the National Committee for Clinical Laboratory Standards (NCCLS) approved procedure.

Interpretation involves correlation of the diameters obtained in the disk test with the minimum inhibitory concentration (MIC) for Cefpodoxime.

Reports from the laboratory giving results of the standardized single disk susceptibility test using a 10 mcg Cefpodoxime disk should be interpreted according to the following criteria:

Zone diameter (mm)	Interpretation
≥ 21	(S) Susceptible
18-20	(I) Intermediate
≤ 17	(R) Resistant

A report of "Susceptible" indicates that the pathogen is likely to be inhibited by generally achievable blood levels. A report of "Intermediate" indicates that the result should be considered equivocal, and, if the organism is not fully susceptible to alternative, clinically feasible drugs, the test should be repeated. This category implies clinical applicability in body sites where the drug is physiologically concentrated or in situations where high dosage of drug can be used. This category provides a buffer zone that prevents small uncontrolled technical factors from causing major discrepancies in interpretation. A report of "Resistant" indicates that achievable concentrations of the antibiotic are unlikely to be inhibitory and other therapy should be selected.

Standardized procedures require the use of laboratory control organisms. The 10 mcg disk should give the following zone diameters:

Organism	Zone diameter (mm)
Escherichia coli ATCC 25922	23-28
Staphylococcus aureus ATCC 25923	19-25

Cephalosporin "class disks" should not be used to test for susceptibility to Cefpodoxime.

Dilution Technique: Use a standardized dilution method[2] (broth, agar, microdilution) or equivalent with Cefpodoxime susceptibility powder. The MIC values should be interpreted according to the following criteria:

MIC (mcg/mL)	Interpretation
≤ 2	(S) Susceptible
4	(I) Intermediate
≥ 8	(R) Resistant

As with standard diffusion methods, dilution procedures require the use of laboratory control organisms. Standard Cefpodoxime susceptibility powder should give the following MIC values:

Organism	MIC range (mcg/mL)
Escherichia coli ATCC 25922	0.25-1
Staphylococcus aureus ATCC 29213	1-8

Note : Susceptibility testing by dilution methods requires the use of Cefpodoxime susceptibility powder.

Cefpodoxime Proxetil granules for oral use should *Not* be used for *in vitro* susceptibility tests.

INDICATIONS AND USAGE

Cefpodoxime Proxetil is indicated for the treatment of patients with mild to moderate infections caused by susceptible strains of the designated microorganisms in the conditions listed below. **Recommended dosages, durations of therapy, and applicable patient populations vary among these infections. Please see "Dosage and Administration" for specific recommendations.**

LOWER RESPIRATORY TRACT

Acute, community-acquired pneumonia caused by *S. pneumoniae* or *H. influenzae* (non-beta-lactamase-producing strains only). Data are insufficient at this time to establish efficacy in patients with pneumonia caused by beta-lactamase-producing strains of *H. influenzae*.

Acute bacterial exacerbation of chronic bronchitis caused by *S. pneumoniae, H. influenzae* (non-beta-lactamase-producing strains only), or *M. catarrhalis*. Data are insufficient at this time to establish efficacy in patients with acute bacterial exacerbations of chronic bronchitis caused by beta-lactamase-producing strains of *H. influenzae*.

SEXUALLY TRANSMITTED DISEASES

Acute, uncomplicated urethral and cervical gonorrhea caused by *Neisseria gonorrhoeae* (including penicillinase-producing strains)

Acute, uncomplicated ano-rectal infections in women due to *Neisseria gonorrhoeae* (including penicillinase-producing strains)
NOTE: The efficacy of Cefpodoxime in treating male patients with rectal infections caused by *N. gonorrhoeae* has not been established. Data do not support the use of Cefpodoxime Proxetil in the treatment of pharyngeal infections due to *N. gonorrhoeae* in men or women.

SKIN AND SKIN STRUCTURES

Uncomplicated skin and skin structure infections caused by *Staphylococcus aureus* (including penicillinase-producing strains) or *Streptococcus pyogenes*. Abscesses should be surgically drained as clinically indicated.

Note: In clinical trials, successful treatment of uncomplicated skin and skin structure infections was dose-related. The effective therapeutic dose for skin infections was higher than those used in other recommended indications. (See *"Dosage and Administration."*)

UPPER RESPIRATORY TRACT
Acute otitis media caused by *Streptococcus pneumoniae*, *Haemophilus influenzae* (including β-lactamase-producing strains), or *Moraxella (Branhamella) catarrhalis*.

Pharyngitis and/or tonsillitis caused by *Streptococcus pyogenes*.

Note: Only penicillin by the intramuscular route of administration has been shown to be effective in the prophylaxis of rheumatic fever. Cefpodoxime Proxetil is generally effective in the eradication of streptococci from the oropharynx. However, data establishing the efficacy of Cefpodoxime Proxetil for the prophylaxis of subsequent rheumatic fever are not available.

URINARY TRACT
Uncomplicated urinary tract infections (cystitis) caused by *Escherichia coli*, *Klebsiella pneumoniae*, *Proteus mirabilis*, or *Staphylococcus saprophyticus*.

Note: In considering the use of Cefpodoxime Proxetil in the treatment of cystitis, Cefpodoxime Proxetil's lower bacterial eradication rates should be weighed against the increased eradication rates and different safety profiles of some other classes of approved agents. (See *"Clinical Studies"* section.)

Appropriate specimens for bacteriological examination should be obtained in order to isolate and identify causative organisms and to determine their susceptibility to Cefpodoxime. Therapy may be instituted while awaiting the results of these studies. Once these results become available, antimicrobial therapy should be adjusted accordingly.

CONTRAINDICATIONS
Cefpodoxime Proxetil is contraindicated in patients with a known allergy to Cefpodoxime or to the cephalosporin group of antibiotics.

WARNINGS
BEFORE THERAPY WITH CEFPODOXIME PROXETIL IS INSTITUTED, CAREFUL INQUIRY SHOULD BE MADE TO DETERMINE WHETHER THE PATIENT HAS HAD PREVIOUS HYPERSENSITIVITY REACTIONS TO CEFPODOXIME, OTHER CEPHALOSPORINS, PENICILLINS, OR OTHER DRUGS. IF CEFPODOXIME IS TO BE ADMINISTERED TO PENICILLIN-SENSITIVE PATIENTS, CAUTION SHOULD BE EXERCISED BECAUSE CROSS HYPERSENSITIVITY AMONG BETA-LACTAM ANTIBIOTICS HAS BEEN CLEARLY DOCUMENTED AND MAY OCCUR IN UP TO 10% OF PATIENTS WITH A HISTORY OF PENICILLIN ALLERGY. IF AN ALLERGIC REACTION TO CEFPODOXIME PROXETIL OCCURS, DISCONTINUE THE DRUG. SERIOUS ACUTE HYPERSENSITIVITY REACTIONS MAY REQUIRE TREATMENT WITH EPINEPHRINE AND OTHER EMERGENCY MEASURES, INCLUDING OXYGEN, INTRAVENOUS FLUIDS, INTRAVENOUS ANTIHISTAMINE, AND AIRWAY MANAGEMENT, AS CLINICALLY INDICATED. PSEUDOMEMBRANOUS COLITIS HAS BEEN REPORTED WITH NEARLY ALL ANTIBACTERIAL AGENTS, INCLUDING CEFPODOXIME, AND MAY RANGE IN SEVERITY FROM MILD TO LIFE-THREATENING. THEREFORE, IT IS IMPORTANT TO CONSIDER THIS DIAGNOSIS IN PATIENTS WHO PRESENT WITH DIARRHEA SUBSEQUENT TO THE ADMINISTRATION OF ANTIBACTERIAL AGENTS.

Extreme caution should be observed when using this product in patients at increased risk for antibiotic-induced, pseudomembranous colitis because of exposure to institutional settings, such as nursing homes or hospitals with endemic *C. difficile*.

Treatment with broad-spectrum antibiotics, including Cefpodoxime Proxetil, alters the normal flora of the colon and may permit overgrowth of clostridia. Studies indicate a toxin produced by *Clostridium difficile* is the primary cause of "antibiotic-associated colitis".

After the diagnosis of pseudomembranous colitis has been established, therapeutic measures should be initiated. Mild cases of pseudomembranous colitis usually respond to drug discontinuation alone. In moderate to severe cases, consideration should be given to management with fluids and electrolytes, protein supplementation, and treatment with an oral antibacterial drug effective against *C. difficile*.

A concerted effort to monitor for *C. difficile* in Cefpodoxime treated patients with diarrhea was undertaken because of an increased incidence of diarrhea associated with *C. difficile* in early trials in normal subjects. *C. difficile* organisms or toxin was reported in 10% of the Cefpodoxime-treated adult patients with diarrhea; however, no specific diagnosis of pseudomembranous colitis was made in these patients.

In post-marketing experience outside the United States, reports of pseudomembranous colitis associated with the use of Cefpodoxime Proxetil have been received.

PRECAUTIONS
GENERAL
In patients with transient or persistent reduction in urinary output due to renal insufficiency, the total daily dose of Cefpodoxime Proxetil should be reduced because high and prolonged serum antibiotic concentrations can occur in such individuals following usual doses. Cefpodoxime, like other cephalosporins, should be administered with caution to patients receiving concurrent treatment with potent diuretics. (See *"Dosage and Administration"*).

As with other antibiotics, prolonged use of Cefpodoxime Proxetil may result in overgrowth of non-susceptible organisms. Repeated evaluation of the patient's condition is essential. If superinfection occurs during therapy, appropriate measures should be taken.

DRUG INTERACTIONS
Antacids: Concomitant administration of high doses of antacids (sodium bicarbonate and aluminum hydroxide) or H$_2$ blockers reduces peak plasma levels by 24% to 42% and the extent of absorption by 27% to 32%, respectively. The rate of absorption is not altered by these concomitant medications. Oral anti-cholinergics

(e.g., propantheline) delay peak plasma levels (47% increase in T$_{max}$), but do not affect the extent of absorption (AUC).

Probenecid: As with other beta-lactam antibiotics, renal excretion of Cefpodoxime was inhibited by probenecid and resulted in an approximately 31% increase in AUC and 20% increase in peak Cefpodoxime plasma levels.

Nephrotoxic Drugs: Although nephrotoxicity has not been noted when Cefpodoxime Proxetil was given alone, close monitoring of renal function is advised when Cefpodoxime Proxetil is administered concomitantly with compounds of known nephrotoxic potential.

DRUG/LABORATORY TEST INTERACTIONS
Cephalosporins, including Cefpodoxime Proxetil, are known to occasionally induce a positive direct Coombs' test.

CARCINOGENESIS, MUTAGENESIS, IMPAIRMENT OF FERTILITY
Long-term animal carcinogenesis studies of Cefpodoxime Proxetil have not been performed. Mutagenesis studies of Cefpodoxime, including the Ames test both with and without metabolic activation, the chromosome aberration test, the unscheduled DNA synthesis assay, mitotic recombination and gene conversion, the forward gene mutation assay and the *in vivo* micronucleus test, were all negative. No untoward effects on fertility or reproduction were noted when 100 mg/kg/day or less (2 times the human dose based on mg/m^2) was administered orally to rats.

PREGNANCY—TERATOGENIC EFFECTS
Pregnancy Category B
Cefpodoxime Proxetil was neither teratogenic nor embryocidal when administered to rats during organogenesis at doses up to 100 mg/kg/day (2 times the human dose based on mg/m^2) or to rabbits at doses up to 30 mg/kg/day (1-2 times the human dose based on mg/m^2).

There are, however, no adequate and well-controlled studies of Cefpodoxime Proxetil use in pregnant women.

Because animal reproduction studies are not always predictive of human response, this drug should be used during pregnancy only if clearly needed.

LABOR AND DELIVERY
Cefpodoxime Proxetil has not been studied for use during labor and delivery. Treatment should only be given if clearly needed.

NURSING MOTHERS
Cefpodoxime is excreted in human milk. In a study of 3 lactating women, levels of Cefpodoxime in human milk were 0%, 2% and 6% of concomitant serum levels at 4 hours following a 200 mg dose of Cefpodoxime Proxetil. At 6 hours post-dosing, levels were 0%, 9% and 16% of concomitant serum levels. Because of the potential for serious reactions in nursing infants, a decision should be made whether to discontinue nursing or to discontinue the drug, taking into account the importance of the drug to the mother.

PEDIATRIC USE
Safety and efficacy in infants less than 6 months of age have not been established.

GERIATRIC USE
Of the 3028 patients in multiple-dose clinical studies of Cefpodoxime Proxetil, 427 (14%) were 65 and over, while 173 (6%) were 75 and over. No overall differences in effectiveness or safety were observed between the elderly and younger patients. In healthy geriatric subjects with normal renal function, Cefpodoxime half-life in plasma averaged 4.2 hours and urinary recovery averaged 21% after a 400 mg dose was given every 12 hours for 15 days. Other pharmacokinetic parameters were unchanged relative to those observed in healthy younger subjects. Dose adjustment in elderly patients with normal renal function is not necessary.

ADVERSE REACTIONS
CLINICAL TRIALS
FILM-COATED TABLETS (MULTIPLE DOSE)
In clinical trials using multiple doses of Cefpodoxime Proxetil film-coated tablets, 3338 patients were treated with the recommended dosages of Cefpodoxime (100 to 400 mg Q 12 hours). There were no deaths or permanent disabilities thought related to drug toxicity. Eighty-one (2.4%) patients discontinued medication due to adverse events thought possibly-or probably-related to drug toxicity. Sixty-six (66%) of the 100 patients who discontinued therapy (whether thought related to drug therapy or not) did so because of gastrointestinal disturbances, usually diarrhea. The percentage of Cefpodoxime Proxetil-treated patients who discontinued study drug because of adverse events was significantly greter at a dose of 800 mg daily than at a dose of 400 mg daily or at a dose of 200 mg daily. Adverse events thought possibly- or probably-related to Cefpodoxime in multiple dose clinical trials (N = 3338 Cefpodoxime-treated patients) were:

INCIDENCE GREATER THAN 1%:
Diarrhea 7.2%

Diarrhea or loose stools were dose related: decreasing from 10.6% of patients receiving 800 mg per day to 5.9% for those receiving 200 mg per day. Of patients with diarrhea, 10% had *C. difficile* organism or toxin in the stool. (See *"Warnings."*)

Nausea 3.8%
Vaginal Fungal Infections 3.1%
Abdominal Pain 1.6%
Rash 1.4%

Headache 1.1%
Vomiting 1.1%

INCIDENCE LESS THAN 1% :
Cardovascular: Chest pain, hypotension.

Dermatologic: Fungal skin infection, skin scaling/peeling.

Endocrine: Menstrual irregularity.

Genital: Pruritus.

Gastrointestinal: Flatulence, decreased salivation, candidiasis, pseudomembranous colitis.

Hypersensitivity: Anaphylactic shock.

Metabolic: Decreased appetite.

Miscellaneous: Malaise, fever.

Central Nervous System: Dizziness, fatigue, anxiety, insomnia, flushing, nightmares, weakness.

Respiratory: Cough, epistaxis.

Special Senses: Taste alteration, eye itching, tinnitus.

GRANULES FOR ORAL SUSPENSION (MULTIPLE DOSE)
In clinical trials using *multiple doses* of Cefpodoxime Proxetil granules for oral suspension, pediatric patients (90% of whom were less than 12 years of age) were treated with the recommended dosages of Cefpodoxime (10 mg/kg/day divided Q 12 hours to a maximum equivalent adult dose). There were no deaths or permanent disabilities in any of the patients in these studies. Seven patients (< 1%) discontinued medication due to adverse events thought possibly- or probably-related to drug toxicity. Primarily, these discontinuations were for gastrointestinal disturbances, usually diarrhea or diaper area rashes.

Adverse events thought possibly- or probably-related to Cefpodoxime Proxetil granules for oral suspension in multiple dose clinical trials (N = 758 Cefpodoxime-treated patients) were:

INCIDENCE GREATER THAN 1%
Diarrhea 7.0%
The incidence of diarrhea ranged from 17.8% in infants and toddlers to 4.1% in 2 to 12 year olds to 6.0% in adolescents.

Diaper Rash 3.5%
Other skin rashes 1.8%
Vomiting 1.7%

INCIDENCE LESS THAN 1%
Central Nervous System: Headache.

Dermatologic: Exacerbation of acne.

Genital: Pruritus or vaginitis.

Gastrointestinal: Nausea, abdominal pain, candidiasis.

Metabolic: Decreased appetite.

Miscellaneous: Fever.

FILM-COATED TABLETS (SINGLE DOSE)
In clinical trials using *a single dose* of Cefpodoxime Proxetil film-coated tablets, 509 patients were treated with the recommended dosage of Cefpodoxime (200 mg). There were no deaths or permanent disabilities thought related to drug toxicity in these studies.

Adverse events thought possibly- or probably-related to Cefpodoxime Podoxime in single dose clinical trials conducted in the United States were:

INCIDENCE GREATER THAN 1%
Nausea 1.4%
Diarrhea 1.2%

INCIDENCE LESS THAN 1%:
Central Nervous System: Dizziness, headache, syncope.

Dermatologic: Rash.

Genital: Vaginitis.

Gastrointestinal: Abdominal pain.

Psychiatric: Anxiety.

LABORATORY CHANGES (ADULT PATIENTS)
Significant laboratory changes that have been reported in adult patients in clinical trials of Cefpodoxime Proxetil, without regard to drug relationship, were:

Hepatic: Transient increases in AST (SGOT), ALT (SGPT), GGT, alkalin phosphatase, bilirubin, and LDH.

Hematologic: Eosinophilia, leukocytosis, lymphocytosis, granulocytosis, basophilia, monocytosis, thrombocytosis, decreased hemoglobin, leukopenia, neutropenia, lymphocytopenia, thrombocytopenia, positive Coombs' test, and prolonged PT, and PTT.

Serum Chemistry: Increases in glucose, decreases in glucose, decreases in serum albumin, decreases in serum total protein.

Renal: Increases in BUN and creatinine.
Most of these abnormalities were transient and not clinically significant.

LABORATORY CHANGES (PEDIATRIC PATIENTS)
Significant laboratory changes that have been reported in pediatric patients in clinical trials of Cefpodoxime Proxetil, without regard to drug relationship, were:

Hematologic: Eosinophilia, decreased hemoglobin, decreased hematocrit.

Hepatic: transiently increased ALT (SGPT)
Most of these abnormalities were transient and not clinically significant.

POSTMARKETING EXPERIENCE
The following serious adverse experiences have been reported in post-marketing surveillance outside the United States: pseudomembranous colitis, bloody diarrhea with abdominal pain, ulcerative colitis, rectorrhagia with hypotension, anaphylactic shock, acute liver injury, *in utero* exposure with miscarriage, purpuric nephritis, pulmonary infiltrate with eosinophilia, and eyelid dermatitis.

One death was attributed to pseudomembranous colitis and disseminated intravascular coagulation.

CEPHALOSPORIN CLASS LABELING
In addition to the adverse reactions listed above which have been observed in patients treated with Cefpodoxime Proxetil, the following adverse reactions and altered laboratory tests have been reported for cephalosporin class antibiotics:

Adverse Reactions and Abnormal Laboratory Tests: Allergic reactions including Stevens-Johnson syndrome, erythema multiforme, toxic epidermal necrolysis, renal dysfunction, toxic nephropathy, hepatic dysfunction including cholestasis, aplastic anemia, hemolytic anemia, hemorrhage; agranulocytosis; and pancytopenia.

Several cephalosporins have been implicated in triggering seizures, particularly in patients with renal impairment when the dosage was not reduced. (See *"Dosage and Administration"* and *"Overdosage."*) If seizures associated with drug therapy occur, the drug should be discontinued. Anticonvulsant therapy can be given if clinically indicated.

OVERDOSAGE
In acute rodent toxicity studies, a single 5 g/kg oral dose produced no adverse effects.

Information on overdosage in humans is not available. In the event of serious toxic reaction from overdosage, hemodialysis or peritoneal dialysis may aid in the removal of Cefpodoxime from the body, particularly if renal function is compromised.

The toxic symptoms following an overdose of β-lactam antibiotics may include nausea, vomiting, epigastric distress, and diarrhea.

DOSAGE AND ADMINISTRATION
(See *"Indications and Usage"* for indicated pathogens.)

FILM-COATED TABLETS
Cefpodoxime Proxetil tablets should be administered orally with food to enhance absorption. (See *"Clinical Pharmacology."*) The recommended dosages, durations of treatment, and applicable patient population are as described in the following chart: (See related table).

GRANULES FOR ORAL SUSPENSION
Cefpodoxime Proxetil Oral Suspension may be given without regard to food. The recommended dosages, durations of treatment, and applicable patient populations are as described in the following chart: (See related table).

CHILDREN (AGE 6 MONTHS THROUGH 12 YEARS) (SEE RELATED TABLE).

PATIENTS WITH RENAL DYSFUNCTION
For patients with severe renal impairment (< 30 mL/min creatinine clearance), the dosing intervals should be increased to Q 24 hours. In patients maintained on hemodialysis, the dose frequency should be 3 times/week after hemodialysis.

When only the serum creatinine level is available, the following formula (based on sex, weight, and age of the patient) may be used to estimate creatinine clearance (mL/min). For this estimate to be valid, the serum creatinine level should represent a steady state of renal function.

Males:
(mL/min) $\dfrac{\text{Weight (kg)} \times (140 - \text{age})}{72 \times \text{serum creatinine (mg/100 mL)}}$
Females: (mL/min) 0.85 × above value

PATIENTS WITH CIRRHOSIS
Cefpodoxime pharmacokinetics in cirrhotic patients (with or without ascites) are similar to those in healthy subjects. Dose adjustment is not necessary in this population.

PREPARATION OF SUSPENSION
Suspend the 50 mg/5 ml strength in a total of 58 mL distilled water. Method: Gently tap the bottle to loosen powder. Add 25 mL distilled water and shake vigorously for 15 seconds to wet powder. Add 33 mL distilled water and shake vigorously for 3 minutes or until all particles are suspended.

Suspend the 100 mg/5 ml strength in a total of 57 mL distilled water. Method: Gently tap the bottle to loosen powder. Add 25 mL distilled water and shake vigorously for 15 seconds to wet powder. Add 32 mL distilled water and shake vigorously for 3 minutes or until all particles are suspended. After mixing, the suspension should be stored in a refrigerator, 2° to 8°C (36° to 46°F). Shake well before using. Keep container tightly closed. The mixture may be used for 14 days. Discard unused portion after 14 days.

FILM-COATED TABLETS

Adults (age 13 years and older):

Type of Infection	Total Daily Dose	Dose Frequency	Duration
Acute community-acquired pneumonia	400 mg	200 mg Q 12 hours	14 days
Acute bacterial exacerbations of chronic bronchitis	400 mg	200 mg Q 12 hours	10 days
Uncomplicated gonorrhea (men and women) and rectal gonococcal infections (women)	200 mg	single dose	
Skin and skin structure	800 mg	400 mg Q 12 hours	7 to 14 days
Pharyngitis and/or tonsillitis	200 mg	100 mg Q 12 hours	10 days
Uncomplicated urinary tract infection	200 mg	100 mg Q 12 hours	7 days

GRANULES FOR ORAL SUSPENSION

Adults (age 13 years and older): Type of Infection

Type of Infection	Total Daily Dose	Dose Frequency	Duration
Acute community-acquired pneumonia	400 mg	200 mg Q 12 hours	14 days
Uncomplicated gonorrhea (men and women) and rectal gonococcal infections (women)	200 mg	single dose	
Skin and skin structure	800 mg	400 mg Q 12 hours	7 to 14 days
Pharyngitis and/or tonsillitis	200 mg	100 mg Q 12 hours	10 days
Uncomplicated urinary tract infection	200 mg	100 mg Q 12 hours	7 days

CHILDREN (age 6 months through 12 years)

Type of Infection	Total Daily Dose	Dose Frequency	Duration
Acute otitis media	10 mg/kg/day divided Q 12 hr (Max 400 mg/day)	5 mg/kg/dose (Max 200 mg/dose)	10 days
Pharyngitis and/or tonsillitis	10 mg/kg/day divided Q 12 hr (Max 200 mg/day)	5 mg/kg/dose (Max 100 mg/dose)	10 days

STORAGE
Tablets: Store tablets between 15° and 30°C (59° to 86°F). Replace cap securely after each opening. Protect unit dose packs from excessive moisture.

Oral Suspension: Store unsuspended granules between 15° and 30°C (59° to 86°F). Directions for mixing are included on the label. After mixing, suspension should be stored in a refrigerator, 2° to 8°C (36° to 46°F). Shake well before using. Keep container tightly closed. The mixture may be used for 14 days. Discard unused portion after 14 days.

REFERENCES
1. National Committee for Clinical Laboratory Standards, Approved Standard: Performance Standards for Antimicrobial Disk Susceptibility Tests, 4th Edition, Vol. 10(7)FD,2-A4, Villanova, PA, April, 1990. 2. National Committee for Clinical Laboratory Standards, Approved Standard: Methods for Dilution Antimicrobial Susceptibility Tests for Bacteria That Grow Aerobically, 2nd Edition, Vol. 10(8)FD,7-A2, Villanova, PA, April, 1990.

CLINICAL TRIALS
CYSTITIS
In two double-blind, 2:1 randomized, comparative trials performed in adults in the United States, Cefpodoxime Proxetil was compared to other beta-lactam antibiotics. In these studies, the following bacterial eradication rates were obtained at 5 to 9 days after therapy:

Organism	Cefpodoxime	Comparators
E. coli	200/243 (82%)	99/123 (80%)
Other pathogens	34/42 (81%)	23/28 (82%)
K. pneumoniae		
P. mirabilis		
S. saprophyticus		
TOTAL	234/285 (82%)	122/151 (81%)

In these studies, clinical cure rates and bacterial eradication rates for Cefpodoxime Proxetil were comparable to the comparator agents; however, the clinical cure rates and bacteriologic eradication rates were lower than those observed with some other classes of approved agents for cystitis.

HOW SUPPLIED
POWDER FOR RECONSTITUTION: 50 MG/5 ML

BRAND/MANUFACTURER	NDC	SIZE	AWP
○ BRAND VANTIN: Upjohn	00009-3531-01	100 ml	$28.38

POWDER FOR RECONSTITUTION: 100 MG/5 ML

BRAND/MANUFACTURER	NDC	SIZE	AWP
○ BRAND VANTIN: Upjohn	00009-3615-01	100 ml	$54.00

TABLETS: 100 MG

BRAND/MANUFACTURER	NDC	SIZE	AWP
○ BRAND VANTIN: Upjohn	00009-3617-01	20s	$34.69
	00009-3617-02	100s	$165.11
	00009-3617-03	100s ud	$169.22

TABLETS: 200 MG

BRAND/MANUFACTURER	NDC	SIZE	AWP
○ BRAND ▶ VANTIN: Upjohn	00009-3618-01	20s	$66.14
	00009-3618-02	100s	$314.50
	00009-3618-03	100s ud	$322.36

Cefprozil

DESCRIPTION
Cefprozil is a semi-synthetic broad-spectrum cephalosporin antibiotic.

Cefprozil is a cis and trans isomeric mixture (≥90% cis). The chemical name for the monohydrate is (6R,7R)-7-[(R)-2-amino-2- (p-hydroxy-phenyl) acetamido]-8-oxo-3-propenyl-5-thia-1-azabicyclo [4.2.0]oct-2-ene-2- carboxylic acid and monohydrate.

Cefprozil is a white to yellowish powder with a molecular formula for the monohydrate of $C_{18}H_{19}N_3O_5 \cdot H_2O$ and a molecular weight of 407.45.

Cefprozil tablets and Cefprozil for oral suspension are intended for oral administration.

Cefprozil tablets contain 250 mg or 500 mg of anhydrous Cefprozil. Certain brands of the 250 mg tablets also contain FD&C Yellow No. 6.

Cefprozil for oral suspension contains 125 mg or 250 mg anhydrous Cefprozil per 5 mL constituted suspension.

Following is its chemical structure:

CLINICAL PHARMACOLOGY
Following oral administration of Cefprozil to fasting subjects, approximately 95% of the dose was absorbed. Using the investigational capsule formulation, no food effect was observed. The food effect on the tablet and on the suspension formulations has not been studied.

The pharmacokinetic data were derived from the capsule dosing; however, bioequivalence has been demonstrated for the oral solution, capsule, tablet and suspension formulations under fasting conditions.

Average peak plasma concentrations after administration of 250 mg, 500 mg, or 1 g doses of Cefprozil to fasting subjects were approximately 6.1, 10.5, and 18.3

◆ RATED THERAPEUTICALLY EQUIVALENT; ◇ THERAPEUTIC EQUIVALENCE UNCONFIRMED; ○ UNRATED

mcg/mL respectively, and were obtained within 1.5 hours after dosing. Urinary recovery accounted for approximately 60% of the administered dose. (See table.)

Dosage mg	Mean Plasma Cefprozil* Concentrations (mcg/mL)			8-hour Urinary Excretion %
	Peak appx. 1.5 hr	4 hr	8 hr	
250 mg	6.1	1.7	0.2	60%
500 mg	10.5	3.2	0.4	62%
1000 mg	18.3	8.4	1.0	54%

* *Data represent mean values of 12 healthy volunteers.*

During the first 4-hour period after drug administration, the average urine concentrations following the 250 mg, 500 mg, and 1 g doses were approximately 700 mcg/mL, 1000 mcg/mL, and 2900 mcg/mL.

Plasma protein binding is approximately 36% and is independent of concentration in the range of 2 mcg/mL to 20 mcg/mL.

The average plasma half-life in normal subjects is 1.3 hours. There was no evidence of accumulation of Cefprozil in the plasma in individuals with normal renal function following multiple oral doses of up to 1000 mg every 8 hours for 10 days.

In patients with reduced renal function, the plasma half-life may be prolonged up to 5.2 hours depending on the degree of the renal dysfunction. In patients with complete absence of renal function the plasma half-life of Cefprozil has been shown to be as long as 5.9 hours. The half-life is shortened during hemodialysis. Excretion pathways in patients with markedly impaired renal function have not been determined. (See *"Precautions"* and *"Dosage and Administration."*)

The average AUC observed in elderly subjects (≥65 years of age) is approximately 35%-60% higher relative to young adults, and the average AUC in females is approximately 15%-20% higher than in males. The magnitude of these age and gender related changes in the pharmacokinetics of Cefprozil are not sufficient to necessitate dosage adjustments. In patients with impaired hepatic function, the half-life increases to approximately 2 hours. The magnitude of the changes does not warrant a dosage adjustment for patients with impaired hepatic function.

Adequate data on CSF levels of Cefprozil are not available.

MICROBIOLOGY

Cefprozil has in vitro activity against a broad range of gram-positive and gram-negative bacteria. The bactericidal action of Cefprozil results from inhibition of cell-wall synthesis. Cefprozil has been shown to be active against most strains of the following organisms both *in vitro* and in clinical infections. (See *"Indications and Usage."*)

AEROBES, GRAM-POSITIVE:
Staphylococcus aureus
    (including penicillinase-producing strains)

Note: Cefprozil is inactive against methicillin-resistant staphylococci

Streptococcus pneumoniae
Streptococcus pyogenes

AEROBES, GRAM-NEGATIVE:
Moraxella (Branhamella) catarrhalis
Haemophilus influenzae (including penicillinase-producing strains)

The following *in vitro* data are available; however, their clinical significance is unknown.

Cefprozil exhibits *in vitro* minimum inhibitory concentrations (MIC) of 8 mcg/mL or less against most strains of the following organisms. The safety and efficacy of Cefprozil in treating infections due to these organisms have not been established in adequate and well-controlled trials.

AEROBES, GRAM-POSITIVE:
Enterococcus durans
Enterococcus faecalis

Note: Cefprozil is inactive against *Enterococcus faecium*.

Listeria monocytogenes
Staphylococcus epidermidis
Staphylococcus saprophyticus
Staphylococcus warneri
Streptococci (Groups C, D, F, and G)
viridans group Streptococci

AEROBES, GRAM-NEGATIVE:
Citrobacter diversus
Escherichia coli
Klebsiella pneumoniae
Neisseria gonorrhoeae (including penicillinase-producing strains)
Proteus mirabilis
Salmonella spp.
Shigella spp.
Vibrio spp.

Note: Cefprozil is inactive against most strains of *Acinetobacter, Enterobacter, Morganella morganii, Proteus vulgaris, Providencia, Pseudomonas,* and *Serratia.*

ANAEROBES:
Bacteroides melaninogenicus

Note: Most strains of the *Bacteroides fragilis* group are resistant to Cefprozil.

Clostridium perfringens
Clostridium difficile
Fusobacterium spp.
Peptostreptococcus spp.
Propionibacterium acnes

SUSCEPTIBILITY TESTS

Diffusion Techniques: Quantitative methods that require measurement of zone diameters give the most precise estimate of the susceptibility of bacteria to antimicrobial agents. One such standardized procedure recommended for use with the 30-mcg Cefprozil disk is the National Committee for Clinical Laboratory Standards (NCCLS) approved procedure.[1] Interpretation involves correlation of the diameter obtained in the disk test with minimum inhibitory concentration (MIC) for Cefprozil.

The class disk for cephalosporin susceptibility testing (the cephalothin disk) is not appropriate because of spectrum differences with Cefprozil. The 30-mcg Cefprozil disk should be used for all *in vitro* testing of isolates.

Reports from the laboratory giving results of the standard single-disk susceptibility test with a 30-mcg Cefprozil disk should be interpreted according to the following criteria:

Zone diameter (mm)	Interpretation
≥18	(S) Susceptible
15-17	(MS) Moderately Susceptible
≤14	(R) Resistant

A report of "Susceptible" indicates that the pathogen is likely to be inhibited by generally achievable blood concentrations. A report of "Moderately Susceptible" indicates that the organism would be susceptible if high dosage is used or if the infection is confined to tissues and fluids (eg, urine) in which high antibiotic levels are attained. A report of "Resistant" indicates that the achievable concentration of the antibiotic is unlikely to be inhibitory and other therapy should be selected.

Standardized procedures require the use of laboratory control organisms. The 30-mcg Cefprozil disk should give the following zone diameters:

Organism	Zone diameter (mm)
Escherichia coli ATCC 25922	21-27
Staphylococcus aureus ATCC 25923	27-33

Dilution Techniques: Use a standardized dilution method[2] (broth, agar, microdilution) or equivalent with Cefprozil powder. The MIC values obtained should be interpreted according to the following criteria:

MIC (mcg/mL)	Interpretation
≤ 8	(S) Susceptible
16	(MS) Moderately Susceptible
≥ 32	(R) Resistant

As with standard diffusion techniques, dilution techniques require the use of laboratory control organisms. Standard Cefprozil powder should give the following MIC values:

Organism	MIC (mcg/mL)
Enterococcus faecalis ATCC 29212	4-16
Escherichia coli ATCC 25922	1-4
Pseudomonas aeruginosa ATCC 27853	> 32
Staphylococcus aureus ATCC 29213	0.25-1

INDICATIONS AND USAGE

Cefprozil is indicated for the treatment of patients with mild to moderate infections caused by susceptible strains of the designated microorganisms in the conditions listed below:

UPPER RESPIRATORY TRACT
Pharyngitis/Tonsillitis caused by *Streptococcus pyogenes.*

Note: The usual drug of choice in the treatment and prevention of streptococcal infections, including the prophylaxis of rheumatic fever, is penicillin given by the intramuscular route. Cefprozil is generally effective in the eradication of *Streptococcus pyogenes* from the nasopharynx; however, substantial data establishing the efficacy of Cefprozil in the subsequent prevention of rheumatic fever are not available at present.

Otitis Media caused by *Streptococcus pneumoniae, Haemophilus influenzae* and *Moraxella (Branhamella) catarrhalis.* (See *"Clinical Studies"* section.)

Note: In the treatment of otitis media due to beta-lactamase producing organisms, Cefprozil had bacteriologic eradication rates somewhat lower than those observed with a product containing a specific beta-lactamase inhibitor. In considering the use of Cefprozil, lower overall eradication rates should be balanced against the susceptibility patterns of the common microbes in a given geographic area and the increased potential for toxicity with products containing beta-lactamase inhibitors.

LOWER RESPIRATORY TRACT
Secondary Bacterial Infection of Acute Bronchitis and Acute Bacterial Exacerbation of Chronic Bronchitis caused by *Streptococcus pneumoniae, Haemophilus influenzae*, (beta-lactamase positive and negative strains), and *Moraxella (Branhamella) catarrhalis.*

SKIN AND SKIN STRUCTURE
Uncomplicated Skin and Skin-Structure Infections caused by *Staphylococcus aureus* (including penicillinase-producing strains) and *Streptococcus pyrogenes.* Abscesses usually require surgical drainage.

Culture and susceptibility testing should be performed when appropriate to determine susceptibility of the causative organism to Cefprozil.

CONTRAINDICATIONS
Cefprozil is contraindicated in patients with known allergy to the cephalosporin class of antibiotics.

WARNINGS
BEFORE THERAPY WITH CEFPROZIL IS INSTITUTED, CAREFUL INQUIRY SHOULD BE MADE TO DETERMINE WHETHER THE PATIENT HAS HAD PREVIOUS HYPERSENSITIVITY REACTIONS TO CEFPROZIL, CEPHALOSPORINS, PENICILLINS, OR OTHER DRUGS. IF THIS PRODUCT IS TO BE GIVEN TO PENICILLIN-SENSITIVE PATIENTS, CAUTION SHOULD BE EXERCISED BECAUSE CROSS-SENSITIVITY AMONG BETA-LACTAM ANTIBIOTICS HAS BEEN CLEARLY DOCUMENTED AND MAY OCCUR IN UP TO 10% OF PATIENTS WITH A HISTORY OF PENICILLIN ALLERGY. IF AN ALLERGIC REACTION TO CEFPROZIL OCCURS, DISCONTINUE THE DRUG. SERIOUS ACUTE HYPERSENSITIVITY REACTIONS MAY REQUIRE TREATMENT WITH EPINEPHRINE AND OTHER EMERGENCY MEASURES, INCLUDING OXYGEN, INTRAVENOUS FLUIDS, INTRAVENOUS ANTIHISTAMINES, CORTICOSTEROIDS, PRESSOR AMINES, AND AIRWAY MANAGEMENT, AS CLINICALLY INDICATED.

Pseudomembranous colitis has been reported with nearly all antibacterial agents, and may range from mild to life-threatening. Therefore, it is important to consider this diagnosis in patients who present with diarrhea subsequent to the administration of antibacterial agents.

Treatment with antibacterial agents alters the normal flora of the colon and may permit overgrowth of clostridia. Studies indicate that a toxin produced by *Clostridium difficile* is a primary cause of "antibiotic-associated colitis".

After the diagnosis of pseudomembranous colitis has been established, therapeutic measures should be initiated. Mild cases of pseudomembranous colitis usually respond to discontinuation of the drug alone. In moderate to severe cases, consideration should be given to management with fluids and electrolytes, protein supplementation and treatment with an antibacterial drug effective against *Clostridium difficile.*

PRECAUTIONS
GENERAL
Evaluation of renal status before and during therapy is recommended, especially in seriously ill patients. In patients with known or suspected renal impairment (see *"Dosage and Administration"*), careful clinical observation and appropriate laboratory studies should be done prior to and during therapy. The total daily dose of Cefprozil should be reduced in these patients because high and/or prolonged plasma antibiotic concentrations can occur in such individuals from usual doses. Cephalosporins, including Cefprozil, should be given with caution to patients receiving concurrent treatment with potent diuretics since these agents are suspected of adversely affecting renal function. Prolonged use of Cefprozil may result in the overgrowth of nonsusceptible organisms. Careful observation of the patient is essential. If superinfection occurs during therapy, appropriate measures should be taken.

Cefprozil should be prescribed with caution in individuals with a history of gastrointestinal disease particularly colitis. Positive direct Coombs' tests have been reported during treatment with cephalosporin antibiotics.

INFORMATION FOR PATIENTS
Phenylketonurics: Cefprozil for oral suspension contains phenylalanine 28 mg per 5 mL (1 teaspoon) constituted suspension.

DRUG INTERACTIONS
Nephrotoxicity has been reported following concomitant administration of aminoglycoside antibiotics and cephalosporin antibiotics. Concomitant administration of probenecid doubled the AUC for Cefprozil.

DRUG/LABORATORY TEST INTERACTIONS
Cephalosporin antibiotics may produce a false positive reaction for glucose in the urine with copper reduction tests (Benedict's or Fehling's solution or with Clinitest®[3] tablets), but not with enzyme-based tests for glycosuria (eg, Tes-Tape®[4]). A false negative reaction may occur in the ferricyanide test for blood glucose. The presence of Cefprozil in the blood does not interfere with the assay of plasma or urine creatinine by the alkaline picrate method.

CARCINOGENESIS, MUTAGENESIS, AND IMPAIRMENT OF FERTILITY
No mutagenic potential of Cefprozil was found in appropriate prokaryotic or eukaryotic cells *in vitro* or *in vivo*. No *in vivo* long-term studies have been performed to evaluate carcinogenic potential.

Reproductive studies revealed no impairment of fertility in animals.

PREGNANCY: TERATOGENIC EFFECTS. PREGNANCY CATEGORY B
Reproduction studies have been performed in mice, rats, and rabbits at doses 14, 7, and 0.7 times the maximum daily human dose (1000 mg) based upon mg/m^2, and have revealed no evidence of harm to the fetus due to Cefprozil. There are, however, no adequate and well-controlled studies in pregnant women. Because animal reproduction studies are not always predictive of human response, this drug should be used during pregnancy only if clearly needed.

LABOR AND DELIVERY
Cefprozil has not been studied for use during labor and delivery. Treatment should only be given if clearly needed.

NURSING MOTHERS
It is not known whether Cefprozil is excreted in human milk. Because many drugs are excreted in human milk, caution should be exercised when Cefprozil is administered to a nursing mother.

PEDIATRIC USE
Safety and effectiveness in children below the age of 6 months have not been established. However, accumulation of other cephalosporin antibiotics in newborn infants (resulting from prolonged drug half-life in this age group) has been reported.

GERIATRIC USE
Healthy geriatric volunteers ($\geq$65 years old) who received a single 1 g dose of Cefprozil had 35%-60% higher AUC and 40% lower renal clearance values when compared to healthy adult volunteers 20-40 years of age. In clinical studies, when geriatric patients received the usual recommended adult doses, clinical efficacy and safety were acceptable and comparable to results in nongeriatric adult patients.

ADVERSE REACTIONS
The adverse reactions to Cefprozil are similar to those observed with other orally administered cephalosporins. Cefprozil was usually well tolerated in controlled clinical trials. Approximately 2% of patients discontinued Cefprozil therapy due to adverse events.

The most common adverse effects observed in patients treated with Cefprozil are:

Gastrointestinal: Diarrhea (2.9%), nausea (3.5%), vomiting (1%) and abdominal pain (1%).

Hepatobiliary: Elevation of AST (SGOT) (2%), ALT (SGPT) (2%), alkaline phosphate (0.2%), and bilirubin values (<0.1%). As with some penicillins and some other cephalosporin antibiotics, cholestatic jaundice has been reported rarely.

Hypersensitivity: Rash (0.9%), urticaria (0.1%). Such reactions have been reported more frequently in children than in adults. Signs and symptoms usually occur a few days after initiation of therapy and subside within a few days after cessation of therapy.

CNS: Dizziness (1%), hyperactivity, headache, nervousness, insomnia, confusion, and somnolence have been reported rarely, (<1%). All were reversible.

Hematopoietic: Decreased leukocyte count (0.2%), eosinophilia (2.3%).

Renal: Elevated BUN (0.1%), serum creatinine (0.1%).

Other: Diaper rash and superinfection (1.5%), genital pruritus and vaginitis (1.6%).

CEPHALOSPORIN CLASS PARAGRAPH
In addition to the adverse reactions listed above which have been observed in patients treated with Cefprozil, the following adverse reactions and altered laboratory tests have been reported for cephalosporin-class antibiotics:

Anaphylaxis, Stevens-Johnson syndrome, erythema multiforme, toxic epidermal necrolysis, serum-sickness like reaction, fever, renal dysfunction, toxic nephropathy, aplastic anemia, hemolytic anemia, hemorrhage, prolonged prothrombin time, positive Coombs' test, elevated LDH, pancytopenia, neutropenia agranulocytosis, thrombocytopenia.

Several cephalosporins have been implicated in triggering seizures, particularly in patients with renal impairment when the dosage was not reduced. (See *"Dosage and Administration"* and *"Overdosage."*) If seizures associated with drug therapy occur, the drug should be discontinued. Anticonvulsant therapy can be given if clinically indicated.

OVERDOSAGE
Cefprozil is eliminated primarily by the kidneys. In case of severe overdosage, especially in patients with comprised renal function, hemodialysis will aid in the removal of Cefprozil from the body.

DOSAGE AND ADMINISTRATION
Cefprozil is administered orally.

Population/Infection	Dosage (mg)	Duration (days)
Adults (13 years and older)		
Upper Respiratory Tract		
Pharyngitis/Tonsillitis	500 q 24h	10*

Population/Infection	Dosage (mg)	Duration (days)
Lower Respiratory Tract		
Secondary Bacterial Infection of Acute Bronchitis and Acute Bacterial Exacerbation of Chronic Bronchitis	500 q 12h	10
Skin and Skin Structure		
Uncomplicated Skin and Skin Structure Infections	250 q 12h or 500 q 24h or 500 q 12h	10
Children (2 years—12 years)		
Upper Respiratory Tract		
Pharyngitis/Tonsillitis	7.5 mg/kg q 12h	10*
Infants & Children (6 months-12 years)		
Upper Respiratory Tract		
Otitis Media	15 mg/kg q 12h	10

(See "Indication and Usage" and "Clinical Studies" sections)

* In the treatment of infections due to Streptococcus pyogenes, Cefprozil should be administered for at least 10 days.

RENAL IMPAIRMENT
Cefprozil may be administered to patients with impaired renal function. The following dosage schedule should be used:

Creatinine Clearance (mL/min)	Dosage (mg)	Dosing Interval
30-120	standard	standard
0-29*	50% of standard	standard

* Cefprozil is in part removed by hemodialysis; therefore, Cefprozil should be administered after the completion of hemodialysis.

HEPATIC IMPAIRMENT
No dosage adjustment is necessary for patients with impaired hepatic function.

STORAGE
Certain brands of the powder formulations for oral suspension contain Cefprozil in a bubble-gum flavored mixture. Directions for mixing are included on the label. After mixing, store in a refrigerator, and discard unused portion after 14 days.
Store at controlled room temperature, 59° to 86°F (15° to 30°C) prior to constitution.

CLINICAL STUDIES
Study One: In a controlled clinical study of acute otitis media performed in the United States, where significant rates of beta-lactamase producing organisms were found, Cefprozil was compared to an oral antimicrobial agent that contained a specific beta-lactamase inhibitor. In this study, using very strict evaluability criteria and microbiologic and clinical response criteria at the 10-16 days post-therapy follow-up, the following presumptive bacterial eradication/clinical cure outcomes (ie, clinical success) and safety results were obtained:

U.S. ACUTE OTITIS MEDIA STUDY CEFPROZIL VS. BETA-LACTAMASE INHIBITOR-CONTAINING CONTROL DRUG

Efficacy Pathogen	% of Cases with Pathogen (n = 155)	Outcome
S. pneumoniae	48.4%	Cefprozil success rate 5% better than control
H. influenzae	35.5%	Cefprozil success rate 17% less than control
M. catarrhalis	13.5%	Cefprozil success rate 12% less than control
S. pyogenes	2.6%	Cefprozil equivalent to control
Overall	100.0%	Cefprozil success rate 5% less than control

Safety: The incidence of adverse events, primarily diarrhea and rash,* were clinically and statistically significantly higher in the control arm versus the Cefprozil arm.

Age Group	Cefprozil	Control
6 months-2 years	21%	41%
3-12 years	10%	19%

* The majority of these involved the diaper area in young children.

Study Two: In a controlled clinical study of acute otitis media performed in Europe, Cefprozil was compared to an oral antimicrobial agent that contained a specific beta-latamase inhibitor. As expected in a European population, this study had a lower incidence of beta-lactamase-producing organisms than usually seen in U.S. trials. In this study, using very strict evaluability criteria and microbiologic and clinical response criteria at the 10-16 day post-therapy follow-up, the following presumptive bacterial eradication/clinical cure outcomes (ie, clinical success) were obtained:

EUROPEAN ACUTE OTITIS MEDIA STUDY CEFPROZIL VS. BETA-LACTAMASE INHIBITOR-CONTAINING CONTROL DRUG

Efficacy Pathogen	% of Cases with Pathogen (n = 47)	Outcome
S. pneumoniae	51.0%	Cefprozil equivalent to control
H. influenzae	29.8%	Cefprozil equivalent to control
M. catarrhalis	6.4%	Cefprozil equivalent to control
S. pyogenes	12.8%	Cefprozil equivalent to control
Overall	100.0%	Cefprozil equivalent to control

Safety: The incidence of adverse events in the Cefprozil arm was comparable to the incidence of adverse events in the control arm (agent that contained a specific beta-lactamase inhibitor).

REFERENCES
1. National Committee for Clinical Laboratory Standards, Performance Standards for Antimicrobial Disk Susceptibility Tests—Fourth Edition. Approved Standard NCCLS Document M2-A4, Vol. 10, No. 7, NCCLS, Villanova, PA, April, 1990. 2. National Committee for Clinical Laboratory Standards, Methods for Dilution Antimicrobial Susceptibility Tests for Bacteria that Grow Aerobically—Second Edition. Approved Standard NCCLS Document M7-A2, Vol. 10, No. 8, NCCLS, Villanova, PA, April, 1990. 3. Clinitest® is registered trademark of Miles Laboratories. Inc. 4. Tes-Tape® is a registered trademark of Eli Lilly and Company.

HOW SUPPLIED
POWDER FOR RECONSTITUTION: 125 MG/5 ML

BRAND/MANUFACTURER	NDC	SIZE	AWP
○ BRAND			
CEFZIL: Bristol Labs	00087-7718-40	50 ml	$13.16
	00087-7718-62	75 ml	$19.65
	00087-7718-64	100 ml	$26.15

POWDER FOR RECONSTITUTION: 250 MG/5 ML

BRAND/MANUFACTURER	NDC	SIZE	AWP
○ BRAND			
CEFZIL: Bristol Labs	00087-7719-40	50 ml	$24.43
	00087-7719-62	75 ml	$35.90
	00087-7719-64	100 ml	$47.40

TABLETS: 250 MG

BRAND/MANUFACTURER	NDC	SIZE	AWP
○ BRAND			
➤ CEFZIL: Bristol Labs	00087-7720-60	100s	$273.75
	00087-7720-66	100s ud	$302.35

TABLETS: 500 MG

BRAND/MANUFACTURER	NDC	SIZE	AWP
○ BRAND			
➤ CEFZIL: Bristol Labs	00087-7721-50	50s	$272.69
	00087-7721-60	100s	$537.94
	00087-7721-66	100s ud	$595.15

Ceftazidime

DESCRIPTION
Ceftazidime is a semisynthetic, broad-spectrum, beta-lactam antibiotic for parenteral administration. It is the pentahydrate of pyridium, 1-[[7-[[(2-amino-4-thiazolyl)[(1-carboxy-1-methylethoxy)imino]acetyl] amino]-2-carboxy-8-oxo-5-thia-1-azabicyclo[4.2.0]oct-2-en-3-yl] methyl]-, hydroxide, inner salt, [6R-[6α,7β(Z)]].

The empirical formula is $C_{22}H_{22}N_6O_7S_2 \cdot 5H_2O$ representing a molecular weight of 636.65.

Ceftazidime for injection is a sterile, dry mixture of Ceftazidime pentahydrate and L-arginine or sodium carbonate. The L-arginine is at a concentration of 349 mg/gm of Ceftazidime activity and facilitates dissolution. The sodium carbonate is at a concentration of 118 mg (18.5 mmol) sodium carbonate/gm of Ceftazidime activity. The total sodium content of the mixture is approximately 54 mg (2.3 mEq)/gm of Ceftazidime activity. It also facilitates dissolution. Ceftazidime dissolves without the evolution of gas. L-arginine contains no sodium ion. Solutions of Ceftazidime range in color from light yellow to amber, depending on the diluent and volume used. The pH of freshly constituted solutions usually ranges from 5 to 7.5 or 8.0.

Following is its chemical structure:

CLINICAL PHARMACOLOGY

After intravenous (IV) administration of 500-mg and 1-g doses of Ceftazidime over 5 minutes to normal adult male volunteers, mean peak serum concentrations of 45 and 90 mcg/mL, respectively, were achieved. After IV infusion of 500-mg, 1-g, and 2-g doses of Ceftazidime over 20 to 30 minutes to normal adult male volunteers, mean peak serum concentrations of 42, 69, and 170 mcg/mL, respectively, were achieved. The average serum concentrations following IV infusion of 500-mg, 1-g, and 2-g doses to these volunteers over an 8-hour interval are given in Table 1.

Table 1

Ceftazidime IV Dose 2-6	Serum Concentrations (mcg/mL)				
	0.5 h	1 h	2 h	4 h	8 h
500 mg	42	25	12	6	2
1 g	60	39	23	11	3
2 g	129	75	42	13	5

The absorption and elimination of Ceftazidime were directly proportional to the size of the dose. The half-life following IV administration was approximately 1.9 hours. Less than 10% of Ceftazidime was protein bound. The degree of protein binding was independent of concentration. There was no evidence of accumulation of Ceftazidime in the serum in individuals with normal renal function following multiple IV doses of 1 and 2 g every 8 hours for 10 days.

Following intramuscular (IM) administration of 500-mg and 1-g doses of Ceftazidime to normal adult volunteers, the mean peak serum concentrations were 17 and 39 mcg/mL, respectively, at approximately 1 hour. Serum concentrations remained above 4 mcg/mL for 6 and 8 hours after the IM administration of 500-mg and 1-g doses, respectively. The half-life of Ceftazidime in these volunteers was approximately 2 hours.

The presence of hepatic dysfunction had no effect on the pharmacokinetics of Ceftazidime in individuals administered 2 g intravenously every 8 hours for 5 days. Therefore, a dosage adjustment from the normal recommended dosage is not required for patients with hepatic dysfunction, provided renal function is not impaired.

Approximately 80% to 90% of an IM or IV dose of Ceftazidime is excreted unchanged by the kidneys over a 24-hour period. After the IV administration of single 500-mg or 1-g doses, approximately 50% of the dose appeared in the urine in the first 2 hours. An additional 20% was excreted between 2 and 4 hours after dosing, and approximately another 12% of the dose appeared in the urine between 4 and 8 hours later. The elimination of Ceftazidime by the kidneys resulted in high therapeutic concentrations in the urine.

The mean renal clearance of Ceftazidime was approximately 100 mL per minute. The calculated plasma clearance of approximately 115 mL per minute indicated nearly complete elimination of Ceftazidime by the renal route. Administration of probenecid before dosing had no effect on the elimination kinetics of Ceftazidime. This suggested that Ceftazidime is eliminated by glomerular filtration and is not actively secreted by renal tabular mechanisms.

Since Ceftazidime is eliminated almost solely by the kidneys, its serum half-life is significantly prolonged in patients with impaired renal function. Consequently, dosage adjustments in such patients as described in the *"Dosage and Administration"* section are suggested.

Ceftazidime concentrations achieved in specific body tissues and fluids are depicted in Table 2.

Table 2
CEFTAZIDIME CONCENTRATIONS IN BODY TISSUES AND FLUIDS

Tissue or Fluid	Dose/Route	No. of Patients	Time of Sample Postdose	Average Tissue or Fluid Level (mcg/mL or mcg/gm)
Urine	500 mg IM	6	0-2 h	2,100.0
	2 g IV	6	0-2 h	12,000.0
Bile	2 g IV	3	90 min	36.4
Synovial fluid	2 g IV	13	2 h	25.6
Peritoneal fluid	2 g IV	8	2 h	48.6
Sputum	1 g IV	8	1 h	9.0

Tissue or Fluid	Dose/Route	No. of Patients	Time of Sample Postdose	Average Tissue or Fluid Level (mcg/mL or mcg/gm)
Cerebrospinal fluid (inflamed meninges)	2 g q8h IV	5	120 min	9.8
	2 g q8h IV	6	180 min	9.4
Aqueous humor	2 g IV	13	1-3 h	11.0
Blister fluid	1 g IV	7	2-3 h	19.7
Lymphatic fluid	1 g IV	7	2-3 h	23.4
Bone	2 g IV	8	0.67 h	31.1
Heart muscle	2 g IV	35	30-280 min	12.7
Skin	2 g IV	22	30-180 min	6.6
Skeletal muscle	2 g IV	35	30-280 min	9.4
Myometrium	2 g IV	31	1-2 h	18.7

MICROBIOLOGY

Ceftazidime is bactericidal in action, exerting its effect by inhibition of enzymes responsible for cell-wall synthesis. A wide range of gram-negative organisms is susceptible to Ceftazidime *in vitro,* including strains resistant to gentamicin and other aminoglycosides. In addition, Ceftazidime has been shown to be active against gram-positive organisms. It is highly stable to most clinically important beta-lactamases, plasmid or chromosomal, which are produced by both gram-negative and gram-positive organisms and, consequently, is active against many strains resistant to ampicillin and other cephalosporins.

Ceftazidime has been shown to be active against the following organisms both *in vitro* and in clinical infections (see *"Indications and Usage"*).

AEROBES, GRAM-NEGATIVE

Citrobacter spp., including *Citrobacter freundii* and *Citrobacter diversus; Enterobacter* spp., including *Enterobacter cloacae* and *Enterobacter aerogenes; Escherichia coli; Haemophilus influenzae,* including ampicillin-resistant strains; *Klebsiella* spp. (including *Klebsiella pneumoniae); Neisseria meningitidis; Proteus mirabilis; Proteus vulgaris; Pseudomonas* spp. (including *Pseudomonas aeruginosa);* and *Serratia* spp.

AEROBES, GRAM-POSITIVE

Staphylococcus aureus, including penicillinase- and non-penicillinase-producing strains; *Streptococcus agalactiae* (group B streptococci); *Streptococcus pneumoniae;* and *Streptococcus pyogenes* (group A beta-hemolytic streptococci).

ANAEROBES

Bacteroides spp. (*Note:* many strains of *Bacteroides fragilis* are resistant).

Ceftazidime has been shown to be active *in vitro* against most strains of the following organisms; however, the clinical significance of this activity is unknown: *Acinetobacter* spp.; *Clostridium* spp. (not including *Clostridium difficile); Haemophilus parainfluenzae; Morganella morganii* (formerly *Proteus morganii); Neisseria gonorrhoeae; Peptococcus* spp., *Peptostreptococcus* spp., *Providencia* spp. (including *Providencia rettgeri,* formerly *Proteus rettgeri); Salmonella* spp.; *Shigella* spp.; *Staphylococcus epidermidis;* and *Yersinia enterocolitica.* Ceftazidime and the aminoglycosides have been shown to be synergistic *in vitro* against some strains of *Pseudomonas aeruginosa* and the enterobacteriaceae. Ceftazidime and carbenicillin have also been shown to be synergistic *in vitro* against *Pseudomonas aeruginosa.*

Ceftazidime is not active *in vitro* against methicillin-resistant staphylococci; *Streptococcus faecalis* and many other enterococci; *Listeria monocytogenes; Campylobacter* spp.; or *Clostridium difficile.*

SUSCEPTIBILITY TESTS

Diffusion Techniques: Quantitative methods that require measurement of zone diameters give the most precise estimate of antibiotic susceptibility. One such procedure[1-3] has been recommended for use with disks to test susceptibility to Ceftazidime.

Reports from the laboratory giving results of the standard single-disk susceptibility test with a 30-mcg Ceftazidime disk should be interpreted according to the following criteria:

Susceptible organisms produce zones of 18 mm or greater, indicating that the test organism is likely to respond to therapy.

Organisms that produce zones of 15 to 17 mm (moderate susceptibility) are expected to be susceptible if high dosage is used or if the infection is confined to tissues and fluids (e.g., urine) in which high antibiotic levels are attained.

Resistant organisms produce zones of 14 mm or less, indicating that other therapy should be selected.

Organisms should be tested with the Ceftazidime disk since Ceftazidime has been shown by *in vitro* tests to be active against certain strains found resistant when other beta-lactam disks are used.

Standardized procedures require the use of laboratory control organisms. The 30-mcg Ceftazidime disk should give zone diameters between 25 and 32 mm for *Escherichia coli* ATCC 25922. For *Pseudomonas aeruginosa* ATCC 27853, the zone diameters should be between 22 and 29 mm. For *Staphylococcus aureus* ATCC 25923, the zone diameters should be between 16 and 20 mm.

Dilution Techniques: In other susceptibility testing procedures, e.g., ICS agar dilution or the equivalent, a bacterial isolate may be considered susceptible if the minimum inhibitory concentration (MIC) value for Ceftazidime is not more than 16 mcg/mL. Organisms are considered resistant to Ceftazidime if the MIC ≥ 64 mcg/mL. Organisms having an MIC value of < 64 mcg/mL but > 16 mcg/mL are expected to be susceptible if high dosage is used or if the infection is confined to tissues and fluids (e.g., urine) in which high antibiotic levels are attained.

As with standard diffusion methods, dilution procedures require the use of laboratory control organisms. Standard Ceftazidime powder should give MIC values in the range of 4 to 16 mcg/mL for *Staphylococcus aureus* ATCC 25923. For *Escherichia coli* ATCC 25922. The MIC range should be between 0.125 and 0.5 mcg/mL. For *Pseudomonas aeruginosa* ATCC 27853, the MIC range should be between 0.5 and 2 mcg/mL.

INDICATIONS AND USAGE
Ceftazidime is indicated for the treatment of patients with infections caused by susceptible strains of the designated organisms in the following diseases:

1. LOWER RESPIRATORY TRACT INFECTIONS
Including pneumonia, caused by *Pseudomonas aeruginosa* and other *Pseudomonas* spp; *Haemophilus influenzae*, including ampicillin-resistant strains; *Klebsiella* spp; *Enterobacter* spp; *Proteus mirabilis*; *Escherichia coli*; *Serratia* spp; *Citrobacter* spp; *Streptococcus pneumoniae*; and *Staphylococcus aureus* (methicillin-susceptible strains).

2. SKIN AND SKIN STRUCTURE INFECTIONS
Caused by *Pseudomonas aeruginosa*; *Klebsiella* spp; *Escherichia coli*; *Proteus* spp., including *Proteus mirabilis* and indole-positive *Proteus*; *Enterobacter* spp.; *Serratia* spp.; *Staphylococcus cureus* (methicillin-susceptible strains); and *Streptococcus pyogenes* (group A beta-hemolytic streptococci).

3. URINARY TRACT INFECTIONS
Both complicated and uncomplicated, caused by *Pseudomonas aeruginosa*; *Enterobacter* spp.; *Proteus* spp., including *Proteus mirabilis* and indole-positive *Proteus*; *Klebsiella* spp.; and *Escherichia coli*.

BACTERIAL SEPTICEMIA
Caused by *Pseudomonas aeruginosa*; *Klebsiella* spp.; *Haemophilus influenzae*; *Escherichia coli*; *Serratia* spp.; *Streptococcus pneumoniae*; and *Staphylococcus aureus* (methicillin-susceptible strains).

5. BONE AND JOINT INFECTIONS
Caused by *Pseudomonas aeruginosa*; *Klebsiella* spp.; *Enterobacter* spp.; and *Staphylococcus aureus* (methicillin-susceptible strains).

6. GYNECOLOGIC INFECTIONS
Including endometritis, pelvic cellulitis, and other infections of the female genital tract caused by *Escherichia coli*.

7. INTRA-ABDOMINAL INFECTIONS
Including peritonitis caused by *Escherichia coli*, *Klebsiella* spp., and *Staphylococcus aureus* (methicillin-susceptible strains) and polymicrobial infections caused by aerobic and anaerobic organisms and *Bacteroides* spp. (many strains of *Bacteroides fragilis* are resistant).

8. CENTRAL NERVOUS SYSTEM INFECTIONS
Including meningitis, caused by *Haemophilus influenzae* and *Neisseria meningitidis*. Ceftazidime has also been used successfully in a limited number of cases of meningitis due to *Pseudomonas aeruginosa* and *Streptococcus pneumoniae*.

Specimens for bacterial cultures should be obtained before therapy in order to isolate and identify causative organisms and to determine their susceptibility to Ceftazidime. Therapy may be instituted before results of susceptibility studies are known; however, once these results become available, the antibiotic treatment should be adjusted accordingly.

As with other extended-spectrum cephalosporins and penicillins, some strains of *Enterobacter* spp. can develop resistance during Ceftazidime therapy due to induced type-1 beta-lactamase production. When clinically appropriate during therapy of *Enterobacter* spp. infections, periodic susceptibility testing should be considered.

Ceftazidime may be used alone in cases of confirmed or suspected sepsis. Ceftazidime has been used successfully in clinical trials as empiric therapy in cases where various concomitant therapies with other antibiotics have been used.

Ceftazidime may also be used concomitantly with other antibiotics such as aminoglycosides, vancomycin, and clindamycin; in severe and life-threatening infections; and in the immunocompromised patient (see *"Compatibility and Stability"*). When such concomitant treatment is appropriate, prescribing information in the labeling for the other antibiotics should be followed. The dosage depends on the severity of the infection and the patient's condition.

UNLABELED USES
Ceftazidime is used alone or as an adjunct in the treatment of pulmonary infections in patients with cystic fibrosis, febrile neutropenia in immunocompromised patients, gram-negative neonatal infections, and nosocomial sepsis.

CONTRAINDICATIONS
Ceftazidime is contraindicated in patients who have shown hypersensitivity to Ceftazidime or the cephalosporin group of antibiotics.

WARNINGS
BEFORE THERAPY WITH CEFTAZIDIME FOR INJECTION IS INSTITUTED, CAREFUL INQUIRY SHOULD BE MADE TO DETERMINE WHETHER THE PATIENT HAS HAD PREVIOUS HYPERSENSITIVITY REACTIONS TO CEFTAZIDIME, CEPHALOSPORINS, PENICILLINS, OR OTHER DRUGS. ANTIBIOTICS SHOULD BE ADMINISTERED WITH CAUTION TO ANY PATIENT WHO HAS DEMONSTRATED SOME FORM OF ALLERGY, PARTICULARLY TO DRUGS. IF THIS PRODUCT IS GIVEN TO PENICILLIN-SENSITIVE PATIENTS, CAUTION SHOULD BE EXERCISED BECAUSE CROSS-HYPERSENSITIVITY AMONG BETA-LACTAM ANTIBIOTICS HAS BEEN CLEARLY DOCUMENTED AND MAY OCCUR IN UP TO 10% OF PATIENTS WITH A HISTORY OF PENICILLIN ALLERGY. IF AN ALLERGIC REACTION TO CEFTAZIDIME OCCURS, DISCONTINUE THE DRUG. SERIOUS ACUTE HYPERSENSITIVITY REACTIONS MAY REQUIRE TREATMENT WITH EPINEPHRINE AND OTHER EMERGENCY MEASURES, INCLUDING OXYGEN, IV FLUIDS, IV ANTIHISTAMINES, CORTICOSTEROIDS, PRESSOR AMINES, AND AIRWAY MANAGEMENT, AS CLINICALLY INDICATED.

Pseudomembranous colitis has been reported with nearly all antibacterial agents, including Ceftazidime, and may range from mild to life threatening. Therefore, it is important to consider this diagnosis in patients who present with diarrhea subsequent to the administration of antibacterial agents.

Treatment with antibacterial agents alters the normal flora of the colon and may permit overgrowth of clostridia. Studies indicate that a toxin produced by *Clostridium difficile* is a primary cause of "antibiotic-associated colitis."

After the diagnosis of pseudomembranous colitis has been established, therapeutic measures should be initiated. Mild cases of pseudomembranous colitis usually respond to discontinuation of the drug alone. In moderate to severe cases, consideration should be given to management with fluids and electrolytes, and protein supplementation. When the colitis does not improve with drug discontinuance or when it is severe, oral vancomycin is the drug of choice for antibiotic-associated pseudomembranous colitis produced by *C. difficile*. Other causes of colitis should be ruled out.

Elevated levels of Ceftazidime in patients with renal insufficiency can lead to seizures, encephalopathy, asterixis, and neuromuscular excitability (see *"Precautions"*).

PRECAUTIONS
General: Ceftazidime has not been shown to be nephrotoxic; however, high and prolonged serum antibiotic concentrations can occur from usual dosages in patients with transient or persistent reduction of urinary output because of renal insufficiency. The total daily dosage should be reduced when Ceftazidime is administered to patients with renal insufficiency (see *"Dosage and Administration"*). Elevated levels of Ceftazidime in these patients can lead to seizures, encephalopathy, asterixis, and neuromuscular excitability. Continued dosage should be determined by degree of renal impairment, severity of infection, and susceptibility of the causative organisms.

As with other antibiotics, prolonged use of Ceftazidime may result in overgrowth of nonsusceptible organisms. Repeated evaluation of the patient's condition is essential. If superinfection occurs during therapy, appropriate measures should be taken.

Cephalosporins may be associated with a fall in prothrombin activity. Those at risk include patients with renal or hepatic impairment, or poor nutritional state, as well as patients receiving a protracted course of antimicrobial therapy. Prothrombin time should be monitored in patients at risk and exogenous vitamin K administered as indicated.

Ceftazidime should be prescribed with caution in individuals with a history of gastrointestinal disease, particularly colitis. Arginine has been shown to alter glucose metabolism and elevate serum potassium transiently when administered at 50 times the recommended dose. The effect of lower dosing is not known.

Intra-arterial administration may lead to arteriospasm and necrosis and should therefore be avoided.

Drug Interactions: Nephrotoxicity has been reported following concomitant administration of cephalosporins with aminoglycoside antibiotics or potent diuretics such as furosemide. Renal function should be carefully monitored, especially if higher dosages of the aminoglycosides are to be administered or if therapy is prolonged, because of the potential nephrotoxicity and ototoxicity of aminoglycosidic antibiotics. Nephrotoxicity and ototoxicity were not noted when Ceftazidime was given alone in clinical trials.

Chloramphenicol has been shown to be antagonistic to beta-lactam antibiotics, including Ceftazidime, based on *in vitro* studies and time kill curves with enteric gram-negative bacilli. Due to the possibility of antagonism *in vivo*, particularly when bactericidal activity is desired, this drug combination should be avoided.

Drug/Laboratory Test Interactions: The administration of Ceftazidime may result in a false-positive reaction for glucose in the urine when using copper reduction tests (Benedict's solution or Fehling's solution). It is recommended that glucose tests based on enzymatic glucose oxidase reactions be used.

Carcinogenesis, Mutagenesis, Impairment of Fertility: Long-term studies in animals have not been performed to evaluate carcinogenic potential. However, a mouse micronucleus test and an Ames test were both negative for mutagenic effects.

Pregnancy: Teratogenic Effects: Pregnancy Category B: Reproduction studies have been performed in mice and rats at doses up to 40 times the human dose and have revealed no evidence of impaired fertility or harm to the fetus due to Ceftazidime.

➤ SHOWN IN PRODUCT IDENTIFICATION GUIDE

Ceftazidime-arginine at 23 times the human dose was not teratogenic or embryotoxic in a rat reproduction study. There are however, no adequate and well-controlled studies in pregnant women. Because animal reproduction studies are not always predictive of human response, this drug should be used during pregnancy only if clearly needed.

Nursing Mothers: Ceftazidime is excreted in human milk in low concentrations. It is not known whether the arginine component of this product is excreted in human milk. Because many drugs are excreted in human milk and because safety of the arginine component of Ceftazidime in nursing infants has not been established, a decision should be made whether to discontinue nursing or to discontinue the drug, taking into account the importance of the drug to the mother.

Pediatric Use: Safety of the arginine component of Ceftazidime in children has not been established. This product is for use in patients 12 years and older. If treatment with Ceftazidime is indicated for pediatric patients, a sodium carbonate formulation should be used.

ADVERSE REACTIONS

Ceftazidime is generally well tolerated. The incidence of adverse reactions associated with the administration of Ceftazidime was low in clinical trials. The following adverse effects from clinical trials were considered to be either related to Ceftazidime therapy or were of uncertain etiology. The most common were local reactions following IV injection and allergic and gastrointestinal reactions. Other adverse reactions were encountered infrequently. No disulfiramlike reactions were reported.

Local Effects, reported in fewer than 2% of patients, were phlebitis and inflammation at the site of injection (1 in 69 patients).

Hypersensitivity Reactions, reported in 2% of patients, were pruritus, rash, and fever. Immediate reactions, generally manifested by rash and/or pruritus, occurred in 1 in 285 patients. Angioedema and anaphylaxis (bronchospasm and/or hypotension) have been reported very rarely.

Gastrointestinal Symptoms, reported in fewer than 2% of patients, were diarrhea (1 in 78), nausea (1 in 156), vomiting (1 in 500), and abdominal pain (1 in 416). The onset of pseudomembranous colitis symptoms may occur during or after treatment (see *"Warnings"*).

Central Nervous System Reactions (fewer than 1%) included headache, dizziness, and paresthesia. Seizures have been reported with several cephalosporins, including Ceftazidime. In addition, encephalopathy, asterixis, and neuromuscular excitability have been reported in renally impaired patients treated with unadjusted dosing regimens of Ceftazidime (see *"Precautions: General"*).

Less Frequent Adverse Events (fewer than 1%) were candidiasis (including oral thrush) and vaginitis.

Hematologic: Exceedingly rare cases of hemolytic anemia have been reported.

Laboratory Test Changes noted during Ceftazidime clinical trials were transient and included: eosinophilia (1 in 13), positive Coombs' test without hemolysis (1 in 23), thrombocytosis (1 in 45), and slight elevations in one or more of the hepatic enzymes, aspartate aminotransferase (AST, SGOT) (1 in 16), alanine aminotransferase (ALT, SGPT) (1 in 15), LDH (1 in 18), GGT (1 in 19), and alkaline phosphatase (1 in 23). As with some other cephalosporins, transient elevations of blood urea, blood urea nitrogen, and/or serum creatinine were observed occasionally. Transient leukopenia, neutropenia, agranulocytosis, thrombocytopenia, and lymphocytosis were seen very rarely. Elevations in hepatic enzymes (SGOT, SGPT, LDH, GGT, alkaline phosphatase) have been reported postmarketing.

In addition to the adverse reactions listed above that have been observed in patients treated with Ceftazidime, the following adverse reactions and altered laboratory tests have been reported for cephalosporin-class antibiotics:

Adverse Reactions: Urticaria, Stevens-Johnson syndrome, erythema multiforme, toxic epidermal necrolysis, colitis, renal dysfunction, toxic nephropathy, hepatic dysfunction including cholestasis, aplastic anemia, hemorrhage.

Altered Laboratory Tests: Prolonged prothrombin time, false-positive test for urinary glucose, elevated bilirubin, pancytopenia.

OVERDOSAGE

Signs and Symptoms: Toxic signs and symptoms following an overdose of Ceftazidime may include pain, inflammation, and phlebitis at the injection site.

The administration of inappropriately large doses of parenteral cephalosporins may cause dizziness, paresthesias, and headaches. Seizures may occur following overdosage with some cephalosporins, particularly in patients with renal impairment where accumulation is likely to occur.

Laboratory abnormalities that may occur after an overdose include elevations in creatinine, BUN, liver enzymes and bilirubin, a positive Coombs' test, thrombocytosis, thrombocytopenia, eosinophilia, leukopenia, and prolongation of the prothrombin time.

The subcutaneous median lethal dose in rats and mice ranged from 5.8 to 20 g/kg, and the intravenous median lethal dose in rabbits was > 2 g/kg.

Ceftazidime overdosage has occurred in patients with renal failure. Reactions have included seizure activity, encephalopathy, asterixis, and neuromuscular excitability.

Treatment: To obtain up-to-date information about the treatment of overdose, a good resource is your certified Regional Poison Control Center. Telephone numbers of certified poison control centers are listed in the *Physicians' Desk*

Reference (PDR). In managing overdosage, consider the possibility of multiple drug overdoses, interaction among drugs, and unusual drug kinetics in your patient. Patients who receive an acute overdosage should be carefully observed and given supportive treatment. In the presence of renal insufficiency, hemodialysis or peritoneal dialysis may aid in the removal of Ceftazidime from the body.

If seizures occur, the drug should be discontinued promptly; anticonvulsant therapy may be administered if clinically indicated. Protect the patient's airway and support ventilation and perfusion. Meticulously monitor and maintain, within acceptable limits, the patient's vital signs, blood gases, serum electrolytes, etc.

In cases of severe overdosage, especially in a patient with renal failure, combined hemodialysis and hemoperfusion may be considered if response to more conservative therapy fails. However, no data supporting such therapy are available.

DOSAGE AND ADMINISTRATION

Dosage: The usual adult dosage is 1 gram administered intravenously or intramuscularly every 8 to 12 hours. The dosage and route should be determined by the susceptibility of the causative organisms, the severity of infection, and the condition and renal function of the patient.

The guidelines for dosage of Ceftazidime for injection are listed in Table 3. The following dosage schedule is recommended:

Table 3
RECOMMENDED DOSAGE SCHEDULE

	Dose	Frequency
Adults 12 years and older*		
Usual recommended dosage	1 g IV or IM	q8-12h
Uncomplicated urinary tract infections	250 mg IV or IM	q12h
Bone and joint infections	2 g IV	q12h
Complicated urinary tract infections	500 mg IV or IM	q8-12h
Uncomplicated pneumonia; mild skin and skin structure infections	500mg-1g IV or IM	q8h
Serious gynecologic and intra-abdominal infections	2 g IV	q8h
Meningitis	2 g IV	q8h
Very severe life-threatening infections, especially in immunocompromised patients	2 g IV	q8h
Lung infections caused by *Pseudomonas* spp. in patients with cystic fibrosis with normal renal function†	30-50 mg/kg IV to a maximum of 6 g per day	q8h
Neonates (0 to 4 weeks)	30 mg/kg IV	q12h
Infants and Children (1 month to 12 years of age)	30-50 mg/kg IV to a maximum of 6 g/day‡	q8h

*   Ceftazidime with arginine is for use in patients 12 years and older. If treatment with Ceftazidime is indicated for pediatric patients, a sodium carbonate formulation should be used.

†   Although clinical improvement has been shown, bacteriologic cures cannot be expected in patients with chronic respiratory disease and cystic fibrosis.

‡   The higher dose should be reserved for immunocompromised children or children with cystic fibrosis or meningitis.

Impaired Hepatic Function: No adjustment in dosage is required for patients with hepatic dysfunction.

Impaired Renal Function: Ceftazidime is excreted by the kidneys, almost exclusively by glomerular filtration. Therefore, in patients with impaired renal function (glomerular filtration rate [GFR] < 50 mL per minute), it is recommended that the dosage of Ceftazidime be reduced to compensate for its slower excretion. In patients with suspected renal insufficiency, an initial loading dose of 1 gm of Ceftazidime may be given. An estimate of GFR should be made to determine the appropriate maintenance dosage. The recommended dosage is presented in Table 4.

Table 4
RECOMMENDED MAINTENANCE DOSAGES OF CEFTAZIDIME IN RENAL INSUFFICIENCY
Note: If the dose recommended in table 3 above is lower than that recommended for patients with renal insufficiency as outlined in table 4, the lower dose should be used.

◆ RATED THERAPEUTICALLY EQUIVALENT; ◇ THERAPEUTIC EQUIVALENCE UNCONFIRMED; ○ UNRATED

Creatinine Clearance (mL/min)	Recommended Unit Dose of Ceftazidime	Frequency of Dosing
50-31	1 gm	q12h
30-16	1 gm	q24h
15-6	500 mg	q24h
<5	500 mg	q48h

When only serum creatinine is available, the following formula (Cockcroft's equation)[4] may be used to estimate creatinine clearance. The serum creatinine should represent a steady state of renal function:

Males:

$$\text{Creatinine clearance (mL/min)} = \frac{\text{Weight (kg)} \times (140 - \text{age})}{72 \times \text{serum creatinine (mg/dL)}}$$

Females: $0.85 \times$ male value

In patients with severe infections who would normally receive 6 g of Ceftazidime daily were it not for renal insufficiency, the unit dose given in the table above may be increased by 50% or the dosing frequency may be increased appropriately. Further dosing should be determined by therapeutic monitoring, severity of the infection, and susceptibility of the causative organism.

In children, as in adults, the creatinine clearance should be adjusted for body surface area or lean body mass, and the dosing frequency should be reduced in cases of renal insufficiency.

In patients undergoing hemodialysis, a loading dose of 1 g is recommended, followed by 1 gram after each hemodialysis period.

Ceftazidime can also be used in patients undergoing intraperitoneal dialysis and continuous ambulatory peritoneal dialysis. In such patients, a loading dose of 1 gram of Ceftazidime may be given, followed by 500 mg every 24 hours. It is not known whether or not Ceftazidime can be safely incorporated into dialysis fluid.

In addition to intravenous use, Ceftazidime sodium carbonate can be incorporated in dialysis fluid at a concentration of 250 mg/2 L of dialysis fluid.

Note: Generally Ceftazidime should be continued for 2 days after the signs and symptoms of infection have disappeared, but in complicated infections longer therapy may be required.

Administration: Ceftazidime may be given intravenously or by deep IM injection into a large muscle mass such as the upper outer quadrant of the gluteus maximus or lateral part of the thigh.

Intramuscular Administration: For IM administration, Ceftazidime should be constituted with one of the following diluents: sterile water for injection, bacteriostatic water for injection, or 0.5% or 1% lidocaine hydrochloride injection. Refer to Table 5.

Intravenous Administration: The IV route is preferable for patients with bacterial septicemia, bacterial meningitis, peritonitis, or other severe or life-threatening infections, or for patients who may be poor risks because of lowered resistance resulting from such debilitating conditions as malnutrition, trauma, surgery, diabetes, heart failure, or malignancy, particularly if shock is present or pending.

For direct intermittent IV administration, constitute Ceftazidime as directed in Table 5 with sterile water for injection, 5% dextrose injection, or 0.9% sodium chloride injection. Slowly inject directly into the vein over a period of 3 to 5 minutes or give through the tubing of an administration set while the patient is also receiving one of the compatible IV fluids (see *"Compatibility and Stability"*).

For IV infusion, constitute the 1- or 2-gram infusion or piggy-back unit with 100 mL of sterile water for injection, sodium chloride injection, or one of the compatible IV fluids listed under the *"Compatibility and Stability"* section. Alternatively, constitute 500 mg, 1- or 2-gram and add an appropriate quantity of the resulting solution to an IV container with one of the compatible IV fluids.

Intermittent IV infusion with a Y-type administration set can be accomplished with compatible solutions. However, during infusion of a solution containing Ceftazidime, it is desirable to discontinue the other solution.

Table 5

PREPARATION OF CEFTAZIDIME SOLUTIONS

Size	Amount of Diluent to Be Added (mL)	Volume to Be Withdrawn (mL)	Approximate Ceftazidime Concentration (mg/mL)
Intramuscular or intravenous direct (bolus) injection			
500 mg	1.5	1.8	280
1 gm	3.0	Total or 3.6	250-280
Intravenous infusion			
500 mg	5	5.3	100
1 gm	10.0	Total or 10.6	90-100
2 gm	10.0	Total or 11.2 or 11.5	170-180
Infusion or piggy-back unit			
1 gm	100*	100	10
2 gm	100*	100	20
Pharmacy bulk package			
6 or 10 gm	26 or 40	Amount needed or 30	200

* *Addition should be in two stages for piggy-back units.*

When Ceftazidime is dissolved, carbon dioxide is released and a positive pressure develops. For ease of use, please follow the recommended techniques of reconstitution described below.

Solutions of Ceftazidime, like those of most beta-lactam antibiotics, should not be added to solutions of aminoglycoside antibiotics because of potential interaction.

However, if concurrent therapy with Ceftazidime and an aminoglycoside is indicated, each of these antibiotics can be administered separately to the same patient.

Instructions for Constitution: Ceftazidime-arginine: No gas-relief needle is required when adding the diluent, except for the infusion unit where it is required during the latter stages of addition (in order to preserve product sterility, a gas-relief needle should not be inserted until an overpressure is produced in the vial). No evolution of carbon dioxide gas occurs on constitution. When the vial contents are dissolved, vials other than infusion units may still be under a reduced pressure. This reduced pressure is particularly noticeable for the 10-g pharmacy bulk package.

For 500 mg IM/IV, 1 g IM/IV, and 2 g IV. containers.

1. Inject the diluent and shake well to dissolve.
2. Carbon dioxide is released as the antibiotic dissolves, generating pressure with the container. The solution will become clear within 1 to 2 minutes.
3. Invert the container, and completely depress the syringe plunger prior to insertion.
4. Insert the needle through the container stopper. Be sure the needle remains within the solution, and withdraw contents of the container in the usual manner. Pressure in the container may aid withdrawal.
5. The withdrawn solution may contain carbon dioxide bubbles which should be expelled from the syringe before injection.

For 1-g and 2-g piggyback containers

1. Inject 10 mL of the diluent and shake to dissolve.
2. Carbon dioxide is released as the antibiotic dissolves, generating pressure with the container. The solution will become clear within 1 to 2 minutes.
3. Insert a vent needle to release pressure before adding additional diluent to the container. Add diluent and then remove the vent needle.
4. After storage, any additional pressure that may develop in the container prior to administration should be released.

COMPATIBILITY AND STABILITY

Intramuscular: Ceftazidime for injection, when constituted as directed with sterile water for injection, bacteriostatic water for injection, or 0.5% or 1% lidocaine hydrochloride injection, maintains satisfactory potency for 18 to 24 hours at room temperature or for 7 days under refrigeration. Solutions in sterile water for injection that are frozen immediately after constitution in the original container are stable for 3 to 6 months when stored at −20°C. Components of the solution may precipitate in the frozen state and will dissolve on reaching room temperature with little or no agitation. Potency is not affected. Frozen solutions should only be thawed at room temperature. Do not force thaw by immersion in water baths or by microwave irradiation. Once thawed, solutions should not be refrozen. Thawed solutions may be stored for up to 8 to 12 hours at room temperature or for 4 to 7 days in a refrigerator.

Intravenous: Ceftazidime concentration greater than 100 mg/mL (2-gm vial or 10-gm pharmacy bulk package): Ceftazidime, when constituted as directed with sterile water for injection, 0.9% sodium chloride injection, or 5% dextrose injection, maintains satisfactory potency for 18 to 24 hours at room temperature or for 7 days under refrigeration. Solutions of a similar concentration in sterile water for injection that are frozen immediately after constitution in the original container are stable for 3 to 6 months when stored at −20°C Components of the solution may precipitate in the frozen state and will dissolve on reaching room temperature with little or no agitation. Potency is not affected. Frozen solutions should only be thawed at room temperature. Do not force thaw by immersion in water baths or by microwave irradiation. For larger volumes where it may be necessary to warm the frozen product (to a maximum of 40°C), care should be taken to avoid heating after thawing is complete. Once thawed, solutions should not be refrozen. Thawed solutions may be stored for up to 8 to 12 hours at room temperature or for 4 to 7 days in a refrigerator.

Ceftazidime concentration of 100 mg/mL or less (1-gm vial or infusion packs): Ceftazidime, when constituted as directed with sterile water for injection, 0.9% sodium chloride injection, or 5% dextrose injection, maintains satisfactory potency for 24 hours at room temperature or for 7 days under refrigeration. Solutions, prepared by a pharmacist, of the approved arginine formulation of Ceftazidime of a similar concentration in sterile water for injection, 0.9% sodium chloride injection, or 5% dextrose injection in the original container or in 0.9% sodium chloride injection in small volume containers that are frozen immediately after constitution by the pharmacist are stable for 3 to 6 months when stored at −20°C. Frozen solutions should only be thawed at room temperature. Do not force thaw by immersion in water baths or by microwave irradiation. For the larger volumes of IV infusion solutions where it may be necessary to warm the frozen product, care should be taken to avoid heating after thawing is complete. Once thawed, solutions should not be refrozen. Thawed solutions may be stored for up to 8 to 18 hours at room temperature or for 4 to 7 days in a refrigerator.

Components of the solution may precipitate in the frozen state and will dissolve upon reaching room temperature with little or no agitation. Potency is not affected. Check for minute leaks in plastic containers by squeezing bag firmly. Discard bag if leaks are found as sterility may be impaired. Do not add supplementary medication to bags. Do not use unless solution is clear and seal is intact.

Use sterile equipment.

Caution: Do not use plastic containers in series connections. Such use could result in air embolism due to residual air being drawn from the primary container before administration of the fluid from the secondary container is complete.

Preparation for Administration:

1. Suspend container from eyelet support.
2. Remove protector from outlet port at bottom of container.
3. Attach administration set. Refer to complete directions accompanying set.

Ceftazidime is compatible with the more commonly used IV infusion fluids. Solutions at concentrations between 1 and 40 mg/mL in 0.9% sodium chloride injection; 1/6 M sodium lactate injection; 5% dextrose injection; 5% dextrose and 0.225% sodium chloride injection; 5% dextrose and 0.45% sodium chloride injection; 5% dextrose and 0.9% sodium chloride injection; 10% dextrose injection; Ringer's injection, USP; lactated Ringer's injection, USP; 10% invert sugar in sterile water for injection; and Normosol®-M in 5% dextrose injection may be stored for up to 24 hours at room temperature or for 7 days if refrigerated.

Ceftazidime is less stable in sodium bicarbonate injection than in other IV fluids. It is not recommended as a diluent. Solutions of Ceftazidime in 5% dextrose injection and 0.9% sodium chloride injection are stable for at least 6 hours at room temperature in plastic tubing, drip chambers, and volume control devices of common IV infusion sets.

Ceftazidime at a concentration of 4 mg/mL has been found compatible for 24 hours at room temperature or for 7 days under refrigeration in 0.9% sodium chloride injection or 5% dextrose injection when admixed with: cefuroxime sodium 3 mg/mL; heparin sodium in concentrations up to 50 U/mL; or potassium chloride in concentrations up to 40 mEq/L. Ceftazidime may be constituted at a concentration of 20 mg/mL with metronidazole injection 5 mg/mL, and the resultant solution may be stored for 24 hours at room temperature or for 7 days under refrigeration. Ceftazidime at a concentration of 20 mg/mL has been found compatible for 24 hours at room temperature or for 7 days under refrigeration in 0.9% sodium chloride injection or 5% dextrose injection when admixed with 6 mg/mL clindamycin (as clindamycin phosphate).

Ceftazidime at a concentration of 20 mg/mL has been found compatible for 18 or 24 hours at room temperature or seven days under refrigeration in sterile water for injection when admixed with: cefazolin sodium 330 mg/mL; heparin 1000 units/mL; and cimetidine HCl 150 mg/mL.

Ceftazidime at a concentration of 20 mg/mL has been found compatible for 18 or 24 hours at room temperature or seven days under refrigeration in 5% dextrose injection when admixed with potassium chloride 40 mEq/l.

Vancomycin solution exhibits a physical incompatibility when mixed with a number of drugs, including Ceftazidime. The likelihood of precipitation with Ceftazidime is dependent on the concentrations of vancomycin and Ceftazidime present. It is therefore recommended, when both drugs are to be administered by intermittent IV infusion, that they be given separately, flushing the IV lines (with one of the compatible IV fluids) between the administration of these two agents.

Note: Parenteral drug products should be inspected visually for particulate matter before administration whenever solution and container permit.

As with other cephalosporins, Ceftazidime powder as well as solutions tend to darken, depending on storage conditions; within the stated recommendations, however, product potency is not adversely affected.

Directions for Dispensing: Pharmacy Bulk Package—Not for Direct Infusion: The pharmacy bulk package is for use in a pharmacy admixture service only under a laminar flow hood. Entry into the vial must be made with a sterile transfer set or other sterile dispensing device, and the contents dispensed in aliquots using aseptic technique. The use of syringe and needle is not recommended as it may cause leakage (see *"Dosage and Administration"*). GOOD PHARMACY PRACTICE DICTATES THAT THE CLOSURE BE PENETRATED ONLY ONE TIME AFTER CONSTITUTION. AFTER INITIAL PENETRATION OF THE CLOSURE, USE ENTIRE CONTENTS OF VIAL PROMPTLY. ANY UNUSED PORTION MUST BE DISCARDED WITHIN 18 HOURS OF CONSTITUTION.

Storage: Before reconstitution, protect from light and store at controlled room temperature, 15° to 30°C (59° to 86°F).

REFERENCES
1. Bauer AW, Kirby WMM, Sherris JC, Turck M. Antibiotic susceptibility testing by a standardized single disk method. *Am J Clin Pathol.* 1966:45:493—496. 2. National Committee for Clinical Laboratory Standards. *Approved Standard: Performance Standards for Antimicrobial Disc Susceptibility Tests.* (M2-A3), December 1984. 3. Certification procedure for antibiotic sensitivity discs (21 CFR 460.1). *Federal Register.* May 30, 1974:39:19182—19184. 4. Cockroft DW, Gault MH. Prediction of creatinine clearance from serum creatinine. *Nephron.* 1976:16:31—41. 5. *Performance standards for antimicrobial disk susceptibility tests,* ed. 4, Tentative Standard: M2-T4. NCCLS, Villanova, PA, 1988.

HOW SUPPLIED
INJECTION: 1 GM/50 ML

BRAND/MANUFACTURER	NDC	SIZE	AWP
◆ **BRAND**			
TAZICEF: SK Beecham Pharm	00007-5088-04	50 ml 24s	$402.00

INJECTION: 1 GM

BRAND/MANUFACTURER	NDC	SIZE	AWP
◆ **BRAND**			
FORTAZ: Glaxo	00173-0434-00	18 ml 25s	$367.68

INJECTION: 1 GM

BRAND/MANUFACTURER	NDC	SIZE	AWP
○ **BRAND**			
FORTAZ: Glaxo	00173-0412-00	50 ml 24s	$406.24

INJECTION: 2 GM/50 ML

BRAND/MANUFACTURER	NDC	SIZE	AWP
◆ **BRAND**			
TAZICEF: SK Beecham Pharm	00007-5089-04	50 ml 24s	$739.89

INJECTION: 2 GM

BRAND/MANUFACTURER	NDC	SIZE	AWP
◆ **BRAND**			
FORTAZ: Glaxo	00173-0435-00	18 ml 10s	$289.34

INJECTION: 2 GM

BRAND/MANUFACTURER	NDC	SIZE	AWP
○ **BRAND**			
FORTAZ: Glaxo	00173-0413-00	50 ml 24s	$747.67

POWDER FOR INJECTION: 500 MG

AVERAGE UNIT PRICE (AVAILABLE SIZES)

BRAND		$7.11	

BRAND/MANUFACTURER	NDC	SIZE	AWP
◆ **BRAND**			
FORTAZ: Glaxo	00173-0377-31	25s	$177.84
TAZIDIME: Lilly	00002-7230-25	25s	$177.85

POWDER FOR INJECTION: 1 GM

AVERAGE UNIT PRICE (AVAILABLE SIZES)

BRAND		$14.91	

BRAND/MANUFACTURER	NDC	SIZE	AWP
◆ **BRAND**			
FORTAZ: Glaxo	00173-0380-32	10s	$145.87
TAZIDIME: Lilly	00002-7238-10	10s	$145.88
TAZICEF: Abbott Hosp	00007-5083-11	10s	$151.95
CEPTAZ: Glaxo	00173-0416-00	10s	$157.52
TAZIDIME: Lilly	00002-7245-24	24s	$375.72
FORTAZ: Glaxo	00173-0378-35	25s	$355.67
TAZIDIME: Lilly	00002-7231-25	25s	$355.68
	00002-7290-25	25s	$367.68
TAZICEF: Abbott Hosp	00007-5082-16	25s	$370.50
CEPTAZ: Glaxo	00173-0414-00	25s	$384.12

POWDER FOR INJECTION: 2 GM

AVERAGE UNIT PRICE (AVAILABLE SIZES)

BRAND		$29.49	

BRAND/MANUFACTURER	NDC	SIZE	AWP
◆ **BRAND**			
FORTAZ: Glaxo	00173-0379-34	10s	$284.53
TAZIDIME: Lilly	00002-7234-10	10s	$284.54
FORTAZ: Glaxo	00173-0381-32	10s	$288.13
TAZIDIME: Lilly	00002-7239-10	10s	$288.14
	00002-7291-10	10s	$289.34
TAZICEF: Abbott Hosp	00007-5084-11	10s	$296.40
	00007-5085-11	10s	$300.15
CEPTAZ: Glaxo	00173-0417-00	10s	$311.17
TAZIDIME: Lilly	00002-7246-24	24s	$717.17
CEPTAZ: Glaxo	00173-0415-00	25s	$768.20

POWDER FOR INJECTION: 6 GM

AVERAGE UNIT PRICE (AVAILABLE SIZES)

BRAND		$84.53	

BRAND/MANUFACTURER	NDC	SIZE	AWP
◆ **BRAND**			
FORTAZ: Glaxo	00173-0382-37	6s	$496.80
TAZICEF: Abbott Hosp	00007-5086-11	10s	$862.50

◆ RATED THERAPEUTICALLY EQUIVALENT; ◇ THERAPEUTIC EQUIVALENCE UNCONFIRMED; ○ UNRATED

POWDER FOR INJECTION: 6 GM

BRAND/MANUFACTURER	NDC	SIZE	AWP
○ BRAND TAZIDIME: Lilly	00002-7241-16	6s	$496.82

POWDER FOR INJECTION: 10 GM

BRAND/MANUFACTURER	NDC	SIZE	AWP
◆ BRAND CEPTAZ: Glaxo	00173-0418-00	6s	$894.24

Ceftin *SEE* CEFUROXIME AXETIL

Ceftizoxime Sodium

DESCRIPTION

Ceftizoxime Sodium is a sterile, semisynthetic, broad-spectrum, beta-lactamase resistant cephalosporin antibiotic for parenteral (I.V., I.M.) administration. It is the sodium salt of [6R-[6a, 7β(Z)]]-7-[[2,3-dihydro-2-imino-4-thiazolyl) (methoxy-imino) acetyl] amino]-8-oxo-5-thia-1-azabicyclo [4.2.0] oct-2-ene-2-carboxylic acid. Its sodium content is approximately 60 mg (2.6 mEq) per gram of Ceftizoxime Sodium activity.

Its empirical formula is $C_{13}H_{12}N_5NaO_5S_2$. Its molecular weight is 405.38.

Sterile Ceftizoxime Sodium is a white to pale yellow crystalline powder.

Ceftizoxime Sodium is supplied in vials equivalent to 500 mg, 1 gram, 2 grams, or 10 grams, and in "Piggyback" Vials for intravenous admixture equivalent to 1 gram or 2 grams.

Ceftizoxime Sodium equivalent to 1 gram or 2 grams, is also supplied as a frozen, sterile, nonpyrogenic solution in an iso-osmotic diluent in plastic containers. After thawing, the solution is intended for intravenous use.

The plastic container is fabricated from specially formulated polyvinyl chloride. Solutions in contact with the plastic container can leach out certain of its chemical components in very small amounts within the expiration period, e.g., di 2-ethylhexyl phthalate (DEHP), up to 5 parts per million. However, the suitability of the plastic has been confirmed in tests in animals according to the USP biological tests for plastic containers as well as by tissue culture toxicity studies.

Following is its chemical structure:

CLINICAL PHARMACOLOGY

The table below demonstrates the serum levels and duration of Ceftizoxime Sodium following intramuscular administration of 500 mg and 1 gram doses, respectively, to normal volunteers.

SERUM CONCENTRATIONS AFTER INTRAMUSCULAR ADMINISTRATION

Serum Concentration (mcg/mL)

Dose	½ hr	1 hr	2 hr	4 hr	6 hr	8 hr
500 mg	13.3	13.7	9.2	4.8	1.9	0.7
1 gram	36.0	39.0	31.0	15.0	6.0	3.0

Following intravenous administration of 1, 2, and 3 gram doses of Ceftizoxime Sodium to normal volunteers, the following serum levels were obtained.

SERUM CONCENTRATIONS AFTER INTRAVENOUS ADMINISTRATION

Serum Concentration (mcg/mL)

Dose	5 min	10 min	30 min	1 hr	2 hr	4 hr	8 hr
1 gram	ND	ND	60.5	38.9	21.5	8.4	1.4
2 grams	131.8	110.9	77.5	53.6	33.1	12.1	2.0
3 grams	221.1	174.0	112.7	83.9	47.4	26.2	4.8

ND = Not Done

A serum half-life of approximately 1.7 hours was observed after intravenous or intramuscular administration.

Ceftizoxime Sodium is 30% protein bound.

Ceftizoxime Sodium is not metabolized, and is excreted virtually unchanged by the kidneys in 24 hours. This provides a high urinary concentration. Concentrations greater than 6000 mcg/mL have been achieved in the urine by 2 hours after a 1 gram dose of Ceftizoxime Sodium intravenously. Probenecid slows tubular secretion and produces even higher serum levels, increasing the duration of measurable serum concentrations.

Ceftizoxime Sodium achieves therapeutic levels in various body fluids, e.g., cerebrospinal fluid (in patients with inflamed meninges), bile, surgical wound fluid, pleural fluid, aqueous humor, ascitic fluid, peritoneal fluid, prostatic fluid and saliva, and in the following body tissues: heart, gallbladder, bone, biliary, peritoneal, prostatic, and uterine.

In clinical experience to date, no disulfiram-like reactions have been reported with Ceftizoxime Sodium.

MICROBIOLOGY

The bacterial action of Ceftizoxime Sodium results from inhibition of cell-wall synthesis. Ceftizoxime Sodium is highly resistant to a broad spectrum of beta-lactamases (penicillinase and cephalosporinase), including Richmond types I, II, III, TEM, and IV, produced by both aerobic and anaerobic gram-positive and gram-negative organisms. Ceftizoxime Sodium is active against a wide range of gram-positive and gram-negative organisms, and is usually active against the following organisms *in vitro* and in clinical situations (See "Indications and Usage")

GRAM-POSITIVE AEROBES

Staphylococcus aureus (including penicillinase- and nonpenicillinase-producing strains)

Note: Methicillin-resistant staphylococci are resistant to cephalosporins, including Ceftizoxime Sodium.

Staphylococcus epidermidis (including penicillinase- and nonpenicillinase-producing strains)
Streptococcus agalactiae
Streptococcus pneumoniae
Streptococcus pyogenes

Note: Ceftizoxime Sodium is usually inactive against most strains of *Enterococcus faecalis* (formerly *S. faecalis*).

GRAM-NEGATIVE AEROBES

Acinetobacter spp.
Enterobacter spp.
Escherichia coli
Haemophilus influenzae (including ampicillin-resistant strains)
Klebsiella pneumoniae
Morganella morganii (formerly *Proteus morganii*)
Neisseria gonorrhoeae
Proteus mirabilis
Proteus vulgaris
Providencia rettgeri (formerly *Proteus rettgeri*)
Pseudomonas aeruginosa
Serratia marcescens

ANAEROBES

Bacteroides spp.
Peptococcus spp.
Peptostreptococcus spp.

Ceftizoxime Sodium is usually active against the following organisms *in vitro,* but the clinical significance of these data is unknown.

GRAM-POSITIVE AEROBES

Corynebacterium diphtheriae

GRAM-NEGATIVE AEROBES

Aeromonas hydrophila
Citrobacter spp.
Moraxella spp.
Neisseria meningitidis
Pasteurella multocida
Providencia stuartii
Salmonella spp.
Shigella spp.
Yersinia enterocolitica

ANAEROBES

Actinomyces spp.
Bifidobacterium spp.
Clostridium spp.

Note: Most strains of *Clostridium difficile* are resistant.

Eubacterium spp.
Fusobacterium spp.
Propionibacterium spp.
Veillonella spp.

SUSCEPTIBILITY TESTING: DIFFUSION TECHNIQUES

Quantitative methods that require measurement of zone diameters give the most precise estimate of susceptibility of bacteria to antimicrobial agents. One such standard procedure[1] has been recommended for use with disks to test susceptibility of organisms to Ceftizoxime Sodium. Interpretation involves the correlation of the diameters obtained in the disk test with the minimum inhibitory concentration (MIC) for Ceftizoxime Sodium.

Organisms should be tested with the Ceftizoxime Sodium disk, since Ceftizoxime Sodium has been shown by *in vitro* tests to be active against certain strains found resistant when other beta-lactam disks are used.

➤ SHOWN IN PRODUCT IDENTIFICATION GUIDE

Reports from the laboratory giving results of the standard single-disk suscepti-bility test with a 30 mcg Ceftizoxime Sodium disk should be interpreted according to the following criteria (with the exception of *Pseudomonas aeruginosa*).

Zone Diameter (mm)	Interpretation
≥20	(S) Susceptible
15-19	(MS) Moderately Susceptible
≤14	(R) Resistant

A report of "Susceptible" indicates that the pathogen is likely to be inhibited by generally achievable blood levels. A report of "Moderately Susceptible" suggests that the organism would be susceptible if high dosage is used or if the infection is confined to tissue and fluids (e.g., urine) in which high antibiotic levels are attained. A report of "Resistant" indicates that achievable concentrations of the antibiotic are unlikely to be inhibitory and other therapy should be selected.

Standardized procedures require the use of laboratory control organisms. The 30 mcg Ceftizoxime Sodium disk should give the following zone diameters:

Organism	ATCC	Zone Diameter (mm)
Escherichia coli	25922	30-36
Pseudomonas aeruginosa	27853	12-17
Staphylococcus aureus	25923	27-35

SUSCEPTIBILITY TESTING FOR PSEUDOMONAS IN URINARY TRACT INFECTIONS

Most strains of Pseudomonas aeruginosa are moderately susceptible to Ceftizox-ime Sodium. Ceftizoxime Sodium achieves high levels in the urine (greater than 6000 mcg/mL at 2 hours with 1 gram IV) and, therefore, the following zone sizes should be used when testing Ceftizoxime Sodium for treatment of urinary tract infections caused by *Pseudomonas aeruginosa*.

Susceptible organisms produce zones of 20 mm or greater, indicating that the test organism is likely to respond to therapy.

Organisms that produce zones of 11 to 19 mm are expected to be susceptible when the infection is confined to the urinary tract (in which high antibiotic levels are attained).

Resistant organisms produce zones of 10 mm or less, indicating that other therapy should be selected.

SUSCEPTIBILITY TESTING: DILUTION TECHNIQUES

When using the NCCLS agar dilution or broth dilution (including microdilution) method[2] or equivalent, the following MIC data should be used in interpretation.

MIC (mcg/mL)	Interpretation
≤8	(S) Susceptible
16-32	(MS) Moderately Susceptible
≥64	(R) Resistant

As with standard disk diffusion methods, dilution procedures require the use of laboratory control organisms. Standard Ceftizoxime Sodium powder should give MIC values in the following ranges.

Organism	ATCC	MIC (mcg/mL)
Escherichia coli	25922	0.03-0.12
Pseudomonas aeruginosa	27853	16-64
Staphylococcus aureus	29213	2-8

INDICATIONS AND USAGE

Ceftizoxime Sodium is indicated in the treatment of infections due to susceptible strains of the microorganisms listed below.

Lower Respiratory Tract Infections caused by *Klebsiella* spp.; *Proteus mirabi-lis; Escherichia coli; Haemophilus influenzae* including ampicillin-resistant strains; *Staphylococcus aureus* (penicillinase- and nonpenicillinase-producing); *Serratia* spp; *Enterobacter* spp.; and *Bacteroides* spp.; and *Streptococcus* spp. including *S. pneumoniae*, but excluding enterococci.

Urinary Tract Infections caused by *Staphylococcus aureus* (penicillinase- and nonpenicillinase-producing); *Escherichia coli; Pseudomonas* spp. including *P. aeruginosa; Proteus mirabilis; P. vulgaris; Providencia rettgeri* (formerly *Proteus rettgeri*) and *Morganella morganii* (formerly *Proteus morganii*); *Klebsiella* spp.; *Serratia* spp. including *S. marcescens;* and *Enterobacter* spp.

Gonorrhea including uncomplicated cervical and urethral gonorrhea caused by *Neisseria gonorrhoeae*.

Pelvic Inflammatory Disease caused by *Neisseria gonorrhoeae, Escherichia coli* or *Streptococcus agalactiae*.

Note: Ceftizoxime Sodium, like other cephalosporins, has no activity against *Chlamydia trachomatis*. Therefore, when cephalosporins are used in the treatment of patients with pelvic inflammatory disease and *C. trachomatis* is one of the suspected pathogens, appropriate anti-chlamydial coverage should be added.

Intra-Abdominal Infections caused by *Escherichia coli; Staphylococcus epider-midis; Streptococcus* spp. (excluding enterococci); *Enterobacter* spp.; *Klebsiella* spp.; *Bacteroides* spp. including *B. fragilis;* and anaerobic cocci, including *Peptococcus* spp. and *Peptostreptococcus* spp.

Septicemia caused by *Streptococcus* spp. including *S. pneumoniae* (but excluding enterococci); *Staphylococcus aureus* (penicillinase- and nonpenicilli-nase-producing); *Escherichia coli; Bacteroides* spp. including *B. fragilis; Klebsiella* spp.; and *Serratia* spp.

Skin and Skin Structure Infections caused by *Staphylococcus aureus* (penicillin-ase- and nonpenicillinase-producing); *Staphylococcus epidermidis; Escherichia coli; Klebsiella* spp.; *Streptococcus* spp. including *Streptococcus pyogenes* (but excluding enterococci); *Proteus mirabilis; Serratia* spp.; *Enterobacter* spp.; *Bacter-oides* spp. including *B. fragilis;* and anaerobic cocci, including *Peptococcus* spp. and *Peptostreptococcus* spp.

Bone and Joint Infections caused by *Staphylococcus aureus* (penicillinase- and nonpenicillinase-producing); *Streptococcus* spp. (excluding enterococci); *Proteus mirabilis; Bacteroides* spp.; and anaerobic cocci, including *Peptococcus* spp. and *Peptostreptococcus* spp.

Meningitis caused by *Haemophilus influenzae*. Ceftizoxime Sodium has also been used successfully in the treatment of a limited number of pediatric and adult cases of meningitis caused by *Streptococcus pneumoniae*.

Ceftizoxime Sodium has been effective in the treatment of seriously ill, compromised patients, including those who were debilitated, immunosuppressed or neutropenic.

Infections caused by aerobic gram-negative and by mixtures of organisms resistant to other cephalosporins, aminoglycosides, or penicillins have responded to treatment with Ceftizoxime Sodium.

Because of the serious nature of some urinary tract infections due to *P. aeruginosa* and because many strains of *Pseudomonas* species are only moderately susceptible to Ceftizoxime Sodium higher dosage is recommended. Other therapy should be instituted if the response is not prompt.

Susceptibility studies on specimens obtained prior to therapy should be used to determine the response of causative organisms to Ceftizoxime Sodium. Therapy with Ceftizoxime Sodium may be initiated pending results of the studies; however, treatment should be adjusted according to study findings. In serious infections, Ceftizoxime Sodium has been used concomitantly with aminoglyco-sides (see *"Precautions"*). Before using Ceftizoxime Sodium concomitantly with other antibiotics, the prescribing information for those agents should be reviewed for contraindications, warnings, precautions, and adverse reactions. Renal function should be carefully monitored.

UNLABELED USES

Ceftizoxime is used alone or as an adjunct in the treatment of bacterial endocarditis, endometritis, pelvic cellulitis, peritonitis, and acute and chronic osteomyelitis secondary to gram-positive organisms.

CONTRAINDICATIONS

Ceftizoxime Sodium is contraindicated in patients who have known allergy to the drug.

WARNINGS

BEFORE THERAPY WITH CEFTIZOXIME SODIUM IS INSTITUTED, CAREFUL INQUIRY SHOULD BE MADE TO DETERMINE WHETHER THE PATIENT HAS HAD PREVIOUS HYPERSENSITIVITY REACTIONS TO CEPHALOSPORINS, PENICILLINS, OR OTHER DRUGS. THIS PROD-UCT SHOULD BE GIVEN CAUTIOUSLY TO PENICILLIN-SENSITIVE PATIENTS. CAUTION SHOULD BE EXERCISED BECAUSE CROSS HY-PERSENSITIVITY AMONG BETA-LACTAM ANTIBIOTICS HAS BEEN CLEARLY DOCUMENTED AND MAY OCCUR IN UP TO 10% OF PA-TIENTS WITH A HISTORY OF PENICILLIN ALLERGY. IF AN ALLERGIC REACTION TO CEFTIZOXIME SODIUM OCCURS, DISCONTINUE THE DRUG. SERIOUS ACUTE HYPERSENSITIVITY REACTIONS MAY RE-QUIRE EPINEPHRINE AND OTHER EMERGENCY MEASURES, INCLUD-ING OXYGEN, INTRAVENOUS FLUIDS, INTRAVENOUS ANTIHISTAMINES, CORTICOSTEROIDS, PRESSOR AMINES, AND AIR-WAY MANAGEMENT, AS CLINICALLY INDICATED.

Pseudomembranous colitis has been reported with the use of cephalosporins (and other broad-spectrum antibiotics); therefore, it is important to consider this diagnosis in patients who develop diarrhea in association with antibiotic use.

Treatment with broad-spectrum antibiotics alters normal flora of the colon and may permit overgrowth of *Clostridia*. Studies indicate a toxin produced by *Clostridium difficile* is one primary cause of antibiotic-associated colitis.

Mild cases of colitis may respond to drug discontinuance alone.

Moderate to severe cases should be managed with fluid, electrolyte, and protein supplementation as indicated.

When the colitis is not relieved by drug discontinuance or when it is severe, oral vancomycin is the treatment of choice for antibiotic-associated pseudomem-branous colitis produced by *C. difficile*. Other causes of colitis should also be considered.

PRECAUTIONS

GENERAL

As with all broad-spectrum antibiotics, Ceftizoxime Sodium should be prescribed with caution in individuals with a history of gastrointestinal disease, particularly colitis.

Although Ceftizoxime Sodium has not been shown to produce an alteration in renal function, renal status should be evaluated, especially in seriously ill patients receiving maximum dose therapy. As with any antibiotic, prolonged use may result in overgrowth of nonsusceptible organisms. Careful observation is essential; appropriate measures should be taken if superinfection occurs.

DRUG INTERACTIONS
Although the occurrence has not been reported with Ceftizoxime Sodium, nephrotoxicity has been reported following concomitant administration of other cephalosporins and aminoglycosides.

CARCINOGENESIS, MUTAGENESIS, IMPAIRMENT OF FERTILITY
Long term studies in animals to evaluate the carcinogenic potential of Ceftizoxime Sodium have not been conducted.

In an *in vitro* bacterial cell assay (i.e., Ames test), there was no evidence of mutagenicity at Ceftizoxime Sodium concentrations of 0.001-0.5 mcg/plate. Ceftizoxime Sodium did not produce increases in micronuclei in the *in vivo* mouse micronucleus test when given to animals at doses up to 7500 mg/kg, approximately six times greater than the maximum human daily dose on a mg/M^2 basis.

Ceftizoxime Sodium had no effect on fertility when administered subcutaneously to rats at daily doses of up to 1000 mg/kg/day, approximately two times the maximum human daily dose on a mg/M^2 basis.

Ceftizoxime Sodium produced no histological changes in the sexual organs of male and female dogs when given intravenously for thirteen weeks at a dose of 1000 mg/kg/day, approximately five times greater than the maximum human daily dose on a mg/M^2 basis.

PREGNANCY: TERATOGENIC EFFECTS: PREGNANCY CATEGORY B.
Reproduction studies performed in rats and rabbits have revealed no evidence of impaired fertility or harm to the fetus due to Ceftizoxime Sodium. There are, however, no adequate and well-controlled studies in pregnant women. Because animal reproduction studies are not always predictive of human effects, this drug should be used during pregnancy only if clearly needed.

LABOR AND DELIVERY
Safety of Ceftizoxime Sodium use during labor and delivery has not been established.

NURSING MOTHERS
Ceftizoxime Sodium is excreted in human milk in low concentrations. Caution should be exercised when Ceftizoxime Sodium is administered to a nursing woman.

PEDIATRIC USE
Safety and efficacy in infants from birth to six months of age have not been established. In children six months of age and older, treatment with Ceftizoxime Sodium has been associated with transient elevated levels of eosinophils, AST (SGOT), ALT (SGPT) and CPK (creatine phosphokinase). The CPK elevation may be related to I.M. administration.

The potential for the toxic effect in children from chemicals that may leach from the single-dose I.V. preparation has not been determined.

ADVERSE REACTIONS
Ceftizoxime Sodium is generally well tolerated. The *most* frequent adverse reactions (*greater than* 1% but *less* than 5%) are:

Hypersensitivity: Rash, pruritus, fever.

Hepatic: Transient elevation in AST (SGOT), ALT (SGPT), and alkaline phosphatase.

Hematologic: Transient eosinophilia, thrombocytosis. Some individuals have developed a positive Coombs test.

Local—Injection site: Burning, cellulitis, phlebitis with I.V. administration, pain, induration, tenderness, paresthesia.

The *less* frequent adverse reactions (*less than* 1%) are:

Hypersensitivity: Numbness and anaphylaxis have rarely been reported.

Hepatic: Elevation of bilirubin has been reported rarely.

Renal: Transient elevations of BUN and creatinine have been occasionally observed with Ceftizoxime Sodium.

Hematologic: Anemia, leukopenia, neutropenia and thrombocytopenia, have been reported rarely.

Urogenital: Vaginitis has occurred rarely.

Gastrointestinal: Diarrhea; nausea and vomiting have been reported occasionally.

Symptoms of pseudomembranous colitis can appear during or after antibiotic treatment (see *"Warnings"*).

In addition to the adverse reactions listed above which have been observed in patients treated with Ceftizoxime Sodium, the following adverse reactions and altered laboratory tests have been reported for cephalosporin-class antibiotics:

Stevens-Johnson syndrome, erythema multiforme, toxic epidermal necrolysis, serum-sickness like reaction, toxic nephropathy, aplastic anemia, hemolytic anemia, hemorrhage, prolonged prothrombin time, elevated LDH, pancytopenia, and agranulocytosis.

Several cephalosporins have been implicated in triggering seizures, particularly in patients with renal impairment, when the dosage was not reduced. (See *"Dosage and Administration"*) If seizures associated with drug therapy occur, the drug should be discontinued. Anticonvulsant therapy can be given if clinically indicated.

DOSAGE AND ADMINISTRATION
The usual adult dosage is 1 or 2 grams of Ceftizoxime Sodium every 8 to 12 hours. Proper dosage and route of administration should be determined by the condition of the patient, severity of the infection, and susceptibility of the causative organisms.

GENERAL GUIDELINES FOR DOSAGE OF CEFTIZOXIME SODIUM

Type of Infection	Daily Dose (Grams)	Frequency and Route
Uncomplicated Urinary Tract	1	500 mg q12h I.M. or I.V.
Other Sites	2-3	1 gram q8-12h, I.M. or I.V.
Severe or Refractory	3-6	1 gram q8h I.M. or I.V. 2 grams q8-12h I.M.[a] or I.V.
PID[b]	6	2 grams q8h I.V.
Life-Threatening[c]	9-12	3-4 grams q8h I.V.

a) When administering 2 gram I.M. doses, the dose should be divided and given in different large muscle masses.
b) If C. trachomatis is a suspected pathogen, appropriate antichlamydial coverage should be added, because Ceftizoxime Sodium has no activity against this organism.
c) In life-threatening infections, dosages up to 2 grams every 4 hours have been given.

Because of the serious nature of urinary tract infections due to *P. aeruginosa* and because many strains of *Pseudomonas* species are only moderately susceptible to Ceftizoxime Sodium, higher dosage is recommended. Other therapy should be instituted if the response is not prompt.

A single, 1 gram I.M. dose is the usual dose for treatment of uncomplicated gonorrhea.

The intravenous route may be preferable for patients with bacterial septicemia, localized parenchymal abscesses (such as intra-abdominal abscess), peritonitis, or other severe or life-threatening infections.

In those with normal renal function, the intravenous dosage for such infections is 2 to 12 grams of Ceftizoxime Sodium. In conditions such as bacterial septicemia, 6 to 12 grams/day may be given initially by the intravenous route for several days, and the dosage may then be gradually reduced according to clinical response and laboratory findings.

PEDIATRIC DOSAGE SCHEDULE

	Unit Dose	Frequency
Children 6 months and older	50 mg/kg	q6-8h

Dosage may be increased to a total daily dose of 200 mg/kg (not to exceed the maximum adult dose for serious infection).

IMPAIRED RENAL FUNCTION
Modification of Ceftizoxime Sodium dosage is necessary in patients with impaired renal function. Following an initial loading dose of 500 mg.-1 gram I.M. or I.V., the maintenance dosing schedule shown below should be followed. Further dosing should be determined by therapeutic monitoring, severity of the infection, and susceptibility of the causative organisms.

When only the serum creatinine level is available, creatinine clearance may be calculated from the following formula. The serum creatinine level should represent current renal function at the steady state.

$$\text{Males} \quad \text{Clcr} = \frac{\text{Weight (kg)} \times (140 - \text{age})}{72 \times \text{serum creatinine (mg/100 mL)}}$$

Females 0.85 of the calculated clearance values for males.

In patients undergoing hemodialysis, no additional supplemental dosing is required following hemodialysis; however, dosing should be timed so that the patient receives the dose (according to the table below) at the end of the dialysis.

DOSAGE IN ADULTS WITH REDUCED RENAL FUNCTION

Creatinine Clearance mL/min	Renal Function	Less Severe Infections	Life-Threatening Infections
79-50	Mild impairment	500 mg q8h	0.75-1.5 grams q8H
49-5	Moderate to severe impairment	250-500 mg q12h	0.5-1 gram q12h
4-0	Dialysis patients	500 mg q48h or 250 mg q24h	0.5-1 gram q48h or 0.5 gram q24h

PREPARATION OF PARENTERAL SOLUTION
Reconstitution:

► SHOWN IN PRODUCT IDENTIFICATION GUIDE

I.M. Administration: Reconstitute with Sterile Water for Injection. SHAKE WELL.

Vial Size	Diluent to Be Added	Approx. Avail. Vol.	Approx. Avg. Concentration
500 mg	1.5 mL	1.8 mL	280 mg/mL
1 gram	3.0 mL	3.7 mL	270 mg/mL
2 grams*	6.0 mL	7.4 mL	270 mg/mL

* *When administering 2 gram I.M. doses, the dose should be divided and given in different large muscle masses.*

I.V. Administration: Reconstitute with Sterile Water for Injection. SHAKE WELL.

Vial Size	Diluent to Be Added	Approx. Avail. Vol.	Approx. Avg. Concentration
500 mg	5 mL	5.3 mL	95 mg/mL
1 gram	10 mL	10.7 mL	95 mg/mL
2 grams	20 mL	21.4 mL	95 mg/mL

These solutions of Ceftizoxime Sodium are stable 24 hours at room temperature or 96 hours if refrigerated (5°C).

Parenteral drug products should be inspected visually for particulate matter prior to administration. If particulate matter is evident in reconstituted fluids, then the drug solution should be discarded. Reconstituted solutions may range from yellow to amber without changes in potency.

Pharmacy Bulk Vials: For I.M. or I.V. direct injection, add Sterile Water for Injection to the 10 gram vial according to table below. SHAKE WELL. For I.V. intermittent or continuous infusion, add Sterile Water for Injection according to table below. SHAKE WELL. Add to parenteral fluids listed below under I.V. Administration.

Vial Size	Diluent to Be Added	Approx. Avail. Vol.	Approx. Avg. Concentration
10 grams	30 mL	37 mL	1 gram/3.5 mL
	45 mL	51 mL	1 gram/5 mL

These reconstituted solutions of Ceftizoxime Sodium are stable 24 hours at room temperature or 96 hours if refrigerated (5°C).

"Piggyback" Vials: Reconstitute with 50 to 100 mL of Sodium Chloride Injection or any other I.V. solution listed below. SHAKE WELL.

Administer with primary I.V. fluids, as a single dose. These solutions of Ceftizoxime Sodium are stable 24 hours at room temperature or 96 hours if refrigerated (5°C).

A solution of 1 gram Ceftizoxime Sodium in 13 mL Sterile Water for Injection is isotonic.

I.M. INJECTION

Inject well within the body of a relatively large muscle. Aspiration is necessary to avoid inadvertent injection into a blood vessel. When administering 2 gram I.M. doses, the dose should be divided and given in different large muscle masses.

IV ADMINISTRATION

Direct (bolus) injection, slowly over 3 to 5 minutes, directly or through tubing for patients receiving parenteral fluids (see list below). Intermittent or continuous infusion, dilute reconstituted Ceftizoxime Sodium in 50 to 100 mL of one of the following solutions:

- Sodium Chloride Injection
- 5% or 10% Dextrose Injection
- 5% Dextrose and 0.9%, 0.45%, or 0.2% Sodium Chloride Injection
- Ringer's Injection
- Lactated Ringer's Injection
- Invert Sugar 10% in Sterile Water for Injection
- 5% Sodium Bicarbonate in Sterile Water for Injection
- 5% Dextrose in Lactated Ringer's Injection (only when reconstituted with 4% Sodium Bicarbonate Injection)

In these fluids, Ceftizoxime Sodium is stable 24 hours at room temperature or 96 hours if refrigerated (5°C).

DIRECTIONS FOR USE OF CEFTIZOXIME SODIUM IN VIAFLEX® PLUS CONTAINERS (PL 146® PLASTIC)

Viaflex and PL 146 are registered trademarks of Baxter International Inc.

Ceftizoxime Sodium in Viaflex® Plus Containers (PL 146® Plastic) is to be administered either as a continuous or intermittent infusion using sterile equipment.

STORAGE

Store in freezer capable of maintaining a temperature of −20°C/−4°F.

THAWING OF PLASTIC CONTAINER

Thaw frozen container at room temperature (25°C/77°F) or under refrigeration (5°C/41°F). DO NOT FORCE THAW BY IMMERSION IN WATER BATHS OR BY MICROWAVE IRRADIATION.

Containers may be thawed individually after separation from the frozen shingle. A shingle consists of stacked frozen containers. Remove frozen shingle from carton and allow to rest at room temperature until the containers can be easily separated (approximately 5 minutes). Then grasp the body of the container (not the ports, corner, or tail flap) to separate individual units.

Promptly return unneeded frozen containers to freezer.

Check for minute leaks by squeezing container firmly. If leaks are detected, discard solution as sterility may be impaired.

Do not add supplementary medication.

The container should be visually inspected. Components of the solution may precipitate in the frozen state and will dissolve upon reaching room temperature with little or no agitation. Potency is not affected. Agitate after solution has reached room temperature. If after visual inspection the solution remains cloudy or if an insoluble precipitate is noted or if any seal or outlet ports are not intact, the container should be discarded.

The thawed solution is stable for 10 days under refrigeration (5°C/41°F) or for 24 hours at room temperature (25°C/77°F). **Do not refreeze thawed antibiotics.**

Caution: Do not use plastic containers in series connections. Air embolism could result due to residual air being drawn from the primary container before administration of the fluid from the secondary container is complete.

Preparation for Intravenous Administration

1. Suspend container from eyelet support.
2. Remove plastic protector from outlet port at bottom of container.
3. Attach administration set. Refer to complete directions accompanying set.

Unreconstituted Ceftizoxime Sodium should be protected from excessive light, and stored at controlled room temperature (59°-86°F) in the original package until used.

REFERENCES
1. National Committee for Clinical Laboratory Standards, Approved Standard. *Performance Standards for Antimicrobial Disk Susceptibility Test,* 4th Edition, Vol. 10(7): M2-A4. Villanova, PA, April 1990. 2. National Committee for Clinical Laboratory Standards, Approved Standard. *Methods for Dilution Antimicrobial Susceptibility Tests for Bacteria that Grow Aerobically,* 2nd Edition, Vol. 10(8): M7-A2. Villanova, PA, April 1990.

HOW SUPPLIED
INJECTION: 500 MG

BRAND/MANUFACTURER	NDC	SIZE	AWP
○ **BRAND**			
CEFIZOX: Fujisawa	57317-0250-01	10 ml	$6.48

INJECTION: 1 GM

BRAND/MANUFACTURER	NDC	SIZE	AWP
○ **BRAND**			
CEFIZOX: Fujisawa	57317-0251-01	20 ml	$11.39
	57317-0220-50	50 ml	$335.52
	57317-0252-01	100 ml	$122.95

INJECTION: 2 GM

BRAND/MANUFACTURER	NDC	SIZE	AWP
○ **BRAND**			
CEFIZOX: Fujisawa	57317-0253-02	20 ml	$21.14
	57317-0221-50	50 ml	$569.66
	57317-0254-02	100 ml	$230.47

INJECTION: 10 GM

BRAND/MANUFACTURER	NDC	SIZE	AWP
○ **BRAND**			
CEFIZOX: Fujisawa	57317-0255-10	100 ml	$1044.44

Ceftriaxone Sodium

DESCRIPTION

Ceftriaxone Sodium is a sterile, semisynthetic, broad-spectrum cephalosporin antibiotic for intravenous or intramuscular administration. Ceftriaxone Sodium is 5-Thia-1-azabicyclo [4.2.0]oct-2-ene-2-carboxylic acid,7-[[(2-amino-4-thiazolyl) (methoxyimino) acetyl]-amino]-8-oxo-3-[[(1, 2, 5, 6-tetrahydro-2-menthyl-5, 6-dioxo-1, 2, 4-triazin-3-yl)thio]methyl]-, disodium salt, [6R-[6α, 7β(Z)]]-.

The chemical formula of Ceftriaxone Sodium is $C_{18}H_{16}N_8Na_2O_7S_33.5H_2O$. It has a calculated molecular weight of 661.59.

Ceftriaxone Sodium is a white to yellowish-orange crystalline powder which is readily soluble in water, sparingly soluble in methanol and very slightly soluble in ethanol. The pH of a 1% aqueous solution is approximately 6.7. The color of Ceftriaxone Sodium solutions ranges from light yellow to amber, depending on the length of storage, concentration and diluent used.

Ceftriaxone Sodium contains approximately 83 mg (3.6 mEq) of Sodium per gram of Ceftriaxone activity.

◆ **RATED THERAPEUTICALLY EQUIVALENT;** ◇ **THERAPEUTIC EQUIVALENCE UNCONFIRMED;** ○ **UNRATED**

Following is its chemical structure:

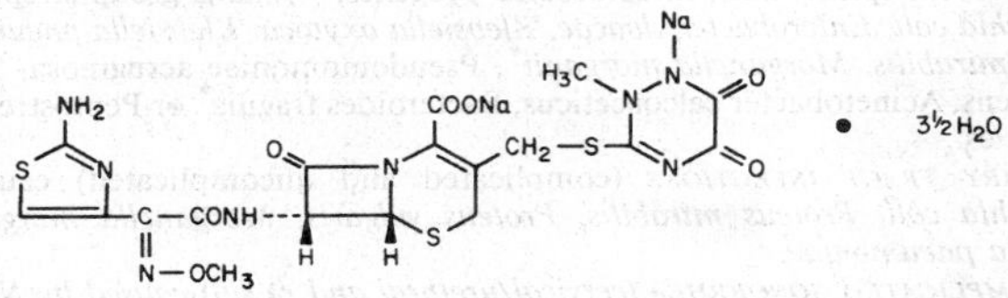

CLINICAL PHARMACOLOGY

Average plasma concentrations of Ceftriaxone following a single 30-minutes intervaneous (I.V.) infusion of a 0.5, 1 or 2 gm dose and intramuscular (I.M.) administration of a single 0.5 or 1 gm dose in healthy subjects are presented in Table 1. (See related table).

Ceftriaxone was completely absorbed following I.M. administration with mean maximum plasma concentrations occurring between two and three hours postdosing. Multiple I.V. or I.M. doses ranging from 0.5 to 2 gm at 12-to 24-hour intervals resulted in 15% to 36% accumulation of Ceftriaxone above single dose values.

Ceftriaxone concentrations in urine are high, as shown in Table 2.

Table 2
URINARY CONCENTRATIONS OF CEFTRIAXONE AFTER SINGLE DOSE ADMINISTRATION

Dose/Route	Average Urinary Concentration (mcg/mL)					
	0-2 hr	2-4 hr	4-8 hr	8-12 hr	12-24 hr	24-48 hr
0.5 gm I.V.	526	366	142	87	70	15
0.5 gm I.M.	115	425	308	127	96	28
1gm I.V.	995	855	293	147	132	32
1 gm I.M.	504	628	418	237	ND*	ND
2 gm I.V.	2692	1976	757	274	198	40

*ND = Not determined.

Thirty-three percent to 67% of a Ceftriaxone dose was excreted in the urine as unchanged drug and the remainder was secreted in the bile and ultimately found in the feces as microbiologically inactive compounds. After a 1 gm I.V. dose, average concentrations of Ceftriaxone, determined from one to three hours after dosing were 581 mcg/mL in the gallbladder bile, 788 mcg/mL in the common duct bile, 898 mcg/mL in the cystic duct bile, 78.2 mcg/gm in the gallbladder wall and 62.1 mcg/mL in the concurrent plasma.

Over a 0.15 to 3 gm dose range in healthy adult subjects, the values of elimination half-life ranged from 5.8 to 8.7 hours; apparent volume of distribution from 5.78 to 13.5 L; plasma clearance from 0.58 to 1.45 L/hour; and renal clearance from 0.32 to 0.73 L/hour. Ceftriaxone is reversibly bound to human plasma proteins, and the binding decreased from a value of 95% bound at plasma concentrations of < 25 mcg/mL to a value of 85% bound at 300 mcg/mL. The average values of maximum plasma concentration, elimination half-life, plasma clearance and volume of distribution after a 50 mg/kg I.V. dose and after a 75 mg/kg I.V. dose in pediatric patients suffering from bacterial meningitis are shown in Table 3. Ceftriaxone penetrated the inflamed meninges of infants and children: CSF concentrations after a 50 mg/kg I.V. dose and after a 75 mg/kg I.V. dose are also shown in Table 3.

Table 3
AVERAGE PHARMACOKINETIC PARAMETERS OF CEFTRIAXONE IN PEDIATRIC PATIENTS WITH MENINGITIS

	50 mg/kg I.V.	75 mg/kg I.V.
Maximum Plasma Concentrations (mcg/mL)	216	275
Elimination Half-life (hr)	4.6	4.3
Plasma Clearance (mL/hr/kg)	49	60
Volume of Distribution (mL/kg)	338	373
CSF Concentration-inflamed meninges (mcg/mL)	5.6	6.4
Range (mcg/mL)	1.3-18.5	1.3-44
Time after dose (hr)	3.7 (± 1.6)	3.3 (± 1.4)

Compared to that in healthy adult subjects, the pharmacokinetics of Ceftriaxone were only minimally altered in elderly subjects and in patients with renal impairment or hepatic dysfunction (Table 4); therefore, dosage adjustments are not necessary for these patients with Ceftriaxone dosages up to 2 gm per day. Ceftriaxone was not removed to any significant extent from the plasma by hemodialysis. In 6 of 26 dialysis patients, the elimination rate of Ceftriaxone was markedly reduced, suggesting that plasma concentrations of Ceftriaxone should be monitored in these patients to determine if dosage adjustments are necessary.

Table 4
AVERAGE PHARMACOKINETIC PARAMETERS OF CEFTRIAXONE IN HUMANS

Subject Group	Elimination Half-Life (hr)	Plasma Clearance (L/hr)	Volume of Distribution (L)
Healthy Subjects	5.8-8.7	0.58-1.45	5.8-13.5
Elderly Subjects (mean age, 70.5 yr)	8.9	0.83	10.7
Patients with renal impairment Hemodialysis patients (0-5 mL/min)*	14.7	0.65	13.7
Severe (5-15 mL/min)	15.7	0.56	12.5
Moderate (16-30 mL/min)	11.4	0.72	11.8
Mild (31-60 mL/min)	12.4	0.70	13.3
Patients with liver disease	8.8	1.1	13.6

* Creatinine clearance

Microbiology: The bactericidal activity of Ceftriaxone results from inhibition of cell wall synthesis. Ceftriaxone has a high degree of stability in the presence of beta-lactamases, both penicillinases and cephalosporinases, of gram-negative and gram-positive bacteria. Ceftriaxone is usually active against the following microorganisms *in vitro* and in clinical infections (see *"Indications and Usage"*).

GRAM-NEGATIVE AEROBES
Acinetobacter calcoaceticus
Enterobacter aerogenes
Enterobacter cloacae
Escherichia coli
Haemophilus influenzae(including ampicillin-resistant strains)
Haemophilus parainfluenzae
Klebsiella oxytoca
Klebsiella pneumoniae
Morganella morganii
Neisseria gonorrhoeae (including penicillinase- and nonpenicillinase-producing strains)
Neisseria meningitidis
Proteus mirabilis
Proteus vulgaris
Serratia marcescens
Ceftriaxone is also active against many strains of *Pseudomonas aeruginosa*.

Note: Many strains of the above organisms that are multiply resistant to other antibiotics, eg, penicillins, cephalosporins and aminoglycosides, are susceptible to Ceftriaxone.

GRAM-POSITIVE AEROBES
Staphylococcus aureus (including penicillinase-producing strains)
Staphylococcus epidermidis
Streptococcus pneumoniae
Streptoccocus pyogenes
Viridans group streptococci

Table 1
CEFTRIAXONE PLASMA CONCENTRATIONS AFTER SINGLE DOSE ADMINISTRATION

Dose/Route	Average Plasma Concentrations mcg/mL								
	0.5 hr	1hr	2 hr	4 hr	6hr	8hr	12	16 hr	24 hr
0.5 gm I.V.*	82	59	48	37	29	23	15	10	5
0.5 gm I.M.	30	41	43	39	31	25	16	ND†	ND
1 gm I.V.*	151	111	88	67	53	43	28	18	9
1 gm I.M.	40	68	76	68	56	44	29	ND	ND
2 gm I.V.*	257	192	154	117	89	74	46	31	15

* I.V. doses were infused at a constant rate over 30 minutes.
† ND = Not determined.

➤ SHOWN IN PRODUCT IDENTIFICATION GUIDE

Note: Methicillin-resistant streptococci are resistant to cephalosporins, including Ceftriaxone. Most strains of Group D streptococci and enterococci, eg, *Enterococcus (Streptococcus) faecalis*, are resistant.

ANAEROBES
Bacteroides fragilis
Clostridium species
Peptostreptococcus species

Note: Most strains of *C. difficile* are resistant. Ceftriaxone also demonstrates *in vitro* activity against most strains of the following microorganisms, although the clinical significance is unknown:

GRAM-NEGATIVE AEROBES
Citrobacter diversus
Citrobacter Freundii
Providencia species (including *Providencia rettgeri*)
Salmonella species (including *S. typhi*)
Shigella species

GRAM-POSITIVE AEROBES
Streptococcus agalactiae

ANAEROBES
Bacteroides bivius
Bacteroides melaninogenicus

Susceptibility Test: Diffusion Techniques: Quantitative methods that require the measurement of zone diameters give the most precise estimate of the susceptibility of bacteria to antimicrobial agents. One such standard procedure[1] which has been recommended for use with disks to test susceptibility of organisms to Ceftriaxone uses a 30 mcg Ceftriaxone disk. Interpretation involves the correlation of the diameters obtained in the disk test with the minimum inhibitory concentration (MIC) for Ceftriaxone.

Reports from the laboratory giving results of the standardized single disk susceptibility test using a 30 mcg Ceftriaxone disk should be interpreted for Ceftriaxone according to the following criteria:

Zone Diameter (mm)	Interpretation
≥ 18	(S) Susceptible
14-17	(MS) Moderately Susceptible
≤ 13	(R) Resistant

A report of "Susceptible" indicates that the pathogen is likely to be inhibited by generally achievable levels. A report of "Moderately Susceptible" suggests that the organism would be susceptible if high dosage (not to exceed 4 gm per day) is used or if the infection is confined to tissues and fluids in which high antimicrobial levels are attained. A report of "Resistant" indicates that achievable concentrations are unlikely to be inhibitory, and other therapy should be selected.

Standardized procedures require the use of laboratory control organisms. The 30 mcg Ceftriaxone disk should give the following zone diameters:

Organism	Zone Diameter (mm)
Staphylococcus aureus ATCC® 25923	22-28
Escherichia coli ATCC® 25922	29-35
Pseudomonas aeruginosa ATCC® 27853	17-23

Dilution Techniques: Use a standardized dilution method[2] (broth, agar, microdilution) or equivalent with Ceftriaxone powder. The MIC values obtained should be interpreted according to the following criteria:

MIC (mcg/mL)	Interpretation
≤ 16	Susceptible
> 16 to < 64	Moderately Susceptible
≥ 64	Resistant

As with standard diffusion techniques, dilution methods require the use of laboratory control organisms. Standard Ceftriaxone powder should provide the following MIC values:

Organism	MIC (mcg/mL)
Staphylococcus aureus ATCC® 29213	1-8
Escherichia coli ATCC® 25922	0.03-0.12
Pseudomonas aeruginosa ATCC® 27853	8-32

INDICATIONS AND USAGE

Ceftriaxone Sodium is indicated for the treatment of the following infections when caused by susceptible organisms:

LOWER RESPIRATORY TRACT INFECTIONS caused by *Streptococcus pneumoniae, Staphylococcus aureus, Haemophilus influenzae, Haemophilus parainfluenzae, Klebsiella pneumoniae, Escherichia coli, Enterobacter aerogenes, Proteus mirabilis* or *Serratia marcescens*.

SKIN AND SKIN STRUCTURE INFECTIONS caused by *Staphylococcus aureus, Staphylococcus epidermidis, Streptococcus pyogenes, Viridans* group streptococci, *Escherichia coli, Enterobacter cloacae, Klebsiella oxytoca, Klebsiella pneumoniae, Proteus mirabilis, Morganella morganii*[*], Pseudomomoniae aeruginosa, Serratia marcescens, Acinetobacter calcoaceticus, Bacteroides fragilis*[*] or Peptostreptococcus species.

URINARY TRACT INFECTIONS (complicated and uncomplicated) caused by *Escherichia coli, Proteus mirabilis, Proteus vulgaris, Morganella morganii* or *Klebsiella pneumoniae*.

UNCOMPLICATED GONORRHEA (cervical/urethral and rectal) caused by *Neisseria gonorrhoeae*, including both penicillinase- and and nonpenicillinase-producing strains, and pharyngeal gonorrhea caused by nonpenicillinase-producing strains of *Neisseria gonorrhoeae*.

PELVIC INFLAMMATORY DISEASE caused by *Neisseria gonorrhoeae*.

BACTERIAL SEPTICEMIA caused by *Staphylococcus aureus, Streptococcus pneumoniae, Escherichia coli, Haemophilus influenzae* or *Klebsiella pneumoniae*.

BONE AND JOINT INFECTIONS caused by *Staphylococcus aureus, Streptococcus pneumoniae, Escherichia coli, Proteus mirabilis, Klebsiella pneumoniae* or *Enterobacter* species.

INTRA-ABDOMINAL INFECTIONS caused by *Escherichia coli, Klebsiello pneumoniae, Bacteroides fragilis, Clostridium* species (Note: most strains of *C. difficile* are resistant) or *Peptostreptococcus* species.

MENINGITIS caused by *Haemophilus influenzae, Neisseria meningitidis* or *Streptococcus pneumoniae*. Ceftriaxone Sodium has also been used successfully in a limited number of cases of meningitis and shunt infection caused by *Staphylococcus epidermidis*[*] and *Escherichia coli.*[*]

Surgical Prophylaxis: The preoperative administration of a single 1 gm dose of Ceftriaxone Sodium may reduce the incidence of postoperative infections in patients undergoing surgical procedures classified as contaminated or potentially contaminated (eg, vaginal or abdominal hysterectomy or cholecystectomy for chronic calculous cholecystitis in high-risk patients, such as those over 70 years of age, with acute cholecystitis not requiring therapeutic antimicrobials, obstructive jaundice or common duct bile stones) and in surgical patients for whom infection at the operative site would present serious risk (eg, during coronary artery bypass surgery). Although Ceftriaxone Sodium has been shown to have been as effective as cefazolin in the prevention of infection following coronary artery bypass surgery, no placebo-controlled trials have been conducted to evaluate any cephalosporin antibiotic in the prevention of infection following coronary artery bypass surgery.

When administered prior to surgical procedures for which it is indicated, a single 1 gm dose of Ceftriaxone Sodium provides protection from most infections due to susceptible organisms throughout the course of the procedure.

Before instituting treatment with Ceftriaxone Sodium, appropriate specimens should be obtained for isolation of the causative organism and for determination of its susceptibility to the drug. Therapy may be instituted prior to obtaining results of susceptibility testing.

UNLABELED USES

Ceftriaxone Sodium is used alone or as an adjunct in the treatment of chancroid, epididymitis, and syphilis. Ceftriaxone Sodium is also used in the treatment of Lyme Disease, typhus fever, and salmonella infections.

CONTRAINDICATIONS

Ceftriaxone Sodium is contraindicated in patients with known allergy to the cephalosporin class of antibiotics.

WARNINGS

BEFORE THERAPY WITH CEFTRIAXONE SODIUM IS INSTITUTED CAREFUL INQUIRY SHOULD BE MADE TO DETERMINE WHETHER THE PATIENT HAS HAD PREVIOUS HYPERSENSITIVITY REACTIONS TO CEPHALOSPORINS, PENICILLINS OR OTHER DRUGS. THIS PRODUCT SHOULD BE GIVEN CAUTIOUSLY TO PENICILLIN-SENSITIVE PATIENTS. ANTIBIOTICS SHOULD BE ADMINISTERED WITH CAUTION TO ANY PATIENT WHO HAS DEMONSTRATED SOME FORM OF ALLERGY, PARTICULARLY TO DRUGS. SERIOUS ACUTE HYPERSENSITIVITY REACTIONS MAY REQUIRE THE USE OF SUBCUTANEOUS EPINEPHRINE AND OTHER EMERGENCY MEASURES.

Pseudomembranous colitis has been reported with nearly all antibacterial agents, including Ceftriaxone, and may range in severity from mild to life-threatening. Therefore, it is important to consider this diagnosis in patients who present with diarrhea subsequent to the administration of antibacterial agents.

Treatment with antibacterial agents alters the normal flora of the colon and may permit overgrowth of clostridia. Studies indicate that a toxin produced by *Clostridium difficile* is one primary cause of "antibiotic-associated colitis."

After the diagnosis of pseudomembranous colitis has been established, therapeutic measures should be initiated. Mild cases of pseudomembranous colitis usually respond to drug discontinuance alone. In moderate to severe cases, consideration should be given to management with fluids and electrolytes, protein supplementation and treatment with an oral antibacterial drug effective against *C. difficile*.

---

[*] Efficacy for this organism in this organ system was studied in fewer than ten infections.

PRECAUTIONS

General: Although transient elevations of BUN and serum creatinine have been observed, at the recommended dosages, the nephrotoxic potential of Ceftriaxone Sodium is similar to that of other cephalosporins.

Ceftriaxone is excreted via both biliary and renal excretion (see *"Clinical Pharmacology"*). Therefore, patients with renal failure normally require no adjustment in dosage when usual doses of Ceftriaxone Sodium are administered, but concentrations of drug in the serum should be monitored periodically. If evidence of accumulation exists, dosage should be decreased accordingly.

Dosage adjustments should not be necessary in patients with hepatic dysfunction; however, in patients with both hepatic dysfunction and significant renal disease, Ceftriaxone Sodium dosage should not exceed 2 gm daily without close monitoring of serum concentrations.

Alterations in prothrombin times have occurred rarely in patients treated with Ceftriaxone Sodium. Patients with impaired vitamin K synthesis or low vitamin K stores (eg, chronic hepatic disease and malnutrition) may require monitoring of prothrombin time during Ceftriaxone Sodium treatment. Vitamin K administration (10 mg weekly) may be necessary if the prothrombin time is prolonged before or during therapy.

Prolonged use of Ceftriaxone Sodium may result in overgrowth of nonsusceptible organisms. Careful observation of the patient is essential. If superinfection occurs during therapy, appropriate measures should be taken.

Ceftriaxone Sodium should be prescribed with caution in individuals with a history of gastrointestinal disease, especially colitis. Rare cases have been reported in which sonographic abnormalities are seen in the gallbladder of patients treated with Ceftriaxone Sodium; these patients may also have symptoms of gallbladder disease. These abnormalities are variously described as sludge, precipitations, echoes with shadows, and may be misinterpreted as concretions. The chemical nature of the sonographically-detected material has not been determined. The condition appears to be transient and reversible when Ceftriaxone Sodium is discontinued and conservative management employed. Therefore, Ceftriaxone Sodium should be discontinued in patients who develop signs and symptoms suggestive of gallbladder disease and/or the sonographic findings described above.

Carcinogenesis, Mutagenesis, Impairment of Fertility: Carcinogenesis: Considering the maximum duration of treatment and the class of the compound, carcinogenicity studies with Ceftriaxone in animals have not been performed. The maximum duration of animal toxicity studies was six months.

Mutagenesis: Genetic toxicology tests included the Ames test, a micronucleus test and a test for chromosomal aberrations in human lymphocytes cultured *in vitro* with Ceftriaxone. Ceftriaxone showed no potential for mutagenic activity in these studies.

Impairment of Fertility: Ceftriaxone produced no impairment of fertility when given intravenously to rats at daily doses up to 586 mg/kg/day, approximately 20 times the recommended clinical dose of 2 gm/day.

Pregnancy: Teratogenic Effects: Pregnancy Category B. Reproductive studies have been performed in mice and rats at doses up to 20 times the usual human dose and have no evidence of embryotoxicity, fetotoxicity or teratogenicity. In primates, no embryotoxicity or teratogenicity was demonstrated at a dose approximately three times the human dose. There are, however, no adequate and well-controlled studies in pregnant women. Because animal reproductive studies are not always predictive of human response, this drug should be used during pregnancy only if clearly needed.

Nonteratogenic Effects: In rats, in the Segment I (fertility and general reproduction) and Segment III (perinatal and postnatal) studies with intravenously administered Ceftriaxone, no adverse effects were noted on various reproductive parameters during gestation and lactation, including postnatal growth, functional behavior and reproductive ability of the offspring, at doses of 586 mg/kg/day or less.

Nursing Mothers: Low concentrations of Ceftriaxone are excreted in human milk. Caution should be exercised when Ceftriaxone Sodium is administered to a nursing woman.

Pediatric Use: Safety and effectiveness of Ceftriaxone Sodium in neonates, infants, and children have been established for the dosages described in the *"Dosage and Administration"* section. *In vitro* studies have shown that Ceftriaxone, like some other cephalosporins, can displace bilirubin from serum albumin. Ceftriaxone Sodium should not be administered to hyperbilirubinemic neonates, especially prematures.

ADVERSE REACTIONS

Ceftriaxone Sodium is generally well tolerated. In clinical trials, the following adverse reactions, which were considered to be related to Ceftriaxone Sodium therapy or of uncertain etiology, were observed:

Local Reactions: pain, induration or tenderness at the site of injection (1%). Less frequently reported (less than 1%) was phlebitis after I.V. administration.

Hypersensitivity: rash (1.7%). Less frequently reported (less than 1%) were pruritus, fever or chills.

Hematologic: eosinophilia (6%), thrombocytosis (5.1%) and leukopenia (2.1%). Less frequently reported (less than 1%) were anemia, hemolytic anemia, neutropenia, lymphopenia, thrombocytopenia and prolongation of the prothrombin time.

Gastrointestinal: diarrhea (2.7%). Less frequently reported (less than 1%) were nausea or vomiting, and dysgeusia. Onset of pseudomembranous colitis symptoms may occur during or after antibiotic treatment (see *"Warnings"*).

Hepatic: elevations of SGOT (3.1%) or SGPT (3.3%). Less frequently reported (less than 1%) were elevations of alkaline phosphatase and bilirubin.

Renal: elevations of the BUN (1.2%). Less frequently reported (less than 1%) were elevations of creatinine and the presence of casts in the urine.

Central Nervous System: headache or dizziness were reported occasionally (less than 1%).

Genitourinary: moniliasis or vaginitis were reported occasionally (less than 1%).

Miscellaneous: diaphoresis and flushing were reported occasionally (less than 1%).

Other rarely observed adverse reactions (less than 0.1%) include leukocytosis, lymphocytosis, monocytosis, basophila, a decrease in the prothrombin time, jaundice, gallbladder sludge, glycosuria, hematuria, anaphylaxis, bronchospasm, serum sickness, abdominal pain, colitis, flatulence, dyspepsia, palpitations and epistaxis.

DOSAGE AND ADMINISTRATION

Ceftriaxone Sodium may be administered intravenously or intramuscularly.

Adults: The usual adult daily dose is 1 to 2 grams given once a day (or in equally divided doses twice a day) depending on the type and severity of infection. The total daily dose should not exceed 4 grams.

For the treatment of uncomplicated gonococcal infections, a single intramuscular dose of 250 mg is recommnended.

For preoperative use (surgical prophylaxis), a single dose of 1 gram administered intravenously ½ to 2 hours before surgery is recommended.

Children: For the treatment of skin and skin structure infections, the recommended total daily dose is 50 to 75 mg/kg given once a day (or in equally divided doses twice a day). The total daily dose should not exceed 2 grams.

For the treatment of serious miscellaneous infections other than meningitis, the recommended total daily dose is 50 to 75 mg/kg, given in divided doses every 12 hours. The total daily dose should not exceed 2 grams.

In the treatment of meningitis, it is recommended that the initial therapeutic dose be 100 mg/kg (not to exceed 4 grams). Thereafter, a total daily dose of 100 mg/kg/day (not to exceed 4 grams daily) is recommended. The daily dose may be administered once a day (or in equally divided doses every 12 hours). The usual duration of therapy is 7 to 14 days.

Generally, Ceftriaxone Sodium therapy should be continued for at least two days after the signs and symptoms of infection have disappeared. The usual duration of therapy is 4 to 14 days; in complicated infections, longer therapy may be required.

When treating infections caused by *Streptococcus pyogenes*, therapy should be continued for at least ten days.

No dosage adjustment is necessary for patients with impairment of renal or hepatic function; however, blood levels should be monitored in patients with severe renal impairment (eg, dialysis patients) and in patients with both renal and hepatic dysfunctions.

DIRECTIONS FOR USE

Intramuscular Administration: Reconstitute Ceftriaxone Sodium powder with the appropriate diluent (see *"Compatibility-Stability"* section).

Vial Dosage Size	Amount of Diluent to be Added
250 mg	0.9 mL
500 mg	1.8 mL
1 gm	3.6 mL
2 gm	7.2 mL

After reconstitution, each 1 mL of solution contains approximately 250 mg equivalent of Ceftriaxone. If required, more dilute solutions could be utilized. As with all intramuscular preparations, Ceftriaxone Sodium should be injected well within the body of a relatively large muscle; aspiration helps to avoid unintentional injection into a blood vessel.

Intravenous Administration: Ceftriaxone Sodium should be administered intravenously by infusion over a period of 30 minutes. Concentrations between 10 mg/mL and 40 mg/mL are recommended; however, lower concentrations may be used if desired. Reconstitute vials or "piggyback" bottles with an appropriate I.V. diluent (see *"Compatibility-Stability"* section).

Vial Dosage Size	Amount of Diluent to be Added
250 mg	2.4 mL
500 mg	4.8 mL
1 gm	9.6 mL
2 gm	19.2 mL

After reconstitution, each 1 mL of solution contains approximately 100 mg equivalent of Ceftriaxone. Withdraw entire contents and dilute to the desired concentration with the appropriate I.V. diluent.

Piggyback Bottle Dosage Size	Amount of Diluent to be Added
1 gm	10 mL
2 gm	20 mL

After reconstitution, further dilute to 50 mL or 100 mL volumes with the appropriate I.V. diluent.

10 gm Bulk Pharmacy Container: This dosage size is *not for direct administration*. Reconstitute powder with 95 mL of an appropriate I.V. diluent. Before parenteral administration, withdraw the required amount, then further dilute to the desired concentration.

Compatibility and Stability: Ceftriaxone Sodium sterile powder should be stored at room temperature—77°F (25°C)—or below and protected from light. After reconstitution, protection from normal light is not necessary. The color of solutions ranges from light yellow to amber, depending on the length of storage, concentration and diluent used.

Ceftriaxone Sodium *intramuscular* solutions remain stable (loss of potency less than 10%) for the following time periods:

Diluent	Concentration mg/mL	Storage Room Temp. (25°C)	Storage Refrigerated (4°C)
Sterile Water for Injection	100	3 days	10 days
	250	24 hours	3 days
0.9% Sodium Chloride Solution	100	3 days	10 days
	250	24 hours	3 days
5% Dextrose Solution	100	3 days	10 days
	250	24 hours	3 days
Bacteriostatic Water + 0.9% Benzyl Alcohol	100	24 hours	10 days
	250	24 hours	10 days
1% Lidocaine Solution (without epinephrine)	100	24 hours	10 days
	250	24 hours	3 days

Ceftriaxone Sodium *intravenous* solutions, at concentrations of 10, 20 and 40 mg/mL, remain stable (loss of potency less than 10%) for the following time periods stored in glass or PVC containers:

Diluent	Storage Room Temp. (25°C)	Storage Refrigerated (4°C)
Sterile Water	3 days	10 days
0.9% Sodium Chloride Solution	3 days	10 days
5% Dextrose Solution	3 days	10 days
10% Dextrose Solution	3 days	10 days
5% Dextrose + 0.9% Sodium Chloride Solution*	3 days	Incompatible
5% Dextrose + 0.45% Sodium Chloride Solution	3 days	Incompatible

*   *Data available for 10-40 mg/mL concentrations in this diluent in PVC containers only.*

Similarly, Ceftriaxone Sodium *intravenous* solutions, at concentrations of 100 mg/mL, remain stable in the I.V. piggyback glass containers for the above specified time periods.

The following *intravenous* Ceftriaxone Sodium solutions are stable at room temperature (25°C) for 24 hours, at concentrations between 10 mg/mL and 40 mg/mL: Sodium Lactate (PVC container), 10% Invert Sugar (glass container), 5% Sodium Bicarbonate (glass container), Freamine III (glass container), Normosol-M in 5% Dextrose (glass and PVC containers), Ionosol-B in 5% Dextrose (glass container), 5% Mannitol (glass container), 10% Mannitol (glass container).

After the indicated stability time periods, unused portions of solutions should be discarded.

Ceftriaxone Sodium reconstituted with 5% Dextrose or 0.9% Sodium Chloride solution at concentrations between 10 mg/mL and 40 mg/mL, and then stored in frozen state (-20°C) in PVC (Viaflex) or polyolefin containers, remains stable for 26 weeks.

Frozen solutions should be thawed at room temperature before use. After thawing, unused portions should be discarded. *Do not refreeze.*

Ceftriaxone Sodium solutions should *not* be physically mixed with or piggybacked into solutions containing other antimicrobial drugs or into diluent solutions other than those listed above, due to possible incompatibility.

Note: Store Ceftriaxone Sodium in the frozen state at or below -20°C/-4°F.

ANIMAL PHARMACOLOGY

Concretions consisting of the precipitated calcium salt of Ceftriaxone have been found in the gallbladder bile of dogs and baboons treated with Ceftriaxone.

These appeared as a gritty sediment in dogs that received 100 mg/kg/day for four weeks. A similar phenomenon has been observed in baboons but only after a protracted dosing period (6 months) at higher dose levels (335 mg/kg/day or

more). The likelihood of this occurrence in humans is considered to be low, since Ceftriaxone has a greater plasma half-life in humans, the calcium salt of Ceftriaxone is more soluble in human gallbladder bile and the calcium content of human gallbladder bile is relatively low.

REFERENCES

1. National Committee for Clinical Standards, *Performance Standards for Antimicrobial Disk Susceptibility Tests.* 4th ed. Villanova, PA:1990. Approved Standard NCCLS Document M2-A4, Vol. 10, No. 7, NCCLS. 2. National Committee for Clinical Laboratory Standards, *Methods for Dilution Antimicrobial Susceptibility Tests for Bacteria That Grow Aerobically*, 2nd ed. Villanova, PA:1990. Approved Standard NCCLS Document M7-A2, Vol. 10, No. 8, NCCLS.

J CODES
Per 250 mg IV,IM—J0696

HOW SUPPLIED
INJECTION: 1 GM

BRAND/MANUFACTURER	NDC	SIZE	AWP
○ **BRAND**			
ROCEPHIN: Baxter	00004-2002-78	50 ml 24s	$964.32

INJECTION: 2 GM

BRAND/MANUFACTURER	NDC	SIZE	AWP
○ **BRAND**			
ROCEPHIN: Baxter	00004-2003-78	50 ml 24s	$1693.68

POWDER FOR INJECTION: 250 MG

BRAND/MANUFACTURER	NDC	SIZE	AWP
○ **BRAND**			
ROCEPHIN: Roche Labs	00004-1962-02	1s	$11.00
	00004-1962-01	10s	$102.96

POWDER FOR INJECTION: 500 MG

BRAND/MANUFACTURER	NDC	SIZE	AWP
○ **BRAND**			
ROCEPHIN: Roche Labs	00004-1963-02	1s	$18.40
	00004-1963-01	10s	$177.15

POWDER FOR INJECTION: 1 GM

BRAND/MANUFACTURER	NDC	SIZE	AWP
○ **BRAND**			
ROCEPHIN: Roche Labs	00004-1964-04	1s	$32.66
	00004-1964-01	10s	$319.53
	00004-1964-05	10s	$323.53
	00004-1964-03	10s	$326.20

POWDER FOR INJECTION: 2 GM

BRAND/MANUFACTURER	NDC	SIZE	AWP
○ **BRAND**			
ROCEPHIN: Roche Labs	00004-1965-01	10s	$635.00
	00004-1965-05	10s	$639.00
	00004-1965-03	10s	$641.64

POWDER FOR INJECTION: 10 GM

BRAND/MANUFACTURER	NDC	SIZE	AWP
○ **BRAND**			
ROCEPHIN: Roche Labs	00004-1971-01	1s	$311.50

Cefuroxime Axetil

DESCRIPTION
Cefuroxime Axetil tablets contain a semisynthetic, broad-spectrum cephalosporin antibiotic for oral administration. Cefuroxime Axetil is the 1-(acetyloxy) ethyl ester of Cefuroxime, which in turn is chemically designated as (6R,7R)-3-carbamoyloxymethyl-7-[Z-2-methoxyimino-2-(fur-2-yl)acetamido] ceph-3-em-4-carboxylate. Cefuroxime Axetil is in the amorphous form.

Each Cefuroxime Axetil tablet contains the equivalent of 125, 250, or 500 mg of Cefuroxime.

Following is its chemical structure:

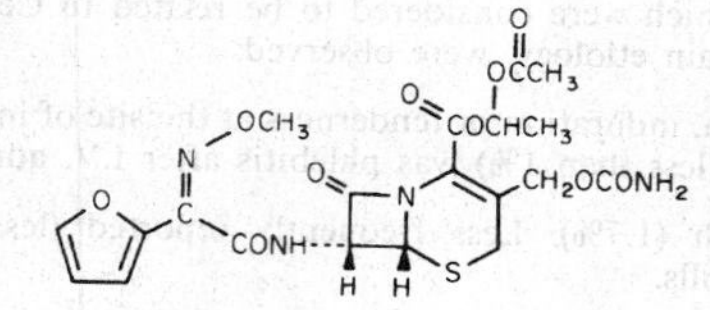

CLINICAL PHARMACOLOGY
After oral administration, Cefuroxime Axetil is absorbed from the gastrointestinal tract and rapidly hydrolyzed by nonspecific esterases in the intestinal mucosa and

blood to release Cefuroxime into the circulation. Cefuroxime is subsequently distributed throughout the extracellular fluids. The axetil moiety is metabolized to acetaldehyde and acetic acid. Cefuroxime is excreted unchanged in the urine.

Serum Cefuroxime concentrations and urinary excretion data are shown in the table below.

BIOAVAILABILITY OF CEFUROXIME ADMINISTERED AS CEFUROXIME AXETIL

Dose* (Cefuroxime Equivalent)	Serum Cefuroxime Concentration† (mcg/mL)		12-h Urinary Excretion † (% of dose)
	Peak	6 h	
125 mg	2.1	0.3	52
250 mg	4.1	0.7	51
500 mg	7.0	2.2	48
1,000 mg	13.6	3.4	43

* Administered immediately after a meal.
† Mean values of 12 normal volunteers. Peak concentrations occurred around 2 hours after the dose.

While Cefuroxime Axetil can be taken after food or on an empty stomach, absorption is greater when taken after food (absolute bioavailability of 52% compared with 37%). Peak serum Cefuroxime concentrations after a 500-mg dose are also greater when taken with food (mean = 7.0 mcg/mL) compared with the fasting state (mean = 4.9 mcg/mL). Despite this difference in absorption, the clinical and bacteriologic responses of patients were independent of food intake at the time of dosing in two studies where this was assessed. Approximately 50% of serum Cefuroxime is bound to protein. The half-life of Cefuroxime after oral administration of Cefuroxime Axetil Tablets is 1.2 hours. Concomitant administration of probenecid increases the area under the serum concentration versus time curve by 50%. Peak serum Cefuroxime concentration after a 1.5-g single dose is greater when taken with 1 g of probenecid (mean = 14.8 mcg/mL) than without probenecid (mean = 12.2 mcg/mL). Concomitant probenecid also increases the time for which serum Cefuroxime concentrations exceed 0.25 mcg/mL from 10.7 hours to 14.0 hours. Because Cefuroxime is renally eliminated, the serum half-life is increased in elderly patients with declining renal function associated with normal aging. In a study of twenty elderly patients (mean age = 83.9 years) having a mean creatinine clearance of 34.9 mL per minute, the mean serum elimination half-life was 3.5 hours (see Geriatric Use subsection under "Precautions").

Microbiology: The *in vivo* bactericidal activity of Cefuroxime Axetil is due to Cefuroxime. Cefuroxime has bactericidal activity against a wide range of common pathogens, including many beta-lactamase-producing strains.

Cefuroxime is highly stable to bacterial beta-lactamases, especially plasmid-mediated enzymes that are commonly found in enterobacteriaceae. The bactericidal action of Cefuroxime results from inhibition of cell-wall synthesis by binding to essential target proteins.

Cefuroxime has been shown to be active against most strains of the following organisms both *in vitro* and in clinical infections (see "Indications and Usage"):

Gram-positive: Staphylococcus aureus, Streptococcus pneumoniae, and Streptococcus pyogenes.

Note: Certain strains of enterococci, e.g., *Enterococcus faecalis* (formerly *Streptococcus faecalis*), are resistant to Cefuroxime. Methicillin-resistant staphylococci are resistant to Cefuroxime.

Gram-negative: Moraxella (Branhamella) catarrhalis, Escherichia coli, Haemophilus influenzae, Haemophilus parainfluenzae, Klebsiella pneumoniae, and Neisseria gonorrhoeae (non-penicillinase-producing strains).

Note: Pseudomonas spp., and Campylobacter spp., Acinetobacter calcoaceticus, and most strains of Serratia spp. and Proteus vulgaris are resistant to most first- and second-generation cephalosporins. Some strains of Morganella morganii, Enterobacter cloacae, and Citrobacter spp. have been shown by *in vitro* tests to be resistant to Cefuroxime and other cephalosporins.

Cefuroxime has been shown to be active *in vitro* against the following micoorganisms; however, the clinical significance of these findings is unknown.

Gram-positive: Staphylococcus epidermidis, Staphylococcus saprophyticus, and Streptococcus agalactiae.

Gram-negative: Citrobacter spp., Enterobacter spp., Klebsiella spp., Morganella morganii, Neisseria gonorrhoeae (including penicillinase- and non-penicillinase-producing strains), Proteus inconstans, Proteus mirabilis, Providencia rettgeri, Salmonella spp., and Shigella spp.

Anaerobes: Bacteroides spp., Colstridium spp., Fusobacterium spp., Peptococcus spp., Peptostreptococcus spp., and Propionibacterium spp.

Note: Most strains of Clostridium difficile and Bacteroides fragilis are resistant to Cefuroxime.

Susceptibility Tests: Diffusion Techniques: Quantitative methods that require measurement of zone diameters give the most precise estimate of antibiotic susceptibility. One such standard procedure[1] that has been recommended for use with disks to test susceptibility of organisms to Cefuroxime uses the 30-mcg Cefuroxime disk. Interpretation involves the correlation of the diameters obtained in the disk test with the minimum inhibitory concentration (MIC) for Cefuroxime.

Reports from the laboratory giving results of the standard single-disk susceptibility test with a 30-mcg Cefuroxime disk should be interpreted according to the following criteria:

Zone diameter (mm)	Interpretation
≥ 23	(S) Susceptible
15-22	(MS) Moderately Susceptible
≤ 14	(R) Resistant

A report of "Susceptible" indicates that the pathogen is likely to be inhibited by generally achievable blood levels. A report of "Moderately Susceptible" suggests that the organism would be susceptible if high dosage is used or if the infection is confined to tissues and fluids in which high antibiotic levels are attained. A report of "Resistant" indicates that achievable concentrations of the antibiotic are unlikely to be inhibitory and other therapy should be selected.

Standardized procedures require the use of laboratory control organisms. The 30-mcg Cefuroxime disk should give the following zone diameters:

Organism	Zone Diameter (mm)
Staphylococcus aureus ATCC 25923	27-35
Escherichia coli ATCC 25922	20-26

Dilution Techniques: Use a standardized dilution method[2] (broth, agar, microdilution) or equivalent with Cefuroxime powder. The MIC values obtained should be interpreted according to the following criteria:

MIC (mcg/mL)	Interpretation
≤ 4	(S) Susceptible
8-16	(MS) Moderately Susceptible
≥ 32	(R) Resistant

As with standard diffusion techniques, dilution methods require the use of laboratory control organisms. Standard Cefuroxime powder should provide the following MIC values:

Organism	MIC (mcg/mL)
Staphylococcus aureus ATCC 29213	0.5-2
Escherichia coli ATCC 25922	2-8

INDICATIONS AND USAGE

Cefuroxime Axetil tablets are indicated for the treatment of patients with infections caused by susceptible strains of the designated organisms in the following diseases:

1. Pharyngitis and Tonsillitis caused by *Streptococcus pyogenes.* (Penicillin is the usual drug of choice in the treatment and prevention of streptococcal infections including the prophylaxis of rheumatic fever. Cefuroxime Axetil tablets are generally effective in the eradication of streptococci from the oropharynx. Cefuroxime Axetil tablets are not indicated for the prophylaxis of subsequent rheumatic fever because data to support such use are not yet available.)

2. Otitis Media caused by *Streptococcus pneumoniae, Haemophilus influenzae* (ampicillin-susceptible and ampicillin-resistant strains), *Moraxella (Branhamella) catarrhalis* and *Streptococcus pyogenes.*

3. Lower Respiratory Tract Infections (bronchitis) caused by *Streptococcus pneumoniae, Haemophilus influenzae* (ampicillin-susceptible strains), and *Haemophilus parainfluenzae* (ampicillin-susceptible strains).

4. Urinary Tract Infections caused by *Escherichia coli* and *Klebsiella pneumoniae* in the absence of urological complications.

5. Skin and Skin Structure Infections caused by *Staphylococcus aureus* and *Streptococcus pyogenes.*

6. Uncomplicated Gonorrhea (urethral and endocervical) caused by non-pencillinase-producing strains of *Neisseria gonorrhoeae.*

Bacteriologic studies to determine the causative organism and its susceptibility to Cefuroxime should be performed. Therapy may be started while awaiting the results of these studies. Once these results become available, antibiotic treatment should be adjusted accordingly.

CONTRAINDICATIONS

Cefuroxime Axetil Tablets are contraindicated in patients with known allergy to the cephalosporin group of antibiotics.

WARNINGS

BEFORE THERAPY WITH CEFUROXIME AXETOL TABLETS IS INSTITUTED, CAREFUL INQUIRY SHOULD BE MADE TO DETERMINE WHETHER THE PATIENT HAS HAD PREVIOUS HYPERSENSITIVITY REACTIONS TO CEPHALOSPORINS, PENCILLINS, OR OTHER DRUGS. IF THIS PRODUCT IS TO BE GIVEN TO PENICILLIN-SENSITIVE PATIENTS, CAUTION SHOULD BE EXERCISED BECAUSE CROSS-HYPERSENSITIVITY AMONG BETA-LACTAM ANTIBIOTICS HAS BEEN CLEARLY DOCUMENTED AND MAY OCCUR IN UP TO 10% OF PATIENTS WITH A HISTORY OF PENICILLIN ALLERGY. ANTIBIOTICS SHOULD BE ADMINISTERED WITH CAUTION TO ANY PATIENT WHO HAS DEMONSTRATED SOME FORM OF ALLERGY, PARTICULARLY TO

► SHOWN IN PRODUCT IDENTIFICATION GUIDE

DRUGS. IF AN ALLERGIC REACTION TO CEFUROXIME AXETIL TAB-LETS OCCURS, DISCONTINUE THE DRUG. SERIOUS ACUTE HYPER-SENSITIVITY REACTIONS MAY REQUIRE TREATMENT WITH EPINEPHRINE AND OTHER EMERGENCY MEASURES, INCLUDING OXYGEN, INTRAVENOUS FLUIDS, INTRAVENOUS ANTIHISTAMINES, CORTICOSTEROIDS, PRESSOR AMINES, AND AIRWAY MANAGEMENT, AS CLINICALLY INDICATED.

Pseudomembranous colitis has been reported with nearly all antibacterial agents, including Cefuroxime, and may range from mild to life-threatening. Therefore, it is important to consider this diagnosis in patients who present with diarrhea subsequent to the administration of antibacterial agents.

Treatment with broad-spectrum antibiotics alters normal flora of the colon and may permit overgrowth of clostridia. Studies indicate that a toxin produced by *Clostridium difficile* is one primary cause of antibiotic-associated colitis. Cholesty-ramine and colestipol resins have been shown to bind the toxin *in vitro*.

Mild cases of colitis may respond to drug discontinuation alone. Moderate to severe cases should be managed with fluid, electrolyte, and protein supplementa-tion as indicated. Elderly patients may be susceptible to fluid losses and should be treated aggressively.

When the colitis is not relieved by drug discontinuation or when it is severe, metronidazole and oral vancomycin have been shown to be beneficial. Oral vancomycin is the treatment of choice for antibiotic-associated pseudomembra-nous colitis produced by *Clostridium difficile*. Other causes of colitis should also be considered.

PRECAUTIONS

General: If an allergic reaction to Cefuroxime Axetil tablets occurs, the drug should be discontinued, and, if necessary, the patient should be treated with appropriate agents, e.g., antihistamines, pressor amines, or corticosteroids.

As with other antibiotics, prolonged use of Cefuroxime Axetil tabets may result in overgrowth of nonsusceptible organisms. If superinfection occurs during therapy, appropriate measures should be taken.

Broad-spectrum antibiotics should be prescribed with caution for individuals with a history of colitis.

Information for Patients: (Pediatric) Cefuroxime Axetil is only available in tablet form. During clinical trials, the tablet was well tolerated by children who could swallow the tablet whole. Children who cannot swallow the tablet whole may have the tablet crushed and mixed with food (e.g., applesauce, ice cream). However, it should be noted that the crushed tablet has a strong, persistent, bitter taste. Discontinuation of therapy due to the taste and/or problems of administering this drug occurred in 13% of children (range, 2%-28% across centers). Thus, the physician and parent should ascertain, preferably while still in the physician's office, that the child can ingest Cefuroxime Axetil tablets reliably. If not, alternative therapy should be considered.

Drug/Laboratory Test Interactions: A false-positive reaction for glucose in the urine may occur with copper reduction tests (Benedict's or Fehling's solution or with Clinitest® tablets), but not with enzyme-based tests for glycosuria (e.g., Clinistix®, Tes-Tape®). As a false-negative result may occur in the ferricyanide test, it is recommended that either the glucose oxidase or hexokinase method be used to determine blood plasma glucose levels in patients recieving Cefuroxime Axetil tablets.

Cefuroxime does not interfere with the assay of serum and urine creatinine by the alkaline picrate method.

Carcinogenesis, Mutagenesis, Impairment of Fertility: Although no long-term studies in animals have been performed to evaluate carcinogenic potential, no mutagenic potential of Cefuroxime was found in standard laboratory tests.

Reproductive studies revealed no impairment of fertility in animals.

Pregnancy: Pregnancy Category B: Reproduction studies have been performed in rats and mice at doses up to 50-160 times the human dose and have revealed no evidence of impaired fertility or harm to the fetus due to Cefuroxime Axetil. There are, however, no adequate and well-controlled studies in pregnant women. Because animal reproduction studies are not always predictive of human response, this drug should be used during pregnancy only if clearly needed.

Nursing Mothers: Since Cefuroxime is excreted in human milk, consideration should be given to discontinuing nursing temporarily during treatment with Cefuroxime Axetil tablets.

Pediatric Use: (see *"Dosage and Administration"*).

Geriatric Use: In clinical trials when 12- to 64-year-old patients and geriatric patients (65 years of age or older) were treated with usual recommended dosages (i.e., 125-500 mg b.i.d., depending on type of infection), no overall differences in effectiveness were observed between the two age-groups. The geriatric patients reported somewhat fewer gastrointestinal events and vaginal candidiasis when compared with adult patients (12-64 years old); however, no clinically significant differences were reported between the two age-groups.

ADVERSE REACTIONS

The adverse reactions to Cefuroxime Axetil tablets are similar to reactions to other orally administered cepbalosporins. Cefuroxime Axetil tablets were usually well tolerated in controlled clinical trials. Pediatric patients taking crushed tablets during clinical trials complained of the bitter taste of Cefuroxime Axetil tablets (see *"Adverse Reactions: Gastrointestinal"* and *"Precautions: Information for Patients: [Pediatric]"*). The majority of adverse events were mild, reversible in nature, and did not require discontinuation of the drug. The incidence of gastrointestinal adverse events increased with the higher recommended doses.

Twenty-five (25) patients have received Cefuroxime Axetil tablets 500 mg twice a day for 1-2.5 months with no increase in frequency or severity of adverse events.

The following adverse reactions have been reported in clinical trials using dosage regimens of 125-500 mg twice a day.

Gastrointestinal: Nausea occurred in 2.4% of patients. Vomiting occurred in 2.0% of patients. Diarrhea occurred in 3.5% of patients. Loose stools occured in 1.3% of patients. Onset of pseudomembranous colitis symptoms may occur during or after antibiotic treatment (see *"Warnings"*).

Crushed tablets have a bitter taste. In pediatric clinical studies conducted with crushed tablets, complaints due to taste ranged from 0/8 (0%) in one center to 47/71 (66%) in another center.

Hypersensitivity: Rash (0.6% of patients), pruritus (0.3% of patients), and urticaria (0.2% of patients) have been observed. One case of severe bronchospasm has been reported among the approximately 1,600 patients treated with Cefuroxime Axetil tablets. Of the patients treated with Cefuroxime Axetil tablets who reported a history of delayed hypersensitivity to a penicillin and not a cephalosporin, 2.9% of patients experienced a delayed hypersensitivity reaction to Cefuroxime Axetil tablets.

Hypersensitivity reactions including Stevens-Johnson syndrome, erythema multiforme, toxic epidermal necrolysis, drug fever, serum sickness-like reactions, and anaphylaxis have been reported.

Central Nervous System: Headache occurred in less than 0.7% of patients, and dizziness occurred in less than 0.2% of patients.

Vaginitis, including vaginal candidiasis, occurred in 1.9% of female patients.

Clinical Laboratory Tests: Transient elevations in AST (SGOT, 2.0% of patients), ALT (SGPT, 1.6% of patients), and LDH (1.0% of patients) have been observed. Eosinophilia (1.1% of patients) and positive Coombs' test (0.4% of patients) have been reported.

Adverse Reactions Following a Single Oral 1-g Dose for the Treatment of Gonorrhea: The incidence of drug-related adverse experiences in patients treated for gonorrhea who received a single 1-g dose of Cefuroxime Axetil was 16%. The most common adverse experiences were diarrhea (4.8%), nausea (4.6%), vomiting (2.5%), abdominal pain (1.2%), and dizziness (1.2%).

In addition to the adverse reactions listed above that have been observed in patients treated with Cefuroxime Axetil tablets, the following adverse reactions and altered laboratory tests have been reported for cephalosporin class antibiotics:

Adverse Reactions: Fever, renal dysfunction, toxic nephropathy, hepatic dysfunc-tion including cholestasis, abdominal pain, superinfection, aplastic anemia, hemolytic anemia, hemorrhage, and pain and/or phlebitis at the injection site.

Several cephalosporins have been implicated in triggering seizures, particularly in patients with renal impairment when the dosage was not reduced. If seizures associated with drug therapy should occur, the drug should be discontinued. Anticonvulsant therapy can be given if clinically indicated.

Altered Laboratory Tests: Increased prothrombin time, increased BUN, increased creatinine, false-positive test for urinary glucose, increased alkaline phosphatase, neutropenia, thrombocytopenia, leukopenia, elevated bilirubin, pancytopenia, and agranulocytosis.

OVERDOSAGE

Overdosage of cephalosporins can cause cerebral irritation leading to convulsions. Serum levels of Cefuroxime can be reduced by hemodialysis and peritoneal dialysis.

DOSAGE AND ADMINISTRATION

Cefuroxime Axetil tablets may be given orally without regard to meals. However, absorption is enhanced when Cefuroxime Axetil tablets are administered with food.

Adults and Children 12 Years of Age and Older: The recommended dosage is 250 mg twice a day. For more severe infections or infections caused by less susceptible organisms, the dosage may be increased to 500 mg twice a day.

For uncomplicated urinary tract infections, the usual recommended dosage is 125 mg twice a day. Dosage may be increased to 250 mg twice a day for some patients with urinary tract infections.

Treatment of Gonorrhea: A single oral 1-g dose is recommended for treating uncomplicated urethral and endocervical gonorrhea.

Geriatric Use: No adjustment of the usual recommended adult dose is usually necessary (see *"Precautions: Geriatric Use"* and *"Clinical Pharmacology"*).

Infants and Children Up to 12 Years of Age: The recommended dosage for children is 125 mg twice a day. For children with otitis media, the recommended dosage is 125 mg twice a day for children less than 2 years of age and 250 mg twice a day for children 2 years of age and older.

Cefuroxime Axetil tablets administered as a crushed tablet have a strong, persistent, bitter taste. Alternative therapy should be considered for children who cannot swallow tablets (see *"Precautions: Information for Patients: [Pediatric]"*).

In the treatment of infections due to *Streptococcus pyogenes,* a therapeutic dosage of Cefuroxime Axetil tablets should be administered for at least 10 days.

Store between 15° and 30° C (59° and 86° F). Replace cap securely after each opening. Protect unit dose packs from excessive moisture.

REFERENCES

1. National Committee for Clinical Laboratory Standards. *Performance Standards for Antimicrobial Disk Susceptibility Tests.* 4th ed. Approved Standards NCCLS Document M2-A4, Vol. 10, No. 7 Villanova, Pa: NCCLS: 1990. 2. National Committee for

---

Clinical Laboratory Standards. *Methods for Dilution. Antimicrobial Susceptibility Tests for Bacteria That Grow Aerobically.* 2nd ed. Approved Standards NCCLS Document M7-A2, Vol. 10, No. 8. Villanova, Pa: NCCLS: 1990

HOW SUPPLIED
POWDER FOR RECONSTITUTION: 125 MG/5 ML

BRAND/MANUFACTURER	NDC	SIZE	AWP
○ BRAND			
CEFTIN: Glaxo	00173-0406-01	50 ml	$14.99
	00173-0406-02	100 ml	$28.58
	00173-0406-04	200 ml	$51.78

TABLETS: 125 MG

BRAND/MANUFACTURER	NDC	SIZE	AWP
○ BRAND			
► CEFTIN: Glaxo	00173-0395-00	20s	$34.86
	00173-0395-01	60s	$99.58
	00173-0395-02	100s ud	$171.07

TABLETS: 250 MG

BRAND/MANUFACTURER	NDC	SIZE	AWP
○ BRAND			
► CEFTIN: Glaxo	00173-0387-00	20s	$65.35
	00173-0387-42	60s	$186.54
	00173-0387-01	100s ud	$316.02

TABLETS: 500 MG

BRAND/MANUFACTURER	NDC	SIZE	AWP
○ BRAND			
► CEFTIN: Glaxo	00173-0394-00	20s	$123.98
	00173-0394-01	50s ud	$308.00
	00173-0394-42	60s	$366.68

Cefuroxime Sodium

DESCRIPTION
Cefuroxime is a semisynthetic, broad-spectrum cephalosporin antibiotic for parenteral administration. It is the sodium salt of (6R, 7R)-3-carbamoyloxyme-thyl-7-[Z-2-methoxyimino-2-(fur-2-yl) acetamido] ceph-3-em-4-carboxylate.

The empirical formula is $C_{16}H_{15}N_4NaO_8S$, representing a molecular weight of 446.4.

Cefuroxime Sodium contains approximately 54.2 mg (2.4 mEq) of sodium per gram of Cefuroxime activity.

Cefuroxime Sodium in sterile crystalline form is supplied in vials equivalent to 750 mg, 1.5 g, or 7.5 g of Cefuroxime as Cefuroxime Sodium. Solutions of Cefuroxime Sodium range in color from light yellow to amber, depending on the concentration and diluent used. The pH of freshly constituted solutions usually ranges from 6-8.5.

Cefuroxime Sodium is available as a frozen, iso-osmotic, sterile, nonpyrogenic solution with 750 mg or 1.5 g of Cefuroxime as Cefuroxime Sodium. Approximately 1.4 g of dextrose hydrous, USP has been added to the 750-mg dose to adjust the osmolality. Sodium citrate hydrous, USP has been added as a buffer (300 mg and 600 mg to the 750-mg and 1.5-g doses, respectively). Cefuroxime Sodium contains approximately 111 mg (4.8 mEq) and 222 mg (9.7 mEq) of sodium in the 750-mg and 1.5-g doses, respectively. The pH has been adjusted with hydrochloric acid and may have been adjusted with sodium hydroxide. Solutions of premixed Cefuroxime Sodium range in color from light yellow to amber. The solution is intended for intravenous (IV) use after thawing to room temperature. The osmolality of the solution is approximately 300 mOsmol/kg, and the pH of thawed solutions ranges from 5-7.5.

The plastic container is fabricated from a specially designed multilayer plastic, PL 2040. Solutions are in contact with the polyethylene layer of this container and can leach out certain chemical components of the plastic in very small amounts within the expiration period. The suitability of the plastic has been confirmed in tests in animals according to USP biological tests for plastic containers as well as by tissue culture toxicity studies.

Following is its chemical structure:

CLINICAL PHARMACOLOGY
After intramuscular (IM) injection of a 750-mg dose of Cefuroxime to normal volunteers, the mean peak serum concentration was 27 mcg/mL. The peak occurred at approximately 45 minutes (range, 15-60 minutes). Following IV doses of 750 mg and 1.5 g, serum concentrations were approximately 50 and 100 mcg/mL, respectively, at 15 minutes. Therapeutic serum concentrations of approximately 2 mcg/mL or more were maintained for 5.3 hours and 8 hours or more, respectively. There was no evidence of accumulation of Cefuroxime in the serum following IV administration of 1.5-g doses every 8 hours to normal volunteers. The serum half-life after either IM or IV injections is approximately 80 minutes.

Approximately 89% of a dose of Cefuroxime is excreted by the kidneys over an 8-hour period, resulting in high urinary concentrations.

Following the IM administration of a 750-mg single dose, urinary concentrations averaged 1,300 mcg/mL during the first 8 hours. Intravenous doses of 750 mg and 1.5 g produced urinary levels averaging 1,150 and 2,500 mcg/mL, respectively, during the first 8-hour period.

The concomitant oral administration of probenecid with Cefuroxime slows tubular secretion, decreases renal clearance by approximately 40%, increases the peak serum level by approximately 30%, and increases the serum half-life by approximately 30%. Cefuroxime is detectable in therapeutic concentrations in pleural fluid, joint fluid, bile, sputum, bone, cerebrospinal fluid (in patients with meningitis), and aqueous humor.

Cefuroxime is approximately 50% bound to serum protein.

Microbiology: Cefuroxime has *in vitro* activity against a wide range of gram-positive and gram-negative organisms, and it is highly stable in the presence of beta-lactamases of certain gram-negative bacteria. The bactericidal action of cefuroxime results from inhibition of cell-wall synthesis. Cefuroxime is usually active against the following organisms *in vitro.*

Aerobes, Gram-positive: Staphylococcus aureus; Staphylococcus epidermidis; Streptococcus pneumoniae; and Streptococcus pyogenes (and other streptococci). *Note:* Most strains of enterococci, e.g., *Enterococcus faecalis* (formerly *Streptococcus faecalis*), are resistant to Cefuroxime. Methicillin-resistant staphylococci and *Listeria monocytogenes* are resistant to cefuroxime.

Aerobes, Gram-negative: Citrobacter spp.; Enterobacter spp.; Escherichia coli; Haemophilus influenzae (including ampicillin-resistant strains); Haemophilus parainfluenzae; Klebsiella spp. (including Klebsiella pneumoniae); Moraxella (Branhamella) catarrhalis (including ampicillin- and cephalothin-resistant strains); Morganella morganii (formerly Proteus morganii); Neisseria gonorrhoeae (including penicillinase- and non-penicillinase-producing strains); Neisseria meningitidis; Proteus mirabilis; Providencia rettgeri (formerly Proteus rettgeri); Salmonella spp.; and Shigella spp.

Note: Some strains of *Morganella morganii, Enterobacter cloacae,* and *Citrobacter* spp. have been shown by *in vitro* tests to be resistant to cefuroxime and other cephalosporins. *Pseudomonas* and *Campylobacter* spp., *Acinetobacter calcoaceticus,* and most strains of *Serratia* spp. and *Proteus vulgaris* are resistant to most first- and second-generation cephalosporins.

Anaerobes: Gram-positive and gram-negative cocci (including *Peptococcus* and *Peptostreptococcus* spp.); gram-positive bacilli (including *Clostridium* spp.); and gram-negative bacilli (including *Bacteroides* and *Fusobacterium* spp.).

Note: Clostridium difficile and most strains of *Bacteroides fragilis* are resistant to Cefuroxime.

Susceptibility Tests: Diffusion Techniques: Quantitative methods that require measurement of zone diameters give an estimate of antibiotic susceptibility. One such standard procedure[1] that has been recommended for use with disks to test susceptibility of organisms to Cefuroxime uses the 30-mcg Cefuroxime disk. Interpretation involves the correlation of the diameters obtained in the disk test with the minimum inhibitory concentration (MIC) for Cefuroxime.

A report of "Susceptible" indicates that the pathogen is likely to be inhibited by generally achievable blood levels. A report of "Moderately Susceptible" suggests that the organism would be susceptible if high dosage is used or if the infection is confined to tissues and fluids in which high antibiotic levels are attained: A report of "Intermediate" suggests an equivocable or indeterminate result. A report of "Resistant" indicates that achievable concentrations of the antibiotic are unlikely to be inhibitory and other therapy should be selected.

Reports from the laboratory giving results of the standard single-disk susceptibility test for organisms other than *Haemophilus* spp. and *Neisseria gonorrhoeae* with a 30-mcg Cefuroxime disk should be interpreted according to the following criteria:

Zone Diameter (mm)	Interpretation
≥ 18	(S) Susceptible
15-17	(MS) Moderately Susceptible
≤ 14	(R) Resistant

Results for *Haemophilus* spp. should be interpreted according to the following criteria:

Zone Diameter (mm)	Interpretation
≥ 24	(S) Susceptible
21-23	(I) Intermediate
≤ 20	(R) Resistant

Results for *Neisseria gonorrhoeae* should be interpreted according to the following criteria:

Zone Diameter (mm)	Interpretation
≥ 31	(S) Susceptible
26-30	(MS) Moderately Susceptible
≤ 25	(R) Resistant

Organisms should be tested with the Cefuroxime disk since Cefuroxime has been shown by *in vitro* tests to be active against certain strains found resistant when

► SHOWN IN PRODUCT IDENTIFICATION GUIDE

other beta-lactam disks are used. The Cefuroxime disk should not be used for testing susceptibility to other cephalosporins.

Standardized procedures require the use of laboratory control organisms. The 30-mcg Cefuroxime disk should give the following zone diameters:

1. Testing for organisms other than *Haemophilus* spp. and *Neisseria gonorrhoeae*:

Organism	Zone Diameter (mm)
Staphylococcus aureus ATCC 25923	27-35
Escherichia coli ATCC 25922	20-26

2. Testing for *Haemophilus* spp.:

Organism	Zone Diameter (mm)
Haemophilus influenzae ATCC 49766	28-36

3. Testing for *Neisseria gonorrhoeae*:

Organism	Zone Diameter (mm)
Neisseria gonorrhoeae ATCC 49226	33-41
Staphylococcus aureus ATCC 25923	29-33

Dilution Techniques: Use a standardized dilution method[1] (broth, agar, microdilution) or equivalent with Cefuroxime powder. The MIC values obtained for bacterial isolates other than *Haemophilus* spp. and *Neisseria gonorrhoeae* should be interpreted according to the following criteria:

MIC (mcg/mL)	Interpretation
≤ 8	(S) Susceptible
16	(MS) Moderately Susceptible
≥ 32	(R) Resistant

MIC values obtained for *Haemophilus* spp. should be interpreted according to the following criteria:

MIC (mcg/mL)	Interpretation
≤ 4	(S) Susceptible
8	(I) Intermediate
≥ 16	(R) Resistant

MIC values obtained for *Neisseria gonorrhoeae* should be interpreted according to the following criteria:

MIC (mcg/mL)	Interpretation
≤ 1	(S) Susceptible
2	(MS) Moderately Susceptible
≥ 4	(R) Resistant

As with standard diffusion techniques, dilution methods require the use of laboratory control organisms. Standard Cefuroxime powder should provide the following MIC values.

1. For organisms other than *Haemophilus* spp. and *Neisseria gonorrhoeae*:

Organism	MIC (mcg/mL)
Staphylococcus aureus ATCC 29213	0.5-2.0
Escherichia coli ATCC 25922	2.0-8.0

2. For *Haemophilus* spp.:

Organism	MIC (mcg/mL)
Haemophilus influenzae ATCC 49766	0.25-1.0

3. For *Neisseria gonorrhoeae*:

Organism	MIC (mcg/mL)
Neisseria gonorrhoeae ATCC 49226	0.25-1.0
Staphylococcus aureus ATCC 29213	0.25-1.0

INDICATIONS AND USAGE

Cefuroxime Sodium is indicated for the treatment of patients with infections caused by susceptible strains of the designated organisms in the following diseases:

1. Lower Respiratory Tract Infections: including pneumonia, caused by *Streptococcus pneumoniae, Haemophilus influenzae* (including ampicillin-resistant strains), *Klebsiella* spp., *Staphylococcus aureus* (penicillinase- and non-penicillinase-producing strains), *Streptococcus pyogenes,* and *Escherichia coli.*

2. Urinary Tract Infections: caused by *Escherichia coli* and *Klebsiella* spp.

3. Skin and Skin Structure Infection: caused by *Staphylococcus aureus* (penicillinase- and non-penicillinase-producing strains), *Streptococcus pyogenes, Escherichia coli, Klebsiella* spp., and *Enterobacter* spp.

4. Septicemia: caused by *Staphylococcus aureus* (penicillinase-and non-penicillinase-producing strains), *Streptococcus pneumoniae, Escherichia coli, Haemophilus influenzae* (including ampicillin-resistant strains), and *Klebsiella* spp.

5. Meningitis: caused by *Streptococcus pneumoniae, Haemophilus influenzae* (including ampicillin-resistant strains), *Neisseria meningitidis,* and *Staphylococcus aureus* (penicillinase- and non-penicillinase-producing).

6. Gonorrhea: Uncomplicated and disseminated gonococcal infections due to *Neisseria gonorrhoeae* (penicillinase- and non-penicillinase-producing strains) in both males and females.

7. Bone and Joint Infections: caused by *Staphyloccus aureus* (including penicillinase- and non-penicillinase-producing strains).

Clinical microbiological studies in skin and skin structure infections frequently reveal the growth of susceptible strains of both aerobic and anaerobic organisms. Cefuroxime Sodium has been used successfully in these mixed infections in which several organisms have been isolated. Appropriate cultures and susceptibility studies should be performed to determine the susceptibility of the causative organisms to Cefuroxime Sodium.

Therapy may be started while awaiting the results of these studies; however, once these results become available, the antibiotic treatment should be adjusted accordingly. In certain cases of confirmed or suspected gram-positive or gram-negative sepsis or in patients with other serious infections in which the causative organism has not been identified, Cefuroxime Sodium may be used concomitantly with an aminoglycoside (See "Precautions"). The recommended doses of both antibiotics may be given depending on the severity of the infection and the patient's condition.

Prevention: The preoperative prophylactic administration of Cefuroxime Sodium may prevent the growth of susceptible disease-causing bacteria and thereby may reduce the incidence of certain postoperative infections in patients undergoing surgical procedures (e.g., vaginal hysterectomy) that are classified as clean-contaminated or potentially contaminated procedures. Effective prophylactic use of antibiotics in surgery depends on the time of administration. Cefuroxime Sodium should usually be given one-half to 1 hour before the operation to allow sufficient time to achieve effective antibiotic concentrations in the wound tissues during the procedure. The dose should be repeated intraoperatively if the surgical procedure is lengthy.

Prophylactic administration is usually not required after the surgical procedure ends and should be stopped within 24 hours. If the majority of surgical procedures, continuing prophylactic administration of any antibiotic does not reduce the incidence of subsequent infections but will increase the possibility of adverse reactions and the development of bacterial resistance.

The perioperative use of Cefuroxime Sodium has also been effective during open heart surgery for surgical patients in whom infections at the operative site would present a serious risk. For these patients it is recommended that Cefuroxime Sodium therapy be continued for at least 48 hours after the surgical procedure ends. If an infection is present, specimens for culture should be obtained for the identification of the causative organism, and appropriate antimicrobial therapy should be instituted.

CONTRAINDICATIONS

Cefuroxime Sodium is contraindicated in patients with known allergy to the cephalosporin group of antibiotics.

WARNINGS

BEFORE THERAPY WITH CEFUROXIME SODIUM IS INSTITUTED, CAREFUL INQUIRY SHOULD BE MADE TO DETERMINE WHETHER THE PATIENT HAS HAD PREVIOUS HYPERSENSITIVITY REACTIONS TO CEPHALOSPORINS, PENICILLINS, OR OTHER DRUGS. THIS PRODUCT SHOULD BE GIVEN CAUTIOUSLY TO PENICILLIN-SENSITIVE PATIENTS. ANTIBIOTICS SHOULD BE ADMINISTERED WITH CAUTION TO ANY PATIENT WHO HAS DEMONSTRATED SOME FORM OF ALLERGY, PARTICULARLY TO DRUGS. IF AN ALLERGIC REACTION TO CEFUROXIME SODIUM OCCURS, DISCONTINUE THE DRUG. SERIOUS ACUTE HYPERSENSITIVITY REACTIONS MAY REQUIRE EPINEPHRINE AND OTHER EMERGENCY MEASURES.

Pseudomembranous colitis has been reported with the use of cephalosporins (and other broad-spectrum antibiotics); therefore, it is important to consider its diagnosis in patients who develop diarrhea in association with antibiotic use.

Treatment with broad-spectrum antibiotics alters the normal flora of the colon and may permit overgrowth of clostridia. Studies indicate that a toxin produced by *Clostridium difficile* is one primary cause of antibiotic-associated colitis. Cholestyramine and colestipol resins have been shown to bind the toxin *in vitro.*

Mild cases of colitis may respond to drug discontinuation alone. Moderate to severe cases should be managed with fluid, electrolyte, and protein supplementation as indicated. When the colitis is not relieved by drug discontinuation or when it is severe, oral vancomycin is the treatment of choice for antibiotic-associated pseudomembranous colitis produced by *Clostridium difficile.* Other causes of colitis should also be considered.

PRECAUTIONS

Although Cefuroxime Sodium rarely produces alterations in kidney function, evaluation of renal status during therapy is recommended, especially in seriously ill patients receiving the maximum doses. Cephalosporins should be given with caution to patients receiving concurrent treatment with potent diuretics as these regimens are suspected of adversely affecting renal function.

The total daily dose of Cefuroxime Sodium should be reduced in patients with transient or persistent renal insufficiency (see "Dosage and Administration"), because high and prolonged serum antibiotic concentrations can occur in such individuals from usual doses.

As with other antibiotics, prolonged use of Cefuroxime Sodium may result in overgrowth of nonsusceptible organisms. Careful observation of the patient is essential. If superinfection occurs during therapy, appropriate measures should be taken.

Broad-spectrum antibiotics should be prescribed with caution in individuals with a history of gastrointestinal disease, particularly colitis.

Nephrotoxicity has been reported following concomitant administration of aminoglycoside antibiotics and cephalosporins.

As with other therapeutic regimens used in the treatment of meningitis, mild-to-moderate hearing loss has been reported in a few pediatric patients treated with Cefuroxime Sodium. Persistence of positive CSF (cerebrospinal fluid) cultures at 18-36 hours has also been noted with Cefuroxime Sodium injection, as well as with other antibiotic therapies; however, the clinical relevance of this is unknown.

Drug/Laboratory Test Interactions: A false-positive reaction for glucose in the urine may occur with copper reduction tests (Benedict's or Fehling's solution or with Clinitest® tablets) but not with enzyme-based tests for glycosuria (e.g., Tes-Tape®). As a false-negative result may occur in the ferricyanide test, it is recommended that either the glucose oxidase or hexokinase method be used to determine blood plasma glucose levels in patients receiving Cefuroxime Sodium.

Cefuroxime does not interfere with the assay of serum and urine creatinine by the alkaline picrate method.

Carcinogenesis, Mutagenesis, Impairment of Fertility: Although no long-term studies in animals have been performed to evaluate carcinogenic potential, no mutagenic potential of Cefuroxime was found in standard laboratory tests. Reproduction studies revealed no impairment of fertility in animals.

Pregnancy: Teratogenic Effects: Pregnancy Category B: Reproduction studies have been performed in mice and rabbits at doses up to 60 times the human dose and have revealed no evidence of impaired fertility or harm to the fetus due to Cefuroxime. There are, however, no adequate and well-controlled studies in pregnant women. Because animal reproduction studies are not always predictive of human response, this drug should be used during pregnancy only if clearly needed.

Nursing Mothers: Since Cefuroxime is excreted in human milk, caution should be exercised when Cefuroxime Sodium is administered to a nursing woman.

Pediatric Use: Safety and effectiveness in children below 3 months of age have not been established. Accumulation of other members of the cephalosporin class in newborn infants (with resulting prolongation of drug half-life) has been reported.

ADVERSE REACTIONS
Cefuroxime Sodium is generally well tolerated. The most common adverse effects have been local reactions following IV administration. Other adverse reactions have been encountered only rarely.

Local Reactions: Thrombophlebitis has occurred with IV administration in 1 in 60 patients.

Gastrointestinal: Gastrointestinal symptoms occurred in 1 in 150 patients and included diarrhea (1 in 220 patients) and nausea (1 in 440 patients). Onset of pseudomembranous colitis symptoms may occur during or after antibiotic treatment (see "Warnings").

Hypersensitivity Reactions: Hypersensitivity reactions have been reported in fewer than 1% of the patients treated with Cefuroxime Sodium and include rash (1 in 125). Pruritus, urticaria, and positive Coombs' test each occurred in fewer than 1 in 250 patients, and, as with other cephalosporins, rare cases of anaphylaxis, drug fever, erythema multiforme, interstitial nephritis, toxic epidermal necrolysis, and Stevens-Johnson syndrome have occurred.

Blood: A decrease in hemoglobin and hematocrit has been observed in 1 in 10 patients and transient eosinophilia in 1 in 14 patients. Less common reactions seen were transient neutropenia (fewer than 1 in 100 patients) and leukopenia (1 in 750 patients). A similar pattern and incidence were seen with other cephalosporins used in controlled studies. As with other cephalosporins, there have been rare reports of thrombocytopenia.

Hepatic: Transient rise in SGOT and SGPT (1 in 25 patients), alkaline phosphatase (1 in 50 patients), LDH (1 in 75 patients), and bilirubin (1 in 500 patients) levels has been noted.

Kidney: Elevations in serum creatinine and/or blood urea nitrogen and a decreased creatinine clearance have been observed, but their relationship to Cefuroxime is unknown.

In addition to the adverse reactions listed above that have been observed in patients treated with Cefuroxime, the following adverse reactions and altered laboratory tests have been reported for cephalosporin-class antibiotics:

Adverse Reactions: Vomiting, abdominal pain, colitis, vaginitis including vaginal candidiasis, toxic nephropathy, hepatic dysfunction including cholestasis, aplastic anemia, hemolytic anemia, hemorrhage.

Several cephalosporins have been implicated in triggering seizures, particularly in patients with renal impairment when the dosage was not reduced (see "Dosage and Administration"). If seizures associated with drug therapy should occur, the

drug should be discontinued. Anticonvulsant therapy can be given if clinically indicated.

Altered Laboratory Tests: Prolonged prothrombin time, pancytopenia, agranulocytosis.

OVERDOSAGE
Overdosage of cephalosporins can cause cerebral irritation leading to convulsions. Serum levels of Cefuroxime can be reduced by hemodialysis and peritoneal dialysis.

DOSAGE AND ADMINISTRATION
Dosage: Adults: The usual adult dosage range for Cefuroxime Sodium is 750 mg to 1.5 grams every 8 hours, usually for 5-10 days. In uncomplicated urinary tract infections, skin and skin structure infections, disseminated gonococcal infections, and uncomplicated pneumonia, a 750-mg dose every 8 hours is recommended. In severe or complicated infections, a 1.5-gram dose every 8 hours is recommended.

In bone and joint infections, a 1.5-gram dose every 8 hours is recommended. In clinical trials, surgical intervention was performed when indicated as an adjunct to Cefuroxime Sodium therapy. A course of oral antibiotics was administered when appropriate following the completion of parenteral administration of Cefuroxime Sodium.

In life-threatening infections or infections due to less susceptible organisms, 1.5 grams every 6 hours may be required. In bacterial meningitis, the dosage should not exceed 3 grams every 8 hours. The recommended dosage for uncomplicated gonococcal infection is 1.5 grams given intramuscularly as a single dosage at two different sites together with 1 gram of oral probenecid. For preventive use for clean-contaminated or potentially contaminated surgical procedures, a 1.5-gram dose administered intravenously just before surgery (approximately one-half to 1 hour before the initial incision) is recommended. Thereafter, give 750 mg intravenously or intramuscularly every 8 hours when the procedure is prolonged.

For preventive use during open heart surgery, a 1.5-gram dose administered intravenously at the induction of anesthesia and every 12 hours thereafter for a total of 6 grams is recommended.

Impaired Renal Function: A reduced dosage must be employed when renal function is impaired. Dosage should be determined by the degree of renal impairment and the susceptibility of the causative organism (see Table 1).

Table 1
DOSAGE OF CEFUROXIME SODIUM IN ADULTS WITH REDUCED RENAL FUNCTION

Creatinine Clearance (mL/min)	Dose	Frequency
> 20	750 mg-1.5 gram	q8h
10-20	750 mg	q12h
> 10	750 mg	q24h*

* Since Cefuroxime Sodium is dialyzable, patients on hemodialysis should be given a further dose at the end of the dialysis.

When only serum creatinine is available, the following formula[2] (based on sex, weight, and age of the patient) may be used to convert this value into creatinine clearance. The serum creatinine should represent a steady state of renal function.

Males:
$$\text{Creatinine Clearance (mL/min)} = \frac{\text{Weight (kg)} \times (140 - \text{age})}{72 \times \text{serum creatinine (mg/dL)}}$$

Females: $0.85 \times$ male value

Note: As with antibiotic therapy in general, administration of Cefuroxime Sodium should be continued for a minimum of 48-72 hours after the patient becomes asymptomatic or after evidence of bacterial eradication has been obtained; a minimum of 10 days of treatment is recommended in infections caused by *Streptococcus pyogenes* in order to guard against the risk of rheumatic fever or glomerulonephritis; frequent bacteriologic and clinical appraisal is necessary during therapy of chronic urinary tract infection and may be required for several months after therapy has been completed; persistent infections may require treatment for several weeks; and doses smaller than those indicated above should not be used. In staphylococcal and other infections involving a collection of pus, surgical drainage should be carried out where indicated.

Infants and Children Above 3 Months of Age: Administration of 50-100 mg/kg per day in equally divided doses every 6-8 hours has been successful for most infections susceptible to Cefuroxime. The higher dosage of 100 mg/kg per day (not to exceed the maximum adult dosage) should be used for the more severe or serious infections.

In bone and joint infections, 150 mg/kg per day (not to exceed the maximum adult dosage) is recommended in equally divided doses every 8 hours. In clinical trials, a course of oral antibiotics was administered to children following the completion of parenteral administration of Cefuroxime Sodium.

In cases of bacterial meningitis, a larger dosage of Cefuroxime Sodium is recommended, 200-240 mg/kg per day intravenously in divided doses every 6-8 hours.

In children with renal insufficiency, the frequency of dosage should be modified consistent with the recommendations for adults.

Preparation of Solution and Suspension: The directions for preparing Zinacef for both IV and IM use are summarized in Table 2.

► SHOWN IN PRODUCT IDENTIFICATION GUIDE

For Intramuscular Use: Each 750-mg vial of Cefuroxime Sodium should be constituted with 3.0 mL of sterile water for injection. Shake gently to disperse and withdraw completely the resulting suspension for injection.

For Intravenous Use: Each 750-mg vial should be constituted with 8.0 mL of sterile water for injection. Withdraw completely the resulting solution for injection.

Each 1.5-gram vial should be constituted with 16.0 mL of sterile water for injection, and the solution should be completely withdrawn for injection.

The 7.5-gram pharmacy bulk vial should be constituted with 77 mL of sterile water for injection; each 8 mL of the resulting solution contains 750 mg of Cefuroxime.

Each 750-mg and 1.5-gram infusion pack should be constituted with 100 mL of sterile water for injection, 5% dextrose injection, 0.9% sodium chloride injection, or any of the solutions listed under the Intravenous portion of the *"Compatibility and Stability"* section.

Table 2
PREPARATION OF SOLUTION AND SUSPENSION

Strength	Amount of Diluent to Be Added (mL)	Volume to Be Withdrawn	Approximate Cefuroxime Concentration (mg/mL)
750-mg Vial	3.0 (IM)	Total*	220
750-mg Vial	8.0 (IV)	Total	90
1.5-gram Vial	16.0 (IV)	Total	90
750-mg Infusion pack	100 (IV)	—	7.5
1.5-gram Infusion pack	100 (IV)	—	15
7.5-gram Pharmacy bulk package	77 (IV)	Amount Needed†	95

* **Note:** *Cefuroxime Sodium is a suspension at IM concentrations.*
† *8 mL of solution contains 750 mg of cefuroxime; 16 mL of solution contains 1.5 grams of cefuroxime.*

Administration: After constitution, Cefuroxime Sodium may be given intravenously or by deep IM injection into a large muscle mass (such as the gluteus or lateral part of the thigh). Before injecting intramuscularly, aspiration is necessary to avoid inadvertent injection into a blood vessel.

Intravenous Administration: The IV route may be preferable for patients with bacterial septicemia or other severe or life-threatening infections or for patients who may be poor risks because of lowered resistance, particularly if shock is present or impending.

For Direct Intermittent IV Administration: slowly inject the solution into a vien over a period of 3-5 minutes or give it through the tubing system by which the patient is also receiving other IV solutions.

For Intermittent IV Infusion with a Y-type Administration Set: dosing can be accomplished through the tubing system by which the patient may be receiving other IV solutions. However, during infusion of the solution containing Cefuroxime Sodium, it is advisable to temporarily discontinue administration of any other solutions at the same site.

ADD-Vantage® vials are to be constituted only with 50 or 100 mL of 5% dextrose injection, 0.9% sodium chloride injection, or 0.45% sodium chloride injection in Abbott ADD-Vantage flexible diluent containers (see Instructions for Constitution section of the package insert). ADD-Vantage vials that have been joined to Abbott ADD-Vantage diluent containers and activated to dissolve the drug are stable for 24 hours at room temperature or for 7 days under refrigeration. Joined vials that have not been activated may be used within a 14-day period; this period corresponds to that for use of Abbott ADD-Vantage containers following removal of the outer packaging (overwrap).

Freezing solutions of Cefuroxime Sodium in the ADD-Vantage system is not recommended.

For Continuous IV Infusion: a solution of Cefuroxime Sodium may be added to an IV infusion pack containing one of the following fluids: 0.9% sodium chloride injection; 5% dextrose injection; 10% dextrose injection; 5% dextrose and 0.9% sodium chloride injection; 5% dextrose and 0.45% sodium chloride injection; or 1/6 M sodium lactate injection.

Solutions of Cefuroxime Sodium, like those of most beta-lactam antibiotics, should not be added to solutions of aminoglycoside antibiotics because of potential interaction.

However, if concurrent therapy with Cefuroxime Sodium and an aminoglycoside is indicated, each of these antibiotics can be administered separately to the same patient.

Directions for Use of Cefuroxime Sodium Frozen in Galaxy® Plastic Containers: Cefuroxime Sodium supplied as a frozen, sterile, iso-osmotic, nonpyrogenic solution in plastic containers is to be administered after thawing either as a continuous or intermittent IV infusion. The thawed solution of the premixed product is stable for 28 days if stored under refrigeration (5° C) or for 24 hours at room temperature (25° C). **Do not Refreeze.**

Thaw container at room temperature (25° C) or under refrigeration (5° C). Do not force thaw by immersion in water baths or by microwave irradiation. Components of the solution may precipitate in the frozen state and will dissolve upon reaching room temperature with little or no agitation. Potency is not affected. Mix after solution has reached room temperature. Check for minute leaks by squeezing bag firmly. Discard bag if leaks are found as sterility may be impaired. Do not add supplementary medication. Do not use unless solution is clear and seal is intact.

Use sterile equipment.

Caution: Do not use plastic containers in series connections. Such use could result in air embolism due to residual air being drawn from the primary container before administration of the fluid from the secondary container is complete.

Preparation for Administration: 1. Suspend container from eyelet support.
2. Remove protector from outlet port at bottom of container.
3. Attach administration set. Refer to complete directions accompanying set.

COMPATIBILITY AND STABILITY
Intramuscular: When constituted as directed with sterile water for injection, suspensions of Cefuroxime Sodium for IM injection maintain satisfactory potency for 24 hours at room temperature and for 48 hours under refrigeration (5° C).

After the periods mentioned above any unused suspensions should be discarded.

Intravenous: When the 750-mg, 1.5-g, and 7.5-g pharmacy bulk vials are constituted as directed with sterile water for injection, the Cefuroxime Sodium solutions for IV administration maintain satisfactory potency for 24 hours at room temperature and for 48 hours (750-mg and 1.5-g vials) or for 7 days (7.5-g pharmacy bulk vial) under refrigeration (5° C). More dilute solutions, such as 750 mg or 1.5 g plus 100 mL of sterile water for injection, 5% dextrose injection, or 0.9% sodium chloride injection, also maintain satisfactory potency for 24 hours at room temperature and for 7 days under refrigeration.

These solutions may be further diluted to concentrations of between 1 and 30 mg/mL in the following solutions and will lose not more than 10% activity for 24 hours at room temperature or for at least 7 days under refrigeration: 0.9% sodium chloride injection; 1/6 M sodium lactate injection; ringer's injection, USP; lactated ringer's injection, USP; 5% dextrose and 0.9% sodium chloride injection; 5% dextrose injection; 5% dextrose and 0.45% sodium chloride injection; 5% dextrose and 0.225% sodium chloride injection; 10% dextrose injection; and 10% invert sugar in water for injection. Unused solutions should be discarded after the time periods mentioned above.

Cefuroxime Sodium has also been found compatible for 24 hours at room temperature when admixed in IV infusion with heparin (10 and 50 U/mL) in 0.9% sodium chloride injection and potassium chloride (10 and 40 mEq/L) in 0.9% sodium chloride injection. Sodium bicarbonate injection, USP is not recommended for the dilution of Cefuroxime Sodium.

The 750-mg and 1.5-g Cefuroxime Sodium ADD-Vantage® vials, when diluted in 50 or 100 mL of 5% dextrose injection, 0.9% sodium chloride injection, or 0.45% sodium chloride injection, may be stored for up to 24 hours at room temperature or for 7 days under refrigeration.

Frozen Stability: Constitute the 750-mg, 1.5-g, or 7.5-g vial as directed for IV administration in Table 2. Immediately withdraw the total contents of the 750-mg or 1.5-g vial or 8 or 16 mL from the 7.5-g bulk vial and add to a Baxter Viaflex® Mini-bag® containing 50 or 100 mL of 0.9% sodium chloride injection or 5% dextrose injection and freeze. Frozen solutions are stable for 6 months when stored at −20°C. Frozen solutions should be thawed at room temperature and not refrozen. Do not force thaw by immersion in water baths or by microwave irradiation. Thawed solutions may be stored for up to 24 hours at room temperature or 7 days in a refrigerator.

Note: Parenteral drug products should be inspected visually for particulate matter and discoloration before administration whenever solution and container permit.

As with other cephalosporins, Cefuroxime Sodium powder as well as solutions and suspensions tend to darken, depending on storage conditions, without adversely affecting product potency.

Directions for Dispensing: Pharmacy Bulk Package—Not for Direct Infusion: The pharmacy bulk package is for use in a pharmacy admixture service only under a laminar flow hood. Entry into the vial must be made with a sterile transfer set or other sterile dispensing device, and the contents dispensed in aliquots using aseptic technique. The use of syringe and needle is not recommended as it may cause leakage (see *"Dosage and Administration"*). AFTER INITIAL WITHDRAWAL USE ENTIRE CONTENTS OF VIAL PROMPTLY. ANY UNUSED PORTION MUST BE DISCARDED WITHIN 24 HOURS.

Sterile Cefuroxime Sodium in the dry state should be stored between 15° and 30°C (59° and 86°F) and protected from light.

Cefuroxime Sodium frozen as a premixed solution of Cefuroxime Sodium should not be stored above −20° C.

REFERENCES
1. National Committee for Clinical Laboratory Standards. *Performance Standards for Antimicrobial Susceptibility Testing.* Third Informational Supplement. NCCLS Document M100-S3, Vol. 11, No. 17. Villanova, Pa: NCCLS: 1991.   2. Cockcroft DW, Gault MH: Prediction of creatinine clearance from serum creatinine. *Nephron.* 1976;16:31-41.

J CODES
Per 750 mg IM,IV—J0697

◆ RATED THERAPEUTICALLY EQUIVALENT; ◇ THERAPEUTIC EQUIVALENCE UNCONFIRMED; ○ UNRATED

HOW SUPPLIED
INJECTION: 7.5 GM

BRAND/MANUFACTURER	NDC	SIZE	AWP
◆ GENERICS			
Geneva	00781-3926-46	100 ml 10s	$593.55

INJECTION: 750 MG

AVERAGE UNIT PRICE (AVAILABLE SIZES)	
BRAND	$0.40
GENERIC	$0.40

BRAND/MANUFACTURER	NDC	SIZE	AWP
◆ BRAND			
ZINACEF: Glaxo	00173-0436-00	18 ml 25s	$181.10
◆ GENERICS			
Geneva	00781-3918-70	10 ml 10s	$73.80
Geneva	00781-3920-46	100 ml 10s	$63.99

INJECTION: 750 MG

BRAND/MANUFACTURER	NDC	SIZE	AWP
○ BRAND			
ZINACEF: Glaxo	00173-0424-00	50 ml 24s	$227.12

INJECTION: 1.5 GM

AVERAGE UNIT PRICE (AVAILABLE SIZES)	
BRAND	$0.77
GENERIC	$0.40

BRAND/MANUFACTURER	NDC	SIZE	AWP
◆ BRAND			
ZINACEF: Glaxo	00173-0437-00	18 ml 10s	$139.39
◆ GENERICS			
Geneva	00781-3922-80	20 ml 10s	$134.01
Geneva	00781-3924-46	100 ml 10s	$124.20

INJECTION: 1.5 GM

BRAND/MANUFACTURER	NDC	SIZE	AWP
○ BRAND			
ZINACEF: Glaxo	00173-0425-00	50 ml 24s	$387.79

POWDER FOR INJECTION: 750 MG

AVERAGE UNIT PRICE (AVAILABLE SIZES)	
BRAND	$7.20

BRAND/MANUFACTURER	NDC	SIZE	AWP
◆ BRAND			
KEFUROX: Lilly	00002-7273-10	10s	$71.09
ZINACEF: Glaxo	00173-0353-32	10s	$71.09
KEFUROX: Lilly	00002-7276-24	24s	$196.71
ZINACEF: Glaxo	00173-0352-31	25s	$169.09
KEFUROX: Lilly	00002-7271-25	25s	$169.10
	00002-7278-25	25s	$181.10

POWDER FOR INJECTION: 1 GM

BRAND/MANUFACTURER	NDC	SIZE	AWP
◆ BRAND			
KEFUROX: Lilly	00002-7272-10	10s	$134.58

POWDER FOR INJECTION: 1.5 GM

AVERAGE UNIT PRICE (AVAILABLE SIZES)	
BRAND	$13.98

BRAND/MANUFACTURER	NDC	SIZE	AWP
◆ BRAND			
KEFUROX: Lilly	00002-7274-10	10s	$138.04
ZINACEF: Glaxo	00173-0356-32	10s	$138.04
KEFUROX: Lilly	00002-7271-10	10s	$139.39
	00002-7277-24	24s	$357.42
ZINACEF: Glaxo	00173-0354-35	25s	$336.44

POWDER FOR INJECTION: 7.5 GM

BRAND/MANUFACTURER	NDC	SIZE	AWP
◆ BRAND			
ZINACEF: Glaxo	00173-0400-00	6s	$395.66

POWDER FOR INJECTION: 7.5 GM

BRAND/MANUFACTURER	NDC	SIZE	AWP
○ BRAND			
KEFUROX: Lilly	00002-7275-16	6s	$395.68

Cefzil SEE CEFPROZIL

Celestone SEE BETAMETHASONE ACETATE AND BETAMETHASONE SODIUM PHOSPHATE

Celestone SEE BETAMETHASONE SODIUM PHOSPHATE

Cellulose Sodium Phosphate

DESCRIPTION
Cellulose Sodium Phosphate (CSP) is a synthetic compound made by phosphorylation of Cellulose.

The molecular weight of the Cellulose Sodium Phosphate monomer is 286.1 and the average molecular weight of the polymer is 858,000.

It has an inorganic Phosphate content of approximately 34% and Sodium content of approximately 11%. It is insoluble in water and nonabsorbable. It has excellent ion exchange properties, the sodium ion exchanging for calcium. When taken orally, Cellulose Sodium Phosphate binds calcium, the complex of calcium and Cellulose Phosphate being excreted in feces. The dosage of Cellulose Sodium Phosphate is powder for oral administration.

CLINICAL PHARMACOLOGY
Cellulose Sodium Phosphate (CSP) alters urinary composition of calcium, Magnesium, Phosphate and oxalate by affecting their absorption in the intestinal tract. When it is given orally with meals, CSP binds dietary and secreted calcium, and reduces urinary calcium by approximately 50 mg/5 grams of CSP. It also binds dietary Magnesium and lowers urinary Magnesium. Oral magnesium supplementation given separately from CSP partly overcomes this effect.

CSP administration increases urinary phosphorus (P) and oxalate. The usual rise in urinary P of 150-250 mg/15 grams CSP largely reflects the hydrolysis of 7-30% of CSP in the intestinal tract and absorption of released P. An increase in urinary oxalate occurs. Since CSP binds divalent cations, the cations are not available to complex oxalate and thereby limit its absorption. The rise in urinary oxalate may be largely prevented by moderate dietary oxalate restriction and the use of a modest dose of CSP (10-15 grams/day).

The marked reduction in urinary calcium with only slightly increased urinary phosphorus and oxalate leads to a reduction in urinary saturation and propensity for spontaneous nucleation of calcium oxalate and calcium phosphate (brushite).

CSP does not apparently alter the metabolism of trace metals, since it does not significantly change the serum concentration of copper, zinc or iron.

INDICATIONS AND USAGE
CSP is indicated only for absorptive hypercalciuria Type I with recurrent calcium oxalate or calcium in phosphate nephrolithiasis. Appropriate use (see *"Dosage and Administration"*) of CSP substantially reduces the incidence of new stone formation in these patients. Causes of hypercalciuria other than hyperabsorption cannot be expected to respond to CSP.[1] Treatment with CSP is not needed for absorptive hypercalciuria Type II because dietary calcium restriction provides adequate treatment. In patients without hyperabsorption of calcium, CSP would be expected to cause excessive parathyroid hormone secretion and possible hyperparathyroid bone disease.

Absorptive hypercalciuria Type I is characterized by (a) recurrent passage or formation of calcium oxalate and/or calcium phosphate renal stones, (b) no evidence of bone disease, (c) normal serum calcium and phosphorus, (d) increased intestinal calcium absorption, (e) hypercalciuria, (f) normal urinary calcium during fasting, (g) normal parathyroid function, and (h) lack of renal "leak" or excessive skeletal mobilization of calculi. **Minimal diagnostic tests include serum calcium and phosphorus, parathyroid hormone (PTH) level obtained before breakfast, 24-hour urinary calcium on a diet restricted in calcium and sodium, and a fasting urinary excretion of calcium.**

The diagnosis of absorptive hypercalciuria Type I can be made if there is: a) recurrent calcium nephrolithiasis without clinical evidence of bone disease, b) normal serum calcium and phosphorus (borderline values should be repeated), c) 24-hour urinary calcium greater than 200 mg/day on a diet of 400 mg calcium and 100 mEq sodium/day, d) normal serum immunoreactive PTH, and e) normal fasting urinary calcium. A definite diagnosis requires, in addition evidence of high intestinal calcium absorption (e.g., urinary calcium > 0.2 mg/mg creatinine after oral load of 1 gram calcium.)

CONTRAINDICATIONS
CSP is contraindicated in (a) primary or secondary hyperparathyroidism, including renal hypercalciuria (renal calcium leak), (b) hypomagnesemic states (serum magnesium < 1.5 mg/dl), (c) bone disease (osteoporosis, osteomalacia, osteitis), (d) hypocalcemic states (e.g., hypoparathyroidism, intestinal malabsorption), (e) normal or low intestinal absorption and renal excretion of calcium, and (f) enteric hyperoxaluria. It should not be used in patients with high fasting urinary calcium or hypophosphatemia, unless a high skeletal mobilization of calcium can be excluded.

► SHOWN IN PRODUCT IDENTIFICATION GUIDE

WARNINGS

In patients with congestive heart failure or ascites, Sodium contained in CSP (35-48 mEq exchangeable sodium/15 grams CSP) may represent a hazard.

PRECAUTIONS

General: By inhibiting intestinal calcium absorption, CSP may stimulate parathyroid function leading to hyperparathyroid hormone levels. CSP treatment has been shown to maintain parathyroid function within normal limits, if it used only in patients with absorptive hypercalciuria Type I (increased intestinal calcium restricted diet), at a dosage just sufficient to restore normal calcium absorption but not sufficient to cause subnormal absorption.

The following additional complications may potentially develop during long-term use of CSP: a) hyperoxaluria and hypomagnesiuria, which would negate the beneficial effect of hypocalciuria on new stone formation, b) magnesium depletion, and c) depletion of trace metals (copper, zinc, iron). All of these effects may be minimized by restricting the use of CSP to absorptive hypercalciuria Type I only (see *"Indications"* for diagnostic criteria), and by taking precautionary measures (see *"Administration and Dosage"*) and by monitoring serum calcium, magnesium, copper, zinc, iron, parathyroid hormone, and complete blood count every 3 to 6 months. Borderline values for parathyroid hormone and calcium should be repeated promptly. Serum PTH should be obtained at least once between the first 2 weeks to 3 months of treatment and the treatment should be adjusted or stopped if a rise in serum PTH above normal appears. If there is an inadequate hypocalciuric response to CSP treatment (a reduction in urinary calcium of less than 30 mg/5 grams of CSP), while patients are maintained on moderate calcium and sodium restriction, the treatment may be considered ineffective and should be stopped. Cessation of treatment may be considered ineffective and should be stopped. Cessation of treatment should be considered if urinary oxalate exceeds 55 mg/day on moderate dietary oxalate restriction.

Carcinogenesis, Mutagenesis, Impairment of Fertility: No longterm studies were conducted to determine the carcinogenic potential of CSP.

Pregnancy: Pregnancy Category C: Animal reproduction studies have not been conducted with CSP. It is also not known whether CSP can cause fetal harm when administered to a pregnant woman or can affect reproduction capacity. However, because of the increased requirement of dietary calcium in pregnant women, CSP should be given to pregnant women only if clearly needed.

Pediatric Use: Because of the increased requirement for dietary calcium in growing children, the use of CSP in children less than 16 years of age is not recommended.

ADVERSE REACTIONS

Some patients may have gastrointestinal complaints, manifested by poor taste of the drug, loose bowel movements, diarrhea or dyspepsia.

DOSAGE AND ADMINISTRATION

The amount of dietary calcium bound depends upon actual mixing of CSP with a meal. Consequently, CSP should be taken with a meal; the amount of dietary calcium bound by CSP is considerably reduced when CSP is administered more than 1 hour after a meal. Both the initial and maintenance doses of CSP are based on measurements of 24-hour urinary calcium excretion. The recommended initial dose of CSP is 15 grams/day (5 grams with each meal) in patients with urinary calcium greater than 300 mg/day (on moderate calcium - restricted diet, i.e., avoidance of dairy products). When urinary calcium declines to less than 150 mg/day, the dosage of CSP should be reduced to 10 grams/day (5 grams with supper, 2.5 grams each with remaining meal). Patients with controlled urinary calcium on moderate calcium - restricted diet of less than 300 mg/day (but greater than 200 mg/day) should begin on CSP 10 grams/day.

The following general measures should be imposed during CSP therapy. A moderate calcium intake is recommended, by avoidance of dairy products. A moderate dietary oxalate restriction should be imposed by discouraging ingestion of spinach (and similar dark greens), rhubarb, chocolate and brewed tea. Vitamin C supplementation should be denied because of its potential metabolism to oxalate. A high sodium intake should be discouraged by advising avoidance of "salty" foods and salt shakers, in an attempt to achieve an intake of less than 150 mEq/day. Fluid intake should be encouraged, to achieve a minimum urine output of 2 liters/day.

The dose of oral Magnesium supplements, given as magnesium gluconate, depends upon the dose of CSP. Those receiving 15 grams of CSP/day should take 1.5 grams of magnesium gluconate before breakfast and again at bedtime (separately from CSP). Those taking 10 grams of CSP/day should take 1 gram of magnesium gluconate twice a day. To avoid binding of Magnesium by CSP, supplemental Magnesium should be given at least 1 hour before or after a dose of CSP.

It is recommended that each dose of CSP (in the powder form) be suspended in a glass of water, soft drink or fruit juice, and ingested within ½ hour of the meal. It should not be given with magnesium gluconate.

Store in a dry place at room temperature, 15° - 30°C (59°-86°F).

HOW SUPPLIED
POWDER:

BRAND/MANUFACTURER	NDC	SIZE	AWP
○ BRAND			
CALCIBIND: Mission	00178-0255-30	300 gm	$93.75

Celontin *SEE* METHSUXIMIDE

Cenolate *SEE* VITAMIN C

Cephalexin

DESCRIPTION

Cephalexin Hydrochloride is a semisynthetic cephalosporin antibiotic intended for oral administration. It is available as capsules, oral suspension, and tablets.

Each capsule contains: Cephalexin Monohydrate equivalent to 250 or 500 mg (720 or 1,439 µmol) Cephalexin

Each 5 ml of oral suspension contains: Cephalexin Monohydrate equivalent to 125 or 250 mg (360 or 720 µmol) Cephalexin

Each tablet contains: Cephalexin Hydrochloride equivalent to 250 or 500 mg (720 or 1,439 µmol) Cephalexin

Chemically, Cephalexin is designated 7-(D-α-amino-α-phenylacetamido)-3-methyl-3-cephem-4-carboxylic acid monohydrate. Cephalexin has the molecular formula $C_{16}H_{17}N_3O_4S \cdot H_2O$ and the molecular weight is 365.4.

Cephalexin Hydrochloride is 7-(D-2-amino-2phenyl-acetamido)-3-methyl-3-cephem-4-carboxylic acid hydrochloride monohydrate, and the chemical formula is $C_{16}H_{17}N_3O_4S \cdot HCl \cdot H_2O$. The molecular weight is 401.86.

The nucleus of Cephalexin is related to that of other cephalosporin antibiotics. The compound is a zwitterion; ie, the molecule contains both a basic and an acidic group. Cephalexin is the hydrochloride salt of Cephalexin. The isoelectric point of Cephalexin in water is approximately 4.5 to 5.

The crystalline form of Cephalexin which is available is a monohydrate. It is a white crystalline solid having a bitter taste. Solubility in water is low at room temperature; 1 or 2 mg/ml may be dissolved readily, but higher concentrations are obtained with increasing difficulty. Solubility of the Hydrochloride salt in water is high at room temperature; greater than 10 mg/mL may be dissolved readily.

The cephalosporins differ from penicillins in the structure of the bicyclic ring system. Cephalexin had a *D*-phenylglycyl group as substituent at the 7-amino position and an unsubstituted methyl group at the 3-position.

Following is its chemical structure:

CLINICAL PHARMACOLOGY

Human Pharmacology: Cephalexin Hydrochloride is acid stable and may be given without regard to meals. It is rapidly absorbed after oral administration. Following doses of 250 mg, 500 mg, and 1 gm, average peak serum levels of approximately 9, 18, and 32 µg/mL respectively were obtained at 1 hour. Following doses of 250 mg, and 500 mg of Cephalexin HCl, average peak serum levels of approximately 9 and 18 µg/mL respectively were obtained at 1 hour and declined to 1.6 and 3.4 µg/mL respectively at 3 hours. Measurable levels of each were present 6 hours after administration. Cephalexin is excreted in the urine by glomerular filtration and tubular secretion. Studies showed that over 90% of the drug was excreted unchanged in the urine within 8 hours. During this period, peak urine concentrations following the 250-mg, 500-mg, and 1-gm doses were approximately 1,000, 2,200, and 5,000 µg/mL respectively. Approximately 70% of the hydrochloride was excreted unchanged in the urine within 12 hours. During the first 6 hours, average urine concentrations following the 250-mg and 500-mg doses were approximately 200 µg/ml (range 54 to 663) and 500 µg/ml (range, 137 to 1,306) respectively. The average serum half-life is 1.1 hours.

Microbiology: In vitro tests demonstrate that the cephalosporins are bactericidal because of their inhibition of cell-wall synthesis. Cephalexin HCl is active against the following organisms *in vitro.*

β-hemolytic streptococci, particularly *Streptococcus pyogenes*
Staphylococcus aureus, including penicillinase-producing strains
Streptococcus pneumoniae
Escherichia coli
Proteus mirabilis
Klebsiella sp., particularly *K. pneumoniae*
Haemophilus influenzae
Moraxella (Branhamella) catarrhalis
Staphylococcus epidermidis (penicillinase-producing strains)

Note: Most strains of enterococci (*Enterococcus faecalis* [formerly *Streptococcus faecalis*]) and a few strains of staphylococci (methicillin-resistant) are resistant to cephalosporins, including Cephalexin. When tested by *in vitro* methods, staphylococci exhibit cross-resistance between Cephalexin HCl and methicillin-type antibiotics. Cephalexin HCl is not active against most strains of *Enterobacter* sp, *Morganella morganii* (formerly *Proteus morganii*), *Serratia* sp, and *Proteus vulgaris.* It has no activity against *Pseudomonas* or *Acinetobacter* sp., particularly *Acinetobacter colcoaceticus.*

◆ RATED THERAPEUTICALLY EQUIVALENT; ◇ THERAPEUTIC EQUIVALENCE UNCONFIRMED; ○ UNRATED

Disk Susceptibility Tests: Quantitative methods that require measurement of zone diameters give the most precise estimates of antibiotic susceptibility. One such procedure has been recommended for use with cephalosporin class (cephalothin) disks for testing susceptibility to Cephalexin, using the 30 μg cephalothin disk. The currently accepted zone diameter interpretations for the cephalothin disks are appropriate for determining susceptibility to Cephalexin. Interpretations correlate zone diameters of the disk test with MIC values for Cephalexin.

Reports from the laboratory giving results of the standard single-disk susceptibility test with a 30-μg cephalothin disk should be interpreted according to the following criteria:

Zone Diameter (mm)	Interpretation
≥18	(S) Susceptible
15-17	(MS) Moderately Susceptible
≤14	(R) Resistant

A report of "Susceptible" indicates that the pathogen is likely to be inhibited by generally achievable blood levels. A report of "Moderately Susceptible" suggests that the organism would be susceptible if high dosage is used or if the infection is confined to tissue and fluids in which high antibiotic levels are obtained. A report of "Resistant" indicates that achievable concentrations of the antibiotic are unlikely to be inhibitory and other therapy should be selected.

Standardized procedures require the use of laboratory control organisms. The 30-μg cephalothin disk should give the following zone diameters:

Organism	Zone Diameter (mm)
E coli ATCC 25922	17-22
S. aureus ATCC 25923	29-37

Dilution Techniques: Use a standardized dilution method† (broth, agar, microdilution) or equivalent with cephalothin powder. The MIC values obtained should be interpreted according to the following criteria:

MIC (μg/mL)	Interpretation
≤8	(S) Susceptible
16	(MS) Moderately Susceptible
≥32	(R) Resistant

As with standard diffusion techniques, dilution methods require the use of laboratory control organisms. Standard cephalothin powder should provide the following MIC values:

Organism	MIC (μg/mL)
E coli ATCC 25922	4.0-16.0
E. faecalis ATCC 29212	8.0-32.0
S. aureus ATCC 29213	0.12-0.5

* Laboratory Standards: Performance standards for antimicrobial disk susceptibility tests—4th ed.
Approved Standard NCCLS Document M2-A4, Vol 10, No 7, NCCLS, Villanova, PA, 1990.
† National Committee for Clinical Laboratory Standards: Methods for dilution antimicrobial susceptibility tests for bacteria that grow aerobically—2nd ed. Approved Standard NCCLS Document M7-A2, Vol 10, No 8, NCCLS, Villanova, PA, 1990. b

INDICATIONS AND USAGE
Cephalexin and Cephalexin HCl are indicated for the treatment of the following infections when caused by susceptible strains of the designated microorganisms:

Respiratory tract infections caused by *S. pneumoniae* and group A β-hemolytic streptococci or *S. pyogenes* (Penicillin is the usual drug of choice in the treatment and prevention of streptococcal infections, including the prophylaxis of rheumatic fever. Cephalexin HCl is generally effective in the eradication of streptococci from the nasopharynx; however, substantial data establishing the efficacy of Cephalexin HCl is the subsequent prevention of rheumatic fever are not available at present.)

Skin and skin structure infections caused by *S. Aureus* and/or β-hemolytic streptococci.

Bone infections caused by *S. aureus* and/or *P. mirabilis.*

Genitourinary tract infections, including acute prostatitis, caused by *E. coli, P. mirabilis,* and *Klebsiella* sp. or *K. pneumoniae.*

Cephalexin is also indicated for otitis media due to *S. pneumoniae, H. influenzae,* staphylococci, streptococci, and *M. catarrhalis.*

Note: Culture and susceptibility tests should be initiated prior to and during therapy. Renal function studies should be performed when indicated.

UNLABELED USES
Cephalexin is used alone or as an adjunct in the treatment of peritonitis.

CONTRAINDICATIONS
Cephalexin Hydrochloride is contraindicated in patients with known allergy to the cephalosporin group of antibiotics.

WARNINGS
BEFORE CEPHALEXIN THERAPY IS INSTITUTED, CAREFUL INQUIRY SHOULD BE MADE CONCERNING PREVIOUS HYPERSENSITIVITY REACTIONS TO CEPHALOSPORINS AND PENICILLIN. CEPHALOSPORIN C DERIVATIVES SHOULD BE GIVEN CAUTIOUSLY TO PENICILLIN-SENSITIVE PATIENTS.

SERIOUS ACUTE HYPERSENSITIVITY REACTIONS MAY REQUIRE EPINEPHRINE AND OTHER EMERGENCY MEASURES.

There is some clinical and laboratory evidence of partial cross-allergenicity of the penicillins and the cephalosporins. Patients have been reported to have had severe reactions (including anaphylaxis) to both drugs.

Any patient who has demonstrated some form of allergy, particularly to drugs, should receive antibiotics cautiously. No exception should be made with regard to Cephalexin Hydrochloride.

Pseudomembranous colitis has been reported with virtually all broad-spectrum antibiotics (including macrolides, semisynthetic penicillins, and cephalosporins); therefore, it is important to consider its diagnosis in patients who develop diarrhea in association with the use of antibiotics. Such colitis may range in severity from mild to life threatening.

Treatment with broad-spectrum antibiotics alters the normal flora of the colon and may permit overgrowth of clostridia. Studies indicate that a toxin produced by *Clostridium difficile* is a primary cause of antibiotic-associated colitis.

Mild cases of pseudomembranous colitis usually respond to drug discontinuance alone. In moderate to severe cases, management should include sigmoidoscopy, appropriate bacteriologic studies, and fluid, electrolyte, and protein supplementation. When the colitis does not improve after the drug has been discontinued or when it is severe, treatment with an oral antibacterial drug effective against *C. difficile* is recommended. Other causes of colitis should be ruled out.

Usage in Pregnancy: Safety of this product for use during pregnancy has not been established.

PRECAUTIONS
General: Patients should be followed carefully so that any side effects or unusual manifestations of drug idiosyncrasy may be detected. If an allergic reaction to Cephalexin Hydrochloride occurs, the drug should be discontinued and the patient treated with the usual agents (eg, epinephrine or other pressor amines, antihistamines, or corticosteroids).

Prolonged use of Cephalexin HCl may result in the overgrowth of nonsusceptible organisms. Careful observation of the patient is essential. If superinfection occurs during therapy, appropriate measures should be taken.

Positive direct Coombs' tests have been reported during treatment with the cephalosporin antibiotics. In hematologic studies or in transfusion cross-matching procedures when antiglobulin tests are performed on the minor side or in Coombs' testing of newborns whose mothers have received cephalosporin antibiotics before parturition, it should be recognized that a positive Coombs' test may be due to the drug.

Cephalexin HCl should be administered with caution in the presence of markedly impaired renal function. Under such conditions, careful clinical observation and laboratory studies should be made because safe dosage may be lower than that usually recommended.

Indicated surgical procedures should be performed in conjunction with antibiotic therapy.

As a result of administration of Cephalexin HCl, a false-positive reaction for glucose in the urine may occur. This has been observed with Benedict's and Fehling's solutions and also with Clinitest® tablets but not with Tes-Tape® (Glucose Enzymatic Test Strip, USP).

Broad-spectrum antibiotics should be prescribed with caution in individuals with a history of gastrointestinal disease, particularly colitis.

Usage in Pregnancy: Pregnancy Category B: The daily oral administration of Cephalexin to rats in doses of 250 or 500 mg/kg prior to and during pregnancy, or to rats and mice during the period of organogenesis only, had no adverse effect on fertility, fetal viability, fetal weight, or litter size. Note that the safety of Cephalexin during pregnancy in humans has not been established.

Cephalexin showed no enhanced toxicity in weanling and newborn rats as compared with adult animals. Nevertheless, because the studies in humans cannot rule out the possibility of harm, Cephalexin should be used during pregnancy only if clearly needed.

Nursing Mothers: The excretion of Cephalexin in the milk increased up to 4 hours after a 500-mg dose; the drug reached a maximum level of 4 μg/mL, then decreased gradually, and had disappeared 8 hours after administration. A decision should be considered to discontinue nursing temporarily during therapy with Cephalexin HCl.

Pediatric Use: Safety and effectiveness in children have not been established.

ADVERSE REACTIONS
Gastrointestinal: Symptoms of pseudomembranous colitis may appear either during or after antibiotic treatment. Nausea and vomiting have been reported rarely. The most frequent side effects has been diarrhea. It was very rarely severe enough to warrant cessation of therapy. Abdominal pain, gastritis, and dyspepsia have also occurred. As with some penicillins and some other cephalosporins, transient hepatitis and cholestatic jaundice have been reported rarely.

Hypersensitivity: Allergic reactions in the form of rash, urticaria, angioedema, and rarely, erythema multiforme, Stevens-Johnson syndrome, or toxic epidermal necrolysis have been observed. These reactions usually subsided upon discontinuation of the drug. In some of these reactions, supportive therapy may be necessary. Anaphylaxis has also been reported.

Other reactions have included genital and anal pruritus, genital moniliasis, vaginitis and vaginal discharge, dizziness, fatigue, headache, agitation, confusion, hallucinations, arthralgia, arthritis, and joint disorder. Reversible interstitial nephritis has been reported rarely. Eosinophilia, neutropenia, thrombocytopenia, slight elevations in aspartate aminotransferase (AST, SGOT) and alanine aminotransferase (ALT, SGPT), and elevated creatinine and BUN have been reported.

In addition to the adverse reactions listed above that have been observed in patients treated with Cephalexin Hydrochloride, the following adverse reactions and altered laboratory tests have been reported for cephalosporin class antibiotics:

Adverse Reactions: Allergic reactions, including fever, colitis, renal dysfunction, toxic nephropathy, and hepatic dysfunction, including cholestasis.

Several cephalosporins have been implicated in triggering seizures, particularly in patients with renal impairment when the dosage was not reduced (see *"Indications and Usage"* and *"Precautions, General"*). If seizures associated with drug therapy should occur, the drug should be discontinued. Anticonvulsant therapy can be given if clinically indicated.

Altered Laboratory Tests: Increased prothrombin time, increased alkaline phosphatase, and leukopenia.

OVERDOSAGE

Signs and Symptoms: Symptoms of oral overdose may include nausea, vomiting, epigastric distress, diarrhea, and hematuria. If other symptoms are present, they are probably secondary to an underlying disease state, an allergic reaction, or toxicity due to ingestion of a second medication.

Treatment: To obtain up-to-date information about the treatment of overdose, a good resource is your certified Regional Poison Control Center. Telephone numbers of certified poison control centers are listed in the *Physician's Desk Reference (PDR)*. In managing overdosage, consider the possibility of multiple drug overdoses, interaction among drugs and unusual drug kinetics in your patient.

Unless 5 to 10 times the normal dose of Cephalexin has been ingested, gastrointestinal decontamination should not be necessary.

Protect the patient's airway and support ventilation and perfusion. Meticulously monitor and maintain, within acceptable limits, the patient's vital signs, blood gases, serum electrolytes, etc. Absorption of drugs from the gastrointestinal tract may be decreased by giving activated charcoal, which, in many cases, is more effective than emesis or lavage; consider charcoal instead of or in addition to gastric emptying. Repeated doses of charcoal over time may hasten elimination of some drugs that have been absorbed. Safeguard the patient's airway when employing gastric emptying or charcoal.

Forced diuresis, peritoneal dialysis, hemodialysis, or charcoal hemoperfusion have not been established as beneficial for an overdose of Cephalexin; however, it would be extremely unlikely that one of these procedures would be indicated. The oral median lethal dose of Cephalexin in rats is 5,000 mg/kg.

DOSAGE AND ADMINISTRATION

Cephalexin Hydrochloride is administered orally. The adult dosage ranges from 1 to 4 gm daily in divided doses. For the following infections, a dosage of 500 mg may be administered every 12 hours: streptococcal pharyngitis, skin and skin structure infections, and uncomplicated cystitis in patients over 15 years of age. Cystitis therapy should be continued for 7 to 14 days. For other infections, the usual dose is 250 mg every 6 hours. For more severe infections or those caused by less susceptible organisms, larger doses may be needed. If daily doses of Cephalexin HCl greater than 4 g are required, parenteral cephalosporins, in appropriate doses, should be considered.

Children: The usual recommended daily dosage for children is 25 to 50 mg/kg in divided doses. For streptococcal pharyngitis in patients over 1 year of age and for skin and skin-structure infections, the total daily dose may be divided and administered every 12 hours.

CEPHALEXIN SUSPENSION

Child's Weight	125 mg/5 mL	250 mg/5 mL
10 kg (22 lb)	½ to 1 tsp q.i.d.	¼ to ½ tsp q.i.d.
20 kg (44 lb)	1 to 2 tsp q.i.d.	½ to 1 tsp q.i.d.
40 kg (88 lb)	2 to 4 tsp q.i.d.	1 to 2 tsp q.i.d.
	or	
Child's Weight	125 mg/5mL	250 mg/5mL
10 kg (22 lb)	1 to 2 tsp b.i.d.	½ to 1 tsp b.i.d.
20 kg (44 lb)	2 to 4 tsp b.i.d.	1 to 2 tsp b.i.d.
40 kg (88 lb)	4 to 8 tsp b.i.d.	2 to 4 tsp b.i.d.

In severe infections, the dosage may be doubled.

In the therapy of otitis media, clinical studies have shown that a dosage of 75 to 100 mg/kg/day in 4 divided doses is required.

In the treatment of β-hemolytic streptococcal infections, a therapeutic dosage of Cephalexin should be administered for at least 10 days.

Store at controlled room temperature, 59° to 86°F (15° to 30°C).

After mixing the oral suspension, store in a refrigerator. May be kept for 14 days without significant loss of potency. Shake well before using. Keep tightly closed.

HOW SUPPLIED

CEPHALEXIN HYDROCHLORIDE
TABLETS: 500 MG

BRAND/MANUFACTURER	NDC	SIZE	AWP
○ BRAND			
▷ KEFTAB: Dista	00777-4143-02	100s	$196.74

CEPHALEXIN MONOHYDRATE
CAPSULE: 250 MG

AVERAGE UNIT PRICE (AVAILABLE SIZES)		GENERIC A-RATED AVERAGE PRICE (GAAP)	
BRAND	$1.32	20s	$12.00
GENERIC	$0.52	100s	$55.09
HCFA FUL (100s ea)	$0.11	500s	$228.91
		1000s	$402.12

BRAND/MANUFACTURER	NDC	SIZE	AWP
◆ BRAND			
▷ KEFLEX: Dista	00777-0869-20	20s	$27.04
	00777-0869-02	100s	$128.78
	00777-0869-33	100s ud	$133.16
◆ GENERICS			
▷ Novopharm	55953-0084-20	20s	$10.77
▷ Biocraft	00332-3145-03	20s	$13.22
UDL	51079-0604-98	60s	$60.00
Raway	00686-3145-09	100s	$16.00
Geneva	00781-2531-01	100s	$42.50
Warner Chilcott	00047-0938-24	100s	$43.39
Jerome Stevens	50564-0470-01	100s	$45.21
Qualitest	00603-2595-21	100s	$47.00
Schein	00364-2161-01	100s	$47.25
Major	00904-3800-60	100s	$49.40
Moore,H.L.	00839-7311-06	100s	$50.07
▷ Zenith	00172-4073-60	100s	$50.20
Mason Dist	11845-0157-01	100s	$50.71
URL	00677-1158-01	100s	$53.10
Novopharm	55953-0084-40	100s	$53.85
Martec	52555-0970-01	100s	$54.92
▷ Rugby	00536-0120-01	100s	$56.86
▷ Apothecon	00003-0749-50	100s	$57.00
Barr	00555-0514-02	100s	$57.70
▷ Lemmon	00093-0541-01	100s	$59.00
Aligen	00405-4152-01	100s	$62.97
Goldline	00182-1278-01	100s	$62.97
▷ Biocraft	00332-3145-09	100s	$62.97
Mylan	00378-6025-01	100s	$63.95
Lederle Std Prod	00005-3413-23	100s	$64.38
Parmed	00349-8651-01	100s	$65.00
Du Pont Multi	00056-0193-70	100s	$69.26
Raway	00686-0604-20	100s ud	$28.00
Major	00904-3800-61	100s ud	$34.95
Novopharm	55953-0084-01	100s ud	$56.35
Vangard	00615-0353-13	100s ud	$62.89
Goldline	00182-1278-89	100s ud	$63.00
Geneva	00781-2531-13	100s ud	$63.50
UDL	51079-0604-20	100s ud	$84.20
Medirex	57480-0468-01	100s ud	$84.20
Major	00904-3800-40	500s	$159.70
▷ Rugby	00536-0120-05	500s	$160.74
Schein	00364-2161-05	500s	$170.55
Warner Chilcott	00047-0938-30	500s	$170.69
Geneva	00781-2531-05	500s	$172.50
Moore,H.L.	00839-7311-12	500s	$178.05
▷ Apothecon	00003-0749-60	500s	$196.08
URL	00677-1158-05	500s	$198.90
Mason Dist	11845-0157-03	500s	$203.40
Jerome Stevens	50564-0470-05	500s	$207.94
▷ Zenith	00172-4073-70	500s	$216.70
Qualitest	00603-2595-28	500s	$220.00
▷ Lemmon	00093-0541-05	500s	$265.00
Novopharm	55953-0084-70	500s	$265.39
Barr	00555-0514-04	500s	$267.62
Martec	52555-0970-04	500s	$268.00
Parmed	00349-8651-05	500s	$270.00
Mylan	00378-6025-05	500s	$283.00
Aligen	00405-4152-02	500s	$283.37
Goldline	00182-1278-05	500s	$283.37
▷ Biocraft	00332-3145-13	500s	$283.37
Du Pont Multi	00056-0193-85	500s	$311.70
Parmed	00349-8651-10	1000s	$300.00
Novopharm	55953-0084-80	1000s	$504.23

◆ RATED THERAPEUTICALLY EQUIVALENT; ◇ THERAPEUTIC EQUIVALENCE UNCONFIRMED; ○ UNRATED

CAPSULE: 500 MG

AVERAGE UNIT PRICE (AVAILABLE SIZES)		GENERIC A-RATED AVERAGE PRICE (GAAP)	
BRAND	$1.94	20s	$22.02
GENERIC	$0.98	100s	$109.09
HCFA FUL (100s ea)	$0.22	250s	$217.06
		500s	$409.53
		1000s	$689.62

BRAND/MANUFACTURER	NDC	SIZE	AWP
◆ BRAND			
▶ KEFLEX: Dista	00777-0871-20	20s	$53.20
ZARTAN: Dartmouth	58869-0871-01	100s	$94.00
▶ KEFLEX: Dista	00777-0871-02	100s	$253.11
	00777-0871-33	100s ud	$257.49
◆ GENERICS			
Schein	00364-2162-40	20s	$18.50
▶ Novopharm	55953-0114-20	20s	$21.54
▶ Biocraft	00332-3147-03	20s	$26.02
UDL	51079-0605-98	60s	$60.00
Raway	00686-3147-09	100s	$25.00
Geneva	00781-2532-01	100s	$83.50
Warner Chilcott	00047-0939-24	100s	$85.23
Jerome Stevens	50564-0469-01	100s	$88.40
Qualitest	00603-2596-21	100s	$90.50
Schein	00364-2162-01	100s	$91.75
Moore,H.L.	00839-7312-06	100s	$96.38
Major	00904-3801-60	100s	$98.60
▶ Zenith	00172-4074-60	100s	$100.10
Mason Dist	11845-0158-01	100s	$100.81
Purepac	00228-2418-10	100s	$104.27
▶ Novopharm	55953-0114-40	100s	$107.69
Martec	52555-0971-01	100s	$108.75
URL	00677-1159-01	100s	$110.65
▶ Rugby	00536-0130-01	100s	$110.70
▶ Apothecon	00003-0874-50	100s	$111.72
▶ Apothecon	00003-0874-51	100s	$111.72
Goldline	00182-1279-01	100s	$112.51
▶ Barr	00555-0515-02	100s	$113.90
▶ Lemmon	00093-0543-01	100s	$118.00
Aligen	00405-4153-01	100s	$123.76
▶ Biocraft	00332-3147-09	100s	$123.76
Parmed	00349-8652-01	100s	$125.00
Mylan	00378-6050-01	100s	$125.95
▶ Lederle Std Prod	00005-3414-23	100s	$126.50
Du Pont Multi	00056-0194-70	100s	$136.13
Raway	00686-0605-20	100s ud	$50.00
▶ Novopharm	55953-0114-01	100s ud	$110.19
Goldline	00182-1279-89	100s ud	$115.00
Vangard	00615-0354-13	100s ud	$123.46
Geneva	00781-2532-13	100s ud	$124.00
UDL	51079-0605-20	100s ud	$173.00
Medirex	57480-0469-01	100s ud	$173.00
Schein	00364-2162-04	250s	$168.73
▶ Novopharm	55953-0114-58	250s	$265.39
Raway	00686-3147-13	500s	$140.00
Major	00904-3801-40	500s	$279.90
▶ Rugby	00536-0130-05	500s	$319.86
Warner Chilcott	00047-0939-30	500s	$332.00
Geneva	00781-2532-05	500s	$335.00
Moore,H.L.	00839-7312-12	500s	$341.40
▶ Novopharm	55953-0114-70	500s	$360.10
Martec	52555-0971-05	500s	$363.70
Aligen	00405-4153-02	500s	$366.74
Mason Dist	11845-0158-03	500s	$370.60
URL	00677-1159-05	500s	$377.55
▶ Apothecon	00003-0874-60	500s	$392.16
Jerome Stevens	50564-0469-05	500s	$420.39
Qualitest	00603-2596-28	500s	$435.00
▶ Zenith	00172-4074-70	500s	$438.90
Parmed	00349-8652-05	500s	$445.00
▶ Barr	00555-0515-04	500s	$478.89
▶ Lemmon	00093-0543-05	500s	$530.00
Mylan	00378-6050-05	500s	$555.95
Goldline	00182-1279-05	500s	$556.93
▶ Biocraft	00332-3147-13	500s	$556.93
Du Pont Multi	00056-0194-85	500s	$612.62
▶ Novopharm	55953-0114-80	1000s	$684.23
Parmed	00349-8652-10	1000s	$695.00

POWDER FOR RECONSTITUTION: 125 MG/5 ML

AVERAGE UNIT PRICE (AVAILABLE SIZES)		GENERIC A-RATED AVERAGE PRICE (GAAP)	
BRAND	$0.13	100 ml	$6.62
GENERIC	$0.06	200 ml	$12.08
HCFA FUL (100 ml)	$0.03		
HCFA FUL (200 ml)	$0.02		

BRAND/MANUFACTURER	NDC	SIZE	AWP
◆ BRAND			
KEFLEX: Dista	00777-2321-48	100 ml	$12.75
	00777-2321-89	200 ml	$25.25

BRAND/MANUFACTURER	NDC	SIZE	AWP
◆ GENERICS			
Raway	00686-4175-32	100 ml	$4.85
Schein	00364-2163-61	100 ml	$5.57
Apothecon	00003-2201-30	100 ml	$5.98
Warner Chilcott	00047-2375-17	100 ml	$5.99
Moore,H.L.	00839-7313-73	100 ml	$6.06
URL	00677-1187-27	100 ml	$6.15
Rugby	00536-0116-82	100 ml	$6.15
Qualitest	00603-6541-64	100 ml	$6.20
Lederle Std Prod	00005-3229-46	100 ml	$6.36
Geneva	00781-7028-46	100 ml	$6.40
Lemmon	00093-0538-73	100 ml	$6.50
Major	00904-3802-04	100 ml	$6.90
Goldline	00182-7020-70	100 ml	$7.08
Biocraft	00332-4175-32	100 ml	$7.08
Parmed	00349-8653-01	100 ml	$7.20
Novopharm	55953-0106-40	100 ml	$7.40
Barr	00555-0525-22	100 ml	$7.67
Aligen	00405-2500-60	100 ml	$7.76
Du Pont Multi	00056-0203-36	100 ml	$8.43
Raway	00686-4175-36	200 ml	$4.65
Schein	00364-2163-63	200 ml	$9.62
Qualitest	00603-6541-68	200 ml	$10.50
Warner Chilcott	00047-2375-20	200 ml	$10.97
Moore,H.L.	00839-7313-78	200 ml	$11.00
Rugby	00536-0116-84	200 ml	$11.10
Barr	00555-0525-23	200 ml	$11.58
Apothecon	00003-2201-30	200 ml	$11.86
URL	00677-1187-29	200 ml	$11.95
Geneva	00781-7028-48	200 ml	$11.99
Lemmon	00093-0538-74	200 ml	$12.00
Lederle Std Prod	00005-3229-60	200 ml	$12.63
Major	00904-3802-08	200 ml	$12.85
Goldline	00182-7020-73	200 ml	$13.09
Biocraft	00332-4175-36	200 ml	$13.09
Parmed	00349-8653-02	200 ml	$13.45
Novopharm	55953-0106-53	200 ml	$13.83
Du Pont Multi	00056-0203-39	200 ml	$15.21
Aligen	00405-2500-70	200 ml	$18.13

POWDER FOR RECONSTITUTION: 250 MG/5 ML

AVERAGE UNIT PRICE (AVAILABLE SIZES)		GENERIC A-RATED AVERAGE PRICE (GAAP)	
BRAND	$0.26	100 ml	$11.68
GENERIC	$0.11	200 ml	$22.15
HCFA FUL (100 ml)	$0.04		
HCFA FUL (200 ml)	$0.04		

BRAND/MANUFACTURER	NDC	SIZE	AWP
◆ BRAND			
KEFLEX: Dista	00777-2368-48	100 ml	$23.99
	00777-2368-89	200 ml	$47.53
	00777-2368-33	5 ml 100s ud	$156.17
◆ GENERICS			
Major	00904-3803-04	100 ml	$6.90
Raway	00686-4177-32	100 ml	$7.95
Schein	00364-2164-61	100 ml	$9.62
Warner Chilcott	00047-2376-17	100 ml	$10.75
Moore,H.L.	00839-7314-73	100 ml	$11.19
Apothecon	00003-2202-30	100 ml	$11.34
Geneva	00781-7029-46	100 ml	$11.39
Qualitest	00603-6542-64	100 ml	$11.50
Rugby	00536-0118-82	100 ml	$11.55
URL	00677-1188-27	100 ml	$11.60
Barr	00555-0526-22	100 ml	$11.73
Lederle Std Prod	00005-3230-46	100 ml	$11.99
Lemmon	00093-0540-73	100 ml	$12.25
Goldline	00182-7021-70	100 ml	$12.62
Biocraft	00332-4177-32	100 ml	$12.62
Aligen	00405-2525-60	100 ml	$13.44
Parmed	00349-8654-01	100 ml	$14.00
Novopharm	55953-0092-40	100 ml	$14.04
Du Pont Multi	00056-0204-36	100 ml	$15.44
Raway	00686-4177-36	200 ml	$8.95
Schein	00364-2164-63	200 ml	$18.15
Warner Chilcott	00047-2376-20	200 ml	$19.76
Qualitest	00603-6542-68	200 ml	$20.00
Barr	00555-0526-23	200 ml	$20.56
Moore,H.L.	00839-7314-78	200 ml	$20.64
Rugby	00536-0118-84	200 ml	$20.85
Lemmon	00093-0540-74	200 ml	$22.50
Geneva	00781-7029-48	200 ml	$22.57
URL	00677-1188-29	200 ml	$22.60
Apothecon	00003-2202-40	200 ml	$22.62
Major	00904-3803-08	200 ml	$23.10
Lederle Std Prod	00005-3230-60	200 ml	$23.76
Parmed	00349-8654-02	200 ml	$24.95
Goldline	00182-7021-73	200 ml	$25.01
Biocraft	00332-4177-36	200 ml	$25.01
Novopharm	55953-0092-53	200 ml	$25.10
Aligen	00405-2525-70	200 ml	$27.02
Du Pont Multi	00056-0204-39	200 ml	$27.61

TABLETS: 250 MG

AVERAGE UNIT PRICE (AVAILABLE SIZES)		GENERIC A-RATED AVERAGE PRICE (GAAP)	
GENERIC	$0.49	100s	$49.12
HCFA FUL (100s ea)	$0.36		

BRAND/MANUFACTURER	NDC	SIZE	AWP
◆ GENERICS			
Moore,H.L.	00839-7461-06	100s	$32.33
Schein	00364-2292-01	100s	$34.11
Major	00904-3795-60	100s	$49.40
Goldline	00182-1886-01	100s	$57.25
Biocraft	00332-2238-09	100s	$57.25
Lederle Std Prod	00005-3331-23	100s	$64.38

TABLETS: 500 MG

AVERAGE UNIT PRICE (AVAILABLE SIZES)		GENERIC A-RATED AVERAGE PRICE (GAAP)	
GENERIC	$0.97	100s	$96.49
HCFA FUL (100s ea)	$0.72		

BRAND/MANUFACTURER	NDC	SIZE	AWP
◆ GENERICS			
Moore,H.L.	00839-7462-06	100s	$64.73
Schein	00364-2293-01	100s	$88.90
Goldline	00182-1887-01	100s	$89.80
Biocraft	00332-2240-09	100s	$112.51
Lederle Std Prod	00005-3332-23	100s	$126.50

Cephalothin Sodium

DESCRIPTION

Cephalothin Sodium, Neutral, is a semisynthetic cephalosporin antibiotic for parenteral use. It is 5-thia-1-azabicyclo[4.2.0]oct-2-ene-2-carboxylic acid, 3-[(acetyloxy)methyl]-8-oxo-7-[(2-thienylacetyl)amino]-, monosodium, salt, (6R-*trans*)-. Cephalothin Sodium, Neutral, contains 30 mg of sodium bicarbonate/g of Cephalothin Sodium to result in reconstituted solutions having a pH ranging between 6.0 and 8.5. Free Cephalothin acid does not form within this range, and the solubility and freezability are thereby enhanced. The total sodium content is approximately 63 mg (2.8 mEq sodium ion) per g of Cephalothin Sodium.

Cephalothin was synthesized in the Lilly Research Laboratories by the reaction of thiophene-2-acetic acid with 7-aminocephalosporanic acid. The cephalosporanic acid nucleus is obtained from cephalosporin C, which is produced by the fungus *Cephalosporium*. Cephalothin is supplied as the sodium salt of 7-(thiophene-2-acetamido) cephalosporanic acid.

Cephalothin is a cream-colored crystalline solid that is stable in the dry state and moderately soluble in distilled water (250 to 300 mg/mL). Calcium disodium edetate, 0.005%, has been added at the time of manufacture.

The molecular weight of Cephalothin Sodium is 418.4 and the molecular formula is $C_{16}H_{15}N_2NaO_6S_2$.

Following is its chemical structure:

CLINICAL PHARMACOLOGY

Human Pharmacology: Cephalothin Sodium is a broad-spectrum antibiotic for parenteral administration. After administration of a 500-mg dose intramuscularly to normal volunteers, the average peak serum antibiotic level at 1/2 hour was 10 µg/mL; with a 1-g dose, the average was about 20 µg/mL. Following a single 1-g intravenous dose of Cephalothin Sodium, blood levels have been about 30 µg/mL at 15 minutes, have ranged from 3 to 12 µg/mL at 1 hour, and have declined to about 1 µg/mL at 4 hours. With continuous infusion at the rate of 500 mg/h, levels have been from 14 to 20 µg/mL of serum. Dosages of 2 g given intravenously over a 30-minute period have produced serum concentrations of 80 to 100 µg/mL 1/2 hour after the infusion; levels ranged from 10 to 40 µg/mL at 1 hour and from 3 to 6 µg/mL at 2 hours and were not assayable after 5 hours.

Sixty percent to 70% of an intramuscular dose is excreted by the kidneys in the first 6 hours; this results in high urine levels, e.g., 800 µg/mL of urine after a 500-mg dose and 2,500 µg/mL following 1 g. Probenecid slows tubular excretion and almost doubles peak blood levels.

Spinal-fluid levels have ranged from 0.4 to 1.4 µg/mL in a child and from 0.15 to 5 µg/mL in adults with meningeal inflammatory states. The antibiotic passes readily into other body fluids, e.g., pleural, joint, and ascitic fluids. Studies of amniotic fluid and cord blood show prompt transfer of Cephalothin Sodium across the placenta.

Following single 1-g intramuscular doses of Cephalothin, peak maternal levels were reached between 31 and 45 minutes after injection; the peak levels in the infants occurred about 15 minutes later. All plasma levels in the infants were far below those of the mothers.

Secondary aqueous-humor levels have averaged 0.5 µg/mL 30 minutes after a single 1-g intravenous dose. The antibiotic has been detected in bile.

Microbiology: The *in vitro* bactericidal action of Cephalothin results from inhibition of cell-wall synthesis. Cephalothin Sodium is usually active against the following organisms *in vitro*:

β-hemolytic and other streptococci (many strains of enterococci, e.g., *Enterococcus* [formerly *Streptococcus*] *faecalis*, are relatively resistant)
Staphylococci, including coagulase-positive, coagulase-negative, and penicillinase-producing strains
Streptococcus pneumoniae
Haemophilus influenzae
Escherichia coli and other coliform bacteria
Klebsiella sp
Proteus mirabilis
Salmonella sp
Shigella sp
Pseudomonas organisms are resistant to Cephalothin Sodium, as are most indole-producing *Proteus* sp and motile *Enterobacter* sp.

Susceptibility Plate Tests: If the Bauer-Kirby-Sherris-Turck method of disk susceptibility testing* is used, a disk containing 30 µg Cephalothin should give a zone of over 17 mm when tested against a Cephalothin-susceptible bacterial strain and a zone of over 14 mm with an organism of intermediate susceptibility.

INDICATIONS AND USAGE

Cephalothin Sodium is indicated for the treatment of serious infections caused by susceptible strains of the designated microorganisms in the diseases listed below. Culture and susceptibility studies should be performed. Therapy may be instituted before results of susceptibility studies are obtained.

Respiratory tract infections caused by *S. pneumoniae*, staphylococci (penicillinase- and non-penicillinase-producing), group A β-hemolytic streptococci, *Klebsiella* sp, and *H. influenzae*

Skin and soft-tissue infections, including peritonitis, caused by staphylococci (penicillinase- and non-penicillinase-producing), group A β-hemolytic steptococci, *E. coli, P. mirabilis,* and *Klebsiella* sp

Genitourinary tract infections caused by *E. coli, P. mirabilis,* and *Klebsiella* sp

Septicemia, including endocarditis, caused by *S. pneumoniae*, staphylococci (penicillinase- and non-penicillinase-producing), group A β-hemolytic streptococci, *Streptococcus viridans, E. coli, P. mirabilis,* and *Klebsiella* sp

Gastrointestinal infections caused by *Salmonella* and *Shigella* sp

Meningitis caused by *S. pneumoniae*, group A β-hemolytic streptococci, and staphylococci (penicillinase- and non-penicillinase-producing)

Note: Inasmuch as only low levels of Cephalothin Sodium are found in the cerebrospinal fluid, the drug is not reliable in the treatment of meningitis and cannot be recommended for that purpose. Cephalothin Sodium has, however, proved to be effective in a number of cases of meningitis and may be considered for unusual circumstances in which other, more reliably effective antibiotics cannot be used.

Bone and joint infections caused by staphylococci (penicillinase- and non-penicillinase-producing)

The prophylactic administration of Cephalothin Sodium preoperatively, intraoperatively, and postoperatively may reduce the incidence of certain postoperative infections in patients undergoing surgical procedures (e.g., vaginal hysterectomy) that are classified as contaminated or potentially contaminated.

The perioperative use of Cephalothin Sodium also may be effective in surgical patients in whom infection at the operative site would present a serious risk, e.g., during open heart surgery and prosthetic arthroplasty.

The prophylactic administration of Cephalothin Sodium should be discontinued within 24 hours after the surgical procedure. If there are signs of infection, specimens for culture should be obtained for the identification of the causative organism so that appropriate therapy may be instituted (see "Dosage and Administration").

Note: If the susceptibility tests show that the causative organism is resistant to Cephalothin Sodium, other appropriate antibiotic therapy should be instituted.

CONTRAINDICATION

Cephalothin Sodium is contraindicated in persons who have shown hypersensitivity to cephalosporin antibiotics.

WARNINGS

BEFORE CEPHALOTHIN THERAPY IS INSTITUTED, CAREFUL INQUIRY SHOULD BE MADE CONCERNING PREVIOUS HYPERSENSITIVITY REACTIONS TO CEPHALOSPORINS AND PENICILLIN. CEPHALOSPORIN C DERIVATIVES SHOULD BE GIVEN CAUTIOUSLY TO PENICILLIN-SENSITIVE PATIENTS.

SERIOUS ACUTE HYPERSENSITIVITY REACTIONS MAY REQUIRE EPINEPHRINE AND OTHER EMERGENCY MEASURES.

There is some clinical and laboratory evidence of partial cross-allergenicity of the penicillins and the cephalosporins. Patients have been reported to have had severe reactions (including anaphylaxis) to both drugs.

Any patient who has demonstrated some form of allergy, particularly to drugs, should receive antibiotics cautiously and then only when absolutely necessary. No exception should be made with regard to Cephalothin Sodium.

---

* Bauer AW, Kirby WMM, Sherris JC, et al: Antibiotic susceptibility testing by a standardized single disk method. *Am Clin Pathol* 1966;45:493; Standardized disk susceptibility test. *Federal Register* 1974;39:19182-19184. National Committee for Clinical Laboratory Standards. Approved Standard: M2-A3 Performance Standards for Antimicrobial Disk Susceptibility Tests—Third Edition, December, 1984.

◆ RATED THERAPEUTICALLY EQUIVALENT; ◇ THERAPEUTIC EQUIVALENCE UNCONFIRMED; ○ UNRATED

Pseudomembranous colitis has been reported with virtually all broad-spectrum antibiotics (including macrolides, semisynthetic penicillins, and cephalosporins); therefore, it is important to consider its diagnosis in patients who develop diarrhea in association with the use of antibiotics. Such colitis may range in severity from mild to life threatening.

Treatment with broad-spectrum antibiotics alters the normal flora of the colon and may permit overgrowth of clostridia. Studies indicate that a toxin produced by *Clostridium difficile* is a primary cause of antibiotic-associated colitis.

Mild cases of pseudomembranous colitis usually respond to drug discontinuance alone. In moderate to severe cases, management should include sigmoidoscopy, appropriate bacteriologic studies, and fluid, electrolyte, and protein supplementation. When the colitis does not improve after the drug has been discontinued, or when it is severe, oral vancomycin is the drug of choice for antibiotic-associated pseudomembranous colitis produced by *C. difficile*. Other causes of colitis should be ruled out.

PRECAUTIONS

General: Patients should be followed carefully so that any side effects or unusual manifestations of drug idiosyncrasy may be detected. If an allergic reaction to Cephalothin Sodium occurs, the drug should be discontinued and the patient treated with the usual agents (e.g., epinephrine or other pressor amines, antihistamines, or corticosteroids).

Although Cephalothin Sodium rarely produces alteration in kidney function, evaluation of renal status is recommended, especially in seriously ill patients receiving maximum doses. Patients with impaired renal function should be placed on the dosage schedule recommended under *"Dosage and Administration"*. Usual doses in such individuals may result in excessive serum concentrations.

When intravenous doses of Cephalothin larger than 6 g daily are given by infusion for periods longer than 3 days, they may be associated with thrombophlebitis, and the veins may have to be alternated. The addition of 10 to 25 mg of hydrocortisone to intravenous solutions containing 4 to 6 g of Cephalothin may reduce the incidence of thrombophlebitis. The use of small IV needles in the larger available veins may be preferred.

Prolonged use of Cephalothin Sodium may result in the overgrowth of nonsusceptible organisms. Constant observation of the patient is essential. If superinfection occurs during therapy, appropriate measures should be taken.

A false-positive reaction for glucose in the urine may occur with Benedict's or Fehling's solution or with Clinitest® tablets but not with Tes-Tape® (Glucose Enzymatic Test Strip.)

An increased incidence of nephrotoxicity has been reported following concomitant administration of cephalosporins and aminoglycoside antibiotics.

Broad-spectrum antibiotics should be prescribed with caution in individuals with a history of gastrointestinal disease, particularly colitis.

Usage in Pregnancy: Pregnancy Category B: Reproduction studies have been performed in rabbits given doses of 200 mg/kg and have revealed no evidence of impaired fertility or harm to the fetus due to Cephalothin Sodium. There are, however, no adequate and well-controlled studies, in pregnant women. Because animal reproduction studies are not always predictive of human response, this drug should be used during pregnancy only if clearly needed.

Nursing Mothers: Caution should be exercised when Cephalothin Sodium is administered to a nursing woman.

ADVERSE REACTIONS

Hypersensitivity: Maculopapular rash, urticaria, reactions resembling serum sickness, and anaphylaxis have been reported. Eosinophilia and drug fever have been observed to be associated with other allergic reactions. These reactions are most likely to occur in patients with a history of allergy, particularly to penicillin.

Blood: Neutropenia, thrombocytopenia, and hemolytic anemia have been reported. Some individuals, particularly those with azotemia, have developed positive direct Coomb's tests during Cephalothin therapy.

Liver: Transient rise in SGOT and alkaline phosphatase has been noted.

Kidney: Rise in BUN and decreased creatinine clearance have been reported, particularly in patients with prior renal impairment. The role of Cephalothin Sodium in renal changes is difficult to assess, because other factors predisposing to prerenal azotemia or to acute renal failure usually have been present.

Local Reactions: Pain, induration, tenderness, and elevation of temperature have been reported following repeated intramuscular injections. Thrombophlebitis has occurred and is usually associated with daily doses of more than 6 g given by infusion for longer than 3 days.

Gastrointestinal: Symptoms of pseudomembranous colitis may appear either during or after antibiotic treatment. Nausea and vomiting have been reported rarely.

OVERDOSAGE

The administration of inappropriately large doses of parenteral cephalosporins may cause seizures, particularly in patients with renal impairment. Dosage reduction is necessary when renal function is impaired (see *"Dosage and Administration"*). If seizures occur, the drug should be promptly discontinued; anticonvulsant therapy may be administered if clinically indicated. Hemodialysis may be considered in cases of overwhelming overdosage.

To obtain up-to-date information about the treatment of overdose, a good resource is your certified regional poison control center. Telephone numbers of certified poison control centers are listed in the *Physicians' Desk Reference (PDR).*

In managing overdosage, consider the possibility of multiple drug overdoses, interaction among drugs, and unusual drug kinetics in your patient.

DOSAGE AND ADMINISTRATION

In adults, the usual dosage range is 500 mg to 1 g of Cephalothin every 4 to 6 hours. A dosage of 500 mg every 6 hours is adequate in uncomplicated pneumonia, furunculosis with cellulitis, and most urinary tract infections. In severe infections, this may be increased by giving the injections every 4 hours or, when the desired response is not obtained, by raising the dose to 1 g. In life-threatening infections, doses up to 2 g every 4 hours may be required.

For perioperative prophylactic use to prevent postoperative infection in contaminated or potentially contaminated surgery in adults, the following doses are recommended:

(a) 1 to 2 g administered IV just prior to surgery (approximately 1/2 to 1 hour before the initial incision);

(b) 1 to 2 g during surgery (administration modified according to the duration of the operative procedure); and

(c) 1 to 2 g q6h postoperatively for 24 hours.

In children, 20 to 30 mg/kg may be given at the times designated above.

Since Cephalothin Sodium has a serum half-life of 30 to 50 minutes, it is important that (1) the preoperative dose be given just prior to the start of surgery so that adequate antibiotic levels are present in the serum and tissues at the time of initial surgical incision; and (2) Cephalothin Sodium be administered, if necessary, at appropriate intervals during surgery to provide sufficient levels of the antibiotic at the anticipated moments of greatest exposure to infective organisms.

When renal function is reduced, an intravenous loading dose of 1 to 2 g may be given. Continued dosage schedule should be determined by degree of renal impairment, severity of infection, and susceptibility of the causative organism. The maximum doses administered should be based on the following recommendations.

DOSAGE OF CEPHALOTHIN SODIUM WHEN RENAL FUNCTION IS IMPAIRED

Status of Renal Function	Maximum Adult Dosage (Maintenance)
Mild Impairment (C_{cr}=80-50 mL/min)	2 g q6h
Moderate Impairment (C_{cr}=50-25 mL/min)	1.5 g q6h
Severe Impairment (C_{cr}=25-10 mL/min)	1 g q6h
Marked Impairment (C_{cr}=10-2 mL/min)	0.5 g q6h
Essentially No Function (C_{cr}=< 2 mL/min)	0.5 g q8h

In infants and children, the dosage should be proportionately less in accordance with age, weight, and severity of infection. Daily administration of 100 mg/kg (80 to 160 mg/kg or 40 to 80 mg/lb) in divided doses has been found effective for most infections susceptible to Cephalothin Sodium.

Antibiotic therapy in β-hemolytic streptococcal infections should continue for at least 10 days. In staphylococcal infections, surgical procedures, such as incision and drainage, should be carried out in all cases when indicated.

Cephalothin Sodium may be given intravenously or by deep intramuscular injection into a large muscle mass, such as the gluteus or lateral aspect of the thigh, to minimize pain and induration.

Intramuscular: Each g of Cephalothin should be diluted with 4 mL of Sterile Water for Injection. If the vial contents do not completely dissolve, an additional small amount of diluent (e.g., 0.2 to 0.4 mL) may be added and the contents warmed slightly.

Intravenous: The intravenous route may be preferable for patients with bacteremia, septicemia, or other severe or life-threatening infections who may be poor risks because of lowered resistance resulting from such debilitating conditions as malnutrition, trauma, surgery, diabetes, heart failure, or malignancy, particularly if shock is present or impending. For these infections in patients with normal renal function, the intravenous dosage is 4 to 12 g of Cephalothin daily. In conditions such as septicemia, 6 to 8 g/day may be given intravenously for several days at the beginning of therapy; then, depending on the clinical response and laboratory findings, the dosage may gradually be reduced.

For intermittent intravenous administration, a solution containing 1 g Cephalothin in 10 mL of diluent may be slowly injected directly into the vein over a period of 3 to 5 minutes or may be given through the tubing when the patient is receiving parenteral solutions.

Intermittent intravenous infusion with a Y-type administration set can also be accomplished while bulk intravenous solutions are being infused. However, during infusion of the solution containing Cephalothin Sodium, it is desirable to discontinue the other solution. When this technique is employed, careful attention should be paid to the volume of the solution containing Cephalothin Sodium so that the calculated dose will be infused.

For continuous intravenous infusion, 1 or 2 g of Cephalothin, diluted and well mixed with at least 10 mL of Sterile Water for Injection, may be added to an IV bottle containing one of the following intravenous solutions: Acetated Ringer's Injection, 5% Dextrose Injection, 5% Dextrose in Lactated Ringer's Injection, Ionosol® B in D5-W, Isolyte® M with 5% Dextrose, Lactated Ringer's Injection, Normosol®-M in D5-W, Plasma-Lyte® Injection, Plasma-Lyte®-M Injection in 5% Dextrose, Ringer's Injection, or 0.9% Sodium Chloride Injection. The choice of solution and the volume to be employed are dictated by fluid and electrolyte management.

▶ SHOWN IN PRODUCT IDENTIFICATION GUIDE

Intraperitoneal: In peritoneal dialysis procedures, Cephalothin has been added to dialysis fluid in concentrations up to 6 mg/100 mL and instilled into the peritoneal space throughout an entire dialysis (16 to 30 hours). Careful assay procedures have shown that 44% of the administered drug was absorbed into the bloodstream. Serum levels of 10 µg/mL were reported, with no evidence of accumulation and no untoward local or systemic reactions.

The intraperitoneal administration of solutions containing 0.1% to 4% Cephalothin Sodium in saline has been used in treating patients with peritonitis or contaminated peritoneal cavities. (The total daily dosage of Cephalothin Sodium should take into account the amount given by the intraperitoneal route.)

STABILITY

While stored under *refrigeration*, the solution has a satisfactory potency for 96 hours after reconstitution. Solutions may precipitate; they can be redissolved by being warmed to room temperature with constant agitation. Kept at *room temperature*, solutions for intramuscular injection should be given within 12 hours after being mixed. Intravenous infusions should be started within 12 hours and completed within 24 hours. For prolonged infusions, replace with a freshly prepared solution at least every 24 hours.

The concentrated solution will darken, especially at room temperature. Slight discoloration of the solution is permissible.

Solutions of Cephalothin Sodium in Sterile Water for Injection, 5% Dextrose Injection, or 0.9% Sodium Chloride Injection that are frozen immediately after reconstitution in the conventional vials in which the drugs are supplied are stable for as long as 12 weeks when stored at −20°C. **If the product is warmed, care should be taken to avoid heating it after the thawing is complete. Once thawed, the solution should not be refrozen.**

J CODES

Up to 1 g IM,IV—J1890

HOW SUPPLIED
POWDER FOR INJECTION: 1 GM

AVERAGE UNIT PRICE (AVAILABLE SIZES)

BRAND		$3.61	

BRAND/MANUFACTURER	NDC	SIZE	AWP
◆ BRAND			
KEFLIN: Lilly	00002-7001-01	1s	$3.42
	00002-7001-25	25s	$85.53
	00002-7260-25	25s	$99.80

POWDER FOR INJECTION: 2 GM

AVERAGE UNIT PRICE (AVAILABLE SIZES)

BRAND		$7.13	

BRAND/MANUFACTURER	NDC	SIZE	AWP
◆ BRAND			
KEFLIN: Lilly	00002-7003-10	10s	$68.42
	00002-7261-10	10s	$74.13

Cephapirin Sodium

DESCRIPTION

Cephapirin Sodium is a cephalosporin antibiotic intended for intramuscular or intravenous administration or for intravenous injection only, depending on the product. Each 500 mg contains 1.18 mEq of sodium; each gram of intravenous (IV) only contains 2.36 mEq of sodium.

Cephapirin Sodium is the sodium salt of 7-α-(4-pyridylthio)-acetamido-cephalosporanic acid. The empirical formula is $C_{17}H_{16}N_3NaO_6S_2$ and the molecular weight is 445.44.

The pharmacy bulk package is a container of a sterile dosage form for parenteral use that contains many single doses. The pharmacy bulk package contains Cephapirin Sodium equivalent to 20 grams Cephapirin. The contents are intended for use in the preparation of admixtures for intravenous infusion. FURTHER DILUTION IS REQUIRED.

Following is its chemical structure:

CLINICAL PHARMACOLOGY

Table 1
DURATION OF BLOOD LEVELS OF CEPHAPIRIN IN NORMAL VOLUNTEERS (FIGURES ARE µg/mL)

	Time After Injection in Hours		
	½	4	6
Cephapirin Sodium 500 mg IM (single dose)	9.0	0.7	0.2
Cephapirin Sodium 1 g IM (single dose)	16.4	1.0	0.3

Cephapirin Sodium and its metabolites were excreted primarily by the kidneys. Antibiotic activity in the urine was equivalent to 35% of a 500 mg dose 6 hours after IM injection, and to 65% of a 500 mg dose 12 hours after injection. Following an IM dose of 500 mg, peak urine levels averaged 900 µg/mL within the first 6 hours.

Table 2
DURATION OF BLOOD LEVELS OF CEPHAPIRIN IN NORMAL VOLUNTEERS (FIGURES ARE µg/mL)

	Time After Injection in Minutes		
	5	30	180
Cephapirin Sodium 500 mg rapid IV	35	6.7	0.27
Cephapirin Sodium 1 g rapid IV	67	14.0	0.61
Cephapirin Sodium 2 g rapid IV	129	31.7	1.11

Seventy percent of the administered dose was recovered in the urine within 6 hours.

Repetitive intravenous administration of 1 g doses over 6 hour periods produced serum levels between 4.5 and 5.5 µg/mL.

At therapeutic drug levels, normal human serum binds Cephapirin Sodium to the extent of 44% to 50%. The average serum half-life of Cephapirin Sodium in patients with normal renal function is approximately 36 minutes.

The major metabolite of Cephapirin is desacetyl Cephapirin which has been shown to contribute to antibacterial activity.

Controlled studies in normal adult volunteers revealed that Cephaprin Sodium was well tolerated intramuscularly. In controlled studies of volunteers and of patients receiving IV Cephapirin Sodium, the incidence of venous irritation was low.

Microbiology: In vitro tests demonstrate that the action of cephalosporins results from inhibition of cell-wall synthesis. Cephapirin Sodium is active against the following organisms *in vitro:*

Beta-hemolytic streptococci and other streptococci. (Many strains of enterococci, eg, *S. faecalis,* are relatively resistant.)

Staphylococcus aureus (penicillinase and nonpenicillinase-producing); *Staphylococcus epidermidis* (methicillin-susceptible strains); *Streptococcus pneumoniae* (formerly *Diplococcus pneumoniae*); *Proteus mirabilis; Haemophilus Influenzae; Escherichia coli;* Klebsiella species.

Most strains of Enterobacter and indole-positive Proteus (*P. vulgaris, P morganii, P rettgeri*) are resistant to Cephapirin Sodium. Methicillin-resistant staphylococci, Serratia, Pseudomonas, Mima, and Herellea species are almost uniformly resistant to Cephapirin Sodium.

Disc Susceptibility Tests: Quantitative methods that require measurement of zone diameters give the most precise estimates of antibiotic susceptibility. One such procedure* has been recommended for use with discs for testing susceptibility to cephalosporin class antibiotics. Interpretations correlate diameters of the disc test with MIC values for Cephapirin Sodium. With this procedure, a report from the laboratory of "susceptible" indicates that the infecting organism is likely to respond to therapy. A report of "resistant" indicates that the infecting organism is not likely to respond to therapy. A report of "intermediate susceptibility" suggests that the organism would be susceptible if high dosage is used, or if the infection is confined to tissues and fluid (eg, urine), in which high antibiotic levels are attained.

INDICATIONS AND USAGE

Cephapirin Sodium is indicated in the treatment of infections caused by susceptible strains of the designated microorganisms in the diseases listed below. Culture and susceptibility studies should be performed. Therapy may be instituted before results of susceptibility studies are obtained.

Respiratory tract infections caused by *S. pneumoniae* (formerly *D. pneumoniae*). *Staphylococcus aureus* (penicillinase and nonpenicillinase-producing), Klebsiella species, *H. influenzae,* and group A beta-hemolytic streptococci.

Skin and skin structure infections caused by *Staphylococcus aureus* (penicillinase and nonpenicillinase-producing), *Staphylococcus epidermidis* (methicillin-susceptible strains), *E. Coli, P. mirabilis,* Klebsiella species, and group A beta-hemolytic streptococci.

Urinary tract infections caused by *Staphylococcus aureus* (penicillinase and nonpenicillinase-producing), *E. coli, P. mirabilis,* and Klebsiella species.

Septicemia caused by *Staphylococcus aureus* (penicillinase and nonpenicillinase-producing), *S. viridans, E. coli,* Klebsiella species and group A beta-hemolytic streptococci.

Endocarditis caused by *Streptococcus viridans* and *Staphylococcus aureus* (penicillinase and nonpenicillinase-producing).

* Bauer, A.W., Kirby, W.M.M., Sherris, J.C. and Turck, M.: Antibiotic Testing by a Standardized Single Disc Method, Am. J. Clin. Pathol., 45:493, 1966; Standardized Disc Susceptibility Test, FEDERAL REGISTER 37:2052729, 1972.

Osteomyelitis caused by *Staphylococcus aureus* (penicillinase and nonpenicillinase-producing), Klebsiella species, *P. mirabilis*, and group A beta-hemolytic streptococci.

Perioperative Prophylaxis: The prophylactic administration of Cephapirin Sodium preoperatively and postoperatively may reduce the incidence of certain postoperative infections in patients undergoing surgical procedures which are classified as contaminated or potentially contaminated, eg, vaginal hysterectomy.

The perioperative use of Cephapirin Sodium may also be effective in surgical patients in whom infection at the operative site would present a serious risk, eg, during open-heart surgery and prosthetic arthroplasty.

The prophylactic administration of Cephapirin Sodium should be discontinued within a 24 hour period after the surgical procedure. In surgery where the occurrence of infection may be particularly devastating, eg, open-heart surgery and prosthetic arthroplasty, the prophylactic administration of Cephapirin Sodium may be continued for 3 to 5 days following completion of surgery. If there are signs of infection, specimens for culture should be obtained for the identification of the causative organism so that appropriate therapy may be instituted. (See *"Dosage and Administration"*.)

Note: If the susceptibility tests show that the causative organism is resistant to Cephapirin Sodium, other appropriate therapy should be instituted.

CONTRAINDICATIONS

Cephapirin Sodium is contraindicated in persons who have shown hypersensitivity to cephalosporin antibiotics.

WARNINGS

IN PENICILLIN-ALLERGIC PATIENTS, CEPHALOSPORINS SHOULD BE USED WITH GREAT CAUTION. THERE IS CLINICAL AND LABORATORY EVIDENCE OF PARTIAL CROSS-ALLERGENICITY OF THE PENICILLINS AND THE CEPHALOSPORINS, AND THERE ARE INSTANCES OF PATIENTS WHO HAVE HAD REACTIONS TO BOTH DRUGS (INCLUDING ANAPHYLAXIS AFTER PARENTERAL USE).

Any patient who has demonstrated some form of allergy, particularly to drugs, should receive antibiotics cautiously and then only when absolutely necessary. No exceptions should be made with regard to Cephapirin Sodium.

Pseudomembranous colitis has been reported with the use of cephalosporins; therefore, it is important to consider its diagnosis in patients who develop diarrhea in association with antibiotic use.

SERIOUS ANAPHYLACTOID REACTIONS REQUIRE IMMEDIATE EMERGENCY TREATMENT WITH EPINEPHRINE. OXYGEN, INTRAVENOUS STEROIDS, AND AIRWAY MANAGE- MENT, INCLUDING INTUBATION, SHOULD ALSO BE ADMINISTERED AS INDICATED.

PRECAUTIONS

Usage in Pregnancy: Pregnancy Category B. Reproduction studies have been performed in rats and mice and have revealed no evidence of impaired fertility or harm to the fetus due to Cephapirin Sodium. There are, however, no well controlled studies in pregnant women. Because animal studies are not always predictive of human response, this drug should be used during pregnancy only if clearly indicated.

Nursing Mothers: Cephapirin Sodium may be present in human milk in small amounts. Caution should be exercised when Cephapirin Sodium is administered to a nursing woman.

The renal status of the patient should be determined prior to and during Cephapirin Sodium therapy, since in patients with impaired renal function, a reduced dose may be appropriate (see *"Dosage, Adults"*). When Cephapirin Sodium was given to patients with marked reduction in renal function and to renal transplant patients, no adverse effects were reported.

Prolonged use of Cephapirin Sodium may result in the overgrowth of nonsusceptible organisms. Careful observation of the patient is essential. If superinfection occurs during therapy, appropriate measures should be taken.

With high urine concentrations of Cephapirin, false-positive glucose reactions may occur if Clinitest, Benedict's Solution, or Fehling's Solution are used. Therefore, it is recommended that glucose tests based on enzymatic glucose oxidase reactions (such as Clinistix or Tes-Tape) be used.

Increased nephrotoxicity has been reported following concomitant administration of cephalosporins and aminoglycoside antibiotics.

ADVERSE REACTIONS

Hypersensitivity: Cephalosporins were reported to produce the following reactions: maculopapular rash, urticaria, reactions resembling serum sickness, and anaphylaxis. Eosinophilia and drug fever have been observed to be associated with other allergic reactions. These reactions are most likely to occur in patients with a history of allergy, particularly to penicillin.

Blood: During large scale clinical trials, rare instances of neutropenia, leukopenia, and anemia were reported. Some individuals, particularly those with azotemia, have developed positive direct Coombs' test during therapy with other cephalosporins.

Liver: Elevations in SGPT or SGOT, alkaline phosphatase, and bilirubin have been reported.

Kidney: Rises in BUN have been observed; their frequency increases in patients over 50 years old.

Gastrointestinal: Symptoms of pseudomembranous colitis can appear during or after antibiotic treatment. (See *"Warnings"*).

DOSAGE AND ADMINISTRATION

Adults: The usual dose is 500 mg to 1 g every 4 to 6 hours intramuscularly or intravenously or, with some products, intravenously only. The lower dose of 500 mg is adequate for certain infections, such as skin and skin structure and most urinary tract infections. However, the higher dose is recommended for more serious infections.

Very serious or life-threatening infections may require doses up to 12 grams daily. The intravenous route is preferable when high doses are indicated.

Depending upon the causative organism and the severity of infection, patients with reduced renal function (moderately severe oliguria or serum creatinine above 5.0 mg/100 mL) may be treated adequately with a lower dose, 7.5 to 15 mg/kg of Cephapirin every 12 hours. Patients with severely reduced renal function and who are to be dialyzed should receive the same dose just prior to dialysis and every 12 hours thereafter.

Perioperative Prophylactic Use: To prevent postoperative infection in contaminated or potentially contaminated surgery. Recommended doses are:

a. 1 to 2 g IM or IV administered ½ hour to 1 hour prior to the start of surgery.
b. 1 to 2 g during surgery (administration modified depending on the duration of the operative procedure).
c. 1 to 2 g IV or IM every 6 hours for 24 hours postoperatively.

It is important (1) the preoperative dose be given just prior to the start of surgery (½ to 1 hour) so that adequate antibiotic levels are present in the serum and tissues at the time of initial surgical incision, and (2) Cephapirin Sodium be administered, if necessary, at appropriate intervals during surgery to provide sufficient levels of the antibiotic at the anticipated moments of greatest exposure to infective organisms.

In surgery where the occurrence of infection may be particularly devastating, eg, open-heart surgery and prosthetic arthroplasty, the prophylactic administration of Cephapirin Sodium may be continued for 3 to 5 days following completion of surgery.

Children: The dosage is in accordance with age, weight, and severity of infection. The recommended total daily dose is 40 to 80 mg/kg (20 to 40 mg/lb) administered in four equally divided doses or administered over a 24-hour period with the ADD-Vantage System.

The drug has not been extensively studied in infants; therefore, in the treatment of children under the age of three months the relative benefit/risk should be considered.

Therapy in beta-hemolytic streptococcal infections should continue for at least 10 days.

Where indicated, surgical procedures should be performed in conjunction with antibiotic therapy.

Cephapirin Sodium may be administered by the intramuscular or the intravenous routes or, with some products, by the intravenous route only. The intent of the pharmacy bulk package is for the preparation of solutions for IV infusion only.

Intramuscular Injection: The 500 mg and 1 g vials should be reconstituted with 1 or 2 mL of Sterile Water for Injection, USP, or Bacteriostatic Water for Injection, USP, respectively. Each 1.2 mL contains 500 mg of Cephapirin. All injections should be deep in the muscle mass.

Intravenous Injection: The intravenous route may be preferable for patients with bacteremia, septicemia, or other severe or life-threatening infections who may be poor risks because of lowered resistance resulting from such debilitating conditions as malnutrition, trauma, surgery, diabetes, heart failure, or malignancy, particularly if shock is present or impending. If patient has impaired renal function, a reduced dose may be indicated (see *"Dosage Adults"*) In conditions such as septicemia, 6 to 8 g per day may be given intravenously for several days at the beginning of therapy, then, depending on the clinical response and laboratory findings, the dosage may gradually be reduced.

When the infection has been refractory to previous forms of treatment and multiple sites have been involved, daily doses up to 12 grams have been used.

Intermittent Intravenous Injection: The contents of the 500 mg, 1 g, or 2 g vial should be diluted with 10 mL or more of the specified diluent and administered slowly over a 3- to 5-minute period or may be given with intravenous infusions.

Intermittent Intravenous Infusion with Y-Tube: Intermittent intravenous infusion with a Y-type administration set can also be accomplished while bulk intravenous solutions are being infused. However, during infusion of the solution containing Cephapirin Sodium it is desirable to discontinue the other solution. When this technique is employed careful attention should be paid to the volume of the solution containing Cephapirin Sodium so that the calculated dose will be infused. When a Y-tube hookup is used, the contents of the 4 g vial of Cephapirin should be diluted by addition of 40 mL of Bacteriostatic Water for Injection, USP, Dextrose Injection, USP, or Sodium Chloride Injection, USP.

STABILITY UTILITY TIME FOR CEPHAPIRIN SODIUM IN VARIOUS DILUENTS AT CONCENTRATIONS RANGING FROM 20 TO 400 MG/ML

Diluent	Approximate Concentration (mg/mL)	25° C	Utility Time 4° C
Water for Injection	50 to 400	12 hours	10 days

Diluent	Approximate Concentration (mg/mL)	Utility Time 25° C	Utility Time 4° C
Bacteriostatic Water for Injection with Benzyl Alcohol or Parabens	250 to 400	48 hours	10 days
Normal Saline	20 to 100	24 hours	10 days
5% Dextrose in Water	20 to 100	24 hours	10 days

This information represents chemical stability only. A pharmacy bulk package should NOT be used after 4 hours of initial entry.

All of the above solutions can be frozen immediately after reconstitution and stored at —15° C for 60 days before use. After thawing, at room temperature (25° C), all of the solutions are stable for at least 12 hours at room temperature or 10 days under refrigeration (4° C).

The pH of the resultant solution ranges from 6.5 to 8.5. During these storage conditions, no precipitation occurs. A change in solution color during this storage time does not affect the potency.

Note: This chemical stability information in no way indicates that it would be acceptable practice to infuse a Cephapirin infusion well after the preparation time. Good professional practice suggests that administration of compounded admixture should be as soon after preparation as is feasible.

Compatibility with the Infusion Solution: Cephapirin Sodium is stable and compatible for 24 hours at room temperature at concentrations between 2 mg/mL and 30 mg/mL in the following solutions:

Sodium Chloride Injection, USP; 5% W/V Dextrose in Water, USP; Sodium Lactate Injection, USP; 5% Dextrose in Normal Saline, USP; 10% Invert Sugar in Normal Saline; 10% Invert Sugar in Water; 5% Dextrose + 0.2% Sodium Chloride Injection, USP; Lactated Ringer's Injection, USP; Lactated Ringer's with 5% Dextrose; 5% Dextrose + 0.45% Sodium Chloride Injection, USP; Ringer's Injection, USP; 10% Dextrose Injection, USP; Sterile Water for Injection, USP; 20% Dextrose Injection, USP; 5% Sodium Chloride in Water; 5% Dextrose in Ringer's Injection; Normosol® R; Normosol® R in 5% Dextrose Injection; Ionosol® D-CM; Ionosol® G in 10% Dextrose Injection.

In addition, Cephapirin Sodium, at a concentration of 4 mg/mL, is stable and compatible for 10 days under refrigeration (4° C) or 14 days in the frozen state (-15° C) followed by 24 hours at room temperature (25° C) in all of the intravenous solutions listed above.

"Piggyback" IV Package: This glass vial contains the labeled quanity of Cephapirin Sodium and is intended for intravenous administration. The diluent and volume are specified on the label.

Parenteral drug products should be inspected visually for particulate matter and discoloration prior to administration, whenever solution and container permit.

Pharmacy Bulk Package: This glass vial contains 20 g Cephapirin Sodium and is designed for use in the pharmacy in preparing IV additives. Add 67 mL of Sodium Chloride Injection, USP or dextrose Injection, USP. The resulting solution will contain 250 mg mL Cephapirin activity per mL.

Directions For Proper Use of Pharmacy Bulk Package: a) The container closure may be penetrated only one time, utilizing a suitable sterile transfer device or other sterile dispensing device which allows measured distribution of the contents. A sterile substance which must be reconstituted prior to use may require a separate closure entry.

b) Use of this product is restricted to a suitable work area, such as a laminar flow hood.

c) After initial entry, the withdrawal of container contents should be accomplished without delay. However, should this not be possible, a maximum time of 4 hours from initial closure entry is permitted to complete fluid transfer operations. This time limit should begin with the introduction of solvent or diluent into the PBP when reconstituting. The prompt use of transferred/admixed fluids is recommended.

J CODES
Up to 1 g IV,IM—J0710

HOW SUPPLIED
POWDER FOR INJECTION: 1 GM

AVERAGE UNIT PRICE (AVAILABLE SIZES)

BRAND		$2.43		

BRAND/MANUFACTURER		NDC	SIZE	AWP
◆ BRAND				
CEFADYL: Apothecon		00015-7628-28	1s	$2.35
		00015-7628-22	1s	$2.51

POWDER FOR INJECTION: 2 GM

BRAND/MANUFACTURER	NDC	SIZE	AWP
◆ BRAND			
CEFADYL: Apothecon	00015-7629-28	1s	$4.84

POWDER FOR INJECTION: 20 GM

BRAND/MANUFACTURER	NDC	SIZE	AWP
◆ BRAND			
CEFADYL: Apothecon	00015-7613-20	1s	$45.07

Cephradine

DESCRIPTION
Cephradine is a semisynthetic cephalosporin antibiotic; oral dosage forms include capsules containing 250 mg and 500 mg Cephradine and Cephradine for oral suspension containing, after constitution, 125 mg and 250 mg per 5 mL dose.

Cephradine is designated chemically as (6R,7R)-7-[(R)-2-amino-2-(1,4-cyclohexadien-1-yl)acetamido]-3-methyl-8-oxo-5-thia-1-azabicyclo[4.2.0]oct-2-ene-2-carboxylic acid. Its empirical formula is $C_{16}H_{19}N_3O_4S$; molecular weight is 349.40 and CAS number is 31828-50.9.

Following is its chemical structure:

CLINICAL PHARMACOLOGY
Cephradine is acid stable. It is rapidly absorbed after oral administration in the fasting state. Following single doses of 250 mg, 500 mg, and 1 g in normal adult volunteers, average peak serum concentrations within one hour were approximately 9 mcg/mL, 16.5 mcg/mL, and 24.2 mcg/mL, respectively. *In vitro* studies by an ultracentrifugation technique show that at therapeutic serum antibiotic concentrations, Cephradine is minimally bound (8 to 17 percent) to normal serum protein. Cephradine does not pass across the blood-brain barrier to any appreciable extent. The presence of food in the gastrointestinal tract delays absorption but does not affect the total amount of Cephradine absorbed. Over 90 percent of the drug is excreted unchanged in the urine within six hours. Peak urine concentrations are approximately 1600 mcg/mL, 3200 mcg/mL, and 4000 mcg/mL following single doses of 250 mg, 500 mg, and 1 g, respectively.

Microbiology: In vitro tests demonstrate that the cephalosporins are bactericidal because of their inhibition of cell-wall synthesis. Cephradine is active against the following organisms *in vitro*:

Group A beta-hemolytic streptococci
Staphylococci, including coagulase-positive, coagulase-negative, and penicillinase-producing strains
Streptococcus pneumoniae (formerly *Diplococcus pneumoniae*)
Escherichia coli
Proteus mirabilis
Klebsiella species
Hemophilus influenzae

Cephradine is not active against most strains of *Enterobacter* species, *P. morganii*, and *P. vulgaris*. It has no activity against *Pseudomonas* or *Herellea* species. When tested by *in vitro* methods, staphylococci exhibit cross-resistance between Cephradine and methicillin-type antibiotics.

Note: Most strains of enterococci (*Streptococcus faecalis*) are resistant to Cephradine.

Disc Susceptibility Tests: Quantitative methods that require measurement of zone diameters give the most precise estimates of antibiotic susceptibility. One recommended procedure (21 CFR § 460.1) uses cephalosporin class discs for testing susceptibility; interpretations correlate zone diameters of this disc test with MIC values for Cephradine. With this procedure, a report from the laboratory of "resistant" indicates that the infecting organism is not likely to respond to therapy. A report of "intermediate susceptibility" suggests that the organism would be susceptible if the infection is confined to the urinary tract, as high antibiotic levels can be obtained in the urine, or if high dosage is used in other types of infection.

INDICATIONS AND USAGE
Cephradine is indicated in the treatment of the following infections when caused by susceptible strains of the designated microorganisms:

Respiratory Tract Infections: e.g., tonsilitis, pharyngitis, and lobar pneumonia) caused by group A beta-hemolytic streptococci and *S. pneumonia* (formerly *D. pneumoniae*).

(Penicillin is the usual drug of choice in the treatment and prevention of streptococcal infections, including the prophylaxis of rheumatic fever. Cephradine is generally effective in the eradication of streptococci from the nasopharynx; substantial data establishing the efficacy of Cephradine in the subsequent prevention of rheumatic fever are not available at present.)

◆ RATED THERAPEUTICALLY EQUIVALENT; ◇ THERAPEUTIC EQUIVALENCE UNCONFIRMED; ○ UNRATED

Ottis Media: caused by group A beta-hemolytic streptococci, *S. pneumoniae* (formerly *D. pneumoniae*) *H. influenzae,* and staphy- lococci.

Skin and Skin Structure Infections: caused by staphylococci (penicillin-susceptible and penicillin-resistant) and beta-hemolytic streptococci.

Urinary Tract Infections: Including prostatitis, caused by *E. coli, P. mirabilis, Klebsiella* species, and enterococci (*S. faecalis*). The high concentrations of Cephradine achievable in the urinary tract will be effective against many strains of enterococci for which disc susceptibility studies indicate relative resistance. It is to be noted that among beta-lactam antibiotics, ampicillin is the drug of choice for enterococcal urinary tract (*S. faecalis*) infection.

Cephradine is also indicated in the treatment of bone infections caused by S. aureus, and septicemia caused by *S. aureus, S. pneumoniae, P. mirabilis* or *E. coli.*

Note: Culture and susceptibility tests should be initiated prior to and during therapy.

Following clinical improvement achieved with parenteral therapy, oral Cephradine may be utilized for continuation of treatment of persistent or severe conditions where prolonged therapy is indicated.

UNLABELED USES
Cephradine is used alone or as an adjunct as an alternative to penicillin in the treatment of syphilis.

CONTRAINDICATIONS
Cephradine is contraindicated in patients with known hypersensitivity to the cephalosporin group of antibiotics.

WARNINGS
In penicillin-sensitive patients, cephalosporin derivatives should be used with great caution. There is clinical and laboratory evidence of partial cross-allergenicity of the penicillins and the cephalosporins, and there are instances of patients who have had reactions to both drug classes (including anaphylaxis after parenteral use).

Any patient who has demonstrated some form of allergy, particularly to drugs, should receive antibiotics, including Cephradine, cautiously and then only when absolutely necessary.

Pseudomembranous colitis has been reported with the use of cephalosporins (and other broad spectrum antibiotics); therefore, it is important to consider its diagnosis in patients who develop diarrhea in association with antibiotic use. Treatment with broad spectrum antibiotics alters normal flora of the colon and may permit overgrowth of clostridia. Studies indicate a toxin produced by *Clostridium difficile* is one primary cause of antibiotic-associated colitis. Cholestyramine and colestipol resins have been shown to bind the toxin *in vitro.* Mild cases of colitis may respond to drug discontinuance alone. Moderate to severe cases should be managed with fluid, electrolyte and protein supplementation as indicated. When the colitis is not relieved by drug discontinuance or when it is severe, oral vancomycin is the treatment of choice for antibiotic-associated pseudomembranous colitis produced by *C. difficile.* Other causes of colitis should also be considered.

PRECAUTIONS
GENERAL
Patients should be followed carefully so that any side effects or unusual manifestations of drug idiosyncrasy may be detected. If a hypersensitivity reaction occurs, the drug should be discontinued and the patient treated with the usual agents, e.g., pressor amines, antihistamines, or corticosteroids.

Administer Cephradine with caution in the presence of markedly impaired renal function. In patients with known or suspected renal impairment, careful clinical observation and appropriate laboratory studies should be made prior to and during therapy as Cephradine accumulates in the serum and tissues. See *"Dosage and Admininstration"* section for information on treatment of patients with impaired renal function.

Cephradine should be prescribed with caution in individuals with a history of gastrointestinal disease, particularly colitis.

Prolonged use of antibiotics may promote the overgrowth of nonsusceptible organisms. Should superinfection occur during therapy, appropriate measures should be taken.

Indicated surgical procedures should be performed in conjunction with antibiotic therapy.

INFORMATION FOR PATIENTS
Caution diabetic patients that false results may occur with urine glucose tests (see *"Precautions, Drug/Laboratory Test Interactions"*).

Advise the patient to comply with the full course of therapy even if he begins to feel better and to take a missed dose as soon as possible. Inform the patient that this medication may be taken with food or milk since gastrointestinal upset may be a factor in compliance with the dosage regimen. The patient should report current use of any medicines and should be cautioned not to take other medications unless the physician knows and approves of their use (see *"Precautions, Drug Interactions"*).

LABORATORY TESTS
In patients with known or suspected renal impairment, it is advisable to monitor renal function (see *"Dosage And Administration"*).

DRUG INTERACTIONS
When administered concurrently, the following drugs may interact with cephalosporins:

Other Antibacterial Agents: Bacteriostats may interfere with the bactericidal action of cephalosporins in acute infection; other agents, e.g., aminoglycosides, colistin, polymyxins, vancomycin, may increase the possibility of nephrotoxicity.

Diuretics: (potent "loop diuretics," e.g., furosemide and ethacrynic acid): Enhanced possibility for renal toxicity.

Probenecid: Increased and prolonged blood levels of cephalosporins, resulting in increased risk of nephrotoxicity.

DRUG/LABORATORY TEST INTERACTIONS
After treatment with Cephradine, a false-positive reaction for glucose in the urine may occur with Benedict's solution, Fehling's solution, or with Clinitest® tablets, but not with enzyme-based tests such as Clinistix® and Tes-Tape®.

False-positive Coombs test results may occur in newborns whose mothers received a cephalosoporin prior to delivery.

Cephalosporins have been reported to cause false-positive reactions in tests for urinary proteins which use sulfosalicylic acid, false elevations of urinary 17-ketosteroid values, and prolonged prothrombin times.

CARCINOGENESIS, MUTAGENESIS
Long-term studies in animals have not been performed to evaluate carcinogenic potential or mutagenesis.

PREGNANCY CATEGORY B
Reproduction studies have been performed in mice and rats at doses up to four times the maximum indicated human dose and have revealed no evidence of impaired fertility or harm to the fetus due to Cephradine. There are, however, no adequate and well-controlled studies in pregnant women. Because animal reproduction studies are not always predictive of human response, this drug should be used during pregnancy only if clearly needed.

NURSING MOTHERS
Since Cephradine is excreted in breast milk during lactation, caution should be exercised when Cephradine is administered to a nursing woman.

PEDIATRIC USE
See *"Dosage and Administration".* Adequate information is unavailable on the efficacy of b.i.d. regimens in children under nine months of age.

ADVERSE REACTIONS
As with other cephalosporins, untoward reactions are limited essentially to gastrointestinal disturbances and, on occasion, to hypersensitivity phenomena. The latter are more likely to occur in individuals who have previously demonstrated hypersensitivity and those with a history of allergy, asthma, hay fever, or urticaria.

The following adverse reactions have been reported following the use of Cephradine:

Gastrointestinal: Symptoms of pseudomembranous colitis can appear during antibiotic treatment. Nausea and vomiting have been reported rarely.

Skin and Hypersensitivity Reactions: Mild urticaria or skin rash, pruritus, and joint pains were reported by very few patients.

Hematologic: Mild, transient eosinophilia, leukopenia, and neutropenia have been reported.

Liver: Transient mild rise of SGOT, SGPT, and total bilirubin have been observed with no evidence of hepatocellular damage.

Renal: Transitory rises in BUN have been observed in some patients treated with cephalosporins; their frequency increases in patients over 50 years old. In adults for whom serum creatinine determinations were performed, the rise in BUN was not accompanied by a rise in serum creatinine.

Other adverse reactions have included dizziness and tightness in the chest and candidal vaginitis.

DOSAGE AND ADMINISTRATION
Cephradine may be given without regard to meals.

Adults: For respiratory tract infections (other than lobar pneumonia) and skin and skin structure infections, the usual dose is 250 mg every 6 hours or 500 mg every 12 hours.

For lobar pneumonia, the usual dose is 500 mg every 6 hours or 1 g every 12 hours.

For uncomplicated urinary tract infections, the usual dose is 500 mg every 12 hours. In more serious urinary tract infections, including prostatitis, 500 mg every 6 hours or 1 g every 12 hours may be administered.

Larger doses (up to 1 g every 6 hours) may be given for severe or chronic infections.

Children: No adequate information is available on the efficacy of b.i.d. regimens in children under nine months of age. The usual dose in children over nine months of age is 25 to 50 mg/kg/day administered in equally divided doses every 6 or 12 hours. For otitis media due to *H. influenzae,* doses are from 75 to 100 mg/kg/day administered in equally divided doses every 6 or 12 hours, but should not exceed 4 g per day. Dosage for children should not exceed dosage recommended for adults.

All patients, regardless of age and weight: Larger doses (up to 1 g q.i.d.) may be given for severe or chronic infections.

As with antibiotic therapy in general, treatment should be continued for a minimum of 48 to 72 hours after the patient becomes asymptomatic or evidence of bacterial eradication has been obtained. In infections caused by group A beta-

► SHOWN IN PRODUCT IDENTIFICATION GUIDE

hemolytic streptococci, a minimum of 10 days of treatment is recommended to guard against the risk of rheumatic fever or glomerulonephritis. In the treatment of chronic urinary tract infection, frequent bacteriologic and clinical appraisal is necessary during therapy and may be necessary for several months afterwards. Persistent infections may require treatment for several weeks. Prolonged intensive therapy is recommended for prostatitis. Doses smaller than those indicated are not recommended.

PATIENTS WITH IMPAIRED RENAL FUNCTION

Not on Dialysis: The following initial dosage schedule is suggested as a guideline based on creatinine clearance. Further modification in the dosage schedule may be required because of individual variations in absorption.

Creatinine Clearance	Dose	Time Interval
> 20 mL/min	500 mg	6 hours
5–20 mL/min	250 mg	6 hours
< 5 mL/min	250 mg	12 hours

On Chronic, Intermittent Hemodialysis:
250 mg Start
250 mg at 12 hours
250 mg 36-48 hours (after start)

Children may require dosage modification proportional to their weight and severity of infection.

STORAGE

Capsules: Keep tightly closed. Do not store above 86°F.

Oral Suspension: Prior to constitution, store at room temperature; avoid excessive heat. After constitution, when stored at room temperature, discard unused portion after seven days; when stored in refrigerator, discard unused portion after 14 days. Keep tightly closed.

HOW SUPPLIED
CAPSULE: 250 MG

AVERAGE UNIT PRICE (AVAILABLE SIZES)		GENERIC A-RATED AVERAGE PRICE (GAAP)	
BRAND	$0.85		
GENERIC	$0.54	24s	$16.38
HCFA FUL (100s ea)	$0.33	100s	$52.42

BRAND/MANUFACTURER	NDC	SIZE	AWP
◆ **BRAND**			
➤ VELOSEF: Apothecon	00003-0113-24	24s	$20.74
	00003-0113-50	100s	$82.55
◆ **GENERICS**			
Schein	00364-2141-24	24s	$16.25
Biocraft	00332-3153-08	24s	$16.50
Raway	00686-3153-09	100s	$30.00
Schein	00364-2141-01	100s	$36.30
Lederle Std Prod	00005-3406-23	100s	$47.46
Warner Chilcott	00047-0808-24	100s	$48.54
Qualitest	00603-2619-21	100s	$53.00
Geneva	00781-2533-01	100s	$53.73
Goldline	00182-1253-01	100s	$54.75
URL	00677-1135-01	100s	$54.95
Rugby	00536-0180-01	100s	$54.98
Major	00904-2837-60	100s	$55.00
Biocraft	00332-3153-09	100s	$55.00
Moore,H.L.	00839-7262-06	100s	$57.90
Aligen	00405-4158-01	100s	$59.51
Parmed	00349-8616-01	100s	$66.34
Raway	00686-0606-20	100s ud	$37.50
Goldline	00182-1253-89	100s	$59.00
UDL	51079-0606-20	100s ud	$67.20
Rugby	00536-0180-05	500s	$260.85

CAPSULE: 500 MG

AVERAGE UNIT PRICE (AVAILABLE SIZES)		GENERIC A-RATED AVERAGE PRICE (GAAP)	
BRAND	$1.66	24s	$26.71
GENERIC	$1.03	100s	$101.61
HCFA FUL (100s ea)	$0.66		

BRAND/MANUFACTURER	NDC	SIZE	AWP
◆ **BRAND**			
➤ VELOSEF: Apothecon	00003-0114-26	24s	$40.81
	00003-0114-50	100s	$162.13
◆ **GENERICS**			
Raway	00686-3155-08	24s	$18.00
Biocraft	00332-3155-08	24s	$26.20
Schein	00364-2142-24	24s	$31.25
Geneva	00781-2534-24	24s	$31.37
Raway	00686-3155-09	100s	$52.00
Lederle Std Prod	00005-3407-23	100s	$93.71
Warner Chilcott	00047-0809-24	100s	$93.99
Qualitest	00603-2620-21	100s	$98.00
Biocraft	00332-3155-09	100s	$102.00

BRAND/MANUFACTURER	NDC	SIZE	AWP
Schein	00364-2142-01	100s	$102.64
Geneva	00781-2534-01	100s	$103.42
Major	00904-2838-60	100s	$104.70
Goldline	00182-1254-01	100s	$104.95
URL	00677-1136-01	100s	$105.35
Moore,H.L.	00839-7263-06	100s	$105.42
Rugby	00536-0185-01	100s	$108.60
Aligen	00405-4159-01	100s	$114.45
Parmed	00349-8617-01	100s	$130.54
Raway	00686-0607-20	100s ud	$65.00
Goldline	00182-1254-89	100s ud	$110.90
UDL	51079-0607-20	100s ud	$131.72
Rugby	00536-0185-05	500s	$488.70

POWDER FOR RECONSTITUTION: 125 MG/5 ML

AVERAGE UNIT PRICE (AVAILABLE SIZES)		GENERIC A-RATED AVERAGE PRICE (GAAP)	
BRAND	$0.09	100 ml	$6.27
GENERIC	$0.06		
HCFA FUL (100 ml)	$0.07		

BRAND/MANUFACTURER	NDC	SIZE	AWP
◆ **BRAND**			
VELOSEF: Apothecon	00003-1193-50	100 ml	$9.05
	00003-1193-80	200 ml	$17.89
◆ **GENERICS**			
Raway	00686-4165-32	100 ml	$4.25
Biocraft	00332-4165-32	100 ml	$7.07
Goldline	00182-7014-70	100 ml	$7.50

POWDER FOR RECONSTITUTION: 250 MG/5 ML

AVERAGE UNIT PRICE (AVAILABLE SIZES)		GENERIC A-RATED AVERAGE PRICE (GAAP)	
BRAND	$0.17	100 ml	$11.56
GENERIC	$0.12		
HCFA FUL (100 ml)	$0.13		

BRAND/MANUFACTURER	NDC	SIZE	AWP
◆ **BRAND**			
VELOSEF: Apothecon	00003-1194-50	100 ml	$16.98
	00003-1194-80	200 ml	$33.62
◆ **GENERICS**			
Raway	00686-4167-32	100 ml	$7.98
Schein	00364-2144-61	100 ml	$12.75
Goldline	00182-7015-70	100 ml	$12.75
Biocraft	00332-4167-32	100 ml	$12.77

Cephulac SEE LACTULOSE

Ceptaz SEE CEFTAZIDIME

Ceredase SEE ALGLUCERASE

Cerezyme SEE IMIGLUCERASE

Cerubidine SEE DAUNORUBICIN HYDROCHLORIDE

Cerumenex SEE TRIETHANOLAMINE POLYPEPTIDE OLEATE-CONDENSATE

Cetacaine SEE BENZOCAINE/BUTAMBEN/TETRACAINE

Cetacort SEE HYDROCORTISONE, TOPICAL

Cetamide SEE SULFACETAMIDE SODIUM, OPHTHALMIC

Cetapred SEE PREDNISOLONE AND SULFACETAMIDE SODIUM

◆ RATED THERAPEUTICALLY EQUIVALENT; ◇ THERAPEUTIC EQUIVALENCE UNCONFIRMED; ○ UNRATED

Chardonna-2 SEE BELLADONNA AND PHENOBARBITAL

Chemet SEE SUCCIMER

Cheracol with Codeine SEE CODEINE PHOSPHATE WITH GUAIFENESIN

Chibroxin SEE NORFLOXACIN, OPHTHALMIC

Children's Advil SEE IBUPROFEN

Chlor-Trimeton SEE CHLORPHENIRAMINE MALEATE, INJECTABLE

Chloral Hydrate

DESCRIPTION

Capsule and Syrup for oral administration:

Each capsule contains:

Chloral Hydrate .... 500 mg
   (**Warning:** *May be habit forming.*)

Syrup available in two strengths as follows:

Each 10 mL delivers:

Chloral Hydrate .... 500 mg
or
Chloral Hydrate .... 1 g
   (**Warning:** *May be habit forming.*)

Chemically, Chloral Hydrate is 1,1-Ethanediol, 2,2,2-trichloro.
   Chloral Hydrate acts as a sedative and hypnotic.

   Following is its chemical structure:

$$CCl_3CH(OH)_2$$

CLINICAL PHARMACOLOGY

Chloral Hydrate is the oldest member of the hypnotic group of drugs. The action of Chloral Hydrate is confined to the cerebral hemispheres. The drug is detoxified in the liver and subsequently eliminated by the kidney.

INDICATIONS AND USAGE

Chloral Hydrate is used primarily as a hypnotic in the treatment of simple insomnia. It is effective as a hypnotic only for short term use. Chloral Hydrate has been found to lose much of its effectiveness for both inducing and maintaining sleep by the end of a 2 week period of drug administration.
   Chloral Hydrate may also be used as a routine sedative. It has been used preoperatively or prior to electroencephalographic evaluation to allay anxiety and produce sedation and/or sleep. Chloral Hydrate, alone or in conjunction with paraldehyde, is effective in preventing alcohol withdrawal symptoms and/or suppressing the syndrome once it develops. The drug may also be effective in reducing anxiety associated with withdrawal of other drugs such as narcotics or barbiturates. Chloral Hydrate is often used in elderly patients, infants, and young children because many clinicians believe that it produces paradoxical excitement less frequently than do barbiturates; however, no well controlled studies have confirmed this clinical impression.

CONTRAINDICATIONS

Chloral Hydrate is contraindicated in patients with marked hepatic or renal impairment and in patients who have previously demonstrated hypersensitivity or an idiosyncratic reaction to the drug.

WARNINGS

Chloral Hydrate may be habit-forming.
   Chloral Hydrate may increase the rate of metabolism of concomitantly administered coumarin anticoagulants, thus reducing their effectiveness. Upon withdrawal of Chloral Hydrate, the rate of metabolism of the anticoagulant drug will decrease and its plasma level will rise, with the possibility of a sudden increase of anticoagulant effects (i.e., development of bleeding tendency and hemorrhage). The prothrombin time of patients on anticoagulant therapy normally must be followed continually; however, when Chloral Hydrate is added to or subtracted from the therapeutic regimen, or when changes in dosage of Chloral Hydrate are contemplated, the effect of the sedative on prothrombin time deserves special attention.

PRECAUTIONS

General: Chloral Hydrate should be used cautiously in patients who are mentally depressed, have suicidal tendencies or a history of drug abuse, or whose history indicates they may increase dosage on their own initiative. Oral administration of Chloral Hydrate should be avoided in patients with esophagitis, gastritis, or gastric or duodenal ulcers. Continued therapeutic doses of Chloral Hydrate have been shown to be without deleterious effect on the heart. Large doses of Chloral Hydrate, however, should not be used in patients with severe cardiac disease. Gastritis, skin eruptions, or parenchymatous renal damage may develop following prolonged administration of Chloral Hydrate. Rarely prolonged use of Chloral Hydrate may produce tolerance and physical and/or psychological dependence. Following chronic administration, Chloral Hydrate should be withdrawn slowly to avoid the possibility of precipitating withdrawal symptoms.

Information for Patients: The patient should be warned that Chloral Hydrate may impair ability to perform hazardous activities requiring mental alertness or physical coordination such as operating machinery or driving a motor vehicle. In addition, the patient should be cautioned against taking other depressant drugs, including alcohol, while using Chloral Hydrate. Chloral Hydrate capsules should be taken with a full glass of water or liquid.

Drug Interactions: Additive central nervous depression may occur when Chloral Hydrate is administered concomitantly with other central nervous system depressants such as paraldehyde, barbiturates or alcohol. In addition, patients receiving Chloral Hydrate may develop a vasodilation reaction characterized by tachycardia, palpitations, facial flushing and dysphoria after ingesting alcohol. If Chloral Hydrate is used concomitantly with other depressant drugs including alcohol, caution should be used to avoid overdosage.
   A reaction characterized by diaphoresis, flushes, variable blood pressure including hypertension, and uneasiness has been reported in some patients with acute myocardial infarction and congestive heart failure who received furosemide (Lasix®) intravenously within 24 hours after administration of an oral hypnotic dose of Chloral Hydrate. Therefore, it may be preferable to use an alternate hypnotic drug, e.g., a benzodiazepine, in patients who require intravenously administered furosemide.
   Although some investigators believe that the clinical significance of the interaction between Chloral Hydrate and coumarin anticoagulants is negligible, some clinical studies have shown that concurrent administration of Chloral Hydrate and warfarin may result in a transient potentiation of warfarin-induced hypoprothrombinemia. Apparently the trichloroacetic acid metabolite of Chloral Hydrate displaces warfarin from its binding sites on plasma albumin resulting in a transient increase in free plasma warfarin. Chloral Hydrate should be used with caution in patients receiving warfarin or other oral anticoagulants and it is preferable to use an alternative hypnotic drug, e.g., a benzodiazepine, which does not alter the anticoagulant response in patients receiving anticoagulants. If Chloral Hydrate is added to the therapeutic regimen of a patient maintained on an oral anticoagulant, reduction in anticoagulant dosage may be required in order to prevent excessive hypoprothrombinemia; conversely, the discontinuation of Chloral Hydrate in patients also taking oral anticoagulants may require increased dosage to maintain adequate anticoagulation.

Drug/Laboratory Test Interactions: Chloral Hydrate may produce false-positive results for urine glucose determinations utilizing cupric sulfate as Benedict's Solution. Apparently, the drug does not interfere with urine glucose tests utilizing cupric sulfate tablets (Clinitest®) or glucose oxidase such as Clinistix® or Testape®. Chloral Hydrate may interfere with fluorometric tests for urine catecholamines, and it has been recommended that the drug not be administered for 48 hours preceding the test. Chloral Hydrate administration may also interfere with the Reddy, Jenkins, Thorn procedure for determining urinary 17-hydroxycorticosteroids.

Pregnancy: Teratogenic Effects-Pregnancy Category C: Animal reproduction studies have not been conducted with Chloral Hydrate. It is also not known whether Chloral Hydrate can cause fetal harm when administered to a pregnant woman or can affect reproduction capacity. Chloral Hydrate should be given to a pregnant woman only if clearly needed (Chloral Hydrate has been shown to cross the placenta and may be found in the amniotic fluid and fetal blood).

Nursing Mothers: Chloral Hydrate is excreted in human milk. Caution should be exercised when Chloral Hydrate is administered to a nursing woman.

ADVERSE REACTIONS

Gastric irritation manifested by nausea, vomiting, and diarrhea is the most frequent side effect of oral Chloral Hydrate administration. This effect may be minimized by administering the capsules with a full glass of water or other liquid. There is no evidence in the published literature to support the claim that the complex, chloral betaine, causes less gastric irritation than does Chloral Hydrate. Residual sedation or "hangover" occurs infrequently following usual hypnotic doses. Cutaneous reactions to Chloral Hydrate are not common but have included scarlatiniform or erythematous rash, urticaria, angioedema, purpura, eczema, bullous lesions, and erythema multiforme. Sometimes these cutaneous reactions have been accompanied by fever. Ataxia and dizziness have also occurred. Rarely, a somnambulistic reaction characterized by disorientation and incoherence has been reported.

DRUG ABUSE AND DEPENDENCE

Controlled Substance: Chloral Hydrate is a schedule IV drug.

Abuse: while Chloral Hydrate may be habit forming, tolerance and addiction are uncommon.

Dependence: Symptoms of Chloral Hydrate dependence are similar to those of chronic alcoholism. Sudden withdrawal of the drug from physically dependent persons may cause delirium tremens and hallucinations. For this reason, Chloral Hydrate should be withdrawn slowly.

OVERDOSAGE

Chloral Hydrate overdosage produces symptoms which are similar to those of barbiturate overdosage and may include coma, hypotension, hypothermia, respiratory depression, and cardiac arrhythmias. Miosis, vomiting, areflexia, and muscle flaccidity may also occur. Esophageal stricture, gastric necrosis and perforation, and gastrointestinal hemorrhage have also been reported. Hepatic and renal function may be impaired and may result in transient jaundice and/or albuminuria. Death may result from respiratory failure or hypotension, ingestion of 4 grams of Chloral Hydrate has caused death, although some patients have survived the ingestion of as much as 30 grams of the drug.

Treatment of Chloral Hydrate intoxication consists of general supportive therapy including maintenance of an adequate airway, assisted respiration, oxygen administration, and maintaining body temperature and circulation. Gastric lavage may be done following oral overdosage if an endotracheal tube with cuff inflated is in place to prevent aspiration of vomitus. Peritoneal dialysis or hemodialysis may be beneficial.

DOSAGE AND ADMINISTRATION

The usual hypnotic dose of Chloral Hydrate for adults is 500 mg to 1 gram 15 to 30 minutes before retiring; the usual sedative dosage is 250 mg 3 times daily after meals. When Chloral Hydrate is administered in the management of alcohol withdrawal symptoms, the usual dosage is 500 mg to 1 gram repeated at 6-hour intervals if needed. Generally, single doses or daily dosage for adults should not exceed 2 grams.

For children, the hypnotic dose of Chloral Hydrate is 50 mg per kg of body weight or 1.5 grams per square meter of body surface area with a maximum single dose of 1 gram. The sedative dosage for children is 8 mg per kg of body weight or 250 mg per square meter of body surface area 3 times a day with a maximum dosage of 500 mg 3 times a day. As a premedication before electroencephalographic evaluation, children have been given Chloral Hydrate in a dosage of 20 to 25 mg per kg of body weight.

HOW SUPPLIED
CAPSULE (C-IV): 500 MG

BRAND/MANUFACTURER	NDC	SIZE	AWP
○ GENERICS			
Phys Total Care	54868-1864-01	30s	$4.07
Allscrips	54569-0897-00	60s	$5.14
Lannett	00527-0557-01	100s	$4.00
Cooper Drug	00779-4147-25	100s	$5.36
Schein	00364-0061-01	100s	$8.15
Mason Dist	11845-0122-01	100s	$8.21
Major	00904-3828-60	100s	$8.25
URL	00677-0225-01	100s	$8.50
Rugby	00536-3477-01	100s	$9.07
Caraco	57664-0204-08	100s	$9.50
Goldline	00182-0297-01	100s	$10.35
Goldline	00182-0324-01	100s	$10.35
Interstate	00814-1625-14	100s	$11.48
Vangard	00615-0413-13	100s ud	$13.89
Roxane	00054-8140-25	100s ud	$17.10
Lannett	00527-0557-05	500s	$17.00

SUPPOSITORY (C-IV): 325 MG

BRAND/MANUFACTURER	NDC	SIZE	AWP
○ BRAND			
AQUACHLORAL SUPPRETTES: Polymedica	00998-6005-75	12s	$26.25

SUPPOSITORY (C-IV): 500 MG

BRAND/MANUFACTURER	NDC	SIZE	AWP
○ GENERICS			
CMC-Cons	00223-5300-01	100s	$125.00
G&W	00713-0122-01	100s ud	$131.25

SUPPOSITORY (C-IV): 650 MG

BRAND/MANUFACTURER	NDC	SIZE	AWP
○ BRAND			
AQUACHLORAL SUPPRETTES: Polymedica	00998-6010-75	12s	$35.31

SYRUP (C-IV): 250 MG/5 ML

BRAND/MANUFACTURER	NDC	SIZE	AWP
○ GENERICS			
Roxane	00054-8139-16	10 ml 40s ud	$23.81
Pharm Assoc	00121-0457-10	10 ml 50s ud	$53.96

SYRUP (C-IV): 500 MG/5 ML

BRAND/MANUFACTURER	NDC	SIZE	AWP
○ GENERICS			
Southwood	58016-0852-06	30 ml	$3.90
Southwood	58016-0852-24	120 ml	$9.75
Liquipharm	54198-0140-16	473 ml	$8.50
Lannett	00527-0832-27	480 ml	$3.40
Geneva	00781-6605-16	480 ml	$6.73
Qualitest	00603-1088-58	480 ml	$8.06
Rugby	00536-0350-85	480 ml	$9.01
Pennex	00832-8533-16	480 ml	$9.60
URL	00677-0517-33	480 ml	$10.45
Goldline	00182-0364-40	480 ml	$10.50
Pennex	00426-8533-16	480 ml	$10.70
Major	00904-1300-16	480 ml	$10.95
Interstate	00814-1627-82	480 ml	$14.25
Lannett	00527-0832-28	3840 ml	$19.80
Roxane	00054-8138-16	10 ml 40s ud	$28.10
UDL	51079-0355-30	5 ml 100s ud	$28.00
Pharm Assoc	00121-0532-05	5 ml 100s ud	$63.76
UDL	51079-0356-30	10 ml 100s ud	$32.00

Chlorambucil

> **WARNING:**
> CHLORAMBUCIL CAN SEVERELY SUPPRESS BONE MARROW FUNCTION. CHLORAMBUCIL IS A CARCINOGEN IN HUMANS. CHLORAMBUCIL IS PROBABLY MUTAGENIC AND TERATOGENIC IN HUMANS. CHLORAMBUCIL PRODUCES HUMAN INFERTILITY. SEE *"WARNINGS" AND "PRECAUTIONS"* SECTIONS.

DESCRIPTION

Chlorambucil was first synthesized by Everett *et al.*[1] It is a bifunctional alkylating agent of the nitrogen mustard type that has been found active against selected human neoplastic diseases. Chlorambucil is known chemically as 4-[bis(2-chloroethyl)amino]benzenebutanoic acid.

Chlorambucil hydrolyzes in water and has a pKa of 5.8.

Chlorambucil is available in tablet form for oral administration. Its molecular weight is 304.2

Following is its chemical structure:

$$(ClCH_2CH_2)_2N \bigcirc CH_2CH_2CH_2COOH$$

CLINICAL PHARMACOLOGY

Chlorambucil is rapidly and completely absorbed from the gastrointestinal tract. After single oral doses of 0.6-1.2 mg/kg, peak plasma Chlorambucil levels are reached within one hour and the terminal half-life of the parent drug is estimated at 1.5 hours. Chlorambucil undergoes rapid metabolism to phenylacetic acid mustard, the major metabolite, and the combined Chlorambucil and phenylacetic acid mustard urinary excretion is extremely low—less than 1% in 24 hours. The peak plasma levels of Chlorambucil and phenylacetic acid mustard are similar, approximating 1 μg/mL; however, the metabolite's half-life is 1.6 times greater than the parent drug.[2,3]

Chlorambucil and its metabolites are extensively bound to plasma and tissue proteins. *In vitro*, Chlorambucil is 99% bound to plasma proteins, specifically albumin.[4] Cerebrospinal fluid levels of Chlorambucil have not been determined. Evidence of human teratogenicity suggests that the drug crosses the placenta.[5,6]

Chlorambucil is extensively metabolized in the liver primarily to phenylacetic acid mustard which has antineoplastic activity.[2,3] Chlorambucil and its major metabolite spontaneously degrade *in vivo* forming monohydroxy and dihydroxy derivatives.[2] After a single dose of radiolabeled Chlorambucil (^{14}C) approximately 15% to 60% of the radioactivity appears in the urine after 24 hours. Again, less than 1% of the urinary radioactivity is in the form of Chlorambucil or phenylacetic acid mustard.[2] In summary, the pharmacokinetic data suggest that oral Chlorambucil undergoes rapid gastrointestinal absorption and plasma clearance and that it is almost completely metabolized, having extremely low urinary excretion.

INDICATIONS AND USAGE

Chlorambucil is indicated in the treatment of chronic lymphatic (lymphocytic) leukemia, malignant lymphomas including lymphosarcoma, giant follicular lymphoma and Hodgkin's disease. It is not curative in any of these disorders but may produce clinically useful palliation.

◆ RATED THERAPEUTICALLY EQUIVALENT; ◇ THERAPEUTIC EQUIVALENCE UNCONFIRMED; ○ UNRATED

UNLABELED USES

Chlorambucil is used alone or as an adjunct in the treatment of Behcet's syndrome, breast cancer, and systemic dermatomyositis. It is also used to treat infiltrated inflammatory lesions of granuloma annulare, hairy cell leukemia, Letterer-Siwe disease, and multiple myeloma. Chlorambucil is also used to prevent Sezary syndrome in mycosis fungoides, biopsy proven "minimal change" nephrotic syndrome in children, ovarian cancer, rheumatoid arthritis, sarcoidosis, and diffuse posterior uveitis.

CONTRAINDICATIONS

Chlorambucil should not be used in patients whose disease has demonstrated a prior resistance to the agent. Patients who have demonstrated hypersensitivity to Chlorambucil should not be given the drug.[7-9] There may be cross-hypersensitivity (skin rash) between Chlorambucil and other alkylating agents.[10]

WARNINGS

Because of its carcinogenic properties, Chlorambucil should not be given to patients with conditions other than chronic lymphatic leukemia or malignant lymphomas. Convulsions,[11] infertility,[12] leukemia[13,14] and secondary malignancies[15] have been observed when Chlorambucil was employed in the therapy of malignant and non-malignant diseases.

There are many reports of acute leukemia arising in patients with both malignant[16] and non-malignant[17] diseases following Chlorambucil treatment. In many instances, these patients also received other chemotherapeutic agents or some form of radiation therapy. The quantitation of the risk of Chlorambucil-induction of leukemia or carcinoma in humans is not possible. Evaluation of published reports of leukemia developing in patients who have received Chlorambucil (and other alkylating agents) suggests that the risk of leukemogenesis increases with both chronicity of treatment and large cumulative doses. However, it has proved impossible to define a cumulative dose below which there is no risk of the induction of secondary malignancy. The potential benefits from Chlorambucil therapy must be weighed on an individual basis against the possible risk of the induction of a secondary malignancy.

Chlorambucil has been shown to cause chromatid or chromosome damage in man.[18,19] Both reversible and permanent sterility have been observed in both sexes receiving Chlorambucil.

A high incidence of sterility has been documented when Chlorambucil is administered to prepubertal and pubertal males.[20] Prolonged or permanent azoospermia has also been observed in adult males.[21] While most reports of gonadal dysfunction secondary to Chlorambucil have related to males, the induction of amenorrhea in females with alkylating agents is well documented and Chlorambucil is capable of producing amenorrhea. Autopsy studies of the ovaries from women with malignant lymphoma treated with combination chemotherapy including Chlorambucil have shown varying degrees of fibrosis, vasculitis, and depletion of primordial follicles.[22,23]

Rare instances of skin rash, progressing to erythema multiforme, toxic epidermal necrolysis, or Stevens-Johnson syndrome have been reported.[8-9] Chlorambucil should be discontinued promptly in patients who develop skin reactions.

Pregnancy: Pregnancy Category D: Chlorambucil can cause fetal harm when administered to a pregnant woman. Unilateral renal agenesis has been observed in two offspring whose mothers received Chlorambucil during the first trimester.[5,6] Urogenital malformations including absence of a kidney were found in fetuses of rats given Chlorambucil.[24] There are no adequate and well-controlled studies in pregnant women. If this drug is used during pregnancy, or if the patient becomes pregnant while taking this drug, the patient should be apprised of the potential hazard to the fetus. Women of childbearing potential should be advised to avoid becoming pregnant.

PRECAUTIONS

General: Many patients develop a slowly progressive lymphopenia during treatment. The lymphocyte count usually rapidly returns to normal levels upon completion of drug therapy. Most patients have some neutropenia after the third week of treatment and this may continue for up to ten days after the last dose. Subsequently, the neutrophil count usually rapidly returns to normal. Severe neutropenia appears to be related to dosage and usually occurs only in patients who have received a total dosage of 6.5 mg/kg or more in one course of therapy with continuous dosing. About one-quarter of all patients receiving the continuous-dose schedule, and one-third of those receiving this dosage in eight weeks or less may be expected to develop severe neutropenia.[25]

While it is not necessary to discontinue Chlorambucil at the first evidence of a fall in neutrophil count, it must be remembered that the fall may continue for ten days after the last dose and that as the total dose approaches 6.5 mg/kg there is a risk of causing irreversible bone marrow damage. The dose of Chlorambucil should be decreased if leukocyte or platelet counts fall below normal values and should be discontinued for more severe depression.

Chlorambucil should **not** be given at full dosages before four weeks after a full course of radiation therapy or chemotherapy because of the vulnerability of the bone marrow to damage under these conditions. If the pretherapy leukocyte or platelet counts are depressed from bone marrow disease process prior to institution of therapy, the treatment should be instituted at a reduced dosage.

Persistently low neutrophil and platelet counts or peripheral lymphocytosis suggest bone marrow infiltration. If confirmed by bone marrow examination, the daily dosage of Chlorambucil appears to be relatively free from gastrointestinal side effects or other evidence of toxicity apart from the bone marrow depressant

action. In humans, single oral doses of 20 mg or more may produce nausea and vomiting.

Children with nephrotic syndrome[11] and patients receiving high pulse doses of Chlorambucil[26] may have an increased risk of seizures. As with any potentially epileptogenic drug, caution should be exercised when administering Chlorambucil to patients with a history of seizure disorder, head trauma or receiving other potentially epileptogenic drugs.

Information for Patients: Patients should be informed that the major toxicities of Chlorambucil are related to hypersensitivity, drug fever, myelosuppression, hepatotoxicity, infertility, seizures, gastrointestinal toxicity, and secondary malignancies. Patients should never be allowed to take the drug without medical supervision and should consult their physician if they experience skin rash, bleeding, fever, jaundice, persistent cough, seizures, nausea, vomiting, amenorrhea, or unusual lumps/masses. Women of childbearing potential should be advised to avoid becoming pregnant.

Laboratory Tests: Patients must be followed carefully to avoid life-endangering damage to the bone marrow during treatment. Weekly examination of the blood should be made to determine hemoglobin levels, total and differential leukocyte counts, and quantitative platelet counts. Also, during the first 3 to 6 weeks of therapy, it is recommended that white blood cell counts be made 3 or 4 days after each of the weekly complete blood counts. Galton *et al*[25] have suggested that in following patients it is helpful to plot the blood counts on a chart at the same time that body weight, temperature, spleen size, etc., are recorded. It is considered dangerous to allow a patient to go more than two weeks without hematological and clinical examination during treatment.

Drug Interactions: There are no known drug/drug interactions with Chlorambucil.

Carcinogenesis, Mutagenesis, Impairment of Fertility: See "Warnings" section for information on carcinogenesis, mutagenesis and impairment of fertility.

Pregnancy: Teratogenic Effects: Pregnancy Category D: See "Warnings" section.

Nursing Mothers: It is not known whether this drug is excreted in human milk. Because many drugs are excreted in human milk and because of the potential for serious adverse reactions in nursing infants from Chlorambucil a decision should be made whether to discontinue nursing or to discontinue the drug, taking into account the importance of the drug to the mother.

Pediatric Use: The safety and effectiveness in children have not been established.

ADVERSE REACTIONS

Hematologic: The most common side effect is bone marrow suppression.[27] Although bone marrow suppression frequently occurs, it is usually reversible if the Chlorambucil is withdrawn early enough. However, irreversible bone marrow failure has been reported.[28,29]

Gastrointestinal: Gastrointestinal disturbances such as nausea and vomiting, diarrhea and oral ulceration occur infrequently.

CNS: Tremors, muscular twitching, confusion, agitation, ataxia, flaccid paresis and hallucinations have been reported as rare adverse experiences to Chlorambucil which resolve upon discontinuation of drug. Rare, focal and/or generalized seizures have been reported to occur in both children[11,30,31] and adults[26,32-35] at both therapeutic daily doses, pulse dosing regimens and in acute overdose (see "Precautions, General").

Dermatologic: Skin hypersensitivity (including rare reports of skin rash progressing to erythema multiforme,[9] toxic epidermal necrolysis,[8] and Stevens-Johnson syndrome) has been reported (see "Warnings").

Miscellaneous: Other reported adverse reactions include; pulmonary fibrosis, hepatotoxicity and jaundice, drug fever, peripheral neuropathy, interstitial pneumonia, sterile cystitis, infertility, leukemia and secondary malignancies (see "Warnings").

OVERDOSAGE

Reversible pancytopenia was the main finding of inadvertent overdoses of Chlorambucil[36,37]. Neurological toxicity ranging from agitated behavior and ataxia to multiple grand mal seizures has also occurred.[30,36] As there is no known antidote, the blood picture should be closely monitored and general supportive measures should be instituted, together with appropriate blood transfusions if necessary. Chlorambucil is not dialyzable.

Oral LD$_{50}$ single doses in mice are 123 mg/kg. In rats, a single intraperitoneal dose of 12.5 mg/kg of Chlorambucil produces typical nitrogen-mustard effects; these include atrophy of the intestinal mucous membrane and lymphoid tissues, severe lymphopenia becoming maximal in four days, anemia and thrombocytopenia. After this dose, the animals begin to recover within three days and appear normal in about a week although the bone marrow may not become completely normal for about three weeks. An intraperitoneal dose of 18.5 mg/kg kills about 50% of the rats within a week with development of convulsions. As much as 50 mg/kg has been given orally to rats as a single dose, with recovery. Such a dose causes bradycardia, excessive salivation, hematuria, convulsions, and respiratory dysfunction.

DOSAGE AND ADMINISTRATION

The usual oral dosage is 0.1 to 0.2 mg/kg body weight daily for three to six weeks as required. This usually amounts to 4 to 10 mg a day for the average patient. The entire daily dose may be given at one time. These dosages are for initiation of therapy or for short courses of treatment. The dosage must be carefully adjusted according to the response of the patient and must be reduced as soon as there is an abrupt fall in the white blood cell count. Patients with Hodgkin's disease usually require 0.2 mg/kg daily whereas patients with other lymphomas or chronic lymphocytic leukemia usually require only 0.1 mg/kg daily. When lymphocytic infiltration of the bone marrow is present, or when the bone marrow is hypoplastic, the daily dose should not exceed 0.1 mg/kg (about 6 mg for the average patient).

Alternate schedules for the treatment of chronic lymphocytic leukemia employing intermittent, biweekly or once monthly pulse doses of Chlorambucil have been reported.[38,39] Intermittent schedules of Chlorambucil begin with an initial single dose of 0.4 mg/kg. Doses are generally increased by 0.1 mg/kg until control of lymphocytosis or toxicity is observed. Subsequent doses are modified to produce mild hematologic toxicity. It is felt that the response rate of chronic lymphocytic leukemia to the biweekly or once monthly schedule of Chlorambucil administration is similar or better to that previously reported with daily administration and that hematologic toxicity was less than or equal to that encountered in studies using daily Chlorambucil.

Radiation and cytotoxic drugs render the bone marrow more vulnerable to damage and Chlorambucil should be used with particular caution within four weeks of a full course of radiation therapy or chemotherapy. However, small doses of palliative radiation over isolated foci remote from the bone marrow will not usually depress the neutrophil and platelet count. In these cases Chlorambucil may be given in the customary dosage.

It is presently felt that short courses of treatment are safer than continuous maintenance therapy although both methods have been effective. It must be recognized that continuous therapy may give the appearance of "maintenance" in patients who are actually in remission and have no immediate need for further drug. If maintenance dosage is used, it should not exceed 0.1 mg/kg daily and may well be as low as 0.03 mg/kg daily. A typical maintenance dose is 2 mg to 4 mg daily, or less, depending on the status of the blood counts. It may, therefore, be desirable to withdraw the drug after maximal control has been achieved since intermittent therapy reinstituted at time of relapse may be as effective as continuous treatment.

Procedures for proper handling and disposal of anticancer drugs should be considered. Several guidelines on this subject have been published.[40-46]

There is no general agreement that all of the procedures recommended in the guidelines are necessary or appropriate.

Store at 15° to 25°C (59° to 77°F) in a dry place.

REFERENCES
1. Everett JL, Roberts JJ, Ross WCJ. Aryl-2-halogenoalkylamines. Pt. XII. Some carboxylic derivatives of NN-Di-2-chloroethylaniline. *J Chem Soc.* 1953;3:2386-2392. 2. Alberts DS, Chang SY, Chen H-SG, Larcom BJ, Jones SE. Pharmacokinetics and metabolism of Chlorambucil in man. *Cancer Treat Rev.* 1979;6 (suppl):9-17. 3. McLean A, Woods RL, Catovsky D, Farmer P. Pharmacokinetics and metabolism of Chlorambucil in patients with malignant disease. *Cancer Treat Rev.* 1979; 6(suppl):33-42. 4. Ehrsson H, Lonroth U, Wallin I, Ehrnebo M, Nilsson SO. Degradation of Chlorambucil in aqueous solution: influence of human albumin binding. *J Pharm Pharmacol.* 1981;33:313-315. Communications. 5. Shotton D, Monie IW. Possible teratogenic effect of Chlorambucil on a human fetus. *JAMA.* 1963;186:74-75. 6. Steege JF, Caldwell DS. Renal agenesis after first trimester exposure to Chlorambucil. *South Med J.* 1980;73:1414-1415. 7. Knisley RE, Settipane GA, Albala MM. Unusual reaction to Chlorambucil in a patient with chronic lymphocytic leukemia. *Arch Dermatol.* 1971;104:77-79. 8. Pietrantonio F. Moriconi L, Torino F, Romano A, Gangovich A. Unusual reaction to Chlorambucil: a case report. *Cancer Lett.* 1990;54:109-111. 9. Hitchins RN, Hocker GA, Thomson DB. Chlorambucil allergy—a series of three cases. *Aust NZ J Med.* 1987;17:600-602. 10. Weiss RB, Bruno S. Hypersensitivity reactions to cancer chemotherapeutic agents. *Ann Intern Med.* 1981; 94:6-72. 11. Williams SA, Makker SP, Grupe WE. Seizures; a significant side effect of Chlorambucil therapy in children. *J Pediatr.* 1978;93:516-518. 12. Freckman HA, Fry HL, Mendez FL, Maurer ER. Chlorambucil-prednisolone therapy for disseminated breast carcinoma. *JAMA.* 1964; 189:23-26. 13. Aymard JP, Frustin J, Witz F, Colomb JN, Lederlin P, Herbeuval R. Acute leukemia after prolonged Chlorambucil treatment for non-malignant disease: a report of a new case and literature survey. *Acta Haematol (Basel).* 1980;63:283-285. 14. Berk PD, Goldberg JD, Silverstein MN, et al. Increased incidence of acute leukemia in polycythemia vera associated with Chlorambucil therapy. *N Engl J Med.* 1981;304:441-447. 15. Lerner HJ. Acute myelogenous leukemia in patients receiving Chlorambucil as long-term adjuvant chemotherapy for stage II breast cancer. *Cancer Treat Rep.* 1978;62:1135-1138. 16. Zarrabi MH, Grunwald HW, Rosner F. Chronic lymphocytic leukemia terminating in acute leukemia. *Arch Intern Med.* 1977;137:1059-1064. 17. Cameron S: Chlorambucil and leukemia. *N Eng J Med.* 1977;296:1065. 18. Lawler SD, Lele KP. Chromosomal damage induced by Chlorambucil in chronic lymphocytic leukemia. *Scand J Haematol* 1972;9:603-612. 19. Stevenson AC, Patel C. Effects of Chlorambucil on human chromosomes. *Mutat Res.* 1973;18:333-351. 20. Guesry P, Lenoir G, Broyer M. Gonadal effects of Chlorambucil given to prepubertal and pubertal boys for nephrotic syndrome. *J Pediatr.* 1978;92:299-303. 21. Richter P, Calamera JC, Morgenfeld MC, Kierszenbaum AL, Lavieri JC, Mancini RE. Effect of Chlorambucil on spermatogenesis in the human with malignant lymphoma. *Cancer.* 1970;25:1026-1030. 22. Morgenfeld MC, Goldberg V, Parisier H, Bugnard SC, Bur GE. Ovarian lesions due to cytostatic agents during the treatment of Hodgkin's disease. *SurgGynecol Obstet.* 1972;134:826-828. 23. Sobrinho LG, Levine RA, DeConti RC. Amenorrhea in patients with Hodgkin's disease treated with antineoplastic agents. *Am J Obstet Gynecol.* 1971;109:135-139. 24. Monie IW. Chlorambucil-induced abnormalities of the urogenital system of rat fetuses. *Anat Rec.* 1961;139:145-153. 25. Galton DAG, Israels LG, Nabarro JDN, Till M. Clinical trials of p-(DI-2-chloroethylamino)-phenylbutyric acid (CB 1348) in malignant lymphoma. *Br Med J.* 1955;2:1172-1176. 26. Ciobanu N, Runowicz C, Gucalp R, et al. Reversible central nervous system toxicity associated with high-dose Chlorambucil in autologous bone marrow transplantation for ovarian carcinoma. *Cancer Treat Rep.* 1987;71:1324-1325. 27. Moore GE, Bross ID, Ausman R, et al. Effects of Chlorambucil (NSC-3088) in 374 patients with advanced cancer. Eastern Clinical Drug Evaluation Program. *Cancer Chemother Rep.* 1968;52(pt 1):661-666. 28. Galton DA, Wiltshaw E, Szur L, Dacie JV. The use of Chlorambucil and steroids in the treatment of chronic lymphocytic leukemia. *Br J Haematol.* 1961;7:73-98. 29. Rudd P, Fries JF, Epstein WV. Irreversible bone marrow failure with Chlorambucil. *J Rheumatol.* 1975;2:421-429. 30. Wolfson S, Olney MB. Accidental ingestion of a toxic dose of Chlorambucil: report of a case in a child. *JAMA.* 1957;165:239-240. 31. Byrne TN, Moseley TAE, Finer MA. Myoclonic seizures following Chlorambucil overdose. *Ann Neurol.* 1981;9:191-194. 32. LaDelfa I, Bayer N, Myers R, Hoffstein V. Chlorambucil-induced myoclonic seizures in an adult. *J Clin Oncol.* 1985;3:1691-1692. 33. Naysmith A, Robson RH: Focal fits during Chlorambucil therapy. *Postgrad Med J.* 1979;55:806-807. 34. Blank DW, Nanji AA, Schreiber DH, Hudman C, Sanders HD. Acute renal failure and seizures associated with Chlorambucil overdose. *J Toxicol Clin Toxicol.* 1983;20:361-365. 35. Ammenti A, Reitter B, Muller-Wiefel DE. Chlorambucil neurotoxicity; report of two cases. *Helv Paediatr Acta.* 1980;35:281-287. 36. Green AA, Naiman JL. Chlorambucil poisoning. *Am J Dis Child.* 1968;116:190-191. 37. Enck RE, Bennett JM. Inadvertent Chlorambucil overdose in adults. *NY State J Med.* 1977;77:1480-1481. 38. Knospe WH, Loeb V Jr, Huguley CM. Bi-weekly Chlorambucil treatment of chronic lymphocytic leukemia. *Cancer.* 1974;33:555-562. 39. Sawitsky A, Rai KR, Glidewell O, et al. Comparison of daily versus intermittent Chlorambucil and prednisone therapy in the treatment of patients with chronic lymphocytic leukemia. *Blood.* 1977;50:1049-1059. 40. Recommendations for the safe handling of parenteral antineoplastic drugs. Washington, DC: Division of Safety; National Institutes of Health; 1983. US Dept of Health and Human Services, Public Health Service publication NIH 83-2621. 41. AMA Council on Scientific Affairs. Guidelines for handling parenteral antineoplastics. *JAMA.* 1985;253: 1590-1591. 42. National Study Commission on Cytotoxic Exposure. Recommendations for handling cytotoxic agents. 1984. Available from Louis P. Jeffrey, ScD, Director of Pharmacy Services, Rhode Island Hospital, 593 Eddy St, Providence, RI 02902. 43. Clinical Oncological Society of Australia. Guidelines and recommendations for safe handling of antineoplastic agents. *Med J Australia.* 1983;1:426-428. 44. Jones RB, Frank R, Mass T. Safe handling of chemotherapeutic agents: a report from the Mount Sinai Medical Center. *CA-A Cancer J for Clin.* 1983;33:258-263. 45. American Society of Hospital Pharmacists. ASHP technical assistance bulletin on handling cytotoxic and hazardous drugs. *Am J Hosp Pharm.* 1990;47:1033-1049. 46. Yodaiken RE, Bennett D. OSHA work-practice guidelines for personnel dealing with cytotoxic (antineoplastic) drugs. *AM J Hosp Pharm.* 1986;43:1193-1204.

HOW SUPPLIED
TABLETS: 2 MG

BRAND/MANUFACTURER	NDC	SIZE	AWP
○ **BRAND** LEUKERAN: Burr Wellcome	00081-0635-35	50s	$54.19

Chloramphenicol

WARNING

SERIOUS AND FATAL BLOOD DYSCRASIAS (APLASTIC ANEMIA, HYPOPLASTIC ANEMIA, THROMBOCYTOPENIA, AND GRANULOCYTOPENIA) ARE KNOWN TO OCCUR AFTER THE ADMINISTRATION OF CHLORAMPHENICOL. IN ADDITION, THERE HAVE BEEN REPORTS OF APLASTIC ANEMIA ATTRIBUTED TO CHLORAMPHENICOL WHICH LATER TERMINATED IN LEUKEMIA. BLOOD DYSCRASIAS HAVE OCCURRED AFTER BOTH SHORT-TERM AND PROLONGED THERAPY WITH THIS DRUG. CHLORAMPHENICOL MUST NOT BE USED WHEN LESS POTENTIALLY DANGEROUS AGENTS WILL BE EFFECTIVE, AS DESCRIBED IN THE INDICATIONS SECTION. *IT MUST NOT BE USED IN THE TREATMENT OF TRIVIAL INFECTIONS OR WHERE IT IS NOT INDICATED, AS IN COLDS, INFLUENZA, INFECTIONS OR OF THE THROAT; OR AS A PROPHYLACTIC AGENT TO PREVENT BACTERIAL INFECTIONS.*

PRECAUTIONS: IT IS ESSENTIAL THAT ADEQUATE BLOOD STUDIES BE MADE DURING TREATMENT WITH THE DRUG. WHILE BLOOD STUDIES MAY DETECT EARLY PERIPHERAL BLOOD CHANGES, SUCH AS LEUKOPENIA, RETICULOCYTOPENIA, OR GRANULOCYTOPENIA, BEFORE THEY BECOME IRREVERSIBLE, SUCH STUDIES CANNOT BE RELIED ON TO DETECT BONE MARROW DEPRESSION PRIOR TO DEVELOPMENT OF APLASTIC ANEMIA. TO FACILITATE APPROPRIATE STUDIES AND OBSERVATION DURING THERAPY, IT IS DESIRABLE THAT PATIENTS BE HOSPITALIZED.

DESCRIPTION

Chloramphenicol is an antibiotic that is clinically useful for, *and should be reserved for,* serious infections caused by organisms susceptible to its antimicrobial effects when less potentially hazardous therapeutic agents are ineffective or contraindicated. Sensitivity testing is essential to determine its indicated use, but may be performed concurrently with therapy initiated on clinical impression that one of the indicated conditions exists (see *"Indications and Usage"* section).

Each capsule contains 250 mg Chloramphenicol.

Following is its chemical structure:

$$O_2N-\underset{}{\bigcirc}-\overset{OH}{\underset{H}{\overset{|}{C}}}-\overset{H}{\underset{NHCOCHCl_2}{\overset{|}{C}}}-CH_2OH$$

CLINICAL PHARMACOLOGY

In vitro Chloramphenicol exerts mainly a bacteriostatic effect on a wide range of gram-negative and gram-positive bacteria and is active *in vitro* against rickettsiae, the lymphogranuloma psittacosis group, and *Vibrio cholerae.* It is particularly active against *Salmonella typhi* and *Hemophilus influenzae*. The mode of action is through interference or inhibition of protein synthesis in intact cells and in cell-free systems.

Chloramphenicol administered orally is absorbed rapidly from the intestinal tract. In controlled studies in adult volunteers using the recommended dosage of 50 mg/kg/day, a dosage of 1 g every 6 hours for 8 doses was given. Using the microbiological assay method, the average peak serum level was 11.2 mcg/ml one hour after the first dose. A cumulative effect gave a peak rise to 18.4 mcg/ml after the fifth dose of 1 g. Mean serum levels ranged from 8 to 14 mcg/ml over the 48-hour period. Total urinary excretion of Chloramphenicol in these studies ranged from a low of 68% to a high of 99% over a three-day period. From 8 to 12% of the antibiotic excreted is in the form of free Chloramphenicol; the remainder consists of microbiologically inactive metabolites, principally the conjugate with glucuronic acid. Since the glucuronide is excreted rapidly, most Chloramphenicol detected in the blood is in the microbiologically active free form. Despite the small proportion of unchanged drug excreted in the urine, the concentration of free Chloramphenicol is relatively high, amounting to several hundred mcg/ml in patients receiving divided doses of 50 mg/kg/day. Small amounts of active drug are found in bile and feces. Chloramphenicol diffuses rapidly, but its distribution is not uniform. Highest concentrations are found in liver and kidney, and lowest concentrations are found in brain and cerebrospinal fluid. Chloramphenicol enters cerebrospinal fluid even in the absence of meningeal inflammation, appearing in concentrations about half of those found in the blood. Measurable levels are also detected in pleural and in ascitic fluids, saliva, milk, and in the aqueous and vitreous humors. Transport across the placental barrier occurs with somewhat lower concentration in cord blood of newborn infants than in maternal blood.

INDICATIONS AND USAGE
In accord with the concepts in the warning box and this indications section, Chloramphenicol must be used only in those serious infections for which less potentially dangerous drugs are ineffective or contraindicated. However, Chloramphenicol may be chosen to initiate antibiotic therapy on the clinical impression that one of the conditions below is believed to be present; *in vitro* sensitivity tests should be performed concurrently so that the drug may be discontinued as soon as possible if less potentially dangerous agents are indicated by such tests. The decision to continue use of Chloramphenicol rather than another antibiotic when both are suggested by *in vitro* studies to be effective against a specific pathogen should be based upon severity of the infection, susceptibility of the pathogen to the various antimicrobial drugs, efficacy of the various drugs in the infection, and the important additional concepts contained in the *"Warning"* box above.

1. Acute infections caused by Salmonella typhi: Chloramphenicol is a drug of choice.* It is not recommended for the routine treatment of the typhoid carrier state.

2. Serious infections caused by susceptible strains in accordance with the concepts expressed above:
    a. *Salmonella* species
    b. *H influenzae*, specifically meningeal infections
    c. Rickettsia
    d. Lymphogranuloma-psittacosis group
    e. Various gram-negative bacteria causing bacteremia, meningitis, or other serious gram-negative infections
    f. Other susceptible organisms which have been demonstrated to be resistant to all other appropriate antimicrobial agents.

3. Cystic fibrosis regimens

CONTRAINDICATIONS
Chloramphenicol is contraindicated in individuals with a history of previous hypersensitivity and/or toxic reaction to it. *It must not be used in the treatment of trivial infections or where it is not indicated, as in colds, influenza, infections of the throat; or as a prophylactic agent to prevent bacterial infections.*

PRECAUTIONS
1. Baseline blood studies should be followed by periodic blood studies approximately every two days during therapy. The drug should be discontinued upon appearance of reticulocytopenia, leukopenia, thrombocytopenia, anemia, or any other blood study findings attributable to Chloramphenicol. However, it should be noted that such studies do not exclude the possible later appearance of the irreversible type of bone marrow depression.

2. Repeated courses of the drug should be avoided if at all possible. Treatment should not be continued longer than required to produce a cure with little or no risk of relapse of the disease.

3. Concurrent therapy with other drugs that may cause bone marrow depression should be avoided.

4. Excessive blood levels may result from administration of the recommended dose to patients with impaired liver or kidney function, including that due to immature metabolic processes in the infant. The dosage should be adjusted accordingly or, preferably, the blood concentration should be determined at appropriate intervals.

5. There are no studies to establish the safety of this drug in pregnancy.

---

* In the treatment of typhoid fever, some authorities recommend that Chloramphenicol be administered at therapeutic levels for 8 to 10 days after the patient has become afebrile to lessen the possibility of relapse.

6. Since Chloramphenicol readily crosses the placental barrier, caution in use of the drug is particularly important during pregnancy at term or during labor because of potential toxic effects on the fetus ("gray syndrome").

7. Precaution should be used in therapy of premature and full-term infants to avoid "gray syndrome" toxicity. (See *"Adverse Reactions".*) Serum drug levels should be carefully followed during therapy of the newborn infant.

8. Precaution should be used in therapy during lactation because of the possibility of toxic effects on the nursing infant.

9. The use of this antibiotic, as with other antibiotics, may result in an overgrowth of nonsusceptible organisms, including fungi. If infections caused by nonsusceptible organisms appear during therapy, appropriate measures should be taken.

ADVERSE REACTIONS
1. Blood Dyscrasias: The most serious adverse effect of Chloramphenicol is bone marrow depression. Serious and fatal blood dyscrasias (aplastic anemia, hypoplastic anemia, thrombocytopenia, and granulocytopenia) are known to occur after the administration of Chloramphenicol. An irreversible type of marrow depression leading to aplastic anemia with a high rate of mortality is characterized by the appearance weeks or months after therapy of bone marrow aplasia or hypoplasia. Peripherally, pancytopenia is most often observed, but in a small number of cases only one or two of the three major cell types (erythrocytes, leukocytes, platelets) may be depressed.

A reversible type of bone marrow depression, which is dose-related, may occur. This type of marrow depression is characterized by vacuolization of the erythroid cells, reduction of reticulocytes, and leukopenia, and responds promptly to the withdrawal of Chloramphenicol.

An exact determination of the risk of serious and fatal blood dyscrasias is not possible because of lack of accurate information regarding (1) the size of the population at risk, (2) the total number of drug-associated dyscrasias, and (3) the total number of nondrug-associated dyscrasias.

In a report to the California State Assembly by the California Medical Association and the State Department of Public Health in January 1967, the risk of fatal aplastic anemia was estimated at 1:24,200 to 1:40,500 based on two dosage levels. There have been reports of aplastic anemia attributed to Chloramphenicol which later terminated in leukemia.

Paroxysmal nocturnal hemoglobinuria has also been reported.

2. Gastrointestinal Reactions: Nausea, vomiting, glossitis and stomatitis, diarrhea, and enterocolitis may occur in low incidence.

3. Neurotoxic Reactions: Headache, mild depression, mental confusion, and delirium have been described in patients receiving Chloramphenicol. Optic and peripheral neuritis have been reported, usually following long-term therapy. If this occurs, the drug should be promptly withdrawn.

4. Hypersensitivity Reactions: Fever, macular and vesicular rashes, angioedema, urticaria, and anaphylaxis may occur. Herxheimer reactions have occurred during therapy for typhoid fever.

5. "Gray Syndrome": Toxic reactions including fatalities have occurred in the premature and newborn; the signs and symptoms associated with these reactions have been referred to as the "gray syndrome". One case of "gray syndrome" has been reported in an infant born to a mother having received Chloramphenicol during labor. One case has been reported in a 3-month-old infant. The following summarizes the clinical and laboratory studies that have been made on these patients:

(a) In most cases, therapy with Chloramphenicol had been instituted within the first 48 hours of life.

(b) Symptoms first appeared after 3 to 4 days of continued treatment with high doses of Chloramphenicol.

(c) The symptoms appeared in the following order:

    (1) abdominal distention with or without emesis;
    (2) progressive pallid cyanosis;
    (3) Vasomotor collapse, frequently accompanied by irregular respiration;
    (4) death within a few hours of onset of these symptoms.

(d) The progression of symptoms from onset to exitus was accelerated with higher dose schedules.

(e) Preliminary blood serum level studies revealed unusually high concentrations of Chloramphenicol (over 90 mcg/ml after repeated doses).

(f) Termination of therapy upon early evidence of the associated symptomatology frequently reversed the process with complete recovery.

DOSAGE AND ADMINISTRATION
DOSAGE RECOMMENDATIONS FOR ORAL CHLORAMPHENICOL PREPARATIONS
The majority of microorganisms susceptible to Chloramphenicol will respond to a concentration between 5 and 20 mcg/ml. The desired concentration of active drug in blood should fall within this range over most of the treatment period. Dosage of 50 mg/kg/day divided into 4 doses at intervals of 6 hours will usually achieve and sustain levels of this magnitude.

Except in certain circumstances (eg, premature and newborn infants and individuals with impairment of hepatic or renal function), lower doses may not achieve these concentrations. Chloramphenicol, like other potent drugs, should be prescribed at recommended doses known to have therapeutic activity. Close observation of the patient should be maintained and in the event of any adverse reactions, dosage should be reduced or the drug discontinued, if other factors in the clinical situation permit.

Adults: Adults should receive 50 mg/kg/day (approximately one 250-mg capsule per each 10 lbs body weight) in divided doses at 6-hour intervals. In exceptional cases, patients with infections due to moderately resistant organisms may require increased dosage up to 100 mg/kg/day to achieve blood levels inhibiting the pathogen, but these high doses should be decreased as soon as possible. Adults with impairment of hepatic or renal function or both may have reduced ability to metabolize and excrete the drug. In instances of impaired metabolic processes, dosages should be adjusted accordingly. (See discussion under "Newborn Infants.") Precise control of concentration of the drug in the blood should be carefully followed in patients with impaired metabolic processes by the available microtechniques (information available on request).

Children: Dosage of 50 mg/kg/day divided into 4 doses at 6-hour intervals yields blood levels in the range effective against most susceptible organisms. Severe infections (eg, bacteremia or meningitis), especially when adequate cerebrospinal fluid concentrations are desired, may require dosage up to 100 mg/kg/day; however, it is recommended that dosage be reduced to 50 ng/kg/day as soon as possible. Children with impaired liver or kidney function may retain excessive amounts of the drug.

Newborn Infants: (see section titled *"Gray Syndrome"* under *"Adverse Reactions"*.)

A total of 25 mg/kg/day in 4 equal doses at 6-hour intervals usually produces and maintains concentrations in blood and tissues adequate to control most infections for which the drug is indicated. Increased dosage in these individuals, demanded by severe infections, should be given only to maintain the blood concentration within a therapeutically effective range. After the first two weeks of life, full-term infants ordinarily may receive up to a total of 50 mg/kg/day equally divided into 4 doses at 6-hour intervals. **These dosage recommendations are extremely important because blood concentration in all premature infants and full-term infants under two weeks of age differs from that of other infants.** This difference is due to variations in the maturity of the metabolic functions of the liver and the kidneys.

When these functions are immature (or seriously impaired in adults), high concentrations of the drug are found which tend to increase with succeeding doses.

Infants and Children with Immature Metabolic Processes: In young infants and other children in whom immature metabolic functions are suspected, a dose of 25 mg/kg/day will usually produce therapeutic concentrations of the drug in the blood. In this group particularly, the concentration of the drug in the blood should be carefully followed by microtechniques. (Information available on request.)

STORAGE
Store at a room temperature below 86°F (30°C). Protect from moisture and excessive heat.

HOW SUPPLIED
CAPSULE: 250 MG

AVERAGE UNIT PRICE (AVAILABLE SIZES)		GENERIC A-RATED AVERAGE PRICE (GAAP)	
BRAND	$1.25	100s	$36.50
GENERIC	$0.35		
HCFA FUL (100s ea)	$0.25		

BRAND/MANUFACTURER		NDC	SIZE	AWP
◆ **BRAND**				
CHLOROMYCETIN: Parke-Davis		00071-0379-24	100s	$125.43
◆ **GENERICS**				
Rugby		00536-0140-01	100s	$32.25
Zenith		00172-2960-60	100s	$36.80
Aligen		00405-4164-01	100s	$40.46

Chloramphenicol/
Desoxyribonuclease/Fibrinolysin

DESCRIPTION
Fibrinolysin and Desoxyribonuclease combined [bovine] is supplied as a lyophilized powder and in an ointment base. The Fibrinolysin component is derived from bovine plasma and the Desoxyribonuclease is isolated in a purified form from choloroform. The Fibrinolysin used in the combination is activated by choloroform.

FIBRINOLYSIN AND DESOXYRIBONUCLEASE WITH CHLORAMPHENICOL
Contains two lytic enzymes, Fibrinolysin and Desoxyribonuclease, combined with chloramphenicol in an ointment base. Chloramphenicol is a broad-spectrum antibiotic originally isolated from *Streptomyces venezuelae.* It is therapeutically active against a wide variety of susceptible organisms, both gram-positive and gram-negative. Chemically, chloramphenicol may be identified as D(-)- *threo-1-p-* nitrophenyl-2-dichloroacetamido-1, 3-propanediol.

ACTION
Combination of these two enzymes is based on the observation that purulent exudates consist largely of fibrinous material and nucleoprotein. Desoxyribonu-

clease attacks the Desoxyribonucleic acid (DNA) and Fibrinolysin attacks principally the fibrin of blood clots and fibrinous exudates.

The activity of Desoxyribonuclease is limited principally to the production of large polynucleotides, which are less likely to be absorbed than the more diffusible protein fractions liberated by certain enzyme preparations obtained from bacteria. The fibrinolytic action is directed mainly against denatured proteins, such as those found in devitalized tissue, while protein elements of living cells remain relatively unaffected.

Fibrinolysin and Desoxyribonuclease combined [bovine] and Fibrinolysin and Desoxyribonuclease combined [bovine] with Chloramphanicol are combinations of active enzymes. This is an important consideration in treating patients suffering from lesions resulting from impaired circulation.

The enzymatic action helps to produce clean surfaces and thus supports healing in a variety of exudative lesions.

DESOXYRIBONUCLEASE WITH CHLORAMPHENICOL OINTMENT
Chloramphenicol is a broad-spectrum antibiotic that is primarily bacteriostatic and acts by inhibition of protein synthesis by interfering with the transfer of activated amino acids from soluble RNA to ribosomes. Development of resistance to chloramphenicol can be regarded as minimal for staphylococci and many other species of bacteria.

INDICATIONS
Fibrinolysin and Desoxyribonuclease, combined [bovine] are indicated for topical use as debriding agents in a variety of inflammatory and infected lesions. These include: (1) general surgical wounds; (2) ulcerative lesions—trophic, decubitus, stasis, arteriosclerotic; (3) second and third-degree burns; (4) circumcision and episiotomy. Fibrinolysin and Desoxyribonuclease, combined [bovine] are used intravaginally in: (1) cervicitis—benign, postpartum, and postconization; (2) vaginitis Fibrinolysin and Desoxyribonuclease, combined [bovine] is used as an irrigating agent in the following conditions: (1) infected wounds—abscesses, fistulae, and sinus tracts; (2) otorhinolaryngologic wounds; (3) superficial hematomas (except when the hematoma is adjacent to or within adipose tissue).

FIBRINOLYSIN AND DESOXYRIBONUCLEASE WITH CHLORAMPHENICOL
Indicated for use in the treatment of infected lesions, such as burns, ulcers, and wounds where the actions of both a debriding agent and a topical antibiotic are desired. This dual-purpose approach is especially useful in the treatment of infections caused by organisms that utilize a process of fibrin deposition as protective device (ie, coagulase and staphylococcus). Appropriate measures should be taken to determine the susceptibility of the pathogen to Chloramphenicol.

CONTRAINDICATIONS
These products are contraindicated in individuals with a history of hypersensitivity reactions to any of their components. Fibrinolysin and Desoxyribonuclease, combined [bovine] is not recommended for parenteral use because the bovine Fibrinolysin may be antigenic.

WARNINGS
FIBRINOLYSIN AND DESOXYRIBONUCLEASE WITH CHLORAMPHENICOL
Bone marrow hypoplasia, including aplastic anemia and death, has been reported following the local application of Chloramphenicol.

PRECAUTIONS
FIBRINOLYSIN AND DESOXYRIBONUCLEASE WITH CHLORAMPHENICOL
The prolonged use of antibiotics may occasionally result in overgrowth of nonsusceptible organisms, including fungi. If new infections appear during medication, the drug should be discontinued and appropriate measures should be taken. In all except very superficial infections, the topical use of Chloramphenicol should be supplemented by appropriate systemic medication.

FIBRINOLYSIN AND DESOXYRIBONUCLEASE;
FIBRINOLYSIN AND DESOXYRIBONUCLEASE WITH CHLORAMPHENICOL
The usual precautions against allergic reactions should be observed, particularly in persons with a history of sensitivity to materials of bovine origin.

FIBRINOLYSIN AND DESOXYRIBONUCLEASE
To be maximally effective, Fibrinolysin and Desoxyribonuclease, combined [bovine] solutions must be freshly prepared before use. The loss in activity is reduced by refrigeration; however, even when stored in a refrigerator, the solution should not be used 24 hours or more after reconstitution.

ADVERSE REACTIONS
Side effects attributable to the enzymes have not been a problem at the dose and for the indications recommended herein. With higher concentrations, side effects have been minimal, consisting of local hyperemia.

Chills and fever attributable to antigenic action of proFibrinolysin activators of bacterial origin are not a problem.

FIBRINOLYSIN AND DESOXYRIBONUCLEASE WITH CHLORAMPHENICOL
Signs of local irritation, with subjective symptoms of itching or burning, angioneurotic edema, urticaria, vesicular and maculopapular dermatitis have

---

◆ RATED THERAPEUTICALLY EQUIVALENT; ◇ THERAPEUTIC EQUIVALENCE UNCONFIRMED; ○ UNRATED

been reported in patients sensitive to Chloramphenicol and are causes for discontinuing the medication. Similar sensitivity reactions to other materials in topical preparations may also occur. Blood dyscrasias have been associated with the use of Chloramphenicol.

PREPARATION OF FIBRINOLYSIN AND DESOXYRIBONUCLEASE SOLUTION

The contents of each vial may be reconstituted with 10 mL of isotonic sodium chloride solution. Higher or lower concentrations can be prepared if desired by varying the amount of the diluent.

DOSAGE AND ADMINISTRATION

Since the conditions for which Fibrinolysin and Desoxyribonuclease, combined [bovine], and Fibrinolysin and Desoxyribonuclease, combined [bovine] with Chloramphenicol are helpful vary considerably in severity, dosage must be adjusted to the individual case; however, the following general recommendations can be made.

Successful use of enzymatic debridement depends on several factors: (1) dense, dry eschar, if present, should be removed surgically before enzymatic debridement is attempted; (2) the enzyme must be in constant contact with the substrate; (3) accumulated necrotic debris must be periodically removed; (4) the enzyme must be replenished at least once daily; and (5) secondary closure or skin grafting must be employed as soon as possible after optimal debridement has been attained. It is further essential that wound-dressing techniques be performed carefully under aseptic conditions and that appropriate systemically acting antibiotics be administered concomitantly if, in the opinion of the physician, they are indicated.

GENERAL TOPICAL USES
FIBRINOLYSIN AND DESOXYRIBONUCLEASE OINTMENT

Local application should be repeated at intervals for as long as enzyme action is desired. After application, Fibrinolysin and Desoxyribonuclease, combined [bovine] becomes rapidly and progressively less active and is probably exhausted for practical purposes at the end of 24 hours. A recommended procedure for application Fibrinolysin and Desoxyribonuclease, combined [bovine] follows.

1. Clean the wound with water, peroxide, or normal saline and dry area gently. If there is a dense, dry eschar present, it should be removed surgically before applying Fibrinolysin and Desoxyribonuclease, combined [bovine].
2. Apply a *thin* layer of Fibrinolysin and Desoxyribonuclease, combined [bovine] ointment.
3. Cover with petrolatum gauze or another type of nonadhering dressing.
4. Change the dressing at least ONCE a day, preferably two or three times daily. Frequency of application is more important than the amount of Fibrinolysin and Desoxyribonuclease, combined [bovine] used. Flush away the necrotic debris and fibrinous exudates with saline, peroxide, or warm water so that newly applied ointment can be in direct contact with the substrate.

FIBRINOLYSIN AND DESOXYRIBONUCLEASE, COMBINED [BOVINE]

Local application should be repeated at intervals for as long as enzyme action is desired. Fibrinolysin and Desoxyribonuclease, combined [bovine] solution may be applied topically as a liquid, spray, or wet dressing. Application of a gentle spray of the solution can be accomplished by using a conventional atomizer. After application, Fibrinolysin and Desoxyribonuclease, combined [bovine], especially in solution, becomes rapidly and progressively less active and is probably exhausted for practical purposes at the end of 24 hours. The dry material for solution is stable at room temperature through the expiration date printed on the package. A recommended procedure for application of a solution of Fibrinolysin and Desoxyribonuclease, combined [bovine] using a Wet-to-Dry method follows.

1. Mix one vial of Fibrinolysin and Desoxyribonuclease, combined [bovine] powder with 10 to 50 mL of saline and saturate strips of fine-mesh gauze or an unfolded sterile gauze sponge with the Fibrinolysin and Desoxyribonuclease, combined [bovine] solution.
2. Pack ulcerated area with the Fibrinolysin and Desoxyribonuclease, combined [bovine]-saturated gauze, making sure the gauze remains in contact with the necrotic substrate (if the lesion is covered with a heavy eschar, it must be removed surgically before wet-to-dry debridement is begun).
3. *Allow Gauze to Dry in Contact with the Ulcerated Lesion* (approximately six to eight hours). As the gauze dries, the necrotic tissues slough and become enmeshed in the gauze.
4. Remove dried gauze. This mechanically debrides the area. Repeat Wet-to-Dry procedure three or four times daily, since frequent dressing changes greatly enhance results. After two, three, or four days, the area becomes clean and starts to fill in with granulation tissue.

INTRAVAGINAL USE
FIBRINOLYSIN AND DESOXYRIBONUCLEASE, OINTMENT

In mild to moderate vaginitis and cervicitis, 5 mL of Fibrinolysin and Desoxyribonuclease, combined [bovine] ointment should be deposited deep in the vagina once nightly at bedtime for approximately five applications, or until the entire contents of one 30-g tube has been used. The patient should be checked by her physician to determine possible need for further therapy. In more severe cervicitis and vaginitis, some physicians prefer to initiate therapy with an application of Fibrinolysin and Desoxyribonuclease, combined, [bovine] in solution.

FIBRINOLYSIN AND DESOXYRIBONUCLEASE SOLUTION

In severe cervicitis and vaginitis, the physician may instill 10 mL of the solution intravaginally, wait one or two minutes for the enzyme to disperse and then insert a cotton tampon in the vaginal canal. The tampon should be removed the next day. Continuing therapy should then be instituted with Fibrinolysin and Desoxyribonuclease, combined [bovine] ointment.

ABSCESSES, EMPYEMA CAVITIES, FISTULAE, SINUS TRACTS, OR SUBCUTANEOUS HEMATOMAS

Despite the contraindication against parenteral use, Fibrinolysin and Desoxyribonuclease, combined [bovine] has been used in irrigating these specific conditions. The Fibrinolysin and Desoxyribonuclease, combined [bovine] solution should be drained and replaced at intervals of six to ten hours to reduce the amount of by-product accumulation and minimize loss of enzyme activity. Traces of blood in the discharge usually indicate active filling in of the cavity.

HOW SUPPLIED

CHLORAMPHENICOL/DESOXYRIBONUCLEASE/ FIBRINOLYSIN
OINTMENT:

BRAND/MANUFACTURER	NDC	SIZE	AWP
○ **BRAND**			
ELASE-CHLOROMYCETIN: Fujisawa	57317-0021-12	10 gm	$17.05
	57317-0023-77	30 gm	$40.80

DESOXYRIBONUCLEASE/FIBRINOLYSIN
OINTMENT:

BRAND/MANUFACTURER	NDC	SIZE	AWP
○ **BRAND**			
ELASE: Fujisawa	57317-0011-12	10 gm	$15.61
	57317-0013-77	30 gm	$37.45

POWDER FOR RECONSTITUTION:

BRAND/MANUFACTURER	NDC	SIZE	AWP
○ **BRAND**			
ELASE: Fujisawa	57317-0030-10	1 ml	$24.22

Chloramphenicol Sodium Succinate

WARNING
SERIOUS AND FATAL BLOOD DYSCRASIAS (APLASTIC ANEMIA, HYPOPLASTIC ANEMIA, THROMBOCYTOPENIA, AND GRANULOCYTOPENIA) ARE KNOWN TO OCCUR AFTER THE ADMINISTRATION OF CHLORAMPHENICOL. IN ADDITION, THERE HAVE BEEN REPORTS OF APLASTIC ANEMIA ATTRIBUTED TO CHLORAMPHENICOL WHICH LATER TERMINATED IN LEUKEMIA. BLOOD DYSCRASIAS HAVE OCCURRED AFTER BOTH SHORT-TERM AND PROLONGED THERAPY WITH THIS DRUG. CHLORAMPHENICOL MUST NOT BE USED WHEN LESS POTENTIALLY DANGEROUS AGENTS WILL BE EFFECTIVE, AS DESCRIBED IN THE INDICATIONS SECTION. *IT MUST NOT BE USED IN THE TREATMENT OF TRIVIAL INFECTIONS OR WHERE IT IS NOT INDICATED, AS IN COLDS, INFLUENZA, INFECTIONS OF THE THROAT; OR AS A PROPHYLACTIC AGENT TO PREVENT BACTERIAL INFECTIONS.*

PRECAUTIONS: IT IS ESSENTIAL THAT ADEQUATE BLOOD STUDIES BE MADE DURING TREATMENT WITH THE DRUG. WHILE BLOOD STUDIES MAY DETECT EARLY PERIPHERAL BLOOD CHANGES, SUCH AS LEUKOPENIA, RETICULOCYTOPENIA, OR GRANULOCYTOPENIA, BEFORE THEY BECOME IRREVERSIBLE, SUCH STUDIES CANNOT BE RELIED ON TO DETECT BONE MARROW DEPRESSION PRIOR TO DEVELOPMENT OF APLASTIC ANEMIA. TO FACILITATE APPROPRIATE STUDIES AND OBSERVATION DURING THERAPY, IT IS DESIRABLE THAT PATIENTS BE HOSPITALIZED.

IMPORTANT CONSIDERATIONS IN PRESCRIBING INJECTABLE CHLORAMPHENICOL SODIUM SUCCINATE: CHLORAMPHENICOL SODIUM SUCCINATE IS INTENDED FOR INTRAVENOUS USE ONLY; IT HAS BEEN DEMONSTRATED TO BE INEFFECTIVE WHEN GIVEN INTRAMUSCULARLY.

1. Chloramphenicol Sodium Succinate must be hydrolyzed to its microbiologically active form and there is a lag in achieving adequate blood levels compared with the base given intravenously.
2. The oral form of Chloramphenicol is readily absorbed and adequate blood levels are achieved and maintained on the recommended dosage.
3. Patients started on intravenous Chloramphenicol Sodium Succinate should be changed to the oral form as soon as practicable.

DESCRIPTION

Chloramphenicol is an antibiotic that is clinically useful for, *and should be reserved for,* serious infections caused by organisms susceptible to its antimicrobial effects when less potentially hazardous therapeutic agents are ineffective or contraindicated. Sensitivity testing is essential to determine its indicated use, but may be performed concurrently with therapy initiated on clinical impression that one of the indicated conditions exists (See *"Indications"* section).

Each gram (10 ml of a 10% solution) of Chloramphenicol Sodium Succinate contains approximately 52 mg (2.25 mEq) of sodium.

Following is its chemical structure:

ACTIONS AND PHARMACOLOGY

In vitro Chloramphenicol exerts mainly a bacteriostatic effect on a wide range of gram-negative and gram-positive bacteria and is active *in vitro* against rickettsiae, the lymphogranuloma-psittacosis group, and *Vibrio cholerae.* It is particularly active against *Salmonella typhi* and *Hemophilus influenzae.* The mode of action is through interference or inhibition of protein synthesis in intact cells and in cell-free systems.

Chloramphenicol administered orally is absorbed rapidly from the intestinal tract. In controlled studies in adult volunteers using the recommended dosage of 50 mg/kg/day, a dosage of 1 g every 6 hours for 8 doses was given. Using the microbiological assay method, the average peak serum level was 11.2 mcg/ml one hour after the first dose. A cumulative effect gave a peak rise to 18.4 mcg/ml after the fifth dose of 1 g. Mean serum levels ranged from 8 to 14 mcg/ml over the 48-hour period. Total urinary excretion of Chloramphenicol in these studies ranged from a low of 68% to a high of 99% over a three-day period. From 8 to 12% of the antibiotic excreted is in the form of free Chloramphenicol, the remainder consists of microbiologically inactive metabolites, principally the conjugate with glucuronic acid. Since the glucuronide is excreted rapidly, most Chloramphenicol detected in the blood is in the microbiologically active free form. Despite the small proportion of unchanged drug excreted in the urine, the concentration of free Chloramphenicol is relatively high, amounting to several hundred mcg/ml in patients receiving divided doses of 50 mg/kg/day. Small amounts of active drug are found in bile and feces. Chloramphenicol diffuses rapidly, but its distribution is not uniform. Highest concentrations are found in liver and kidney, and lowest concentrations are found in brain and cerebrospinal fluid. Chloramphenicol enters cerebrospinal fluid even in the absence of meningeal inflammation, appearing in concentrations about half of those found in the blood. Measurable levels are also detected in pleural and in ascitic fluids, saliva, milk, and in the aqueous and vitreous humors. Transport across the placental barrier occurs with somewhat lower concentration in cord blood of newborn infants than in maternal blood.

INDICATIONS

In accord with the concepts in the warning box and this indications section Chloramphenicol must be used only in those serious infections for which less potentially dangerous drugs are ineffective or contraindicated. However, Chloramphenicol may be chosen to initiate antibiotic therapy on the clinical impression that one of the conditions below is believed to be present; *in vitro* sensitivity tests should be performed concurrently so that the drug may be discontinued as soon as possible if less potentially dangerous agents are indicated by such tests. The decision to continue use of Chloramphenicol rather than another antibiotic when both are suggested by *in vitro* studies to be effective against a specific pathogen should be based upon severity of the infection, susceptibility of the pathogen to the various antimicrobial drugs, efficacy of the various drugs in the infection, and the important additional concepts contained in the *"Warning"* box above:

1. ACUTE INFECTIONS CAUSED BY *S TYPHI**
It is not recommended for the routine treatment of the typhoid carrier state.

2. SERIOUS INFECTIONS CAUSED BY SUSCEPTIBLE STRAINS IN ACCORDANCE WITH THE CONCEPTS EXPRESSED ABOVE
a. *Salmonella* species
b. *H influenzae,* specifically meningeal infections
c. Rickettsia
d. Lymphogranuloma-psittacosis group
e. Various gram-negative bacteria causing bacteremia, meningitis, or other serious gram-negative infections
f. Other susceptible organisms which have been demonstrated to be resistant to all other appropriate antimicrobial agents.

3. CYSTIC FIBROSIS REGIMENS

UNLABELED USES

Chloramphenicol Sodium Succinate is used alone or as an adjunct in the treatment of stage II or III Lyme disease, campylobacter enteritis, and Rocky Mountain Spotted fever.

---

* In the treatment of typhoid fever, some authorities recommend that Chloramphenicol be administered at therapeutic levels for 8 to 10 days after the patient has become afebrile to lessen the possibility of relapse.

CONTRAINDICATIONS

Chloramphenicol is contraindicated in individuals with a history of previous hypersensitivity and/or toxic reaction to it. *It must not be used in the treatment of trivial infections or where it is not indicated, as in colds, influenza, infections of the throat; or as a prophylactic agent to prevent bacterial infection.*

PRECAUTIONS

1. Baseline blood studies should be followed by periodic blood studies approximately every two days during therapy. The drug should be discontinued upon appearance of reticulocytopenia, leukopenia, thrombocytopenia, anemia, or any other blood study findings attributable to Chloramphenicol. However, it should be noted that such studies do not exclude the possible later appearance of the irreversible type of bone marrow depression.
2. Repeated courses of the drug should be avoided if at all possible. Treatment should not be continued longer than required to produce a cure with little or no risk of relapse of the disease.
3. Concurrent therapy with other drugs that may cause bone marrow depression should be avoided.
4. Excessive blood levels may result from administration of the recommended dosage to patients with impaired liver or kidney function, including that due to immature metabolic processes in the infant. The dosage should be adjusted accordingly or, preferably, the blood concentration should be determined at appropriate intervals.
5. There are no studies to establish the safety of this drug in pregnancy.
6. Since Chloramphenicol readily crosses the placental barrier, caution in use of the drug is particularly important during pregnancy at term or during labor because of potential toxic effects on the fetus (gray syndrome).
7. Precaution should be used in therapy of premature and full-term infants to avoid gray syndrome toxicity (see *"Adverse Reactions"*). Serum drug levels should be carefully followed during therapy of the newborn infant.
8. Precaution should be used in therapy during lactation because of the possibility of toxic effects on the nursing infant.
9. The use of this antibiotic, as with other antibiotics, may result in an overgrowth of nonsusceptible organisms, including fungi. If infections caused by nonsusceptible organisms appear during therapy, appropriate measures should be taken.

ADVERSE REACTIONS

1. BLOOD DYSCRASIAS

The most serious adverse effect of Chloramphenicol is bone marrow depression. Serious and fatal blood dyscrasias (aplastic anemia, hypoplastic anemia, thrombocytopenia, and granulocytopenia) are known to occur after the administration of Chloramphenicol. An irreversible type of marrow depression leading to aplastic anemia with a high rate of mortality is characterized by the appearance weeks or months after therapy of bone marrow aplasia or hypoplasia. Peripherally, pancytopenia is most often observed, but in a small number of cases only one or two of the three major cell types (erythrocytes, leukocytes, platelets) may be depressed.

A reversible type of bone marrow depression, which is dose-related, may occur. This type of marrow depression is characterized by vacuolization of the erythroid cells, reduction of reticulocytes, and leukopenia, and responds promptly to the withdrawal of chloramphenicol.

An exact determination of the risk of serious and fatal blood dyscrasias is not possible because of lack of accurate information regarding (1) the size of the population at risk, (2) the total number of drug-associated dyscrasias, and (3) the total number of nondrug-associated dyscrasias.

In a report to the California State Assembly by the California Medical Association and the State Department of Public Health in January 1967, the risk of fatal aplastic anemia was estimated at 1:24,200 to 1:40,500 based on two dosage levels. There have been reports of aplastic anemia attributed to Chloramphenicol which later terminated in leukemia.

Paroxysmal nocturnal hemoglobinuria has also been reported.

2. GASTROINTESTINAL REACTIONS

Nausea vomiting, glossitis and stomatitis, diarrhea, and enterocolitis may occur in low incidence.

3. NEUROTOXIC REACTIONS

Headache, mild depression, mental confusion, and delirium have been described in patients receiving Chloramphenicol Sodium Succinate. Optic and peripheral neuritis have been reported, usually following long-term therapy. If this occurs, the drug should be promptly withdrawn.

4. HYPERSENSITIVITY REACTIONS

Fever, macular and vesicular rashes, angio-edema, urticaria, and anaphylaxis may occur. Herxheimer reactions have occurred during therapy for typhoid fever.

5. "GRAY SYNDROME"

Toxic reactions including fatalities have occurred in the premature and newborn; the signs and symptoms associated with these reactions have been referred to as the gray syndrome. One case of gray syndrome has been reported in an infant born to a mother having received Chloramphenicol during labor. One case has been reported in a 3-month-old infant. The following summarizes the clinical and laboratory studies that have been made on these patients:

a) In most cases, therapy with Chloramphenicol had been instituted within the first 48 hours of life.
b) Symptoms first appeared after 3 to 4 days of continued treatment with high doses of Chloramphenicol.

---

c) The symptoms appeared in the following order:
  (1) abdominal distention with or without emesis;
  (2) progressive pallid cyanosis;
  (3) vasomotor collapse, frequently accompanied by irregular respiration;
  (4) death within a few hours of onset of these symptoms.
d) The progression of symptoms from onset to exitus was accelerated with higher dose schedules.
e) Preliminary blood serum level studies revealed unusually high concentrations of Chloramphenicol (over 90 mcg/ml after repeated doses).
f) Termination of therapy upon early evidence of the associated symptomatology frequently reversed the process with complete recovery.

ADMINISTRATION

Chloramphenicol, like other potent drugs, should be prescribed at recommended doses known to have therapeutic activity. Administration of 50 mg/kg/day in divided doses will produce blood levels of the magnitude to which the majority of susceptible microorganisms will respond.

As soon as feasible, an oral dosage form of Chloramphenicol should be substituted for the intravenous form because adequate blood levels are achieved with Chloramphenicol by mouth.

The following method of administration is recommended: Intravenously as a 10% (100 mg/ml) solution to be injected over at least a one-minute interval. This is prepared by the addition of 10 ml of an aqueous diluent, such as water for injection or 5% dextrose injection.

DOSAGE
ADULTS

Adults should receive 50 mg/kg/day in divided doses at 6-hour intervals. In exceptional cases, patients with infections due to moderately resistant organisms may require increased dosage up to 100 mg/kg/day to achieve blood levels inhibiting the pathogen, but these high doses should be decreased as soon as possible. Adults with impairment of hepatic or renal function or both may have reduced ability to metabolize and excrete the drug. In instances of impaired metabolic processes, dosages should be adjusted accordingly. (See discussion under "Newborn Infants.") Precise control of concentration of the drug in the blood should be carefully followed in patients with impaired metabolic processes by the available microtechniques (information available on request).

CHILDREN

Dosage of 50 mg/kg/day divided into 4 doses at 6-hour intervals yields blood levels in the range effective against most susceptible organisms. Severe infections (e.g., bacteremia or meningitis), especially when adequate cerebrospinal fluid concentrations are desired, may require dosage up to 100 mg/kg/day; however, it is recommended that dosage be reduced to 50 mg/kg/day as soon as possible. Children with impaired liver or kidney function may retain excessive amounts of the drug.

NEWBORN INFANTS

(See section titled "Gray Syndrome" under "Adverse Reactions".) A total of 25 mg/kg/day in 4 equal doses at 6-hour intervals usually produces and maintains concentrations in blood and tissues adequate to control most infections for which the drug is indicated. Increased dosage in these individuals, demanded by severe infections, should be given only to maintain the blood concentration within a therapeutically effective range. After the first two weeks of life, full-term infants ordinarily may receive up to a total of 50 mg/kg/day equally divided into 4 doses at 6-hour intervals. *These dosage recommendations are extremely important because blood concentration in all premature infants and full-term infants under two weeks of age differs from that of other infants.* This difference is due to variations in the maturity of the metabolic functions of the liver and the kidneys.

When these functions are immature (or seriously impaired in adults), high concentrations of the drug are found which tend to increase with succeeding doses.

INFANTS AND CHILDREN WITH IMMATURE METABOLIC PROCESSES

In young infants and other children in whom immature metabolic functions are suspected, a dose of 25 mg/kg/day will usually produce therapeutic concentrations of the drug in the blood. In this group particularly, the concentration of the drug in the blood should be carefully followed by microtechniques. (Information available on request.)

J CODES
Up to 1 g IV—J0720

HOW SUPPLIED
POWDER FOR INJECTION: 1 GM

BRAND/MANUFACTURER	NDC	SIZE	AWP
◆ BRAND			
CHLOROMYCETIN SODIUM SUCCINATE: Parke-Davis	00071-4057-03	10s	$41.48
◆ GENERICS			
Fujisawa	00469-1100-90	1s	$6.65

Chloramphenicol with Hydrocortisone Acetate

> **WARNING**
> BONE MARROW HYPOPLASIA INCLUDING APLASTIC ANEMIA AND DEATH HAS BEEN REPORTED FOLLOWING LOCAL APPLICATION OF CHLORAMPHENICOL. CHLORAMPHENICOL SHOULD NOT BE USED WHEN LESS POTENTIALLY DANGEROUS AGENTS WOULD BE EXPECTED TO PROVIDE EFFECTIVE TREATMENT.

DESCRIPTION

Chloramphenicol and Hydrocortisone Acetate for Suspension is a sterile, buffered antibiotic/anti-inflammatory dry mixture for suspension for ophthalmic administration. Each vial of Chloramphenicol/Hydrocortisone Ophthalmic contains 12.5 mg Chloramphenicol and 25 mg Hydrocortisone Acetate per mL, in the suspension when prepared as directed. A 5 ml vial of Sterile Distilled Water is included in each package for use as a diluent in the preparation of a suspension of Chloramphenicol/Hydrocortisone suitable for ophthalmic use.

The chemical names for Chloramphenicol are:
  (1) Acetamide,2,2-dichloro-N-[2-hydroxy-1-(hydroxymethyl)-2-(4-nitrophenyl) ethyl]-, and
  (2) D-threo-(−)-2,2-Dichloro-N-[β-hydroxy-α-(hydroxymethyl) -p-nitrophenethyl] acetamide.
Its empirical formula is $C_{11}H_{12}Cl_2N_2O_5$ and molecular weight is 323.13.
The chemical names for Hydrocortisone Acetate are:
  (1) Pregn-4-ene-3,20-dione,21-(acetyloxy)-11, 17-dihydroxy-,(11β)-, and
  (2) 17-Hydroxycorticosterone 21-acetate
Its empirical formula is $C_{23}H_{32}O_6$ and molecular weight is 404.50.

CLINICAL PHARMACOLOGY

Corticoids suppress the inflammatory response to a variety of agents and they probably delay or slow healing. Since corticoids may inhibit the body's defense mechanism against infection, a concomitant antimicrobial drug may be used when this inhibition is considered to be clinically significant in a particular case.

The anti-inefective component in this combination is included to provide action against specific organisms susceptible to it. Chloramphenicol is considered active against a wide spectrum of gram-negative and gram-positive organisms such as *Escherichia coli, Hemophilus influenzae, Staphylococcus aureus, Streptococcus hemolyticus,* and *Moraxella lacunata* (Morax-Axenfeld bacillus). Development of resistance to Chloramphenicol can be regarded as minimal for staphylococci and many other species of bacteria. Chloramphenicol is primarily bacteriostatic and acts by inhibition of protein synthesis by interfering with the transfer of activated amino acids from soluble RNA to ribosomes. It has been noted that Chloramphenicol is found in measurable amounts in the aqueous humor following local application to the eye.

When a decision to administer both a corticoid and an antimicrobial is made, the administration of such drugs in combination has the advantage of greater patient compliance and convenience, with the added assurance that the appropriate dosage of both drugs is administered, plus assured compatibility of ingredients when both types of drug are in the same formulation and, particularly, that the correct volume of drug is delivered and retained.

The relative potency of corticosteroids depends on the molecular structure, concentration, and release from the vehicle.

INDICATIONS AND USAGE

Chloramphenicol should be used only in those serious infections for which less potentially dangerous drugs are ineffective or contraindicated. Bacteriological studies should be performed to determine the causative organisms and their sensitivity to Chloramphenicol (See box *"Warning"*).

For steroid-responsive inflammatory ocular conditions for which a corticosteroid is indicated and where bacterial infection or a risk of bacterial ocular infection exists.

Ocular steroids are indicated in inflammatory conditions of the palpebral and bulbar conjunctiva, cornea, and anterior segment of the globe where the inherent risk of steroid use in certain infective conjunctivitides is accepted to obtain a diminution in edema and inflammation. They are also indicated in chronic anterior uveitis and corneal injury from chemical radiation, thermal burns, or penetration of foreign bodies.

The use of a combination drug with antiinefective component is indicated where the risk of infection is high or where there is an expectation that potentially dangerous numbers of bacteria will be present in the eye.

The particular anti-infective drug in this product is active against the following common bacterial eye pathogens:

Staphylococcus aureus
Streptococci, including *Streptococcus pneumoniae*
Escherichia coli

Hemophilus influenzae
Klebsiella/Enterobacter species
Moraxella lacunata (Morax-Axenfeld bacillus)
Neisseria species

The product does not provide adequate coverage against:

Pseudomonas aeruginosa
Serratia marcescens

CONTRAINDICATIONS

Epithelial herpes simplex keratitis (dendritic keratitis), vaccinia, varicella, and many other viral diseases of the cornea and conjunctiva. Mycobacterial infection of the eye. Fungal diseases of ocular structures. Hypersensitivity to a component of the medication. (Hypersensitivity to the antibiotic component occurs at a higher rate than for other components.)

The use of these combinations is always contraindicated after uncomplicated removal of a corneal foreign body.

WARNINGS

See box *"Warning"*.

Prolonged use of steroids may result in glaucoma, with damage to the optic nerve, defects in visual acuity and fields of vision, and posterior subcapsular cataract formation.

Prolonged use may suppress the host response and thus increase the hazard of secondary ocular infections. In those diseases causing thinning of the cornea or sclera, perforations have been known to occur with the use of topical steroids. In acute purulent conditions of the eye, steroids may mask infection or enhance existing infection. If these products are used for 10 days or longer, intraocular pressure should be routinely monitored even though it may be difficult in children and uncooperative patients.

Employment of steroid medication in the treatment of herpes simplex requires great caution.

PRECAUTIONS

The initial prescription and renewal of the medication order beyond 20 milliliters should be made by a physician only after examination of the patient with the aid of magnification, such as slit lamp biomicroscopy and, where appropriate, fluorescein staining.

The possibility of persistent fungal infections of the cornea should be considered after prolonged steroid dosing.

The prolonged use of antibiotics may occasionally result in overgrowth of nonsusceptible organisms, including fungi. If new infections appear during medication, the drug should be discontinued and appropriate measures should be taken.

In all serious infections the topical use of Chloramphenicol should be supplemented by appropriate systemic medication.

ADVERSE REACTIONS

Blood dyscrasias have been reported in association with the use of Chloramphenicol. (See *"Warnings"*).

Adverse reactions have occurred with steroid/antiinfective combination drugs which can be attributed to the steriod component, the antiinefective component, or the combination.

Exact incidence figures are not available since no denominator of treated patients is available.

Reactions occurring most often from the presence of the antiinfective ingredient are allergic sensitizations. The reactions due to the steroid component in decreasing order of frequency are: elevation of intraocular pressure (IOP) with possible development of glaucoma, and infrequent optic nerve damage; posterior subcapsular cataract formation; and delayed wound healing.

Secondary Infection: The development of secondary infection has occurred after use of combinations containing steroids and antimicrobials. Fungal infections of the cornea are particularly prone to develop coincidentally with long-term applications of steroid. The possibility of fungal invasion must be considered in any persistent corneal ulceration where steroid treatment has been used.

Secondary bacterial ocular infection following suppression of host responses also occurs.

DOSAGE AND ADMINISTRATION

Two drops applied to the affected eye every three hours, or more frequently if deemed advisable by the prescribing physician. Administration should be continued day and night for the first 48 hours, after which the interval between applications may be increased. Treatment should be continued for at least 48 hours after the eye appears normal.

Directions for Dispensing: Add 5 ml sterile distilled water to contents of vial under aseptic conditions. Shake to make uniform suspension. Place sterile dropper in vial. Each ml of suspension prepared as directed contains 2.5 mg Chloramphenicol and 5 mg Hydrocortisone Acetate.

Not more than 20 milliliters should be prescribed initially and the prescription should not be refilled without further evaluation as outlined in *"Precautions"* above.

After dispensing, the product may be stored at room temperature for a period of not more than 10 days.

HOW SUPPLIED

DROP:

BRAND/MANUFACTURER	NDC	SIZE	AWP
○ **BRAND**			
CHLOROMYCETIN W/HYDROCORTISONE: Parke-Davis	00071-3228-36	5 ml	$23.74

Chloramphenicol/Hydrocortisone Acetate/Polymyxin B Sulfate

> **WARNING**
> BONE MARROW HYPOPLASIA INCLUDING APLASTIC ANEMIA AND DEATH HAS BEEN REPORTED FOLLOWING LOCAL APPLICATION OF CHLORAMPHENICOL. CHLORAMPHENICOL SHOULD NOT BE USED WHEN LESS POTENTIALLY DANGEROUS AGENTS WOULD BE EXPECTED TO PROVIDE EFFECTIVE TREATMENT.

DESCRIPTION

Chloramphenicol, Polymyxin B Sulfate, and Hydrocortisone Acetate Ophthalmic Ointment, USP is a sterile antibiotic/antiinflammatory ointment for ophthalmic administration. Each gram of Chloramphenicol/Polymyxin B Sulfate, Hydrocortisone Acetate contains 10 mg Chloramphenicol, 10,000 units Polymyxim B (as the Sulfate), and 5 mg Hydrocortisone Acetate. It contains no preservatives.

The chemical names for Chloramphenicol are: (1) Acetamide, 2,2-dichloro-N-[2-hydroxy-1-(hydroxymethyl)-2-(4-nitrophenyl) ethyl]-, and (2) D-*threo*-(—)-2,2-dichloro-N-[B-hydroxy-α-(hydroxymethyl)-p- nitrophenethyl] acetamide.

Chloramphenicol has the following empirical formula and molecular weight. $C_{11}H_{12}Cl_2N_2O_5$, Mol Wt 323.13.

The chemical names for Hydrocortisone Acetate are: (1) Pregn-4-ene-3,20-dione,21-(acetyloxy)-11,17-dihydroxy-,(11β)-, and (2) 17-Hydroxycorticosterone 21-acetate.

Hydrocortisone Acetate has the following empirical formulae and molecular weight. $C_{23}H_{32}O_6$, Mol Wt 404.50.

Polymyxin B Sulfate is the Sulfate salt of an antibiotic substance elaborated by various strains of *Bacillus polymyxa*.

Polymyxin B_1:R = (+)-6-Methyloctanoyl
Polymyxin B_2:R = 6-Methylhepatanoyl
DAB = α, γ-Diaminobutyric Acid

CLINICAL PHARMACOLOGY

Corticoids suppress the inflammatory response to a variety of agents and they probably delay or slow healing. Since corticoids may inhibit the body's defense mechanism against infection, a concomitant antimicrobial drug may be used when this inhibition is considered to be clinically significant in a particular case.

The antiinfective components in this combination are included to provide action against specific organisms susceptible to them. Chloramphenicol is considered active against a wide spectrum of gram-negative and gram-positive organisms such as *Escherichia coli, Hemophilus influenzae, Staphylococcus aureus, Streptococcus hemolyticus,* and *Moraxella lacunata* (Morax-Axenfeld bacillus). Development of resistance to chloramphenicol can be regarded as minimal for staphylococci and many other species of bacteria. Chloramphenicol is primarily bacteriostatic and acts by inhibition of protein synthesis by interfering with the transfer of activated amino acids from soluble RNA to ribosomes. It has been noted that Chloramphenicol is found in measurable amounts in the aqueous humor following local application to the eye.

Polymyxin B Sulfate has a bactericidal action against almost all gram-negative bacilli except the *Proteus* group. All gram-positive bacteria, fungi, and the gram-negative cocci, *Neisseria gonorrhoeae* and *N meningitidis,* are resistant.

When a decision to administer both a corticoid and an antimicrobial is made, the administration of such drugs in combination has the advantage of greater patient compliance and convenience, with the added assurance that the appropriate dosage of both drugs is administered, plus assured compatibility of ingredients when both types of drug are in the same formulation and, particularly, that the correct volume of drug is delivered and retained.

The relative potency of corticosteroids depends on the molecular structure, concentration, and release from the vehicle.

INDICATIONS AND USAGE

Chloramphenicol should be used only in those serious infections for which less potentially dangerous drugs are ineffective or contraindicated. Bacteriological studies should be performed to determine the causative organisms and their sensitivity to chloramphenicol (See box *"Warning"*).

For steroid-responsive inflammatory ocular conditions for which a corticosteroid is indicated and where bacterial infection or a risk of bacterial ocular infection exists.

Ocular steroids are indicated in inflammatory conditions of the palpebral and bulbar conjunctiva, cornea, and anterior segment of the globe where the inherent risk of steroid use in certain infective conjunctivities is accepted to obtain a diminution in edema and inflammation. They are also indicated in chronic anterior uveitis and corneal injury from chemical radiation, thermal burns, or penetration of foreign bodies.

The use of a combination of drug with an anti-infective component is indicated where the risk of infection is high or where there is an expectation that potentially dangerous numbers of bacteria will be present in the eye.

The particular anti-infective drugs in this product are active against the following common bacterial eye pathogens:

Staphylococcus aureus
Streptococci, including *Streptococcus pneumoniae*
Escherichia coli
Hemophilus influenzae
Klebsiella/Enterobacter species
Neisseria species
Moraxella lacunata
(Morax-Axenfeld bacillus)
Pseudomonas aeruginosa

The product does not provide adequate coverage against: *Serratia marcescens*

CONTRAINDICATIONS
Epithelial herpes simplex keratitis (dendritic keratitis), vaccinia, varicella, and many other viral diseases of the cornea and conjunctive. Mycobacterial infection of the eye. Fungal diseases of ocular structures. Hypersensitivity to a component of the medication. (Hypersensitivity to the antibiotic component occurs at a higher rate than for other components.)

The use of these combinations is always contraindicated after uncomplicated removal of a corneal foreign body.

WARNINGS
See box *"Warning"*

Prolonged use of steroids may result in glaucoma, with damage to the optic nerve, defects in visual acuity and fields of vision, and posterior subcapsular cataract formation. Prolonged use may suppress the host response and thus increase the hazard of secondary ocular infections. In those diseases causing thinning of the cornea or sclera, perforations have been known to occur with the use of topical steroids. In acute purulent conditions of the eye, steroids may mask infection or enhance existing infection. If these products are used for 10 days or longer, intraocular pressure should be routinely monitored even though it may be difficult in children and uncooperative patients.

Employment of steroid medication in the treatment of herpes simplex requires great caution.

Ophthalmic ointments may retard corneal wound healing.

PRECAUTIONS
The initial prescription and renewal of the medication order beyond 8 grams should be made by a physician only after examination of the patient with the aid of magnification, such as slit lamp biomicroscopy and, where appropriate, fluorescein staining.

The possibility of persistent fungal infections of the cornea should be considered after prolonged steroid dosing.

The prolonged use of antibiotics may occasionally result in overgrowth of nonsusceptible organisms, including fungi. If new infections appear during medication, the drug should be discontinued and appropriate measures should be taken.

In all serious infections the topical use of Chloramphenicol should be supplemented by appropriate systemic medication.

ADVERSE REACTIONS
There have been reports of punctate staining of the cornea following intensive treatment (every one to two hours during the waking day) or corneal ulcers with Chloramphenicol/Hydrocortisone Acetate/Polymyxin B Sulfate. In each reported case, the staining has disappeared after discontinuation of the medication.

Blood dyscrasias have been reported in association with the use of Chloramphenicol. (See *"Warnings"*.)

Adverse reactions have occurred with steroid/antiinfective combination drugs which can be attributed to the steroid component, the antiinfective component, or the combination. Exact incidence figures are not available since no denominator of treated patients is available.

Reactions occurring most often from the presence of the anti-infective ingredient are allergic sensitizations. The reactions due to the steroid component in decreasing order of frequency are: elevation of intraocular pressure (IOP) with possible development of glaucoma, and infrequent optic nerve damage; posterior subcapsular cataract formation; and delayed wound healing.

Secondary Infection: The development of secondary infection has occurred after use of combinations containing steroids and antimicrobials. Fungal infections of the cornea are particularly prone to develop coincidentally with long-term applications of steroid. The possibility of fungal invasion must be considered in any persistent corneal ulceration where steroid treatment has been used.

Secondary bacterial ocular infection following suppression of host responses also occurs.

DOSAGE AND ADMINISTRATION
Application of a small amount of ointment, placed in the lower conjunctival sac, is made to the affected eye every three hours, or more frequently if deemed advisable by the prescribing physician. Administration should be continued day and night for the first 48 hours, after which the interval between applications may be increased. Treatment should be continued for at least 48 hours after the eye appears normal.

Not more than 8 grams should be prescribed initially and the prescription should be refilled without further evaluation as outlined in Precautions above.

WARNING: May be manufactured with CFC-12, a substance which harms public health and environment by destroying ozone in the upper atmosphere.

HOW SUPPLIED
OINTMENT:

BRAND/MANUFACTURER	NDC	SIZE	AWP
○ BRAND OPHTHOCORT: Parke-Davis	00071-3079-07	3.5 gm	$15.21

Chlorcyclizine Hydrochloride and Hydrocortisone Acetate

DESCRIPTION
Chlorcyclizine Hydrochloride and Hydrocortisone Acetate Cream contains the antihistamine Chlorcyclizine Hydrochloride 2% and the corticosteroid Hydrocortisone Acetate 0.5%.

Chlorcyclizine Hydrochloride and Hydrocortisone Acetate Cream is an antipruritic-anti-inflammatory-anesthetic for topical administration.

Chlorcyclizine Hydrochloride is known chemically as 1-[(4-chlorophenyl)phenylmethyl]-4-methylpiperazine monohydrochloride.

Hydrocortisone Acetate is the Acetate ester of cortisol, known chemically as 21-(acetyloxy)-11β,17-dihydroxypregn-4-ene-3,20-dione.

The pH of this product is approximately 4.5.

CLINICAL PHARMACOLOGY
Chlorcyclizine Hydrochloride is an H_1 histamine-receptor antagonist that will occupy receptor sites in effector cells to the exclusion of histamine. It blocks most of the effects of histamine mediated by H_1 receptors, including contraction of smooth muscle and increased capillary permeability. Absorption of Chlorcyclizine Hydrochloride into the skin is rapid following topical application, whereas systemic absorption from the skin is minimal. Chlorcyclizine Hydrochloride prevents local edema and provides local anesthetic and antipruritic action in the skin.

Hydrocortisone Acetate administered topically suppresses most inflammatory and allergic responses in the skin. Following topical application, it is absorbed rapidly into the skin, where it reduces local heat, redness, swelling, and tenderness. A small part of the dose applied to broken skin is absorbed systemically and metabolized by the liver.

INDICATIONS AND USAGE
Chlorcyclizine Hydrochloride and Hydrocortisone Acetate Cream is indicated for the treatment of pruritic skin eruptions and other dermatoses including: eczema (allergic, nuchal and nummular); dermatitis (atopic, lichenoid and seborrheic); contact dermatitis including poison ivy, poison oak and poison sumac; localized neurodermatitis; insect bites; sunburn; intertrigo; and anogenital pruritus.

CONTRAINDICATIONS
This preparation is contraindicated in patients who are hypersensitive to any of its components; in tuberculosis of the skin, vaccinia, varicella, and herpes simplex. As with other topical products containing hydrocortisone, the cream should not be used in bacterial infections of the skin unless antibacterial therapy is concomitant.

Not for ophthalmic use.

WARNINGS
Oral Chlorcyclizine is teratogenic in animals. Long-term reproduction studies of topical Chlorcyclizine have not been conducted in humans.

PRECAUTIONS
General: If signs of irritation develop with use of this cream, treatment should be discontinued and appropriate therapy instituted.

Any of the side effects reported following systemic use of corticosteroids, including adrenal suppression, may also occur following their topical use, especially in infants and children. Systemic absorption of topically applied steroids will be increased if extensive body surface areas are treated or if the occlusive technique is used. Under these circumstances, suitable precautions should be taken when long-term use is anticipated, particularly in infants and children.

Carcinogenesis, Mutagenesis, Impairment of Fertility: Oral Chlorcyclizine is teratogenic in animals. Long-term reproduction studies of topical Chlorcyclizine have not been conducted. It is poorly absorbed percutaneously.

Pregnancy: Teratogenic Effects: Pregnancy Category C. Animal reproduction studies have not been conducted with Chlorcyclizine and HC Cream. It is also not known whether Chlorcyclizine and HC Cream can cause fetal harm when administered to a pregnant woman or can affect reproduction capacity. Chlorcyclizine and HC Cream should be given to a pregnant woman only if clearly needed.

Nursing Mothers: Hydrocortisone Acetate appears in human milk following oral administration of the drug.

Caution should be exercised when Hydrocortisone Acetate is administered to a nursing woman.

It is not known whether Chlorcyclizine Hydrochloride is excreted in human milk. Because many drugs are excreted in human milk, caution should be exercised when Chlorcyclizine Hydrochloride is administered to a nursing woman.

ADVERSE REACTIONS

Allergic contact dermatitis may occur with topical application of Chlorcyclizine Hydrochloride. Systemic side effects have been reported after topical application of antihistamines to large areas of skin.

The following local adverse reactions have been reported with topical corticosteroids, especially under occlusive dressings; irritation, folliculitis, hypertrichosis, acneiform eruptions, hypopigmentation, allergic contact dermatitis, secondary infection, skin atrophy; striae and miliaria.

OVERDOSAGE

With continued application of topical corticosteroid on large areas of damaged skin and under occlusion, there is a remote possibility that sufficient absorption could occur to produce Cushing's syndrome. This is more likely in children.

Systemic toxicity following topical application of Chlorcyclizine has never been reported.

The oral LD_{50} of Chlorcyclizine Hydrochloride in the mouse is 300 mg/kg.

DOSAGE AND ADMINISTRATION

Apply to the skin two to five times daily. If the condition of the skin will permit, the cream should be well rubbed in.

Store at 15° to 25°C (59° to 77°F).

HOW SUPPLIED
CREAM: 2%-0.5%

BRAND/MANUFACTURER	NDC	SIZE	AWP
○ BRAND			
MANTADIL: Burr Wellcome	00081-0650-94	15 gm	$17.66

Chlordiazepoxide

DESCRIPTION

Chlordiazepoxide is a versatile therapeutic agent of proven value for the relief of anxiety. Chlordiazepoxide is among the safer of the effective psychopharmacologic compounds available, as demonstrated by extensive clinical evidence.

Chlordiazepoxide is available as capsules or tablets containing 5 mg, 10 mg or 25 mg Chlordiazepoxide and in injectable form containing 100 mg Chlordiazepoxide per ampul.

Chlordiazepoxide 7-chloro-2-(methylamino)-5-phenyl-3H-1,4-benzodiazepine 4-oxide. The powder must be protected from light.

Following is its chemical structure:

ACTIONS

Chlordiazepoxide has antianxiety, sedative, appetite-stimulating and weak analgesic actions. The precise mechanism of action is not known. The drug blocks EEG arousal from stimulation of the brain stem reticular formation. It takes several hours for peak blood levels to be reached and the half-life of the drug is between 24 and 48 hours. After the drug is discontinued plasma levels decline slowly over a period of several days. Chlordiazepoxide is excreted in the urine, with 1% to 2% unchanged and 3% to 6% as a conjugate.

Animal Pharmacology: The drug has been studied extensively in many species of animals and these studies are suggestive of action on the limbic system of the brain, which recent evidence indicates is involved in emotional responses. Hostile monkeys were made tame by oral drug doses which did not cause sedation. Chlordiazepoxide HCl revealed a "taming" action with the elimination of fear and aggression. The taming effect of Chlordiazepoxide HCl was further demonstrated in rats made vicious by lesions in the septal area of the brain. The drug dosage which effectively blocked the vicious reaction was well below the dose which caused sedation in these animals.

The LD_{50} of parenterally administered Chlordiazepoxide HCl was determined in mice (72 hours) and rats (5 days), and calculated according to the method of Miller and Tainter, with the following results: mice, IV, 123 ± 12 mg/kg; mice, IM. 366 ± 7 mg/kg; rats, IV, 120 ± 7 mg/kg; rats, IM, > 160 mg/kg.

Effects on Reproduction: Reproduction studies in rats fed 10, 20 and 80 mg/kg daily and bred through one or two matings showed no congenital anomalies, nor were there adverse effects on lactation of the dams or growth of the newborn. However, in another study at 100 mg/kg daily there was noted a significant decrease in the fertilization rate and a marked decrease in the viability and body weight of offspring which may be attributable to sedative activity, thus resulting in lack of interest in mating and lessened maternal nursing and care of the young. One neonate in each of the first and second matings in the rat reproduction study at the 100 mg/kg dose exhibited major skeletal defects. Further studies are in progress to determine the significance of these findings.

INDICATIONS

Chlordiazepoxide is indicated for the management of anxiety disorders or for the short-term relief of symptoms of anxiety, withdrawal symptoms of acute alcoholism, and preoperative apprehension and anxiety. Anxiety or tension associated with the stress of everyday life usually does not require treatment with an anxiolytic.

The effectiveness of Chlordiazepoxide in long-term use, that is, more than 4 months, has not been assessed by systematic clinical studies. The physician should periodically reassess the usefulness of the drug for the individual patient.

CONTRAINDICATIONS

Chlordiazepoxide is contraindicated in patients with known hypersensitivity to the drug.

WARNINGS

Chlordiazepoxide may impair the mental and/or physical abilities required for the performance of potentially hazardous tasks such as driving a vehicle or operating machinery. Similarly, it may impair mental alertness in children. The concomitant use of alcohol or other central nervous system depressants may have an additive effect. PATIENTS SHOULD BE WARNED ACCORDINGLY.

Usage in Pregnancy: An increased risk of congenital malformations associated with the use of minor tranquilizers (Chlordiazepoxide, diazepam and meprobamate) during the first trimester of pregnancy has been suggested in several studies. Because use of these drugs is rarely a matter of urgency, their use during this period should almost always be avoided. The possibility that a woman of childbearing potential may be pregnant at the time of institution of therapy should be considered. Patients should be advised that if they become pregnant during therapy or intend to become pregnant they should communicate with their physicians about the desirability of discontinuing the drug.

Withdrawal symptoms of the barbiturate type have occurred after the discontinuation of benzodiazepines. (See *"Drug Abuse and Dependence"* section.)

PRECAUTIONS

In elderly and debilitated patients, it is recommended that the dosage be limited to the smallest effective amount to preclude the development of ataxia or oversedation (10 mg or less per day initially, to be increased gradually as needed and tolerated). Injectable Chlordiazepoxide (intramuscular or intravenous) is indicated primarily in acute states, and patients receiving this form of therapy should be kept under observation, preferably in bed, for a period of up to 3 hours. Ambulatory patients should not be permitted to operate a vehicle following an injection. Injectable Chlordiazepoxide should not be given to patients in shock or comatose states. Reduced dosage (usually 25 to 50 mg) should be used for elderly or debilitated patients, and for children age 12 or older. In general, the concomitant administration of Chlordiazepoxide and other psychotropic agents is not recommended. If such combination therapy seems indicated, careful consideration should be given to the pharmacology of the agents to be employed — particularly when the known potentiating compounds such as the MAO inhibitors and phenothiazines are to be used. The usual precautions in treating patients with impaired renal or hepatic function should be observed. Paradoxical reactions, eg, excitement, stimulation and acute rage, have been reported in psychiatric patients and in hyperactive aggressive children, and should be watched for during Chlordiazepoxide therapy. The usual precautions are indicated when Chlordiazepoxide is used in the treatment of anxiety states where there is any evidence of impending depression; it should be borne in mind that suicidal tendencies may be present and protective measures may be necessary. Although clinical studies have not established a cause and effect relationship, physicians should be aware that variable effects on blood coagulation have been reported very rarely in patients receiving oral anticoagulants and Chlordiazepoxide. In view of isolated reports associating Chlordiazepoxide with exacerbation of porphyria, caution should be exercised in prescribing Chlordiazepoxide to patients suffering from this disease.

Information for Patients: To assure the safe and effective use of benzodiazepines, patients should be informed that, since benzodiazepines may produce psychological and physical dependence it is advisable that they consult with their physician before either increasing the dose or abruptly discontinuing this drug.

ADVERSE REACTIONS

The necessity of discontinuing therapy because of undesirable effects has been rare. Drowsiness, ataxia and confusion have been reported in some patients — particularly the elderly and debilitated. While these effects can be avoided in almost all instances by proper dosage adjustment, they have occasionally been observed at the lower dosage ranges. In a few instances syncope has been reported.

Other adverse reactions reported during therapy include isolated instances of skin eruptions, edema, minor menstrual irregularities, nausea and constipation, extrapyramidal symptoms, as well as increased and decreased libido; additional adverse reactions from Injectable Chlordiazepoxide are: hypotension, tachycardia, and blurred vision. Such side effects have been infrequent and are generally controlled with reduction of dosage. Similarly, with Injectable Chlordiazepoxide hypotension associated with spinal anesthesia has occurred. Pain following intramuscular injection has been reported. Changes in EEG patterns (low-voltage fast activity) have been observed in patients during and after Chlordiazepoxide treatment.

Blood dyscrasias (including agranulocytosis), jaundice and hepatic dysfunction have occasionally been reported during therapy. When Chlordiazepoxide treatment is protracted, periodic blood counts and liver function tests are advisable.

DRUG ABUSE AND DEPENDENCE

Chlordiazepoxide capsules, tablets, and injectable are classified by the Drug Enforcement Administration as a Schedule IV controlled substance.

◆ RATED THERAPEUTICALLY EQUIVALENT; ◇ THERAPEUTIC EQUIVALENCE UNCONFIRMED; ○ UNRATED

Withdrawal symptoms, similar in character to those noted with barbiturates and alcohol (convulsions, tremor, abdominal and muscle cramps, vomiting and sweating), have occurred following abrupt discontinuance of Chlordiazepoxide. The more severe withdrawal symptoms have usually been limited to those patients who had received excessive doses over an extended period of time. Generally milder withdrawal symptoms (eg, dysphoria and insomnia) have been reported following abrupt discontinuance of benzodiazepines taken continuously at therapeutic levels for several months. Consequently, after extended therapy, abrupt discontinuation should generally be avoided and a gradual dosage tapering schedule followed. Addiction-prone individuals (such as drug addicts or alcoholics) should be under careful surveillance when receiving Chlordiazepoxide or other psychotropic agents because of the predisposition of such patients to habituation and dependence.

OVERDOSAGE

Manifestations of Chlordiazepoxide overdosage include somnolence, confusion, coma and diminished reflexes. Respiration, pulse and blood pressure should be monitored, as in all cases of drug overdosage, although in general, these effects have been minimal following Chlordiazepoxide overdosage. General supportive measures should be employed, along with immediate gastric lavage. Intravenous fluids should be administered and an adequate airway maintained. Hypotension may be combated by the use of norepinephrine or metaraminol. Dialysis is of limited value. There have been occasional reports of excitation in patients following Chlordiazepoxide overdosage; if this occurs barbiturates should not be used. As with the management of intentional overdosage with any drug, it should be borne in mind that multiple agents may have been ingested.

Flumazenil, a specific benzodiazepine-receptor antagonist, is indicated for the complete or partial reversal of the sedative effects of benzodiazepines and may be used in situations when an overdose with a benzodiazepine is known or suspected. Prior to the administration of flumazenil, necessary measures should be instituted to secure airway, ventilation and intravenous access. Flumazenil is intended as an adjunct to, not as a substitute for, proper management of benzodiazepine overdose. Patients treated with flumazenil should be monitored for resedation, respiratory depression and other residual benzodiazepine effects for an appropriate period after treatment. **The prescriber should be aware of a risk of seizure in association with flumazenil treatment, particularly in long-term benzodiazepine users and in cyclic antidepressant overdose.** The complete flumazenil package insert, including "Contraindications, Warnings" and "Precautions", should be consulted prior to use.

DOSAGE AND ADMINISTRATION

Because of the wide range of clinical indications for Chlordiazepoxide, the optimum dosage varies with the diagnosis and response of the individual patient. The dosage, therefore, should be individualized for maximum beneficial effects.

Adults	Usual Daily Dose
Relief of Mild and Moderate Anxiety Disorders and Symptoms of Anxiety	5 mg or 10 mg, 3 or 4 times daily
Relief of Severe Anxiety Disorders and Symptoms of Anxiety	20 mg or 25 mg, 3 or 4 times daily
Geriatric Patients, or in the presence of debilitating disease	5 mg, 2 to 4 times daily

PREOPERATIVE APPREHENSION AND ANXIETY

On days preceding surgery, 5 to 10 mg orally, 3 or 4 times daily. If used as preoperative medication, 50 to 100 mg IM 1 hour prior to surgery.

Children	Usual Daily Dose
Because of the varied response of children to CNS-acting drugs, therapy should be initiated with the lowest dose and increased as required.	5 mg, 2 to 4 times daily (may be increased in some children to 10 mg, 2 or 3 times daily)
Since clinical experience in children under 6 years of age is limited, the use of the drug in this age group is not recommended.	

For the relief of withdrawal symptoms of acute alcoholism, the parenteral form is usually used initially. If the drug is administered orally, the suggested initial dose is 50 to 100 mg, to be followed by repeated doses as needed until agitation is controlled — up to 300 mg per day. Dosage should then be reduced to maintenance levels.

INJECTABLE CHLORDIAZEPOXIDE
PREPARATION AND ADMINISTRATION OF SOLUTIONS

Solutions of Chlordiazepoxide for intramuscular or intravenous use should be prepared aseptically. Sterilization by heating should not be attempted.

Intramuscular: Add 2 mL of *intramuscular diluent* to contents of 5-mL dry-filled amber ampul of Chlordiazepoxide sterile powder (100 mg). Avoid excessive pressure in injecting the diluent into the ampul containing the powder since bubbles will form on the surface of the solution. Agitate gently until completely dissolved. Solution should be prepared immediately before administration. Any unused solution should be discarded. Deep intramuscular injection should be given *slowly* into the upper outer quadrant of the gluteus muscle.

Caution: Chlordiazepoxide solution made with the Special Intramuscular Diluent should not be given intravenously because of the air bubbles which form when the intramuscular diluent is added to the Chlordiazepoxide powder. Do not use diluent solution if it is opalescent or hazy.

Intravenous: In most cases, intramuscular injection is the preferred route of administration of Injectable Chlordiazepoxide since beneficial effects are usually seen within 15 to 30 minutes. When, in the judgment of the physician, even more rapid action is mandatory, Injectable Chlordiazepoxide may be administered intravenously. A suitable solution for intravenous administration may be prepared as follows: Add 5 mL of *sterile physiological saline* or *sterile water for injection* to contents of 5-mL dry-filled amber ampul of Chlordiazepoxide sterile powder (100 mg). Agitate gently until thoroughly dissolved. Solution should be prepared immediately before administration. Any unused portion should be discarded. *Intravenous injection should be given slowly over a 1-minute period.*

Caution: Chlordiazepoxide solution made with physiological saline or sterile water for injection should not be given intramuscularly because of pain on injection.

DOSAGE

Dosage should be individualized according to the diagnosis and the response of the patient. While 300 mg may be given during a 6-hour period, this dose should not be exceeded in any 24-hour period.

Indication	Adult Dosage*
Withdrawal Symptoms of Acute Alcoholism	50 to 100 mg IM or IV initially; repeat in 2 to 4 hours, if necessary
Acute or Severe Anxiety Disorders or Symptoms of Anxiety	50 to 100 mg IM or IV initially; then 25 to 50 mg 3 or 4 times daily, if necessary
Preoperative Apprehension and Anxiety	50 to 100 mg IM 1 hour prior to surgery

* *Lower doses (usually 25 to 50 mg) should be used for elderly or debilitated patients, and for older children. Since clinical experience in children under 12 years of age is limited, the use of the drug in this age group is not recommended.*

In most cases, acute symptoms may be rapidly controlled by parenteral administration so that subsequent treatment, if necessary, may be given orally.

J CODES
Up to 100 mg IM,IV—J1990

HOW SUPPLIED
CAPSULE (C-IV): 5 MG

AVERAGE UNIT PRICE (AVAILABLE SIZES)		GENERIC A-RATED AVERAGE PRICE (GAAP)	
BRAND	$0.35	100s	$5.82
GENERIC	$0.05	500s	$22.13
HCFA FUL (100s ea)	$0.03	1000s	$33.49

BRAND/MANUFACTURER	NDC	SIZE	AWP
◆ BRAND			
➤ LIBRIUM: Roche Prod	00140-0001-01	100s	$33.71
	00140-0001-49	100s ud	$35.75
	00140-0001-50	100s ud	$36.26
	00140-0001-14	500s	$167.44
◆ GENERICS			
Richlyn	00115-2758-01	100s	$2.42
Parmed	00349-2032-01	100s	$3.77
Moore,H.L.	00839-1130-06	100s	$5.60
Goldline	00182-0977-01	100s	$5.70
Aligen	00405-0040-01	100s	$5.84
Barr	00555-0158-02	100s	$6.01
Rosemont	00832-0305-00	100s	$6.04
Major	00904-0090-60	100s	$6.15
Geneva	00781-2080-01	100s	$6.19
URL	00677-0457-01	100s	$6.20
➤ Rugby	00536-3487-01	100s	$6.26
Qualitest	00603-2666-21	100s	$6.90
UDL	51079-0374-20	100s ud	$6.44
UDL	51079-0374-21	100s ud	$6.44
Auro	55829-0844-10	100s ud	$6.56
Goldline	00182-0977-89	100s ud	$6.56
Parmed	00349-2032-05	500s	$13.84
Major	00904-0090-40	500s	$19.65
URL	00677-0457-05	500s	$23.00
➤ Rugby	00536-3487-05	500s	$23.06
Barr	00555-0158-04	500s	$23.98
Geneva	00781-2080-05	500s	$24.10
Rosemont	00832-0305-50	500s	$24.19
Aligen	00405-0040-02	500s	$25.24
Richlyn	00115-2758-03	1000s	$18.60
Major	00904-0090-80	1000s	$18.75
Rosemont	00832-0305-10	1000s	$31.54
Geneva	00781-2080-10	1000s	$39.05
Moore,H.L.	00839-1130-16	1000s	$39.14
➤ Rugby	00536-3487-10	1000s	$39.20
Qualitest	00603-2666-32	1000s	$48.12

CAPSULE (C-IV): 10 MG

AVERAGE UNIT PRICE (AVAILABLE SIZES)		GENERIC A-RATED AVERAGE PRICE (GAAP)	
BRAND	$0.50	100s	$7.00
GENERIC	$0.05	500s	$20.40
HCFA FUL (100s ea)	$0.04	1000s	$34.95

BRAND/MANUFACTURER	NDC	SIZE	AWP
◆ BRAND			
➤ LIBRIUM: Roche Prod	00140-0002-01	100s	$49.08
	00140-0002-49	100s ud	$51.11
	00140-0002-50	100s ud	$51.63
	00140-0002-14	500s	$244.30
◆ GENERICS			
Richlyn	00115-2760-01	100s	$3.08
Parmed	00349-2033-01	100s	$3.94
Aligen	00405-0041-01	100s	$5.52
Goldline	00182-0978-01	100s	$6.00
Barr	00555-0033-02	100s	$6.08
Rosemont	00832-0306-00	100s	$6.16
URL	00677-0458-01	100s	$6.35
Qualitest	00603-2667-21	100s	$6.40
Geneva	00781-2082-01	100s	$6.49
Major	00904-0091-60	100s	$6.60
Moore,H.L.	00839-1131-06	100s	$6.68
➤ Rugby	00536-3488-01	100s	$7.04
POXI: Seneca	47028-0012-01	100s	$19.92
Goldline	00182-0978-89	100s ud	$6.70
UDL	51079-0375-20	100s ud	$7.36
UDL	51079-0375-21	100s ud	$7.36
Auro	55829-0845-10	100s ud	$7.36
Major	00904-0091-40	500s	$15.50
Rosemont	00832-0306-50	500s	$18.36
Goldline	00182-0978-05	500s	$21.00
URL	00677-0458-05	500s	$22.10
Geneva	00781-2082-05	500s	$22.49
➤ Rugby	00536-3488-05	500s	$22.97
Richlyn	00115-2760-03	1000s	$23.70
Parmed	00349-2033-10	1000s	$23.94
Major	00904-0091-80	1000s	$27.85
Goldline	00182-0978-10	1000s	$31.45
Barr	00555-0033-05	1000s	$31.62
Rosemont	00832-0306-10	1000s	$33.26
Aligen	00405-0041-03	1000s	$36.23
Geneva	00781-2082-10	1000s	$39.98
URL	00677-0458-10	1000s	$40.10
Qualitest	00603-2667-32	1000s	$41.11
➤ Rugby	00536-3488-10	1000s	$44.55
Moore,H.L.	00839-1131-16	1000s	$45.56

CAPSULE (C-IV): 25 MG

AVERAGE UNIT PRICE (AVAILABLE SIZES)		GENERIC A-RATED AVERAGE PRICE (GAAP)	
BRAND	$0.85	100s	$6.78
GENERIC	$0.06	500s	$24.27
HCFA FUL (100s ea)	$0.05	1000s	$37.80

BRAND/MANUFACTURER	NDC	SIZE	AWP
◆ BRAND			
➤ LIBRIUM: Roche Prod	00140-0003-01	100s	$84.15
	00140-0003-49	100s ud	$86.19
	00140-0003-50	100s ud	$86.70
	00140-0003-14	500s	$419.68
◆ GENERICS			
Richlyn	00115-2762-01	100s	$4.00
Parmed	00349-2034-01	100s	$4.10
Major	00904-0092-60	100s	$5.70
Aligen	00405-0042-01	100s	$6.24
Goldline	00182-0979-01	100s	$6.70
Moore,H.L.	00839-1132-06	100s	$6.95
Barr	00555-0159-02	100s	$6.96
Geneva	00781-2084-01	100s	$6.98
Rosemont	00832-0307-00	100s	$7.02
URL	00677-0459-01	100s	$7.50
➤ Rugby	00536-3489-01	100s	$7.58
Qualitest	00603-2668-21	100s	$7.80
Goldline	00182-0979-89	100s ud	$7.50
UDL	51079-0141-20	100s ud	$7.58
UDL	51079-0141-21	100s ud	$7.58
Auro	55829-0846-01	100s ud	$8.35
Parmed	00349-2034-05	500s	$17.07
Moore,H.L.	00839-1132-12	500s	$18.21
Major	00904-0092-40	500s	$20.10
Rosemont	00832-0307-50	500s	$21.68
Geneva	00781-2084-05	500s	$22.50
Aligen	00405-0042-02	500s	$22.71
Barr	00555-0159-04	500s	$25.25
URL	00677-0459-05	500s	$27.00
➤ Rugby	00536-3489-05	500s	$27.06
Qualitest	00603-2668-28	500s	$41.12

Chlordiazepoxide Hydrochloride with Clidinium Bromide

DESCRIPTION

Each capsule contains 5 mg Chlordiazepoxide Hydrochloride and 2.5 mg Clidinium Bromide.

Chlordiazepoxide Hydrochloride/Clindium Bromide combines in a single capsule formulation the antianxiety action of Chlordiazepoxide Hydrochloride and the anticholinergic/spasmolytic effects of Clidinium Bromide.

Each capsule contains 5 mg Chlordiazepoxide Hydrochloride and 2.5 mg Clidinium Bromide. Chlordiazepoxide Hydrochloride is a versatile therapeutic agent of proven value for the relief of anxiety and tension. It is indicated when anxiety, tension or apprehension are significant components of the clinical profile. It is among the safer of the effective psychopharmacologic compounds.

Chlordiazepoxide Hydrochloride is 7-chloro-2-methyl-amino-5-phenyl-3H-1, 4-benzodiazepine 4-oxide Hydrochloride. A colorless, crystalline substance, it is soluble in water. It is unstable in solution and the powder must be protected from light. The molecular weight is 336.22.

Clidinium Bromide is a synthetic anticholinergic agent which has been shown in experimental and clinical studies to have a pronounced antispasmodic and antisecretory effect on the gastrointestinal tract.

ANIMAL PHARMACOLOGY

Chlordiazepoxide Hydrochloride has been studied extensively in many species of animals and these studies are suggestive of action on the limbic system of the brain,[1,2,3] which recent evidence indicates is involved in emotional responses.[4,5]

Hostile monkeys were made tame by oral drug dose which did not cause sedation. Chlordiazepoxide Hydrochloride revealed a 'taming' action with the elimination of fear and aggression.[6] The taming effect of Chlordiazepoxide Hydrochloride was further demonstrated in rats made vicious by lesions in the septal area of the brain. The drug dosage which effectively blocked the vicious reaction was well below the dose which caused sedation in these animals.[6]

The oral LD_{50} of single doses of Chlordiazepoxide Hydrochloride, calculated according to the method of Miller and Tainter,[7] is 720 ± 51 mg/kg as determined in mice observed over a period of five days following dosage. Clidinium Bromide is an effective anticholinergic agent with activity approximating that of atropine sulfate against acetylcholine-induced spasms in isolated intestinal strips. On oral administration in mice it proved an effective antisialagogue in preventing pilocarpine-induced salivation. Spontaneous intestinal motility in both rats and dogs is reduced following oral dosing with 0.1 to 0.25 mg/kg. Potent cholinergic ganglionic blocking effects (vagal) are produced with intravenous usage in anesthetized dogs.

Oral doses of 2.5 mg/kg to dogs produced signs of nasal dryness and slight pupillary dilation. In two other species, monkeys and rabbits, doses of 5 mg/kg, p.o., given three times daily for 5 days did not produce apparent secretory or visual changes.

The oral LD_{50} of single doses of Clidinium Bromide is 860 ± 57 mg/kg as determined in mice observed over a period of 5 days following dosage: the calculations were made according to the method of Miller and Tainter.[7]

Effects on Reproduction: Reproduction studies in rats fed Chlordiazepoxide Hydrochloride, 10, 20 and 80 mg/kg daily, and bred through one or two matings showed no congenital anomalies, nor were there adverse effects on lactation of the dams or growth of the newborn. However, in another study at 100 mg/kg daily there was noted a significant decrease in the fertilization rate and a marked decrease in the viability and body weight of offspring which may be attributable to sedative activity, thus resulting in lack of interest in mating and lessened maternal nursing and care of the young.[8,9] One neonate in each of the first and second matings in the rat reproduction study at the 100 mg/kg dose exhibited major skeletal defects. Further studies are in progress to determine the significance of these findings.

Two series of reproduction experiments with Clidinium Bromide were carried out in rats, employing dosages of 2.5 and 10 mg/kg daily in each experiment. In the first experiment Clidinium Bromide was administered for a 9-week interval prior to mating; no untoward effect on fertilization or gestation was noted. The offspring were taken by caesarean section and did not show a significant incidence of congenital anomalies when compared to control animals. In the second experiment adult animals were given Clidinium Bromide for ten days prior to and through two mating cycles. No significant effects were observed on fertility, gestation, viability of offspring or lactation, as compared to control animals, nor was there a significant incidence of congenital anomalies in the offspring derived from these experiments.

A reproduction study of Chlordiazepoxide Hydrochloride/Clidinium Bromide was carried out in rats through two successive matings. Oral daily doses were administered in two concentrations: 2.5 mg/kg Chlordiazepoxide Hydrochloride with 1.25 mg/kg Clidinium Bromide, or 25 mg/kg Chlordiazepoxide Hydrochloride with 12.5 mg/kg Clidinium Bromide. In the first mating no significant differences were noted between the control or the treated groups, with the exception of a slight decrease in the number of animals surviving during lactation among those receiving the highest dosage. As with all anticholinergic drugs, an inhibiting effect on lactation may occur. In the second mating similar results were obtained except for a slight decrease in the number of pregnant females and in the percentage of offspring surviving until weaning. No congenital anomalies were

---

◆ RATED THERAPEUTICALLY EQUIVALENT; ◇ THERAPEUTIC EQUIVALENCE UNCONFIRMED; ○ UNRATED

observed in both matings in either the control or treated groups. Additional animal reproduction studies are in progress.

INDICATIONS

BASED ON A REVIEW OF THIS DRUG BY THE NATIONAL ACADEMY OF SCIENCES—NATIONAL RESEARCH COUNCIL AND/OR OTHER INFORMATION, FDA HAS CLASSIFIED THE INDICATIONS AS FOLLOWS:
"POSSIBLY" EFFECTIVE: AS ADJUNCTIVE THERAPY IN THE TREATMENT OF PEPTIC ULCER AND IN THE TREATMENT OF THE IRRITABLE BOWEL SYNDROME (IRRITABLE COLON, SPASTIC COLON, MUCOUS COLITIS) AND ACUTE ENTEROCOLITIS.
FINAL CLASSIFICATION OF THE LESS-THAN-EFFECTIVE INDICATIONS REQUIRES FURTHER INVESTIGATION.

CONTRAINDICATIONS

Chlordiazepoxide Hydrochloride/Clidinium Bromide is contraindicated in the presence of glaucoma (since the anticholinergic component may produce some degree of mydriasis) and in patients with prostatic hypertrophy and benign bladder neck obstruction. It is contraindicated in patients with known hypersensitivity to Chlordiazepoxide Hydrochloride and/or Clidinium Bromide.

WARNINGS

As in the case of other preparations containing CNS-acting drugs, patients receiving Chlordiazepoxide Hydrochloride/Clidinium Bromide should be cautioned about possible combined effects with alcohol and other CNS depressants. For the same reason, they should be cautioned against hazardous occupations requiring complete mental alertness such as operating machinery or driving a motor vehicle.

Usage in Pregnancy: An increased risk of congenital malformations associated with the use of minor tranquilizers (Chlordiazepoxide, diazepam and meprobamate) during the first trimester of pregnancy has been suggested in several studies. Because use of these drugs is rarely a matter of urgency, their use during this period should almost always be avoided. The possibility that a woman of childbearing potential may be pregnant at the time of institution of therapy should be considered. Patients should be advised that if they become pregnant during therapy or intend to become pregnant they should communicate with their physicians about the desirability of discontinuing the drug.

As with all anticholinergic drugs, an inhibiting effect on lactation may occur. (See "Animal Pharmacology.")

Management of Overdosage: Manifestations of Chlordiazepoxide Hydrochloride overdosage include somnolence, confusion, coma and diminished reflexes. Respiration, pulse and blood pressure should be monitored, as in all cases of drug overdosage, although, in general, these effects have been minimal following Chlordiazepoxide Hydrochloride overdosage.

While the signs and symptoms of Chlordiazepoxide Hydrochloride/Clidinium Bromide overdosage may be produced by either of its components, usually such symptoms will be overshadowed by the anticholinergic actions of Clidinium Bromide. The symptoms of overdosage of Clidinium Bromide are excessive dryness of mouth, blurring of vision, urinary hesitancy and constipation.

General supportive measures should be employed, along with immediate gastric lavage. Administer physostigmine (Antilirium) 0.5 to 2 mg at a rate of no more than 1 mg per minute. This may be repeated in 1 to 4 mg doses if arrhythmias, convulsions or deep coma recur. Intravenous fluids should be administered and an adequate airway maintenance. Hypotension may be combated by the use of levarterenol or metaraminol. Methylphenidate or caffeine and sodium benzoate may be given to combat CNS-depressive effects. Dialysis is of limited value. Should excitation occur, barbiturates should not be used. As with the management of intentional overdosage with any drug, it should be borne in mind that multiple agents may have been ingested.

Withdrawal symptoms of the barbiturate type have occurred after the discontinuation of benzodiazepines. (See *"Drug Abuse and Dependence"* section.)

PRECAUTIONS

In elderly and debilitated patients, it is recommended that the dosage be limited to the smallest effective amount to preclude the development of ataxia, oversedation, or confusion (not more than two Chlordiazepoxide Hydrochloride/Clidinium Bromide capsules per day initially, to be increased gradually as needed and tolerated). In general, the concomitant administration of Chlordiazepoxide Hydrochloride/Clidinium Bromide and other psychotropic agents is not recommended. If such combination therapy seems indicated, careful consideration should be given to the pharmacology of the agents to be employed—particularly when the known potentiating compounds such as the MAO inhibitors and phenothiazines are to be used. The usual precautions in treating patients with impaired renal or hepatic function should be observed.

Paradoxical reactions to Chlordiazepoxide Hydrochloride, e.g., excitement, stimulation and acute rage, have been reported in psychiatric patients and should be watched for during Chlordiazepoxide Hydrochloride/Clidinium Bromide therapy. The usual precautions are indicated when Chlordiazepoxide Hydrochloride is used in the treatment of anxiety states where there is any evidence of impending depression; it should be borne in mind that suicidal tendencies may be present and protective measures may be necessary. Although clinical studies have not established a cause and effect relationship, physicians should be aware that

variable effects on blood coagulation have been reported very rarely in patients receiving oral anticoagulants and Chlordiazepoxide Hydrochloride.

Information for Patients: To assure the safe and effective use of benzodiazepines, patients should be informed that, since benzodiazepines may produce psychological and physical dependence, it is advisable that they consult with their physician before either increasing the dose or abruptly discontinuing this drug.

ADVERSE REACTIONS[10]

No side effects or manifestations not seen with either compound alone have been reported with the administration of Chlordiazepoxide Hydrochloride/Clidinium Bromide. However, since Chlordiazepoxide Hydrochloride/Clidinium Bromide contains Chlordiazepoxide Hydrochloride and Clidinium Bromide, the possibility of untoward effects which may be seen with either of these two compounds cannot be excluded.

When Chlordiazepoxide Hydrochloride has been used alone the necessity of discontinuing therapy because of undesirable effects has been rare.[11] Drowsiness,[12] ataxia[13] and confusion[9] have been reported in some patients—particularly the elderly and debilitated.[9] While these effects can be avoided in almost all instances by proper dosage adjustment, they have occasionally been observed at the lower dosage ranges. In a few instances syncope has been reported.[14]

Other adverse reactions reported during therapy with Chlordiazepoxide Hydrochloride include isolated instances of skin eruptions,[12] edema,[15] minor menstrual irregularities,[12] nausea and constipation,[16] extrapyramidal symptoms,[9] as well as increased and decreased libido. Such side effects have been infrequent and are generally controlled with reduction of dosage. Changes in EEG patterns (low-voltage fast activity) have been observed in patients during and after Chlordiazepoxide Hydrochloride treatment.[17]

Blood dyscrasias,[10] including agranulocytosis,[18] jaundice and hepatic dysfunction[19] have occasionally been reported during therapy with Chlordiazepoxide Hydrochloride. When Chlordiazepoxide Hydrochloride treatment is protracted, periodic blood counts and liver function tests are advisable.

Adverse effects reported with use of Chlordiazepoxide Hydrochloride/Clidinium Bromide are those typical of anticholinergic agents, *i.e.*, dryness of the mouth, blurring of vision, urinary hesitancy and constipation. Constipation has occurred most often when Chlordiazepoxide Hydrochloride/Clidinium Bromide therapy has been combined with other spasmolytic agents and/or a low residue diet.

DRUG ABUSE AND DEPENDENCE

Withdrawal symptoms, similar in character to those noted with barbiturates and alcohol (convulsions, tremor, abdominal and muscle cramps, vomiting and sweating), have occurred following abrupt discontinuance of Chlordiazepoxide. The more severe withdrawal symptoms have usually been limited to those patients who had received excessive doses over an extended period of time. Generally milder withdrawal symptoms (*e.g.*, dysphoria and insomnia) have been reported following abrupt discontinuance of benzodiazepines taken continuously at therapeutic levels for several months. Consequently, after extended therapy, abrupt discontinuation should generally be avoided and a gradual dosage tapering schedule followed. Addiction-prone individuals (such as drug addicts or alcoholics) should be under careful surveillance when receiving Chlordiazepoxide or other psychotropic agents because of the predisposition of such patients to habituation and dependence.

DOSAGE

Because of the varied individual responses to tranquilizers and anticholinergics, the optimum dosage of Chlordiazepoxide Hydrochloride/Clidinium Bromide varies with the diagnosis and response of the individual patient. The dosage, therefore, should be individualized for maximum beneficial effects. The usual maintenance dose is 1 or 2 capsules, 3 or 4 times a day administered before meals and at bedtime.

REFERENCES

1. Schallek, W., *et al*: Arch. Int. Pharmacodyn. 149:467-483. 1964. 2. Himwich, H. E., *et al*: J. Neuropsych. 3 (Suppl. 1):S15-S26, August 1962. 3. Morillo, A., *et al*: Psychopharmacologia 3 (No. 5):386-394, 1962. 4. MacLean, P. D.: Psychosomatic Med. 17:355-366, September 1955. 5. Morgan, C. T.: Physiological Psychology, 3rd Ed.; New York, McGraw-Hill, 1965. 6. Randall, L. O. *et al*: J. Pharm. Exper. Therap. 129:163-171, June 1960. 7. Miller, L. C. and Tainter, M. C.: Proc. Soc. Exp. Biol. & Med. 57:261, 1944. 8. Zbinden, G., *et al*: Toxicology and Applied Pharmacology 3:619-637, November 1961. 9. Data on file, Hoffmann-La Roche Inc., Nutley, New Jersey. 10. Bibliography and References available on request from Roche Laboratories. 11. Rickels, K. *et al*: Med. Times 93:238-245, March 1965. 12. Tobin, J. M. *et al*: J. Amer. Med. Assoc. 174:1242-1249. November 1960. 13. Jenner, F. A., *et al*: J. Ment. Sci. 107:575-582, May 1961. 14. Robinson, R. C. V.: Dis. Nerv. System 21:43-45, March 1960. 15. Rose, J. T.: Amer. J. Psychiat. 120:899-900, March 1964. 16. Hines, L. R.: Curr. Therap. Res. 2:227-236, June 1960. 17. Gibbs, F. A. and Gibbs, E. L.: J. Neuropsych., 3 (Suppl. 1)PS,73-S78, August 1962. 18. Kaelbling, R., *et al*: J. Amer. Med. Assoc. 174:1863-1865, December 1960. 19. Cacioppo, J., *et al*: Amer. J. Psychiat. 117:1040-1041, May 1961.

HOW SUPPLIED
CAPSULE: 5 MG-2.5 MG

BRAND/MANUFACTURER	NDC	SIZE	AWP
○ **BRAND**			
▶ LIBRAX: Roche Prod	00140-0007-01	100s	$66.02
	00140-0007-49	100s ud	$68.09
	00140-0007-14	500s	$329.01

For additional alternatives, turn to the section beginning on page 2859.

Chlorhexidine Gluconate

DESCRIPTION

Chlorhexidine Gluconate is an oral rinse containing 0.12% Chlorhexidine Gluconate (1,1′-hexamethylene bis [5-(p-chlorophenyl) biguanide] di-D-Gluconate). Chlorhexidine Gluconate is a near-neutral solution (pH range 5-7). Chlorhexidine Gluconate is a salt of Chlorohexidine and Gluconic acid.

Following is its chemical structure:

CLINICAL PHARMACOLOGY

Chlorhexidine Gluconate provides microbicidal activity during oral rinsing. The clinical significance of Chlorhexidine Gluconate antimicrobial activities is not clear. Microbiological sampling of plaque has shown a general reduction of counts of certain assayed bacteria, both aerobic and anaerobic, ranging from 54-97% through six months' use.

Use of Chlorhexidine Gluconate in a six-month clinical study did not result in any significant changes in bacterial resistance, overgrowth of potentially opportunistic organisms or other adverse changes in the oral microbial ecosystem. Three months after Chlorhexidine Gluconate use was discontinued the number of bacteria in plaque had returned to baseline levels and resistance of plaque bacteria to Chlorehexidine Gluconate was equal to that at baseline.

PHARMACOKINETICS

Pharmacokinetic studies with Chlorhexidine Gluconate indicate approximately 30% of the active ingredient, Chlorhexidine Gluconate, is retained in the oral cavity following rinsing. This retained drug is slowly released into the oral fluids. Studies conducted on human subjects and animals demonstrate that any ingested Chlorhexidine Gluconate is poorly absorbed from the gastrointestinal tract. The mean plasma level of Chlorhexidine Gluconate reached a peak of 0.206 µg/g in humans 30 minutes after they ingested a 300-mg dose of the drug. Detectable levels of Chlorhexidine Gluconate were not present in the plasma of these subjects 12 hours after the compound was administered. Excretion of Chlorhexidine Gluconate occurred primarily through the feces (~ 90%). Less than 1% of the Chlorhexidine Gluconate ingested by these subjects was excreted in the urine.

INDICATION

Chlorhexidine Gluconate is indicated for use between dental visits as part of a professional program for the treatment of gingivitis as characterized by redness and swelling of the gingivae, including gingival bleeding upon probing. Chlorhoxidine Gluconate has not been tested among patients with acute necrotizing ulcerative gingivitis (ANUG). For patients having coexisting gingivitis and periodonitis, see *"Precautions"*.

CONTRAINDICATIONS

Chlorhexidine Gluconate should not be used by persons who are known to be hypersensitive to Chlorhexidine Gluconate.

WARNINGS

The effect of Chlorhexidine Gluconate on periodontitis has not been determined. An increase in supragingival calculus was noted in clinical testing in Chlorhexidine Gluconate users compared with control users. It is not known if Chlorhexidine Gluconate use results in an increase in subgingival calculus. Calculus deposits should be removed by a dental prophylaxis at intervals no greater than six months. Rare hypersensitivity and generalized allergic reactions have also been reported. Chlorhexidine Gluconate should not be used by persons who have a sensitivity to it or its components.

PRECAUTIONS

GENERAL

1. For patients having coexisting gingivitis and periodontitis, the presence or absence of gingival inflammation following treatment with Chlorhexidine Gluconate should not be used as a major indicator of underlying periodontitis.

2. Chlorhexidine Gluconate can cause staining of oral surfaces, such as tooth surfaces, restorations, and the dorsum of the tongue. Not all patients will experience a visually significant increase in toothstaining. In clinical testing, 56% of Chlorhexidine Gluconate users exhibited a measurable increase in facial anterior stain, compared to 35% of control users after six months: 15% of Chlorhexidine Gluconate users developed what was judged to be heavy stain, compared to 1% of control users after six months. Stain will be more pronounced in patients who have heavier accumulations of unremoved plaque.

Stain resulting from use of Chlorhexidine Gluconate does not adversely affect health of the gingivae or other oral tissues. Stain can be removed from most tooth surfaces by conventional professional prophylactic techniques. Additional time may be required to complete the prophylaxis.

Discretion should be used when prescribing to patients with anterior facial restorations with rough surfaces or margins. If natural stain cannot be removed from these surfaces by a dental prophylaxis, patients should be excluded from Chlorhexidine Gluconate treatment if permanent discoloration is unacceptable. Stain in these areas may be difficult to remove by dental prophylaxis and on rare occasions may necessitate replacement of these restorations.

3. Some patients may experience an alteration in taste perception while undergoing treatment with Chlorhexidine Gluconate. Most patients accommodate to this effect with continued use of Chlorhexidine Gluconate. No instances of permanent taste alteration due to Chlorhexidine Gluconate have been reported.

Usage in Pregnancy: Pregnancy Category B. Reproduction and fertility studies with Chlorhexidine Gluconate have been conducted. No evidence of impaired fertility was observed in rats at doses up to 100 mg/kg/day, and no evidence of harm to the fetus was observed in rats and rabbits at doses up to 300 mg/kg/day and 40 mg/kg/day, respectively. These doses are approximately 100, 300, and 40 times that which would result from a person's ingesting 30 ml (2 capfuls) of Chlorhexidine Gluconate per day. Since controlled studies in pregnant women have not been conducted, the benefits of the drug in pregnant women should be weighed against possible risk to the fetus.

Nursing Mothers: It is not known whether this drug is excreted in human milk. Because many drugs are excreted in human milk, caution should be exercised when Chlorhexidine Gluconate is administered to a nursing woman.

In parturition and lactation studies with rats, no evidence of impaired parturition or of toxic effects to suckling pups was observed when Chlorhexidine Gluconate was administered to dams at doses what were over 100 times greater than that which would result from a person's ingesting 30 ml (2 capfuls) of Chlorhexidine Gluconate per day.

Pediatric use: Clinical effectiveness and safety of Chlorhexidine Gluconate have not been established in children under the age of 18.

Carcinogenesis, Mutagenesis: In a drinking water study in rats, carcinogenesis was not observed. The highest dose of Chlorhexidine Gluconate used in this study, 38 mg/kg/day, is at least 500 times the amount that would be ingested from the recommended daily dose of Chlorhexidine Gluconate.

In two mammalian *in vivo* mutagenic studies with Chlorhexidatine Gluconate, mutagenesis was not observed. The highest dose of Chlorhexidine Gluconate used in a mouse dominant lethal assay was 1000 mg/kg/day and in a hamster cytogenetics test was 250 mg/kg/day, i.e. > 3200 times the amount that would be ingested from the recommended daily dose of Chlorhexidine Gluconate.

ADVERSE REACTIONS

The most common side effects associated with Chlorhexidine Gluconate oral rinses are (1) an increase in staining of teeth and other oral surfaces, (2) an increase in calculus formation, and (3) an alteration in taste perception: see *"Warnings"* and *"Precautions"*. No serious systemic adverse reactions associated with use of Chlorhexidine Gluconate were observed in clinical testing.

Minor irritation and superficial desquamation of the oral mucosa have been noted in patients using Chlorhexidine Gluconate, particularly among chilldren.

Although there have been no reports of parotitis (inflammation or swelling of salivary glands) among Chlorhexidine Gluconate users in controlled clinical studies, transient parotitis has been reported in research studies with Chlorhexidine-containing mouthrinses.

OVERDOSAGE

Ingestion of 1 or 2 ounces of Chlorhexidine Gluconate by a small child (~ 10 kg body weight) might result in gastric distress, including nausea, or signs of alcohol intoxication. Medical attention should be sought if more than 4 ounces of Chlorhexidine Gluconate is ingested by a small child or if signs of alcohol intoxication develop.

DOSAGE AND ADMINISTRATION

Chlorhexidine Gluconate therapy should be initiated directly following a dental prophylaxis and periodontal examination. Patients using Chlorhexidine Gluconate should be reevaluated and given a thorough prophylaxis at intervals no longer than six months.

Recommended use is twice daily oral rinsing for 30 seconds, morning and evening after toothbrushing. Usual dosage is ½ fl. oz. (marked in cap) of undiluted Chlorhexidine Gluconate. Chlorhexidine Gluconate is not intended for ingestion and should be expectorated after rinsing.

Store above freezing (32°F).

HOW SUPPLIED
LIQUID: 0.12%

BRAND/MANUFACTURER	NDC	SIZE	AWP
○ **BRAND**			
PERIOGARD: Colgate Oral	00126-0271-16	480 ml	$11.82
PERIDEX: P&G Company	37000-0007-01	480 ml 3s	$35.46

Chlormezanone

DESCRIPTION

Chlormezanone is [2-(p-Chlorophenyl)tetrahydro-3-methyl-4H-1, 3-thiazin-4-one 1, 1-dioxide], a white, virtually tasteless, crystalline powder with a solubility of less than 0.25 percent w/v in water.

Following is its chemical structure:

CLINICAL PHARMACOLOGY

Chlormezanone improves the emotional state by allaying mild anxiety, usually without impairing clarity of consciousness. The relief of symptoms is often apparent in fifteen to thirty minutes after administration and may last up to six hours or longer.

INDICATIONS AND USAGE

Chlormezanone is indicated for the treatment of mild anxiety and tension states.

The effectiveness of Chlormezanone in long-term use, that is, more than 4 months, has not been assessed by systematic clinical studies. The physician should periodically reassess the usefulness of the drug for the individual patient.

CONTRAINDICATION

Contraindicated in patients with a history of a previous hypersensitivity reaction to Chlormezanone.

WARNINGS

Should drowsiness occur, the dose should be reduced. As with other CNS-acting drugs, patients receiving Chlormezanone should be warned against performing potentially hazardous tasks which require complete mental alertness, such as operating a motor vehicle or dangerous machinery. Patients should also be warned of the possible additive effects which may occur when the drug is taken with alcohol or other CNS-acting drugs.

Usage in Pregnancy: Safe use of this preparation in pregnancy or lactation has not been established, as no animal reproduction studies have been performed; therefore, use of the drug in pregnancy, lactation, or in women of childbearing age requires that the potential benefit of the drug be weighed against its possible hazards to the mother and fetus.

ADVERSE REACTIONS

Adverse effects reported to occur with Chlormezanone include drowsiness, drug rash, dizziness, flushing, nausea, depression, edema, inability to void, weakness, excitement, tremor, confusion, and headache. Rare instances of erythema multiforme, Stevens-Johnson syndrome, and toxic epidermal necrolysis have been reported. Medication should be discontinued or modified as the case demands.

Jaundice, apparently of the cholestatic type, has been reported as occurring rarely during the use of Chlormezanone, but was reversible on discontinuance of therapy.

OVERDOSAGE

Overdose with amounts as low as 7 g has resulted in coma, hypotension, absence of reflexes, and flaccidity. Ingestion of higher doses may also result in alternation between coma and excitement.

DOSAGE AND ADMINISTRATION

The usual **adult** dosage is 200 mg orally three or four times daily but in some patients 100 mg may suffice. The dosage for *children from 5 to 12 years* is 50 mg to 100 mg three or four times daily. Since the effect of CNS-acting drugs varies, treatment, particularly in children, should begin with the lowest dosage which may be increased as needed.

HOW SUPPLIED
TABLETS: 100 MG

BRAND/MANUFACTURER	NDC	SIZE	AWP
○ BRAND TRANCOPAL: Sanofi Winthrop	00024-1973-04	100s	$90.94

TABLETS: 200 MG

BRAND/MANUFACTURER	NDC	SIZE	AWP
○ BRAND TRANCOPAL: Sanofi Winthrop	00024-1974-04	100s	$104.22

Chloromycetin *SEE* CHLORAMPHENICOL

Chloromycetin Sodium Succinate
SEE CHLORAMPHENICOL SODIUM SUCCINATE

Chloromycetin W/Hydrocortisone
SEE CHLORAMPHENICOL WITH HYDROCORTISONE ACETATE

Chlorophyllin Copper Complex/Papain/Urea

DESCRIPTION

Chlorophyllin Copper Complex Papain/ Urea Ointment is an enzymatic debriding-healing ointment which contans standardized Papain 10%, Urea USP 10% and Chlorophyllin Copper Complex 0.5% in a hydrophilic base. Papain/Urea Ointment is an enzymatic debriding ointment containing standardized Papain (10,000 Rystan Units of enzyme activity per gm of ointment) and Urea USP 10% in a hydrophilic base. One Rystan Unit is that quantity which under specified conditions will clot 10 microliters of milk substrate in 1 minute at 40°C.

CLINICAL PHARMACOLOGY

Papain, the proteolytic enzyme derived from the fruit of carica papaya, is a potent digestant of nonviable protein matter, but is harmless to viable tissue. It has the unique advantage of being active over a wide pH range, 3 to 12. Despite its recognized value as a digestive agent, Papain is relatively ineffective when used alone as a debriding agent, primarily because it requires the presence of activators to exert its digestive function.

In Chlorophyllin Coppr Complex/Papain/Urea Ointment: Urea is combined with Papain to provide two supplementary chemical actions: 1) to expose by solvent action the activators of Papain (sulfhydryl groups) which are always present, but not necessarily accessible, in the nonviable tissue or debris of lesions, and 2) to denature the nonviable protein matter in lesions and thereby render it more susceptible to enzymatic digestion. In pharmacologic studies involving digestion of beef powder, Miller[1] showed that the combination of Papain and Urea produced twice as much digestion as Papain alone.

Chlorophyllin Copper Complex adds healing action to the cleansing action of the proteolytic Papain/Urea combination. The basic wound-healing properties of Chlorophyllin Copper Complex are promotion of healthy granulations, control of local inflammation and reduction of wound odors.[2] Specifically, Chlorophyllin Copper Complex inhibits the hemag-glutinating and inflammatory properties of protein degradation products in the wound, including the products of enzymatic digestion, thus providing an additional protective factor.[1,3] The incorporation of Chlorophyllin Copper Complex in Chlorophyllin Copper Complex/Papain/Urea Ointment permits its continuous use for as long as desired to help produce and then maintain a clean wound base and to promote healing.

INDICATIONS AND USES

Chlorophyllin Copper Complex/Papain/Urea Ointment and Papain/Urea Ointments are suggested for treatment of acute and chronic lesions such as varicose, diabetic and decubitus ulcers, burns, postoperative wounds, pilonidal cyst wounds, carbuncles and miscellaneous traumatic or infected wounds. Chlorophyllin Copper Complex/Papain/Urea and Papain/Urea Ointments are applied continuously throughout treatment of these conditions (1) for enzymatic debridement of necrotic tissue and liquefaction of fibrinous, purulent debris, (2) to *keep* the wound clean, and simultaneously (3) to promote normal healing.

CONTRAINDICATIONS

None known.

PRECAUTIONS

See *"Dosage and Administration"*.
Not to be used in eyes.

ADVERSE REACTIONS

Chlorophyllin Copper Complex/Papain/Urea and Papain/Urea Ointment are generally well tolerated and nonirritating. A small percentage of patients may experience a transient "burning" sensation on application of the ointment. Occasionally, the profuse exudate resulting from enzymatic digestion may cause irritation. In such cases, more frequent changes of dressings until exudate diminishes will alleviate discomfort.

DOSAGE AND ADMINISTRATION

Apply Chlorophyllin Copper Complex/Papain/Urea or Papain/Urea Ointment directly to lesion and cover with appropriate dressing. When practicable, daily or twice daily changes of dressings are preferred. Longer intervals between redressings (two or three days) have proved satisfactory, and Chlorophyllin Copper Complex/Papain/Urea or Papain/Urea Ointment may be applied under pressure dressings. At each redressing, the lesion should be irrigated with isotonic saline solution or other mild cleansing solution (except hydrogen peroxide solution, which may inactivate the Papain) to remove any accumulation of liquefied necrotic material.

NOTE

Papain may also be inactivated by the salts of heavy metals (lead, silver, mercury, etc.) Contact with medications containing these metals should be avoided.

► SHOWN IN PRODUCT IDENTIFICATION GUIDE

HOW SUPPLIED
OINTMENT:

BRAND/MANUFACTURER	NDC	SIZE	AWP
○ **BRAND**			
PANAFIL-WHITE: Rystan	00263-5148-01	30 gm	$28.13
PANAFIL: Rystan	00263-5145-01	30 gm	$28.19
	00263-5145-16	454 gm	$186.37

Chloroprocaine Hydrochloride

DESCRIPTION

Chloroprocaine Hydrochloride Injections are sterile nonpyrogenic local anesthetics. The active ingredient is Chloroprocaine HCl (benzoic acid, 4-amino-2-chloro-2-(diethylamino) ethyl ester, monohydrochloride).

Following is its chemical structure:

$$NH_2 - - COOCH_2CH_2N(C_2H_5)_2 \cdot HCl$$
$$Cl$$

CLINICAL PHARMACOLOGY

Chloroprocaine, like other local anesthetics, blocks the generation and the conduction of nerve impulses, presumably by increasing the threshold for electrical excitation in the nerve, by slowing the propagation of the nerve impulse and by reducing the rate of rise of the action potential. In general, the progression of anesthesia is related to the diameter, myelination and conduction velocity of affected nerve fibers. Clinically, the order of loss of nerve function is as follows: (1) pain, (2) temperature, (3) touch, (4) proprioception, and (5) skeletal muscle tone.

Systemic absorption of local anesthetics produces effects on the cardiovascular and central nervous systems. At blood concentrations achieved with normal therapeutic doses, changes in cardiac conduction, excitability, refractoriness, contractility, and peripheral vascular resistance are minimal. However, toxic blood concentrations depress cardiac conduction and excitability, which may lead to atrioventricular block and ultimately to cardiac arrest. In addition, with toxic blood concentrations myocardial contractility may be depressed and peripheral vasodilation may occur, leading to decreased cardiac output and arterial blood pressure.

Following systemic absorption, toxic blood concentrations of local anesthetics can produce central nervous system stimulation, depression, or both. Apparent central stimulation may be manifested as restlessness, tremors and shivering, which may progress to convulsions. Depression and coma may occur, possibly progressing ultimately to respiratory arrest.

However, the local anesthetics have a primary depressant effect on the medulla and on higher centers. The depressed stage may occur without a prior stage of central nervous system stimulation.

PHARMACOKINETICS

The rate of systemic absorption of local anesthetic drugs is dependent upon the total dose and concentration of drug administered, the route of administration, the vascularity of the administration site, and the presence or absence of epinephrine in the anesthetic injection. Epinephrine usually reduces the rate of absorption and plasma concentration of local anesthetics and is sometimes added to local anesthetic injections in order to prolong the duration of action.

The onset of action with Chloroprocaine is rapid (usually within 6 to 12 minutes), and the duration of anesthesia, depending upon the amount used and the route of administration, may be up to 60 minutes.

Local anesthetics appear to cross the placenta by passive diffusion. However, the rate and degree of diffusion varies considerably among the different drugs as governed by: (1) the degree of plasma protein binding, (2) the degree of ionization, and (3) the degree of lipid solubility. Fetal/maternal ratios of local anesthetics appear to be inversely related to the degree of plasma protein binding, since only the free, unbound drug is available for placental transfer. Thus, drugs with the highest protein binding capacity may have the lowest fetal/maternal ratios. The extent of placental transfer is also determined by the degree of ionization and lipid solubility of the drug. Lipid soluble, nonionized drugs readily enter the fetal blood from the maternal circulation.

Depending upon the route of administration, local anesthetics are distributed to some extent to all body tissues, with high concentrations found in highly perfused organs such as the liver, lungs, heart and brain.

Various pharmacokinetic parameters of the local anesthetics can be significantly altered by the presence of hepatic or renal disease, addition of epinephrine, factors affecting urinary pH, renal blood flow, the route of administration, and the age of the patient. The *in vitro* plasma half-life of Chloroprocaine in adults is 21 ± 2 seconds for males and 25 ± 1 seconds for females. The *in vitro* plasma half-life in neonates is 43 ± 2 seconds.

Chloroprocaine is rapidly metabolized in plasma by hydrolysis of the ester linkage by pseudocholinesterase. The hydrolysis of Chloroprocaine results in the production of β-diethylaminoethanol and 2-chloro-4-aminobenzoic acid, which inhibits the action of the sulfonamides (see "Precautions"). The kidney is the main excretory organ for most local anesthetics and their metabolites. Urinary excretion is affected by urinary perfusion and factors affecting urinary pH.

INDICATIONS AND USAGE

Chloroprocaine Hydrochloride 1% and 2% Injections, in multidose vials with methylparaben as preservative, are indicated for the production of local anesthesia by infiltration and peripheral nerve block. They are not to be used for lumbar or caudal epidural anesthesia.

Chloroprocaine Hydrochloride for Infiltration and Nerve Block 2% and 3% Injections, in single-dose vials without preservative, are indicated for the production of local anesthesia by infiltration, peripheral and central nerve block, including lumbar and caudal epidural blocks.

Chloroprocaine Hydrochloride Injections, are not to be used for subarachnoid administration.

CONTRAINDICATIONS

Chloroprocaine Hydrochloride Injections are contraindicated in patients hypersensitive (allergic) to drugs of the PABA ester group.

Lumbar and caudal epidural anesthesia should be used with extreme caution in persons with the following conditions: existing neurological disease, spinal deformities, septicemia and severe hypertension.

WARNINGS

LOCAL ANESTHETICS SHOULD ONLY BE EMPLOYED BY CLINICIANS WHO ARE WELL VERSED IN DIAGNOSIS AND MANAGEMENT OF DOSE RELATED TOXICITY AND OTHER ACUTE EMERGENCIES WHICH MIGHT ARISE FROM THE BLOCK TO BE EMPLOYED, AND THEN ONLY AFTER ENSURING THE *IMMEDIATE* AVAILABILITY OF OXYGEN, OTHER RESUSCITATIVE DRUGS, CARDIOPULMONARY RESUSCITATIVE EQUIPMENT, AND THE PERSONNEL RESOURCES NEEDED FOR PROPER MANAGEMENT OF TOXIC REACTIONS AND RELATED EMERGENCIES. (See also "Adverse Reactions" and "Precautions".) DELAY IN PROPER MANAGEMENT OF DOSE RELATED TOXICITY, UNDERVENTILATION FROM ANY CAUSE AND/OR ALTERED SENSITIVITY MAY LEAD TO THE DEVELOPMENT OF ACIDOSIS, CARDIAC ARREST AND, POSSIBLY, DEATH. CHLOROPROCAINE HYDROCHLORIDE contains methylparaben and should not be used for lumbar or caudal epidural anesthesia because safety of this antimicrobial preservative has not been established with regard to intrathecal injection, either intentional or unintentional. Chloroprocaine Hydrochloride for Infiltration and Nerve Block Injection contains no preservative; discard unused injection remaining in vial after initial use.

Vasopressors should not be used in the presence of ergot-type oxytocic drugs, since a severe persistent hypertension may occur.

To avoid intravascular injection, aspiration should be performed before the anesthetic solution is injected. The needle must be repositioned until no blood return can be elicited. However, the absence of blood in the syringe does not guarantee that intravascular injection has been avoided.

Mixtures of local anesthetics are sometimes employed to compensate for the slower onset of one drug and the shorter duration of action of the second drug. Experiments in primates suggest that toxicity is probably additive when mixtures of local anesthetics are employed, but some experiments in rodents suggest synergism. Caution regarding toxic equivalence should be exercised when mixtures of local anesthetics are employed.

PRECAUTIONS

General: The safety and effective use of Chloroprocaine depend on proper dosage, correct technique, adequate precautions and readiness for emergencies. Resuscitative equipment, oxygen and other resuscitative drugs should be available for immediate use (see "Warnings" and "Adverse Reactions"). The lowest dosage that results in effective anesthesia should be used to avoid high plasma levels and serious adverse effects. Injections should be made slowly, with frequent aspirations before and during the injection to avoid intravascular injection. Syringe aspirations should also be performed before and during each supplemental injection in continuous (intermittent) catheter techniques. During the administration of epidural anesthesia, it is recommended that a test dose be administered (3 mL of 3% or 5 mL of 2% Chloroprocaine Hydrochloride for Infiltration and Nerve Block Injection) initially and that the patient be monitored for central nervous system toxicity and cardiovascular toxicity, as well as for signs of unintended intrathecal administration, before proceeding. When clinical conditions permit, consideration should be given to employing a chloroprocaine solution that contains epinephrine for the test dose because circulatory changes characteristic of epinephrine may also serve as a warning sign of unintended intravascular injection. An intravascular injection is still possible even if aspirations for blood are negative. With the use of continuous catheter techniques, it is recommended that a fraction of each supplemental dose be administered as a test dose in order to verify proper location of the catheter. Injection of repeated doses of local anesthetics may cause significant increases in plasma levels with each repeated dose due to slow accumulation of the drug or its metabolites. Tolerance to elevated blood levels varies with the physical condition of the patient. Debilitated, elderly patients, acutely ill patients, and children should be given reduced doses commensurate with their age and physical status. Local anesthetics should also be used with caution in patients with hypotension or heart block.

Careful and constant monitoring of cardiovascular and respiratory (adequacy of ventilation) vital signs and the patient's state of consciousness should be accomplished after each local anesthetic injection. It should be kept in mind at such times that restlessness, anxiety, tinnitus, dizziness, blurred vision, tremors, depression or drowsiness may be early warning signs of central nervous system toxicity.

Local anesthetic injections containing a vasoconstrictor should be used cautiously and in carefully circumscribed quantities in areas of the body supplied by end arteries or having otherwise compromised blood supply. Patients with peripheral vascular disease and those with hypertensive vascular disease may exhibit exaggerated vasoconstrictor response. Ischemic injury or necrosis may result.

Since ester-type local anesthetics are hydrolyzed by plasma cholinesterase produced by the liver, chloroprocaine should be used cautiously in patients with hepatic disease.

Local anesthetics should also be used with caution in patients with impaired cardiovascular function since they may be less able to compensate for functional changes associated with the prolongation of A-V conduction produced by these drugs.

Use in Ophthalmic Surgery: When local anesthetic injections are employed for retrobulbar block, lack of corneal sensation should not be relied upon to determine whether or not the patient is ready for surgery. This is because complete lack of corneal sensation usually precedes clinically acceptable external ocular muscle akinesia.

INFORMATION FOR PATIENTS
When appropriate, patients should be informed in advance that they may experience temporary loss of sensation and motor activity, usually in the lower half of the body, following proper administration of epidural anesthesia.

Clinically Significant Drug Interactions: The administration of local anesthetic solutions containing epinephrine or norepinephrine to patients receiving mono-amine oxidase inhibitors, tricyclic antidepressants or phenothiazines may produce severe, prolonged hypotension or hypertension. Concurrent use of these agents should generally be avoided. In situations when concurrent therapy is necessary, careful patient monitoring is essential.

Concurrent administration of vasopressor drugs (for the treatment of hypotension related to obstetric blocks) and ergot-type oxytocic drugs may cause severe, persistent hypertension or cerebrovascular accidents.

The para-aminobenzoic acid metabolite of chloroprocaine inhibits the action of sulfonamides. Therefore, chloroprocaine should not be used in any condition in which a sulfonamide drug is being employed.

Carcinogenesis, Mutagenesis, Impairment of Fertility: Long-term studies in animals to evaluate carcinogenic potential and reproduction studies to evaluate mutagenesis or impairment of fertility have not been conducted with Chloroprocaine.

Pregnancy Category C: Animal reproduction studies have not been conducted with Chloroprocaine. It is also not known whether Chloroprocaine can cause fetal harm when administered to a pregnant woman or can affect reproduction capacity. Chloroprocaine should be given to a pregnant woman only if clearly needed. This does not preclude the use of chloroprocaine at term for the production of obstetrical anesthesia.

Labor and Delivery: Local anesthetics rapidly cross the placenta, and when used for epidural, paracervical, pudendal or caudal block anesthesia, can cause varying degrees of maternal, fetal and neonatal toxicity. (See *"Clinical Pharmacology"* and *"Pharmacokinetics".*)

The incidence and degree of toxicity depend upon the procedure performed, the type and amount of drug used, and the technique of drug administration. Adverse reactions in the parturient, fetus and neonate involve alterations of the central nervous system, peripheral vascular tone and cardiac function.

Maternal hypotension has resulted from regional anesthesia. Local anesthetics produce vasodilation by blocking sympathetic nerves. Elevating the patient's legs and positioning her on her left side will help prevent decreases in blood pressure. The fetal heart rate also should be monitored continuously, and electronic fetal monitoring is highly advisable.

Epidural, paracervical, or pudendal anesthesia may alter the forces of parturition through changes in uterine contractility or maternal expulsive efforts. In one study, paracervical block anesthesia was associated with a decrease in the mean duration of first stage labor and facilitation of cervical dilation. However, epidural anesthesia has also been reported to prolong the second stage of labor by removing the parturient's reflex urge to bear down or by interfering with motor function. The use of obstetrical anesthesia may increase the need for forceps assistance.

The use of some local anesthetic drug products during labor and delivery may be followed by diminished muscle strength and tone for the first day or two of life. The long-term significance of these observations is unknown.

Careful adherence to recommended dosage is of the utmost importance in obstetrical paracervical block. Failure to achieve adequate analgesia with recommended doses should arouse suspicion of intravascular or fetal intracranial injection. Cases compatible with unintended fetal intracranial injection of local anesthetic injection have been reported following intended paracervical or pudendal block or both. Babies so affected present with unexplained neonatal depression at birth which correlates with high local anesthetic serum levels and usually manifest seizures within six hours. Prompt use of supportive measures combined with forced urinary excretion of the local anesthetic has been used successfully to manage this complication.

Case reports of maternal convulsions and cardiovascular collapse following use of some local anesthetics for paracervical block in early pregnancy (as anesthesia for elective abortion) suggest that systemic absorption under these circumstances may be rapid. The recommended maximum dose of each drug should not be exceeded. Injection should be made slowly and with frequent aspiration. Allow a 5-minute interval between sides.

There are no data concerning use of Chloroprocaine for obstetrical paracervical block when toxemia of pregnancy is present or when fetal distress or prematurity is anticipated in advance of the block; such use is, therefore, not recommended.

The following information should be considered by clinicians who select Chloroprocaine for obstetrical paracervical block anesthesia: 1) Fetal bradycardia (generally a heart rate of less than 120 per minute for more than 2 minutes) has been noted by electronic monitoring in about 5 to 10 percent of the cases (various studies) where initial total doses of 120 mg to 400 mg of chloroprocaine were employed. The incidence of bradycardia, within this dose range, might not be dose related. 2) Fetal acidosis has not been demonstrated by blood gas monitoring around the time of bradycardia or afterwards. These data are limited and generally restricted to nontoxemic cases where fetal distress or prematurity was not anticipated in advance of the block. 3) No intact Chloroprocaine and only trace quantities of a hydrolysis product, 2-chloro-4-aminobenzoic acid, have been demonstrated in umbilical cord arterial or venous plasma following properly administered paracervical block with Chloroprocaine. 4) The role of drug factors and non-drug factors associated with fetal bradycardia following paracervical block are unexplained at this time.

Nursing Mothers: It is not known whether this drug is excreted in human milk. Because many drugs are excreted in human milk, caution should be exercised when chloroprocaine is administered to a nursing woman.

Pediatric Use: Guidelines for the administration of Chloroprocaine Hydrochloride Injections to children are presented in *"Dosage and Administration".*

ADVERSE REACTIONS
Systemic: The most commonly encountered acute adverse experiences that demand immediate countermeasures are related to the central nervous system and the cardiovascular system. These adverse experiences are generally dose-related and may result from rapid absorption from the injection site, diminished tolerance, or from unintentional intravascular injection of the local anesthetic solution. In addition to systemic dose-related toxicity, unintentional subarachnoid injection of drug during the intended performance of caudal or lumbar epidural block or nerve blocks near the vertebral column (especially in the head and neck region) may result in underventilation or apnea ("Total Spinal"). Factors influencing plasma protein binding, such as acidosis, systemic diseases that alter protein production, or competition of other drugs for protein binding sites, may diminish individual tolerance. Plasma cholinesterase deficiency may also account for diminished tolerance to ester type local anesthetics.

Central Nervous System Reactions: These are characterized by excitation and/or depression. Restlessness, anxiety, dizziness, tinnitus, blurred vision or tremors may occur, possibly proceeding to convulsions. However, excitement may be transient or absent, with depression being the first manifestation of an adverse reaction. This may quickly be followed by drowsiness merging into unconsciousness and respiratory arrest.

The incidence of convulsions associated with the use of local anesthetics varies with the procedure used and the total dose administered. In a survey of studies of epidural anesthesia, overt toxicity progressing to convulsions occurred in approximately 0.1 percent of local anesthetic administrations.

Cardiovascular System Reactions: High doses, or unintended intravascular injection, may lead to high plasma levels and related depression of the myocardium, hypotension, bradycardia, ventricular arrhythmias and, possibly, cardiac arrest.

Allergic: Allergic type reactions are rare and may occur as a result of sensitivity to the local anesthetic or to other formulation ingredients, such as the antimicrobial preservative methylparaben, contained in multiple dose vials. These reactions are characterized by signs such as urticaria, pruritis, erythema, angioneurotic edema (including laryngeal edema), tachycardia, sneezing, nausea, vomiting, dizziness, syncope, excessive sweating, elevated temperature, and possibly, anaphylactoid type symptomatology (including severe hypotension). Cross sensitivity among members of the ester-type local anesthetic group has been reported. The usefulness of screening for sensitivity has not been definitely established.

Neurologic: In the practice of caudal or lumbar epidural block, occasional unintentional penetration of the subarachnoid space by the catheter may occur (see *"Precautions"*). Subsequent adverse observations may depend partially on the amount of drug administered intrathecally. These observations may include spinal block of varying magnitude (including total spinal block), hypotension secondary to spinal block, loss of bladder, and bowel control, and loss of perineal sensation and sexual function. Arachnoiditis, persistent motor, sensory and/or autonomic (sphincter control) deficit of some lower spinal segments with slow recovery (several months) or incomplete recovery have been reported in rare instances. (See *"Dosage and Administration"* discussion of *"Caudal and Lumbar Epidural Block"*). Backache and headache have also been noted following lumbar epidural or caudal block.

OVERDOSAGE
Acute emergencies from local anesthetics are generally related to high plasma levels encountered during therapeutic use of local anesthetics or to unintended subarachnoid injection of local anesthetic solution (See *"Adverse Reactions,"* *"Warnings,"* and *"Precautions"*).

In mice, the intravenous LD_{50} of Chloroprocaine Hydrochloride is 97 mg/kg and the subcutaneous LD_{50} of Chloroprocaine Hydrochloride is 950 mg/kg.

Management of Local Anesthetic Emergencies: The first consideration is prevention, best accomplished by careful and constant monitoring of cardiovascular and respiratory vital signs and the patient's state of consciousness after each local anesthetic injection. At the first sign of change, oxygen should be administered.

The first step in the management of convulsions, as well as underventilation or apnea due to unintentional subarachnoid injection of drug solution, consists of immediate attention to the maintenance of a patent airway and assisted or controlled ventilation with oxygen and a delivery system capable of permitting immediate positive airway pressure by mask. Immediately after the institution of these ventilatory measures, the adequacy of the circulation should be evaluated, keeping in mind that drugs used to treat convulsions sometimes depress the circulation when administered intravenously. Should convulsions persist despite adequate respiratory support, and if the status of the circulation permits, small increments of an ultra-short acting barbiturate (such as thiopental or thiamylal) or a benzodiazepine (such as diazepam) may be administered intravenously; the clinician should be familiar, prior to the use of local anesthetics, with these anticonvulsant drugs. Supportive treatment of circulatory depression may require administration of intravenous fluids and, when appropriate, a vasopressor dictated by the clinical situation (such as ephedrine to enhance myocardial contractile force).

If not treated immediately, both convulsions and cardiovascular depression can result in hypoxia, acidosis, bradycardia, arrhythmias and cardiac arrest. Underventilation or apnea due to unintentional subarachnoid injection of local anesthetic solution may produce these same signs and also lead to cardiac arrest if ventilatory support is not instituted. If cardiac arrest should occur, standard cardiopulmonary resuscitative measures should be instituted. Recovery has been reported after prolonged resuscitative efforts.

Endotracheal intubation, employing drugs and techniques familiar to the clinician, may be indicated, after initial administration of oxygen by mask, if difficulty is encountered in the maintenance of a patent airway or if prolonged ventilatory support (assisted or controlled) is indicated.

DOSAGE AND ADMINISTRATION

Chloroprocaine may be administered as a single injection or continuously through an indwelling catheter. As with all local anesthetics, the dose administered varies with the anesthetic procedure, the vascularity of the tissues, the depth of anesthesia and degree of muscle relaxation required, the duration of anesthesia desired, and the physical condition of the patient. The smallest dose and concentration required to produce the desired result should be used. Dosage should be reduced for children, elderly and debilitated patients and patients with cardiac and/or liver disease. The maximum single recommended doses of Chloroprocaine in adults are: without epinephrine. 11 mg/kg, not to exceed a maximum total dose of 800 mg; with epinephrine (1:200,000), 14 mg/kg, not to exceed a maximum total dose of 1000 mg. For specific techniques and procedures, refer to standard textbooks.

Caudal and Lumbar Epidural Block: In order to guard against adverse experiences sometimes noted following unintended penetration of the subarachnoid space, the following procedure modifications are recommended: 1. Use an adequate test dose (3 mL of Chloroprocaine Hydrochloride for Infiltration and Nerve Block 3% Injection or 5 mL of Chloroprocaine Hydrochloride for Infiltration and Nerve Block 2% Injection) prior to induction of complete block. This test dose should be repeated if the patient is moved in such a fashion as to have displaced the epidural catheter. Allow adequate time for onset of anesthesia following administration of each test dose. 2. Avoid the rapid injection of a large volume of local anesthetic injection through the catheter. Consider fractional doses, when feasible. 3. In the event of the known injection of a large volume of local anesthetic injection into the subarachnoid space, after suitable resuscitation and if the catheter is in place, consider attempting the recovery of drug by draining a moderate amount of cerebrospinal fluid (such as 10 mL) through the epidural catheter.

As a guide for some routine procedures, suggested doses are given below:
1. Infiltration and Peripheral Nerve Block: Chloroprocaine Hydrochloride Injections

Anesthetic Procedure	Solution Concentration %	Volume (mL)	Total Dose (mg)
Mandibular	2	2-3	40-60
Infraorbital	2	0.5-1	10-20
Brachial plexus	2	30-40	600-800
Digital (without epinephrine)	1	3-4	30-40
Pudendal	2	10 each side	400
Paracervical (see also "Precautions")	1	3 per each of 4 sites	up to 120

2. Caudal and Lumbar Epidural Block: Chloroprocaine Hydrochloride Injection for Infiltration and Nerve Block. For caudal anesthesia, the initial dose is 15 to 25 mL of a 2% or 3% solution. Repeated doses may be given at 40 to 60 minutes intervals.

For lumbar epidural anesthesia, 2 to 2.5 mL per segment of a 2% or 3% solution can be used. The usual total volume of Chloroprocaine Hydrochloride Injection for Infiltration and Nerve Block is from 15 to 25 mL. Repeated doses 2 to 6 mL less than the original dose may be given at 40 to 50 minutes intervals.

The above dosages are recommended as a guide for use in the average adult. Maximum dosages of all local anesthetics must be individualized after evaluating the size and physical condition of the patient and the rate of systemic absorption from a particular injection site.

Pediatric Dosage: It is difficult to recommend a maximum dose of any drug for children, since this varies as a function of age and weight. For children over 3 years of age who have a normal lean body mass and normal body development, the maximum dose is determined by the child's age and weight and should not exceed 11 mg/kg (5 mg/lb). For example, in a child of 5 years weighing 50 lbs (23 kg), the dose of Chloroprocaine HCl without epinephrine would be 250 mg. Concentrations of 0.5-1.0% are suggested for infiltration and 1.0-1.5% for nerve block. In order to guard against systemic toxicity, the lowest effective concentration and lowest effective dose should be used at all times. Some of the lower concentrations for use in infants and smaller children are not available in pre-packaged containers; it will be necessary to dilute available concentrations with the amount of 0.9% sodium chloride injectin necessary to obtain the required final concentration of chloroprocaine solution.

Preparation of Epinephrine Injections: To prepare a 1:200,000 epinephrine-Chloroprocaine HCl injection, add 0.15 mL of a 1 to 1000 Epinephrine Injection USP to 30 mL of Chloroprocaine Hydrochloride Injection for Infiltration and Nerve Block.

Chloroprocaine is incompatible with caustic alkalis and their carbonates, soaps, silver salts, iodine and iodides.

Parental drug products should be inspected visually for particulate matter and discoloration prior to administration, whenever injection and container permit. As with other anesthetics having a free aromatic amino group, Chloroprocaine Hydrochloride Injections are slightly photosensitive and may become discolored after prolonged exposure to light. It is recommended that these vials be stored in the original outer containers, protected from direct sunlight. Discolored injection should not be administered. If exposed to low temperatures, Chloroprocaine Hydrochloride Injection may deposit crystals of Chloroprocaine HCl which will redissolve with shaking when returned to room temperature. The product should not be used if it contains undissolved (e.g., particulate) material.

Storage: Keep from freezing. Protect from light. Store at controlled room temperature: 15°-30°C (59°-86°F).

J CODES
VAR—J2400

HOW SUPPLIED
INJECTION: 1%

BRAND/MANUFACTURER	NDC	SIZE	AWP
○ BRAND			
NESACAINE: Astra	00186-0971-66	30 ml	$14.63

INJECTION: 2%

AVERAGE UNIT PRICE (AVAILABLE SIZES)			
BRAND	$0.53		

BRAND/MANUFACTURER	NDC	SIZE	AWP
◆ BRAND			
NESACAINE: Astra	00186-0972-66	30 ml	$14.99
NESACAINE-MPF: Astra	00186-0993-66	30 ml	$16.95
◆ GENERICS			
Abbott Hosp	00074-4169-01	30 ml 25s	$197.13

INJECTION: 3%

BRAND/MANUFACTURER	NDC	SIZE	AWP
◆ BRAND			
NESACAINE-MPF: Astra	00186-0994-66	30 ml	$17.80
◆ GENERICS			
Abbott Hosp	00074-4170-01	30 ml 25s	$240.17

Chloroquine

> **WARNING**
> PHYSICIANS SHOULD COMPLETELY FAMILIARIZE THEMSELVES WITH THE COMPLETE CONTENTS OF THIS MONOGRAPH BEFORE PRESCRIBING CHLOROQUINE.

DESCRIPTION

Chloroquine is an antimalarial and amebicidal agent. Chloroquine is a 4-aminoquinoline compound for oral administration. It is a white, odorless, bitter tasting, crystalline substance, freely soluble in water.

◆ RATED THERAPEUTICALLY EQUIVALENT; ◇ THERAPEUTIC EQUIVALENCE UNCONFIRMED; ○ UNRATED

Chemically, Chloroquine phosphate is 7-chloro- 4-[[4- (diethylamino) -1-methylbutyl]amino] quinoline phosphate (1:2).

Chloroquine hydrochloride, a 4-aminoquinoline compound for parenteral administration, is chemically 7-chloro-4-[[4-(diethylamino)-1-methylbutyl]amino]-quinoline dihydrochloride, a white, crystalline substance, freely soluble in water. Each mL contains 50 mg of the dihydrochloride salt equivalent to 40 mg of Chloroquine base.

Following is its chemical structure:

CLINICAL PHARMACOLOGY
Chloroquine Phosphate and Hydrochloride have been found to be highly active against the erythrocytic forms of *Plasmodium vivax* and *Plasmodium malariae* and most strains of *Plasmodium falciparum* (but not the gametocytes of *P. falciparum*).

The mechanism of plasmodicidal action of Chloroquine is not completely certain. While the drug can inhibit certain enzymes, its effect is believed to result, at least in part, from its interaction with DNA.

Chloroquine is rapidly and almost completely absorbed from the gastrointestinal tract, and only a small proportion of the administered dose is found in the stools. Approximately 55% of the drug in the plasma is bound to nondiffusible plasma constituents. Excretion of Chloroquine is quite slow, but is increased by acidification of the urine. Chloroquine is deposited in the tissues in considerable amounts. In animals, from 200 to 700 times the plasma concentration may be found in the liver, spleen, kidney, and lung; leukocytes also concentrate the drug. The brain and spinal cord, in contrast, contain only 10 to 30 times the amount present in plasma.

Chloroquine undergoes appreciable degradation in the body. The main metabolite is desethylchloroquine, which accounts for one fourth of the total material appearing in the urine; bisdesethylchloroquine, a carboxylic acid derivative, and other metabolic products as yet uncharacterized are found in small amounts. Slightly more than half of the urinary drug products can be accounted for as unchanged Chloroquine.

MICROBIOLOGY
Chloroquine has been found to be highly active against the erythrocytic forms of *Plasmodium vivax* and *malariae* and most strains of *Plasmodium falciparum* (but not the gametocytes of *P. falciparum*). The precise mechanism of action of the drug is not known.

In vitro studies with trophozoites of *Entamoeba histolytica* have demonstrated that Chloroquine also possesses amebicidal activity comparable to that of emetine.

INDICATIONS AND USAGE
Chloroquine is indicated for the suppressive treatment and for acute attacks of malaria due to *P. vivax*, *P. malariae*, *P. ovale*, and susceptible strains of *P. falciparum*. The drug is also indicated for the treatment of extraintestinal amebiasis.

Chloroquine does not prevent relapses in patients with vivax or malariae malaria because it is not effective against exoerythrocytic forms of the parasite, nor will it prevent vivax or malariae infection when administered as a prophylactic. It is highly effective as a suppressive agent in patients with vivax or malariae malaria, in terminating acute attacks, and significantly lengthening the interval between treatment and relapse. In patients with falciparum malaria it abolishes the acute attack and effects complete cure of the infection, unless due to a resistant strain of *P. falciparum*.

UNLABELED USES
Chloroquine is used alone or as an adjunct in the treatment of rheumatoid arthritis, sarcoidosis, and porphyria cutanea tarda.

CONTRAINDICATIONS
Use of this drug is contraindicated in the presence of retinal or visual field changes either attributable to 4-aminoquinoline compounds or to any other etiology, and in patients with known hypersensitivity to 4-aminoquinoline compounds. However, in the treatment of acute attacks of malaria caused by susceptible strains of plasmodia, the physician may elect to use this drug after carefully weighing the possible benefits and risks to the patient.

WARNINGS
Children and infants are extremely susceptible to adverse effects from an overdose of parenteral Chloroquine Hydrochloride and sudden deaths have been recorded after such administration. In no instance should the single dose of parenteral Chloroquine Hydrochloride administered to infants or children exceed 5 mg base per kg.

In recent years it has been found that certain strains of *P. falciparum* have become resistant to 4-aminoquinoline compounds (including Chloroquine and hydroxychloroquine) as shown by the fact that normally adequate doses have failed to prevent or cure clinical malaria or parasitemia. Treatment with quinine or other specific forms of therapy is therefore advised for patients infected with a resistant strain of parasites.

Irreversible retinal damage has been observed in some patients who had received long-term or high-dosage 4-aminoquinoline therapy. Retinopathy has been reported to be dose related.

When prolonged therapy with any antimalarial compound is contemplated, initial (base line) and periodic ophthalmologic examinations (including visual acuity, expert slit-lamp, funduscopic, and visual field tests) should be performed.

If there is any indication (past or present) of abnormality in the visual acuity, visual field, or retinal macular areas (such as pigmentary changes, loss of foveal reflex), or any visual symptoms (such as light flashes and streaks) which are not fully explainable by difficulties of accommodation or corneal opacities, the drug should be discontinued immediately and the patient closely observed for possible progression. Retinal changes (and visual disturbances) may progress even after cessation of therapy.

All patients on long-term therapy with this preparation should be questioned and examined periodically, including testing knee and ankle reflexes, to detect any evidence of muscular weakness. If weakness occurs, discontinue the drug.

A number of fatalities have been reported following the accidental ingestion of Chloroquine, sometimes in relatively small doses (0.75 g or 1 g Chloroquine phosphate in one 3-year-old child). Patients should be strongly warned to keep this drug out of the reach of children because they are especially sensitive to the 4-aminoquinoline compounds.

Use of Chloroquine in patients with psoriasis may precipitate a severe attack of psoriasis. When used in patients with porphyria the condition may be exacerbated. The drug should not be used in these conditions unless in the judgment of the physician the benefit to the patient outweighs the possible hazard.

PRECAUTIONS
GENERAL
If any severe blood disorder appears which is not attributable to the disease under treatment, discontinuance of the drug should be considered.

Since this drug is known to concentrate in the liver, it should be used with caution in patients with hepatic disease or alcoholism or in conjunction with known hepatotoxic drugs.

The drug should be administered with caution to patients having G-6-PD (glucose-6-phosphate dehydrogenase) deficiency.

LABORATORY TESTS
Complete blood cell counts should be made periodically if patients are given prolonged therapy.

USAGE IN PREGNANCY
Usage of this drug during pregnancy should be avoided except in the suppression or treatment of malaria when in the judgment of the physician the benefit outweighs the possible hazard. It should be noted that radioactively tagged Chloroquine administered intravenously to pregnant pigmented CBA mice passed rapidly across the placenta, accumulated selectively in the melanin structures of the fetal eyes and was retained in the ocular tissues for five months after the drug had been eliminated from the rest of the body.[1]

NURSING MOTHERS
Because of the potential for serious adverse reactions in nursing infants from Chloroquine, a decision should be made whether to discontinue nursing or to discontinue the drug, taking into account the importance of the drug to the mother.

PEDIATRIC USE
See *"Warnings"* and *"Dosage and Administration"*.

ADVERSE REACTIONS
Respiratory depression, cardiovascular collapse, shock, convulsions, and death have been reported with overdoses of Chloroquine Hydrochloride, especially in infants and children.

Ocular reactions: Irreversible retinal damage in patients receiving long-term or high-dosage 4-aminoquinoline therapy; visual disturbances (blurring of vision and difficulty of focusing or accommodation); nyctalopia; scotomatous vision with field defects of paracentral, pericentral ring types, and typically temporal scotomas, eg, difficulty in reading with words tending to disappear, seeing half an object, misty vision, and fog before the eyes. Rarely, scotomatous vision may occur without observable retinal changes.

Neuromuscular reactions: Convulsive seizures associated with oral Chloroquine therapy in patients with extraintestinal amebiasis.

Auditory reactions: Nerve type deafness; tinnitus, reduced hearing in patients with preexisting auditory damage.

Gastrointestinal reactions: Anorexia, nausea, vomiting, diarrhea, abdominal cramps.

Dermatologic reactions: Pleomorphic skin eruptions, skin and mucosal pigmentary changes; lichen planus-like eruptions, pruritus, and hair loss.

CNS reactions: Mild and transient headache, psychic stimulation.

Cardiovascular reactions: Rarely, hypotension, electrocardiographic changes (particularly inversion or depression of the T-wave, widening of the QRS complex).

OVERDOSAGE

Symptoms: Chloroquine is very rapidly and completely absorbed after ingestion. Toxic doses of Chloroquine can be fatal. As little as 1 g may be fatal in children. Toxic symptoms can occur within minutes. These consist of headache, drowsiness, visual disturbances, nausea and vomiting, cardiovascular collapse, and convulsions followed by sudden and early respiratory and cardiac arrest. The electrocardiogram may reveal atrial standstill, nodal rhythm, prolonged intraventricular conduction time, and progressive bradycardia leading to ventricular fibrillation and/or arrest.

Inadvertent toxic doses of Chloroquine Hydrochloride Injection may produce respiratory depression or shock with hypotension. Respiratory depression is treated by artificial respiration and administration of oxygen.

Treatment: Treatment is symptomatic and must be prompt with immediate evacuation of the stomach by emesis (at home, before transportation to the hospital) or gastric lavage until the stomach is completely emptied. If finely powdered, activated charcoal is introduced by stomach tube, after lavage, and within 30 minutes after ingestion of the antimalarial, it may inhibit further intestinal absorption of the drug. To be effective, the dose of activated charcoal should be at least five times the estimated dose of Chloroquine ingested.

Convulsions, if present, should be controlled before attempting gastric lavage. If due to cerebral stimulation, cautious administration of an ultra short-acting barbiturate may be tried but, if due to anoxia, it should be corrected by oxygen administration and artificial respiration. In shock with hypotension, a potent vasopressor such as phenylephrine hydrochloride should be administered intramuscularly in doses of 2 mg to 5 mg. Because of the importance of supporting respiration, tracheal intubation or tracheostomy, followed by gastric lavage, may also be necessary. Peritoneal dialysis and exchange transfusions have also been suggested to reduce the level of the drug in the blood.

A patient who survives the acute phase and is asymptomatic should be closely observed for at least six hours. Fluids may be forced, and sufficient ammonium chloride (8 g daily in divided doses for adults) may be administered for a few days to acidify the urine to help promote urinary excretion in cases of both overdosage or sensitivity.

DOSAGE AND ADMINISTRATION

The dosage of Chloroquine Phosphate is often expressed or calculated as the base. Each 500 mg tablet of Chloroquine Phosphate is equivalent to 300 mg base. In infants and children the dosage is preferably calculated on the body weight.

MALARIA

Adult Dose, Chloroquine Phosphate: For suppression, 500 mg (= 300 mg base) on exactly the same day of each week.

Adult Dose, Chloroquine Hydrochloride: An initial dose of 4 mL or 5 mL of Chloroquine Hydrochloride Injection (160 mg to 200 mg Chloroquine base) may be injected intramuscularly and repeated in 6 hours if necessary. The total parenteral dosage in the first 24 hours should not exceed 800 mg Chloroquine base. Treatment by mouth should be started as soon as practicable and continued until a course of approximately 1.5 g of base in 3 days is completed.

Pediatric Dose, Chloroquine Phosphate: The weekly suppressive dosage is 5 mg calculated as base, per kg of body weight, but should not exceed the adult dose regardless of weight.

If circumstances permit, suppressive therapy should begin two weeks prior to exposure. However, failing this in adults, an initial double (loading) dose of 1 g (= 600 mg base), or in children 10 mg base/kg may be taken in two divided doses, six hours apart. The suppressive therapy should be continued for eight weeks after leaving the endemic area.

Pediatric Dose, Chloroquine Hydrochloride: Infants and children are extremely susceptible to overdosage of parenteral Chloroquine Hydrochloride. Severe reactions and deaths have occurred. In the pediatric age range, parenteral Chloroquine Hydrochloride dosage should be calculated in proportion to the adult dose based upon body weight. The recommended single dose in infants and children is 5 mg base per kg. This dose may be repeated in 6 hours; however, the total dose in any 24 hour period should not exceed 10 mg base per kg of body weight. Parenteral administration should be terminated and oral therapy instituted as soon as possible.

FOR TREATMENT OF ACUTE ATTACK

Adults, Chloroquine Phosphate: An initial dose of 1 g (= 600 mg base) followed by an additional 500 mg (= 300 mg base) after six to eight hours and a single dose of 500 mg (= 300 mg base) on each of two consecutive days. This represents a total dose of 2.5 g Chloroquine Phosphate or 1.5 g base in three days.

The dosage for adults may also be calculated on the basis of body weight; this method is preferred for infants and children. A total dose representing 25 mg of base per kg of body weight is administered in three days, as follows:

First dose: 10 mg base per kg (but not exceeding a single dose of 600 mg base). Second dose: 5 mg base per kg (but not exceeding a single dose of 300 mg base) 6 hours after first dose.
Third dose: 5 mg base per kg 18 hours after second dose.
Fourth dose: 5 mg base per kg 24 hours after third dose.

For radical cure of *vivax* and *malariae* malaria concomitant therapy with an 8-aminoquinoline compound is necessary.

EXTRAINTESTINAL AMEBIASIS

Adults, Chloroquine Phosphate: 1 g (600 mg base) daily for two days, followed by 500 mg (300 mg base) daily for at least two to three weeks. Treatment is usually combined with an effective intestinal amebicide.

Chloroquine Hydrochloride: In adult patients not able to tolerate oral therapy, from 4 mL to 5 mL (160 mg to 200 mg Chloroquine base) of Chloroquine Hydrochloride may be injected daily for 10 to 12 days. Oral administration should be substituted or resumed as soon as possible.

REFERENCE

1. Ullberg S. Lindquist N G, Sjostrand S E: Accumulation of chorio-retinotoxic drugs in the foetal eye. *Nature* 1970; 227:1257.

J CODES

Up to 50 mg IM—J0390

HOW SUPPLIED

CHLOROQUINE HYDROCHLORIDE
INJECTION: 50 MG/ML

BRAND/MANUFACTURER	NDC	SIZE	AWP
○ BRAND			
ARALEN HYDROCHLORIDE: Sanofi Winthrop	00024-0074-01	5 ml 5s	$70.07

CHLOROQUINE PHOSPHATE
TABLETS: 250 MG

AVERAGE UNIT PRICE (AVAILABLE SIZES)	
GENERIC	$0.07

BRAND/MANUFACTURER	NDC	SIZE	AWP
◆ GENERICS			
Richlyn	00115-2790-01	100s	$7.78
Richlyn	00115-2790-03	1000s	$59.85

TABLETS: 500 MG

BRAND/MANUFACTURER	NDC	SIZE	AWP
◆ BRAND			
ARALEN PHOSPHATE: Sanofi Winthrop	00024-0084-01	25s	$88.93

Chlorothiazide

DESCRIPTION

Chlorothiazide is a diuretic and antihypertensive. Chlorothiazide for oral administration is 6-chloro-2*H*-1,2,4-benzothiadiazine-7-sulfonamide 1,1-dioxide. Its empirical formula is $C_7H_6ClN_3O_4S_2$.

It is a white, or practically white, crystalline powder with a molecular weight of 295.72, which is very slightly soluble in water, but readily soluble in dilute aqueous sodium hydroxide. It is soluble in urine to the extent of about 150 mg per 100 mL at pH 7.

Chlorothiazide Sodium for intravenous administration is 6-chloro-2*H*-1,2,4-benzothiadiazine-7-sulfonamide 1,1-dioxide monosodium salt and its molecular weight is 317.70. Its empirical formula is $C_7H_5ClN_3NaO_4S_2$.

Chlorothiazide is supplied as: tablets 250 mg/500 mg.
Chlorothiazide Oral Suspension contains: Chlorothiazide 250 mg/5mL.
Intravenous Chlorothiazide Sodium, a sterile lyophilized white powder supplied in a vial, contains 0.5g Chlorothiazide Sodium equivalent to Chlorothiazide.

Following is its chemical structure:

CLINICAL PHARMACOLOGY

The mechanism of the antihypertensive effect of thiazides is unknown. Chlorothiazide does not usually affect normal blood pressure.

Chlorothiazide affects the distal renal tubular mechanism of electrolyte reabsorption. At maximal therapeutic dosage all thiazides are approximately equal in their diuretic efficacy.

Chlorothiazide increases excretion of sodium and chloride in approximately equivalent amounts. Natriuresis may be accompanied by some loss of potassium and bicarbonate.

After oral use diuresis begins within 2 hours, peaks in about 4 hours and lasts about 6 to 12 hours.

Following intravenous use of Chlorothiazide Sodium, onset of the diuretic action occurs in 15 minutes and the maximal action in 30 minutes.

PHARMACOKINETICS AND METABOLISM

Chlorothiazide is not metabolized but is eliminated rapidly by the kidney. The plasma half-life of Chlorothiazide is 45-120 minutes. After oral doses, 10-15 percent of the dose is excreted unchanged in the urine; 96 percent of an intravenous dose is excreted unchanged in the urine within 23 hours. Chlorothiazide crosses the placental but not the blood-brain barrier and is excreted in breast milk.

INDICATIONS AND USAGE
Chlorothiazide is indicated as adjunctive therapy in edema associated with congestive heart failure, hepatic cirrhosis, and corticosteroid and estrogen therapy.

Chlorothiazide has also been found useful in edema due to various forms of renal dysfunction such as nephrotic syndrome, acute glomerulonephritis, and chronic renal failure.

Oral Chlorothiazide is indicated in the management of hypertension either as the sole therapeutic agent or to enhance the effectiveness of other antihypertensive drugs in the more severe forms of hypertension.

Use in Pregnancy: Routine use of diuretics during normal pregnancy is inappropriate and exposes mother and fetus to unnecessary hazard. Diuretics do not prevent development of toxemia of pregnancy and there is no satisfactory evidence that they are useful in the treatment of toxemia.

Edema during pregnancy may arise from pathologic causes or from the physiologic and mechanical consequences of pregnancy. Thiazides are indicated in pregnancy when edema is due to pathologic causes, just as they are in the absence of pregnancy (see *"Precautions, Pregnancy"*). Dependent edema in pregnancy, resulting from restriction of venous return by the gravid uterus, is properly treated through elevation of the lower extremities and use of support stockings. Use of diuretics to lower intravascular volume in this instance is illogical and unnecessary. During normal pregnancy there is hypervolemia which is not harmful to the fetus or the mother in the absence of cardiovascular disease. However, it may be associated with edema, rarely generalized edema. If such edema causes discomfort, increased recumbency will often provide relief. Rarely this edema may cause extreme discomfort which is not relieved by rest. In these instances, a short course of diuretic therapy may provide relief and be appropriate.

UNLABELED USES
Chlorothiazide is used alone or as an adjunct in the treatment of osteoporosis.

CONTRAINDICATIONS
Anuria.
Hypersensitivity to this product or to other sulfonamide-derived drugs.

WARNINGS
Intravenous use in infants and children has been limited and is not generally recommended.

Use with caution in severe renal disease. In patients with renal disease, thiazides may precipitate azotemia. Cumulative effects of the drug may develop in patients with impaired renal function.

Thiazides should be used with caution in patients with impaired hepatic function or progressive liver disease, since minor alterations of fluid and electrolyte balance may precipitate hepatic coma.

Thiazides may add to or potentiate the action of other antihypertensive drugs.

Sensitivity reactions may occur in patients with or without a history of allergy or bronchial asthma.

The possibility of exacerbation or activation of systemic lupus erythematosus has been reported.

Lithium generally should not be given with diuretics (see *"Precautions, Drug Interactions"*).

PRECAUTIONS
GENERAL
All patients receiving diuretic therapy should be observed for evidence of fluid or electrolyte imbalance: namely, hyponatremia, hypochloremic alkalosis, and hypokalemia. Serum and urine electrolyte determinations are particularly important when the patient is vomiting excessively or receiving parenteral fluids. Warning signs or symptoms of fluid and electrolyte imbalance, irrespective of cause, include dryness of mouth, thirst, weakness, lethargy, drowsiness, restlessness, confusion, seizures, muscle pains or cramps, muscular fatigue, hypotension, oliguria, tachycardia, and gastrointestinal disturbances such as nausea and vomiting.

Hypokalemia may develop, especially with brisk diuresis, when severe cirrhosis is present or after prolonged therapy. Interference with adequate oral electrolyte intake will also contribute to hypokalemia. Hypokalemia may cause cardiac arrhythmias and may also sensitize or exaggerate the response of the heart to the toxic effects of digitalis (e.g., increased ventricular irritability). Hypokalemia may be avoided or treated by use of potassium sparing diuretics or potassium supplements such as foods with a high potassium content.

Although any chloride deficit is generally mild and usually does not require specific treatment except under extraordinary circumstances (as in liver disease or renal disease), chloride replacement may be required in the treatment of metabolic alkalosis.

Dilutional hyponatremia may occur in edematous patients in hot weather; appropriate therapy is water restriction, rather than administration of salt, except in rare instances when the hyponatremia is life-threatening. In actual salt depletion, appropriate replacement is the therapy of choice. Hyperuricemia may occur or acute gout may be precipitated in certain patients receiving thiazides.

In diabetic patients dosage adjustments of insulin or oral hypoglycemic agents may be required. Hyperglycemia may occur with thiazide diuretics. Thus latent diabetes mellitus may become manifest during thiazide therapy.

The antihypertensive effects of the drug may be enhanced in the post-sympathectomy patient.

If progressive renal impairment becomes evident, consider withholding or discontinuing diuretic therapy.

Thiazides have been shown to increase the urinary excretion of magnesium; this may result in hypomagnesemia.

Thiazides may decrease urinary calcium excretion. Thiazides may cause intermittent and slight elevation of serum calcium in the absence of known disorders of calcium metabolism. Marked hypercalcemia may be evidence of hidden hyperparathyroidism. Thiazides should be discontinued before carrying out tests for parathyroid function.

Increases in cholesterol and triglyceride levels may be associated with thiazide diuretic therapy.

LABORATORY TESTS
Periodic determination of serum electrolytes to detect possible electrolyte imbalance should be done at appropriate intervals.

DRUG INTERACTIONS
When given concurrently the following drugs may interact with thiazide diuretics.

Alcohol, Barbiturates, or Narcotics: potentiation of orthostatic hypotension may occur.

Antidiabetic Drugs (Oral Agents and Insulin): dosage adjustment of the antidiabetic drug may be required.

Other Antihypertensive Drugs: additive effect or potentiation.

Cholestyramine and Colestipol Resins: Both cholestyramine and colestipol resins have the potential of binding oral thiazide diuretics and reducing diuretic absorption from the gastrointestinal tract.

Corticosteroids, ACTH: intensified electrolyte depletion, particularly hypokalemia.

Pressor Amines (e.g., Norepinephrine): possible decreased response to pressor amines but not sufficient to preclude their use.

Skeletal Muscle Relaxants, Nondepolarizing (e.g., Tubocurarine): possible increased responsiveness to the muscle relaxant.

Lithium: generally should not be given with diuretics. Diuretic agents reduce the renal clearance of lithium and add a high risk of lithium toxicity. Refer to the package insert for lithium preparations before use of such preparations with Chlorothiazide.

Nonsteroidal Anti-inflammatory Drugs: In some patients, the administration of a non-steroidal anti-inflammatory agent can reduce the diuretic, natriuretic, and antihypertensive effects of loop, potassium-sparing and thiazide diuretics. Therefore, when Chlorothiazide and non-steroidal anti-inflammatory agents are used concomitantly, the patient should be observed closely to determine if the desired effect of the diuretic is obtained.

DRUG/LABORATORY TEST INTERACTIONS
Thiazides should be discontinued before carrying out tests for parathyroid function (see *"Precautions, General"*).

CARCINOGENESIS, MUTAGENESIS, IMPAIRMENT OF FERTILITY
Carcinogenicity studies have not been done with Chlorothiazide.

Chlorothiazide was not mutagenic *in vitro* in the Ames microbial mutagen test (using a maximum concentration of 5 mg/plate) and *Salmonella typhimurium* strains TA98 and TA100) and was not mutagenic and did not induce mitotic nondisjunction in diploid-strains of *Aspergillus nidulans.*

Chlorothiazide had no adverse effects on fertility in female rats at doses up to 60 mg/kg/day and no adverse effects on fertility in male rats at doses up to 40 mg/kg/day. These doses are 1.5 and 1.0 times* the recommended maximum human dose, respectively, when compared on a body weight basis.

PREGNANCY
Teratogenic Effects—Pregnancy Category C: Although reproduction studies performed with Chlorothiazide doses of 50 mg/kg/day in rabbits, 60 mg/kg/day in rats and 500 mg/kg/day in mice revealed no external abnormalities of the fetus or impairment of growth and survival of the fetus due to Chlorothiazide, such studies did not include complete examinations for visceral and skeletal abnormalities. It is not known whether Chlorothiazide can cause fetal harm when administered to a pregnant woman; however, thiazides cross the placental barrier and appear in cord blood. Chlorothiazide should be used during pregnancy only if clearly needed (see *"Indications and Usage"*).

Nonteratogenic Effects: These may include fetal or neonatal jaundice, thrombocytopenia, and possibly other adverse reactions which have occurred in the adult.

NURSING MOTHERS
Because of the potential for serious adverse reactions in nursing infants from Chlorothiazide, a decision should be made whether to discontinue nursing or to discontinue the drug, taking into account the importance of the drug to the mother.

PEDIATRIC USE
Safety and effectiveness of Intravenous Chlorothiazide Sodium in children has not been established.

---

* Calculations based on a human body weight of 50 kg

ADVERSE REACTIONS

The following adverse reactions have been reported and, within each category, are listed in order of decreasing severity.

Body as a Whole: Weakness.

Cardiovascular: Hypotension including orthostatic hypotension (may be aggravated by alcohol, barbiturates, narcotics or antihypertensive drugs).

Digestive: Pancreatitis, jaundice (intrahepatic cholestatic jaundice), diarrhea, vomiting, sialadenitis, cramping, constipation, gastric irritation, nausea, anorexia.

Hematologic: Aplastic anemia, agranulocytosis, leukopenia, hemolytic anemia, thrombocytopenia.

Hypersensitivity: Anaphylactic reactions, necrotizing angiitis (vasculitis and cutaneous vasculitis), respiratory distress including pneumonitis and pulmonary edema, photosensitivity, fever, urticaria, rash, purpura.

Metabolic: Electrolyte imbalance (see *"Precautions"*), hyperglycemia, glycosuria, hyperuricemia.

Musculoskeletal: Muscle spasm.

Nervous System/Psychiatric: Vertigo, paresthesias, dizziness, headache, restlessness.

Renal: Renal failure, renal dysfunction, interstitial nephritis (see *"Warnings"*); hematuria (following intravenous use).

Skin: Erythema multiforme including Stevens-Johnson syndrome, exfoliative dermatitis including toxic epidermal necrolysis, alopecia.

Special Senses: Transient blurred vision, xanthopsia.

Urogenital: Impotence.

Whenever adverse reactions are moderate or severe, thiazide dosage should be reduced or therapy withdrawn.

OVERDOSAGE

The most common signs and symptoms observed are those caused by electrolyte depletion (hypokalemia, hypochloremia, hyponatremia) and dehydration resulting from excessive diuresis. If digitalis has also been administered, hypokalemia may accentuate cardiac arrhythmias.

In the event of overdosage, symptomatic and supportive measures should be employed. With oral Chlorothiazide, emesis should be induced or gastric lavage performed. Correct dehydration, electrolyte imbalance, hepatic coma and hypotension by established procedures. If required, give oxygen or artificial respiration for respiratory impairment. The degree to which Chlorothiazide Sodium is removed by hemodialysis has not been established.

The oral LD_{50} of Chlorothiazide is 8.5 g/kg, greater than 10 g/kg, and greater than 1 g/kg, in the mouse, rat and dog respectively. The intravenous LD_{50} of Chlorothiazide in the mouse is 1.1 g/kg.

DOSAGE AND ADMINISTRATION

Therapy should be individualized according to patient response. Use the smallest dosage necessary to achieve the required response.

ADULTS

For Edema (Oral and Intravenous): The usual adult dosage is 0.5 to 1.0 g once or twice a day. Many patients with edema respond to intermittent therapy, i.e., administration on alternate days or on three to five days each week. With an intermittent schedule, excessive response and the resulting undesirable electrolyte imbalance are less likely to occur.

For Control of Hypertension (Oral): The usual adult starting dosage is 0.5 or 1.0 g a day as a single or divided dose. Dosage is increased or decreased according to blood pressure response. Rarely some patients may require up to 2.0 g a day in divided doses.

INFANTS AND CHILDREN

For Diuresis and For Control of Hypertension (Oral): The usual pediatric dosage is 5 to 10 mg per pound (10 to 20 mg/kg) per day in single or two divided doses, not to exceed 375 mg per day (2.5 to 7.5 mL or 1/2 to 1 1/2 teaspoonfuls of the oral suspension daily) in infants up to 2 years of age or 1 g per day in children 2 to 12 years of age. In infants less than 6 months of age, doses up to 15 mg per pound (30 mg/kg) per day in two divided doses may be required.

Intravenous Chlorothiazide Sodium should be reserved for patients unable to take oral medication or for emergency situations. Intravenous use in infants and children has been limited and is not generally recommended.

Intravenous Chlorothiazide Sodium may be given slowly by direct intravenous injection or by intravenous infusion.

Add 18 mL of Sterile Water for Injection to the vial to form an isotonic solution for intravenous injection. Never add less than 18 mL. When reconstituted with 18 mL of Sterile Water, the final concentration of Intravenous Chlorothiazide Sodium is 28 mg/mL. Unused solution may be stored at room temperature for 24 hours, after which it must be discarded. Parenteral drug products should be inspected visually for particulate matter and discoloration prior to use whenever solution and container permit. The solution is compatible with dextrose or sodium chloride solutions for intravenous infusion. Avoid simultaneous administration of solutions of Chlorothiazide with whole blood or its derivatives.

Extravasation must be rigidly avoided. Do not give subcutaneously or intramuscularly.

STORAGE:

Intravenous Chlorothiazide Sodium: Store lyophilized powder between 2-25°C (36-77° F).

Store reconstituted solution at room temperature, 15-30°C (59-86°F), and discard unused portion after 24 hours.

Tablets Chlorothiazide: Keep container tightly closed. Protect from moisture, freezing, -20°C (-4°F) and store at room temperature, 15-30°C (59-86°F).

Oral Suspension Chlorothiazide: Keep container tightly closed. Protect from freezing, -20°C(-4°F) and store at room temperature, 15-30°C (59-86°F).

J CODES
IV—J1205

HOW SUPPLIED
POWDER FOR INJECTION: 0.5 GM

BRAND/MANUFACTURER	NDC	SIZE	AWP
○ **BRAND**			
DIURIL SODIUM: Merck	00006-3250-32	1s	$8.59

SUSPENSION: 250 MG/5 ML

BRAND/MANUFACTURER	NDC	SIZE	AWP
○ **BRAND**			
DIURIL: Merck	00006-3239-66	237 ml	$9.53

TABLETS: 250 MG

AVERAGE UNIT PRICE (AVAILABLE SIZES)		GENERIC A-RATED AVERAGE PRICE (GAAP)	
BRAND	$0.13	100s	$6.14
GENERIC	$0.05	1000s	$43.32
HCFA FUL (100s ea)	$0.05		

BRAND/MANUFACTURER	NDC	SIZE	AWP
◆ **BRAND**			
DIURIL: Merck	00006-0214-68	100s	$13.06
	00006-0214-82	1000s	$122.71
◆ **GENERICS**			
Parmed	00349-2016-01	100s dozdoz	$9.36
Major	00904-0183-60	100s	$4.75
Rugby	00536-3460-01	100s	$5.00
Mylan	00378-0150-01	100s	$5.62
West-Ward	00143-1209-01	100s	$5.67
Moore,H.L.	00839-5967-06	100s	$6.08
Qualitest	00603-2737-21	100s	$6.18
URL	00677-0439-01	100s	$6.20
Schein	00364-0389-01	100s	$7.25
UDL	51079-0060-20	100s ud	$7.12
Raway	00686-0060-20	100s ud	$7.50
Major	00904-0183-70	250s	$13.15
West-Ward	00143-1209-10	1000s	$38.50
Moore,H.L.	00839-5967-16	1000s	$39.14
Parmed	00349-2016-10	1000s	$39.16
Major	00904-0183-80	1000s	$46.90
Rugby	00536-3460-10	1000s	$52.88

TABLETS: 500 MG

AVERAGE UNIT PRICE (AVAILABLE SIZES)		GENERIC A-RATED AVERAGE PRICE (GAAP)	
BRAND	$0.19	100s	$10.66
GENERIC	$0.10	1000s	$82.42
HCFA FUL (100s ea)	$0.09		

BRAND/MANUFACTURER	NDC	SIZE	AWP
◆ **BRAND**			
DIURIL: Merck	00006-0432-68	100s	$20.70
	00006-0432-82	1000s	$191.69
	00006-0432-86	5000s	$923.55
◆ **GENERICS**			
West-Ward	00143-1210-01	100s	$8.75
Rugby	00536-3461-01	100s	$9.30
Mylan	00378-0162-01	100s	$9.50
Qualitest	00603-2738-21	100s	$10.40
URL	00677-0438-01	100s	$10.48
Schein	00364-0390-01	100s	$10.50
Aligen	00405-4180-01	100s	$10.50
CHLOROTHIAZIDE: Goldline	00182-0790-01	100s	$10.50
Moore,H.L.	00839-7695-06	100s	$10.79
Major	00904-0184-60	100s	$10.90
Parmed	00349-2023-01	100s	$11.95
Raway	00686-0061-20	100s ud	$11.50
UDL	51079-0061-20	100s ud	$13.57
URL	00677-0438-10	1000s	$64.45
Parmed	00349-2023-10	1000s	$72.04
West-Ward	00143-1210-10	1000s	$72.07
Rugby	00536-3461-10	1000s	$78.15
Qualitest	00603-2738-32	1000s	$80.53
Mylan	00378-0162-10	1000s	$83.38
Moore,H.L.	00839-7695-16	1000s	$99.08
Moore,H.L.	00839-5930-16	1000s	$109.69

◆ RATED THERAPEUTICALLY EQUIVALENT; ◇ THERAPEUTIC EQUIVALENCE UNCONFIRMED; ○ UNRATED

Chlorothiazide and Methyldopa

WARNING

THIS FIXED COMBINATION DRUG IS NOT INDICATED FOR INITIAL THERAPY OF HYPERTENSION. HYPERTENSION REQUIRES THERAPY TITRATED TO THE INDIVIDUAL PATIENT. IF THE FIXED COMBINATION REPRESENTS THE DOSAGE SO DETERMINED, ITS USE MAY BE MORE CONVENIENT IN PATIENT MANAGEMENT. THE TREATMENT OF HYPERTENSION IS NOT STATIC, BUT MUST BE RE-EVALUATED AS CONDITIONS IN EACH PATIENT WARRANT.

DESCRIPTION

Chlorothiazide/Methyldopa combines two antihypertensives: Methyldopa and Chlorothiazide.

Each tablet contains:

Chlorothiazide/Methyldopa 150
- Chlorothiazide .... 150 mg
- Methyldopa .... 250 mg

Chlorothiazide/Methyldopa 250
- Chlorothiazide .... 250 mg
- Methyldopa .... 250 mg

METHYLDOPA

Methyldopa is an antihypertensive and is the *L*-isomer of alpha-methyldopa. It is levo-3-(3,4-dihydroxyphenyl)-2-methylalanine. Its empirical formula is $C_{10}H_{13}NO_4$, with a molecular weight of 211.22.

Methyldopa is a white to yellowish white, odorless fine powder, and is soluble in water.

CHLOROTHIAZIDE

Chlorothiazide is a diuretic and antihypertensive. It is 6-chloro-2*H*-1,2,4-benzothiadiazine-7-sulfonamide 1,1-dioxide. Its empirical formula is $C_7H_6ClN_3O_4S_2$.

It is a white, or practically white crystalline powder with a molecular weight of 295.72, which is very slightly soluble in water, but readily soluble in dilute aqueous sodium hydroxide. It is soluble in urine to the extent of about 150 mg per 100 mL at pH 7.

CLINICAL PHARMACOLOGY

METHYLDOPA

Methyldopa is an aromatic-amino-acid decarboxylase inhibitor in animals and in man. Although the mechanism of action has yet to be conclusively demonstrated, the antihypertensive effect of Methyldopa probably is due to its metabolism to alpha-methylnorepinephrine, which then lowers arterial pressure by stimulation of central inhibitory alpha-adrenergic receptors, false neurotransmission, and/or reduction of plasma renin activity. Methyldopa has been shown to cause a net reduction in the tissue concentration of serotonin, dopamine, norepinephrine, and epinephrine.

Only Methyldopa, the *L*-isomer of alpha-methyldopa, has the ability to inhibit dopa decarboxylase and to deplete animal tissues of norepinephrine. In man, the antihypertensive activity appears to be due solely to the *L*-isomer. About twice the dose of the racemate (*DL*-alpha-methyldopa) is required for equal antihypertensive effect.

Methyldopa has no direct effect on cardiac function and usually does not reduce glomerular filtration rate, renal blood flow, or filtration fraction. Cardiac output usually is maintained without cardiac acceleration. In some patients the heart rate is slowed.

Normal or elevated plasma renin activity may decrease in the course of Methyldopa therapy.

Methyldopa reduces both supine and standing blood pressure. It usually produces highly effective lowering of the supine pressure with infrequent symptomatic postural hypotension. Exercise hypotension and diurnal blood pressure variations rarely occur.

CHLOROTHIAZIDE

The mechanism of the antihypertensive effect of thiazides is unknown. Chlorothiazide does not usually affect normal blood pressure.

Chlorothiazide affects the distal renal tubular mechanism of electrolyte reabsorption. At maximal therapeutic dosage all thiazides are approximately equal in their diuretic efficacy. Chlorothiazide increases excretion of sodium and chloride in approximately equivalent amounts. Natriuresis may be accompanied by some loss of potassium and bicarbonate. After oral use diuresis begins within 2 hours, peaks in about 4 hours and lasts about 6 to 12 hours.

PHARMACOKINETICS AND METABOLISM

METHYLDOPA

The maximum decrease in blood pressure occurs four to six hours after oral dosage. After withdrawal, blood pressure usually returns to pretreatment levels within 24-48 hours. Methyldopa is extensively metabolized. The known urinary metabolites are: α-methyldopa mono-0-sulfate; 3-0 methyl-α-methyldopa; 3,4,-dihydroxyphenylacetone; α-methyldopamine; 3-0-methyl-α-methyldopamine and their conjugates. Approximately 70 percent of the drug which is absorbed is excreted in the urine as Methyldopa and its mono-0-sulfate conjugate. The renal clearance is about 130 mL/min in normal subjects and is diminished in renal insufficiency. The plasma half-life of Methyldopa is 105 minutes. After oral doses, excretion is essentially complete in 36 hours.

Methyldopa crosses the placental barrier, appears in cord blood, and appears in breast milk.

CHLOROTHIAZIDE

Chlorothiazide is not metabolized but is eliminated rapidly by the kidney. The plasma half-life is 45-120 minutes. After oral doses, 20-24 percent of the dose is excreted unchanged in the urine. Chlorothiazide crosses the placental but not the blood-brain barrier and is excreted in breast milk.

INDICATION AND USAGE

Hypertension (see box *"Warning"*).

CONTRAINDICATIONS

Active hepatic disease, such as acute hepatitis and active cirrhosis.

If previous methyldopa therapy has been associated with liver disorders (see *"Warnings"*).

Anuria.

Hypersensitivity to Methyldopa, or to Chlorothiazide or other sulfonamide-derived drugs.

WARNINGS

METHYLDOPA

It is important to recognize that a positive Coombs test, hemolytic anemia, and liver disorders may occur with Methyldopa therapy. The rare occurrences of hemolytic anemia or liver disorders could lead to potentially fatal complications unless properly recognized and managed. Read this section carefully to understand these reactions.

With prolonged Methyldopa therapy, 10 to 20 percent of patients develop a positive direct Coombs test which usually occurs between 6 and 12 months of Methyldopa therapy. Lowest incidence is at daily dosage of 1 g or less. This on rare occasions may be associated with hemolytic anemia, which could lead to potentially fatal complications. One cannot predict which patients with a positive direct Coombs test may develop hemolytic anemia.

Prior existence or development of a positive direct Coombs test is not in itself a contraindication to use of Methyldopa. If a positive Coombs test develops during Methyldopa therapy, the physician should determine whether hemolytic anemia exists and whether the positive Coombs test may be a problem. For example, in addition to a positive direct Coombs test there is less often a positive indirect Coombs test which may interfere with cross matching of blood.

Before treatment is started, it is desirable to do a blood count (hematocrit, hemoglobin, or red cell count) for a baseline or to establish whether there is anemia. Periodic blood counts should be done during therapy to detect hemolytic anemia. It may be useful to do a direct Coombs test before therapy and at 6 and 12 months after the start of therapy.

If Coombs-positive hemolytic anemia occurs, the cause may be Methyldopa and the drug should be discontinued. Usually the anemia remits promptly. If not, corticosteroids may be given and other causes of anemia should be considered. If the hemolytic anemia is related to Methyldopa, the drug should not be reinstituted.

When Methyldopa causes Coombs positivity alone or with hemolytic anemia, the red cell is usually coated with gamma globulin of the IgG (gamma G) class only. The positive Coombs test may not revert to normal until weeks to months after Methyldopa is stopped.

Should the need for transfusion arise in a patient receiving Methyldopa, both a direct and an indirect Coombs test should be performed. In the absence of hemolytic anemia, usually only the direct Coombs test will be positive. A positive direct Coombs test alone will not interfere with typing or cross matching. If the indirect Coombs test is also positive, problems may arise in the major cross match and the assistance of a hematologist or transfusion expert will be needed.

Occasionally, fever has occurred within the first three weeks of Methyldopa therapy, associated in some cases with eosinophilia or abnormalities in one or more liver function tests, such as serum alkaline phosphatase, serum transaminases (SGOT, SGPT), bilirubin, and prothrombin time. Jaundice, with or without fever, may occur with onset usually within the first two to three months of therapy. In some patients the findings are consistent with those of cholestasis. In others the findings are consistent with hepatitis and hepatocellular injury.

Rarely fatal hepatic necrosis has been reported after use of Methyldopa. These hepatic changes may represent hypersensitivity reactions. Periodic determination of hepatic function should be done particularly during the first 6 to 12 weeks of therapy or whenever an unexplained fever occurs. If fever, abnormalities in liver function tests, or jaundice appear, stop therapy with Methyldopa. If caused by Methyldopa, the temperature and abnormalities in liver function characteristically have reverted to normal when the drug was discontinued. Methyldopa should not be reinstituted in such patients.

Rarely, a reversible reduction of the white blood cell count with a primary effect on the granulocytes has been seen. The granulocyte count returned promptly to normal on discontinuance of the drug. Rare cases of granulocytopenia have been reported. In each instance, upon stopping the drug, the white cell count returned to normal. Reversible thrombocytopenia has occurred rarely.

CHLOROTHIAZIDE

Use with caution in severe renal disease. In patients with renal disease, thiazides may precipitate azotemia. Cumulative effects of the drug may develop in patients with impaired renal function.

Thiazides should be used with caution in patients with impaired hepatic function or progressive liver disease, since minor alterations of fluid and electrolyte balance may precipitate hepatic coma.

Thiazides may add to or potentiate the action of other antihypertensive drugs.

Sensitivity reactions may occur in patients with or without a history of allergy or bronchial asthma.

The possibility of exacerbation or activation of systemic lupus erythematosus has been reported.

Lithium generally should not be given with diuretics (see "Precautions, Drug Interactions").

PRECAUTIONS
GENERAL
Methyldopa: Methyldopa should be used with caution in patients with a history of previous liver disease or dysfunction (see "Warnings").

Some patients taking Methyldopa experience clinical edema or weight gain which may be controlled by use of a diuretic. Methyldopa should not be continued if edema progresses or signs of heart failure appear.

Hypertension has recurred occasionally after dialysis in patients given Methyldopa because the drug is removed by this procedure.

Rarely involuntary choreoathetotic movements have been observed during therapy with methyldopa in patients with severe bilateral cerebrovascular disease. Should these movements occur, stop therapy.

Chlorothiazide: All patients receiving diuretic therapy should be observed for evidence of fluid or electrolyte imbalance: namely, hyponatremia, hypochloremic alkalosis, and hypokalemia. Serum and urine electrolyte determinations are particularly important when the patient is vomiting excessively or receiving parenteral fluids. Warning signs or symptoms of fluid and electrolyte imbalance, irrespective of cause include dryness of mouth, thirst, weakness, lethargy, drowsiness, restlessness, confusion, seizures, muscle pains or cramps, muscular fatigue, hypotension, oliguria, tachycardia, and gastrointestinal disturbances such as nausea and vomiting. Hypokalemia may develop, especially after prolonged therapy or when severe cirrhosis is present (see "Contraindications" and "Warnings").

Interference with adequate oral electrolyte intake will also contribute to hypokalemia. Hypokalemia may cause cardiac arrhythmia and may also sensitize or exaggerate the response of the heart to the toxic effects of digitalis (e.g., increased ventricular irritability). Hypokalemia may be avoided or treated by use of potassium sparing diuretics or potassium supplements such as foods with a high potassium content.

Although any chloride deficit is generally mild and usually does not require specific treatment except under extraordinary circumstances (as in liver disease or renal disease), chloride replacement may be required in the treatment of metabolic alkalosis.

Dilutional hyponatremia may occur in edematous patients in hot weather; appropriate therapy is water restriction, rather than administration of salt, except in rare instances when the hyponatremia is life threatening. In actual salt depletion, appropriate replacement is the therapy of choice. Hyperuricemia may occur or acute gout may be precipitated in certain patients receiving thiazides.

In diabetic patients dosage adjustments of insulin or oral hypoglycemic agents may be required. Hyperglycemia may occur with thiazide diuretics. Thus latent diabetes mellitus may become manifest during thiazide therapy.

The antihypertensive effects of the drug may be enhanced in the postsympathectomy patient.

If progressive renal impairment becomes evident, consider withholding or discontinuing diuretic therapy.

Thiazides have been shown to increase the urinary excretion of magnesium; this may result in hypomagnesemia.

Thiazides may decrease urinary calcium excretion. Thiazides may cause intermittent and slight elevation of serum calcium in the absence of known disorders of calcium metabolism. Marked hypercalcemia may be evidence of hidden hyperparathyroidism. Thiazides should be discontinued before carrying out tests for parathyroid function.

Increases in cholesterol and triglyceride levels may be associated with thiazide diuretic therapy.

LABORATORY TESTS
Methyldopa: Blood count, Coombs test and liver function tests are recommended before initiating therapy and at periodic intervals (see "Warnings").

Chlorothiazide: Periodic determination of serum electrolytes to detect possible electrolyte imbalance should be done at appropriate intervals.

DRUG INTERACTIONS
METHYLDOPA
When Methyldopa is used with other antihypertensive drugs, potentiation of antihypertensive effect may occur. Patients should be followed carefully to detect side reactions or unusual manifestations of drug idiosyncrasy.

Patients may require reduced doses of anesthetics when on Methyldopa. If hypotension does occur during anesthesia, it usually can be controlled by vasopressors. The adrenergic receptors remain sensitive during treatment with Methyldopa.

CHLOROTHIAZIDE
When given concurrently the following drugs may interact with thiazide diuretics.

Alcohol, Barbiturates, or Narcotics: potentiation of orthostatic hypotension may occur.

Antidiabetic Drugs (Oral Agents and Insulin): dosage adjustment of the antidiabetic drug may be required.

Other Antihypertensive Drugs: additive effect or potentiation.

Cholestyramine and Colestipol Resins: Cholestyramine and colestipol resins bind chlorothiazide and reduce its absorption from the gastrointestinal tract, with cholestyramine producing greater binding *in vitro*. Thiazides should be administered two to four hours before the resin when the two drugs are used concomitantly.

Corticosteroids, ACTH: intensified electrolyte depletion, particularly hypokalemia.

Pressor Amines (e.g., Norepinephrine): possible decreased response to pressor amines but not sufficient to preclude their use.

Skeletal Muscle Relaxants, Nondepolarizing (e.g., Tubocurarine): possible increased responsiveness to the muscle relaxant.

Lithium: generally should not be given with diuretics. Diuretic agents reduce the renal clearance of lithium and add a high risk of lithium toxicity. Refer to the package insert for lithium preparations before use of such preparations with Chlorothiazide/Methyldopa.

CHLOROTHIAZIDE/METHYLDOPA
Nonsteroidal Anti-inflammatory Drugs: In some patients, the administration of a non-steroidal anti-inflammatory agent can reduce the diuretic, natriuretic, and antihypertensive effects of loop, potassium sparing and thiazide diuretics. Therefore, when Chlorothiazide/Methyldopa and non-steroidal anti-inflammatory agents are used concomitantly, the patient should be observed closely to determine if the desired effect of the diuretic is obtained.

DRUG/LABORATORY TEST INTERACTIONS
Methyldopa: Methyldopa may interfere with measurement of: urinary uric acid by the phosphotungstate method, serum creatinine by the alkaline picrate method, and SGOT by colorimetric methods. Interference with spectrophotometric methods for SGOT analysis has not been reported.

Since methylopa causes fluorescence in urine samples at the same wave lengths as catecholamines, falsely high levels of urinary catecholamines may be reported. This will interfere with the diagnosis of pheochromocytoma. It is important to recognize this phenomenon before a patient with a possible pheochromocytoma is subjected to surgery. Methyldopa does not interfere with measurement of VMA (vanillylmandelic acid), a test for pheochromocytoma, by those methods which convert VMA to vanillin. Methyldopa is not recommended for the treatment of patients with pheochromocytoma. Rarely, when urine is exposed to air after voiding, it may darken because of breakdown of Methyldopa or its metabolites.

Chlorothiazide: Thiazides should be discontinued before carrying out tests for parathyroid function (see "Precautions, General").

CARCINOGENESIS, MUTAGENESIS, IMPAIRMENT OF FERTILITY
Long-term studies in animals have not been performed to evaluate the effects upon fertility, mutagenic or carcinogenic potential of the combination.

Methyldopa: Methyldopa is currently under study in the U.S. Carcinogensis Testing Program.

Methyldopa did not have mutagenic activity *in vitro* in the Ames microbial mutagen test with or without metabolic activation.

Methyldopa given in a two-litter study in rats at approximately three to six times the usual daily dose did not impair fertility.

Chlorothiazide: Carcinogenic studies have not been done with chlorothiazide.

Chlorothiazide was not mutagenic *in vitro* in the Ames mutagenicity assay of *Salmonella typhimurium* strains TA98 and TA100 at a maximum concentration of 5 mg/plate. Chlorothiazide did not produce any significant mutagenicity in the dominant lethal assay in the mouse after 8 oral doses of 50 mg/kg or single intraperitoneal doses of 525 or 644 mg/kg, although early fetal deaths and preimplantation losses were increased beyond control values. It was not mutagenic and did not induce disjunction in diploid strains of *Aspergillus nidulans*.

Chlorothiazide had no adverse effects on fertility in a two-litter study in rats at doses two times the maximum recommended dose (60 mg/kg, assumed body weight of 50 kg).

PREGNANCY
Use of diuretics during normal pregnancy is inappropriate and exposes mother and fetus to unnecessary hazard. Diuretics do not prevent development of toxemia of pregnancy and there is no satisfactory evidence that they are useful in treatment of toxemia.

Teratogenic Effects—Pregnancy Category B: Reproduction studies in the rat, at doses up to 40 mg/kg/day (3-4 times the maximum recommended human dose), did not impair fertility or cause abnormalities of the fetus due to Chlorothiazide/Methyldopa. There are no adequate and well-controlled studies with Chlorothiazide/Methyldopa in pregnant women. Because animal reproduction studies are not always predictive of human response, this drug should be used during pregnancy only if clearly needed.

Chlorothiazide: Thiazides cross the placental barrier and appear in cord blood.

Reproduction studies in the rabbit, the mouse and the rat at doses up to 500 mg/kg/day (25 times the maximum recommended human dose) showed no evidence of external abnormalities of the fetus due to Chlorothiazide. Chlorothiazide given in a two-litter study in rats at doses up to 60 mg/kg/day (2 times the maximum recommended human dose) did not impair fertility or produce birth abnormalities in the offspring.

Methyldopa: Reproduction studies have been performed in the rabbit, the mouse, and the rat at doses up to 1000 mg/kg/day (16.6 times the maximum recommended human dose) and have revealed no evidence of impaired fertility or harm to the fetus due to Methyldopa. There are, however, no adequate and well-controlled studies in pregnant women in the first trimester of pregnancy. Because animal reproduction studies are not always predictive of human response, Methyldopa should be used during pregnancy only if clearly needed.

Published reports of the use of Methyldopa during all trimesters indicate that if this drug is used during pregnancy the possibility of fetal harm appears remote. In five studies, three of which were controlled, involving 332 pregnant hypertensive women, treatment with Methyldopa was associated with an improved fetal outcome. The majority of these women were in the third trimester when Methyldopa therapy was begun.

In one study, women who had begun Methyldopa treatment between weeks 16 and 20 of pregnancy gave birth to infants whose average head circumference was reduced by a small amount (34.2 ± 1.7 cm vs. 34.6 ± 1.3 cm [mean ± 1 S.D.]). Long-term follow up of 195 (97.5%) of the children born to Methyldopa-treated pregnant women (including those who began treatment between weeks 16 and 20) failed to uncover any significant adverse effect on the children. At four years of age, the developmental delay commonly seen in children born to hypertensive mothers was less evident in those whose mothers were treated with Methyldopa during pregnancy than those whose mothers were untreated. The children of the treated group scored consistently higher than the children of the untreated group on five major indices of intellectual and motor development. At age seven and one-half developmental scores and intelligence indices showed no significant differences in children of treated or untreated hypertensive women.

Nonteratogenic Effects: These may include fetal or neonatal jaundice, thrombocytopenia, and possibly other adverse reactions which have occurred in the adult.

NURSING MOTHERS
Methyldopa and thiazides appear in breast milk. Therefore, because of the potential for serious adverse reactions in nursing infants from chlorothiazide, a decision should be made whether to discontinue nursing or to discontinue the drug, taking into account the importance of the drug to the mother.

PEDIATRIC USE
Safety and effectiveness of Chlorothiazide/Methyldopa in children has not been established.

ADVERSE REACTIONS
The following adverse reactions have been reported and, within each category, are listed in order of decreasing severity.

METHYLDOPA
Sedation, usually transient, may occur during the initial period of therapy or whenever the dose is increased. Headache, asthenia, or weakness may be noted as early and transient symptoms. However, significant adverse effects due to Methyldopa have been infrequent and this agent usually is well tolerated.

Cardiovascular: Aggravation of angina pectoris, congestive heart failure, prolonged carotid sinus hypersensitivity, orthostatic hypotension (decrease daily dosage), edema or weight gain, bradycardia.

Digestive: Pancreatitis, colitis, vomiting, diarrhea, sialadenitis, sore or "black" tongue, nausea, constipation, distension, flatus, dryness of mouth.

Endocrine: Hyperprolactinemia.

Hematologic: Bone marrow depression, leukopenia, granulocytopenia, thrombocytopenia, hemolytic anemia; positive tests for antinuclear antibody, LE cells, and rheumatoid factor, positive Coombs test.

Hepatic: Liver disorders including hepatitis, jaundice, abnormal liver function tests (see *"Warnings"*).

Hypersensitivity: Myocarditis pericarditis, vasculitis, lupus-like syndrome, drug-related fever.

Nervous System/Psychiatric: Parkinsonism, Bell's palsy, decreased mental acuity, involuntary choreoathetotic movements, symptoms of cerebrovascular insufficiency, pschic disturbances including nightmares and reversible mild psychoses or depression, headache, sedation, asthenia or weakness, dizziness, lightheadedness, paresthesias.

Metabolic: Rise in BUN.

Musculoskeletal: Arthralgia, with or without joint swelling; myalgia.

Respiratory: Nasal stuffness.

Skin: Toxic epidermal necrolysis, rash.

Urogenital: Amenorrhea, breast enlargement, gynecomastia, lactation, impotence, decreased libido.

CHLOROTHIAZIDE
Body as a Whole: Weakness.

Cardiovascular: Hypotension including orthostatic hypotension (may be aggravated by alcohol, barbiturates, narcotics or antihypertensive drugs).

Digestive: Pancreatitis, jaundice (intrahepatic cholestatic jaundice), diarrhea, vomiting, sialadenitis, cramping, constipation, gastric irritation, nausea, anorexia.

Hematologic: Aplastic anemia, agranulocytosis, leukopenia, hemolytic anemia, thrombocytopenia.

Hypersensitivity: Anaphylactic reactions, necrotizing angiitis (vasculitis and cutaneous vasculitis), respiratory distress including pneumonitis and pulmonary edema, photosensitivity, fever, urticaria, rash, purpura.

Metabolic: Electrolyte imbalance (see *"Precautions"*), hyperglycemia, glycosuria, hyperuricemia.

Musculoskeletal: Muscle spasm.

Nervous System/Psychiatric: Vertigo, paresthesias, dizziness, headache, restlessness.

Renal: renal failure, renal dysfunction, interstitial nephritis. (see *"Warnings"*).

Skin: Erythema multiforme including Stevens-Johnson syndrome, exfoliative dermatitis including toxic epidermal necrolysis, alopecia.

Special Senses: Transient blurred vision, xanthopsia.

Urogenital: Impotence.

OVERDOSAGE
Acute overdosage may produce acute hypotension with other responses attributable to brain and gastrointestinal malfunction (excessive sedation, weakness, bradycardia, dizziness, lightheadedness, constipation, distention, flatus, diarrhea, nausea, vomiting).

In the event of overdosage, symptomatic and supportive measures should be employed. When ingestion is recent, gastric lavage or emesis may reduce absorption. Otherwise, management includes special attention to cardiac rate and output, blood volume, electrolyte imbalance, paralytic ileus, urinary function and cerebral activity.

Sympathomimetic drugs (e.g. levarterenol, epinephrine, metaraminol bitartrate) may be indicated. Methytlopa is dialyzable. The degree to which Chlorothiazide is removed by hemodialysis has not been established. The oral LD_{50} of Methyldopa is greater than 1.5 g/kg in both the mouse and the rat. The oral LD_{50} of Chlorothiazide is 8.5 g/kg, greater than 10 g/kg, and greater than 1 g/kg in the mouse, rat, and dog respectively.

DOSAGE AND ADMINISTRATION
DOSAGE MUST BE INDIVIDUALIZED, AS DETERMINED BY TITRATION OF THE INDIVIDUAL COMPONENTS (see box *"Warning"*). Once the patient has been successfully titrated, Chlorothiazide/Methylodopa may be substituted if the previously determined titrated doses are the same as in the combination. The usual starting dosage is one tablet of Chlorothiazide/Methyldopa 150 or one tablet of Chlorothiazide/Methyldopa 250 two or three times a day.

When administered individually, the usual daily dosage of Chlorothiazide is 0.5 g to 1.0 g in single or divided doses and that of Methyldopa is 500 mg to 2 g. To minimize the sedation associated with Methyldopa, start dosage increases in the evening.

Occasionally tolerance to Methyldopa may occur, usually between the second and third month of therapy. Additional separate doses of Methyldopa or replacement of Chlorothiazide/Methyldopa with single entity agents is necessary until the new effective dose ratio is re-established by titration. The maximum recommended daily dose of Methyldopa is 3 g. When Chlorothiazide/Methyldopa 150 is used to provide 1 g of Methyldopa, 0.6 g of Chlorothiazide is delivered. When Chlorothiazide/Methyldopa 250 is used to provide 1 g to Methyldopa, 1 g of Chlorothiazide is delivered. It is prudent, if greater than 1 g of Methyldopa per day is required, to provide the additional Methyldopa as Methyldopa alone.

If Chlorothiazide/Methyldopa does not adequately control blood pressure, additional doses of other agents may be given. When Chlorothiazide/Methyldopa is given with antihypertensives other than thiazides, the initial dosage of Methyldopa should be limited to 500 mg daily in divided doses and the dose of these other agents may need to be adjusted to effect a smooth transition. Since both components of Chlorothiazide/Methyldopa have a relatively short duration of action, withdrawal is followed by return of hypertension usually within 48 hours. This is not complicated by an overshoot of blood pressure.

Since Methyldopa is largely excreted by the kidney, patients with impaired renal function may respond to smaller doses. Syncope in older patients may be related to an increased sensitivity and advanced arteriosclerotic vascular disease. This may be avoided by lower doses.

Protect from moisture; freezing, −20°C (−4°F) and excessive heat, 40°C (104°F).

HOW SUPPLIED
TABLETS: 150 MG-250 MG

BRAND/MANUFACTURER	NDC	SIZE	AWP
◆ BRAND ALDOCLOR-150: Merck	00006-0612-68	100s	$46.25

TABLETS: 250 MG-250 MG

BRAND/MANUFACTURER	NDC	SIZE	AWP
◆ BRAND ALDOCLOR-250: Merck	00006-0634-68	100s	$52.39

➤ SHOWN IN PRODUCT IDENTIFICATION GUIDE

BRAND/MANUFACTURER	NDC	SIZE	AWP
◆ **GENERICS**			
Rugby	00536-4053-01	100s	$28.17

Chlorothiazide with Reserpine

> **WARNING**
>
> THIS FIXED COMBINATION DRUG IS NOT INDICATED FOR INITIAL THERAPY OF HYPERTENSION. HYPERTENSION REQUIRES THERAPY TITRATED TO THE INDIVIDUAL PATIENT. IF THE FIXED COMBINATION REPRESENTS THE DOSAGE SO DETERMINED, ITS USE MAY BE MORE CONVENIENT IN PATIENT MANAGEMENT. THE TREATMENT OF HYPERTENSION IS NOT STATIC, BUT MUST BE RE-EVALUATED AS CONDITIONS IN EACH PATIENT WARRANT.

DESCRIPTION

Chlorothiazide/Reserpine combines two antihypertensives: Chlorothiazide and Reserpine.

CHLOROTHIAZIDE

Chlorothiazide is a diuretic and antihypertensive. Its chemical name is 6-chloro-2H-1,2,4-benzothiadiazine-7-sulfonamide1,1-dioxide. Its empirical formula is Chlorothiazide $C_7H_6ClN_3O_4S_2$.

Chlorothiazide is a white, or practically white, crystalline powder with a molecular weight of 295.72, which is very slightly soluble in water, but readily soluble in dilute aqueous sodium hydroxide. It is soluble in urine to the extent of about 150 mg per 100 mL at pH 7.

RESERPINE

The chemical name of Reserpine is 11,17α-dimethoxy-18β-[(3, 4, 5-trimethoxybenzoyl)oxy] -3β,20α-yohimban- 16β-carboxylic acid methylester. It is a crystalline alkaloid derived from Rauwolfia serpentina. Its empirical formula is $C_{33}H_{40}N_2O_9$.

Reserpine is a white or pale buff to slightly yellowish, odorless, crystalline powder with a molecular weight of 608.69, is insoluble in water and freely soluble in glacial acetic acid.

Each tablet contains:

1. Chlorothiazide .... 250 mg
   Reserpine .... 0.125 mg
2. Chlorothiazide .... 500 mg
   Reserpine .... 0.125 mg

CLINICAL PHARMACOLOGY

CHLOROTHIAZIDE

The mechanism of the antihypertensive effect of thiazides is unknown. Chlorothiazide does not usually affect normal blood pressure.

Chlorothiazide affects the distal renal tubular mechanism of electrolyte reabsorption. At maximal therapeutic dosage all thiazides are approximately equal in their diuretic efficacy.

Chlorothiazide increases excretion of sodium and chloride in approximately equivalent amounts. Natriuresis may be accompanied by some loss of potassium and bicarbonate.

After oral use diuresis begins within 2 hours, peaks in about 4 hours and lasts about 6 to 12 hours.

RESERPINE

Reserpine has antihypertensive, bradycardic, and tranquilizing properties. It lowers arterial blood pressure by depletion of catecholamines. Reserpine is beneficial in relieving anxiety, tension, and headache in the hypertensive patient. It acts at the hypothalamic level of the central nervous system to promote relaxation without hypnosis or analgesia. The sleep pattern shown by the electroencephalogram following barbiturates does not occur with this drug. In laboratory animals spontaneous activity and response to external stimuli are decreased, but confusion or difficulty of movement is not evident.

The bradycardic action of Reserpine promotes relaxation and may eliminate sinus tachycardia. It is most pronounced in subjects with sinus tachycardia and usually is not prominent in persons with a normal pulse rate.

Miosis, relaxation of the nictitating membrane, ptosis, hypothermia, and increased gastrointestinal activity are noted in animals given Reserpine, sometimes in subclinical doses. None of these effects, except increased gastrointestinal activity, has been found to be clinically significant in man with therapeutic doses.

PHARMACOKINETICS AND METABOLISM

CHLOROTHIAZIDE

Chlorothiazide is not metabolized but is eliminated rapidly by the kidney. The plasma half-life of Chlorothiazide is 45-120 minutes. After oral doses, 10-15 percent is excreted unchanged in the urine. Chlorothiazide crosses the placental but not the blood-brain barrier and is excreted in breast milk.

RESERPINE

Oral Reserpine is rapidly absorbed from the gastrointestinal tract. Methylreserpate and trimethoxybenzoic acid are the primary metabolites which result from the hydrolytic cleavage of Reserpine. Maximal blood levels are achieved approximately 2 hours after the oral dosage of ^{3}H-Reserpine to six normal volunteers; within 96 hours approximately 8 percent was excreted in urine and 62 percent in feces. Reserpine appears in human breast milk. Reserpine crosses the placental barrier in guinea pigs.

INDICATION AND USAGE

HYPERTENSION (SEE *"BOX WARNING"*).

Use in Pregnancy: Routine use of diuretics during normal pregnancy is inappropriate and exposes mother and fetus to unnecessary hazard. Diuretics do not prevent development of toxemia of pregnancy and there is no satisfactory evidence that they are useful in the treatment of toxemia.

Edema during pregnancy may arise from pathologic causes or from the physiologic and mechanical consequences of pregnancy. Thiazides are indicated in pregnancy when edema is due to pathologic causes, just as they are in the absence of pregnancy (see *"Precautions Pregnancy"*).

Dependent edema in pregnancy, resulting from restriction of venous return by the gravid uterus, is properly treated through elevation of the lower extremities and use of support stockings. Use of diuretics to lower intravascular volume in this instance is illogical and unnecessary. During normal pregnancy there is hypervolemia which is not harmful to the fetus or the mother in the absence of cardiovascular disease. However, it may be associated with edema, rarely generalized edema. If such edema causes discomfort, increased recumbency will often provide relief. Rarely this edema may cause extreme discomfort which is not relieved by rest. In these instances, a short course of diuretic therapy may provide relief and be appropriate.

CONTRAINDICATIONS

Chlorothiazide is contraindicated in anuria.

Chlorothiazide/Reserpine is contraindicated in hypersensitivity to Chlorothiazide or other sulfonamide-derived drugs or to Reserpine.

Electroshock therapy should not be given to patients while on Reserpine, as severe and even fatal reactions have been reported with minimal convulsive electroshock dosage. After discontinuing Reserpine, allow at least seven days before starting electroshock therapy.

Active peptic ulcer, ulcerative colitis, and active mental depression, especially suicidal tendencies, are contraindications to Reserpine therapy.

WARNINGS

CHLOROTHIAZIDE

Use with caution in severe renal disease. In patients with renal disease, thiazides may precipitate azotemia. Cumulative effects of the drug may develop in patients with impaired renal function.

Thiazides should be used with caution in patients with impaired hepatic function or progressive liver disease, since minor alterations of fluid and electrolyte balance may precipitate hepatic coma.

Thiazides may add to or potentiate the action of other antihypertensive drugs.

Sensitivity reactions may occur in patients with or without a history of allergy or bronchial asthma.

The possibility of exacerbation or activation of systemic lupus erythematosus has been reported.

Lithium generally should not be given with diuretics (see *"Precautions, Drug Interactions"*).

RESERPINE

The occurrence of mental depression due to Reserpine in doses of 0.25 mg daily or less is unusual. In any event, Chlorothiazide/Reserpine should be discontinued at the first sign of depression.

PRECAUTIONS

GENERAL

CHLOROTHIAZIDE

All patients receiving diuretic therapy should be observed for evidence of fluid or electrolyte imbalance: namely, hyponatremia, hypochloremic alkalosis, and hypokalemia. Serum and urine electrolyte determinations are particularly important when the patient is vomiting excessively or receiving parenteral fluids. Warning signs or symptoms of fluid and electrolyte imbalance, irrespective of cause, include dryness of mouth, thirst, weakness, lethargy, drowsiness, restlessness, confusion, seizures, muscle pains or cramps, muscular fatigue, hypotension, oliguria, tachycardia, and gastrointestinal disturbances such as nausea and vomiting.

Hypokalemia may develop, especially with brisk diuresis, when severe cirrhosis is present or after prolonged therapy. Interference with adequate oral electrolyte intake will contribute to hypokalemia. Hypokalemia may cause cardiac arrhythmia and may also sensitize or exaggerate the response of the heart to the toxic effects of digitalis (e.g., increased ventricular irritability). Hypokalemia may be avoided or treated by use of potassium sparing diuretics or potassium supplements such as foods with a high potassium content.

Although any chloride deficit is generally mild and usually does not require specific treatment except under extraordinary circumstances (as in liver disease or renal disease), chloride replacement may be required in the treatment of metabolic alkalosis.

Dilutional hyponatremia may occur in edematous patients in hot weather. Appropriate therapy is water restriction, rather than administration of salt, except in rare instances when the hyponatremia is life threatening. In actual salt depletion, appropriate replacement is the therapy of choice. Hyperuricemia may occur or acute gout may be precipitated in certain patients receiving thiazides.

In diabetic patients dosage adjustments of insulin or oral hypoglycemic agents may be required. Hyperglycemia may occur with thiazide diuretics. Thus latent diabetes mellitus may become manifest during thiazide therapy.

The antihypertensive effect of the drug may be enhanced in the postsympathectomy patient.

If progressive renal impairment becomes evident, consider withholding or discontinuing diuretic therapy.

Thiazides have been shown to increase the urinary excretion of magnesium; this may result in hypomagnesemia.

Thiazides may decrease urinary calcium excretion. Thiazides may cause intermittent and slight elevation of serum calcium in the absence of known disorders of calcium metabolism. Marked hypercalcemia may be evidence of hidden hyperparathyroidism. Thiazides should be discontinued before carrying out tests for parathyroid function.

Increases in cholesterol and triglyceride levels may be associated with thiazide diuretic therapy.

RESERPINE

Since Reserpine may increase gastric secretion and motility, it should be used cautiously in patients with a history of peptic ulcer, ulcerative colitis, or other gastrointestinal disorder. This compound may precipitate biliary colic in patients with gallstones, or bronchial asthma in susceptible persons. Reserpine may cause hypotension including orthostatic hypotension.

Anxiety or depression, as well as psychosis, may develop during Reserpine therapy. If depression is present when therapy is begun, it may be aggravated. Mental depression is unusual with Reserpine doses of 0.25 mg daily or less. In any case, Chlorothiazide/Reserpine should be discontinued at the first sign of depression. Extreme caution should be used in treating patients with a history of mental depression, and the possibility of suicide should be kept in mind.

As with most antihypertensive therapy, caution should be exercised when treating hypertensive patients with renal insufficiency, since they adjust poorly to lowered blood pressure.

When two or more antihypertensives are given, the individual dosages may have to be reduced to prevent excessive drop in blood pressure. In hypertensive patients with coronary artery disease, it is important to avoid a precipitous drop in blood pressure.

LABORATORY TESTS
Periodic determination of serum electrolytes to detect possible electrolyte imbalance should be done at appropriate intervals.

DRUG INTERACTIONS
CHLOROTHIAZIDE
When given concurrently the following drugs may interact with thiazide diuretics.

Alcohol, Barbiturates, or Narcotics: potentiation of orthostatic hypotension may occur.

Antidiabetic Drugs (Oral Agents and Insulin): dosage adjustment of the antidiabetic drug may be required.

Other Antihypertensive Drugs: additive effect or potentiation.

Cholestyramine and Colestipol Resins: Both cholestyramine and colestipol resins have the potential of binding thiazide diuretics and reducing diuretic absorption from the gastrointestinal tract.

Corticosteroids, ACTH: intensified electrolyte depletion, particularly hypokalemia.

Pressor Amines (e.g., Norepinephrine): possible decreased response to pressor amines but not sufficient to preclude their use.

Skeletal Muscle Relaxants, Nondepolarizing (e.g., Tubocurarine): possible increased responsiveness to the muscle relaxant.

Lithium: generally should not be given with diuretics. Diuretic agents reduce the renal clearance of lithium and add a high risk of lithium toxicity. Refer to the package insert for lithium preparations before use of such preparations with Chlorothiazide/Reserpine.

Nonsteroidal Anti-inflammatory Drugs: In some patients, the administration of a nonsteroidal anti-inflammatory agent can reduce the diuretic, natriuretic, and antihypertensive effects of loop, potassium-sparing and thiazide diuretics. Therefore, when Chlorothiazide/Reserpine and nonsteroidal anti-inflammatory agents are used concomitantly, the patient should be observed closely to determine if the desired effect of the diuretic is obtained.

RESERPINE
In hypertensive patients on Reserpine therapy significant hypotension and bradycardia may develop during surgical anesthesia. The anesthesiologist should be aware that Reserpine has been taken, since it may be necessary to give vagal blocking agents parenterally to prevent or reverse hypotension and/or bradycardia.

Use Reserpine cautiously with digitalis and quinidine; cardiac arrhythmias have occurred with Reserpine preparations.

Barbiturates enhance the central nervous system depressant effects of Reserpine.

DRUG/LABORATORY TEST INTERACTIONS
Thiazides should be discontinued before carrying out tests for parathyroid function (see "Precautions, General").

CARCINOGENESIS, MUTAGENESIS, IMPAIRMENT OF FERTILITY
Long-term carcinogenic or mutagenic studies have not been done with Chlorothiazide/Reserpine.

In a two-litter study in the rat at an oral dose of 50.0/0.25 mg/kg, the combination of Chlorothiazide/Reserpine did not impair fertility or produce abnormalities in the fetus.

CHLOROTHIAZIDE
Carcinogenic studies have not been done with Chlorothiazide.

Chlorothiazide was not mutagenic *in vitro*, in the Ames microbial mutagen test at a maximum concentration of 5 mg/plate using Strains TA98 and TA100. Chlorothiazide did not produce any significant mutagenicity in the dominant lethal assay in the mouse after 8 oral doses of 50 mg/kg or single intraperitoneal doses of 525 or 644 mg/kg, although early fetal deaths and preimplantation losses were increased beyond control values. In the test using *Aspergillus nidulans*, Chlorothiazide was negative and did not induce disjunction. Chlorothiazide had no effect on fertility in a two-litter study in rats at doses up to 60 mg/kg/day (2 times the maximum recommended human dose).

RESERPINE
Reserpine at a concentration of 1 to 5000 mcg/plate had no mutagenic activity against four strains of *S. typhimurium in vitro* in the Ames microbial mutagen test with or without metabolic activation. Reserpine did not induce malignant transformation of mouse fibroblasts *in vitro* at concentrations of 0.3 to 10 mcg/mL.

A few chromosomal aberrations were induced by Reserpine *in vitro* in cultured mouse mammary carcinoma cells but were considered negative in this study. The drug did not produce chromosomal aberrations in human peripheral leucocyte cultures although an increase in mitotic figures occurred. One study reported chromosomal aberrations and dominant lethal mutations in mice at doses up to 10 mg/kg of Reserpine in the form of a pharmaceutical preparation. Another study did not show dominant lethal mutations in mice at IP doses of 0.92 and 4.6 mg/kg of Reserpine.

Reserpine did not impair fertility in a two-litter study in the rat at an oral dose of 0.25 mg/kg (35 times the maximum recommended human dose).

Rodent studies have shown that Reserpine is an animal tumorigen, causing an increased incidence of mammary fibroadenomas in female mice, malignant tumors of the seminal vesicle in male mice, and malignant adrenal medullary tumors in male rats. These findings arose in two year studies in which the drug was administered in the feed at concentrations of 5 and 10 ppm—about 100 to 300 times the usual human dose. The breast neoplasms are thought to be related to Reserpine's prolactin-elevating effect. Several other prolactin-elevating drugs have also been associated with an increased incidence of mammary neoplasia in rodents.

The extent to which these findings indicate a risk to humans is uncertain. Tissue culture experiments shows that about one-third of human breast tumors are prolactin-dependent *in vitro*, a factor of considerable importance if the use of the drug is contemplated in a patient with previously detected breast cancer. The possibility of an increased risk of breast cancer in Reserpine users has been studied extensively; however, no firm conclusion has emerged. Although a few epidemiologic studies have suggested a slightly increased risk (less than twofold in all studies except one) in women who have used Reserpine, other studies of generally similar design have not confirmed this. Epidemiologic studies conducted using other drugs (neuroleptic agents) that, like Reserpine, increase prolactin levels and therefore would be considered rodent mammary carcinogens, have not shown an association between chronic administration of the drug and human mammary tumorigenesis. While long-term clinical observation has not suggested such an association, the available evidence is considered too limited to be conclusive at this time. An association of Reserpine intake with pheochromocytoma or tumors of the seminal vesicles has not been explored.

PREGNANCY—TERATOGENIC EFFECTS
Pregnancy Category C: There are no adequate and well-controlled studies in pregnant women. Chlorothiazide/Reserpine may cause fetal harm when given to a pregnant woman. Chlorothiazide/Reserpine should be used during pregnancy only if the potential benefit justifies the potential risk to the fetus. (See "Indications and Usage".).

Reserpine: Reproduction studies in rats have shown that Reserpine is teratogenic at doses of 1-2 mg/kg (125-250 times the maximum recommended human dose) IM or IP given early in pregnancy. A variety of abnormalities was produced including anophthalmia, absence of the axial skeleton, hydronephrosis, etc. Pregnancy in rabbits was interrupted when doses as low as 0.04 mg/kg (10 times the maximum recommended human dose) were given early or late in pregnancy.

Chlorothiazide: Thiazides cross the placental barrier and appear in cord blood.

Reproduction studies in the rabbit, the mouse and the rat at doses up to 500 mg/kg/day (25 times the maximum recommended human dose) showed no evidence of external abnormalities of the fetus due to Chlorothiazide. Chlorothiazide given in a two-litter study in rats at doses up to 60 mg/kg/day (2 times the maximum recommended human dose) did not impair fertility or produce birth abnormalities in the offspring.

NONTERATOGENIC EFFECTS

Reserpine: Reserpine has been demonstrated to cross the placental barrier in guinea pig with depression of adrenal catecholamine stores in the newborn. There is some evidence that side effects such as nasal congestion, lethargy, depressed Moro reflex, and bradycardia may appear in infants born of Reserpine-treated mothers.

Chlorothiazide: These may include fetal or neonatal jaundice, thrombocytopenia, and possibly other adverse reactions which have occurred in the adult.

NURSING MOTHERS

Thiazides and Reserpine appear in breast milk. Because of the potential for serious adverse reactions in nursing infants from Chlorothiazide/Reserpine, a decision should be made whether to discontinue nursing or to discontinue the drug, taking into account the imortance of the drug to the mother.

PEDIATRIC USE

Safety and effectiveness of Chlorthiazide/Reserpine in children had not been established.

ADVERSE REACTIONS

The following adverse reactions have been reported and, within each category, are listed in order of decreasing severity.

CHLOROTHIAZIDE

Body as a Whole: Weakness.

Cardiovascular: Hypotension including orthostatic hypotension (may be aggravated by alcohol, barbiturates, narcotics or antihypertensive drugs.

Digestive: Pancreatitis, jaundice (intrahepatic cholestatic jaundice), diarrhea, vomiting, sialadenitis, cramping, constipation, gastric inrriation, nausea, anorexia.

Hematologic: Aplastic anemia, agranulocytosis, leukopnia, hemolytic anemia, thrombocytopenia.

Hypersensitivity: Anaphylactic reactions, necrotizing angitis (vasculitis and cutaneous vasculitis), respiratory distress including pneumonitis and pulmonary edema, photosensitivity, fever, urticarcia, rash, purpura.

Metabolic: Electrolyte inbalance (See *"Precautions"*), hyperglycemia, glycosuria, hyperuricemia.

Musculoskeletal: Muscle spasm.

Nervous System Psychiatric: Vertigo, paresthesias, dizziness, headache, restlessness.

Renal: Renal failure, renal dysfunction, intersititial nephritis. (See *"Warnings"*.)

Skin: Erythema multiforme including Stevens-Johnson syndrome, exfoliative dermatitis including toxic epidermal necrolysis, alopecia.

Special Senses: Transient blurred vision, xanthopsia.

Urogenital: Impotence.

Whenever adverse reactions are moderate or severe, thiazide dosage should be reduced or therapy withdrawn.

RESERPINE

Cardiovascular: Angina pectoris, arrhythmia, premature ventricular contractions, other direct cardiac effects (e.g., fluid retention, congestive heart failure), bradycardia.

Digestive: Vomiting, diarrhea, nausea, hypersecretion and increased motility, anorexia, dryness of mouth, increased salivation.

Hematologic: Thrombocytopenic purpura, excessive bleeding following prostatic surgery.

Hypersensitivity: Pruritis, rash, flushing of skin.

Metabolic: Weight gain.

Musculoskeletal: Muscular aches.

Nervous System/Psychiatric: Mental depression, dull sensorium, syncope, paradoxical anxiety, excessive sedation, nightmares, headache, dizziness, nervousness, parkinsonism (usually reversible with decreased dosage or discontinuance of therapy).

Respiratory: Dyspnea,expistaxis, nasal congestion, enhanced suceptibility to colds.

Special Senses: Optic trophy, uveitis, deafness, glaucoma, conjunctival injection, blurred vision.

Urogenital: Dysuria, impotence, decreased libido, nonpuerperal lactation.

OVERDOSAGE

Overdosage may lead to excessive sedation, mental depression, sever hypotension, extrapyramidal reactions.

There is no specific antidote. In the event of overdosage, symptomatic and supportive measures should be employed. Emesis should be induced or gastric lavage performed. Correct dehydration, electrolyte imbalance, hepatic coma and hypotension by established procedures. If required, give oxygen or artificial respiration for respiratory impairment. In the even of severe hypotension from the Reserpine component, intravenous use of a vasopressor is indicated (e.g., metaraminol bitartrate, levarternol, phenylephrine). Anticholingergis may be needed to relieve gastrointestinal distresss from Reserpine. Because the effects of the rauwolfia alkaloids are prolonged, the patients should be closely observed for at least 72 hours.

The oral LD$_{50}$ or Chlorothiazide is 8.5 g/kg, greater than 10 g/kg, and greater than 1 g/kg, in the mouse, rat and dog, respectively. The oral LD$_{50}$ of Reserpine in the mouse is 390 mg/kg.

DOSAGE AND ADMINSTRATION

The initial dosages of Chlorothiazide/Reserpine should conform to the dosages of the individual components established during titration (see *"box warning"*).

The usual adult dosage of Chlorothiazide 250 mg/Reserpine 0.125 mg is 1 or 2 tablets once or twice a day; that of Chlorothiazide 500 mg/Reserpine 0.125 mg is 1 tablet once or twice a day. Dosage may require adjustment according to the blood pressure response of the patient.

Keep container tightly closed. Protect from light.

HOW SUPPLIED

TABLETS: 250 MG-0.125 MG

BRAND/MANUFACTURER	NDC	SIZE	AWP
◇ **BRAND**			
DIUPRES-250: Merck	00006-0230-68	100s	$27.26
	00006-0230-82	1000s	$252.40
◇ **GENERICS**			
Mylan	00378-0175-01	100s	$8.00
Moore,H.L.	00839-7941-06	100s	$12.05

TABLETS: 500 MG-0.125 MG

BRAND/MANUFACTURER	NDC	SIZE	AWP
◇ **BRAND**			
DIUPRES-500: Merck	00006-0405-68	100s	$42.51
	00006-0405-82	1000s	$391.06
◇ **GENERICS**			
Mylan	00378-0176-01	100s	$12.30
Moore,H.L.	00839-7942-06	100s	$21.98

Chlorotrianisene

DESCRIPTION

Chlorotrianisene USP is available in capsule form suitable for oral administration. Each capsule contains 12 mg or 25 mg of Chlorotrianisene.

Chlorotrianisene is a long-acting, synthetic estrogen with the chemical name 1,1',1"-(1-chloro-1-ethenyl-2-ylidene)-tris[4-methoxy]-be nzene. Chlorotrianisene occurs as small, white crystals or as a crystalline powder. It is odorless. It is slightly soluble in alcohol and very slightly soluble in water.

Following is its chemical structure:

INDICATIONS AND USAGE

Chlorotrianisene is indicated in the treatment of:

1. Advanced androgen-dependent carcinoma of the prostate (for palliation only).

2. Moderate to severe vasomotor symptoms associated with the menopause. There is no adequate evidence that estrogens are effective for nervous symptoms or depression which might occur during menopause and they should not be used to treat these conditions.

3. Atrophic vaginitis.

4. Kraurosis vulvae.

5. Hypoestrogenism due to hypogonadism, castration, or primary ovarian failure.

CONTRAINDICATIONS

Chlorotrianisene is contraindicated in patients with a known hypersensitivity to Chlorotrianisene or other ingredients of the formulation.

Chlorotrianisene should not be used in women or men with any of the following conditions:

1. Known or suspected pregnancy. (See boxed *"Warning."*) Estrogen may cause fetal harm when administered to a pregnant woman.

2. Known or suspected cancer of the breast except in appropriately selected patients being treated for metastatic disease.

3. Known or suspected estrogen-dependent neoplasia.

4. Undiagnosed abnormal genital bleeding.

5. Active thrombophlebitis or thromboembolic disorders—Women on estrogen replacement therapy have not been reported to have an increased risk of thrombophlebitis and/or thromboembolic disease. However, there is insufficient information regarding women who have had previous thromboembolic disease.

WARNINGS

1. Induction of malignant neoplasms: Some studies have suggested a possible increased incidence of breast cancer in those women on estrogen therapy taking higher doses for prolonged periods of time. The majority of studies, however, have not shown an association with the usual doses used for estrogen replacement therapy. Women on this therapy should have regular breast examinations and should be instructed in breast self-examination. The reported endometrial cancer risk among estrogen users was about fourfold or greater than in non-users, and appears dependent on duration of treatment and on estrogen dose. There is no significantly increased risk associated with the use of estrogens for less than one year. The greatest risk appears associated with prolonged use—five years or more. In one study, persistence of risk was demonstrated for 10 years after cessation of estrogen treatment. In another study, a significant decrease in the incidence of endometrial cancer occurred six months after estrogen withdrawal.

Estrogen therapy during pregnancy is associated with an increased risk of fetal congenital reproductive tract disorders. In females, there is an increased risk of vaginal adenosis, squamous cell dysplasia of the cervix, and cancer later in life; in the male, urogenital abnormalities. Although some of these changes are benign, it is not known whether they are precursors of malignancy.

2. Gallbladder disease: The risk of surgically confirmed gallbladder disease has been reported to be 2.5 times higher in women receiving postmenopausal estrogens.

3. Cardiovascular disease: Large doses of estrogen (5 mg conjugated estrogens per day), comparable to those used to treat cancer of the prostate and breast, have been shown in a large prospective clinical trial in men to increase the risk of non-fatal myocardial infarction, pulmonary embolism, and thrombophlebitis. It cannot necessarily be extrapolated from men to women. However, to avoid the theoretical cardiovascular risk caused by high estrogen doses, the doses for estrogen replacement therapy should not exceed the recommended dose.

4. Elevated blood pressure: There is no evidence that this may occur with use of estrogens in the menopause. However, blood pressure should be monitored with estrogen use, especially if high doses are used.

5. Hypercalcemia: Administration of estrogens may lead to severe hypercalcemia in patients with breast cancer and bone metastases. If this occurs, the drug should be stopped and appropriate measures taken to reduce the serum calcium level.

PRECAUTIONS
GENERAL

1. Addition of a progestin: Studies of the addition of a progestin for seven or more days of a cycle of estrogen administration have reported a lowered incidence of endometrial hyperplasia. Morphological and biochemical studies of the endometrium suggest that 10 to 13 days of progestin are needed to provide maximal maturation of the endometrium and to eliminate any hyperplastic changes. Whether this will provide protection from endometrial carcinoma has not been clearly established. There are possible additional risks which may be associated with the inclusion of progestin in estrogen replacement regimens. The potential

risks include adverse effects on carbohydrate and lipid metabolism. The choice of progestin and dosage may be important in minimizing these adverse effects.

2. Physical examination: A complete medical and family history should be taken prior to the initiation of any estrogen therapy. The pretreatment and periodic physical examinations should include special reference to blood pressure, breasts, abdomen, and pelvic organs, and should include a Papanicolaou smear. As a general rule, estrogen should not be prescribed for longer than 1 year without another physical examination being performed.

3. Fluid retention: Because estrogens may cause some degree of fluid retention, conditions which might be influenced by this factor such as asthma, epilepsy, migraine, and cardiac or renal dysfunction, require careful observation.

4. Uterine bleeding and mastodynia: Certain patients may develop undesirable manifestations of estrogenic stimulation, such as abnormal uterine bleeding and mastodynia.

5. Uterine fibroids: Pre-existing uterine leiomyomata may increase in size during prolonged high-dose estrogen use.

6. Impaired liver function: Estrogens may be poorly metabolized in patients with impaired liver function and should be administered with caution.

7. Hypercalcemia (and renal insufficiency): Prolonged use of estrogens can influence the metabolism of calcium and phosphorus. Estrogens should be used with caution in patients with metabolic bone disease or in patients with renal insufficiency.

Information for the Patient: See text of Patient Package Insert which accompanies this drug product.

Laboratory Tests: Clinical response at the smallest dose should generally be the guide to estrogen administration for relief of symptoms for those indications in which symptoms are observable. Tests used to measure adequacy of estrogen replacement therapy include serum estrone and estradiol levels and suppression of serum gonadotropin levels.

Drug/Laboratory Test Interactions: Some of these drug/laboratory test interactions have been observed only with estrogen-progestin combinations (oral contraceptives):

1. Increased prothrombin and factors VII, VIII, IX, and X; decreased antithrombin 3; increased norepinephrine-induced platelet aggregability, decreased fibrinolysis.

2. Increased thyroid-binding globulin (TBG) leading to increased circulating total thyroid hormone, as measured by T_4 levels determined either by column or by radioimmunoassay. Free T_3 resin uptake is decreased, reflecting the elevated TBG; free T_4 concentrations is unaltered.

3. Impaired glucose tolerance.

4. Reduced response to metyrapone test.

5. Reduced serum folate concentration.

Note: Certain brands of Chlorotrianisene contain FD&C Yellow No. 5 (tartrazine), which may cause allergic-type reactions (including bronchial asthma) in certain susceptible individuals. Although the overall incidence of FD&C Yellow No. 5 (tartrazine) sensitivity in the general population is low, it is frequently seen in patients who also have aspirin hypersensitivity.

Mutagenesis and Carcinogenesis: Long-term continuous administration of natural and synthetic estrogens in certain animal species increases the frequency of carcinomas of the breast, cervix, vagina, and liver.

Pregnancy Category X: Estrogens should not be used during pregnancy. (See *"Contraindications"* and boxed *"Warning".*)

Nursing Mothers: As a general principle, the administration of any drug to nursing mothers should be done only when clearly necessary since many drugs are excreted in human milk.

ADVERSE REACTIONS

(See *"Warnings"* regarding induction of neoplasia, adverse effects on the fetus, increased incidence of gallbladder disease). The following additional adverse reactions have been reported with estrogen therapy:

1. Genitourinary system: Changes in vaginal bleeding pattern and abnormal withdrawal bleeding or flow; breakthrough bleeding, spotting; increase in size of uterine fibromyomata; vaginal candidiasis; change in amount of cervical secretion.

2. Breasts: Tenderness, enlargement.

3 Gastrointestinal: Nausea, vomiting; abdominal cramps, bloating; cholestatic jaundice.

4. Skin: Chloasma or melasma, that may persist when drug is discontinued; erythema multiforme; erythema nodosum; urticaria; hemorrhagic eruption; loss of scalp hair; hirsutism.

5. Eyes: Steepening of corneal curvature; intolerance of contact lenses.

6. CNS: Headache, migraine, dizziness; mental depression; chorea.

7. Miscellaneous: Increase or decrease in weight; reduced carbohydrate tolerance; aggravation of porphyria; edema; changes in libido.

ACUTE OVERDOSAGE

Numerous reports of ingestion of large doses of estrogen-containing oral contraceptives by young children indicate that acute serious ill effects do not occur. Overdosage of estrogen may cause nausea and vomiting.

DOSAGE AND ADMINISTRATION

1. Advanced androgen-dependent carcinoma of the prostate, for palliation only. The usual dosage is 12 to 25 mg daily (one or two 12 mg capsules or one 25 mg capsule).

2. For treatment of moderate to severe vasomotor symptoms, atrophic vaginitis, or kraurosis vulvae associated with the menopause. The lowest dose that will control symptoms should be chosen and medication should be discontinued as promptly as possible. Administration should be cyclic (e.g., 3 weeks on and 1 week off).

Attempts to discontinue or taper medication should be made at 3-month to 6-month intervals.

The usual dosage range for vasomotor symptoms, atrophic vaginitis, or kraurosis vulvae associated with the menopause is 12 to 25 mg daily (one or two 12 mg capsules or one 25 mg capsule) for 30 days; one or more courses may be prescribed.

3. Female hypogonadism; primary ovarian failure.

The usual dosage is 12 to 25 mg daily (one or two 12 mg capsules or one 25 mg capsule) for 21 days. This course may, if desired, be followed immediately by the intramuscular injection of 100 mg of progesterone; alternatively, an oral progesterone such as medroxyprogesterone may be given during the last 5 days of Chlorotrianisene therapy. The next course may begin on the 5th day of the induced uterine bleeding.

Treated patients with an intact uterus should be monitored closely for signs of endometrial cancer, and appropriate diagnostic measures should be taken to rule out malignancy in the event of persistent or recurrent abnormal vaginal bleeding.

INFORMATION FOR PATIENTS

CHLOROTRIANISENE IS A SYNTHETIC ESTROGEN SUPPLIED IN 12 MG AND 25 MG CAPSULES.

This leaflet describes when and how to use estrogens and the risks of estrogen treatment.

ESTROGEN DRUGS

Estrogens have several important uses but also some risks. You must decide, with your doctor, whether the risks of estrogens are acceptable in view of their benefits. If you decide to start taking estrogens, check with your doctor to make sure you are using the lowest possible effective dose. The length of treatment with estrogens will depend upon the reason for use. This should also be discussed with your doctor.

USES OF ESTROGEN

1. *To reduce menopausal symptoms:* Estrogens are hormones produced by the ovaries. The decrease in the amount of estrogen that occurs in all women, usually between ages 45 and 55, causes the menopause. Sometimes the ovaries are removed by an operation, causing "surgical menopause." When the amount of estrogen begins to decrease, some women develop very uncomfortable symptoms, such as feelings of warmth in the face, neck and chest or sudden intense episodes of heat and sweating ("hot flashes"). The use of drugs containing estrogens can help the body adjust to lower estrogen levels.

Most women have none or only mild menopausal symptoms and do not need estrogens. Other women may need estrogens for a few months while their bodies adjust to lower estrogen levels. The majority of women do not need estrogen replacement for longer than six months for these symptoms.

2. *To treat atrophic vaginitis:* (itching, burning, dryness in or around the vagina) and *kraurosis vulvae* (which may cause chronic irritation of the vagina and vulva).

3. *To treat certain cancers*

WHEN ESTROGENS SHOULD NOT BE USED

Estrogens should not be used:

1. *During Pregnancy*

Although the possibility is fairly small, there is a greater risk of having a child born with a birth defect if you take estrogens during pregnancy. A male child may have an increased risk of developing abnormalities of the urinary system and sex organs. A female child may have an increased risk of developing cancer of the vagina or cervix in her teens or twenties. Estrogen is not effective in preventing miscarriage (abortion).

2. *If You Have Had Any Heart or Circulation Problems*

Estrogen therapy should be used only after consultation with your physician and only in recommended doses. Patients with a tendency for abnormal blood clotting should avoid estrogen use (see below).

3. *If You Have Had Cancer*

Since estrogens increase the risk of certain cancers, you should not take estrogens if you have ever had cancer of the breast or uterus. In certain situations, your doctor may choose to use estrogen in the treatment of breast cancer or prostate cancer.

4. *When They Are Ineffective*

Sometimes women experience nervous symptoms or depression during menopause. There is no evidence that estrogens are effective for such symptoms. You may have heard that taking estrogens for long periods (years) after menopause will keep your skin soft and supple and keep you feeling young. There is no evidence that this is so and such long-term treatment may carry serious risks.

DANGERS OF ESTROGENS

1. *Cancer of the Uterus*

The risk of cancer of the uterus increases the longer estrogens are used and when larger doses are taken. One study showed that when estrogens are discontinued, this increased risk of cancer seems to fall off quickly. In another study, the persistence of risk was demonstrated for 10 years after stopping estrogen treatment. Because of this risk, *it is important to take the lowest dose of estrogen that will control your symptoms and to take it only as long as you need it.* There is a higher risk of cancer of the uterus if you are overweight, diabetic, or have high blood pressure.

If you have had your uterus removed (total hysterectomy), there is no danger of developing cancer of the uterus.

2. *Cancer of the Breast*

The majority of studies have shown no association with the usual doses used for estrogen replacement therapy and breast cancer. Some studies have suggested a possible increased incidence of breast cancer in those women taking estrogens for prolonged periods of time and especially if higher doses are used.

Regular breast examinations by a health professional and self-examination are recommended for women receiving estrogen therapy, as they are for all women.

3. *Gallbladder Disease*

Women who use estrogens after menopause are more likely to develop gallbladder disease needing surgery than women who do not use estrogens.

4. *Abnormal Blood Clotting*

Taking estrogens may increase the risk of blood clots. This can cause a stroke, heart attack or pulmonary embolus, any of which may be fatal.

SIDE EFFECTS

In addition to the risk of estrogens described above, the following side effects have been reported with estrogen use:

1. Nausea and vomiting
2. Breast tenderness or enlargement
3. Enlargement of benign tumors of the uterus
4. Retention of excess fluid This may make some conditions worsen, such as asthma, epilepsy, migraine, heart disease, or kidney disease.
5. A spotty darkening of the skin, particularly on the face.

Note: Certain brands of Chlorotrianisene 12 and 25 mg capsules contain a dye (FD&C Yellow No. 5 or tartrazine), which may cause allergic-type reactions (including asthma) in certain susceptible individuals. Although the over-all frequency of tartrazine sensitivity in the general population is low, it is frequently seen in patients who also have aspirin hypersensitivity.

REDUCING RISK OF ESTROGEN USE

If you decide to take estrogens, you can reduce your risks by carefully monitoring your treatment.

1. *See Your Doctor Regularly*

While you are taking estrogens, it is important that you visit your doctor at least once a year for a physical examination. If members of your family have had breast cancer or if you have ever had breast nodules or an abnormal mammogram (breast x-ray), you may need to have more frequent breast examinations.

2. *Reevaluate Your Need For Estrogens*

You and your doctor should reevaluate your need for estrogens at least every six months.

3. *Be Alert For Signs of Trouble*

Report these or any other unusual side effects to your doctor immediately:

1. Abnormal bleeding from the vagina
2. Pains in the calves or chest, a sudden shortness of breath or coughing blood (indicating possible clots in the legs, heart, or lungs)
3. Severe headache, dizziness, faintness, or changes in vision, indicating possible clots in the brain or eye
4. Breast lumps
5. Yellowing of the skin
6. Pain, swelling, or tenderness in the abdomen.

OTHER INFORMATION

Some physicians may choose to prescribe another hormonal drug to be used in association with estrogen treatment.

These drugs, progestins, have been reported to lower the frequency of occurrence of a possible precancerous condition of the uterine lining. Whether this will provide protection from uterine cancer has not been clearly established. There are possible additional risks that may be associated with the inclusion of a progestin in estrogen treatment. The possible risks include unfavorable effects on blood fats and sugars.

The choice of progestin and its dosage may be important in minimizing these effects.

Your doctor has prescribed this drug for you and you alone.

Do not give the drug to anyone else.

Keep this and all drugs out of the reach of children. In case of overdose, call your doctor, hospital, or poison control center immediately.

This leaflet provides the most important information about estrogens. If you want to read more, ask your doctor or pharmacist to let you read the professional labeling.

◆ RATED THERAPEUTICALLY EQUIVALENT; ◇ THERAPEUTIC EQUIVALENCE UNCONFIRMED; ○ UNRATED

HOW SUPPLIED
CAPSULE: 12 MG

BRAND/MANUFACTURER	NDC	SIZE	AWP
◆ BRAND TACE: Marion Merrell Dow	00068-0690-61	100s	$98.46

CAPSULE: 25 MG

BRAND/MANUFACTURER	NDC	SIZE	AWP
◆ BRAND TACE: Marion Merrell Dow	00068-0691-60	60s	$113.64

Chloroxine

DESCRIPTION
Chloroxine is an antibacterial shampoo containing 2% (w/w) Chloroxine (each gram contains 20 mg Chloroxine).

Chloroxine is a synthetic antibacterial compound that is effective in the treatment of dandruff and seborrheic dermatitis when incorporated in a shampoo.

The chemical name of chloroxine is 5,7-dichloro-8-hydroxyquinoline.

Following is its chemical structure:

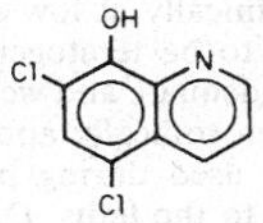

CLINICAL PHARMACOLOGY
Well controlled studies demonstrate Chloroxine effectively reduces the excess scaling in patients with dandruff or seborheic dermatitis. Though the cause of dandruff is not known, it is thought to be the result of accelerated mitotic activity in the epidermis. The presumed mechanism of action to reduce scaling would be to slow down the mitotic activity.

The role of microbes in seborrheic dermatitis is not known; however, *Staphylococcus aureus* and *Pityrosporon* species are often present in increased numbers during the course of the disease. Chloroxine is antibacterial, inhibiting the growth of Gram-positive as well as some Gram-negative organisms. Antifungal activity against some dermatophytes and yeasts also has been shown.

The absorption, metabolism and pharmacokinetics of Chloroxine in humans have not been studied.

INDICATIONS AND USAGE
Chloroxine is indicated in the treatment of dandruff and mild-to-moderately severe seborrheic dermatitis of the scalp. Clinical studies indicate that improvement may be observed after 14 days of therapy.

CONTRAINDICATIONS
Chloroxine is contraindicated in those patients with a history of hypersensitivity to any of the listed ingredients.

WARNINGS
Chloroxine should not be used on acutely inflamed (exudative) lesions of the scalp.

PRECAUTIONS
Information for patients: Exercise care to prevent Chloroxine from entering the eyes. If contact occurs, the patient should flush eyes with cool water. Discoloration of light-colored hair (e.g. blond, gray or bleached) may follow use of this preparation.

Irritation and a burning sensation on the scalp and adjacent areas have been reported.

Drug/Laboratory Test Interactions: There is no known interference of Chloroxine with laboratory tests.

Carcinogenesis, Mutagenesis: No long term studies in animals have been performed to evaluate the carcinogenic potential of Chloroxine.

Results of the *in vitro* Ames Salmonella/Microsome Plate test show that Chloroxine does not demonstrate genetic activity and is considered non-mutagenic.

Pregnancy Category C: Animal reproduction studies have not be conducted with Chloroxine. It is also not known whether Chloroxine can cause fetal harm when administered to a pregnant woman or can affect reproduction capacity. Chloroxine should be given to a pregnant woman only if clearly needed.

Nursing Mothers: It is not known whether this drug is excreted in human milk. Because many drugs are excreted in human milk, caution should be exercised when Chloroxine is administered to a nursing woman.

Pediatric Use: Specific studies to demonstrate the safety and effectiveness for use of Chloroxine in children have not been conducted.

ADVERSE REACTION
One patient out of 225 in clinical studies was reported to have contact dermatitis.

OVERDOSAGE
The acute oral LD_{50} in mice was found to be 200 mg/kg and in rats 450 mg/kg. On the basis of these animal studies, Chloroxine may be considered practically nontoxic.

DOSAGE AND ADMINISTRATION
Chloroxine should be massaged thoroughly onto the wet scalp, avoiding contact with the eyes. Lather should remain on the scalp for approximately three minutes, then rinsed. The application should be repeated and the scalp rinsed thoroughly. Two treatments per week are usually sufficient.

Store at room temperature.

HOW SUPPLIED
SHAMPOO: 2%

BRAND/MANUFACTURER	NDC	SIZE	AWP
○ BRAND CAPITROL: Westwood-Squibb	00072-6850-04	120 ml	$15.88

Chloroxylenol and Undecylenic Acid

DESCRIPTION
Chloroxylenol/Undecylenic Acid is an antifungal solution for topical use containing 25% Undecylenic Acid and 3% Chloroxylenol as its active ingredients in a penetrating oil base. Undecylenic Acid is chemically 10-hendecenoic acid having the empirical formula $C_{11}H_{20}O_2$ and the chemical bond structure $CH_2 = CH(CH_2)_8CO_2H$.

Undecylenic Acid is a colorless to pale yellow liquid. It is soluble in water and soluble in alcohol, chloroform and ether.

Chloroxylenol is chemically 2-chloro-5-hydroxy-1,3-dimethylbenzene having the empirical formula C_8H_9ClO.

CLINICAL PHARMACOLOGY
Undecylenic Acid is a fungistatic agent employed in the treatment of tinea pedis, tinea capitis, ringworm and dermatophytosis.

Chloroxylenol is a topical antiseptic, germicide and antifungal agent effective against a wide variety of causitive fungi and yeast organisms. Among those affected by chloroxylenol are candida albicans, aspergillus niger, aspergillus flavus, trychophyton rubrum, tricophyton mentagrophytes, penicillum luteum and epidermophyton floccosum.

The penetrating oil base vehicle serves as a delivery system, enhancing the impregnation of Undecylenic Acid and Chloroxylenol as antimicrobial agents in the treatment of onychomycosis.

INDICATIONS
Chloroxylenol/Undecylenic Acid is indicated in the treatment and prevention of onychomycosis, cutaneous fungus infections, as well as a softener for callous nail grooves.

CONTRAINDICATIONS
Chloroxylenol/Undecylenic Acid is contraindicated in patients who are sensitive to Undecylenic Acid or Chloroxylenol.

WARNINGS
FOR EXTERNAL USE ONLY. Not for ophthalmic or optic use. Avoid inhaling and contact with eyes or other mucous membranes. Not to be applied over blistered, raw or oozing areas of skin or over deep puncture wounds.

PRECAUTIONS
If a reaction suggesting sensitivity or chemical irritation should occur with the use of Chloroxylenol/Undecylenic Acid, treatment should be discontinued. Use of Chloroxylenol/Undecylenic Acid in pregnancy has not been established.

ADVERSE REACTIONS
No significant adverse reactions have been reported. However, attention should be paid to localized hypersensitivity.

DOSAGE AND ADMINISTRATION
Cleanse the affected area thoroughly. Paint on affected area twice daily, morning and evening. As a precaution against relapse of the condition, continue therapy for several weeks after the condition has cleared.

Store at controlled room temperatures (59°-86°F).

For external use only.

Keep out of reach of children.

HOW SUPPLIED
SOLUTION:

BRAND/MANUFACTURER	NDC	SIZE	AWP
○ **BRAND**			
GORDOCHOM: Gordon	10481-3010-02	30 ml doz	$92.50

Chloroxylenol/Hydrocortisone/ Pramoxine Hydrochloride

DESCRIPTION

Each 1 ml for otic administration contains:

Chloroxylenol	1 mg
Hydrocortisone	10 mg
Pramoxine Hydrochloride	10 mg

Chloroxylenol: 4-chloro-3,5-dimethyl-phenol is a broad spectrum bactericidal agent which occurs as white crystals with a phenolic odor. It is soluble in alcohol, ether, and alkali hydroxides.

Hydrocortisone: Pregn-4-ene-3, 20-dione,11,17, 21-trihydroxy-, (11 β)-; is an anti-inflammatory and antipruritic agent. It occurs as a white to practically white, odorless, crystalline powder which melts at about 215°C with decomposition. It is very slightly soluble in water and in ether; sparingly soluble in acetone and in alcohol; slightly soluble in chloroform.

Pramoxine Hydrochloride: Morpholine, 4-[3-(4-butoxyphenoxy) propyl]-, Hydrochloride is a topical anesthetic proven to be safe and effective in hospital tests. It occurs as white to practically white, crystalline powder, having a numbing taste and it may have a slight aromatic odor. It is freely soluble in water and in alcohol: soluble in chloroform; and very slightly soluble in ether.

CLINICAL PHARMACOLOGY
Chloroxylenol/Hydrocortisone/Pramoxine Hydrochloride Otic Ear Drops are effective both as an antibacterial and antifungal agent.

Chloroxylenol is a halogenated phenol and is a germicide with a high phenol coefficient. It is nontoxic, noncorrosive, nonstaining, and may be applied directly to the ear canal.

Hydrocortisone is a topical corticosteroid which has anti-inflammatory, antipruritic and vasoconstrictive actions. The mechanism of anti-inflammatory activity of the topical corticosteroids is unclear. Various laboratory methods, including vasoconstrictor assays are used to compare and predict potencies and/or clinical efficacies of the topical corticosteroids. There is some evidence to suggest that a recognizable correlation exists between vasoconstrictor potency and therapeutic efficacy in man. The extent of percutaneous absorption of topical corticosteroids is determined by many factors including the vehicle and the integrity of the epidermal barrier. Topical corticosteroids can be absorbed from normal intact skin. Inflammation and/or other disease processes in the skin increase percutaneous absorption. Once absorbed through the skin, topical corticosteroids are handled through pharmacokinetic pathways similar to systemically administered corticosteroids. Corticosteroids are bound to plasma proteins in varying degrees. Corticosteroids are metabolized primarily in the liver and are then excreted by the kidneys. Some of the topical corticosteroids and their metabolites are also excreted into the bile.

Pramoxine Hydrochloride is a topical anesthetic agent which provides temporary relief from itching and pain. It acts by stabilizing the neuronal membranes of nerve endings with which it comes into contact.

Certain brands of Chloroxylenol/Hydrocortisone/Pramoxine Hydrochloride Otic Drops contain benzalkonium chloride which lowers surface tension, permitting better penetration to the auditory meatal skin. It is also a cationic germicide of high bactericidal and bacteriostatic potency.

INDICATIONS AND USAGE
For the treatment of superficial infections of the external auditory canal complicated by inflammation caused by organisms and susceptible to the action of the antimicrobial, or to control itching.

CONTRAINDICATIONS
Topical steroids are contraindicated in varicella, vaccinia and in patients sensitive to any of the components of this preparation. This or any medication should not be applied in the external auditory canal of patients with perforated eardrums.

WARNINGS
This preparation is not intended for ophthalmic or oral use. If accidental ingestion occurs, seek professional help.

PRECAUTIONS
General: If a favorable response does not occur promptly, discontinue the use of this preparation until the infection is controlled by other appropriate measures. Although systemic side effects are not common with topical corticosteroids, the possibility of occurrence must be kept in mind particularly when used for an extended period of time.

Systemic absorption of topical corticosteroids has produced reversible hypothalamic-pituitary-adrenal (HPA) axis suppression, manifestations of Cushing's syndrome, hyperglycemia and glycosuria in some patients. Conditions which augment systemic absorption include the application of more potent steroids. Recovery of HPA axis function is generally prompt and complete upon discontinuation of the drug. Infrequently, signs and symptoms of steroid withdrawal may occur, requiring supplemental corticosteroids. Children may absorb proportionately larger amounts of topical corticosteroids and thus be more susceptible to systemic toxicity (see *"Precautions—Pediatric Use"*).

WARNING
If irritation or sensitization occurs, promptly discontinue use of this preparation and institute other measures.

Information for the Patient: Patients using topical corticosteroids should receive the following information and instructions:

1. This medication is to be used as directed by the physician. It is for external use only. Avoid contact with the eyes.
2. Patients should be advised not to use this medication for any disorder other than for which it was prescribed.
3. Patients should report any signs of local adverse reactions.

Laboratory Tests: The urinary free cortisol test and the ACTH stimulation test may be helpful in evaluating the HPA axis suppression.

Carcinogenesis, Mutagenesis, Impairment of Fertility: Long-term animal studies have not been performed to evaluate the carcinogenic potential or the effect of topical corticosteroids on fertility. Studies to determine mutagenicity with prednisolone and hydrocortisone have revealed negative results.

Pregnancy Category C: Corticosteroids are generally teratogenic in laboratory animals when administered systemically at low dosage levels. The more potent corticosteroids have been shown to be teratogenic after dermal application in laboratory animals. There are no adequate and well-controlled studies in pregnant women on teratogenic effects from topically applied corticosteroids. Therefore, topical corticosteroids should be used during pregnancy only if the potential benefit justifies the potential risk to the fetus. Drugs of this class should not be used extensively on pregnant patients, in large amounts, or for prolonged periods of time.

Nursing Mothers: It is not known whether topical administration of corticosteroids could result in sufficient systemic absorption to produce detectable quantities in breast milk. Systemically administered corticosteroids are secreted into breast milk in quantities not likely to have a deleterious effect on the infant. Nevertheless, caution should be exercised when topical corticosteroids are administered to a nursing woman.

Pediatric Use: Pediatric patients may demonstrate greater susceptibility to topical corticosteroid-induced HPA axis suppression and Cushing's Syndrome than mature patients because of a larger skin surface area to body weight ratio. Hypothalamic-pituitary-adrenal (HPA) axis suppression, Cushing's Syndrome, and intracranial hypertension have been reported in children receiving topical corticosteroids. Manifestations of adrenal suppression in children include linear growth retardation, delayed weight gain, low plasma cortisol levels and absence of response to ACTH stimulation. Manifestations of intracranial hypertension include bulging fontanelles, headaches and bilateral papilledema. Administration of topical corticosteroids to children should be limited to the least amount compatible with an effective therapeutic regimen. Chronic corticosteroids therapy may interfere with the growth and development of children.

Drug Interactions: Interaction of other drugs with the Hydrocortisone component of this product is possible. Inform your physician of other medication you are currently taking.

ADVERSE REACTIONS
The following adverse reactions with topical corticosteroids have been observed: itching, burning, irritation, dryness, folliculitis, hypertrichosis, acneform eruptions, hypopigmentation, perioral dermatitis, allergic contact dermatitis, maceration of the skin, secondary infection, skin atrophy, striae and miliaria.

OVERDOSAGE
Topically applied corticosteroids can be absorbed in sufficient amount to produce systemic effects.

DOSAGE AND ADMINISTRATION
The external auditory canal should be thoroughly cleansed and dried with a sterile cotton applicator. For adults, 4 to 5 drops of the solution should be instilled into the affected ear 3 or 4 times daily.

For infants and small children, 3 drops are suggested because of the smaller capacity of the ear canal.

The patient should lie with the affected ear upward to instill the drops and this position should be maintained for 5 minutes to facilitate penetration of the drops into the ear canal. Repeat, if necessary, for the opposite ear.

If preferred, a wick may be inserted into the canal *after* the drops have been applied. More drops may be applied to saturate the wick with solution. Instruct the patient to add a few drops to the wick every four hours. Remove the wick after the first 24 hours and continue to instill 5 drops 3 or 4 times daily thereafter. This product may be used in the unaffected ear 3 times daily as a preventive.

HOW SUPPLIED
DROP:

BRAND/MANUFACTURER	NDC	SIZE	AWP
○ **BRAND**			
CORTANE B-OTIC: Blansett	51674-0116-01	10 ml	$15.95

◆ RATED THERAPEUTICALLY EQUIVALENT; ◇ THERAPEUTIC EQUIVALENCE UNCONFIRMED; ○ UNRATED

BRAND/MANUFACTURER	NDC	SIZE	AWP
○ GENERICS			
OTOZONE: McNeil,R.A.	12830-0781-10	10 ml	$19.50
TRI-OTIC: Pharmics	00813-0393-11	10 ml	$19.95

DROP: 1 MG-10 MG-10 MG

BRAND/MANUFACTURER	NDC	SIZE	AWP
○ GENERICS			
ZOTO-HC: Horizon Pharm	59630-0130-01	10 ml	$17.95

DROP: 10 MG-10 MG-1 MG

BRAND/MANUFACTURER	NDC	SIZE	AWP
○ BRAND			
CORTIC: Everett	00642-0011-01	10 ml	$19.95

LIQUID:

BRAND/MANUFACTURER	NDC	SIZE	AWP
○ GENERICS			
OTOMAR HC: Marnel	00682-9090-10	10 ml	$19.90

Chlorphenesin Carbamate

DESCRIPTION
Each tablet contains Chlorphenesin Carbamate which is a white to off-white crystalline solid, almost insoluble in cold water, benzene or cyclohexane, fairly readily soluble in dioxane, and readily soluble in ethyl acetate, 95% ethanol and acetone.

The chemical name for Chlorphenesin Carbamate is 3-(p-chlorophenoxy)-2-hydroxypropyl carbamate.

Each tablet for oral use contains 400 mg of Chlorphenesin Carbamate.

Following is its chemical structure:

$$Cl-C_6H_4-OCH_2CHCH_2OCONH_2$$
$$|$$
$$OH$$

ACTIONS
The mode of therapeutic action in man has not been identified, but may be related to its sedative properties. It has no direct action on the contractile mechanism of striated muscle, the motor end plate, or the nerve fiber.

INDICATIONS AND USAGE
Chlorphenesin Carbamate Tablets are indicated as an adjunct to rest, physical therapy and other measures for the relief of discomfort associated with acute, painful musculoskeletal conditions. The mode of action of this drug has not been completely identified, but may be related to its sedative properties. Chlorphenesin Carbamate does not directly relax skeletal muscles in man.

UNLABELED USES
Chlorphenesin Carbamate is used alone or as an adjunct in the treatment of trigeminal neuralgia.

CONTRAINDICATIONS
Patients who have demonstrated evidence of hypersensitivity to Chlorphenesin Carbamate Tablets, such as skin rash, should not receive further treatment with it.

WARNINGS
Use in Pregnancy: The safe use of Chlorphenesin Carbamate Tablets in pregnancy has not been established. Therefore, its use during pregnancy, lactation or in women who may become pregnant is not recommended, unless, in the opinion of the physician, potential benefits outweigh possible hazards. Adequate animal reproduction studies have not been done.

Use in Children: The safety and effectiveness of this drug in children have not been established; therefore, Chlorphenesin Carbamate is not recommended for use in the pediatric age group.

Chlorphenesin Carbamate may impair the mental and/or physical abilities required for the performance of potentially hazardous tasks, such as driving a motor vehicle or operating machinery. The patient should be warned accordingly.

PRECAUTIONS
The safe use of Chlorphenesin Carbamate Tablets for periods exceeding eight weeks has not been established. Chlorphenesin Carbamate should be used with caution in patients with pre-existing liver disease or impaired hepatic function.

Certain formulations of this product contain FD&C Yellow No. 5 (tartrazine) which may cause allergic-type reactions (including bronchial asthma) in certain susceptible individuals. Although the overall incidence of FD&C Yellow No. 5 (tartrazine) sensitivity in the general population is low, it is frequently seen in patients who also have aspirin hypersensitivity.

ADVERSE REACTIONS
Hematopoietic: Rare cases of leukopenia, thrombocytopenia, agranulocytosis and pancytopenia have been reported.

Hypersensitivity: Anaphylactoid reactions and drug fever have been observed occasionally. The possibility of other allergic phenomena should be borne in mind. Such reactions are an indication for discontinuing the medication.

Drowsiness, dizziness, confusion, nausea and epigastric distress have been infrequently reported. While not established as drug related, two cases of gastrointestinal bleeding have been reported.

Occasionally, paradoxical stimulation, insomnia, increased nervousness and headache have been reported. Dose reduction will usually control these symptoms.

OVERDOSAGE
One patient has been reported who attempted suicide by ingesting 12 grams of Chlorphenesin Carbamate. He was slightly nauseated and drowsy for about six hours but recovered with only routine supportive therapy.

In treating accidental or intentional overdosage, vomiting may be induced or gastric lavage and/or saline catharsis may be employed. Supportive therapy should suffice in most instances of excessive dosage.

DOSAGE AND ADMINISTRATION
Initial dosage of two tablets three times daily is recommended until the desired effect is obtained. For maintenance, dosage may then be reduced to one tablet four times daily, or less as required.

Store at controlled room temperature 15° to 30° C (59° to 86° F).

ANIMAL TOXICITY
In toxicity studies in rats and dogs, comparison of treated and untreated (control) animals revealed no meaningful changes attributable to Chlorphenesin Carbamate. Nevertheless, it should be noted that at the high dosage levels (100-300 mg/kg in rats and 260-300 mg/kg in dogs) liver weight:body weight ratios increased.

No hepatocellular changes were noted in the rats, but in dogs, one of three given 300 mg/kg of Chlorphenesin Carbamate for 28 days and one of four given 260 mg/kg of Chlorphenesin Carbamate for 174 days showed nonspecific hepatocellular degeneration on microscopic examination. However, attention should be called to the fact that at the high dosage levels the dogs involved were markedly obtunded and ate poorly.

HOW SUPPLIED
TABLETS: 400 MG

BRAND/MANUFACTURER	NDC	SIZE	AWP
○ BRAND			
MAOLATE: Upjohn	00009-0412-01	50s	$36.38

Chlorpheniramine Maleate and Epinephrine Hydrochloride

DESCRIPTION
Each Chlorpheniramine/Epinephrine Anaphylaxis Emergency Treatment Kit contains:

Epinephrine Injection, USP, (1:1000), contained in a sterile, 1 mL syringe, designed to deliver 2 doses of 0.3 mL each. Product is intended for subcutaneous or intramuscular use. Each mL of Epinephrine Injection, USP, (1:1000) contains 1 mg *l*-Epinephrine as the Hydrochloride.

Epinephrine is a sympathomimetic catecholamine. Its naturally occurring levo isomer, which is twenty times as active as the *d* isomer, is now obtained in pure form by separation from the synthetically produced racemate.

Chemically, Epinephrine is 1-(3,4-dihydroxyphenyl)-2-(methyl amino)ethanol.

Chlorpheniramine Maleate Tablets: 4 chewable tablets, each containing 2 mg Chlorpheniramine Maleate, USP, for oral administration. Chlorpheniramine Maleate is an antihistamine having the chemical name 2-(4-chlorophenyl)-N,N-dimethyl-2-pyridinepropanamine. (Z)-2-butenedioate(1:1):

DEVICES: 2 sterile pads containing isopropyl alcohol 70% by volume. One tourniquet.

CLINICAL PHARMACOLOGY
Epinephrine: The most valuable drug for the emergency treatment of severe allergic reactions is Epinephrine. The vasoconstrictor effect of Epinephrine on the capillary directly antagonizes the generalized vasodilation produced by histamine. Epinephrine reverses the increased permeability of dilated capillaries to plasma. The shock of severe allergic reactions is due to the loss of circulating blood volume by pooling in the dilated capillary beds and loss of plasma into the tissues. Epinephrine quickly restores circulating blood volume and blood pressure by constricting the capillary bed. The itching during episodes of hives or angioedema is promptly relieved by Epinephrine. Epinephrine is a powerful relaxer of the smooth muscle of the bronchioles, stomach, intestine, pregnant uterus and urinary bladder wall. The bronchospasm, wheezing and dyspnea of the acute allergic reactions are relieved. Where abdominal cramping, defecation or involuntary urination have occurred during severe allergic attacks, Epinephrine rapidly produces relief. Subcutaneously or intramuscularly administered Epinephrine has a rapid onset and short duration of action. Subcutaneous administration during asthmatic attacks may produce bronchodilation within 5 to 10 minutes, and maximal effects may occur within 20 minutes.

➤ SHOWN IN PRODUCT IDENTIFICATION GUIDE

Chlorpheniramine Maleate: Chlorpheniramine Maleate is an effective agent in nullifying the characteristic effects of histamine and is especially valuable in the prophylaxis and relief of many allergic symptoms. It is readily absorbed from the intestinal tract and released into the tissues from the bloodstream. This action is both prompt and sustained. Elimination of the drug is such that there is a low incidence of side effects.

INDICATIONS AND USAGE

Chlorpheniramine/Epinephrine Anaphylaxis Emergency Treatment Kit is indicated for use by adult and pediatric patients under the following situations:

1. Allergic reactions including anaphylactic shock due to stinging insects (primarily of the Hymenoptera order, which includes bees, wasps, hornets, yellow jackets, bumble bees, and fire ants.)

2. Severe allergic or anaphylactoid reactions due to allergy injections, exposures to pollens, dusts, molds, foods, drugs, and exercise or unknown substances (so-called idiopathic anaphylaxis).

3. Severe, life-threatening asthma attacks characterized by wheezing, dyspnea and inability to breathe.

In the sensitive patient, severe allergic reactions and anaphylactic shock may occur within minutes of the insect sting or exposure to an allergenic substance.

Symptoms may include bronchoconstriction, wheezing, sneezing, hoarseness, urticaria, angioedema, erythema, pruritis, tachycardia, thready pulse, falling blood pressure, sense of oppression or impending doom, disorientation, cramping abdominal pain, incontinance, faintness, loss of consciousness.

The Chlorpheniramine/Epinephrine Kit is compactly designed to be carried and used by patients when severe symptoms arise, and the patient is out of reach of immediate attention by a doctor or hospital.

CONTRAINDICATIONS

Epinephrine: Epinephrine must not be given intra-arterially as marked vasoconstriction may result in gangrene. *This unit is not intended for intravenous use.* Further dilution would be necessary and is not practical with this emergency syringe.

Epinephrine Injection, USP, (1:1000) must not be used if there is hypersensitivity to any of the components.

Epinephrine is contraindicated in narrow-angle glaucoma; cardiogenic, traumatic, or hemorrhagic shock; cardiac dilation; cerebral arteriosclerosis; and organic brain damage.

Epinephrine should not be used to counteract circulatory collapse or hypotension due to phenothiazines, since such agents may reverse the pressor effect of Epinephrine, leading to a further lowering of blood pressure.

Epinephrine should not be administered concomitantly with other sympathomimetic agents, since the effects are additive and may be detrimental to the patient.

Chlorpheniramine Maleate: No known contraindications.

WARNINGS

Epinephrine: Overdosage or accidental intravenous administration of conventional subcutaneous doses may induce severe or fatal hypertension, or cerebrovascular hemorrhage. Fatalities may also occur from pulmonary edema resulting from peripheral constriction and cardiac stimulation. The marked pressor effects may be counteracted by use of rapidly acting vasodilators, such as the nitrites and alpha-adrenergic blockers.

Deaths have been reported in asthmatics treated with Epinephrine following the use of isoproterenol or orciprenaline. Epinephrine is the preferred treatment for serious allergic or other emergency situations even though this product contains sodium bisulfite, a sulfite that may in other products cause allergic-type reactions including anaphylactic symptoms or life-threatening or less severe asthmatic episodes in certain susceptible persons. The alternatives to using Epinephrine in a life-threatening situation may not be satisfactory. The presence of a sulfite(s) in this product should not deter administration of the drug for treatment of serious allergic or other emergency situations.

Epinephrine must be administered with great caution, if at all, in patients with cardiac arrhythmias, coronary artery or organic heart disease, and hypertension. In patients with coronary insufficiency or ischemic heart disease, Epinephrine may precipitate or aggravate angina pectoris as well as produce potentially fatal ventricular arrhythmias. Epinephrine should be administered only with great caution to elderly patients, those with diabetes mellitus, hyperthyroidism or psychoneurotic disorders; also to those with long-standing bronchial asthma and emphysema if such individuals may also have degenerative heart disease, and to pregnant women (see *"Pregnancy"*).

Chlorpheniramine Maleate: Chlorpheniramine Maleate should be used with extreme caution in patients with stenosing peptic ulcer, pyloroduodenal obstruction, prostatic hypertrophy, or bladder neck obstruction. These compounds have an atropine-like action and therefore should be used with caution in patients with a history of increased intraocular pressure, cardiovascular disease, or hypertension. The asthmatic patient should take the Chlorpheniramine Maleate tablets with caution.

PRECAUTIONS

General: Chlorpheniramine/Epinephrine is not intended to be a substitute for medical attention or hospital care. The kit is designed to be compact and easy to carry, and to provide emergency treatment when medical care is not immediately available. Highly sensitive individuals should have the kit readily available at all times. Because of its small size it can be carried by outdoor sportsmen, golfers, gardeners, or any sensitive individual who may be exposed to stinging insects

(wasps, hornets, yellow jackets, fire ants or bees) or other potentially life-threatening allergens. The drugs in the Chlorpheniramine/Epinephrine Kit, when used as directed immediately following exposure to an allergen, may prove life-saving. Certain changes in the emergency instructions and in the kit itself may be made by the doctor according to the needs of the patient. IN ALL CASES THE PHYSICIAN SHOULD INSTRUCT THE PATIENT, AND/OR ANY OTHER PERSON WHO MIGHT BE IN A POSITION TO ADMINISTER THE EPINEPHRINE IN THE PROPER USE OF THE SYRINGE AND THE OTHER COMPONENTS OF THIS KIT.

Information for Patients: Complete patient information, including dosage, directions for proper administration, and precautions, can be found at the end of this monograph, as well as inside each Chlorpheniramine/Epinephrine kit.

Since Epinephrine injection may produce disturbing or frightening reactions, it may be desirable to forewarn patients. Reactions commonly include an increase in pulse rate, a more forceful heartbeat, palpitations, a throbbing headache, pallor, feelings of overstimulation, anxiety, weakness, shakiness, dizziness, or nausea. Symptoms not involving an overdose generally do not indicate anything serious and usually subside rapidly with rest, quiet, and recumbency. Patients with hypertension or hyperthyroidism are prone to more severe or persistent effects, as are patients with coronary-artery disease, who may experience angina. Psychoneurotic patients may experience a worsening of symptoms. Diabetic patients may require an increased dose of insulin or other antidiabetic medication. Patients with Parkinson's disease may notice a temporary worsening of symptoms.

DRUG INTERACTIONS

Caution is indicated in patients receiving cardiac glycosides or mercurial diuretics, since these agents may sensitize the myocardium to beta-adrenergic stimulation and make cardiac arrhythmias more likely.

The effects of Epinephrine may be potentiated by tricyclic antidepressants, sodium levothyroxine, and certain antihistamines, notably Chlorpheniramine, tripelennamine and diphenhydramine.

The cardiostimulating and bronchodialating effects of Epinephrine are antagonized by beta-adrenergic blocking drugs, such as propranolol. The vasoconstricting and hypertensive effects are antagonized by alpha-adrenergic blocking drugs, such as phentolamine. Ergot alkaloids and phenothiazines may also reverse the pressor effects of Epinephrine.

Diabetic patients receiving Epinephrine may require an increased dose of insulin or oral hypoglycemic drugs.

Carcinogenesis, Mutagenesis, Impairment of Fertility: There are no data from either animal or human studies regarding the carcinogenicity or mutagenicity of Epinephrine or Chlorpheniramine Maleate, and no studies have been conducted to determine their potential for the impairment of fertility.

Pregnancy: Teratogenic Effects. Pregnancy Category C—Epinephrine has been shown to be teratogenic in rats and hamsters at dose levels hundreds of times as high as the maximal human dose. Although there are no adequate or well-controlled studies in pregnant women, Epinephrine crosses the placenta and its use during pregnancy may cause anoxia in the fetus. Epinephrine should be used in pregnancy only if the potential benefit justifies the potential risk to the fetus.

Pediatric Use: Administer Epinephrine or Chlorpheniramine Maleate with caution to infants and children (see *"Dosage and Administration"*). Syncope has occurred following the administration of Epinephrine to asthmatic children.

ADVERSE REACTIONS

Epinephrine: Adverse reactions include transient, moderate anxiety, apprehensiveness, restlessness, tremor, weakness, dizziness, sweating, palpitations, pallor, nausea and vomiting, headache, and respiratory difficulties. These symptoms occur in some persons receiving therapeutic doses of Epinephrine, but are more likely to occur, or to occur in exaggerated form, in those with hypertension or hyperthyroidism. Excessive doses cause acute hypertension. Arrhythmias, including fatal ventricular fibrillation, have been reported, particularly in patients with underlying cardiac disease or those receiving certain drugs (see *"Drug Interactions"*).

Rapid rise in blood pressure has produced cerebral hemorrhage, particularly in elderly patients with cerebrovascular disease. Angina may occur in patients with coronary-artery disease.

Chlorpheniramine Maleate: Drowsiness, dizziness, blurred vision, dry mouth and gastrointestinal upsets may occur. Patients should not drive or operate machinery after taking the drug. Large doses produce central nervous system depression and occasionally tremors or convulsions. Reports of hematological disorders are rare.

OVERDOSAGE

Epinephrine: Epinephrine is rapidly inactivated in the body, and treatment is primarily supportive. If necessary, pressor effects may be counteracted by rapidly acting vasodilators or alpha-adrenergic blocking drugs. If prolonged hypotension follows such measures, it may be necessary to administer another pressor drug, such as levarterenol.

Overdosage of Epinephrine may produce extremely elevated arterial pressure, which may result in cerebrovascular hemorrhage, particularly in elderly patients.

If an Epinephrine overdose induces pulmonary edema that interferes with respiration, treatment consists of a rapidly acting alpha-adrenergic blocking drug such as phentolamine and/or intermittent positive-pressure respiration.

Epinephrine overdosage can also cause transient bradycardia followed by tachycardia, and these may be accompanied by potentially fatal cardiac arrhythmias. Ventricular premature contractions may appear within one minute after injection and may be followed by multilocal ventricular tachycardia (prefibrillation rhythm). Subsidence of the ventricular effects may be followed by atrial tachycardia and occasionally by atrioventricular block. Treatment of arrhythmias consists of administration of a beta-adrenergic blocking drug such as propranolol.

Overdosage sometimes also results in extreme pallor and coldness of the skin, metabolic acidosis, and kidney failure. Suitable corrective measures must be taken.

Chlorpheniramine Maleate: Overdose symptoms may be sedation, apnea, cardiovascular collapse to stimulation, insomnia, hallucinations, tremors or convulsions. Also there may be dizziness, tinnitus, ataxia, blurred vision, hypotension, dry mouth, flushing, and abdominal symptoms.

Treatment: The patient should be induced to vomit, preferably with ipecac syrup—and large amounts of water. Prevent aspiration of vomitus. Gastric lavage may be necessary using activated charcoal and saline. Hypersomotic cathartics such as Milk of Magnesia may hasten elimination of residual cling. Vasopressors can be used to correct hypotension. Diazepan may be used to control seizures. Hyperpyrexia can be treated with cool sponges or a hypothermic blanket.

DOSAGE AND ADMINISTRATION
Parenteral drug products should be inspected visually for particulate matter and discoloration prior to administration, whenever solution and container permit. Do not use Epinephrine Injection, USP, if it has a pinkish or darker than slightly yellow color or contains a precipitate.

The physician who prescribes the Chlorpheniramine/Epinephrine Kit should review the package insert in detail with the patient. This review should include the proper use of the 2-dose Epinephrine syringe to insure that subcutaneous or intramuscular injections are given into the deltoid region of the arm or the anteriolateral aspect of the thigh. See also the *"Patient Directions For Use"*.

Epinephrine: For subcutaneous or intramuscular injection only.

Adults and children over 12 years: 0.3 mL; 6-12 years: 0.2 mL; 2-6 years: 0.15 mL; Infants to 2 years: 0.05 to 0.1 mL. When syringe is properly set up, as directed in the Patient Instruction Sheet, a 0.3 mL dose is administered when plunger is pushed until it stops. Syringe barrel has 0.1 mL graduations so that smaller doses can be measured. (Operation of syringe is explained in the *"Patient Directions For Use"* section at the end of this monograph.)

If after 10 minutes from the first injection symptoms are not noticeably improved, administer a second dose of Epinephrine from the syringe.

Chlorpheniramine Maleate: Tablets are chewable antihistamines. Adults and children over 12 years: 4 tablets; children 6-12 years: 2 tablets; children under 6 years: 1 tablet.

Protect from light. Store at room temperature, approx. 25° C (77° F). Protect from freezing.

PATIENT DIRECTIONS FOR USE
Chlorpheniramine/Epinephrine Anaphylaxis Emergency Treatment Kit
(Please read entire direction sheet before an emergency arises.)

The Chlorpheniramine/Epinephrine Kit IS TO BE USED ONLY WHEN PRESCRIBED BY A PHYSICIAN, for patients who are highly allergic to pollens, foods, dusts, insect stings, and drugs which may produce a life-threatening anaphylactic reaction, or have severe asthma attacks.

IN THE EVENT OF A LIFE-THREATENING SITUATION, FOLLOW THESE STEPS IMMEDIATELY TO ADMINISTER THE EPINEPHRINE.

1. REMOVE RED RUBBER NEEDLE COVER. HOLD SYRINGE UPRIGHT AND PUSH PLUNGER TO EXPEL AIR AND EXCESS EPINEPHRINE (PLUNGER WILL STOP).

2. ROTATE RECTANGULAR PLUNGER ¼ TURN TO THE RIGHT. PLUNGER WILL ALIGN WITH SLOT IN BARREL OF SYRINGE. WIPE INJECTION SITE WITH ALCOHOL SWAB.

3. INSERT NEEDLE STRAIGHT INTO ARM OR THIGH AS ILLUSTRATED.

4. PUSH PLUNGER UNTIL IT STOPS. SYRINGE WILL INJECT A 0.3 ML DOSE FOR ADULTS AND CHILDREN OVER 12 YEARS.

CHILDREN: SYRINGE BARREL HAS 0.1 ML GRADUATIONS SO THAT SMALLER DOSES CAN BE MEASURED. ADMINISTER TO INFANTS TO 2 YEARS: 0.05 TO 0.1 ML; 2-6 YEARS: 0.15 ML; AND 6-12 YEARS: 0.2 ML.

ONCE THE INITIAL EPINEPHRINE INJECTION HAS BEEN ADMINISTERED, FOLLOW THESE ADDITIONAL STEPS.
1. CONTACT PHYSICIAN, IF POSSIBLE.
2. REMOVE STINGER if stung by insect. (Use fingernails. DO NOT push, pinch or squeeze, or further imbed the stinger into the skin as this may cause further venom to be injected.)
3. APPLY TOURNIQUET. If exposure to life-threatening agent was by injection (allergic extract, drug) or insect sting on an arm or leg, place tourniquet between injection or sting site and body. (If exposure is elsewhere—neck, face, or body—proceed immediately to Step 5.)
4. TIGHTEN TOURNIQUET. To tighten, pull on the end of ONE STRING. Then, at least every ten minutes, loosen the tourniquet by pulling on the small metal ring.
5. CHEW AND SWALLOW CHLORPHENIRAMINE MALEATE TABLETS. For adults and children over 12 years, take 4 tablets; children 6-12 years take 2

tablets; children under 6 years take 1 tablet. These tablets are chewable antihistamine which is generally tolerated.
6. PREPARE SYRINGE FOR A POSSIBLE SECOND INJECTION. Turn the rectangular plunger ¼ turn to the right to line up with rectangular slot in the syringe. (A slight wiggling may aid the turning and alignment of the plunger.)
7. THE SECOND INJECTION. If after 10 minutes from the first injection symptoms are not noticeably improved, a second injection is required. Cleanse skin area with alcohol swab and make second injection as in STEPS 3 and 4 for the first Epinephrine injection. (A small amount of Epinephrine will remain in syringe after the second dose and cannot be expelled.) **Note: Dispose of syringe and remaining contents if second injection is not required.**
8. APPLY ICE PACKS IF AVAILABLE, AT THE SITE OF THE DRUG OR ALLERGY INJECTION, OR INSECT STING (if applicable).
9. KEEP PATIENT WARM AND AVOID EXERTION.

PRECAUTIONS
Epinephrine: For subcutaneous or intramuscular injection only. **Not intended for intravenous use.**

Epinephrine Injection, USP, contains sodium bisulfite. Patients with a suspected sulfite sensitivity should consult their physician well in advance before the need to use this product becomes critical.

Epinephrine is light sensitive and should be stored in box provided. STORE AT ROOM TEMPERATURE, approximately 25°C (77°F). Protect from freezing. Any Epinephrine solution in contact with the needle may cause rusting of the metal. **Do not try to force air out of the syringe until you are ready to use the Epinephrine.** This may rupture the seal and allow the Epinephrine solution to contact the metal promoting deterioration. **Never remove rubber protector over needle until ready to use syringe** as this may cause needle and contents to become contaminated.

Parenteral drug products should be inspected visually for particulate matter and discloration prior to administration, whenever solution and container permit. Do not use Epinephrine Injection, USP, if it has a pinkish or darker than slightly yellow color or contains a precipitate. Obtain replacement syringe from physician. Periodically check expiration date on syringe. If expiration date is near, re-order new syringe and discard outdated syringe after new syringe has been received.

Chlorpheniramine Maleate: As with any drug, if you are pregnant or nursing a baby, seek the advice of a health professional before using this product.

Patients should not drive or operate machinery after taking Chlorpheniramine Maleate. Drowsiness, dizziness, blurred vision, dry mouth and gastrointestinal upsets may occur. Keep out of reach of children.

The asthmatic patient should take the Chloropheniramine Maleate tablets with caution.

HOW SUPPLIED
KIT:

BRAND/MANUFACTURER	NDC	SIZE	AWP
○ **BRAND**			
ANA-KIT: Miles Allergy	00118-9988-01	1s	$18.92
	00118-9988-06	6s	$113.49

Chlorpheniramine Maleate and Phenylephrine Hydrochloride

DESCRIPTION
Each capsule contains:

Chlorpheniramine Maleate . . . . .8 mg
Phenylephrine Hydrochloride . . . . .20 mg

This product contains ingredients in the following therapeutic classes: antihistamine, decongestant.

CLINICAL PHARMACOLOGY
Chlorpheniramine Maleate is an alkylamine-type antihistamine. This group of antihistamines are among the most active histamine antagonists and are generally effective in relatively low doses. The drugs are not so prone to produce drowsiness and are among the most suitable agents for daytime use; but again, a significant proportion of patients do experience this effect. Phenylephrine Hydrochloride is a sympathomimetic which acts predominantly on alpha receptors and has little action on beta receptors. It therefore functions as an oral nasal decongestant with minimal Central nervous system (CNS) stimulation.

INDICATIONS
For the temporary relief of symptoms of the common cold, allergic rhinitis (hay fever) and sinusitis.

CONTRAINDICATIONS
Hypersensitivity to any of the ingredients. Also contraindicated in patients with severe hypertension, severe coronary artery disease, patients on MAO inhibitor therapy, patients with narrow-angle glaucoma, urinary retention, peptic ulcer and during an asthmatic attack.

Should not be used in children under 12 years or in nursing mothers.

WARNINGS

Considerable caution should be exercised in patients with hypertension, diabetes mellitus, ischemic heart disease, hyperthyroidism, asthma, glaucoma, chronic pulmonary disease, difficulty in breathing, increased intraocular pressure and prostatic hypertrophy. The elderly (60 years or older) are more likely to exhibit adverse reactions.

Antihistamines may cause excitability, especially in children. At dosages higher than the recommended dose, nervousness, dizziness or sleeplessness may occur. Alcholic beverages may increase the drowsiness effect. Caution should be exercised in operating motor vehicle or machinery.

PRECAUTIONS

General: Caution should be exercised in patients with high blood pressure, heart disease, diabetes or thyroid disease. The antihistamine in this product may exhibit additive effects with other CNS depressants, including alcohol.

Information for Patients: Antihistamine may cause drowsiness and ambulatory patients who operate machinery or motor vehicles should be cautioned accordingly.

Drug Interactions: MAO inhibitors and beta adrenergic blockers increase the effects of sympathomimetics. Sympathomimetics may reduce the antihypertensive effects of methyldopa, mecamylamine, reserpine and veratrum alkaloids. Concomitant use of antihistamines with alcohol and other CNS depressants may have an additive effect.

Pregnancy: The safety of use of this product in pregnancy has not been established.

ADVERSE REACTIONS

Adverse reactions include drowsiness, lassitude, nausea, giddiness, dryness of mouth, blurred vision, cardiac palpitations, flushing, increased irritability, or excitement (especially in children).

DOSAGE AND ADMINISTRATION

Adults and children over 12 years of age - 1 capsule orally every 12 hours.

Store and Dispense in a Tight Container as Defined in USP/NF with Child-Resistant Closure.

Store Between 15°-30°C (59°-86°F).

HOW SUPPLIED
CAPSULE, EXTENDED RELEASE:

BRAND/MANUFACTURER	NDC	SIZE	AWP
○ GENERICS			
ALERSULE: Misemer	00276-3101-01	100s	$22.00
PREHIST: Marnel	00682-0101-01	100s	$24.20

CAPSULE, EXTENDED RELEASE: 12 MG-75 MG

BRAND/MANUFACTURER	NDC	SIZE	AWP
○ GENERICS			
Allscrips	54569-1672-02	12s	$5.15
Allscrips	54569-1672-04	14s	$5.25
Allscrips	54569-1672-03	20s	$5.80
Allscrips	54569-1672-05	30s	$6.50
Allscrips	54569-1672-00	50s	$7.95
Allscrips	54569-1672-01	100s	$11.20
Allscrips	54569-1672-06	1000s	$74.55

ELIXIR:

BRAND/MANUFACTURER	NDC	SIZE	AWP
○ GENERICS			
CHEM-TUSS: Norton,HN	50732-0102-16	480 ml	$32.37

LIQUID: 4 MG-10 MG/5 ML

BRAND/MANUFACTURER	NDC	SIZE	AWP
○ GENERICS			
ED A-HIST: Edwards	00485-0055-16	480 ml	$19.00

TABLETS:

BRAND/MANUFACTURER	NDC	SIZE	AWP
○ GENERICS			
TUSS DELAY: Norton,HN	50732-0609-01	100s	$17.28
PRO-TUSS: Econolab	55053-0073-01	100s	$19.80
TUSS DELAY: Norton,HN	50732-0609-05	500s	$79.19
TUSS DELAY: Norton,HN	50732-0609-10	1000s	$150.23
PRO-TUSS: Econolab	55053-0073-10	1000s	$188.00

TABLETS: 8 MG-20 MG

BRAND/MANUFACTURER	NDC	SIZE	AWP
○ GENERICS			
ED A-HIST: Edwards	00485-0054-01	100s	$32.00

Chlorpheniramine Maleate and Pseudoephedrine Hydrochloride

DESCRIPTION

Each capsule for oral use contains 120 mg Pseudoephedrine Hydrochloride and 8 mg Chlorpheniramine Maleate. The specially formulated pellets in each capsule are designed to provide continuous therapeutic effect for 12 hours. About one-half of the active ingredients is released soon after administration and the remainder is released slowly over the remaining time period.

Pseudoephedrine Hydrochloride is a nasal decongestant. Chemically it is α-[1-(methylamino)ethyl]-[*S*-(*R**, *R**)]-benzenemethanol hydrochloride.

Chlorpheniramine Maleate is an antihistamine. Chemically it is α-(4-chlorophenyl)-N,N-dimethyl-2-pyridinepropanamine.

CLINICAL PHARMACOLOGY

Pseudoephedrine is an orally active sympathomimetic amine and exerts a decongestant action on the nasal mucosa. Pseudoephedrine produces peripheral effects similar to those of ephedrine and central effects similar to, but less intense than amphetamines. It has the potential for excitatory side effects. At the recommended oral dosages it has little or no pressor effect in normotensive adults. The serum half-life (T ½) of Pseudoephedrine is approximately 4 to 6 hours. T ½ is decreased with increased excretion of drug at urine pH lower than 6 and may be increased with decreased excretion at urine pH higher than 8.

Chlorpheniramine is an antihistaminic that possesses anticholinergic and sedative effects. It is considered one of the most effective and least toxic of the histamine antagonists. Chlorpheniramine is an H₁ receptor antagonist. It antagonizes many of the pharmacologic actions of histamine. It prevents released histamine from dilating capillaries and causing edema of the respiratory mucosa. Chlorpheniramine has a duration of action of 4 to 6 hours in clinical studies. Its half-life in serum, however, is 12 to 16 hours.

INDICATIONS AND USAGE

Relief of nasal congestion and eustachian tube congestion associated with the common cold, sinusitis and acute upper respiratory infections. It is also indicated for perennial and seasonal allergic rhinitis, vasomotor rhinitis, allergic conjunctivitis due to inhalant allergens and foods and for mild, uncomplicated allergic skin manifestations of urticaria and angioedema. Decongestants in combination with antihistamines have been used for many years to relieve eustachian tube congestion associated with acute eustachian salpingitis, aerotitis media, acute otitis media and serous otitis media. May be given concomitantly with analgesics and antibiotics.

CONTRAINDICATIONS

Patients with severe hypertension, severe coronary artery disease, and in patients on MAO inhibitor therapy. Antihistamines are contraindicated in patients with narrow-angle glaucoma, urinary retention, peptic ulcer, during an asthmatic attack, and in patients receiving MAO inhibitors.

HYPERSENSITIVITY

Contraindicated in patients with hypersensitivity or idiosyncrasy to sympathomimetic amines or phenanthrene derivatives.

NURSING MOTHERS

Contraindicated because of the higher than usual risk for infants from sympathomimetic amines.

WARNINGS

Sympathomimetic amines should be used judiciously and sparingly in patients with hypertension, diabetes mellitus ischemic heart disease, increased intraocular pressure, hyperthyroidism, or prostatic hypertrophy (see *"Contraindications"*). Sympathomimetics may produce CNS stimulation and convulsions or cardiovascular collapse with accompanying hypotension.

Chlorpheniramine Maleate has an atropine-like action and should be used with caution in patients with increased intraocular pressure, cardiovascular disease, hypertension or in patients with a history of bronchial asthma (see *"Contraindications"*). Do not exceed recommended dose.

USE IN ELDERLY

The elderly (60 years and older) are more likely to have adverse reactions to sympathomimetics. Overdosage of sympathomimetics in this age group may cause hallucinations, convulsions, CNS depression and death.

PRECAUTIONS
GENERAL

Should be used with caution in patients with diabetes, hypertension, cardiovascular disease and hyperreactivity to ephedrine. The antihistaminic may cause drowsiness and ambulatory patients who operate machinery or motor vehicles should be cautioned accordingly.

◆ RATED THERAPEUTICALLY EQUIVALENT; ◇ THERAPEUTIC EQUIVALENCE UNCONFIRMED; ○ UNRATED

INFORMATION FOR PATIENTS
Antihistamines may impaire mental and physical abilities required for the performance of potentially hazardous tasks, such as driving a vehicle or operating machinery and mental alertness in children.

DRUG INTERACTIONS
MAO inhibitors and beta adrenergic blockers increase the effect of sympathomimetics. Sympathomimetics may reduce the antihypertensive effects of methyldopa, mecamylamine, reserpine and veratrum alkaloids. Concomitant use of antihistamines with alcohol, tricyclic antidepressants, barbiturates and other CNS depressants may have an additive effect.

PREGNANCY CATEGORY C
Animal reproduction studies have not been conducted with Chlorpheniramine Maleate/Pseudoephedrine Hydrochloride capsules. It is also not known whether Chlorpheniramine Maleate/Pseudoephedrine Hydrochloride capsules can cause fetal harm when administered to a pregnant woman or can affect reproduction capacity. Chlorpheniramine Maleate/Pseudoephedrine Hydrochloride capsules may be given to a pregnant woman only if clearly needed.

NURSING MOTHERS
Pseudoephedrine is contraindicated in nursing mothers because of the higher than usual risk for infants from sympathomimetic amines.

ADVERSE REACTIONS
Hyperreactive individuals may display ephedrine-like reactions such as tachycardia, palpitations, headache, dizziness, or nausea. Patients sensitive to antihistamines may experience mild sedation. Sympathomimetic drugs have been associated with certain untoward reactions including fear, anxiety, tenseness, restlessness, tremor, weakness, pallor, respiratory difficulty, dysuria, insomnia, hallucinations, convulsions, CNS depression, arrhythmias, and cardiovascular collapse with hypotension.

Possible side effects of antihistamines are drowsiness, restlessness, dizziness, weakness, dry mouth, anorexia, nausea, headache, nervousness, blurring of vision, heartburn, dysuria and very rarely dermatitis. Patient idiosyncrasy to adrenergic agents may be manifested by insomnia, dizziness, weakness, tremor or arrhythmias.

OVERDOSAGE
Acute overdosage with Chlorpheniramine Maleate/Pseudoephedrine Hydrochloride capsules may produce clinical signs of CNS stimulation and variable cardiovascular effects. Pressor amines should be used with great caution in the presence of Pseudoephedrine. Patients with signs of stimulation should be treated conservatively.

DOSAGE AND ADMINISTRATION
One capsule every 12 hours. Do not give to children under 12 years of age.

HOW SUPPLIED
CAPSULE: 8 MG-120 MG

BRAND/MANUFACTURER	NDC	SIZE	AWP
○ BRAND			
CLORFED: Stewart Jackson	45985-0542-01	100s	$32.45

CAPSULE, EXTENDED RELEASE: 4 MG-60 MG

BRAND/MANUFACTURER	NDC	SIZE	AWP
○ BRAND			
ATROHIST SPRINKLE: Adams	53014-0028-10	100s	$38.77

CAPSULE, EXTENDED RELEASE: 8 MG-120 MG

BRAND/MANUFACTURER	NDC	SIZE	AWP
○ BRAND			
FEDAHIST TIMECAPS: Schwarz	00091-0055-01	100s	$52.21
NOVAFED A: Marion Merrell Dow	00068-0106-61	100s	$52.80

CAPSULE, EXTENDED RELEASE: 10 MG-65 MG

BRAND/MANUFACTURER	NDC	SIZE	AWP
○ BRAND			
FEDAHIST GYROCAPS: Schwarz	00091-1053-01	100s	$52.21

CAPSULE, EXTENDED RELEASE: 12 MG-120 MG

AVERAGE UNIT PRICE (AVAILABLE SIZES)			
GENERIC	$0.27		

BRAND/MANUFACTURER	NDC	SIZE	AWP
○ GENERICS			
COPHENE NO. 2: Dunhall	00217-0409-01	100s	$28.00
COPHENE NO. 2: Dunhall	00217-0409-03	500s	$126.00

SYRUP:

BRAND/MANUFACTURER	NDC	SIZE	AWP
○ BRAND			
HISTALET: Solvay	00032-1035-78	480 ml	$30.73

TABLETS: 4 MG-60 MG

BRAND/MANUFACTURER	NDC	SIZE	AWP
○ BRAND			
CLORFED II: Stewart Jackson	45985-0575-01	100s	$21.95

Chlorpheniramine Maleate with Phenylpropanolamine Hydrochloride

DESCRIPTION
Chlorpheniramine Maleate/Phenylpropanolamine Hydrochloride is a combination of an oral nasal decongestant and an antihistamine.

Each capsule contains Phenylpropanolamine Hydrochloride, 75 mg and Chlorpheniramine Maleate, 12 mg.

Each capsule is so prepared that an initial dose is released promptly and the remaining medication is released gradually over a prolonged period.

Chlorpheniramine Maleate is 2-[p-Chloro-α-[2-(dimethylamino) ethyl] benzyl] pyridine maleate (1:1), an antihistamine. M.W. 390.87

Phenylpropanolamine Hydrochloride is benzenemethanol, α-(1-aminoethyl)-, Hydrochloride, (R*, S*)-, (±), an adrenergic agent. M.W. 187.67

CLINICAL PHARMACOLOGY
PHENYLPROPANOLAMINE HYDROCHLORIDE
Phenylpropanolamine Hydrochloride is a sympathomimetic agent which is closely related to ephedrine in chemical structure and pharmacologic action, but produces less central nervous system stimulation than ephedrine. It is a vasoconstrictor with decongestant action on nasal and upper respiratory tract mucosal membranes.

The drug may directly stimulate adrenergic receptors but probably indirectly stimulates both alpha (α) and beta (β) adrenergic receptors by releasing norepinephrine from its storage sites. Phenylpropanolamine increases heart rate, force of contraction and cardiac output, and excitability. It acts on alpha receptors in the mucosa of the respiratory tract, producing vasoconstriction which results in shrinkage of swollen mucous membranes, reduction of tissue, hyeremia, edema and nasal congestion, and an increase in nasal airway patency. Phenylpropanolamine causes CNS stimulation and reportedly has an anorexigenic effect.

CHLORPHENIRAMINE MALEATE
Chlorpheniramine Maleate is an antihistamine with anti-cholinergic (drying) and sedative side effects. Antihistamines appear to compete with histamine for H_1 cell receptor sites on effector cells.

Chlorpheniramine Maleate is a member of the alkylamine class of antihistamines which are among the least sedating antihistamines.

PHARMACOKINETICS
A single Chlorpheniramine/Phenylpropanolamine capsule produces blood levels comparable to those produced by administration of three 25 mg doses of Phenylpropanolamine Hydrochloride and three 4 mg doses of Chlorpheniramine Maleate in conventional release form given at 4-hour intervals or of two liquid doses containing 6 mg of Chlorpheniramine Maleate and 37.5 mg of Phenylpropanolamine Hydrochloride taken at six hour intervals. The absorption half-life of the drugs from a non-timed liquid is appreciably more rapid than from the slow-release formulation. At steady-state conditions, the following peak levels are reached after the oral administration of a Chlorpheniramine/Phenylpropanolamine capsule: 21 ng/mL Chlorpheniramine in 7.7 hours; 173 ng/mL Phenylpropanolamine Hydrochloride in 6.1 hours; under these circumstances, the half-lives are approximately 21 and 7 hours, respectively.

When studied under controlled conditions, the peak Chlorpheniramine serum level occurs about 5.5 hours after administration and the peak Phenylpropanolamine level occurs after about 3.5 hours. The average half-life of elimination is about 17.5 hours for Chlorpheniramine and 5.0 hours for Phenylpropanolamine.

INDICATIONS AND USAGE
For the treatment of the symptoms of seasonal and perennial allergic rhinitis and vasomotor rhinitis, including nasal obstruction (congestion); also for the treatment of runny nose, sneezing and nasal congestion associated with the common cold.

CONTRAINDICATIONS
Hypersensitivity to either Phenylpropanolamine Hydrochloride or Chlorpheniramine Maleate and other antihistamines of similar chemical structure: severe hypertension; coronary artery disease; stenosing peptic ulcer; pyoroduodenal or bladder neck obstruction.

This drug should NOT be used in newborn or premature infants.

Because of the higher risk of antihistamines for infants generally, and for newborns and prematures in particular, antihistamine therapy is contraindicated in nursing mothers.

As with any product containing a sympathomimetic Chlorpheniramine/Phenylpropanolamine capsules should NOT be used in patients taking monoamine oxidase (MAO) inhibitors.

These capsules should NOT be used to treat lower respiratory tract conditions, including asthma.

WARNINGS

Chlorpheniramine/Phenylpropanolamine capsules may potentiate the effects of alcohol and other CNS depressants. Also this product should not be taken simultaneously with other products containing Phenylpropanolamine Hydrochloride or amphetamines.

Chlorpheniramine/Phenylpropanolamine capsules should be used with considerable caution in patients with narrow-angle glaucoma, stenosing peptic ulcer, pyloroduodenal obstruction, symptomatic prostatic hypertrophy, or bladder neck obstruction.

Use in Children: In infants and children, especially, antihistamines in *overdosage* may cause hallucinations, convulsions, or death. As in adults, antihistamines may diminish mental alertness in children. In the young child, particularly, they may produce excitation.

Use in the Elderly: (approximately 60 years or older): Antihistamines are more likely to cause dizziness, sedation and hypotension in elderly patients.

PRECAUTIONS

General: Use with caution in patients with lower respiratory disease including asthma, hypertension, cardiovascular disease, hyperthyroidism, increased intraocular pressure, or diabetes.

Information for Patients: Caution patients about activities requiring alertness (e.g., operating vehicles or machinery). Also caution patients about the possible additive effects of alcohol and other CNS depressants (hypnotics, sedatives, tranquilizers, etc.), and not to take simultaneously other products containing Phenylpropanolamine Hydrochloride or amphetamines. Patients should not take Chlorpheniramine/Phenylpropanolamine capsules in conjunction with a monoamine oxidase inhibitor or an oral anticoagulant.

Drug Interactions: Chlorpheniramine/Phenylpropanolamine capsules may interact with alcohol and other CNS depressants to potentiate their effects.

This product may have additive effects when taken simultaneously with other products containing Phenylpropanolamine Hydrochloride or amphetamines.

MAO inhibitors prolong and intensify the anticholinergic (drying) effects of antihistamines and potentiate the pressor effects of sympathomimetics such as Phenylpropanolamine Hydrochloride (see *"Contraindications"*).

Phenylpropanolamine Hydrochloride should not be used with ganglionic blocking drugs—such as mecamylamine—which potentiate reactions of sympathomimetics. It also should not be used with adrenergic blocking drugs, such as guanethidine sulfate or bethanidine, since it antagonizes the hypotensive action of these drugs.

The action of oral anticoagulants may be inhibited by antihistamines.

The CNS depressant and atropine-like effects of anticholinergics may be potentiated by concomitant administration of antihistamines. Concomitant administration of anticholinergics such as trihexyphenidyl, and other drugs with anticholinergic action (such as imipramine), with antihistamines may result in xerostomia.

β-ardrenergic blockers may be antagonized by antihistamines.

Concomitant administration of corticosteroids and antihistamines may decrease the effects of the corticosteroids by enzyme induction.

Antihistamines inhibit norepinephrine reuptake by tissues and therefore potentiate the cardiovascular effects of norepinephrine.

Concomitant use of antihistamines with phenothiazines may produce an additive CNS depressant effect; concomitant use also may cause urinary retention or glaucoma.

Carcinogenesis, Mutagenesis, Impairment of Fertility: A long-term oncogenic study in rats with the Chlorpheniramine Maleate component of Chlorpheniramine/Phenylpropanolamine capsules did not produce an increase in the incidence of tumors in the drug-treated groups, as compared with the controls. No evidence of mutagenicity was found when Chlorpheniramine Maleate was evaluated in a battery of mutagenic studies, including the Ames test.

In an early study in rats with Chlorpheniramine Maleate a reduction in fertility was observed in female rats at doses approximately 67 times the human dose. More recent studies in rabbits and rats, using more appropriate methodology and doses up to approximately 50 and 85 times the human dose, showed no reduction in fertility.

There are no studies available which indicate whether Phenylpropanolamine Hydrochloride has carcinogenic or mutagenic effects or impairs fertility.

Pregnancy, Teratogenic Effects, Pregnancy Category B: Reproduction studies have been performed with the components of Chlorpheniramine/Phenylpropanolamine capsules. Studies with Chlorpheniramine Maleate in rabbits and rats at doses up to 50 times and 85 times the human dose, respectively, revealed no evidence of harm to the fetus. A study with Phenylpropanolamine Hydrochloride in rats at doses up to 7 times the human dose revealed no evidence of harm to the fetus. There are, however, no adequate and well-controlled studies in pregnant women. Because animal reproduction studies are not always predictive of human response, Chlorpheniramine/Phenylpropanolamine capsules should be used during pregnancy only if clearly needed.

Nonteratogenic Effects: Studies of Chlorpheniramine Maleate in rats showed a decrease in the postnatal survival rate of offspring of animals dosed with 33 and 67 times the human dose.

Nursing Mothers: Small amounts of antihistamines are excreted in breast milk. Because of the higher risk with antihistamines in infants generally, and for newborns and prematures in particular, Chlorpheniramine/Phenylpropanolamine capsules should not be administered to a nursing mother (see *"Contraindications"*).

Pediatric Use: The safety and effectiveness of Chlorpheniramine/Phenylpropanolamine capsules in children under 12 years of age have not been established.

In infants and children, especially, antihistamines in *overdosage* may cause hallucinations, convulsions, or death.

As in adults, antihistamines may diminish mental alertness in children. In the young child, particularly, they may produce excitation. (See *"Warnings"*).

ADVERSE REACTIONS

The following adverse reactions have been reported following the use of antihistamines and/or sympathomimetic amines:

General: Anaphylactic shock; chills; drug rash; excessive dryness of mouth, nose and throat; increased intraocular pressure; excessive perspiration; photosensitivity; urticaria; weakness.

Cardiovascular System: Angina pain; extrasystoles; headache; hypertension; hypotension; palpitations; tachycardia.

Hematologic: Agranulocytosis; hemolytic anemia; leukopenia; thrombocytopenia.

Nervous System: Blurred vision; confusion; convulsions; diplopia; disturbed coordination; dizziness; drowsiness; euphoria: excitation; fatigue; hysteria; insomnia; irritability; acute labyrinthitis; nervousness; neuritis; paresthesia; restlessness; sedation; tinnitus; tremor; vertigo.

GI System: Abdominal pain; anorexia; constipation; diarrhea; epigastric distress; nausea; vomiting.

GU System: Dysuria; early menses; urinary frequency; urinary retention.

Respiratory System: Thickening of bronchial secretions; tightness of chest and wheezing; nasal stuffiness.

OVERDOSAGE

In the event of overdosage, emergency treatment should be started immediately.

Symptoms: Effects of antihistamine overdosage may vary from central nervous system depression (sedation, apnea, diminished mental alertness, cardiovascular collapse) to stimulation (insomnia, hallucinations, tremors, or convulsions) to death.

Other signs and symptoms may be dizziness, tinnitus, ataxia, blurred vision and hypotension or hypertension. Stimulation is particularly likely in children, as are atropine-like signs and symptoms (dry mouth; fixed, dilated pupils; flushing; hyperthermia; and gastrointestinal symptoms). In large doses, sympathomimetics may cause giddiness, headache, nausea, vomiting, sweating, thirst, tachycardia, precordial pain, palpitations, difficulty in micturition, muscular weakness and tenseness, anxiety, restlessness and insomnia. Many patients can present a toxic psychosis with delusions and hallucinations. Some may develop cardiac arrhythmias, circulatory collapse, convulsions, coma and respiratory failure.

Toxicity: In acute oral toxicity tests in rats, the LD_{50} for the ratio of 75 mg Phenylpropanolamine Hydrochloride and 12 mg Chlorpheniramine Maleate was 774.2 mg/kg; in mice, the LD_{50} for the formulation was 757.4 mg/kg.

Treatment: The patient should be induced to vomit even if emesis has occurred spontaneously. Pharmacologically induced vomiting by the administration of ipecac syrup is a preferred method. But vomiting should not be induced in patients with impaired consciousness. The action of ipecac is facilitated by physical activity and by the administration of 8 to 12 fluid ounces of water. If emesis does not occur within 15 minutes, the dose of ipecac should be repeated. Precautions against aspiration must be taken, especially in infants and children.

Following emesis, any drug remaining in the stomach may be adsorbed by activated charcoal administered as a slurry with water. If vomiting is unsuccessful or contraindicated, gastric lavage should be performed. Isotonic and one-half isotonic saline are the lavage solutions of choice. Since much of the capsule medication is coated for gradual release, saline cathartics should be administered to hasten evacuation of pellets that have not already released medication. Saline cathartics, such as milk of magnesia, draw water into the bowel by osmosis and therefore may be valuable for their action in rapid dilution of bowel content. Dialysis has not been reported to be effective in the treatment of Phenylpropanolamine Hydrochloride and Chlorpheniramine Maleate overdosage. After emergency treatment, the patient should continue to be medically monitored.

Treatment of the signs and symptoms of overdosage is symptomatic and supportive. *Stimulants* (analeptic agents), which might precipitate convulsions, should *not* be used. Vasopressors may be used to treat hypotension. Short-acting barbiturates, diazepam, or paraldehyde may be administered to control seizures. Hyperpyrexia, especially in children, may require treatment with tepid water sponge baths or a hypothermic blanket. Apnea is treated with ventilatory support.

DOSAGE AND ADMINISTRATION

Adults and children 12 years of age and over—one capsule every 12 hours.

Chlorpheniramine/Phenylpropanolamine capsules are not recommended in children under 12.

Capsules should be stored at controlled room temperature (59° to 86°F); protect from moisture and light.

◆ RATED THERAPEUTICALLY EQUIVALENT; ◇ THERAPEUTIC EQUIVALENCE UNCONFIRMED; ○ UNRATED

HOW SUPPLIED
CAPSULE:

BRAND/MANUFACTURER	NDC	SIZE	AWP
◆ GENERICS			
ORAGEST-TD: Major	00904-2132-60	100s	$9.10

CAPSULE, EXTENDED RELEASE: 12 MG-75 MG

AVERAGE UNIT PRICE (AVAILABLE SIZES)	
BRAND	$0.80
GENERIC	$0.72

BRAND/MANUFACTURER	NDC	SIZE	AWP
◆ BRAND			
ORNADE SPANSULES: SK Beecham Pharm	00007-4421-15	50s	$40.55
	00007-4421-25	500s	$392.35
◆ GENERICS			
RESAID: Geneva	00781-2427-01	100s	$72.91
RESAID: Geneva	00781-2427-10	1000s	$705.45

ELIXIR (C-V):

AVERAGE UNIT PRICE (AVAILABLE SIZES)	
GENERIC	$0.007

BRAND/MANUFACTURER	NDC	SIZE	AWP
◆ GENERICS			
PHENYLHISTINE: Cenci,H.R.	00556-0331-16	480 ml	$4.20
PHENYLHISTINE: Cenci,H.R.	00556-0331-28	3840 ml	$23.58

LIQUID (C-V):

AVERAGE UNIT PRICE (AVAILABLE SIZES)	
GENERIC	$0.02

BRAND/MANUFACTURER	NDC	SIZE	AWP
◆ GENERICS			
PHENYLHISTINE: Cenci,H.R.	00556-0333-04	120 ml	$2.90
PHENYLHISTINE: Cenci,H.R.	00556-0333-16	480 ml	$9.50
PHENYLHISTINE: Cenci,H.R.	00556-0333-28	3840 ml	$58.60

SYRUP:

BRAND/MANUFACTURER	NDC	SIZE	AWP
○ BRAND			
TUSSANIL PLAIN: Misemer	00276-1620-16	480 ml	$14.00

Chlorpheniramine Maleate, Injectable

DESCRIPTION
Chlorpheniramine Maleate Injection is a sterile solution of Chlorpheniramine Maleate, an antihistamine, in Water for Injection.

Chlorpheniramine Maleate Injection is supplied in two concentrations: 10 mg/mL and 100 mg/mL for intramuscular or subcutaneous injection.

The 10 mg/mL concentration may also be administered by intravenous injection.

Each mL contains: Chlorpheniramine Maleate 10 mg or 100 mg, with benzyl alcohol 1.5% as preservative in Water for Injection q.s. Sodium hydroxide and/or hydrochloric acid may have been used to adjust pH. pH range is 4.0 to 5.2.

Chlorpheniramine Maleate occurs as a white, odorless, crystalline powder. It is freely soluble in water; and soluble in alcohol.

Following is its chemical structure:

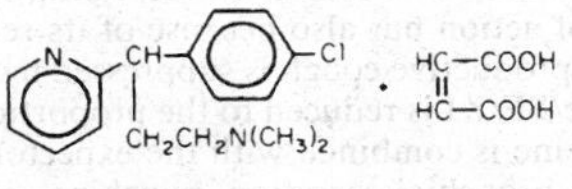

CLINICAL PHARMACOLOGY
Chlorpheniramine Maleate is an antihistamine, with anticholinergic (drying) and sedative side effects.

Antihistamines competitively antagonize those pharmacological effects of histamine which are mediated through activation of histamine H_1-receptor sites on effector cells. Histamine-related allergic reactions and tissue injury are blocked or diminished in intensity. Antihistamines antagonize the vasodilator effect of endogenously released histamine, especially in small vessels, and mitigate the effect of histamine which causes increased capillary permeability and edema formation. As consequences of these actions, antihistamines antagonize the physiological manifestations of histamine release in the nose following antigen-antibody interaction, such as congestion related to vascular engorgement, mucosal edema, and profuse watery secretions, and irritation and sneezing resulting from histamine action on afferent nerve terminals.

Chlorpheniramine Maleate is readily absorbed from the gastrointestinal tract and from the site of injection.

Following a single dose of tritium-labeled Chlorpheniramine Maleate to human adults, the drug was found to be extensively metabolized whether given orally or intravenously. The drug and its metabolites were excreted primarily in the urine. Chlorpheniramine Maleate is bound (about 70%) to plasma protein. While the antihistamines have not been studied for passage through the blood-brain and placental barriers, the occurrence of pharmacologic effects in the central nervous system and in the newborn indicate presence of the drug.

INDICATIONS AND USAGE
Chlorpheniramine Maleate Injection is indicated for use in the following conditions when use of the oral form of the drug is impractical:

Amelioration of allergic reactions to blood and plasma.

In anaphylaxis as an adjunct to epinephrine and other standard measures after the acute symptoms have been controlled.

For other uncomplicated allergic conditions of the immediate type when oral therapy is impossible or contraindicated.

CONTRAINDICATIONS
Antihistamines, including Chlorpheniramine Maleate, are contraindicated in patients hypersensitive to this medication and to other antihistamines of similar chemical structure.

WARNINGS
Antihistamines should be used with caution in patients with: narrow angle glaucoma; stenosing peptic ulcer; pyloroduodenal obstruction; and urinary bladder obstruction due to symptomatic prostatic hypertrophy or narrowing of the bladder neck.

Use in Patients Approximately 60 Years or Older: Antihistamines are more likely to cause dizziness, sedation, and hypotension in patients over 60 years of age.

Use in Children: In infants and children, especially, antihistamines in *overdosage* may cause hallucinations, convulsions, or death. (See "Overdosage".)

As in adults, antihistamines may diminish mental alertness in children. In the young child, particularly, they may produce excitation.

PRECAUTIONS
General: Chlorpheniramine Maleate has an atropine-like action and, therefore, should be used with caution in patients with a history of bronchial asthma; increased intraocular pressure; hyperthyroidism; cardiovascular disease; hypertension.

Chlorpheniramine Maleate Injection should be administered as recommended in *"Dosage And Administration"*. It should be used only as adjunctive therapy to epinephrine and other standard measures in anaphylaxis after acute symptoms have been controlled.

Information for Patients: Patients being treated with Chlorpheniramine Maleate Injection should receive the following information and instructions. This information is intended to aid in the safe and effective use of this medication: It is not a disclosure of all possible adverse or intended effects.

1. Antihistamines may cause drowsiness.
2. Patients taking antihistamines should not engage in activities requiring mental alertness, such as driving a car or operating machinery, certain appliances, etc., until their response to this medication has been determined.
3. Antihistamines have additive effects with alcohol and other CNS depressants (hypnotics, sedatives, barbiturates, tranquilizers, etc.).
4. This medication should not be administered to patients if they are receiving oral anticoagulants.
5. This medication should not be given to children less than 12 years of age.

Drug Interactions: (See "Warnings" section.) Additive CNS depression may occur when antihistamines are administered concomitantly with other CNS depressants including barbiturates, tranquilizers, and alcohol. Patients should be advised against the concurrent use of other CNS depressant drugs. The action of oral anticoagulants may be diminished by antihistamines. (See also *"Dosage And Administration"*.)

Drug/Laboratory Test Interaction: Antihistamines should be discontinued about four days prior to skin testing procedures since these drugs may prevent or diminish otherwise positive reactions to dermal reactivity indicators.

Carcinogenesis, Mutagenesis, and Impairment of Fertility: Long-term oral dosing of rats with Chlorpheniramine Maleate showed no evidence of carcinogenesis. Ames mutagenicity tests of Chlorpheniramine and its nitrosation product were negative. The oral administration of Chlorpheniramine Maleate to male rats before mating and to female rats before, during and after pregnancy at doses up to 67 times the human dose did not affect fecundity, pregnancy, or prenatal survival of the offspring.

Pregnancy Category B: Reproduction studies have been performed in rats and rabbits at doses up to 50 times and 30 times the oral human dose, respectively, and have revealed no evidence of impaired fertility or harm to the fetus due to Chlorpheniramine Maleate. There are, however, no adequate and well-controlled studies in pregnant women. Because animal reproduction studies are not always predictive of human response, this drug should be used during pregnancy only if clearly needed. (See *"Nonteratogenic Effects"*.)

Nonteratogenic Effects: Antihistamines should not be used in the third trimester of pregnancy because newborns and premature infants may have severe reactions, such as convulsions, to them.

Nursing Mothers: It is not known whether this drug is excreted in human milk. However, certain antihistamines are known to be excreted in human milk in low concentration. Because of the higher risk of antihistamines for infants generally and for newborns and prematures in particular, a decision should be made whether to discontinue nursing or to discontinue the drug, taking into account the importance of the drug to the mother.

Pediatric Use: Safety and effectiveness in children below the age of 12 years have not been established. (See *"Warnings - Use in Children".*) Overdosage of antihistamines may also produce in infants and children fixed, dilated pupils, flushed face, dry mouth, fever, excitation, athetoses, tonic-clonic convulsions and post-ictal depression.

ADVERSE REACTIONS
Slight to moderate drowsiness may occur with Chlorpheniramine Maleate. Other possible side effects common to antihistamines in general include (the most frequent are italicized):

General: Urticaria, drug rash, anaphylactic shock, photosensitivity, excessive perspiration, chills, dryness of mouth, nose, and throat.

Cardiovascular: Hypotension, headache, palpitations, tachycardia, extrasystoles.

Hematologic: Hemolytic anemia, hypoplastic anemia, thrombocytopenia, agranulocytosis.

Nervous: Sedation, dizziness, disturbed coordination, fatigue, confusion, restlessness, excitation, nervousness, tremor, irritability, insomnia, euphoria, paresthesias, blurred vision, diplopia, vertigo, tinnitus, acute labyrinthitis, hysteria, neuritis, convulsions.

Gastrointestinal: Epigastric distress, anorexia, nausea, vomiting, diarrhea, constipation.

Ganitourinary: Urinary frequency, difficult urination, urinary retention, early menses.

Respiratory: Thickening of bronchial secretions, tightness of chest and wheezing, nasal stuffiness.

DRUG ABUSE AND DEPENDENCE
There is no information to indicate that abuse or dependency occurs with Chlorpheniramine Maleate.

OVERDOSAGE
In the event of overdosage, emergency treatment should be started immediately.

Manifestations: Antihistamine overdosage effects may vary from central nervous system depression (sedation, apnea, diminished mental alertness, cyanosis, hyperreflexia, cardiovascular collapse) to stimulation (insomnia, hallucinations, tremors, or convulsions) to death. Other signs and symptoms may be dizziness, tinnitus, ataxia, blurred vision, and hypotension. Stimulation is particularly likely in children (see "Pediatric Usage") as are atropine-like signs and symptoms (dry mouth; fixed, dilated pupils; flushing; hyperthemia; and gastrointestinal symptoms).

Treatment: The patients should be induced to vomit, even if emesis has occurred spontaneously. Pharmacologic vomiting by the administration of ipecac syrup is a preferred method. However, vomiting should not be induced in patients with impaired consciousness. The action of ipecac is facilitated by physical activity and by the administration of 8 to 12 fluid ounces of water. If emesis does not occur within 15 minutes, the dose of ipecac should be repeated. Precautions against aspiration must be taken, especially in infants and children. Following emesis, any drug remaining in the stomach may be adsorbed by activated charcoal administered as a slurry with water. If vomiting is unsuccessful or contraindicated, gastric lavage should be performed. Physiologic saline solution is the lavage solution of choice, particularly in children. In adults, tap water can be used; however, as much as possible of the amount administered should be removed before the next instillation. Saline cathartics, such as milk of magnesia, draw water into the bowel by osmosis and, therefore, may be valuable for their action in rapid dilution of bowel content. Dialysis is of little value in antihistamine poisoning. After emergency treatment the patient should continue to be medically monitored.

Treatment of the signs and symptoms of overdosage is symptomatic and supportive. *Stimulants* (analeptic agents) *should not* be used. Vasopressors may be used to treat hypotension. Short-acting barbiturates, diazepam, or paraldehyde may be administered to control seizures. Hyperpyrexia, especially in children, may require treatment with tepid water sponge baths of a hypothermic blanket. Apnea is treated with ventilatory support.

DOSAGE AND ADMINISTRATION
Dosage should be individualized according to the needs and response of the patient.

CHLORIDHENIRAMINE MALEATE INJECTION
Adults and Children 12 Years of Age or Older: For amelioration of allergic reactions to blood or plasma: 10 to 20 mg administered as a single dose; the maximum recommended dose in a 24-hour period is 40 mg.

In anaphylaxis, as an adjunct to epinephrine and other standard measures after the acute symptoms have been controlled 10 to 20 mg administered intravenously as a single dose.

For other uncomplicated allergic conditions of the immediate type when oral therapy is impossible or contraindicated: 5 to 20 mg administered as a single dose.

Note: Chlorpheniramine Maleate Injection, 100 mg/mL, is intended for intramuscular or subcutaneous use only and is not to be used when intravenous administration is indicated. Intradermal administration is not recommended.

Chlorpheniramine Maleate Injection, 10 mg/mL, is intended for intravenous, intramuscular, or subcutaneous administration.

Parenteral drug products should be inspected visually for particulate matter and discoloration whenever solution and container permit.

It should not be mixed with other parenteral therapeutic medications or with diagnostic agents.

Protect from light. Store in carton until contents are used. Store at controlled room temperature 15°-30°C (59°-86°F). Cooling below 32°F may produce Chlorpheniramine crystals. If present, dissolve by warming to 85°F before using.

J CODES
Up to 200 mg IV,IM,SC—J0730

HOW SUPPLIED
INJECTION: 10 MG/ML

AVERAGE UNIT PRICE (AVAILABLE SIZES)		GENERIC A-RATED AVERAGE PRICE (GAAP)	
BRAND	$2.34	30 ml	$6.44
GENERIC	$0.22		

BRAND/MANUFACTURER	NDC	SIZE	AWP
◆ BRAND			
CHLOR-TRIMETON: Schering	00085-0200-06	1 ml 100s	$234.28
◆ GENERICS			
Moore,H.L.	00839-5161-36	30 ml	$6.20
Steris	00402-0178-30	30 ml	$6.68

Chlorpheniramine Maleate/ Codeine Phosphate/ Phenylephrine Hydrochloride/ Potassium Iodide

DESCRIPTION
Each teaspoon (5 mL) contains:

Codeine Phosphate, USP	5.0 mg
(Warning: May be habit forming.)	
Phenylephrine Hydrochloride, USP	2.5 mg
Chlorpheniramine Maleate, USP	0.75 mg
Potassium Iodide, USP	75.0 mg

Chlorpheniramine Maleate/Codeine Phosphate/Phenylephrine Hydrochloride/ Potassium Iodide (CPM/Codeine/PE/KI) is a pleasant-tasting, raspberry-flavored cough syrup. It contains four active ingredients in proper proportion for children. Codeine Phosphate is a white crystalline, odorless powder which is freely soluble in water. It is a narcotic analgesic.

Codeine Phosphate is 7,8-Didehydro-4,5α-epoxy-3-methoxy-17-methylmorphinan-6α-ol phosphate.

Phenylephrine Hydrochloride is a vasoconstrictor and pressor drug chemically related to epinephrine and ephedrine. It is a synthetic sympathomimetic agent. Chemically, Phenylephrine Hydrochloride is (−)-*m*-Hydroxy-α-[(methylamino)methyl]-benzyl alcohol hydrochloride.

Chlorpheniramine Maleate is an alkylamine H_1-blocking agent (antihistamine) which is chemically 2-Pyridinepropanamine, γ-(4-chlorphenyl)-*N,N*-dimethyl-, (*Z*)-2-butenedioate.

Potassium Iodide is an expectorant.

CLINICAL PHARMACOLOGY
Codeine Phosphate is an antitussive that is well recognized not only because of its efficiency and rapidity of action but also because of its relative safety in clinical use. Thus, irritating, nonproductive cough is suppressed by Codeine. The Codeine content of CPM/Codeine/PE/KI is reduced to the proportion that is most suitable for children. When Codeine is combined with the expectorant Potassium Iodide, which tends to increase bronchial secretion, coughing, although minimized, is more productive when it does occur. The continuous fatiguing effect of useless coughing is thereby avoided. Codeine is a narcotic analgesic and antitussive which resembles morphine pharmacologically. Codeine is metabolized by the liver and excreted chiefly in the urine, largely in inactive forms. A small fraction (10%) of administered Codeine is demethylated to form morphine, and both free and conjugated morphine can be found in the urine after therapeutic doses of Codeine. When administered subcutaneously, 120 mg of Codeine is approximately equivalent to 10 mg of morphine. The abuse liability of Codeine is generally considered to be much lower than that of morphine.

The half-life of Codeine in plasma is 2.5 to 3.0 hours.

Codeine has diverse additional actions. It depresses the respiratory center, stimulates the vomiting center, depresses the cough reflex, constricts the pupils, increases the tone of the gastrointestinal and genitourinary tracts, and produces mild vasolidation.

Phenylephrine Hydrochloride, produces effective decongestion of the mucous membranes of the respiratory tract via its powerful postsynaptic α-receptor stimulant action. It has little effect on cardiac β-receptors. Most of its effects are due to direct action on receptors and only a small part is due to norepinephrine release. Central stimulant activity is minimal.

Chlorpheniramine Maleate helps control allergic coughs and mucosal congestion. The mild anticholinergic action of Chlorpheniramine Maleate may aid in reducing rhinorrhea, and its mild sedative action may also be beneficial to patients whose excessive coughing has caused them to lose sleep.

Clinical experience with CPM/Codeine/PE/KI has shown it to be a dependable medication for the relief of cough and the reduction of nasal congestion in children.

INDICATIONS AND USAGE

Coughs due to colds as well as coughs and congestive symptoms associated with upper respiratory tract infections such as tracheobronchitis or laryngobronchitis, croup, pharyngitis, allergic bronchitis, and infectious bronchitis, when accompanied by disturbing and fatiguing cough, have been treated successfully with CPM/Codeine/PE/KI in children.

CONTRAINDICATIONS

CPM/Codeine/PE/KI is contraindicated in patients who are hypersensitive to any of its ingredients. Due to the component Phenylephrine, CPM/Codeine/PE/KI is contraindicated in patients with ventricular tachycardia or severe hypertension.

WARNINGS

Respiratory Depression: Codeine produces dose-related respiratory depression by acting directly on brain stem respiratory centers. Codeine also affects centers that control respiratory rhythm and may produce irregular and periodic breathing. If significant respiratory depression occurs, it may be antagonized by the use of naloxone hydrochloride. (See *"Overdosage"*).

Head Injury and Increased Intracranial Pressure: The respiratory depressant effects of narcotics and their capacity to elevate cerebrospinal fluid pressure may be markedly exaggerated in the presence of head injury, other intracranial lesions, or a preexisting increase in intracranial pressure. Furthermore, narcotics can produce adverse reactions which may obscure the clinical course of patients with head injuries.

Acute Abdominal Conditions: The administration of narcotics may obscure the diagnosis or clinical course of patients with acute abdominal conditions.

PRECAUTIONS

Caution should be exercised if CPM/Codeine/PE/KI is administered to patients with cardiac disorders other than ventricular tachycardia, which is contraindicated; mild hypertension and hyperthyroidism.

SPECIAL RISK PATIENTS

Codeine: should be used with caution in patients with impaired renal or hepatic function, hypothyroidism, Addison's disease, or urethral stricture.

In asthma, the indiscriminate use of Codeine may, due to its drying action upon the mucosa of the respiratory tract, precipitate severe respiratory insufficiency resulting from increased viscosity of the bronchial secretions and suppression of the cough reflex. As with any narcotic analgesic agent, the usual precautions should be observed and the possibility of respiratory depression should be kept in mind.

Phenylephrine Hydrochloride: should be employed only with extreme caution in patients with hyperthyroidism, bradycardia, partial heart block, and myocardial disease.

Chlorpheniramine Maleate: should be used with considerable caution in patients with narrow angle glaucoma, pyloroduodenal obstruction, and bladder neck obstruction. Chlorpheniramine Maleate has an atropine-like action and therefore should be used with caution in patients with a history of bronchial asthma, increased intraocular pressure, hyperthyroidism, cardiovascular disease, and hypertension.

Drug Interactions: Patients receiving other narcotic analgesics, general anesthetics, phenothiazines, tranquilizers, sedative-hypnotics, MAO inhibitors, tricyclic antidepressants, or other CNS depressants (including alcohol) concomitantly with codeine may exhibit an additive CNS depression. When such combined therapy is contemplated, the dose of one or both agents should be reduced.

Carcinogenesis, Mutagenesis, Impairment of Fertility: No long-term animal studies have been performed to evaluate the potential of CPM/Codeine/PE/KI in the areas.

Nonteratogenic Effects: Dependence has been reported in newborns whose mothers received opiates regularly during pregnancy. Withdrawal signs include irritability, excessive crying, tremors, hyperreflexia, fever, vomiting, and diarrhea. Signs usually appear during the first few days of life.

ADVERSE REACTIONS

The only significant untoward effects that have occurred are mild anorexia and an occasional tendency to constipation. However, discontinuance of CPM/Codeine/PE/KI has seldom been required. Mild drowsiness occurs in some patients but, when cough is relieved, the quieting effect of CPM/Codeine/PE/KI is considered beneficial in many instances. Because of its iodide content CPM/Codeine/PE/KI may cause elevation of the protein-bound iodine. Adverse reactions to codeine include:

Central Nervous System: Sedation, drowsiness, mental clouding, dizziness, lethargy, impairment of mental and physical performance, anxiety, convulsions, fear, miosis, dysphoria, psychic dependence, mood changes, and respiratory depression.

Gastrointestinal System: Nausea, vomiting, increased pressure in the biliary tract, and constipation.

Cardiovascular System: Orthosatic hypotension, fainting, and tachycardia.

Genitourinary System: Ureteral spasm, spasm of vesical sphincters and urinary retention have been reported.

Other: Flushing, sweating, pruritus, allergic reactions, and suppressed cough reflex.

Adverse reactions to Phenylephrine Hydrochloride include headache, reflex bradycardia, excitability restlessness and, rarely, arrhythmias.

Adverse reactions to Chlorpheniramine Maleate include slight to moderate drowsiness. Other possible side effects common to antihistamines in general include:

General: Urticaria, drug rash, anaphylactic shock, photosensitivity, excessive perspiration, chills, dryness of mouth, nose, and throat.

Cardiovascular System: Hypotension, headache, palpitations, tachycardia, and extrasystoles.

Hematologic System: Hemolytic anemia, thrombocytopenia, and agranulocytosis.

Nervous System: Sedation, dizziness, disturbed coordination, fatigue, confusion, restlessness, excitation, nervousness, tremor, irritability, insomnia, euphoria, paresthesias, blurred vision, diplopia, vertigo, tinnitus, acute labyrinthitis, hysteria, neuritis, and convulsions.

Gastrointestinal System: Epigastric distress, anorexia, nausea, vomiting, diarrhea, and constipation.

Genitourinary System: Urinary frequency, difficult urination, urinary retention, and early menses.

Respiratory System: Thickening of bronchial secretions, tightness of chest and wheezing, and nasal stuffiness.

OVERDOSAGE

CODEINE

Signs and Symptoms: Overdosage with codeine is characterized by respiratory depression (a decrease in respiratory rate and/or tidal volume, Cheyne-stokes respiration, cyanosis), pinpoint pupils, extreme somnolence progressing to stupor or coma, skeletal muscle flaccidity, cold and clammy skin, and sometimes bradycardia and hypotension. In severe overdosage, particularly by the intravenous route, apnea, circulatory collapse, cardiac arrest, and death may occur.

Treatment: Primary attention should be given to the reestablishment of adequate respiratory exchange through provision of a patent airway and institution of assisted or controlled ventilation. Naloxone hydrochloride is a specific and effective antagonist for respiratory depression which may result from overdosage. If the desired degree of counteraction and improvement in respiratory function is not obtained immediately following IV administration, it may be repeated intravenously at 2 to 3 minute intervals. Failure to obtain significant improvement after 2 or 3 doses suggests that the condition may be due partly or completely to other disease processes or nonopioid drugs. The usual initial pediatric dose is 0.01 mg/kg body weight given IV, IM, or SC. If necessary, naloxone can be diluted with Sterile Water for Injection, USP. Oxygen, intravenous fluids, vasopressors, and other supportive measures should be employed as indicated.

Oral LD_{50} in the mouse is 693 mg/kg. Codeine is not dialyzable.

PHENYLEPHRINE HYDROCHLORIDE

Signs and Symptoms: Overdosage may induce ventricular extrasystoles and short paroxysms of ventricular tachycardia, a sensation of fullness in the head, and tingling of the extremities.

Treatment: Should an excessive elevation of blood pressure occur, it may be immediately relieved by an α-adrenergic blocking agent, eg, phentolamine. The oral LD_{50} in the rat: 350 mg/kg; mouse: 120 mg/kg.

CHLORPHENIRAMINE MALEATE

Signs and Symptoms: Antihistamine overdosage may vary from central nervous system depression (sedation, apnea, and cardiovascular collapse) to stimulation (insomnia, hallucinations, tremors or convulsions). Other signs and symptoms may be dizziness, tinnitus, ataxia, blurred vision, and hypotension. Stimulation and atropine-like signs and symptoms (dry mouth; fixed, dilated pupils; flushing; hyperthermia; and gastrointestinal symptoms) are particularly likely in children.

Treatment: Emergency treatment should be started immediately. Vomiting should be induced, even if it has occurred spontaneously. Vomiting by the administration of ipecac syrup is preferred. Vomiting should *not* be induced in patients with impaired consciousness. The action of ipecac is facilitated by physical activity and by the administration of eight to twelve fluid ounces of water. If emesis does not occur within fifteen minutes, the dose of ipecac should be repeated. Precautions against aspiration must be taken, especially in infants and children. Following emesis, any drug remaining in the stomach may be absorbed by activated charcoal administered as a slurry with water. If vomiting is unsuccessful or contraindicated, gastric lavage should be performed. Isotonic and one-half isotonic saline are the lavage solutions of choice. Saline cathartics, such as milk of magnesia, draw water into the bowel by osmosis and, therefore, may be valuable for their action in rapid dilution of bowel content. After emergency treatment the patient should continue to be medically monitored. Treatment of the signs and symptoms of overdosage is symptomatic and supportive.

Stimulants (analeptic agents) should *not* be used. Vasopressors may be used to treat hypotension. Short-acting barbiturates, diazepam, or paraldehyde may be administered to control seizures. Hyperpyrexia, especially in children, may require treatment with tepid water sponge baths or a hypothermic blanket. Apnea is treated with ventilatory support.

DOSAGE AND ADMINISTRATION

CPM/Codeine/PE/KI should be given in accordance with the needs and age of the patient. Frequency of administration may be adjusted as cough is brought under control. The following doses, to be given at 4 to 6 hour intervals, are suggested for patients under 12 years of age: *from 6 months to 1 year,* 1/4 teaspoon; *from 1 to 3 years,* 1/2 to 1 teaspoon; *from 3 to 6 years,* 1 to 2 teaspoons; and *from 6 to 12 years,* 2 teaspoons.

HOW SUPPLIED
SYRUP (C-V):

BRAND/MANUFACTURER	NDC	SIZE	AWP
○ **BRAND**			
PEDIACOF: Sanofi Winthrop	00024-1509-06	480 ml	$42.84
○ **GENERICS**			
PEDITUSS: Major	00904-1239-16	480 ml	$23.25
DEMI-COF: Econolab	55053-0610-16	480 ml	$29.95
PEDITUSS: Major	00904-1239-28	3840 ml	$124.00

Chlorpheniramine Maleate/ Codeine Phosphate/ Pseudoephedrine Hydrochloride

DESCRIPTION

Each 5 ml teaspoonful contains Codeine Phosphate, 10 mg (Warning: may be habit forming), Pseudoephedrine Hydrochloride, 30 mg, Chlorpheniramine Maleate, 2 mg.

ACTIONS

Antitussive, decongestant and antihistaminic actions. Codeine, at the recommended dose, causes suppression of the cough reflex by a direct effect on the cough center in the medulla of the brain. Codeine has antitussive, mild analgesic and sedative effects.

Pseudoephedrine Hydrochloride, an orally effective nasal decongestant, is a sympathomimetic amine with peripheral effects similar to epinephrine and central effects similar to, but less intense than, amphetamines. Therefore, it has the potential for excitatory side effects. Pseudoephedrine at the recommended oral dosage has little or no pressor effect in normotensive adults. Patients taking Pseudoephedrine orally have not been reported to experience the rebound congestion sometimes experienced with frequent, repeated use of topical decongestants. Pseudoephedrine is not known to produce drowsiness.

Chlorpheniramine possesses antihistaminic, mild anticholinergic and sedative effects. It antagonizes many of the pharmacologic actions of histamine. It prevents released histamine from dilating capillaries and causing edema of the respiratory mucosa.

INDICATIONS

For the temporary relief of cough associated with minor throat and bronchial irritation or nasal congestion due to the common cold, sinusitis, and hay fever (allergic rhinitis).

A minimum dosage of Codeine is provided for the symptomatic relief of nonproductive cough. Decongestants have been used to relieve eustachian salpingitis, aerotitis, otitis, and serous otitis media. Chlorpheniramine Maleate provides temporary relief from runny nose, sneezing, itching of nose or throat, and itchy and watery eyes as may occur in hay fever (allergic rhinitis).

May be used as supportive therapy for acute otitis media and relief of mild otalgia.

May be given concomitantly, when indicated, with analgesics and antibiotics.

CONTRAINDICATIONS

Patients with severe hypertension, severe coronary artery disease, and in patients on MAO inhibitor therapy.

Nursing Mothers: Pseudoephedrine is contraindicated in nursing mothers because of the higher than usual risk for infants from sympathomimetic amines.

Hypersensitivity: This drug is contraindicated in patients with hypersensitivity or idiosyncrasy to its ingredients. Patient idiosyncrasy to adrenergic agents may be manifested by insomnia, dizziness, weakness, tremor or arrhythmias.

WARNINGS

Codeine should be prescribed and administered with the same degree of caution as all oral medications containing a narcotic analgesic. Codeine appears in the milk of nursing mothers.

If sympathomimetic amines are used in patients with hypertension, diabetes mellitus, ischemic heart disease, hyperthyroidism, increased intraocular pressure or prostatic hypertrophy, judicious caution should be exercised. See, however, *"Contraindications".* Sympathomimetics may produce CNS stimulation with convulsions or cardiovascular collapse with accompanying hypotension. Do not exceed recommended dosage.

The elderly (60 years and older) are more likely to have adverse reactions to sympathomimetics. Safety for use during pregnancy has not been established.

Antihistamines may cause excitability, especially in children.

PRECAUTIONS

If cough persists for more than one week, tends to recur or is accompanied by fever, rash or headache, discontinue treatment. Other medications containing a narcotic analgesic, phenothiazines, tranquilizers, sedatives, hypnotics and other CNS depressants, including alcohol, may have an additive CNS depressant effect when used concomitantly. The dose should be reduced when such combined therapy is contemplated.

Caution should be exercised if used in patients with high blood pressure, heart disease, asthma, emphysema, diabetes, thyroid disease and hyperreactivity to ephedrine.

The antihistamine may cause drowsiness, and ambulatory patients who operate machinery or motor vehicles should be cautioned accordingly.

ADVERSE REACTIONS

Nausea, vomiting, constipation, dizziness, sedation, palpitations or pruritus may occur. More frequent or higher than recommended dosage may cause respiratory depression, especially in patients with respiratory disease associated with carbon dioxide retention.

Drugs containing sympathomimetic amines have been associated with certain untoward reactions including fear, anxiety, tenseness, restlessness, tremor, weakness, pallor, respiratory difficulty, dysuria, insomnia, hallucinations, convulsions, CNS depression, arrhythmias and cardiovascular collapse with hypotension.

Patients sensitive to antihistamine drugs may experience mild sedation. Other side effects from antihistamines may include dry mouth, dizziness, weakness, anorexia, nausea, vomiting, headache, nervousness, polyuria, heartburn, diplopia, dysuria, and very rarely, dermatitis.

DRUG INTERACTIONS

Codeine may potentiate the effects of other narcotics, general anesthetics, tranquilizers, sedatives and hypnotics, tricyclic antidepressants, MAO inhibitors, alcohol and other CNS depressants.

Beta adrenergic blockers and MAO inhibitors potentiate the sympathomimetic effects of Pseudoephedrine. Sympathomimetics may reduce the antihypertensive effects of methyldopa, mecamylamine, reserpine and veratrum alkaloids. Antihistamines have been shown to enhance one or more of the effects of alcohol, tricyclic antidepressants, barbiturates and other CNS depressants.

DOSAGE

Adults, 2 teaspoonfuls; children 50-90 lbs, ½ to 1 teaspoonful; 25-50 lbs, ¼ to ½ teaspoonful. Repeat every 4 to 6 hours. May be given to children under 2 at the discretion of the physician. *Do not exceed 4 doses in a 24-hour period.*

Product label dosage is as follows: Adults and children 12 years and older, 2 teaspoonfuls every 4 to 6 hours. Children 6 to under 12 years, 1 teaspoonfuls every 4 to 6 hours. Do not exceed 4 doses in 24 hours. For children under 6 years, give only as directed by a physician.

HOW SUPPLIED
ELIXIR (C-V): 2 MG-10 MG-30 MG/5 ML

BRAND/MANUFACTURER	NDC	SIZE	AWP
○ **GENERICS**			
DIHISTINE DH: Moore,H.L.	00839-6694-65	120 ml	$2.42
PHENYLHISTINE DH: Aligen	00405-0075-76	120 ml	$2.80
PHENYLHISTINE DH: Cenci,H.R.	00556-0332-04	120 ml	$2.80
DIHISTINE DH: Barre	00472-1639-04	120 ml	$2.94
DECOHISTINE DH: Morton Grove	60432-0584-04	120 ml	$3.00
CODEHIST DH: Geneva	00781-6760-04	120 ml	$4.93
PHENYLHISTINE DH: Aligen	00405-0075-16	473 ml	$8.80
DIHISTINE DH: Moore,H.L.	00839-6694-69	480 ml	$6.74
PHENYLHISTINE DH EXPECTORANT: Qualitest	00603-1520-58	480 ml	$7.65
PHENYLHISTINE DH: URL	00677-0820-33	480 ml	$7.85
DECOHISTINE DH: Morton Grove	60432-0584-16	480 ml	$8.03
PHENYLHISTINE DH: Cenci,H.R.	00556-0332-16	480 ml	$8.10
DIHISTINE DH: Barre	00472-1639-16	480 ml	$8.61
CODEHIST DH: Geneva	00781-6760-16	480 ml	$16.40
DIHISTINE DH: Moore,H.L.	00839-6694-70	3840 ml	$49.80
DIHISTINE DH: Barre	00472-1639-28	3840 ml	$58.59
PHENYLHISTINE DH: Cenci,H.R.	00556-0332-28	3840 ml	$59.86

For additional alternatives, turn to the section beginning on page 2859.

Chlorpheniramine Maleate/ Dextromethorphan Hydrobromide/Guaifenesin/ Phenylephrine Hydrochloride

DESCRIPTION

Each 5 mL (teaspoonful), contains:

Dextromethorphan Hydrobromide	7.5 mg
Chlorpheniramine Maleate	2 mg
Phenylephrine Hydrochloride	10 mg
Guaifenesin	100 mg

◆ RATED THERAPEUTICALLY EQUIVALENT; ◇ THERAPEUTIC EQUIVALENCE UNCONFIRMED; ○ UNRATED

Chlorpheniramine Maleate/Dextromethorphan Hydrobromide/Guaifenesin/Phenylephrine Hydrochloride (CPM/DM/GG/PE) Syrup contains ingredients of the following therapeutic classes: cough suppressant, antihistamine, nasal decongestant, and expectorant.

CLINICAL PHARMACOLOGY

Dextromethorphan acts centrally to elevate the threshold for coughing. It has no analgesic or addictive properties. The onset of antitussive action occurs in 15 to 30 minutes after administration and is of long duration.

Chlorpheniramine Maleate competitively antagonizes most of the smooth muscle stimulating actions of histamine on the H1 receptors of the GI tract, uterus, large blood vessels and bronchial muscle. It also antagonizes the action of histamine that results in increased capillary permeability and the formation of edema.

Phenylephrine acts predominantly by a direct action on alpha adrenergic receptors. In therapeutic doses, the drug has no significant stimulant effect on the beta adrenergic receptors of the heart. Following oral administration, constriction of blood vessels in the nasal mucosa may relieve nasal congestion. In therapeutic doses, the drug causes little, if any, central nervous system stimulation.

Guaifenesin promotes lower respiratory tract drainage by thinning bronchial secretions, lubricates irritated respiratory tract membranes through increased mucous flow, and facilitates removal of viscous, inspissated mucous. As a result, sinus and bronchial drainage is improved, and dry, nonproductive coughs become more productive and less frequent.

INDICATIONS AND USAGE

Cough suppressant, antihistamine, nasal decongestant, and expectorant as an aid in the management of cough and mucosal congestion or edema of the respiratory tract, or nasal passages due to the common cold, bronchitis, laryngitis, tracheitis, pharyngitis, pertussis, influenza, measles, or chronic paranasal sinusitis.

CONTRAINDICATIONS

Hypersensitivity to any of the ingredients. Also contraindicated in patients with hypertension, hyperthyroidism, prostatic hypertrophy, and patients on MAO inhibitor therapy.

WARNINGS

Pediatric Use: Safety and effectiveness of CPM/DM/GG/PE syrup in children below the age of 2 have not been established.

Use with caution in the presence of cardiac disorders, diabetes or peripheral vascular disease.

PRECAUTIONS

Pregnancy: Pregnancy Category C; It is not known whether CPM/DM/GG/PE syrup can cause fetal harm when administered to a pregnant woman or can affect reproduction capacity CPM/DM/GG/PE syrup should be given to a pregnant woman only if clearly needed.

Nursing Mothers: It is not known whether this drug is excreted in human milk. Because many drugs are excreted in human milk, caution should be exercised when CPM/DM/GG/PE syrup is administered to a nursing woman.

ADVERSE REACTIONS

May include drowsiness, dizziness, nervousness, insomnia, headache, palpitation, dysuria.

Note: Guaifenesin has been shown to produce a color interference with certain clinical laboratory determinations of 5-hydroxyindoleacetic acid (5-HIAA) and vanillylmandelic acid (VMA).

OVERDOSAGE

In all cases of suspected overdose, immediately call your regional poison center and/or contact a physician immediately.

DOSAGE AND ADMINISTRATION

Adults and children 12 years and older, 1 teaspoonful; children 6 to under 12 years, 1/2 teaspoonful; children 2 to under 6 years, 1/4 teaspoonful. May be repeated in 4 to 6 hours if required for relief. Not to exceed 6 doses in 24 hours. Children under 2, at discretion of physician.

Store at controlled room temperature, 15°-30°C (59°-86°F).

Dispense in a tight, light-resistant container as defined in the USP/NF with a child-resistant closure.

HOW SUPPLIED
SYRUP:

BRAND/MANUFACTURER	NDC	SIZE	AWP
○ GENERICS			
BRONCOPECTOL: Med Prod	00576-0131-08	240 ml	$7.48
DONATUSSIN: Laser	00277-0139-41	480 ml	$18.22
DONATUSSIN: Laser	00277-0139-42	3840 ml	$134.09

Chlorpheniramine Maleate/ Dextromethorphan Hydrobromide/Guaifenesin/ Phenylpropanolamine Hydrochloride/Potassium Guaiacolsulfonate/ Pseudoephedrine Hydrochloride

DESCRIPTION

Each 5 mL contains:

Dextromethorphan HBr	7.5 mg
Guaifenesin	50 mg
Potassium Guaiacolsulfonate	50 mg
Pseudoephedrine HCl	10 mg
Phenylpropanolamine HCl	5 mg
Chlorpheniramine Maleate	2 mg

These ingredients are in the following therapeutic classes: cough suppressant, expectorant, nasal decongestant and antihistamine.

CLINICAL PHARMACOLOGY

Dextromethorphan HBr acts centrally to elevate the threshold for coughing. It has no analgesic or addictive properties. The onset of antitussive action occurs in 15 to 30 minutes after administration and is of long duration.

Guaifenesin promotes lower respiratory tract drainage by thinning bronchial secretions, lubricates irritated respiratory tract membranes through increased mucous flow, and facilitates removal of viscous, inspissated mucous. As a result, sinus and bronchial drainage is improved, and dry, nonproductive coughs become more productive and less frequent.

Potassium Guaiacolsulfonate has been used empirically for many decades as an expectorant.

Pseudoephedrine Hydrochloride acts on α-adrenergic receptors in the mucosa of the respiratory tract producing vasoconstriction. The medication shrinks swollen nasal mucous membranes; reduces tissue hyperemia, edema, and nasal congestion; and increases nasal airway patency. Also, drainage of sinus secretions may be increased and obstructed eustachian ostia may be opened.

Phenylpropanolamine Hydrochloride acts on α-adrenergic receptors in the mucosa of the respiratory tract to produce vasoconstriction, which temporarily reduces the swelling associated with inflammation of the mucous membranes lining the nasal passages.

Chlorpheniramine Maleate competitively antagonizes most of the smooth muscle stimulating actions of histamine on the H1 receptors of the GI tract, uterus, large blood vessels and bronchial muscle. It also antagonizes the action of histamine that results in increased capillary permeability and the formation of edema.

INDICATIONS AND USAGE

Antihistamine, antitussive, cough suppressant, expectorant, and nasal decongestant as an aid in the management of cough and mucosal congestion or edema of the respiratory tract, or nasal passages due to the common cold, bronchitis, laryngitis, tracheitis, pharyngitis, pertussis, influenza, measles, chronic paranasal sinusitis, or tobacco irritation.

CONTRAINDICATIONS

Hypersensitivity to any of the ingredients. Also contraindicated in patients with hypertension, coronary artery disease, glaucoma, hyperthyroidism, glaucoma, prostatic hypertrophy, and patients on Monoamine oxidase inhibitor (MAOI) therapy.

WARNINGS

A persistent cough may be a sign of a serious condition. If cough persists for more than 1 week, tends to recur, or is accompanied by fever, rash, or persistent headache, consult a doctor.

Avoid or use with caution in patients with hypertension, hyperthyroidism, diabetes mellitus, ischemic heart disease, cardiovascular disease, narrow angle glaucoma, peptic ulcer, pyloroduodenal obstruction, sympathomatic prostatic hypertrophy, asthmatic attack, bladder neck obstruction, or chronic pulmonary disease.

May cause drowsiness; alcohol, sedatives, and tranquilizers may increase the drowsiness effect. Avoid alcoholic beverages while taking this product. Do not take this product if you are taking sedatives or tranquilizers, without first consulting your doctor. Use caution when driving a motor vehicle or operating machinery.

► SHOWN IN PRODUCT IDENTIFICATION GUIDE

Do not exceed recommended dosage because at higher doses nervousness, dizziness, or sleeplessness may occur.

Usage in respiratory disease: Do not use for persistent or chronic cough (ie, smoking, asthma, emphysema) or where cough is accompanied by excessive secretions. Persons with a high fever, rash, persistent headache, nausea or vomiting should use only under medical supervision.

Usage in Children: Antihistamine overdosage may cause hallucinations, convulsions and death. Antihistamines may diminish mental alertness. In the young child, they may produce paradoxical excitation.

Use in the Elderly (approximately 60 years or older): More likely to cause dizziness, sedation and hypertension in elderly patients. Overdosage may cause hallucinations, convulsions, CNS depression or death.

Usage in Pregnancy: Pregnancy Category B; it is not known whether this product can cause fetal harm when administered to a pregnant woman or can affect reproduction capacity. This product should be given to a pregnant woman only if clearly needed.

Usage in Lactation: It is not known whether this drug is excreted in human milk. Because many drugs are excreted in human milk, caution should be exercised when this product is administered to a nursing woman.

PRECAUTIONS

Hazardous Tasks: May cause drowsiness; patients should observe caution while driving or performing other tasks requiring alertness.

Drug Interactions: Do not take this product if you are presently taking a prescription drug for high blood pressure or depression, without first consulting your doctor.

Alcohol and Other CNS Depressants: (hypnotics, sedatives, tranquilizers, anti-anxiety agents, narcotic analgesics) have additive effects with antihistamines. Dosage adjustment of CNS depressants may be necessary to avoid profound CNS depression.

Oral Anticoagulant action may be diminished by antihistamines.

Furazolidone and MAOI Inhibitors prolong and intensify the anticholinergic (drying) effects of antihistamines and increase the α-adrenergic effects of sympathomimetics. Interaction may occur several weeks after discontinuing furazolidone or MAOIs. Headache, hyperpyrexia, hypertension, hypertensive crisis and intracranial hemorrhage may occur.

Heparin: Antihistamines may partially counteract the anticoagulant action of heparin.

Guanethidine, Tricyclic Antidepressants and Rauwolfia Alkaloids: Alpha-adrenergic effects of sympathomimetics (phenylpropanolamine) and the effects of the direct-acting sympathomimetics (ephedrine, phenylephrine) may be increased. Dose adjustment may be necessary.

Methyldopa may potentiate the α-adrenergic (pressor) effects of sympathomimetics and may lead to hypertension.

Phenothiazines may block the α-adrenergic effects of epinephrine, producing hypotension and tachycardia. One fatality due to ventricular arrhythmias has been attributed to a nasal decongestant containing Phenylpropanolamine.

Urinary Alkalinization increases the half-life and prolongs the duration of action of Pseudoephedrine.

ADVERSE REACTIONS

Cardiovascular: Arrhythmias and cardiovascular collapse with hypotension. Palpitations, tachycardia, precordial pain, transient hypertension, bradycardia, and extrasystoles.

Hematologic: Hemolytic anemia, hypoplastic anemia, thrombocytopenia, leukopenia, agranulocytosis, and pancytopenia.

CNS: Most frequent: Drowsiness, sedation, dizziness and disturbed coordination. *Others:* Fear, tenseness, fatigue, confusion, restlessness, light-headedness, excitation, nervousness, tremor, headache, irritability, insomnia, euphoria, paresthesias, blurred vision, diplopia, vertigo, tinnitus, acute labyrinthitis, hysteria, neuritis, hallucinations, psychological disturbances, prolonged psychosis (paranoia, terror, delusions), convulsions, CNS depression; weakness. Paradoxical excitation, especially in children and in the elderly.

Ocular: Blepharospasm (ocular irritation, tearing, photophobia).

GI: Most frequent: Epigastric distress. *Others:* Anorexia, increased appetite, and weight gain, nausea, vomiting, diarrhea and constipation.

GU: Urinary frequency, dysuria, urinary retention, early menses, decreased libido, impotence.

Respiratory: Most frequent: Thickening of bronchial secretions. Other: Chest tightness, wheezing, and nasal stuffiness. Dry mouth, nose and throat; sore throat; respiratory depression.

Other: Tingling, heaviness and weakness of the hands; urticaria; rash; anaphylactic shock; excessive perspiration; chills; pallor; respiratory difficulty; orofacial dystonia.

Note: Guaifenesin has been shown to produce a color interference with certain clinical laboratory determinations of 5-hydroxyindolacetic acid (5-HIAA) and vanillylmandelic acid (VMA).

Patient Information: Do not exceed recommended dosage; higher doses may cause nervousness, dizziness or sleeplessness.

If symptoms do not improve within 7 days or are accompanied by high fever, consult a physician before continuing use.

Patients with hypertension, or other cardiovascular disease, hyperthyroidism, diabetes mellitus or prostatic hypertrophy should use this product only with medical advice.

May cause drowsiness or dizziness; patients should observe caution while driving or performing other tasks requiring alertness. Avoid alcohol and other CNS depressants (sedatives, hypnotics, tranquilizers, etc).

May cause dry mouth. May cause GI upset; take with food.

OVERDOSAGE

In all cases of suspected overdosage, immediately call your regional poison center and/or contact a physician.

DOSAGE AND ADMINISTRATION

Adults and children 12 years and older: 1 or 2 teaspoonfuls; children 4 to 12 years: 1/2 to 1 teaspoonful; children 2 to 4 years: 1/4 teaspoonful. Not recommended for children under 2 years. May be repeated in 6 to 8 hours if required for relief. Store in tight, light-resistant containers, as defined in the USP, between 15°-30°C(59°-86°F).

Dispense in child resistant containers.

HOW SUPPLIED
LIQUID:

BRAND/MANUFACTURER	NDC	SIZE	AWP
○ BRAND			
LEMOTUSSIN DM: Seneca	47028-0015-16	480 ml	$25.52

Chlorpheniramine Maleate/ Ephedrine Sulfate/Guaifenesin/ Hydriodic Acid

DESCRIPTION

Each 5 mL (1 teaspoonful) for oral administration contains:

Chlorpheniramine Maleate	4 mg
Guaifenesin	100 mg
Ephedrine Sulfate	8.216 mg
Hydriodic Acid Syrup	1.67 mL
Alcohol (Ethyl)	5%

Chlorpheniramine Maleate: $C_{16}H_{19}CIN_2.C_4H_4O_4$, 2-pyridine propanamine, lambda-(4-chlorophenyl)-N,N,-dimethyl-,(Z)-2-butenedioate (1:1), is an antihistaminic that exists as a white, odorless, crystalline powder. Its solutions have a pH between 4 and 5. It is freely soluble in water, soluble in alcohol and chloroform, and slightly soluble in ether and benzene.

Guaifenesin: $C_{10}H_{14}O_4$, 1,2-Propanediol, 3-(2-methoxyphenoxy)-, is an expectorant. It occurs as a white to slightly gray, crystalline powder, having a bitter taste. It may have a slight characteristic odor. It is soluble in water, alcohol, chloroform, glycerin and propylene glycol.

Ephedrine Sulfate: $(C_{10}H_{15}NO)_2.H_2SO_4$, benzenemethanol, alpha-[1-(methylamino) ethyl]-,[R-(R*,S*)]-,sulfate (2:1) (salt), is an adrenergic which exists as fine, white, odorless crystals or powder. Darkens on exposure to light. It is freely soluble in water and sparingly soluble in alcohol.

Hydriodic Acid: (HI) Colorless or not more than pale yellow, odorless liquid with a specific gravity of about 1.1. It is miscible with water or alcohol.

CLINICAL PHARMACOLOGY

Chlorpheniramine Maleate: Chlorpheniramine is an antihistamine belonging to the alkylamine class. It possesses anticholinergic and sedative effects. Antihistamines appear to compete with histamine for H1 cell receptor sites on effector cells, thereby counteracting the effects of histamine release associated with allergic manifestations of upper respiratory tract inflammatory disorders. Chlorpheniramine Maleate does not prevent the release of histamine in response to injury, drugs, or antigens. Antihistamines effectively block most smooth muscle responses to histamine and act as an antagonist of the constrictor action of histamine on respiratory smooth muscle. Antihistamines counteract edema formation and whealing in response to injury, antigens, or histamine-liberating drugs. Chlorpheniramine is readily absorbed from the gastrointestinal tract and has a duration of 4 to 6 hours. Plasma half-life is approximately 22 hours. Degradation products of Chlorpheniramine's metabolic transformation by the liver are almost completely excreted in 24 hours via the kidney. The alkylamines of which Chlorpheniramine is the prototype, are among the most potent H1 blockers. Although not so prone as others to cause drowsiness, a significant proportion of patients do experience this effect. CNS stimulation is more common in Chlorpheniramine than in other groups of H1 blockers.

◆ RATED THERAPEUTICALLY EQUIVALENT; ◇ THERAPEUTIC EQUIVALENCE UNCONFIRMED; ○ UNRATED

Guaifenesin: Guaifenesin has an expectorant action which increases the output of respiratory tract fluid by reducing adhesiveness and surface tension. The increased flow of less viscid secretions promotes ciliary action, lubricating irritated respiratory tract membranes, and facilitates removal of viscous inspissated mucus. As a result, sinus and bronchial drainage is improved and dry, nonproductive coughs become more productive and less frequent. Guaifenesin is readily absorbed from the gastrointestinal tract and is rapidly metabolized and excreted in the urine. It has a plasma half-life of one hour. The major urinary metabolite is beta- (2-methoxyphenoxy) lactic acid.

Ephedrine Sulfate: In ordinary doses Ephedrine acts indirectly through release of norepinephrine from adrenergic nerves. In higher doses it has a more direct sympathomimetic action. It penetrates membranes and into the brain, and hence has central nervous actions, which, however, are not as prominent as those of amphetamines. Although Ephedrine mainly acts indirectly through the release of norepinephrine, its peripheral effects are as though it possessed weak alpha-agonist activity, except that it acts rather strongly on the trigone sphincter, and has moderate beta 1- and beta 2-agonist activity, except that the beta 2- activity being limited to the bronchioles; its weak hyperglycemic effect results mainly from central nervous actions. Its most important use has been that as a bronchodilator. It is also used in various drug combinations with central depressants to counteract sedative effects. Ephedrine is resistant to monoamine oxidase (MAO) and is thus orally efficacious. By the oral route, its duration of action is 2 to 3 hours. The half-life is about 6 hours, but when the urine is alkaline, it is longer, and, when acidic, it is shorter. Although it is not a substrate of MAO, it is said that MAO inhibitors may cause a hypertensive crisis in response to otherwise safe doses; therefore, caution is indicated. As a rule, salts of Ephedrine are employed instead of the free base.

INDICATIONS
For temporary symptomatic relief of cough, particularly when associated with thick tenacious mucus.

CONTRAINDICATIONS
Sensitivity to any of the components, iodides, antihistamines, cases of active or dormant tuberculosis. Antihistamines such as Chlorpheniramine Maleate should not be administered to premature or newborn infants or be used to treat lower respiratory tract symptoms. Because of the Ephedrine, Chlorpheniramine Maleate/Ephedrine Sulfate/Guaifenesin/Hydriodic Acid is contraindicated in cardiovascular disease, hyperthyroidism and hypertension.

WARNINGS
Do Not Exceed Recommended Dosage: Keep this and all drugs out of the reach of children. As with any drug, if the patient is pregnant or nursing a baby, a health care professional should be notified before using this product.

Antihistamines may impair mental and physical abilities required for the performance of potentially hazardous tasks such as driving a vehicle or operating machinery, and may impair mental alertness in children. Chlorpheniramine has an atropine-like action and should be used with caution in patients with increased intraocular pressure, cardiovascular disease, hypertension or in patients with a history of bronchial asthma. Guaifenesin should be prescribed with caution in patients with persistent or chronic cough due to smoking, asthma, or emphysema, or where cough is accompanied by excessive secretions. In patients with chronic pulmonary disease or shortness of breath, this product should be administered with caution.

PRECAUTIONS
General: Before prescribing medication to suppress or modify cough, it is important to ascertain that the underlying cause of cough is identified, that modification of cough does not increase the risk of clinical or physiological complications, and that appropriate therapy for the primary disease is instituted. Because of the Ephedrine component, this drug should be used with caution in elderly males or those with known prostatic hypertrophy.

Information for Patients: Antihistamines may impair mental and physical abilities required for the performance of potentially hazardous tasks such as driving a vehicle or operating machinery. Patients should also be warned about possible additive effects with alcohol and other central nervous system depressants (hypnotics, sedatives, and tranquilizers).

Drugs/Laboratory Test Interactions: Concomitant use of antihistamines with alcohol, tricyclic depressants, barbiturates and other CNS depressants may have an additive effect. Guaifenesin may increase renal clearance for urate and thereby lower serum uric acid levels. Guaifenesin may produce an increase in urinary 5-hydroxyindoleacetic acid and may therefore interfere with the interpretation of this test for the diagnosis of carcinoid syndrome. It may also falsely elevate the VMA test for catechols. Administration of this drug should be discontinued 48 hours prior to the collection of urine specimens for such tests.

Carcinogenesis, Mutagenesis, and Impairment of Fertility: No long term studies have been performed using Chlorpheniramine Maleate/Ephedrine Sulfate/Guaifenesin/Hydriodic Acid to determine the long term potential for carcinogenesis, mutagenesis, and impairment of fertility.

Usage in Pregnancy: Pregnancy Category C: Animal reproduction studies have not been conducted with the ingredients in Chlorpheniramine Maleate/Ephedrine Sulfate/Guaifenesin/Hydriodic Acid. Chlorpheniramine Maleate/Ephedrine Sulfate/Guaifenesin/Hydriodic Acid should be used in pregnant women only if the potential benefits outweigh the possible risk to the fetus.

Nursing Mothers: It is not known whether the components of Chlorpheniramine Maleate/Ephedrine Sulfate/Guaifenesin/Hydriodic Acid are excreted in human milk. Because many drugs are excreted in human milk, caution should be exercised when Chlorpheniramine Maleate/Ephedrine Sulfate/Guaifenesin/Hydriodic Acid is administered to a nursing woman and a decision should be made whether to discontinue nursing or to discontinue the drug, taking into account the importance of the drug to the mother.

Pediatric Use: In infants and children especially, antihistamines in overdosage may cause hallucinations, convulsions or death. As in adults, antihistamines may diminish mental alertness in children. In the young child particularly, they produce excitation.

Geriatric Use: Antihistamines are more likely to cause dizziness, sedation, and hypotension in elderly patients.

ADVERSE REACTIONS
Chlorpheniramine Maleate may cause slight to moderate drowsiness. Less frequent side effects of antihistamines in general include: urticaria, drug rash, anaphylactic shock, photosensitivity, excessive perspiration, chills, dryness of mouth, nose, and throat; cardiovascular effects (hypotension, headache, palpitation, tachycardia, extrasystoles); hematological effects (hemolytic anemia, thrombocytopenia, agranulocytosis); CNS disturbances (sedation, dizziness, disturbed coordination, fatigue, confusion, restlessness, excitation, nervousness, tremor, irritability, insomnia, euphoria, paresthesia, blurred vision, diplopia, vertigo, tinnitus, hysteria, neuritis, convulsions); gastrointestinal effects (epigastric distress, anorexia, nausea, vomiting, diarrhea, constipation); genitourinary effects (urinary frequency, difficult urination, urinary retention, early menses); and respiratory effects (thickening of bronchial secretions, tightening of chest, wheezing, and nasal stuffiness).

With large doses of Ephedrine, excitation, tremulousness, insomnia, nervousness, palpitation, tachycardia, precordial pain, cardiac arrhythmias, vertigo, dryness of the nose and throat, headache, sweating, and warmth may occur. Because Ephedrine is a sympathomimetic agent, some patients may develop vesical sphincter spasm and resultant urinary hesitation, and occasionally acute urinary retention. This should be borne in mind when administering preparations containing Ephedrine to elderly males or those with known prostatic hypertrophy. A side effect occasionally reported is palpitation, and this can be controlled with dosage adjustment, or discontinuation of the medication. When Ephedrine is given three or more times daily, patients may develop tolerance after several weeks of therapy.

OVERDOSAGE
SIGNS AND SYMPTOMS
Chlorpheniramine Maleate: Manifestations of antihistamine overdosage may vary from central nervous system depression (sedation, apnea, cardiovascular collapse) to stimulation (insomnia, hallucinations, tremors or convulsions). Other signs and symptoms may be dizziness, tinnitus, ataxia, blurred vision and hypotension. Stimulation is particularly likely in children, as are atropine-like signs and symptoms (dry mouth; fixed, dilated pupils; flushing, hyperthermia and gastrointestinal symptoms).

Guaifenesin: Overdosage with Guaifenesin is unlikely to produce toxic effects since its toxicity is low. Guaifenesin, when administered by stomach tube to test animals in doses up to 5 grams/kg, produced no signs of toxicity.

TREATMENT
The patient should be induced to vomit, even if emesis has occurred spontaneously. Pharmacologic vomiting by the administration of ipecac syrup is a preferred method. However, vomiting should not be induced in patients with impaired consciousness. The action of ipecac is facilitated by physical activity and by the administration of eight to twelve fluid ounces of water. If emesis does not occur within fifteen minutes, the dose of ipecac should be repeated. Precautions against aspiration must be taken, especially in infants and children. Following emesis, any drug remaining in the stomach may be absorbed by activated charcoal administered as a slurry with water. If vomiting is unsuccessful or contraindicated, gastric lavage should be performed. Isotonic and one-half isotonic saline are the lavage solutions of choice. Saline cathartics, such as milk of magnesia, draw water into the bowel by osmosis and, therefore, may be valuable for their action in rapid dilution of bowel content. After emergency treatment, the patient should continue to be medically monitored. Treatment of the signs and symptoms of overdosage is symptomatic and supportive. Only in cases of extreme overdosage or individual sensitivity do vital signs including respiration, pulse, blood pressure, temperature and EKG need to be monitored.

DOSAGE AND ADMINISTRATION
Adults and children over 12 years of age: 1 teaspoonful taken orally. Children 6 to 12 years of age: 1/2 teaspoonful taken orally. Dosage may be repeated in 3 to 4 hours if required for relief.

Preserve and dispense in tight, light-resistant containers. Store at controlled room temperature 15-30°C (59-86°F).

HOW SUPPLIED
LIQUID:

BRAND/MANUFACTURER	NDC	SIZE	AWP
○ **BRAND**			
BRONKOTUSS: Hyrex	00314-0001-16	480 ml	$21.50
	00314-0001-28	3840 ml	$138.00

Chlorpheniramine Maleate/ Hydrocodone Bitartrate/ Phenylephrine Hydrochloride

DESCRIPTION

Each teaspoon (5 mL) of Chlorpheniramine Maleate/Hydrocodone Bitartrate/ Phenylephrine Hydrochloride contains:

Hydrocodone Bitartrate ....1.6 mg or 2.5 mg
(WARNING: May be habit forming)
Phenylephrine Hydrochloride ....5 mg or 10 mg
Chlorpheniramine Maleate ....2 mg or 4 mg
Alcohol 5%

CLINICAL PHARMACOLOGY

Chlorpheniramine Maleate/Hydrocodone Bitartrate/Phenylephrine Hydrochloride (CPM/Hydrocodone/Phenylephrine) combines the centrally acting antitussive activity of Hydrocodone Bitartrate with the nasal decongestant action of Phenylephrine Hydrochloride with the antihistaminic activity of Chlorpheniramine Maleate.

Chlorpheniramine Maleate is an alkylamine type antihistamine. This group of antihistamines are among the most active histamine antagonists and are generally effective in relatively low doses. The drugs are not so prone to produce drowsiness and are among the most suitable agents for daytime use; but a significant proportion of patients do experience this effect.

Phenylephrine HCl is a sympathomimetic which acts predominantly on alpha receptors and has little action on beta receptors. It therefore functions as an oral nasal decongestant with minimal CNS stimulation.

Hydrocodone Bitartrate is a potent antitussive which causes suppression of the cough reflex by direct action on the cough center. Hydrocodone is approximately six times as potent as codeine on a weight basis and has a higher addiction potential also.

INDICATIONS AND USAGE

To control cough and provide for the temporary symptomatic relief from congestion in the upper respiratory tract due to the common cold, pertussis or influenza.

CONTRAINDICATIONS

Hypersensitivity to any component of the drug. CPM/Hydrocodone/Phenylephrine is also contraindicated in patients with bronchial asthma or pulmonary emphysema and pregnant women and nursing mothers and is also contraindicated in patients with severe hypertension, severe coronary artery disease, patients on MAO inhibitor therapy, patients with narrow-angle glaucoma, urinary retention, peptic ulcer and during an asthmatic attack.

WARNINGS

Hydrocodone can produce drug dependence and, therefore, has the potential for being abused. This product should be prescribed and administered with the appropriate degree of caution.

Considerable caution should be exercised in patients with hypertension, diabetes mellitus, ischemic heart disease, hyperthyroidism, increased intraocular pressure and prostatic hypertrophy. The elderly (60 years and older) are more likely to exhibit adverse reactions. Antihistamines may cause excitability, especially in children. At dosages higher than the recommended dose nervousness, dizziness, or sleeplessness may occur.

PRECAUTIONS

Use CPM/Hydrocodone/Phenylephrine with caution in patients with diabetes, hyperthyroidism, hypertension, cardiovascular disease, who are debilitated, or who have undergone thoracotomies or laparotomies. Patients should be cautioned about participating in activities which require alertness, since drowsiness and dizziness may occur. *Note*: Before prescribing medication to suppress or modify cough, it is important to determine the primary cause of the cough and that modification of the cough does not increase the risk of clinical or physiologic complications, and that appropriate concomitant therapy for the primary condition is provided.

The Hydrocodone and antihistamine in this product may exhibit additive effects with other CNS depressants, including alcohol.

Respiratory depression can be a real hazard so caution should be used, especially in patients with chronic obstructive pulmonary disease.

Information For Patients: Antihistamines and Hydrocodone may cause drowsiness and ambulatory patients who operate machinery or motor vehicles should be cautioned accordingly.

Drug Interactions: MAO inhibitors and beta adrenergic blockers increase the effects of sympathomimetics. Sympathomimetics may reduce the antihypertensive effects of methyldope, mecamylamine, reserpine and veratrum alkaloids. Concomitant use of narcotics and antihistamines with alcohol and other CNS depressants may have an additive effect.

Pregnancy: Pregnancy Category C: Animal reproduction studies have not been conducted with this product. It is also not known whether it can cause fetal harm when administered to a pregnant woman or can affect reproduction capacity. This product should be given to a pregnant woman only if clearly needed.

Nursing Mothers: Due to the possible passage of the ingredients into breast milk, this product should not be given to nursing mothers.

ADVERSE REACTIONS

Occasional drowsiness, cardiac palpitations, dizziness, nervousness, gastrointestinal upset, lassitude, nausea, constipation, respiratory depression, addiction, dryness of mouth, blurred vision, flushing, and increased irritability or excitement (especially in children).

DRUG ABUSE AND DEPENDENCE

This product is a schedule III Controlled Substance. Because of the Hydrocodone content, some abuse might be expected. Psychic dependence, physical dependence and tolerance may develop upon repeated administration. It should be prescribed and administered with appropriate caution.

OVERDOSAGE

Symptoms of overdosage include respiratory depression, extreme somnolence progressing to stupor or coma, skeletal muscle flaccidity, cold and clammy skin and other symptoms common with narcotic overdosage.

Primary treatment consists of insuring adequate respiration through provision of a patent airway and the institution of assisted or controlled ventilation. Naloxone hydrochloride should be administered in small intravenous doses (consult specific product labeling before use). In addition, oxygen, intravenous fluids, vasopressors and other supportive measures should be employed as indicated.

Gastric emptying may be useful in removing unabsorbed drug. Activated charcoal may also be of benefit.

DOSAGE AND ADMINISTRATION

Adults: 2 teaspoonfuls (10 ml) 3 or 4 times daily.

Children 6 to 12 years old: 1 teaspoonful (5 ml) 3 or 4 times daily.

DOSAGE FOR THE PRODUCT CONTAINING 2.5 MG OF HYDROCODONE BITARTRATE PER 5 ML
Adults and children over 12 years: 1 teaspoon.

Children, 6 to 12 years of age: ½ teaspoonful.

Children, 2 to 6 years of age: ¼ teaspoonful.

These doses may be given four times daily as needed. Not recommended for children under 2 years of age.

STORAGE

Store and dispense in tight containers as defined in USP/NF.
Store at controlled room temperature 15°-30°C (59°-86°F).
Dispense in child-resistant containers.

HOW SUPPLIED
LIQUID (C-III):

BRAND/MANUFACTURER	NDC	SIZE	AWP
○ **GENERICS**			
CHEMDAL HD: Norton,HN	50732-0855-16	480 ml	$15.34
QUENDAL HD: Qualitest	00603-1621-58	480 ml	$15.80
CHEMDAL HD PLUS: Norton,HN	50732-0895-16	480 ml	$16.50
EFASIN-HD: Major	00904-3542-16	480 ml	$17.05
GUIAPHEN HD: Rugby	00536-2650-85	480 ml	$23.15
QUENDAL HD PLUS: Qualitest	00603-1622-58	480 ml	$24.90
MED-HIST-HC: Med-Tek	52349-0400-16	480 ml	$29.45
POLY-TUSSIN: Poly	50991-0727-16	480 ml	$30.10
CHEMDAL HD: Norton,HN	50732-0855-28	3840 ml	$101.71

LIQUID (C-III): 2 MG-1.67 MG-5 MG/5 ML

BRAND/MANUFACTURER	NDC	SIZE	AWP
○ **GENERICS**			
ENDAGEN-HD: Abana	12463-0200-16	480 ml	$9.15
ED-TLC: Edwards	00485-0052-16	480 ml	$16.00
PARA-HIST HD: Pharmics	00813-0050-16	480 ml	$21.00
VANEX-HD: Abana	12463-0300-16	480 ml	$22.21

LIQUID (C-III): 2 MG-1.7 MG-5 MG/5 ML

BRAND/MANUFACTURER	NDC	SIZE	AWP
○ **GENERICS**			
ENDAL-HD: Forest Pharm	00785-6200-16	480 ml	$28.50

◆ RATED THERAPEUTICALLY EQUIVALENT; ◇ THERAPEUTIC EQUIVALENCE UNCONFIRMED; ○ UNRATED

LIQUID (C-III): 2 MG-2.5 MG-5 MG/5 ML

BRAND/MANUFACTURER	NDC	SIZE	AWP
○ GENERICS			
ENDAL-HD PLUS: Forest Pharm	00785-6283-16	473 ml	$33.59

LIQUID (C-III): 2 MG-5 MG-2.5 MG/5 ML

BRAND/MANUFACTURER	NDC	SIZE	AWP
○ GENERICS			
EFASIN-HD PLUS: Major	00904-7886-16	480 ml	$20.95

LIQUID (C-III): 2.5 MG-5 MG-2 MG/5 ML

BRAND/MANUFACTURER	NDC	SIZE	AWP
○ GENERICS			
ATUSS HD: Atley	59702-0025-16	480 ml	$15.60

LIQUID (C-III): 4 MG-1.67 MG-5 MG

BRAND/MANUFACTURER	NDC	SIZE	AWP
○ GENERICS			
CHLORGEST HD: Great Southern	51301-0542-16	480 ml	$13.49
CHLORGEST HD: Great Southern	51301-0542-28	3840 ml	$89.00

LIQUID (C-III): 4 MG-2.5 MG-10 MG/5 ML

BRAND/MANUFACTURER	NDC	SIZE	AWP
○ GENERICS			
ED-TUSS HC: Edwards	00485-0053-16	480 ml	$22.00

LIQUID (C-III): 12 MG-10 MG-30 MG/30 ML

BRAND/MANUFACTURER	NDC	SIZE	AWP
○ GENERICS			
RINDAL-HD: Econolab	55053-0670-16	480 ml	$15.95

LIQUID (C-III): 12 MG-30 MG-10 MG

BRAND/MANUFACTURER	NDC	SIZE	AWP
○ GENERICS			
Goldline	00182-0272-40	480 ml	$16.80

SYRUP (C-III):

BRAND/MANUFACTURER	NDC	SIZE	AWP
○ GENERICS			
MAXI-TUSS HC: MCR/Amer Pharm, Inc.	58605-0507-01	480 ml	$19.97
UNI-TUSS HC: URL	00677-1491-33	480 ml	$27.19

SYRUP (C-III): 2 MG-1.7 MG-5 MG/5 ML

BRAND/MANUFACTURER	NDC	SIZE	AWP
○ GENERICS			
ANAPLEX HD: ECR	59010-0130-04	120 ml	$5.75
ANAPLEX HD: ECR	59010-0130-16	480 ml	$15.75

SYRUP (C-III): 2 MG-2.5 MG-5 MG/5 ML

BRAND/MANUFACTURER	NDC	SIZE	AWP
○ GENERICS			
UNI TUSS HC: URL	00677-1512-33	480 ml	$27.19
COMTUSSIN HC: Rugby	00536-2701-85	480 ml	$29.43
COMTUSSIN HC: Rugby	00536-2901-85	480 ml	$29.43
HISTUSSIN-HC: Bock	00563-0860-16	480 ml	$32.71

SYRUP (C-III): 2 MG-5 MG-2.5 MG/5 ML

BRAND/MANUFACTURER	NDC	SIZE	AWP
○ GENERICS			
CHEMTUSSIN HC: Norton,HN	50732-0919-16	480 ml	$16.50
ENPLUS-HD: Alphagen	59743-0008-16	480 ml	$17.90
HISTINEX HC: Ethex	58177-0877-07	480 ml	$25.16
COMTUSSIN HC: Econolab	55053-0810-16	480 ml	$27.95

SYRUP (C-III): 2.5 MG/5 ML

BRAND/MANUFACTURER	NDC	SIZE	AWP
○ GENERICS			
VENTUSS SYRUP: Venture	59785-0301-16	480 ml	$19.50

SYRUP (C-III): 2.5 MG-5 MG-2 MG/5 ML

BRAND/MANUFACTURER	NDC	SIZE	AWP
○ GENERICS			
COMTUSSIN HC: Moore,H.L.	00839-7845-69	480 ml	$18.89
COTUSS-V: Alphagen	59743-0020-16	480 ml	$32.00

SYRUP (C-III): 2.5 MG-5 MG-2 MG

BRAND/MANUFACTURER	NDC	SIZE	AWP
○ GENERICS			
CYTUSS HC: Aligen	00405-0058-16	480 ml	$17.37

SYRUP (C-III): 12 MG-10 MG-30 MG/30 ML

BRAND/MANUFACTURER	NDC	SIZE	AWP
○ GENERICS			
HYPHEN-HD: Alphagen	59743-0012-16	480 ml	$16.95

Chlorpheniramine Maleate/ Hydrocodone Bitartrate/ Pseudoephedrine Hydrochloride

DESCRIPTION

Each 5 ml (one teaspoonful) contains:

Chlorpheniramine Maleate ....2 mg
Hydrocodone Bitartrate ....2.5 mg
(*WARNING: May be habit forming)
Pseudoephedrine Hydrochloride ....30 mg

Chlorpheniramine Maleate is an antihistaminic that occurs as a white, odorless, crystalline powder. Its solutions have a pH between 4 and 5. It is freely soluble in water, soluble in alcohol and in chloroform, and slightly soluble in ether and benzene. The chemical name is 2-pyridinepropanamine, α-(4-chlorophenyl) - N, N-dimentyl-(Z)-2-Butene-dioate (1:1). Its empirical formula is $C_{16}H_{19}CIN_2 \cdot C_4H_4O_4$, and its molecular weight 390.87.

Hydrocodone Bitartrate is an opioid analgesic and antitussive and occurs as fine, white crystals or as a crystalline powder. It is affected by light. The chemical name is 4,5 α-expoxy-3-methoxy-17-methylmorphinan-6-one-tar-trade (1:1) hydrate (2:5). Its empirical formula is $C_{18}H_{21}NO_3 \cdot C_4H_6O_6 2$ ½ H_2O, and its molecular weight 494.50.

Pseudoephedrine Hydrochloride (HCl) is an adrenergic (vasoconstrictor) which occurs as fine, white to off-white crystals or powder, having a faint characteristic odor. It is very soluble in water, freely soluble in alcohol, and sparingly soluble in chloroform. The chemical name is benzenemethanol, α-(1-methylamino)ethyl)-, [S-(R*,R*)]-hydrochloride. Its empirical formula is $C_{10}H_{15}NO \cdot HC1$, and its molecular weight 201.70.

CLINICAL PHARMACOLOGY

Chlorpheniramine is an antihistamine that possesses anticholinergic and sedative effects. It is considered one of the most effective and least toxic of the histamine antagonists. Chlorpheniramine is a H_1 receptor antagonist. It antagonizes many of the pharmacologic actions of histamine. It prevents released histamine from dilating capillaries and causing edema of the respiratory mucosa. Chlorpheniramine is well absorbed and has a duration of action 4 to 6 hours. Its half-life in serum is 12 to 16 hours. Degradation products of Chlorpheniramine's metabolic transformation by the liver are almost completely excreted in 24 hours.

Hydrocodone is a semisynthetic narcotic antitussive with multiple actions qualitatively similar to those of codeine. Most of these involve the central nervous system and smooth muscle. The precise mechanism of action of Hydrocodone and other opiates is not known; however, Hydrocodone is believed to act directly on the cough center. In excessive doses, Hydrocodone, like other opium derivatives, will depress respiration. The effects of Hydrocodone in therapeutic doses on the cardiovascular system are insignificant. Hydrocodone can produce miosis, euphoria, physical and physiological dependence.

Following a 10 mg oral dose of Hydrocodone administered to five adult male subjects, the mean peak concentration was 23.6 ± 5.2 mg/mL. Maximum serum levels were achieved at 1.3 ± 0.3 hours and the half-life was determined to be 3.8 ± 0.3 hours. Hydrocodone exhibits a complex pattern of metabolism including O-demethylation, N-demethylation and 6-keto reduction to the corresponding 6-α- and 6-β-hydroxy metabolites.

Pseudoephedrine acts as an indirect sympathomimetic agent by stimulating sympathetic (adrenergic) nerve endings to release norepinephrine. Norepinephrine in turn stimulates alpha and beta receptors throughout the body. The action of Pseudoephedrine HCl is apparently more specific for the blood vessels of the upper respiratory tract and less specific for the blood vessels of the systemic circulation. The vasconstriction elicited at these sites results in the shrinkage of swollen tissues in the sinuses and nasal passages. Pseudoephedrine is rapidly and almost completely absorbed from the gastrointestinal tract. Considerable variation in half-life has been observed (from about 4.5 to 10 hours) which is attributed to differences in absorption and excretion. Excretion rates are also altered by urine pH, increasing with acidification and decreasing with alkalinization. As a result, mean half-life falls to about 4 hours at pH 5 and increases to 12 to 13 hours at pH 8. After administration of a 60 mg tablet, 87 to 97% of the Pseudoephedrine is cleared from the body within 24 hours. The drug is distributed to body tissues and fluids, including fetal tissue, breast milk, and the central nervous system. About 55 to 75% of an administered dose is excreted unchanged in the urine; the remainder is apparently metabolized in the liver to inactive compounds by N-demethylation, parahydroxylation, and oxidative deamination.

INDICATIONS

Chlorpheniramine Maleate/Hydrocodone Bitartrate/Pseudoephedrine HCl syrup is indicated for relief of cough and congestion due to colds, acute respiratory infections, laryngeal and pulmonary tuberculosis, acute and chronic bronchitis and hay fever. In addition Chlorpheniramine Maleate/Hydrocodone Bitartrate/Pseudoephedrine HCl syrup helps relieve the sneezing and itching associated with hay fever.

CONTRAINDICATIONS

Hypersensitivity to any of the ingredients.

Patients known to be hypersensitive to other sympathomimetic amines may exhibit cross sensitivity with Pseudoephedrine. Sympathomimetic amines are contraindicated in patients with severe hypertension, severe coronary artery disease, and patients on monoamine oxidase (MAO) inhibitor therapy.

Antihistamines are contraindicated in patients with narrow-angle glaucoma, urinary retention, peptic ulcer, during an asthmatic attack and in patients receiving MAO inhibitors.

Chlorpheniramine Maleate/Hydrocodone Bitartrate/Pseudoephedrine HCl syrup should not be administered to premature or full-term infants.

Chlorpheniramine Maleate/Hydrocodone Bitartrate/Pseudoephedrine HCl syrup is contraindicated in nursing mothers because of the higher than usual risk for infants from sympathomimetic amines.

WARNINGS

General: Sympathomimetic amines should be used with caution in patients with hypertension, ischemic heart disease, diabetes mellitus, increased intraocular pressure, hyperthyroidism, or prostatic hypertrophy. Sympathomimetics may produce central nervous system stimulation with convulsions or cardiovascular collapse with accompanying hypotension. DO NOT EXCEED RECOMMENDED DOSAGE.

Hypertensive crises can occur with concurrent use of Pseudoephedrine and monoamine oxidase (MAO) inhibitors, indomethacin, or with betablockers and methyldopa. If a hypertensive crisis occurs, these drugs should be discontinued immediately and therapy to lower blood pressure should be instituted. Fever should be managed by means of external cooling.

Chlorpheniramine has an atropine-like action and should be used with caution in patients with increased intraocular pressure, cardiovascular disease, hypertension or in patients with a history of bronchial asthma.

Head Injury and Increased Intracranial Pressure: The respiratory depressant effects of narcotics and their capacity to elevate cerebrospinal fluid pressure may be markedly exaggerated in the presence of head injury, other intracranial lesions or a preexisting increase in intracranial pressure. Furthermore, narcotics produce adverse reactions which may obscure the clinical course of patients with head injuries.

Acute Abdominal Conditions: The administration of narcotics may obscure the diagnosis or clinical course of patients with acute abdominal conditions.

PRECAUTIONS

Special Risk Patients: As with any narcotic, Chlorpheniramine Maleate/Hydrocodone Bitartrate/Pseudoephedrine HCl syrup should be used with caution in elderly or debilitated patients and those with severe impairment of hepatic or renal function, hypothyroidism, Addison's disease, prostatic hypertrophy or urethral stricture. The usual precautions should be observed and the possibility of respiratory depression should be kept in mind.

Information for Patients: Narcotics and antihistamines may impair the mental and physical abilities required for the performance of potentially hazardous tasks, such as driving a vehicle or operating machinery. Patients should also be warned about the possible additive effects with alcohol and other central nervous system depressants (hypnotics, sedatives, tranquilizers).

Drug Interactions: Patients receiving other narcotics, antipsychotics, antianxiety agents, or other CNS depressants (including alcohol) concomitantly with Chlorpheniramine Maleate/Hydrocodone Bitartrate/Pseudoephedrine HCl syrup may exhibit an additive CNS depression. When combined therapy is contemplated, the dose of one or both agents should be reduced.

The use of MAO inhibitors or tricyclic antidepressants with Hydrocodone preparations may increase the effect of either the antidepressant or Hydrocodone.

The concurrent use of anticholinergics with Hydrocodone may produce paralytic ileus.

Beta-adrenergic blockers and MAO inhibitors may potentiate the pressor effects of Pseudoephedrine. Concurrent use of digitalis glycosides may increase the possibility of cardiac arrhythmias. Sympathomimetics may reduce the hypotensive effects of guanethidine, mecamylamine, methyldopa, reserpine, and veratrum alkaloids. Concurrent use of tricyclic antidepressants may antagonize the effects of Pseudoephedrine.

Laboratory Test Interactions: Antihistamines may suppress the wheal and flare reactions to antigen skin testing. Considerable interindividual variation in the extent and duration of suppression have been reported, depending on the antigen and test technique, antihistamine and dosage regimen, time since last dose and individual response to testing. In one study, usual oral dosages of Chlorpheniramine suppressed the wheal response for about 2 days after the last dose. Whenever possible, antihistamines should be discontinued about 4 days prior to skin testing

procedures since they may prevent otherwise positive reactions to dermal reactivity indicators.

Carcinogenesis, Mutagenesis and Impairment of Fertility: No long-term or reproduction studies in animals have been performed with Chlorpheniramine Maleate/Hydrocodone Bitartrate/Pseudoephedrine HCl syrup to evaluate its carcinogenic, mutagenic and impairment of fertility potential.

Usage in Pregnancy

Teratogenic Effects: Pregnancy Category C. Hydrocodone has been shown to be teratogenic in hamsters when given in doses 700 times the human dose. There are no adequate and well-controlled studies in pregnant women. Chlorpheniramine Maleate/Hydrocodone Bitartate/Pseudoephedrine HCl syrup should be used during pregnancy only if the potential benefit justifies the potential risk to the fetus.

Nonteratogenic Effects: Babies born to mothers who have been taking opioids regularly prior to delivery will be physically dependent. The withdrawal signs include irritability and excessive crying, tremors, hyperactive reflexes, increased respiratory rate, increased stools, sneezing, yawning, vomiting and fever. The intensity of the syndrome does not always correlate with the duration of maternal opioid use or dose. There is no concensus on the best method of managing withdrawal. Chlorpromazine 0.7 to 1 mg/kg q6h, and paregoric 2 to 4 drops q4h, have been used to treat withdrawal symptoms in infants. The duration of therapy is 4 to 28 days, with the dosage decreased as tolerated.

Labor and Delivery: As with all narcotics, adminstration of Chlorpheniramine Maleate/Hydrocodone Bitartrate/Pseudoephedrine HCl syrup to the mother shortly before delivery may result in some degree of respiratory depression in the newborn, especially if higher doses are used.

Nursing Mothers: Chlorpheniramine Maleate/Hydrocodone Bitartrate/Pseudoephedrine HCl syrup is contraindicated in nursing mothers because of the higher than usual risk for infants with sympathomimetic amines.

Pediatric Use: Antihistamines may cause excitability, especially in children. Do not exceed recommended dosage because at higher doses nervousness, dizziness, or sleeplessness may occur.

In young children, as well as adults, the respiratory center is sensitive to the depressant action of narcotic cough suppressants in a dose-dependent manner. Benefit to risk ratio should be carefully considered, especially in children with respiratory embarrassment (e.g., croup).

Use in the Elderly: The elderly (60 years and older) are more likely to have adverse reactions to sympathomimetics. Overdosage of sympathomimetics in this age group may cause hallucinations, convulsions, CNS depression and death.

ADVERSE REACTIONS

CHLORPHENIRAMINE MALEATE

Slight to moderate drowsiness may occur and is the most frequent side effect. Other possible side effects of antihistamines in general include:

General: Urticaria, drug rash, anaphylactic shock, photosensitivity, excessive perspiration, chills, dryness of mouth, nose and throat.

Cardiovascular: Hypotension, headache, palpitation, tachycardia, extrasystoles.

Hematological: Hemolytic anemia, thrombocytopenia, agranulocytosis.

CNS: Sedation, dizziness, disturbed coordination, fatigue, confusion, restlessness, excitation, nervousness, tremor, irritability, insomnia, euphoria, paresthesia, blurred vision, diplopia, vertigo, tinnitus, hysteria, neuritis, convulsion.

Gastrointestinal: Epigastric distress, anorexia, nausea, vomiting, diarrhea, constipation.

Genitourinary: Urinary frequency, difficult urination, urinary retention, early menses.

Respiratory: Thickening of bronchial secretions, tightness of chest, wheezing and nasal stiffness.

HYDROCODONE BITARTRATE

The most frequently observed adverse reactions include lightheadedness, dizziness, sedation, nausea and vomiting. These effects seem to be more prominent in ambulatory patients than in nonambulatory patients and some of these adverse reactions may be alleviated if the patient lies down.

Other adverse reactions include:

Central Nervous System: Drowsiness, mental clouding, lethargy, impairment of mental and physical performance, anxiety, fear, dysphoria, psychic dependence, mood changes.

Gastrointestinal System: Prolonged administration may produce constipation.

Genitourinary System: Ureteral spasm, spasm of vesical sphincters and urinary retention have been reported.

PSEUDOEPHEDRINE HYDROCHLORIDE

Pseudoephedrine may cause mild central nervous system stimulation, especially in those patients who are hypersensitive to sympathomimetic drugs. Nervousness, excitability, restlessness, dizziness, weakness and insomnia may also occur. Headache and drowsiness have also been reported. Large doses may cause lightheadedness, nausea and/or vomiting. Sympathomimetic drugs have also been associated with certain untoward reactions including fear, anxiety, tenseness, restlessness, tremor, weakness, pallor, respiratory difficulty, dysuria, insomnia, hallucination, convulsion, CNS depression, arrhythmias and cardiovascular collapse with hypotension.

DRUG ABUSE AND DEPENDENCE

Chlorpheniramine Maleate/Hydrocodone Bitartrate/Pseudoephedrine HCl syrup is subject to the Federal Controlled Substances Act (Schedule III).

Psychic dependence, physical dependence, and tolerance may develop upon repeated administration of narcotics; therefore, Chlorpheniramine Maleate/Hydrocodone Bitartrate/Pseudoephedrine HCl syrup should be prescribed and administered with caution. However, psychic dependence is unlikely to develop when Chlorpheniramine Maleate/Hydrocodone Bitartrate/Pseudoephedrine HCl syrup is used for a short time.

Physical dependence, the condition in which continued administration of the drug is required to prevent the appearance of a withdrawal syndrome, assumes clinically significant proportions only after several weeks of continued narcotic use, although some mild degree of physical dependence may develop after a few days of narcotic therapy. Tolerance, in which increasingly large doses are required to produce the same degree of effectiveness, is manifested initially by a shortened duration of effect, and subsequently by decreases in the intensity of effect. The rate of development of tolerance varies among patients.

OVERDOSAGE

SIGNS AND SYMPTOMS

Chlorpheniramine: Manifestations of antihistamine overdosage may vary from central nervous system depression (sedation, apnea, cardiovascular collapse) to stimulation (insomnia, hallucinations, tremors or convulsions). Other signs and symptoms may be dizziness, tinnitus, ataxia, blurred vision and hypotension. Stimulation is particularly likely in children, as are atropine-like signs and symptoms (dry mouth, dilated pupils, flushing, hyperthermia), and gastrointestinal symptoms.

Hydrocodone: Serious overdosage with Hydrocodone is characterized by respiratory depression (a decrease in respiratory rate and/or tidal volume, Cheyne-Stokes respiration, cyanosis), extreme somnolence progressing to stupor or coma, skeletal muscle flaccidity, cold and clammy skin, and sometimes bradycardia and hypotension. In severe overdosage, apnea, circulatory collapse, cardiac arrest and death may occur.

Pseudoephedrine: Overdosage with Pseudoephedrine can cause excessive central nervous system stimulation resulting in excitement, nervousness, anxiety, tremor, restlessness, and insomnia. Other effects include tachycardia, hypertension, pallor, mydriasis, hyperglycemia, and urinary retention. Severe overdosage may cause tachypnea, or hyperpnea, hallucinations, convulsions, or delirium, but in some individuals there may be central nervous system depression with somnolence, stupor, or respiratory depression. Arrhythmias (including ventricular fibrillation) may lead to hypotension and circulatory collapse. Severe hypokalemia can occur, probably due to compartmental shift rather than depletion of potassium. No organ damage or significant metabolic arrangement is associated with Pseudoephedrine overdosage. The toxic and lethal concentration in human biologic fluids are not known. Excretion rates increase with urine acidification and decrease with alkalinization. Few reports of toxicity due to Pseudoephedrine have been published, and no case of fatal overdosage is known.

TREATMENT

Primary attention should be given to the reestablishment of adequate respiratory exchange through provision of a patent airway and the institution of assisted or controlled ventilation. The narcotic antagonist naloxone is a specific antidote against respiratory depression which may result from overdosage or unusual sensitivity to narcotics, including Hydrocodone. Therefore, an appropriate dose of naloxone HCl (see package insert) should be administered, preferably by the intravenous route and simultaneously with efforts at respiratory resuscitation. Since the duration of action of Hydrocodone may exceed that of the antagonist, the patient should be kept under continued surveillance and repeated doses of the antagonist should be administered as needed to maintain adequate respiration.

An antagonist should not be administered in the absence of clinically significant respiratory or cardiovascular depression. Oxygen, intravenous fluids, vasopressors and other supportive measures should be employed as indicated.

Gastric emptying may be useful in removing unabsorbed drug.

The patient should be induced to vomit even if emesis has occurred spontaneously; however, vomiting should not be induced in patients with impaired consciousness. Precautions against aspiration should be taken, especially in infants and children.

Ipecac syrup is the preferred method for inducing vomiting. The action of ipecac is facilitated by physical activity and the administration of eight to twelve fluid ounces of water. If emesis does not occur within fifteen minutes, the dose of ipecac should be repeated. Following emesis, any drug remaining in the stomach may be absorbed by activated charcoal administered as a slurry with water.

If vomiting is unsuccessful or contraindicated, gastric lavage should be performed. Isotonic and one-half isotonic saline are the lavage solution of choice. Saline cathartics, such as milk of magnesia, draw water into the bowel by osmosis and, therefore, may be valuable for their action in rapid dilution of bowel content.

Treatment of the signs and symptoms of overdosage is symptomatic and supportive. Vasopressors may be used to treat hypotension. Short-acting barbiturates diazepam or paraldehyde may be administered to control seizures. Hyperpyrexia, especially in children, may require treatment with tepid water sponge baths or a hypothermic blanket. Apnea is treated with ventilatory support. Stimulants (analeptic agents) should not be used.

DOSAGE AND ADMINISTRATION

Adults, 2 teaspoonfuls every 4 to 6 hours. *Children,* 6 to 12 years, 1 teaspoonful every 4 to 6 hours. *Children,* 2 to 6 years, 1/2 teaspoonful every 4 to 6 hours. Do not exceed four doses in a 24 hour period.

Storage: Store at controlled room temperature, 15°-30°C (59°-86°F). Dispense in a tight, light-resistant container with a child-resistant closure. A Schedule CIII Controlled Substance.

HOW SUPPLIED

LIQUID (C-III): 2 MG-2.5 MG-30 MG/5 ML

BRAND/MANUFACTURER	NDC	SIZE	AWP
○ BRAND			
NOTUSS: Stewart Jackson	45985-0621-16	480 ml	$21.19
PANCOF HC: Pan Amer	00525-0744-16	480 ml	$30.40
○ GENERICS			
M-END: McNeil,R.A.	12830-0722-16	480 ml	$14.80

SYRUP (C-III): 2 MG-2.5 MG-30 MG/5 ML

BRAND/MANUFACTURER	NDC	SIZE	AWP
○ BRAND			
P-V-TUSSIN: Solvay	00032-1083-78	480 ml	$50.73
	00032-1083-79	3840 ml	$384.49
○ GENERICS			
HEXATUSSIN: Moore,H.L.	00839-7483-69	480 ml	$14.84
HYPHED: Aligen	00405-0099-16	480 ml	$26.32
TUSSIN-V: Alphagen	59743-0001-16	480 ml	$28.00
Q-V TUSSIN: Qualitest	00603-1609-58	480 ml	$28.00
AMTUSSIN: Econolab	55053-0940-16	480 ml	$38.75
HISTINEX PV: Ethex	58177-0883-07	480 ml	$38.84

Chlorpheniramine Maleate/ Methscopolamine/Phenylephrine Hydrochloride

DESCRIPTION

Each timed action SR capsule contains Phenylephrine Hydrochloride 20 mg; Methscopolamine Nitrate 2.5 mg; Chlorpheniramine Maleate 8 mg. The JR potency is exactly half-strength. Green/red color for both. Each 5 cc of root beer flavored syrup and tablet contains: Phenylephrine Hydrochloride 10 mg; Methscopolamine Nitrate 1.25 mg; Chlorpheniramine Maleate 2 mg.

ACTION AND USES

Antihistaminic-decongestant for relief of respiratory congestion; allergic rhinitis; allergic skin reactions of urticaria and angioedema.

ADMINISTRATION AND DOSAGE

Capsules—one every 12 hours of the SR for adults; one JR every 12 hours for children 6-12 years. Syrup—two teaspoonfuls every 4 hours for adults; children 1 teaspoonful every 4 hours. Tablets—adults two and children one every 4 hours. Do not exceed 4 doses in 24 hours.

Children under 6 years as recommended by a physician.

PRECAUTIONS

Withdraw therapy if drowsiness occurs. Patients are cautioned against driving or operating mechanical devices.

CONTRAINDICATIONS

Glaucoma, cardiac disease, hyperthyroidism and hypertension.

HOW SUPPLIED
CAPSULE:

BRAND/MANUFACTURER	NDC	SIZE	AWP
○ GENERICS			
SINODEC: Primedics	00684-0170-01	100s	$15.90
SINODEC: Primedics	00684-0170-05	500s	$50.00

CAPSULE, EXTENDED RELEASE: 4 MG-1.25 MG-10 MG

BRAND/MANUFACTURER	NDC	SIZE	AWP
○ BRAND			
EXTENDRYL JR.: Fleming	00256-0177-01	100s	$24.50
	00256-0177-02	1000s	$222.50

CAPSULE, EXTENDED RELEASE: 8 MG-2.5 MG-20 MG

BRAND/MANUFACTURER	NDC	SIZE	AWP
○ GENERICS			
EXTENDRYL SR.: Fleming	00256-0111-01	100s	$26.50
PREHIST D: Marnel	00682-0100-01	100s	$28.20
HISTOR-D TIMECELLES: Roberts/Hauck	59441-0147-01	100s	$40.00
EXTENDRYL SR.: Fleming	00256-0111-02	1000s	$244.50
DALLERGY: Laser	00277-0101-03	1000s	$307.37

CHEW TABLET:

BRAND/MANUFACTURER	NDC	SIZE	AWP
○ GENERICS			
D.A. CHEWABLE: Dura	51479-0013-01	100s	$43.51

CHEW TABLET: 2 MG-1.25 MG-10 MG

BRAND/MANUFACTURER	NDC	SIZE	AWP
○ BRAND			
EXTENDRYL CHEWS: Fleming	00256-0133-01	100s	$20.20
	00256-0133-02	1000s	$184.10
○ GENERICS			
AH-CHEW: WE Pharm	59196-0003-01	100s	$33.75

SYRUP: 2 MG-0.625 MG-10 MG

BRAND/MANUFACTURER	NDC	SIZE	AWP
○ GENERICS			
DALLERGY: Laser	00277-0156-01	480 ml	$18.07
DALLERGY: Laser	00277-0156-02	3840 ml	$132.92

SYRUP: 2 MG-1.25 MG-10 MG/5 ML

BRAND/MANUFACTURER	NDC	SIZE	AWP
○ BRAND			
EXTENDRYL SYRUP: Fleming	00256-0127-01	480 ml	$14.10
	00256-0127-02	3840 ml	$102.90

SYRUP: 2 MG-5 MG

BRAND/MANUFACTURER	NDC	SIZE	AWP
○ GENERICS			
HISTOR-D: Roberts/Hauck	59441-0445-16	480 ml	$17.76

TABLET, EXTENDED RELEASE:

BRAND/MANUFACTURER	NDC	SIZE	AWP
○ GENERICS			
DURA-VENT/DA: Dura	51479-0008-01	100s	$59.85

TABLET, EXTENDED RELEASE: 8 MG-2.5 MG-20 MG

BRAND/MANUFACTURER	NDC	SIZE	AWP
○ GENERICS			
OMNIHIST L.A.: WE Pharm	59196-0002-01	100s	$43.75

TABLETS: 4 MG-1.25 MG-10 MG

BRAND/MANUFACTURER	NDC	SIZE	AWP
○ GENERICS			
DALLERGY: Laser	00277-0160-01	100s	$19.38
DALLERGY: Laser	00277-0180-01	100s	$39.98

Chlorpheniramine Maleate/ Phenindamine Tartrate/ Phenylpropanolamine Hydrochloride

DESCRIPTION

Each timed-release tablet contains:

Chlorpheniramine Maleate ....4 mg
Phenindamine Tartrate ....24 mg
Phenylpropanolamine Hydrochloride ....50 mg
Formulated to provide 8 to 12 hours of continuous relief.

INDICATIONS

As a nasal decongestant associated with the common cold, sinusitis, hay fever and other allergies.

CONTRAINDICATIONS

Hypersensitivity to any of the components. Contraindicated in concurrent MAO inhibitor therapy.

SIDE EFFECTS

Nervousness, insomnia, tremors, dizziness and drowsiness may occur occasionally.

PRECAUTIONS

Antihistamines may cause drowsiness and should be used with caution in patients who operate motor vehicles or dangerous machinery. Use with caution in patients with hypertension, cardiovascular disease, diabetes or hyperthyroidism. This product should be used with caution in patients with prostatic hypertrophy or glaucoma.

DOSAGE

Usual adult dose: Orally, one tablet every 8 hours. In mild cases, one tablet every 10 to 12 hours.

Store at controlled room temperature, 15°-30°C (59°-86°F) and keep away from light.

HOW SUPPLIED
LIQUID (C-V):

BRAND/MANUFACTURER	NDC	SIZE	AWP
○ GENERICS			
EFASIN EXPECTORANT SF: Major	00904-3541-16	480 ml	$17.95

TABLET, EXTENDED RELEASE:

BRAND/MANUFACTURER	NDC	SIZE	AWP
○ GENERICS			
AMILON: Moore,H.L.	00839-7710-06	100s	$11.48

TABLET, EXTENDED RELEASE: 4 MG-24 MG-50 MG

BRAND/MANUFACTURER	NDC	SIZE	AWP
○ BRAND			
NOLAMINE: Carnrick	00086-0204-10	100s	$24.65
	00086-0204-25	250s	$49.15

TABLETS:

BRAND/MANUFACTURER	NDC	SIZE	AWP
○ GENERICS			
NORPHENAMINE: Major	00904-2226-60	100s	$14.40
NORPHENAMINE: Major	00904-2226-40	500s	$64.30

Chlorpheniramine Maleate/ Phenylephrine Hydrochloride/ Phenylpropanolamine Hydrochloride/Phenyltoloxamine Citrate

DESCRIPTION

This preparation contains: (1) Phenylpropanolamine Hydrochloride—Benzenemethanol, α-(1-aminoethyl)- hydrochloride, (2) Phenylephrine Hydrochloride—1-m-hydroxy-α-[(methylamino)methyl]benzyl alcohol hydrochloride, (3) Phenyltoloxamine Citrate—N, N-dimethyl-2(alpha phenyl-ortho-toloxy)-ethylamine citrate, (4) Chlorpheniramine Maleate—2-[p-chloro-α-[2-(dimethylamino)ethyl]benzyl] pyridine maleate.

Each sustained-action tablet contains:	For immediate action	For delayed action	Total contents
Phenylpropanolamine Hydrochloride	20.0 mg	20.0 mg	40.0 mg
Phenylephrine Hydrochloride	5.0 mg	5.0 mg	10.0 mg
Phenyltoloxamine Citrate	7.5 mg	7.5 mg	15.0 mg
Chlorpheniramine Maleate ...	2.5 mg	2.5 mg	5.0 mg

Each teaspoonful (5 mL) of syrup contains:

Phenylpropanolamine Hydrochloride ....20.0 mg	
Phenylephrine Hydrochloride ....5.0 mg	
Phenyltoloxamine Citrate ....7.5 mg	
Chlorpheniramine Maleate ....2.5 mg	

Each pediatric formulation contains the following ingredients:	Pediatric Syrup each 5 mL contains:	Pediatric Drops each 1 mL contains:
Phenylpropanolamine Hydrochloride .	5.0 mg	5.0 mg
Phenylephrine Hydrochloride	1.25 mg	1.25 mg
Phenyltoloxamine Citrate	2.0 mg	2.0 mg
Chlorpheniramine Maleate	0.5 mg	0.5 mg

◆ RATED THERAPEUTICALLY EQUIVALENT; ◇ THERAPEUTIC EQUIVALENCE UNCONFIRMED; ○ UNRATED

CLINICAL PHARMACOLOGY

PHENYLPROPANOLAMINE HYDROCHLORIDE

The drug may directly stimulate adrenergic receptors but probably indirectly stimulates both alpha (α) and beta (β) adrenergic receptors by releasing norepinephrine from its storage sites. Phenylpropanolamine increases heart rate, force of contraction and cardiac output, and excitability. It acts on α receptors in the mucosa of the respiratory tract, producing vasoconstriction which results in shrinkage of swollen mucous membranes, reduction of tissue hyperemia, edema and nasal congestion, and an increase in nasal airway patency. Phenylpropanolamine causes CNS stimulation and reportedly has an anorexigenic effect.

PHENYLEPHRINE HYDROCHLORIDE

Phenylephrine acts predominantly by a direct action on alpha (α) adrenergic receptors. In therapeutic doses, the drug has no significant stimulant effect on the beta (β) adrenergic receptors of the heart. Following oral administration, construction of blood vessels in the nasal mucosa may relieve nasal congestion. In therapeutic doses the drug causes little, if any, central nervous system stimulation.

PHENYLTOLOXAMINE CITRATE

Phenyltoloxamine is an H_1 blocking agent which interferes with the action of histamine primarily in capillaries surrounding mucous tissues and sensory nerves of nasal and adjacent areas. It has the ability to interfere with certain actions of acetylcholine-inhibiting secretions in the nose, mouth and pharynx. It commonly causes CNS depression.

CHLORPHENIRAMINE MALEATE

Chlorpheniramine competitively antagonizes most of the smooth muscle stimulating actions of histamine on the H_1 receptors of the GI tract, uterus, large blood vessels and bronchial muscle. It also antagonizes the action of histamine that results in increased capillary permeability and the formation of edema.

INDICATIONS AND USAGE

For the relief of nasal congestion and eustachian tube congestion associated with the common cold, sinusitis and acute upper respiratory infections. Also indicated for symptomatic relief of perennial and seasonal allergic rhinitis, vasomotor rhinitis.

Decongestants in combination with antihistamines have been used to relieve eustachian tube congestion associated with acute eustachian salpingitis, aerotitis and serous otitis media.

CONTRAINDICATIONS

Patients with severe hypertension, severe coronary artery disease, patients on MAO inhibitor therapy; patients with narrow angle glaucoma, urinary retention, peptic ulcer and during an asthmatic attack. Also contraindicated in patients with hypersensitivity or idiosyncrasy to sympathominetic amines or antihistamines.

WARNINGS

Sympathomimetic amines should be used judiciously and sparingly in patients with hypertension, diabetes mellitus, ischemic heart disease, increased intraocular pressure, hyperthyroidism or prostatic hypertrophy. See, however, *"Contraindications"*. Sympathomimetics may produce central nervous system stimulation with convulsions or cardiovascular collapse with accompanying hypotension.

Antihistamines may impair mental and physical abilities required for the performance of potentially hazardous tasks, such as driving a vehicle or operating machinery, and may impair mental alertness in children. Chlorpheniramine and Phenyltoloxamine have an atropine-like action and should be used with caution in patients with increased intraocular pressure, cardiovascular disease, hypertension or in patients with a history of bronchial asthma. See, however, *"Contraindications"*.

Do not exceed recommended dosage.

PRECAUTIONS

Patients with diabetes, hypertension, cardiovascular disease and hyperreactivity to ephedrine. The antihistaminics may cause drowsiness and ambulatory patients who operate machinery or motor vehicles should be cautioned accordingly.

DRUG INTERACTIONS

MAO inhibitors and beta adrenergic blockers increase the effect of sympathomimetics. Sympathomimetics may reduce the antihypertensive effects of methyldopa, mecamylamine, reserpine and veratrum alkaloids. Concomitant use of antihistamines with alcohol, tricyclic antidepressants, barbiturates and other CNS depressants may have an additive effect.

PREGNANCY CATEGORY C

Animal reproduction studies have not been conducted with this combination drug. It is also not known whether it can cause fetal harm when administered to a pregnant woman or can affect reproductive capacity. It should be given to a pregnant woman only if clearly needed.

NURSING MOTHERS

Caution should be exercised when this drug is given to nursing mothers due to the higher than usual risk of the sympathomimetic amines in infants.

ADVERSE REACTIONS

Hyperreactive individuals may display ephedrine-like reactions such as tachycardia, palpitations, headache, dizziness or nausea. Patients sensitive to antihistamines may experience mild sedation. Sympathomimetics have been associated with certain untoward reactions including restlessness, tremor, weakness, pallor, respiratory difficulty, dysuria, insomnia, hallucinations, convulsions, CNS depression, arrhythmias and cardiovascular collapse with hypotension. Possible side effects of antihistamines are drowsiness, restlessness, dizziness, weakness, dry mouth, anorexia, nausea, vomiting, headache, nervousness, blurring of vision, polyuria, heartburn, dysuria and, very rarely, dermatitis.

OVERDOSAGE

In the event of overdosage, emergency treatment should be started immediately.

Symptoms: Overdosage symptoms may vary from central nervous system depression to stimulation. Symptoms may include: nervousness, dry mouth, possible convulsions, respiratory failure, acute hypertension. In both children and adults, coma and cardiovascular collapse may occur.

Management: It is suggested that the management principles (consistent with the clinical status of the patient when first seen) outlined below be instituted and that simultaneous contact with a Regional Poison Control Center be established. In this way both updated information and individualization regarding required therapy may be provided.

Induction of emesis and gastric lavage may be performed if the patient is alert and seen within early hours after ingestion. Drug remaining in the stomach may be adsorbed by the administration of activated charcoal.

Respiratory distress should be treated promptly. *Stimulants* (analeptic agents) should not be used because they may precipitate convulsions. Use of a short-acting barbiturate is recommended if convulsions or marked CNS excitement occur.

DOSAGE AND ADMINISTRATION

This chart represents single dosages for the products listed below. Usual dosage schedule for pediatric drops, pediatric syrup and syrup is every 3 to 4 hours, not to exceed four doses in a 24-hour period. For sustained-action tablets, doses should be administered on arising, in midafternoon, and at bedtime. (See related table).

HOW SUPPLIED
CAPSULE, EXTENDED RELEASE:

BRAND/MANUFACTURER	NDC	SIZE	AWP
○ GENERICS			
Jerome Stevens	50564-0510-01	100s	$22.38

DROP:

BRAND/MANUFACTURER	NDC	SIZE	AWP
○ BRAND			
NALDECON PEDIATRIC: Apothecon	00015-5615-30	30 ml	$19.34
○ GENERICS			
Goldline	00182-6091-66	30 ml	$7.50
NALDELATE PEDIATRIC: Moore,H.L.	00839-7648-63	30 ml	$8.09
NALPHEN PEDIATRIC: Hi-Tech	50383-0765-01	30 ml	$10.00
NALDA-RELIEF PEDIATRIC: Liquipharm	54198-0134-30	30 ml	$10.00
NALGEST PEDIATRIC: Major	00904-1011-30	30 ml	$10.10
TRI-PHEN-CHLOR PEDIATRIC: Rugby	00536-2195-75	30 ml	$10.32
NALDELATE PEDIATRIC: Barre	00472-0809-31	30 ml	$11.48
TRI-PHEN-MINE: Goldline	00182-6123-66	30 ml	$12.30
NALDELATE PEDIATRIC: Qualitest	00603-1465-45	30 ml	$12.50
SINUCON PEDIATRIC: Norton,HN	50732-0865-30	30 ml	$13.75

SYRUP:

BRAND/MANUFACTURER	NDC	SIZE	AWP
○ BRAND			
NALDECON PEDIATRIC: Apothecon	00015-5616-60	480 ml	$45.80
NALDECON: Apothecon	00015-5601-60	480 ml	$49.27
○ GENERICS			
SINUCON PEDIATRIC: Norton,HN	50732-0831-04	118 ml	$8.48
NALPHEN PEDIATRIC: Hi-Tech	50383-0764-04	120 ml	$2.30
NALDELATE PEDIATRIC: Barre	00472-1007-04	120 ml	$2.77
NALDELATE PEDIATRIC: Phys Formlry	53261-0531-91	120 ml	$4.69
SINUCON PEDIATRIC: Norton,HN	50732-0831-16	473 ml	$24.52
SINUCON: Norton,HN	50732-0832-16	473 ml	$27.61
Goldline	00182-1495-40	480 ml	$6.00
QUADRAHIST PEDIATRIC: Schein	00364-7332-16	480 ml	$6.30
NALDELATE PEDIATRIC: Moore,H.L.	00839-7033-69	480 ml	$6.68
NALPHEN PEDIATRIC: Hi-Tech	50383-0764-16	480 ml	$6.80
NALGEST: Major	00904-1004-16	480 ml	$6.90
NALGEST PEDIATRIC: Major	00904-1010-16	480 ml	$6.90
NALPHEN: Hi-Tech	50383-0763-16	480 ml	$7.20
NALDELATE PEDIATRIC: Barre	00472-1007-16	480 ml	$7.48
NALDELATE: Qualitest	00603-1464-58	480 ml	$7.55

➤ SHOWN IN PRODUCT IDENTIFICATION GUIDE

Single Dosage for...	Pediatric Drops	Pediatric Syrup	Syrup	Tablets
3 to 6 months (12.17 lbs)	¼ mL			
6 to 12 months (17.24 lbs)	½ mL	½ teaspoonful		
1 to 6 years (24.50 lbs)	1 mL	1 teaspoonful		
6 to 12 years (over 50 lbs)		2 teaspoonfuls	½ teaspoonful	½ tablet
over 12 years			1 teaspoonful	1 tablet

BRAND/MANUFACTURER	NDC	SIZE	AWP
NALDELATE PEDIATRIC: Qualitest	00603-1466-58	480 ml	$7.55
NALDELATE: URL	00677-0770-33	480 ml	$7.90
NALDELATE: Moore,H.L.	00839-6055-69	480 ml	$8.00
NALDELATE PEDIATRIC: URL	00677-0776-33	480 ml	$8.05
NALDELATE: Barre	00472-0801-16	480 ml	$8.20
TRI-PHEN-CHLOR: Rugby	00536-2190-85	480 ml	$8.93
TRI-PHEN-CHLOR PEDIATRIC: Rugby	00536-2180-85	480 ml	$9.30
SINUCON PEDIATRIC: Norton,HN	50732-0831-28	3785 ml	$79.30
SINUCON: Norton,HN	50732-0832-28	3785 ml	$91.99
NALGEST PEDIATRIC: Major	00904-1010-28	3840 ml	$37.45
NALPHEN PEDIATRIC: Hi-Tech	50383-0764-28	3840 ml	$38.00
NALPHEN: Hi-Tech	50383-0763-28	3840 ml	$40.00
NALDELATE PEDIATRIC: Barre	00472-1007-28	3840 ml	$42.23
NALDELATE: Barre	00472-0801-28	3840 ml	$46.95

TABLET, EXTENDED RELEASE:

BRAND/MANUFACTURER	NDC	SIZE	AWP
○ **BRAND**			
NALDECON: Apothecon	00015-5600-60	100s	$85.68
	00015-5600-80	500s	$416.94
○ **GENERICS**			
DECONGESTABS: Parmed	00349-2315-01	100s	$4.02
Qualitest	00603-3120-21	100s	$5.41
DECONGESTABS: Moore,H.L.	00839-1430-06	100s	$5.66
WEST-DECON: West-Ward	00143-1279-01	100s	$5.70
Geneva	00781-1576-01	100s	$5.75
NALGEST: Major	00904-1003-60	100s	$6.85
TRI-PHEN-MINE: Goldline	00182-1094-01	100s	$6.90
NALSPAN: Rosemont	00832-1086-00	100s	$7.75
UNI DECON: URL	00677-0472-01	100s	$9.16
TRI-PHEN-CHLOR: Rugby	00536-5655-01	100s	$9.29
PROP-A-HIST: Bolan	44437-0248-01	100s	$44.65
WEST-DECON: West-Ward	00143-1279-05	500s	$25.60
TRI-PHEN-CHLOR: Rugby	00536-5655-05	500s	$31.80
DECONGESTABS: Parmed	00349-2315-10	1000s	$28.84
WEST-DECON: West-Ward	00143-1279-10	1000s	$33.00
Qualitest	00603-3120-32	1000s	$38.40
UNI DECON: URL	00677-0472-10	1000s	$41.34
DECONGESTABS: Moore,H.L.	00839-1430-16	1000s	$43.19
Geneva	00781-1576-10	1000s	$44.75
TRI-PHEN-CHLOR: Rugby	00536-5655-10	1000s	$45.38
NALGEST: Major	00904-1003-80	1000s	$53.85
TRI-PHEN-MINE: Goldline	00182-1094-10	1000s	$57.75
NALSPAN: Rosemont	00832-1086-10	1000s	$77.50

Chlorpheniramine Maleate/ Phenylephrine Hydrochloride/ Phenylpropanolamine Hydrochloride/Pyrilamine Maleate

DESCRIPTION

Each Chlorpheniramine Maleate/Phenylephrine Hydrochloride/ Phenylpropanolamine Hydrochloride/Pyrilamine Maleate tablet contains:

Phenylpropanolamine HCl	50 mg
Pyrilamine Maleate	25 mg
Chlorpheniramine Maleate	4 mg
Phenylephrine HCl	10 mg

CLINICAL PHARMACOLOGY

PHENYLPROPANOLAMINE HYDROCHLORIDE

The drug may directly stimulate adrenergic receptors, but probably indirectly stimulates both alpha (α) and beta (β) adrenergic receptors by releasing norepinephrine from its storage sites. Phenylpropanolamine increases heart rate, force of contraction and cardiac output, and excitability. It acts on alpha receptors in the mucosa of the respiratory tract, producing vasoconstriction which results in shrinkage of swollen mucous membranes, reduction of tissue, hyperemia, edema

and nasal congestion, and an increase in nasal airway patency. Phenylpropanolamine causes CNS stimulation and reportedly has an anorexigenic effect.

PHENYLEPHRINE HYDROCHLORIDE

Phenylephrine acts predominantly by a direct action on alpha (α) adrenergic receptors. In therapeutic doses the drug has no significant stimulant effect on the beta (β) adrenergic receptors of the heart. Following oral administration, constriction of blood vessels in the nasal mucosa may relieve nasal congestion. In therapeutic doses the drug causes little, if any, central nervous system stimulation.

CHLORPHENIRAMINE MALEATE

Chlorpheniramine is an antihistamine belonging to the alkylamine class. It possesses anticholinergic and sedative effects. It is considered one of the most effective and least toxic of the histamine antagonists. Chlorpheniramine is an H_1 receptor antagonist. It antagonizes many of the pharmacologic actions of histamine. It prevents released histamine from dilating capillaries and causing edema of the respiratory mucosa. Chlorpheniramine has a duration of action of 4 to 6 hours in clinical studies.

PYRILAMINE MALEATE

Pyrilamine is an antihistamine belonging to the ethylenediamine class. Pyrilamine is a highly effective H_1 blocker. Pyrilamine is an especially active H_1 blocking drug which possesses local anesthetic activity. Pyrilamine antagonizes most of the smooth muscle stimulating actions of histamine on the H_1 receptors of the gastro-intestinal tract, blood vessels and bronchial muscle. It also antagonizes the actions of histamine that results in increased capillary permeability and the formation of edema. Pyrilamine has a duration of action of 4 to 6 hours in clinical studies.

INDICATIONS AND USAGE

This combination is indicated for symptomatic relief in allergic rhinitis, allergic bronchitis, bronchospasm, hay fever, common cold, sinusitis and skin allergies.

CONTRAINDICATIONS

This preparation is contraindicated for individuals sensitive to Phenylephrine HCl and antihistamines.

PRECAUTIONS

GENERAL PRECAUTIONS

Administer with caution to patients with hypertension, cardiac or peripheral vascular disease, hyperthyroidism or diabetes.

INFORMATION FOR PATIENTS

This medication may cause drowsiness. Patients should be advised not to drive a car or operate dangerous machinery while taking this medication.

USAGE IN PREGNANCY

Pregnancy Category C. Animal reproduction studies have not been conducted with this combination. It is also not known whether this combination can cause fetal harm when administered to a pregnant woman or can affect reproductive capacity. This combination should be given to a pregnant woman only if clearly needed.

DOSAGE AND ADMINISTRATION

Adults and children over 12, one tablet 2-3 times daily. Children 6-12, 1/2 tablet 2-3 times daily. Children under 6, only as directed by physician.
   Do not exceed recommended dosage.
   Store at controlled room temperature, 15°C-30°C (59°-86°F).

HOW SUPPLIED
SUSPENSION:

BRAND/MANUFACTURER	NDC	SIZE	AWP
○ **GENERICS**			
TRIPLE TANNATE PEDIATRIC: Hi-Tech	50383-0808-16	480 ml	$22.00

TABLET, EXTENDED RELEASE:

BRAND/MANUFACTURER	NDC	SIZE	AWP
○ **GENERICS**			
DUOHIST FORTE L.A.:	52765-1371-03	30s	$19.95
VANEX FORTE: Abana	12463-0125-01	100s	$51.24
DUOHIST FORTE L.A.:	52765-1371-02	250s	$129.95

◆ RATED THERAPEUTICALLY EQUIVALENT; ◇ THERAPEUTIC EQUIVALENCE UNCONFIRMED; ○ UNRATED

TABLETS:

BRAND/MANUFACTURER	NDC	SIZE	AWP
○ **BRAND**			
POLY HIST FORTE: Poly	50991-0101-01	100s	$35.75
HISTALET FORTE: Solvay	00032-1039-01	100s	$72.45
	00032-1039-07	250s	$176.02
○ **GENERICS**			
LANTUSS FORTE: Columbia Drug	11735-0026-11	100s	$17.00
HISTATIME FORTE: Major	00904-3466-60	100s	$22.35
LANTUSS FORTE: Columbia Drug	11735-0026-12	500s	$72.00

Chlorpheniramine Maleate/ Phenylephrine Hydrochloride/ Phenyltoloxamine Citrate

DESCRIPTION

Each yellow and clear capsule for oral administration contains:

Chlorpheniramine Maleate ....4 mg
Phenyltoloxamine Citrate ....50 mg
Phenylephrine Hydrochloride ....20 mg

in a special base to provide a prolonged therapeutic effect. This product contains ingredients of the following therapeutic classes: antihistamine and decongestant.

Chlorpheniramine Maleate is an antihistamine having the chemical name γ-(4-chlorophenyl)-N,N-dimethyl-2-pyridine-propanamine, (Z)-2-butenedioate(1:1).

Phenyltoloxamine Citrate is an antihistamine having the chemical name N,N-dimethyl-2-(α-phenyl-o-tolyloxy) ethylamine dihydrogen Citrate.

Phenylephrine Hydrochloride is a decongestant having the chemical name 3-hydroxy-α[(methylamino)methyl]benzene-methanol   Hydrochloride.

CLINICAL PHARMACOLOGY

Chlorpheniramine Maleate is an alkylamine-type antihistamine while phenyltoloxamine Citrate belongs to the ethanolamine chemical class. The antihistamines in Chlorpheniramine/Phenylephrine/Phenyltoloxamine act by competing with histamine for H_1 histamine receptor sites, thereby preventing the action of histamine on the cell. Clinically, chlorpheniramine and phenyltoloxamine suppress the histamine-mediated symptoms of allergic rhinitis, relieving sneezing, rhinorrhea, and itching of the eyes, nose, and throat.

Phenylephrine Hydrochloride is an α-adrenergic receptor agonist (sympathomimetic) which produces vasoconstriction by stimulating α-receptors within the mucosa of the respiratory tract. Clinically, Phenylephrine shrinks swollen mucous membranes, reduces tissue hyperemia, edema, and nasal congestion, and increases nasal airway patency.

INDICATIONS AND USAGE

Chlorpheniramine/Phenylephrine/Phenyltoloxamine is indicated for the relief of rhinorrhea and congestion associated with seasonal and/or perennial allergic rhinitis and vasomotor rhinitis.

CONTRAINDICATIONS

Chlorpheniramine/Phenylephrine/Phenyltoloxamine is contraindicated in persons hypersensitive to any of its components. It should not be administered to children under 12 years of age, patients with severe hypertension, narrow angle glaucoma, or asthmatic symptoms, or patients taking monoamine oxidase inhibitors.

WARNINGS

Chlorpheniramine Maleate and Phenyltoloxamine Citrate should be used with extreme caution in patients with stenosing peptic ulcer, pyloroduodenal obstruction, prostatic hypertrophy, or bladder neck obstruction. These compounds have an atropine-like action and therefore should be used with caution in patients with a history of bronchial asthma, increased intraocular pressure, cardiovascular disease, or hypertension. Sympathomimetic amines should be used with caution in patients with hypertension, diabetes mellitus, heart disease, increased intraocular pressure, hyperthyroidism, or prostatic hypertrophy.

PRECAUTIONS

Information for Patients: This product may cause sedation. Patients should be cautioned against engaging in activities requiring mental alertness, such as driving a car or operating machinery.

Drug Interactions: The sedative effects of Chlorpheniramine Maleate and Phenyltoloxamine Citrate are additive to the CNS depressant effects of alcohol, hypnotics, sedatives, and tranquilizers. Chlorpheniramine/Phenylephrine/Phenyltoloxamine should not be used in patients taking monoamine oxidase inhibitors.

Pregnancy: Pregnancy Category C. Animal reproduction studies have not been conducted with Chlorpheniramine/Phenylephrine/Phenyltoloxamine. It is also not known whether Chlorpheniramine/Phenylephrine/Phenyltoloxamine can cause fetal harm when administered to a pregnant woman or can affect reproduction capacity Chlorpheniramine/Phenylephrine/Phenyltolaxamine should be given to pregnant women only if clearly needed.

Nursing Mothers: It is not known whether the drugs in Chlorpheniramine/Phenylephrine/Phenyltoloxamine are excreted in human milk. Because many drugs are excreted in human milk and because of the potential for serious adverse reactions in nursing infants, a decision should be made whether to discontinue nursing or to discontinue the product, taking into account the importance of the drug to the mother.

Pediatric Use: Safety and effectiveness of Chlorpheniramine/Phenylephrine/Phenyltoloxamine in children below the age of 12 have not been established.

ADVERSE REACTIONS

General: Urticaria, drug rash, dryness of mouth, nose, and throat.

Cardiovascular System: Hypotension, headache, palpitations.

Hematologic System: Thrombocytopenia, agranulocytosis, leukopenia.

Nervous System: Sedation, dizziness, excitation (especially in children), nervousness, insomnia, blurred vision, convulsions.

Gastrointestinal System: Epigastric distress, anorexia, nausea, vomiting, diarrhea, constipation.

Genitourinary System: Urinary frequency, urinary retention.

Respiratory System: Thickening of bronchial secretions, tightness of chest and wheezing, nasal stuffiness.

OVERDOSAGE

The treatment of overdosage should provide symptomatic and supportive care. If the amount ingested is considered dangerous or excessive, induce vomiting with ipecac syrup unless the patient is convulsing, comatose, or has lost the gag reflex, in which case perform gastric lavage using a largebore tube. If indicated, follow with activated charcoal and a saline cathartic. Since the effects of Chlorpheniramine/Phenylephrine/Phenyltoloxamine may last up to 12 hours, treatment should be continued for at least that length of time.

DOSAGE AND ADMINISTRATION

Adults and children 12 years of age and older—1 capsule every 8 to 12 hours; not recommended for children under 12 years of age.

HOW SUPPLIED
CAPSULE: 4 MG-20 MG-50 MG

BRAND/MANUFACTURER	NDC	SIZE	AWP
○ **GENERICS**			
Q-HIST LA: Qualitest	00603-5537-21	100s	$26.91
Goldline	00182-1574-01	100s	$33.00

CAPSULE, EXTENDED RELEASE:

BRAND/MANUFACTURER	NDC	SIZE	AWP
○ **GENERICS**			
CHLORTOX: Major	00904-3545-60	100s	$29.25
LINHIST-L.A.: Rugby	00536-3975-01	100s	$30.39

CAPSULE, EXTENDED RELEASE: 4 MG-20 MG-50 MG

BRAND/MANUFACTURER	NDC	SIZE	AWP
○ **BRAND**			
COMHIST LA: Roberts Pharm	54092-0065-01	100s	$69.35
○ **GENERICS**			
LINHIST-L.A.: Econolab	55053-0524-01	100s	$29.95
C-HIST-SR: Alphagen	59743-0057-01	100s	$30.50

TABLETS:

BRAND/MANUFACTURER	NDC	SIZE	AWP
○ **BRAND**			
NALEX-A: Blansett	51674-0008-01	100s	$41.95

TABLETS: 2 MG-10 MG-25 MG

BRAND/MANUFACTURER	NDC	SIZE	AWP
○ **BRAND**			
COMHIST: Roberts Pharm	54092-0066-01	100s	$54.82

Chlorpheniramine Polistirex with Hydrocodone Polistirex

DESCRIPTION

Each teaspoonful (5 mL) of Chlorpheniramine Polistirex/Hydrocodone Polistirex Extended-Release Suspension contains Hydrocodone Polistirex equivalent to 10 mg of Hydrocodone bitartrate (Warning: May be habit-forming) and Chlorpheniramine Polistirex equivalent to 8 mg of Chlorpheniramine maleate. Chlorpheni-rame Polistirex/Hydrocone Polistirex (CPM/Hydrocodone) Extended-Release Suspension provides up to 12-hour relief per dose. Hydrocodone is a centrally-acting narcotic antitussive. Chlorpheniramine is an antihistamine. CPM/Hydrocodone Extended-Release Suspension is for oral use only.

Hydrocodone Polistirex: sulfonated styrene-divinylbenzene copolymer complex with 4,5α-epoxy-3-methoxy-17-methyl-morphinan-6-one.

Chlorpheniramine Polistirex: sulfonated styrene-divinyl-benzene copolymer complex with 2-[*p*-chloro-α-[2-(dimethylamino)ethyl]-benzyl]pyridine.

CLINICAL PHARMACOLOGY

Hydrocodone is a semisynthetic narcotic antitussive and analgesic with multiple actions qualitatively similar to those of codeine. The precise mechanism of action of Hydrocodone and other opiates is not known; however, Hydrocodone is believed to act directly on the cough center. In excessive doses, Hydrocodone, like other opium derivatives, will depress respiration. The effects of Hydrocodone in therapeutic doses on the cardiovascular system are insignificant. Hydrocodone can produce miosis, euphoria, physical and psychological dependence.

Chlorpheniramine is an antihistamine drug (H_1 receptor antagonist) that also possesses anticholinergic and sedative activity. It prevents released histamine from dilating capillaries and causing edema of the respiratory mucosa.

Hydrocodone release from CPM/Hydrocodone Extended-Release Suspension is controlled by an extended-release drug delivery system which combines an ion-exchange polymer matrix with a diffusion rate-limiting permeable coating. Chlorpheniramine release is prolonged by use of an ion-exchange polymer system.

Following multiple dosing with CPM/Hydrocodone Extended-Release Suspension, Hydrocodone mean (S.D.) peak plasma concentrations of 22.8 (5.9) ng/mL occurred at 3.4 hours. Chlorpheniramine mean (S.D.) peak plasma concentrations of 58.4 (14.7) ng/mL occurred at 6.3 hours following multiple dosing. Peak plasma levels obtained with an immediate-release syrup occurred at approximately 1.5 hours for Hydrocodone and 2.8 hours for Chlorpheniramine. The plasma half-lives of Hydrocodone and Chlorpheniramine have been reported to be approximately 4 and 16 hours, respectively.

INDICATIONS AND USAGE

CPM/Hydrocodone Extended-Release Suspension is indicated for relief of cough and upper respiratory symptoms associated with allergy or a cold.

CONTRAINDICATIONS

Known allergy or sensitivity to Hydrocodone or Chlorpheniramine.

WARNINGS

Respiratory Depression: As with all narcotics, CPM/Hydrocodone Extended-Release Suspension produces dose-related respiratory depression by directly acting on brain stem respiratory centers. Hydrocodone affects the center that controls respiratory rhythm, and may produce irregular and periodic breathing. Caution should be exercised when CPM/Hydrocodone Extended-Release Suspension is used postoperatively and in patients with pulmonary disease or whenever ventilatory function is depressed. If respiratory depression occurs, it may be antagonized by the use of naloxone hydrochloride and other supportive measures when indicated (see *"Overdosage"*).

Head Injury and Increased Intracranial Pressure: The respiratory depressant effects of narcotics and their capacity to elevate cerebrospinal fluid pressure may be markedly exaggerated in the presence of head injury, other intracranial lesions or a pre-existing increase in intracranial pressure. Furthermore, narcotics produce adverse reactions which may obscure the clinical course of patients with head injuries.

Acute Abdominal Conditions: The administration of narcotics may obscure the diagnosis or clinical course of patients with acute abdominal conditions.

Obstructive Bowel Disease: Chronic use of narcotics may result in obstructive bowel disease especially in patients with underlying intestinal motility disorder.

Pediatric Use: In young children, as well as adults, the respiratory center is sensitive to the depressant action of narcotic cough suppressants in a dose-dependent manner. Benefit to risk ratio should be carefully considered especially in children with respiratory embarrassment (e.g., croup) (see *"Precautions"*).

PRECAUTIONS

General: Caution is advised when prescribing this drug to patients with narrow-angle glaucoma, asthma or prostatic hypertrophy.

Special Risk Patients: As with any narcotic agent CPM/Hydrocodone Extended-Release Suspension should be used with caution in elderly or debilitated patients and those with severe impairment of hepatic or renal function, hypothyroidism, Addison's disease, prostatic hypertrophy or urethral stricture. The usual precautions should be observed and the possibility of respiratory depression should be kept in mind.

Information for Patients: As with all narcotics, CPM/Hydrocodone Extended-Release Suspension may produce marked drowsiness and impair the mental and/or physical abilities required for the performance of potentially hazardous tasks such as driving a car or operating machinery; patients should be cautioned accordingly. CPM/Hydrocodone Extended-Release Suspension must not be diluted with fluids or mixed with other drugs as this may alter the resin-binding and change the absorption rate, possibly increasing the toxicity.

Keep out of the reach of children.

Cough Reflex: Hydrocodone suppresses the cough reflex; as with all narcotics, caution should be exercised when CPM/Hydrocodone Extended-Release Suspension is used postoperatively, and in patients with pulmonary disease.

Drug Interactions: Patients receiving narcotics, antihistaminics, antipsychotics, antianxiety agents or other CNS depressants (including alcohol) concomitantly with CPM/Hydrocodone Extended-Release Suspension may exhibit an additive CNS depression. When combined therapy is contemplated, the dose of one or both agents should be reduced.

The use of MAO inhibitors or tricyclic antidepressants with Hydrocodone preparations may increase the effect of either the antidepressant or Hydrocodone.

The concurrent use of other anticholinergics with Hydrocodone may produce paralytic ileus.

Carcinogenesis, Mutagenesis, Impairment of Fertility: Carcinogenicity, mutagenicity and reproductive studies have not been conducted with CPM/Hydrocodone Extended-Release Suspension.

PREGNANCY

Teratogenic Effects—Pregnancy Category C: Hydrocodone has been shown to be teratogenic in hamsters when given in doses 700 times the human dose. There are no adequate and well-controlled studies in pregnant women. CPM/Hydrocodone Extended-Release Suspension should be used during pregnancy only if the potential benefit justifies the potential risk to the fetus.

Nonteratogenic Effects: Babies born to mothers who have been taking opioids regularly prior to delivery will be physically dependent. The withdrawal signs include irritability and excessive crying, tremors, hyperactive reflexes, increased respiratory rate, increased stools, sneezing, yawning, vomiting and fever. The intensity of the syndrome does not always correlate with the duration of maternal opioid use or dose.

Labor and Delivery: As with all narcotics, administration of CPM/Hydrocodone Extended-Release Suspension to the mother shortly before delivery may result in some degree of respiratory depression in the newborn, especially if higher doses are used.

Nursing Mothers: It is not known whether this drug is excreted in human milk. Because many drugs are excreted in human milk and because of the potential for serious adverse reactions in nursing infants from CPM/Hydrocodone Extended-Release Suspension, a decision should be made whether to discontinue nursing or to discontinue the drug, taking into account the importance of the drug to the mother.

Pediatric Use: Safety and effectiveness of CPM/Hydrocodone Extended-Release Suspension in children under six have not been established.

ADVERSE REACTIONS

Central Nervous System: Sedation, drowsiness, mental clouding, lethargy, impairment of mental and physical performance, anxiety, fear, dysphoria, euphoria, dizziness, psychic dependence, mood changes.

Dermatologic System: Rash, pruritus.

Gastrointestinal System: Nausea and vomiting may occur; they are more frequent in ambulatory than in recumbent patients. Prolonged administration of CPM/Hydrocodone Extended-Release Suspension may produce constipation.

Genitourinary System: Ureteral spasm, spasm of vesicle sphincters and urinary retention have been reported with opiates.

Respiratory Depression: CPM/Hydrocodone Extended-Release Suspension may produce dose-related respiratory depression by acting directly on brain stem respiratory centers (see *"Overdosage"*).

Respiratory System: Dryness of the pharynx, occasional tightness of the chest.

DRUG ABUSE AND DEPENDENCE

CPM/Hydrocodone Extended-Release Suspension is a Schedule III narcotic. Psychic dependence, physical dependence and tolerance may develop upon repeated administration of narcotics; therefore CPM/Hydrocodone. Extended-Release Suspension should be prescribed and administered with caution. However, psychic dependence is unlikely to develop when CPM/Hydrocodone Extended-Release Suspension is used for a short time for the treatment of cough. Physical dependence, the condition in which continued administration of the drug is required to prevent the appearance of a withdrawal syndrome, assumes clinically significant proportions only after several weeks of continued oral narcotic use, although some mild degree of physical dependence may develop after a few days of narcotic therapy.

OVERDOSAGE

Signs and Symptoms: Serious overdosage with Hydrocodone is characterized by respiratory depression (a decrease in respiratory rate and/or tidal volume, Cheyne-Stokes respiration, cyanosis), extreme somnolence progressing to stupor or coma, skeletal muscle flaccidity, cold and clammy skin, and sometimes bradycardia and hypotension. Although miosis is characteristic of narcotic overdose, mydriasis may occur in terminal narcosis or severe hypoxia. In severe overdosage apnea, circulatory collapse, cardiac arrest and death may occur. The manifestations of chlorpheniramine overdosage may vary from central nervous system depression to stimulation.

Treatment: Primary attention should be given to the reestablishment of adequate respiratory exchange through provision of a patent airway and the institution of assisted or controlled ventilation. The narcotic antagonist naloxone hydrochloride is a specific antidote for respiratory depression which may result from overdosage or unusual sensitivity to narcotics including Hydrocodone. Therefore, an appropriate dose of naloxone hydrochloride should be administered preferably by the intravenous route, simultaneously with efforts at respiratory resuscitation. Since the duration of action of Hydrocodone in this formulation may exceed that of the antagonist, the patient should be kept under continued surveillance and repeated doses of the antagonist should be administered as needed to maintain

---

adequate respiration. For further information, see full prescribing information for naloxone hydrochloride. An antagonist should not be administered in the absence of clinically significant respiratory depression. Oxygen, intravenous fluids, vasopressors and other supportive measures should be employed as indicated. Gastric emptying may be useful in removing unabsorbed drug.

DOSAGE AND ADMINISTRATION
Shake well before using.

Adults: 1 teaspoonful (5 mL) every 12 hours; do not exceed 2 teaspoonfuls in 24 hours.

Children 6-12: 1/2 teaspoonful every 12 hours; do not exceed 1 teaspoonful in 24 hours.
Not recommended for children under 6 years of age (see *"Precautions"*).
Shake well. Dispense in a well-closed container. Store at 59°-86°F (15°-30°C).

HOW SUPPLIED
SUSPENSION, EXTENDED RELEASE (C-III): 2.5 MG-2 MG/5 ML

BRAND/MANUFACTURER	NDC	SIZE	AWP
○ BRAND			
S-T FORTE 2: Scot-Tussin	00372-0048-08	240 ml	$12.35
	00372-0048-16	480 ml	$24.70
	00372-0048-28	3840 ml	$176.82

SUSPENSION, EXTENDED RELEASE (C-III): 8 MG-10 MG/5 ML

BRAND/MANUFACTURER	NDC	SIZE	AWP
○ BRAND			
TUSSIONEX PENNKINETIC: Fisons Presc	00585-0548-67	480 ml	$75.71
	00585-0548-91	900 ml	$136.54

Chlorpheniramine Tannate with Pseudoephedrine Tannate

DESCRIPTION
Each 5 mL contains:

Chlorpheniramine tannate . . . . 4.5 mg.
Pseudoephedrine tannate . . . . 75.0 mg.

CLINICAL PHARMACOLOGY
Chlorpheniramine Tannate antagonizes the physiological action of histamine by acting as an H1 receptor blocking agent.

Pseudoephedrine Tannate is an orally active sympathomimetic amine and exerts a decongestant action on the nasal mucosa. It does this by vasoconstriction, which results in reduction of tissue hyperemia, edema, nasal congestion and an increase in nasal airway patency. The vasoconstrictive action of Pseudoephedrine is similar to that of ephedrine. In the usual dose it has minimal vasopressor effects.

INDICATIONS
For relief of nasal congestion associated with the common cold, hay fever and other allergies, sinusitis, eustachian tube blockage, and vasomotor and allergic rhinitis.

CONTRAINDICATIONS
Patients with severe hypertension, severe coronary artery disease and patients on MAO inhibitor therapy.

This product is also contraindicated in patients sensitive to antihistamines or sympathomimetic agents.

WARNINGS
Chlorpheniramine Tannate should be used with extreme caution in patients with narrow angle glaucoma; stenosing peptic ulcer; pyloroduodenal obstruction; sympathomatic prostatic hypertrophy; or bladder neck obstruction. Due to its mild atropine-like action, Chlorpheniramine Tannate should be used cautiously in patients with bronchial asthma.

Sympathomimetic amines should be used with caution in patients with hypertension, ischemic heart disease, diabetes mellitis, increased intraocular pressure, hyperthyroidism and prostatic hypertrophy. Sympathomimetics may produce central nervous system stimulation with convulsions or cardiovascular collapse with accompanying hypotension.

PRECAUTIONS
INFORMATION FOR PATIENTS
Antihistamines may impair mental and physical abilities required for the performance of potentially hazardous tasks, such as driving a vehicle or operating machinery. Patients should also be warned about possible additive effects with alcohol and other central nervous system depressants (hypnotics, sedatives, tranquilizers).

DRUG INTERACTIONS
Pseudoephedrine containing drugs should not be given to patients treated with monoamine oxidase (MAO) inhibitors because of the possibility of precipitating a hypertensive crisis. MAO inhibitors also prolong and intensify the anticholinergic effects of antihistamines. Sympathomimetics may reduce the antihypertensive effect of methyldopa, reserpine, veratrum alkaloids and mecamylamine. Alcohol and other sedative drugs will potentiate the sedative effects of chlorpheniramine. Care should be taken in administering this product concomitantly with other sympathomimetic amines since their combined affects on the cardiovascular system may be harmful to the patient.

PREGNANCY
Pregnancy Category C: Animal reproduction studies have not been conducted with this product. It is not known whether this medication can cause fetal harm when administered to a pregnant woman or can affect reproduction capacity. This product should be given to a pregnant woman only if clearly needed.

Nursing Mothers: Due to the possible passage of Pseudoephedrine and Chlorpheniramine into breast milk, and, because of the higher than usual risk for infants from sympathomimetic amines and antihistamines, the benefit to the mother versus the potential risk should be considered and a decision should be made whether to discontinue nursing or to discontinue the drug.

ADVERSE REACTIONS
CHLORPHENIRAMINE TANNATE
Slight to moderate drowsiness may occur and is the most frequent side effect. Other possible side effects of antihistamines in general include:

General: urticaria, drug rash, anaphylactic shock, photosensitivity, excessive perspiration, chills, dryness of mouth, nose and throat;

Cardiovascular: hypotension, headache, palpitation, tachycardia, extrasystoles;

Hematologic: hemolytic anemia, thrombocytopenia, agranulocytosis;

CNS: sedation, dizzyness, disturbed coordination, fatigue, confusion, restlessness, excitation, nervousness, tremor, irritability, insomnia, euphoria, paresthesia, blurred vision, diplopia, vertigo, tinnitus, hysteria, neuritis, convulsion;

Gastrointestinal: epigastric distress, anorexia, nausea, vomiting, diarrhea, constipation;

Genitourinary: urinary frequency, difficult urination, urinary retention, early menses;

Respiratory: thickening of bronchial secretions, tightness of chest, wheezing and nasal stuffiness.

PSEUDOEPHEDRINE TANNATE
Pseudoephedrine may cause mild central nervous system stimulation, especially in those patients who are hypersensitive to sympathomimetic drugs. Nervousness, excitability, restlessness, dizziness, weakness and insomnia may also occur. Headache and drowsiness have also been reported. Large doses may cause lightheadedness, nausea and/or vomiting. Sympathomimetic drugs have also been associated with certain un-toward reactions including fear, anxiety, tenseness, restlessness, tremor, weakness, pallor, respiratory difficulty, dysuria, insomnia, hallucination, convulsion, CNS depression, arrhythmias and cardiovascular collapse with hypotension.

OVERDOSAGE
Signs & Symptoms: may vary from CNS depression to stimulation (restlessness to convulsions). Antihistamine overdosage in young children may lead to convulsions and death. Atropine-like signs and symptoms may be prominent.

Treatment: Induce vomiting if it has not occurred spontaneously. Precautions must be taken against aspiration especially in infants, children and comatose patients. If gastric lavage is indicated, isotonic or half-isotonic saline solution is preferred. Stimulants should not be used. If hypotension is a problem, vasopressor agents may be considered.

DOSAGE AND ADMINISTRATION
Administer the recommended dose every 12 hours.
Adults and children over 12 years - 10 to 20 mL (2 to 4 teaspoonfuls).
Children 6 to 12 years - 5 to 10 mL (1 to 2 teaspoonfuls) not to exceed 4 teaspoonfuls in 24 hours.
Children 2 to 6 years: - 2.5 to 5 mL (1/2 to 1 teaspoonful) not to exceed 2 teaspoonfuls in 24 hours.

Note: While, at first glance, it may appear that the suggested dosage is on the high side, the rational for dosing is derived from the fact that the tannate molecules are so large. This accounts for their slow breakdown in the body which manifests itself in a naturally occurring long lasting therapeutic effect. The percentage of Pseudoephedrine in Pseudoephedrine Tannate is only 32.6% while in the frequently used Pseudoephedrine HCl, the Pseudoephedrine is 82.3%. Similarly, the percentage of Chlorpheniramine in Chlorpheniramine Tannate is 47.2% while the Chlorpheniramine percentage in the frequently used Chlorpheniramine Maleate is 70.4%.

Dispense in a tight, light-resistant container with a child-resistant closure. Shake well before use.

Store at controlled room temperature, 15°-30°C (59°-86°F). Protect from freezing.

➤ SHOWN IN PRODUCT IDENTIFICATION GUIDE

HOW SUPPLIED
SUSPENSION:

BRAND/MANUFACTURER	NDC	SIZE	AWP
○ **BRAND**			
TANAFED: Horizon Pharm	59630-0120-04	120 ml	$14.50
	59630-0120-16	480 ml	$49.95

Chlorpheniramine Tannate/ Phenylephrine Tannate/ Pyrilamine Tannate

DESCRIPTION
Chlorpheniramine Tannate/Phenylephrine Tannate/Pyrilamine Tannate is an antihistamine/nasal decongestant combination available for oral administration as **Tablets** and as **Pediatric Suspension**.

Each tablet contains:

Phenylephrine Tannate	.25 mg
Chlorpheniramine Tannate	.8 mg
Pyrilamine Tannate	.25 mg

Each 5 mL (teaspoonful) of the Pediatric Suspension contains:

Phenylephrine Tannate	.5 mg
Chlorpheniramine Tannate	.2 mg
Pyrilamine Tannate	.12.5 mg

CLINICAL PHARMACOLOGY
Chlorpheniramine/Phenylephrine/Pyrilamine combines the sympathomimetic decongestant effect of Phenylephrine with the antihistaminic actions of Chlorpheniramine and Pyrilamine.

INDICATIONS AND USAGE
Chlorpheniramine/Phenylephrine/Pyrilamine is indicated for symptomatic relief of the coryza and nasal congestion associated with the common cold, sinusitis, allergic rhinitis and other upper respiratory tract conditions. Appropriate therapy should be provided for the primary disease.

CONTRAINDICATIONS
Chlorpheniramine/Phenylephrine/Pyrilamine is contraindicated for newborns, nursing mothers and patients sensitive to any of the ingredients or related compounds.

WARNINGS
Use with caution in patients with hypertension, cardiovascular disease, hyperthyroidism, diabetes, narrow angle glaucoma or prostatic hypertrophy. Use with caution or avoid use in patients taking monoamine oxidase (MAO) inhibitors. This product contains antihistamines which may cause drowsiness and may have additive central nervous system (CNS) effects with alcohol or other CNS depressants (e.g., hypnotics, sedatives, tranquilizers).

PRECAUTIONS
General: Antihistamines are more likely to cause dizziness, sedation and hypotension in elderly patients. Antihistamines may cause excitation, particularly in children, but their combination with sympathomimetics may cause either mild stimulation or mild sedation.

Information for Patients: Caution patients against drinking alcoholic beverages or engaging in potentially hazardous activities requiring alertness, such as driving a car or operating machinery while using this product.

Drug Interactions: MAO inhibitors may prolong and intensify the anticholinergic effects of antihistamines and the overall effects of sympathomimetic agents.

Carcinogenesis, Mutagenesis, Impairment of Fertility: No long-term animal studies have been performed with Chlorpheniramine/Phenylephrine/Pyrilamine.

Pregnancy: Teratogenic Effects: Pregnancy Category C. Animal reproduction studies have not been conducted with Chlorpheniramine/Phenylephrine/Pyrilamine. It is also not known whether Chlorpheniramine/Phenylephrine/Pyrilamine can cause fetal harm when administered to a pregnant woman or can affect reproduction capacity. Chlorpheniramine/Phenylephrine/Pyrilamine should be given to a pregnant woman only if clearly needed.

Nursing Mothers: Chlorpheniramine/Phenylephrine/Pyrilamine should not be administered to a nursing woman.

ADVERSE REACTIONS
Adverse effects associated with Chlorpheniramine/Phenylephrine/Pyrilamine at recommended doses have been minimal. The most common have been drowsiness, sedation, dryness of mucous membranes, and gastrointestinal effects. Serious side effects with oral antihistamines or sympathomimetics have been rare.

OVERDOSAGE
Signs and Symptoms: May vary from CNS depression to stimulation (restlessness to convulsions). Antihistamine overdosage in young children may lead to convulsions and death. Atropine-like signs and symptoms may be prominent.

Treatment: Induce vomiting if it has not occurred spontaneously. Precautions must be taken against aspiration especially in infants, children and comatose patients. If gastric lavage is indicated, isotonic or half-isotonic saline solution is preferred. Stimulants should not be used. If hypotension is a problem, vasopressor agents may be considered.

DOSAGE AND ADMINISTRATION
Administer the recommended dose every 12 hours.

Tablets: Adults—1 or 2 tablets.

Pediatric Suspension: **Children over six years of age**—5 to 10 mL (1 to 2 teaspoonfuls); **Children two to six years of age**—2.5 to 5 mL (½ to 1 teaspoonful); **Children under two years of age**—Titrate dose individually.

Storage: Tablets—Store at controlled room temperature 15-30°C (59°-86°F).
   Pediatric Suspension—Store at controlled room temperature 15°-30°C (59°-86°F). Protect from freezing.
   Dispense in a tight container.

HOW SUPPLIED
SUSPENSION:

BRAND/MANUFACTURER	NDC	SIZE	AWP
○ **BRAND**			
RYNATAN PEDIATRIC: Wallace	00037-0715-68	480 ml	$99.13
RYNATAN-S PEDIATRIC: Wallace	00037-0715-67	120 ml 4s	$92.47

SUSPENSION: 2 MG-5 MG-12.5 MG/5 ML

BRAND/MANUFACTURER	NDC	SIZE	AWP
◆ **GENERICS**			
R-TANNATE PEDIATRIC: Warner Chilcott	00047-2885-23	480 ml	$42.66

TABLETS:

BRAND/MANUFACTURER	NDC	SIZE	AWP
◇ **GENERICS**			
TRITAN: Aligen	00405-4806-01	100s	$29.80

TABLETS:

BRAND/MANUFACTURER	NDC	SIZE	AWP
○ **BRAND**			
RYNATAN: Wallace	00037-0713-92	100s	$117.41
	00037-0713-96	500s	$570.22
	00037-0713-95	2000s	$2060.42

TABLETS: 8 MG-25 MG-25 MG

BRAND/MANUFACTURER	NDC	SIZE	AWP
◆ **GENERICS**			
R-TANNATE: Warner Chilcott	00047-0940-24	100s	$52.42

Chlorpromazine

DESCRIPTION
Chlorpromazine is 10-(3-dimethylaminopropyl)-2-chlorphenothiazine, a dimethylamine derivative of Phenothiazine. It is present in oral and injectable forms as the hydrochloride salt, and in the suppositories as the base.

Tablets: Each tablet contains Chlorpromazine Hydrochloride as follows: 10 mg, 25 mg, 50 mg, 100 mg, 200 mg.

Sustained Release Capsules: Each Chlorpromazine sustained release capsule is so prepared that an initial dose is released promptly and the remaining medication is released gradually over a prolonged period.
   Each capsule contains Chlorpromazine Hydrochloride as follows: 30 mg, 75 mg, 150 mg.

Ampuls: Each mL contains, in aqueous solution, Chlorpromazine hydrochloride, 25 mg; ascorbic acid, 2 mg; sodium bisulfite, 1 mg; sodium chloride, 6 mg; sodium sulfite, 1 mg.

Multidose Vials: Each mL contains, in aqueous solution, Chlorpromazine Hydrochloride, 25 mg; ascorbic acid, 2 mg; sodium bisulfite, 1 mg; sodium chloride, 1 mg; sodium sulfite, 1 mg; benzyl alcohol, 2%, as a preservative.

Syrup: Each 5 mL (one teaspoonful) of liquid contains Chlorpromazine Hydrochloride, 10 mg.

Suppositories: Each suppository contains Chlorpromazine, 25 or 100 mg, glycerin, glyceryl monopalmitate, glyceryl monostearate, hydrogenated coconut oil fatty acids, and hydrogenated palm kernel oil fatty acids.

Concentrate: Each mL contains Chlorpromazine hydrochloride, 30 or 100 mg.

◆ RATED THERAPEUTICALLY EQUIVALENT; ◇ THERAPEUTIC EQUIVALENCE UNCONFIRMED; ○ UNRATED

Following is its chemical structure:

$CH_2CH_2CH_2N(CH_3)_2$

ACTIONS

The precise mechanism whereby the therapeutic effects of Chlorpromazine are produced is not known. The principal pharmacological actions are psychotropic. It also exerts sedative and antiemetic activity. Chlorpromazine has actions at all levels of the central nervous system—primarily at subcortical levels—as well as on multiple organ systems. Chlorpromazine has strong antiadrenergic and weaker peripheral anticholinergic activity; ganglionic blocking action is relatively slight. It also possesses slight antihistaminic and antiserotonin activity.

INDICATIONS

For the management of manifestations of psychotic disorders.

To control nausea and vomiting.

For relief of restlessness and apprehension before surgery.

For acute intermittent porphyria.

As an adjunct in the treatment of tetanus.

To control the manifestations of the manic type of manic-depressive illness.

For relief of intractable hiccups.

For the treatment of severe behavioral problems in children marked by combativeness and/or explosive hyperexcitable behavior (out of proportion to immediate provocations), and in the short-term treatment of hyperactive children who show excessive motor activity with accompanying conduct disorders consisting of some or all of the following symptoms: impulsivity, difficulty sustaining attention, aggressivity, mood lability and poor frustration tolerance.

UNLABELED USES

Chlorpromazine is used alone or as an adjunct in the treatment of migraine headache, postoperative paralytic ileus, and fluid loss due to cholera. It is also used to decrease motor manifestations of Sydenham's chorea.

CONTRAINDICATIONS

Do not use in patients with known hypersensitivity to phenothiazines.

Do not use in comatose states or in the presence of large amounts of central nervous system depressants (alcohol, barbiturates, narcotics, etc.).

WARNINGS

The extrapyramidal symptoms which can occur secondary to Chlorpromazine may be confused with the central nervous system signs of an undiagnosed primary disease responsible for the vomiting, e.g., Reye's syndrome or other encephalopathy. The use of Chlorpromazine and other potential hepatotoxins should be avoided in children and adolescents whose signs and symptoms suggest Reye's syndrome.

Tardive Dyskinesia: Tardive dyskinesia, a syndrome consisting of potentially irreversible, involuntary, dyskinetic movements, may develop in patients treated with neuroleptic (antipsychotic) drugs. Although the prevalence of the syndrome appears to be highest among the elderly, especially elderly women, it is impossible to rely upon prevalence estimates to predict, at the inception of neuroleptic treatment, which patients are likely to develop the syndrome. Whether neuroleptic drug products differ in their potential to cause tardive dyskinesia is unknown.

Both the risk of developing the syndrome and the likelihood that it will become irreversible are believed to increase as the duration of treatment and the total cumulative dose of neuroleptic drugs administered to the patient increase. However, the syndrome can develop, although much less commonly; after relatively brief treatment periods at low doses. There is no known treatment for established cases of tardive dyskinesia, although the syndrome may remit, partially or completely, if neuroleptic treatment is withdrawn. Neuroleptic treatment itself, however, may suppress (or partially suppress) the signs and symptoms of the syndrome and thereby possibly mask the underlying disease process. The effect that symptomatic suppression has upon the long-term course of the syndrome is unknown.

Given these considerations, neuroleptics should be prescribed in a manner that is most likely to minimize the occurrence of tardive dyskinesia. Chronic neuroleptic treatment should generally be reserved for patients who suffer from a chronic illness that, 1) is known to respond to neuroleptic drugs, and, 2) for whom alternative, equally effective, but potentially less harmful treatments are *not* available or appropriate. In patients who do require chronic treatment, the smallest dose and the shortest duration of treatment producing a satisfactory clinical response should be sought. The need for continued treatment should be reassessed periodically.

If signs and symptoms of tardive dyskinesia appear in a patient on neuroleptics, drug discontinuation should be considered. However, some patients may require treatment despite the presence of the syndrome.

For further information about the description of tardive dyskinesia and its clinical detection, please refer to the sections on Precautions and Adverse Reactions.

Neuroleptic Malignant Syndrome (NMS): A potentially fatal symptom complex sometimes referred to as Neuroleptic Malignant Syndrome (NMS) has been reported in association with antipsychotic drugs. Clinical manifestations of NMS are hyperpyrexia, muscle rigidity, altered mental status and evidence of autonomic instability (irregular pulse or blood pressure, tachycardia, diaphoresis, and cardiac dysrhythmias).

The diagnostic evaluation of patients with this syndrome is complicated. In arriving at a diagnosis, it is important to identify cases where the clinical presentation includes both serious medical illness (e.g., pneumonia, systemic infection, etc.) and untreated or inadequately treated extrapyramidal signs and symptoms (EPS). Other important considerations in the differential diagnosis include central anticholinergic toxicity, heat stroke, drug fever and primary central nervous system (CNS) pathology.

The management of NMS should include 1) immediate discontinuation of antipsychotic drugs and other drugs not essential to concurrent therapy, 2) intensive symptomatic treatment and medical monitoring, and 3) treatment of any concomitant serious medical problems for which specific treatments are available. There is no general agreement about specific pharmacological treatment regimens for uncomplicated NMS.

If a patient requires antipsychotic drug treatment after recovery from NMS, the potential reintroduction of drug therapy should be carefully considered. The patient should be carefully monitored, since recurrences of NMS have been reported.

Chlorpromazine ampuls and multidose vials contain sodium bisulfite and sodium sulfite, sulfites that may cause allergic-type reactions including anaphylactic symptoms and life-threatening or less severe asthmatic episodes in certain susceptible people. The overall prevalence of sulfite sensitivity in the general population is unknown and probably low. Sulfite sensitivity is seen more frequently in asthmatic than in nonasthmatic people.

Patients with bone marrow depression or who have previously demonstrated a hypersensitivity reaction (e.g., blood dyscrasias, jaundice) with a phenothiazine should not receive any phenothiazine, including Chlorpromazine, unless in the judgment of the physician the potential benefits of treatment outweigh the possible hazard.

Chlorpromazine may impair mental and/or physical abilities, especially during the first few days of therapy. Therefore, caution patients about activities requiring alertness (e.g., operating vehicles or machinery).

The use of alcohol with this drug should be avoided due to possible additive effects and hypotension.

Chlorpromazine may counteract the antihypertensive effect of guanethidine and related compounds.

Usage in Pregnancy: Safety for the use of Chlorpromazine during pregnancy has not been established. Therefore, it is not recommended that the drug be given to pregnant patients except when, in the judgment of the physician, it is essential. The potential benefits should clearly outweigh possible hazards. There are reported instances of prolonged jaundice, extrapyramidal signs, hyperreflexia or hyporeflexia in newborn infants whose mothers received phenothiazines.

Reproductive studies in rodents have demonstrated potential for embryotoxicity, increased neonatal mortality and nursing transfer of the drug. Tests in the offspring of the drug-treated rodents demonstrate decreased performance. The possibility of permanent neurological damage cannot be excluded.

Nursing Mothers: There is evidence that Chlorpromazine is excreted in the breast milk of nursing mothers. Because of the potential for serious adverse reactions in nursing infants from Chlorpromazine, a decision should be made whether to discontinue nursing or to discontinue the drug, taking into account the importance of the drug to the mother.

PRECAUTIONS

GENERAL

Given the likelihood that some patients exposed chronically to neuroleptics will develop tardive dyskinesia, it is advised that all patients in whom chronic use is contemplated be given, if possible, full information about this risk. The decision to inform patients and/or their guardians must obviously take into account the clinical circumstances and the competency of the patient to understand the information provided.

Chlorpromazine should be administered cautiously to persons with cardiovascular, liver or renal disease. There is evidence that patients with a history of hepatic encephalopathy due to cirrhosis have increased sensitivity to the C.N.S. effects of Chlorpromazine (i.e., impaired cerebration and abnormal slowing of the EEG).

Because of its C.N.S. depressant effect, Chlorpromazine should be used with caution in patients with chronic respiratory disorders such as severe asthma, emphysema and acute respiratory infections, particularly in children.

Because Chlorpromazine can suppress the cough reflex, aspiration of vomitus is possible.

Chlorpromazine prolongs and intensifies the action of C.N.S. depressants such as anesthetics, barbiturates and narcotics. When Chlorpromazine is administered concomitantly, about ¼ to ½ the usual dosage of such agents is required. When Chlorpromazine is not being administered to reduce requirements of C.N.S. depressants, it is best to stop such depressants before starting Chlorpromazine treatment. These agents may subsequently be reinstated at low doses and increased as needed.

Note: Chlorpromazine does *not* intensify the anticonvulsant action of barbiturates. Therefore, dosage of anticonvulsants, including barbiturates, should *not* be reduced if Chlorpromazine is started. Instead, start Chlorpromazine at low doses and increase as needed.

Use with caution in persons who will be exposed to extreme heat, organophosphorus insecticides, and in persons receiving atropine or related drugs.

Neuroleptic drugs elevate prolactin levels; the elevation persists during chronic administration. Tissue culture experiments indicate that approximately one third of human breast cancers are prolactin-dependent *in vitro*, a factor of potential

BRAND/MANUFACTURER	NDC	SIZE	AWP
◆ GENERICS			
Rugby	00536-3485-01	100s	$5.25
Major	00904-7663-60	100s	$5.50
Goldline	00182-1434-01	100s	$6.00
Schein	00364-0564-01	100s	$6.20
URL	00677-0682-01	100s	$6.25
Mutual	53489-0111-01	100s	$6.25
Parmed	00349-2356-01	100s	$6.30
Zenith	00172-2974-60	100s	$6.35
Geneva	00781-1726-01	100s	$6.55
Qualitest	00603-2860-21	100s	$6.58
Mylan	00378-0222-01	100s	$7.95
Moore,H.L.	00839-6488-06	100s	$7.95
Sidmak	50111-0362-01	100s	$8.53
Martec	52555-0372-01	100s	$8.80
Aligen	00405-4211-01	100s	$8.98
Major	00904-1349-61	100s ud	$8.27
Raway	00686-0528-20	100s ud	$8.95
Auro	55829-0200-10	100s ud	$13.79
UDL	51079-0058-20	100s ud	$14.50
Rugby	00536-3485-05	500s	$21.32
Rugby	00536-3485-10	1000s	$38.48
Schein	00364-0564-02	1000s	$39.40
Goldline	00182-1434-10	1000s	$40.00
Mutual	53489-0111-10	1000s	$40.25
Parmed	00349-2356-10	1000s	$40.95
URL	00677-0682-10	1000s	$41.05
Major	00904-1349-80	1000s	$41.55
Major	00904-7663-80	1000s	$41.55
Zenith	00172-2974-80	1000s	$43.15
Moore,H.L.	00839-6488-16	1000s	$49.75
Mylan	00378-0222-10	1000s	$51.20
Qualitest	00603-2860-32	1000s	$54.70
Sidmak	50111-0362-03	1000s	$60.89
Martec	52555-0372-10	1000s	$62.70
Aligen	00405-4211-03	1000s	$64.09

TABLETS: 25 MG

BRAND/MANUFACTURER	NDC	SIZE	AWP
◇ BRAND			
THALITONE: Horus Therapeutics	59229-0076-01	100s	$69.60

TABLETS: 50 MG

	AVERAGE UNIT PRICE (AVAILABLE SIZES)		GENERIC A-RATED AVERAGE PRICE (GAAP)	
BRAND	$0.78		100s	$9.25
GENERIC	$0.08		1000s	$62.35
HCFA FUL (100s ea)	$0.03			

BRAND/MANUFACTURER	NDC	SIZE	AWP
◆ BRAND			
HYGROTON: RPR	00075-0020-00	100s	$77.88
◆ GENERICS			
Goldline	00182-1435-01	100s	$6.40
Major	00904-7665-60	100s	$6.45
Schein	00364-0528-01	100s	$6.72
Rugby	00536-5644-01	100s	$7.12
Geneva	00781-1728-01	100s	$7.42
Zenith	00172-2999-60	100s	$7.45
Qualitest	00603-2861-21	100s	$7.98
URL	00677-0683-01	100s	$8.00
Mutual	53489-0112-01	100s	$8.00
Mylan	00378-0213-01	100s	$9.50
Sidmak	50111-0363-01	100s	$9.54
Aligen	00405-4212-01	100s	$9.58
Martec	52555-0373-01	100s	$9.85
Moore,H.L.	00839-6369-06	100s	$10.11
Raway	00686-0059-20	100s ud	$9.50
Auro	55829-0201-10	100s ud	$15.70
UDL	51079-0059-20	100s ud	$18.00
HYLIDONE: Major	00904-1350-70	250s	$15.89
Schein	00364-0528-02	1000s	$44.73
Major	00904-1350-80	1000s	$54.90
Major	00904-7665-80	1000s	$54.90
Zenith	00172-2999-80	1000s	$56.65
Mutual	53489-0112-10	1000s	$59.50
Qualitest	00603-2861-32	1000s	$59.60
URL	00677-0683-10	1000s	$59.90
Geneva	00781-1728-10	1000s	$59.95
Aligen	00405-4212-10	1000s	$66.93
Sidmak	50111-0363-03	1000s	$69.93
Martec	52555-0373-10	1000s	$71.35
Moore,H.L.	00839-6369-16	1000s	$71.82
Mylan	00378-0213-10	1000s	$80.45

TABLETS: 100 MG

	AVERAGE UNIT PRICE (AVAILABLE SIZES)		GENERIC A-RATED AVERAGE PRICE (GAAP)	
BRAND	$1.30		100s	$10.86
GENERIC	$0.10		1000s	$92.23

BRAND/MANUFACTURER	NDC	SIZE	AWP
◆ BRAND			
HYGROTON: RPR	00075-0021-00	100s	$130.20
◆ GENERICS			
Qualitest	00603-2862-21	100s	$9.35
Schein	00364-0787-01	100s	$10.00
Major	00904-1351-60	100s	$10.40
Martec	52555-0374-01	100s	$10.60
Zenith	00172-2904-60	100s	$10.90
Moore,H.L.	00839-6370-06	100s	$11.46
Parmed	00349-7025-01	100s	$11.50
Aligen	00405-4213-01	100s	$12.70
Parmed	00349-7025-10	1000s	$90.95
Zenith	00172-2904-80	1000s	$92.35
Moore,H.L.	00839-6370-16	1000s	$93.39

Chlorthalidone with Clonidine Hydrochloride

DESCRIPTION

Clonidine Hydrochloride is a centrally acting antihypertensive agent and Chlorthalidone a diuretic. Chlorthalidone/Clonidine Hydrochloride is available as tablets for oral administration in three dosage strengths: 0.1/15 mg, 0.2/15 mg and 0.3/15 mg of Clonidine Hydrochloride/Chlorthalidone, respectively.

CLONIDINE HYDROCHLORIDE:
Clonidine Hydrochloride is an imidazoline derivative and exists as a mesomeric compound. The chemical name is 2-(2,6-dichlorophenylamino)-2-imidazoline Hydrochloride.

The molecular formula of Clonidine is $C_9H_9Cl_2N_3 \cdot HCl$ and the molecular weight is 266.56.

Clonidine Hydrochloride is an odorless, bitter, white crystalline substance soluble in water and alcohol.

CHLORTHALIDONE
Chlorthalidone is a monosulfamyl diuretic that differs chemically from thiazide diuretics in that a double ring system is incorporated in its structure. It is a racemic mixture of 2-chloro-5-(1- hydroxy-3-oxo-1-isoindolinyl) benzenesulfonamide.

The molecular formula of Chlorthalidone is $C_{14}H_{11}ClN_2O_4S$ and the molecular weight is 338.76.

Chlorthalidone is practically insoluble in water, in ether and in chloroform; soluble in methanol; slightly soluble in alcohol.

CLINICAL PHARMACOLOGY

CHLORTHALIDONE/CLONIDINE HYDROCHLORIDE
Chlorthalidone/Clonidine Hydrochloride produces a more pronounced antihypertensive response than occurs after either Clonidine Hydrochloride or Chlorthalidone in equivalent doses.

CLONIDINE HYDROCHLORIDE
Clonidine Hydrochloride acts relatively rapidly. The patient's blood pressure declines within 30 to 60 minutes after an oral dose, the maximum decrease occurring within 2 to 4 hours. The plasma level of Clonidine Hydrochloride peaks in approximately 3 to 5 hours and the plasma half-life ranges from 12 to 16 hours. The half-life increases up to 41 hours in patients with severe impairment of renal function. Following oral administration about 40-60% of the absorbed dose is recovered in the urine as unchanged drug in 24 hours. About 50% of the absorbed dose is metabolized in the liver.

Clonidine Hydrochloride stimulates alpha-adrenoreceptors in the brain stem, resulting in reduced sympathetic outflow from the central nervous system and a decrease in peripheral resistance, renal vascular resistance, heart rate, and blood pressure. Renal blood flow and glomerular filtration rate remain essentially unchanged. Normal postural reflexes are intact and therefore orthostatic symptoms are mild and infrequent. Acute studies with Clonidine Hydrochloride in humans have demonstrated a moderate reduction (15 to 20%) of cardiac output in the supine position with no change in the peripheral resistance; at a 45° tilt there is a smaller reduction in cardiac output and a decrease of peripheral resistance. During long-term therapy, cardiac output tends to return to control values, while peripheral resistance remains decreased. Slowing of the pulse rate has been observed in most patients given Clonidine but the drug does not alter normal hemodynamic response to exercise.

Other studies in patients have provided evidence of a reduction in plasma renin activity and in the excretion of aldosterone and catecholamines, but the exact relationship of these pharmacologic actions to the antihypertensive effect has not been fully elucidated.

Clonidine Hydrochloride acutely stimulates growth hormone release in both children and adults, but does not produce a chronic elevation of growth hormone with long-term use.

◆ RATED THERAPEUTICALLY EQUIVALENT; ◇ THERAPEUTIC EQUIVALENCE UNCONFIRMED; ○ UNRATED

Tolerance may develop in some patients, necessitating a reevaluation of therapy.

CHLORTHALIDONE

Chlorthalidone is a long-acting oral diuretic with antihypertensive activity. Its diuretic action commences a mean of 2.6 hours after dosing and continues for up to 72 hours. The drug produces diuresis with increased excretion of sodium and chloride. The diuretic effects of Chlorthalidone and the benzothiadiazine (thiazide) diuretics appear to arise from similar mechanisms and the maximal effect of Chlorthalidone and the thiazides appears to be similar. The site of action appears to be the distal convoluted tubule of the nephron. The diuretic effects of Chlorthalidone lead to decreased extracellular fluid volume, plasma volume, cardiac output, total exchangeable sodium, glomerular filtration rate, and renal plasma flow. Although the mechanism of action of Chlorthalidone and related drugs is not wholly clear, sodium and water depletion appear to provide a basis for its antihypertensive effect. Like the thiazide diuretics, Chlorthalidone produces dose-related reductions in serum potassium levels, elevations in serum uric acid and blood glucose, and it can lead to decreased sodium and chloride levels.

The mean plasma half-life of Chlorthalidone is about 40 to 60 hours. It is eliminated primarily as unchanged drug in the urine. Non-renal routes of elimination have yet to be clarified. In the blood, approximately 75% of the drug is bound to plasma proteins.

INDICATIONS AND USAGE

Clonidine Hydrochloride USP Chlorthalidone USP is indicated in the treatment of hypertension. **This fixed combination drug is not indicated for initial therapy of hypertension. Hypertension requires therapy titrated to the individual patient. If the fixed combination represents the dosage so determined, its use may be more convenient in patient management. The treatment of hypertension is not static, but must be reevaluated as conditions in each patient warrant.**

CONTRAINDICATIONS

Anuria. Chlorthalidone/Clonidine Hydrochloride is containdicated in patients with known hypersensitivity to Chlorthalidone or other sulfonamide-derived drugs.

WARNINGS

Chlorthalidone should be used with caution in severe renal disease. In patients with renal disease, Chlorthalidone or related drugs may precipitate azotemia. Cumulative effects of the drug may develop in patients with impaired renal function. Chlorthalidone should be used with caution in patients with impaired hepatic function or progressive liver disease, because minor alterations of fluid and electrolyte balance may precipitate hepatic coma.

Sensitivity reactions may occur in patients with a history of allergy or bronchial asthma. The possibility of exacerbation or activation of systemic lupus erythematosus has been reported with thiazide diuretics which are structurally related to Chlorthalidone. However, systemic lupus erythematosus has not been reported following Chlorthalidone administration.

PRECAUTIONS

CLONIDINE HYDROCHLORIDE

General: In patients who have developed localized contact sensitization to Catapress-TTS® Clonidine), substitution of oral Clonidine Hydrochloride therapy may be associated with the development of a generalized skin rash.

In patients who develop an allergic reaction from Catapres-TTS® Clonidine) that extends beyond the local patch site (such as generalized skin rash, urticaria, or angioedema), oral Clonidine Hydrochloride substitution may elicit a similar reaction.

As with all antihypertensive therapy, Clonidine Hydrochloride should be used with caution in patients with severe coronary insufficiency, recent myocardial infarction, cerebrovascular disease or chronic renal failure.

Withdrawal: Patients should be instructed not to discontinue therapy without consulting their physician. Sudden cessation of Clonidine treatment has resulted in subjective symptoms such as nervousness, agitation and headache, accompanied or followed by a rapid rise in blood pressure and elevated catecholamine concentrations in the plasma, but such occurrences have usually been associated with previous administration of high oral doses (exceeding 1.2 mg/day) and/or with continuation of concomitant beta-blocker therapy. Rare instances of hypertensive encephalopathy and death have been reported. When discontinuing therapy with Clonidine Hydrochloride, the physician should reduce the dose gradually over 2 to 4 days to avoid withdrawal symptomatology.

An excessive rise in blood pressure following Conidine Hydrochloride discontinuance can be reversed by administration of oral Clonidine or by intravenous phentolamine. If therapy is to be discontinued in patients receiving beta-blockers and Clonidine concurrently, beta-blockers should be discontinued several days before the gradual withdrawal of Clonidine Hydrochloride.

Perioperative Use: Administration of Clonidine Hydrochloride should be continued to within four hours of surgery and resumed as soon as possible thereafter. The blood pressure should be carefully monitored and appropriate measures instituted to control it as necessary.

Information for Patients: Patients who engage in potentially hazardous activities, such as operating machinery or driving, should be advised of a potential sedative effect of Clonidine. Patients should be cautioned against interruption of Clonidine Hydrochloride therapy without a physician's advice.

Drug Interactions: If a patient receiving Clonidine Hydrochloride is also taking tricyclic antidepressants, the effect of Clonidine may be reduced, thus necessitating an increase in dosage. Clonidine Hydrochloride may enhance the CNS-depressive effects of alcohol, barbiturates or other sedatives. Amitriptyline in combination with Clonidine enhances the manifestation of corneal lesions in rats (see *"Ocular Toxicity"*).

OCULAR TOXICITY

In several studies, oral Clonidine Hydrochloride produced a dose-dependent increase in the incidence and severity of spontaneously occurring retinal degeneration in albino rats treated for six months or longer. Tissue distribution studies in dogs and monkeys revealed that Clonidine Hydrochloride was concentrated in the choroid of the eye. In view of the retinal degeneration observed in rats, eye examinations were performed in 908 patients prior to the start of Clonidine Hydrochloride therapy, who were then examined periodically thereafter. In 353 of these 908 patients, examinations were performed for periods of 24 months or longer. Except for some dryness of the eyes, no drug-related abnormal ophthalmologic findings were recorded and Clonidine Hydrochloride did not alter retinal function as shown by specialized tests such as the electroretinogram and macular dazzle.

In rats, Clonidine Hydrochloride in combination with amitriptyline produced corneal lesions within 5 days.

Carcinogenesis, Mutagenesis, Impairment of Fertility: In a 132-week (fixed concentration) dietary administration study in rats, Clonidine Hydrochloride administered at 32 to 46 times the maximum recommended daily human oral dose was unassociated with evidence of carcinogenic potential. Fertility of male or female rats was unaffected by Clonidine Hydrochloride doses as high as 150 mcg/kg or about 3 times the maximum recommended daily human oral dose (MRDHD). Fertility of female rats did, however, appear to be affected (in another experiment) at dose levels of 500 to 2000 mcg/kg or 10 to 40 times the MRDHD.

USAGE IN PREGNANCY

Teratogenic Effects: Pregnancy Category C. Reproduction studies performed in rabbits at doses up to approximately 3 times the maximum recommended daily human dose (MRDHD) of Clonidine Hydrochloride have revealed no evidence of teratogenic or embryotoxic potential. In rats however, doses as low as ⅓ the MRDHD were associated with increased resorptions in a study in which dams were treated continuously from 2 months prior to mating. Increased resorptions were not associated with treatment at the same or at higher dose levels (up to 3 times the MRDHD) when dams were treated days 6-15 of gestation. Increased resorptions were observed at much higher levels (40 times the MRDHD) in rats and mice treated days 1-14 of gestation (lowest dose employed in that study was 500 mcg/kg). There are, however, no adequate and well-controlled studies in pregnant women. Because animal reproduction studies are not always predictive of human response, this drug should be used during pregnancy only if clearly needed.

Nursing Mothers: As Clonidine Hydrochloride is excreted in human milk, caution should be exercised when it is administered to a nursing woman.

Pediatric Use: Safety and effectiveness in children have not been established.

CHLORTHALIDONE

General: Hypokalemia and other electrolyte abnormalities, including hyponatremia and hypochloremic alkalosis, are common in patients receiving Chlorthalidone. These abnormalities are dose-related but may occur even at the lowest marketed doses of Chlorthalidone. Serum electrolytes should be determined before initiating therapy and at periodic intervals during therapy. Serum and urine electrolyte determinations are particularly important when the patient is vomiting excessively or receiving parenteral fluids. All patients taking Chlorthalidone should be observed for clinical signs of electrolyte imbalance, including dryness of mouth, thirst, weakness, lethargy, drowsiness, restlessness, muscle pains or cramps, muscular fatigue, hypotension, oliguria, tachycardia, palpitations and gastrointestinal disturbances, such as nausea and vomiting. Digitalis therapy may exaggerate metabolic effects of hypokalemia especially with reference to myocardial activity.

Any chloride deficit is generally mild and usually does not require specific treatment except under extraordinary circumstances (as in liver disease or renal disease). Dilutional hyponatremia may occur in edematous patients in hot weather: appropriate therapy is water restriction, rather than administration of salt, except in rare instances when the hyponatremia is life-threatening. In cases of actual salt depletion, appropriate replacement is the therapy of choice.

Uric Acid: Hyperuricemia may occur or frank gout may be precipitated in certain patients receiving Chlorthalidone.

Other: Increases in serum glucose may occur and latent diabetes mellitus may become manifest during Chlorthalidone therapy (see *"Precautions, Drug Interactions"*). Chlorthalidone and related drugs may decrease serum PBI levels without signs of thyroid disturbance.

Information for Patients: Patients should inform their doctor if they have: 1) had an allergic reaction to Chlorthalidone or other diuretics or have asthma 2) kidney disease 3) liver disease 4) gout 5) systemic lupus erythematosus, or 6) been taking other drugs such as cortisone, digitalis, lithium carbonate, or drugs for diabetes.

Patients should be cautioned to contact their physician if they experience any of the following symptoms of potassium loss: excess thirst, tiredness, drowsiness, restlessness, muscle pains or cramps, nausea, vomiting or increased heart rate or pulse.

Patients should also be cautioned that taking alcohol can increase the chance of dizziness occurring.

Laboratory Tests: Periodic determination of serum electrolytes to detect possible electrolyte imbalance should be performed at appropriate intervals.

All patients receiving Chlorthalidone should be observed for clinical signs of fluid or electrolyte imbalance: namely, hyponatremia, hypochloremic alkalosis and hypokalemia. Serum and urine electrolyte determinations are particularly important when the patient is vomiting excessively or receiving parenteral fluids.

Drug Interactions: Chlorthalidone may add to or potentiate the action of other antihypertensive drugs. Insulin requirements in diabetic patients may be increased, decreased or unchanged. Higher dosage of oral hypoglycemic agents may be required. Chlorthlidone and related drugs may increase the responsiveness to tubocurarine. Chlorthalidone and related drugs may decrease arterial responsiveness to norepinephrine. This diminution is not sufficient to preclude effectiveness of the pressor agent for therapeutic use. Lithium renal clearance is reduced by Chlorthalidone, increasing the risk of lithium toxicity.

Drug/Laboratory Test Interactions: Chlorthalidone and related drugs may decrease serum PBI levels without signs of thyroid disturbance.

Carcinogenesis, Mutagenesis, Impairment of Fertility: No information is available.

USAGE IN PREGNANCY

Teratogenic effects: Pregnancy Category B. Reproduction studies have been performed in the rat and the rabbit at doses up to 420 times the human dose and have revealed no evidence of harm to the fetus due to Chlorthalidone. There are, however, no adequate and well-controlled studies in pregnant women. Because animal reproduction studies are not always predictive of human response, this drug should be used during pregnancy only if clearly needed.

Nonteratogenic Effects: Thiazides cross the placental barrier and appear in cord blood. The use of Chlorthalidone and related drugs in pregnant women requires that the anticipated benefits of the drug be weighed aganist possible hazards to the fetus. These hazards include fetal or neonatal jaundice, thrombocytopenia, and possibly other adverse reactions that have occurred in the adult.

Nursing Mothers: Thiazides are excreted in human milk. Because of the potential for serious adverse reactions in nursing infants from Chlorthalidone, a decision should be made whether to discontinue nursing or to discontinue the drug, taking into account the importance of the drug to the mother.

Pediatric Use: Safety and effectiveness in children have not been established.

ADVERSE REACTIONS

Chlorthalidone/Clonidine Hydrochloride is generally well tolerated. Most adverse effects are mild and tend to diminish with continued therapy. The most frequent (which appear to be dose-related) are dry mouth, occurring in about 40 in 100 patients; drowsiness, about 33 in 100; dizziness, about 16 in 100; constipation and sedation, each about 10 in 100.

In addition to the reactions listed above, certain less frequent adverse experiences, which are shown below, have also been reported in patients receiving the component drugs of Chlorthalidone/Clonidine Hydrochloride but in many cases patients were receiving concomitant medication and a causal relationship has not been established:

CLONIDINE HYDROCHLORIDE:
Gastrointestinal: Nausea and vomiting, about 5 in 100 patients; anorexia and malaise, each about 1 in 100: mild transient abnormalities in liver function tests, about 1 in 100; rare reports of hepatitis; parotitis, rarely.

Metabolic: Weight gain, about 1 in 100 patients; gynecomastia, about 1 in 1000, transient elevation of blood glucose or serum creatine phosphokinase, rarely.

Central Nervous System: Nervousness and agitation, about 3 in 100 patients; mental depression, about 1 in 100; headache, about 1 in 100; insomnia, about 5 in 1000. Vivid dreams or nightmares, other behavioral changes, restlessness, anxiety, visual and auditory hallucinations and delirium have been reported.

Cardiovascular: Orthostatic symptoms, about 3 in 100 patients; palpitations and tachycardia, and bradycardia, about 5 in 1000. Raynaud's phenomenon, congestive heart failure, and electrocardiographic abnormalities i.e. conduction disturbances and arrhythmias have been reported rarely. Rare cases of sinus bradycardia and atrioventricular block have been reported, both with and without the use of concomitant digitals.

Dermatological: Rash, about 1 in 100 patients; pruritus, about 7 in 1000; hives, angioneurotic edema and urticaria, about 5 in 1000, alopecia, about 2 in 1000.

Genitourinary: Decreased sexual activity, impotence and loss of libido, about 3 in 100 patients; nocturia, about 1 in 100; difficulty in micturition, about 2 in 1000; urinary retention, about 1 in 1000.

Other: Weakness, about 10 in 100 patients; fatigue, about 4 in 100; discontinuation syndrome, about 1 in 100; muscle or joint pain, about 6 in 1000 and cramps of the lower limbs, about 3 in 1000. Dryness, burning of the eyes, blurred vision, dryness of the nasal mucosa, pallor, weakly positive Coombs' test, increased sensitivity to alcohol and fever have been reported.

CHLORTHALIDONE
Gastrointestinal: Anorexia, gastric irritation, nausea, vomiting, cramping, diarrhea, constipation, jaundice (intrahepatic cholestatic jaundice), pancreatitis.

Central Nervous System: Dizziness, vertigo, paresthesias, headache, xanthopsia.

Hematologic: Leukopenia, agranulocytosis, thrombocytopenia, aplastic anemia.

Dermatologic-Hypersensitivity: Purpura, photosensitivity, rash, urticaria, necrotizing angiitis (vasculitis) (cutaneous vasculitis), Lyell's syndrome (toxic epidermal necrolysis).

Cardiovascular: Orthostatic hypotension may occur and may be aggravated by alcohol, barbiturates or narcotics.

Other adverse reactions: Hyperglycemia, glycosuria, hyperuricemia, muscle spasm, weakness, restlessness, impotence. Whenever adverse reactions are moderate or severe, Chlorthalidone dosage should be reduced or therapy withdrawn.

OVERDOSAGE

CLONIDINE HYDROCHLORIDE
The signs and symptoms of Clonidine Hydrochloride overdosage include hypotension, bradycardia, lethargy, irritability, weakness, somnolence, diminished or absent reflexes, miosis, vomiting and hypoventilation. With large overdoses, reversible cardiac conduction defects or arrhythmias, apnea, seizures and transient hypertension have been reported. The oral LD_{50} of Clonidine in rats was 465 mg/kg, and in mice 206 mg/kg.

The general treatment of Clonidine Hydrochloride overdosage may include intravenous fluids as indicated. Bradycardia can be treated with intravenous atropine sulfate and hypotension with dopamine infusion in addition to intravenous fluids. Hypertension, associated with overdosage, has been treated with intravenous furosemide or diazoxide or alpha-blocking agents such as phentolamine. Tolazoline, an alpha-blocker, in intravenous doses of 10 mg at 30-minute intervals, may reverse Clonidine's effects if other efforts fail. Routine hemodialysis is of limited benefit, since a maximum of 5% of circulating Clonidine is removed.

In a patient who ingested 100 mg Clonidine Hydrochloride, plasma Clonidine levels were 60 ng/ml (one hour), 190 ng/ml (1.5 hours), 370 ng/ml (two hours) and 120 ng/ml (5.5 and 6.5 hours). This patient developed hypertension followed by hypotension, bradycardia, apnea, hallucinations, semicoma, and premature ventricular contractions. The patient fully recovered after intensive treatment.

CHLORTHALIDONE
Symptoms of acute overdosage include nausea, weakness, dizziness and disturbances of electrolyte balance. The oral LD_{50} of the drug in the mouse and the rat is more than 25,000 mg/kg body weight. The minimum lethal dose (MLD) in humans has not been established. There is no specific antidote but gastric lavage is recommended, followed by supportive treatment. Where necessary, this may include intravenous dextrose-saline with potassium, administered with caution.

DOSAGE AND ADMINISTRATION

The dosage must be determined by individual titration. (See *"Indications and Usage"*.)

Chlorthalidone is usually initiated at a dose of 25 mg once daily and may be increased to 50 mg if the response is insufficient after a suitable trial.

Clonidine Hydrochloride is usually initiated at a dose of 0.1 mg twice daily. Elderly patients may benefit from a lower initial dose. Further increments of 0.1 mg/day may be made if necessary until the desired response is achieved. The therapeutic doses most commonly employed have ranged from 0.2 to 0.6 mg per day in divided doses.

One Clonidine Hydrochloride Chlorthalidone Tablet administered once or twice daily can be used to administer a minimum of 0.1 mg Clonidine Hydrochloride and 15 mg Chlorthalidone to a maximum of 0.6 mg Clonidine Hydrochloride and 30 mg Chlorthalidone.

Store below 86°F (30°C). Avoid excess humidity.

Dispense in tight, light-resistant container.

HOW SUPPLIED
TABLETS: 0.2 MG-15 MG

BRAND/MANUFACTURER	NDC	SIZE	AWP
◆ GENERICS			
Rugby	00536-3535-01	100s	$43.42

TABLETS: 15 MG-0.1 MG

AVERAGE UNIT PRICE (AVAILABLE SIZES)		GENERIC A-RATED AVERAGE PRICE (GAAP)	
BRAND	$0.70	100s	$33.15
GENERIC	$0.33		
HCFA FUL (100s ea)	$0.22		

BRAND/MANUFACTURER	NDC	SIZE	AWP
◆ BRAND			
COMBIPRES: Boehr Ingelheim	00597-0008-01	100s	$70.25
◆ GENERICS			
Schein	00364-2174-01	100s	$28.50
Goldline	00182-1275-01	100s	$28.50
Qualitest	00603-2978-21	100s	$31.43
Mylan	00378-0001-01	100s	$32.15
Moore,H.L.	00839-7285-06	100s	$33.21
URL	00677-1146-01	100s	$33.80
Rugby	00536-3533-01	100s	$33.83
Par	49884-0113-01	100s	$37.50
Aligen	00405-4248-01	100s	$39.47

◆ RATED THERAPEUTICALLY EQUIVALENT; ◇ THERAPEUTIC EQUIVALENCE UNCONFIRMED; ○ UNRATED

TABLETS: 15 MG-0.2 MG

AVERAGE UNIT PRICE (AVAILABLE SIZES)		GENERIC A-RATED AVERAGE PRICE (GAAP)	
BRAND	$0.94	100s	$43.86
GENERIC	$0.44		
HCFA FUL (100s ea)	$0.26		

BRAND/MANUFACTURER	NDC	SIZE	AWP
◆ BRAND			
COMBIPRES: Boehr Ingelheim	00597-0009-01	100s	$94.00
◆ GENERICS			
Goldline	00182-1276-01	100s	$37.50
Schein	00364-2175-01	100s	$39.50
Qualitest	00603-2979-21	100s	$39.84
Mylan	00378-0027-01	100s	$42.90
URL	00677-1147-01	100s	$43.75
Moore,H.L.	00839-7286-06	100s	$45.75
Par	49884-0115-01	100s	$49.50
Aligen	00405-4249-01	100s	$52.11

TABLETS: 15 MG-0.3 MG

AVERAGE UNIT PRICE (AVAILABLE SIZES)		GENERIC A-RATED AVERAGE PRICE (GAAP)	
BRAND	$1.13	100s	$52.39
GENERIC	$0.52		
HCFA FUL (100s ea)	$0.32		

BRAND/MANUFACTURER	NDC	SIZE	AWP
◆ BRAND			
COMBIPRES: Boehr Ingelheim	00597-0010-01	100s	$113.40
◆ GENERICS			
Qualitest	00603-2980-21	100s	$41.00
Goldline	00182-1277-01	100s	$45.75
Moore,H.L.	00839-7943-06	100s	$49.49
Mylan	00378-0072-01	100s	$51.85
Par	49884-0116-01	100s	$61.50
Aligen	00405-4250-01	100s	$64.73

Chlorthalidone with Reserpine

DESCRIPTION
Chlorthalidone/Reserpine is a drug combination of two well-known antihypertensive agents, Chlorthalidone and Reserpine. Chemistry: A monosulfamyl diuretic, Chlorthalidone differs from thiazide diuretics in that a double-ring system is incorporated in its structure. Chemically it is 2-Chloro-5-(1-hydroxy-3-oxo-1-isoindolinyl) benzenesulfonamide:

Chlorthalidone is practically insoluble in water, in ether, and in chloroform; soluble in methanol; slightly soluble in alcohol.

Reserpine is a pure crystalline alkaloid from the root of Rauwolfia serpentina.

Reserpine is insoluble in water, freely soluble in acetic acid and in chloroform, slightly soluble in benzene; very slightly soluble in alcohol and in ether.

ACTIONS
The pharmacologic effects are those of the constituent drugs. Chlorthalidone produces a saluretic effect in humans, beginning within two hours after an oral dose and continuing for as long as 72 hours. Copious diuresis is produced, with greatly increased excretion of sodium and chloride.

Reserpine, because it reduces arterial blood pressure and exerts a sedative effect, is particularly useful in the therapy of hypertension with related emotional disturbance. Reserpine is characterized by slow onset of action and sustained effect. Both its cardiovascular and central nervous system effects may persist following withdrawal of the drug (See *"Precautions"*.)

Both Chlorthalidone and Reserpine have prolonged action, and the combination is thus able to exert a smooth and concerted effect over a long period. The two drugs appear to enhance each other, and this gives the combination a high degree of effectiveness. When considered necessary the combination may be prescribed together with other antihypertensive agents which may then be given in lower dosage with lessened chance of side reactions.

ANIMAL PHARMACOLOGY
In animal biochemical studies, Chlorthalidone is absorbed slowly from the gastrointestinal tract, due to low solubility. After passage to the liver some of the drug enters the general circulation, while some is excreted in the bile to be reabsorbed later. In the general circulation, the drug is distributed widely to the tissues, but is taken up in the highest concentrations in the kidneys, where amounts have been found 72 hours after ingestion, long after it has disappeared from other tissues. The drug is excreted unchanged in the urine. The high renal concentration of Chlorthalidone may be casually associated with the prolonged saluretic effect of the drug. Chlorthalidone appears to inhibit sodium and chloride reabsorption in the cortical diluting segment of ascending limb of Henle's loop. The reduction of plasma volume following diuresis is a probable mechanism in the initial antihypertensive action of the drug.

Reserpine probably produces its sedative and hypotensive effects through a depletion in tissue stores of catecholamines. The antihypertensive action of Reserpine is probably due to loss of epinephrine and norepinephrine from peripheral sites. By contrast, its sedative and tranquilizing properties are thought to be related to depletion of 5-hydroxytryptamine from the brain.

INDICATION
Treatment of hypertension. (See box *"Warning"*.)

CONTRAINDICATIONS
Patients with a history of mental depression, demonstrated hypersensitivity, and most cases of severe renal or hepatic diseases are the only contraindications.

WARNINGS

> THESE FIXED COMBINATION DRUGS ARE NOT INDICATED FOR INITIAL THERAPY OF HYPERTENSION. HYPERTENSION REQUIRES THERAPY TITRATED TO THE INDIVIDUAL PATIENT. IF THE FIXED COMBINATION REPRESENTS THE DOSAGE SO DETERMINED, ITS USE MAY BE MORE CONVENIENT IN PATIENT MANAGEMENT. THE TREATMENT OF HYPERTENSION IS NOT STATIC, BUT MUST BE REEVALUATED AS CONDITIONS IN EACH PATIENT WARRANT.

These drugs should be used with caution in severe renal disease, since products containing Chlorthalidone or similar drugs may precipitate azolemia. Cumulative effects of the drug may develop in patients with impaired renal function.

They should be used with caution in patients with impaired hepatic function or progressive liver disease, since minor alterations of fluid and electrolyte balance may precipitate hepatic coma.

Chlorthalidone/Reserpine may add to or potentiate the action of other antihypertensive drugs. Potentiation occurs with ganglionic or peripheral adrenergic-blocking drugs.

Sensitivity reactions may occur in patients with a history of allergy or bronchial asthma.

Reserpine may cause mental depression. Recognition of depression may be difficult because this condition may often be disguised by somatic complaints (masked depression). The drug should be discontinued at first signs of depression such as despondency, early morning insomnia, loss of appetite, impotence, or self-depreciation. Drug induced depression may persist for several months after drug withdrawal and may be severe enough to result in suicide. In patients who have had depression, the drug should not be started. Electroschock therapy should not be given to patients taking Reserpine, since severe and even fatal reactions have occurred. The drug should be stopped at least seven days before giving electroshock therapy.

In susceptible patients, peptic ulcer may be precipitated or activated, in which case the drug should be discontinued.

Usage in Pregnancy: Reproduction studies with Chlorthalidone in various animal species at multiples of the human dose showed no significant level of teratogenicity, no fetal or congenital abnormalities were observed. Animal data should not be extrapolated for clinical application.

Thiazides cross the placental barrier and appear in cord blood. The use of Chlorthalidone and related drugs in pregnant women requires that the anticipated benefits of the drug be weighed against possible hazards to the fetus. These hazards include fetal or neonatal jaundice, thrombocytopenia and possibly other adverse reactions which have occurred in the adult.

Nursing Mothers: Thiazides and Reserpine cross the placental barrier and appear in cord blood and breast milk increased respiratory secretions, nasal congestion, cyanosis and anorexia may occur in infants born to reserpine-treated mothers. If use of the drug is deemed essential the patient should stop nursing.

PRECAUTIONS
Antihypertensive therapy with Chlorthalidone/Reserpine combinations should always be initiated cautiously in postsympathectomy patients and in those receiving ganglionic blocking agents, other potent antihypertensive drugs, or curare. At least a one-half reduction in the usual dosage of such agents may be advisable. Careful and continuous supervision of patients on such multiple-drug regimens is necessary.

Since some patients receiving Rauwolfia preparations have experienced hypotension when undergoing surgery, it may be advisable to discontinue Chlorthalidone/Reserpine combination drugs therapy about two weeks prior to elective surgical procedures. Emergency surgery may be carried out by using if necessary, anticholinergic or adrenergic drugs to prevent vagocirculatory responses, other supportive measures may be used as indicated.

Because of the possibility of progression of renal damage periodic kidney function tests are indicated. In case of a rising BUN, the drug should be stopped.

The drug should be discontinued in cases of aggravated liver dysfunction (hepatic coma may be precipitated).

Periodic determination of serum electrolytes to detect possible electrolyte imbalance should be performed at appropriate intervals.

All patients receiving Chlorthalidone should be observed for clinical signs of fluid or electrolyte imbalance; namely, hyponatremia, hypochloremic alkalosis, and hypokalemia. Serum and urine electrolyte determinations are particularly important when the patient is vomiting excessively or receiving parenteral fluids. Medication such as digitalis may also influence serum electrolytes. Warning signs, irrespective of cause, are: dryness of mouth, thirst, weakness, lethargy, drowsiness, restlessness, muscle pains or cramps, muscular fatigue, hypotension, oliguria, tachycardia and gastrointestinal disturbances such as nausea and vomiting.

➤ SHOWN IN PRODUCT IDENTIFICATION GUIDE

Hypokalemia may develop with Chlorthalidone as with any other potent diuretic, especially with brisk diuresis, when severe cirrhosis is present, or during concomitant use of corticosteroids or ACTH.

Interference with adequate oral electrolyte intake will also contribute to hypokalemia. Digitalis therapy may exaggerate metabolic effects of hypokalemia especially with reference to myocardial activity.

Any chloride deficit is generally mild and usually does not require specific treatment except under extraordinary circumstances (as in liver disease or renal disease). Dilutional hyponatremia may occur in edematous patients in hot weather. Appropriate therapy is water restriction rather than administration of salt except in rare instances when the hyponatremia is life threatening. In actual salt depletion, appropriate replacement is the therapy of choice.

Hyperuncemia may occur or frank gout may be precipitated in certain patients receiving Chlorthalidone.

Insulin requirements in diabetic patients may be increased, decreased or unchanged. Latent diabetes mellitus may become manifest during Chlorthalidone administration.

Chlorthalidone and related drugs may decrease arterial responsiveness to norepinephrine. This diminution is not sufficient to preclude effectiveness of the pressor agent for therapeutic use.

Chlorthalidone and related drugs may decrease serum PBI levels without signs of thyroid disturbance.

Because Reserpine increases gastrointestinal motility and secretion, Chlorthalidone/Reserpine should be used cautiously in patients with ulcerative colitis or gallstones. Where biliary colic may be precipitated in susceptible patients, bronchial asthma may occur.

Animal Tumongenicity: Rodent studies have shown that Reserpine is an animal tumongen, causing an increased incidence of mammary fibroadenomas in female mice, malignant tumors of the seminal vesicles in male mice, and malignant adrenal medullary tumors in male rats. These findings arose in 2-year studies in which the drug was administered in the feed at concentrations of 5 and 10 ppm- about 100 to 300 times the usual human dose. The breast neoplasms are thought to be related to Reserpine's prolactin-elevating effect. Several other prolactin-elevating drugs have also been associated with an increased incidence of mammary neoplasia in rodents.

The extent to which these findings indicate a risk to humans is uncertain. Tissue culture experiments show that about one-third of human breast tumors are prolactin-dependent *in vitro*, a factor of considerable importance if the use of the drug is contemplated in a patient with previously detected breast cancer. The possibility of an increased risk of breast cancer in Reserpine users has been studied extensively, however, no firm conclusion has emerged. Although a few epidemiologic studies have suggested a slightly increased risk (less than twofold in all studies except one) in women who have used Reserpine, other studies of generally similar design have not confirmed this. Epidemiologic studies conducted using other drugs (neuroleptic agents) that, like Reserpine, increase prolactin levels and, therefore, would be considered rodent mammary carcinogens, have not shown an association between chronic administration of the drug and human mammary tumorigenesis. While long-term clinical observation has not suggested such an association, the available evidence is considered too limited to be conclusive at this time. An association of Reserpine intake with pheochromocytoma or tumors of the serminal vesicles has not been explored.

ADVERSE REACTIONS

Clinical trials indicate that the combination of Chlorthalidone with Reserpine is generally well tolerated. The adverse reactions most frequently seen include anorexia, gastric irritation, nausea, vomiting, diarrhea, constipation, nasal congestion, muscle cramps, dizziness, weakness, headache, drowsiness, and mental depression. Skin rashes, urticaria, and a case of ecchymosis have been reported. (Other dermatologic manifestations may occur—see below.)

A decreased glucose tolerance evidenced by hyperglycemia and glycosuria may develop inconsistently. This condition—usually reversible on discontinuation of therapy—responds to control with antidiabetic treatment. Diabetics and those predisposed should be checked regularly.

Hyperuricemia may be observed on occation and acute attacks of gout have been precipitated in cases where prolonged and significant elevation of blood uric acid concentration is considered potentially deleterious. Concomitant use of a uricosuric agent is effective in reversing hyperuricemia without loss of diuretic and/or antihypertensive activity.

In addition to the reactions listed above, certain adverse reactions attributable to the drugs components are shown below. Since combinations of Chlorthalidone and Reserpine are in relatively small doses, such reactions may be less than when those drugs are used in full dosage.

Chlorthalidone: Idiosyncratic drug reactions such as apiastic anema, purpura, thrombocytopenia, leukopenia, agranulocytosis, necrotizing angiitis and Lyell's syndrome (toxic epidermal necrolysis) have occurred, but are rare.

The remote possibility of pancreatitis should be considered when epigastric pain or unexplained gastrointestinal symptoms develop after prolonged administration.

Other reported reactions include restlessness, transient myopia, impotence or dysuria, and orthostatic hypotension, which may be potentiated when Chlorthalidone is combined with alcohol, barbiturates or narcotics. Since jaundice, xanthopsia paresthesia and photosensitization have been documented in related compounds, the possibility of these reactions should be kept in mind.

Reserpine: The sedative effect of Reserpine may lead to drowsiness or lessitude in some patients. Frequently, this effect disappears with continued administration.

Nasal stuffiness sometimes occurs. Gastrointestinal reactions include increased gastric secretions, loose stools, or increased bowel frequency.

Symptoms of mental depression may occur in a small percentage of patients, although the recommended dosage of Chlorthalidone/Reserpine contains substantially less Reserpine than that usually implicated in such reactions. The same is true of other rare side effects recorded for Reserpine, which include bradycardia and ectopic cardiac rhythms (especially when used with digitalis), pruritus eruptions and/or flushing of skin, angina pectoris, headache, dizziness, paradoxical anxiety, nightmare, dull sensorium, muscular aches, a reversible paralysis agitans-like syndrome, blurred vision, conjunctival infection, uveitis, optic atrophy and glaucoma, increased susceptibility to colds, dyspnea, weight gain, decreased libido or impotence dryness of the mouth, deafness, and anorexia.

OVERDOSAGE

Adverse reactions resulting from accidental acute overdosage may include nausea, weakness, dizziness, syncope, and disturbances of electrolyte balance. There is no specific antidote. However, the following is recommended. Gastric lavage followed by supportive treatment, including intravenous dextrose-saline with potassium chloride if necessary to be given with the usual caution. If marked hypotension results from overdosage, it can be trusted with vasopressor drugs.

DOSAGE AND ADMINISTRATION

Selection of drug and dosage should be determined by individual titration. (See box *"Warning"*). According to the requirement, the recommended dose of Chlorthalidone/Reserpine is usually one tablet once a day. Some patients may require two tablets once a day. Divided doses are unnecessary, and a single dose given in the morning with food is recommended.

Maintenance: Maintenance dosage must be individually adjusted. Mild cases may be adequately controlled with one Chlorthalidone/Reserpine tablet daily. Optimal lowering of elevated blood pressure may require two weeks or more in some cases because of the slow onset of action of Reserpine.

Combination with Other Drugs: In more severe cases, if the response to a Chlorthalidone/Reserpine combination alone is inadequate, potent antihypertensives may be added gradually in dosages at least 50% lower than those usually employed. Such patients should be supervised carefully and continuously. As soon as desired blood pressure levels have been attained the lowest effective maintenance dosage should be followed.

Store at controlled room temperature between 15°-30°C (59°-86°F). Dispense in tight, light-resistant containers as defined in USP.

HOW SUPPLIED
TABLETS: 25 MG-0.125 MG

BRAND/MANUFACTURER	NDC	SIZE	AWP
○ BRAND DEMI-REGROTON: RPR	00075-0032-00	100s	$128.55

TABLETS: 50 MG-0.25 MG

BRAND/MANUFACTURER	NDC	SIZE	AWP
○ BRAND REGROTON: RPR	00075-0031-00	100s	$146.48

Chlorzoxazone

DESCRIPTION

Each caplet contains:

Chlorzoxazone * ....500 mg
* 5-chlorobenzoxazolinone

Following is its chemical structure:

ACTIONS

Chlorzoxazone is a centrally-acting agent for painful musculoskeletal conditions. Data available from animal experiments as well as human study indicate that Chlorzoxazone acts primarily at the level of the spinal cord and subcortical areas of the brain where it inhibits multisynaptic reflex arcs involved in producing and maintaining skeletal muscle spasm of varied etiology. The clinical result is a reduction of the skeletal muscle spasm with relief of pain and increased mobility of the involved muscles. Blood levels of Chlorzoxazone can be detected in people during the first 30 minutes and peak levels may be reached, in the majority of the subjects, in about 1 to 2 hours after oral administration of Chlorzoxazone. Chlorzoxazone is rapidly metabolized and is excreted in the urine, primarily in a conjugated form as the glucuronide. Less than one percent of a dose of Chlorzoxazone is excreted unchanged in the urine in 24 hours.

INDICATIONS

Chlorzoxazone is indicated as an adjunct to rest, physical therapy, and other measures for the relief of discomfort associated with acute, painful musculoskeletal conditions. The mode of action of this drug has not been clearly identified, but

---

◆ RATED THERAPEUTICALLY EQUIVALENT; ◇ THERAPEUTIC EQUIVALENCE UNCONFIRMED; ○ UNRATED

may be related to its sedative properties. Chlorzoxazone does not directly relax tense skeletal muscles in man.

CONTRAINDICATIONS

Chlorzoxazone is contraindicated in patients with known intolerance to the drug.

WARNINGS

The concomitant use of alcohol or other central nervous system depressants may have an additive effect.

Usage in Pregnancy: The safe use of Chlorzoxazone has not been established with respect to the possible adverse effects upon fetal development. Therefore, it should be used in women of childbearing potential only when, in the judgment of the physician, the potential benefits outweigh the possible risks.

PRECAUTIONS

Chlorzoxazone should be used with caution in patients with known allergies or with a history of allergic reactions to drugs. If a sensitivity reaction occurs such as urticaria, redness, or itching of the skin, the drug should be stopped.

If any signs or symptoms suggestive of liver dysfunction are observed, the drug should be discontinued.

ADVERSE REACTIONS

After more than twenty-six years of extensive clinical use of Chlorzoxazone-containing products in an estimated thirty-two million patients, it is apparent that the drug is well tolerated and seldom produces undesirable side effects. Occasional patients may develop gastrointestinal disturbances. It is possible in rare instances that Chlorzoxazone may have been associated with gastrointestinal bleeding. Drowsiness, dizziness, light-headedness, malaise, or overstimulation may be noted by an occasional patient. Rarely, allergic-type skin rashes, petechiae, or ecchymoses may develop during treatment. Angioneurotic edema or anaphylactic reactions are extremely rare. There is no evidence that the drug will cause renal damage. Rarely, a patient may note discoloration of the urine resulting from a phenolic metabolite of Chlorzoxazone. This finding is of no known clinical significance.

Approximately thirty-six patients have been reported in whom the administration of Chlorzoxazone-containing products was suspected as being the cause of liver damage. In one case, the jaundice was subsequently considered to be due to a carcinoma of the head of the pancreas rather than to the drug. In a second case, there was no jaundice but an elevated alkaline phosphatase and BSP retention. In this patient there was a malignancy with bony and liver metastases. The role of the drug was difficult to determine. A third and fourth case had cholelithiasis. Diagnosis in a fifth case was submassive hepatic necrosis possibly due to abusive use of the drug for approximately one year. The remaining cases had a clinical picture compatible with either a viral hepatitis or a drug-induced hepatitis. In all these latter cases, the drug was stopped, and, with one exception, the patients recovered. It is not possible to state that the hepatitis in these patients was or was not drug-induced.

OVERDOSAGE

Symptoms: Initially, gastrointestinal disturbances such as nausea, vomiting, or diarrhea together with drowsiness, dizziness, light-headedness or headache may occur. Early in the course there may be malaise or sluggishness followed by marked loss of muscle tone, making voluntary movement impossible. The deep tendon reflexes may be decreased or absent. The sensorium remains intact, and there is no peripheral loss of sensation. Respiratory depression may occur with rapid, irregular respiration and intercostal and substernal retraction. The blood pressure is lowered, but shock has not been observed.

Treatment: Gastric lavage or induction of emesis should be carried out, followed by administration of activated charcoal. Thereafter, treatment is entirely supportive. If respirations are depressed, oxygen and artificial respiration should be employed and a patent airway assured by use of an oropharyngeal airway or endotracheal tube. Hypotension may be counteracted by use of dextran, plasma, concentrated albumin or a vasopressor agent such as norepinephrine. Cholinergic drugs or analeptic drugs are of no value and should not be used.

DOSAGE AND ADMINISTRATION

Usual Adult Dosage: One caplet three or four times daily. If adequate response is not obtained with this dose, it may be increased to 1½ caplets (750 mg) three or four times daily. As improvement occurs dosage can usually be reduced.

STORAGE

Dispense in a tight container as defined in the official compendium.
Store at room temperature.

HOW SUPPLIED
TABLETS: 250 MG

AVERAGE UNIT PRICE (AVAILABLE SIZES)		GENERIC A-RATED AVERAGE PRICE (GAAP)	
BRAND	$0.55	100s	$7.54
GENERIC	$0.07	1000s	$67.13
HCFA FUL (100s ea)	$0.06		

BRAND/MANUFACTURER	NDC	SIZE	AWP
◆ BRAND			
PARAFLEX: McNeil Pharm	00045-0317-60	100s	$55.06

BRAND/MANUFACTURER	NDC	SIZE	AWP
◆ GENERICS			
Pioneer	60104-6012-02	100s	$4.29
Goldline	00182-1780-01	100s	$6.00
Amide	52152-0053-02	100s	$6.95
Par	49884-0016-01	100s	$9.50
Geneva	00781-1303-01	100s	$10.95
Pioneer	60104-6012-06	500s	$17.60
Pioneer	60104-6012-08	1000s	$33.44
Amide	52152-0053-05	1000s	$62.95
Par	49884-0016-10	1000s	$105.00

TABLETS: 500 MG

AVERAGE UNIT PRICE (AVAILABLE SIZES)		GENERIC A-RATED AVERAGE PRICE (GAAP)	
BRAND	$0.95	100s	$43.14
GENERIC	$0.40	500s	$187.75
HCFA FUL (100s ea)	$0.11		

BRAND/MANUFACTURER	NDC	SIZE	AWP
◆ BRAND			
▶ PARAFON FORTE DSC: McNeil Pharm	00045-0325-60	100s	$94.74
	00045-0325-10	100s ud	$99.07
	00045-0325-70	500s	$453.58
◆ GENERICS			
Ferndale	00496-1055-02	100s	$9.06
STRIFON FORTE DSC: Ferndale	00496-1039-02	100s	$18.00
EZE-DS: Seneca	47028-0052-01	100s	$29.95
▶ Lemmon	00093-0542-01	100s	$44.21
Major	00904-0302-60	100s	$44.25
Aligen	00405-4219-01	100s	$44.32
Qualitest	00603-2886-21	100s	$44.35
Rugby	00536-3444-01	100s	$44.40
Mutual	53489-0193-01	100s	$44.50
Goldline	00182-1189-01	100s	$45.00
Mason Dist	11845-0380-01	100s	$45.12
Geneva	00781-1304-01	100s	$45.25
Royce	51875-0239-01	100s	$45.40
URL	00677-1221-01	100s	$45.60
Schein	00364-2255-01	100s	$45.64
Pioneer	60104-6048-02	100s	$45.65
Caraco	57664-0122-08	100s	$45.75
Martec	52555-0263-01	100s	$46.30
Moore,H.L.	00839-7445-06	100s	$46.97
Moore,H.L.	00839-7725-06	100s	$46.97
Econolab	55053-0787-01	100s	$48.00
Barr	00555-0585-02	100s	$48.98
Parmed	00349-8778-01	100s	$49.33
Raway	00686-0476-20	100s ud	$42.00
UDL	51079-0476-20	100s ud	$49.48
Geneva	00781-1304-13	100s ud	$49.95
Medirex	57480-0431-01	100s ud	$50.25
Ferndale	00496-1055-10	500s	$40.00
STRIFON FORTE DSC: Ferndale	00496-1039-10	500s	$60.00
Goldline	00182-1189-05	500s	$150.00
Major	00904-0302-40	500s	$155.05
Martec	52555-0263-05	500s	$175.70
Mutual	53489-0193-05	500s	$195.00
Moore,H.L.	00839-7445-12	500s	$195.74
Qualitest	00603-2886-28	500s	$198.70
Rugby	00536-3444-05	500s	$210.90
Royce	51875-0239-02	500s	$211.75
Caraco	57664-0122-13	500s	$211.95
Barr	00555-0585-04	500s	$215.81
Parmed	00349-8778-05	500s	$217.30
▶ Lemmon	00093-0542-05	500s	$217.74
Aligen	00405-4219-02	500s	$217.80
Geneva	00781-1304-05	500s	$217.95
Pioneer	60104-6048-06	500s	$219.90
Econolab	55053-0787-05	500s	$228.00
Mason Dist	11845-0380-03	500s	$228.00
STRIFON FORTE DSC: Ferndale	00496-1039-11	1000s	$112.50

Choledyl *SEE* OXTRIPHYLLINE

Cholera Vaccine

DESCRIPTION

Cholera Vaccine, is a sterile suspension of equal parts of Ogawa and Inaba serotypes of killed *Vibrio Cholerae (V. comma)* in buffered sodium chloride injection. The Inaba and Ogawa strains of *V. cholarae* are grown on trypticase soy agar medium, removed from the medium with buffered sodium chloride injection and killed by the addition of 0.5 percent phenol. Phenol in a concentration of 0.5 percent is also used as the preservative in the finished vaccine. The vaccine contains 8 units of each serotype antigen (Ogawa and Inaba) per milliliter.

Cholera Vaccine may be injected intracutaneously (intradermally), subcutaneously or intramuscularly.

CLINICAL PHARMACOLOGY

Cholera Vaccine is used for active immunization against Cholera. Field studies carried out in endemic Cholera areas have shown Cholera Vaccines to be approximately 50% effective in reducing incidence of disease and for only 3 to 6 months. Use of Cholera Vaccine does not prevent transmission of infection.

INDICATION AND USAGE

Active immunization against Cholera is indicated only for individuals traveling to or residing in countries where Cholera is endemic or epidemic.

CONTRAINDICATIONS

Use of Cholera Vaccine should be postponed in the presence of any acute illness.

A history of severe systemic reaction or allergic response following a prior dose of Cholera Vaccine is a contraindication to further use.

WARNINGS

DO NOT INJECT INTRAVENOUSLY.

Cholera Vaccine should not be administered intramuscularly to persons with thrombocytopenia or any coagulation disorder that would contraindicate intramuscular injection.

PRECAUTIONS

GENERAL

A separate, sterilized syringe and needle should be use for each patient to prevent transmission of hepatitis B virus and other infectious agents from one person to another.

Before delivering the dose intramuscularly or subcutaneously, aspirate to help avoid inadvertent injection into a blood vessel.

Before the injection of any biological, the physician should take all precautions known for prevention of allergic or other side reactions. This should include: a review of the patient's history regarding possible sensitivity: and a knowledge of the recent literature pertaining to the use of the biological concerned.

Epinephrine (1:1000) should be available for immediate use when this product is injected.

Some data suggest that administration of Cholera and yellow fever Vaccines within three weeks of each other may result in decreased levels of antibody response to both vaccines as compared with administration at longer intervals. However, there is no evidence that protection to either disease is diminished following simultaneous administration.[1] It is currently recommended that, when feasible, Cholera and yellow fever Vaccines should be administered at a minimal interval of three weeks, unless time constraints preclude this. If the vaccines cannot be administered at least three weeks apart, they should be given simultaneously.[2]

PREGNANCY

Pregnancy Category C. Animal reproduction studies have not been conducted with Cholera Vaccine. It is also not known whether Cholera Vaccine can cause fetal harm when administered to a pregnant woman or can affect reproductive capacity. However, as with other inactivated bacterial vaccines, its use is not contraindicated during pregnancy unless the intended recipient has manifested significant systemic or allergic reaction following administration of prior doses. Use of Cholera Vaccine during pregnancy should be individualized to reflect actual need.[1,3]

ADVERSE REACTIONS

Local reactions manifested by erythema, induration, pain, and tenderness at the site of injection occur in most recipients, and such local reactions may persist for a few days. Recipients frequently develop malaise, headache, and mild-to-moderate temperature elevations which may persist for 1 to 2 days.[1,4]

DOSAGE AND ADMINISTRATION

SHAKE VIAL VIGOROUSLY BEFORE WITHDRAWING EACH DOSE.

Parenteral drug products should be inspected visually for presence of particulate matter and discoloration prior to use. The primary immunizing course consists of two doses administered one week to one month or more apart. The table below summarizes the recommended doses for both primary and booster immunizations by age, volume (mL), and route of administration.[3,5] The intracutaneous (intradermal) route is satisfactory for person 5 years of age and older, but higher levels of antibody may be achieved in children less than 5 years old by the subcutaneous or intramuscular routes.

Route & Age

Dose Number	Intradermal		Subcutaneous or Intramuscular	
	5 years and over	6 mos- 4 years	5-10 years	Over 10 years
1 & 2	0.2 mL	0.2 mL	0.3 mL	0.5 mL
Booster	0.2 mL	0.2 mL	0.3 mL	0.5 mL

In areas where Cholera is epidemic or endemic, booster doses should be given every six months.

The primary immunizing series need never be repeated for booster doses to be effective.

Before injection, the rubber diaphragm of the vial and the skin over the site to be injected should be cleansed and prepared with a suitable germicide.

Keep between 2 and 8°C (35 and 46°F). Keep from freezing.

REFERENCES

1. Recommendation of the Immunization Practices Advisory Committee (ACIP). General recommendations on immunization. MMWR 32(1):1, 1983. 2. Recommendations of the Immunization Practices Advisory Committee (ACIP). yellow fever vaccine. MMWR 32(52):679, 1984. 3. Recommendation of the Public Health Service Advisory Committee on Immunization Practices—Cholera Vaccine. MMWR 27(20):173, 1978. 4. GANGAROSA. E. and FAICH, G.: Cholera: The risk to American travelers. Ann. Int. Med. 74:412, 1971. 5. Report of the Committee on Infectious Diseases, American Academy of Pediatrics, 1982 (Red Book).

HOW SUPPLIED

INJECTION:

BRAND/MANUFACTURER	NDC	SIZE	AWP
○ GENERICS			
Wyeth-Ayerst	00008-0342-02	1.5 ml	$9.10
Wyeth-Ayerst	00008-0342-01	20 ml	$32.53

Cholestyramine

DESCRIPTION

Cholestyramine, the chloride salt of a basic anion exchange resin, a cholesterol lowering agent, is intended for oral administration. Cholestyramine resin is quite hydrophilic, but insoluble in water. The Cholestyramine resin is not absorbed from the digestive tract. One packet or one level scoopful of Cholestyramine Powder contains 4 grams of anhydrous Cholestyramine resin; each tablet contains 1 gram of anhydrous Cholestyramine resin.*

CLINICAL PHARMACOLOGY

Cholesterol is probably the sole precursor of bile acids. During normal digestion, bile acids are secreted into the intestines. A major portion of the bile acids is absorbed from the intestinal tract and returned to the liver via the enterohepatic circulation. Only very small amounts of bile acids are found in normal serum.

Cholestyramine resin adsorbs and combines with the bile acids in the intestine to form an insoluble complex which is excreted in the feces. This results in a partial removal of bile acids from the enterohepatic circulation by preventing their absorption.

The increased fecal loss of bile acids due to Cholestyramine administration leads to an increased oxidation of cholesterol to bile acids, a decrease in beta lipoprotein or low density lipoprotein plasma levels and a decrease in serum cholesterol levels. Although in man, Cholestyramine produces an increase in hepatic synthesis of cholesterol, plasma cholesterol levels fall.

In patients with partial biliary obstruction, the reduction of serum bile acid levels by Cholestyramine reduces excess bile acids deposited in the dermal tissue with resultant decrease in pruritus.

INDICATIONS AND USAGE

1) Cholestyramine is indicated as adjunctive therapy to diet for the reduction of elevated serum cholesterol in patients with primary hypercholesterolemia (elevated low density lipoprotein [LDL] cholesterol) who do not respond adequately to diet. Cholestyramine may be useful to lower LDL cholesterol in patients who also have hypertriglyceridemia, but it is not indicated where hypertriglyceridemia is the abnormality of most concern.

In a large, placebo-controlled, multi-clinic study, the LRC-CPPT[a], hypercholesterolemic subjects treated with Cholestyramine had significant reductions in total and low-density lipoprotein cholesterol (LDL-C). Over the 7-year study period the Cholestyramine group experienced a 19% reduction in the combined rate of coronary heart disease death plus nonfatal myocardial infarction (cumulative incidences of 7% Cholestyramine and 8.6% placebo). The subjects included in the study were middle-aged men (age 35-59) with serum cholesterol levels above 265 mg/dL and no previous history of heart disease. It is not clear to what extent these findings can be extrapolated to other segments of the hypercholesterolemic population not studied.

Dietary therapy specific for the type of hyperlipoproteinemia is the initial treatment of choice. Excess body weight may be an important factor and caloric restriction for weight normalization should be addressed prior to drug therapy in the overweight. The use of drugs should be considered only when reasonable attempts have been made to obtain satisfactory result with nondrug methods. If the decision ultimately is to use drugs, the patient should be instructed that this does not reduce the importance of adhering to diet.

2) Cholestyramine is indicated for the relief of pruritus associated with partial biliary obstruction. Cholestyramine has been shown to have a variable effect on serum cholesterol in these patients. Patients with primary biliary cirrhosis may exhibit an elevated cholesterol as part of their disease.

CONTRAINDICATIONS

Cholestyramine is contraindicated in patients with complete biliary obstruction where bile is not secreted into the intestine and in those individuals who have shown hypersensitivity to any of its components.

---

* As this book went to press, the tablet form was withdrawn from the market.

◆ RATED THERAPEUTICALLY EQUIVALENT; ◇ THERAPEUTIC EQUIVALENCE UNCONFIRMED; ○ UNRATED

WARNING

Phenylketonurics: Some forms of Cholestyramine contain phenylalanine.

PRECAUTIONS

General: Before instituting therapy with Cholestyramine, diseases contributing to increased blood cholesterol such as hypothyroidism, diabetes mellitus, nephrotic syndrome, dysproteinemias and obstructive liver disease should be looked for and specifically treated. A favorable trend in cholesterol reduction should occur during the first month of Cholestyramine therapy. The therapy should be continued to sustain cholesterol reduction. If adequate cholesterol reduction is not attained, Cholestyramine therapy should be discontinued.

Chronic use of Cholestyramine may be associated with increased bleeding tendency due to hypoprothrombinemia associated with Vitamin K deficiency. This will usually respond promptly to parenteral Vitamin K_1 and recurrences can be prevented by oral administration of Vitamin K_1. Reduction of serum or red cell folate has been reported over long term administration of Cholestyramine. Supplementation with folic acid should be considered in these cases.

There is a possibility that prolonged use of Cholestyramine, since it is a chloride form of anion exchange resin, may produce hyperchloremic acidosis. This would especially be true in younger and smaller patients where the relative dosage may be higher.

Cholestyramine may produce or worsen preexisting constipation. Dosage should be reduced or discontinued in such cases. Fecal impaction and aggravation of hemorrhoids may occur. Every effort should be made to avert severe constipation and its inherent problems in those patients with clinically symptomatic coronary artery disease.

Information for Patients: Inform your physician if you are pregnant or plan to become pregnant or are breastfeeding. Drink plenty of fluids while taking Cholestyramine. Mix each dose of Cholestyramine Powder in at least 2 to 6 ounces of fluid before taking. When taking the daily prescribed dosage of Cholestyramine tablets, drink a minimum of one ounce (i.e., a mouthful) of water or other fluid with or following each tablet. Each tablet should be swallowed promptly, one tablet at a time.

Laboratory Tests: Serum cholesterol levels should be determined frequently during the first few months of therapy and periodically thereafter. Serum triglyceride levels should be measured periodically to detect whether significant changes have occurred.

The LRC-CPPT showed a dose-related increase in serum triglycerides of 10.7%-17.1% in the Cholestyramine-treated group, compared with an increase of 7.9%-11.7% in the placebo group. Based on the mean values and adjusting for the placebo group, the Cholestyramine-treated group showed an increase of 5% over pre-entry levels the first year of the study and an increase of 4.3% the seventh year.

Drug Interactions: Cholestyramine may delay or reduce the absorption of concomitant oral medication such as phenylbutazone, warfarin, chlorothiazide (acidic) or propranolol (basic), as well as tetracycline, penicillin G, phenobarbital, thyroid and thyroxine preparations, and digitalis. Interference with the absorption of oral phosphate supplements has been observed with another positively-charged bile acid sequestrant. The discontinuance of Cholestyramine could pose a hazard to health if a potentially toxic drug such as digitalis has been titrated to a maintenance level while the patient was taking Cholestyramine.

Because Cholestyramine binds bile acids, Cholestyramine may interfere with normal fat digestion and absorption and thus may prevent absorption of fat soluble vitamins such as A, D and K. When Cholestyramine is given for long periods of time, concomitant supplementation with water-miscible (or parenteral) form of vitamins A and D should be considered.

SINCE CHOLESTYRAMINE MAY BIND OTHER DRUGS GIVEN CONCURRENTLY, PATIENTS SHOULD TAKE OTHER DRUGS AT LEAST 1 HOUR BEFORE OR 4 TO 6 HOURS AFTER CHOLESTYRAMINE (OR AT AS GREAT AN INTERVAL AS POSSIBLE) TO AVOID IMPEDING THEIR ABSORPTION.

Carcinogenesis, Mutagenesis and Impairment of Fertility: In studies conducted in rats in which Cholestyramine resin was used as a tool to investigate the role of various intestinal factors, such as fat, bile salts and microbial flora, in the development of intestinal tumors induced by potent carcinogens, the incidence of such tumors was observed to be greater in Cholestyramine resin-treated rats than in control rats.

The relevance of this laboratory observation from studies in rats to the clinical use of Cholestyramine is not known. In the LRC-CPPT study referred to above, the total incidence of fatal and nonfatal neoplasms was similar in both treatment groups. When the many different categories of tumors are examined, various alimentary system cancers were somewhat more prevalent in the Cholestyramine group. The small numbers and the multiple categories prevent conclusions from being drawn. However, in view of the fact that Cholestyramine resin is confined to the GI tract and not absorbed, and in light of the animal experiments referred to above, further follow-up of the LRC-CPPT participants is planned for cause-specific mortality and cancer morbidity.

Pregnancy: Since Cholestyramine is not absorbed systemically, it is not expected to cause fetal harm when administered during pregnancy in recommended dosages. There are, however, no adequate and well-controlled studies in pregnant women, and the known interference with absorption of fat-soluble vitamins may be detrimental even in the presence of supplementation.

Nursing Mothers: Caution should be exercised when Cholestyramine is administered to a nursing mother. The possible lack of proper vitamin absorption described in the *"Pregnancy"* section may have an effect on nursing infants.

Pediatric Use: As experience in infants and children is limited, a practical dosage schedule has not been established. In calculating pediatric dosages, 44.4 mg or 80 mg of anhydrous Cholestyramine resin are contained in 100 mg of Cholestyramine. The effects of long-term drug administration, as well as its effect in maintaining lowered cholesterol levels in pediatric patients, are unknown.

ADVERSE REACTIONS

The most common adverse reaction is constipation. When used as a cholesterol-lowering agent, predisposing factors for most complaints of constipation are high dose and increased age (more than 60 years old). Most instances of constipation are mild, transient, and controlled with conventional therapy. Some patients require a temporary decrease in dosage or discontinuation of therapy.

Less Frequent Adverse Reactions: Abdominal discomfort and/or pain, flatulence, nausea, vomiting, diarrhea, dyspepsia, eructation, anorexia, and steatorrhea, bleeding tendencies due to hypoprothrombinemia (Vitamin K deficiency) as well as Vitamin A (one case of night blindness reported) and D deficiencies, hyperchloremic acidosis in children, osteoporosis, rash and irritation of the skin, tongue and perianal area. One 10-month-old baby with biliary atresia had an impaction presumed to be due to Cholestyramine after 3 days administration of 9 grams daily. She developed acute intestinal sepsis and died.

Occasional calcified material has been observed in the biliary tree, including calcification of the gallbladder, in patients to whom Cholestyramine resin has been given. However, this may be a manifestation of the liver disease and not drug related.

One patient experienced biliary colic on each of three occasions on which he took Cholestyramine. One patient diagnosed as acute abdominal symptom complex was found to have a "pasty mass" in the transverse colon on x-ray.

Other events (not necessarily drug related) reported in patients taking Cholestyramine include:

Gastrointestinal: GI-rectal bleeding, black stools, hemorrhoidal bleeding, bleeding from known duodenal ulcer, dysphagia, hiccups, ulcer attack, sour taste, pancreatitis, rectal pain, diverticulitis.

Laboratory Test Changes: Liver function abnormalties.

Hematologic: Prolonged prothrombin time, ecohymosis, anemia.

Hypersensitivity: Urticaria, asthma, wheezing, shortness of breath.

Musculoskeletal: Backache, muscle and joint pains, arthritis.

Neurologic: Headache, anxiety, vertigo, dizziness, fatigue, tinnitus, syncope, drowsiness, femoral nerve pain, paresthesia.

Eye: Uveitis.

Renal: Hematuria, dysuria, burnt odor to urine, diuresis.

Miscellaneous: Weight loss, weight gain, increased libido, swollen glands, edema, dental bleeding, dental caries.

OVERDOSAGE

Overdosage with Cholestyramine has been reported in a patient taking 150% of the maximum recommended daily dosage for a period of several weeks. No ill effects were reported. Should overdosage occur, the chief potential harm would be obstruction of the gastrointestinal tract. The location of such potential obstruction, the degree of obstruction, and the presence or absence of normal gut motility would determine treatment.

DOSAGE AND ADMINISTRATION

The recommended starting adult dose for Cholestyramine is 1 packet, 1 level scoopful, or 4 tablets Cholestyramine (4 grams of anhydrous Cholestyramine resin) once or twice a day. The recommended maintenance dose for Cholestyramine is 2 to 4 packets or scoopfuls or 8 to 16 tablets daily (8-16 grams anhydrous Cholestyramine resin) divided into two doses. It is recommended that increases in dose be gradual with periodic assessment of lipid/lipoprotein levels at intervals of not less than 4 weeks. The maximum recommended daily dose is 6 packets or scoopfuls or 24 tablets of Cholestyramine (24 grams of anhydrous Cholestyramine resin). The suggested time of administration is at mealtime but may be modified to avoid interference with absorption of other medications. Although the recommended dosing schedule is twice daily, Cholestyramine may be administered in 1 to 6 doses per day.

Cholestyramine powder should not be taken in its dry form. Always mix Cholestyramine powder with water or other fluids before ingesting. (See *"Preparation Instructions"*.)

At least 4 ounces of water or other fluid should be taken with or following each 4 tablet dose. It is recommended that each tablet be swallowed promptly, 1 at a time, with a minimum of 1 ounce (i.e., a mouthful) of fluid.

CONCOMITANT THERAPY

Preliminary evidence suggests that the lipid-lowering effects of Cholestyramine on total and LDL-cholesterol are enhanced when combined with a HMG-CoA reductase inhibitor, e.g., pravastatin, lovastatin, and simvastatin. Additive effects on LDL-cholesterol are also seen with combined nicotinic acid/Cholestyramine therapy. See the Drug Interactions subsection of the *"Precautions"* section for recommendations on administering concomitant therapy.

➤ SHOWN IN PRODUCT IDENTIFICATION GUIDE

PREPARATION OF POWDER

The color of Cholestyramine may vary somewhat from batch to batch but this variation does not affect the performance of the product. Place the contents of one single-dose packet or one level scoopful of Cholestyramine in a glass or cup. Add at least 2 to 6 ounces of water or the beverage of your choice. Stir to a uniform consistency.

Cholestyramine may also be mixed with highly fluid soups or pulpy fruits with a high moisture content such as applesauce or crushed pineapple.

Store at room temperature.

CLINICAL STUDIES

The NIH has concluded a 10-year randomized double-blind placebo-controlled study[a] in 12 lipid research clinics on the effect of lowering plasma cholesterol on coronary heart disease (CHD) risk (the risk of either coronary death or nonfatal myocardial infarction). Plasma cholesterol was lowered by a combination of a modest cholesterol-lowering diet and Cholestyramine. The dose response relationship between the amount of Cholestyramine ingested daily, the lowering of total plasma cholesterol, and the reduction in CHD risk is summarized below:

RELATION OF REDUCTION IN CHOLESTEROL TO REDUCTION IN CORONARY HEART DISEASE RISK

Packet Count	Grams of Cholestyramine Resin	No.	Total Cholesterol Lowering	Reduction in CHD Risk
0-2	0-8	439	4.4%	10.9%
2-5	8-20	496	11.5%	26.1%
5-6	20-24	965	19.0%	39.3%

REFERENCE

[a] Anon: The Lipid Research Clinics Coronary Primary Prevention Trial Results: (1) Reduction in Incidence of Coronary Heart Disease; (II) The Relationship of Reduction in Incidence of Coronary Heart Disease to Cholesterol Lowering. *JAMA.* 1984: 251:351-374.

HOW SUPPLIED
POWDER FOR RECONSTITUTION: 4 GM/9 GM

BRAND/MANUFACTURER	NDC	SIZE	AWP
○ **BRAND**			
QUESTRAN: Bristol Labs	00087-0580-11	60s	$79.41
	00087-0580-05	378 gm	$34.79

POWDER FOR RECONSTITUTION: 4 GM/5 GM

BRAND/MANUFACTURER	NDC	SIZE	AWP
○ **BRAND**			
QUESTRAN LIGHT: Bristol Labs	00087-0589-03	60s	$79.41
	00087-0589-01	210 gm	$34.79

TABLETS: 1 GM

BRAND/MANUFACTURER	NDC	SIZE	AWP
○ **BRAND**			
QUESTRAN: Bristol Labs	00087-5003-41	240s	$71.47

Choline Bitartrate and Dexpanthenol

DESCRIPTION

Each tablet contains Choline Bitartrate 25 mg and Dexpanthenol 50 mg. Choline Bitartrate/Dexpanthenol tablets are indicated for use as an antiflatulent. Choline is chemically 2-hydroxy-N,N,N-trimethylethanaminium hydroxide. Dexpanthenol is a derivative of pantothenic acid, a member of the B complex vitamins. The chemical name is D(+)-2,4-dihydroxy-N-(3-hydroxypropyl)-3,3-dimethylbutyramide.

The empirical formula for Choline Bitartrate is $C_9H_{19}NO_7$ and the empirical formula for Dexpanthenol is $C_9H_{19}NO_4$.

CLINICAL PHARMACOLOGY

Pantothenic acid is a precursor of coenzyme A which serves as a cofactor for a variety of enzyme-catalyzed reactions involving transfer of acetyl groups. The final step in the synthesis of acetylcholine consists of Choline acetylase transfer of an acetyl group from acetylcoenzyme A to Choline. Acetylcholine is the neurohumoral transmitter in the parasympathetic system and as such maintains the normal functions of the intestine. Decrease in acetylcholine content would result in decreased peristalsis and in extreme cases adynamic ileus. The pharmacological mode of action of the drug is unknown.

In addition to being the precursor for acetylcholine, Choline is essential for normal transport of fat, as a constituent of the phospholipid lecithin. It can also serve as a methyl donor in intermediary metabolism. Choline qualitatively has the same pharmacological actions as acetylcholine, but is much less active. Single oral doses of 10 g produce no obvious pharmacodynamic response.

A study in humans found that urinary concentrations of pantothenic acid increased ten to fifty-fold above baseline during a four hour period following ingestion of 100 mg Dexpanthenol. Within 24 hours urinary levels were only slightly above baseline. One subject excreted 38 mg during the 24 hours following the oral administration of 100 mg.

Choline is fairly readily absorbed from the gastrointestinal tract. However, a proportion of Choline administered orally to human subjects appears to be converted to trimethylamine and its oxide by intestinal bacteria before absorption takes place. On ingestion of 2 to 8 g of Choline (as bicarbonate) by humans less than 0.3 percent of the dose was found in the urine, while two-thirds of the ingested Choline nitrogen appeared in the urine as trimethylamine or its oxide. Following intravenous infusion of 1 or 2 g of Choline base in 500 or 1000 mL of 5 percent dextrose solution about 9 percent of the Choline was found in the urine with no significant increase in urinary trimethylamine.

INDICATIONS AND USAGE

May be helpful in relieving patients with gas retention associated with the splenic flexure syndrome, cholecystitis, gastritis, gastric hyper-acidity, irritable colon, regional ileitis, postantibiotic and postoperative gas retention or during laxative withdrawal.

CONTRAINDICATIONS

There are no known contraindications to the use of Choline Bitartrate/Dexpanthenol.

WARNINGS

There have been rare instances of allergic reactions of unknown cause during the concomitant use of Dexpanthenol with drugs such as antibiotics, narcotics and barbiturates.

If any signs of a hypersensitivity reaction appear, Choline Bitartrate/Dexpanthenol should be discontinued.

Choline Bitartrate/Dexpanthenol should not be administered within one hour of succinylcholine.

PRECAUTIONS

Drug Interactions: The effects of succinylcholine appeared to have been prolonged in a woman administered Dexpanthenol.

Carcinogenicity, Mutagenicity, and Impairment of Fertility: There have been no studies in animals to evaluate the carcinogenic, mutagenic, or impairment of fertility potential of Choline Bitartrate/Dexpanthenol.

Pregnancy: Category C. Animal reproduction studies have not been conducted with Choline Bitartrate/Dexpanthenol. It is also not known whether Choline Bitartrate/Dexpanthenol can cause fetal harm when administered to a pregnant woman or can affect reproduction capacity. Choline Bitartrate/Dexpanthenol should be given to a pregnant woman only if clearly needed.

Nursing Mothers: It is not known whether Choline or Dexpanthenol are excreted in human milk. Because many drugs are excreted in human milk, caution should be exercised when Choline Bitartrate/Dexpanthenol is administered to a nursing woman.

Pediatric Use: Safety and effectiveness in children have not been established.

ADVERSE REACTIONS

There have been reports of generalized dermatitis in two patients, urticaria in one patient and a dull headache in one patient treated with Choline Bitartrate/Dexpanthenol. A causal relationship is uncertain.

DOSAGE AND ADMINISTRATION

Adult dosage—2 to 3 tablets three times daily.

Store at controlled room temperature, 15°-30°C (59°-86°F).

Protect from light.

HOW SUPPLIED
TABLETS:

BRAND/MANUFACTURER	NDC	SIZE	AWP
○ **BRAND**			
ILOPAN CHOLINE: Savage	00281-2311-17	100s	$72.12
	00281-2311-21	500s	$334.64

Choline Magnesium Trisalicylate

DESCRIPTION

Choline Magnesium Trisalicylate is a nonsteroidal, anti-inflammatory preparation which is freely soluble in water. The absolute structure of Choline Magnesium Trisalicylate is not known at this time. Choline Magnesium Trisalicylate has a molecular formula of $C_{26}H_{29}O_{10}NMg$ and a molecular weight of 539.8. Choline Magnesium Trisalicylate is available as tablets and as a liquid.

Each 500-mg tablet contains:

Choline Salicylate	293 mg
Magnesium Salicylate	362 mg
(500 mg Salicylate content)	

Each 750-mg tablet contains:

Choline Salicylate	440 mg
Magnesium Salicylate	544 mg
(750 mg Salicylate content)	

◆ RATED THERAPEUTICALLY EQUIVALENT; ◇ THERAPEUTIC EQUIVALENCE UNCONFIRMED; ○ UNRATED

Each 1000-mg tablet contains:

Choline Salicylate	587 mg
Magnesium Salicylate	725 mg
(1000 mg Salicylate content)	

Each teaspoonful (5 ml) of liquid contains:

Choline Salicylate	293 mg
Magnesium Salicylate	362 mg
(500 mg Salicylate content)	

Following is its chemical structure:

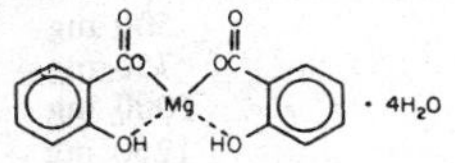

CLINICAL PHARMACOLOGY

Choline Magnesium Trisalicylate tablets and liquid contain Salicylate with anti-inflammatory analgesic and antipyretic action. On ingestion of Choline Magnesium Trisalicylate tablets and liquid, the Salicylate moiety is absorbed rapidly and reaches peak blood levels within an average of one to two hours after single doses of the tablets or liquid. The primary route of excretion is renal: the excretion products are chiefly the glycine and glucuronide conjugates. At higher serum Salicylate concentrations, the glycine conjugation pathway becomes rapidly saturated. Thus, the slower glucuronide conjugation pathway becomes the rate limiting step for Salicylate excretion. In addition, Salicylate excreted in the bile as glucuronide conjugate may be reabsorbed. These factors account for the prolongation of Salicylate half-life and the nonlinear increase in plasma Salicylate level as the Salicylate dose is increased. The serum concentration of Salicylate is increased by conditions that decrease glomerular filtration rate or proximal tubular secretion.

The bioequivalence of Choline Magnesium Trisalicylate liquid and tablets 500 mg/750 mg/100 mg has been established. With the tablets, a steady-state condition is usually reached after 4 to 5 doses, and the half-life of elimination, on repeated administration of tablets, is 9 to 17 hours. This permits a maintenance dosage schedule of once or twice daily. Unlike aspirin and certain other non-steroidal anti-inflammatory agents, such as arylpropionic acid derivatives and arylacetic acid derivatives, Choline Magnesium Trisalicylate, at therapeutic dosage levels, does not affect platelet aggregation, as shown by *in vitro* and *in vivo* studies.

INDICATIONS AND USAGE

Osteoarthritis, Rheumatoid Arthritis and Acute Painful Shoulder: Salicylates are considered the base therapy of choice in the arthritides; and Choline Magnesium Trisalicylate preparations are indicated for the relief of the signs and symptoms of rheumatoid arthritis, osteoarthritis and other arthritides. Choline Magnesium Trisalicylate tablets and liquid are indicated in the long-term management of these diseases and especially in the acute flare of rheumatoid arthritis. Choline Magnesium Trisalicylate tablets and liquid are also indicated for the treatment of acute painful shoulder.

Choline Magnesium Trisalicylate preparations are effective and generally well tolerated, and are logical choices whenever Salicylate treatment is indicated. They are particularly suitable when a once-a-day or b.i.d. dosage regimen is important to patient compliance; when gastrointestinal intolerance to aspirin is encountered; when gastrointestinal microbleeding or hematologic effects of aspirin are considered a patient hazard; and when interference (or the risk of interference) with normal platelet function by aspirin or by propionic acid derivatives is considered to be clinically undesirable. Use of Choline Magnesium Trisalicylate liquid is appropriate when a liquid dosage form is preferred, as in the elderly patient.

The efficacy of Choline Magnesium Trisalicylate preparations has not been studied in those patients who are designated by the American Rheumatism Association as belonging in Functional Class IV (incapacitated, largely or wholly bedridden or confined to a wheelchair, with little or no self-care). Analgesic and Antipyretic Action: Choline Magnesium Trisalicylate tablets and liquid are also indicated for the relief of mild to moderate pain and for antipyresis. *In children,* Choline Magnesium Trisalicylate preparations are indicated for conditions requiring anti-inflammatory or analgesic action—such as juvenile rheumatoid arthritis and other appropriate conditions.

CONTRAINDICATIONS

Patients who are hypersensitive to non-acetylated Salicylates should not take Choline Magnesium Trisalicylate tablets or liquid.

WARNINGS

Reye Syndrome is a rare but serious disease which may develop in children and teenagers who have chicken pox, influenza, or flu symptoms. While the cause of Reye Syndrome is unknown, some studies suggest a possible association between the development of Reye Syndrome and the use of medicines containing acetylated Salicylates or aspirin. Choline Magnesium Trisalicylate tablets and liquid are a combination of Choline Salicylate and Magnesium Salicylate, which are nonacetylated Salicylates, and there have been no reported cases associating Choline Magnesium Trisalicylate with Reye Syndrome. Nevertheless, Choline Magnesium Trisalicylate as a Salicylate-containing product, is not recommended for use in children and teenagers with chicken pox, influenza or flu symptoms.

PRECAUTIONS

General Precautions: As with other Salicylates and non-steroidal anti-inflammatory drugs, Choline Magnesium Trisalicylate preparations should be used with caution in patients with acute or chronic renal insufficincy, with acute or chronic hepatic dysfunction, or with gastritis or peptic ulcer disease.

Although reports exist of cross reactivity, including bronchospasm, with the use of non-acetylated Salicylate products in aspirin-sensitive patients, Choline Magnesium Trisalicylate preparations were found to be well tolerated with regard to pulmonary function and respiratory symptoms when these parameters were monitored in a group of documented aspirin-sensitive asthmatics dosed with Choline Magnesium Trisalicylate in both controlled and open label studies.[1]

Concurrent use of other Salicylate-containing products and Choline Magnesium Trisalicylate preparations can lead to an increase in plasma Salicylate concentration and may result in potentially toxic Salicylate levels.

Laboratory Tests: Plasma Salicylate levels can be periodically assessed during treatment with Choline Magnesium Trisalicylate preparations to determine whether a therapeutically effective anti-inflammatory concentration of 15 to 30 mg/100 ml (150-300 micrograms/ml) is being maintained. Manifestations of systemic Salicylate intoxication are usually not seen until the concentration exceeds 30 mg/100 ml. However, such tests rarely differentiate between the active free and inactive protein bound Salicylate components. Since protein binding of Salicylate is affected by age, nutritional status, competitive binding of other drugs, and underlying disease (e.g. rheumatoid arthritis), plasma Salicylate level determinations may not always accurately reflect efficacious or toxic levels of active free Salicylate. Acidification of the urine can significantly diminish the renal clearance of Salicylate and increase plasma Salicylate concentrations.

Drug Interactions: Foods and drugs that alter urine pH may affect renal clearance of Salicylate and plasma Salicylate concentrations. Raising urine pH, as with chronic antacid use, can enhance renal Salicylate clearance and diminish plasma Salicylate concentration; urine acidification can decrease urinary Salicylate excretion and increase plasma levels.

When Salicylate drug products are concurrently dosed with other plasma protein bound drug products, adverse effects may result. Although Choline Magnesium Trisalicylate preparations are a rational choice for anti-inflammatory and analgesic therapy in patients on oral anticoagulants due to their demonstrated lack of effect *in vivo* and *in vitro* on platelet aggregation, bleeding time, platelet count, prothrombin time, and serum thromboxane B2 generation[1-7], the potential exists for increased levels of unbound warfarin with their concurrent use. Prothrombin time should be closely monitored and warfarin dose appropriately adjusted when therapy with Choline Magnesium Trisalicylate preparations is initiated. The effect of Choline Magnesium Trisalicylate on blood prothrombin levels has not been established. Salicylates may increase the therapeutic as well as toxic effects of methotrexate, particularly when administered in chemotherapeutic doses, by inhibition of renal methotrexate excretion and by displacement of plasma protein bound methotrexate. Caution should be exercised in administering Choline Magnesium Trisalicylate to rheumatoid arthritis patients on methotrexate. When sulfonylurea oral hypoglycemic agents are co-administered with Salicylates, the hypoglycemic effect may be enhanced via increased insulin secretion or by displacement of sulfonylurea agents from binding sites. Insulin-treated diabetics on high doses of Salicylates should also be closely monitored for a similar hypoglycemic response. Other drugs with which Salicylate competes for protein binding sites, and whose plasma concentration or free fraction may be altered by concurrent Salicylate administration, include the following: phenytoin, valproic acid, and carbonic anhydrase inhibitors.

The efficacy of uricosuric agents may be decreased when administered with Salicylate products. Although low doses of Salicylate (1 to 2 grams per day) have been reported to decrease urate excretion and elevate plasma urate concentrations, intermediate doses (2 to 3 grams per day) usually do not alter urate excretion. Larger Salicylate doses (over 5 grams per day) can induce uricosuria and lower plasma urate levels.

Corticosteroids can reduce plasma Salicylate levels by increasing renal elimination and perhaps by also stimulating hepatic metabolism of Salicylates. By monitoring plasma Salicylate levels, Salicylate dosage may be titrated to accommodate changes in corticosteroid dose or to avoid Salicylate toxicity during corticosteroid taper.

Drug/Laboratory Test Interactions: Free T4 values may be increased in patients on Salicylate drug products due to competitive plasma protein binding; a concurrent decrease in total plasma T4 may be observed. Thyroid function is not affected.

Carcinogenesis: No long-term animal studies have been performed with Choline Magnesium Trisalicylate to evaluate its carcinogenic potential.

Use in Pregnancy: Pregnancy Category C. Animal reproduction studies have not been conducted with Choline Magnesium Trisalicylate preparations. It is also not known whether Choline Magnesium Trisalicylate can cause fetal harm when administered to a pregnant woman or can affect reproduction capacity. Choline Magnesium Trisalicylate should be given to a pregnant woman only if clearly needed. Because of the known effects of other Salicylate drug products on the fetal cardiovascular system (closure of ductus arteriosus), use during late pregnancy should be avoided.

Labor and Delivery: The effects of Choline Magnesium Trisalicylate on labor and delivery in pregnant women are unknown. Since prolonged gestation and prolonged labor due to prostaglandin inhibition have been reported with the use of other Salicylate products, the use of Choline Magnesium Trisalicylate preparations near term is not recommended. Other Salicylate products have also been associated with alterations in maternal and neonatal hemostasis mechanisms and with perinatal mortality.

Nursing Mothers: Salicylate is excreted in human milk. Peak milk Salicylate levels are delayed, occurring as long as 9 to 12 hours post dose, and the milk: plasma ratio has been reported to be as high as 0.34. Because of the potential for significant Salicylate absorption by the nursing infant, caution should be exercised when Choline Magnesium Sulfate is administered to a nursing woman.

Pediatric Use: In a four-week open label pilot study of patients with juvenile rheumatoid arthritis, children from 6 to 16 years of age previously on aspirin received weight adjusted doses (50-60 mg/kg) of Choline Magnesium Sulfate 500 mg tablets on a divided BID schedule with subsequent dose titration to achieve therapeutic serum Salicylate levels. Eighty-three percent (83%) of the patients rated the therapeutic effect of Choline Magnesium Sulfate as good or excellent. Tinnitus was reported by one patient and elevated SGOT levels at Week 1, which decreased during the trial, were detected in two patients. (See *"Warning"* section.)

ADVERSE REACTIONS

The most frequent adverse reactions observed with Choline Magnesium Sulfate preparations in clinical trials[7-12] are tinnitus and gastrointestinal complaints (including nausea, vomiting, gastric upset, indigestion, heartburn, diarrhea, constipation and epigastric pain). These occur in less than twenty percent (20%) of patients. Should tinnitus develop, reduction of daily dosage is recommended until the tinnitus is resolved. Less frequent adverse reactions, occurring in less than two percent (2%) of patients, are: hearing impairment, headache, light-headedness, dizziness, drowsiness, and lethargy. Adverse reactions occurring in less than one percent (1%) of patients are: gastric ulceration, positive fecal occult blood, elevation in serum BUN and creatinine, rash, pruritus, anorexia, weight gain, edema, epistaxis and dysgeusia.

Spontaneous reporting has yielded isolated or rare reports of the following adverse experiences: duodenal ulceration, elevated hepatic transaminases, hepatitis, esophagitis, asthma, erythema multiforme, urticaria, ecchymoses, irreversible hearing loss and/or tinnitus, mental confusion, hallucinations.

DRUG ABUSE AND DEPENDENCE

Drug abuse and dependence have not been reported with Choline Magnesium Trisalicylate preparations.

OVERDOSAGE

Death in adults has been reported following ingestion of doses from 10 to 30 grams of Salicylate; however, larger doses have been taken without resulting fatality.

Symptoms: Salicylate intoxication, known as salicylism, may occur with large doses or extended therapy. Common symptoms of salicylism include headache, dizziness, tinnitus, hearing impairment, confusion, drowsiness, sweating, vomiting, diarrhea, and hyperventilation. A more severe degree of Salicylate intoxication can lead to CNS disturbances, alteration in electrolyte balance, respiratory and metabolic acidosis, hyperthermia, and dehydration.

Treatment: Reduction of further absorption of Salicylate from the gastrointestinal tract can be achieved via emesis, gastric lavage, use of activated charcoal, or a combination of the above. Appropriate I.V. fluids should be administered to correct dehydration, electrolyte imbalance, and acidosis and to maintain adequate renal function. To accelerate Salicylate excretion, forced diuresis with alkalinizing solution is recommended. In extreme cases, peritoneal dialysis or hemodialysis should be considered for effective Salicylate removal.

DOSAGE AND ADMINISTRATION

Adults: In rheumatoid arthritis, osteoarthritis, the more severe arthritides, and acute painful shoulder, the recommended starting dosage is 1500 mg given b.i.d.. Some patients may be treated with 3000 mg given once per day (h.s.). In the elderly patient, a daily dosage of 2250 mg given as 750 mg t.i.d. may be efficacious and well tolerated. Dosage should be adjusted in accordance with the patient's response. In patients with renal dysfunction, monitor Salicylate levels and adjust dose accordingly.

For mild to moderate pain or for antipyresis, the usual dosage is 2000 mg to 3000 mg daily in divided doses (b.i.d.). Based on patient response or Salicylate blood levels, dosage may be adjusted to achieve optimum therapeutic effect. Salicylate blood levels should be in the range of 15 to 30 mg/100 ml for anti-inflammatory effect and 5 to 15 mg/100 ml for analgesia and antipyresis.

Each 500 mg tablet or teaspoonful is equivalent in Salicylate content to 10 gr of aspirin; each 750 mg tablet, to 15 gr of aspirin, and each 1000 mg tablet, to 20 gr of aspirin.

If the physician prefers, the recommended daily dosage may be administered on a t.i.d. schedule.

As with other therapeutic agents, individual dosage adjustment is advisable, and a number of patients may require higher or lower dosages than those recommended. Certain patients require 2 to 3 weeks of therapy for optimal effect.

Children: Usual daily dose for children for anti-inflammatory or analgesic action: Choline Magnesium Trisalicylate 500 mg tablets/liquid and Choline Magnesium Trisalicylate 750 mg and 1000 mg tablets, 50 mg/kg/day.

Weight (kg)	Total daily dose
12-13	500 mg
14-17	750 mg
18-22	1000 mg
23-27	1250 mg
28-32	1500 mg
33-37	1750 mg

Total daily doses should be administered in divided doses (b.i.d.). Doses of Choline Magnesium Trisalicylate preparations are calculated as the total daily dose of 50 mg/kg/day for children of 37 kg body weight or less and 2250 mg/day for heavier children. Choline Magnesium Trisalicylate liquid is available for greater convenience in treating younger patients and those adult patients unable to swallow a solid dosage form.

Storage: Store at controlled room temperature, 59° to 86°F (15° to 30°C).

REFERENCES
1. Szczeklik, A et al; Choline magnesium trisalicylate in patients with aspirin-induced asthma; *Eur Respir F*, 3:535-539, 1990. 2. Zucker, MB and Rothwell KB; Differential influences of salicylate compounds on platelet aggregation and serotonin release: *Current Therapeutic Research*; 23(2), Feb 1987. 3. Stuart, JJ and Pisko, EJ: Choline magnesium trisalicylate does not impair platelet aggregation: *Pharmatherapeutica*; 2(8):547, 1981. 4. Danesh, BJZ, Saniabadi, AR, Russel, RI et al: Therapeutic potential of choline magnesium trisalicylate as an alternative to aspirin for patients with bleeding tendencies: *Scottish Medical Journal*; 32:167-168, 1987. 5. Danesh, BJZ, McLaren, M. Russell, RI et al: Does nonacetylated salicylate inhibit thromboxane biosynthesis in human platelets? *Scottish Medical Journal*; 33: 315-316, 1988. 6. Danesh, BJZ, McLaren, M, Russeli, RI et al; Comparison of the effect of aspirin and choline magnesium trisalicylate on thromboxane biosynthesis in human platelets: role of the acetyl moiety; *Haemostasis*, 19:169-173, 1989. 7. Data on file, Medical Department. The Purdue Frederick Company, 1989. 8. Blechman, WJ, and Lechner, BL; Clinical comparative evaluation of choline magnesium trisalicylate and acetylsalicylic acid in rheumatoid arthritis: *Rheumatology and Rehabilitation*; 18:119-124, 1979. 9. McLaughlin, G; Choline magnesium trisalicylate vs. naproxen in rheumatoid arthritis; *Current Therapeutic Research*; 32(4):579-585, 1982. 10. Ehrlich, GE; Miller, SB; and Zeiders, RS; Choline magnesium trisalicylate vs. ibuprofen in rheumatoid arthritis; *Rheumatology and Rehabilitation*; 19:30-41, 1980. 11. Goldenberg, A; Rudnicki, RD, and Koonce, ML; Clinical comparison of efficacy and safety of choline magnesium trisalicylate and indomethacin in treating osteoarthritis: *Current Therapeutic Research*; 24(3):245-260, 1978. 12. Guerin, BK and Burnstein, SL; Conservative therapy of acute painful shoulder; *Orthopedic Review*, XI(7):29-37, 1982.

HOW SUPPLIED
LIQUID: 500 MG/5 ML

BRAND/MANUFACTURER	NDC	SIZE	AWP
○ BRAND			
TRILISATE: Purdue Frederick	00034-0520-80	240 ml	$28.67

TABLET: 500 MG

BRAND/MANUFACTURER	NDC	SIZE	AWP
○ BRAND			
TRILISATE: Purdue Frederick	00034-0500-80	100s	$60.31
	00034-0500-10	100s ud	$62.92
	00034-0500-50	500s	$301.72
○ GENERICS			
Medirex	57480-0401-06	30s	$9.60
Apotex USA	60999-0150-10	100s	$11.22
TRICOSAL: Duramed	51285-0832-02	100s	$27.70
Invamed	52189-0241-24	100s	$27.70
Geneva	00781-1637-01	100s	$28.56
Goldline	00182-1894-01	100s	$29.49
URL	00677-1390-01	100s	$29.90
CMT: Moore,H.L.	00839-7499-06	100s	$32.52
Sidmak	50111-0528-01	100s	$33.00
Goldline	00182-1899-01	100s	$33.00
Aligen	00405-4229-01	100s	$33.43
Martec	52555-0528-01	100s	$34.65
TRICOSAL: Qualitest	00603-6215-21	100s	$34.90
Major	00904-3395-60	100s	$34.95
Rugby	00536-3452-01	100s	$41.09
Barre	00472-0140-10	100s	$48.55
Medirex	57480-0401-01	100s ud	$32.00

For additional alternatives, turn to the section beginning on page 2859.

◆ RATED THERAPEUTICALLY EQUIVALENT; ◇ THERAPEUTIC EQUIVALENCE UNCONFIRMED; ○ UNRATED

Cholografin Meglumine SEE IODIPAMIDE
MEGLUMINE

Choloxin SEE DEXTROTHYROXINE SODIUM

Chroma-Pak SEE CHROMIC CHLORIDE

Chromic Chloride

DESCRIPTION
Chromic Chloride Injection, USP is a sterile, nonpyrogenic solution intended for use as an additive to intravenous solutions for total parenteral nutrition. Each mL of solution contains 20.5 mcg chromic chloride, hexahydrate and 9 mg sodium chloride. The pH is 2.0 (1.5 to 2.5); solution may contain hydrochloric acid and/or sodium hydroxide for pH adjustment. The osmolarity is 0.308 mOsmol/mL (calc.); specific gravity is 1.003.

The Pharmacy Bulk Package is a sterile dosage form which contains multiple single doses for use only in a pharmacy bulk admixture program. Each vial contains Chromic Chloride 30 mL (4 mcg/mL).

Chromic Chloride, USP is chemically designated Chromic Chloride, hexahydrate $CrCl_3 \cdot 6H_2O$, a crystalline compound soluble in water.

Sodium chloride, USP is chemically designated NaCl, a white, crystalline compound freely soluble in water.

The Pharmacy Bulk Package is designed for use with manual, gravity flow operations and automated compounding devices for preparing sterile parenteral nutrient admixtures. The Pharmacy Bulk Package contains no bacteriostat or antimicrobial agent. Multiple single doses may be dispensed during continual aliquoting operations. The entire contents should be dispensed within 24 hours.

CLINICAL PHARMACOLOGY
Trivalent chromium is part of glucose tolerance factor, an essential activator of insulin-mediated reactions. Chromic Chloride helps to maintain normal glucose metabolism and peripheral nerve function.

Providing chromium during total parenteral nutrition (TPN) helps prevent deficiency symptoms including impaired glucose tolerance, ataxia, peripheral neuropathy and a confusional state similar to mild/moderate hepatic encephalopathy.

Serum chromium is bound to transferrin (siderophilin) in the beta globulin fraction. Typical blood levels for chromium range from 1 to 5 mcg/liter, but blood levels are not considered a meaningful index of tissue stores. Administration of chromium supplements to chromium-deficient patients can result in normalization of the glucose tolerance curve from the diabetic-like curve typical of chromium deficiency. This response is viewed as a more meaningful indicator of chromium nutriture than serum chromium levels.

Excretion of chromium is via the kidneys, ranging from 3 to 50 mcg/day. Biliary excretion via the small intestine may be an ancillary route, but only small amounts of chromium are believed to be excreted in this manner.

INDICATIONS AND USAGE
Chromic Chloride is indicated for use as a supplement to intravenous solutions given for TPN. Administration helps to maintain chromium serum levels and to prevent depletion of endogenous stores and subsequent deficiency symptoms.

CONTRAINDICATIONS
None known.

WARNINGS
Direct intramuscular or intravenous injection of Chromic Chloride is contraindicated, as the acidic pH of the solution (2) may cause considerable tissue irritation.

Severe kidney disease may make it necessary to reduce or omit chromium and zinc doses because these elements are primarily eliminated in the urine.

PRECAUTIONS
GENERAL
Do not use unless solution is clear and seal is intact.

Chromic Chloride should only be used in conjunction with a pharmacy directed admixture program using aseptic technique in a laminar flow environment; it should be used promptly and in a single operation without any repeated penetrations. Solution contains no preservatives; discard unused portion immediately after admixture procedure is completed.

In assessing the contribution of chromium supplements to maintenance of glucose homeostasis, consideration should be given to the possibility that the patient may be diabetic.

LABORATORY TESTS
Because chromium is present in the bloodstream in microgram quantities, routine measurement is impractical. If necessary, samples can be sent to a reference laboratory for assay.

CARCINOGENESIS, MUTAGENESIS, AND IMPAIRMENT OF FERTILITY
Long-term animal studies to evaluate the carcinogenic potential of Chromic Chloride have not been performed, nor have studies been done to assess mutagenesis or impairment of fertility.

NURSING MOTHERS
It is not known whether this drug is excreted in human milk. Because many drugs are excreted in human milk, caution should be exercised when Chromic Chloride is administered to a nursing woman.

PEDIATRIC USE
See "Dosage and Administration" section. Safety and effectiveness in children have not been established.

Pregnancy Category C: Animal reproduction studies have not been conducted with Chromic Chloride. It is also not known whether Chromic Chloride can cause fetal harm when administered to a pregnant woman or can affect reproductive capacity. Chromic Chloride should be given to a pregnant woman only if clearly needed.

ADVERSE REACTIONS
None known.

DRUG ABUSE AND DEPENDENCE
None known.

OVERDOSAGE
Trivalent chromium administered intravenously to TPN patients has been shown to be nontoxic when given at dosage levels of up to 250 mcg/day for two consecutive weeks.

Reported toxic reactions to chromium include nausea, vomiting, ulcers of the gastrointestinal tract, renal and hepatic damage, convulsions and coma. The acute LD_{50} for intravenous trivalent chromium in rats was reported as 10 to 18 mg/kg.

DOSAGE AND ADMINISTRATION
Chromic Chloride contains 4 mcg chromium/mL and is administered intravenously only after dilution. The additive should be administered in a volume of fluid not less than 100 mL. For the adult receiving TPN, the suggested additive dosage is 10 to 15 mcg chromium/day (2.5 to 3.75 mL/day). The metabolically stable adult with intestinal fluid loss may require 20 mcg chromium/day (5 mL/day), with frequent monitoring of blood levels as a guideline for subsequent administration. For pediatric patients, the suggested additive dosage is 0.14 to 0.20 mcg/kg/day (0.035 to 0.05 mL/kg/day).

Chromic Chloride in the Pharmacy Bulk Package is designed for use with manual, gravity flow operations and automated compounding devices for preparing intravenous nutritional admixtures.

Parenteral drug products should be inspected visually for particulate matter and discloration prior to administration, whenever solution and container permit. See "Precautions".

RECOMMENDED DIRECTIONS FOR USE OF THE PHARMACY BULK PACKAGE USE ASEPTIC TECHNIQUE LST
1. During use, container must be stored, and all manipulations performed, in an appropriate laminar flow hood.
2. Remove fliptop from vial and cleanse stopper with antiseptic.
3. Pierce stopper with transfer device. Insertion of transfer device into stopper should be performed only once in a Pharmacy Bulk Package solution without antimicrobial preservative. The time frame permitted for container withdrawals should be as brief as possible, usually no longer than needed to systematically complete aliquoting operations without interruption. Discard container within 24 hours after penetration.
4. Sequentially dispense aliquots of Chromic Chloride into pooling containers using appropriate transfer device. During fluid transfer operations, the Pharmacy Bulk Package should be maintained under the recommended storage conditions.

Store at controlled room temperature, 15° to 30°C (59° to 86°F).

HOW SUPPLIED
INJECTION: 4 MCG/ML

BRAND/MANUFACTURER	NDC	SIZE	AWP
◆ GENERICS			
Abbott Hosp	00074-4093-01	10 ml 25s	$146.95

INJECTION: 4 MCG/ML

BRAND/MANUFACTURER	NDC	SIZE	AWP
○ BRAND			
CHROMA-PAK: Solo Pak	39769-0049-10	10 ml 25s	$59.69

Chromic Phosphate

DESCRIPTION
Therapeutic: For Interstitial or Intracavitary Use Only
Chromic Phosphate P-32 is supplied as a sterile, nonpyrogenic aqueous suspension in a 30% dextrose solution. 2% benzyl alcohol added as preservative.

ACTIONS

Local irradiation by beta emission.

INDICATIONS

Chromic Phosphate P-32 is employed by intracavitary instillation for the treatment of peritoneal or pleural effusions caused by metastatic disease, and may be injected interstitially for the treatment of cancer.

CONTRAINDICATIONS

Chromic Phosphate P-32 therapy should not be used in the presence of ulcerative tumors.

Administration should not be made in exposed cavities or where there is evidence of loculation unless the extent of loculation is determined.

WARNINGS

Not for intravascular use.

This radiopharmaceutical should not be administered to patients who are pregnant or during lactation unless the therapeutic benefits outweigh the potential hazards.

Radiopharmaceuticals should be used only by physicians who are qualified by specific training in the safe use and handling of radionuclides produced by nuclear reactor or particle accelerator and whose experience and training have been approved by the appropriate government agency authorized to license the use of radionuclides.

PRECAUTIONS

As in the use of any other radioactive material care should be taken to insure minimum radiation exposure to the patient, consistent with proper patient management, and to insure minimum radiation exposure to occupational workers.

Careful intracavitary instillation is required to avoid placing the dose of Chromic Phosphate P-32 into intrapleural or intraperitoneal loculations, bowel lumen or into the body wall. Intestinal fibrosis or necrosis and chronic fibrosis of the body wall have been reported to result from unrecognized misplacement of the therapeutic agent.

The presence of large tumor masses indicates the need for other forms of treatment. However, when other forms of treatment fail to control the effusion, Chromic Phosphate P-32 may be useful. In bloody effusion, treatment may be less effective.

ADVERSE REACTIONS

Untoward effects may be associated with use of Chromic Phosphate P-32. These include transitory radiation sickness, bone marrow depression, pleuritis, peritonitis, nausea and abdominal cramping. Radiation damage may occur if accidentally injected intersitially or into a loculation.

DOSAGE AND ADMINISTRATION

The suggested dose range employed in the average patient (70 kg) is:

Intraperitoneal instillation: 370 to 740 megabecquerels (10 to 20 millicuries)
Intrapleural instillation: 222 to 444 megabecquerels (6 to 12 millicuries)

Doses for interstitial use should be based on estimated gram weight of tumor, about 3.7 to 18.5 MBq/gm (0.1 to 0.5 mCi/gm).

The patient dose should be measured by a suitable radioactivity calibration system immediately prior to administration.

PHYSICAL CHARACTERISTICS

Phosphorus-32 decays by beta emission with a physical half-life of 14.3 days.[1] The mean energy of the beta particle is 695 keV.

Table 1
PRINCIPAL RADIATION EMISSION DATA

Radiation	Mean Percent/ Disintegration	Mean Energy (keV)
Beta-1	100.0	694.9

The range of the phosphorus-32 beta particle, which has a maximum energy of 1.71 MeV, is 2.8 mm of aluminum.

To correct for physical decay of this radionuclide, the percentages that remain at selected time intervals before and after the day of calibration are shown in Table 2.

Table 2
PHYSICAL DECAY CHART; PHOSPHORUS-32, HALF-LIFE 14.3 DAYS

Days	Fraction Remaining	Days	Fraction Remaining	Days	Fraction Remaining
-15	2.07	2	0.908	35	0.183
-10	1.62	5	0.785	40	0.144
-5	1.28	10	0.616	45	0.113
-2	1.10	15	0.483	50	0.089
-1	1.05	20	0.379	55	0.070
0*	1.00	25	0.297	60	0.055
1	0.953	30	0.233	65	0.043

* *Calibration Day*

RADIATION DOSIMETRY

The effective half-life of phosphorus-32 is considered to be equal to its physical half-life, with a residence time of 495 hours.

The radiation dose from a uniformly distributed concentration of 37 kilobecquerels (1 microcurie) per gram within a 16-gram prostate is estimated to be equivalent to about 7.3 grays (730 rads). Table 3 shows the estimated radiation doses to the prostate and the pleural or peritoneal surfaces of an average patient (70 kg) from a dose of 740 megabecquerels (20 millicuries) of phosphorus-32.

In comparison to the distribution in the prostate, the distribution of phosphorus-32 on the pleural and peritoneal surfaces is non-uniform, with great extremes in local doses. To obtain an estimate of the average dose, the surface area of the pleural and peritoneal cavities can be assumed to amount to 4,000 and 5,000 cm^2, respectively. The estimated[2] radiation doses to an average patient (70 kg) with 90% retention of a dose of 740 megabecquerels (20 millicuries) of phosphorus-32 distributed uniformly over these areas are shown in Table 3. The decreases of the averaged radiation doses at various tissue depths away from the surfaces of the pleural and peritoneal cavities are also tabulated.

Table 3
ESTIMATED RADIATION DOSES

Surface/Organ		Pleural		Peritoneal		Prostate	
% Retention Area/wt		90 4000 cm2		90 5000 cm2		100 16 gm	
Dose rate*				Tissue Dose/740 MBq (20mCi)			
Depth in tissue (cm)	(rads/ hr)	(mGy/ hr)	rads	grays	rads	grays	rads	grays
0.004	10.2	102	23000	230	18000	180	910000	9100
0.008	8.58	85.8	19000	190	15000	150		
0.012	7.61	76.1	17000	170	14000	140		
0.016	6.91	69.1	15000	150	12000	120		
0.020	6.36	63.6	14000	140	11000	110		
0.10	2.41	24.1	5400	54	4300	43		
0.20	0.94	9.4	2100	21	1700	17		

* *For surface deposition of 37 kBq(1 μCi)/ cm2*

REFERENCES

1. Kocher, David C., "Radioactive Decay Data Tables," DOE/TIC 11026, page 70 (1981). 2. Estimated radiation doses shown in Table 3 are based on compilations by Cross, William G., Table of Beta Dose Distribution, Report AECL 2793 Chalk River, Ontario, November 1967.

HOW SUPPLIED

Current prices are unavailable. Check wholesaler for further information.

HOW SUPPLIED INJECTION:

BRAND/MANUFACTURER	NDC	SIZE	AWP
○ BRAND			
PHOSPHOCOL P32: Mallinckrodt Medical	(Not Available)	5mci/ml	$1,985.00

Chronulac *SEE* LACTULOSE

Chymex *SEE* BENTIROMIDE

Chymodiactin *SEE* CHYMOPAPAIN

Chymopapain

WARNINGS

CHYMOPAPAIN SHOULD ONLY BE USED IN A HOSPITAL SETTING BY PHYSICIANS EXPERIENCED AND TRAINED IN THE DIAGNOSIS OF LUMBAR DISC DISEASE AND ALL STANDARD TREATMENT METHODS, INCLUDING SURGERY. ADDITIONALLY, THESE PHYSICIANS AND THEIR SUPPORT PERSONNEL SHOULD BE COMPETENT IN THE DIAGNOSIS AND MANAGEMENT OF ALL POTENTIAL COMPLICATIONS FROM THE USE OF CHYMOPAPAIN.

ANAPHYLAXIS, WHICH CAN BE FATAL, IS INDEPENDENT OF THE TYPE OF ANESTHESIA USED, AND OCCURS IN APPROXIMATELY 0.5% OF PATIENTS RECEIVING CHYMOPAPAIN.

PARAPLEGIA/PARAPARESIS, CENTRAL NERVOUS SYSTEM HEMORRHAGE, AND OTHER SERIOUS NEUROLOGIC ADVERSE EVENTS HAVE BEEN OBSERVED WITHIN HOURS OR DAYS FOLLOWING

CHYMOPAPAIN INJECTION AT A RATE OF LESS THAN 1 IN 2,000. ONSET OF PARAPLEGIA/PARAPARESIS HAS ALSO BEEN REPORTED 2 TO 3 WEEKS AFTER CHYMOPAPAIN INJECTION AT A MUCH LOWER RATE OF LESS THAN 1 IN 20,000. A CAUSE AND EFFECT RELATIONSHIP BETWEEN THESE NEUROLOGIC EVENTS AND CHYMOPAPAIN WHEN PROPERLY INJECTED HAS NOT BEEN ESTABLISHED.

CHYMOPAPAIN IS EXTREMELY TOXIC WHEN INJECTED INTRATHECALLY, AS ARE SOME RADIOPAQUE CONTRAST MEDIA USED FOR DISCOGRAPHY. IN MANY OF THE REPORTED CASES OF SERIOUS NEUROLOGIC ADVERSE EVENTS, DISCOGRAPHY WAS PERFORMED AS PART OF THE PROCEDURE. GREAT CARE MUST BE TAKEN TO ASSURE THAT THE DURA IS NOT PENETRATED AND THAT CHYMOPAPAIN, OR CONTRAST MEDIUM IF USED, DOES NOT ENTER THE SUBARACHNOID SPACE. IF THERE IS ANY QUESTION REGARDING NEEDLE TIP LOCATION WITHIN THE NUCLEUS OF THE DISC OR IF CONTRAST MEDIUM IS USED AND IT EXTRAVASATES INTO THE SUBARACHNOID SPACE, THE PROCEDURE SHOULD BE ABANDONED AND CHYMOPAPAIN SHOULD NOT BE INJECTED.

CHEMONUCLEOLYSIS USING SUPPLEMENTED LOCAL ANESTHESIA WHENEVER POSSIBLE SHOULD BE LIMITED TO THE DISC(S) PRODUCING THE PATIENT'S SIGNS AND SYMPTOMS.

DESCRIPTION

Chymopapain is a proteolytic enzyme in the form of a sterile, nonpyrogenic, lyophilized powder. The unit of Chymopapain activity is the picoKatal (pKat). One unit (pKat) of enzyme, under the conditions of assay, forms 1 picomole of p-nitroaniline per second from DL-benzoyl arginine-p-nitroanilide (BAPNA) substrate. In general, 1 mg of Chymopapain contains approximately 500 pKat units.

Chymopapain is available in 2 mL vials and is accompanied by a vial of Sterile Water for Injection, USP, which is to be used as diluent. The 2 mL vial, which is to be reconstituted with 2 mL of diluent, contains 4,000 pKat units of Chymopapain and 1.4 mg of sodium L-cysteine hydrochloride. The concentration of the solution in a reconstituted vial is 2,000 pKat units of active drug per mL. The vial contains no preservatives.

The proteolytic enzyme Chymopapain is derived from the crude latex of *Carica papaya*. Sodium L-cysteine hydrochloride is added as a reducing agent for this sulphur-containing enzyme to maintain the sulphur in the sulphydryl form. The pH of the reconstituted drug is 5.5 to 6.5.

CLINICAL PHARMACOLOGY

When injected into the herniated nucleus pulposus of the lumbar intervertebral disc, Chymopapain causes rapid hydrolysis of the noncollagenous polypeptides or proteins that maintain the tertiary structure of the chondromucoprotein of the nucleus pulposus. By causing degradation of the chondromucoprotein, the intradiscal osmotic activity is lessened, thereby decreasing fluid absorption and reducing intradiscal pressure. The foregoing mechanism of action is based on animal *in vitro* and *in vivo* data. Although the mechanism of action in the human has not been established directly, operative findings in patients who have had surgery following injection have usually revealed the nucleus pulposus to be reduced in size. A temporary increase in urinary mucopolysaccharide occurs in humans following intradiscal injection of Chymopapain, it appears that the inhibitory activity of the alpha2-macroglobulin prevents expression of any significant proteolytic activity outside the disc.

As Chymopapain is injected directly into the herniated lumbar intervertebral disc, absorption, distribution, and metabolism are not necessary for it to achieve its intended purpose. Pharmacological activity has been demonstrated by direct observation *in vivo* and *in vitro* in animals, *in vitro* in human tissue, and pharmacokinetically in the human by observation of increases in urinary excretion of substances known to be in high concentration in the disc.

After injection into the central portion of human lumbar intervertebral discs (*in vivo*), there is an increase in the urinary excretion of glycosaminoglycans of the type known to occur in human intervertebral discs. Chymopapain or its immunologically reactive fragments (CIP) are also detectable by radioimmunoassay in plasma at 30 minutes and are declining at 24 hours. Small amounts of CIP are also detected in the urine. These findings indicate that, after intradiscal injection of Chymopapain, CIP diffuses rapidly into plasma. Due to the inhibitory activity of the alpha2-macroglobulin and the low concentration of CIP, it is unlikely that any proteolytic activity is expressed outside the disc.

In a randomized, double-blind clinical comparison, approximately 75% of patients responded successfully to Chymopapain compared to approximately 45% receiving placebo. When those failing to respond to placebo were then treated with Chymopapain, 90% responded with partial or total relief of symptoms. In a multicenter, open-label study involving approximately 1,500 patients, the results were also favorable, with success rates ranging from 80% to 89% depending on the criteria used to determine outcome.

INDICATIONS AND USAGE

Chymopapain intradiscal injection is indicated for the treatment of patients with documented herniated lumbar intervertebral discs whose symptoms and signs, particularly sciatica, have not responded to an adequate period or periods of conservative therapy. Chymopapain has not been studied in the treatment of herniated discs in areas other than the lumbar spine.

Chymopapain should only be used by physicians who are qualified by training and experience to perform laminectomy, discectomy, or other spinal procedures, and who have received specialized training in chemonucleolysis. Appropriate use of Chymopapain requires experience and training in the use of all appropriate diagnostic and treatment methods, including surgical intervention (laminectomy/discectomy), and knowledge of all aspects of pre- and post-operative patient management. Proper selection of patients for chemonucleolysis requires extensive training and experience in the diagnosis and management of all spinal disorders and diseases since there are circumstances in which nerve root compression resulting from conditions other than a herniated disc can produce similar signs and symptoms.

Chymopapain should be used only in hospitals. Support personnel, as well as physicians, must be trained and experienced in the diagnosis and management of all potential complications of the use of Chymopapain.

CONTRAINDICATIONS

Chymopapain is contraindicated in patients with a known sensitivity to Chymopapain, papaya or papaya derivatives such as certain papain-containing contact lens cleaners and meat tenderizer preparations. Other contraindications are severe spondylolisthesis; significant spinal stenosis; severe, progressing paralysis as indicated by rapidly progressing neurologic dysfunction; and evidence of spinal cord tumor or other lesions producing spinal motor or sensory dysfunction (e.g. cauda equina lesion).

Chymopapain, a foreign protein, has the potential for generating an immunologic response. Therefore, its use is contraindicated in patients who have been previously injected with any form of Chymopapain. It is contraindicated for any patient shown to have circulating Chymopapain specific IgE antibodies.

Chymopapain has only been studied in the lumber spine; therefore, its use is contraindicated in other regions of the spine.

WARNINGS

(1) Anaphylaxis has been observed after injection of Chymopapain in about 0.5% of patients and may be life threatening if not treated promptly and correctly. *At least one open intravenous line must always be in place to permit rapid management.* This reaction can be immediate or delayed up to two hours after injection and can last for minutes to several hours or longer. The patient may present with almost immediate hypotension and/or bronchospasm (the former being more common), laryngeal edema or cardiac arrhythmia possibly progressing to cardiac arrest, coma and death. Speed in diagnosis and treatment is essential since the clinical signs, severity, progression and duration of an anaphylactic reaction are very unpredictable. The patient must also be observed for development of other allergic signs such as erythema, pilomotor erection, rash, urticaria, conjunctivitis, vasomotor rhinitis, angioedema, or various gastrointestinal disturbances.

Postmarketing surveillance of more than 38,200 patients for whom data are available demonstrate that the incidence of anaphylaxis secondary to Chymopapain injection varies with gender and race.

	White	Black	Hispanic	Other
Male	0.2%	0.3%	0.3%	0.2%
Female	0.6%	1.7%	0.7%	0.7%

The overall anaphylaxis rate is significantly higher in females (0.7%) than in males (0.2%), black females being particularly at risk (1.7%).

Although clinical judgment, choice and speed of therapy enter into the treatment of anaphylaxis, *epinephrine is the definitive therapeutic agent in the immediate treatment of anaphylaxis.* Substitution of other agents such as steroids should be reserved for cases where epinephrine is not appropriate.

(2) Paraplegia/paraparesis, other serious neurologic adverse events (e.g. the cauda equina syndrome), subarachnoid/cerebral hemorrhage and seizures have been observed within hours or days following Chymopapain injection at a rate of less than 1 in 2,000. Delayed rapid onset of paraplegia/paraparesis has also been reported 2 to 3 weeks after injection of Chymopapain at a lower rate of less than 1 in 20,000. Causal relationships to the drug when properly administered have not been established. Needle trauma and/or injection of Chymopapain and/or contrast media into the spinal fluid may have been responsible in some of these cases. Other less severe neurologic reactions have included burning sacral or leg pain, hypalgesia, leg weakness, foot drop, cramping in both calves, pain in the opposite leg, paresthesia, tingling in legs and numbness in the legs/toes.

Regarding serious neurologic adverse events, the following should be noted:

(a) In many of the reported cases of serious neurologic adverse events, discography was performed as part of the procedure. Some contrast media approved for use in discography are neurotoxic when introduced intrathecally and such toxicity may be enhanced by intrathecal bleeding. Also, as shown in experimental animals intrathecal Chymopapain is highly toxic (see *"Animal Pharmacology and Toxicology"*). Based on this information and to avoid introduction of contrast medium and Chymopapain into the spinal fluid, great care should be taken before injection to ensure that the tip of the injection needle is in the center of the nucleus pulposus and that the dura has not been pierced. The transdural or posterior approach for needle placement must be avoided.

(b) Patients receiving injections at two or more disc spaces appear to be at increased risk of serious neurologic adverse events. *Chemonucleolysis should be limited to the disc or discs responsible for the patient's symptoms.*

(c) Nearly all of the patients who experienced a serious neurologic adverse event had the procedure performed under general anesthesia. Local anesthesia provides an awake patient, more likely to experience pain and complain if the needle impinges on nerve tissue. Also, it is unlikely that a patient under local anesthesia will tolerate an excessive number of attempts to place the needle. Although the final choice of anesthetic rests with the patient's physician, *it is recommended that local or supplemental local anesthesia be used for chemonucleolysis whenever possible.*

(d) Patients who have had prior surgery of the lumbar spine appear to be at increased risk of experiencing a serious neurologic adverse event. Therefore, it is recommended that such patients be selected for chemonucleolysis only after careful consideration of the risk/benefit ratio.

(e) A number of patients with a history of hypertension, known or suspected cerebrovascular anomaly, previous cerebrovascular accident, or a strong family history of cerebrovascular accident have experienced severe, or fatal central nervous system hemorrhage following chemonucleolysis.

(3) Chymopapain is extremely toxic intrathecally in animals. If Chymopapain is introduced intrathecally, capillaries can be disrupted potentially resulting in subarachnoid/cerebral hemorrhage, severe neurological injury and/or death. Great caution must be exercised in assuring that Chymopapain does not enter the intrathecal space. The transdural or posterior approach for needle placement must be avoided.

(4) Certain radiopaque contrast media used for discography are neurotoxic when injected intrathecally. The toxicity of these materials may be enhanced by intrathecal bleeding. If Chymopapain is inadvertently administered intrathecally, disruption of the capillaries may occur resulting in intrathecal bleeding.

PRECAUTIONS

PATIENT SELECTION

(1) A careful history should be obtained to determine if the patient has multiple allergies, especially a known allergy to papaya or papaya derivatives or iodine. Absorbable iodine should not be used during myelography (or discography, if performed—see *"Warnings"*) in patients allergic to iodine.

The use of a preoperative screening test for Chymopapain-specific IgE antibody should be considered to identify patients at risk for anaphylaxis.

(2) A number of patients with a history of prior surgery of the lumbar spine, hypertension, known or suspected cerebrovascular anomaly, previous cerebrovascular accident, or strong family history of cerebrovascular accident have experienced a serious neurologic adverse event following chemonucleolysis. (See *"Warnings."*)

(3) Females, particularly black females, are more likely to develop anaphylactic reactions secondary to Chymopapain. (See *"Warnings."*)

(4) In case of anaphylaxis, beta-blocker therapy may block the action of epinephrine.

PRETREATMENT

(1) It is recommended that patients be pretreated prior to the injection of Chymopapain with histamine receptor (H_1 and H_2) antagonists to lessen the severity of an anaphylactic reaction.

(2) Because of the abrupt decrease in intravascular volume during anaphylaxis, patients should be well hydrated by oral or intravenous fluids prior to chemonucleolysis. *At least one open intravenous line must always be in place to permit rapid and adequate management of such an occurrence.*

PROCEDURE

(1) The choice of anesthetic for a specific patient should be made by the attending surgeon and anesthesiologist; however, local or supplemental local anesthetic is recommended whenever possible.

The advantages of local or supplemental local anesthesia include possible early recognition of anaphylaxis, possible recognition of evoked sciatic pain with a specific nerve root, and possible decreased risk of a serious neurologic adverse event secondary to difficult needle placement (see *"Warning"*).

The advantages of general anesthesia include more precise patient positioning for injection, less patient discomfort and ease of airway management if anaphylaxis should develop. If halothane anesthesia is used, epinephrine used in the treatment of any anaphylactic reaction could induce cardiac arrhythmia.

(2) Needle placement for the intradiscal administration of Chymopapain should be made by physicians experienced in needle placement via the lateral approach to avoid puncture of the dura mater. Clinical trials have not been conducted using the posterior approach for needle placement and serious neurologic toxicity has been reported using a posterior transdural approach; therefore, this method of needle placement must be avoided. Prior to injection of Chymopapain, visualization of the needle tip position in the disc must be confirmed using x-ray image intensifier for both the anteroposterior and lateral views. *If high quality x-ray equipment including an image intensifier is not available, chemonucleolysis should not be performed.*

(3) If discography is deemed essential at the time of the chemonucleolysis procedure (see *"Warnings"*), at least 15 minutes should elapse after the administration of radiopaque contrast medium to be sure there has been no reaction from the contrast agent.

(4) For 3 minutes prior to Chymopapain injection, 100% O_2 may be administered to the patient by the anesthesiologist to maximize oxygenation in case of anaphylaxis.

(5) A test dose injection of 0.2 mL of Chymopapain followed by a 10 to 15 minute wait is recommended prior to the injection of the full therapeutic dose. The purpose of the test dose is to help identify those patients who are most sensitive to Chymopapain, and patients who develop signs and/or symptoms of anaphylaxis following the test dose must not receive the therapeutic dose. However, some patients have been reported who failed to react to the test dose,

but developed anaphylaxis to the therapeutic dose, suggesting that sensitivity to Chymopapain may be dose related.

PATIENT INSTRUCTIONS

(1) Patients should be instructed that after injection they may experience back pain or involuntary muscle spasm in the lower area of the back for several days. This is not uncommon nor is a residual stiffness or soreness of the low back which may persist for several months.

(2) Patients should be instructed to anticipate the possibility of any of the following delayed allergic reactions which may occur as late as 15 days after injection: rash of any type, urticaria, or itching. If any of these occur, patients should contact their physician.

Pregnancy: Pregnancy Category C. Animal reproduction studies have not been conducted with Chymopapain. It is also not known whether Chymopapain can cause fetal harm when administered to a pregnant woman or can affect reproductive capacity. Chymopapain should be given to a pregnant woman only if the potential benefits outweigh the possible risks.

Pediatric Use: Safety and effectiveness of Chymopapain has not been studied in pediatric patients; therefore, the drug should not be used in children.

ADVERSE REACTIONS

Based on postmarketing surveillance reports, the overall frequency of anaphylaxis is 0.5% or about 1 in 200 patients. The frequency in females is approximately 0.8% and in males approximately 0.3%.

Fatalities have been reported after injection of Chymopapain. Some, such as those due to anaphylaxis or its complications, to disc space infection, or to central nervous system hemorrhage, may be associated with the drug or the procedure. Others appear to be coincidental. The overall mortality rate after Chymopapain injection has been reported to be approximately 0.025% compared with approximately 0.1% mortality reported following surgery.

Paraplegia/paraparesis, other serious neurologic adverse events (e.g. the cauda equina syndrome), subarachnoid/cerebral hemorrhage and seizures have been observed within hours or days following Chymopapain injection at a rate of less than 1 in 2,000. Delayed rapid onset of paraplegia/paraparesis has also been reported 2 to 3 weeks after injection of Chymopapain at a lower rate of less than 1 in 20,000. Causal relationships to the drug when properly administered have not been established. Needle trauma and/or injection of Chymopapain and/or contrast media into the spinal fluid may have been responsible in some of these cases. Other less severe neurologic reactions have included burning sacral or leg pain, hypalgesia, leg weakness, foot drop, cramping in both calves, pain in the opposite leg, paresthesia, tingling in the legs, and numbness of the legs/toes.

Discitis, probably due to bacteria, has been reported.

Less severe, but more frequent adverse reactions include back pain/stiffness/soreness in approximately 50% of treated patients and/or back spasm in approximately 30%. Less frequent adverse reactions, occurring in less than 1% of patients studied include rash, itching, urticaria, nausea, paralytic ileus, urinary retention, headache, and dizziness.

DRUG ABUSE AND DEPENDENCE

Chymopapain injection does not lend itself to drug abuse and dependence.

OVERDOSAGE

Overdosage has not been reported in clinical trials of Chymopapain or subsequently.

DOSAGE AND ADMINISTRATION

Each vial of Chymopapain contains 4,000 pKat units of enzyme and should be reconstituted with 2.0 mL Sterile Water for Injection, USP. The concentration of solution in the reconstituted vial is 2,000 pKat units of Chymopapain per mL, with a pH of 5.5 to 6.5. Recommended dosage is 2,000 to 4,000 pKat units per disc, usually 3,000 pKat units per disc, or a volume of injection of 1 to 2 mL, usually 1.5 mL per disc. If more than one disc is to be injected (see *"Warnings"*), an individual patient should not receive more than 8,000 pKat units.

A 5 mL vial of Sterile Water for Injection, USP, is supplied with each vial of Chymopapain. *This is the only diluent which should be used to reconstitute the drug. Bacteriostatic Water for Injection, USP, must not be used* because it may inactivate the enzyme.

Alcohol should be used to cleanse the vial stopper prior to insertion of needles into the vial. However, since residual alcohol may inactivate the enzyme, it should be allowed to air dry before continuing with the reconstitution process. Parenteral drug products should be inspected visually for particulate matter and discoloration prior to administration. Care should be exercised in the selection of proper size and use of needles inserted into the vials in the reconstitution process to reduce the possibility of coring the stopper. The manufacturing process results in a residual vacuum in the vial; therefore, the use of automatic filling syringes is not recommended.

The drug must be used within two hours of its reconstitution with Sterile Water for Injection, USP. Unused drug must be promptly discarded and not stored for future use.

Appropriate use of Chymopapain requires precise diagnosis, experience and training in the use of all appropriate diagnostic and treatment methods, including surgical intervention (laminectomy/discectomy) and knowledge of all aspects of pre- and postoperative patient management.

The proper selection of patients for chemonucleolysis requires extensive training and experience in the diagnosis and management of all spinal disorders and diseases, since there are circumstances in which nerve root compression

---

◆ RATED THERAPEUTICALLY EQUIVALENT; ◇ THERAPEUTIC EQUIVALENCE UNCONFIRMED; ○ UNRATED

resulting from conditions other than a herniated disc can produce similar signs and symptoms.

The use of Chymopapain therefore, should be limited to physicians who are trained not only in chemonucleolysis but who are qualified by training and experience to care routinely for such patients in other ways.

Chymopapain should be used only in a hospital setting with the assistance of trained personnel, and in such a manner as to ensure immediate and proper management of all potential complications.

Chymopapain can be shipped unrefrigerated; however, it should be stored refrigerated (36° to 46°F or 2° to 8°C) until reconstituted for use.

ANIMAL PHARMACOLOGY AND TOXICOLOGY

Injection of Chymopapain into the lumbar intervertebral disc of mature beagle dogs revealed narrowing of the intervertebral space noted on radiographs obtained at 48 hours and at 14 days. In dogs sacrificed at 14 days following injection, cavitation of the nucleus pulposus was observed, but the endplates were unaffected.

Chymopapain has previously been shown to dissolve the nucleus pulposus of dogs and rabbits at doses as low as 100 pKat units/disc and 50 pKat units/disc, respectively. Doses of 3,000 pKat units/disc cause thinning of only the inner portion of the annulus in rabbits but do not penetrate the entire structure, while doses as high as 24,000 pKat units/disc in dogs resulted in no apparent significant change in the peripheral portion of the annulus. *In vitro* studies demonstrated that Chymopapain solubilized the mucopolysaccharide protein complex of human nucleus pulposus, but did not attack the collagen of this structure.

When Chymopapain is injected into dogs, doses up to 100 times greater than that required to remove the nucleus pulposus were well tolerated when injected intravenously, intradiscally, and epidurally. The drug is extremely toxic when injected intrathecally; the approximate LD_{50} is 15 pKat units/kg in rabbits, 150 pKat units/kg in dogs and 200 pKat units/kg in baboons. Therefore, great caution must be exercised in assuring that Chymopapain is not injected intrathecally.

In baboons the serial injection into the spinal fluid of contrast agents Renografin®, Conray or Amipaque® followed by Chymopapain 15 minutes later produced serious neurotoxicity, including weakness, paralysis and death. When administered singly at the same doses, Conray, Amipaque, and Chymopapain were not toxic; Renografin® was less toxic singly than in combination with Chymopapain. This information supports the clinical observation that the documented entry of contrast agent and presumed entry of Chymopapain into the spinal fluid can produce serious neurotoxicity including paraplegia and central nervous system hemorrhage.

HOW SUPPLIED
POWDER FOR INJECTION: 4000 U/ML

BRAND/MANUFACTURER	NDC	SIZE	AWP
○ BRAND CHYMODIACTIN: Boots Pharm	00048-0110-02	1s	$1395.75

Chymotrypsin

DESCRIPTION

Each vial contains:
Chymotrypsin for ophthalmic solution ....300 units

When reconstituted yields a clear, colorless, 1:5,000 dilution of Chymotrypsin in an isotonic sodium chloride solution.

CLINICAL PHARMACOLOGY

The proteolytic enzyme, Chymotrypsin, dissolves the zonular fibers attached to the lens when inserted into the posterior chamber.

INDICATIONS AND USAGE

For enzymatic zonulysis prior to intracapsular lens extraction.

CONTRAINDICATIONS

High vitreous pressure and gaping incisional wound.
Congenital cataracts.
Patients under 20 years of age.
Hypersensitivity to any of the components.

WARNINGS

If blister or peelable backing is damaged or broken, sterility of the enclosed bottle cannot be assured. Open under aseptic conditions only.

PRECAUTIONS

General: The enzyme will not lyse the synechiae that may exist between the lens and other eye structures.

Note: The enzyme solution should be freshly prepared. Discard any solution which is not clear and colorless or has not been used.

PEDIATRIC USE

Use of Chymotrypsin is contraindicated in patients under 20 years of age.

ADVERSE REACTIONS

Transient increases in intraocular pressure, moderate uveitis, corneal edema and striation have been reported. Delayed healing of incisions has been reported but not confirmed.

DOSAGE AND ADMINISTRATION

Zonular strength and the surgeon's experience determine the dilution and volume of Chymotrypsin required to produce zonulysis. The following dosing instructions are applicable to Chymotrypsin 1:5,000.

Note: Syringes and instruments should be free of alcohol or disinfectants which may inactivate the enzyme.

Inspect prepared solution visually for particulate matter and discoloration prior to administration. At the appropriate time, irrigate the posterior chamber with about 1 to 2 mL of Chymotrypsin 1:5,000. Wait 2 to 4 minutes, then irrigate anterior chamber with suitable irrigating solution, if desired. If zonules are still intact, irrigate the posterior chamber with an additional 0.5 to 2 mL of Chymotrypsin. Wait an additional 2 to 4 minutes, then irrigate with suitable irrigating solution, if desired. Extract lens.

Note: The enzyme solution should be freshly prepared. Discard any solution which is not clear and colorless or has not been used. DO NOT RESTERILIZE.
Keep from freezing.
Refrigerate at 2°-8°C (36°-46°F).

HOW SUPPLIED
SOLUTION: 1:5,000

BRAND/MANUFACTURER	NDC	SIZE	AWP
○ BRAND CATARASE: Iolab	00058-2010-45	2 ml	$28.32

Ciclopirox Olamine

DESCRIPTION

Ciclopirox Olamine Cream 1% is for topical use. Each gram of Ciclopirox Olamine Cream 1% contains 10 mg Ciclopirox Olamine in a water miscible vanishing cream base.

Ciclopirox Olamine Cream 1% contains synthetic, broad-spectrum, antifungal agent Ciclopirox Olamine. The chemical name is 6-cyclohexyl-1-hydroxy-4-methyl-2(1*H*).pyridone, 2-aminoethanol salt.

Ciclopirox Olamine Cream 1% has a pH of 7.

Following is its chemical structure:

CLINICAL PHARMACOLOGY

Ciclopirox Olamine is a broad-spectrum, antifungal agent that inhibits the growth of pathogenic dermatophytes, yeasts, and *Malassezia furfur*. Ciclopirox Olamine exhibits fungicidal activity *in vitro* against isolates of *Trichophyton rubrum*, *Trichophyton mentagrophytes*, *Epidermophyton floccosum*, *Microsporum cunis*, and *Candida albicans*.

Pharmacokinetic studies in men with tagged 1% Ciclopirox Olamine solution in polyethylene glycol 400 showed an average of 1.3% absorption of the dose when it was applied topically to 750 cm^2 on the back followed by occlusion for 6 hours. The biological half-life was 1.7 hours and excretion occurred via the kidney. Two days after application only 0.01% of the dose applied could be found in the urine. Fecal excretion was negligible.

Penetration studies in human cadaverous skin from the back, with Ciclopirox Olamine Cream 1% with tagged Ciclopirox Olamine showed the presence of 0.8 to 1.6% of the dose in stratum corneum 1.5 to 6 hours after application. The levels in the dermis were still 10 to 15 times above the minimum inhibitory concentrations.

Autoradiographic studies with human cadaverous skin showed that Ciclopirox Olamine penetrates into the hair and through the epidermis and hair follicles into the sebaceous glands and dermis, while a portion of the drug remains in the stratum corneum.

Draize Human Sensitization Assay, 21-Day Cumulative Irritancy study, Phototoxicity study, and Photo-Draize study conducted in a total of 142 healthy male subjects showed no contact sensitization of the delayed hypersensitivity type, no irritation, no phototoxicity, and no photo-contact sensitization due to Ciclopirox Olamine Cream 1%.

INDICATIONS AND USAGE

Ciclopirox Olamine Cream 1% is indicated for the topical treatment of the following dermal infections: tinea pedis, tinea cruris and tinea corporis due to *Trichophyton rubrum, Trichophyton mentagrophytes, Epidermophyton floccosum*, and *Microsporum canis*; candidiasis (moniliasis) due to *Candida albicans*; and tinea (pityriasis) versicolor due to *Malassezia furfur*.

UNLABELED USES

Ciclopirox Olamine is used alone in the treatment of vaginal candidiasis and onychomycosis.

CONTRAINDICATIONS

Ciclopirox Olamine Cream 1% is contraindicated in individuals who have shown hypersensitivity to any of its components.

WARNINGS

General: Ciclopirox Olamine Cream 1% is not for ophthalmic use.

PRECAUTIONS

If a reaction suggesting sensitivity or chemical irritation should occur with the use Ciclopirox Olamine Cream 1%, treatment should be discontinued and appropriate therapy instituted.

INFORMATION FOR PATIENTS

The patient should be told to:

1. Use the medication for the full treatment time even though symptoms may have improved and notify the physician if there is no improvement after four weeks.
2. Inform the physician if the area of application shows signs of increased irritation (redness, itching, burning, blistering, swelling, oozing) indicative of possible sensitization.
3. Avoid the use of occlusive wrappings or dressings.

CARCINOGENESIS, MUTAGENESIS, IMPAIRMENT OF FERTILITY

A carcinogenicity study in female mice dosed cutaneously twice per week for 50 weeks followed by a 6-month drug-free observation period prior to necropsy revealed no evidence of tumors at the application site. Several mutagenicity tests with Ciclopirox Olamine indicated no potential for mutagenesis, in a battery of *in vitro* genotoxicity tests with Ciclopirox free acid, one assay was positive: however, the positive findings were not substantiated by *in vivo* testing.

PREGNANCY CATEOGRY B

Reproduction studies have been performed in the mouse, rat, rabbit, and monkey, (via various routes of administration) at doses 10 times or more the topical human dose and have revealed no significant evidence of impaired fertility or harm to the fetus due to Ciclopirox Olamine. There are, however, no adequate or well-controlled studies in pregnant women. Because animal reproduction studies are not always predictive of human response this drug should be used during pregnancy only if clearly needed.

NURSING MOTHERS

It is not known whether this drug is excreted in human milk. Because many drugs are excreted in human milk, caution should be exercised when Ciclopirox Olamine Cream 1% is administered to a nursing woman.

PEDIATRIC USE

Safety and effectiveness in children below the age of 10 years have not been established.

ADVERSE REACTIONS

In all controlled clinical studies with 514 patients using Ciclopirox Olamine Cream 1% and in 296 patients using the vehicle cream, the incidence of adverse reactions was low. This included pruritus at the site of application in one patient and worsening of the clinical signs and symptoms in Ciclopirox Olamine Cream 1% and burning in one patient and worsening of the clinical signs and symptoms in another patient using the vehicle cream.

DOSAGE AND ADMINISTRATION

Gently massage Ciclopirox Olamine Cream 1% into the affected and surrounding skin areas twice daily, in the morning and evening. Clinical improvement with relief of pruritus and other symptoms usually occurs within the first week of treatment. If a patient shows no clinical improvement after four weeks of treatment with Ciclopirox Olamine Cream 1%, the diagnosis should be redetermined. Patients with tinea versicolor usually exhibit clinical and mycological clearing after two weeks of treatment.

Shake Lotion vigorously before each use.
Store at controlled room temperature (59° - 86°F)

HOW SUPPLIED
CREM: 1%

BRAND/MANUFACTURER	NDC	SIZE	AWP
○ BRAND			
LOPROX: Hoechst Derm	00039-0009-15	15 gm	$10.18
	00039-0009-30	30 gm	$18.20
	00039-0009-90	90 gm	$32.76

LOTION: 1%

BRAND/MANUFACTURER	NDC	SIZE	AWP
○ BRAND			
LOPROX: Hoechst Derm	00039-0008-30	30 ml	$20.00
	00039-0008-06	60 ml	$37.98

Cilastatin Sodium and Imipenem

DESCRIPTION

Cilastatin Sodium/Imipenem is a sterile formulation of Imipenem, a thienamycin antibiotic, and Cilastatin Sodium, the inhibitor of the renal dipeptidase, dehydropeptidase I. Cilastatin Sodium/Imipenem is a potent broad spectrum antibacterial agent available for intravenous (IV) or intramuscular (IM) administration. Imipenem (N-formimidoylthienamycin monohydrate) is a crystalline derivative of thienamycin, which is produced by *Streptomyces cattleya*. Its chemical name is [5R-[5 α, 6α (R*)]]-6(1-hydroxyethyl)-3-[[2-[(iminomethyl)amino] ethyl] thio]-7-oxo-1-azabicyclo [3.20] hept-2-ene-2-carboxylic acid monohydrate. It is an off-white, nonhygroscopic crystalline compound with a molecular weight of 317.37. It is sparingly soluble in water, and slightly soluble in methanol. Its empirical formula is $C_{12}H_{17}N_3O_4S \cdot H_2O$.

Cilastatin Sodium is the sodium salt of a derivatized heptenoic acid. Its chemical name is [R-[R*S*- (Z)]]-7-[(2-amino-2-carboxyethyl)thio]-2-[[(2, 2-dimethylcyclopropyl) carbonyl]amino]-2-heptenoic acid, monosodium salt. It is an off-white to yellowish-white, hygroscopic, amorphous compound with a molecular weight of 380.43. It is very soluble in water and in methanol. Its empirical formula is $C_{16}H_{25}N_2O_5S$ Na.

Cilastatin Sodium/Imipenem IV is buffered to provide solutions in the pH range of 6.5 to 7.5. There is no significant change in pH when solutions are prepared and used as directed. (See *"Compatibility and Stability"*.) Cilastatin Sodium/Imipenem IV 250 contains 18.8 mg of sodium (0.8 mEq) and Cilastatin Sodium/Imipenem IV 500 contains 37.5 mg of sodium (1.6 mEq). Cilastatin Sodium/Imipenem IM 500 contains 32 mg of sodium (1.4 mEq) and Solutions of Cilastatin Sodium/Imipenem IV range from colorless to yellow. Solutions of Cilastatin Sodium/Imipenem Suspension range from white to light tan in color. Variations of color within this range do not affect the potency of the product.

CLINICAL PHARMACOLOGY
INTRAVENOUS ADMINISTRATION

Intravenous infusion of Cilastatin Sodium/Imipenem over 20 minutes results in peak plasma levels of Imipenem antimicrobial activity that range from 14 to 24 mcg/mL for the 250 mg dose, from 21 to 58 mcg/mL for the 500 mg dose and from 41 to 83 mcg/mL for the 1000 mg dose. At these doses, plasma levels of Imipenem antimicrobial activity decline to below 1 mcg/mL or less in 4 to 6 hours. Peak plasma levels of Cilastatin following a 20-minute intravenous infusion of Cilastatin Sodium/Imipenem, range from 15 to 25 mcg/mL for the 250 mg dose, from 31 to 49 mcg/mL for the 500 mg dose and from 56 to 88 mcg/mL for the 1000 mg dose.

GENERAL

Following intramuscular administrations of 500 or 750 mg doses of Cilastatin Sodium/Imipenem in a 1:1 ratio with 1% lidocaine, peak plasma levels of Imipenem antimicrobial activity occur within 2 hours and average 10 and 12 mcg/mL, respectively. For Cilastatin, peak plasma levels average 24 and 33 mcg/mL, respectively, and occur within 1 hour. When compared to intravenous administration of Cilastatin Sodium/Imipenem, Imipenem is approximately 75% bioavailable following intramuscular administration while Cilastatin is approximately 95% bioavailable.

The plasma half-life of each component is approximately 1 hour. The binding of Imipenem to human serum proteins is approximately 20% and that of Cilastatin is approximately 40%. The absorption of Imipenem from the IM injection site continues for 6 to 8 hours while that for Cilastatin is essentially complete within 4 hours. This prolonged absorption of Imipenem following the administration of the intramuscular formulation of Cilastatin Sodium/Imipenem results in an effective plasma half-life of Imipenem of approximately 2 to 3 hours and plasma levels of the antibiotic which remain above 2 mcg/mL for at least 6 or 8 hours, following a 500 mg or 750 mg dose, respectively. This plasma profile for Imipenem permits IM administration of the intramuscular formulation of Cilastatin Sodium/Imipenem every 12 hours with no accumulation of Cilastatin and only slight accumulation of Imipenem. A comparison of plasma levels of Imipenem after a single dose of 500 mg or 750 mg of Cilastatin Sodium/Imipenem (intravenous formulation) administered intravenously or of Cilastatin Sodium/Imipenem (intramuscular formulation) diluted with 1% lidocaine and administered intramuscularly is as follows:

PLASMA CONCENTRATIONS OF IMIPENEM (mcg/mL)

Time	500 MG		750 MG	
	IV	IM	IV	IM
25 min	45.1	6.0	57.0	6.7
1 hr	21.6	9.4	28.1	10.0
2 hr	10.0	9.9	12.0	11.4
4 hr	2.6	5.6	3.4	7.3
6 hr	0.6	2.5	1.1	3.8
12 hr	ND†	0.5	NS†	0.8

† ND: Not Detectable (< 0.3 mcg/mL)

Approximately 70% of the IV administered Imipenem is recovered in the urine within 10 hours after which no further urinary excretion is detectable. Urine concentrations of Imipenem in excess of 10 mcg/mL can be maintained for up to 8 hours with Cilastatin Sodium/Imipenem IV at the 500 mg dose. Approximately 70% of the Cilastatin Sodium dose is recovered in the urine within 10 hours of administration of Cilastatin Sodium/Imipenem IV. No accumulation of Cilastatin Sodium/Imipenem IV in plasma or urine is observed with regimens administered as frequently as every 6 hours in patients with normal renal function.

Imipenem urine levels remain above 10 mcg/mL for the 12 hour dosing interval following the administration of 500 mg or 750 mg doses of the intramuscular formulation of Cilastatin Sodium/Imipenem. Total urinary excretion of Imipenem averages 50% while that for Cilastatin averages 75% following either dose of the intramuscular formulation of Cilastatin Sodium/Imipenem.

Imipenem, when administered alone, is metabolized in the kidneys by dehydropeptidase I resulting in relatively low levels in urine. Cilastatin Sodium,

---

an inhibitor of this enzyme, effectively prevents renal metabolism of Imipenem so that when Imipenem and Cilastatin Sodium are given concomitantly fully adequate antibacterial levels of Imipenem are achieved in the urine.

After a 1 gram dose of Cilastatin Sodium/Imipenem IV, the following average levels of Imipenem were measured (usually at 1 hour post-dose except where indicated) in the tissues and fluids listed: (See related table).

In a clinical study in which a 500 mg dose of the intramuscular formulation of Cilastatin Sodium/Imipenem was administered to healthy subjects, the average peak level of Imipenem in interstitial fluid (skin blister fluid) was approximately 5.0 mcg/mL within 3.5 hours after administration. Cilastatin Sodium/Imipenem is hemodialyzable. However, usefulness of this procedure in the overdosage setting is questionable (see "Overdosage").

MICROBIOLOGY

The bactericidal activity of Imipenem results from the inhition of cell wall synthesis. Its greatest affinity is for penicillin binding proteins (PBP) 1A, 1B, 2, 4, 5, and 6 of *Escherichia coli*, and 1A, 1B, 2, 4 and 5 of *Pseudomonas aeruginosa*. The lethal effect is related to binding to PBP 2 and PBP 1B. Imipenen has *in vitro* activity against a wide range of gram-positive and gram-negative organisms.

Imipenem has a high degree of stability in the presence of beta-lactamases, both penicillinases and cephalosporinases produced by gram-negative and gram-positive bacteria. It is a potent inhibitor of beta-lactamases from certain gram-negative bacteria which are inherently resistant to most beta-lactam antibiotics, e.g., *Pseudomonas aeruginosa*, *Serratia spp.*, and *Enterobacter spp.*

Imipenem has *in vitro* activity against a wide range of gram-positive and gram-negative organisms.

In vitro, Imipenem is active against most strains of clinical isolates of the following microorganisms and in clinical infections treated with the intramuscular formulation of C S/I (see "Indications and Usage").

GRAM-POSITIVE

Group D streptococci, including enterococci e.g., Enterococcus faecalis (formerly *Streptococcus faecalis*)

Note: Imipenem is inactive against Enterococcus faecium (formerly *Streptococcus faecium*).

Streptococcus pyogenes (Group A streptococci)
Streptococcus agalactiae (Group B streptococci)
Group C streptococci
Group G streptococci
Viridans streptococci
Streptococcus pneumoniae (formerly *Diplococcus pneumoniae*)
Staphylococcus aureus including penicillinase producing strains
Staphylococcus epidermidis including penicillinase producing strains

Note: Many strains of methicillin-resistant staphylococci are resistant to Imipenem.

GRAM-NEGATIVE

Escherichia coli
Proteus mirabilis
Proteus vulgaris
Morganella morganii
Providencia rettgeri
Providencia stuartii
Citrobacter spp.
Klebsiella spp. including *K. pneumoniae* and *K. oxytoca*
Enterobacter cloacae
Enterobacter spp.
Hafnia spp. including *H. alvei*
Serratia marcescens
Serratia spp: including *S. liquefaciens*
Haemophilus parainfluenzae
H. influenzae
Gardnerella vaginalis
Acinetobacter spp., including *A. calcoaceticus*
Pseudomonas aeruginosa

Note: Imipenem is inactive in vitro against *P. maltophilia* and some strains of *P. cepacia*.

ANAEROBES

Bacteroides spp. including *Bacteroides bivius*, Bacterades distasonis, *Bacteroides fragilis*, *Bacteroides melaninogenicus* intermedius, Bacteroides thetaiotaomicron
Clostridium spp. including *C. perfringens*
Eubacterium spp.
Fusobacterium spp.
Peptococcus spp.
Peptostreptococcus spp.
Propionibacterium spp. including *P. acnes*
Actinomyces spp.
Veillonella spp.

Imipenem has been shown to be active *in vitro* against the following microorganisms; however, clinical efficacy has not yet been established.

GRAM-POSITIVE AEROBES

Listeria monocytogenes
Nocardia spp.
Staphylococcus epidermidis including penicillinase-producing strains.

Note: Methicillin-resistant staphylococci should be reported as resistant to Imipenem.

Streptococcus agalactiae (Group B streptococcus)
Group C streptococcus
Group G streptococcus

GRAM-NEGATIVE AEROBES

Salmonella spp.
Shigella spp.
Yersinia spp. including *Yersinia enterocolitica*, *Yersinia pseudotuberculosis*
Bordetella bronchiseptica
Campylobacter spp.
Achromobacter spp.
Alcaligenes spp.
Moraxella spp.
Pasteurella multocida
Aeromonas hydrophila
Plesiomonas shigelloides
Neisseria gonorrhoeae (including penicillinase-producing strains)
Enterobacter spp.
Gardnerella vaginalis
Haemophilus parainfluenzae
Hafnia spp., including *H. alvei*
Klebsiella spp., including *K. oxytoca*
Moraxella spp.
Morganella morganii
Gram-positive anaerobes:
Actinomyces spp.
Clostridium spp., including *C. perfringens*
Eubacterium spp.
Peptococcus niger
Propionibacterium spp., including *P. acnes*
Gram-negative anaerobes:
Bacteroides bivius
Bacteroides asaccharolyticus
Bacteroides disiens
Bacteroides distasonis
Bacteroides ovatus
Bacteroides thetaiotaomicron
Bacteroides vulgatus
Porphyromonas asaccharolytica (formerly *Bacteroides asaecharolyticus*)
Veillonella spp.

Tissue or Fluid	n	Imipenem Level mcg/mL or mcg/g	Range
Vitreous Humor	3	3.4 (3.5 hours post dose)	2.88-3.6
Aqueous Humor	5	2.99 (2 hours post dose)	2.4-3.9
Lung Tissue	8	5.6 (median)	3.5-15.5
Sputum	1	2.1	-
Pleural	1	22.0	-
Peritoneal	12	23.9 S.D. ± 5.3 (2 hours post dose)	-
Bile	2	5.3 (2.25 hours post dose)	4.6 to 6.0
CSF (uninflamed)	5	1.0 (4 hours post dose)	0.26-2.0
CSF (inflamed)	7	2.6 (2 hours post dose)	0.5-5.5
Fallopian Tubes	1	13.6	-
Endometrium	1	11.1	-
Myometrium	1	5.0	-
Bone	10	2.6	0.4-5.4
Interstitial Fluid	12	16.4	10.0-22.6
Skin	12	4.4	NA
Fascia	12	4.4	NA

In vitro tests show Imipenem to act synergistically with aminoglycoside antibiotics against some isolates of *Pseudomonas aeruginosa*.

SUSCEPTIBILITY TESTING

Diffusion Techniques: Quantitative methods that require measurement of zone diameters give the most precise estimate of antibiotic susceptibility. One such standard procedure, which has been recommended for use with disks to test susceptibility of organisms to Imipenem, uses the 10-mcg Imipenem disk. Interpretation involves the correlation of the diameters obtained in the disk test with the minimum inhibitory concentration (MIC) for Imipenem.

Reports from the laboratory giving results of the standard single-disc susceptibility test with a 10 mcg Imipenem disc should be interpreted according to the following criteria.

Fully susceptible organisms produce zones of 16 mm or greater, indicating that the test organism is likely to respond to doses of 2 g per day or less (see *"Dosage and Administration"*).

Moderately susceptible organisms produce zones of 14 to 15 mm and are expected to be susceptible if the maximum recommended dosage is used or if infection is confined to tissues and fluids in which high antibiotic levels are attained.

Resistant organisms produce zones of 13 mm or less, indicating that other therapy should be selected.

Dilution Techniques: Use a standardized dilution method[2] (broth, agar, microdilution) or equivalent with Imipenem powder. The MIC values obtained should be interpreted according to the following criteria:

A bacterial isolate may be considered fully susceptible if the MIC value for Imipenem is equal to or less than 4 mcg/mL. Organisms are considered moderately susceptible if the MIC value is 8 mcg/mL. Organisms are considered resistant if the MIC is equal to or greater than 16 mcg/mL.

The standardized quality control procedure requires use of control organisms. The 10 mcg Imipenem disc should give the zone diameters listed below for the quality control strains.

Organism	ATCC	Zone Size Range
E. coli	25922	26-32 mm
Ps. aeruginosa	27853	20-28 mm

Dilution susceptibility tests should give MICs between the ranges listed below for the quality control strains.

Organism	ATCC	MIC (mcg/mL)
E. coli	25922	0.06-0.25
S. aureus	29213	0.015-0.06
S. faecalis	29212	0.5-2.0
Ps. aeruginosa	27853	1.0-4.0

For anaerobic bacteria, the MIC of Imipenem can be determined by agar or broth dilution (including microdilution) techniques.[3]

Based on blood levels of Imipenem achieved in man, breakpoint criteria have been adopted for Imipenem.

Category	Zone Diameter (mm)	Recommended MIC Breakpoint (mcg/mL)
Fully Susceptible	≥ 16	≤ 4
Moderately Susceptible	14-15	8
Resistant	≤ 13	≥ 16

INDICATIONS AND USAGE

Cilastatin Sodium/Imipenem IV is indicated for the treatment of serious infections caused by susceptible strains of the designated microorganisms in the diseases listed below:

(1) Lower respiratory tract infections: Staphylococcus aureus (penicillinase producing strains), *Escherichia coli, Klebsiella* species, *Enterobacter* species, *Haemophilus influenzae, Haemophilus parainfluenzae**, Acinetobacter species, Serratia marcescens.

(2) Urinary tract infections: Complicated and uncomplicated). *Staphylococcus aureus* (penicillinase producing strains)*, Group D streptococci (enterococci), *Escherichia coli, Klebsiella* species, *Enterobacter* species. *Proteus vulgaris**, *Providencia rettgeri**, *Morganella morganii**, *Pseudomonas aeruginosa.*

(3) Intra-abdominal infections: Staphylococcus aureus (penicillinase producing strains)*, *Staphylococcus epidermidis*, Group D streptococci (enterococci), *Escherichia coli, Klebsiella* species, *Enterobacter* species, *Proteus* species (indole positive and indole negative), *Morganella morganii**, *Pseudomonas aeruginosa, Citrobacter* species, *Clostridium* species, Gram-positive anaerobes, including *Peptococcus* species*, *Peptostreptococcus* species, *Eubacterium* species, *Propionibacterium* species*, *Bifidobacterium* species, *Bacteroides* species, including *B. fragilis, Fusobacterium* species.

(4) Gynecologic infections: Staphylococcus aureus (penicillinase producing strains)*, *Staphylococcus epidermidis*, Group B streptococci, Group D streptococci

---

* Efficacy for this organism in this organ system was studied in fewer than 10 infections.

(enterococci), *Escherichia coli, Klebsiella* species*, *Proteus* species (indole positive and indole negative), *Enterobacter* species*, Gram-positive anaerobes, including *Peptococcus* species*, *Peptostreptococcus* species, *Propionibacterium* species*, *Bifidobacterium* species*, *Bacteroides* species, *B. fragilis**, *Gerdnerella vaginalis*.

(5) Bacterial septicemia: Staphylococcus aureus (penicillinase producing strains), Group D streptococci (enterococci), *Escherichia coli, Klebsiella* species, *Pseudomonas aeruginosa, Serratia* species*, *Enterobacter* species, *Bacteroides* species, *B. fragilis**.

(6) Bone and joint infections: Staphylococcus aureus (penicillinase producing strains), *Staphylococcus epidermidis*, Group D streptococci (enterococci), *Enterobacter* species, *Pseudomonas aeruginosa*.

(7) Skin and skin structure infections: Staphylococcus aureus (penicillinase producing strains), *Staphylococcus epidermidis*, Group D streptococci (enterococci), *Escherichia coli, Klebsiella* species, *Enterobacter* species, *Proteus vulgaris, Providencia rettgeri**, *Morganella morganii**, *Pseudomonas aeruginosa, Serratia* species, *Citrobacter* species, *Acinetobacter* species, Gram-positive anaerobes, including *Peptococcus* species and *Peptostreptococcus* species, *Bacteroides* species, including *B. fragilis, Fusobacterium* species*.

(8) Endocarditis: Staphylococcus aureus (penicillinase producing strains).

(9) Polymicrobic infections: Cilastatin Sodium/Imipenem IV is indicated for polymicrobic infections including those in which *S. pneumoniae* (pneumonia, septicemia), Group A beta-hemolytic streptococcus (skin and skin structure), or nonpenicillinase-producing *S. aureus* is one of the causative organisms. However, monobacterial infections due to these organisms are usually treated with narrower spectrum antibiotics, such as penicillin G.

Cilastatin Sodium/Imipenem IM is indicated for the treatment of infections caused by susceptible strains of the designated microorganisms in the conditions listed below:

(1) Lower respiratory tract infections: including pneumonia and bronchitis as an exacerbation of COPD, caused by *Streptococcus pneumoniae* and *Haemophilus influenzae.*

(2) Intra-abdominal infections: including acute gangrenous or perforated appendicitis and appendicitis with peritonitis, caused by Group D streptococcus including *Enterococcus faecalis**; *Streptococcus viridans* group*; *Escherichia coli; Klebsiella pneumoniae**; *Pseudomonas aeruginosa**; *Bacteroides* species including *B. fragilis, B. distasonis**, *B. intermedius** and *B. thetaiotaomicron**; *Fusobacterium* species and *Peptostreptococcus** species.

(3) Skin and skin structure infections: including abscesses, cellulitis, infected skin ulcers and wound infections caused by *Staphylococcus aureus* including penicillinase-producing strains; *Streptococcus pyogenes**; Group D streptococcus including *Enterococcus faecalis; Acinetobacter* species* including *A. calcoaceticus**; *Citrobacter* species*; *Escherichia coli; Enterobacter cloacae; Klebsiella pneumoniae**; *Pseudomonas aeruginosa** and *Bacteroides* species* including *B. fragilis**.

(4) Gynecologic infections: including postpartum endomyometritis, caused by Group D streptococcus including *Enterococcus faecalis**; *Escherichia coli; Klebsiella pneumoniae**; *Bacteroides intermedius**; and *Peptostreptococcus* species*.

Cilastatin Sodium/Imipenem IV is not indicated in patients with meningitis because safety and efficacy have not been established.

Because of its broad spectrum of bactericidal activity against gram-positive and gram-negative aerobic and anaerobic bacteria, Cilastatin Sodium/Imipenem IV is useful for the treatment of mixed infections and as presumptive therapy prior to the identification of the causative organisms.

Although clinical improvement has been observed in patients with cystic fibrosis, chronic pulmonary disease, and lower respiratory tract infections caused by *Pseudomonas aeruginosa*, bacterial eradication may not necessarily be achieved.

As with other beta-lactam antibiotics, some strains of *Pseudomonas aeruginosa* may develop resistance fairly rapidly on treatment with Cilastatin Sodium/ Imipenem. When clinically appropriate during therapy of *Pseudomonas aeruginosa* infections, periodic susceptibility testing should be done.

Infections resistant to other antibiotics, for example, cephalosporins, penicillin, and aminoglycosides, have been shown to respond to treatment with Cilastatin Sodium/Imipenem IV.

Cilastatin Sodium/Imipenem IM is not intended for the therapy of severe or life-threatening infections, including bacterial sepsis or endocarditis, or in instances of major physiological impairments such as shock.

UNLABELED USES

Cilastatin Sodium/Imipenem is used alone or as an adjunct in the treatment of febrile neotropenia, uncomplicated gonococcal infections, and in Legionnaires' Disease.

CONTRAINDICATIONS

Cilastatin Sodium/Imipenem is contraindicated in patients who have shown hypersensitivity to any component of this product.

Due to the use of lidocaine hydrochloride diluent in the IM preparation, this product is contraindicated in patients with a known hypersensitivity to local anesthetics of the amide type and in patients with severe shock or heart block. (Refer to the package circular for lidocaine hydrochloride.)

---

* Efficacy for this organism in this organ system was studied in fewer than 10 infections.

WARNINGS

SERIOUS AND OCCASIONALLY FATAL HYPERSENSITIVITY (anaphylactic) REACTIONS HAVE BEEN REPORTED IN PATIENTS RECEIVING THERAPY WITH BETA-LACTAMS. THESE REACTIONS ARE MORE APT TO OCCUR IN PERSONS WITH A HISTORY OF SENSITIVITY TO MULTIPLE ALLERGENS.

THERE HAVE BEEN REPORTS OF PATIENTS WITH A HISTORY OF PENICILLIN HYPERSENSITIVITY WHO HAVE EXPERIENCED SEVERE HYPERSENSITIVITY REACTIONS WHEN TREATED WITH ANOTHER BETA-LACTAM. BEFORE INITIATING THERAPY WITH CILASTATIN SODIUM/IMIPENEM, CAREFUL INQUIRY SHOULD BE MADE CONCERNING PREVIOUS HYPERSENSITIVITY REACTIONS TO PENICILLINS, CEPHALOSPORINS, OTHER BETA-LACTAMS, AND OTHER ALLERGENS. IF AN ALLERGIC REACTION TO CILASTATIN SODIUM/IMIPENEM OCCURS, DISCONTINUE THE DRUG, SERIOUS ANAPHYLACTIC REACTIONS REQUIRE IMMEDIATE EMERGENCY TREATMENT WITH EPINEPHRINE. OXYGEN, IV STEROIDS, AND AIRWAY MANAGEMENT, INCLUDING INTUBATION MAY ALSO BE ADMINISTERED AS INDICATED.

Treatment with antibacterial agents alters the normal flora of the colon and may permit overgrowth of clostridia. Studies indicate that a toxin produced by *Clostridium difficile* is one primary cause of "antibiotic-associated colitis".

Pseudomembranous colitis has been reported with virtually all antibiotics, including Cilastatin Sodium/Imipenem, therefore it is important to consider its diagnosis in patients who develop diarrhea in association with antibiotic use. This colitis may range in severity from mild to life threatening.

After the diagnosis of pseudomembranous colitis has been established, therapeutic measures should be initiated.

Mild cases of pseudomembranous colitis may respond to drug discontinuance alone. In more severe cases, management may include sigmoidoscopy, appropriate bacteriological studies, fluid, electrolyte and protein supplementation, and the use of a drug effective against C. difficile, such as oral vancomycin, as indicated. Isolation of the patient may be advisable. Other causes of colitis should also be considered.

PRECAUTIONS

GENERAL

CNS adverse experiences such as confusional states, myoclonic activity, and seizures have been reported during treatment with Cilastatin Sodium/Imipenem IV, especially when recommended dosages were exceeded. These experiences have occurred most commonly in patients with CNS disorders (e.g., brain lesions or history of seizures) and/or compromised renal function. However, there have been reports of CNS adverse experiences in patients who had no recognized or documented underlying CNS disorder or compromised renal function. These adverse CNS effects have not been seen with Cilastatin Sodium/Imipenem IM: however, should they occur during treatment, Cilastatin Sodium/Imipenem IM should be discontinued. Anticonvulsant therapy should be continued in patients with a known seizure disorder.

Patients with severe or marked impairment of renal function, whether or not undergoing hemodialysis, had a higher risk of seizure activity when receiving maximum recommended doses than those with no impairment of renal function; therefore, maximum recommended doses should be used only where clearly indicated (see *"Dosage and Administration"*).

Patients with creatinine clearances of ≤ 5 mL/min/1.73 m^2 should not receive Cilastatin Sodium/Imipenem unless hemodialysis is instituted within 48 hours.

For patients on hemodialysis, Cilastatin Sodium/Imipenem is recommended only when the benefit outweighs the potential risk of seizures.

Close adherence to the recommended dosage and dosage schedules is urged, especially in patients with known factors that predispose to convulsive activity. Anticonvulsant therapy should be continued in patients with known seizure disorders. If focal tremors, myoclonus, or seizures occur, patients should be evaluated neurologically, placed on anticonvulsant therapy if not already instituted, and the dosage of Cilastatin Sodium/Imipenem re-examined to determine whether it should be decreased or the antibiotic discontinued.

As with other antibiotics, prolonged use of Cilastatin Sodium/Imipenem may result in overgrowth of nonsusceptible organisms. Repeated evaluation of the patient's condition is essential. If superinfection occurs during therapy, appropriate measures should be taken.

While Cilastatin Sodium/Imipenem possesses the characteristic low toxicity of the beta-lactam group of antibiotics, periodic assessment of organ system function during prolonged therapy is advisable.

For intramuscular injection, caution should be taken to avoid inadvertent injection into a blood vessel (see *"Dosage and Administration"*). For additional precautions, refer to the package circular for lidocaine HCl.

DRUG INTERACTIONS

Generalized seizures have been reported in patients who received ganciclovir and Cilastatin Sodium/Imipenem. These drugs should not be used concomitantly unless the potential benefits outweigh the risks.

Since concomitant administration of Cilastatin Sodium/Imipenem and probenecid results in only minimal increases in plasma levels of Imipenem and plasma half-life, it is not recommended that probenecid be given with Cilastatin Sodium/Imipenem.

Cilastatin Sodium/Imipenem should not be mixed with or physically added to other antibiotics. However Cilastatin Sodium/Imipenem may be administered concomitantly with other antibiotics, such as aminoglycosides.

CARCINOGENESIS, MUTAGENESIS, IMPAIRMENT OF FERTILITY

Long term studies in animals have not been performed to evaluate carcinogenic potential of Cilastatin Sodium/Imipenem.

Gene toxicity studies were performed in a variety of bacterial and mammalian tests *in vivo* and *in vitro*. The tests were: V79 mammalian cell mutation assay Cilastatin Sodium/Imipenem alone and Imipenem alone), Ames test (Cilastatin Sodium alone and Imipenem alone), unscheduled DNA synthesis assay Cilastatin Sodium/Imipenem and *in vivo* mouse cytogenicity test Cilastatin Sodium/Imipenem. None of these tests showed any evidence of genetic damage.

Reproduction tests in male and female rats were performed with Cilastatin Sodium/Imipenem at dosage levels up to 8 times (IV) or 11 times (IM) (based on patient weight of 50 kg) the usual human dose. Slight decreases in live fetal body weight were restricted to the highest dosage level. No other adverse effects were observed on fertility, reproductive performance, fetal viability, growth or postnatal development of pups. Similarly, no adverse effects on the fetus or on lactation were observed when Cilastatin Sodium/Imipenem was administered to rats late in gestation.

PREGNANCY

Pregnancy Category C: Teratogenicity studies with Cilastatin Sodium in rabbits and rats at 10 and 33 times the usual human dose, respectively, showed no evidence of adverse effect on the fetus. No evidence of teratogenicity or adverse effect on postnatal growth or behavior was observed in rats given Imipenem at dosage levels up to 30 times the usual human dose. Similarly, no evidence of adverse effect on the fetus was observed in teratology studies in rabbits with Imipenem at dosage levels at (IV) or up to 2 times (IM) the usual human dose.

Teratology studies with Cilastatin Sodium/Imipenem at doses up to 11 times the usual human dose in pregnant mice and rats during the period of major organogenesis revealed no evidence of teratogenicity.

Data from preliminary studies suggests an apparent intolerance to Cilastatin Sodium/Imipenem IV (including emesis, inappetence, body weight loss, diarrhea and death) at doses equivalent to the average human dose in pregnant rabbits. In other studies, Cilastatin Sodium/Imipenem IV, was well tolerated in equivalent or higher doses (up to 11 times the average human dose) in pregnant rats and mice. Further studies are underway to evaluate these findings.

Cilastatin Sodium/Imipenem IM, when administered to pregnant rabbits at dosages above the usual human dose of the intramuscular formulation (1000-1500 mg/day), caused body weight loss, diarrhea, and maternal deaths. When comparable doses of Cilastatin Sodium/Imipenem IM, were given to non-pregnant rabbits, body weight loss, diarrhea, and deaths were also observed. This intolerance is not unlike that seen with other beta-lactam antibiotics in this species and is probably due to alteration of gut flora.

A teratology study in pregnant cynomolgus monkeys given Cilastatin Sodium/Imipenem at doses of 40 mg/kg/day (bolus intravenous injection) or 160 mg/kg/day (subcutaneous injection) resulted in maternal toxicity including emesis, inappetence, body weight loss, diarrhea, abortion and death in some cases. In contrast, no significant toxicity was observed when nonpregnant cynomolgus monkeys were given doses of Cilastatin Sodium/Imipenem up to 180 mg/kg/day (subcutaneous injection). When doses of Cilastatin Sodium/Imipenem (approximately 100 mg/kg/day or approximately 3 times† the maximum daily recommended human dose of the intramuscular formulation) were administered to pregnant cynomolgus monkeys at an intravenous infusion rate which mimics human clinical use, there was minimal maternal intolerance (occasional emesis), no maternal deaths, no evidence of teratogenicity, but an increase in embryonic loss relative to the control groups.

There are, however, no adequate and well-controlled studies in pregnant women. Cilastatin Sodium/Imipenem IV should be used during pregnancy only if the potential benefit justifies the potential risk to the fetus.

NURSING MOTHERS

It is not known whether this drug is excreted in human milk. Because many drugs are excreted in human milk, caution should be exercised when Cilastatin Sodium/Imipenem IV, is administered to a nursing woman.

PEDIATRIC USE

Safety and effectiveness in infants and children below 12 years of age have not yet been established.

ADVERSE REACTIONS

CILASTIN SODIUM/IMIPENEM IV

Cilastatin Sodium/Imipenem IV is generally well tolerated. Many of the 1,723 patients treated in clinical trials were severely ill and had multiple background diseases and physiological impairments, making it difficult to determine causal relationship of adverse experiences to therapy with Cilastatin Sodium/Imipenem IV.

LOCAL ADVERSE REACTIONS

Adverse local clinical reactions that were reported as possibly, probably or definitely related to therapy with Cilastatin Sodium/Imipenem IV were:

Phlebitis/thrombophlebitis—3.1%
Pain at the injection site—0.7%
Erythema at the injection site—0.4%
Vein induration—0.2%
Infused vein infection—0.1%

---

† Based on patient weight of 50 kg.

SYSTEMIC ADVERSE REACTIONS

The most frequently reported systemic adverse clinical reactions that were reported as possibly, probably, or definitely related to Cilastatin Sodium/Imipenem IV were nausea (2.0%) (see "Granulocytopenic Patients" below), diarrhea (1.8%), vomiting (1.5%), rash (0.9%), fever (0.5%), hypotension (0.4%), seizures (0.4%) (see "Precautions"), dizziness (0.3%), pruritus (0.3%), urticaria (0.2%), somnolence (0.2%).

Additional adverse systemic clinical reactions reported as possibly, probably or definitely drug related occurring in less than 0.2% of the patients or reported since the drug was marketed are listed within each body system in order of decreasing severity.

Gastrointestinal: pseudomembranous colitis (see "Warnings"), hemorrhagic colitis, hepatitis (rarely), jaundice, gastroenteritis, abdominal pain, glossitis, tongue papillar hypertrophy, staining of the teeth, heartburn, pharyngeal pain, increased salivation

Hematologic: agranulocytosis, thrombocytopenia, neutropenia, leukopenia

CNS: encephalopathy, tremor, confusion, myoclonus, paresthesia, vertigo, headache, psychic disturbances

Special Senses: hearing loss, tinnitus, taste perversion

Respiratory: chest discomfort, dyspnea, hyperventilation, thoracic spine pain

Cardiovascular: palpitations, tachycardia

Skin: toxic epidermal necrolysis (rarely), erythema multiforme, angioneurotic edema, flushing, cyanosis, hyperhidrosis, skin texture changes, candidiasis, pruritus vulvae

Body as a Whole: polyarthralgia, asthenia/weakness

Renal: acute renal failure (rarely), oliguria/anuria, polyuria, urine discoloration

The role of Cilastatin Sodium/Imipenem IV in changes in renal function is difficult to assess, since factors predisposing to pre-renal azotemia or to impaired renal function usually have been present.

GRANULOCYTOPENIC PATIENTS

Drug-related nausea and/or vomiting appear to occur more frequently in granulocytopenic patients than in nongranulocytopenic patients treated with Cilastatin Sodium/Imipenem IV.

ADVERSE LABORATORY CHANGES

Adverse laboratory changes without regard to drug relationship that were reported during clinical trials or reported since the drug was marketed were:

Hepatic: Increased SGPT, SGOT, alkaline phosphatase, bilirubin and LDH.

Hemic: Increased eosinophils, positive Coombs test, increased WBC, increased platelets, decreased hemoglobin and hematocrit, increased monocytes, abnormal prothrombin time, increased lymphocytes, increased basophils.

Electrolytes: Decreased serum sodium, increased potassium, increased chloride.

Renal: Increased BUN, creatinine.

Urinalysis: Presence of urine protein, urine red blood cells, urine white blood cells, urine casts, urine bilirubin, and urine urobilinogen.

CILASTATIN SODIUM/IMIPENEM IM

In 686 patients in multiple dose clinical trials of Cilastatin Sodium/Imipenem IM, the following adverse reactions were reported:

LOCAL ADVERSE REACTIONS

The most frequent adverse local clinical reaction that was reported as possibly, probably or definitely related to therapy with Cilastatin Sodium/Imipenem IM was pain at the injection site (1.2%).

SYSTEMIC ADVERSE REACTIONS

The most frequently reported systemic adverse clinical reactions that were reported as possibly, probably or definitely related to Cilastatin Sodium/Imipenem IM were nausea (0.6%), diarrhea (0.6%), vomiting (0.3%) and rash (0.4%).

ADVERSE LABORATORY CHANGES

Adverse laboratory changes without regard to drug relationship that were reported during clinical trials were:

Hemic: decreased hemoglobin and hematocrit, eosinophilia, increased and decreased WBC, increased and decreased platelets, decreased erythrocytes, and increased prothrombin time.

Hepatic: increased AST, ALT, alkaline phosphatase, and bilirubin.

Renal: increased BUN and creatinine.

Urinalysis: presence of red blood cells, white blood cells, casts, and bacteria in the urine.

OVERDOSAGE

The intravenous LD_{50} of Imipenem is greater than 2000 mg/kg in the rat and approximately 1500 mg/kg in the mouse. The intravenous LD_{50} of Cilastatin Sodium is approximately 5000 mg/kg in the rat and approximately 8700 mg/kg in the mouse.

The intravenous LD_{50} of Cilastatin Sodium/Imipenem IV is approximately 1000 mg/kg in the rat and approximately 1100 mg/kg in the mouse.

The acute intravenous toxicity of Cilastatin Sodium/Imipenem in a ratio of 1:1 was studied in mice at doses of 751 to 1359 mg/kg. Following drug administration, ataxia was rapidly produced and clonic convulsions were noted in about 45 minutes. Deaths occurred within 4-56 minutes at all doses. The acute intravenous

toxicity of Cilastatin Sodium/Imipenem was produced within 5-10 minutes in rats at doses of 771 to 1583 mg/kg. In all dosage groups, females had decreased activity, bradypnea and ptosis with clonic convulsions preceding death: in males, ptosis was seen at all dose levels while tremors and clonic convulsions were seen at all but the lowest dose (771 mg/kg). In another rat study, female rats showed ataxia, bradypnea and decreased activity in all but the lowest dose (550 mg/kg): deaths were preceded by clonic convulsions. Male rats showed tremors at all doses and clonic convulsions and ptosis were seen at the two highest doses (1130 and 1734 mg/kg). Deaths occurred between 6 and 88 minutes with doses of 771 to 1734 mg/kg.

In the case of overdosage, discontinue Cilastatin Sodium/Imipenem, treat symptomatically, and institute supportive measures as required. Imipenem-Cilastatin Sodium is hemodialyzable. However, usefulness of this procedure in the overdosage setting is questionable.

Information on overdosage in humans is not available.

DOSAGE AND ADMINISTRATION

The dosage recommendations for Cilastatin Sodium/Imipenem IV represent the quantity of Imipenem to be administered. An equivalent amount of Cilastatin is also present in the solution. Each 250 mg or 500 mg dose should be given by intravenous administration over 20 to 30 minutes. Each 1000 mg dose should be infused over 40 to 60 minutes. In patients who develop nausea during the infusion, the rate of infusion may be slowed. The total daily dosage for Cilastatin Sodium/Imipenem IV should be based on the type or severity of infection and given in equally divided doses based on consideration of degree of susceptibility of the pathogen(s), renal function and body weight. Patients with impaired renal function, as judged by creatinine clearance $\leq$ 70 mL/min/1.73 m^2, require adjustment of dosage as described in the succeeding section of these guidelines.

Dosage regimens in column A in the Table for Adults with Normal Renal Function are recommended for infections caused by fully susceptible organisms which represent the majority of pathogenic species. Dosage regimens in column B of this Table are recommended for infections caused by organisms with moderate susceptibility to Imipenem, primarily some strains of *Ps. aeruginosa.*

Doses cited in the Table below are based on a body weight of 70 kg. A further proportionate reduction in dose administered must be made for patients with a body weight less than 70 kg by multiplying the selected dose by the patient's weight in kg divided by 70.

INTRAVENOUS DOSAGE SCHEDULE FOR ADULTS WITH NORMAL RENAL FUNCTION

Type or Severity of Infection	A Fully susceptible organisms including gram-positive and gram-negative aerobes and anaerobes	B Moderately susceptible organisms, primarily some strains of Ps. aeruginosa
Mild	250 mg q6h	500 mg q6h
Moderate	500 mg q8h 500 mg q6h	500 mg q6h 1 g q8h
Severe, life threatening	500 mg q6h	1 g q8h 1 g q6h
Uncomplicated urinary tract infection	250 mg q6h	250 mg q6h
Complicated urinary tract infection	500 mg q6h	500 mg q6h

Due to the high antimicrobial activity of Cilastatin Sodium/Imipenem IV, it is recommended that the maximum total daily dosage not exceed 50 mg/kg/day or 4.0 g/day, whichever is lower.

There is no evidence that higher doses provide greater efficacy. However, patients over twelve years of age with cystic fibrosis and normal renal function have been treated with Cilastatin Sodium/Imipenem IV at doses up to 90 mg/kg/day in divided doses, not exceeding 4.0 g/day.

INTRAVENOUS DOSAGE SCHEDULE FOR ADULTS WITH IMPAIRED RENAL FUNCTION

Patients with creatinine clearance of $\leq$ 70 mL/min/1.73m^2 require adjustment of the dosage of Cilastatin Sodium/Imipenem IV as indicated in the table below. Creatinine clearance may be calculated from serum creatinine concentration by the following equation:

$$T_{cc} \text{ (Males)} = \frac{(\text{wt in kg}) (140 - \text{age})}{(72) (\text{creatinine in mg/dL})}$$

$$T_{cc} \text{ (Females)} = 0.85 \times \text{above value}$$

Column A of the following Table shows maximum dosages recommended in each category of impaired renal function for infections caused by fully susceptible organisms which represent the majority of pathogenic species. The maximum dosages in column B are recommended only for infections caused by organisms with moderate susceptibility to Imipenem, primarily some strains of *Ps. aeruginosa.* Doses cited are based on a body weight of 70 kg. A further proportionate reduction in dose administered must be made for patients with a body weight less than 70 kg by multiplying the selected dose by the patient's weight in kg divided by 70.

Patients with creatinine clearance ≤ 5 mL/min/1.73 m² should not receive Cilastatin Sodium/Imipenem IV unless hemodialysis is instituted within 48 hours. There is inadequate information to recommend usage of Cilastatin Sodium/ Imipenem IV for patients undergoing peritoneal dialysis.

MAXIMUM RECOMMENDED INTRAVENOUS DOSAGE OF CILASTATIN SODIUM/IMIPENEM IV IN ADULTS WITH IMPAIRED RENAL FUNCTION

Creatinine Clearance (mL/min/ 1.73 m²)	Renal Function	A Fully susceptible organisms including gram-positive and gram-negative aerobes and anaerobes	B Moderately susceptible organisms, primarily some strains of Ps. aeruginosa
31-70	Mild Impairment	500 mg q8h	500 mg q6h
21-30	Moderate Impairment	500 mg q12h	500 mg q8h
6-20	Severe to Marked Impairment	250 mg q12h, See Text Below	500 mg q12h, See Text Below
0-5	None, but on Hemodialysis		

Patients with *creatinine clearances of 6 to 20 mL/min/1.73 m₂* should be treated with 250 mg (or 3.5 mg/kg whichever is lower) every 12 hours for most pathogens. When the 500 mg dose is used in these patients, there may be an increased risk of seizures.

Similar dosage and safety considerations apply in the treatment of patients with *creatinine clearances of ≤ 5 mL/min/1.73m² who are undergoing hemodialysis.* Both Imipenem and Cilastatin are cleared from the circulation during hemodialysis. The patient should receive Cilastatin Sodium/Imipenem IV after hemodialysis and at 12 hour intervals timed from the end of that hemodialysis session. Dialysis patients, especially those with background CNS disease, should be carefully monitored; for patients on hemodialysis, Cilastatin Sodium/Imipenem IV, is recommended only when the benefit outweights the potential risk of seizures (see *"Precautions"*).

PREPARATION OF SOLUTION
Infusion Bottles: Contents of the infusion bottles of Cilastatin Sodium/Imipenem IV. Powder should be restored with 100 mL of diluent (see list of diluents under *"Compatibility and Stability"*) and shaken until a clear solution is obtained.

Vials: Contents of the vials must be suspended and transferred to 100 mL of an appropriate infusion solution.

A suggested procedure is to add approximately 10 mL from the appropriate infusion solution (see list of diluents under *"Compatibility and Stability"*) to the vial. Shake well and transfer the resulting suspension to the infusion solution container.

Caution: THE SUSPENSION IS NOT FOR DIRECT INFUSION.

Repeat with an additional 10 mL of infusion solution to ensure complete transfer of vial contents to the infusion solution. *The resulting mixture should be agitated until clear.*

COMPATIBILITY AND STABILITY
Before reconstitution: The dry powder should be stored at a temperature below 30°C.

Reconstituted solutions: Solutions Cilastatin Sodium/Imipenem IV range from colorless to yellow. Variations of color within this range do not affect the potency of the product.

Cilastatin Sodium/Imipenem IV, as supplied in infusion bottles and vials and reconstituted as above with the following diluents, maintains satisfactory potency for four hours at room temperature or for 24 hours under refrigeration (5°C) (note exception below). Solutions of Cilastatin Sodium/Imipenem IV should not be frozen.

0.9% Sodium Chloride Injection*
5% or 10% Dextrose Injection
5% Dextrose Injection with 0.02% sodium bicarbonate solution
5% Dextrose and 0.9% Sodium Chloride Injection
5% Dextrose Injection with 0.225% or 0.45% saline solution
NORMOSOL†-M in D5-W**
5% Dextrose Injection with 0.15% potassium chloride solution
Mannitol 2.5%, 5% and 10%

Cilastatin Sodium/Imipenem IV is supplied in single dose ADD-Vantage® vials and should be prepared as directed in the accompanying INSTRUCTIONS FOR USE OF Cilastatin Sodium/Imipenem IV. IN ADD-Vantage® VIALS using ADD-Vantage® diluent containers containing 100 mL of either 0.9% Sodium Chloride Injection or 5% Dextrose Injection. When prepared with either of these diluents, Cilastatin Sodium/Imipenem IV maintains satisfactory potency for 8 hours at room temperature.

* Cilastatin Sodium/Imipenem IV has been found to be stable in 0.9% Sodium Chloride Injection for 10 hours at room temperature or 48 hours under refrigeration.
** Cilastatin Sodium/Imipenem IV has been found to be stable in Normosol-M in D5-W for 2 hours at room temperature or 9 hours under refrigeration.

Cilastatin Sodium/Imipenem IV should not be mixed with or physically added to other antibiotics. However, Cilastatin Sodium/Imipenem IV may be administered concomitantly with other antibiotics, such as aminoglycosides.

CILASTATIN SODIUM/IMIPENEM IM
Cilastatin Sodium/Imipenem IM is for intramuscular use only.

The dosage recommendations for Cilastatin Sodium/Imipenem IM represent the quantity of Imipenem to be administered. An equivalent amount of Cilastatin is also present.

Patients with lower respiratory tract infections, skin and skin structure infections, and gynecologic infections of mild to moderate severity may be treated with 500 mg or 750 mg administered every 12 hours depending on the severity of the infection.

Intra-abdominal infection may be treated with 750 mg every 12 hours. [See table below.]

DOSAGE GUIDELINES

Type†/Location of Infection	Severity	Dosage Regimen
Lower respiratory tract Skin and skin structure * Gynecologic	Mild/Moderate	500 or 750 mg q12h depending on the severity of infection
Intra-abdominal	Mild/ Moderate	750 mg q12h

† See "Indications and Usage" section.

Total daily IM dosages greater than 1500 mg per day are not recommended.

The dosage for any particular patient should be based on the location of and severity of the infection, the susceptibility of the infecting pathogen(s), and renal function.

The duration of therapy depends upon the type and severity of the infection. Generally, Cilastatin Sodium/Imipenem IM should be continued for at least two days after the signs and symptoms of infection have resolved. Safety and efficacy of treatment beyond fourteen days have not been established.

Cilastatin Sodium/Imipenem IM should be administered by deep intramuscular injection into a large muscle mass (such as the gluteal muscles or lateral part of the thigh) with a 21 gauge 2' needle. Aspiration is necessary to avoid inadvertent injection into a blood vessel.

ADULTS WITH IMPAIRED RENAL FUNCTION
The safety and efficacy of Cilastatin Sodium/Imipenem IM have not been studied in patients with creatinine clearance of less than 20 mL/min/1.73m². Serum creatinine alone may not be a sufficiently accurate measure of renal function. Creatinine clearance (T_{cc}) may be estimated from the following equation:

$$T_{cc} \text{ (Males)} = \frac{\text{(wt. in kg) (140-age)}}{\text{(72) (creatinine in mg/dL)}}$$

$$T_{cc} \text{ (Females)} = 0.85 \times \text{above value}$$

PREPARATION FOR ADMINISTRATION
Cilastatin Sodium/Imipenem IM should be prepared for use with 1.0% lidocaine HCl solution† (without epinephrine). Cilastatin Sodium/Imigenem IM 500 should be prepared with 2 mL of Cilastatin Sodium/Imipenem IM 750 with 3 mL of lidocaine HCl. Agitate to form a suspension then withdraw and inject the entire contents of vial intramuscularly. The suspension of Cilastatin Sodium/Imipenem IM in lidocaine HCl should be used within one hour after preparation. *Note: The IM formulation is not for IV use.*

COMPATIBILITY AND STABILITY
Before reconsition: The dry powder should be stored at a temperature below 30°C (86°F).

Suspensions for IM Administration: Suspensions of Cilastatin Sodium/Imipenem IM are white to light tan in color. Variations of color within this range do not affect the potency of the product.

The suspension of Cilastatin Sodium/Imipenem IM in lidocaine HCl should be used within one hour after preparation.

Cilastatin Sodium/Imipenem IM should not be mixed with or physically added to other antibiotics. However, Cilastatin Sodium/Imipenem IM may be administered concomitantly but at separate sites with other antibiotics, such as aminoglycosides.

J CODES
Per 250 mg IV,IM—J0743

HOW SUPPLIED
POWDER FOR INJECTION: 250 MG-250 MG

BRAND/MANUFACTURER	NDC	SIZE	AWP
○ **BRAND**			
PRIMAXIN: Merck	00006-3515-74	10s	$140.99
	00006-3514-58	25s	$320.54
	00006-3551-58	25s	$332.81

† Refer to the package circular for lidocaine HCl for detailed information concerning *"Contraindications, Warnings, Precautions,"* and *"Adverse Reactions".*

POWDER FOR INJECTION: 500 MG-500 MG

BRAND/MANUFACTURER	NDC	SIZE	AWP
○ BRAND			
PRIMAXIN: Merck	00006-3582-75	10s	$241.33
	00006-3517-75	10s	$254.13
	00006-3516-59	25s	$603.26
	00006-3552-59	25s	$615.14

POWDER FOR INJECTION: 750 MG-750 MG

BRAND/MANUFACTURER	NDC	SIZE	AWP
○ BRAND			
PRIMAXIN: Merck	00006-3583-76	10s	$362.00

Ciloxan *SEE* CIPROFLOXACIN HYDROCHLORIDE, OPHTHALMIC

Cimetidine

DESCRIPTION

Cimetidine is a histamine H_2-receptor antagonist. Chemically it is N''-cyano-N-methyl-N'-[2-[[(5-methyl-1H- imidazol-4-yl)methyl] thio]-ethyl]-guanidine.

The empirical formula for Cimetidine is $C_{10}H_{16}N_6S$ and for Cimetidine hydrochloride, $C_{10}H_{16}N_6SHCl$; these represent molecular weights of 252.34 and 288.80, respectively.

Cimetidine contains an imidazole ring, and is chemically related to histamine. (The liquid and injection dosage forms contain Cimetidine as the hydrochloride.)

Cimetidine has a bitter taste and characteristic odor.

Solubility Characteristics: Cimetidine is soluble in alcohol, slightly soluble in water, very slightly soluble in chloroform and insoluble in ether. Cimetidine hydrochloride is freely soluble in water, soluble in alcohol, very slightly soluble in chloroform and practically insoluble in ether.

Tablets for Oral Administration: Available in strengths of 200 mg, 300 mg, and 400 mg.

Liquid for Oral Administration: Each 5 mL (1 teaspoonful) of clear liquid contains Cimetidine hydrochloride equivalent to Cimetidine, 300 mg; alcohol, 2.8%. Each 6.67 mL is equivalent to 400 mg of Cimetidine; alcohol, 28%.

INJECTION

Single-Dose Vials for Intramuscular or Intravenous Administration: Each 2 mL contains, in sterile aqueous solution (pH range 3.8 to 6), Cimetidine hydrochloride equivalent to Cimetidine, 300 mg; phenol, 10 mg.

Multi-Dose Vials for Intramuscular or Intravenous Administration: 8 mL (300 mg/ 2 mL): Each 2 mL contains, in sterile aqueous solution (pH range 3.8 to 6), Cimetidine hydrochloride equivalent to Cimetidine, 300 mg; phenol, 10 mg.

Single-Dose Premixed Plastic Containers for Intravenous Administration: Each 50 mL of sterile aqueous solution (pH range 5 to 7) contains Cimetidine hydrochloride equivalent to 300 mg Cimetidine and 0.45 grams sodium chloride.

No preservative has been added.

The plastic container is fabricated from specially formulated polyvinyl chloride. The amount of water that can permeate from inside the container into the overwrap is insufficient to affect the solution significantly. Solutions in contact with the plastic container can leach out certain of its chemical components in very small amounts within the expiration period, e.g., di 2-ethylhexyl phthalate (DEHP), up to 5 parts per million. However, the safety of the plastic has been confirmed in tests in animals according to the USP biological tests for plastic containers as well as by tissue culture toxicity studies.

Vials for Intravenous Administration: Each 2 mL contains, in sterile aqueous solution (pH range 3.8 to 6), Cimetidine hydrochloride equivalent to Cimetidine, 300 mg; phenol, 10 mg.

All of the above injection formulations are pyrogen free, and sodium hydroxide N.F. is used as an ingredient to adjust the pH.

Following is its chemical structure:

CLINICAL PHARMACOLOGY

Cimetidine competitively inhibits the action of histamine at the histamine H_2 receptors of the parietal cells and thus is a histamine H_2-receptor antagonist.

Cimetidine is not an anticholinergic agent. Studies have shown that Cimetidine inhibits both daytime and nocturnal basal gastric acid secretion. Cimetidine also inhibits gastric acid secretion stimulated by food, histamine, pentagastrin, caffeine and insulin.

ANTISECRETORY ACTIVITY

(1) Acid Secretion: Nocturnal: Cimetidine 800 mg orally at bedtime reduces mean hourly H^+ activity by greater than 85% over an 8-hour period in duodenal ulcer patients, with no effect on daytime acid secretion. Cimetidine 1600 mg orally h.s. produces 100% inhibition of mean hourly H^+ activity over an 8-hour period in duodenal ulcer patients, but also reduces H^+ activity by 35% for an additional 5 hours into the following morning. Cimetidine 400 mg b.i.d. and 300 mg q.i.d. decrease nocturnal acid secretion in a dose-related manner, i.e., 47% to 83% over a 6- to 8-hour period and 54% over a 9-hour period, respectively.

Food Stimulated: During the first hour after a standard experimental meal, oral Cimetidine 300 mg inhibited gastric acid secretion in duodenal ulcer patients by at least 50%. During the subsequent 2 hours Cimetidine inhibited gastric acid secretion by at least 75%.

The effect of a 300 mg breakfast dose of Cimetidine continued for at least 4 hours and there was partial suppression of the rise in gastric acid secretion following the luncheon meal in duodenal ulcer patients. This suppression of gastric acid output was enhanced and could be maintained by another 300 mg dose of Cimetidine given with lunch.

In another study, Cimetidine 300 mg given with the meal increased gastric pH as compared with placebo.

	Mean Gastric pH	
	Cimetidine	Placebo
1 hour	3.5	2.6
2 hours	3.1	1.6
3 hours	3.8	1.9
4 hours	6.1	2.2

24-Hour Mean H^+ Activity: Cimetidine 800 mg h.s., 400 mg b.i.d. and 300 mg q.i.d. all provide a similar, moderate (less than 60%) level of 24-hour acid suppression. However, the 800 mg h.s. regimen exerts its entire effect on nocturnal acid, and does not affect daytime gastric physiology.

Chemically Stimulated: Oral Cimetidine significantly inhibited gastric acid secretion stimulated by betazole (an isomer of histamine), pentagastrin, caffeine and insulin as follows:

Stimulant	Stimulant Dose	Cimetidine	% Inhibition
Betazole	1.5 mg/kg (sc)	300 mg (po)	85% at 2 1/2 hours
Pentagastrin	6mcg/kg/hr (iv)	100mg/hr (iv)	60% at 1 hour
Caffeine	5mg/kg/hr (iv)	300mg (po)	100% at 1 hour
Insulin	0.03 units/kg/hr (iv)	100mg/hr (iv)	82% at 1 hour

When food and betazole were used to stimulate secretion, inhibition of hydrogen ion concentration usually ranged from 45% to 75% and the inhibition of volume ranged from 30% to 65%.

Parenteral administration also significantly inhibits gastric acid secretion. In a crossover study involving patients with active or healed duodenal or gastric ulcers, either continuous I.V. infusion of Cimetidine 37.5 mg/hour (900 mg/day) or intermittent injection of Cimetidine 300 mg q6h (1200 mg/day) maintained gastric pH above 4.0 for more than 50% of the time under steady-state conditions.

2) Pepsin: Oral Cimetidine 300 mg reduced total pepsin output as a result of the decrease in volume of gastric juice.

3) Intrinsic Factor: Intrinsic factor secretion was studied with betazole as a stimulant. Oral Cimetidine 300 mg inhibited the rise in intrinsic factor concentration produced by betazole, but some intrinsic factor was secreted at all times.

OTHER

Lower Esophageal Sphincter Pressure and Gastric Emptying: Cimetidine has no effect on lower esophageal sphincter (LES) pressure or the rate of gastric emptying.

PHARMACOKINETICS

Cimetidine is rapidly absorbed after oral administration and peak levels occur in 45 to 90 minutes. The half-life of Cimetidine is approximately 2 hours. Both oral and parenteral (I.V. or I.M.) administration provide comparable periods of therapeutically effective blood levels; blood concentrations remain above that required to provide 80% inhibition of basal gastric acid secretion for 4 to 5 hours following a dose of 300 mg.

Steady-state blood concentrations of Cimetidine with continuous infusion of Cimetidine are determined by the infusion rate and clearance of the drug in the individual patient. In a study of peptic ulcer patients with normal renal function, an infusion rate of 37.5 mg/hour produced average steady-state plasma Cimetidine concentrations of about 0.9 mcg/mL. Blood levels with other infusion rates will vary in direct proportion to the infusion rate.

The principal route of excretion of Cimetidine is the urine. Following parenteral administration, most of the drug is excreted as the parent compound; following oral administration, the drug is more extensively metabolized, the sulfoxide being the major metabolite. Following a single oral dose, 48% of the drug is recovered from the urine after 24 hours as the parent compound.

◆ RATED THERAPEUTICALLY EQUIVALENT; ◇ THERAPEUTIC EQUIVALENCE UNCONFIRMED; ○ UNRATED

Following I.V. or I.M. administration, approximately 75% of the drug is recovered from the urine after 24 hours as the parent compound.

CLINICAL TRIALS

Duodenal Ulcer: Cimetidine has been shown to be effective in the treatment of active duodenal ulcer and, at reduced dosage, in maintenance therapy following healing of active ulcers.

Active Duodenal Ulcer: Cimetidine accelerates the rate of duodenal ulcer healing. Healing rates reported in U.S. and foreign controlled trials with Cimetidine are summarized below, beginning with the regimen providing the lowest nocturnal dose.

DUODENAL ULCER HEALING RATES WITH VARIOUS CIMETIDINE DOSAGE REGIMENS*

Regimen	300 mg q.i.d.	400 mg b.i.d.	800 mg h.s.	1600 mg h.s.
week 4	68%	73%	80%	86%
week 6	80%	80%	89%	—
week 8	—	92%	94%	—

* *Averages from controlled clinical trials.*

A U.S., double-blind, placebo-controlled, dose-ranging study demonstrated that all once-daily at bedtime (h.s.) Cimetidine regimens were superior to placebo in ulcer healing and that Cimetidine 800 mg h.s. healed 75% of patients at 4 weeks. The healing rate with 800 mg h.s. was significantly superior to 400 mg h.s. (66%) and not significantly different from 1600 mg h.s. (81%).

In the U.S. dose-ranging trial, over 80% of patients receiving Cimetidine 800 mg h.s. experienced nocturnal pain relief after 1 day. Relief from daytime pain was reported in approximately 70% of patients after 2 days. As with ulcer healing, the 800 mg h.s. dose was superior to 400 mg h.s. and not different from 1600 mg h.s.

In foreign, double-blind studies with Cimetidine 800 mg h.s., 79% to 85% of patients were healed at four weeks.

While short-term treatment with Cimetidine can result in complete healing of the duodenal ulcer, acute therapy will not prevent ulcer recurrence after Cimetidine has been discontinued. Some follow-up studies have reported that the rate of recurrence once therapy was discontinued was slightly higher for patients healed on Cimetidine than for patients healed on other forms of therapy; however, the Cimetidine-treated patients generally had more severe disease.

Maintenance Therapy in Duodenal Ulcer: Treatment with a reduced dose of Cimetidine has been proven effective as maintenance therapy following healing of active duodenal ulcers.

In numerous placebo-controlled studies conducted worldwide, the percent of patients with observed ulcers at the end of 1 year's therapy with Cimetidine 400 mg h.s. was significantly lower (10% to 45%) than in patients receiving placebo (44% to 70%). Thus, from 55% to 90% of patients were maintained free of observed ulcers at the end of 1 year with Cimetidine 400 mg h.s.

Factors such as smoking, duration and severity of disease, gender, and genetic traits may contribute to variations in actual percentages.

Trials of other antiulcer therapy, whether placebo-controlled, positive-controlled or open, have demonstrated a range of results similar to that seen with Cimetidine.

Active Benign Gastric Ulcer: Cimetidine has been shown to be effective in the short-term treatment of active benign gastric ulcer.

In a multicenter, double-blind U.S. study, patients with endoscopically confirmed benign gastric ulcer were treated with Cimetidine 300 mg four times a day or with placebo for 6 weeks. Patients were limited to those with ulcers ranging from 0.5 to 2.5 cm in size. Endoscopically confirmed healing at 6 weeks was seen in significantly* more Cimetidine-treated patients than in patients receiving placebo, as shown below:

	Cimetidine	Placebo
week 2	14/63 (22%)	7/63 (11%)
total at week 6	43/65 (66%)*	30/67 (45%)

* *p < 0.05*

In a similar multicenter U.S. study of the 800 mg h.s. oral regimen, the endoscopically confirmed healing rates were:

	Cimetidine	Placebo
total at week 6	63/83 (76%)*	44/80 (55%)

* *p = 0.005*

Similarly, in worldwide double-blind clinical studies, endoscopically evaluated benign gastric ulcer healing rates were consistently higher with Cimetidine than with placebo.

Gastroesophageal Reflux Disease: in two multicenter, double-blind, placebo-controlled studies in patients with gastroesophageal reflux disease (GERD) and endoscopically proven erosions and/or ulcers, Cimetidine was significantly more effective than placebo in healing lesions. The endoscopically confirmed healing rates were:

Trial	Cimetidine (800 mg b.i.d.)	Cimetidine (400 mg q.i.d.)	Placebo	p-Value (800 mg b.i.d. vs placebo)
1 Week 6	45%	52%	26%	0.02
Week 12	60%	66%	42%	0.02
2 Week 6	50%		20%	< 0.01
Week 12	67%		36%	< 0.01

In these trials Cimetidine was superior to placebo by most measures in improving symptoms of day- and night-time heartburn, with many of the differences statistically significant. The q.i.d. regimen was generally somewhat better than the b.i.d. regimen where these were compared.

Prevention of Upper Gastrointestinal Bleeding in Critically Ill Patients: A double-blind, placebo-controlled randomized study of continuous infusion Cimetidine was performed in 131 critically ill patients (mean APACHE II score = 15.99) to compare the incidence of upper gastrointestinal bleeding, manifested as hematemesis or bright red blood which did not clear after adjustment of the nasogastric tube and a 5 to 10 minute lavage, persistent Gastroccult® positive coffee grounds for 8 consecutive hours which did not clear with 100 cc lavage and/or which were accompanied by a drop in hematocrit of 5 percentage points, or melena, with an endoscopically documented upper gastrointestinal source of bleed. 14% (9/65) of patients treated with Cimetidine continuous infusion developed bleeding compared to 33% (22/66) of the placebo group. Coffee grounds was the manifestation of bleeding that accounted for the difference between groups. Another randomized, double-blind placebo-controlled study confirmed these results for an end point of upper gastrointestinal bleeding with a confirmed upper gastrointestinal source noted on endoscopy, and by post hoc analyses of bleeding episodes between groups.

Pathological Hypersecretory Conditions (such as Zollinger-Ellison Syndrome): Cimetidine significantly inhibited gastric acid secretion and reduced occurrence of diarrhea, anorexia and pain in patients with pathological hypersecretion associated with Zollinger-Ellison Syndrome, systemic mastocytosis and multiple endocrine adenomas. Use of Cimetidine was also followed by healing of intractable ulcers.

INDICATIONS AND USAGE

Cimetidine is indicated in:

(1) Short-term treatment of active duodenal ulcer: Most patients heal within 4 weeks and there is rarely reason to use Cimetidine at full dosage for longer than 6 to 8 weeks (see *"Dosage and Administration—Duodenal Ulcer"*). Concomitant antacids should be given as needed for relief of pain. However, simultaneous administration of Cimetidine and antacids is not recommended, since antacids have been reported to interfere with the absorption of Cimetidine.

(2) Maintenance therapy for duodenal ulcer patients at reduced dosage after healing of active ulcer: Patients have been maintained on continued treatment with Cimetidine 400 mg h.s. for periods of up to 5 years.

(3) Short-term treatment of active benign gastric ulcer: There is no information concerning usefulness of treatment periods of longer than 8 weeks.

(4) Erosive gastroesophageal reflux disease (GERD): Erosive esophagitis diagnosed by endoscopy. Treatment is indicated for 12 weeks for healing of lesions and control of symptoms. The use of Cimetidine beyond 12 weeks has not been established (see *"Dosage and Administration—GERD"*).

(5) Prevention of upper gastrointestinal bleeding in critically ill patients.

(6) The treatment of pathological hypersecretory conditions: (i.e., Zollinger-Ellison Syndrome, systemic mastocytosis, multiple endocrine adenomas).

UNLABELED USES

Cimetidine is used alone or as an adjunct in the treatment of Mendelson's syndrome (for prophylaxis of aspiration pneumonitis), drug-induced gastritis, and acne vulgaris. It is also used in alopecia androgenetica and Barrett's esophagus.

CONTRAINDICATIONS

Cimetidine is contraindicated for patients known to have hypersensitivity to the product.

PRECAUTIONS

General: Rare instances of cardiac arrhythmias and hypotension have been reported following the rapid administration of Cimetidine hydrochloride Injection by intravenous bolus.

Symptomatic response to Cimetidine therapy does not preclude the presence of a gastric malignancy. There have been rare reports of transient healing of gastric ulcers despite subsequently documented malignancy.

Reversible confusional states (see *"Adverse Reactions"*) have been observed on occasion, predominantly, but not exclusively, in severely ill patients. Advancing age (50 or more years) and preexisting liver and/or renal disease appear to be contributing factors. In some patients these confusional states have been mild and have not required discontinuation of Cimetidine therapy. In cases where discontinuation was judged necessary, the condition usually cleared within 3 to 4 days of drug withdrawal.

Drug Interactions: Cimetidine, apparently through an effect on certain microsomal enzyme systems, has been reported to reduce the hepatic metabolism of warfarin-type anticoagulants, phenytoin, propranolol, nifedipine, chlordiazepoxide, diazepam, certain tricyclic antidepressants, lidocaine, theophylline and metronidazole, thereby delaying elimination and increasing blood levels of these drugs.

Clinically significant effects have been reported with the warfarin anticoagulants; therefore, close monitoring of prothrombin time is recommended, and adjustment of the anticoagulant dose may be necessary when Cimetidine is administered concomitantly. Interaction with phenytoin, lidocaine and theophylline has also been reported to produce adverse clinical effects.

However, a crossover study in healthy subjects receiving either Cimetidine 300 mg q.i.d. or 800 mg h.s. concomitantly with a 300 mg b.i.d. dosage of theophylline demonstrated less alteration in steady-state theophylline peak serum levels with the 800 mg h.s. regimen, particularly in subjects aged 54 years and older. Data beyond 10 days are not available. (Note: All patients receiving theophylline should be monitored appropriately, regardless of concomitant drug therapy.)

Dosage of the drugs mentioned above and other similarly metabolized drugs, particularly those of low therapeutic ratio or in patients with renal and/or hepatic impairment, may require adjustment when starting or stopping concomitantly administered Cimetidine to maintain optimum therapeutic blood levels.

Additional clinical experience may reveal other drugs affected by the concomitant administration of Cimetidine.

Carcinogenesis, Mutagenesis, Impairment of Fertility: In a 24-month toxicity study conducted in rats, at dose levels of 150, 378 and 950 mg/kg/day (approximately 8 to 48 times the recommended human dose), there was a small increase in the incidence of benign Leydig cell tumors in each dose group; when the combined drug-treated groups and control groups were compared, this increase reached statistical significance. In a subsequent 24-month study, there were no differences between the rats receiving 150 mg/kg/day and the untreated controls. However, a statistically significant increase in benign Leydig cell tumor incidence was seen in the rats that received 378 and 950 mg/kg/day. These tumors were common in control groups as well as treated groups and the difference became apparent only in aged rats.

Cimetidine has demonstrated a weak antiandrogenic effect. In animal studies this was manifested as reduced prostate and seminal vesicle weights. However, there was no impairment of mating performance or fertility, nor any harm to the fetus in these animals at doses 8 to 48 times the full therapeutic dose of Cimetidine, as compared with controls. The cases of gynecomastia seen in patients treated for 1 month or longer may be related to this effect.

In human studies Cimetidine has been shown to have no effect on spermatogenesis, sperm count, motility, morphology or *in vitro* fertilizing capacity.

Pregnancy: Teratogenic Effects. Pregnancy Category B: Reproduction studies have been performed in rats, rabbits and mice at doses up to 40 times the normal human dose and have revealed no evidence of impaired fertility or harm to the fetus due to Cimetidine. There are, however, no adequate and well-controlled studies in pregnant women. Because animal reproductive studies are not always predictive of human response, this drug should be used during pregnancy only if clearly needed.

Nursing Mothers: Cimetidine is secreted in human milk and, as a general rule, nursing should not be undertaken while a patient is on a drug.

Pediatric Use: Clinical experience in children is limited. Therefore, Cimetidine therapy cannot be recommended for children under 16, unless, in the judgment of the physician, anticipated benefits outweigh the potential risks. In very limited experience, doses of 20 to 40 mg/kg per day have been used.

ADVERSE REACTIONS

Adverse effects reported in patients taking Cimetidine are described below by body system. Incidence figures of 1 in 100 and greater are generally derived from controlled clinical studies.

Gastrointestinal: Diarrhea (usually mild) has been reported in approximately 1 in 100 patients.

CNS: Headaches, ranging from mild to severe, have been reported in 3.5% of 924 patients taking 1600 mg/day, 2.1% of 2,225 patients taking 800 mg/day and 2.3% of 1,897 patients taking placebo. Dizziness and somnolence (usually mild) have been reported in approximately 1 in 100 patients on either 1600 mg/day or 800 mg/day.

Reversible confusional states, e.g., mental confusion, agitation, psychosis, depression, anxiety, hallucinations, disorientation, have been reported predominantly, but not exclusively, in severely ill patients. They have usually developed within 2 to 3 days of initiation of Cimetidine therapy and have cleared within 3 to 4 days of discontinuation of the drug.

Endocrine: Gynecomastia has been reported in patients treated for 1 month or longer. In patients being treated for pathological hypersecretory states, this occurred in about 4% of cases while in all others the incidence was 0.3% to 1% in various studies. No evidence of induced endocrine dysfunction was found, and the condition remained unchanged or returned toward normal with continuing Cimetidine treatment.

Reversible impotence has been reported in patients with pathological hypersecretory disorders, e.g., Zollinger-Ellison Syndrome, receiving Cimetidine, particularly in high doses, for at least 12 months (range 12 to 79 months, mean 38 months). However, in large-scale surveillance studies at regular dosage, the incidence has not exceeded that commonly reported in the general population.

Hematologic: Decreased white blood cell counts in Cimetidine-treated patients (approximately 1 per 100,000 patients), including agranulocytosis (approximately 3 per million patients), have been reported, including a few reports of recurrence

on rechallenge. Most of these reports were in patients who had serious concomitant illnesses and received drugs and/or treatment known to produce neutropenia. Thrombocytopenia (approximately 3 per million patients) and, very rarely, cases of pancytopenia or aplastic anemia have also been reported. As with some other H_2-receptor antagonists, there have been extremely rare reports of immune hemolytic anemia.

Hepatobiliary: Dose-related increases in serum transaminase have been reported. In most cases they did not progress with continued therapy and returned to normal at the end of therapy. There have been rare reports of cholestatic or mixed cholestatic-hepatocellular effects. These were usually reversible. Because of the predominance of cholestatic features, severe parenchymal injury is considered highly unlikely. However, as in the occasional liver injury with other H_2-receptor antagonists, in exceedingly rare circumstances fatal outcomes have been reported.

There has been reported a single case of biopsy-proven periportal hepatic fibrosis in a patient receiving Cimetidine.

Rare cases of pancreatitis, which cleared on withdrawal of the drug, have been reported.

Hypersensitivity: Rare cases of fever and allergic reactions including anaphylaxis and hypersensitivity vasculitis, which cleared on withdrawal of the drug, have been reported.

Renal: Small, possibly dose-related increases in plasma creatinine, presumably due to competition for renal tubular secretion, are not uncommon and do not signify deteriorating renal function. Rare cases of interstitial nephritis and urinary retention, which cleared on withdrawal of the drug, have been reported.

Cardiovascular: Rare cases of bradycardia, tachycardia and A-V heart block have been reported with H_2-receptor antagonists.

Musculoskeletal: There have been rare reports of reversible arthralgia and myalgia: exacerbation of joint symptoms in patients with preexisting arthritis has also been reported. Such symptoms have usually been alleviated by a reduction in Cimetidine dosage. Rare cases of polymyositis have been reported, but no causal relationship has been established.

Integumental: Mild rash and, very rarely, cases of severe generalized skin reactions including Stevens-Johnson syndrome, epidermal necrolysis, erythema multiforme, exfoliative dermatitis and generalized exfoliative erythroderma have been reported with H_2-receptor antagonists. Reversible alopecia has been reported very rarely.

OVERDOSAGE

Studies in animals indicate that toxic doses are associated with respiratory failure and tachycardia that may be controlled by assisted respiration and the administration of a beta-blocker.

Reported acute ingestions orally of up to 20 grams have been associated with transient adverse effects similar to those encountered in normal clinical experience. The usual measures to remove unabsorbed material from the gastrointestinal tract, clinical monitoring and supportive therapy should be employed.

There have been reports of severe CNS symptoms, including unresponsiveness, following ingestion of between 20 and 40 grams of Cimetidine, and extremely rare reports following concomitant use of multiple CNS-active medications and ingestion of Cimetidine at doses less than 20 grams. An elderly, terminally ill dehydrated patient with organic brain syndrome receiving concomitant antipsychotic agents and Cimetidine 4800 mg intravenously over a 24-hour period experienced mental deterioration with reversal on Cimetidine discontinuation.

There have been two deaths in adults who were reported to have ingested over 40 grams orally on a single occasion.

DOSAGE AND ADMINISTRATION
DUODENAL ULCER

Active Duodenal Ulcer: Clinical studies have indicated that suppression of nocturnal acid is the most important factor in duodenal ulcer healing (see *"Clinical Pharmacology—Acid Secretion"*). This is supported by recent clinical trials (see *"Clinical Trials—Active Duodenal Ulcer"*). Therefore, there is no apparent rationale, except for familiarity with use, for treating with anything other than a once-daily at bedtime dosage regimen (h.s.).

In a U.S. dose-ranging study of 400 mg h.s., 800 mg h.s. and 1600 mg h.s., a continuous dose response relationship for ulcer healing was demonstrated.

However, 800 mg h.s. is the dose of choice for most patients, as it provides a high healing rate (the difference between 800 mg h.s. and 1600 mg h.s. being small), maximal pain relief, a decreased potential for drug interactions (see *"Precautions—Drug Interactions"*) and maximal patient convenience. Patients unhealed at 4 weeks, or those with persistent symptoms, have been shown to benefit from 2 to 4 weeks of continued therapy.

It has been shown that patients who both have an endoscopically demonstrated ulcer larger than 1.0 cm and are also heavy smokers (i.e., smoke one pack of cigarettes or more per day) are more difficult to heal. There is some evidence which suggests that more rapid healing can be achieved in this subpopulation with Cimetidine 1600 mg at bedtime. While early pain relief with either 800 mg h.s. or 1600 mg h.s. is equivalent in all patients, 1600 mg h.s. provides an appropriate alternative when it is important to ensure healing within 4 weeks for this subpopulation. Alternatively, approximately 94% of all patients will also heal in 8 weeks with Cimetidine 800 mg h.s.

Other Cimetidine regimens in the U.S. which have been shown to be effective are: 300 mg four times daily, with meals and at bedtime, the original regimen with which U.S. physicians have the most experience, and 400 mg twice daily, in the morning and at bedtime (see *"Clinical Trials—Active Duodenal Ulcer"*).

◆ RATED THERAPEUTICALLY EQUIVALENT; ◇ THERAPEUTIC EQUIVALENCE UNCONFIRMED; ○ UNRATED

Concomitant antacids should be given as needed for relief of pain. However, simultaneous administration of Cimetidine and antacids is not recommended, since antacids have been reported to interfere with the absorption of Cimetidine.

While healing with Cimetidine often occurs during the first week or two, treatment should be continued for 4 to 6 weeks unless healing has been demonstrated by endoscopic examination.

Maintenance Therapy for Duodenal Ulcer: In those patients requiring maintenance therapy, the recommended adult oral dose is 400 mg at bedtime.

ACTIVE BENIGN GASTRIC ULCER
The recommended adult oral dosage for short-term treatment of active benign gastric ulcer is 800 mg h.s., or 300 mg four times a day with meals and at bedtime. Controlled clinical studies were limited to 6 weeks of treatment (see *"Clinical Trials"*). 800 mg h.s. is the preferred regimen for most patients based upon convenience and reduced potential for drug interactions. Symptomatic response to Cimetidine does not preclude the presence of a gastric malignancy. It is important to follow gastric ulcer patients to assure rapid progress to complete healing.

EROSIVE GASTROESOPHAGEAL REFLUX DISEASE (GERD)
The recommended adult oral dosage for the treatment of erosive esophagitis that has been diagnosed by endoscopy is 1600 mg daily in divided doses (800 mg b.i.d. or 400 mg q.i.d.) for 12 weeks. The use of Cimetidine beyond 12 weeks has not been established.

PREVENTION OF UPPER GASTROINTESTINAL BLEEDING
The recommended adult dosing regimen is continous I.V. infusion of 50 mg/hour. Patients with creatinine clearance less than 30 cc/min. should receive half the recommended dose. Treatment beyond 7 days has not been studied.

PATHOLOGICAL HYPERSECRETORY CONDITIONS
(SUCH AS ZOLLINGER-ELLISON SYNDROME)
Recommended adult oral dosage: 300 mg four times a day with meals and at bedtime. In some patients it may be necessary to administer higher doses more frequently. Doses should be adjusted to individual patient needs, but should not usually exceed 2400 mg per day and should continue as long as clinically indicated.

PARENTERAL ADMINISTRATION
In hospitalized patients with pathological hypersecretory conditions or intractable ulcers or in patients who are unable to take oral medication, Cimetidine may be administered parenterally.

The doses and regimen for parenteral administration in patients with GERD have not been established.

All parenteral drug products should be inspected visually for particulate matter and discoloration prior to administration.

RECOMMENDATIONS FOR PARENTERAL ADMINISTRATION
Intramuscular Injection: 300 mg q 6 to 8 hours (no dilution necessary). Transient pain at the site of injection has been reported.

Intravenous Injection: 300 mg q 6 to 8 hours. In some patients it may be necessary to increase dosage. When this is necessary, the increases should be made by more frequent administration of a 300 mg dose, but should not exceed 2400 mg per day. Dilute Cimetidine hydrochloride Injection, 300 mg, in Sodium Chloride Injection (0.9%) or another compatible I.V. solution (see *"Stability of Cimetidine Injection"*) to a total voluime of 20 mL and inject over a period of not less than 5 minutes (see *"Precautions"*).

Intermittent Intravenous Infusion: 300 mg q 6 to 8 hours infused over 15 to 20 minutes. In some patients it may be necessary to increase dosage. When this is necessary, the increases should be made by more frequent administration of a 300 mg dose, but should not exceed 2400 mg per day. *Vials:* Dilute Cimetidine injection, 300 mg, in at least 50 mL of 5% Dextrose Injection, or another compatible I.V. solution (see *"Stability of Cimetidine Injection"*). *Plastic containers:* Use premixed Cimetidine Injection, 300 mg, in 0.9% Sodium Chloride in 50 mL plastic containers. *ADD-Vantage® Vials:* Dilute contents of one vial in an ADD-Vantage® Diluent Container, available in 50 mL and 100 mL sizes of 0.9% Sodium Chloride Injection, and 5% Dextrose Injection.

Continuous Intravenous Infusion: 37.5 mg/hour (900 mg/day). For patients requiring a more rapid elevation of gastric pH, continuous infusion may be preceded by a 150 mg loading dose administered by I.V. infusion as described above. Dilute 900 mg Cimetidine Injection in a compatible I.V. fluid (see *"Stability of Cimetidine Injection"*) for constant rate infusion over a 24-hour period. *Note:* Cimetidine may be diluted in 100 to 1000 mL: however, a volumetric pump is recommended if the volume for 24-hour infusion is less than 250 mL. In one study in patients with pathological hypersecretory states, the mean infused dose of Cimetidine was 160 mg/hour with a range of 40 to 600 mg/hour.

These doses maintained the intragastric acid secretory rate at 10 mEq/hour or less. The infusion rate should be adjusted to individual patient requirements.

DIRECTIONS FOR USE OF CIMETIDINE HYDROCHLORIDE INJECTION IN PLASTIC CONTAINERS
To open: Tear overwrap down side at slit and remove solution containers.

Some opacity of the plastic due to moisture absorption during the sterilization process may be observed. This is normal and does not affect solution quality or safety. The opacity will diminish gradually.

Do not add other drugs to premixed Cimetidine injection in plastic containers.

Caution: Check for minute leaks by squeezing inner bag firmly. If leaks are found, discard solution as sterility may be impaired. Additives should not be introduced into this solution. Do not use if the solution is cloudy or precipitated or if the seal is not intact.

Do not use plastic containers in series connections. Such use could result in air embolism due to residual air being drawn from the primary container before administration of the fluid from the secondary container is complete. Use sterile equipment.

Preparation for Administration:
1. Suspend container from eyelet support.
2. Remove plastic protector from outlet port at bottom of container.
3. Attach administration set. Refer to complete directions accompanying set.
Directions for use of Cimetidine Injection in ADD-Vantage® Vials are enclosed in ADD-Vantage® Vial packaging.

STABILITY OF CIMETIDINE INJECTION
When added to or diluted with most commonly used intravenous solutions, e.g., Sodium Chloride Injection (0.9%), Dextrose Injection (5% or 10%), Lactated Ringer's Solution, 5% Sodium Bicarbonate Injection, Cimetidine hydrochloride injection should not be used after more than 48 hours of storage at room temperature.

Cimetidine injection premixed in plastic containers is stable through the labeled expiration date when stored under the recommended conditions.

DOSAGE ADJUSTMENT FOR PATIENTS WITH IMPAIRED RENAL FUNCTION
Patients with severely impaired renal function have been treated with Cimetidine. However, such usage has been very limited. On the basis of this experience the recommended dosage is 300 mg q 12 hours orally or by intravenous injection. Should the patient's condition require, the frequency of dosing may be increased to q 8 hours or even further with caution. In severe renal failure, accumulation may occur and the lowest frequency of dosing compatible with an adequate patient response should be used. When liver impairment is also present, further reductions in dosage may be necessary. Hemodialysis reduces the level of circulating Cimetidine. Ideally, the dosage schedule should be adjusted so that the timing of a scheduled dose coincides with the end of hemodialysis.

Patients with creatinine clearance less than 30 cc/min. who are being treated for prevention of upper gastrointestinal bleeding should receive half the recommended dose.

STORAGE
Store at controlled room temperature (15° to 30°C; 59° to 86°F); do not refrigerate.

Liquid: Store at controlled room temperature (15° to 30°C; 59° to 86°F); dispense in a tight, light-resistant container.

Single-Dose Premixed Plastic Containers: Exposure of the premixed product to excessive heat should be avoided. It is recommended the product be stored at controlled room temperature (15° to 30°C; 59° to 86°F). Brief exposure up to 40°C does not adversely affect the premixed product.

HOW SUPPLIED
INJECTION: 150 MG/ML

AVERAGE UNIT PRICE (AVAILABLE SIZES)				
GENERIC	$0.77			

BRAND/MANUFACTURER		NDC	SIZE	AWP
◆ BRAND				
TAGAMET: SK Beecham Pharm		00108-5022-11	8 ml 10s	$128.60
		00108-5017-16	2 ml 25s	$99.05
		00108-5031-16	2 ml 25s	$109.70
		00108-5022-16	8 ml 25s	$306.25
		00108-5029-04	50 ml 48s	$267.60
◆ GENERICS				
Endo		60951-0637-53	2 ml 10s	$18.12
Endo		60951-0637-69	8 ml 10s	$54.37
Endo		60951-0637-57	2 ml 25s	$44.37
Endo		60951-0637-27	8 ml 25s	$120.62

SOLUTION: 300 MG/5 ML

AVERAGE UNIT PRICE (AVAILABLE SIZES)		GENERIC A-RATED AVERAGE PRICE (GAAP)	
BRAND	$0.45	240 ml	$87.12
GENERIC	$0.36	240 ml	$88.81

BRAND/MANUFACTURER		NDC	SIZE	AWP
◆ BRAND				
TAGAMET: SK Beecham Pharm		00108-5014-48	240 ml	$99.75
		00108-5014-10	5 ml 10s ud	$24.60
◆ GENERICS				
Qualitest		00603-1092-56	240 ml	$86.20
Goldline		00182-6164-44	240 ml	$86.25
Barre		00472-0514-08	240 ml	$86.25

BRAND/MANUFACTURER	NDC	SIZE	AWP
Schein	00364-2602-76	240 ml	$87.00
Geneva	00781-6527-08	240 ml	$89.68
Major	00904-7897-97	240 ml	$89.75
Rugby	00536-2975-59	240 ml	$89.77
Barre	00472-0514-16	480 ml	$140.95
Moore,H.L.	00839-7923-69	480 ml	$173.00

TABLETS: 200 MG

AVERAGE UNIT PRICE (AVAILABLE SIZES)		GENERIC A-RATED AVERAGE PRICE (GAAP)	
BRAND	$0.85	100s	$74.79
GENERIC	$0.74	500s	$356.85
		1000s	$674.30

BRAND/MANUFACTURER	NDC	SIZE	AWP
◆ BRAND			
➤ TAGAMET: SK Beecham Pharm	00108-5012-20	100s	$84.70
◆ GENERICS			
Rosemont	00832-0101-00	100s	$72.40
Qualitest	00603-2890-21	100s	$72.48
URL	00677-1527-01	100s	$73.20
Schein	00364-2591-01	100s	$73.25
Rugby	00536-5661-01	100s	$73.31
Novopharm	55953-0181-40	100s	$73.40
West Point	59591-0259-68	100s	$73.49
Endo	60951-0630-70	100s	$74.50
Aligen	00405-5370-01	100s	$75.42
Mylan	00378-0053-01	100s	$75.80
Geneva	00781-1447-01	100s	$76.15
Major	00904-7866-60	100s	$76.20
Moore,H.L.	00839-7906-06	100s	$76.21
Goldline	00182-1983-01	100s	$76.23
Martec	52555-0515-01	100s	$76.30
Novopharm	55953-3416-01	100s ud	$75.15
Goldline	00182-1983-89	100s ud	$77.90
Novopharm	55953-0181-70	500s	$348.65
Geneva	00781-1447-05	500s	$359.79
Major	00904-7866-40	500s	$362.10
Novopharm	55953-0181-80	1000s	$662.44
Major	00904-7866-80	1000s	$686.15

TABLETS: 300 MG

AVERAGE UNIT PRICE (AVAILABLE SIZES)		GENERIC A-RATED AVERAGE PRICE (GAAP)	
BRAND	$0.89	30s	$24.23
GENERIC	$0.77	100s	$78.31
		500s	$375.95
		1000s	$731.51

BRAND/MANUFACTURER	NDC	SIZE	AWP
◆ BRAND			
TAGAMET: SK Beecham Pharm	00108-5013-20	100s	$88.65
	00108-5013-21	100s ud	$90.10
	00108-5013-25	500s	$443.25
	00108-5013-38	5000s	$4432.50
◆ GENERICS			
Allscrips	54569-3837-04	8s	$6.20
Allscrips	54569-3837-01	12s	$9.30
Allscrips	54569-3837-02	21s	$16.27
Allscrips	54569-3837-00	30s	$23.25
Medirex	57480-0813-06	30s	$25.20
Rosemont	00832-0102-00	100s	$75.78
Qualitest	00603-2891-21	100s	$75.85
URL	00677-1528-01	100s	$76.40
Schein	00364-2592-01	100s	$76.50
Warner Chilcott	00047-0768-24	100s	$76.50
Rugby	00536-5662-01	100s	$76.73
Novopharm	55953-0192-40	100s	$76.80
West Point	59591-0260-68	100s	$76.87
Aligen	00405-5371-01	100s	$77.20
Lederle Std Prod	00005-3416-23	100s	$77.50
Endo	60951-0631-70	100s	$78.20
➤ Mylan	00378-0317-01	100s	$79.34
Geneva	00781-1448-01	100s	$79.70
Major	00904-7867-60	100s	$79.75
Goldline	00182-1984-01	100s	$79.78
Moore,H.L.	00839-7907-06	100s	$79.79
Martec	52555-0516-01	100s	$79.80
Novopharm	55953-0192-01	100s ud	$78.55
Goldline	00182-1984-89	100s ud	$81.09
Medirex	57480-0813-01	100s ud	$84.00
Allscrips	54569-3837-03	120s	$92.99
Rosemont	00832-0102-50	500s	$359.98
Qualitest	00603-2891-28	500s	$360.40
URL	00677-1528-05	500s	$363.00
Schein	00364-2592-05	500s	$363.35
Novopharm	55953-0192-70	500s	$364.80
Major	00904-7867-40	500s	$376.30
Geneva	00781-1448-05	500s	$376.57
➤ Mylan	00378-0317-05	500s	$376.91
Aligen	00405-5371-02	500s	$396.32
Goldline	00182-1984-05	500s	$398.90

BRAND/MANUFACTURER	NDC	SIZE	AWP
Martec	52555-0516-05	500s	$398.95
Novopharm	55953-0192-80	1000s	$693.12
Major	00904-7867-80	1000s	$717.00
Moore,H.L.	00839-7907-16	1000s	$718.13
Goldline	00182-1984-10	1000s	$797.80

TABLETS: 400 MG

AVERAGE UNIT PRICE (AVAILABLE SIZES)		GENERIC A-RATED AVERAGE PRICE (GAAP)	
BRAND	$1.48	30s	$40.07
GENERIC	$1.28	60s	$77.35
		100s	$130.33
		500s	$627.75
		1000s	$1222.84

BRAND/MANUFACTURER	NDC	SIZE	AWP
◆ BRAND			
➤ TAGAMET: SK Beecham Pharm	00108-5026-18	60s	$88.25
	00108-5026-21	100s ud	$148.90
	00108-5026-25	500s	$735.40
➤ TAGAMET: SK Beecham Pharm	00108-5026-38	5000s	$7354.15
◆ GENERICS			
Allscrips	54569-3838-00	30s	$38.73
Medirex	57480-0814-06	30s	$41.40
Lederle Std Prod	00005-3417-32	60s	$77.25
Allscrips	54569-3838-01	60s	$77.45
Rosemont	00832-0103-00	100s	$125.72
Qualitest	00603-2892-21	100s	$125.85
URL	00677-1529-01	100s	$126.00
Schein	00364-2593-01	100s	$126.75
Warner Chilcott	00047-0765-24	100s	$126.75
West Point	59591-0261-68	100s	$126.86
Rugby	00536-5663-01	100s	$127.53
Novopharm	55953-0204-40	100s	$127.65
Endo	60951-0632-70	100s	$129.50
➤ Mylan	00378-0372-01	100s	$131.63
Geneva	00781-1449-01	100s	$132.22
Moore,H.L.	00839-7908-06	100s	$132.37
Aligen	00405-5372-01	100s	$133.10
Major	00904-7868-60	100s	$134.00
Goldline	00182-1985-01	100s	$134.01
Martec	52555-0517-01	100s	$134.01
Novopharm	55953-0204-01	100s ud	$129.40
Endo	60951-0632-75	100s ud	$131.05
Goldline	00182-1985-89	100s ud	$134.01
Medirex	57480-0814-01	100s ud	$138.00
Rosemont	00832-0103-50	500s	$597.14
Qualitest	00603-2892-28	500s	$597.80
URL	00677-1529-05	500s	$602.00
Schein	00364-2593-05	500s	$602.05
Novopharm	55953-0204-70	500s	$606.34
Geneva	00781-1449-05	500s	$624.76
➤ Mylan	00378-0372-05	500s	$625.24
Major	00904-7868-40	500s	$640.60
Aligen	00405-5372-02	500s	$668.20
Goldline	00182-1985-05	500s	$670.05
Martec	52555-0517-05	500s	$671.10
Novopharm	55953-0204-80	1000s	$1152.05
Moore,H.L.	00839-7908-16	1000s	$1191.31
Major	00904-7868-80	1000s	$1207.90
Goldline	00182-1985-10	1000s	$1340.10

TABLETS: 400 MG

BRAND/MANUFACTURER	NDC	SIZE	AWP
◇ GENERICS			
Warrick	59930-1802-03	1000s	$1172.44

TABLETS: 800 MG

AVERAGE UNIT PRICE (AVAILABLE SIZES)		GENERIC A-RATED AVERAGE PRICE (GAAP)	
BRAND	$2.61	30s	$71.09
GENERIC	$2.37	100s	$238.21
		500s	$1160.84
		1000s	$2284.37

BRAND/MANUFACTURER	NDC	SIZE	AWP
◆ BRAND			
➤ TAGAMET: SK Beecham Pharm	00108-5027-13	30s	$78.20
	00108-5027-21	100s ud	$262.80
	00108-5027-25	500s	$1303.35
◆ GENERICS			
Allscrips	54569-3839-01	15s	$39.56
Rugby	00536-5664-07	30s	$67.68
West Point	59591-0264-31	30s	$67.93
Endo	60951-0633-30	30s	$68.80
Lederle Std Prod	00005-3418-38	30s	$69.50
Medirex	57480-0815-06	30s	$73.50
Allscrips	54569-3839-00	30s	$79.13
Rosemont	00832-0104-00	100s	$222.83
Qualitest	00603-2893-21	100s	$223.08

◆ **RATED THERAPEUTICALLY EQUIVALENT**; ◇ **THERAPEUTIC EQUIVALENCE UNCONFIRMED**; ○ **UNRATED**

BRAND/MANUFACTURER	NDC	SIZE	AWP
URL	00677-1530-01	100s	$224.00
Schein	00364-2594-01	100s	$224.50
Warner Chilcott	00047-0508-24	100s	$224.50
Mylan	00378-0541-01	100s	$233.29
Geneva	00781-1444-01	100s	$234.34
Major	00904-7869-60	100s	$236.50
Martec	52555-0518-01	100s	$236.50
Goldline	00182-1986-01	100s	$236.52
Moore,H.L.	00839-7909-06	100s	$260.67
Novopharm	55953-0235-40	100s	$263.75
Aligen	00405-5373-01	100s	$264.20
Goldline	00182-1986-89	100s ud	$236.52
Medirex	57480-0815-01	100s ud	$245.00
Novopharm	55953-0235-01	100s ud	$245.10
Geneva	00781-1444-05	500s	$1107.27
Major	00904-7869-40	500s	$1122.35
Novopharm	55953-0235-70	500s	$1252.89
Major	00904-7869-80	1000s	$2126.60
Moore,H.L.	00839-7909-16	1000s	$2346.03
Novopharm	55953-0235-80	1000s	$2380.48

Cin-Quin SEE QUINIDINE SULFATE

Cinobac SEE CINOXACIN

Cinoxacin

DESCRIPTION
Cinoxacin, is a synthetic antibacterial agent for oral administration. Cinoxacin, a quinolone, is 1-ethyl-1,4-dihydro-4-oxo-[1,3] dioxolo [4,5-g] cinnoline-3-carboxylic acid and occurs as white or very light yellow, needle-shaped crystals. Cinoxacin is available as 250- (0.95 mmol) and 500-mg (1.9 mmol) capsules.

The molecular formula is $C_{12}H_{10}N_2O_5$ and the molecular weight is 262.22.

Following is its chemical structure:

CLINICAL PHARMACOLOGY
Cinoxacin is rapidly absorbed after oral administration. In fluorometric assay, a 500-mg dose produced a peak serum concentration of 15 μ g/mL, which declined to approximately 1 to 2 μg/mL 6 hours after administration. A 500-mg dose produced an average urine concentration of approximately 300 μg/mL during the first 4 hours and approximately 100 μg/mL during the second 4-hour period. These urine concentrations are many times greater than the minimal inhibitory concentration (MIC) of Cinoxacin for most gram-negative organisms commonly found in urinary tract infections.

Ninety-seven percent of a 500-mg oral dose of radiolabeled Cinoxacin was recovered in the urine within 24 hours, 60% of which was present as unaltered Cinoxacin and the remainder as inactive metabolic products.

The presence of food did not affect the total absorption of Cinoxacin. Peak serum concentrations were reduced by 30%, but the 24-hour urinary recovery of antibacterial activity was unaltered. The mean serum half-life is 1.5 hours.

Microbiology: Cinoxacin has in *vitro* activity against many gram negative aerobic bacteria, particularly strains of *Enterobacteriaceae.* Cinoxacin inhibits bacterial deoxyribonucleic acid (DNA) synthesis, is bactericidal, and is active over the entire urinary pH range. Cross-resistance with nalidixic acid has been demonstrated.

Conventional chromosomal resistance to Cinoxacin taken at recommended doses has been reported to emerge in approximately 4% of patients during treatment; however, bacterial resistance to Cinoxacin has not been shown to be transferable via R-factor. Cinoxacin has been shown to be active against most strains of the following organisms both *in vitro* and in clinical infections (see "*Indications and Usage*").

GRAM-NEGATIVE AEROBES:
Enterobacter species
Escherichia coli
Klebsiella species
Proteus mirabilis
Proteus vulgaris

Note: *Enterococcus* species, *Pseudomonas* species, and *Staphyloccus* species are resistant.

SUSCEPTIBILITY TESTS
Diffusion Techiques: Quantitative methods that require measurement of zone diameters give an estimate of bacterial susceptibility. One such procedure is the

National Committee for Clinical Laboratory Standards (NCCLS) approved procedure (M2-A4—Performance Standards for Antimicrobial Disk Susceptibility Tests 1990). This method has been recommended for use with the 100-μg Cinoxacin disk to test susceptibility to Cinoxacin.

Interpretation involves correlation of the diameters obtained in the disk test with minimum inhibitory concentrations (MIC) for Cinoxacin. Reports from the laboratory giving results of the standard single-disk susceptibility test with a 100-μg Cinoxacin disk should be interpreted according to the following criteria (**these criteria only apply to isolates from urinary tract infections**):

Zone diameter (mm)	Interpretation
≥ 19	(S) Susceptible
15-18	(I) Intermediate
≤ 14	(R) Resistant

A report of "susceptible" indicates that the pathogen is likely to be inhibited by generally achievable urine levels. A report of "intermediate" indicates that the test results be considered equivocal or indeterminate. A report of "resistant" indicates that achievable concentrations of the antibiotic are unlikely to be inhibitory and other therapy should be selected.

Certain strains of *Enterobacteriaceae* exhibit heterogeneity of resistance to Cinoxacin. These strains produce isolated colonies within the inhibition zone. When such strains are encountered, the clear inhibition zone should be measured within the isolated colonies.

Standardized procedures require the use of laboratory control organisms. The 100-μg Cinoxacin disk should give the following zone diameter:

Organism	Zone diameter (mm)
E. coli ATCC 25922	26-32

Other quinolone antibacterial disks should not be substituted when performing susceptibility tests for Cinoxacin because of spectrum differences between Cinoxacin and other quinolones. The 100-μg Cinoxacin disk should be used for all *in vitro* testing of isolates.

Dilution Techniques: Broth and agar dilution methods, such as those recommended by the NCCLS (M7-A2—Methods for Dilution Antimicrobial Susceptibility Tests for Bacteria that Grow Aerobically 1990) may be used to determine the MIC of Cinoxacin. MIC test results should be interpreted according to the following criteria (**these criteria only apply to isolates from urinary tract infections**):

MIC (μg/mL)	Interpretation
≤ 16	(S) Susceptible
32	(I) Intermediate
≥ 64	(R) Resistant

As with standard diffusion methods, dilution procedures require the use of laboratory control organisms. Standard Cinoxacin powder should give the following MIC values:

Organism	MIC range (μg/mL)
E. coli ATCC 25922	2.0-8.0

INDICATIONS AND USAGE
Cinoxacin is indicated for the treatment of initial and recurrent urinary tract infections in adults caused by the following susceptible microorganisms: *Escherichia coli, Proteus mirabilis, Proteus vulgaris, Klebsiella species* (including *K. pneumoniae*), and *Enterobacter species.*

Cinoxacin is effective preventing urinary tract infections for up to 5 months in women with a history of recurrent urinary tract infections.

In vitro susceptibility testing should be performed prior to administration of the drug and, when clinically indicated, during treatment.

CONTRAINDICATION
Cinoxacin is contraindicated in patients with a history of hypersensitivity to Cinoxacin or other quinolones.

WARNINGS
THE SAFETY AND EFFECTIVENESS OF CINOXACIN IN CHILDREN, ADOLESCENTS (UNDER THE AGE OF 18 YEARS), PREGNANT WOMEN, AND LACTATING WOMEN HAVE NOT BEEN ESTABLISHED. (SEE "PEDIATRIC USE," "PREGNANCY," AND "NURSING MOTHERS" SUBSECTIONS IN THE "PRECAUTIONS" SECTIONS) The oral administration of a single 250-mg/kg dose of Cinoxacin causes lameness in immature dogs. Histopathological examination of the weight-bearing joints of these dogs revealed lesions of the cartilage. Other quinolones also produce erosions of cartilage of weight-bearing joints and other signs of arthropathy in immature animals of various species.

Serious and occasionally fatal hypersensitivity (anaphylactic) reactions, some following the first dose, have been reported in patients receiving quinolone class antimicrobials. Some reactions were accompanied by cardiovascular collapse, loss of consciousness, tingling, pharyngeal or facial edema, dyspnea, urticaria, and itching. Only a few patients had a history of previous hypersensitivity reactions. If an allergic reaction to Cinoxacin occurs, discontinue the drug. Serious acute hypersensitivity reactions may require treatment with epinephrine and other resuscitative measures, including oxygen, intravenous fluids, intravenous antihistamines, corticosteroids, pressor amines, and airway management as clinically indicated.

Convulsions and abnormal electroencephalograms have been reported in a few patients receiving quinolone class antimicrobials. No causal relationship has been established. Convulsions, increased intracranial pressure, and toxic psychoses have also been reported in patients receiving other drugs in this class.

Quinolones may also cause central nervous system (CNS) stimulation with tremors, restlessness, light-headedness, confusion, or hallucinations. If these reactions occur in patients receiving Cinoxacin, the drug should be discontinued and appropriate measures instituted. As with all quinolones, Cinoxacin should be used with caution in patients with known or suspected CNS disorders, such as severe cerebral arteriosclerosis, epilepsy, and other factors that predispose to seizures (see "Adverse Reactions").

PRECAUTIONS

General: Since Cinoxacin is eliminated primarily by the kidney, the usual dosage should be lower in patients with reduced renal function (see "Dosage and Administration"). Administration of Cinoxacin is not recommended for anuric patients.

In clinical trials with large doses of quinolones, crystalluria was reported in some volunteers. Although crystalluria is not expected to occur with the usually recommended dosages of Cinoxacin, patients should be well hydrated, and alkalinization of urine should be avoided.

Moderate to severe phototoxicity reactions have been observed in patients who were exposed to direct sunlight while receiving some members of this drug class. Excessive sunlight should be avoided. Therapy should be discontinued if phototoxicity occurs.

As with any potent drug, periodic assessment of organ system function, including renal, hepatic, and hematopoietic function, is advisable during prolonged therapy.

Information for Patients: Patients should be advised that Cinoxacin may be taken with or without meals. Patients should drink fluids liberally. Since sucralfate or antacids affect the absorption of certain quinolones, patients should not take sucralfate or antacids within 2 hours of the administration of Cinoxacin.

Patients should be advised to avoid excessive sunlight during Cinoxacin therapy. If phototoxicity occurs, therapy should be discontinued.

Cinoxacin may be associated with hypersensitivity reactions following even a single dose. The drug should be discontinued at the first sign of skin rash or allergic reaction.

Cinoxacin can cause dizziness and light-headedness; therefore, patients should know how they react to the drug before operating an automobile or machinery or engaging in an activity requiring mental alertness or coordination.

Patients should be advised that Cinoxacin may increase the effects of theophylline and caffeine. There is a possibility of caffeine accumulation when products containing caffeine are consumed during Cinoxacin therapy.

Drug Interactions: Elevated plasma levels of theophylline have been reported with concomitant use of some quinolones. There have been reports of theophylline-related side-effects in patients on concomitant theophylline-quinolone therapy. Therefore, monitoring of theophylline plasma levels should be considered and dosage of theophylline adjusted as required.

Quinolones have also been shown to interfere with the metabolism of caffeine. This may lead to reduce clearance of caffeine and a prolongation of its plasma half-life. Although this interaction has not been reported with Cinoxacin, caution should be exercised when Cinoxacin is given concomitantly with caffeine-containing products.

Antacids or sucralfate substantially interfere with the absorption of some quinolones, resulting in low urine levels.

Also, concomitant administration of quinolones with products containing iron or multivitamins containing zinc may result in low urine levels.

Quinolones, including Cinoxacin, may enhance the effect of oral anticoagulants, such as warfarin or its derivatives. When these products are administered concomitantly, prothrombin time or other suitable coagulation tests should be closely monitored.

Seizures have been reported in patients taking another quinolone class antimicrobial and the nonsteroidal anti-inflammatory drug fenbufen concurrently. Animal studies also suggest an increase potential for seizures when these 2 drugs are given concomitantly. Fenbufen is not approved in the United States at this time. Physicians are provided this information to increase awareness of the potential for serious interactions when Cinoxacin and certain nonsteroidal anti-inflammatory agents are administered concomitantly. Elevated cyclosporine serum levels have been reported with the concomitant use of quinolones and cyclosporine.

Pregnancy—Teratogenic Effects—Pregnancy Category C: Reproduction studies have been performed in rats and rabbits at doses up to 10 times the daily human dose and have revealed no evidence of impaired fertility or harm to the fetus due to Cinoxacin. There are, however, no adequate and well-controlled studies in pregnant women. Cinoxacin should be used during pregnancy only if the potential benefit justifies the potential risk to the fetus (see "Warnings").

Nursing Mothers: It is not known whether Cinoxacin is excreted in human milk. Because other drugs in this class are excreted in human milk and because of the potential for serious adverse reactions from Cinoxacin in nursing infants, a decision should be made whether to discontinue nursing or to discontinue the drug, taking into account the importance of the drug to the mother.

Pediatric Use: Safety and effectiveness in children and adolescents below the age of 18 years have not been established. Cinoxacin causes arthropathy in juvenile animals (see "Warnings").

ADVERSE REACTIONS

In clinical studies involving 1,118 patients, the following adverse effects were considered to be related to Cinoxacin therapy:

Gastrointestinal: Nausea was reported most commonly and occurred in less than 3 in 100 patients. Other side effects, occurring less frequently (1 in 100), were anorexia, vomiting, abdominal cramps/pain, perverse taste, and diarrhea.

Central Nervous System: The most frequent side effects were headache and dizziness reported by 1 in 100 patients. Other adverse reactions possibly related to Cinoxacin include insomnia, drowsiness, tingling sensation, perineal burning, photophobia, and tinnitus. These were reported by less than 1 in 100 patients.

Hypersensitivity: Rash, urticaria, pruritus, edema, angioedema, and eosinophilia were reported by less than 3 in 100 patients. Rare cases of anaphylactic reactions have been reported. Toxic epidermal necrolysis has been reported very rarely. Erythema multiforme and Stevens-Johnson syndrome have been reported with Cinoxacin and other drugs in this class.

Hematologic: Rare reports of thrombocytopenia.

Laboratory values reported to be abnormal were, in descending order of frequency, elevation of BUN (1 in 100), AST (SCOT), ALT (SCPT), serum creatinine, and alkaline phosphatase; reduction in hematocrit/hemoglobin (each less than 1 in 100).

Although not observed in the 1,118 patients treated with Cinoxacin, the following side effects have been reported for other drugs in the same pharmacologically active and chemically related class: restlessness, nervousness, change in color perception, difficulty in focusing, decrease in visual acuity, double vision, weakness, constipation, erythema and bullae, feelings of disorientation or agitation or acute anxiety, palpitation, soreness of the gums, joint stiffness, swelling of the extremities, and toxic psychosis or convulsions (rare). All adverse reactions observed with drugs in this class were reversible.

The most frequently reported adverse events in postmarketing surveillance of Cinoxacin have been rash and anaphylactic reactions. Other frequently reported reactions have been pruritus, urticaria, allergic reactions, nausea, abdominal pain, and headache.

OVERDOSAGE

Signs and Symptoms: Symptoms following an overdose of Cinoxacin may include anorexia, nausea, vomiting, epigastric distress, and diarrhea. The severity of the epigastric distress and the diarrhea are dose related. Headache, dizziness, insomnia, photophobia, tinnitus, and a tingling sensation have been reported in some patients. If other symptoms are present, they are probably secondary to an underlying disease state, an allergic reaction, or the ingestion of a second medication with toxicity.

Treatment: In all cases of suspected overdosage, call your regional Poison Control Center to obtain the most up-to-date information about the treatment of overdose. This recommendation is made because, in general, information regarding the treatment of overdosage may change more rapidly than do package inserts.

In managing overdosage, consider the possibility of multiple drug overdoses interaction among drugs, and unusual drug kinetics in your patient.

Patients who have ingested an overdose of Cinoxacin should be kept well hydrated to prevent crystalluria.

Protect the patient's airway and support ventilation and perfusion. Meticulously monitor and maintain, within acceptable limits, the patient's vital signs, blood gases, serum electrolytes, etc. Absorption of drugs from the gastrointestinal tract may be decreased by given activated charcoal, which, in many cases, is more effective than emesis or lavage; consider charcoal instead of, or in addition to, gastric emptying. Repeated doses of charcoal over time may hasten elimination of some drugs that have been absorbed. Safeguard the patient's airway when employing gastric emptying or charcoal.

Forced diuresis, peritoneal dialysis, hemodialysis, or charcoal hemoperfusion have not been established as beneficial for an overdose of Cinoxacin.

DOSAGE AND ADMINISTRATION

The usual adult dosage for the treatment of urinary tract infections is 1 g daily, administered orally in 2 or 4 divided doses (500 mg b.i.d. or 250 mg q.i.d. respectively) for 7 to 14 days. Although susceptible organisms may be eradicated within a few days after therapy has begun, the full treatment course is recommended.

Impaired Renal Function: When renal function is impaired, a reduced dosage must be employed. After an initial dose of 500 mg, a maintenance dosage schedule should be used (see "Table").

MAINTENANCE DOSAGE GUIDE FOR PATIENTS WITH RENAL IMPAIRMENT

Creatinine Clearance	Renal Function	Dosage
mL/min/1.73m^2		
> 80	Normal	500 mg b.i.d.
80-50	Mild Impairment	250 mg t.i.d.
50-20	Moderate Impairment	250 mg b.i.d.
< 20	Marked Impairment	250 mg q.d.

Administration of Cinoxacin to anuric patients is not recommended. When only serum creatinine is available, the following formula (based on sex, weight, and age of patient) may be used to convert this value into creatinine clearance. The serum creatinine should represent a steady state of renal function.

Males: $\dfrac{\text{Weight (kg)} \times (140 - \text{age})}{72 \times \text{serum creatinine}}$

Females: $0.9 \times$ male value

Preventive Therapy: A single dose of 250 mg at bedtime for up to 5 months has been shown to be effective in women with a history of recurrent urinary tract infections.

Store at controlled room temperature, 59° to 86°F (15° to 30°C).

ANIMAL PHARMACOLOGY

Crystalluria, sometimes associated with secondary urinary tract pathology, occurs in laboratory animals treated orally with Cinoxacin. In the rhesus monkey, crystalluria (without urinary tract pathology) has been noted at doses as low as 50 mg/kg/day (lowest dose tested). Cinoxacin-related crystalluria has not been observed in humans receiving twice the recommended daily dosage.

Cinoxacin and other quinolones have been shown to cause arthropathy in immature animals of most species tested (see *"Warnings"*).

Some drugs of this class have been shown to have oculotoxic potential. Cinoxacin administered to cats at high dosages (200 mg/kg/day) resulted in retinal degeneration and other ocular changes. The dog appeared to be somewhat resistant to these effects, but high dosages (500 mg/kg/day) resulted in mild retinal atrophy. No Cinoxacin-related ocular changes were noted in rabbit, rat, monkey, or human studies. (In one of the studies involving the monkey Cinoxacin was administered for 1 year at 10 times the recommended clinical dose.)

HOW SUPPLIED
CAPSULE: 250 MG

BRAND/MANUFACTURER	NDC	SIZE	AWP
◆ **BRAND**			
CINOBAC: Oclassen	55515-0055-02	40s	$43.85

CAPSULE: 500 MG

AVERAGE UNIT PRICE (AVAILABLE SIZES)		GENERIC A-RATED AVERAGE PRICE (GAAP)	
BRAND	$1.91	**50s**	$82.53
GENERIC	$1.65		

BRAND/MANUFACTURER	NDC	SIZE	AWP
◆ **BRAND**			
CINOBAC: Oclassen	55515-0056-04	50s	$95.31
◆ **GENERICS**			
Biocraft	00332-3181-07	50s	$77.60
Moore, H.L.	00839-7757-04	50s	$84.98
Goldline	00182-1957-19	50s	$85.00

Cipro *SEE* CIPROFLOXACIN, SYSTEMIC

Ciprofloxacin Hydrochloride, Ophthalmic

DESCRIPTION

Ciprofloxacin Hydrochloride Ophthalmic solution is a synthetic, sterile, multiple dose, antimicrobial for topical ophthalmic use. Ciprofloxacin is a fluoroquinolone antibacterial active against a broad spectrum of gram-positive and gram-negative ocular pathogens. It is available as the monohydrochloride monohydrate salt of 1-cyclopropyl-6-fluoro-1,4-dihydro-4-oxo-7- (1-piperazinyl)-3-quinoline-carboxylic acid. It is a faint to light yellow crystalline powder with a molecular weight of 385.8. Its empirical formula is $C_{17}H_{18}FN_3O_3 \cdot HCl \cdot H_2O$.

Ciprofloxacin differs from other quinolones in that it has a fluorine atom at the 6-position, a piperazine moiety at the 7-position, and a cyclopropyl ring at the 1-position.

Following is its chemical structure:

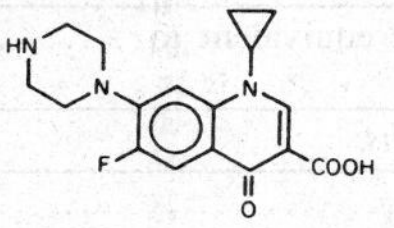

CLINICAL PHARMACOLOGY

Systemic Absorption. A systemic absorption study was performed in which Ciprofloxacin Hydrochloride Ophthalmic solution was administered in each eye every two hours while awake for two days followed by every four hours while awake for an additional 5 days. The maximum reported plasma concentration of Ciprofloxacin was less than 5 ng/mL. The mean concentration was usually less than 2.5 ng/mL.

Microbiology: Ciprofloxacin Hydrochloride has *in vitro* activity against a wide range of gram-negative and gram-positive organisms. The bactericidal action of Ciprofloxacin results from interference with the enzyme DNA gyrase which is needed for the synthesis of bacterial DNA.

Ciprofloxacin Hydrochloride has been shown to be active against most strains of the following organisms both *in vitro* and in clinical infections. (See *"Indications and Usage"* section).

GRAM-POSITIVE
Staphylococcus aureus (including methicillin-susceptible and methicillin-resistant strains)
Staphylococcus epidermidis
Streptococcus pneumoniae
Streptococcus (Viridans Group)

GRAM-NEGATIVE
Pseudomonas aeruginosa
Serratia marcescens

Ciprofloxacin Hydrochloride has been shown to be active *in vitro* against most strains of the following organisms, however, *the clinical significance of these data is unknown:*

GRAM-POSITIVE
Enterococcus faecalis (Many strains are only moderately susceptible)
Staphylococcus haemolyticus
Staphylococcus hominis
Staphylococcus saprophyticus
Streptococcus pyogenes

GRAM-NEGATIVE
Acinetobacter calcoaceticus subsp anitratus
Aeromonas caviae
Aeromonas hydrophila
Brucella melitensis
Campylobacter coli
Campylobacter jujuni
Citrobacter diversus
Citrobacter freundii
Edwardsiella tarda
Enterobacter aerogenes
Enterobacter cloacae
Escherichia coli
Haemophilus ducreyi
Haemophilus influenzae
Haemophilus parainfluenzae
Klebsiella pneumoniae
Klebsiella oxytoca
Legionella pneumophila
Moraxella (Branhamella) catarrhalis
Morganella morganii
Neisseria gonorrhoeae
Neisseria meningitidis
Pasteurella multocida
Proteus mirabilis
Proteus vulgaris
Providencia rettgeri
Providencia stuartii
Salmonella enteritidis
Salmonella typhi
Shigella sonneii
Shigella flexneri
Vibrio cholerae
Vibrio parahaemolyticus
Vibrio vulnificus
Yersinia enterocolitica

Other Organisms: Chalamydia trachomatis (only moderately susceptible) and *Mycobacterium tuberculosis* (only moderately susceptible).

Most strains of *Pseudomonas cepacia* and some strains of *Pseudomonas maltophilia* are resistant to Ciprofloxacin as are most anaerobic bacteria, including *Bacteroides fragilis* and *Clostridium difficile.*

The minimal bactericidal concentration (MBC) generally does not exceed the minimal inhibitory concentration (MIC) by more than a factor of 2. Resistance to Ciprofloxacin *in vitro* usually develops slowly (multiple-step mutation).

Ciprofloxacin Hydrochloride does not cross-react with other antimicrobial agents such as beta-lactams or aminoglycosides; therefore, organisms resistant to these drugs may be susceptible to Ciprofloxacin.

Clinical Studies: Following therapy with Ciprofloxacin Hydrochloride Ophthalmic Solution, 76% of the patients with corneal ulcers and positive bacterial cultures were clinically cured and complete re-epithelialization occurred in about 92% of the ulcers.

In 3 and 7 day multicenter clinical trials, 52% of the patients with conjunctivitis and positive conjunctival cultures were clinically cured and 70-80% had all causative pathogens eradicated by the end of treatment.

INDICATIONS AND USAGE

Ciprofloxacin Hydrochloride Ophthalmic solution is indicated for the treatment of infections caused by susceptible strains of the designated microorganisms in the conditions listed below:

CORNEAL ULCERS
Pseudomonas aeruginosa, Serratia marcescens, Staphylococcus aureus, Staphylococcus epidermidis, Streptococcus pneumoniae, Streptococcus* (Viridans Group)*
*Efficacy for this organism was studied in fewer than 10 infections.

CONJUNCTIVITIS
*Staphylococcus aureus, Staphylococcus epidermidis, Streptococcus pneumoniae**

CONTRAINDICATIONS
A history of hypersensitivity to Ciprofloxacin Hydrochloride or any other component of the medication is a contraindication to its use. A history of hypersensitivity to other quinolones may also contraindicate the use of Ciprofloxacin.

WARNINGS
NOT FOR INJECTION INTO THE EYE.
Serious and occasionally fatal hypersensitivity (anaphylactic) reactions, some following the first dose, have been reported in patients receiving systemic quinolone therapy. Some reactions were accompanied by cardiovascular collapse, loss of consciousness, tingling, pharyngeal or facial edema, dyspnea, urticaria, and itching. Only a few patients had a history of hypersensitivity reactions. Serious anaphylactic reactions require immediate emergency treatment with epinephrine and other resuscitation measures, including oxygen, intravenous fluids, intravenous antihistamines, corticosteroids, pressor amines and airway management, as clinically indicated.

PRECAUTIONS
General: As with other antibacterial preparations, prolonged use of Ciprofloxacin Hydrochloride may result in overgrowth of non-susceptible organisms, including fungi. If superinfection occurs, appropriate therapy should be initiated. Whenever clinical judgment dictates, the patient should be examined with the aid of magnification, such as slit lamp biomicroscopy and, where appropriate, fluorescein staining.

Ciprofloxacin Hydrochloride should be discontinued at the first appearance of a skin rash or any other sign of hypersensitivity reaction. In clinical studies of patients with bacterial corneal ulcer, a white crystalline precipitate located in the superficial portion of the corneal defect was observed in 35 (16.6%) of 210 patients. The onset of the precipitate was within 24 hours to 7 days after starting therapy. In one patient, the precipitate was immediately irrigated out upon its appearance. In 17 patients, resolution of the precipitate was seen in 1 to 8 days (seven within the first 24-72 hours): in five patients, resolution was noted in 10-13 days. In nine patients, exact resolution days were unavailable; however, at follow-up examinations, 18-44 days after onset of the event, complete resolution of the precipitate was noted. In three patients, outcome information was unavailable. The precipitate did not preclude continued use of Ciprofloxacin, nor did it adversely affect the clinical course of the ulcer or visual outcome. (See *"Adverse Reactions"*.)

Drug Interactions: Specific drug interaction studies have not been conducted with ophthalmic Ciprofloxacin. However, the systemic administration of some quinolones has been shown to elevate plasma concentrations of theophylline, interfere with the metabolism of caffeine, enhance the effects of the oral anticoagulant, warfarin, and its derivatives and have been associated with transient elevations in serum creatinine in patients receiving cyclosporine concomitantly.

Carcinogenesis, Mutagenesis, Impairment of Fertility: Eight *in vitro* mutagenicity tests have been conducted with Ciprofloxacin and the test results are listed below:
   Salmonella/Microsome Test (Negative)
   E. coli DNA Repair Assay (Negative)
   Mouse Lymphoma Cell Forward Mutation Assay (Positive)
   Chinese Hamster V₇₉ Cell HGPRT Test (Negative)
   Syrian Hamster Embryo Cell Transformation Assay (Negative)
   Saccharomyces cerevisiae Point Mutation Assay (Negative)
   Saccharomyces cerevisiae Mitotic Crossover and Gene Conversion Assay (Negative)
   Rat Hepatocyte DNA Repair Assay (Positive)
   Thus, two of the eight tests were positive, but the results of the following three *in vivo* test systems gave negative results:
   Rat Hepatocyte DNA Repair Assay
   Micronucleus Test (Mice)
   Dominant Lethal Test (Mice)
   Long term carcinogenicity studies in mice and rats have been completed. After daily oral dosing for up to two years, there is no evidence that Ciprofloxacin had any carcinogenic or tumorigenic effects in these species.

Pregnancy—Pregnancy Category C: Reproduction studies have been performed in rats and mice at doses up to six times the usual daily human oral dose and have revealed no evidence of impaired fertility or harm to the fetus due to Ciprofloxacin. In rabbits, as with most antimicrobial agents, Ciprofloxacin (30 and 100 mg/kg orally) produced gastrointestinal disturbances resulting in maternal weight loss and an increased incidence of abortion. No teratogenicity was observed at either dose. After intravenous administration, at doses up to 20 mg/kg, no maternal toxicity was produced and no embryotoxicity or teratogenicity was observed. There are no adequate and well controlled studies in pregnant women. Ciprofloxacin Hydrochloride Ophthalmic Solution should be used during pregnancy only if the potential benefit justifies the potential risk to the fetus.

Nursing Mothers: It is not known whether topically applied Ciprofloxacin is excreted in human milk: however, it is known that orally administered Ciprofloxacin is excreted in the milk of lactating rats and oral Ciprofloxacin has been reported in human breast milk after a single 500 mg dose. Caution should be exercised when Ciprofloxacin Hydrochloride Ophthalmic Solution is administered to a nursing mother.

Pediatric Use: Safety and effectiveness in children below the age of 12 have not been established.

Although Ciprofloxacin Hydrochloride and other quinolones cause arthropathy in immature animals after oral administration, topical ocular administration of Ciprofloxacin Hydrochloride to immature animals did not cause any arthropathy and there is no evidence that the ophthalmic dosage form has any effect on the weight bearing joints.

ADVERSE REACTIONS
The most frequently reported drug related adverse reaction was local burning or discomfort. In corneal ulcer studies with frequent administration of the drug, white crystalline precipitates were seen in approximately 17% of patients (See *"Precautions"*). Other reactions occurring in less than 10% of patients included lid margin crusting, crystals/scales, foreign body sensation, itching, conjunctival hyperemia and a bad taste following instillation. Additional events occurring in less than 1% of patients included corneal staining, keratopathy/keratitis, allergic reactions, lid edema, tearing, photophobia, corneal infiltrates, nausea and decreased vision.

OVERDOSAGE
A topical overdose of Ciprofloxacin Hydrochloride Ophthalmic solution may be flushed from the eye(s) with warm tap water.

DOSAGE AND ADMINISTRATION
The recommended dosage regimen for the treatment of **corneal ulcers** is: Two drops into the affected eye every 15 minutes for the first six hours and then two drops into the affected eye every 30 minutes for the remainder of the first day. On the second day, instill two drops in the affected eye hourly. On the third through the fourteenth day, place two drops in the affected eye every four hours. Treatment may be continued after 14 days if corneal re-epithelialization has not occurred.

The recommended dosage regimen for the treatment of **bacterial conjunctivitis** is: One or two drops instilled into the conjunctival sac(s) every two hours while awake for two days and one or two drops every four hours while awake for the next five days.

Store at 2° to 30°C (36° to 86°F). Protect from light.

ANIMAL PHARMACOLOGY
Ciprofloxacin and related drugs have been shown to cause arthropathy in immature animals of most species tested following oral administration. However, a one-month topical ocular study using immature beagle dogs did not demonstrate any articular lesions.

HOW SUPPLIED
DROP: 0.3%

BRAND/MANUFACTURER	NDC	SIZE	AWP
○ **BRAND**			
CILOXAN: Alcon Labs	00065-0656-25	2.5 ml	$10.31
	00065-0656-05	5 ml	$20.63

Ciprofloxacin, Systemic

DESCRIPTION
Ciprofloxacin, Systemic is a synthetic broadspectrum antibacterial agent available as tablets for oral administration and as a solution for intravenous (IV) infusion. Ciprofloxacin as the monohydrochloride monohydrate salt has a molecular weight of 385.8. Its empirical formula is $C_{17}H_{18}FN_3O_3 \cdot HCl \cdot H_2O$.

Each tablet contains:
Ciprofloxacin Hydrochloride equivalent to ....250, 500, or 750 mg Ciprofloxacin

The infusion solution contains:
Ciprofloxacin in ....1% and 0.2% strengths

Ciprofloxacin, a fluoroquinolone, is 1-cyclopropyl-6-fluoro-1, 4-dihydro-4-oxo-7-(1-piperazinyl)-3-quinolinecarboxylic acid. Its empirical formula is $C_{17}H_{18}FN_3O_3$.

Ciprofloxacin is a faint to light yellow crystalline powder with a molecular weight of 331.4. It is soluble in dilute (0.1N) hydrochloric acid and is practically insoluble in water and ethanol. Ciprofloxacin differs from other quinolones in that it has a fluorine atom at the 6-position, a piperazine moiety at the 7-position, and a cyclopropyl ring at the 1-position.

The pharmacy bulk package is a single-entry container of a sterile preparation for parenteral use that contains many single doses. The contents are intended for use in a pharmacy admixture program and are restricted to the preparation of admixtures for intravenous infusion.

Following is its chemical structure:

CLINICAL PHARMACOLOGY

Ciprofloxacin Hydrochloride tablets are rapidly and well absorbed from the gastrointestinal tract after oral administration. The absolute bioavailability is approximately 70% with no substantial loss by first pass metabolism. Serum concentrations increase proportionately with the dose as shown:

Dose (mg)	Maximum Serum Concentration (µg/mL)	Area Under Curve (AUC) (µg - hr/mL)
250	1.2	4.8
500	2.4	11.6
750	4.3	20.2
1000	5.4	30.8

Maximum serum concentrations are attained 1 to 2 hours after oral dosing. Mean concentrations 12 hours after dosing with 250, 500, or 750 mg are 0.1, 0.2, and 0.4 µg/mL, respectively. The serum elimination half-life in subjects with normal renal function is approximately 4 hours.

Following 60-minute intravenous infusions of 200 mg and 400 mg Ciprofloxacin to normal volunteers, the mean maximum serum concentrations achieved were 2.1 and 4.6 µg/mL, respectively; the concentrations at 12 hours were 0.1 and 0.2 µg/mL, respectively.

STEADY-STATE CIPROFLOXACIN SERUM CONCENTRATIONS (µg/mL) AFTER 60-MINUTE IV INFUSIONS Q 12 H.

Dose	Time after starting the infusion					
	30 min.	1 hr.	3 hr.	6 hr.	8 hr.	12 hr.
200 mg	1.7	2.1	0.6	0.3	0.2	0.1
400 mg	3.7	4.6	1.3	0.7	0.5	0.2

The pharmacokinetics of Ciprofloxacin are linear over the dose range of 200 to 400 mg administered intravenously. The serum elimination half-life is approximately 5-6 hours and the total clearance is around 35 L/hr. Comparison of the pharmacokinetic parameters following the 1st and 5th IV dose on a q 12 h regimen indicates no evidence of drug accumulation.

The absolute bioavailability of oral Ciprofloxacin is within a range of 70—80% with no substantial loss by first pass metabolism. An intravenous infusion of 400 mg Ciprofloxacin given over 60 minutes every 12 hours has been shown to produce an area under the serum concentration time curve (AUC) equivalent to that produced by a 500 mg oral dose given every 12 hours. A 400 mg IV dose administered over 60 minutes every 12 hours results in a C_{max} similar to that observed with a 750 mg oral dose. An infusion of 200 mg Ciprofloxacin every 12 hours produces an AUC equivalent to that produced by a 250 mg oral dose given every 12 hours.

Approximately 40 to 50% of an orally administered dose is excreted in the urine as unchanged drug. After a 250 mg oral dose, urine concentrations of Ciprofloxacin usually exceed 200 µg/mL during the first two hours and are approximately 30 µg/mL at 8 to 12 hours after dosing. The urinary excretion of Ciprofloxacin is virtually complete within 24 hours after dosing. The renal clearance of Ciprofloxacin, which is approximately 300 mL/minute, exceeds the normal glomerular filtration rate of 120 mL/minute. Thus, active tubular secretion would seem to play a significant role in its elimination.

After intravenous administration, approximately 50% to 70% of the dose is excreted to the urine as unchanged drug. Following a 200 mg IV dose, concentrations in the urine usually exceed 200 µg/mL 0-2 hours after dosing and are generally greater than 15 µg/mL 8-12 hours after dosing. Following a 400 mg IV dose, urine concentrations generally exceed 400 µg/mL 0-2 hours after dosing and are usually greater than 30 µg/mL 8-12 hours after dosing. The renal clearance is approximately 22 L/hr. The urinary excretion of Ciprofloxacin is virtually complete by 24 hours after dosing.

Co-administration of probenecid with Ciprofloxacin results in about a 50% reduction in the Ciprofloxacin renal clearance and a 50% increase in its concentration in the systemic circulation. Although bile concentrations of Ciprofloxacin are several fold higher than serum concentrations after oral or IV dosing, only a small amount of the dose administered is recovered from the bile as unchanged drug. An additional 1-2% of the dose is recovered from the bile in the form of metabolites. Approximately 20 to 35% of an oral dose and 15% of an IV dose is recovered from the feces within 5 days after dosing. This may arise from either biliary clearance or transintestinal elimination. Four metabolites have been identified in human urine which together account for approximately 15% of an oral dose. After IV administration, three metabolites of Ciprofloxacin have been identified in human urine which together account for approximately 10% of the intravenous dose. The metabolites have antimicrobial activity, but are less active than unchanged Ciprofloxacin.

When oral Ciprofloxacin is given concomitantly with food, there is a delay in the absorption of the drug, resulting in peak concentrations that are closer to 2 hours after dosing rather than 1 hour. The overall absorption, however, is not substantially affected. Concurrent administration of antacids containing magnesium hydroxide or aluminum hydroxide may reduce the bioavailability of Ciprofloxacin by as much as 90% (see "Precautions").

Concomitant administration of Ciprofloxacin with theophylline decreases the clearance of theophylline resulting in elevated serum theophylline levels, and increased risk of a patient developing CNS or other adverse reactions. Ciprofloxacin also decreases caffeine clearance and inhibits the formation of paraxanthine after caffeine administration. (See "Precautions.")

In patients with reduced renal function, the half-life of Ciprofloxacin is slightly prolonged. Dosage adjustments may be required (see "Dosage and Administration").

In preliminary studies in patients with stable chronic liver cirrhosis, no significant changes in Ciprofloxacin pharmacokinetics have been observed. The kinetics of Ciprofloxacin in patients with acute hepatic insufficiency, however, have not been fully elucidated.

The binding of Ciprofloxacin to serum proteins is 20 to 40% which is not likely to be high enough to cause significant protein binding interactions with other drugs.

After oral or IV administration Ciprofloxacin is widely distributed throughout the body. Tissue concentrations often exceed serum concentrations in both men and women, particularly in genital tissue including the prostate. Ciprofloxacin is present in active form in the saliva, nasal and bronchial secretions, sputum, skin blister fluid, lymph, peritoneal fluid, bile and prostatic secretions. Ciprofloxacin has also been detected in lung, skin, fat, muscle, cartilage, and bone. The drug diffuses into the cerebrospinal fluid (CSF); however, CSF concentrations are generally less than 10% of peak serum concentrations. Low levels of the drug have been detected in the aqueous and vitreous humors of the eye.

Microbiology: Ciprofloxacin has *in vitro* activity against a wide range of gram-negative and gram-positive organisms. The bactericidal action of Ciprofloxacin results from interference with the enzyme DNA gyrase which is needed for the synthesis of bacterial DNA.

Ciprofloxacin has been shown to be active against most strains of the following organisms both *in vitro* and in clinical infections (see "Indications and Usage" section):

GRAM-POSITIVE BACTERIA
Enterococcus faecalis (Many strains are only moderately susceptible)
Staphylococcus aureus
Staphylococcus epidermidis
Streptococcus pneumoniae
Streptococcus pyogenes

GRAM-NEGATIVE BACTERIA
Campylobacter jejuni
Citrobacter diversus
Citrobacter freundii
Enterobacter cloacae
Escherichia coli
Haemophilus influenzae
Haemophilus parainfluenzae
Klebsiella pneumoniae
Morganella morganii
Proteus mirabilis
Proteus vulgaris
Providencia rettgeri
Providencia stuartii
Pseudomonas aeruginosa
Serratia marcescens
Shigella flexneri
Shigella sonnei

Ciprofloxacin has been shown to be active *in vitro* against most strains of the following organisms; however, *the clinical significance of these data is unknown.*

GRAM-POSITIVE BACTERIA
Staphylococcus haemolyticus
Staphylococcus hominis
Staphylococcus saprophyticus

GRAM-NEGATIVE BACTERIA
Acinetobacter calcoaceticus subs. *antiratus*
Acinetobacter calcoaceticus subs. *Iwoffi*
Aeromonas caviae
Aeromonas hydrophilia
Brucella melitensis
Campylobacter coli
Edwardsiella tarda
Enterobacter aerogenes
Haemophilus ducreyi
Klebsiella oxytoca
Legionella pneumophila
Moraxella (Branhamella) catarrhalis
Neisseria gonorrhoeae
Neisseria meningitidis

Pasteurella multocida
Salmonella enteritidis
Salmonella typhi
Vibrio cholerae
Vibrio parahaemolyticus
Vibrio vulnificus
Yersinia enterocolitica

OTHER ORGANISMS
Chlamydia trachomatis (only moderately susceptible)
   Mycobacterium tuberculosis (only moderately susceptible)
   Most strains of *Pseudomonas cepacia* and some strains of *Xanthomonas (Pseudomonas) maltophilia* are resistant to Ciprofloxacin as are most anaerobic bacteria, including *Bacteroides fragilis* and *Clostridium difficile*.
   Ciprofloxacin is slightly less active when tested at acidic pH. The inoculum size has little effect when tested *in vitro*. The minimum bactericidal concentration (MBC) generally does not exceed the minimum inhibitory concentration (MIC) by more than a factor of 2. Resistance to Ciprofloxacin *in vitro* develops slowly (multiple-step mutation).
   Ciprofloxacin does not cross-react with other antimicrobial agents such as beta-lactams or aminoglycosides; therefore, organisms resistant to these drugs may be susceptible to Ciprofloxacin.
   In vitro studies have shown that additive activity often results when Ciprofloxacin is combined with other antimicrobial agents such as beta-lactams, aminoglycosides, clindamycin, or metronidazole. Synergy has been reported particularly with the combination of Ciprofloxacin and a beta-lactam; antagonism is observed only rarely.

SUSCEPTIBILITY TESTS
Diffusion Techniques: Quantitative methods that require measurement of zone diameters give the most precise estimates of susceptibility of bacteria to antimicrobial agents. One such standardized procedure[1] which has been recommended for use with disks to test susceptibility of organisms to Ciprofloxacin uses the 5-μg Ciprofloxacin disk. Interpretation involves correlation of the diameters obtained in the disk test with minimum inhibitory concentrations (MICs) for Ciprofloxacin. Only a 5-μg Ciprofloxacin disk should be used, and it should not be used for testing susceptibility to less active quinolones; there are no suitable surrogate disks.
   Reports from the laboratory giving results of the standard single-disk susceptibility test with a 5-μg Ciprofloxacin disk should be interpreted according to the following criteria:

Zone Diameter (mm)	Interpretation
≥ 21	(S) Susceptible
	(I) Intermediate (Moderately
16-20	Susceptible)
≥ 15	(R) Resistant

A report of "Susceptible" indicates that the pathogen is likely to be inhibited by generally achievable blood levels. A report of "Intermediate (Moderately Susceptible)" suggests that the organism would be susceptible if high dosage is used or if the infection is confined to tissues and fluids in which high antimicrobial levels are attained. A report of "Resistant" indicates that achievable drug concentrations are unlikely to be inhibitory and other therapy should be selected.

Dilution Techniques: Use a standardized dilution method[2] (broth, agar, microdilution) or equivalent with ciprofloxacin powder. The MIC values obtained should be interpreted according to the following criteria:

MIC (μg/mL)	Interpretation
≤ 1	(S) Susceptible
2	(I) Intermediate (Moderately
	Susceptible)
≥ 4	(R) Resistant

Standardized procedures require the use of laboratory control organisms. This is true for both standardized diffusion techniques and standardized dilution techniques. The 5-μg Ciprofloxacin disk should give the following zone diameters and the standard Ciprofloxacin powder should provide the following MIC values:

OC Strains	Disk Zone Diameter (mm)	MIC (μg/mL)
S. aureus (ATCC 25923)	22-30	—
S. aureus (ATCC 29213)	—	0.12-0.5
E. coli (ATCC 25922)	30-40	0.004-0.015
P. aeruginosa (ATCC 27853)	25-33	0.25-1.0
E. faecalis (ATCC 29212)	—	0.25-2.0

For anaerobic bacteria the MIC of ciprofloxacin can be determined by agar or broth dilution (including microdilution) techniques.[3]

INDICATIONS AND USAGE
Ciprofloxacin, Systemic, oral, is indicated for the treatment of infections caused by susceptible strains of the designated microorganisms in the conditions listed below. Please see *"Dosage and Administration"* for specific recommendations.

LOWER RESPIRATORY INFECTIONS
Caused by *Escherichia coli, Klebsiella pneumoniae, Enterobacter cloacae, Proteus mirabilis, Pseudomonas aeruginosa, Haemophilus influenzae, Haemophilus parainfluenzae,* or *Streptococcus pneumoniae.*

SKIN AND SKIN STRUCTURE INFECTIONS
Caused by *Escherichia coli, Klebsiella pneumoniae, Enterobacter cloacae, Proteus mirabilis, Proteus vulgaris, Providencia stuartii, Morganella morganii, Citrobacter freundii, Pseudomonas aeruginosa, Staphylococcus aureus, Staphylococcus epidermidis,* or *Streptococcus pyogenes.*

BONE AND JOINT INFECTIONS
Caused by *Enterobacter cloacae, Serratia marcescens,* or *Pseudomonas aeruginosa.*

URINARY TRACT INFECTIONS
Caused by *Escherichia coli, Klebsiella pneumoniae, Enterobacter cloacae, Serratia marcescens, Proteus mirabilis, Providencia rettgeri, Morganella morganii, Citrobacter diversus, Citrobacter freundii, Pseudomonas aeruginosa, Staphylococcus epidermidis,* or *Enterococcus faecalis.*

INFECTIOUS DIARRHEA
Caused by *Escherichia coli* (enterotoxigenic strains), *Campylobacter jejuni, Shigella flexneri** or *Shigella sonnei** when antibacterial therapy is indicated.
   Ciprofloxacin, Systemic, IV, is indicated for the treatment of infections caused by susceptible strains of the designated microorganisms in the conditions listed below when the intravenous administration offers a route of administration advantageous to the patient:

URINARY TRACT INFECTIONS—MILD, MODERATE, SEVERE AND COMPLICATED INFECTIONS
Caused by *Escherichia coli,* (including cases with secondary bacteremia), *Klebsiella pneumoniae* subspecies *pneumoniae, Enterobacter cloacae, Serratia marcescens, Proteus mirabilis, Providencia rettgeri, Morganella morganii, Citrobacter diversus, Citrobacter freundii, Pseudomonas aeruginosa, Staphylococcus epidermidis,* and *Enterococcus faecalis.*
   Ciprofloxacin, Systemic, IV, is also indicated for the treatment of mild to moderate lower respiratory tract infections, skin and skin structure infections and bone and joint infections due to the organisms listed in each section below. In severe and complicated lower respiratory tract infections, skin and skin structure infections and bone and joint infections, safety and effectiveness of the IV formulation have not been established.

LOWER RESPIRATORY INFECTIONS—MILD TO MODERATE INFECTIONS
Caused by *Escherichia coli, Klebsiella pneumoniae* subspecies *pneumoniae, Enterobacter cloacoa, Proteus mirabilis, Pseudomonas aeruginosa, Haemophilus influenzae, Haemophilus parainfluenzae,* and *Streptococcus pneumoniae.*

SKIN AND SKIN STRUCTURE INFECTIONS—MILD TO MODERATE INFECTIONS
Caused by *Escherichia coli, Klebsiella pneumoniae* subspecies *pneumoniae, Enterobacter cloacae, Proteus mirabilis, Proteus vulgaris, Providencia stuartii, Morganella morganii, Citrobacter freundii, Pseudomonas aeruginosa, Staphylococcus aureus, Staphylococcus epidermidis,* and *Streptococcus pyogenes.*

BONE AND JOINT INFECTIONS—MILD TO MODERATE INFECTIONS
Caused by *Enterobacter cloacae, Serratia marcescens,* and *Pseudomonas aeruginosa.*
   If anaerobic organisms are suspected of contributing to the infection, appropriate therapy should be administered.
   Appropriate culture and susceptibility tests should be performed before treatment in order to isolate and identify organisms causing infection and to determine their susceptibility to Ciprofloxacin. Therapy with Ciprofloxacin, Systemic, may be initiated before results of these tests are known; once results become available, appropriate therapy should be continued. As with other drugs, some strains of *Pseudomonas aeruginosa* may develop resistance fairly rapidly during treatment with Ciprofloxacin. Culture and susceptibility testing performed periodically during therapy will provide information not only on the therapeutic effect of the antimicrobial agent but also on the possible emergence of bacterial resistance.

UNLABELED USES
Ciprofloxacin is used alone or as an adjunct in the treatment of selective decontamination of the alimentary tract in leukemic patients during remission induction treatment, severe biliary tract infections, and chancroid. It is also used in the treatment of cholera, pseudomembranous colitis, *Pseudomonas Aeruginosa* pulmonary infections in cystic fibrosis, and febrile neutropenia in immunocompromised patients. Ciprofloxacin is also used in the treatment of gonorrhea, uncomplicated gonococcal infections, and urethral, cervical, rectal, or pharyngeal

---

* Although treatment of infections due to this organism in this organ system demonstrated a clinically significant outcome, efficacy was studied in fewer than 10 patients.

gonococcal infections. In addition, it is also used in treating *Mycobacterium Avium* infection, nasopharyngeal carriage of Neisseria Meningitidis, chronic otorrhea, prostatitis, *Salmonella Typhi* infection, and as prophylaxis for transurethral resection of the prostate, traveler's diarrhea, and typhoid fever.

CONTRAINDICATIONS

Ciprofloxacin, Systemic, is contraindicated in persons with a history of hypersensitivity to Ciprofloxacin or any member of the quinolone class of antimicrobial agents.

WARNINGS

THIS SAFETY AND EFFECTIVENESS OF CIPROFLOXACIN IN CHILDREN, ADOLESCENTS (LESS THAN 18 YEARS OF AGE), PREGNANT WOMEN, AND LACTATING WOMEN HAVE NOT BEEN ESTABLISHED (SEE *"Precautions—Pediatric Use'*, *"Pregnancy"* AND *"Nursing Mothers"* SUBSECTIONS). Ciprofloxacin caused lameness in immature dogs. Histopathological examination of the weight-bearing joints of these dogs revealed permanent lesions of the cartilage. Related quinolone-class drugs also produce erosions of cartilage of weight-bearing joints and other signs of arthropathy in immature animals of various species. (See *"Animal Pharmacology"*.)

Convulsions have been reported in patients receiving Ciprofloxacin. Convulsions, increased intracranial pressure, and toxic psychosis have been reported in patients receiving Ciprofloxacin and other drugs in this case. Quinolones may also cause central nervous system (CNS) stimulation which may lead to tremors, restlessness, light-headedness, confusion and hallucinations. If these reactions occur in patients receiving Ciprofloxacin, the drug should be discontinued and appropriate measures instituted. As with all quinolones, Ciprofloxacin should be used with caution in patients with known or suspected CNS disorders, such as severe cerebral arteriosclerosis, epilepsy, and other factors that predispose to seizures. (See *"Adverse Reactions"*.)

SERIOUS AND FATAL REACTIONS HAVE BEEN REPORTED IN PATIENTS RECEIVING CONCURRENT ADMINISTRATION OF CIPROFLOXACIN AND THEOPHYLLINE. These reactions have included cardiac arrest, seizure, status epilepticus and respiratory failure. Although similar serious adverse events have been reported in patients receiving theophylline alone, the possibility that these reactions may be potentiated by Ciprofloxacin cannot be eliminated. If concomitant use cannot be avoided, serum levels of theophylline should be monitored and dosage adjustments made as appropriate.

Serious and occasionally fatal hypersensitivity (anaphylactic) reactions, some following the first dose, have been reported in patients receiving quinolone therapy. Some reactions were accompanied by cardiovascular collapse, loss of consciousness, tingling, pharyngeal or facial edema, dyspnea, urticaria, and itching. Only a few patients had a history of hypersensitivity reactions. Serious anaphylactic reactions require immediate emergency treatment with epinephrine. Oxygen, intravenous fluids, intravenous antihistamines, corticosteroids, pressor amines, and airway management, including intubation, should be administered as indicated. Severe hypersensitivity reactions characterized by rash, fever, eosinophilia, jaundice, and hepatic necrosis with fatal outcome have also been rarely reported in patients receiving Ciprofloxacin along with other drugs. The possibility that these reactions were related to Ciprofloxacin cannot be excluded. Ciprofloxacin should be discontinued at the first appearance of a skin rash or any other sign of hypersensitivity.

Pseudomembranous colitis has been reported with nearly all antibacterial agents, including Ciprofloxacin, and may range in severity from mild to life-threatening. Therefore, it is important to consider this diagnosis in patients who present with diarrhea subsequent to the administration of antibacterial agents.

Treatment with antibacterial agents alters the normal flora of the colon and may permit overgrowth of clostridia. Studies indicate that a toxin produced by *Clostridium difficile* is one primary cause of "antibiotic-associated colitis".

After the diagnosis of pseudomembranous colitis has been established, therapeutic measures should be initiated. Mild cases of pseudomembranous colitis usually respond to drug discontinuation alone. In moderate to severe cases, consideration should be given to management with fluids and electrolytes, protein supplementation and treatment with an antibacterial drug clinically effective against *C. difficile* colitis.

PRECAUTIONS

General: Crystals of Ciprofloxacin have been observed rarely in the urine of human subjects but more frequently in the urine of laboratory animals, which is usually alkaline. (See *"Animal Pharmacology"*.) Crystalluria related to Ciprofloxacin has been reported only rarely in humans because human urine is usually acidic. Alkalinity of the urine should be avoided in patients receiving Ciprofloxacin.

Patients should be well hydrated to prevent the formation of highly concentrated urine.

Alteration of the dosage regimen is necessary for patients with impairment of renal function. (See *"Dosage and Administration"*.)

Moderate to severe phototoxicity manifested by an exaggerated sunburn reaction has been observed in patients who are exposed to direct sunlight while receiving some members of the quinolone class of drugs. Excessive sunlight should be avoided. Therapy should be discontinued if phototoxicity occurs.

As with any potent drug, periodic assessment of organ system functions, including renal, hepatic, and hematopoietic function, is advisable during prolonged therapy.

Intravenous Ciprofloxacin should be administered by slow infusion over a period of 60 minutes. Local IV site reactions have been reported with the intravenous administration of Ciprofloxacin. These reactions are more frequent if infusion time is 30 minutes or less or if small veins of the hand are used. (See *"Adverse Reactions"*.)

Information for Patients: Patients should be advised that oral Ciprofloxacin may be taken with or without meals. The preferred time of dosing is two hours after a meal. Patients should also be advised to drink fluids liberally and not take antacids containing magnesium, aluminum, or calcium, products containing iron, or multivitamins containing zinc. However, usual dietary intake of calcium has not been shown to alter the absorption of Ciprofloxacin.

Patients should be advised that Ciprofloxacin may be associated with hypersensitivity reactions, even following a single dose, and to discontinue the drug at the first sign of a skin rash or other allergic reaction.

Patients should be advised to avoid excessive sunlight or artificial ultraviolet light while receiving Ciprofloxacin and to discontinue therapy if phototoxicity occurs.

Ciprofloxacin may cause dizziness and lightheadedness; therefore patients should know how they react to this drug before they operate an automobile or machinery or engage in activities requiring mental alertness or coordination.

Patients should be advised that Ciprofloxacin may increase the effects of theophylline and caffeine. There is a possibility of caffeine accumulation when products containing caffeine are consumed while taking quinolones.

Drug Interactions: As with some other quinolones, concurrent administration of Ciprofloxacin with theophylline may lead to elevated serum concentrations of theophylline and prolongation of its elimination half-life. This may result in increased risk of theophylline-related adverse reactions. (See *"Warnings"*.) If concomitant use cannot be avoided, serum levels of theophylline should be monitored and dosage adjustments made as appropriate.

Some quinolones, including Ciprofloxacin, have also been shown to interfere with the metabolism of caffeine. This may lead to reduced clearance of caffeine and a prolongation of its serum half-life.

Concurrent administration of oral Ciprofloxacin with antacids containing magnesium, aluminum, or calcium; with sucralfate or divalent and trivalent cations such as iron may substantially interfere with the absorption of Ciprofloxacin, resulting in serum and urine levels considerably lower than desired. To a lesser extent this effect is demonstrated with zinc containing multivitamins. (See *"Dosage and Administration"* for concurrent administration of these agents with Ciprofloxacin.)

Some quinolones, including Ciprofloxacin, have been associated with transient elevations in serum creatinine in patients receiving cyclosporine concomitantly.

Quinolones have been reported to enhance the effects of the oral anticoagulant warfarin or its derivatives. When these products are administered concomitantly, prothrombin time or other suitable coagulation tests should be closely monitored.

Probenecid interferes with renal tubular secretion of Ciprofloxacin and produces an increase in the level of Ciprofloxacin in the serum. This should be considered if patients are receiving both drugs concomitantly.

As with other broad spectrum antimicrobial agents, prolonged use of Ciprofloxacin may result in overgrowth of nonsusceptible organisms. Repeated evaluation of the patient's condition and microbial susceptibility testing is essential. If superinfection occurs during therapy, appropriate measures should be taken.

Carcinogenesis, Mutagenesis, Impairment of Fertility: Eight *in vitro* mutagenicity tests have been conducted with Ciprofloxacin and the test results are listed below:

Salmonella/Microsome Test (Negative)
E. coli DNA Repair Assay (Negative)
Mouse Lymphoma Cell Forward Mutation Assay (Positive)
Chinese Hamster V_{79} Cell HGPRT Test (Negative)
Syrian Hamster Embryo Cell Transformation Assay (Negative)
Saccharomyces cerevisiae Point Mutation Assay (Negative)
Saccharomyces cerevisiae Mitotic Crossover and Gene Conversion Assay (Negative)
Rat Hepatocyte DNA Repair Assay (Positive)

Thus 2 of the 8 tests were positive but results of the following 3 *in vivo* test systems gave negative results:

Rat Hepatocyte DNA Repair Assay
Micronucleus Test (Mice)
Dominant Lethal Test (Mice)

Long term carcinogenicity studies in mice and rats have been completed. After daily oral dosing for up to 2 years, there is no evidence that Ciprofloxacin had any carcinogenic or tumorigenic effects in these species.

Pregnancy: Teratogenic Effects. Pregnancy Category C: Reproduction studies have been performed in rats and mice at doses up to 6 times the usual daily human dose and have revealed no evidence of impaired fertility or harm to the fetus due to Ciprofloxacin. In rabbits, as with most antimicrobial agents, Ciprofloxacin (30 and 100 mg/kg orally) produced gastrointestinal disturbances resulting in maternal weight loss and an increased incidence of abortion. No teratogenicity was observed at either dose. After intravenous administration, at doses up to 20 mg/kg, no maternal toxicity was produced, and no embryotoxicity or teratogenicity was observed. There are, however, no adequate and well-controlled studies in pregnant women. Ciprofloxacin should be used during pregnancy only if the potential benefit justifies the potential risk to the fetus. (See *"Warnings"*.)

Nursing Mothers: Ciprofloxacin is excreted in human milk. Because of the potential for serious adverse reactions in infants nursing from mothers taking Ciprofloxacin, a decision should be made either to discontinue nursing or to discontinue the drug, taking into account the importance of the drug to the mother.

Pediatric Use: Safety and effectiveness in children and adolescents less than 18 years of age have not been established. Ciprofloxacin causes arthropathy in juvenile animals. (See *"Warnings".*)

ADVERSE REACTIONS

Oral: During clinical investigation, 2,799 patients received 2,868 courses of the drug. Adverse events that were considered likely to be drug related occurred in 7.3% of patients treated, possibly related in 9.2%, (total of 16.5% thought to be possibly or probably related to drug therapy), and remotely related in 3.0%. Ciprofloxacin was discontinued because of an adverse event in 3.5% of patients treated, primarily involving the gastrointestinal system (1.5%), skin (0.6%), and central nervous system (0.4%).

The most frequently reported events, drug related or not, were nausea (5.2%), diarrhea (2.3%), vomiting (2.0%), abdominal pain/discomfort (1.7%), headache (1.2%), restlessness (1.1%), and rash (1.1%).

IV: The most frequently reported events, without regard to drug relationship, among patients treated with intravenous Ciprofloxacin were nausea, diarrhea, central nervous system disturbance, local IV site reactions, abnormalities of liver associated enzymes (hepatic enzymes) and eosinophilia. Headache, restlessness and rash were also noted in greater than 1% of patients treated with the most common doses of Ciprofloxacin.

Local IV site reactions have been reported with the intravenous administration of Ciprofloxacin. These reactions are more frequent if the infusion time is 30 minutes or less. These may appear as local skin reactions which resolve rapidly upon completion of the infusion. Subsequent intravenous administration is not contraindicated unless the reactions recur or worsen.

Additional events, without regard to drug relationship or route of administration, that occurred in 1% or less of Ciprofloxacin courses are listed below:

Gastrointestinal: ileus; jaundice; gastrointestinal bleeding; *C. difficile* associated diarrhea; pseudomembranous colitis; pancreatitis; hepatic necrosis; intestinal perforation; dyspepsia; epigastric or abdominal pain; vomiting; constipation; oral ulceration; painful oral mucosa; oral candidiasis; mouth dryness; anorexia; dysphagia; flatulence.

Central Nervous System: convulsive seizures; paranoia; toxic psychosis; depression; dysphasia; phobia; depersonalization; manic reaction; unresponsiveness; ataxia; confusion; hallucinations; dizziness; light-headedness; paresthesia; anxiety; tremor; insomnia; nightmares; weakness; drowsiness; irritability; malaise; lethargy.

Skin/Hypersensitivity: anaphylactic reactions; erythema multiforme/Stevens-Johnson syndrome; exfoliative dermatitis; toxic epidermal necrolysis; vasculitis; angioedema; edema of the lips, face, neck; conjunctivae; hands or lower extremities; purpura; fever; chills; flushing; pruritus; urticaria; cutaneous candidiasis; vesicles; increased perspiration; hyperpigmentation; erythema nodosum; photosensitivity.

Allergic reactions ranging from urticaria to anaphylactic reactions have been reported. (See *"Warnings".*)

Special Senses: decreased visual acuity; blurred vision; disturbed vision (flashing lights; change in color perception; overbrightness of lights; diplopia); eye pain; anosmia; hearing loss; tinnitus; nystagmus; a bad taste.

Musculoskeletal: joint pain; jaw, arm or back pain; joint stiffness; neck and chest pain; achiness; flare up of gout.

Renal/Urogenital: renal failure; interstitial nephritis; hemorrhagic cystitis; renal calculi; frequent urination; nephritis; acidosis; urethral bleeding; polyuria; urinary retention; gynecomastia; candiduria; vaginitis; Crystalluria; cylindruria; hematuria; and albuminuria have also been reported.

Cardiovascular: cardiovascular collapse; cardiopulmonary arrest; myocardial infarction; arrhythmia; tachycardia; palpitation; cerebral thrombosis; syncope; cardiac murmur; hypertension; hypotension; angina pectoris; atrial flutter; ventricular ectopy.

Respiratory: respiratory arrest; pulmonary embolism; dyspnea; laryngeal or pulmonary edema; respiratory distress; pleural effusion; hemoptysis; epistaxis; hiccough, bronchospasm.

IV Infusion Site: thrombophlebitis; burning; pain; pruritus; paresthesia; erythema; swelling.

Also reported were agranulocytosis, prolongation of prothrombin time and possible exacerbation of myasthenia gravis.

Most of the adverse events reported were described as only mild or moderate in severity, abated soon after the drug was discontinued, and required no treatment.

In several instances nausea, vomiting, tremor, irritability or palpitation were judged by investigators to be related to elevated serum levels of theophylline possibly as a result of drug interaction with Ciprofloxacin.

Other adverse events reported in the postmarketing phase include hepatic necrosis and postural hypotension. Also reported were hemolytic anemia; elevation of serum triglycerides, serum cholesterol, blood glucose, serum potassium; vaginal candidiasis; and change in serum phenytoin. (See *"Precautions".*)

Adverse Laboratory Changes: Changes in laboratory parameters listed as adverse events without regard to drug relationship:

Hepatic—Elevations of: ALT (SGPT) 1.9%, AST (SGOT) (1.7%), alkaline phosphate (0.8%), LDH (0.4%), serum bilirubin (0.3%).

Hematologic—Eosinophilia (0.6%), leukopenia (0.4%), decreased blood platelets (0.1%), hemoglobin, and/or hematocrit, elevated blood platelets (0.1%), pancytopenia (0.1%).

Renal—Elevations of: Serum creatinine (1.1%), BUN (0.9%), uricacid. *Crystalluria, Cylinduria and Hematuria* have been reported.

Other—Elevations of serum creatine phosphokinase, serum theophylline (in patients receiving theophylline concomitantly), blood glucose, and triglycerides.

Other changes occurring infrequently were: decreased leukocyte count, elevated atypical lymphocyte count, immature WBC's elevated serum calcium, elevation of serum gammaglutamyl, transferase or transpeptidase (γ GT), decreased BUN, decreased uric acid, decreased total serum protein, decreased serum albumin, decreased serum potassium, elevated serum potassium, elevated serum cholesterol.

Other changes occurring rarely during administration of Ciprofloxacin were: elevation of serum amylase, decrease of blood glucose, pancytopenia, leukocytosis, increase in blood monocytes, elevated sedimentation rate, change in serum phenytoin, decreased prothrombin time, hemolytic anemia, and bleeding diathesis.

OVERDOSAGE

In the event of acute overdosage, the stomach should be emptied by inducing vomiting or by gastric lavage (oral ingestion). The patient should be carefully observed and given supportive treatment. Adequate hydration must be maintained. Only a small amount of Ciprofloxacin (< 10%) is removed from the body after hemodialysis *or* peritoneal dialysis.

DOSAGE AND ADMINISTRATION

Oral: The usual adult dosage for patients with urinary tract infections is 250 mg every 12 hours. For patients with complicated infections caused by organisms not highly susceptible, 500 mg may be administered every 12 hours.

Lower respiratory tract infections, skin and skin structure infections, and bone and joint infections may be treated with 500 mg every 12 hours. For more severe or complicated infections, a dosage of 750 mg may be given every 12 hours.

The recommended dosage for infectious diarrhea is 500 mg every 12 hours. (See related table).

The determination of dosage for any particular patient must take into consideration the severity and nature of the infection, the susceptibility of the causative organism, the integrity of the patient's host-defense mechanisms, and the status of renal function and hepatic function.

The duration of treatment depends upon the severity of infection. Generally Ciprofloxacin should be continued for at least 2 days after the signs and symptoms of infection have disappeared. The usual duration is 7 to 14 days; however, for severe and complicated infections more prolonged therapy may be required. Bone and joint infections may require treatment for 4 to 6 weeks or longer. Infectious diarrhea may be treated for 5-7 days.

Concurrent Use With Antacids or Multivalent Cations: Concurrent administration of Ciprofloxacin with sucralfate or divalent and trivalent cations such as iron or antacids containing magnesium, aluminum, or calcium may substantially interfere with the absorption of Ciprofloxacin, resulting in serum and urine levels considerably lower than desired. Therefore, concurrent administration of these agents with Ciprofloxacin should be avoided. However, usual dietary intake of calcium has not been shown to alter the bioavailability of Ciprofloxacin. Single dose bioavailability studies have shown that antacids may be administered either 2 hours after or 6 hours before Ciprofloxacin dosing without a significant decrease in bioavailability. Histamine H_2-receptor antagonists appear to have no significant effect on the bioavailability of Ciprofloxacin.

Impaired Renal Function: Ciprofloxacin is eliminated primarily by renal excretion; however, the drug is also metabolized and partially cleared through the

DOSAGE GUIDELINES

Location of Infection	Type or Severity	Unit Dose	Frequency	Daily Dose
Urinary Tract	Mild/Moderate	250 mg	q 12 h	500 mg
	Severe/Complicated	500 mg	q 12 h	1000 mg
Lower Respiratory Tract; Bone and Joint;	Mild/Moderate	500 mg	q 12 h	1000 mg
Skin & Skin Structure	Severe/Complicated	750 mg	q 12 h	1500 mg
Infectious Diarrhea	Mild/Moderate/Severe	500 mg	q 12 h	1000 mg

biliary system of the liver and through the intestine. These alternate pathways of drug elimination appear to compensate for the reduced renal excretion in patients with renal impairment. Nonetheless, some modification of dosage is recommended, particularly for patients with severe renal dysfunction. The following table provides dosage guidelines for use in patients with renal impairment; however, monitoring of serum drug levels provides the most reliable basis for dosage adjustment:

RECOMMENDED STARTING AND MAINTENANCE DOSES FOR PATIENTS WITH IMPAIRED RENAL FUNCTION

Creatinine Clearance (mL/min)	Dose
> 50	See Usual Dosage
30-50	250-500 mg q 12 h
5-29	250-500 mg q 18 h
Patients on hemodialysis or Peritoneal dialysis	250-500 mg q 24 h (after dialysis)

When only the serum creatinine concentration is known, the following formula may be used to estimate creatinine clearance.

Men: Creatinine clearance

$$(mL/min) = \frac{Weight\ (kg) \times (140 - age)}{72 \times serum\ creatinine\ (mg/dL)}$$

Women: 0.85 + the value calculated for men.

The serum creatinine should represent a steady state of renal function.

In patients with severe infections and severe renal impairment, a unit dose of 750 mg may be administered at the intervals noted above; however, patients should be carefully monitored and the serum Ciprofloxacin concentration should be measured periodically. Peak concentrations (1-2 hours after dosing) should generally range from 2 to 4 µg/mL. For patients with changing renal function or for patients with renal impairment and hepatic insufficiency, measurement of serum concentrations of Ciprofloxacin will provide additional guidance for adjusting dosage.

Intravenous: The recommended adult dosage for urinary tract infections of mild to moderate severity is 200 mg every 12 hours. For severe or complicated urinary tract infections the recommended dosage is 400 mg every 12 hours.

The recommended adult dosage for lower respiratory tract infections, skin and skin structure infections and bone and joint infections of mild to moderate severity is 400 mg every 12 hours.

The determination of dosage for any particular patient must take into consideration the severity and nature of the infection, the susceptibility of the causative organism, the integrity of the patient's host-defense mechanisms and the status of renal and hepatic function. (See related table).

Ciprofloxacin, Systemic, IV, should be administered by intravenous infusion over a period of 60 minutes.

The duration of treatment depends upon the severity of infection. Generally, Ciprofloxacin should be continued for at least 2 days after the signs and symptoms of infection have disappeared. The usual duration is 7 to 14 days. Bone and joint infections may require treatment for 4 to 6 weeks or longer.

Parenteral therapy may be changed to Ciprofloxacin, Systemic, oral tablets when the condition warrants, at the discretion of the physician.

Impaired Renal Function: The following table provides dosage guidelines for use in patients with renal impairment; however, monitoring of serum drug levels provides the most reliable basis for dosage adjustment.

RECOMMENDED STARTING AND MAINTENANCE DOSES FOR PATIENTS WITH IMPAIRED RENAL FUNCTION

Creatinine Clearance (mL/min)	Dosage
≥ 30	See usual dosage
5-29	200-400 mg q 18-24 hr

When only the serum creatinine concentration is known, the following formula may be used to estimate creatinine clearance.

Men: Creatinine clearance

$$(mL/min) = \frac{Weight\ (kg) \times (140 - age)}{72 \times serum\ creatinine\ (mg/dL)}$$

Women: 0.85 + the value calculated for men.

The serum creatinine should represent a steady state of renal function.

For patients with changing renal function or for patients with renal impairment and hepatic insufficiency, measurement of serum concentrations of Ciprofloxacin will provide additional guidance for adjusting dosage.

INTRAVENOUS ADMINISTRATION

Ciprofloxacin, Systemic, IV, should be administered by intravenous infusion over a period of 60 minutes. Slow infusion of a dilute solution into a large vein will minimize patient discomfort and reduce the risk of venous irritation.

Some Formulations Must Be Diluted Before Use: The intravenous dose should be prepared by aseptically withdrawing the appropriate volume of concentrate. This should be diluted with a suitable intravenous solution to a final concentration of 0.5-2 mg/mL. (See *"Compatibility and Stability."*) The resulting solution should be infused over a period of 60 minutes by direct infusion or through a Y-type intravenous infusion set which may already be in place. If this method or the "piggyback" method of administration is used, it is advisable to discontinue temporarily the administration of any other solutions during the infusion of Ciprofloxacin, Systemic.

Some formulations are available as a premixed solution that may be infused as described above.

COMPATIBILITY AND STABILITY

Ciprofloxacin injection 1% (10 mg/mL), when diluted with the following intravenous solution to concentrations of 0.5 to 2.0 mg/mL, is stable for up to 14 days at refrigerated or room temperature storage.

0.9% Sodium Chloride Injection, USP
5% Dextrose Injection, USP

If Ciprofloxacin, Systemic, IV, is to be given concomitantly with another drug, each drug should be given separately in accordance with the recommended dosage and route of administration for each drug.

Pharmacy Bulk Package: The pharmacy bulk package is a single-entry container of a sterile preparation for parenteral use that contains many single doses. The contents are intended for use in a pharmacy admixture program and are restricted to the preparation of admixtures for intravenous infusion. *The closure shall be penetrated only one time* with a suitable sterile transfer set or dispensing device which allows measured dispensing of the contents.

The pharmacy bulk package is to be used only in a suitable work area such as laminar flow hood or an equivalent clean air or compounding area.

Storage: Store tablets below 86°F (30°C). Store solution between 41° and 86°F (5° and 30°C); store premixed solution between 41° and 77°F (5° and 25°C).

ANIMAL PHARMACOLOGY

Ciprofloxacin and other quinolones have been shown to cause arthropathy in immature animals of most species tested (See *"Warnings"*). Damage of weight bearing joints was observed in juvenile dogs and rats. In young beagles 100 mg/kg Ciprofloxacin given daily for 4 weeks, caused degenerative articular changes of the knee joint. At 30 mg/kg the effect on the joint was minimal. In a subsequent study in beagles removal of weight bearing from the joint reduced the lesions but did not totally prevent them.

Crystalluria, sometimes associated with secondary nephropathy, occurs in laboratory animals dosed with Ciprofloxacin. This is primarily related to the reduced solubility of Ciprofloxacin under alkaline conditions, which predominate in the urine of test animals; in man, crystalluria is rare since human urine is typically acidic. In rhesus monkeys, crystalluria without nephropathy has been noted after single oral or IV doses as low as 5 mg/kg. After 6 months of intravenous dosage at 10 mg/kg/day, no nephropathological changes were noted; however, nephropathy was observed after dosing at 20 mg/kg/day for the same duration.

In dogs, Ciprofloxacin at 3 and 10 mg/kg by rapid IV injection (15 sec.) produces pronounced hypotensive effects. These effects are considered to be related to histamine release since they are partially antagonized by pyrilamine, an antihistamine. In rhesus monkeys, rapid IV injection also produces hypotension but the effect in this species is inconsistent and less pronounced.

In mice, concomitant administration of nonsteroidal anti-inflammatory drugs such as fenbufen, phenylbutazone and indomethacin with quinolones has been reported to enhance the CNS stimulatory effect of quinolones.

Ocular toxicity seen with some related drugs has not been observed in Ciprofloxacin-treated animals.

REFERENCES

1. National Committee for Clinical Laboratory Standards, *Performance Standards for Antimicrobial Disk Susceptibility Tests*—Fourth Edition. Approved Standard NCCLS Document M2-A4, Vol. 10, No. 7, NCCLS, Villanova, PA, April 1990. 2. National Committee for Clinical Laboratory Standards, *Methods for Dilution Antimicrobial Susceptibility Tests for Bacteria that Grow Aerobically*—Second Edition. Approved

DOSAGE GUIDELINES

Location of Infection	Type or Severity	Intravenous Unit Dose	Frequency	Daily Dose
Urinary Tract	Mild/Moderate	200 mg	q 12 h	400 mg
	Severe/Complicated	400 mg	q 12 h	800 mg
Lower Respiratory Tract: Skin and Skin Structure: Bone and Joint	Mild/Moderate	400 mg	q 12 h	800 mg

Standard NCCLS Document M7-A2, Vol. 10, No. 8, NCCLS, Villanova, PA, April 1990. 3. National Committee for Clinical Laboratory Standards, *Methods for Antimicrobial Susceptibility Testing of Anaerobic Bacteria*—Second Edition. Approved Standard NCCLS Document M11-A2, Vol. 10, No. 15, NCCLS, Villanova, PA, December, 1990.

HOW SUPPLIED
INJECTION: 200 MG/ML

BRAND/MANUFACTURER	NDC	SIZE	AWP
○ BRAND			
CIPRO I.V.: Miles Pharm	00026-8562-20	20 ml 10s	$144.06
	00026-8552-36	100 ml 24s	$374.55

INJECTION: 400 MG/ML

BRAND/MANUFACTURER	NDC	SIZE	AWP
○ BRAND			
CIPRO I.V.: Miles Pharm	00026-8564-64	40 ml 10s	$288.12
	00026-8554-63	200 ml 24s	$720.29

INJECTION: 1200 MG/ML

BRAND/MANUFACTURER	NDC	SIZE	AWP
○ BRAND			
CIPRO I.V.: Miles Pharm	00026-8566-65	120 ml 6s	$466.36

TABLETS: 250 MG

BRAND/MANUFACTURER	NDC	SIZE	AWP
○ BRAND			
▶ CIPRO: Miles Pharm	00026-8512-51	100s	$261.38
	00026-8512-48	100s ud	$270.76

TABLETS: 500 MG

BRAND/MANUFACTURER	NDC	SIZE	AWP
○ BRAND			
▶ CIPRO: Miles Pharm	00026-8513-51	100s	$302.48
	00026-8513-48	100s ud	$312.56

TABLETS: 750 MG

BRAND/MANUFACTURER	NDC	SIZE	AWP
○ BRAND			
▶ CIPRO: Miles Pharm	00026-8514-50	50s	$262.32
	00026-8514-48	100s ud	$533.65

Cisapride

DESCRIPTION
Cisapride Tablets contain Cisapride as the monohydrate, which is an oral gastrointestinal prokinetic agent chemically designated as (±)-cis-4-amino-5-chloro-N-[1-[3-(4-fluorophenoxy)proyl]-3-methoxy-4-piperidinyl]-2- methoxybenzamide monohydrate. Its empirical formula is $C_{23}H_{29}ClFN_3O_4 \cdot H_2O$. The molecular weight is 483.97.

Cisapride as the monohydrate is a white to slightly beige odorless powder. It is practically insoluble in water, sparingly soluble in methanol, and soluble in acetone. Each 1.04 mg of Cisapride as the monohydrate is equivalent to one mg of Cisapride.

Cisapride is available for oral use in tablets containing Cisapride as the monohydrate equivalent to 10 mg of Cisapride.

Following is its chemical structure:

CLINICAL PHARMACOLOGY
PHARMACOKINETICS
Cisapride is rapidly absorbed after oral administration; peak plasma concentrations are reached 1 to 1.5 hr after dosing. The absolute bioavailability of Cisapride is 35-40%. When gastric acidity was reduced by high dose histamine H_2 receptor blocker and sodium bicarbonate in fasting subjects, there was a decrease in the rate, and to a lesser degree the extent, of Cisapride absorption. Cisapride binds to an extent of 97.5-98% to plasma proteins, mainly to albumin. The volume of distribution of Cisapride is about 180 L, indicating extensive tissue distribution.

The plasma clearance of Cisapride is about 100 mL/min. The mean terminal half-life reported for Cisapride ranges from 6 to 12 hr; longer half-lives, up to 20 hr, have been reported following intravenous (IV) administration. Cisapride is extensively metabolized; unchanged drug accounts for less than 10% of urinary and fecal recovery following oral administration. Norcisapride, formed by N-dealkylation, is the principal metabolite in plasma, feces and urine.

There was no unusual drug accumulation due to time-dependent or non-linear changes in PK. After cessation of the repeated dosing, the elimination half-lives (8 to 10 hr) were in the same order as after single dosing. There is some evidence that the degree of accumulation of Cisapride and/or its metabolites may be somewhat higher in patients with hepatic or renal impairment and in elderly patients compared to young healthy volunteers, but the differences are not consistent and do not require dosage adjustment.

PHARMACODYNAMICS
The onset of pharmacological action in Cisapride is approximately 30 to 60 minutes after oral administration.

The mechanism of action of Cisapride is thought to be primarily enhancement of release of acetycholine at the myenteric plexus. Cisapride does not induce muscarinic or nicotinic receptor stimulation, nor does it inhibit acetycholinesterase activity. It is less potent than metoclopramide in dopamine receptor-blocking effects in rats. It does not increase or decrease basal or pentagastrin-induced gastric acid secretion.

In vitro studies have shown that Cisapride is serotonin-4 (5-HT$_4$) receptor agonist. This agonistic action may result in increased gastrointestinal motility and cardiac rate.

Esophagus: Single doses of Cisapride (4 to 10 mg IV) increased the lower esophageal sphincter pressure (LESP) and lower esophageal peristalsis compared to placebo and/or metoclopramide. In patients with gastroesophageal reflux disease (GERD) and a LESP of < 10 mm Hg Cisapride dose-dependently increased the strength of esophageal peristalsis and more than doubled LESP, raising it to normal values. The increase in LESP was partially reversed by atropine, suggesting that the effect is partly, but not exclusively, cholinergically-mediated. Twenty mg oral Cisapride given once to healthy volunteers similarly increased LESP, starting 45 minutes after dosing, with a peak response at 75 minutes. The full duration of the effect was not monitored, and doses smaller than 20 mg were ineffective. Ten mg oral Cisapride, administered 3 times daily for several days to patients with GERD, resulted in a significant increase in LESP, and an increased esophageal acid clearance.

Stomach: Cisapride (single 10 mg doses IV or oral or 10 mg given orally 3 times daily up to six weeks) significantly accelerated gastric emptying of both liquids and solids. Acceleration of gastric emptying, measured over a four hour period following a radio-labeled test meal given at lunch time, was greatest when 10 mg Cisapride was given both in the morning and again before the test meal, intermediate when 20 mg was given as a single administration in the morning and least when only 10 mg was given on the morning of the test meal. The increases in gastric emptying were proportional to the plasma levels of Cisapride measured in these subjects over the same 4 hours that the gastric emptying test was conducted.

CLINICAL TRIALS
Clinical trials have shown that Cisapride can reduce the symptoms of nocturnal heartburn associated with gastroesophageal reflux disease. Two placebo-controlled studies, one using a dose of 10 mg QID, the other both 10 and 20 mg QID, showed effects on nighttime heartburn, although the 10 mg dose in the second study was only marginally effective. There were no consistent effects on daytime heartburn, symptoms of regurgitation, or histopathology of the esophagus. Use of antacids was only infrequently affected and slightly decreased. In a third controlled trial of similar design to the others, neither 10 mg nor 20 mg taken 4 times was superior to placebo.

These clinical trials did not show a significant effect on LESP, perhaps because the majority of these patients had normal LESP's at the beginning and end of the study period.

In a clinical trial comparing 10 mg Cisapride to placebo, pH probe evaluation, in a relatively small number of patients, did not reveal a significant difference in pH.

INDICATIONS
Cisapride is indicated for the symptomatic treatment of patients with nocturnal heartburn due to gastroesophageal reflux disease.

UNLABELED USES
Cisapride is used alone or as an adjunct in gatroparesis.

CONTRAINDICATIONS
Cisapride should not be used in patients in whom an increase in gastrointestinal motility could be harmful, e.g., in the presence of gastrointestinal hemorrhage, mechanical obstruction, or perforation. Cisapride is contraindicated in patients with known sensitivity or intolerance to the drug.

PRECAUTIONS
Information for Patients: Although Cisapride does not affect psycomotor function nor does it induce sedation or drowsiness when used alone, patients should be advised that the sedative effects of benzodiazepines and of alcohol may be accelerated by Cisapride.

Drug Interactions: Concurrent administration of anticho-linergic compounds would be expected to compromise the beneficial effects of Cisapride.

The acceleration of gastric emptying by Cisapride could effect the rate of absorption of other drugs. Patients receiving narrow therapeutic ratio drugs or other drugs that require careful titration should be followed closely; if plasma levels are being monitored, they should be reassessed.

In patients receiving oral anticoagulants, the coagulation times were increased in some cases. It is advisable to check coagulation time within the first few days after the start and discontinuation of Cisapride therapy, with an appropriate adjustment of the anticoagulant dose, if necessary.

◆ RATED THERAPEUTICALLY EQUIVALENT; ◇ THERAPEUTIC EQUIVALENCE UNCONFIRMED; ○ UNRATED

Cimetidine coadministration leads to an increased peak plasma concentration and AUC of Cisapride, there is no effect on Cisapride absorption when it is coadministered with ranitidine. The gastrointestinal absorption of cimetidine and ranitidine is accelerated when they are coadministered with Cisapride.

Carcinogenesis, Mutagenesis, Impairment of Fertility: In a twenty-five month oral carcinogenicity study in rats, Cisapride at daily doses up to 80 mg/kg was not tumorigenic. For a 50 kg person of average height (1.46 m^2 body surface area), this dose represents 50 times the maximum recommended human dose (1.6 mg/kg/day) on a mg/kg basis and 7 times the maximum recommended human dose (54.4 mg/m^2) on a body surface area basis. In a nineteen-month oral carcinogenicity study in mice, Cisapride at daily doses up to 80 mg/kg was not tumorigenic. This dose represents 50 times the maximum recommended human dose on a mg/kg basis and about 4 times the maximum recommended human dose on a body surface area basis.

Cisapride was not mutagenic in the *in vitro* Ames test, human lymphocyte chromosomal aberration test, mouse lymphoma cell forward mutation test, and rat hepatocyte UDS test and *in vitro* rat micronucleus test, male and female mouse dominant lethal mutations tests, and sex linked recessive lethal test in male *Drosophila melanogaster.*

Fertility and reproductive performance studies were conducted in male and female rats. Cisapride was found to have no effect on fertility and reproductive performance of male rats at oral doses up to 160 mg/kg/day (100 times the maximum recommended human dose on a mg/kg basis and 14 times the maximum recommended human dose on a mg/m^2 basis.) In the female rats, Cisapride at oral doses of 40 mg/kg/day and higher prolonged the breeding interval required for impregnation. Similar effects were also observed at maturity in the female offspring (F_1) of the female rats (F_0) treated with oral doses of Cisapride at 10 mg/kg/day or higher. Cisapride at an oral dose of 160 mg/kg/day also exerted contragestational/pregnancy disrupting effects in female rats (F_0).

Pregnancy: Teratogenic Effects: Pregnancy Category C: Oral teratology studies have been conducted in rats (doses up to 160 mg/kg/day) and rabbits (doses up to 40 mg/kg/day). There was no evidence of a teratogenic potential of Cisapride in rats or rabbits. Cisapride was embryotoxic and fetotoxic in rats at a dose of 160 mg/kg/day (100 times the maximum recommended human dose on a mg/kg basis and 14 times the maximum recommended human dose on a mg/m^2 basis) and in rabbits at a dose of 20 mg/kg/day (approximately 12 times the maximum recommended human dose on a mg/kg basis) or higher. It also produced reduced birth weights of pups in rats at 40 and 160 mg/kg/day and adversely affected the pup survival. There are no adequate and well-controlled studies in pregnant women. Cisapride should be used during pregnancy only if the potential benefit justifies the potential risk to the fetus.

Nursing Mothers: Cisapride is excreted in human milk at concentrations approximately one twentieth of those observed in plasma. Caution should be exercised when Cisapride is administered to a nursing woman.

Pediatric Use: Safety and effectiveness in children have not been established.

Geriatric Use: Steady-state plasma levels are generally higher in older than in younger patients, due to a moderate prolongation of the elimination half-life. Therapeutic doses, however, are similar to those used in younger adults. The rate of adverse experiences in patients greater that 65 years of age was similar to that in younger adults.

ADVERSE REACTIONS

In the U.S. clinical trial population of 1728 patients (comprising 506 with gastroesophageal reflux disorders, and the remainder with other motility disorders) the following adverse experiences were reported in more than 1% of patients treated with Cisapride and at least as often on Cisapride as on placebo. The percent of patients who discontinued treatment is displayed in parenthesis.

System/Adverse Event	Cisapride N = 1042	Placebo N = 686
Central & Peripheral		
Nervous Systems		
Headache	19.3% (1.1%)	17.1% (0.4%)
Gastrointestinal		
Diarrhea	14.2 (0.7)	10.3 (0.1)
Abdominal pain	10.2 (1.2)	7.7 (0.9)
Nausea	7.6 (1.0)	7.6 (0.3)
Constipation	6.7 (0.1)	3.4 (0.0)
Flatulence	3.5 (0.4)	3.1 (0.4)
Dyspepsia	2.7 (0.1)	1.0 (0.0)
Respiratory System		
Rhinitis	7.3 (0.1)	5.7 (0.1)
Sinusitis	3.6 (0.0)	3.5 (0.0)
Coughing	1.5 (0.2)	1.2 (0.0)
Resistance Mechanism		
Viral infection	3.6 (0.2)	3.2 (0.0)
Upper respiratory tract infection	3.1 (0.0)	2.8 (0.0)
Body as a Whole		
Pain	3.4 (0.0)	2.3 (0.0)
Fever	2.2 (0.1)	1.5 (0.0)
Urinary System		
Urinary tract infection	2.4 (0.0)	1.9 (0.0)

System/Adverse Event	Cisapride N = 1042	Placebo N = 686
Micturition frequency	1.2 (0.1)	0.6 (0.0)
Psychiatric		
Insomnia	1.9 (0.3)	1.3 (0.4)
Anxiety	1.4 (0.1)	1.0 (0.1)
Nervousness	1.4 (0.2)	0.7 (0.0)
Skin & Appendages		
Rash	1.6 (0.0)	1.6 (0.3)
Pruritus	1.2 (0.1)	1.0 (0.0)
Musculoskeletal System		
Arthralgia	1.4 (0.1)	1.2 (0.0)
Vision		
Abnormal vision	1.4 (0.2)	0.3 (0.0)
Reproductive Female		
Vaginitis	1.2 (0.0)	0.9 (0.0)

The following adverse events also reported in more than 1% of Cisapride patients were more frequently reported on placebo: dizziness, vomiting, pharyngitis, chest pain, fatigue, back pain, depression, dehydration, and myalgia. Diarrhea, abdominal pain, constipation, flatulence, and rhinitis all occurred more frequently in patients using 20 mg of Cisapride than in patients using 10 mg.

Additional adverse experiences reported to occur in 1% or less of patients in the U.S. clinical studies are: dry mouth, somnolence, palpitation, migraine, tremor, and edema.

In other U.S. and international trials and in foreign marketing experience, there have been rare reports of seizures and extrapyramidal effects, tachycardia, elevated liver enzymes, hepatitis, thrombocytopenia, leukopenia, aplastic anemia, pancytopenia and granulocytopenia. The relationship of Cisapride to the event was not clear in these cases. There have been rare cases of sinus tachycardia reported. Rechallenge precipitated relapse in some of those patients.

OVERDOSAGE

Reports of overdosage with Cisapride include an adult who took 540 mg and for 2 hours experienced retching, borborymi, flatulence, stool frequency and urinary frequency. Treatment should include gastric lavage and/or activated charcoal, close observation and general supportive measures.

Single oral doses of Cisapride at 4000 mg/kg, 160 mg/kg, 1280 mg/kg and 640 mg/kg were lethal in adult rats, neonatal rats, mice and dogs, respectively. Symptoms of acute toxicity were ptosis, tremors, convulsions, dyspnea, loss of righting reflex, catalepsy, catatonia, hypotonia and diarrhea.

DOSAGE AND ADMINISTRATION

Adults: Initiate therapy with 10 mg of Cisapride 4 times daily at least 15 minutes before meals and at bedtime. In some patients the dosage will need to be increased to 20 mg, given as above, to obtain a satisfactory result.

In elderly patients, steady-state plasma levels are generally higher due to a moderate prolongation of the elimination half-life. Therapeutic doses however, are similar to those used in younger adults.

Store at controlled room temperature, 15°-30°C (59°-86°F). Protect from moisture. The 20 mg tablets should also be protected from light.

HOW SUPPLIED
TABLETS: 10 MG

BRAND/MANUFACTURER	NDC	SIZE	AWP
○ BRAND			
➤ PROPULSID: Janssen	50458-0430-10	100s	$60.00
	50458-0430-01	100s ud	$66.00

TABLETS: 20 MG

BRAND/MANUFACTURER	NDC	SIZE	AWP
○ BRAND			
➤ PROPULSID: Janssen	50458-0440-10	100s	$116.40

Cisplatin

WARNING

CISPLATIN SHOULD BE ADMINISTERED UNDER THE SUPERVISION OF A QUALIFIED PHYSICIAN EXPERIENCED IN THE USE OF CANCER CHEMOTHERAPEUTIC AGENTS. APPROPRIATE MANAGEMENT OF THERAPY AND COMPLICATIONS IS POSSIBLE ONLY WHEN ADEQUATE DIAGNOSTIC AND TREATMENT FACILITIES ARE READILY AVAILABLE.

CUMULATIVE RENAL TOXICITY ASSOCIATED WITH CISPLATIN IS SEVERE. OTHER MAJOR DOSE-RELATED TOXICITIES ARE MYELOSUPPRESSION, NAUSEA, AND VOMITING.

OTOTOXICITY, WHICH MAY BE MORE PRONOUNCED IN CHILDREN, AND IS MANIFESTED BY TINNITUS, AND/OR LOSS OF HIGH FREQUENCY HEARING AND OCCASIONALLY DEAFNESS, IS SIGNIFICANT.

➤ SHOWN IN PRODUCT IDENTIFICATION GUIDE

ANAPHYLACTIC-LIKE REACTIONS TO CISPLATIN HAVE BEEN REPORTED. FACIAL EDEMA, BRONCHOCONSTRICTION, TACHYCARDIA, AND HYPOTENSION MAY OCCUR WITHIN MINUTES OF CISPLATIN ADMINISTRATION. EPINEPHRINE, CORTICOSTEROIDS, AND ANTIHISTAMINES HAVE BEEN EFFECTIVELY EMPLOYED TO ALLEVIATE SYMPTOMS (SEE "WARNINGS" AND "ADVERSE REACTIONS" SECTIONS).

DESCRIPTION

Cisplatin (cis-diamminedichloroplatinum) is a heavy metal complex containing a central atom of platinum surrounded by two chloride atoms and two ammonia molecules in the cis position. It is a white lyophilized powder with the molecular formula Pt $Cl_2H_6N_2$, and a molecular weight of 300.1. It is soluble in water or saline at 1 mg/mL and in dimethylformamide at 24 mg/mL. It has a melting point of 207°C.

Cisplatin Aqueous is a sterile aqueous solution, each mL containing 1 mg Cisplatin and 9 mg sodium chloride. HCl and/or sodium hydroxide added to adjust pH..

Each vial of Cisplatin contains: Cisplatin 10 or 50 mg

Each vial of Cisplatin Aqueous contains: Cisplatin 10, 50, or 100 mg

Following is its chemical structure:

$$Cl \quad \overset{Pt^{2+}}{\underset{}{}} \quad NH_3$$
$$Cl \qquad\qquad NH_3$$

CLINICAL PHARMACOLOGY

Plasma concentrations of the parent compound, Cisplatin, decay monoexponentially with a half-life of about 20 to 30 minutes following bolus administrations of 50 or 100 mg/m^2 doses. Monoexponential decay and plasma half-lives of about 0.5 hour are also seen following two hour or seven hour infusions of 100 mg/m^2. After the latter, the total-body clearances and volumes of distribution at steady-state for Cisplatin are about 15 to 16 L/h/m^2 and 11 to 12 L/m^2.

Due to its unique chemical structure, the chlorine atoms of Cisplatin are more subject to chemical displacement reactions by nucleophiles, such as water or sulfhydryl groups, than to enzyme-catalyzed metabolism. At physiological pH in the presence of 0.1M NaCl, the predominant molecular species are Cisplatin and monohydroxymonochloro *cis*-diammine platinum (II) in nearly equal concentrations. The latter, combined with the possible direct displacement of the chlorine atoms by sulfhydryl groups of amino acids or proteins, accounts for the instability of Cisplatin in biological matrices. The ratios of Cisplatin to total free (ultrafilterable) platinum in the plasma vary considerably between patients and range from 0.5 to 1.1 after a dose of 100 mg/m^2.

Cisplatin does not undergo the instantaneous and reversible binding to plasma proteins that is characteristic of normal drug-protein binding. However, the platinum from Cisplatin, but not Cisplatin itself, becomes bound to several plasma proteins including albumin, transferrin, and gamma globulin. Three hours after a bolus injection and two hours after the end of a three-hour infusion, 90% of the plasma platinum is protein bound. The complexes between albumin and the platinum from Cisplatin do not dissociate to a significant extent are slowly eliminated with a minimum half-life of five days or more.

Following Cisplatin doses of 20 to 120 mg/m^2, the concentrations of platinum are highest in liver, prostate, and kidney, somewhat lower in bladder, muscle, testicle, pancreas, and spleen and lowest in bowel, adrenal, heart, lung, cerebrum, and cerebellum. Platinum is present in tissues for as long as 180 days after the last administration. With the exception of intracerebral tumors, platinum concentrations in tumors are generally somewhat lower than the concentrations in the organ where the tumor is located. Different metastatic sites in the same patient may have different platinum concentrations. Hepatic metastases have the highest platinum concentrations, but these are similar to the platinum concentrations in normal liver. Maximum red blood cell concentrations of platinum are reached within 90 to 150 minutes after a 100 mg/m^2 dose of Cisplatin and decline in a biphasic manner with a terminal half-life to 36 to 47 days.

Over a dose range of 40 to 140 mg Cisplatin/m^2 given as a bolus injection or as infusions varying in length from 1 hour to 24 hours, from 10% to about 40% of the administered platinum is excreted in the urine in 24 hours. Over five days following administration of 40 to 100 mg/m^2 doses given as rapid, 2 to 3 hours, or 6 to 8 hour infusions, a mean of 35% to 51% of the dosed platinum is excreted in the urine. Similar mean urinary recoveries of platinum of about 14% to 30% of the dose are found following five daily administrations of 20, 30, or 40 mg/m^2 day. Only a small percentage of the administered platinum is excreted beyond 24 hours post infusion and most of the platinum excreted in the urine in 24 hours is excreted within the first few hours. Platinum-containing species excreted in the urine are the same as those found following the incubation of Cisplatin with urine from healthy subjects, except that the proportions are different.

The parent compound, Cisplatin, is excreted in the urine and accounts for 13% to 17% of the dose excreted within one hour after administration of 50 mg/m^2. The mean renal clearance of Cisplatin exceeds creatinine clearance and is 62 and 50 mL/min/m^2 following administration of 100 mg/m^2 as 2 hour or 6 to 7 hour infusions, respectively.

The renal clearance of free (ultrafilterable) platinum also exceeds the glomerular filtration rate indicating that Cisplatin or other platinum-containing molecules are actively secreted by the kidneys. The renal clearance of free platinum is nonlinear and variable and is dependent on dose, urine flow rate, and individual variability in the extent of active secretion and possible tubular reabsorption.

There is a potential for accumulation of ultrafilterable platinum plasma concentrations whenever Cisplatin is administered on a daily basis but not when dosed on an intermittent basis.

No significant relationships exist between the renal clearance of either free platinium or Cisplatin and creatinine clearance.

Although small amounts of platinum are present in the bile and large intestine after administration of Cisplatin, the fecal excretion of platinum appears to be insignificant.

INDICATIONS

Cisplatin is indicated as therapy to be employed as follows:

Metastatic Testicular Tumors: In established combination therapy with other approved chemotherapeutic agents in patients with metastatic testicular tumors who have already received appropriate surgical and/or radiotherapeutic procedures.

Metastatic Ovarian Tumors: In established combination therapy with other approved chemotherapeutic agents in patients with metastatic ovarian tumors who have already received appropriate surgical and/or radiotherapeutic procedures. An established combination consists of Cisplatin and cyclophosphamide. Cisplatin, as a single agent, is indicated as secondary therapy in patients with metastatic ovarian tumors refractory to standard chemotherapy who have not previously received Cisplatin therapy.

Advanced Bladder Cancer: Cisplatin is indicated as a single agent for patients with transitional cell bladder cancer which is no longer amenable to local treatments such as surgery and/or radiotherapy.

UNLABELED USES

Cisplatin is used alone or as an adjunct in the treatment of central nervous system cancer, including gliomas, neuroblastomas, and ependymomas. It is also used in metastatic breast cancer, cervical cancer, esophageal cancer, gastric cancer, head and neck squamous cell carcinomas, hypercalcemia of malignancy, pancreatic cancer, and small cell lung cancer.

CONTRAINDICATIONS

Cisplatin is contraindicated in patients with preexisting renal impairment. Cisplatin should not be employed in myelosuppressed patients, or patients with hearing impairment.

Cisplatin is contraindicated in patients with a history of allergic reactions to Cisplatin or other platinum-containing compounds.

WARNINGS

Cisplatin produces cumulative nephrotoxicity which is potentiated by aminoglycoside antibiotics. The serum creatinine, BUN, creatinine clearance, and magnesium, sodium, potassium and calcium levels should be measured prior to initiating therapy, and prior to each subsequent course. At the recommended dosage, Cisplatin should not be given more frequently than once every 3 to 4 weeks (see "Adverse Reactions").

There are reports of severe neuropathies in patients in whom regimens are employed using higher doses of Cisplatin or greater dose frequencies than those recommended. These neuropathies may be irreversible and are seen as paresthesias in a stocking-glove distribution, areflexia, and loss of proprioception and vibratory sensation.

Anaphylactic-like reactions to Cisplatin have been reported. These reactions have occurred within minutes of administration to patients with prior exposure to Cisplatin, and have been alleviated by administration of epinephrine, corticosteroids, and antihistamines.

Since ototoxicity of Cisplatin is cumulative, audiometric testing should be performed prior to initiating therapy and prior to each subsequent dose of drug (see "Adverse Reactions").

Cisplatin can cause fetal harm when administered to a pregnant woman. Cisplatin is mutagenic in bacteria and produces chromosome aberrations in animal cells in tissue culture. In mice Cisplatin is teratogenic and embryotoxic. If this drug is used during pregnancy or if the patient becomes pregnant while taking this drug, the patient should be apprised of the potential hazard to the fetus. Patients should be advised to avoid becoming pregnant.

The carcinogenic effect of Cisplatin was studied in BD IX rats. Cisplatin was administered i.p. to 50 BD IX rats for 3 weeks, 3 X 1 mg/kg body weight per week. Four hundred and fifty-five days after the first application, 33 animals died, 13 of them related to malignancies: 12 leukemias and 1 renal fibrosarcoma.

The development of acute leukemia coincident with the use of Cisplatin has rarely been reported in humans. In these reports, Cisplatin was generally given in combination with other leukemogenic agents.

PRECAUTIONS

Peripheral blood counts should be monitored weekly. Liver function should be monitored periodically. Neurologic examination should also be performed regularly (see "Adverse Reactions").

Drug Interactions: Plasma levels of anticonvulsant agents may become subtherapeutic during cisplatin therapy.

Carcinogenesis, Mutagenesis, Impairment of Fertility: see "Warnings" section.

Pregnancy: Category D, see "Warnings" section.

◆ RATED THERAPEUTICALLY EQUIVALENT; ◇ THERAPEUTIC EQUIVALENCE UNCONFIRMED; ○ UNRATED

ADVERSE REACTIONS

Nephrotoxicity: Dose-related and cumulative renal insufficiency is the major dose-limiting toxicity of Cisplatin for injection. Renal toxicity has been noted in 28% to 36% of patients treated with a single dose of 50 mg/m². It is first noted during the second week after a dose and is manifested by elevations in BUN and creatinine, serum uric acid and/or a decrease in creatinine clearance.

Renal toxicity becomes more prolonged and severe with repeated courses of the drug. Renal function must return to normal before another dose of Cisplatin can be given.

Impairment of renal function has been associated with renal tubular damage. The administration of Cisplatin using a 6- to 8-hour infusion with intravenous hydration, and mannitol has been used to reduce nephrotoxicity. However, renal toxicity still can occur after utilization of these procedures.

Ototoxicity: Ototoxicity has been observed in up to 31% of patients treated with a single dose of Cisplatin 50 mg/m², and is manifested by tinnitus and/or hearing loss in the high frequency range (4,000 to 8,000 Hz). Decreased ability to hear normal conversational tones may occur occasionally. Deafness after the initial dose of Cisplatin has been reported rarely. Ototoxic effects may be more severe in children receiving Cisplatin. Hearing loss can be unilateral or bilateral and tends to become more frequent and severe with repeated doses. Ototoxicity may be enhanced with prior or simultaneous cranial irradiation. It is unclear whether Cisplatin-induced ototoxicity is reversible. Ototoxic effects may be related to the peak plasma concentration of Cisplatin. Careful monitoring of audiometry should be performed prior to initiation of therapy and prior to subsequent doses of Cisplatin.

Vestibular toxicity has also been reported.

Ototoxicity may become more severe in patients being treated with other drugs with nephrotoxic potential.

Hematologic: Myelosuppression occurs in 25% to 30% of patients treated with Cisplatin. The nadirs in circulating platelets and leukocytes occur between days 18 to 23 (range 7.5 to 45) with most patients recovering by day 39 (range 13 to 62). Leukopenia and thrombocytopenia are more pronounced at higher doses (> 50 mg/m²). Anemia (decrease of 2 g hemoglobin/100 mL) occurs at approximately the same frequency and with the same timing as leukopenia and thrombocytopenia.

In addition to anemia secondary to myelosuppression, a Coombs' positive hemolytic anemia has been reported. In the presence of cisplatin hemolytic anemia, a further course of treatment may be accompanied by increased hemolysis and this risk should be weighed by the treating physician.

The development of acute leukemia coincident with the use of Cisplatin has rarely been reported in humans. In these reports, Cisplatin was generally given in combination with other leukemogenic agents.

Gastrointestinal: Marked nausea and vomiting occur in almost all patients treated with Cisplatin and are occasionally so severe that the drug must be discontinued. Nausea and vomiting usually begin within 1 to 4 hours after treatment and last up to 24 hours. Various degrees of vomiting, nausea and/or anorexia may persist for up to 1 week after treatment.

Delayed nausea and vomiting (begins or persists 24 hours or more after chemotherapy) has occurred in patients attaining complete emetic control on the day of Cisplatin therapy. Diarrhea has also been reported.

OTHER TOXICITIES

Vascular toxicities coincident with the use of Cisplatin in combination with other antineoplastic agents have been reported rarely. The events are clinically heterogeneous and may include myocardial infarction, cerebrovascular accident, thrombotic microangiopathy (HUS), or cerebral arteritis. Various mechanisms have been proposed for these vascular complications. There are also reports of Raynaud's phenomenon occurring in patients treated with the combination of bleomycin, vinblastine with or without Cisplatin. It has been suggested that hypomagnesemia developing coincident with the use of Cisplatin may be an added, although not essential, factor associated with this event. However, it is currently unknown if the cause of Raynaud's phenomenon in these cases is the disease, underlying vascular compromise, bleomycin, vinblastine, hypomagnesemia, or a combination of any of these factors.

Serum Electrolyte Disturbances: Hypomagnesemia, hypocalcemia, hyponatremia, hypokalemia and hypophosphatemia have been reported to occur in patients treated with Cisplatin and are probably related to renal tubular damage. Tetany has occasionally been reported in those patients with hypocalcemia and hypomagnesemia. Generally, normal serum electrolyte levels are restored by administering supplemental electrolytes and discontinuing Cisplatin. Inappropriate antidiuretic hormone syndrome has also been reported.

Hyperuricemia: Hyperuricemia has been reported to occur at approximately the same frequency as the increases in BUN and serum creatinine.

It is more pronounced after doses greater than 50 mg/m², and peak levels of uric acid generally occur between 3 to 5 days after the dose. Allopurinol therapy for hyperuricemia effectively reduces uric acid levels.

Neurotoxicity: (see "Warnings" section): Neurotoxicity, usually characterized by peripheral neuropathies, has been reported. The neuropathies usually occur after prolonged therapy (4 to 7 months); however, neurologic symptoms have been reported to occur after a single dose. Although symptoms and signs of Cisplatin neuropathy usually develop during treatment, symptoms of neuropathy may begin 3 to 8 weeks after the last dose of Cisplatin, although this is rare. Cisplatin therapy should be discontinued when the symptoms are first observed. The neuropathy, however, may progress further even after stopping treatment. Preliminary evidence suggests peripheral neuropathy may be irreversible in some patients.

Lhermitte's sign, dorsal column myelopathy, and autonomic neuropathy have also been reported.

Loss of taste and seizures have also been reported.

Muscle cramps, defined as localized, painful, involuntary skeletal muscle contractions of sudden onset and short duration, have been reported and were usually associated in patients receiving a relatively high cumulative dose of Cisplatin and with a relatively advanced symptomatic stage of peripheral neuropathy.

Ocular Toxicity: Optic neuritis, papilledema, and cerebral blindness have been reported infrequently in patients receiving standard recommended doses of Cisplatin. Improvement and/or total recovery usually occurs after discontinuing Cisplatin. Steroids with or without mannitol have been used; however, efficacy has not been established.

Blurred vision and altered color perception have been reported after the use of regimens with higher doses of Cisplatin or greater dose frequencies than those recommended in the package insert. The altered color perception manifests as a loss of color discrimination, particularly in the blue-yellow axis. The only finding on funduscopic exam is irregular retinal pigmentation of the macular area.

Anaphylactic-like Reactions: Anaphylactic-like reactions have been occasionally reported in patients previously exposed to Cisplatin. The reactions consist of facial edema, wheezing, tachycardia, and hypotension within a few minutes of drug administration. Reactions may be controlled by intravenous epinephrine with corticosteroids and/or antihistamines as indicated. Patients receiving Cisplatin should be observed carefully for possible anaphylactic-like reactions and supportive equipment and medication should be available to treat such a complication.

Hepatotoxicity: Transient elevations of liver enzymes, especially SGOT, as well as bilirubin, have been reported to be associated with Cisplatin administration at the recommended doses.

Other Events: Other toxicities reported to occur infrequently are cardiac abnormalities, hiccups, elevated serum amylase, and rash. Alopecia has also been reported.

Local soft tissue toxicity has rarely been reported following extravasation of Cisplatin. Severity of the local tissue toxicity appears to be related to the concentration of the Cisplatin solution. Infusion of solutions with a Cisplatin concentration greater than 0.5 mg/mL may result in tissue cellulitis, fibrosis, and necrosis.

OVERDOSAGE

Caution should be exercised to prevent inadvertent overdosage with Cisplatin.

Acute overdosage with this drug may result in kidney failure, liver failure, deafness, ocular toxicity (including detachment of the retina), significant myelosuppression, intractable nausea and vomiting and/or neuritis. In addition, death can occur following overdosage.

No proven antidotes have been established for Cisplatin overdosage. Hemodialysis, even when initiated four hours after the overdosage, appears to have little effect on removing platinum from the body because of Cisplatin's rapid and high degree of protein binding. Management of overdosage should include general supportive measures to sustain the patient through any period of toxicity that may occur.

DOSAGE AND ADMINISTRATION

Note: **Needles or intravenous sets containing aluminum parts that may come in contact with Cisplatin should not be used for preparation or administration. Aluminum reacts with Cisplatin, causing precipitate formation and a loss of potency.**

Metastatic Testicular Tumors: The usual Cisplatin dose for the treatment of testicular cancer in combination with other approved chemotherapeutic agents is 20 mg/m² IV daily for 5 days.

Metastatic Ovarian Tumors: The usual Cisplatin dose for the treatment of metastatic ovarian tumors in combination with cyclophosphamide or other approved chemotherapeutic agents is 75-100 mg/m² IV once every 4 weeks, (Day 1).[1,2]

The dose of cyclophosphamide when used in combination with Cisplatin is 600 mg/m² IV once every 4 weeks, (Day 1).[1,2]

For directions for the administration of cyclophosphamide refer to the cyclophosphamide package insert.

In combination therapy, Cisplatin and cyclophosphamide are administered sequentially.

As a single agent, Cisplatin should be administered at a dose of 100 mg/m² IV once every 4 weeks.

Advanced Bladder Cancer: Cisplatin should be administered as a single agent at a dose of 50 to 70 mg/m² IV once every 3 to 4 weeks depending on the extent of prior exposure to radiation therapy and/or prior chemotherapy. For heavily pretreated patients an initial dose of 50 mg/m² repeated every 4 weeks is recommended.

Pretreatment hydration with 1 to 2 liters of fluid infused for 8 to 12 hours prior to a Cisplatin dose is recommended. The drug is then diluted in 2 liters of 5% Dextrose in ½ or ⅓ normal saline containing 37.5 g of mannitol, and infused over a 6- to 8-hour period. If diluted solution is not to be used within 6 hours, protect solution from light. Do not dilute Cisplatin in just 5% Dextrose injection. Adequate hydration and urinary output must be maintained during the following 24 hours.

A repeat course of Cisplatin should not be given until the serum creatinine is below 1.5 mg/100 mL, and/or the BUN is below 25 mg/100 mL. A repeat course should not be given until circulating blood elements are at an acceptable level (platelets $\geq$ 100,000/mm^3, WBC $\geq$ 4,000/mm^3). Subsequent doses of Cisplatin should not be given until an audiometric analysis indicates that auditory acuity is within normal limits.

As with other potentially toxic compounds, caution should be exercised in handling the powder and preparing the solution of Cisplatin and in handling the aqueous solution. Skin reactions associated with accidental exposure to Cisplatin may occur. The use of gloves is recommended. If Cisplatin powder or solution contacts the skin or mucosae, immediately wash the skin or mucosae thoroughly with soap and water.

PREPARATION OF INTRAVENOUS SOLUTIONS

The 10 and 50 mg vials should be reconstituted with 10 mL or 50 mL of sterile water for injection, USP, respectively. Each mL of the resulting solution will contain 1 mg of Cisplatin. Reconstitution as recommended results in a clear, colorless solution.

The reconstituted solution and the aqueous solution should be used intravenously only and should be administered by IV infusion over a 6- to 8-hour period. (See "Dosage and Administration".)

STABILITY

Unopened vials of dry powder are stable for the lot life indicated on the package when stored at room temperature (27°C).

The reconstituted solution is stable for 20 hours at room temperature (27°C). Solution removed from the amber vial should be protected from light if it is not to be used within 6 hours.

Important note: Once reconstituted, the solution should be kept at room temperature (27°C). If the reconstituted solution is refrigerated, a precipitate will form.

STABILITY

Cisplatin Aqueous is a sterile, multidose vial without preservatives. Store at 15°C-25°C. Do not refrigerate. Protect unopened container from light.

The Cisplatin remaining in the amber vial following initial entry is stable for 28 days protected from light or for seven days under fluorescent room light.

Procedures for proper handling and disposal: of anticancer drugs should be considered. Several guidelines on this subject have been published.[3-9] There is no general agreement that all of the procedures recommended in the guidelines are necessary or appropriate.

REFERENCES

1. Alberts DS, et al: Improved Therapeutic Index of Carboplatin Plus Cyclophosphamide versus Cisplatin Plus Cyclophosphamide: Final Report by the Southwest Oncology Group of a Phase III Randomized Trial in Stages III and IV Ovarian Cancer. *J Clin Oncol.* 1992; 10:706-717. 2. Swenerton K, et al: Cisplatin-Cyclophosphamide versus Carboplatin-Cyclophosphamide in Advanced Ovarian Cancer: A Randomized Phase III Study of the National Cancer Institute of Canada Clinical Trials Group. *J Clin Oncol.* 1992; 10:718-726. 3. Recommendations for the Safe Handling of Parenteral Antineoplastic Drugs. NIH Publication No. 83-2621. For sale by the Superintendent of Documents. US Government Printing Office, Washington, D.C. 20402. 4. AMA Council Report. Guidelines for Handling Parenteral Antineoplastics. *JAMA.* 1985; 253(II):1590-1592. 5. National Study Commission on Cytotoxic Exposure—Recommendations for Handling Cytotoxic Agents. Available from Louis P. Jeffrey, ScD, Chairman, National Study Commission on Cytotoxic Exposure, Massachusetts College of Pharmacy and Allied Health Sciences, 179 Longwood Avenue, Boston, Massachusetts 02115. 6. Clinical Oncological Society of Australia. Guidelines and Recommendations for Safe Handling of Antineoplastic Agents. *Med J Australia.* 1983;1:426-428. 7. Jones RB, et al: Safe Handling of Chemotherapeutic Agents: A Report from the Mount Sinai Medical Center. *CA—A Cancer Journal for Clinicians.* 1983; (Sept/Oct);258-263. 8. American Society of Hospital Pharmacists Technical Assistance Bulletin on Handling Cytotoxic and Hazardous Drugs. *Am J Hosp Pharm.* 1990;47: 1033-1049. 9. OSHA Work-Practice Guidelines for Personnel Dealing with Cytotoxic (Antineoplastic) Drugs. *Am J Hosp Pharm.* 1986;43:1193-1204.

J CODES

50 mg IV—J9062
Per 10 mg IV—J9060

HOW SUPPLIED
INJECTION: 50 MG

BRAND/MANUFACTURER	NDC	SIZE	AWP
○ BRAND			
PLATINOL-AQ: Bristol-Myer Onc/Hiv	00015-3220-22	50 ml	$162.75

INJECTION: 100 MG

BRAND/MANUFACTURER	NDC	SIZE	AWP
○ BRAND			
PLATINOL-AQ: Bristol-Myer Onc/Hiv	00015-3221-22	100 ml	$325.48

POWDER FOR INJECTION: 10 MG

BRAND/MANUFACTURER	NDC	SIZE	AWP
○ BRAND			
PLATINOL: Bristol-Myer Onc/Hiv	00015-3070-20	1s	$32.85

POWDER FOR INJECTION: 50 MG

BRAND/MANUFACTURER	NDC	SIZE	AWP
○ BRAND			
PLATINOL: Bristol-Myer Onc/Hiv	00015-3072-20	1s	$153.54

Citanest HCl *SEE* PRILOCAINE HYDROCHLORIDE AND PRILOCAINE WITH EPINEPHRINE

Citric Acid and Potassium Bicarbonate

DESCRIPTION

An oral potassium supplement. Each effervescent tablet in solution provides 25 mEq of Potassium as supplied by 2.5 g Potassium Bicarbonate, with 2 g Citric Acid.

CLINICAL PHARMACOLOGY

Potassium ion is the principal intracellular cation of most body tissues. Potassium ions participate in many essential physiological processes, such as the maintenance of intracellular tonicity, nerve impulse transmission, enzymatic reactions in intermediary metabolism, cardiac, skeletal and smooth muscle function, and the maintenance of normal renal function.

Potassium depletion may occur whenever the rate of potassium loss through renal excretion and/or loss from the gastrointestinal tract exceeds the rate of potassium intake. Potassium depletion usually develops slowly as a result of lengthy therapy with oral diuretics, primary or secondary hyperaldosteronism, diabetic ketoacidosis, or inadequate replacement of potassium in patients on prolonged parenteral nutrition. Depletion is additionally associated with severe diarrhea, accompanied by vomiting. Potassium depletion due to these causes is usually accompanied by a concomitant loss of chloride and is manifested by hypokalemia and metabolic alkalosis. Potassium depletion may result in fatigue, weakness, nausea, drowsiness, loss of appetite, edema, oliguria, and chronic ileus with distention. Potassium deficiency may be manifested by shallow breathing, lowered blood pressure, disturbances of cardiac rhythm (primarily ectopic beats), prominent U-waves in the electrocardiogram, or other ECG changes, such as lengthened Q-T interval, depressed S-T segment, and depressed or inverted T wave. In advanced cases of potassium deficiency, flaccid paralysis and/or impaired ability to concentrate urine may be evident.

INDICATIONS AND USAGE

1. For therapeutic use in patients with hypokalemia with or without metabolic alkalosis; digitalis intoxication and in patients with hypokalemic familial periodic paralysis.
2. For prevention of potassium depletion when the dietary intake of potassium is inadequate in the following conditions: patients receiving digitalis and diuretics for congestive heart failure; hepatic cirrhosis with ascites; states of aldosterone excess with normal renal function; potassium-losing nephropathy, and certain diarrheal states.
3. The use of potassium salts in patients receiving diuretics for uncomplicated essential hypertension is often unnecessary when such patients have a normal dietary pattern. Serum potassium should be checked periodically, however, and, if hypokalemia occurs, dietary supplementation with potassium-containing foods may be adequate to control milder cases. In more severe cases supplementation with potassium salts may be indicated.

CONTRAINDICATIONS

Potassium supplements are contraindicated for patients having hyperkalemia, since a further increase in serum potassium level in these patients can result in cardiac arrest. Hyperkalemia may complicate any of the following conditions: chronic renal failure; systemic acidosis, such as diabetic acidosis; acute dehydration; extensive tissue breakdown, as in severe burns; adrenal insufficiency. Hypokalemia should not be treated by the simultaneous use of potassium salts and a potassium-sparing diuretic, such as spironolactone or triamterene, since the concomitant use of these medications can result in severe hyperkalemia.

WARNINGS

The administration of Potassium salts can produce hyperkalemia and cardiac arrest in patients with impaired mechanisms for Potassium excretion. These reactions most commonly occur in patients receiving potassium intravenously, but may also occur in patients receiving oral potassium. Potentially fatal hyperkalemia can develop quickly and be asymptomatic. Patients using potassium salts with chronic renal disease, or any other condition which impairs the excretion of potassium, require especially careful monitoring of serum potassium concentration and appropriate adjustment of dosage.

PRECAUTIONS

General Precautions: The diagnosis of potassium depletion is ordinarily made by demonstrating hypokalemia in a patient with a clinical history suggesting a cause for potassium depletion. When interpreting the serum Potassium concentration, the physician should be aware that acute alkalosis can cause hypokalemia without showing a deficit in total body potassium. Acute acidosis can increase the serum

◆ RATED THERAPEUTICALLY EQUIVALENT; ◇ THERAPEUTIC EQUIVALENCE UNCONFIRMED; ○ UNRATED

Potassium level to normal even with a reduced total body potassium. Thus close attention to acid-base balance, serum electrolytes, the clinical status of the patient, and the ECG is required in the treatment of potassium depletion.

Information for Patients: Patients should be instructed to dissolve each tablet completely in the required amount of water to reduce the risk of gastrointestinal irritation associated with the oral use of concentrated potassium salt products.

Laboratory Tests: Serum potassium determinations and ECG should be a part of the frequent clinical evaluation of the patient.

Drug Interactions: Severe hyperkalemia can be produced by the simultaneous administration of potassium supplements and a potassium-sparing diuretic (see *"Contraindications"*). Potassium supplements should be used carefully by patients who are using salt substitutes, because many of these substitutes contain large amounts of potassium. This simultaneous use could produce hyperkalemia.

Usage in Pregnancy: Pregnancy Category C: Animal reproduction studies have not been conducted with this effervescent potassium product. It is unknown whether this product can cause fetal harm when given to a pregnant woman or if it can affect reproduction capacity. Pregnant women should be given this product only if it is clearly needed.

Nursing Mothers: Because many drugs are excreted in human milk, there exists the potential for serious adverse reactions in nursing infants from oral potassium supplements. Therefore, it should be decided whether to discontinue nursing or to discontinue the drug, considering the importance of the drug to the mother.

Pediatric Use: Safety and effectiveness in children have not been established.

ADVERSE REACTIONS

Abdominal discomfort, diarrhea, vomiting, and nausea are the most common adverse reactions to oral potassium supplements. These adverse reactions occur most frequently when the preparation is not taken with food, is not properly diluted, or not completely dissolved.

Hyperkalemia occurs infrequently in patients with normal renal function who receive oral potassium supplements. The following are symptoms of hyperkalemia: mental confusion, unexplained anxiety, cardiac arrhythmias, numbness or tingling in lips, feet, or hands, difficult breathing or shortness of breath, weakness or heaviness of legs, and unusual fatigue or weakness. (See *"Contraindications"*, *"Warnings"*, and *"Overdosage."*)

OVERDOSAGE

The use of oral potassium salts by persons with normal renal function rarely results in serious hyperkalemia. However, if excretory mechanisms are impaired or if potassium is administered too rapidly intravenously, potentially fatal hyperkalemia can result. (See *"Contraindications"* and *"Warnings."*) The earliest clinical signs of hyperkalemia may be only increased serum potassium concentrations and characteristic ECG changes, such as depression of S-T segment, prolongation of the QT interval, peaking of T-waves and the loss of P-wave. The above mentioned changes in the ECG most frequently occur when the serum potassium level gets to 7 or 8 mEq per liter. At a level of 9 to 10 mEq per liter, other clinical manifestations may occur, such as muscle paralysis and death due to cardiac arrest.

The focus of the treatment of severe hyperkalemia should be on the reduction of the serum potassium level by furthering the transfer of potassium from the extracellular to the intracellular space. The treatment may include the following: a) intravenous administration of 1 liter of a 10 per cent glucose solution which contains 30 to 40 units of insulin; b) in the acidolic patient, 150 mEq to 300 mEq of sodium bicarbonate administered intravenously. Other actions should include the discontinuing of potassium-sparing diuretics and potassium-containing drugs and often the oral use of a cation exchange resin (such as sodium polystyrene sulfonate) in order to eliminate gastrointestinal potassium. To make sure that the resin moves rapidly through the gastrointestinal tract, a nonabsorbable polyhydric alcohol such as sorbitol should be administered in sufficient amounts to cause a soft to semiliquid bowel movement to occur every few hours.

Hemodialysis can also be used as an effective alternative means to remove excess Potassium.

DOSAGE AND ADMINISTRATION

Adults: One effervescent tablet (25 mEq potassium) completely dissolved in three to four ounces or more of cold water and taken two to four times daily, or as directed by physician. It is suggested this Potassium solution be taken with meals and sipped slowly over a five to ten minute period.

HOW SUPPLIED
TABLET, EFFERVESCENT: 25 MEQ

BRAND/MANUFACTURER	NDC	SIZE	AWP
○ **BRAND**			
K-LYTE: Apothecon	00087-0760-01	30s	$26.44
	00087-0761-01	30s	$26.44
	00087-0760-43	100s	$83.65
	00087-0761-43	100s	$83.65
	00087-0761-02	250s	$198.02
○ **GENERICS**			
EFFER-K: Nomax	51801-0001-30	30s	$5.31
EFFER-K: Nomax	51801-0002-30	30s	$5.31
Geneva	00781-1525-31	30s	$7.25
Goldline	00182-1497-17	30s	$9.15
KLOR-CON/EF: Upsher-Smith	00245-0039-30	30s	$9.81
EFFER-K: Nomax	51801-0001-40	100s	$17.50

BRAND/MANUFACTURER	NDC	SIZE	AWP
KLOR-CON/EF: Upsher-Smith	00245-0039-01	100s	$30.74
EFFER-K: Nomax	51801-0001-18	250s	$40.00

TABLET, EFFERVESCENT: 50 MEQ

BRAND/MANUFACTURER	NDC	SIZE	AWP
○ **BRAND**			
K-LYTE DS: Apothecon	00087-0771-41	30s	$47.59
	00087-0771-42	100s	$142.73

Citric Acid and Potassium Citrate

DESCRIPTION

Citric Acid/Potassium Citrate is a stable and pleasant-tasting oral systemic alkalizer containing Potassium Citrate and Citric Acid in a nonalcoholic base.

COMPOSITION

Citric Acid/Potassium Citrate Oral Solution contains in each teaspoonful (5 mL):

Potassium Citrate Monohydrate	1100 mg
Citric Acid Monohydrate	334 mg

Each mL contains 2 mEq Potassium ion and is equivalent to 2 mEq bicarbonate (HCO_3).

Citric Acid/Potassium Citrate Crystals. Each unit dose packet contains:

Potassium Citrate Monohydrate	3300 mg
Citric Acid Monohydrate	1002 mg

Each unit dose packet, when reconstituted, supplies the same amount of active ingredients as is contained in 15 mL (one tablespoonful) Citric Acid/Potassium Citrate Oral Solution and provides 30 mEq Potassium ion and is equivalent to 30 mEq bicarbonate (HCO_3).

ACTIONS

Potassium Citrate is absorbed and metabolized to Potassium bicarbonate, thus acting as a systemic alkalizer. The effects are essentially those of chlorides before absorption and those of bicarbonates, subsequently. Oxidation is virtually complete so that less than 5% of the Potassium Citrate is excreted in the urine unchanged.

INDICATIONS AND ADVANTAGES

Citric Acid/Potassium Citrate is an effective alkalinizing agent useful in those conditions where long-term maintenance of an alkaline urine is desirable, such as in patients with uric acid and cystine calculi of the urinary tract, especially when the administration of sodium salts is undesirable or contraindicated. In addition, it is a valuable adjuvant when administered with uricosuric agents in gout therapy, since urates tend to crystallize out of an acid urine. It is also effective in correcting the acidosis of certain renal tubular disorders, where the administration of Potassium Citrate may be preferable. Citric Acid/Potassium Citrate is highly concentrated, and when administered after meals and before bedtime, allows one to maintain an alkaline urinary pH around the clock, usually without the necessity of a 2 A.M. dose. Citric Acid/Potassium Citrate alkalinizes the urine without producing a systemic alkalosis in recommended dosage. It is highly palatable, pleasant tasting, and tolerable even when administered for long periods. Potassium Citrate does not neutralize the gastric juice or disturb digestion.

CONTRAINDICATIONS

Severe renal impairment with oliguria or azotemia, untreated Addison's disease, adynamia episodica hereditaria, acute dehydration, heat cramps, anuria, severe myocardial damage, and hyperkalemia from any cause.

WARNING

Large doses may cause hyperkalemia and alkalosis, especially in the presence of renal disease. Concurrent administration of Potassium-containing medication, Potassium-sparing diuretics, angiotensin-converting enzyme (ACE) inhibitors, or cardiac glycosides may lead to toxicity.

PRECAUTIONS

Should be used with caution by patients with low urinary output unless under the supervision of a physician. As with all liquids containing a high concentration of Potassium, patients should be directed to dilute adequately with water or other liquids to minimize the possibility of gastrointestinal injury associated with the oral ingestion of concentrated potassium salt preparations; and preferably, to take each dose after meals to avoid saline laxative effect.

ADVERSE REACTIONS

Citric Acid/Potassium Citrate Oral Solution and Citric Acid/Potassium Citrate Crystals are generally well tolerated without any unpleasant side effects when given in recommended doses to patients with normal renal function and urinary output. However, as with any alkalinizing agent, caution must be used in certain patients with abnormal renal mechanisms to avoid development of hyperkalemia or alkalosis. Potassium intoxication causes listlessness, weakness, mental confusion, tingling of extremities, and other symptoms associated with a high concentration of Potassium in the serum. Periodic determinations of serum electrolytes should be carried out in those patients with renal disease in order to avoid these complications. Hyperkalemia may exhibit the following electrocardiographic abnormalities: Disappearance of the P wave, widening and slurring of QRS complex, changes of the S-T segment, tall peaked T waves, etc.

OVERDOSAGE

The administration of oral Potassium salts to persons with normal excretory mechanisms for Potassium rarely causes serious hyperkalemia. However, if excretory mechanisms are impaired, hyperkalemia can result (see "Contraindications" and "Warnings"). Hyperkalemia, when detected, must be treated immediately because lethal levels can be reached in a few hours.

TREATMENT OF HYPERKALEMIA

Should hyperkalemia occur, treatment measures include the following: (1) Elimination of foods or medications containing Potassium. (2) The intravenous administration of 300 to 500 mL/hr of dextrose solution (10 to 25%), containing 10 units of insulin/20 g dextrose. (3) The use of exchange resins, hemodialysis, or peritoneal dialysis. In treating hyperkalemia, it should be recalled that in patients who have been stabilized on digitalis, too rapid a lowering of the plasma Potassium concentration can produce digitalis toxicity.

DOSAGE AND ADMINISTRATION

Citric Acid/Potassium Citrate should be taken diluted in water according to directions, followed by additional water, if desired. Palatability is enhanced if chilled before taking.

Usual Adult Dose: Citric Acid/Potassium Citrate Oral Solution—3 to 6 teaspoonfuls (15 to 30 mL), diluted with 1 glass of water, after meals and at bedtime, or as directed by physician.

Citric Acid/Potassium Citrate Crystals—Contents of 1 packet reconstituted with at least 6 ounces of cool water or juice, after meals and at bedtime, or as directed by physician.

Usual Pediatric Dose: Citric Acid/Potassium Citrate Oral Solution—1 to 3 teaspoonfuls (5 to 15 mL), diluted with ½ glass of water, after meals and at bedtime or as directed by physician. Citric Acid/Potassium Citrate is not recommended for pediatric use. Dosage can be more easily regulated using Citric Acid/Potassium Citrate Oral Solution.

Usual Dosage Range: 2 to 3 teaspoonfuls (10 to 15 mL) Citric Acid/Potassium Citrate Oral Solution, diluted with a glassful of water, taken four times a day, or contents of 1 packet Citric Acid/Potassium Citrate Crystals reconstituted as directed and taken four times a day, will usually maintain a urinary pH of 6.5 to 7.4. 3 to 4 teaspoonfuls (15 to 20 mL). Citric Acid/Potassium Citrate Oral Solution, diluted with a glassful of water, taken four times a day, will usually maintain a urinary pH of 7.0-7.6 throughout most of the 24 hours without unpleasant side effects. To check urinary pH, Hydrion Paper (pH 6.0-8.0) or Nitrazine Paper (pH 4.5-7.5) are available and easy to use.

Keep tightly closed and protect from excessive heat or freezing.

HOW SUPPLIED
LIQUID:

BRAND/MANUFACTURER	NDC	SIZE	AWP
○ BRAND			
POLYCITRA-K: Baker Norton	00575-0222-01	480 ml	$15.10

POWDER FOR RECONSTITUTION:

BRAND/MANUFACTURER	NDC	SIZE	AWP
○ BRAND			
POLYCITRA-K CRYSTALS: Baker Norton	00575-0221-01	100s ud	$51.29

Citric Acid and Sodium Citrate

DESCRIPTION

Citric Acid/Sodium Citrate Oral Solution is a stable and pleasant-tasting oral systemic alkalizer in a sugar-free base. Citric Acid/Sodium Citrate is the USP formula for Shohl's solution.

COMPOSITION

Each teaspoonful (5mL) contains:

Citric Acid Monohydrate ....334 mg (0.32 Molar)
Sodium Citrate Dihydrate ....500 mg (0.34 Molar)

Each mL contains 1 mEq Sodium ion and is equivalent to 1 mEq bicarbonate (HCO_3).

ACTIONS

Sodium Citrate is absorbed and metabolized to sodium bicarbonate, thus acting as a systemic alkalizer. The effects are essentially those of chlorides before absorption and those of bicarbonates subsequently. Oxidation is virtually complete so that less than 5% of Sodium Citrate is excreted in the urine unchanged.

INDICATIONS AND ADVANTAGES

Citric Acid/Sodium Citrate is an effective alkalinizing agent and a nonparticulate neutralizing buffer. It is useful in those conditions where long-term maintenance of an alkaline urine is desirable, and is of value in the alleviation of chronic metabolic acidosis, such as results from chronic renal insufficiency or the syndrome of renal tubular acidosis, especially when the administration of potassium salts is undesirable or contraindicated. Citric Acid/Sodium Citrate is also useful for buffering and neutralizing gastric hydrochloric acid quickly and effectively.

Citric Acid/Sodium Citrate is concentrated, and when administered after meals and before bedtime, allows one to maintain an alkaline urinary pH around the clock, usually without the necessity of a 2 A.M. dose. Citric Acid/Sodium Citrate alkalinizes the urine without producing a systemic alkalosis in the recommended dosage. Citric Acid/Sodium Citrate is a highly palatable, pleasant tasting, and tolerable, even when administered for long periods, and offers these advantages over Shohl's solution, while supplying the equivalent sodium content. Citric Acid/Sodium Citrate is sugar-free.

CONTRAINDICATIONS

Patients on Sodium-restricted diets or with severe renal impairment. In certain situations, potassium citrate solution may be preferable.

PRECAUTIONS

Should be used with caution by patients with low urinary output unless under the supervision of a physician Citric Acid/Sodium Citrate should not be administered concurrently with aluminum-based antacids. Patients should be directed to dilute adequately with water and, preferably, to take each dose after meals to avoid saline laxative effect. Sodium salts should be used cautiously in patients with cardiac failure, hypertension, impaired renal function, peripheral and pulmonary edema, and toxemia of pregnancy. Periodic examinations and determinations of serum electrolytes, particularly serum bicarbonate level, should be carried out in those patients with renal disease in order to avoid these complications.

ADVERSE REACTIONS

Citric Acid/Sodium Citrate is generally well tolerated, without any unpleasant side effects, when given in recommended doses to patients with normal renal function and urinary output. However, as with any alkalinizing agent, caution must be used in certain patients with abnormal renal mechanisms to avoid development of alkalosis, especially in the presence of hypocalcemia.

OVERDOSAGE

Overdosage with sodium salts may cause diarrhea, nausea and vomiting, hypernoia, and convulsions.

DOSAGE AND ADMINISTRATION

Citric Acid/Sodium Citrate should be taken diluted in water, followed by additional water, if desired. Palatability is enhanced if chilled before taking.

FOR SYSTEMIC ALKALIZATION
Usual Adult Dose: 2 to 6 teaspoonfuls (10 to 30 mL), diluted in 1 to 3 ounces of water, after meals and at bedtime, or as directed by physician.

Usual Adult Prescribing Limits: Up to 150 mL daily.

Usual Pediatric Dose: 1 to 3 teaspoonfuls (5 to 15 mL), diluted in 1 to 3 ounces of water, after meals and at bedtime, or as directed by physician.

As a Neutralizing Buffer: 3 teaspoonfuls (15 mL), diluted with 15 mL water, taken as a single dose, or as directed by physician.

Occasional patients will require more or less to achieve the desired alkalizing effect, and since 1 mEq sodium ion is supplied per each mL, dosage is easy to regulate. To check urinary pH, Hydrion paper (pH 6.0-8.0) or Nitrazine paper (pH 4.5-7.5) are available and easy to use.

Keep tightly closed and protect from excessive heat or freezing.

HOW SUPPLIED
SOLUTION:

BRAND/MANUFACTURER	NDC	SIZE	AWP
○ BRAND			
BICITRA: Baker Norton	00575-0225-01	480 ml	$8.33
	00575-0225-04	120 ml 36s	$176.41
	00575-0225-15	15 ml 100s ud	$61.36
	00575-0225-30	30 ml 100s ud	$82.23
○ GENERICS			
Emerson	00802-3962-94	120 ml	$4.04
Emerson	00802-3962-16	480 ml	$4.47
ORACIT: Carolina	46287-0014-01	480 ml	$4.79
Emerson	00802-3962-28	3840 ml	$17.06
ORACIT: Carolina	46287-0014-99	3840 ml	$18.75
ORACIT: Carolina	46287-0014-15	15 ml 100s ud	$68.75
ORACIT: Carolina	46287-0014-30	30 ml 100s ud	$87.50

◆ RATED THERAPEUTICALLY EQUIVALENT; ◇ THERAPEUTIC EQUIVALENCE UNCONFIRMED; ○ UNRATED

SOLUTION: 1002 MG-1500 MG/15 ML

BRAND/MANUFACTURER	NDC	SIZE	AWP
○ **GENERICS**			
Pharm Assoc	00121-0595-16	480 ml	$6.15
Pharm Assoc	00121-0595-15	15 ml 100s ud	$45.22
Pharm Assoc	00121-0595-30	30 ml 100s ud	$60.70

Citric Acid/Glucono-delta-lactone/ Magnesium Carbonate

DESCRIPTION

Citric Acid/Glucono-delta-lactone/Magnesium Carbonate irrigation is a sterile, nonpyrogenic irrigation for use within the urinary tract in the prevention and dissolution of calculi.

Each 100mL contains:

Citric Acid (anhydrous) . . . . .6.602 gm
(Empirical formula $C_6H_8O_7$)
Glucono-delta-lactone . . . . .0.198 gm
(Empirical formula $C_6H_{10}O_6$)
Magnesium Carbonate, USP . . . . .3.177 gm
(Empirical formula $(MgCO_3)_4 \cdot Mg(OH)_2 \cdot 3H_2O$)

CLINICAL PHARMACOLOGY

Citric Acid/Glucono-delta-lactone/Magnesium Carbonate irrigation's action on susceptible apatite calculi results from an exchange of Magnesium from the irrigating solution for calcium contained in the stone matrix. The Magnesium salts thereby formed are soluble in the gluconocitrate irrigating solution resulting in the dissolution of the calculus. Struvite calculi are composed mainly of Magnesium ammonium phosphates which are solubilized by Citric Acid/Glucono-delta-lactone/Magnesium Carbonate irrigation due to its acidic pH.

Citric Acid/Glucono-delta-lactone/Magnesium Carbonate irrigation is not effective for dissolution of calcium oxalate, uric acid or cysteine stones.

INDICATIONS AND USAGE

Citric Acid/Glucono-delta-lactone/Magnesium Carbonate irrigation is indicated for use by local irrigation in the dissolution of renal calculi composed of apatite (a calcium carbonate phosphate compound) or struvite (Magnesium ammonium phosphates) in patients who are not candidates for surgical removal of the calculi.

It may also be used as adjunctive therapy to dissolve residual apatite or struvite calculi and fragments after surgery or to achieve partial dissolution of renal calculi to facilitate surgical removal.

Citric Acid/Glucono-delta-lactone/Magnesium Carbonate irrigation is also indicated for dissolution of bladder calculi of the struvite or apatite variety by local intermittent irrigation through a urethral catheter or cystostomy catheter as an alternative or adjunct to surgical procedures.

Citric Acid/Glucono-delta-lactone/Magnesium Carbonate irrigation is also indicated for use as an intermittent irrigating solution to prevent or minimize encrustations of indwelling urinary tract catheters.

Since many complications are experienced by patients receiving infusions of Citric Acid/Glucono-delta-lactone/Magnesium Carbonate irrigation into the renal pelvis, considerable caution must be employed. Additionally, hospitalization is prolonged for days to weeks when chemolytic therapy is used in lieu of, or following surgery. For these reasons, use of this therapy should be reserved for selected patients.

Citric Acid/Glucono-delta-lactone/Magnesium Carbonate irrigation is not indicated for dissolution of calcium oxalate, uric acid or cysteine calculi.

CONTRAINDICATIONS

The use of Citric Acid/Glucono-delta-lactone/Magnesium Carbonate irrigation in the treatment of renal calculi is contraindicated in patients with urinary tract infections. Urea splitting bacteria reside within struvite and apatite stones which therefore serve as a source of infection. Dissolution therapy with Citric Acid/Glucono-delta-lactone/Magnesium Carbonate irrigation in the presence of an infected urinary tract may lead to sepsis and death. Urine specimens should be obtained for culture prior to initiating chemolytic therapy of the renal pelvis. Appropriate antibiotic therapy should be instituted to treat any infection detected. A sterile urine must be present prior to initiating therapy. An infected stone can serve as a continual source for infection and, therefore, antibiotic therapy should be continued throughout the course of dissolution therapy.

Citric Acid/Glucono-delta-lactone/Magnesium Carbonate irrigation is contraindicated in the presence of demonstrable urinary tract extravasation.

WARNINGS

Citric Acid/Glucono-delta-lactone/Magnesium Carbonate irrigation use should be stopped immediately if the patient develops fever, urinary tract infection, signs and symptoms consistent with urinary tract infection, or persistent flank pain. Irrigation should be stopped if hypermagnesemia or elevated serum creatinine develops.

Severe hypermagnesemia has been reported with Citric Acid/Glucono-delta-lactone/Magnesium Carbonate irrigation. Caution should be employed when irrigating the renal pelvis of patients with impaired renal function. Patients should be observed for early signs and symptoms of hypermagnesemia including

nausea, lethargy, confusion and hypotension. Severe hypermagnesemia may result in hyporeflexia, dyspnea, apnea, coma, cardiac arrest and subsequent death. Serum magnesium levels should be monitored and deep tendon reflexes should be evaluated. Treatment of hypermagnesemia should include discontinuation of Citric Acid/Glucono-delta-lactone/Magnesium Carbonate irrigation followed by medical therapy with intravenous calcium gluconate, fluids and diuresis in severe cases.

PRECAUTIONS

Care must be taken during chemolysis of renal calculi with Citric Acid/Glucono-delta-lactone/Magnesium Carbonate irrigation to maintain the patency of the irrigating catheter. Calculus fragments and debris may obstruct the outflow catheter. Continued irrigation under those circumstances leads to increased intrapelvic pressure with a danger of tissue damage or absorption of the irrigating solution. Catheter outflow blockage may be prevented by flushing the catheter with saline and repositioning of the catheter. Frequent monitoring of the system should be performed by a nurse, an aide or any person with sufficient skills to be able to detect any problems with the patency of the catheter. At the first sign of obstruction, irrigation should be discontinued and the system disconnected.

Intrapelvic pressures must be maintained at or below 25 cm of water. The preferred method of pressure control is the insertion of an open Y connection pop-off valve into the infusion line allowing immediate decompression if pressure exceeds 25 cm of water. An alternative method has been proposed to direct or stop the flow of the irrigating solution to prevent increased intrapelvic pressure: placement of a pinch clamp on the inflow line which can be used by the patient or nurse to stop the irrigation at the first sign of flank pain. However, extreme caution must be taken when relying on cooperation of the patient. Patients may not be sufficiently alert to detect signs and symptoms of outflow obstruction. This is especially true in elderly patients or patients who have been sedated or who have severe neurological dysfunction with varying degrees of sensory loss and/or motor paralysis.

Patients with indwelling urethral or cystostomy catheters frequently have vesicoureteral reflux. Cystogram prior to initiation of Citric Acid/Glucono-delta-lactone/Magnesium Carbonate irrigation is essential for such patients. If reflux is demonstrated, all precautions recommended for renal pelvis irrigation must be taken.

Throughout the course of therapy, patients should be monitored to assure safety. Serum creatinine, phosphate and Magnesium should be obtained every several days. Urine specimens should be collected for culture and antibacterial sensitivity every three days or less and at the first sign of fever. The irrigation should be stopped if any culture exhibits growth and appropriate antibacterial therapy should be initiated. The irrigation may be started again after a course of antibacterial therapy upon demonstration of a sterile urine. Struvite calculi frequently contain bacteria within the stone and antibacterial therapy should therefore be continued throughout the course of dissolution therapy. Hypermagnesemia or an elevated serum creatinine level are indications to halt the irrigation until they return to pre-irrigation levels. Evidence of severe urothelial edema on x-ray is also an indication for temporarily halting the irrigation until the complication resolves.

Concurrent use of Magnesium-containing medications may contribute to production of hypermagnesemia and is not recommended.

Carcinogenesis, Mutagenesis Impairment of Fertility: Long term studies to evaluate carcinogenic potential of Citric Acid/Glucono-delta-lactone/Magnesium Carbonate irrigation in animals have not been conducted. Mutagenicity studies have not been conducted.

Pregnancy Category C: Animal reproduction studies have not been conducted with Citric Acid/Glucono-delta-lactone/Magnesium Carbonate irrigation. It is also not known whether Citric Acid/Glucono-delta-lactone/Magnesium Carbonate irrigation can cause fetal harm when administered to a pregnant women or can affect reproduction capacity. Citric Acid/Glucono-delta-lactone/Magnesium Carbonate irrigation should be given to a pregnant woman only if clearly needed.

Nursing Mothers: Magnesium is known to be excreted into human milk. It is not known whether Citric Acid/Glucono-delta-lactone/Magnesium Carbonate irrigation is excreted in human milk. Because many drugs are excreted in human milk, caution should be exercised when Citric Acid/Glucono-delta-lactone/Magnesium Carbonate irrigation is administered to a nursing woman.

ADVERSE REACTIONS

The most common adverse reaction in selected case series is transient flank pain which occurs in most patients. Additional common reactions include urothelial ulceration and/or edema (13%) or fever (20% but up to 40% in some case series). Other adverse reactions which occur in 1-10% of cases include: urinary tract infection, back pain, dysuria, transient hematuria, nausea, hypermagnesemia, hyperphosphatemia, elevated serum creatinine, candidiasis, and bladder irritability. Adverse reactions which occur in less than 1% of patients include: septicemia, ileus, vomiting and thrombophlebitis. Death from sepsis has been reported.

OVERDOSAGE:

See *"Warning."*

DOSAGE AND ADMINISTRATION

Citric Acid/Glucono-delta-lactone/Magnesium Carbonate irrigation (sterile, nonpyrogenic) in water for local irrigation within the urinary tract.

The action of Citric Acid/Glucono-delta-lactone/Magnesium Carbonate irrigation in the prevention and dissolution of calculi results from an ion exchange mechanism or solvent action. (See "Clinical Pharmacology.")

Parenteral drug products should be inspected visually for particulate matter and discoloration prior to administration whenever solution and container permit.

Renal Calculi: See "Precautions." It is essential that patients be free from urinary tract infections prior to initiating chemolytic therapy. Urine specimens should be collected for culture and appropriate antibiotic therapy should be initiated for any bacteria identified. A nephrostomy tube is placed at surgery or percutaneously to permit lavage of the calculi. A single catheter may be sufficient if the calculus is not obstructing the ureter or ureteropelvic junction. In patients with an obstructed ureter, a retrograde catheter can be placed through the ureter to the renal pelvis via a cystoscope. This second catheter is used to irrigate the calculus while the percutaneous nephrostomy tube is used for drainage.

Plain radiographs and nephrostomograms are performed to assure proper placement of the catheter(s). Pressure measurements are made under fluoroscopy to assure that 2-3 mL/min can be infused without causing pain, pyelovenous or pyelotubular backflow or manometric evidence of elevated pressure within the collecting system.

For postoperative patients irrigation should not be started before the fourth or fifth postoperative day. Irrigation of the renal pelvis is begun with sterile saline only after a sterile urine has been demonstrated. The saline is infused at a rate of 60 mL/hr initially and the rate is increased until pain or an elevated pressure (25 cm H_2O) appears, or until a maximum flow-rate of 120 mL/hr is achieved. The site of insertion should be inspected for leakage. If leakage occurs, the irrigation is discontinued temporarily to allow for complete healing around the nephrostomy tube.

If no leakage or flank pain occur, irrigation is then started with Citric Acid/ Glucono-delta-lactone/Magnesium Carbonate irrigation with a flow rate equal to the maximum rate achieved with the saline solution. A clamp should be placed on the inflow tube and patients (see "Precautions") and nursing personnel should be instructed to stop the irrigating solution whenever pain develops. Nursing personnel who are responsible for performing the irrigation must be instructed concerning the location of the nephrostomy tube(s) and the direction of flow of the irrigating solution to insure against misconnection of the inflowing and egress tubes. Nephrostomograms should be performed periodically to assure proper placement of the catheter tip and to assess efficacy. If stones fail to change size after several days of adequate irrigation, the procedure should be discontinued.

Upon demonstration of complete dissolution of the calculus the inflow tube is clamped and left in place for a few days to ensure that no obstruction exists, after which time the nephrostomy tube is removed.

Bladder Calculi: Chemolysis of bladder calculi is used as an alternative to cystoscopic or surgical removal of the stones in patients who refuse surgery or cystoscopic removal or in whom these procedures constitute an unwarranted risk. Following appropriate studies to evaluate possible vesicoureteral reflux, 30 mL of Citric Acid/Glucono-delta-lactone/Magnesium Carbonate irrigation is instilled through a urinary catheter into the bladder and the catheter is clamped for 30-60 minutes. The clamp is then released and the bladder is drained. This is repeated 4-6 times a day. A continuous drip through a 3-way Foley catheter is an alternative means of dissolving bladder stones. In the presence of bladder spasm and associated high pressure reflux, all precautions required for irrigation of the renal pelvis must be observed.

Indwelling Urinary Tract Catheter Encrustation: Periodic instillation of Citric Acid/Glucono-delta-lactone/Magnesium Carbonate irrigation is indicated to minimize or prevent encrustation of indwelling catheters which frequently results in plugging of the catheter and discomfort to the patient. This is accomplished by instilling 30 mL of the solution through the catheter and then clamping the catheter for 10 minutes, after which the clamp is removed to allow drainage of the bladder. This process is repeated 3 times a day.

Storage: Exposure of Citric Acid/Glucono-delta-lactone/Magnesium Carbonate irrigation to heat or cold should be minimized. Citric Acid/Glucono-delta-lactone/Magnesium Carbonate irrigation should be stored at controlled room temperature, 59° to 86°F (15° to 30°C). Avoid excessive heat or cold (keep from freezing). Brief exposure to temperatures of up to 40°C or temperatures down to 5°C does not adversely affect the product.

HOW SUPPLIED
POWDER FOR RECONSTITUTION:

BRAND/MANUFACTURER	NDC	SIZE	AWP
○ BRAND			
RENACIDIN: Guardian	00327-0007-03	300 gm	$32.10
	00327-0007-06	25 gm 6s	$32.10
	00327-0011-05	500 ml	$23.60

Citric Acid/Magnesium Oxide/ Sodium Carbonate

DESCRIPTION
Citric Acid/Magnesium Oxide/Sodium Carbonate is a sterile, nonpyrogenic solution of the ingredients listed below, in water for irrigation.

The solution is administered only by transurethral irrigation for dissolving phosphatic calculi in the urinary bladder. It must not be used for transurethral surgical procedures involving electrical instrumentation.

Each 100 mL of Citric Acid/Magnesium Oxide/Sodium Carbonate contains:

Citric Acid, hydrous	3.24 g
Sodium Carbonate, anhydrous	0.43 g
Magnesium Oxide, anhydrous	0.38 g

pH 4.0 (3.8 - 4.2).

It contains no bacteriostat, antimicrobial agent or added buffer.

Citric Acid, USP, hydrous (monohydrate) is chemically designated $C_6H_8O_7 \cdot H_2O$, colorless, translucent crystals or white crystalline powder very soluble in water.

Sodium Carbonate, NF, anhydrous is chemically designated Na_2CO_3, odorless hygroscopic powder freely soluble in water.

Magnesium Oxide, USP, anhydrous is chemically designated MgO, white powder soluble in dilute acids.

Water for Injection, USP is chemically designated H_2O.

The semi-rigid container is fabricated from a specially formulated polyolefin.

CLINICAL PHARMACOLOGY
The dissolution of urinary calculi by Citric Acid/Magnesium Oxide/Sodium Carbonate Irrigation derives primarily from the ability of the citrate ion to complex with calcium in the calculi, forming soluble calcium citrates. This effect provided by Citric Acid in the formula is limited to urinary bladder stones composed of calcium phosphate, with or without magnesium ammonium phosphate and/or calcium carbonate.

Sodium Carbonate in the formula serves as a mild alkali to control acidity of the solution.

Magnesium Oxide in the formula serves to diminish irritation of the bladder mucosa caused by the Citric Acid.

INDICATIONS AND USAGE
Citric Acid/Magnesium Oxide/Sodium Carbonate is indicated for use as an irrigating solution to help dissolve calculi of phosphatic origin in the urinary bladder in patients for whom other methods of treatment are impractical or contraindicated.

CONTRAINDICATIONS
Not for injection into body tissue.

Contraindicated for irrigation during transurethral surgical procedures. This solution is conductive and should not be used in the presence of electrical instrumentation.

WARNINGS
FOR IRRIGATION ONLY: NOT FOR INJECTION
Citric Acid/Magnesium Oxide/Sodium Carbonate Irrigation is not recommended for dissolving phosphatic calculi in the renal pelvis because of the risk of creating back pressure that may reactivate an existing pyelonephritis.

This solution should not be used to replace other indicated measures, including correction of underlying metabolic disorders, surgical intervention and treatment of infection.

The contents of an opened container should be used promptly to minimize the possibility of bacterial growth or pyrogen formation.

Do not heat over 66°C (150°F).

PRECAUTIONS
Do not open container until ready to use. Dilute aqueous solutions of citric acid not kept in tightly closed containers are susceptible to fermentation, fungus growth and/or bacterial contamination on standing.

Do not use unless solution is clear and seal is intact. Discard unused portion.

Pregnancy Category C: Animal reproduction studies have not been conducted with Citric Acid/Magnesium Oxide/Sodium Carbonate Irrigation. It is also not known whether this irrigation solution can cause fetal harm when given to a pregnant women or can affect reproduction capacity. This irrigation solution should be given to a pregnant woman only if clearly needed.

ADVERSE REACTIONS
Patients may complain of some discomfort or pain due to bladder irritation during irrigation, or irrigation may initiate bleeding from the bladder in the presence of undetected mucosal lesions. In such cases the physician should re-evaluate the basis for irrigation therapy versus other indicated methods of treatment.

Hypermagnesemia, causing severe respiratory depression, has been reported following extended continuous irrigation with a Magnesium containing urologic irrigating solution.

DOSAGE AND ADMINISTRATION
Citric Acid/Magnesium Oxide/Sodium Carbonate Irrigation may be administered by intermittent irrigation or by tidal instillation and drainage to allow continuous irrigation of the bladder for periods of several hours. The usual dose is one to three liters daily.

Intermittent irrigation of the bladder (after the manner of intermittent peritoneal dialysis) may be preferred to promote more prolonged contact of the irrigation with bladder stones; tidal (continuous in and out flow) irrigation may be less efficient and require larger amounts of irrigation fluid.

◆ RATED THERAPEUTICALLY EQUIVALENT; ◇ THERAPEUTIC EQUIVALENCE UNCONFIRMED; ○ UNRATED

The LD_{50} intraperitoneal dose of citric acid in rats is 975 mg/kg.

Parenteral drug products should be inspected visually for particulate matter and discoloration prior to administration, whenever container and solution permit. (See "Precautions").

Exposure of pharmaceutical products to heat should be minimized. Avoid excessive heat. Protect from freezing. It is recommended that the product be stored at room temperature (25°C); however, brief exposure up to 40°C does not adversely affect the product.

HOW SUPPLIED
SOLUTION:

AVERAGE UNIT PRICE (AVAILABLE SIZES)		GENERIC A-RATED AVERAGE PRICE (GAAP)	
BRAND	$0.02	1000 ml 6s	$43.35
GENERIC	$0.01		

BRAND/MANUFACTURER	NDC	SIZE	AWP
◆ **BRAND**			
IRRIGATING SOLUTION G: Baxter	00338-0286-04	1000 ml 12s	$200.08
◆ **GENERICS**			
UROLOGIC G: Baxter	00338-0287-04	1000 ml 6s	$35.04
UROLOGIC G: Baxter	00338-0287-44	1000 ml 6s	$51.66
UROLOGIC G: Abbott Hosp	00074-7168-09	1000 ml 12s	$345.85

Citric Acid/Potassium Citrate/ Sodium Citrate

DESCRIPTION
These products are stable, pleasant-tasting oral systemic alkalizers containing Potassium Citrate, Sodium Citrate, and Citric Acid. The syrup is available with or without sugar. Both products are nonalcoholic and contain identical amounts of active ingredients.

COMPOSITION
Each teaspoonful (5 mL) contains:

Potassium Citrate Monohydrate . . . . .550 mg
Sodium Citrate Dihydrate . . . . .500 mg
Citric Acid Monohydrate . . . . .334 mg

Each mL contains 1 mEq Potassium and 1 mEq Sodium ion and is equivalent to 2 mEq bicarbonate (HCO_3).

ACTIONS
Potassium Citrate and Sodium Citrate are absorbed and metabolized to potassium bicarbonate and sodium bicarbonate, thus acting as systemic alkalizers. The effects are essentially those of chlorides before absorption and those of bicarbonates subsequently. Oxidation is virtually complete so that less than 5% of the citrates are excreted in the urine unchanged.

INDICATIONS
These syrups are effective alkalinizing agents useful in those conditions where long-term maintenance of an alkaline urine is desirable, such as in patients with uric acid and cystine calculi of the urinary tract. In addition, they are valuable adjuvants when administered with uricosuric agents in gout therapy, since urates tend to crystallize out of an acid urine. They are also effective in correcting the acidosis of certain renal tubular disorders. The syrups are highly concentrated, and when administered after meals and before bedtime, allow one to maintain an alkaline urine pH around the clock, usually without the necessity of a 2 A.M. dose. The syrups alkalinize the urine without producing a systemic alkalosis in recommended dosage. They are highly palatable, pleasant tasting, and tolerable, even when administered for long periods. Potassium Citrate and Sodium Citrate do not neutralize the gastric juice or disturb digestion.

CONTRAINDICATIONS
Severe renal impairment with oliguria or azotemia, untreated Addison's disease, or severe myocardial damage.

PRECAUTIONS AND WARNINGS
Should be used with caution by patients with low urinary output or reduced glomerular filtration rates unless under the supervision of a physician. Aluminum-based antacids should be avoided in these patients. Patients should be directed to dilute adequately with water and, preferably, to take each dose after meals, to minimize the possibility of gastrointestinal injury associated with oral ingestion of potassium salt preparations and to avoid saline laxative effect. Sodium salts should be used cautiously in patients with cardiac failure, hypertension, peripheral and pulmonary edema, and toxemia of pregnancy.

Concurrent administration of potassium-containing medication, potassium-sparing diuretics, angiotensin-converting enzyme (ACE) inhibitors, or cardiac glycosides may lead to toxicity. Periodic examination and determinations of serum electrolytes, particularly serum bicarbonate level, should be carried out in those patients with renal disease in order to avoid these complications.

ADVERSE REACTIONS
Citric Acid/Potassium Citrate/Sodium Citrate is generally well tolerated without any unpleasant side effects when given in recommended doses to patients with normal renal function and urinary output. However, as with any alkalinizing agent, caution must be used in certain patients with abnormal renal mechanisms to avoid development of hyperkalemia or alkalosis, especially in the presence of hypocalcemia. Potassium intoxication causes listlessness, weakness, mental confusion and tingling of extremities.

OVERDOSAGE
Overdosage with sodium salts may cause diarrhea, nausea and vomiting, hypernoia, and convulsions. Overdosage with potassium salts may cause hyperkalemia and alkalosis, especially in the presence of renal disease.

DOSAGE AND ADMINISTRATION
The syrup should be taken diluted in water, followed by additional water if desired. Palatability is enhanced if chilled before taking.

Usual Adult Dose: 3 to 6 teaspoonfuls (15 to 30 mL), diluted in water, four times a day, after meals and at bedtime, or as directed by physician.

Usual Pediatric Dose: 1 to 3 teaspoonfuls (10 to 15 mL), diluted in water, for times a day, after meals and at bedtime, or as directed by physician.

Usual Dosage Range: 2 to 3 teaspoonfuls (10 to 15 mL), diluted with water, taken four times a day, will usually maintain a urine pH of 6.5-7.4. 3 to 4 teaspoonfuls (15 to 20 mL), diluted with water, taken four times a day, will usually maintain a urine pH of 7.0-7.6 throughout most of the 24 hours without unpleasant side effects. To check urine pH, Hydrion Paper (pH 6.0-8.0) or Nitrazine Paper (pH 4.5-7.5) are available and easy to use.

Storage: Keep tightly closed and protect from excessive heat and freezing.

HOW SUPPLIED
CITRIC ACID/POTASSIUM CITRATE/SODIUM CITRATE
LIQUID:

BRAND/MANUFACTURER	NDC	SIZE	AWP
○ **BRAND**			
POLYCITRA-LC: Baker Norton	00575-0224-01	480 ml	$15.23

SYRUP:

BRAND/MANUFACTURER	NDC	SIZE	AWP
○ **BRAND**			
POLYCITRA: Baker Norton	00575-0223-01	480 ml	$15.16

POTASSIUM ACETATE
INJECTION: 2 MEQ/ML

AVERAGE UNIT PRICE (AVAILABLE SIZES)	
GENERIC	$0.14

BRAND/MANUFACTURER	NDC	SIZE	AWP
◆ **GENERICS**			
Fujisawa	00469-7600-40	20 ml	$2.01
Fujisawa	00469-7600-60	50 ml	$3.90
Fujisawa	00469-7601-00	100 ml	$10.45
Abbott Hosp	00074-8183-01	20 ml 25s	$115.19
Abbott Hosp	00074-3294-51	50 ml 25s	$227.11
Abbott Hosp	00074-3294-06	100 ml 25s	$380.59

INJECTION: 4 MEQ/ML

BRAND/MANUFACTURER	NDC	SIZE	AWP
◆ **GENERICS**			
Fujisawa	00469-3300-60	50 ml	$6.46

Citrolith SEE POTASSIUM CITRATE AND SODIUM CITRATE

Cladribine

WARNING

CLADRIBINE INJECTION SHOULD BE ADMINISTERED UNDER THE SUPERVISION OF A QUALIFIED PHYSICIAN EXPERIENCED IN THE USE OF ANTINEOPLASTIC THERAPY. SUPPRESSION OF BONE MARROW FUNCTION SHOULD BE ANTICIPATED. THIS IS USUALLY REVERSIBLE AND APPEARS TO BE DOSE DEPENDENT. HIGH DOSES (4 TO 9 TIMES THE RECOMMENDED DOSE FOR HAIRY CELL LEUKEMIA), IN CONJUNCTION WITH CYCLOPHOSPHAMIDE AND TOTAL BODY IRRADIATION AS PREPARATION FOR BONE MARROW TRANSPLANTATION, HAVE BEEN ASSOCIATED WITH SEVERE, IRREVERSIBLE, NEUROLOGIC TOXICITY (PARAPARESIS/QUADRIPARESIS) AND/OR ACUTE RENAL INSUFFICIENCY IN 45% OF PATIENTS TREATED FOR 7-14 DAYS.

➤ SHOWN IN PRODUCT IDENTIFICATION GUIDE

DESCRIPTION

Cladribine Injection (also commonly known as 2-chloro-2'-deoxy-β-D-adenosine) is a synthetic antineoplastic agent for continuous intravenous infusion. It is a clear, colorless, sterile, preservative-free, isotonic solution. Cladribine Injection is available in single-use vials containing 10 mg (1 mg/mL) of Cladribine, a chlorinated purine nucleoside analog. Each milliliter of Cladribine Injection contains 1 mg of the active ingredient and 9 mg (0.15 mEq) of sodium chloride as an inactive ingredient. The solution has a pH range of 5.5 to 8.0. Phosphoric acid and/or dibasic sodium phosphate may have been added to adjust the pH to 6.3 ± 0.6.

The chemical name for Cladribine is 2-chloro-6-amino-9-(2-deoxy-β-D-erythropento-furanosyl) purine.

Following is its chemical structure:

CLINICAL PHARMACOLOGY

CELLULAR RESISTANCE AND SENSITIVITY

The selective toxicity of 2-chloro-2'-deoxy-β-D-adenosine towards certain normal and malignant lymphocyte and monocyte populations is based on the relative activities of deoxycytidine kinase, deoxynucleotidase and adenosine deaminase. In cells with a high ratio of deoxycytidine kinase to deoxynucleotidase, 2-chloro-2'-deoxy-β-D-adenosine, a purine nucleoside analog, passively crosses the cell membrane. It is phosphorylated by deoxycytidine kinase to 2-chloro-2'-deoxy-β-D-adenosine monophosphate (2-CdAMP). Since 2-chloro-2'-deoxy-β-D-adenosine is resistant to deamination by adenosine deaminase and there is little deoxynucleotide deaminase in lymphocytes and monocytes, 2-CdAMP accumulates intracellularly and is subsequently converted into the active triphosphate deoxynucleotide, 2-chloro-2'-deoxy-β-D-adenosine triphosphate (2-CdATP). It is postulated that cells with high deoxycytidine kinase and low deoxynucleotidase activities will be selectively killed by 2-chloro-2'-deoxy-β-D-adenosine as toxic deoxynucleotides accumulate intracellularly.

Cells containing high concentrations of deoxynucleotides are unable to properly repair single-strand DNA breaks. The broken ends of DNA activate the enzyme poly (ADP-ribose) polymerase resulting in NAD and ATP depletion and disruption of cellular metabolism. There is evidence, also, that 2-CdATP is incorporated into the DNA of dividing cells, resulting in impairment of DNA synthesis. Thus, 2-chloro-2'-deoxy-β-D-adenosine can be distinguished from other chemotherapeutic agents affecting purine metabolism in that it is cytotoxic to both actively dividing and quiescent lymphocytes and monocytes, inhibiting both DNA synthesis and repair.

HUMAN PHARMACOLOGY

In a clinical investigation, 17 patients with Hairy Cell Leukemia (HCL) and normal renal function were treated for 7 days with the recommended treatment regimen of Cladribine Injection (0.09 mg/kg/day) by continuous intravenous infusion. The mean steady-state serm concentration was estimated to be 5.7 ng/mL with an estimated systemic clearance of 663.5 mL/h/kg when Cladribine was given by continuous infusion over 7 days. Accumulation of Cladribine over the seven day treatment period was not noted. In Hairy Cell Leukemia patients, there does not appear to be a relationship between serum concentrations and ultimate clinical outcome.

In another study, 8 patients with hematologic malignancies received a two (2) hour infusion of Cladribine Injection (0.12 mg/kg). The mean end-of-infusion plasma Cladribine concentration was 48 ± 19 ng/mL. For 5 of these patients, the disappearance of Cladribine could be described by either a biphasic or triphasic decline. For these patients with normal renal function, the mean terminal half-life was 5.4 hours. Mean values for clearance and steady-state volume of distribution were 978 ± 422 mL/h/kg and 4.5 ± 2.8 L/kg, respectively.

Cladribine is bound approximately 20% to plasma proteins.

Except for some understanding of the mechanism of cellular toxicity, no other information is available on the metabolism or route of excretion of Cladribine in humans. In a pilot study in rats treated with radiolabeled Cladribine, approximately 41% to 44% of the administered label was recovered in the urine in the first 6 hours from a 1 mg/kg bolus or infusion. Only small amounts of radioactivity were recovered after 6 hours. Less than 1% of the administered radioactivity was excreted in the feces following a bolus dose to rats. The effect of renal and hepatic impairment on the elimination of Cladribine has not been investigated in humans.

Two single-center open label studies of Cladribine have been conducted in patients with Hairy Cell Leukemia with evidence of active disease requiring therapy. In the study conducted at the Scripps Clinic and Research Foundation (Study A), 89 patients were treated with a single course of Cladribine Injection given by continuous intravenous infusion for 7 days at a dose of 0.09 mg/kg/day. In the study conducted at the M.D. Anderson Cancer Center (Study B), 35 patients were treated with a 7-day continuous intravenous infusion of Cladribine Injection at a comparable dose of 3.6 mg/m²/day. A complete response (CR) required clearing of the peripheral blood and bone marrow of hairy cells and recovery of the hemoglobin to 12 g/dL, platelet count to 100 x 10⁹/L, and absolute neutrophil count to 1500 x 10⁶/L. A good partial response (GPR) required the same hematologic parameters as a complete response, and that fewer than 5% hairy cells remain in the bone marrow. A partial response (PR) required that hairy cells in the bone marrow be decreased by at least 50% from baseline and the same response for hematologic parameters as for complete response. A pathologic elapse was defined as an increase in bone marrow hairy cells to 25% of pretreatment levels. A clinical relapse was defined as the recurrence of cytopenias, specifically, decreases in hemoglobin ≥ 2 g/dL, ANC ≥ 25% or platelet counts ≥ 50,000. Patients who met the criteria for a complete response but subsequently were found to have evidence of bone marrow hairy cells (< 25% of pretreatment levels) were reclassified as partial responses and were not considered to be complete responses with relapse.

Among patients evaluable for efficacy (N = 106), using the hematologic and bone marrow response criteria described above, the complete response rates in patients treated with Cladribine Injection were 65% and 68% for Study A and Study B, respectively, yielding a combined complete response rate of 66%. Overall response rates (i.e. Complete plus Good Partial plus Partial Responses) were 89% and 86% in Study A and Study B, respectively, for a combined overall response rate of 88% in evaluable patients treated with Cladribine Injection.

Using an intent-to-treat analysis (N = 123) and further requiring no evidence of splenomegaly as a criterion for CR (i.e., no palpable spleen on physical examination and ≤ 13 cm on CT scan), the complete response rates for Study A and Study B were 54% and 53%, respectively, giving a combined CR rate of 54%. The overall response rates (CR + GPR + PR) were 90% and 85%, for Studies A and B respectively, yielding a combined overall response rate of 89%.

RESPONSE RATES TO CLADRIBINE TREATMENT IN PATIENTS WITH HAIRY CELL LEUKEMIA

	CR	Overall
Evaluable Patients N = 106	66%	88%
Intent-to-treat Population N = 123	54%	89%

In these studies, 60% of the patients had not received prior chemotherapy for HCL or had undergone spienectomy as the only prior treatment and were receiving Cladribine as a first-line treatment. The remaining 40% of the patients received Cladribine as a second-line treatment, having been treated previously with other agents, including α-interferon and/or deoxycoformycin. The overall response rate for patients without prior chemotherapy was 92%, compared with 84% for previously treated patients. Cladribine is active in previously treated patients; however, retrospective analysis suggests that the overall response rate is decreased in patients previously treated with splenectomy or deoxycoformycin and in patients refractory to α-interferon.

OVERALL RESPONSE RATES (CR + GPR + PR) TO CLADRIBINE TREATMENT IN PATIENTS WITH HAIRY CELL LEUKEMIA

	Overall Response (N = 123)	NR + Relapse
No Prior Chemotherapy	68/74 92%	6 + 4 14%
Any Prior Chemotherapy	41/49 84%	8 + 3 22%
Previous Splenectomy	32/41* 78%	9 + 1 24%
Previous Interferon	40/48 83%	8 + 3 23%
Interferon Refractory	6/11* 55%	5 + 2 64%
Previous Deoxycoformycin	3/6* 50%	3 + 1 66%

NR = No Response
* P < 0.05

After a reversible decline, normalization of peripheral blood counts (Hemoglobin > 12.0 g/dL, Platelets > 100 x 10⁹/L, Absolute Neutrophil Count (ANC) > 1500 x 10⁶/L) was achieved by 92% of evaluable patients. The median time to normalization of peripheral counts was 9 weeks from the start of treatment (Range: 2 to 72). The median time to normalization of Platelet Count was 2 weeks, the median time to normalization of ANC was 5 weeks and the median time to normalization of Hemoglobin was 8 weeks. With normalization of Platelet Count and Hemoglobin, requirements for platelet and RBC transfusion were abolished after Months 1 and 2, respectively, in those patients with complete response. Platelet recovery may be delayed in a minority of patients with severe baseline thrombocytopenia. Corresponding to normalization of ANC, a trend toward a reduced incidence of infection was seen after the third month when compared to the months immediately preceding Cladribine therapy (see also *"Warnings," "Precautions"* and *"Adverse Reactions"*).

◆ RATED THERAPEUTICALLY EQUIVALENT; ◇ THERAPEUTIC EQUIVALENCE UNCONFIRMED; ○ UNRATED

CLADRIBINE TREATMENT IN PATIENTS WITH HAIRY CELL LEUKEMIA
TIME TO NORMALIZATION OF PERIPHERAL BLOOD COUNTS

Parameter	Median Time to Normalization of Count*
Platelet Count	2 weeks
Absolute Neutrophil Count	5 weeks
Hemoglobin	8 weeks
ANC, Hemoglobin and Platelet Count	9 weeks

*Day 1 = First day of infusion

For patients achieving a complete response, the median time to response (i.e., absence of hairy cells in bone marrow and peripheral blood together with normalization of peripheral blood parameters), measured from treatment start, was approximately 4 months. Since bone marrow aspiration and biopsy were frequently not performed at the time of peripheral blood normalization, the median time to complete response may actually be shorter than that which was recorded. At the time of data cut-off, the median duration of complete response was greater than 8 months and ranged to 25 + months. Among 93 responding patients, seven had shown evidence of disease progression at the time of the data cut-off. In four of these patients, disease was limited to the bone marrow without peripheral blood abnormalities (pathologic progression), while in three patients there were also peripheral blood abnormalities (clinical progression). Seven patients who did not respond to a first course of Cladribine received a second course of therapy. In the five patients who had adequate followup, additional courses did not appear to improve their overall response.

INDICATIONS FOR USE
Cladribine Injection is indicated for the treatment of active Hairy Cell Leukemia as defined by clinically significant anemia, neutropenia, thrombocytopenia or disease-related symptoms.

UNLABELED USES
Cladribine is used alone or as an adjunct in the treatment of acute leukemia including acute myeloid leukemia, chronic leukemia including chronic lymphocytic leukemia, lymphocytic lymphoma, and Waldenstrom's macroglobulinemia.

CONTRAINDICATIONS
Cladribine Injection is contraindicated in those patients who are hypersensitive to this drug or any of its components.

WARNINGS
Severe bone marrow suppression, including neutropenia, anemia and thrombocytopenia, has been commonly observed in patients treated with Cladribine, especially at high doses. At initiation of treatment, most patients in the clinical studies had hematologic impairment as a manifestation of active Hairy Cell Leukemia. Following treatment with Cladribine, further hematologic impairment occurred before recovery of peripheral blood counts began. During the first two weeks after treatment initiation, mean Platelet Count, ANC, and Hemoglobin concentration declined and subsequently increased with normalization of mean counts by Day 12, Week 5 and Week 8, respectively. The myelosuppressive effects of Cladribine were most notable during the first month following treatment. Forty-four percent (44%) of patients received transfusions with RBCs and 14% received transfusions with platelets during Month 1. Careful hematologic monitoring, especially during the first 4 to 8 weeks after treatment with Cladribine Injection, is recommended (see "Precautions").

Fever (T > 100°F) was associated with the use of Cladribine in approximately two-thirds of patients (131/196) in the first month of therapy. Virtually all of these patients were treated empirically with parenteral antibiotics. Overall, 47% (93/196) of all patients had fever in the setting of neutropenia (ANC ≤ 1000), including 62 patients (32%) with severe neutropenia (i.e., ANC ≤ 500).

In a Phase I investigational study using Cladribine in high doses (4 to 9 times the recommended dose for Hairy Cell Leukemia) as part of a bone marrow transplant conditioning regimen, which also included high dose cyclophosphamide and total body irradiation, acute nephrotoxicity and delayed onset neurotoxicity were observed. Thirty-one (31) poor-risk patients with drug-resistant acute leukemia in relapse (29 cases) or nonHodgkins Lymphoma (2 cases) received Cladribine for 7 to 14 days prior to bone marrow transplantation. During infusion, 8 patients experienced gastrointestinal symptoms. While the bone marrow was initially cleared of all hematopoietic elements, including tumor cells, leukemia eventually recurred in all treated patients. Within 7 to 13 days after starting treatment with Cladribine, 6 patients (19%) developed manifestations of renal dysfunction (e.g., acidosis, anuria, elevated serum creatinine, etc.) and 5 required dialysis. Several of these patients were also being treated with other medications having known nephrotoxic potential. Renal dysfunction was reversible in 2 of these patients. In the 4 patients whose renal function had not recovered at the time of death, autopsies were performed: in 2 of these, evidence of tubular damage was noted. Eleven (11) patients (35%) experienced delayed onset neurologic toxicity. In the majority, this was characterized by progressive irreversible motor weakness (paraparesis/quadriparesis) of the upper and/or lower extremities, first noted 35 to 84 days after starting high dose therapy with Cladribine. Non-invasive testing (electromyography and nerve conduction studies) was consistent with demyelinating disease. Severe neurologic toxicity has also been noted with high doses of another drug in this class.

In patients with Hairy Cell Leukemia treated with the recommended treatment regimen (0.09 mg/kg/day for 7 consecutive days), there have been no reports of similar nephro- or neurologic toxicities. Mild neurologic toxicities, specifically paresthesias and dizziness, have been reported rarely.

Of the 196 Hairy Cell Leukemia patients entered in the two trials, there were 8 deaths following treatment. Of these, 6 were of infectious etiology, including 3 pneumonias, and 2 occurred in the first month following Cladribine therapy. Of the 8 deaths, 6 occurred in previously treated patients who were refractory to α-interferon.

Benzyl alcohol is a constituent of the recommended diluent for the 7-day infusion solution. Benzyl alcohol has been reported to be associated with a fatal "Gasping Syndrome" in premature infants (see "Dosage and Administration").

Pregnancy category D: Cladribine is teratogenic in mice and rabbits and consequently has the potential to cause fetal harm when administered to a pregnant woman. A significant increase in fetal variations was observed in mice receiving 1.5 mg/kg/day (4.5 mg m^2) and increased resorptions, reduced litter size and increased fetal malformations were observed when mice received 3.0 mg/kg/day (9 mg/m^2). Fetal death and malformations were observed in rabbits that received 3.0 mg/kg/day (33.0 mg/m^2). No fetal effects were seen in mice at 0.5 mg/kg/day (1.5 mg/m^2) or in rabbits at 1.0 mg/kg/day (11.0 mg/m^2).

Although there is no evidence of teratogenicity in humans due to Cladribine, other drugs which inhibit DNA synthesis (e.g. methotrexate and aminopterin) have been reported to be teratogenic in humans. Cladribine has been shown to be embryotoxic in mice when given at doses equivalent to the recommended dose. If Cladribine is used during pregnancy, or if the patient becomes pregnant while taking this drug, the patient should be apprised of the potential hazard to the fetus. Women of childbearing age should be advised to avoid becoming pregnant. Cladribine should be used during pregnancy only if the potential benefit justifies the potential risk to the fetus.

PRECAUTIONS
General: Cladribine Injection is a potent antineoplastic agent with potentially significant toxic side effects. It should be administered only under the supervision of a physician experienced with the use of cancer chemotherapeutic agents. Patients undergoing therapy should be closely observed for signs of hematologic and non-hematologic toxicity. Periodic assessment of peripheral blood counts, particularly during the first 4 to 8 weeks post-treatment, is recommended to detect the development of anemia, neutropenia and thrombocytopenia and for early detection of any potential sequelae (e.g. infection or bleeding). As with other potent chemotherapeutic agents, monitoring of renal and hepatic function is also recommended, especially in patients with underlying kidney or liver dysfunction. (See "Warnings" and "Adverse Reactions.")

Fever was a frequently observed side effect during the first month on study. Since the majority of fevers occurred in neutropenic patients, patients should be closely monitored during the first month of treatment and empiric antibiotics should be initiated as clinically indicated. Although 69% of patients developed fevers, less than ⅓ of febrile events were associated with documented infection. Given the known myelosuppressive effects of Cladribine, practitioners should carefully evaluate the risks and benefits of administering this drug to patients with active infections. (See "Warnings" and "Adverse Reactions.")

The kidney has not been established as the organ of excretion for Cladribine. There are inadequate data on dosing of patients with renal or hepatic insufficiency. Development of acute renal insufficiency in some patients receiving high doses of Cladribine has been described. Until more information is available, caution is advised when administering the drug to patients with known or suspected renal or hepatic insufficiency. (See "Warnings.")

While hyperuricemia and tumor lysis syndrome is always possible in patients with large tumor burdens, patients in these studies were treated empirically with allopurinol and no episodes of tumor lysis were reported.

Cladribine Injection must be diluted in designated intravenous solutions prior to administration. (See "Dosage and Administration.")

Laboratory Tests: During and following treatment, the patient's hematologic profile should be monitored regularly to determine the degree of hematopoietic suppression. In the clinical studies, following reversible declines in all cell counts, the mean Platelet Count reached 100×10^9/L by Day 12, the mean Absolute Neutrophil Count reached 1500×10^6/L by Week 5 and the mean Hemoglobin reached 12 g/dL by Week 8. After peripheral counts have normalized, bone marrow aspiration and biopsy should be performed to confirm response to treatment with Cladribine. Febrile events should be investigated with appropriate laboratory and radiologic studies. Periodic assessment of renal function and hepatic function should be performed as clinically indicated.

Drug Interactions: There are no known drug interactions with Cladribine Injection. Caution should be exercised if Cladribine Injection is administered following or in conjunction with other drugs known to cause myelosuppression.

Carcinogenesis: No animal carcinogenicity studies have been conducted with Cladribine.

Mutagenesis: As expected for compounds in this class, the actions of Cladribine have been shown to yield DNA damage. In mammalian cells in culture, Cladribine has been shown to cause an imbalance of intracellular deoxyribonucleotide triphosphate pools. This imbalance results in the inhibition of DNA synthesis and DNA repair, yielding DNA strand breaks and subsequently cell death. Inhibition of thymidine incorporation into human lymphoblastic cells was 90% at concentrations of 0.3µM. Cladribine was also incorporated into DNA of these cells. Cladribine was not mutagenic to bacteria and did not induce unscheduled DNA synthesis in primary rat hepatocyte cultures.

Impairment of Fertility: When administered intravenously to Cynomolgus monkeys, Cladribine has been shown to cause suppression of rapidly generating cells, including testicular cells. The effect on human fertility is unknown.

Pregnancy: Pregnancy Category D: (See *"Warnings."*)

Nursing Mothers: It is not known whether this drug is excreted in human milk. Because many drugs are excreted in human milk and because of the potential for serious adverse reactions in nursing infants from Cladribine, a decision should be made whether to discontinue nursing or discontinue the drug, taking into account the importance of the drug for the mother.

Pediatric Use: Safety and effectiveness in children has not been established. In a Phase 1 study involving patients 1-21 years old with relapsed acute leukemia, Cladribine was given by continuous intravenous infusion in doses ranging from 3 to 10.7 mg/m²/day for 5 days (one-half to twice the dose recommended in Hairy Cell Leukemia). In this study, the dose-limiting toxicity was severe myelosuppression with profound neutropenia and thrombocytopenia. At the highest dose (10.7 mg/m²/day), 3 of 7 patients developed irreversible myelosuppression and fatal systemic bacterial or fungal infections. No unique toxicities were noted in this study.[1] (See *"Warnings"* and *"Adverse Reactions."*)

ADVERSE REACTIONS

Safety data are based on 196 patients with HCL: the original cohort of 124 patients plus an additional 72 patients enrolled at the same 2 centers after the original enrollment cutoff. In Month 1 of the Hairy Cell Leukemia clinical trials, severe neutropenia was noted in 70% of patients, fever in 69%, and infection was documented in 28%. Other adverse experiences reported frequently during the first 14 days after initiating treatment included: fatigue (45%), nausea (28%), rash (27%), headache (22%) and injection site reactions (19%). Most nonhematologic adverse experiences were mild to moderate in severity.

Myelosuppression was frequently observed during the first month after starting treatment. Neutropenia (ANC < 500×10^6/L) was noted in 70% of patients, compared with 26% in whom it was present initially. Severe anemia (Hemoglobin < 8.5 g/dL) developed in 37% of patients, compared with 10% initially and thrombocytopenia (Platelets < 20×10^9/L) developed in 12% of patients, compared to 4% in whom it was noted initially.

During the first month, 54 of 196 patients (28%) exhibited documented evidence of infection. Serious infections (e.g. septicemia, pneumonia) were reported in 6% of all patients: the remainder were mild or moderate. Several deaths were attributable to infection and/or complications related to the underlying disease. During the second month, the overall rate of documented infection was 6%; these infections were mild to moderate and no severe systemic infections were seen. After the third month, the monthly incidence of infection was either less than or equal to that of the months immediately preceding Cladribine therapy.

During the first month, 11% of patients experienced severe fever (i.e. ≥ 104°F). Documented infections were noted in fewer than one-third of febrile episodes. Of the 196 patients studied, 19 were noted to have a documented infection in the month prior to treatment. In the month following treatment, there were 54 episodes of documented infection: 23 (42%) were bacterial, 11 (20%) were viral and 11 (20%) were fungal. Seven (7) of 8 documented episodes of herpes zoster occurred during the month following treatment. Fourteen (14) of 16 episodes of documented fungal infections occurred in the first two months following treatment. Virtually all of these patients were treated empirically with antibiotics. (See *"Warnings"* and *"Precautions."*)

Analysis of lymphocyte subsets indicates that treatment with Cladribine is associated with prolonged depression of the CD4 counts. Prior to treatment, the mean CD4 count was 766/μl. The mean CD4 count nadir, which occurred 4 to 6 months following treatment, was 272/μl. Fifteen (15) months after treatment, mean CD4 counts remained below 500/μl. CD8 counts behaved similarly, though increasing counts were observed after 9 months. There were no associated opportunistic infections reported during this time.

Another event of unknown clinical significance includes the observation of prolonged bone marrow hypocellularity. Bone marrow cellularity of < 35% was noted after 4 months in 42 of 124 patients (34%) treated in the two pivotal trials. This hypocellularity was noted as late as Day 1010. It is not known whether the hypocellularity is the result of disease related marrow fibrosis or if it is the result of Cladribine toxicity. There was no apparent clinical effect on the peripheral blood counts.

The vast majority of rashes were mild and occurred in patients who were receiving or had recently been treated with other medications (e.g. allopurinol or antibiotics) known to cause rash.

Most episodes of nausea were mild, not accompanied by vomiting, and did not require treatment with antiemetics. In patients requiring antiemetics, nausea was easily controlled, most frequently with chlorpromazine.

Adverse reactions reported during the first 2 weeks following treatment initiation (regardless of relationship to drug) by > 5% of patients included:

Body as a Whole: fever (69%), fatigue (45%), chills (9%), asthenia (9%), diaphoresis (9%), malaise (7%), trunk pain (6%)

Gastrointestinal: nausea (28%), decreased appetite (17%), vomiting (13%), diarrhea (10%), constipation (9%), abdominal pain (6%)

Hemic/Lymphatic: purpura (10%), petechiae (8%), epistaxis (5%)

Nervous System: headache (22%), dizziness (9%), insomnia (7%)

Cardiovascular System: edema (6%), tachycardia (6%)

Respiratory System: abnormal breath sounds (11%), cough (10%), abnormal chest sounds (9%), shortness of breath (7%)

Skin/Subcutaneous Tissue: rash (27%), injection site reactions (19%), pruritis (6%), pain (6%), erythema (6%)

Musculoskeletal System: myalgia (7%), arthralgia (5%)

Adverse experiences related to intravenous administration included: injection site reaction (9%) (i.e. redness, swelling, pain), thrombosis (2%), phlebitis (2%) and a broken catheter (1%). These appear to be related to the infusion procedure and/or indwelling catheter, rather than the medication or the vehicle.

From Day 15 to the last follow-up visit, the only events reported by > 5% of patients were: fatigue (11%), rash (10%), headache (7%), cough (7%), and malaise (5%).

For a description of adverse reactions associated with use of high doses in non-Hairy Cell Leukemia patients, see *"Warnings."*

OVERDOSAGE

High doses of Cladribine have been associated with: irreversible neurologic toxicity (paraparesis/quadriparesis), acute nephrotoxicity, and severe bone marrow suppression resulting in neutropenia, anemia and thrombocytopenia (see *"Warnings"*). There is no known specific antidote to overdosage. Treatment of overdosage consists of discontinuation of Cladribine, careful observation and appropriate supportive measures. It is not known whether the drug can be removed from the circulation by dialysis or hemofiltration.

DOSAGE AND ADMINISTRATION

Usual Dose: The recommended dose and schedule of Cladribine Injection for active Hairy Cell Leukemia is as a single course given by continuous infusion for 7 consecutive days at a dose of 0.09 mg/kg/day. Deviations from this dosage regimen are not advised. Physicians should consider delaying or discontinuing the drug if neurotoxicity or renal toxicity occurs (see *"Warnings"*).

Specific risk factors predisposing to increased toxicity from Cladribine have not been defined. In view of the known toxicities of agents of this class, it would be prudent to proceed carefully in patients with known or suspected renal insufficiency of severe bone marrow impairment of any etiology. Patients should be monitored closely for hematologic and non-hematologic toxicity (see *"Warnings"* and *"Precautions"*).

Preparation and Administration of Intravenous Solutions: Cladribine injection must be diluted with the designated diluent prior to administration. Since the drug product does not contain any anti-microbial preservative or bacteriostatic agent, **aseptic technique and proper environmental precautions must be observed in preparation of Cladribine injection solutions.**

To prepare a single daily dose: Add the calculated dose (0.09 mg/kg or 0.09 mL/kg) of Cladribine Injection to an infusion bag containing 500 mL of 0.9% Sodium Chloride Injection, USP. Infuse continuously over 24 hours. Repeat daily for a total of 7 consecutive days. **The use of 5% dextrose as a diluent is not recommended because of increased degradation of Cladribine.** Admixtures of Cladribine Injection are chemically and physically stable for at least 24 hours at room temperature under normal room fluorescent light in Baxter Viaflex † PVC infusion containers. **Since limited compatibility data are available, adherence to the recommended diluents and infusion systems is advised.**

	Dose of Cladribine Injection	Recommended Diluent	Quantity of Diluent
24 hour infusion method	1 (day) × 0.09 mg/kg	0.9% Sodium Chloride Injection, USP	500 mL

To prepare a 7-day infusion: The 7-day infusion solution should only be prepared with Bacteriostatic 0.9% Sodium Chloride Injection, USP (0.9% benzyl alcohol preserved). In order to minimize the risk of microbial contamination, both Cladribine Injection and the diluent should be passed through a sterile 0.22μ disposable hydrophilic syringe filter as each solution is being introduced into the infusion reservoir. First add the calculated dose of Cladribine Injection (7 days × 0.09 mg/kg or mL/kg) to the infusion reservoir through the sterile filter. Then add a calculated amount of Bacteriostatic 0.9% Sodium Chloride Injection, USP (0.9% benzyl alcohol preserved) also through the filter to bring the total volume of the solution to 100 mL. After completing solution preparation, clamp off the line, disconnect and discard the filter. Aseptically aspirate air bubbles from the reservoir as necessary using the syringe and a dry second sterile filter or a sterile vent filter assembly. Reclamp the line and discard the syringe and filter assembly. Infuse continuously over 7 days. Solutions prepared with Bacteriostatic Sodium Chloride Injection for individuals weighing more than 85 kg may have reduced preservative effectiveness due to greater dilution of the benzyl alcohol preservative. Admixtures for the 7-day infusion have demonstrated acceptable chemical and physical stability for at least 7 days in Pharmacia Deltec MEDICATION CASSETTES. ‡

† Viaflex® containers, manufactured by Baxter Healthcare Corporation—Code No. 2B8013 (tested in 1991)

‡ MEDICATION CASSETTE® Reservoir, manufactured by Pharmacia Deltec, Inc.— Model No. 602100A (tested in 1991)

	Dose of Cladribine Injection		Recommended Diluent	Quantity of Diluent
7-day infusion method (use sterile 0.22 µ filter when preparing infusion solution)	7 (days) 0.09 mg/kg	×	Bacteriostatic 0.9% Sodium Chloride Injection, USP (0.9% benzyl alcohol)	q.s. to 10 mL

Since limited compatibility data are available, adherence to the recommended diluents and infusion systems is advised. Solutions containing Cladribine Injection should not be mixed with other intravenous drugs or additives or infused simultaneously via a common intravenous line, since compatibility testing has not been performed. Preparations containing benzyl alcohol should not be used in neonates (see *"Warnings"*).

Care must be taken to assure the sterility of prepared solutions. Once diluted, solutions of Cladribine injection should be administered promptly or stored in the refrigerator (2° to 8°C) for no more than 8 hours prior to start of administration. Vials of Cladribine Injection are for single-use only. Any unused portion should be discarded in an appropriate manner (see "Handling and Disposal").

Parenteral drug products should be inspected visually for particulate matter and discoloration prior to administration, whenever solution and container permit. A precipitate may occur during the exposure of Cladribine Injection to low temperatures; it may be resolubilized by allowing the solution to warm naturally to room temperature and by shaking vigorously. **DO NOT HEAT OR MICROWAVE.**

Chemical Stability of Vials: When stored in refrigerated conditions between 2° to 8°C (36° to 46°F) protected from light, unopened vials of Cladribine Injection are stable until the expiration date indicated on the package. Freezing does not adversely affect the solution. If freezing occurs, thaw naturally to room temperature. DO NOT heat or microwave. Once thawed, the vial of Cladribine Injection is stable until expiry if refrigerated. DO NOT refreeze. Once diluted, solutions containing Cladribine Injection should be administered promptly or stored in the refrigerator (2° to 8°C) for no more than 8 hours prior to administration.

Handling and Disposal: The potential hazards associated with cytotoxic agents are well established and proper precautions should be taken when handling, preparing, and administering Cladribine Injection. The use of disposable gloves and protective garments is recommended. If Cladribine Injection contacts the skin or mucous membranes, wash the involved surface immediately with copious amounts of water. Several guidelines on this subject have been published.[2-8] There is no general agreement that all of the procedures recommended in the guidelines are necessary or appropriate. Refer to your institution's guidelines and all applicable state/local regulations for disposal of cytotoxic waste.

Storage: Store refrigerated 2° to 8°C (36° to 46°F). Protect from light during storage.

REFERENCES:
1. Santana VM, Mirro J, Harwood FC, *et al*: A phase 1 clinical trial of 2-Chlorodeoxyadenosine in pediatric patients with acute leukemia. *J. Clin. Onc.*, **9**:416 (1991). 2. Recommendations for the Safe Handling of Parenteral Antineoplastic Drugs. NIH Publication No. 83-2621. For sale by the Superintendent of Documents, U.S. Government Printing Office, Washington, D.C. 20402. 3. AMA Council Report Guidelines for Handling Parenteral Antineoplastics, *JAMA*, March 15 (1985). 4. National Study Commission on Cytotoxic Exposure—Recommendations for Handling Cytotoxic Agents. Available from Louis P. Jeffrey, Sc.D., Chairman, National Study Commission on Cytotoxic Exposure, Massachusetts College of Pharmacy and Allied Health Sciences, 179 Longwood Avenue, Boston, Massachusetts 02115. 5. Clinical Oncological Society of Australia: Guidelines and Recommendations for Safe Handling of Antineoplastic Agents. *Med. J. Australia* **1**:425 (1983). 6. Jones RB, *et al*. Safe Handling of Chemotherapeutic Agents: A Report from the Mount Sinai Medical Center. *Ca-A Cancer Journal for Clinicians*, Sept/Oct. 258-263 (1983). 7. American Society of Hospital Pharmacists Technical Assistance Bulletin on Handling Cytotoxic Drugs in Hospitals. *Am.J. Hosp. Pharm.*, **42**:131 (1985). 8. OSHA Work-Practice Guidelines for Personnel Dealing with Cytotoxic (antineoplastic) Drugs, *Am. J. Hosp. Pharm.*, **43**:1193 (1986).

HOW SUPPLIED
INJECTION: 1 MG/ML

BRAND/MANUFACTURER	NDC	SIZE	AWP
○ **BRAND** LEUSTATIN: Ortho Biotech	59676-0201-01	10 ml	$480.00

Claforan *SEE* **CEFOTAXIME SODIUM**

Clarithromycin

DESCRIPTION
Clarithromycin is a semi-synthetic macrolide antibiotic. Chemically, it is 6-0-Methylerythromycin. The molecular formula is $C_{38}H_{69}NO_{13}$, and the molecular weight is 747.96. Clarithromycin is a white to off-white crystalline powder. It is soluble in acetone, slightly soluble in methanol, ethanol and acetonitrile, and practically insoluble in water.

Each Clarithromycin is available as tablets and granules for oral suspension. Clarithromycin tablet contains 250 mg or 500 mg of Clarithromycin for oral administration.

After constitution, each 5 mL of Clarithromycin suspension contains 125 mg or 250 mg Clarithromycin. Each bottle of Clarithromycin granules contains 2500 mg (100 mL size) or 5000 mg (100 and 200 mL sizes) of Clarithromycin.

Following is its chemical structure:

CLINICAL PHARMACOLOGY
Clarithromycin is rapidly absorbed from the gastrointestinal tract after oral administration. The absolute bioavailability of 250 mg Clarithromycin tablets was approximately 50%. Food slightly delays both the onset of Clarithromycin absorption and the formation of the antimicrobially active metabolite, 14-OH Clarithromycin, but does not affect the extent of bioavailability. Therefore, Clarithromycin tablets may be given without regard to meals.

In fasting healthy human subjects, peak serum concentrations were attained within 2 hours after oral dosing. Steady-state peak serum Clarithromycin concentrations were attained in 2 to 3 days and were approximately 1 µg/mL with a 250 mg dose administered every 12 hours and 2 to 3 µg/mL with a 500 mg dose administered every 12 hours. The elimination half-life of Clarithromycin was about 3 to 4 hours with 250 mg administered every 12 hours but increased to 5 to 7 hours with 500 mg administered every 12 hours. The nonlinearity of Clarithromycin pharmacokinetics is slight at the recommended doses of 250 mg and 500 mg administered every 12 hours. With a 250 mg every 12 hours dosing, the principal metabolite, 14-OH Clarithromycin, attains a peak steady-state concentration about 0.6 µg/mL and has an elimination half-life of 5 to 6 hours. With a 500 mg every 12 hours, the peak steady-state concentrations of 14-OH Clarithromycin are slightly higher (up to 1 mcg/mL), and its elimination half-life is about 7 hours. With either dose, the steady-state concentration of this metabolite is generally attained within 2 to 3 days.

After a 250 mg tablet every 12 hours, approximately 20% of the dose is excreted in the urine as Clarithromycin, while after a 500 mg tablet every 12 hours dosing, the urinary excretion of Clarithromycin is somewhat greater, approximately 30%. In comparison, after an oral dose of 250 mg (125 mg/5 mL) suspension every 12 hours approximately 40% is excreted in urine as Clarithromycin. The renal clearance of Clarithromycin is, however, relatively independent of the dose size and approximates the normal glomerular filtration rate. The major metabolite found in the urine is 14-OH Clarithromycin which accounts for an additional 10% to 15% of the dose with either 250 mg or 500 mg tablet administered every 12 hours.

Steady-state concentrations of Clarithromycin and 14-OH Clarithromycin observed following administration of 500 mg doses of Clarithromycin every 12 hours to adult patients with HIV infection were similar to those observed in healthy volunteers. In adult HIV-infected patients taking 500 and 1000 mg doses of Clarithromycin every 12 hours, steady-state Clarithromycin C_{max} values ranged from 2-4 µg/mL and 5-10 µg/mL respectively.

The steady-state concentrations of Clarithromycin in subjects with impaired hepatic function did not differ from those in normal subjects; however, the 14-OH Clarithromycin concentrations were lower in the hepatically impaired subjects. The decreased formation of 14-OH Clarithromycin was at least partially offset by an increase in renal clearance of Clarithromycin in the subjects with impaired hepatic function when compared to healthy subjects.

The pharmacokinetics of Clarithromycin were also altered in subjects with impaired renal function. (See *"Precautions"* and *"Dosage and Administration."*)

Clarithromycin and the 14-OH Clarithromycin metabolite distribute readily into body tissues and fluids. There are no data available on cerebrospinal fluid penetration. Because of high intracellular concentrations, tissue concentrations are higher than serum concentrations. Examples from tissue and serum concentrations are presented below.

CONCENTRATION (AFTER 250 MG Q 12H)

Tissue Type	Tissue (µg/g)	Serum (µg/mL)
Tonsil	1.6	0.8
Lung	8.8	1.7

When 250 mg doses of Clarithromycin suspension were administered to fasting healthy adult subjects, peak plasma concentrations were attained around 3 hours after dosing. Steady-state peak plasma concentrations were attained in 2 to 3 days and were approximately 2 µg/mL for Clarithromycin and 0.7 µg/mL for 14-OH Clarithromycin when 250 mg doses of the Clarithromycin suspension were administered every 12 hours. Elimination half-lives for Clarithromycin (3 to 4 hours) and 14-OH Clarithromycin (5 to 7 hours) were similar to those observed at steady-state following administration of equivalent doses of Clarithromycin tablets. For adult patients the bioavailability of 10 mL of the 125 mg/5 mL suspension or 10 mL of the 250 mg/5 mL suspension is similar to a 250 mg or 500 mg tablet, respectively.

In children requiring antibiotic therapy, administration of 7.5 mg/kg BID doses of Clarithromycin as the suspension generally resulted in steady-state peak plasma concentrations of 3 to 7 µg/mL for Clarithromycin and 1 to 2 µg/mL for 14-OH Clarithromycin.

In HIV-infected children taking 15 mg/kg every 12 hours, steady-state Clarithromycin peak concentrations generally ranged from 6-15 µg/mL.

In adults given 250 mg Clarithromycin as the suspension (n = 22), food appeared to decrease mean peak plasma Clarithromycin concentration by 23% and the extent of absorption by 10%. When children (n = 10) were administered a single oral dose of 7.5 mg/kg suspension, food appeared to increase mean peak plasma Clarithromycin concentrations by 27% and the extent of absorption by 42%.

MICROBIOLOGY

Clarithromycin exerts its antibacterial action by binding to the 50S ribosomal subunit of susceptible organisms and inhibiting protein synthesis.

Clarithromycin is active *in vitro* against a variety of aerobic and anaerobic gram-positive and gram-negative organisms as well as most *Mycobacterium avium* complex (MAC) organisms. Additionally, the 14-OH Clarithromycin metabolite also has clinically significant antimicrobial activity. Against *Haemophilus influenzae* organisms, 14-OH Clarithromycin is twice as active as the parent compound. However, for *Mycobacterium avium* complex (MAC) isolates the 14-OH metabolite was 4 to 7 times less active than Clarithromycin. The clinical significance of this activity against *Mycobacterium avium* complex is unknown.

Clarithromycin has been shown to be active against most strains of the following organisms both *in vitro* and in clinical infections: (See *"Indications and Usage."*)

GRAM-POSITIVE AEROBES
Staphylococcus aureus
Streptococcus pneumoniae
Streptococcus pyogenes

GRAM-NEGATIVE AEROBES
Haemophilus influenzae
Moraxella (Branhamella) catarrhalis

OTHER AEROBES
Mycoplasma pneumoniae

MYCOBACTERIE
Mycobacterium avium complex (MAC) consisting of:
   Mycobacterium avium
   Mycobacterium intracellulare

Beta-lactamase production should have no effect on clarithromycin activity.

Note: Most strains of methicillin-resistant and oxacillin-resistant staphylococci are resistant to Clarithromycin.

Clarithromycin has been shown to be active *in vitro* against most strains of the following organisms. The following *in vitro* data are available; however, their clinical significance is unknown.

GRAM-POSITIVE AEROBES
Listeria monocytogenes
Streptococcus agalactiae
Streptococci (Groups C, F, G)
Viridans group streptococci

GRAM-NEGATIVE AEROBES
Bordetella pertussis
Campylobacter jejuni
Legionella pneumophila
Neisseria gonorrhoeae
Pasteurella multocida

OTHER AEROBES
Chlamydia trachomatis

GRAM-POSITIVE ANAEROBES
Clostridium perfringens
Peptococcus niger
Propionibacterium acnes

GRAM-NEGATIVE ANAEROBES
Bacteroides melaninogenicus

SUSCEPTIBILITY TESTING EXCLUDING MYCOBACTERIA
Diffusion Techniques: Quantitative methods that require measurement of zone diameters give the most precise estimate of the susceptibility of bacteria to antimicrobial agents. One such standard procedure[1] which has been recommended for use with disks to test susceptibility of organisms to Clarithromycin, uses the 15-µg disk. Interpretation involves the correlation of the diameter obtained in the disk test with minimum inhibitory concentration (MIC) for Clarithromycin.

Reports from the laboratory giving results of the standard single-disk susceptibility test with a 15-µg Clarithromycin disk should be interpreted according to the following criteria:

Zone Diameter (mm)	Interpretation
≥ 18	(S) Susceptible
14-17	(I) Intermediate
≤ 13	(R) Resistant

A report of "Susceptible" indicates that the pathogen is likely to respond to monotherapy with Clarithromycin.

A report of "Intermediate" indicates that the result be considered equivocal and, if the organism is not fully susceptible to alternative clinically feasible drugs, the test should be repeated. This category provides a buffer zone which prevents small uncontrolled technical factors from causing major discrepancies in interpretations.

However, standardized diffusion methods for routine *in vitro* susceptibility testing, using the 15-µg Clarithromycin disk, do not measure the additive antimicrobial activity of the 14-OH metabolite and thus may underestimate the drug's potential activity against *Haemophilus influenzae*, *Haemophilus influenzae* isolates falling into the "Intermediate" category often respond to treatment.

A report of "Resistant" indicates that achievable drug concentrations are unlikely to be inhibitory, and other therapy should be selected.

Standardized procedures require the use of laboratory control organisms. The 15-µg Clarithromycin disk should give the following zone diameters:

Organism	Zone Diameter (mm)
S. aureus ATCC 25933	23-30

Dilution Techniques: Use a standardized dilution method[2] (broth, agar, microdilution) or equivalent with Clarithromycin powder. The MIC values obtained should be interpreted according to the following criteria:

MIC (µg/mL)	Interpretation
≤ 2.0	(S) Susceptible
4.0	(I) Intermediate
≥ 8.0	(R) Resistant

As with standard diffusion techniques, dilution methods require the use of laboratory control organisms. Standard Clarithromycin powder should provide the following MIC values:

Organism	MIC (µg/mL)
S. aureus ATCC 29213	0.06-0.25
E. faecalis ATCC 29212	0.25-1.0

In vitro Activity of Clarithromycin against Mycobacteria: Clarithromycin has demonstrated *in vitro* activity against *Mycobacterium avium* complex (MAC) organisms isolated from both AIDS and non-AIDS patients. While gene probe techniques may be used to distinguish *M. avium* species from *M. intracellulare*, many studies only reported results on *M. avium* complex (MAC) isolates.

Various *in vitro* methodologies employing broth or solid media at different pHs, with and without oleic acid-albumin-dextrose-catalose (OADC), have been used to determine Clarithromycin MIC values for mycobacterial species. In general, MIC values decreased more than 16 fold as the pH of Middlebrook 7H12 broth media increased from 5.0 to 7.4. At pH 7.4, MIC values determined with Mueller-Hinton agar were 4-8 fold higher than that observed with Middlebrook 7H12 media. Utilization of oleic acid-albumin-dextrose-catalose (OADC) in these assays has been shown to further alter MIC values.

Clarithromycin activity against 80 MAC isolates from AIDS patients and 211 MAC isolates from non-AIDS patients was evaluated using a microdilution method with Middlebrook 7H9 broth. Results showed an MIC value of ≤ 4.0 µg/mL in 81% and 89% of the AIDS and non-AIDS MAC isolates, respectively. Twelve percent of the non-AIDS isolates had an MIC value ≤ 0.5 µg/mL. Clarithromycin was also shown to be active against phagocytized *M. avium* complex (MAC) in mouse and human macrophage cell cultures as well as in the beige mouse infection model.

Clarithromycin activity was evaluated against *Mycobacterium tuberculosis* organisms. In one study, utilizing the agar dilution method with Middlebrook 7H10 media, 3 of 30 clinical isolates had an MIC of 2.5 µg/mL. Clarithromycin inhibited all isolates at > 10.0 µg/mL.

Susceptibility Testing for Mycobacterium Avium Complex (MAC): The disk diffusion techniques and dilution methods for susceptibility testing against gram-positive and gram-negative bacteria should not be used for determining Clarithromycin MIC values against mycobacteria. *In vitro* susceptibility testing methods and diagnostic products currently available for determining minimum inhibitory concentration (MIC) values against *Mycobacterium avium* complex (MAC) organisms have not been standardized or validated. Clarithromycin MIC values will vary depending on the susceptibility testing method employed, composition and pH of media, and the utilization of nutritional supplements. Breakpoints to determine whether clinical isolates of *M. avium* or *M. intracelulare* are susceptibile or resistant to Clarithromycin have not been established.

INDICATIONS AND USAGE
Clarithromycin is indicated for the treatment of mild to moderate infections caused by susceptible strains of the designated microorganisms in the conditions listed below:
Upper Respiratory Tract Infections
 Pharyngitis/Tonsillitis due to *Streptococcus pyogenes*
 Acute maxillary sinusitis due to *Streptococcus pneumoniae*
Lower Respiratory Tract Infections
 Acute bacterial exacerbation of chronic bronchitis due to *Haemophilus influenzae*, *Moraxella catarrhalis*, or *Streptococcus pneumoniae*
Pneumonia due to *Myocoplasma pneumoniae*, or *Streptococcus pneumoniae*
Uncomplicated Skin and Skin Structure Infections due to *Straphylococcus aureus*, or *Streptococcus pyogenes*. Abscesses usually require surgical drainage.
Clarithromycin is indicated for the treatment of disseminated mycobacterial infections due to *Mycobacterium avium* and *Mycobacterium intracellulare*.

UNLABELED USES
Clarithiromycin is used alone or as an adjunct in the treatment of pertussis.

CONTRAINDICATIONS
Clarithromycin is contraindicated in patients with known hypersensitivity to Clarithromycin, erythromycin, or any of the macrolide antibiotics.

WARNINGS
CLARITHROMYCIN SHOULD NOT BE USED IN PREGNANT WOMEN EXCEPT IN CLINICAL CIRCUMSTANCES WHERE NO ALTERNATIVE THERAPY IS APPROPRIATE. IF PREGNANCY OCCURS WHILE TAKING THIS DRUG, THE PATIENT SHOULD BE APPRISED OF THE POTENTIAL HAZARD TO THE FETUS. CLARITHROMYCIN HAS DEMONSTRATED ADVERSE EFFECTS ON PREGNANCY OUTCOME AND/OR EMBRYO-FETAL DEVELOPMENT IN MONKEYS, RATS, MICE, AND RABBITS AT DOSES THAT PRODUCED PLASMA LEVELS 2 TO 17 TIMES THE SERUM LEVELS ACHIEVED IN HUMANS TREATED AT THE MAXIMUM RECOMMENDED HUMAN DOSES. (SEE "PREGNANCY.")
Pseudomembranous colitis has been reported with nearly all antibacterial agents, including macrolides, and may range in severity from mild to life threatening. Therefore, it is important to consider this diagnosis in patients who present with diarrhea subsequent to the administration of antibacterial agents.
Treatment with antibacterial agents alters the normal flora of the colon and may permit overgrowth of clostridia. Studies indicate that a toxin produced by *Clostridium difficile* is a primary cause of "antibiotic-associated colitis."
After the diagnosis of pseudomembranous colitis has been established, therapeutic measures should be initiated. Mild cases of pseudomembranous colitis usually respond to discontinuation of the drug alone. In moderate to severe cases, consideration should be given to management with fluids and electrolyes, protein supplementation, and treatment with an antibacterial drug effective against *Clostridium difficile*.

PRECAUTIONS
General: Clarithiromycin is principally excreted via the liver and kidney. Clarithromycin may be administered without dosage adjustment to patients with hepatic impairment and normal renal function. However, in the presence of severe renal impairment with or without coexisting hepatic impairment, decreased dosage or prolonged dosing intervals may be appropriate.

Drug Interactions: Clarithromycin use in patients who are receiving theophylline may be associated with an increase of serum theophylline concentrations. Monitoring of serum theophylline concentrations should be considered for patients receiving high doses of theophylline or with baseline concentrations in the upper therapeutic range. In two studies in which theophylline was administered with Clarithromycin (a theophylline sustained-release formulation was dosed at either 6.5 mg/kg or 12 mg/kg together with 250 mg or 500 mg q 12 h Clarithromycin), the steady-state levels of C_{max}, C_{min}, and the area under the serum concentration time curve (AUC) increased about 20%.
Single-dose administration of Clarithromycin has been shown to result in increased concentrations of carbamazepine. Blood level monitoring of carbamazepine may be considered.
When Clarithromycin and terfenadine were coadministered, plasma concentrations of the active acid metabolite of terfenadine, were three-fold higher, on average, than the values observed when terfenadine was administered alone. The pharmacokinetics of Clarithromycin and 14(R)-hydroxy-clarithromycin were not significantly affected by coadministration of terfenadine once Clarithromycin reached steady-state conditions.
Simultaneous oral administration of Clarithroycin tablets and zidovudine to HIV-infected adult patients resulted in decreased steady-state zidovudine concentrations. When 500 mg of Clarithromycin was administered twice daily, steady state zidovudine AUC was reduced by a mean of 12% (n=4). Individual values ranged from a decrease of 34% to an increase of 14%.
The following drug interactions, other than increased serum concentrations of carbamazepine and active acid metabolite of terfenadine, have not been reported

in clinical trials with Clarithromycin; however, they have been observed with erythromycin products:
Concomitant administration of erythromycin and digoxin has been reported to result in elevated digoxin levels.
There have been reports of increased anticoagulant effects when erythromycin and oral anticoagulants were used concomitantly.
Concurrent use of erythromycin and ergotamine or dihydroergotamine has been associated in some patients with acute ergot toxicity characterized by severe peripheral vasospasm and dysesthesia.
The use of erythromycin in patients concurrently taking drugs metabolized by the cytochrome P450 system may be associated with elevations in serum levels of these other drugs. There have been reports of interactions of erythromycin with carbamazepine, cyclosporine, hexobarbital, and phenytoin. Serum concentrations of drugs metabolized by the cytochrome P450 system should be monitored closely in patients concurrently receiving erythromycin.

Carcinogenesis, Mutagenesis, Impairment of Fertility: The following *in vitro* mutagenicity tests have been conducted with Clarithromycin:

Salmonella/Mammalian Microsomes Test
Bacterial Induced Mutation Frequency Test
In vitro Chromosome Aberration Test
Rat Hepatocyte DNA Synthesis Assay
Mouse Lymphoma Assay
Mouse Dominant Lethal Study
Mouse Micronucleus Test

All tests had negative results except the *In Vitro* Chromosome Aberration Test which was weakly positive in one test and negative in another.
In addition, a Bacterial Reserve-Mutation Test (Ames Test) has been performed on Clarithromycin metabolites with negative results.
Fertility and reproduction studies have shown that daily doses of 150-160 mg/kg/day to male and female rats caused no adverse effects on the estrous cycle, fertility, parturition, or number and viability of offspring. Plasma levels in rats after 150 mg/kg/day were 2 times the human serum levels. In the 150 mg/kg/day monkey studies, plasma levels were 3 times the human serum levels. When given orally at 150 mg/kg/day, Clarithromycin was shown to produce embryonic loss in monkeys. This effect has been attributed to marked maternal toxicity of the drug at this high dose.
In rabbits, *in utero* fetal loss occurred at an intravenous dose of 33 mg/m^2, which is 17 times less than the maximum proposed human oral daily dose of 618 mg/m^2.
Long-term studies in animals have not been performed to evaluate carcinogenic potential.

Pregnancy: Teratogenic Effects: Pregnancy Category C. Four teratogenicity studies in rats (three with oral doses and one with intravenous doses up to 160 mg/kg/day administered during the period of major organogenesis) and two in rabbits (at oral doses up to 125 mg/kg/day or intravenous doses of 30 mg/kg/day administered during gestation days 6 to 18) failed to demonstrate any teratogenicity from Clarithromycin. Two additional oral studies in a different rat strain at similar doses and similar conditions demonstrated a low incidence of cardiovascular anomalies at doses of 150 mg/kg/day administered during gestation days 6 to 15. Plasma levels after 150 mg/kg/day were 2 times the human serum levels. Four studies in mice revealed a variable incidence of cleft palate following oral doses of 1000 mg/kg/day during gestation days 6 to 15. Cleft palate was also seen at 500 mg/kg/day. The 1000 mg/kg/day exposure resulted in plasma levels 17 times the human serum levels. In monkeys, an oral dose of 70 mg/kg/day produced fetal growth retardation at plasma levels that were 2 times the human serum levels.
There are no adequate and well-controlled studies in pregnant women. Clarithromycin should be used during pregnancy only if the potential benefit justifies the potential risk to the fetus. (See "Warnings.")

Nursing Mothers: It is not known whether Clarithromycin is excreted in human milk. Because many drugs are excreted in human milk, caution should be exercised when Clarithromycin is administered to a nursing woman. It is known that Clarithromycin is excreted in the milk of lactating animals and that other drugs of this class are excreted in human milk.
Preweaned rats, exposed indirectly via consumption of milk from dams treated with 150 mg/kg/day for 3 weeks, were not adversely affected, despite data indicating higher drug levels in milk than in plasma.

Pediatric Use: Safety and effectiveness of Clarithromycin in children under 6-months of age have not been established.
The safety of Clarithromycin has not been studied in MAC patients under the age of 20 months. Neonatal and juvenile animals tolerated Clarithromytcin in a manner similar to adult animals. Young animals were slightly more intolerant to acute overdosage and to subtle reductions in erythrocytes, platelets and leukocytes, but were less sensitive to toxicity in the liver, kidney, thymus and genitalia.

Geriatric Use: In a steady-state study in which healthy elderly subjects (age 65 to 81 years old) were given 500 mg every 12 hours, the maximum concentrations of Clarithromycin and 14-OH Clarithromycin were increased. The AUC was also increased. These changes in pharmacokinetics parallel known age-related decreases in renal function. In clinical trials, elderly patients did not have an increased incidence of adverse events when compared to younger patients. Dosage adjustment should be considered in the elderly patients with severe renal impairment.

ADVERSE REACTIONS

The majority of side effects observed in clinical trials were of a mild and transient nature. Fewer than 3% of adult patients without mycobacterial infections discontinued therapy because of drug-related side effects.

The most frequently reported events in adults, whether drug-related or not, were diarrhea (3%), nausea (3%), abnormal taste (3%), dyspepsia (2%), abdominal pain/discomfort (2%), and headache (2%). Most of these events were described as mild or moderate in severity. Of the reported adverse events, only 1% were described as severe.

In studies of pneumonia comparing Clarithromycin to erythromycin base or erythromycin stearate, there were fewer adverse events involving the digestive system in Clarithromycin-treated patients compared to erythyromycin-treated patients (13% vs 32%; p < 0.01). Twenty percent of erythromycin-treated patients discontinued therapy due to adverse events compared to 4% of Clarithromycin-treated patients. The following adverse events have been reported with erythromycin products but not in clinical trials of Clarithromycin: Rarely, erythromycin has been associated with ventricular arrhythmias, including ventricular tachycardia, and torsades de pointes, in individuals with prolonged QT intervals.

Changes in Laboratory Values: Changes in laboratory values with possible clinical significance were as follows:

Hepatic—Elevated SGPT (ALT) < 1%, SGOT (AST) < 1%, GGT < 1%, alkaline phosphatase < 1%, LDH < 1%, and total billirubin < 1%.
Hematologic—Decreased WBC < 1%, and elevated prothrombin time 1%.
Renal—Elevated BUN 4%, and elevated serum creatinine < 1%.

DOSAGE AND ADMINISTRATION

Clarithromycin tablets or suspension may be given with or without meals.

ADULT DOSAGE GUIDELINES

Infection	Dosage (q 12 h)	Normal Duration (days)
Upper respiratory tract	250-500 mg	10-14
Pharyngitis/Tonsillitis	250 mg	10
Acute maxillary sinusitis	500 mg	14
Lower respiratory tract	250-500 mg	7-14
Acute exacerbation of chronic bronchitis due to:		
S. pneumoniae	250 mg	7-14
M. catarrhalis	250 mg	7-14
H. influenzae	500 mg	7-14
Pneumonia due to:		
S. pneumoniae	250 mg	7-14
M. pneumoniae	250 mg	7-14
Uncomplicated skin and skin structure	250 mg	7-14

Beta-lactamase production should have no effect on Clarithromycin activity.

Clarithromycin may be administered without dosage adjustment in the presence of hepatic impairment if there is normal renal function. However, in the presence of severe renal impairment with or without coexisting hepatic impairment, decreased doses or prolongation of dosing intervals may be appropriate.

Mycobacterial Infections: Clarithromycin is recommended as the primary agent for the treatment of disseminated infection due to *Mycobacterium avium* complex. Clarithromycin should be used in combination with other antimycobacterial drugs which have shown in vitro activity against MAC, including ethambutol, clofazimine, and rifampin. Although no controlled clinical trial information is available for combination therapy with Clarithromycin, the U.S. Public Health Service Task Force has provided recommendations for the treatment of MAC.[4] The recommended dose for mycobacterial infections in adults is 500 mg BID. In children, the recommended dose is 7.5 mg/kg BID up to 500 mg BID. Dosing recommendations for children are in the table below.

PEDIATRIC DOSAGE GUIDELINES FOR MYCOBACTERIAL INFECTIONS ONLY

	Based on Body Weight			
		Dosing Calculated on 7.5 mg/kg BID		
Weight		Dose (BID)	125 mg/ 5 mL	250 mg/ 5 mL
kg	lbs			
9	20	62.5 mg	2.5 mL BID	1.25 mL BID
17	37	125 mg	5 mL BID	2.5 mL BID
25	55	187.5 mg	7.5 mL BID	3.75 mL BID
33	73	250 mg	10 mL BID	5 mL BID

Clarithromycin therapy should continue for life if clinical and mycobacterial improvement are observed.

CONSTITUTING INSTRUCTIONS
The table below indicates the volume of water to be added when constituting:

Total volume after constitution	Clarithromycin concentration after constitution	Amount of water to be added*
100 mL	125 mg/5 mL	56 mL
200 mL	125 mg/5 mL	113 mL
100 mL	250 mg/5 mL	55 mL

* *See instructions below.*

Add half the volume of water to the bottle and shake vigorously. Add the remainder of water to the bottle and shake. Shake well before each use. Keep tightly closed.

Do not refrigerate. After mixing, store at 15° to 30°C (59° to 86°F) and use within 14 days. Store tablets at controlled room temperature 15° to 30°C (59° to 86°F) in a well-closed container. Protect from light.

INFORMATION TO PATIENTS
Clarithromycin suspension can be taken with or without meals, and can be taken with milk. Do **NOT** refrigerate the suspension.

CLINICAL STUDIES
MYCOBACTERIAL INFECTIONS
Three randomized studies (500, 577, and 521) compared different dosages of Clarithromycin in patients with CDC-defined AIDS and CD4 counts < 100 cells/μL. These studies accrued patients from May 1991 to March 1992. Study 500 was randomized, double-blind; Study 577 was open-label compassionate use. Both studies used 500 and 1000 mg BID doses; Study 500 also had a 2000 mg BID group. Study 521 was a pediatric study at 3.75, 7.5 and 15 mg/kg BID. Study 500 enrolled 154 adult patients, Study 577 enrolled 469 adult patients, and Study 521 enrolled 25 patients between the ages of 1-20. The majority of patients had CD4 cell counts < 50/μL at study entry. The studies were designed to evaluate the following end points: 1. Change in MAC bacteremia or blood cultures negative for *M. avium.*

2. Change in clinical signs and symptoms of MAC infection including one or more of the following: fever, night sweats, weight loss, diarrhea, splenomegaly, and hepatomegaly.

The results for the 500 study are described below. The 577 study results were similar to the results of the 500 study. Results with the 7.5 mg/kg BID dose in the pediatric study were comparable to those for the 500 mg BID regimen in the adult studies.

MAC BACTEREMIA
Decreases in MAC bacteremia or negative blood cultures were seen in the majority of patients in all dose groups. Mean reductions in colony forming units (CFU) are shown below. Included in the table are results from a separate study with a four drug regimen[3] (ciprofloxacin, ethambutol, rifampicin, and clofazimine). Since patient populations and study procedures may vary between these two studies, comparisons between the Clarithromycin results and the combination therapy results should be interpreted cautiously.

MEAN REDUCTIONS IN LOG CFU FROM BASELINE (AFTER 4 WEEKS OF THERAPY)

500 mg BID (N = 35)	1000 mg BID (N = 32)	2000 mg BID (N = 26)	Four Drug Regimen (N = 24)
1.5	2.3	2.3	1.4

Although the 1000 mg and 2000 mg BID doses showed significantly better control of bacteremia during the first four weeks of therapy, no significant differences were seen beyond that point. The percent of patients whose blood was sterilized as shown by one or more negative cultures at any time during acute therapy was 61% (30/49) for the 500 mg BID group and 59% (29/49) and 52% (25/48) for the 1000 and 2000 mg BID groups, respectively. The percent of patients who had 2 or more negative cultures during acute therapy which were sustained through study Day 84 was 25% (12/49) in both the 500 and 1000 mg BID groups and 8% (4/48) for the 2000 mg BID group. By Day 84, 23% (11/49), 37% (18/ 49), and 56% (27/48) of patients had died or discontinued from the study, and 14% (7/49), 12% (6/49), and 13% (6/48) of patients had relapsed in the 500, 1000, and 2000 mg BID dose groups, respectively. All of the isolates had an MIC < 8 μg/mL at pretreatment. Relapse was almost always accompanied by an increase in MIC. The median time to first negative culture was 54, 41, and 29 days with the 500, 1000, and 2000 mg BID groups, respectively. The time to first decrease of at least 1 log in CFU count was significantly shorter with the 1000 and 2000 mg BID doses (median equal to 16 and 15 days respectively) in comparison to the 500 mg BID group (median equal to 29 days). The median time to first positive culture or study discontinuation following the first negative culture was 43, 59 and 43 days for the 500, 1000, and 2000 mg BID groups respectively.

CLINICALLY SIGNIFICANT DISSEMINATED MAC DISEASE
Among patients experiencing night sweats prior to therapy, 84% showed resolution or improvement at some point during the 12 weeks of Clarithromycin at 500-2000 mg BID doses. Similarly, 77% of patients reported resolution or improvement in fevers at some point. Response rates for clinical signs of MAC are given below:

◆ RATED THERAPEUTICALLY EQUIVALENT; ◇ THERAPEUTIC EQUIVALENCE UNCONFIRMED; ○ UNRATED

Resolution of Fever			Resolution of Night Sweats		
BID Dose (mg)	% ever afebrile	% afebrile ≥ 6 weeks	BID Dose (mg)	% ever resolving	% resolving ≥ 6 weeks
500	67%	23%	500	85%	42%
1000	67%	12%	1000	70%	33%
2000	62%	22%	2000	72%	36%

Weight Gain > 3%			Hemoglobin Increase > 1 gm		
BID Dose (mg)	% ever gaining	% gaining ≥ 6 weeks	BID Dose (mg)	% ever increasing	% increasing ≥ 6 weeks
500	33%	14%	500	58%	26%
1000	26%	17%	1000	37%	6%
2000	26%	12%	2000	62%	18%

The median duration of response, defined as improvement or resolution of clinical signs and symptoms, was 2-6 weeks. Since the study was not designed to determine the benefit of monotherapy beyond 12 weeks, the duration of response may be underestimated for the 25-33% of patients who continued to show clinical response after 12 weeks.

SURVIVAL
Median survival time from study entry (study 500) was 249 days at the 500 mg BID dose compared to 215 days with the 1000 mg BID dose. However, during the first 12 weeks of therapy there were 2 deaths in 53 patients in the 500 mg BID group versus 13 deaths in 51 patients in the 1000 mg BID group. The reason for this apparent mortality difference is not known. Survival in the two groups was similar beyond 12 weeks. The median survival times for these dosages were similar to recent historical controls with MAC when treated with combination therapies.[3]

Median survival time from study entry in Study 577 was 199 days for the 500 mg BID dose and 179 days for the 1000 mg BID dose. During the first 4 weeks of therapy, while patients were maintained on their originally assigned dose, there were 11 deaths in 255 patients taking 500 mg BID and 18 deaths in 214 patients taking 1000 mg BID.

SAFETY
The adverse event profiles showed that both the 500 and 1000 mg BID doses were well tolerated. The 2000 mg BID dose was poorly tolerated and resulted in a higher proportion of premature discontinuations.

In AIDS and other immunocomprised patients treated with the higher doses of Clarithromycin over long periods of time for mycobacterial infections, it was often difficult to distinguish adverse events possibly associated with Clarithromycin administration from underlying signs of HIV disease or intercurrent illness.

The following analyses summarize experience during the first 12 weeks of therapy with Clarithromycin. Data are reported separately for Study 500 (randomized, double-blind) and Study 577 (open-label, compassionate use) and also combined. Adverse events were reported less frequently in Study 577, which may be due in part to differences in monitoring between the two studies. In adult patients receiving Clarithromycin 500 mg BID, the most frequently reported adverse events, considered possibly or probably related to study drug, with an incidence of 5% or greater are listed below. Most of these events were mild to moderate in severity, although 5% (Study 500: 8%; Study 577: 4%) of patients receiving 500 mg BID and 5% (Study 500: 4%; Study 577: 6%) of patients receiving 1000 mg BID reported severe adverse events. Excluding those patients who discontinued therapy or died due to complications of their underlying non-mycobacterial disease, approximately 8% (Study 500: 15%; Study 577: 7%) of the patients who received 500 mg BID and 12% (Study 500: 14%; Study 577: 12%) of the patients who received 1000 mg BID discontinued therapy due to drug-related events during the first 12 weeks of therapy. Overall, the 500 and 1000 mg BID doses had similar adverse event profiles.

TREATMENT-RELATED* ADVERSE EVENT INCIDENCE RATES IN IMMUNOCOMPRISED ADULT PATIENTS DURING THE FIRST 12 WEEKS OF THERAPY WITH 500 MG BID CLARITHROMYCIN DOSE

Adverse Event	Study 500 (n = 53)	Study 577 (n = 255)	Combined (n = 308)
Abdominal Pain	7.5	2.4	3.2
Diarrhea	9.4	1.6	2.9
Flatulence	7.5	0.0	1.3
Headache	7.5	0.4	1.6
Nausea	28.3	9.0	12.3
Rash	9.4	2.0	3.2
Taste Perversion	18.9	0.4	3.6
Vomiting	24.5	3.9	7.5

* Includes those events possibly or probably related to study drug and excludes concurrent conditions.

A limited number of pediatric AIDS patients have been treated with Clarithromycin suspension for mycobacterial infections. The most frequently reported adverse events, excluding those due to the patient's concurrent condition, were consistent with those observed in adult patients.

CHANGES IN LABORATORY VALUES
In immunocompromised patients with Clarithromycin for mycobacterial infections, evaluations of laboratory values were made by analyzing those values outside the seriously abnormal level (i.e., the extreme high or low limit) for the specified test.

PERCENTAGE OF PATIENTS(A) EXCEEDING EXTREME LABORATORY VALUE LIMITS DURING FIRST 12 WEEKS OF TREATMENT 500 MG BID DOSE(B)

		Study 500	Study 577	Combined
BUN	> 50 mg/dL	0%	< 1%	< 1%
Platelet Count	< 50 × 10⁹/L	0%	< 1%	< 1%
SGOT	> 5 × ULN[c]	0%	3%	2%
SGPT	> 5 × ULN[c]	0%	2%	1%
WBC	< 1 × 10⁹/L	0%	1%	1%

[a] Includes only patients with baseline values within the normal range or borderline high (hematology variables) and within the normal range or borderline low (chemistry variables).
[b] Includes all values within first 12 weeks for patients who start on 500 mg BID
[c] ULN = Upper Limit of Normal

ANIMAL PHARMACOLOGY AND TOXICOLOGY
Clarithromycin is rapidly and well-absorbed with dose-linear kinetics, low protein binding, and a high volume of distribution. Plasma half-life ranged from 1-6 hours and was species dependent. High tissue concentrations were achieved, but negligible accumulation was observed. Fecal clearance predominated. Hepatotoxicity occurred in all species tested (i.e., in rats and monkeys at doses 2 times greater than and in dogs at doses comparable to the maximum human daily dose, based on a mg/m^2 basis). Renal tubular degeneration (calculated on a mg/m^2 basis) occurred in rats at doses 2 times, in monkeys at doses 8 times, and in dogs at doses 12 times greater than the maximum human daily dose. Testicular atrophy (on a mg/m^2 basis) occurred in rats at doses 7 times, in dogs at doses 3 times, and in monkeys at doses 8 times greater than the maximum human daily dose. Corneal opacity (on a mg/m^2 basis) occurred in dogs at doses 12 times and in monkeys at doses 8 times greater than the maximum human daily dose. Lymphoid depletion (on a mg/m^2 basis) occurred in dogs at doses 3 times greater than and in monkeys at doses 2 times greater than the maximum human daily dose. These adverse events were absent during clinical trials.

REFERENCES
1. National Committee for Clinical Laboratory Standards. Performance Standards for Antimicrobial Disk Susceptibility Tests—Fourth Edition. Approved Standard NCCLS Document M2-A4, Vol. 10, No. 7, NCCLS, Villanova, PA, 1990. 2. National Committee for Clinical Laboratory Standards. Methods for Dilution Antimicrobial Susceptibility Tests for Bacteria that Grow Aerobically—Second Edition. Approved Standard NCCLS Document M7-A2, Vol. 10, No. 8, NCCLS, Villanova, PA, 1990. 3. Kemper CA, et al. Treatment of Mycobacterium avium Complex Bacteremia in AIDS with a Four-Drug Oral Regimen. Ann Intern Med. 1992; 116:466-472. 4. Public Health Service Task Force on Prophylaxis and Therapy for Mycobacterium avium complex. Recommendations on Prophylaxis and Therapy for Disseminated Mycobacterium avium Complex Disease in Patients Infected With The Human Immunodeficiency Virus. NEJM. 1993; 329:898-904.

HOW SUPPLIED
GRANULE FOR RECONSTITUTION: 125 MG/5 ML

BRAND/MANUFACTURER	NDC	SIZE	AWP
BRAND BIAXIN: Abbott Pharm	00074-3163-13	100 ml	$24.93

GRANULE FOR RECONSTITUTION: 250 MG/5 ML

BRAND/MANUFACTURER	NDC	SIZE	AWP
BRAND BIAXIN: Abbott Pharm	00074-3188-13	100 ml	$47.48

TABLETS: 250 MG

BRAND/MANUFACTURER	NDC	SIZE	AWP
BRAND BIAXIN FILMTAB: Abbott Pharm	00074-3368-60	60s	$178.30
	00074-3368-11	100s ud	$314.69

TABLETS: 500 MG

BRAND/MANUFACTURER	NDC	SIZE	AWP
BRAND BIAXIN FILMTAB: Abbott Pharm	00074-2586-60	60s	$178.30
	00074-2586-11	100s ud	$314.69

Claritin SEE LORATADINE

➤ SHOWN IN PRODUCT IDENTIFICATION GUIDE

Clavulanate Potassium with Ticarcillin Disodium

DESCRIPTION

Clavulanate Potassium/Ticarcillin Disodium is an injectable antibacterial combination consisting of the semisynthetic antibiotic, Ticarcillin Disodium, and the β-lactamase inhibitor, Clavulanate Potassium (the potassium salt of clavulanic acid), for intravenous administration. Ticarcillin is derived from the basic penicillin nucleus, 6-amino-penicillanic acid.

Chemically, it is 4-Thia-1-azabicyclo[3.2.0]heptane-2-carboxylic acid, 6-[(carboxy-3-thienylacetyl)amino]-3,3-dimethyl-7-oxo-, disodium salt, [2S-[2α,5α,6β(S*)]]-.

Clavulanic acid is produced by the fermentation of Streptomyces clavuligerus. It is a β-lactam structurally related to the penicillins and possesses the ability to inactivate a wide variety of β-lactamases by blocking the active sites of these enzymes. Clavulanic acid is particularly active against the clinically important plasmid-mediated β-lactamases frequently responsible for transferred drug resistance to penicillins and cephalosporins.

Chemically, Clavulanate Potassium is Potassium 4-Oxa-1-azabicyclo[3.2.0]heptane-2-carboxylic acid, 3-(2-hydroxyethylidene)-7-oxo-, monopotassium salt [2R-(2α, 3Z,5α)]-.

Clavulanate Potassium/Ticarcillin Disodium is supplied as a white to pale yellow powder for reconstitution. Clavulanate Potassium/Ticarcillin Disodium is very soluble in water, its solubility being greater than 600 mg/mL. The reconstituted solution is clear, colorless or pale yellow, having a pH of 5.5 to 7.5. For the Clavulanate Potassium/Ticarcillin Disodium 3.1 gram and 3.2 gram dosages, the theoretical sodium content is 4.75 mEq (109 mg) per gram of Clavulanate Potassium/Ticarcillin Disodium. The theoretical potassium content is 0.15 mEq (6 mg) and 0.3 mEq (11.9 mg) per gram of Clavulanate Potassium/Ticarcillin Disodium for the 3.1 gram and 3.2 gram dosages, respectively.

CLINICAL PHARMACOLOGY

After an intravenous infusion (30 min.) of 3.1 grams or 3.2 grams Clavulanate Potassium/Ticarcillin Disodium peak serum concentrations of both Ticarcillin Disodium and clavulanic acid are attained immediately after completion of infusion. Ticarcillin Disodium serum levels are similar to those produced by the administration of equivalent amounts of Ticarcillin Disodium alone with a mean peak serum level of 330 mcg/mL for the 3.1 gram and 3.2 gram formulations. The corresponding mean peak serum levels for clavulanic acid were 8 mcg/mL and 16 mcg/mL for the 3.1 gram and 3.2 gram formulations, respectively. (See following table).

The mean area under the serum concentration curves for Ticarcillin Disodium was 485 mcg/mL. hr. for the Clavulanate Potassium/Ticarcillin Disodium 3.1 gram and 3.2 gram formulations. The corresponding areas under the serum concentration curves for clavulanic acid were 8.2 mcg/mL.hr. and 15.6 mcg/mL.hr. for the Clavulanate Potassium/Ticarcillin Disodium 8.1 gram and 3.2 gram formulations, respectively.

The mean serum half-lives of Ticarcillin Disodium and clavulanic acid in healthy volunteers are 68 minutes and 64 minutes, respectively, following administration of 3.1 grams or 3.2 grams of Clavulanate Potassium/Ticarcillin Disodium.

Approximately 60% to 70% of Ticarcillin Disodium and approximately 35% to 45% of clavulanic acid are excreted unchanged in urine during the first 6 hours after administration of a single dose of Clavulanate Potassium/Ticarcillin Disodium to normal volunteers with normal renal function. Two hours after an intravenous injection of 3.1 grams or 3.2 grams Clavulanate Potassium/Ticarcillin Disodium concentrations of Ticarcillin Disodium in urine generally exceed 1500 mcg/mL. The corresponding concentrations of clavulanic acid in urine generally exceed 40 mcg/mL and 70 mcg/mL following administration of the 3.1 gram and 3.2 gram doses, respectively. By 4 to 6 hours after injection, the urine concentrations of Ticarcillin Disodium and clavulanic acid usually decline to approximately 190 mcg/mL and 2 mcg/mL, respectively, for both doses.

Neither component of Clavulanate Potassium/Ticarcillin Disodium is highly protein bound; Ticarcillin Disodium has been found to be approximately 45% bound to human serum protein and clavulanic acid approximately 9% bound.

Somewhat higher and more prolonged serum levels or Ticarcillin Disodium can be achieved with the concurrent administration of probenecid; however, probenecid does not enhance the serum levels of clavulanic acid.

Ticarcillin Disodium can be detected in tissues and interstitial fluid following parenteral administration.

Penetration of Ticarcillin Disodium into the bile, pleural fluid and cerebrospinal fluid with inflamed meninges has been demonstrated. The results of experiments involving the administration of clavulanic acid to animals suggest that this compound, like Ticarcillin Disodium, is well distributed in body tissues. An inverse relationship exists between the serum half-life of Ticarcillin Disodium and creatinine clearance. The dosage of Clavulanate Potassium/Ticarcillin Disodium need only be adjusted in cases of severe renal impairment (see "Dosage and Administration").

Ticarcillin Disodium may be removed from patients undergoing dialysis; the actual amount removed depends on the duration and type of dialysis.

Microbiology: Ticarcillin Disodium is a semisynthetic antibiotic with a broad spectrum of bactericidal activity against many gram-positive and gram-negative aerobic and anaerobic bacteria.

Ticarcillin Disodium is, however, susceptible to degradation by β-lactamases and therefore the spectrum of activity does not normally include organisms which produce these enzymes.

Clavulanic acid is a β-lactam, structurally related to the penicillins, which possesses the ability to inactivate a wide range of β-lactamase enzymes commonly found in microorganisms resistant to penicillins and cephalosporins. In particular, it has good activity against the clinically important plasmid-mediated β-lactamases frequently responsible for transferred drug resistance.

The formation of Ticarcillin Disodium with clavulanic acid in Clavulanate Potassium/Ticarcillin Disodium protects Ticarcillin from degradation by β-lactamase enzymes and effectively extends the antibiotic spectrum of Ticarcillin to include many bacteria normally resistant to Ticarcillin and other β-lactam antibiotics. Thus Clavulanate Potassium/Ticarcillin Disodium possesses the distinctive properties of a broad-spectrum antibiotic and a β-lactamase inhibitor.

While in vitro studies have demonstrated the susceptibility of most strains of the following organisms, clinical efficacy for infections other than those included in the "Indications and Usage" section has not been documented.

GRAM-NEGATIVE BACTERIA

Pseudomonas aeruginosa (β-lactamase and non-β-lactamase producing), Pseudomonas species including P. maltophilia (β-lactamase and non-β-lactamase producing), Escherichia coli (β-lactamase and non-β-lactamase producing), Proteus mirabilis (β-lactamase and non-β-lactamase producing), Proteus vulgaris (β-lactamase and non-β-lactamase producing), Providencia rettgeri (formerly Proteus rettgeri) (β-lactamase and non-β-lactamase producing), Providencia stuartii (β-lactamase and non-β-lactamase producing), Morganella morganii (formerly Proteus morganii) (β-lactamase and non-β-lactamase producing), Enterobacter species (Although most strains of Enterobacter species are resistant in vitro, clinical efficacy has been demonstrated with Clavulanate Potassium/Ticarcillin Disodium in urinary tract infections caused by these organisms.), Acinetobacter species (β-lactamase and non-β-lactamase producing), Hemophilus influenzae (β-lactamase and non-β-lactamase producing), Branhamella catarrhalis (β-lactamase and non-β-lactamase producing), Serratia species including S. marcescens (β-lactamase and non-β-lactamase producing), Neisseria gonorrhoeae (β-lactamase and non-β-lactamase producing), Neisseria meningitidis*, Salmonella species (β-lactamase and non-β-lactamase producing), Klebsiella species including K. pneumoniae (β-lactamase and non-β-lactamase producing), Citrobacter species including C. freundii, C. diversus and C. amalonaticus (β-lactamase and non-β-lactamase producing).

GRAM-POSITIVE BACTERIA

Staphylococcus aureus (β-lactamase and non-β-lactamase producing), Staphylococcus saprophyticus, Staphylococcus epidermidis (coagulase-negative staphylococci) (β-lactamase and non-β-lactamase producing), Streptococcus pneumoniae* (D. pneumoniae), Streptococcus bovis*, Streptococcus agalactiae* (Group B), Strepto-

SERUM LEVELS IN ADULTS AFTER A 30-MINUTE I.V. INFUSION OF CLAVULANATE POTASSIUM/TICARCILLIN DISODIUM

TICARCILLIN SERUM LEVELS (MCG/ML)

Dose	0	15 min.	30 min.	1 hr.	1.5 hr.	3.5 hr.	5.5 hr.
3.1 gram	324 (293 to 388)	223 (184 to 293)	176 (135 to 235)	131 (102 to 195)	90 (65 to 119)	27 (19 to 37)	6 (5 to 7)
3.2 gram	336 (301 to 386)	214 (180 to 258)	186 (160 to 218)	122 (108 to 136)	78 (33 to 113)	29 (19 to 44)	10 (5 to 15)

CLAVULANIC ACID SERUM LEVELS (MCG/ML)

Dose	0	15 min.	30 min.	1 hr.	1.5 hr.	3.5 hr.	5.5 hr.
3.1 gram	8.0 (5.3 to 10.3)	4.6 (3.0 to 7.6)	2.6 (1.8 to 3.4)	1.8 (1.6 to 2.2)	1.2 (0.8 to 1.6)	0.3 (0.2 to 0.3)	0
3.2 gram	15.8 (11.7 to 21.0)	8.3 (6.4 to 10.0)	5.2 (3.5 to 6.3)	3.4 (1.9 to 4.0)	2.5 (1.3 to 3.4)	0.5 (0.2 to 0.8)	0

◆ RATED THERAPEUTICALLY EQUIVALENT; ◇ THERAPEUTIC EQUIVALENCE UNCONFIRMED; ○ UNRATED

coccus faecalis* (Enterococcus), Streptococcus pyogenes* (Group A, β-hemolytic), Viridans group streptococci*.

ANAEROBIC BACTERIA
Bacteroides species, including B. fragilis group (B. fragilis, B. vulgatus) (β-lactamase and non-β-lactamase producing), non-B. fragilis (β-melaninogenicus) (β-lactamase and non-β-lactamase producing), B. thetaiotaomicron, B. ovatus, B. distasonis, (β-lactamase and non-β-lactamase producing), Clostridium species including C. perfringens, C. difficile, C. sporogenes, C. ramosum and C. bifermentans*, Eubacterium species, Fusobacterium species including F. nucleatum and F. necrophorum*, Peptococcus species*, Peptostreptococcus species*, Veillonella species.

In vitro synergism between Clavulanate Potassium/Ticarcillin Disodium and gentamicin, tobramycin or amikacin against multiresistant strains of Pseudomonas aeruginosa has been demonstrated.

* These are non-β-lactamase-producing strains and therefore are susceptible to Ticarcillin Disodium alone. Some of the β-lactamase-producing strains are also susceptible to Ticarcillin Disodium alone.

SUSCEPTIBILITY TESTING
Diffusion Technique: An 85 mcg Clavulanate Potassium/Ticarcillin Disodium (75 mcg Ticarcillin Disodium plus 10 mcg clavulanic acid) diffusion disk is available for use with the Kirby-Bauer method. Based on the zone sizes given below, a report of "Susceptible" indicates that the infecting organism is likely to respond to Clavulanate Potassium/Ticarcillin Disodium therapy, while a report of "Resistant" indicates that the organism is not likely to respond to therapy with this antibiotic. A report of "Intermediate" susceptibility indicates that the organism would be susceptible to Clavulanate Potassium/Ticarcillin Disodium at a higher dosage or if the infection is confined to tissues or fluids (e.g., urine) in which high antibiotic levels are attained.

Dilution Technique: Broth or agar dilution methods may be used to determine the minimal inhibitory concentration (MIC) values for bacterial isolates to Clavulanate Potassium/Ticarcillin Disodium Tubes should be inoculated with the test culture containing 10^4 to 10^5 CFU/mL or plates spotted with a test solution containing 10^3 to 10^4 CFU/mL.

The recommended dilution pattern utilizes a constant level of clavulanic acid, 2 mcg/mL, in all tubes together with varying amounts of Ticarcillin Disodium. MICs are expressed in terms of the Ticarcillin Disodium concentration in the presence of 2 mcg/mL clavulanic acid.

RECOMMENDED RANGES FOR CLAVULANATE POTASSIUM/ TICARCILLIN DISODIUM SUSCEPTIBILITY TESTING[1-3]

Diffusion Method Disk Zone Size, mm		
Res	Inter.	Susc.
≤ 11	12 to 14	≥ 15

Dilution Method MIC Correlates[4], mcg/mL	
Res.	Susc.
≥ 128	≤ 64

[1] The non-β-lactamase-producing organisms which are normally susceptible to Ticarcillin Disodium will have similar zone sizes as for Ticarcillin Disodium.

[2] Staphylococci which are susceptible to Clavulanate Potassium/Ticarcillin Disodium but resistant to methicillin, oxacillin or nafcillin must be considered as resistant.

[3] The quality control cultures should have the following assigned daily ranges for Clavulanate Potassium/Ticarcillin Disodium.

	Disks	MIC Range (mcg/mL)
E. coli (ATCC 25922)	24 to 30 mm	2/2 to 8/2
S. aureus (ATCC 25923)	32 to 40 mm	-
Ps. aeruginosa (ATCC 27853)	20 to 28 mm	8/2 to 32/2
E. coli (ATCC 35218)	21 to 25 mm	4/2 to 16/2
S. aureus (ATCC 29213)	—	0.5/2 to 2/2

[4] Expressed as concentration of Ticarcillin Disodium in the presence of a constant 2.0 mcg/mL concentration of clavulanic acid.

INDICATIONS AND USAGE
Clavulanate Potassium/Ticarcillin Disodium is indicated in the treatment of infections caused by susceptible strains of the designated organisms in the conditions listed below:

Septicemia: including bacteremia, caused by β-lactamase-producing strains of Klebsiella spp.*, E. coli Staphylococcus aureus*, or Pseudomonas aeruginosa*, (or other Pseudomonas species*).

Lower Respiratory Infections: caused by β-lactamase-producing strains of Staphylococcus aureus, Hemophilus influenzae* or Klebsiella spp.*

Bone and Joint Infections: caused by β-lactamase-producing strains of Staphylococcus aureus.

Skin and Skin Structure Infections: caused by β-lactamase-producing strains of Staphylococcus aureus, Klebsiella spp.* or E. coli*.

Urinary Tract Infections (complicated and uncomplicated): caused by β-lactamase-producing strains of E. coli, Klebsiella spp., Pseudomonas aeruginosa* (or other Pseudomonas spp.*), Citrobacter spp.*, Enterobacter cloacae*, Serratia marcescens* or Staphylococcus aureus*.

Gynecologic Infections: endometritis caused by β-lactamase-producing strains of B. melaninogenicus*, Enterobacter spp. (including E. cloacae*), Escherichia coli, Klebsiella pneumoniae*, Staphylococcus aureus or Staphylococcus epidermidis.

Intra-abdominal Infections: peritonitis caused by β-lactamase-producing stains of Escherichia coli, Klebsiella pneumoniae or Bacteroides fragilis* group.

While Clavulanate Potassium/Ticarcillin Disodium is indicated only for the conditions listed above, infections caused by Ticarcillin-susceptible organisms are also amenable to Clavulanate Potassium/Ticarcillin Disodium treatment due to its Ticarcillin Disodium content. Therefore, mixed infections caused by Ticarcillin Disodium-susceptible organisms and β-lactamase-producing organisms susceptible to Clavulanate Potassium/Ticarcillin Disodium should not require the addition of another antibiotic.

Appropriate culture and susceptibility tests should be performed before treatment in order to isolate and identify organisms causing infection and to determine their susceptibility to Clavulanate Potassium/Ticarcillin Disodium. Because of its broad spectrum of bactericidal activity against gram-positive and gram-negative bacteria, Clavulanate Potassium/Ticarcillin Disodium is particularly useful for the treatment of mixed infections and for presumptive therapy prior to the identification of the causative organisms. Clavulanate Potassium/ Ticarcillin Disodium has been shown to be effective as single drug therapy in the treatment of some serious infections where normally combination antibiotic therapy might be employed. Therapy with Clavulanate Potassium/Ticarcillin Disodium may be initiated before results of such tests are known when there is reason to believe the infection may involve any of the β-lactamase-producing organisms listed above; however, once these results become available, appropriate therapy should be continued.

Based on the in vitro synergism between Clavulanate Potassium/Ticarcillin Disodium and aminoglycosides against certain strains of Pseudomonas aeruginosa, combined therapy has been successful, especially in patients with impaired host defenses. Both drugs should be used in full therapeutic doses. As soon as results of culture and susceptibility tests become available, antimicrobial therapy should be adjusted as indicated.

CONTRAINDICATIONS
Clavulanate Potassium/Ticarcillin Disodium is contraindicated in patients with a history of hypersensitivity reactions to any of the penicillins.

WARNINGS
SERIOUS AND OCCASIONALLY FATAL HYPERSENSITIVITY (ANAPHYLACTOID) REACTIONS HAVE BEEN REPORTED IN PATIENTS ON PENICILLIN THERAPY. THESE REACTIONS ARE MORE LIKELY TO OCCUR IN INDIVIDUALS WITH A HISTORY OF PENICILLIN HYPERSENSITIVITY AND/OR A HISTORY OF SENSITIVITY TO MULTIPLE ALLERGENS. THERE HAVE BEEN REPORTS OF INDIVIDUALS WITH A HISTORY OF PENICILLIN HYPERSENSITIVITY WHO HAVE EXPERIENCED SEVERE REACTIONS WHEN TREATED WITH CEPHALOSPORINS. BEFORE INITIATING THERAPY WITH CLAVULANATE POTASSIUM/TICARCILLIN DISODIUM, CAREFUL INQUIRY SHOULD BE MADE CONCERNING PREVIOUS HYPERSENSITIVITY REACTIONS TO PENICILLINS, CEPHALOSPORINS OR OTHER DRUGS. IF AN ALLERGIC REACTION OCCURS, CLAVULANATE POTASSIUM/TICARCILLIN DISODIUM SHOULD BE DISCONTINUED AND THE APPROPRIATE THERAPY INSTITUTED.

SERIOUS ANAPHYLACTOID REACTIONS REQUIRE IMMEDIATE EMERGENCY TREATMENT WITH EPINEPHRINE. OXYGEN, INTRAVENOUS STEROIDS AND AIRWAY MANAGEMENT, INCLUDING INTUBATION, SHOULD ALSO BE PROVIDED AS INDICATED.

Pseudomembranous colitis has been reported with nearly all antibacterial agents, including Clavulanate Potassium/Ticarcillin Disodium and has ranged in severity from mild to life-threatening. Therefore, it is important to consider this diagnosis in patients who present with diarrhea subsequent to the administration of antibacterial agents.

Treatment with antibacterial agents alters the normal flora of the colon and may permit overgrowth of clostridia. Studies indicate that a toxin produced by Clostridium difficile is one primary cause of "antibiotic-associated colitis."

Mild cases of pseudomembranous colitis usually respond to drug discontinuation alone. In moderate to severe cases, consideration should be given to management with fluids and electrolytes, protein supplementation and treatment with an antibacterial drug effective against C. difficile.

PRECAUTIONS
General: While Clavulanate Potassium/Ticarcillin Disodium possesses the characteristic low toxicity of the penicillin group of antibiotics, periodic assessment of organ system functions, including renal, hepatic and hematopoietic function is advisable during prolonged therapy.

Bleeding manifestations have occurred in some patients receiving β-lactam antibiotics. These reactions have been associated with abnormalities of coagulation tests such as clotting time, platelet aggregation and prothrombin time and are more likely to occur in patients with renal impairment. If bleeding manifestations

* Efficacy for this organism in this organ system was studied in fewer than 10 infections.

appear, Clavulanate Potassium/Ticarcillin Disodium treatment should be discontinued and appropriate therapy instituted.

Clavulanate Potassium/Ticarcillin Disodium has only rarely been reported to cause hypokalemia; however, the possibility of this occurring should be kept in mind particularly when treating patients with fluid and electrolyte imbalance. Periodic monitoring of serum potassium may be advisable in patients receiving prolonged therapy.

The theoretical sodium content is 4.75 mEq (109 mg) per gram of Clavulanate Potassium/Ticarcillin Disodium. This should be considered when treating patients requiring restricted salt intake.

As with any penicillin, an allergic reaction, including anaphylaxis, may occur during Clavulanate Potassium/Ticarcillin Disodium administration, particularly in a hypersensitive individual.

The possibility of superinfections with mycotic or bacterial pathogens should be kept in mind, particularly during prolonged treatment. If superinfections occur, appropriate measures should be taken.

Drug/Laboratory Test Interactions: As with other penicillins, the mixing of Clavulanate Potassium/Ticarcillin Disodium with an aminoglycoside in solutions for parenteral administration can result in substantial inactivation of the aminoglycoside.

Probenecid interferes with the renal tubular secretion of Ticarcillin, thereby increasing serum concentrations and prolonging serum half-life of the antibiotic.

High urine concentrations of Ticarcillin Disodium may produce false-positive protein reactions (pseudoproteinuria) with the following methods: sulfosalicylic acid and boiling test, acetic acid test, biuret reaction and nitric acid test. The bromphenol blue (Multi-stix®) reagent strip test has been reported to be reliable.

The presence of clavulanic acid in Clavulanate Potassium/Ticarcillin Disodium may cause a nonspecific binding of IgG and albumin by red cell membranes leading to a false-positive Coombs test.

Carcinogenesis, Mutagenesis, Impairment of Fertility: Long-term studies in animals have not been performed to evaluate carcinogenic potential. Results of studies performed with Clavulanate Potassium/Ticarcillin Disodium *in vitro* and *in vivo* did not indicate a potential for mutagenicity.

Pregnancy (Category B): Reproduction studies have been performed in rats given doses up to 1050 mg/kg/day and have revealed no evidence of impaired fertility or harm to the fetus due to Clavulanate Potassium/Ticarcillin Disodium. There are, however, no adequate and well-controlled studies in pregnant women. Because animal reproduction studies are not always predictive of human response, this drug should be used during pregnancy only if clearly needed.

Nursing Mothers: Caution should be exercised when Clavulanate Potassium/Ticarcillin Disodium is administered to a nursing woman.

Pediatric Use: The efficacy and safety of Clavulanate Potassium/Ticarcillin Disodium have not been established in infants and children under the age of 12.

Drug Abuse and Dependence: Neither Clavulanate Potassium/Ticarcillin Disodium abuse nor Clavulanate Potassium/Ticarcillin Disodium dependence has been reported.

ADVERSE REACTIONS

As with other penicillins, the following adverse reactions may occur:

Hypersensitivity Reactions: skin rash, pruritus, urticaria, arthralgia, myalgia, drug fever, chills, chest discomfort and anaphylactic reactions.

Central Nervous System: headache, giddiness, neuromuscular hyperirritability or convulsive seizures.

Gastrointestinal Disturbances: disturbances of taste and smell, stomatitis, flatulence, nausea, vomiting and diarrhea, epigastric pain and pseudomembranous colitis. Onset of pseudomembranous colitis symptoms may occur during or after antibiotic treatment (see *"Warnings"*).

Hemic and Lymphatic Systems: thrombocytopenia, leukopenia, neutropenia, eosinophilia and reduction of hemoglobin or hematocrit. Prolongation of prothrombin time and bleeding time.

Abnormalities of Hepatic and Renal Function Tests: elevation of serum aspartate aminotransferase (SGOT), serum alanine aminotransferase (SGPT), serum alkaline phosphatase, serum LDH, serum bilirubin. Rarely, transient hepatitis and cholestatic jaundice—as with some other penicillins and some cephalosporins. Elevation of serum creatinine and/or BUN, hypernatremia. Reduction in serum potassium and uric acid.

Local Reactions: pain, burning, swelling and induration at the injection site and thrombophlebitis with intravenous administration.

OVERDOSAGE

As with other penicillins, Clavulanate Potassium/Ticarcillin Disodium in overdosage has the potential to cause neuromuscular hyperirritability or convulsive seizures. Ticarcillin Disodium may be removed from circulation by hemodialysis. The molecular weight, degree of protein binding and pharmacokinetic profile of Clavulanic acid together with information from a single patient with renal insufficiency all suggest that this compound may also be removed by hemodialysis.

DOSAGE AND ADMINISTRATION

Clavulanate Potassium/Ticarcillin Disodium should be administered by intravenous infusion (30 min.).

Adults: The usual recommended dosage for systemic and urinary tract infections for average (60 kg) adults is 3.1 grams Clavulanate Potassium Ticarcillin Disodium (3.1 gram vial containing 3 grams Ticarcillin Disodium and 100 mg clavulanic acid) given every 4 to 6 hours. For gynecologic infections, Clavulanate Potassium/Ticarcillin Disodium should be administered as follows: Moderate infections 200 mg/kg/day in divided doses every 6 hours and for severe infections 300 mg/kg/day in divided doses every 4 hours. For patients weighing less than 60 kg, the recommended dosage is 200 to 300 mg/kg/day, based on Ticarcillin Disodium content, given in divided doses every 4 to 6 hours.

In urinary tract infections, a dosage of 3.2 grams Clavulanate Potassium/Ticarcillin Disodium (3.2 gram vial containing 3 grams Ticarcillin Disodium and 200 mg clavulanic acid) given every 8 hours is adequate.

For infections complicated by renal insufficiency,[1] an initial loading dose of 3.1 grams should be followed by doses based on creatinine clearance and type of dialysis as indicated below:

Creatinine clearance mL/min.	Dosage
over 60	3.1 grams every 4 hrs.
30 to 60	2 grams every 4 hrs.
10 to 30	2 grams every 8 hrs.
less than 10	2 grams every 12 hrs.
less than 10 with hepatic dysfunction	2 grams every 24 hrs.
patients on peritoneal dialysis	3.1 grams every 12 hrs.
patients on hemodialysis	2 grams every 12 hrs. supplemented with 3.1 grams after each dialysis

To calculate creatinine clearance* from a serum creatinine value use the following formula.

$$C_{cr} = \frac{(140 - Age)\ (wt.\ in\ kg)}{72 \times S_{cr}(mg/100\ mL)}$$

This is the calculated creatinine clearance for adult males; for females it is 15% less.

Dosage for any individual patient must take into consideration the site and severity of infection, the susceptibility of the organisms causing infection and the status of the patient's host defense mechanisms.

The duration of therapy depends upon the severity of infection. Generally, Clavulanate Potassium/Ticarcillin Disodium should be continued for at least 2 days after the signs and symptoms of infection have disappeared. The usual duration is 10 to 14 days; however, in difficult and complicated infections, more prolonged therapy may be required.

Frequent bacteriologic and clinical appraisal is necessary during therapy of chronic urinary tract infection and may be required for several months after therapy has been completed; persistent infections may require treatment for several weeks and doses smaller than those indicated above should not be used.

In certain infections, involving abscess formation, appropriate surgical drainage should be performed in conjunction with antimicrobial therapy.

INTRAVENOUS ADMINISTRATION
DIRECTIONS FOR USE

3.1 Gram and 3.2 Gram Vials and Piggyback Bottles: The 3.1 gram or 3.2 gram vial should be reconstituted by adding approximately 13 mL of Sterile Water for Injection, USP, or Sodium Chloride Injection, USP, and shaking well. When dissolved, the concentration of Ticarcillin Disodium will be approximately 200 mg/mL with corresponding concentrations of 6.7 mg/mL and 13.4 mg/mL clavulanic acid for the 3.1 gram and 3.2 gram respective doses. Conversely, each 5.0 mL of the 3.1 gram dose reconstituted with approximately 13 mL of diluent will contain approximately 1 gram of Ticarcillin Disodium and 33 mg of clavulanic acid. For the 3.2 gram dose reconstituted with 13 mL of diluent, each 5.0 mL will contain 1 gram of Ticarcillin Disodium and 66 mg of clavulanic acid.

Intravenous Infusion: The dissolved drug should be further diluted to desired volume using the recommended solution listed in the *"Compatibility And Stability Section (Stability Period")* to a concentration between 10 mg/mL to 100 mg/mL. The solution of reconstituted drug may then be administered over a period of 30 minutes by direct infusion or through a Y-type intravenous infusion set. If this method or the "piggyback" method of administration is used, it is advisable to discontinue temporarily the administration of any other solutions during the infusion of Clavulanate Potassium/Ticarcillin Disodium.

Stability: For I.V. solutions, see *"Stability Period"* below.

When Clavulanate Potassium/Ticarcillin Disodium is given in combination with another antimicrobial, such as an aminoglycoside, each drug should be given separately in accordance with the recommended dosage and routes of administration for each drug.

After reconstitution and prior to administration, Clavulanate Potassium/Ticarcillin Disodium, as with other parenteral drugs, should be inspected visually for particulate matter. If this condition is evident, the solution should be discarded.

---

1 The half-life of Ticarcillin in patients with renal failure is approximately 13 hours.
* Cockcroft, D. W., et al: Prediction of Creatinine Clearance from Serum Creatinine. *Nephron* 16:31-41, 1976.

The color of reconstituted solutions of Clavulanate Potassium/Ticarcillin Disodium normally ranges from light to dark yellow depending on concentration, duration and temperature of storage while maintaining label claim characteristics.

COMPATIBILITY AND STABILITY

3.1 Gram and 3.2 Gram Vials and Piggyback Bottles (Dilutions Derived from a Stock Solution of 200 mg/ml): The concentrated stock solution at 200 mg/mL is stable for up to 6 hours at room temperature 21° to 24°C (70° to 75°F) or up to 72 hours under refrigeration 4°C (40°F).

If the concentrated stock solution (200 mg/mL) is held for up to 6 hours at room temperature 21° to 24°C (70° to 75°F) or up to 72 hours under refrigeration 4°C (40°F) and further diluted to a concentration between 10 mg/mL and 100 mg/mL with any of the diluents listed below, then the following stability periods apply.

STABILITY PERIOD
(3.1 GRAM AND 3.2 GRAM VIALS AND PIGGYBACK BOTTLES)

Intravenous Solution Ticarcillin concentrations of 10 mg/mL to 100 mg/mL)	Room Temperature 21° to 24°C (70° to 75°F)	Refrigerated 4°C (40°F)
Dextrose Injection 5%, USP	24 hours	3 days
Sodium Chloride Injection, USP	24 hours	7 days
Lactated Ringer's Injection, USP	24 hours	7 days

If the concentrated stock solution (200 mg/mL) is stored for up to 6 hours at room temperature and then further diluted to a concentration between 10 mg/mL and 100 mg/mL, solutions of Sodium Chloride Injection USP, and Lactated Ringer's Injection, USP, may be stored frozen -18°C (0°F) for up to 30 days. Solutions prepared with Dextrose Injection 5%, USP, may be stored frozen -18°C (0°F) for up to 7 days. All thawed solutions should be used within 8 hours or discarded. Once thawed, solutions should not be refrozen.

Note: Clavalanate Potassium/Ticarcillin Disodium is incompatible with sodium bicarbonate.

Unused solutions must be discarded after the time periods listed above.

STORAGE
Clavulanate Potassium/Ticarcillin Disodium vials should be stored at room temperature 21° to 24°C (70° to 75°F) or below.

HOW SUPPLIED
POWDER FOR INJECTION: 3 GM-100 MG

BRAND/MANUFACTURER	NDC	SIZE	AWP
○ **BRAND**			
TIMENTIN: SK Beecham Pharm	00029-6571-26	1s	$13.35
	00029-6571-40	1s	$13.65
	00029-6571-21	1s	$14.20
	00029-6571-31	12s	$188.70

POWDER FOR INJECTION: 30 GM-1 GM

BRAND/MANUFACTURER	NDC	SIZE	AWP
○ **BRAND**			
TIMENTIN: SK Beecham Pharm	00029-6579-21	1s	$133.50

Clemastine Fumarate

DESCRIPTION
Each teaspoonful (5 ml) of Clemastine Fumarate Syrup for oral administration contains Clemastine 0.5 mg (present as Clemastine Fumarate 0.67 mg). Clemastine Fumarate is also available for oral administration as tablets of 1.34 mg and 2.68 mg.

Clemastine Fumarate belongs to the benzhydryl ether group of antihistaminic compounds. The chemical name is (+)-(2R)-2[2- [[(R)-p-Chloro-α-methyl -α-phenylbenzyl]-oxy]ethyl]-1-methylopyrrolidine Fumarate.*

Clemastine Fumarate occurs as a colorless to faintly yellow, practically odorless, crystalline powder. Clemastine Fumarate Syrup has an approximate pH of 6.2.

Following is its chemical structure:

CLINICAL PHARMACOLOGY
Clemastine Fumarate is an antihistamine with anticholinergic (drying) and sedative side effects. Antihistamines competitively antagonize various physiological effects of histamine including increased capillary permeability and dilatation, the formation of edema, the "flare" and "itch" response, and gastrointestinal and respiratory smooth muscle constriction. Within the vascular tree, H_1-receptor

* U.S. Patent No. 3,097,212.

antagonists inhibit both the vasoconstrictor and vasodilator effects of histamine. Depending on the dose, H_1-receptor antagonists can produce CNS stimulation or depression. Most antihistamines exhibit central and/or peripheral anticholinergic activity. Antihistamines act by competitively blocking H_1-receptor sites. Antihistamines do not pharmacologically antagonize or chemically inactivate histamine, nor do they prevent the release of histamine.

PHARMACOKINETICS
Antihistamines are well-absorbed following oral administration. Chlorpheniramine maleate, Clemastine Fumarate, and diphenhydramine hydrochloride achieve peak blood levels within 2-5 hours following oral administration. The absorption of antihistamines is often partially delayed by the use of controlled release dosage forms. In these instances, plasma concentrations from identical doses of the immediate and controlled release dosage forms will not be similar.

Tissue distribution of the antihistamines in humans has not been established.

Antihistamines appear to be metabolized in the liver chiefly via mono- and didemethylation and glucuronide conjugation. Antihistamine metabolites and small amounts of unchanged drug are excreted in the urine. Small amounts of the drugs may also be excreted in breast milk.

In normal human subjects who received histamine injections over a 24 hour period, the antihistaminic activity of Clemastine Fumarate reached a peak at 5-7 hours, persisted for 10-12 hours and, in some cases, for as long as 24 hours. Pharmacokinetic studies in man utilizing ^3H and ^{14}C labeled compound demonstrates that Clemastine Fumarate is rapidly absorbed from the gastrointestinal tract, peak plasma concentrations are attained in 2-4 hours, and urinary excretion is the major mode of elimination.

INDICATIONS AND USAGE
Clemastine Fumarate Syrup and Tablets are indicated for the relief of symptoms associated with allergic rhinitis such as sneezing, rhinorrhea, pruritus and lacrimation. Clemastine Fumarate Syrup is indicated for use in pediatric populations (age 6 years through 12) and adults (see *"Dosage and Administration"*).

It should be noted that Clemastine Fumarate is indicated for the relief of mild uncomplicated allergic skin manifestations of urticaria and angioedema at the 2 mg dosage level only. Clemastine Fumarate Tablets 2.68 mg are also indicated for the relief of mild, uncomplicated allergic skin manifestations of urticaria and angioedema. It should be noted that Clemastine Fumarate is indicated for the dermatologic indications at the 2.68 mg dosage level only.

UNLABELED USES
Clemastine Fumarate is used alone or as an adjunct in the treatment of various allergic dermatoses such as eczema, exanthema and angioneurotic edema.

CONTRAINDICATIONS
Antihistamines are contraindicated in patients hypersensitive to the drug or to other antihistamines of similar chemical structure (see *"Precautions—Drug Interactions"*).

Antihistamines *should not* be used *in newborn or premature infants.* Because of the higher risk of antihistamines for infants generally and for newborns and prematures in particular, antihistamine therapy is contraindicated *in nursing mothers* (see *"Precautions—Nursing Mothers"*).

Antihistamines *should not* be used to treat lower respiratory tract symptoms including asthma.

Antihistamines are also contraindicated in monamine oxidase inhibitor therapy. (See *"Drug Interaction"* section.)

WARNINGS
Antihistamines should be used with considerable caution in patients with: narrow angle glaucoma, stenosing peptic ulcer, pyloroduodenal obstruction, symptomatic prostatic hypertrophy, and bladder neck obstruction.

Use with CNS Depressants: Clemastine Fumarate has additive effects with alcohol and other CNS depressants (hypnotics, sedatives, tranquilizers, etc.)

Use in Activities Requiring Mental Alertness: Patients should be warned about engaging in activities requiring mental alertness such as driving a car or operating appliances, machinery, etc.

Use in the Elderly (approximately 60 years or older): Antihistamines are more likely to cause dizziness, sedation, and hypotension in elderly patients.

PRECAUTIONS
GENERAL
Clemastine Fumarate should be used with caution in patients with: history of bronchial asthma, increased intraocular pressure, hyperthyroidism, cardiovascular disease, and hypertension.

INFORMATION FOR PATIENTS
Patients taking antihistamines should receive the following information and instructions:
1. Antihistamines are prescribed to reduce allergic symptoms.
2. Patients should be questioned regarding a history of glaucoma, peptic ulcer, urinary retention, or pregnancy before starting antihistamine therapy.
3. Patients should be told not to take alcohol, sleeping pills, sedatives, or tranquilizers while taking antihistamines.
4. Antihistamines may cause drowsiness, dizziness, dry mouth, blurred vision, weakness, nausea, headache, or nervousness in some patients.
5. Patients should avoid driving a car or working with hazardous machinery until they assess the effects of this medicine.

➤ SHOWN IN PRODUCT IDENTIFICATION GUIDE

6. Patients should be told to store this medicine in a tightly closed container in a dry, cool place away from heat or direct sunlight and out of the reach of children.

DRUG INTERACTIONS
Addictive CNS depression may occur when antihistamines are administered concomitantly with other CNS depressants including barbiturates, tranquilizers, and alcohol. Patients receiving antihistamines should be advised against the concurrent use of other CNS depressant drugs.

Monoamine oxidase (MAO) inhibitors prolong and intensify the anticholinergic effects of antihistamines.

CARCINOGENESIS, MUTAGENESIS, IMPAIRMENT OF FERTILITY
Carcinogenesis and Mutagenesis: In a 2-year oral study in the rat at a dose of 84 mg/kg (about 500 times the adult human dose) and an 85-week oral study in the mouse at 206 mg/kg (about 1300 times the adult human dose), Clemastine Fumarate showed no evidence of carcinogenesis. No mutagenic studies have been conducted with Clemastine Fumarate.

Impairment of Fertility: Oral doses of Clemastine Fumarate in the rat produced a decrease in mating ability of the male at 312 times the adult human dose. This effect was not found at 156 times the adult human dose.

PREGNANCY
Pregnancy Category B: Oral reproduction studies performed with Clemastine Fumarate in rats and rabbits at doses up to 312 and 188 times the adult human doses respectively, have revealed no evidence of teratogenic effects.

Experience with this drug in pregnant women is inadequate to determine whether there exists a potential for harm to the developing fetus.

There are no adequate and well-controlled studies of Clemastine Fumarate in pregnant women. Because animal reproduction studies are not always predictive of human response, this drug should be used in pregnancy only if clearly needed.

NURSING MOTHERS
Although quantitative determinations of antihistaminic drugs in breast milk have not been reported, qualitative tests have documented the excretion of diphenhydramine, pyrilamine, and tripelennamine in human milk.

Because of the potential for adverse reactions in nursing infants from antihistamines, a decision should be made whether to discontinue nursing or to discontinue the drug.

PEDIATRIC USE
The safety and efficacy of Clemastine Fumarate Syrup has been confirmed in the pediatric population (age 6 years through 12). Safety and dose tolerance studies have confirmed children 6 through 11 years tolerated dosage ranges of 0.75 to 2.25 mg Clemastine. Infants and children particularly, antihistamines in overdosage may produce hallucinations, convulsions, and death. Symptoms of antihistamine toxicity in children may include fixed dilated pupils, flushed face, dry mouth, fever, excitation, hallucinations, ataxia, incoordination, athetosis, tonic clonic convulsions, and postictal depression (see *"Overdosage"*).

Safety and efficacy of Clemastine Fumarate Tablets have not been established in children under the age of 12.

ADVERSE REACTIONS
Transient drowsiness, the most common adverse reaction associated with Clemastine Fumarate, occurs relatively frequently and may require discontinuation of therapy in some instances.

The most frequent adverse reactions are italicized:

Nervous System: Sedation, sleepiness, dizziness, disturbed coordination, fatigue, confusion, restlessness, excitation, nervousness, tremor, irritability, insomnia, euphoria, paresthesia, blurred vision, diplopia, vertigo, tinnitus, acute labyrinthitis, hysteria, neuritis, convulsions.

Gastrointestinal System: Epigastric distress, anorexia, nausea, vomiting, diarrhea, constipation.

Respiratory System: Thickening of bronchial secretions, tightness of chest and wheezing, nasal stuffiness.

Cardiovascular System: Hypotension, headache, palpitations, tachycardia, extrasystoles.

Hematologic System: Hemolytic anemia, thrombocytopenia, agranulocytosis.

Genitourinary System: Urinary frequency, difficult urination, urinary retention, early menses.

ANTIHISTAMINIC COMPOUNDS
It should be noted that the following reactions have occurred with one or more antihistamines and, therefore, should be kept in mind when prescribing drugs belonging to this class, including Clemastine Fumarate. The most frequent adverse reactions are italicized.

1. General: Urticaria, drug rash, anaphylactic shock, photosensitivity, excessive perspiration, chills, dryness of mouth, nose, and throat.

2. Cardiovascular System: Hypotension, headache, palpitations, tachycardia, extrasystoles.

3. Hematologic System: Hemolytic anemia, thrombocytopenia, agranulocytosis.

4. Nervous System: Sedation, sleepiness, dizziness, disturbed coordination, fatigue, confusion, restlessness, excitation, nervousness, tremor, irritability, insomnia,

euphoria, parasthesias, blurred vision, diplopia, vertigo, tinnitus, acute labyrinthitis, hysteria, neuritis, convulsions.

5. GI System: Epigastric distress, anorexia, nausea, vomiting, diarrhea, constipation.

6. GU System: Urinary frequency, difficult urination, urinary retention, early menses.

7. Respiratory System: Thickening of bronchial secretions, tightness of chest and wheezing, nasal stuffiness.

OVERDOSAGE
Antihistamine overdosage reactions may vary from central nervous system depression to stimulation. In children, stimulation predominates initially in a syndrome which may include excitement, hallucinations, ataxia, incoordination, muscle twitching, athetosis, hyperthermia, cyanosis convulsions, tremors, and hyperreflexia followed by postictal depression and cardio-respiratory arrest. Convulsions in children may be preceded by mild depression. Dry mouth, fixed dilated pupils, flushing of the face, and fever are common. In adults, CNS depression, ranging from drowsiness to coma, is more common. The convulsant dose of antihistamines lies near the lethal dose. Convulsions indicate a poor prognosis. In both children and adults, coma and cardiovascular collapse may occur. Deaths are reported especially in infants and children.

There is no specific therapy for acute overdosage with antihistamines. The latent period from ingestion to appearance of toxic effects is characteristically short (½-2 hours). General symptomatic and supportive measures should be instituted promptly and maintained for as long as necessary.

Since overdoses of other classes of drugs (i.e., tricyclic anti-depressants) may also present anticholinergic symptomatology, appropriate toxicological analysis should be performed as soon as possible to identify the causative agent.

If vomiting has not occurred spontaneously the conscious patient should be induced to vomit. This is best done by having him drink a glass of water or milk after which he should be made to gag. Precautions against aspiration must be taken, especially in infants and children.

If vomiting cannot be induced, gastric lavage is indicated within 3 hours after ingestion and even later if large amounts of milk or cream were given beforehand. Isotonic and ½ isotonic saline is the lavage solution of choice. Adequate precautions must be taken to protect against aspiration, especially in infants and children. Charcoal slurry or other suitable agents should be instilled into the stomach after vomiting or lavage. Saline cathartics or milk of magnesia may be of additional benefit.

In the unconscious patient, the airway should be secured with a cuffed endotracheal tube before attempting to evacuate the gastric contents. Intensive supportive and nursing care is indicated, as for any comatose patient.

If breathing is significantly impaired, maintenance of an adequate airway and mechanical support of respiration is the most effective means of providing adequate oxygenation.

Hypotension is an early sign of impending cardiovascular collapse and should be treated vigorously. Although general supportive measures are important, specific treatment with intravenous infusion of a vasopressor titrated to maintain adequate blood pressure may be necessary.

Do not use with CNS stimulants.

Convulsions should be controlled by careful administration of diazepam or a short-acting barbiturate, repeated as necessary. Physostigmine may also be considered for use in controlling centrally mediated convulsions.

Ice packs and cooling sponge baths, not alcohol, can aid in reducing the fever commonly seen in children. A more detailed review of antihistamine toxicology and overdose management is available in Gosselin, R.E. et al., "Clinical Toxicology of Commercial Products."

DOSAGE AND ADMINISTRATION
DOSAGE SHOULD BE INDIVIDUALIZED ACCORDING TO THE NEEDS AND RESPONSE OF THE PATIENT.

CLEMASTINE FUMARATE SYRUP
PEDIATRIC (CHILDREN AGED 6 TO 12 YEARS).
For Symptoms of Allergic Rhinitis: The starting dose is 1 teaspoonful (0.5 mg Clemastine) twice daily. Since single doses of up to 2.25 mg Clemastine were well tolerated by this age group, dosage may be increased as required, but not to exceed 6 teaspoonsful daily (3 mg Clemastine).

For Urticaria and Angioedema: The starting dose is 2 teaspoonsful (1 mg Clemastine) twice daily, not to exceed 6 teaspoonsful daily (3 mg Clemastine).

ADULTS AND CHILDREN 12 YEARS AND OVER
For Symptoms of Allergic Rhinitis: The starting dose is 2 teaspoonsful (1.0 mg Clemastine) twice daily. Dosage may be increased as required, but not to exceed 12 teaspoonsful daily (6 mg Clemastine).

For Urticaria and Angioedema: The starting dose is 4 teaspoonsful (2 mg Clemastine) twice daily, not to exceed 12 teaspoonsful daily (6 mg Clemastine).

Clemastine Fumarate Tablets 1.34 mg: The recommended starting dose is one tablet twice daily. Dosage may be increased as required, but not to exceed six tablets daily.

Clemastine Fumarate Tablets 2.68 mg: The maximum recommended dosage is one tablet three times daily. Many patients respond favorably to a single dose which may be repeated as required, but not to exceed three tablets daily.

◆ RATED THERAPEUTICALLY EQUIVALENT; ◇ THERAPEUTIC EQUIVALENCE UNCONFIRMED; ○ UNRATED

STORE AND DISPENSE
Below 77°F (25°C), tight, amber glass bottle. Store in an upright position.

TABLETS
Store at controlled room temperature between 15°-30°C (59°-86°F), in tight, light-resistant container.

HOW SUPPLIED
SYRUP: 0.5 MG/5 ML

AVERAGE UNIT PRICE (AVAILABLE SIZES)		GENERIC A-RATED AVERAGE PRICE (GAAP)		
BRAND	$0.19	120 ml		$17.61
GENERIC	$0.15	120 ml		$18.72

BRAND/MANUFACTURER	NDC	SIZE	AWP
◆ BRAND			
TAVIST: Sandoz Pharm	00078-0222-31	120 ml	$22.68
◆ GENERICS			
Copley	38245-0268-14	120 ml	$16.50
Qualitest	00603-1096-54	120 ml	$16.50
Geneva	00781-6128-04	120 ml	$16.58
Barre	00472-0857-04	120 ml	$17.50
Rugby	00536-0735-97	120 ml	$17.50
Schein	00364-2445-77	120 ml	$17.50
URL	00677-1441-41	120 ml	$18.37
Goldline	00182-6036-37	120 ml	$18.50
Moore,H.L.	00839-7625-65	120 ml	$18.89
Aligen	00405-2529-76	120 ml	$20.10
Major	00904-1524-20	120 ml	$22.45

TABLETS: 1.34 MG

AVERAGE UNIT PRICE (AVAILABLE SIZES)		GENERIC A-RATED AVERAGE PRICE (GAAP)	
GENERIC	$0.48	100s	$47.56

BRAND/MANUFACTURER	NDC	SIZE	AWP
◆ GENERICS			
Lemmon	00093-0307-01	100s	$31.17
Major	00904-7678-60	100s	$31.25
Schein	00364-2520-01	100s	$33.00
Moore,H.L.	00839-7739-06	100s	$36.44
Goldline	00182-1935-01	100s	$57.50
Medirex	57480-0448-01	100s ud	$96.00

TABLETS: 2.68 MG

AVERAGE UNIT PRICE (AVAILABLE SIZES)		GENERIC A-RATED AVERAGE PRICE (GAAP)	
BRAND	$0.99	100s	$80.97
GENERIC	$0.81		
HCFA FUL (100s ea)	$0.82		

BRAND/MANUFACTURER	NDC	SIZE	AWP
◆ BRAND			
▶ TAVIST: Sandoz Pharm	00078-0072-05	100s	$99.06
◆ GENERICS			
Lemmon	00093-0308-01	100s	$72.50
Aligen	00405-5356-01	100s	$72.50
Qualitest	00603-2900-21	100s	$74.20
Goldline	00182-1936-01	100s	$76.50
Rugby	00536-3506-01	100s	$76.95
Schein	00364-2521-01	100s	$76.95
Moore,H.L.	00839-7740-06	100s	$76.95
Geneva	00781-1359-01	100s	$76.96
URL	00677-1443-01	100s	$77.06
Major	00904-7679-60	100s	$82.10
Medirex	57480-0449-01	100s ud	$128.00

Cleocin SEE CLINDAMYCIN, TOPICAL

Cleocin SEE CLINDAMYCIN, SYSTEMIC AND CLINDAMYCIN, VAGINAL

Clidinium Bromide

DESCRIPTION
Clidinium Bromide is 3-hydroxy-1-methylquinuclidinium bromide benzilate. A white or nearly white crystalline compound, it is soluble in water and has a calculated molecular weight of 432.36.

Clidinium Bromide is a quaternary ammonium compound with anticholinergic and antispasmodic activity available in 2.5 mg and 5 mg capsules.

Following is its chemical structure:

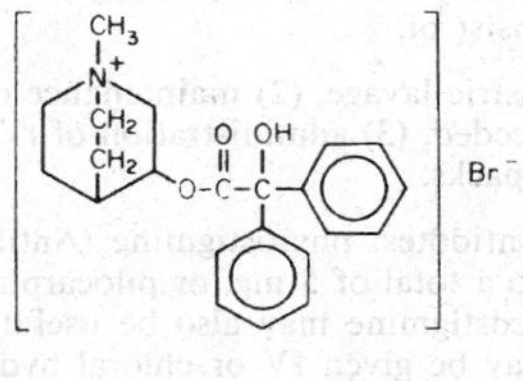

ACTIONS
Clidinium Bromide inhibits gastrointestinal motility and diminishes gastric acid secretion. Its anticholinergic activity approximates that of atropine sulfate and propantheline bromide.

INDICATIONS
Clidinium Bromide is effective as adjunctive therapy in peptic ulcer disease. Clidinium Bromide has not been shown to be effective in contributing to the healing of peptic ulcer, decreasing the rate of recurrence or preventing complications.

UNLABELED USES
Clidinium Bromide is used alone or as an adjunct in the treatment of irritable bowel syndrome and as an adjunct for symptomatic relief in other gastrointestinal disorders.

CONTRAINDICATIONS
Known hypersensitivity to clidinium bromide or to other anticholinergic drugs, glaucoma, obstructive uropathy (for example, bladder neck obstruction due to prostatic hypertrophy), obstructive disease of the gastrointestinal tract (for example, pyloroduodenal stenosis), paralytic ileus, intestinal atony of the elderly or debilitated patient, unstable cardiovascular status in acute hemorrhage, severe ulcerative colitis, "toxic megacolon" complicating ulcerative colitis, myasthenia gravis.

WARNINGS
Clidinium Bromide may produce drowsiness or blurred vision. The patient should be cautioned regarding activities requiring mental alertness such as operating a motor vehicle or other machinery or performing hazardous work while taking this drug. In the presence of high environmental temperature, heat prostration (fever and heat stroke) may occur with the use of anticholinergics due to decreased sweating. Diarrhea may be an early symptom of incomplete intestinal obstruction, especially in patients with ileostomy or colostomy. Use of anticholinergics in patients with suspected intestinal obstruction would be inappropriate and possibly harmful. With overdosage, a curare-like action may occur, i.e., neuromuscular blockade leading to muscular weakness and possible paralysis.

Usage in Pregnancy: No controlled studies in humans have been performed to establish the safety of the drug in pregnancy. Uncontrolled data derived from clinical usage have failed to show abnormalities attributable to its use. Reproduction studies in rats have failed to show any impaired fertility or abnormality in the fetuses that might be associated with the use of Clidinium Bromide. Use of any drug in pregnancy or in women of childbearing potential requires that the potential benefit of the drug be weighed against the possible hazards to mother and fetus.

Nursing Mothers: As with all anticholinergic drugs, Clidinium Bromide may be secreted in human milk and may inhibit lactation. As a general rule, nursing should not be undertaken while a patient is on Clidinium Bromide, or the drug should not be used by nursing mothers.

Pediatric Use: Since there is no adequate experience in children who have received this drug, safety and efficacy in children have not been established.

PRECAUTIONS
Use Clidinium Bromide with caution in the elderly and in all patients with autonomic neuropathy, hepatic or renal disease, ulcerative colitis—large doses may suppress intestinal motility to the point of producing a paralytic ileus and for this reason precipitate or aggravate "toxic megacolon," a serious complication of the disease: hyperthyroidism; coronary heart disease: congestive heart failure; cardiac tachy-arrhythmias; tachycardia; hypertension; prostatic hypertrophy; hiatal hernia associated with reflux esophagitis, since anticholinergic drugs may aggravate this condition.

ADVERSE REACTIONS
As with other anticholinergic drugs, the most frequently reported adverse effects are dryness of mouth, blurring of vision, urinary hesitancy and constipation. Other adverse effects reported with the use of anticholinergic drugs include decreased sweating, urinary retention, tachycardia, palpitations, dilatation of the pupils, cycloplegia, increased ocular tension, loss of taste, headaches, nervousness, mental confusion, drowsiness, weakness, dizziness, insomnia, nausea, vomiting, bloated feeling, impotence, suppression of lactation and severe allergic reactions or drug idiosyncrasies including anaphylaxis, urticaria and other dermal manifestations.

OVERDOSAGE
The symptoms of overdosage with Clidinium Bromide progress from an intensification of the usual side effects to CNS disturbances (from restlessness and

excitement to psychotic behavior), circulatory changes (flushing, tachycardia, fall in blood pressure, circulatory failure), respiratory failure, paralysis and coma.
Treatment should consist of:

General measures: (1) gastric lavage, (2) maintenance of adequate airway, using artificial respiration if needed, (3) administration of IV fluids, and (4) for fever: alcohol sponging or ice packs.

Specific measures: (1) Antidotes: physostigmine (Antilirium) 0.5 to 2 mg, IV, repeated as needed up to a total of 5 mg; or pilocarpine, 5 mg, s.c. at intervals until mouth is moist; neostigmine may also be useful, (2) Against excitement; sodium pentothal 2% may be given IV or chloral hydrate (100 to 200 ml, 2% solution) *rectally,* (3) Against hypotension and circulatory collapse: levarterenol or metaraminol infusions. (4) Against CNS depression; caffeine and sodium benzoate.
The usefulness of dialysis is not known.

DOSAGE AND ADMINISTRATION
For maximum efficacy, dosage should be individualized according to severity of symptoms and occurrence of side effects. The usual dosage is 2.5 to 5 mg three or four times daily before meals and at bedtime. Dosage in excess of 20 mg daily is usually not required to obtain maximum effectiveness. For the aged or debilitated, one 2.5-mg capsule three times daily before meals is recommended. The desired pharmacological effect of the drug is unlikely to be attained without occasional side effects.

DRUG INTERACTIONS
No specific drug interactions are known.

HOW SUPPLIED
CAPSULE: 2.5 MG

BRAND/MANUFACTURER	NDC	SIZE	AWP
○ BRAND			
QUARZAN: Roche Prod	00140-0119-01	100s	$19.22

CAPSULE: 5 MG

BRAND/MANUFACTURER	NDC	SIZE	AWP
○ BRAND			
QUARZAN: Roche Prod	00140-0120-01	100s	$26.20

Clindamycin, Systemic

WARNING

CLINDAMYCIN THERAPY HAS BEEN ASSOCIATED WITH SEVERE COLITIS WHICH MAY END FATALLY. THEREFORE, IT SHOULD BE RESERVED FOR SERIOUS INFECTIONS WHERE LESS TOXIC ANTIMICROBIAL AGENTS ARE INAPPROPRIATE, AS DESCRIBED IN THE INDICATIONS AND USAGE SECTION. IT SHOULD NOT BE USED IN PATIENTS WITH NONBACTERIAL INFECTIONS, SUCH AS MOST UPPER RESPIRATORY TRACT INFECTIONS. STUDIES INDICATE A TOXIN(S) PRODUCED BY *CLOSTRIDIA* IS ONE PRIMARY CAUSE OF ANTIBIOTIC-ASSOCIATED COLITIS. CHOLESTYRAMINE AND COLESTIPOL RESINS HAVE BEEN SHOWN TO BIND THE TOXIN *IN VITRO.* SEE "WARNINGS" SECTION. THE COLITIS IS USUALLY CHARACTERIZED BY SEVERE, PERSISTENT DIARRHEA AND SEVERE ABDOMINAL CRAMPS AND MAY BE ASSOCIATED WITH THE PASSAGE OF BLOOD AND MUCUS. ENDOSCOPIC EXAMINATION MAY REVEAL PSEUDOMEMBRANOUS COLITIS. STOOL CULTURE FOR *CLOSTRIDIUM DIFFICILE* AND STOOL ASSAY FOR *C. DIFFICILE* TOXIN MAY BE HELPFUL DIAGNOSTICALLY.

WHEN SIGNIFICANT DIARRHEA OCCURS, THE DRUG SHOULD BE DISCONTINUED OR, IF NECESSARY, CONTINUED ONLY WITH CLOSE OBSERVATION OF THE PATIENT. LARGE BOWEL ENDOSCOPY HAS BEEN RECOMMENDED.

ANTIPERISTALTIC AGENTS SUCH AS OPIATES AND DIPHENOXYLATE WITH ATROPINE MAY PROLONG AND/OR WORSEN THE CONDITION. VANCOMYCIN HAS BEEN FOUND TO BE EFFECTIVE IN THE TREATMENT OF ANTIBIOTIC ASSOCIATED PSEUDOMEMBRANOUS COLITIS PRODUCED BY *CLOSTRIDIUM DIFFICILE.* THE USUAL ADULT DOSAGE IS 500 MG TO 2 GM OF VANCOMYCIN ORALLY PER DAY IN THREE TO FOUR DIVIDED DOSES ADMINISTERED FOR 7 TO 10 DAYS. CHOLESTYRAMINE OR COLESTIPOL RESINS BIND VANCOMYCIN *IN VITRO.* IF BOTH A RESIN AND VANCOMYCIN ARE TO BE ADMINISTERED CONCURRENTLY, IT MAY BE ADVISABLE TO SEPARATE THE TIME OF ADMINISTRATION OF EACH DRUG.

DIARRHEA, COLITIS, AND PSEUDOMEMBRANOUS COLITIS HAVE BEEN OBSERVED TO BEGIN UP TO SEVERAL WEEKS FOLLOWING CESSATION OF THERAPY WITH CLINDAMYCIN.

DESCRIPTION
Clindamycin is a semisynthetic antibiotic produced by a 7(S)-chloro-substitution of the 7(R)-hydroxyl group of the parent compound lincomycin. Clindamycin, Systemic, is available as a solution for injection, oral solution, and capsules.

Each ml of solution for injection contains:
Clindamycin Phosphate equivalent to ....150 mg Clindamycin

Premixed solution for intravenous use contains:
Clindamycin Phosphate equivalent to ....300, 600, or 900 mg Clindamycin

Each 5 ml of oral solution contains:
Clindamycin Palmitate Hydrochloride equivalent to ....75 mg Clindamycin

Each capsule contains:
Clindamycin Hydrochloride equivalent to ....75, 150, or 300 mg Clindamycin

Clindamycin phosphate is a water soluble ester of Clindamycin and phosphoric acid. The chemical name of Clindamycin phosphate is L-*threo*-α-D-*galacto*-Octopyranoside, methyl 7-chloro-6,7,8-trideoxy-6-[[(1-methyl-4-propyl-2-pyrrolidinyl) cabonyl] amino]-1-thio-, 2 (dihydrogen phosphate), (2S-*trans)*-.
The molecular formula is $C_{18}H_{34}ClN_2O_8PS$ and the molecular weight is 504.96.
Clindamycin palmitate hydrochloride is a water soluble hydrochloride salt of the ester of Clindamycin and palmitic acid.
The chemical name for Clindamycin palmitate hydrochloride is Methyl 7-chloro-6,7,8-trideoxy-6(1-methyl-*trans*-4-propyl- L-2-pyrrolindinecarboxamido)-1-thio-L-*threo*-α-D-*galacto*-octopyranoside 2-palmitate monohydrochloride.
Clindamycin hydrochloride is the hydrated hydrochloride salt of Clindamycin.
The chemical name for Clindamycin hydrochloride is Methyl 7-chloro-6,7,8-trideoxy-6-(1-methyl-*trans*-4-propyl-L-2- pyrrolindinecarboxamido)-1-thio-L-*threo*-α-D-*galacto*-octopyranoside monohydrochloride.

Following is its chemical structure:

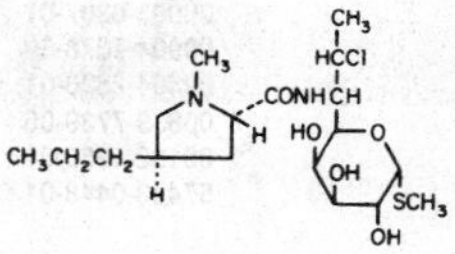

CLINICAL PHARMACOLOGY
Biologically inactive Clindamycin phosphate is rapidly converted to active Clindamycin.
By the end of short-term intravenous infusion, peak serum levels of active Clindamycin are reached. Biologically inactive Clindamycin phosphate disappears rapidly from the serum; the average disappearance half-life is 6 minutes; however, the serum disappearance half-life of active Clindamycin is about 3 hours in adults and 2 1/2 hours in children.
After intramuscular injection of Clindamycin phosphate, peak levels of active Clindamycin are reached within 3 hours in adults and 1 hour in children. Serum level curves may be constructed from IV peak serum levels as given in Table 1 by application of disappearance half-lives listed above.
Serum levels of Clindamycin can be maintained above the *in vitro* minimum inhibitory concentrations for most indicated organisms by administration of Clindamycin phosphate every 8-12 hours in adults and every 6-8 hours in children, or by continuous intravenous infusion. An equilibrium state is reached by the third dose.

Human Pharmacology: Blood level studies comparing Clindamycin Palmitate HCl with Clindamycin HCl show that both products reach their peak active serum levels at the same time, indicating a rapid hydrolysis of the palmitate to the Clindamycin.
Clindamycin is widely distributed in body fluids and tissues (including bones). Approximately 10% of the biological activity is excreted in the urine and 3.6% in the feces; the remainder is excreted as biologically inactive metabolites. The average biological half-life after doses of Clindamycin is approximately two hours in children.
Doses of up to 2 grams of Clindamycin per day for 14 days have been well tolerated by healthy volunteers, except that the incidence of gastrointestinal side effects is greater with the higher doses.
Serum level studies with Clindamycin palmitate HCl in normal children weighing 50-100 lbs given 2, 3 or 4 mg/kg every 6 hours (8, 12 or 16 mg/kg/day) demonstrated mean peak Clindamycin serum levels of 1.24, 2.25 and 2.44 mcg/mL respectively, one hour after the first dose. By the fifth dose, the 6-hour serum concentration had reached equilibrium. Peak serum concentration after this time would be about 2.46, 2.98 and 3.79 mcg/mL with doses of 8, 12, 16 mg/kg/day, respectively. Serum levels have been uniform and predictable from person to person and dose to dose. Multiple-dose studies in newborns and infants up to 6 months of age show that the drug does not accumulate in the serum and is excreted rapidly. Serum levels exceed the MICs for most indicated organisms for at least six hours following administration of the usually recommended doses of Clindamycin palmitite HCl in adults and children.

◆ RATED THERAPEUTICALLY EQUIVALENT; ◇ THERAPEUTIC EQUIVALENCE UNCONFIRMED; ○ UNRATED

Serum level studies with a 150 mg oral dose of Clindamycin HCl in 24 normal adult volunteers showed that Clindamycin was rapidly absorbed after oral administration. An average peak serum level of 2.50 mcg/mL was reached in 45 minutes; serum levels averaged 1.51 mcg/mL at 3 hours and 0.70 mcg/mL at 6 hours. Absorption of an oral dose is virtually complete (90%), and the concomitant administration of food does not appreciably modify the serum concentrations; serum levels have been uniform and predictable from person to person and dose to dose. Serum level studies following multiple doses of Clindamycin HCl capsules for up to 14 days show no evidence of accumulation or altered metabolism of drug.

The disappearance half-life of Clindamycin is increased slightly in patients with markedly reduced renal or hepatic function. Hemodialysis and peritoneal dialysis do not appreciably affect the half-life of Clindamycin in the serum and are not effective in removing Clindamycin from the serum. Dosage schedules need not be modified in the presence of mild or moderate renal or hepatic disease.

No significant levels of Clindamycin are attained in the cerebrospinal fluid, even in the presence of inflamed meninges. Serum assays for active Clindamycin require an inhibitor to prevent *in vitro* hydrolysis of Clindamycin phosphate.

Table 1

AVERAGE PEAK SERUM CONCENTRATIONS AFTER DOSING WITH CLINDAMYCIN PHOSPHATE

Clindamycin Phosphate Dosage Regimen	Clindamycin > mcg/ml	Clindamycin Phosphate mcg/ml
Healthy Adult Males (Post equilibrium)		
300 mg IV in 10 min, q8h	7	15
600 mg IV in 20 min, q8h	10	23
900 mg IV in 30 min, q12h	11	29
1200 mg IV in 45 min, q12h	14	49
300 mg IM q8h	6	3
600 mg IM q12h*	9	3
Children (first dose)*		
5-7 mg/kg IV in 1 hr	10	
3-5 mg/kg IM	4	
5-7 mg/kg IM	8	

Data in this group from patients being treated for infection

Microbiology: Although Clindamycin phosphate and Clindamycin phosphate hydrochloride are inactive *in vitro*, rapid *in vivo* hydrolysis converts these compounds to the antibacterially active Clindamycin.

Clindamycin has been shown to have *in vitro* activity against isolates of the following organisms:

AEROBIC GRAM POSITIVE COCCI
Including:
Staphylococcus aureus
Staphylococcus epidermidis (penicillinase and nonpenicillinase producing strains).

When tested by *in vitro* methods some staphylococcal strains originally resistant to erythromycin rapidly develop resistance to Clindamycin.

Streptococci (except *Streptococcus faecalis*)
Pneumococci

ANAEROBIC GRAM NEGATIVE BACILLI
Including:
Bacteroides species (including *Bacteroides fragilis* group and *Bacteroides melaninogenicus* group)
Fusobacterium species

ANAEROBIC GRAM POSITIVE NONSPOREFORMING BACILLI
Including:
Propionibacterium
Eubacterium
Acticomyces species

ANAEROBIC AND MICROAEROPHILIC GRAM POSITIVE COCCI
Including:
Peptococcus species
Peptostreptococcus species
Microaerophilic streptococci

Clostridia: Clostridia are more resistant than most anaerobes to Clindamycin. Most *Clostridium perfringens* are susceptible, but other species, eg, *Clostridium sporogenes* and *Clostridium tertium* are frequently resistant to Clindamycin. Susceptibility testing should be done.

Cross resistance has been demonstrated between Clindamycin and lincomycin. Antagonism has been demonstrated between Clindamycin and erythromycin.

IN VITRO SUSCEPTIBILITY TESTING
Disk Diffusion Technique: Quantitative methods that require measurement of zone diameters give the most precise estimates of antibiotic susceptibility. One such procedure[1] has been recommended for use with disks to test susceptibility to Clindamycin.

Reports from a laboratory using the standardized single-disk susceptibility test[1] with a 2 mcg Clindamycin disk should be interpreted according to the following criteria:

Susceptible organisms produce zones of 17 mm or greater, indicating that the tested organism is likely to respond to therapy.

Organisms of intermediate susceptibility produce zones of 15-16 mm, indicating that the tested organism would be susceptible if a high dosage is used or if the infection is confined to tissues and fluids (e.g., urine), in which high antibiotic levels are attained.

Resistant organisms produce zones of 14 mm or less, indicating that other therapy should be selected.

Standardized procedures require the use of control organisms. The 2 mcg Clindamycin disk should give a zone diameter between 24 and 30 mm for *S. aureus* ATCC 25923.

Dilution techniques: A bacterial isolate may be considered susceptible if the minimum inhibitory concentration (MIC) for Clindamycin is not more than 1.6 mcg/mL. Organisms are considered moderately susceptible if the MIC is greater than 1.6 mcg/mL and less than or equal to 4.8 mcg/mL. Organisms are considered resistant if the MIC is greater than 4.8 mcg per mL.

The range of MIC's for the control strains are as follows:

S. aureus ATCC 29213, 0.06-0.25 mcg/mL.
E. faecalis ATCC 29212, 4.0-16 mcg/mL.

For anaerobic bacteria the minimum inhibitory concentration (MIC) of Clindamycin can be determined by agar dilution and broth dilution (including microdilution) techniques.[2] If MICs are not determined routinely, the disk broth method is recommended for routine use. *The Kirby-Bauer disk diffusion method and its interpretive standards are not recommended for anaerobes.*

INDICATIONS AND USAGE
Clindamycin phosphate products are indicated in the treatment of serious infections caused by susceptible anaerobic bacteria.

Clindamycin phosphate products are also indicated in the treatment of serious infections due to susceptible strains of streptococci, pneumococci, and staphylococci. Its use should be reserved for penicillin-allergic patients or other patients for whom, in the judgment of the physician, a penicillin is inappropriate. Because of the risk of antibiotic-associated pseudomembranous colitis, as described in the *"Warning"* box, before selecting Clindamycin the physician should consider the nature of the infection and the suitability of less toxic alternatives (e.g., erythromycin).

Bacteriologic studies should be performed to determine the causative organisms and their susceptibility to Clindamycin. Indicated surgical procedures should be performed in conjunction with antibiotic therapy.

Clindamycin phosphate is indicated in the treatment of serious infections caused by susceptible strains of the designated organisms in the conditions listed below:

Lower respiratory tract infections including pneumonia, empyema, and lung abscess caused by anaerobes, *Streptococcus pneumoniae*, other streptococci (except *E. faecalis*), pneumococci, and *Staphylococcus aureus.*

Skin and skin structure infections caused by *Streptococcus pyogenes, Staphylococcus aureus*, and anaerobes.

Gynecological infections including endometritis, nongonococcal tube ovarian abscess, pelvic cellulitis, and postsurgical vaginal cuff infection caused by susceptible anaerobes.

Intra-abdominal infections including peritonitis and intra-abdominal abscess caused by susceptible anaerobic organisms—typically organisms resident in the normal gastrointestinal tract.

Septicemia caused by *Staphylococcus aureus,* streptococci (except *Enterococcus faecalis*), and susceptible anaerobes. Bone and joint infections including acute hematogenous osteomyelitis caused by *Staphylococcus aureus* and as adjunctive therapy in the surgical treatment of chronic bone and joint infections due to susceptible organisms.

UNLABELED USES
Clindamycin is used alone or as an adjunct in the treatment of babesiosis, endometritis, malaria due to chloroquine-resistant *Plasmodium Falciparum,* and in pediatric patients with chronic recurrent suppurative otitis media. It is also used to control the rate of disease progression in refractory peridonitis in adult patients, in the treatment and prevention of *Pneumocystis Carinii* pneumonia (PCP) associated with acquired immunodeficiency syndrome (AIDS), and as an treatment adjunct in toxoplasmosis. In addition, oral Clindamycin is used as an alternative to metronidazole for treating bacterial vaginosis.

CONTRAINDICATIONS
This drug is contraindicated in individuals with a history of hypersensitivity to preparations containing Clindamycin or lincomycin.

WARNINGS
See *"Warning"* box. Studies indicate a toxin(s) produced by *Clostridia* is one primary cause of antibiotic associated colitis.[3-7] Cholestyramine and colestipol resins have been shown to bind the toxin *in vitro*. Mild cases of colitis may respond to drug discontinuance alone. Moderate to severe cases should be managed promptly with fluid, electrolyte and protein supplementation as indicated. Vancomycin has been found to be effective in the treatment of antibiotic-associated pseudomembranous colitis produced by *Clostridium difficile*. The usual adult dosage is 500 milligrams to 2 grams of vancomycin orally per day in three to four divided doses administered for 7 to 10 days. Cholestyramine or colestipol resins bind vancomycin *in vitro*. If both a resin and vancomycin are to be administered concurrently, it may be advisable to separate the time of

administration of each drug. Systemic corticoids and corticoid retention enemas may help relieve the colitis. Other causes of colitis should also be considered.

A careful inquiry should be made concerning previous sensitivities to drugs and other allergens.

Some brands contain benzyl alcohol as a preservative. Benzyl alcohol has been associated with a fatal "Gasping Syndrome" in premature infants. (See *"Precautions—Pediatric Use."*)

Usage in Meningitis: Since clindamycin does not diffuse adequately into the cerebrospinal fluid, the drug should not be used in the treatment of meningitis.

SERIOUS ANAPHYLACTOID REACTIONS REQUIRE IMMEDIATE EMERGENCY TREATMENT WITH EPINEPHRINE, OXYGEN AND INTRAVENOUS CORTICOSTEROIDS SHOULD ALSO BE ADMINISTERED AS INDICATED.

PRECAUTIONS
GENERAL
Review of experience to date suggests that a subgroup of older patients with associated severe illness may tolerate diarrhea less well. When Clindamycin is indicated in these patients, they should be carefully monitored for change in bowel frequency.

Clindamycin phosphate products should be prescribed with caution in individuals with a history of gastrointestinal disease, particularly colitis.

Clindamycin phosphate should be prescribed with caution in atopic individuals.

Certain infections may require incision and drainage or other indicated surgical procedures in addition to antibiotic therapy.

The use of Clindamycin phosphate may result in overgrowth of nonsusceptible organisms—particularly yeasts. Should superinfections occur, appropriate measures should be taken as indicated by the clinical situation.

Clindamycin phosphate should not be injected intravenously undiluted as a bolus, but should be infused over at least 10-60 minutes as directed in the *"Dosage and Administration"* section.

Patients with very severe renal disease and/or very severe hepatic disease accompanied by severe metabolic aberrations should be dosed with caution, and serum Clindamycin levels monitored during high-dose therapy (see *"Overdosage"*).

LABORATORY TESTS
During prolonged therapy periodic liver and kidney function tests and blood counts should be performed.

DRUG INTERACTIONS
Clindamycin has been shown to have neuromuscular blocking properties that may enhance the action of other neuro-muscular blocking agents. Therefore, it should be used with caution in patients receiving such agents.

Antagonism has been demonstrated between Clindamycin and erythromycin *in vitro.* Because of possible clinical significance, the two drugs should not be administered concurrently.

USAGE IN PREGNANCY
Safety for use in pregnancy has not been established.

NURSING MOTHERS
Clindamycin has been reported to appear in breast milk in the range of 0.7 to 3.8 mcg/ml at dosages of 150 mg orally to 600 mg intravenously. Because of the potential for adverse reactions due to Clindamycin in neonates (see *"Pediatric Use"*), the decision to discontinue the drug should be made, taking into account the importance of the drug to the mother.

PEDIATRIC USE
When Clindamycin phosphate is administered to newborns, infants, and children, appropriate monitoring of organ system functions is desirable.

USAGE IN NEWBORNS AND INFANTS
Some brands contain benzyl alcohol as a preservative. Benzyl alcohol has been associated with a fatal "Gasping Syndrome" in premature infants.

When Clindamycin palmitate HCl oral solution is administered to newborns and infants, appropriate monitoring of organ system functions is desirable.

The potential for the toxic effect in children from chemicals that may leach from the single dose premixed IV preparation in plastic has not been evaluated.

Some formulations of some brands contain FD&C Yellow No. 5 (tartrazine) which may cause allergic-type reactions (including bronchial asthma) in certain susceptible individuals. Although the overall incidence of FD&C Yellow No. 5 (tartrazine) sensitivity in the general population is low, it is frequently seen in patients who also have aspirin hypersensitivity.

ADVERSE REACTIONS
The following reactions have been reported with the use of clindamycin.

Gastrointestinal: Abdominal pain, esophagitis, nausea, vomiting and diarrhea (see *"Warnings"*). An unpleasant or metallic taste occasionally has been reported after intravenous administration of the higher doses of Clindamycin phosphate.

Hypersensitivity Reactions: Maculopapular rash and urticaria have been observed during drug therapy. Generalized mild to moderate morbilliform-like skin rashes are the most frequently reported of all adverse reactions. Rare instances of erythema multiforme, some resembling Stevens-Johnson syndrome, have been associated with Clindamycin. A few cases of anaphylactoid reactions have been reported.

If a hypersensitivity reaction occurs, the drug should be discontinued. The usual agents (epinephrine, corticosteroids, antihistamines) should be available for emergency treatment of serious reactions.

Liver: Jaundice and abnormalities in liver function tests have been observed during Clindamycin therapy.

Renal: Although no direct relationship of Clindamycin to renal damage has been established, renal dysfunction as evidenced by azotemia, oliguria, and/or proteinuria has been observed in rare instances.

Hematopoietic: Transient neutropenia (leukopenia) and eosinophilia have been reported. Reports of agranulocytosis and thrombocytopenia have been made. No direct etiologic relationship to concurrent Clindamycin therapy could be made in any of the foregoing.

Local Reactions: Pain, induration and sterile abscess have been reported after intramuscular injection and thrombophlebitis after intravenous infusion. Reactions can be minimized or avoided by giving deep intramuscular injections and avoiding prolonged use of indwelling intravenous catheters.

Musculoskeletal: Rare instances of polyarthritis have been reported.

Cardiovascular: Rare instances of cardiopulmonary arrest and hypotension have been reported following too rapid intravenous administration. (See *"Dosage and Administration"* section.)

OVERDOSAGE
Hemodialysis and peritoneal dialysis are not effective in removing Clindamycin from the serum.

DOSAGE AND ADMINISTRATION
If diarrhea occurs during therapy, this antibiotic should be discontinued. (See *"Warning"* box).

PARENTERAL (IM OR IV ADMINISTRATION)
Adults: Serious infections due to aerobic gram-positive cocci and the more susceptible anaerobes (NOT generally including *Bacteroides fragilis, Peptococcus* species and *Clostridium* species other than *Clostridium perfringens*):
  600-1200 mg/day in 2, 3 or 4 equal doses.
More severe infections, particularly those due to proven or suspected *Bacteroides fragilis Peptococcus* species, or *Clostridium* species other than *Clostridium perfringens:*
  1200-2700 mg/day in 2, 3 or 4 equal doses.
For more serious infections, these doses may have to be increased. In life threatening situations due to aerobes or anaerobes, these doses may be increased. Doses of as much as 4800 mg daily have been given intravenously to adults. See *"Dilution and Infusion Rates"* section below.

Single intramuscular injections of greater than 600 mg are not recommended.

Alternatively, drug may be administered in the form of a single rapid infusion of the first dose followed by continuous IV infusion as follows:

Clindamycin Phosphate To maintain serum Clindamycin levels	Rapid infusion rate	Maintenance infusion rate
Above 4 mcg/ml	10 mg/min for 30 min	0.75 mg/min
Above 5 mcg/ml	15 mg/min for 30 min	1.00 mg/min
Above 6 mcg/ml	20 mg/min for 30 min	1.25 mg/min

Neonates (less than 1 month): 15 to 20 mg/kg/day in 3 to 4 equal doses. The lower dosage may be adequate for small prematures.

Children (over 1 month of age): 20 to 40 mg/kg/day in 3 or 4 equal doses. The higher doses would be used for more severe infections. As an alternative to dosing on a body weight basis, children may be dosed on the basis of square meters body surface: 350 mg/m^2/day for serious infections and 450 mg/m^2/day for more severe infections.

Parenteral therapy may be changed to oral Clindamycin palmitate HCl pediatric granules or Clindamycin HCl capsules when the condition warrants and at the discretion of the physician.

In cases of β-hemolytic streptococcal infections, treatment should be continued for at least 10 days.

DILUTION AND INFUSION RATES
Clindamycin phosphate must be diluted prior to IV administration. The concentration of Clindamycin in diluent for infusion should not exceed 18 mg per mL. Infusion rates should not exceed 30 mg per minute. The usual infusion dilutions and rates are as follows:

Dose	Diluent	Time
300 mg	50 mL	10 min
600 mg	50 mL	20 min
900 mg	100 mL	30 min
1200 mg	100 mL	40 min

Administration of more than 1200 mg in a single 1-hour infusion is not recommended.

Parenteral drug products should be inspected visually for particulate matter and discoloration prior to administration, whenever solution and container permit.

Dilution and Compatibility: Physical and biological compatibility studies monitored for 24 hours at room temperature have demonstrated no inactivation or incompatibility with the use of Clindamycin phosphate solution in IV solutions containing sodium chloride, glucose, calcium or potassium, and solutions containing vitamin B complex in concentrations usually used clinically. No incompatibility has been demonstrated with the antibiotics cephalothin, kanamycin, gentamicin, penicillin or carbenicillin.

The following drugs are physically incompatible with Clindamycin phosphate: ampicllin sodium, phenytoin sodium, barbiturates, aminophylline, calcium gluconate, and magnesium sulfate.

The compatibility and duration of stability of drug admixtures will vary depending on concentration and other conditions.

PHYSICO-CHEMICAL STABILITY OF DILUTED SOLUTIONS OF CLINDAMYCIN PHOSPHATE

Room temperature: 6, 9, and 12 mg/mL (equivalent to Clindamycin base) in dextrose 5% in water, sodium chloride 0.9%, or Lactated Ringer's in glass bottles or minibags, demonstrated physical and chemical stability for at least 16 days at 25℃. Also, 18 mg/mL (equivalent to Clindamycin base) in dextrose 5% in water, in minibags, demonstrated physical and chemical stability for at least 16 days at 25℃.

Refrigeration: 6, 9 and 12 mg/ml (equivalent to Clindamycin base) in dextrose 5% in water, sodium chloride 0.9%, or Lactated Ringer's in glass bottles or minibags, demonstrated physical and chemical stability for at least 32 days at 4℃. Frozen: 6, 9 and 12 mg/ml equivalent to Clindamycin base) in dextrose 5% in water, sodium chloride 0.9%, or Lactated Ringer's in minibags demonstrated physical and chemical stability for at least eight weeks at −10℃.

Frozen solutions should be thawed at room temperature and not refrozen.

DIRECTIONS FOR DISPENSING

Pharmacy Bulk Package: Not for Direct Infusion.

The Pharmacy Bulk Package is for use in a Pharmacy Admixture Service only under a laminar flow hood. Entry into the vial should be made with a small diameter sterile transfer set or other small diameter sterile dispensing device, and contents dispensed in aliquots using aseptic technique. Multiple entries with a needle and syringe are not recommended. *After entry use entire contents of vial promptly. Any unused portion must be discarded within 24 hours after initial entry.*

DIRECTIONS FOR USE

PREMIXED CLINDAMYCIN, PHOSPHATE IV SOLUTION

Premixed Clindamycin phosphate IV solution is for intravenous administration using sterile equipment. Check for minute leaks prior to use by squeezing bag firmly. If leaks are found, discard solution as sterility may be impaired. Do not add supplementary medication. Parenteral drug products should be inspected visually for particulate matter and discoloration prior to administration whenever solution and container permit. Do not use unless solution is clear and seal is intact.

Caution: Do not use plastic containers in series connections. Such use could result in air embolism due to residual air being drawn from the primary container before administration of the fluid from the secondary container is complete.

Preparation for Administration:

1. Suspend container from eyelet support.
2. Remove protector from outlet port at bottom of container.
3. Attach administration set. Refer to complete directions accompanying set.

Preparation of Clindamycin phosphate in ADD-Vantage‡Ssystem-For IV Only. Clindamycin phosphate 600 mg and 900 mg may be reconstituted in 50 mg or 100 ml, respectively, of 5% Dextrose or 0.9% Sodium Chloride in the ADD-diluent container. Refer to separate instructions for ADD-Vantage System.

ORAL SOLUTION

Concomitant administration of food does not adversely affect the absorption of Clindamycin palmitate HCl contained in Clindamycin pediatric granules for oral solution.

Serious infections: 8-12 mg/kg/day (4-6 mg/lb/day) divided into 3 or 4 equal doses.

Severe infections: 13-16 mg/kg/day (6.5-8 mg/lb/day) divided into 3 or 4 equal doses.

More severe infections: 17-25 mg/kg/day (8.5-12.5 mg/lb/day) divided into 3 or 4 equal doses.

In children weighing 10 kg or less, 1/2 teaspoon (37.5 mg) three times a day should be considered the minimum recommended dose.

Serious infections due to anaerobic bacteria are usually treated with Clindamycin phosphate regular solution. However, in clinically appropriate circumstances, the physician may elect to initiate treatment or continue treatment with the pediatric solution.

Note: In cases of β-hemolytic streptococcal infections, treatment should be continued for at least 10 days.

RECONSTITUTION INSTRUCTIONS

When reconstituted with water as follows, each 5 mL (teaspoon) of solution contains Clindamycin Palmitate HCl equivalent to 75 mg Clindamycin.

Reconstitute bottles of 100 mL with **75 mL** of water. Add a large portion of the water and shake vigorously; add the remainder of the water and shake until the solution is uniform.

STORAGE CONDITIONS

Store unreconstituted product at controlled room temperature 15°-30°C (59°-86°F).

Do *not* refrigerate the reconstituted solution; when chilled, the solution may thicken and be difficult to pour. The solution is stable for 2 weeks at room temperature.

CAPSULES

Adults

Serious infections: 150 to 300 mg every 6 hours.

More severe infections: 300 to 450 mg every 6 hours.

Children

Serious infections: 8 to 16 mg/kg/day (4 to 8 mg/lb/day) divided into three or four equal doses.

More severe infections: 16 to 20 mg/kg/day (8 to 10 mg/lb/day) divided into three or four equal doses.

To avoid the possibility of esophageal irritation, Clindamycin HCl capsules should be taken with a full glass of water.

Serious infections due to anaerobic bacteria are usually treated with Clindamycin Phosphate solution. However, in clinically appropriate circumstances, the physician may elect to initiate treatment or continue treatment with Clindamycin HCl capsules.

In cases of β-hemolytic streptococcal infections, treatment should continue for at least 10 days.

Exposure of pharmaceutical products to heat should be minimized. It is recommended that Galaxy plastic containers be stored at room temperature (25° C). Avoid temperatures above 30°C.

REFERENCES

1. Bauer, AW. Kirby, WMM, Sherris, JC. Turck, M: Antibiotic susceptibility testing by a standardized single disc method. *Am J Clin Path,* 45:493-496, 1966. Standardized Disc Susceptibility Test, *Federal Register 37:20527-29, 1972.* 2. National Committee for Clinical Lab. Standards. Methods for Antimicrobial Susceptibility Testing of Anaerobic Bacteria—Second Edition; Tentative Standard. NCCLS publication M11-T2. Villanova, PA; NCCLS: 1988. 3. Bartlett JG, et al: Antibiotic associated pseudomembranous colitis due to toxin-producing *Clostridia. N Engl J Med* 298(10):531-534, 1978. 4. George RH, et al: Identification of *Clostridium difficile* as a cause of pseudomembranous colitis. *Br Med J* 6114:669-671, 1978. 5. Larson HE, Price AB: Pseudomembranous colitis presence of clostridial toxin. *Lancet* 8052/3:1312-1314, 1977. 6. Rifkin GD, Fekety FR, Silva J: Antibiotic-induced colitis implication of a toxin neutralized by *Clostridium sordellii* antitoxin. *Lancet* 8048:1103-1106, 1977. 7. Bailey WR, Scott EG: Diagnostic Microbiology. The CV Mosby Company, St. Louis, 1978.

HOW SUPPLIED

CLINDAMYCIN HYDROCHLORIDE
CAPSULE: 75 MG

BRAND/MANUFACTURER	NDC	SIZE	AWP
◆ BRAND			
▶ CLEOCIN HCL: Upjohn	00009-0331-02	100s	$60.14

CAPSULE: 150 MG

AVERAGE UNIT PRICE (AVAILABLE SIZES)		GENERIC A-RATED AVERAGE PRICE (GAAP)	
BRAND	$1.15	100s	$89.98
GENERIC	$0.90		
HCFA FUL (100s ea)	$0.75		

BRAND/MANUFACTURER	NDC	SIZE	AWP
◆ BRAND			
▶ CLEOCIN HCL: Upjohn	00009-0225-01	16s	$18.89
	00009-0225-02	100s	$111.01
	00009-0225-03	100s ud	$114.50
◆ GENERICS			
Allscrips	54569-3456-01	15s	$14.04
Allscrips	54569-3456-00	30s	$28.08
Raway	00686-3171-09	100s	$59.00
Biocraft	00332-3171-09	100s	$85.00
Mason Dist	11845-0461-01	100s	$86.00
Goldline	00182-1202-01	100s	$87.99
Schein	00364-2337-01	100s	$91.25
Geneva	00781-2937-01	100s	$93.38
Aligen	00405-4233-01	100s	$96.20
Qualitest	00603-2909-21	100s	$96.43
Moore,H.L.	00839-7534-06	100s	$97.19
URL	00677-1333-01	100s	$97.20
Major	00904-3838-60	100s	$97.90
Rugby	00536-0155-01	100s	$103.73
U.S. Trading	56126-0418-11	100s ud	$83.76
UDL	51079-0598-20	100s ud	$85.40
Raway	00686-0598-20	100s ud	$89.30

CAPSULE: 300 MG

AVERAGE UNIT PRICE (AVAILABLE SIZES)			
BRAND	$2.28		

BRAND/MANUFACTURER	NDC	SIZE	AWP
◆ BRAND			
➤ CLEOCIN HCL: Upjohn	00009-0395-13	16s	$37.65
	00009-0395-14	100s	$221.26
	00009-0395-02	100s ud	$225.79

INJECTION: 150 MG/ML

BRAND/MANUFACTURER	NDC	SIZE	AWP
◆ GENERICS			
Raway	00686-9102-04	2 ml 25s	$60.00

CLINDAMYCIN PALMITATE HYDROCHLORIDE
GRANULE FOR RECONSTITUTION: 75 MG/5 ML

BRAND/MANUFACTURER	NDC	SIZE	AWP
◆ BRAND			
CLEOCIN PEDIATRIC: Upjohn	00009-0760-04	100 ml	$12.34

CLINDAMYCIN PHOSPHATE
INJECTION: 9 GM

BRAND/MANUFACTURER	NDC	SIZE	AWP
◆ BRAND			
CLEOCIN PHOSPHATE: Upjohn	00009-0728-05	60 ml	$181.18

INJECTION: 150 MG/ML

AVERAGE UNIT PRICE (AVAILABLE SIZES)		GENERIC A-RATED AVERAGE PRICE (GAAP)	
BRAND	$3.45	2 ml 25s	$189.07
GENERIC	$3.31	4 ml 25s	$344.40
		6 ml 25s	$468.37

BRAND/MANUFACTURER	NDC	SIZE	AWP
◆ BRAND			
CLEOCIN PHOSPHATE: Upjohn	00009-0870-21	2 ml	$7.58
	00009-0775-20	4 ml	$13.86
	00009-3124-01	4 ml	$14.70
	00009-0902-11	6 ml	$18.49
	00009-3447-01	6 ml	$19.41
◆ GENERICS			
Abbott Hosp	00074-4197-01	60 ml	$206.82
Astra	00186-1453-01	60 ml 5s	$343.75
Lederle Std Prod	00205-2801-24	60 ml 10s	$1743.75
Astra	00186-1450-04	2 ml 25s	$140.63
Solo Pak	39769-0226-02	2 ml 25s	$140.63
Gensia	00703-9102-04	2 ml 25s	$156.88
Lederle Std Prod	00205-2801-83	2 ml 25s	$180.31
Abbott Hosp	00074-4050-01	2 ml 25s	$256.80
Abbott Hosp	00074-4053-03	2 ml 25s	$259.17
Astra	00186-1451-04	4 ml 25s	$250.00
Solo Pak	39769-0226-04	4 ml 25s	$260.94
Gensia	00703-9110-04	4 ml 25s	$280.00
Lederle Std Prod	00205-2801-93	4 ml 25s	$328.13
Abbott Hosp	00074-4051-01	4 ml 25s	$471.14
Abbott Hosp	00074-4054-03	4 ml 25s	$476.19
Astra	00186-1452-04	6 ml 25s	$328.13
Solo Pak	39769-0226-06	6 ml 25s	$346.88
Gensia	00703-9120-04	6 ml 25s	$366.25
Lederle Std Prod	00205-2801-47	6 ml 25s	$501.88
Abbott Hosp	00074-4052-01	6 ml 25s	$630.56
Abbott Hosp	00074-4055-03	6 ml 25s	$636.50

INJECTION: 300 MG/50 ML

BRAND/MANUFACTURER	NDC	SIZE	AWP
◆ BRAND			
CLEOCIN PHOSPHATE: Upjohn	00009-3381-01	50 ml	$4.11

INJECTION: 600 MG/50 ML

BRAND/MANUFACTURER	NDC	SIZE	AWP
◆ BRAND			
CLEOCIN PHOSPHATE: Upjohn	00009-3375-01	50 ml	$5.80

INJECTION: 900 MG/50 ML

BRAND/MANUFACTURER	NDC	SIZE	AWP
◆ BRAND			
CLEOCIN PHOSPHATE: Upjohn	00009-3382-01	50 ml	$6.06

Clindamycin, Topical

DESCRIPTION
Clindamycin topical solution, gel and lotion contain Clindamycin phosphate, USP, at a concentration equivalent to 10 mg Clindamycin per milliliter.

Clindamycin phosphate is a water soluble ester of the semisynthetic antibiotic produced by a 7(S)-chloro-substitution of the 7(R)-hydroxyl group of the parent antibiotic lincomycin.

The chemical name for Clindamycin phosphate is 7(S)-chloro-7-deoxylincomycin-2-phosphate. (MW = 504.96).

Following is its chemical structure:

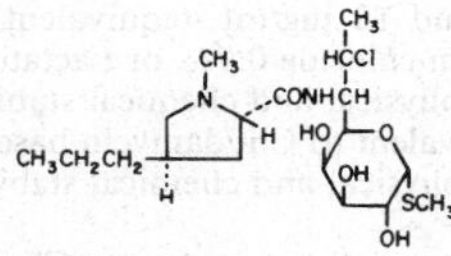

CLINICAL PHARMACOLOGY
Although Clindamycin phosphate is inactive *in vitro,* rapid *in vivo* hydrolysis converts this compound to the antibacterially active Clindamycin.

Clindamycin has been shown to have *in vivo* activity against isolates of *Propionibacterium acnes.* This may account for its usefulness in acne.

Cross resistance has been demonstrated between Clindamycin and lincomycin. Antagonism has been demonstrated between Clindamycin and erythromycin.

Following multiple topical applications of Clindamycin phosphate at a concentration equivalent to 10 mg Clindamycin per mL in an isopropyl alcohol and water solution, very low levels of Clindamycin are present in the serum (0-3 ng/mL) and less than 0.2% of the dose is recovered in urine as Clindamycin.

Clindamycin activity has been demonstrated in comedones from acne patients. The mean concentration of antibiotic activity in extracted comedones after application of Clindamycin topical solution for 4 weeks was 597 mcg/g of comedonal material (range 0-1490). Clindamycin *in vitro* inhibits all *Propionibacterium acnes* cultures tested (MICs 0.4 mcg/mL). Free fatty acids on the skin surface have been decreased from approximately 14% to 2% following application of Clindamycin.

INDICATIONS AND USAGE
Clindamycin topical solution, gel and lotion are indicated in the treatment of acne vulgaris. In view of the potential for diarrhea, bloody diarrhea and pseudomembranous colitis, the physician should consider whether other agents are more appropriate. (See *"Contraindications," "Warnings"* and *"Adverse Reactions".*)

CONTRAINDICATIONS
Clindamycin topical solution, gel and lotion are contraindicated in individuals with a history of hypersensitivity to preparations containing Clindamycin or lincomycin, a history of regional enteritis or ulcerative colitis, or a history of antibiotic-associated colitis.

WARNINGS
Orally and parenterally administered Clindamycin has been associated with severe colitis which may end fatally. Use of the topical formulation results in absorption of the antibiotic from the skin surface. Diarrhea, bloody diarrhea, and colitis (including pseudomembranous colitis) have been reported with the use of topical and systemic Clindamycin. Symptoms can occur after a few days, weeks or months following initiation of Clindamycin therapy. They have also been observed to begin up to several weeks after cessation of therapy with Clindamycin. Studies indicate a toxin(s) produced by *Clostridium difficile* is one primary cause of antibiotic-associated colitis. The colitis is usually characterized by severe persistent diarrhea and severe abdominal cramps and may be associated with the passage of blood and mucus. Endoscopic examination may reveal pseudomembranous colitis.

When significant diarrhea occurs, the drug should be discontinued. Large bowel endoscopy should be considered in cases of severe diarrhea.

Antiperistaltic agents such as opiates and diphenoxylate with atropine may prolong and/or worsen the condition. Vancomycin has been found to be effective in the treatment of antibiotic-associated pseudomembranous colitis produced by *Clostridium difficile.* The usual adult dosage is 500 mg to 2 grams of vancomycin orally per day in three to four divided doses administered for 7 to 10 days.

Mild cases of colitis may respond to discontinuance of Clindamycin. Moderate to severe cases should be managed promptly with fluid, electrolyte, and protein supplementation as indicated. Cholestyramine and colestipol resins have been shown to bind the toxin *in vitro.* If both a resin and vancomycin are to be administered concurrently, it may be advisable to separate the time of administration of each drug. Systemic corticoids and corticoid retention enemas may help relieve the colitis. Other causes of colitis should also be considered. A careful inquiry should be made concerning previous sensitivities to drugs and other allergens.

◆ RATED THERAPEUTICALLY EQUIVALENT; ◇ THERAPEUTIC EQUIVALENCE UNCONFIRMED; ○ UNRATED

PRECAUTIONS

Clindamycin topical solution contains an alcohol base which will cause burning and irritation of the eye. In the event of accidental contact with sensitive surfaces (eye, abraded skin, mucous membranes), bathe with copious amounts of cool tap water. The solution has an unpleasant taste and caution should be exercised when applying medication around the mouth.

Clindamycin, Topical should be prescribed with caution in atopic individuals.

PREGNANCY CATEGORY B

Reproduction studies have been performed in rats and mice using subcutaneous and oral doses of Clindamycin ranging from 100 to 600 mg/kg/day and have revealed no evidence of impaired fertility or harm to the fetus due to Clindamycin. There are, however, no adequate and well-controlled studies in pregnant women. Because animal reproduction studies are not always predictive of human response, this drug should be used during pregnancy only if clearly needed.

NURSING MOTHERS

It is not known whether Clindamycin is excreted in human milk following use of Clindamycin, Topical. However, orally and parenterally administered Clindamycin has been reported to appear in breast milk. As a general rule, nursing should not be undertaken while a patient is on a drug since many drugs are excreted in human milk.

PEDIATRIC USE

Safety and effectiveness in children under the age of 12 has not been established.

ADVERSE REACTIONS

Skin dryness is the most common adverse reaction seen with the solution.

Clindamycin has been associated with severe colitis which may end fatally (see "Warnings").

Cases of diarrhea, bloody diarrhea and colitis (including pseudomembranous colitis) have been reported as adverse reactions in patients treated with topical formulations of Clindamycin.

Other effects which have been reported in association with the use of topical formulations of Clindamycin include:

Local Effects	Systemic Effects
Contact dermatitis	Abdominal pain
Irrigation (e.g., erythema, peeling, and burning)	Gastrointestinal disturbances
Oily skin	
Gram-negative folliculitis	

DOSAGE AND ADMINISTRATION

Apply a thin film of Clindamycin topical solution, lotion or gel twice daily to affected area.

Store at controlled room temperature 15°-30°C (59°-86°F).

Protect from freezing.

Lotion: Shake well immediately before using. Keep all dosage form containers tightly closed.

HOW SUPPLIED

GEL: 1%

BRAND/MANUFACTURER	NDC	SIZE	AWP
○ BRAND			
CLEOCIN T: Upjohn	00009-3331-02	30 gm	$19.15

LOTION: 1%

BRAND/MANUFACTURER	NDC	SIZE	AWP
○ BRAND			
CLEOCIN T: Upjohn	00009-3329-01	60 ml	$26.61

SOLUTION: 1%

AVERAGE UNIT PRICE (AVAILABLE SIZES)		GENERIC A-RATED AVERAGE PRICE (GAAP)	
GENERIC	$0.33	30 ml	$10.02
		60 ml	$19.58

BRAND/MANUFACTURER	NDC	SIZE	AWP
◆ GENERICS			
Qualitest	00603-1098-45	30 ml	$9.17
Barre	00472-0987-91	30 ml	$9.74
Aligen	00405-2540-53	30 ml	$10.20
Major	00904-7733-30	30 ml	$10.95
Qualitest	00603-1098-49	60 ml	$17.94
Barre	00472-0987-92	60 ml	$19.04
Aligen	00405-2540-56	60 ml	$19.80
Major	00904-7733-03	60 ml	$21.55

SOLUTION: 1%

BRAND/MANUFACTURER	NDC	SIZE	AWP
○ BRAND			
C/T/S: Hoechst Derm	00039-0115-30	30 ml	$10.35
CLEOCIN T: Upjohn	00009-3116-01	30 ml	$11.81
C/T/S: Hoechst Derm	00039-0115-60	60 ml	$20.23

BRAND/MANUFACTURER	NDC	SIZE	AWP
CLEOCIN T: Upjohn	00009-3116-02	60 ml	$23.10

SOLUTION: 10 MG

AVERAGE UNIT PRICE (AVAILABLE SIZES)	
GENERIC	$0.33

BRAND/MANUFACTURER	NDC	SIZE	AWP
◆ GENERICS			
Goldline	00182-6028-66	30 ml	$10.80
Goldline	00182-6028-68	60 ml	$18.00

SWAB: 1%

BRAND/MANUFACTURER	NDC	SIZE	AWP
○ BRAND			
CLEOCIN T: Upjohn	00009-3116-14	60s	$27.48

Clindamycin, Vaginal

DESCRIPTION

Clindamycin phosphate is a water soluble ester of the semisynthetic antibiotic produced by a 7(S)-chloro-substitution of the 7(R)-hydroxyl group of the parent antibiotic lincomycin. The chemical name for Clindamycin phosphate is methyl 7-chloro-6,7,8-trideoxy-6-(1-methyl-*trans*-4-propyl-L-2-pyrro-lidinecarboxami-do)-1-thio-L-*threo*-α-D-galacto-octopyrano-side 2-(dihydrogen phosphate). It has a molecular weight of 504.96, and the molecular formula is $C_{18}H_{34}ClN_2O_8PS$.

Clindamycin vaginal cream 2%, is a semisolid, white cream, which contains 2% Clindamycin phosphate, USP, at a concentration equivalent to 20 mg Clindamycin per gram. The pH of the cream is between 3.0 and 6.0.

Each applicatorful of 5 grams of vaginal cream contains approximately 100 mg of Clindamycin phosphate.

Following is its chemical structure:

CLINICAL PHARMACOLOGY

Following a once a day intravaginal dose of 100 mg of Clindamycin phosphate vaginal cream 2%, administered to 6 healthy female volunteers for 7 days, approximately 5% (range 0.6% to 11%) of the administered dose was absorbed systemically. The peak serum Clindamycin concentration observed on the first day averaged 18 ng/mL (range 4 to 47 ng/mL) and averaged 25 ng/mL (range 6 to 61 ng/mL) on day 7. These peak concentrations were attained in approximately 10 hours post-dosing (range 4-24 hours).

Following a once a day intravaginal dose of 100 mg of Clindamycin phosphate vaginal cream 2%, administered for 7 consecutive days to 5 women with bacterial vaginosis, absorption was slower and less variable than that observed in healthy females. Approximately, 5% (range 2% to 8%) of the dose was absorbed systemically. The peak serum Clindamycin concentration observed on the first day averaged 13 ng/mL (range 3 to 34 ng/mL) and averaged 16 ng/mL (range 7 to 26 ng/mL) on day 7. These peak concentrations were attained in approximately 16 hours postdosing (range 8-24 hours).

There was little or no systemic accumulation of Clindamycin after repeated vaginal dosing of Clindamycin phosphate vaginal cream 2%. The systemic $t_{1/2}$ was 1.5 to 2.6 hours.

MICROBIOLOGY

Clindamycin inhibits bacterial protein synthesis by its action at the bacterial ribosome. The antibiotic binds preferentially to the 50S ribosomal subunit and affects the process of peptide chain initiation. Although Clindamycin phosphate is inactive *in vitro*, rapid *in vivo* hydrolysis converts this compound to the antibacterially active Clindamycin.

Culture and sensitivity testing of bacteria are not routinely performed to establish the diagnosis of bacterial vaginosis. (See *Indications and Usage*".) Standard methodology for the susceptibility testing of the potential bacterial vaginosis pathogens, *Gardnerella vaginalis*, *Mobiluncus* spp., or *Mycoplasma hominis*, has not been defined.

Nonetheless, Clindamycin is an antimicrobial agent active *in vitro* against most strains of the following organisms that have been reported to be associated with bacterial vaginosis:

Bacteroides spp.
Mycoplasma hominis
Gardnerella vaginalis
Peptostreptococcus spp.
Mobiluncus spp.

➤ SHOWN IN PRODUCT IDENTIFICATION GUIDE

INDICATIONS AND USAGE

Clindamycin vaginal cream 2%, is indicated in the treatment of bacterial vaginosis (formerly referred to as *Haemophilus* vaginitis, *Gardnerella* vaginitis, nonspecific vaginitis, *Corynebacterium* vaginitis, or anaerobic vaginosis).

Note: For purposes of this indication, a clinical diagnosis of bacterial vaginosis is usually defined by the presence of a homogeneous vaginal discharge that (a) has a pH of greater than 4.5, (b) emits a "fishy" amino odor when mixed with a 10% KOH solution, and (c) contains consistent clue cells on microscopic examination. Gram's stain results consistent with a diagnosis of bacterial vaginosis include (a) markedly reduced or absent *Lactobacillus* morphology, (b) predominance of *Gardnerella* morphotype, and (c) absent or few white blood cells.

Other pathogens commonly associated with vulvovaginitis, e.g., *Trichomonas vaginalis, Chlamydia trachomatis, N. gonorrhoeae, Candida albicans,* and *Herpes simplex* virus should be ruled out.

CONTRAINDICATIONS

Clindamycin vaginal cream 2%, is contraindicated in individuals with a history of hypersensitivity to Clindamycin, lincomycin, or any of the components of this vaginal cream.

Clindamycin vaginal cream 2%, is also contraindicated in individuals with a history of regional enteritis, ulcerative colitis, or a history of "antibiotic-associated" colitis.

WARNINGS

Pseudomembranous colitis has been reported with nearly all antibacterial agents, including Clindamycin, and may range in severity from mild to life-threatening. Orally and parenterally administered Clindamycin has been associated with severe colitis which may end fatally. Diarrhea, bloody diarrhea, and colitis (including pseudomembranous colitis) have been reported with the use of orally and parenterally administered Clindamycin, as well as with topical (dermal) formulations of Clindamycin. Therefore, it is important to consider this diagnosis in patients who present with diarrhea subsequent to the administration of Clindamycin, even when administered by the vaginal route, because approximately 5% of the Clindamycin dose is systemically absorbed from the vagina.

Treatment with antibacterial agents alter the normal flora of the colon and may permit overgrowth of clostridia. Studies indicate that a toxin produced by *Clostridium difficile* is a primary cause of "antibiotic-associated colitis".

After the diagnosis of pseudomembranous colitis has been established, therapeutic measures should be initiated. Mild cases of pseudomembranous colitis usually respond to discontinuation of the drug alone. In moderate to severe cases, consideration should be given to management with fluids and electrolytes, protein supplementation, and treatment with an antibacterial drug clinically effective against *Clostridium difficile* colitis.

Onset of pseudomembranous colitis symptoms may occur during or after antimicrobial treatment.

This cream contains mineral oil. Mineral oil may weaken latex or rubber products such as condoms or vaginal contraceptive diaphragms; therefore, use of such products within 72 hours following treatment with Clindamycin vaginal cream 2% is not recommended.

PRECAUTIONS

GENERAL

Clindamycin vaginal cream 2%, contains ingredients that will cause burning and irritation of the eye. In the event of accidental contact with the eye, rinse the eye with copious amounts of cool tap water.

The use of Clindamycin phosphate vaginal cream may result in the overgrowth of nonsusceptible organisms—particularly yeasts—in the vagina. Approximately 16% of patients treated with Clindamycin phosphate vaginal cream developed symptomatic cervicitis/vaginitis with 11% of patients developing cervicitis/vaginitis secondary to *C. albicans.*

INFORMATION FOR THE PATIENT

The patient should be instructed not to engage in vaginal intercourse during treatment with this product.

DRUG INTERACTIONS

Clindamycin has been shown to have neuromuscular blocking properties that may enhance the action of other neuromuscular blocking agents. Therefore, it should be used with caution in patients receiving such agents.

CARCINOGENESIS, MUTAGENESIS, IMPAIRMENT OF FERTILITY

Long term studies in animals have not been performed with Clindamycin to evaluate carcinogenic potential. Genotoxicity tests performed included a rat micronucleus test and an Ames test. Both tests were negative. Fertility studies in rats treated orally with up to 300 mg/kg/day (31 times the human exposure based on mg/m^2) revealed no effects on fertility or mating ability.

PREGNANCY: TERATOGENIC EFFECTS

Pregnancy Category B: Reproduction studies have been performed in rats and mice using oral and parenteral doses of Clindamycin up to 600 mg/kg/day (62 and 25 times, respectively, the maximum human exposure based on mg/m^2) and have revealed no evidence of harm to the fetus due to Clindamycin. In one mouse strain, cleft palates were observed in treated fetuses; this outcome was not produced in other mouse strains or in other species and is, therefore, considered to be a strain specific effect.

There are, however, no adequate and well-controlled studies in pregnant women. Because animal reproduction studies are not always predictive of human response, this drug should be used during pregnancy only if clearly needed.

NURSING MOTHERS

It is not known if Clindamycin is excreted in human milk following the use of vaginally administered Clindamycin phosphate. However, after oral or parenteral administration, Clindamycin has been detected in human milk.

Because of the potential for serious adverse reactions in nursing infants from Clindamycin phosphate, a decision should be made whether to discontinue nursing or to discontinue the drug, taking into account the importance of the drug to the mother.

PEDIATRIC USE

Safety and effectiveness in children have not been established.

ADVERSE REACTIONS

CLINICAL TRIALS

In clinical trials, approximately 4% of non-pregnant patients treated with Clindamycin vaginal cream 2%, discontinue therapy due to drug-related adverse events. Medical events judged to be related, probably related, or possibly related to vaginally administered Clindamycin phosphate vaginal cream 2%, were reported for 249/1020 (24%) non-pregnant patients. Unless percentages are otherwise stipulated, the incidence of individual adverse reactions listed below was less than 1%:

Genital tract: Cervicitis/vaginitis, symptomatic (16%), *Candida albicans* (11%), *Trichomonas vaginalis* (1%), Vulvar irritation (6%)

Central Nervous System: Dizziness, headache, vertigo

Dermatologic: Rash

Gastrointestinal: Heartburn, nausea, vomiting, diarrhea, constipation, abdominal pain

Hypersensitivity: Urticaria

OTHER CLINDAMYCIN FORMULATIONS

Other effects that have been reported in association with the use of topical (dermal) formulations of Clindamycin include severe colitis (include pseudomembranous colitis), contact dermatitis, skin irritation (*e.g.,* erythema, peeling and burning), oily skin, gram-negative folliculitis, abdominal pain, and gastrointestinal disturbances.

Clindamycin vaginal cream affords minimal peak serum levels and systemic exposure (A.U.C.'s) of Clindamycin compared to 100 mg oral Clindamycin dosing. Although these lower levels of exposure are less likely to produce the common reactions seen with oral Clindamycin, the possibility of these and other reactions cannot be excluded presently. Data from well-controlled trials directly comparing Clindamycin administered orally to Clindamycin administered vaginally are not available.

The following adverse reactions and altered laboratory tests have been reported with the oral or parenteral use of Clindamycin:

Gastrointestinal: Abdominal pain, esophagitis, nausea, vomiting, and diarrhea. (See *"Warnings."*)

Hematopoietic: Transient neutropenia (leukopenia), eosinophilia, agranulocytosis, and thrombocytopenia have been reported. No direct etiologic relationship to concurrent Clindamycin therapy could be made in any of these reports.

Hypersensitivity Reactions: Maculopapular rash and urticaria have been observed during drug therapy. Generalized mild to moderate morbilliform-like skin rashes are the most frequently reported of all adverse reactions. Rare instances of erythema multiforme, some resembling Stevens-Johnson syndrome, have been associated with Clindamycin. A few cases of anaphylactoid reactions have been reported. If a hypersensitivity reaction occurs, the drug should be discontinued.

Liver: Jaundice and abnormalities in liver function tests have been observed during Clindamycin therapy.

Musculoskeletal: Rare instances of polyarthritis have been reported.

Renal: Although no direct relationship of Clindamycin to renal damage has been established, renal dysfunction as evidenced by azotemia, oliguria and/or proteinuria has been observed in rare instances.

OVERDOSAGE

Vaginally applied Clindamycin phosphate vaginal cream 2%, could be absorbed in sufficient amounts to produce systemic effects. (See *"Warnings".*)

DOSAGE AND ADMINISTRATION

The recommended dose is one applicatorful of Clindamycin phosphate vaginal cream 2%, (5 grams containing approximately 100 mg of Clindamycin phosphate) intravaginally, preferably at bedtime, for seven consecutive days.

Store at controlled room temperature 15° to 30°C (59° to 86°F). Protect from freezing.

HOW SUPPLIED

CREAM: 2%

BRAND/MANUFACTURER	NDC	SIZE	AWP
○ BRAND			
CLEOCIN VAGINAL: Upjohn	00009-3448-01	40 gm	$28.03

Clinoril *SEE SULINDAC*

◆ RATED THERAPEUTICALLY EQUIVALENT; ◇ THERAPEUTIC EQUIVALENCE UNCONFIRMED; ○ UNRATED

Clioquinol with Hydrocortisone

DESCRIPTION
Clioquinol with Hydrocortisone, a topical compound for dermatologic use, combines the antifungal and antibacterial actions of Clioquinol and the anti-inflammatory and antipruritic effects of Hydrocortisone to provide broad control of acute and chronic dermatosis. Clioquinol is 5-chloro-7-iodo-8 quinolinol. Hydrocortisone is 11β, 17, 21-tri-hydroxy- pregn-4-ene-3, 20-dione.

ACTIONS
In vitro studies have demonstrated that Clioquinol effectively inhibits the growth of various mycotic organisms such as Microsporons, Trichophytons, and *Candida albicans* and gram positive cocci such as staphylococci and enterococci. The role of steroids in alleviating the inflammation pruritus associated with many dermatoses has been well established.

INDICATIONS
Based on a review of this drug by the National Academy of Science-National Research Council and/or other information, FDA has classified the indications as follows: "Possibly" effective: Contact or atopic dermatitis; Impetiginized eczema; nummular eczema; infantile eczema; endogenous chronic infectious dermatitis; stasis dermatitis; pyoderma; nuchal eczema and chronic eczematoid otitis externa; acne urticata; localized or disseminated neurodermatitis; lichen simplex chronicus; anogenital pruritus (vulvae, scroti, ani); folliculitis; bacterial dermatoses; mycotic dermatoses such as tinea (capitis, cruris, corporis, pedis); miliasis; intertrigo. Final classification of the less-than-effective indications require further investigation.

CONTRAINDICATIONS
Hypersensitivity to Clioquinol with Hydrocortisone or any of its ingredients or related compounds; lesions of the eye; tuberculosis of the skin; most viral skin lesions (including herpes simplex, vaccinia, and varicella).

WARNINGS
This product is not for ophthalmic use. In the presence of systemic infections, appropriate systemic antibiotics should be used.

Usage in Pregnancy: Although topical steroids have not been reported to have an adverse effect on pregnancy, the safety of their use in pregnant women has not been absolutely established. In laboratory animals, increases in incidence of fetal abnormalities have been associated with exposure of gestating females to topical corticosteroids, in some cases at rather low dosage levels. Therefore, drugs of this class should not be used extensively on pregnant patients in large amounts or for prolonged periods of time.

PRECAUTIONS
May prove irritating to sensitized skin in rare cases. If irritation occurs, discontinue therapy. Staining of skin and fabrics may occur. Additionally, there are rare reports of discoloration of hair and nails. Signs and symptoms of systemic toxicity, electrolyte imbalance, or adrenal suppression have not been reported with Clioquinol with Hydrocortisone. Nevertheless, the possibility of suppression of the pituitary-adrenal axis during therapy should be kept in mind, especially when the drug is used under occlusive dressings, for a prolonged period, or for treating extensive cutaneous areas since significant absorption of corticosteroid may occur under these conditions, particularly in children and infants.

Clioquinol may be absorbed through the skin and interfere with thyroid function tests. If such tests are contemplated, wait at least one month between discontinuation of therapy and performance of these tests. The ferric chloride test for phenylketonuria (PKU) can yield a false-positive result if Clioquinol is present in the diaper or urine. Prolonged use may result in overgrowth of nonsusceptible organisms requiring appropriate therapy.

ADVERSE REACTIONS
There have been a few reports of rash and hypersensitivity. The following local adverse reactions have been reported with topical corticosteroids, especially under occlusive dressings; burning, itching, irritation; dryness; folliculitis; hypertrichosis; acneiform eruptions; hypopigmentation; perioral dermatitis; allergic contact dermatitis; maceration of the skin; secondary infection; skin atrophy; striae; miliaria. Discontinue therapy if any unknown reaction occurs.

DOSAGE AND ADMINISTRATION
Apply a thin layer to the affected parts 3 or 4 times daily. The cream, because of its slight drying effect, is primarily useful for moist, weeping lesions.

HOW SUPPLIED
CREAM: 3%-1%

BRAND/MANUFACTURER	NDC	SIZE	AWP
GENERICS			
Southwood	58016-3101-01	20 gm	$5.64
HCV: Saron	00834-7036-78	15 gm	$6.50
TOPIC FORM HC:	52765-0104-07	20 gm	$5.75

CREAM: 1%-3%

BRAND/MANUFACTURER	NDC	SIZE	AWP
GENERICS			
Major	00904-0753-36	15 gm	$1.73
Moore,H.L.	00839-5508-45	20 gm	$2.01
LANVISONE: Lannett	00527-0438-20	20 gm	$2.10
Thames	49158-0104-07	20 gm	$2.10
Clay-Park	45802-0006-02	20 gm	$2.16
CMC-Cons	00223-4128-20	20 gm	$2.40
Qualitest	00603-7801-76	20 gm	$2.43
URL	00677-0726-38	20 gm	$2.75
CORQUE: Geneva	00781-7007-22	20 gm	$2.79
NMC	23317-0341-20	20 gm	$2.82
Major	00904-0753-29	20 gm	$2.85
STEROFORM: Legere	25332-2007-01	20 gm	$2.95
DEK-QUIN: Truxton	00463-8003-20	20 gm	$3.00
Goldline	00182-0875-48	20 gm	$3.00
Allscrips	54569-2992-00	20 gm	$3.29
Med-Derm	45565-0505-07	20 gm	$3.95
Allscrips	54569-1119-00	20 gm	$6.20
PEDI-CORT V: Pedinol	00884-1171-20	20 gm	$6.50
Thames	49158-0105-16	30 gm	$2.00
IODO-HC: Veratex	17022-5588-03	30 gm	$2.10
Thames	49158-0104-08	30 gm	$2.80
Clay-Park	45802-0006-03	30 gm	$3.24
CMC-Cons	00223-4128-30	30 gm	$3.60
Goldline	00182-0875-34	30 gm	$4.00
Thames	49158-0104-16	454 gm	$25.00
Clay-Park	45802-0006-05	454 gm	$32.94
CMC-Cons	00223-4128-01	454 gm	$34.00

CREAM: 0.5%-3%

BRAND/MANUFACTURER	NDC	SIZE	AWP
GENERICS			
Moore,H.L.	00839-5513-49	30 gm	$1.88
Clay-Park	45802-0005-03	30 gm	$2.26
CMC-Cons	00223-4127-30	30 gm	$3.00
ALA-QUIN: Del-Ray	00316-0123-01	30 gm	$6.14
Clay-Park	45802-0005-05	454 gm	$21.60

CREAM:

BRAND/MANUFACTURER	NDC	SIZE	AWP
GENERICS			
IODO-HC: Veratex	17022-5588-01	20 gm	$1.50

OINTMENT: 1%-3%

BRAND/MANUFACTURER	NDC	SIZE	AWP
GENERICS			
Moore,H.L.	00839-5509-45	20 gm	$2.01
Clay-Park	45802-0016-02	20 gm	$2.16
Major	00904-2680-29	20 gm	$2.35
Rugby	00536-1001-99	20 gm	$4.28
Clay-Park	45802-0016-03	30 gm	$3.24
Clay-Park	45802-0016-05	454 gm	$32.94

OINTMENT:

BRAND/MANUFACTURER	NDC	SIZE	AWP
GENERICS			
HYSONE: Mallard	59441-0315-20	20 gm	$4.25

Clobetasol Propionate

DESCRIPTION
Clobetasol Propionate cream, ointment, and scalp application contain the active compound Clobetasol Propionate a synthetic corticosteroid, for topical dermatologic use. Clobetasol, an analog of prednisolone, has a high degree of glucocorticoid activity and a slight degree of mineralocorticoid activity.

Chemically, Clobetasol Propionate is (11β,16β)-21-chloro-9-fluoro-11-hydroxy-16-methyl-17-(1-oxopropoxy)-pregna-1,4-diene-3,20-dione, and it has the following structural formula:

Clobetasol Propionate has the empirical formula $C_{25}H_{32}ClFO_5$ and a molecular weight of 467. It is a white to cream-colored crystalline powder insoluble in water.

Clobetasol Propionate Cream contains Clobetasol Propionate 0.5 mg/g in a cream base Clobetasol Propionate.

Clobetasol Propionate Ointment contains Clobetasol Propionate 0.5 mg/g in a base.

Clobetasol Propionate Scalp Application contains Clobetasol Propionate 0.5 mg/g in a base.

Clobetasol Propionate Emollient Cream contains clobetasol propionate 0.05 mg/g in an emollient base.

Clobetasol Propionate Gel contains clobetasol propionate 0.05 mg/g in a base.

► SHOWN IN PRODUCT IDENTIFICATION GUIDE

Following is its chemical structure:

CLINICAL PHARMACOLOGY

The corticosteroids are a class of compounds comprising steroid hormones secreted by the adrenal cortex and their synthetic analogs. In pharmacologic doses, corticosteroids are used primarily for their anti-inflammatory and/or immunosuppressive effects. Topical corticosteroids such as Clobetasol Propionate are effective in the treatment of corticosteroid-responsive dermatoses primarily because of their anti-inflammatory, antipruritic, and vasoconstrictive actions. However, while the physiologic, pharmacologic, and clinical effects of the corticosteroids are well known, the exact mechanisms of their actions in each disease are uncertain.

Clobetasol Propionate, a corticosteroid, has been shown to have topical (dermatologic) and systemic pharmacologic and metabolic effects characteristic of this class of drugs.

Pharmacokinetics: The extent of percutaneous absorption of topical corticosteroids, including Clobetasol Propionate, is determined by many factors, including the vehicle, the integrity of the epidermal barrier, and the use of occlusive dressings (see *"Dosage and Administration"*).

As with all topical corticosteroids, Clobetasol Propionate can be absorbed from normal intact skin. Inflammation and/or other disease processes in the skin may increase percutaneous absorption. Occlusive dressings substantially increase the percutaneous absorption of topical corticosteroids (see *"Dosage and Administration"*).

Once absorbed through the skin, topical corticosteroids enter pharmacokinetic pathways similarly to systemically administered corticosteroids. Corticosteroids are bound to plasma proteins in varying degrees. Corticosteroids are metabolized primarily in the liver and are then excreted by the kidneys. Some of the topical corticosteroids, including Clobetasol Propionate and its metabolites, are also excreted into the bile. Clobetasol Propionate cream and ointment have been shown to depress the plasma levels of adrenal cortical hormones following repeated nonocclusive application to diseased skin in patients with psoriasis and eczematous dermatitis. These effects have been shown to be transient and reversible upon completion of a 2-week course of treatment.

Following repeated nonocclusive application in the treatment of scalp psoriasis, there is some evidence that Clobetasol Propionate Scalp Application has the potential to depress plasma cortisol levels in some patients. However, hypothalamic-pituitary-adrenal (HPA) axis effects produced by systematically absorbed Clobetasol Propionate have been shown to be transient and reversible upon completion of a 2-week course of treatment.

Clobetasol Propionate Emollient Cream and Clobetasol Propionate Gel: Like other topical corticosteroids, clobetasol propionate has anti-inflammatory, antipruritic, and vasoconstrictive properties. The mechanism of the anti-inflammatory activity of the topical steroids, in general, is unclear. However, corticosteroids are thought to act by the induction of phospholipase A_2 inhibitory proteins, collectively called lipocortins. It is postulated that these proteins control the biosynthesis of potent mediators of inflammation such as prostaglandins and leukotrienes by inhibiting the release of their common precursor, arachidonic acid. Arachidonic acid is released from membrane phospholipids by phospholipase A_2.

Pharmacokinetics: The extent of percutaneous absorption of topical corticosteroids is determined by many factors, including the vehicle and the integrity of the epidermal barrier. Occlusive dressing with hyrocortisone for up to 24 hours has not been demonstrated to increase penetration; however, occlusion of hydrocortisone for 96 hours markedly enhances penetration. Topical corticosteroids can be absorbed from normal intact skin, while inflammation and/or other disease processes in the skin may increase percutaneous absorption. Greater absorption was observed for the Clobetasol Propionate gel formulation as compared to the cream formulation in *in vitro* human skin penetration studies.

Studies performed with Clobetasol Propionate Emollient Cream and Gel indicate that they are in the super-high range of potency as compared with other topical corticosteroids.

INDICATIONS AND USAGE

Clobetasol Propionate Cream, Ointment, and Scalp Application are indicated for short-term treatment of inflammatory and pruritic manifestations of moderate to severe corticosteroid-responsive dermatoses.

Clobetasol Propionate Emollient Cream and Clobetasol Propionate Gel are super-high potency corticosteroid formulations indicated for the relief of the inflammatory and pruritic manifestations of corticosteroid-responsive dermatoses.

Treatment beyond 2 consecutive weeks is not recommended, and the total dosage should not exceed 50 g per week of cream and ointment and 50 mL per week of scalp application because of the potential for the drug to suppress the HPA axis.

These products are not recommended for use in children under 12 years of age.

UNLABELED USES
Clobetasol Propionate is used alone or as an adjunct in the treatment of vitiligo.

CONTRAINDICATIONS

Clobetasol Propionate cream, ointment, and scalp application are contraindicated in patients who are hypersensitive to Clobetasol Propionate, to other corticosteroids, or to any ingredient in these preparations. Clobetasol Propionate scalp application is also contraindicated in patients with primary infections of the scalp.

Clobetasol Propionate Emollient Cream and Clobetasol Propionate Gel are contraindicated in those patients with a history of hypersensitivity to any of the components of the preparation.

PRECAUTIONS

CLOBETASOL PROPIONATE CREAM, OINTMENT, AND SCALP APPLICATION

General: **Clobetasol Propionate is a highly potent topical corticosteroid that has been shown to suppress the HPA axis at doses as low as 2 g (of ointment) per day.** Systemic absorption of topical corticosteroids has resulted in reversible HPA axis suppression, manifestations of Cushing's syndrome, hyperglycemia, and glucosuria in some patients.

Conditions that augment systemic absorption include the implication of the more potent corticosteroids, use over large surface areas, prolonged use, and the addition of occlusive dressings. Therefore, patients receiving a large dose of a potent topical steroid applied to a large surface area should be evaluated periodically for evidence of HPA axis suppression by using the urinary free cortisol and ACTH stimulation tests. If HPA axis suppression is noted, an attempt should be made to withdraw the drug, to reduce the frequency of application, or to substitute a less potent steroid.

Recovery of HPA axis function is generally prompt and complete upon discontinuation of the drug. Infrequently, signs and symptoms of steroid withdrawal may occur, requiring supplemental systemic corticosteroids.

Children may absorb proportionally larger amounts of topical corticosteroids and thus be more susceptible to systemic toxicity (see *"Precautions: Pediatric Use"*).

If irritation develops, topical corticosteroids should be discontinued and appropriate therapy instituted. Irritation is possible if Clobetasol Propionate scalp application contacts the eye. If that should occur, immediate flushing of the eye with a large volume of water is recommended. In the presence of dermatologic infections, the use of an appropriate antifungal or antibacterial agent should be instituted. If a favorable response does not occur promptly, the corticosteroid should be discontinued until the infection has been adequately controlled.

Certain areas of the body, such as the face, groin, and axillae, are more prone to atrophic changes than other areas of the body following treatment with corticosteroids, although Clobetasol Propionate scalp application is intended for the treatment of inflammatory conditions of the scalp. Frequent observation of the patient is important if these areas are to be treated. As with other potent topical corticosteroids, Clobetasol Propionate cream, ointment, and scalp application should not be used in the treatment of rosacea and perioral dermatitis. Topical corticosteroids in general should not be used in the treatment of acne or as sole therapy in widespread plaque psoriasis.

Information for Patients: Patients using Clobetasol Propionate cream, ointment, and scalp application should receive the following information and instructions:

1. This medication is to be used as directed by the physician and should not be used longer than the prescribed time period. It is for external use only. Avoid contact with the eyes.
2. This medication should not be used for any disorder other than that for which it was prescribed.
3. The treated skin area should not be bandaged or otherwise covered or wrapped so as to be occlusive.
4. Patients should report any signs of local adverse reactions to the physician.

Laboratory Tests: The following tests may be helpful in evaluating HPA axis suppression:
   Urinary free cortisol test
   ACTH stimulation test

Carcinogenesis, Mutagenesis, Impairment of Fertility: Long-term animal studies have not been performed to evaluate the carcinogenic potential or the effect on fertility of topical corticosteroids.

Studies to determine mutagenicity with prednisolone have revealed negative results.

Pregnancy: Teratogenic Effects: Pregnancy Category C: The more potent corticosteroids have been shown to be teratogenic in animals after dermal application. Clobetasol Propionate has not been tested for teratogenicity by this route; however, it is absorbed percutaneously, and when administered subcutaneously it was a significant teratogen in both the rabbit and the mouse. Clobetasol Propionate has greater teratogenic potential than steroids that are less potent.

There are no adequate and well-controlled studies of the teratogenic effects of topically applied corticosteroids including Clobetasol, in pregnant women. Therefore, Clobetasol and other topical corticosteroids should be used during pregnancy only if the potential benefit justifies the potential risk to the fetus, and they should not be used extensively on pregnant patients, in large amounts, or for prolonged periods of time.

Nursing Mothers: It is not known whether topical administration of corticosteroids could result in sufficient systemic absorption to produce detectable quantities in breast milk. Systemically administered corticosteroids are secreted into breast milk in quantities not likely to have a deleterious effect on the infant. Nevertheless, caution should be exercised when topical corticosteroids are prescribed for a nursing woman.

Pediatric Use: Use of Clobetasol Propionate cream, ointment, and scalp application in children under 12 years of age is not recommended.

Pediatric patients may demonstrate greater susceptibility to topical corticosteroid-induced HPA axis suppression and Cushing's syndrome than mature patients because of a larger skin surface area to body weight ratio.

HPA axis suppression, Cushing's syndrome, and intracranial hypertension have been reported in children receiving topical corticosteroids. Manifestations of adrenal suppression in children include linear growth retardation, delayed weight gain, low plasma cortisol levels, and absence of response to ACTH stimulation. Manifestations of intracranial hypertension include bulging fontanelles, headaches, and bilateral papilledema.

CLOBETASOL PROPIONATE EMOLLIENT CREAM AND CLOBETASOL PROPIONATE GEL

General: **Clobetasol propionate is a highly potent topical corticosteroid that has been shown to suppress the HPA axis at doses as low as 2 g per day.**

Systemic absorption of topical corticosteroids can produce reversible HPA axis suppression with the potential for glucocorticosteroid insufficency after withdrawal from treatment. Manifestations of Cushing's syndrome, hyperglycemia, and glucosuria can also be produced in some patients by systemic absorption of topical corticosteroids while on therapy.

Patients receiving a large dose applied to a large surface area or under an occlusive dressing should be evaluated periodically for evidence of HPA axis suppression. This may be done by using the ACTH stimulation, a.m. plasma cortisol, and urinary free cortisol tests. Patients receiving super-potent corticosteroids should not be treated for more than 2 weeks at a time, and only small areas should be treated at any one time due to the increased risk of HPA suppression.

If HPA axis suppression is noted, an attempt should be made to withdraw the drug, to reduce the frequency of application, or to substitute a less potent corticosteroid. Recovery of HPA axis function is generally prompt and complete upon discontinuation of topical corticosteroids. Infrequently, signs and symptoms of glucocorticosteroid insufficency may occur that require supplemental systemic corticosteroids. For information on systemic supplementation, see prescribing infotmation for those products.

Children may be more susceptible to systemic toxicity from equivalent doses due to their larger skin surface to body mass ratios (see *"Precautions: Pediatric Use".)*

If irritation develops, Clobetasol Propionate Emollient Cream and Gel should be discontinued and appropiate therapy instituted. Allergic contact dermatitis with corticosteroids is usually diagnosed by observing *failure to heal* rather than noting a clinical exacerbation as with most topical products not containing corticosteroids. Such an observation should be corroborated with appropiate diagnostic patch testing.

If concomitant skin infections are present or develop, an appropiate antifungal or antibacterial agent should be used. If a favorable response does not occur promptly, use of Clobetasol Propionate Emollient Cream and Gel should be discontinued until the infection has been adequately controlled.

Clobetasol Propionate Emollient Cream and Gel should not be used in the treatment of rosacea or perioral dermatitis, and should not be used on the face, groin, or axillae.

Information for Patients: Patients using topical corticosteroids should receive the following information and instructions:
1. This medication is to be used as directed by the physician.
2. This medication should not be used for any disorder other than that for which it was prescribed.
3. The treated skin area should not be used bandaged or otherwise covered or wrapped so as to be occlusive unless directed by the physician.
4. Patients should report any signs of local adverse reactions to the physician.
5. Patients should inform their physicians that they are using Clobetasol Propionate if surgery is contemplated.

Laboratory Tests: The following tests may be helpful in evaluating patients for HPA axis suppression:
ACTH stimulation test
A.M. plasma cortisol test
Urinary free cortisol test

Carcinogenesis, Mutagenesis, Impairment of Fertility: Long-term animal studies have not been performed to evaluate the carcinogenic potential of Clobetasol Propionate.

Studies in the rat following oral administration at dosage levels up to 50 mg/kg per day revealed no significant effect on the males. The females exhibited an increase in the number of resorbed embryos and a decrease in the number of living fetuses at the highest dose.

Clobetasol Propionate was nonmutagenic in three different test systems: the Ames test, the *Saccharomyces cerevisiae* gene conversion assay, and the E. *coli* B WP2 fluctuation test.

Pregnancy: Teratogenic Effects: Pregnancy Category C: Corticosteroids have been shown to be teratogenic in laboratory animals when administered systemically at relatively low dosage levels. Some corticosteroids have been shown to be teratogenic after dermal application to laboratory animals.

Clobetasol Propionate has not been tested for teratogenicity by this route; however, it is absorbed percutaneously, and when administered subcutaneously it was a significant teratogen in both the rabbit and mouse. Clobetasol Propionate has greater teratogenic potential than steroids that are less potent.

Teratogenicity studies in mice using the subcutaneous route resulted in fetotoxicity at the highest dose tested (1 mg/kg) and teratogenicity at all dose levels tested down to 0.03 mg/kg. These doses are approximately 0.33 and 0.01 times, respectively, the human topical dose of Clobetasol Propionate Emollient Cream and Gel. Abnormalities seen included cleft palate and skeletal abnormalities.

In rabbits, Clobetasol Propionate given by the same route was teratogenic at doses of 3 and 10 mcg/kg. These doses are approximately 0.0001 and 0.003 times, respectively, the human topical dose of Clobetasol Propionate Emollient Cream and Gel. Abnormalities seen included cleft palate, cranioschisis, and other skeletal abnormalities.

There are no adequate or well-controlled studies of the teratogenic potential of Clobetasol Propionate in pregnant women. Clobetasol Propionate Emollient Cream and Gel should be used during pregnancy only if the potential benefit justifies the potential risk to the fetus.

Nursing Mothers: Systemically administered corticosteroids appear in human milk and could suppress growth, interfere with endogenous corticosteroid production, or cause other untoward effects. It is not known whether topical administration of corticosteroids could result in sufficient systemic absorption to produce detectable quantities in human milk. Because many drugs are excreted in human milk, caution should be exercised when Clobetasol Propionate Gel is administered to a nursing woman.

Pediatric Use: **Safety and effectiveness of Clobetasol Propionate Emollient Cream and Gel in children and infants have not been established; therefore, use in children under 12 years of age is not recommended. Because of a higher ratio of skin surface area to body mass, children are at a greater risk than adults of HPA axis suppression when they are treated with topical corticosteroids. They are therefore also at greater risk of glucocorticosteroid insuffiency after withdrawal of treatment and of Cushing's syndrome while on treatment. Adverse effects including striae have been reported with inappropriate use of topical corticosteroids in infants and children (see *"Precautions"*).**

HPA axis suppression, Cushing's syndrome, and intracranial hypertension have been reported in children receiving topical corticosteroids. Manifestations of adrenal suppression in children include linear growth retardation, delayed weight gain, low plasma cortisol levels, and absence of response of ACTH stimulation. Manifestations of intracranial hypertension include bulging fontanelles, headaches, and bilateral papilledema.

ADVERSE REACTIONS

Clobetasol Propionate Cream, Ointment, and Scalp Application are generally well tolerated when used for 2-week treatment periods.

The most frequent adverse reactions reported for Clobetasol Propionate Cream have been local and have included burning sensation in 4 of 421 patients and stinging sensation in 3 of 421 patients. Less frequent adverse reactions were itching, skin atrophy, and cracking and fissuring of the skin, which occurred in 1 of 421 patients.

The most frequent adverse events reported for Clobetasol Propionate Ointment have been local and have included burning sensation, irritation, and itching. These occurred in 2 of 366 patients. Less frequent adverse reactions were stinging, cracking, erythema, folliculitis, numbness of fingers, skin atrophy, and telangiectasia, which occurred in 1 of 366 patients.

The most frequent adverse events reported for Clobetasol Propionate Scalp Application have been local and have included burning and/or stinging sensation, which occurred in 29 of 294 patients; scalp pustules, which occurred in 3 of 294 patients; and tingling and folliculitis, each of which occurred in 2 of 294 patients. Less frequent adverse events were itching and tightness of the scalp, dermatitis, tenderness, headache, hair loss, and eye irritation, each of which occurred in 1 of 294 patients.

The following local adverse reactions are reported infrequently when topical corticosteroids are used as recommended. These reactions are listed in an approximately decreasing order of occurrence: burning, itching, irritation, dryness, folliculitis, hypertrichosis, acneiform eruptions, hypopigmentation, perioral dermatitis, allergic contact dermatitis, maceration of the skin, secondary infection, skin atrophy, striae, and miliaria. Systemic absorption of topical corticosteroids has produced reversible HPA axis suppression, manifestations of Cushing's syndrome, hyperglycemia, and glucosuria in some patients. In rare instances, treatment (or withdrawal of treatment) of psoriasis with corticosteroids is thought to have exacerbated the disease or provoked the pustular form of the disease, so careful patient supervision is recommended.

Clobetasol Propionate Emollient Cream and Clobetasol Propionate Gel: In controlled trials with Clobetasol Propionate Emollient Cream and Gel, the only reported adverse reaction that was considered to be drug related was a report of burning sensation (1.9% and 1.8%, respectively, of treated patients).

In larger controlled clinical trials with other Clobetasol Propionate formulations, the most frequently reported adverse reactions have included burning, stinging, irritation, pruritus, erythema, folliculitis, cracking and fissuring of the skin, numbness of the fingers, skin atrophy, and telangiectasia (all less than 2%).

Cushing's syndrome has been reported in infants and adults as a result of prolonged use of topical Clobetasol Propionate formulations.

The following additional local adverse reactions are reported infrequently with topical corticosteroids, but may occur more frequently with super-high potency corticosteroids, such as Clobetasol Propionate Emollient Cream and Gel. These reactions are listed in approximate decreasing order of occurrence: dryness, hypertrichosis, acneiform eruptions, hypopigmentation, perioral dermatitis, allergic contact dermatitis, secondary infection, irritation, striae, and miliaria.

OVERDOSAGE

Topically applied Clobetasol Propionate cream, ointment, and scalp application; Clobetasol Propionate Emollient Cream; and Clobetasol Propionate Gel can be absorbed in sufficient amounts to produce systemic effects (see *"Precautions"*).

DOSAGE AND ADMINISTRATION

A thin layer of Clobetasol Propionate cream or ointment should be applied with gentle rubbing to the affected skin areas twice daily, once in the morning and once at night. Clobetasol Propionate cream and ointment are potent; therefore, treatment must be limited to 2 consecutive weeks, and amounts greater than 50 g per week should not be used. Clobetasol Propionate cream and ointment are not to be used with occlusive dressings.

Clobetasol Propionate scalp application should be applied to the affected scalp areas twice daily, once in the morning and once at night. Clobetasol Propionate Scalp Application is potent; therefore, treatment must be limited to 2 consecutive weeks, and amounts greater than 50 mL per week should not be used. Clobetasol Propionate scalp application is not to be used with occlusive dressings.

Clobetasol Propionate Emollient Cream and Clobetasol Propionate Gel: Apply a thin layer of Clobetasol Propionate Emollient Cream or Gel to the affected skin areas twice daily and rub in gently and completely (see *"Indications and Usage"*).

Clobetasol Propionate Emollient Cream and Gel are super-high potency topical corticosteroids; therefore, **treatment should be limited to 2 consecutive weeks, and amounts greater than 50 g per week should not be used.**

As with other highly active corticosteroids, therapy should be discontinued when control has been achieved. If no improvement is seen within 2 weeks, reassessment of diagnosis may be necessary.

Clobetasol Propionate Emollient Cream and Gel should not be used with occlusive dressings.

Store cream and ointment at between 15° and 30°C (59° and 86°F). Clobetasol Propionate Cream should not be refrigerated.

Store scalp application at between 4° and 25°C (39° and 77°F). Do not use near an open flame.

HOW SUPPLIED
CREAM: 0.05%

AVERAGE UNIT PRICE (AVAILABLE SIZES)		GENERIC A-RATED AVERAGE PRICE (GAAP)	
BRAND	$1.03	15 gm	$18.38
GENERIC	$0.97	30 gm	$25.43
		45 gm	$37.03

BRAND/MANUFACTURER	NDC	SIZE	AWP
◆ BRAND			
TEMOVATE: Glaxo Derm	00173-0375-73	15 gm	$20.45
TEMOVATE EMOLLIENT: Glaxo Derm	00173-0454-01	15 gm	$20.45
TEMOVATE: Glaxo Derm	00173-0375-72	30 gm	$28.28
TEMOVATE EMOLLIENT: Glaxo Derm	00173-0454-02	30 gm	$28.28
TEMOVATE: Glaxo Derm	00173-0375-01	45 gm	$41.15
	00173-0375-02	60 gm	$51.36
TEMOVATE EMOLLIENT: Glaxo Derm	00173-0454-03	60 gm	$51.36
◆ GENERICS			
Copley	38245-0650-70	15 gm	$18.35
NMC	23317-0400-15	15 gm	$18.40
Copley	38245-0650-71	30 gm	$25.40
NMC	23317-0400-30	30 gm	$25.45
Copley	38245-0650-72	45 gm	$37.00
NMC	23317-0400-45	45 gm	$37.05

GEL: 0.05%

BRAND/MANUFACTURER	NDC	SIZE	AWP
○ BRAND			
TEMOVATE: Glaxo Derm	00173-0455-01	15 gm	$20.45
	00173-0455-02	30 gm	$28.28
	00173-0455-03	60 gm	$51.36

OINTMENT: 0.05%

AVERAGE UNIT PRICE (AVAILABLE SIZES)		GENERIC A-RATED AVERAGE PRICE (GAAP)	
BRAND	$1.02	15 gm	$18.38
GENERIC	$0.97	30 gm	$25.43
		45 gm	$37.03

BRAND/MANUFACTURER	NDC	SIZE	AWP
◆ BRAND			
TEMOVATE: Glaxo Derm	00173-0376-73	15 gm	$20.44
	00173-0376-72	30 gm	$28.28
	00173-0376-01	45 gm	$41.15
	00173-0376-02	60 gm	$51.36
◆ GENERICS			
Copley	38245-0128-70	15 gm	$18.35
NMC	23317-0401-15	15 gm	$18.40
Copley	38245-0128-71	30 gm	$25.40
NMC	23317-0401-30	30 gm	$25.45
Copley	38245-0128-72	45 gm	$37.00
NMC	23317-0401-45	45 gm	$37.05

SOLUTION: 0.05%

BRAND/MANUFACTURER	NDC	SIZE	AWP
○ BRAND			
TEMOVATE: Glaxo Derm	00173-0432-00	25 ml	$23.40
	00173-0432-01	50 ml	$45.02

Clocortolone Pivalate

DESCRIPTION

Clocortolone Pivalate Cream 0.1% contains the medium potency topical corticosteroid, Clocortolone Pivalate, in a specially formulated water-washable emollient cream base.

Chemically, Clocortolone Pivalate is 9-chloro-6α-fluoro-11β,21-dihydroxy-16α-methylpregna-1,4-diene-3,20-dione 21-pivalate.

Following is its chemical structure:

CLINICAL PHARMACOLOGY

Topical corticosteroids share anti-inflammatory, antipruritic and vasoconstrictive actions.

The mechanism of anti-inflammatory activity of the topical corticosteroids is unclear. Various laboratory methods, including vasoconstrictor assays, are used to compare and predict potencies and/or clinical efficacies of the topical corticosteroids. There is some evidence to suggest that a recognizable correlation exists between vasoconstrictor potency and therapeutic efficacy in man.

Pharmacokinetics: The extent of percutaneous absorption of topical corticosteroids is determined by many factors including the vehicle, the integrity of the epidermal barrier, and the use of occlusive dressings.

Topical corticosteroids can be absorbed from normal intact skin. Inflammation and/or other disease processes in the skin increase percutaneous absorption. Occlusive dressings substantially increase the percutaneous absorption of topical corticosteroids. Thus, occlusive dressings may be a valuable therapeutic adjunct for treatment of resistant dermatoses. (See *"Dosage and Administration"*.)

Once absorbed through the skin, topical corticosteroids are handled through pharmacokinetic pathways similar to systemically administered corticosteroids. Corticosteroids are bound to plasma proteins in varying degrees. Corticosteroids are metabolized primarily in the liver and are then excreted by the kidneys. Some of the topical corticosteroids and their metabolites are also excreted into the bile.

INDICATIONS AND USAGE

Topical corticosteroids are indicated for the relief of the inflammatory and pruritic manifestations of corticosteroid-responsive dermatoses.

CONTRAINDICATIONS

Topical corticosteroids are contraindicated in those patients with a history of hypersensitivity to any of the components of the preparation.

PRECAUTIONS

General: Systemic absorption of topical corticosteroids has produced reversible hypothalamic-pituitary-adrenal (HPA) axis suppression, manifestations of Cushing's syndrome, hyperglycemia, and glucosuria in some patients.

Conditions which augment systemic absorption include the application of the more potent steroids, use over large surface areas, prolonged use, and the addition of occlusive dressings.

Therefore, patients receiving a large dose of a potent topical steroid applied to a large surface area or under an occlusive dressing should be evaluated periodically for evidence of HPA axis suppression by using the urinary free cortisol and ACTH stimulation tests. If HPA axis suppression is noted, an attempt should be made to withdraw the drug, to reduce the frequency of application, or to substitute a less potent steroid.

Recovery of HPA axis function is generally prompt and complete upon discontinuation of the drug. Infrequently, signs and symptoms of steroid withdrawal may occur, requiring supplemental systemic corticosteroids.

Children may absorb proportionally larger amounts of topical corticosteroids and thus be more susceptible to systemic toxicity (see *"Precautions—Pediatric Use"*).

If irritation develops, topical corticosteroids should be discontinued and appropriate therapy instituted.

In the presence of dermatological infections, the use of an appropriate antifungal or antibacterial agent should be instituted. If a favorable response does

◆ RATED THERAPEUTICALLY EQUIVALENT; ◇ THERAPEUTIC EQUIVALENCE UNCONFIRMED; ○ UNRATED

not occur promptly, the corticosteroid should be discontinued until the infection has been adequately controlled.

Information for the Patient: Patients using topical corticosteroids should receive the following information and instructions:

1. This medication is to be used as directed by the physician. It is for external use only. Avoid contact with the eyes.
2. Patients should be advised not to use this medication for any disorder other than for which it was prescribed.
3. The treated skin area should not be bandaged or otherwise covered or wrapped as to be occlusive unless directed by the physician.
4. Patients should report any signs of local adverse reactions especially under occlusive dressing.
5. Parents of pediatric patients should be advised not to use tight-fitting diapers or plastic pants on a child being treated in the diaper area, as these garments may constitute occlusive dressings.

Laboratory Tests: The following tests may be helpful in evaluating the HPA axis suppression:
    Urinary free cortisol test
    ACTH stimulation test

Carcinogenesis, Mutagenesis, and Impairment of Fertility: Long-term animal studies have not been performed to evaluate the carcinogenic potential or the effect on fertility of topical corticosteroids.

Studies to determine mutagenicity with prednisolone and hydrocortisone have revealed negative results. ·

Pregnancy Category C: Corticosteroids are generally teratogenic in laboratory animals when administered systemically at relatively low dosage levels. The more potent corticosteroids have been shown to be teratogenic after dermal application in laboratory animals. There are no adequate and well-controlled studies in pregnant women on teratogenic effects from topically applied corticosteroids. Therefore, topical corticosteroids should be used during pregnancy only if the potential benefit justifies the potential risk to the fetus. Drugs of this class should not be used extensively on pregnant patients, in large amounts, or for prolonged periods of time.

Nursing Mothers: It is not known whether topical administration of corticosteroids could result in sufficient systemic absorption to produce detectable quantities in breast milk. Systemically administered corticosteroids are secreted into breast milk in quantities not likely to have a deleterious effect on the infant. Nevertheless, caution should be exercised when topical corticosteroids are administered to a nursing woman.

Pediatric Use: Pediatric patients may demonstrate greater susceptibility to topical corticosteroid-induced HPA axis suppression and Cushing's syndrome than mature patients because of a larger skin surface area to body weight ratio.

Hypothalamic-pituitary-adrenal (HPA) axis suppression, Cushing's syndrome, and intracranial hypertension have been reported in children receiving topical corticosteroids. Manifestations of adrenal suppression in children include linear growth retardation, delayed weight gain, low plasma cortisol levels, and absence of response to ACTH stimulation. Manifestations of intracranial hypertension include bulging fontanelles, headaches, and bilateral papilledema.

Administration of topical corticosteroids to children should be limited to the least amount compatible with an effective therapeutic regimen. Chronic corticosteroid therapy may interfere with the growth and development of children.

ADVERSE REACTIONS

The following local adverse reactions are reported infrequently with topical corticosteroids, but may occur more frequently with the use of occlusive dressings. These reactions are listed in an approximate decreasing order of occurrence:

    Burning
    Itching
    Irritation
    Dryness
    Folliculitis
    Hypertrichosis
    Acneform eruptions
    Hypopigmentation
    Perioral dermatitis
    Allergic contact dermatitis
    Maceration of the skin
    Secondary infection
    Skin atrophy
    Striae
    Miliaria

OVERDOSAGE

Topically applied corticosteroids can be absorbed in sufficient amounts to produce systemic effects (see *"Precautions"*).

DOSAGE AND ADMINISTRATION

Apply Clocortolone Pivalate Cream 0.1% sparingly to the affected areas three times a day and rub in gently.

Occlusive dressings may be used for the management of psoriasis or recalcitrant conditions.

If an infection develops, the use of occlusive dressings should be discontinued and appropriate antimicrobial therapy instituted.

Store Clocortolone Pivalate Cream between 15° and 30° C (59° and 86°F). Avoid freezing.

HOW SUPPLIED
CREAM: 0.1%

AVERAGE UNIT PRICE (AVAILABLE SIZES)

GENERIC	$0.68		
BRAND/MANUFACTURER	NDC	SIZE	AWP
◆ GENERICS			
CLODERM: Hermal	48017-1375-02	15 gm	$12.25
CLODERM: Hermal	48017-1375-06	45 gm	$24.50

Clofazimine

DESCRIPTION

Clofazimine is an antileprosy agent available as capsules for oral administration. Each capsule contains 50 mg or 100 mg of micronized Clofazimine suspended in an oil-wax base. Clofazimine is a substituted iminophenazine bright-red dye. Its chemical name is 3-(p-chloroani lino)-10-(p-chlorophenyl)-2, 10-dihydro-2-isopropyliminophenazine. Clofazimine is a reddish-brown powder. It is readily soluble in benzene; soluble in chloroform; poorly soluble in acetone and in ethyl acetate; sparingly soluble in methanol and in ethanol; and virtually insoluble in water. Its molecular weight is 473.4.

Following is its chemical structure:

CLINICAL PHARMACOLOGY

Clofazimine exerts a slow bactericidal effect on *Mycobacterium leprae* (Hansen's bacillus). Clofazimine inhibits mycobacterial growth and binds preferentially to mycobacterial DNA. Clofazimine also exerts anti-inflammatory properties in controlling erythema nodosum leprosum reactions. However, its precise mechanisms of action are unknown.

PHARMACOKINETICS

Clofazimine as a variable absorption rate in leprosy patients, ranging from 45-62% after oral administration. The average serum concentrations in leprosy patients treated with 100 mg and 300 mg daily were 0.7 µg/ml and 1.0 µg/ml, respectively. After ingestion of a single dose of 300 mg, elimination of unchanged Clofazimine and its metabolites in a 24-hour urine collection was negligible. Clofazimine is retained in the human body for a long time. The half-life of Clofazimine following repeated oral doses is estimated to be at least 70 days. Part of the ingested drug recovered from the feces may represent excretion via the bile. A small amount is also eliminated in the sputum, sebum, and sweat.

Clofazimine is highly lipophilic and tends to be deposited predominantly in fatty tissue and in cells of the reticuloendothelial system. It is taken up by macrophages throughout the body. In autopsies performed on leprosy patients Clofazimine crystals were found predominantly in the mesenteric lymph nodes, adrenals, subcutaneous fat, liver, bile, gall bladder, spleen, small intestine, muscles, bones, and skin.

MICROBIOLOGY

Measurement of the minimum inhibitory concentration (MIC) of Clofazimine against leprosy bacilli *in vitro* is not yet feasible. In the mouse footpad system, the multiplication of *M. leprae* is inhibited by introducing 0.0001-0.001% Clofazimine in the diet. Although bacterial killing may begin shortly after starting the drug, it cannot be measured in biopsy tissues taken from patients for mouse footpad studies until approximately 50 days after the start of therapy.

Clofazimine does not show cross-resistance with dapsone or rifampin.

The following *in vitro* data are available, but their clinical significance is unknown Clofazimine has been shown *in vitro* to inhibit *M. avium* and *M. bovis* at concentrations of approximately 0.1-1.0 µg/ml. The MIC for *M. avium-intracellulare* isolated from patients with acquired immuno-deficiency syndrome (AIDS) ranged from 1.0 to 5.0 µg/ml. With a few exceptions, microorganisms other than mycobacteria are not inhibited by Clofazimine.

INDICATIONS AND USAGE

Clofazimine is indicated in the treatment of lepromatous leprosy, including dapsone-resistant lepromatous leprosy and lepromatous leprosy complicated by erythema nodosum leprosum. Clofazimine has not been demonstrated to be effective in the treatment of other leprosy-associated inflammatory reactions.

➤ SHOWN IN PRODUCT IDENTIFICATION GUIDE

Combination drug therapy has been recommended for initial treatment of multibacillary leprosy to prevent the development of drug resistance.

UNLABELED USES
Clofazimine has been used alone or as an adjunct in the treatment of mycobacterium avium infection, pyoderma gangunosum, and systemic lupus erythematosus.

CONTRAINDICATIONS
There are no known contraindications.

WARNINGS
Severe abdominal symptoms (see below) have necessitated exploratory laparotomies in some patients receiving Clofazimine. Rare reports have included splenic infarction, bowel obstruction, and gastrointestinal bleeding. There have also been reports of death following severe abdominal symptoms. Autopsies have revealed crystalline deposits of Clofazimine in various tissues including the intestinal mucosa, liver, spleen, and mesenteric lymph nodes.

Clofazimine should be used with caution in patients who have gastrointestinal problems such as abdominal pain and diarrhea. Dosages of Clofazimine of more than 100 mg daily should be given for as short a period as possible and only under close medical supervision. If a patient complains of colicky or burning pain in the abdomen, nausea, vomiting, or diarrhea, the dose should be reduced, and if necessary, the interval between doses should be increased, or the drug should be discontinued.

PRECAUTIONS
GENERAL
Physicians should be aware that skin discoloration due to Clofazimine may result in depression. Two suicides have been reported in patients receiving Clofazimine. For skin dryness and ichthyosis, oil can be applied to the skin.

INFORMATION FOR PATIENTS
Patients should be warned that Clofazimine may cause a discoloration of the skin from red to brownish black, as well as discoloration of the conjunctivae, lacrimal fluid, sweat, sputum, urine, and feces. Patients should be advised that skin discoloration, although reversible, may take several months or years to disappear after the conclusion of therapy with Clofazimine.

Patients should be told to take Clofazimine with meals.

DRUG INTERACTIONS
Preliminary data which suggest that dapsone may inhibit the anti-inflammatory activity of Clofazimine have not been confirmed. If leprosy-associated inflammatory reactions develop in patients being treated with dapsone and Clofazimine, it is still advisable to continue treatment with both drugs.

CARCINOGENESIS, MUTAGENESIS, IMPAIRMENT OF FERTILITY
Long-term carcinogenicity studies in animals have not been conducted with Clofazimine. Results of mutagenicity studies (Ames test) were negative. There was some evidence of impaired fertility in one study in rats treated at a dose 25 times the usual human dose; the number of offspring was reduced and there was a lower proportion of implantations.

PREGNANCY CATEGORY C
Clofazimine was not teratogenic in laboratory animals at dose levels equivalent to 8 times (rabbit) and 25 times (rat) the usual human daily dose. However, there was evidence of fetotoxicity in the mouse at 12-25 times the human dose, i.e., retardation of fetal skull ossification, increased incidence of abortions and stillbirths, and impaired neonatal survival. The skin and fatty tissue of offspring became discolored approximately 3 days after birth, which was attributed to the presence of Clofazimine in the maternal milk.

It has been found that Clofazimine crosses the human placenta. The skin of infants born to women who had received the drug during pregnancy was found to be deeply pigmented at birth. No evidence of teratogenicity was found in these infants. There are no adequate and well-controlled studies in pregnant women. Clofazimine should be used during pregnancy only if the potential benefit justifies the risk to the fetus.

NURSING MOTHERS
Clofazimine is excreted in the milk of nursing mothers. Clofazimine should not be administered to a nursing woman unless clearly indicated.

PEDIATRIC USE
Safety and effectiveness in children have not been established. Several cases of children treated with Clofazimine have been reported in the literature.

ADVERSE REACTIONS
In general Clofazimine is well tolerated when administered in dosages no greater than 100 mg daily. The most consistent adverse reactions are usually dose related and are usually reversible when Clofazimine is discontinued.

ADVERSE REACTIONS OCCURRING IN MORE THAN 1% OF PATIENTS
Skin: Pigmentation from pink to brownish-black in 75-100% of the patients within a few weeks of treatment; ichthyosis and dryness (8-28%); rash and pruritus (1-5%).

Gastrointestinal: Abdominal and epigastric pain, diarrhea, nausea, vomiting, gastrointestinal intolerance (40-50%).

Ocular: Conjunctival and corneal pigmentation due to Clofazimine crystal deposits; dryness; burning; itching; irritation.

Other: Discoloration of urine, feces, sputum, sweat; elevated blood sugar; elevated ESR.

ADVERSE REACTIONS OCCURRING IN LESS THAN 1% OF PATIENTS
Skin: Phototoxicity, erythroderma, acneiform eruptions, monilial cheilosis.

Gastrointestinal: Bowel obstruction (see *"Warnings"*), gastrointestinal bleeding (see *"Warnings"*), anorexia, constipation, weight loss, hepatitis, jaundice, eosinophilic enteritis, enlarged liver.

Ocular: Diminished vision.

Nervous: Dizziness, drowsiness, fatigue, headache, giddiness, neuralgia, taste disorder.

Psychiatric: Depression secondary to skin discoloration; two suicides have been reported.

Laboratory: Elevated levels of albumin, serum bilirubin, and AST (SGOT); eosinophilia; hypokalemia.

Other: Splenic infarction (see *"Warnings"*), thromboembolism, anemia, cystitis, bone pain, edema, fever, lymphadenopathy, vascular pain.

OVERDOSAGE
No specific data are available on the treatment of overdosage with Clofazimine. However, in case of overdose, the stomach should be emptied by inducing vomiting or by gastric lavage, and supportive symptomatic treatment should be employed.

DOSAGE AND ADMINISTRATION
Clofazimine should be taken with meals.

Clofazimine should be used preferably in combination with one or more other antileprosy agents to prevent the emergence of drug resistance.

For the treatment of proven dapsone-resistant leprosy, Clofazimine should be given at a dosage of 100 mg daily in combination with one or more other antileprosy drugs for 3 years, followed by monotherapy with 100 mg of Clofazimine daily. Clinical improvement usually can be detected between the first and third months of treatment and is usually clearly evident by the sixth month.

For dapsone-sensitive multibacillary leprosy, a combination therapy with two other antileprosy drugs is recommended. The triple-drug regimen should be given for at least 2 years and continued, if possible, until negative skin smears are obtained. At this time, monotherapy with an appropriate antileprosy drug can be instituted.

The treatment of erythema nodosum leprosum reactions depends on the severity of symptoms. In general, the basic antileprosy treatment should be continued, and if nerve injury or skin ulceration is threatened, corticosteroids should be given. Where prolonged corticosteroid therapy becomes necessary Clofazimine administered at dosages of 100 mg to 200 mg daily for up to 3 months may be useful in eliminating or reducing corticosteroid requirements. Dosages above 200 mg daily are not recommended, and the dosage should be tapered to 100 mg daily as quickly as possible after the reactive episode is controlled. The patient must remain under medical surveillance.

For advice about combination drug regimens, contact the USPHS Gillis W. Long Hansen's Disease Center, Carville, LA (504-642-7771).

Do not store above 86°F. Protect from moisture.

Dispense in tight container (USP).

HOW SUPPLIED
CAPSULE: 50 MG

BRAND/MANUFACTURER	NDC	SIZE	AWP
○ BRAND LAMPRENE: Geigy	00028-0108-01	100s	$12.52

CAPSULE: 100 MG

BRAND/MANUFACTURER	NDC	SIZE	AWP
○ BRAND LAMPRENE: Geigy	00028-0109-01	100s	$23.19

Clofibrate

DESCRIPTION
Clofibrate is ethyl 2-(p-chlorophenoxy)-2-methyl-propionate, and antilipidemic agent.

Its molecular formula is $C_{12}H_{15}O_3Cl$, molecular weight 242.7, and boiling point 148-150°C at 25 mm Hg. It is a stable, colorless to pale-yellow liquid with a faint odor and characteristic taste, soluble in common solvents but not in water. Each Clofibrate capsule contains 500 mg Clofibrate for oral administration.

Following is its chemical structure:

$$CH_3$$
$$CH_3CCOOCH_2CH_3$$

Cl

CLINICAL PHARMACOLOGY

Clofibrate is an antilipidemic agent. It acts to lower elevated serum lipids by reducing the very low-density lipoprotein fraction (S_f20-400) rich in triglycerides. Serum cholesterol may be decreased, particularly in those patients whose cholesterol elevation is due to the presence of IDL as a result of Type III hyperlipoproteinemia.

The mechanism of action has not been established definitively. Clofibrate may inhibit the hepatic release of lipoproteins (particularly VLDL), potentiate the action of lipoprotein lipase, and increase the fecal excretion of neutral sterols.

Between 95% and 99% of an oral dose of Clofibrate is excreted in the urine as free and conjugated clofibric acid: thus, the absorption of Clofibrate is virtually complete. The half-life of clofibric acid in normal volunteers averages 18 to 22 hours (range 14 to 35 hours) but can vary by up to 7 hours in the same subject at different times. Clofibric acid is highly protein-bound (95% to 97%). In subjects undergoing continuous Clofibrate treatment, 1 g q12h, plasma concentrations of clofibric acid range from 120 to 125 mcg/mL to an approximate peak of 200 mcg/mL.

Several investigators have observed in their studies that Clofibrate may produce a decrease in cholesterol linoleate but an increase in palmitoleate and oleate, the latter being considered atherogenic in experimental animals. The significance of this finding is unknown at this time.

Reduction of triglycerides in some patients treated with Clofibrate or certain of its chemically and clinically similar analogs may be associated with an increase in LDL cholesterol. Increase in LDL cholesterol has been observed in patients whose cholesterol is initially normal.

Animal studies suggest that Clofibrate interrupts cholesterol biosynthesis prior to mevalonate formation.

INDICATIONS AND USAGE

The initial treatment of choice for hyperlipidemia is dietary therapy specific for the type of hyperlipidemia.[1]

Excess body weight and alcoholic intake may be important factors in hypertriglyceridemia and should be addressed prior to any drug therapy. Physical exercise can be an important ancillary measure. Estrogen therapy, some beta-blockers, and thiazide diuretics may also be associated with increases in plasma triglycerides. Discontinuation of such products may obviate the need for specific antilipidemic therapy. Contributory diseases such as hypothyroidism or diabetes mellitus should be looked for and adequately treated. The use of drugs should be considered only when reasonable attempts have been made to obtain satisfactory results with non-drug methods. If the decision ultimately is to use drugs, the patient should be instructed that this does not reduce the importance of adhering to diet.

Because Clofibrate is associated with certain serious adverse findings reported in two large clinical trials (see "Warnings"), agents other than Clofibrate may be more suitable for a particular patient.

Clofibrate is indicated for Primary Dysbetalipoproteinemia (Type III hyperlipidemia) that does not respond adequately to diet.

Clofibrate may be considered for the treatment of adult patients with very high serum-triglyceride levels (Types IV and V hyperlipidemia) who present a risk of abdominal pain and pancreatitis and who do not respond adequately to a determined dietary effort to control them. Patients who present such risk typically have serum triglycerides over 2000 mg/dl and have elevations of VLDL-cholesterol as well as fasting chylomicrons (Type V hyperlipidemia). Subjects who consistently have total serum or plasma triglycerides below 1000 mg/dl are unlikely to present a risk of pancreatitis. Clofibrate therapy may be considered for those subjects with triglyceride elevations between 1000 and 2000 mg/dl who have a history of pancreatitis or of recurrent abdominal pain typical of pancreatitis. It is recognized that some Type IV patients with triglycerides under 1000 mg/dl may, through dietary or alcoholic indiscretion, convert to a Type V pattern with massive triglyceride elevations accompanying fasting chylomicronemia, but the influence of Clofibrate therapy on the risk of pancreatitis in such situations has not been adequately studied.

Clofibrate is not useful for the hypertriglyceridemia of Type I hyperlipidemia, where elevations of chylomicrons and plasma triglycerides are accompanied by normal levels of very low-density lipoprotein (VLDL). Inspection of plasma refrigerated for 12 to 14 hours is helpful in distinguishing Types I, IV, and V hyperlipoproteinemia.[2]

Clofibrate has not been shown to be effective for prevention of coronary heart disease.

The biochemical response to Clofibrate is variable, and it is not always possible to predict from the lipoprotein type or other factors which patients will obtain favorable results. LDL cholesterol, as well as triglycerides, should be re-checked during the first several months of therapy in order to detect rises in LDL cholesterol that often accompany fibric-acid-type drug-induced reductions in elevated triglycerides. It is essential that lipid levels be reassessed periodically and that the drug be discontinued in any patient in whom lipids do not show significant improvement.

UNLABELED USES

Clofibrate has been used alone or as an adjunct in the treatment of neonatal jaundice.

CONTRAINDICATIONS

Clofibrate is contraindicated in pregnant women. While teratogenic studies have not demonstrated any effect attributable to Clofibrate, it is known that serum of the rabbit fetus accumulates a higher concentration of Clofibrate than that found in maternal serum, and it is possible that the fetus may not have developed the enzyme system required for the excretion of Clofibrate.

It is contraindicated in patients with clinically significant hepatic or renal dysfunction. Rhabdomyolysis and severe hyperkalemia have been reported in association with preexisting renal insufficiency.

It is contraindicated in patients with primary biliary cirrhosis, since it may raise the already elevated cholesterol in these cases.

It is contraindicated in patients with a known hypersensitivity to Clofibrate.

It is contraindicated in nursing women (see "Precautions").

WARNINGS

IN A LARGE STUDY INVOLVING 5,000 PATIENTS IN A CLOFIBRATE TREATED GROUP AND 5,000 IN A PLACEBO-TREATED GROUP FOLLOWED FOR AN AVERAGE OF FIVE YEARS ON DRUG OR PLACEBO AND ONE YEAR BEYOND (THE *WHO* STUDY), THERE WAS A STATISTICALLY SIGNIFICANT 44% HIGHER AGE-ADJUSTED TOTAL MORTALITY IN THE CLOFIBRATE-TREATED GROUP THAN IN A COMPARABLE PLACEBO GROUP. THE EXCESS DEATHS WERE DUE TO NON-CARDIOVASCULAR CAUSES: HALF OF THIS DIFFERENCE WAS DUE TO MALIGNANCY; OTHER CAUSES OF DEATH INCLUDED POSTCHOLECYSTECTOMY COMPLICATIONS AND PANCREATITIS.[3] IN ANOTHER PROSPECTIVE STUDY INVOLVING 1,000 CLOFIBRATE- AND 3,000 PLACEBO-TREATED PATIENTS FOLLOWED FOR AN AVERAGE OF SIX YEARS ON DRUG OR PLACEBO (THE CORONARY DRUG PROJECT STUDY), THE NONCARDIOVASCULAR MORTALITY RATE, INCLUDING THAT OF MALIGNANCY, WAS NOT SIGNIFICANTLY DIFFERENT IN THE CLOFIBRATE- AND PLACEBO-TREATED GROUPS.[4] THIS SHOULD NOT BE INTERPRETED TO MEAN THAT CLOFIBRATE IS NOT ASSOCIATED WITH AN INCREASED RISK OF NONCARDIOVASCULAR DEATH, BECAUSE THE PATIENTS IN THE CORONARY DRUG PROJECT WERE MUCH OLDER THAN THOSE IN THE *WHO* STUDY AND THEY ALL HAD HAD A PREVIOUS MYOCARDIAL INFARCTION, SO THAT THE DEATHS IN THE CORONARY DRUG PROJECT WERE OVERWHELMINGLY DUE TO CARDIOVASCULAR CAUSES, AND IT WOULD HAVE BEEN VERY DIFFICULT TO DISCERN CLOFIBRATE-ASSOCIATED RISK OF DEATH DUE TO NONCARDIOVASCULAR CAUSES IF IT EXISTED. BOTH STUDIES DEMONSTRATED THAT CLOFIBRATE USERS HAVE TWICE THE RISK OF DEVELOPING CHOLELITHIASIS AND CHOLECYSTITIS REQUIRING SURGERY AS DO NONUSERS.

A POTENTIAL BENEFIT OF CLOFIBRATE WAS, HOWEVER, REPORTED IN THE *WHO* STUDY WHICH INVOLVED PATIENTS WITH HYPERCHOLESTEROLEMIA AND NO HISTORY OF MYOCARDIAL INFARCTION OR ANGINA PECTORIS. IN THIS STUDY, THERE WAS A STATISTICALLY SIGNIFICANT 25% DECREASE IN SUBSEQUENT NONFATAL MYOCARDIAL INFARCTIONS IN THE CLOFIBRATE-TREATED GROUP WHEN COMPARED WITH THE PLACEBO GROUP. THERE WAS NO DIFFERENCE IN INCIDENCE OF FATAL MYOCARDIAL INFARCTION IN THE TWO GROUPS. IN THE CORONARY DRUG PROJECT STUDY, WHICH INVOLVED PATIENTS WITH OR WITHOUT HYPERCHOLESTEROLEMIA AND/OR HYPERTRIGLYCERIDEMIA AND WITH A HISTORY OF PREVIOUS MYOCARDIAL INFARCTION, THERE WAS NO SIGNIFICANT DIFFERENCE IN INCIDENCE OF EITHER NONFATAL OR FATAL MYOCARDIAL INFARCTION BETWEEN THE CLOFIBRATE AND PLACEBO-TREATED GROUPS.[3]

AS A RESULT OF THESE AND OTHER STUDIES, THE FOLLOWING CAN BE STATED.

1. CLOFIBRATE, IN GENERAL, CAUSES A RELATIVELY MODEST REDUCTION OF SERUM CHOLESTEROL AND A SOMEWHAT GREATER REDUCTION OF SERUM TRIGLYCERIDES. IN TYPE III HYPERLIPIDEMIA, HOWEVER, SUBSTANTIAL REDUCTIONS OF BOTH CHOLESTEROL AND TRIGLYCERIDES CAN OCCUR WITH CLOFIBRATE USE.

2. NO STUDY TO DATE HAS SHOWN A CONVINCING REDUCTION IN INCIDENCE OF *FATAL* MYOCARDIAL INFARCTION.

3. A SIGNIFICANTLY INCREASED INCIDENCE OF CHOLELITHIASIS HAS BEEN DEMONSTRATED CONSISTENTLY IN CLOFIBRATE-TREATED GROUPS, AND AN INCREASE IN MORBIDITY FROM THIS COMPLICATION AND MORTALITY FROM CHOLECYSTECTOMY MUST BE ANTICIPATED DURING CLOFIBRATE TREATMENT.

4. SEVERAL TYPES OF OTHER UNDESIRABLE EVENTS HAVE BEEN ASSOCIATED IN A STATISTICALLY SIGNIFICANT WAY WITH CLOFIBRATE ADMINISTRATION IN THE *WHO* AND THE CORONARY DRUG PROJECT STUDIES. THERE WAS AN INCREASE IN INCIDENCE OF NONCARDIOVASCULAR DEATHS REPORTED IN THE *WHO* STUDY. THERE WAS AN INCREASE IN CARDIAC ARRHYTHMIAS, INTERMITTENT CLAUDICATION, AND DEFINITE OR SUSPECTED THROMBOEMBOLIC EVENTS, AND ANGINA REPORTED IN THE CORONARY DRUG PROJECT, WHICH WAS NOT, HOWEVER, REPORTED IN THE *WHO* STUDY.

5. ADMINISTRATION OF CLOFIBRATE TO MICE AND RATS IN LONG-TERM STUDIES AT EIGHT TIMES THE HUMAN DOSE, AND TO RATS AT

FIVE TIMES THE HUMAN DOSE, RESULTED IN A HIGHER INCIDENCE OF BENIGN AND MALIGNANT LIVER TUMORS THAN IN CONTROLS. LOWER DOSES WERE NOT INCLUDED IN THESE STUDIES.

AN INCREASE IN BENIGN LEYDIG-CELL TUMORS IN MALE RATS TREATED AT 400 MG/KG (10 TIMES THE ESTIMATED HUMAN DOSE) WAS OBSERVED IN A SINGLE STUDY WITH CLOFIBRATE; SIMILAR INCREASES WERE NOT OBSERVED IN OTHER STUDIES CONDUCTED WITH CLOFIBRATE ALTHOUGH THEY HAVE BEEN OBSERVED WITH OTHER FIBRIC-ACID DERIVATIVES.

6. ADMINISTRATION OF CLOFIBRATE TO MALE MONKEYS AT DOSAGES OF 2 TO 6 TIMES THE HUMAN DOSE RESULTED IN INCREASES IN MORTALITY OF 2 - TO 5- FOLD. AS IN THE CASE OF MEN IN THE *WHO* STUDY, NO SINGLE CAUSE OF DEATH WAS IDENTIFIED.

BECAUSE OF THE TUMORIGENICITY OF CLOFIBRATE IN RODENTS AND THE POSSIBLE INCREASED RISK OF MALIGNANCY ASSOCIATED WITH CLOFIBRATE IN THE HUMAN, AS WELL AS THE INCREASED RISK OF CHOLELITHIASIS, AND BECAUSE THERE IS NOT, TO DATE, SUBSTANTIAL EVIDENCE OF A BENEFICIAL EFFECT ON CARDIOVASCULAR MORTALITY FROM CLOFIBRATE, THIS DRUG SHOULD BE UTILIZED ONLY FOR THOSE PATIENTS DESCRIBED IN THE "INDICATIONS AND USAGE" SECTION, AND SHOULD BE DISCONTINUED IF SIGNIFICANT LIPID RESPONSE IS NOT OBTAINED.

CONCOMITANT ANTICOAGULANTS

CAUTION SHOULD BE EXERCISED WHEN ANTICOAGULANTS ARE GIVEN IN CONJUNCTION WITH CLOFIBRATE. THE DOSAGE OF THE ANTICOAGULANT SHOULD BE REDUCED USUALLY BY ONE-HALF (DEPENDING ON THE INDIVIDUAL CASE) TO MAINTAIN THE PROTHROMBIN TIME AT THE DESIRED LEVEL TO PREVENT BLEEDING COMPLICATIONS. FREQUENT PROTHROMBIN DETERMINATIONS ARE ADVISABLE UNTIL IT HAS BEEN DEFINITELY DETERMINED THAT THE PROTHROMBIN LEVEL HAS BEEN STABILIZED.

SKELETAL MUSCLE

Myalgia, myositis, myopathy, and rhabdomyolysis with or without elevation of CPK have been associated with Clofibrate therapy. Consideration should be given to withholding or discontinuing drug therapy in any patient with a risk factor predisposing to the development of renal failure secondary to rhabdomyolysis, including: severe acute infection: hypotension; major surgery; trauma; severe acute metabolic, endocrine or electrolyte disorders; and uncontrolled seizures. Clofibrate therapy should be discontinued if markedly elevated CPK levels occur or myositis is diagnosed.

AVOIDANCE OF PREGNANCY

Strict birth control procedures must be exercised by women of child-bearing potential. In patients who plan to become pregnant, Clofibrate should be withdrawn several months before conception. Because of the possibility of pregnancy occurring despite birth control precautions in patients taking Clofibrate the possible benefits of the drug to the patient must be weighed against possible hazards to the fetus. (See *"Pregnancy"* section).

PRECAUTIONS
GENERAL

Before instituting therapy with Clofibrate, attempts should be made to control serum lipids with appropriate dietary regimens, weight loss in obese patients, control of diabetes mellitus, etc.

Because of the long-term administration of a drug of this nature, adequate baseline studies should be performed to determine that the patient has significantly elevated serum lipid levels. Frequent determinations of serum lipids should be obtained during the first few months of Clofibrate administration and periodic determinations thereafter. The drug should be withdrawn after three months if response is inadequate. However, in the case of xanthoma tuberosum, the drug should be employed for longer periods (even up to one year) provided that there is a reduction in the size and/or number of the xanthomata.

Since cholelithiasis is a possible side effect of Clofibrate therapy, appropriate diagnostic procedures should be performed if signs and symptoms related to disease of the biliary system should occur.

Clofibrate may produce "flu-like" symptoms (muscular aching, soreness, cramping) associated with increased creatine kinase levels. The physician should differentiate this from actual viral and/or bacterial disease.

Use with caution in patients with peptic ulcer since reactivation has been reported. Whether this is drug related is unknown.

Various cardiac arrhythmias have been reported with the use of Clofibrate.

LABORATORY TESTS

Subsequent serum lipid determinations should be done to detect a paradoxical rise in serum cholesterol or triglyceride levels. Clofibrate will not alter the seasonal variations of serum cholesterol: peak elevations in midwinter and late summer and decreases in fall and spring. If the drug is discontinued, the patient should be continued on an appropriate hypolipidemic diet, and serum lipids should be monitored until stabilized, as a rise in these values to or above the original baseline may occur.

During Clofibrate therapy, frequent serum-transaminase determinations and other liver-function tests should be performed, since the drug may produce abnormalities in these parameters. These effects are usually reversible when the drug is discontinued. Hepatic biopsies are usually within normal limits. If the hepatic-function tests steadily rise or show excessive abnormalities, the drug should be withdrawn. Therefore, use with caution in those patients with a past history of jaundice or hepatic disease.

Complete blood counts should be done periodically since anemia, and more frequently, leukopenia have been reported in patients who have been taking Clofibrate.

DRUG INTERACTIONS

Caution should be exercised when anticoagulants are given in conjunction with Clofibrate. Usually, the dosage of the anticoagulant should be reduced by one-half (depending on the individual case) to maintain the prothrombin time at the desired level to prevent bleeding complications. Frequent prothrombin determinations are advisable until it has been determined definitely that the prothrombin level has been stabilized.

Clofibrate may displace acidic drugs such as phenytoin or tolbutamide from their binding sites. Caution should be exercised when treating patients with either of these drugs or other highly protein-bound drugs and Clofibrate. The hypoglycemic effect of tolbutamide has been reported to increase when Clofibrate is given concurrently.

Fulminant rhabdomyolysis has been seen as early as three weeks after initiation of combined therapy with another fibrate and lovastatin but may be seen after several months. For these reasons, it is felt that, in most subjects who have had an unsatisfactory lipid response to either drug alone, the possible benefits of combined therapy with lovastatin and a fibrate do not outweigh the risks of severe myopathy, rhabdomyolysis, and acute renal failure. While it is not known whether this interaction occurs with fibrates other than gemfibrozil, myopathy and rhabdomyolysis have occasionally been associated with the use of fibrates alone including Clofibrate. Therefore, the combined use of lovastatin with fibrates should generally be avoided.

CARCINOGENESIS, MUTAGENESIS, IMPAIRMENT OF FERTILITY

See *"Warnings"* section for information on carcinogenesis and mutagenesis.

Arrest of spermatogenesis has been seen in both dogs and monkeys at doses approximately 4 to 6 times the human therapeutic dose.

PREGNANCY
TERATOGENIC EFFECTS

Pregnancy Category C. Animal reproduction studies have not been conducted with Clofibrate. It is also not known whether Clofibrate can cause fetal harm when administered to a pregnant woman or can affect reproductive capacity. However, animal reproduction studies with Clofibrate plus androsterone showed increases in neonatal deaths and pup mortality during lactation.

NURSING MOTHERS

Clofibrate is contraindicated in lactating women, since an active metabolite (CPIB) has been measured in breast milk.

PEDIATRIC USE

Safety and efficacy in children have not been established.

ADVERSE REACTIONS

The most common is nausea. Less frequently encountered gastrointestinal reactions are vomiting, loose stools, dyspepsia, flatulence, and abdominal distress. Reactions reported less often than gastrointestinal ones are headache, dizziness, and fatigue; muscle cramping, aching, and weakness; skin rash, urticaria, and pruritus; dry brittle hair, and alopecia. The following reported adverse reactions are listed alphabetically by systems:

Cardiovascular: Increased or decreased angina
   Cardiac arrhythmias
   Both swelling and phlebitis at site of xanthomas

Dermatologic: Allergic reactions including urticaria
   Skin rash
   Pruritus
   Dry skin and dry, brittle hair
   Alopecia
   Toxic epidermal necrolysis

Gastrointestinal: Gallstones
   Nausea
   Vomiting
   Diarrhea
   Gastrointestinal upset (bloating, flatulence, abdominal distress)
   Hepatomegaly (not associated with hepatotoxicity)
   Stomatitis and gastritis

Genitourinary: Findings consistent with renal dysfunction as evidenced by dysuria, hematuria, proteinuria, decreased urine output. One patient's renal biopsy suggested "allergic reaction."
   Impotence and decreased libido

Hematologic: Leukopenia
   Potentiation of anticoagulant effect
   Anemia
   Eosinophilia
   Agranulocytosis

Musculoskeletal: Myalgia (muscle cramping, aching, weakness)
   "Flu-like" symptoms

Myositis
Myopathy
Rhabdomyolysis in the setting of preexisting renal insufficiency
Arthralgia

Neurologic: Fatigue, weakness, drowsiness
Dizziness
Headache

Miscellaneous: Weight gain
Polyphagia

LABORATORY FINDINGS

Abnormal liver-function tests as evidenced by increased transaminase (SGOT and SGPT), BSP retention, and increased thymol turbidity
Proteinuria
Increased creatine phosphokinase
Hyperkalemia in association with renal insufficiency and continuous ambulatory peritoneal dialysis treatment

Reported adverse reactions whose direct relationship with the drug has not been established: peptic ulcer, gastrointestinal hemorrhage, rheumatoid arthritis, tremors, increased perspiration, systemic lupus erythematosus, blurred vision, gynecomastia, thrombocytopenic purpura.

OVERDOSAGE

While there has been no reported case of overdosage, should it occur, symptomatic supportive measures should be taken.

DOSAGE AND ADMINISTRATION

Initial: The recommended dosage for adults is 2 g daily in divided doses. Some patients may respond to a lower dosage.

Maintenance: Same as for initial dosage.

Storage: Store at room temperature (approximately 25°C).
Dispense in a well-closed, light-resistant container as defined in the USP.
Avoid freezing and excessive heat.

REFERENCES

1. Coronary Risk Handbook (1973). American Heart Association. 2. Nikkila, EA: Familial lipoprotein lipase deficiency and related disorders of chylomicron metabolism. In Stanbury JB et al (eds): The Metabolic Basis of Inherited Disease, 5th ed., Mcgraw-Hill, 1983, Chap. 30. p.622-642. 3. Report from the Committee of Principal Investigators: A cooperative trial in the primary prevention of ischaemic heart disease using clofibrate. Br Heart J 40:1069, 1978. 4. The Coronary Drug Project Research Group: Clofibrate and niacin in coronary heart disease. JAMA 231:360, 1975.

HOW SUPPLIED
CAPSULE: 500 MG

AVERAGE UNIT PRICE (AVAILABLE SIZES)		GENERIC A-RATED AVERAGE PRICE (GAAP)	
BRAND	$0.80	100s	$25.28
GENERIC	$0.25		
HCFA FUL (100s ea)	$0.15		

BRAND/MANUFACTURER	NDC	SIZE	AWP
◆ BRAND			
ATROMID-S: Wyeth-Ayerst	00046-0243-81	100s	$79.51
◆ GENERICS			
Chase	54429-3148-01	100s	$20.00
Qualitest	00603-2932-21	100s	$23.31
Schein	00364-2136-01	100s	$24.50
Aligen	00405-4236-01	100s	$24.50
Caremark	00339-5651-12	100s	$25.12
Moore,H.L.	00839-7228-06	100s	$25.23
Goldline	00182-1269-01	100s	$25.45
Novopharm	55953-0382-40	100s	$25.48
Rosemont	00832-0413-00	100s	$25.50
Mason Dist	11845-0187-01	100s	$25.50
URL	00677-1111-01	100s	$26.00
Geneva	00781-2600-01	100s	$26.08
Rugby	00536-3466-01	100s	$26.24
Major	00904-2916-60	100s	$26.40
Parmed	00349-8604-01	100s	$26.70
Martec	52555-0111-01	100s	$28.43

Clomid *SEE* CLOMIPHENE CITRATE

Clomiphene Citrate

DESCRIPTION

Clomiphene Citrate is designated chemically as 2-[p-(2-chloro-1,2-diphenylvinyl) phenoxy] triethylamine dihydrogen citrate.

As shown, one molecule of citric acid is chemically bound with one molecule of the organic base, Clomiphene.

Clomiphene Citrate is a chemical analog of other triarylethylene compounds such as chlorotrianisene and the cholesterol inhibitor, triparanol.

Following is its chemical structure:

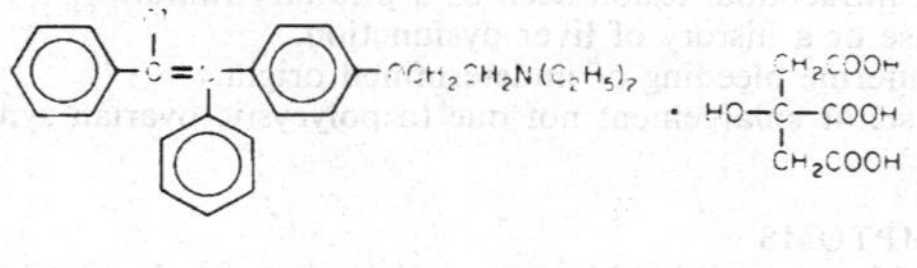

ACTIONS

Clomiphene Citrate, an orally-administered, nonsteroidal agent, may induce ovulation in selected anovulatory women. It is a drug of considerable pharmacologic potency. Careful evaluation and selection of the patient and close attention to the timing of the dose is mandatory prior to treatment with Clomiphene Citrate. Conservative selection and management of the patient contribute to successful therapy of anovulation. Clomiphene Citrate induces ovulation in most selected anovulatory patients. The various criteria for ovulation include: an ovulation peak of estrogen excretion followed by a biphasic basal body temperature curve, urinary excretion of pregnanediol at postovulatory levels, and endometrial histologic findings characteristic of the luteal phase.

A review of eleven publications appearing between 1964 and 1978 showed that pregnancy occurred in 35% of 5154 patients with ovulatory dysfunction who received Clomiphene Citrate.

PREGNANCIES FOLLOWING CLOMIPHENE CITRATE, USP[a]

		(Range)
Number of Patients	= 5154	
Percent of Patients Ovulating[b]	= 75	(50-94%)
Percent of Ovulatory Cycles	= 53	(33-69%)
Percent of Patients Pregnant	= 35	(11-52%)
Percent Patients Pregnant	= 46	(22-61%)
Percent Patients Ovulating		
Percent Live Births	= 86	(74-99.8%)
Percent Abortions	= 14	(0.2-26%)
Percent of Single Births	= 90	(67-100%)
Percent Surviving	= 99	(98.2-100%)
Percent of Multiple Births	= 10	(0-33%)
Percent Surviving	= 96	(82-100%)

a) includes patients receiving other than recommended dosage regimen.
b) average from studies.

Clomiphene Citrate therapy appears to mediate ovulation through increased output of pituitary gonadotropins. These stimulate the maturation and endocrine activity of the ovarian follicle which is followed by the development and function of the corpus luteum. Increased urinary excretion of gonadotropins and estrogen suggests involvement of the pituitary.

Studies with ^{14}C labeled Clomiphene Citrate have shown that it is readily absorbed orally in humans and is excreted principally in the feces. An average of 51% of the administered dose was excreted after 5 days. After intravenous administration, 37% was excreted in 5 days. The appearance of ^{14}C in the feces six weeks after administration suggests that the remaining drug and/or metabolites are slowly excreted from a sequestered enterohepatic recirculation pool.

INDICATIONS

Clomiphene Citrate is indicated for the treatment of ovulatory failure in patients desiring pregnancy and whose husbands are fertile and potent. Impediments to this goal must be excluded or adequately treated before beginning therapy. Administration of Clomiphene Citrate is indicated only in patients with demonstrated ovulatory dysfunction and in whom the following conditions apply:
1. Normal liver function.
2. Physiologic indications of normal endogenous estrogen (as estimated from vaginal smears, endometrial biopsy, assay of serum [or urinary] estrogen, or from bleeding in response to progesterone). Reduced estrogen levels, while less favorable, do not prevent successful therapy.
3. Clomiphene Citrate therapy is not effective for those patients with primary pituitary or ovarian failure. It cannot substitute for appropriate therapy of other disturbances leading to ovulatory dysfunction, e.g., diseases of the thyroid or adrenals.
4. Particularly careful evaluation prior to Clomiphene Citrate therapy should be done in patients with abnormal uterine bleeding. It is most important that neoplastic lesions are detected.

CONTRAINDICATIONS

PREGNANCY

Although no direct effect of Clomiphene Citrate therapy on the human fetus has been seen established, Clomiphene Citrate should not be administered in cases of suspected pregnancy as such effects have been reported in animals. To prevent inadvertent Clomiphene Citrate administration during early pregnancy, the basal body temperature should be recorded throughout all treatment cycles, and therapy should be discontinued if pregnancy is suspected. If the basal body temperature following Clomiphene Citrate is biphasic and is not followed by menses, the possibility of an ovarian cyst and/or pregnancy should be excluded. Until the correct diagnosis has been determined, the next course of therapy should be delayed.

Clomiphene Citrate is also contraindicated in patients who have:

1. Uncontrolled thyroid or adrenal dysfunction.
2. An organic intracranial lesion such as a pituitary tumor.
3. Liver disease or a history of liver dysfunction.
4. Abnormal uterine bleeding of undetermined origin.
5. Ovarian cysts or enlargement not due to polycystic ovarian syndrome.

WARNINGS

VISUAL SYMPTOMS
Patients should be warned that blurring and/or other visual symptoms may occur occasionally with Clomiphene Citrates therapy. These may make activities such as driving or operating machinery more hazardous than usual, particularly under conditions of variable lighting. While their significance is not yet understood (see *"Adverse Reactions"*), patients having any visual symptoms should discontinue treatment and have a complete ophthalmologic evaluation.

OVARIAN HYPERSTIMULATION SYNDROME
The Ovarian Hyperstimulation Syndrome (OHSS) has been reported to occur in patients receiving drug therapy for ovulation induction, including in rare cases patients receiving Clomiphene Citrate therapy. OHSS is a medical event distinct from uncomplicated ovarian enlargement. OHSS may progress rapidly (within 24 hours to several days) to become a serious medical event. It is characterized by an apparent dramatic increase in vascular permeability which can result in a rapid accumulation of fluid in the peritoneal cavity, thorax, and potentially, the pericardium. The early warning signs of development of OHSS are severe pelvic pain, nausea, vomiting, and weight gain. The following symptomatology has been seen with cases of OHSS: abdominal pain, abdominal distension, gastrointestinal symptoms including nausea, vomiting and diarrhea, severe ovarian enlargement, weight gain, dyspnea, and oliguria. Clinical evaluation may reveal hypovolemia, hemoconcentration, electrolyte imbalances, ascites, hemoperitoneum, pleural effusions, hydrothorax, acute pulmonary distress, and thromboembolic phenomena. Transient liver function test abnormalities, suggestive of hepatic dysfunction, which may be accompanied by morphologic changes on liver biopsy, have been reported in association with the Ovarian Hyperstimulation Syndrome (OHSS).

PRECAUTIONS

DIAGNOSIS PRIOR TO CLOMIPHENE CITRATE THERAPY
Careful evaluation should be given to candidates for Clomiphene Citrate therapy. A complete pelvic examination should be performed prior to treatment and repeated before each subsequent course. Clomiphene Citrate should not be given to patients with an ovarian cyst, as further ovarian enlargement may result.

Since the incidence of endometrial carcinoma and of ovulatory disorders increases with age, endometrial biopsy should always exclude the former as causative in such patients. If abnormal uterine bleeding is present, full diagnostic measures are necessary.

OVARIAN OVERSTIMULATION DURING TREATMENT WITH CLOMIPHENE CITRATE
To minimize the hazard associated with the occasional abnormal ovarian enlargement during Clomiphene Citrate therapy (see *"Adverse Reactions"*), the lowest dose producing good results should be chosen. Some patients with polycystic ovarian syndrome are unusually sensitive to gonadotropins and may have an exaggerated response to usual doses of Clomiphene Citrate. Maximal enlargement of the ovary, whether abnormal or physiologic, does not occur until several days after discontinuation of Clomiphene Citrate. The patient complaining of pelvic pains after receiving Clomiphene Citrate should be examined carefully. If enlargement of the ovary occurs, Clomiphene Citrate therapy should be withheld until the ovaries have returned to pretreatment size, and the dosage or duration of the next course should be reduced. The ovarian enlargement and cyst formation following Clomiphene Citrate therapy regress spontaneously within a few days or weeks after discontinuing treatment. Therefore, unless a strong indication for laparoscopy (or laparotomy) exists, such cystic enlargement always should be managed conservatively.

MULTIPLE PREGNANCY
In the reviewed publications, the incidence of multiple pregnancies was increased during those cycles in which Clomiphene Citrate was given. Among the 1,803 pregnancies on which the outcome was reported, 90% were single and 10% twins. Less than 1% of the reported deliveries resulted in triplets or more.

Of these multiple pregnancies, 96-99% resulted in the births of live infants. The patient and her husband should be advised of the frequency and potential hazards of multiple pregnancy before starting treatment.

ADVERSE REACTIONS
At the recommended dosage of Clomiphene Citrate side effects occur infrequently and generally do not interfere with treatment. Adverse reactions tend to occur more frequently at higher doses and in the longer treatment courses used in some early studies.

The most frequent adverse reactions to Clomiphene Citrate include ovarian enlargement (approximately 1 in 7 patients), vasomotor flushes resembling menopausal symptoms which are not usually severe and promptly disappear after treatment is discontinued (approximately 1 in 10 patients), and abdominal discomfort (approximately 1 in 15 patients). Adverse reactions which occur less frequently (approximately 1 in 50 patients or more) include breast tenderness, nausea and vomiting, nervousness, insomnia, and visual disturbances. Other side effects which occur in less than 1 in 100 patients include headache, dizziness and light-headedness, increased urination, depression, fatigue, urticaria and allergic dermatitis, abnormal uterine bleeding, weight gain, ovarian cysts (ovarian enlargement or cysts could, as such, be complicated by adnexal torsion), and reversible hair loss. Thromboembolic events, such as pulmonary embolism, arterial occlusion, and phlebitis, have been reported rarely in patients treated with Clomiphene Citrate. It is not clear what, if any, relationship these events have to Clomiphene Citrate therapy.

When Clomiphene Citrate is administered at the recommended dose, abnormal ovarian enlargement (see *"Precautions"*) is infrequent, although the usual cyclic variation in ovarian size may be exaggerated. Similarly, mid-cycle ovarian pain (mittelschmerz) may be accentuated.

With prolonged or higher dosage, ovarian enlargement and cyst formation (usually luteal) may occur more often, and the luteal phase of the cycle may be prolonged. Patients with polycystic ovarian syndrome may be unusually sensitive to Clomiphene therapy. Rare occurrences of massive ovarian enlargement have been reported, for example, in a patient with polycystic ovarian syndrome whose Clomiphene Citrate therapy consisted of 100 mg daily for 14 days. Since abnromal ovarian enlargement usually regresses spontaneously, most of these patients should be treated conservatively. The Ovarian Hyperstimulation Syndrome has been reported to occur in rare cases in patients receiving Clomiphene Citrate therapy (see *"Warnings"*).

The incidence of visual symptoms (see *"Warnings"* for further recommendations), usually described as "blurring" or spots or flashes (scintillating scotomata), correlates with increasing total dose. Other visual symptoms which may occur include diplopia, phosphenes, photophobia, decreased visual acuity, loss of peripheral vision, and spatial distortion. The symptoms disappear usually within a few days or weeks after Clomiphene Citrate is discontinued. This may be due to intensification and/or prolongation of after-images. Symptoms often appear first, or are accentuated, upon exposure to a more brightly lit environment.

While measured visual acuity generally has not been affected, in one patient taking 200 mg daily, visual blurring developed on the seventh day of treatment and progressed to severe diminution of visual acuity by the tenth day. No other abnormality was coincident, and the visual acuity was normal by the third day after treatment was stopped. Ophthalmologically definable scotomata and electroretinographic retinal function changes have also been reported.

BSP LABORATORY STUDIES
Greater than 5% retention of sulfobromophthalein (BSP) has been reported in approximately 10% to 20% of patients in whom it was measured. Retention was usually minimal but was elevated during prolonged Clomiphene Citrate administration or with apparently unrelated liver disease. In some patients, pre-existing BSP retention decreased even though Clomiphene Citrate therapy was continued. Other liver function tests were usually normal.

OTHER LABORATORY STUDIES
Clomiphene Citrate has not been reported to cause a significant abnormality in hematologic or renal tests, in protein bound iodine, or in serum cholesterol levels.

BIRTH DEFECTS
The following medical events have been reported subsequent to pregnancies following ovulation induction therapy with Clomiphene Citrate: ectopic pregnancy and congenital abnormalities such as syndactyly, polydactyly, congenital heart defects, retinal aplasia, hypospadias, ovarian dysplasia, cleft lip/palate, microencephaly and neural tube defects, including anencephaly. Some medical literature reports have implied an increased occurrence of neural tube defects, while others indicate that an increased incidence over that found in the general population does not exist. One case of a congenital abnormality (adactyly) in an infant exposed to Clomiphene Citrate in utero has been reported.

Of 1,803 births following Clomiphene Citrate administration, 45 infants with birth defects were reported for a cumulative rate of 2.5%.

Six cases of Down's syndrome, one neonatal death with multiple malformations, and one case of each of the following were reported: club-foot, tibial torsion, blocked tear duct, and hemangioma. The other congenital abnormalities were not described. The investigators did not report that these were presumed to be due to therapy. The cumulative rate of congenital abnormalities does not exceed that reported in the general population.

DOSAGE AND ADMINISTRATION

GENERAL CONSIDERATIONS
Physicians experienced in managing gynecologic or endocrine disorders should supervise the work-up and treatment of candidate patients for Clomiphene Citrate therapy. Patients should be chosen for Clomiphene Citrate therapy only after careful diagnostic evaluations (see *"Indications"*). The plan of therapy should be outlined in advance. Impediments to achieving the goal of therapy must be excluded or adequately treated before beginning Clomiphene Citrate.

In determining a starting dose schedule, efficacy must be balanced against potential side effects. For example, the available data so far suggest that ovulation and pregnancy are slightly more attainable with 100 mg/day for 5 days than with 50 mg/day for 5 days. As the dosage is increased, however, ovarian overstimulation and other side effects may be expected to increase. Although the data do not yet establish a relationship between dose level and multiple births, it is reasonable that such a correlation exists on pharmacologic grounds.

For these reasons, treatment of the usual patient should initiate with a 50 mg daily dose for 5 days. The dose may be increased only in those patients who do not respond to the first course (see *"Recommended Dosage"*). Special treatment with lower dosage over shorter duration is particularly recommended if unusual sensitivity to pituitary gonadotropin is suspected, including patients with polycystic ovarian syndrome (see *"Precautions"*).

◆ RATED THERAPEUTICALLY EQUIVALENT; ◇ THERAPEUTIC EQUIVALENCE UNCONFIRMED; ○ UNRATED

RECOMMENDED DOSAGE

The recommended dosage for the first course of Clomiphene Citrate is 50 mg (1 tablet) daily for 5 days. Therapy may be started at any time if the patient has had no recent uterine bleeding. If progestin-induced bleeding is intended, or if spontaneous uterine bleeding occurs prior to therapy, the regimen of 50 mg daily for 5 days should be started on or about the fifth day of the cycle. When ovulation occurs at this dosage, there is no advantage to increasing the dose in subsequent cycles of treatment. If ovulation does not appear to have occurred after the first course of therapy, a second course of 100 mg daily (two 50 mg tablets given as a single daily dose) for 5 days may be started. This course may begin as early as 30 days after the previous one. It is recommended that the patient be examined for pregnancy, ovarian enlargement, or cyst formation between each treatment cycle. Increasing the dosage or duration of therapy beyond 100 mg/day for 5 days should not be undertaken.

The majority of patients who respond do so during the first course of therapy, and 3 courses constitute an adequate therapeutic trial. If ovulatory menses do not occur, the diagnosis should be re-evaluated. Treatment beyond this is not recommended in the patient who does not exhibit evidence of ovulation.

PREGNANCY

Properly timed coitus is very important for good results. For regularity of cyclic ovulatory response, it is also important that each course of Clomiphene Citrate be started on or about the fifth day of the cycle, once ovulation has been established. As with other therapeutic modalities, Clomiphene Citrate therapy follows the rule of diminishing returns, such that the likelihood of conception diminishes with each succeeding course of therapy. If pregnancy has not been achieved after 3 ovulatory responses to Clomiphene Citrate further treatment generally is not recommended. Before starting treatment, patients should be advised of the possibility and potential hazards of multiple pregnancy if conception occurs following Clomiphene Citrate therapy.

LONG-TERM CYCLIC THERAPY—NOT RECOMMENDED

Since the relative safety of long-term cyclic therapy has not yet been demonstrated conclusively, and since the majority of patients will ovulate following 3 courses, long-term cyclic therapy is not recommended.

Protect from light, moisture, and excessive heat. Dispense in well-closed, light resistant container as defined in the USP, with child resistant closure. Store at room temperature (15°-30°C/59°-86°F).

HOW SUPPLIED
TABLETS: 50 MG

AVERAGE UNIT PRICE (AVAILABLE SIZES)		GENERIC A-RATED AVERAGE PRICE (GAAP)	
BRAND	$6.55	30s	$163.78
GENERIC	$5.55		

BRAND/MANUFACTURER	NDC	SIZE	AWP
◆ BRAND			
SEROPHENE: Serono	44087-8090-06	10s	$63.32
	44087-8090-01	30s	$181.44
CLOMID: Marion Merrell Dow	00068-0226-30	30s	$217.92
◆ GENERICS			
Lemmon	00093-0041-03	10s	$57.32
Rugby	00536-3109-07	30s	$163.29
Lemmon	00093-0041-56	30s	$164.27

Clomipramine Hydrochloride

DESCRIPTION

Clomipramine Hydrochloride is an antiobsessional drug that belongs to the class (dibenzazepine) of pharmacologic agents known as tricyclic antidepressants. Clomipramine Hydrochloride is available as capsules of 25 50 and 75 mg for oral administration.

Clomipramine Hydrochloride is 3-chloro-5-[3-(dimethyl-amino)propyl]- 10,11-dihydro-5H-dibenz[b,f]azepine monohydrochloride.

Clomipramine Hydrochloride is a white to off-white crystalline powder. It is freely soluble in water, in methanol, and in methylene chloride, and insoluble in ethyl ether and in hexane. Its molecular weight is 351.3.

Following is its chemical structure:

$CH_2CH_2CH_2N(CH_3)_2$ · HCl

CLINICAL PHARMACOLOGY

PHARMACODYNAMICS

Clomipramine Hydrochloride is presumed to influence obsessive and compulsive behaviors through its effects on serotonergic neuronal transmission. The actual neurochemical mechanism is unknown, but Clomipramine Hydrochloride's capacity to inhibit the reuptake of serotonin (5-HT) is thought to be important.

PHARMACOKINETICS

Absorption/Bioavailability: Clomipramine Hydrochloride from capsules is as bioavailable as Clomipramine Hydrochloride from a solution. The bioavailability of Clomipramine Hydrochloride from capsules is not significantly affected by food. In a dose proportionality study involving multiple Clomipramine Hydrochloride doses, steady-state plasma concentrations (C_{ss}) and area-under-plasma-concentration-time curves (AUC) of Clomipramine Hydrochloride and Clomipramine Hydrochloride major active metabolite, desmethylclomipramine were not proportional to dose over the ranges evaluated, i.e., between 25-100 mg/day and between 25-150 mg/day, although C_{ss} and AUC are approximately linearly related to dose between 100-150 mg/day. The relationship between dose and Clomipramine Hydrochloride/desmethylclomipramine concentrations at higher daily doses has not been systematically assessed, but if there is significant dose dependency at doses above 150 mg/day, there is the potential for dramatically higher C_{ss} and AUC even for patients dosed within the recommended range. This may pose a potential risk to some patients (see *"Warnings and Precautions, Drug Interactions"*).

After a single 50-mg oral dose, maximum plasma concentrations of Clomipramine Hydrochloride occur within 2-6 hours (mean, 4.7 hr) and range from 56 ng/ml to 154 ng/ml (mean, 92 ng/ml). After multiple daily doses of 150 mg of Clomipramine Hydrochloride, steady-state maximum plasma concentrations range from 94 ng/ml to 339 ng/ml (mean, 218 ng/ml) for Clomipramine Hydrochloride and from 134 ng/ml to 532 ng/ml (mean, 274 ng/ml) for DM1. No pharmacokinetic information is available for doses ranging from 150 mg/day to 250 mg/day, the maximum recommended daily dose.

Distribution: Clomipramine Hydrochloride distributes into cerebrospinal fluid (CSF) and brain and into breast milk. desmethylclomipramine also distributes into CSF, with a mean CSF/plasma ratio of 2.6. The protein binding of Clomipramine Hydrochloride is approximately 97%, principally to albumin, and is independent of Clomipramine Hydrochloride concentration. The interaction between Clomipramine Hydrochloride and other highly protein-bound drugs has not been fully evaulated, but may be important (see *"Precautions, Drug Interactions"*).

Metabolism: Clomipramine Hydrochloride is extensively biotransformed to desmethylclomipramine and other metabolites and their glucuronide conjugates. Desmethylclomipramine is pharmacologically active, but its effects on OCD behaviors are unknown. These metabolites are excreted in urine and feces, following biliary elimination. After a 25-mg radiolabeled dose of Clomipramine Hydrochloride in two subjects, 60% and 51%, respectively, of the dose were recovered in the urine and 32% and 24%, respectively, in feces. In the same study, the combined urinary recoveries of Clomipramine Hydrochloride and desmethylchlomipramine were only about 0.8-1.3% of the dose administered. Clomipramine Hydrochloride does not induce drug-metabolizing enzymes, as measured by antipyrine half-life.

Elimination: Evidence that the C_{ss} and AUC for Clomipramine Hydrochloride and desmethylchlomipramine may increase disproportionately with increasing oral doses suggests that the metabolism of Clomipramine Hydrochloride and desmethylchlomipramine may be capacity limited. This fact must be considered in assessing the estimates of the pharmacokinetic parameters presented below, as these were obtained in individuals exposed to doses of 150 mg. If the pharmacokinetics of Clomipramine Hydrochloride and desmethylchlomipramine are nonlinear at doses above 150 mg, their elimination half-lives may be considerably lengthened at doses near the upper end of the recommended dosing range (i.e., 200 mg/day to 250 mg/day). Consequently, Clomipramine Hydrochloride and desmethylchlomipramine may accumulate, and this accumulation may increase the incidence of any dose- or plasma-concentration-dependent adverse reactions, in particular seizures (see *"Warnings"*).

After a 150-mg dose, the half-life of Clomipramine Hydrochloride ranges from 19 hours to 37 hours (mean, 32 hr) and that of desmethylchlomipramine ranges from 54 hours to 77 hours (mean, 69 hr). Steady-state levels after multiple dosing are typically reached within 7-14 days for Clomipramine Hydrochloride. Plasma concentrations of the metabolite exceed the parent drug on multiple dosing. After multiple dosing with 150 mg/day, the accumulation factor for Clomipramine Hydrochloride is approximately 2.5 and for desmethylchlomipramine is 4.6. Importantly, it may take two weeks or longer to achieve this extent of accumulation at constant dosing because of the relatively long elimination half-lives of Clomipramine Hydrochloride and desmethylchlomipramine (see *"Dosage and Administration"*). The effects of hepatic and renal impairment on the disposition of Clomipramine Hydrochloride have not been determined.

Interactions: Coadministration of haloperidol with Clomipramine Hydrochloride increases plasma concentrations of Clomipramine Hydrochloride. Coadministration of Clomipramine Hydrochloride with phenobarbital increases plasma concentrations of phenobarbital (see *"Precautions, Drug Interactions"*). Younger subjects (18-40 years of age) tolerated Clomipramine Hydrochloride better and had significantly lower steady-state plasma concentrations, compared with subjects over 65 years of age. Children under 15 years of age had significantly lower plasma concentration/dose ratios, compared with adults. Plasma concentrations of Clomipramine Hydrochloride were significantly lower in smokers than in nonsmokers.

INDICATIONS AND USAGE

Clomipramine Hydrochloride is indicated for the treatment of obsessions and compulsions in patients with Obsessive-Compulsive Disorder (OCD). The obsessions or compulsions must cause marked distress, be time-consuming, or significantly interfere with social or occupational functioning, in order to meet the DSM-III-R (circa 1989) diagnosis of OCD.

Obsessions are recurrent, persistent ideas, thoughts, images, or impulses that are ego-dystonic. Compulsions are repetitive, purposeful, and intentional behaviors performed in response to an obsession or in a stereotyped fashion, and are recognized by the person as excessive or unreasonable.

The effectiveness of Clomipramine Hydrochloride for the treatment of OCD was demonstrated in multicenter, placebo-controlled, parallel-group studies, including two 10-week studies in adults and one 8-week study in children and adolescents 10-17 years of age. Patients in all studies had moderate-to-severe OCD (DSM-III), with mean baseline ratings on the Yale-Brown Obsessive Compulsive Scale (YBOCS) ranging from 26 to 28 and a mean baseline rating of 10 on the NIMH Clinical Global Obsessive Compulsive Scale (NIMH-OC). Patients taking Clomipramine Hydrochloride experienced a mean reduction of approximately 10 on the YBOCS, representing an average improvement on this scale of 35% to 42% among adults and 37% among children and adolescents. Clomipramine Hydrochloride treated patients experienced a 3.5 unit decrement on the NIMH-OC. Patients on placebo showed no important clinical response on either scale. The maximum dose was 250 mg/day for most adults and 3 mg/kg/day (up to 200 mg) for all children and adolscents. The effectiveness of Clomipramine Hydrochloride for long-term use (i.e., for more than 10 weeks) has not been systematically evaluated in placebo-controlled trials. The physician who elects to use Clomipramine Hydrochloride for extended periods should periodically reevaluate the long-term usefulness of the drug for the individual patient (see *"Dosage and Administration"*).

UNLABELED USES
Clomipramine is used alone or as an adjunct in the treatment of agoraphobia, panic anxiety, and depression. It is also used in diabetic neuropathy and myotonic dystrophy, and is prescribed in the management of premenstrual syndrome, retrograde ejaculation, trichotillomania, and onychophagia.

CONTRAINDICATIONS
Clomipramine Hydrochloride is contraindicated in patients with a history of hypersensitivity to Clomipramine Hydrochloride or other tricyclic antidepressants.

Clomipramine Hydrochloride should not be given in combination, or within 14 days before or after treatment, with a monoamine oxidase (MAO) inhibitor. Hyperpyretic crisis, seizures, coma, and death have been reported in patients receiving such combinations.

Clomipramine Hydrochloride is contraindicated during the acute recovery period after a myocardial infarction.

WARNINGS
SEIZURES
During premarket evaluation seizure was identified as the most significant risk of Clomipramine Hydrochloride use.

The observed cumulative incidence of seizures among patients exposed to Clomipramine Hydrochloride at doses up to 300 mg/day was 0.64% at 90 days, 1.12% at 180 days, and 1.45% at 365 days. The cumulative rates correct the crude rate of 0.7% (25 of the 3519 patients) for the variable duration of exposure in clinical trials.

Although dose appears to be a predictor of seizures, there is a confounding of dose and duration of exposure, making it difficult to assess independently the effect of either factor alone. The ability to predict the occurrence of seizures in subjects exposed to doses of Clomipramine Hydrochloride greater than 250 mg is limited, given that the plasma concentration of Clomipramine Hydrochloride may be dose-dependent and may vary among subjects given the same dose. Nevertheless, prescribers are advised to limit the daily dose to a maximum of 250 mg in adults and 3 mg/kg (or 200 mg) in children and adolescents (See *"Dosage And Administration"*).

Caution should be used in administering Clomipramine Hydrochloride to patients with a history of seizures or other predisposing factors, e.g., brain damage of varying etiology, alcoholism, and concomitant use with other drugs that lower the seizure threshold.

Rare reports of fatalities in association with seizures have been reported by foreign post-marketing surveillance, but not in U.S. clinical trials. In some of these cases, Clomipramine Hydrochloride had been administered with other epileptogenic agents; in others, the patients involved had possibly predisposing medical conditions. Thus a causal association between Clomipramine Hydrochloride treatment and these fatalities has not been established.

Physicians should discuss with patients the risk of taking Clomipramine Hydrochloride while engaging in activities in which sudden loss of consciousness could result in serious injury to the patient or others, e.g., the operation of complex machinery, driving, swimming, climbing.

PRECAUTIONS
GENERAL
Suicide: Since depression is a commonly associated feature of OCD, the risk of suicide must be considered. Prescriptions for Clomipramine Hydrochloride should be written for the smallest quantity of capsules consistent with good patient management, in order to reduce the risk of overdose.

Cardiovascular Effects: Modest orthostatic decreases in blood pressure and modest tachycardia were each seen in approximately 20% of patients taking Clomipramine Hydrochloride in clinical trials; but patients were frequently asymptomatic. Among approximately 1400 patients treated with Clomipramine Hydrochloride in the premarketing experience who had ECGs, 1.5% developed abnormalities during treatment, compared with 3.1% of patients receiving active control drugs and 0.7% of patients receiving placebo. The most common ECG changes were PVCs, ST-T wave changes, and intraventricular conduction abnormalities. These changes were rarely associated with significant clinical

symptoms. Nevertheless, caution is necessary in treating patients with known cardiovascular disease, and gradual dose titration is recommended.

Psychosis, Confusion, and Other Neuropsychiatric Phenomena: Patients treated with Anafranil have been reported to show a variety of neuropsychiatric signs and symptoms including delusions, hallucinations, psychotic episodes, confusion, and paranoia. Because of the uncontrolled nature of many of the studies, it is impossible to provide a precise estimate of the extent of risk imposed by treatment with Clomipramine Hydrochloride. As with tricyclic antidepressants to which it is closely related, Clomipramine Hydrochloride may precipitate an acute psychotic episode in patients with unrecognized schizophrenia.

Mania/Hypomania: During premarketing testing of Clomipramine Hydrochloride in patients with affective disorder, hypomania or mania was precipitated in several patients. Activation of mania or hypomania has also been reported in a small proportion of patients with affective disorder treated with marketed tricyclic antidepressants, which are closely related to Clomipramine Hydrochloride.

Hepatic Changes: During premarketing testing, Clomipramine Hydrochloride was occasionally associated with elevations in SGOT and SGPT (pooled incidence of approximately 1% and 3%, respectively) of potential clinical importance (i.e., values greater than 3 times the upper limit of normal). In the vast majority of instances these enzyme increases were not associated with other clinical findings suggestive of hepatic injury; moreover, none were jaundiced. Rare reports of more severe liver injury, some fatal, have been recorded in foreign post-marketing experience. Caution is indicated in treating patients with known liver disease, and periodic monitoring of hepatic enzyme levels is recommended in such patients.

Hematologic Changes: Although no instances of severe hematologic toxicity were seen in the premarketing experience with Clomipramine Hydrochloride, there have been post-marketing reports of leukopenia, agranulocytosis, thrombocytopenia, anemia, and pancytopenia in association with Clomipramine Hydrochloride use. As is the case with tricyclic antidepressants to which Clomipramine Hydrochloride is closely related, leukocyte and differential blood counts should be obtained in patients who develop fever and sore throat during treatment with Clomipramine Hydrochloride.

Central Nervous System: More than 30 cases of hyperthermia have been recorded by nondomestic post-marketing surveillance systems. Most cases occurred when Clomipramine Hydrochloride was used in combination with other drugs when Clomipramine Hydrochloride and a neuroleptic were used concomitantly, the cases were sometimes considered to be examples of a neuroleptic malignant syndrome.

Sexual Dysfunction: The rate of sexual dysfunction in male patients with OCD who were treated with Clomipramine Hydrochloride in the premarketing experience was markedly increased compared with placebo controls (i.e., 42% experienced ejaculatory failure and 20% experienced impotence, compared with 2.0% and 2.6%, respectively, in the placebo group). Approximately 85% of males with sexual dysfunction chose to continue treatment.

Weight Changes: In controlled studies of OCD, weight gain was reported in 18% of patients receiving Clomipramine Hydrochloride, compared with 1% of patients receiving placebo. In these studies, 28% of patients receiving Clomipramine Hydrochloride had a weight gain of at least 7% of their initial body weight, compared with 4% of patients receiving placebo. Several patients had weight gains in excess of 25% of their initial body weight. Conversely, 5% of patients receiving Clomipramine Hydrochloride and 1% receiving placebo had weight losses of at least 7% of their initial body weight.

Electroconvulsive Therapy: As with closely related tricyclic antidepressants, concurrent administration of Clomipramine Hydrochloride with electroconvulsive therapy may increase the risks; such treatment should be limited to those patients for whom it is essential, since there is limited clinical experience.

Surgery: Prior to elective surgery with general anesthetics, therapy with Chlomipramine Hydrochloride should be discontinued for as long as is clinically feasible, and the anesthetist should be advised.

Use in Concomitant Illness: As with closely related tricyclic antidepressants, Clomipramine Hydrochloride should be used with caution in the following:
1. Hyperthyroid patients or patients receiving thyroid medication, because of the possibility of cardiac toxicity.
2. Patients with increased intraocular pressure, a history of narrow-angle glaucoma, or urinary retention, because of the anticholinergic properties of the drug.
3. Patients with tumors of the adrenal medulla (e.g., pheochromocytoma, neuroblastoma) in whom the drug may provoke hypertensive crises.
4. Patients with significantly impaired renal function.

Withdrawal Symptoms: A variety of withdrawal symptoms have been reported in association with abrupt discontinuation of Clomipramine Hydrochloride, including dizziness, nausea, vomiting, headache, malaise, sleep disturbance, hyperthermia, and irritability. In addition, such patients may experience a worsening of psychiatric status. While the withdrawal effects of Clomipramine Hydrochloride have not been systematically evaluated in controlled trials, they are well known with closely related tricyclic antidepressants, and it is recommended that the dosage be tapered gradually and the patient monitored carefully during discontinuation (see *"Drug Abuse and Dependence"*).

INFORMATION FOR PATIENTS
Physicians are advised to discuss the following issues with patients for whom they prescribed Clomipramine Hydrochloride:

1. The risk of seizure (see *"Warnings"*);

2. The relatively high incidence of sexual dysfunction among males (see *"Precautions, Sexual Dysfunction"*);

3. Since Clomipramine Hydrochloride may impair the mental and/or physical abilities required for the performance of complex tasks, and since Clomipramine Hydrochloride is associated with a risk of seizures, patients should be cautioned about the performance of complex and hazardous tasks (see *"Warnings"*);

4. Patients should be cautioned about using alcohol, barbiturates, or other CNS depressants concurrently, since Clomipramine Hydrochloride may exaggerate their response to these drugs;

5. Patients should notify their physician if they become pregnant or intend to become pregnant during therapy;

6. Patients should notify their physician if they are breast feeding.

DRUG INTERACTIONS
The risks of using Clomipramine Hydrochloride in combination with other drugs have not been systematically evaluated. Given the primary CNS effects of Clomipramine Hydrochloride, caution is advised in using it concomitantly with other CNS-active drugs (see *"Information for Patients"*). Clomipramine Hydrochloride should *not be* used with MAO inhibitors (see *"Contraindications"*).

Close supervision and careful adjustment of dosage are required when Clomipramine Hydrochloride is administered with anticholinergic or sympathomimetic drugs.

Several tricyclic antidepressants have been reported to block the pharmacologic effects of guanethidine, clonidine, or similar agents, and such an effect may be anticipated with Clomipramine Hydrochloride because of its structural similarity to other tricyclic antidepressants.

The plasma concentration of Clomipramine Hydrochloride has been reported to be increased by the concomitant administration of haloperidol; plasma levels of several closely related tricyclic antidepressants have been reported to be increased by the concomitant administration of methylphenidate or hepatic enzyme inhibitors (e.g., cimetidine, fluoxetine) and decreased by the concomitant administration of hepatic enzyme inducers (e.g., barbiturates, phenytoin), and such an effect may be anticipated with Clomipramine Hydrochloride as well. Administration of Clomipramine Hydrochloride has been reported to increase the plasma levels of phenobarbital, if given concomitantly (see *"Clinical Pharmacology, Interactions"*).

Because Clomipramine Hydrochloride is highly bound to serum protein, the administration of Clomipramine Hydrochloride to patients taking other drugs that are highly bound to protein (e.g., warfarin, digoxin) may cause an increase in plasma concentrations of these drugs, potentially resulting in adverse effects. Conversely, adverse effects may result from displacement of protein-bound Clomipramine Hydrochloride by other highly bound drugs (see *"Clinical Pharmacology, Distribution"*).

CARCINOGENESIS, MUTAGENESIS, IMPAIRMENT OF FERTILITY
In a 2-year bioassay, no clear evidence of carcinogenicity was found in rats given doses 20 times the maximum daily human dose. Three out of 235 treated rats had a rare tumor (hemangioendothelioma); it is unknown if these neoplasms are compound related.

In reproduction studies, no effects on fertility were found in rats given doses approximately 5 times the maximum daily human dose.

PREGNANCY CATEGORY C
No teratogenic effects were observed in studies performed in rats and mice at doses up to 20 times the maximum daily human dose. Slight nonspecific fetotoxic effects were seen in the offspring of pregnant mice given doses 10 times the maximum daily human dose. Slight nonspecific embryotoxicity was observed in rats given doses 5-10 times the maximum daily human dose.

There are no adequate or well-controlled studies in pregnant women. Withdrawal symptoms, including jitteriness, tremor, and seizures, have been reported in neonates whose mothers had taken Clomipramine Hydrochloride until delivery. Clomipramine Hydrochloride should be used during pregnancy only if the potential benefit justifies the potential risk to the fetus.

NURSING MOTHERS
Clomipramine Hydrochloride has been found in human milk. Because of the potential for adverse reactions, a decision should be made whether to discontinue nursing or to discontinue the drug, taking into account the importance of the drug to the mother.

PEDIATRIC USE
In a controlled clinical trial in children and adolescents (10-17 years of age), 46 outpatients received Clomipramine Hydrochloride for up to 8 weeks. In addition, 150 adolescent patients have received Clomipramine Hydrochloride in open-label protocols for periods of several months to several years. Of the 196 adolescents studied, 50 were 13 years of age or less and 146 were 14-17 years of age. While the adverse reaction profile in this age group (see *"Adverse Reactions"*) is similar to that in adults, it is unknown what, if any, effects long-term treatment with Clomipramine Hydrochloride may have on the growth and development of children. The safety and effectiveness in children below the age of 10 have not been established. Therefore, specific recommendations cannot be made for the use of Clomipramine Hydrochloride in children under the age of 10.

USE IN ELDERLY
Clomipramine Hydrochloride has not been systematically studied in older patients; but 152 patients at least 60 years of age participating in U.S. clinical trials received Clomipramine Hydrochloride for periods of several months to several years. No unusual age-related adverse events have been identified in this elderly population, but these data are insufficient to rule out possible age-related differences, particularly in elderly patients who have concomitant systemic illnesses or who are receiving other drugs concomitantly.

ADVERSE REACTIONS
COMMONLY OBSERVED
The most commonly observed adverse events associated with the use of Clomipramine Hydrochloride and not seen at an equivalent incidence among placebo-treated patients were gastrointestinal complaints, including dry mouth, constipation, nausea, dyspepsia, and anorexia; nervous system complaints, including somnolence, tremor, dizziness, nervousness, and myoclonus; genitourinary complaints, including changed libido; ejaculatory failure, impotence, and micturition disorder; and other miscellaneous complaints, including fatigue, sweating, increased appetite, weight gain, and visual changes.

LEADING TO DISCONTINUATION OF TREATMENT
Approximately 20% of 3616 patients who received Clomipramine Hydrochloride in U.S. premarketing clinical trials discontinued treatment because of an adverse event. Approximately one-half of the patients who discontinued (9% of the total) had multiple complaints, none of which could be classified as primary. Where a primary reason for discontinuation could be identified, most patients discontinued because of nervous system complaints (5.4%), primarily somnolence. The second-most-frequent reason for discontinuation was digestive system complaints (1.3%), primarily vomiting and nausea.

INCIDENCE IN CONTROLLED CLINICAL TRIALS
The following table enumerates adverse events that occurred at an incidence of 1% or greater among patients with OCD who received Clomipramine Hydrochloride in adult or pediatric placebo-controlled clinical trials. The frequencies were obtained from pooled data of clinical trials involving either adults receiving Clomipramine Hydrochloride (N = 322) or placebo (N = 319) or children treated with Clomipramine Hydrochloride (N = 46) or placebo (N = 44). The prescriber should be aware that these figures cannot be used to predict the incidence of side effects in the course of usual medical practice, in which patient characteristics and other factors differ from those which prevailed in the clinical trials. Similarly, the cited frequencies cannot be compared with figures obtained from other clinical investigations involving different treatment, uses, and investigators. The cited figures, however, provide the physician with a basis for estimating the relative contribution of drug and nondrug factors to the incidence of side effects in the populations studied. (See related tables.)

OTHER EVENTS OBSERVED DURING THE PREMARKETING EVALUATION OF CLOMIPRAMINE HYDROCHLORIDE
During clinical testing in the U.S., multiple doses of Clomipramine Hydrochloride were administered to approximately 3600 subjects. Untoward events associated with this exposure were recorded by clinical investigators using terminology of their own choosing. Consequently, it is not possible to provide a meaningful estimate of the proportion of individuals experiencing adverse events without first grouping similar types of untoward events into a smaller number of standardized event categories.

In the tabulations that follow, a modified World Health Organization dictionary of terminology has been used to classify reported adverse events. The frequencies presented, therefore, represent the proportion of the 3525 individuals exposed to Clomipramine Hydrochloride who experienced an event of the type cited on at least one occasion while receiving Clomipramine Hydrochloride. All events are included except those already listed in the previous table, those reported in terms so general as to be uninformative, and those in which an association with the drug was remote. It is important to emphasize that although the events reported occurred during treatment with Clomipramine Hydrochloride, they were not necessarily caused by it.

Events are further categorized by body system and listed in order of decreasing frequency according to the following definitions: frequent adverse events are those occurring on one or more occasions in at least 1/100 patients; infrequent adverse events are those occurring in 1/100 to 1/1000 patients; rare events are those occurring in less than 1/1000 patients.

Body as a Whole: Infrequent—general edema, increased susceptibility to infection, malaise. *Rare*—dependent edema, withdrawal syndrome.

Cardiovascular System: Infrequent—abnormal ECG, arrhythmia, bradycardia, cardiac arrest, extrasystoles, pallor. *Rare*—aneurysm, atrial flutter, bundle branch block, cardiac failure, cerebral hemorrhage, heart block, myocardial infarction, myocardial ischemia, peripheral ischemia, thrombophlebitis, vasospasm, ventricular tachycardia.

Digestive System: Infrequent—abnormal hepatic function, blood in stool, colitis, duodenitis, gastric ulcer, gastritis, gastroesophageal reflux, gingivitis, glossitis, hemorrhoids, hepatitis, increased saliva, irritable bowel syndrome, peptic ulcer, rectal hemorrhage, tongue ulceration, tooth caries. *Rare*—cheilitis, chronic enteritis, discolored feces, gastric dilatation, gingival bleeding, hiccup, intestinal obstruction, oral/pharyngeal edema, paralytic ileus, salivary gland enlargement.

Endocrine System: Infrequent—hypothyroidism. *Rare*—goiter, gynecomastia, hyperthyroidism.

Hemic and Lymphatic System: Infrequent—lymphadenopathy. *Rare*—leukemoid reaction, lymphoma-like disorder, marrow depression.

Metabolic and Nutritional Disorder: Infrequent—dehydration, diabetes mellitus, gout, hypercholesterolemia, hyperglycemia, hyperuricemia, hypokalemia. *Rare*—fat intolerance, glycosuria.

Musculoskeletal System: Infrequent—arthrosis. *Rare*—dystonia, exostosis, lupus erythematosus rash, bruising, myopathy, myositis, polyarteritis nodosa, torticollis.

Nervous System: Frequent—abnormal thinking, vertigo. *Infrequent*—abnormal coordination, abnormal EEG, abnormal gait, apathy, ataxia, coma, convulsions, delirium, delusion, dyskinesia, dysphonia, encephalopathy, euphoria, extrapyramidal disorder, hallucinations, hostility, hyperkinesia, hypnagogic hallucinations, hypokinesia, leg cramps, manic reaction, neuralgia, paranoia, phobic disorder, psychosis, sensory distubance, somnambulism, stimulation, suicidal ideation, suicide attempt, teeth-grinding. *Rare*—anticholinergic syndrome, aphasia, apraxia, catalepsy, cholinergic syndrome, choreoathetosis, generalized spasm, hemiparesis, hyperesthesia, hyperreflexia, hypoesthesia, illusion, impaired impulse control, indecisiveness, mutism, neuropathy, nystagmus, oculogyric crisis, oculomotor nerve paralysis, schizophrenic reaction, stupor, suicide.

Respiratory System: Infrequent—bronchitis, hyperventilation, increased sputum, pneumonia. *Rare*—cyanosis, hemoptysis, hypoventilation, laryngismus.

Skin and Appendages: Infrequent—alopecia, cellulitis, cyst, eczema, erythematous rash, genital pruritus, maculopapular rash, photosensitivity reaction, psoriasis, pustular rash, skin discoloration. *Rare*—chloasma, folliculitis, hypertrichosis, piloerection, seborrhea, skin hypertrophy, skin ulceration.

Special Senses: Infrequent—abnormal accommodation, deafness, diplopia, earache, eye pain, foreign body sensation, hyperacusis, parosmia, photophobia, scleritis, taste loss. *Rare*—blepharitis, chromatopsia, conjunctival hemorrhage, exophthalmos, glaucoma, keratitis, labyrinth disorder, night blindness, retinal disorder, strabismus, visual field defect.

Urogenital System: Infrequent—endometriosis, epididymitis, hematuria, nocturia, oliguria, ovarian cyst, perineal pain, polyuria, prostatic disorder, renal calculus, renal pain, urethral disorder, urinary incontinence, uterine hemorrhage, vaginal hemorrhage. *Rare*—albuminuria, anorgasmy, breast engorgement, breast fibroadenosis, cervical dysplasia, endometrial hyperplasia, premature ejaculation, pyelonephritis, pyuria renal cyst, uterine inflammation, vulvar disorder.

DRUG ABUSE AND DEPENDENCE
Clomipramine Hydrochloride has not been systematically studied in animals or humans for its potential for abuse, tolerance, or physical dependence. While a variety of withdrawal symptoms have been described in association with Clomipramine Hydrochloride discontinuation (see *"Precautions, Withdrawal Symptoms"*), there is no evidence for drug-seeking behavior, except for a single report of potential Clomipramine Hydrochloride abuse by a patient with a history of dependence on codeine, benzodiazepines, and multiple psychoactive drugs. The patient received Clomipramine Hydrochloride for depression and panic attacks and appeared to become dependent after hospital discharge.

Despite the lack of evidence suggesting an abuse liability for Clomipramine Hydrochloride in foreign marketing, it is not possible to predict the extent to which Clomipramine Hydrochloride might be misused or abused once marketed in the U.S. Consequently, physicians should carefully evaluate patients for a history of drug abuse and follow such patients closely.

OVERDOSAGE
HUMAN EXPERIENCE
In U.S. clinical trials, 2 deaths occurred in 12 reported cases of acute overdosage with Clomipramine Hydrochloride either alone or in combination with other drugs. One death involved a patient suspected of ingesting a dose of 7000 mg. The second death involved a patient suspected of ingesting a dose of 5750 mg. The 10 nonfatal cases involved doses of up to 5000 mg, accompanied by plasma levels of up to 1010 ng/ml. All 10 patients completely recovered. Among reports from other countries of Clomipramine Hydrochloride overdose, the lowest dose associated with a fatality was 750 mg. Based upon post-marketing reports in the United Kingdom, Clomipramine Hydrochloride lethality in overdose is considered to be similar to that reported for closely related tricyclic compounds marketed as antidepressants.

INCIDENCE OF TREATMENT-EMERGENT ADVERSE EXPERIENCE IN PLACEBO-CONTROLLED CLINICAL TRIALS

Body System/ Adverse Event*	(Percentage of Patients Reporting Event)			
	Adults		Children and Adolescents	
	Clomipramine Hydrochloride (N = 322)	Placebo (N = 319)	Clomipramine Hydrochloride (N = 46)	(Placebo (N = 44)
Nervous System				
Somnolence	54	16	46	11
Tremor	54	2	33	2
Dizziness	54	14	41	14
Headache	52	41	28	34
Insomnia	25	15	11	7
Libido change	21	3	-	-
Nervousness	18	2	4	2
Myoclonus	13	-	2	-
Increased appetite	11	2	-	2
Paresthesia	9	3	2	2
Memory impairment	9	1	7	2
Anxiety	9	4	2	-
Twitching	7	1	4	5
Impaired concentration	5	2	-	-
Depression	5	1	-	-
Hypertonia	4	1	-	-
Sleep disorder	4	-	9	5
Psychosomatic disorder	3	-	-	-
Yawning	3	-	-	-
Confusion	3	-	2	-
Speech disorder	3	-	-	-
Abnormal dreaming	3	-	-	2
Agitation	3	-	-	-
Migraine	3	-	-	-
Depersonalization	2	-	-	-
Irritability	2	2	-	-
Emotional lability	2	-	-	2
Panic reaction	1	-	2	-
Aggressive reaction	-	-	2	-
Paresis	-	-	2	-
Skin and Appendages				
Increased sweating	29	3	9	-
Rash	8	1	4	2
Pruritis	6	-	2	2
Dermatitis	2	-	-	2
Acne	2	2	-	5
Dry Skin	2	-	-	5
Urticaria	1	-	-	-
Abnormal skin odor	-	-	2	-

◆ RATED THERAPEUTICALLY EQUIVALENT; ◇ THERAPEUTIC EQUIVALENCE UNCONFIRMED; ○ UNRATED

SIGNS AND SYMPTOMS

Signs and symptoms vary in severity depending upon factors such as the amount of drug absorbed, the age of the patient, and the time elapsed since drug ingestion. Blood and urine levels of Clomipramine Hydrochloride may not reflect the severity of poisoning: they have chiefly a qualitative rather than quantitative value, and they are unreliable indicators in the clinical management of the patient. The first signs and symptoms of poisoning with tricyclic antidepressants are generally severe anticholinergic reactions. CNS abnormalities may include drowsiness, stupor, coma, ataxia, restlessness, agitation, delirium, severe perspiration, hyperactive reflexes, muscle rigidity, athetoid and choreiform movements, and convulsions. Cardiac abnormalities may include arrhythmia, tachycardia, ECG evidence of impaired conduction, and signs of congestive heart failure, and in very rare cases, cardiac arrest. Respiratory depression, cyanosis, hypotension, shock, vomiting, hyperpyrexia, mydriasis, oliguria or anuria, and diaphoresis may also be present.

TREATMENT

The recommended treatment for tricyclic overdose may change periodically. Therefore, it is recommended that the physician contact a poison control center for current information on treatment.

Because CNS involvement, respiratory depression, and cardiac arrhythmia can occur suddenly, hospitalization and close observation may be necessary, even when the amount ingested is thought to be small or the initial degree of intoxication appears slight or moderate. All patients with ECG abnormalities should have continuous cardiac monitoring and be closely observed until well after the cardiac status has returned to normal; relapses may occur after apparent recovery.

In the alert patient, the stomach should be emptied promptly by lavage. In the obtunded patient, the airway should be secured with a cuffed endotracheal tube before beginning lavage (do not induce emesis). Instillation of activated charocal slurry may help reduce absorption of Clomipramine Hydrochloride.

External stimulation should be minimized to reduce the tendency for convulsions. If anticonvulsants are necessary, diazepam and phenytoin may be useful. Adequate respiratory exchange should be maintained, including intubation and artificial respiration, if necessary. Respiratory stimulants should not be used.

In severe hypotension or shock, the patient should be placed in an appropriate position and given a plasma expander, and, if necessary, a vasopressor agent by intravenous drip. The use of corticosteroids in shock is controversial and may be contraindicated in cases of overdosage with tricyclic antidepressants. Digitalis may increase conduction abnormalities and further irritate an already sensitized myocardium. If congestive heart failure necessitates rapid digitalization, particular care must be exercised. Hyperpyrexia should be controlled by whatever external means are available, including ice packs and cooling sponge baths, if necessary. Hemodialysis, peritoneal dialysis, exchange transfusions, and forced diuresis have generally been reported as ineffective because of the rapid fixation of Clomipramine Hydrochloride tissues.

The slow intravenous administration of physostigmine salicylate has been used as a last resort to reverse severe CNS anticholinergic manifestations of overdosage with tricyclic antidepressants; however, it should not be used routinely, since it may induce seizures and cholinergic crises.

DOSAGE AND ADMINISTRATION

The treatment regimens described below are based on those used in controlled clinical trials of Clomipramine Hydrochloride in 520 adults, and 91 children and adolescents with OCD. During initial titration, Clomipramine Hydrochloride should be given in divided doses with meals to reduce gastrointestinal side effects. The goal of this initial titration phase is to minimize side effects by permitting tolerance to side effects to develop or allowing the patient time to adapt if tolerance does not develop.

Because both Clomipramine Hydrochloride and its active metabolite desmethylclomipramine have long elimination half-lives, the prescriber should take into consideration the fact that steady-state plasma levels may not be achieved

INCIDENCE OF TREATMENT-EMERGENT ADVERSE EXPERIENCE IN PLACEBO-CONTROLLED CLINICAL TRIALS

Body System/ Adverse Event*	Adults		Children and Adolescents	
	Clomipramine Hydrochloride (N = 322)	Placebo (N = 319)	Clomipramine Hydrochloride (N = 46)	Placebo (N = 44)
Digestive System				
Dry mouth	84	17	63	16
Constipation	47	11	22	9
Nausea	33	14	9	11
Dyspepsia	22	10	13	2
Diarrhea	13	9	7	5
Anorexia	12	-	22	2
Abdominal pain	11	9	13	16
Vomiting	7	2	7	-
Flatulence	6	3	-	2
Tooth disorder	5	-	-	-
Gastrointestinal disorder	2	-	-	2
Dysphagia	2	-	-	-
Esophagitis	1	-	-	-
Eructation	-	-	2	2
Ulcerative stomatitis	-	-	2	-
Body as a Whole				
Fatigue	39	18	35	9
Weight increase	18	1	2	-
Flushing	8	-	7	-
Hot flushes	5	-	2	-
Chest pain	4	4	7	-
Fever	4	-	2	7
Allergy	3	3	7	5
Pain	3	2	4	2
Local edema	2	4	-	-
Chills	2	1	-	-
Weight decrease	-	-	7	-
Otitis media	-	-	4	5
Asthenia	-	-	2	-
Halitosis	-	-	2	-
Cardiovascular System				
Postural hypotension	6	-	4	-
Palpitation	4	2	4	-
Tachycardia	4	-	2	-
Syncope	-	-	2	-
Respiratory System				
Pharyngitis	14	9	-	5
Rhinitis	12	10	7	9
Sinusitis	6	4	2	5
Coughing	6	6	4	5
Bronchospasm	2	-	7	2
Epistaxis	2	-	-	2
Dyspnea	-	-	2	-
Laryngitis	-	1	2	-

➤ SHOWN IN PRODUCT IDENTIFICATION GUIDE

until 2-3 weeks after dosage change (see "Clinical Pharmacology"). Therefore, after initial titration, it may be appropriate to wait 2-3 weeks between further dosage adjustments.

INITIAL TREATMENT/DOSE ADJUSTMENT (ADULTS)
Treatment with Clomipramine Hydrochloride should be initiated at a dosage of 25 mg daily and gradually increased, as tolerated, to approximately 100 mg during the first 2 weeks. During initial titration, Clomipramine Hydrochloride should be given in divided doses with meals to reduce gastrointestinal side effects. Thereafter, the dosage may be increased gradually over the next several weeks, up to a maximum of 250 mg daily. After titration, the total daily dose may be given once daily at bedtime to minimize daytime sedation.

INITIAL TREATMENT/DOSE ADJUSTMENT (CHILDREN AND ADOLESCENTS)
As with adults, the starting dose is 25 mg daily and should be gradually increased (also given in divided doses with meals to reduce gastrointestinal side effects) during the first 2 weeks, as tolerated, up to a daily maximum of 3 mg/kg or 100 mg, whichever is smaller. Thereafter, the dosage may be increased gradually over the next several weeks up to a daily maximum of 3 mg/kg or 200 mg, whichever is smaller (see "Precautions, Pediatric Use"). As with adults, after titration, the total daily dose may be given once daily at bedtime to minimize daytime sedation.

MAINTENANCE/CONTINUATION TREATMENT (ADULTS, CHILDREN, AND ADOLESCENTS)
While there are no systematic studies that answer the question of how long to continue Clomipramine Hydrochloride, OCD is a chronic condition and it is reasonable to consider continuation for a responding patient. Although the efficacy of Clomipramine Hydrochloride after 10 weeks has not been documented in controlled trials, patients have been continued in therapy under double-blind conditions for up to 1 year without loss of benefit. However, dosage adjustments should be made to maintain the patient on the lowest effective dosage, and patients should be periodically reassessed to determine the need for treatment. During maintenance, the total daily dose may be given once daily at bedtime.

Do not store above 86°F (30°C). Protect from moisture. Dispense in tight container (USP).

ANIMAL TOXICOLOGY
Testicular and lung changes commonly associated with tricyclic compounds have been observed with Clomipramine Hydrochloride. In 1- and 2-year studies in rats, changes in the testes (atrophy, aspermatogenesis, and calcification) and drug-induced phospholipidosis in the lungs were observed at doses 4 times the maximum daily human dose. Testicular atrophy was also observed in a 1-year oral toxicity study in dogs at 10 times the maximum daily human dose.

HOW SUPPLIED
CAPSULE: 25 MG

BRAND/MANUFACTURER	NDC	SIZE	AWP
○ BRAND			
▶ ANAFRANIL: Basel	58887-0115-30	100s	$76.01
	58887-0115-32	100s ud	$79.24

CAPSULE: 50 MG

BRAND/MANUFACTURER	NDC	SIZE	AWP
○ BRAND			
▶ ANAFRANIL: Basel	58887-0116-30	100s	$102.50
	58887-0116-32	100s ud	$106.27

CAPSULE: 75 MG

BRAND/MANUFACTURER	NDC	SIZE	AWP
○ BRAND			
▶ ANAFRANIL: Basel	58887-0117-30	100s	$134.92
	58887-0117-32	100s	$141.06

INCIDENCE OF TREATMENT-EMERGENT ADVERSE EXPERIENCE IN PLACEBO-CONTROLLED CLINICAL TRIALS

	(Percentage of Patients Reporting Event)			
	Adults		Children and Adolescents	
Body System/ Adverse Event*	Clomipramine Hydrochloride (N = 322)	Placebo (N = 319)	Clomipramine Hydrochloride (N = 46)	Placebo (N = 44)
Urogenital System				
Male and Female Patients Combined				
Micturition disorder	14	2	4	2
Urinary tract infection	6	1	-	-
Micturition frequency	5	3	-	-
Urinary retention	2	-	7	-
Dysuria	2	2	-	-
Cystitis	2	-	-	-
Female Patients Only	(N = 182)	(N = 167)	(N = 10)	(N = 21)
Dysmenorrhea	12	14	10	10
Lactation (nonpuerperal)	4	-	-	-
Menstrual disorder	4	2	-	-
Vaginitis	2	-	-	-
Leukorrhea	2	-	-	-
Breast enlargement	2	-	-	-
Breast pain	1	-	-	-
Amenorrhea	1	-	-	-
Male Patients Only	(N = 140)	(N = 152)	(N = 36)	(N = 23)
Ejaculation failure	42	2	6	-
Impotence	20	3	-	-
Special Senses				
Abnormal vision	18	4	7	2
Taste perversion	8	-	4	-
Tinnitus	6	-	4	-
Abnormal lacrimation	3	2	-	-
Mydriasis	2	-	-	-
Conjunctivitis	1	-	-	-
Anisocoria	-	-	2	-
Blepharospasm	-	-	2	-
Ocular allergy	-	-	2	-
Vestibular disorder	-	-	2	2
Musculoskeletal				
Myalgia	13	9	-	-
Back pain	6	6	-	-
Arthralgia	3	5	-	-
Muscle weakness	1	-	2	-
Hemic and Lymphatic				
Purpura	3	-	-	-
Anemia	-	-	2	2
Metabolic and Nutritional				
Thirst	2	2	-	2

*Events reported by at least 1% of Clomipramine Hydrochloride patients are included.

◆ RATED THERAPEUTICALLY EQUIVALENT; ◇ THERAPEUTIC EQUIVALENCE UNCONFIRMED; ○ UNRATED

Clonazepam

DESCRIPTION

Clonazepam is available as scored tablets containing 0.5 mg, 1 mg or 2 mg Clonazepam. Chemically, Clonazepam is 5-(2-chlorophenyl)-1,3-dihydro-7-nitro-2H-1,4-benzodiazepin-2-one. It is a light yellow crystalline powder. It has a molecular weight of 315.7.

Following is its chemical structure:

ACTIONS

In laboratory animals, Clonazepam exhibits several pharmacologic properties which are characteristic of the benzodiazepine class of drugs. Convulsions produced in rodents by pentylenetetrazol or electrical stimulation are antagonized, as are convulsions produced by photic stimulation in susceptible baboons. A taming effect in aggressive primates, muscle weakness and hypnosis are likewise produced by Clonazepam. In humans it is capable of suppressing the spike and wave discharge in absence seizures (petit mal) and decreasing the frequency, amplitude, duration and spread of discharge in minor motor seizures.

Single oral dose administration of Clonazepam to humans gave maximum blood levels of drug, in most cases, within one to two hours. The half-life of the parent compound varied from approximately 18 to 50 hours, and the major route of excretion was in the urine. In humans, five metabolites have been identified. In general, the biotransformation of Clonazepam followed two pathways: oxidative hydroxylation at the C-3 position and reduction of the 7-nitro function to form 7-amino and/or 7-acetyl-amino derivatives.

INDICATIONS

Clonazepam is useful alone or as an adjunct in the treatment of the Lennox-Gastaut syndrome (petit mal variant), akinetic and myoclonic seizures. In patients with absence seizures (petit mal) who have failed to respond to succinimides, Clonazepam may be useful.

In some studies, up to 30% of patients have shown a loss of anticonvulsant activity, often within three months of administration. In some cases, dosage adjustment may reestablish efficacy.

CONTRAINDICATIONS

Clonazepam should not be used in patients with a history of sensitivity to benzodiazepines, nor in patients with clinical or biochemical evidence of significant liver disease. It may be used in patients with open angle glaucoma who are receiving appropriate therapy, but is contraindicated in acute narrow angle glaucoma.

WARNINGS

Since Clonazepam produces CNS depression, patients receiving this drug should be cautioned against engaging in hazardous occupations requiring mental alertness, such as operating machinery or driving a motor vehicle. They should also be warned about the concomitant use of alcohol or other CNS-depressant drugs during Clonazepam therapy (see "Drug Interactions").

Usage in Pregnancy: The effects of Clonazepam in human pregnancy and nursing infants are unknown.

Recent reports suggest an association between the use of anticonvulsant drugs by women with epilepsy and an elevated incidence of birth defects in children born to these women. Data are more extensive with respect to diphenylhydantoin and phenobarbital, but these are also the most commonly prescribed anticonvulsants; less systematic or anecdotal reports suggest a possible similar association with the use of all known anticonvulsant drugs.

The reports suggesting an elevated incidence of birth defects in children of drug-treated epileptic women cannot be regarded as adequate to prove a definite cause and effect relationship. There are intrinsic methodologic problems in obtaining adequate data on drug teratogenicity in humans; the possibility also exists that other factors, *e.g.*, genetic factors or the epileptic condition itself, may be more important than drug therapy in leading to birth defects. The great majority of mothers on anticonvulsant medication deliver normal infants. It is important to note that anticonvulsant drugs should not be discontinued in patients in whom the drug is administered to prevent seizures because of the strong possibility of precipitating status epilepticus with attendant hypoxia and threat to life. In individual cases where the severity and frequency of the seizure disorder are such that the removal of medication does not pose a serious threat to the patient, discontinuation of the drug may be considered prior to and during

pregnancy, although it cannot be said with any confidence that even mild seizures do not pose some hazards to the developing embryo or fetus.

These considerations should be weighed in treating or counseling epileptic women of childbearing potential.

Use of Clonazepam in women of childbearing potential should be considered only when the clinical situation warrants the risk. Mothers receiving Clonazepam should not breast feed their infants.

In a two-generation reproduction study with Clonazepam given orally to rats at 10 or 100 mg/kg/day, there was a decrease in the number of pregnancies and a decrease in the number of offspring surviving until weaning. When Clonazepam was administered orally to pregnant rabbits at 0.2, 1.0, 5.0 or 10.0 mg/kg/day, a nondose-related incidence of cleft palates, open eyelids, fused sternebrae and limb defects was observed at the 0.2 and 5.0 mg/kg/day levels. Nearly all of the malformations were seen from one dam in each of the affected dosages.

Usage in Children: Because of the possibility that adverse effects on physical or mental development could become apparent only after many years, a benefit-risk consideration of the long-term use of Clonazepam is important in pediatric patients.

Withdrawal symptoms of the barbiturate type have occurred after the discontinuation of benzodiazepines. (See "Drug Abuse and Dependence" section.)

PRECAUTIONS

When used in patients in whom several different types of seizure disorders coexist, Clonazepam may increase the incidence or precipitate the onset of generalized tonic-clonic seizures (grand mal). This may require the addition of appropriate anticonvulsants or an increase in their dosages. The concomitant use of valproic acid and Clonazepam may produce absence status.

Periodic blood counts and liver function tests are advisable during long-term therapy with Clonazepam.

The abrupt withdrawal of Clonazepam, particularly in those patients on long-term, high-dose therapy, may precipitate status epilepticus. Therefore, when discontinuing Clonazepam gradual withdrawal is essential. While Clonazepam is being gradually withdrawn, the simultaneous substitution of another anticonvulsant may be indicated. Metabolites of Clonazepam are excreted by the kidneys; to avoid their excess accumulation, caution should be exercised in the administration of the drug to patients with impaired renal function.

Clonazepam may produce an increase in salivation. This should be considered before giving the drug to patients who have difficulty handling secretions. Because of this and the possibility of respiratory depression, Clonazepam should be used with caution in patients with chronic respiratory diseases.

Information for Patients: To assure the safe and effective use of benzodiazepines, patients should be informed that, since benzodiazepines may produce psychological and physical dependence, it is advisable that they consult with their physician before either increasing the dose or abruptly discontinuing this drug.

ADVERSE REACTIONS

The most frequently occurring side effects of Clonazepam are referable to CNS depression. Experience to date has shown that drowsiness has occurred in approximately 50% of patients and ataxia in approximately 30%. In some cases, these may diminish with time; behavior problems have been noted in approximately 25% of patients. Others, listed by system, are:

Neurologic: Abnormal eye movements, aphonia, choreiform movements, coma, diplopia, dysarthria, dysdiadochokinesis, "glassy-eyed" appearance, headache, hemiparesis, hypotonia, nystagmus, respiratory depression, slurred speech, tremor, vertigo.

Psychiatric: Confusion, depression, amnesia, hallucinations, hysteria, increased libido, insomnia, psychosis, suicidal attempt (the behavior effects are more likely to occur in patients with a history of psychiatric disturbances).

Respiratory: Chest congestion, rhinorrhea, shortness of breath, hypersecretion in upper respiratory passages.

Cardiovascular: Palpitations.

Dermatologic: Hair loss, hirsutism, skin rash, ankle and facial edema.

Gastrointestinal: Anorexia, coated tongue, constipation, diarrhea, dry mouth, encopresis, gastritis, hepatomegaly, increased appetite, nausea, sore gums.

Genitourinary: Dysuria, enuresis, nocturia, urinary retention.

Musculoskeletal: Muscle weakness, pains.

Miscellaneous: Dehydration, general deterioration, fever, lymphadenopathy, weight loss or gain.

Hematopoietic: Anemia, leukopenia, thrombocytopenia, eosinophilia.

Hepatic: Transient elevations of serum transaminases and alkaline phosphatase.

DRUG ABUSE AND DEPENDENCE

Withdrawal symptoms, similar in character to those noted with barbiturates and alcohol (e.g., convulsions, psychosis, hallucinations, behavioral disorder, tremor, abdominal and muscle cramps) have occurred following abrupt discontinuance of Clonazepam. The more severe withdrawal symptoms have usually been limited to those patients who received excessive doses over an extended period of time. Generally milder withdrawal symptoms (e.g., dysphoria and insomnia) have been reported following abrupt discontinuance of benzodiazepines taken continuously at therapeutic levels for several months. Consequently, after extended therapy, abrupt discontinuation should generally be avoided and a gradual dosage tapering schedule followed. Addiction-prone individuals (such as drug addicts or alcoholics) should be under careful surveillance when receiving Clonazepam or other psychotropic agents because of the predisposition of such patients to habituation and dependence.

DRUG INTERACTIONS

The CNS-depressant action of the benzodiazepine class of drugs may be potentiated by alcohol, narcotics, barbiturates, nonbarbiturate hypnotics, antianxiety agents, the phenothiazines, thioxanthene and butyrophenone classes of antipsychotic agents, monoamine oxidase inhibitors and the tricyclic antidepressants, and by other anticonvulsant drugs.

OVERDOSAGE

Symptoms of Clonazepam overdosage, like those produced by other CNS depressants, include somnolence, confusion, coma and diminished reflexes. Treatment includes monitoring of respiration, pulse and blood pressure, general supportive measures and immediate gastric lavage. Intravenous fluids should be administered and an adequate airway maintained. Hypotension may be combated by the use of levarterenol or metaraminol. Methylphenidate or caffeine and sodium benzoate may be given to combat CNS depression. Dialysis is of no known value.

DOSAGE AND ADMINISTRATION

Infants and Children: Clonazepam is administered orally. In order to minimize drowsiness, the initial dose for infants and children (up to 10 years of age or 30 kg of body weight) should be between 0.01 and 0.03 mg/kg/day but not to exceed 0.05 mg/kg/day given in two or three divided doses. Dosage should be increased by no more than 0.25 to 0.5 mg every third day until a daily maintenance dose of 0.1 to 0.2 mg/kg of body weight has been reached unless seizures are controlled or side effects preclude further increase. Whenever possible, the daily dose should be divided into three equal doses. If doses are not equally divided, the largest dose should be given before retiring.

Adults: The initial dose for adults should not exceed 1.5 mg/day divided into three doses. Dosage may be increased in increments of 0.5 to 1 mg every three days until seizures are adequately controlled or until side effects preclude any further increase. Maintenance dosage must be individualized for each patient depending upon response. Maximum recommended daily dose is 20 mg.

The use of multiple anticonvulsants may result in an increase of depressant adverse effects. This should be considered before adding Clonazepam to an existing anticonvulsant regimen.

HOW SUPPLIED
TABLETS (C-IV): 0.5 MG

BRAND/MANUFACTURER	NDC	SIZE	AWP
○ BRAND			
➤ KLONOPIN: Roche Labs	00004-0068-01	100s	$66.83
	00004-0068-50	100s ud	$69.99

TABLETS (C-IV): 1 MG

BRAND/MANUFACTURER	NDC	SIZE	AWP
○ BRAND			
➤ KLONOPIN: Roche Labs	00004-0058-01	100s	$76.23
	00004-0058-50	100s ud	$79.43

TABLETS (C-IV): 2 MG

BRAND/MANUFACTURER	NDC	SIZE	AWP
○ BRAND			
➤ KLONOPIN: Roche Labs	00004-0098-01	100s	$105.64
	00004-0098-50	100s ud	$108.81

Clonidine

DESCRIPTION

Clonidine is available as a tablet (Clonidine Hydrochloride) and as a transdermal system providing continuous systemic delivery of Clonidine for 7 days at an approximately constant rate. *Each tablet contains:* Clonidine HCl 0.1, 0.2, and 0.3 mg.

	Programmed Delivery Clonidine In Vitro Per Day Over 1 Week	Clonidine Content
Clonidine transdermal system	0.1 mg	2.5 mg
Clonidine transdermal system	0.2 mg	5.0 mg
Clonidine transdermal system	0.3 mg	7.5 mg

Clonidine and Clonidine Hydrochloride are centrally acting alpha agonists and antihypertensive agents. They are imidazoline derivatives whose chemical names are, respectively, 2,6-dichloro-N-2-imidazolidinylidenebenzenamine and 2-(2,6-dichlorophenylamino)-2-imidazoline hydrochloride.

Clonidine HCl is an odorless, bitter, white crystalline substance soluble in water and alcohol. Its empirical formula is $C_9H_9Cl_2N_3 \cdot HCl$ and its molecular weight is 266.56.

Clonidine transdermal system releases Clonidine at an approximately constant rate for 7 days. The energy source for drug release derives from the concentration gradient existing between a saturated solution of drug in the system and the much lower concentration prevailing in the skin. Clonidine flows in the direction of the lower concentration at a constant rate.

Therapeutic plasma Clonidine levels are achieved 2 to 3 days after initial application of Clonidine transdermal system.

The Clonidine transdermal system delivers 0.1, 0.2, or 0.3 mg Clonidine per day. To ensure constant release of drug over 7 days, the total drug content of the system is greater than the total amount of drug delivered. Application of a new system to a fresh skin site at weekly intervals continuously maintains therapeutic plasma concentrations of Clonidine. If the Clonidine transdermal system is removed and not replaced with a new system, therapeutic plasma Clonidine levels will persist for about 8 hours and then decline slowly over several days. Over this time period, blood pressure returns gradually to pretreatment levels. If the patient experiences localized skin irritation before completing 7 days of use, the system may be removed and replaced with a new one applied on a fresh skin site.

CLINICAL PHARMACOLOGY

Clonidine Hydrochloride USP acts relatively rapidly. The patient's blood pressure declines within 30 to 60 minutes after an oral dose, the maximum decrease occuring within 2 to 4 hours. The plasma level of Clonidine HCl peaks in approximately 3 to 5 hours and the plasma half-life ranges from 12 to 16 hours. The half-life increases up to 41 hours in patients with severe impairment of renal function. Following oral administration about 40-60% of the absorbed dose is recovered in the urine as unchanged drug in 24 hours. About 50% of the absorbed dose is metabolized in the liver. The plasma half-life of Clonidine is 12.7 ± 7 hours.

Clonidine stimulates alpha-adrenoreceptors in the brain stem, resulting in reduced sympathetic outflow from the central nervous system and a decrease in peripheral resistance, renal vascular resistance, heart rate, and blood pressure. Renal blood flow and glomerular filtration rate remain essentially unchanged. Normal postural reflexes are intact, and therefore orthostatic symptoms are mild and infrequent. Acute studies with Clonidine HCl in humans have demonstrated a moderate reduction (15% to 20%) of cardiac output in the supine position with no change in the peripheral resistance; at a 45° tilt there is a smaller reduction in cardiac output and a decrease of peripheral resistance. During long-term therapy, cardiac output tends to return to control values, while peripheral resistance remains decreased. Slowing of the pulse rate has been observed in most patients given Clonidine, but the drug does not alter normal hemodynamic response to exercise.

Other studies in patients have provided evidence of a reduction in plasma renin activity and in the excretion of aldosterone and catecholamines, but the exact relationship of these pharmacologic actions to the antihypertensive effect has not been fully elucidated.

Clonidine acutely stimulates growth hormone release in both children and adults, but does not produce a chronic elevation of growth hormone with long-term use.

Tolerance may develop in some patients, necessitating a reevaluation of therapy.

INDICATIONS FOR USE

Clonidine is indicated in the treatment of hypertension. They may be employed alone or concomitantly with other antihypertensive agents.

UNLABELED USES

Clonidine is used alone or as an adjunct in the treatment of atrial fibrillation, angina pectoris, congestive heart failure, and malignant hypertension (hypertensive urgencies). It is also used in migraine headache, reflex sympathetic dystrophy, neuroleptic-induced akathisia, generalized anxiety disorders or panic disorders, and social phobia. Clonidine is also prescribed in the treatment of attention deficit disorder, bipolar disorders, including mania, schizophrenia, tardive dyskinesia, Tourette's syndrome, and in children with aggressive and disruptive behavior disorders. Additionally, Clonidine is also used to control alcohol and opiates withdrawal symptoms, as an adjunctive therapy in nicotine cessation programs, paroxysmal localized hyperhidrosis, vasomotor symptoms of menopause (hot flashes), growth hormone stimulation test, diagnosis of pheochromocytoma, diarrhea, chemotherapy induced nausea and vomiting, proctalgia fugax, and sialorrhea, including clozapine-induced sialorrhea. It is also used in neurogenic bladder disease, portal hypertension, spasticity due to spinal cord injury, chronic glaucoma (when administered intraocular), dysmenorrhea, and premenstrual syndrome.

CONTRAINDICATIONS

Clonidine should not be used in patients with known hypersensitivity to Clonidine or to any other component of the adhesive layer of the therapeutic system. There are no known contraindications to the use of Clonidine HCl.

PRECAUTIONS

General: In patients who have developed localized contact sensitization to Clonidine transdermal system, substitution of oral Clonidine HCl therapy may be associated with development of a generalized skin rash.

In patients who develop an allergic reaction to Clonidine transdermal system that extends beyond the local patch site (such as generalized skin rash, urticaria, or angioedema) oral Clonidine HCl substitution may elicit a similar reaction.

◆ RATED THERAPEUTICALLY EQUIVALENT; ◇ THERAPEUTIC EQUIVALENCE UNCONFIRMED; ○ UNRATED

As with all antihypertensive therapy, Clonidine should be used with caution in patients with severe coronary insufficiency, recent myocardial infarction, cerebrovascular disease, or chronic renal failure.

Transdermal Clonidine systems should be removed before attempting defibrillation or cardioversion because of the potential for altered electrical conductivity which may enhance the possibility of arcing, a phenomenon associated with the use of defibrillators.

Withdrawal: Patients should be instructed not to discontinue therapy without consulting their physician. Sudden cessation of Clonidine treatment has resulted in subjective symptoms such as nervousness, agitation and headache, accompanied or followed by a rapid rise in blood pressure and elevated catecholamine concentrations in the plasma, but such occurrences have usually been associated with previous administration of high oral doses (exceeding 1.2 mg/day) and/or with continuation of concomitant beta-blocker therapy. Rare instances of hypertensive encephalopathy and death have been reported.

When discontinuing therapy with Clonidine HCl tablets, the physician should reduce the dose gradually over 2 to 4 days to avoid withdrawal symptomatology.

An excessive rise in blood pressure following Clonidine discontinuance can be reversed by administration of oral Clonidine or by intravenous phentolamine. If therapy is to be discontinued in patients receiving beta-blockers and Clonidine concurrently, beta-blockers should be discontinued several days before cessation of Clonidine administration or gradual withdrawal of Clonidine HCl.

Perioperative Use: Administration of Clonidine HCl should be continued to within four hours of surgery and resumed as soon as possible thereafter. Clonidine therapy should not be interrupted during the surgical period. Blood pressure should be carefully monitored during surgery and additional measures to control blood pressure should be available if required. Physicians considering starting Clonidine transdermal system therapy during the perioperative period must be aware that therapeutic plasma Clonidine levels are not achieved until 2 to 3 days after initial application of Clonidine transdermal system (see *"Dosage and Administration"*).

Information for Patients: Patients who engage in potentially hazardous activities, such as operating machinery or driving, should be advised of a potential sedative effect of Clonidine. Patients should be cautioned against interruption of Clonidine therapy without a physician's advice. Patients should be advised that if the Clonidine transdermal system begins to loosen from the skin after application, the adhesive overlay should be applied directly over the system to ensure good adhesion over its 7-day lifetime. Patients who develop moderate or severe erythema and/or localized vesicle formation at the site of application, or a generalized skin rash, should consult their physician promptly about the possible need to remove the patch.

Drug Interactions: If a patient receiving Clonidine is also taking tricyclic antidepressants, the effect of Clonidine may be reduced, thus necessitating an increase in dosage. Clonidine may enhance the CNS-depressive effects of alcohol, barbiturates or other sedatives. Amitriptyline in combination with Clonidine enhances the manifestation of corneal lesions in rats. (See *"Toxicology"* section.)

Carcinogenesis, Mutagenesis, Impairment of Fertility: In a 132-week (fixed concentration) dietary administration study in rats, Clonidine HCl administered at 32 to 46 times the oral maximum recommended daily human dose (MRDHD) was unassociated with evidence of carcinogenic potential. Results from the Ames test with Clonidine HCl revealed no evidence of mutagenesis. Fertility of male or female rats was unaffected by Clonidine HCl doses as high as 150 mcg/kg or about 3 times the oral MRDHD. Fertility of female rats did, however, appear to be affected (in another experiment) at the dose levels of 500 to 2000 mcg/kg or 10 to 40 times the oral MRDHD.

Pregnancy/Teratogenic Effects: Pregnancy Category C: Reproduction studies performed in rabbits at doses up to approximately 3 times the oral maximum recommended daily human dose (MRDHD) of Clonidine HCl have revealed no evidence of teratogenic or embryotoxic potential in rabbits. In rats, however, doses as low as 1/3 the oral MRDHD of Clonidine were associated with increased resorptions in a study in which dams were treated continuously from 2 months prior to mating. Increased resorptions were not associated with treatment at the same or at higher dose levels (up to 3 times the oral MRDHD) when dams were treated days 6-15 of gestation. Increased resorptions were observed at much higher levels (40 times the oral MRDHD) in rats and mice treated days 1-14 of gestation (lowest dose employed in the study was 500 mcg/kg). There are, however, no adequate and well-controlled studies in pregnant women. Because animal reproduction studies are not always predictive of human response, this drug should be used during pregnancy only if clearly needed.

Nursing Mothers: As Clonidine is excreted in human milk, caution should be exercised when Clonidine transdermal system or Clonidine HCl tablets are administered to a nursing woman.

Pediatric Use: Safety and effectiveness of the Clonidine transdermal system in children below the age of twelve have not been established. Safety and effectiveness of Clonidine HCl tablets in children have not been established.

ADVERSE REACTIONS
CLONIDINE TRANSDERMAL SYSTEM
Most systemic adverse effects during therapy with Clonidine transdermal system have been mild and have tended to diminish with continued therapy. In a 3-month, multiclinic trial of Clonidine transdermal system in 101 hypertensive patients, the most frequent systemic reactions were dry mouth (25 patients) and drowsiness (12 patients).

Transient localized skin reactions, primarily localized pruritus, occurred in 51 patients. Twenty-six patients experienced localized erythema. This erythema and pruritus were more common in patients utilizing an adhesive overlay for the entire 7-day treatment period. Allergic contact sensitization to Clonidine transdermal system was observed in 5 patients.

In additional clinical experience contact dermatitis resulting in treatment discontinuation was observed in 128 of 673 patients (about 19 in 100) after a mean duration of treatment of 37 weeks. The incidence in white females was about 34 in 100; in white males about 18 in 100; in black females about 14 in 100; and in black males about 8 in 100.

The following less frequent adverse experiences were also reported in patients involved in the multiclinical trial with Clonidine transdermal system.

Gastrointestinal: Constipation (1 patient); nausea (1); and change in taste (1).

Central Nervous System: Fatigue (6 patients); headache (5); lethargy (3); sedation (3); insomnia (2); dizziness (2); and nervousness (1).

Genitourinary: Impotence/sexual dysfunction (2 patients).

Dermatological: Localized vesiculation (7 patients); hyperpigmentation (5); edema (3); excoriation (3); burning (3); papules (1); throbbing (1); blanching (1); and generalized macular rash (1).

In additional clinical experience involving 3539 patients, less common dermatologic reactions have occurred, where a causal relationship to Clonidine transdermal system was not established: maculopapular skin rash (10 cases); urticaria (2 cases); angioedema involving the face (2 cases), one of which also involved the tongue.

Oro-otolaryngeal: Dry throat (2 patients).

CLONIDINE HCL TABLETS
Most adverse effects are mild and tend to diminish with continued therapy. The most frequent (which appear to be dose-related) are dry mouth, occurring in about 40 of 100 patients; drowsiness, about 33 in 100; dizziness, about 16 in 100; constipation and sedation, each about 10 in 100.

The following less frequent adverse experiences have also been reported in patients receiving Clonidine HCl, but in many cases patients were receiving concomitant medication and a causal relationship has not been established.

Gastrointestinal: Nausea and vomiting, about 5 in 100 patients; anorexia and malaise, each about 1 in 100; mild transient abnormalities in liver function tests, about 1 in 100; rare reports of hepatitis; parotitis, rarely.

Metabolic: Weight gain, about 1 in 100 patients; gynecomastia, about 1 in 1000; transient elevation of blood glucose or serum creatine phosphokinase, rarely.

Central Nervous System: Nervousness and agitation, about 3 in 100 patients; mental depression, about 1 in 100; headache, about 1 in 100; insomnia, about 5 in 1000. Vivid dreams or nightmares, other behavioral changes, restlessness, anxiety, visual and auditory hallucinations and delirium have been reported.

Cardiovascular: Orthostatic symptoms, about 3 in 100 patients; palpitations and tachycardia, and bradycardia, each about 5 in 1000. Raynaud's phenomenon, congestive heart failure, and electrocardiographic abnormalities (i.e. conduction disturbances and arrhythmias) have been reported rarely. Rare cases of sinus bradycardia and atrioventricular block have been reported, both with and without the use of concomitant digitalis.

Dermatological: Rash, about 1 in 100 patients; pruritus, about 7 in 1000; hives, angioneurotic edema and urticaria, about 5 in 1000; alopecia, about 2 in 1000.

Genitourinary: Decreased sexual activity, impotence and loss of libido, about 3 in 100 patients; nocturia, about 1 in 100; difficulty in micturition, about 2 in 1000; urinary retention, about 1 in 1000.

Other: Weakness, about 10 in 100 patients; fatigue, about 4 in 100; discontinuation syndrome, about 1 in 100; muscle or joint pain, about 6 in 1000 and cramps of the lower limbs, about 3 in 1000. Dryness, burning of the eyes, blurred vision, dryness of the nasal mucosa, pallor, weakly positive Coombs' test, increased sensitivity to alcohol and fever have been reported.

OVERDOSAGE
If symptoms of overdosage occur, remove all Clonidine transdermal systems. The signs and symptoms of Clonidine overdosage include hypotension, bradycardia, lethargy, irritability, weakness, somnolence, diminished or absent reflexes, miosis, vomiting and hypoventilation. With large overdoses, reversible cardiac conduction defects or arrhythmias, apnea, seizures and transient hypertension have been reported. The oral LD_{50} of Clonidine in rats was 465 mg/kg, and in mice 206 mg/kg.

The general treatment of Clonidine overdosage may include intravenous fluids as indicated. Bradycardia can be treated with intravenous atropine sulfate and hypotension with dopamine infusion in addition to intravenous fluids. Hypertension associated with overdosage has been treated with intravenous furosemide or diazoxide or alpha-blocking agents such as phentolamine. Tolazoline, an alpha-blocker, in intravenous doses of 10 mg at 30-minute intervals, may reverse Clonidine's effects if other efforts fail. Routine hemodialysis is of limited benefit, since a maximum of 5% of circulating Clonidine is removed.

In a patient who ingested 100 mg Clonidine HCl, plasma Clonidine levels were 60 ng/ml (1 hour), 190 ng/ml (1.5 hours), 370 ng/ml (2 hours) and 120 ng/ml (5.5 and 6.5 hours). This patient developed hypertension followed by hypotension, bradycardia, apnea, hallucinations, semicoma, and premature ventricular contractions. The patient fully recovered after intensive treatment.

DOSAGE AND ADMINISTRATION

CLONIDINE HCL TABLETS

Adults: The dose of Clonidine HCl must be adjusted according to the patient's individual blood pressure response. The following is a general guide to its administration.

Initial Dose: 0.1 mg tablet twice daily (morning and bed-time). Elderly patients may benefit from a lower initial dose.

Maintenance Dose: Further increments of 0.1 mg per day may be made if necessary until the desired response is achieved. Taking the larger portion of the total daily dose at bedtime may minimize transient adjustment effects of dry mouth and drowsiness. The therapeutic doses most commonly employed have ranged from 0.2 mg to 0.6 mg per day given in divided doses. Studies have indicated that 2.4 mg is the maximum effective daily dose, but doses as high as this have rarely been employed.

Renal Impairment: Dosage must be adjusted according to the degree of impairment, and patients should be carefully monitored. Since only a minimal amount of Clonidine is removed during routine hemodialysis, there is no need to give supplemental Clonidine following dialysis.

CLONIDINE TRANSDERMAL SYSTEM

Apply Clonidine transdermal system to a hairless area of intact skin on the upper arm or torso, once every 7 days. Each new application of Clonidine transdermal system should be on a different skin site from the previous location. If the system loosens during 7-day wearing, the adhesive overlay should be applied directly over the system to ensure good adhesion.

To initiate therapy, Clonidine transdermal system dosage should be titrated according to individual therapeutic requirements, starting with Clonidine transdermal system 0.1 mg. If after one or two weeks the desired reduction in blood pressure is not achieved, increase the dosage by adding an additional Clonidine transdermal system 0.1 mg or changing to a larger system. An increase in dosage above two Clonidine transdermal systems 0.3 mg is usually not associated with additional efficacy.

When substituting Clonidine transdermal system in patients on prior antihypertensive therapy, physicians should be aware that the antihypertensive effect of Clonidine transdermal system may not commence until 2 to 3 days after initial application. Therefore, gradual reduction of prior drug dosage is advised. Some or all previous antihypertensive treatment may have to be continued, particularly in patients with more severe forms of hypertension.

STORAGE AND HANDLING

Store below 86°F (30°C). Dispense tablets in tight, light-resistant container.

TOXICOLOGY

In several studies, oral Clonidine HCl produced a dose-dependent increase in the incidence and severity of spontaneously occurring retinal degeneration in albino rats treated for six months or longer. Tissue distribution studies in dogs and monkeys revealed that Clonidine HCl was concentrated in the choroid of the eye. In view of the retinal degeneration observed in rats, eye examinations were performed in 908 patients prior to the start of Clonidine HCl therapy, who were then examined periodically thereafter. In 353 of these 908 patients, examinations were performed for periods of 24 months or longer. Except for some dryness of the eyes, no drug-related abnormal ophthalmologic findings were recorded and Clonidine HCl did not alter retinal function as shown by specialized tests such as the electroretinogram and macular dazzle.

In rats, Clonidine HCl in combination with amitriptyline produced corneal lesions within 5 days.

HOW SUPPLIED

CLONIDINE

FILM, EXTENDED RELEASE: 0.1 MG

BRAND/MANUFACTURER	NDC	SIZE	AWP
○ **BRAND**			
CATAPRES-TTS-1: Boehr Ingelheim	00597-0031-12	12s	$87.58

FILM, EXTENDED RELEASE: 0.2 MG

BRAND/MANUFACTURER	NDC	SIZE	AWP
○ **BRAND**			
CATAPRES-TTS-2: Boehr Ingelheim	00597-0032-12	12s	$147.43

FILM, EXTENDED RELEASE: 0.3 MG

BRAND/MANUFACTURER	NDC	SIZE	AWP
○ **BRAND**			
CATAPRES-TTS-3: Boehr Ingelheim	00597-0033-34	4s	$68.10

CLONIDINE HYDROCHLORIDE

TABLETS: 0.1 MG

AVERAGE UNIT PRICE (AVAILABLE SIZES)		GENERIC A-RATED AVERAGE PRICE (GAAP)	
BRAND	$0.55	100s	$11.09
GENERIC	$0.10	500s	$38.61
HCFA FUL (100s ea)	$0.02	750s	$142.88
		1000s	$72.43

BRAND/MANUFACTURER	NDC	SIZE	AWP
◆ **BRAND**			
➤ CATAPRES: Boehr Ingelheim	00597-0006-01	100s	$54.22
	00597-0006-61	100s ud	$58.25
	00597-0006-10	1000s	$525.65
◆ **GENERICS**			
Raway	00686-0299-20	100s	$4.50
Vangard	00615-2572-01	100s	$4.75
Schein	00364-0820-01	100s	$5.80
Goldline	00182-1250-01	100s	$5.95
Goldline	00182-1767-01	100s	$5.95
Rugby	00536-5621-01	100s	$6.13
Qualitest	00603-2954-21	100s	$6.30
Geneva	00781-1471-01	100s	$6.45
Moore,H.L.	00839-7182-06	100s	$7.63
Purepac	00228-2127-10	100s	$10.43
➤ Mylan	00378-0152-01	100s	$10.45
Aligen	00405-4241-01	100s	$10.98
Lederle Std Prod	00005-3180-23	100s	$17.10
Parmed	00349-8921-01	100s	$18.00
U.S. Trading	56126-0110-11	100s ud	$3.41
Auro	55829-0211-10	100s ud	$10.50
Major	00904-1025-61	100s ud	$11.19
Schein	00364-0820-90	100s ud	$15.00
Goldline	00182-1767-89	100s ud	$15.00
Vangard	00615-2572-13	100s ud	$19.05
UDL	51079-0299-20	100s ud	$23.62
Medirex	57480-0309-01	100s ud	$25.80
Goldline	00182-1250-05	500s	$22.45
Goldline	00182-1767-05	500s	$22.45
Rugby	00536-5621-05	500s	$27.38
Qualitest	00603-2954-28	500s	$28.60
Aligen	00405-4241-02	500s	$47.70
Purepac	00228-2127-50	500s	$52.15
Parmed	00349-8921-05	500s	$69.55
Glasgow	60809-0114-55	750s ud	$142.88
Glasgow	60809-0114-72	750s ud	$142.88
Mason Dist	11845-0191-04	1000s	$46.60
Schein	00364-0820-02	1000s	$48.50
Major	00904-1025-80	1000s	$51.50
Geneva	00781-1471-10	1000s	$51.60
Moore,H.L.	00839-7182-16	1000s	$73.29
➤ Mylan	00378-0152-10	1000s	$73.95
Lederle Std Prod	00005-3180-34	1000s	$161.60

TABLETS: 0.2 MG

AVERAGE UNIT PRICE (AVAILABLE SIZES)		GENERIC A-RATED AVERAGE PRICE (GAAP)	
BRAND	$0.83	100s	$14.32
GENERIC	$0.12	500s	$48.91
HCFA FUL (100s ea)	$0.02	1000s	$87.92

BRAND/MANUFACTURER	NDC	SIZE	AWP
◆ **BRAND**			
➤ CATAPRES: Boehr Ingelheim	00597-0007-01	100s	$82.87
	00597-0007-61	100s ud	$86.99
	00597-0007-10	1000s	$803.83
◆ **GENERICS**			
Vangard	00615-2573-01	100s	$5.00
Raway	00686-0300-20	100s	$5.50
Goldline	00182-1251-01	100s	$7.45
Goldline	00182-1768-01	100s	$7.45
Schein	00364-0821-01	100s	$7.90
Geneva	00781-1472-01	100s	$7.95
Qualitest	00603-2955-21	100s	$9.80
Rugby	00536-5622-01	100s	$9.87
Moore,H.L.	00839-7183-06	100s	$10.92
Purepac	00228-2128-10	100s	$14.33
Mylan	00378-0186-01	100s	$14.35
Aligen	00405-4242-01	100s	$15.08
Parmed	00349-8922-01	100s	$20.00
Lederle Std Prod	00005-3181-23	100s	$26.86
U.S. Trading	56126-0111-11	100s ud	$3.57
Auro	55829-0212-10	100s ud	$12.16
Major	00904-1026-61	100s ud	$12.85
Goldline	00182-1768-89	100s ud	$18.75
Schein	00364-0821-90	100s ud	$20.00
Vangard	00615-2573-13	100s ud	$23.01
UDL	51079-0300-20	100s ud	$31.10

◆ RATED THERAPEUTICALLY EQUIVALENT; ◇ THERAPEUTIC EQUIVALENCE UNCONFIRMED; ○ UNRATED

BRAND/MANUFACTURER	NDC	SIZE	AWP
Medirex	57480-0310-01	100s ud	$31.10
Goldline	00182-1251-05	500s	$26.95
Goldline	00182-1768-05	500s	$26.95
Rugby	00536-5622-05	500s	$33.63
Qualitest	00603-2955-28	500s	$38.80
Aligen	00405-4242-02	500s	$64.14
Purepac	00228-2128-50	500s	$71.65
Parmed	00349-8922-05	500s	$80.25
Aligen	00405-4242-03	1000s	$50.95
Mason Dist	11845-0192-04	1000s	$57.45
URL	00677-1078-10	1000s	$62.48
Schein	00364-0821-02	1000s	$62.50
Goldline	00182-1768-10	1000s	$62.50
Geneva	00781-1472-10	1000s	$63.60
Moore,H.L.	00839-7183-16	1000s	$86.79
Mylan	00378-0186-10	1000s	$87.25
Lederle Std Prod	00005-3181-34	1000s	$257.80

TABLETS: 0.3 MG

AVERAGE UNIT PRICE (AVAILABLE SIZES)		GENERIC A-RATED AVERAGE PRICE (GAAP)	
BRAND	$1.04	100s	$17.71
GENERIC	$0.17		
HCFA FUL (100s ea)	$0.03		

BRAND/MANUFACTURER	NDC	SIZE	AWP
◆ BRAND			
➤ CATAPRES: Boehr Ingelheim	00597-0011-01	100s	$104.12
◆ GENERICS			
Vangard	00615-2574-01	100s	$5.77
Goldline	00182-1252-01	100s	$8.95
Goldline	00182-1769-01	100s	$8.95
Raway	00686-0301-20	100s	$9.50
Mason Dist	11845-0193-01	100s	$9.50
Schein	00364-0824-01	100s	$9.80
Rugby	00536-5623-01	100s	$10.00
Qualitest	00603-2956-21	100s	$10.00
URL	00677-1114-01	100s	$10.90
Geneva	00781-1473-01	100s	$10.95

Clorazepate Dipotassium

DESCRIPTION

Chemically, Clorazepate Dipotassium is a benzodiazepine. The empirical formula is $C_{16}H_{11}ClK_2N_2O_4$; the molecular weight is 408.92.

The compound occurs as a fine, light yellow, practically odorless powder. It is insoluble in the common organic solvents, but very soluble in water. Aqueous solutions are unstable, clear, light yellow, and alkaline.

Clorazepate Dipotassium tablets contain either 3.75 mg, 7.5 mg or 15 mg of Clorazepate Dipotassium for oral administration. The sustained release tablets contain 11.25 and 22.5 mg of Clorazepate Dipotassium. These tablets gradually release Clorazepate and are designed for once a day administration in patients already stabilized on Clorazepate Dipotassium tablets.

Following is its chemical structure:

CLINICAL PHARMACOLOGY

Pharmacologically, Clorazepate Dipotassium has the characteristics of the benzodiazepines. It has depressant effects on the central nervous system. The primary metabolite, nordiazepam, quickly appears in the blood stream. The serum half-life is about 2 days. The drug is metabolized in the liver and excreted primarily in the urine. (See "Animal and Clinical Pharmacology" section).

Studies in healthy men have shown that Clorazepate Dipotassium has depressant effects on the central nervous system. Prolonged administration of single daily doses as high as 120 mg was without toxic effects. Abrupt cessation of high doses was followed in some patients by nervousness, insomnia, irritability, diarrhea, muscle aches, or memory impairment. Since orally administered Clorazepate Dipotassium is rapidly decarboxylated to form nordiazepam, there is essentially no circulating parent drug. Nordiazepam, the primary metabolite, quickly appears in the blood and is eliminated from the plasma with an apparent half-life of about 40 to 50 hours. Plasma levels of nordiazepam increase proportionally with Clorazepate Dipotassium dose and show moderate accumulation with repeated administration. The protein binding of nordiazepam in plasma is high (97-98%).

Within 10 days after oral administration of a 15 mg (50μCi) dose of ^{14}C-Clorazepate Dipotassium to two volunteers, 62-67% of the radioactivity was excreted in the urine and 15-19% was eliminated in the feces. Both subjects were still excreting measurable amounts of radioactivity in the urine (about 1% of the ^{14}C-dose) on day ten.

Nordiazepam is further metabolized by hydroxylation. The major urinary metabolite is conjugated oxazepam (3-hydroxynordiazepam), and smaller amounts of conjugated p-hydroxynordiazepam and nordiazepam are also found in the urine.

INDICATIONS

Clorazepate Dipotassium is indicated for the management of anxiety disorders or for the short-term relief of the symptoms of anxiety. Anxiety or tension associated with the stress of everyday life usually does not require treatment with an anxiolytic.

Clorazepate Dipotassium is indicated as adjunctive therapy in the management of partial seizures.

The effectiveness of Clorazepate Dipotassium in long-term management of anxiety, that is, more than 4 months, has not been assessed by systematic clinical studies. Long-term studies in epileptic patients, however, have shown continued therapeutic activity. The physician should reassess periodically the usefulness of the drug for the individual patient.

Clorazepate Dipotassium is indicated for the symptomatic relief of acute alcohol withdrawal.

CONTRAINDICATIONS

Clorazepate Dipotassium is contraindicated in patients with a known hypersensitivity to the drug, and in those with acute narrow angle glaucoma.

WARNINGS

Clorazepate Dipotassium is not recommended for use in depressive neuroses or in psychotic reactions.

Patients on Clorazepate Dipotassium should be cautioned against engaging in hazardous occupations requiring mental alertness, such as operating dangerous machinery including motor vehicles.

Since Clorazepate Dipotassium has a central nervous system depressant effect, patients should be advised against the simultaneous use of other CNS-depressant drugs, and cautioned that the effects of alcohol may be increased.

Because of the lack of sufficient clinical experience, Clorazepate Dipotassium is not recommended for use in patients less than 9 years of age.

Physical and Psychological Dependence: Withdrawal symptoms (similar in character to those noted with barbiturates and alcohol) have occurred following abrupt discontinuance of Clorazepate Dipotassium. Withdrawal symptoms associated with the abrupt discontinuation of benzodiazepines have included convulsions, delirium, hallucinations, tremor, abdominal and muscle aches or cramps, vomiting, sweating, nervousness, insomnia, irritability, diarrhea, and memory impairment. The more severe withdrawal symptoms have usually been limited to those patients who had received excessive doses over an extended period of time. Generally milder withdrawal symptoms have been reported following abrupt discontinuance of benzodiazepines taken continuously at therapeutic levels for several months. Consequently, after extended therapy, abrupt discontinuation of clorazepate should generally be avoided and a gradual dosage tapering schedule followed.

Caution should be observed in patients who are considered to have a psychological potential for drug dependence.

Evidence of drug dependence has been observed in dogs and rabbits which was characterized by convulsive seizures when the drug was abruptly withdrawn or the dose was reduced; the syndrome in dogs could be abolished by administration of Clorazepate Dipotassium.

Usage in Pregnancy: **An increased risk of congenital malformations associated with the use of minor tranquilizers (chlordiazepoxide, diazepam, and meprobamate) during the first trimester of pregnancy has been suggested in several studies. Clorazepate Dipotassium, a benzodiazepine derivative, has not been studied adequately to determine whether it, too, may be associated with an increased risk of fetal abnormality. Because use of these drugs is rarely a matter of urgency, their use during this period should almost always be avoided. The possibility that a woman of childbearing potential may be pregnant at the time of institution of therapy should be considered. Patients should be advised that if they become pregnant during therapy or intend to become pregnant they should communicate with their physician about the desirability of discontinuing the drug.**

Usage during Lactation: Clorazepate Dipotassium should not be given to nursing mothers since it has been reported that nordiazepam is excreted in human breast milk.

PRECAUTIONS

In those patients in which a degree of depression accompanies the anxiety, suicidal tendencies may be present and protective measures may be required. The least amount of drug that is feasible should be available to the patient.

Patients on Clorazepate Dipotassium for prolonged periods should have blood counts and liver function tests periodically. The usual precautions in treating patients with impaired renal or hepatic function should also be observed.

In elderly or debilitated patients, the initial dose should be small, and increments should be made gradually, in accordance with the response of the patient, to preclude ataxia or excessive sedation.

Information for Patients: To assure the safe and effective use of benzodiazepines, patients should be informed that, since benzodiazepines may produce psychological and physical dependence, it is essential that they consult with their physician before either increasing the dose or abruptly discontinuing this drug.

ADVERSE REACTIONS

The side effect most frequently reported was drowsiness. Less commonly reported (in descending order of occurrence) were: dizziness, various gastrointestinal complaints, nervousness, blurred vision, dry mouth, headache, and mental confusion. Other side effects included insomnia, transient skin rashes, fatigue, ataxia, genitourinary complaints, irritability, diplopia, depression, tremor, and slurred speech.

There have been reports of abnormal liver and kidney function tests and of decrease in hematocrit.

Decrease in systolic blood pressure has been observed.

DRUG INTERACTIONS

If Clorazepate Dipotassium is to be combined with other drugs acting on the central nervous system, careful consideration should be given to the pharmacology of the agents to be employed. Animal experience indicates that Clorazepate Dipotassium prolongs the sleeping time after hexobarbital or after ethyl alcohol, increases the inhibitory effects of chlorpromazine, but does not exhibit monoamine oxidase inhibition. Clinical studies have shown increased sedation with concurrent hypnotic medications. The actions of the benzodiazepines may be potentiated by barbiturates, narcotics, phenothiazines, monoamine oxidase inhibitors or other antidepressants.

If Clorazepate Dipotassium is used to treat anxiety associated with somatic disease states, careful attention must be paid to possible drug interaction with concomitant medication.

In bioavailability studies with normal subjects, the concurrent administration of antacids at therapeutic levels did not significantly influence the bioavailability of Clorazepate Dipotassium.

OVERDOSAGE

Overdosage is usually manifested by varying degrees of CNS depression ranging from slight sedation to coma. As in the management of overdosage with any drug, it should be borne in mind that multiple agents may have been taken.

The treatment of overdosage should consist of the general measures employed in the management of overdosage of any CNS depressant. Gastric evacuation either by the induction of emesis, lavage, or both, should be performed immediately. General supportive care, including frequent monitoring of the vital signs and close observation of the patient, is indicated. Hypotension, though rarely reported, may occur with large overdoses. In such cases the use of agents such as norepinephrine bitartrate injection, USP or metaraminol bitartrate injection, USP should be considered.

While reports indicate that individuals have survived overdoses of Clorazepate Dipotassium as high as 450 to 675 mg, these doses are not necessarily an accurate indication of the amount of drug absorbed since the time interval between ingestion and the institution of treatment was not always known. Sedation in varying degrees was the most common physiological manifestation of Clorazepate Dipotassium overdosage. Deep coma when it occurred was usually associated with the ingestion of other drugs in addition to Clorazepate Dipotassium.

Flumazenil, a specific benzodiazepine receptor antagonist, is indicated for the complete or partial reversal of the sedative effects of benzodiazepines and may be used in situations when an overdose with a benzodiazepine is known or suspected. Prior to the administration of flumazenil, necessary measures should be instituted to secure airway, ventilation, and intravenous access. Flumazenil is intended as an adjunct to, not as a substitute for, proper management of benzodiazepine overdose. Patients treated with flumazenil should be monitored for resedation, respiratory depression, and other residual benzodiazepine effects for an appropriate period after treatment. *The prescriber should be aware of a risk of seizure in association with flumazenil treatment, particularly in long-term benzodiazepine users and in cyclic antidepressant overdose.* The complete flumazenil package insert including *"Contraindications"*, *"Warnings"*, and *"Precautions"* should be consulted prior to use.

DOSAGE AND ADMINISTRATION

For the Symptomatic Relief of Anxiety: Clorazepate Dipotassium tablets are administered orally in divided doses. The usual daily dose is 30 mg. The dose should be adjusted gradually within the range of 15 to 60 mg daily in accordance with the response of the patient. In elderly or debilitated patients it is advisable to initiate treatment at a daily dose of 7.5 to 15 mg.

Clorazepate Dipotassium may also be administered in a single dose daily at bedtime; the recommended initial dose is 15 mg. After the initial dose, the response of the patient may require adjustment of subsequent dosage. Lower doses may be indicated in the elderly patient. Drowsiness may occur at the initiation of treatment and with dosage increment.

Clorazepate Dipotassium (22.5 mg) sustained-release tablets may be administered as a single dose every 24 hours. This tablet is intended as an alternate dosage form for the convenience of patients stabilized on a dose of 7.5 mg tablets three times a day. Clorazepate Dipotassium sustained-release tablets (22.5 mg) should not be used to initiate therapy.

Clorazepate Dipotassium (11.25 mg) sustained-release tablets may be administered as a single dose every 24 hours. This tablet is intended as an alternate dosage form for the convenience of patients stabilized on a dose of 3.75 mg tablets three times a day. Clorazepate Dipotassium sustained-release (11.25 mg) should not be used to initiate therapy.

For the Symptomatic Relief of Acute Alcohol Withdrawal: The following dosage schedule is recommended:

1st 24 hours (Day 1)	30 mg Clorazepate Dipotassium initially: followed by 30 to 60 mg in divided doses
2nd 24 hours (Day 2)	45 to 90 mg in divided doses
3rd 24 hours (Day 3)	22.5 to 45 mg in divided doses
Day 4	15 to 30 mg in divided doses

Thereafter, gradually reduce the daily dose to 7.5 to 15 mg. Discontinue drug therapy as soon as patient's condition is stable.

The maximum recommended total daily dose is 90 mg. Avoid excessive reductions in the total amount of drug administered on successive days.

As an Adjunct to Antiepileptic Drugs: In order to minimize drowsiness, the recommended initial dosages and dosage increments should not be exceeded.

Adults: The maximum recommended initial dose in patients over 12 years old is 7.5 mg three times a day. Dosage should be increased by no more than 7.5 mg every week and should not exceed 90 mg/day.

Children (9-12 years): The maximum recommended initial dose is 7.5 mg two times a day. Dosage should be increased by no more than 7.5 mg every week and should not exceed 60 mg/day.

Storage: Store below 77°F (25°C).

ANIMAL AND CLINICAL PHARMACOLOGY

Studies in rats and monkeys have shown a substantial difference between doses producing tranquilizing, sedative and toxic effects. In rats, conditioned avoidance response was inhibited at an oral dose of 10 mg/kg; sedation was induced at 32 mg/kg; the LD_{50} was 1320 mg/kg. In monkeys aggressive behavior was reduced at an oral dose of 0.25 mg/kg; sedation (ataxia) was induced at 7.5 mg/kg; the LD_{50} could not be determined because of the emetic effect of large doses, but the LD_{50} exceeds 1600 mg/kg.

Twenty-four dogs were given Clorazepate Dipotassium orally in a 22-month toxicity study; doses up to 75 mg/kg were given. Drug-related changes occurred in the liver; weight was increased and cholestasis with minimal hepatocellular damage was found, but lobular architecture remained well preserved.

Eighteen rhesus monkeys were given oral doses of Clorazepate Dipotassium from 3 to 36 mg/kg daily for 52 weeks. All treated animals remained similar to control animals. Although total leucocyte count remained within normal limits it tended to fall in the female animals on the highest doses.

Examination of all organs revealed no alterations attributable to Clorazepate Dipotassium. There was no damage to liver function or structure.

Reproduction Studies: Standard fertility, reproduction, and teratology studies were conducted in rats and rabbits. Oral doses in rats up to 150 mg/kg and in rabbits up to 15 mg/kg produced no abnormalities in the fetuses. Clorazepate Dipotassium did not alter the fertility indices or reproductive capacity of adult animals. As expected, the sedative effect of high doses interfered with care of the young by their mothers (see *"Usage in Pregnancy"*).

HOW SUPPLIED
TABLETS (C-IV): 3.75 MG

AVERAGE UNIT PRICE (AVAILABLE SIZES)		GENERIC A-RATED AVERAGE PRICE (GAAP)	
BRAND	$1.14		
GENERIC	$0.31	100s	$32.03
HCFA FUL (100s ea)	$0.04	500s	$140.15

BRAND/MANUFACTURER	NDC	SIZE	AWP
◆ **BRAND**			
► TRANXENE T-TAB: Abbott Pharm	00074-4389-13	100s	$111.76
	00074-4389-11	100s ud	$120.15
	00074-4389-53	500s	$547.66
◆ **GENERICS**			
GEN-XENE: Alra	51641-0242-03	30s	$11.02
Schein	00364-2201-01	100s	$20.00
GEN-XENE: Alra	51641-0242-01	100s	$22.16
Purepac	00228-2078-10	100s	$22.31
Geneva	00781-1865-01	100s	$22.60
Qualitest	00603-3004-21	100s	$24.18
URL	00677-1175-01	100s	$24.55
Rugby	00536-4940-01	100s	$24.56
Major	00904-3970-60	100s	$24.60
Goldline	00182-0009-01	100s	$24.65
Watson	52544-0363-01	100s	$24.95
Martec	52555-0986-01	100s	$24.95
Warner Chilcott	00047-0451-24	100s	$24.98
Moore,H.L.	00839-7335-06	100s	$25.18
Mason Dist	11845-0363-01	100s	$25.33
► Mylan	00378-0030-01	100s	$25.95
Parmed	00349-8960-01	100s	$31.46
Parmed	00349-8984-01	100s	$31.46
Barre	00472-0047-10	100s	$78.47
Aligen	00405-0050-01	100s	$78.47
UDL	51079-0633-20	100s ud	$34.16
GEN-XENE: Alra	51641-0242-11	100s ud	$57.64
Schein	00364-2201-05	500s	$54.25
Rugby	00536-4940-05	500s	$59.13
Major	00904-3970-40	500s	$69.45
GEN-XENE: Alra	51641-0242-05	500s	$94.60
Mason Dist	11845-0363-03	500s	$107.03

◆ RATED THERAPEUTICALLY EQUIVALENT; ◇ THERAPEUTIC EQUIVALENCE UNCONFIRMED; ○ UNRATED

BRAND/MANUFACTURER	NDC	SIZE	AWP
Geneva	00781-1865-05	500s	$107.35
Warner Chilcott	00047-0451-30	500s	$114.74
Goldline	00182-0009-05	500s	$115.00
Qualitest	00603-3004-28	500s	$115.12
Moore,H.L.	00839-7335-12	500s	$118.73
Watson	52544-0363-05	500s	$119.95
Martec	52555-0986-05	500s	$119.95
Mylan	00378-0030-05	500s	$120.95
Parmed	00349-8960-05	500s	$157.20
Barre	00472-0047-50	500s	$384.51
Aligen	00405-0050-02	500s	$384.51

TABLETS (C-IV): 7.5 MG

AVERAGE UNIT PRICE (AVAILABLE SIZES)		GENERIC A-RATED AVERAGE PRICE (GAAP)	
BRAND	$1.41	100s	$40.27
GENERIC	$0.38	500s	$171.26
HCFA FUL (100s ea)	$0.04		

BRAND/MANUFACTURER	NDC	SIZE	AWP
◆ BRAND			
➤ TRANXENE T-TAB: Abbott Pharm	00074-4390-13	100s	$139.10
	00074-4390-11	100s ud	$148.84
	00074-4390-53	500s	$681.20
◆ GENERICS			
GEN-XENE: Alra	51641-0243-03	30s	$13.12
Schein	00364-2202-01	100s	$25.75
GEN-XENE: Alra	51641-0243-01	100s	$27.10
Purepac	00228-2081-10	100s	$28.03
Geneva	00781-1866-01	100s	$28.15
Qualitest	00603-3005-21	100s	$31.00
Rugby	00536-4941-01	100s	$31.31
URL	00677-1176-01	100s	$31.35
Goldline	00182-0010-01	100s	$31.40
Warner Chilcott	00047-0452-24	100s	$31.40
Major	00904-3971-60	100s	$31.45
Watson	52544-0364-01	100s	$31.95
Martec	52555-0987-01	100s	$31.95
Moore,H.L.	00839-7336-06	100s	$31.98
Mason Dist	11845-0364-01	100s	$32.00
➤ Mylan	00378-0040-01	100s	$32.95
Parmed	00349-8961-01	100s	$39.27
Parmed	00349-8985-01	100s	$39.27
Barre	00472-0049-10	100s	$97.61
Aligen	00405-0051-01	100s	$97.61
UDL	51079-0634-20	100s ud	$38.46
GEN-XENE: Alra	51641-0243-11	100s ud	$75.62
Schein	00364-2202-05	500s	$65.75
Rugby	00536-4941-05	500s	$66.50
Major	00904-3971-40	500s	$69.10
GEN-XENE: Alra	51641-0243-05	500s	$118.70
Mason Dist	11845-0364-03	500s	$128.94
Purepac	00228-2081-50	500s	$134.83
Geneva	00781-1866-05	500s	$138.96
Warner Chilcott	00047-0452-30	500s	$143.50
Qualitest	00603-3005-28	500s	$144.12
Moore,H.L.	00839-7336-12	500s	$145.06
Goldline	00182-0010-05	500s	$150.00
Watson	52544-0364-05	500s	$151.95
Martec	52555-0987-05	500s	$151.95
➤ Mylan	00378-0040-05	500s	$152.95
Parmed	00349-8961-05	500s	$192.51
Barre	00472-0049-50	500s	$478.26
Aligen	00405-0051-02	500s	$478.26

TABLETS (C-IV): 15 MG

AVERAGE UNIT PRICE (AVAILABLE SIZES)		GENERIC A-RATED AVERAGE PRICE (GAAP)	
BRAND	$1.92	100s	$57.35
GENERIC	$0.56	500s	$196.62
HCFA FUL (100s ea)	$0.05		

BRAND/MANUFACTURER	NDC	SIZE	AWP
◆ BRAND			
➤ TRANXENE T-TAB: Abbott Pharm	00074-4391-13	100s	$188.64
	00074-4391-11	100s ud	$201.06
	00074-4391-53	500s	$924.31
◆ GENERICS			
GEN-XENE: Alra	51641-0244-03	30s	$21.68
Schein	00364-2203-01	100s	$33.50
GEN-XENE: Alra	51641-0244-01	100s	$39.00
Purepac	00228-2083-10	100s	$40.46
Qualitest	00603-3006-21	100s	$41.77
Geneva	00781-1867-01	100s	$41.88
Rugby	00536-5595-01	100s	$45.06
URL	00677-1177-01	100s	$45.14
Goldline	00182-0014-01	100s	$45.15
Moore,H.L.	00839-7337-06	100s	$45.35
Major	00904-3973-60	100s	$45.75
Warner Chilcott	00047-0453-24	100s	$46.19
Watson	52544-0365-01	100s	$46.95
Martec	52555-0988-01	100s	$46.95
Mylan	00378-0070-01	100s	$47.95
Mason Dist	11845-0365-01	100s	$47.99

TABLETS (C-IV): 11.25 MG

BRAND/MANUFACTURER	NDC	SIZE	AWP
◆ BRAND			
➤ TRANXENE-SD	00074-2699-13	100s	$295.74

TABLETS (C-IV): 22.5 MG

BRAND/MANUFACTURER	NDC	SIZE	AWP
◆ BRAND			
➤ TRANXENE	00074-2997-13	100s	$378.74

Clorfed *SEE* CHLORPHENIRAMINE MALEATE AND PSEUDOEPHEDRINE HYDROCHLORIDE

Clotrimazole

DESCRIPTION

Clotrimazole, is a synthetic antifungal agent having the chemical name [1-(o-Chloro-α,α-diphenylbenzyl)imidazole]; the empirical formula, $C_{22}H_{17}ClN_2$: a molecular weight of 344.84.

Clotrimazole is an odorless, white crystalline substance. It is practically insoluble in water, sparingly soluble in ether and very soluble in polyethylene glycol 400, ethanol and chloroform.

Each gram of Clotrimazole Cream contains:
Clotrimazole ....10 mg.

Each gram of Clotrimazole Lotion contains:
Clotrimazole ....10 mg.

Each mL of Clotrimazole Topical Solution contains:
Clotrimazole ....10 mg.

Each troche for topical oral administration contains:
Clotrimazole ....10 mg.

Each vaginal tablet contains:
Clotrimazole ....500 mg.

Following is its chemical structure:

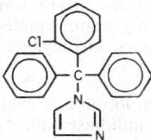

CLINICAL PHARMACOLOGY

Clotrimazole is a broad-spectrum antifungal agent that is used for the treatment of dermal infections caused by various species of pathogenic dermatophytes, yeasts, and *Malassezia furfur*. The primary action of Clotrimazole is against dividing and growing organisms.

In vitro, Clotrimazole exhibits fungistatic and fungicidal activity against isolates of *Trichophyton rubrum, Trichophyton mentagrophytes, Epidermophyton floccosum, Microsporum canis*, and *Candida* species, including *Candida albicans*. The action of Clotrimazole Troches is fungistatic at concentrations of drug up to 20 mcg/mL and may be fungicidal *in vitro* against *Candida albicans* and other species of the genus *Candida* at higher concentrations. At concentrations as low as 2-5 μg/mL Vaginal Clotrimazole exhibits fungicidal activity *in vitro* against *Candida albicans* and other species of the genus *Candida*. In general, the *in vitro* activity of Clotrimazole corresponds to that of tolnaftate and griseofulvin against the mycelia of dermatophytes (*Trichophyton, Microsporum*, and *Epidermophyton*), and to that of the polyenes (amphotericin B and nystatin) against budding fungi (*Candida*). Using an *in vivo* (mouse) and an *in vitro* (mouse kidney homogenate) testing system, Clotrimazole and miconazole were equally effective in preventing the growth of the pseudomycelia and mycelia of *Candida albicans*.

Strains of fungi having a natural resistance to Clotrimazole are rare. Only a single isolate of *Candida guilliermondi* had been reported to have primary resistance to Clotrimazole.

No single-step or multiple-step resistance to Clotrimazole has developed during successive passages of *Candida albicans* and *Trichophyton mentagrophytes*. No appreciable change in sensitivity was detected after successive passages of isolates of *C. albicans, C. krusei*, or *C pseudotropicalis* in liquid or solid media containing Clotrimazole. Also, resistance could not be developed in chemically induced mutant strains of polyene-resistant isolates of *C. albicans*. Slight, reversible resistance was noted in three isolates of *C. albicans* tested by one investigator. There is a single report that records the clinical emergence of a *C. albicans* strain with considerable resistance to flucytosine and miconazole, and with cross-resistance to Clotrimazole; the strain remained sensitive to nystatin and amphotericin B.

In studies of the mechanism of action, the minimum fungicidal concentration of Clotrimazole caused leakage of intracellular phosphorus compounds into the ambient medium with concomitant breakdown of cellular nucleic acids and accelerated potassium efflux. Both these events began rapidly and extensively after addition of the drug.

Clotrimazole appears to be well absorbed in humans following oral administration and is eliminated mainly as inactive metabolites. Following topical and vaginal administration, however, Clotrimazole appears to be minimally absorbed.

After oral administration of a 10 mg Clotrimazole troche to healthy volunteers, concentrations sufficient to inhibit most species of *Candida* persist in saliva for up to three hours following the approximately 30 minutes needed for a troche to dissolve. The long term persistence of drug in saliva appears to be related to the slow release of Clotrimazole from the oral mucosa to which the drug is apparently bound. Repetitive dosing at three hour intervals maintains salivary levels above the minimum inhibitory concentrations of most strains of *Candida:* however, the relationship between *in vitro* susceptibility of pathogenic fungi to Clotrimazole and prophylaxis or cure of infections in humans has not been established.

In another study, the mean serum concentrations were 4.98 ± 3.7 and 3.23 ± 1.4 nanograms/mL of Clotrimazole at 30 and 60 minutes, respectively, after administration as a troche.

Six hours after the application of radioactive Clotrimazole 1% cream and 1% solution onto intact and acutely inflamed skin, the concentration of Clotrimazole varied from 100 mcg/cm^3 in the stratum corneum to 0.5 to 1 mcg/cm^3 in the stratum reticulare, and 0.1 mcg/cm^3 in the subcutis. No measurable amount of radioactivity (≤ 0.001 mcg/mL) was found in the serum within 48 hours after application under occlusive dressing of 0.5 mL of the solution or 0.8 g of the cream. Only 0.5% or less of the applied radioactivity was excreted in the urine.

Following intravaginal administration of 100 mg ^{14}C-Clotrimazole vaginal tablets to nine adult females, an average peak serum level, corresponding to only 0.03 μg equivalents/mL of Clotrimazole, was reached one to two days after application. After intravaginal administration of 5 g of 1% ^{14}C-Clotrimazole vaginal cream containing 50 mg active drug, to five subjects (one with candidal colpitis), serum levels corresponding to approximately 0.01 μg equivalents/mL were reached between 8 and 24 hours after application.

Serum levels and levels in vaginal secretions of Clotrimazole were measured in six healthy volunteers who had one 500 mg vaginal tablet inserted. Although serum levels of Clotrimazole were higher than those in other volunteers given 100 mg and 200 mg vaginal tablets these levels did not exceed 10 nanograms/mL. It has been estimated that three to ten percent of a vaginal dose of Clotrimazole may be absorbed, but the drug rapidly and efficiently degrades to microbiologically inactive metabolites. The Clotrimazole concentrations remaining in vaginal secretions were still in the mg/mL range for 48 hours and in two of the six subjects at 72 hours.

The findings of high Clotrimazole concentrations in vaginal secretions for up to 72 hours and low concentrations in the serum suggest that nearly all the Clotrimazole given in the 500 mg vaginal tablet remains in the vagina for 48 hours, and in some cases 72 hours, in fungicidal concentrations.

INDICATIONS AND USAGE

Prescription Clotrimazole cream, lotion and solution 1% products are indicated for the topical treatment of candidiasis due to *Candida albicans* and tinea versicolor due to *Malassezia furfur.*

These formulations are also available as the Clotrimazole cream, lotion and solution 1% line of nonprescription products which are indicated for the topical treatment of the following dermal infections: tinea pedis, tinea cruris, and tinea corporis due to *Trichophyton rubrum, Trichophyton mentagrophytes, Epidermophyton floccosum,* and *Microsporum canis.*

Clotrimazole Troches are indicated for the local treatment of oropharyngeal candidiasis. The diagnosis should be confirmed by a KOH smear and/or culture prior to treatment. Clotrimazole Troches are also indicated prophylactically to reduce the incidence of oropharyngeal candidiasis in patients immunocompromised by conditions that include chemotherapy, radiotherapy, or steroid therapy utilized in the treatment of leukemia, solid tumors, or renal transplantation. There are no data from adequate and well-controlled trials to establish the safety and efficacy of this product for prophylactic use in patients immunocompromised by etiologies other than those listed in the previous sentence. (See "Dosage and Administration".)

Clotrimazole Vaginal Tablets are indicated for the local treatment of vulvovaginal candidiasis when one day therapy is felt warranted. In the case of severe vulvovaginitis due to candidiasis, longer antimycotic therapy is recommended. The diagnosis should be confirmed by KOH smears and/or cultures. Other pathogens commonly associated with vulvovaginitis, *Trichomonas* and *Gardnerella (Haemophilus) vaginalis,* should be ruled out by appropriate laboratory methods.

CONTRAINDICATIONS

Clotrimazole products are contraindicated in individuals who have shown hypersensitivity to any of their components.

WARNINGS

Clotrimazole products are not for ophthalmic use.

Clotrimazole Troches are not indicated for the treatment of systemic mycoses including systemic candidiasis.

PRECAUTIONS

General: If irritation or sensitivity develops with the use of Clotrimazole, treatment should be discontinued and appropriate therapy instituted.

Abnormal liver function tests have been reported in patients treated with Clotrimazole Troches; elevated SGOT levels were reported in about 15% of patients in the clinical trials. In most cases the elevations were minimal and it was

often impossible to distinguish effects of Clotrimazole from those of other therapy and the underlying disease (malignancy in most cases). Periodic assessment of hepatic function is advisable particularly in patients with pre-existing hepatic impairment.

Since patients must be instructed to allow each troche to dissolve slowly in the mouth in order to achieve maximum effect of the medication, they must be of such an age and physical and/or mental condition to comprehend such instructions.

If there is a lack of response to Clotrimazole Vaginal Tablets, appropriate microbiological studies should be repeated to confirm the diagnosis and rule out other pathogens before instituting another course of antimycotic therapy.

Information For Patients: This information is intended to aid in the safe and effective use of this medication. It is not a disclosure of all possible adverse or intended effects.

The patient should be advised to:

1. Use the medication for the full treatment time even though the symptoms may have improved. Notify the physician if there is no improvement after four weeks of treatment.

2. Inform the physician if the area of application shows signs of increased irritation (redness, itching, burning, blistering, swelling, oozing) indicative of possible sensitization.

3. Avoid sources of infection or reinfection.

Laboratory Tests: If there is lack of response to Clotrimazole, appropriate microbiological studies should be repeated to confirm the diagnosis and rule out other pathogens before instituting another course of antimycotic therapy.

Drug Interactions: Synergism of antagonism between Clotrimazole and nystatin, or amphotericin B, or flucytosine against strains of *C. albicans* has not been reported.

Carcinogenesis, Mutagenesis, Impairment of Fertility: An 18-month oral dosing study with Clotrimazole in rats has not revealed any carcinogenic effect.

No long term studies in animals have been performed to evaluate the carcinogenic potential of Clotrimazole Vaginal Tablets intravaginally. A long term study in rats (Wistar strains) where Clotrimazole was administered orally provided no indication of carcinogenicity.

In tests for mutagenesis, chromosomes of the spermatophores of Chinese hamsters which had been exposed to Clotrimazole were examined for structural changes during the metaphase. Prior to testing, the hamsters had received five *oral* Clotrimazole doses of 100 mg/kg body weight. The results of this study showed that Clotrimazole had no mutagenic effect.

Usage in Pregnancy: Pregnancy Category B (Topical and Vaginal Clotrimazole): The disposition of ^{14}C-Clotrimazole has been studied in humans and animals. Clotrimazole is very poorly absorbed following dermal application or intravaginal administration to humans. (See "Clinical Pharmacology".)

In clinical trials, use of vaginally applied Clotrimazole in pregnant women in their second and third trimesters has not been associated with ill effects. There are, however, no adequate and well-controlled studies in pregnant women during the first trimester of pregnancy.

Studies in pregnant rats with *intravaginal* doses up to 100 mg/kg have revealed no evidence of harm to the fetus due to Clotrimazole.

High *oral* doses to Clotrimazole in rats and mice ranging from 50 to 120 mg/kg resulted in embryotoxicity (possibly secondary to maternal toxicity), impairment of mating, decreased litter size and number of viable young and decreased pup survival to weaning. However, Clotrimazole was *not* teratogenic in mice, rabbits and rats at oral doses up to 200, 180 and 100 mg/kg, respectively. Oral absorption in the rat amounts to approximately 90% of the administered dose. Because animal reproduction studies are not always predictive of human response, this drug should be used only if clearly indicated during the first trimester of pregnancy.

Pregnancy Category C (Clotrimazole Troches): Clotrimazole given orally to mice from nine weeks before mating through weaning at a dose 120 times the human dose was associated with impairment of mating, decreased number of viable young, and decreased survival to weaning. No effects were observed at 60 times the human dose. When the drug was given to rats during a similar time period at 50 times the human dose, there was a slight decrease in the number of pups per litter and decreased pup viability.

There are no adequate and well controlled studies in pregnant women. Clotrimazole troches should be used during pregnancy only if the potential benefit justifies the potential risk to the fetus.

Nursing Mothers: It is not known whether this drug is excreted in human milk. Because many drugs are excreted in human milk, caution should be exercised when Clotrimazole is used by a nursing woman.

Pediatric Use: Safety and effectiveness in children have been established for Topical Clotrimazole when used as indicated and in the recommended dosage.

Safety and effectiveness of Clotrimazole Troches in children below the age of 3 years have not been established; therefore, its use in such patients is not recommended.

The safety and efficacy of the prophylactic use of Clotrimazole Troches in children have not been established.

ADVERSE REACTIONS

The following adverse reactions have been reported in connection with the use of Topical Clotrimazole: erythema, stinging, blistering, peeling, edema, pruritus, urticaria, burning, and general irritation of the skin.

◆ RATED THERAPEUTICALLY EQUIVALENT; ◇ THERAPEUTIC EQUIVALENCE UNCONFIRMED; ○ UNRATED

Abnormal liver function tests have been reported in patients treated with Clotrimazole Troches; elevated SGOT levels were reported in about 15% of patients in the clinical trials (See *"Precautions"* section). Nausea, vomiting, unpleasant mouth sensations and pruritus have also been reported with the use of the troche.

Of 297 patients in double-blind studies with the 500 mg vaginal tablet, 3 of 149 patients treated with active drug and 3 of 148 patients treated with placebo reported complaints during therapy that were possibly drug related. In the active drug group, vomiting occurred in one patient, vaginal soreness with coitus in another, and complaints of vaginal irritation, itching, burning and dyspareunia in the third patient. In the placebo group, clitoral irritation occurred in one patient and dysuria, described as remotely related to drug, in the other. A third patient in the placebo group developed bacterial vaginitis which the investigator classed as possibly related to drug.

Eighteen (1.6%) of the 1116 patients treated with Clotrimazole in other formulations in double blind studies reported complaints during therapy that were possibly drug-related. Mild burning occurred in six patients while other complaints such as skin rash, itching, vulval irritation, lower abdominal cramps and bloating, slight cramping, slight urinary frequency, and burning or irritation in the sexual partner, occurred rarely.

OVERDOSAGE
Acute overdosage with topical application of Clotrimazole is unlikely and would not be expected to lead to a life-threatening situation.

DOSAGE AND ADMINISTRATION
Clotrimazole Cream, Lotion, Topical Solution: Gently massage sufficient Clotrimazole into the affected and surrounding skin areas twice a day, in the morning and evening.

Clinical improvement, with relief of pruritus, usually occurs within the first week of treatment with Clotrimazole. If the patient shows no clinical improvement after four weeks of treatment with Clotrimazole, the diagnosis should be reviewed.

Clotrimazole Troches are administered only as a lozenge that must be slowly dissolved in the mouth. The recommended dose is one troche five times a day for fourteen consecutive days. Only limited data are available on the safety and effectiveness of the Clotrimazole Troche after prolonged administration; therefore, therapy should be limited to short term use, if possible.

For prophylaxis to reduce the incidence of oropharyngeal candidiasis in patients immunocompromised by conditions that include chemotherapy, radiotherapy, or steroid therapy utilized in the treatment of leukemia, solid tumors, or renal transplantation, the recommended dose is one troche three times daily for the duration of chemotherapy or until steroids are reduced to maintenance levels.

Clotrimazole Vaginal Tablets: The recommended dose is one tablet inserted intravaginally one time only, preferably at bedtime. In the event of treatment failure, that is, persistence of signs and symptoms of vaginitis after five days, other pathogens commonly responsible for vaginitis should be ruled out before instituting another course of antimycotic therapy.

Shake Clotrimazole Lotion well before using.
Store Topical Clotrimazole between 2° and 30°C (36° and 86°F).
Store Clotrimazole Troches below 86°F; avoid freezing.
Store Clotrimazole Vaginal Tablets below 86°F.

HOW SUPPLIED
CREAM: 1%

AVERAGE UNIT PRICE (AVAILABLE SIZES)			
BRAND	$1.85		
GENERIC	$0.40		

BRAND/MANUFACTURER	NDC	SIZE	AWP
◆ **BRAND**			
MYCELEX: Miles Pharm	00026-3098-22	1s	$14.45
	00026-3091-61	15 gm	$8.86
LOTRIMIN: Schering	00085-0613-02	15 gm	$10.42
MYCELEX: Miles Pharm	00026-3091-59	30 gm	$15.13
LOTRIMIN: Schering	00085-0613-05	30 gm	$17.68
MYCELEX-G: Miles Pharm	00026-3094-45	45 gm	$14.00
LOTRIMIN: Schering	00085-0613-04	45 gm	$21.44
MYCELEX-G: Miles Pharm	00026-3094-46	90 gm	$24.44
MYCELEX: Miles Pharm	00026-3091-67	90 gm	$25.30
LOTRIMIN: Schering	00085-0613-03	90 gm	$29.38
◆ **GENERICS**			
Taro	51672-1275-01	15 gm	$7.85
Taro	51672-1275-02	30 gm	$13.40
Taro	51672-1275-06	45 gm	$16.25
Taro	51672-1275-07	45 gm 2s	$22.25

LOTION: 1%

BRAND/MANUFACTURER	NDC	SIZE	AWP
○ **BRAND**			
LOTRIMIN: Schering	00085-0707-02	30 ml	$19.97

LOZENGE/TROCHE: 10 MG

BRAND/MANUFACTURER	NDC	SIZE	AWP
○ **BRAND**			
MYCELEX TROCHE: Miles Pharm	00026-3095-55	70s	$52.59
	00026-3095-38	70s ud	$56.18
	00026-3095-56	140s	$95.52

SOLUTION: 1%

AVERAGE UNIT PRICE (AVAILABLE SIZES)			
BRAND	$0.72		

BRAND/MANUFACTURER	NDC	SIZE	AWP
◆ **BRAND**			
MYCELEX: Miles Pharm	00026-3092-10	10 ml	$7.82
LOTRIMIN: Schering	00085-0182-02	10 ml	$9.17
MYCELEX: Miles Pharm	00026-3092-30	30 ml	$16.42
LOTRIMIN: Schering	00085-0182-04	30 ml	$19.08

TABLETS: 100 MG

BRAND/MANUFACTURER	NDC	SIZE	AWP
◆ **BRAND**			
MYCELEX-G: Miles Pharm	00026-3093-17	7s	$14.71

TABLETS: 500 MG

BRAND/MANUFACTURER	NDC	SIZE	AWP
○ **BRAND**			
MYCELEX-G: Miles Pharm	00026-3097-01	1s	$12.71

Cloxacillin Sodium

DESCRIPTION
Cloxacillin Sodium is an antibacterial agent of the isoxazolyl penicillin series. It is a penicillinase-resistant, acid-resistant semisynthetic penicillin suitable for oral administration.

Chemically, Cloxacillin Sodium is 4-Thia-1-azabicyclo [3.2.0]heptane-2-carboxylic acid, 6[[[3-(2-chlorophenyl)-5-methyl-4-isoxazolyl]-carbonyl]amino]-3,3-dimethyl-7-oxo-, monosodium salt, monohydrate, [2S-(2α5α,6β)]-; $C_{19}H_{17}ClN_3NaO_5S \cdot H_2O$. 475.88 [CAS-7081-44-9].

Following is its chemical structure:

CLINICAL PHARMACOLOGY
Microbiology: Penicillinase-resistant penicillins exert a bactericidal action against penicillin-susceptible microorganisms during the state of active multiplication. All penicillins inhibit the biosynthesis of the bacterial cell wall.

The drugs in this class are highly resistant to inactivation by staphylococcal penicillinase and are active against penicillinase-producing and nonpenicillinase-producing strains of *Staphylococcus aureus*. The penicillinase-resistant penicillins are active *in vitro* against a variety of other bacteria.

Susceptibility Plate Testing: Quantitative methods of susceptibility testing that require measurement of zone diameters or minimal inhibitory concentrations (MIC's) give the most precise estimates of antibiotic susceptibility. One such procedure has been recommended for use with discs to test susceptibility to this class of drugs.

Interpretations correlate diameters on the disc test with MIC values. A penicillinase-resistant class disc may be used to determine microbial susceptibility to cloxacillin, dicloxacillin, methicillin, nafcillin, and oxacillin. With this procedure, employing a 5 microgram methicillin sodium disc, a report from the laboratory of "susceptible" (zone of at least 14 mm) indicates that the infecting organism is likely to respond to therapy. A report of "resistant" (zone of less than 10 mm) indicates that the infecting organism is not likely to respond to therapy. A report of "intermediate susceptibility" (zone of 10 to 13 mm) suggests that the organism might be susceptible if high doses of the antibiotic are used, or if the infection is confined to tissues and fluids (eg, urine), in which high antibiotic levels are attained.

In general, all staphylococci should be tested against the penicillin G disc and against the methicillin disc. Routine methods of antibiotic susceptibility testing may fail to detect strains of organisms resistant to the penicillinase-resistant penicillins. For this reason, the use of large inocula and 48-hour incubation periods may be necessary to obtain accurate susceptibility studies with these antibiotics. Bacterial strains which are resistant to one of the penicillinase-resistant penicillins should be considered resistant to all of the drugs in the class.

Pharmacokinetics: Cloxacillin Sodium is resistant to destruction by acid. Absorption of Cloxacillin Sodium after oral administration is rapid but incomplete. Studies with an oral dose of 1 gram gave average serum levels at 60 minutes of 14.4 µg/mL. At four hours, average levels were 2 µ/mL. In one study, single oral doses of 500 mg produced peak serum concentrations of 7.5 to 14.4 µg/mL at 1 to 1.5 hours.

Once absorbed, Cloxacillin Sodium binds to serum protein, mainly albumin. The degree of protein binding reported varies with the method of study and the investigator, but generally has been found to be 95.2 ± 0.5%. Oral absorption of Cloxacillin is delayed when the drug is administered after meals.

Cloxacillin Sodium, with normal doses, has insignificant concentrations in the cerebrospinal and ascitic fluids. It is found in therapeutic concentrations in the pleural, bile, and amniotic fluids. Cloxacillin Sodium is rapidly excreted as unchanged drug in the urine by glomerular filtration and active tubular secretion.

INDICATIONS AND USAGE

The penicillinase-resistant penicillins are indicated in the treatment of infections caused by penicillinase-producing staphylococci which have demonstrated susceptibility to the drugs. Cultures and susceptibility tests should be performed initially to determine the causative organism and their sensitivity to the drug (see *"Clinical Pharmacology—Susceptibility Plate Testing"*).

The penicillinase-resistant penicillins may be used to initiate therapy in suspected cases of resistant staphylococcal infections prior to the availability of laboratory test results. The penicillinase-resistant penicillins should not be used in infections caused by organisms susceptible to penicillin G. If the susceptibility tests indicate that the infection is due to an organism other than a resistant staphylococcus, therapy should not be continued with a penicillinase-resistant penicillin.

CONTRAINDICATIONS

A history of a hypersensitivity (anaphylactic) reaction to any penicillin is a contraindication.

WARNINGS

Serious and occasionally fatal hypersensitivity (anaphylactic shock with collapse) reactions have occurred in patients receiving penicillin. The incidence of anaphylactic shock in all penicillin-treated patients is between 0.015 and 0.04 percent. Anaphylactic shock resulting in death has occurred in approximately 0.002 percent of the patients treated. Although anaphylaxis is more frequent following a parenteral administration, it has occurred in patients receiving oral penicillins.

When penicillin therapy is indicated, it should be initiated only after a comprehensive patient drug and allergy history has been obtained. If an allergic reaction occurs, the drug should be discontinued and the patient should receive supportive treatment, eg, artificial maintenance of ventilation, pressor amines, antihistamines, and corticosteroids. Individuals with a history of penicillin hypersensitivity may also experience allergic reactions when treated with a cephalosporin.

PRECAUTIONS

General: Penicillinase-resistant penicillins should generally not be administered to patients with a history of sensitivity to any penicillin.

Penicillin should be used with caution in individuals with histories of significant allergies and/or asthma. Whenever allergic reactions occur, penicillin should be withdrawn unless, in the opinion of the physician, the condition being treated is life-threatening and amenable only to penicillin therapy.

The oral route of administration should not be relied upon in patients with severe illness, or with nausea, vomiting, gastric dilation, cardiospasm, or intestinal hypermotility. Occasionally patients will not absorb therapeutic amounts of orally administered penicillin.

The use of antibiotics may result in overgrowth of nonsusceptible organisms. If new infections due to bacteria or fungi occur, the drug should be discontinued and appropriate measures taken.

Information for the Patient: Patients receiving penicillins should be given the following information and instructions by the physician:

1. Patients should be told that penicillin is an antibacterial agent which will work with the body's natural defenses to control certain types of infections. They should be told that the drug should not be taken if they have had an allergic reaction to any form of penicillin previously, and to inform the physician of any allergies or previous allergic reactions to any drugs they may have had (see *"Warnings"*).
2. Patients who have previously experienced an anaphylactic reaction to penicillin should be instructed to wear a medical identification tag or bracelet.
3. Because most antibacterial drugs taken by mouth are best absorbed on an empty stomach, patients should be directed, unless circumstances warrant otherwise, to take penicillin one hour before meals or two hours after eating (see *"Clinical Pharmacology—Pharmacokinetics"*).
4. Patients should be told to take the entire course of therapy prescribed, even if fever and other symptoms have stopped (see *"Precautions—General"*).
5. If any of the following reactions occur, stop taking your prescription and notify the physician: shortness of breath, wheezing, skin rash, mouth irritation, black tongue, sore throat, nausea, vomiting, diarrhea, fever, swollen joints, or any unusual bleeding or bruising (see *"Adverse Reactions"*).
6. Do not take any additional medications without physician approval, including non-prescription drugs such as antacids, laxatives, or vitamins.

Laboratory Tests: Bacteriologic studies to determine the causative organisms and their susceptibility to the penicillinase-resistant penicillins should be performed (see *"Clinical Pharmacology—Microbiology"*). In the treatment of suspected staphylococcal infections, therapy should be changed to another active agent if culture tests fail to demonstrate the presence of staphylococci.

Periodic assessment of organ system function including renal, hepatic, and hematopoietic should be made during prolonged therapy with the penicillinase-resistant penicillins.

Blood cultures, white blood cell, and differential cell counts should be obtained prior to initiation of therapy and at least weekly during therapy with penicillinase-resistant penicillins.

Periodic urinalysis, blood urea nitrogen, and creatinine determinations should be performed during therapy with the penicillinase-resistant penicillins and dosage alterations should be considered if these values become elevated. If any impairment of renal function is suspected or known to exist, a reduction in the total dosage should be considered and blood levels monitored to avoid possible neurotoxic reactions (see *"Dosage and Administration"*).

SGOT and SGPT values should be obtained periodically during therapy to monitor for possible liver function abnormalities.

Drug Interactions: Tetracycline, a bacteriostatic antibiotic, may antagonize the bactericidal effect of penicillin and concurrent use of these drugs should be avoided.

Carcinogenesis, Mutagenesis, Impairment of Fertility: No long-term animal studies have been conducted with these drugs.

Studies on reproduction (nafcillin) in rats and rabbits reveal no fetal or maternal abnormalities before conception and continuously through weaning (one generation).

Pregnancy Category B: Reproduction studies performed in the mouse, rat, and rabbit have revealed no evidence of impaired fertility or harm to the fetus due to the penicillinase-resistant penicillins. Human experience with the penicillins during pregnancy has not shown any positive evidence of adverse effects on the fetus. There are, however, no adequate or well-controlled studies in pregnant women showing conclusively that harmful effects of these drugs on the fetus can be excluded. Because animal reproduction studies are not always predictive of human response, this drug should be used during pregnancy only if clearly needed.

Nursing Mothers: Penicillins are excreted in breast milk. Caution should be exercised when penicillins are administered to a nursing woman.

Pediatric Use: Because of incompletely developed renal function in newborns, penicillinase-resistant penicillins (especially methicillin) may not be completely excreted, with abnormally high blood levels resulting. Frequent blood levels are advisable in this group with dosage adjustments when necessary. All newborns treated with penicillin should be monitored closely for clinical and laboratory evidence of toxic or adverse effects (see *"Dosage and Administration"*).

ADVERSE REACTIONS

Body as a Whole: The reported incidence of allergic reactions to penicillin ranges from 0.7 to 10 percent (see *"Warnings"*). Sensitization is usually the result of treatment but some individuals have had immediate reactions to penicillin when first treated. In such cases, it is thought that the patients may have had prior exposure to the drug via trace amounts present in milk and vaccines.

Two types of allergic reactions to penicillin are noted clinically, immediate and delayed.

Immediate reactions usually occur within 20 minutes of administration and range in severity from urticaria and pruritus to angioneurotic edema, laryngospasm, bronchospasm, hypotension, vascular collapse, and death. Such immediate anaphylactic reactions are very rare (see *"Warnings"*) and usually occur after parenteral therapy but have occurred in patients receiving oral therapy. Another type of immediate reaction, an accelerated reaction, may occur between 20 minutes and 48 hours after administration and may include urticaria, pruritus, and fever. Although laryngeal edema, laryngospasm, and hypotension occasionally occur, fatality is uncommon.

Delayed allergic reactions to penicillin therapy usually occur after 48 hours and sometimes as late as 2 to 4 weeks after initiation of therapy. Manifestations of this type of reaction include serum sickness-like symptoms (ie, fever, malaise, urticaria, myalgia, arthralgia, abdominal pain) and various skin rashes. Nausea, vomiting, diarrhea, stomatitis, black or hairy tongue, and other symptoms of gastrointestinal irritation may occur, especially during oral penicillin therapy.

Nervous System Reactions: Neurotoxic reactions similar to those observed with penicillin G may occur with large intravenous doses of the penicillinase-resistant penicillins especially in patients with renal insufficiency.

Urogenital Reactions: Renal tubular damage and interstitial nephritis have been associated with the administration of methicillin sodium and infrequently with the administration of nafcillin and oxacillin. Manifestations of this reaction may include rash, fever, eosinophilia, hematuria, proteinuria, and renal insufficiency. Methicillin-induced nephropathy does not appear to be dose-related and is generally reversible upon prompt discontinuation of therapy.

Metabolic Reactions: Agranulocytosis, neutropenia, and bone marrow depression have been associated with the use of methicillin sodium, nafcillin, oxacillin, and Cloxacillin. Hepatotoxicity, characterized by fever, nausea, and vomiting associated with abnormal liver function tests, mainly elevated SGOT levels, has been associated with the use of oxacillin and Cloxacillin.

DOSAGE AND ADMINISTRATION

The penicillinase-resistant penicillins are available for oral administration and for intramuscular and intravenous injection. The sodium salts of methicillin, oxacillin, and nafcillin may be administered parenterally and the sodium salts of Cloxacillin, dicloxacillin, oxacillin, and nafcillin are available for oral use.

Bacteriologic studies to determine the causative organisms and their sensitivity to the penicillinase-resistant penicillins should always be performed. Duration of therapy varies with the type and severity of infection as well as the overall condition of the patient, therefore, it should be determined by the clinical and bacteriological response of the patient. In severe staphylococcal infections, therapy with penicillinase-resistant penicillins should be continued for at least 14 days. Therapy should be continued for at least 48 hours after the patient has become afebrile, asymptomatic, and cultures are negative. The treatment of endocarditis and osteomyelitis may require a longer term of therapy.

Concurrent administration of the penicillinase-resistant penicillins and probenecid increases and prolongs serum penicillin levels. Probenecid decreases the apparent volume of distribution and slows the rate of excretion by competitively inhibiting renal tubular secretion of penicillin. Penicillin-probenecid therapy is generally limited to those infections where very high serum levels of penicillin are necessary.

Oral preparations of the penicillinase-resistant penicillins should not be used as initial therapy in serious, life-threatening infections (see *"Precautions—General"*). Oral therapy with the penicillinase-resistant penicillins may be used to follow-up the previous use of a parenteral agent as soon as the clinical condition warrants. For intramuscular gluteal injections, care should be taken to avoid sciatic nerve injury. With intravenous administration, particularly in elderly patients, care should be taken because of the possibility of thrombophlebitis.

RECOMMENDED DOSAGES FOR CLOXACILLIN SODIUM IN MILD TO MODERATE AND SEVERE INFECTIONS

Drug	Adults		Children	
	Mild to Moderate	Severe	Mild to Moderate	Severe
Cloxacillin	250 mg every 6 hours	500 mg or higher every 6 hours	50 mg/kg/day[a] in equally divided doses every 6 hours	100 mg/kg/day[a] or higher in equally divided doses every 6 hours

[a] Patients weighing less than 20 kg (44 lbs).

Dispense in a tight container, as defined by USP.

HOW SUPPLIED
CAPSULE: 250 MG

AVERAGE UNIT PRICE (AVAILABLE SIZES)		GENERIC A-RATED AVERAGE PRICE (GAAP)	
GENERIC	$0.35		
HCFA FUL (100s ea)	$0.22	100s	$34.87

BRAND/MANUFACTURER	NDC	SIZE	AWP
◆ GENERICS			
Raway	00686-3119-09	100s	$22.95
Apothecon	57783-5028-01	100s	$32.87
Warner Chilcott	00047-0949-24	100s	$34.15
Geneva	00781-2034-01	100s	$34.90
Moore,H.L.	00839-6436-06	100s	$35.49
Aligen	00405-4255-01	100s	$35.52
Goldline	00182-1358-01	100s	$36.50
CLOXAPEN: SK Beecham Pharm	00029-6250-30	100s	$36.60
URL	00677-0928-01	100s	$36.75
Rugby	00536-1130-01	100s	$36.83
Biocraft	00332-3119-09	100s	$37.96
Qualitest	00603-3029-21	100s	$37.96

CAPSULE: 500 MG

AVERAGE UNIT PRICE (AVAILABLE SIZES)		GENERIC A-RATED AVERAGE PRICE (GAAP)	
GENERIC	$0.65	100s	$64.99
HCFA FUL (100s ea)	$0.39		

BRAND/MANUFACTURER	NDC	SIZE	AWP
◆ GENERICS			
Raway	00686-3121-09	100s	$40.00
Qualitest	00603-3030-21	100s	$61.40
Warner Chilcott	00047-0950-24	100s	$62.60
Moore,H.L.	00839-6437-06	100s	$63.71
Goldline	00182-1359-01	100s	$64.00
URL	00677-0929-01	100s	$64.05
Rugby	00536-1140-01	100s	$64.12
Apothecon	57783-6038-01	100s	$65.57
Geneva	00781-2036-01	100s	$66.50
CLOXAPEN: SK Beecham Pharm	00029-6255-30	100s	$72.65
Biocraft	00332-3121-09	100s	$75.65
Aligen	00405-4256-01	100s	$79.63

POWDER FOR RECONSTITUTION: 125 MG/5 ML

AVERAGE UNIT PRICE (AVAILABLE SIZES)		GENERIC A-RATED AVERAGE PRICE (GAAP)	
BRAND	$0.11	100 ml	$5.50
GENERIC	$0.05	200 ml	$9.67
HCFA FUL (100 ml)	$0.05		
HCFA FUL (200 ml)	$0.05		

BRAND/MANUFACTURER	NDC	SIZE	AWP
◆ BRAND			
TEGOPEN: Apothecon	00015-7941-40	100 ml	$10.80
	00015-7941-64	200 ml	$20.89

BRAND/MANUFACTURER	NDC	SIZE	AWP
◆ GENERICS			
Major	00904-1619-04	100 ml	$4.90
Warner Chilcott	00047-2995-17	100 ml	$5.23
Goldline	00182-1720-70	100 ml	$5.35
Biocraft	00332-4159-32	100 ml	$5.43
Raway	00686-4159-32	100 ml	$5.50
Aligen	00405-2530-60	100 ml	$5.72
Rugby	00536-1110-82	100 ml	$6.38
Raway	00686-4159-36	200 ml	$7.75
Major	00904-1619-08	200 ml	$8.75
Goldline	00182-1720-73	200 ml	$9.40
Rugby	00536-1120-84	200 ml	$9.82
Warner Chilcott	00047-2995-20	200 ml	$10.46
Biocraft	00332-4159-36	200 ml	$10.49
Aligen	00405-2530-70	200 ml	$11.04

Clozapine

DESCRIPTION

Clozapine an atypical antipsychotic drug, is a tricyclic dibenzodiazepine derivative, 8-chloro-11-(4-methyl-1-piperazinyl)-5*H*-dibenzo [*b*,*e*] [1,4] diazepine.

Clozapine is a yellow crystalline powder, very slightly soluble in water.

Following is its chemical structure:

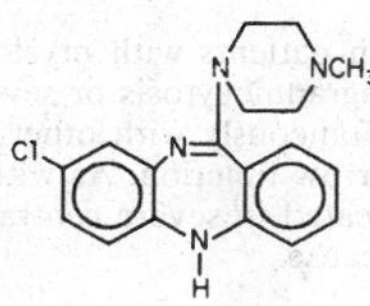

CLINICAL PHARMACOLOGY

PHARMACODYNAMICS

Clozapine is classified as an 'atypical' antipsychotic drug because its profile of binding to dopamine receptors and its effects on various dopamine mediated behaviors differ from those exhibited by more typical antipsychotic drug products. In particular, although Clozapine does interfere with the binding of dopamine at both D-1 and D-2 receptors, it does not induce catalepsy nor inhibit apomorphine-induced stereotypy. This evidence consistent with the view that Clozapine is preferentially more active at limbic than at striatal dopamine receptors, may explain the relative freedom of Clozapine from extrapyramidal side effects. Clozapine also acts as an antagonist at adrenergic, cholinergic, histaminergic and serotonergic receptors.

ABSORPTION, DISTRIBUTION, METABOLISM AND EXCRETION

In man Clozapine tablets (25 mg and 100 mg) are equally bioavailable relative to a Clozapine solution. Following a dosage of 100 mg b.i.d., the average steady state peak plasma concentration was 319 ng/mL (range: 102-771 ng/mL), occurring at the average of 2.5 hours (range: 1-6 hours) after dosing. The average minimum concentration at steady state was 122 ng/mL (range: 41-343 ng/mL), after 100 mg b.i.d. dosing. Food does not appear to affect the systemic bioavailability of Clozapine. Thus Clozapine may be administered with or without food.

Clozapine is approximately 95% bound to serum proteins. The interaction between Clozapine and other highly protein-bound drugs has not been fully evaluated but may be important. (See *"Precautions".*)

Clozapine is almost completely metabolized prior to excretion and only trace amounts of unchanged drug are detected in the urine and feces. Approximately 50% of the administered dose is excreted in the urine and 30% in the feces. The demethylated, hydroxylated and N-oxide derivatives are components in both urine and feces. Pharmacological testing has shown the desmethyl metabolite to have only limited activity, while the hydroxylated and N-oxide derivatives were inactive.

The mean elimination half-life of Clozapine after a single 75 mg dose was 8 hours (range: 4-12 hours), compared to a mean elimination half-life, after achieving steady state with 100 mg b.i.d. dosing, of 12 hours (range: 4-66 hours). A comparison of single-dose and multiple-dose administration of Clozapine showed that the elimination half-life increased significantly after multiple dosing relative to that after single-dose administration, suggesting the possibility of concentration dependent pharmacokinetics. However, at steady state, linearly dose-proportional changes with respect to AUC (area under the curve), peak and minimum Clozapine plasma concentrations were observed after administration of 37.5 mg, 75 mg, and 150 mg b.i.d.

HUMAN PHARMACOLOGY

In contrast to more typical antipsychotic drugs, Clozapine, therapy produces little or no prolactin elevation.

As is true of more typical antipsychotic drugs, clinical EEG studies have shown that Clozapine increases delta and theta activity and slows dominant alpha frequencies. Enhanced synchronization occurs, and sharp wave activity and spike and wave complexes may also develop. Patients on rare occasions may report an intensification of dream activity during Clozapine therapy. REM sleep was found to be increased to 85% of the total sleep time. In these patients, the onset of REM sleep occurred almost immediately after falling asleep.

INDICATIONS AND USAGE

Clozapine is indicated for the management of severely ill schizophrenic patients who fail to respond adequately to standard antipsychotic drug treatment. Because of the significant risk of agranulocytosis and seizure associated with its use, Clozapine should be used only in patients who have failed to respond adequately to treatment with appropriate courses of standard antipsychotic drugs, either because of insufficient effectiveness or the inability to achieve an effective dose due to intolerable adverse effects from those drugs. (See *"Warning"*.)

The effectiveness of Clozapine in a treatment resistant schizophrenic population was demonstrated in a 6-week study comparing Clozapine and chlorpromazine. Patients meeting DSM-III criteria for schizophrenia and having a mean BPRS total score of 61 were demonstrated to be treatment resistant by history and by open, prospective treatment with haloperidol before entering into the double-blind phase of the study. The superiority of Clozapine to chlorpromazine was documented in statistical analyses employing both categorical and continuous measures of treatment effect.

Because of the significant risk of agranulocytosis and seizure, events which both present a continuing risk over time, the extended treatment of patients failing to show an acceptable level of clinical response should ordinarily be avoided. In addition, the need for continuing treatment in patients exhibiting beneficial clinical responses should be periodically re-evaluated.

UNLABELED USES
Clozapine is used alone or as adjunct in the treatment of bipolar disorder, including manic depressive episodes, and in the treatment of Parkinson's disease.

CONTRAINDICATIONS

Clozapine is contraindicated in patients with myeloproliferative disorders, or a history of Clozapine induced agranulocytosis or severe granulocytopenia. Clozapine should not be used simultaneously with other agents having a well-known potential to suppress bone marrow function. As with more typical antipsychotic drugs, Clozapine is contraindicated in severe central nervous system depression or comatose states from any cause.

WARNINGS
GENERAL
BECAUSE OF THE SIGNIFICANT RISK OF AGRANULOCYTOSIS, A POTENTIALLY LIFE-THREATENING ADVERSE EVENT (SEE *Following*), CLOZAPINE SHOULD BE RESERVED FOR USE IN THE TREATMENT OF SEVERELY ILL SCHIZOPHRENIC PATIENTS WHO FAIL TO SHOW AN ACCEPTABLE RESPONSE TO ADEQUATE COURSES OF STANDARD ANTIPSYCHOTIC DRUG TREATMENT, EITHER BECAUSE OF INSUFFICIENT EFFECTIVENESS OR THE INABILITY TO ACHIEVE AN EFFECTIVE DOSE DUE TO INTOLERABLE ADVERSE EFFECTS FROM THOSE DRUGS. CONSEQUENTLY, BEFORE INITIATING TREATMENT WITH CLOZAPINE IT IS STRONGLY RECOMMENDED THAT A PATIENT BE GIVEN AT LEAST 2 TRIALS, EACH WITH A DIFFERENT STANDARD ANTIPSYCHOTIC DRUG PRODUCT, AT AN ADEQUATE DOSE, AND FOR AN ADEQUATE DURATION.

PATIENTS WHO ARE BEING TREATED WITH CLOZAPINE MUST HAVE A BASELINE WHITE BLOOD CELL (WBC) AND DIFFERENTIAL COUNT BEFORE INITIATION OF TREATMENT, AND A WBC COUNT EVERY WEEK THROUGHOUT TREATMENT, AND FOR 4 WEEKS AFTER THE DISCONTINUATION OF CLOZAPINE. CLOZAPINE IS AVAILABLE ONLY THROUGH A DISTRIBUTION SYSTEM THAT ENSURES WEEKLY WBC TESTING PRIOR TO DELIVERY OF THE NEXT WEEK'S SUPPLY OF MEDICATION.

AGRANULOCYTOSIS
AGRANULOCYTOSIS, DEFINED AS A GRANULOCYTE COUNT (POLYS — BANDS) OF LESS THAN 500/mm^3 HAS BEEN ESTIMATED TO OCCUR IN ASSOCIATION WITH CLOZAPINE USE AT A CUMULATIVE INCIDENCE AT 1 YEAR OF APPROXIMATELY 1.3%, BASED ON THE OCCURRENCE OF 15 US CASES OUT OF 1743 PATIENTS EXPOSED TO CLOZAPINE DURING ITS CLINICAL TESTING PRIOR TO DOMESTIC MARKETING.

ALL OF THESE CASES OCCURRED AT A TIME WHEN THE NEED FOR CLOSE MONITORING OF WBC COUNTS WAS ALREADY RECOGNIZED. THIS REACTION COULD PROVE FATAL IF NOT DETECTED EARLY AND THERAPY INTERRUPTED. OF THE 149 CASES OF AGRANULOCYTOSIS REPORTED WORLDWIDE IN ASSOCIATION WITH CLOZAPINE USE AS OF DECEMBER 31, 1989, 32% WERE FATAL. HOWEVER, FEW OF THESE DEATHS OCCURRED SINCE 1977, AT WHICH TIME THE KNOWLEDGE OF CLOZAPINE INDUCED AGRANULOCYTOSIS BECAME MORE WIDESPREAD, AND CLOSE MONITORING OF WBC COUNTS MORE WIDELY PRACTICED. NEVERTHELESS, IT IS UNKNOWN AT PRESENT WHAT THE CASE FATALITY RATE WILL BE FOR CLOZAPINE INDUCED AGRANULOCYTOSIS, DESPITE STRICT ADHERENCE TO THE RECOMMENDATION FOR WEEKLY MONITORING OF WBC COUNTS. IN THE US, UNDER A WEEKLY WBC MONITORING SYSTEM IN PREMARKETING STUDIES AND IN POSTMARKETING EXPERIENCE WITH CLOZAPINE THERE HAVE BEEN 68 CASES OF AGARANULOCYTOSIS AND ONE ASSOCIATED FATALITY AS OF JANUARY 1, 1991.

BECAUSE OF THE SUBSTANTIAL RISK OF AGRANULOCYTOSIS IN ASSOCIATION WITH CLOZAPINE USE, WHICH MAY PERSIST OVER AN EXTENDED PERIOD OF TIME, PATIENTS MUST HAVE A BLOOD SAMPLE DRAWN FOR A WBC COUNT BEFORE INITIATION OF TREATMENT WITH CLOZAPINE AND MUST HAVE SUBSEQUENT WBC COUNTS DONE AT LEAST WEEKLY FOR THE DURATION OF THERAPY, AS WELL AS FOR 4

WEEKS THEREAFTER. THE DISTRIBUTION OF CLOZAPINE IS CONTINGENT UPON PERFORMANCE OF THE REQUIRED BLOOD TESTS.

TREATMENT SHOULD NOT BE INITIATED IF THE WBC COUNT IS LESS THAN 3500/mm^3, OR IF THE PATIENTS HAS A HISTORY OF A MYELOPROLIFERATIVE DISORDER, OR PREVIOUS CLOZAPINE INDUCED AGRANULOCYTOSIS OR GRANULOCYTOPENIA. PATIENTS SHOULD BE ADVISED TO REPORT IMMEDIATELY THE APPEARANCE OF LETHARGY, WEAKNESS, FEVER, SORE THROAT OR ANY OTHER SIGNS OF INFECTION. IF, AFTER THE INITIATION OF TREATMENT, THE TOTAL WBC COUNT HAS DROPPED BELOW 3500/mm^3 OR IT HAS DROPPED BY A SUBSTANTIAL AMOUNT FROM BASELINE, EVEN IF THE COUNT IS ABOVE 3500/ mm^3, OR IF IMMATURE FORMS ARE PRESENT, A REPEAT WBC COUNT AND A DIFFERENTIAL COUNT SHOULD BE DONE. IF SUBSEQUENT WBC COUNTS AND THE DIFFERENTIAL COUNT REVEAL A TOTAL WBC COUNT BETWEEN 3000 AND 3500/mm^3 AND A GRANULOCYTE COUNT ABOVE 1500/ mm^3, TWICE WEEKLY WBC COUNTS AND DIFFERENTIAL COUNTS SHOULD BE PERFORMED.

IF THE TOTAL WBC COUNT FALLS BELOW 3000/mm^3 OR THE GRANULOCYTE COUNT BELOW 15000/mm^3, CLOZAPINE THERAPY SHOULD BE INTERRUPTED, WBC COUNT AND DIFFERENTIAL SHOULD BE PERFORMED DAILY, AND PATIENTS SHOULD BE CAREFULLY MONITORED FOR FLU-LIKE SYMPTOMS OR OTHER SYMPTOMS SUGGESTIVE OF INFECTION. CLOZAPINE THERAPY MAY BE RESUMED IF NO SYMPTOMS OF INFECTION DEVELOP, AND IF THE TOTAL WBC COUNT RETURNS TO LEVELS ABOVE 3000/mm^3 AND THE GRANULOCYTE COUNT RETURNS TO LEVELS ABOVE 1500/mm^3. HOWEVER, IN THIS EVENT, TWICE-WEEKLY WBC COUNTS AND DIFFERENTIAL COUNTS SHOULD CONTINUE UNTIL TOTAL WBC COUNTS RETURN TO LEVELS ABOVE 3500/mm^3.

IF THE TOTAL WBC COUNT FALLS BELOW 2000/mm^3 OR THE GRANULOCYTE COUNT FALLS BELOW 1000/mm^3, BONE MARROW ASPIRATION SHOULD BE CONSIDERED TO ASCERTAIN GRANULOPOIETIC STATUS. PROTECTIVE ISOLATION WITH CLOSE OBSERVATION MAY BE INDICATED IF GRANULOPOIESIS IS DETERMINED TO BE DEFICIENT. SHOULD EVIDENCE OF INFECTION DEVELOP, THE PATIENT SHOULD HAVE APPROPRIATE CULTURES PERFORMED AND AN APPROPRIATE ANTIBIOTIC REGIMEN INSTITUTED.

PATIENTS WHOSE TOTAL WBC COUNTS FALL BELOW 2000/mm^3, OR GRANULOCYTE COUNTS BELOW 1000/mm^3 DURING CLOZAPINE THERAPY SHOULD HAVE DAILY WBC COUNT AND DIFFERENTIAL. THESE PATIENTS SHOULD NOT BE RE-CHALLENGED WITH CLOZAPINE. PATIENTS DISCONTINUED FROM CLOZAPINE THERAPY DUE TO SIGNIFICANT WBC SUPPRESSION HAVE BEEN FOUND TO DEVELOP AGRANULOCYTOSIS UPON RE-CHALLENGE, OFTEN WITH A SHORTER LATENCY ON RE-EXSPOSURE. TO REDUCE THE CHANCES OF RE-CHALLENGE OCCURRING IN PATIENTS WHO HAVE EXPERIENCED SIGNIFICANT BONE MARROW SUPPRESSION DURING CLOZAPINE THERAPY, A SINGLE, NATIONAL MASTER FILE WILL BE MAINTAINED CONFIDENTIALLY.

EXCEPT FOR EVIDENCE OF SIGNIFICANT BONE MARROW SUPPRESSION DURING INITIAL CLOZAPINE THERAPY, THERE ARE NO ESTABLISHED RISK FACTORS, BASED ON WORLD-WIDE EXPERIENCE, FOR THE DEVELOPMENT OF AGRANULOCYTOSIS IN ASSOCIATION WITH CLOZAPINE USE. HOWEVER, A DISPROPORTIONATE NUMBER OF THE US CASES OF AGRANULOCYTOSIS OCCURRED IN PATIENTS OF JEWISH BACKGROUND COMPARED TO THE OVERALL PROPORTION OF SUCH PATIENTS EXPOSED DURING DOMESTIC DEVELOPEMENT OF CLOZAPINE. MOST OF THE US CASES OCCURED WITHIN 4-10 WEEKS OF EXPOSURE, BUT NEITHER DOSE NOR DURATION IS A RELIABLE PREDICTOR OF THIS PROBLEM. NO PATIENT CHARACTERISTICS HAVE BEEN CLEARLY LINKED TO THE DEVELOPMENT OF AGRANULOCYTOSIS IN ASSOCIATION WITH CLOZAPINE USE, BUT AGRANULOCYTOSIS ASSOCIATED WITH OTHER ANTIPSYCHOTIC DRUGS HAS BEEN REPORTED TO OCCUR WITH A GREATER FREQUENCY IN WOMEN, THE ELDERLY AND IN PATIENTS WHO ARE CACHECTIC OR HAVE SERIOUS UNDERLYING MEDICAL ILLNESS; SUCH PATIENTS MAY ALSO BE AT PARTICULAR RISK WITH CLOZAPINE.

TO REDUCE THE RISK OF AGRANULOCYTOSIS DEVELOPING UNDETECTED, CLOZAPINE IS AVAILABLE ONLY THROUGH A DISTRIBUTION SYSTEM THAT ENSURES WEEKLY WBC TESTING PRIOR TO DELIVERY OF THE NEXT WEEK'S SUPPLY OF MEDICATION.

SEIZURES
SEIZURE HAS BEEN ESTIMATED TO OCCUR IN ASSOCIATION WITH CLOZAPINE USE AT A CUMULATIVE INCIDENCE AT ONE YEAR OF APPROXIMATELY 5%, BASED ON THE OCCURRENCE OF ONE OR MORE

SEIZURES IN 61 OF 1743 PATIENTS EXPOSED CLOZAPINE DURING ITS CLINICAL TESTING PRIOR TO DOMESTIC MARKETING (I.E., A CRUDE RATE OF 3.5%). DOSE APPEARS TO BE AN IMPORTANT PREDICTOR OF SEIZURE, WITH A GREATER LIKELIHOOD OF SEIZURE AT THE HIGHER CLOZAPINE DOSES USED.

CAUTION SHOULD BE USED IN ADMINISTERING CLOZAPINE TO PATIENTS HAVING A HISTORY OF SEIZURES OR OTHER PREDISPOSING FACTORS. BECAUSE OF THE SUBSTANTIAL RISK OF SEIZURE ASSOCIATED WITH CLOZAPINE USE, PATIENTS SHOULD BE ADVISED NOT TO ENGAGE IN ANY ACTIVITY WHERE SUDDEN LOSS OF CONSCIOUSNESS COULD CAUSE SERIOUS RISK TO THEMSELVES OR OTHERS, E.G., THE OPERATION OF COMPLEX MACHINERY, DRIVING AN AUTOMOBILE, SWIMMING, CLIMBING, ETC.

ADVERSE CARDIOVASCULAR AND RESPIRATORY EFFECTS

ORTHOSTATIC HYPOTENSION WITH OR WITHOUT SYNCOPE CAN OCCUR WITH CLOZAPINE TREATMENT AND MAY REPRESENT A CONTINUING RISK IN SOME PATIENTS. RARELY (APPROXIMATELY 1 CASE PER 3,000 PATIENTS), COLLAPSE CAN BE PROFOUND AND BE ACCOMPANIED BY RESPIRATORY AND/OR CARDIAC ARREST. ORTHOSTATIC HYPOTENSION IS MORE LIKELY TO OCCUR DURING INITIAL TITRATION IN ASSOCIATION WITH RAPID DOSE ESCALATION AND MAY EVEN OCCUR ON FIRST DOSE. IN ONE REPORT, INITIAL DOSES AS LOW AS 12.5 mg WERE ASSOCIATED WITH COLLAPSE AND RESPIRATORY ARREST. WHEN RESTARTING PATIENTS WHO HAVE HAD EVEN A BRIEF INTERVAL OFF CLOZAPINE, I.E., 2 DAYS OR MORE SINCE THE LAST DOSE, IT IS RECOMMENDED THAT TREATMENT BE REINITIATED WITH ONE-HALF OF A 25 mg TABLET (12.5 mg) ONCE OR TWICE DAILY (SEE *DOSAGE AND ADMINISTRATION*).

SOME OF THE CASES OF COLLAPSE/RESPIRATORY ARREST/CARDIAC ARREST DURING INITIAL TREATMENT OCCURRED IN PATIENTS WHO WERE BEING ADMINISTERED BENZODIAZEPINES; SIMILAR EVENTS HAVE BEEN REPORTED IN PATIENTS TAKING OTHER PSYCHOTROPIC DRUGS OR EVEN CLOZAPINE BY ITSELF. ALTHOUGH IT HAS NOT BEEN ESTABLISHED THAT THERE IS AN INTERACTION BETWEEN CLOZAPINE AND BENZODIAZEPINES OR OTHER PSYCHOTROPICS, CAUTION IS ADVISED WHEN CLOZAPINE IS INITIATED IN PATIENTS TAKING A BENZODIAZEPINE OR ANY OTHER PSYCHOTROPIC DRUG.

Tachycardia, which may be sustained, has also been observed in approximately 25% of patients taking Clozapine with patients having an average increase in pulse rate of 10-15 bpm. The sustained tachycardia is not simply a reflex response to hypotension, and is present in all positions monitored. Either tachycardia or hypotension may pose a serious risk for an individual with compromised cardiovascular function.

A minority of Clozapine treated patients experience ECG repolarization changes similar to those seen with other antipsychotic drugs, including S-T segment depression and flattening or inversion of T waves, which all normalize after discontinuation of Clozapine. The clinical significance of these changes is unclear. However, in clinical trials with Clozapine, several patients experienced significant cardiac events, including ischemic changes, myocardial infarction, nonfatal arrhythmias and sudden unexplained death. In addition there have been postmarketing reports of congestive heart failure and myocarditis in association with Clozapine use. Causality assessment was difficult in many of these cases because of serious preexisting cardiac disease and plausible alternative causes. Rare instances of sudden, unexplained death have been reported in psychiatric patients, with or without associated antipsychotic drug treatment, and the relationship of these events to antipsychotic drug use is unknown.

Clozapine should be used with caution in patients with known cardiovascular and/or pulmonary disease, and the recommendation for gradual titration of dose should be carefully observed.

NEUROLEPTIC MALIGNANT SYNDROME (NMS)

A potentially fatal symptom complex sometimes referred to as Neuroleptic Malignant Syndrome (NMS) has been reported in association with antipsychotic drugs. Clinical manifestations of NMS are hyperpyrexia, muscle rigidity, altered mental status and evidence of autonomic instability (irregular pulse or blood pressure, tachycardia, diaphoresis, and cardiac dysrhythmias).

The diagnostic evaluation of patients with this syndrome is complicated. In arriving at a diagnosis, it is important to identify cases where the clinical presentation includes both serious medical illness (e.g., pneumonia, systemic infection, etc.) and untreated or inadequately treated extrapyramidal signs and symptoms (EPS). Other important considerations in the differential diagnosis include central anticholinergic toxicity, heat stroke, drug fever and primary central nervous system (CNS) pathology.

The management of NMS should include 1) immediate discontinuation of antipsychotic drugs and other drugs not essential to concurrent therapy, 2) intensive symptomatic treatment and medical monitoring, and 3) treatment of any concomitant serious medical problems for which specific treatments are available. There is no general agreement about specific pharmacological treatment regimens for uncomplicated NMS.

If a patient requires antipsychotic drug treatment after recovery from NMS, the potential reintroduction of drug therapy should be carefully considered. The patient should be carefully monitored, since recurrences of NMS have been reported.

There have been several reported cases of NMS in patients receiving Clozapine usually in combination with lithium or other CNS-active agents.

TARDIVE DYSKINESIA

A syndrome consisting of potentially irreversible, involuntary, dyskinetic movements may develop in patients treated with antipsychotic drugs. Although the prevalence of the syndrome appears to be highest among the elderly, especially elderly women, it is impossible to rely upon prevalence estimates to predict, at the inception of treatment, which patients are likely to develop the syndrome.

There are several reasons for predicting that Clozapine may be different from other antipsychotic drugs in its potential for inducing tardive dyskinesia, including the preclinical finding that it has a relatively weak dopamine blocking effect and the clinical finding of a virtual absence of certain acute extrapyramidal symptoms, e.g. dystonia. A few cases of tardive dyskinesia have been reported in patients on Clozapine who had been previously treated with other antipsychotic agents, so that a causal relationship cannot be established. There have been no reports of tardive dyskinesia directly attributable to Clozapine alone. Nevertheless, it cannot be concluded, without more extended experience, that Clozapine is incapable of inducing this syndrome.

Both the risk of developing the syndrome and the likelihood that it will become irreversible are believed to increase as the duration of treatment and the total cumulative dose of antipsychotic drugs administered to the patient increase. However, the syndrome can develop, although much less commonly, after relatively brief treatment periods at low doses. There is no known treatment for established cases of tardive dyskinesia, although the syndrome may remit, partially or completely, if antipsychotic drug treatment is withdrawn. Antipsychotic drug treatment, itself, however, may suppress (or partially suppress) the signs and symptoms of the syndrome and thereby may possibly mask the underlying process. The effect that symptom suppression has upon the long-term course of the syndrome is unknown.

Given these considerations, Clozapine should be prescribed in a manner that is most likely to minimize the occurrence of tardive dyskinesia. As with any antipsychotic drug, chronic Clozapine use should be reserved for patients who appear to be obtaining substantial benefit from the drug. In such patients, the smallest dose and the shortest duration of treatment should be sought. The need for continued treatment should be reassessed periodically.

If signs and symptoms of tardive dyskinesia appear in a patient on Clozapine drug discontinuation should be considered. However, some patients may require treatment with Clozapine despite the presence of the syndrome.

PRECAUTIONS
GENERAL

Because of the significant risk of agranulocytosis and seizure, both of which present a continuing risk over time, the extended treatment of patients failing to show an acceptable level of clinical response should ordinarily be avoided. In addition, the need for continuing treatment in patients exhibiting beneficial clinical responses should be periodically re-evaluated.

The mechanism Clozapine induced agranulocytosis is unknown: nonetheless, the possibility that causative factors may interact synergistically to increase the risk and/or severity of bone marrow suppression warrants consideration. Therefore, Clozapine should not be used with other agents having a well-known potential to suppress bone marrow function.

FEVER

During Clozapine therapy, patients may experience transient temperature elevations above 100.4°F (38°C), with the peak incidence within the first 3 weeks of treatment. While this fever is generally benign and self limiting, it may necessitate discontinuing patients from treatment. On occasion, there may be an associated increase or decrease in WBC count. Patients with fever should be carefully evaluated to rule out the possibility of an underlying infectious process or the development of agranulocytosis. In the presence of high fever, the possibility of Neuroleptic Malignant Syndrome (NMS) must be considered. There have been several reports of NMS in patients receiving Clozapine usually in combination with lithium or other CNS-active drugs (see *"Neuroleptic Malignant Syndrome [NMS]"*, under *"Warnings"*).

ANTICHOLINERGIC TOXICITY

Clozapine has very potent anticholinergic effects and great care should be exercised in using this drug in the presence of prostatic enlargement or narrow angle glaucoma.

INTERFERENCE WITH COGNITIVE AND MOTOR PERFORMANCE

Because of initial sedation, Clozapine may impair mental and/or physical abilities, especially during the first few days of therapy. The recommendations for gradual dose escalation should be carefully adhered to, and patients cautioned about activities requiring alertness.

USE IN PATIENTS WITH CONCOMITANT ILLNESS

Clinical experience with Clozapine in patients with concomitant systemic diseases is limited. Nevertheless, caution is advisable in using Clozapine in patients with hepatic, renal or cardiac disease.

INFORMATION FOR PATIENTS

Physicians are advised to discuss the following issues with patients for whom they prescribe Clozapine:

—Patients who are to receive Clozapine should be warned about the significant risk of developing agranulocytosis. They should be informed that weekly blood tests are required to monitor for the occurrence of agranulocytosis, and that Clozapine tablets will be made available only through a special program designed to ensure the required blood monitoring. Patients should be advised to report immediately the appearance of lethargy, weakness, fever, sore throat, malaise, mucous membrane ulceration or other possible signs of infection. Particular attention should be paid to any flu-like complaints or other symptoms that might suggest infection.

—Patients should be informed of the significant risk of seizure during Clozapine treatment, and they should be advised to avoid driving and any other potentially hazardous activity while taking Clozapine.

—Patients should be advised of the risk of orthostatic hypotension, especially during the period of initial dose titration.

—Patients should be informed that if they stop taking Clozapine for more than 2 days, they should not restart their medication at the same dosage, but should contact their physician for dosing instructions.

—Patients should notify their physician if they are taking, or plan to take, any prescription or over-the-counter drugs or alcohol.

—Patients should notify their physician if they become pregnant or intend to become pregnant during therapy.

—Patients should not breast feed an infant if they are taking Clozapine.

DRUG INTERACTIONS

The risks of using Clozapine in combination with other drugs have not been systematically evaluated.

The mechanism Clozapine-induced agranulocytosis is unknown: nonetheless, the possibility that causative factors may interact synergistically to increase the risk and/or severity or bone marrow suppression warrants consideration. Therefore, Clozapine should not be used with other agents having a well-known potential to suppress bone marrow function.

Given the primary CNS effects of Clozapine, caution is advised in using it concomitantly with other CNS-active drugs.

Orthostatic hypotension in patients taking Clozapine can, in rare cases (approximately 1 case per 3,000 patients), be accompanied by profound collapse and respiratory and/or cardiac arrest. Some of the cases of collapse/respiratory arrest/cardiac arrest during initial treatment occurred in patients who were being administered benzodiazepines; similar events have been reported in patients taking other psychotropic drugs or even Clozapine by itself. Although it has not been established that there is an interaction between Clozapine and benzodiazepines or other psychotropics, caution is advised when Clozapine is initiated in patients taking a benzodiazepine or any other psychotropic drug.

Because Clozapine is highly bound to serum protein, the administration of Clozapine to a patient taking another drug which is highly bound to protein (e.g., warfarin, digitoxin) may cause an increase in plasma concentrations of these drugs, potentially resulting in adverse effects. Conversely, adverse effects may result from displacement of protein-bound Clozapine by other highly bound drugs.

Cimetidine may increase plasma levels of Clozapine, potentially resulting in adverse effects. Phenytoin may decrease Clozapine plasma levels, resulting in a decrease in effectiveness of a previously effective Clozapine dose.

Clozapine may also potentiate the hypotensive effects of antihypertensive drugs and the anticholinergic effects of atropine-type drugs. The administration of epinephrine should be avoided in the treatment of drug-induced hypotension because of a possible reverse epinephrine effect.

CARCINOGENESIS, MUTAGENESIS, IMPAIRMENT OF FERTILITY

No carcinogenic potential was demonstrated in long-term studies in mice and rats at doses approximately 7 times the typical human dose on a mg/kg basis. Fertility in male and female rats was not adversely affected by Clozapine. Clozapine did not produce genotoxic or mutagenic effects when assayed in appropriate bacterial and mammalian tests.

PREGNANCY CATEGORY B

Reproduction studies have been performed in rats and rabbits at doses of approximately 2-4 times the human dose and have revealed no evidence of impaired fertility or harm to the fetus due to Clozapine. There are, however, no adequate and well-controlled studies in pregnant women. Because animal reproduction studies are not always predictive of human response, and in view of the desirability of keeping the administration of all drugs to a minimum during pregnancy, this drug should be used only if clearly needed.

NURSING MOTHERS

Animal studies suggest that Clozapine may be excreted in breast milk and have an effect on the nursing infant. Therefore, women receiving Clozapine should not breast feed.

PEDIATRIC USE

Safety and effectiveness in children below age 16 have not been established.

ADVERSE REACTIONS

ASSOCIATED WITH DISCONTINUATION OF TREATMENT

Sixteen percent of 1080 patients who receive Clozapine in premarketing clinical trials discontinued treatment due to an adverse event, including both those that could be reasonably attributed to Clozapine treatment and those that might more appropriately be considered intercurrent illness. The more common events considered to be causes of discontinuation included: CNS, primarily drowsiness/sedation, seizures, dizziness/syncope; cardiovascular, primarily tachycardia, hypotension and ECG changes; gastrointestinal, primarily nausea/vomiting; hematologic, primarily leukopenia/granulocytopenia/agranulocytosis; and fever. None of the events enumerated accounts for more than 1.7% of all discontinuations attributed to adverse clinical events.

COMMONLY OBSERVED

Adverse events observed in association with the use of Clozapine in clinical trials at an incidence of greater than 5% were; central nervous system complaints, including drowsiness/sedation, dizziness/vertigo, headache and tremor; autonomic nervous system complaints, including salivation, sweating, dry mouth and visual disturbances; cardiovascular findings, including tachycardia, hypotension and syncope; and gastrointestinal complaints, including constipation and nausea; and fever. Complaints of drowsiness/sedation tend to subside with continued therapy or dose reduction. Salivation may be profuse, especially during sleep, but may be diminished with dose reduction.

INCIDENCE IN CLINICAL TRIALS

The following table enumerates adverse events that occurred at a frequency of 1% or greater among Clozapine patients who participated in clinical trials. These rates are not adjusted for duration of exposure.

TREATMENT-EMERGENT ADVERSE EXPERIENCE INCIDENCE AMONG PATIENTS TAKING CLOZAPINE IN CLINICAL TRIALS
(N = 842)
(PERCENTAGE OF PATIENTS REPORTING)

Body System Adverse Event[a]	Percent
Central Nervous System	
Drowsiness/Sedation	39
Dizziness/Vertigo	19
Headache	7
Tremor	6
Syncope	6
Disturbed sleep/Nightmares	4
Restlessness	4
Hypokinesia/Akinesia	4
Agitation	4
Seizures (convulsions)	3[b]
Rigidity	3
Akathisia	3
Confusion	3
Fatigue	2
Insomnia	2
Hyperkinesia	1
Weakness	1
Lethargy	1
Ataxia	1
Slurred speech	1
Depression	1
Epileptiform movements/Myoclonic jerks	1
Anxiety	1
Cardiovascular	
Tachycardia	25[b]
Hypotension	9
Hypertension	4
Chest pain/Angina	1
ECG change/Cardiac abnormality	1
Gastrointestinal	
Constipation	14
Nausea	5
Abdominal discomfort/Heartburn	4
Nausea/Vomiting	3
Vomiting	3
Diarrhea	2
Liver test abnormality	1
Anorexia	1
Urogenital	
Urinary abnormalities	2
Incontinence	1
Abnormal ejaculation	1
Urinary urgency/frequency	1
Urinary retention	1
Autonomic Nervous System	
Salivation	31
Sweating	6
Dry mouth	6
Visual disturbances	5
Integumentary (Skin)	
Rash	2

◆ RATED THERAPEUTICALLY EQUIVALENT; ◇ THERAPEUTIC EQUIVALENCE UNCONFIRMED; ○ UNRATED

Body System Adverse Event[a]	Percent
Musculoskeletal	
Muscle weakness	1
Pain (back, neck, legs)	1
Muscle spasm	1
Muscle pain, ache	1
Respiratory	
Throat discomfort	1
Dyspnea, shortness of breath	1
Nasal congestion	1
Hemic/Lymphatic	
Leukopenia/Decreased WBC/	
Neutropenia	3
Agranulocytosis	1[b]
Esoniophilia	1
Miscellaneous	
Fever	5
Weight gain	4
Tongue numb/sore	1

[a] Events reported by at least 1% of Clozapine patients are included.
[b] Rate based on population of approximately 1700 exposed during premarket clinical evaluation of Clozapine.

OTHER EVENTS OBSERVED DURING THE PREMARKETING EVALUATION OF CLOZAPINE

This section reports additional, less frequent adverse events which occurred among the patients taking Clozapine in clinical trials. Various adverse events were reported as part of the total experience in these clinical studies; a causal relationship to Clozapine treatment cannot be determined in the absence of appropriate controls in some of the studies. The table above enumerates adverse events that occurred at a frequency of at least 1% of patients treated with Clozapine. The list below includes all additional adverse experiences reported as being temporally associated with the use of the drug which occurred at a frequency less than 1%, enumerated by organ system.

Central Nervous System: loss of speech, amentia, tics, poor coordination, delusions/hallucinations, involuntary movement, stuttering, dysarthria, amnesia/memory loss, histrionic movements, libido increase or decrease, paranoia, shakiness, Parkinsonism, and irritability.

Cardiovascular System: edema, palpitations, phlebitis/ thrombophlebitis, cyanosis, premature ventricular contraction, bradycardia, and nose bleed.

Gastrointestinal System: abdominal distention, gastroenteritis, rectal bleeding, nervous stomach, abnormal stools, hematemesis, gastric ulcer, bitter taste, and eructation.

Urogenital System: dysmenorrhea, impotence, breast pain/discomfort, and vaginal itch/infection.

Autonomic Nervous System: numbness, polydypsia, hot flashes, dry throat, and mydriasis.

Integumentary (Skin): pruritus, pallor, eczema, erythema, bruise, dermatitis, petechiae, and urticaria.

Musculoskeletal System: twitching and joint pain.

Respiratory System: coughing, pneumonia/pneumonia-like symptoms, rhinorrhea, hyperventilation, wheezing, bronchitis, laryngitis, and sneezing.

Hemic and Lymphatic System: anemia and leukocytosis.

Miscellaneous: chills/chills with fever, malaise, appetite increase, ear disorder, hypothermia, eyelid disorder, bloodshot eyes, and nystagmus.

POSTMARKETING CLINICAL EXPERIENCE

Postmarketing experience has shown an adverse experience profile similar to that presented above. Reports of adverse events temporally associated with Clozapine that may have no causal relationship with the drug include the following: salivary gland swelling, periorbital edema, paralytic ileus, atrial fibrillation, hyperuricemia, hyperglycemia, priapism, pleural effusion, myasthenic syndrome, cholestasis and possible mild cataplexy.

DRUG ABUSE AND DEPENDENCE

Physical and psychological dependence have not been reported or observed in patients taking Clozapine.

OVERDOSAGE

HUMAN EXPERIENCE

The most commonly signs and symptoms associated with Clozapine overdose are: altered states of consciousness, including drowsiness, delirium and coma: tachycardial: hypotension; respiratory depression or failure: hypersalivation. Seizures have occurred in a minority of reported cases. Fetal overdoses have been reported with Clozapine, generally at doses above 2500 mgs. There have also been reports of patients recovering from overdoses well in excess of 4 gms.

MANAGEMENT OF OVERDOSE

Establish and maintain an airway; ensure adequate oxygenation and ventilation. Activated charcoal, which may be used with sorbitol, may be as or more effective than emesis or lavage, and should be considered in treating overdosage. Cardiac and vital signs monitoring is recommended along with general symptomatic and supportive measures. Additional surveillance should be continued for several days because of the risk of delayed effects. Avoid epinephrine and derivatives when treating hypotension, and quinidine and procainamide when treating cardiac arrhythmia.

There are no specific antidotes for Clozapine. Forced diuresis, dialysis, hemoperfusion and exchange transfusion are unlikely to be of benefit.

In managing overdosage, the physician should consider the possibility of multiple drug involvement.

Up-to-date information about the treatment of overdose can often be obtained from a certified Regional Poison Control Center. Telephone numbers of certified Poison Control Centers are listed in the *Physicians' Desk Reference* (PDR).

DOSAGE AND ADMINISTRATION

In order to minimize the risk of agranulocytosis. Clozapine is available only through a distribution system that ensures weekly WBC testing prior to delivery of the next week's supply of medication. Upon initiation of Clozapine therapy, up to a 1 week supply of additional Clozapine tablets may be provided to the patient to be held for emergencies (e.g., weather, holidays).

INITIAL TREATMENT

It is recommended that treatment with Clozapine begin with one-half of a 25 mg tablet (12.5 mg) once or twice daily and then be continued with daily dosage increments of 25-50 mg/day, if well-tolerated, to achieve a target dose of 300-450 mg/day by the end of 2 weeks. Subsequent dosage increments should be made no more than once or twice-weekly, in increments not to exceed 100 mg. Cautious titration and a divided dosage schedule are necessary to minimize the risk of hypotension, seizure, and sedation.

In the multicenter study that provides primary support for the effectiveness of Clozapine in patients resistant to standard antipsychotic drug treatment, patients were titrated during the first 2 weeks up to a maximum dose of 500 mg/day, on a t.i.d. basis, and were then dosed in a total daily dose range of 100-900 mg/day, on a t.i.d. basis thereafter, with clinical response and adverse effects as guides to correct dosing.

THERAPEUTIC DOSE ADJUSTMENT

Daily dosing should continue on a divided basis as an effective and tolerable dose level is sought. While many patients may respond adequately at doses between 300-600 mg/day, it may be necessary to raise the dose to the 600-900 mg/day range to obtain an acceptable response. [Note: In the multicenter study providing the primary support for the superiority of Clozapine in treatment resistant patients, the mean and median Clozapine doses were both approximately 600 mg/day.]

Because of the possibility of increased adverse reactions at higher doses, particularly seizures, patients should ordinarily be given adequate time to respond to a given dose level before escalation to a higher dose is contemplated.

Dosing should not exceed 900 mg/day. Because of the significant risk of agranulocytosis and seizure, events which both present a continuing risk over time, the extended treatment of patients failing to show an acceptable level of clinical response should ordinarily be avoided.

MAINTENANCE TREATMENT

While the maintenance effectiveness of Clozapine in schizophrenia is still under study, the effectiveness of maintenance treatment is well established for many other antipsychotic drugs. It is recommended that responding patients be continued on Clozapine, but at the lowest level needed to maintain remission. Because of the significant risk associated with the use of Clozapine, patients should be periodically reassessed to determine the need for maintenance treatment.

DISCONTINUATION OF TREATMENT

In the event of planned termination of Clozapine therapy, gradual reduction in dose is recommended over a 1-2 week period. However, should a patient's medical condition require abrupt discontinuation (e.g., leukopenia), the patient should be carefully observed for the recurrence of psychotic symptoms.

RE-INITIATION OF TREATMENT IN PATIENTS PREVIOUSLY DISCONTINUED

When restarting patients who have had even a brief interval off Clozapine, i.e., 2 days or more since the last dose, it is recommended that treatment be reinitiated with one-half of a 25 mg tablet (12.5 mg) once or twice daily (see *"Warnings"*). If that dose is well tolerated, it may be feasible to titrate patients back to a therapeutic dose more quickly than is recommended for initial treatment. However, any patient who has previously experienced respiratory or cardiac arrest with initial dosing, but was then able to be successfully titrated to a therapeutic dose, should be retitrated with extreme caution after even 24 hours of discontinuation.

Certain additional precautions seem prudent when re-initiating treatment. The mechanisms underlying Clozapine induced adverse reactions are unknown. It is conceivable, however, that re-exposure of a patient might enhance the risk of an untoward event's occurrence and increase its severity. Such phenomena, for example, occur when immune mediated mechanisms are responsible. Consequently, during the re-initiation of treatment, additional caution is advised. Patients discontinued for WBC counts below 2000/mm^3 or a granulocyte count below 1000/mm^3 must *not* be restarted on Clozapine. (See *"Warnings"*.)

► SHOWN IN PRODUCT IDENTIFICATION GUIDE

STORE AND DISPENSE
Storage temperature should not exceed 86°F (30°C). Drug dispensing should not ordinarily exceed a weekly supply. Dispensing should be contingent upon the results of a WBC count.

HOW SUPPLIED
TABLETS: 25 MG

BRAND/MANUFACTURER	NDC	SIZE	AWP
○ BRAND			
► CLOZARIL: Sandoz Pharm	00078-0126-05	100s	$132.00
	00078-0126-06	100s ud	$132.00

TABLETS: 100 MG

BRAND/MANUFACTURER	NDC	SIZE	AWP
○ BRAND			
► CLOZARIL: Sandoz Pharm	00078-0127-05	100s	$342.00
	00078-0127-06	100s ud	$342.00

Clozaril *SEE* CLOZAPINE

Cocaine Hydrochloride

DESCRIPTION

Each mL contains:

Cocaine Hydrochloride ....40 mg or 100 mg

(*Warning: May be habit forming.*) An aqueous solution.

> **NOT FOR INJECTION OR OPHTHALMIC USE**

NOTE (for Glass Bottle): Do not steam autoclave. Cocaine Hydrochloride USP is a crystalline, granular, or powder substance having a saline, slightly bitter taste that numbs tongue and lips. Cocaine Hydrochloride is a local anesthetic.

Following is its chemical structure:

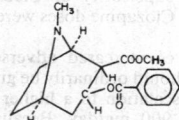

CLINICAL PHARMACOLOGY
Cocaine blocks the initiation or conduction of the nerve impulse following local application, thereby effecting local anesthetic action.

Cocaine is absorbed from all sites of application, including mucous membranes and the gastrointestinal mucosa. Cocaine is degraded by plasma esterases, with the half-life in the plasma being approximately one hour.

INDICATIONS AND USAGE
Cocaine Hydrochloride Topical Solution is indicated for the introduction of local (topical) anesthesia of accessible mucous membranes of the oral, laryngeal and nasal cavities.

CONTRAINDICATIONS
Cocaine Hydrochloride is contraindicated in patients with a known history of hypersensitivity to the drug or to the components of the topical solution.

WARNINGS
RESUSCITATIVE EQUIPMENT AND DRUGS SHOULD BE IMMEDIATELY AVAILABLE WHEN ANY LOCAL ANESTHETIC IS USED.

CARCINOGENESIS, MUTAGENESIS
Long-term studies to determine the carcinogenic and mutagenic potential of cocaine are not available.

PREGNANCY: TERATOGENIC EFFECTS—PREGNANCY CATEGORY C
Animal reproduction studies have not been conducted with Cocaine. It is also not known whether cocaine can cause fetal harm when administered to a pregnant woman or can affect reproduction capacity. Cocaine should be given to a pregnant woman only if needed.

PRECAUTIONS
GENERAL
The safety and effectiveness of Cocaine Hydrochloride Topical Solution depends on proper dosage, correct technique, adequate precautions, and readiness for emergencies. Standard textbooks should be consulted for specific techniques and precautions for various anesthetic procedures.

The lowest dosage that results in effective anesthesia should be used to avoid high plasma levels and serious adverse effects. Debilitated, elderly patients,

acutely ill patients, and children should be given reduced doses commensurate with their age and physical status.

Cocaine Hydrochloride Topical Solution should be used with caution in patients with severely traumatized mucosa and sepsis in the region of the proposed application. Use with caution in persons with known drug sensitivities.

ADVERSE REACTIONS
Adverse reactions may be due to high plasma levels as a result of excessive and rapid absorption of the drug. Reactions are systemic in nature and involve the central nervous system and/or the cardiovascular system. A small number of reactions may result from hypersensitivity, idiosyncrasy or diminished tolerance on the part of the patient.

CNS reactions are excitatory and/or depressant and may be characterized by nervousness, restlessness, and excitement. Tremors and eventually clonictonic convulsions may result. Emesis may occur. Central stimulation is followed by depression, with death resulting from respiratory failure.

Small doses of cocaine slow the heart rate, but after moderate doses, the rate is increased due to central sympathetic stimulation.

Cocaine is pyrogenic, augmenting heat production in stimulating muscular activity and causing vasoconstriction which decreases heat loss. Cocaine is known to interfere with the uptake of norepinephrine by adrenergic nerve terminals, producing sensitization to catecholamines, causing vasoconstriction and mydriasis.

Cocaine causes sloughing of the corneal epithelium, causing clouding, pitting, and occasionally ulceration of the cornea. The drug is not meant for ophthalmic use.

OVERDOSAGE
The fatal dose of Cocaine has been approximated at 1.2 g although severe toxic effects have been reported from doses as low as 20 mg.

SYMPTOMS
The symptoms of Cocaine poisoning are referable to the CNS, namely the patient becomes excited, restless, garrulous, anxious, and confused. Enhanced reflexes, headache, rapid pulse, irregular respiration, chills, rise in body temperature, mydriasis, exothalmos, nausea, vomiting and abdominal pain are noticed. In severe overdoses, delirium. Cheyne-Stoke respiration, convulsions, unconsciousness, and death from respiratory arrest result. Acute poisoning by cocaine is rapid in developing.

TREATMENT
The specific treatment of acute Cocaine poisoning is the intravenous administration of a short-acting barbiturate or diazepam. Artificial respiration may be necessary. It is important to limit absorption of the drug. If entrance of the drug into circulation can be checked, and respiratory exchange maintained, the prognosis is favorable since cocaine is eliminated fairly rapidly.

DOSAGE AND ADMINISTRATION
The dosage varies and depends upon the area to be anesthetized, vascularity of the tissues, individual tolerance, and the technique of anesthesia. The lowest dosage needed to provide effective anesthesia should be administered. Dosages should be reduced for children and for elderly and debilitated patients. Cocaine Hydrochloride Topical Solution can be administered by means of cotton applicators or packs, instilled into a cavity, or as a spray.

Store at controlled room temperature: 15°-30°C (59°-86°F)

HOW SUPPLIED
INJECTION (C-II): 4%

BRAND/MANUFACTURER	NDC	SIZE	AWP
○ GENERICS			
Astra	00186-1790-78	4 ml 5s	$117.85
Astra	00186-1791-13	10 ml 5s	$291.31

INJECTION (C-II): 10%

BRAND/MANUFACTURER	NDC	SIZE	AWP
○ GENERICS			
Astra	00186-1792-78	4 ml 5s	$201.31
Astra	00186-1793-13	10 ml 5s	$499.69

POWDER (C-II):

BRAND/MANUFACTURER	NDC	SIZE	AWP
○ GENERICS			
Mallinckrodt-II	00406-1520-53	5 gm	$293.50
Mallinckrodt-II	00406-1520-55	25 gm	$1467.50

SOLUTION (C-II): 4%

BRAND/MANUFACTURER	NDC	SIZE	AWP
○ GENERICS			
Roxane	00054-3110-40	10 ml	$48.88
Roxane	00054-3154-40	10 ml	$48.88
Schein	00364-3023-54	10 ml	$55.35
Roxane	00054-8163-03	4 ml 5s	$98.88
Roxane	00054-8110-03	4 ml 5s	$98.88
Schein	00364-3023-26	4 ml 5s	$113.55

◆ RATED THERAPEUTICALLY EQUIVALENT; ◇ THERAPEUTIC EQUIVALENCE UNCONFIRMED; ○ UNRATED

SOLUTION (C-II): 10%

BRAND/MANUFACTURER	NDC	SIZE	AWP
GENERICS			
Roxane	00054-3111-40	10 ml	$83.85
Roxane	00054-3155-40	10 ml	$83.85
Schein	00364-3024-54	10 ml	$98.10
Roxane	00054-8164-03	4 ml 5s	$168.92
Roxane	00054-8111-03	4 ml 5s	$168.92
Schein	00364-3024-26	4 ml 5s	$195.30

Codeine

DESCRIPTION

Codeine is an alkaloid obtained from opium or prepared from morphine by methylation and occurs as white crystals. Codeine effloresces slowly in dry air and is affected by light.

It is available as Codeine sulfate tablets for oral use and soluble tablets for the preparation of solutions for parenteral administration; and Codeine phosphate soluble tablets and injection.

Codeine phosphate injection is intended for subcutaneous or intramuscular injection; some brands are also intended for intravenous use. The chemical name of Codeine sulfate is 7,8-Didehydro-4,5α-epoxy-3-methoxy-17-methylmorphinan-6α-ol sulfate (2:1) (salt) trihydrate; it has the empirical formula of $(C_{18}H_{21}NO_3)_2 \cdot H_2SO_4 \cdot 3H_2O$. Its molecular weight is 750.9.

The chemical name of Codeine phosphate is 7,8-Didehydro-4,5α-epoxy-3-methoxy-17-methylmorphinan-6α-ol phosphate (1:1) (salt) hemihydrate; and it has the empirical formula of $C_{18}H_{21}NO_3 \cdot H_3PO_4 \cdot \frac{1}{2}H_2O$. Its molecular weight is 406.4.

Each soluble tablet contains:
Codeine sulfate 15 mg (0.02 mmol), 30 mg (0.04 mmol), or 60 mg (0.08 mmol)
or
Codeine phosphate 30 mg (0.074 mmol) or 60 mg (0.15 mmol)

Each ml of injection contains:
Codeine phosphate 30 or 60 mg

Each tablet for oral use contains:
Codeine sulfate 15 mg (0.02 mmol), 30 mg (0.04 mmol), or 60 mg (0.08 mmol).

Codeine is classified pharmacologically as a narcotic analgesic. Codeine Sulfate is an analgesic and antitussive; Codeine phosphate is an analgesic.

The phosphate salt of Codeine occurs as white, needle-shaped crystals or white crystalline powder. Codeine phosphate is freely soluble in water and slightly soluble in alcohol.

Following is its chemical structure:

CLINICAL PHARMACOLOGY

Narcotic analgesics, including Codeine, exert their primary effects on the central nervous system and gastrointestinal tract. The analgesic effects of Codeine are due to its central action; however, the precise sites of action have not been determined and the mechanisms involved appear to be quite complex. Codeine resembles morphine both structurally and pharmacologically, but its actions at the doses of Codeine used therapeutically are milder, with less sedation, respiratory depression, and gastrointestinal, urinary, and pupillary effects. Codeine produces an increase in biliary-tract pressure, but less than morphine or meperidine. Codeine is less constipating than morphine.

When administered parenterally, 120 mg of Codeine sulfate or phosphate produces an analgesic response equivalent to that from 10 mg of morphine. Other actions of Codeine sulfate and phosphate include respiratory depression; depression of the cough center; release of antidiuretic hormone; activation of the vomiting center; pupillary constriction; a decrease in gastric, pancreatic, and biliary secretion; a reduction in intestinal motility; an increase in biliary tract pressure; and an increased amplitude of ureteral contractions.

The onset of analgesia following intramuscular, subcutaneous, or oral administration occurs within 10 to 30 minutes. The effect persists for 4 to 6 hours.

Codeine and its salts are well absorbed following both oral and parenteral administration.

Codeine is about 2/3 as effective orally as parenterally. Codeine is metabolized primarily in the liver by enzymes of the endoplasmic reticulum, where it undergoes O-demethylation, N-demethylation, and partial conjugation with glucuronic acid. The drug is excreted primarily in the urine, largely as inactive metabolites and small amounts of free and conjugated morphine. Negligible amounts of Codeine and its metabolites are found in the feces. Most of a dose of Codeine is excreted within 24 hours, 5% to 15% as unchanged Codeine and the remainder as the products of glucuronide conjugation of Codeine and its metabolites.

Codeine in therapeutic dosage does not usually exert major effects on the cardiovascular system. However, particularly after larger parenteral dosage, some patients may exhibit a propensity to develop orthostatic hypotension and fainting. Rapid intravenous injection is more likely to precipitate a fall in blood pressure than are intramuscular or subcutaneous injections.

Narcotic analgesics may cause nausea and vomiting by stimulating the chemoreceptor trigger zone (CTZ); however, they also depress the vomiting center, so that subsequent doses are unlikely to produce vomiting. Nausea is minimal after usual oral doses of Codeine. Codeine has good antitussive activity, although less than that of morphine on a weight basis. It is used in preference to morphine because side effects are infrequent at the usual antitussive dose of Codeine.

Narcotic analgesics cause histamine release, which appears to be responsible for wheals or urticaria sometimes seen at the site of injection. Histamine release may also produce dilation of cutaneous blood vessels, with resultant flushing of the face and neck, pruritus, and sweating.

INDICATIONS AND USAGE

Codeine sulfate and phosphate are analgesics indicated for the relief of mild to moderate pain. The injection can also be useful in mild to moderate pain that does not respond to an orally administered analgesic.

UNLABELED USES
Codeine sulfate is used alone or as an adjunct in the treatment of migraine headache.

CONTRAINDICATION

Hypersensitivity to codeine. Narcotic analgesics, including Codeine, are contraindicated in premature infants or during labor when delivery of a premature infant is anticipated.

WARNINGS

CODEINE MAY BE HABIT FORMING. DO NOT USE THE INJECTION IF IT IS MORE THAN SLIGHTLY DISCOLORED OR CONTAINS A PRECIPITATE.

Some brands contain sodium metabisulfite, a sulfite that may cause allergic-type reactions, including anaphylactic symptoms and life-threatening or less severe asthmatic episodes, in certain susceptible people. The overall prevalence of sulfite sensitivity in the general population is unknown and probably low. Sulfite sensitivity is seen more frequently in asthmatic than in nonesthmatic people.

PRECAUTIONS

GENERAL

Head Injury and Increased Intracranial Pressure: The respiratory depressant effects of narcotics and their capacity to elevate cerebrospinal-fluid pressure may be markedly exaggerated in the presence of head injury, other intracranial lesions, or a preexisting increase in intracranial pressure. Usual oral doses of Codeine produce little respiratory depression; however, caution should be exercised, particularly with larger doses and parenteral administration. Furthermore, narcotics produce adverse reactions that may obscure the clinical course in patients with head injuries.

While usual oral doses of Codeine produce little sedation or other CNS effects, caution is recommended in these patients.

Acute Abdominal Conditions: The administration of Codeine or other narcotics may obscure the diagnosis or clinical course in patients with acute abdominal conditions.

Special-Risk Patients: Codeine should be given with caution and the initial dose reduced in certain patients, such as the elderly or debilitated and those with acute abdominal conditions, convulsive disorders, severe impairment of hepatic or renal function, fever, hypothyroidism, Addison's disease, ulcerative colitis, and prostatic hypertrophy or urethral stricture, and in those who have had recent gastrointestinal or urinary tract surgery.

Kidney or Liver Dysfunction: Codeine sulfate or phosphate may have a prolonged cumulative effect in patients with kidney or liver dysfunction.

Information for Patients: Codeine may impair the mental and/or physical abilities required for the performance of potentially hazardous tasks, such as driving a car or operating machinery. Codeine in combination with other narcotic analgesics, phenothiazines, sedative/hypnotics, tranquilizers, antihistamines, and alcohol has additive depressant effects. Codeine, like other narcotic analgesics, may produce orthostatic hypotension in some ambulatory patients. Patients should be cautioned accordingly.

Drug Interactions: Codeine in combination with other narcotic analgesics, general anesthetics, phenothiazines, tranquilizers, sedative/hypnotics, or other CNS depressants (including alcohol) has additive depressant effects. When such combination therapy is contemplated, the dosage of one or both agents should be reduced.

Virtually all drug interactions involving MAO inhibitors and narcotic analgesics have been reported with meperidine, which is contraindicated in such patients. In patients receiving MAO inhibitors, therefore, before initiating therapy with other narcotic analgesics, including Codeine, an initial small test dose is advisable to allow observation of excessive narcotic effects or MAO interaction.

Drug/Laboratory Test Interactions: Because narcotic analgesics may increase biliary-tract pressure, with resultant increases in plasma amylase or lipase levels, determination of these enzyme levels may be unreliable for 24 hours after a narcotic analgesic has been given.

Carcinogenesis, Mutagenesis, Impairment of Fertility: Long-term animal studies have not been performed to assess the carcinogenic potential of codeine. Codeine has been reported to show no evidence of carcinogenicity or mutagenicity in a variety of test systems, including the micronucleus and sperm abnormality assays and the *Salmonella* assay.

Usage in Pregnancy: Pregnancy Category C: Animal reproduction studies have not been conducted with Codeine sulfate or phosphate. It is also not known whether Codeine sulfate or phosphate can cause fetal harm when administered to a pregnant woman or can affect reproduction capacity. On the basis of the historical use of Codeine sulfate and Codeine phosphate during all stages of pregnancy, there is no known risk of fetal abnormality.

Teratogenic Effects: A study in rats and rabbits reported no teratogenic effect of Codeine administered during the period of organogenesis in doses ranging from 5 to 120 mg/kg. In the rat, doses at the 120 mg/kg level, in the toxic range for the adult animal, were associated with an increase in embryo resorption at the time of implantation. In another study, a single 100 mg/kg dose of Codeine administered to pregnant mice reportedly resulted in delayed ossification in the offspring. There are no studies in humans, and the significance of these findings to humans, if any, is not known. Codeine should be used in pregnancy only if the potential benefit justifies the potential risk to the fetus.

Nonteratogenic Effects: Dependence has been reported in newborns whose mothers took opiates regularly during pregnancy. Withdrawal signs include irritability, excessive crying, tremors, hyperreflexia, fever, vomiting, and diarrhea. Signs usually appear during the first few days of life.

Labor and Delivery: The use of Codeine sulfate or phosphate in obstetrics may prolong labor. Narcotic analgesics cross the placental barrier. The closer to delivery and the larger the dose used, the greater the possibility of respiratory depression in the newborn. Narcotic analgesics should be avoided during labor if delivery of a premature infant is anticipated. If the mother has received narcotic analgesics during labor, newborn infants should be observed closely for signs of respiratory depression. Resuscitation and, in severe depression, the administration of naloxone may be required. The effect of Codeine, if any, on the later growth, development, and functional maturation of the child is unknown.

Nursing Mothers: Some studies, but not others, have reported detectable amounts of Codeine in breast milk. The levels are probably not clinically significant after usual therapeutic dosage. The possibility of clinically important amounts being excreted in breast milk in individuals abusing Codeine should be considered. Caution should be exercised when it is administered to a nursing woman.

Asthma and Other Respiratory Conditions: Narcotic analgesics, including Codeine, should be used with extreme caution in patients having an acute asthmatic attack, patients with chronic obstructive pulmonary disease or cor pulmonale, patients having a substantially decreased respiratory reserve, and patients with preexisting respiratory depression, hypoxia, or hypercapnia. In such patients, even usual therapeutic doses of narcotics may decrease respiratory drive while simultaneously increasing airway resistance to the point of apnea. While usual oral doses of Codeine produce little respiratory depression, caution is advised in these patients, particularly with larger parenteral doses. In asthma and pulmonary emphysema, the indiscriminate use of Codeine may, due to its drying action upon the mucosa of the respiratory tract, precipitate severe respiratory insufficiency resulting from increased viscosity of the bronchial secretions and suppression of the cough reflex. If any of the above effects occur, the drug should be discontinued promptly. If respiratory depression occurs, a suitable narcotic antagonist, such as naloxone, should be administered.

Intravenous Use: If necessary, Codeine may be given intravenously, but the injection should be given very slowly. Rapid intravenous injection of narcotic analgesics, including Codeine, increases the incidence of adverse reactions; severe respiratory depression, apnea, hypotension, peripheral circulatory collapse, cardiac arrest, as well as anaphylactoid reactions, have occurred with various narcotic analgesics. Codeine should not be administered intravenously unless a narcotic antagonist and facilities for resuscitation and assisted or controlled respiration are immediately available. The patient should be lying down when Codeine is administered intravenously.

Hypotensive Effect: The administration of narcotic analgesics, including Codeine, particularly in larger parenteral doses, may result in severe hypotension in an individual whose ability to maintain his blood pressure has already been compromised by a depleted blood volume or concurrent administration of drugs such as certain phenothiazines or anesthetics. Codeine may produce orthostatic hypotension in ambulatory patients.

Caution must be used when injecting any opioid subcutaneously or intramuscularly into chilled areas or in patients with hypotension or shock, since impaired perfusion may prevent complete absorption; if repeated injections are administered, an excessive amount may be suddenly absorbed if normal circulation is reestablished.

Pediatric Use: Narcotic analgesics, including Codeine, should not be used in premature infants (see "Contraindications"). Narcotics are reported to cross the immature blood-brain barrier to a greater extent, thereby producing disproportionate respiratory depression. Narcotic analgesics should be administered to infants and small children only with great caution and in carefully monitored

dosage. Safety and effectiveness of Codeine in newborn infants have not been established.

ADVERSE REACTIONS

In usual oral dosage Codeine has minimal side effects, nausea, vomiting, sedation, lightheadedness, dizziness, and constipation being reported most commonly.

Rarely, anaphylactoid reactions have been reported when Codeine or other phenanthrene alkaloids of opium are administered intravenously.

Other adverse reactions include:

Central Nervous System: The major hazards of Codeine, as with other narcotic analgesics, involve CNS depression, particularly respiratory depression, and to a lesser extent, circulatory depression. Respiratory arrest, shock, and cardiac arrest have occurred, particularly with overdosage or with rapid intravenous administration. Other CNS effects of narcotic analgesics include light-headedness, dizziness, sedation, euphoria, dysphoria, weakness, headache, transient hallucinations, disorientation, visual disturbances, and convulsions.

These effects are more common with larger parenteral doses, in ambulatory patients, and in those who are not experiencing severe pain. Some adverse reactions in ambulatory patients may be alleviated if the patient lies down.

Gastrointestinal: Codeine may produce nausea, vomiting, constipation, and biliary-tract spasm. Patients with chronic ulcerative colitis may experience increased colonic motility; in patients with acute ulcerative colitis, toxic dilation has been reported.

Cardiovascular: Narcotic analgesics may produce tachycardia, bradycardia, palpitation, faintness, syncope, and orthostatic hypotension.

Genitourinary: Narcotic analgesics may cause oliguria and urinary retention; an antidiuretic effect has been reported.

Allergic: Allergic reactions to opiates occur infrequently; pruritus, giant urticaria, angioneurotic edema and laryngeal edema have been reported with Codeine. Rarely, anaphylactoid reactions have been reported following intravenous administration.

Other: Opiate-induced histamine release may be responsible for the flushing of the face, sweating, and pruritus often seen with these drugs. Wheals and urticaria at the site of injection are probably related to histamine release. Local tissue irritation, pain, and induration have been reported following repeated subcutaneous injection.

DRUG ABUSE AND DEPENDENCE

Controlled Substance: Codeine sulfate and phosphate are Schedule II narcotics.

Codeine is known to be subject to abuse; however, the abuse potential of oral Codeine appears to be quite low. Even parenteral Codeine does not appear to offer the psychic effects sought by addicts to the same degree as heroin or morphine, so that addicts generally use Codeine only when other narcotics are unavailable.

Personality characteristics play a major role in determining which patients are likely to abuse drugs. The overwhelming majority of patients who receive opiates for medical indications do not develop drug-seeking behavior or compulsive drug use. Considering its widespread use, the record of Codeine is very good in this respect. However, Codeine must be administered only under close supervision to patients with a history of drug abuse or dependence.

Dependence: Psychological dependence, physical dependence, and tolerance are known to occur with Codeine.

Patients given 60 mg of Codeine every 6 hours for 2 months usually show some tolerance and mild withdrawal symptoms. Development of the dependent state is recognizable by an increased tolerance to the analgesic effect and the appearance of purposive phenomena (complaints, pleas, demands, or manipulative actions) shortly before the time of the next scheduled dose. The severity of the abstinence syndrome is related to the degree of dependence, the abruptness of withdrawal, and the drug used. If the abstinence syndrome is precipitated by administration of a narcotic antagonist, symptoms appear within a few minutes and are maximal within thirty minutes. Administration of a narcotic antagonist as a means of detecting dependence is not usually recommended.

While Codeine can partially suppress the symptoms of morphine withdrawal, the Codeine withdrawal syndrome (after 1200 to 1800 mg of Codeine per day), though qualitatively similar to that seen with morphine, is considerably less intense. Withdrawal symptoms in patients dependent on Codeine include yawning, sweating, lacrimation, rhinorrhea, a restless, tossing sleep, dilated pupils, gooseflesh, irritability, tremor, nausea, vomiting, and diarrhea. A patient in withdrawal should be treated in a hospital environment. Usually, it is necessary only to provide supportive care, including maintenance of proper fluid and eletrolyte balance, with administration of a tranquilizer to suppress anxiety. Severe symptoms of withdrawal may require administration of a replacement narcotic.

OVERDOSAGE

Signs and Symptoms: Codeine is metabolized to morphine and its effects are similar to those of morphine and other opiate analgesics. Respiratory depression (a decrease in respiratory rate and/or tidal volume, Cheyne-Stokes respiration, cyanosis), extreme somnolence progressing to stupor or coma, and miosis are common symptoms of overdose. Other symptoms include nausea, vomiting, skeletal muscle flaccidity, bradycardia, hypotension, and cool, clammy skin. The triad of coma, pinpoint pupils, and respiratory depression is strongly suggestive of opiate poisoning. In severe overdosage, particularly by the intravenous route, apnea, circulatory collapse, cardiac arrest, and death may occur.

It is difficult to determine what constitutes a standard toxic or lethal dose. However, the lethal oral dose of Codeine in an adult is reported to be in the range of 0.5 to 1.0 gram. Infants and children are believed to be relatively more sensitive to opiates on a body-weight basis.

Children have had apnea after doses as small as 5 mg/kg. Elderly patients are also comparatively intolerant to opiates. Noncardiac pulmonary edema may develop after opioid overdose, and monitoring of heart filling pressure may be helpful.

Treatment: To obtain up-to-date information about the treatment of overdose, a good resource is your certified Regional Poison Control Center. Telephone numbers of certified poison control centers are listed in the *Physicians' Desk Reference (PDR).* In managing overdosage, consider the possibility of multiple drug overdoses, interaction among drugs, and unusual drug kinetics in your patient.

Primary attention should be given to the reestablishment of adequate respiratory exchange through provision of a patient airway and institution of assisted or controlled ventilation. The narcotic antagonist, naloxone hydrochloride, is a specific antidote against respiratory depression which may result from overdosage or unusual sensitivity to narcotics. Therefore, an appropriate dose of naloxone hydrochloride should be administered, preferably by the intravenous route, simultaneously with efforts at respiratory resuscitation.

An antagonist should only be administered in the presence of clinically significant respiratory or cardiovascular depression induced by a narcotic. Oxygen, intravenous fluids, vasopressors, and other supportive measures should be employed as indicated.

Protect the airway as naloxone may induce vomiting. Naloxone has a shorter duration of action than Codeine; repeated doses may be needed. In patients who abuse opioids chronically, a withdrawal syndrome may be manifest on administration of naloxone. This may include yawning, tearing, restlessness, sweating, dilated pupils, piloerection, vomiting, diarrhea, and abdominal cramps. This syndrome usually abates quickly as the effect of naloxone dissipates. The severity of this syndrome will depend on the degree of physical dependence and the dose of antagonist administered. The use of narcotic antagonists in such individuals should be avoided if possible. If a narcotic antagonist must be used to treat serious respiratory depression in the physically dependent patient, the antagonist should be administered with extreme care and only one-tenth to one-fifth the usual initial dose administered.

Meticulously monitor and maintain, within acceptable limits, the patient's vital signs, blood gases, serum electrolytes, etc. Gastric lavage may be indicated even several hours after ingestion of an overdosage of oral Codeine, since the drug often induces pylorospasm. A saline cathartic may then be left in the stomach. Absorption of drugs from the gastrointestinal tract may be decreased by giving activated charcoal, which, in many cases, is more effective than emesis or lavage; consider charcoal instead of or in addition to gastric emptying. Repeated doses of charcoal over time may hasten elimination of some drugs that have been absorbed. Safeguard the patient's airway when employing gastric emptying or charcoal.

The patient should be closely observed for a rise in temperature or pulmonary complications that may signal the need for institution of antibiotic therapy.

Forced diuresis, peritoneal dialysis, hemodialysis, or charcoal hemoperfusion have not been established as beneficial for an overdose of Codeine sulfate or phosphate.

DOSAGE AND ADMINISTRATION

FOR ANALGESIA

Dosage should be adjusted according to the severity of the pain and the response of the patient.

Adults: 15 to 60 mg every 4 to 6 hours (usual adult dose, 30 mg).

Children: 1 Year of Age or Older — 0.5 mg/kg of body weight or 15 mg/m^2 of body surface every 4 to 6 hours. Doses for injection also range from 0.5 mg/kg or 16.7 mg/m^2 every 4 hours, IM or SC, to 3 mg/kg/24 hours or 100 mg/m^2/24 hours, divided into 6 doses, IM or SC. Do not use in premature infants (see "Contraindications"). Safety and effectiveness in newborn infants have not been established.

Tablets Codeine sulfate are given orally. Soluble tablets Codeine sulfate or phosphate are administered subcutaneously or intramuscularly.

Codeine phosphate injection has been reported to be chemically or physically incompatible with a variety of other injectable medications. Before diluting with any intravenous solution or combining with any other medication, consult specialized references. Do not use if there is any indication of precipitation or other signs of incompatibility.

Solutions for injection should be prepared with sterile water and filtered through a 0.22 μ membrane filter.

Note: Parenteral drug products should be inspected visually for particulate matter and discoloration prior to administration, whenever solution and container permit. Do not use the solution if it is more than slightly discolored or contains a precipitate.

Store injection at room temperature, approximately 25°C (77°F).
Protect from light. Avoid freezing.
Use carton to protect contents from light.

J CODES
IM,IV,SC—J0745

HOW SUPPLIED
INJECTION (C-II): 30 MG/ML

BRAND/MANUFACTURER	NDC	SIZE	AWP
GENERICS			
Wyeth-Ayerst	00008-0728-01	1 ml 10s	$8.24
Sanofi Winthrop	00024-0272-02	2 ml 10s	$8.21
Elkins-Sinn	00641-0100-25	1 ml 25s	$15.00
Elkins-Sinn	00641-0100-26	1 ml 100s ud	$60.00

INJECTION (C-II): 60 MG/ML

BRAND/MANUFACTURER	NDC	SIZE	AWP
GENERICS			
Wyeth-Ayerst	00008-0729-01	1 ml 10s	$9.14
Sanofi Winthrop	00024-0274-02	2 ml 10s	$9.04
Elkins-Sinn	00641-0110-25	1 ml 25s	$17.50
Elkins-Sinn	00641-0110-26	1 ml 100s ud	$70.00

TABLETS (C-II): 15 MG

BRAND/MANUFACTURER	NDC	SIZE	AWP
GENERICS			
Roxane	00054-8155-24	100s ud	$31.45

TABLETS (C-II): 30 MG

BRAND/MANUFACTURER	NDC	SIZE	AWP
GENERICS			
Halsey Pharm	00879-0002-01	100s	$27.25
Roxane	00054-4156-25	100s	$33.85
Lilly	00002-1010-02	100s	$42.39
Knoll	00044-0623-02	100s	$43.64
Lilly	00002-2557-02	100s	$50.34
Roxane	00054-8156-24	100s ud	$37.49
Halsey Pharm	00879-0002-10	1000s	$205.50

TABLETS (C-II): 60 MG

BRAND/MANUFACTURER	NDC	SIZE	AWP
GENERICS			
Roxane	00054-4157-25	100s	$62.01
Lilly	00002-1011-02	100s	$80.97
Knoll	00044-0626-02	100s	$83.20
Lilly	00002-2558-02	100s	$96.20
Roxane	00054-8157-24	100s ud	$68.07

Codeine Phosphate and Promethazine Hydrochloride

DESCRIPTION
Each teaspoon (5 mL) of Codeine Phosphate/Promethazine Hydrochloride contains 10 mg Codeine Phosphate (Warning—may be habit-forming) and 6.25 mg Promethazine Hydrochloride in a flavored syrup base with a pH between 4.7 and 5.2. Alcohol 7%.

Codeine is one of the naturally occurring phenanthrene alkaloids of opium derived from the opium poppy; it is classified pharmacologically as a narcotic analgesic. Codeine Phosphate may be chemically named as (5α,6α)-7,8-didehydro-4,5-epoxy-3-methoxy-17-methylmorphinan- 6-ol phosphate (1:1) (salt) hemihydrate.

The Phosphate salt of Codeine occurs as white, needle-shaped crystals or white crystalline powder. Codeine Phosphate is freely soluble in water and slightly soluble in alcohol, with a molecular weight of 406.37. The empirical formula is $C_{18}H_{21}NO_3 \cdot H_3PO_4 \cdot \frac{1}{2}H_2O$, and the stereochemistry is 5α, 6α isomer as indicated in the structure.

Promethazine Hydrochloride (Promethazine HCl) is a racemic compound; the empirical formula is $C_{17}H_{20}N_2S \cdot HCl$ and its molecular weight is 320.88.

Promethazine HCl, a phenothiazine derivative, is designated chemically as N,N,α-trimethyl-10H-phenothiazine-10-ethanamine monohydrochloride.

Promethazine HCl occurs as a white to faint yellow, practically odorless, crystalline powder which slowly oxidizes and turns blue on prolonged exposure to air. It is soluble in water and freely soluble in alcohol.

CLINICAL PHARMACOLOGY
CODEINE

Narcotic analgesics, including Codeine, exert their primary effects on the central nervous system and gastrointestinal tract. The analgesic effects of Codeine are due to its central action; however, the precise sites of action have not been determined, and the mechanisms involved appear to be quite complex. Codeine resembles morphine both structurally and pharmacologically, but its actions at the doses of Codeine used therapeutically are milder, with less sedation, respiratory depression, and gastrointestinal, urinary, and pupillary effects. Codeine produces an increase in biliary tract pressure, but less than morphine or meperidine. Codeine is less constipating than morphine.

➤ SHOWN IN PRODUCT IDENTIFICATION GUIDE

Codeine has good antitussive activity, although less than that of morphine at equal doses. It is used in preference to morphine, because side effects are infrequent at the usual antitussive dose of codeine.

Codeine in oral therapeutic dosage does not usually exert major effects on the cardiovascular system.

Narcotic analgesics may cause nausea and vomiting by stimulating the chemoreceptor trigger zone (CTZ); however, they also depress the vomiting center, so that subsequent doses are unlikely to produce vomiting. Nausea is minimal after usual oral doses of Codeine.

Narcotic analgesics cause histamine release, which appears to be responsible for wheals or urticaria sometimes seen at the site of injection on parenteral administration. Histamine release may also produce dilation of cutaneous blood vessels, with resultant flushing of the face and neck, pruritus, and sweating.

Codeine and its salts are well absorbed following both oral and parenteral administration. Codeine is about ⅔ as effective orally as parenterally. Codeine is metabolized primarily in the liver by enzymes of the endoplasmic reticulum, where it undergoes O-demethylation, N-demethylation, and partial conjugation with glucuronic acid. The drug is excreted primarily in the urine, largely as inactive metabolites and small amounts of free and conjugated morphine. Negligible amounts of Codeine and its metabolites are found in the feces. Following oral or subcutaneous administration of Codeine, the onset of analgesia occurs within 15 to 30 minutes and lasts for four to six hours.

The cough-depressing action, in animal studies, was observed to occur 15 minutes after oral administration of Codeine, peak action at 45 to 60 minutes after ingestion. The duration of action, which is dose-dependent, usually did not exceed 3 hours.

PROMETHAZINE

Promethazine HCl is a phenothiazine derivative which differs structurally from the antipsychotic phenothiazines by the presence of a branched side chain and no ring substitution. It is thought that this configuration is responsible for its lack (1/10 that of chlorpromazine) of dopaminergic (CNS) action. Promethazine HCl is an H_1 receptor blocking agent. In addition to its antihistaminic action, it provides clinically useful sedative and antiemetic effects. In therapeutic dosages, promethazine produces no significant effects on the cardiovascular system.

Promethazine HCl is well absorbed from the gastrointestinal tract. Clinical effects are apparent within 20 minutes after oral administration and generally last four to six hours, although they may persist as long as 12 hours. Promethazine HCl is metabolized by the liver to a variety of compounds; the sulfoxides of Promethazine and N-demethylpromethazine are the predominant metabolites appearing in the urine.

INDICATIONS AND USAGE

Codeine Phosphate/Promethazine HCl is indicated for the temporary relief of coughs and upper respiratory symptoms associated with allergy or the common cold.

CONTRAINDICATIONS

Codeine is contraindicated in patients with a known hypersensitivity to the drug.

Promethazine is contraindicated in individuals known to be hypersensitive or to have had an idiosyncratic reaction to Promethazine or to other phenothiazines.

Antihistamines and Codeine are both contraindicated for use in the treatment of lower respiratory tract symptoms, including asthma.

WARNINGS
CODEINE PHOSPHATE
Dosage of Codeine SHOULD NOT BE INCREASED if cough fails to respond; an unresponsive cough should be reevaluated in 5 days or sooner for possible underlying pathology, such as foreign body or lower respiratory tract disease.

Codeine may cause or aggravate constipation.

Respiratory depression leading to arrest, coma, and death has occurred with the use of Codeine antitussives in young children, particularly in the under-one-year infants whose ability to deactivate the drug is not fully developed.

Administration of Codeine may be accompanied by histamine release and should be used with caution in atopic children.

Head Injury and Increased Intracranial Pressure: The respiratory-depressant effects of narcotic analgesics and their capacity to elevate cerebrospinal fluid pressure may be markedly exaggerated in the presence of head injury, intracranial lesions, or a preexisting increase in intracranial pressure. Narcotics may produce adverse reactions which may obscure the clinical course of patients with head injuries.

Asthma and Other Respiratory Conditions: Narcotic analgesics or cough suppressants, including Codeine, should not be used in asthmatic patients (see "Contraindications"). Nor should they be used in acute febrile illness associated with productive cough or in chronic respiratory disease where interference with ability to clear the tracheobronchial tree of secretions would have a deleterious effect on the patient's respiratory function.

Hypotensive Effect: Codeine may produce orthostatic hypotension in ambulatory patients.

PROMETHAZINE
Promethazine may cause marked drowsiness. Ambulatory patients should be cautioned against such activities as driving or operating dangerous machinery until it is known that they do not become drowsy or dizzy from Promethazine therapy.

The sedative action of Promethazine HCl is additive to the sedative effects of central nervous system depressants; therefore, agents such as alcohol, narcotic analgesics, sedatives, hypnotics, and tranquilizers should either be eliminated or given in reduced dosage in the presence of Promethazine. When given concomitantly with Promethazine, the dose of barbiturates should be reduced by at least one-half, and the dose of analgesic depressants, such as morphine or meperidine, should be reduced by one-quarter to one-half.

Promethazine may lower seizure threshold. This should be taken into consideration when administering to persons with known seizure disorders or when giving in combination with narcotics or local anesthetics which may also affect seizure threshold.

Sedative drugs or CNS depressants should be avoided in patients with a history of sleep apnea.

Antihistamines should be used with caution in patients with narrow-angle glaucoma, stenosing peptic ulcer, pyloroduodenal obstruction, and urinary bladder obstruction due to symptomatic prostatic hypertrophy and narrowing of the bladder neck.

Administration of Promethazine has been associated with reported cholestatic jaundice.

PRECAUTIONS
Animal reproduction studies have not been conducted with the drug combination—Promethazine and Codeine. It is not known whether this drug combination can cause fetal harm when administered to a pregnant woman or can affect reproduction capacity. Codeine Phosphate/Promethazine HCl should be given to a pregnant woman only if clearly needed.

GENERAL
Narcotic analgesics, including Codeine, should be administered with caution and the initial dose reduced in patients with acute abdominal conditions, convulsive disorders, significant hepatic or renal impairment, fever, hypothyroidism, Addison's disease, ulcerative colitis, prostatic hypertrophy, in patients with recent gastrointestinal or urinary tract surgery, and in the very young or elderly or debilitated patients. Promethazine HCl should be used cautiously in persons with cardiovascular disease or with impairment of liver function.

INFORMATION FOR PATIENTS
Codeine Phosphate/Promethazine HCl may cause marked drowsiness or may impair the mental and/or physical abilities required for the performance of potentially hazardous tasks, such as driving a vehicle or operating machinery. Ambulatory patients should be told to avoid engaging in such activities until it is known that they do not become drowsy or dizzy from Codeine Phosphate/Promethazine HCl therapy. Children should be supervised to avoid potential harm in bike riding or in other hazardous activities.

The concomitant use of alcohol or other central nervous system depressants, including narcotic analgesics, sedatives, hypnotics, and tranquilizers, may have an additive effect and should be avoided or their dosage reduced.

Patients should be advised to report any involuntary muscle movements or unusual sensitivity to sunlight.

Codeine like other narcotic analgesics, may produce orthostatic hypotension in some ambulatory patients. Patients should be cautioned accordingly.

DRUG INTERACTIONS
CODEINE
In patients receiving MAO inhibitors, an initial small test dose is advisable to allow observation of any excessive narcotic effects or MAOI interaction.

PROMETHAZINE
The sedative action of Promethazine is additive to the effects of other central nervous system depressants, including alcohol, narcotic analgesics, sedatives, hypnotics, tricyclic antidepressants, and tranquilizers; therefore, these agents should be avoided or administered in reduced dosage to patients receiving Promethazine.

DRUG/LABORATORY TEST INTERACTIONS
Because narcotic analgesics may increase biliary tract pressure, with resultant increase in plasma amylase or lipase levels, determination of these enzyme levels may be unreliable for 24 hours after a narcotic analgesic has been given. The following laboratory tests may be affected in patients who are receiving therapy with Promethazine.

Pregnancy Tests: Diagnostic pregnancy tests based on immunological reactions between HCG and anti-HCG may result in false-negative or false-positive interpretations.

Glucose Tolerance Test: An increase in blood glucose has been reported in patients receiving Promethazine.

CARCINOGENESIS, MUTAGENESIS, IMPAIRMENT OF FERTILITY
Long-term animal studies have not been performed to assess the carcinogenic potential of Codeine or of Promethazine, nor are there other animal or human data concerning carcinogenicity, mutagenicity, or impairment of fertility with these agents. Codeine has been reported to show no evidence of carcinogenicity or mutagenicity in a variety of test systems, including the micronucleus and sperm abnormality assays and the *Salmonella* assay. Promethazine was nonmutagenic in the *Salmonella* test system of Ames.

PREGNANCY
Teratogenic Effects—Pregnancy Category C

◆ RATED THERAPEUTICALLY EQUIVALENT; ◇ THERAPEUTIC EQUIVALENCE UNCONFIRMED; ○ UNRATED

CODEINE

A study in rats and rabbits reported no teratogenic effect of Codeine administered during the period of organogenesis in doses ranging from 5 to 120 mg/kg. In the rat, doses at the 120-mg/kg level, in the toxic range for the adult animal, were associated with an increase in embryo resorption at the time of implantation. In another study a single 100-mg/kg dose of Codeine administered to pregnant mice reportedly resulted in delayed ossification in the offspring.

There are no studies in humans, and the significance of these findings to humans, if any, is not known.

PROMETHAZINE

Teratogenic effects have not been demonstrated in rat-feeding studies at doses of 6.25 and 12.5 mg/kg of Promethazine. These doses are 8.3 and 16.7 times the maximum recommended total daily dose of Promethazine for a 50-kg subject. Specific studies to test the action of the drug on parturition, lactation, and development of the animal neonate were not done, but a general preliminary study in rats indicated no effect on these parameters. Although antihistamines, including Promethazine, have been found to produce fetal mortality in rodents, the pharmacological effects of histamine in the rodent do not parallel those in man. There are no adequate and well-controlled studies of Promethazine in pregnant women.

Codeine Phosphate/Promethazine HCl should be used during pregnancy only if the potential benefit justifies the potential risk to the fetus.

Nonteratogenic Effects: Dependence has been reported in newborns whose mothers took opiates regularly during pregnancy. Withdrawal signs include irritability, excessive crying, tremors, hyperreflexia, fever, vomiting, and diarrhea. Signs usually appear during the first few days of life.

Promethazine taken within two weeks of delivery may inhibit platelet aggregation in the newborn.

LABOR AND DELIVERY

Narcotic analgesics cross the placental barrier. The closer to delivery and the larger the dose used, the greater the possibility of respiratory depression in the newborn. Narcotic analgesics should be avoided during labor if delivery of a premature infant is anticipated. If the mother has received narcotic analgesics during labor, newborn infants should be observed closely for signs of respiratory depression. Resuscitation may be required (see *"Overdosage"*). The effect of Codeine, if any, on the later growth, development, and functional maturation of the child is unknown. See also *"Nonteratogenic Effects"*.

NURSING MOTHERS

Some studies, but not others, have reported detectable amounts of Codeine in breast milk. The levels are probably not clinically significant after usual therapeutic dosage. The possibility of clinically important amounts being excreted in breast milk in individuals abusing Codeine should be considered.

It is not known whether Promethazine is excreted in human milk.

Caution should be exercised when Codeine Phosphate/Promethazine HCl is administered to a nursing woman.

PEDIATRIC USE

This product should not be used in children under 2 years of age because safety for such use has not been established.

ADVERSE REACTIONS

CODEINE

Nervous System: CNS depression, particularly respiratory depression, and to a lesser extent circulatory depression; light-headedness, dizziness, sedation, euphoria, dysphoria, headache, transient hallucination, disorientation, visual disturbances, and convulsions.

Cardiovascular: Tachycardia, bradycardia, palpitation, faintness, syncope, orthostatic hypotension (common to narcotic analgesics).

Gastrointestinal: Nausea, vomiting, constipation, and biliary tract spasm. Patients with chronic ulcerative colitis may experience increased colonic motility; in patients with acute ulcerative colitis, toxic dilation has been reported.

Genitourinary: Oliguria, urinary retention; antidiuretic effect has been reported (common to narcotic analgesics).

Allergic: Infrequent pruritus, giant urticaria, angioneurotic edema, and laryngeal edema.

Other: Flushing of the face, sweating and pruritus (due to opiate induced histamine release); weakness.

PROMETHAZINE

Nervous System: Sedation, sleepiness, occasional blurred vision, dryness of mouth, dizziness; rarely confusion, disorientation, and extrapyramidal symptoms such as oculogyric crisis, torticollis, and tongue protrusion (usually in association with parenteral injection or excessive dosage).

Cardiovascular: Increased or decreased blood pressure.

Dermatologic: Rash, rarely photosensitivity.

Hematologic: Rarely leukopenia, thrombocytopenia; agranulocytosis (1 case).

Gastrointestinal: Nausea and vomiting.

DRUG ABUSE AND DEPENDENCE

CONTROLLED SUBSTANCE

Codeine/Promethazine HCl is a Schedule V Controlled Substance.

ABUSE

Codeine is known to be subject to abuse; however, the abuse potential of oral Codeine appears to be quite low. Even parenteral Codeine does not appear to offer the psychic effects sought by addicts to the same degree as heroin or morphine. However, Codeine must be administered only under close supervision to patients with a history of drug abuse or dependence.

DEPENDENCE

Psychological dependence, physical dependence, and tolerance are known to occur with Codeine.

OVERDOSAGE

CODEINE

Serious overdose with Codeine is characterized by respiratory depression (a decrease in respiratory rate and/or tidal volume, Cheyne-Stokes respiration, cyanosis), extreme somnolence progressing to stupor or coma, skeletal muscle flaccidity, cold and clammy skin, and sometimes bradycardia and hypotension. The triad of coma, pinpoint pupils, and respiratory depression is strongly suggestive of opiate poisoning. In severe overdosage, particularly by the intravenous route, apnea, circulatory collapse, cardiac arrest, and death may occur. Promethazine HCl is additive to the depressant effects of Codeine.

It is difficult to determine what constitutes a standard toxic or lethal dose. However, the lethal oral dose of Codeine in an adult is reported to be in the range of 0.5 to 1.0 gram. Infants and children are believed to be relatively more sensitive to opiates on a body-weight basis. Elderly patients are also comparatively intolerant to opiates.

PROMETHAZINE

Signs and symptoms of overdosage with Promethazine HCl range from mild depression of the central nervous system and cardiovascular system to profound hypotension, respiratory depression, and unconsciousness.

Stimulation may be evident, especially in children and geriatric patients. Convulsions may rarely occur. A paradoxical reaction has been reported in children receiving single doses of 75 mg to 125 mg orally, characterized by hyperexcitability and nightmares.

Atropine-like signs and symptoms—dry mouth, fixed, dilated pupils, flushing, as well as gastrointestinal symptoms, may occur.

TREATMENT

The treatment of overdosage with Codeine Phosphate/Promethazine HCl is essentially symptomatic and supportive. Only in cases of extreme overdosage or individual sensitivity do vital signs including respiration, pulse, blood pressure, temperature, and EKG need to be monitored. Activated charcoal orally or by lavage may be given, or sodium or magnesium sulfate orally as a cathartic. Attention should be given to the reestablishment of adequate respiratory exchange through provision of a patent airway and institution of assisted or controlled ventilation. The narcotic antagonist, naloxone hydrochloride, may be administered when significant respiratory depression occurs with Codeine Phosphate/Promethazine HCl; any depressant effects of Promethazine HCl are not reversed with naloxone. Diazepam may be used to control convulsions. Avoid analeptics, which may cause convulsions. Acidosis and electrolyte losses should be corrected. A rise in temperature or pulmonary complications may signal the need for institution of antibiotic therapy.

Severe hypotension usually responds to the administration of norepinephrine or phenylephrine. *Epinephrine should not be used,* since its use in a patient with partial adrenergic blockade may further lower the blood pressure.

Limited experience with dialysis indicates that it is not helpful.

DOSAGE AND ADMINISTRATION

The average effective dose is given in the following table: (See related table).

Keep bottles tightly closed—store at room temperature, between 15° C and 25°C and (59°F and 77°F).
  Protect from light.
  Dispense in light-resistant, glass, tight container.

HOW SUPPLIED
SYRUP: 10 MG-6.25 MG

BRAND/MANUFACTURER	NDC	SIZE	AWP
◆ GENERICS			
Goldline	00182-0346-37	120 ml	$18.00

➤ SHOWN IN PRODUCT IDENTIFICATION GUIDE

CODEINE PHOSPHATE/PROMETHAZINE HCL

Adults | 1 teaspoon (5 mL) every 4 to 6 hours, not to exceed 30.0 mL in 24 hours.

Children 6 years to under 12 years | ½ to 1 teaspoon (2.5 to 5 mL) every 4 to 6 hours, not to exceed 30.0 mL in 24 hours.

Children under 6 years (weight: 18 kg or 40 lbs) | ¼ to ½ teaspoon (1.25 to 2.5 mL) every 4 to 6 hours, not to exceed 9.0 mL in 24 hours.

Children under 6 years (weight: 16 kg or 35 lbs) | ¼ to ½ teaspoon (1.25 to 2.5 mL) every 4 to 6 hours, not to exceed 8.0 mL in 24 hours.

Children under 6 years (weight: 14 kg or 30 lbs) | ¼ to ½ teaspoon (1.25 to 2.5 mL) every 4 to 6 hours, not to exceed 7.0 mL in 24 hours.

Children under 6 years (weight: 12 kg or 25 lbs) | ¼ to ½ teaspoon (1.25 to 2.5 mL) every 4 to 6 hours, not to exceed 6.0 mL in 24 hours.

Codeine Phosphate/Promethazine HCl is not recommended for children under 2 years of age.

SYRUP (C-V): 10 MG-6.25 MG/5 ML

AVERAGE UNIT PRICE (AVAILABLE SIZES)		GENERIC A-RATED AVERAGE PRICE (GAAP)	
BRAND	$0.06	480 ml	$29.15
GENERIC	$0.02	3840 ml	$29.15
HCFA FUL (480 ml)	$0.01	120 ml	$2.72
		480 ml	$7.43
		3840 ml	$49.88

BRAND/MANUFACTURER	NDC	SIZE	AWP
◆ BRAND			
PHENERGAN W/CODEINE: Wyeth-Ayerst	00008-0550-01	120 ml	$6.65
	00008-0550-03	480 ml	$28.63
	00008-0550-02	120 ml 24s	$190.46
◆ GENERICS			
Major	00904-1510-00	120 ml	$2.50
Cenci,H.R.	00556-0343-04	120 ml	$2.50
Barre	00472-1627-04	120 ml	$2.55
Halsey Pharm	00879-0513-04	120 ml	$2.55
Major	00904-1510-20	120 ml	$2.60
Qualitest	00603-1578-54	120 ml	$2.71
Aligen	00405-0166-76	120 ml	$2.77
Moore,H.L.	00839-7059-65	120 ml	$2.77
Goldline	00182-1712-37	120 ml	$3.00
Rugby	00536-1805-97	120 ml	$3.14
Geneva	00781-6930-04	120 ml	$3.27
Schein	00364-7390-16	480 ml	$6.75
Cenci,H.R.	00556-0343-16	480 ml	$7.10
Barre	00472-1627-16	480 ml	$7.20
Aligen	00405-0166-16	480 ml	$7.30
Qualitest	00603-1578-58	480 ml	$7.30
URL	00677-0963-33	480 ml	$7.36
Halsey Pharm	00879-0513-16	480 ml	$7.45
Major	00904-1510-16	480 ml	$7.50
Goldline	00182-1712-40	480 ml	$7.80
Rugby	00536-1805-85	480 ml	$7.82
Moore,H.L.	00839-7059-69	480 ml	$7.82
Geneva	00781-6930-16	480 ml	$8.15
Major	00904-1510-28	3840 ml	$42.70
Moore,H.L.	00839-7059-70	3840 ml	$44.54
Cenci,H.R.	00556-0343-28	3840 ml	$49.50
Rugby	00536-1805-90	3840 ml	$50.48
Barre	00472-1627-28	3840 ml	$52.20
Halsey Pharm	00879-0513-28	3840 ml	$52.25
Goldline	00182-1712-41	3840 ml	$52.50
Geneva	00781-6930-28	3840 ml	$55.47
Pharm Assoc	00121-0547-05	5 ml 100s ud	$58.76
Pharm Assoc	00121-0547-10	10 ml 100s ud	$70.62

Codeine Phosphate with Guaifenesin

Each 5 mL (1 teaspoonful) contains:

Guaifenesin, USP ....100 mg
Codeine Phosphate, USP ....10 mg
(Warning: May be habit forming)

ACTIONS

Codeine/Guaifenesin combines the expectorant, Guaifenesin, with the cough suppresant, Codeine. Guaifenesin enhances the output of lower respiratory tract fluid. The enhanced flow of less viscid secretions promotes and facilitates the removal of mucus. Codeine is a centrally acting agent which elevates the threshold for cough.

As a result, dry, unproductive coughs become more productive and less frequent.

Under Federal law, Codeine/Guaifenesin is available without a prescription. Certain state laws may differ. The container label contains the following indications, warnings and drug interaction precaution statements and directions:

INDICATIONS

Temporarily controls cough due to minor throat and bronchial irritation as may occur with the common cold or inhaled irritants. Helps loosen phlegm (mucus) and thin bronchial secretions to make coughs more productive.

WARNINGS

A persistent cough may be a sign of a serious condition. If cough persists for more than 1 week, tends to recur, or is accompanied by fever, rash, or persistent headache, consult a doctor. Do not take this product for persistent or chronic cough such as occurs with smoking, asthma, chronic bronchitis, emphysema, or if cough is accompanied by excessive phlegm (mucus) unless directed by a doctor. Adults and children who have a chronic pulmonary disease or shortness of breath, or children who are taking other drugs, should not take this product unless directed by a doctor. May cause or aggravate constipation. As with any drug, if you are pregnant or nursing a baby, seek the advice of a health professional before using this product.

Professional Note: Guaifenesin has been shown to produce a color interference with certain clinical laboratory determinations of 5-hydroxyindoleacetic acid (5-HIAA) and vanillylmandelic acid (VMA).

DRUG INTERACTION PRECAUTION

Caution should be used when taking this product with sedatives, tranquilizers and drugs used for depression, especially monoamine oxidase inhibitors (MAOIs). These combinations may cause greater sedation (drowsiness) than is caused by the products used alone.

DIRECTIONS

Take orally as stated below or use as directed by a doctor.

Adults and children 12 years of age and over; 2 teaspoonfuls every 4 hours, not to exceed 12 teaspoonfuls in a 24-hour period; children 6 to under 12 years: 1 teaspoonful every 4 hours, not to exceed 6 teaspoonfuls in a 24-hour period; children under 6 years: consult a doctor. A special measuring device should be used to give an accurate dose of this product to children under 6 years of age. Giving a higher dose than recommended by a doctor could result in serious side effects for a child. Use of Codeine-containing preparations is not recommended for children under 2 years of age. Do not exceed recommended dosage.

HOW SUPPLIED
LIQUID (C-V): 2.5 MG-75 MG/5 ML

BRAND/MANUFACTURER	NDC	SIZE	AWP
○ BRAND			
BRONTEX: P&G Pharm	00149-0441-16	473 ml	$28.37

SYRUP (C-V): 10 MG-100 MG/5 ML

BRAND/MANUFACTURER	NDC	SIZE	AWP
○ BRAND			
CHERACOL W/CODEINE: Roberts Pharm	54092-0402-60	60 ml	$3.37
ROBITUSSIN-AC: Robins Pharm	00031-8674-05	60 ml	$6.68
CHERACOL W/CODEINE: Roberts Pharm	54092-0402-04	120 ml	$5.59
ROBITUSSIN-AC: Robins Pharm	00031-8674-12	120 ml	$11.15
CHERACOL W/CODEINE: Roberts Pharm	54092-0402-16	480 ml	$21.07
ROBITUSSIN-AC: Robins Pharm	00031-8674-25	480 ml	$37.66
	00031-8674-29	3840 ml	$268.08

For additional alternatives, turn to the section beginning on page 2859.

◆ RATED THERAPEUTICALLY EQUIVALENT; ◇ THERAPEUTIC EQUIVALENCE UNCONFIRMED; ○ UNRATED

Codeine Phosphate with Pseudoephedrine Hydrochloride

DESCRIPTION

Codeine Phosphate/Pseudoephedrine Hydrochloride Syrup and Capsules is an antitussive-decongestant containing in each 5 ml (teaspoonful) and each capsule: Codeine Phosphate, 20 mg (Warning: May Be Habit Forming); Pseudoephedrine Hydrochloride, 60 mg.

Chemically, Codeine is 7,8-didehydro-4,5α-epoxy-3-methoxy-17-methylmorphinan-6αol phosphate (1:1) salt hemihydrate.

Chemically, Pseudoephedrine is [S-(R*.R*)]-a-[1- (methylamino) ethyl]benzenemethanol hydrochloride.

CLINICAL PHARMACOLOGY

The clinical pharmacology of this formulated product is thought to be due to the action of its ingredients, Codeine Phosphate and Pseudoephedrine Hydrochloride.

Codeine Phosphate: Codeine causes suppression of the cough reflex by a direct effect on the cough center in the medulla and appears to exert a drying effect on respiratory tract mucosa and to increase viscosity of bronchial secretions.

Codeine is well absorbed from the gastrointestinal tract. Following oral administration, peak antitussive effects usually can be expected to occur within 1-2 hours and may persist for a period of four hours. Codeine is metabolized in the liver.

The drug undergoes O-demethylation, N-demethylation, and partial conjugation with glucuronic acid, and is excreted mainly in the urine as norcodeine and morphine in the free and conjugated forms.

Codeine appears in breast milk of nursing mothers and has been reported to cross the placental barrier.

Pseudoephedrine Hydrochloride: Pseudoephedrine is a physiologically active stereoisomer of ephedrine which acts directly on alpha, and, to a lesser degree, beta-adrenergic receptors. The alpha-adrenergic effects are believed to result from the reduced production of cyclic adenosine-3′,5′ monophosphate (cyclic 3′,5′-AMP) by inhibition of the enzyme adenyl cyclase, where beta-adrenergic effects appear to be caused by the stimulation of adenyl cyclase activity.

Pseudoephedrine acts directly on alpha-adrenergic receptors in the respiratory tract mucosa producing vasoconstriction resulting in shrinkage of swollen nasal mucous membranes, reduction of tissue hyperemia, edema, and nasal congestion, and an increase in nasal airway patency. Drainage of sinus secretions is increased and obstructed eustachian ostia may be opened. Relaxation of bronchial smooth muscle by stimulation of beta$_2$ adrenergic receptors may also occur. Following oral administration, significant bronchodilation has not been demonstrated consistently.

Nasal decongestion with Codeine Phosphate/Pseudoephedine Hydrochloride (Codeine/Pseudoephedrine) Syrup and Capsules usually occurs within 30 minutes and persists for 4-6 hours after oral administration of 60 mg of Pseudoephedrine Hydrochloride.

INDICATIONS AND USAGE

Codeine/Pseudoephedrine is indicated for symptomatic relief when both coughing and congestion are associated with upper respiratory infections and related conditions such as common cold, bronchitis, influenza, and sinusitis.

CONTRAINDICATIONS

Hypersensitivity to product's active ingredients.

WARNINGS

Persons with persistent cough such as occurs with smoking, asthma, emphysema, or where cough is accompanied by excessive secretions should not take this product except under the advice and supervision of a physician.

May cause or aggravate constipation.

Do not give this product to children taking other drugs except under the advice and supervision of a physician.

Persons with a chronic pulmonary disease or shortness of breath, high blood pressure, heart disease, diabetes, or thyroid diseases should not take this product except under the advice and supervision of a physician.

Do not exceed recommended dosage because at higher doses nervousness, dizziness, or sleeplessness may occur.

If symptoms do not improve within 7 days or are accompanied by fever, consult a physician before continuing use.

PRECAUTIONS

General: Inasmuch as the active ingredients consist of Codeine Phosphate/Pseudoephedrine Hydrochloride, this medication should be used with caution in the presence of the following:

- Cardiovascular disease (of any etiology)
- Diabetes mellitus
- Hypertension (of any severity)
- Abnormal thyroid function
- Prostatic hypertrophy
- Addison's disease
- Chronic ulcerative colitis
- History of drug abuse or dependence
- Chronic respiratory disease or impairment
- Functional impairment of the liver or kidney

Patients taking Codeine/Pseudoephedrine should be cautioned when driving or doing jobs requiring alertness and to get up slowly from a lying or sitting position, or to lie down if nausea occurs.

Possible Drug Interactions: Because of the potential for drug interactions, persons currently taking any of the following medications should take Codeine/Pseudoephedrine Syrup and Capsules on the advice and under the supervision of a physician.

- Beta adrenergic blockers—concurrent use may increase the possibility of cardiac arrhythmias.
- Digitalis glycosides—concurrent use with Pseudoephedrine may increase the possibility of cardiac arrhythmias.
- Antihypertensive agents including Veratrum alkaloids—hypotensive effects may be decreased by the concurrent use of Pseudoephedrine.
- Monoamine oxidase (MAO) inhibitors—these agents may potentiate the pressor effect of Pseudoephedrine and may result in a hypertensive crisis; Pseudoephedrine should not be administered during or within 14 days of MAO inhibitors.
- Sympathomimetics, other—sympathomimetics used concurrently may increase the effects either of these agents or of Pseudoephedrine, thereby increasing the potential for side effects.
- Tricyclic antidepressants—the concurrent use of tricyclic antidepressants themselves or of the codeine component.
- CNS depressants
- Alcohol
- General anesthetics
- Anticholinergics—concurrent use may result in paralytic ileus.

Drug/Laboratory Test Interactions: Codeine may cause an elevation in serum amylase levels due to the spasm producing potential of narcotic analgesics on the sphincter of Oddi.

Pregnancy: Category C: Animal reproduction studies of the components of Codeine/Pseudoephedrine Syrup and Capsules have not been conducted. Thus, it is not known whether these agents can cause fetal harm when administered to pregnant women only where clearly needed.

Nursing Mothers: Codeine/Pseudoephedrine are excreted in breast milk; therefore, caution should be exercised when this medication is prescribed for a nursing mother.

Pediatric Use

Do not give Codeine/Pseudoephedrine Syrup and Capsules to children under two years of age except on the advice and under the supervision of a physician.

ADVERSE REACTIONS

Based on the composition of Codeine/Pseudoephedrine Syrup and Capsules, the following side effects may occur: nervousness, restlessness, trouble in sleeping, drowsiness, difficult or painful urination, dizziness or light-headedness, headache, nausea and vomiting, constipation, trembling, troubled breathing, increase in sweating, unusual paleness, weakness, and changes in heart rate.

DRUG ABUSE AND DEPENDENCE

Codeine/Pseudoephedrine Syrup and Capsules are placed in Schedule III of the Controlled Substances Act.

OVERDOSAGE

Codeine/Pseudoephedrine Syrup and Capsules contain Codeine Phosphate and Pseudoephedrine Hydrochloride. Overdosage as a result of these products should be treated based upon the symptomatology of the patient as it relates to the individual ingredient. Treatment of acute overdosage would probably be based upon treating the patient for codeine toxicity which may be manifested as:

- Gradual drowsiness, dizziness, heaviness of the head, weariness, diminution of sensibility, and loss of pain and other modalities of sensation.
- Nausea and vomiting.
- A transient excitement stage, characterized by extreme restlessness, delirium, and rarely epileptiform convulsions, is sometimes seen in children and rarely in adult women.
- Bilateral miosis, progressing to pinpoint pupils, which do not react to light or accommodation. The pupils may dilate during terminal asphyxia.
- Itching of the skin and nose, sometimes with skin rashes and urticaria.
- Coma, with muscular relaxation and depressed or absent superficial and deep reflexes. A Babinski toe sign may appear.
- Marked slowing of the respiratory rate with inadequate pulmonary ventilation and consequent cyanosis. Breathing becomes stertorous and irregular (Cheyne-Stokes or Biot).
- The pulse is slow and the blood pressure gradually falls to shock levels. Urine formation ceases or is reduced to a very slow rate.

➤ SHOWN IN PRODUCT IDENTIFICATION GUIDE

CODEINE/PSEUDOEPHEDRINE SYRUP AND CAPSULES
The lethal dose of Codeine for an adult is about 0.5-1.0 g. Treatment is as recommended for narcotics.

DOSAGE AND ADMINISTRATION
CODEINE/PSEUDOEPHEDRINE SYRUP AND CAPSULES
RECOMMENDED DOSAGE: CAPSULE
Adults: 1 capsule every 6 hours, not to exceed 4 capsules in 24 hours.

RECOMMENDED DOSAGE: SYRUP
Adults: 1 teaspoonful every 6 hours, not to exceed 4 teaspoonfuls in 24 hours.

Children: 6 to under 12 years: ½ teaspoonful every 6 hours, not to exceed 2 teaspoonfuls in 24 hours.

2 to under 6 years: ¼ teaspoonful every 6 hours, not to exceed 1 teaspoonful in 24 hours.

Do not give this product to children under 2 years, except under the advice and supervision of a physician.

HOW SUPPLIED
CAPSULE (C-III): 60 MG-20 MG

BRAND/MANUFACTURER	NDC	SIZE	AWP
○ **BRAND**			
NUCOFED: Roberts Pharm	54092-0005-60	60s	$28.03

SYRUP (C-III): 20 MG-60 MG/5 ML

BRAND/MANUFACTURER	NDC	SIZE	AWP
○ **GENERICS**			
Aligen	00405-0054-16	480 ml	$27.90

SYRUP (C-III): 60 MG-20 MG/5 ML

BRAND/MANUFACTURER	NDC	SIZE	AWP
○ **BRAND**			
NUCOFED: Roberts Pharm	54092-0403-16	473 ml	$37.74

Codeine Phosphate/Guaifenesin/Phenylpropanolamine Hydrochloride

DESCRIPTION
Each 5mL contains:

Codeine Phosphate ....10 mg
Phenylpropanolamine Hydrochloride ....12.5 mg
Guaifenesin ....100 mg

INDICATIONS
For prompt, temporary relief of coughs and nasal congestion due to the common cold. Helps loosen bronchial secretions to drain bronchial tubes.

WARNINGS
A persistent cough may be a sign of a serious condition. If cough persists for more than 1 week, tends to recur, or is accompanied by fever, rash, or persistent headache, consult a physician. Do not take this product for more than 7 days. If symptoms do not improve or are accompanied by fever consult a physician. Do not take this product for persistent or chronic cough such as occurs with smoking, asthma, chronic bronchitis, or emphysema, or where cough is accompanied by excessive phlegm (sputum) unless directed by a physician. Adults and children who have a chronic pulmonary disease or shortness of breath, or children who are taking other drugs, should not take this product unless directed by a physician. This product may cause or aggravate constipation. Do not take this product if you have heart disease, high blood pressure, thyroid disease, diabetes, or difficulty in urination due to enlargement of the prostate gland unless directed by a physician. As with any drug if you are pregnant or nursing a baby, seek the advice of a health professional before using this product. Keep this and all drugs out of the reach of children. In case of accidental overdose, seek professional assistance or contact a Poison Control Center immediately.

DRUG INTERACTION PRECAUTION
Do not take this product if you are presently taking a prescription drug for high blood pressure or depression, without first consulting a physician.

DOSAGE
Adults and children 12 years of age and over: 2 teaspoonfuls every 4 hours. Children 6 to under 12 years of age: 1 teaspoonful every 4 hours. Unless directed by a physician, do not exceed 6 doses in 24 hours. Children under 6 years of age: Consult a physician.

A dispensing device (such as a dropper calibrated for age or weight) should be dispensed along with the product when it is intended for use in children 2 to

under 6 years of age to prevent possible overdose due to improper measuring of the dose.

Parents should be instructed to obtain and use a calibrated measuring device for administering the drug to the child, to use extreme care in measuring the dosage, and not to exceed the recommended daily dosage.

Codeine is not recommended for use in children under 2 years of age. Children under 2 years may be more susceptible to the respiratory depressant effects of codeine, including respiratory arrest, coma, and death.

HOW SUPPLIED
LIQUID (C-V): 10 MG-100 MG-12.5 MG/5ML

BRAND/MANUFACTURER	NDC	SIZE	AWP
○ **GENERICS**			
EFASIN EXPECTORANT SF: Major	00904-3541-16	480 ml	$17.95
ALPHEN EXPECTORANT: Alphagen	59743-0112-16	480 ml	$18.25
Aligen	00405-0059-16	480 ml	$20.95

LIQUID (C-V): 10 MG-200 MG-12.5 MG/5ML

BRAND/MANUFACTURER	NDC	SIZE	AWP
○ **BRAND**			
NALDECON-CX ADULT: Apothecon	00015-5661-40	120 ml	$6.52
	00015-5661-60	480 ml	$23.39
TRIAMINIC EXP W/CODEINE: Sandoz Consumer	00043-0528-16	480 ml	$33.04
○ **GENERICS**			
CONEX W/CODEINE: Forest Pharm	00456-0612-04	120 ml	$4.00
MEDI-TUSS W/CODEINE: Medi-Plex	59010-0150-04	120 ml	$6.60
ENDITUSSIN EXPECTORANT: Southwood	58016-4176-04	120 ml	$11.95
CHEMDAL EXPECTORANT: Norton,HN	50732-0854-16	473 ml	$17.73
CODEGEST EXPECTORANT: Great Southern	51301-0540-16	480 ml	$15.49
QUENDAL EXPECTORANT: Qualitest	00603-1620-58	480 ml	$15.80
Goldline	00182-0153-40	480 ml	$22.95
STATUSS: Huckaby	58407-0376-16	480 ml	$26.81
ENDAL EXPECTORANT: Forest Pharm	00785-6226-16	480 ml	$36.60
ENDITUSSIN EXPECTORANT: Southwood	58016-4176-16	480 ml	$45.50
CHEMDAL EXPECTORANT: Norton,HN	50732-0854-28	3785 ml	$108.17
CODEGEST EXPECTORANT: Great Southern	51301-0540-28	3840 ml	$99.00

SYRUP (C-V): 10 MG-200 MG-12.5 MG/5ML

BRAND/MANUFACTURER	NDC	SIZE	AWP
○ **GENERICS**			
C-TUSSIN: Century	00436-0920-04	3600 ml	$1.60
C-TUSSIN: Century	00436-0920-28	3840 ml	$42.00

Codeine Phosphate/Guaifenesin/Pseudoephedrine Hydrochloride

DESCRIPTION
Each 5 ml teaspoonful contains Codeine Phosphate, 10 mg (Warning: may be habit forming), Pseudoephedrine Hydrochloride, 30 mg, Guaifenesin, 100 mg.

ACTIONS
Expectorant, antitussive and decongestant actions. Codeine, at the recommended dose, causes suppression of the cough reflex by a direct effect on the cough center in the medulla of the brain. Codeine has antitussive and mild analgesics and sedative effects.

Pseudoephedrine Hydrochloride, an orally effective nasal decongestant, is a sympathomimetic amine with peripheral effects similar to epinephrine and central effects similar to, but less intense than, amphetamines. Therefore, it has the potential for excitatory side effects. Pseudoephedrine at the recommended oral dosage has little or no pressor effect in normotensive adults. Patients taking pseudoephedrine orally have not been reported to experience the rebound congestion sometimes experienced with frequent, repeated use of topical decongestants. Pseudoephedrine is not known to produce drowsiness.

Guaifenesin helps drainage of bronchial tubes by thinning the mucus, and facilitates expectoration by loosening phlegm and bronchial secretions.

◆ RATED THERAPEUTICALLY EQUIVALENT; ◇ THERAPEUTIC EQUIVALENCE UNCONFIRMED; ○ UNRATED

INDICATIONS

For loosening tenacious pulmonary secretions associated with cough and respiratory congestion.

A minimum dosage of codeine phosphate is provided for the symptomatic relief of nonproductive cough. Decongestants have been used to relieve eustachian tube congestion associated with acute eustachian salpingitis, aerotitis, otitis and serous otitis media. Guaifenesin helps loosen phlegm (sputum) and bronchial secretions.

May be used as supportive therapy for acute otitis media and relief of mild otalgia.

May be given concomitantly when indicated, with analgesics and antibiotics.

CONTRAINDICATIONS

Patients with severe hypertension, severe coronary artery disease, and in patients on MAO inhibitor therapy.

Nursing Mothers: Pseudoephedrine is contraindicated in nursing mothers because of the higher than usual risk for infants from sympathomimetic amines.

Hypersensitivity: This drug is contraindicated in patients with hypersensitivity or idiosyncrasy to its ingredients. Patient idiosyncrasy to adrenergic agents may be manifested by insomnia, dizziness, weakness, tremor or arrhythmias.

WARNINGS

Codeine should be prescribed and administered with the same degree of caution as all oral medications containing a narcotic analgesic. Codeine appears in the milk of nursing mothers.

If sympathomimetic amines are used in patients with hypertension, diabetes mellitus, ischemic heart disease, hyperthyroidism, increased intraocular pressure and prostatic hypertrophy, judicious caution should be exercised. See, however, *"Contraindications."* Sympathomimetics may produce CNS stimulation with convulsions or cardiovascular collapse with accompanying hypotension. Do not exceed recommended dosage.

The elderly (60 years and older) are more likely to have adverse reactions to sympathomimetics. Safety for use during pregnancy has not been established.

PRECAUTIONS

If cough persists for more than one week, tends to recur or is accompanied by fever, rash or headache, discontinue treatment.

Other medications containing a narcotic analgesic, phenothiazines, tranquilizers, sedatives, hypnotics, and other CNS depressants, including alcohol, may have an additive CNS depressant effect when used concomitantly. The dose should be reduced when such combined therapy is contemplated. Caution should be exercised if used in patients with high blood pressure, heart disease, asthma, emphysema, diabetes, thyroid disease and hyperreactivity to ephedrine.

ADVERSE REACTIONS

Nausea, vomiting, constipation, dizziness, sedation, palpitations, or pruritus may occur. More frequent or higher than recommended dosage may cause respiratory depression, especially in patients with respiratory disease associated with carbon dioxide retention.

Drugs containing sympathomimetic amines have been associated with certain untoward reactions including fear, anxiety, tenseness, restlessness, tremor, weakness, pallor, respiratory difficulty, dysuria, insomnia, hallucinations, convulsions, CNS depression, arrhythmias and cardiovascular collapse with hypotension.

Note: Guaifenesin interferes with the colorimetric determination of 5-hydroxyindoleacetic acid (5-HIAA) and vanillymandelic acid (VMA).

DRUG INTERACTIONS

Codeine may potentiate the effects of other narcotics, general anesthetics, tranquilizers, sedatives and hypnotics, tricyclic antidepressants, MAO inhibitors, alcohol and other CNS depressants.

Beta adrenergic blockers and MAO inhibitors potentiate the sympathomimetic effects of pseudoephedrine. Sympathomimetics may reduce the antihypertensive effects of methyldopa, mecamylamine reserpine and veratrum alkaloids.

DOSAGE

Adults: 2 teaspoonfuls; children 50-90 lbs, 1/2 to 1 teaspoonful; 25-50 lbs, 1/4 to 1/2 teaspoonful. Repeat every 4 hours. May be given to children under 2 at the discretion of the physician. *Do not exceed 4 doses in a 24-hour period.*

Product Label Dosage is as Follows: Adults and children 12 years and older, 2 teaspoonfuls every 4 hours. Children 6 to under 12 years, 1 teaspoonful every 4 hours. Do not exceed 4 doses in 24 hours. For children under 6 years, give only as directed by a physician.

HOW SUPPLIED
LIQUID (C-V): 10 MG-100 MG-30 MG/5 ML

AVERAGE UNIT PRICE (AVAILABLE SIZES)

GENERIC			$0.02
BRAND/MANUFACTURER	NDC	SIZE	AWP
◆ GENERICS			
PHENYLHISTINE: Cenci,H.R.	00556-0333-04	120 ml	$2.90
PHENYLHISTINE: Cenci,H.R.	00556-0333-16	480 ml	$9.50
PHENYLHISTINE: Cenci,H.R.	00556-0333-28	3840 ml	$58.60

For additional alternatives, turn to the section beginning on page 2859.

Codeine Phosphate/ Phenylephrine Hydrochloride/ Promethazine Hydrochloride

DESCRIPTION

Each teaspoon (5 mL) of Codeine Phosphate/Phenylephrine Hydrochloride/Promethazine Hydrochloride contains 10 mg Codeine, phosphate (Warning—may be habit-forming), 6.25 Promethazine and 5 mg Hydrochloride and 5 mg Phenylephrine Hydrochloride in a flavored syrup base with a pH between 4.7 and 5.2.

Codeine is one of the naturally occurring phenanthrene alkaloids of opium derived from the opium poppy; it is classified pharmacologically as a narcotic analgesic. Codeine may be chemically named as (5α, 6α)-7,8-didehydro-4, 5-epoxy-3-methoxy-17-methylmorphianan-6-01 phosphate (1:1) (salt) hemihydrate.

The Phosphate salt of Codeine occurs as white, needle-shaped crystals or white crystalline power. Codeine Phosphate is freely soluble in water and slightly souble in alcohol, with a molecular weight of 406.37. The empirical formula is $C_{18}H_{21}NO_3 \cdot H_3PO_4 \cdot \frac{1}{2}H_2O$, and the stereochemistry is 5α, 6α isomer is indicated in the structure.

Promethazine Hydrochloride is a racemic compound; the empirical formula is $C_{17}H_{20}N_2 \cdot HCl$ and its molecular weight is 320.88

Promethazine Hydrochloride, a phenothiazine derivative, is designated chemically as N,N,α-trimethyl-1OH-phenothiazine-10-ethanamine monohydrochloride.

Promethazine Hydrochloride occurs as a white to faint yellow, practically odorless, crystalline powder which slowly oxidizes and turns blue on prolonged exposure to air. It is soluble in water and freely soluble in alcohol.

Phenylephrine Hydrochloride is a sympathomimetic amine salt. It may be chemially named as 3-hydroxy-α-[(methylamino) methyl]-benzenemethanol hydrochloride.

Phenylephrine occurs as white or nearly white crystals, having a bitter taste. It is freely soluble in water and alcohol, with a molecular weight of 203.67. The empirical formula is $C_9H_{13}NO_2 \cdot HCl$, and the stereochemistry is R-isomer as indicated in the structure; Specific Rotation—between −42° and Phenylephrine is subject to oxidation and must be protected from light and air.

CLINICAL PHARMACOLOGY

Codeine Narcotic analgesics, including Codeine, exert their primary effects on the central nervous system and gastrointestinal tract. The analgesic effects of Codeine are due to its central action: however, the precise sites of action have not been determined, and the mechanism involved appear to be quite complex. Codeine resembles morphine both structurally and pharmacologically, but its actions at the doses of Codeine used therapeutically are milder, with less sedation, respiratory depression, and gastrointestinal, urinary, and pupillary effects. Codeine produces an increase in biliary tract pressure, but less than morphine or meperidine. Codeine is less constipating than morphine.

Codeine has good antitussive activity, although less than that of morphine at equal doses. It is used in preference to morphine, because side effects are infrequent at the usual antitussive doses of Codeine.

Codeine in oral therapeutic dosage does not usually exert major effects on the cardiovascular system.

Narcotic analgesics may cause nausea and vomiting by stimulating the chemoreceptor trigger zone (CTZ); however, they also depress the vomiting center, so that subsequent doses are unlikely to produce vomiting. Nausea is minimal after usual oral doses of Codeine.

Narcotic analgesics cause histamine release, which appears to be responsible for wheals or urticaria sometimes seen at the site of injection on parenteral administration, Histamine release may also produce dilation of cutaneous blood vessels, with resultant flushing of the face and neck, pruritus, and sweating.

Codeine and its salts are well absorbed following both oral and parenteral administration. Codeine is about ⅔ as effective orally as parenterally. Codeine is metabolized primarily in the liver by enzymes of the endoplasmic reticulum, where it undergoes O-demethylation, N-demethylation, and partial conjugation with glucuronic acid. The drug is excreted primarily in the urine, largely as

➤ SHOWN IN PRODUCT IDENTIFICATION GUIDE

inactive metabolites and small amounts of free and conjugated morphine. Negligible amounts of Codeine and its metabolites are found in the feces.

Following oral or subcutaneous administration of Codeine the onset of analgesia occurs within 15 to 80 minutes and lasts for four to six hours.

The cough-depressing action, in animal studies, was observed to occur 15 minutes after oral administration of Codeine; peak action at 45 to 60 minutes after ingestion. The duration of action, which is dose-dependent, usually did not exceed 3 hours.

Promethazine: Promethazine is a phenothiazine derivative which differs structurally from the antipsychotic phenothiazines by the presence of a branched side chain and no ring substitution. It is thought that this configuration is responsible for its relative lack (1/10 that of chlorpromazine) of dopaminergic (CNS) action.

Promethazine is an H_1 receptor blocking agent. In addition to its antihistaminic action, it provides clinically useful sedative and antiemetic effects. In therapeutic dosages Promethazine produces no significant effects on the cardiovascular system.

Promethazine is well absorbed from the gastrointestinal tract. Clinical effects are apparent within 20 minutes after oral administration and generally last four to six hours, although they may persist as long as 12 hours. Promethazine is metabolized by the liver to a variety of compounds; the sulfoxides of Promethazine and N-demethylpromethazine are the predominant metabolites appearing in the urine.

Phenylephrine: Phenylephrine is a potent postsynaptic α-receptor agonist with little effect on β receptors of the heart. Phenylephrine has no effect on β-adrenergic receptors of the bronchi or peripheral blood vessels. A direct action at receptors accounts for the greater part of its effects, only a small part being due to its ability to release norepinephrine.

Therapeutic doses of Phenylephrine mainly cause vasoconstriction. Phenylephrine increases resistance and, to a lesser extent, decreases capacitance of blood vessels. Total peripheral resistance is increased, resulting in increased systolic and diastolic blood pressure. Pulmonary arterial pressure is usually increased, and renal blood flow is usually decreased. Local vasoconstriction and hemostasis occur following topical application or infiltration of Phenylephrine into tissues. The main effect of Phenylephrine on the heart is bradycardia; it produces a positive inotropic effect on the myocardium in doses greater than those usually used therapeutically. Rarely, the drug may increase the irritability of the heart, causing arrhythmias. Cardiac output is decreased slightly. Phenylephrine increases the work of the heart by increasing peripheral arterial resistance.

Phenylephrine has a mild central stimulant effect.

Following oral administration or topical application of Phenylephrine to the mucosa, constriction of blood vessels in the nasal mucosa relieves nasal congestion associated with allergy or head colds. Following oral administration, nasal decongestion may occur within 15 or 20 minutes and may persist for up to 4 hours.

Phenylephrine is irregularly absorbed from and readily metabolized in the gastrointestinal tract. Phenylephrine is metabolized in the liver and intestine by monoamine oxidase. The metabolites and their route and rate of excretion have not been identified. The pharmacologic action of Phenylephrine is terminated at least partially by uptake of the drug into tissues.

INDICATIONS AND USAGE

Codeine Phosphate/Phenylephrine HCl/Promethazine HCl is indicated for the temporary relief of coughs and upper respiratory symptoms, including nasal congestion, associated with allergy or the common cold.

CONTRAINDICATIONS

Codeine is contraindicated in patients with a known hypersensitivity to the drug.

Promethazine is contraindicated in individuals known to be hypersensitive or to have had an idiosyncratic reaction to promethazine or to other phenothiazines.

Phenylephrine is contraindicated in patients with hypertension or with peripheral vascular insufficiency (ischemia may result with risk of gangrene or thrombosis of compromised vascular beds). Phenylephrine should not be used in patients known to be hypersensitive to the drug or in those receiving a monoamine oxidase inhibitor (MAOI).

Antihistamines and Codeine are both contraindicated for use in the treatment of lower respiratory tract symptoms, including asthma.

WARNINGS

Codeine: Dosage of Codeine SHOULD NOT BE INCREASED if cough fails to respond; an unresponsive cough should be reevaluated in 5 days or sooner for possible underlying pathology, such as foreign body or lower respiratory tract disease.

Codeine may cause or aggravate constipation. Respiratory depression leading to arrest, coma, and death has occurred with the use of Codeine antitussives in young children, particularly in the under-one-year infants whose ability to deactivate the drug is not fully developed.

Administration of Codeine may be accompanied by histamine release and should be used with caution in atopic children.

Head Injury and Increased Intracranial Pressure: The respiratory-depressant effects of narcotic analgesics and their capacity to elevate cerebrospinal fluid pressure may be markedly exaggerated in the presence of head injury, intracranial lesions, or a preexisting increase in intracranial pressure. Narcotics may produce adverse reactions which may obscure the clinical course of patients with head injuries.

Asthma and Other Respiratory Conditions: Narcotic analgesics or cough suppressants, including Codeine should not be used in asthmatic patients (see ''Contraindications''). Nor should they be used in acute febrile illness associated with productive cough or in chronic respiratory disease where interference with ability to clear the tracheobronchial tree of secretions would have a deleterious effect on the patient's respiratory function.

Hypotensive Effect: Codeine may produce orthostatic hypotension in ambulatory patients.

Promethazine: Promethazine may cause marked drowsiness. Ambulatory patients should be cautioned against such activities as driving or operating dangerous machinery until it is known that they do not become drowsy or dizzy from Promethazine therapy.

The sedative action of Promethazine is additive to the sedative effects of central nervous system depressants; therefore, agents such as alcohol, narcotic analgesics, sedatives, hypnotics, and tranquilizers should either be eliminated or given in reduced dosage in the presence of Promethazine Hydrochloride. When given concomitantly with Promethazine Hydrochloride, the dose of barbiturates should be reduced by at least one-half, and the dose of analgesic depressants, such as morphine or meperidine, should be reduced by one-quarter to one-half.

Promethazine may lower seizure threshold. This should be taken into consideration when administering to persons with known seizure disorders or when giving in combination with narcotics or local anesthetics which may also affect seizure threshold.

Sedative drugs or CNS depressants should be avoided in patients with a history of sleep apnea. Antihistamines should be used with caution in patients with narrow-angle glaucoma, stenosing peptic ulcer, pyloroduodenal obstruction, and urinary bladder obstruction due to symptomatic prostatic hypertrophy and narrowing of the bladder neck.

Administration of Promethazine has been associated with reported cholestatic jaundice.

Phenylephrine: Because Phenylephrine is an adrenergic agent, it should be given with caution to patients with thyroid diseases, diabetes mellitus, and heart diseases or those receiving tricyclic antidepressants.

Men with symptomatic, benign prostatic hypertrophy can experience urinary retention when given oral nasal decongestants.

Phenylephrine can cause a decrease in cardiac output, and extreme caution should be used when administering the drug, parenterally or orally, to patients with arteriosclerosis, to elderly individuals, and/or to patients with initially poor cerebral or coronary circulation.

Phenylephrine should be used with caution in patients taking diet preparations, such as amphetamines or phenylpropanolamine, because synergistic adrenergic effects could result in serious hypertensive response and possible stroke.

PRECAUTIONS

Animal reproduction studies have not been conducted with the drug combination Codeine/Phenylephrine HCl/Promethazine HCl. It is not known whether this drug combination can cause fetal harm when administered to a pregnant woman or can affect reproduction capacity. Codeine/Phenylephrine HCl/Promethazine HCl should be given to a pregnant woman only if clearly needed.

GENERAL

Narcotic analgesics, including Codeine should be administered with caution and the initial dose reduced in patients with acute abdominal conditions, convulsive disorders, significant hepatic or renal impairment, fever, hypothyroidism, Addison's disease, ulcerative colitis, prostatic hypertrophy, in patients with recent gastrointestinal or urinary tract surgery, and in the very young or elderly or debilitated patients. Promethazine should be used cautiously in persons with cardiovascular disease or with impairment of liver function. Phenylephrine should be used with caution in patients with cardiovascular disease, particularly hypertension.

INFORMATION FOR PATIENTS

Codeine/Phenylephrine HCl/Promethazine HCl may cause marked drowsiness or impair the mental and/or physical abilities required for the performance of potentially hazardous tasks, such as driving a vehicle or operating machinery. Ambulatory patients should be told to avoid engaging in such activities until it is known that they do not become drowsy or dizzy from Codeine Phosphate/Phenylephrine HCl/Promethazine HCl therapy. Children should be supervised to avoid potential harm in bike riding or in other hazardous activities.

The concomitant use of alcohol or other central nervous system depressants, including narcotic analgesics, sedatives, hypnotics, and tranquilizers, may have an additive effect and should be avoided or their dosage reduced.

Patients should be advised to report any involuntary muscle movements or unusual sensitivity to sunlight.

Codeine, like other narcotic analgesics, may produce orthostatic hypotension in some ambulatory patients. Patients should be cautioned accordingly.

DRUG INTERACTIONS

Codeine: In patients receiving MAO inhibitors, an initial small test dose is advisable to allow observation of any excessive narcotic effects or MAOI interaction.

Promethazine: The sedative action of Promethazine is additive to the effects of other central nervous system depressants, including alcohol, narcotic analgesics, sedatives, hypnotics, tricyclic antidepressants, and tranquilizers; therefore, these agents should be avoided or administered in reduced dosage to patients receiving Promethazine HCl.

◆ RATED THERAPEUTICALLY EQUIVALENT; ◇ THERAPEUTIC EQUIVALENCE UNCONFIRMED; ○ UNRATED

CODEINE PHOSPHATE/PHENYLEPHRINE HCL/PROMETHAZINE HCL

PHENYLEPHRINE Drug	EFFECT
Phenylephrine with prior administration of monoamine oxidase inhibitors (MAOI).	Cardiac pressor response potentiated. May cause acute hypertensive crisis.
Phenylephrine with tricyclic antidepressants.	Pressor response increased.
Phenylephrine with ergot alkaloids.	Excessive rise in blood pressure.
Phenylephrine with bronchodilator sympathomimetic agents and with epinephrine or other sympathomimetics.	Tachycardia or other arrhythmias may occur.
Phenylephrine with prior administration of propranolol or other β-adrenergic blockers.	Cardiostimulating effects blocked.
Phenylephrine with atropine sulfate.	Reflex bradycardia blocked; pressor response enhanced.
Phenylephrine with prior administration of phentolamine or other α-adrenergic blockers.	Pressor response decreased.
Phenylephrine with diet preparations, such as amphetamines or phenylpropanolamine.	Synergistic adrenergic response.

DRUG/LABORATORY TEST INTERACTIONS
Because narcotic analgesics may increase biliary tract pressure, with resultant increases in plasma amylase or lipase levels, determination of these enzyme levels may be unreliable for 24 hours after a narcotic analgesic has been given. The following laboratory tests may be affected in patients who are receiving therapy with Promethazine.

Pregnancy Tests: Diagnostic pregnancy tests based on immunological reactions between HCG and anti-HCG may result in false-negative or false-positive interpretations.

Glucose Tolerance Test: An increase in blood glucose has been reported in patients receiving Promethazine.

CARCINOGENESIS, MUTAGENESIS, IMPAIRMENT OF FERTILITY
Codeine and Promethazine: Long-term animals studies have not been performed to assess the carcinogenic potential of Codeine or Promethazine nor are there other animal or human data concerning carcinogenicity, mutagenicity, or impairment of fertility with these agents. Codeine has been reported to show no evidence of carcinogenicity or mutagenicity in a variety of test systems, including the micronucleus and sperm abnormality assays and the *Salmonella* assay. Promethazine was nonmutagenic in the *Salmonella* test system of Ames.

Phenylephrine: A study which followed the development of cancer in 143,574 patients over a four-year period indicated that in 11,981 patients who received Phenylephrine (systemic or topical), there was no statistically significant association between the drug and cancer at any or all sites.

Long-term animal studies have not been performed to assess the carcinogenic potential of Phenylephrine nor are there other animal or human data concerning mutagenicity.

A study of the effects of adrenergic drugs on ovum transport in rabbits indicated that treatment with Phenylephrine did not alter incidence of pregnancy; the number of implantations was significantly reduced when high doses of the drug were used.

PREGNANCY
Teratogenic Effects: Pregnancy Category C

Codeine: A study in rats and rabbits reported no teratogenic effect of Codeine administered during the period of organogenesis in doses ranging from 5 to 120 mg/kg. In the rat, doses at the 120 mg/kg level, in the toxic range for the adult animal, were associated with an increase in embryo resorption at the time of implantation. In another study a single 100 mg/kg dose of Codeine administered to pregnant mice reportedly resulted in delayed ossification in the offspring.

There are no studies in humans, and the significance of these findings to humans, if any, is not known.

Promethazine: Teratogenic effects have not been demonstrated in rat-feeding studies at doses of 6.25 and 12.5 mg/kg of Promethazine. These doses are 8.3 and 16.7 times the maximum recommended total daily dose for a 50-kg subject. Specific studies to test the action of the drug on parturition, lactation, and development of the animal neonate were not done, but a general preliminary study in rats indicated no effect on these parameters. Although antihistamines, including Promethazine, have been found to produce fetal mortality in rodents, the pharmacological effects of histamine in the rodent do not parallel those in man. There are no adequate and well-controlled studies of Promethazine in pregnant women.

Phenylephrine: A study in rabbits indicated that continued moderate overexposure to Phenylephrine (3 mg/day) during the second half of pregnancy (22nd day of gestation to delivery) may contribute to perinatal wastage, prematurity, premature labor, and possibly fetal anomalies; when Phenylephrine (3 mg/day) was given to rabbits during the first half of pregnancy (3rd day after mating for seven days), a significant number gave birth to litters of low birth weight. Another

study showed that Phenylephrine was associated with anomalies of aortic arch and with ventricular septal defect in the chick embryo.

Codeine Phosphate/Phenylephrine HCl/Promethazine HCl should be used during pregnancy only if the potential benefit justifies the potential risk to the fetus.

Nonteratogenic Effects: Dependence has been reported in newborns whose mothers took opiates regularly during pregnancy. Withdrawal signs include irritability, excessive crying, tremors, hyperreflexia, fever, vomiting, and diarrhea. Signs usually appear during the first few days of life.

Promethazine taken within two weeks of delivery may inhibit platelet aggregation in the newborn.

LABOR AND DELIVERY
Narcotic analgesics cross the placental barrier. The closer to delivery and the larger the dose used, the greater the possibility of respiratory depression in the newborn. Narcotic analgesics should be avoided during labor if delivery of a premature infant is anticipated. If the mother has received narcotic analgesics during labor, newborn infants should be observed closely for signs of respiratory depression. Resuscitation may be required (see *"Overdosage"*). The effect of Codeine if any, on the later growth, development, and functional maturation of the child is unknown.

Administration of Phenylephrine to patients in late pregnancy or labor may cause fetal anoxia or bradycardia by increasing contractility of the uterus and decreasing uterine blood flow.

See also *"Nonteratogenic Effects"*.

NURSING MOTHERS
Some studies, but not others, have reported detectable amounts of Codeine in breast milk. The levels are probably not clinically significant after usual therapeutic dosage. The possibility of clinically important amounts being excreted in breast milk in individuals abusing Codeine should be considered.

It is not known whether either Phenylephrine or Promethazine is excreted in human milk.

Caution should be exercised when Codeine Phosphate/Phenylephrine HCl/ Promethazine HCl is administered to a nursing woman.

PEDIATRIC USE
This product should not be used in children under 2 years of age because safety for such use has not been established.

ADVERSE REACTIONS
CODEINE
Nervous System: CNS depression, particularly respiratory depression, and to a lesser extent circulatory depression; light-headedness, dizziness, sedation, euphoria, dysphoria, headache, transient hallucinations, disorientation, visual disturbances, and convulsions.

Cardiovascular: Tachycardia, bradycardia, palpitation, faintness, syncope, orthostatic hypotension (common to narcotic analgesics).

Gastrointestinal: Nausea, vomiting, constipation, and biliary tract spasm. Patients with chronic ulcerative colitis may experience increased colonic motility; in patients with acute ulcerative colitis, toxic dilation has been reported.

Genitourinary: Oliguria, urinary retention; antidiuretic effect has been reported (common to narcotic analgesics).

Allergic: Infrequent pruritus, giant urticaria, angioneurotic edema, and laryngeal edema.

Other: Flushing of the face, sweating and pruritus (due to opiate-induced histamine release); weakness.

PROMETHAZINE
Nervous System: Sedation, sleepiness, occasional blurred vision, dryness of mouth, dizziness; rarely confusion, disorientation, and extrapyramidal symptoms such as oculogyric crisis, torticollis, and tongue protrusion (usually in association with parenteral injection or excessive dosage.)

Cardiovascular: Increased or decreased blood pressure.

Dermatologic: Rash, rarely photosensitivity.

Hematologic: Rarely leukopenia, thrombocytopenia; agranulocytosis (1 case).

Gastrointestinal: Nausea and vomiting.

PHENYLEPHRINE
Nervous System: Restlessness, anxiety, nervousness, and dizziness.

Cardiovascular: Hypertension (see *"Warnings"*).

Other: Precordial pain, respiratory distress, tremor, and weakness.

DRUG ABUSE AND DEPENDENCE
CONTROLLED SUBSTANCE
Codeine Phosphate/Phenylephrine HCl/Promethazine HCl is a Schedule V Controlled Substance.

ABUSE
Codeine is known to be subject to abuse; however, the abuse potential of oral Codeine appears to be quite low. Even parenteral codeine does not appear to offer the psychic effects sought by addicts to the same degree as heroin or morphine. However, Codeine must be administered only under close supervision to patients with a history of drug abuse or dependence.

DEPENDENCE

Psychological dependence, physical dependence, and tolerance are known to occur with Codeine.

OVERDOSAGE

Codeine: Serious overdose with Codeine is characterized by respiratory depression (a decrease in respiratory rate and or tidal volume, Cheyne-Stokes respiration cyanosis), extreme somnolence progressing to stupor or coma, skeletal muscle flaccidity, cold and clammy skin, and sometimes bradycardia and hypotension. The triad of coma, pinpoint pupils, and respiratory depression is strongly suggestive of opiate poisoning. In severe overdosage, particularly by the intravenous route, apnea, circulatory collapse, cardiac arrest, and death may occur. Promethazine is additive to the depressant effects of Codeine.

It is difficult to determine what constitutes a standard toxic or lethal dose. However, the lethal oral dose of Codeine in an adult is reported to be in the range of 0.5 to 1.0 gram. Infants and children are believed to be relatively more sensitive to opiates on a body-weight basis. Elderly patients are also comparatively intolerant to opiates.

Promethazine: Signs and symptoms of overdosage with Promethazine range from mild depression of the central nervous system and cardiovascular system to profound hypotension, respiratory depression, and unconsciousness.

Stimulation may be evident, especially in children and geriatric patients. Convulsions may rarely occur. A paradoxical reaction has been reported in children receiving single doses of 75 mg to 125 mg orally, characterized by hyperexcitability and nightmares.

Atropine-like signs and symptoms—dry mouth, fixed, dilated pupils, flushing, as well as gastrointestinal symptoms, may occur.

Phenylephrine: Signs and symptoms of overdosage with Phenylephrine include hypertension, headache, convulsions, cerebral hemorrhage, and vomiting. Ventricular premature beats and short paroxysms of ventricular tachycardia may also occur. Headache may be a symptom of hypertension. Bradycardia may also be seen early in phenylephrine overdosage through stimulation of baroreceptors.

Treatment: Treatment of overdosage with Codeine Phosphate/Phenylephrine HCl/Promethazine HCl is essentially symptomatic and supportive. Only in cases of extreme overdosage or individual sensitivity do vital signs including respiration, pulse, blood pressure, temperature, and EKG need to be monitored. Activated charcoal orally or by lavage may be given, or sodium or magnesium sulfate orally as a cathartic. Attention should be given to the reestablishment of adequate respiratory exchange through provision of a patent airway and institution of assisted or controlled ventilation. The narcotic antagonist, naloxone hydrochloride, may be administered when significant respiratory depression occurs with Codeine Phosphate/Phenylephrine HCl/Promethazine HCl any depressant effects of Promethazine are not reversed by naloxone. Diazepam may be used to control convulsions. Avoid analeptics, which may cause convulsions. Acidosis and electrolyte losses should be corrected. A rise in temperature or pulmonary complications may signal the need for institution of antibiotic therapy.

Severe hypotension usually responds to the administration of norepinephrine or phenylephrine. EPINEPHRINE SHOULD NOT BE USED, since its use in a patient with partial adrenergic blockade may further lower the blood pressure. Limited experience with dialysis indicates that it is not helpful.

DOSAGE AND ADMINISTRATION

The average effective dose is given in the following table:

CODEINE PHOSPHATE/PHENYLEPHRINE HCL/ PROMETHAZINE HCL

Adults	1 teaspoon (5 mL) every 4 to 6 hours, not to exceed 30.0 mL in 24 hours.
Children 6 years to under 12 years	½ to teaspoon (2.5 to 5 mL) every 4 to 6 hours, not to exceed 30.0 mL in 24 hours.
Children under 6 years (weight: 18 kg or 40 lbs)	¼ to ½ teaspoon (1.25 to 2.5 mL) every 4 to 6 hours, not to exceed 9.0 mL in 24 hours.
Children under 6 years (weight: 16 kg or 35 lbs)	¼ to ½ teaspoon (1.25 to 2.5 mL) every 4 to 6 hours, not to exceed 8.0 mL in 24 hours.
Children under 6 years (weight: 14 kg or 30 lbs)	¼ to ½ teaspoon (1.25 to 2.5 mL) every 4 to 6 hours, not to exceed 7.0 mL in 24 hours.
Children under 6 years (weight: 12 kg or 25 lbs)	¼ to ½ teaspoon (1.25 to 2.5 mL) every 4 to 6 hours, not to exceed 6.0 mL in 24 hours.

Codeine Phosphate/Phenylephrine HCl/ Promethazine HCl is not recommended for children under 2 years of age.

Keep bottles tightly closed—Stored at room temperature, between 15°C and 25°C (59°F and 77°F).
Protect from light.
Dispense in light-resistant, glass, tight container.

HOW SUPPLIED
SYRUP (C-V): 10 MG-5 MG-6.25 MG/5 ML

		GENERIC A-RATED AVERAGE PRICE (GAAP)	
		480 ml	$31.60
		3840 ml	$31.60
AVERAGE UNIT PRICE (AVAILABLE SIZES)		120 ml	$2.80
BRAND	$0.06	120 ml	$2.87
GENERIC	$0.02	480 ml	$8.85
HCFA FUL (480 ml)	$0.01	3840 ml	$59.65

BRAND/MANUFACTURER	NDC	SIZE	AWP
◆ **BRAND**			
PHENERGAN VC W/CODEINE: Wyeth-Ayerst	00008-0552-01	120 ml	$5.33
	00008-0552-03	480 ml	$30.90
	00008-0552-02	120 ml 24s	$205.40
◆ **GENERICS**			
Cenci,H.R.	00556-0345-04	120 ml	$2.60
Moore,H.L.	00839-7061-65	120 ml	$2.69
Barre	00472-1629-04	120 ml	$2.70
Halsey Pharm	00879-0515-04	120 ml	$2.70
Major	00904-1514-00	120 ml	$2.75
Rugby	00536-1872-97	120 ml	$2.85
Major	00904-1514-20	120 ml	$2.85
Qualitest	00603-1581-54	120 ml	$2.88
Geneva	00781-6950-04	120 ml	$3.65
Qualitest	00603-1581-58	480 ml	$7.18
Schein	00364-7389-16	480 ml	$7.75
URL	00677-0965-33	480 ml	$8.25
Cenci,H.R.	00556-0345-16	480 ml	$8.30
Moore,H.L.	00839-7061-69	480 ml	$8.49
Rugby	00536-1872-85	480 ml	$8.90
Major	00904-1514-16	480 ml	$8.95
Barre	00472-1629-16	480 ml	$9.15
Halsey Pharm	00879-0515-16	480 ml	$9.20
Goldline	00182-1713-40	480 ml	$10.50
Geneva	00781-6950-16	480 ml	$10.75
Major	00904-1514-28	3840 ml	$51.40
Rugby	00536-1872-90	3840 ml	$54.29
Moore,H.L.	00839-7061-70	3840 ml	$54.93
Cenci,H.R.	00556-0345-28	3840 ml	$59.00
Goldline	00182-1713-41	3840 ml	$61.50
Barre	00472-1629-28	3840 ml	$63.20
Halsey Pharm	00879-0515-28	3840 ml	$63.25
Geneva	00781-6950-28	3840 ml	$64.27

Codeine Phosphate/ Pseudoephedrine Hydrochloride/ Triprolidine Hydrochloride

DESCRIPTION

Each 5 mL (1 teaspoonful) contains: Codeine Phosphate 10 mg (Warning—may be habit-forming), Triprolidine Hydrochloride 1.25 mg, Pseudoephedrine Hydrochloride 30 mg. This medication is intended for oral administration.

Codeine Phosphate/Pseudoephedrine Hydrochloride/Triprolidine Hydrochloride Cough Syrup has antitussive, antihistaminic and nasal decongestant effects. The components of Codeine Phosphate/Pseudoephedrine Hydrochloride/Triprolidine Hydrochloride Cough Syrup have the following chemical names.

Codeine Phosphate, U.S.P.: 7,8-didehydro-4,5α-epoxy-3-methoxy-17-methylmorphinan-6α-ol phosphate (1:1) (salt) hemihydrate

Triprolidine Hydrochloride Monohydrate: (E)-2-[3-(1-pyrrolidinyl)-1-(p-tolyl) propenyl]pyridine monohydrochloride monohydrate

Pseudoephedrine Hydrochloride: [S-(R*,R*)]-α-[1-(methylamino)ethyl] benzenemethanol hydrochloride.

CLINICAL PHARMACOLOGY

Codeine: Codeine probably exerts its antitussive activity by depressing the medullary (brain) cough center, thereby raising its threshold for incoming cough impulses.

Codeine is readily absorbed from the gastrointestinal tract, with a therapeutic dose reaching peak antitussive effectiveness in about 2 hours and persisting for 4 to 6 hours. Codeine is rapidly distributed from blood to body tissues and taken up preferentially by parenchymatous organs such as liver, spleen and kidney. It passes the blood brain barrier and is found in fetal tissue and breast milk.

The drug is not bound by plasma proteins nor is it accumulated in body tissues. Codeine is metabolized in the liver to morphine and norcodeine, each representing about 10 percent of the administered Codeine dose. About 90 percent of the dose is excreted within 24 hours, primarily through the kidneys. Urinary excretion products are free and glucuronide-conjugated Codeine (about 70%), free and conjugated norcodeine (about 10%), free and conjugated morphine (about 10%), normorphine (under 4%) and hydrocodone (< 1%). The remainder of the dose appears in the feces.

Triprolidine: Antihistamines such as Triprolidine Hydrochloride act as antagonists of the H₁ histamine receptor. Consequently, they prevent histamine from eliciting typical immediate hypersensitivity responses in the nose, eyes, lungs and skin.

Animal distribution studies have shown localization of Triprolidine in lung, spleen and kidney tissue. Liver microsome studies have revealed the presence of several metabolites with an oxidized product of the toluene methyl group predominating.

Pseudoephedrine: Pseudoephedrine acts as an indirect sympathomimetic agent by stimulating sympathetic (adrenergic) nerve endings to release norepinephrine. Norepinephrine in turn stimulates alpha and beta receptors throughout the body. The action of Pseudoephedrine Hydrochloride is apparently more specific for the blood vessels of the upper respiratory tract and less specific for the blood vessels of the systemic circulation. The vasoconstriction elicited at these sites results in the shrinkage of swollen tissues in the sinuses and nasal passages.

Pseudoephedrine is rapidly and almost completely absorbed from the gastrointestinal tract. Considerable variation in half-life has been observed (from about 4½ to 10 hours), which is attributed to individual differences in absorption and excretion. Excretion rates are also altered by urine pH, increasing with acidification and decreasing with alkalinization. As a result, mean half-life falls to about 4 hours at pH 5 and increases to 12 to 13 hours at pH 8.

After administration of a 60 mg tablet, 87 to 96% of the Pseudoephedrine is cleared from the body within 24 hours. The drug is distributed to body tissues and fluids, including fetal tissue, breast milk and the central nervous system (CNS). About 55 to 75% of an administered dose is excreted unchanged in the urine; the remainder is apparently metabolized in the liver to inactive compounds by N-demethylation, parahydroxylation and oxidative deamination.

The pharmacokinetic properties of 10 mL of Codeine Phosphate/Pseudoephedrine Hydrochloride/Triprolidine Hydrochloride Cough Syrup were investigated compared to a reference preparation of equal component doses in 18 healthy adults. The results of this study showed that Codeine Phosphate/Pseudoephedrine Hydrochloride/Triprolidine Hydrochloride Cough Syrup and the reference preparation were bioequivalent.

Pharmacokinetic parameters for Codeine Phosphate/Pseudoephedrine Hydrochloride/Triprolidine Hydrochloride Cough Syrup are as follows: (See related table).

INDICATIONS AND USAGE

Codeine Phosphate/Pseudoephedrine Hydrochloride/Triprolidine Hydrochloride Cough Syrup is indicated for temporary relief of coughs and upper respiratory symptoms, including nasal congestion, associated with allergy or the common cold.

CONTRAINDICATIONS

Codeine Phosphate/Pseudoephedrine Hydrochloride/Triprolidine Hydrochloride Cough Syrup is contraindicated under the following conditions:

Use in Newborn or Premature Infants: This drug should *not* be used in newborn or premature infants.

Use in Lower Respiratory Disease: Antihistamines should *not* be used to treat lower respiratory tract symptoms, including asthma.

Hypersensitivity to: 1) Codeine Phosphate or other narcotics; 2) Triprolidine Hydrochloride or other antihistamines of similar chemical structure; or 3) sympathomimetic amines, including Pseudoephedrine.

Sympathomimetic amines are contraindicated in patients with severe hypertension, severe coronary artery disease and in patients on monoamine oxidase (MAO) inhibitor therapy (see *"Drug Interaction"* section).

WARNINGS

Codeine Phosphate/Pseudoephedrine Hydrochloride/Triprolidine Hydrochloride Cough Syrup should be used with considerable caution in patients with increased intraocular pressure (narrow angle glaucoma), stenosing peptic ulcer, pyloroduodenal obstruction, symptomatic prostatic hypertrophy, bladder neck obstruction, hypertension, diabetes mellitus, ischemic heart disease, and hyperthyroidism.

In the presence of head injury or other intracranial lesions, the respiratory depressant effects of Codeine and other narcotics may be markedly enhanced, as well as their capacity for elevating cerebrospinal fluid pressure.

Narcotics also produce other CNS depressant effects, such as drowsiness, that may further obscure the clinical course of patients with head injuries.

Codeine or other narcotics may obscure signs on which to judge the diagnosis or clinical course of patients with acute abdominal conditions.

PRECAUTIONS

General: Codeine Phosphate/Pseudoephedrine Hydrochloride/Triprolidine Hydrochloride Cough Syrup should be prescribed with caution for certain special-risk patients, such as the elderly or debilitated, and for those with severe impairment of renal or hepatic function, gallbladder disease or gallstones, respiratory impairment, cardiac arrhythmias, history of bronchial asthma, prostatic hypertrophy or urethral stricture, and in patients known to be taking other antitussive, antihistamine or decongestant medications. Patient's self-medication habits should be investigated to determine their use of such medications. Codeine Phosphate/Pseudoephedrine Hydrochloride/Triprolidine Hydrochloride Cough Syrup is intended for short-term use only.

Information for Patients:
1. Patients should be warned about engaging in activities requiring mental alertness such as driving a car, operating dangerous machinery or hazardous appliances.
2. Patients with a history of glaucoma, peptic ulcer, urinary retention or pregnancy should be cautioned before starting Pseudoephedrine Hydrochloride/Triprolidine Hydrochloride.
3. Patients should be told not to take alcohol, sleeping pills, sedatives or tranquilizers while taking Pseudoephedrine Hydrochloride/Triprolidine Hydrochloride.
4. Antihistamines as in Pseudoephedrine Hydrochloride/Triprolidine Hydrochloride may cause dizziness, drowsiness, dry mouth, blurred vision, weakness, nausea, headache or nervousness in some patients.
5. Patients should be told to store this medicine in a tightly closed container in a dry, cool place away from heat or direct sunlight and out of the reach of children.
6. For information on nursing mothers, refer to the section below.

Codeine Phosphate/Pseudoephedrine Hydrochloride/Triprolidine Hydrochloride Cough Syrup should not be used by persons intolerant to sympathomimetics used for the relief of nasal or sinus congestion. Such drugs include ephedrine, epinephrine, phenylpropanolamine, and phenylephrine. Symptoms of intolerance include drowsiness, dizziness, weakness, difficulty in breathing, tenseness, muscle tremors or palpitations.

Codeine may be habit-forming when used over long periods or in high doses. Patients should take the drug only for as long, in the amounts, and as frequently as prescribed.

Drug Interactions: Codeine Phosphate/Pseudoephedrine Hydrochloride/Triprolidine Hydrochloride Cough Syrup may *enhance* the effects of:

1. monoamine oxidase (MAO) inhibitors;
2. other narcotic analgesics, alcohol, general anesthetics, tranquilizers, sedative-hypnotics, surgical skeletal muscle relaxants, or other CNS depressants, by causing increased CNS depression.

Codeine Phosphate/Pseudoephedrine Hydrochloride/Triprolidine Hydrochloride Cough Syrup may *diminish:* the antihypertensive effects of guanethidine, bethanidine, methyldopa, and reserpine.

Drug/Laboratory Test Interactions: Codeine: Narcotic administration may increase serum amylase levels.

Carcinogenesis, Mutagenesis, Impairment of Fertility: No adequate studies have been conducted in animals to determine whether the components of Codeine Phosphate/Pseudoephedrine Hydrochloride/Triprolidine Hydrochloride Cough Syrup have a potential for carcinogenesis, mutagenesis or impairment of fertility.

Pregnancy: Teratogenic Effects: Pregnancy Category C. Animal reproduction studies have not been conducted with Codeine Phosphate/Pseudoephedrine Hydrochloride/Triprolidine Hydrochloride Cough Syrup. It is also not known whether Codeine Phosphate/Pseudoephedrine Hydrochloride/Triprolidine Hydrochloride Cough Syrup can cause fetal harm when administered to a pregnant woman or can affect reproduction capacity. Codeine Phosphate/Pseudoephedrine Hydrochloride/Triprolidine Hydrochloride Cough Syrup should be given to a pregnant woman only if clearly needed. Teratology studies have been conducted with three ingredients of Codeine Phosphate/Pseudoephedrine Hydrochloride/Triprolidine Hydrochloride Cough Syrup. Pseudoephedrine studies were conducted in rats at doses up to 150 times the human dose; Triprolidine was studied in rats and rabbits at doses up to 125 times the human dose, and Codeine studies were conducted in rats and rabbits at doses up to 150 times the human dose. No evidence of teratogenic harm to the fetus was revealed in any of these studies. However, overt signs of toxicity were observed in the dams which received Pseudoephedrine. This was reflected in reduced average weight and length and rate of skeletal ossification in their fetuses.

Nursing Mothers: The components of Codeine Phosphate/Pseudoephedrine Hydrochloride/Triprolidine Hydrochloride Cough Syrup are excreted in breast milk in small amounts, but the significance of their effects on nursing infants is not known. Because of the potential for serious adverse reactions in nursing

Parameter	Codeine*	Triprolidine†	Pseudoephedrine‡
Elimination Half Life (hr)	2.7 ± 0.4§	4.0 ± 2.2	5.5 ± 0.9
Time to Maximum Concentration (hr)	1.2 ± 0.5	1.8 ± 0.7	2.6 ± 1.0
Maximum Plasma Concentration (ng/mL)	44.8 ± 11.7	4.9 ± 1.8	189 ± 44
Area Under Plasma Curve from t = 0 to t = ∞ (ng/mL·hr)	226 ± 41	42.5 ± 34.0	1938 ± 440

* 20 mg Codeine Phosphate hemihydrate (equivalent to 14.7 mg free base)
† 2.5 mg Triprolidine HCl monohydrate (equivalent to 2.1 mg free base)
‡ 60 mg Pseudoephedrine HCl (equivalent to 49.1 mg free base)
§ Means ± S.D.

infants from maternal ingestion of Codeine Phosphate/Pseudoephedrine Hydrochloride/Triprolidine Hydrochloride Cough Syrup, a decision should be made whether to discontinue nursing or to discontinue the drug, taking into account the importance of the drug to the mother.

Pediatric Use: As in adults, the combination of an antihistamine, sympathomimetic amine and Codeine can elicit either mild stimulation or mild sedation in children. In infants and children particularly, the ingredients in this drug product *in overdosage* may produce hallucinations, convulsions and death. Symptoms of toxicity in children may include fixed dilated pupils, flushed face, dry mouth, fever, excitation, hallucinations, ataxia, incoordination, athetosis, tonic clonic convulsions and postictal depression (see *"Contraindications"* and *"Overdosage"* sections).

Use in Elderly (approximately 60 years or older): The ingredients in Codeine Phosphate/Pseudoephedrine Hydrochloride/Triprolidine Hydrochloride Cough Syrup are more likely to cause adverse reactions in elderly patients.

ADVERSE REACTIONS
(The most frequent adverse reactions are italicized:)

General: Dryness of mouth, dryness of nose, dryness of throat, urticaria, drug rash, anaphylactic shock, photosensitivity, excessive perspiration and chills.

Cardiovascular System: Hypotension, headache, palpitations, tachycardia, extrasystoles.

Hematologic System: Hemolytic anemia, thrombocytopenia, agranulocytosis.

Nervous System: Sedation, sleepiness, dizziness, disturbed coordination, fatigue, confusion, restlessness, excitation, anxiety, nervousness, tremor, irritability, insomnia, euphoria, paresthesias, blurred vision, diplopia, vertigo, tinnitus, acute labyrinthitis, hysteria, neuritis, convulsions, CNS depression, hallucination.

G.I. System: Epigastric distress, anorexia, nausea, vomiting, diarrhea, constipation.

G.U. System: Urinary frequency, difficult urination, urinary retention, early menses.

Respiratory System: Thickening of bronchial secretions, tightness of chest and wheezing, nasal stuffiness, respiratory depression.

DRUG ABUSE AND DEPENDENCE
Like other medications containing a narcotic, Codeine Phosphate/Pseudoephedrine Hydrochloride/Triprolidine Hydrochloride Cough Syrup is controlled by the Drug Enforcement Administration. It is classified under Schedule V.

Codeine Phosphate/Pseudoephedrine Hydrochloride/Triprolidine Hydrochloride Cough Syrup can produce drug dependence of the morphine type, and therefore it has a potential for being abused. Psychic dependence, physical dependence and tolerance may develop on repeated administration.

The dependence liability of Codeine has been found to be too small to permit a full definition of its characteristics. Studies indicate that addiction to Codeine is extremely uncommon and requires very high parenteral doses.

When dependence on Codeine occurs at therapeutic doses, it appears to require from one to two months to develop, and withdrawal symptoms are mild. Most patients on long-term oral Codeine therapy show no signs of physical dependence upon abrupt withdrawal.

OVERDOSAGE
Since Codeine Phosphate/Pseudoephedrine Hydrochloride/Triprolidine Hydrochloride Cough Syrup is comprised of three pharmacologically different compounds it is difficult to predict the exact manifestation of symptoms in a given individual. Reaction to an overdosage of Codeine Phosphate/Pseudoephedrine Hydrochloride/Triprolidine Hydrochloride Cough Syrup may vary from CNS depression to stimulation. A detailed description of symptoms which are likely to appear after ingestion of an excess of the individual components follows:

Overdosage with Codeine can cause transient euphoria, drowsiness, dizziness, weariness, diminution of sensibility, loss of sensation, vomiting, transient excitement in children and occasionally in adult women, miosis progressing to non-reactive pinpoint pupils, itching sometimes with skin rashes and urticaria, and clammy skin with mottled cyanosis. In more severe cases, muscular relaxation with depressed or absent superficial and deep reflexes and a positive Babinski sign may appear. Marked slowing of the respiratory rate with inadequate pulmonary ventilation and consequent cyanosis may occur. Terminal signs include shock, pulmonary arrest, with death occurring within 6-12 hours following ingestion.

Overdoses of antihistamines may cause hallucinations, convulsions, or possibly death, especially in infants and children. Antihistamines are more likely to cause dizziness, sedation, and hypotension in elderly patients.

Overdosage with Triprolidine may produce reactions varying from depression to stimulation of the Central Nervous System (CNS); the latter is particularly likely in children. Atropine-like signs and symptoms (dry mouth, fixed dilated pupils, flushing, tachycardia, hallucinations, convulsions, urinary retention, cardiac arrhythmias and coma) may occur.

Overdosage with Pseudoephedrine can cause excessive CNS stimulation resulting in excitement, nervousness, anxiety, tremor, restlessness and insomnia. Other effects include tachycardia, hypertension, pallor, mydriasis, hyperglycemia and urinary retention. Severe overdosage may cause tachypnea or hyperpnea, hallucinations, convulsions, or delirium, but in some individuals there may be CNS depression with somnolence, stupor or respiratory depression. Arrhythmias (including ventricular fibrillation) may lead to hypotension and circulatory

collapse. Severe hypokalemia can occur, probably due to compartmental shift rather than depletion of potassium. No organ damage or significant metabolic derangement is associated with Pseudoephedrine overdosage.

The toxic plasma concentration of Codeine is not known with certainty. Experimental production of mild to moderate CNS depression in healthy, nontolerant subjects occurs at plasma concentrations of 0.5-1.9 µg/mL when Codeine is given by intravenous infusion. The single lethal dose of Codeine in adults is estimated to be from 0.5 to 1.0 gram. It is also estimated that 5 mg/kg could be fatal in children.

The LD_{50} (single, oral dose) of Triprolidine is 163 to 308 mg/kg in the mouse (depending upon strain) and 840 mg/kg in the rat.

Insufficient data are available to estimate the toxic and lethal doses of Triprolidine in humans. No reports of acute poisoning with Triprolidine have appeared.

The Ld_{50} (single, oral dose) of Pseudoephedrine is 726 mg/kg in the mouse, 2206 mg/kg in the rat and 1177 mg/kg in the rabbit. The toxic and lethal concentrations in human biologic fluids are not known. Excretion rates increase with urine acidification and decrease with alkalinization. Few reports of toxicity due to Pseudoephedrine have been published and no case of fatal overdosage is known.

Therapy, if instituted within 4 hours of overdosage, is aimed at reducing further absorption of the drug. In the conscious patient, vomiting should be induced even though it may have occurred spontaneously. If vomiting cannot be induced, gastric lavage is indicated. Adequate precautions must be taken to protect against aspiration, especially in infants and children. Charcoal slurry or other suitable agents should be instilled into the stomach after vomiting or lavage. Saline cathartics or milk of magnesia may be of additional benefit.

In the unconscious patient, the airway should be secured with a cuffed endotracheal tube before attempting to evacuate the gastric contents. Intensive supportive and nursing care is indicated, as for any comatose patient.

If breathing is significantly impaired, maintenance of an adequate airway and mechanical support of respiration is the most effective means of providing adequate oxygenation. Hypotension is an early sign of impending cardiovascular collapse and should be treated vigorously.

Do not use CNS stimulants. Convulsions should be controlled by careful administration of diazepam or short-acting barbiturate, repeated as necessary. Physostigmine may be also considered for use in controlling centrally mediated convulsions.

Ice packs and cooling sponge baths, not alcohol, can aid in reducing the fever commonly seen in children.

For Codeine, continuous stimulation that arouses, but does not exhaust, the patient is useful in preventing coma. Continuous or intermittent oxygen therapy is usually indicated, while Naloxone is useful as a Codeine antidote. Close nursing care is essential.

Saline cathartics, such as milk of magnesia, help to dilute the concentration of the drugs in the bowel by drawing water into the gut, thereby hastening drug elimination.

Adrenergic receptor blocking agents are antidotes to Pseudoephedrine. In practice, the most useful is the beta-blocker propranolol, which is indicated when there are signs of cardiac toxicity.

There are no specific antidotes to Triprolidine. Histamine should not be given.

Pseudoephedrine and Codeine are theoretically dialyzable, but the procedures have not been clinically established.

In severe cases of overdosage, it is essential to monitor both the heart (by electrocardiograph) and plasma electrolytes and to give intravenous potassium as indicated by these continuous controls. Vasopressors may be used to treat hypotension, and excessive CNS stimulation may be counteracted with parenteral diazepam. Stimulants should not be used.

DOSAGE AND ADMINISTRATION
Dosage should be individualized according to the needs and response of the patient.

Usual Dose:		Teaspoonfuls (5 mL)
Adults and children 12 years and older	2	every 4-6 hours not to exceed
Children 6 to under 12 years	1	4 doses in a 24-hour period
Children 2 to under 6 years	½	

Store at 15° to 25°C (59° to 77°F) and protect from light.

HOW SUPPLIED
SYRUP (C-V): 10 MG-30 MG-1.25 MG

AVERAGE UNIT PRICE (AVAILABLE SIZES)		GENERIC A-RATED AVERAGE PRICE (GAAP)	
BRAND	$0.10	120 ml	$3.22
GENERIC	$0.02	480 ml	$11.45
HCFA FUL (480 ml)	$0.01	3840 ml	$67.16

BRAND/MANUFACTURER	NDC	SIZE	AWP
◆ BRAND			
ACTIFED W/CODEINE: Burr Wellcome	00081-0025-96	480 ml	$46.07

◆ RATED THERAPEUTICALLY EQUIVALENT; ◇ THERAPEUTIC EQUIVALENCE UNCONFIRMED; ○ UNRATED

BRAND/MANUFACTURER	NDC	SIZE	AWP
◆ GENERICS			
Pennex	00426-8462-04	120 ml	$3.04
Pennex	00832-8462-04	120 ml	$3.04
TRIACIN C: Barre	00472-1633-04	120 ml	$3.57
ALLERFRIN W/CODEINE: Rugby	00536-0065-85	480 ml	$7.25
Major	00904-1579-16	480 ml	$9.15
TRIACIN C: Barre	00472-1633-16	480 ml	$9.20
Pennex	00426-8462-16	480 ml	$9.70
Pennex	00832-8462-16	480 ml	$9.70
ACTAGEN-C: Goldline	00182-1710-40	480 ml	$10.50
TRIAFED CODEINE: Schein	00364-7385-16	480 ml	$13.00
TRIFED C: Geneva	00781-6550-16	480 ml	$23.09
ALLERFRIN W/CODEINE: Rugby	00536-0065-90	3840 ml	$63.53
Pennex	00426-8462-28	3840 ml	$65.70
Pennex	00832-8462-28	3840 ml	$65.70
Major	00904-1579-28	3840 ml	$67.45
TRIACIN C: Barre	00472-1633-28	3840 ml	$68.60
ACTAGEN-C: Goldline	00182-1710-41	3840 ml	$72.00

Codiclear DH *SEE* GUAIFENESIN AND HYDROCODONE BITARTRATE

Codimal DH *SEE* HYDROCODONE BITARTRATE/ PHENYLEPHRINE HYDROCHLORIDE/PYRILAMINE MALEATE

Cogentin *SEE* BENZTROPINE MESYLATE

Cognex *SEE* TACRINE HYDROCHLORIDE

ColBENEMID *SEE* COLCHICINE WITH PROBENECID

Colchicine

DESCRIPTION
A phenanthrene derivative, Colchicine is the active alkaloidal principle derived from the dried corns and seeds of Colchicum autumnale, the autumn crocus or meadow saffron. It appears as pale-yellow amorphous scales or powder that darkens on exposure to light. One g dissolves in 25 mL of water and in 220 mL of ether. Colchicine is freely soluble in alcohol and chloroform.

Chemically, it is acetamide, N-(5,6,7,9-tetrahydro- 1,2,3,10-tetramethoxy-9-oxobenzo[α]heptalen-7-yl)-, (S)-. The molecular weight is 399.44, the empirical formula is $C_{22}H_{25}NO_6$.

Colchicine, an acetyltrimethylcolchicinic acid, is hydrolyzed in the presence of dilute acids or alkalies, with cleavage of a methyl group as methanol and formation of *colchiceine*, which has very little therapeutic activity. On hydrolysis with strong acids. Colchicine is converted to trimethylcolchicinic acid.

Colchicine Tablets, USP are oral anti-inflammatory agents supplied in two dosage strengths 0.5 mg (1/120 g) and 0.6 mg (1/100 gr).

Ampoules Colchicine Injection, USP, provide a sterile aqueous solution of Colchicine for intravenous use. Each ampoule contains 1 mg (2.5 μmol) of Colchicine in 2 mL of solution. Sodium hydroxide may have been added during manufacture to adjust the pH.

Following is its chemical structure:

CLINICAL PHARMACOLOGY
The mechanism of the relief afforded by Colchicine in acute attacks of gouty arthritis is not completely known, but studies on the processes involved in precipitation of an acute attack have helped elucidate how this drug may exert its effects. The mechanism of action of Colchicine involves (1) a reduction in lactic acid production by leukocytes which results in a decrease in uric acid deposition, and (2) a reduction in phagocytosis, with abatement of the inflammatory response. The drug is not an analgesic, does not relieve other types of pain or inflammation, and is of no value in other types of arthritis. It is not a diuretic and does not influence the renal excretion of uric acid or its level in the blood or the magnitude of the "miscible pool" of uric acid. It also does not alter the solubility of urate in the plasma.

Colchicine is not a uricosuric agent and will not prevent progression of gout to chronic gouty arthritis. It does have a prophylactic, suppressive effect that helps to reduce the incidence of acute attacks and to relieve the residual pain and mild discomfort that patients with gout occasionally feel. An acute attack of gout apparently occurs as a result of an inflammatory reaction to crystals of monosodium urate that are deposited in the joint tissue from hyperuric body fluids; the reaction is aggravated as more urate crystals accumulate. The initial inflammatory response involves local infiltration of granulocytes that phagocytize the urate crystals. Interference with these processes will prevent the development of an acute attack. Colchicine apparently exerts its effect by reducing the inflammatory response to the deposited crystals and also by diminishing phagocytosis. The deposition of uric acid is favored by an acid pH. In synovial tissues and in leukocytes associated with inflammatory processes, lactic acid production is high; this favors a local decrease in pH that enhances uric acid deposition. Colchicine diminishes lactic acid production by leukocytes both directly and by diminishing phagocytosis, thereby interrupting the cycle of urate crystal deposition and inflammatory response that sustains the acute attack. The oxidation of glucose in phagocytizing as well as in non-phagocytizing leukocytes *in vitro* is suppressed by Colchicine; this suppression may explain the diminished lactic acid production. The precise biochemical step that is affected by Colchicine is not yet known. The antimitotic activity of Colchicine is unrelated to its effectiveness in the treatment of acute gout, as indicated by the fact that trimethylcolchicinic acid, an analog of Colchicine, has no antimitotic activity except in extremely high doses.

In man and certain other animals, Colchicine can produce a temporary leukopenia that is followed by leukocytosis.

Colchicine has other pharmacologic actions in animals: it alters neuromuscular function, intensifies gastrointestinal activity by neurogenic stimulation, increases sensitivity to central depressants, heightens response to sympathomimetic compounds, depresses the respiratory center, constricts blood vessels, causes hypertension by central vasomotor stimulation, and lowers body temperature.

Colchicine is rapidly absorbed after oral administration. Large amounts of the drug and metabolites enter the intestinal tract in bile and intestinal secretions. High concentrations of Colchicine are found in the kidney, liver, and spleen, as well. Colchicine does not appear to be tightly bound to serum protein, hence the drug rapidly leaves the blood stream. Excretion occurs primarily by biliary and renal routes.

INDICATIONS AND USAGE
Colchicine is indicated for the treatment of gout. It is effective in relieving the pain of acute attacks, especially if therapy is begun early in the attack and in adequate dosage. Many therapists use Colchicine as interval therapy to prevent acute attacks of gout at the first sign of articular discomfort. It has no effect on nongouty arthritis or on uric acid metabolism.

The intravenous use of Colchicine is advantageous when a rapid response is desired or when gastrointestinal side effects interfere with oral administration of the medication. Occasionally, intravenous Colchicine is effective when the oral preparation is not. After the acute attack has subsided, the patient can usually be given Colchicine tablets by mouth.

UNLABELED USES
Colchicine is used alone or as an adjunct in the treatment of bronchial asthma, Behcet's disease, and primary biliary cirrhosis. It is also used to arrest the progression of neurological disability caused by chronic progressive multiple sclerosis. Colchicine is also used in the treatment of familial Mediterranean fever (recurrent polyserositis), pustulosis palmaris et plantaris, and Sweet's syndrome.

CONTRAINDICATIONS
Colchicine is contraindicated in patients with gout who also have serious gastrointestinal, renal, hepatic, or cardiac disorders. Colchicine should not be given in the presence of combined renal and hepatic disease. Colchicine is also contraindicated in patients with a known hypersensitivity to the drug and in those with blood dyscrasias.

WARNINGS
Colchicine can cause fetal harm when administered to a pregnant woman. If this drug is used during pregnancy, or if the patient becomes pregnant while taking it, the woman should be apprised of the potential hazard to the fetus.

Colchicine arrests cell division in animals and plants. It has adversely affected spermatogenesis in humans and in some animal species under certain conditions.

Mortality Related to Overdosage: **Cumulative intravenous doses of Colchicine above 4 mg have resulted in irreversible multiple organ failure and death (see *"Overdosage"* and *"Dosage and Administration"*) or discontinuation of therapy.**

PRECAUTIONS
General: Reduction in dosage or discontinuation of therapy is indicated if weakness, anorexia, nausea, vomiting or diarrhea occurs. Rarely, thrombophlebitis occurs at the site of injection. Colchicine should be administered with great caution to aged and debilitated patients, especially those with renal, hepatic, gastrointestinal, or heart disease.

Laboratory Tests: In patients receiving long-term therapy, periodic blood counts should be done.

Drug Interactions: Colchicine has been shown to induce reversible malabsorption of vitamin B_{12}, apparently by altering the function of ileal mucosa. The possibility that Colchicine may increase response to central nervous system depressants and to sympathomimetic agents is suggested by the results of experiments on animals.

Colchicine is inhibited by *acidifying agents*.

The action of Colchicine is potentiated by *alkalinizing agents*.

Laboratory Test Interactions: Colchicine therapy may cause elevated alkaline phosphatase and SGOT values.

Decreased thrombocyte values may be obtained during Colchicine therapy. Colchicine may cause false positive results when testing urine for RBC or hemoglobin.

Carcinogenesis: Data in the literature does not indicate Colchicine as a carcinogenic agent.

Fertility: see "*Warnings*" section for information on impairment of fertility.

Colchicine has been shown to be teratogenic in mice when given doses of 1.25 and 1.5 mg/kg and in hamsters when given 10 mg/kg. There are no adequate and well-controlled studies in pregnant women. Colchicine should be used during pregnancy only if the potential benefit justifies the potential risk to the fetus.

Usage in Pregnancy—Pregnancy Category D: (see "*Warnings*") Colchicine has been shown to be teratogenic in mice when given doses of 1.25 and 1.5 mg/kg and in hamsters when given 10 mg/kg. There are no adequate and well-controlled studies in pregnant women. Colchicine should be used during pregnancy only if the potential benefit justifies the potential risk to the fetus.

Nursing Mothers: It is not known whether this drug is excreted in human milk. Because many drugs are excreted in human milk, caution should be exercised when Colchicine is administered to a nursing woman.

Usage in Children: Safety and effectiveness in children have not been established.

ADVERSE REACTIONS

Adverse reactions in decreasing order of severity are: bone marrow depression, with aplastic anemia, with agranulocytosis or with thrombocytopenia may occur in patients receiving long-term therapy. Peripheral neuritis, purpura, myopathy, loss of hair, and reversible azoospermia have also been reported.

With oral dosing, vomiting, diarrhea, abdominal pain and nausea may occur with Colchicine therapy, especially when maximal doses are necessary for a therapeutic effect. The diarrhea may be severe. To avoid more serious toxicity, the drug should be discontinued when these symptoms appear, regardless of whether or not joint pain has been relieved.

The gastrointestinal symptoms may occur even though the drug is given intravenously; however, such symptoms are unusual unless the recommended dose is exceeded.

Prolonged administration may cause bone marrow depression, with agranulocytosis, thrombocytopenia, and aplastic anemia. Peripheral neuritis and depilation have also been reported.

Myopathy may occur in patients on usual maintenance doses, especially in the presence of renal impairment.

Dermatoses have been reported. Hypersensitivity reactions may occur infrequently.

OVERDOSAGE

Signs and Symptoms: Symptoms, the onset of which may be delayed, include nausea, vomiting, diarrhea, abdominal pain, hemorrhagic gastroenteritis, and burning pain in the throat, stomach, and skin. The diarrhea may be severe and bloody owing to hemorrhagic gastroenteritis. To control the diarrhea and cramps, paregoric is usually administered. Fluid extravasation may lead to shock. Myocardial injury may be accompanied by ST-segment elevation, decreased contractility, and profound shock.

Kidney damage, evidenced by hematuria and oliguria, may occur. Severe dehydration and hypotension may develop. Muscular weakness may be marked, and ascending paralysis of the central nervous system may develop; the patient usually remains conscious. Delirium and convulsions may occur. Death due to respiratory arrest may result. Hepatocellular damage, renal failure, and lung parenchymal infiltrates may occur and, by the fifth day after overdose, leukopenia, thrombocytopenia, and coagulopathy may also occur. If the patient survives, alopecia and stomatitis may be experienced. There is no clear separation of nontoxic, toxic, and lethal doses of Colchicine. The lethal dose of Colchicine has been estimated to be 65 mg; however, *death has resulted from intravenous doses as small as 7 mg acutely* (see "*Warnings*" and "*Dosage and Administration*") or oral doses of 8 mg, although higher doses have been taken without fatal results. Serum concentrations that may be toxic or lethal are not defined. The intravenous median lethal dose in rats is 1.7 mg/kg.

Treatment: To obtain up-to-date information about the treatment of overdose, a good resource is your certified Regional Poison Control Center. Telephone numbers of certified poison control centers are listed in the *Physicians' Desk Reference (PDR)*. In managing overdosage, consider the possibility of multiple drug overdoses, interaction among drugs, and unusual drug kinetics in your patient.

Protect the patient's airway and support ventilation and perfusion. Meticulously monitor and maintain, within acceptable limits, the patient's vital signs, blood gases, serum electrolytes, etc. Use measures to prevent shock. If Colchicine was recently ingested and vomiting has not occurred, perform gastric lavage once the patient is stabilized. Absorption of drugs from the gastrointestinal tract may be decreased by giving activated charcoal, which, in many cases, is more effective than emesis or lavage; consider charcoal instead of or in addition to gastric emptying. Repeated doses of charcoal over time may hasten elimination of some drugs that have been absorbed. Safeguard the patient's airway when employing gastric emptying or charcoal.

Recent studies appear to support the use of hemodialysis or peritoneal dialysis as part of the treatment of acute overdosage in addition to gastric lavage. Symptomatic and supportive treatment may include atropine and morphine for the relief of abdominal pain, and artificial respiration with oxygen to combat respiratory distress. No specific antidote is known.

DOSAGE AND ADMINISTRATION

COLCHICINE TABLETS

For Acute Gouty Arthritis: The usual dose to relieve or abort an attack is 1 to 1.2 mg (two 0.5 mg granules or two 0.6 mg tablets). This dose may be followed by one unit of either preparation (granule or tablet) every hour, or two units every two hours, until pain is relieved or until diarrhea ensues. Each patient should learn the dose needed and should keep the drug at hand for use at the first sign of an attack; a delay of a few hours impairs its effectiveness. After the initial dose, it is sometimes sufficient to take 0.5 or 0.6 mg every two or three hours. The drug should be stopped if there is gastrointestinal discomfort or diarrhea. (Opiates may be needed to control diarrhea.) In subsequent attacks, the patient should be able to judge his medication requirement accurately enough to stop short of his "diarrheal dose." The total amount of Colchicine needed to control pain and inflammation during an attack usually ranges from 4 to 8 mg. Articular pain and swelling typically abate within 12 hours and are usually gone in 24 to 48 hours. An interval of three days between Colchicine courses is advised in order to minimize the possibility of cumulative toxicity.

If corticotropin (ACTH) is administered for treatment of an attack of gouty arthritis, it is recommended that Colchicine also be given in doses of at least 1 mg per day, and that the latter be continued for a few days after the hormone is withdrawn.

For Prophylaxis During Intercritical Periods: To reduce the frequency of paroxysms and lessen their severity, Colchicine may be administered continuously. In patients who have less than one attack per year, the usual dose is 0.5 or 0.6 mg per day, three or four days a week. For cases involving more than one attack per year, the usual dose is 0.5 or 0.6 mg daily; severe cases may require two or three 0.5 mg granules or 0.6 mg tablets daily.

For Prophylaxis Against Attacks of Gout in Patients Undergoing Surgery: In patients with gout, an attack may be precipitated by even a minor surgical procedure. Colchicine, one 0.5 mg granule three times a day or one 0.6 mg tablet three times daily, should be administered for three days before and three days after surgery.

COLCHICINE INJECTION

Colchicine Injection is for intravenous use only. Severe local irritation occurs if it is administered subcutaneously or intramuscularly.

It is extremely important that the needle be properly positioned in the vein before Colchicine is injected. If leakage into surrounding tissue or outside the vein along its course should occur during intravenous administration, considerable irritation and possible tissue damage may follow. There is no specific antidote for the prevention of this irritation. Local application of heat or cold, as well as the administration of analgesics, may afford relief.

The injection should take 2 to 5 minutes for completion. To minimize the risk of extravasation, it is recommended that the injection be made into an established intravenous line into a large vein using normal saline as the intravenous fluid. Colchicine Injection should not be diluted with 5% Dextrose in Water. If a decrease in concentration of Colchicine in solution is required, 0.9% Sodium Chloride Injection, which does not contain a bacteriostatic agent, should be used. Solutions that become turbid should not be used.

In the treatment of acute gouty arthritis, the average initial dose of Colchicine Injection is 2 mg (4 mL). This may be followed by 0.5 mg (1 mL) every 6 hours until a satisfactory response is achieved. In general, the total dosage for the first 24-hour period should not exceed 4 mg (8 mL). Cumulative doses of Colchicine above 4 mg have resulted in irreversible multiple organ failure and death. The total dosage for a single course of treatment should not exceed 4 mg. Some clinicians recommend a single intravenous dose of 3 mg, whereas others recommend an initial dose of not more than 1 mg of Colchicine intravenously, followed by 0.5 mg once or twice daily if needed.

If pain recurs, it may be necessary to administer a daily dose of 1 to 2 mg (2 to 4 mL) for several days; however, *no more Colchicine should be given by any route for at least 7 days after a full course of IV therapy (4 mg).*[1,2] Many patients can be transferred to oral Colchicine at a dosage similar to that being given intravenously.

In the prophylactic or maintenance therapy of recurrent or chronic gouty arthritis, a dosage of 0.5 to 1 mg (1 to 2 mL) once or twice daily may be used. However, in these cases, oral administration of Colchicine is preferable, usually taken in conjunction with a uricosuric agent. If an acute attack of gout accurs while the patient is taking Colchicine as maintenance therapy, an alternative drug should be instituted in preference to increasing the dose of Colchicine.

Parenteral drug products should be inspected visually for particulate matter and discoloration prior to administration, whenever solution and container permit.

STORAGE

Store at controlled room temperature, 59° to 86°F (15° to 30°C). Protect from light and moisture.

Dispense in a tight, light-resistant container as defined in the USP using a child-resistant closure.

Colchicine is extremely poisonous.

REFERENCES
1. Wallace SL, Singer JZ: Review: Systemic toxicity associated with the intravenous administration of colchicine—guidelines for use. *J. Rheumatol* 1988 15:495-499. 2. Simons RJ, Kingma DW: Fatal colchicine toxicity *Am J Med* 1989; 86:356-357.

J CODES
Up to 2 mg IV—J0760

HOW SUPPLIED
INJECTION: 0.5 MG/ML

BRAND/MANUFACTURER	NDC	SIZE	AWP
○ GENERICS			
Lilly	00002-1443-16	2 ml 6s	$19.55

For additional alternatives, turn to the section beginning on page 2859.

Colchicine with Probenecid

DESCRIPTION
Tablet: Contains Probenecid, which is a uricosuric agent, and Colchicine, which has antigout activity, the mechanism of which is unknown.

Probenecid is the generic name for 4-[(dispropylamino) sulfonyl] benzoic acid (molecular weight 285.36).

Probenecid is a white or nearly white, fine, crystalline powder. It is soluble in dilute alkali, in alcohol, in chloroform, and in acetone; it is practically insoluble in water and in dilute acids.

Colchicine is an alkaloid obtained from various species of colchicum. The chemical name for Colchicine is (S)-N-(5,6,7,9-tetrahydro-1,2,3,10-tetramethoxy-9-oxobenzo [a] heptalen-7-yl) acetamide (molecular weight 399.43).

Colchicine consists of pale yellow scales or powder; it darkens on exposure to light. Colchicine is soluble in water, freely soluble in alcohol and in chloroform, and slightly soluble in ether.

Each tablet contains 0.5 g Probenecid and 0.5 mg Colchicine.

ACTIONS
Probenecid is a uricosuric and renal tubular blocking agent. It inhibits the tubular reabsorption of urate, thus increasing the urinary excretion of uric acid and decreasing serum urate levels. Effective urisocuria reduces the miscible urate pool, retards urate deposition, and promotes resorption of urate deposits.

Probenecid inhibits the tubular secretion of penicillin and usually increases penicillin plasma levels by any route the antibiotic is given. A 2-fold to 4-fold elevation has been demonstrated for various penicillins.

Probenecid also has been reported to inhibit the renal transport of many other compounds including aminohippuric acid (PAH), aminosalicylic acid (PAS), indomethacin, sodium iodomethamate and related iodinated organic acids, 17-ketosteroids, pantothenic acid, phenolsulfonphthalein (PSP), sulfonamides, and sulfonylureas. See also *"Drug Interactions"*.

Probenecid decreases both hepatic and renal excretion of sulfobromophthalein (BSP). The tubular reabsorption of phosphorus is inhibited in hypoparathyroid but not in euparathyroid individuals.

Probenecid does not influence plasma concentrations of salicylates, nor the excretion of streptomycin, chloramphenicol, chlortetracycline, oxytetracycline, or neomycin.

The mode of action of Colchicine in gout is unknown. It is not an analgesic, though it relieves pain in acute attacks of gout. It is not a uricosuric agent and will not prevent progression of gout to chronic gouty arthritis. It does have a prophylactic, suppressive effect that helps to reduce the incidence of acute attacks and to relieve the residual pain and mild discomfort that patients with gout occasionally feel.

In man and certain other animals, Colchicine can produce a temporary leukopenia that is followed by leukocytosis.

Colchicine has other pharmacologic actions in animals: It alters neuromuscular function, intensifies gastrointestinal activity by neurogenic stimulation, increases sensitivity to central depressants, heightens response to sympathomimetic compounds, depresses the respiratory center, constricts blood vessels, causes hypertension by central vasomotor stimulation, and lowers body temperature.

INDICATIONS
For the treatment of chronic gouty arthritis when complicated by frequent, recurrent acute attacks of gout.

CONTRAINDICATIONS
Hypersensitivity to this product or to Probenecid or Colchicine.

Children under 2 years of age.

Not recommended in persons with known blood dyscrasias or uric acid kidney stones.

Therapy with Colchicine/Probenecid should not be started until an acute gouty attack has subsided.

Pregnancy: Probenecid crosses the placental barrier and appears in cord blood. Colchicine can arrest cell division in animals and plants. In certain species of animal under certain conditions, Colchicine has produced teratogenic effects. The possibility of such effects in humans also has been reported. Because of the Colchicine component Colchicine/Probenecid is contraindicated in pregnant patients. The use of any drug in women of childbearing potential requires that the anticipated benefit be weighed against possible hazards.

WARNINGS
Exacerbation of gout following therapy with Colchicine/Probenecid may occur; in such cases additional Colchicine or other appropriate therapy is advisable.

Probenecid increases plasma concentrations of methotrexate in both animals and humans. In animal studies, increased methotrexate toxicity has been reported. If Colchicine/Probenecid is given with methotrexate, the dosage of methotrexate should be reduced and serum levels may need to be monitored.

In patients on Colchicine/Probenecid the use of salicylates in either small or large doses is contraindicated because it antagonizes the uricosuric action of Probenecid. The biphasic action of salicylates in the renal tubules accounts for the so-called "paradoxical effect" of uricosuric agents. In patients on Colchicine/Probenecid who require a mild analgesic agent the use of acetaminophen rather than small doses of salicylates would be preferred.

Rarely, severe allergic reactions and anaphylaxis have been reported with the use of Colchicine/Probenecid. Most of these have been reported to occur within several hours after readministration following prior usage of the drug.

The appearance of hypersensitivity reactions requires cessation of therapy with Colchicine/Probenecid.

Colchicine has been reported to adversely affect spermatogenesis in animals. Reversible azoospermia has been reported in one patient.

PRECAUTIONS
GENERAL
Hematuria, renal colic, costovertebral pain, and formation of uric acid stones associated with the use of Colchicine/Probenecid in gouty patients may be prevented by alkalization of the urine and a liberal fluid intake (see *"Dosage and Administration"*). In these cases when alkali is administered, the acid-base balance of the patient should be watched.

Use with caution in patients with a history of peptic ulcer. Colchicine/Probenecid has been used in patients with some renal impairment but dosage requirements may be increased. Colchicine/Probenecid may not be effective in chronic renal insufficiency particularly when the glomerular filtration rate is 30 mL/minute or less.

A reducing substance may appear in the urine of patients receiving Probenecid. This disappears with discontinuance of therapy. Suspected glycosuria should be confirmed by using a test specific for glucose.

Adequate animal studies have not been conducted to determine the carcinogenicity potential of Probenecid or this drug combination. Since Colchicine is an established mutagen, its ability to act as a carcinogen must be suspected and administration of Colchicine/Probenecid should involve a weighing of the benefit-vs-risk when long-term administration is contemplated.

DRUG INTERACTIONS
When Probenecid is used to elevate plasma concentrations of penicillin, or other beta-lactams, or when such drugs are given to patients taking Probenecid therapeutically, high plasma concentrations of the other drug may increase the incidence of adverse reactions associated with that drug. In the case of penicillin, or other beta-lactams, psychic disturbances have been reported.

The use of salicylates antagonizes the uricosuric action of Probenecid (see *"Warnings"*). The uricosuric action of Probenecid is also antagonized by pyrazinamide.

Probenecid produces an insignificant increase in free sulfonamide plasma concentrations but a significant increase in total sulfonamide plasma levels. Since Probenecid decreases the renal excretion of conjugated sulfonamides, plasma concentrations of the latter should be determined from time to time when a sulfonamide and Colchicine/Probenecid are coadministered for prolonged periods. Probenecid may prolong or enhance the action of oral sulfonylureas and thereby increase the risk of hypoglycemia.

It has been reported that patients receiving Probenecid require significantly less thiopental for induction of anesthesia. In addition, ketamine and thiopental anesthesia were significantly prolonged in rats receiving Probenecid.

The concomitant administration of Probenecid increases the mean plasma elimination half-life of a number of drugs which can lead to increased plasma concentrations. These include agents such as indomethacin, acetaminophen, naproxen, ketoprofen, meclofenamate, lorazepam, and rifampin. Although the clinical significance of this observation has not been established, a lower dosage of the drug may be required to produce a therapeutic effect, and increases in dosage of the drug in question should be made cautiously and in small increments when Probenecid is being co-administrated. Although specific instances of toxicity due to this potential interaction have not been observed to date, physicians should be alert to this possibility.

Probenecid given concomitantly with sulindac had only a slight effect on plasma sulfide levels, while plasma levels of sulindac and sulfone were increased. Sulindac was shown to produce a modest reduction in the uricosuric action of Probenecid, which probably is not significant under most circumstances.

In animals and in humans, Probenecid has been reported to increase plasma concentrations of methotrexate (see *"Warnings"*).

Falsely high readings for theophylline have been reported in an *in vitro* study, using the Schack and Waxler technic, when therapeutic concentrations of theophylline and Probenecid were added to human plasma.

ADVERSE REACTIONS
The following adverse reactions have been observed and within each category are listed in order of decreasing severity.

PROBENECID
Central Nervous System: headache, dizziness.

Metabolic: precipitation of acute gouty arthritis.

Gastrointestinal: hepatic necrosis, vomiting, nausea, anorexia, sore gums.

Genitourinary: nephrotic syndrome, uric acid stones with or without hematuria, renal colic, costovertebral pain, urinary frequency.

Hypersensitivity: anaphylaxis, fever, urticaria, pruritus.

Hematologic: aplastic anemia, leukopenia, hemolytic anemia which in some patients could be related to genetic deficiency of glucose -6- phosphate dehydrogenase in red blood cells, anemia.

Integumentary: dermatitis, alopecia, flushing.

COLCHICINE

Side effects due to Colchicine appear to be a function of dosage. The possibility of increased Colchicine toxicity in the presence of hepatic dysfunction should be considered. The appearance of any of the following symptoms may require reduction of dosage or discontinuance of the drug.

Central Nervous System: peripheral neuritis.

Musculoskeletal: muscular weakness.

Gastrointestinal: nausea, vomiting, abdominal pain, or diarrhea may be particularly troublesome in the presence of peptic ulcer or spastic colon.

Hypersensitivity: urticaria.

Hematologic: aplastic anemia, agranulocytosis.

Integumentary: dermatitis, purpura, alopecia.

At toxic doses, Colchicine may cause severe diarrhea, generalized vascular damage, and renal damage with hematuria and oliguria.

DOSAGE AND ADMINISTRATION

Therapy with Colchicine/Probenecid should not be *started* until an acute gouty attack has subsided. However, if an acute attack is precipitated *during* therapy, Colchicine/Probenecid may be continued without changing the dosage, and additional Colchicine or other appropriate therapy should be given to control the acute attack.

The recommended adult dosage is 1 tablet of Colchicine/Probenecid daily for one week, followed by 1 tablet twice a day thereafter.

Some degree of renal impairment may be present in patients with gout. A daily dosage of 2 tablets may be adequate. However, if necessary, the daily dosage may be increased by 1 tablet every four weeks within tolerance (and usually not above 4 tablets per day) if symptoms of gouty arthritis are not controlled or the 24 hour uric acid excretion is not above 700 mg. As noted, Probenecid may not be effective in chronic renal insufficiency particularly when the glomerular filtration rate is 30 mL/minute or less.

Gastric intolerance may be indicative of overdosage, and may be corrected by decreasing the dosage.

As uric acid tends to crystallize out of an acid urine, a liberal fluid intake is recommended, as well as sufficient sodium bicarbonate (3 to 7.5 g daily) or potassium citrate (7.5 g daily) to maintain an alkaline urine (see *"Precautions"*).

Alkalization of the urine is recommended until the serum urate level returns to normal limits and tophaceous deposits disappear, i.e., during the period when urinary excretion of uric acid is at a high level. Thereafter, alkalization of the urine and the usual restriction of purine-producing foods may be somewhat relaxed.

Colchicine/Probenecid (or Probenecid) should be continued at the dosage that will maintain normal serum urate levels. When acute attacks have been absent for six months or more and serum urate levels remain within normal limits, the daily dosage of Colchicine/Probenecid may be decreased by 1 tablet every six months. The maintenance dosage should not be reduced to the point where serum urate levels tend to rise.

Protect from light.

HOW SUPPLIED
TABLETS: 0.5 MG-500 MG

BRAND/MANUFACTURER	NDC	SIZE	AWP
◇ **BRAND**			
COLBENEMID: Merck	00006-0614-68	100s	$35.63
◇ **GENERICS**			
Richlyn	00115-4302-01	100s	$14.41
Moore,H.L.	00839-1172-06	100s	$14.43
Goldline	00182-0478-01	100s	$15.75
URL	00677-0339-01	100s	$16.60
PROBEN-C: Rugby	00536-4365-01	100s	$16.65
Major	00904-2193-60	100s	$16.70
Qualitest	00603-5382-21	100s	$17.10
Zenith	00172-2193-60	100s	$17.45
Geneva	00781-1023-01	100s	$17.45
Schein	00364-0315-01	100s	$17.47
Aligen	00405-4846-01	100s	$17.50
Parmed	00349-8875-01	100s	$18.50
Richlyn	00115-4302-03	1000s	$110.85
Schein	00364-0315-02	1000s	$119.36
PROBEN-C: Rugby	00536-4365-10	1000s	$134.33

BRAND/MANUFACTURER	NDC	SIZE	AWP
Parmed	00349-8875-10	1000s	$158.36
Zenith	00172-2193-80	1000s	$160.70

Colestid *SEE* COLESTIPOL HYDROCHLORIDE

Colestipol Hydrochloride

DESCRIPTION

Colestipol HCl Granules consist of Colestipol Hydrochloride, which is a lipid lowering agent for oral use. Colestipol HCl is an insoluble, high molecular weight basic anion-exchange copolymer of diethylenetriamine and 1-chloro-2,3-epoxy-propane, with approximately 1 out of 5 amine nitrogens protonated (chloride form). It is a light yellow resin which is hygroscopic and swells when placed in water or aqueous fluids. Colestipol Hydrochloride is tasteless and odorless.

CLINICAL PHARMACOLOGY

Cholesterol is the major, and probably the sole precursor of bile acids. During normal digestion, bile acids are secreted via the bile from the liver and gall bladder into the intestines. Bile acids emulsify the fat and lipid materials present in food, thus facilitating absorption. A major portion of the bile acids secreted is reabsorbed from the intestines and returned via the portal circulation to the liver, thus completing the enterohepatic cycle. Only very small amounts of bile acids are found in normal serum.

Colestipol HCl Granules bind bile acids in the intestine forming a complex that is excreted in the feces. This nonsystemic action results in a partial removal of the bile acids from the enterohepatic circulation, preventing their reabsorption. Since Colestipol Hydrochloride is an anion exchange resin, the chloride anions of the resin can be replaced by other anions, usually those with a greater affinity for the resin than chloride ion.

Colestipol HCl is hydrophilic, but it is virtually water insoluble (99.75%) and it is not hydrolyzed by digestive enzymes. The high molecular weight polymer in Colestipol HCl apparently is not absorbed. Less than 0.05% of ^{14}C-labeled Colestipol Hydrochloride is excreted in the urine.

The increased fecal loss of bile acids due to administration of Colestipol HCl leads to an increased oxidation of cholesterol to bile acids. This results in an increase in the number of LDL receptors, increased hepatic uptake of LDL and a decrease in beta lipoprotein or low density lipoprotein serum levels, and a decrease in serum cholesterol levels. Although Colestipol HCl produces an increase in the hepatic synthesis of cholesterol in man, serum cholesterol levels fall.

There is evidence to show that this fall in cholesterol is secondary to an increased rate of cholesterol rich lipoproteins (beta or low density lipoproteins) from the plasma. Serum triglyceride levels may increase or remain unchanged in colestipol treated patients.

The decline in serum cholesterol levels with treatment with Colestipol HCl is usually evident by one month. When Colestipol HCl is discontinued, serum cholesterol levels usually return to baseline levels within one month. Periodic determinations of serum cholesterol levels as outlined in the National Cholesterol Education Program (NCEP) guidelines should be done to confirm a favorable initial and long-term response.[1]

In patients with heterozygous familial hypercholesterolemia who have not obtained an optimal response to Colestipol Hydrochloride alone in maximal doses, the combination of Colestipol Hydrochloride and nicotinic acid has been shown to provide effective further lowering of serum cholesterol, triglyceride, and LDL cholesterol values. Simultaneously, HDL cholesterol values increased significantly. In many such patients it is possible to normalize serum lipid values.[1-3]

Preliminary evidence suggests that the cholesterol-lowering effects of lovastatin and the bile acid sequestrant, Colestipol, are additive.

The effect of intensive lipid-lowering therapy on coronary atherosclerosis has been assessed by arteriography in hyperlipidemic patients. In these randomized, controlled clinical trials, patients were treated for two to four years by either conventional measures (diet, placebo, or in some cases low-dose resin) or with intensive combination therapy using diet plus Colestipol HCl Granules plus either nicotinic acid or lovastatin. When compared to conventional measures, intensive lipid-lowering combination therapy significantly reduced the frequency of progression and increased the frequency of regression of coronary atherosclerotic lesions in patients with or at risk for coronary artery disease.[5-8]

INDICATIONS AND USAGE

Since no drug is innocuous, strict attention should be paid to the indications and contraindications, particularly when selecting drugs for chronic long-term use.

Colestipol HCl Granules are indicated as adjunctive therapy to diet for the reduction of elevated serum total and low-density lipoprotein (LDL) cholesterol in patients with primary hypercholesterolemia (elevated low density lipoproteins [LDL] cholesterol) who do not respond adequately to diet. Generally, Colestipol HCl has no clinically significant effect on serum triglycerides, but with its use triglyceride levels may be raised in some patients.

In a large, placebo-controlled, multiclinic study, the LRC-CPPT[4], hypercholesterolemic subjects treated with cholestyramine, a bile acid sequestrant with a mechanism of action and an effect on serum cholesterol similar to that of

---

◆ RATED THERAPEUTICALLY EQUIVALENT; ◇ THERAPEUTIC EQUIVALENCE UNCONFIRMED; ○ UNRATED

Colestipol HCl had reductions in total and low-density lipoprotein cholesterol (LDL-C). Over the seven-year study period the cholestyramine group experienced a 19% reduction in the combined rate of coronary heart disease death plus non-fatal myocardial infarction (cumulative incidences of 7% cholestyramine and 8.6% placebo). The subjects included in the study were middle-aged men (age 35-59) with serum cholesterol levels above 265 mg/dl, LDL-C above 175 mg/dL on a moderate cholesterol lowering diet, and no history of heart disease. It is not clear to what extent these findings can be extrapolated to other segments of the hypercholesterolemic population not studied.

Treatment for elevated serum cholesterol (> 200 mg/dL) should begin with dietary therapy and be carried out in two steps (i.e., Step-One and Step-Two Diets). A minimum of six months of intensive dietary therapy and counseling should be carried out prior to initiation of drug therapy. Shorter periods can be considered in patients with severe elevations of LDL-cholesterol (> 225 mg/dL) or with definite CHD.

CONTRAINDICATIONS
Colestipol HCl Granules are contraindicated in those individuals who have shown hypersensitivity to any of its components.

WARNINGS
TO AVOID ACCIDENTAL INHALATION OR ESOPHAGEAL DISTRESS, COLESTIPOL HCl GRANULES SHOULD NOT BE TAKEN IN ITS DRY FORM. ALWAYS MIX COLESTIPOL HCl WITH WATER OR OTHER FLUIDS BEFORE INGESTING.

PRECAUTIONS
Before instituting therapy with Colestipol HCl Granules, diseases contributing to increased blood cholesterol such as hypothyroidism, diabetes mellitus, nephrotic syndrome, dysproteinemias and obstructive liver disease should be looked for and specifically treated. The patient's current medications should be reviewed for their potential to increase serum LDL-cholesterol or total cholesterol. It should be verified that an elevated LDL-C level is responsible for high total cholesterol, especially in those patients with marked elevations of high density lipoprotein (HDL) cholesterol and those with triglycerides over 400 mg/dL whose total cholesterol elevation may be due to very low density lipoprotein (VLDL) cholesterol rather than LDL-C. In most patients, LDL-C may be estimated according to the following equation:

$$LDL\text{-}C = total\ cholesterol - [0.16 \times (triglycerides) + HDL\text{-}C]$$

When the total triglycerides are greater than 400, this equation is less accurate.

Because it sequesters bile acids, Colestipol HCl may interfere with normal fat absorption and thus may prevent absorption of fat soluble vitamins such as A, D, and K.

Chronic use of Colestipol HCl may be associated with an increased bleeding tendency due to hypoprothrombinemia from vitamin K deficiency. This will usually respond promptly to parenteral vitamin K_1 and recurrences can be prevented by oral administration of vitamin K_1.

Serum cholesterol and triglyceride levels should be determined periodically based on NCEP guidelines to confirm a favorable initial and adequate long-term response.

Colestipol HCl may produce or severely worsen pre-existing constipation. The dosage should be increased gradually in patients to minimize the risk of developing fecal impaction. In patients with preexisting constipation, the starting dose should be 5 grams (1 packet or 1 scoop) once daily for 5-7 days, increasing to 5 grams twice daily with monitoring of constipation and of serum lipoproteins, at least twice, 4-6 weeks apart. Increased fluid and fiber intake should be encouraged to alleviate constipation and a stool softener may occasionally be indicated. If the initial dose is well tolerated, the dose may be increased as needed by a further 5 grams/ day (at monthly intervals) with periodic monitoring of serum lipoproteins. If constipation worsens or the desired therapeutic response is not achieved at 5-30 grams/day, combination therapy or alternate therapy should be considered. Particular effort should be made to avoid constipation in patients with symptomatic coronary artery disease. Constipation associated with Colestipol HCl may aggravate hemorrhoids.

While there have been no reports of hypothyroidism induced in individuals with normal thyroid function, the theoretical possibility exists, particularly in patients with limited thyroid reserve.

Since Colestipol HCl is a chloride form of an anion exchange resin, there is a possibility that prolonged use may lead to development of hyperchloremic acidosis.

CARCINOGENESIS, MUTAGENESIS AND IMPAIRMENT OF FERTILITY
In studies conducted in rats in which cholestyramine resin (a bile acid sequestering agent similar to Colestipol Hydrochloride) was used as a tool to investigate the role of various intestinal factors, such as fat, bile salts and microbial flora, in the development of intestinal tumors induced by potent carcinogens, the incidence of such tumors was observed to be greater in cholestyramine resin treated rats than in control rats.

The relevance of this laboratory observation from studies in rats with cholestyramine resin to the clinical use of Colestipol HCl is not known. In the LRC-CPPT study referred to above, the total incidence of fatal and non-fatal neoplasms was similar in both treatment groups. When the many different categories of tumors are examined, various alimentary system cancers were somewhat more prevalent in the cholestyramine group. The small numbers and the multiple categories prevent conclusions from being drawn. Further follow-up

of the LRC-CPPT participants by the sponsors of that study is planned for cause-specific mortality and cancer morbidity.

When Colestipol HCl was administered in the diet to rats for 18 months, there was no evidence of any drug related intestinal tumor formation. In the Ames assay Colestipol HCl was not mutagenic.

USE IN PREGNANCY
The use of Colestipol HCl in pregnancy or lactation or by women of childbearing age requires that the potential benefits of drug therapy be weighed against the possible hazards to the mother and child. The safe use of the resin in Colestipol HCl by pregnant women has not been established.

USE IN CHILDREN
Safety and effectiveness in children have not been established.

DRUG INTERACTIONS
Since Colestipol Hydrochloride is an anion exchange resin, it may have a strong affinity for anions other than the bile acids. Therefore Colestipol Hydrochloride resin may delay or reduce the absorption of concomitant oral medication. The interval between the administration of Colestipol HCl and any other medication should be as long as possible. Patients should take other drugs at least one hour before or four hours after Colestipol HCl to avoid impeding their absorption. Human studies have demonstrated that Colestipol HCl may decrease propranolol absorption. Effects on the absorption of other beta-blockers have not been determined. Therefore, patients on propranolol should be observed when Colestipol HCl is either added or deleted from a therapeutic regimen.

In vitro studies have indicated that Colestipol HCl binds a number of drugs. Studies in humans show that the absorption of chlorothiazide as reflected in urinary excretion is markedly decreased even when administered one hour before Colestipol HCl. The absorption of tetracycline, furosemide, penicillin G and gemfibrozil were significantly decreased when given simultaneously with Colestipol HCl, these drugs were not tested to determine the effect of administration one hour before Colestipol HCl.

No depressant effect on blood levels in humans was noted when Colestipol HCl was administered with any of the following drugs: aspirin, clindamycin, clofibrate, methyldopa, tolbutamide, phenytoin or warfarin. Particular caution should be observed with digitalis preparations since there are conflicting results for the effect of Colestipol HCl on the availability of digoxin and digitoxin. The potential for binding of these drugs if given concomitantly is present. Discontinuing Colestipol HCl could pose a hazard to health if a potentially toxic drug that is significantly bound to the resin has been titrated to a maintenance level while the patient was taking Colestipol HCl.

Bile acid binding resins may interfere with the absorption of oral phosphate supplements.

ADVERSE REACTIONS
1. GASTROINTESTINAL
The most common adverse reactions are confined to the gastrointestinal tract. To achieve minimal GI disturbance with an optimal LDL-cholesterol lowering effect, a gradual increase of dosage starting with 5 grams once daily is recommended. Constipation, reported by about one patient in 10, is the major single complaint and at times is severe and occasionally accompanied by impaction. Most instances of constipation are mild, transient, and controlled with standard treatment. Increased fluid intake and inclusion of additional dietary fiber should be the first step; a stool softener may be added if needed. Some patients require decreased dosage or discontinuation of therapy. Hemorrhoids may be aggravated.

Less frequent gastrointestinal complaints occurring in about one in 30 to one in 100 patients, are abdominal discomfort (abdominal pain and distention), belching, flatulence, nausea, vomiting, and diarrhea. Peptic ulceration, gastrointestinal irritation and bleeding, cholecystitis, and cholelithiasis have been reported by fewer than one in 500 patients and are not necessarily drug related.

2. HYPERSENSITIVITY
Urticaria and dermatitis were noted in fewer than one in 1,000 patients. Asthma and wheezing were not reported in the studies with Colestipol HCl but have been noted during treatment with other cholesterol-lowering agents.

3. MUSCULOSKELETAL
Muscle and joint pains, and arthritis have had a reported incidence of less than one in 1,000 patients.

4. NEUROLOGIC
Headache and dizziness were noted in about one in 300 patients; anxiety, vertigo, and drowsiness were reported in fewer than one in 1,000.

5. MISCELLANEOUS
Anorexia, fatigue, weakness, and shortness of breath have been seen in 1-3 patients in 1,000. Transient and modest elevations of serum glutamic oxaloacetic transaminase and of alkaline phosphatase were observed in one or more occasions in various patients treated with Colestipol HCl Granules. Some patients have shown an increase in serum phosphorus and chloride with a decrease in sodium and potassium.

OVERDOSE
Overdosage of Colestipol HCl Granules has not been reported. Should overdosage occur, however, the chief potential harm would be obstruction of the gastrointestinal tract. The location of such potential obstruction, the degree of obstruction and the presence or absence of normal gut motility would determine treatment.

➤ SHOWN IN PRODUCT IDENTIFICATION GUIDE

DOSAGE AND ADMINISTRATION

For adults Colestipol HCl Granules are recommended in doses of 5-30 grams/day given once or in divided doses. The starting dose should be 5 grams once or twice daily with a daily increment of 5 grams at one- or two-month intervals. Appropriate use of lipid profiles as per NCEP guidelines including LDL-cholesterol and trigycerides is advised so that optimal, but not excessive doses are used to obtain the desired therapeutic effect on LDL-cholesterol level. If the desired therapeutic effect is not obtained at a dose of 5-30 grams/day with good compliance and acceptable side effects, combined therapy or alternate treatment should be considered.

To avoid accidental inhalation or esophageal distress, Colestipol HCl should not be taken in its dry form. Colestipol HCl should always be mixed with water or other fluids before ingesting. Patients should take other drugs at least one hour before or four hours after Colestipol HCl to minimize possible interference with their absorption. (See "Drug Interactions".)

BEFORE ADMINISTRATION OF COLESTIPOL HCL
1. Define the type of hyperlipoproteinemia, as described in NCEP guidelines.
2. Institute a trial of diet and weight reduction.
3. Establish baseline serum total and LDL-cholesterol and triglyceride levels.

DURING ADMINISTRATION OF COLESTIPOL HCL
1. The patient should be carefully monitored clinically, including serum cholesterol and triglyceride levels. Periodic determinations of serum cholesterol levels is outlined in the NCEP guidelines should be done to confirm a favorable initial and long-term response.
2. Failure of total or LDL-cholesterol to fall within the desired range should lead one to first examine dietary and drug compliance. If these are deemed acceptable, combined therapy or alternate treatment should be considered.
3. Significant rise in triglyceride level should be considered as indication for dose reduction, drug discontinuation, or combined or alternate therapy.

MIXING AND ADMINISTRATION GUIDE
Colestipol HCl Granules should always be taken mixed in a liquid such as orange or tomato juice, milk, carbonated beverage, or water. It may also be taken in soups or with cereals or pulpy fruits. Colestipol HCl *should never be taken in its dry form.*

WITH BEVERAGES
1. Add the prescribed amount of Colestipol HCl to a glassful (three ounces or more) of water, milk, flavored drink, or a favorite juice (orange, tomato, pineapple, or other fruit juice). A heavy or pulpy juice may minimize complaints relative to consistency. An unsweetened juice may improve palatability.
2. Stir the mixture until the medication is completely mixed. (Colestipol HCl will not dissolve in the liquid.) Colestipol HCl may also be mixed with carbonated beverages, slowly stirred in a large glass; however, this mixture may be associated with GI complaints.

Rinse the glass with a small amount of additional beverage to make sure all the medication is taken.

WITH CEREALS, SOUPS, AND FRUITS
Colestipol HCl may be taken mixed with milk in hot or regular breakfast cereals, or even mixed in soups that have a high fluid content (tomato or chicken noodle soup). It may also be added to fruits that are pulpy such as crushed pineapple, pears, peaches, or fruit cocktail.

Store at controlled room temperature 15°-30°C (59°-86°F).

REFERENCES
1. National Cholesterol Education Program (NCEP), The Expert Panel. Report of the National Cholesterol Education Program Expert Panel on Detection, Evaluation, and Treatment of High Blood Cholesterol in Adults. *Arch Intern Med* 148:36-69, 1988. 2. Kane JP, Malloy MJ, Tun P et al: Normalization of low-density-lipoprotein levels in heterozygous familial hypercholesterolemia with a combined drug regimen. *N. Engl J. Med* 304:251-258, 1981. 3. Illingworth DR, Phillipson BE, JH Rapp et al. Colestipol plus nicotinic acid in treatment of heterozygous familial hypercholesterolemia, *Lancet* 1:296-298, 1981. 4. Kuo PT, Kostis JB, Moreyra AE et al: Familial type II hyperlipoproteinemia with coronary heart disease: Effect of diet-colestipol-nicotinic acid treatment. *Chest* 79:286-291, 1981. 5. Blankenhorn DH, et al. Beneficial Effects of Combined Colestipol-Niacin Therapy on Coronary Atherosclerosis and Coronary Venous Bypass Grafts. *JAMA* 257(23):3233-3240, 1987. 6. Cashin-Hemphill L, et al. Beneficial Effects of Colestipol-Niacin on Coronary Atherosclerosis: A 4-Year Follow-up. *JAMA* 264:3013-3017, 1990. 7. Brown G, et al. Regression of Coronary Artery Disease as a Result of Intensive Lipid-Lowering Therapy in Men with High Levels of Apolipoprotein B. *N Engl. J. Med* 323:1289-1298, 1990. 8. Kane JP, Malloy MJ, et al. Regression of Coronary Atherosclerosis During Treatment of Familial Hypercholesterolemia with Combined Drug Regimens. *JAMA* 264:3007-3012, 1990. 9. Lipid Metabolism-Atherogenesis Branch. National Heart, Lung, and Blood Institute, Bethesda, MD: The Lipid Research Clinics Coronary Primary Prevention Trial Results. I. Reduction in Incidence of Coronary Heart Disease, *JAMA* 251:351-364, 1984.

HOW SUPPLIED
GRANULE FOR RECONSTITUTION:

BRAND/MANUFACTURER	NDC	SIZE	AWP
○ **BRAND**			
COLESTID: Upjohn	00009-0260-01	30s	$35.69
COLESTID FLAVORED: Upjohn	00009-0370-03	60s	$69.94
COLESTID: Upjohn	00009-0260-04	90s	$104.91
	00009-0260-17	300 gm	$44.64
	00009-0260-05	450 gm	$44.64
COLESTID FLAVORED: Upjohn			
COLESTID: Upjohn	00009-0260-02	500 gm	$74.40

TABLETS: 1 GM

BRAND/MANUFACTURER	NDC	SIZE	AWP
○ **BRAND**			
COLESTID: Upjohn	00009-0450-03	120s	$34.38

Colfosceril Palmitate

DESCRIPTION
Colfosceril Palmitate for Intratracheal Suspension is a protein-free synthetic lung surfactant stored under vacuum as a sterile lyophilized powder. Colfosceril Palmitate is reconstituted with preservative-free Sterile Water for Injection prior to administration by intratracheal instillation. Each 10 mL vial contains 108 mg Colfosceril Palmitate, commonly known as dipalmitoylphosphatidylcholine (DPPC), 12 mg cetyl alcohol, 8 mg tyloxapol, and 47 mg sodium chloride. Sodium hydroxide or hydrochloric acid may have been added to adjust pH. When reconstituted with 8 mL Sterile Water for Injection, the Colfosceril Palmitate suspension contains 13.5 mg/mL Colfosceril Palmitate, 1.5mg/mL cetyl alcohol, and 1 mg/mL tyloxapol in 0.1 N NaCl. The suspension appears milky white with a pH of 5 to 7 and an osmolality of 185 mOsm/L.

The chemical names of Colfosceril Palmitate for Intratracheal Suspension are **Colfosceril Palmitate** (1,2-dipalmitoyl-*sn*-3-phosphoglycerocholine), **cetyl alcohol** (1-hexadecanol), and **tyloxapol** (formaldehyde polymer with oxirane and 4-(1,1,3,3-tetramethylbutyl)-phenol).

Following is its chemical structure:

$$
\begin{array}{c}
O \\
\| \\
CH_2OC(CH_2)_{14}CH_3 \\
| \\
CH_3(CH_2)_{14}CO\!\!-\!\!C\!\!-\!\!H \\
| \quad\quad | \\
O \quad\quad CH_2\!\!-\!\!O\!\!-\!\!\overset{+}{P}\!\!-\!\!OCH_2CH_2\overset{+}{N}(CH_3)_3 \\
| \\
O^-
\end{array}
$$

CLINICAL PHARMACOLOGY
Surfactant deficiency is an important factor in the development of the neonatal respiratory distress syndrome (RDS). Thus, surfactant replacement therapy early in the course of RDS should ameliorate the disease and improve symptoms. Natural surfactant, a combination of lipids and apoproteins, exhibits not only surface tension reducing properties (conferred by the lipids), but also rapid spreading and adsorption (conferred by the apoproteins). The major fraction of the lipid component of natural surfactant is DPPC, which comprises up to 70% of natural surfactant by weight.

Although DPPC reduces surface tension, DPPC alone is ineffective in RDS because DPPC spreads and adsorbs poorly. In Colfosceril Palmitate which is protein free, cetyl alcohol acts as the spreading agent for the DPPC on the air-fluid interface. Tyloxapol, a polymeric long-chain repeating alcohol, is a nonionic surfactant which acts to disperse both DPPC and cetyl alcohol. Sodium chloride is added to adjust osmolality.

Pharmacokinetics: Colfosceril Palmitate is administered directly into the trachea. Human pharmacokinetic studies of the absorption, biotransformation, and excretion of the components of Colfosceril Palmitate have not been performed. Nonclinical studies, however, have shown that DPPC can be absorbed from the alveolous into lung tissue where it can be catabolized extensively and reutilized for further phospholipid synthesis and secretion. In the developing rabbit, 90% of alveolar phospholipids are recycled. In premature rabbits, the alveolar half-life of intratracheally administered H^3-labeled phosphatidylcholine is approximately 12 hours.

Animal Studies: In animal models of RDS, treatment with Colfosceril Palmitate significantly improved lung volume, compliance and gas exchange in premature rabbits and lambs. The amount and distribution of lung water were not affected by Colfosceril Palmitate treatment of premature rabbit pups. The extent of lung injury in premature rabbit pups undergoing mechanical ventilation was reduced significantly by Colfosceril Palmitate treatment. In premature lambs, neither systemic blood flow nor flow through the ductus arteriosus were affected by Colfosceril Palmitate treatment. Survival was significantly better in both premature rabbits and premature lambs treated with Colfosceril Palmitate.

Clinical Studies: Colfosceril Palmitate has been studied in the U.S. and Canada in controlled clinical trials involving more than 4400 infants. Over 10,000 infants have received Colfosceril Palmitate through an open, uncontrolled, North American study designed to provide the drug to premature infants who might benefit and to obtain additional safety information.

Prophylactic Treatment: The efficacy of a single dose of Colfosceril Palmitate in prophylactic treatment of infants at risk of developing respiratory distress syndrome (RDS) was examined in three double-blind, placebo-controlled studies, one involving 215 infants weighing 500 to 700 grams, one involving 385 infants weighing 700 to 1350 grams, and one involving 446 infants weighing 700 to 1100 grams. The infants were intubated and placed on mechanical ventilation, and received 5 mL/kg Colfosceril Palmitate or placebo (air) within 30 minutes of birth.

The efficacy of one versus three doses of Colfosceril Palmitate in prophylactic treatment of infants at risk of developing RDS was examined in a double-blind, placebo-controlled study of 823 infants weighing 700 to 1100 grams. The infants were intubated and placed on mechanical ventilation, and received a first 5 mL/kg dose of Colfosceril Palmitate within 30 minutes. Repeat 5 mL/kg doses of Colfosceril Palmitate or placebo (air) were given to all infants who remained on mechanical ventilation at approximately 12 and 24 hours of age. An initial analysis of 716 infants is available.

The major efficacy parameters from these studies are presented in Table 1. (See related table).

Rescue Treatment: The efficacy of Colfosceril Palmitate in the rescue treatment of infants with RDS was examined in two double-blind, placebo-controlled studies. One study enrolled 419 infants weighing 700 to 1350 grams; the second enrolled 1237 infants weighing 1250 grams and above. In the rescue treatment studies, infants received an initial dose (5 mL/kg) of Colfosceril Palmitate or placebo (air) between 2 and 24 hours of life followed by a second dose (5 mL/kg) approximately 12 hours later to infants who remained on mechanical ventilation. The major efficacy parameters from these studies are presented in Table 2. (See related table).

Clinical Results: In these six controlled clinical studies, infants in the Colfosceril Palmitate group showed significant improvements in FiO_2 and ventilator settings which persisted for at least 7 days. Pulmonary air leaks were significantly reduced in each study. Five of these studies also showed a significant reduction in death from RDS. Further, overall mortality was reduced for all infants weighing > 700 grams. The one versus three-dose prophylactic treatment study in 700 to 1100 gram infants showed a further reduction in overall mortality with two additional doses.

Safety information is presented in Tables 3 and 4 (see *"Adverse Reactions"*). Beneficial effects in the Colfosceril Palmitate group were observed for some safety assessments. Various forms of pulmonary air leak and use of pancuronium were reduced in infants receiving Colfosceril Palmitate in all six studies.

Follow-up data at one year adjusted age are available on 1094 of 2470 surviving infants. Growth and development of infants who received Colfosceril Palmitate in this sample were comparable to infants who received placebo.

INDICATIONS AND USAGE
Colfosceril Palmitate is indicated for:
Prophylactic treatment of infants with birth weights of less than 1350 grams who are at risk of developing RDS (see *"Precautions"*),
Prophylactic treatment of infants with birth weights greater than 1350 grams who have evidence of pulmonary immaturity, and
Rescue treatment of infants who have developed RDS.
For prophylactic treatment, the first dose of Colfosceril Palmitate should be administered as soon as possible after birth (see *"Dosage and Administration: General Guidelines for Administration"*).
Infants considered as candidate for rescue treatment with Colfosceril Palmitate should be on mechanical ventilation and have a diagnosis of RDS by both of the following criteria:
1. Respiratory distress not attributable to causes other than RDS, based on clinical and laboratory assessments.
2. Chest radiographic findings consistent with the diagnosis of RDS.
During the clinical development of Colfosceril Palmitate, all infants who received the drug were intubated and on mechanical ventilation. For three-dose prophylactic treatment with Colfosceril Palmitate, the first dose of drug was administered as soon as possible after birth and repeat doses were given at approximately 12 and 24 hours after birth if infants remained on mechanical ventilation at those times. For rescue treatment, two doses were given; one

Table 1
EFFICACY ASSESSMENTS—PROPHYLACTIC TREATMENT

Number of Doses: Birth Weight Range:	*Single Dose* *500 to 700 grams*		*Single Dose* *700 to 1350 grams*		*Single Dose* *700 to 1100 grams*		*Three Doses* *700 to 1100 grams*	
Treatment Group: Number of Infants:	Placebo (Air) N = 106	Colfosceril Palmitate N = 109	Placebo (Air) N = 185	Colfosceril Palmitate N = 176	Placebo (Air) N = 222	Colfosceril Palmitate N = 224	One Colfosceril Palmitate Dose N = 356	Three Colfosceril Palmitate Doses N = 360
	% of Infants		*% of Infants*		*% of Infants*		*% of Infants*	
Death ≤ Day 28[a]	53	50	11	6	21	15	16	9*
Death through 1 Year[a]	59	60	14	11	30	20**	17	12*
Death from RDS[b]	25	13*	4	3	10	5§	17	2
Intact Cardiopulmonary Survival[a,c]	29	25	69	78*	65	68	74	78
Bronchopulmonary Dysplasia (BPD)[a,d]	43	44	23	18	19	21	8	12
RDS Incidence[b]	73	81	46	42	55	55	63	68

[a] *"Intent-to-treat" analyses (as randomized) except for the 700 to 1350 gram, single dose study in which infants with congenital infections and anomalies were excluded*
[b] *"As-treated" analyses*
[c] *Defined by survival through 28 days of life without bronchopulmonary dysplasia*
[d] *Defined by a combination of clinical and radiographic criteria*
* < 0.05
** < 0.01
§ *p = 0.051*

Table 2
EFFICACY ASSESSMENTS-RESCUE TREATMENT

Number of Doses: Birth Weight Range:	*Two Doses* *700 to 1350 grams*		*Two Doses* *1250 grams and above*	
Treatment Group Number of Infants:	Placebo (Air) N = 213	Colfosceril Palmitate N = 206	Placebo (Air) N = 623	Colfosceril Palmitate N = 614
	% of Infants		*% of Infants*	
Death ≤ Day 28[a]	23	11***	7	4*
Death through 1 Year[a]	27	15***	9	6§
Death from RDS[b]	10	3**	3	1*
Intact Cardiopulmonary Survival[a,c]	62	75**	88	93**
Bronchopulmonary Dysplasia (BPD)[a,d]	18	15	6	3*

[a] *"Intent-to-treat" analyses (as randomized)*
[b] *"As-treated" analyses*
[c] *Defined by survival through 28 days of life without bronchopulmonary dysplasia*
[d] *Defined by a combination of clinical and radiographic criteria*
* *p < 0.05*
** *p < 0.01*
*** *p < 0.001*
§ *p = 0.067*

between 2 and 24 hours of life, and a second approximately 12 hours later if infants remained on mechanical ventilation. Infants who received rescue treatment with Colfosceril Palmitate had a documented arterial to alveolar oxygen tension ratio (a/A) < 0.22.

CONTRAINDICATIONS

There are no known contraindications to treatment with Colfosceril Palmitate.

WARNINGS

Intratracheal Administration Only: Colfosceril Palmitate should be administered only by instillation into the trachea (see *"Dosage and Administration"*).

GENERAL

The use of Colfosceril Palmitate requires expert clinical care by experienced neonatologists and other clinicians who are accomplished at neonatal intubation and ventilatory management. Adequate personnel, facilities, equipment, and medications are required to optimize perinatal outcome in premature infants.

Instillation of Colfosceril Palmitate should be performed **only** by trained medical personal experienced in airway and clinical management of unstable premature infants. Vigilant clinical attention should be given to all infants prior to, during, and after administration of Colfosceril Palmitate.

Acute Effects: Colfosceril Palmitate can rapidly affect oxygenation and lung compliance.

Lung Compliance: If chest expansion improves substantially after dosing peak ventilator inspiratory pressures should be reduced immediately, without waiting for confirmation of respiratory improvement by blood gas assessment. Failure to reduce inspiratory ventilator pressures rapidly in such instances can result in lung overdistention and fatal pulmonary air leak.

Hyperoxia: If the infant becomes pink and transcutaneous oxygen saturation is in excess of 95%, FiO_2 should be reduced in small but repeated steps (until saturation is 90 to 95%) without waiting for confirmation of elevated arterial pO_2 by blood gas assessment. Failure to reduce FiO_2 in such instances can result in hyperoxia.

Hypocarbia: If arterial or transcutaneous CO_2 measurements are < 30 torr, the ventilator rate should be reduced at once. Failure to reduce ventilator rates in such instances can result in marked hypocarbia, which is known to reduce brain blood flow.

Pulmonary Hemorrhage: In the single study conducted in infants weighing < 700 grams at birth, the incidence of pulmonary hemorrhage (10% vs 2% in the placebo group) was significantly increased in the Colfosceril Palmitate group. None of the five studies involving infants with birth weights > 700 grams showed a significant increase in pulmonary hemorrhage in the Colfosceril Palmitate group. In a cross-study analysis of these five studies, pulmonary hemorrhage was reported for 1% (14/1420) of infants in the placebo group and 2% (27/1411) of infants in the Colfosceril Palmitate group. Fatal pulmonary hemorrhage occurred in three infants; two in the Colfosceril Palmitate group and one in the placebo group. Mortality from all causes among infants who developed pulmonary hemorrhage was 43% in the placebo group and 37% in the Colfosceril Palmitate group.

Pulmonary hemorrhage in both Colfosceril Palmitate and placebo infants was more frequent in infants who were younger, smaller, male, or who had a patent ductus arteriosus. Pulmonary hemorrhage typically occurred in the first 2 days of life in both treatment groups.

In more than 7700 infants in the open, uncontrolled study, pulmonary hemorrhage was reported in 4%, but fatal pulmonary hemorrhage was reported rarely (0.4%).

In the controlled clinical studies Colfosceril Palmitate treated infants who received steriods more than 24 hours prior to delivery or indomethacin postnatally had a lower rate of pulmonary hemorrhage than other Colfosceril Palmitate treated infants. Attention should be paid to early and aggressive diagnosis and treatment (unless contraindicated) of patent ductus arteriosus during the first 2 days of life (while the ductus arteriosus is often clinically silent). Other potentially protective measures include attempting to decrease FiO_2 preferentially over ventilator pressures during the first 24 to 48 hours after dosing, and attempting to decrease PEEP minimally for at least 48 hours after dosing.

Mucous Plugs: Infants whose ventilation becomes markedly impaired during or shortly after dosing may have mucous plugging of the endotracheal tube, particularly if pulmonary secretions were prominent prior to drug administration. Suctioning of all infants prior to dosing may lessen the chance of mucous plugs obstructing the endotracheal tube. If endotracheal tube obstruction from such plugs is suspected, and suctioning is unsuccessful in removing the obstruction, the blocked endotracheal tube should be replaced immediately.

PRECAUTIONS

General: In the controlled clinical studies, infants known prenatally or postnatally to have major congenital anomalies, or who were suspected of having congenital infection, were excluded from entry. However, these disorders cannot be recognized early in life in all cases, and a few infants with these conditions were entered. The benefits of Colfosceril Palmitate in the affected infants who received drug appeared to be similar to the benefits observed in infants without anomalies or occult infection.

Prophylactic Treatment—Infants < 700 Grams: In infants weighing 500 to 700 grams a single prophylactic dose of Colfosceril Palmitate significantly: improved FiO_2 and ventilator settings, reduced pneumothorax, and reduced death from RDS, but increased pulmonary hemorrhage (see *"Warnings"*). Overall mortality

did not differ significantly between the placebo and Colfosceril Palmitate groups (see Table 1). Data on multiple doses in infants in this weight class are not yet available. Accordingly, clinicians should carefully evaluate the potential risks and benefits of Colfosceril Palmitate administration in these infants.

Rescue Treatment—Number of Doses: A small number of infants with RDS have received more than two doses of Colfosceril Palmitate as rescue treatment. Definitive data on the safety and efficacy of these additional doses are not available.

Carcinogenesis, Mutagenesis, Impairment of Fertility: Colfosceril Palmitate at concentrations up to 10,000 µg/plate was not mutagenic in the Ames Salmonella assay.

Long-term studies have not been performed in animals to evaluate the carcinogenic potential of Colfosceril Palmitate. The effects of Colfosceril Palmitate on fertility have not been studied.

ADVERSE REACTIONS

General: Premature birth is associated with a high incidence of morbidity and mortality. Despite significant reductions in overall mortality associated with Colfosceril Palmitate, some infants who received Colfosceril Palmitate developed severe complications and either survived with permanent handicaps or died.

In controlled clinical studies evaluating the safety and efficacy of Colfosceril Palmitate, numerous safety assessments were made. In infants receiving Colfosceril Palmitate, pulmonary hemorrhage, apnea and use of methylxanthines were increased. A number of other adverse events were significantly reduced in the Colfosceril Palmitate group, particularly various forms of pulmonary air leak and use of pancuronium. (See *"Clinical Pharmacology, Clinical Results."*) Tables 3 and 4 summarize the results of the major safety evaluations from the controlled clinical studies. (See related tables).

Pulmonary Hemorrhage: See *"Warnings."*

Abnormal Laboratory Values: Abnormal laboratory values are common in critically ill, mechanically ventilated, premature infants. A higher incidence of abnormal laboratory values in the Colfosceril Palmitate group was not reported.

Events During Dosing: Data on events during dosing are available from more than 8800 infants in the open, uncontrolled clinical study (Table 5).

Table 5
EVENTS DURING DOSING IN THE OPEN, UNCONTROLLED STUDY[a]

Treatment Type: Number of Infants:	Prophylactic Treatment N = 1127 % of Infants	Rescue Treatment N = 7711 % of Infants
Reflux of Colfosceril Palmitate	20	31
Drop in O_2 saturation ($\geq$ 20%)	6	22
Rise in O_2 saturation ($\geq$ 10%)	5	6
Drop in transcutaneous pO_2 ($\geq$ 20 mm Hg)	1	8
Rise in transcutaneous pO_2 ($\geq$ 20 mm Hg)	2	5
Drop in transcutaneous pCO_2 ($\geq$ 20 mm Hg)	< 1	1
Rise in transcutaneous pCO_2 ($\geq$ 20 mm Hg)	1	3
Bradycardia (< 60 beats/min)	1	3
Tachycardia (> 200 beats/min)	< 1	< 1
Gagging	1	5
Mucous Plugs	< 1	< 1

a Infants may have experienced more than one event. Investigators were prohibited from adjusting FiO_2 and/or ventilator settings during dosing unless significant clinical deterioration occurred.

Reflux: Reflux of Colfosceril Palmitate into the endotracheal tube during dosing has been observed and may be associated with rapid drug administration. If reflux occurs, drug administration should be halted and, if necessary, peak inspiratory pressure on the ventilator should be increased by 4 to 5 cm H_2O until the endotrachealtube clears.

> 20% Drop in Transcutaneous Oxygen Saturation: If transcutaneous oxygen saturation declines during dosing, drug administration should be halted and, if necessary, peak inspiratory pressure on the ventilator should be increased by 4 to 5 cm H_2O for 1 to 2 minutes. In addition, increases of FiO_2 may be required for 1 to 2 minutes.

Mucous Plugs: See *"Warnings."*

OVERDOSAGE

There have been no reports of massive overdosage with Colfosceril Palmitate.

DOSAGE AND ADMINISTRATION

Preparation of Suspension: Colfosceril Palmitate is best reconstituted immediately before use because it does not contain antibacterial preservatives. However, the reconstituted suspension is chemically and physically stable and remains sterile (when reconstituted using aseptic techniques) when stored at 2° to 30°C (36° to 86°F) for up to 12 hours following reconstitution.

Solutions containing buffers or preservatives should not be used for reconstitution. *Do Not Use Bacteriostatic Water for Injection, USP.* Each vial of Colfosceril

Palmitate should be reconstituted only with *8 mL* of the accompanying diluent (preservative-free Sterile Water for Injection) as follows:

1. Fill a 10 mL or 12 mL syringe with 8 mL preservative-free Sterile Water for Injection using an 18 or 19 gauge needle;
2. Allow the vacuum in the vial to draw the sterile water into the vial;
3. Aspirate as much as possible of the 8 mL out of the vial into the syringe (while maintaining the vacuum), then *Suddenly* release the syringe plunger.

Step 3 should be repeated three or four times to assure adequate mixing of the vial contents. If vacuum is not present the vial of Colfosceril Palmitate should not be used.

The appropriate dosage volume for the entire dose (5 mL/kg) should then be drawn into the syringe from *below* the froth in the vial (again maintaining the vacuum). If the infant weighs less than 1600 grams, unused Colfosceril Palmitate suspension will remain in the vial after the entire dose is drawn into the syringe. If the infant weighs more than 1600 grams, at least two vials will be required for each dose.

Reconstituted Colfosceril Palmitate is a milky white suspension with a total volume of 8 mL per vial. Each mL of reconstituted Colfosceril Palmitate contains 13.5 mg Colfosceril Palmitate, 1.5 mg cetyl alcohol, 1 mg tyloxapol, and sodium chloride to provide a 0.1 N concentration. If the suspension appears to separate, gently shake or swirl the vial to resuspend the preparation. The reconstituted product should be inspected visually for homogeneity immediately before administration; if persistent large flakes or particles are present, the vial should not be used.

Dosage: **Accurate determination of weight at birth is the key to accurate dosing.**

Prophylactic Treatment: The first dose of Colfosceril Palmitate should be administered as a single 5 mL/kg dose as soon as possible after birth. Second and third doses should be administered approximately 12 and 24 hours later to all infants who remain on mechanical ventilation at those times.

Rescue Treatment: Colfosceril Palmitate should be administered in two 5 mL/kg doses. The initial dose should be administered as soon as possible after the diagnosis of RDS is confirmed. The second dose should be administered approximately 12 hours following the first dose, provided the infant remains on mechanical ventilation. A small number of infants with RDS have received more than two doses of Colfosceril Palmitate as rescue treatment. Definitive data on the safety and efficacy of these additional doses are not available (see *"Precautions"*).

Use of Special Endotrachear Tube Adapter: With each vial of Colfosceril Palmitate for Intratracheal Suspension, five different sized endotracheal tube adapters each with a special right angle Luer®-lock sideport are supplied. The adapters are clean but not sterile. The adapters should be used as follows:

1. Select an adapter size which corresponds to the inside diameter of the endotracheal tube.
2. Insert the adapter into the endotracheal tube with a firm push-twist motion.
3. Connect the breathing circuit wye to the adapter.
4. Remove the cap from the sideport on the adapter. Attach the syringe containing drug to the sideport.
5. After completion of dosing, remove the syringe and RECAP THE SIDEPORT.

Administration: The infant should be suctioned prior to administration of Colfosceril Palmitate.

Colfosceril Palmitate suspension is administered via the sideport on the special endotracheal tube adapter *Without Interrupting Mechanical Ventilation.*

Each Colfosceril Palmitate dose is administered in two 2.5 mL/kg half-doses. Each half-dose is instilled slowly over 1 to 2 minutes (30 to 50 mechanical

Table 3
SAFETY ASSESSMENTS[a]—PROPHYLACTIC TREATMENT

Number of Doses: Birth Weight Range: Treatment Group: Number of Infants:	Single Dose 500 to 700 grams		Single Dose 700 to 1350 grams		Single Dose 700 to 1100 grams		One Versus Three Doses 700 to 1100 grams	
	Placebo (Air) N = 108	Colfosceril Palmitate N = 107	Placebo (Air) N = 193	Colfosceril Palmitate N = 192	Placebo (Air) N = 222	Colfosceril Palmitate N = 224	One Colfosceril Palmitate Dose N = 356	Three Colfosceril Palmitate Doses N = 360
	% of Infants		% of Infants		% of Infants		% of Infants	
Intraventricular Hemorrhage (IVH)								
Overall	51	57	31	27	36	36	38	35
Severe IVH	26	25	10	8	13	14	9	9
Pulmonary Air Leak (PAL)								
Overall	52	48	16	11	32	25	29	27
Pneumothorax	23	10*	5	6	19	11*	14	12
Pneumopericardium	1	4	2	0	< 1	1	1	1
Pneumomediastinum	2	1	2	3	7	1**	3	2
Pulmonary Interstitial								
Emphysema	43	44	13	7*	26	20	23	22
Death from PAL	4	6	< 1	< 1	2	1	2	1
Patent Ductus Arteriosus	49	53	66	70	50	55	59	57
Necrotizing Entercoolitis	2	4	11	13	3	4	6	2*
Pulmonary Hemorrhage	2	10**	2	4	1	4	4	6
Congenital								
Pneumonia	4	4	2	4	2	2	1	1
Nosocomial Pneumonia	10	10	2	4	4	7	14	15
Non-Pulmonary Infections	33	35	34	39	28	29	35	34
Sepsis	30	34	30	34	23	24	30	27
Death From Sepsis	4	4	3	3	1	2	3	2
Meningtis	4	6	3	1	2	3	1	2
Other Infections	7	4	5	3	6	10	10	11
Major Anomalies	3	1	2	4	7	4	4	4
Hypotension	70	77	52	47	59	62	54	50
Hyperbilirubinemia	22	21	63	61	27	31	20	21
Exchange Transfusion	4	3	1	2	2	2	3	1
Thrombocytopenia[b]	21	25	not available		9	8	12	10
Persistent Fetal Circulation	0	1	1	1	0	2*	1	< 1
Seizures	11	8	2	2	11	9	6	5
Apnea	34	33	76	73	55	65*	62	68
Drug Therapy								
Antibiotics	96	99	98	96	98	99	> 99	99
Diuretics	55	60	39	37	59	63	64	65
Anticonvulsants	14	18	23	24	20	16	9	8
Inotropes	46	40	20	20	26	20	28	27
Sedatives	62	71	65	64	63	57	52	52
Pancuronium	19	11	22	14*	19	13*	15	11
Methylxanthines	38	43	77	77	61	72*	75	82*

[a] All parameters were examined with "as-treated" analyses.
[b] Thrombocytopenia requiring platelet transfusion.
* p <
** p < 0.01

breaths) in small bursts timed with inspiration. After the first 2.5 mL/kg half-dose is administered in the midline position, the infant's head and torso are turned 45° to the *right* for 30 seconds while mechanical ventilation is continued. After the infant is returned to the midline position, the second 2.5 mL/kg half-dose is given in an identical fashion over another 1 to 2 minutes. The infant's head and torso are then turned 45° to the *left* for 30 seconds while mechanical ventilation is continued, and the infant is then turned back to the middle position. These maneuvers allow gravity to assist in the distribution of Colfosceril Palmitate in the lungs.

During dosing, heart rate, color, chest expansion, facial expressions, the oximeter, and the endotracheal tube patency and position should be monitored. If heart rate slows, the infant becomes dusky or agitated, transcutaneous oxygen saturation falls more than 15%, or Colfosceril Palmitate backs up in the endotracheal tube, dosing should be slowed or halted, and, if necessary, the peak inspiratory pressure, ventilator rate, and/or FiO₂ turned up. On the other hand, rapid improvements in lung function may require immediate reductions in peak inspiratory pressure, ventilator rate, and/or FiO₂. (See *"Warnings"* and see below for additional information concerning administration.)

Suctioning should not be performed for two hours after Colfosceril Palmitate is administered, except when dictated by clinical necessity.

General Guidelines for Administration: Administration of Colfosceril Palmitate should not take precedence over clinical assessment and stabilization of critically ill infants.

Intubation: Prior to dosing with Colfosceril Palmitate it is important to ensure that the endotracheal tube tip is in the trachea and not in the esophagus or right or left mainstem bronchus. Brisk and symmetrical chest movement with each mechanical inspiration should be confirmed prior to dosing, as should equal breath sounds in the two axillae. In prophylactic treatment, dosing with Colfosceril Palmitate need not be delayed for radiographic confirmation of the endotracheal tube tip position. In rescue treatment, bedside confirmation of endotracheal tube tip position is usually sufficient, if at least one chest radiograph subsequent to the last intubation confirmed proper position of the endotracheal tube tip. Some lung areas will remain undosed if the endotracheal tube tip is too low.

Monitoring: Continuous ECG and transcutaneous oxygen saturation monitoring during dosing are essential. In most infants treated prophylactically, it should be possible to initiate such monitoring prior to administration of the first dose of Colfosceril Palmitate. For subsequent prophylactic and all rescue doses, arterial blood pressure monitoring during dosing is also highly desirable. After both prophylactic and rescue dosing, frequent arterial blood gas sampling is required to prevent post-dosing hyperoxia and hypocarbia (see *"Warnings"*).

Ventilatory Support During Dosing: The 5 mL/kg dosage volume may cause transient impairment of gas exchange by physical blockage of the airway, particularly in infants on low ventilator settings. As a result, infants may exhibit a drop in oxygen saturation during dosing, especially if they are on low ventilator settings prior to dosing. These transient effects are easily overcome by increasing peak inspiratory pressure on the ventilator by 4 to 5 cm H₂O for 1 to 2 minutes during dosing. FiO₂ can also be increased if necessary. In infants who are particularly fragile or reactive to external stimuli, increasing peak inspiratory pressure by 4 to 5 cm H₂O and/or FiO₂ 20% prior to dosing may minimize any transient deterioration in oxygenation. However, in virtually all cases it should be possible to return the infant to pre-dose settings within a very short time of dose completion.

Post-Dosing: At the end of dosing, position of the endotracheal tube should be confirmed by listening for equal breath sounds in the two axillae. Attention should be paid to chest expansion, color, transcutaneous saturation, and arterial blood gases. Infants who receive Colfosceril Palmitate and other surfactants respond with rapid improvements in pulmonary compliance, minute ventilation, and gas exchange (see *"Warnings"*). Constant bedside attention of an experienced clinician for at least 30 minutes after dosing is essential. Frequent blood gas sampling also is absolutely essential. Rapid changes in lung function require immediate changes in peak inspiratory pressure, ventilator rate, and/or FiO₂.

Store Colfosceril Palmitate for Intratracheal Suspension at 15° to 30°C (59° to 86°F) in a dry place.

Table 4
SAFETY ASSESSMENTS[a]—RESCUE TREATMENT

Number of Doses: Birth Weight Range:	Two Doses 700 to 1350 grams		Two Doses 1250 grams and above	
Treatment Group: Number of Infants:	Placebo (Air) N = 213	Colfosceril Palmitate N = 206	Placebo (Air) N = 622	Colfosceril Palmitate N = 615
	% of Infants		% of Infants	
Intraventricular Hemorrhage (IVH)				
Overall	48	52	23	18*
Severe IVH	13	9	5	4
Pulmonary Air Leak (PAL)				
Overall	54	34***	30	18***
Pneumothorax	29	20*	20	10***
Pneumopericardium	4	1	1	2
Pneumomediastinum	8	4	5	2**
Pulmonary Interstitial Emphysema	48	25***	24	13***
Death from PAL	7	3	< 1	1
Patent Ductus Arteriosus	66	57	54	45*
Necrotizing Enterocolitis	3	3	1	2
Pulmonary Hemorrhage	3	1	< 1	1
Congenital Pneumonia	2	3	2	2
Nosocomial Pneumonia	5	7	2	2
Non-Pulmonary Infections	19	22	13	13
Sepsis	15	17	8	8
Death From Sepsis	< 1	< 1	1	< 1
Meningitis	1	< 1	1	< 1*
Other Infections	5	8	5	6
Major Anomalies	3	3	4	4
Hypotension	62	57	50	39**
Hyperbilirubinemia	17	19	12	10
Exchange Transfusion	3	4	1	2
Thrombocytopenia[b]	10	11	4	< 1**
Persistent Fetal Circulation	1	1	6	2**
Seizures	10	10	6	3*
Apnea	48	65**	37	44*
Drug Therapy				
Antibiotics	100	99	98	98
Diuretics	60	65	45	34***
Anticonvulsants	17	17	10	5**
Inotropes	36	31	27	16***
Sedatives	72	68	76	64***
Pancuronium	34	17**	33	15***
Methylxanthines	62	74**	49	53

[a]   All parameters were examined with "as-treated" analyses.
[b]   Thrombocytopenia requiring platelet transfusion.
* $p < 0.05$
** $p < 0.01$
*** $p < 0.001$

Colistimethate Sodium

DESCRIPTION
Colistimethate Sodium contains the sodium salt of Colistimethate. Colistimethate Sodium is a polypeptide antibiotic with an approximate molecular weight of 1750; the empirical formula is $C_{58}H_{105}N_{16}Na_5O_{28}S_5$.

CLINICAL PHARMACOLOGY
MICROBIOLOGY
Colistimethate Sodium has bactericidal activity against the following gram-negative bacilli: *Enterobacter aerogenes, Escherichia coli, Klebsiella pneumoniae*, and *Pseudomonas aeruginosa*.

HUMAN PHARMACOLOGY
Typical serum and urine levels following a single 150 mg dose of Colistimethate Sodium IM or IV in normal adult subjects are shown in Figure 1.

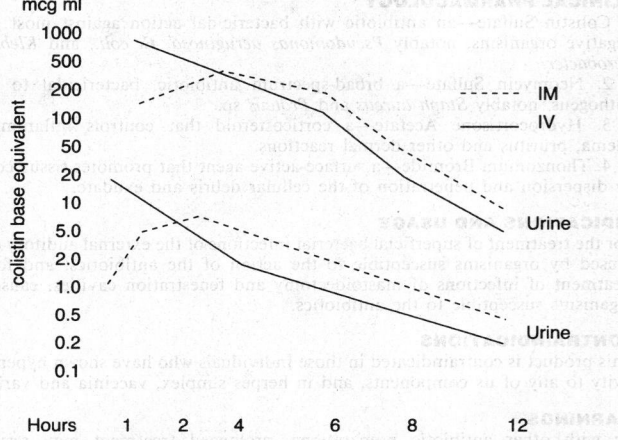

Figure 1. Urine and serum values in adults following parenteral (IM or IV) administration of Colistimethate Sodium

Higher serum levels were obtained at 10 minutes following IV administration. Serum concentration declined with a half-life of 2-3 hours following either intravenous or intramuscular administration in adults and children, including premature infants.

Colistimethate Sodium is transferred across the placental barrier, and blood levels of about 1 mcg/ml are obtained in the fetus following intravenous administration to the mother.

Average urine levels ranged from about 270 mcg/ml at 2 hours to about 15 mcg/ml at 8 hours after intravenous administration and from about 200 to about 25 mcg/ml during a similar period following intramuscular administration.

INDICATIONS AND USAGE
Colistimethate Sodium is indicated for the treatment of acute or chronic infections due to sensitive strains of certain gram-negative bacilli. It is particularly indicated when the infection is caused by sensitive strains of *Pseudomonas aeruginosa*. This antibiotic is not indicated for infections due to *Proteus* or *Neisseria*. Colistimethate Sodium arenteral has proven clinically effective in treatment of infections due to the following gram-negative organisms: *Enterobacter aerogenes, Escherichia coli, Klebsiella pneumoniae*, and *Pseudomonas aeruginosa*.

Pending results of appropriate bacteriologic cultures and sensitivity tests, Colistimethate Sodium may be used to initiate therapy in serious infections that are suspected to be due to gram-negative organisms.

CONTRAINDICATIONS
The use of Colistimethate Sodium is contraindicated for patients with a history of sensitivity to the drug.

WARNING
Maximum daily dose should not exceed 5 mg/kg/day (2.3 mg/lb) with normal renal function.

Transient neurological disturbances may occur. These include circumoral paresthesias or numbness, tingling or formication of the extremities, generalized pruritus, vertigo, dizziness, and slurring of speech. For these reasons, patients should be warned not to drive vehicles or use hazardous machinery while on therapy. Reduction of dosage may alleviate symptoms. Therapy need not be discontinued, but such patients should be observed with particular care. Overdosage can result in renal insufficiency, muscle weakness and apnea. See

"Precautions" for use concomitantly with curariform drugs, and see "Dosage and Administration" section for use in renal impairment.

PRECAUTIONS
Since Colistimethate Sodium is eliminated mainly by renal excretion, it should be used with caution when the possibility of impaired renal function exists. The decline in renal function with advanced age should be considered.

When actual renal impairment is present Colistimethate Sodium may be used, but the greatest caution should be exercised and the dosage should be reduced in proportion to the extent of the impairment. Administration of amounts of Colistimethate Sodium in excess of renal excretory capacity will lead to high serum levels and can result in further impairment of renal function, initiating a cycle which, if not recognized, can lead to acute renal insufficiency, renal shutdown and further concentration of the antibiotic to toxic levels in the body. At this point, interference of nerve transmission at neuromuscular junctions may occur and result in muscle weakness and apnea.

Easily recognized signs indicating the development of impaired renal function are diminishing urine output, rising BUN and serum creatinine. If present, therapy with Colistimethate Sodium should be discontinued immediately.

If a life-threatening situation exists, therapy may be reinstated at a lower dosage after blood levels have fallen.

Certain other antibiotics (kanamycin, streptomycin, dihydrostreptomycin, polymyxin, neomycin) have also been reported to interfere with the nerve transmission at the neuromuscular junction. Based on this reported activity, they should not be given concomitantly with Colistimethate Sodium except with the greatest caution. The antibiotics with a gram-positive antimicrobial spectrum, e.g., penicillin, tetracycline, Sodium cephalothin, have not been reported to interfere with nerve transmission and, accordingly, would not be expected to potentiate this activity of Colistimethate Sodium.

Other drugs, including curariform muscle relaxants (ether, tubocurarine, succinylcholine, gallamine, decamethonium and Sodium citrate), potentiate the neuromuscular blocking effect and should be used with extreme caution in patients being treated with Colistimethate Sodium.

If apnea occurs, it may be treated with assisted respiration, oxygen, and calcium chloride injections.

USE IN PREGNANCY
The safety of Colistimethate Sodium during human pregnancy has not been established.

ADVERSE REACTIONS
Respiratory arrest has been reported following intramuscular administration of Colistimethate Sodium. Impaired renal function increases the possibility of apnea and neuromuscular blockade following administration of Colistimethate Sodium. This has been generally due to failure to follow recommended guidelines, usually overdosage, failure to reduce dose commensurate with degree of renal impairment, and/or concomitant use of other antibiotics or drugs with neuromuscular blocking potential.

A decrease in urine output or increase in blood urea nitrogen or serum creatinine can be interpreted as signs of nephrotoxicity, which is probably a dose-dependent effect of Colistimethate Sodium. These manifestations of nephrotoxicity are reversible following discontinuation of the antibiotic.

Increases of blood urea nitrogen have been reported for patients receiving Colistimethate Sodium at dose levels of 1.6-5 mg/kg per day. The BUN values returned to normal following cessation of Colistimethate Sodium administration.

Paresthesia, tingling of the extremities or tingling of the tongue and generalized itching or urticaria have been reported by patients who received Colistimethate Sodium by intravenous or intramuscular injection. In addition, the following adverse reactions have been reported for Colistimethate Sodium: drug fever and gastrointestinal upset, vertigo, and slurring of speech. The subjective symptoms reported by the adult may not be manifest in infants or young children, thus requiring close attention to renal function.

DOSAGE AND ADMINISTRATION
Important: Colistimethate Sodium is supplied in vials containing Colistimethate Sodium equivalent to 150 mg colistin base activity per vial.

Reconstitution: The *150-mg* vial should be reconstituted with *2.0 ml* Sterile Water for Injection USP. The reconstituted solution provides Colistimethate Sodium at a concentration of 75 mg/ml.

During reconstitution swirl *gently* to avoid frothing.

DOSAGE
Adults and children—intravenous or intramuscular administration: Colistimethate Sodium should be given in 2 to 4 divided doses at dose levels of 2.5 to 5 mg/kg per day for patients with normal renal function, depending on the severity of the infection.

The daily dose should be reduced in the presence of any renal impairment, which can often be anticipated from the history.

Modifications of dosage in the presence of renal impairment are presented in Table 1. (See related table).

INTRAVENOUS ADMINISTRATION
1. DIRECT INTERMITTENT ADMINISTRATION—SLOWLY INJECT ONE-HALF OF THE TOTAL DAILY DOSE OVER A PERIOD OF 3 TO 5 MINUTES EVERY 12 HOURS.

➤ SHOWN IN PRODUCT IDENTIFICATION GUIDE

Table 1
SUGGESTED MODIFICATION OF DOSAGE SCHEDULES OF COLISTIMETHATE SODIUM FOR ADULTS WITH IMPAIRED RENAL FUNCTION

Renal Function	Degree Of Impairment			
	Normal	*Mild*	*Moderate*	*Considerable*
Plasma creatinine, (mg/100 ml)	0.7-1.2	1.3-1.5	1.6-2.5	2.6-4.0
Urea clearance, % of normal	80-100	40-70	25-40	10-25
Dosage				
Unit dose of Colistimethate Sodium, mg	100-150	75-115	66-150	100-150
Frequency, times/day	4 to 2	2	2 or 1	every 36 hr
Total daily dose, mg	300	150-230	133-150	100
Approximate daily dose, mg/kg/day	5.0	2.5-3.8	2.5	1.5

Note: The suggested unit dose is 2.5-5 mg/kg; however, the time INTERVAL between injections should be increased in the presence of impaired renal function.

2. CONTINUOUS INFUSION—SLOWLY INJECT ONE-HALF THE TOTAL DAILY DOSE OVER 3 TO 5 MINUTES. ADD THE REMAINING HALF OF THE TOTAL DAILY DOSE OF COLISTIMETHATE SODIUM TO ONE OF THE FOLLOWING: 0.9% NaCL; 5% DEXTROSE IN 0.9% NaCL; 5% DEXTROSE IN WATER; 5% DEXTROSE IN 0.45% NaCL; 5% DEXTROSE IN 0.225% NaCL; LACTATED RINGER'S SOLUTION, OR 10% INVERT SUGAR SOLUTION. THERE ARE NOT SUFFICIENT DATA TO RECOMMEND USAGE OF COLISTIMETHATE SODIUM WITH OTHER DRUGS OR WITH OTHER THAN THE ABOVE LISTED INFUSION SOLUTIONS.

ADMINISTER BY SLOW INTRAVENOUS INFUSION STARTING 1 TO 2 HOURS AFTER THE INITIAL DOSE AT A RATE OF 5-6 MG/HR IN THE PRESENCE OF NORMAL RENAL FUNCTION. IN THE PRESENCE OF IMPAIRED RENAL FUNCTION, REDUCE THE INFUSION RATE DEPENDING ON THE DEGREE OF RENAL IMPAIRMENT.

THE CHOICE OF INTRAVENOUS SOLUTION AND THE VOLUME TO BE EMPLOYED ARE DICTATED BY THE REQUIREMENTS OF FLUID AND ELECTROLYTE MANAGEMENT.

ANY INFUSION SOLUTION CONTAINING COLISTIMETHATE SODIUM SHOULD BE FRESHLY PREPARED AND USED FOR NO LONGER THAN 24 HOURS.

Store at controlled room temperature (15° to 30°C) (59° to 86°F).
Store reconstituted solution in refrigerator (2° to 8°C) (36° to 46°F) or at controlled room temperature (15° to 30°C) (59° to 86°F), and use within 7 days.

TOXICOLOGY AND ANIMAL PHARMACOLOGY:
Acute Toxicity: The intravenous LD_{50} was 41.5 mg/kg in the dog and 739 mg/kg in the mouse; intramuscular toxicity was 42 mg/kg in the dog and 267 mg/kg in the mouse.

Subacute Toxicity: In albino rabbits and beagle dogs, IV doses of 5, 10 and 20 mg/kg/day for 28 days resulted in elevated blood urea nitrogen in the dog (10 mg/kg dose group) and in both 20 mg/kg dose groups.

Clinically Studies: Clinically Colistimethate Sodium has been of particular therapeutic value in acute and chronic urinary tract infections caused by sensitive strains of *Pseudomonas aeruginosa*. Colistimethate Sodium is clinically effective in the treatment of infections due to other sensitive gram-negative pathogenic bacilli that have become resistant to broad-spectrum antibiotics.

Colistimethate Sodium has been used to treat bacteriuria and overt urinary infections in pregnant women during the third trimester. However, in view of the evidence of possible embryotoxic and teratogenic effects of Colistimethate Sodium in pregnant rabbits, caution should be exercised in use of this drug in women of childbearing potential.

J CODES
Up to 150 mg IM,IV—J0770

HOW SUPPLIED
POWDER FOR INJECTION:

BRAND/MANUFACTURER	NDC	SIZE	AWP
○ BRAND			
COLY-MYCIN M: Parke-Davis	00071-4145-01	1s	$31.01

Colistin Sulfate/Hydrocortisone/ Neomycin Sulfate/Thonzonium Bromide

DESCRIPTION
Colistin Sulfate/Hydrocortisme/Neomycin Sulfate/Thonzonium Bromide otic suspension is a sterile aqueous suspension containing in each ml: Colistin base

activity, 3 mg (as the Sulfate): Neomycin base activity, 3.3 mg (as the Sulfate); Hydrocortisone Acetate, 10 mg (1%); Thonzonium Bromide, 0.5 mg (0.05%); It is a non-viscous liquid, buffered at pH 5, for instillation into the canal of the external ear or direct application to the affected aural skin.

CLINICAL PHARMACOLOGY
1. Colistin Sulfate—an antibiotic with bactericidal action against most gram-negative organisms, notably *Pseudomonas aeruginosa, E. coli.,* and *Klebsiella-Aerobacter.*
2. Neomycin Sulfate—a broad-spectrum antibiotic, bactericidal to many pathogens, notably *Staph aureus* and *Proteus* sp.
3. Hydrocortisone Acetate—a corticosteroid that controls inflammation, edema, pruritus and other dermal reactions.
4. Thonzonium Bromide—a surface-active agent that promotes tissue contact by dispersion and penetration of the cellular debris and exudate.

INDICATIONS AND USAGE
For the treatment of superficial bacterial infections of the external auditory canal, caused by organisms susceptible to the action of the antibiotics; and for the treatment of infections of mastoidectomy and fenestration cavities, caused by organisms susceptible to the antibiotics.

CONTRAINDICATIONS
This product is contraindicated in those individuals who have shown hypersensitivity to any of its components, and in herpes simplex, vaccinia and varicella.

WARNINGS
As with other antibiotic preparations, prolonged treatment may result in overgrowth of nonsusceptible organisms and fungi.

If the infection is not improved after one week, cultures and susceptibility tests should be repeated to verify the identify of the organism and to determine whether therapy should be changed.

Patients who prefer to warm the medication before using should be cautioned against heating the solution above body temperature, in order to avoid loss of potency.

PRECAUTIONS
General: If sensitization or irritation occurs, medication should be discontinued promptly.

This drug should be used with care in cases of perforated eardrum and in longstanding cases of chronic otitis media because of the possibility of ototoxicity caused by neomycin. Treatment should not be continued for longer than ten days. Allergic cross-reactions may occur which could prevent the use of any or all of the following antibiotics for the treatment of future infections: kanamycin, paromomycin, streptomycin, and possibly gentamicin.

ADVERSE REACTIONS
Neomycin is a not uncommon cutaneous sensitizer. There are articles in the current literature that indicate an increase in the prevalence of persons sensitive to neomycin.

DOSAGE AND ADMINISTRATION
The external auditory canal should be thoroughly cleansed and dried with a sterile cotton applicator.

When using the calibrated dropper:
For adults, 5 drops of the suspension should be instilled into the affected ear 3 or 4 times daily. For infants and children, 4 drops are suggested because of the smaller capacity of the ear canal.

This dosage correlates to the 4 drops (for adults) and 3 drops (for children) recommended when using the dropper-bottle container for this product.

The patient should lie with the affected ear upward and then the drops should be instilled. This position should be maintained for 5 minutes to facilitate penetration of the drops into the ear canal. Repeat, if necessary, for the opposite ear. If preferred, a cotton wick may be inserted into the canal and then the cotton may be saturated with the solution. This wick should be kept moist by adding further solution every 4 hours. The wick should be replaced at least once every 24 hours.

◆ RATED THERAPEUTICALLY EQUIVALENT; ◇ THERAPEUTIC EQUIVALENCE UNCONFIRMED; ○ UNRATED

Shake well before using.
Store at controlled room temperature 15°-30°C (59°-86°F).

Stable for 18 months at room temperature; prolonged exposure to higher temperatures should be avoided.

HOW SUPPLIED
DROP: 3 MG-1%-3.3 MG/ML

BRAND/MANUFACTURER	NDC	SIZE	AWP
BRAND			
COLY-MYCIN S OTIC: Parke-Davis	00071-3141-35	5 ml	$13.30
	00071-3141-36	10 ml	$21.33

Collagen Hemostat

DESCRIPTION

Collagen Absorbable Hemostat is a purified and lyophilized bovine dermal collagen. The material, prepared as a sponge-like pad, is lightly cross-linked, sterile, nonpyrogenic, and absorbable. Microfibrillar Collagen Hemostat is a dry, white absorbent hemostatic agent in a microfibrillar form. The raw material for Microfibrillar Collagen Hemostat is obtained from bovine deep flexor tendon (achilles tendon), known to be one of the purest sources of collagen that can be readily processed in commercial amounts. Further purification during processing ensures that Microfibrillar Collagen Hemostat is a consistent material with uniform behavior.

Hemostatic activity, which is an inherent property of collagen, is largely dependent on the basic helical structure of this protein. The helical structure of native collagen is preserved during the manufacture of Collagen Absorbable Hemostat. When collagen comes into contact with blood, platelets aggregate on the collagen and release coagulation factors which, together with plasma factors results in the formation of fibrin, and finally in the formation of a clot.

The microfibrillar form of the product allows the surgeon to grasp with forceps any amount of Microfibrillar Collagen Hemostat needed to achieve hemostasis at a particular bleeding site. The microfibrillar form may be more convenient than the sponge form for hard to reach or irregularly shaped bleeding sites. Although it is easy to pull the desired amount of Microfibrillar Collagen Hemostat from the entire supply, the group of selected fibers continue to cohere to one another and application to the bleeding site is easily controlled. Unwanted dispersal over the operative site does not occur. The microfibrillar structure of Collagen Hemostat provides for the additional strengthening of the clot.

Topical application of Collagen Hemostat effectively controls bleeding, usually within 2 to 4 minutes, when applied directly to the bleeding site. Collagen Hemostat is designed to be completely absorbable if left *in situ* after hemostasis. In contact with blood, the fibers expand to become a coherent gelatinous mass that conforms to the shape of the bleeding area. If desired, recovery of this mass is easily accomplished.

Absorption of a collagen hemostatic agent was evaluated after subcutaneous and intraheptic implantation in rats. In 1 out of 5 animals, complete subcutaneous absorption was observed by day 14; and by day 56, 3 out of 4 had complete absorption. Complete intraperitoneal absorption was not observed by day 56. Tissue reactions elicited by the collagen hemostatic agent during implantation are similar to tissue reactions caused by other hemostatic agents.

The collagen hemostatic agent has been evaluated *in vitro* for the enhancement of bacterial growth of *Staphylococcus aureus* and *Escherichia coli*. Enhancement of bacterial growth did not occur for either organism.

In vivo studies using guinea pigs showed that incidence of infection (abscess) of incision sites inoculated with *Staphylococcus aureus* was not enhanced by the presence of the collagen material when compared to another collagen hemostatic agent. However, extent of wound infection tended to be greater than control with the collagen material as was the case with another collagen hemostatic agent tested. This tendency is observed with many foreign substances.

The collagen hemostatic agent was evaluated for potential allergenic sensitivity. A guinea pig maximization study showed that the collagen material did not produce irritation or contact sensitization. A chemical assay of the collagen material compared to one other collagen hemostat showed significantly less specific glycoprotein immunoreactive substances in the collagen material. A hemoagglutination study was conducted evaluating the collagen material as the antigen. There was no agglutination observed.

INDICATIONS

Collagen Absorbable Hemostat and Microfibrillar Collagen Hemostat are indicated in surgical procedures (other than in neurosurgical, and ophthalmological surgery; Microfibrillar Collagen Hemostat is also not to be used in urological surgery) for use as an adjunct to hemostasis when control of bleeding by ligature or other conventional methods is ineffective or impractical.

CONTRAINDICATIONS

Collagen Hemostat should not be used in the closure of skin incisions as it may interfere with the healing of skin edges. This interference is due to simple mechanical interposition of dry collagen and not due to any intrinsic interference with wound healing. It has been reported with one absorbable collagen hemostat that, in filling porosities of cancellous bone, collagen may reduce the bonding strength of methylmethacrylate. Therefore, Collagen Absorable Hemostat should not be applied on bone surfaces to which prosthetic materials are to be attached with methylmethacrylate adhesives.

WARNINGS

Collagen Hemostat is inactivated by autoclaving. It should not be resterilized. As with any foreign substance, use in contaminated wounds may enhance infection.

Collagen Absorbable Hemostat should not be used in instances of pumping arterial hemorrhage.

Collagen Absorbable Hemostat should not be used where blood or other fluids have pooled or in cases where the point of hemorrhage is submerged. Collagen Absorbable Hemostat will not act as a tampon or plug in a bleeding site nor will it close off an area of blood collecting behind a tampon.

Only the amount of Collagen Absorbable Hemostat necessary to provide hemostasis should be used. The long-term effects of leaving Collagen Absorbable Hemostat *in situ* are unknown. Opened, unused Collagen Absorbable Hemostat should be discarded because it cannot be resterilized.

PRECAUTIONS

As with other hemostatic agents, it is not recommended that Collagen Hemostat be left in an infected or contaminated space, nor it is recommended for use in persons known to be sensitive to materials of bovine origin. When placed into cavities or closed spaces, care should be exercised to avoid overpacking Collagen Hemostat as it may absorb fluid and expand and press against neighboring structures. In urological procedures, Collagen Absorbable Hemostat should not be left in the renal pelvis or ureters to eliminate the potential foci for calculus formation.

Safety of this product has not been established in children and pregnant women; therefore Collagen Hemostat should only be used when benefit to risk clearly warrants its use. Microfibrillar collagen agent has been reported to cause interference with the healing of skin edges when used in the closure of skin incisions. Collagen Hemostat is not intended to be used to treat systemic coagulation disorders.

ADVERSE REACTIONS

Collagen Hemostat is a collagen product. Although several types of post-operative complications were observed in patients treated with Collagen Hemostat, none were attributed to Collagen Hemostat except one case of fibrotic reaction where Collagen Hemostat involvement could not be ruled out. Adverse reactions reported for collagen hemostats include hematoma, potentiation of infection, wound dehiscence, inflammation and edema. Other reported adverse reactions that may be related to the use of collagen hemostats include adhesion formation, allergic reaction, foreign body reaction and subgaleal seroma (in a single case). The use of microfibrillar collagen in dental extraction sockets has been reported to increase the incidence of alveolalgia.

ADMINISTRATION

Collagen Absorbable Hemostat is applied directly to the bleeding surface with pressure. Collagen Absorbable Hemostat can be cut to size. The amount needed and the period of time necessary to apply pressure will vary with the type and amount of bleeding to be controlled. Hemostasis time depends upon the type of surgery and degree of pretreatment bleeding. It usually occurred between 2 to 5 minutes with Collagen Absorbable Hemostat.

Collagen Absorbable Hemostat maintains its integrity in the presence of blood and is not dispersed when wet. It is easily removed from the site following hemostasis. It is most effective when used dry.

Collagen Absorbable Hemostat may be left *in situ* whenever necessary. However, the surgeon, at his discretion, should remove any excess of Collagen Absorbable Hemostat prior to wound closure. Animal implant studies have demonstrated that absorption and tissue reaction to Collagen Absorbable Hemostat are similar those observed with another absorbable collagen hemostatic agent. In these studies, on visual examination, most of Collagen Absorbable Hemostat was found to be absorbed in 8 to 10 weeks after implantation.

Using forceps, the desired amount of Microfibrillar Collagen Hemostat can be easily selected from the entire supply. The coherent fibers should then be applied directly to the bleeding surface using some pressure. The period of time pressure is needed and the amount of Microfibrillar Collagen Hemostat necessary to achieve hemostasis will be dependent upon the nature and amount of bleeding to be controlled. It has been shown that hemostasis usually occurs within 2-4 minutes. In contact with blood, Microfibrillar Collagen Hemostat becomes a coherent gelatinuous unit that is completely absorbed if left *in situ*. However, it is suggested that the surgeon simply remove the collagen mass prior to wound closure.

STORAGE

Store at controlled room temperature 15°-30°C (59°-86°F). Do not resterilize.

CLINICAL STUDIES

The safety, effectiveness and handling characteristics of Collagen Absorbable Hemostat were evaluated in a variety of surgical procedures. The median time to hemostasis for Collagen Absorbable Hemostat was 3 minutes. Passive Hemagglutination Assay (PHA) and Enzyme-Linked Immunoabsorbent Assay (ELISA) methods have been used to evaluate the immunologic potential for Collagen Absorbable Hemostat to produce antibodies in patients. These assays revealed mild elevation of antibody titers in both Collagen Absorbable Hemostat treated patients and patients treated with a collagen control hemostat, confirming that Collagen Hemostat is a weak antigen.

HOW SUPPLIED

PAD:

BRAND/MANUFACTURER	NDC	SIZE	AWP
○ **BRAND**			
HEMO-PAD: Astra	00186-2001-00	10s	$457.50
	00186-2002-00	10s	$997.50
	00186-2003-00	10s	$1795.00
HEMOTENE: Astra	00186-2005-02	1 gm 5s	$423.75

SPONGE:

BRAND/MANUFACTURER	NDC	SIZE	AWP
○ **GENERICS**			
COLLASTAT: Genesis Bio-Pharm	21101-1204-20	5s	$1025.00
COLLASTAT: Genesis Bio-Pharm	21101-1204-04	10s	$185.00
COLLASTAT: Genesis Bio-Pharm	21101-1204-10	10s	$370.00

Collagenase

DESCRIPTION
Collagenase is a sterile enzymatic debriding ointment which contains 250 Collagenase units per gram of white petrolatum USP. The enzyme Collagenase is derived from the fermentation by *Clostridium histolyticum*. It possesses the unique ability to digest native and denatured collagen in necrotic tissue.

CLINICAL PHARMACOLOGY
Since collagen accounts for 75% of the dry weight of skin tissue, the ability of Collagenase to digest collagen in the physiological pH range and temperature makes it particularly effective in the removal of detritus.[1] Collagenase thus contributes towards the formation of granulation tissue and subsequent epithelization of dermal ulcers and severely burned areas.[2,3,4,5,6] Collagen in healthy tissue or in newly formed granulation tissue is not attacked.[2,3,4,5,6,7,8]

INDICATIONS
Collagenase is indicated for debriding chronic dermal ulcers[2,3,4,5,6,8,9,10,11,12,13,14,15,16,17,18] and severely burned areas.[3,4,5,7,16,19,20,21]

CONTRAINDICATIONS
Collagenase is contraindicated in patients who have shown local or systemic hypersensitivity to Collagenase.

PRECAUTIONS
The optimal pH range of Collagenase is 6 to 8. Higher or lower pH conditions will decrease the enzyme's activity and appropriate precautions should be taken. The enzymatic activity is also adversely affected by detergents, hexachlorophene and heavy metal ions such as mercury and silver which are used in some antiseptics. When it is suspected such materials have been used, the site should be carefully cleansed by repeated washings with normal saline before Collagenase is applied. Soaks containing metal ions or acidic solutions such as Burow's solution should be avoided because of the metal ion and low pH. Cleansing materials such as hydrogen peroxide, Dakin's solution, and sterile saline are compatible with Collagenase.

Debilitated patients should be closely monitored for systemic bacterial infections because of the theoretical possibility that debriding enzymes may increase the risk of bacteremia. A slight transient erythema has been noted occasionally in the surrounding tissue, particularly when Collagenase was not confined to the lesion. Therefore, the ointment should be applied carefully within the area of the lesion.

ADVERSE REACTIONS
No allergic sensitivity or toxic reactions have been noted in the recorded clinical investigations. However, one case of systemic manifestations of hypersensitivity to Collagenase in a patient treated for more than one year with a combination of Collagenase and cortisone has been reported to us.

OVERDOSAGE
Action of the enzyme may be stopped, should this be desired, by the application of Burow's solution USP (pH 3.6-4.4) to the lesion.

DOSAGE AND ADMINISTRATION
Collagenase should be applied once daily (or more frequently if the dressing becomes soiled, as from incontinence) in the following manner:

(1) Prior to application the lesion should be cleansed of debris and digested material by gently rubbing with a gauze pad saturated with hydrogen peroxide or Dakin's solution followed by sterile normal saline.
(2) Whenever infection is present it is desirable to use an appropriate topical antibiotic powder. The antibiotic should be applied to the lesion prior to the application of Collagenase. Should the infection not respond, therapy with Collagenase should be discontinued until remission of the infection.
(3) Collagenase should be applied directly to deep lesions with a wooden tongue depressor or spatula. For shallow lesions, Collagenase may be applied to a sterile gauze pad which is then applied to the wound and properly secured.
(4) Crosshatching thick eschar with a #10 blade allows Collagenase more surface contact with necrotic debris. It is also desirable to remove, with forceps and scissors, as much loosened detritus as can be done readily.

(5) All excess ointment should be removed each time dressing is changed.
(6) Use of Collagenase should be terminated when debridement of necrotic tissue is complete and granulation tissue is well established.

REFERENCES
1. Mandl, I., Adv. Enzymol. 23:163, 1961. 2. Boxer, A.M., Gottesman, N., Bernstein, H., & Mandl, I., Geriatrics 24:75, 1969. 3. Mazurek, I., Med. Welt 22:150, 1971. 4. Zimmerman, W.E., in "Collagenase," I. Mandl, ed., Gordon & Breach, Science Publishers, New York, 1971, p. 131, p. 185. 5. Vetra, H., & Whittaker, D., Geriatrics 30:53, 1975. 6. Rao, D.B., Sane, P.G., & Georgiev, E.L., J. Am. Geriatrics Soc. 23:22, 1975. 7. Vrabec, R., Moserova, J., Konickova, Z., Behounkova, E., & Blaha, J., J. Hyg. Epidemiol. Microbiol. Immunol. 18:496, 1974. 8. Lippmann, H.I., Arch. Phys. Med. Rehabil. 54:588, 1973. 9. German, F.M., in "Collagenase," I. Mandl. ed. Gordon & Breach, Science Publishers, New York, 1971, p. 165. 10. Lee, L.K., & Ambrus, J.L., Geriatrics 30:91, 1975. 11. Haimovici, H. & Strauch, B., in "Collagenase," I. Mandl, ed., Gordon & Breach, Science Publishers, New York, 1971, p. 177. 11. Lee, L.K., & Ambrus, J.L., Geriatrics 30:91, 1975. 12. Locke, R.K., & Heifitz, N.M., J. AM. Pod. Assoc. 65:242, 1975. 13. Varma, A.O., Bugatch, E., & German, F.M., Surg. Gynecol. Obstet. 136:281, 1973. 14. Barrett, D., Jr., & Klibanski, A., Am. J. Nurs. 73:849, 1973. 15. Bardfeld, L.A., J. Pod. Ed. 1:41, 1970. 16. Blum, G., Schweiz, Rundschau Med. Praxis 62:820, 1973. Abstr. in Dermatology Digest, Feb. 1974, p. 36. 17. Zaruba, F., Lettl, A., Brozkova, L., Skrdlantova, H., & Krs, V., J. Hyg. Epidemiol. Microbiol. Immunol. 18:499, 1974. 18. Altman, M.I., Goldstein, L., Horowitz, S., J. Am. Pod. Assoc. 68:11, 1978. 19. Rehn, V.J., Med. Klin. 58:799, 1963. 20. Krauss, H., Koslowski, L., & Zimmermann, W.E., Langenbecks Arch. Klin. Chir. 303:23, 1963. 21. Gruenagel, H.H., Med. Klin. 58:442, 1963.

HOW SUPPLIED
OINTMENT: 250 U/GM

BRAND/MANUFACTURER	NDC	SIZE	AWP
○ **BRAND**			
SANTYL: Knoll	00044-5270-02	15 gm	$27.89
	00044-5270-03	30 gm	$53.03

Colovage SEE ELECTROLYTES AND POLYETHYLENE GLYCOL 3350

Colrex Compound SEE ACETAMINOPHEN/ CHLORPHENIRAMINE MALEATE/CODEINE PHOSPHATE/ PHENYLEPHRINE HYDROCHLORIDE

Coly-Mycin M SEE COLISTIMETHATE SODIUM

Coly-Mycin S SEE COLISTIN SULFATE/ HYDROCORTISONE/NEOMYCIN SULFATE/THONZONIUM BROMIDE

Colyte SEE ELECTROLYTES AND POLYETHYLENE GLYCOL 3350

Combipres SEE CHLORTHALIDONE WITH CLONIDINE HYDROCHLORIDE

Comhist SEE CHLORPHENIRAMINE MALEATE/ PHENYLEPHRINE HYDROCHLORIDE/PHENYLTOLOXAMINE CITRATE

Compazine SEE PROCHLORPERAZINE

Condylox SEE PODOFILOX

Conray SEE IOTHALAMATE AND IOTHALAMATE MEGLUMINE

Cordarone SEE AMIODARONE HYDROCHLORIDE

Cordran SEE FLURANDRENOLIDE

Corgard SEE NADOLOL

Cort-Dome SEE HYDROCORTISONE, RECTAL AND HYDROCORTISONE, TOPICAL

Cortane B-Otic SEE CHLOROXYLENOL/ HYDROCORTISONE/PRAMOXINE HYDROCHLORIDE

Cortef SEE HYDROCORTISONE CYPIONATE AND HYDROCORTISONE, SYSTEMIC

Cortenema SEE HYDROCORTISONE, RECTAL

Cortic SEE CHLOROXYLENOL/HYDROCORTISONE/PRAMOXINE HYDROCHLORIDE

Corticotropin

DESCRIPTION
Corticotropin is a sterile lyophilized ACTH which in dry form is stable at room temperature. Each vial contains 25 or 40 Units of Corticotropin USP and approximately 9 and 14 milligrams of hydrolyzed gelatin respectively. After reconstitution, this product is administered in the intravenous, intramuscular, or subcutaneous route.

ACTH is a 39 amino acid peptide.

CLINICAL PHARMACOLOGY
ACTH stimulates the adrenal cortex to secrete cortisol, corticosterone, aldosterone, and a number of weakly androgenic substances. Although ACTH does stimulate secretion of aldosterone, the rate is relatively independent. Prolonged administration of large doses of ACTH induces hyperplasia and hypertrophy of the adrenal cortex and continuous high output of cortisol, corticosterone and weak androgens. The release of ACTH is under the influence of the nervous system via the corticotropin regulatory hormone released from the hypothalamus and by a negative corticosteroid feedback mechanism. Elevated plasma cortisol suppresses ACTH release.

The trophic effects of ACTH on the adrenal cortex are not understood beyond the fact that they appear to be mediated by cyclic AMP.

ACTH rapidly disappears from the circulation following its intravenous administration; in man the plasma half-life is about 15 minutes.

The maximal effects of a trophic hormone on a target organ are achieved when optimal amounts of hormone are acting continuously. Thus, a fixed dose of ACTH will demonstrate a linear increase in adrenocortical secretion with increasing duration for the infusion.

INDICATIONS AND USAGE
Corticotropin is indicated for diagnostic testing of adrenocortical function.

Corticotropin has limited therapeutic value in those conditions responsive to corticosteroid therapy; in such cases, corticosteroid therapy is considered to be the treatment of choice. Corticotropin may be employed in the following disorders:

Endocrine Disorders: Nonsuppurative thyroiditis: Hypercalcemia associated with cancer.

Nervous System Diseases: Acute exacerbations of multiple sclerosis.

Rheumatic Disorders: As adjunctive therapy for short-term administration (to tide the patient over an acute episode or exacerbation) in:
Psoriatic arthritis; Rheumatoid arthritis, including juvenile rheumatoid arthritis (selected cases may require low-dose maintenance therapy); ankylosing spondylitis: Acute and subacute bursitis. Acute nonspecific tenosynovitis. Acute gouty arthritis; Post-traumatic arthritis; Synovitis of osteoarthritis; Epicondylitis.

Collagen Diseases: During an exacerbation or as maintenance therapy in selected cases of:
Systemic lupus erythematosus: Systemic dermatomyositis (polymyositis). Acute rheumatic carditis.

Dermatologic Diseases: Pemphigus: Bullous dermatitis herpetiforms: Severe erythema multiforme (Stevens-Johnson syndrome); Exfoliative dermatitis: Severe psoriasis; Severe seborrheic dermatitis; Mycosis fungoides.

Allergic States: Control of severe or incapacitating allergic conditions intractable to adequate trials of conventional treatment.

Seasonal or perennial allergic rhinitis: Bronchial asthma; Contact dermatitis; Atopic dermatitis: Serum sickness.

Ophthalmic Diseases: Severe acute and chronic allergic and inflammatory processes involving the eye and its adnexa such as:

Allergic conjunctivitis: Keratitis; Herpes zoster ophthalmicus: Iritis and iridocyclitis; Diffuse posterior uveitis and choroiditis: Optic neuritis; Sympathetic ophthalmia; Chorioretinitis; Anterior segment inflammation; Allergic corneal marginal ulcers.

Respiratory Diseases: Symptomatic sarcoidosis: Loefflers syndrome not manageable by other means; Berylliosis; Fulminating or disseminated pulmonary tuberculosis when used concurrently with antituberculous chemotherapy; Aspiration pneumonitis.

Hematologic Disorders: Acquired (autoimmune) hemolytic anemia; Secondary thrombocytopenia in adults: Erythroblastopenia (RBC anemia); Congenital (erythroid) hypoplastic anemia.

Neoplastic Diseases: For palliative management of: Leukemias and lymphomas in adults; Acute leukemia of childhood.

Edematous State: To induce a diuresis or a remission of proteinuria in the nephrotic syndrome without uremia of the idiopathic type or that due to lupus erythematosus.

Gastrointestinal Diseases: To tide the patient over a critical period of the disease in: Ulcerative colitis: Regional enteritis.

Miscellaneous: Tuberculous meningitis with subarachnoid block or impending block when used concurrently with appropriate anti-tuberculous chemotherapy; Trichinosis with neurologic or myocardial involvement.

UNLABELED USES
Corticotropin, is used alone or as an adjunct in the treatment of Bell's Palsy, acute gout, Guillian-Barré syndrome, and infantile spasms.

Corticotropin, is also used for treatment of hypopigmentation of the skin (vitiligo) and as an aid in smoking cessation.

CONTRAINDICATIONS
Corticotropin is contraindicated in patients with scleroderma, osteoporosis, systemic fungal infections, ocular herpes simplex, recent surgery, history of or the presence of a peptic ulcer, congestive heart failure, hypertension, or sensitivity to proteins of porcine origin.

Treatment of conditions listed within the *"Indications"* section (see above) is contraindicated when they are accompanied by primary adrenocortical insufficiency or adrenocortical hyperfunction.

Intravenous administration of Corticotropin is contraindicated for treatment of conditions listed within the *"Indications"* section, but Corticotropin is used intravenously for diagnostic purposes (see *"Dosage and Administration"*).

WARNINGS
Chronic administration of Corticotropin may lead to adverse effects which are not reversible. Corticotropin may only suppress symptoms and signs of chronic diseases without altering the natural course of the disease. Corticotropin should be administered for treatment until adrenal responsiveness has been verified with the route of administration which will be utilized during treatment, intramuscularly or subcutaneously. A rise in urinary and plasma corticosteroid values provides direct evidence of a stimulatory effect. Prolonged administration of Corticotropin increases the risk of hypersensitivity reactions. Although the action of Corticotropin is similar to that of exogenous adrenocortical steroids, the quantity of adrenocorticoid may be variable. In patients who receive prolonged Corticotropin therapy the additional use of rapidly acting corticosteroids before, during, and after an unusual stressful situation is indicated.

Prolonged use of Corticotropin may produce posterior subcapsular cataracts and glaucoma with possible damage to the optic nerves.

Corticotropin may mask some signs of infection, and new infections including those of the eye due to fungi or viruses may appear during its use. There may be decreased resistance and inability to localize infection when Corticotropin is used.

Corticotropin can cause elevation of blood pressure, salt and water retention, and increased excretion of potassium. Dietary salt restriction and potassium supplementation may be necessary. Corticotropin increases calcium excretion.

While on Corticotropin therapy, patients should not be vaccinated against smallpox. Other immunization procedures should be undertaken with caution in patients who are receiving Corticotropin, especially when high doses are administered because of the possible hazards of neurological complications and lack of antibody response.

PRECAUTIONS
1. GENERAL
Corticotropin injection should be used in the lowest dose for the shortest period of time to accomplish the therapeutic goal. Corticotropin should be used for treatment only when the disease is intractable to non-steroid treatment.

There is an enhanced effect in patients with hypothyroidism and in those with cirrhosis of the liver. Sensitivity to porcine protein should be considered before starting therapy and during the course of treatment should symptoms arise.

When an infection is present, appropriate antibiotic therapy should be given. Patients with latent tuberculosis should be observed closely, and if therapy is prolonged, chemoprophylaxis should be instituted.

Psychic symptoms may appear with use of Corticotropin or pre-existing symptoms may be enhanced. These may range from mood alteration to a psychotic state.

Patients with a secondary disease may have that disease worsened. Caution should be used when prescribing Corticotropin in patients with diabetes, renal insufficiency, diverticulitis, and myasthenia gravis.

Corticotropin often acts by suppressing symptoms without altering the course of the underlying disease. Since complications with Corticotropin use are dependent on the dose and duration of treatment, a risk/benefit decision must be made in each case.

Suppression of the pituitary adrenal axis occurs following prolonged therapy which may be slow in returning to normal. Patients should be protected from the stress of trauma or surgery by the use of corticosteroids during the period of stress.

Since maximal Corticotropin stimulation of the adrenals may be limited during the first few days of treatment, other drugs should be administered when an immediate therapeutic effect is desirable.

Although controlled clinical trials have shown ACTH to be effective in speeding the resolution of acute exacerbations of multiple sclerosis, they do not show that it affects the ultimate outcome or natural history of the disease. The studies do show that relatively high doses of ACTH are necessary to demonstrate a significant effect. (See *"Dosage and Administration"* section.)

Treatment of acute gouty arthritis should be limited to a few days. Since rebound attacks may occur when Corticotropin is discontinued, conventional concomitant therapy should be administered during Corticotropin treatment and for several days after it is stopped.

Aspirin should be used cautiously in conjunction with Corticotropin in hypoprothrombinemia.

2. DRUG INTERACTIONS
Corticotropin may accentuate the electrolyte loss associated with diuretic therapy.

3. CARCINOGENESIS, MUTAGENESIS, IMPAIRMENT OF FERTILITY
Adequate and well-controlled studies have not been done in animals. Human use has not been associated with an increase in malignant disease. See *"Pregnancy"* warning below.

4. PREGNANCY
Pregnancy Class C: Corticotropin has been shown to have an embryocidal effect. There are no adequate and well-controlled studies in pregnant women. Corticotropin should be used during pregnancy only if the potential benefit justifies the potential risk to the fetus.

5. NURSING MOTHERS
It is not known whether this drug is excreted in human milk. Because many drugs are excreted in human milk and because of the potential for serious adverse reactions in nursing infants from Corticotropin, a decision should be made whether to discontinue nursing or to discontinue the drug, taking into account the importance of the drug to the mother.

6. PEDIATRIC USE
Prolonged use of Corticotropin in children will inhibit skeletal growth. If use is necessary, it should be given intermittently and the child carefully observed.

ADVERSE REACTIONS
Fluid and electrolyte disturbances: Sodium retention; fluid retention; potassium loss; hypokalemic alkalosis; calcium loss.

Musculoskeletal: Muscle weakness; steroid myopathy; loss of muscle mass; osteoporosis; vertebral compression fractures; aseptic necrosis of femoral and humeral heads; pathologic fracture of long bones.

Gastrointestinal: Peptic ulcer with possible perforation and hemorrhage; pancreatitis; abdominal distention; ulcerative esophagitis.

Dermatologic: Impaired wound healing; thin fragile skin; petechiae and ecchymoses; facial erythema; increased sweating; suppression of skin test reactions; acne; hyperpigmentation.

Cardiovascular: Hypertension; necrotizing angitis; congestive heart failure.

Neurological: Convulsions; increased intracranial pressure with papilledema, (pseudo-tumor cerebri) usually after treatment; headache, vertigo.

Endocrine: Menstrual irregularities; development of Cushingoid state: suppression of growth in children; secondary adrenocortical and pituitary unresponsiveness, particularly in times of stress, as in trauma, surgery or illness; decreased carbohydrate tolerance; manifestations of latent diabetes mellitus; increased requirements for insulin or oral hypoglycemic agents in diabetics; hirsutism.

Ophthalmic: Posterior subcapsular cataracts; increased intraocular pressure; glaucoma with possible damage to optic nerve; exophthalmos.

Metabolic: Negative nitrogen balance due to protein catabolism.

Allergic reactions: Especially in patients with allergic responses to proteins manifesting as dizziness, nausea and vomiting, shock, skin reactions.

Miscellaneous: Abscess; prolonged use of ACTH may result in antibodies to it and resulting loss of stimulatory effect.

DRUG ABUSE AND DEPENDENCE
Although drug dependence does not occur, sudden withdrawal of Corticotropin after prolonged use may lead to recurrent symptoms which make it difficult to stop. It may be necessary to taper the dose and increase the injection interval to gradually discontinue the medication.

OVERDOSE
An acute overdose would present no different adverse reactions.

DOSAGE AND ADMINISTRATION
Standard tests for verification of adrenal responsiveness to Corticotropin may utilize as much as 80 units as a single injection or one or more injections of a lesser dosage. Verification tests should be performed prior to treatment with Corticotropins. The test should utilize the route(s) of administration proposed for treatment. Following verification, dosage should be individualized according to the disease under treatment and the general medical condition of each patient. Frequency and dose of the drug should be determined by considering severity of the disease, plasma and urine corticosteroid levels and the initial response of the patient. Only gradual change in dosage schedules should be attempted, after full drug effects have become apparent.

The chronic administration of more than 40 units daily may be associated with uncontrollable adverse effects.

When reduction in dosage is indicated this should be done gradually by either reducing the amount of each injection, administering injections at longer intervals or by a combination of both of the above. During reduction of dosage careful consideration should be given to the disease being treated, the general medical conditions of the patient and the duration over which Corticotropin was administered.

Corticotropin must be reconstituted at the time of use by dissolving in a convenient volume of Sterile Water for Injection or Sodium Chloride Injection in such a manner that the individual dose will be contained in 1—2mL of solution. The reconstituted solution should be refrigerated and used within 24 hours.

Corticotropin may be administered intramuscularly or subcutaneously.

The usual intramuscular or subcutaneous dose of Corticotropin is 20 units four times a day.

In the treatment of acute exacerbations of multiple sclerosis daily intramuscular doses of 80—120 units for 2—3 weeks may be administered.

For diagnostic purposes Corticotropin may be given intravenously in doses of 10—25 units dissolved in 500 mL of 5% glucose infused over an 8-hour period.

Corticotropin is stable for the period indicated on the label when stored at controlled room temperature, 15°—30° C (59°—86° F).

J CODES
Up to 40 units IV,IM,SC—J0800

HOW SUPPLIED

CORTICOTROPIN
POWDER FOR INJECTION: 25 U

BRAND/MANUFACTURER	NDC	SIZE	AWP
◆ **BRAND**			
ACTHAR: RPR	00075-1025-01	1s	$19.56

POWDER FOR INJECTION: 40 U

BRAND/MANUFACTURER	NDC	SIZE	AWP
◆ **BRAND**			
ACTHAR: RPR	00075-1040-01	1s	$28.78
◆ **GENERICS**			
Parke-Davis	00071-4198-01	1s	$17.38

CORTICOTROPIN, REPOSITORY
INJECTION: 40 U/ML

BRAND/MANUFACTURER	NDC	SIZE	AWP
◇ **BRAND**			
ACTHAR GEL, H.P.: RPR	00075-1330-02	1 ml 10s	$141.62

INJECTION: 80 U/ML

BRAND/MANUFACTURER	NDC	SIZE	AWP
◇ **BRAND**			
ACTHAR GEL, H.P.: RPR	00075-1350-01	5 ml	$39.85
	00075-1350-02	1 ml 10s	$243.43

POWDER FOR INJECTION: 40 U/ML

BRAND/MANUFACTURER	NDC	SIZE	AWP
◇ **BRAND**			
ACTHAR GEL, H.P.: RPR	00075-1330-01	1s	$20.08

Cortifoam *SEE* HYDROCORTISONE, RECTAL

Cortisone Acetate

DESCRIPTION
Glucocorticoids are adrenocortical steroids, both naturally occurring and synthetic, which are readily absorbed from the gastrointestinal tract.

Cortisone Acetate is a white or practically white, odorless, crystalline powder. It is stable in air. It is insoluble in water. The molecular weight is 402.49. It is designated chemically as 21-(acetyloxy)-17-hydroxypregn-4-ene-3,11,20-trione. The empirical formula is $C_{23}H_{30}O_6$.

◆ RATED THERAPEUTICALLY EQUIVALENT; ◇ THERAPEUTIC EQUIVALENCE UNCONFIRMED; ○ UNRATED

Cortisone Acetate tablets contain 25 mg of Cortisone Acetate in each tablet.

Cortisone Acetate sterile suspension is a sterile suspension containing 50 mg per milliliter of Cortisone Acetate. No attempt should be made to alter Cortisone Acetate sterile suspension. Diluting it or mixing it with other substances may affect the state of suspension or change the rate of absorption and reduce its effectiveness.

Following is its chemical structure:

ACTIONS

Naturally occurring glucocorticoids (hydrocortisone and Cortisone), which also have salt-retaining properties, are used as replacement therapy in adrenocortical deficiency states. They are also used for their potent anti-inflammatory effects in disorders of many organ systems.

Glucocorticoids cause profound and varied metabolic effects. In addition, they modify the body's immune responses to diverse stimuli.

Cortisone Acetate sterile suspension has a slow onset but long duration of action when compared with more soluble preparations. When daily corticosteroid therapy is required and oral therapy is not feasible, the required daily dosage may be given in a single intramuscular injection of this preparation.

INDICATIONS

1. ENDOCRINE DISORDERS

Primary or secondary adrenocortical insufficiency (hydro-Cortisone or Cortisone is the first choice; synthetic analogs may be used in conjunction with mineralocorticoids where applicable; in infancy mineralocorticoid supplementation is of particular importance)

Acute adrenocortical insufficiency (hydrocortisone or Cortisone is the drug of choice; mineralocorticoid supplementation may be necessary, particularly when synthetic analogs are used)

Preoperatively, and in the event of serious trauma or illness, in patients with known adrenal insufficiency or when adrenocortical reserve is doubtful

Shock unresponsive to conventional therapy if adrenocortical insufficiency exists or is suspected

Congential adrenal hyperplasia
Nonsuppurative thyroiditis
Hypercalcemia associated with cancer

2. RHEUMATIC DISORDERS

As adjunctive therapy for short-term administration (to tide the patient over an acute episode or exacerbation) in:

Psoriatic arthritis
Rheumatoid arthritis, including juvenile rheumatoid arithitis (selected cases may require low-dose maintenance therapy).
Ankylosing spondylitis
Acute and subacute bursitis
Acute nonspecific tenosynovitis
Acute gouty arthritis
Post-traumatic osteoarthritis
Synovitis of osteoarthritis
Epicondylitis
Psoriatic arthritis

3. COLLAGEN DISEASES

During an exacerbation or as maintenance therapy in selected cases of—

Systemic lupus erythematosus
Acute rheumatic carditis
Systemic dermatomyositis (polymyositis)

4. DERMATOLOGIC DISEASES

Pemphigus
Bullous dermatitis herpetiformis
Severe erythema multiforme (Stevens-Johnson syndrome)
Exfoliative dermatitis
Mycosis fungoides
Severe psoriasis
Severe seborrheic dermatitis

5. ALLERGIC STATES

Control of severe or incapacitating allergic conditions intractable to adequate trials of conventional treatment:

Seasonal or perennial allergic rhinitis
Bronchial asthma
Contact dermatitis
Atopic dermatitis
Serum sickness
Drug hypersensitivity reactions
Urticarial transfusion reactions
Acute noninfectious laryngeal edema

6. OPHTHALMIC DISEASES

Severe acute and chronic allergic and inflammatory processes involving the eye and its adnexa, such as:

Allergic conjunctivitis
Keratitis
Allergic corneal marginal ulcers
Herpes-zoster ophthalmicus
Iritis and iridocyclitis
Chorioretinitis
Anterior segment inflammation
Diffuse posterior uveitis and choroiditis
Optic neuritis
Sympathetic ophthalmia

7. RESPIRATORY DISEASES

Symptomatic sarcoidosis
Loeffler's syndrome not manageable by other means
Berylliosis
Fulminating or disseminated pulmonary tuberculosis when used concurrently with appropriate antituberculous chemotherapy
Aspiration pneumonitis

8. HEMATOLOGIC DISORDERS

Idiopathic thrombocytopenic purpura in adults
Secondary thrombocytopenia in adults
Acquired (autoimmune) hemolytic anemia
Erythoblastopenia (RBC anemia)
Congenital (erythroid) hypoplastic anemia

9. NEOPLASTIC DISEASES

For palliative management of:

Leukemias and lymphomas in adults
Acute leukemia of childhood

10. EDEMATOUS STATES

To induce a diuresis or remission of proteinuria in the nephrotic syndrome, without uremia, of the idiopathic type or that due to lupus erythematosus

11. GASTROINTESTINAL DISEASES

To tide the patient over a critical period of the disease in:

Ulcerative colitis
Regional enteritis

12. MISCELLANEOUS

Tuberculous meningitis with subarachnoid block or impending block when used concurrently with appropriate antituberculous chemotherapy

Trichinosis with neurologic or myocardial involvement

CONTRAINDICATIONS

Systemic fungal infections
Hypersensitivity to this product

WARNINGS

In patients on corticosteroid therapy subjected to unusual stress, increased dosage of rapidly acting corticosteroids before, during, and after the stressful situation is indicated. Drug-induced secondary adrenocortical insufficiency may result from too rapid withdrawal of corticosteroids and may be minimized by gradual reduction of dosage. This type of relative insufficiency may persist for months after discontinuation of therapy; therefore, in any situation of stress occurring during that period, hormone therapy should be reinstituted. If the patient is receiving steroids already, dosage may have to be increased. Since mineralocorticoid secretion may be impaired, salt and/or a mineralocorticoid should be administered concurrently.

Corticosteroids may mask some signs of infection, and new infections may appear during their use. There may be decreased resistance and inability to localize infection when corticosteroids are used. Moreover, corticosteroids may affect the nitroblue-tetrazolium test for bacterial infection and produce false negative results.

In cerebral malaria, a double-blind trial has shown that the use of corticosteroids is associated with prolongation of coma and a higher incidence of pneumonia and gastrointestinal bleeding.

Corticosteroids may activate latent amebiasis. Therefore, it is recommended that latent or active amebiasis be ruled out before initiating corticosteroid therapy in any patient who has spent time in the tropics or any patient with unexplained diarrhea.

Prolonged use of corticosteroids may produce posterior subcapsular cataracts, glaucoma with possible damage to the optic nerves, and may enhance the establishment of secondary ocular infections due to fungi or viruses.

Usage in pregnancy: Since adequate human reproduction studies have not been done with corticosteroids, use of these drugs in pregnancy or in women of childbearing potential requires that the anticipated benefits be weighed against the possible hazards to the mother and embryo or fetus. Infants born of mothers who have received substantial doses of corticosteroids during pregnancy should be carefully observed for signs of hypoadrenalism.

Corticosteroids appear in breast milk and could suppress growth, interfere with endogenous corticosteroid production, or cause other unwanted effects. Mothers taking pharmacologic doses of corticosteroids should be advised not to nurse.

Average and large doses of hydrocortisone or Cortisone can cause elevation of blood pressure, salt and water retention, and increased excretion of potassium. These effects are less likely to occur with the synthetic derivatives except when used in large doses. Dietary salt restriction and potassium supplementation may be necessary. All corticosteroids increase calcium excretion.

Administration of live virus vaccines, including smallpox, is contraindicated in individuals receiving immunosuppressive doses of corticosteroids. If inactivated viral or bacterial vaccines are administered to individuals receiving immunosuppressive doses of corticosteroids, the expected serum antibody response may not be obtained. However, immunization procedures may be undertaken in patients who are receiving corticosteroids as replacement therapy, e.g., for Addison's disease.

Patients who are on drugs which suppress the immune system are more susceptible to infections than healthy individuals. Chickenpox and measles, for example, can have a more serious or even fatal course in non-immune children or adults on corticosteroids. In such children or adults who have not had these diseases, particular care should be taken to avoid exposure. The risk of developing a disseminated infection varies among individuals and can be related to the dose, route and duration of corticosteroid administration as well as to the underlying disease. If exposed to chickenpox, prophylaxis with varicella zoster immune globulin (VZIG) may be indicated. If chickenpox develops, treatment with antiviral agents may be considered. If exposed to measles, prophylaxis with immune globulin (IG) may be indicated. (See the respective package inserts for VZIG and IG for complete prescribing information.)

The use of Cortisone Acetate tablets in active tuberculosis should be restricted to those cases of fulminating or disseminated tuberculosis in which the corticosteroid is used for the management of the disease in conjunction with an appropriate antituberculous regimen.

If corticosteroids are indicated in patients with latent tuberculosis or tuberculin reactivity, close observation is necessary as reactivation of the disease may occur. During prolonged corticosteroid therapy, these patients should receive chemoprophylaxis.

Literature reports suggest an apparent association between use of corticosteroids and left ventricular free wall rupture after a recent myocardial infarction; therefore, therapy with corticosteroids should be used with great caution in these patients.

PRECAUTIONS

Following prolonged therapy, withdrawal of corticosteroids may result in symptoms of the corticosteroid withdrawal syndrome including fever, myalgia, arthralgia, and malaise. This may occur in patients even without evidence of adrenal insufficiency.

There is an enhanced effect of corticosteroids in patients with hypothyroidism and in those with cirrhosis.

Corticosteroids should be used cautiously in patients with ocular herpes simplex because of possible corneal perforation.

The lowest possible dose of corticosteroid should be used to control the condition under treatment, and when reduction in dosage is possible, the reduction should be gradual.

Psychic derangements may appear when corticosteroids are used, ranging from euphoria, insomnia, mood swings, personality changes, and severe depression, to frank psychotic manifestations. Also, existing emotional instability or psychotic tendencies may be aggravated by corticosteroids. Aspirin should be used cautiously in conjunction with corticosteroids in hypoprothrombinemia.

Steroids should be used with caution in nonspecific ulcerative colitis, if there is a probability of impending perforation, abscess, or other pyogenic infection, diverticulitis, fresh intestinal anastomoses, active or latent peptic ulcer, renal insufficiency, hypertension, osteoporosis, and myasthenia gravis. Signs of peritoneal irritation following gastrointestinal perforation in patients receiving large doses of corticosteroids may be minimal or absent. Fat embolism has been reported as a possible complication of hypercortisonism.

When large doses are given, some authorities advise that corticosteroids be taken with meals and antacids taken between meals to help to prevent peptic ulcer.

Growth and development of infants and children on prolonged corticosteroid therapy should be carefully observed. Steroids may increase or decrease motility and number of spermatozoa in some patients.

Phenytoin, phenobarbital, ephedrine, and rifampin may enhance the metabolic clearance of corticosteroids, resulting in decreased blood levels and lessened physiologic activity, thus requiring adjustment in corticosteroid dosage.

The prothrombin time should be checked frequently in patients who are receiving corticosteroids and coumarin anticoagulants at the same time because of reports that corticosteroids have altered the response to these anticoagulants. Studies have shown that the usual effect produced by adding corticosteroids is inhibition of response to coumarins, although there have been some conflicting reports of potentiation not substantiated by studies.

When corticosteroids are administered concomitantly with potassium-depleting diuretics, patients should be observed closely for development of hypokalemia.

INFORMATION FOR PATIENTS

Susceptible patients who are on immunosuppressant doses of corticosteroids should be warned to avoid exposure to chickenpox or measles. Patients should also be advised that if they are exposed, medical advice should be sought without delay.

ADVERSE REACTIONS

FLUID AND ELECTROLYTE DISTURBANCES
Sodium retention
Fluid retention
Congestive heart failure in susceptible patients
Potassium loss
Hypokalemic alkalosis
Hypertension

MUSCULOSKELETAL
Muscle weakness
Steroid myopathy
Loss of muscle mass
Osteoporosis
Vertebral compression fractures
Aseptic necrosis of femoral and humeral heads
Pathologic fracture of long bones
Tendon rupture

GASTROINTESTINAL
Peptic ulcer with possible perforation and hemorrhage
Perforation of the small and large bowel, particularly in patients with inflammatory bowel disease
Pancreatitis
Abdominal distention
Ulcerative esophagitis

DERMATOLOGIC
Impaired wound healing
Thin fragile skin
Petechiae and ecchymoses
Erythema
Increased sweating
May suppress reactions to skin tests
Other cutaneous reactions, such as allergic dermatitis, urticaria, angioneurotic edema

NEUROLOGIC
Convulsions
Increased intracranial pressure with papilledema
(pseudotumor cerebri), usually after treatment
Vertigo
Headache
Psychic disturbances

ENDOCRINE
Menstrual irregularities
Development of cushingoid state
Suppression of growth in children
Secondary adrenocortical and pituitary unresponsiveness, particularly in times of stress, as in trauma, surgery, or illness
Decreased carbohydrate tolerance
Manifestations of latent diabetes mellitus
Increased requirements for insulin or oral hypoglycemic agents in diabetics
Hirsutism

OPHTHALMIC
Posterior subcapsular cataracts
Increased intraocular pressure
Glaucoma
Exophthalmos

METABOLIC
Negative nitrogen balance due to protein catabolism

CARDIOVASCULAR
Myocardial rupture following recent myocardial infarction (see "Warnings").

OTHER
Hypersensitivity
Thromboembolism
Weight gain
Increased appetite
Nausea
Malaise

OVERDOSAGE

Reports of acute toxicity and/or death following overdosage of glucocorticoids are rare. In the event of overdosage, no specific antidote is available; treatment is supportive and symptomatic.

The intraperitoneal LD_{50} of Cortisone Acetate in female mice was 1405 mg/kg.

◆ RATED THERAPEUTICALLY EQUIVALENT; ◇ THERAPEUTIC EQUIVALENCE UNCONFIRMED; ○ UNRATED

DOSAGE AND ADMINISTRATION

FOR ORAL ADMINISTRATION

DOSAGE REQUIREMENTS ARE VARIABLE AND MUST BE INDIVIDUALIZED ON THE BASIS OF THE DISEASE AND THE RESPONSE OF THE PATIENT.

The initial dosage varies from 25 to 300 mg a day depending on the disease being treated. In less severe diseases doses lower than 25 mg may suffice, while in severe diseases doses higher than 300 mg may be required. The initial dosage should be maintained or adjusted until the patient's response is satisfactory. If satisfactory clinical response does not occur after a reasonable period of time, discontinue Cortisone Acetate tablets and transfer the patient to other therapy.

After a favorable initial response, the proper maintenance dosage should be determined by decreasing the initial dosage in small amounts to the lowest dosage that maintains an adequate clinical response.

Patients should be observed closely for signs that might require dosage adjustment, including changes in clinical status resulting from remissions or exacerbations of the disease, individual drug responsiveness, and the effect of stress (e.g., surgery, infection, trauma). During stress it may be necessary to increase dosage temporarily.

If the drug is to be stopped after more than a few days of treatment, it usually should be withdrawn gradually.

FOR INTRAMUSCULAR INJECTION ONLY

NOT FOR INTRAVENOUS USE

DOSAGE REQUIREMENTS ARE VARIABLE AND MUST BE INDIVIDUALIZED ON THE BASIS OF THE DISEASE AND THE RESPONSE OF THE PATIENT.

The initial dosage varies from 20 to 300 mg a day depending on the disease being treated. In less severe diseases doses lower than 20 mg may suffice, while in severe diseases doses higher than 300 mg may be required. The initial dosage should be maintained or adjusted until the patient's response is satisfactory. If satisfactory clinical response does not occur after a reasonable period of time, discontinue Cortise Acetate sterile suspension and transfer the patient to other therapy.

After a favorable initial response, the proper maintenance dosage should be determined by decreasing the initial dosage in small amounts to the lowest dosage that maintains an adequate clinical response.

Patients should be observed closely for signs that might require dosage adjustment, including changes in clinical status resulting from remissions or exacerabations of the disease, individual drug responsiveness, and the effect of stress (e.g., surgery, infection, trauma). During stress it may be necessary to increase dosage temporarily.

If the drug is to be stopped after more than a few days of treatment, it usually should be withdrawn gradually.

J CODES

Up to 50 mg IM—J0810

HOW SUPPLIED
INJECTION: 50 MG/ML

BRAND/MANUFACTURER	NDC	SIZE	AWP
◇ BRAND			
CORTONE ACETATE: Merck	00006-7069-10	10 ml	$24.55

TABLETS: 5 MG

BRAND/MANUFACTURER	NDC	SIZE	AWP
◇ GENERICS			
Upjohn	00009-0015-01	50s	$6.23

TABLETS: 10 MG

BRAND/MANUFACTURER	NDC	SIZE	AWP
◇ GENERICS			
Upjohn	00009-0023-01	100s	$22.95

TABLETS: 25 MG

BRAND/MANUFACTURER	NDC	SIZE	AWP
◇ BRAND			
CORTONE ACETATE: Merck	00006-0219-68	100s	$60.41
◇ GENERICS			
Richlyn	00115-2920-01	100s	$11.66
West-Ward	00143-1202-01	100s	$42.50
Qualitest	00603-3062-21	100s	$42.50
Major	00904-2043-60	100s	$43.50
Moore,H.L.	00839-5084-06	100s	$45.48
URL	00677-0046-01	100s	$47.95
Goldline	00182-1648-01	100s	$48.00
Rugby	00536-3530-01	100s	$50.48
Upjohn	00009-0034-01	100s	$55.49

BRAND/MANUFACTURER	NDC	SIZE	AWP
Raway	00686-1202-01	100s ud	$41.00
Rugby	00536-3530-05	500s	$235.90
Richlyn	00115-2920-03	1000s	$89.70

Cortisporin SEE BACITRACIN ZINC/HYDROCORTISONE/NEOMYCIN SULFATE/POLYMYXIN B SULFATE AND HYDROCORTISONE/NEOMYCIN SULFATE/POLYMYXIN B SULFATE

Cortone Acetate SEE CORTISONE ACETATE

Cortrosyn SEE COSYNTROPIN

Corzide SEE BENDROFLUMETHIAZIDE AND NADOLOL

Cosmegen SEE DACTINOMYCIN

Cosyntropin

DESCRIPTION

Cosyntropin for injection is a sterile lyophilized powder in vials containing 0.25 mg of Cosyntropin and 10 mg of mannitol to be reconstituted with 1 mL sodium chloride for injection, USP as solvent. Administration is by intravenous or intramuscular injection. Cosyntropin is α 1-24 corticotropin, a synthetic subunit of ACTH. It is an open chain polypeptide containing, from the N terminus, the first 24 of the 39 amino acids of natural ACTH.

Following is its chemical structure:

Ser-Tyr-Ser-Met-Glu-His-Phe-Arg-Trp-Gly-Lys-Pro-Val-Gly-Lys-Lys-Arg-Arg-Pro-Val-Lys-Val-Tyr-Pro
1   2   3   4   5   6   7   8   9 10 11 12 13 14 15 16 17 18 19 20 21 22 23 24

CLINICAL PHARMACOLOGY

Cosyntropin exhibits the full corticosteroidogenic activity of natural ACTH. Various studies have shown that the biologic activity of ACTH resides in the N-terminal portion of the molecule and that the 1-20 amino acid residue is the minimal sequence retaining full activity. Partial or complete loss of activity is noted with progressive shortening of the chain beyond 20 amino acid residue. For example, the decrement from 20 to 19 results in a 70% loss of potency.

The pharmacologic profile of Cosyntropin is similar to that of purified natural ACTH. It has been established that 0.25 mg of Cosyntropin will stimulate the adrenal cortex maximally and to the same extent as 25 units of natural ACTH. This dose of Cosyntropin will produce maximal secretion of 17-OH corticosteroids, 17-ketosteroids and/or 17-ketogenic steroids.

The extra-adrenal effects which natural ACTH and Cosyntropin have in common include increased melanotropic activity, increased growth hormone secretion and an adipokinetic effect. These are considered to be without physiological or clinical significance.

Animal, human and synthetic ACTH (1-39), which all contain 39 amino acids, exhibit similar immunologic activity. This activity resides in the C-terminal portion of the molecule and the 22-39 amino acid residues exhibit the greatest degree of antigenicity. In contrast, synthetic polypeptides containing 1-19 or fewer amino acids have no detectable immunologic activity. Those containing 1-26, 1-24 or 1-23 amino acids have very little immunologic although full biologic activity. This property of Cosyntropin assumes added importance in view of the known antigenicity of natural ACTH.

INDICATIONS AND USAGE

Cosyntropin is intended for use as a diagnostic agent in the screening of patients presumed to have adrenocortical insufficiency. Because of its rapid effect on the adrenal cortex it may be utilized to perform a 30-minute test of adrenal function (plasma cortisol response) as an office or outpatient procedure, using only 2 venipunctures. (See *"Dosage and Administration"* section for details.)

Severe hypofunction of the pituitary-adrenal axis is usually associated with subnormal plasma cortisol values but a low basal level is not per se evidence of adrenal insufficiency and does not suffice to make the diagnosis. Many patients with proven insufficiency will have normal basal levels and will develop signs of insufficiency only when stressed. For this reason the only criterion which should be used in establishing the diagnosis is the failure to respond to adequate corticotropin stimulation as provided by 0.25 mg of Cosyntropin for injection. When presumptive adrenal insufficiency is diagnosed by a subnormal Cosyntropin test, further studies are indicated to determine if it is primary or secondary.

Primary adrenal insufficiency (Addison's disease) is the result of an intrinsic disease process, such as tuberculosis within the gland. The production of adrenocortical hormones is deficient despite high ACTH levels (feedback mechanism). Secondary or relative insufficiency arises as the result of defective production of ACTH leading in turn to disuse atrophy of the adrenal cortex. It is commonly seen, for example, as a result of corticosteroid therapy, Sheehan's syndrome and pituitary tumors or ablation.

The differentiation of both types is based on the premise that a primarily defective gland cannot be stimulated by ACTH whereas a secondarily defective gland is potentially functional and will respond to adequate stimulation with ACTH. Patients selected for further study as the result of a subnormal Cosyntropin test should be given a 3 or 4 day course of treatment with Repository Corticotropin Injection USP and then retested. Suggested doses are 40 USP units twice daily for 4 days or 60 USP units twice daily for 3 days. Under these conditions little or no increase in plasma cortisol levels will be seen in Addison's disease whereas higher or even normal levels will be seen in cases with secondary adrenal insufficiency.

UNLABELED USES
Cosyntropin is used alone or as an adjunct in the treatment of infantile spasms (West's syndrome) and in symptomatic treatment of multiple sclerosis and ulcerative colitis. It is also used in acute gout, Bell's palsy, and peripheral neuropathy.

CONTRAINDICATIONS
The only contraindication to Cosyntropin is a history of a previous adverse reaction to it.

PRECAUTIONS
General: Cosyntropin exhibits slight immunologic activity, does not contain foreign animal protein and is therefore less risky to use than natural ACTH. Patients known to be sensitized to natural ACTH with markedly positive skin tests will, with few exceptions, react negatively when tested intradermally with Cosyntropin. Further, most patients with a history of a previous hypersensitivity reaction to natural ACTH or a pre-existing allergic disease will tolerate Cosyntropin without incident. Despite this, however, Cosyntropin is not completely devoid of immunologic activity and hypersensitivity reactions are possible, at least in susceptible patients. Therefore, the physician should be prepared, prior to injection, to treat any possible acute hypersensitivity reaction.

Drug Interactions: Corticotropin may accentuate the electrolyte loss associated with diuretic therapy.

Carcinogenesis, Mutagenesis, Impairment of Fertility: Long term studies in animals have not been performed to evaluate carcinogenic or mutagenic potential or impairment of fertility. A study in rats noted inhibition of reproductive function like natural ACTH.

Pregnancy: Pregnancy Category C. Animal reproduction studies have not been conducted with Cosyntropin. It is also not known whether Cosyntropin can cause fetal harm when administered to a pregnant woman or can affect reproduction capacity. Cosyntropin should be given to a pregnant woman only if clearly needed.

Nursing Mothers: It is not known whether this drug is excreted in human milk. Because many drugs are excreted in human milk, caution should be exercised when Cosyntropin is administered to a nursing woman.

Pediatric Usage: (See *"Dosage and Administration"* section for details.)

ADVERSE REACTIONS
Since Cosyntropin for injection is intended for diagnostic and not therapeutic use, adverse reactions other than a rare hypersensitivity reaction are not anticipated. To date only 3 such reactions have been reported in the literature and in each instance the patient had a pre-existing allergic disease and/or a previous reaction to natural ACTH. One investigator reported a single instance of slight whealing with splotchy erythema at the injection site. A similar but more marked reaction was also noted in the same patient following an injection of natural ACTH.

DOSAGE AND ADMINISTRATION
Cosyntropin may be administered intramuscularly or as a direct intravenous injection when used as a rapid screening test of adrenal function. It may also be given as an intravenous infusion over a 4 to 8 hour period to provide a greater stimulus to the adrenal glands. Doses of Cosyntropin 0.25 to 0.75 mg have been used in clinical studies and a maximal response noted with the smallest dose.

A suggested method for a rapid screening test of adrenal function has been described by Wood and associates.[1] A control blood sample of 6 to 7 mL is collected in a heparinized tube. Reconstitute 0.25 mg of Cosyntropin in solvent (ampul of 1 mL sodium chloride injection USP—0.9%) and inject intramuscularly. In children, aged 2 years or less, a dose of 0.125 mg will often suffice. A second blood sample is collected exactly 30 minutes later. Both blood samples should be refrigerated until sent to the laboratory for determination of the plasma cortisol response by some appropriate method. If it is not possible to send them to the laboratory or perform the fluorimetric procedure within 12 hours, then the plasma should be separated and refrigerated or frozen according to need.

The usual normal response in most cases is an approximate doubling of the basal level, provided that the basal level does not exceed the normal range. Patients taking inadvertent doses of cortisone or hydrocortisone on the test day and patients taking spironolactone or women taking drugs which contain estrogen may exhibit abnormally high basal plasma cortisol levels. A paradoxical response may be noted in the former group as seen in a decrease in plasma cortisol values following a stimulating dose of Cosyntropin. In the latter group only a normal incremental response is to be expected. Many patients with normal adrenal function, however, do not respond to the expected degree so that the following criteria have been established to denote a normal response:
1. The control plasma cortisol level should exceed 5 mcg/100 mL.
2. The 30-minute level should show an increment of at least 7 mcg/100 mL above the basal level.
3. The 30-minute level should exceed 18 mcg/100 mL. Comparable figures have been reported by Greig and co-workers.[2] These criteria also apply when the drug is injected intravenously in 2 to 5 mL of saline over a 2-minute period.

Plasma cortisol levels usually peak about 45 to 60 minutes after an injection of Cosyntropin for injection and some prefer the 60-minute interval for testing for this reason. While it is true that the 60-minute values are usually higher than the 30-minute values, the difference may not be significant enough in most cases to outweigh the disadvantage of a longer testing period. If the 60-minute test period is used, the criterion for a normal response is an approximate doubling of the basal plasma cortisol value.

When given as an intravenous infusion: Cosyntropin, 0.25 mg may be added to glucose or saline solutions and given at the rate of approximately 40 mcg per hour over a 6-hour period. It should not be added to blood or plasma as it is apt to be inactivated by enzymes. Adrenal response may be measured in the usual manner by determining urinary steroid excretion before and after treatment or by measuring plasma cortisol levels before and at the end of the infusion. The latter is preferable because the urinary steroid excretion does not always accurately reflect the adrenal or plasma cortisol response to ACTH. Patients receiving cortisone, hydrocortisone or spironolactone should omit their pre-test doses on the day selected for testing. In patients with a raised plasma bilirubin or in patients where the plasma contains free hemoglobin, falsely high fluorescence measurements will result. The test may be performed at any time during the day but because of the physiological diurnal variation of plasma cortisol the criteria listed by Wood cannot apply. It has been shown that basal plasma cortisol levels and the post Cosyntropin increment exhibit diurnal changes. However, the 30 minute plasma cortisol level remains unchanged throughout the day so that only this single criterion should be used.[3]

Parenteral drug products should be inspected visually for particulate matter and discoloration whenever solution and container permit. Reconstituted Cosyntropin should not be retained.

REFERENCES:
1. Wood, J.B. et al. LANCET 1.243, 1965. 2. Greig, W.R. et al. J. ENDOCR 34.411, 1966. 3. McGill, P.E. et al. ANN RHEUM DIS 26. 123, 1967.

HOW SUPPLIED
POWDER FOR INJECTION: 0.25 MG

BRAND/MANUFACTURER	NDC	SIZE	AWP
○ **BRAND**			
CORTROSYN: Organon	00052-0731-10	10s	$120.85

Cotazym *SEE* PANCRELIPASE

Coumadin *SEE* WARFARIN SODIUM

Creon *SEE* PANCRELIPASE

Cromolyn Sodium

DESCRIPTION
Cromolyn Sodium is the disodium salt of 1,3-bis (2-carboxychromon-5-yloxy)-2-hydroxypropane. The empirical formula is $C_{23}H_{14}Na_2O_{11}$; the molecular weight is 512.34. Cromolyn Sodium is a water-soluble, odorless, white, hydrated crystaline powder. It is tasteless at first, but leaves a slightly bitter aftertaste.

Each 2 mL ampule Cromolyn Sodium Nebulizer Solution contains:
Cromolyn Sodium . . . . .20 mg.

Each metered inhalation of Cromolyn Sodium Inhalation Aerosol delivers:
Approximately 800 mcg Cromolyn Sodium through the mouthpiece.

Each Cromolyn Sodium Capsule for Inhalation contains:
Cromolyn Sodium . . . . .20 mg.

Each mL of Cromolyn Sodium Nasal Solution contains:
Cromolyn Sodium . . . . .40 mg.

Each actuation delivers:
A metered spray containing 5.2 mg Cromolyn Sodium.

Pharmacologic Category: Mast cell stabilizer/antiallergic.
Therapeutic Category: Antiasthmatic; reduces bronchial hyper- reactivity.

Following is its chemical structure:

CLINICAL PHARMACOLOGY

In vitro and *in vivo* animal studies have shown that Cromolyn Sodium inhibits sensitized mast cell degranulation which occurs after exposure to specific antigens. Cromolyn Sodium acts by inhibiting the release of mediators from mast cells. Studies show that Cromolyn Sodium indirectly blocks calcium ions from entering the mast cell, thereby preventing mediator release.

Rhinitis induced by the inhalation of specific antigens can be inhibited to varying degrees by pretreatment with Cromolyn Sodium Nasal Solution.

Cromolyn Sodium inhibits both the immediate and nonimmediate broncho-constrictive reactions to inhaled antigen. Cromolyn Sodium also attenuates bronchospasm caused by exercise, toluene diisocyanate, aspirin, cold air, sulphur dioxide and environmental pollutants.

Another activity demonstrated *in vitro* is the capacity of Cromolyn Sodium to inhibit the degranulation of non-sensitized rat mast cells by phospholipase A and the subsequent release of chemical mediators. An additional *in vitro* study showed that Cromolyn Sodium did not inhibit the enzymatic activity of released phospholipase A on its specific substrate.

Cromolyn Sodium has no intrinsic bronchodilator, antihistaminic or anti-inflammatory activity.

After administration by inhalation, approximately 8% of the total Cromolyn Sodium dose administered is absorbed and rapidly excreted unchanged, approximately equally divided between urine and bile. The remainder of the dose is either exhaled or deposited in the oropharynx, swallowed and excreted via the alimentary tract.

Cromolyn Sodium is poorly absorbed from the gastrointestinal tract. After instillation of Cromolyn Sodium Nasal Solution, less than 7% of the total dose administered is absorbed and is rapidly excreted unchanged in the bile and urine. The remainder of the dose is expelled from the nose, or swallowed and excreted via the alimentary tract.

INDICATIONS AND USAGE

Cromolyn Sodium is a prophylactic agent indicated in the management of patients with bronchial asthma.

In patients whose symptoms are sufficiently frequent to require a continuous program of medication, Cromolyn Sodium is given by inhalation on a regular daily basis (see *"Dosage and Administration"*). The effect of Cromolyn Sodium is usually evident after several weeks of treatment, although some patients show an almost immediate response.

If improvement occurs, it will ordinarily occur within the first 4 weeks of administration as manifested by a decrease in the severity of clinical symptoms of asthma, or in the need for concomitant therapy, or both.

In patients who develop acute bronchoconstriction in response to exposure to exercise, toluene diisocyanate, environmental pollutants, etc. Cromolyn Sodium should be given shortly before exposure to the precipitating factor, i.e., within 10-15 minutes but not more than 60 minutes (see *"Dosage and Administration"*). Cromolyn Sodium Inhaler may be effective in relieving bronchospasm in some, but not all, patients with exercise induced bronchospasm.

Cromolyn Sodium Nasal Solution is indicated for the prevention and treatment of the symptoms of allergic rhinitis.

CONTRAINDICATIONS

Cromolyn Sodium is contraindicated in those patients who have shown hypersensitivity to Cromolyn Sodium.

WARNINGS

Cromolyn Sodium Inhaler has no role in the treatment of an acute attack of asthma, especially status asthmaticus. Severe anaphylactic reactions can occur after Cromolyn Sodium administration. The recommended dosage should be decreased in patients with decreased renal or hepatic function. Cromolyn Sodium Inhaler should be discontinued if the patient develops eosinophilic pneumonia (or pulmonary infiltrates with eosinophilia). Because of the propellants in this preparation, it should be used with caution in patients with coronary artery disease or a history of cardiac arrhythmias.

PRECAUTIONS

General: In view of the biliary and renal routes of excretion for Cromolyn Sodium, consideration should be given to decreasing the dosage or discontinuing the administration of the drug in patients with impaired renal or hepatic function. Occasionally, patients may experience cough and/or bronchospasm following Cromolyn Sodium inhalation. At times, patients who develop bronchospasm may not be able to continue Cromolyn Sodium administration despite prior bronchodilator administration. Some patients may experience transient nasal stinging and/or sneezing immediately following instillation of Cromolyn Sodium Nasal Solution. Except in rare occurrences, these experiences have not caused discontinuation of therapy. Rarely, very severe bronchospasm has been encountered.

Symptoms of asthma may recur if Cromolyn Sodium is reduced below the recommended dosage or discontinued.

INFORMATION FOR PATIENTS

Cromolyn Sodium is to be taken as directed by the physician. Because it is preventive medication, it may take up to four weeks before the patient experiences maximum benefit.

Cromolyn Sodium Nebulizer Solution should be used in a power-driven nebulizer with an adequate airflow rate equipped with a suitable face mask or mouthpiece.

The glass is an easy-break ampule. The glass is weakened at both ends so that they will break off easily by hand. As with all glass ampules, use caution when opening the ampule. Keep well away from nebulizer unit and face.

To open you should hold the ampule at an angle and break off the lower end (no solution will come out). Turn the ampule so the open end faces upward. Place your forefinger carefully over the open end of the ampule and now break off the other end.

To empty you should hold the ampule over the solution container and release your forefinger. The solution will flow out.

Patients may experience irritation of the throat or coughing after inhalation of the powder. In some cases, rinsing the mouth or taking a drink of water immediately before and/or after using the Cromolyn Sodium Inhaler will eliminate the throat irritation or cough.

If the patient experiences difficulty in emptying the capsule, which may require several deep inhalations, check to make certain the patient is following the directions carefully. A light dusting of powder remaining in the capsule is normal, and is not an indication that the Cromolyn Sodium Inhaler or capsule is faulty or that the proper dose was not delivered. The Cromolyn Sodium Inhaler should be washed in clean, warm water at least once a week, and dried thoroughly before use.

CARCINOGENESIS, MUTAGENESIS, AND IMPAIRMENT OF FERTILITY

Long term studies in mice (12 months intraperitoneal treatment followed by 6 months observation), hamsters (12 months intraperitoneal treatment followed by 12 months observation), and rats (18 months subcutaneous treatment) showed no neoplastic effect of Cromolyn Sodium.

No evidence of chromosomal damage or cytotoxicity was obtained in various mutagenesis studies.

No evidence of impaired fertility was shown in laboratory animal reproduction studies.

PREGNANCY

Pregnancy Category B. Reproduction studies with Cromolyn Sodium administered parenterally to pregnant mice, rats, and rabbits in doses up to 338 times the human clinical dose produced no evidence of fetal malformations. Adverse fetal effects (increased resorptions and decreased fetal weight) were noted only at the very high parenteral doses that produced maternal toxicity. There are, however, no adequate and well-controlled studies in pregnant women. Because animal reproduction studies are not always predictive of human response, this drug should be used during pregnancy only if clearly needed.

DRUG INTERACTION DURING PREGNANCY

Cromolyn Sodium and isoproterenol were studied following subcutaneous injections in pregnant mice. Cromolyn Sodium alone in doses of 60 to 540 mg/kg (38 to 338 times the human dose) did not cause significant increases in resorptions or major malformations. Isoproterenol alone at a dose of 2.7 mg/kg (90 times the human dose) increased both resorptions and malformations. The addition of Cromolyn Sodium (338 times the human dose) to isoproterenol (90 times the human dose) appears to have increased the incidence of both resorptions and malformations.

NURSING MOTHERS

It is not known whether this drug is excreted in human milk. Because many drugs are excreted in human milk, caution should be exercised when Cromolyn Sodium is administered to a nursing woman, and the attending physician must make a benefit/risk assessment in regarding to its use in this situation.

PEDIATRIC USE

Safety and effectiveness in children below the age of 2 years (Cromolyn Sodium Inhaler—5 years, Cromolyn Sodium Nasal Solution—6 years) have not been established.

For young children unable to utilize the Inhaler or Cromolyn Sodium Capsules for Inhalation, Cromolyn Sodium Nebulizer Solution is recommended. Because of the possibility that adverse effects of this drug could become apparent only after many years, a benefit/risk consideration of the long-term use of Cromolyn Sodium Inhaler is particularly important in pediatric patients.

ADVERSE REACTIONS

Clinical experience with the use of Cromolyn Sodium suggests that adverse reactions are rare events. The following adverse reactions have been associated with Cromolyn Sodium Nebulizer Solution: cough, nasal congestion, nausea, sneezing and wheezing.

Other reactions have been reported in clinical trials; however, a causal relationship could not be established: drowsiness, nasal itching, nose bleed, nose burning, serum sickness, and stomachache.

In addition, adverse reactions have been reported with Cromolyn Sodium Inhalation Capsules USP. The most common side effects are associated with inhalation of the powder and include transient cough (1 in 5 patients) and mild wheezing (1 in 25 patients). These effects rarely require treatment or discontinuation of the drug.

Information on the incidence of adverse reactions to Cromolyn Sodium Capsules has been derived from U.S. postmarketing surveillance experience. The following adverse reactions attributed to Cromolyn Sodium, based upon recurrence following readministration, have been reported in less than 1 in 10,000 patients: laryngeal edema, swollen parotid gland, angiodema, bronchospasm, joint swelling and pain, dizziness, dysuria and urinary frequency, nausea, cough, wheezing, headache, nasal congestion, rash, urticaria and lacrimation.

Other adverse reactions have been reported in less than 1 in 100,000 patients, and it is unclear whether these are attributable to the drug: anaphylaxis, nephrosis, periarteritic vasculitis, pericarditis, peripheral neuritis, pulmonary infiltrates with eosinophilia, polymyositis, exfoliative dermatitis, hemotypsis, anemia, myalgia, hoarseness, photodermatitis and vertigo.

In controlled clinical studies of Cromolyn Sodium Inhaler, the most frequently reported adverse reactions attributed to cromolyn sodium treatment were: Throat irritation or dryness, bad taste, cough, wheeze, nausea.

The most frequently reported adverse reactions attributed to other forms of Cromolyn Sodium (on the basis of reoccurrence following readministration) involve the respiratory tract and are: bronchospasm [sometimes severe, associated with a precipitous fall in pulmonary function (FEV_1)], cough, laryngeal edema (rare), nasal congestion (sometimes severe), pharyngeal irritation and wheezing.

Adverse reactions which occur infrequently and are associated with administration of the drug are: anaphylaxis, angio-edema, dizziness, dysuria and urinary frequency, joint swelling and pain, lacrimation, nausea and headache, rash, swollen parotid gland, urticaria, pulmonary infiltrates with eosinophilia, substernal burning, and myopathy.

The following adverse reactions have been reported as rare events and it is unclear whether they are attributable to the drug: anemia, exfoliative dermatitis, hemoptysis, hoarseness, myalgia, nephrosis, periarteritic vasculitis, pericarditis, nasal itching, nasal bleeding, nasal burning, serum sickness, stomach ache, polymyositis, vertigo, and liver disease.

The following adverse effects have been reported in less than 1 in 10,000 patients, and are a consequence of the Cromolyn Sodium Inhaler delivery system: inhalation of (capsule) gelatin particles and inhalation of mouthpiece or propeller.

The most frequent adverse reactions occurring in the 430 patients included in the clinical trials with Cromolyn Sodium Nasal Solution were sneezing (1 in 10 patients), nasal stinging (1 in 20). Headaches and bad taste were reported in about 1 in 50 patients. Epistaxis. postnasal drip, and rash were reported in less than one percent of the patients. One patient in the clinical trials developed anaphylaxis.

Adverse reactions which have occurred in the use of other Cromolyn Sodium formulations for inhalation include angioedema, joint pain and swelling, urticaria, cough, and wheezing. Other reactions reported rarely are serum sickness, periarteritic vasculitis, polymyositis, pericarditis, photodermatitis, exfoliative dermatitis, peripheral neuritis, and nephrosis.

OVERDOSAGE

There is no clinical syndrome associated with an overdosage or Cromolyn Sodium. Acute toxicity testing in a wide variety of species has demonstrated an extremely low order of toxicity for Cromolyn Sodium, regardless of whether administration was parenteral, oral or by inhalation. Parenteral administration in mice, rats, guinea pigs, hamsters and rabbits demonstrated an LD_{50} in the region of 4000 mg/kg. Intravenous administration in monkeys also indicated a similar order of toxicity. The highest dose administered by the oral route in rats and mice was 8000 mg/kg, and at this dose level no deaths occurred. By inhalation, even in long term studies, it proved impossible to achieve toxic dose levels of Cromolyn Sodium in a range of mammalian species.

DOSAGE AND ADMINISTRATION

For management of bronchial asthma in adults and children (two years of age and over), the usual starting dosage is the contents of one ampule administered by nebulization four times a day at regular intervals.

Patients with chronic asthma should be advised that the effect of Cromolyn Sodium therapy is dependent upon its administration at regular intervals, as directed. Cromolyn Sodium should be introduced into the patient's therapeutic regimen when the acute episode has been controlled, the airway has been cleared and the patient is able to inhale adequately.

For the prevention of acute bronchospasm which follows exercise or exposure to cold dry air, environmental agents (e.g., animal danders, toluene diisocyanate, pollutants), etc., the usual dose is the contents of one ampule administered by nebulization shortly before exposure to the precipitating factor.

It should be emphasized to the patient that the drug is poorly absorbed when swallowed and is not effective by this route of administration.

CROMOLYN SODIUM THERAPY IN RELATION TO OTHER TREATMENTS FOR ASTHMA:

NONSTEROIDAL AGENTS

Cromolyn Sodium should be *added* to the patient's existing treatment regimen (e.g., bronchodilators). When a clinical response to Cromolyn Sodium is evident, usually within two to four weeks, and if the asthma is under good control, an attempt may be made to decrease concomitant medication usage gradually.

If concomitant medications are eliminated or required on no more than a prn basis, the frequency of administration of Cromolyn Sodium may be titrated downward to the lowest level consistent with the desired effect. The usual decrease is from four to three ampules per day, from two metered inhalations four times daily to three times daily to twice daily (Cromolyn Sodium Inhaler), or from four to three to two capsules per day (Cromolyn Sodium Capsules for Inhalation). It is important that the dosage be reduced gradually to avoid exacerbation of asthma. It is emphasized that in patients whose dosage has been titrated to fewer than four ampules, four inhalations, or four capsules per day, an increase in the dose of Cromolyn Sodium and the introduction of, or increase in, symptomatic medications may be needed if the patient's clinical condition deteriorates.

For management of bronchial asthma in adults and children (5 years of age and over) who are able to use the Inhaler, the usual starting dosage is two metered inhalations four times daily at regular intervals. This dose should not be exceeded

Not all patients will respond to the recommended dose and there is evidence to suggest, at least in younger patients, that a lower dose may provide efficacy.

Patients with chronic asthma should be advised that the effect of Cromolyn Sodium Inhaler therapy is dependent upon its administration at regular intervals, as directed. Cromolyn Sodium Inhaler should be introduced into the patient's therapeutic regimen when the acute episode has been controlled, the airway has been cleared, and the patient is able to inhale adequately.

For the prevention of acute bronchospasm which follows exercise, exposure to cold dry air or environmental agents, the usual dose is two metered inhalations shortly, i.e., 10-15 minutes but not more than 60 minutes, before exposure to the precipitating factor.

Cromolyn Sodium Inhaler should be *added* to the patient's existing treatment regimen (e.g., bronchodilators). When a clinical response to Cromolyn Sodium Inhaler is evident, usually within two to four weeks, and if the asthma is under good control, an attempt may be made to decrease concomitant medication usage gradually.

If concomitant medications are eliminated or required on no more than a prn basis the frequency of administration of Cromolyn Sodium Inhaler may be titrated downward to the lowest level consistent with the desired effect.

For management of bronchial asthma in adults and children (two years of age and over) who are able to use the Cromolyn Sodium turbo-inhaler, the usual starting dosage is the contents of one Cromolyn Sodium Capsule inhaled four times daily at regular intervals.

Patients with chronic asthma should be advised that the effect of Cromolyn Sodium therapy is dependent upon its administration at regular intervals, as directed. Cromolyn Sodium should be introduced into the patient's therapeutic regimen when the acute episode has been controlled, the airway has been cleared and the patient is able to inhale adequately.

For the prevention of acute bronchospam which follows exercise or exposure to cold dry air, environmental agents, (e.g., animal danders, toluene diisocyanate, pollutants), etc., the usual dose is the contents of one Cromolyn Sodium Capsule inhaled shortly before exposure to the precipitating factor.

CORTICOSTEROIDS

In patients chronically receiving corticosteroids for the management of bronchial asthma, the dosage should be maintained following the introduction of Cromolyn Sodium. If the patient improves, an attempt to decrease corticosteroids should be made. Even if the corticosteroid-dependent patient fails to show symptomatic improvement following Cromolyn Sodium administration, the potential to reduce corticosteroids may nonetheless be present. Thus, gradual tapering of corticosteroid dosage may be attempted. It is important that the dose be reduced slowly, maintaining close supervision of the patient to avoid an exacerbation of asthma.

It should be borne in mind that prolonged corticosteriod therapy frequently causes an impairment in the activity of the hypothalamic-pituitary-adrenal axis and a reduction in the size of the adrenal cortex. A potentially critical degree of impairment or insufficiency may persist asymptomatically for some time even after gradual discontinuation of adrenocortical steroids. Therefore, if a patient is subjected to significant stress, such as a severe asthmatic attack, surgery, trauma or severe illness while being treated or within one year (occasionally up to two years) after corticosteroid treatment has been terminated, consideration should be given to reinstituting corticosteroid therapy. When respiratory function is impaired, as may occur in severe exacerbation of asthma, a temporary increase in the amount of corticosteroids may be required to regain control of the patient's asthma.

It is particularly important that great care be exercised if, for any reason, Cromolyn Sodium is withdrawn in cases where its use has permitted a reduction in the maintenance dose of corticosteroids. In such cases, continued close supervision of the patient is essential since there may be sudden reappearance of severe manifestations of asthma which will require immediate therapy and possible reintroduction of corticosteroids.

The dose Cromolyn Sodium Nasal Solution for adults and children 6 years and older is *one spray in each nostril* 3-4 times daily at regular intervals. If needed, this dose may be increased to one spray to each nostril 6 times daily. The patient should be instructed to clear the nasal passages before administering the spray and should inhale through the nose during administration.

In the management of seasonal (pollenotic) rhinitis, and for prevention of rhinitis caused by exposure to other types of specific inhalant allergens, treatment with Cromolyn Sodium Nasal Solution will be more effective if started prior to expected contact with the offending allergen. Treatment should be continued throughout the period of exposure, i.e., until the pollen season is over or until exposure to the offending allergen is terminated.

In the management of perennial allergic rhinitis, the effects of treatment with Cromolyn Sodium Nasal Solution may become apparent only after two to four weeks of treatment. The concomitant use of antihistamines and/or nasal decongestants may be necessary during the initial phase of treatment, but the need for this type of medication should diminish and may be eliminated when the full benefit of Cromolyn Sodium Nasal Solution is achieved.

Nebulizer Solution: Store between 15°C and 25°C (59°F and 77°F) and protected from light. Do not use if it contains a precipitate.

Cromolyn Solution Inhaler: Store between 15°-30°C (59°-86°F). Contents under pressure.

Do not puncture, incinerate, or place near sources of heat.

◆ RATED THERAPEUTICALLY EQUIVALENT; ◇ THERAPEUTIC EQUIVALENCE UNCONFIRMED; ○ UNRATED

Keep out of the reach of children.

Cromolyn Sodium Capsules each contain 20 mg Cromolyn Sodium. Store capsules between 15°C and 30°C (59°F and 86°F). Keep out of the reach of children. Turbo-inhalers are supplied separately in individual containers. The Inhaler should be replaced after 6 months of use.

Cromolyn Sodium Nasal Solution should be stored between 15° and 25°C (59°F and 77°F) and protected from light.

J CODES
Per 20 mg INH—J7630

HOW SUPPLIED
AEROSOL LIQUID W/ADAPTER: 0.8 MG/INH

BRAND/MANUFACTURER	NDC	SIZE	AWP
○ **BRAND**			
INTAL INHALER: Fisons Presc	00585-0675-02	8.1 ml	$37.98
	00585-0675-01	14.2 ml	$60.43

SOLUTION: 10 MG/ML

BRAND/MANUFACTURER	NDC	SIZE	AWP
○ **BRAND**			
NASALCROM: Fisons Presc	00585-0671-03	13 ml	$21.43
	00585-0671-04	26 ml	$39.25
INTAL: Fisons Presc	00585-0673-02	2 ml 60s	$48.25
	00585-0673-03	2 ml 120s	$90.13
○ **GENERICS**			
Dey	49502-0689-02	2 ml 60s	$42.00
Dey	49502-0689-12	2 ml 120s	$84.00

Cromolyn Sodium, Oral

DESCRIPTION
Each Cromolyn Sodium Capsule contains 100 mg of Cromolyn Sodium. Cromolyn Sodium is a hygroscopic, white powder having little odor. Cromolyn Sodium may leave a slighty bitter aftertaste. It is soluble in water (1 part in 20) and the resulting solution is neutral. It is intended for oral use.

Chemically, Cromolyn Sodium is the diSodium salt of 1,3-bis (2-carboxychromon-5-yloxy)-2-hydroxypropane. The empirical formula is $C_{23}H_{14}Na_2O_{11}$: the molecular weights is 512.34.

Following is its chemical structure:

CLINICAL PHARMACOLOGY
In vitro and *in vivo* animal studies have shown that Cromolyn Sodium inhibits the release of mediators from sensitized mast cells. Cromolyn Sodium acts by inhibiting the release of histamine and leukotrienes (SRS-A) from the mast cell. Cromolyn Sodium has no intrinsic vasoconstrictor, antihistaminic or anti-inflammatory activity.

Cromolyn Sodium is poorly absorbed from the gastrointestinal tract. No more than 1% of an administered dose is absorbed by humans after oral administration, the remainder being excreted in the feces. Very little absorption of Cromolyn Sodium was seen after oral administration of 500 mg by mouth to each of 12 volunteers. From 0.28 to 0.50% of the administered dose was recovered in the first 24 hours of urinary excretion in 3 subjects. The mean urinary excretion of an administered dose over 24 hours in the remaining 9 subjects was 0.45%.

INDICATIONS AND USAGE
Cromolyn Sodium is indicated in the management of patients with mastocytosis. Use of this product has been associated with improvement in diarrhea, flushing, headaches, vomiting, urticaria, abdominal pain, nausea, and itching in some patients.

CONTRAINDICATIONS
Cromolyn Sodium is contraindicated in those patients who have shown hypersensitivity to Cromolyn Sodium.

WARNINGS
The recommended dosage should be decreased in patients with decreased renal or hepatic function. Severe anaphylactic reactions may occur rarely in association with Cromolyn Sodium administration.

PRECAUTIONS
In view of the biliary and renal routes of excretion of Cromolyn Sodium consideration should be given to decreasing the dosage of the drug in patients with impaired renal or hepatic function.

Carcinogenesis, Mutagenesis, and Impairment of Fertility: Long-term studies in mice (12 months intraperitoneal treatment followed by six months observation), hamsters (12 months intraperitoneal treatment followed by 12 months observation), and rats (18 months subcutaneous treatment) showed no neoplastic effect of Cromolyn Sodium.

No evidence of chromosomal damage or cytotoxicity was obtained in various mutagenesis studies.

No evidence of impaired fertility was shown in laboratory animal reproduction studies.

Pregnancy: Pregnancy Category B. Reproduction studies with Cromolyn Sodium administered parenterally to pregnant mice, rats, and rabbits in doses up to 338 times the human clinical dose produced no evidence of fetal malformations. Adverse fetal effects (increased resorption and decreased fetal weight) were noted only at the very high parenteral doses that produced maternal toxicity. There are, however, no adequate and well controlled studies in pregnant women.

Because animal reproduction studies are not always predictive of human response, this drug should be used during pregnancy only if clearly needed.

Drug Interaction During Pregnancy: Cromolyn Sodium and isoproterenol were studied following subcutaneous injections in pregnant mice. Cromolyn Sodium alone in doses of 60 to 540 mg/kg (38 to 338 times the human dose) did not cause significant increases in resorptions or major malformations. Isoproterenol alone at a dose of 2.7 mg/kg (90 times the human dose) increased both resorptions and malformations. The addition of Cromolyn Sodium (338 times the human dose) to isoproterenol (90 times the human dose) appears to have increased the incidence of both resorptions and malformations.

Nursing Mothers: It is not known whether this drug is excreted in human milk. Because many drugs are excreted in human milk, caution should be exercised when Cromolyn Sodium is administered to a nursing woman.

Pediatric Use: Animal studies suggest increased risk of toxicity in premature animals when given doses much higher than clinically recommended. In term infants up to six months of age, available clinical data suggest that the dose should not exceed 20 mg/kg/day. The use of this product in children less than two years should be reserved for patients with severe disease in which the potential benefits clearly outweigh the risks.

ADVERSE REACTIONS
Most of the adverse events reported in mastocytosis patients have been transient and could represent symptoms of the disease. The most frequently reported adverse events in mastocytosis patients who have received Cromolyn Sodium during clinical studies were headache and diarrhea. Each occurred in 4 of the 87 patients. Pruritus, nausea, and myalgia were each reported in 3 patients and abdominal pain, rash, and irritability in 2 patients each. One report of malaise was also recorded.

A generally similar profile of adverse events has been reported during studies in other clinical conditions. Additional reports which have been received during the course of these studies and spontaneous reports during foreign marketing include: flushing, urticaria/angioedema, arthralgia, dizziness, fatigue, paresthesia, taste perversion, migraine, psychosis, anxiety, depression, insomnia, behavior change, esophagospasm, flatulence, dysphagia, hepatic function test abnormal, edema, dyspnea, polycythemia, neutropenia, dysuria, hallucinations, skin erythema and burning, burning mouth and throat, stiffness and weakness of the legs, and postprandial light-headedness and lethargy. These events are infrequent, the majority representing only a single report, and in many cases the causal relationship to Cromolyn Sodium is uncertain.

DOSAGE AND ADMINISTRATION
NOT FOR INHALATION. SEE DIRECTIONS FOR USE.
The usual starting dose is as follows:

Adults: Two capsules four times daily one-half hour before meals and at bedtime.

Premature to Term Infants: Not recommended.

Term to 2 years: 20 mg/kg/day in four divided doses. Use of this product in children less than 2 years is not recommended and should be attempted only in those patients with severe incapacitating diseases where the benefits clearly outweigh the risks.

Children 2-12 years: One capsule four times daily one-half hour before meals and bedtime.

If satisfactory control of symptoms is not achieved within two to three weeks the dosage may be increased but should not exceed 40 mg/kg/day (30 mg/kg/day for children six months to two years).

Patients should be advised that the effect of Cromolyn Sodium therapy is dependent upon its administration at regular intervals, as directed.

Maintenance Dose: Once a therapeutic response has been achieved the dose may be reduced to the minimum required to maintain the patient with a lower degree of symptomatology. To prevent relapses, the dosage should be maintained.

Administration: Cromolyn Sodium should be administered as a solution in water at least ½ hour before meals after preparation according to the following directions:

1. Open capsule(s) and pour powder contents of capsule(s) into ½ glass of hot water.
2. Stir until completely dissolved (clear solution).
3. Add equal quantity of cold water while stirring.
4. DO NOT MIX WITH FRUIT JUICE, MILK OR FOODS.
5. Drink all of the liquid.
Keep tightly closed and out of the reach of children. Store between 15°-30°C (59°-86°F).

➤ SHOWN IN PRODUCT IDENTIFICATION GUIDE

HOW SUPPLIED
CAPSULE: 100 MG

BRAND/MANUFACTURER	NDC	SIZE	AWP
○ **BRAND**			
GASTROCROM: Fisons Presc	00585-0677-01	100s	$94.10

Crotamiton

DESCRIPTION

Crotamiton USP is a scabicidal and antipruitic agent available as a cream or lotion for topical use only. Crotamiton provides 10% (w/w) of the synthetic, Crotamiton USP, in a vanishing-cream or emollient-lotion base containing: water, petrolatum, propylene glycol, steareth-2, cetyl alcohol, dimethicone, laureth-23, fragrance, magnesium aluminum silicate, carbomer-934, sodium hydroxide, diazolidinyl urea, methylchloroisothiazolinone, methylisothiazolinone and magnesium nitrate. In addition, the cream contains glyceryl stearate. Crotamiton is N-ethyl-N-(o-methylphenyl)-2-butenamide.

Crotamiton is a colorless to slightly yellowish oil, having a faint amine-like odor. It is miscible with alcohol and with methanol. Crotamiton is a mixture of the *cis* and *trans* isomers. Its molecular weight is 203.28.

Following is its chemical structure:

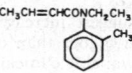

CLINICAL PHARMACOLOGY

Crotamiton has scabicidal and antipruritic actions. The mechanisms of these actions are not known.

INDICATIONS AND USAGE

For eradication of scabies (*Sarcoptes scabiei*) and for symptomatic treatment of pruritic skin.

CONTRAINDICATIONS

Crotamitin should not be applied topically to patients who develop a sensitivity or are allergic to it or who manifest a primary irritation response to topical medications.

WARNINGS

If severe irritation or sensitization develops, treatment with this product should be discontinued and appropriate therapy instituted.

PRECAUTIONS

General: Crotamiton should not be applied in the eyes or mouth because it may cause irritation. It should not be applied to acutely inflamed skin or raw or weeping surfaces until the acute inflammation has subsided.

Information for Patients: See "Directions for patients with scabies."

Drug Interactions: None known.

Carcinogenesis, Mutagenesis, Impairment of Fertility: Long-term carcinogenicity studies in animals have not been conducted.

Pregnancy (Category C): Animal reproduction studies have not been conducted with Crotamiton. It is also not known whether Crotamiton can cause fetal harm when applied topically to a pregnant woman or can affect reproduction capacity. Crotamiton should be given to a pregnant woman only if clearly needed.

Pediatric Use: Safety and effectiveness in children have not been established.

ADVERSE REACTIONS

Allergic sensitivity or primary irritation reactions may occur in some patients.

OVERDOSAGE

There is no specific information on the effect of overtreatment with repeated topical applications in humans. Acute toxicity (after accidental oral administration in children): Highest known doses ingested: Cream: children—2 g (age 1½ years); Lotion: 1 ounce (age 2 years). A death was reported but cause was not confirmed.

Oral LD_{50} in animals (mg/kg): rats, 2212; mice, 2011.

Signs and Symptoms (of Oral Ingestion): Burning sensation in the mouth, irritation of the buccal, esophageal and gastric mucosa, nausea, vomiting, abdominal pain.

Treatment: There is no specific antidote if taken orally. General measures to eliminate the drug and reduce its absorption, combined with symptomatic treatment, are recommended.

DOSAGE AND ADMINISTRATION

LOTION: Shake well before using— *In Scabies*: Thoroughly massage into the skin of the whole body from the chin down, paying particular attention to all folds and creases. A second application is advisable 24 hours later. Clothing and bed linen should be changed the next morning. A cleansing bath should be taken 48 hours after the last application. *In Pruritis*: Massage gently into affected areas until medication is completely absorbed. Repeat as needed.

Store at room temperature.

DIRECTIONS FOR PATIENTS WITH SCABIES

1. Take a routine bath or shower. Thoroughly massage Crotamiton cream or lotion into the skin from the chin to the toes including folds and creases.
   2. A second application is advisable 24 hours later.
   3. This 60 gram tube or bottle is sufficient for two applications.
   4. Clothing and bed linen should be changed the next day. Contaminated clothing and bed linen may be dry-cleaned, or washed in the hot cycle of the washing machine.
   5. A cleansing bath should be taken 48 hours after the last application.

HOW SUPPLIED
CREAM: 10%

BRAND/MANUFACTURER	NDC	SIZE	AWP
◆ **BRAND**			
EURAX: Westwood-Squibb	00072-2103-60	60 gm	$9.91

LOTION: 10%

AVERAGE UNIT PRICE (AVAILABLE SIZES)			
BRAND	$0.16		

BRAND/MANUFACTURER	NDC	SIZE	AWP
◆ **BRAND**			
EURAX: Westwood-Squibb	00072-2203-60	60 ml	$10.57
	00072-2203-16	480 ml	$68.86

Crystodigin SEE DIGITOXIN

C-Solve-2 SEE ERYTHROMYCIN, TOPICAL

C/T/S SEE CLINDAMYCIN, TOPICAL

Cuprimine SEE PENICILLAMINE

Curretab SEE MEDROXYPROGESTERONE ACETATE, ORAL

Cutivate SEE FLUTICASONE PROPIONATE

CVC Heparin Flush SEE HEPARIN

Cyclandelate

DESCRIPTION

Each 200 mg capsule contains 200 mg of Cyclandelate. Each 400 mg capsule contains 400 mg Cyclandelate. Cyclandelate is a white amorphous powder having a faint menthol-like odor.

Following is its chemical structure:

ACTIONS

Cyclandelate is an orally acting vasodilator. The activity of this drug, as measured by pharmacological tests against various types of smooth-muscle spasm produced by acetylcholine, histamine, and barium chloride, exceeds that of papaverine, particularly in regards to the neurotropic component produced by acetylcholine. Cyclandelate is musculotropic, acting directly on vascular smooth muscle with no significant adrenergic simulating or blocking actions. The drug is not intended to substitute for other appropriate medical or surgical programs in the treatment of peripheral or cerebral vascular disease.

INDICATIONS

Based on a review of this drug by National Academy of Sciences-National Research Council and/or other information, FDA has classified the indications as follows: *"Possibly" effective*: Cyclandelate is indicated for adjunctive therapy in intermittent claudication; arteriosclerosis obliterans; thrombophlebitis (to control associated vasospasm and muscular ischemia); nocturnal leg cramps; Raynaud's phenomenon, and for selected cases of ischemic cerebral-vascular disease.

Final classification of the less-than-effective indications requires further investigation.

CONTRAINDICATIONS
Cyclandelate is contraindicated in cases of known hypersensitivity to the drug.

WARNINGS
1. In patients with severe obliterative coronary-artery or cerebral-vascular disease, Cyclandelate should be used with extreme caution since there is a possibility that these diseased areas may be compromised by the vasodilatory effects of Cyclandelate elsewhere.

2. Use in Pregnancy: The safety of Cyclandelate for use in pregnancy or lactation has not been established; therefore, it should not be used in pregnant women or in women of child bearing age unless in the judgment of the physician, its use is deemed absolutely essential to the welfare of the patient.

3. Although no prolongation of bleeding time has been demonstrated in humans in therapeutic dosages, it has been demonstrated in animals at very large doses. Therefore, the hazard of a prolonged bleeding time should be carefully considered when administering Cyclandelate to a patient with active bleeding or a bleeding tendency.

PRECAUTIONS
Since Cyclandelate is a vasodilator, it should be used with caution in patients having glaucoma.

ADVERSE REACTIONS
Gastrointestinal distress (pyrosis, pain and eructation) may occur with Cyclandelate. These symptoms occur infrequently and are usually mild. Relief can often be obtained by taking the medication with meals or by the concommitant use of antacids.

Mild flush, headache, feeling of weakness, or tachycardia may occur, especially during the first week of administration.

DOSAGE AND ADMINISTRATION
It is often advantageous to initiate therapy at higher dosage; e.g.: 1200 mg to 1600 mg per day, given in divided dosage before meals and at bedtime. When a clinical response is noted, the dosage can be decreased by 200 mg decrements until the maintenance dosage is reached. The usual maintenance dosage of cyclandelate is between 400 mg and 800 mg per day given in two to four divided doses.

Although objective signs of therapeutic benefit may be rapid and dramatic, more often, this improvement occurs gradually over weeks of therapy. It is strongly recommended that the patient be educated to the fact that prolonged use of Cyclandelate may be necessary. Short-term use of Cyclandelate is rarely beneficial, nor is it likely to be of any permanent value.

Keep tightly closed. Protect from light.

Dispense in tight, light-resistant container.

HOW SUPPLIED
CAPSULE: 200 MG

BRAND/MANUFACTURER	NDC	SIZE	AWP
○ **BRAND**			
CYCLOSPASMOL: Wyeth-Ayerst	00008-4124-01	100s	$49.24
○ **GENERICS**			
Lannett	00527-0534-01	100s	$3.68
CMC-Cons	00223-0706-01	100s	$5.25
Parmed	00349-8915-01	100s	$5.76
Major	00904-0238-60	100s	$5.90
Pioneer	60104-4001-02	100s	$5.94
Goldline	00182-1540-01	100s	$13.50
Qualitest	00603-3075-21	100s	$13.50
Rugby	00536-3531-01	100s	$13.52
Amide	52152-0082-02	100s	$14.00
Aligen	00405-4284-01	100s	$14.21
Moore,H.L.	00839-1217-06	100s	$14.30
Major	00904-0238-61	100s ud	$12.93
Auro	55829-0622-10	100s ud	$16.25
Pioneer	60104-4001-06	500s	$24.75
Lannett	00527-0534-10	1000s	$29.00
Major	00904-0238-80	1000s	$39.80
Pioneer	60104-4001-08	1000s	$41.25
CMC-Cons	00223-0706-02	1000s	$50.00
Amide	52152-0082-05	1000s	$121.80
Moore,H.L.	00839-1217-16	1000s	$122.03

CAPSULE: 400 MG

BRAND/MANUFACTURER	NDC	SIZE	AWP
○ **BRAND**			
CYCLOSPASMOL: Wyeth-Ayerst	00008-4148-04	100s	$89.03
○ **GENERICS**			
Lannett	00527-0563-01	100s	$6.20
Major	00904-0239-60	100s	$7.00
Pioneer	60104-4002-02	100s	$7.70
CMC-Cons	00223-0707-01	100s	$8.00
Parmed	00349-8916-01	100s	$10.50
Goldline	00182-1541-01	100s	$17.55

BRAND/MANUFACTURER	NDC	SIZE	AWP
Qualitest	00603-3076-21	100s	$17.75
Aligen	00405-4285-01	100s	$17.80
Rugby	00536-3529-01	100s	$17.87
Amide	52152-0083-02	100s	$18.60
Moore,H.L.	00839-6027-06	100s	$18.89
Major	00904-0239-61	100s ud	$14.15
Auro	55829-0623-10	100s ud	$20.95
Pioneer	60104-4002-06	500s	$31.02
Lannett	00527-0563-10	1000s	$49.20
Major	00904-0239-80	1000s	$50.95
Pioneer	60104-4002-08	1000s	$52.69
Parmed	00349-2310-10	1000s	$55.00
CMC-Cons	00223-0707-02	1000s	$77.50
Amide	52152-0083-05	1000s	$162.75
Moore,H.L.	00839-6027-16	1000s	$163.07

Cyclobenzaprine Hydrochloride

DESCRIPTION
Cyclobenzaprine Hydrochloride is a white, crystalline tricyclic amine salt with the empirical formula $C_{20}H_{21}N \cdot HCl$ and a molecular weight of 311.9. It has a melting point of 217°C, and a pK_a of 8.47 at 25°C. It is freely soluble in water and alcohol, sparingly soluble in isopropanol, and insoluble in hydrocarbon solvents. If aqueous solutions are made alkaline, the free base separates. Cyclobenzaprine Hydrochloride is designated chemically as 3-(5H-dibenzo[a,d]cyclohepten-5-ylidene)-N,N-dimethyl-1-propanamine hydrochloride.

Cyclobenzaprine is supplied as 10 mg tablets for oral administration.

Following is its chemical structure:

$$CHCH_2CH_2N(CH_3)_2 \qquad \cdot \ HCl$$

CLINICAL PHARMACOLOGY
Cyclobenzaprine Hydrochloride relieves skeletal muscle spasm of local origin without interfering with muscle function. It is ineffective in muscle spasm due to central nervous system disease. Cyclobenzaprine reduced or abolished skeletal muscle hyperactivity in several animal models. Animal studies indicate that Cyclobenzaprine does not act at the neuromuscular junction or directly on skeletal muscle. Such studies show that Cyclobenzaprine acts primarily within the central nervous system at brain stem as opposed to spinal cord levels, although its action on the latter may contribute to its overall skeletal muscle relaxant activity. Evidence suggests that the net effect of Cyclobenzaprine is a reduction of tonic somatic motor activity, influencing both gamma (γ) and alpha (α) motor systems.

Pharmacological studies in animals showed a similarity between the effects of Cyclobenzaprine and the structurally related tricyclic antidepressants, including reserpine antagonism, norepinephrine potentiation, potent peripheral and central anticholinergic effects, and sedation. Cyclobenzaprine caused slight to moderate increase in heart rate in animals.

Cyclobenzaprine is well absorbed after oral administration, but there is a large intersubject variation in plasma levels. Cyclobenzaprine is eliminated quite slowly with a half-life as long as one to three days. It is highly bound to plasma proteins, is extensively metabolized primarily to glucuronide-like conjugates, and is excreted primarily via the kidneys. No significant effect on plasma levels or bioavailability of Cyclobenzaprine or aspirin was noted when single or multiple doses of the two drugs were administered concomitantly. Concomitant administration of Cyclobenzaprine and aspirin is usually well tolerated and no unexpected or serious clinical or laboratory adverse effects have been observed. No studies have been performed to indicate whether Cyclobenzaprine enhances the clinical effect of aspirin or other analgesics, or whether analgesics enhance the clinical effect of Cyclobenzaprine in acute musculoskeletal conditions.

CLINICAL STUDIES
Controlled clinical studies show that Cyclobenzaprine significantly improves the signs and symptoms of skeletal muscle spasm as compared with placebo. The clinical responses include improvement in muscle spasm as determined by palpation, reduction in local pain and tenderness, increased range of motion, and less restriction in activities of daily living. When daily observations were made, clinical improvement was observed as early as the first day of therapy.

Eight double-blind controlled clinical studies were performed in 642 patients comparing Cyclobenzaprine, diazepam, and placebo. Muscle spasm, local pain and tenderness, limitation of motion, and restriction in activities of daily living were evaluated. In three of these studies there was a significantly greater improvement with Cyclobenzaprine than with diazepam, while in the other studies the improvement following both treatments was comparable.

Although the frequency and severity of adverse reactions observed in patients treated with Cyclobenzaprine were comparable to those observed in patients treated with diazepam, dry mouth was observed more frequently in patients treated with Cyclobenzaprine and dizziness more frequently in those treated with diazepam. The incidence of drowsiness, the most frequent adverse reaction, was similar with both drugs. Analysis of the data from controlled studies shows that Cyclobenzaprine produces clinical improvement whether or not sedation occurs.

➤ **SHOWN IN PRODUCT IDENTIFICATION GUIDE**

INDICATIONS AND USAGE

Cyclobenzaprine is indicated as an adjunct to rest and physical therapy for relief of muscle spasm associated with acute, painful musculoskeletal conditions.

Improvement is manifested by relief of muscle spasm and its associated signs and symptoms, namely, pain, tenderness, limitation of motion, and restriction in activities of daily living.

Cyclobenzaprine should be used only for short periods (up to two or three weeks) because adequate evidence of effectiveness for more prolonged use is not available and because muscle spasm associated with acute, painful musculoskeletal conditions is generally of short duration and specific therapy for longer periods is seldom warranted.

Cyclobenzaprine has not been found effective in the treatment of spasticity associated with cerebral or spinal cord disease, or in children with cerebral palsy.

CONTRAINDICATIONS

Hypersensitivity to the drug.

Concomitant use of monoamine oxidase inhibitors or within 14 days after their discontinuation.

Acute recovery phase of myocardial infarction, and patients with arrhythmias, heart block or conduction disturbances, or congestive heart failure.

Hyperthyroidism.

WARNINGS

Cyclobenzaprine is closely related to the tricyclic antidepressants, e.g., amitriptyline and imipramine. In short term studies for indications other than muscle spasm associated with acute musculoskeletal conditions, and usually at doses somewhat greater than those recommended for skeletal muscle spasm, some of the more serious central nervous system reactions noted with the tricyclic antidepressants have occurred (see *"Warnings"*, below, and *"Adverse Reactions"*).

Cyclobenzaprine may interact with monoamine oxidase (MAO) inhibitors. Hyperpyretic crisis, severe convulsions, and deaths have occurred in patients receiving tricyclic antidepressants and MAO inhibitor drugs.

Tricyclic antidepressants have been reported to produce arrhythmias, sinus tachycardia, prolongation of the conduction time leading to myocardial infarction and stroke. Cyclobenzaprine may enhance the effects of alcohol, barbiturates, and other CNS depressants.

PRECAUTIONS

GENERAL

Because of its atropine-like action Cyclobenzaprine should be used with caution in patients with a history of urinary retention, angle-closure glaucoma, increased intraocular pressure, and in patients taking anticholinergic medication.

INFORMATION FOR PATIENTS

Cyclobenzaprine may impair mental and/or physical abilities required for performance of hazardous tasks, such as operating machinery or driving a motor vehicle.

DRUG INTERACTIONS

Cyclobenzaprine may enhance the effects of alcohol, barbiturates, and other CNS depressants.

Tricyclic antidepressants may block the antihypertensive action of guanethidine and similarly acting compounds.

CARCINOGENESIS, MUTAGENESIS, IMPAIRMENT OF FERTILITY

In rats treated with Cyclobenzaprine for up to 67 weeks at doses of approximately 5 to 40 times the maximum recommended human dose, pale, sometimes enlarged, livers were noted and there was a dose-related hepatocyte vacuolation with lipidosis. In the higher dose groups this microscopic change was seen after 26 weeks and even earlier in rats which died prior to 26 weeks; at lower doses, the change was not seen until after 26 weeks.

Cyclobenzaprine did not affect the onset, incidence or distribution of neoplasia in an 81-week study in the mouse or in a 105-week study in the rat.

At oral doses of up to 10 times the human dose, Cyclobenzaprine did not adversely affect the reproductive performance or fertility of male or female rats. Cyclobenzaprine did not demonstrate mutagenic activity in the male mouse at dose levels of up to 20 times the human dose.

PREGNANCY

Pregnancy Category B: Reproduction studies have been performed in rats, mice and rabbits at doses up to 20 times the human dose, and have revealed no evidence of impaired fertility or harm to the fetus due to Cyclobenzaprine. There are, however, no adequate and well-controlled studies in pregnant women. Because animal reproduction studies are not always predictive of human response, this drug should be used during pregnancy only if clearly needed.

NURSING MOTHERS

It is not known whether this drug is excreted in human milk. Because Cyclobenzaprine is closely related to the tricyclic antidepressants, some of which are known to be excreted in human milk, caution should be exercised when Cyclobenzaprine is administered to a nursing woman.

PEDIATRIC USE

Safety and effectiveness of Cyclobenzaprine in children below the age of 15 have not been established.

ADVERSE REACTIONS

The following list of adverse reactions is based on the experience in 473 patients treated with Cyclobenzaprine in controlled clinical studies, 7607 patients in the post-marketing surveillance program, and reports received since the drug was marketed. The overall incidence of adverse reactions among patients in the surveillance program was less than the incidence in the controlled clinical studies.

The adverse reactions reported most frequently with Cyclobenzaprine were drowsiness, dry mouth and dizziness. The incidence of these common adverse reactions was lower in the surveillance program than in the controlled clinical studies:

	Clinical Studies	Surveillance Program
drowsiness	39%	16%
dry mouth	27%	7%
dizziness	11%	3%

Among the less frequent adverse reactions, there was no appreciable difference in incidence in controlled clinical studies or in the surveillance program. Adverse reactions which were reported in 1% to 3% of the patients were: fatigue/tiredness, asthenia, nausea, constipation, dyspepsia, unpleasant taste, blurred vision, headache, nervousness, and confusion.

INCIDENCE LESS THAN 1 IN 100

The following adverse reactions have been reported at an incidence of less than 1 in 100:

Body as a Whole: Syncope; malaise.

Cardiovascular: Tachycardia; arrhythmia; vasodilatation; palpitation; hypotension.

Digestive: Vomiting; anorexia; diarrhea; gastrointestinal pain; gastritis; thirst; flatulence; edema of the tongue; abnormal liver function and rare reports of hepatitis, jaundice and cholestasis.

Hypersensitivity: Anaphylaxis; angioedema; pruritus; facial edema; urticaria; rash.

Musculoskeletal: Local weakness.

Nervous System and Psychiatric: Ataxia; vertigo; dysarthria; tremors; hypertonia; convulsions; muscle twitching; disorientation; insomnia; depressed mood; abnormal sensations; anxiety; agitation; abnormal thinking and dreaming; hallucinations; excitement; paresthesia; diplopia.

Skin: Sweating.

Special Senses: Ageusia; tinnitus.

Urogenital: Urinary frequency and/or retention.

CAUSAL RELATIONSHIP UNKNOWN

Other reactions, reported rarely for Cyclobenzaprine under circumstances where a causal relationship could not be established or reported for other tricyclic drugs, are listed to serve as alerting information to physicians:

Body as a Whole: Chest pain; edema.

Cardiovascular: Hypertension; myocardial infarction; heart block; stroke.

Digestive: Paralytic ileus; tongue discoloration; stomatitis; parotid swelling.

Endocrine: Inappropriate ADH syndrome.

Hematic and Lymphatic: Purpura; bone marrow depression; leukopenia; eosinophilia; thrombocytopenia.

Metabolic, Nutritional and Immune: Elevation and lowering of blood sugar levels; weight gain or loss.

Musculoskeletal: Myalgia.

Nervous System and Psychiatric: Decreased or increased libido; abnormal gait; delusions; peripheral neuropathy; Bell's palsy; alteration in EEG patterns; extrapyramidal symptoms.

Respiratory: Dyspnea.

Skin: Photosensitization; alopecia.

Urogenital: Impaired urination; dilatation of urinary tract; impotence; testicular swelling; gynecomastia; breast enlargement; galactorrhea.

DRUG ABUSE AND DEPENDENCE

Pharmacologic similarities among the tricyclic drugs require that certain withdrawal symptoms be considered when Cyclobenzaprine is administered, even though they have not been reported to occur with this drug. Abrupt cessation of treatment after prolonged administration may produce nausea, headache, and malaise. These are not indicative of addiction.

OVERDOSAGE

Manifestations: High doses may cause temporary confusion, disturbed concentration, transient visual hallucinations, agitation, hyperactive reflexes, muscle rigidity, vomiting, or hyperpyrexia, in addition to anything listed under *"Adverse Reactions"*. Based on the known pharmacologic actions of the drug, overdosage may cause drowsiness, hypothermia, tachycardia and other cardiac rhythm abnormalities such as bundle branch block, ECG evidence of impaired conduction, and congestive heart failure. Other manifestations may be dilated pupils, convulsions, severe hypotension, stupor, and coma.

The acute oral LD_{50} of Cyclobenzaprine is approximately 338 and 425 mg/kg in mice and rats, respectively.

Treatment: Treatment is symptomatic and supportive. Empty the stomach as quickly as possible by emesis, followed by gastric lavage. After gastric lavage, activated charcoal may be administered. Twenty to 30 g of activated charcoal may be given every four to six hours during the first 24 to 48 hours after ingestion. An

---

◆ RATED THERAPEUTICALLY EQUIVALENT; ◇ THERAPEUTIC EQUIVALENCE UNCONFIRMED; ○ UNRATED

ECG should be taken and close monitoring of cardiac function must be instituted if there is any evidence of dysrhythmia. Maintenance of an open airway, adequate fluid intake, and regulation of body temperature are necessary.

The intravenous administration of 1-3 mg of physostigmine salicylate is reported to reverse symptoms of poisoning by atropine and other drugs with anticholinergic activity. Physostigmine may be helpful in the treatment of Cyclobenzaprine overdose. Because physostigmine is rapidly metabolized, the dosage of physostigmine should be repeated as required, particularly if life-threatening signs such as arrhythmias, convulsions, and deep coma recur or persist after the initial dosage of physostigmine. Because physostigmine itself may be toxic, it is not recommended for routine use. Standard medical measures should be used to manage circulatory shock and metabolic acidosis. Cardiac arrhythmias may be treated with neostigmine, pyridostigmine, or propranolol. When signs of cardiac failure occur, the use of a short-acting digitalis preparation should be considered. Close monitoring of cardiac function for not less than five days is advisable.

Anticonvulsants may be given to control seizures.

Dialysis is probably of no value because of low plasma concentrations of the drug.

Since overdosage is often deliberate, patients may attempt suicide by other means during the recovery phase. Deaths by deliberate or accidental overdosage have occurred with this class of drugs.

DOSAGE AND ADMINISTRATION

The usual dosage of Cyclobenzaprine is 10 mg three times a day, with a range of 20 to 40 mg a day in divided doses. Dosage should not exceed 60 mg a day. Use of Cyclobenzaprine for periods longer than two or three weeks is not recommended. (See "Indications and Usage".)

HOW SUPPLIED
TABLETS: 10 MG

AVERAGE UNIT PRICE (AVAILABLE SIZES)		GENERIC A-RATED AVERAGE PRICE (GAAP)	
BRAND	$0.95	100s	$81.00
GENERIC	$0.77	500s	$361.10
HCFA FUL (100s ea)	$0.27	1000s	$673.82

BRAND/MANUFACTURER	NDC	SIZE	AWP
◆ BRAND			
➤ FLEXERIL: Merck	00006-0931-68	100s	$92.93
	00006-0931-28	100s ud	$97.35
◆ GENERICS			
Schein	00364-2348-30	30s	$24.95
UDL	51079-0644-97	45s	$60.00
Qualitest	00603-3077-21	100s	$70.66
Duramed	51285-0852-02	100s	$73.00
Watson	52544-0418-01	100s	$73.99
Schein	00364-2348-01	100s	$74.00
Goldline	00182-1919-01	100s	$74.00
➤ West Point	59591-0156-68	100s	$75.90
Martec	52555-0441-01	100s	$76.20
Aligen	00405-4290-01	100s	$78.20
Warner Chilcott	00047-0057-24	100s	$78.25
URL	00677-1429-01	100s	$78.35
Rugby	00536-4840-01	100s	$78.39
Moore,H.L.	00839-7711-06	100s	$78.64
Major	00904-2221-60	100s	$79.25
Major	00904-7586-60	100s	$79.25
Major	00904-7809-60	100s	$79.25
➤ Mylan	00378-0751-01	100s	$79.95
Geneva	00781-1324-01	100s	$79.97
Geneva	00781-1324-13	100s	$83.94
Invamed	52189-0252-24	100s	$87.10
Major	00904-7586-61	100s	$88.42
Raway	00686-0644-20	100s ud	$78.00
Schein	00364-2348-90	100s ud	$80.00
Vangard	00615-3520-13	100s ud	$85.00
Major	00904-2221-61	100s ud	$88.42
Goldline	00182-1919-89	100s ud	$96.00
Medirex	57480-0461-01	100s ud	$96.25
UDL	51079-0644-20	100s ud	$96.90
Schein	00364-2348-05	500s	$336.75
Goldline	00182-1919-05	500s	$350.00
Major	00904-2221-40	500s	$352.25
Major	00904-7586-40	500s	$352.25
Major	00904-7809-40	500s	$352.25
Martec	52555-0441-05	500s	$356.80
URL	00677-1429-05	500s	$359.00
Watson	52544-0418-05	500s	$365.08
Qualitest	00603-3077-28	500s	$365.08
Rugby	00536-4840-05	500s	$372.60
Geneva	00781-1324-05	500s	$379.86
Warner Chilcott	00047-0057-30	500s	$391.25
Major	00904-7586-80	1000s	$528.40
Major	00904-7809-80	1000s	$528.40
Aligen	00405-4290-03	1000s	$602.00
Schein	00364-2348-02	1000s	$639.75
Qualitest	00603-3077-32	1000s	$670.43
Rugby	00536-4840-10	1000s	$670.68
➤ West Point	59591-0156-82	1000s	$683.00
Watson	52544-0418-10	1000s	$725.00
Duramed	51285-0852-05	1000s	$727.00
Invamed	52189-0252-30	1000s	$727.00

BRAND/MANUFACTURER	NDC	SIZE	AWP
➤ Mylan	00378-0751-10	1000s	$727.99
Moore,H.L.	00839-7566-16	1000s	$764.99
Moore,H.L.	00839-7711-16	1000s	$764.99

Cyclocort SEE AMCINONIDE

Cyclogyl SEE CYCLOPENTOLATE HYDROCHLORIDE

Cyclomydril SEE CYCLOPENTOLATE HYDROCHLORIDE WITH PHENYLEPHRINE HYDROCHLORIDE

Cyclopentolate Hydrochloride

DESCRIPTION
Cyclopentolate Hydrochoride is an anticholinergic prepared as a sterile, borate buffered solution for topical ocular use. It is supplied in three strengths.

Its molecular formula is $C_{17}H_{25}NO_3.HCl$ and molecular weight is 327.85.

Established name: Cyclopentolate Hydrochloride

Chemical name: 2-(Dimethylamino)ethyl 1-hydroxy-α-phenylcyclopentaneacetate hydrochloride

Each mL contains: Cyclopentolate Hydrochloride 0.5%, 1% or 2%.

Following is its chemical structure:

$$\text{CH—COOCH}_2\text{CH}_2\text{N(CH}_3)_2 \cdot \text{HCl}$$

CLINICAL PHARMACOLOGY
This anticholinergic preparation blocks the responses of the sphincter muscle of the iris and the accommodative muscle of the ciliary body to cholinergic stimulation, producing pupillary dilation (mydriasis) and paralysis of accommodation (cycloplegia). It acts rapidly, but has a shorter duration than atropine. Maximal cycloplegia occurs within 25 to 75 minutes after instillation. Complete recovery of accommodation usually takes 6 to 24 hours. Complete recovery from mydriasis in some individuals may require several days.

INDICATIONS AND USAGE
Cyclopentolate Hydrochloride is used to produce mydriasis and cycloplegia.

CONTRAINDICATIONS
Should not be used when narrow-angle glaucoma or anatomical narrow angles are present, or where there is hypersensitivity to any component of this preparation.

WARNINGS
For topical use only—not for injection. This preparation may cause CNS disturbances. This is especially true in younger age groups, but may occur at any age, especially with the stronger solutions. Premature and small infants are especially prone to CNS and cardiopulmonary side effects from systemic absorption of Cyclopentolate. To minimize absorption, use only 1 drop of 0.5% Cyclopentolate Hydrochloride solution per eye, followed by pressure applied over the nasolacrimal sac for two to three minutes. Observe infants closely for at least 30 minutes following instillation.

PRECAUTIONS
General: To avoid inducing angle closure glaucoma, an estimation of the depth of the angle of the anterior chamber should be made. The lacrimal sac should be compressed by digital pressure for two to three minutes after instillation to avoid excessive systemic absorption. Caution should be observed when considering use of this medication in the presence of Down's syndrome and in those predisposed to angle-closure glaucoma.

Information for Patients: Do not touch dropper tip to any surface as this may contaminate the solution. A transient burning sensation may occur upon instillation. Patients should be advised not to drive or engage in other hazardous activities while pupils are dilated. Patients may experience sensitivity to light and should protect eyes in bright illumination during dilation. Parents should be warned not to get this preparation in their child's mouth and to wash their own hands and the child's hands following administration.

Drug Interactions: Cyclopentolate may interfere with the anti-glaucoma action of carbachol or pilocarpine; also, concurrent use of these medications may antagonize the antiglaucoma and miotic actions of ophthalmic cholinesterase inhibitors.

Carcinogenesis, Mutagenesis, and Impairment of Fertility: Studies in animals or humans have not been conducted to evaluate the potential of these effects.

➤ **SHOWN IN PRODUCT IDENTIFICATION GUIDE**

Pregnancy Category C: Animal reproduction studies have not been conducted with Cyclopentolate. It is also not known whether Cyclopentolate can cause fetal harm when administered to a pregnant woman or can affect reproduction capacity. Cyclopentolate should be administered to a pregnant woman only if clearly needed.

Nursing Mothers: It is not known whether this drug is excreted in human milk. Because many drugs are excreted in human milk, caution should be exercised when Cyclopentolate Hydrochloride is administered to a nursing woman.

Pediatrics: Increased susceptibility to Cyclopentolate has been reported in infants, young children, and in children with spastic paralysis or brain damage. Therefore, Cyclopentolate should be used with great caution in these patients. Feeding intolerance may follow ophthalmic use of this product in neonates. It is recommended that feeding be withheld for four (4) hours after examination. Do not use in concentrations higher than 0.5% in small infants (see *"Warnings"*).

Geriatrics: In the elderly and others where increased intraocular pressure may be encountered, mydriatics and cycloplegics should be used cautiously.

ADVERSE REACTIONS
Ocular: Increased intraocular pressure, burning, photophobia, blurred vision, irritation, hyperemia, conjunctivitis, blepharoconjunctivitis, punctate keratitis, synechiae.

Systemic: Use of Cyclopentolate has been associated with psychotic reactions and behavioral disturbances, usually in children, especially with 2% concentration. These disturbances include ataxia, incoherent speech, restlessness, hallucinations, hyperactivity, seizures, disorientation as to time and place, and failure to recognize people. This drug produces reactions similar to those of other anticholinergic drugs, but the central nervous system manifestations as noted above are more common. Other toxic manifestations of anticholinergic drugs are skin rash, abdominal distention in infants, unusual drowsiness, tachycardia, hyperpyrexia, vasodilation, urinary retention, diminished gastrointestinal motility and decreased secretion in salivary and sweat glands, pharynx, bronchii and nasal passages. Severe manifestations of toxicity include coma, medullary paralysis and death.

OVERDOSAGE
Excessive dosage may produce exaggerated symptoms as noted in *"Adverse Reactions."* When administration of the drug product is discontinued, the patient usually recovers spontaneously. In case of severe manifestations of toxicity the antidote of choice is physostigmine salicylate.

Pediatric Dose: As an antidote, slowly inject intravenously 0.5 mg physostigmine salicylate. If toxic symptoms persist and no cholinergic symptoms are produced, repeat at five minute intervals to a maximum cumulative dose of 2 mg.

Adolescent and Adult: As an antidote, slowly inject 2 mg physostigmine salicylate intravenously. A second dose of 1 to 2 mg may be given after 20 minutes if no reversal of toxic manifestations has occurred.[1,2,3]

DOSAGE AND ADMINISTRATION
Adults: One or two drops of 0.5%, 1% or 2% solution in the eye which may be repeated in five to ten minutes if necessary. Complete recovery usually occurs in 24 hours.

Children: One or two drops of 0.5%, 1% or 2% solution in the eye which may be repeated five to ten minutes later by a second application of 0.5% or 1% solution if necessary.

Small Infants: A single instillation of one drop of 0.5% Cyclopentolate Hydrochloride in the eye. To minimize absorption, apply pressure over the nasolacrimal sac for two to three minutes. Observe infant closely for at least 30 minutes following instillation. Individuals with heavily pigmented irides may require higher strengths.

Storage: Store at 8°-27°C (46°-80°F).

REFERENCES
1. Rumack, B. H.: Anticholinergic Poisoning: Treatment with Physostigmine. *Pediatrics* 52(6):449-51, 1973. 2. Duvoisin, R. C. and Katz, R.: Reversal of Central Anticholinergic Syndromes in Man by Physostigmine, *J. Am. Med. Assn.* 206(9): 1963-65, 1968. 3. Grant, W. M.: *Toxicology of the Eye.* Second Edition. Volume 1. Springfield, Illinois, Charles C. Thomas: 1974.

HOW SUPPLIED
DROP: 0.5%

AVERAGE UNIT PRICE (AVAILABLE SIZES)			
BRAND		$2.14	

BRAND/MANUFACTURER	NDC	SIZE	AWP
◆ BRAND			
CYCLOGYL: Alcon Ophthalmic	00065-0395-02	2 ml	$5.69
	00065-0395-05	5 ml	$10.88
	00065-0395-15	15 ml	$20.75

DROP: 1%

AVERAGE UNIT PRICE (AVAILABLE SIZES)		GENERIC A-RATED AVERAGE PRICE (GAAP)	
BRAND	$2.44	15 ml	$7.99
GENERIC	$1.03		

BRAND/MANUFACTURER	NDC	SIZE	AWP
◆ BRAND			
CYCLOGYL: Alcon Ophthalmic	00065-0396-02	2 ml	$6.75
	00065-0396-05	5 ml	$12.44
	00065-0396-15	15 ml	$22.00
◆ GENERICS			
AK-PENTOLATE: Akorn	17478-0100-20	2 ml	$4.38
Bausch&Lomb Pharm	24208-0735-60	5 ml	$4.11
Schein	00364-7362-72	15 ml	$6.50
Steris	00402-0777-15	15 ml	$6.50
Bausch&Lomb Pharm	24208-0735-06	15 ml	$6.76
AK-PENTOLATE: Akorn	17478-0100-12	15 ml	$12.19
Bausch&Lomb Pharm	24208-0735-01	2 ml 12s	$49.68

DROP: 2%

BRAND/MANUFACTURER	NDC	SIZE	AWP
○ BRAND			
CYCLOGYL: Alcon Ophthalmic	00065-0397-02	2 ml	$9.31
	00065-0397-05	5 ml	$15.25
	00065-0397-15	15 ml	$25.88

Cyclopentolate Hydrochloride with Phenylephrine Hydrochloride

DESCRIPTION
Cyclopentolate Hydrochloride/Phenylephrine Hydrochloride is a mydriatic prepared as a sterile topical ophthalmic solution.

The chemical name of Cyclopentolate Hydrochloride is 2-(Dimethylamino)ethyl 1-hydroxy-α-phenylcyclepentaneacetate hydrochloride. The chemical name of Phenylephrine hydrochloride is 3-hydroxy- α[(methylamino)-methyl]-, Benzenemethanol, hydrochloride (R)-.

Each ml contains: Cyclopentolate Hydrochloride 0.2%, Phenylephrine Hydrochloride 1%.

CLINICAL PHARMACOLOGY
Cyclopentolate HCl is an anticholinergic drug and Phenylephrine HCl is an adrenergic drug. This combination induces mydriasis that is considerably greater than that of either drug alone. The concentrations of Cyclopentolate HCl and of Phenylephrine HCl have been selected to induce safe and rapid mydriasis with little or no accompanying cycloplegia.

INDICATIONS AND USAGE
For the production of mydriasis.

CONTRAINDICATION
Do not use in patients with narrow angle glaucoma or with anatomically narrow angles or where there is hypersensitivity to any component of this preparation.

WARNING
Do not touch dropper tip to any surface, as this may contaminate the solution. For topical use only—not for injection. The use of this combination may have an adverse effect on individuals suffering from cardiovascular disease, hypertension, and hyperthyroidism; and it may cause CNS disturbances. Small infants are especially prone to CNS and cardiopulmonary side effects from systemic absorption of Cyclopentolate.

PRECAUTIONS
To avoid inducing angle closure glaucoma, an estimation of the depth of the angle of the anterior chamber should be made. The lacrimal sac should be compressed by digital pressure for two to three minutes after instillation to avoid excessive systemic absorption. The effect of long-term use of this preparation has not been established, therefore it should be restricted to short-term use.

PATIENT WARNING
Patients should be advised not to drive or engage in other hazardous activities while pupils are dilated. Patient may experience sensitivity to light and should protect eyes in bright illumination during dilation. Parents should be warned not to get this preparation in their child's mouth and to wash their own hands and the child's hands following administration. Feeding intolerance may follow ophthalmic use of this product in neonates. It is recommended that feeding be withheld for four (4) hours after examination.

ADVERSE REACTIONS
Increased intraocular pressure. Use of Cyclopentolate has been associated with psychotic reactions and behavioral disturbances in children, especially with 2% concentration. These disturbances include ataxia, incoherent speech, restlessness, hallucinations, hyperactivity, seizures, disorientation as to time and place, and failure to recognize people. This drug produces reactions similar to those of other anticholinergic drugs; however, the central nervous system manifestations as noted above are more common. Other toxic manifestations of anticholinergic

drugs are tachycardia, hyperpyrexia, vasodilation, urinary retention, diminished gastrointestinal motility and decreased secretion in salivary and sweat glands, pharynx, bronchii and nasal passages. Severe manifestations of toxicity include coma, medullary paralysis and death.

OVERDOSAGE

When administration of the drug product is discontinued, the patient usually recovers spontaneously. In case of severe manifestations of toxicity, the antidote of choice is physostigmine salicylate.

Pediatric Dose: As an antidote, slowly inject intravenously 0.5 mg of physostigmine salicylate. If toxic symptoms persist and no cholinergic symptoms are produced repeat at five minute intervals to a maximum dose of 2.0 mg.

Adolescent and Adult Dose: As an antidote, slowly inject intravenously 2.0 mg of physostigmine salicylate. A second dose of 1-2 mg may be given after 20 minutes if no reversal of toxic manifestations has occurred.[1,2,3]

DOSAGE AND ADMINISTRATION

For funduscopy, instill one drop in each eye every five to ten minutes, not to exceed three times, to produce rapid mydriasis, permitting ready visual access to the fundus. Heavily pigmented irides may require larger doses. To minimize absorption in premature and small infants, apply pressure over the nasolacrimal sac for two to three minutes following instillation. Observe infants closely for at least 30 minutes.

Storage: Store at 46° to 80° F.

REFERENCE

1. Rumack. B. H.: Anticholinergic Poisoning: Treatment with Physostigmine. PEDIATRICS 52(6):449-51, 1973. 2. Duvoisin, R. C. and Katz, R.: Reversal of Central Anticholinergic Syndromes in Man by Physostigmine. J. AM. MED. ASSN. 206(9):1963-65, 1968. 3. Grant. W. M.: *Toxicology of the Eye.* Second Edition, Volume 1, Springfield, Illinois, Charles C. Thomas; 1974.

HOW SUPPLIED
DROP: 0.2%-1%

BRAND/MANUFACTURER	NDC	SIZE	AWP
○ BRAND			
CYCLOMYDRIL: Alcon Labs	00065-0359-02	2 ml	$6.75
	00065-0359-05	5 ml	$12.19

Cyclophosphamide

DESCRIPTION

Cyclophosphamide is a synthetic antineoplastic drug chemically related to the nitrogen mustards. Cyclophosphamide is available as a sterile powder for injection, a sterile, lyophilized powder for injection, and tablets for oral administration.

Each vial of powder or lyophilized powder contains:
Cyclophosphamide ....100 mg, 200 mg, 500 mg, 1 gm, or 2 gm

Each tablet contains:
Cyclophosphamide ....25 mg or 50 mg

Cyclophosphamide is a white crystalline powder with the molecular formula $C_7H_{15}Cl_2N_2O_2P\cdot H_2O$ and a molecular weight of 279.1. The chemical name of Cyclophosphamide is 2-[bis(2-chloroethyl)amino]tetrahydro-2H-1,3,2-oxazaphosphorine 2-oxide monohydrate. Cyclophosphamide is soluble in water, saline, or ethanol.

Following is its chemical structure:

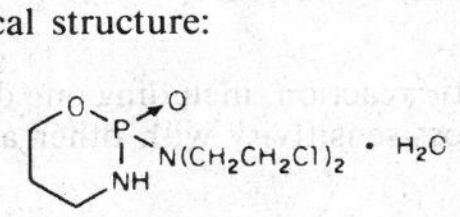

CLINICAL PHARMACOLOGY

Cyclophosphamide is biotransformed principally in the liver to active alkylating metabolites by a mixed function microsomal oxidase system. These metabolites interfere with the growth of susceptible rapidly proliferating malignant cells. The mechanism of action is thought to involve cross-linking of tumor cell DNA.

Cyclophosphamide is well absorbed after oral administration with a bioavailability greater than 75%. The unchanged drug has an elimination half-life of 3 to 12 hours. It is eliminated primarily in the form of metabolites, but from 5 to 25% of the dose is excreted in urine as unchanged drug. Several cytotoxic and noncytotoxic metabolites have been identified in urine and in plasma. Concentrations of metabolites reach a maximum in plasma 2 to 3 hours after an intravenous dose. Plasma protein binding of unchanged drug is low but some metabolites are bound to an extent greater than 60%. It has not been demonstrated that any single metabolite is responsible for either the therapeutic or toxic effects of Cyclophosphamide. Although elevated levels of metabolites of Cyclophosphamide have been observed in patients with renal failure, increased clinical toxicity in such patients has not been demonstrated.

INDICATIONS AND USAGE
MALIGNANT DISEASES
Cyclophosphamide, although effective alone in susceptible malignancies, is more frequently used concurrently or sequentially with other antineoplastic drugs. The following malignancies are often susceptible to Cyclophosphamide treatment:
1. Malignant lymphomas (Stages III and IV of the Ann Arbor staging system), Hodgkin's disease, lymphocytic lymphoma (nodular or diffuse), mixed-cell type lymphoma, histiocytic lymphoma, Burkitt's lymphoma.
2. Multiple myeloma.
3. Leukemias: Chronic lymphocytic leukemia, chronic granulocytic leukemia (it is usually ineffective in acute blastic crisis), acute myelogenous and monocytic leukemia, acute lymphoblastic (stem cell) leukemia in children (Cyclophosphamide given during remission is effective in prolonging its duration).
4. Cutaneous T-cell lymphoma Mycosis fungoides—(advanced disease).
5. Neuroblastoma (disseminated disease).
6. Adenocarcinoma of the ovary.
7. Retinoblastoma.
8. Carcinoma of the breast.

UNLABELED USES
Cyclophosphamide is used alone or as an adjunct in the treatment of Graves' ophthalmopathy, lupus nephritis, multiple sclerosis, and pemphigus vulgaris. It is also used as an adjunct in the treatment of malignant pheochromocytoma, metastatic prostate cancer, rheumatoid arthritis, and stomach carcinoma.

NON-MALIGNANT DISEASE: BIOPSY PROVEN ''MINIMAL CHANGE'' NEPHROTIC SYNDROME IN CHILDREN
Cyclophosphamide is useful in carefully selected cases of biopsy proven "minimal change" nephrotic syndrome in children but should not be used as primary therapy. In children whose disease fails to respond adequately to appropriate adrenocorticosteroid therapy or in whom the adrenocorticosteroid therapy produces or threatens to produce intolerable side effects, Cyclophosphamide may induce a remission. Cyclophosphamide is not indicated for the nephrotic syndrome in adults or for any other renal disease.

CONTRAINDICATIONS
Continued use of Cyclophosphamide is contraindicated in patients with severely depressed bone marrow function. Cyclophosphamide is contraindicated in patients who have demonstrated a previous hypersensitivity to it. See *"Warnings"* and *"Precautions"* sections.

WARNINGS
CARCINOGENESIS, MUTAGENESIS, IMPAIRMENT OF FERTILITY
Second malignancies have developed in some patients treated with Cyclophosphamide used alone or in association with other antineoplastic drugs and/or modalities. Most frequently, they have been urinary bladder, myeloproliferative, or lymphoproliferative malignancies. Second malignancies most frequently were detected in patients treated for primary myeloproliferative or lymphoproliferative malignancies or nonmalignant disease in which immune processes are believed to be involved pathologically. In some cases, the second malignancy developed several years after Cyclophosphamide treatment had been discontinued. Urinary bladder malignancies generally have occurred in patients who previously had hemorrhagic cystitis. One case of carcinoma of the renal pelvis was reported in a patient receiving long-term Cyclophosphamide therapy for cerebral vasculitis. The possibility of Cyclophosphamide-induced malignancy should be considered in any benefit-to-risk assessment for use of the drug.

Cyclophosphamide can cause fetal harm when administered to a pregnant woman and such abnormalities have been reported following Cyclophosphamide therapy in pregnant women. Abnormalities were found in two infants and a six-month-old fetus born to women treated with Cyclophosphamide. Ectrodactylia was found in two of the three cases. Normal infants have also been born to women treated with Cyclophosphamide during pregnancy, including the first trimester. If this drug is used during pregnancy, or if the patient becomes pregnant while taking (receiving) this drug, the patient should be apprised of the potential hazard to the fetus. Women of childbearing potential should be advised to avoid becoming pregnant.

Cyclophosphamide interferes with oogenesis and spermatogenesis. It may cause sterility in both sexes. Development of sterility appears to depend on the dose of Cyclophosphamide, duration of therapy, and the state of gonadal function at the time of treatment. Cyclophosphamide-induced sterility may be irreversible in some patients.

Amenorrhea associated with decreased estrogen and increased gonadotropin secretion develops in a significant proportion of women treated with Cyclophosphamide. Affected patients generally resume regular menses within a few months after cessation of therapy. Girls treated with Cyclophosphamide during prepubescence generally develop secondary sexual characteristics normally and have regular menses. Ovarian fibrosis with apparently complete loss of germ cells after prolonged Cyclophosphamide treatment in late prepubescence has been reported. Girls treated with Cyclophosphamide during prepubescence subsequently have conceived.

Men treated with Cyclophosphamide may develop oligospermia or azoospermia associated with increased gonadotropin but normal testosterone secretion. Sexual potency and libido are unimpaired in these patients. Boys treated with Cyclophosphamide during prepubescence develop secondary sexual characteristics normally, but may have oligospermia or azoospermia and increased gonadotropin secretion. Some degree of testicular atrophy may occur. Cyclophosphamide-induced azoospermia is reversible in some patients, though the reversibility may not occur for several years after cessation of therapy. Men temporarily rendered sterile by Cyclophosphamide have subsequently fathered normal children.

URINARY SYSTEM

Hemorrhagic cystitis may develop in patients treated with Cyclophosphamide. Rarely, this condition can be severe and even fatal. Fibrosis of the urinary bladder, sometimes extensive, also may develop with or without accompanying cystitis. Atypical urinary bladder epithelial cells may appear in the urine. These adverse effects appear to depend on the dose of Cyclophosphamide and the duration of therapy. Such bladder injury is thought to be due to Cyclophosphamide metabolites excreted in the urine. Forced fluid intake helps to assure an ample output of urine, necessitates frequent voiding, and reduces the time the drug remains in the bladder. This helps to prevent cystitis. Hematuria usually resolves in a few days after cyclophosphamide treatment is stopped, but it may persist. Medical and/or surgical supportive treatment may be required, rarely, to treat protracted cases of severe hemorrhagic cystitis. It is usually necessary to discontinue Cyclophosphamide therapy in instances of severe hemorrhagic cystitis.

CARDIAC TOXICITY

Although a few instances of cardiac dysfunction have been reported following use of recommended doses of Cyclophosphamide, no causal relationship has been established. Cardiotoxicity has been observed in some patients receiving high doses of Cyclophosphamide ranging from 120 to 270 mg/kg administered over a period of a few days, usually as a portion of an intensive antineoplastic multi-drug regimen or in conjunction with transplantation procedures. In a few instances with high doses of Cyclophosphamide, severe, and sometimes fatal, congestive heart failure has occurred within a few days after the first Cyclophosphamide dose. Histopathologic examination has primarily shown hemorrhagic myocarditis. Hemopericardium has occurred secondary to hemorrhagic myocarditis and myocardial necrosis. Pericarditis has been reported independent of any hemopericardiums.

No residual cardiac abnormalities, as evidenced by electrocardiogram or echocardiogram appear to be present in patients surviving episodes of apparent cardiac toxicity associated with high doses of Cyclophosphamide.

Cyclophosphamide has been reported to potentiate doxorubicin-induced cardiotoxicity.

INFECTIONS

Treatment with Cyclophosphamide may cause significant suppression of immune responses. Serious, sometimes fatal, infections may develop in severely immuno-suppressed patients. Cyclophosphamide treatment may not be indicated or should be interrupted or the dose reduced in patients who have or who develop viral, bacterial, fungal, protozoan, or helminthic infections.

OTHER

Rare instances of anaphylactic reaction, including one death, have been reported. One instance of possible cross-sensitivity with other alkylating agents has been reported.

PRECAUTIONS

GENERAL

Special attention to the possible development of toxicity should be exercised in patients being treated with Cyclophosphamide if any of the following conditions are present.

1. Leukopenia
2. Thrombocytopenia
3. Tumor cell infiltration of bone marrow
4. Previous x-ray therapy
5. Previous therapy with other cytotoxic agents
6. Impaired hepatic function
7. Impaired renal function

LABORATORY TESTS

During treatment, the patient's hematologic profile (particularly neutrophils and platelets) should be monitored regularly to determine the degree of hematopoietic suppression. Urine should also be examined regularly for red cells which may precede hemorrhagic cystitis.

DRUG INTERACTIONS

The rate of metabolism and the leukopenic activity of Cyclophosphamide reportedly are increased by chronic administration of high doses of phenobarbital.

The physician should be alert for possible combined-drug actions, desirable or undesirable, involving Cyclophosphamide, even though Cyclophosphamide has been used successfully concurrently with other drugs, including other cytotoxic drugs.

Cyclophosphamide treatment, which causes a marked and persistent inhibition of cholinesterase activity, potentiates the effects of succinylcholine chloride.

If a patient has been treated with Cyclophosphamide within 10 days of general anesthesia, the anesthesiologist should be alerted.

ADRENALECTOMY

Since Cyclophosphamide has been reported to be more toxic in adrenalectomized dogs, adjustment of the doses of both replacement steroids and Cyclophosphamide may be necessary for the adrenalectomized patient.

WOUND HEALING

Cyclophosphamide may interfere with normal wound healing.

CARCINOGENESIS, MUTAGENESIS, IMPAIRMENT OF FERTILITY

See "Warnings" section for information on carcinogenesis, mutagenesis, and impairment of fertility.

PREGNANCY

Pregnancy Category D — See "Warnings" section.

NURSING MOTHERS

Cyclophosphamide is excreted in breast milk. Because of the potential for serious adverse reactions and the potential for tumorigenicity shown for Cyclophosphamide in humans, a decision should be made whether to discontinue nursing or to discontinue the drug, taking into account the importance of the drug to the mother.

ADVERSE REACTIONS

Information on adverse reactions associated with the use of Cyclophosphamide is arranged according to body system affected or type of reaction. The adverse reactions are listed in order of decreasing incidence. The most serious adverse reactions are described in the See "Warnings" section.

REPRODUCTIVE SYSTEM

See "Warnings" section for imformation on impairment of fertility.

DIGESTIVE SYSTEM

Nausea and vomiting commonly occur with Cyclophosphamide therapy. Anorexia and, less frequently, abdominal discomfort or pain and diarrhea may occur. There are isolated reports of hemorrhagic colitis, oral mucosal ulceration and jaundice occurring during therapy. These adverse drug effects generally remit when Cyclophosphamide treatment is stopped.

SKIN AND ITS STRUCTURES

Alopecia occurs commonly in patients treated with Cyclophosphamide. The hair can be expected to grow back after treatment with the drug or even during continued drug treatment, though it may be different in texture or color. Skin rash occurs occasionally in patients receiving the drug. Pigmentation of the skin and changes in nails can occur.

HEMATOPOIETIC SYSTEM

Leukopenia occurs in patients treated with Cylophosphamide, is related to the dose of the drug, and can be used as a dosage guide. Leukopenia of less than 200 cells/mm^3 develops commonly in patients treated with an initial loading dose of the drug, and less frequently in patients maintained on smaller doses. The degree of neutropenia is particularly important because it correlates with a reduction in resistance to infections.

Thrombocytopenia or anemia develop occasionally in patients treated with Cyclophosphamide. These hematologic effects usually can be reversed by reducing the drug dose or by interrupting treatment. Recovery from leukopenia usually begins in 7 to 10 days after cessation of therapy.

URINARY SYSTEM

See "Warnings" section for information on cystitis and urinary bladder fibrosis.

Hemorrhagic ureteritis and renal tubular necrosis have been reported to occur in patients treated with Cyclophosphamide. Such lesions usually resolve following cessation of therapy.

INFECTIONS

See "Warnings" section for information on reduced host resistance to infections.

CARCINOGENESIS SEE "WARNINGS" SECTION FOR INFORMATION ON CARCINOGENESIS.

RESPIRATORY SYSTEM

Interstitial pulmonary fibrosis has been reported in patients receiving high doses of Cyclophosphamide over a prolonged period.

OTHER

Rare instances of anaphylactic reaction, including one death, have been reported. One instance of possible cross-sensitivity with other alkylating agents has been reported.

OVERDOSAGE

No specific antidote for Cyclophosphamide is known. Overdosage should be managed with supportive measures, including appropriate treatment for any concurrent infection, myelosuppression, or cardiac toxicity should it occur.

DOSAGE AND ADMINISTRATION

TREATMENT OF MALIGNANT DISEASES: ADULTS AND CHILDREN

When used as the only oncolytic drug therapy, the initial course of Cyclophosphamide for patients with no hematologic deficiency usually consists of 40 to 50 mg/kg given intravenously in divided doses over a period of 2 to 5 days. Other intravenous regimens include 10 to 15 mg/kg given every 7 to 10 days or 3 to 5 mg/kg twice weekly.

Oral Cyclophosphamide dosing is usually in the range of 1 to 5 mg/kg/day for both initial and maintenance dosing.

Many other regimens of intravenous and oral Cyclophosphamide have been reported. Dosages must be adjusted in accord with evidence of antitumor activity and/or leukopenia. The total leukocyte count is a good, objective guide for regulating dosage. Transient decreases in the total white blood cell count to 2000

---

cells/mm^3 (following short courses) or more persistent reduction to 300 cells/mm^3 (with continuing therapy) are tolerated without serious risk of infection if there is no marked granulocytopenia.

When Cyclophosphamide is included in combined cytotoxic regimens, it may be necessary to reduce the dose of Cyclophosphamide as well as that of the other drugs.

Cyclophosphamide and its metabolites are dialyzable although there are probably quantitative differences depending upon the dialysis system being used. Patients with compromised renal function may show some measurable changes in pharmacokinetic parameters of Cyclophosphamide metabolism, but there is no consistent evidence indicating a need for Cyclophosphamide dosage modification in patients with renal function impairment.

TREATMENT OF NONMALIGNANT DISEASES: BIOPSY PROVEN "MINIMAL CHANGE" NEPHROTIC SYNDROME IN CHILDREN
An oral dose of 2.5 to 3 mg/kg daily for a period of 60 to 90 days is recommended. In males, the incidence of oligospermia and azoospermia increases if the duration of Cyclophosphamide treatment exceeds 60 days. Treatment beyond 90 days increases the probability of sterility. Adrenocorticosteroid therapy may be tapered and discontinued during the course of Cyclophosphamide therapy. See "Precautions" section concerning hematologic monitoring.

PREPARATION AND HANDLING OF SOLUTIONS
Parenteral drug products should be inspected visually for particulate matter and discoloration prior to administration, whenever solution and container permit.

Lyophilized and Cyclophosphamide for injection should be prepared for parenteral use by adding Bacteriostatic Water for Injection, USP, (paraben preserved only) or Sterile Water for Injection, USP to the vial and shaking to dissolve. Use the quantity of diluent shown below to reconstitute the product.

Dosage Strength	Quantity of Diluent	Lyophilized Cyclophosphamide Quantity of Diluent
100 mg	5 mL	5 mL
200 mg	10 mL	10 mL
500 mg	25 mL	20-25 mL
1g	50 mL	50 mL
2g	100 mL	80-100 mL

Solutions of lyophilized Cyclophosphamide for injection and may be injected intravenously, intramuscularly, intraperitoneally, or intrapleurally or they may be infused intravenously in the following:
Dextrose Injection, USP (5% dextrose)
Dextrose and Sodium Chloride Injection, USP (5% dextrose and 0.9% sodium chloride)
5% Dextrose and Ringer's Injection
Lactated Ringer's Injection, USP
Sodium Chloride Injection, USP (0.45% sodium chloride)
Sodium Lactate Injection, USP ($^1/_6$ molar sodium lactate)
Reconstituted lyophilized Cyclophosphamide for injection and are chemically and physically stable for 24 hours at room temperature or for six days in the refrigerator; they do not contain any antimicrobial preservative and thus care must be taken to assure the sterility of prepared solutions.

Lyophilized Cyclophosphamide for injection and prepared by adding Bacteriostatic Water for Injection, USP (paraben preserved only) should be used within 24 hours if stored at room temperature or within 6 days if stored under refrigeration.

If lyophilized Cyclophosphamide for injection are not prepared by adding Bacteriostatic Water for Injection, USP (paraben-preserved only), it is recommended that the solution be used promptly (preferably within six hours).

The osmolarities of solutions of lyophilized Cyclophosphamide for injection and normal saline are compared in the following table:

	mOsm/L
Lyophilized Cyclophosphamide for injection	431
Cyclophosphamide for injection	219 (4 mL diluent/100 mg Cyclophosphamide)
	172 (5 mL diluent/100 mg Cyclophosphamide)
	352
Normal saline	287

Lyophilized Cyclophosphamide and Cyclophosphamide are hypertonic with respect to normal saline.

Extemporaneous liquid preparations of Cyclophosphamide for oral administration may be prepared by dissolving lyophilized Cyclophosphamide for injection or Cyclophosphamide for injection in Aromatic Elixir, NF. Such preparations should be stored under refrigeration in glass containers and used within 14 days.

HANDLING AND DISPOSAL
Procedures for proper handling and disposal of anticancer drugs should be considered. Several guidelines on this subject have been pub-lished.[1-7] There is no general agreement that all the procedures recommended in the guidelines are necessary or appropriate.

STORAGE
Storage at temperatures not exceeding 25°C (77°F) is recommended. It will withstand brief exposure to temperatures up to 30°C (86°F), but it is to be protected from temperatures above 30°C (86°F).

REFERENCES
1. Recommendations for the Safe Handling of Parenteral Antineoplastic Drugs. NIH Publication No. 83-2621. For sale by the Superintendent of Documents, US Government Printing Office, Washington, DC 20402. 2. AMA Council Report. Guidelines for Handling Parenteral Antineoplastics, JAMA, 1985; 253(11):1590-1592. 3. National Study Commission on Cytotoxic Exposure—Recommendations for Handling Cytotoxic Agents. Available from Louis P. Jeffrey, Sc.D., Chairman, National Study Commission on Cytotoxic Exposure, Massachusetts College of Pharmacy and Allied Health Sciences, 179 Longwood Avenue, Boston, Massachusetts 02115. 4. Clinical Oncological Society of Australia. Guidelines and Recommendations for Safe Handling of Antineoplastic Agents. Med J Australia 1983 1:426-428. 5. Jones RB, et al: Safe handling of chemotherapeutic agents: A report from the Mount Sinai Medical Center, CA-A Cancer J for Clinicians 1983; (Sept/Oct) 258-263. 6. American Society of Hospital Pharmacists Technical Assistance Bulletin on Handling Cytotoxic and Hazardous Drugs. Am J. Hosp. Pharm 1990: 47:1033-1049. 7. American Society of Hospital Pharmacists technical assistance bulletin on handling cytotoxic drugs in hospitals. Am J Hosp Pharm 42:131-137, 1985. 8. OSHA Work-practice Guidelines for Personal Dealing with Cytotoxic (Antineoplastic) Drugs, AM J Hosp Pharm 1986; 43:1193-1204.

J CODES
2 g IV—J9097
200 mg IV—J9094
500 mg IV—J9095
100 mg IV—J9093
1 g IV—J9096

HOW SUPPLIED
POWDER FOR INJECTION: 100 MG

AVERAGE UNIT PRICE (AVAILABLE SIZES)	
BRAND	$5.72

BRAND/MANUFACTURER	NDC	SIZE	AWP
◆ BRAND			
CYTOXAN: Bristol-Myer Onc/Hiv	00015-0500-41	1s	$5.31
NEOSAR: Pharmacia	00013-5606-93	1s	$5.39
CYTOXAN LYOPHILIZED: Bristol-Myer Onc/Hiv	00015-0539-41	1s	$6.45

POWDER FOR INJECTION: 200 MG

AVERAGE UNIT PRICE (AVAILABLE SIZES)	
BRAND	$10.87

BRAND/MANUFACTURER	NDC	SIZE	AWP
◆ BRAND			
CYTOXAN: Bristol-Myer Onc/Hiv	00015-0501-41	1s	$10.11
NEOSAR: Pharmacia	00013-5606-93	1s	$10.24
CYTOXAN LYOPHILIZED: Bristol-Myer Onc/Hiv	00015-0546-41	1s	$12.25

POWDER FOR INJECTION: 500 MG

AVERAGE UNIT PRICE (AVAILABLE SIZES)	
BRAND	$22.82

BRAND/MANUFACTURER	NDC	SIZE	AWP
◆ BRAND			
CYTOXAN: Bristol-Myer Onc/Hiv	00015-0502-41	1s	$21.24
NEOSAR: Pharmacia	00013-5626-93	1s	$21.50
CYTOXAN LYOPHILIZED: Bristol-Myer Onc/Hiv	00015-0547-41	1s	$25.71

POWDER FOR INJECTION: 1 GM

AVERAGE UNIT PRICE (AVAILABLE SIZES)	
BRAND	$45.64

BRAND/MANUFACTURER	NDC	SIZE	AWP
◆ BRAND			
CYTOXAN: Bristol-Myer Onc/Hiv	00015-0505-41	1s	$42.49
NEOSAR: Pharmacia	00013-5636-70	1s	$43.01
CYTOXAN LYOPHILIZED: Bristol-Myer Onc/Hiv	00015-0548-41	1s	$51.43

POWDER FOR INJECTION: 2 GM

AVERAGE UNIT PRICE (AVAILABLE SIZES)	
BRAND	$91.30

BRAND/MANUFACTURER	NDC	SIZE	AWP
◆ BRAND			
CYTOXAN: Bristol-Myer Onc/Hiv	00015-0506-41	1s	$85.00
NEOSAR: Pharmacia	00013-5646-70	1s	$86.00
CYTOXAN LYOPHILIZED: Bristol-Myer Onc/Hiv	00015-0549-41	1s	$102.89

TABLETS: 25 MG

BRAND/MANUFACTURER	NDC	SIZE	AWP
○ BRAND			
▶ CYTOXAN: Bristol-Myer Onc/Hiv	00015-0504-01	100s	$150.35

▶ SHOWN IN PRODUCT IDENTIFICATION GUIDE

TABLETS: 50 MG

BRAND/MANUFACTURER	NDC	SIZE	AWP
○ **BRAND**			
▶ CYTOXAN: Bristol-Myer Onc/Hiv	00015-0503-01	100s	$275.95
	00015-0503-02	1000s	$2628.19

Cycloserine

DESCRIPTION
Cycloserine 3-isoxazolidinone, 4-amino-, (R)-, is a broad-spectrum antibiotic that is produced by a strain of *Streptomyces orchidaceus* and has also been synthesized. Cycloserine is a white to off-white powder that is soluble in water and stable in alkaline solution. It is rapidly destroyed at a neutral or acid pH.

Cycloserine has a pH between 5.5 and 6.5 in a solution containing 100 mg/mL. The molecular weight of Cycloserine is 102.09, and it has an empirical formula of $C_3H_6N_2O_2$.

Each Pulvule® contains Cycloserine, 250 mg (2.45 mmol).

Following is its chemical structure:

CLINICAL PHARMACOLOGY
After oral administration, Cycloserine is readily absorbed from the gastrointestinal tract, with peak blood levels occurring in 4 to 8 hours. Blood levels of 25 to 30 µg/mL can generally be maintained with the usual dosage of 250 mg twice a day, although the relationship of plasma levels to dosage is not always consistent. Concentrations in the cerebrospinal fluid, pleural fluid, fetal blood, and mother's milk approach those found in the serum. Detectable amounts are found in ascitic fluid, bile, sputum, amniotic fluid, and lung and lymph tissues. Approximately 65% of a single dose of Cycloserine can be recovered in the urine within 72 hours after oral administration. The remaining 35% is apparently metabolized to unknown substances. The maximum excretion rate occurs 2 to 6 hours after administration, with 50% of the drug eliminated in 12 hours.

Microbiology: Cycloserine inhibits cell-wall synthesis in susceptible strains of gram-positive and gram-negative bacteria and in *Mycobacterium tuberculosis.*

Susceptibility Tests: Cycloserine clinical laboratory standard powder is available for both direct and indirect methods[1] of determining the susceptibility of strains of mycobacteria. Cycloserine MICs for susceptible strains are 25 µg/mL or lower.

INDICATIONS AND USAGE
Cycloserine is indicated in the treatment of active pulmonary and extrapulmonary tuberculosis (including renal disease) when the causative organisms are susceptible to this drug and when treatment with the primary medications (streptomycin, isoniazid, rifampin, and ethambutol) has proved inadequate. Like all antituberculosis drugs, Cycloserine should be administered in conjunction with other effective chemotherapy and not as the sole therapeutic agent.

Cycloserine may be effective in the treatment of acute urinary tract infections caused by susceptible strains of gram-positive and gram-negative bacteria, especially *Enterobacter* sp. and *Escherichia coli.* It is generally no more and is usually less effective than other antimicrobial agents in the treatment of urinary tract infections caused by bacteria other than mycobacteria. Use of Cycloserine in these infections should be considered only when more conventional therapy has failed and when the organism has been demonstrated to be susceptible to the drug.

CONTRAINDICATIONS
Administration is contraindicated in patients with any of the following:

Hypersensitivity to Cycloserine
Epilepsy
Depression, severe anxiety, or psychosis
Severe renal insufficiency
Excessive concurrent use of alcohol

WARNINGS
Administration of Cycloserine should be discontinued or the dosage reduced if the patient develops allergic dermatitis or symptoms of CNS toxicity, such as convulsions, psychosis, somnolence, depression, confusion, hyperreflexia, headache, tremor, vertigo, paresis, or dysarthria.

The toxicity of Cycloserine is closely related to excessive blood levels (above 30 µg/mL), as determined by high dosage or inadequate renal clearance. The ratio of toxic dose to effective dose in tuberculosis is small.

The risk of convulsions is increased in chronic alcoholics. Patients should be monitored by hematologic, renal excretion, blood level, and liver function studies.

PRECAUTIONS
General: Before treatment with Cycloserine is initiated, cultures should be taken and the organism's susceptibility to the drug should be established. In tuberculous infections, the organism's susceptibility to the other antituberculosis agents in the regimen should also be demonstrated.

Anticonvulsant drugs or sedatives may be effective in controlling symptoms of CNS toxicity, such as convulsions, anxiety, and tremor. Patients receiving more than 500 mg of Cycloserine daily should be closely observed for such symptoms. The value of pyridoxine in preventing CNS toxicity from Cycloserine has not been proved.

Administration of Cycloserine and other antituberculosis drugs has been associated in a few instances with vitamin B_{12} and/or folic acid deficiency, megaloblastic anemia, and sideroblastic anemia. If evidence of anemia develops during treatment, appropriate studies and therapy should be instituted.

Laboratory Tests: Blood levels should be determined at least weekly for patients with reduced renal function, for individuals receiving a daily dosage of more than 500 mg, and for those showing signs and symptoms suggestive of toxicity. The dosage should be adjusted to keep the blood level below 30 µg/mL.

Drug Interactions: Concurrent administration of ethionamide has been reported to potentiate neurotoxic side effects.

Alcohol and Cycloserine are incompatible, especially during a regimen calling for large doses of the latter. Alcohol increases the possibility and risk of epileptic episodes.

Concurrent administration of isoniazid may result in increased incidence of CNS effects, such as dizziness or drowsiness. Dosage adjustments may be necessary and patients should be monitored closely for signs of CNS toxicity.

Carcinogenesis, Mutagenicity, and Impairment of Fertility: Studies have not been performed to determine potential for carcinogenicity. The Ames test and unscheduled DNA repair test were negative. A study in 2 generations of rats showed no impairment of fertility relative to controls for the first mating but somewhat lower fertility in the second mating.

Pregnancy Category C: A study in 2 generations of rats given doses up to 100 mg/kg/day demonstrated no teratogenic effect in offspring. It is not known whether Cycloserine can cause fetal harm when administered to a pregnant woman or can affect reproduction capacity. Cycloserine should be given to a pregnant woman only if clearly needed.

Nursing Mothers: Because of the potential for serious adverse reactions in nursing infants from Cycloserine a decision should be made whether to discontinue nursing or to discontinue the drug, taking into account the importance of the drug to the mother.

Usage in Children: Safety and dosage have not been established for pediatric use.

ADVERSE REACTIONS
Most adverse reactions occurring during therapy with Cycloserine involve the nervous system or are manifestations of drug hypersensitivity. The following side effects have been observed in patients receiving Cycloserine:

Nervous System Symptoms: (which appear to be related to higher dosages of the drug, ie, more than 500 mg daily)

Convulsions
Drowsiness and somnolence
Headache
Tremor
Dysarthria
Vertigo
Confusion and disorientation with loss of memory
Psychoses, possibly with suicidal tendencies
   Character changes
   Hyperirritability
   Aggression
Paresis
Hyperreflexia
Paresthesia
Major and minor (localized) clonic seizures
Coma

Cardiovascular: Sudden development of congestive heart failure in patients receiving 1 to 1.5 g of Cycloserine daily has been reported.

Allergy: (apparently not related to dosage)

Skin rash

Miscellaneous: Elevated serum transaminase, especially in patients with preexisting liver disease.

OVERDOSAGE
Signs and Symptoms: Acute toxicity from Cycloserine can occur if more than 1 g is ingested by an adult. Chronic toxicity from Cycloserine is dose related and can occur if more than 500 mg is administered daily. Patients with renal impairment will accumulate Cycloserine and may develop toxicity if the dosing regimen is not modified. Patients with severe renal impairment should not receive the drug. The central nervous system is the most common organ system involved with toxicity. Toxic effects may include headache, vertigo, confusion, drowsiness, hyperirritability, paresthesias, dysarthria, and psychosis. Following larger ingestions, paresis, convulsions, and coma often occur. Ethyl alcohol may increase the risk of seizures in patients receiving Cycloserine.

The oral median lethal dose in mice is 5,290 mg/kg.

Treatment: To obtain up-to-date information about the treatment of overdose, a good resource is your certified regional poison control center. Telephone numbers of certified poison control centers are listed in the *Physicians' Desk Reference (PDR).* In managing overdosage, consider the possibility of multiple drug overdoses, interaction among drugs, and unusual drug kinetics in your patient.

◆ RATED THERAPEUTICALLY EQUIVALENT; ◇ THERAPEUTIC EQUIVALENCE UNCONFIRMED; ○ UNRATED

Overdoses of Cycloserine have been reported rarely. The following is provided to serve as a guide should such an overdose be encountered.

Protect the patient's airway and support ventilation and perfusion. Meticulously monitor and maintain, within acceptable limits, the patient's vital signs, blood gases, serum electrolytes, etc. Absorption of drugs from the gastrointestinal tract may be decreased by giving activated charcoal, which, in many cases, is more effective than emesis or lavage; consider charcoal instead of or in addition to gastric emptying. Repeated doses of charcoal over time may hasten elimination of some drugs that have been absorbed. Safeguard the patient's airway when employing gastric emptying or charcoal.

In adults, many of the neurotoxic effects of Cycloserine can be both treated and prevented with the administration of 200 to 300 mg of pyridoxine daily.

The use of hemodialysis has been shown to remove Cycloserine from the bloodstream. This procedure should be reserved for patients with life-threatening toxicity that is unresponsive to less invasive therapy.

DOSAGE AND ADMINISTRATION

Cycloserine is effective orally and is currently administered only by this route. The usual dosage is 500 mg to 1 g daily in divided doses monitored by blood levels.[2] The initial adult dosage most frequently given is 250 mg twice daily at 12-hour intervals for the first 2 weeks. A daily dosage of 1 g should not be exceeded.

REFERENCES

1. Kubica GP, Dye WE: Laboratory methods for clinical and public health—mycobacteriology. US Department of Health, Education and Welfare, Public Health Service, 1967, pp. 47-55, 66-70. 2. Jones LR: Colorimetric determination of cycloserine, a new antibiotic. *Anal Chem* 1956; 28:39.

HOW SUPPLIED
CAPSULE: 250 MG

BRAND/MANUFACTURER	NDC	SIZE	AWP
○ BRAND SEROMYCIN: Lilly	00002-0604-40	40s	$131.21

Cyclospasmol SEE CYCLANDELATE

Cyclosporine

WARNING

ONLY PHYSICIANS EXPERIENCED IN IMMUNOSUPPRESSIVE THERAPY AND MANAGEMENT OF ORGAN TRANSPLANT PATIENTS SHOULD PRESCRIBE CYCLOSPORINE. PATIENTS RECEIVING THE DRUG SHOULD BE MANAGED IN FACILITIES EQUIPPED AND STAFFED WITH ADEQUATE LABORATORY AND SUPPORTIVE MEDICAL RESOURCES. THE PHYSICIAN RESPONSIBLE FOR MAINTENANCE THERAPY SHOULD HAVE COMPLETE INFORMATION REQUISITE FOR THE FOLLOW-UP OF THE PATIENT.

CYCLOSPORINE SHOULD BE ADMINISTERED WITH ADRENAL CORTICOSTEROIDS BUT NOT WITH OTHER IMMUNOSUPPRESSIVE AGENTS. INCREASED SUSCEPTIBILITY TO INFECTION AND THE POSSIBLE DEVELOPMENT OF LYMPHOMA MAY RESULT FROM IMMUNOSUPPRESSION.

THE ABSORPTION OF CYCLOSPORINE DURING CHRONIC ADMINISTRATION OF CYCLOSPORINE CAPSULES AND ORAL SOLUTION WAS FOUND TO BE ERRATIC. IT IS RECOMMENDED THAT PATIENTS TAKING THE CAPSULES OR ORAL SOLUTION OVER A PERIOD OF TIME BE MONITORED AT REPEATED INTERVALS FOR CYCLOSPORINE BLOOD LEVELS, AND SUBSEQUENT DOSE ADJUSTMENTS BE MADE IN ORDER TO AVOID TOXICITY DUE TO HIGH LEVELS AND POSSIBLE ORGAN REJECTION DUE TO LOW ABSORPTION OF CYCLOSPORINE. THIS IS OF SPECIAL IMPORTANCE IN LIVER TRANSPLANTS. NUMEROUS ASSAYS ARE BEING DEVELOPED TO MEASURE BLOOD LEVELS OF CYCLOSPORINE. COMPARISON OF LEVELS IN PUBLISHED LITERATURE TO PATIENT LEVELS USING CURRENT ASSAYS MUST BE DONE WITH DETAILED KNOWLEDGE OF THE ASSAY METHODS EMPLOYED. (SEE BLOOD LEVEL MONITORING UNDER *"DOSAGE AND ADMINISTRATION"*)

DESCRIPTION

Cyclosporine is a cyclic polypeptide immunosuppressant agent consisting of 11 amino acids. It is produced as a metabolite by the fungus species Tolypocladium inflatum Gams.

Chemically, Cyclosporine is designated as [R-[R,*R*-(E)]]-cyclic(L-alanyl-D-alanyl-N-methyl-L-leucyl-N-methyl-L- leucyl-N-methyl-L-valyl-3-hyroxy-N,4-dimethyl-L-2-amino-6-octenoyl-L-α- amino-butyrl-N-methylglycyl-N-methyl-L-leucyl-L-valyl-N-methyl-L-leucyl).

Cyclosporine is available as tablets, oral solution, and concentrate for injection.

Each capsule contains:
Cyclosporine ....25, 50, or 100 mg

Each ml of oral solution contains:
Cyclosporine ....100 mg

Each ml of concentrate for injection contains:
Cyclosporine ....50 mg

The empirical formula is $C_{62}H_{111}N_{11}O_{12}$ and the molecular weight 1202.63.

Following is its chemical structure:

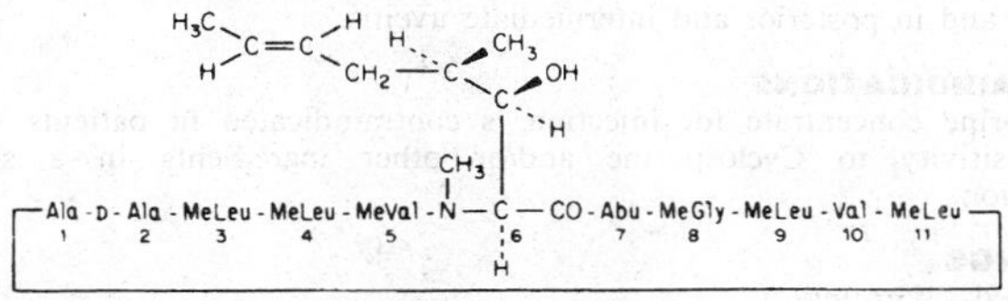

CLINICAL PHARMACOLOGY

Cyclosporine is a potent immunosuppressive agent which in animals prolongs survival of allogeneic transplants involving skin, heart, kidney, pancreas, bone marrow, small intestine, and lung. Cyclosporine has been demonstrated to suppress some humoral immunity and, to a greater extent, cell-mediated reactions such as allograft rejection, delayed hypersensitivity, experimental allergic encephalomyelitis, Freund's adjuvant arthritis, and graft vs. host disease in many animal species for a variety of organs.

Successful kidney, liver, and heart allogeneic transplants have been performed in man using Cyclosporine.

The exact mechanism of action of Cyclosporine is not known. Experimental evidence suggests that the effectiveness of Cyclosporine is due to specific and reversible inhibition of immunocompetent lymphocytes in the G_0- or G_1-phase of the cell cycle. T-lymphocytes are preferentially inhibited. The T-helper cell is the main target, although the T-suppressor cell may also be suppressed. Cyclosporine also inhibits lymphokine production and release including interleukin-2 or T-cell growth factor (TCGF).

No functional effects on phagocytic (changes in enzyme secretions not altered, chemotactic migration of granulocytes, macrophage migration, carbon clearance *in vivo*) or tumor cells (growth rate, metastasis) can be detected in animals. Cyclosporine does not cause bone marrow suppression in animal models or man.

The absorption of Cyclosporine from the gastrointestinal tract is incomplete and variable. Peak concentrations (C_{max}) in blood and plasma are achieved at about 3.5 hours. C_{max} and area under the plasma or blood concentration/time curve (AUC) increase with the administered dose; for blood the relationship is curvilinear (parabolic) between 0 and 1400 mg. As determined by a specific assay, C_{max} is approximately 1.0 ng/mL/mg of dose for plasma and 2.7-1.4 ng/mL/mg of dose for blood (for low to high doses). Compared to an intravenous infusion, the absolute bioavailability of the oral solution is approximately 30% based upon the results in 2 patients. The bioavailability of Cyclosporine capsules is equivalent to Cyclosporine oral solution.

Cyclosporine is distributed largely outside the blood volume. In blood the distribution is concentration dependent. Approximately 33%-47% is in plasma, 4%-9% in lymphocytes, 5%-12% in granulocytes, and 41%-58% in erythrocytes. At high concentrations, the uptake by leukocytes and erythrocytes becomes saturated. In plasma, approximately 90% is bound to proteins, primarily lipoproteins.

The disposition of Cyclosporine from blood is biphasic with a terminal half-life of approximately 19 hours (range: 10-27 hours). Elimination is primarily biliary with only 6% of the dose excreted in the urine.

Cyclosporine is extensively metabolized but there is no major metabolic pathway. Only 0.1% of the dose is excreted in the urine as unchanged drug. Of 15 metabolites characterized in human urine, 9 have been assigned structures. The major pathways consist of hydroxylation of the Cλ-carbon of 2 of the leucine residues, C -carbon hydroxylation, and cyclic ether formation (with oxidation of the double bond) in the side chain of the amino acid 3-hydroxyl-N,4-dimethyl-L-2-amino-6-octenoic acid and N-demethylation of N-methyl leucine residues. Hydrolysis of the cyclic peptide chain or conjugation of the aforementioned metabolites do not appear to be important biotransformation pathways.

INDICATIONS AND USAGE

Cyclosporine is indicated for the prophylaxis of organ rejection in kidney, liver, and heart allogeneic transplants. It is always to be used with adrenal corticosteroids. The drug may also be used in the treatment of chronic rejection in patients previously treated with other immunosuppressive agents.

Because of the risk of anaphylaxis, Cyclosporine concentrate for injection should be reserved for patients who are unable to take the capsules or oral solution.

UNLABELED USES

Cyclosporine is used alone or as an adjunct in the treatment of male pattern baldness, alopecia, alopecia areata, alopecia universalis, and alopecia totalis. It is also used to decrease proteinuria in patients with Alport's syndrome, amyotrophic lateral sclerosis, arthous stomatitis, red cell aplasia, Diamond-Blackfan anemia, aplastic anemia, and asthma. Cyclosporine is also prescribed to treat atopic dermatitis, Behcet's syndrome, Crohn's disease, dermatomyositis, polymyositis, type-1 diabetes mellitus, Felty's syndrome, epidermolysis bullosa, erythema nodosum leprosum, and Graves' Ophthalmopathy. It is also used in the treatment of vernal keratoconjunctivitis (with ophthalmic administration), lichen planus, severe keratoconjunctivitis sicca associated with Sjogren's syndrome, for use in corneal

---

► SHOWN IN PRODUCT IDENTIFICATION GUIDE

melting syndromes of known or presumed immunologic etiopathogenesis, including Mooren's ulcer, and treatment of patients at high risk of graft rejection following pentrating keratoplasty. Cyclosporine is also used in the treatment of progressively worsening generalized myasthenia gravis, IGA nephropathy, palmoplantar pustulosis, pemphigus vulgaris, pemphigus foliaceus, pemphigus erythematosus, severe psoriasis, psoriatic arthritis, rheumatoid arthritis, sarcoidosis, scleritis, nonnecrotising scleritis, severe scleroderma, Sjogren's syndrome, Sweet's syndrome, to prevent graft-versus-host-disease (GVHD) in recipients of bone marrow transplant, to prevent graft rejection in high-risk cornea transplant patients, and in posterior and intermediate uveitis.

CONTRAINDICATIONS
Cyclosporine concentrate for injection is contraindicated in patients with a hypersensitivity to Cyclosporine and/or other ingredients in a specific formulation.

WARNINGS
(See boxed "Warnings").

Cyclosporine, when used in high doses, can cause hepatotoxicity and nephrotoxicity.

It is not unusual for serum creatinine and BUN levels to be elevated during Cyclosporine therapy. These elevations in renal transplant patients do not necessarily indicate rejection, and each patient must be fully evaluated before dosage adjustment is initiated.

Nephrotoxicity has been noted in 25% of cases of renal transplantation, 38% of cases of cardiac transplantation, and 37% of cases of liver transplantation. Mild nephrotoxicity was generally noted 2-3 months after transplant and consisted of an arrest in the fall of the preoperative elevations of BUN and creatinine at a range of 35-45 mg/dl and 2.0-2.5 mg/dl respectively. These elevations were often responsive to dosage reduction.

More overt nephrotoxicity was seen early after transplantation and was characterized by a rapidly rising BUN and creatinine. Since these events are similar to rejection episodes care must be taken to differentiate between them. This form of nephrotoxicity is usually responsive to Cyclosporine dosage reduction.

Although specific diagnostic criteria which reliably differentiate renal graft rejection from drug toxicity have not been found, a number of parameters have been significantly associated with one or the other. It should be noted however, that up to 20% of patients may have simultaneous nephrotoxicity and rejection. (See related table).

A form of chronic progressive Cyclosporine-associated nephrotoxicity is characterized by serial deterioration in renal function and morphologic changes in the kidneys. From 5%-15% of transplant recipients will fail to show a reduction in a rising serum creatinine despite a decrease or discontinuation of Cyclosporine therapy. Renal biopsies from these patients will demonstrate an interstitial fibrosis with tubular atrophy. In addition, toxic tubulopathy, peritubular capillary congestion, arteriolopathy, and a striped form of interstitial fibrosis with tubular atrophy may be present. Though none of these morphologic changes is entirely specific, a histologic diagnosis of chronic progressive Cyclosporine-associated nephrotoxicity requires evidence of these.

When considering the development of chronic nephrotoxicity it is noteworthy that several authors have reported an association between the appearance of interstitial fibrosis and higher cumulative doses or persistently high circulating trough levels of Cyclosporine. This is particularly true during the first 6 posttransplant months when the dosage tends to be highest and when, in kidney recipients, the organ appears to be most vulnerable to the toxic effects of Cyclosporine. Among other contributing factors to the development of interstitial fibrosis in these patients must be included, prolonged perfusion time, warm ischemia time, as well as episodes of acute toxicity, and acute and chronic rejection. The reversibility of interstitial fibrosis and its correlation to renal function have not yet been determined.

Impaired renal function at any time requires close monitoring, and frequent dosage adjustment may be indicated. In patients with persistently high elevations of BUN and creatinine who are unresponsive to dosage adjustments, consideration should be given to switching to other immunosuppressive therapy. In the event of severe and unremitting rejection, it is preferable to allow the kidney transplant to be rejected and removed rather than increase the Cyclosporine dosage to a very high level in an attempt to reverse the rejection.

Occasionally patients have developed a syndrome of thrombocytopenia and microangiopathic hemolytic anemia which may result in graft failure. The vasculopathy can occur in the absence of rejection and is accompanied by avid platelet consumption within the graft as demonstrated by Indium 111-labeled platelet studies. Neither the pathogenesis nor the management of this syndrome is clear. Though resolution has occurred after reduction or discontinuation of Cyclosporine and 1) administration of streptokinase and heparin or 2) plasmapheresis, this appears to depend upon early detection with Indium 111-labeled platelet scans. (See "Adverse Reactions").

Significant hyperkalemia (sometimes associated with hyperchloremic metabolic acidosis) and hyperuricemia have been seen occasionally in individual patients.

Hepatotoxicity has been noted in 4% of cases of renal transplantation, 7% of cases of cardiac transplantation, and 4% of cases of liver transplantation. This was usually noted during the first month of therapy when high doses of Cyclosporine were used and consisted of elevations of hepatic enzymes and bilirubin. The chemistry elevations usually decreased with a reduction in dosage.

As in patients receiving other immunosuppressants, those patients receiving Cyclosporine are at increased risk for development of lymphomas and other malignancies, particularly those of the skin. The increased risk appears related to the intensity and duration of immunosuppression rather than to the use of specific agents. Because of the danger of oversuppression of the immune system, which can also increase susceptibility to infection, Cyclosporine should not be administered with other immunosuppressive agents except adrenal corticosteroids. The efficacy and safety of Cyclosporine in combination with other immunosuppressive agents has not been determined.

There have been reports of convulsions in adult and pediatric patients receiving Cyclosporine, particularly in combination with high dose methylprednisolone.

Rarely (approximately 1 in 1000), patients receiving certain brands of Cyclosporine concentrate for injection, have experienced anaphylactic reactions. Although the exact cause of these reactions is unknown, it is believed to be due to the polyoxyethylated castor oil used as the vehicle for the intravenous formulation in these brands. These reactions have consisted of flushing of the face and upper thorax, acute respiratory distress with dyspnea and wheezing, blood pressure changes, and tachycardia. One patient died after respiratory arrest and aspiration pneumonia. In some cases, the reaction subsided after the infusion was stopped.

Patients receiving those brands of Cyclosporine concentrate for injection should be under continuous observation for at least the first 30 minutes following the start of the infusion and at frequent intervals thereafter. If anaphylaxis occurs, the infusion should be stopped. An aqueous solution of epinephrine 1:1000 should be available at the bedside as well as a source of oxygen.

Anaphylactic reactions have not been reported with capsules or oral solution which lack polyoxyethylated castor oil. In fact, patients experiencing anaphylactic reactions have been treated subsequently with the capsules or oral solution without incident. Care should be taken in using cyclosporine with nephrotoxic drugs. (See "Precautions.")

PRECAUTIONS
GENERAL
Patients with malabsorption may have difficulty in achieving therapeutic levels with Cyclosporine capsules or oral solution.

Hypertension is a common side effect of Cyclosporine therapy. (See "Adverse Reactions".) Mild or moderate hypertension is more frequently encountered than severe hypertension and the incidence decreases over time. Antihypertensive therapy may be required. Control of blood pressure can be accomplished with any of the common antihypertensive agents. However, since Cyclosporine may cause hyperkalemia, potassium-sparing diuretics should not be used. While calcium antagonists can be effective agents in treating Cyclosporine-associated hypertension, care should be taken since interference with Cyclosporine metabolism may require a dosage adjustment. (See "Drug Interactions.")

During treatment with Cyclosporine, vaccination may be less effective; and the use of live attenuated vaccines should be avoided.

INFORMATION FOR PATIENTS
Patients should be informed of the necessity of repeated laboratory tests while they are receiving the drug. They should be given careful dosage instruction, advised of the potential risks during pregnancy, and informed of the increased risk of neoplasia.

LABORATORY TESTS
Renal and liver functions should be assessed repeatedly by measurements of BUN, serum creatinine, serum bilirubin, and liver enzymes.

DRUG INTERACTIONS
All of the individual drugs cited below are well substantiated to interact with Cyclosporine.

Drugs That Exhibit Nephrotoxic Synergy:

gentamicin	cimetidine
tobramycin	ranitidine
vancomycin	diclofenac
amphotericin B	trimethoprim with
ketoconazole	sulfamethoxazole
melphalan	azapropazon

Careful monitoring of renal function should be practiced when Cyclosporine is used with nephrotoxic drugs.

Drugs That Alter Cyclosporine Levels: Cyclosporine is extensively metabolized by the liver. Therefore, circulating Cyclosporine levels may be influenced by drugs that affect hepatic microsomal enzymes, particularly the cytochrome P-450 system. Substances known to inhibit these enzymes will decrease heptic metabolism and increase Cyclosporine levels. Substances that are inducers of cytochrome P-450 activity will increase hepatic metabolism and decrease Cyclosporine levels. Monitoring of circulating Cyclosporine levels and appropriate Cyclosporine dosage adjustment are essential when these drugs are used concomitantly (see "Blood Level Monitoring").

Drugs That Increase Cyclosporine Levels:

diltazem
nicardipine
verapamil
ketoconazole
fluconazole
itraconazole
danazol
bromocriptine
metoclopramide

erythromycin
methylprednisolone

Drugs That Decrease Cyclosporine Levels:

rifampin
phenytoin
phenobarbital
carbamazepine

Other Drug Interactions: Reduced clearance of prednisolone, digoxin and lovastatin have been observed when these drugs are administered with Cyclosporine. In addition, a decrease in the apparent volume of distribution of digoxin has been reported after Cyclosporine administration. Severe digitalis toxicity has been seen within days of starting Cyclosporine in several patients taking digoxin. Cyclosporine should not be used with potassium-sparing diuretics because hyperkalemia can occur. During treatment with Cyclosporine, vaccination may be less effective; and the use of live vaccines should be avoided. Myositis has occurred with concomitant lovastatin, frequent gingival hyperplasia with nifedipine, and convulsions with high dose methylprednisolone.

CARCINOGENESIS, MUTAGENESIS, AND IMPAIRMENT OF FERTILITY

Cyclosporine gave no evidence of mutagenic or teratogenic effects in appropriate test systems. Only at dose levels toxic to dams, were adverse effects seen in reproduction studies in rats. (See "Pregnancy").

Carcinogenicity studies were carried out in male and female rats and mice. In the 78-week mouse study, at doses of 1, 4, and 16 mg/kg/day, evidence of a statistically significant trend was found for lymphocytic lymphomas in females, and the incidence of hepatocellular carcinomas in mid-dose males significantly exceeded the control value. In the 24-month rat study, conducted at 0.5, 2, and 8 mg/kg/day, pancreatic islet cell adenomas significantly exceeded the control rate in the low dose level. The hepatocellular carcinomas and pancreatic islet cell adenomas were not dose related. No impairment in fertility was demonstrated in studies in male and female rats.

Cyclosporine has not been found mutagenic/genotoxic in the Ames Test, the V79-HGPRT Test, the micronucleus test in mice and Chinese hamsters, the chromosome-aberration tests in Chinese hamster bone-marrow, the mouse dominant lethal assay, and the DNA-repair test in sperm from treated mice. A recent study analyzing sister chromatid exchange (SCE) induction by Cyclosporine using human lymphocytes *in vitro* gave indication of a positive effect (i.e., induction of SCE), at high concentrations in this system.

An increased incidence of malignancy is a recognized complication of immunosuppression in recipients of organ transplants. The most common forms of neoplasms are non-Hodgkin's lymphoma and carcinomas of the skin. The risk of malignancies in Cyclosporine recipients is higher than in the normal, healthy population but similar to that in patients receiving other immunosuppressive therapies. It has been reported that reduction or discontinuance of immunosuppression may cause the lesions to regress.

PREGNANCY

Pregnancy Category C: Cyclosporine oral solution has been shown to be embryo- and fetotoxic in rats and rabbits when given in doses 2-5 times the human dose. At toxic doses (rats at 30 mg/kg/day and rabbits at 100 mg/kg/day), Cyclosporine oral solution was embryo- and fetotoxic as indicated by increased pre- and postnatal mortality and reduced fetal weight, together with related skeletal retardations. In the well-tolerated dose range (rats at up to 17 mg/kg/day and rabbits at up to 30 mg/kg/day). Cyclosporine oral solution proved to be without any embryolethal or teratogenic effects.

There are no adequate and well-controlled studies in pregnant women. Cyclosporine should be used during pregnancy only if the potential benefit justifies the potential risk to the fetus.

The following data represent the reported outcomes of 116 pregnancies in women receiving Cyclosporine during pregnancy, 90% of whom were transplant patients and most of whom received Cyclosporine throughout the entire

NEPHROTOXICITY VS REJECTION

Parameter	Nephrotoxicity	Rejection
History	Donor > 50 years old or hypotensive Prolonged kidney preservation Prolonged anastamosis time Concomitant nephrotoxic drugs	Antidonor immune response Retransplant patient
Clinical	Often > 6 weeks postop[b] Prolonged initial nonfunction (acute tubular necrosis)	Often < 4 weeks postop[b] Fever > 37.5° C Weight gain > 0.5 Kg Graft swelling and tenderness Decrease in daily urine volume > 500 mL (or 50%)
Laboratory	CyA serum trough level > 200 ng/mL Gradual rise in Cr (< 0.15 mg/dl/day)[a] Cr plateau < 25% above baseline BUN/Cr ≥ 20	CyA serum trough level < 150 ng/mL Rapid rise in Cr (> 0.3 mg/dl/day)[a] Cr > 25% above baseline BUN/Cr < 20
Biopsy	Arteriolopathy (medial hypertrophy[a], hyalinosis, nodular deposits, intimal thickening, endothelial vacuolization, progressive scarring) Tubular atrophy, isometric vacuolization, isolated calcifications Minimal edema Mild focal infiltrates[c] Diffuse interstitial fibrosis, often striped form	Endovasculitis[c] (proliferation[a], intimal arteritis[b], necrosis, sclerosis) Tubulitis with RBC[b] and WBC[b] casts, some irregular vacuolization Interstitial edema[c] and hemorrhage[b] Diffuse moderate to severe mononuclear infiltrates[d] Glomerulitis (mononuclear cells)[c]
Aspiration Cytology	CyA deposits in tubular and endothelial cells Fine isometric vacuolization of tubular cells	Inflammatory infiltrate with mononuclear phagocytes, macrophages, lymphoblastoid cells, and activated T-cells These strongly express HLA-DR antigens
Urine Cytology	Tubular cells with vacuolization and granularization	Degenerative tubular cells, plasma cells, and lymphocyturia > 20% of sediment
Manometry	Intracapsular pressure < 40 mm Hg[b]	Intracapsular pressure > 40 mm Hg[b]
Ultrasonography	Unchanged graft cross sectional area	Increase in graft cross sectional area AP diameter ≥ Transverse diameter
Magnetic Resonance Imagery	Normal appearance	Loss of distinct corticomedullary junction, swelling image intensity of parachyma approaching that of psoas, loss of hilar fat
Radionuclide Scan	Normal or generally decreased perfusion Decrease in tubular function (^{191}1-hippuran) > decrease in perfusion (^{99m} Tc DTPA)	Patchy arterial flow Decrease in perfusion > decrease in tubular function Increased uptake of Indium 111 labeled platelets or Tc-99m in colloid
Therapy	Responds to decreased Cyclosporine	Responds to increased steroids or antilymphocyte globulin

$^a p < 0.05$, $^b p < 0.01$, $^c p < 0.001$, $^d p < 0.0001$

► SHOWN IN PRODUCT IDENTIFICATION GUIDE

gestational period. Since most of the patients were not prospectively identified, the results are likely to be biased toward negative outcomes. The only consistent patterns of abnormality were premature birth (gestational period of 28 to 36 weeks) and low birth weight for gestational age. It is not possible to separate the effects of Cyclosporine on these pregnancies from the effects of the other immunosuppressants, the underlying maternal disorders, or other aspects of the transplantation milieu. Sixteen fetal losses occurred. Most of the pregnancies (85 to 100) were complicated by disorders; including pre-eclampsia, eclampsia, premature labor, abruptio placentae, oligohydramnios, Rh incompatibility and fetoplacental dysfunction. Preterm delivery occurred in 47%. Seven malformations were reported in 5 viable infants and in 2 cases of fetal loss. Twenty-eight percent of the infants were small for gestational age. Neonatal complications occurred in 27%. In a report of 23 children followed up to 4 years, postnatal development was said to be normal.

NURSING MOTHERS
Since Cyclosporine is excreted in human milk, nursing should be avoided.

Pediatric Use: Although no adequate and well-controlled studies have been conducted in children, patients as young as 6 months of age have received the drug with no unusual adverse effects.

ADVERSE REACTIONS
The principal adverse reactions of Cyclosporine therapy are renal dysfunction, tremor, hirsultism, hypertension, and gum hyperplasia.

Hypertension, which is usually mild-to-moderate, may occur in approximately 50% of patients following renal transplantation and in most cardiac-transplant patients.

Glomerular capillary thrombosis has been found in patients treated with Cyclosporine and may progress to graft failure. The pathologic changes resemble those seen in the hemolytic-uremic syndrome and include thrombosis of the renal microvasculature, with platelet-fibrin thrombi occluding glomerular capillaries and afferent arterioles, microangiopathic hemolytic anemia, thrombocytopenia, and decreased renal function. Similar findings have been observed when other immunosuppressives have been employed post-transplantation.

Hypomagnesemia has been reported in some, but not all, patients exhibiting convulsions while on Cyclosporine therapy. Although magnesium-depletion studies in normal subjects suggest that hypomagnesemia is associated with neurologic disorders, multiple factors, including hypertension, high dose methyl-prednisolone, hypocholesterolemia, and nephrotoxicity associated with high plasma concentrations of Cyclosporine appear to be related to the neurological manifestations of Cyclosporine toxicity.

The following reactions occurred in 3% or greater of 892 patients involved in clinical trials of kidney, heart, and liver tranplants: (See related table).

The following reactions occurred in 2% or less of patients: allergic reactions, anemia, anorexia, confusion, conjunctivitis, edema, fever, brittle fingernails, gastritis, hearing loss, hiccups, hyperglycemia, muscle pain, peptic ulcer, thrombocytopenia, tinnitus.

The following reactions occurred rarely: anxiety, chest pain, constipation, depression, hair breaking, hematuria, joint pain, lethargy, mouth sores, myocardial infarction, night sweats, pancreatitis, pruritus, swallowing difficulty, tingling, upper GI bleeding, visual disturbance, weakness, weight loss.

| | Randomized Patients | | All Cyclosporine Patients |
Reason for Discontinuation	Cyclosporine (N = 227) %	Azathioprine (N = 228) %	(N = 705) %
Renal Toxicity	5.7	0	5.4
Infection	0	0.4	0.9
Lack of Efficacy	2.6	0.9	1.4
Acute Tubular Necrosis	2.6	0	1.0
Lymphoma/ Lymphoproliferative Disease	0.4	0	0.3
Hypertension	0	0	0.3
Hematological Abnormalities	0	0.4	0
Other	0	0	0.7

Cyclosporine was discontinued on a temporary basis and then restarted in 18 additional patients.

INFECTIOUS COMPLICATIONS IN THE RANDOMIZED RENAL TRANSPLANT PATIENTS

Complication	Cyclosporine Treatment (N = 227) % of Complications	Standard Treatment* (N = 228) % of Complications
Septicemia	5.3	4.8
Abscesses	4.4	5.3
Systemic Fungal Infection	2.2	3.9
Local Fungal Infection	7.5	9.6
Cytomegalovirus	4.8	12.3
Other Viral Infections	15.9	18.4
Urinary Tract Infections	21.1	20.2
Wound and Skin Infections	7.0	10.1
Pneumonia	6.2	9.2

*   *Some patients also received ALG.*

Polyoxyethylated castor oil, contained in some brands, is known to cause hyperlipemia and electrophoretic abnormalities of lipoproteins. These effects are reversible upon discontinuation of treatment but are usually not a reason to stop treatment.

OVERDOSAGE
There is a minimal experience with overdosage. Because of the slow absorption of Cyclosporine capsules or oral solution, forced emesis would be of value up to 2

| | Randomized Kidney Patients | | All Cyclosporine Patients | | |
Body System/ Adverse Reactions	Cyclosporine (N = 227) %	Azathioprine (N = 228) %	Kidney (N = 705) %	Heart (N = 112) %	Liver (N = 75) %
Genitourinary					
Renal Dysfunction	32	6	25	38	37
Cardiovascular					
Hypertension	26	18	13	53	27
Cramps	4	< 1	2	< 1	0
Skin					
Hirsutism	21	< 1	21	28	45
Acne	6	8	2	2	1
Central Nervous System					
Tremor	12	0	21	31	55
Convulsions	3	1	1	4	5
Headache	2	< 1	2	15	4
Gastrointestinal					
Gum Hyperplasia	4	0	9	5	16
Diarrhea	3	< 1	3	4	8
Nausea/Vomiting	2	< 1	4	10	4
Hepatotoxicity	< 1	< 1	4	7	4
Abdominal Discomfort	< 1	0	< 1	7	0
Autonomic Nervous System					
Paresthesia	3	0	1	2	1
Flushing	< 1	0	4	0	4
Hematopoietic					
Leukopenia	2	19	< 1	6	0
Lymphoma	< 1	0	1	6	
Respiratory					
Sinusitis	< 1	0	4	3	7
Miscellaneous					
Gynecomastia	< 1	0	< 1	4	3

◆ RATED THERAPEUTICALLY EQUIVALENT; ◇ THERAPEUTIC EQUIVALENCE UNCONFIRMED; ○ UNRATED

hours after administration. Transient hepatoxicity and nephrotoxicity may occur which should resolve following drug withdrawal. General supportive measures and symptomatic treatment should be followed in all cases of overdosage. Cyclosporine is not dialyzable to any great extent, nor is it cleared well by charcoal hemoperfusion. The oral LD_{50} is 2329 mg/kg in mice, 1480 mg/kg in rats, and > 1000 mg/kg in rabbits. The intravenous LD_{50} is 148 mg/kg in mice, 104 mg/kg in rats, and 46 mg/kg in rabbits.

DOSAGE AND ADMINISTRATION
CYCLOSPORINE CAPSULES AND CYCLOSPORINE ORAL SOLUTION
The initial oral dose of Cyclosporine should be given 4-12 hours prior to transplantation as a single dose of 15 mg/kg. Although a daily single dose of 14-18 mg/kg was used in most clinical trials, few centers continue to use the highest dose, most favoring the lower end of the scale. There is a trend towards use of even lower initial doses for renal transplantation in the ranges of 10-14 mg/kg/ day. The initial single daily dose is continued postoperatively for 1-2 weeks and then tapered by 5% per week to a maintenance dose of 5-10 mg/kg/day. Some centers have successfully tapered the maintenance dose to as low as 3 mg/kg/day in selected *renal* transplant patients without an apparent rise in rejection rate.

(See "Blood-Level Monitoring" below)

In pediatric usage, the same dose and dosing regimen may be used as in adults, although in several studies, children have required and tolerated higher doses than those used in adults.

Adjunctive therapy with adrenal corticosteroids is recommended. Different tapering dosage schedules of prednisone appear to achieve similar results. A dosage schedule based on the patient's weight started with 2.0 mg/kg/day for the first 4 days tapered to 1.0 mg/kg/day by 1 week, 0.6 mg/kg/day by 2 weeks, 0.3 mg/kg/day by 1 month, and 0.15 mg/kg/day by 2 months and thereafter as a maintenance dose. Another center started with an initial dose of 200 mg tapered by 40 mg/day until reaching 20 mg/day. After 2 months at this dose, a further reduction to 10 mg/day was made. Adjustments in dosage of prednisone must be made according to the clinical situation.

To make Cyclosporine oral solution more palatable, the oral solution may be diluted with milk, chocolate milk, or orange juice preferably at room temperature. Patients should avoid switching diluents frequently. Cyclosporine capsules and oral solution should be administered on a consistent schedule with regard to time of day and relation to meals.

Take the prescribed amount of Cyclosporine from the container using the dosage syringe supplied. Transfer the solution to a glass of milk, chocolate milk, or orange juice. Stir well and drink at once. Do not allow to stand before drinking. It is best to use a glass container and rinse it with more diluent to ensure that the total dose is taken. After use, replace the dosage syringe in the protective cover, if one is supplied. To avoid cloudiness, do not rinse the dosage syringe with water or other cleaning agents. If the dosage syringe requires cleaning, it must be completely dry before resuming use.

CYCLOSPORINE CONCENTRATE FOR INJECTION
FOR INFUSION ONLY
Note: Anaphylactic reactions have occurred with Cyclosporine concentrate for injection. (See "Warnings")

Patients unable to take Cyclosporine capsules or oral solution pre- or postoperatively may be treated with the intravenous concentrate. **Cyclosporine concentrate for injection, is administered at ⅓ the oral dose.** The initial dose of Cyclosporine concentrate for injection, should be given 4-12 hours prior to transplantation as a single intravenous dose of 5-6 mg/kg/day. This daily single dose is continued postoperatively until the patient can tolerate the capsules or oral solution. Patients should be switched to Cyclosporine capsules or oral solution as soon as possible after surgery. In pediatric usage, the same dose and dosing regimen may be used, although higher doses may be required.

Adjunct steroid therapy is to be used. (*See aforementioned*) Immediately before use, the intravenous concentrate should be diluted 1 mL Cyclosporine concentrate for injection in 20 mL-100 mL 0.9% Sodium Chloride Injection or 5% Dextrose Injection and given in a slow intravenous infusion over approximately 2-6 hours.

Diluted infusion solutions should be discarded after 24 hours.

The polyoxyethylated castor oil contained in some concentrates for intravenous infusion can cause phthalate stripping from PVC.

Parenteral drug products should be inspected visually for particulate matter and discoloration prior to administration, whenever solution and container permit.

BLOOD LEVEL MONITORING
Several study centers have found blood level monitoring of Cyclosporine useful in patient management. While no fixed relationships have yet been established, in one series of 375 consecutive cadaveric renal transplant recipients, dosage was adjusted to achieve specific whole blood 24-hour trough levels of 100-200 ng/mL as determined by high-pressure liquid chromatography (HPLC).

Of major importance to blood level analysis is the type of assay used. The above levels are specific to the parent Cyclosporine molecule and correlate directly to the new monoclonal specific radioimmunoassays (mRIA-sp). Nonspecific assays are also available which detect the parent compound molecule and various of its metabolites. Older studies often cited levels using a nonspecific assay which were roughly twice those of specific assays. Assay results are not interchangeable and their use should be guided by their approved labeling. If plasma specimens are employed, levels will vary with the temperature at the time of separation from whole blood. Plasma levels may range from $1/2$ to $1/5$ of whole blood levels. Refer to individual assay labeling for complete instructions. In addition, *Transplantation Proceedings* (June 1990) contains position papers and a broad consensus generated at the Cyclosporine-Therapeutic Drug Monitoring conference that year. Blood level monitoring is not a replacement for renal function monitoring or tissue biopsies.

STORAGE
Store capsules in the original unit-dose container at temperatures below 86°F (30°C). Store oral solution in the original container at temperatures below 86°F (30°C). Do not store in the refrigerator. Once opened, the contents must be used within 2 months. Store concentrate for injection at temperatures below 86°F (30°C) and protected from light. Protect from freezing.

J CODES
250 mg IV K0122
25 mg ORAL K0121
Amp,250 mg, 5 ml, 10s ea UD IV—J7503
Sol;100 mg/ml, 50 ml, ea ORAL—J7502

HOW SUPPLIED
CAPSULE: 25 MG

BRAND/MANUFACTURER	NDC	SIZE	AWP
○ **BRAND**			
SANDIMMUNE: Sandoz Pharm	00078-0240-15	30s ud	$37.50

CAPSULE: 50 MG

BRAND/MANUFACTURER	NDC	SIZE	AWP
○ **BRAND**			
SANDIMMUNE: Sandoz Pharm	00078-0242-15	30s ud	$74.94

CAPSULE: 100 MG

BRAND/MANUFACTURER	NDC	SIZE	AWP
○ **BRAND**			
SANDIMMUNE: Sandoz Pharm	00078-0241-15	30s ud	$149.88

INJECTION: 50 MG/ML

BRAND/MANUFACTURER	NDC	SIZE	AWP
○ **BRAND**			
SANDIMMUNE: Sandoz Pharm	00078-0109-01	5 ml 10s ud	$222.78

SOLUTION: 100 MG/ML

BRAND/MANUFACTURER	NDC	SIZE	AWP
○ **BRAND**			
SANDIMMUNE: Sandoz Pharm	00078-0110-22	50 ml	$249.66

Cyclothiazide

DESCRIPTION
Cyclothiazide is 6-chloro-3,4-dihydro-3-(5-norbornen-2-yl)-2H-1,2,4- benzothiadiazine-7-sulfonamide 1,1-dioxide.

Cyclothiazide is a white crystalline solid with a melting point of approximately 220°C. It is moderately soluble in hot ethyl alcohol and hot dilute alcohol, very soluble in cold ethyl acetate (an ethyl acetate solvate is formed), and relatively insoluble in ether, benzene, or chloroform.

Cyclothiazide is an orally effective diuretic-antihypertensive agent. It is available in 2-mg (5-µmol) tablets.

Following is its chemical structure:

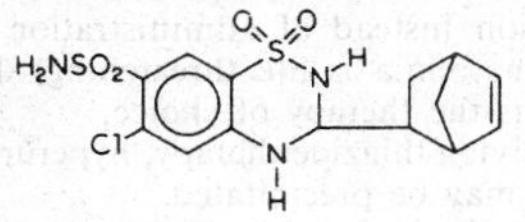

CLINICAL PHARMACOLOGY
The diuretic effect of Cyclothiazide results from inhibition of renal tubular reabsorption of sodium and chloride in the distal portion of the nephron. Cyclothiazide increases the urinary excretion of sodium and chloride in approximately equal proportion. The excretion of potassium is generally increased to a lesser extent than that of sodium. The excretion of bicarbonate is slightly increased by Cyclothiazide although not enough to change urinary pH. At maximum therapeutic dosage, all thiazides have approximately equal diuretic efficacy.

Like other benzothiazides, Cyclothiazide also has antihypertensive properties. The mechanism of the antihypertensive effect of benzothiazides is not known.

During chronic administration of Cyclothiazide, as with other benzothiazides, some patients develop hypokalemia, hyperuricemia, and hyperglycemia. Hyponatremia and hypochloremia also occur, particularly in edematous patients, and appear to be related to positive water balance.

Thiazides are rapidly absorbed from the gastrointestinal tract. All thiazides probably undergo active secretion in the proximal tubule. The renal clearance of thiazides is high. Most compounds are rapidly excreted within 3 to 6 hours.

The diuretic effect of Cyclothiazide starts within 2 to 4 hours, peaks between 7 and 12 hours, and has a total duration of 18 to 24 hours following the administration of a single dose.

INDICATIONS AND USAGE

Cyclothiazide is indicated as adjunctive therapy in edema associated with congestive heart failure, hepatic cirrhosis, and corticosteroid and estrogen therapy.

Cyclothiazide has also been found useful in edema due to various forms of renal dysfunction, such as nephrotic syndrome, acute glomerulonephritis, and chronic renal failure.

Cyclothiazide is indicated in the management of hypertension either as the sole therapeutic agent or to enhance the effectiveness of other antihypertensive drugs in the more severe forms of hypertension.

Usage in Pregnancy: The routine use of diuretics in an otherwise healthy woman is inappropriate and exposes mother and fetus to unnecessary hazard. Diuretics do not prevent development of toxemia of pregnancy, and there is no satisfactory evidence that they are useful in the treatment of developed toxemia.

Edema during pregnancy may arise from pathologic causes or from the physiologic and mechanical consequences of pregnancy. Thiazides are indicated in pregnancy, as in the absence of pregnancy, when edema is due to pathologic causes (however, see *"Pregnancy"* under *"Precautions"* below). Dependent edema in pregnancy, resulting from restriction of venous return caused by the expanded uterus, is properly treated through elevation of the lower extremities and use of support hose; in such cases, use of diuretics to lower intravascular volume is illogical and unnecessary. In the majority of pregnant women, hypervolemia occurs during normal pregnancy and is not harmful to either the fetus or the mother (in the absence of cardiovascular disease) but is associated with edema, including generalized edema. If this edema produces discomfort, increased recumbency will often provide relief. In rare instances, such edema may cause extreme discomfort that is not relieved by rest. In these cases, a short course of diuretics may provide relief and may be appropriate.

CONTRAINDICATIONS

Cyclothiazide is contraindicated in anuria and in patients who are hypersensitive to Cyclothiazide or other sulfonamide-derived drugs.

WARNINGS

Thiazides should be used with caution in severe renal disease. In patients with renal disease, thiazides may precipitate azotemia. Cumulative effects of the drug may develop in patients with impaired renal function.

Thiazides should be used with caution in patients with impaired hepatic function or progressive liver disease, since minor alterations of fluid and electrolyte balance may precipitate hepatic coma.

PRECAUTIONS

General: All patients receiving thiazides should be observed for clinical signs of fluid or electrolyte imbalance, eg, hyponatremia, hypochloremic alkalosis, and hypokalemia. Serum and urine electrolyte determinations are particularly important when the patient is vomiting excessively or receiving parenteral fluids. Medication such as digitalis may also influence serum electrolytes. Warning signs, irrespective of cause, are dryness of mouth, thirst, weakness, lethargy, drowsiness, restlessness, muscle pains or cramps, muscular fatigue, hypotension oliguria, tachycardia, and gastrointestinal disturbances, such as nausea and vomiting.

Hypokalemia may develop with use of thiazides, as with any other potent diuretic, especially with brisk diuresis, in the presence of severe cirrhosis, or during concomitant use of corticosteroids or ACTH. Interference with adequate oral electrolyte intake will also contribute to hypokalemia.

Any chloride deficit is generally mild and does not require specific treatment except under extraordinary circumstances (as in liver or renal disease). Dilutional hyponatremia may occur in edematous patients in hot weather. The appropriate therapy is water restriction instead of administration of salt (except in rare instances when the hyponatremia is life threatening). In actual salt depletion, appropriate replacement is the therapy of choice.

In certain patients receiving thiazide therapy, hyperuricemia or hypercalcemia may occur or frank gout may be precipitated.

Hypomagnesemia may also occur in some patients, especially the elderly, during thiazide therapy.

The antihypertensive effects of the drug may be enhanced in postsympathectomy patients.

Thiazides may decrease arterial responsiveness to norepinephrine. This diminution is not sufficient to preclude effectiveness of the pressor agent for therapeutic use.

If progressive renal impairment becomes evident, as indicated by a rising nonprotein nitrogen or blood urea nitrogen, therapy should be carefully reappraised, because it may be necessary to withhold or discontinue diuretic therapy.

Sensitivity reactions may occur in patients with a history of allergy or bronchial asthma.

The possibility of exacerbation or activation of systemic lupus erythematosus has been reported.

Information for Patients: Patients should be informed about the possible additive effects of treatment with corticosteroids, excessive gastrointestinal fluid losses (vomiting, diarrhea), and the effect of treatment with thiazides on potassium depletion. Patients should also be informed about the potential risks of drug-related potassium depletion and hypokalemia with regard to the enhancement of digitalis toxicity. When the weather is hot, diuretic-receiving patients, especially the elderly, should be warned of the increased risk of heatstroke.

Laboratory Test: Determination of serum electrolytes to detect possible imbalance should be performed at appropriate intervals.

Drug Interactions: Thiazides may add to or potentiate the action of other antihypertensive drugs. Potentiation occurs with ganglionic or peripheral adrenergic blocking drugs.

The concurrent use of ACTH or corticosteroids and thiazide diuretics may enhance urinary potassium loss.

Potassium depletion and hypokalemia secondary to the use of thiazide diuretics may potentiate the effects of digitalis on the heart, thus enhancing the possibility of digitalis toxicity.

Insulin requirements in diabetic patients may be increased, decreased, or unchanged. Latent diabetes mellitus may become manifest during thiazide administration.

Thiazide drugs may increase the responsiveness of tubocurarine.

The renal clearance of lithium may be reduced during administration of thiazide derivatives, thus enhancing lithium toxicity.

Concurrent administration of some nonsteroidal anti-inflammatory agents may reduce the diuretic, natriuretic, and antihypertensive effects of thiazide diuretics.

Drug/Laboratory Test Interactions: Thiazides may decrease serum PBI levels without signs of thyroid disturbance.

Carcinogenesis, Mutagenesis, Impairment of Fertility: No studies have been performed in animals to evaluate the carcinogenic or mutagenic potential of Cyclothiazide. No animal studies have been conducted to determine whether Cyclothiazide has the potential to impair fertility.

Pregnancy: Teratogenic Effects: Pregnancy Category C: Animal reproduction studies have not been conducted with Cyclothiazide. It is also not known whether this drug can cause fetal harm when administered to a pregnant woman or can affect reproduction capacity. Cyclothiazide should be given to a pregnant woman only if clearly needed (see *"Indications and Usage"*).

Nonteratogenic Effects: Thiazides cross the placental barrier and appear in cord blood. The use of thiazides in pregnant women requires that the anticipated benefit be weighed against possible hazards to the fetus. These hazards include fetal or neonatal jaundice, thrombocytopenia, and possibly other adverse reactions that have occurred in the adult.

Nursing Mothers: Thiazides appear in breast milk. If use of the drug is deemed essential, the patient should stop nursing.

Pediatric Use: Safety and effectiveness in children have not been established.

ADVERSE REACTIONS

The following adverse reactions have been observed, but there is not enough systematic collection of data to support an estimate of their frequency.

Gastrointestinal: Anorexia, gastric irritation, nausea, vomiting, cramping, diarrhea, constipation, jaundice (intrahepatic cholestatic jaundice), pancreatitis.

Central Nervous System: Dizziness, vertigo, paresthesias, headache, xanthopsia.

Hematologic: Leukopenia, agranulocytosis, thrombocytopenia, aplastic anemia.

Dermatologic and Hypersensitivity: Purpura, photosensitivity, rash, urticaria, necrotizing angiitis (vasculitis or cutaneous vasculitis).

Cardiovascular: Orthostatic hypotension may occur and may be aggravated by alcohol, barbiturates, or narcotics.

Other: Hyperglycemia, glycosuria, hyperuricemia, muscle spasm, weakness, restlessness.

Whenever adverse reactions are moderate or severe, thiazide dosage should be reduced or therapy withdrawn.

OVERDOSAGE

Signs and Symptoms: Symptoms of overdose from Cyclothiazide are often related to hypovolemia, hypokalemia, and other types of electrolyte imbalance. Symptoms may also include orthostatic hypotension, weakness, confusion dizziness, hyporeflexia, impaired urinary concentrating ability, and cardiac arrhythmias. Cyclothiazide may also cause hyperglycemia, hypercalcemia, and hyperuricemia.

Treatment: To obtain up-to-date information about the treatment of overdose, a good resource is your certified Regional Poison Control Center. Telephone numbers of certified poison control centers are listed in the *Physicians' Desk Reference (PDR)*. In managing overdosage, consider the possibility of multiple drug overdoses, interaction among drugs, and unusual drug kinetics in your patients.

For small overdoses, correct fluid and electrolyte balance and monitor electrolytes frequently.

Protect the patient's airway and support ventilation and perfusion. Meticulously monitor and maintain, within acceptable limits, the patient's vital signs, blood gases, serum electrolytes, etc. Absorption of drugs from the gut may be decreased by giving activated charcoal, which, in many cases, is more effective than emesis or lavage; consider charcoal instead of or in addition to gastric emptying. Repeated doses of charcoal over time may hasten elimination of some drugs that have been absorbed. Safeguard the patient's airway when employing gastric emptying or charcoal.

◆ RATED THERAPEUTICALLY EQUIVALENT; ◇ THERAPEUTIC EQUIVALENCE UNCONFIRMED; ○ UNRATED

DOSAGE AND ADMINISTRATION

Therapy should be individualized according to patient response. This therapy should be titrated to gain maximum therapeutic response with the minimum dose possible to maintain that response.

For Diuretic Effect: The usual adult dosage of Cyclothiazide is ½ or 1 tablet (1 or 2 mg) once a day, preferably given early in the morning in order to obtain diuresis predominantly during the day and avoid disturbing the patient's rest at night. After the edema is eliminated, the dosage should be reduced according to the patient's need; body weight is usually a very helpful guide. For maintenance therapy, ½ to 1 tablet given on alternate days or 2 or 3 times a week may be sufficient. Such an intermittent dosage schedule reduces the possibility of excessive depletion of body sodium and chloride or of potassium deficiency.

For Antihypertensive Effect: The dosage of Cyclothiazide, like that of other thiazides, is often greater than that required for diuresis. The usual dosage of Cyclothiazide is 1 tablet (2 mg) once a day; in some cases, it may be necessary to give 1 tablet 2 or 3 times a day.

Since Cyclothiazide augments the action of other antihypertensive drugs, dosage of the latter should be reduced—perhaps to 50% of the usually recommended dosage—at the start of treatment and carefully readjusted upward or downward according to the patient's response and need.

Store at controlled room temperature, 59° to 86°F (15° to 30°C).

Dispense in well-closed container.

HOW SUPPLIED

Current prices are unavailable. Check wholesaler for further information.

Cyklokapron *SEE* TRANEXAMIC ACID

Cylert *SEE* PEMOLINE

Cyproheptadine Hydrochloride

DESCRIPTION

Cyproheptadine Hydrochloride is an antithistaminic and antiserotonergic agent.

Cyproheptadine Hydrochloride is a white to slightly yellowish, crystalline solid, with a molecular weight of 350.89, which is soluble in water, freely soluble in methanol, sparingly soluble in ethanol, soluble in chloroform, and practically insoluble in ether. It is the sesquihydrate of 4-(5*H*-dibenzo[*a,b*]cyclohepten-5-ylidene)-1-methylpiperidine hydrochloride. The empirical formula of the anhydrous salt is $C_{21}H_{21}N \cdot HCl$.

Cyproheptadine is available in tablets, containing 4 mg of Cyproheptadine Hydrochloride, and as a syrup in which 5 mL contains 2 mg of Cyproheptadine Hydrochloride, with a pH range of 3.5 to 4.5.

Following is its chemical structure:

• HCl • 1.5H$_2$O

CLINICAL PHARMACOLOGY

Cyproheptadine is a serotonin and histamine antagonist with anticholinergic and sedative effects. Antiserotonin and antihistamine drugs appear to compete with serotonin and histamine, respectively, for receptor sites.

PHARMACOKINETICS AND METABOLISM

After a single 4 mg oral dose of ^{14}C-labelled Cyproheptadine HCl in normal subjects, given as tablets or syrup, 2-20% of the radioactivity was excreted in the stools. Only about 34% of the stool radioactivity was unchanged drug, corresponding to less than 5.7% of the dose. At least 40% of the administered radioactivity was excreted in the urine. No significant difference in the mean urinary excretion exists between the tablet and syrup formulations. No detectable amounts of unchanged drugs were present in the urine of patients on chronic 12-20 mg daily doses of Cyproheptadine Syrup. The principle metabolite found in human urine has been identified as a quaternary ammonium glucuronide conjugate of Cyproheptadine. Elimination is diminished in renal insufficiency.

INDICATIONS AND USAGE

Perennial and seasonal allergic rhinitis

Vasomotor rhinitis

Allergic conjunctivitis due to inhalant allergens and foods

Mild, uncomplicated allergic skin manifestations of urticaria and angioedema

Amelioration of allergic reactions to blood or plasma

Cold urticaria

Dermatographism

As therapy for anaphylactic reactions *adjunctive* to epinephrine and other standard measures after the acute manifestations have been controlled.

UNLABELED USES

Cyproheptadine is used alone or as an adjunct in the treatment of Cushing's Disease, as an appetite stimulant during treatment of anorexia nervosa, and as prophylaxis for migraine headache.

CONTRAINDICATIONS

NEWBORN OR PREMATURE INFANTS

This drug should *not* be used in newborn or premature infants.

NURSING MOTHERS

Because of the higher risk of antihistamines for infants generally and for newborns and prematures in particular, antihistamine therapy is contraindicated in nursing mothers.

OTHER CONDITIONS

Hypersensitivity to Cyproheptadine and other drugs of similar chemical structure:

Monoamine oxidase inhibitor therapy (see *"Drug Interactions"*)

Angle-closure glaucoma

Stenosing peptic ulcer

Symptomatic prostatic hypertrophy

Bladder neck obstruction

Pyloroduodenal obstruction

Elderly, debilitated patients

WARNINGS

CHILDREN

Overdosage of antihistamines, particularly in infants and children, may produce hallucinations, central nervous system depression, convulsions, and death.

Antihistamines may diminish mental alertness; conversely, particularly, in the young child, they may occasionally produce excitation.

CNS DEPRESSANTS

Antihistamines may have additive effects with alcohol and other CNS depressants, e.g., hypnotics, sedatives, tranquilizers, antianxiety agents.

ACTIVITIES REQUIRING MENTAL ALERTNESS

Patients should be warned about engaging in activities requiring mental alertness and motor coordination, such as driving a car or operating machinery.

Antihistamines are more likely to cause dizziness, sedation, and hypotension in elderly patients.

PRECAUTIONS

GENERAL

Cyproheptadine has an atropine-like action and, therefore, should be used with caution in patients with:

History of bronchial asthma

Increased intraocular pressure

Hyperthyroidism

Cardiovascular disease

Hypertension

INFORMATION FOR PATIENTS

Antihistamines may diminish mental alertness; conversely, particularly, in the young child, they may occasionally produce excitation.

Patients should be warned about engaging in activities requiring mental alertness and motor coordination, such as driving a car or operating machinery.

DRUG INTERACTIONS

MAO inhibitors prolong and intensify the anticholinergic effects of antihistamines.

Antihistamines may have additive effects with alcohol and other CNS depressants, e.g., hypnotics, sedatives, tranquilizers, antianxiety agents.

CARCINOGENESIS, MUTAGENESIS, IMPAIRMENT OF FERTILITY

Long-term carcinogenic studies have not been done with Cyproheptadine.

Cyproheptadine had no effect on fertility in a two-litter study in rats or a two generation study in mice at about 10 times the human dose.

Cyproheptadine did not produce chromosome damage in human lymphocytes or fibroblasts *in vitro*; high doses (10^{-4} M) were cytotoxic. Cyproheptadine did not have any mutagenic effect in the Ames microbial mutagen test; concentrations of above 500 mcg/plate inhibited bacterial growth.

PREGNANCY

Pregnancy Category B: Reproduction studies have been performed in rabbits, mice, and rats at oral or subcutaneous doses up to 32 times the maximum recommended human oral dose and have revealed no evidence of impaired fertility or harm to the fetus due to Cyproheptadine. Cyproheptadine has been shown to be fetotoxic in rats when given by intraperitoneal injection in doses four times the maximum recommended human oral dose. Two studies in pregnant women, however, have not shown that Cyproheptadine increases the risk of abnormalities when administered during the first, second and third trimesters of pregnancy. No teratogenic effects were observed in any of the newborns. Nevertheless, because the studies in humans cannot rule out the possibility of harm, Cyproheptadine should be used during pregnancy only if clearly needed.

► SHOWN IN PRODUCT IDENTIFICATION GUIDE

NURSING MOTHERS

It is not known whether this drug is excreted in human milk. Because many drugs are excreted in human milk, and because of the potential for serious adverse reactions in nursing infants from Cyproheptadine, a decision should be made whether to discontinue nursing or to discontinue the drug, taking into account the importance of the drug to the mother (see "Contraindications").

PEDIATRIC USE

Safety and effectiveness in children below the age of two have not been established. See "Contraindications, Newborn Premature Infants," and "Warnings, Children."

ADVERSE REACTIONS

Adverse reactions which have been reported with the use of antihistamines are as follows:

Central Nervous System: Sedation and sleepiness (often transient), dizziness, disturbed coordination, confusion, restlessness, excitation, nervousness, tremor, irritability, insomnia, paresthesias, neuritis, convulsions, euphoria, hallucinations, hysteria, faintness.

Integumentary: Allergic manifestation of rash and edema, excessive perspiration, urticaria, photosensitivity.

Special Senses: Acute labyrinthitis, blurred vision, diplopia, vetigo, tinnitus.

Cardiovascular: Hypotension, palpitation, tachycardia, extrasystoles, anaphylactic shock.

Hematologic: Hemolytic anemia, leukopenia, agranulocytosis, thrombocytopenia.

Digestive System: Dryness of mouth, epigastric distress, anorexia, nausea, vomiting, diarrhea, constipation, jaundice.

Genitourinary: Urinary frequency, difficult urination, urinary retention, early menses.

Respiratory: Dryness of nose and throat, thickening of bronchial secretions, tightness of chest and wheezing, nasal stuffiness.

Miscellaneous: Fatigue, chills, headache.

OVERDOSAGE

Antihistamine overdosage reactions may vary from central nervous system depression to stimulation especially in children. Also, atropine-like signs and symptoms (dry mouth; fixed, dilated pupils; flushing, etc.) as well as gastrointestinal symptoms may occur.

If vomiting has not occurred spontaneously the patient should be induced to vomit with syrup of ipecac.

If the patient is unable to vomit, perform gastric lavage followed by activated charcoal. Isotonic or ½ isotonic saline is the lavage of choice. Precautions against aspiration must be taken especially in infants and children.

When life threatening CNS signs and symptoms are present, intravenous physostigmine salicylate may be considered. Dosage and frequency of administration are dependent on age, clinical response, and recurrence after response. (See package circulars for physostigmine products.)

Saline cathartics, as milk of magnesia, by osmosis draw water into the bowel and, therefore, are valuable for their action in rapid dilution of bowel content.

Stimulants should *not* be used.

Vasopressors may be used to treat hypotension.

The oral LD$_{50}$ of Cyproheptadine is 123 mg/kg, and 295 mg/kg in the mouse and rat, respectively.

DOSAGE AND ADMINISTRATION

DOSAGE SHOULD BE INDIVIDUALIZED ACCORDING TO THE NEEDS AND THE RESPONSE OF THE PATIENT. Each Cyproheptadine tablet contains 4 mg of Cyproheptadine Hydrochloride. Each 5 mL of Cyproheptadine syrup contains 2 mg of Cyproheptadine Hydrochloride.

Although intended primarily for administration to children, the syrup is also useful for administration to adults who cannot swallow tablets.

CHILDREN

The total daily dosage for children may be calculated on the basis of body weight or body area using approximately 0.25 mg/kg/day (0.11 mg/lb/day) or 8 mg per square meter of body surface (8 mg/M^2). In small children for whom the calculation of dosage based upon body size is most important, it may be necessary to use Cyproheptadine syrup to permit accurate dosage.

AGE 2 TO 6 YEARS

The usual dose is 2 mg (½ tablet or 1 teaspoon) two or three times a day, adjusted as necessary to the size and response of the patient. The dose is not to exceed 12 mg a day.

AGE 7 TO 14 YEARS

The usual dose is 4 mg (1 tablet or 2 teaspoons) two or three times a day, adjusted as necessary to the size and response of the patient. The dose is not to exceed 16 mg a day.

ADULTS

The total daily dose for adults should not exceed 0.5 mg/kg/day (0.23 mg/lb/day).

The therapeutic range is 4 to 20 mg a day, with the majority of patients requiring 12 to 16 mg a day. An occasional patient may require as much as 32 mg a day for adequate relief. It is suggested that dosage be initiated with 4 mg (1

tablet or 2 teaspoons) three times a day and adjusted according to the size and response of the patient.

STORAGE

Store Tablets in a well-closed container. Avoid storage at temperatures above 40°C (104°F).

Store Syrup in a container which is kept tightly closed. Avoid storage at temperatures below −20°C (−4°F) and above 40°C (104°F).

HOW SUPPLIED
SYRUP: 2 MG/5 ML

AVERAGE UNIT PRICE (AVAILABLE SIZES)		GENERIC A-RATED AVERAGE PRICE (GAAP)	
BRAND	$0.06	480 ml	$9.48
GENERIC	$0.02		
HCFA FUL (480 ml)	$0.01		

BRAND/MANUFACTURER	NDC	SIZE	AWP
◆ **BRAND**			
PERIACTIN: Merck	00006-3289-74	480 ml	$30.16
◆ **GENERICS**			
Moore,H.L.	00839-6493-69	480 ml	$6.74
Schein	00364-7272-16	480 ml	$8.50
Qualitest	00603-1117-58	480 ml	$8.65
Rugby	00536-1930-85	480 ml	$8.69
Major	00904-1146-16	480 ml	$8.90
Goldline	00182-1355-40	480 ml	$9.00
Halsey Pharm	00879-0473-16	480 ml	$10.50
Barre	00472-0755-16	480 ml	$10.71
Aligen	00405-2600-16	480 ml	$12.65
Halsey Pharm	00879-0473-28	3840 ml	$61.90

TABLETS: 4 MG

AVERAGE UNIT PRICE (AVAILABLE SIZES)		GENERIC A-RATED AVERAGE PRICE (GAAP)	
BRAND	$0.39	100s	$7.11
GENERIC	$0.06	500s	$13.62
HCFA FUL (100s ea)	$0.02	1000s	$34.38

BRAND/MANUFACTURER	NDC	SIZE	AWP
◆ **BRAND**			
PERIACTIN: Merck	00006-0062-68	100s	$39.43
◆ **GENERICS**			
Schein	00364-0499-01	100s	$3.50
Camall	00147-0236-10	100s	$3.55
Goldline	00182-1132-01	100s	$4.00
Rugby	00536-3515-01	100s	$4.13
URL	00677-0623-01	100s	$4.20
Major	00904-1145-60	100s	$4.25
Zenith	00172-2929-60	100s	$4.25
Qualitest	00603-3098-21	100s	$4.31
Martec	52555-0043-01	100s	$4.45
Moore,H.L.	00839-6300-06	100s	$4.71
Moore,H.L.	00839-7866-06	100s	$4.71
Par	49884-0043-01	100s	$5.05
Aligen	00405-4295-01	100s	$6.55
Sidmak	50111-0314-01	100s	$6.55
U.S. Trading	56126-0043-11	100s ud	$3.59
Raway	00686-0159-20	100s ud	$9.00
Major	00904-1145-61	100s ud	$9.29
Goldline	00182-1132-89	100s ud	$10.85
Vangard	00615-1536-13	100s ud	$11.33
Auro	55829-0220-10	100s ud	$11.40
UDL	51079-0159-20	100s ud	$18.40
Medirex	57480-0428-01	100s ud	$18.45
Camall	00147-0236-05	500s	$10.34
Rugby	00536-3515-05	500s	$14.93
Schein	00364-0499-05	500s	$15.60
Camall	00147-0236-20	1000s	$18.53
Zenith	00172-2929-80	1000s	$22.70
Rugby	00536-3515-10	1000s	$29.25
URL	00677-0623-10	1000s	$29.40
Goldline	00182-1132-10	1000s	$30.00
Major	00904-1145-90	1000s	$30.10
Moore,H.L.	00839-6300-16	1000s	$30.50
Moore,H.L.	00839-7866-16	1000s	$30.50
Martec	52555-0043-10	1000s	$41.50
Qualitest	00603-3098-32	1000s	$42.85
Aligen	00405-4295-03	1000s	$44.28
Sidmak	50111-0314-03	1000s	$44.28
Par	49884-0043-10	1000s	$53.03

Cysteine Hydrochloride

DESCRIPTION

Cysteine Hydrochloride is a sterile, nonpyrogenic solution containing 0.5 gram of Cysteine Hydrochloride, monohydrate in 10 ml of water for injection. Cysteine is a sulfur-containing amino acid. In premixed solutions of crystalline amino acids, cysteine is relatively unstable over time, eventually converting to insoluble cystine. To avoid such precipitation, Cysteine Hydrochloride Injection, USP is

---

◆ RATED THERAPEUTICALLY EQUIVALENT; ◇ THERAPEUTIC EQUIVALENCE UNCONFIRMED; ○ UNRATED

provided as an additive for use with crystalline amino acid solutions immediately prior to administration to the patient.

Cysteine Hydrochloride, monohydrate is chemically designated $C_3H_7NO_2S \cdot HCl \cdot H_2O$, a white crystalline powder soluble in water.

Following is its chemical structure:

$$HSCH_2 - \underset{\underset{NH_2}{|}}{\overset{\overset{H}{|}}{C}} - COOH \cdot HCl \cdot H_2O$$

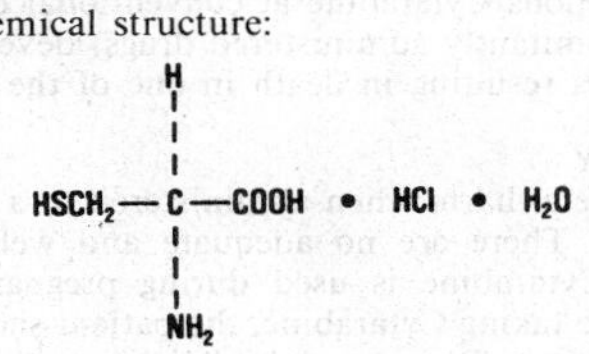

CLINICAL PHARMACOLOGY

Cysteine is synthesized from methionine via the trans-sulfuration pathway in the adult, but newborn infants lack the enzyme, cystathionase, necessary to effect this conversion. Therefore, Cysteine Hydrochloride is generally considered to be an essential amino acid in infants.

Metabolism of cysteine produces pyruvate and inorganic sulfate as end products. Cysteine is introduced directly into the pathway of carbohydrate metabolism at the pyruvate stage with all three carbons convertible to glucose. The sulfur is primarily transformed to inorganic sulfate, which is introduced into complex polysaccharides among other structural components.

INDICATIONS AND USAGE

Cysteine Hydrochloride is indicated for use only after dilution as an additive to Aminosyn (a crystalline amino acid solution) to meet the intravenous amino acid nutritional requirements of infants receiving total parenteral nutrition.

CONTRAINDICATIONS, WARNINGS, PRECAUTIONS AND ADVERSE REACTIONS

The contraindications, warnings, precautions and adverse reactions associated with Cysteine Hydrochloride amino acids, injectable, additive are the same as those cited for, given as part of a total parenteral nutrition program, as defined in the accompanying amino acids, injectable, package insert.

Pregnancy Category C: Animal reproduction studies have not been conducted with Cysteine Hydrochloride. It is also not known whether this additive can cause fetal harm when administered to pregnant women or can affect reproductive capacity. This additive should be given to a pregnant woman only if clearly indicated.

OVERDOSAGE

In the event of overhydration or solute overload, re-evaluate the patient and institute appropriate corrective measures. See *"Warning"* and *"Precautions"* appearing in accompanying amino acids, injectable, package insert.

DOSAGE AND ADMINISTRATION

Cysteine Hydrochloride is intended for use in a crystalline, amino acid solution. Each 10 ml of Cysteine Hydrochloride 0.5 gram should be combined aseptically with 12.5 grams of amino acids, such as that present in 250 ml of amino acids, injectable 5%. The admixture is then diluted with 250 ml of dextrose 50% or such lesser volume as indicated. Equal volumes of amino acids, injectable 5% and dextrose 50% produce a final solution which contains amino acids, injectable 2.5% in dextrose 25%, which is suitable for administration by central venous infusion. Administration of the final admixture should begin within one hour of mixing. Otherwise, the admixture should be refrigerated immediately and used within 24 hours of the time of mixing. For the recommended rate of administration, see the Aminosyn package insert.

Parenteral drug products should be inspected visually for particulate matter and discoloration prior to administration whenever solution and container permit.

Exposure of pharmaceutical products to heat should be minimized. Avoid excessive heat. Protect from freezing. It is recommended that the product be stored at room temperature (25° C); however, brief exposure up to 40° C does not adversely affect the product.

HOW SUPPLIED
INJECTION: 50 MG/ML

BRAND/MANUFACTURER	NDC	SIZE	AWP
◆ GENERICS			
Abbott Hosp	00074-8975-02	10 ml 25s	$431.06

Cysto-Conray *SEE* IOTHALAMATE MEGLUMINE

Cystografin *SEE* DIATRIZOATE MEGLUMINE

Cystospaz *SEE* HYOSCYAMINE SULFATE

Cytadren *SEE* AMINOGLUTETHIMIDE

Cytarabine

<hr>

WARNING

ONLY PHYSICIANS EXPERIENCED IN CANCER CHEMOTHERAPY SHOULD USE CYTARABINE STERILE POWDER.

FOR INDUCTION THERAPY PATIENTS SHOULD BE TREATED IN A FACILITY WITH LABORATORY AND SUPPORTIVE RESOURCES SUFFICIENT TO MONITOR DRUG TOLERANCE AND PROTECT AND MAINTAIN A PATIENT COMPROMISED BY DRUG TOXICITY. THE MAIN TOXIC EFFECT OF CYTARABINE IS BONE MARROW SUPPRESSION WITH LEUKOPENIA, THROMBOCYTOPENIA AND ANEMIA. LESS SERIOUS TOXICITY INCLUDES NAUSEA, VOMITING, DIARRHEA AND ABDOMINAL PAIN, ORAL ULCERATION, AND HEPATIC DYSFUNCTION.

THE PHYSICIAN MUST JUDGE POSSIBLE BENEFIT TO THE PATIENT AGAINST KNOWN TOXIC EFFECTS OF THIS DRUG IN CONSIDERING THE ADVISABILITY OF THERAPY WITH CYTARABINE. BEFORE MAKING THIS JUDGMENT OR BEGINNING TREATMENT, THE PHYSICIAN SHOULD BE FAMILIAR WITH THE FOLLOWING TEXT.

<hr>

DESCRIPTION

Cytarabine Sterile Powder, commonly known as ara-C, an antineoplastic, is a sterile lyophilized material for reconstitution and intravenous, intrathecal or subcutaneous administration. It is available in multidose vials containing 100 mg, 500 mg, 1 g or 2 g sterile Cytarabine. The pH of Cytarabine was adjusted, when necessary, with hydrochloric acid and/or sodium hydroxide.

Cytarabine is chemically 4-amina-1-β-D-arabinofuranosyl-2 (1H)-pyrimidinone.

Cytarabine is an odorless, white to off-white, crystalline powder which is freely soluble in water and slightly soluble in alcohol and in chloroform.

Following is its chemical structure:

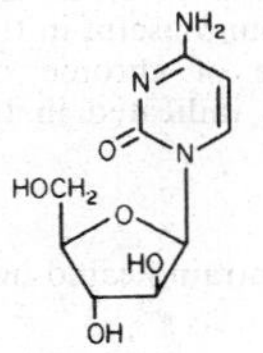

PHARMACOLOGY
CELL CULTURE STUDIES

Cytarabine is cytotoxic to a wide variety of proliferating mammalian cells in culture. It exhibits cell phase specificity, primarily killing cells undergoing DNA synthesis (S-phase) and under certain conditions blocking the progression of cells from the G_1 phase to the S-phase. Although the mechanism of action is not completely understood, it appears that Cytarabine acts through the inhibition of DNA polymerase. A limited, but significant, incorporation of Cytarabine into both DNA and RNA has also been reported. Extensive chromosomal damage, including chromatoid breaks, have been produced by Cytarabine and malignant transformation of rodent cells in culture has been reported. Deoxycytidine prevents or delays (but does not reverse) the cytotoxic activity.

Cell culture studies have shown an antiviral effect.[1] However, efficacy against herpes zoster or smallpox could not be demonstrated in controlled clinical trials.[2-4]

CELLULAR RESISTANCE AND SENSITIVITY

Cytarabine is metabolized by deoxycytidine kinase and other nucleotide kinases to the nucleotide triphosphate, and effective inhibitor of DNA polymerase; it is inactivated by a pyrimidine nucleoside deaminase which converts it to the nontoxic uracil derivative. It appears that the balance of kinase and deaminase levels may be an important factor in determining sensitivity or resistance of the cell to Cytarabine.

ANIMAL STUDIES

In experimental studies with mouse tumors, Cytarabine was most effective in those tumors with a high growth fraction. The effect was dependent on the treatment schedule; optimal effects were achieved when the schedule (multiple closely spaced doses or constant infusion) ensured contact of the drug with the tumor cells when the maximum number of cells were in the susceptible S-phase. The best results were obtained when courses of therapy were separated by intervals sufficient to permit adequate host recovery.

HUMAN PHARMACOLOGY

Cytarabine is rapidly metabolized and is not effective orally; less than 20 percent of the orally administered dose is absorbed from the gastrointestinal tract.

<hr>

➤ SHOWN IN PRODUCT IDENTIFICATION GUIDE

Following rapid intravenous injection of Cytarabine with tritium, the disappearance from plasma is biphasic. There is an initial distributive phase with a half-life of about 10 minutes, followed by a second elimination phase with a half-life of about 1 to 3 hours. After the distributive phase, more than 80 percent of plasma radioactivity can be accounted for by the inactive metabolite 1-β-D-arabinofuranosyluracil (ara-U). Within 24 hours about 80 percent of the administered radioactivity can be recovered in the urine, approximately 90 percent of which is excreted as ara-U.

Relatively constant plasma levels can be achieved by continuous intravenous infusion.

After subcutaneous or intramuscular administration of Cytarabine labeled with tritium, peak-plasma levels of radio-activity are achieved about 20 to 60 minutes after injection and are considerably lower than those after intravenous administration.

Cerebrospinal fluid levels of Cytarabine are low in comparison to plasma levels after single intravenous injection. However, in one patient in whom cerebrospinal levels were examined after 2 hours of constant intravenous infusion, levels approached 40 percent of the steady state plasma level. With intrathecal administration, levels of Cytarabine in the cerebrospinal fluid declined with a first order half-life of about 2 hours. Because cerebrospinal fluid levels of deaminase are low, little conversion to ara-U was observed.

IMMUNOSUPPRESSIVE ACTION

Cytarabine Sterile Powder is capable of obliterating immune responses in man during administration with little or no accompanying toxicity.[5,6] Suppression of antibody responses to E-coli-VI antigen and tetanus toxoid have been demonstrated. This suppression was obtained during both primary and secondary antibody responses.

Cytarabine also suppressed the development of cell-mediated immune responses such as delayed hypersensitivity skin reaction to dinitrochlorobenzene. However, it had no effect on already established delayed hypersensitivity reactions.

Following 5-day courses of intensive therapy with Cytarabine the immune response was suppressed, as indicated by the following parameters: macrophage ingress into skin windows; circulating antibody response following primary antigenic stimulation; lymphocyte blastogenesis with phytohemagglutinin. A few days after termination of therapy there was a rapid return to normal.[7]

INDICATIONS AND USAGE

Cytarabine Sterile Powder in combination with other approved anticancer drugs is indicated for remission induction in acute non-lymphocytic leukemia of adults and children. It has also been found useful in the treatment of acute lymphocytic leukemia and the blast phase of chronic myelocytic leukemia. Intrathecal administration of cytarabine is indicated in the prophylaxis and treatment of meningeal leukemia.

CONTRAINDICATIONS

Cytarabine Sterile Powder is contraindicated in those patients who are hypersensitive to the drug.

WARNINGS

(SEE BOXED "WARNING")

Cytarabine is a potent bone marrow suppressant. Therapy should be started cautiously in patients with pre-existing drug-induced bone marrow suppression. Patients receiving this drug must be under close medical supervision and, during induction therapy, should have leukocyte and platelet counts performed daily. Bone marrow examinations should be performed frequently after blasts have disappeared from the peripheral blood. Facilities should be available for management of complications, possibly fatal, of bone marrow suppression (infection resulting from granulocytopenia and other impaired body defenses, and hemorrhage secondary to thrombocytopenia). One case of anaphylaxis that resulted in acute cardiopulmonary arrest and required resuscitation has been reported. This occurred immediately after the intravenous administration of Cytarabine Sterile Powder.

Severe and at times fatal CNS, GI and pulmonary toxicity (different from that seen with conventional therapy regimens of Cytarabine) has been reported following some experimental dose schedules of Cytarabine.[8-11] These reactions include reversible corneal toxicity, and hemorrhagic conjunctivitis, which may be prevented or diminished by prophylaxis with a local corticosteroid eye drop; cerebral and cerebellar dysfunction, including personality changes, somnolence and coma, usually reversible; severe gastrointestinal ulceration, including pneumatosis cystoides intestinalis leading to peritonitis; sepsis and liver abscess; pulmonary edema, liver damage with increased hyperbilirubinemia; bowel necrosis; and necrotizing colitis. Rarely, severe skin rash, leading to desquamation has been reported. Complete alopecia is more commonly seen with experimental high dose therapy than with standard treatment programs for Cytarabine. If experimental high dose therapy is used, do not use a diluent containing benzyl alcohol.

An increase in cardiomyopathy with subsequent death has been reported following experimental high dose therapy with Cytarabine in combination with cyclophosphamide when used for bone marrow transplant preparation.[12]

A syndrome of sudden respiratory distress, rapidly progressing to pulmonary edema and radiographically pronounced cardiomegaly has been reported following experimental high dose therapy with Cytarabine used for the treatment of relapsed leukemia from one institution in 16/72 patients. The outcome of this syndrome can be fatal.[13]

Certain brands of Cytarabine contain benzyl alcohol in the diluent. Benzyl alcohol has been reported to be associated with a fatal "Gasping Syndrome" in premature infants.

Two patients with childhood acute myelogenous leukemia who received intrathecal and intravenous Cytarabine at conventional doses (in addition to a number of other concomitantly administered drugs) developed delayed progressive ascending paralysis resulting in death in one of the two patients.[14]

USE IN PREGNANCY

Cytarabine can cause fetal harm when administered to a pregnant woman. (See "Animal Toxicology".) There are no adequate and well-controlled studies in pregnant women. If Cytarabine is used during pregnancy, or if the patient becomes pregnant while taking Cytarabine, the patient should be apprised of the potential hazard to the fetus. Women of childbearing potential should be advised to avoid becoming pregnant.

PRECAUTIONS

1. GENERAL PRECAUTIONS

Patients receiving Cytarabine Sterile Powder must be monitored closely. Frequent platelet and leukocyte counts and bone marrow examinations are mandatory. Consider suspending or modifying therapy when drug-induced marrow depression has resulted in a platelet count under 50,000 or a polymorphonuclear granulocyte count under 1000/mm³. Counts of formed elements in the peripheral blood may continue to fall after the drug is stopped and reach lowest values after drug-free intervals of 12 to 24 days. When indicated, restart therapy when definite signs of marrow recovery appear (on successive bone marrow studies). Patients whose drug is withheld until "normal" peripheral blood values are attained may escape from control.

When large intravenous doses are given quickly, patients are frequently nauseated and may vomit for several hours postinjection. This problem tends to be less severe when the drug is infused.

The human liver apparently detoxifies a substantial fraction of an administered dose. Use the drug with caution and at reduced dose in patients whose liver function is poor.

Periodic checks of bone marrow, liver and kidney functions should be performed in patients receiving Cytarabine.

Like other cytotoxic drugs, Cytarabine may induce hyperuricemia secondary to rapid lysis of neoplastic cells. The clinician should monitor the patient's blood uric acid level and be prepared to use such supportive and pharmacologic measures as might be necessary to control this problem.

Acute pancreatitis has been reported to occur in patients being treated with Cytarabine who have had prior treatment with L-asparaginase.[15]

2. INFORMATION FOR PATIENT

Not applicable.

3. LABORATORY TESTS

See "General Precautions".

4. DRUG INTERACTIONS

Reversible decreases in steady-state plasma digoxin concentrations and renal glycoside excretion were observed in patients receiving beta-acetyldigoxin and chemotherapy regimens containing cyclophosphamide, vincristine and prednisone with or without Cytarabine or procarbazine.[39] Steady-state plasma digitoxin concentrations did not appear to change. Therefore, monitoring of plasma digoxin levels may be indicated in patients receiving similar combination chemotherapy regimens. The utilization of digitoxin for such patients may be considered as an alternative.

An *in vitro* interaction study between gentamicin and Cytarabine showed a Cytarabine related antagonism for the susceptibility of *K. pneumoniae* strains. This study suggests that in patients on Cytarabine being treated with gentamicin for a *K. pneumoniae* infection, the lack of a prompt therapeutic response may indicate the need for reevaluation of antibacterial therapy.[40]

Clinical evidence in one patient showed possible inhibition of fluorocytosine efficacy during therapy with Cytarabine.[41] This may be due to potential competitive inhibition of its uptake.[42]

5. CARCINOGENESIS, MUTAGENESIS, IMPAIRMENT OF FERTILITY

Extensive chromosomal damage, including chromatoid breaks have been produced by Cytarabine and malignant transformation of rodent cells in culture has been reported.

6. PREGNANCY

Pregnancy Category D. See "Warnings".

A review of the literature has shown 32 reported cases were Cytarabine was given during pregnancy, either alone or in combination with other cytotoxic agents:

Eighteen normal infants were delivered. Four of these had first trimester exposure. Five infants were premature or low birth weight. Twelve of the 18 normal infants were followed up at ages ranging from six weeks to seven years, and showed no abnormalities. One apparently normal infant died at 90 days of gastroenteritis.

Two cases of congenital abnormalities have been reported, one with upper and lower distal limb defects,[16] and the other with extremity and ear deformities.[17] Both of these cases had first trimester exposure.

There were seven infants with various problems in the neonatal period, including pancytopenia; transient depression of WBC, hematocrit or platelets; electrolyte abnormalities; transient eosinophilia; and one case of increased IgM levels and hyperpyrexia possibly due to sepsis. Six of the seven infants were also premature. The child with pancytopenia died at 21 days of sepsis.

Therapeutic abortions were done in five cases. Four fetuses were grossly normal, but one had an enlarged spleen and another showed Trisomy C chromosome abnormality in the chorionic tissue.

Because of the potential for abnormalities with cytotoxic therapy, particularly during the first trimester, a patient who is or who may become pregnant while on Cytarabine should be apprised of the potential risk to the fetus and the advisability of pregnancy continuation. There is a definite, but considerably reduced risk if therapy is initiated during the second or third trimester. Although normal infants have been delivered to patients treated in all three trimesters of pregnancy, follow-up of such infants would be advisable.

7. LABOR AND DELIVERY
Not applicable

8. NURSING MOTHERS
It is not known whether this drug is excreted in human milk. Because many drugs are excreted in human milk and because of the potential for serious adverse reactions in nursing infants from Cytarabine, a decision should be made whether to discontinue nursing or to discontinue the drug, taking into account the importance of the drug to the mother.

9. PEDIATRIC USE
See *"Indications and Usage"*.

ADVERSE REACTIONS
EXPECTED REACTIONS
Because Cytarabine is a bone marrow suppressant, anemia, leukopenia, thrombocytopenia, megaloblastosis and reduced reticulocytes can be expected as a result of administration with Cytarabine Sterile Powder. The severity of these reactions are dose and schedule dependent.[18] Cellular changes in the morphology of bone marrow and peripheral smears can be expected.[19]

Following 5-day constant infusions or acute injections of 50 mg/m^2 to 600 mg/m^2, white cell depression follows a biphasic course. Regardless of initial count, dosage level, or schedule, there is an initial fall starting the first 24 hours with a nadir at days 7-9. This is followed by a brief rise which peaks around the twelfth day. A second and deeper fall reaches nadir at days 15-24. Then there is rapid rise to above baseline in the next 10 days. Platelet depression is noticeable at 5 days with a peak depression occurring between days 12-15. Thereupon, a rapid rise to above baseline occurs in the next 10 days.[20]

INFECTIOUS COMPLICATIONS
Infection: Viral, bacterial, fungal, parasitic, or saprophytic infections, in any location in the body may be associated with the use of Cytarabine alone or in combination with other immunosuppressive agents following immunosuppressant doses that affect cellular or humoral immunity. The infections may be mild, but can be severe and at times fatal.

THE CYTARABINE (ARA-C) SYNDROME
A Cytarabine syndrome has been described by Castleberry.[21] It is characterized by fever, myalgia, bone pain, occasionally chest pain, maculopapular rash, conjunctivitis and malaise. It usually occurs 6-12 hours following drug administration. Corticosteroids have been shown to be beneficial in treating or preventing this syndrome. If the symptoms of the syndrome are deemed treatable, corticosteroids should be contemplated as well as continuation of therapy with Cytarabine.

MOST FREQUENT ADVERSE REACTIONS
anorexia
nausea
vomiting
diarrhea
oral and anal inflammation or ulceration
hepatic dysfunction
fever
rash
thrombophlebitis
bleeding (all sites)

Nausea and vomiting are most frequent following rapid intravenous injection.

LESS FREQUENT ADVERSE REACTIONS
sepsis
pneumonia
cellulitis at injection site
skin ulceration
urinary retention
renal dysfunction
neuritis
neural toxicity
sore throat
esophageal ulceration
esophagitis
chest pain
bowel necrosis
abdominal pain
freckling
jaundice
conjunctivitis (may occur with rash)

dizziness
alopecia
anaphylaxis (See *"Warnings"*)
allergic edema
pruritus
shortness of breath
urticaria
headache

EXPERIMENTAL DOSES
Severe and at times fatal CNS, GI and pulmonary toxicity (different from that seen with conventional therapy regimens of Cytarabine) has been reported following some experimental dose schedules of Cytarabine.[8-11] These reactions include reversible corneal toxicity and hemorrhagic conjunctivitis, which may be prevented or diminished by prophylaxis with a local corticosteroid eye drop; cerebral and cerebellar dysfunction, including personality changes, somnolence and coma, usually reversible; severe gastrointestinal ulceration, including pneumatosis cystoides intestinalis leading to peritonitis; sepsis and liver abscess; pulmonary edema, liver damage with increased hyperbilirubinemia; bowel necrosis; and necrotizing colitis. Rarely, severe skin rash, leading to desquamation has been reported. Complete alopecia is more commonly seen with experimental high dose therapy than with standard treatment programs of Cytarabine. If experimental high dose therapy is used, do not use a diluent containing benzyl alcohol.

An increase in cardiomyopathy with subsequent death has been reported following experimental high dose therapy with Cytarabine in combination with cyclophosphamide when used for bone marrow transplant preparation.[12] **This cardiac toxicity may be schedule dependent[45].**

A syndrome of sudden respiratory distress, rapidly progressing to pulmonary edema and radiographically pronounced cardiomegaly has been reported following experimental high dose therapy with Cytarabine used for the treatment of relapsed leukemia from one institution in 16/72 patients. The outcome of this syndrome can be fatal.[13]

Two patients with adult acute non-lymphocytic leukemia developed peripheral motor and sensory neuropathies after consolidation with high-dose Cytarabine, daunorubicin, and asparaginase. Patients treated with high-dose Cytarabine should be observed for neuropathy since dose schedule alterations may be needed to avoid irreversible neurologic disorders.[22]

Ten patients treated with experimental intermediate doses of Cytarabine (1 g/m^2) with and without other chemotherapeutic agents (meta-AMSA, daunorubicin, etoposide) at various dose regimes developed a diffuse interstitial pneumonitis without clear cause that may have been related to the Cytarabine.[45]

Two cases of pancreatitis have been reported following experimental doses of Cytarabine and numerous other drugs. Cytarabine could have been the causative agent.[46]

OVERDOSAGE
There is no antidote for overdosage of Cytarabine. Doses of 4.5 g/m^2 by intravenous infusion over 1 hour every 12 hours for 12 doses has caused an unacceptable increase in irreversible CNS toxicity and death.[9].

Single doses as high as 3 g/m^2 have been administered by rapid intravenous infusion without apparent toxicity.[23]

DOSAGE AND ADMINISTRATION
Cytarabine Sterile Powder is not active orally. The schedule and method of administration varies with the program of therapy to be used. Cytarabine may be given by intravenous infusion or injection, subcutaneously or intrathecally. Thrombophlebitis has occurred at the site of drug injection or infusion in some patients, and rarely patients have noted pain and inflammation at subcutaneous injection sites. In most instances, however, the drug has been well tolerated.

Patients can tolerate higher total doses when they receive the drug by rapid intravenous injection as compared with slow infusion. This phenomenon is related to the drug's rapid inactivation and brief exposure of susceptible normal and neoplastic cells to significant levels after rapid injection. Normal and neoplastic cells seem to respond in somewhat parallel fashion to these different modes of administration and no clear-cut clinical advantage has been demonstrated for either.

In the induction therapy of acute non-lymphocytic leukemia, the usual Cytarabine dose in combination with other anti-cancer drugs is 100 mg/m^2 day by continuous IV infusion (Days 1-7) or 100 mg/m^2 IV every 12 hours (Days 1-7).

The literature should be consulted for the current recommendations for use in acute lymphocytic leukemia.

INTRATHECAL USE IN MENINGEAL LEUKEMIA
Cytarabine has been used intrathecally in acute leukemia in doses ranging from 5 mg/m^2 to 75 mg/m^2 of body surface area. The frequency of administration varied from once a day for 4 days to once every 4 days. The most frequently used dose was 30 mg/m^2 every 4 days until cerebrospinal fluid findings were normal, followed by one additional treatment.[24-28] The dosage schedule is usually governed by the type and severity of central nervous system manifestations and the response to previous therapy.

If used intrathecally, do not use a diluent containing benzyl alcohol. Many clinicians reconstitute with autologous spinal fluid or preservative-free 0.9% Sodium Chloride, USP, for Injection and use immediately.

Cytarabine given intrathecally may cause systemic toxicity and careful monitoring of the hemopoietic system is indicated. Modification of other antileukemia therapy may be necessary. Major toxicity is rare. The most frequently reported reactions after intrathecal administration were nausea, vomiting and fever; these reactions are mild and self-limiting. Paraplegia has been reported.[29] Necrotizing leukoencephalopathy occurred in 5 children; these patients had also been treated with intrathecal methotrexate and hydrocortisone, as well as by central nervous system radiation.[30] Isolated neurotoxicity has been reported.[31] Blindness occurred in two patients in remission whose treatment had consisted of combination systemic chemotherapy, prophylactic central nervous system radiation and intrathecal Cytarabine.[32]

Focal leukemic involvement of the central nervous system may not respond to intrathecal Cytarabine and may better be treated with radiotherapy.

The 100 mg vial may be reconstituted with 5 ml of Bacteriostatic Water for Injection with Benzyl Alcohol 0.945% w/v added as preservative. The resulting solution contains 20 mg of Cytarabine per ml. (Do not use Bacteriostatic Water for Injection with Benzyl Alcohol 0.945% w/v as a diluent for intrathecal use. See *"Warnings".*)

The 500 mg vial may be reconstituted with 10 ml Bacteriostatic Water for Injection with Benzyl Alcohol 0.945% w/v added as preservative. The resulting solution contains 50 mg of Cytarabine per ml. (Do not use Bacteriostatic Water for Injection with Benzyl Alcohol 0.945% w/v as a diluent for intrathecal use. See *"Warnings".*)

The 1 gram vial may be reconstituted with 10 ml of Bacteriostatic Water for Injection with Benzyl Alcohol 0.945% w/v added as preservative. The resulting solution contains 100 mg of Cytarabine per ml. (Do not use Bacteriostatic Water for Injection with Benzyl Alcohol 0.945% w/v as a dilient for intrathecal use. See *"Warnings".*)

The 2 gram vial may be reconstituted with 20 ml of Bacteriostatic Water for Injection with Benzyl Alcohol 0.945% w/v added as preservative. The resulting solution contains 100 mg of Cytarabine per ml. (Do not use Bacteriostatic Water for Injection with Benzyl Alcohol 0.945% w/v as a diluent for intrathecal use. See *"Warnings".*)

If used intrathecally many clinicians reconstitute with preservative-free 0.9% Sodium Chloride for Injection and use immediately.

The pH of the reconstituted solutions is about 5. Solutions reconstituted with Bacteriostatic Water for Injection with Benzyl Alcohol 0.945% w/v may be stored at controlled room temperature, 15°-30°C (59°-86°F) for 48 hours. Discard any solutions in which a slight haze develops.

Solutions reconstituted without a preservative should be used immediately.

CHEMICAL STABILITY OF INFUSION SOLUTIONS

Chemical stability studies were performed by ultraviolet assay on infusion solutions of Cytarabine. These studies showed that when reconstituted Cytarabine was added to Water for Injection, 5% Dextrose in Water or Sodium Chloride Injection, 94 to 96 percent of the Cytarabine was present after 192 hours storage at room temperature.

Parenteral drugs should be inspected visually for particulate matter and discoloration, prior to administration, whenever solution and container permit.

Procedures for proper handling and disposal of anticancer drugs should be considered. Several guidelines on this subject have been published.[33-38] There is no general agreement that all of the procedures recommended in the guidelines are necessary or appropriate.

Store the product at controlled room temperature 15°-30°C (59°-86°F.)

REFERENCES

1. Zaky DA, Betts RF, Douglas RG, et al: Varicella-Zoster Virus and Subcutaneous Cytarabine: Correlation of In Vitro Sensitivities to Blood Levels, *Antimicrob Agents Chemother* 1975; *7*:229-232 2. Davis CM. VanDersarl JV, Coltman CA Jr: Failure of Cytarabine in Varicella-Zoster Infections, *JAMA* 1973; *224*:122-123 3. Betts RF, Zaky DA, Douglas RG, et al: Ineffectiveness of Subcutaneous Cytosine Arabinoside in Localized Herpes Zoster, *Ann Intern Med* 1975; *82*:778-783 4. Dennis DT, Doberstyn EB, Awoke S, et al: Failure of Cytosine Arabinoside in Treatment Smallpox; A Double-blind Study, *Lancet* 1974; *2*:377-379 5. Gray GD: ARA-C and Derivatives as Examples of Immunosuppressive Nucleoside Analogs, *Ann NY Acad Sci* 1975; *255*:372-379 6. Mitchell MS, Wade ME, DeConti RC, et al: Immunosuppressive Effects of Cytosine Arabinoside and Methotrexate in Man, *Ann Intern Med* 1969; *70*:535-547 7. Frei E, Ho DHW, Bodey GP, et al: Pharmacologic and Cytokinetic Studies of Arabinosyl Cytosine. In *Unifying Concepts of Leukemia, Bibl. Hematol.* No. 39. Karger, Basel 1973, pp 1085-1097 8. Hopen G, Mondino BJ, Johnson BL, et al: Corneal Toxicity with Systemic Cytarabine, *Am J Ophthalmol* 1981; *91*:500-504 9. Lazarus HM, Herzig RH, Herzig GP, et al; Central Nervous System Toxicity of High-Dose Systemic Cytosine Arabinoside, *Cancer* 1981; *48*:2577-2582 10. Slavin RE, Dias MA, Soral R: Cytosine Arabinoside Induced Gastrointestinal Toxic Alterations in Sequential Chemotherapeutic Protocols—A Clinical Pathologic Study of 33 Patients, *Cancer* 1978; *42*:1747-1759 11. Haupt HM, Hutchins GM, Moore GW; Ara-C-Lung: Noncardiogenic Pulmonary Edema Complicating Cytosine Arabinoside Therapy of Leukemia, *Am J Med* 1981; *70*:256-261. 12. Takvorian T. Anderson K. Ritz J: A Fatal Cardiomyopathy Associated with High Dosage Ara-C (HIDAC) and Cyclophosphamide (CTX) in Bone Marrow Transplantation (BMTx). (Abstract submitted for 1985 AACR Meetings in Houston, Texas.) 13. Anderson BS, Cogan B, Keating MJ, Estey EH, et al: Subacute Pulmonary Failure Complicating Therapy with High-Dose Ara-C in Acute Leukemia, *Cancer* 1985; *56*:2181-2184 14. Dunton SF, Ruprecht N, Spruce W, et al: Progressive Ascending Paralysis Following Administration of Intrathecal and Intravenous Cytosine Arabinoside, *Cancer* 1986; *57*:1083-1088 15. Altman AJ, Dinndorf P, Quinn JJ: Acute Pancreatitis in Association with cytosine Arabinoside Therayp, *Cancer* 1982; *49*:1384-1386 16. Shafer AI: Teratogenic Effects of Antileukemic Chemotherapy, *Arch Intern Med* 1981, *141*:514-515 17. Wagner VM, et al: Congenital Abnormalities in Baby Born to Cytarabine Treated Mother, *Lancet* 1980; *2*:98-99 18. Frei E III, Bickers JN, Hewlett JS, et al: Dose Schedule and Antitumor Studies of Arabinosyl Cytosine (NSC 63878), *Cancer Res* 1969; *29*:1325-1332 19. Bell WR, Wang JJ, Carbone PP, et al: Cytogenetic and Morphologic Abnormalities in Human Bone Marrow Cells during Cytosine Arabinoside Therapy, *J Hematol* 1966; *27*:771-781 20. Burke PJ, Serpick AA, Carbone PP, et al: The Clinical Evaluation of Dose and Schedule of Administration of Cytosine Arabinoside (NSC 63878), *Cancer Res* 1968; *28*:274-279 21. Castleberry RP, Crist WM, Holbrook T, et al: The Cytosine Arabinoside (Ara-C) Syndrome, *Med Pediatr Oncol* 1981: *9*:257-264 22. Powell BL, Capizzi RL, Lyerly EW, et al: Peripheral Neuropathy After High-Dose Cytosine Arabinoside, Daunorubicin, and Asparaginase Consolidation for Acute Nonlymphocytic Leukemia, *J Clin Oncol* 1986; *4*(1):95-97 23. Rudnick SA, et al: High Dose Cytosine Arabinoside (HDARAC) in Refractory Acute Leukemia, *Cancer* 1979; *44*:1189-1193 24. Proceedings of the Chemotherapy Conference on ARA-C: Development and Application (Cytosine Arabinoside Hydrochloride—NSC 63878), Oct. 10. 1969 25. Lay HN, Colebatch JH, Ekert H: Experiences with Cytosine Arabinoside in Childhood Leukaemia and Lymphoma, *Med J Aust* 1971; *2*:187-192 26. Halikowski B, Cyklis R, Armata J, et al: Cytosine Arabinoside Administered Intrathecally in Cerebromeningeal Leukemia, *Acta Paediat Scand* 1970; *59*:164-168 27. Wang JJ, Pratt CB: Intrathecal Arabinosyl Cytosine in Meningeal Leukemia, *Cancer* 1970; *25*:531-534 28. BandPR, Holland JF, Bernard J, et al: Treatment of Central Nervous System Leukemia with Intrathecal Cytosine Arabinoside, *Cancer* 1973; *32*:744-748 29. Saiki JH, Thompson S, Smith F, et al: Paraplegia Following Intrathecal Chemotherapy, *Cancer* 1972; *29*:370-374 30. Rubinstein LJ, Herman MM, Long TF, et al: Disseminated Necrotizing Leukoencephalopathy: A Complication of Treated Central System Leukemia and Lymphoma, *Cancer* 1975; *35*:291-305 31. Marmont A.M. Damasio EE: Neurotoxicity of Intrathecal Chemotherapy for Leukaemia, *Brit Med J* 1973; *4*:47 32. Margileth DA, Poplack DG, Pizzo PA, et al: Blindness During Remission in Two Patients with Acute Lymphoblastic Leukemia, *Cancer* 1977; *39*:58-61 33. Recommendations for the Safe Handling of Parenteral Antineoplastic Drugs. NIH Publication No. 83-2621. For sale by the Superintendent of Documents, US Government Printing Office, Washington, DC 20402. 34. AMA Council Report. Guidelines for Handling Parenteral Antineoplastics. *JAMA,* March 15, 1985. 35. National Study Commission on Cytotoxic Exposure-Recommendations for Handling Cytotoxic Agents. Available from Louis P. Jeffrey, ScD, Director of Pharmacy Services, Rhode Island Hospital, 593 Eddy Street, Providence, Rhode Island 02902. 36. Clinical Oncological Society of Australia: Guidelines and recommendations for safe handling of antineoplastic agents. *Med J Australia* 1983; *1*:426-428. 37. Jones, RB, et al. Safe handling of chemotherapeutic agents: A report from the Mount Sinai Medical Center CA-A *Cancer Journal for Clinicians* Sept/Oct., 1983, pp. 258-263. 38. American Society of Hospital Pharmacists Technical assistance bulletin on handling cytotoxic drugs in hospitals. *Am J Hosp Pharm* 1985; *42*:131-137. 39. Kuhlman J: Inhibition of Digoxin Absorption but not of Digitoxin During Cytostatic Drug Therapy. *Arzneim Forsch* 1982; *32*:698-704. 40. Moody MR, Morris JJ, Yang VM, et al: Effect of Two Cancer Chemotherapeutic Agents on the Antibacterial Activity of Three Antimicrobial Agents. *Antimicrob Agents Chemother* 1978; *14*:737-742. 41. Holt RJ: Clinical Problems with 5-Fluorocytosine. *Mykosen* 1978; *21*(11):363-369. 42. Polak A, Grenson M: Interference Between the Uptake of Pyrimidines and Purines in Yeasts. *Path Microbiol* 1973; *39*:37-38. 43. Peters WG, Willemze R, Colly LP: Results of Induction and Consolidation Treatment with Intermediate and High-Dose Ara-C and m-AMSA Containing Regimens in Patients with Primarily Failed or Relapsed Acute Leukemia and Non-Hodgkin's Lymphoma. *Scan J Hemat* 1986; *36* (Suppl 44):7-16. 44. Siemers RF, Friedenberg WR. Norfleet RG: High-Dose Cytosine Arabinoside-Associated Pancreatitis. *Cancer* 1985; *56*:1940-1942. 45. Paul S, et al: "High Dose Ara-C Does Not Increase the Cardiotoxicity of cyclophosphamide—Total Body Irradiation Conditioning Regimes for Bone Marrow Transplation". *Proceeding of ASCO* 1989; 8:16, abstract 60.

ANIMAL TOXICOLOGY

Toxicity of Cytarabine in experimental animals, as well as activity, is markedly influenced by the schedule of administration. For example, in mice the LD_{10} for single intraperitoneal administration is greater than 6000 mg/m^2. However, when administered in 8 doses, each separated by 3 hours, the LD^{10} is less than 750 mg/m^2 total dose. Similarly, although a total dose of 1920 mg/m^2 administered as 12 injections at 6-hour intervals was lethal to beagle dogs (severe bone marrow hypoplasia with evidence of liver and kidney damage), dogs receiving the same total dose administered in 8 injections (again at 6-hour intervals) over a 48-hour period survived with minimal signs of toxicity. The most consistent observation in surviving dogs was elevated transaminase levels. In all experimental species the primary limiting toxic effect is marrow suppression with leukopenia. In addition, Cytarabine causes abnormal cerebellar development in the neonatal hamster and is teratogenic to the rat fetus.

J CODES

100 mg SC,IV—J9100
500 mg SC,IV—J9110

HOW SUPPLIED

POWDER FOR INJECTION: 100 MG

AVERAGE UNIT PRICE (AVAILABLE SIZES)	
BRAND	$6.72
GENERIC	$5.88

BRAND/MANUFACTURER	NDC	SIZE	AWP
◆ **BRAND**			
CYTOSAR-U: Upjohn	00009-0373-01	1s	$6.72
◆ **GENERICS**			
Schein	00364-2467-53	1s	$5.50
Chiron Therapeutics	53905-0131-10	10s	$62.50

POWDER FOR INJECTION: 500 MG

AVERAGE UNIT PRICE (AVAILABLE SIZES)	
BRAND	$26.73
GENERIC	$23.000

BRAND/MANUFACTURER	NDC	SIZE	AWP
◆ **BRAND**			
CYTOSAR-U: Upjohn	00009-0473-01	1s	$26.73

◆ RATED THERAPEUTICALLY EQUIVALENT; ◇ THERAPEUTIC EQUIVALENCE UNCONFIRMED; ○ UNRATED

BRAND/MANUFACTURER	NDC	SIZE	AWP
◆ GENERICS			
Schein	00364-2468-54	1s	$21.00
Chiron Therapeutics	53905-0132-10	10s	$250.00

POWDER FOR INJECTION: 1 GM

BRAND/MANUFACTURER	NDC	SIZE	AWP
◆ BRAND			
CYTOSAR-U: Upjohn	00009-3295-01	1s	$50.79

POWDER FOR INJECTION: 2 GM

BRAND/MANUFACTURER	NDC	SIZE	AWP
◆ BRAND			
CYTOSAR-U: Upjohn	00009-3296-01	1s	$99.43

Cytomel SEE LIOTHYRONINE SODIUM

Cytosar-U SEE CYTARABINE

Cytotec SEE MISOPROSTOL

Cytovene SEE GANCICLOVIR SODIUM

Cytoxan SEE CYCLOPHOSPHAMIDE

Dacarbazine

WARNING

IT IS RECOMMENDED THAT DACARBAZINE BE ADMINISTERED UNDER THE SUPERVISION OF A QUALIFIED PHYSICIAN EXPERIENCED IN THE USE OF CANCER CHEMOTHERAPEUTIC AGENTS.

1. HEMOPOIETIC DEPRESSION IS THE MOST COMMON TOXICITY WITH DACARBAZINE (SEE "WARNINGS").

2. HEPATIC NECROSIS HAS BEEN REPORTED (SEE "WARNINGS").

3. STUDIES HAVE DEMONSTRATED THIS AGENT TO HAVE A CARCINOGENIC AND TERATOGENIC EFFECT WHEN USED IN ANIMALS.

4. IN TREATMENT OF EACH PATIENT, THE PHYSICIAN MUST WEIGH CAREFULLY THE POSSIBILITY OF ACHIEVING THERAPEUTIC BENEFIT AGAINST THE RISK OF TOXICITY.

DESCRIPTION

Sterile Dacarbazine is a colorless to an ivory colored solid which is light sensitive. Each vial contains 100 mg of Dacarbazine, or 200 mg of Dacarbazine (the active ingredient), anhydrous citric acid and mannitol. Dacarbazine is reconstituted and administered intravenously (pH 3-4). Dacarbazine is an anticancer agent. Chemically, Dacarbazine is 5-(3,3-dimethyl-1-triazeno)-imidazole-4-carboxamide.

Following is its chemical structure:

$$(CH_3)_2NN=N \quad H_2NC \quad O \quad N \quad N \quad H$$

CLINICAL PHARMACOLOGY

After intravenous administration Dacarbazine, the volume of distribution exceeds total body water content suggesting localization in some body tissue, probably the liver. Its disappearance from the plasma is biphasic with initial half-life of 19 minutes and a terminal half-life of 5 hours.[1] In a patient with renal and hepatic dysfunctions, the half lives were lengthened to 55 minutes and 7.2 hours.[1] The average cumulative excretion of unchanged Dacarbazine in the urine is 40% of the injected dose in 6 hours.[1] Dacarbazine is subject to renal tubular secretion rather than glomerular filtration. At therapeutic concentrations Dacarbazine is not appreciably bound to human plasma protein.

In man, Dacarbazine is extensively degraded. Besides unchanged Dacarbazine, 5-aminoimidazole -4 carboxamide (AIC) is a major metabolite of Dacarbazine excreted in the urine. AIC is not derived endogenously but from the injected Dacarbazine, because the administration of radioactive Dacarbazine labeled with

^{14}C in the imidazole portion of the molecule (Dacarbazine-2-^{14}C) gives rise to AIC-2-^{14}C.[1]

Although the exact mechanism of action of Dacarbazine is not known, three hypotheses have been offered:

1. inhibition of DNA synthesis by acting as a purine analog
2. action as an alkylating agent
3. interaction with SH groups

INDICATIONS AND USAGE

Dacarbazine is indicated in the treatment of metastatic malignant melanoma. In addition, Dacarbazine is also indicated for Hodgkin's disease as a secondary-line therapy when used in combination with other effective agents.

UNLABELED USES

Dacarbazine is used as an adjunct in the treatment of bronchogenic carcinoma, malignant pheochromocytoma, lymphosarcoma, and small cell lung cancer.

CONTRAINDICATIONS

Dacarbazine is contraindicated in patients who have demonstrated a hypersensitivity to it in the past.

WARNINGS

Hemopoietic depression is the most common toxicity with Dacarbazine and involves primarily the leukocytes and platelets, although, anemia may sometimes occur. Leukopenia and thrombocytopenia may be severe enough to cause death. The possible bone marrow depression requires careful monitoring of white blood cells, red blood cells, and platelet levels. Hemopoietic toxicity may warrant temporary suspension or cessation of therapy with Dacarbazine.

Hepatic toxicity accompanied by hepatic vein thrombosis and hepatocellular necrosis resulting in death, has been reported. The incidence of such reactions has been low; approximately 0.01% of patients treated. This toxicity has been observed mostly when Dacarbazine has been administered concomitantly with other anti-neoplastic drugs; however, it has also been reported in some patients treated with Dacarbazine alone.

Anaphylaxis can occur following the administration of Dacarbazine.

PRECAUTIONS

Hospitalization is not always necessary but adequate laboratory study capability must be available. Extravasation of the drug subcutaneously during intravenous administration may result in tissue damage and severe pain. Local pain, burning sensation, and irritation at the site of injection may be relieved by locally applied hot packs.

Carcinogenicity of Dacarbazine was studied in rats and mice. Proliferative endocardial lesions, including fibrosarcomas and sarcomas were induced by Dacarbazine in rats. In mice, administration of Dacarbazine resulted in the induction of angiosarcomas of the spleen.

Pregnancy Category C. Dacarbazine has been shown to be teratogenic in rats when given in doses 20 times the human daily dose on day 12 of gestation. Dacarbazine when administered in 10 times the human daily dose to male rats (twice weekly for 9 weeks) did not affect the male libido, although female rats mated to male rats had higher incidence of resorptions than controls. In rabbits, Dacarbazine daily dose 7 times the human daily dose given on Days 6-15 of gestation resulted in fetal skeletal anomalies. There are no adequate and well controlled studies in pregnant women. Dacarbazine should be used during pregnancy only if the potential benefit justifies the potential risk to the fetus.

It is not known whether this drug is excreted in human milk. Because many drugs are excreted in human milk and because of the potential for tumorigenicity shown for Dacarbazine in animal studies, a decision should be made whether to discontinue nursing or to discontinue the drug, taking into account the importance of the drug to the mother.

ADVERSE REACTIONS

Symptoms of anorexia, nausea, and vomiting are the most frequently noted of all toxic reactions. Over 90% of patients are affected with the initial few doses. The vomiting lasts 1-12 hours and is incompletely and unpredictably palliated with phenobarbital and/or prochlorperazine. Rarely, intractable nausea and vomiting have necessitated discontinuance of therapy with Dacarbazine. Rarely, Dacarbazine has caused diarrhea. Some helpful suggestions include restricting the patient's oral intake of food for 4-6 hours prior to treatment. The rapid toleration of these symptoms suggests that a central nervous system mechanism may be involved, and usually these symptoms subside after the first 1 or 2 days.

There are a number of minor toxicities that are infrequently noted. Patients have experienced an influenza-like syndrome of fever to 39°C, myalgias and malaise. These symptoms occur usually after large single doses, may last for several days, and they may occur with successive treatments. Alopecia has been noted as has facial flushing and facial paresthesia. There have been few reports of significant liver or renal function test abnormalities in man. However, these abnormalities have been observed more frequently in animal studies.

Erythematous and urticarial rashes have been observed infrequently after administration of Dacarbazine. Rarely, photosensitivity reactions may occur.

OVERDOSAGE

Give supportive treatment and monitor blood cell counts.

DOSAGE AND ADMINISTRATION

Malignant Melanoma: The recommended dosage is 2 to 4.5mg/kg/day for 10 days. Treatment may be repeated at 4 week intervals.[2]

▶ SHOWN IN PRODUCT IDENTIFICATION GUIDE

An alternate recommended dosage is 250mg/square meter body surface/day I.V. for 5 days. Treatment may be repeated every 3 weeks.[3,4]

Hodgkin's Disease: The recommended dosage of Dacarbazine in the treatment of Hodgkin's Disease is 150mg/square meter body surface/day for 5 days, in combination with other effective drugs. Treatment may be repeated every 4 weeks.[5] An alternative recommended dosage is 375mg/square meter body surface on day 1, in combination with other effective drugs, to be repeated every 15 days.[6]

Dacarbazine 100mg/vial and 200mg/vial are reconstituted with 9.9 mL and 19.7 mL, respectively, of Sterile Water for Injection, U.S.P. The resulting solution contains 10mg/mL of Dacarbazine having a pH of 3.0 to 4.0. The calculated dose of the resulting solution is drawn into a syringe and administered *only* intravenously.

The reconstituted solution may be further diluted with 5% dextrose injection, U.S.P. or sodium chloride injection, U.S.P. and administered as an intravenous infusion.

After reconstitution and prior to use, the solution in the vial may be stored at 4°C for up to 72 hours or at normal room conditions (temperature and light) for up to 8 hours. If the reconstituted solution is further diluted in 5% dextrose injection, U.S.P. or sodium chloride injection, U.S.P., the resulting solution may be stored at 4°C for up to 24 hours or at normal room conditions for up to 8 hours.

Procedures for proper handling and disposal of anticancer drugs should be considered. Several guidelines on this subject have been published.[7-12] There is no general agreement that all of the procedures recommended in the guidelines are necessary or appropriate.

Storage: Store in a refrigerator 2°C to 8°C (36°F to 46°F).

REFERENCES

1. Loo, T.J., *et al.*: Mechanism of action and pharmacology studies with DTIC (NSC-45388). Cancer Treatment Reports 60: 149-152, 1976.   2. Nathanson, L., *et al.*: Characteristics of prognosis and response to an imidazole carboxamide in malignant melanoma. Clinical Pharmacology and Therapeutics 12:955-962, 1971.   3. Costanza, M.E., *et al.*: Therapy of malignant melanoma with an imidazole carboxamide and bischloroethyl nitrosourea. Cancer 30: 1457-1461, 1972.   4. Luce, J.K., *et al.*: Clinical trials with the antitumor agent 5-(3, 3-dimethyl-l-triazeno) imidazole-4-carboxamide (NSC-45388). Cancer Chemotherapy Reports 54:119-124, 1970.   5. Bonadonna, G., *et al.*: Combined Chemotherapy (MOPP or ABVD)—radiotherapy approach in advanced Hodgkin's disease. Cancer Treatment Reports 61: 769-777, 1977.   6. Santoro, A., and Bonadonna, G.: Prolonged disease-free survival in MOPP-resistant Hodgkin's disease after treatment with adriamycin, bleomycin, vinblastine and decarbazine (ABVD). Cancer Chemotherapy Pharmacol. 2: 101-105, 1979.   7. Recommendations for the Safe Handling of Parenteral Antineoplastic Drugs. NIH Publication No. 83-2621. For sale by the Superintendent of Documents, U.S. Government Printing Office, Washington, D.C. 20402.   8. AMA Council Report. Guidelines for Handling Parenteral Antineoplastics. JAMA, March 15, 1985.   9. National Study Commission on Cytotoxic Exposure—Recommendations for Handling Cytotoxic Agents. Available from Louis P. Jeffrey, Sc. D., Director of Pharmacy Services, Rhode Island Hospital, 593 Eddy Street, Providence, Rhode Island 02902.   10. Clinical Oncological Society of Australia: Guidelines and recommendations for safe handling of antineoplastic agents. Med. J. Australia 1: 426-428, 1983.   11. Jones, R.B., *et al.*: Safe handling of chemotherapeutic agents: A report from the Mount Sinai Medical Center. Ca-A Cancer Journal for Clinicians Sept./Oct. 258-263, 1983.   12. American Society of Hospital Pharmacists technical assistance bulletin on handling cytotoxic drugs in hospitals. Am. J. Hosp. Pharm. 42: 131-137, 1985.

J CODES

100 mg IV—J9130
200 mg IV—J9140

HOW SUPPLIED
POWDER FOR INJECTION: 100 MG

BRAND/MANUFACTURER	NDC	SIZE	AWP
◆ BRAND			
DTIC-DOME: Miles Pharm	00026-8151-10	12s	$158.02

POWDER FOR INJECTION: 200 MG

BRAND/MANUFACTURER	NDC	SIZE	AWP
◆ BRAND			
DTIC-DOME: Miles Pharm	00026-8151-20	12s	$254.00

Dactinomycin

WARNING
DACTINOMYCIN IS EXTREMELY CORROSIVE TO SOFT TISSUE. IF EXTRAVASATION OCCURS DURING INTRAVENOUS USE, SEVERE DAMAGE TO SOFT TISSUES WILL OCCUR. IN AT LEAST ONE INSTANCE, THIS HAS LED TO CONTRACTURE OF THE ARMS.

DOSAGE
THE DOSAGE OF (DACTINOMYCIN) IS CALCULATED IN MICROGRAMS (MCG). THE USUAL ADULT DOSAGE IS 500 MICROGRAMS (0.5 MG) DAILY INTRAVENOUSLY FOR A MAXIMUM OF FIVE DAYS. THE DOSAGE FOR ADULTS OR CHILDREN SHOULD NOT EXCEED 15 MCG/KG OR 400-600 MCG/SQUARE METER OF BODY SURFACE DAILY INTRAVENOUSLY FOR

FIVE DAYS. CALCULATION OF THE DOSAGE FOR OBESE OR EDEMATOUS PATIENTS SHOULD BE ON THE BASIS OF SURFACE AREA IN AN EFFORT TO RELATE DOSAGE TO LEAN BODY MASS.

DESCRIPTION
Dactinomycin is one of the actinomycins, a group of antibiotics produced by various species of *Streptomyces*. Dactinomycin is the principal component of the mixture of actinomycins produced by *Streptomyces parvullus*. Unlike other species of *Streptomyces*, this organism yields an essentially pure substance that contains only traces of similar compounds differing in the amino acid content of the peptide side chains. The empirical formula is $C_{62}H_{86}N_{12}O_{16}$.

Dactinomycin is a sterile, yellow lyophilized powder for injection by the intravenous route or by regional perfusion after reconstitution. Each vial contains 0.5 mg (500 mcg) of Dactinomycin and 20.0 mg of mannitol.

Following is its chemical structure:

CLINICAL PHARMACOLOGY
ACTION
Generally, the actinomycins exert an inhibitory effect on gram-positive and gram-negative bacteria and on some fungi. However, the toxic properties of the actinomycins (including Dactinomycin) in relation to antibacterial activity are such as to preclude their use as antibiotics in the treatment of infectious diseases.

Because the actinomycins are cytotoxic, they have an anti-neoplastic effect which has been demonstrated in experimental animals with various types of tumor implant. This cytotoxic action is the basis for their use in the palliative treatment of certain types of cancer.

PHARMACOKINETICS AND METABOLISM
Results of a study in patients with malignant melanoma indicate that Dactinomycin (^{3}H actinomycin D) is minimally metabolized, is concentrated in nucleated cells, and does not penetrate the blood brain barrier. Approximately 30% of the dose was recovered in urine and feces in one week. The terminal plasma half-life for radioactivity was approximately 36 hours.

INDICATIONS AND USAGE
WILMS' TUMOR
The neoplasm responding most frequently to Dactinomycin is Wilms' tumor. With low doses of both Dactinomycin and radiotherapy, temporary objective improvement may be as good as and may last longer than with higher doses of each given alone. In the National Wilms' Tumor study, combination therapy with Dactinomycin and vincristine together with surgery and radiotherapy, was shown to have significantly improved the prognosis of patients in groups II and III. Dactinomycin and vincristine were given for a total of seven cycles, so that maintenance therapy continued for approximately 15 months.

Postoperative radiotherapy in group I patients and optimal combination chemotherapy for those in group IV are unsettled issues. About 70 percent of lung metastases have disappeared with an appropriate combination of radiation, Dactinomycin and vincristine.

RHABDOMYOSARCOMA
Temporary regression of the tumor and beneficial subjective results have occurred with Dactinomycin in rhabdomyosarcoma which, like most soft tissue sarcomas, is comparatively radio-resistant.

Several groups have reported successful use of cyclophosphamide, vincristine Dactinomycin and doxorubicin hydrochloride in various combinations. Effective combinations have included vincristine and Dactinomycin; vincristine, Dactinomycin and cyclophosphamide (VAC therapy) and all four drugs in sequence. At present, the most effective treatment for children with inoperable or metastatic rhabdomyosarcoma has been VAC chemotherapy. Two-thirds of these children were doing well without evidence of disease at a median time of three years after diagnosis.

CARCINOMA OF TESTIS AND UTERUS
The sequential use of Dactinomycin and methotrexate, along with meticulous monitoring of human chorionic gonadotropin levels until normal, has resulted in survival in the majority of women with metastatic choriocarcinoma. Sequential therapy is used if there is:

1. Stability in gonadotropin titers following two successive courses of an agent.
2. Rising gonadotropin titers during treatment.
3. Severe toxicity preventing adequate therapy.

In patients with nonmetastatic choriocarcinoma, Dactinomycin or methotrexate or both, have been used successfully, with or without surgery.

Dactinomycin has been beneficial as a single agent in the treatment of metastatic nonseminomatour testicular carcinoma when used in cycles of 500 mcg/day for five consecutive days, every 6-8 weeks for periods of four months or longer.

OTHER NEOPLASMS
Dactinomycin has been given intravenously or by regional perfusion, either alone or with other antineoplastic compounds or x-ray therapy, in the palliative treatment of Ewing's sarcoma and sarcoma botryoides. For nonmetastatic Ewing's sarcoma, promising results were obtained when Dactinomycin (45 mcg/m^2) and cyclophosphamide (1200 mg/m^2) were given sequentially and with radiotherapy, over an 18 month period. Those with metastatic disease remain the subject of continued investigation with a more aggressive chemotherapeutic regimen employed initially.

Temporary objective improvement and relief of pain and discomfort have followed the use of Dactinomycin usually in conjunction with radiotherapy for sarcoma botryoides. This palliative effect ranges from transitory inhibition of tumor growth to a considerable but temporary regression in tumor size.

DACTINOMYCIN AND RADIATION THERAPY
Much evidence suggests that Dactinomycin potentiates the effects of x-ray therapy. The converse also appears likely; i.e., Dactinomycin may be more effective when radiation therapy also is given.

With combined Dactinomycin-radiation therapy, the normal skin, as well as the buccal and pharyngeal mucosa, show early erythema. A smaller than usual x-ray dose when given with Dactinomycin causes erythema and vesiculation, which progress more rapidly through the stages of tanning and desquamation. Healing may occur in four to six weeks rather than two to three months. Erythema from previous x-ray therapy may be reactivated by Dactinomycin alone, even when irradiation occurred many months earlier, and especially when the interval between the two forms of therapy is brief. This potentiation of radiation effect represents a special problem when the irradiation treatment area includes the mucous membrane. When irradiation is directed toward the nasopharynx, the combination may produce severe oropharyngeal mucositis. *Severe reactions may ensure if high doses of both Dactinomycin and radiation therapy are used or if the patient is particularly sensitive to such combined therapy.*

Because of this potentiating effect Dactinomycin may be tried in radiosensitive tumors not responding to doses of x-ray therapy that can be tolerated. Objective improvement in tumor size and activity may be observed when lower, better tolerated doses of both types of therapy are employed.

DACTINOMYCIN AND PERFUSION TECHNIC
Dactinomycin alone or with other antineoplastic agents has also been given by the isolation-perfusion technic, either as palliative treatment or as an adjunct to resection of a tumor. Some tumors considered resistant to chemotherapy and radiation therapy may respond when the drug is given by the perfusion technic. Neoplasms in which Dactinomycin has been tried by this technic include various types of sarcoma, carcinoma, and adenocarcinoma.

In some instances tumors regressed, pain was relieved for variable periods, and surgery made possible. On other occasions, however, the outcome has been less favorable. Nevertheless, in selected cases, the drug by perfusion may provide more effective palliation than when given systemically.

Dactinomycin by the isolation-perfusion technic offers certain advantages, provided leakage of the drug through the general circulation into other areas of the body is minimal. By this technic the drug is in continuous contact with the tumor for the duration of treatment. The dose may be increased well over that used by the systemic route, usually without adding to the danger of toxic effects. If the agent is confined to an isolated part, it should not interfere with the patient's defense mechanism. Systemic absorption of toxic products from neoplastic tissue can be minimized by removing the perfusate when the procedure is finished.

UNLABELED USES
Dactinomycin is used alone or as an adjunct in the treatment of melanoma and ovarian carcinoma.

CONTRAINDICATIONS
If Dactinomycin is given at or about the time of infection with chicken pox or herpes zoster, a severe generalized disease, which may result in death, may occur.

PRECAUTIONS
GENERAL
Dactinomycin should be administered only under the supervision of a physician who is experienced in the use of cancer chemotherapeutic agents.

This drug is highly toxic and both powder and solution must be handled and administered with care. Inhalation of dust or vapors and contact with skin or mucous membranes, especially those of the eyes, must be avoided. Should accidental eye contact occur, copious irrigation with water should be instituted immediately, followed by prompt ophthalmologic consultation. Should accidental skin contact occur, the affected part must be irrigated immediately with copious amounts of water for at least 15 minutes.

As with all antineoplastic agents, Dactinomycin is a toxic drug and very careful and frequent observation of the patient for adverse reactions is necessary. These reactions may involve any tissue of the body. The possibility of an anaphylactoid reaction should be borne in mind.

Increased incidence of gastrointestinal toxicity and marrow suppression has been reported when Dactinomycin was given with x-ray therapy.

Particular caution is necessary when administering Dactinomycin within two months of irradiation for the treatment of right-sided Wilms' tumor, since hepatomegaly and elevated SGOT levels have been noted.

Nausea and vomiting due to Dactinomycin make it necessary to give this drug intermittently. It is extremely important to observe the patient daily for toxic side effects when multiple chemotherapy is employed, since a full course of therapy occasionally is not tolerated. If stomatitis, diarrhea, or severe hemopoietic depression appear during therapy, these drugs should be discontinued until the patient has recovered. Recent reports indicate an increased incidence of second primary tumors following treatment with radiation and antineoplastic agents, such as Dactinomycin. Multimodal therapy creates the need for careful, long-term observation of cancer survivors.

LABORATORY TESTS
Many abnormalities of renal, hepatic, and bone marrow function have been reported in patients with neoplatic disease and receiving Dactinomycin. It is advisable to check renal, hepatic, and bone marrow functions frequently.

DRUG/LABORATORY TEST INTERACTIONS
It has been reported that Dactinomycin may interfere with bioassay procedures for the determination of antibacterial drug levels.

CARCINOGENESIS, MUTAGENESIS, IMPAIRMENT OF FERTILITY
The International Agency on Research on Cancer has judged that Dactinomycin is a positive carcinogen in animals. Local sarcomas were produced in mice and rats after repeated subcutaneous or intraperitoneal injection. Mesenchymal tumors occurred in male F344 rats given intraperitoneal injections of 0.05 mg/kg, 2 to 5 times per week for 18 weeks. The first tumor appeared at 23 weeks.

Dactinomycin has been shown to be mutagenic in a number of test systems *in vitro* and *in vivo* including human fibroblasts and leucocytes, and HELA cells. DNA damage and cytogenetic effects have been demonstrated in the mouse and the rat.

Adequate fertility studies have not been reported.

PREGNANCY
Pregnancy Category C. Dactinomycin has been shown to cause malformations and embryotoxicity in the rat, rabbit and hamster when given in doses of 50-100 mcg/kg intravenously (3-7 times the maximum recommended human dose). There are no adequate and well-controlled studies in pregnant women. Dactinomycin should be used during pregnancy only if the potential benefit justifies the potential risk to the fetus.

NURSING MOTHERS
It is not known whether this drug is excreted in human milk. Because many drugs are excreted in human milk and because of the potential for serious adverse reactions in nursing infants from Dactinomycin a decision should be made whether to discontinue nursing or to discontinue the drug, taking into account the importance of the drug to the mother.

PEDIATRIC USE
The greater frequency of toxic effects of Dactinomycin in infants suggest that this drug should be given to infants only over the age of 6 to 12 months.

ADVERSE REACTIONS
Toxic effects (excepting nausea and vomiting) usually do not become apparent until one to four days after a course of therapy is stopped, and may not be maximal before one to two weeks have elapsed. Deaths have been reported. However, adverse reactions are usually reversible on discontinuance of therapy. They include the following:

Miscellaneous: malaise, fatigue, lethargy, fever, myalgia, proctitis, hypocalcemia.

Oral: cheilitis, dysphagia, esophagitis, ulcerative stomatitis, pharyngitis.

Gastrointestinal: anorexia, nausea, vomiting abdominal pain, diarrhea, gastrointestinal ulceration, liver toxicity including ascites, hepatomegaly, hepatitis, and liver function test abnormalities. Nausea and vomiting, which occur early during the first few hours after administration, may be alleviated by giving antiemetics.

Hematologic: anemia, even to the point of aplastic anemia, agranulocytosis, leukopenia, thrombopenia, pancytopenia, reticulopenia. Platelet and white cell counts should be done *daily* to detect severe hemopoietic depression. If either count markedly decreases, the drug should be withheld to allow marrow recovery. This often takes up to three weeks.

Dermatologic: alopecia, skin eruptions, acne, flare-up of erythema or increased pigmentation of previously irradiated skin.

Soft Tissues: Dactinomycin is extremely corrosive. If extravastion occurs during intravenous use, severe damage to soft tissues will occur. In at least one instance, this has led to contracture of the arms.

OVERDOSAGE
The intravenous LD$_{50}$ of Dactinomycin in the rat is 460 mcg/kg.

DOSAGE AND ADMINISTRATION
Toxic reactions due to Dactinomycin are frequent and may be severe (see *"Adverse Reactions"*), thus limiting in many instances the amount that may be given. However, the severity of toxicity varies markedly and is only partly dependent on the dose employed. The drug must be given in short courses.

INTRAVENOUS USE
The dosage of Dactinomycin varies depending on the tolerance of the patient, the size and location of the neoplasm, and the use of other forms of therapy. It may be necessary to decrease the usual dosages suggested below when other chemotherapy or x-ray therapy is used concomitantly or has been used previously.

The dosage for adults or children should not exceed 15 mcg/kg or 400-600 mcg/square meter of body surface daily intravenously for five days. Calculation of the dosage for obese or edematous patients should be on the basis of surface area in an effort to relate dosage to lean body mass.

Adults: The usual adult dosage is 500 mcg (0.5 mg) daily intravenously for a maximum of five days.

Children: In children 15 mcg (0.015 mg) per kilogram of body weight is given intravenously daily for five days. An alternative schedule is a total dosage of 2500 mcg (2.5 mg) per square meter of body surface given intravenously over a one week period.

In both adults and children, a second course may be given after at least three weeks have elapsed, provided all signs of toxicity have disappeared.

Reconstitute Dactinomycin by adding 1.1 ml of **Sterile Water for Injection (without preservative)** using aseptic precautions. The resulting solution of Dactinomycin will contain approximately 500 mcg or 0.5 mg per ml.

Parenteral drug products should be inspected visually for particulate matter and discoloration prior to administration, whenever solution and container permit. When reconstituted, Dactinomycin is a clear, gold-colored solution.

Once reconstituted, the solution of Dactinomycin can be added to infusion solutions of Dextrose Injection 5 percent or Sodium Chloride Injection either directly or to the tubing of a running intravenous infusion.

Although reconstituted Dactinomycin is chemically stable, the product does not contain a preservative and accidental microbial contamination might result. Any unused portion should be discarded. Use of water containing preservatives (benzyl alcohol or parabens) to reconstitute Dactinomycin for injection, results in the formation of a precipitate.

Partial removal of Dactinomycin from intravenous solutions by cellulose ester membrane filters used in some intravenous in-line filters has been reported.

Since Dactinomycin is extremely corrosive to soft tissue, precautions for materials of this nature should be observed.

If the drug is given directly into the vein without the use of an infusion, the "two-needle technic" should be used. Reconstitute and withdraw the calculated dose from the vial with one sterile needle. Use another sterile needle for direct injection into the vein.

Discard any unused portion of the Dactinomycin solution.

ISOLATION-PERFUSION TECHNIC

The dosage schedules and the technic itself vary from one investigator to another; the published literature, therefore, should be consulted for details. In general, the following doses are suggested:

50 mcg (0.05 mg) per kilogram of body weight for lower extremity or pelvis.
35 mcg (0.035 mg) per kilogram of body weight for upper extremity.

It may be advisable to use lower doses in obese patients, or when previous chemotherapy or radiation therapy has been employed.

Complications of the perfusion technic are related mainly to the amount of drug that escapes into the systemic circulation and may consist of hemopoietic depression, absorption of toxic products from massive destruction of neoplastic tissue, increased susceptibility to infection, impaired wound healing, and superficial ulceration of the gastric mucosa. Other side effects may include edema of the extremity involved, damage to soft tissues of the perfused area, and (potentially) venous thrombosis.

Protect from light. Store in a dry place below 30°C (86°F); transient temperatures (i.e., for a period not exceeding two weeks) of up to 50°C (122°F) are permissible.

SPECIAL HANDLING

Due to the drug's toxic and mutagenic properties, appropriate precautions including the use of appropriate safety equipment are recommended for the preparation of Dactinomycin for parenteral administration. The National Institutes of Health presently recommends that the preparation of injectable antineoplastic drugs should be performed in a Class II laminar flow biological safety cabinet and that personnel preparing drugs of this class should wear surgical gloves and a closed front surgical-type gown with knit cuffs.

J CODES
0.5 mg IV—J9120

HOW SUPPLIED
POWDER FOR INJECTION: 0.5 MG

BRAND/MANUFACTURER	NDC	SIZE	AWP
○ **BRAND**			
COSMEGEN: Merck	00006-3298-22	1s	$11.34

Dalgan *SEE* DEZOCINE

Dalmane *SEE* FLURAZEPAM HYDROCHLORIDE

Damason-P *SEE* ASPIRIN WITH HYDROCODONE
BITARTRATE

Danazol

DESCRIPTION
Danazol, is a synthetic steroid derived from ethisterone. Chemically, Danazol is 17α-Pregna-2,4-dien-20-yno[2,3-*d*]-isoxazol-17-ol.

Following is its chemical structure:

CLINICAL PHARMACOLOGY
Danazol suppresses the pituitary-ovarian axis. This suppression is probably a combination of depressed hypothalamic-pituitary response to lowered estrogen production, the alteration of sex steroid metabolism, and interaction of Danazol with sex hormone receptors. The only other demonstrable hormonal effect is weak androgenic activity.

Danazol depresses the output of both follicle-stimulating hormone (FSH) and luteinizing hormone (LH).

Recent evidence suggests a direct inhibitory effect at gonadal sites and a binding of Danazol to receptors of gonadal steroids at target organs.

Bioavailability studies indicate that blood levels do not increase proportionally with increases in the administered dose. When the dose of Danazol is doubled, the increase in plasma levels is only about 35% to 40%.

Separate single dosing of 100 mg and 200 mg capsules of Danazol to female volunteers showed that both the extent of availability and the maximum plasma concentration increased by three-to-four fold, respectively, following a meal (>30 grams of fat), when compared to the fasted state. Further, food also delayed mean time to peak concentration of Danazol by about 30 minutes.

In the treatment of endometriosis Danazol alters the normal and ectopic endometrial tissue so that it becomes inactive and atrophic. Complete resolution of endometrial lesions occurs in the majority of cases.

Changes in vaginal cytology and cervical mucus reflect the suppressive effect of Danazol on the pituitary-ovarian axis.

In the treatment of fibrocystic breast disease, Danazol usually produces partial to complete disappearance of nodularity and complete relief of pain and tenderness. Changes in the menstrual pattern may occur.

Generally, the pituitary-suppressive action of Danazol is reversible. Ovulation and cyclic bleeding usually return within 60 to 90 days when therapy with Danazol is discontinued.

In the treatment of hereditary angioedema, Danazol at effective doses prevents attacks of the disease characterized by episodic edema of the abdominal viscera, extremities, face, and airway which may be disabling and, if the airway is involved, fatal. In addition, Danazol corrects partially or completely the primary biochemical abnormality of hereditary angioedema by increasing the levels of the deficient C1 esterase inhibitor (C1E1). As a result of this action the serum levels of the C4 component of the complement system are also increased.

INDICATIONS AND USAGE
Endometriosis: Danazol is indicated for the treatment of endometriosis amenable to hormonal management.

Fibrocystic Breast Disease: Most cases of symptomatic fibrocystic breast disease may be treated by simple measures (eg, padded brassieres and analgesics).

In infrequent patients, symptoms of pain and tenderness may be severe enough to warrant treatment by suppression of ovarian function. Danazol is usually effective in decreasing nodularity, pain, and tenderness. It should be stressed to the patient that this treatment is not innocuous in that it involves considerable alterations of hormone levels and that recurrence of symptoms is very common after cessation of therapy.

Hereditary Angioedema: Danazol is indicated for the prevention of attacks of angioedema of all types (cutaneous, abdominal, laryngeal) in males and females.

UNLABELED USES
Danazol is used alone or as an adjunct in the treatment of autoimmune hemolytic anemia, hemophilia, premenstrual syndrome, systemic lupus erythematosus, and idiopathic thrombocytopenic purpura.

CONTRAINDICATIONS
Danazol should not be administered to patients with:

1. Undiagnosed abnormal genital bleeding.
2. Markedly impaired hepatic, renal, or cardiac function.
3. Pregnancy. (See *"Warnings"*.)
4. Breast feeding.
5. Porphyria—Danazol can induce ALA synthetase activity and hence porphyrin metabolism.

WARNINGS
USE OF DANAZOL IN PREGNANCY IS CONTRAINDICATED. A SENSITIVE TEST (EG, BETA SUBUNIT TEST IF AVAILABLE) CAPABLE OF DETERMINING EARLY PREGNANCY IS RECOMMENDED IMMEDIATELY PRIOR TO START OF THERAPY. ADDITIONAL-

---

◆ RATED THERAPEUTICALLY EQUIVALENT; ◇ THERAPEUTIC EQUIVALENCE UNCONFIRMED; ○ UNRATED

LY A NONHORMONAL METHOD OF CONTRACEPTION SHOULD BE USED DURING THERAPY. IF A PATIENT BECOMES PREGNANT WHILE TAKING DANAZOL, ADMINISTRATION OF THE DRUG SHOULD BE DISCONTINUED AND THE PATIENTS SHOULD BE APPRISED OF THE POTENTIAL RISK TO THE FETUS. EXPOSURE TO DANAZOL IN UTERO MAY RESULT IN ANDROGENIC EFFECTS ON THE FEMALE FETUS; REPORTS OF CLITORAL HYPERTROPHY, LABIAL FUSION, UROGENITAL SINUS DEFECT, VAGINAL ATRESIA, AND AMBIGUOUS GENITALIA HAVE BEEN RECEIVED. (SEE *"PRECAUTIONS: PREGNANCY, TERATOGENIC EFFECTS"*.)

THROMBOEMBOLISM, THROMBOTIC AND THROMBOPHLEBITIC EVENTS INCLUDING SAGITTAL SINUS THROMBOSIS AND LIFE-THREATENING OR FATAL STROKES HAVE BEEN REPORTED.

EXPERIENCE WITH LONG-TERM THERAPY WITH DANAZOL IS LIMITED. PELIOSIS HEPATIS AND BENIGN HEPATIC ADENOMA HAVE BEEN OBSERVED WITH LONG-TERM USE. PELIOSIS HEPATIS AND HEPATIC ADENOMA MAY BE SILENT UNTIL COMPLICATED BY ACUTE, POTENTIALLY LIFE-THREATENING INTRA-ABDOMINAL HEMORRHAGE. THE PHYSICIAN THEREFORE SHOULD BE ALERT TO THIS POSSIBILITY. ATTEMPTS SHOULD BE MADE TO DETERMINE THE LOWEST DOSE THAT WILL PROVIDE ADEQUATE PROTECTION. IF THE DRUG WAS BEGUN AT A TIME OF EXACERBATION OF HEREDITARY ANGIONEUROTIC EDEMA DUE TO TRAUMA, STRESS OR OTHER CAUSE, PERIODIC ATTEMPTS TO DECREASE OR WITHDRAW THERAPY SHOULD BE CONSIDERED.

DANAZOL HAS BEEN ASSOCIATED WITH SEVERAL CASES OF BENIGN INTRACRANIAL HYPERTENSION ALSO KNOWN AS PSEUDOTUMOR CEREBRI. EARLY SIGNS AND SYMPTOMS OF BENIGN INTRACRANIAL HYPERTENSION INCLUDE PAPILLEDEMA, HEADACHE, NAUSEA AND VOMITING, AND VISUAL DISTURBANCES. PATIENTS WITH THESE SYMPTOMS SHOULD BE SCREENED FOR PAPILLEDEMA AND, IF PRESENT, THE PATIENTS SHOULD BE ADVISED TO DISCONTINUE DANAZOL IMMEDIATELY AND BE REFERRED TO A NEUROLOGIST FOR FURTHER DIAGNOSIS AND CARE.

A temporary alteration of lipoprotein in the form of decreased high density lipoproteins and possibly increased low density lipoproteins has been reported during Danazol therapy. These alterations may be marked, and prescribers should consider the potential impact on the risk of atherosclerosis and coronary artery disease in accordance with the potential benefit of the therapy to the patient.

Before initiating therapy of fibrocystic breast disease with Danazol, carcinoma of the breast should be excluded. However, nodularity, pain, tenderness due to fibrocystic breast disease may prevent recognition of underlying carcinoma before treatment is begun. Therefore, if any nodule persists or enlarges during treatment, carcinoma should be considered and ruled out.

Patients should be watched closely for signs of androgenic effects some of which may not be reversible even when drug administration is stopped.

PRECAUTIONS

Because Danazol may cause some degree of fluid retention, conditions that might be influenced by this factor, such as epilepsy, migraine, or cardiac or renal dysfunction, require careful observation.

Since hepatic dysfunction manifested by modest increases in serum transaminase levels has been reported in patients treated with Danazol, periodic liver function tests should be performed (see *"Warnings"* and *"Adverse Reactions"*).

Administration of Danazol has been reported to cause exacerbation of the manifestations of acute intermittent porphyria. (See *"Contraindications"*.)

Drug Interactions: Prolongation of prothrombin time occurs in patients stabilized on warfarin. Therapy with Danazol may cause an increase in carbamazepine levels in patients taking both drugs.

Laboratory Tests: Danazol treatment may interfere with laboratory determinations of testosterone, androstenedione, and dehydroepiandrosterone.

Carcinogenesis, Mutagenesis, Impairment of Fertility: No valid studies have been performed to assess the carcinogenicity of Danazol.

Pregnancy, Teratogenic Effects: (See *"Contraindications"*.) Pregnancy Category X. Danazol administered orally to pregnant rats from the 6th through the 15th day of gestation at doses up to 250 mg/kg/day (7-15 times the human dose) did not result in drug-induced embryotoxicity or teratogenicity, nor difference in litter size, viability or weight of offspring compared to controls. In rabbits, the administration of Danazol on days 6-18 of gestation at doses of 60 mg/kg/day and above (2-4 times the human dose) resulted in inhibition of fetal development.

Nursing Mothers: (See *"Contraindications"*.)

Pediatric Use: Safety and effectiveness in children have not been established.

ADVERSE REACTIONS

The following events have been reported in association with the use of Danazol:

Andogen-like effects include weight gain, acne, and seborrhea. Mild hirsutism, edema, hair loss, voice change, which may take the form of hoarseness, sore throat, or of instability or deepening of pitch, may occur and may persist after cessation of therapy. Hypertrophy of the clitoris is rare.

Other possible endocrine effects include menstrual disturbances in the form of spotting, alteration of the timing of the cycle and amenorrhea. Although cyclical bleeding and ovulation usually return within 60 to 90 days after discontinuation of therapy with Danazol persistent amenorrhea has occasionally been reported.

Flushing, sweating, vaginal dryness and irritation, and reduction in breast size may reflect lowering of estrogen. Nervousness and emotional lability have been reported. In the male a modest reduction in spermatogenesis may be evident during treatment. Abnormalities in semen volume, viscosity, sperm count, and motility may occur in patients receiving long-term therapy.

Hepatic dysfunction, as evidenced by reversible elevated serum enzymes and/or jaundice has been reported in patients receiving a daily dosage of Danazol of 400 mg or more. It is recommended that patients receiving Danazol be monitored for hepatic dysfunction by laboratory tests and clinical observation. Serious hepatic toxicity including cholestatic jaundice, peliosis hepatis, and hepatic adenoma have been reported. (See *"Warnings"* and *"Precautions"*.)

Abnormalities in laboratory tests may occur during therapy with Danazol including CPK, glucose tolerance, glucagon, thyroid binding globulin, sex hormone binding globulin, other plasma proteins, lipids and lipoproteins.

The following reactions have been reported, a causal relationship to the administration of Danazol has neither been confirmed nor refuted:

Allergic: urticaria, pruritus and rarely, nasal congestion;

CNS effects: headache, nervousness and emotional lability, dizziness and fainting, depression, fatigue, sleep disorders, tremor, paresthesias, weakness, visual disturbances, and rarely, benign intracranial hypertension, anxiety, changes in appetite, chills, and rarely convulsions, Guillain-Barré syndrome;

Gastrointestinal: gastroenteritis, nausea vomiting, constipation, and rarely, pancreatitis;

Musculoskeletal: muscle cramps or spasms, or pains, joint pain, joint lockup, joint swelling, pain in back, neck, or extremities, and rarely, carpal tunnel syndrome which may be secondary to fluid retention;

Genitourinary: hematuria, prolonged posttherapy amenorrhea;

Hematologic: an increase in red cell and platelet count. Reversible erythrocytosis, leukocytosis or polycythemia may be provoked. Eosinophilia, leukopenia or thrombocytopenia have also been noted.

Skin: rashes (maculopapular, vesicular, papular, purpuric, petechial), and rarely, sun sensitivity, Stevens-Johnson syndrome;

Other: increased insulin requirements in diabetic patients, changes in libido, elevation in blood pressure, and rarely, cataracts, bleeding gums, fever, pelvic pain, nipple discharge. Malignant liver tumors have been reported in rare instances, after long-term use.

DOSAGE AND ADMINISTRATION

Endometriosis: In moderate to severe disease, or in patients infertile due to endometriosis, a starting dose of 800 mg given in two divided doses is recommended. Amenorrhea and rapid response to painful symptoms is best achieved at this dosage level. Gradual downward titration to a dose sufficient to maintain amenorrhea may be considered depending upon patient response. For mild cases, an initial daily dose of 200 mg to 400 mg given in two divided doses is recommended and may be adjusted depending on patient response. **Therapy should begin during menstruation. Otherwise, appropriate tests should be performed to ensure that the patient is not pregnant while on therapy with Danazol. (See *"Contraindications"* and *"Warnings"*.) It is essential that therapy continue uninterrupted for 3 to 6 months but may be extended to 9 months if necessary.** After termination of therapy, if symptoms recur, treatment can be reinstituted.

Fibrocystic Breast Disease: The total daily dosage of Danazol for fibrocystic breast disease ranges from 100 mg to 400 mg given in two divided doses depending upon patient response. **Therapy should begin during menstruation. Otherwise, appropriate tests should be performed to ensure that the patient is not pregnant while on therapy with Danazol.** A nonhormonal method of contraception is recommended when Danazol is administered at this dose, since ovulation may not be suppressed.

In most instances, breast pain and tenderness are significantly relieved by the first month and eliminated in 2 to 3 months. Usually elimination of nodularity requires 4 to 6 months of uninterrupted therapy. Regular menstrual patterns, irregular menstrual patterns, and amenorrhea each occur in approximately one-third of patients treated with 100 mg of Danazol. Irregular menstrual patterns and amenorrhea are observed more frequently with higher doses. Clinical studies have demonstrated that 50% of patients may show evidence of recurrence of symptoms within one year. In this event, treatment may be reinstated.

Hereditary Angioedema: The dosage requirements for continuous treatment of hereditary angioedema with Danazol, should be individualized on the basis of the clinical response of the patient. It is recommended that the patient be started on 200 mg, two or three times a day. After a favorable initial response is obtained in terms of prevention of episodes of edematous attacks, the proper continuing dosage should be determined by decreasing the dosage by 50% or less at intervals of one to three months or longer if frequency of attacks prior to treatment dictates. If an attack occurs, the daily dosage may be increased by up to 200 mg. During the dose adjusting phase, close monitoring of the patient's response is indicated, particularly if the patient has a history of airway involvement.

HOW SUPPLIED
CAPSULE: 50 MG

BRAND/MANUFACTURER	NDC	SIZE	AWP
◆ BRAND			
DANOCRINE: Sanofi Winthrop	00024-0303-06	100s	$114.69

CAPSULE: 100 MG

BRAND/MANUFACTURER	NDC	SIZE	AWP
◆ **BRAND** DANOCRINE: Sanofi Winthrop	00024-0304-06	100s	$172.09

CAPSULE: 200 MG

AVERAGE UNIT PRICE (AVAILABLE SIZES)			
BRAND	$3.07		

BRAND/MANUFACTURER	NDC	SIZE	AWP
◆ **BRAND** DANOCRINE: Sanofi Winthrop	00024-0304-60	60s	$185.82
	00024-0305-60	60s	$195.12
	00024-0305-06	100s	$286.78

Danocrine *SEE* DANAZOL

Dantrium *SEE* DANTROLENE SODIUM

Dantrolene Sodium

DANTROLENE SODIUM HAS A POTENTIAL FOR HEPATOTOXICITY, AND SHOULD NOT BE USED IN CONDITIONS OTHER THAN THOSE RECOMMENDED. SYMPTOMATIC HEPATITIS (FATAL AND NON-FATAL) HAS BEEN REPORTED AT VARIOUS DOSE LEVELS OF THE DRUG. THE INCIDENCE REPORTED IN PATIENTS TAKING UP TO 400 MG/DAY IS MUCH LOWER THAN IN THOSE TAKING DOSES OF 800 MG OR MORE PER DAY. EVEN SPORADIC SHORT COURSES OF THESE HIGHER DOSE LEVELS WITHIN A TREATMENT REGIMEN MARKEDLY INCREASED THE RISK OF SERIOUS HEPATIC INJURY. LIVER DYSFUNCTION AS EVIDENCED BY BLOOD CHEMICAL ABNORMALITIES ALONE (LIVER ENZYME ELEVATIONS) HAS BEEN OBSERVED IN PATIENTS EXPOSED TO DANTROLENE SODIUM FOR VARYING PERIODS OF TIME. OVERT HEPATITIS HAS OCCURRED AT VARYING INTERVALS AFTER INITIATION OF THERAPY, BUT HAS BEEN MOST FREQUENTLY OBSERVED BETWEEN THE THIRD AND TWELFTH MONTH OF THERAPY. THE RISK OF HEPATIC INJURY APPEARS TO BE GREATER IN FEMALES, IN PATIENTS OVER 35 YEARS OF AGE, AND IN PATIENTS TAKING OTHER MEDICATION(S) IN ADDITION TO DANTROLENE SODIUM. DANTROLENE SODIUM SHOULD BE USED ONLY IN CONJUNCTION WITH APPROPRIATE MONITORING OF HEPATIC FUNCTION INCLUDING FREQUENT DETERMINATION OF SGOT OR SGPT. IF NO OBSERVABLE BENEFIT IS DERIVED FROM THE ADMINISTRATION OF DANTROLENE SODIUM AFTER A TOTAL OF 45 DAYS, THERAPY SHOULD BE DISCONTINUED. THE LOWEST POSSIBLE EFFECTIVE DOSE FOR THE INDIVIDUAL PATIENT SHOULD BE PRESCRIBED.

DESCRIPTION

The chemical formula of Dantrolene Sodium is hydrated 1-[[[5-(4-nitrophenyl)-2-furanyl]methylene]amino]-2, 4-imidazolidinedione sodium salt. It is slightly soluble in water, but due to its slightly acidic nature the solubility increases somewhat in alkaline solution. The anhydrous salt has a molecular weight of 336. The hydrated salt contains approximately 15% water (3-½ moles) and has a molecular weight of 399.

Following is its chemical structure:

$$O_2N\text{---}\bigcirc\text{---}\bigcirc\text{---}CH=N\text{---}N\begin{matrix}\\ \end{matrix}$$

CLINICAL PHARMACOLOGY

In isolated nerve-muscle preparation, Dantrolene Sodium has been shown to produce relaxation by affecting the contractile response of the skeletal muscle at a site beyond the myoneural junction, directly on the muscle itself. In skeletal muscle, Dantrolene Sodium dissociates the excitation-contraction coupling, probably by interfering with the release of Ca^{++} from the sarcoplasmic reticulum. This effect appears to be more pronounced in fast muscle fibers as compared to slow ones, but generally affects both. A central nervous system effect occurs, with drowsiness, dizziness, and generalized weakness occasionally present. Although Dantrolene Sodium does not appear to directly affect the CNS, the extent of its indirect effect is unknown. The administration of intravenous Dantrolene Sodium to human volunteers is associated with loss of grip strength and weakness in the legs, as well as subjective CNS complaints (see also *"Precautions, Information for Patients"*). Information concerning the passage of Dantrolene Sodium across the blood-brain barrier is not available. The absorption of Dantrolene Sodium after oral administration in humans is incomplete and slow but consistent, and dose-related blood levels are obtained. The duration and intensity of skeletal muscle relaxation is related to the dosage and blood levels. The mean biologic half-life of Dantrolene Sodium in adults is 8.7 hours after a 100-mg dose, 4 to 8 hours after intravenous administration. Based on assays of whole blood and plasma, slightly greater amounts of Dantrolene are associated with red blood cells than with the plasma fraction of blood. Significant amounts of Dantrolene are bound to plasma proteins, mostly albumin, and this binding is readily reversible. Specific metabolic pathways in the degradation and elimination of Dantrolene Sodium in human subjects have been established. Metabolic patterns are similar in adults and children. In addition to the parent compound, Dantrolene, which is found in measurable amounts in blood and urine, the major metabolites noted in body fluids are the 5 hydroxy analog and the acetamido analog. Dantrolene Sodium may also undergo hydrolysis and subsequent oxidation forming nitrophenylfuroic acid. Since Dantrolene Sodium is probably metabolized by hepatic microsomal enzymes, enhancement of its metabolism by other drugs is possible. However, neither, phenobarbital nor diazepam appears to affect Dantrolene Sodium metabolism.

Clinical experience in the management of fulminant human malignant hyperthermia, as well as experiments conducted in malignant hyperthermia susceptible swine, have revealed that the administration of intravenous Dantrolene, combined with indicated supportive measures, is effective in reversing the hypermetabolic process of malignant hyperthermia. Known differences between human and swine malignant hyperthermia are minor. The prophylactic administration of oral or intravenous Dantrolene to malignant hyperthermia susceptible swine will attenuate or prevent the development of signs of malignant hyperthermia in a manner dependent upon the dosage of Dantrolene administered and the intensity of the malignant hyperthermia triggering stimulus. Limited clinical experience with the administration of oral Dantrolene to patients judged malignant hyperthermia susceptible, when combined with clinical experience in the use of intravenous Dantrolene for the treatment of malignant hyperthermia and data derived from the above cited animal model experiments, suggests that oral Dantrolene will also attenuate or prevent the development of signs of human malignant hyperthermia, provided that currently accepted practices in the management of such patients are adhered to (see *"Indications and Usage"*): intravenous Dantrolene should also be available for use should the signs of malignant hyperthermia appear.

Cardiopulmonary depression has not been observed in MHS swine following the administration of up to 7.5 mg/kg i.v. Dantrolene. This is twice the amount needed to maximally diminish twitch response to single supramaximal peripheral nerve stimulation (95% inhibition). A transient, inconsistent, depressant effect on gastrointestinal smooth muscles has been observed at high doses.

INDICATIONS AND USAGE

IN CHRONIC SPASTICITY

Dantrolene Sodium is indicated in controlling the manifestations of clinical spasticity resulting from upper motor neuron disorders (*e.g.*, spinal cord injury, stroke, cerebral palsy, or multiple sclerosis). It is of particular benefit to the patient whose functional rehabilitation has been retarded by the sequelae of spasticity. Such patients must have presumably reversible spasticity where relief of spasticity will aid in restoring residual function. Dantrolene Sodium is not indicated in the treatment of skeletal muscle spasm resulting from rheumatic disorders. If improvement occurs, it will ordinarily occur within the dosage titration (see *"Dosage and Administration"*), and will be manifested by a decrease in the severity of spasticity and the ability to resume a daily function not quite attainable without Dantrolene Sodium.

Occasionally, subtle but meaningful improvement in spasticity may occur with Dantrolene Sodium therapy. In such instances, information regarding improvement should be solicited from the patient and those who are in constant daily contact and attendance with him. Brief withdrawal of Dantrolene Sodium for a period of 2 to 4 days will frequently demonstrate exacerbation of the manifestations of spasticity and may serve to confirm a clinical impression.

A decision to continue the administration of Dantrolene Sodium on a long-term basis is justified if introduction of the drug into the patient's regimen:

produces a significant reduction in painful and/or disabling spasticity such as clonus, or

permits a significant reduction in the intensity and/or degree of nursing care required, or

rids the patient of any annoying manifestation of spasticity considered important by the patient himself.

IN MALIGNANT HYPERTHERMIA

Oral Dantrolene Sodium is also indicated preoperatively to prevent or attenuate the development of signs of malignant hyperthermia in known, or strongly suspect, malignant hyperthermia susceptible patients who require anesthesia and/or surgery. Currently accepted clinical practices in the management of such patients must still be adhered to (careful monitoring for early signs of malignant hyperthermia, minimizing exposure to triggering mechanisms and prompt use of intravenous Dantrolene Sodium and indicated supportive measures should signs of malignant hyperthermia appear.

Dantrolene Sodium Intravenous is indicated, along with appropriate supportive measures, for the management of the fulminant hypermetabolism of skeletal muscle characteristic of MH crisis in patients of all ages. Dantrolene Sodium

Intravenous should be administered by continuous rapid intravenous push as soon as the MH reaction is recognized (*i.e.*, tachycardia, tachypnea, central venous desaturation, hypercarbia, metabolic acidosis, skeletal muscle rigidity, increased utilization of anesthesia circuit carbon dioxide absorber, cyanosis and mottling of the skin, and, in many cases, fever).

Dantrolene Sodium Intravenous is also indicated preoperatively, and sometimes postoperatively, to prevent or attenuate the development of clinical and laboratory signs of malignant hyperthermia in individuals judged to be malignant hyperthermia susceptible.

Oral Dantrolene Sodium should be administered following a malignant hyperthermic crisis to prevent recurrence of the signs of malignant hyperthermia.

UNLABELED USES

Dantrolene Sodium is also used alone or as an adjunct in the treatment of heat stroke, neuroleptic malignant syndrome, and posttraumatic muscle contracture. It is also used in Parkinson's disease, muscular dystrophy, and tetanus.

CONTRAINDICATIONS

Active hepatic disease, such as hepatitis and cirrhosis, is a contraindication for use of oral Dantrolene Sodium. Oral Dantrolene Sodium is contraindicated where spasticity is utilized to sustain upright posture and balance in locomotion or whenever spasticity is utilized to obtain or maintain increased function.

There are no contraindications to use of Intravenous Dantrolene Sodium.

WARNINGS

It is important to recognize that fatal and non-fatal liver disorders of an idiosyncratic or hypersensitivity type may occur with Dantrolene Sodium therapy.

At the start of Oral Dantrolene Sodium therapy, it is desirable to do liver function studies (SGOT, SGPT, alkaline phosphatase, total bilirubin) for a baseline or to establish whether there is preexisting liver disease. If baseline liver abnormalities exist and are confirmed, there is a clear possibility that the potential for Dantrolene Sodium hepatotoxicity could be enhanced, although such a possibility has not yet been established.

Liver function studies (*e.g.*, SGOT or SGPT), should be performed at appropriate intervals during Oral Dantrolene Sodium therapy. If such studies reveal abnormal values, therapy should generally be discontinued. Only where benefits of the drug have been of major importance to the patient, should reinitiation or continuation of therapy be considered. Some patients have revealed a return to normal laboratory values in the face of continued therapy while others have not.

If symptoms compatible with hepatitis, accompanied by abnormalities in liver function tests or jaundice appear, Oral Dantrolene Sodium should be discontinued. If caused by Oral Dantrolene Sodium and detected early, the abnormalities in liver function characteristically have reverted to normal when the drug was discontinued.

Oral Dantrolene Sodium therapy has been reinstituted in a few patients who have developed clinical and/or laboratory evidence of hepatocellular injury. If such reinstitution of therapy is done, it should be attempted only in patients who clearly need Oral Dantrolene Sodium and only after previous symptoms and laboratory abnormalities have cleared. The patient should be hospitalized and the drug should be restarted in very small and gradually increasing doses. Laboratory monitoring should be frequent and the drug should be withdrawn immediately if there is any indication of recurrent liver involvement. Some patients have reacted with unmistakable signs of liver abnormality upon administration of a challenge dose, while others have not.

Oral Dantrolene Sodium should be used with particular caution in females and in patients over 35 years of age in view of apparent greater likelihood of drug-induced, potentially fatal, hepatocellular disease in these groups.

Long-term safety of Oral Dantrolene Sodium in humans has not been established. Chronic studies in rats, dogs, and monkeys at dosages greater than 30 mg/kg/day showed growth or weight depression and signs of hepatopathy and possible occlusion nephropathy, all of which were reversible upon cessation of treatment. Sprague-Dawley female rats fed Oral Dantrolene Sodium for 18 months at dosage levels of 15, 30, and 60 mg/kg/day showed an increased incidence of benign and malignant mammary tumors compared with concurrent controls and, at the highest dosage, an increase in the incidence of hepatic lymphangiomas and hepatic angiosarcomas. These effects were not seen in 2-½-year studies in Sprague-Dawley or Fischer 344 rats or in 2-year studies in mice of the HaM/ICR strain. Carcinogenicity in humans cannot be fully excluded, so that this possible risk of chronic administration must be weighed against the benefits of the drug (*i.e.*, after a brief trial) for the individual patient.

The use of Dantrolene Sodium Intravenous in the management of MH crisis is not a substitute for previously known supportive measures. These measures must be individualized, but it will usually be necessary to discontinue the suspect triggering agents, attend to increased oxygen requirements, manage the metabolic acidosis, institute cooling when necessary, monitor urinary output, and monitor for electrolyte imbalance.

Since the effect of disease state and other drugs on the consequences of Dantrolene Sodium related skeletal muscle weakness, including possible respiratory depression, cannot be predicted, patients who receive i.v. Dantrolene Sodium preoperatively should have vital signs monitored.

If patients judged malignant hyperthermia susceptible are administered intravenous or oral Dantrolene Sodium preoperatively, anesthetic preparation must still follow a standard MHS regimen, including the avoidance of known triggering agents. Monitoring for early clinical and metabolic signs of MH is indicated because attenuation of MH, rather than prevention, is possible. These signs usually call for the administration of additional IV Dantrolene.

CARCINOGENESIS, MUTAGENESIS, AND IMPAIRMENT OF FERTILITY

Studies of Dantrolene Sodium in animals to evaluate mutagenic potential and the effect on fertility have not been conducted. Sprague-Dawley female rats fed Dantrolene Sodium for 18 months at dosage levels of 15, 30, and 60 mg/kg/day showed an increased incidence of benign and malignant mammary tumors compared with concurrent controls. At the highest dosage, there was an increase in the incidence of hepatic lymphangiomas and hepatic angiosarcomas. These effects were not seen in 30-month studies in Sprague-Dawley or Fisher-344 rats or in 24-month studies in mice of the HaM/ICR strain. Although the possibility that the drug may be carcinogenic in humans cannot be fully excluded, the risks associated with administration of Dantrolene Sodium Intravenous in a life-threatening crisis would appear to be minimal.

USAGE IN PREGNANCY

The safety of Dantrolene Sodium for use in women who are or who may become pregnant has not been established. Dantrolene Sodium should be used during pregnancy only if the potential benefit justifies the potential risk to the fetus. Dantrolene Sodium should not be used in nursing mothers.

LABOR AND DELIVERY

In one uncontrolled study, 100 mg per day of prophylactic oral Dantrolene Sodium was administered to term pregnant patients awaiting labor and delivery. Dantrolene readily crossed the placenta, with maternal and fetal whole blood levels approximately equal at delivery; neonatal levels then fell approximately 50% per day for 2 days before declining sharply. No neonatal respiratory and neuromuscular side effects were detected at low dose. More data, at higher doses, are needed before more definitive conclusions can be made.

Usage in Children: The long-term safety of Dantrolene Sodium in children under the age of 5 years has not been established. Because of the possibility that adverse effects of the drug could become apparent only after many years, a benefit-risk consideration of the long-term use of Dantrolene Sodium is particularly important in pediatric patients.

Drug Interactions: While a definite drug interaction with estrogen therapy has not yet been established, caution should be observed if the two drugs are to be given concomitantly. Hepatotoxicity has occurred more often in women over 35 years of age receiving concomitant estrogen therapy.

Dantrolene Sodium is metabolized by the liver, and it is theoretically possible that its metabolism may be enhanced by drugs known to induce hepatic microsomal enzymes. However, neither phenobarbital nor diazepam appears to affect Dantrolene Sodium metabolism. Binding to plasma protein is not significantly altered by diazepam, diphenylhydantoin, or phenylbutazone. Binding to plasma proteins is reduced by warfarin and clofibrate and increased by tolbutamide.

There are very rare reports of cardiovascular collapse in patients treated simultaneously with verapamil and Dantrolene Sodium. The combination of therapeutic doses of intravenous Dantrolene Sodium and verapamil in halothane/α-chloralose anesthetized swine has resulted in ventricular fibrillation and cardiovascular collapse in association with marked hyperkalemia. Until the relevance of these findings to humans is established, the combination of Dantrolene Sodium and verapamil is not recommended during the management of malignant hyperthermia.

PRECAUTIONS

Dantrolene Sodium should be used with caution in patients with impaired pulmonary function, particularly those with obstructive pulmonary disease, and in patients with severely impaired cardiac function due to myocardial disease. It should be used with caution in patients with a history of previous liver disease or dysfunction (see *"Warnings"*).

Patients should be cautioned against driving a motor vehicle or participating in hazardous occupations while taking Dantrolene Sodium. Caution should be exercised in the concomitant administration of tranquilizing agents.

Dantrolene Sodium might possibly evoke a photosensitivity reaction; patients should be cautioned about exposure to sunlight while taking it.

Care must be taken to prevent extravasation of Dantrolene Sodium Intravenous solution into the surrounding tissues due to the high pH of the intravenous formulation.

When mannitol is used for prevention or treatment of late renal complications of MH, the 3 g of mannitol needed to dissolve each 20 mg vial of IV Dantrolene Sodium should be taken into consideration.

Information for Patients: Based upon data in human volunteers, it will sometimes be appropriate to tell patients who receive Dantrolene Sodium Intravenous that decrease in grip strength and weakness of leg muscles, especially walking down stairs, can be expected postoperatively. In addition, symptoms such as "light-headedness" may be noted. Since some of these symptoms may persist for up to 48 hours, patients must not operate an automobile or engage in other hazardous activity during this time. Caution is also indicated at meals on the day of administration because difficulty swallowing and choking has been reported.

ADVERSE REACTIONS

The most frequently occurring side effects of Dantrolene Sodium have been drowsiness, dizziness, weakness, general malaise, fatigue, and diarrhea. These are generally transient, occurring early in treatment, and can often be obviated by beginning with a low dose and increasing dosage gradually until an optimal regimen is established. Diarrhea may be severe and may necessitate temporary withdrawal of Dantrolene Sodium therapy. If diarrhea recurs upon readministration of Dantrolene Sodium, therapy should probably be withdrawn permanently.

Other less frequent side effects, listed according to system, are:

Gastrointestinal: Constipation, GI bleeding, anorexia, swallowing difficulty, gastric irritation, abdominal cramps.

Hepatobiliary: Hepatitis (see *"Warnings"*).

Neurologic: Speech disturbance, seizure, headache, light-headedness, visual disturbance, diplopia, alteration of taste, insomnia.

Cardiovascular: Tachycardia, erratic blood pressure, phlebitis.

Psychiatric: Mental depression, mental confusion, increased nervousness.

Urogenital: Increased urinary frequency, crystalluria, hematuria, difficult erection, urinary incontinence and/or nocturia, difficult urination and/or urinary retention.

Integumentary: Abnormal hair growth, acne-like rash, pruritus, urticaria, eczematoid eruption, sweating.

Musculoskeletal: Myalgia, backache.

Respiratory: Feeling of suffocation.

Special Senses: Excessive tearing.

Hypersensitivity: Pleural effusion with pericarditis.

Other: Chills and fever.

There have been occasional reports of death following MH crisis even when treated with Intravenous Dantrolene; incidence figures are not available (the pre-Dantrolene mortality of MH crisis was approximately 50%). Most of these deaths can be accounted for by late recognition, delayed treatment, inadequate dosage, lack of supportive therapy, intercurrent disease and/or the development of delayed complications such as renal failure or disseminated intravascular coagulopathy. In some cases there are insufficient data to completely rule out therapeutic failure of Dantrolene.

There are rare reports of fatality in MH crisis, despite initial satisfactory response to i.v. Dantrolene, which involve patients who could not be weaned from Dantrolene after initial treatment.

The following adverse reactions are in approximate order of severity:

There are rare reports of pulmonary edema developing during the treatment of MH crisis in which the diluent volume and mannitol needed to deliver i.v. Dantrolene possibly contributed.

There have been reports of thrombophlebitis following administration of Intravenous Dantrolene; actual incidence figures are not available.

There have been rare reports of urticaria and erythema possibly associated with the administration of i.v. Dantrolene Sodium. There has been one case of anaphylaxis.

None of the serious reactions occasionally reported with long-term oral Dantrolene Sodium use, such as hepatitis, seizures, and pleural effusion with pericarditis, have been reasonably associated with short-term Dantrolene Sodium Intravenous therapy. The following events have been reported in patients receiving Oral Dantrolene: aplastic anemia, leukopenia, lymphocytic lymphoma, and heart failure.

The published literature has included some reports of Dantrolene Sodium use in patients with Neuroleptic Malignant Syndrome (NMS). Dantrolene Sodium Intravenous is not indicated for the treatment of NMS and patients may expire despite treatment with Dantrolene Sodium Intravenous.

OVERDOSAGE

For acute overdosage, general supportive measures should be employed along with immediate gastric lavage.

Intravenous fluids should be administered in fairly large quantities to avert the possibility of crystalluria. An adequate airway should be maintained and artificial resuscitation equipment should be at hand. Electrocardiographic monitoring should be instituted, and the patient carefully observed. To date, no experience has been reported with dialysis and its value in Dantrolene Sodium overdosage is not known.

Because Dantrolene Sodium Intravenous must be administered at a low concentration in a large volume of fluid, acute toxicity of Dantrolene Sodium could not be assessed in animals. In 14-day (subacute) studies, the intravenous formulation of Dantrolene Sodium was relatively non-toxic to rats at doses of 10 mg/kg/day and 20 mg/kg/day. While 10 mg/kg/day in dogs for 14 days evoked little toxicity, 20 mg/kg/day for 14 days caused hepatic changes of questionable biologic significance.

No data are available to define the symptomatology of an overdose of Dantrolene Sodium Intravenous. If an overdose is suspected, treatment is symptomatic and supportive. There is no known antidote.

DOSAGE AND ADMINISTRATION

For Use in Chronic Spasticity: Prior to the administration of Dantrolene Sodium, consideration should be given to the potential response to treatment. A decrease in spasticity sufficient to allow a daily function not otherwise attainable should be the therapeutic goal of treatment with Dantrolene Sodium. Refer to *"Indications and Usage"* section for description of response to be anticipated.

It is important to establish a therapeutic goal (regain and maintain a specific function such as therapeutic exercise program, utilization of braces, transfer maneuvers, etc.) before beginning Dantrolene Sodium therapy. Dosage should be

increased until the maximum performance compatible with the dysfunction due to underlying disease in achieved. No further increase in dosage is then indicated.

Usual Dosage: It is important that the dosage be titrated and individualized for maximum effect. The lowest dose compatible with optimal response is recommended.

In view of the potential for liver damage in long-term Dantrolene Sodium *use, therapy should be stopped if benefits are not evident within 45 days.*

Adults: Begin therapy with 25 mg once daily; increase to 25 mg two, three, or four times daily and then by increments of 25 mg up to as high as 100 mg two, three, or four times daily if necessary. As most patients will respond to a dose of 400 mg/day or less, rarely should doses higher than 400 mg/day be used (see Box *"Warning"*).

Each dosage level should be maintained for four to seven days to determine the patient's response. The dose should not be increased beyond, and may even have to be reduced to, the amount at which the patient received maximal benefit without adverse effects.

Children: A similar approach should be utilized starting with 0.5 mg/kg of body weight twice daily; this is increased to 0.5 mg/kg three or four times daily and then by increments of 0.5 mg/kg up to as high as 3 mg/kg two, three, or four times daily, if necessary. Doses higher than 100 mg four times daily should not be used in children.

For Malignant Hyperthermia: As soon as the MH reaction is recognized, all anesthetic agents should be discontinued; the administration of 100% oxygen is recommended. Dantrolene Sodium Intravenous should be administered by continuous rapid intravenous push beginning at a minimum dose of 1 mg/kg, and continuing until symptoms subside or the maximum cumulative dose of 10 mg/kg has been reached.

If the physiologic and metabolic abnormalities reappear, the regimen may be repeated. It is important to note that administration of Dantrolene Sodium Intravenous should be continuous until symptoms subside. The effective dose to reverse the crisis is directly dependent upon the individual's degree of susceptibility to MH, the amount and time of exposure to the triggering agent, and the time elapsed between onset of the crisis and initiation of treatment.

CHILDREN'S DOSE

Experience to date indicates that the dose of Dantrolene Sodium Intravenous for children is the same as for adults.

Preoperatively: Dantrolene Sodium Intravenous and/or Dantrolene Sodium Capsules may be administered preoperatively to patients judged MH susceptible as part of the overall patient management to prevent or attenuate the development of clinical and laboratory signs of MH.

Dantrolene Sodium Intravenous: The recommended prophylactic dose of Dantrolene Sodium Intravenous is 2.5 mg/kg, starting approximately 1 1/4 hours before anticipated anesthesia and infused over approximately 1 hour. This dose should prevent or attenuate the development of clinical and laboratory signs of MH provided that the usual precautions, such as avoidance of established MH triggering agents, are followed.

Additional Dantrolene Sodium Intravenous may be indicated during anesthesia and surgery because of the appearance of early clinical and/or blood gas signs of MH or because of prolonged surgery (see also *"Clinical Pharmacology"*, *"Warnings"*, and *"Precautions"*). Additional doses must be individualized.

Administer 4 to 8 mg/kg/day of oral Dantrolene Sodium in 3 or 4 divided doses for one or two days prior to surgery, with the last dose being given approximately 3 to 4 hours before scheduled surgery with a minimum of water. This dosage will usually be associated with skeletal muscle weakness and sedation (sleepiness or drowsiness); adjustment can usually be made within the recommended dosage range to avoid incapacitation or excessive gastrointestinal irritation (including nausea and/or vomiting).

Post-Crisis Follow-up: Oral Dantrolene Sodium should also be administered following a malignant hyperthermia crisis, in doses of 4 to 8 mg/kg per day in four divided doses, for a one to three day period to prevent recurrence of the manifestations of malignant hyperthermia.

Intravenous Dantrolene Sodium may be used postoperatively to prevent or attenuate the recurrence of signs of MH when oral Dantrolene Sodium administration is not practical. The i.v. dose of Dantrolene Sodium in the postoperative period must be individualized, starting with 1 mg/kg or more as the clinical situation dictates.

PREPARATION OF DANTROLENE SODIUM INTRAVENOUS

Each vial of Dantrolene Sodium Intravenous should be reconstituted by adding 60 mL of *sterile water for injection USP (without a bacteriostatic agent), and the vial shaken until the solution is clear.* 5% Dextrose Injection USP, 0.9% Sodium Chloride Injection USP, and other acidic solutions are not compatible with Dantrolene Sodium Intravenous and should not be used. The contents of the vial must be *protected from direct light* and *used within 6 hours* after reconstitution. Store reconstituted solutions at controlled room temperature (59°F to 86°F or 15°C to 30°C).

Reconstituted Dantrolene Sodium Intravenous should *not* be transferred to large glass bottles for prophylactic infusion due to precipitate formation observed with the use of some glass bottles as reservoirs.

For prophylactic infusion, the required number of individual vials of Dantrolene Sodium Intravenous should be reconstituted as outlined above. The contents of individual vials are then transferred to a larger volume sterile intravenous plastic bag. Stability data indicate commercially available sterile

---

plastic bags are acceptable drug delivery devices. However, it is recommended that the prepared infusion be inspected carefully for cloudiness and/or precipitation prior to dispensing and administration. Such solutions should not be used. While stable for 6 hours, it is recommended that the infusion be prepared immediately prior to the anticipated dosage administration time.

Parenteral drug products should be inspected visually for particulate matter and discoloration prior to administration.

Oral Dantrolene Sodium: Avoid excessive heat (over 104°F or 40°C).

Store unreconstituted Dantrolene Sodium Intravenous at controlled room temperature (59°F to 86°F or 15°C to 30°C) and avoid prolonged exposure to light.

HOW SUPPLIED
CAPSULE: 25 MG

BRAND/MANUFACTURER	NDC	SIZE	AWP
○ **BRAND**			
DANTRIUM: P&G Pharm	00149-0030-05	100s	$69.40
	00149-0030-77	100s ud	$76.26
	00149-0030-66	500s	$336.56

CAPSULE: 50 MG

BRAND/MANUFACTURER	NDC	SIZE	AWP
○ **BRAND**			
DANTRIUM: P&G Pharm	00149-0031-05	100s	$103.96

CAPSULE: 100 MG

BRAND/MANUFACTURER	NDC	SIZE	AWP
○ **BRAND**			
DANTRIUM: P&G Pharm	00149-0033-05	100s	$129.29
	00149-0033-77	100s ud	$135.98

POWDER FOR INJECTION: 20 MG

BRAND/MANUFACTURER	NDC	SIZE	AWP
○ **BRAND**			
DANTRIUM INTRAVENOUS: P&G Pharm	00149-0734-02	1s	$55.21

Dapiprazole Hydrochloride

DESCRIPTION
For ophthalmic use only.

Dapiprazole is an alpha-adrenergic blocking agent.

Dapiprazole Hydrochloride is 5,6,7,8-tetrahydro-3-[2-(4-o-tolyl-1- piperazinyl)ethyl]-s-triazolo[4,3-a]pyridine hydrochloride.

Dapiprazole Hydrochloride has the empirical formula $C_{19}H_{27}N_5HCl$ and a molecular weight of 361.93.

Dapiprazole Hydrochloride is a sterile, white, lyophilized powder soluble in water.

Hydrochloride eyedrops is a clear, colorless, slightly viscous solution for topical application. Each mL (when reconstituted as directed) contains 5 mg of dapiprazole hydrochloride as the active ingredient.

The reconstituted solution has a pH of approximately 6.6 and an osmolarity of approximately 415 mOsm.

Hydrochloride eyedrops, 0.5% is supplied in a kit consisting of one vial of dapiprazole hydrochloride (25 mg), one vial of diluent (5 mL) and one dropper for dispensing.

Following is its chemical structure:

CLINICAL PHARMACOLOGY
Dapiprazole acts through blocking the alpha-adrenergic receptors in smooth muscle. Dapiprazole produces miosis through an effect on the dilator muscle of the iris.

Dapiprazole does not have any significant activity on ciliary muscle contraction and, therefore, does not induce a significant change in the anterior chamber depth or the thickness of the lens.

Dapiprazole has demonstrated safe and rapid reversal of mydriasis produced by phenylephrine and to a lesser degree tropicamide. In patients with decreased accommodative amplitude due to treatment with tropicamide, dapiprazole partially restores the accommodative amplitude. This activity is not only due to its miotic effect but also to a direct effect on accommodation.

Eye color affects the rate of pupillary constriction. In individuals with brown irides, the rate of pupillary constriction may be slightly slower than in individuals with blue or green irides. Eye color does not appear to affect the final pupil size.

Dapiprazole does not significantly alter intraocular pressure in normotensive or in eyes with elevated intraocular pressure.

INDICATIONS AND USAGE
Dapiprazole is indicated in the treatment of iatrogenically induced mydriasis produced by adrenergic (phenylephrine) or parasympatholytic (tropicamide)

agents. Dapiprazole is not indicated for the reduction of intraocular pressure or in the treatment of open angle glaucoma.

CONTRAINDICATIONS
Miotics are contraindicated where constriction is undesirable, such as acute iritis, and in those subjects showing hypersensitivity to any component of this preparation.

WARNING
For Topical Ophthalmic Use Only.

NOT FOR INJECTION. Do not touch the dropper up to lids or any surface, as this may contaminate the solution. Dapiprazole should not be used in the same patient more frequently than once a week.

PRECAUTIONS
Information to Patients: Miosis may cause difficulty in dark adaptation and may reduce the field of vision. Patients should exercise caution when involved in night driving or other activities in poor illumination.

Carcinogenesis, Mutagenesis, Impairment of Fertility: Dapiprazole has been shown to significantly increase the incidence of liver tumors in rats after continuous dietary administration for 104 weeks. This effect was found only in male rats treated with the highest dose administered in the study, ie, 300 mg/kg/day (80,000 times the human dose) and was not observed in male and female rats at doses of 30 and 100 mg/kg/day and female rats at doses of 300 mg/kg/day.

Negative results have been reported on the mutagenicity and impairment of fertility studies with Dapiprazole.

Pregnancy: Pregnancy Category B: Reproduction studies have been performed in rats and rabbits at doses up to 128,000 (rat) and 27,000 (rabbit) times the human ophthalmic dose and revealed no evidence of impaired fertility or harm to the fetus due to Dapiprazole. There are, however, no adequate and well-controlled studies in pregnant women. Because animal reproduction studies are not always predictive of human response, this drug should be used during pregnancy only if clearly needed.

Nursing Mothers: It is not known whether this drug is excreted in human milk. Because many drugs are excreted in human milk, caution should be exercised when Dapiprazole is administered to a nursing woman.

Pediatric Use: Safety and effectiveness in children have not been established.

ADVERSE REACTIONS
In controlled studies the most frequent reaction to Dapiprazole was conjunctival injection lasting 20 minutes in over 80% of patients. Burning on instillation of Dapiprazole was reported in approximately half of all patients. Reactions occurring in 10% to 40% of patients included ptosis, lid erythema, lid edema, chemosis, itching, punctate keratitis, corneal edema, brow ache, photophobia and headaches. Other reactions reported less frequently included dryness of eyes, tearing, and blurring of vision.

DOSAGE AND ADMINISTRATION
Two drops followed 5 minutes later by an additional 2 drops applied topically to the conjunctiva of each eye should be administered after the ophthalmic examination to reverse the diagnostic mydriasis. Dapiprazole should not be used in the same patient more frequently than once per week.

Directions for Preparing Eyedrops:
1. Use aseptic technique
2. Tear off aluminum seals, remove and discard rubber plugs from both drug and diluent vials.
3. Pour diluent into drug vial.
4. Remove dropper assembly from its sterile wrapping and attach to the drug vial.
5. Shake container for several minutes to ensure mixing.

Storage and Stability of Eyedrops: Once the eyedrops have been reconstituted they may be stored at room temperature 15°-30°C (59°-86°F) for 21 days. Discard any solution that is not clear and colorless.

HOW SUPPLIED
POWDER FOR RECONSTITUTION: 0.5%

BRAND/MANUFACTURER	NDC	SIZE	AWP
○ **BRAND**			
REV-EYES: Storz/Lederle	57706-0761-62	5 ml	$31.19

Dapsone

DESCRIPTION
Dapsone-USP, 4-4' diaminodiphenylsulfone (DDS) is a primary treatment for Dermatitis herpetiformis. It is an antibacterial drug for susceptible cases of leprosy. It is a white, odorless crystalline powder, practically insoluble in water and insoluble in fixed and vegetable oils.

Following is its chemical structure:

➤ SHOWN IN PRODUCT IDENTIFICATION GUIDE

CLINICAL PHARMACOLOGY

Actions: The mechanism of action in Dermatitis herpetiformis has not been established. By the kinetic method in mice, Dapsone is bactericidal as well as bacteriostatic against *Mycobacterium leprae.*

Absorption and Excretion: Dapsone, when given orally, is rapidly and almost completely absorbed. About 85 percent of the daily intake is recoverable from the urine mainly in the form of water-soluble metabolites. Excretion of the drug is slow and a constant blood level can be maintained with the usual dosage.

Blood Levels: Detected a few minutes after ingestion, the drug reaches peak concentration in 4-8 hours. Daily administration for at least eight days is necessary to achieve a plateau level. With doses of 200 mg daily, this level averaged 2.3 µg/mL with a range of 0.1-7.0 µg/mL. The half-life in the plasma in different individuals varies from ten hours to fifty hours and averages twenty-eight hours. Repeat tests in the same individual are constant. Daily administration (50-100 mg) in leprosy patients will provide blood levels in excess of the usual minimum inhibitory concentration even for patients with a short Dapsone half-life.

INDICATIONS AND USAGE

Dermatitis herpetiformis (D.H.). All forms of leprosy except for cases of proven Dapsone resistance.

UNLABELED USES

Dapsone is used alone or as an adjunct in the treatment of rheumatoid arthritis.

CONTRAINDICATION

Hypersensitivity to Dapsone and/or its derivatives.

WARNINGS

The patient should be warned to respond to the presence of clinical signs such as sore throat, fever, pallor, purpura or jaundice. Deaths associated with the administration of Dapsone have been reported from agranulocytosis, aplastic anemia and other blood dyscrasias. Complete blood counts should be done frequently in patients receiving Dapsone. The FDA Dermatology Advisory Committee recommended that, when feasible counts should be done weekly for the first month, monthly for six months and semi-annually thereafter. If a significant reduction in leucocytes, platelets or hemopoiesis is noted. Dapsone should be discontinued and the patient followed intensively. Folic acid antagonists have similar effects and may increase the incidence of hematologic reactions; if co-administered with Dapsone the patient should be monitored more frequently. Patients on weekly Pyrimethamine and Dapsone have developed agranulocytosis during the second and third month of therapy.

Severe anemia should be treated prior to initiation of therapy and hemoglobin monitored. Hemolysis and methemoglobin may be poorly tolerated by patients with severe cardio-pulmonary disease.

Carcinogenesis, mutagenesis: Dapsone has been found carcinogenic (sarcomagenic) for male rats and female mice causing mesenchymal tumors in the spleen and peritoneum, and thyroid carcinoma in female rats. Dapsone is not mutagenic with or without microsomal activation in *S. typhimurium* tester strains 1535, 1537, 1538, 98, or 100.

Cutaneous reactions, especially bullous, include exfoliative dermatitis and are probably one of the most serious, though rare, complications of sulfone therapy. They are directly due to drug sensitization. Such reactions include toxic erythema, erythema multiforme, toxic epidermal necrolysis, morbilliform and scariatiniform reactions, urticaria and erythema nodosum. If new or toxic dermatologic reactions occur, sulfone therapy must be promptly discontinued and appropriate therapy instituted.

Leprosy reactional states, including cutaneous, are not hypersensitivity reactions to Dapsone and do not require discontinuation. See special section.

PRECAUTIONS

General: Hemolysis and Heinz body formation may be exaggerated in individuals with a glucose-6-phosphate dehydrogenase (G6PD) deficiency, or methemoglobin reductase deficiency, or hemoglobin M. This reaction is frequently dose-related. Dapsone should be given with caution to these patients or if the patient is exposed to other agents or conditions such as infection or diabetic ketosis capable of producing hemolysis. Drugs or chemicals which have produced significant hemolysis in G6PD or methemoglobin reductase deficient patients include Dapsone, sulfanilamide, nitrite, aniline, phenylhydrazine, napthalene, niridazole, nitrofurantoin and 8-amino-antimalarials such as primaquine.

Toxic hepatitis and cholestatic jaundice have been reported early in therapy. Hyperbilirubinemia may occur more often in G6PD deficient patients. When feasible, baseline and subsequent monitoring of liver function is recommended. If abnormal, Dapsone should be discontinued until the source of the abnormality is established.

Drug Interactions: Rifampin lowers Dapsone levels 7 to 10-fold by accelerating plasma clearance; in leprosy this reduction has not required a change in dosage.

Folic acid antagonists such as pyrimethamine may increase the likelihood of hematologic reactions.

Pregnancy Category C: Animal reproduction studies have not been conducted with Dapsone. Extensive, but uncontrolled experience and two published surveys on the use of Dapsone in pregnant women have not shown that Dapsone increases the risk of fetal abnormalities if administered during all trimesters of pregnancy or can affect reproduction capacity. Because of the lack of animal studies or controlled human experience, Dapsone should be given to a pregnant woman only

if clearly needed. In general, for leprosy, USPHS at Carville recommends maintenance of Dapsone.

Dapsone has been important for the management of some pregnant D.H. patients.

Nursing Mothers: Dapsone is excreted in breast milk in substantial amounts. Hemolytic reactions can occur in neonates. See section on hemolysis. Because of the potential for tumorgenicity shown for Dapsone in animal studies a decision should be made whether to discontinue nursing or discontinue the drug taking into account the importance of the drug to the mother.

Pediatric Use: Children are treated on the same schedule as adults but with correspondingly smaller doses. Dapsone is generally not considered to have an effect on the later growth development and functional development of the child.

ADVERSE REACTIONS

In addition to the warnings listed above, the following syndromes and serious reactions have been reported in patients on Dapsone.

Hematologic Effects: Dose-related hemolysis is the most common adverse effect and is seen in patients with or without G6PD deficiency. Almost all patients demonstrate the interrelated changes of a loss of 1-2g of HB, an increase in the reticulocytes (2-12%), a shortened red cell life span and a rise in methemoglobin. G6PD deficient patients have greater responses.

Nervous System Effects: Peripheral neuropathy is a definite but unusual complication of Dapsone therapy in non-leprosy patients. Motor loss is predominent. If muscle weakness appears, Dapsone should be withdrawn. Recovery on withdrawal is usually substantially complete. The mechanism of recovery is reportedly by axonal regeneration. Some recovered patients have tolerated retreatment at reduced dosage. In leprosy this complication may be difficult to distinguish from a leprosy reactional state.

Body As A Whole: In addition to the warnings and adverse effects reported above, additional adverse reactions include: nausea, vomiting, abdominal pains, pancreatitis, vertigo, blurred vision, tinnitus, insomnia, fever, headache, psychosis, phototoxicity, tachycardia, albuminuria, the nephrotic syndrome, hypoalbuminemia without proteinuria, renal papillary necrosis, male infertility, drug-induced Lupus erythematosus and an infectious mononucleosis-like syndrome. In general, with the exception of the complications of severe anoxia from overdosage (retinal and optic nerve damage, etc.) these adverse reactions have regressed off drug.

OVERDOSAGE

Nausea, vomiting, hyperexcitability can appear a few minutes up to 24 hours after ingestion or an overdose. Methemoglobin induced depression, convulsions and severe cyanosis requires prompt treatment. In normal and methemoglobin reductase deficient patients, methylene blue, 1-2 mg/kg of body weight, given slowly intravenously is the treatment of choice. The effect is complete in 30 minutes, but may have to be repeated if methemoglobin reaccumulates. For non-emergencies, if treatment is needed, methylene blue may be given orally in doses of 3-5 mg/kg every 4-6 hours.

Methylene blue reduction depends on G6PD and should not be given to fully expressed G6PD deficient patients.

DOSAGE AND ADMINISTRATION

Dermatitis herpetiformis: The dosage should be individually titrated starting in adults with 50 mg daily and correspondingly smaller doses in children. If full control is not achieved within the range of 50-300 mg daily, higher doses may be tried. Dosage should be reduced to a minimum maintenance level as soon as possible. In responsive patients there is a prompt reduction in pruritus followed by clearance of skin lesions. There is no effect on the gastrointestinal component of the disease.

Dapsone levels are influenced by acetylation rates. Patients with high acetylation rates, or who are receiving treatment affecting acetylation may require an adjustment in dosage. A strict gluten free diet is an option for the patient to elect, permitting many to reduce or eliminate the need for Dapsone; the average time for dosage reduction is 8 months with a range of 4 months to 2½ years and for dosage elimination 29 months with a range of 6 months to 9 years.

Leprosy: In order to reduce secondary Dapsone resistance, the WHO Expert Committee on Leprosy and the USPHS at Carville, LA, recommend that Dapsone should be commenced in combination with one or more anti-leprosy drugs. In the multi-drug program Dapsone should be maintained at the full dosage of 100 mg daily without interruption (with correspondingly smaller doses for children) and provided to all patients who have sensitive organisms with new or recrudescent disease or who have not yet completed a two year course of Dapsone monotherapy. For advice and other drugs, the USPHS at Carville, LA, (1 800-642-2477) should be contacted. Before using other drugs consult appropriate product labeling.

In bacteriologically negative tuberculoid and indeterminate disease, the recommendation is the coadministration of Dapsone 100 mg daily with six months of rifampin 600 mg daily. Under WHO, daily rifampin may be replaced by 600 mg rifampin monthlty, if supervised. The Dapsone is continued until all signs of clinical activity are controlled—usually after an additional six months. Then Dapsone should be continued for an additional three years for tuberculoid and indeterminate patients and for five years for borderline tuberculoid patients.

In lepromatous and borderline lepromatous patients, the recommendation is the coadministration of Dapsone 100 mg daily with two years of rifampin 600 mg daily. Under WHO, daily rifampin may be replaced by 600 mg rifampin monthly, if supervised. One may elect the concurrent administration of a third anti-leprosy

---

drug, usually either clofazamine 50-100 mg daily or ethionamide 250-500 mg daily. Dapsone 100 mg daily is continued 3-10 years until all signs of clinical activity are controlled with skin scrapings and biopsies negative for one year. Dapsone should then be continued for an additional 10 years for borderline patients and for life for lepromatous patients.

Secondary Dapsone resistance should be suspected whenever a lepromatous or borderline lepromatous patient receiving Dapsone treatment relapses clinically and bacteriologically, solid staining bacilli being found in the smears taken from the new active lesions. If such cases show no response to regular and supervised Dapsone therapy within three to six months or good compliance for the past 3-6 months can be assured, Dapsone resistance should be considered confirmed clinically. Determination of drug sensitivity using the mouse footpad method is recommended and, after prior arrangement, is available without charge from the USPHS, Carville, LA. Patients with proven Dapsone resistance should be treated with other drugs.

Leprosy Reactional States: Abrupt changes in clinical activity occur in leprosy with any effective treatment and are known as reactional states. The majority can be classified into two groups.

The "Reversal" reaction (Type 1) may occur in borderline or tuberculoid leprosy patients often soon after chemotherapy is started. The mechanism is presumed to result from a reduction in the antigenic load: the patient is able to mount an enhanced delayed hypersensitivity response to residual infection leading to swelling ("Reversal") of existing skin and nerve lesions. If severe, or if neuritis is present, large doses of steroids should *always* be used. If severe, the patient should be hospitalized. In general anti-leprosy treatment is continued and therapy to suppress the reaction is indicated such as analgesics, steroids, or surgical decompression of swollen nerve trunks. USPHS at Carville, LA should be contacted for advice in management.

Erythema nodosum leprosum (ENL) (lepromatous lepra reaction) (Type 2 reaction) occurs mainly in lepromatous patients and small numbers of borderline patients. Approximately 50% of treated patients show this reaction in the first year. The principal clinical features are fever and tender erythematous skin nodules sometimes associated with malaise, neuritis, orchitis, albuminuria, joint swelling, iritis, epistaxis or depression. Skin lesions can become pustular and/or ulcerate. Histologically there is a vasculitis with an intense polymorphonuclear infiltrate. Elevated circulating immune complexes are considered to be the mechanism of the reaction. If severe, patients should be hospitalized. In general, anti-leprosy treatment is continued. Analgesics, steroids, and other agents available from USPHS, Carville, LA, are used to suppress the reaction.

Dispense this product in a well-closed child-resistant container.

HOW SUPPLIED
TABLETS: 25 MG

BRAND/MANUFACTURER	NDC	SIZE	AWP
○ **BRAND**			
DAPSONE: Jacobus	49938-0102-01	100s	$17.20
○ **GENERICS**			
DAPSONE: Allscrips	54569-4040-00	60s	$14.45

TABLETS: 100 MG

BRAND/MANUFACTURER	NDC	SIZE	AWP
○ **BRAND**			
DAPSONE: Jacobus	49938-0101-01	100s	$18.00
○ **GENERICS**			
DAPSONE: Allscrips	54569-2015-02	14s	$2.52
DAPSONE: Allscrips	54569-2016-02	14s	$5.25
DAPSONE: Allscrips	54569-2015-00	100s	$22.20

Dapsone *SEE* DAPSONE

Daranide *SEE* DICHLORPHENAMIDE

Daraprim *SEE* PYRIMETHAMINE

Darvocet-N *SEE* ACETAMINOPHEN AND PROPOXYPHENE NAPSYLATE

Darvon *SEE* PROPOXYPHENE HYDROCHLORIDE

Darvon Compound-65 *SEE* ASPIRIN/ CAFFEINE/PROPOXYPHENE HYDROCHLORIDE

Darvon-N *SEE* PROPOXYPHENE NAPSYLATE

Daunorubicin Hydrochloride

WARNINGS

1. DAUNORUBICIN HYDROCHLORIDE MUST BE GIVEN INTO A RAPIDLY FLOWING INTRAVENOUS INFUSION. IT MUST *NEVER* BE GIVEN BY THE INTRAMUSCULAR OR SUBCUTANEOUS ROUTE. SEVERE LOCAL TISSUE NECROSIS WILL OCCUR IF THERE IS EXTRAVASATION DURING ADMINISTRATION.

2. MYOCARDIAL TOXICITY MANIFESTED IN ITS MOST SEVERE FORM BY POTENTIALLY FATAL CONGESTIVE HEART FAILURE MAY OCCUR EITHER DURING THERAPY OR MONTHS TO YEARS AFTER TERMINATION OF THERAPY. THE INCIDENCE OF MYOCARDIAL TOXICITY INCREASES AFTER A TOTAL CUMULATIVE DOSE EXCEEDING 400-550 MG/M^2 IN ADULTS, 300 MG/M^2 IN CHILDREN MORE THAN 2 YEARS OF AGE, OR 10 MG/KG IN CHILDREN LESS THAN 2 YEARS OF AGE.

3. SEVERE MYELOSUPPRESSION OCCURS WHEN USED IN THERAPEUTIC DOSES.

4. IT IS RECOMMENDED THAT DAUNORUBICIN HYDROCHLORIDE BE ADMINISTERED ONLY BY PHYSICIANS WHO ARE EXPERIENCED IN LEUKEMIA CHEMOTHERAPY AND IN FACILITIES WITH LABORATORY AND SUPPORTIVE RESOURCES ADEQUATE TO MONITOR DRUG TOLERANCE AND PROTECT AND MAINTAIN A PATIENT COMPROMISED BY DRUG TOXICITY. THE PHYSICIAN AND INSTITUTION MUST BE CAPABLE OF RESPONDING RAPIDLY AND COMPLETELY TO SEVERE HEMORRHAGIC CONDITIONS AND/OR OVERWHELMING INFECTION.

5. DOSAGE SHOULD BE REDUCED IN PATIENTS WITH IMPAIRED HEPATIC OR RENAL FUNCTION.

DESCRIPTION
Daunorubicin Hydrochloride is the hydrochloride salt of an anthracycline cytotoxic antibiotic produced by a strain of *Streptomyces coeruleorubidus*. It is provided as a sterile reddish lyophilized powder in vials for intravenous administration only. Each vial contain 20 mg of base activity (21.4 mg as the hydrochloride salt) and 100 mg of mannitol. It is soluble in water when adequately agitated and produces a reddish solution. It has the following structural formula which may be described with the chemical name of 7-(3-amino-2,3,6-trideoxy-L-iyxohexo- syloxy)-9acetyl-7,8,9,10-tetrahydro-6,9,11 -trihy-droxy-4-methoxy-5,12-naphthacenequinone hydrochloride. Its empirical formula is $C_{27}H_{29}NO_{10}HCl$ with a molecular weight of 563.99. It is a hygroscopic crystalline powder. The pH of a 5 mg/mL aqueous solution is 4.5 to 6.5.

Following is its chemical structure:

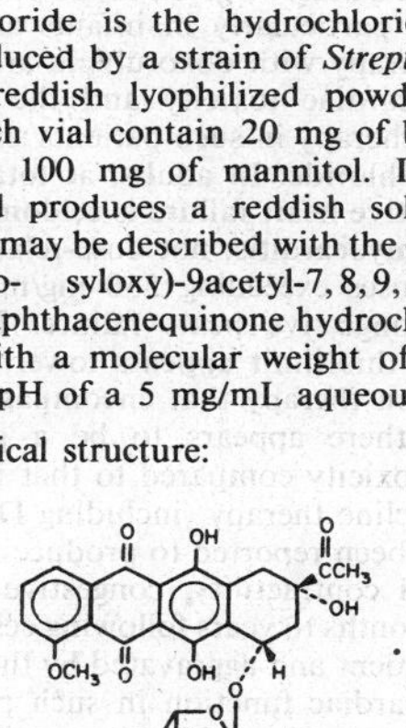

ACTION
Daunorubicin Hydrochloride inhibits the synthesis of nucleic acids: its effect on deoxyribonucleic acid is particularly rapid and marked. Daunorubicin Hydrochloride has antimitotic and cytotoxic activity although the precise mode of action is unknown. Daunorubicin Hydrochloride displays an immunosuppressive effect. It has been shown to inhibit the production of heterohemagglutinins in mice. *In vitro*, it inhibits blast-cell transformation of canine lymphocytes at 0.01 mcg/mL.

Daunorubicin Hydrochloride possesses a potent antitumor effect against a wide spectrum of animal tumors either grafted or spontaneous.

CLINICAL PHARMACOLOGY
Following intravenous injection of Daunorubicin Hydrochloride, plasma levels of Daunorubicin decline rapidly, indicating rapid tissue uptake and concentration. Thereafter, plasma levels decline slowly with a half-life of 18.5 hours. By one hour after drug administration, the predominant plasma species is daunorubicinol, an active metabolite, which disappears with a half-life of 26.7 hours. Further metabolism via reduction cleavage of the glycosidic bond, 4-0 demethylation, and conjugation with both sulfate and glucuronide have been demonstrated. Simple glycosidic cleavage of Daunorubicin Hydrochloride or daunorubicinol is not a significant metabolic pathway in man. Twenty-five percent of an administered dose of Daunorubicin Hydrochloride is eliminated in an active form by urinary excretion and an estimated 40% by biliary excretion.

➤ SHOWN IN PRODUCT IDENTIFICATION GUIDE

There is no evidence that Daunorubicin Hydrochloride crosses the blood-brain barrier.

In the treatment of adult acute nonlymphocytic leukemia, Daunorubicin Hydrochloride, used as a single agent, has produced complete remission rates of 40 to 50%, and in combination with cytarabine, has produced complete remission rates of 53 to 65%.

The addition of Daunorubicin Hydrochloride to the two-drug induction regimen of vincristine-prednisone in the treatment of childhood acute lymphocytic leukemia does not increase the rate of complete remission. In children receiving identical CNS prophylaxis and maintenance therapy (without consolidation), there is prolongation of complete remission duration (statistically significant, $p <$ 0.02) in those children induced with the three-drug (Cerubidine-vincristine-prednisone) regimen as compared to two drugs. There is no evidence of any impact of Daunorubicin Hydrochloride on the duration of complete remission when a consolidated (intensification) phase is employed as part of a total treatment program.

In adult acute lymphocytic leukemia, in contrast to childhood acute lymphocytic leukemia, Daunorubicin Hydrochloride during induction significantly increases the rate of complete remission, but not remission duration, compared to that obtained with vincristine, prednisone, and L-asparaginase alone. The use of Daunorubicin Hydrochloride in combination with vincristine, prednisone, and L-asparaginase has produced complete remission rates of 83% in contrast to a 47% remission in patients not receiving Daunorubicin Hydrochloride.

INDICATIONS AND USAGE
Daunorubicin Hydrochloride in combination with other approved anticancer drugs is indicated for remission induction in acute nonlymphocytic leukemia (myelogenous, monocytic, erythroid) of adults and for remission induction in acute lymphocytic leukemia of children and adults.

UNLABELED USES
Daunorubicin Hydrochloride is used alone or as an adjunct in the treatment of AIDS-related Kaposi's Sarcoma.

WARNINGS
Bone Marrow: Daunorubicin Hydrochloride is a potent bone-marrow suppressant. Suppression will occur in all patients given a therapeutic dose of this drug. Therapy with Daunorubicin Hydrochloride should not be started in patients with preexisting drug-induced bone-marrow suppression unless the benefit from such treatment warrants the risk.

Cardiac Effects: Special attention must be given to the potential cardiac toxicity of Daunorubicin Hydrochloride, particularly in infants and children. Preexisting heart disease and previous therapy with doxorubicin are co-factors of increased risk of Cerubidine-induced cardiac toxicity and the benefit-to-risk ratio of Daunorubicin Hydrochloride therapy in such patients should be weighted before starting Daunorubicin Hydrochloride. In adults, at total cumulative doses less than 550 mg/m^2, acute congestive heart failure is seldom encountered. However, rare instances of pericarditis-myocarditis, not dose-related, have been reported.

In adults, at cumulative doses exceeding 550 mg/m^2, there is an increased incidence of drug-induced congestive heart failure. Based on prior clinical experience with doxorubicin, this limit appears lower, namely 400 mg/m^2, in patients who received radiation therapy that encompassed the heart.[1]

In infants and children, there appears to be a greater susceptibility to anthracycline-induced cardiotoxicity compared to that in adults, which is more clearly dose-related. Anthracycline therapy (including Daunorubicin Hydrochloride) in pediatric patients has been reported to produce impaired left ventricular systolic performance, reduced contractility, congestive heart failure or death. These conditions may occur months to years following cessation of chemotherapy. This appears to be dose-dependent and aggravated by thoracic irradiation. Long-term periodic evaluation of cardiac function in such patients should, thus, be performed.[2-7] In both children and adults, the total dose of Daunorubicin Hydrochloride administered should also take into account any previous or concomitant therapy with other potentially cardiotoxic agents or related compounds such as doxorubicin.

There is no absolutely reliable method of predicting the patients in whom acute congestive heart failure will develop as a result of the cardiac toxic effect of Daunorubicin Hydrochloride. However, certain changes in the electrocardiogram and a decrease in the systolic ejection fraction from pretreatment baseline may help to recognize those patients at greatest risk to develop congestive heart failure. On the basis of the electrocardiogram, a decrease equal to or greater than 30% in limb lead QRS voltage has been associated with a significant risk of drug-induced cardiomyopathy. Therefore, an electrocardiogram and/or determination of systolic ejection fraction should be performed before each course of Daunorubicin Hydrochloride. In the event that one or the other of these predictive parameters should occur, the benefit of continued therapy must be weighed against the risk of producing cardiac damage.

Early clinical diagnosis of drug-induced congestive heart failure appears to be essential for successful treatment with digitalis, diuretics, sodium restriction, and bed rest.

Evaluation of Hepatic and Renal Function: Significant hepatic or renal impairment can enhance the toxicity of the recommended doses of Daunorubicin Hydrochloride; therefore, prior to administration, evaluation of hepatic function and renal function using conventional clinical laboratory tests is recommended (see "Dosage and Administration").

Pregnancy: Daunorubicin Hydrochloride may cause fetal harm when administered to a pregnant woman because of its teratogenic potential. An increased incidence of fetal abnormalities (parieto-occipital cranioschisis, umbilical hernias, or rachischisis) and abortions was reported in rabbits. Decreases in fetal birth weight and postdelivery growth rate were observed in mice. There are no adequate and well-controlled studies in pregnant women. If this drug is used during pregnancy, or if the patient becomes pregnant while taking this drug, the patient should be apprised of the potential hazard to the fetus. Women of childbearing potential should be advised to avoid becoming pregnant.

Extravasation at Injection Site: Extravasation of Daunorubicin Hydrochloride at the site of intravenous administration can cause severe local tissue necrosis.

PRECAUTIONS
Therapy with Daunorubicin Hydrochloride requires close patient observation and frequent complete blood-count determinations. Cardiac, renal, and hepatic function should be evaluated prior to each course of treatment.

Daunorubicin Hydrochloride may induce hyperuricemia secondary to rapid lysis of leukemic cells. As a precaution, allopurinol administration is usually begun prior to initiating antileukemic therapy. Blood uric acid levels should be monitored and appropriate therapy initiated in the event that hyperuricemia develops.

Appropriate measures must be taken to control any systemic infection before beginning therapy with Daunorubicin Hydrochloride.

Daunorubicin Hydrochloride may transiently impart a red coloration to the urine after administration, and patients should be advised to expect this.

Carcinogenesis, Mutagenesis, Impairment of Fertility: Daunorubicin Hydrochloride, when injected subcutaneously into mice, causes fibrosarcomas to develop at the injection site. When administered to mice orally or intraperitoneally, no carcinogenic effect was noted after 22 months of observation.

In male dogs at a daily dose of 0.25 mg/kg administered intravenously, testicular atrophy was noted at autopsy. Histologic examination revealed total aplasia of the spermatocyte series in the seminiferous tubules with complete aspermatogenesis.

Pregnancy Category D: (see "Warnings" section).

ADVERSE REACTIONS
Dose-limiting toxicity includes myelosuppression and cardiotoxicity (see "Warnings"). Other reactions include:

Cutaneous: Reversible alopecia occurs in most patients.

Gastrointestinal: Acute nausea and vomiting occur but are usually mild. Antiemetic therapy may be of some help. Mucositis may occur three to seven days after administration. Diarrhea has occasionally been reported.

Local: If extravasation occurs during administration, tissue necrosis can result at the site.

Acute Reactions: Rarely, anaphylactoid reaction, fever, chills, and skin rash can occur.

DOSAGE AND ADMINISTRATION
Parenteral drug products should be inspected visually for particulate matter and discoloration prior to administration, whenever solution and container permit.

Principles: In order to eradicate the leukemic cells and induce a complete remission, a profound suppression of the bone marrow is usually required. Evaluation of both the peripheral blood and bone marrow are mandatory in the formulation of appropriate treatment plans.

It is recommended that the dosage of Daunorubicin Hydrochloride be reduced in instances of hepatic or renal impairment. For example, using serum bilirubin and serum creatinine as indicators of liver and kidney function, the following dose modifications are recommended:

Serum Bilirubin	Serum Creatine	Recommended Dose
1.2 to 3.0 mg%		¾ normal dose
> 3 mg%	> 3 mg%	½ normal dose

REPRESENTATIVE DOSE SCHEDULES AND COMBINATION FOR THE APPROVED INDICATION OF REMISSION INDUCTION IN ADULT ACUTE NONLYMPHOCYTIC LEUKEMIA

In Combination[8,9]: For patients under age 60, Daunorubicin Hydrochloride 45 mg/m^2/day IV on days 1, 2, 3 of the first course and on days 1, 2 of subsequent courses AND cytosine arabinoside 100 mg/m^2/day IV infusion daily for 7 days for the first course and for 5 days for subsequent courses.

For patients 60 years of age and above, Daunorubicin Hydrochloride 80 mg/m^2/day IV on days 1, 2, 3 of the first course and on days 1, 2 of subsequent courses AND cytosine arabinoside 100 mg/m^2/day IV infusion daily for 7 days for the first course and for 5 days for subsequent courses.[9] This Daunorubicin Hydrochloride dose-reduction is based on a single study and may not be appropriate if optimal supportive care is available.

The attainment of a normal-appearing bone marrow may require up to three courses of induction therapy. Evaluation of the bone marrow following recovery from the previous course of induction therapy determines whether a further course of induction treatment is required.

REPRESENTATIVE DOSE SCHEDULE AND COMBINATION FOR THE APPROVED INDICATION OF REMISSION INDUCTION IN PEDIATRIC ACUTE LYMPHOCYTIC LEUKEMIA

In Combination: Daunorubicin Hydrochloride 25 mg/m^2 IV on day 1 every week, vincristine 1.5 mg/m^2 IV on day 1 every week, prednisone 40 mg/m^2 PO daily. Generally, a complete remission will be obtained within four such courses of therapy; however, if after four courses the patient is in partial remission, an additional one or, if necessary, two courses may be given in an effort to obtain a complete remission.

In children less than 2 years of age or below 0.5 m^2 body surface area, it has been recommended that the Daunorubicin Hydrochloride dosage calculation should be based on weight (1.0 mg/kg) instead of body surface area.[17]

REPRESENTATIVE DOSE SCHEDULES AND COMBINATION FOR THE APPROVED INDICATION OF REMISSION INDUCTION IN ADULT ACUTE LYMPHOCYTIC LEUKEMIA

In Combination[10]: Daunorubicin Hydrochloride 45 mg/m^2/day IV on days 1,2, and 3 AND vincristine 2 mg IV on days 1, 8, and 15: prednisone 40 mg/m^2/day PO on days 1 thru 22, then tapered between days 22 to 29; L-asparaginase 500 IU/kg/day × 10 days IV on days 22 thru 32.

The contents of a vial should be reconstituted with 4 mL of Sterile Water for Injection. USP, and agitated gently until the material has completely dissolved. The withdrawable vial contents provide 20 mg of Daunorubicin Hydrochloride activity, with 5 mg of Daunorubicin Hydrochloride activity per mL. The desired dose is withdrawn into a syringe containing 10 mL to 15 mL of normal saline and then injected into the tubing or sidearm of a rapidly flowing IV infusion of 5 percent glucose or normal saline solution. Daunorubicin Hydrochloride should not be administered mixed with other drugs or heparin. The reconstituted solution is stable for 24 hours at room temperature and 48 hours under refrigeration. It should be protected from exposure to sunlight.

Procedures for proper handling and disposal of anticancer drugs should be considered. Several guidelines on this subject have been published.[11-16] There is no general agreement that all of the procedures recommended in the guidelines are necessary or appropriate.

STORAGE
Store at 15° to 25°C.

REFERENCES
1. Gilladoga AC, Manuel C, Tan CTC, et al: The cardiotoxicity of Adriamycin and daunomycin in children. Cancer 37:1070-1078, 1976. 2. Bleyer WA: Delayed toxicities of chemotherapy on childhood tissues. Front Radiat. Ther One 16:40-54, 1982. 3. Isner JM, Ferrans VJ, Cohen SR, et al: Clinical and morphological cardiac findings after anthracycline chemotherapy. Am J Cardiol 51:1167-1174, 1983. 4. Rhoden WE, Jenny M, Beton DC, et al: Long term effects on left ventricular function of treatment for childhood malignancy. Br Heart J 66:59, 1991. 5. Steinherz LJ, Steinherz PG, Tan CTC, et al: Cardiac toxicity 4 to 20 years after completing anthracycline therapy JAMA 266:1672-1677, 1991. 6. Lipshultz SE, Colan SD, Gelber RD, et al: Late cardiac effects of doxorubicin therapy for acute lymphoblastic leukemia in childhood. N Engl J Med 324:808-815, 1991. 7. Steinherz L. Steinherz P: Delayed cardiac toxicity from anthracycline therapy. Pediatrician 18:49-52, 1991. 8. Rai KR, Holland JF, Glidewell O, et al: Treatment of acute myelocytic leukemia: a study by Cancer and Leukemia Group B. Blood 58:1203-1212, 1981. 9. Yates J, Glidewell O. Wiernik P, et al: Cytosine arabinoside with daunorubicin or Adriamycin for therapy of acute myelocytic leukemia: a CALGB study. Blood 60:454-462, 1982. 10. Gottlieb AJ, Weinberg V. Ellison RR: Efficacy of daunorubicin in the therapy of adult acute lymphocytic leukemia: a prospective randomized trial by Cancer and Leukemia Group B. Blood 64:267-274, 1984. 11. Recommendations for the Safe Handling of Parenteral Antineoplastic Drugs. NIH Publication No. 83-2621. For sale by the Superintendent of Documents. U.S. Government Printing Office, Washington, D.C. 20402. 12. AMA Council Report. Guidelines for Handling Parenteral Antineoplastics. JAMA, March 15, 1985. 13. National Study Commission on Cytotoxic Exposure—Recommendations for Handling Cytotoxic Agents. Available from Louis P. Jeffrey, Sc. D., Director of Pharmacy Services, Rhode Island Hospital, 593 Eddy Street, Providence, Rhode Island 02902. 14. Clinical Oncological Society of Australia: Guidelines and recommendations for safe handling of antineoplastic agents. Med J Australia 1:426-428, 1983. 15. Jones RB, et al: Safe handling of chemotherapeutic agents: A report from the Mount Sinai Medical Center, Ca-A Cancer Journal for Clinicians Sept/Oct, 258-263, 1983. 16. American Society of Hospital Pharmacists technical assistance bulletin on handling cytotoxic drugs in hospitals. Am J Hosp Pharm 42:131-137, 1985. 17. Sallan SE: Personal Communication, 1981.

J CODES
10 mg IV—J9150

HOW SUPPLIED
POWDER FOR INJECTION: 20 MG

BRAND/MANUFACTURER	NDC	SIZE	AWP
◆ BRAND			
CERUBIDINE: Wyeth-Ayerst	00008-4155-01	10s	$1550.41

Daypro *SEE* **OXAPROZIN**

DDAVP *SEE* **DESMOPRESSIN ACETATE**

Deca-Durabolin *SEE* **NANDROLONE**

Decadron *SEE* **DEXAMETHASONE, INJECTABLE, DEXAMETHASONE, OPHTHALMIC, DEXAMETHASONE, ORAL** *AND* **DEXAMETHASONE, TOPICAL**

Decadron with Xylocaine *SEE* **DEXAMETHASONE SODIUM PHOSPHATE WITH LIDOCAINE HYDROCHLORIDE**

Decaspray *SEE* **DEXAMETHASONE, TOPICAL**

Declomycin *SEE* **DEMECLOCYCLINE HYDROCHLORIDE**

Deconsal *SEE* **GUAIFENESIN AND PHENYLEPHRINE HYDROCHLORIDE** *AND* **GUAIFENESIN AND PSEUDOEPHEDRINE HYDROCHLORIDE**

Deferoxamine Mesylate

DESCRIPTION
Deferoxamine Mesylate is an iron-chelating agent, available in vials for intramuscular, subcutaneous, and intravenous administration. Each vial contains 500 mg of Deferoxamine Mesylate USP in sterile, lyophilized form. Deferoxamine Mesylate is N-[5-[3-[(5-aminopentyl)-hydroxycarbamoyl] propionamido]-pentyl]-3-[[5-(N-hydroxyacetamido) pentyl]carbamoyl] propionohydroxamic acid monomethane-sulfonate (salt).

Deferoxamine Mesylate USP is a white to off-white powder. It is freely soluble in water and slightly soluble in methanol. Its molecular weight is 656.79.

Following is its chemical structure:

$$H_2N(CH_2)_5N-C(CH_2)_2CNH(CH_2)_5N-C(CH_2)_2CNH(CH_2)_5N-CCH_3$$

CLINICAL PHARMACOLOGY
Deferoxamine Mesylate chelates iron by forming a stable complex that prevents the iron from entering into further chemical reactions. It readily chelates iron from ferritin and hemosiderin but not readily from transferrin; it does not combine with the iron from cytochromes and hemoglobin. Deferoxamine Mesylate does not cause any demonstrable increase in the excretion of electrolytes or trace metals. Theoretically, 100 parts by weight of Deferoxamine Mesylate is capable of binding approximately 8.5 parts by weight of ferric iron.

Deferoxamine Mesylate is metabolized principally by plasma enzymes, but the pathways have not yet been defined. The chelate is readily soluble in water and passes easily through the kidney, giving the urine a characteristic reddish color. Some is also excreted in the feces via the bile.

INDICATIONS AND USAGE
Deferoxamine Mesylate is indicated for the treatment of acute iron intoxication and of chronic iron overload due to transfusion-dependent anemias.

ACUTE IRON INTOXICATION
Deferoxamine Mesylate is an adjunct to, and not a substitute for, standard measures used in treating acute iron intoxication, which may include the following: induction of emesis with syrup of ipecac; gastric lavage; suction and maintenance of a clear airway; control of shock with intravenous fluids, blood, oxygen, and vasopressors; and correction of acidosis.

CHRONIC IRON OVERLOAD
Deferoxamine Mesylate can promote iron excretion in patients with secondary iron overload from multiple transfusions (as may occur in the treatment of some chronic anemias, including thalassemia). Long-term therapy with Deferoxamine Mesylate slows accumulation of hepatic iron and retards or eliminates progression of hepatic fibrosis.

Iron mobilization with Deferoxamine Mesylate is relatively poor in patients under the age of 3 years with relatively little iron overload. The drug should ordinarily not be given to such patients unless significant iron mobilization (e.g., 1 mg or more of iron per day) can be demonstrated.

Deferoxamine Mesylate is not indicated for the treatment of primary hemochromatosis, since phlebotomy is the method of choice for removing excess iron in this disorder.

UNLABELED USES
Deferoxamine Mesylate is used alone or as an adjunct in the treatment of Cooley's Anemia.

CONTRAINDICATIONS
Deferoxamine Mesylate is contraindicated in patients with severe renal disease or anuria, since the drug and the iron chelate are excreted primarily by the kidney.

WARNINGS
Ocular and auditory disturbances have been reported when Deferoxamine Mesylate was administered over prolonged periods of time, at high doses, or in patients with low ferritin levels. The ocular disturbances observed have been blurring of vision; cataracts after prolonged administration in chronic iron overload; decreased visual acuity including visual loss; impaired peripheral, color, and night vision; and retinal pigmentary abnormalities. The auditory abnormalities reported have been tinnitus and hearing loss including high frequency sensorineural hearing loss. In most cases, both ocular and auditory disturbances were reversible upon immediate cessation of treatment. Slit-lamp examinations performed in patients treated with Deferoxamine Mesylate for acute iron intoxication have not revealed cataracts.

Visual acuity tests, slit-lamp examinations, funduscopy and audiometry are recommended periodically in patients treated for prolonged periods of time. Toxicity is more likely to be reversed if symptoms or test abnormalities are detected early.

PRECAUTIONS
GENERAL
Flushing of the skin, urticaria, hypotension, and shock have occurred in a few patients when Deferoxamine Mesylate was administered by rapid intravenous injection. THEREFORE, DEFEROXAMINE MESYLATE SHOULD BE GIVEN INTRAMUSCULARLY OR BY SLOW SUBCUTANEOUS OR INTRAVENOUS INFUSION.

Iron overload increases susceptibility of patients to Yersinia enterocolitica infections. In some rare cases, treatment with Deferoxamine Mesylate has enhanced this susceptibility, resulting in generalized infections by providing this bacteria with a siderophore otherwise missing. In such cases, Deferoxamine Mesylate treatment should be discontinued until the infection is resolved.

In patients undergoing hemodialysis while receiving Deferoxamine Mesylate, there have been rare reports of fungal infections (i.e., mucormycosis) that have sometimes been fatal; however, a causal relationship to the drug has not been established.

INFORMATION FOR PATIENTS
Patients should be informed that occasionally their urine may show a reddish discoloration.

CARCINOGENESIS, MUTAGENESIS, IMPAIRMENT OF FERTILITY
Long-term carcinogenicity studies in animals have not been performed with Deferoxamine Mesylate.

Cytotoxicity may occur, since Deferoxamine Mesylate has been shown to inhibit DNA synthesis *in vitro*.

PREGNANCY CATEGORY C
Delayed ossification in mice and skeletal anomalies in rabbits were observed after Deferoxamine Mesylate was administered in daily doses up to 4.5 times the maximum daily human dose. No adverse effects were observed in similar studies in rats.

There are no adequate and well-controlled studies in pregnant women. Deferoxamine Mesylate should be used during pregnancy only if the potential benefit justifies the potential risk to the fetus.

NURSING MOTHERS
It is not known whether this drug is excreted in human milk. Because many drugs are excreted in human milk, caution should be exercised when Deferoxamine Mesylate is administered to a nursing woman.

PEDIATRIC USE
Safety and effectiveness in children under the age of 3 years have not been established (see *"Indications and Usage"*).

ADVERSE REACTIONS
The following adverse reactions have been observed, but there are not enough data to support an estimate of their frequency.

Skin: Localized irritation and pain, swelling and induration, pruritus, erythema, wheal formation.

Hypersensitive Reactions: Generalized erythema (rash), urticaria, anaphylactic reaction.

Cardiovascular: Tachycardia, hypotension, shock.

Digestive: Abdominal discomfort, diarrhea.

Special Senses: Ocular and auditory disturbances (see *"Warnings"*).

Other: Dysuria, leg cramps, fever.

OVERDOSAGE
ACUTE TOXICITY
Intravenous LD_{50}'s (mg/kg): mice, 287; rats, 329.

SIGNS AND SYMPTOMS
Since Deferoxamine Mesylate is available only for parenteral administration, acute poisoning is unlikely to occur. However, tachycardia, hypotension, and gastrointestinal symptoms have occasionally developed in patients who received overdoses of Deferoxamine Mesylate.

TREATMENT
There is no specific antidote.
  Signs and symptoms of overdosage may be eliminated by reducing the dosage.
  Deferoxamine Mesylate is readily dialyzable.

DOSAGE AND ADMINISTRATION
ACUTE IRON INTOXICATION
Intramuscular Administration: This route is preferred and should be used for ALL PATIENTS NOT IN SHOCK.
  Dosage. A dose of 1.0 g should be administered initially. This may be followed by 500 mg (one vial) every 4 hours for two doses. Depending upon the clinical response, subsequent doses of 500 mg may be administered every 4-12 hours. The total amount administered should not exceed 6.0 g in 24 hours.
  Preparation of Solution. Deferoxamine Mesylate is dissolved by adding 2 mL of Sterile Water for Injection to each vial, resulting in a solution of 250 mg/mL. The drug should be completely dissolved before the solution is withdrawn. Deferoxamine Mesylate is then administered intramuscularly. See *Note* below.

Intravenous Administration: THIS ROUTE SHOULD BE USED ONLY FOR PATIENTS IN A STATE OF CARDIOVASCULAR COLLAPSE AND THEN ONLY BY SLOW INFUSION. THE RATE OF INFUSION SHOULD NOT EXCEED 15 MG/KG PER HOUR.
  Dosage. An initial dose of 1.0 g should be administered at a rate NOT TO EXCEED 15 mg/kg per hour. This may be followed by 500 mg every 4 hours for two doses. Depending upon the clinical response, subsequent doses of 500 mg may be administered every 4-12 hours. The total amount administered should not exceed 6.0 g in 24 hours.
  As soon as the clinical condition of the patient permits, intravenous administration should be discontinued and the drug should be administered intramuscularly.

Preparation of Solution: Deferoxamine Mesylate is dissolved by adding 2 mL of Sterile Water for Injection to each vial, resulting in a solution of 250 mg/mL. The drug should be completely dissolved before the solution is withdrawn. The solution is then added to physiologic saline, glucose in water, or Ringer's lactate solution and administered at a rate NOT TO EXCEED 15 mg/kg per hour. See *Note* below.

CHRONIC IRON OVERLOAD
The more effective of the following routes of administration must be chosen on an individual basis for each patient.

Intramuscular Administration: A daily dose of 0.5-1.0 g should be administered intramuscularly. In addition, 2.0 g should be administered intravenously with each unit of blood transfused; however, Deferoxamine Mesylate should be administered separately from the blood. The rate of intravenous infusion must not exceed 15 mg/kg per hour.

Subcutaneous Administration: A daily dose of 1.0-2.0 g (20-40 mg/kg per day) should be administered over 8-24 hours, utilizing a small portable pump capable of providing continuous mini-infusion. The duration of infusion must be individualized. In some patients, as much iron will be excreted after a short infusion of 8-12 hours as with the same dose given over 24 hours.

Preparation of Solution for Subcutaneous or Intramuscular Administration: Deferoxamine Mesylate is dissolved by adding 2.0 mL of Sterile Water for Injection to each vial, resulting in a solution of 250 mg/mL. The drug should be completely dissolved before the solution is withdrawn into the syringe to be used for administration. See *Note* below.
  Note: Parenteral drug products should be inspected visually for particulate matter and discoloration prior to administration, whenever solution and container permit.
  Deferoxamine Mesylate reconstituted with Sterile Water for Injection may be stored under sterile conditions and protected from light at room temperature for not longer than 1 week.
  Reconstituting Deferoxamine Mesylate in solvents or under conditions other than indicated may result in precipitation. Turbid solutions should not be used.
  Do not store above 86°F (30°C).

J CODES
500 mg per 5 cc IM,SC,IV—J0895

HOW SUPPLIED
POWDER FOR INJECTION: 500 MG

BRAND/MANUFACTURER	NDC	SIZE	AWP
○ BRAND			
DESFERAL: Ciba Pharm	00083-3801-04	4s	$37.91

Dehydrocholic Acid

DESCRIPTION

Dehydrocholic Acid, an oxidation product of cholic acid (a natural bile acid), occurs as a white, odorless, bitter powder. It is practically insoluble in water, and soluble in solutions of alkali hydroxides.

It is available in white, compressed tablets, each containing 250 mg. (3 3/4 grains) of Dehydrocholic Acid.

Following is its chemical structure:

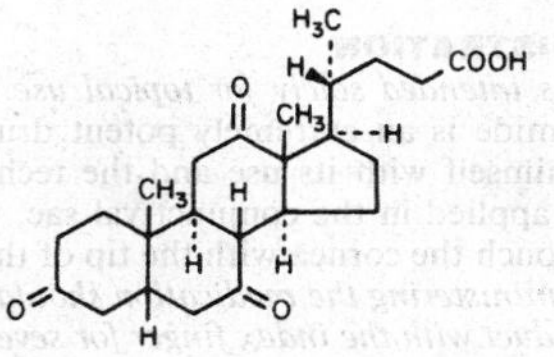

ACTIONS

At recommended dosage levels, Dehydrocholic Acid exerts laxative and hydrocholeretic (increased volume and water content of bile) actions. The mechanisms of actions are unknown. Unlike the natural bile acids and their conjugates, Dehydrocholic Acid does not readily form micelles (small aggregates of bile acids, fats, and phospholipids necessary for normal fat absorption).

INDICATIONS

Temporary relief of constipation. Also as adjunctive therapy of biliary stasis, without complete mechanical obstruction of the common or hepatic bile ducts, where hydrocholeresis is desired.

CONTRAINDICATIONS

Significant cholelithiasis; presence of jaundice; marked hepatic insufficiency; complete obstruction of the common or hepatic bile ducts or of the G.I. or G.U. tracts; hypersensitivity to bile acids or their conjugates. Not for use as a diuretic or as an adjunct thereto.

WARNINGS

No data supporting a recommended pediatric dose are available. Thus, this drug should not be used in children under 12 years of age.

PRECAUTIONS

Use with caution in elderly persons. If promotion of true bile flow is desired, a cholagogue should be used.

ADVERSE REACTIONS

Hypersensitivity (pruritus, dermatitis).

DOSAGE & ADMINISTRATION

One or two tablets three times daily after meals. Thereafter, titrate dosage to individual patient's needs.

HOW SUPPLIED
TABLETS: 250 MG

BRAND/MANUFACTURER	NDC	SIZE	AWP
○ GENERICS			
Richlyn	00115-3030-01	100s	$11.43
Goldline	00182-0489-01	100s	$21.00
Richlyn	00115-3030-03	1000s	$87.90

Delatestryl SEE TESTOSTERONE, INJECTABLE

Delestrogen SEE ESTRADIOL, INJECTABLE

Demadex SEE TORSEMIDE

Demecarium Bromide

DESCRIPTION

Ophthalmic Solution Demecarium Bromide is a sterile solution supplied in two dosage strengths: 0.125 percent and 0.25 percent. Demecarium Bromide is a quaternary ammonium compound with a molecular weight of 716.60. Its chemical name is 3,3′-[1,10-decanediylbis [(methylimino) carbonyloxy]] bis [N,N,N-trimethylbenzenaminium] dibromide. Its empirical formula is $C_{32}H_{52}Br_2N_4O_4$.

Following is its chemical structure:

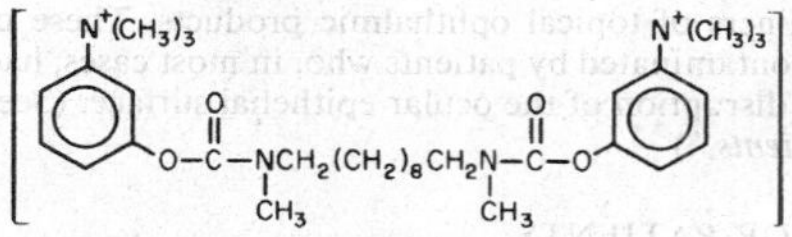

CLINICAL PHARMACOLOGY

Demecarium Bromide is a cholinesterase inhibitor with sustained activity. It acts mainly on true (erythrocyte) cholinesterase. Application of Demecarium Bromide to the eye produces intense miosis and ciliary muscle contraction due to inhibition of cholinesterase, allowing acetylcholine to accumulate at sites of cholinergic transmission. These effects are accompanied by increased capillary permeability of the ciliary body and iris, increased permeability of the blood-aqueous barrier, and vasodilation. Myopia may be induced or, if present, may be augmented by the increased refractive power of the lens that results from the accommodative effect of the drug. Demecarium Bromide indirectly produces some of the muscarinic and nicotinic effects of acetylcholine as quantities of the latter accumulate.

INDICATIONS AND USAGE

Open-angle glaucoma (Demecarium Bromide should be used in glaucoma only when shorter-acting miotics have proved inadequate.)

Conditions obstructing aqueous outflow, such as synechial formation, that are amenable to miotic therapy

Following iridectomy

Accommodative estropia (accommodative convergent strabismus)

CONTRAINDICATIONS

Hypersensitivity to any component of this product.

Because of the toxicity of cholinesterase inhibitors in general, Demecarium Bromide is contraindicated in women who are or who may become pregnant. If this drug is used during pregnancy, or if the patient becomes pregnant while taking this drug, the patient should be apprised of the potential hazard to the fetus.

Because miotics may aggravate inflammation, Demecarium Bromide should not be used in active uveal inflammation and/or glaucoma associated with iridocyclitis.

WARNINGS

In patients receiving cholinesterase inhibitors such as Demecarium Bromide, succinylcholine should be administered with extreme caution before and during general anesthesia.

Because of possible adverse additive effects, Demecarium Bromide should be administered only with extreme caution to patients with myasthenia gravis who are receiving systemic anticholinesterase therapy; conversely, extreme caution should be exercised in the use of an anticholinesterase drug for the treatment of myasthenia gravis patients who are already undergoing topical therapy with cholinesterase inhibitors.

PRECAUTIONS

GENERAL

Gonioscopy is recommended prior to medication with Demecarium Bromide.

Demecarium Bromide should be used with caution in patients with chronic angle-closure (narrow-angle) glaucoma or in patients with narrow angles, because of the possibility of producing pupillary block and increasing angle blockage.

When an intraocular inflammatory process is present, the intensity and persistence of miosis and ciliary muscle contraction that result from anticholinesterase therapy require abstention from, or cautious use of, Demecarium Bromide. Systemic effects are infrequent when Demecarium Bromide is instilled carefully. Compression of the lacrimal duct for several seconds immediately following instillation minimizes drainage into the nasal chamber with its extensive absorption surface. Wash the hands immediately after instillation. Discontinue Demecarium Bromide if salivation, urinary incontinence, diarrhea, profuse sweating, muscle weakness, respiratory difficulties, shock, or cardiac irregularities occur.

Persons receiving cholinesterase inhibitors who are exposed to organophosphate-type insecticides and pesticides (gardeners, organophosphate plant or warehouse workers, farmers, residents of communities which are undergoing insecticide spraying or dusting, etc.) should be warned of the added systemic effects possible from absorption through the respiratory tract or skin. Wearing of respiratory masks, frequent washing, and clothing changes may be advisable.

Anticholinesterase drugs should be used with extreme caution, if at all, in patients with marked vagotonia, bronchial asthma, spastic gastrointestinal disturbances, peptic ulcer, pronounced bradycardia and hypotension, recent myocardial infarction, epilepsy, parkinsonism, and other disorders that may respond adversely to vagotonic effects.

After long-term use of Demecarium Bromide dilation of blood vessels and resulting greater permeability increase the possibility of hyphema during ophthalmic surgery. Therefore, this drug should be discontinued before surgery.

Despite observance of all precautions and the use of only the recommended dose, there is some evidence that repeated administration may cause depression of the concentration of cholinesterase in the serium and erythrocytes, with resultant systemic effects.

There have been reports of bacterial keratitis associated with the use of multiple dose containers of topical ophthalmic products. These containers had been inadvertently contaminated by patients who, in most cases, had a concurrent corneal disease or a disruption of the ocular epithelial surface. (See *"Precautions, Information for Patients"*.)

INFORMATION FOR PATIENTS

Patients should be instructed to avoid allowing the tip of the dispensing container to contact the eye or surrounding structures.

Patients should also be instructed that ocular solutions, if handled improperly, can become contaminated by common bacteria known to cause ocular infections. Serious damage to the eye and subsequent loss of vision may result from using contaminated solutions. (See *"Precautions, General"*.)

Patients should also be advised that if they develop an intercurrent ocular condition (e.g., trauma, ocular surgery or infection), they should immediately seek their physician's advice concerning the continued use of the present multidose container.

The preservative in Demecarium Bromide benzalkonium chloride, may be absorbed by soft contact lenses. Patients wearing soft contact lenses should be instructed to wait at least 15 minutes after instilling Demecarium Bromide before they insert their lenses.

DRUG INTERACTIONS

See *"Warnings"* regarding possible drug interactions of Demecarium Bromide with succinylcholine or with other anticholinesterase agents.

CARCINOGENESIS, MUTAGENESIS, IMPAIRMENT OF FERTILITY

Long-term studies in animals have not been performed to evaluate the effects of Demecarium Bromide on fertility or carcinogenic potential.

PREGNANCY

Pregnancy Category X: (See *"Contraindications."*)

NURSING MOTHERS

It is not known whether this drug is excreted in human milk. Because of the potential for serious adverse reactions in nursing infants from Demecarium Bromide, a decision should be made whether to discontinue nursing or to discontinue the drug, taking into account the importance of the drug to the mother.

PEDIATRIC USE

The occurrence of iris cysts is more frequent in children. (See *"Adverse Reactions"* and *"Dosage and Administration"*.)

Extreme caution should be exercised in children receiving Demecarium Bromide who may require general anesthesia (see *"Warnings"*).

Since Demecarium Bromide is a potent cholinesterase inhibitor it should be kept out of the reach of children.

ADVERSE REACTIONS

Stinging, burning, lacrimation, lid muscle twitching, conjunctival and ciliary redness, brow ache, headache, and induced myopia with visual blurring may occur.

Activation of latent iritis or uveitis may occur.

As with all miotic therapy, retinal detachment has been reported occasionally.

Iris cysts may form, enlarge, and obscure vision. Occurrence is more frequent in children. The iris cyst usually shrinks upon discontinuance of the miotic. Rarely, the cyst may rupture or break free into the aqueous. Frequent examination for this occurrence is advised.

Lens opacities have been reported in patients on miotic therapy. Routine slit-lamp examinations, including the lens, should accompany prolonged use.

Paradoxical increase in intraocular pressure may follow anticholinesterase instillation. This may be alleviated by pupil-dilating medication.

Prolonged use may cause conjunctival thickening and obstruction of nasolacrimal canals.

Systemic effects, which occur rarely, are suggestive of increased cholinergic activity. Such effects may include nausea, vomiting, abdominal cramps, diarrhea, urinary incontinence, salivation, sweating, difficulty in breathing, bradycardia, or cardiac irregularities. Medical management of systemic effects may be indicated (see *"Treatment of Adverse Effects"*).

TREATMENT OF ADVERSE EFFECTS

Demecarium Bromide is taken systemically by accident, or if systemic effects occur after topical application in the eye or from accidental skin contact, administer atropine sulfate parenterally (intravenously if necessary) in a dose (for adults) of 0.4 to 0.6 mg or more. The recommended dosage of atropine in infants and children up to 12 years of age is 0.01 mg/kg repeated every two hours as needed until the desired effect is obtained, or adverse effects of atropine preclude further usage. The maximum single dose should not exceed 0.4 mg.

The use of much larger doses of atropine in treating anticholinesterase intoxication in adults has been reported in the literature. Initially 2 to 6 mg may be given followed by 2 mg every hour or more often, as long as muscarinic effects continue. The greater possibility of atropinization with large doses, particularly in sensitive individuals, should be borne in mind.

Pralidoxime Chloride has been reported to be useful in treating systemic effects due to cholinesterase inhibitors. However, its use is recommended in addition to and not as substitute for atropine.

A short-acting barbiturate is indicated if convulsions occur that are not entirely relieved by atropine. Barbiturate dosage should be carefully adjusted to avoid central respiratory depression. Marked weakness or paralysis of muscles of respiration should be treated promptly by artificial respiration and maintenance of a clear airway.

The oral LD_{50} of Demecarium Bromide is 2.96 mg/kg in the mouse.

DOSAGE AND ADMINISTRATION

Demecarium Bromide *is intended solely for topical use in the conjunctival sac.*

As Demecarium Bromide is an extremely potent drug, the physician should thoroughly familiarize himself with its use and the technic of instillation.

The required dose is applied in the conjunctival sac, with the patient supine, care being taken not to touch the cornea with the tip of the ophthalmic dispenser. *The patient or person administering the medication should apply continuous gentle pressure on the lacrimal duct with the index finger for several seconds immediately following instillation of the drops. This is to prevent drainage overflow of solution into the nasal and pharyngeal spaces, which might cause systemic absorption. Wash the hands immediately after administration.*

Demecarium Bromide *should not be used more often than directed. Caution is necessary to avoid overdosage.*

Initial titration and dosage adjustments with Demecarium Bromide must be individualized to obtain maximal therapeutic effect. The patient must be closely observed during the initial period. If the response is not adequate within the first 24 hours, other measures should be considered.

Keep frequency of use to a minimum in all patients, but especially in children, to reduce the chance of iris cyst development (see *"Adverse Reactions"*).

GLAUCOMA

For initial therapy with Demecarium Bromide (0.125 percent or 0.25 percent) place 1 drop (children) or 1 or 2 drops (adults) in the glaucomatous eye. A decrease in intraocular pressure should occur within a few hours. During this period, keep the patient under supervision and make tonometric examinations at least hourly for 3 or 4 hours to be sure that no immediate rise in pressure occurs (see *"Adverse Reactions"*).

Duration of effect varies with the individual. The usual dosage can vary from as much as 1 or 2 drops twice a day to as little as 1 or 2 drops twice a week. The 0.125 percent strength used twice a day usually results in smooth control of the physiologic diurnal variation in intraocular pressure. This is probably the preferred dosage for most wide (open) angle glaucoma patients.

STRABISMUS

Essentially equal visual acuity of both eyes is a prerequisite to the successful treatment of esotropia with Demecarium Bromide. For initial evaluation it may be used as a diagnostic aid to determine if an accommodative factor exists. This is especially useful preoperatively in young children and in patients with normal hypermetropic refractive errors. One drop is given daily for 2 weeks, then 1 drop every 2 days for 2 to 3 weeks. If the eyes become straighter, an accommodative factor is demonstrated. This technic may supplement or complement standard testing with atropine and trial with glasses for the accommodative factor.

In esotropia uncomplicated by amblyopia or anisometropia, Demecarium Bromide may be instilled in both eyes, *not more than 1 drop at a time every day for 2 to 3 weeks*, as too severe a degree of miosis may interfere with vision. Then reduce the dosage to 1 drop every other day for 3 to 4 weeks and reevaluate the patient's status.

Demecarium Bromide may be continued in a dosage of 1 drop every 2 days to 1 drop twice a week. (The latter dosage may be maintained for several months.) Evaluate the patient's condition every 4 to 12 weeks. If improvement continues, change the schedule to 1 drop once a week and eventually to a trial without medication. However, if after 4 months, control of the condition still requires 1 drop every 2 days, therapy with Demecarium Bromide should be stopped.

STORAGE

Protect from freezing and excessive heat.

HOW SUPPLIED
DROP: 0.125%

BRAND/MANUFACTURER	NDC	SIZE	AWP
○ BRAND			
HUMORSOL OCUMETER: Merck	00006-3255-03	5 ml	$14.23

◆ RATED THERAPEUTICALLY EQUIVALENT; ◇ THERAPEUTIC EQUIVALENCE UNCONFIRMED; ○ UNRATED

DROP: 0.25%

BRAND/MANUFACTURER	NDC	SIZE	AWP
○ **BRAND** HUMORSOL OCUMETER: Merck	00006-3267-03	5 ml	$15.25

Demeclocycline Hydrochloride

DESCRIPTION

Demeclocycline Hydrochloride is an antibiotic isolated from a mutant strain of *Streptomyces aureofaciens*. Chemically it is 7-Chloro-4-(dimethylamino)-1,4,4a,5,5a,6,11,12a-octahydro-3,6,10, 12, 12a- pentahydroxy - 1,11-dioxo -2-naphthacenecarboxamide monohydrochloride.

Following is its chemical structure:

CLINICAL PHARMACOLOGY

The tetracyclines are primarily bacteriostatic and are thought to exert their antimicrobial effect by the inhibition of protein synthesis. Tetracyclines are active against a wide range of gram-negative and gram-positive organisms.

The drugs in the tetracycline class have closely similar antimicrobial spectra, and cross-resistance among them is common. Microorganisms may be considered susceptible if the MIC (minimum inhibitory concentration) is not more than 4 mcg/mL and intermediate if the MIC is 4 to 12.5 mcg/mL. Susceptibility plate testing: A tetracycline disc may be used to determine microbial susceptibility to drugs in the tetracycline class. If the Kirby-Bauer method of disc susceptibility testing is used, a 30 mcg tetracycline disc should give a zone of at least 19 mm when tested against a tetracycline-susceptible bacterial strain.

Tetracyclines are readily absorbed and are bound to plasma proteins in varying degrees. They are concentrated by the liver in the bile and excreted in the urine and feces at high concentrations and in a biologically active form.

INDICATIONS AND USAGE

Demeclocycline Hydrochloride is indicated in infections caused by the following microorganisms:

Rickettsiae: (Rocky Mountain spotted fever, typhus fever and the typhus group, Q fever, rickettsialpox, tick fevers).

Mycoplasma pneumoniae (PPLO, Eaton agent).

Agents of psittacosis and ornithosis.

Agents of lymphogranuloma venereum and granuloma inguinale.

The spirochetal agent of relapsing fever (*Borrelia recurrentis*).

The following gram-negative microorganisms:

Haemophilus ducreyi (chancroid),

Yersinia pestis and *Francisella tularensis*, formerly *Pasteurella pestis* and *Pasteurella tularensis*,

Bartonella bacilliformis,

Bacteroides species,

Vibrio comma and *Vibrio fetus*.

Brucella species (in conjunction with streptomycin).

Because many strains of the following groups of microorganisms have been shown to be resistant to tetracyclines, culture and susceptibility testing are recommended.

Demeclocycline Hydrochloride is indicated for treatment of infections caused by the following gram-negative microorganisms, when bacteriologic testing indicates appropriate susceptibility to the drug:

Escherichia coli,

Enterobacter aerogenes (formerly *Aerobacter aerogenes*),

Shigella species,

Mima species and *Herellea* species,

Haemophilus influenzae (respiratory infections),

Klebsiella species (respiratory and urinary infections).

Demeclocycline Hydrochloride is indicated for treatment of infections caused by the following gram-positive microorganisms when bacteriologic testing indicates appropriate susceptibility to the drug:

Streptococcus species:

Up to 44% of strains of *Streptococcus pyogenes* and 74% of *Streptococcus faecalis* have been found to be resistant to tetracycline drugs. Therefore, tetracyclines should not be used for streptococcal disease unless the organism has been demonstrated to be sensitive.

For upper respiratory infections due to Group A beta-hemolytic streptococci, penicillin is the usual drug of choice, including prophylaxis of rheumatic fever.

Streptococcus pneumoniae,

Staphylococcus aureus, skin and soft tissue infections. Tetracyclines are not the drugs of choice in the treatment of any type of staphylococcal infection.

When penicillin is contraindicated, tetracyclines are alternative drugs in the treatment of infections due to:

Neisseria gonorrhoeae,

Treponema pallidum and *Treponema pertenue* (syphilis and yaws),

Listeria monocytogenes,

Clostridium species,

Bacillus anthracis,

Fusobacterium fusiforme (Vincent's infection),

Actinomyces species.

In acute intestinal amebiasis, the tetracyclines may be a useful adjunct to amebicides.

Demeclocycline Hydrochloride is indicated in the treatment of trachoma, although the infectious agent is not always eliminated, as judged by immunofluorescence.

Inclusion conjunctivitis may be treated with oral tetracyclines or with a combination of oral and topical agents.

UNLABELED USES

Demeclocycline Hydrochloride is used alone or as an adjunct in the treatment of acne.

CONTRAINDICATIONS

This drug is contraindicated in persons who have shown hypersensitivity to any of the tetracyclines.

WARNINGS

THE USE OF DRUGS OF THE TETRACYCLINE CLASS DURING TOOTH DEVELOPMENT (LAST HALF OF PREGNANCY, INFANCY, AND CHILDHOOD TO THE AGE OF 8 YEARS) MAY CAUSE PERMANENT DISCOLORATION OF THE TEETH (YELLOW-GRAY-BROWN).

This adverse reaction is more common during long-term use of the drugs but has been observed following repeated short-term courses. Enamel hypoplasia has also been reported. TETRACYCLINE DRUGS, THEREFORE, SHOULD NOT BE USED IN THIS AGE GROUP UNLESS OTHER DRUGS ARE NOT LIKELY TO BE EFFECTIVE OR ARE CONTRAINDICATED.

If renal impairment exists, even usual oral or parenteral doses may lead to excessive systemic accumulation of the drug and possible liver toxicity. Under such conditions, lower than usual total doses are indicated and, if therapy is prolonged, serum level determinations of the drug may be advisable.

Phototoxic reactions can occur in individuals taking Demeclocycline Hydrochloride, and are characterized by severe burns of exposed surfaces resulting from direct exposure of patients to sunlight during therapy with moderate or large doses of Demeclocycline Hydrochloride. Patients apt to be exposed to direct sunlight or ultraviolet light should be advised that this reaction can occur, and treatment should be discontinued at the first evidence of skin erythema.

The anti-anabolic action of the tetracyclines may cause an increase in BUN. While this is not a problem in those with normal renal function, in patients with significantly impaired function, higher serum levels of tetracycline may lead to azotemia, hyperphosphatemia, and acidosis.

Administration of Demeclocycline Hydrochloride has resulted in appearance of the diabetes insipidus syndrome (polyuria, polydipsia, and weakness) in some patients on long-term therapy. The syndrome has been shown to be nephrogenic, dose-dependent, and reversible on discontinuance of therapy.

Usage in Pregnancy: (See above "Warnings" about use during tooth development.) Results of animal studies indicate that tetracyclines cross the placenta, are found in fetal tissues and can have toxic effects on the developing fetus (often related to retardation of skeletal development). Evidence of embryotoxicity has also been noted in animals treated early in pregnancy.

Usage in Newborns, Infants, and Children: (See above "Warnings" about use during tooth development.)

All tetracyclines form a stable calcium complex in any bone forming tissue. A decrease in the fibula growth rate has been observed in prematures given oral tetracycline in doses of 25 mg/kg every 6 hours. This reaction was shown to be reversible when the drug was discontinued.

Tetracyclines are present in the milk of lactating women who are taking a drug in this class.

PRECAUTIONS

General: Pseudotumor cerebri (benign intracranial hypertension) in adults has been associated with the use of tetracyclines. The usual clinical manifestations are headache and blurred vision. Bulging fontanels have been associated with the use of tetracyclines in infants. While both of these conditions and related symptoms usually resolve soon after discontinuation of the tetracycline, the possibility for permanent sequelae exists.

As with other antibiotic preparations, use of this drug may result in overgrowth of nonsusceptible organisms, including fungi. If superinfection occurs, the antibiotic should be discontinued and appropriate therapy should be instituted.

In venereal diseases when coexistent syphilis is suspected, darkfield examination should be done before treatment is started and the blood serology repeated monthly for at least 4 months.

In long-term therapy, periodic laboratory evaluation of organ systems, including hematopoietic, renal and hepatic studies should be performed.

All infections due to Group A beta-hemolytic streptococci should be treated for at least 10 days.

Interpretation of Bacteriologic Studies: Following a course of therapy, persistence for several days in both urine and blood of bacterio-suppressive levels of

➤ **SHOWN IN PRODUCT IDENTIFICATION GUIDE**

Demeclocycline Hydrochloride may interfere with culture studies. These levels should not be considered therapeutic.

Drug Interactions: Because the tetracyclines have been shown to depress plasma prothrombin activity, patients who are on anticoagulant therapy may require downward adjustment of their anticoagulant dosage.

Since bacteriostatic drugs, such as the tetracycline class of antibiotics, may interfere with the bactericidal action of penicillins, it is not advisable to administer these drugs concomitantly.

Concurrent use of tetracyclines with oral contraceptives may render oral contraceptives less effective. Breakthrough bleeding has been reported.

ADVERSE REACTIONS

Gastrointestinal: Anorexia, nausea, vomiting, diarrhea, glossitis, dysphagia, enterocolitis, pancreatitis, and inflammatory lesions (with monilial overgrowth) in the anogenital region, increases in liver enzymes, and hepatic toxicity has been reported rarely. Rare instances of esophagitis and esophageal ulcerations have been reported in patients taking the tetracycline-class antibiotics in capsule and tablet form. Most of these patients took the medication immediately before going to bed. (See *"Dosage and Administration".*)

Skin: Maculopapular and erythematous rashes. Exfoliative dermatitis has been reported but is uncommon. Photosensitivity is discussed above. (See *"Warnings".*)

Renal Toxicity: Rise in BUN has been reported and is apparently dose related. Nephrogenic diabetes insipidus. (See *"Warnings".*)

Hypersensitivity Reactions: Urticaria, angioneurotic edema, anaphylaxis, anaphylactoid purpura, pericarditis, and exacerbation of systemic lupus erythematosus.

Blood: Hemolytic anemia, thrombocytopenia, neutropenia, and eosinophilia have been reported.

CNS: Pseudotumor cerebri (benign intracranial hypertension) in adults and bulging fontanels in infants (see *"Precautions—General"*). Dizziness, tinnitus, and visual disturbances have been reported. Myasthenic syndrome has been reported rarely.

Other: When given over prolonged periods, tetracyclines have been reported to produce brown-black microscopic discoloration of thyroid glands. No abnormalities of thyroid function studies are known to occur.

DOSAGE AND ADMINISTRATION

Therapy should be continued for at least 24 to 48 hours after symptoms and fever have subsided.

Concomitant therapy: Antacids containing aluminum, calcium, or magnesium impair absorption and should not be given to patients taking oral tetracycline.

Foods and some dairy products also interfere with absorption. Oral forms of tetracycline should be given 1 hour before or 2 hours after meals.

In patients with renal impairment: (See *"Warnings".*) Total dosage should be decreased by reduction of recommended individual doses and/or by extending time intervals between doses.

In the treatment of streptococcal infections, a therapeutic dose of Demeclocycline Hydrochloride should be administered for at least 10 days.

Adults: Usual daily dose—Four divided doses of 150 mg each or two divided doses of 300 mg each.

For children above 8 years of age: Usual daily dose, 3 to 6 mg per pound body weight per day, depending upon the severity of the disease, divided into two to four doses.

Gonorrhea patients sensitive to penicillin may be treated with Demeclocycline Hydrochloride administered as an initial oral dose of 600 mg followed by 300 mg every 12 hours for 4 days to a total of 3 grams.

Store at controlled room temperature 15°-30°C (59°-86°F).

HOW SUPPLIED
TABLETS: 150 MG

BRAND/MANUFACTURER	NDC	SIZE	AWP
○ BRAND			
DECLOMYCIN: Lederle Labs	00005-9218-23	100s	$327.56

TABLETS: 300 MG

BRAND/MANUFACTURER	NDC	SIZE	AWP
○ BRAND			
DECLOMYCIN: Lederle Labs	00005-9270-29	48s	$286.10

Demerol HCl *SEE* MEPERIDINE HYDROCHLORIDE

Demi-Regroton *SEE* CHLORTHALIDONE WITH RESERPINE

Demser *SEE* METYROSINE

Demulen *SEE* ETHINYL ESTRADIOL WITH ETHYNODIOL DIACETATE

Depakene *SEE* VALPROIC ACID

Depakote *SEE* DIVALPROEX SODIUM

Depen *SEE* PENICILLAMINE

Depo-Estradiol *SEE* ESTRADIOL, INJECTABLE

Depo-Medrol *SEE* METHYLPREDNISOLONE

Depo-Provera *SEE* MEDROXYPROGESTERONE ACETATE, CONTRACEPTIVE *AND* MEDROXYPROGESTERONE ACETATE, INJECTABLE

Depo-Testadiol *SEE* ESTRADIOL CYPIONATE AND TESTOSTERONE CYPIONATE

Depo-Testosterone *SEE* TESTOSTERONE, INJECTABLE

Deponit *SEE* NITROGLYCERIN

Derma-Smoothe/FS *SEE* FLUOCINOLONE ACETONIDE

Dermacin *SEE* FLUOCINONIDE

Dermacort *SEE* HYDROCORTISONE, TOPICAL

Dermatop *SEE* PREDNICARBATE

Deserpidine

DESCRIPTION

Deserpidine is a purified rauwolfia alkaloid which occurs as a white to light yellow crystalline powder. Deserpidine is insoluble in water and very slightly soluble in alcohol. Chemically, Deserpidine is identified as 17α-methoxy-18β-[(3,4,5-trimethoxybenzoyl)oxy]-3β, 20α-yohimban-16β-carboxylic acid methyl ester.

Deserpidine is an oral antihypertensive and antipsychotic agent available as tablets containing 0.25 mg of Deserpidine.

Following is its chemical structure:

CLINICAL PHARMACOLOGY

The pharmacologic actions of Deserpidine are essentially the same as those of other active rauwolfia alkaloids. Deserpidine probably produces its antihypertensive effects through depletion of tissue stores of catecholamines (epinephrine and norepinephrine) from peripheral sites. By contrast, its sedative and tranquilizing properties are thought to be related to depletion of 5-hydroxytryptamine from the brain.

The antihypertensive effect is often accompanied by bradycardia. There is no significant alteration in cardiac output or renal blood flow. The carotoid sinus reflex is inhibited, but postural hypotension is rarely seen with the use of conventional doses of Deserpidine alone.

Deserpidine, like other rauwolfia alkaloids, is characterized by slow onset of action and sustained effect which may persist following withdrawal of the drug.

Information is limited on the human pharmacokinetics of the rauwolfia alkaloids. Rauwolfia alkaloids appear to be widely distributed in body tissues, especially adipose tissue. They also cross the blood-brain barrier. Rauwolfia alkaloids are extensively metabolized. The unchanged alkaloid and the metabolites are excreted slowly in urine and feces.

INDICATIONS AND USAGE

Deserpidine is indicated for the treatment of mild essential hypertension. It is also useful as adjunctive therapy with other antihypertensive agents in the more severe forms of hypertension.

The drug is also indicated for the relief of symptoms in agitated psychotic states, e.g., schizophrenia — primarily in those individuals unable to tolerate phenothiazine derivatives or those who also require antihypertensive medication.

CONTRAINDICATIONS

Deserpidine is contraindicated in patients with known hypertensivity, history of mental depression especially with suicidal tendencies, active peptic ulcer, and ulcerative colitis. It is also contraindicated in patients receiving electroconvulsive therapy.

WARNINGS

Deserpidine differs slightly in chemical structure from reserpine, however, its actions, indications, cautions and adverse reactions are common to the class of rauwolfia alkaloids. Reserpine may cause mental depression. Recognition of depression may be difficult because this condition may often be disguised by somatic complaints (masked depression). The drug should be discontinued at first signs of depression such as despondency, early morning insomnia, loss of appetite, impotence, or self-deprecation. Drug-induced depression may persist for several months after drug withdrawal and may be severe enough to result in suicide.

PRECAUTIONS

General: Because rauwolfia preparations increase gastrointestinal motility and secretion, this drug should be used cautiously in patients with a history of peptic ulcer, ulcerative colitis, or gallstones, where biliary colic may be precipitated.

Caution should be exercised when treating hypertensive patients with renal insufficiency since they adjust poorly to lowered blood pressure levels.

Preoperative withdrawal of Deserpidine does not assure that circulatory instability will not occur. It is important that the anesthesiologist be aware of the patient's drug intake and consider this in the overall management, since hypotension has occurred in patients receiving rauwolfia preparations. Anticholinergic and/or adrenergic drugs (metaraminol, norepinephrine) have been employed to treat adverse vagocirculatory effects.

Information for Patients: The patient and his family should be warned of the possibility of depression. If signs of despondency, early morning insomnia, loss of appetite, impotence, or self-deprecation appear, the drug should be discontinued and the physician consulted.

Patients who engage in potentially hazardous activities such as operating machinery or driving motor vehicles should be warned about possible central nervous system (CNS) side effects.

The physician should inform patients of other possible side effects and advise patients to take this medication every day as directed.

Concomitant use of alcohol with Deserpidine may cause additive CNS-depressant effects.

Drug Interactions: Use Deserpidine cautiously with *digitalis* and *quinidine* since cardiac arrhythmias have occurred with rauwolfia preparations.

Hypotensive effects of rauwolfia alkaloids may be enhanced when used concurrently with other *antihypertensive agents, diuretics,* or *phenothiazine derivatives,* therefore, careful titration of dosage is necessary.

Additive CNS-depressant effects can occur when rauwolfia alkaloids are taken concomitantly with other CNS-*depressant agents* or *alcohol.*

Monoamine oxidase inhibitors should be avoided or used with extreme caution.

Drug/Laboratory Test Interactions: Rauwolfia alkaloids have been reported to interfere with assay procedures for the determination of urinary 17-hydroxycorticosteroids and 17-ketosteroids.

Carcinogenesis, Mutagenesis, Impairment of Fertility: No long-term Deserpidine data are available concerning the potential for carcinogenicity. Adequate studies for determination of mutagenic potential of Deserpidine and its effects on fertility have not been done.

Animal Tumorigenicity: Although there are no studies demonstrating that Deserpidine is an animal tumorigen, it is a prolactin stimulator and structurally related to reserpine. Rodent studies have shown that reserpine is an animal

tumorigen, causing an increased incidence of mammary fibroadenomas in female mice, malignant tumors of the seminal vesicles in male mice, and malignant adrenal medulary tumors in male rats. These findings rose in 2 year studies in which the drug was administrered in the feed at concentrations of 5 and 10 ppm — about 100 to 300 times the usual human dose. The breast neoplasms are thought to be related to reserpine's prolactin-elevating effect. Several other prolactin-elevating drugs have also been associated with an increased incidence of mammary neoplasia in rodents.

The extent to which these findings indicate a risk to humans is uncertain. Tissue culture experiments show that about one-third of human breast tumors are prolactin-dependent *in vitro,* a factor of considerable importance if the use of the drug is contemplated in a patient with previously detected breast cancer. The possibility of an increased risk of breast cancer in reserpine users has been studied extensively; however, no firm conclusion has emerged. Although a few epidemiologic studies have suggested a slightly increased risk (less than twofold in all studies except one) in women who have used reserpine, other studies of generally similar design have not confirmed this. Epidemiologic studies conducted using other drugs (neuroleptic agents) that, like reserpine, increase prolactin levels and, therefore, would be considered rodent mammary carcinogens, have not shown an association between chronic administration of the drug and human mammary tumorigenesis. While long-term clinical observation has not suggested such an association, the available evidence is considered too limited to be conclusive at this time. An association of reserpine intake with pheochromocytoma or tumors of the seminal vesicles has not been explored.

Pregnancy Category C: Animal reproduction studies have not been conducted with Deserpidine. It is also not known whether Deserpidine can cause fetal harm when administered to a pregnant woman or can affect reproduction capacity. Deserpidine should be given to a pregnant woman only if clearly needed.

Nonteratogenic Effects: Rauwolfia alkaloids are known to cross the placental barrier, to enter the fetal circulation, and to appear in cord blood. Increased respiratory secretions, nasal congestion, cyanosis, and anorexia may occur in neonates of rauwolfia alkaloid-treated mothers.

Nursing Mothers: Deserpidine is excreted in human milk. Because of the potential for serious adverse reactions in nursing infants from Deserpidine, a decision should be made whether to discontinue nursing or to discontinue the drug, taking into account the importance of the drug to the mother.

Pediatric Use: Safety and effectiveness in children have not been established.

ADVERSE REACTIONS

The following adverse reactions have been observed with rauwolfia preparations, but there has not been enough systematic collection of data to support an estimate of their frequency. Consequently the reactions are categorized by organ system and are listed in decreasing order of severity and not frequency.

Body as a Whole: Headache.

Cardiovascular System: Arrhythmias (particularly when used concurrently with digitalis or quinidine), syncope, angina-like symptoms, bradycardia, fluid retention.

Digestive System: Vomiting, diarrhea, nausea, anorexia, dryness of mouth, hypersecretion, increased motility, increased salivation.

Hemic and Lymphatic System: Thrombocytopenic purpura.

Metabolic and Nutritional Disorders: Weight gain.

Musculoskeletal System: Muscular aches.

Nervous System: Rare parkinsonian syndrome and other extrapyramidal tract symptoms, dizziness, paradoxical anxiety, depression, nervousness, nightmares, dull sensorium, drowsiness, decreased libido.

Respiratory System: Asthma in asthmatic patients, dyspnea, epistaxis, nasal congestion.

Skin and Appendages: Rash, pruritus, flushing of skin.

Special Senses: Deafness, optic atropy, glaucoma, uveitis, conjunctival injection.

Urogenital System: Nonpuerperal lactation, impotence, dysuria, gynecomastia, breast engorgement.

OVERDOSAGE

An overdosage of Deserpidine is characterized by flushing of the skin, conjunctival injection, and pupillary constriction. Sedation ranging from drowsiness to coma may occur. Hypotension, hypothermia, central respiratory depression and bradycardia may develop in cases of severe overdosage.

Treatment consists of the careful evacuation of stomach contents followed by the usual procedures for the symptomatic management of CNS depressant overdosage. If severe hypotension occurs, it should be treated with a direct-acting vasopressor (e.g., norepinephrine). If bradycardia becomes marked, especially with cardiac arrhythmia, consider use of atropine or other anticholinergic drug. Because of prolonged effects of Deserpidine, the patient should be closely observed for at least 72 hours.

DOSAGE AND ADMINISTRATION

Deserpidine is administered orally. For the management of mild essential hypertension in the average patient not receiving other antihypertensive agents, the usual initial adult dose is 0.75 to 1 mg daily. Debilitated and elderly patients may require lower doses. Because 10 to 14 days are required to produce the full effects of the drug, adjustments in dosage should not be made more frequently. If the therapeutic response is not adequate, it is generally advisable to add another antihypertensive agent to the regimen. For maintenance, dosage should be reduced. A single daily dose of 0.25 mg of Deserpidine may suffice for some patients.

Concomitant use of Deserpidine with ganglionic blocking agents, guanethidine, veratrum, hydralazine, methyldopa, chlorthalidone, or thiazides necessitates careful titration of dosage with each agent.

For Psychiatric Disorders: The average initial oral dose is 0.5 mg daily with a range of 0.125 to 1 mg. Adjust dosage upward or downward according to the patient's response.

Recommended Storage: Store at controlled room temperature 59°—86°F (15°—30°C).

HOW SUPPLIED
TABLETS: 0.25 MG

BRAND/MANUFACTURER	NDC	SIZE	AWP
○ **BRAND**			
HARMONYL: Abbott Pharm	00074-6906-07	100s	$17.61

Deserpidine and Hydrochlorothiazide

> **WARNING:**
> THIS FIXED COMBINATION DRUG IS NOT INDICATED FOR INITIAL THERAPY OF HYPERTENSION. HYPERTENSION REQUIRES THERAPY TITRATED TO THE INDIVIDUAL PATIENT. IF THE FIXED COMBINATION REPRESENTS THE DOSAGE SO DETERMINED, ITS USE MAY BE MORE CONVENIENT IN PATIENT MANAGEMENT. THE TREATMENT OF HYPERTENSION IS NOT STATIC, BUT MUST BE REEVALUATED AS CONDITIONS IN EACH PATIENT WARRANT.

DESCRIPTION
Deserpidine/Hydrochlorothiazide tablets are an orally administered combination of Hydrochlorothiazide and Deserpidine. Hydrochlorothiazide is a diuretic-antihypertensive agent of the benzothiadiazine (thiazide) class. Deserpidine is a purified rauwolfia alkaloid, chemically identified as 11-desmethoxyreserpine, which produces antihypertensive effects.

ACTIONS
The combined antihypertensive actions of Hydrochlorothiazide and Deserpidine result in a total clinical antihypertensive effect which is greater than can ordinarily be achieved by either drug given individually.

The diuretic and saluretic effects of Hydrochlorothiazide result from a drug-induced inhibition of the renal tubular reabsorption of electrolytes. The excretion of sodium and chloride is greatly enhanced. Potassium excretion is also enhanced to a variable degree, as it is with the other thiazides. Although urinary excretion of bicarbonate is increased slightly, there is usually no significant change in urinary pH. Hydrochlorothiazide has a per mg natriuretic activity approximately 10 times that of the prototype thiazide, chlorothiazide. At maximal therapeutic dosages, all thiazides are approximately equal in their diuretic/natriuretic effects.

There is significant natriuresis and diuresis within two hours after administration of a single oral dose of Hydrochlorothiazide. These effects reach a peak in about 6 hours and persist for about 12 hours following oral administration of a single dose.

Like other benzothiadiazines, Hydrochlorothiazide also has antihypertensive properties, and may be used for this purpose either alone or to enhance the antihypertensive action of other drugs. The mechanism by which the benzothiadiazines, including Hydrochlorothiazide, produce a reduction of elevated blood pressure is not known. However, sodium depletion appears to be involved.

Hydrochlorothiazide is readily absorbed from the gastrointestinal tract and is excreted unchanged by the kidneys.

The pharmacologic actions of Deserpidine are essentially the same as those of other active rauwolfia alkaloids. Deserpidine probably produces its antihypertensive effects through depletion of tissue stores of catecholamines (epinephrine and norepinephrine) from peripheral sites. The antihypertensive effect is often accompanied by bradycardia. There is no significant alteration in cardiac output or renal blood flow. The carotid sinus reflex is inhibited, but postural hypotension is rarely seen with the use of conventional doses of Deserpidine alone.

Deserpidine, like other rauwolfia alkaloids, is characterized by slow onset of action and sustained effect which may persist following withdrawal of the drug.

INDICATIONS
Hydrochlorothiazide and Deserpidine is indicated in the treatment of patients with mild to moderately severe hypertension (see boxed warning). It may be used alone for this purpose or added to other antihypertensive agents for the management of more severe hypertension. When administered with Deserpidine/Hydrochlorothiazide tablets, more potent agents can be given at reduced dosage to minimize undesirable side effects.

CONTRAINDICATIONS
Hydrochlorothiazide is contraindicated in patients with renal decompensation and in those who are hypersensitive to this or other sulfonamide-derived drugs.

Deserpidine is contraindicated in patients with known hypersensitivity, history of mental depression especially with suicidal tendencies, active peptic ulcer, and ulcerative colitis. It is also contraindicated in patients receiving electroconvulsive therapy.

WARNINGS
HYDROCHLOROTHIAZIDE
Hydrochlorothiazide shares with other thiazides the propensity to deplete potassium reserves to an unpredictable degree.

Thiazides should be used with caution in patients with renal disease or significant impairment of renal function, since azotemia may be precipitated and cumulative drug effects may occur.

Thiazides should be used with caution in patients with impaired hepatic function or progressive liver disease, since minor alterations of fluid and electrolyte balance may precipitate hepatic coma.

Thiazides may be additive or potentiative of the action of other antihypertensive drugs. Potentiation occurs with ganglionic or peripheral adrenergic blocking drugs.

Sensitivity reactions may occur in patients with a history of allergy or bronchial asthma.

The possibility of exacerbation or activation of systemic lupus erythematosus has been reported.

DESERPIDINE
Deserpidine differs slightly in chemical structure from reserpine, however, its actions, indications, cautions and adverse reactions are common to the class of rauwolfia alkaloids. Reserpine may cause mental depression. Recognition of depression may be difficult because this condition may often be disguised by somatic complaints (masked depression). The drug should be discontinued at first signs of depression such as despondency, early morning insomnia, loss of appetite, impotence, or self-deprecation. Drug-induced depression may persist for several months after drug withdrawal and may be severe enough to result in suicide.

USAGE IN PREGNANCY AND LACTATION
HYDROCHLOROTHIAZIDE
Thiazides cross the placental barrier and appear in cord blood. The use of thiazides in pregnant women requires that the anticipated benefit be weighed against possible hazards to the fetus. These hazards include fetal or neonatal jaundice, thrombocytopenia, and possible other adverse reactions that have occurred in the adult.

Thiazides appear in breast milk. If use of the drug is deemed essential, the patient should stop nursing.

DESERPIDINE
The safety of Deserpidine for use during pregnancy or lactation has not been established; therefore, it should be used in pregnant women or in women of childbearing potential only when in the judgment of the physician its use is deemed essential to the welfare of the patient. Increased respiratory secretions, nasal congestion, cyanosis, and anorexia may occur in infants born to rauwolfia alkaloid-treated mothers, since these preparations are known to cross the placental barrier to enter the fetal circulation and appear in cord blood. They also are secreted by nursing mothers into breast milk.

Reproductive and teratology studies in rats reduced the mating index and neonatal survival indices; the no-effect dosage has not been established.

PRECAUTIONS
Periodic determinations of serum electrolytes should be performed at appropriate intervals for the purpose of detecting possible electrolyte imbalances such as hyponatremia, hypochloremic alkalosis, and hypokalemia. Serum and urine electrolyte determinations are particularly important when a patient is vomiting excessively or receiving parenteral fluids. All patients should be observed for other clinical signs of electrolyte imbalances such as dryness of mouth, thirst, weakness, lethargy, drowsiness, restlessness, muscle pains or cramps, muscular fatigue, hypotension, oliguria, tachycardia, and gastrointestinal disturbances such as nausea and vomiting.

Hypokalemia may develop with thiazides as with any other potent diuretic, especially when brisk diuresis occurs, severe cirrhosis is present, or when corticosteroids or ACTH are given concomitantly. Interference with the adequate oral intake of electrolytes will also contribute to the possible development of hypokalemia. Potassium depletion, even of a mild degree, resulting from thiazide use, may sensitize a patient to the effects of cardiac glycosides such as digitalis.

Any chloride deficit is generally mild and usually does not require specific treatment except under extraordinary circumstances (as in liver disease or renal disease). Dilutional hyponatremia may occur in edematous patients in hot weather; appropriate therapy is water restriction rather than administration of salt, except in rare instances when the hyponatremia is life threatening.

In actual salt depletion, appropriate replacement is the therapy of choice.

Hyperuricemia may occur or frank gout may be precipitated in certain patients receiving thiazide therapy.

Insulin requirements in diabetic patients may be increased, decreased, or unchanged. Latent diabetes mellitus may become manifest during thiazide administration.

Thiazide drugs may increase the responsiveness to tubocurarine.

◆ RATED THERAPEUTICALLY EQUIVALENT; ◇ THERAPEUTIC EQUIVALENCE UNCONFIRMED; ○ UNRATED

The antihypertensive effects of the drug may be enhanced in the postsympathectomy patient.

Thiazides may decrease arterial responsiveness to norepinephrine. This diminution is not sufficient to preclude effectiveness of the pressor agent for therapeutic use.

If progressive renal impairment becomes evident as indicated by a rising nonprotein nitrogen or blood urea nitrogen, a careful reappraisal of therapy is necessary with consideration given to withholding or discontinuing diuretic therapy.

Thiazides may decrease serum protein bound iodine levels without signs of thyroid disturbance.

Thiazides have been reported, on rare occasions, to have elevated serum calcium to hypercalcemic levels. The serum calcium levels have returned to normal when the medication has been stopped. This phenomenon may be related to the ability of the thiazide diuretics to lower the amount of calcium excreted in the urine.

Because rauwolfia preparations increase gastrointestinal motility and secretion, this drug should be used cautiously in patients with a history of peptic ulcer, ulcerative colitis, or gallstones, where biliary colic may be precipitated.

Caution should be exercised when treating hypertensive patients with renal insufficiency since they adjust poorly to lowered blood pressure levels.

Use Deserpidine cautiously with digitalis and quinidine since cardiac arrhythmias have occurred with rauwolfia preparations.

Preoperative withdrawal of Deserpidine does not assure that circulatory instability will not occur. It is important that the anesthesiologist be aware of the patient's drug intake and consider this in the overall management, since hypotension has occurred in patients receiving rauwolfia preparations. Anticholinergic and/or adrenergic drugs (metaraminol, norepinephrine) have been employed to treat adverse vagocirculatory effects.

Animal Tumorigenicity: There are no studies demonstrating that Deserpidine is an animal tumorigen, although it is a prolactin stimulator and structurally related to reserpine. Rodent studies with reserpine, however, have shown that reserpine is an animal tumorigen, causing an increased incidence of mammary fibroadenomas in female mice, malignant tumors of the seminal vesicles in male mice, and malignant adrenal medullary tumors in male rats. These findings arose in 2 year studies in which the drug was administered in the feed at concentrations of 5 and 10 ppm-about 100 to 300 times the usual human dose. The breast neoplasms are thought to be related to reserpine's prolactin-elevating effect. Several other prolactin-elevating drugs have also been associated with an increased incidence of mammary neoplasia in rodents.

The extent to which these findings indicate a risk to humans is uncertain. Tissue culture experiments show that about one-third of human breast tumors are prolactin-dependent *in vitro,* a factor of considerable importance if the use of the drug is contemplated in a patient with previously detected breast cancer. The possibility of an increased risk of breast cancer in reserpine users has been studied extensively; however, no firm conclusion has emerged. Although a few epidemiologic studies have suggested a slightly increased risk (less than twofold in all studies except one) in women who have used reserpine, other studies of generally similar design have not confirmed this. Epidemiologic studies conducted using other drugs (neuroleptic agents) that, like reserpine, increase prolactin levels and, therefore, would be considered rodent mammary carcinogens, have not shown an association between chronic administration of the drug and human mammary tumorigenesis. While long-term clinical observation has not suggested such an association, the available evidence is considered too limited to be conclusive at this time. An association of reserpine intake with pheochromocytoma or tumors of the seminal vesicles has not been explored.

ADVERSE REACTIONS

HYDROCHLOROTHIAZIDE

Gastrointestinal System Reactions: Anorexia, gastric irritation, nausea, vomiting, cramping, diarrhea, constipation, jaundice (intrahepatic cholestatic jaundice), pancreatitis.

Central Nervous System Reactions: Dizziness, vertigo, paresthesias, headache, xanthopsia.

Hematologic Reactions: Leukopenia, agranulocytosis, thrombocytopenia, aplastic anemia.

Dermatologic - Hypersensitivity Reactions: Purpura, photosensitivity, rash, urticaria, necrotizing angiitis (vasculitis) (cutaneous vasculitis).

Cardiovascular Reaction: Orthostatic hypotension may occur and may be aggravated by alcohol, barbiturates, or narcotics.

Other: Hyperglycemia, glycosuria, hypercalcemia, hyperuricemia, muscle spasm, weakness, restlessness, respiratory distress including pneumonitis and pulmonary edema.

There have been isolated reports that certain nonedematous individuals developed severe fluid and electrolyte derangements after only brief exposure to normal doses of thiazide and non-thiazide diuretics. The condition is usually manifested as severe dilutional hyponatremia, hypokalemia, and hypochloremia. It has been reported to be due to inappropriately increased ADH secretion and appears to be idiosyncratic. Potassium replacement is apparently the most important therapy in the treatment of this syndrome along with removal of the offending drug.

Whenever adverse reactions are severe, treatment should be discontinued.

DESERPIDINE

The following adverse reactions have been reported with rauwolfia preparations. These reactions are usually reversible and disappear when the drug is discontinued.

Gastrointestinal: Including hypersecretion, anorexia, diarrhea, nausea, and vomiting.

Cardiovascular: Including angina-like symptoms, arrhythmias (particularly when used concurrently with digitalis or quinidine), and bradycardia.

Central Nervous System: Including drowsiness, depression, nervousness, paradoxical anxiety, nightmares, extrapyramidal tract symptoms, CNS sensitization manifested by dull sensorium, and deafness.

Dermatologic - Hypersensitivity: Including pruritus, rash, and asthma in asthmatic patients.

Ophthalmologic: Including glaucoma, uveitis, optic atrophy, and conjunctival injection.

Hematologic: Thrombocytopenic purpura.

Miscellaneous: Nasal congestion, weight gain, impotence or decreased libido, dysuria, dyspnea, muscular aches, dryness of mouth, dizziness, and headache.

OVERDOSAGE

Symptoms of thiazide overdosage include electrolyte imbalance and signs of potassium deficiency such as confusion, dizziness, muscular weakness, and gastrointestinal disturbances. General supportive measures including replacement of fluids and electrolytes may be indicated in treatment of overdosage.

An overdosage of Deserpidine is characterized by flushing of the skin, conjunctival injection, and pupillary constriction. Sedation ranging from drowsiness to coma may occur. Hypotension, hypothermia, central respiratory depression and bradycardia may develop in cases of severe overdosage. Treatment consists of the careful evacuation of stomach contents followed by the usual procedures for the symptomatic management of CNS depressant overdosage. If severe hypotension occurs it should be treated with a direct acting vasopressor such as norepinephrine bitartrate injection.

DOSAGE AND ADMINISTRATION

Dosage should be determined by individual titration of ingredients (see boxed warning). Dosage of both components should be carefully adjusted to the needs of the individual patients. Since at least 10 days to 2 weeks may elapse before the full effects of the drugs become manifest, the dosage should not be adjusted more frequently.

Three tablet strengths, Hydrochlorothiazide 25 mg, Deserpidine 0.125 mg; Hydrochlorothiazide 50 mg, Deserpidine 0.125 mg; and Hydrochlorothiazide 25 mg, Deserpidine 0.25 mg, all grooved, are provided to permit considerable latitude in meeting the dosage requirements of individual patients.

The table below will help in determining which dose of Deserpidine/Hydrochlorothiazide best represents the equivalent of the titrated dose.

	Hydro-chlorothiazide	Deserpidine
1 tablet bid	25.0 mg bid	0.125 mg bid
1 1/2 tablet bid	37.5 mg bid	0.188 mg bid
2 tablets bid	50.0 mg bid	0.250 mg bid

	Hydro-chlorothiazide	Deserpidine
1 tablet bid	50 mg bid	0.125 mg bid
1 1/2 tablet bid	75 mg bid	0.188 mg bid
2 tablets bid	100 mg bid	0.250 mg bid

	Hydro-chlorothiazide	Deserpidine
1 tablet bid	25.0 mg bid	0.250 mg bid
1 1/2 tablet bid	37.5 mg bid	0.375 mg bid
2 tablets bid	50.0 mg bid	0.500 mg bid

The usual adult dosage is one Deserpidine/Hydrochlorothiazide (50 mg) tablet two times daily.

When other antihypertensive agents are to be added to the regimen, this should be accomplished gradually. Ganglionic blocking agents should be given at only half the usual dose since their effect is potentiated by pretreatment with Hydrochlorothiazide and Deserpidine. Store below 86°F (30°C).

► SHOWN IN PRODUCT IDENTIFICATION GUIDE

HOW SUPPLIED
TABLETS:

BRAND/MANUFACTURER	NDC	SIZE	AWP
○ **BRAND**			
ORETICYL 25: Abbott Pharm	00074-6922-01	100s	$24.74
ORETICYL FORTE: Abbott Pharm	00074-6927-01	100s	$34.75
ORETICYL 50: Abbott Pharm	00074-6931-01	100s	$36.74

Deserpidine and Methyclothiazide

> **WARNING**
> THIS FIXED COMBINATION DRUG IS NOT INDICATED FOR INITIAL THERAPY OF HYPERTENSION. HYPERTENSION REQUIRES THERAPY TITRATED TO THE INDIVIDUAL PATIENT. IF THE FIXED COMBINATION REPRESENTS THE DOSAGE SO DETERMINED, ITS USE MAY BE MORE CONVENIENT IN PATIENT MANAGEMENT. THE TREATMENT OF HYPERTENSION IS NOT STATIC, BUT MUST BE REEVALUATED AS CONDITIONS IN EACH PATIENT WARRANT.

DESCRIPTION
Deserpidine/Methyclothiazide is an orally-administered combination of Methyclothiazide and Deserpidine. Methylclothiazide is an oral diuretic-antihypertensive of the benzothiadiazine (thiazide) class. Deserpidine is a purified rauwolfia alkaloid, chemically identified as 11-desmethoxyreserpine, which produces antihypertensive effects.

ACTIONS
The combined antihypertensive actions of Methyclothiazide and Deserpidine result in a total clinical antihypertensive effect which is greater than can ordinarily be achieved by either drug given individually.

The diuretic and saluretic effects of Methyclothiazide result from a drug-induced inhibition of the renal tubular reabsorption of electrolytes. The excretion of sodium and chloride is greatly enhanced. Potassium excretion is also enhanced to a variable degree, as it is with the other thiazides. Although urinary excretion of bicarbonate is increased slightly, there is usually no significant change in urinary pH. Methyclothiazide has a per mg natriuretic activity approximately 100 times that of the prototype thiazide, chlorothiazide. At maximal therapeutic dosages, all thiazides are approximately equal in their diuretic/natriuretic effects.

There is significant natriuresis and diuresis within two hours after administration of a single dose of Methyclothiazide. These effects reach a peak in about six hours and persist for 24 hours following oral administration of a single dose.

Like other benzothiadiazines, Methyclothiazide also has antihypertensive properties, and may be used for this purpose either alone or to enhance the antihypertensive action of other drugs. The mechanism by which the benzothiadiazines, including Methyclothiazide, produce a reduction of elevated blood pressure is not known. However, sodium depletion appears to be involved.

Methyclothiazide is rapidly absorbed and slowly eliminated by the kidney as both intact drug and as a metabolite showing no diuretic activity in a rat model.

The pharmacologic actions of Deserpidine are essentially the same as those of other active rauwolfia alkaloids. Deserpidine probably produces its antihypertensive effects through depletion of tissue stores of catecholamines (epinephrine and norepinephrine) from peripheral sites. The antihypertensive effect is often accompanied by bradycardia. There is no significant alteration in cardiac output or renal blood flow. The carotid sinus reflex is inhibited, but postural hypotension is rarely seen with the use of conventional doses of Deserpidine alone.

Deserpidine, like other rauwolfia alkaloids, is characterized by slow onset of action and sustained effect which may persist following withdrawal of the drug.

INDICATIONS
Deserpidine/Methyclothiazide is indicated in the treatment of mild to moderately severe hypertension (see boxed warning). In many cases Deserpidine/Methyclothiazide alone produces an adequate reduction of blood pressure. In resistant or unusually severe cases Deserpidine/Methyclothiazide also may be supplemented by more potent antihypertensive agents. When administered with Deserpidine/Methyclothiazide, more potent agents can be given at reduced dosage to minimize undesirable side effects.

CONTRAINDICATIONS
Methyclothiazide is contraindicated in patients with renal decompensation and in those who are hypersensitive to this or other sulfonamide-derived drugs.

Deserpidine is contraindicated in patients with known hypersensitivity, history of mental depression especially with suicidal tendencies, active peptic ulcer, and ulcerative colitis. It is also contraindicated in patients receiving electroconvulsive therapy.

WARNINGS
Methyclothiazide: Methyclothiazide shares with other thiazides the propensity to deplete potassium reserves to an unpredictable degree.

Thiazides should be used with caution in patients with renal disease or significant impairment of renal function, since azotemia may be precipitated and cumulative drug effects may occur.

Thiazides should be used with caution in patients with impaired hepatic function or progressive liver disease, since minor alterations of fluid and electrolyte balance may precipitate hepatic coma.

Thiazides may be additive or potentiative of the action of other antihypertensive drugs. Potentiation occurs with ganglionic or peripheral adrenergic blocking drugs.

Sensitivity reactions may occur in patients with a history of allergy or bronchial asthma.

The possibility of exacerbation or activation of systemic lupus erythematosus has been reported.

Deserpidine: Deserpidine differs slightly in chemical structure from reserpine, however, its actions, indications, cautions and adverse reactions are common to the class of rauwolfia alkaloids. Reserpine may cause mental depression. Recognition of depression may be difficult because this condition may often be disguised by somatic complaints (Masked Depression). The drug should be discontinued at first signs of depression such as despondency, early morning insomnia, loss of appetite, impotence, or self-deprecation. Drug-induced depression may persist for several months after drug withdrawal and may be severe enough to result in suicide.

USAGE IN PREGNANCY AND LACTATION
Methyclothiazide: Thiazides cross the placental barrier and appear in cord blood. The use of thiazides in pregnant women requires that the anticipated benefit be weighed against possible hazards to the fetus. These hazards include fetal or neonatal jaundice, thrombocytopenia, and possible other adverse reactions that have occurred in the adult.

Thiazides appear in breast milk. If use of the drug is deemed essential, the patient should stop nursing.

Deserpidine: The safety of Deserpidine for use during pregnancy or lactation has not been established; therefore, it should be used in pregnant women or in women of childbearing potential only when in the judgment of the physician its use is deemed essential to the welfare of the patient. Increased respiratory secretions, nasal congestion, cyanosis, and anorexia may occur in infants born to rauwolfia alkaloid-treated mothers, since these preparations are known to cross the placental barrier to enter the fetal circulation and appear in cord blood. They also are secreted by nursing mothers into breast milk.

Reproductive and teratology studies in rats reduced the mating index and neonatal survival indices; the no-effect dosage has not been established.

PRECAUTIONS
Periodic determinations of serum electrolytes should be performed at appropriate intervals for the purpose of detecting possible electrolyte imbalances such as hyponatremia, hypochloremic alkalosis, and hypokalemia. Serum and urine electrolyte determinations are particularly important when a patient is vomiting excessively or receiving parenteral fluids. All patients should be observed for other clinical signs of electrolyte imbalances such as dryness of mouth, thirst, weakness, lethargy, drowsiness, restlessness, muscle pains or cramps, muscular fatigue, hypotension, oliguria, tachycardia, and gastrointestinal disturbances such as nausea and vomiting.

Hypokalemia may develop with thiazides as with any other potent diuretic, especially when brisk diuresis occurs, severe cirrhosis is present, or when corticosteroids or ACTH are given concomitantly. Interference with the adequate oral intake of electrolytes will also contribute to the possible development of hypokalemia. Potassium depletion, even of a mild degree, resulting from thiazide use, may sensitize a patient to the effects of cardiac glycosides such as digitalis.

Any chloride deficit is generally mild and usually does not require specific treatment except under extraordinary circumstances (as in liver disease or renal disease). Dilutional hyponatremia may occur in edematous patients in hot weather; appropriate therapy is water restriction rather than administration of salt, except in rare instances when the hyponatremia is life threatening.

In actual salt depletion, appropriate replacement is the therapy of choice.

Hyperuricemia may occur or frank gout may be precipitated in certain patients receiving thiazide therapy.

Insulin requirements in diabetic patients may be increased, decreased, or unchanged. Latent diabetes mellitus may become manifest during thiazide administration.

Thiazide drugs may increase the responsiveness to tubocurarine.

The antihypertensive effects of the drug may be enhanced in the postsympathectomy patient.

Thiazides may decrease arterial responsiveness to norepinephrine. This diminution is not sufficient to preclude effectiveness of the pressor agent for therapeutic use.

If progressive renal impairment becomes evident as indicated by a rising-nonprotein nitrogen or blood urea nitrogen, a careful reappraisal of therapy is necessary with consideration given to withholding or discontinuing diuretic therapy.

Thiazides may decrease serum PBI levels without signs of thyroid disturbance.

Thiazides have been reported, on rare occasions, to have elevated serum calcium to hypercalcemic levels. The serum calcium levels have returned to normal when the medication has been stopped. This phenomenon may be related to the ability of the thiazide diuretics to lower the amount of calcium excreted in the urine.

Because rauwolfia preparations increase gastrointestinal motility and secretion, this drug should be used cautiously in patients with a history of peptic ulcer, ulcerative colitis, or gallstones, where biliary colic may be precipitated.

◆ RATED THERAPEUTICALLY EQUIVALENT; ◇ THERAPEUTIC EQUIVALENCE UNCONFIRMED; ○ UNRATED

Caution should be exercised when treating hypertensive patients with renal insufficiency since they adjust poorly to lowered blood pressure levels.

Use Deserpidine cautiously with digitalis and quinidine since cardiac arrhythmias have occurred with rauwolfia preparations.

Preoperative withdrawal of Deserpidine does not assure that circulatory instability will not occur. It is important that the anesthesiologist be aware of the patient's drug intake and consider this in the overall management, since hypotension has occurred in patients receiving rauwolfia preparations. Anticholinergic and/or adrenergic drugs (metaraminol, norepinephrine) have been employed to treat adverse vagocirculatory effects.

Animal Tumorigenicity: There are no studies demonstrating that Deserpidine is an animal tumorigen, although it is a prolactin stimulator and structurally related to reserpine. Rodent studies with reserpine, however, have shown that reserpine is an animal tumorigen, causing an increased incidence of mammary fibroadenomas in female mice, malignant tumors of the seminal vesicles in male mice, and malignant adrenal medullary tumors in male rats. These findings arose in 2 year studies in which the drug was administered in the feed at concentrations of 5 and 10 ppm - about 100 to 300 times the usual human dose. The breast neoplasms are thought to be related to reserpine's prolactin-elevating effect. Several other prolactin-elevating drugs have also been associated with an increased incidence of mammary neoplasia in rodents.

The extent to which these findings indicate a risk to humans is uncertain. Tissue culture experiments show that about one-third of human breast tumors are prolactin-dependent *in vitro*, a factor of considerable importance if the use of the drug is contemplated in a patient with previously detected breast cancer. The possibility of an increased risk of breast cancer in reserpine users has been studied extensively; however, no firm conclusion has emerged. Although a few epidemiologic studies have suggested a slightly increased risk (less than twofold in all studies except one) in women who have used reserpine, other studies of generally similar design have not confirmed this. Epidemiologic studies conducted using other drugs (neuroleptic agents) that, like reserpine, increase prolactin levels and, therefore, would be considered rodent mammary carcinogens, have not shown an association between chronic administration of the drug and human mammary tumorigenesis. While long-term clinical observation has not suggested such an association, the available evidence is considered too limited to be conclusive at this time. An association of reserpine intake with pheochromocytoma or tumors of the seminal vesicles has not been explored.

ADVERSE REACTIONS
METHYCLOTHIAZIDE
Gastrointestinal System Reactions: Anorexia, gastric irritation, nausea, vomiting, cramping, diarrhea, constipation, jaundice (intrahepatic cholestatic jaundice), pancreatitis.

Central Nervous System Reactions: Dizziness, vertigo, paresthesias, headache, xanthopsia.

Hematologic Reactions: Leukopenia, agranulocytosis, thrombocytopenia, aplastic anemia.

Dermatologic—Hypersensitivity Reactions: Purpura, photosensitivity, rash, urticaria, necrotizing angiitis (vasculitis) (cutaneous vasculitis).

Cardiovascular Reaction: Orthostatic hypotension may occur and may be aggravated by alcohol, barbiturates, or narcotics.

Other: Hyperglycemia, glycosuria, hypercalcemia, hyperuricemia, muscle spasm, weakness, restlessness.

There have been isolated reports that certain nonedematous individuals developed severe fluid and electrolyte derangements after only brief exposure to normal doses of thiazide and non-thiazide diuretics. The condition is usually manifested as severe dilutional hyponatremia, hypokalemia, and hypochloremia. It has been reported to be due to inappropriately increased ADH secretion and appears to be idiosyncratic. Potassium replacement is apparently the most important therapy in the treatment of this syndrome along with removal of the offending drug.

Whenever adverse reactions are severe, treatment should be discontinued.

DESERPIDINE
The following adverse reactions have been reported with rauwolfia preparations. These reactions are usually reversible and disappear when the drug is discontinued.

Gastrointestinal: Including hypersecretion, anorexia, diarrhea, nausea, and vomiting.

Cardiovascular: Including angina-like symptoms, arrhythmias (particularly when used concurrently with digitalis or quinidine), and bradycardia.

Central Nervous System: Including drowsiness, depression, nervousness, paradoxical anxiety, nightmares, extrapyramidal tract symptoms, CNS sensitization manifested by dull sensorium, and deafness.

Dermatologic—Hypersensitivity: Including pruritus, rash, and asthma in asthmatic patients.

Ophthalmologic: Including glaucoma, uveitis, optic atrophy, and conjunctival injection.

Hematologic: Thrombocytopenic purpura.

Miscellaneous: Nasal congestion, weight gain, impotence or decreased libido, dysuria, dyspnea, muscular aches, dryness of mouth, dizziness, and headache.

DOSAGE AND ADMINISTRATION
Dosage should be determined by individual titration of ingredients (see boxed warning). Dosage of both components should be carefully adjusted to the needs of the individual patient. Since at least ten days to two weeks may elapse before the full effects of the drugs become manifest, the dosage of the drugs should not be adjusted more frequently.

Two tablet strengths, Deserpidine 0.25mg/Methyclothiazide 5mg and Deserpidine 0.5mg/Methyclothiazide 5mg each grooved, are provided to permit considerable latitude in meeting the dosage requirements of individual patients.

The following table will help in determining which dose of Deserpidine 0.25mg/Methyclothiazide 5mg or Deserpidine 0.5mg/Methyclothiazide 5mg best represents the equivalent of the titrated dose.

Daily Dosage of Deserpidine 0.25mg/ Methyclothiazide 5mg	Methyclothiazide	Deserpidine
½ tablet	2.5 mg	0.125 mg
1 tablet	5.0 mg	0.250 mg
1 ½ tablets	7.5 mg	0.375 mg
2 tablets	10.0 mg	0.500 mg

Daily Dosage of Deserpidine 0.5mg/ Methyclothiazide 5mg	Methyclothiazide	Deserpidine
½ tablet	2.5 mg	0.250 mg
1 tablet	5.0 mg	0.500 mg
1 ½ tablets	7.5 mg	0.750 mg
2 tablets	10.0 mg	1.000 mg

The appropriate dose of Deserpidine/Methyclothiazide is administered orally, once daily. The usual adult dosage is one lower-strength Deserpidine/Methyclothiazide tablet daily.

There is no contraindication to combining the administration of Deserpidine/Methyclothiazide with other antihypertensive agents. When other antihypertensive agents are to be added to the regimen, this should be accomplished gradually. Ganglionic blocking agents should be given at only half the usual dose since their effect is potentiated by pretreatment with Deserpidine/Methyclothiazide.

Store below 86°F (30°C).

OVERDOSAGE
Symptoms of thiazide overdosage include electrolyte imbalance and signs of potassium deficiency such as confusion, dizziness, muscular weakness and gastrointestinal disturbances. General supportive measures including replacement of fluids and electrolytes may be indicated in treatment of overdosage.

An overdosage of Deserpidine is characterized by flushing of the skin, conjunctival injection and pupillary constriction. Sedation ranging from drowsiness to coma may occur. Hypotension, hypothermia, central respiratory depression and bradycardia may develop in cases of severe overdosage. Treatment consists of the careful evacuation of stomach contents followed by the usual procedures for the symptomatic management of CNS depressant overdosage. If severe hypotension occurs it should be treated with a direct acting vasopressor such as norepinephrine bitartrate injection.

HOW SUPPLIED
TABLETS: 0.25 MG-5 MG

BRAND/MANUFACTURER	NDC	SIZE	AWP
◇ **BRAND**			
ENDURONYL: Abbott Pharm	00074-6838-01	100s	$113.63
	00074-6838-06	100s ud	$121.48
	00074-6838-02	1000s	$1102.13

TABLETS: 0.5 MG-5 MG

BRAND/MANUFACTURER	NDC	SIZE	AWP
◇ **BRAND**			
ENDURONYL FORTE: Abbott Pharm	00074-6854-01	100s	$129.85

Desferal *SEE* DEFEROXAMINE MESYLATE

Desflurane

INDICATIONS AND USAGE
Desflurane is indicated as an inhalation agent for induction and/or maintenance of anesthesia for inpatient and outpatient surgery in adults (see *"Precautions"*).

Desflurane is not recommended for induction of anesthesia in pediatric patients because of a high incidence of moderate to severe upper airways adverse events (see *"Warnings"*). After induction of anesthesia with agents other than Desflurane and tracheal intubation, Desflurane is indicated for maintenance of anesthesia in infants and children.

Following is its chemical structure:

$$F-\underset{\underset{F}{|}}{\overset{\overset{H}{|}}{C}}-\underset{\underset{F}{|}}{\overset{\overset{H}{|}}{C}}-O-\underset{\underset{F}{|}}{\overset{\overset{H}{|}}{C}}-H$$

CONTRAINDICATIONS

Desflurane should not be used in patients with a known or suspected genetic susceptibility to malignant hyperthermia.

WARNINGS

Pediatric Use: Desflurane is not recommended for induction of general anesthesia via mask in infants or children because of the high incidence of moderate to severe laryngospasm in 50% of patients, coughing 72%, breathholding 68%, increase in secretions 21% and oxyhemoglobin desaturation 26%.

Desflurane should be administered only by persons trained in the administration of general anesthesia, using a vaporizer specifically designed and designated for use with Desflurane. Facilities for maintenance of a patent airway, artificial ventilation, oxygen enrichment, and circulatory resuscitation must be immediately available. Hypotension and respiratory depression increase as anesthesia is deepened.

Desflurane may present an increased risk in patients with a known sensitivity to halogenated anesthetic agents.

PRECAUTIONS

During the maintenance of anesthesia, increasing concentrations of Desflurane produce dose-dependent decreases in blood pressure. Excessive decreases in blood pressure may be related to depth of anesthesia and in such instances may be corrected by decreasing the inspired concentration of Desflurane.

Concentrations of Desflurane exceeding 1 MAC may increase heart rate. Thus an increased heart rate may not be a sign of inadequate anesthesia.

In patients with intracranial space occupying lesions, Desflurane should be administered at 0.8 MAC or less, in conjunction with a barbiturate induction and hyperventilation (hypocapnia). Appropriate measures should be taken to maintain cerebral perfusion pressure (see *"Clinical Studies, Neurosurgery"*).

In patients with coronary artery disease, maintenance of normal hemodynamics is important to the avoidance of myocardial ischemia. Desflurane should not be used as the sole agent for anesthetic induction in patients with coronary artery disease or patients where increases in heart rate or blood pressure are undesirable. It should be used with other medications, preferably intravenous opioids and hypnotics (see *"Clinical Studies, Cardiovascular Surgery"*).

Inspired concentrations of Desflurane greater than 12% have been safely administered to patients, particularly during induction of anesthesia. Such concentrations will proportionately dilute the concentration of oxygen; therefore, maintenance of an adequate concentration of oxygen may require a reduction of nitrous oxide or air if these gases are used concurrently.

The recovery from general anesthesia should be assessed carefully before patients are discharged from the post anesthesia care unit (PACU).

DRUG INTERACTIONS

No clinically significant adverse interactions with commonly used preanesthetic drugs, or drugs used during anesthesia (muscle relaxants, intravenous agents, and local anesthetic agents) were reported in clinical trials. The effect of Desflurane on the disposition of other drugs has not been determined.

Like isoflurane, Desflurane does not predispose to premature ventricular arrhythmias in the presence of exogenously infused epinephrine in swine.
BENZIODIAZEPINES and OPIOIDS (MAC Reduction):
Benzodiazepines (midazolam 25-50 µg/kg) decrease the MAC of Desflurane by 16% as do the opioids (fentanyl 3-6 µg/kg by 50% (see *"Dosage and Administration"*).
NEUROMUSCULAR BLOCKING AGENTS:
Anesthetic concentrations of Desflurane at equilibrium (administered for 15 or more minutes before testing) reduced the ED₉₅ of succinylcholine by approximately 30% and that of atracurium and pancuronium by approximately 50% compared to N₂O/opioid anesthesia. The effect of Desflurane on duration of nondepolarizing neuromuscular blockade has not been studied.

DOSAGE OF MUSCLE RELAXANT CAUSING 95% DEPRESSION IN NEUROMUSCULAR BLOCKADE

Desflurane Concentration	Mean ED₉₅ Pancuronium	(1 µg/kg) Atracurium	Succinylcholine
0.65 MAC 60% N₂O/O₂	26	123	—
1.25 MAC 60% N₂O/O₂	18	91	—
1.25 MAC O₂	22	120	362

Dosage reduction of neuromuscular blocking agents during induction of anesthesia may result in delayed onset of conditions suitable for endotracheal intubation or inadequate muscle relaxation, because potentiation of neuromuscular blocking agents requires equilibration of muscle with the delivered partial pressure of Desflurane.

Among nondepolarizing drugs, only pancuronium and atracurium interactions have been studied. In the absence of specific guidelines:

1. For endotracheal intubation, do not reduce the dose of nondepolarizing muscle relaxants or succinylcholine.

2. During maintenance of anesthesia, the dose of nondepolarizing muscle relaxants is likely to be reduced compared to that during N₂O/opioid anesthesia. Administration of supplemental doses of muscle relaxants should be guided by the response to nerve stimulation.

Malignant Hyperthermia: In susceptible individuals, potent inhalation anesthetic agents may trigger a skeletal muscle hypermetabolic state leading to high oxygen demand and the clinical syndrome known as malignant hyperthermia. In genetically susceptible pigs, Desflurane induced malignant hyperthermia. The clinical syndrome is signalled by hypercapnia, and may include muscle rigidity, tachycardia, tachypnea, cyanosis, arrhythmias, and/or unstable blood pressure. Some of these nonspecific signs may also appear during light anesthesia, acute hypoxia, hypercapnia, and hypovolemia.

Treatment of malignant hyperthermia includes discontinuation of triggering agents, administration of intravenous dantrolene sodium, and application of supportive therapy. (Consult prescribing information for dantrolene sodium intravenous for additional information on patient management.) Renal failure may appear later, and urine flow should be monitored and sustained if possible.

RENAL OR HEPATIC INSUFFICIENCY

Nine patients receiving Desflurane (N = 9) were compared to 9 patients receiving isoflurane, all with, chronic renal insufficiency (serum creatinine 1.5-6.9 mg/dL). No differences in hematological or biochemical tests, including renal function evaluation, were seen between the two groups. Similarly, no differences were found in a comparison of patients receiving either Desflurane (N = 28) or isoflurane (N = 30) undergoing renal transplant. Eight patients receiving Desflurane were compared to six patients receiving isoflurane, all with chronic hepatic disease (viral hepatitis, alcoholic hepatitis, or cirrhosis). No differences in hematological or biochemical tests, including hepatic enzymes and hepatic function evaluation, were seen.

CARCINOGENESIS, MUTAGENESIS, IMPAIRMENT OF FERTILITY

Animal carcinogenicity studies have not been performed with Desflurane. *In vitro* and *in vivo* genotoxicity studies did not demonstrate mutagenicity or chromosomal damage by Desflurane. Tests for genotoxicity included the Ames mutation assay, the metaphase analysis of human lymphocytes, and the mouse micronucleus assay.

Fertility was not affected after 1 MAC-Hour per day exposure (cumulative 63 and 14 MAC-Hours for males and females, respectively). At higher doses, parental toxicity (mortalities and reduced weight gain) was observed which could affect fertility.

Teratogenic Effects: No teratogenic effect was observed at approximately 10 and 13 cumulative MAC-Hour exposures at 1 MAC-Hour per day during organogenesis in rats or rabbits. At higher doses increased incidences of post-implantation loss and maternal toxicity were observed. However, at 10 MAC-Hours cumulative exposure in rats, about 6% decrease in the weight of male pups was observed at preterm caesarean delivery.

Pregnancy Category B: There are no adequate and well-controlled studies in pregnant women. Desflurane should be used during pregnancy only if the potential benefit justifies the potential risk to the fetus.

Rats exposed to Desflurane at 1 MAC-hour per day from gestation day 15 to lactation day 21, did not show signs of dystocia. Body weight of pups delivered by these dams at birth and during lactation were comparable to that of control pups. No treatment related behavioral changes were reported in these pups during lactation.

Labor and Delivery: The safety of Desflurane during labor or delivery has not been demonstrated.

Nursing Mothers: The concentrations of Desflurane in milk are probably of no clinical importance 24 hours after anesthesia. Because of rapid washout, Desflurane concentrations in milk are predicted to be below those found with other volatile potent anesthetics.

Geriatric Use: The average MAC for Desflurane in a 70 year old patient is two-thirds the MAC for a 20 year old patient (see *"Dosage and Administration"*).

Pediatric Use: Desflurane is not recommended for induction of general anesthesia via mask in infants or children because of the high incidence of moderate to severe laryngospasm, coughing, breathholding and increase in secretions and oxyhemoglobin desaturation (see *"Warnings"*).

Neurosurgical Use: Desflurane may produce a dose-dependent increase in cerebrospinal fluid pressure (CSFP) when administered to patients with intracranial space occupying lesions. Desflurane should be administered at 0.8 MAC or less, and in conjunction with a barbiturate induction and hyperventilation (hypocapnia) until cerebral decompression in patients with known or suspected increases in CSFP. Appropriate attention must be paid to maintain cerebral perfusion pressure (see *"Clinical Studies, Neurosurgery"*).

ADVERSE REACTIONS

Adverse event information is derived from controlled clinical trials, the majority of which were conducted in the United States. The studies were conducted using a variety of premedications, other anesthetics, and surgical procedures of varying length. Most adverse events reported were mild and transient, and may reflect the surgical procedures, patient characteristics (including disease) and/or medications administered.

Of the 1,843 patients exposed to Desflurane in clinical trials, 370 adults and 152 children were induced with Desflurane alone and 687 patients were maintained principally with Desflurane. The frequencies given reflect the percent of patients with the event. Each patient was counted once for each type of adverse event. They are presented in alphabetical order according to body system. **PROBABLY CAUSALLY RELATED: INCIDENCE GREATER THAN 1%.**

INDUCTION (USE AS A MASK INHALATION AGENT):

Adult patients (N=370): Coughing 34%, breathholding 30%*, apnea 15%, increased secretions*, laryngospasm*, oxyhemoglobin desaturation (SpO₂ 90%)*, pharyngitis*.

Pediatric patients (N=152): Coughing 72%, breathholding 68%, laryngospasm 50%, oxyhemoglobin desaturation (SpO₂ 90%) 26%, increased secretions 21%, broncho-spasm*. (See *"Warnings"*)

MAINTENANCE OR RECOVERY
Adult and pediatric patients (N=687):

Body as a Whole:	Headache.
Cardiovascular:	Bradycardia, hypertension, nodal arrhythmia, tachycardia.
Digestive:	Nausea 27%, vomiting 16%.
Nervous system:	Increased Salivation.
Respiratory:	Apnea*, breathholding, cough increased*, laryngospasm*, pharyngitis.
Special Senses:	Conjunctivitis (conjunctival hyperemia)

* *Incidence of events: 3%-10%*

PROBABLY CAUSALLY RELATED: INCIDENCE LESS THAN 1% AND REPORTED IN 3 OR MORE PATIENTS, REGARDLESS OF SEVERITY (N=1,843)

Cardiovascular:	Arrhythmia, bigeminy, electrocardiogram abnormal, myocardial ischemia, vasodilation.
Nervous System:	Agitation, dizziness.
Respiratory:	Asthma, dyspnea, hypoxia.

CAUSAL RELATIONSHIP UNKNOWN: INCIDENCE LESS THAN 1% AND REPORTED IN 3 OR MORE PATIENTS, REGARDLESS OF SEVERITY (N=1,843)

Body as a Whole:	Fever.
Cardiovascular:	Hemorrhage, myocardial infarct.
Metabolic and Nutrition:	Increased creatinine phosphokinase.
Musculoskeletal System:	Myalgia.
Skin and Appendages:	Pruritus.

See *"Precautions"* for information regarding pediatric use and malignant hyperthermia.

Laboratory Findings: Transient elevations in glucose and white blood cell count may occur as with use of other anesthetic agents.

OVERDOSAGE
In the event of overdosage, or suspected overdosage, take the following actions: discontinue administration of Desflurane, maintain a patent airway, initiate assisted or controlled ventilation with oxygen, and maintain adequate cardiovascular function.

SAFETY AND HANDLING
Occupational Caution: There is no specific work exposure limit established for Desflurane. However, the National Institute for Occupational Safety and Health Administration has recommended an 8-hr, time-weighted average limit of 2 ppm for halogenated anesthetic agents in general (0.5 ppm when coupled with exposure to N₂O).

The predicted effects of acute overexposure by inhalation of Desflurane include headache, dizziness or (in extreme cases) unconsciousness.

There are no documented adverse effects of chronic exposure to halogenated anesthetic vapors (*Waste Anesthetic Gases* or *WAGs*) in the workplace. Although results of some epidemiological studies suggest a link between exposure to halogenated anesthetics and increased health problems (particularly spontaneous abortion), the relationship is not conclusive. Since exposure to WAGs is one possible factor in the findings for these studies, operating room personnel, and pregnant women in particular, should minimize exposure. Precautions include adequate general ventilation in the operating room, the use of a well-designed and well-maintained scavenging system, work practices to minimize leaks and spills while the anesthetic agent is in use, and routine equipment maintenance to minimize leaks.

HOW SUPPLIED
LIQUID: 99.9%

BRAND/MANUFACTURER	NDC	SIZE	AWP
○ **BRAND**			
SUPRANE: Ohmeda	10019-0641-24	240 ml 6s	$70.00

Desipramine Hydrochloride

DESCRIPTION
Desipramine Hydrochloride is an antidepressant drug of the tricyclic type, and is chemically:

5*H*-Dibenz[*b,f*]azepine-5-propanamine, 10,11-dihydro-*N*-methyl-, monohydrochloride.

Following is its chemical structure:

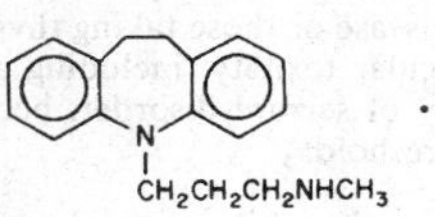

CLINICAL PHARMACOLOGY
MECHANISM OF ACTION
Available evidence suggests that many depressions have a biochemical basis in the form of a relative deficiency of neurotransmitters such as norepinephrine and serotonin. Norepinephrine deficiency may be associated with relatively low urinary 3-methoxy-4-hydroxyphenyl glycol (MHPG) levels, while serotonin deficiencies may be associated with low spinal fluid levels of 5-hydroxyindoleacetic acid.

While the precise mechanism of action of the tricyclic antidepressants is unknown, a leading theory suggests that they restore normal levels of neurotransmitters by blocking the re-uptake of these substances from the synapse in the central nervous system. Evidence indicates that the secondary amine tricyclic antidepressants, including Desipramine HCl, may have greater activity in blocking the re-uptake of norepinephrine. Tertiary amine tricyclic antidepressants, such as amitriptyline, may have greater effect on serotonin re-uptake.

Desipramine HCl is not a monoamine oxidase (MAO) inhibitor and does not act primarily as a central nervous system stimulant. It has been found in some studies to have a more rapid onset of action than Imipramine. Earliest therapeutic effects may occasionally be seen in 2 to 5 days, but full treatment benefit usually requires 2 to 3 weeks to obtain.

METABOLISM
Tricyclic antidepressants, such as Desipramine Hydrochloride, are rapidly absorbed from the gastrointestinal tract. Tricyclic antidepressants or their metabolites are to some extent excreted through the gastric mucosa and reabsorbed from the gastrointestinal tract. Desipramine is metabolized in the liver and approximately 70% is excreted in the urine. The rate of metabolism of tricyclic antidepressants varies widely from individual to individual, chiefly on a genetically determined basis. Up to a thirty-six-fold difference in plasma level may be noted among individuals taking the same oral dose of Desipramine. In general, the elderly metabolize tricyclic antidepressants more slowly than do younger adults.

Certain drugs, particularly the psychostimulants and the phenothiazines, increase plasma levels of concomitantly administered tricyclic antidepressants through competition for the same metabolic enzyme systems. Concurrent administration of cimetidine and tricyclic antidepressants can produce clinically significant increases in the plasma concentrations of the tricyclic antidepressants. Conversely, decreases in plasma levels of the tricyclic antidepressants have been reported upon discontinuation of cimetidine which may result in the loss of the therapeutic efficacy of the tricyclic antidepressant. Other substances, particularly barbiturates and alcohol, induce liver enzyme activity and thereby reduce tricyclic antidepressant plasma levels. Similar effects have been reported with tobacco smoke.

Research on the relationship of plasma level to therapeutic response with the tricyclic antidepressants has produced conflicting results. While some studies report no correlation, many studies cite therapeutic levels for most tricyclics in the range of 50 to 300 nanograms per milliliter. The therapeutic range is different for each tricyclic antidepressant. For Desipramine, an optimal range of therapeutic plasma levels has not been established.

INDICATIONS
Desipramine HCl is indicated for relief of symptoms in various depressive syndromes, especially endogenous depression.

UNLABELED USES
Desipramine Hydrochloride is used alone or as an adjunct in the treatment of attention deficit disorders with hyperactivity, bulimia nervosa, refractory depression, and diabetic neuropathy. It is also used in the treatment of agoraphobia, postherpetic neuralgia, and drug-induced extrapyramidal reactions, and is prescribed as adjunctive therapy for enuresis.

CONTRAINDICATIONS
Desipramine Hydrochloride should not be given in conjunction with, or within 2 weeks of, treatment with an MAO inhibitor drug; hyperpyretic crises, severe

convulsions, and death have occurred in patients taking MAO inhibitors and tricyclic antidepressants. When Desipramine HCl is substituted for an MAO inhibitor, at least 2 weeks should elapse between treatments. Desipramine HCl should then be started cautiously and should be increased gradually.

The drug is contraindicated in the acute recovery period following myocardial infarction. It should not be used in those who have shown prior hypersensitivity to the drug. Cross sensitivity between this and other dibenzazepines is a possibility.

WARNINGS

1. Extreme caution should be used when this drug is given in the following situations:

a. In patients with cardiovascular disease, because of the possibility of conduction defects, arrhythmias, tachycardias, strokes, and acute myocardial infarction.

b. In patients with a history of urinary retention or glaucoma, because of the anticholinergic properties of the drug.

c. In patients with thyroid disease or those taking thyroid medication, because of the possibility of cardiovascular toxicity, including arrhythmias.

d. In patients with a history of seizure disorder, because this drug has been shown to lower the seizure threshold.

2. This drug is capable of blocking the antihypertensive effect of guanethidine and similarly acting compounds.

3. USE IN PREGNANCY
Safe use of Desipramine Hydrochloride during pregnancy and lactation has not been established; therefore, if it is to be given to pregnant patients, nursing mothers, or women of childbearing potential, the possible benefits must be weighed against the possible hazards to mother and child. Animal reproductive studies have been inconclusive.

4. USE IN CHILDREN
Desipramine HCl is not recommended for use in children since safety and effectiveness in the pediatric age group have not been established. (See "Adverse Reactions", "Cardiovascular").

5. The patient should be cautioned that this drug may impair the mental and/or physical abilities required for the performance of potentially hazardous tasks such as driving a car or operating machinery.

6. In patients who may use alcohol excessively, it should be borne in mind that the potentiation may increase the danger inherent in any suicide attempt or overdosage.

PRECAUTIONS

1. It is important that this drug be dispensed in the least possible quantities to depressed outpatients, since suicide has been accomplished with this class of drug. Ordinary prudence requires that children not have access to this drug or to potent drugs of any kind; if possible, this drug should be dispensed in containers with child-resistant safety closures. Storage of this drug in the home must be supervised responsibly.

2. If serious adverse effects occur, dosage should be reduced or treatment should be altered.

3. Desipramine HCl therapy in patients with manic-depressive illness may induce a hypomanic state after the depression phase terminates.

4. The drug may cause exacerbation of psychosis in schizophrenic patients.

5. Close supervision and careful adjustment of dosage are required when this drug is given concomitantly with anticholinergic or sympathomimetic drugs.

6. Patients should be warned that while taking this drug their response to alcoholic beverages may be exaggerated.

7. Clinical experience in the concurrent administration of ECT and antidepressant drugs is limited. Thus, if such treatment is essential, the possibility of increased risk relative to benefits should be considered.

8. If Desipramine HCl is to be combined with other psychotropic agents such as tranquilizers or sedative/hypnotics, careful consideration should be given to the pharmacology of the agents employed since the sedative effects of Desipramine HCl and benzodiazepines (e.g., chlordiazepoxide or diazepam) are additive. Both the sedative and anticholinergic effects of the major tranquilizers are also additive to those of Desipramine HCl.

9. Concurrent administration of cimetidine and tricyclic antidepressants can produce clinically significant increases in the plasma levels of the tricyclic antidepressants (see "Clinical Pharmacology, Metabolism"). Conversely, decreases in plasma levels of the tricyclic antidepressants have been reported upon discontinuation of Cimetidine which may result in the loss of the therapeutic efficacy of the tricyclic antidepressant.

10. There have been greater than twofold increases of previously stable plasma levels of tricyclic antidepressants when Fluoxetine has been administered in combination with these agents.

11. This drug should be discontinued as soon as possible prior to elective surgery because of the possible cardiovascular effects. Hypertensive episodes have been observed during surgery in patients taking Desipramine Hydrochloride.

12. Both elevation and lowering of blood sugar levels have been reported.

13. Leukocyte and differential counts should be performed in any patient who develops fever and sore throat during therapy; the drug should be discontinued if there is evidence of pathologic neutrophil depression.

ADVERSE REACTIONS

Note: Included in the following listing are a few adverse reactions that have not been reported with this specific drug. However, the pharmacologic similarities among the tricyclic antidepressant drugs require that each of the reactions be considered when Desipramine HCl is given.

Cardiovascular: hypotension, hypertension, palpitations, heart block, myocardial infarction, stroke, arrhythmias, premature ventricular contractions, tachycardia, ventricular tachycardia, ventricular fibrillation, sudden death.

There has been a report of an "acute collapse" and "sudden death" in an eight-year old (18 kg) male, treated for two years for hyperactivity. There have been additional reports of sudden death in children. (See "Warnings, Use in Children").

Psychiatric: confusional states (especially in the elderly) with hallucinations, disorientation, delusions; anxiety, restlessness, agitation; insomnia and nightmares; hypomania; exacerbation of psychosis.

Neurologic: numbness, tingling, paresthesias of extremities; incoordination, ataxia, tremors; peripheral neuropathy; extrapyramidal symptoms; seizures; alteration in EEG patterns; tinnitus.

Anticholinergic: dry mouth, and rarely associated sublingual adenitis; blurred vision, disturbance of accommodation, mydriasis, increased intraocular pressure; constipation, paralytic ileus; urinary retention, delayed micturition, dilation of urinary tract.

Allergic: skin rash, petechiae, urticaria, itching, photosensitization (avoid excessive exposure to sunlight); edema (of face and tongue or general), drug fever, cross sensitivity with other tricyclic drugs.

Hematologic: bone marrow depressions including agranulocytosis, eosinophilia, purpura, thrombocytopenia.

Gastrointestinal: anorexia, nausea and vomiting, epigastric distress, peculiar taste, abdominal cramps, diarrhea, stomatitis, black tongue, hepatitis, jaundice (simulating obstructive), altered liver function, elevated liver function tests, increased pancreatic enzymes.

Endocrine: gynecomastia in the male, breast enlargement and galactorrhea in the female; increased or decreased libido, impotence, painful ejaculation, testicular swelling; elevation or depression of blood sugar levels; syndrome of inappropriate antidiuretic hormone secretion (SIADH).

Other: weight gain or loss; perspiration, flushing, urinary frequency, nocturia; parotid swelling; drowsiness, dizziness, weakness and fatigue, headache; fever; alopecia; elevated alkaline phosphatase.

Withdrawal Symptoms: Though not indicative of addiction, abrupt cessation of treatment after prolonged therapy may produce nausea, headache, and malaise.

OVERDOSAGE

SIGNS, SYMPTOMS, AND LABORATORY FINDINGS
Signs and symptoms of toxicity with tricyclic antidepressants most often involve the cardiovascular and central nervous systems. Overdosage with this class of drugs has resulted in death. Within a few hours of ingestion, the patient may become agitated, restless, confused, delirious or stuporous, and then comatose. Mydriasis, dry mucous membranes, vomiting, urinary retention, and diminished bowel sounds may occur. Hypotension, shock, respiratory depression, and renal shutdown may ensue. Generalized seizures, both early and later after ingestion, have been reported. Hyperactive reflexes, hyperpyrexia, and muscle rigidity can occur. ECG evidence of impaired conduction and serious disturbances of cardiac rate, rhythm, and output may occur. The duration of the QRS complex on ECG may be a helpful guide to the severity of tricyclic overdose. Physicians should be aware that relapses may occur after apparent recovery.

ORAL LD$_{50}$
The oral LD$_{50}$ of Desipramine is 290 mg/kg in male mice and 320 mg/kg in female rats.

TOXIC AND LETHAL DOSES/PLASMA LEVELS
In humans, doses at 10-30 times the usual daily dosage have been considered within the lethal range. The lethal dose for children and geriatric patients would be lower than that for the general adult population. Serious adverse events in general are more frequently associated with plasma levels in excess of 1000 ng/mL.

DIALYSIS
After overdosage, low plasma desipramine concentrations are found because of the drug's large volume of distribution in the body. Forced diuresis and hemodialysis are, therefore, ineffective in removing tricyclic antidepressants.

◆ RATED THERAPEUTICALLY EQUIVALENT; ◇ THERAPEUTIC EQUIVALENCE UNCONFIRMED; ○ UNRATED

TREATMENT

There is no specific antidote for desipramine overdosage, nor are there specific phenomena of diagnostic value characterizing poisoning by the drug.

Because CNS involvement, respiratory depression, and cardiac arrhythmia can occur suddenly, hospitalization and close observation are generally advisable, even when the amount ingested is thought to be small or the initial degree of intoxication appears slight or moderate. Aggressive supportive therapy of cardiac, neurologic, or acid base disturbances may be necessary.

The initial phase of therapy in a tricyclic antidepressant overdose should be devoted to protection of the patient's airway, stabilization of the vital signs, establishing an intravenous line, obtaining an ECG, and initiating continuous cardiac monitoring, and maintaining renal output. It should be remembered that rapid deterioration of vital signs, seizures, respiratory failure, and ventricular arrhythmias are common during the first twenty-four hours after ingestion.

Ventricular arrhythmias and intraventricular conduction abnormalities may respond to administration of sodium bicarbonate to correct the metabolic acidosis. During alkalinization, the patient's electrolytes and renal function must be closely monitored with frequent laboratory determinations. Arrhythmias may be treated with standard antiarrhythmic therapy (e.g., lidocaine). Physostigmine may be used with caution to reverse severe cardiovascular abnormalities or coma; too rapid administration may result in seizures.

If the patient is hypotensive, supportive measures (e.g., intravenous fluids) should be used. Vasopressor agents may be used with caution if necessary.

If the patient develops seizures, intravenous diazepam may be used. In addition, longer acting anticonvulsants (e.g., barbiturates) may be necessary for repetitive seizures.

Once the patient is stabilized, gastric lavage with a large bore orogastic tube should be used to evacuate the stomach. The physician must be prepared to protect the airway by endotracheal intubation if seizures or loss of consciousness occur prior to completion of the lavage procedure. Because of the potential for rapid onset of life-threatening events, emesis should not be used to empty the stomach. Activated charcoal (as single or repeated doses) in a water slurry should be given by mouth or instilled through the lavage tube.

Additional information regarding treatment of overdosage may be available from poison control centers.

DOSAGE AND ADMINISTRATION

Not recommended for use in children.

Lower dosages are recommended for elderly patients and adolescents. Lower dosages are also recommended for outpatients compared to hospitalized patients, who are closely supervised. Dosage should be initiated at a low level and increased according to clinical response and any evidence of intolerance. Following remission, maintenance medication may be required for a period of time and should be at the lowest dose that will maintain remission.

USUAL ADULT DOSE

The usual adult dose is 100 to 200 mg per day. In more severely ill patients, dosage may be further increased gradually to 300 mg/day if necessary. Dosages above 300 mg/day are not recommended.

Dosage should be initiated at a lower level and increased according to tolerance and clinical response.

Treatment of patients requiring as much as 300 mg should generally be initiated in hospitals, where regular visits by the physician, skilled nursing care, and frequent electrocardiograms (ECG's) are available.

The best available evidence of impending toxicity from very high doses of Norpramin is prolongation of the QRS or QT intervals on the ECG. Prolongation of the PR interval is also significant, but less closely correlated with plasma levels. Clinical symptoms of intolerance, especially drowsiness, dizziness, and postural hypotension, should also alert the physician to the need for reduction in dosage. Plasma Desipramine measurement would constitute the optimal guide to dosage monitoring.

Initial therapy may be administered in divided doses or a single daily dose.

Maintenance therapy may be given on a once-daily schedule for patient convenience and compliance.

ADOLESCENT AND GERIATRIC DOSE

The usual adolescent and geriatric dose is 25 to 100 mg daily. Dosage should be initiated at a lower level and increased according to tolerance and clinical response to a usual maximum of 100 mg daily. In more severely ill patients, dosage may be further increased to 150 mg/day. Doses above 150 mg/day are not recommended in these age groups.

Initial therapy may be administered in divided doses or a single daily dose.

Maintenance therapy may be given on a once-daily schedule for patient convenience and compliance.

Desipramine HCl tablets should be stored at room temperature, preferably below 86°F (30°C). Protect from excessive heat.

HOW SUPPLIED
TABLET: 10 MG

HCFA FUL (100s ea)			$0.15

BRAND/MANUFACTURER	NDC	SIZE	AWP
◆ BRAND			
NORPRAMIN: Marion Merrell Dow	00068-0007-01	100s	$49.44
◆ GENERICS			
Geneva	00781-1971-01	100s	$25.19

TABLET: 25 MG

AVERAGE UNIT PRICE (AVAILABLE SIZES)		GENERIC A-RATED AVERAGE PRICE (GAAP)	
BRAND	$0.62	100s	$27.59
GENERIC	$0.25	500s	$102.86
HCFA FUL (100s ea)	$0.10	1000s	$188.05

BRAND/MANUFACTURER	NDC	SIZE	AWP
◆ BRAND			
NORPRAMIN: Marion Merrell Dow	00068-0011-01	100s	$59.46
	00068-0011-61	100s ud	$63.84
◆ GENERICS			
Eon	00185-0019-01	100s	$19.95
Warner Chilcott	00047-0594-24	100s	$21.04
Qualitest	00603-3166-21	100s	$23.48
Sidmak	50111-0436-01	100s	$23.50
Mason Dist	11845-0308-01	100s	$23.68
Major	00904-1570-60	100s	$23.90
Major	00904-1581-60	100s	$23.90
Rugby	00536-4774-01	100s	$23.92
Rugby	00536-4881-01	100s	$23.92
Goldline	00182-1332-01	100s	$24.00
Martec	52555-0564-01	100s	$24.20
Lemmon	00093-0325-01	100s	$25.18
URL	00677-1198-01	100s	$25.25
Schein	00364-2209-01	100s	$25.50
Moore,H.L.	00839-7551-06	100s	$26.72
Geneva	00781-1972-01	100s	$26.75
Aligen	00405-4305-01	100s	$27.37
Parmed	00349-8728-01	100s	$32.25
U.S. Trading	56126-0376-11	100s ud	$12.63
Raway	00686-0489-20	100s ud	$18.00
Major	00904-1581-61	100s ud	$23.06
Vangard	00615-3509-13	100s ud	$41.94
Medirex	57480-0318-01	100s ud	$44.00
UDL	51079-0489-20	100s ud	$44.15
Geneva	00781-1972-13	100s ud	$44.15
Goldline	00182-1332-89	100s ud	$45.00
Eon	00185-0019-05	500s	$92.50
Major	00904-1570-40	500s	$101.60
Rugby	00536-4774-05	500s	$108.67
Rugby	00536-4881-05	500s	$108.67
Sidmak	50111-0436-03	1000s	$147.40
Goldline	00182-1332-10	1000s	$150.00
Major	00904-1570-80	1000s	$186.40
Major	00904-1581-80	1000s	$186.40
Geneva	00781-1972-10	1000s	$186.50
Eon	00185-0019-10	1000s	$189.50
Qualitest	00603-3166-32	1000s	$214.30
Parmed	00349-8728-10	1000s	$215.25
Moore,H.L.	00839-7551-16	1000s	$216.66

TABLET: 50 MG

AVERAGE UNIT PRICE (AVAILABLE SIZES)		GENERIC A-RATED AVERAGE PRICE (GAAP)	
BRAND	$1.16	100s	$47.32
GENERIC	$0.44	500s	$193.51
HCFA FUL (100s ea)	$0.15	1000s	$350.87

BRAND/MANUFACTURER	NDC	SIZE	AWP
◆ BRAND			
NORPRAMIN: Marion Merrell Dow	00068-0015-01	100s	$111.72
	00068-0015-61	100s ud	$120.66
◆ GENERICS			
Eon	00185-0721-01	100s	$37.50
Warner Chilcott	00047-0595-24	100s	$38.61
Aligen	00405-4306-01	100s	$42.56
Major	00904-1582-60	100s	$45.15
Schein	00364-2210-01	100s	$46.50
Rugby	00536-4775-01	100s	$47.02
Rugby	00536-4882-01	100s	$47.02
Major	00904-1571-60	100s	$47.50
URL	00677-1199-01	100s	$48.05
Qualitest	00603-3167-21	100s	$48.10
Sidmak	50111-0437-01	100s	$48.20
Goldline	00182-1333-01	100s	$48.20
Lemmon	00093-0326-01	100s	$49.53
Geneva	00781-1973-01	100s	$49.55
Martec	52555-0565-01	100s	$49.65
Moore,H.L.	00839-7552-06	100s	$52.72
Parmed	00349-8729-01	100s	$59.45
U.S. Trading	56126-0377-11	100s ud	$17.19
Raway	00686-0490-20	100s ud	$30.00
Major	00904-1582-61	100s ud	$43.19
Vangard	00615-3510-13	100s ud	$49.22
Geneva	00781-1973-13	100s ud	$50.95
Medirex	57480-0319-01	100s ud	$62.00
UDL	51079-0490-20	100s ud	$62.12
Goldline	00182-1333-89	100s ud	$63.00
Major	00904-1571-40	500s	$169.30
Eon	00185-0721-05	500s	$179.95
Rugby	00536-4775-05	500s	$212.40
Rugby	00536-4882-05	500s	$212.40
Sidmak	50111-0437-03	1000s	$277.20
Goldline	00182-1333-10	1000s	$277.20
Major	00904-1571-80	1000s	$316.00
Major	00904-1582-80	1000s	$316.00

➤ SHOWN IN PRODUCT IDENTIFICATION GUIDE

BRAND/MANUFACTURER	NDC	SIZE	AWP
Geneva	00781-1973-10	1000s	$316.25
Eon	00185-0721-10	1000s	$369.00
Parmed	00349-8729-10	1000s	$417.80
Moore,H.L.	00839-7552-16	1000s	$427.53
Qualitest	00603-3167-32	1000s	$440.81

TABLET: 75 MG

AVERAGE UNIT PRICE (AVAILABLE SIZES)		GENERIC A-RATED AVERAGE PRICE (GAAP)	
BRAND	$1.42	100s	$58.23
GENERIC	$0.57		
HCFA FUL (100s ea)	$0.19		

BRAND/MANUFACTURER	NDC	SIZE	AWP
◆ BRAND			
NORPRAMIN: Marion Merrell Dow	00068-0019-01	100s	$142.26
◆ GENERICS			
Eon	00185-0722-01	100s	$45.00
Schein	00364-2243-01	100s	$49.00
Warner Chilcott	00047-0596-24	100s	$49.85
Major	00904-1583-60	100s	$53.15
Aligen	00405-4307-01	100s	$54.15
Sidmak	50111-0438-01	100s	$58.10
Goldline	00182-1335-01	100s	$58.10
Qualitest	00603-3168-21	100s	$58.15
Geneva	00781-1974-01	100s	$58.85
URL	00677-1210-01	100s	$59.80
Rugby	00536-4776-01	100s	$59.85
Rugby	00536-4883-01	100s	$59.85
Martec	52555-0288-01	100s	$59.85
Major	00904-1572-60	100s	$59.90
Lemmon	00093-0327-01	100s	$61.15
Moore,H.L.	00839-7553-06	100s	$62.84
Parmed	00349-8764-01	100s	$72.15
Raway	00686-0491-20	100s ud	$50.00
Medirex	57480-0320-01	100s ud	$64.00
UDL	51079-0491-20	100s ud	$64.12
Goldline	00182-1335-89	100s ud	$65.00
Eon	00185-0722-05	500s	$215.00
Sidmak	50111-0438-03	1000s	$407.00

For additional alternatives, turn to the section beginning on page 2859.

Desmopressin Acetate

DESCRIPTION
Desmopressin Acetate is an antidiuretic hormone affecting renal water conservation and is a synthetic analogue of 8-arginine vasopressin. It is chemically defined as follows:

Molecular Weight: 1183.2

Empirical Formula: $C_{48}H_{74}N_{14}O_{17}S_2$

SCH_2CH_2CO-Tyr-Phe-Gln-Asn-Cys-Pro-D-Arg-Gly-NH_2.

$C_2H_4O_2 \cdot 3H_2O$

1-(3-mercaptopropionic acid)-8-D-arginine vasopressin monoacetate (salt) trihydrate

Desmopressin Acetate Injection is provided as a sterile, aqueous solution for injection.

Each mL provides:

Desmopressin Acetate	4.0 mcg
Sodium chloride	9.0 mg
Hydrochloric acid to adjust pH to 4.0	

The 10 mL vial contains chlorobutanol as a preservative (5.0 mg/mL).

Desmopressin Acetate Nasal Spray and Desmopressin Acetate Rhinal Tube are each provided as a sterile, aqueous solution for intranasal use.

Each mL contains:

Desmopressin Acetate	0.1 mg
Chlorobutanol	5.0 mg
Sodium Chloride	9.0 mg

Hydrochloric acid to adjust pH to approximately 4. The Desmopressin Acetate Nasal Spray compression pump delivers 0.1 mL (10 mcg) of Desmopressin Acetate per spray.

Following is its chemical structure:

SCH_2CH_2C-Tyr-Phe-Gln-Asn-Cys-Pro-D-Arg-Gly-NH_2 • CH_3COOH • $3H_2O$
1   2   3   4   5   6   7   8   9

CLINICAL PHARMACOLOGY
Desmopressin Acetate contains as active substance, 1-(3-mercaptopropionic acid)-8-D-arginine vasopressin, a synthetic analogue of the natural hormone arginine vasopressin. One mL (4 mcg) of Desmopressin Acetate solution has an antidiuretic activity of about 16 IU and 1 mL (0.1 mg) of Nasal Spray or Rhinal Tube has an antidiuretic activity of about 400 IU; 1 mcg of Desmopressin Acetate is equivalent to 4 IU.

Desmopressin Acetate has been shown to be more potent than arginine vasopressin in increasing plasma levels of factor VIII activity in patients with hemophilia and von Willebrand's disease Type I.

Dose-response studies were performed in healthy persons, using doses of 0.1 to 0.4 mcg/kg body weight, infused over a 10-minute period. Maximal dose response occurred at 0.3 to 0.4 mcg/kg. The response to Desmopressin Acetate of factor VIII activity and plasminogen activator is dose-related, with maximal plasma levels of 300 to 400 percent of initial concentrations obtained after infusion of 0.4 mcg/kg body weight. The increase is rapid and evident within 30 minutes, reaching a maximum at a point ranging from 90 minutes to two hours. The factor VIII related antigen and ristocetin cofactor activity were also increased to a smaller degree, but still are dose-dependent.

1. The biphasic half-lives of Desmopressin Acetate were 7.8 and 75.5 minutes for the fast and slow phases, respectively, compared with 2.5 and 14.5 minutes for lysine vasopressin, another form of the hormone. As a result, Desmopressin Acetate provides a prompt onset of antidiuretic action with a long duration after each administration.

2. The change in structure of arginine vasopressin to Desmopressin Acetate has resulted in a decreased vasopressor action and decreased actions on visceral smooth muscle relative to the enhanced antidiuretic activity, so that clinically effective antidiuretic doses are usually below threshold levels for effects on vascular or visceral smooth muscle.

3. When administered by injection, Desmopressin Acetate has an antidiuretic effect about ten times that of an equivalent dose administered intranasally.

4. The bioavailability of the subcutaneous route of administration was determined qualitatively using urine output data. The exact fraction of drug absorbed by that route of administration has not been quantitatively determined.

5. The percentage increase of factor VIII levels in patients with mild hemophilia A and von Willebrand's disease was not significantly different from that observed in normal healthy individuals when treated with 0.3 mcg/kg of Desmopressin Acetate infused over 10 minutes.

6. Plasminogen activator activity increases rapidly after Desmopressin Acetate infusion, but there has been no clinically significant fibrinolysis in patients treated with Desmopressin Acetate.

7. The effect of repeated Desmopressin Acetate administration when doses were given every 12 to 24 hours has generally shown a gradual diminution of the factor VIII activity increase noted with a single dose. The initial response is reproducible in any particular patient if there are 2 or 3 days between administrations.

INDICATIONS AND USAGE
HEMOPHILIA A
Desmopressin Acetate Injection is indicated for patients with hemophilia A with factor VIII coagulant activity levels greater than 5%. Desmopressin Acetate will often maintain hemostasis in patients with hemophilia A during surgical procedures and postoperatively when administered 30 minutes prior to scheduled procedure.

Desmopressin Acetate will also stop bleeding in hemophilia A patients with episodes of spontaneous or trauma-induced injuries such as hemarthroses, intramuscular hematomas or mucosal bleeding.

Desmopressin Acetate is not indicated for the treatment of hemophilia A with factor VIII coagulant activity levels equal to or less than 5%, or for the treatment of hemophilia B, or in patients who have factor VIII antibodies.

In certain clinical situations, it may be justified to try Desmopressin Acetate in patients with factor VIII levels between 2%-5%; however, these patients should be carefully monitored.

VON WILLEBRAND'S DISEASE (TYPE I)
Desmopressin Acetate Injection is indicated for patients with mild to moderate classic von Willebrand's disease (Type I) with factor VIII levels greater than 5%. Desmopressin Acetate will often maintain hemostasis in patients with mild to moderate von Willebrand's disease during surgical procedures and postoperatively when administered 30 minutes prior to the scheduled procedure.

Desmopressin Acetate will usually stop bleeding in mild to moderate von Willebrand's patients with episodes of spontaneous or trauma-induced injuries such as hemarthroses, intramuscular hematomas or mucosal bleeding.

Those von Willebrand's disease patients who are least likely to respond are those with severe homozygous von Willebrand's disease with factor VIII coagulant activity and factor VIII von Willebrand factor antigen levels less than 1%. Other patients may respond in a variable fashion depending on the type of molecular defect they have. Bleeding time and factor VIII coagulant activity, ristocetin cofactor activity, and von Willebrand factor antigen should all be checked during administration of Desmopressin Acetate to ensure that adequate levels are being achieved.

Desmopressin Acetate is not indicated for the treatment of severe classic von Willebrand's disease (Type I) and when there is evidence of an abnormal molecular form of factor VIII antigen. See *"Warnings"*.

DIABETES INSIPIDUS
Desmopressin Acetate Injection, Nasal Spray, and Rhinal Tube are indicated as antidiuretic replacement therapy in the management of central (cranial) diabetes insipidus and for the management of the temporary polyuria and polydipsia following head trauma or surgery in the pituitary region. Desmopressin Acetate is ineffective for the treatment of nephrogenic diabetes insipidus.

The use of Desmopressin Acetate Nasal Spray or Desmopressin Acetate Rhinal Tube in patients with an established diagnosis will result in a reduction in urinary output with increase in urine osmolality and a decrease in plasma osmolality. This will allow the resumption of a more normal life style with a decrease in urinary frequency and nocturia.

There are reports of an occasional change in response to Desmopressin Acetate Nasal Spray or Desmopressin Acetate Rhinal Tube with time usually greater than 6 months. Some patients may show a decreased responsiveness, others a shortened duration of effect. There is no evidence this effect is due to the development of binding antibodies but may be due to a local inactivation of the peptide.

Patients are selected for therapy establishing the diagnosis by means of the water deprivation test, the hypertonic saline infusion test, and/or the response to antidiuretic hormone. Continued response to Desmopressin Acetate can be monitored by urine volume and osmolality.

The injection should be used when the intranasal route may be compromised. These situations include nasal congestion and blockage, nasal discharge, atrophy of nasal mucosa, and severe atrophic rhinitis. Intranasal delivery may also be inappropriate where there is an impaired level of consciousness. In addition, cranial surgical procedures, such as transphenoidal hypophysectomy create situations where an alternative route of administration is needed as in cases of nasal packing or recovery from surgery.

PRIMARY NOCTURNAL ENURESIS

Desmopressin Acetate Nasal Spray and Desmopressin Acetate Rhinal Tube are indicated for the management of primary nocturnal enuresis. It may be used alone or adjunctive to behavioral conditioning or other nonpharmacological intervention. It has been shown to be effective in some cases that are refractory to conventional therapies.

CONTRAINDICATION

Known hypersensitivity to Desmopressin Acetate.

WARNINGS

Patients who do not have need of antidiuretic hormone for its antidiuretic effect, in particular those who are young or elderly, should be cautioned to ingest only enough fluid to satisfy thirst, in order to decrease the potential occurrence of water intoxication and hyponatremia.

Fluid intake should be adjusted, particularly in very young and elderly patients, in order to decrease the potential occurrence of water intoxication and hyponatremia.

Particular attention should be paid to the possibility of the rare occurrence of an extreme decrease in plasma osmolality and resulting seizures.

Desmopressin Acetate should not be used to treat patients with Type IIB von Willebrand's disease since platelet aggregation may be induced.

Desmopressin Acetate Nasal Spray and Rhinal Tube are for intranasal use only. The intranasal preparation can be compromised by poor intranasal absorption.

PRECAUTIONS

GENERAL

Desmopressin Acetate Injection has infrequently produced changes in blood pressure causing either a slight elevation in blood pressure or a transient fall in blood pressure and a compensatory increase in heart rate. The Nasal Spray and Rhinal Tube at high dosages have also infrequently produced a slight elevation of blood pressure, which disappeared with a reduction in dosage. The drug should be used with caution in patients with coronary artery insufficiency and/or hypertensive cardiovascular disease.

Desmopressin Acetate should be used with caution in patients with conditions associated with fluid and electrolyte imbalance, such as cystic fibrosis, because these patients are prone to hyponatremia.

There have been rare reports of thrombotic events following Desmopressin Acetate Injection in patients predisposed to thrombus formation. No causality has been determined, however, the drug should be used with caution in these patients.

Severe allergic reactions have been reported with Desmopressin Acetate Injection. It is not known whether antibodies to Desmopressin Acetate Injection are produced after repeated injections.

HEMOPHILIA A

Laboratory tests for assessing patient status include levels of factor VIII coagulant, factor VIII antigen and factor VIII ristocetin cofactor (von Willebrand factor) as well as activated partial thromboplastin time. Factor VIII coagulant activity should be determined before giving Desmopressin Acetate for hemostasis. If factor VIII coagulant activity is present at less than 5% of normal, Desmopressin Acetate should not be relied on.

VON WILLEBRAND'S DISEASE

Laboratory tests for assessing patient status include levels of factor VIII coagulant activity, factor VIII ristocetin cofactor activity, and factor VIII von Willebrand factor antigen. The skin bleeding time may be helpful in following these patients.

DIABETES INSIPIDUS

Laboratory tests for monitoring the patient with central cranial diabetes insipidus or postsurgical or head trauma-related polyuria and polydipsia include urine volume and osmolality. In some cases, plasma osmolality may be required.

With the intranasal route, changes in the nasal mucosa such as scarring, edema, or other disease may cause erratic, unreliable absorption in which case intranasal Desmopressin Acetate should not be used.

PRIMARY NOCTURNAL ENURESIS

If changes in the nasal mucosa have occurred, unreliable absorption may result. Desmopressin Acetate intranasal solution should be discontinued until the nasal problems resolve.

For the healthy patient with primary nocturnal enuresis, serum electrolytes should be checked at least once if therapy is continued beyond 7 days.

DRUG INTERACTIONS

Although the pressor activity of Desmopressin Acetate is very low compared with the antidiuretic activity, use of doses as large as 0.3 mcg/kg of Desmopressin Acetate with other pressor agents should be done only with careful patient monitoring.

Desmopressin Acetate has been used with epsilon aminocaproic acid without adverse effects.

INFORMATION FOR PATIENTS

Patients should be informed that the Desmopressin Acetate Nasal Spray bottle accurately delivers 50 doses of 10 mcg each. Any solution remaining after 50 doses should be discarded since the amount delivered thereafter may be substantially less than 10 mcg of drug. No attempt should be made to transfer remaining solution to another bottle. Patients should be instructed to read accompanying directions on use of the spray pump carefully before use.

CARCINOGENICITY, MUTAGENICITY, IMPAIRMENT OF FERTILITY

Teratology studies in rats have shown no abnormalities. No further data are available.

PREGNANCY

Category B: Reproduction studies performed in rats and rabbits with doses up to 12.5 times the human dose when used for factor VIII stimulation and 125 times the human dose when used in diabetes insipidus have revealed no evidence of harm to the fetus due to Desmopressin Acetate. There are several publications of management of diabetes insipidus in pregnant women with no harm to the fetus reported; however, there are no adequate and well-controlled studies in pregnant women. Published reports stress that, as opposed to preparations containing the natural hormones Desmopressin Acetate in antidiuretic doses has no uterotonic action, but the physician will have to weigh possible therapeutic advantages against possible danger in each case.

NURSING MOTHERS

It is not known whether this drug is excreted in human milk. A single study in a postpartum woman demonstrated a marked change in plasma, but little if any change in assayable Desmopressin Acetate in breast milk following an intranasal dose of 10 mcg. Because many drugs are excreted in human milk, caution should be exercised when Desmopressin Acetate is administered to a nursing woman.

PEDIATRIC USE

Use of the injectable form of Desmopressin Acetate in infants and children will require careful fluid intake restriction to prevent possible hyponatremia and water intoxication. *Desmopressin Acetate Injection should not be used in infants younger than three months* in the treatment of hemophilia A or von Willebrand's disease; safety and effectiveness in children under 12 years of age with diabetes insipidus have not been established.

Primary Nocturnal Enuresis: Desmopressin Acetate has been used in childhood nocturnal enuresis. Short-term (4-8 weeks) Desmopressin Acetate administration has been shown to be safe and modestly effective in children aged 6 years or older with severe childhood nocturnal enuresis. Adequately controlled studies with intranasal Desmopressin Acetate in primary nocturnal enuresis have not been conducted beyond 4-8 weeks. The dose should be individually adjusted to achieve the best results.

Central Cranial Diabetes Insipidus: Desmopressin Acetate Nasal Spray and Desmopressin Acetate Rhinal Tube have been used in children with diabetes insipidus. The dose must be individually adjusted to the patient with attention in the very young to the danger of an extreme decrease in plasma osmolality with resulting convulsions. Dose should start at 0.05 mL or less.

Since the spray cannot deliver less than 0.1 mL (10 mcg), smaller doses should be administered using the rhinal tube delivery system. Do not use the nasal spray in pediatric patients requiring less than 0.1 mL (10 mcg) per dose.

There are reports of an occasional change in response to Desmopressin Acetate Nasal Spray or Desmopressin Acetate Rhinal Tube with time, usually greater than 6 months. Some patients may show a decreased responsiveness, others a shortened duration of effect. There is no evidence this effect is due to the development of binding antibodies but may be due to a local inactivation of the peptide.

ADVERSE REACTIONS

Infrequently, Desmopressin Acetate Injection has produced transient headache, nausea, mild abdominal cramps and vulval pain. These symptoms disappeared with reduction in dosage. Occasionally, Desmopressin Acetate has produced local erythema, swelling or burning pain. Occasional facial flushing has been reported with the administration of Desmopressin Acetate.

Desmopressin Acetate Injection has infrequently produced changes in blood pressure causing either a slight elevation or a transient fall and a compensatory increase in heart rate. See *"Warning"* for the possibility of water intoxication and hyponatremia.

➤ SHOWN IN PRODUCT IDENTIFICATION GUIDE

There have been rare reports of thrombotic events (acute cerebrovascular thrombosis, acute myocardial infarction) following Demopressin Acetate Injection in patients predisposed to thrombus formation.

Infrequently, high dosages of Desmopressin Acetate Nasal Spray or Desmopressin Acetate Rhinal Tube have also produced transient headache and nausea. Nasal congestion, rhinitis and flushing have also been reported occasionally. These symptoms disappeared with reduction in dosage. Nosebleed, sore throat, cough and upper respiratory infections have also been reported with the nasal route.

The following table lists the percent of patients having adverse experiences without regard to relationship to study drug from the pooled pivotal study data for nocturnal enuresis.

DESMOPRESSIN ACETATE INTRANASAL

Adverse Reaction	Placebo (N=59) %	20 mcg (N=60) %	40 mcg (N=61) %
Body as a Whole			
Abdominal Pain	0	2	0
Asthenia	0	0	2
Chills	0	0	2
Headache	0	2	5
Throat Pain	2	0	0
Nervous System			
Depression	2	0	0
Dizziness	0	0	3
Respiratory System			
Epistaxis	2	3	0
Nostril Pain	0	2	0
Respiratory Infection	2	0	0
Rhinitis	2	8	3
Cardiovascular System			
Vasodilation	2	0	0
Digestive System			
Gastrointestinal Disorder	0	2	0
Nausea	0	0	2
Skin & Appendages			
Leg Rash	2	0	0
Rash	2	0	0
Special Senses			
Conjunctivitis	0	2	0
Edema Eyes	0	2	0
Lacrymation Disorder	0	0	2

OVERDOSAGE

See *"Adverse Reactions"* above. In case of overdosage, the dosage should be reduced, frequency of administration decreased, or the drug withdrawn according to the severity of the condition.

There is no known specific antidote for Desmopressin Acetate.

An oral LD$_{50}$ has not been established. An intravenous dose of 2 mg/kg in mice demonstrated no effect.

DOSAGE AND ADMINISTRATION

HEMOPHILIA A AND VON WILLEBRAND'S DISEASE (TYPE I)

Desmopressin Acetate Injection is administered as an intravenous infusion at a dose of 0.3 mcg Desmopressin Acetate/kg body weight diluted in sterile physiological saline and infused slowly over 15 to 30 minutes. In adults and children weighing more than 10 kg, 50 mL of diluent is used; in children weighing 10 kg or less, 10 mL of diluent is used. Blood pressure and pulse should be monitored during infusion. If Desmopressin Acetate Injection is used preoperatively, it should be administered 30 minutes prior to the scheduled procedure.

The necessity for repeat administration of Desmopressin Acetate or use of any blood products for hemostasis should be determined by laboratory response as well as the clinical condition of the patient. The tendency toward tachyphylaxis (lessening of response) with repeated administration given more frequently than every 48 hours should be considered in treating each patient.

DIABETES INSIPIDUS

This formulation is administered subcutaneously or by direct intravenous injection. Desmopressin Acetate Injection dosage must be determined for each patient and adjusted according to the pattern of response. Response should be estimated by two parameters: adequate duration of sleep and adequate, not excessive, water turnover.

The usual dosage range in adults is 0.5 mL (2.0 mcg) to 1 mL (4.0 mcg) daily, administered intravenously or subcutaneously, usually in two divided doses. The morning and evening doses should be separately adjusted for an adequate diurnal rhythm of water turnover. For patients who have been controlled on intranasal Desmopressin Acetate and who must be switched to the injection form, either because of poor intranasal absorption or because of the need for surgery, the comparable antidiuretic dose of the injection is about one-tenth the intranasal dose. Patients with nasal congestion and blockage have often responded well to Desmopressin Acetate. The nasal spray pump can only deliver doses of 0.1 mL (10 mcg) or multiples of 0.1 mL. If doses other than these are required, the rhinal tube delivery system may be used. Desmopressin Acetate Rhinal Tube is administered into the nose through a soft, flexible plastic rhinal tube that has four

graduation marks on it that measure 0.2, 0.15, 0.1, and 0.05 mL. The usual dosage range in adults is 0.1 to 0.4 mL daily, either as a single dose or divided into two or three doses. Most adults require 0.2 mL daily in two divided doses. The morning and evening doses should be separately adjusted for an adequate diurnal rhythm of water turnover. For children aged 3 months to 12 years, the usual dosage range is 0.05 to 0.3 mL daily, either as a single dose or divided into two doses.

About ¼ to ⅓ of patients can be controlled by a single daily dose of Desmopressin Acetate administered intranasally.

Parenteral drug products should be inspected visually for particulate matter and discoloration prior to administration whenever solution and container permit.

PRIMARY NOCTURNAL ENURESIS

Dosage should be adjusted according to the individual. The recommended initial dose for those 6 years of age and older is 20 mcg or 0.2 mL solution intranasally at bedtime. Adjustment up to 40 mcg is suggested if the patient does not respond. Some patients may respond to 10 mcg and adjustment to that lower dose may be done if the patient has shown a response to 20 mcg. It is recommended that one-half of the dose be administered per nostril. Adequately controlled studies with intranasal Desmopressin Acetate in primary nocturnal enuresis have not been conducted beyond 4-8 weeks.

STORAGE

Injection: Keep refrigerated at about 4°C (39°F).

Nasal Spray: Keep refrigerated at 2°-8°C (36-46°F). When traveling, product will maintain stability for up to 3 weeks when stored at room temperature, 22°C (72°F).

Rhinal Tube: Keep refrigerated at about 4°C (39°F). When traveling—controlled room temperature 22°C (72°F) closed sterile bottles will maintain stability for 3 weeks.

HOW SUPPLIED

INJECTION: 4 MCG/ML

BRAND/MANUFACTURER	NDC	SIZE	AWP
◇ BRAND			
DDAVP: RPR	00075-2451-53	10 ml	$231.48
	00075-2451-01	1 ml 10s	$228.64

SOLUTION: 0.01%

BRAND/MANUFACTURER	NDC	SIZE	AWP
◇ BRAND			
DDAVP RHINAL TUBE: RPR	00075-2450-01	2.5 ml	$65.53

SPRAY: 1.5 MG/ML

BRAND/MANUFACTURER	NDC	SIZE	AWP
◇ BRAND			
DDAVP: RPR	00075-2450-02	5 ml	$107.70

SPRAY: 1.5 MG/ML

BRAND/MANUFACTURER	NDC	SIZE	AWP
○ BRAND			
STIMATE: Armour	00053-2453-00	2.5 ml	$525.00

Desogen *SEE* DESOGESTREL AND ETHINYL ESTRADIOL

Desogestrel and Ethinyl Estradiol

DESCRIPTION

Desogestrel/Ethinyl Estradiol (21 and 28-day) Tablets provide an oral contraceptive regimen of 21 tablets each containing 0.15 mg Desogestrel (13-ethyl-11-methylene-18,19-dinor-17 alpha-pregen-4-en-20-yn-17-ol) and 0.03 mg Ethinyl Estradiol (19-nor-17 alpha-pregna-1,3,5 (10)-trien-20-yne-3,17,diol).

CLINICAL PHARMACOLOGY

PHARMACODYNAMICS

Combination oral contraceptives act by suppression of gonadotropins. Although the primary mechanism of this action is inhibition of ovulation, other alterations include changes in the cervical mucus, which increase the difficulty of sperm entry into the uterus, and changes in the endometrium which reduce the likelihood of implantation.

Receptor binding studies, as well as studies in animals and humans, have shown that 3-keto-Desogestrel, the biologically active metabolite of Desogestrel, combines high progestational activity with minimal intrinsic androgenicity[91,92]. Desogestrel, in combination with Ethinyl Estradiol, does not counteract the estrogen-induced increases in SHBG, resulting in lower serum levels of free testosterone[96-99].

PHARMACOKINETICS

Desogestrel is rapidly and almost completely absorbed and converted into 3-keto-Desogestrel, its biologically active metabolite. Following oral administration, the relative bioavailability of Desogestrel, as measured by serum levels of 3-keto-Desogestrel, is approximately 84%.

In the third cycle of use after a single dose of Desogestrel/Ethinyl Estradiol, maximum concentrtions of 3-keto-Desogestrel of $2,805 \pm 1,203$ pg/mL (mean $\pm$ SD) are reached at 1.4 ± 0.8 hours. The area under the curve ($AUC_{0-\infty}$) is 33,858 $\pm$ 11,043 pg/mL·hr after a single dose. At steady-state, attained from at least day 19 onwards, maximum concentrations of $5,840 \pm 1,667$ pg/mL are reached at 1.4 ± 0.9 hours. The minimum plasma levels of 3-keto-Desogestrel at steady state are $1,400 \pm 560$ pg/mL. The AUC_{0-24} at steady state is $52,299 \pm 17,878$ pg/mL·hr. The mean $AUC_{0-\infty}$ for 3-keto-Desogestrel at single dose is significantly lower than the mean AUC_{0-24} at steady state. This indicates that the kinetics of 3-keto-Desogestrel are nonlinear due to an increase in binding of 3-keto-Desogestrel to sex hormone-binding globulin in the cycle, attributed to increased sex hormone-binding globulin levels which are induced by the daily administration of Ethinyl Estradiol. Sex hormone-binding globulin levels increased significantly in the third treatment cycle from day 1 (150 ± 64 nmol/L) to day 21 (230 ± 59 nmol/L).

The elimination half-life for 3-keto-Desogestrel is approximately 38 ± 20 hours at steady state. In addition to 3-keto-Desogestrel, other phase I metabolites are 3α-OH-Desogestrel, 3β-OH-Desogestrel, and 3α-OH-5α-H-Desogestrel. These other metabolites are not known to have any pharmacologic effects, and are further converted in part by conjugation (phase II metabolism) into polar metabolites, mainly sulfates and glucuronides.

Ethinyl Estradiol is rapidly and almost completely absorbed. In the third cycle of use after a single dose of Desogestrel/Ethinyl Estradiol, the relative bioavailability is approximately 83%.

In the third cycle of use after a single dose of Desogestrel/Ethinyl Estradiol, maximum concentrations of Ethinyl Estradiol of 95 ± 34 pg/mL are reached at 1.5 ± 0.8 hours. The $AUC_{0-\infty}$ is $1,471 \pm 268$ pg/mL+b•hr after a single dose. At steady state, attained from at least day 19 onwards, maximum Ethinyl Estradiol concentrations of 141 ± 48 pg/mL are reached at about 1.4 ± 0.7 hours. The minimum serum levels of Ethinyl Estradiol at steady state are 24 ± 8.3 pg/mL. The AUC_{0-24}, at steady state is $1,117 \pm 302$ pg/mL•hr. The mean $AUC_{0-\infty}$ for Ethinyl Estradiol following a single dose during treatment cycle 3 does not significantly differ from the mean AUC_{0-24} at steady state. This finding indicates linear kinetics for Ethinyl Estradiol.

The elimination half-life is 26 ± 6.8 hours at steady state. Ethinyl Estradiol is subject to a significant degree of presystemic conjugation (phase II metabolism). Ethinyl Estradiol escaping gut wall conjugation undergoes phase I metabolism and hepatic conjugation (phase II metabolism). Major phase I metabolites are 2-OH-Ethinyl Estradiol and 2-methoxyEthinyl Estradiol. Sulfate and glucuronide conjugates of both Ethinyl Estradiol and phase I metabolites, which are excreted in bile, can undergo enterohepatic circulation.

INDICATIONS AND USAGE
Desogestrel/Ethinyl Estradiol Tablets are indicated for the prevention of pregnancy in women who elect to use oral contraceptive as a method of contraception.

Oral contraceptives are highly effective. Table 1 lists the typical accidental pregnancy rates for users of combination oral contraceptives and other methods of contraception. The efficacy of these contraceptive methods, except sterilization, depends upon the reliability with which they are used. Correct and consistent use of these methods can result in lower failure rates.

Table 1
LOWEST EXPECTED AND TYPICAL FAILURE RATES (%) DURING THE FIRST YEAR OF USE OF A CONTRACEPTIVE METHOD

Method	Lowest Expected*	Typical**
Oral Contraceptives		3
combined	0.1	N/A
progestin only	0.5	N/A
Diaphragm with		
spermicidal cream or		
jelly	6	18
Spermicides alone		
(foam, creams, jellies		
and vaginal		
suppositories)	3	21
Vaginal Sponge		
nulliparous	6	18
parous	9	28
IUD (medicated)	2	3
Implant		
capsules	0.04	0.04
rods	0.03	0.03
Condom without		
spermicide	2	12
Cervical Cap	6	18
Periodic abstinence		
(all methods)	1–9	20
Female sterilization	0.2	0.4
Male sterilization	0.1	0.15
No contraception		
(planned pregnancy)	85	85

Adapted from J. Trussell, et al. Table 1, ref. #1.
N/A—Data not available.

* *The author's best estimate of the percentage of women expected to experience an accidental pregnancy among couples who initiate a method (not necessarily for the first time) and who use it consistently and correctly during the first year, if they do not stop for any other reason.*

** *This term represents 'typical' couples who initiate use of a method (not necessarily for the first time), who experience an accidental pregnancy during the first year, if they do not stop use for any other reason.*

In a clinical trial with Desogestrel/Ethinyl Estradiol, 1,195 subjects completed 11,656 cycles and a total of 10 pregnancies were reported. This represents an overall user-efficacy (typical user-efficacy) pregnancy rate of 1.12 per 100 women-years. This rate includes patients who did not take the drug correctly.

CONTRAINDICATIONS
Oral contraceptives should not be used in women who currently have the following conditions:

- Thrombophlebitis or thromboembolic disorders
- A past history of deep vein thrombophlebitis or thromboembolic disorders
- Cerebral vascular or coronary artery disease
- Known or suspected carcinoma of the breast
- Carcinoma of the endometrium or other known or suspected estrogen-dependent neoplasia
- Undiagnosed abnormal genital bleeding
- Cholestatic jaundice of pregnancy or jaundice with prior pill use
- Hepatic adenomas or carcinomas
- Known or suspected pregnancy.

WARNINGS

> CIGARETTE SMOKING INCREASES THE RISK OF SERIOUS CARDIOVASCULAR SIDE EFFECTS FROM ORAL CONTRACEPTIVE USE. THIS RISK INCREASES WITH AGE AND WITH HEAVY SMOKING (15 OR MORE CIGARETTES PER DAY) AND IS QUITE MARKED IN WOMEN OVER 35 YEARS OF AGE. WOMEN WHO USE ORAL CONTRACEPTIVES SHOULD BE STRONGLY ADVISED NOT TO SMOKE.

The use of oral contraceptives is associated with increased risks of several serious conditions including myocardial infarction, thromboembolism, stroke, hepatic neoplasia, and gallbladder disease, although the risk of serious morbidity or mortality is very small in healthy women without underlying risk factors. The risk of morbidity and mortality increases significantly in the presence of other underlying risk factors such as hypertension, hyperlipidemias, obesity and diabetes.

Practitioners prescribing oral contraceptives should be familiar with the following information relating to these risks. The information contained in this package insert is principally based on studies carried out in patients who used oral contraceptives with formulations of higher doses of estrogens and progestogens than those in common use today. The effect of long term use of the oral contraceptives with formulations of lower doses of both estrogens and progestogens remains to be determined.

Throughout this labeling, epidemiological studies reported are of two types: retrospective or case control studies and prospective or cohort studies. Case control studies provide a measure of the relative risk of a disease, namely, *a ratio* of the incidence of a disease among oral contraceptive users to that among nonusers. The relative risk does not provide information on the actual clinical occurrence of a disease. Cohort studies provide a measure of attributable risk, which is the *difference* in the incidence of disease between oral contraceptive users and nonusers. The attributable risk does provide information about the actual occurrence of a disease in the population (adapted from refs. 2 and 3 with the author's permission). For further information, the reader is referred to a text on epidemiological methods.

1. THROMBOEMBOLIC DISORDERS AND OTHER VASCULAR PROBLEMS
a. Myocardial infarction
An increased risk of myocardial infarction has been attributed to oral contraceptive use. This risk is primarily in smokers or women with other underlying risk factors for coronary artery disease such as hypertension, hypercholesterolemia, morbid obesity, and diabetes. The relative risk of heart attack for current oral contraceptive users has been estimated to be two to six[4-10]. The risk is very low in women under the age of 30.

Smoking in combination with oral contraceptive use has been shown to contribute substantially to the incidence of myocardial infarctions in women in their mid-thirties or older with smoking accounting for the majority of excess cases[11]. Mortality rates associated with circulatory disease have been shown to increase substantially in smokers, especially in those 35 years of age and older among women who use oral contraceptives. (See Table 2)

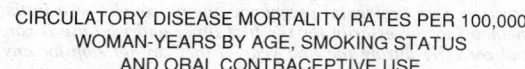

CIRCULATORY DISEASE MORTALITY RATES PER 100,000
WOMAN-YEARS BY AGE, SMOKING STATUS
AND ORAL CONTRACEPTIVE USE

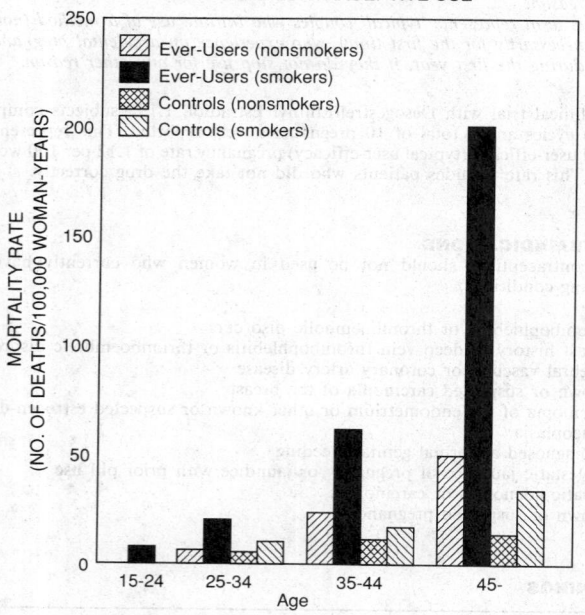

Table 2. (Adapted from P.M. Layde and V. Beral, ref. #12.)

Oral contraceptives may compound the effects of well-know risk factors, such as hypertension, diabetes, hyperlipidemias, age and obesity.[13] In particular, some progestogens are known to decrease HDL cholesterol and cause glucose intolerance, while estrogens may create a state of hyperinsulinism[14-18]. Oral contraceptives have been shown to increase blood pressure among users (see section 9 in Warnings). Similar effects on risk factors have been associated with an increased risk of heart disease. Oral contraceptives must be used with caution in women with cardiovascular disease risk factors.

b. Thromboembolism

An increased risk of thromboembolic and thrombotic disease associated with the use of oral contraceptives is well established. Case control studies have found the relative risk of users compared to nonusers to be 3 for the first episode of superficial venous thrombosis, 4 to 11 for deep vein thrombosis or pulmonary embolism, and 1.5 to 6 for women with predisposing conditions for venous thromboembolic disease[2,3,19-24]. Cohort studies have shown the relative risk to be somewhat lower, about 3 for new cases and about 4.5 for new cases requiring hospitalization[25]. The risk of thromboembolic disease associated with oral contraceptives is not related to length of use and disappears after pill use is stopped.[2].

A two- to four-fold increase in relative risk of post-operative thromboembolic complications has been reported with the use of oral contraceptives[9]. The relative risk of venous thrombosis in women who have predisposing conditions is twice that of women without such medical conditions[26]. If feasible oral contraceptives should be discontinued at least four weeks prior to and for two weeks after elective surgery of a type associated with an increase in risk of thromboembolism and during and following prolonged immobilization. Since the immediate postpartum period is also associated with an increased risk of thromboembolism, oral contraceptives should be started no earlier than four weeks after delivery in women who elect not to breast feed.

c. Cerebrovascular diseases

Oral contraceptives have been shown to increase both the relative and attributable risks of cerebrovascular events (thrombotic and hemorrhagic strokes), although, in genera, the risk is greatest among older (> 35 years), hypertensive women who also smoke. Hypertension was found to be a risk factor for both users and nonusers, for both types of strokes, and smoking interacted to increase the risk of stroke[27-29].

In a large study, the relative risk of thrombotic strokes has been shown to range from 3 for normotensive users to 14 for users with severe hypertension[30]. The relative risk of hemorrhagic stroke is reported to be 1.2 for non-smokers who used oral contraceptives, 2.6 for smokers who did not use oral contraceptives, 7.6 for smokers who used oral contraceptives, 1.8 for normotensive users and 25.7 for users with severe hypertension[30]. The attributable risk is also greater in older women[3].

d. Dose-related risk of vascular disease from oral contraceptives

A positive association has been observed between the amount of estrogen and progestogen in oral contraceptives and the risk of vascular disease[31-33]. A decline

in serum high density lipoproteins (HDL) has been reported with many progestational agents[14-16]. A decline in serum high density lipoproteins has been associated with an increased incidence of ischemic heart disease. Because estrogens increase HDL cholesterol, the net effect of an oral contraceptive depends on a balance achieved between doses of estrogen and progestogen and the nature and absolute amount of progestogens used in the contraceptives. The amount of both hormones should be considered in the choice of an oral contraceptive. Minimizing exposure to estrogen and progestogen is in keeping with good principles of therapeutics. For any particular estrogen/progestogen combination, the dosage regimen prescribed should be one which contains the least amount of estrogen and progestogen that is compatible with a low failure rate and the needs of the individual patient. New acceptors or oral contraceptive agents should be started on preparations containing 0.035 mg or less of estrogen.

e. Persistence of risk of vascular disease

There are two studies which have shown persistence of risk of vascular disease for ever-users of oral contraceptives. In a study in the United States, the risk of developing myocardial infarction after discontinuing oral contraceptives persists for at least 9 years for women 40-49 years old who had used oral contraceptives for five or more years, but this increased risk was not demonstrated in other age groups.[8] In another study in Great Britain, the risk of developing cerebrovascular disease persisted for at least 6 years after discontinuation of oral contraceptives, although excess risk was very small[34].

However, both studies were performed with oral contraceptive formulations containing 0.050 mg or higher of estrogens.

2. ESTIMATES OF MORTALITY FROM CONTRACEPTIVE USE

One study gathered data from a variety of sources which have estimated the mortality rate associated with different methods of contraception at different ages (Table 3). These estimates include the combined risk of death associated with contraceptive methods plus the risk attributable to pregnancy in the event of method failure. Each method of contraception has its specific benefits and risks. The study concluded that with the exception of oral contraceptive users 35 and older who smoke and 40 and older who do not smoke, mortality associated with all methods of birth control is low and below that associated with childbirth.

The observation of an increase in risk of mortality with age for oral contraceptive users is based on data gathered in the 1970's[35]. Current clinical recommendation involves the use of lower estrogen dose formulations and a careful consideration of risk factors. In 1989, the Fertility and Maternal Health Drugs Advisory committee was asked to review the use of oral contraceptives in women 40 years of age and over. The committee concluded that although cardiovascular disease risk may be increased with oral contraceptive use after age 40 in healthy non-smoking women (even with the newer low-dose formulations), there are also greater potential health risks associated with pregnancy in older women and with the alternative surgical and medical procedures which may be necessary if such women do not have access to effective and acceptable means of contraception. The committee recommended that the benefits of low-dose oral contraceptive use by healthy non-smoking women over 40 may outweigh the possible risks.

Of course, older women, as all women who take oral contraceptives, should take an oral contraceptive which contains the least amount of estrogen and progestogen that is compatible with a low failure rate and individual patient needs. (See related table).

3. CARCINOMA OF THE REPRODUCTIVE ORGANS AND BREASTS

Numerous epidemiological studies have been performed on the incidence of breast, endometrial, ovarian and cervical cancer in women using oral contraceptives. While there are conflicting reports most studies suggest that the use of oral contraceptives is not associated with an overall increase in the risk of developing breast cancer. Some studies have reported an increased relative risk of developing breast cancer, particularly at a younger age. This increased relative risk appears to be related to duration of use[36-43,79-89].

Some studies suggest that oral contraceptive use has been associated with an increase in the risk of cervical intraepithelial neoplasia in some populations of women[45-48]. However, there continues to be controversy about the extent to which such findings may be due to differences in sexual behavior and other factors.

4. HEPATIC NEOPLASIA

Benign hepatic adenomas are associated with oral contraceptive use, although the incidence of benign tumors is rare in the United States. Indirect calculations have estimated the attributable risk to be in the range of 3.3 cases/100,000 for users, a risk that increases after four or more years of use especially with oral contraceptives of higher dose[49]. Rupture of rare, benign, hepatic adenomas may cause death through intra-abdominal hemorrhage[50,51].

Studies from Britain have shown an increased risk of developing hepatocellular carcinoma[52-54] in long-term (> 8 years) oral contraceptive users. However, these cancers are rare in the U.S. and the attributable risk (the excess incidence) of liver cancers in oral contraceptive users approaches less than one per million users.

5. OCULAR LESIONS

There have been clinical case reports of retinal thrombosis associated with the use of oral contraceptives. Oral contraceptives should be discontinued if there is unexplained partial or complete loss of vision; onset of proptosis or diplopia; papilledema; or retinal vascular lesions. Appropriate diagnostic and therapeutic measures should be undertaken immediately.

6. ORAL CONTRACEPTIVE USE BEFORE OR DURING EARLY PREGNANCY

Extensive epidemiological studies have revealed no increased risk of birth defects in women who have used oral contraceptives prior to pregnancy[56-57]. The majority of recent studies also do not indicate a teratogenic effect, particularly in so far as cardiac anomalies and limb reduction defects are concerned[55,56,58,59], when oral contraceptives are taken inadvertently during early pregnancy.

The administration of oral contraceptives to induce withdrawal bleeding should not be used as a test for pregnancy. Oral contraceptives should not be used during pregnancy to treat threatened or habitual abortion.

It is recommended that for any patient who has missed two consecutive periods, pregnancy should be ruled out before continuing oral contraceptive use. If the patient has not adhered to the prescribed schedule, the possibility of pregnancy should be considered at the time of the first missed period. Oral contraceptive use should be discontinued until pregnancy is ruled out.

7. GALLBLADDER DISEASE

Earlier studies have reported an increased lifetime relative risk of gallbladder surgery in users of oral contraceptives and estrogens[60,61]. More recent studies, however, have shown that the relative risk of developing gallbladder disease among oral contraceptive users may be minimal[62-64]. The recent findings of minimal risk may be related to the use of oral contraceptive formulations containing lower hormonal doses of estrogens and pregestogens.

8. CARBOHYDRATE AND LIPID METABOLIC EFFECTS

Oral contraceptives have been shown to cause a decrease in glucose tolerance in a significant percentage of users[17]. This effect has been shown to be directly related to estrogen dose[65]. In general, progestogens increase insulin secretion and create insulin resistance, this effect varying with different progestational agents[17,66]. In the nondiabetic woman, oral contraceptives appear to have no effect on fasting blood glucose[67]. Because of these demonstrated effects, prediabetic and diabetic women should be carefully monitored while taking oral contraceptives.

A small proportion of women will have persistent hypertriglyceridemia while on the pill. As discussed earlier (see *"Warnings 1.a"* and *"1.d."*), changes in serum triglycerides and lipoprotein levels have been reported in oral contraceptive users.

9. ELEVATED BLOOD PRESSURE

An increase in blood pressure has been reported in women taking oral contraceptives[68] and this increase is more likely in older oral contraceptive users[69] and with extended duration of use[61]. Data from the Royal College of General Practitioners[12] and subsequent randomized trials have shown that the incidence of hypertension increases with increasing progestational activity.

Women with a history of hypertension or hypertension-related diseases, or renal disease[70] should be encouraged to use another method of contraception. If women elect to use oral contraceptives, they should be monitored closely and if significant elevation of blood pressure occurs, oral contraceptives should be discontinued. For most women, elevated blood pressure will return to normal after stopping oral contraceptives[69], and there is no difference in the occurrence of hypertension among former and never users[68,70,71].

10. HEADACHE

The onset or exacerbation of migraine or development of headache with a new pattern which is recurrent, persistent or severe requires discontinuation of oral contraceptives and evaluation of the cause.

11. BLEEDING IRREGULARITIES

Breakthrough bleeding and spotting are sometimes encountered in patients on oral contraceptives, especially during the first three months of use. Nonhormonal causes should be considered and adequate diagnostic measures taken to rule out malignancy or pregnancy in the event of breakthrough bleeding, as in the case of any abnormal vaginal bleeding. If pathology has been excluded, time or a change to another formulation may solve the problem. In the event of amenorrhea, pregnancy should be ruled out.

Some women may encounter post-pill amenorrhea or oligomenorrhea, especially when such a condition was pre-existent.

12. ECTOPIC PREGNANCY

Ectopic as well as intrauterine pregnancy may occur in contraceptive failures.

PRECAUTIONS

1. PHYSICAL EXAMINATION AND FOLLOW UP

A complete medical history and physical examination should be taken prior to the initiation or reinstitution of oral contraceptives and at least annually during use of oral contraceptives. These physical examinations should include special reference to blood pressure, breasts, abdomen and pelvic organs, including cervical cytology, and relevant laboratory tests. In case of undiagnosed, persistent or recurrent abnormal vaginal bleeding, appropriate diagnostic measures should be conducted to rule out malignancy. Women with a strong family history of breast cancer or who have breast nodules should be monitored with particular care.

2. LIPID DISORDERS

Women who are being treated for hyperlipidemias should be followed closely if they elect to use oral contraceptives. Some progestogens may elevate LDL levels and may render the control of hyperlipidemias more difficult.

3. LIVER FUNCTION

If jaundice develops in any woman receiving such drugs, the medication should be discontinued. Steroid hormones may be poorly metabolized in patients with impaired liver function.

4. FLUID RETENTION

Oral contraceptives may cause some degree of fluid retention. They should be prescribed with caution, and only with careful monitoring, in patients with conditions which might be aggravated by fluid retention.

5. EMOTIONAL DISORDERS

Women with a history of depression should be carefully observed and the drug discontinued if depression recurs to a serious degree.

6. CONTACT LENSES

Contact lens wearers who develop visual changes or changes in lens tolerance should be assessed by an ophthalmologist.

7. DRUG INTERACTIONS

Reduced efficacy and increased incidence of breakthrough bleeding and menstrual irregularities have been associated with concomitant use of rifampin. A similar association, though less marked, has been suggested with barbiturates, phenylbutazone, phenytoin sodium, carbamazepine and possibly with griseofulvin, ampicillin and tetracyclines[72].

8. INTERACTIONS WITH LABORATORY TESTS

Certain endocrine and liver function tests and blood components may be affected by oral contraceptives:

a. Increased prothrombin and factors VII, VIII, IX and X; decreased antithrombin 3; increased norepinephrine-induced platelet aggregability.

b. Increased thyroid binding globulin (TBG) leading to increased circulating total thyroid hormone, as measured by protein-bound iodine (PBI), T4 by column or by radioimmunoassay. Free T3 resin uptake is decreased, reflecting the elevated TBG; free T4 concentration is unaltered.

c. Other binding proteins may be elevated in serum.

d. Sex hormone binding globulins are increased and result in elevated levels of total circulating sex steroids however, free or biologically active levels either decrease or remain unchanged.

e. High-density lipoprotein (HDL-C) and triglycerides may be increased, while low-density lipoprotein cholesterol (LDL-C) and total cholesterol (Total-C) may be decreased or unchanged.

f. Glucose tolerance may be decreased.

g. Serum folate levels may be depressed by oral contraceptive therapy. This may be of clinical significance if a woman becomes pregnant shortly after discontinuing oral contraceptives.

9. CARCINOGENESIS

See *"Warnings"* section.

10. PREGNANCY

Pregnancy Category X. See *"Contraindications"* and *"Warnings"* sections.

Table 3
ANNUAL NUMBER OF BIRTH-RELATED OR METHOD-RELATED DEATHS ASSOCIATED WITH CONTROL OF FERTILITY PER 100,000 NON-STERILE WOMEN, BY FERTILITY CONTROL METHOD ACCORDING TO AGE

Method of control and outcome	15-19	20-24	25-29	30-34	35-39	40-44
No fertility control methods*	7.0	7.4	9.1	14.8	25.7	28.2
Oral contraceptives non-smoker**	0.3	0.5	0.9	1.9	13.8	31.6
Oral contraceptives smoker**	2.2	3.4	6.6	13.5	51.1	117.2
IUD**	0.8	0.8	1.0	1.0	1.4	1.4
Condom*	1.1	1.6	0.7	0.2	0.3	0.4
Diaphragm/spermicide*	1.9	1.2	1.2	1.3	2.2	2.8
Periodic abstinence*	2.5	1.6	1.6	1.7	2.9	3.6

* *Deaths are birth-related*
** *Deaths are method-related*
Adapted from H.W. Ory, ref. #35.

11. NURSING MOTHERS

Small amounts of oral contraceptive steroids have been identified in the milk of nursing mothers and a few adverse effects on the child have been reported, including jaundice and breast enlargement. In addition, oral contraceptives given in the postpartum period may interfere with lactation by decreasing the quantity and quality of breast milk. If possible, the nursing mother should be advised not to use oral contraceptives but to use other forms of contraception until she has completely weaned her child.

INFORMATION FOR THE PATIENT

See manufacturer's patient information.

ADVERSE REACTIONS

An increased risk of the following serious adverse reactions has been associated with the use of oral contraceptives (see *"Warnings"* section).

- Thrombophlebitis and venous thrombosis with or without embolism
- Arterial thromboembolism
- Pulmonary embolism
- Myocardial infarction
- Cerebral hemorrhage
- Cerebral thrombosis
- Hypertension
- Gall bladder disease
- Hepatic adenomas or benign liver tumors

The following adverse reactions have been reported in patients receiving oral contraceptives and are believed to be drug-related:

- Nausea
- Vomiting
- Gastrointestinal symptoms (such as abdominal cramps and bloating)
- Breakthrough bleeding
- Spotting
- Change in menstrual flow
- Amenorrhea
- Temporary infertility after discontinuation of treatment
- Edema
- Melasma which may persist
- Breast changes: tenderness, enlargement, secretion
- Change in weight (increase or decrease)
- Change in cervical erosion and secretion
- Diminution in lactation when given immediately postpartum
- Cholestatic jaundice
- Migraine
- Rash (allergic)
- Mental depression
- Reduced tolerance to carbohydrates
- Vaginal candidiasis
- Change in corneal curvature (steepening)
- Intolerance to contact lenses

The following adverse reactions have been reported in users of oral contraceptives and the association has been neither confirmed nor refuted:

- Pre-menstrual syndrome
- Cataracts
- Changes in appetite
- Cystitis-like syndrome
- Headache
- Nervousness
- Dizziness
- Hirsutism
- Loss of scalp hair
- Erythema multiforme
- Erythema nodosum
- Hemorrhagic eruption
- Vaginitis
- Porphyria
- Impaired renal function
- Hemolytic uremic syndrome
- Acne
- Changes in libido
- Colitis
- Budd-Chiari Syndrome

OVERDOSAGE

Serious ill effects have not been reported following acute ingestion of large doses of oral contraceptives by young children. Overdosage may cause nausea, and withdrawal bleeding may occur in females.

NONCONTRACEPTIVE HEALTH BENEFITS

The following non-contraceptive health benefits related to the use of oral contraceptives are supported by epidemiological studies which largely utilized oral contraceptive formulations containing estrogen doses exceeding 0.035 mg of Ethinyl Estradiol or 0.05 mg of mestranol[73-78].

Effects on menses:

- increased menstrual cycle regularity
- decreased blood loss and decreased incidence of iron deficiency anemia
- decreased incidence of dysmenorrhea

Effects related to inhibition of ovulation:

- decreased incidence of functional ovarian cysts
- decreased incidence of ectopic pregnancies

Effects from long-term use:

- decreased incidence of fibroadenomas and fibrocystic disease of the breast
- decreased incidence of acute pelvic inflammatory disease
- decreased incidence of endometrial cancer
- decreased incidence of ovarian cancer

DOSAGE AND ADMINISTRATION

To achieve maximum contraceptive effectiveness. Desogestrel/Ethinyl Estradiol must be taken exactly as directed and at intervals not exceeding 24 hours. Desogestrel/Ethinyl Estradiol is available in a tablet dispenser which is present for a Sunday start. Day 1 start is also provided.

21-DAY REGIMEN (DAY 1 START)

The dosage of Desogestrel/Ethinyl Estradiol 21 for the initial cycle of therapy is one tablet administered daily from the 1st day through the 21st day of the menstrual cycle, counting the first day of menstrual flow as "Day 1". For subsequent cycles, no tablets are taken for 7 days, then a new course is started of one tablet a day for 21 days. The dosage regimen then continues with 7 days of no medication, followed by 21 days of medication, instituting a three-weeks-on, one-week-off dosage regimen.

The use of Desogestrel/Ethinyl Estradiol 21 for contraception may be initiated 4 weeks postpartum in women who elect not to breast feed. When the tablets are administered during the postpartum period, the increased risk of thromboembolic disease associated with the postpartum period must be considered. (See *"Contraindications"* and *"Warnings"* concerning thromboembolic disease. See also *"Precautions"* for *"Nursing Mothers".*) If the patient starts on Desogestrel/Ethinyl Estradiol postpartum, and has not yet had a period, she should be instructed to use another method of contraception until a tablet has been taken daily for 7 days. The possibility of ovulation and conception prior to initiation of medication should be considered. If the patient misses one (1) active tablet in Weeks 1, 2, or 3, the tablet should be taken as soon as she remembers. If the patient misses two (2) active tablets in Week 1 or Week 2, the patient should take two (2) tablets the day she remembers and two (2) tablets the next day; and then continue taking one (1) tablet a day until she finishes the pack. The patient should be instructed to use a back-up method of birth control if she has sex in the seven (7) days after missing pills. If the patient misses two (2) active tablets in the third week or misses three (3) or more active tablets in a row, the patient should throw out the rest of the pack and start a new pack that same day. The patient should be instructed to use a back-up method of birth control if she has sex in the seven (7) days after missing pills.

21-DAY REGIMEN (SUNDAY START)

When taking Desogestrel/Ethingl Estradiol 21, the first tablet should be taken on the first Sunday after menstruation begins. If period begins on Sunday, the first tablet is taken on that day. If switching directly from another oral contraceptive, the first tablet should be taken on the first Sunday after the last ACTIVE tablet of the previous product. One tablet is taken daily for 21 days. For subsequent cycles, no tablets are taken for seven days, then a new course is started of one tablet a day for 21 days instituting a 3-weeks-on, one-week-off dosage regimen. When initiating a Sunday start regimen, another method of contraception should be used until after the first 7 consecutive days of administration.

The use of Desogestrel/Ethinyl Estradiol 21 for contraception may be initiated 4 weeks postpartum in women who elect not to breast feed. When the tablets are administered during the postpartum period, the increased risk of thromboembolic disease associated with the postpartum period must be considered. (See *"Contraindications"* and *"Warnings"* concerning thromboembolic disease. See also *"Precautions"* for *"Nursing Mothers".*) If the patient starts on Desogestrel/Ethinyl Estradiol postpartum, and has not yet had a period, she should be instructed to use another method of contraception until a tablet has been taken daily for 7 days. The possibility of ovulation and conception prior to initiation of medication should be considered. If the patient misses one (1) active tablet in Weeks 1, 2, or 3, the tablet should be taken as soon as she remembers. If the patient misses two (2) active tablets in Week 1 or Week 2, the patient should take two (2) tablets the day she remembers and two (2) tablets the next day; and then continue taking one (1) tablet a day until she finishes the pack. The patient should be instructed to use a back-up method of birth control if she has sex in the seven (7) days after missing pills. If the patient misses two (2) active tablets in the third week or misses three (3) or more tablets in a row, the patient should continue taking one tablet every day until Sunday. On Sunday the patient should throw out the rest of the pack and start a new pack that same day. The patient should be instructed to use a back-up method of birth control if she has sex in the seven (7) days after missing pills.

28-DAY REGIMEN (DAY 1 START)

The dosage of Desogestrel/Ethinyl Estradiol 28 for the initial cycle of therapy is one tablet administered daily from the 1st day through 21st day of the menstrual cycle, counting the first day of menstrual flow as "Day 1". Tablets are taken without interruption as follows: one tablet daily for 21 days, then one tablet daily for 7 days. Certain brands of Desogestrel/Ethinyl Estradiol have 21 orange tablets and 7 green tablets. After 28 tablets have been taken, a new course is started and an orange tablet is taken the next day.

The use of Desogestrel/Ethinyl Estradiol 28 for contraception may be initiate 4 weeks postpartum in women who elect not to breast feed. When the tablets are administered during the postpartum period, the increased risk of thromboembolic

---

♦ RATED THERAPEUTICALLY EQUIVALENT; ◇ THERAPEUTIC EQUIVALENCE UNCONFIRMED; ○ UNRATED

disease associated with the postpartum period must be considered (See *"Contraindications"* and *"Warnings"* concerning thromboembolic disease. See *"Precautions"* for *"Nursing Mothers"*. If the patient starts on Desogestrel/Ethinyl Estradiol postpartum, and has not yet had a period, she should be instructed to use another method of contraception until a tablet has been taken daily for 7 days. The possibility of ovulation and conception prior to initiation of medication should be considered. If the patient misses one (1) active tablet in Weeks 1, 2, or 3, the tablet should be taken as soon as she remembers. If the patient misses two (2) active tablets in Week 1 or Week 2, the patient should take two (2) tablets the day she remembers and two (2) tablets the next day; and then continue taking one (1) tablet a day until she finishes the pack. The patient should be instructed to use a back-up method of birth control if she has sex in the seven (7) days after missing pills. If the patient misses two (2) active tablets in the third week or misses three (3) or more active tablets in a row, the patient should throw out the rest of the pack and start a new pack that same day. The patient should be instructed to use a back-up method of birth control if she has sex in the seven (7) days after missing pills.

28-DAY REGIMEN (SUNDAY START)

When taking Desogestrel/Ethinyl Estradiol 28, the first tablet should be taken on the first Sunday after menstruation begins. If period begins on Sunday, the first tablet is taken on that day. If switching directly from another oral contraceptive, the first tablet should be taken on the first Sunday after the last ACTIVE tablet of the previous product. Tablets are taken without interruption as follows: One tablet daily for 21 days, then one tablet daily for 7 days. Certain brands of Desogestrel/Ethinyl Estradiol have 21 orange tablets and 7 green tablets. After 28 tablets have been taken, a new course is started and an orange tablet is taken the next day (Sunday). When initiating a Sundary start regimen, another method of contraception should be used until after the first 7 consecutive days of adminstration.

The use of Desogestrel/Ethinyl Estradiol 28 for contraception may be initiated 4 weeks postpartum. When the tablets are administered during the postpartum period, the increased risk of thromboembolic disease associated with the postpartum period must be considered. (see *"Contraindications"* and *"Warnings"* concerning thromboembolic disease. See also *"Precautions"* for *"Nursing Mothers"*.) If the patient starts on Desogestrel/Ethinyl Estradiol postpartum, and has not yet had a period, she should be instructed to use another method of contraception until a tablet has been taken daily for 7 days. The possibility of ovulation and conception prior to initiation of medication should be considered. If the patient misses one (1) active tablet in Weeks 1, 2, or 3, the tablet should be taken as soon as she remembers. If the patient misses two (2) active tablets in Week 1 or Week 2, the patient should take two (2) tablets the day she remembers and two (2) tablets the next day; and then continue taking one (1) tablet a day until she finishes the pack. The patient should be instructed to use a back-up method of birth control if she has sex in the seven (7) days after missing pills. If the patient misses two (2) active tablets in the third week or misses three (3) or more tablets in a row, the patient should continue taking one tablet every day until Sunday. On Sunday the patient should throw out the rest of the pack and start a new pack that same day. The patient should be instructed to use a back-up method of birth control if she has sex in the seven (7) days after missing pills.

ALL ORAL CONTRACEPTIVES

Breakthrough bleeding, spotting, and amenorrhea are frequent reasons for patients discontinuing oral contraceptives. In breakthrough bleeding, as in all cases of irregular bleeding from the vagina, nonfunctional causes should be borne in mind. In undiagnosed persistent or recurrent abnormal bleeding from the vagina, adequate diagnostic measures are indicated to rule out pregnancy or malignancy. If pathology has been excluded, time or a change to another formulation may solve the problem. Changing to an oral contraceptive with a higher estrogen content, while potentially useful in minimizing menstrual irregularity, should be done only if necessary since this may increase the risk of thromboembolic disease.

Use of oral contraceptives in the event of a missed menstrual period:

1. If the patient has not adhered to the prescribed schedule, the possibility of pregnancy should be considered at the time of the first missed period and oral contraceptive use should be discontinued until pregnancy is ruled out.

2. If the patient has adhered to the prescribed regimen and misses two consecutive periods, pregnancy should be ruled out before continuing oral contraceptive use.

REFERENCES

1. Reproduced with permission of the Population Council from J. Trussel et al. Contraceptive failure in the United States: An update. Studies in Family Planning, 21 (1), January/February 1990. 2. Stadel BV. Oral contraceptives and cardiovascular disease. (Pt. 1). N Engl J Med 1981; 305:612-618. 3. Stadel BV. Oral contraceptives and cardiovascular disease. (Pt. 2). N Engl J Med 1981; 305:672-677. 4. Adam SA, Thorogood M. Oral contraception and myocardial infarction revisited: the effects of new preparations and prescribing patterns. Br J Obstet and Gynecol 1981; 88:838-845. 5. Mann JI, Inman WH. Oral contraceptives and death from myocardial infarction. Br Med J 1975; 2(5965):245-248. 6. Mann JI, Vessey MP, Thorogood M. Doll R. Myocardial infarction in young women with special reference to oral contraceptive practice. Br Med J 1975; 2(5956):241-245. 7. Royal College of General Practitioners' Oral Contraception Study: Further analyses of mortality in oral contraceptive users. Lancet 1981;1:541-546. 8. Slone D, Shapiro S, Kaufman DW, Rosenberg L, Miettinen OS, Stolley PD. Risk of myocardial infarction in relation to current and discontinued use of oral contraceptives. N Engl J Med 1981; 305:420-424. 9. Vessey MP. Female hormones and vascular disease—an epidemiological overview. Br J Fam Plann 1980; 6:1-12. 10. Russell-Briefel RG, Ezzati TM. Fulwood R, Perlman JA, Murphy RS. Cardiovascular risk status and oral contraceptive use, United States, 1976-80. Prevent Med 1986; 15:352-362. 11. Goldbaum GM, Kendrick JS, Hogelin GC, Gentry EM. The relative impact of smoking and oral contraceptive use on women in the United States. JAMA 1987;258:1339-1342. 12. Layde PM, Beral V. Further analyses of mortality in oral contraceptive users: Royal College General Practitioners' Oral Contraception Study. (Table 5) Lancet 1981; 1:541-546. 13. Knopp RH. Arteriosclerosis risk: the roles of oral contraceptives and postmenopausal estrogens. J Reprod Med 1986; 31(9) (Supplement):913-921. 14. Krauss RM, Roy S, Mishell DR, Casagrande J, Pike MC. Effects of two low-dose oral contraceptives on serum lipids and lipoproteins: Differential changes in high-density lipoprotein subclasses. Am J Obstet 1983; 145:446-452. 15. Wahl P, Walden C, Knopp R, Hoover J. Wallace R, Heiss G, Rifkind B. Effect of estrogen/progestin potency on lipid/lipoprotein cholesterol. N Engl J Med 1983; 308:862-867. 16. Wynn V, Niththyanathan R. The effect of progestin in combined oral contraceptives on serum lipids with special reference to high-density lipoproteins. Am J Obstet Gynecol 1982; 142:766-771. 17. Wynn V, Godsland I. Effects of oral contraceptives and carbohydrate metabolism. J Reprod Med 1986; 31 (9) (Supplement):892-897. 18. LaRosa JC, Atherosclerotic risk factors in cardiovascular disease. J Reprod Med 1986:31 (9) (Supplement):906-912. 19. Inman WH, Vessey MP. Investigation of death from pulmonary, coronary, and cerebral thrombosis and embolism in women of childbearing age. Br Med J 1968; 2 (5599):193-199. 20. Maguire MG, Tonascia J, Sartwell PE, Stolley PD, Tockman MS. Increased risk of thrombosis due to oral contraceptives: a further report. Am J Epidemiol 1979; 110(2):188-195. 21. Pettiti DB, Wingerd J, Pellegrin F, Ramacharan S. Risk of vascular disease in women: smoking, oral contraceptives, noncontraceptive estrogens, and other factors. JAMA 1979; 242:1150-1154. 22. Vessey MP, Doll R. Investigation of relation between use of oral contraceptives and thromboembolic disease. Br Med J 1968; 2(5599):199-205. 23. Vessey MP, Doll R. Investigation of relation between use of oral contraceptives and thromboembolic disease. A further report. Br Med J 1969; 2 (5658):651-657. 24. Porter JB, Hunter JR, Danielson DA, Jick H, Stergachis A. Oral contraceptives and non-fatal vascular disease—recent experience. Obstet Gynecol 1982; 59 (3):299-302. 25. Vessey M. Doll R, Peto R. Johnson B, Wiggins P. A long-term follow-up study of women using different methods of contraception: an interim report. J Biosocial Sci 1976; 8:375-427. 26. Royal College of General Practitioners: Oral contraceptives, venous thrombosis, and varicose veins. J Royal Coll Gen Pract 1978; 28:393-399. 27. Collaborative Group for the Study of Stroke in Young Women: Oral contraception and increased risk of cerebral ischemia or thrombosis. N Engl J Med 1973; 288:871-878. 28. Petitti DB, Wingerd J. Use of oral contraceptives, cigarette smoking, and risk of subarachnoid hemorrhage, Lancet 1978; 2:234-236. 29. Inman WH. Oral contraceptives and fatal subarachnoid hemorrhage. Br Med J 1979; 2 (6203):1468-70. 30. Collaborative Group for the study of Stroke in Young Women: Oral contraceptives and stroke in young women: associated risk factors. JAMA 1975; 231:718-722. 31. Inman WH, Vessey MP, Westerholm B, Engelund A. Thromboembolic disease and the steroidal content of oral contraceptives. A report to the Committee on Safety of Drugs. Br Med J 1970; 2:203-209. 32. Meade TW, Greenberg G, Thompson SG. Progestogens and cardiovascular reactions associated with oral contraceptives and a comparison of the safety of 50- and 35-mcg oestrogen preparations. Br Med J 1980; 280 (6224):1157-1161. 33. Kay, CR. Progestogens and arterial disease—evidence from the Royal College of General Practitioners' Study. Am J Obstet Gynecol 1982; 142:762-765. 34. Royal College of General Practitioners: Incidence of arterial disease among oral contraceptive users. J Royal Coll Gen Pract 1983; 33:75-82. 35. Ory HW. Mortality associated with fertility and fertility control: 1983. Family Planning Perspectives 1983; 15:50-56. 36. The Cancer and Steroid Hormone Study of the Centers for Disease Control and the National Institute of Child Health and Human Development: Oral-contraceptive use and the risk of breast cancer. N Engl J Med 1986; 315:405-411. 37. Pike MC, Henderson BE, Krailo MD, Duke A, Roy S. Breast cancer risk in young women and use of oral contraceptives: possible modifying effect of formulation and age at use. Lancet 1983; 2:926-929. 38. Paul C. Skegg DG, Spears GFS, Kaldor JM. Oral contraceptives and breast cancer: A national study, Br Med J 1986; 293:723-725. 39. Miller DR, Rosenberg L, Kaufman DW, Schottenfeld D, Stolley PD, Shapiro S. Breast cancer risk in relation to early oral contraceptive use. Obstet Gynecol 1986; 68:863-868. 40. Olson H, Olson KL, Moller TR, Ranstam J, Holm P. Oral contraceptive use and breast cancer in young women in Sweden (letter). Lancet 1985; 2:748-749. 41. McPherson K, Vessey M, Neil A, Doll R. Jones L, Roberts M. Early contraceptive use and breast cancer: Results of another case-control study. Br J Cancer 1987; 56:653-660. 42. Huggins GR, Zucker PF. Oral contraceptives and neoplasia: 1987 update. Fertil Steril 1987; 47:733-761. 43. McPherson K, Drife JO. The pill and breast cancer: why the uncertainty? Br Med J 1986; 293:709-710. 44. Shapiro S. Oral contraceptives—time to take stock. N Engl J Med 1987; 315:450-451. 45. Ory H, Naib Z, Conger SB, Hatcher RA, Tyler CW. Contraceptive choice and prevalence of cervical dysplasia and carcinoma in situ. Am J Obstet Gynecol 1976;124:573-577. 46. Vessey MP, Lawless M. McPherson K, Yeates D. Neoplasia of the cervix uteri and contraception: a possible adverse effect of the pill. Lancet 1983; 2:930. 47. Brinton LA, Huggins GR, Lehman HF, Malli K, Savitz DA, Trapido E, Rosenthal J, Hoover R. Long term use of oral contraceptives and risk of invasive cervical cancer. Int J Cancer 1986; 38:339-344. 48. WHO Collaborative Study of Neoplasia and Steroid Contraceptives: Invasive cervical cancer and combined oral contraceptives. Br Med J 1985; 290:961-965. 49. Rooks JB, Ory HW, Ishak KG, Strauss LT, Greenspan JR, Hill AP, Tyler CW. Epidemiology of hepatocellular adenoma: the role of oral contraceptive use. JAMA 1979: 242:644-648. 50. Bein NN, Goldsmith HS. Recurrent massive hemorrhage from benign hepatic tumors secondary to oral contraceptives. Br J Surg 1977; 64:433-435. 51. Klatskin G. Hepatic tumors: possible relationship to use of oral contraceptives. Gastroenterology 1977; 73:386-394. 52. Henderson BE, Preston-Martin S. Edmondson HA, Peters RL, Pike MC. Hepatocellular carcinoma and oral contraceptives. Br J Cancer 1983; 48:437-440. 53. Neuberger J. Forman D, Doll R, Williams R. Oral contraceptives and hepatocellular carcinoma. Br Med J 1986; 292:1355-1357. 54. Forman D, Vincent TJ, Doll R. Cancer of the liver and oral contraceptives, Br Med J 1986; 292:1357-1361. 55. Harlap S, Eldor J. Births following oral contraceptive failures. Obstet Gynecol 1980; 55:447-452. 56. Salvolainen E, Saksela E, Saxen L. Teratogenic hazards of oral national malformation register. Am J Obstet Gynecol 1981; 140:521-524. 57. Janerich DT, Piper JM, Glebatis DM. Oral contraceptives and birth defects. Am J Epidemiol 1980; 112:73-79. 58. Ferencz C, Matanoski GM, Wilson PD, Rubin JD, Neil CA, Gutberlet R. Maternal hormone therapy and congenital heart disease. Teratology 1980; 21:225-239. 59. Rothman KJ, Fyler DC, Goldblatt A, Kreidberg MB. Exogenous hormones and other drug exposures of children with congenital heart disease. Am J Epidemiol 1979; 109:433-439. 60. Boston Collaborative Drug Surveillance Program: Oral contraceptives and venous thromboembolic disease, surgically confirmed gall-bladder disease, and breast tumors. Lancet 1973: 1:1399-1404. 61. Royal College of General Practitioners: Oral contraceptives and health. New York, Pittman, 1974. 62. Layde

PM, Vessey MP, Yeates D. Risk of gall bladder disease: a cohort study of young women attending family planning clinics. J Epidemiol Community Health 1982; 36:274-278. 63. Rome Group for the Epidemiology and Prevention of Cholelithiasis (GREPCO): Prevalence of gallstone disease in an Italian adult female population. Am J Epidemiol 1984; 119:796-805. 64. Strom BL, Tamragouri RT, Morse ML, Lazar EL, West SL, Stolley PD, Jones JK. Oral contraceptives and other risk factors for gall bladder disease. Clin Pharmacol Ther 1986; 39:335-341. 65. Wynn V, Adams PW, Godsland IF, Melrose J, Niththyananthan R, Oakley NW, Seedj A. Comparison of effects of different combined oral-contraceptive formulations on carbohydrate and lipid metabolism. Lancet 1979; 1:1045-1049. 66. Wynn V. effect of progesterone and progestins on carbohydrate metabolism. In Progesterone and Progestin. Edited by Bardin CW, Milgrom E, Mauvis-Jarvis P. New York, Raven Press, 1983 pp. 395-410. 67. Perlman JA, Rousell-Briefel RG, Ezzati TM, Lieberknecht G. Oral glucose tolerance and the potency of oral contraceptive progesterone. J Chronic Dis 1985; 38:857-864. 68. Royal College of General Practitioners' Oral Contraception Study: Effect on hypertension and benign breast disease of progestogen component in combined oral contraceptives. Lancet 1977; 1:624. 69. Fisch IR, Frank J. Oral contraceptives and blood pressure. JAMA 1977; 237:2499-2503. 70. Laragh AJ. Oral contraceptive induced hypertension—nine years later. Am J Obstet Gynecol 1976; 126:141-147. 71. Ramcharan S. Peritz E, Pellegrin FA, Williams WT. Incidence of hypertension in the Walnut Creek Contraceptive Drug Study cohort. In Pharmacology of Steroid Contraceptive Drugs. Garattini S, Berendes HW. Eds. New York, Raven Press, 1977 pp. 277-278. (Monographs of the Mario Negri Institute for Pharmacological Research, Milan). 72. Stockley I. Interactions with oral contraceptives. J Pharm 1976; 216:140-143. 73. The Cancer and Steroid Hormone Study of the Centers for Disease Control and the National Institute of Child Health and Human Development: Oral contraceptive use and the risk of ovarian cancer. JAMA 1983; 249:1596-1599. 74. The Cancer and Steroid Hormone Study of the Centers for Disease Control and the National Institute of Child Health and Human Development: Combination oral contraceptive use and the risk of endometrial cancer. JAMA 1987; 257:796-800. 75. Ory HW. Functional ovarian cysts and oral contraceptives: negative association confirmed surgically. JAMA 1974; 228:68-69. 76. Ory HW, Cole P, Macmahon B, Hoover R. Oral contraceptives and reduced risk of benign breast disease. N Engl J Med 1976; 294:419-422. 77. Ory HW. The noncontraceptive health benefits from oral contraceptive use. Fam Plann Perspect 1982; 14:182-184. 78. Ory HW, Forrest JD, Lincoln R. Making Choices: Evaluating the health risks and benefits of birth control methods. New York, The Alan Guttmacher Institute, 1983; p. 1. 79. Schlesselman J, Stadel BV, Murray P, Lai S. Breast Cancer in relation to early use of oral contraceptives 1988; 259:1828-1833. 80. Hennekens CH, Speizer FE, Lipnick RJ, Rosner B, Bain C, Belanger C, Stampfer MJ, Willett W, Peto R. A case-controlled study of oral contraceptive use and breast cancer. JNCI 1984;72:39-42. 81. LaVecchia C, Decarli A, Fasoli M, Franceschi S, Gentile A, Negri E. Parazini F, Tognoni G. Oral contraceptives and cancers of the breast and of the female genital tract. Interim results from a case-control study. Br J Cancer 1986; 54:311-317. 82. Meirik O, Lund E. Adami H, Bergstrom R, Christoffersen T, Bergsjo P. Oral contraceptive use in breast cancer in young women. A Joint National Case-control study in Sweden and Norway. Lancet 1986; 11:650-654. 83. Kay CR, Hannaford PC. Breast cancer and the pill—A further report from the Royal College of General Practitioners' oral contraception study. Br J Cancer 1988; 58:675-680. 84. Stadel BV, Lai S, Schlesselman JJ, Murray P. Oral contraceptives and premenopausal breast cancer in nulliparous women. Contraception 1988; 38:287-299. 85. Miller DR, Rosenberg L, Kaufman DW, Stolley P, Warshauer ME, Shapiro S. Breast cancer before age 45 and oral contraceptive use: New Findings. Am J Epidemiol 1989; 129:269-280. 86. The UK National Case-Control Study Group, Oral contraceptive use and breast cancer risk in young women. Lancet 1989; 1:973-982. 87. Schlesselman JJ. Cancer of the breast and reproductive tract in relation to use of oral contraceptives. Contraception 1989; 40:1-38. 88. Vessey MP, McPherson K, Villard-Mackintosh L, Yeates D. Oral contraceptives and breast cancer: latest findings in a large cohort study. Br J Cancer 1989; 59:613-617. 89. Jick SS, Walker AM, Stergachis A, Jick H. Oral contraceptives and breast cancer. Br J Cancer 1989; 59:618-621. 90. Godsland, I et al. The effects of different formulations of oral contraceptive agents on lipid and carbohydrate metabolism. N Engl J Med 1990;323:1375-81. 91. Kloosterboer, HJ et al. Selectivity in progesterone and androgen receptor binding of progestogens used in oral contraception. Contraception, 1988;38:325-32. 92. Van der Vies, J and de Visser, J. Endocrinological studies with Desogestrel. Arzneim. Forsch./ Drug Res., 1983;33(1),2:231-6. 93. Data on file, Organon Inc. 94. Fotherby, K. Oral contraceptives, lipids and cardiovascular diseases. Contraception, 1985; Vol. 31; 4:367-94. 95. Lawrence, DM et al. Reduced sex hormone binding globulin and derived free testosterone levels in women with severe acne. Clinical Endocrinology, 1981; 15:87-91. 96. Cullberg, G et al. Effects of a low-dose Desogestrel-Ethinyl Estradiol combination on hirsutism, androgens and sex hormone binding globulin in women with a polycystic ovary syndrome. Acta Obstet Gynecol Scand, 1985;64:195-202. 97. Jung-Hoffmann, C and Kuhl, H. Divergent effects of two low-dose oral contraceptives on sex hormone-binding of globulin and free testosterone. AJOG, 1987; 156:199-203. 98. Hammond, G et al. Serum steroid binding protein concentrations, distribution of progestogens, and bioavailability of testosterone during treatment with contraceptives containing Desogestrel or levonorgestrel. Fertil Steril, 1984;42:44-51. 99. Palatsi, R et al. Serum total and unbound testosterone and sex hormone binding globulin (SHBG) in female acne patients treated with two different oral contraceptives. Acta Derm Venereol, 1984; 64:517-23.

HOW SUPPLIED
TABLETS: 0.15 MG-30 MCG

BRAND/MANUFACTURER	NDC	SIZE	AWP
○ BRAND			
▶ ORTHO-CEPT: Ortho Pharm	00062-1795-15	21s	$22.20
	00062-1796-15	28s	$22.31
DESOGEN: Organon	00052-0261-06	168s	$117.31

Desonide

DESCRIPTION
Desonide, is a nonfluorinated corticosteroid for topical use. It has the chemical name: Pregna-1,4-diene-3,20-dione,11,21-dihydroxy-16,17- [(1-methylethyli-dene)bis(oxy)]-,(11β, 16α)-; the molecular formula: $C_{24}H_{32}O_6$; molecular weight: 416.51.

Desonide is available as a cream, an ointment, and a lotion.

Each gram of cream, ointment, or lotion contains:

Desonide . . . . 0.5 mg

Following is its chemical structure:

CLINICAL PHARMACOLOGY
Topical corticosteroids share anti-inflammatory, anti-pruritic, and vasoconstrictive actions.

The mechanism of anti-inflammatory activity of the topical corticosteroids is unclear. Various laboratory methods, including vasoconstrictor assays, are used to compare and predict potencies and/or clinical efficacies of the topical corticosteroids. There is some evidence to suggest that a recognizable correlation exists between vasoconstrictor potency and therapeutic efficacy in man.

Pharmacokinetics: The extent of percutaneous absorption of topical corticosteroids is determined by many factors including the vehicle, the integrity of the epidermal barrier, and the use of occlusive dressings.

Topical corticosteroids can be absorbed from normal intact skin. Inflammation and/or other disease processes in the skin increase percutaneous absorption. Occlusive dressings substantially increase the percutaneous absorption of topical corticosteroids. Thus, occlusive dressings may be a valuable therapeutic adjunct for treatment of resistant dermatoses. (See *"Dosage and Administration"*.)

Once absorbed through the skin, topical corticosteroids are handled through pharmacokinetic pathways similar to systemically administered corticosteroids. Corticosteroids are bound to plasma proteins in varying degrees. Corticosteroids are metabolized primarily in the liver and are then excreted by the kidneys. Some of the topical corticosteroids and their metabolites are also excreted into the bile.

INDICATIONS AND USAGE
Desonide cream, ointment, and lotion are indicated for the relief of the inflammatory and pruritic manifestations of corticosteroid-responsive dermatoses.

CONTRAINDICATIONS
Topical corticosteroids are contraindicated in those patients with a history of hypersensitivity to any of the components of the preparation.

PRECAUTIONS
General: Systemic absorption of topical corticosteroids has produced reversible hypothalamic-pituitary-adrenal (HPA) axis suppression, manifestations of Cushing's syndrome, hyperglycemia, and glucosuria in some patients.

Conditions which augment systemic absorption include the application of the more potent steroids, use over large surface areas, prolonged use, and the addition of occlusive dressings.

Therefore, patients receiving a large dose of a potent topical steroid applied to a large surface area or under an occlusive dressing should be evaluated periodically for evidence of HPA axis suppression by using the urinary free cortisol and ACTH stimulation tests. If HPA axis suppression is noted, an attempt should be made to withdraw the drug, to reduce the frequency of application, or to substitute a less potent steroid.

Recovery of HPA axis function is generally prompt and complete upon discontinuation of the drug. Infrequently, signs and symptoms of steroid withdrawal may occur, requiring supplemental systemic corticosteroids.

Children may absorb proportionally larger amounts of topical corticosteroids and thus be more susceptible to systemic toxicity (see *"Precautions—Pediatric Use"*).

If irritation develops, topical corticosteroids should be discontinued and appropriate therapy instituted.

In the presence of dermatological infections, the use of an appropriate antifungal or antibacterial agent should be instituted. If a favorable response does not occur promptly, the corticosteroids should be discontinued until the infection has been adequately controlled.

Information for the Patient: Patients using topical corticosteroids should receive the following information and instructions:

1. This medication is to be used as directed by the physician. It is for external use only. Avoid contact with the eyes.
2. Patients should be advised not to use this medication for any disorder other than for which it was prescribed.
3. The treated skin area should not be bandaged or otherwise covered or wrapped as to be occlusive unless directed by the physician.
4. Patients should report any signs of local adverse reactions especially under occlusive dressing.

5. Parents of pediatric patients should be advised not to use tight-fitting diapers or plastic pants on a child being treated in the diaper area, as these garments may constitute occlusive dressings.

Laboratory Tests: The following tests may be helpful in evaluating the HPA axis suppression:
   Urinary free cortisol test
   ACTH stimulation test

Carcinogenesis, Mutagenesis, and Impairment of Fertility: Long-term animal studies have not been performed to evaluate the carcinogenic potential or the effect on fertility of topical corticosteroids.

Studies to determine mutagenicity with prednisolone and hydrocortisone have revealed negative results.

Pregnancy Category C: Corticosteroids are generally teratogenic in laboratory animals when administered systemically at relatively low dosage levels. The more potent corticosteroids have been shown to be teratogenic after dermal application in laboratory animals. There are no adequate and well controlled studies in pregnant women on teratogenic effects from topically applied corticosteroids. Therefore, topical corticosteroids should be used during pregnancy only if the potential benefit justifies the potential risk to the fetus. Drugs of this class should not be used extensively on pregnant patients, in large amounts, or for prolonged periods of time.

Nursing Mothers: It is not known whether topical administration of corticosteroids could result in sufficient systemic absorption to produce detectable quantities in breast milk. Systemically administered corticosteroids are secreted into breast milk, in quantities *not* likely to have a deleterious effect on the infant. Nevertheless, caution should be exercised when topical corticosteroids are administered to a nursing woman.

Pediatric Use: Pediatric patients may demonstrate greater susceptibility to topical corticosteroid-induced HPA axis suppression and Cushing's syndrome than mature patients because of a larger skin surface area to body weight ratio.

Hypothalamic-pituitary-adrenal (HPA) axis suppression, Cushing's syndrome, and intracranial hypertension have been reported in children receiving topical corticosteroids. Manifestations of adrenal suppression in children include linear growth retardation, delayed weight gain, low plasma cortisol levels, and absence of response to ACTH stimulation. Manifestations of intracranial hypertension include bulging fontanelles, headaches, and bilateral papilledema.

Administration of topical corticosteroids to children should be limited to the least amount compatible with an effective therapeutic regimen. Chronic corticosteroid therapy may interfere with the growth and development of children.

ADVERSE REACTIONS
The following local adverse reactions are reported infrequently with topical corticosteroids, but may occur more frequently with the use of occlusive dressings. These reactions are listed in an approximate decreasing order of occurrence: burning, itching, irritation, dryness, folliculitis, hypertrichosis, acneiform eruptions, hypopigmentation, perioral dermatitis, allergic contact dermatitis, maceration of the skin, secondary infection, skin atrophy, striae and miliaria.

OVERDOSAGE
Topically applied corticosteroids can be absorbed in sufficient amounts to produce systemic effects (see *"Precautions"*).

DOSAGE AND ADMINISTRATION
Desonide cream, ointment, or lotion should be applied to the affected area as a thin film two or three times daily depending on the severity of the condition. SHAKE LOTION WELL BEFORE USING.

Occlusive dressings may be used for the management of psoriasis or recalcitrant conditions.

If an infection develops, the use of occlusive dressings should be discontinued and appropriate antimicrobial therapy instituted.

Store below 86°F (30°C). Avoid freezing.

HOW SUPPLIED
CREAM: 0.05%

AVERAGE UNIT PRICE (AVAILABLE SIZES)		GENERIC A-RATED AVERAGE PRICE (GAAP)	
BRAND	$0.51	15 gm	$8.97
GENERIC	$0.50	60 gm	$24.51
HCFA FUL (15 gm)	$0.58		
HCFA FUL (60 gm)	$0.40		

BRAND/MANUFACTURER	NDC	SIZE	AWP
◆ BRAND			
TRIDESILON: Miles Pharm	00026-5561-61	15 gm	$10.29
DESOWEN: Galderma	00299-5770-15	15 gm	$12.06
TRIDESILON: Miles Pharm	00026-5561-62	60 gm	$29.46
DESOWEN: Galderma	00299-5770-60	60 gm	$30.81
	00299-5770-90	90 gm	$33.75
TRIDESILON: Miles Pharm	00026-5561-92	2270 gm	$432.56
◆ GENERICS			
Taro	51672-1280-01	15 gm	$7.58
Copley	38245-0184-70	15 gm	$7.96
Geneva	00781-7230-27	15 gm	$8.82
Major	00904-7724-36	15 gm	$8.95
Goldline	00182-5066-51	15 gm	$9.15
Moore,H.L.	00839-7135-47	15 gm	$11.33

BRAND/MANUFACTURER	NDC	SIZE	AWP
Taro	51672-1280-03	60 gm	$21.69
Copley	38245-0184-73	60 gm	$22.78
Geneva	00781-7230-35	60 gm	$25.25
Major	00904-7724-02	60 gm	$25.50
Goldline	00182-5066-52	60 gm	$25.50
Moore,H.L.	00839-7135-50	60 gm	$26.31

LOTION: 0.05%

BRAND/MANUFACTURER	NDC	SIZE	AWP
○ BRAND			
DESOWEN: Galderma	00299-5765-02	60 ml	$21.63
	00299-5765-04	120 ml	$31.50

OINTMENT: 0.05%

AVERAGE UNIT PRICE (AVAILABLE SIZES)	
BRAND	$0.62
GENERIC	$0.43

BRAND/MANUFACTURER	NDC	SIZE	AWP
◆ BRAND			
TRIDESILON: Miles Pharm	00026-5591-61	15 gm	$10.29
DESOWEN: Galderma	00299-5775-15	15 gm	$12.06
TRIDESILON: Miles Pharm	00026-5591-62	60 gm	$29.46
DESOWEN: Galderma	00299-5775-60	60 gm	$30.81
◆ GENERICS			
Taro	51672-1281-01	15 gm	$7.58
Taro	51672-1281-03	60 gm	$21.69

DesOwen *SEE* DESONIDE

Desoximetasone

DESCRIPTION
Desoximetasone Emollient Cream 0.25%, and 0.05%, is a synthetic corticosteroid. The topical corticosteroids constitute a class of primarily synthetic steroids used as anti-inflammatory and anti-pruritic agents. Each gram of the Emollient Cream 0.25% contains 2.5 mg of Desoximetasone in an emollient cream.

Each gram of the Emollient Cream 0.05% contains 0.5 mg of Desoximetasone in an emollient cream.

The chemical name of Desoximetasone is Pregna-1,4-diene-3, 20-dione, 9-fluoro-11, 21-dihydroxy-16-methyl-, (11β, 16α)-. Desoximetasone has the empirical formula $C_{22}H_{29}FO_4$ and a molecular weight of 376.47.

Following is its chemical structure:

CLINICAL PHARMACOLOGY
Topical corticosteroids share antiinflammatory, antipruritic and vasoconstrictive actions.

The mechanism of anti-inflammatory activity of the topical corticosteroids is unclear. Various laboratory methods, including vasoconstrictor assays, are used to compare and predict potencies and/or clinical efficacies of the topical corticosteroids. There is some evidence to suggest that a recognizable correlation exists between vasoconstrictor potency and therapeutic efficacy in man.

PHARMACOKINETICS
The extent of percutaneous absorption of topical corticosteroids is determined by many factors including the vehicle, the integrity of the epidermal barrier, and the use of occlusive dressings.

Topical corticosteroids can be absorbed from normal intact skin. Inflammation and/or other disease processes in the skin increase percutaneous absorption. Occlusive dressings substantially increase the percutaneous absorption of topical corticosteroids. Thus, occlusive dressings may be a valuable therapeutic adjunct for treatment of resistant dermatoses.

Once absorbed through the skin, topical corticosteroids are handled through pharmacokinetic pathways similar to systemically administered corticosteroids. Corticosteroids are bound to plasma proteins in varying degrees. Corticosteroids are metabolized primarily in the liver and are then excreted by the kidneys. Some of the topical corticosteroids and their metabolites are also excreted into the bile.

Pharmacokinetic studies in men with Desoximetasone Emollient Cream 0.25% with tagged Desoximetasone showed a total of 5.2% ± 2.9% excretion in urine (4.1% ± 2.3%) and feces (1.1% ± 0.6%) and no detectable level (limit of sensitivity: 0.005 µg/mL) in the blood when it was applied topically on the back followed by occlusion for 24 hours. Seven days after application, no further radioactivity was detected in urine or feces. The half-life of the material was 15 ± 2 hours (for urine) and 17 ± 2 hours (for feces) between the third and fifth trial day.

Studies with other similarly structured steroids have shown that predominant metabolite reaction occurs through conjugation to form the glucuronide and sulfate ester.

INDICATIONS AND USAGE

Desoximetasone Emollient Cream 0.25% and 0.05% are indicated for the relief of the inflammatory and pruritic manifestations of corticosteroid-responsive dermatoses.

CONTRAINDICATIONS

Topical corticosteroids are contraindicated in those patients with a history of hypersensitivity to any of the components of the preparation.

PRECAUTIONS

GENERAL

Systemic absorption of topical corticosteroids has produced reversible hypothalamic-pituitary-adrenal (HPA) axis suppression, manifestations of Cushing's syndrome, hyperglycemia, and glucosuria in some patients.

Conditions which augment systemic absorption include the application of the more potent steroids, use over large surface areas, prolonged use, and the addition of occlusive dressings.

Therefore, patients receiving a large dose of a potent topical steroid applied to a large surface area or under an occlusive dressing should be evaluated periodically for evidence of HPA axis suppression by using the urinary free cortisol and ACTH stimulation tests. If HPA axis suppression is noted, an attempt should be made to withdraw the drug, to reduce the frequency of application, or to substitute a less potent steroid.

Recovery of HPA axis function is generally prompt and complete upon discontinuation of the drug. Infrequently, signs and symptoms of steroid withdrawal may occur, requiring supplemental systemic corticosteroids.

Children may absorb proportionally larger amounts of topical corticosteroids and thus be more susceptible to systemic toxicity. (See "Precautions: Pediatric Use".)

If irritation develops, topical corticosteroids should be discontinued and appropriate therapy instituted.

In the presence of dermatological infections, the use of an appropriate antifungal or antibacterial agent should be instituted. If a favorable response does not occur promptly, the corticosteroid should be discontinued until the infection has been adequately controlled.

INFORMATION FOR THE PATIENT

Patients using topical corticosteroids should receive the following information and instructions:

1. This medication is to be used as directed by the physician. It is for external use only. Avoid contact with the eyes.
2. Patients should be advised not to use this medication for any disorder other than for which it was prescribed.
3. The treated skin area should not be bandaged or otherwise covered or wrapped as to be occlusive unless directed by the physician.
4. Patients should report any signs of local adverse reactions especially under occlusive dressing.
5. Parents of pediatric patients should be advised not to use tight-fitting diapers or plastic pants on a child being treated in the diaper area, as these garments may constitute occlusive dressings.

LABORATORY TESTS

The following tests may be helpful in evaluating the HPA axis suppression:
Urinary free cortisol test
ACTH stimulation test

CARCINOGENESIS, MUTAGENESIS, AND IMPAIRMENT OF FERTILITY

Long-term animal studies have not been performed to evaluate the carcinogenic potential or the effect on fertility of topical corticosteroids.

Studies to determine mutagenicity with prednisolone and hydrocortisone have revealed negative results. Desoximetasone did not show potential for mutagenic activity *in vitro* in the Ames microbial mutagen test with or without metabolic activation.

PREGNANCY CATEGORY C

Corticosteroids are generally teratogenic in laboratory animals when administered systemically at relatively low dosage levels. The more potent corticosteroids have been shown to be teratogenic after dermal application in laboratory animals.

Desoximetasone has been shown to be teratogenic and embryotoxic in mice, rats, and rabbits when given by subcutaneous or dermal routes of administration in doses 3 to 30 times the human dose of Desoximetasone Emollient Cream 0.25% or 15 to 150 times the human dose of Desoximetasone Emollient Cream 0.05%.

There are no adequate and well-controlled studies in pregnant women on teratogenic effects from topically applied corticosteroids. Therefore, Desoximetasone Emollient Cream 0.25% and 0.05% should be used during pregnancy only if the potential benefit justifies the potential risk to the fetus. Drugs of this class should not be used extensively on pregnant patients, in large amounts, or for prolonged periods of time.

NURSING MOTHERS

It is not known whether topical administration of corticosteroids could result in sufficient systemic absorption to produce detectable quantities in breast milk. Systemically administered corticosteroids are secreted into breast milk in quantities not likely to have a deleterious effect on the infant. Nevertheless, caution should be exercised when topical corticosteroids are administered to a nursing woman.

PEDIATRIC USE

Pediatric patients may demonstrate greater susceptibility to topical corticosteroid-induced HPA axis suppression and Cushing's syndrome than mature patients because of a larger skin surface area to body weight ratio.

Hypothalamic-pituitary-adrenal (HPA) axis suppression, Cushing's syndrome, and intracranial hypertension have been reported in children receiving topical corticosteroids. Manifestations of adrenal suppression in children include linear growth retardation, delayed weight gain, low plasma cortisol levels, and absence of response to ACTH stimulation. Manifestations of intracranial hypertension include bulging fontanelles, headaches, and bilateral papilledema.

Administration of topical corticosteroids to children should be limited to the least amount compatible with an effective therapeutic regimen. Chronic corticosteroid therapy may interfere with the growth and development of children.

ADVERSE REACTIONS

The following local adverse reactions are reported infrequently with topical corticosteroids, but may occur more frequently with the use of occlusive dressings. These reactions are listed in an approximate decreasing order of occurrence: Burning, Itching, Irritation, Dryness, Folliculitis, Hypertrichosis, Acneiform eruptions, Hypopigmentation, Perioral dermatitis, Allergic contact dermatitis, Maceration of the skin, Secondary infection, Skin Atrophy, Striae, Miliaria.

In controlled clinical studies the incidence of adverse reactions was low (0.8%) for Desoximetasone Emollient Cream 0.25% and included burning, folliculitis and folliculo-pustular lesions. The incidence of adverse reactions was also 0.8% for Desoximetasone Emollient Cream 0.05% and included pruritus, erythema, vesiculation and burning sensation.

OVERDOSAGE

Topically applied corticosteroids can be absorbed in sufficient amounts to produce systemic effects. (See "Precautions".)

DOSAGE AND ADMINISTRATION

Apply a thin film of Desoximetasone Emollient Cream 0.25% or 0.05% to the affected skin areas twice daily. Rub in gently.

Store at controlled room temperature (59°—86°F).

HOW SUPPLIED
CREAM: 0.05%

AVERAGE UNIT PRICE (AVAILABLE SIZES)		GENERIC A-RATED AVERAGE PRICE (GAAP)	
BRAND	$0.66	15 gm	$9.45
GENERIC	$0.50	60 gm	$22.72
HCFA FUL (15 gm)	$0.52		
HCFA FUL (60 gm)	$0.34		

BRAND/MANUFACTURER	NDC	SIZE	AWP
◆ **BRAND**			
TOPICORT LP: Hoechst Derm	00039-0012-23	15 gm	$12.33
	00039-0012-60	60 gm	$29.84
◆ **GENERICS**			
Geneva	00781-7185-27	15 gm	$8.25
Taro	51672-1271-01	15 gm	$9.32
Rugby	00536-4228-20	15 gm	$9.88
Major	00904-0765-36	15 gm	$9.90
Goldline	00182-5057-51	15 gm	$9.90
Geneva	00781-7185-35	60 gm	$19.99
Taro	51672-1271-03	60 gm	$22.56
Major	00904-0765-02	60 gm	$23.55
Rugby	00536-4228-25	60 gm	$23.58
Goldline	00182-5057-52	60 gm	$23.90

CREAM: 0.25%

AVERAGE UNIT PRICE (AVAILABLE SIZES)		GENERIC A-RATED AVERAGE PRICE (GAAP)	
BRAND	$0.76	15 gm	$11.57
GENERIC	$0.61	60 gm	$27.00
HCFA FUL (15 gm)	$0.69		
HCFA FUL (60 gm)	$0.41		

BRAND/MANUFACTURER	NDC	SIZE	AWP
◆ **BRAND**			
TOPICORT: Hoechst Derm	00039-0011-23	15 gm	$16.40
	00039-0011-60	60 gm	$39.35
	00039-0011-04	120 gm	$63.85
◆ **GENERICS**			
Moore,H.L.	00839-7665-47	15 gm	$10.38
Geneva	00781-7085-27	15 gm	$10.99
URL	00677-1413-40	15 gm	$11.50
Major	00904-0764-36	15 gm	$11.85
Rugby	00536-4229-20	15 gm	$11.90
Goldline	00182-5054-51	15 gm	$11.90

◆ RATED THERAPEUTICALLY EQUIVALENT; ◇ THERAPEUTIC EQUIVALENCE UNCONFIRMED; ○ UNRATED

BRAND/MANUFACTURER	NDC	SIZE	AWP
Taro	51672-1270-01	15 gm	$12.45
Goldline	00182-5054-52	60 gm	$24.50
Moore,H.L.	00839-7665-50	60 gm	$25.23
Geneva	00781-7085-35	60 gm	$26.36
URL	00677-1413-43	60 gm	$27.30
Rugby	00536-4229-25	60 gm	$27.48
Major	00904-0764-02	60 gm	$28.35
Taro	51672-1270-03	60 gm	$29.75

GEL: 0.05%

BRAND/MANUFACTURER	NDC	SIZE	AWP
BRAND			
TOPICORT: Hoechst Derm	00039-0014-23	15 gm	$14.25
	00039-0014-60	60 gm	$34.90

OINTMENT: 0.25%

BRAND/MANUFACTURER	NDC	SIZE	AWP
BRAND			
TOPICORT: Hoechst Derm	00039-0025-15	15 gm	$16.30
	00039-0025-60	60 gm	$39.05

Desoxyn SEE METHAMPHETAMINE HYDROCHLORIDE

Desquam SEE BENZOYL PEROXIDE

Desyrel SEE TRAZODONE HYDROCHLORIDE

Dexacidin SEE DEXAMETHASONE/NEOMYCIN SULFATE/ POLYMYXIN B SULFATE

Dexacort In Turbinaire SEE DEXAMETHASONE SODIUM PHOSPHATE, INHALATION

Dexamethasone and Tobramycin

DESCRIPTION

Dexamethasone/Tobramycin Ophthalmic Suspension and Ointment are sterile, multiple dose antibiotic and steroid combinations for topical ophthalmic use.

Empirical formula for Tobramycin is $C_{18}H_{37}N_5O_9$ and chemical name is O-3-Amino-3-deoxy-α-D-glucopyranosyl-(1→4)-O-[2,6-diamino-2,3,6-trideoxy-α-D-ribo-hexopyranosyl-(1→6)]-2-deoxy-L-strepta- mine.

Empirical formula for Dexamethasone is $C_{22}H_{29}FO_5$ and the chemical name is 9-Fluoro-11β,17,21-trihydroxy-16α-methylpregna-1,4-diene-3,20-dione.

Each mL of Dexamethasone/Tobramycin Suspension contains: Active: Tobramycin 0.3% (3 mg) and Dexamethasone 0.1% (1 mg).

CLINICAL PHARMACOLOGY

Corticoids suppress the inflammatory response to a variety of agents and they probably delay or slow healing. Since corticoids may inhibit the body's defense mechanism against infection, a concomitant antimicrobial drug may be used when this inhibition is considered to be clinically significant. Dexamethasone is a potent corticoid.

The antibiotic component in the combination (Tobramycin) is included to provide action against susceptible organisms. In vitro studies have demonstrated that Tobramycin is active against susceptible strains of the following microorganisms: Staphylococci, including S. aureus and S. epidermidis (coagulase-positive and coagulase-negative), including penicillin-resistant strains.

Streptococci, including some of the Group A beta-hemolytic species, some nonhemolytic species, and some Streptococcus pneumoniae.

Pseudomonas aeruginosa, Escherichia coli, Klebsiella pneumoniae, Enterobacter aerogenes, Proteus mirabilis, Morganella morganii, most Proteus vulgaris strains, Haemophilus influenzae and H. aegyptius, Moraxella lacunata, and Acinetobacter calcoaceticus and some Neisseria species.

Bacterial susceptibility studies demonstrate that in some cases microorganisms resistant to gentamicin remain susceptible to Tobramycin. A significant bacterial population resistant to Tobramycin has not yet emerged; however, bacterial resistance may develop upon prolonged use.

No data are available on the extent of systemic absorption from Dexamethasone/Tobramycin Ophthalmic Suspension or Ointment; however, it is known that some systemic absorption can occur with ocularly applied drugs. If the maximum dose of Dexamethasone/Tobramycin Ophthalmic Suspension is given for the first 48 hours (two drops in each eye every 2 hours) and complete systemic absorption occurs, which is highly unlikely, the daily dose of Dexamethasone would be 2.4 mg. The usual physiologic replacement dose is 0.75 mg daily. If Dexamethasone/Tobramycin Ophthalmic Suspension is given after the first 48 hours as two drops in each eye every 4 hours, the administered dose of Dexamethasone would be 1.2 mg daily. The administered dose for Dexamethasone/Tobramycin Ophthalmic Ointment in both eyes four times daily would be 0.4 mg of Dexamethasone daily.

INDICATIONS AND USAGE

Dexamethasone/Tobramycin Ophthalmic Suspension and Ointment are indicated for steroid-responsive inflammatory ocular conditions for which a corticosteroid is indicated and where superficial bacterial ocular infection or a risk of bacterial ocular infection exists.

Ocular steroids are indicated in inflammatory conditions of the palpebral and bulbar conjunctiva, cornea and anterior segment of the globe where the inherent risk of steroid use in certain infective conjunctivides is accepted to obtain a diminution in edema and inflammation. They are also indicated in chronic anterior uveitis and corneal injury from chemical, radiation or thermal burns, or penetration of foreign bodies. The use of a combination drug with an anti-infective component is indicated where the risk of superficial ocular infection is high or where there is an expectation that potentially dangerous numbers of bacteria will be present in the eye. The particular anti-infective drug in this product is active against the following common bacterial eye pathogens:

Staphylococci, including S. aureus and S. epidermidis (coagulase-positive and coagulase-negative), including penicillin-resistant strains.

Streptococci, including some of the Group A beta-hemolytic species, some nonhemolytic species, and some Streptococcus pneumoniae.

Pseudomonas aeruginosa, Escherichia coli, Klebsiella pneumoniae, Enterobacter aerogenes, Proteus mirabilis, Morganella morganii, most Proteus vulgaris strains, Haemophilus influenzae and H. aegyptius, Moraxella lacunata, and Acinetobacter calcoaceticus and some Neisseria species.

CONTRAINDICATIONS

Epithelial herpes simplex keratitis (dendritic keratitis), vaccinia, varicella, and many other viral diseases of the cornea and conjunctiva. Mycobacterial infection of the eye. Fungal diseases of ocular structures. Hypersensitivity to a component of the medication.

The use of this combination is always contraindicated after uncomplicated removal of a corneal foreign body.

WARNINGS

Not for Injection into the Eye: Sensitivity to topically applied aminoglycosides may occur in some patients. If a sensitivity reaction does occur, discontinue use. Prolonged use of steroids may result in glaucoma, with damage to the optic nerve, defects in visual acuity and fields of vision, and posterior subcapsular cataract formation. Intraocular pressure should be routinely monitored even though it may be difficult in children and uncooperative patients. Prolonged use may suppress the host response and thus increase the hazard of secondary ocular infections. In those diseases causing thinning of the cornea or sclera, perforations have been known to occur with the use of topical steroids. In acute purulent conditions of the eye, steroids may mask infection or enhance existing infection.

PRECAUTIONS

General: The possibility of fungal infections of the cornea should be considered after long-term steroid dosing. As with other antibiotic preparations, prolonged use may result in overgrowth of nonsusceptible organisms, including fungi. If superinfection occurs, appropriate therapy should be initiated. When multiple prescriptions are required, or whenever clinical judgement dictates, the patient should be examined with the aid of magnification, such as slit lamp biomicroscopy and, where appropriate, fluorescein staining.

Information for Patients: Do not touch dropper or tube tip to any surface as this may contaminate the contents.

Carcinogenesis, Mutagenesis, Impairment of Fertility: No studies have been conducted to evaluate the carcinogenic or mutagenic potential. No impairment of fertility was noted in studies of subcutaneous Tobramycin in rats at doses of 50 and 100 mg/kg/day.

Pregnancy Category C: Corticosteroids have been found to be teratogenic in animal studies. Ocular administration of 0.1% Dexamethasone resulted in 15.6% and 32.3% incidence of fetal anomalies in two groups of pregnant rabbits. Fetal growth retardation and increased mortality rates have been observed in rats with chronic Dexamethasone therapy. Reproduction studies have been performed in rats and rabbits with Tobramycin at doses up to 100 mg/kg/day parenterally and have revealed no evidence of impaired fertility or harm to the fetus. There are no adequate and well-controlled studies in pregnant women. Dexamethasone/Tobramycin Ophthalmic Suspension and Ointment should be used during pregnancy only if the potential benefit justifies the potential risk to the fetus.

Nursing Mothers: It is not known whether this drug is excreted in human milk. Because many drugs are excreted in human milk, a decision should be considered to discontinue nursing temporarily while using Dexamethasone/Tobramycin Ophthalmic Suspension or Ointment.

Pediatric Use: Safety and effectiveness in children have not been established.

ADVERSE REACTIONS

Adverse reactions have occurred with steroid/anti-infective combination drugs which can be attributed to the steroid component, the anti-infective component, or the combination. Exact incidence figures are not available. The most frequent adverse reactions to topical ocular tobramycin Demethasone/Tobramycin are hypersensitivity and localized ocular toxicity, including lid itching and swelling, and conjunctival erythema. These reactions occur in less than 4% of patients. Similar reactions may occur with the topical use of other aminoglycoside antibiotics. Other adverse reactions have not been reported; however, if topical ocular Tobramycin is administered concomitantly with systemic aminoglycoside antibiotics, care should be taken to monitor the total serum concentration. The reactions due to the steroid component are: elevation of intraocular pressure (IOP) with possible development of glaucoma, and infrequent optic nerve damage; posterior subcapsular cataract formation; and delayed wound healing.

Secondary Infection: The development of secondary infection has occurred after use of combinations containing steroids and antimicrobials. Fungal infections of the cornea are particularly prone to develop coincidentally with long-term applications of steroids. The possibility of fungal invasion must be considered in any persistent corneal ulceration where steroid treatment has been used. Secondary bacterial ocular infection following suppression of host responses also occurs.

DOSAGE AND ADMINISTRATION

Suspension: One or two drops instilled into the conjunctival sac(s) every four to six hours. During the initial 24 to 48 hours, the dosage may be increased to one or two drops every two (2) hours. Frequency should be decreased gradually as warranted by improvement in clinical signs. Care should be taken not to discontinue therapy prematurely.

Ointment: Apply a small amount (approximately 1/2 inch ribbon) into the conjunctival sac(s) up to three or four times daily.

Dexamethasone/Tobramycin Ophthalmic Ointment may be used at bedtime in conjunction with Dexamethasone/Tobramycin Ophthalmic Suspension used during the day. Not more than 20 mL or 8 g should be prescribed initially and the prescription should not be refilled without further evaluation as outlined in *"Precautions"* above.

STORAGE
Store at 46° to 80°F (8° to 27°C).
Store suspension upright and shake well before using.

HOW SUPPLIED
DROP: 0.3%-0.1%

BRAND/MANUFACTURER	NDC	SIZE	AWP
○ **BRAND**			
TOBRADEX: Alcon Labs	00065-0647-25	2.5 ml	$10.63
	00065-0647-05	5 ml	$21.25

OINTMENT: 0.3%-0.1%

BRAND/MANUFACTURER	NDC	SIZE	AWP
○ **BRAND**			
TOBRADEX: Alcon Labs	00065-0648-35	3.5 gm	$21.25

Dexamethasone Sodium Phosphate and Neomycin Sulfate, Topical

DESCRIPTION
Dexamethasone Sodium Phosphate/Neomycin Sulfate, Topical Cream is a topical steroid-antibiotic preparation.

Dexamethasone Sodium Phosphate/Neomycin Sulfate, Topical Cream contains in each gram: Dexamethasone Sodium Phosphate equivalent to 1 mg (0.1%) Dexamethasone Phosphate, and Neomycin Sulfate equivalent to 3.5 mg Neomycin base, in a greaseless bland base.

Dexamethasone Sodium Phosphate is 9-fluoro-11β,17-dihydroxy-16α-methyl-21-(phosphonooxy)pregna- 1,4-diene-3,20- dione disodium salt. Its empirical formula is $C_{22}H_{28}FNa_2O_8P$. Dexamethasone Sodium Phosphate has a molecular weight of 516.41.

Glucocorticoids are adrenocortical steroids, both naturally occurring and synthetic. Dexamethasone is a synthetic analog of naturally occurring glucocorticoids (hydrocortisone and cortisone).

Neomycin Sulfate is a mixture of the sulfate salts of Neomycin, an antibacterial substance produced by the growth of *Streptomyces fradiae* Waksman (Fam. Streptomycetaceae). Neomycin is a complex typically containing 8-13% Neomycin C, less than 0.2% Neomycin A and the rest, Neomycin B. The empirical formulas and molecular weights for the three components are: Neomycin B, $C_{23}H_{46}N_6O_{13}$, molecular weight 614.65: Neomycin C, $C_{23}H_{46}N_6O_{13}$, molecular weight 614.65: Neomycin A, (also referred to as neamine), $C_{12}H_{26}N_4O_6$, molecular weight 322.36.

CLINICAL PHARMACOLOGY
Topical corticosteroids share anti-inflammatory, antipruritic, and vasoconstrictive actions.

The mechanism of anti-inflammatory activity of the topical corticosteroids is unclear. Various laboratory methods, including vasoconstrictor assays, are used to compare and predict potencies and/or clinical efficacies of the topical corticosteroids. There is some evidence to suggest that a recognizable correlation exists between vasoconstrictor potency and therapeutic efficacy in man.

PHARMACOKINETICS
The extent of percutaneous absorption of topical corticosteroids is determined by many factors including the vehicle, the integrity of the epidermal barrier, and the use of occlusive dressings.

Topical corticosteroids can be absorbed from normal intact skin. Inflammation and/or other disease processes in the skin increase percutaneous absorption. Occlusive dressings substantially increase the percutaneous absorption of topical corticosteroids. Thus, occlusive dressings may be a valuable therapeutic adjunct for treatment of resistant dermatoses. (See *"Dosage and Administration"*.)

Once absorbed through the skin, topical corticosteroids are handled through pharmacokinetic pathways similar to systemically administered corticosteroids. Corticosteroids are bound to plasma proteins in varying degrees. Corticosteroids are metabolized primarily in the liver and are then excreted by the kidneys. Some of the topical corticosteroids and their metabolites are also excreted into the bile.

The antibiotic component, Neomycin, is bactericidal to many gram-positive and gram-negative bacteria.

INDICATIONS AND USAGE
For the treatment of corticosteroid-responsive dermatoses with secondary infection. It has not been demonstrated that this steroid-antibiotic combination provides greater benefit than the steroid component alone after 7 days of treatment (see *"Warnings"*).

CONTRAINDICATIONS
Hypersensitivity to any component of this product, including sulfites (see *"Warnings"*).

WARNINGS
Dexamethasone Sodium Phosphate/Neomycin Sulfate, Topical Cream contains sodium bisulfite, a sulfite that may cause allergic-type reactions including anaphylactic symptoms and life-threatening or less severe asthmatic episodes in certain susceptible people. The overall prevalence of sulfite sensitivity in the general population is unknown and probably low. Sulfite sensitivity is seen more frequently in asthmatic than in nonasthmatic people.

Because of the concern of nephrotoxicity and ototoxicity associated with Neomycin, this combination product should not be used over a wide area or for extended periods of time. Topically applied steroids are absorbed systemically. There may be rare instances in which this absorption results in immunosuppression. Patients who are on drugs which suppress the immune system are more susceptible to infections than healthy individuals. Chickenpox and measles, for example, can have a more serious or even fatal course in nonimmune children or adults on corticosteroids. In such children or adults who have not had these diseases, particular care should be taken to avoid exposure. The risk of developing a disseminated infection varies among individuals and can be related to the dose, route and duration of corticosteroid administration as well as to the underlying disease. If exposed to chickenpox, prophylaxis with varicella zoster immune globulin (VZIG) may be indicated. If chickenpox develops, treatment with antiviral agents may be considered. If exposed to measles, prophylaxis with immune globulin (IG) may be indicated. (See the respective package inserts for VZIG and IG for complete prescribing information.)

PRECAUTIONS
GENERAL
Systemic absorption of topical corticosteroids has produced reversible hypothalamic-pituitary-adrenal (HPA) axis suppression, manifestations of Cushing's syndrome, hyperglycemia, and glycosuria in some patients.

Conditions which augment systemic absorption include the application of the more potent corticosteroids, use over large surface areas, prolonged use, and the addition of occlusive dressings.

Therefore, patients receiving a large dose of a potent topical corticosteroid applied to a large surface area or under an occlusive dressing should be evaluated periodically for evidence of HPA axis suppression by using urinary free cortisol and ACTH stimulation tests. If HPA axis suppression is noted, an attempt should be made to withdraw the drug, to reduce the frequency of application, or to substitute a less potent corticosteroid.

Recovery of HPA axis function is generally prompt and complete upon discontinuation of the drug. Infrequently, signs and symptoms of corticosteroid withdrawal may occur, requiring supplemental systemic corticosteroids.

Children may absorb proportionally larger amounts of topical corticosteroids and thus be more susceptible to systemic toxicity (see *"Precautions, Pediatric Use"*).

Corticosteroids may mask some signs of infection, and new infections may appear during their use. There may be decreased resistance and inability to localize infection when corticosteroids are used. Therefore, patients with bacterial infections should also be given appropriate antibiotic therapy if Dexamethasone Sodium Phosphate/Neomycin Sulfate, Topical is used. Moreover, corticosteroids may affect the nitroblue-tetrazolium test for bacterial infection and produce false-negative results.

Corticosteroid therapy exerts its major immunosuppressive effects by impairing the normal function of the T-lymphocyte population and macrophages. When T-cell and/or macrophage function is impaired, latent disease may be activated or there may be an exacerbation of intercurrent infections due to pathogens, including those caused by Candida, Mycobacterium, Ameba, Toxoplasma,

---

◆ RATED THERAPEUTICALLY EQUIVALENT; ◇ THERAPEUTIC EQUIVALENCE UNCONFIRMED; ○ UNRATED

Strongyloides, Pneumocystis, Cryptococcus, Nocardia, etc. Products containing steroids should be used with caution in patients with impaired T-cell function or in patients receiving other immunosuppressive therapy.

In the presence of dermatological infections, the use of an appropriate antifungal or antibacterial agent should be instituted. If a favorable response does not occur promptly, the corticosteroid should be discontinued until the infection has been adequately controlled.

If irritation develops, topical corticosteroids should be discontinued and appropriate therapy instituted.

This product is not for ophthalmic use. However, if applied to the eyelids or skin near the eyes, the drug may enter the eyes. In patients with a history of herpes simplex keratitis, ocular exposure to corticosteroids may lead to a recurrence. Prolonged ocular exposure may cause steroid glaucoma.

A few individuals may be sensitive to one or more of the components of this product. Sensitivity to Neomycin may occasionally develop, especially when it is applied to abraded skin. If any reaction indicating sensitivity is observed, discontinue use. There are reports in the current medical literature that indicate an increase in the prevalence of persons sensitive to Neomycin.

Generally, occlusive dressings should not be used on weeping or exudative lesions.

If the occlusive dressing technique is employed, caution should be exercised with regard to the use of plastic films which are often inflammable and may pose a suffocation hazard for children.

When large areas of the body are covered with an occlusive dressing, thermal homeostasis may be impaired. If elevation of body temperature occurs, use of the occlusive dressing should be discontinued.

INFORMATION FOR THE PATIENT
Patients using topical corticosteroids should receive the following information and instructions:

1. This medication is to be used as directed by the physician. It is for external use only. Avoid contact with the eyes.

2. Patients should be advised not to use this medication for any disorder other than that for which it was prescribed.

3. The treated skin area should not be bandaged or otherwise covered or wrapped so as to be occlusive unless directed by the physician.

4. Patients should report any signs of local adverse reactions, especially under occlusive dressings.

5. Parents of pediatric patients should be advised not to use tight-fitting diapers or plastic pants on a child being treated in the diaper area, as these garments may constitute occlusive dressings.

6. Susceptible patients who are on immunosuppressant doses of corticosteroids should be warned to avoid exposure to chickenpox or measles. Patients should also be advised that if they are exposed, medical advice should be sought without delay.

LABORATORY TESTS
The following tests may be helpful in evaluating the HPA axis suppression:

- Urinary free cortisol test
- ACTH stimulation test

CARCINOGENESIS, MUTAGENESIS AND IMPAIRMENT OF FERTILITY
Long-term animal studies have not been performed to evaluate the carcinogenic potential or the effect on fertility of Dexamethasane Sodium Phosphate/Neomycin Sulfate, Topical.

Studies to determine mutagenicity with prednisolone and hydrocortisone have revealed negative results.

PREGNANCY
PREGNANCY CATEGORY C:
Corticosteroids are generally teratogenic in laboratory animals when administered systemically at relatively low dosage levels. The more potent corticosteroids have been shown to be teratogenic after dermal application in laboratory animals. There are no adequate and well controlled studies in pregnant women on teratogenic effects from topically applied corticosteroids. Therefore, topical corticosteroids should be used during pregnancy only if the potential benefit justifies the potential risk to the fetus. Drugs of this class should not be used extensively on pregnant patients, in large amounts, or for prolonged periods of time.

NURSING MOTHERS
It is not known whether topical administration of corticosteroids could result in sufficient systemic absorption to produce detectable quantities in breast milk. Systemically administered corticosteroids are secreted into breast milk in quantities *not* likely to have a deleterious effect on the infant. Nevertheless, caution should be exercised when topical corticosteroids are administered to a nursing woman.

PEDIATRIC USE
Pediatric patients may demonstrate greater susceptibility to topical corticosteroid-induced HPA axis suppression and Cushing's syndrome than mature patients because of a larger skin surface to body weight ratio.

Hypothalamic-pituitary-adrenal (HPA) axis suppression, Cushing's syndrome, and intracranial hypertension have been reported in children receiving topical corticosteroids. Manifestations of adrenal suppression in children include linear growth retardation, delayed weight gain, low plasma cortisol levels, and absence of response to ACTH stimulation. Manifestations of intracranial hypertension include bulging fontanelles, headaches, and bilateral papilledema.

Administration of topical corticosteroids to children should be limited to the least amount compatible with an effective therapeutic regimen. Chronic corticosteroid therapy may interfere with the growth and development of children.

ADVERSE REACTIONS
The following adverse reactions are reported infrequently with topical corticosteroids, but may occur more frequently with the use of occlusive dressings. These reactions are listed in an approximate decreasing order of occurrence:

Burning
Itching
Irritation
Dryness
Folliculitis
Hypertrichosis
Acneiform eruptions
Hypopigmentation
Perioral dermatitis
Allergic contact dermatitis
Maceration of the skin
Secondary infection
Skin atrophy
Striae
Miliaria

Prevalence of Neomycin hypersensitivity is increasing. Ototoxicity and nephrotoxicity have been reported with prolonged use or use of large amounts of topical Neomycin preparations.

OVERDOSAGE
Topically applied corticosteroids can be absorbed in sufficient amounts to produce systemic effects (see *"Precautions"*).

DOSAGE AND ADMINISTRATION
Apply to the affected area as a thin film three or four times daily.

Before using Dexamethasone Sodium Phosphate/Neomycin Sulfate, Topical Cream in the *ear*, clean the aural canal thoroughly and sponge dry. Confirm that the eardrum is intact. With a cotton-tipped applicator, apply a thin coating of the cream to the affected canal area two or three times a day. When a favorable response is obtained, reduce the number of daily applications to one or two, and eventually discontinue.

HOW SUPPLIED
CREAM: 0.1%-3.5 MG/GM

BRAND/MANUFACTURER	NDC	SIZE	AWP
○ **BRAND**			
NEO-DECADRON CREAM: Merck	00006-7607-12	15 gm	$11.39
	00006-7607-24	30 gm	$17.04

Dexamethasone Sodium Phosphate with Lidocaine Hydrochloride

DESCRIPTION
Dexamethasone Sodium Phosphate is a white or slightly yellow, crystalline powder. It is freely soluble in water and is exceedingly hygroscopic. The molecular weight is 516.41. It is designated chemically as 9-fluoro-11β, 17-dihydroxy-16α-methyl-21-(phosphonooxy)pregna-1,4-diene-3,20-dione disodium salt. The empirical formula is $C_{22}H_{28}FNa_2O_8P$.

Lidocaine Hydrochloride is a white, crystalline powder that is very soluble in water and alcohol, soluble in chloroform, and insoluble in ether. The molecular weight is 288.82. It is designated chemically as 2-(diethylamino)-N-(2,6-dimethylphenyl)acetamide, monohydrochloride, monohydrate. The empirical formula is $C_{14}H_{22}N_2O \cdot HCl \cdot H_2O$.

Dexamethasone Sodium Phosphate/Lidocaine Hydrochloride injection is provided as a sterile solution (pH 6.5 to 6.9), sealed under nitrogen, for the convenience of physicians who prefer to treat patients with simultaneous administration of a corticosteroid and a local anesthetic.

Each milliliter contains Dexamethasone Sodium Phosphate equivalent to Dexamethasone Phosphate, 4 mg; and Lidocaine Hydrochloride, 10 mg.

Methylparaben, 1.5 mg, and propylparaben, 0.2 mg, added as preservatives.

ACTIONS
Dexamethasone Sodium Phosphate is a synthetic glucocorticoid used primarily for its potent anti-inflammatory effects in disorders of many organ systems. Glucocorticoids cause profound and varied metabolic effects. In addition, they modify the body's immune responses to diverse stimuli.

Lidocaine Hydrochloride is a local anesthetic with a rapid onset and moderate duration of action.

Local anesthesia appears within a few minutes after injection of Dexamethasone Sodium Phosphate/Lidocaine Hydrochloride and lasts 45 minutes to one hour. By the time the anesthesia wears off, steroid activity usually has begun. If the anesthesia wears off before full steroid effect appears, there may be some discomfort beginning about an hour after injection and relief of pain may be delayed for a short time.

INDICATIONS
Acute and subacute bursitis
Acute and subacute nonspecific tenosynovitis

CONTRAINDICATIONS
Hypersensitivity to any component of this product, including sulfites (see "Warnings").

DEXAMETHASONE SODIUM PHOSPHATE
Systemic fungal infections

LIDOCAINE HYDROCHLORIDE
Patients with known history of hypersensitivity to local anesthetics of the amide type (e.g., mepivacaine, prilocaine)
  Severe shock
  Heart block

WARNINGS
Because rare instances of anaphylactoid reactions have occurred in patients receiving parenteral corticosteroid therapy, appropriate precautionary measures should be taken prior to administration, especially when the patient has a history of allergy to any drug. Anaphylactoid and hypersensitivity reactions have been reported for Injection Dexamethasone Sodium Phosphate/Lidocaine Hydrochloride (see "Adverse Reactions").

Certain brands of injection contain sodium bisulfite, a sulfite that may cause allergic-type reactions including anaphylactic symptoms and life-threatening or less severe asthmatic episodes in certain susceptible people. The overall prevalence of sulfite sensitivity in the general population is unknown and probably low. Sulfite sensitivity is seen more frequently in asthmatic than in nonasthmatic people.

LIDOCAINE HYDROCHLORIDE
RESUSCITATIVE EQUIPMENT AND DRUGS SHOULD BE IMMEDIATELY AVAILABLE WHEN ANY LOCAL ANESTHETIC IS USED.

Usage in Pregnancy: The safe use of Lidocaine Hydrochloride has not been established with respect to adverse effects upon fetal development. Careful consideration should be given to this fact before administering this drug to women of childbearing potential, particularly during early pregnancy.

DEXAMETHASONE SODIUM PHOSPHATE
In patients on corticosteroid therapy subjected to unusual stress, increased dosage of rapidly acting corticosteroids before, during, and after the stressful situation is indicated. Drug-induced secondary adrenocortical insufficiency may result from too rapid withdrawal of corticosteroids and may be minimized by gradual reduction of dosage. This type of relative insufficiency may persist for months after discontinuation of therapy: therefore, in any situation of stress occurring during that period, hormone therapy should be reinstituted. If the patient is receiving steroids already, dosage may have to be increased. Since mineralocorticoid secretion may be impaired, salt and/or a mineralocorticoid should be administered concurrently.

Corticosteroids may mask some signs of infection, and new infections may appear during their use. There may be decreased resistance and inability to localize infection when corticosteroids are used. Moreover, corticosteroids may affect the nitroblue-tetrazolium test for bacterial infection and produce false negative results.

Corticosteroids may activate latent amebiasis. Therefore, it is recommended that latent or active amebiasis be ruled out before initiating corticosteroid therapy in any patient who has spent time in the tropics or any patient with unexplained diarrhea.

Prolonged use of corticosteroids may produce posterior subcapsular cataracts, glaucoma with possible damage to the optic nerves, and may enhance the establishment of secondary ocular infections due to fungi or viruses.

Usage in Pregnancy: Since adequate human reproduction studies have not been done with corticosteroids, use of these drugs in pregnancy or in women of childbearing potential requires that the anticipated benefits be weighed against the possible hazards to the mother and embryo or fetus. Infants born of mothers who have received substantial doses of corticosteroids during pregnancy should be carefully observed for signs of hypoadrenalism.

Corticosteroids appear in breast milk and could suppress growth, interfere with endogenous corticosteroid production, or cause other unwanted effects. Mothers taking pharmacologic doses of corticosteroids should be advised not to nurse. Average and large doses of cortisone or hydrocortisone can cause elevation of blood pressure, salt and water retention, and increased excretion of potassium. These effects are less likely to occur with the synthetic derivatives except when used in large doses. Dietary salt restriction and potassium supplementation may be necessary. All corticosteroids increase calcium excretion.

Administration of live virus vaccines, including smallpox, is contraindicated in individuals receiving immunosuppressive doses of corticosteroids. If inactivated viral or bacterial vaccines are administered to individuals receiving immunosuppressive doses of corticosteroids, the expected serum antibody response may not be obtained.

Patients who are on drugs which suppress the immune system are more susceptible to infections than healthy individuals. Chickenpox and measles, for example, can have a more serious or even fatal course in non-immune children or adults on corticosteroids. In such children or adults who have not had these diseases, particular care should be taken to avoid exposure. The risk of developing a disseminated infection varies among individuals and can be related to the dose, route and duration of corticosteroid administration as well as to the underlying disease. If exposed to chickenpox, prophylaxis with varicella zoster immune globulin (VZIG) may be indicated. If chickenpox develops, treatment with antiviral agents may be considered. If exposed to measles, prophylaxis with immune globulin (IG) may be indicated. (See the respective package inserts for VZIG and IG for complete prescribing information.)

If corticosteroids are indicated in patients with latent tuberculosis or tuberculin reactivity, close observation is necessary as reactivation of the disease may occur. During prolonged corticosteroid therapy, these patients should receive chemoprophylaxis.

Literature reports suggest an apparent association between use of corticosteroids and left ventricular free wall rupture after a recent myocardial infarction; therefore, therapy with corticosteroids should be used with great caution in these patients.

PRECAUTIONS
This product, like many other steroid formulations, is sensitive to heat. Therefore, it should not be autoclaved when it is desirable to sterilize the exterior of the vial.

Therapy with this preparation does not eliminate the need for conventional supportive measures. Although capable of ameliorating symptoms, and even suppressing them completely in some patients, it is not a cure. Neither the hormone nor the anesthetic has any effect on the basic cause of inflammation.

Supportive measures, such as analgesics, pertinent orthopedic procedures, heat or cold, rest, rehabilitation, and physiotherapy must be used as applicable. If physiotherapy is applied immediately following injection, it may cause severe pain.

In some patients, a single injection fully restores mobility. Patients should be strongly impressed with the importance of not overusing the affected part as long as the inflammatory process remains active.

Injection into an infected site is to be avoided.

DEXAMETHASONE SODIUM PHOSPHATE
Following prolonged therapy, withdrawal of corticosteroids may result in symptoms of the corticosteroid withdrawal syndrome including fever, myalgia, arthralgia, and malaise. This may occur in patients even without evidence of adrenal insufficiency.

There is an enhanced effect of corticosteroids in patients with hypothyroidism and in those with cirrhosis.

Corticosteroids should be used cautiously in patients with ocular herpes simplex for fear of corneal perforation.

Psychic derangements may appear when corticosteroids are used, ranging from euphoria, insomnia, mood swings, personality changes, and severe depression to frank psychotic manifestations. Also, existing emotional instability or psychotic tendencies may be aggravated by corticosteroids.

Aspirin should be used cautiously in conjunction with corticosteroids in hypoprothrombinemia.

Steroids should be used with caution in non-specific ulcerative colitis, if there is a probability of impending perforation, abscess, or other pyogenic infection, also in diverticulitis, fresh intestinal anastomoses, active or latent peptic ulcer, renal insufficiency, hypertension, osteoporosis, and myasthenia gravis. Signs of peritoneal irritation following gastrointestinal perforation in patients receiving large doses of corticosteroids may be minimal or absent. Fat embolism has been reported as a possible complication of hypercortisonism.

When large doses are given, some authorities advise that antacids be administered between meals to help to prevent peptic ulcer.

Growth and development of infants and children on prolonged corticosteroid therapy should be carefully followed. Steroids may increase or decrease motility and number of spermatozoa in some patients.

Phenytoin, phenobarbital, ephedrine, and rifampin may enhance the metabolic clearance of corticosteroids, resulting in decreased blood levels and lessened physiologic activity, thus requiring adjustment in corticosteroid dosage.

The prothrombin time should be checked frequently in patients who are receiving corticosteroids and coumarin anticoagulants at the same time because of reports that corticosteroids have altered the response to these anticoagulants. Studies have shown that the usual effect produced by adding corticosteroids is inhibition of response to coumarins, although there have been some conflicting reports of potentiation not substantiated by studies.

When corticosteroids are administered concomitantly with potassium-depleting diuretics, patients should be observed closely for development of hypokalemia.

LIDOCAINE HYDROCHLORIDE
The safety and effectiveness of Lidocaine Hydrochloride depend on proper dosage, correct technique, adequate precautions, and readiness for emergencies.

Injection of repeated doses may cause significant increases in blood levels with each repeated dose due to slow accumulation of the drug or its metabolites. Tolerance varies with the status of the patient. Debilitated, elderly patients, acutely ill patients, and children should be given reduced doses commensurate with their age and physical status. INJECTIONS SHOULD ALWAYS BE MADE SLOWLY AND WITH FREQUENT ASPIRATIONS. Aspiration is advisable since it reduces the possibility of intravascular injection, thereby keeping the incidence of side effects and anesthetic failures to a minimum. Consult standard textbooks for specific techniques and precautions for various local anesthetic procedures.

Lidocaine Hydrochloride should be used with caution in persons with known drug sensitivities. Patients allergic to para-aminobenzoic acid derivatives (procaine, tetracaine, benzocaine, etc.) have not shown cross sensitivity to Lidocaine Hydrochloride.

Local anesthetics react with certain metals and cause the release of their respective ions which, if injected, may cause severe local irritation. Adequate precaution should be taken to avoid this type of interaction.

INFORMATION FOR PATIENTS

Susceptible patients who are on immunosuppressant doses of corticosteroids should be warned to avoid exposure to chickenpox or measles. Patients should also be advised that if they are exposed, medical advice should be sought without delay.

ADVERSE REACTIONS

DEXAMETHASONE SODIUM PHOSPHATE FLUID AND ELECTROLYTE DISTURBANCES

Sodium retention
Fluid retention
Congestive heart failure in susceptible patients
Potassium loss
Hypokalemic alkalosis
Hypertension

MUSCULOSKELETAL

Muscle weakness
Steroid myopathy
Loss of muscle mass
Osteoporosis
Vertebral compression fractures
Aseptic necrosis of femoral and humeral heads
Pathologic fracture of long bones
Tendon rupture

GASTROINTESTINAL

Peptic ulcer with possible subsequent perforation and hemorrhage
Perforation of the small and large bowel, particularly in patients with inflammatory bowel disease
Pancreatitis
Abdominal distention
Ulcerative esophagitis

DERMATOLOGIC

Impaired wound healing
Thin fragile skin
Petechiae and ecchymoses
Erythema
Increased sweating
May suppress reactions to skin tests
Other cutaneous reactions, such as allergic dermatitis, urticaria, angioneurotic edema

NEUROLOGIC

Convulsions
Increased intracranial pressure with papilledema (pseudotumor cerebri) usually after treatment
Vertigo
Headache
Psychic disturbances

ENDOCRINE

Menstrual irregularities
Development of cushingoid state
Suppression of growth in children
Secondary adrenocortical and pituitary unresponsiveness, particularly in times of stress, as in trauma, surgery, or illness
Decreased carbohydrate tolerance
Manifestations of latent diabetes mellitus
Increased requirements for insulin or oral hypoglycemic agents in diabetics
Hirsutism.

OPHTHALMIC

Posterior subcapsular cataracts
Increased intraocular pressure
Glaucoma
Exophthalmos

METABOLIC

Negative nitrogen balance due to protein catabolism

CARDIOVASCULAR

Myocardial rupture following recent myocardial infarction (see *"Warnings"*).

OTHER

Anaphylactoid or hypersensitivity reactions
Thromboembolism
Weight gain

Increased appetite
Nausea
Malaise
Hiccups

The following *additional* adverse reactions are related to parenteral corticosteroid therapy:

Rare instances of blindness associated with intralesional therapy around the face and head
Hyperpigmentation or hypopigmentation
Subcutaneous and cutaneous atrophy
Sterile abscess
Charcot-like arthropathy

LIDOCAINE HYDROCHLORIDE

Adverse reactions may result from high plasma levels due to excessive dosage, rapid absorption or inadvertent intravascular injection, or may result from a hypersensitivity, idiosyncrasy or diminished tolerance on the part of the patient. Such reactions are systemic in nature and involve the central nervous system and/or the cardiovascular system. CNS reactions are excitatory and/or depressant, and may be characterized by nervousness, dizziness, blurred vision, and tremors followed by drowsiness, convulsions, unconsciousness, and possibly respiratory arrest. The excitatory reactions may be very brief or may not occur at all, in which case the first manifestations of toxicity may be drowsiness merging into unconsciousness and respiratory arrest.

Cardiovascular reactions are depressant, and may be characterized by hypotension, myocardial depression, bradycardia and possibly cardiac arrest.

Treatment of a patient with toxic manifestations consists of assuring and maintaining a patent airway and supporting ventilation using oxygen and assisted or controlled respiration as required. This usually will be sufficient in the management of most reactions. Should circulatory depression occur, vasopressors, such as ephedrine or metaraminol, and intravenous fluids may be used. Should a convulsion persist despite oxygen therapy, small increments of an ultrashort acting barbiturate (thiopental or thiamylal) or a short acting barbiturate (pentobarbital or secobarbital) may be given intravenously.

Allergic reactions are characterized by cutaneous lesions, urticaria, edema or anaphylactoid reactions. The detection of sensitivity by skin testing is of doubtful value.

DOSAGE AND ADMINISTRATION

FOR LOCAL INJECTION ONLY

NOT FOR INTRAVENOUS USE

DOSAGE AND FREQUENCY OF INJECTION ARE VARIABLE AND MUST BE INDIVIDUALIZED ON THE BASIS OF THE DISEASE AND THE RESPONSE OF THE PATIENT.

Injections should always be made slowly and with frequent aspiration.

The initial dose ranges from 0.1 to 0.75 mL depending on the disease being treated and the size of the area to be injected. Frequency of injection depends on symptomatic response. In some patients, acute conditions are controlled adequately by a single injection. In others, additional injections are required, usually at intervals of four to seven days. If satisfactory clinical response does not occur after a reasonable period of time, discontinue Dexamethasone Sodium Phosphate/Lidocaine Hydrochloride Injection and transfer the patient to other therapy.

Patients should be observed closely for signs that might require dosage adjustment, including changes in clinical status resulting from remissions or exacerbations of the disease, and individual drug responsiveness.

The usual doses are:

	Acute and Subacute Bursitis	Acute and Subacute Nonspecific Tenosynovitis
Amount of injection (mL)	0.5 to 0.75	0.1 to 0.25
Amount of Dexamethasone Sodium Phosphate (mg)	2 to 3	0.4 to 1
Amount of Lidocaine Hydrochloride (mg)	5 to 7.5	1 to 2.5

Dexamethasone Sodium Phosphate/Lidocaine Hydrochloride may be given undiluted directly from the vial, or it may be diluted with Sterile Water for Injection or Sodium Chloride Injection, using up to five parts of diluent to each part of injection. Dilutions should be used within one hour, since there is a possibility of change in pH, and this may adversely affect the stability or activity of the components.
Sensitive to heat. Do not autoclave.
Protect from freezing.

HOW SUPPLIED
INJECTION:

BRAND/MANUFACTURER	NDC	SIZE	AWP
○ BRAND			
DECADRON W/XYLOCAINE: Merck	00006-7625-03	5 ml	$30.74

Dexamethasone Sodium Phosphate with Neomycin Sulfate, Ophthalmic

DESCRIPTION
Ophthalmic Solution Dexamethasone Sodium Phosphate/Neomycin Sulfate is a topical corticosteroid antibiotic solution for use in certain disorders of the anterior segment of the eye.

Each milliliter of buffered Dexamethasone Sodium Phosphate/Neomycin Sulfate ophthalmic solution contains: Dexamethasone Sodium Phosphate equivalent to 1 mg (0.1%), Dexamethasone Phosphate, and Neomycin Sulfate equivalent to 3.5 mg Neomycin base.

Dexamethasone Sodium Phosphate is a water soluble, inorganic ester of Dexamethasone. Its empirical formula is $C_{22}H_{28}FNa_2O_8P$. It is approximately three thousand times more soluble in water at 25°C than hydrocortisone.

Neomycin Sulfate is the sulfate salt of Neomycin, an antibacterial substance produced by the growth of *Streptomyces fradiae* Waksman (Fam. Streptomycetaceae).

CLINICAL PHARMACOLOGY
Dexamethasone Sodium Phosphate, a corticosteroid, suppresses the inflammatory response to a variety of agents, and it probably delays or slows healing. Since corticosteroids may inhibit the body's defense mechanism against infection, a concomitant antimicrobial drug may be used when this inhibition is considered to be clinically significant in a particular case.

Neomycin Sulfate, the anti-infective component in the combination, is included to provide action against specific organisms susceptible to it. Neomycin Sulfate is considered active mainly against gram-negative organisms, except *Bacteroides* spp. and *Pseudomonas aeruginosa*, which are resistant. Gram-positive organisms except for *Staphylococcus aureus* are usually resistant.

When a decision to administer both a corticosteroid and an antimicrobial is made, the administration of such drugs in combination has the advantage of greater patient compliance and convenience, with the added assurance that the appropriate dosage of both drugs is administered, plus assured compatibility of ingredients when both types of drug are in the same formulation and, particularly, that the correct volume of drug is delivered and retained.

The relative potency of corticosteroids depends on the molecular structure, concentration, and release from the vehicle.

INDICATIONS AND USAGE
For steroid-responsive inflammatory ocular conditions for which a corticosteroid is indicated and where bacterial infection or a risk of bacterial ocular infection exists.

Ocular steroids are indicated in inflammatory conditions of the palpebral and bulbar conjunctiva, cornea, and anterior segment of the globe where the inherent risk of steroid use in certain infective conjunctivitides is accepted to obtain a diminution in edema and inflammation. They are also indicated in chronic anterior uveitis and corneal injury from chemical, radiation, or thermal burns, or penetration of foreign bodies. The use of a combination drug with an anti-infective component is indicated where the risk of infection is high or where there is an expectation that potentially dangerous numbers of bacteria will be present in the eye.

The particular anti-infective drug in this product is active against the following common bacterial eye pathogens:
Staphylococcus aureus
Echerichia coli
Haemophilus influenzae
Klebsiella/Enterobacter species
Neisseria species
The product does not provide adequate coverage against:
Pseudomonas aeruginosa
Serratia marcescens
Streptococci, including *Streptococcus pneumoniae*

CONTRAINDICATIONS
Epithelial herpes simplex keratitis (dendritic keratitis), acute infectious stages of vaccinia, varicella, and many other viral diseases of the cornea and conjunctiva. Mycobacterial infection of the eye. Fungal diseases of ocular structures. Hypersensitivity to any component of this product, including sulfites (see *"Warnings"*). (Hypersensitivity to the antibiotic component occurs at a higher rate than for other components.)

The use of these combinations is always contraindicated after uncomplicated removal of a corneal foreign body.

WARNINGS
Prolonged use may result in glaucoma, with damage to the optic nerve, defects in visual acuity and fields of vision, and posterior subcapsular cataract formation. Prolonged use may suppress the host response and thus increase the hazard of secondary ocular infections. In those diseases causing thinning of the cornea or sclera, perforations have been known to occur with the use of topical corticosteroids. In acute purulent conditions of the eye, corticosteroids may mask infection or enhance existing infection. If these products are used for 10 days or longer, intraocular pressure should be routinely monitored even though it may be difficult in children and uncooperative patients.

Employment of corticosteroid medication in the treatment of herpes simplex requires great caution: periodic slit-lamp microscopy is recommended.

Any substance (e.g., Neomycin Sulfate) may occasionally cause cutaneous sensitization. If any reaction indicating such sensitivity is observed, discontinue use.

Ophthalmic Solution Dexamethasone Sodium Phosphate/Neomycin Sulfate contains sodium bisulfite, a sulfite that may cause allergic-type reactions including anaphylactic symptoms and life-threatening or less severe asthmatic episodes in certain susceptible people. The overall prevalence of sulfite sensitivity in the general population is unknown and probably low. Sulfite sensitivity is seen more frequently in asthmatic than in nonasthmatic people.

PRECAUTIONS
The initial prescription and renewal of the medication order beyond 20 milliliters should be made by a physician only after examination of the patient with the aid of magnification, such as slit-lamp biomicroscopy and, where appropriate, fluorescein staining.

The possibility of persistent fungal infections of the cornea should be considered after prolonged corticosteroid dosing.

Information for Patients: One of the preservatives in Ophthalmic Solution Dexamethasone Sodium Phosphate/Neomycin Sulfate, benzalkonium chloride, may be absorbed by soft contact lenses. Patients wearing soft contact lenses should be instructed to wait at least 15 minutes after instilling Ophthalmic Solution Dexamethasone Sodium Phosphate/Neomycin Sulfate before they insert their lenses.

Usage in Pregnancy: Safety of intensive or protracted use of topical corticosteroids during pregnancy has not been substantiated.

ADVERSE REACTIONS
Adverse reactions have occurred with corticosteroid/anti-infective combination drugs which can be attributed to the corticosteroid component, the anti-infective component, the combination, or any other component of the product. Exact incidence figures are not available since no denominator of treated patients is available.

Reactions occurring most often from the presence of the anti-infective ingredient are allergic sensitizations. The reactions due to the corticosteroid component in decreasing order of frequency are: elevation of intraocular pressure (IOP) with possible development of glaucoma, and infrequent optic nerve damage: posterior subcapsular cataract formation: and delayed wound healing.

Secondary Infection: The development of secondary infection has occurred after use of combinations containing corticosteroids and antimicrobials. Fungal infections of the cornea are particularly prone to develop coincidentally with long-term applications of corticosteroid. The possibility of fungal invasion must be considered in any persistent corneal ulceration where corticosteroid treatment has been used. Secondary bacterial ocular infection following suppression of host responses also occurs.

DOSAGE AND ADMINISTRATION
The duration of treatment will vary with the type of lesion and may extend from a few days to several weeks, according to therapeutic response. Relapses, more common in chronic active lesions than in self-limited conditions, usually respond to retreatment.

Instil one or two drops of Ophthalmic Solution Dexamethasone Sodium Phosphate/Neomycin Sulfate into the conjunctival sac every hour during the day and every two hours during the night as initial therapy. When a favorable response is observed, reduce dosage to one drop every four hours. Later, further reduction in dosage to one drop three or four times daily may suffice to control symptoms.

Not more than 20 milliliters should be prescribed initially and the prescription should not be refilled without further evaluation as outlined in *"Precautions"* above.

HOW SUPPLIED
DROP: 0.1%-3.5 MG/GM

AVERAGE UNIT PRICE (AVAILABLE SIZES)		GENERIC A-RATED AVERAGE PRICE (GAAP)	
BRAND	$2.26	5 ml	$7.90
GENERIC	$1.58		

BRAND/MANUFACTURER	NDC	SIZE	AWP
◆ BRAND			
AK-NEO-DEX: Akorn	17478-0277-10	5 ml	$7.50
NEO-DECADRON OCUMETER: Merck	00006-7639-03	5 ml	$15.09

◆ RATED THERAPEUTICALLY EQUIVALENT; ◇ THERAPEUTIC EQUIVALENCE UNCONFIRMED; ○ UNRATED

BRAND/MANUFACTURER	NDC	SIZE	AWP
◆ GENERICS			
Schein	00364-0762-53	5 ml	$6.90
Steris	00402-0775-05	5 ml	$6.90
NEODEXAIR: Bausch&Lomb Pharm	24208-0955-60	5 ml	$6.92
Aligen	00405-6090-05	5 ml	$7.10
Moore,H.L.	00839-7111-25	5 ml	$7.90
Goldline	00182-1794-62	5 ml	$8.10
NEO-DEX: Qualitest	00603-7204-37	5 ml	$8.50
NEO DEXAIR: Major	00904-3007-05	5 ml	$8.95
Rugby	00536-1905-65	5 ml	$9.82

OINTMENT: 0.1%-3.5 MG/GM

BRAND/MANUFACTURER	NDC	SIZE	AWP
○ BRAND			
NEO-DECADRON: Merck	00006-7617-04	3.5 gm	$6.15

Dexamethasone Sodium Phosphate, Inhalation

DESCRIPTION
Dexamethasone Sodium Phosphate is an inorganic ester of Dexamethasone, a synthetic adrenocortical steroid with basic glucocorticoid actions and effects. It is available as an aersol for oral and nasal inhalation.

Dexamethasone Sodium Phosphate equivalent to approximately 0.1 mg of Dexamethasone Phosphate or approximately 0.084 mg of Dexamethasone is dispensed by oral inhalation with each activation. On a regimen of 12 inhalations daily, it has been determined that the patient absorbs approximately 0.4-0.6 mg of Dexamethasone. Each spray of the nasal inhalation contains Dexamethasone Sodium Phosphate equivalent to approximately 0.1 mg Dexamethasone Phosphate or to approximately 0.084 mg Dexamethasone. Twelve sprays deliver a theoretical maximum of 1.0 mg Dexamethasone.

Dexamethasone Sodium Phosphate, a synthetic adrenocortical steroid, is a white or slightly yellow, crystalline powder. It is freely soluble in water and is exceedingly hygroscopic. The molecular weight is 516.41. It is designated chemically as 9-fluoro-11β,17-dihydroxy-16α-methyl-21-(phosphono-oxy)pregna - 1, 4-diene-3, 20-dione disodium salt. The empirical formula is $C_{22}H_{28}FNa_2O_8P$.

Following is its chemical structure:

ACTIONS
Because of the high water solubility of orally administered Sodium Phosphate, the aerosolized particles dissolve readily in the secretions of the bronchial and bronchiolar mucous membrane. The nasal inhalation acts to inhibition inflammatory response to inciting agents of mechanical, chemical or immunological nature.

INDICATIONS
Dexamethasone Sodium Phosphate oral inhalation is indicated for the treatment of bronchial asthma and related corticosteroid responsive bronchospastic states intractable to adequate trial of conventional therapy. Dexamethasone Sodium Phosphate nasal inhalation is indicated for the treatment of allergic or inflammatory nasal conditions, and nasal polyps (excluding polyps originating within the sinuses).

CONTRAINDICATIONS
Systemic fungal infections.
Hypersensitivity to any component of this medication.
Persistently positive cultures of the sputum for *Candida albicans (oral)*.
Tuberculous, viral and fungal nasal conditions, ocular herpes simplex (nasal).

WARNINGS
Rare instances of laryngeal and pharyngeal fungal infections have been observed in patients using Dexamethasone Sodium Phosphate oral inhalation. These have usually responded promptly to discontinuation of therapy and institution of antifungal treatment.

In patients on therapy with Dexamethasone Sodium Phosphate oral or nasal inhalation subjected to unusual stress, increased dosage of rapidly acting corticosteroids before, during, and after the stressful situation is indicated.

Drug-induced secondary adrenocortical insufficiency may result from too rapid withdrawal of corticosteroids and may be minimized by gradual reduction of dosage. This type of relative insufficiency may persist for months after discontinuation of therapy; therefore, in any situation of stress occurring during that period, hormone therapy should be reinstituted. If the patient is receiving steroids already, dosage may have to be increased. Since mineralocorticoid

secretion may be impaired, salt and/or a mineralocorticoid should be administered concurrently.

Dexamethasone may mask some signs of infection, and new infections may appear during its use. There may be decreased resistance and inability to localize infection when corticosteroids are used. Therefore, patients with bacterial infections should also be given appropriate antibiotic therapy if Dexamethasone Sodium Phosphate nasal inhalation is used. Moreover, Dexamethasone may affect the nitroblue-tetrazolium test for bacterial infection and produce false negative results.

Corticosteroids may activate latent amebiasis. Therefore, it is recommended that latent or active amebiasis be ruled out before initiating corticosteroid therapy in any patient who has spent time in the tropics or any patient with unexplained diarrhea.

Prolonged use of Dexamethasone Sodium Phosphate oral or nasal inhalation may produce posterior subcapsular cataracts, glaucoma with possible damage to the optic nerves, and may enhance the establishment of secondary ocular infections due to fungi or viruses.

Usage in Pregnancy: Since adequate human reproduction studies have not been done with Dexamethasone Sodium Phosphate oral or nasal inhalation, use of this drug in pregnancy or in women of childbearing potential requires that the anticipated benefits be weighed against the possible hazards to the mother and embryo or fetus. Infants born of mothers who have received substantial doses of Dexamethasone during pregnancy, should be carefully observed for signs of hypoadrenalism.

Dexamethasone appears in breast milk and could suppress growth, interfere with endogenous corticosteroid production, or cause other unwanted effects. Mothers taking pharmacologic doses of Dexamethasone should be advised not to nurse.

Average and large doses of hydrocortisone or cortisone can cause elevation of blood pressure, salt and water retention, and increased excretion of potassium. These effects are less likely to occur with the synthetic derivatives and with Dexamethasone Sodium Phosphate oral or nasal inhalation except when used in large doses. Dietary salt restriction and potassium supplementation may be necessary. All corticosteroids increase calcium excretion.

Administration of live virus vaccines, including smallpox, is contraindicated in individuals receiving immunosuppressive doses of corticosteroids. If inactivated viral or bacterial vaccines are administered to individuals receiving immunosuppressive doses of corticosteroids, the expected serum antibody response may not be obtained.

Patients who are on drugs which suppress the immune system are more susceptible to infections than healthy individuals. Chickenpox and measles, for example, can have a more serious or even fatal course in non-immune children or adults on corticosteroids. In such children or adults who have not had these diseases, particular care should be taken to avoid exposure. The risk of developing a disseminated infection varies among individuals and can be related to the dose, route and duration of corticosteroid administration as well as to the underlying disease. If exposed to chickenpox, prophylaxis with varicella zoster immune globulin (VZIG) may be indicated. If chickenpox develops, treatment with antiviral agents may be considered. If exposed to measles, prophylaxis with immune globulin (IG) may be indicated. (See the respective package inserts for VZIG and IG for complete prescribing information.)

If Dexamethasone Sodium Phosphate oral or nasal inhalation is indicated in patients with latent tuberculosis or tuberculin reactivity, close observation is necessary as reactivation of the disease may occur. During prolonged therapy with Dexamethasone Sodium Phosphate oral or nasal inhalation, these patients should receive chemoprophylaxis.

Literature reports suggest an apparent association between use of corticosteroids and left ventricular free wall rupture after a recent myocardial infarction; therefore, therapy with corticosteroids should be used with great caution in these patients.

Keep out of reach of children.

PRECAUTIONS
During local corticosteroid therapy, the possibility of pharyngeal candidiasis should be kept in mind.

Dexamethasone Sodium Phosphate oral inhalation is *not* indicated for relief of the occasional mild and isolated attack of asthma which is readily responsive to the immediate, though short-lived, action of epinephrine, isoproterenol, aminophylline, etc. Nor should it be employed for the treatment of severe status asthmaticus where intensive measures are required. Dexamethasone Sodium Phosphate oral inhalation should be considered only for the following classes of patients: patients not on corticosteroid therapy who have not responded adequately to other treatment; patients already on systemic corticosteroid therapy—in an attempt to reduce or eliminate systemic administration.

Although systemic absorption is low when Dexamethasone Sodium Phosphate oral or nasal inhalation is used in the recommended dosage, adrenal suppression may occur. In addition, other systemic effects of steroid administration must be considered as a possibility.

Following prolonged therapy, withdrawal of corticosteroids may result in symptoms of the corticosteroid withdrawal syndrome including fever, myalgia, arthralgia, and malaise. This may occur in patients even without evidence of adrenal insufficiency. Replacement of systemic steroid with Dexamethasone Sodium Phosphate nasal inhalation should be gradual and carefully monitored by the physician.

There is an enhanced effect of Dexamethasone in patients with hypothyroidism and in those with cirrhosis.

Dexamethasone Sodium Phosphate oral or nasal inhalation should be used cautiously in patients with ocular herpes simplex for fear of corneal perforation.

The lowest possible dose of Dexamethasone Sodium Phosphate oral or nasal inhalation should be used to control the condition under treatment, and when reduction in dosage is possible, the reduction must be gradual. If beneficial effect is not evident within 7 days after initiation of therapy, the patient should be re-evaluated.

Psychic derangements may appear when Dexamethasone is used, ranging from euphoria, insomnia, mood swings, personality changes, and severe depression, to frank psychotic manifestations. Also, existing emotional instability or psychotic tendencies may be aggravated.

Aspirin should be used cautiously in conjunction with Dexamethasone Sodium Phosphate oral or nasal inhalation in hypoprothrombinemia.

Dexamethasone Sodium Phosphate oral or nasal inhalation should be used with caution in nonspecific ulcerative colitis, if there is a probability of impending perforation, abscess or other pyogenic infection: also in diverticulitis; fresh intestinal anastomoses; active or latent peptic ulcer; renal insufficiency; hypertension; osteoporosis; and myasthenia gravis. Signs of peritoneal irritation following gastrointestinal perforation in patients receiving large doses of corticosteroids may be minimal or absent. Fat embolism has been reported as a possible complication of hypercortisonism.

Growth and development of infants and children on prolonged therapy with Dexamethasone Sodium Phosphate oral or nasal inhalation should be carefully followed. Because clinical studies have not been done, the use of Dexamethasone Sodium Phosphate nasal inhalation in children under the age of 6 years is not recommended.

Dexamethasone may increase or decrease motility and number of spermatozoa in some patients.

Phenytoin, phenobarbital, ephedrine and rifampin may enhance the metabolic clearance of Dexamethasone, resulting in decreased blood levels and lessened physiologic activity, thus requiring adjustment in Dexamethasone dosage.

The prothrombin time should be checked frequently in patients who are receiving Dexamethasone Sodium Phosphate oral or nasal inhalation and coumarin anticoagulants at the same time because of reports that corticosteroids have altered the response to these anticoagulants. Studies have shown that the usual effect produced by adding corticosteroids is inhibition of response to coumarins, although there have been some conflicting reports of potentiation, not substantiated by studies.

When Dexamethasone Sodium Phosphate oral or nasal inhalation is used concomitantly with potassium-depleting diuretics, patients should be observed closely for development of hypokalemia. Since the contents of Dexamethasone Sodium Phosphate oral or nasal inhalation are under pressure, the container should not be broken, stored in extreme heat, or incinerated. It should be stored at a temperature below 120°F.

Information for Patients: Susceptible patients who are on immunosuppressant doses of corticosteroids should be warned to avoid exposure to chickenpox or measles. Patients should also be advised that if they are exposed, medical advice should be sought without delay.

ADVERSE REACTIONS

Side effects which may occur in patients treated with Dexamethasone Sodium Phosphate oral inhalation include throat irritation, hoarseness, coughing, and laryngeal and pharyngeal fungal infections.

Patients should be observed for the hormonal effects described below.

Nasal irritation and dryness are the most common adverse reactions to Dexamethasone Sodium Phosphate nasal inhalation. The following have been reported: headache, lightheadedness, urticaria, nausea, epistaxis, rebound congestion, bronchial asthma, perforation of the nasal septum, and anosmia. Signs of adrenal hypercorticism may occur in some patients, especially with overdosage.

Systemic effects from therapy with Dexamethasone Sodium Phosphate nasal inhalation are less likely to occur than with oral or parenteral corticosteroid therapy because of a lower total dose administered. Nevertheless, patients should be observed for the hormonal effects described below because of absorption of Dexamethasone from the nasal mucosa.

Fluid and Electrolyte Disturbances:
Sodium retention
Fluid retention
Congestive heart failure in susceptible patients
Potassium loss
Hypokalemic alkalosis
Hypertension

Musculoskeletal:
Muscle weakness
Steroid myopathy
Loss of muscle mass
Osteoporosis
Vertebral compression fractures
Aseptic necrosis of femoral and humeral heads
Pathologic fracture of long bones
Tendon rupture

Gastrointestinal:
Peptic ulcer with possible subsequent perforation and hemorrhage
Perforation of the small and large bowel, particularly in patients with inflammatory bowel disease
Pancreatitis

Abdominal distention
Ulcerative esophagitis

Dermatologic:
Impaired wound healing
Thin fragile skin
Petechiae and ecchymoses
Erythema
Increased sweating
May suppress reactions to skin tests
Other cutaneous reactions, such as allergic dermatitis, urticaria, angioneurotic edema

Neurologic:
Convulsions
Increased intracranial pressure with papilledema (pseudotumor cerebri) usually after treatment
Vertigo
Headache
Psychic disturbances

Endocrine:
Menstrual irregularities
Development of cushingoid state
Suppression of growth in children
Secondary adrenocortical and pituitary unresponsiveness, particularly in times of stress, as in trauma, surgery, or illness
Decreased carbohydrate tolerance
Manifestations of latent diabetes mellitus
Increased requirements for insulin or oral hypoglycemic agents in diabetics
Hirsutism

Ophthalmic:
Posterior subcapsular cataracts
Increased intraocular pressure
Glaucoma
Exophthalmos

Metabolic:
Negative nitrogen balance due to protein catabolism

Cardiovascular:
Myocardial rupture following recent myocardial infarction (see *"Warnings"*).

Other:
Hypersensitivity
Thromboembolism
Weight gain
Increased appetite
Nausea
Malaise
Hiccups

OVERDOSAGE

Reports of acute toxicity and/or death following overdosage of glucocorticoids are rare. In the event of overdosage, no specific antidote is available; treatment is supportive and symptomatic.

The oral LD_{50} of Dexamethasone in female mice was 6.5 g/kg. The intravenous LD_{50} of Dexamethasone Sodium Phosphate in female mice was 794 mg/kg.

DOSAGE AND ADMINISTRATION
ORAL INHALATION
Recommended initial dosage:

Adults —3 inhalations 3 or 4 times per day.
Children —2 inhalations 3 or 4 times per day.

Maximum dosage:

Adults —3 inhalations *per dose*; 12 inhalations *per day*.
Children —2 inhalations *per dose*; 8 inhalations *per day*.

When a favorable response is attained, the dose may be gradually reduced. In patients on systemic corticosteroids, it is recommended that systemic therapy be reduced or eliminated before reduction of Dexamethasone Sodium Phosphate oral inhalation dosage is begun. Gradual reduction of systemic corticosteroid therapy must be emphasized to avoid withdrawal symptoms.

NASAL INHALATION
DO NOT EXCEED THE RECOMMENDED DOSAGE
The usual initial dosage of Dexamethasone Sodium Phosphate nasal inhalation is:

Adults—2 sprays in each nostril 2 or 3 times a day.
Children (6 to 12 years of age)—1 or 2 sprays in each nostril 2 times a day depending on age.

When improvement occurs the dosage should be gradually reduced. Some patients will be symptom-free on one spray in each nostril 2 times a day. The maximum daily dosage for adults is 12 sprays, and for children, 8 sprays. Therapy should be discontinued as soon as feasible. It may be reinstituted if recurrence of symptoms occurs.

STORAGE
Store at a temperature below 49°C (120°F).

◆ RATED THERAPEUTICALLY EQUIVALENT; ◇ THERAPEUTIC EQUIVALENCE UNCONFIRMED; ○ UNRATED

HOW SUPPLIED
AEROSOL SOLID W/ADAPTER: 0.1 MG/INH

BRAND/MANUFACTURER	NDC	SIZE	AWP
○ **BRAND**			
DEXACORT IN TURBINAIRE: Adams	53014-0201-13	12.6 gm	$31.45

Dexamethasone, Injectable

DESCRIPTION

Dexamethasone Sodium Phosphate, a synthetic adrenocortical steroid, is a white or slightly yellow, crystalline powder. It is freely soluble in water and is exceedingly hygroscopic. The molecular weight is 516.41. It is designated chemically as 9-fluoro-11β, 17-dihydroxy-16α-methyl-21-(phosphonooxy)pregna-1, 4-diene-3, 20-dione disodium salt. The empirical formula is $C_{22}H_{28}FNa_2O_8P$.

Dexamethasone acetate, a synthetic adrenocortical steroid, is a white to practically white, odorless powder. It is a practically insoluble ester of Dexamethasone.

It has a molecular weight of 434.5 and its empirical formula is $C_{24}H_{31}FO_6$. As the monohydrate, its empirical formula is $C_{24}H_{31}FO_6 \cdot H_2O$, and its molecular weight, 452.52. Dexamethasone acetate is designated chemically as 21-(acetyloxy)-9-fluoro-11β,17-dihydroxy-16α-methylpregna-1,4- diene-3,20-dione.

Dexamethasone, Injectable injection is a sterile solution (pH 7.0 to 8.5) of Dexamethasone sodium phosphate in two concentrations, 4 mg/mL and 24 mg/mL, or a sterile white suspension (pH 5.0 to 7.5) of Dexamethasone Acetate that settles on standing, but is easily resuspended by mild shaking.

Each ml of Dexamethasone, Injectable contains: Dexamethasone Sodium Phosphate equivalent to 3.33 mg or 20 mg Dexamethasone (solution) or Dexamethasone acetate equivalent to 8 or 16 mg Dexamethasone (suspension).

Following is its chemical structure:

ACTIONS

Dexamethasone Sodium Phosphate has a rapid onset but short duration of action when compared with less soluble preparations. Because of this, it is suitable for the treatment of acute disorders responsive to adrenocortical steroid therapy.

Dexamethasone Acetate sterile suspension is a long-acting, repository adrenocorticosteroid preparation with a prompt onset of action. It is suitable for intramuscular or local injection, but not when an immediate effect of short duration is desired.

Naturally occurring glucocorticoids (hydrocortisone and cortisone), which also have salt-retaining properties, are used as replacement therapy in adrenocortical deficiency states. Their synthetic analogs, including dexamethasone, are primarily used for their potent anti-inflammatory effects in disorders of many organ systems.

Glucocorticoids cause profound and varied metabolic effects. In addition, they modify the body's immune responses to diverse stimuli.

At equipotent anti-inflammatory doses, Dexamethasone almost completely lacks the sodium-retaining property of hydrocortisone and closely related derivatives of hydrocortisone.

INDICATIONS

A. BY INTRAVENOUS OR INTRAMUSCULAR INJECTION (when oral therapy is not feasible and the strength, dosage form, and route of administration of the drug reasonably lend the preparation to the treatment of the condition):

1. Endocrine Disorders: Primary or secondary adrenocortical insufficiency (hydrocortisone or cortisone is the drug of choice; synthetic analogs may be used in conjunction with mineralocorticoids where applicable; in infancy, mineralocorticoid supplementation is of particular importance)

Acute adrenocortical insufficiency (hydrocortisone or cortisone is the drug of choice; mineralocorticoid supplementation may be necessary, particularly when synthetic analogs are used)

Preoperatively, and in the event of serious trauma or illness, in patients with known adrenal insufficiency or when adrenocortical reserve is doubtful

Shock unresponsive to conventional therapy if adrenocortical insufficiency exists or is suspected

Congenital adrenal hyperplasia
Nonsuppurative thyroiditis
Hypercalcemia associated with cancer

2. Rheumatic Disorders: As adjunctive therapy for short-term administration (to tide the patient over an acute episode or exacerbation) in:

Post-traumatic osteoarthritis
Synovitis of osteoarthritis
Rheumatoid arthritis, including juvenile rheumatoid arthritis (selected cases may require low-dose maintenance therapy)
Acute and subacute bursitis
Epicondylitis

Acute nonspecific tenosynovitis
Acute gouty arthritis
Psoriatic arthritis
Ankylosing spondylitis

3. Collagen Diseases: During an exacerbation or as maintenance therapy in selected cases of:

Systemic lupus erythematosus
Acute rheumatic carditis

4. Dermatologic Diseases:

Pemphigus
Severe erythema multiforme (Stevens-Johnson syndrome)
Exfoliative dermatitis
Bullous dermatitis herpetiformis
Severe seborrheic dermatitis
Severe psoriasis
Mycosis fungoides

5. Allergic States: Control of severe or incapacitating allergic conditions intractable to adequate trials of conventional treatment in:

Bronchial asthma
Contact dermatitis
Atopic dermatitis
Serum sickness
Seasonal or perennial allergic rhinitis
Drug hypersensitivity reactions
Urticarial transfusion reactions
Acute noninfectious laryngeal edema (epinephrine is the drug of first choice)

6. Ophthalmic Diseases: Severe acute and chronic allergic and inflammatory processes involving the eye, such as:

Herpes zoster ophthalmicus
Iritis, iridocyclitis
Chorioretinitis
Diffuse posterior uveitis and choroiditis
Optic neuritis
Sympathetic ophthalmia
Anterior segment inflammation
Allergic conjunctivitis
Keratitis
Allergic corneal marginal ulcers

7. Gastrointestinal Diseases: To tide the patient over a critical period of the disease in:

Ulcerative colitis (Systemic therapy)
Regional enteritis (Systemic therapy)

8. Respiratory Diseases:

Symptomatic sarcoidosis
Berylliosis
Fulminating or disseminated pulmonary tuberculosis when used concurrently with appropriate antituberculous chemotherapy
Loeffler's syndrome not manageable by other means
Aspiration pneumonitis

9. Hematologic Disorders:

Acquired (autoimmune) hemolytic anemia
Idiopathic thrombocytopenic purpura in adults (I.V. only; I.M. administration is contraindicated)
Secondary thrombocytopenia in adults
Erythroblastopenia (RBC anemia)
Congenital (erythroid) hypoplastic anemia

10. Neoplastic Diseases: For palliative management of:

Leukemias and lymphomas in adults
Acute leukemia of childhood

11. Edematous States: To induce diuresis or remission of proteinuria in the nephrotic syndrome, without uremia, of the idiopathic type, or that due to lupus erythematosus

12. Miscellaneous:

Tuberculous meningitis with subarachnoid block or impending block when used concurrently with appropriate antituberculous chemotherapy
Trichinosis with neurologic or myocardial involvement

13. Diagnostic testing of adrenocortical hyperfunction

14. Cerebral Edema: associated with primary or metastatic brain tumor, craniotomy, or head injury (Dexamethasone, Sodium Phosphate only). Use in cerebral edema is not a substitute for careful neurosurgical evaluation and definitive management such as neurosurgery or other specific therapy.

B. BY INTRA-ARTICULAR OR SOFT TISSUE INJECTION
As adjunctive therapy for short-term administration (to tide the patient over an acute episode or exacerbation) in:

Synovitis of osteoarthritis
Rheumatoid arthritis
Acute and subacute bursitis
Acute gouty arthritis
Epicondylitis
Acute nonspecific tenosynovitis
Post-traumatic osteoarthritis

C. BY INTRALESIONAL INJECTION
Keloids
Localized hypertrophic, infiltrated, inflammatory lesions of: lichen planus, psoriatic plaques, granuloma annulare, and lichen simplex chronicus (neurodermatitis)
Discoid lupus erythematosus
Necrobiosis lipoidica diabeticorum
Alopecia areata
May also be useful in cystic tumors of an aponeurosis or tendon (ganglia).

UNLABELED USES
Dexamethasone is used alone or as an adjunct in the treatment of cystic acne, congenital adrenal hyperplasia, bronchopulmonary dysplasia, and to control symptoms of acute laryngotracheitis (croup). It is also used in the treatment of depression, insulin lipodystrophy, acute mountain sickness, and oligomenorrhea. It is also prescribed as an adjunct in pemphigus vulgaris and pemphigus foliaceus, and is used in the diagnosis of affective disorders (Dexamethasone suppression test). The drug is also used in Peyronie's disease, respiratory distress syndrome, chemotherapy-induced vomiting, and temporal arteritis.

CONTRAINDICATIONS
Systemic fungal infections. (See *"Warnings"* regarding amphotericin B.)
Hypersensitivity to any component of this product, including sulfites (see *"Warnings"*).

WARNINGS
DO NOT INJECT DEXAMETHASONE, INJECTABLE CONTAINING DEXAMETHASONE ACETATE SUSPENSION INTRAVENOUSLY
Because rare instances of anaphylactoid reactions have occurred in patients receiving parenteral corticosteroid therapy, appropriate precautionary measures should be taken prior to administration, especially when the patient has a history of allergy to any drug. Anaphylactoid and hypersensitivity reactions have been reported for Dexamethasone, Injectable (see *"Adverse Reactions"*). Corticosteroids may suppress reaction to skin tests.

Some brands of Dexamethasone, Injectable contain sodium bisulfite or metabisulfite, a sulfite that may cause allergic-type reactions including anaphylactic symptoms and life-threatening or less severe asthmatic episodes in certain susceptible people. The overall prevalence of sulfite sensitivity in the general population is unknown and probably low. Sulfite sensitivity is seen more frequently in asthmatic than in nonasthmatic people.

Corticosteroids may exacerbate systemic fungal infections and therefore should not be used in the presence of such infections unless they are needed to control drug reactions due to amphotericin B. Moreover, there have been cases reported in which concomitant use of amphotericin B and hydrocortisone was followed by cardiac enlargement and congestive failure.

In patients on corticosteroid therapy subjected to any unusual stress, increased dosage of rapidly acting corticosteroids before, during, and after the stressful situation is indicated.

Drug-induced secondary adrenocortical insufficiency may result from too rapid withdrawal of corticosteroids and may be minimized by gradual reduction of dosage. This type of relative insufficiency may persist for months after discontinuation of therapy; therefore, in any situation of stress occurring during that period, hormone therapy should be reinstituted. If the patient is receiving steroids already, dosage may have to be increased. Since mineralocorticoid secretion may be impaired, salt and/or a mineralocorticoid should be administered concurrently.

Corticosteroids may mask some signs of infection, and new infections may appear during their use. There may be decreased resistance and inability to localize infection when corticosteroids are used. Moreover, corticosteroids may affect the nitroblue-tetrazolium test for bacterial infection and produce false negative results.

In cerebral malaria, a double-blind trial has shown that the use of corticosteroids is associated with prolongation of coma and a higher incidence of pneumonia and gastrointestinal bleeding.

Corticosteroids may activate latent amebiasis. Therefore, it is recommended that latent or active amebiasis be ruled out before initiating corticosteroid therapy in any patient who has spent time in the tropics or any patient with unexplained diarrhea.

Prolonged use of corticosteroids may produce posterior subcapsular cataracts, glaucoma with possible damage to the optic nerves, and may enhance the establishment of secondary ocular infections due to fungi or viruses.

Usage in Pregnancy: Since adequate human reproduction studies have not been done with corticosteroids, use of these drugs in pregnancy or in women of childbearing potential requires that the anticipated benefits be weighed against the possible hazards to the mother and embryo or fetus. Infants born of mothers who have received substantial doses of corticosteroids during pregnancy should be carefully observed for signs of hypoadrenalism.

Corticosteroids appear in breast milk and could suppress growth, interfere with endogenous corticosteroid production, or cause other unwanted effects. Mothers taking pharmacologic doses of corticosteroids should be advised not to nurse.

Average and large doses of cortisone or hydrocortisone can cause elevation of blood pressure, salt and water retention, and increased excretion of potassium. These effects are less likely to occur with the synthetic derivatives except when used in large doses. Dietary salt restriction and potassium supplementation may be necessary. All corticosteroids increase calcium excretion.

Administration of live virus vaccines, including smallpox, is contraindicated in individuals receiving immunosuppressive doses of corticosteroids. If inactivated viral or bacterial vaccines are administered to individuals receiving immunosuppressive doses of corticosteroids, the expected serum antibody response may not be obtained and there is a risk of neurologic complications. However, immunization procedures may be undertaken in patients who are receiving corticosteroids as replacement therapy, e.g., for Addison's disease.

Patients who are on drugs which suppress the immune system are more susceptible to infections that healthy individuals. Chickenpox and measles, for example, can have a more serious or even fatal course in non-immune children or adults on corticosteroids. In such children or adults who have not had these diseases, particular care should be taken to avoid exposure. The risk of developing a disseminated infection varies among individuals and can be related to the dose, route and duration of corticosteroid administration as well as to the underlying disease. If exposed to chickenpox, prophylaxis with varicella zoster immune globulin (VZIG) may be indicated. If chickenpox develops, treatment with antiviral agents may be considered. If exposed to measles, prophylaxis with immune globulin (IG) may be indicated. (See the respective package inserts for VZIG and IG for complete prescribing information.)

The use of Dexamethasone, Injectable in active tuberculosis should be restricted to those cases of fulminating or disseminated tuberculosis in which the corticosteroid is used for the management of the disease in conjunction with an appropriate antituberculous regimen.

If corticosteroids are indicated in patients with latent tuberculosis or tuberculin reactivity, close observation is necessary as reactivation of the disease may occur. During prolonged corticosteroid therapy, these patients should receive chemoprophylaxis.

Literature reports suggest an apparent association between use of corticosteroids and left ventricular free wall rupture after a recent myocardial infarction; therefore, therapy with corticosteroids should be used with great caution in these patients.

Respository adrenocorticosteroid preparations may cause atrophy at the site of injection. To minimize the likelihood and/or severity of atrophy, do not inject subcutaneously, avoid injection into the deltoid muscle, and avoid repeated intramuscular injections into the same site if possible.

Dosage in children under 12 has not been established.

PRECAUTIONS
Dexamethasone, Injectable sterile suspension is not recommended as initial therapy in acute, life-threatening situations.

This product, like many other steroid formulations, is sensitive to heat. Therefore, it should not be autoclaved when it is desirable to sterilize the exterior of the vial.

Following prolonged therapy, withdrawal of corticosteroids may result in symptoms of the corticosteroid withdrawal syndrome including fever, myalgia, arthralgia, and malaise. This may occur in patients even without evidence of adrenal insufficiency.

There is an enhanced effect of corticosteroids in patients with hypothyroidism and in those with cirrhosis.

Corticosteroids should be used cautiously in patients with ocular herpes simplex for fear of corneal ulceration and perforation.

The lowest possible dose of corticosteroid should be used to control the condition under treatment, and when reduction in dosage is possible, the reduction must be gradual.

Psychic derangements may appear when corticosteroids are used, ranging from euphoria, insomnia, mood swings, personality changes, and severe depression to frank psychotic manifestations. Also, existing emotional instability or psychotic tendencies may be aggravated by corticosteroids.

Aspirin should be used cautiously in conjunction with corticosteroids in hypoprothrombinemia.

Steroids should be used with caution in nonspecific ulcerative colitis, if there is a probability of impending perforation, abscess, or other pyogenic infection; also in diverticulitis, fresh intestinal anastomoses, active or latent peptic ulcer, renal insufficiency, hypertension, osteoporosis, and myasthenia gravis. Signs of peritoneal irritation following gastrointestinal perforation in patients receiving large doses of corticosteroids may be minimal or absent. Fat embolism has been reported as a possible complication of hypercortisonism.

When large doses are given, some authorities advise that antacids be administered between meals to help to prevent peptic ulcer. An ulcer regimen including an antacid should be considered as a prophylactic measure during prolonged therapy.

Growth and development of infants and children on prolonged corticosteroid therapy should be carefully followed.

Steroids may increase or decrease motility and number of spermatozoa in some patients.

Phenytoin, phenobarbital, ephedrine, and rifampin may enhance the metabolic clearance of corticosteroids, resulting in decreased blood levels and lessened physiologic activity, thus requiring adjustment in corticosteroid dosage. These interactions may interfere with Dexamethasone suppression tests which should be interpreted with caution during administration of these drugs.

False negative results in the dexamethasone suppression test (DST) in patients being treated with indomethacin have been reported. Thus, results of the DST should be interpreted with caution in these patients.

The prothrombin time should be checked frequently in patients who are receiving corticosteroids and coumarin anticoagulants at the same time because of reports that corticosteroids have altered the response to these anticoagulants.

Studies have shown that the usual effect produced by adding corticosteroids is inhibition of response to coumarins, although there have been some conflicting reports of potentiation not substantiated by studies.

When corticosteroids are administered concomitantly with potassium-depleting diuretics, patients should be observed closely for development of hypokalemia.

Intra-articular injection of a corticosteroid may produce systemic as well as local effects.

Appropriate examination of any joint fluid present is necessary to exclude a septic process.

A marked increase in pain accompanied by local swelling, further restriction of joint motion, fever, and malaise is suggestive of septic arthritis. If this complication occurs and the diagnosis of sepsis is confirmed, appropriate antimicrobial therapy should be instituted.

Injection of a steroid into an infected site is to be avoided. Corticosteroids should not be injected into unstable joints. Patients should be impressed strongly with the importance of not overusing joints in which symptomatic benefit has been obtained as long as the inflammatory process remains active.

Frequent intra-articular injection may result in damage to joint tissues.

The slower rate of absorption by intramuscular administration should be recognized.

Information for Patients: Susceptible patients who are on immunosuppressant doses of corticosteroids should be warned to avoid exposure to chickenpox or measles. Patients should also be advised that if they are exposed, medical advice should be sought without delay.

ADVERSE REACTIONS
Fluid and Electrolyte Disturbances:
Sodium retention
Fluid retention
Congestive heart failure in susceptible patients
Potassium loss
Hypokalemic alkalosis
Hypertension
Hypotensive or shock-like reaction

Musculoskeletal:
Muscle weakness
Steroid myopathy
Loss of muscle mass
Osteoporosis
Vertebral compression fractures
Aseptic necrosis of femoral and humeral heads
Pathologic fracture of long bones
Tendon rupture

Gastrointestinal:
Peptic ulcer with possible subsequent perforation and hemorrhage
Perforation of the small and large bowel, particularly in patients with inflammatory bowel disease
Pancreatitis
Abdominal distention
Ulcerative esophagitis

Dermatologic:
Impaired wound healing
Thin fragile skin
Petechiae and ecchymoses
Erythema
Increased sweating
May suppress reactions to skin tests
Burning or tingling, especially in the perineal area (after I.V. injection) (Dexamethasone sodium phosphate)
Other cutaneous reactions, such as allergic dermatitis, urticaria, angioneurotic edema

Neurologic:
Convulsions
Increased intracranial pressure with papilledema (pseudotumor cerebri) usually after treatment
Vertigo
Headache
Psychic disturbances

Endocrine:
Menstrual irregularities
Development of cushingoid state
Suppression of growth in children
Secondary adrenocortical and pituitary unresponsiveness, particularly in times of stress, as in trauma, surgery, or illness
Decreased carbohydrate tolerance
Manifestations of latent diabetes mellitus
Increased requirements for insulin or oral hypoglycemic agents in diabetics
Hirsutism

Ophthalmic:
Posterior subcapsular cataracts
Increased intraocular pressure

Glaucoma
Exophthalmos

Metabolic:
Negative nitrogen balance due to protein catabolism

Cardiovascular:
Myocardial rupture following recent myocardial infarction (see *"Warnings"*).

Other:
Anaphylactoid or hypersensitivity reactions
Thromboembolism
Weight gain
Increased appetite
Nausea
Malaise
Hiccups

The following *additional* adverse reactions are related to parenteral corticosteroid therapy:
Rare instances of blindness associated with intralesional therapy around the face and head
Hyperpigmentation or hypopigmentation
Subcutaneous and cutaneous atrophy
Sterile abscess
Postinjection flare (following intra-articular use)
Charcot-like arthropathy
Scarring
Induration
Inflammation
Paresthesia
Ecchymosis
Delayed pain or soreness

Muscle twitching, ataxia, hiccups, and nystagmus have been reported in low incidence after injection of Dexamethasone, Injectable sterile suspension.

OVERDOSAGE
Reports of acute toxicity and/or death following overdosage of glucocorticoids are rare. In the event of overdosage, no specific antidote is available; treatment is supportive and symptomatic.

The oral LD_{50} of Dexamethasone in female mice was 6.5 g/kg. The intravenous LD_{50} of Dexamethasone sodium phosphate in female mice was 794 mg/kg. The intraperitoneal LD_{50} of Dexamethasone acetate in female mice was 424 mg/kg.

DOSAGE AND ADMINISTRATION
DEXAMETHASONE SODIUM PHOSPHATE
Dexamethasone Sodium Phosphate 4 mg/mL—*For intravenous, intramuscular, intra-articular, intralesional, and soft tissue injection.*

Dexamethasone Sodium Phosphate, 24 mg/mL—*For intravenous injection only.*

Dexamethasone Sodium Phosphate can be given directly from the vial, or it can be added to Sodium Chloride Injection or Dextrose Injection and administered by intravenous drip. Solutions used for intravenous administration or further dilution of this product should be preservative-free when used in the neonate, especially the premature infant.

When it is mixed with an infusion solution, sterile precautions should be observed. Since infusion solutions generally do not contain preservatives, mixtures should be used within 24 hours.

Dosage requirements are variable and must be individualized on the basis of the disease and the response of the patient.

INTRAVENOUS AND INTRAMUSCULAR INJECTION
The initial dosage of Dexamethasone Sodium Phosphate varies from 0.5 to 9 mg a day depending on the disease being treated. In less severe diseases doses lower than 0.5 mg may suffice, while in severe diseases doses higher than 9 mg may be required.

The initial dosage should be maintained or adjusted until the patient's response is satisfactory. If a satisfactory clinical response does not occur after a reasonable period of time, discontinue Dexamethasone Sodium Phosphate and transfer the patient to other therapy.

After a favorable initial response, the proper maintenance dosage should be determined by decreasing the initial dosage in small amounts to the lowest dosage that maintains an adequate clinical response.

Patients should be observed closely for signs that might require dosage adjustment, including changes in clinical status resulting from remissions or exacerbations of the disease, individual drug responsiveness, and the effect of stress (e.g., surgery, infection, trauma). During stress it may be necessary to increase dosage temporarily.

If the drug is to be stopped after more than a few days of treatment, it usually should be withdrawn gradually.

When the intravenous route of administration is used, dosage usually should be the same as the oral dosage. In certain overwhelming, acute, life-threatening situations, however, administration in dosages exceeding the usual dosages may be justified and may be in multiples of the oral dosages. The slower rate of absorption by intramuscular administration should be recognized.

Shock: There is a tendency in current medical practice to use high (pharmacologic) doses of corticosteroids for the treatment of unresponsive shock. The following dosages of Dexamethasone Sodium Phosphate have been suggested by various authors:

Author*	Dosage
Cavanagh[1]	3 mg/kg of body weight per 24 hours by constant intravenous infusion after an initial intravenous injection of 20 mg
Dietzman[2]	2 to 6 mg/kg of body weight as a single intravenous injection
Frank[3]	40 mg initially followed by repeat intravenous injection every 4 to 6 hours while shock persists
Oaks[4]	40 mg initially followed by repeat intravenous injection every 2 to 6 hours while shock persists
Schumer[5]	1 mg/kg of body weight as a single intravenous injection

Administration of high dose corticosteroid therapy should be continued only until the patient's condition has stabilized and usually not longer than 48 to 72 hours.

Although adverse reactions associated with high dose, short term corticosteroid therapy are uncommon, peptic ulceration may occur.

Cerebral Edema: Dexamethasone, Sodium Phosphate is generally administered initially in a dosage of 10 mg intravenously followed by 4 mg every six hours intramuscularly until the symptoms of cerebral edema subside. Response is usually noted within 12 to 24 hours and dosage may be reduced after two to four days and gradually discontinued over a period of five to seven days. For palliative management of patients with recurrent or inoperable brain tumors, maintenance therapy with two mg two or three times a day may be effective.

Acute Allergic Disorders: In acute, self-limited allergic disorders or acute exacerbations of chronic allergic disorders, the following dosage schedule combining parenteral and oral therapy is suggested:

Dexamethasone Sodium Phosphate 4 mg/mL: *first day,* 1 or 2 mL (4 or 8 mg), intramuscularly.

Dexamethasone tablets, 0.75 mg: *second and third days,* 4 tablets in two divided doses each day; *fourth day,* 2 tablets in two divided doses; *fifth and sixth days,* 1 tablet each day; *seventh day,* no treatment; *eighth day,* follow-up visit.

This schedule is designed to ensure adequate therapy during acute episodes, while minimizing the risk of overdosage in chronic cases.

INTRA-ARTICULAR, INTRALESIONAL, AND SOFT TISSUE INJECTION
Intra-articular, intralesional, and soft tissue injections are generally employed when the affected joints or areas are limited to one or two sites. Dosage and frequency of injection varies depending on the condition and the site of injection. The usual dose is from 0.2 to 6 mg. The frequency usually ranges from once every three to five days to once every two to three weeks. Frequent intra-articular injection may result in damage to joint tissues.

Some of the usual single doses are:

Site of Injection	Amount of Dexamethasone Phosphate (mg)
Large Joints (e.g., Knee)	2 to 4
Small Joints (e.g., Interphalangeal, Temporomandibular)	0.8 to 1
Bursae	2 to 3
Tendon Sheaths	0.4 to 1
Soft Tissue Infiltration	2 to 6
Ganglia	1 to 2

Dexamethasone Sodium Phosphate is particularly recommended for use in conjunction with one of the less soluble, longer-acting steroids for intra-articular and soft tissue injection.

DEXAMETHASONE ACETATE
For intramuscular, intralesional, intra-articular, and soft tissue injection.

Dosage requirements are variable and must be individualized on the basis of the disease and the response of the patient.

Dosage in children under 12 has not been established.

Intramuscular Injection: Dosage ranges from 0.5 to 1 ml or 1 to 2 mL, equivalent to 8 to 16 mg of Dexamethasone. If further treatment is needed, dosage may be repeated at intervals of 1 to 3 weeks.

Intralesional Injection: The usual dose is 0.1 to 0.2 mL, equivalent to 0.8 to 1.6 mg of Dexamethasone, per injection site.

Intra-articular and Soft Tissue Injection: The dose varies, depending on the location and the severity of inflammation. The usual dose is 0.25 to 1 ml or 0.5 to 2 mL, equivalent to 4 to 16 mg of Dexamethasone. If further treatment is needed,

*1. Cavanagh, D.; Singh, K. B.: Endotoxin shock in pregnancy and abortion, in "Corticosteroids in the Treatment of Shock", Schumer, W.; Nyhus, L. M., Editors, Urbana, University of Illinois Press, 1970, pp. 86-96.
2. Dietzman, R. H.; Ersek, R. A.; Bloch, J. M.; Lillehei, R. C.: High-output, low-resistance gram-negative septic shock in man, Angiology 20:691-700, Dec. 1969.
3. Frank, E.: Clinical observations in shock and management (In: Shields, T. F., ed.: Symposium on current concepts and management of shock), J. Maine Med. Ass. 59:195-200, Oct. 1968.
4. Oaks, W. W.; Cohen, H. E.: Endotoxin shock in the geriatric patient, Geriat. 22:120-130, Mar. 1967.
5. Schumer, W.; Nyhus, L. M.: Corticosteroid effect on biochemical parameters of human oligemic shock, Arch. Surg. 100:405-408, Apr. 1970.

dosage may be repeated at intervals of 1 to 3 weeks. Frequent intra-articular injection may result in damage to joint tissues.

Parenteral drug products should be inspected visually for particulate matter and discoloration prior to administration, whenever the solution and container permit.

STORAGE
Store at controlled room temperature, 59°-86°F (15°-30°C).
Sensitive to heat. Do not autoclave.
Protect from freezing.
Protect from light. Store container in carton until contents have been used.

J CODES
Up to 4 mg/ml IM,IV,OTH—J1100

HOW SUPPLIED

DEXAMETHASONE ACETATE
INJECTION: 8 MG/ML

BRAND/MANUFACTURER	NDC	SIZE	AWP
◆ GENERICS			
Insource	58441-7644-03	5 ml	$32.93

INJECTION: 8 MG/ML

BRAND/MANUFACTURER	NDC	SIZE	AWP
◇ BRAND			
DECADRON-LA: Merck	00006-7644-01	1 ml	$11.35
	00006-7644-03	5 ml	$45.70
◇ GENERICS			
SOLUREX LA: Hyrex	00314-0897-75	5 ml	$16.50
URL	00677-0822-20	5 ml	$18.00
Major	00904-0906-05	5 ml	$22.50
Goldline	00182-0928-62	5 ml	$24.45
Rugby	00536-4163-65	5 ml	$27.88
Schein	00364-6699-53	5 ml	$29.93
Steris	00402-0092-05	5 ml	$29.93
DECAJECT-L.A.: Mayrand	00259-0328-05	5 ml	$32.00
King Pharm	60793-0108-05	5 ml	$32.93
Genl Inject	52584-0092-05	5 ml	$32.93

INJECTION: 8 MG/5 ML

BRAND/MANUFACTURER	NDC	SIZE	AWP
◆ GENERICS			
Geneva	00781-3008-75	5 ml	$25.71

DEXAMETHASONE SODIUM PHOSPHATE
INJECTION: 4 MG/ML

AVERAGE UNIT PRICE (AVAILABLE SIZES)		GENERIC A-RATED AVERAGE PRICE (GAAP)	
BRAND	$5.44	5 ml	$3.66
GENERIC	$0.63	10 ml	$6.92
		30 ml	$9.37
		1 ml 25s	$25.83
		5 ml 25s	$70.25

BRAND/MANUFACTURER	NDC	SIZE	AWP
◆ BRAND			
DECADRON PHOSPHATE: Merck	00006-7628-03	5 ml	$28.55
	00006-7628-25	25 ml	$110.80
	00006-7628-66	1 ml 25s	$154.71
◆ GENERICS			
Fujisawa	00469-1650-00	1 ml	$1.04
Elkins-Sinn	00641-2273-41	5 ml	$1.38
Moore,H.L.	00839-5160-25	5 ml	$1.74
Steris	00402-0807-05	5 ml	$2.47
Fujisawa	00469-1650-25	5 ml	$2.66
SOLUREX: Hyrex	00314-0896-75	5 ml	$3.20
Insource	58441-1126-05	5 ml	$3.20
URL	00677-0385-20	5 ml	$3.50
HEXADROL PHOSPHATE: Organon	00052-0796-05	5 ml	$4.70
Rugby	00536-4151-65	5 ml	$6.00
DECAJECT: Mayrand	00259-0297-05	5 ml	$7.70
Schein	00364-6681-54	10 ml	$3.38
Steris	00402-0807-10	10 ml	$3.38
SOLUREX: Hyrex	00314-0896-70	10 ml	$4.95
DEXACEN-4: Central	00131-1230-05	10 ml	$9.50
DECAJECT: Mayrand	00259-0297-10	10 ml	$13.40
Moore,H.L.	00839-5160-30	30 ml	$5.39
Schein	00364-6681-56	30 ml	$6.00
Steris	00402-0807-30	30 ml	$6.00
Insource	58441-1103-03	30 ml	$6.43
SOLUREX: Hyrex	00314-0896-30	30 ml	$11.50
Rugby	00536-4151-75	30 ml	$13.62
Elkins-Sinn	00641-2276-41	30 ml	$16.66
Fujisawa	00469-1650-30	30 ml	$15.96
Elkins-Sinn	00641-0372-25	1 ml 25s	$11.19
Amer Regent	00517-4901-25	1 ml 25s	$27.19
HEXADROL PHOSPHATE: Organon	00052-0796-26	1 ml 25s	$39.10

BRAND/MANUFACTURER	NDC	SIZE	AWP
Amer Regent	00517-4905-25	5 ml 25s	$54.69
Schein	00364-6681-32	5 ml 25s	$61.65
HEXADROL PHOSPHATE: Organon	00052-0796-27	5 ml 25s	94.40
Amer Regent	00517-4930-25	30 ml 25s	$195.94

INJECTION: 4 MG/ML

BRAND/MANUFACTURER	NDC	SIZE	AWP
◇ GENERICS			
Major	00904-0905-05	5 ml	$3.60
Major	00904-0905-10	10 ml	$5.80
Major	00904-0905-30	30 ml	$9.24

INJECTION: 4 MG

AVERAGE UNIT PRICE (AVAILABLE SIZES)	
GENERIC	$0.42

BRAND/MANUFACTURER	NDC	SIZE	AWP
◆ GENERICS			
Goldline	00182-3007-62	5 ml	$2.70
Goldline	00182-3007-66	30 ml	$9.00

INJECTION: 10 MG/ML

AVERAGE UNIT PRICE (AVAILABLE SIZES)		GENERIC A-RATED AVERAGE PRICE (GAAP)	
GENERIC	$1.47	10 ml	$12.22
		1 ml 25s	$60.73

BRAND/MANUFACTURER	NDC	SIZE	AWP
◆ GENERICS			
Schein	00364-2360-54	10 ml	$4.13
Steris	00402-0661-10	10 ml	$4.13
Elkins-Sinn	00641-2277-41	10 ml	$15.38
HEXADROL PHOSPHATE: Organon	00052-0797-10	10 ml	$25.25
Gensia	00703-3524-01	10 ml	$5.20
Elkins-Sinn	00641-0367-25	1 ml 25s	$58.21
HEXADROL PHOSPHATE: Organon	00052-0797-26	1 ml 25s	$63.25

INJECTION: 24 MG/ML

AVERAGE UNIT PRICE (AVAILABLE SIZES)	
BRAND	$21.78

BRAND/MANUFACTURER	NDC	SIZE	AWP
◆ BRAND			
DECADRON PHOSPHATE: Merck	00006-7646-03	5 ml	$110.00
	00006-7646-10	10 ml	$215.50

Dexamethasone, Ophthalmic

DESCRIPTION
Dexamethasone, Ophthalmic is an adrenocortical steroid prepared as a sterile topical ophthalmic suspension, ointment, and solution.

Established names:
Dexamethasone
Dexamethasone Sodium Phosphate

Chemical names:
Pregna-1,4-diene-3,20-dione, 9-fluoro-11,17,21-trihydroxy-16-methyl-, (11β,16α)-.

Pregn-4-ene-3,20-dione, 9-fluoro-11,17-dihydroxy-16-methyl-21- (phosphono-oxy)-, disodium salt, (11β,16α)-.

Each gram of ointment contains: Dexamethasone sodium phosphate equivalent to Dexamethasone phosphate 0.5mg (0.05%).

Each mL of suspension contains: Dexamethasone 0.1%.

Each mL of solution contains: Dexamethasone sodium phosphate equivalent to 1 mg (0.1%) Dexamethasone phosphate.

Dexamethasone is a synthetic analog of naturally occurring glucocorticoids (hydrocortisone and cortisone). Dexamethasone sodium phosphate is a water soluble, inorganic ester of Dexamethasone. It is approximately three thousand times more soluble in water at 25°C than hydrocortisone.

Following is its chemical structure:

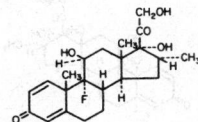

CLINICAL PHARMACOLOGY
Dexamethasone and Dexamethasone sodium phosphate suppress the inflammatory response to a variety of agents and it probably delays or slows healing. No generally accepted explanation of these steroid properties has been advanced.

INDICATIONS AND USAGE
Steroid responsive inflammatory conditions of the palpebral and bulbar conjunctiva, cornea, and anterior segment of the globe such as allergic conjunctivitis, acne rosacea, superficial punctate keratitis, herpes zoster keratitis, iritis, cyclitis, selected infective conjunctivitides when the inherent hazard of steroid use is accepted to obtain an advisable diminution in edema and inflammation; corneal injury from chemical, radiation or thermal burns, or penetration of foreign bodies.

Dexamethasone sodium phosphate solution is also indicated in steroid responsive inflammatory conditions of the external auditory meatus, such as allergic otitis externa, selected purulent and nonpurulent infective otitis externa when the hazard of steroid use is accepted to obtain an advisable diminution in edema and inflammation.

CONTRAINDICATIONS
Contraindicated in epithelial herpes simplex keratitis (dendritic keratitis), acute infections stages of vaccinia, varicella, and most other viral diseases of the cornea and conjunctiva; tuberculosis of the eye; fungal disease of ocular or auricular (solution) structures; mycobacterial infection of the eye; perforation of a drum membrane (solution); and in those persons who have shown hypersensitivity to any component of this preparation. Steroids should not be used after uncomplicated removal of a corneal foreign body.

WARNINGS
Prolonged use may result in ocular hypertension and/or glaucoma, with damage to the optic nerve, defects in visual acuity and fields of vision, and posterior subcapsular cataract formation. Prolonged use may suppress the host response and thus increase the hazard of secondary ocular infections. In those diseases causing thinning of the cornea or sclera, perforations have been known to occur with the use of topical corticosteroids. In acute purulent conditions of the eye or ear, corticosteroids may mask infection or enhance existing infection. If these products are used for 10 days or longer, intraocular pressure should be routinely monitored even though it may be difficult in children and uncooperative patients. Employment of corticosteroid medication in the treatment of herpes simplex other than epithelial herpes simplex keratitis, in which it is contraindicated, requires great caution; periodic slit-lamp microscopy is essential.

Some brands and/or formulations contain sodium bisulfite, a sulfite that may cause allergic-type reactions including anaphylactic symptoms and life-threatening or less severe asthmatic episodes in certain susceptible people. The overall prevalence of sulfite sensitivity in the general population is unknown and probably low. Sulfite sensitivity is seen more frequently in asthmatic than in nonasthmatic people.

PRECAUTIONS
General: The possibility of persistent fungal infections of the cornea should be considered after prolonged corticosteroid dosing.

The possibility of persistent fungal infections of the cornea should be considered after prolonged corticosteroid dosing. There have been reports of bacterial keratitis associated with the use of multiple dose containers of topical ophthalmic products. These containers had been inadvertently contaminated by patients who, in most cases, had a concurrent corneal disease or a disruption of the ocular epithelial surface. (See "Precautions, Information for Patients".)

Information for Patients: Do not touch the tip of the dispensing container including the eye or surrounding structures to any surface, as this may contaminate the contents.

Patients should also be instructed that ocular preparations, if handled improperly, can become contaminated by common bacteria known to cause ocular infections. Serious damage to the eye and subsequent loss of vision may result from using contaminated preparations. (See "Precautions, General".) Patients should also be advised that if they develop an intercurrent ocular condition condition (e.g., trauma, ocular surgery or infection), they should immediately seek their physician's advice concerning the continued use of the present multidose container.

A preservative contained in some brands, benzalkonium chloride, may be absorbed by soft contact lenses. Patients wearing soft contact lenses should be instructed to wait at least 15 minutes after instilling Dexamethasone, Ophthalmic before they insert their lenses.

Carcinogenesis, Mutagenesis, Impairment of Fertility: Long-term animal studies have not been performed to evaluate the carcinogenic potential or the effect on fertility of Dexamethasone, Ophthalmic.

Pregnancy: Pregnancy Category C. Dexamethasone has been shown to be teratogenic in mice and rabbits following topical ophthalmic application in multiples of the therapeutic dose.

In the mouse, corticosteroids produce fetal resorptions and a specific abnormality, cleft palate. In the rabbit, corticosteroids have produced fetal resorptions and multiple abnormalities involving the head, ears, limbs, palate, etc.

There are no adequate or well controlled studies in pregnant women. Dexamethasone, Ophthalmic should be used during pregnancy only if the potential benefit to the mother justifies the potential risk to the embryo or fetus. Infants born to mothers who have received substantial doses of corticosteroids during pregnancy should be observed carefully for signs of hypoadrenalism.

➤ SHOWN IN PRODUCT IDENTIFICATION GUIDE

Nursing Mothers: Topically applied steroids are absorbed systemically. Therefore, because of the potential for serious adverse reactions in nursing infants from Dexamethasone and Dexamethasone sodium phosphate a decision should be made whether to discontinue nursing or discontinue the drug, taking into account the importance of the drug to the mother.

Pediatric Use: Safety and effectiveness in children have not been established.

ADVERSE REACTIONS

Glaucoma with optic nerve damage, visual acuity and field defects; posterior subcapsular cataract formation; secondary ocular infection following suppression of host response from pathogens including herpes simplex; and perforation of the globe may occur.

Rarely, filtering blebs have been reported when topical steroids have been used following cataract surgery.

Rarely, stinging or burning may occur.

DOSAGE AND ADMINISTRATION

SUSPENSION

Shake well before using. One or two drops topically in the conjunctival sac(s). In severe disease, drops may be used hourly, being tapered to discontinuation as the inflammation subsides. In mild disease, drops may be used up to four to six times daily.

OINTMENT

The duration of treatment will vary with the type of lesion and may extend from a few days to several weeks, according to therapeutic response. Relapses, more common in chronic active lesions than in self-limited conditions, usually respond to treatment.

Apply a one-half to one inch ribbon of ointment into the conjunctival sac(s) up to four times daily. When a favorable response is observed, dosage may be reduced gradually to once a day application for several days. Dexamethasone Ophthalmic Ointment may be used in conjunction with Dexamethasone Ophthalmic Suspension.

Dexamethasone sodium phosphate ointment is particularly convenient when an eye pad is used. It may also be the preparation of choice for patients in whom therapeutic benefit depends on prolonged contact of the active ingredients with ocular tissues.

How To Apply Dexamethasone Ophthalmic Ointment:
1. Tilt your head back.
2. Place a finger on your cheek just under your eye and gently pull down until a 'V' pocket is formed between your eyeball and your lower lid.
3. Place a small amount (about ½ inch) of Dexamethasone Ophthalmic in the 'V' pocket. Do not let the tip of the tube touch your eye.
4. Look downward before closing your eye.

SOLUTION

The duration of treatment will vary with the type of lesion and may extend from a few days to several weeks, according to therapeutic response. Relapses, more common in chronic active lesions than in self-limited conditions, usually respond to retreatment.

Eye: Instill one or two drops of solution into the conjunctival sac every hour during the day and every two hours during the night as initial therapy. When a favorable response is observed, reduce dosage to one drop every four hours. Later, further reduction in dosage to one drop three or four times daily may suffice to control symptoms.

Ear: Clean the aural canal thoroughly and sponge dry. Instill the solution directly into the aural canal. A suggested initial dosage is three or four drops two or three times a day. When a favorable response is obtained, reduce dosage gradually and eventually discontinue.

If preferred, the aural canal may be packed with a gauze wick saturated with solution. Keep the wick moist with the preparation and remove from the ear after 12 to 24 hours. Treatment may be repeated as often as necessary at the discretion of the physician.

STORAGE

Store at 8°-27°C (46°-80°F). Keep suspension upright.

HOW SUPPLIED

DEXAMETHASONE
DROP: 0.1%

AVERAGE UNIT PRICE (AVAILABLE SIZES)

BRAND	$2.75

BRAND/MANUFACTURER	NDC	SIZE	AWP
◆ **BRAND**			
MAXIDEX: Alcon Ophthalmic	00998-0615-05	5 ml	$17.50
	00998-0615-15	15 ml	$30.00
◆ **GENERICS**			
DEXAIR: Qualitest	00603-7105-37	5 ml	$2.88

OINTMENT: 0.05%

AVERAGE UNIT PRICE (AVAILABLE SIZES)

GENERIC	$0.98

BRAND/MANUFACTURER	NDC	SIZE	AWP
◆ **GENERICS**			
DEXAIR: Qualitest	00603-7104-70	3.75 gm	$3.60
Goldline	00182-5071-31	3.75 gm	$3.75

DEXAMETHASONE SODIUM PHOSPHATE
DROP: 0.1%

AVERAGE UNIT PRICE (AVAILABLE SIZES)		*GENERIC A-RATED AVERAGE PRICE (GAAP)*	
BRAND	$3.02	5 ml	$3.43
GENERIC	$0.69		

BRAND/MANUFACTURER	NDC	SIZE	AWP
◆ **BRAND**			
DECADRON PHOSPHATE OCUMETER: Merck	00006-7643-03	5 ml	$15.09
◆ **GENERICS**			
Moore,H.L.	00839-6663-25	5 ml	$2.42
Rugby	00536-0800-65	5 ml	$2.56
URL	00677-0898-20	5 ml	$2.90
Bausch&Lomb Pharm	24208-0720-02	5 ml	$3.01
Schein	00364-7237-53	5 ml	$3.10
Steris	00402-0748-05	5 ml	$3.10
Aligen	00405-6050-05	5 ml	$3.53
Major	00904-3006-05	5 ml	$3.75
DEXASOL: Ocusoft	54799-0525-05	5 ml	$4.95
AK-DEX: Akorn	17478-0279-10	5 ml	$5.00

OINTMENT: 0.05%

AVERAGE UNIT PRICE (AVAILABLE SIZES)		*GENERIC A-RATED AVERAGE PRICE (GAAP)*	
BRAND	$1.76	3.5 gm	$3.58
GENERIC	$1.04		
HCFA FUL (3.5 gm)	$0.71		

BRAND/MANUFACTURER	NDC	SIZE	AWP
◆ **BRAND**			
DECADRON PHOSPHATE: Merck	00006-7615-04	3.5 gm	$6.15
◆ **GENERICS**			
Moore,H.L.	00839-6680-43	3.5 gm	$2.96
Bausch&Lomb Pharm	24208-0640-55	3.5 gm	$3.06
Aligen	00405-0935-08	3.5 gm	$3.12
Major	00904-3008-38	3.5 gm	$4.00
AK-DEX: Akorn	17478-0278-35	3.5 gm	$4.06
Schein	00364-2551-70	3.5 gm	$4.29
Rugby	00536-6475-91	3.75 gm 12s	$51.48

OINTMENT: 0.5%

BRAND/MANUFACTURER	NDC	SIZE	AWP
◆ **GENERICS**			
DEXASOL: Ocusoft	54799-0526-35	3.5 gm	$4.95

Dexamethasone, Oral

DESCRIPTION

Glucocorticoids are adrenocortical steroids, both naturally occurring and synthetic, which are readily absorbed from the gastrointestinal tract.

Dexamethasone, a synthetic adrenocortical steroid, is a white to practically white, odorless, crystalline powder. It is stable in air. It is practically insoluble in water. The molecular weight is 392.47. It is designated chemically as 9-fluoro-11β, 17, 21-trihydroxy-16α-methylpregna-1, 4-diene-3,20-dione. The empirical formula is $C_{22}H_{29}FO_5$.

Dexamethasone, Oral, is available as tablets and elixir.

Each tablet contains:
Dexamethasone ....0.25 mg, 0.5 mg, 0.75 mg, 1.5 mg, 4 mg, or 6 mg
Each 5 mL of elixir contains:
Dexamethasone ....0.5 mg

Following is its chemical structure:

ACTIONS

Naturally occurring glucocorticoids (hydrocortisone and cortisone), which also have salt-retaining properties, are used as replacement therapy in adrenocortical deficiency states. Their synthetic analogs including Dexamethasone are primarily used for their potent anti-inflammatory effects in disorders of many organ systems.

Glucocorticoids cause profound and varied metabolic effects. In addition, they modify the body's immune responses to diverse stimuli.

At equipotent anti-inflammatory doses, Dexamethasone almost completely lacks the sodium-retaining property of hydrocortisone and closely related derivatives of hydrocortisone.

INDICATIONS

1. *Endocrine Disorders:* Primary or secondary adrenocortical insufficiency (hydrocortisone or cortisone is the first choice; synthetic analogs may be used in conjunction with mineralocorticoids where applicable; in infancy mineralocorticoid supplementation is of particular importance)
   Congenital adrenal hyperplasia
   Nonsuppurative thyroiditis
   Hypercalcemia associated with cancer

2. *Rheumatic Disorders:* As adjunctive therapy for short-term administration (to tide the patient over an acute episode or exacerbation) in:
   Psoriatic arthritis
   Rheumatoid arthritis, including juvenile rheumatoid arthritis (selected cases may require low-dose maintenance therapy).
   Ankylosing spondylitis
   Acute and subacute bursitis
   Acute nonspecific tenosynovitis
   Acute gouty arthritis
   Post-traumatic osteoarthritis
   Synovitis of osteoarthritis
   Epicondylitis

3. *Collagen Diseases:* During an exacerbation or as maintenance therapy in selected cases of—
   Systemic lupus erythematosus
   Acute rheumatic carditis

4. *Dermatologic Diseases:*
   Pemphigus
   Bullous dermatitis herpetiformis
   Severe erythema multiforme (Stevens-Johnson syndrome)
   Exfoliative dermatitis
   Mycosis fungoides
   Severe psoriasis
   Severe seborrheic dermatitis

5. *Allergic States:* Control of severe or incapacitating allergic conditions intractable to adequate trials of conventional treatment:
   Seasonal or perennial allergic rhinitis
   Bronchial asthma
   Contact dermatitis
   Atopic dermatitis
   Serum sickness
   Drug hypersensitivity reactions

6. *Ophthalmic Diseases:* Severe acute and chronic allergic and inflammatory processes involving the eye and its adnexa, such as—
   Allergic conjunctivitis
   Keratitis
   Allergic corneal marginal ulcers
   Herpes zoster ophthalmicus
   Iritis and iridocyclitis
   Chorioretinitis
   Anterior segment inflammation
   Diffuse posterior uveitis and choroiditis
   Optic neuritis
   Sympathetic ophthalmia

7. *Respiratory Diseases:*
   Symptomatic sarcoidosis
   Loeffler's syndrome not manageable by other means
   Berylliosis
   Fulminating or disseminated pulmonary tuberculosis when used concurrently with appropriate antituberculous chemotherapy
   Aspiration pneumonitis

8. *Hematologic Disorders:*
   Idiopathic thrombocytopenic purpura in adults
   Secondary thrombocytopenia in adults
   Acquired (autoimmune) hemolytic anemia
   Erythroblastopenia (RBC anemia)
   Congenital (erythroid) hypoplastic anemia

9. *Neoplastic Diseases:* For palliative management of:
   Leukemias and lymphomas in adults
   Acute leukemia of childhood

10. *Edematous States:* To induce a diuresis or remission of proteinuria in the nephrotic syndrome, without uremia, of the idiopathic type or that due to lupus erythematosus

11. *Gastrointestinal Diseases:* To tide the patient over a critical period of the disease in:
    Ulcerative colitis
    Regional enteritis

12. *Cerebral Edema:* associated with primary or metastatic brain tumor, craniotomy, or head injury (tablets only). Use in cerebral edema is not a substitute for careful neurosurgical evaluation and definitive management such as neurosurgery or other specific therapy.

13. *Miscellaneous:* Tuberculous meningitis with subarachnoid block or impending block when used concurrently with appropriate antituberculous chemotherapy
    Trichinosis with neurologic or myocardial involvement

14. *Diagnostic testing of adrenocortical hyperfunction.*

UNLABELED USES

Dexamethasone is used alone or as an adjunct in the treatment of cystic acne, congenital adrenal hyperplasia, and bronchopulmonary dysplasia. It is prescribed to control symptoms of acute laryngotracheitis (croup), and is used in the treatment of depression, insulin lipodystrophy, acute mountain sickness, oligomenorrhea, and, adjunctively, in pemphigus vulgaris and pemphigus foliaceous. Dexamethasone is also used in the diagnosis of affective disorders (Dexamethasone suppression test), and in Peyronie's disease, respiratory distress syndrome, chemotherapy-induced vomiting, and temporal arteritis.

CONTRAINDICATIONS

Systemic fungal infections
   Hypersensitivity to this drug

WARNINGS

In patients on corticosteroid therapy subjected to unusual stress, increased dosage of rapidly acting corticosteroids before, during, and after the stressful situation is indicated.

Drug-induced secondary adrenocortical insufficiency may result from too rapid withdrawal of corticosteroids and may be minimized by gradual reduction of dosage. This type of relative insufficiency may persist for months after discontinuation of therapy; therefore, in any situation of stress occurring during that period, hormone therapy should be reinstituted. If the patient is receiving steroids already, dosage may have to be increased. Since mineralocorticoid secretion may be impaired, salt and/or a mineralocorticoid should be administered concurrently.

Corticosteroids may mask some signs of infection, and new infections may appear during their use. There may be decreased resistance and inability to localize infection when corticosteroids are used. Moreover, corticosteroids may affect the nitroblue-tetrazolium test for bacterial infection and produce false negative results.

In cerebral malaria, a double-blind trial has shown that the use of corticosteroids is associated with prolongation of coma and a higher incidence of pneumonia and gastrointestinal bleeding.

Corticosteroids may activate latent amebiasis. Therefore, it is recommended that latent or active amebiasis be ruled out before initiating corticosteroid therapy in any patient who has spent time in the tropics or any patient with unexplained diarrhea.

Prolonged use of corticosteroids may produce posterior subcapsular cataracts, glaucoma with possible damage to the optic nerves, and may enhance the establishment of secondary ocular infections due to fungi or viruses.

Usage in Pregnancy: Since adequate human reproduction studies have not been done with corticosteroids, use of these drugs in pregnancy or in women of childbearing potential requires that the anticipated benefits be weighed against the possible hazards to the mother and embryo or fetus. Infants born of mothers who have received substantial doses of corticosteroids during pregnancy should be carefully observed for signs of hypoadrenalism.

Corticosteroids appear in breast milk and could suppress growth, interfere with endogenous corticosteroid production, or cause other unwanted effects. Mothers taking pharmacologic doses of corticosteroids should be advised not to nurse. Average and large doses of hydrocortisone or cortisone can cause elevation of blood pressure, salt and water retention, and increased excretion of potassium. These effects are less likely to occur with the synthetic derivatives except when used in large doses. Dietary salt restriction and potassium supplementation may be necessary. All corticosteroids increase calcium excretion.

Administration of live virus vaccines, including smallpox, is contraindicated in individuals receiving immunosuppressive doses of corticosteroids. If inactivated viral or bacterial vaccines are administered to individuals receiving immunosuppressive doses of corticosteroids, the expected serum antibody response may not be obtained. However, immunization procedures may be undertaken in patients who are receiving corticosteroids as replacement therapy, e.g., for Addison's disease.

Patients who are on drugs which suppress the immune system are more susceptible to infections than healthy individuals. Chickenpox and measles, for example, can have a more serious or even fatal course in non-immune children or adults on corticosteroids. In such children or adults who have not had these diseases, particular care should be taken to avoid exposure. The risk of developing a disseminated infection varies among individuals and can be related to the dose, route and duration of corticosteroid administration as well as to the underlying disease. If exposed to chickenpox, prophylaxis with varicella zoster immune globulin (VZIG) may be indicated. If chickenpox develops, treatment with antiviral agents may be considered. If exposed to measles, prophylaxis with immune globulin (IG) may be indicated. (See the respective package inserts for VZIG and IG for complete prescribing information.)

The use of Dexamethasone, Oral, in active tuberculosis should be restricted to those cases of fulminating or disseminated tuberculosis in which the corticosteroid is used for the management of the disease in conjunction with an appropriate antituberculous regimen.

If corticosteroids are indicated in patients with latent tuberculosis or tuberculin reactivity, close observation is necessary as reactivation of the disease may occur. During prolonged corticosteroid therapy, these patients should receive chemoprophylaxis.

Literature reports suggest an apparent association between use of corticosteroids and left ventricular free wall rupture after a recent myocardial infarction; therefore, therapy with corticosteroids should be used with great caution in these patients.

PRECAUTIONS

Following prolonged therapy, withdrawal of corticosteroids may result in symptoms of the corticosteroid withdrawal syndrome including fever, myalgia, arthralgia, and malaise. This may occur in patients even without evidence of adrenal insufficiency.

There is an enhanced effect of corticosteroids in patients with hypothyroidism and in those with cirrhosis.

Corticosteroids should be used cautiously in patients with ocular herpes simplex because of possible corneal perforation.

The lowest possible dose of corticosteroid should be used to control the condition under treatment, and when reduction in dosage is possible, the reduction should be gradual.

Psychic derangements may appear when corticosteroids are used, ranging from euphoria, insomnia, mood swings, personality changes, and severe depression, to frank psychotic manifestations. Also, existing emotional instability or psychotic tendencies may be aggravated by corticosteroids.

Aspirin should be used cautiously in conjunction with corticosteroids in hypoprothrombinemia.

Steroids should be used with caution in nonspecific ulcerative colitis, if there is a probability of impending perforation, abscess, or other pyogenic infection, diverticulitis, fresh intestinal anastomoses, active or latent peptic ulcer, renal insufficiency, hypertension, osteoporosis, and myasthenia gravis. Signs of peritoneal irritation following gastrointestinal perforation in patients receiving large doses of corticosteroids may be minimal or absent. Fat embolism has been reported as a possible complication of hypercortisonism.

When large doses are given, some authorities advise that corticosteroids be taken with meals and antacids taken between meals to help to prevent peptic ulcer.

Growth and development of infants and children on prolonged corticosteroid therapy should be carefully observed. Steroids may increase or decrease motility and number of spermatozoa in some patients.

Phenytoin, phenobarbital, ephedrine, and rifampin may enhance the metabolic clearance of corticosteroids, resulting in decreased blood levels and lessened physiologic activity, thus requiring adjustment in corticosteriod dosage. These interactions may interfere with Dexamethasone suppression tests which should be interpreted with caution during administration of these drugs.

False-negative results in the Dexamethasone suppression test (DST) in patients being treated with indomethacin have been reported. Thus, results of the DST should be interpreted with caution in these patients.

The prothrombin time should be checked frequently in patients who are receiving corticosteroids and coumarin anticoagulants at the same time because of reports that corticosteroids have altered the response to these anticoagulants. Studies have shown that the usual effect produced by adding corticosteroids is inhibition of response to coumarins, although there have been some conflicting reports of potentiation not substantiated by studies.

When corticosteroids are administered concomitantly with potassium-depleting diuretics, patients should be observed closely for development of hypokalemia.

Information for Patients: Susceptible patients who are on immunosuppressant doses of corticosteroids should be warned to avoid exposure to chickenpox or measles. Patients should also be advised that if they are exposed, medical advice should be sought without delay.

ADVERSE REACTIONS

Fluid and Electrolyte Disturbances:
Sodium retention
Fluid retention
Congestive heart failure in susceptible patients
Potassium loss
Hypokalemic alkalosis
Hypertension

Musculoskeletal:
Muscle weakness
Steroid myopathy
Loss of muscle mass
Osteoporosis
Vertebral compression fractures
Aseptic necrosis of femoral and humeral heads
Pathologic fracture of long bones
Tendon rupture

Gastrointestinal:
Peptic ulcer with possible perforation and hemorrhage
Perforation of the small and large bowel, particularly in patients with inflammatory bowel disease
Pancreatitis
Abdominal distention
Ulcerative esophagitis

Dermatologic:
Impaired wound healing
Thin fragile skin
Petechiae and ecchymoses
Erythema
Increased sweating
May suppress reactions to skin tests
Other cutaneous reactions, such as allergic dermatitis, urticaria, angioneurotic edema.

Neurologic:
Convulsions
Increased intracranial pressure with papilledema (pseudo-tumor cerebri) usually after treatment
Vertigo
Headache
Psychic disturbances

Endocrine:
Menstrual irregularities
Development of cushingoid state
Suppression of growth in children
Secondary adrenocortical and pituitary unresponsiveness, particularly in times of stress, as in trauma, surgery, or illness
Decreased carbohydrate tolerance
Manifestations of latent diabetes mellitus
Increased requirements for insulin or oral hypoglycemic agents in diabetics
Hirsutism

Ophthalmic:
Posterior subcapsular cataracts
Increased intraocular pressure
Glaucoma
Exophthalmos

Metabolic: Negative nitrogen balance due to protein catabolism

Cardiovascular: Myocardial rupture following recent myocardial infarction (see "Warnings")

Other:
Hypersensitivity
Thromboembolism
Weight gain
Increased appetite
Nausea
Malaise
Hiccups

OVERDOSAGE

Reports of acute toxicity and/or death following overdosage of glucocorticoids are rare. In the event of overdosage, no specific antidote is available; treatment is supportive and symptomatic.

The oral LD_{50} of Dexamethasone in female mice was 6.5 g/kg.

DOSAGE AND ADMINISTRATION

FOR ORAL ADMINISTRATION

Dosage Requirements are Variable and Must be Individualized on the Basis of the Disease and the Response of the Patient: The initial dosage varies from 0.75 to 9 mg a day depending on the disease being treated. In less severe diseases doses lower than 0.75 mg may suffice, while in severe diseases doses higher than 9 mg may be required. The initial dosage should be maintained or adjusted until the patient's response is satisfactory. If satisfactory clinical response does not occur after a reasonable period of time, discontinue Dexamethasone, Oral and transfer the patient to other therapy. After a favorable initial response, the proper maintenance dosage should be determined by decreasing the initial dosage in small amounts to the lowest dosage that maintains an adequate clinical response.

Patients should be observed closely for signs that might require dosage adjustment, including changes in clinical status resulting from remissions or exacerbations of the disease, individual drug responsiveness, and the effect of stress (e.g., surgery, infection, trauma). During stress it may be necessary to increase dosage temporarily.

If the drug is to be stopped after more than a few days of treatment, it usually should be withdrawn gradually.

The following milligram equivalents facilitate changing to Dexamethasone, Oral from other glucocorticoids:

DEXAMETHASONE, ORAL

	Methylprednisolone and Triamcinolone		Hydrocortisone Prednisolone and Prednisone	Cortisone
0.75 mg =	4 mg =	5 mg =	20 mg =	25 mg

In *acute, self-limited allergic disorders or acute exacerbations of chronic allergic disorders*, the following dosage schedule combining parenteral and oral therapy is suggested:

Dexamethasone Sodium Phosphate injection, 4 mg per mL:

First Day: 1 or 2 mL, intramuscularly
Dexamethasone, Oral, tablets, 0.75 mg:

Second Day: 4 tablets in two divided doses

Third Day: 4 tablets in two divided doses

Fourth Day: 2 tablets in two divided doses

Fifth Day: 1 tablet

Sixth Day: 1 tablet

Seventh Day: No treatment

Eighth Day: Follow-up visit

This schedule is designed to ensure adequate therapy during acute episodes, while minimizing the risk of overdosage in chronic cases.

In *cerebral edema*, Dexamethasone Sodium Phosphate injection is generally administered initially in a dosage of 10 mg intravenously followed by 4 mg every six hours intramuscularly until the symptoms of cerebral edema subside. Response is usually noted within 12 to 24 hours and dosage may be reduced after two to four days and gradually discontinued over a period of five to seven days. For palliative management of patients with recurrent or inoperable brain tumors, maintenance therapy with either Dexamethasone Sodium Phosphate injection or Dexamethasone, Oral tablets in a dosage of two mg two or three times daily may be effective.

DEXAMETHASONE SUPPRESSION TESTS
1. Tests for Cushing's syndrome
   Give 1.0 mg of Dexamethasone, Oral, orally at 11:00 p.m. Blood is drawn for plasma cortisol determination at 8:00 a.m. the following morning.
   For greater accuracy, give 0.5 mg of Dexamethasone, Oral, orally every 6 hours for 48 hours. Twenty-four hour urine collections are made for determination of 17-hydroxycorticosteroid excretion.
2. Test to distinguish Cushing's syndrome due to pituitary ACTH excess from Cushing's syndrome due to other causes
   Give 2.0 mg of Dexamethasone, Oral, orally every 6 hours for 48 hours. Twenty-four hour urine collections are made for determination of 17-hydroxycorticosteroid excretion.

STORAGE
Keep container tightly closed.

HOW SUPPLIED
ELIXIR:

AVERAGE UNIT PRICE (AVAILABLE SIZES)		GENERIC A-RATED AVERAGE PRICE (GAAP)	
GENERIC	$0.05	240 ml	$10.75

BRAND/MANUFACTURER	NDC	SIZE	AWP
◆ GENERICS			
Pennex	00832-8466-08	240 ml	$10.00
Pennex	00426-8466-08	240 ml	$11.50

ELIXIR: 0.5 MG/5 ML

AVERAGE UNIT PRICE (AVAILABLE SIZES)		GENERIC A-RATED AVERAGE PRICE (GAAP)	
BRAND	$0.12	100 ml	$8.64
GENERIC	$0.07	240 ml	$14.41
HCFA FUL (100 ml)	$0.08		

BRAND/MANUFACTURER	NDC	SIZE	AWP
◆ BRAND			
DECADRON: Merck	00006-7622-55	100 ml	$16.44
HEXADROL: Organon	00052-0793-04	120 ml	$7.05
DECADRON: Merck	00006-7622-66	237 ml	$30.65
◆ GENERICS			
Schein	00364-7182-61	100 ml	$6.50
Pennex	00832-8466-00	100 ml	$7.26
Major	00904-0972-04	100 ml	$7.45
Pennex	00426-8466-00	100 ml	$8.00
Barre	00472-0972-33	100 ml	$14.00
Qualitest	00603-1145-56	240 ml	$11.70
Goldline	00182-1013-44	240 ml	$12.45
Moore,H.L.	00839-6044-66	240 ml	$12.49
Rugby	00536-0452-59	240 ml	$12.67
URL	00677-0601-42	240 ml	$12.75
Geneva	00781-6400-08	240 ml	$12.75
Major	00904-0972-09	240 ml	$12.95

BRAND/MANUFACTURER	NDC	SIZE	AWP
Schein	00364-7182-76	240 ml	$15.00
Barre	00472-0972-08	240 ml	$26.95

TABLETS: 0.25 MG

BRAND/MANUFACTURER	NDC	SIZE	AWP
◆ BRAND			
➤ DECADRON: Merck	00006-0020-68	100s	$27.96

TABLETS: 0.25 MG

BRAND/MANUFACTURER	NDC	SIZE	AWP
◇ GENERICS			
Rugby	00536-3581-01	100s	$3.56
Par	49884-0083-01	100s	$4.10
Schein	00364-0397-01	100s	$4.20
Aligen	00405-4313-01	100s	$4.20
Moore,H.L.	00839-6019-06	100s	$4.25
Schein	00364-0397-02	1000s	$36.50
Par	49884-0083-10	1000s	$41.00

TABLETS: 0.5 MG

AVERAGE UNIT PRICE (AVAILABLE SIZES)		GENERIC A-RATED AVERAGE PRICE (GAAP)	
BRAND	$0.50	100s	$13.50
GENERIC	$0.13		

BRAND/MANUFACTURER	NDC	SIZE	AWP
◆ BRAND			
➤ DECADRON: Merck	00006-0041-68	100s	$50.26
◆ GENERICS			
Roxane	00054-4179-25	100s	$12.01
Roxane	00054-8179-25	100s ud	$14.99
Roxane	00054-4179-31	1000s	$117.87

TABLETS: 0.5 MG

BRAND/MANUFACTURER	NDC	SIZE	AWP
◇ GENERICS			
Rugby	00536-3582-01	100s	$4.56
Major	00904-0243-60	100s	$5.99
Goldline	00182-1612-01	100s	$6.40
Qualitest	00603-3190-21	100s	$6.45
Par	49884-0084-01	100s	$6.50
Schein	00364-0398-01	100s	$6.50
Aligen	00405-4314-01	100s	$6.72
Moore,H.L.	00839-6020-06	100s	$6.82
DEXONE 0.5: Solvay	00032-3205-01	100s	$7.14
Par	49884-0084-10	1000s	$65.00

TABLETS: 0.75 MG

AVERAGE UNIT PRICE (AVAILABLE SIZES)		GENERIC A-RATED AVERAGE PRICE (GAAP)	
BRAND	$0.64	100s	$15.92
GENERIC	$0.16		

BRAND/MANUFACTURER	NDC	SIZE	AWP
◆ BRAND			
➤ DECADRON: Merck	00006-0063-12	12s	$7.91
	00006-0063-68	100s	$62.84
◆ GENERICS			
Roxane	00054-4180-25	100s	$14.61
Roxane	00054-8180-25	100s ud	$17.22

TABLETS: 0.75 MG

BRAND/MANUFACTURER	NDC	SIZE	AWP
◇ GENERICS			
Moore,H.L.	00839-1228-03	12s	$3.04
Qualitest	00603-3191-11	12s	$3.50
Major	00904-0244-12	12s	$3.55
Horizon Pharm Inc	60904-0085-27	12s	$5.45
Goldline	00182-0488-01	100s	$5.95
Rugby	00536-3583-01	100s	$6.44
URL	00677-0340-01	100s	$6.60
Major	00904-0244-60	100s	$6.65
Par	49884-0085-01	100s	$7.50
Qualitest	00603-3191-21	100s	$7.55
Aligen	00405-4315-01	100s	$7.64
Martec	52555-0064-01	100s	$7.65
Schein	00364-0098-01	100s	$7.75
Moore,H.L.	00839-1228-06	100s	$7.90
DEXONE 0.75: Solvay	00032-3210-01	100s	$7.97
Par	49884-0085-05	500s	$37.50
Rugby	00536-3583-10	1000s	$46.19
Schein	00364-0098-02	1000s	$62.50
Par	49884-0085-10	1000s	$75.00

TABLES: 1.5 MG

AVERAGE UNIT PRICE (AVAILABLE SIZES)		GENERIC A-RATED AVERAGE PRICE (GAAP)	
BRAND	$1.13	100s	$28.11
GENERIC	$0.28		

BRAND/MANUFACTURER	NDC	SIZE	AWP
◆ BRAND			
▶ DECADRON: Merck	00006-0095-50	50s	$56.59
◆ GENERICS			
Roxane	00054-4182-25	100s	$27.14
Roxane	00054-8181-25	100s ud	$29.08

TABLES: 1.5 MG

BRAND/MANUFACTURER	NDC	SIZE	AWP
◇ GENERICS			
Goldline	00182-1613-19	50s	$9.40
Par	49884-0086-03	50s	$10.40
Rugby	00536-3584-01	100s	$8.25
Qualitest	00603-3192-21	100s	$13.50
DEXONE 1.5: Solvay	00032-3215-01	100s	$14.50
Schein	00364-0399-01	100s	$14.50
Major	00904-0245-60	100s	$15.90
Par	49884-0086-01	100s	$20.00
Par	49884-0086-05	500s	$100.00
Par	49884-0086-10	1000s	$197.00

TABLES: 4 MG

AVERAGE UNIT PRICE (AVAILABLE SIZES)		GENERIC A-RATED AVERAGE PRICE (GAAP)	
BRAND	$1.82	100s	$57.41
GENERIC	$0.57		

BRAND/MANUFACTURER	NDC	SIZE	AWP
◆ BRAND			
▶ DECADRON: Merck	00006-0097-50	50s	$90.94
	00006-0097-28	100s ud	$181.90
◆ GENERICS			
Roxane	00054-4184-25	100s	$58.41
Roxane	00054-8175-25	100s ud	$56.41

TABLES: 4 MG

BRAND/MANUFACTURER	NDC	SIZE	AWP
◇ BRAND			
HEXADROL: Organon	00052-0798-91	100s	$47.25
	00052-0798-90	100s	$50.80
◇ GENERICS			
Major	00904-0246-51	50s	$8.50
Rugby	00536-3580-06	50s	$11.81
Goldline	00182-1614-19	50s	$16.50
Par	49884-0087-03	50s	$19.00
Major	00904-0246-60	100s	$22.54
Qualitest	00603-3194-21	100s	$22.55
URL	00677-0849-01	100s	$24.45
Goldline	00182-1614-01	100s	$28.50
DEXONE 4: Solvay	00032-3220-01	100s	$30.60
Par	49884-0087-01	100s	$32.00
Martec	52555-0066-01	100s	$32.65
Moore,H.L.	00839-6734-06	100s	$34.09
Par	49884-0087-05	500s	$160.00
Par	49884-0087-10	1000s	$320.00

TABLES: 6 MG

BRAND/MANUFACTURER	NDC	SIZE	AWP
◇ BRAND			
▶ DECADRON: Merck	00006-0147-50	50s	$134.90
◇ GENERICS			
Par	49884-0129-03	50s	$31.00
Par	49884-0129-01	100s	$57.00
Roxane	00054-4186-25	100s	$98.88
Roxane	00054-8183-25	100s ud	$88.49

Dexamethasone, Topical

DESCRIPTION

Dexamethasone, Topical, is a topical steroid preparation available as a cream and an aerosol.

Each gram of cream contains: Dexamethasone Sodium Phosphate equivalent to 1 mg Dexamethasone Phosphate.

Each 25 grams of aerosol contain: Dexamethasone 10 mg. Each second of spray dispenses approximately 0.075 Dexamethasone.

The topical corticosteroids constitute a class of primarily synthetic steroids used as anti-inflammatory and antipruritic agents.

Dexamethasone sodium phosphate is 9-fluoro-11β,17-dihydroxy-16α-methyl-21-(phosphonooxy)pregna-1,4-diene-3,20-dione disodium salt. Its empirical formula is $C_{22}H_{28}FNa_2O_8P$. Dexamethasone is 9-fluoro-11β,17,21-trihydroxy-16α-methylpregna-1, 4-diene-3, 20 dione. Its empirical formula is $C_{22}H_{29}FO_5$. Dexamethasone Sodium Phosphate has a molecular weight of 516.41; Dexamethasone, 392.47.

Following is its chemical structure:

CLINICAL PHARMACOLOGY

Topical corticosteroids share anti-inflammatory, anti-pruritic and vasoconstrictive actions.

The mechanism of anti-inflammatory activity of the topical corticosteroids is unclear. Various laboratory methods, including vasoconstrictor assays, are used to compare and predict potencies and/or clinical efficacies of the topical corticosteroids. There is some evidence to suggest that a recognizable correlation exists between vasoconstrictor potency and therapeutic efficacy in man.

PHARMACOKINETICS

The extent of percutaneous absorption of topical corticosteroids is determined by many factors including the vehicle, the integrity of the epidermal barrier, and the use of occlusive dressings.

Topical corticosteroids can be absorbed from normal intact skin. Inflammation and/or other disease processes in the skin increase percutaneous absorption. Occlusive dressings substantially increase the percutaneous absorption of topical corticosteroids. Thus, occlusive dressings may be a valuable therapeutic adjunct for treatment of resistant dermatoses. (See *"Dosage and Administration"*.)

Once absorbed through the skin, topical corticosteroids are handled through pharmacokinetic pathways similar to systemically administered corticosteroids. Corticosteroids are bound to plasma proteins in varying degrees. Corticosteroids are metabolized primarily in the liver and are then excreted by the kidneys. Some of the topical corticosteroids and their metabolites are also excreted into the bile.

INDICATIONS AND USAGE

Dexamethasone, Topical, is indicated for relief of the inflammatory and pruritic manifestations of corticosteroid-responsive dermatoses.

CONTRAINDICATIONS

Topical corticosteroids are contraindicated in those patients with a history of hypersensitivity to any of the components of the preparation.

WARNING

Topically applied steroids are absorbed systemically. There may be rare instances in which this absorption results in immunosuppression. Patients who are on drugs which suppress the immune system are more susceptible to infections than healthy individuals. Chickenpox and measles, for example, can have a more serious or even fatal course in non-immune children (see *"Precautions, Pediatric Use"*) or adults on corticosteroids. In such children or adults who have not had these diseases, particular care should be taken to avoid exposure. The risk of developing a disseminated infection varies among individuals and can be related to the dose, route and duration of corticosteroid administration as well as to the underlying disease. If exposed to chickenpox, prophylaxis with varicella zoster immune globulin (VZIG) may be indicated. If chickenpox develops, treatment with antiviral agents may be considered. If exposed to measles, prophylaxis with immune globulin (IG) may be indicated. (See the respective package inserts for VZIG and IG for complete prescribing information.)

Avoid spraying the aerosol in eyes or nose. Contents under pressure. Do not puncture or burn. Keep out of reach of children. Use only as directed. Intentional misuse by deliberately concentrating and inhaling the contents can be harmful or fatal.

PRECAUTIONS

GENERAL

Systemic absorption of topical corticosteroids has produced reversible hypothalamic-pituitary-adrenal (HPA) axis suppression, manifestations of Cushing's syndrome, hyperglycemia, and glycosuria in some patients.

Conditions which augment systemic absorption include the application of the more potent corticosteroids, use over large surface areas, prolonged use, and the addition of occlusive dressings.

Therefore, patients receiving a large dose of a potent topical corticosteroid applied to a large surface area or under an occlusive dressing should be evaluated periodically for evidence of HPA axis suppression by using urinary free cortisol and ACTH stimulation tests. If HPA axis suppression is noted, an attempt should be made to withdraw the drug, to reduce the frequency of application, or to substitute a less potent corticosteroid.

Recovery of HPA axis function is generally prompt and complete upon discontinuation of the drug. Infrequently, signs and symptoms of corticosteroid withdrawal may occur, requiring supplemental systemic corticosteroids.

Children may absorb proportionally larger amounts of topical corticosteroids and thus be more susceptible to systemic toxicity (See *"Precautions, Pediatric Use"*).

If irritation develops, topical corticosteroids should be discontinued and appropriate therapy instituted.

◆ RATED THERAPEUTICALLY EQUIVALENT; ◇ THERAPEUTIC EQUIVALENCE UNCONFIRMED; ○ UNRATED

In the presence of dermatological infections, the use of an appropriate antifungal or antibacterial agent should be instituted. If a favorable response does not occur promptly, the corticosteroid should be discontinued until the infection has been adequately controlled.

This product is not for ophthalmic use. However, if applied to the eyelids or skin near the eyes, the drug may enter the eyes. In patients with a history of herpes simplex keratitis, ocular exposure to corticosteroids may lead to a recurrence. Prolonged ocular exposure may cause steroid glaucoma.

Generally, occlusive dressings should not be used on weeping or exudative lesions.

If occlusive dressing therapy is used, inspect lesions between dressings for development of infection. If infection develops, the technique should be discontinued and appropriate anti-microbial therapy instituted.

When large areas of the body are covered with an occlusive dressing, thermal homeostasis may be impaired. If elevation of body temperature occurs, use of the occlusive dressing should be discontinued.

A few individuals may be sensitive to one or more of the components of the aerosol. If any reaction indicating sensitivity is observed, discontinue use.

Caution: The aerosol is flammable. Do not use around open flame or while smoking.

INFORMATION FOR THE PATIENT
Patients using topical corticosteroids should receive the following information and instructions:

1. This medication is to be used as directed by the physician. It is for external use only. Avoid contact with the eyes.
2. Patients should be advised not to use this medication for any disorder other than that for which it was prescribed.
3. The treated skin area should not be bandaged or otherwise covered or wrapped so as to be occlusive unless directed by the physician.
4. Patients should report any signs of local adverse reactions, especially under occlusive dressing.
5. Parents of pediatric patients should be advised not to use tight-fitting diapers or plastic pants on a child being treated in the diaper area, as these garments may constitute occlusive dressings.
6. Susceptible patients who are on immunosuppressant doses of corticosteroids should be warned to avoid exposure to chickenpox or measles. Patients should also be advised that if they are exposed, medical advice should be sought without delay.

LABORATORY TESTS
The following tests may be helpful in evaluating the HPA axis suppression:
- Urinary free cortisol test
- ACTH stimulation test

CARCINOGENESIS, MUTAGENESIS, AND IMPAIRMENT OF FERTILITY
Long-term animal studies have not been performed to evaluate the carcinogenic potential or the effect on fertility of topical corticosteroids.

Studies to determine mutagenicity with prednisolone and hydrocortisone have revealed negative results.

PREGNANCY
Pregnancy Category C: Corticosteroids are generally teratogenic in laboratory animals when administered systemically at relatively low dosage levels. The more potent corticosteroids have been shown to be teratogenic after dermal application in laboratory animals. There are no adequate and well-controlled studies in pregnant women on teratogenic effects from topically applied corticosteroids. Therefore, topical corticosteroids should be used during pregnancy only if the potential benefit justifies the potential risk to the fetus. Drugs of this class should not be used extensively on pregnant patients, in large amounts, or for prolonged periods of time.

NURSING MOTHERS
It is not known whether topical administration of corticosteroids could result in sufficient systemic absorption to produce detectable quantities in breast milk. Systemically administered corticosteroids are secreted into breast milk in quantities *not* likely to have a deleterious effect on the infant. Nevertheless, caution should be exercised when topical corticosteroids are administered to a nursing woman.

PEDIATRIC USE
Pediatric patients may demonstrate greater susceptibility to topical corticosteroid-induced HPA axis suppression and Cushing's syndrome than mature patients because of a larger skin surface area to body weight ratio.

Hypothalamic-pituitary-adrenal (HPA) axis suppression, Cushing's syndrome, and intracranial hypertension have been reported in children receiving topical corticosteroids. Manifestations of adrenal suppression in children include linear growth retardation, delayed weight gain, low plasma cortisol levels, and absence of response to ACTH stimulation. Manifestations of intracranial hypertension include bulging fontanelles, headaches, and bilateral papilledema.

Administration of topical corticosteroids to children should be limited to the least amount compatible with an effective therapeutic regimen. Chronic corticosteroid therapy may interfere with the growth and development of children.

ADVERSE REACTIONS
The following adverse reactions are reported infrequently with topical corticosteroids, but may occur more frequently with the use of occlusive dressings. These reactions are listed in an approximate decreasing order of occurrence:

Burning
Itching
Irritation
Dryness
Folliculitis
Hypertrichosis
Acneiform eruptions
Hypopigmentation
Perioral dermatitis
Allergic contact dermatitis
Maceration of the skin
Secondary infection
Skin atrophy
Striae
Miliaria

OVERDOSAGE
Topically applied corticosteroids can be absorbed in sufficient amounts to produce systemic effects. (See *"Precautions"*.)

DOSAGE AND ADMINISTRATION
Cream: Apply to the affected area as a thin film three or four times daily.

Occlusive dressings may be used for the management of psoriasis or recalcitrant conditions.

Before using this preparation in the *ear*, clean the aural canal thoroughly and sponge dry. Confirm that the eardrum is intact. With a cotton-tipped applicator, apply a thin coating of the cream to the affected canal area three or four times a day.

Aerosol: Patients should be instructed in the correct way to use Dexamethasone, Topical, Spray. The preparation is readily applied, even on hairy areas. It does not have to be rubbed into the skin.

Optimal effects will be obtained with Dexamethasone, Topical, Spray when these directions are followed:

1. Keep the affected area clean to reduce the possibility of infection.
2. Shake the container *gently* once or twice each time before using. Hold it about six inches from the area to be treated. Effective medication may be obtained with the container held either upright or inverted, since it is fitted with a special valve that dispenses approximately the same dosage in either position.
3. Spray each four inch square of affected area for one or two seconds three or four times a day, depending on the nature of the condition and the response to therapy.
4. When a favorable response is obtained, reduce dosage gradually and eventually discontinue.
5. Occlusive dressings may be used for the management of psoriasis or recalcitrant conditions.

HOW SUPPLIED

DEXAMETHASONE
AEROSOL SOLID INGREDIENTS: 0.01%

BRAND/MANUFACTURER	NDC	SIZE	AWP
○ BRAND			
AEROSEB-DEX: Allergan Inc	00023-0852-90	58 gm	$17.58

AEROSOL SOLID INGREDIENTS: 0.04%

BRAND/MANUFACTURER	NDC	SIZE	AWP
○ BRAND			
DECASPRAY: Merck	00006-7623-25	25 gm	$14.28

DEXAMETHASONE SODIUM PHOSPHATE
CREAM: 0.1%

BRAND/MANUFACTURER	NDC	SIZE	AWP
○ BRAND			
DECADRON PHOSPHATE: Merck	00006-7616-12	15 gm	$11.39
	00006-7616-24	30 gm	$17.04

Dexamethasone/Neomycin Sulfate/Polymyxin B Sulfate

DESCRIPTION
Dexamethasone/Neomycin Sulfate/Polymyxin B Sulfate is a multiple dose anti-infective steroid combination in sterile suspension and sterile ointment forms for topical application.

The chemical name of Dexamethasone is Pregna-1, 4-diene-3, 20-dione, 9-fluoro-11,17, 21-trihydroxy-16-methyl-, (11β, 16α)-.

Each mL of suspension contains: Dexamethasone 0.1%, Neomycin Sulfate equivalent to Neomycin 3.5 mg, Polymyxin B Sulfate 10,000 units.

Each gram of ointment contains: Dexamethasone 0.1%, Neomycin Sulfate equivalent to Neomycin 3.5 mg, Polymyxin B Sulfate 10,000 units.

CLINICAL PHARMACOLOGY

Corticoids suppress the inflammatory response to a variety of agents and they probably delay or slow healing. Since corticoids may inhibit the body's defense mechanism against infection, a concomitant antimicrobial drug may be used when this inhibition is considered to be clinically significant in a particular case.

When a decision to administer both a corticoid and an antimicrobial is made, the administration of such drugs in combination has the advantage of greater patient compliance and convenience, with the added assurance that the appropriate dosage of both drugs is administered, plus assured compatibility of ingredients when both types of drugs are in the same formulation and, particularly, that the correct volume of drug is delivered and retained.

The relative potency of corticosteroids depends on the molecular structure, concentration and release from the vehicle.

INDICATIONS AND USAGE

For steroid-responsive inflammatory ocular conditions for which a corticosteroid is indicated and where bacterial infection or a risk of bacterial ocular infection exists.

Ocular steroids are indicated in inflammatory conditions of the palpebral and bulbar conjunctiva, cornea, and anterior segment of the globe where the inherent risk of steroid use in certain infective conjunctivitises is accepted to obtain a diminution in edema and inflammation. They are also indicated in chronic anterior uveitis and corneal injury from chemical, radiation or thermal burns; or penetration of foreign bodies.

The use of a combination drug with an anti-infective component is indicated where the risk of infection is high or where there is an expectation that potentially dangerous numbers of bacteria will be present in the eye.

The particular anti-infective drug in this product is active against the following common bacterial eye pathogens: *Staphyloccus, aureus, Escherichia coli, Haemophilus influenzae, Klebsiella Enterobacter species, Neisseria species,* and *Pseudomonas aeruginosa.*

This product does not provide adequate coverage against: *Serratia marcescens* and Streptococci, including *Streptococcus pneumoniae.*

CONTRAINDICATIONS

Epithelial herpes simplex keratitis (dendritic keratitis), vaccinia, varicella, and many other viral diseases of the cornea and conjunctiva. Mycobacterial infection of the eye. Fungal diseases of ocular structures. Hypersensitivity to a component of the medication. (Hypersensitivity to the *antibiotic* component occurs at a higher rate than for other components.)

The use of these combinations is always contraindicated after uncomplicated removal of a corneal foreign body.

WARNINGS

NOT FOR INJECTION. Do not touch dropper or tube tip to any surface, as this may contaminate the contents. Prolonged use may result in glaucoma, with damage to the optic nerve, defects in visual acuity and fields of vision, and posterior subcapsular cataract formation. Prolonged use may suppress the host response and thus increase the hazard of secondary ocular infections. In those diseases causing thinning of the cornea or sclera, perforations have been known to occur with the use of topical steroids. In acute purulent conditions of the eye, steroids may mask infection or enhance existing infection. If these products are used for 10 days or longer, intraocular pressure should be routinely monitored even though it may be difficult in children and uncooperative patients.

Products containing Neomycin Sulfate may cause cutaneous sensitization.

Employment of steroid medication in the treatment of herpes simplex requires great caution.

PRECAUTIONS

The initial prescription and renewal of the medication order beyond 20 mL or 8 g should be made by a physician only after examination of the patient with the aid of magnification, such as a slit lamp biomicroscopy and, where appropriate, fluorescein staining.

The possibility of persistent fungal infections of the cornea should be considered after prolonged steroid dosing.

USAGE IN PREGNANCY

The safety of intensive or protracted use of topical steroids in pregnancy has not been studied.

ADVERSE REACTIONS

Adverse reactions have occurred with steroid/anti-infective combination drugs which can be attributed to the steroid component, the anti-infective component, or the combination. Exact incidence figures are not available since no denominator of treated patients is available.

Reactions occurring most often from the presence of the anti-infective ingredient are allergic sensitizations. The reactions due to the steroid component are: elevation of intraocular pressure (IOP) with possible development of glaucoma, and infrequent optic nerve damage; posterior subcapsular cataract formation; and delayed wound healing.

Secondary Infection: The development of secondary infection has occurred after use of combinations containing steroids and antimicrobials. Fungal infections of

the cornea are particularly prone to develop coincidentally with long-term applications of steroid. The possibility of fungal invasion must be considered in any persistent corneal ulceration where steroid treatment has been used.

Secondary bacterial ocular infection following suppression of host responses also occurs.

DOSAGE AND ADMINISTRATION

Dexamethasone/Neomycin Sulfate/Polymyxin B Sulfate Suspension: One to two drops topically in the conjunctival sac(s). In severe disease, drops may be used hourly, being tapered to discontinuation as the inflammation subsides. In mild disease, drops may be used up to four to six times daily. Dexamethasone/ Neomycin Sulfate/Polymyxin B Sulfate *Ointment:* Apply a small amount into the conjunctival sac(s) up to three or four times daily or, may be used adjunctively with drops at bedtime.

Not more than 20 mL or 8 g should be prescribed initially and the prescription should not be refilled without further evaluation as outlined in *"Precautions"* above.

Store at 46° - 80°F.

HOW SUPPLIED
DROP: 0.35%, 0.1%, 10,000 U/ML

BRAND/MANUFACTURER	NDC	SIZE	AWP
◆ GENERICS			
STORZ-N-P-D: Storz/Lederle	57706-0867-31	5 ml	$4.68

DROP:

AVERAGE UNIT PRICE (AVAILABLE SIZES)		GENERIC A-RATED AVERAGE PRICE (GAAP)	
BRAND	$2.74	5 ml	$6.86
GENERIC	$1.37		

BRAND/MANUFACTURER	NDC	SIZE	AWP
◆ BRAND			
DEXACIDIN: Iolab	00058-2250-05	5 ml	$8.04
MAXITROL: Alcon Ophthalmic	00998-0630-06	5 ml	$19.38
◆ GENERICS			
Schein	00364-7394-53	5 ml	$5.50
DEXASPORIN: Bausch&Lomb Pharm	24208-0830-60	5 ml	$5.59
DEXASPORIN: URL	00677-0900-20	5 ml	$6.17
Moore,H.L.	00839-6709-25	5 ml	$7.28
Rugby	00536-0830-65	5 ml	$7.46
METHADEX: Major	00904-3003-05	5 ml	$7.50
Goldline	00182-7023-62	5 ml	$7.50
POLY-DEX: Ocusoft	54799-0520-05	5 ml	$7.85

DROP: 0.1%

BRAND/MANUFACTURER	NDC	SIZE	AWP
◆ GENERICS			
AK-TROL: Akorn	17478-0239-10	5 ml	$6.88

DROP: 3.5 MG/10 ML

BRAND/MANUFACTURER	NDC	SIZE	AWP
◆ GENERICS			
Aligen	00405-6100-05	5 ml	$7.18

OINTMENT:

AVERAGE UNIT PRICE (AVAILABLE SIZES)		GENERIC A-RATED AVERAGE PRICE (GAAP)	
BRAND	$3.87	3.5 gm	$6.76
GENERIC	$1.93		
HCFA FUL (3.5 gm)	$2.54		

BRAND/MANUFACTURER	NDC	SIZE	AWP
◆ BRAND			
DEXACIDIN: Iolab	00058-2255-01	3.5 gm	$7.68
MAXITROL: Alcon Ophthalmic	00065-0631-36	3.5 gm	$19.38
◆ GENERICS			
DEXASPORIN: Bausch&Lomb Pharm	24208-0795-55	3.5 gm	$5.84
Fougera	00168-0221-38	3.5 gm	$6.43
DEXASPORIN: Bausch&Lomb Pharm	24208-0796-35	3.5 gm	$7.13
POLY-DEX: Ocusoft	54799-0520-35	3.5 gm	$7.85

Dexchlorpheniramine Maleate

DESCRIPTION

These products contain Dexchlorpheniramine Maleate, an antihistamine having the formula, $C_{16}H_{19}ClN_2 \cdot C_4H_4O_4$, and a molecular weight of 390.87. Chemically, it is (+)-2-[ρ-Chloro-α-+-(dimethylamino) ethyl] benzyl] pyridine maleate (1:1).

Tablets contain 2 mg Dexchlorpheniramine Maleate.

Syrup contains 2 mg dexchlorpheniramine Maleate, USP per 5 ml.

Dexchlorpheniramine Maleate is a white, odorless, crystalline powder which in aqueous solution has a pH of between 4 and 5. It is freely soluble in water, soluble in alcohol and in chloroform, but only slightly soluble in benzene or ether.

◆ RATED THERAPEUTICALLY EQUIVALENT; ◇ THERAPEUTIC EQUIVALENCE UNCONFIRMED; ○ UNRATED

Following is its chemical structure:

CLINICAL PHARMACOLOGY
Is an antihistamine with anticholinergic properties. It is capable of producing a slight-to-moderate sedative effect. Antihistamines appear to compete with histamine for receptor sites on effector cells and are of value clinically in the prevention and relief of many allergic manifestations.

In vitro and *in vivo* assays of the antihistamine potencies of the optically active isomers of chlorpheniramine demonstrate that the predominant activity is in the dextro-isomer. The dextro-isomer is approximately two times more active than the racemic compound. Since Dexchlorpheniramine is the dextro-isomer and active moiety of chlorpheniramine, it can be assumed that experience with Chlorpheniramine also applies to Dexchlorpheniramine.

Chlorpheniramine Maleate 4 mg given to fasting human volunteers produced prompt blood levels after oral administration. Peak blood levels were approximately 7 ng/ml at an average time of 3 hours after administration. The half-life of chlorpheniramine maleate ranged from 20 to 24 hours. Following a single dose of tritium-labeled Chlorpheniramine Maleate to humans, the drug was found to be extensively metabolized whether given orally or by intravenous administration. The drug and metabolites were primarily excreted in the urine, with 19% of the dose appearing in 24 hours and a total of 34% in 48 hours.

In a study in normal volunteers, a high flow rate of acidic urine resulted in a high excretion rate of chlorpheniramine maleate. Over a concentration range of 0.28 to 1.24 mcg/ml of plasma, chlorpheniramine maleate was 72 to 69% bound to plasma protein, respectively.

INDICATIONS AND USAGE
Dexchlorpheniramine Maleate Tablets and Syrup are indicated for the treatment of perennial and seasonal allergic rhinitis; vasomotor rhinitis; allergic conjunctivitis; mild uncomplicated allergic skin manifestations of urticarla and angioedema; amelioration of allergic reactions to blood or plasma; and dermographism. They are also indicated as therapy for anaphylactic reactions adjunctive to epinephrine and other standard measures after the acute manifestations have been controlled.

CONTRAINDICATIONS
Hypersensitivity to Dexchlorpheniramine Maleate of other antihistamines of similar chemical structure contraindicates the use of Dexchlorpheniramine Maleate Tablets or Syrup.

Drug products containing Dexchlorpheniramine Maleate should not be used in newborn or premature infants because of the possibility of severe reactions, such as convulsions.

Antihistamines *should not* be used to treat lower respiratory tract symptoms. Antihistamines are also contraindicated for use in conjunction with monoamine oxidase inhibitor therapy.

WARNINGS
Dexchlorpheniramine, as with all antihistamines, should be used with caution in patients with narrow-angle glaucoma, stenosing peptic ulcer, pyloroduodenal obstruction, symptomatic prostatic hypertrophy, and bladder neck obstruction.

Overdoses of antihistamines may cause hallucinations, convulsions, or death, especially in infants and children.

Products containing Dexchlorpheniramine Maleate have additive effects with alcohol and other CNS depressants (hypnotics, sedatives, tranquilizers, etc.). Patients should not engage in activities requiring mental alertness, such as driving a car or operating machinery.

Antihistamines are more likely to cause dizziness, sedation, and hypotension in elderly patients (approximately 60 years or older).

PRECAUTIONS
General: Dexcholoropheniramine Mediate has an atropine-like action and therefore products containing it should be used with caution in patients with: a history of bronchial asthma; increased intraocular pressure; hyperthyroidism; cardiovascular disease; hypertension.

Information for Patients:
1. Dexchlorpheniramine may cause slight-to-moderate drowsiness.
2. Patients should not engage in activities requiring mental alertness, such as driving or operating machinery.
3. Alcohol or other sedative drugs may enhance the drowsiness caused by antihistamines.
4. Patients should not take Dexchlorpheniramine Maleate Taromar or Tablets or Syrup in conjunction with a monoamine oxidase inhibitor or oral anticoagulant.

Drug Interactions: Dexchlorpheniramine Maleate may cause severe hypotension when given in conjunction with a monoamine oxidase inhibitor.

Alcohol and other sedative drugs will potentiate the sedative effects of Dexchlorpheniramine. (See *"Warnings".*)

The action of oral anticoagulants may be inhibited by antihistamines.

Carcinogenesis, Mutagenesis, Impairment of Fertility: Although there have been no oncogenic or mutagenic studies on Dexchlorpheniramine, a 103-week oncogenic study in rats on the racemic mixture, chlorpheniramine, did not produce an increase in the incidence of tumors in the drug-treated groups, as compared with the controls.

An Ames mutagenicity test performed on chlorpheniramine and its nitrosation product was negative. An early study in rats with chlorpheniramine maleate revealed a reduction in fertility in female rats at doses approximately 67 times the human dose. More recent studies in rabbits and rats, using more appropriate methodology and doses up to approximately 50 and 85 times the human dose, showed no reduction in fertility in the animals.

Pregnancy Category B: Reproduction studies have been performed in rabbits and rats at doses up to 50 times and 85 times the human dose, respectively, and have revealed no evidence of harm to the fetus due to chlorpheniramine maleate. (See above, *"Impairment of Fertility".*) There are, however, no adequate and well-controlled studies in pregnant women. Because animal reproduction studies are not always predictive of human response, this drug should be used during the first two trimesters of pregnancy only if clearly needed. Dexchlorpheniramine Maleate should not be used in the third trimester of pregnancy because newborn and premature infants may have severe reactions to anti-histamines. (See *"Contraindications".*)

Nonteratogenic Effects: Studies of chlorpheniramine maleate done in rats revealed a decrease in the postnatal survival rate of pups of animals dosed with 33 and 67 times the human dose.

Nursing Mothers: It is not known whether this drug is excreted in human milk. Because certain other antihistamines are known to be excreted in human milk, and because Dexchlorpheniramine Maleate is contraindicated in newborn and premature infants, caution should be exercised when it is administered to a nursing woman.

Pediatric Use: Safety and effectiveness in children below the age of 2 years have not been established.

ADVERSE REACTIONS
Slight-to-moderate drowsiness is the most frequent side effect of Dexchlorpheniramine Maleate. Other possible side effects of antihistamines include:

General: urticaria, drug rash, anaphylactic shock, photosensitivity, excessive perspiration, chills, dryness of mouth, nose, and throat.

Cardiovascular System: headache, palpitations, tachycardia, extrasysoles, hypotension.

Hematologic System: hemolytic anemia, hypoplastic anema, thrombocytopenia, agranulocytosis.

Nervous System: sedation, dizziness, vertigo, tinnitus, acute labyrinthitis, disturbed coordination, fatigue, confusion, restlessness, excitation, nervousness, tremor irritability, insomnia, euphoria, paresthesias, blurred vision, hysteria, neuritis, convulsions.

Gastrointestinal System: epigastric distress, anorexia, nausea, vomiting, diarrhea, constipation.

Genitourinary System: urinary frequency, difficult urination, urinary retention, early menses.

Respiratory System: thickening of bronchial secretions, tightness of chest, wheezing, nasal stuffiness.

OVERDOSAGE
In the event of overdosage, emergency treatment should be started immediately.

Manifestations of antihistamine overdosage may vary from central nervous system depression (sedation, apnea, diminished mental alertness, cardiovascular collapse) to stimulation (insomnia, hallucinations, tremors, or convulsions) to death. Other signs and symptoms may be dizziness, tinnitus, ataxia, blurred vision, and hypotension. Stimulation is particularly likely in children, as are atropine-like signs and symptoms (dry mouth; fixed, dilated pupils; flushing; hyperthermia; and gastrointestinal symptoms).

Treatment: The patient should be induced to vomit, even if emesis has occurred spontaneously. Pharmacologic vomiting by the administration of ipecac syrup is a preferred method. However, vomiting should not be induced in patients with impaired consciousness. The action of ipecac is facilitated by physical activity and by the administration of eight to twelve fluid ounces of water. If emesis does not occur within fifteen minutes, the dose of ipecac should be repeated. Precautions against aspiration must be taken, especially in infants and children. Following emesis, any drug remaining in the stomach may be absorbed by activated charcoal administered as a slurry with water. If vomiting is unsuccessful or contraindicated, gastric lavage should be performed. Isotonic and one-half isotonic saline are the lavage solutions of choice. Saline cathartics, such as milk of magnesia, draw water into the bowel by osmosis and therefore may be valuable for their action in rapid dilution of bowel content. Dialysis is of little value in antihistamine poisoning. After emergency treatment, the patient should continue to be medically monitored.

Treatment of the signs and symptoms of overdosage is symptomatic and supportive. *Stimulants* (analeptic agents) *should not* be used. Vasopressors may be used to treat hypotension. Short-acting barbiturates, diazepam, or paraldehyde may be administered to control seizures. Hyperpyrexia, especially in children, may require treatment with tepid water sponge baths or a hypothermic blanket. Apnea is treated with ventilatory support.

➤ **SHOWN IN PRODUCT IDENTIFICATION GUIDE**

In mice, the oral LD$_{50}$ of Dexchlorpheniramine is 258 mg/kg. In humans, the estimated lethal dose of racemic chlorpheniramine is 5 to 10 mg/kg. Thus a dose of 2.5 to 5 mg/kg of Dexchlorpheniramine should be similarly regarded.

DOSAGE AND ADMINISTRATION
DOSAGE SHOULD BE INDIVIDUALIZED ACCORDING TO THE NEEDS AND RESPONSE OF THE PATIENT.

Dexchlorpheniramine Maleate Tablets: Adults and children 12 years of age and over: one tablet every 4 to 6 hours. Children 6 through 11 years: one-half tablet every 4 to 6 hours. Children 2 through 5 years: one-quarter tablet every 4 to 6 hours.

Dexchlorpheniramine Maleate Syrup: Adults and children 12 years of age and over: one teaspoonful (2 mg) every 4 to 6 hours. Children 6 through 11 years: one-half teaspoonful (1 mg) every 4 to 6 hours. Children 2 through 5 years: one-quarter teaspoonful (½ mg) every 4 to 6 hours.

Store Dexchlorpheniramine Maleate Tablets and Syrup between 2° and 30°C (36° and 86°F).

HOW SUPPLIED
SYRUP:

AVERAGE UNIT PRICE (AVAILABLE SIZES)		GENERIC A-RATED AVERAGE PRICE (GAAP)	
GENERIC	$0.02	480 ml	$12.48
		3840 ml	$86.97

BRAND/MANUFACTURER	NDC	SIZE	AWP
◆ GENERICS			
Pennex	00832-8539-16	480 ml	$11.46
Pennex	00426-8539-16	480 ml	$13.50
Pennex	00832-8539-28	3840 ml	$82.93
Pennex	00426-8539-28	3840 ml	$91.00

SYRUP: 2 MG/5 ML

AVERAGE UNIT PRICE (AVAILABLE SIZES)		GENERIC A-RATED AVERAGE PRICE (GAAP)	
BRAND	$0.08	480 ml	$12.95
GENERIC	$0.03		

BRAND/MANUFACTURER	NDC	SIZE	AWP
◆ BRAND			
POLARAMINE: Schering	00085-0016-05	480 ml	$37.34
◆ GENERICS			
Rugby	00536-0460-85	480 ml	$12.75
Major	00904-0624-16	480 ml	$13.15
Major	00904-0624-28	3840 ml	$101.90

TABLET, EXTENDED RELEASE: 4 MG

BRAND/MANUFACTURER	NDC	SIZE	AWP
○ BRAND			
POLARAMINE REPETABS: Schering	00085-0095-03	100s	$60.06

TABLET, EXTENDED RELEASE: 6 MG

BRAND/MANUFACTURER	NDC	SIZE	AWP
○ BRAND			
POLARAMINE REPETABS: Schering	00085-0148-03	100s	$83.94

TABLETS: 2 MG

BRAND/MANUFACTURER	NDC	SIZE	AWP
◆ BRAND			
POLARAMINE: Schering	00085-0820-03	100s	$35.21

Dexchlorpheniramine Maleate/ Guaifenesin/Pseudoephedrine Sulfate

DESCRIPTION
Dexchlorpheniramine/Guaifenesin/Pseudoephedrine in each 5 ml (one teaspoonful) contains 2 mg Dexchlorpheniramine Maleate, USP: 20 mg Pseudoephedrine Sulfate, USP: and 100 mg Guaifenesin, USP.

Dexchlorpheniramine Maleate is an antihistamine having the chemical formula $C_{16}H_{10}ClN_2 \cdot C_2H_2O_2$, and a molecular weight of 390.87. Chemically, it is (+)-2-[p-Chloro-α-[2-(dimethyl-amino)ethyl]benzyl] pyridine maleate (1:1).

Dexchlorpheniramine Maleate is a white, odorless, crystalline powder which in aqueous solution has a pH between 4 and 5. It is freely soluble in water, soluble in alcohol and in chloroform, but only slightly soluble in benzene or in ether.

Pseudoephedrine, an adrenergic agent, is one of the naturally occurring alkaloids obtained from various species of the plant *Ephedra*. The chemical name of Pseudoephedrine Sulfate is benzenemethanol, α-[1-(methylamino)ethyl]-, [S-(R*,R*)]-, sulfate (2:1) (salt): it is $(C_{10}H_{12}NO)_2 \cdot H_2SO_4$. The compound is a white to off-white crystal or powder with a molecular weight of 428.6. It is very soluble in water, freely soluble in alcohol, and sparingly soluble in chloroform.

Guaifenesin, an expectorant, is the glyceryl ether of guaiacol having the chemical formula, $C_{10}H_{14}O_4$. It is a white to slightly gray crystalline powder with a molecular weight of 198.22. One gram dissolves in 15 ml of water. The drug is soluble in alcohol, in chloroform, in glycerin, and in propylene glycol. The chemical name is 1.2-Propanediol, 3-(2-methoxyphenoxy).

CLINICAL PHARMACOLOGY
Dexchlorpheniramine/Guaifenesin/Pseudoephedrine combines the antihistaminic actions of Dexchlorpheniramine Maleate with the nasal vasoconstrictive properties of Pseudoephedrine Sulfate: Guaifenesin increases respiratory tract fluid output and eases expectoration.

Dexchlorpheniramine Maleate is an antihistamine with anticholinergic properties. It is capable of producing a mild to moderate sedative effect. Antihistamines appear to compete with histamine for receptor sites on effector cells and are of value clinically in the prevention and relief of many allergic manifestations.

In vitro and *in vivo* assays of the antihistamine potencies of the optically active isomers of chlorpheniramine demonstrate that the predominant activity is in the dextro-isomer. The dextro-isomer is approximately two times more active than the racemic compound. Since Dexchlorpheniramine is the dextro-isomer and active moiety of chlorpheniramine, it can be assumed that experience with chlorpheniramine also applies to Dexchlorpheniramine.

Chlorpheniramine maleate 4 mg given to fasting human volunteers produced prompt blood levels after oral administration. Peak blood levels were approximately 7 ng/ml at an average time of 3 hours after administration. The half-life of chlorpheniramine maleate ranged from 20 to 24 hours. Following a single dose of tritium-labeled chlorpheniramine maleate to humans, the drug was found to be extensively metabolized whether given orally or by intravenous administration. The drug and metabolites were primarily excreted in the urine, with 19% of the dose appearing in 24 hours and a total of 34% in 48 hours.

In a study in normal volunteers, a high flow rate of acidic urine resulted in a high excretion rate of chlorpheniramine maleate. Over a concentration range of 0.28 to 1.24 mcg/ml of plasma, chlorpheniramine maleate was 72 to 69% bound to plasma protein, respectively.

Guaifenesin increases sputum volume and decreases sputum tenaciousness. It has been claimed that guaifenesin acts reflexly by stimulating receptors in the gastric mucosa which, in turn, stimulate respiratory secretions. This allows ciliary motion and coughing to move the loosened secretions toward the pharynx, thus promoting the expulsion of secretions from the respiratory tract. As a result, unproductive coughs become more productive and less frequent.

Pseudoephedrine Sulfate appears to exert its sympathomimetic effect predominantly through indirect means by releasing adrenergic mediators from postganglionic nerve terminals. The clinical action is primarily as a nasal decongestant due to vasoconstriction of nasal blood vessels. At recommended doses other sympathomimetic effects, such as pressor activity and CNS stimulation, are minimal.

It has been reported that excretion of Pseudoephedrine was directly related to urinary pH: the more alkaline the urine, the greater the rate of excretion of the drug. Further studies done in rats with ^{14}C-labeled Pseudoephedrine revealed that the drug was distributed in the tissues in the following organs in decreasing order of magnitude: kidneys, lungs, spleen, adrenals, liver, intestine, heart, and plasma.

Pseudoephedrine passes through the blood-brain barrier. Wakefulness may occasionally be observed. Fetal-placental transfer and plasma protein binding of Pseudoephedrine have not been studied.

The half-life of Pseudoephedrine is 5.2 to 8 hours.

INDICATIONS AND USAGE
Dexchlorpheniramine/Guaifenesin/Pseudoephedrine is indicated for relief of coughs and complications associated with allergic disorders and allergic manifestations of respiratory illnesses, such as hay fever and vasomotor rhinitis.

CONTRAINDICATIONS
Hypersensitivity to Dexchlorpheniramine Maleate or other antihistamines of similar chemical structure, Guaifenesin, or Pseudoephedrine contraindicates the use of this product.

Drug products containing Dexchlorpheniramine Maleate should not be used in newborn or premature infants because of the possibility of severe reactions, such as convulsions. Antihistamines *should not* be used to treat lower respiratory tract symptoms. Antihistamines are also contraindicated for use in conjunction with monoamine oxidase (MAO) inhibitor therapy.

Pseudoephedrine Sulfate is contraindicated in patients who have shown hypersensitivity or idiosyncrasy to adrenergic agents, which may be manifested by insomnia, dizziness, weakness, tremor, or arrhythmias. In patients with severe hypertension, severe coronary artery disease, hyperthyroidism, and in those receiving monoamine oxidase (MAO) inhibitor therapy or within 10 days of stopping such treatment; sympathomimetic amines are contraindicated.

WARNINGS
Dexchlorpheniramine, as with all antihistamines, should be used with caution in patients with narrow angle glaucoma, stenosing peptic ulcer, pyloroduodenal obstruction, symptomatic prostatic hypertrophy, and bladder neck obstruction. Overdosage of antihistamines may cause hallucinations, convulsions, or death, especially in infants and children.

Products containing Dexchlorpheniramine Maleate have additive effects with alcohol and other CNS depressants (hypnotics, sedatives, tranquilizers, etc.). Patients should not engage in activities requiring mental alertness, such as driving a car or operating machinery.

◆ RATED THERAPEUTICALLY EQUIVALENT; ◇ THERAPEUTIC EQUIVALENCE UNCONFIRMED; ○ UNRATED

Antihistamines are more likely to cause dizziness, sedation, and hypotension in elderly patients (approximately 60 years or older).

In patients with prostatic enlargement, Pseudoephedrine may increase difficulty in micturition. In patients with narrow angle glaucoma, it may precipitate angle closure. It should also be used with caution and at a lower dosage in the elderly who are more sensitive to the CNS stimulating effects of the drug which may result in confusion, delirium, hallucinations, and convulsions.

PRECAUTIONS

General: Dexchlorpheniramine Maleate has an atropine-like action and therefore products containing it should be used with caution in patients with: a history of bronchial asthma; increased intraocular pressure; hyperthyroidism; cardiovascular disease; hypertension.

Pseudoephedrine should be used with caution in patients with hypertension, diabetes mellitus, ischemic heart disease, angina, or in patients receiving digitalis.

Information for Patients:
1. Products containing antihistamines may cause drowsiness.
2. Patients should not engage in activities requiring mental alertness, such as driving or operating machinery.
3. Alcohol or other sedative drugs may enhance the drowsiness caused by antihistamines.
4. Patients should not take Dexchlorpheniramine/Guaifenesin/Pseudoephedrine if they are receiving a monoamine oxidase (MAO) inhibitor or within ten days of stopping such treatment, or if they are receiving oral anticoagulants.

Drug Interactions: Dexchlorpheniramine Maleate may cause severe hypotension when given in conjunction with a monoamine oxidase inhibitor.

Alcohol and other sedative drugs will potentiate the sedative effects of Dexchlorpheniramine. (See *"Warnings".*)

Pseudoephedrine-containing drugs should not be given to patients treated with monoamine oxidase (MAO) inhibitors or within ten days of stopping such treatment because of the possibility of precipitating a hypertensive crisis, potentially resulting in intracranial hemorrhage, convulsions, coma, and in some cases, death.

Pseudoephedrine should not be used with ganglionic blocking drugs, such as mecamylamine hydrochloride, which potentiates reactions of sympathomimetics. Also, it should not be used with adrenergic blocking drugs, such as guanethidine sulfate or bethanidine, since it antagonizes the hypotensive action of these drugs. Increased ectopic pacemaker activity can occur when Pseudoephedrine is used concomitantly with digitalis. Antacids increase the rate of absorption of Pseudoephedrine, while kaolin decreases it.

Drug/Laboratory Test Interactions: Guaifenesin has been shown to produce a color interference with certain clinical laboratory determinations of 5-hydroxyindole-acetic acid (5-HIAA) and vanillylmandelic acid (VMA).

The *in vitro* addition of Pseudoephedrine to sera containing the cardiac isoenzyme MB of serum creatine phosphokinase progressively inhibits the activity of the enzyme. The inhibition becomes complete over six hours.

Carcinogenesis, Mutagenesis, Impairment of Fertility: Although there have been no oncogenic or mutagenic studies on Dexchlorpheniramine, a 103-week oncogenic study in rats on the racemate, chlorpheniramine, did not produce an increase in the incidence of tumors in the drug-treated groups, as compared with the controls. An Ames mutagenicity test performed on chlorpheniramine and its nitrosation product was negative. An early study in rats with chlorpheniramine maleate revealed a reduction in fertility in female rats at doses approximately 67 times the human dose. More recent studies in rabbits and rats, using more appropriate methodology and doses up to approximately 50 and 85 times the human dose, showed no reduction in fertility in the animals.

Pseudoephedrine and Guaifenesin have not been evaluated for oncogenic or mutagenic potential. Their effects on fertility are not known.

Pregnancy Category C: (See statements on *"Guaifenesin"* below.) Reproduction studies have been performed in rabbits and rats at doses up to 50 times and 85 times the human dose, respectively, and have revealed no evidence of harm to the fetus due to chlorpheniramine maleate. (See above *"Impairment of Fertility."*) Animal reproduction studies have not been conducted with Guaifenesin. It is also not known whether Guaifenesin can cause fetal harm when administered to a pregnant woman or can affect reproduction capacity. Reproduction studies have been done in rats receiving up to 50 times the therapeutic dose and have revealed no evidence of harm to the fetus due to Pseudoephedrine. There are, however, no adequate and well-controlled studies of Dexchlorpheniramine Maleate, Guaifenesin, or Pseudoephedrine in pregnant women. Because animal reproduction studies are not always predictive of human response Dexchlorpheniramine/Guaifenesin/Pseudoephedrine should be used during the first two trimesters of pregnancy only if clearly needed. Dexchlorpheniramine Maleate should not be used in the third trimester of pregnancy because newborn and premature infants may have severe reactions to antihistamines. (See *"Contraindications".*)

Nonteratogenic Effects: Studies of chlorpheniramine maleate done in rats revealed a decrease in the postnatal survival rate of pups of animals dosed with 33 and 67 times the human dose.

Nursing Mothers: It is not known whether this drug is excreted in human milk. Because certain antihistamines are known to be excreted in human milk, because Dexchlorpheniramine Maleate is contraindicated in newborn and premature infants, and because of a report of irritability, excessive crying, and disturbed sleeping patterns in a nursing infant whose mother had taken a product containing an antihistamine and Pseudoephedrine, caution should be exercised when Dexchlorpheniramine/Guaifenesin/Pseudoephedrine is administered to a nursing woman.

Pediatric Use: Safety and effectiveness in children below the age of 2 years have not been established.

ADVERSE REACTIONS

DEXCHLORPHENIRAMINE MALEATE

Slight to moderate drowsiness is the most frequent side effect of Dexchlorpheniramine Maleate. Other possible side effects of antihistamines include:

General: urticaria, drug rash, anaphylactic shock, photosensitivity, excessive perspiration, chills, dryness of mouth, nose, and throat.

Cardiovascular System: headache, palpitations, tachycardia, extrasystoles, hypotension.

Hematologic System: hemolytic anemia, hypoplastic anemia, thrombocytopenia, agranulocytosis.

Nervous System: sedation, dizziness, vertigo, tinnitus, acute labyrinthitis, disturbed coordination, fatigue, confusion, restlessness, excitation, nervousness, tremor, irritability, insomnia, euphoria, paresthesias, blurred vision, hysteria, neuritis, convulsions.

Gastrointestinal System: epigastric distress, anorexia, nausea, vomiting, diarrhea, constipation.

Genitourinary System: urinary frequency, difficult urination, urinary retention, early menses.

Respiratory System: thickening of bronchial secretions, tightness of chest, wheezing, nasal stuffiness.

GUAIFENESIN

No serious adverse reactions have been reported with Guaifenesin. Nausea, gastrointestinal disturbances, and drowsiness have been reported infrequently.

PSEUDOEPHEDRINE SULFATE

Pseudoephedrine, like other sympathomimetic amines, may cause disturbing reactions, such as fear, anxiety, excessive perspiration, tenseness, restlessness, throbbing headache, tremor, weakness, dizziness, nausea, pallor, dysuria, respiratory difficulty, palpitations, tachycardia, and insomnia. Hyperthyroid and hypertensive individuals are particularly susceptible to the untoward and pressor responses of Pseudoephedrine, which may also induce angina, hypertension, and cardiac arrhythmias. Sympathomimetics have also produced CNS depression and cardiovascular collapse with accompanying hypotension. In psychoneurotic individuals, existing symptoms are often markedly exaggerated by the drug. The elderly are particularly sensitive to the CNS stimulating effects, and hallucinations and convulsions have occurred. Symptoms of unusual sensitivity to the effects of Pseudoephedrine have been reported in an infant with phenylketonuria.

DRUG ABUSE AND DEPENDENCE

There is no information to indicate abuse or dependency with Dexchlorpheniramine or Guaifenesin.

Pseudoephedrine, like other CNS stimulants, has been abused. At elevated dosages, subjects commonly experience an elevation of mood, a sense of increased energy and alertness, and decreased appetite. Some individuals become anxious, irritable, and loquacious. In addition to the marked euphoria, the user experiences a sense of markedly enhanced physical strength and mental capacity. With continued use, tolerance develops and toxic signs and symptoms appear. Depression may follow rapid withdrawal.

OVERDOSAGE

In the event of overdosage, emergency treatment should be started immediately.

Manifestations: Antihistamine overdosage may vary from central nervous system depression (sedation, apnea, diminished mental alertness, cardiovascular collapse) to stimulation (insomnia, hallucinations, tremors, or convulsions) to death. Other signs and symptoms may be dizziness, tinnitus, ataxia, blurred vision, and hypotension. Stimulation is particularly likely in children, as are atropine-like signs and symptoms (dry mouth; fixed, dilated pupils; flushing; hyperthermia; and gastrointestinal symptoms).

In large doses sympathomimetics may give rise to giddiness, headache, nausea, vomiting, sweating, thirst, tachycardia, precordial pain, palpitations, difficulty in micturition, muscular weakness and tenseness, anxiety, restlessness, and insomnia. Many patients can show a full-blown toxic psychosis with delusions and hallucinations. Some may develop cardiac arrhythmias, circulatory collapse, convulsions, coma, and respiratory failure.

Treatment: The patient should be induced to vomit, even if emesis has occurred spontaneously. Pharmacologic vomiting by the administration of ipecac syrup is a preferred method. However, vomiting should not be induced in patients with impaired consciousness. The action of ipecac is facilitated by physical activity and by the administration of 8 to 12 fluid ounces of water. If emesis does not occur within 15 minutes, the dose of ipecac should be repeated. Precautions against aspiration must be taken, especially in infants and children. Following emesis, any drug remaining in the stomach may be adsorbed by activated charcoal administered as a slurry with water. If vomiting is unsuccessful or contraindicated, gastric lavage should be performed. Isotonic and one-half isotonic saline are the lavage solutions of choice. Saline cathartics, such as milk of magnesia, draw water into the bowel by osmosis and therefore may be valuable for their action in rapid dilution of bowel content. Dialysis is of little value in antihistamine poisoning.

► SHOWN IN PRODUCT IDENTIFICATION GUIDE

After emergency treatment, the patient should continue to be medically monitored.

Treatment of the signs and symptoms of overdosage is symptomatic and supportive. *Stimulants* (analeptic agents) should *not* be used. Vasopressors may be used to treat hypotension. Short-acting barbiturates, diazepam, or paraldehyde may be administered to control seizures. Hyperpyrexia, especially in children, may require treatment with tepid water sponge baths or a hypothermic blanket. Apnea is treated with ventilatory support.

In humans, the estimated lethal dose of chlorpheniramine maleate is 5 to 10 mg/kg. Thus, a dose of 2.5 to 5 mg/kg of Dexchlorpheniramine should be similarly regarded.

The oral $LD_{50}S$ of the active components of Dexchlorpheniramine/Guaifenesin/Pseudoephedrine were established in mice as follows:

Dexchlorpheniramine 330 = 71 mg/kg
Pseudoephedrine sulfate 300 = 60 mg/kg
Guaifenesin 1200 = 175 mg/kg

Doses of Dexchlorpheniramine/Guaifenesin/Pseudoephedrine up to 32 ml/kg in rats and mice were not lethal to any animal; thus, the LD_{50} could not be determined on the basis of this study.

DOSAGE AND ADMINISTRATION

Adults and children 12 years and older: one or two teaspoonfuls 3 or 4 times daily.

Children 6 through 11 years: one-half to one teaspoonful 3 or 4 times daily.

Children 2 through 5 years: one-quarter to one-half teaspoonful 3 or 4 times daily.

Store between 2° to 30° C (36° to 86°F).

HOW SUPPLIED
SYRUP:

BRAND/MANUFACTURER	NDC	SIZE	AWP
○ **BRAND**			
POLARAMINE EXPECTORANT: Schering	00085-0268-05	480 ml	$48.14

Dexedrine SEE DEXTROAMPHETAMINE SULFATE

Dexol SEE DEXPANTHENOL

Dexpanthenol

DESCRIPTION

Dexpanthenol is a derivative of pantothenic acid, a B complex vitamin. Dexpanthenol is a sterile aqueous solution indicated for use as a gastrointestinal stimulant.

Each mL contains dexpanthenol 250 mg in water for injection.

Following is its chemical structure:

$$HOCH_2 - \overset{\overset{CH_3}{|}}{\underset{\underset{CH_3}{|}}{C}} - \overset{\overset{OH}{|}}{\underset{\underset{H}{|}}{C}} - CONHCH_2CH_2CH_2OH$$

CLINICAL PHARMACOLOGY

Pantothenic acid is a precursor of coenzyme A, which serves as a cofactor for a variety of enzyme-catalyzed reactions involving transfer of acetyl groups. The final step in the synthesis of acetylcholine consists of the choline acetylase transfer of an acetyl group from acetylcoenzyme A to choline. Acetylcholine is the neurohumoral transmitter in the parasympathetic system and as such maintains the normal functions of the intestine. Decrease in acetylcholine content would result in decreased peristalsis and in extreme cases adynamic ileus. The pharmacological mode of action of the drug is unknown. Pharmacokinetic data in humans are unavailable.

INDICATIONS AND USAGE

Prophylactic use immediately after major abdominal surgery to minimize the possibility of paralytic ileus. Intestinal atony causing abdominal distention; postoperative or postpartum retention of flatus, or postoperative delay in resumption of intestinal motility; paralytic ileus.

CONTRAINDICATIONS

There are no known contraindications to the use of Dexpanthenol.

WARNINGS

There have been rare instances of allergic reactions of unknown cause during the concomitant use of Dexpanthenol with drugs such as antibiotics, narcotics and barbiturates.

Administration of Dexpanthenol directly into the vein is not advised (see *"Dosage and Administration"*).

Dexpanthenol should not be administered within one hour of succnylcholine.

PRECAUTIONS

General: If any signs of a hypersensitivity reaction appear, Dexpanthenol should be discontinued. If ileus is a secondary consequence of mechanical obstruction, primary afternoon should be directed to the obstruction.

The management of adynamic ileus includes the correction of any fluid and electrolyte imbalances (especially hypokalemia), anemia and hypoproteinemia, treatment of infection, avoidance where possible of drugs which are known to decrease gastrointestinal motility and decompression of the gastrointestinal tract when considerably distended by nasogastric action or use of a long intestinal tube.

Drug Interactions: The effects of succinylcholine appeared to have been prolonged in a woman administered Dexpanthenol.

Carcinogenicity, Mutagenicity, and Impairment of Fertility: There have been no studies in animals to evaluate the carcinogenic, mutagenic, or impairment of fertility potential of Dexpanthenol.

Pregnancy: Teratogenic Effects: Pregnancy category C: Animal reproduction studies have not been conducted with Dexpanthenol. It is also not known whether Dexpanthenol can cause fetal harm when administered to a pregnant women or can affect reproduction capacity. Dexpanthenol should be given to a pregnant woman only if clearly needed.

Nursing Mothers: It is not known whether this drug is excreted in human milk. Because many drugs are excreted in human milk, caution should be exercised when Dexpanthenol is administered to a nursing woman.

Pediatric Use: Safety and effectiveness in children have not been established.

ADVERSE REACTIONS

There have been a few reports of allergic reactions and single reports of several other adverse events in association with the administration of Dexpanthenol. A causal relationship is uncertain. One patient experienced itching, tingling, difficulty in breathing. Another patient had red patches of skin. Two patients had generalized dermatitis and one patient urticaria.

One patient experienced temporary respiratory difficulty following administration of Dexpanthenol 5 minutes after succinylcholine was discontinued.

One patient experienced a noticeable but slight drop in blood pressure after administration of Dexpanthenol while in the recovery room.

One patient experienced intestinal colic one-half hour after the drug was administered.

Two patients vomited following administration and two patients had diarrhea 10 days post-surgery and after Dexpanthenol.

One elderly patient became agitated after administration of the drug.

DOSAGE AND ADMINISTRATION

Prevention of Post-Operative Adynamic Ileus: 250 mg (1 mL) or 500 (2 mL) intramuscularly. Repeat in 2 hours and then every 6 hours until all danger of adynamic ileus has passed. For 250 mg dose use ampul.

Treatment of Adynamic Ileus: 500 mg (2 mL) intramuscularly. Repeat in 2 hours and then every 6 hours as needed.

Intravenous Administration: Dexpanthenol 2 mL (500 mg) may be mixed with bulk I.V. solutions such as glucose or Lactated Ringer's and slowly infused intravenously.

Parenteral drug products should be inspected visually for particulate matter and discoloration prior to administration, whenever solution and container permit.

Storage: Protect from freezing or excessive heat. Store at controlled room temperature 15° - 30° C (50° - 86°F).

HOW SUPPLIED
INJECTION: 250 MG/ML

BRAND/MANUFACTURER	NDC	SIZE	AWP
○ **BRAND**			
DEXOL: Legere	25332-0107-10	10 ml	$12.95
○ **GENERICS**			
Schein	00364-2179-54	10 ml	$3.55
Steris	00402-0260-10	10 ml	$3.55
CMC-Cons	00223-7414-10	10 ml	$3.75
McGuff	49072-0161-10	10 ml	$3.79
Torrance	00389-0260-10	10 ml	$3.99
D-PAN: Merit	30727-0316-70	10 ml	$8.85
Pasadena	00418-1250-10	10 ml	$11.06
D-PAN: Merit	30727-0316-80	30 ml	$12.75
Amer Regent	00517-0131-25	2 ml 25s	$101.56
Schein	00364-2179-48	2 ml 25s	$131.25

INJECTION: 250 MG/2 ML

BRAND/MANUFACTURER	NDC	SIZE	AWP
○ **BRAND**			
ILOPAN: Savage	00281-2356-95	2 ml 25s	$270.05

Dextran 40

DESCRIPTION

Dextran 40 is a sterile, colloid solution for intravenous infusion. Each 100 ml consists of 10 g Dextran 40, in either 5 g dextrose or 0.9 g sodium chloride and water for injection. Dextran 40 is a plasma-volume expander.

Dextran is a branched polysaccharide composed of glucose units, formed by the action of a bacterium, *Leuconostoc mesenteroides*, on sucrose. This crude, high molecular weight dextran is then hydrolyzed and differentially fractionated to obtain Dextran fractions of varying molecular size.

The degree of branching of the Dextran fraction present in Dextran 40 is relatively low, with more than 90% of the glycosidic linkages being the 1-6 alpha type. Its weight-average molecular weight is 40,000 with more than 90% being within the range of 10,000 to 75,000. Its empirical formula is $(C_6H_{10}O_5)n$.

CLINICAL PHARMACOLOGY

ADJUNCTIVE THERAPY IN SHOCK

Regardless of the cause, shock is recognized as a failure of the circulatory system to perfuse adequately the vital tissues. Failure may result from a deficit in blood volume, an increase in capacity of the vascular bed, depression of myocardial function or, usually, a combination of these factors. Their occurrence initiates a series of functional alterations and compensatory homeostatic responses which constitute the syndrome recognized as shock.

Treatment will vary according to the cause and duration of the shock syndrome, but the aim of all therapy is to improve tissue perfusion, thereby preventing further progression of the shock state. When used in combination with other forms of therapy, Dextran 40 can contribute significantly to the improvement of circulatory function. As a hyperoncotic solution, the drug produces an immediate and short-lived expansion of plasma volume, and the low molecular weight of Dextran 40 acts to prevent or reverse the increased erythrocyte aggregation known to occur in many cases of shock. Together, these two properties of the drug act to correct the ultimate deficiency in shock, the decreased perfusion of the peripheral vascular bed.

In its adjunctive role, Dextran 40 has shown important clinical advantages for patients in shock. These include:

1. Rapid, short-lived plasma volume expansion to increase venous return to the heart.

2. Increase in arterial pressure, pulse pressure, cardiac output, and central venous pressure to help restore normal circulatory dynamics.

3. Prevention or reversal of erythrocyte aggregation, to improve microcirculatory flow, decrease resistance to flow, and increase venous return to the heart.

4. Increase in urinary output, resulting from increased renal perfusion.

Plasma Volume Expansion: The concentration of Dextran 40 equivalent in colloid osmotic pressure to normal plasma is approximately 2.5%. Since one gram of Dextran 40 will "bind" about 40 ml of water, a 10% Dextran 40 solution will cause a rapid expansion of plasma volume. The extent and duration of volume expansion produced will be dependent upon the pre-existing blood volume, the rate of infusion and the rate of Dextran clearance by the kidney. Since the renal threshold for Dextran is about 50,000 daltons, molecules with a size below that are rapidly cleared from the blood. If the excretion of the lower molecular weight portion of Dextran is considered *in vivo*, then a water retaining capacity of 20-25 ml g Dextran in circulation can be assumed for clinical application. Generally, plasma volume is increased by one to two times the volume of Dextran 40 infused and decreases from this maximum over the succeeding 12 hours.

The intense, but relatively short-lived, expansion of plasma volume produced by Dextran 40 has been found advantageous in the treatment of early shock since it acts rapidly to correct hypovolemia while allowing control of the plasma volume. Should signs of over-expansion occur, the discontinuation of the infusion will result in a decline in plasma volume due to loss of Dextran from the intravascular space.

Circulatory Dynamics: Intravenous infusion Dextran 40 into patients in shock usually results in an increase in arterial pressure, pulse pressure, cardiac output, and central venous pressure. Mean transit time, heart rate, and peripheral resistance usually are reduced. Urinary output usually increases soon after initiation of the infusion. Hematocrit is lowered in proportion to the volume of the infusion, but seldom does it fall more than 5 to 10 vol. % after 1,000 ml of Dextran 40 administered over 12 hours.

Microcirculatory Flow: Numerous animal studies have shown conclusively that small vessel flow, principally in the capillaries and post-capillary venules, is often decreased or halted in shock. Aggregates of erythrocytes are commonly observed in these vessels. Clinical confirmation of these events has been difficult to achieve, but one study using labeled erythrocytes has shown a delayed mixing of the radioactive-labeled cells with the total red cell mass in shock patients. This is believed to be due to the presence of red cell aggregates sequestered in the venous channels.

Dextran 40 has been shown to prevent or reduce cellular aggregation in both animals and humans in shock. In animal studies, it has been observed that an improvement in microcirculatory flow paralleled this effect upon cellular aggregation. This improvement is probably a result of three actions of the drug; namely, an increase in perfusion due to the increased cardiac output, a decrease in blood viscosity due to the lowered hematocrit, and a decrease in the number of erythrocyte aggregates which hinder small vessel perfusion.

Prophylaxis Against Venous Thrombosis and Thromboembolism: The infusion of Dextran 40 during and after surgical trauma reduces the incidence of deep venous thrombosis (DVT) and pulmonary embolism (PE) in patients subject to surgical procedures with a high incidence of thromboembolic complication. Unlike antithrombogenic agents of the anti-coagulant type, Dextran 40 does not achieve its effect so much by blocking the conversion of fibrinogen to fibrin but acts by simultaneously inhibiting other mechanisms essential to thrombus formation such as vascular stasis and platelet adhesiveness and by altering the structure and,

thereby, the lysability of fibrin clots. Vascular stasis has long been recognized as one of the most important conditions predisposing to thrombus formation. Dextran 40 has a number of profound effects on blood flow. Dextran 40 increases cardiac output, arterial, venous and microcirculatory flow and reduces mean transit time, chiefly by expanding plasma volume and by reducing red cell aggregation. Histopathological studies have shown that the development of a mural platelet thrombus is the first stage of thrombus formation in both the arterial and the venous system. A number of studies have demonstrated that many patients who develop thromboembolic complications also show an abnormally high-platelet adhesiveness. Infusion of Dextran 40 has been shown to reduce platelet adhesiveness as measured by various *in vitro* tests on blood samples obtained from humans and to inhibit the growth of a mural platelet thrombus at the site of experimental (laser beam) injury in the rabbit ear chamber.

Studies have shown an increase in the lysability of thrombi formed in the presence of Dextran. A consistent and characteristic alteration in fibrin structure has been observed when fibrin is formed in the presence of Dextran. Further experiments demonstrated such fibrin to be more susceptible to plasmin digestion. Other studies have shown that Dextran infused into patients during surgery increases the lysability of *ex vitro* thrombi. Controlled clinical trials have shown that thrombi in patients treated with Dextran have a more pronounced tendency to undergo lysis as determined by phlebography.

In controlled studies in which venography, lung scanning techniques, and/or clinical diagnosis were employed to determine the results of prophylaxis with Dextran 40 the incidence of DVT observed in patients undergoing elective hip surgery was substantially reduced compared to the incidence observed in untreated control patients.

The antithrombogenic action of Dextran 40 has been extensively documented in experimental investigations involving patients, healthy volunteers, and laboratory animals.

It has been shown in patients that the rise in platelet adhesiveness that normally occurs postoperatively, can be prevented and even reversed by the infusion of dextran.

Experimental studies in healthy volunteers have shown that:

1. Dextran 40, when infused at a dose of 15 ml/kg, reduces platelet adhesiveness in whole blood without simultaneously reducing the number of circulating platelets.

2. Dextran 40, when infused at a dose of 1-10 ml/kg, reduces platelet adhesiveness induced *in vitro* by the addition of ADP to platelet rich plasma. The Dextran-induced reduction in platelet adhesiveness becomes more pronounced with increasing dosages. Maximum depression of platelet adhesiveness is reached between two and five hours after infusion.

3. Unlike antithrombogenic agents of the anticoagulant type, Dextran 40 in health subjects, in doses of up to 15 ml/kg of body weight, usually produces no overall inhibition of the hemostatic system, as determined by bleeding time.

Investigations in a variety of experimental animal models (dogs, hamsters, rabbits, etc.) have produced objective evidence to show that Dextran 40:

1. Reduces the number of platelet aggregates leaving the site of laser induced injury to small vessels. This effect reaches a maximum between two and four hours after infusion and becomes more pronounced over a dosage range of 5-20 ml/kg of body weight.

2. Increases the thrombogenic threshold in blood vessels.

3. Increases the patency rate of arteries and veins that have been subjected to electrical or surgical trauma of the type that causes thrombus formation.

4. Prevents deposits of platelets and fibrin from forming on the surface of synthetic prostheses (heart valves, vascular grafts, etc.).

5. Protects platelets from thrombin induced morphological changes *in vitro*.

6. Exerts these antithrombogenic effects at doses that do not significantly alter the coagulation system.

Pharmacokinetic Information: During an infusion of Dextran 40, Dextran is evenly distributed in the vascular system. The concentration of Dextran in plasma will, therefore, depend upon:

1. Total amount infused
2. Rate of infusion
3. Clearance from plasma

A large portion of the Dextran is eliminated via the kidneys and excreted in the urine. After intravenous infusion of 500 ml of Dextran 40 in normovolemic persons, approximately 60% of the Dextran is excreted within 6 hours and about 70% within 24 hours. Tubular reabsorption of Dextran is negligible.

Of the Dextran that is not excreted via the kidneys, about 70 mg/kg of body weight is removed from the circulation per 24 hours. The main part of this is taken up by the liver where it is metabolized to CO_2 and water.

Most clinical studies and animal experiments indicate that Dextran does not cross the placental or the blood brain barrier.

INDICATIONS AND USAGE

Dextran 40 is indicated for adjunctive use in the treatment of shock, but should not replace other forms of therapy known to be of value in the treatment of shock.

Dextran 40 is indicated for use as a priming fluid, either as sole primer or as an additive, in pump oxygenators during extracorporeal circulation.

Dextran 40 is indicated for use in prophylaxis against venous thrombosis and pulmonary embolism in patients undergoing procedures known to be associated with a high incidence of thromboembolic complications, such as hip surgery.

Since Dextran has no oxygen-carrying capacity, Dextran 40 is not indicated as a replacement for whole blood or blood components if they are available.

UNLABELED USES

Dextran 40 is used alone or as an adjunct in the treatment of thrombotic thrombocytopenic purpura, intermittent claudication, to prevent postoperative thrombosis following vascular surgery or elective hip surgery or knee reconstruction. It is also used in the treatment of traumatic shock and preventing trauma-induced adult respiratory distress syndrome.

CONTRAINDICATIONS

Known hypersensitivity to Dextran: marked hemostatic defects of all types (thrombocytopenia, hypofibrinogenemia, etc.), including those caused by drugs (heparin, warfarin, etc.): marked cardiac decompensation; renal disease with severe oliguria or anuria. Decreased urinary output, secondary to shock, is not a contraindication unless there is no improvement in urine output after the initial dose of Dextran 40 (see *"Precautions"*).

WARNINGS

Although infrequent, all colloid plasma volume substitutes have the ability to cause severe and potentially fatal anaphylactic reactions (see figure). These reactions consist of severe hypotension (bp < 60 mmHg), hypotension and bradycardia (< 60 bpm), cardiac and/or respiratory arrest, and death. Hypersensitivity reactions can occur regardless of whether or not the patient had previously received a clinical Dextran solution, and they occur early in the infusion period. Since the administration of less than 1 ml of clinical dextran can cause severe reactions, a test dose is NOT recommended.

INCIDENCE OF SEVERE ANAPHYLACTIC REACTIONS CAUSED BY COLLOID VOLUME SUBSTITUTES

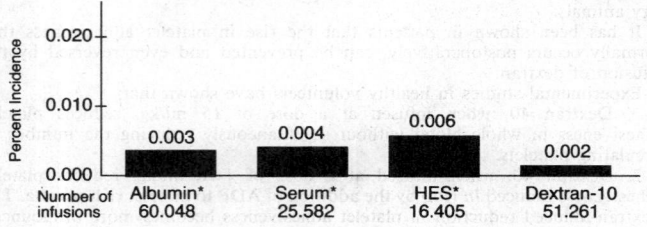

* Ring and Messmer. *Lancet* 1977.

It has been demonstrated that patients exhibiting severe hypersensitivity reactions have high titres of preformed Dextran-reactive antibodies (DRA) of the IgG type. These antibodies evidently arise in response to dietary or bacterial polysaccharides and not as the result of previous dextran administration; clinical Dextran is not immunogenic.

Dextran-induced anaphylactic reactions (DIAR) are considered to be of the immune complex anaphylaxis type, the immune complex consisting of Dextran and DRA. It has been demonstrated that a low molecular weight fraction of Dextran (MW = 1000), available under the name of Promit, can act as a monovalent hapten. A monovalent hapten can only bind to a single binding site of the bivalent antibody, thereby eliminating the prerequisite for immune complex formation and the occurrence of anaphylaxis.

To impede hypersensitivity reactions, 20 ml of Dextran 1 (Promit) is injected intravenously 1-2 minutes before the start of a Dextran 40 infusion. The time interval between the administration of Dextran 1 and Dextran 40 should not exceed 15 minutes; if a longer period has elapsed, another dose of Dextran 1 should be given. It is necessary to repeat the injection of Dextran 1 if more than 48 hours have elapsed since the last infusion of Dextran 40, was stopped. In order to assure compliance, Dextran 1 may be administered 1-2 minutes before every unit of Dextran 40.

It is strongly recommended that patients be observed closely during the early part of the infusion period. Infusion must be stopped immediately if in the judgment of the physician a hypersensitivity reaction is imminent. Resuscitative measures should be readily available for emergency administration in the event such a reaction occurs. In circulatory collapse due to anaphylaxis, rapid volume substitution with an agent other than Dextran should be initiated.

As Dextran 40 is a hypertonic colloid solution, it will attract water from the extravascular space. This fluid shift should be considered when the drug is administered intravenously to poorly hydrated patients. Noncolloidal solutions should be administered as required in order to prevent extravascular dehydration and to maintain adequate urine flow.

Renal excretion of Dextran produces an elevation in urine viscosity and specific gravity proportional to the urine Dextran concentration. In the presence of adequate urine flow only minor elevations occur, but in patients with diminished urine flow, urine viscosity and specific gravity can be increased markedly. As osmolarity is only slightly affected by the presence of Dextran molecules, it is recommended that, when desired, a patient's state of hydration be assessed by determination of urine or serum osmolarity. If signs of dehydration are noted, additional fluids should be administered. An osmotic diuretic such as mannitol has been found useful in maintaining adequate urine flow.

Renal failure, sometimes irreversible, has been reported to occur following the use of Dextran 40. While the pre-existing clinical condition of these patients could account for their oliguria and/or anuria, it is possible that the administration of Dextran 40 may have contributed to their development. Evidence of tubular vacuolization (osmotic nephrosis) has been found following Dextran 40 adminis-

tration in animals and man. While these changes appear to be reversible experimentally in animals and to be a consequence of high urine concentration of Dextran, this has not been shown in clinical use and the exact clinical significance is unknown at present.

Occasional abnormal renal and hepatic function values have been reported following intravenous administration of Dextran 40. However, the specific effect of Dextran 40 on renal and hepatic function could not be determined since most of these patients had also undergone surgery or cardiac catheterization. In a large study comparing Dextran 40 and 5% dextrose in water as pump primers in open heart surgery, one investigator reported similar elevations of SGOT (AST) and SGPT (ALT) values in both groups.

Caution should be employed when Dextran 40 is administered to patients with active hemorrhage as the resulting increase in perfusion pressure and improved microcirculatory flow may result in additional blood loss.

Administering infusions of Dextran 40 that exceed the recommended dose should be avoided, since a dose related increase in the incidence of wound hematoma, wound seroma, wound bleeding, distant bleeding (hematuria and melena), and pulmonary edema has been observed. Recommended doses should never be exceeded in patients with advanced renal disease, since excessive doses may precipitate renal failure.

PRECAUTIONS

In individuals with normal hemostatis, dosages of Dextran 40 up to 15 ml/kg body weight may produces slight changes in coagulation or bleeding time. At these dosages, slight decreases in platelet adhesiveness occur, and decreases in fibrinogen. Factor V and Factor IX are usually only slightly greater than might be expected from hemodilution alone. Although doses in this range markedly decrease Factor VIII, they generally do not prolong bleeding time significantly. Since changes in coagulation and hemostasis tend to be more pronounced following trauma or major surgery, all patients should be observed for early signs of bleeding complications.

It is recommended that close attention be paid to the hemostatic integrity of the patients who receive Dextran in the presence of other drugs known to affect coagulation, such as heparin or warfarin.

It is strongly recommended that central venous pressure be monitored frequently during the initial infusion of the drug. With monitoring, the first 500 ml may be administered rapidly but should be abruptly discontinued should there be a precipitous rise in central venous pressure. If central venous pressure is not monitored, intravenous infusion of the drug should be slower and the patient should be carefully observed for signs of circulatory overloading.

Urine output should be carefully observed. Usually, an increase in urine output occurs in oliguric patients after the administration of Dextran 40. If no increase is observed after the infusion of 500 ml of Dextran 40, the drug should be discontinued until adequate diuresis develops spontaneously or can be provoked by other means. Care should be taken to prevent a depression of the hematocrit below 30%.

In patients who have received Dextran 40, blood sugar determinations that employ high concentrations of acid may result in hydrolysis of Dextran yielding falsely elevated glucose assay results. This has been observed with both sulfuric acid and acetic acid. In other laboratory tests the presence of Dextran may result in the development of turbidity, which can interfere with the assay. This has been observed in bilirubin assays in which alcohol has been employed, in total protein assays employing biuret reagent, and in blood sugar determinations with the ortho-toluidine method. Blood typing and cross-matching procedures employing enzyme techniques may give unreliable readings if the samples are taken after infusion of Dextran 40. Other blood typing and cross-matching procedures are not affected.

It is recommended, therefore, that whenever possible, blood samples for the above determinations be drawn prior to initiating infusion of Dextran 40 or, alternatively, the laboratory be informed that the patient has received Dextran 40 so that suitable assay methods can be applied.

Since extensive use in man has not given evidence that Dextran 40 may be carcinogenic or mutagenic, no long-term studies to evaluate carcinogenic potential or mutagenic effect have been performed.

Pregnancy Category C: Animal reproduction studies have not been conducted with Dextran 40. It is also not known whether Dextran 40 can cause fetal harm when administered to a pregnant woman or can affect reproduction capacity. Dextran 40 should be given to a pregnant woman only if clearly needed, and only after preinjection of Promit (see *"Warnings"*).

Three studies (1,2,3) have shown that the administration of Dextran to women in the second and third trimester did not result in passage of Dextran through the placental barrier. In one study (4), maternal plasma concentrations of Dextran exceeding 0.25 g/100 ml resulted in some passage of Dextran into the fetal circulation. However, the other studies could not demonstrate any passage of Dextran across the placental barrier even with maternal concentration of Dextran as high as 0.74 g/100 ml plasma. No harmful effects to the fetuses from the Dextran administration were found in any of the four studies.

During labor and delivery. Dextran 40 has reportedly been used for adjunctive therapy in states of shock. A number of papers have been published about this use, but there is no information about any adverse effects from Dextran 40 on mothers or fetuses. Anaphylactic reactions in the mother, however, have been reported to cause anoxic brain damage and or death in the fetus.

It is not known whether this drug is excreted in human milk; because many drugs are excreted in human milk, caution should be exercised when Dextran 40 is administered to a nursing woman.

◆ RATED THERAPEUTICALLY EQUIVALENT; ◇ THERAPEUTIC EQUIVALENCE UNCONFIRMED; ○ UNRATED

ADVERSE REACTIONS

When Dextran 40 is used in connection with surgery, a tendency to increased bleeding complications can be expected. From clinical studies using Dextran 40 as prophylactic therapy against venous thrombosis and thromboembolism, the frequency of bleeding with any clinical consequence varies between 1 and 10%. Dextran 40 does not appear to cause more bleeding complications than other anti-thrombotic agents such as heparin, warfarin or aspirin.

Dextran 40 is relatively free of antigenic effect. However, due to cross-reacting antibodies (DRA) in some patients, immune complexes between these antibodies and dextran may form and very rarely lead to a dextran-induced anaphylactic reaction (DIAR). In two studies (5,6) the frequency of severe DIAR has been reported to be between 0.002% and 0.013% per unit of Dextran 40 given.

An extensive study (7) has shown that this incidence is reduced by a factor of 15 to 20 by pre-injection of 20 ml Dextran 1 intravenously (see "Warnings"). However, Dextran-induced anaphylactoid (allergic) reactions are not prevented by Dextran 1.

If a severe DIAR occurs, it will usually develop in the first few minutes following initiation of therapy. Therefore, the patients should be observed closely for the symptoms, generalized urticaria, nausea, vomiting, headache, fever, tightness of chest, wheezing and shock. If any of these symptoms occur, the infusion should be stopped immediately. Appropriate therapy, including epinephrine, steroids, and antihistamines, and in the case of shock, rapid volume substitution with an agent other than Dextran should be started promptly.

OVERDOSAGE

If the dosage recommendations are followed, overdosage should normally not occur. However, some individuals with borderline cardiac function sometimes cannot compensate for the increase in circulating blood volume.

If central venous pressure is monitored, the first 500 ml may be administered rapidly, but should be discontinued immediately if there is a rapid rise in venous pressure. If central venous pressure is not monitored, the infusion of Dextran 40 should be slower and the patient carefully observed for signs of circulatory overloading.

DOSAGE AND ADMINISTRATION

Infusion of Dextran 40 for any indication should begin 1-2 minutes after the intravenous administration of one vial of Dextran 1.

ADJUNCTIVE THERAPY IN SHOCK

Total dosage during the first 24 hours should not exceed 20 ml/kg of body weight. The first 500 ml should be infused rapidly (see above) with the remaining dose being administered more slowly. Should therapy continue beyond 24 hours, total daily dosage should not exceed 10 ml kg of body weight, and therapy should not continue beyond five days.

HEMODILUENT IN EXTRACORPOREAL CIRCULATION

The dosage of Dextran 40 employed in the priming fluid will vary with the volume of the pump oxygenator employed. It may be added as the sole primer or as an additive. Generally, 10 to 20 ml/kg of body weight are added to the pertusion circuit. Total dosage of Dextran 40 should not exceed 20 ml/kg of body weight.

PROPHYLACTIC THERAPY OF VENOUS THROMBOSIS AND THROMBOEMBOLISM

The dosage of Dextran 40 should be chosen according to the risk of thromboembolic complications, e.g., type of surgery and duration of immobilization. In general, treatment with Dextran 40 should be initiated during surgery; 500 to 1,000 ml (approximately 10 ml/kg body weight) should be administered on the day of operation. Treatment should be continued at a dose of 500 ml daily for an additional two to three days. Thereafter, and depending on the risk of complications, 500 ml Dextran 40 may be administered every second or third day during the period of risk for up to two weeks.

In children, the best guide to dosage is the body weight or surface area of the patient, total dosing should not exceed 15 ml/kg of body weight.

Dextran 40 is a parenteral drug product and should be inspected visually for particulate matter and discoloration prior to administration.

STORAGE

Store at 20 - 25°C (68 - 77°F).
Protect from cold.

REFERENCES

1. Kivikoski, J. Lundbom, S., and Airaksinen, J.T. The dextran concentration in the umbilical cord of a newborn infant. European Congress of Anesthesiology, Vol. 2, Copenhagen, 1966. 2. Ricketts, C.R., Cope, E., and Thomlinson, J. Dextran and the placental barrier, Br Med J 256 (5494): 1050, 1966. 3. Falk, V., Forkman. B., and Arfors, K. The permeability of the placenta to dextrans. Acta Obstet Gynecol Scand 46: 414-418, 1967. 4. Borell, U. and Aberg, B. Studies on the placental passage and excretion rate of Macrodex in pregnant women. Acta Obstet Gynecol Scand 34: 75-79, 1955. 5. Ring, J. and Messmer, K. Incidence and severity of anaphylactoid reactions to colloid volume substitutes. Lancet I: 466-469, 1977. 6. Ljungstrom, K.G., Renck, H., Strandberg, K., Hedin. H., Richter, W., and Widerlov, E. Adverse reactions to dextran in Sweden 1970-1979. Acta Chir Scand 149: 253-262, 1983. 7. Renck, H., Ljungstrom, K.G., Hedin, H., and Richter, W. Prevention of dextran-induced anaphylactic reactions by hapten inhibition. A Scandinavian multicenter study on the effects of 20 ml Dextran 1, 15%, administered before Dextran 70 or Dextran 40, Acta Chir Scand 149: 355-360, 1983.

HOW SUPPLIED

INJECTION:

AVERAGE UNIT PRICE (AVAILABLE SIZES)

BRAND	$0.17

BRAND/MANUFACTURER	NDC	SIZE	AWP
◆ BRAND			
GENTRAN 75: Baxter	00338-0265-03	500 ml 24s	$1762.92
GENTRAN 40: Baxter	00338-0270-03	500 ml 24s	$2386.32

INJECTION:

BRAND/MANUFACTURER	NDC	SIZE	AWP
○ BRAND			
RHEOMACRODEX: Pharmacia	00016-0211-65	500 ml 6s	$170.63

Dextran and Dextrose

DESCRIPTION

Dextran 40 and Dextrose is a sterile, nonpyrogenic preparation of low molecular weight Dextran (average mol. wt. 40,000) in 5% Dextrose Injection. It is also available as a 0.9% Sodium Chloride Injection. It is administered by intravenous infusion.

Also described as low viscous or low viscosity Dextran, Dextran 40 is prepared by acid hydrolysis and differential fractionation of a crude macromolecular polysaccharide produced from the fermentation of sucrose by the bacterium, Leuconostoc mesenteroides (strain B-512). The crude material is composed of linked glucose units. In the fraction represented by Dextran 40, 80% of the molecules have a molecular weight ranging from 10,000 to 90,000 (average approximately 40,000) when measured by a light scattering method. More than 90% of the linkages are of the 1,6 alpha glucosidic, straight chain type.

Each 100 mL of 10% Dextran 40 in 5% Dextrose Injection contains 10 g Dextran 40 and 5 g Dextrose hydrous in water for injection. Total osmolar concentration is 255 mOsmol/liter (calc.); pH is 3.7 (3.0—7.0).

Each 100 mL of 10% Dextran 40 in 0.9% Sodium Chloride Injection contains 10 g Dextran 40 and 0.9 g sodium chloride in water for injection. Total osmolar concentration is 310 mOsmol/liter (calc.); pH is 4.5 (3.5—7.0) (may contain sodium hydroxide and/or hydrochloric acid for pH adjustment). Electrolyte concentration per liter: Na^+ 154 mEq; Cl^- 154 mEq (not including ions for pH adjustment).

The solutions contain no bacteriostat, antimicrobial agent or added buffers (except for pH adjustment) and are intended only for single-dose injection. When smaller doses are required the unused portion should be discarded.

10% Dextran 40 is an artificial colloid pharmacologically classified as a plasma volume expander; 5% Dextrose Injection is a fluid and nutrient replenisher; 0.9% Sodium Chloride Injection is a fluid and electrolyte replenisher.

Dextran 40 is a linear glucose polymer (polysaccharide) chemically designated $(C_6H_{10}O_5)_n$.

Dextrose, USP is chemically designated D-glucose monohydrate $(C_6H_{12}O_6 \cdot H_2O)$, a hexose sugar freely soluble in water.

Sodium Chloride, USP is chemically designated NaCl, a white crystalline powder freely soluble in water.

Water for Injection, USP, is chemically designated H_2O.

The flexible plastic container is fabricated from a specially formulated polyvinylchloride. Water can permeate from inside the container into the overwrap but not in amounts sufficient to affect the solution significantly. Solutions inside the plastic container also can leach out certain of the chemical components of the plastic in very small amounts before the expiration period is attained. However, safety of the plastic has been confirmed by tests in animals according to USP biological standards for plastic containers.

Dextran HM 32% is a nonpyrogenic clear, viscid, sterile, solution of Dextran 70 (32% W/V) in Dextrose (10% W/V). Dextran 70 is that fraction of Dextran, a branched polysaccharide composed of glucose units, having a weight average molecular weight of 70,000. The fluid is electrolyte-free and non-conductive. At room temperature Dextran HM 32% has a viscosity of 220 cS.

Each 100 mL of Dextran HM 32% contains Dextran 70, 32 g and Dextrose hydrous, 10 g in water for injection. Total osmolar concentration is 509 mOsmol/liter (calc.). pH is 4.2 (3.0 to 5.5).

CLINICAL PHARMACOLOGY

The fundamental action of Dextran 40 is the enhancement of blood flow, particularly in the microcirculation. This enhancement is due to:

1. Its primary effect of volume expansion with resultant hemodilution;
2. Maintenance of the electronegativity of red blood cells;
3. Coating of red blood cells and platelets;
4. Increase in the suspension stability of blood;
5. Decrease in the viscosity of blood.

It should be emphasized that the above effects are not exerted separately, but conjointly they result in the enhancement of blood flow.

Dextran used in the treatment of shock, produces significant increases in blood volume, central venous pressure, cardiac output, stroke volume, blood pressure and urinary output. It reduces blood viscosity, peripheral resistance and improves peripheral blood flow with the release of sequestered blood cells, thereby increasing venous return to the heart.

When used as part of the pump prime for extracorporeal procedures, Dextran, as compared to whole blood, albumin 5%, or whole blood plus 5% dextrose and water, leads to less destruction of red blood cells and platelets, reduces intravascular hemagglutination and maintains erythrocyte electronegativity.

The infusion of Dextran 40 during and after surgical trauma reduces the incidence of deep venous thrombosis (DVT) and pulmonary embolism (PE) in patients subject to surgical procedures with a high incidence of thromboembolic complication. Unlike antithrombogenic agents of the anticoagulant type, Dextran does not achieve its effect so much by blocking fibrinogen-fibrin conversion but acts by simultaneously inhibiting other mechanisms essential to thrombus formation such as vascular stasis and platelet adhesiveness and by altering the structure and thereby the lysability of fibrin clots.

Histopathological studies have shown that the development of a mural platelet thrombus is the first stage of thrombus formation not only in the arterial, but also in the venous system. A number of studies have further shown that many patients who develop thromboembolic complications show an abnormally high platelet adhesiveness. Infusion of Dextran has been shown to reduce platelet adhesiveness as measured by various in vitro tests on blood samples obtained from humans and to inhibit the growth of a mural platelet thrombus at the site of experimental (laser beam) injury in the rabbit's ear chamber.

Studies have shown an increase in the lysability of thrombi formed in the presence of Dextran. A consistent and characteristic alteration in fibrin structure has been observed when fibrin is formed in the presence of Dextran, and further experiments demonstrated such fibrin to be more susceptible to plasmin digestion. Other studies have shown that Dextran infused into patients during surgery increases the lysability of ex vivo thrombi. Controlled clinical trials have shown that thrombi in patients treated with Dextran have a more pronounced tendency to undergo lysis as determined by phlebography.

Dextran is evenly distributed in the vascular system. Its distribution according to molecular weight shifts toward higher molecular weights as the smaller molecules are excreted by the kidney. In normovolemic subjects, approximately 50% is excreted within 3 hours, 60% is excreted within 6 hours and about 75% within 24 hours. Reabsorption of Dextran by the renal tubules is negligible. The unexcreted molecules of Dextran diffuse into the extravascular compartment and are temporarily taken up by the reticuloendothelial system. Some of these molecules are returned to the intravascular compartment via the lymphatics. Dextran is slowly degraded by the enzyme dextranase to glucose.

Solutions containing carbohydrate in the form of Dextrose restore blood glucose levels and provide calories. Carbohydrate in the form of Dextrose may aid in minimizing liver glycogen depletion and exerts a protein sparing action. Dextrose injected parenterally undergoes oxidation to carbon dioxide and water.

Sodium chloride in water dissociates to provide sodium (Na$^+$) and chloride (Cl$^-$) ions. Sodium (Na$^+$) is the principal cation of the extracellular fluid and plays a large part in the therapy of fluid and electrolyte disturbances. Chloride (Cl$^-$) has an integral role in buffering action when oxygen and carbon dioxide exchange occurs in red blood cells. The distribution and excretion of sodium (Na$^+$) and chloride (Cl$^-$) are largely under the control of the kidney, which maintains a balance between intake and output.

Water is an essential constituent of all body tissues and accounts for approximately 70% of total body weight. Average normal adult daily requirement ranges from two to three liters (1.0 to 1.5 liters each for insensible water loss by perspiration and urine production).

Water balance is maintained by various regulatory mechanisms. Water distribution depends primarily on the concentration of electrolytes in the body compartments and sodium (Na$^+$) plays a major role in maintaining physiologic equilibrium.

INDICATIONS AND USAGE

Dextran 40 is indicated for use in the adjunctive treatment of shock or impending shock due to hemorrhage, burns, surgery or other trauma. It is not indicated as a replacement for whole blood or blood components if they are available. It should not replace other forms of therapy known to be of value in the treatment of shock.

Dextran is also indicated for use as a priming fluid, either as a sole prime or as an additive, in pump oxygenators during extracorporeal circulation.

Dextran is also indicated for use in prophylaxis of venous thrombosis and pulmonary embolism in patients undergoing procedures known to be associated with a high incidence of thromboembolic complications, such as hip surgery.

Dextran HM 32% is indicated for use with the hysteroscope as an aid in distending the uterine cavity and in irrigating and visualizing its surfaces.

CONTRAINDICATIONS

Dextran 40 is contraindicated in patients with known hypersensitivity to Dextran, in those with marked hemostatic defects of all types (thrombocytopenia, hypofibrinogenemia, etc.) including those caused by drugs (heparin, warfarin, etc.), marked cardiac decompensation and in renal disease with severe oliguria or anuria.

NOT FOR INJECTION BY USUAL PARENTERAL ROUTES.

Dextran HM 32% should not be instilled in patients known to be hypersensitive to Dextran. All other contraindications are those related to the hysteroscopic procedure itself, such as pregnancy, endometrial carcinoma, etc.

WARNINGS

Although infrequent, severe and fatal anaphylactoid reactions consisting of marked hypotension or cardiac and respiratory arrest have been reported, most of these reactions have occurred in patients not previously exposed to intravenous Dextran and early in the infusion period. It is strongly recommended, therefore,

that patients not previously exposed to Dextran be observed closely during the first minutes of the infusion period.

Because of the seriousness of anaphylactoid reactions, it is recommended that the infusion of intravenous Dextran be stopped at the first sign of an allergic reaction provided that other means of sustaining the circulation are available. Resuscitative measures should be readily available for emergency administration in the event such a reaction occurs. In circulatory collapse due to anaphylaxis, rapid volume substitutions with an agent other than Dextran should be instituted.

Because Dextran 40 is a hypertonic colloid solution, it attracts water from the extravascular space. This shift of fluid should be considered if the drug is used for poorly hydrated patients where additional fluid therapy will be needed. If Dextran is given in excess, vascular overload could occur. The latter possibility can be avoided with careful clinical monitoring, preferably by central venous pressure.

Renal excretion of Dextran causes elevations of the specific gravity of the urine. In the presence of adequate urine flow only minor elevation will occur, whereas in patients with reduced urine output, urine viscosity and specific gravity can be increased markedly. Since urine osmolarity is only slightly increased by the presence of Dextran molecules, it is recommended that, when desired, a patient's state of hydration be assessed by determination of urine or serum osmolarity. If signs of dehydration are present, additional fluid should be administered. An osmotic diuretic such as mannitol also can be used to maintain an adequate urine flow.

Although numerous studies attest to the "nephrotonic" effect of Dextran, renal failure has been reported to occur after the use of Dextran.

Evidence of tubular vacuolization (osmotic nephrosis) has been found following Dextran administration in animals and man. While this appears to be reversible experimentally in animals and to be a consequence of high urine concentration of the drug, its exact clinical significance is presently unknown.

Occasional abnormal renal and hepatic function values have been reported following administration of Dextran. However, the specific effect of Dextran on renal and hepatic function could not be determined because most of the patients also had undergone surgery or cardiac catheterization. A comparative study of Dextran 40 and 5% Dextrose in water as pump-priming fluids in open-heart surgery has shown similar elevations of serum glutamic oxaloacetic transaminase (SGOT), aspartate aminotransferase and serum glutamic pyruvic transaminase (SGPT), alanine aminotransferase values in both groups.

Caution should be employed when Dextran is administered to patients with active hemorrhage as the resulting increase in perfusion pressure and improved microcirculatory flow may result in additional blood loss.

Administering infusions of Dextran that exceed the recommended dose should be avoided, since a dose-related increase in the incidence of wound hematoma, wound seroma, wound bleeding, distant bleeding (hematuria and melena) and pulmonary edema has been observed. Recommended doses should never be exceeded in patients with advanced renal disease, since excessive doses may precipitate renal failure.

Dextran may interfere to some extent with platelet function and should be used with caution in cases with thrombocytopenia. Transient prolongation of bleeding time and/or slightly increased bleeding tendency may occur with the administration of doses greater than 1000 mL. Care should be taken to prevent a depression of hematocrit below 30% by volume. When large volumes of Dextran are administered, plasma protein levels will be decreased.

Solutions containing sodium ions should be used with great care, if at all, in patients with congestive heart failure, severe renal insufficiency and in clinical states in which there exists edema with sodium retention.

The intravenous administration of this solution can cause fluid and/or solute overloading resulting in dilution of serum electrolyte concentrations, overhydration, congested states or pulmonary edema. The risk of dilutional states is inversely proportional to the electrolyte concentrations of administered parenteral solutions.

The risk of solute overload causing congested states with peripheral and pulmonary edema is directly proportional to the electrolyte concentrations of such solutions.

In patients with diminished renal function, administration of solutions containing sodium ions may result in sodium retention.

FOR IRRIGATION ONLY
NOT FOR INJECTION
It is possible that during hysteroscopy Dextran may leak into the peritoneal cavity, the precise amount depending on the volume of Dextran HM 32% used and the infusion pressure. Slow absorption from the peritoneal cavity (peak blood levels are reached in 3–4 days) may result in systemic effects varying from simple plasma volume expansion or a transient prolongation of the bleeding time, to severe, fatal anaphylactic reactions. It is also reported that Dextran may enter the pleural cavity through a pathway that has yet to be defined. When Dextran HM 32% is employed during diagnostic hysteroscopy adverse effects are rare. In hysteroscopic surgery greater volumes of Dextran HM 32% are infused over a longer period of time and the exposed blood vessels of the freshly traumatized endometrium allow the Dextran direct access to the systemic circulation.

There is, therefore, the potential for these patients to rapidly develop adverse systemic effects, in particular pulmonary edema. Patients are considered at increased risk of developing pulmonary edema if:
1. They undergo a surgical procedure lasting more than 45 minutes when Dextran HM 32% is being used to distend the uterus.
2. Greater than 500 mL of Dextran HM 32% are infused.
3. Large areas of endometrium are traumatized during surgery.

PRECAUTIONS

The possibility of circulatory overload should be kept in mind. Special care should be exercised in patients with impaired renal clearance of Dextran. When the risk of pulmonary edema and/or congestive heart failure may be increased, Dextran should be used with caution.

In patients with normal hemostasis, dosage of Dextran 40 approximating 15 mL/kg of body weight may prolong bleeding time and depress platelet function. Dosages in this range also markedly decrease factor VIII, and decrease factors V and IX to a greater degree than would be expected to occur from hemodilution alone. Since these changes tend to be more pronounced following trauma or major surgery, patients should be observed for early signs of bleeding complications.

Since increased rouleaux formation may occur in the presence of Dextran, it is recommended that blood samples be drawn for typing and cross-matching prior to the infusion of Dextran and reserved for subsequent use if necessary. If blood is drawn after infusion of Dextran, the saline agglutination and indirect antiglobulin methods may be used for typing and cross-matching. Difficulty may be encountered when proteolytic enzyme techniques are used to match blood.

Consideration should be given to withdrawal of blood for chemical laboratory tests prior to initiating therapy with Dextran because of the following:

1. Blood sugar determinations that employ high concentrations of acid may result in hydrolysis of Dextran, yielding falsely elevated glucose assay results. This has been observed both with sulfuric acid and with acetic acid.

2. In other laboratory tests, the presence of Dextran in the blood may result in the development of turbidity, which can interfere with the assay. This has been observed in bilirubin assays in which alcohol is employed and in total protein assays employing biuret reagent.

Solutions containing Dextrose should be used with caution in patients with known subclinical or overt diabetes mellitus.

Caution must be exercised in the administration of parenteral fluids, especially those containing sodium ions, to patients receiving corticosteroids or corticotropin.

Do not administer unless solution is clear and container is undamaged. Discard unused portion.

Pregnancy Category C: Animal reproduction studies have not been conducted with Dextran 40 in Dextrose or sodium chloride. It is also not known whether Dextran 40 in Dextrose or sodium chloride can cause fetal harm when administered to a pregnant woman or can affect reproduction capacity. 10% Dextran 40 in Dextrose or sodium chloride should be given to a pregnant woman only if clearly needed.

Nursing Mothers: It is not known whether this drug is excreted in human milk. Because many drugs are excreted in human milk, caution should be exercised when 10% Dextran 40 in Dextrose or sodium chloride is administered to a nursing woman.

Drug Interactions: Additive medications should not be delivered via plasma volume expanders.

ADVERSE REACTIONS

Antigenicity of Dextrans is directly related to their degree of branching. Since Dextran 40 has a low degree of branching, it is relatively free of antigenic effect. However, a few individuals have experienced mild urticarial reactions. More severe reactions, consisting of severe anaphylactoid reaction, generalized urticaria, tightness of the chest, wheezing, hypotension, nausea and vomiting may occur in rare instances. Symptoms and signs of adverse systemic reaction may be relieved by parenteral administration of antihistamines, ephedrine or epinephrine, while other means of shock therapy are instituted. The route of administration and dosages of the therapeutic agent selected will depend upon the severity and rapidity of progression of the reaction.

Reactions which may occur because of the solution or the technique of administration include febrile response, infection at the site of injection, venous thrombosis or phlebitis extending from the site of injection, extravasation and hypervolemia.

If an adverse reaction does occur, discontinue the infusion, evaluate the patient, institute appropriate therapeutic countermeasures, and save the remainder of the fluid for examination if deemed necessary (see *"Warnings"* for treatment of anaphylactic shock). The following adverse reactions, although rare, have been reported for Dextran HM 32%: fatal anaphylactic reaction, generalized itching, macular rash, urticaria, nasal congestion, flushing, hypotension, dyspnea, tightness of chest, cyanosis, wheezing, coughing, peripheral edema, pulmonary edema, pleural effusion, ascites, nausea, vomiting, fever, joint pains, oliguria, convulsions and increased clotting time.

Should any adverse reaction occur, discontinue the irrigant, evaluate the patient, institute appropriate therapeutic countermeasures and save the remainder of the fluid for examination if deemed necessary.

DOSAGE AND ADMINISTRATION

Dextran 40 is administered by I.V. infusion only.

1. *In shock,* it is suggested that total dosage not exceed 20 mL/kg during the first 24 hours. The first 10 mL/kg may be infused as rapidly as necessary to effect improvement. It is strongly recommended that central venous pressure be monitored frequently during the initial infusion of the drug. Should therapy continue beyond 24 hours, subsequent dosage should not exceed 10 mL/kg per day and therapy should not continue beyond five days.

2. *In extracorporeal perfusion,* the dosage of Dextran used will vary with the volume of the pump oxygenator. Dextran can serve as a sole primer or as an additive to other priming fluids. Generally 10 to 20 mL of a 10% solution (1 to 2

g) of Dextran per kilogram of body weight are added to the perfusion circuit. Usually total dosage should not exceed 2 g/kg of body weight.

3. *In prophylaxis of venous thrombosis and thromboembolism,* the dosage of Dextran should be chosen according to the risk of thromboembolic complications, e.g., type of surgery and duration of immobilization. In general, treatment should be initiated during surgery; 500 to 1000 mL (approximately 10 mL/kg of body weight) should be administered on the day of operation. Treatment should be continued at a dose of 500 mL daily for an additional two to three days; then, according to the risk of complications, 500 mL may be given every second or third day during the period of risk, for up to two weeks.

4. Infants may be given 5 mL per kg body weight and children 10 mL per kg. Parenteral drug products should be inspected visually for particulate matter and discoloration prior to administration, whenever solution and container permit. See *"Precautions"*.

Note: When infusing concentrated Dextran, the administration set should include a filter.

INSTRUCTIONS FOR USE

To Open

Tear outer wrap at notch and remove solution container. Some opacity of the plastic due to moisture absorption during the sterilization process may be observed. This is normal and does not affect solution quality or safety. The opacity will diminish gradually.

PREPARATION FOR ADMINISTRATION

(Use aseptic technique)

1. Close flow control clamp of administration set.
2. Remove cover from outlet port at bottom of container.
3. Insert piercing pin of administration set into port with a twisting motion until the set is firmly seated. *Note:* See full directions on administration set carton.
4. Suspend container from hanger.
5. Squeeze and release drip chamber to establish proper fluid level in drip chamber.
6. Open flow control clamp and clear air from set. Close clamp.
7. Attach set to venipuncture device. If device is not indwelling, prime and make venipuncture.
8. Regulate rate of administration with flow control clamp.

The amount of Dextran HM 32% required depends on a number of factors, including the type and length of the procedure and whether manipulation or surgery is performed. Usually the amount of Dextran HM 32% instilled into the uterus for diagnosis will be between 50 mL and 100 mL. Dextran HM 32% should be introduced into the uterine cavity through the cannula of a hysteroscope under low pressure (approximately 100 mm Hg) until the uterus is sufficiently distended to permit adequate visualization. During the hysteroscopic examination, Dextran HM 32% should be infused at a rate that keeps the cavity suitably distended. To avoid injection of the fluid into the tissues of the uterus and parametria and to prevent unnecessary amounts of the fluid leaking into the peritoneal cavity and backwards along the side of the hysteroscope, infusion pressures should not exceed 150 mm Hg.

Note: Dextran HM 32% has as tendency to crystallize when subjected to temperature variations or when stored for long periods. If flakes are present, heat at 100—110° C until complete dissolution is achieved.

WARNING: Do not use flexible container in series connections.

Do not use if crystallization has occurred.

STORAGE

Exposure of pharmaceutical products to heat should be minimized. Avoid excessive heat. Protect from freezing. It is recommended that the product be stored at room temperature 25°C (77°F); however, brief exposure up to 40°C (104°F) does not adversely affect the product.

J CODES

500 ml IV—J7110
500 ml IV—J7100

HOW SUPPLIED

INJECTION: 10%

BRAND/MANUFACTURER	NDC	SIZE	AWP
○ **BRAND**			
LMD W/5% DEXTROSE: Abbott Hosp	00074-7418-03	500 ml 12s	$1432.98
LMD W/0.9% SODIUM CHLORIDE: Abbott Hosp	00074-7419-03	500 ml 12s	$1432.98

INJECTION: 32%

BRAND/MANUFACTURER	NDC	SIZE	AWP
○ **GENERICS**			
Abbott Hosp	00074-8085-01	100 ml 5s	$178.01

Dextran-1

DESCRIPTION

Dextran-1 is a sterile, nonpyrogenic solution for intravenous injection. Each mL contains 150 mg Dextran-1, 6 mg sodium chloride, hydrochloric acid adjusted to pH 4.5 and water for injection.

➤ SHOWN IN PRODUCT IDENTIFICATION GUIDE

Dextran-1 is an alpha 1-6 linked glucose polymer having a weight average molecular weight of 1,000. Dextran-1 is formed, as are the other Dextrans, by the action of a bacterium. Leuconostoc mesenteroides, on sucrose. The crude Dextrans produced are then hydrolyzed and differentially fractionated to obtain Dextran fractions of desired molecular weights.

The empirical formula of Dextran-1 is $(C_6H_{10}O_5)n$.

CLINICAL PHARMACOLOGY

Dextran-1 behaves as a monovalent hapten. It reacts with dextran-reactive immunoglobulin (IgG) without bridge formation and, therefore, with no tendency for the formation of large immune complexes. A polyvalent hapten may form complexes with antibodies as an antigen does, but a monovalent hapten can only bind to individual combining sites of antibodies, thereby eliminating the prerequisite for immune complex formation. In this way, a molar excess of monovalent hapten given just prior to the I.V. administration of a clinical dextran solution competitively prevents the formation of immune complexes with the polyvalent clinical dextrans, and thus, impedes occurrence of anaphylaxis. From an immunological viewpoint, protection against anaphylactic dextran reactions is provided in two ways. During the initial phase of the infusion of clinical dextrans, protection is effected by hapten inhibition with Dextran-1.

During the later phase of the dextran infusion and on the following day, protection is exerted by the dextran molecules in the clinical Dextran solutions due to the fact that an antigen excess (higher concentration of dextran compared to Dextran-reactive antibodies) develops in the circulation and only small non-anaphylactogenic immune complexes can be formed. Forty-eight (48) hours after the infusion of one unit of clinical dextran, the concentration of clinical Dextran in the serum has decreased and the concentration of free Dextran-reactive antibodies may increase so that the risk of formation of large anaphylactogenic immune complexes arises again upon infusion of another dose of clinical Dextran. An additional injection of Dextran-1 is therefore recommended if 48 hours or more has elapsed since the previous infusion of clinical Dextran.

Because of its low molecular weight, Dextran-1 is rapidly and completely excreted by glomerular filtration. After I.V. injection of a single dose of 20 ml, about 50 percent of the original concentration is cleared from the blood within 30 minutes. The mean urinary elimination half-life was found to be 41 ± 11 minutes in 12 normal healthy individuals.

Dextran-induced anaphylactic reactions (DIAR) are reactions involving formation of immune complexes between circulating dextran-reactive antibodies of the IgG class and clinical dextran. Two large retrospective studies [1,2] have shown the incidence of severe DIAR to be in the range of 0.002-0.025% per unit used (0.002-0.013% for Dextran 40 and 0.017-0.025% for Dextran 60/75). In a smaller prospective study involving the preoperative use of low-dose heparin and Dextran 70 the incidence of severe DIAR was 0.25% per patient treated[3]. By means of hapten (Dextran-1) inhibition, the incidence of these reactions has been calculated to be 15 to 20 times lower.[4]

INDICATIONS AND USAGE

Dextran-1 is indicated for the prophylaxis of serious anaphylactic reactions in connection with the I.V. infusion of clinical dextran solutions. By means of hapten (Dextran-1) inhibition, the incidence of these reactions is significantly reduced[4]. (See "Clinical Pharmacology").

Mild dextran-induced anaphylactic (allergic) reactions are not prevented by Dextran-1.

CONTRAINDICATIONS

There are no known contraindications to Dextran-1.

If the I.V. administration of clinical Dextran solutions is contraindicated, Dextran-1 should not be given.

Contraindications for clinical Dextran solutions include marked hemostatic defects of all types or hemorrhagic tendencies, marked cardiac decompensation and renal disease with severe oliguria or anuria.

WARNINGS

In a population of more than 70,000 patients[4,5,6] receiving Dextran-1, two severe adverse reactions were noted. One patient experienced severe hypotension (systolic B.P. < 60 mmHg) and one experienced bradycardia with severe hypotension after Dextran-1 administration. The routine clinical use of Dextran-1 to date has involved only one severe and fatal reaction, which was reported in a patient with pre-existing cardiac disease (see "Contraindications").

PRECAUTIONS

If any reaction to Dextran-1 occurs, clinical dextran solutions should not be administered.

Pregnancy: Teratogenic Effects

Pregnancy Category B: Reproduction studies have been performed in the mouse and rabbit at doses up to 70 times the human dose. The studies in the mouse revealed no evidence of impaired fertility or harm to the fetus due to Dextran-1. At high doses i.e., 35 times the human dose or higher, there was increased incidence of fetal resorption and post-implantation fetal loss in the rabbit. At 70 times the human dose, there was also retardation of fetal long-bone ossification and marginal retardation of fetal growth in the rabbit, but fetal morphology was unaffected by the treatment. There are, however, no adequate and well controlled studies in pregnant women. Because animal reproduction studies are not always predictive of human response, this drug should be used during pregnancy only if clearly needed.

Pregnancy: Nonteratogenic Effects

It is not known whether Dextran-1 is excreted in human milk. Because many drugs are excreted in human milk, caution should be exercised when Dextran-1 is administered to a nursing woman.

ADVERSE REACTIONS

The potential of Dextran-1 to cause adverse reactions was investigated in three trials[4,5,6] involving a total of 70,351 patients. Effects observed following the injection of Dextran-1 consisted of: cutaneous reactions in eleven (0.016%) patients; moderate hypotension (systolic b.p. > 60 mm Hg) in ten (0.014%) patients; severe hypotension (systolic b.p. < 60 mm Hg) in one (0.001%) patient; bradycardia (> 60 bpm) and moderate hypotension in nine (0.013%) patients; bradycardia and severe hypotension in one (0.001%) patient; and bradycardia alone in 3 (0.004%) patients. In the same studies, eight (0.011%) patients reacted to Dextran-1 with nausea, pallor and shivering. In routine clinical use to date, Dextran-1 has not been attended by adverse reactions that differ in either character or frequency from those already reported in these three studies. However, its use in one patient with pre-existing coronary atherosclerosis and left ventricular hypertrophy may have resulted in fatal circulatory collapse. A subsequent infusion of clinical dextran should not be administered if an adverse reaction to Dextran-1 is observed.

OVERDOSAGE

Human data concerning overdosage with Dextran-1 are unavailable. Dextran-1 is rapidly cleared by renal excretion and any overdosage, therefore, should be of short duration and of minimal consequence.

The acute I.V. injection of Dextran-1 at a dose of 50 ml/kg (approximately 170 times the human therapeutic dose) was tolerated without effect in mice and rabbits.

Repeated dose studies in which dogs and rabbits received doses of Dextran-1 I.V. for two weeks at 22 and 60 times, respectively, the human therapeutic dose demonstrated a very low potential for toxicity. Toxicity was not demonstrated in the dog, and in the rabbit only osmotic nephrosis was found.

DOSAGE AND ADMINISTRATION

Adults: Administer 20 ml of Dextran-1 intravenously 1-2 minutes before the I.V. infusion of clinical dextran solutions.

Children: 0.3 ml per kg body weight in a corresponding manner.

Dextran-1 should be injected before starting an infusion of clinical dextran. Dextran-1 must NOT be diluted or admixed with clinical dextran.

The time interval between the administration of Dextran-1 and clinical dextran solutions should not exceed 15 minutes; if a longer period has elapsed, another dose of Dextran-1 should be given.

It is necessary to repeat the injection of Dextran-1 if more than 48 hours have elapsed since the last infusion of clinical dextran solution was stopped. In order to insure compliance, Dextran-1 may be administered 1-2 minutes before every I.V. clinical dextran infusion.

I. Utilizing Needle and Syringe

If using a needle and syringe, 20 ml of Dextran-1 should be administered by rapid intravenous injection 1-2 minutes before the infusion of clinical dextran solutions.

II. Utilizing Y Injection Site or Gum Rubber Injection Site of an Existing I.V.

As an alternative, Dextran-1 may be administered I.V. through a Y or gum rubber injection site, providing that there is minimal dilution of Dextran-1 with the primary solution. Dextran-1 should not be administered through an I.V. set that has been used to infuse clinical dextran solutions.

III. Other Hospital Accepted I.V. Procedures

Other hospital accepted procedures may be used providing that Dextran-1 is administered in a manner corresponding to the procedures outlined in Sections I and II.

Parenteral drug products should be inspected visually for particulate matter and discoloration prior to administration, whenever solution and container permit.

Storage: Store at room temperature, preferably not exceeding 25° C. Protect from freezing.

REFERENCES
1. Ring, J. and Messmer, K. Incidence and Severity of Anaphylactoid Reactions of Colloid Volume Substitutes Lancet I: 466-469, 1977. 2. Ljungstroem, K.G., Renck, H. Strandberg, K., Hedin, H. Richter, W. and Widerloev, E. Adverse Reactions to Dextran in Sweden 1970-1979. Acts Chir Scan 149:253-262, 1983. 3. Gruber, U.F., Saldeen, T., Brokop, T., et al. Incidences of fatal postoperative pulmonary embolism after prophylaxis with dextran 70 and low-dose heparin: an international multicentre study. Br Med J 10: 69-77, 1980. 4. Renck, H., Ljungstroem, K.G., Hedin., and Richter, W. Prevention of Dextran Induced-Anaphylactic Reactions by Hapten Inhibition. A Scandinavian Multicenter Study of the Effects of 20 ml Dextran 1, 15%, Administered before Dextran 70 or Dextran 40. Acts Chir Scand 149: 355-360, 1983. 5. Ljungstroem, K.G., Renck, H., Hedin., H., Richter, W. and Roseberg, B. Prevention of Dextran Induced-Anaphylactic Reactions by Hapten Inhibition. A Scandinavian Multicenter Study on the Effects of 10 ml Dextran 1, 15%, Administered before Dextran 70 or Dextran 40. Acts Chir Scand 149: 341-348, 1983. 6. Renck, H., Ljungstroem, K.G., Roseberg, B., Dhuner, K.G., and Dahl, S. Prevention of Dextran Induced-Anaphylactic Reactions by Hapten Inhibition. A Comparison of the Effects of 20 ml Dextran 1, 15%. Administered either Admixed to or before Dextran 70 or Dextran 40. Acts Chir Scand 149: 349-353, 1983.

◆ RATED THERAPEUTICALLY EQUIVALENT; ◇ THERAPEUTIC EQUIVALENCE UNCONFIRMED; ○ UNRATED

BRAND/MANUFACTURER	NDC	SIZE	AWP
○ GENERICS			
PROMIT: Pharmacia	00016-0200-20	20 ml 6s	$51.00

BRAND/MANUFACTURER	NDC	SIZE	AWP
○ BRAND			
HYSKON: Pharmacia	00016-0231-62	250 ml 6s	$408.78
	00016-0231-61	100 ml 12s	$349.56

Dextran-70 in Dextrose

DESCRIPTION
Dextran-70/Dextrose Hysteroscopy Fluid is a clear, viscid, sterile, non-pyrogenic solution of dextran-70 (32% W/V) in dextrose (10% W/V). Dextran-70 is that fraction of Dextran, a branched polysaccharide composed of glucose units, having a weight average molecular weight of 70,000. The fluid is electrolyte-free and non-conductive. At room temperature Dextran-70/Dextrose Hysteroscopy Fluid has a viscosity of 220 cS.

Dextran-70/Dextrose has a tendency to crystalize when subjected to temperature variations or when stored for long periods. If flakes of dextran are present, heat at 100°-110° C until complete dissolution is achieved.

INDICATIONS
Dextran-70/Dextrose Hysteroscopy Fluid is indicated for use with the hysteroscope as an aid in distending the uterine cavity and in irrigating and visualizing its surfaces.

CONTRAINDICATIONS
Dextran-70/Dextrose Hysteroscopy Fluid should not be instilled in patients known to hypersensitive to Dextran. All other contraindications are those related to the hysteroscopic procedure itself, such as pregnancy, endometrial carcinoma, etc.

WARNINGS
It is possible that during hysteroscopy dextran may leak into the peritoneal cavity, the precise amount depending on the volume of Dextran-70/Dextrose used and the infusion pressure. Slow absorption from the peritoneal cavity (peak blood levels are reached in 3-4 days) (1) may result in systemic effects varying from simple plasma volume expansion or a transient prolongation of the bleeding time, to severe, fatal anaphylactic reactions. It is also reported that dextran may enter the pleural cavity through a pathway that has yet to be defined (2). When Dextran-70/Dextrose is employed during diagnostic hysteroscopy adverse effects are rare. In hysteroscopic surgery greater volumes of Dextran-70/Dextrose are infused over a longer period of time and the exposed blood vessels of the freshly traumatized endometrium allow the dextran direct access to the systemic circulation.

There is therefore, the potential for these patients to rapidly develop adverse systemic effects, in particular pulmonary edema (3). Patients are considered at increased risk of developing pulmonary edema if:
1. They undergo a surgical procedure lasting more than 45 minutes when Dextran-70/Dextrose is being used to distend the uterus.
2. Greater than 500 ml of Dextran-70/Dextrose are infused.
3. Large areas of endometrium are traumatized during surgery.

ADVERSE REACTIONS
The following adverse reactions, although rare, have been reported for Dextran-70/Dextrose: fatal anaphylactic reaction, generalized itching, macular rash, urticaria, nasal congestion, flushing, hypotension, dyspnea, tightness of chest, cyanosis, wheezing, coughing, peripheral edema, pulmonary edema, pleural effusion, ascites, nausea, vomiting, fever, joint pains, oliguria, convulsions and increased clotting time.

DOSAGE AND ADMINISTRATION
The amount of Dextran-70/Dextroscopy Fluid required depends on a number of factors, including the type and length of the procedure and whether manipulation or surgery is performed. Usually, the amount of Dextran-70/Dextrose instilled into the uterus will be between 50 mL and 100 mL.

Dextran-70/Dextrose should be introduced into the uterine cavity through the cannula of a hysteroscope under low pressure (approximately 100 mm Hg) until the uterus is sufficiently distended to permit adequate visualization. During the hysteroscopic examination, Dextran-70/Dextrose should be infused at a rate that keeps the cavity suitably distended. To avoid injection of the fluid into the tissues of the uterus and parametria and to prevent unnecessary amounts of the fluid leaking into the peritoneal cavity and backwards along the side of the hysteroscope, infusion pressures should not exceed 150 mm Hg.

Store at 20-25°C (68-77°F). Protect from cold.

REFERENCES
1. Cleary R.E., Howard T., diZerega G.S.: Plasma dextran levels after abdominal instillation of 32% dextran 70: Evidence for prolonged intraperitoneal retention. Submitted for publication, 1984. 2. Adoni A., Adatto-Levy R., Mogle P., Palti Z.: Post-operative pleural effusion caused by dextran. Int J Gyn Obs 18:243, 1980. 3. Flores E., Neuwirth R.S.: Acute pulmonary edema occurring after a hysteroscopic surgical procedure using Dextran-70/Dextrose as the distending medium. Submitted for publication, 1984.

Dextroamphetamine Sulfate

> **WARNING**
> AMPHETAMINES HAVE A HIGH POTENTIAL FOR ABUSE. THEY SHOULD THUS BE TRIED ONLY IN WEIGHT REDUCTION PROGRAMS FOR PATIENTS IN WHOM ALTERNATIVE THERAPY HAS BEEN INEFFECTIVE. ADMINISTRATION OF AMPHETAMINES FOR PROLONGED PERIODS OF TIME IN OBESITY MAY LEAD TO DRUG DEPENDENCE AND MUST BE AVOIDED. PARTICULAR ATTENTION SHOULD BE PAID TO THE POSSIBILITY OF SUBJECTS OBTAINING AMPHETAMINES FOR NONTHERAPEUTIC USE OR DISTRIBUTION TO OTHERS, AND THE DRUGS SHOULD BE PRESCRIBED OR DISPENSED SPARINGLY.

DESCRIPTION
Dextroamphetamine Sulfate is the dextro isomer of the compound d,l-amphetamine sulfate, a sympathomimetic amine of the amphetamine group. Chemically, Dextroamphetamine Sulfate is d-alpha-methylphenethylamine, and is present in all forms as the neutral sulfate.

CAPSULES
Each sustained release capsule is so prepared that an initial dose is released promptly and the remaining medication is released gradually over a prolonged period.

Each capsule, contains Dextroamphetamine Sulfate as follows: 5 mg, 10 mg, 15 mg.

TABLETS
Each tablet contains Dextroamphetamine Sulfate, 5 mg.

Following is its chemical structure:

CLINICAL PHARMACOLOGY
Amphetamines are noncatecholamine, sympathomimetic amines with CNS stimulant activity. Peripheral actions include elevations of systolic and diastolic blood pressures and weak bronchodilator and respiratory stimulant action.

There is neither specific evidence which clearly establishes the mechanism whereby amphetamines produce mental and behavioral effects in children, nor conclusive evidence regarding how these effects relate to the condition of the central nervous system.

Drugs of this class used in obesity are commonly known as "anorectics" or "anorexigenics." It has not been established, however, that the action of such drugs in treating obesity is primarily one of appetite suppression. Other central nervous system actions, or metabolic effects, may be involved, for example.

Adult obese subjects instructed in dietary management and treated with "anorectic" drugs lose more weight on the average than those treated with placebo and diet, as determined in relatively short-term clinical trials.

The magnitude of increased weight loss of drug-treated patients over placebo-treated patients is only a fraction of a pound a week. The rate of weight loss is greatest in the first weeks of therapy for both drug and placebo subjects and tends to decrease in succeeding weeks. The origins of the increased weight loss due to the various possible drug effects are not established. The amount of weight loss associated with the use of an "anorectic" drug varies from trial to trial, and the increased weight loss appears to be related in part to variables other than the drug prescribed, such as the physician-investigator, the population treated and the diet prescribed. Studies do not permit conclusions as to the relative importance of the drug and nondrug factors on weight loss. The natural history of obesity is measured in years, whereas the studies cited are restricted to a few weeks' duration; thus, the total impact of drug-induced weight loss over that of diet alone must be considered clinically limited.

Dextroamphetamine Sulfate capsules are formulated to release the active drug substance *in vivo* in a more gradual fashion than the standard formulation, as demonstrated by blood levels. The formulation has not been shown superior in effectiveness over the same dosage of the standard, noncontrolled-release formulations given in divided doses.

PHARMACOKINETICS
Tablet—The single ingestion of two 5 mg tablets by healthy volunteers produced an average peak Dextroamphetamine Sulfate blood level of 29.2 ng/mL at 2 hours post-administration. The average half-life was 10.25 hours. The average urinary recovery was 45% in 48 hours.

➤ SHOWN IN PRODUCT IDENTIFICATION GUIDE

Capsule—Ingestion of a capsule containing 15 mg radiolabeled Dextroamphetamine Sulfate by healthy volunteers produced a peak blood level of radioactivity, on the average, at 8 to 10 hours post-administration with peak urinary recovery seen at 12 to 24 hours.

INDICATIONS AND USAGE
Dextroamphetamine Sulfate is indicated:

1. In Narcolepsy.

2. In Attention Deficit Disorder with Hyperactivity, as an integral part of a total treatment program which typically includes other remedial measures (psychological, educational, social) for a stabilizing effect in children with a behavioral syndrome characterized by the following group of developmentally inappropriate symptoms: moderate to severe distractibility, short attention span, hyperactivity, emotional lability, and impulsivity. The diagnosis of this syndrome should not be made with finality when these symptoms are only of comparatively recent origin. Nonlocalizing (soft) neurological signs, learning disability, and abnormal EEG may or may not be present, and a diagnosis of central nervous system dysfunction may or may not be warranted.

CONTRAINDICATIONS
Advanced arteriosclerosis, symptomatic cardiovascular disease, moderate to severe hypertension, hyperthyroidism, known hypersensitivity or idiosyncrasy to the sympathomimetic amines, glaucoma.

Agitated states.

Patients with a history of drug abuse.

During or within 14 days following the administration of monoamine oxidase inhibitors (hypertensive crises may result).

WARNING
When tolerance to the "anorectic" effect develops, the recommended dose should not be exceeded in an attempt to increase the effect; rather, the drug should be discontinued.

PRECAUTIONS
General: Caution is to be exercised in prescribing amphetamines for patients with even mild hypertension.

The least amount feasible should be prescribed or dispensed at one time in order to minimize the possibility of overdosage.

Certain brands of Dextroamphetamine Sulfate contain FD&C Yellow No. 5 (tartrazine), which may cause allergic-type reactions (including bronchial asthma) in certain susceptible individuals. Although the overall incidence of FD&C Yellow No. 5 (tartrazine) sensitivity in the general population is low, it is frequently seen in patients who also have aspirin hypersensitivity.

Information for Patients: Amphetamines may impair the ability of the patient to engage in potentially hazardous activities such as operating machinery or vehicles; the patient should therefore be cautioned accordingly.

DRUG INTERACTIONS
Acidifying agents—Gastrointestinal acidifying agents (guanethidine, reserpine, glutamic acid HCl, ascorbic acid, fruit juices, etc.) lower absorption of amphetamines. Urinary acidifying agents (ammonium chloride, sodium acid phosphate, etc.) increase the concentration of the ionized species of the amphetamine molecule, thereby increasing urinary excretion. Both groups of agents lower blood levels and efficacy of amphetamines.

Adrenergic blockers—Adrenergic blockers are inhibited by amphetamines.

Alkalinizing agents—Gastrointestinal alkalinizing agents (sodium bicarbonate, etc.) increase absorption of amphetamines. Urinary alkalinizing agents (acetazolamide, some thiazides) increase the concentration of the non-ionized species of the amphetamine molecule, thereby decreasing urinary excretion. Both groups of agents increase blood levels and therefore potentiate the actions of amphetamines.

Antidepressants, tricyclic—Amphetamines may enhance the activity of tricyclic or sympathomimetic agents Dextroamphetamine Sulfate with desipramine or protriptyline and possibly other tricyclics cause striking and sustained increases in the concentration of Dextroamphetamine Sulfate in the brain; cardiovascular effects can be potentiated.

MAO inhibitors—MAOI antidepressants, as well as a metabolite of furazolidone, slow amphetamine metabolism. This slowing potentiates amphetamines, increasing their effect on the release of norepinephrine and other monoamines from adrenergic nerve endings; this can cause headaches and other signs of hypertensive crisis. A variety of neurological toxic effects and malignant hyperpyrexia can occur, sometimes with fatal results.

Antihistamines—Amphetamines may counteract the sedative effect of antihistamines.

Antihypertensives—Amphetamines may antagonize the hypotensive effects of antihypertensives.

Chlorpromazine—Chlorpromazine blocks dopamine and norepinephrine reuptake, thus inhibiting the central stimulant effects of amphetamines, and can be used to treat amphetamine poisoning.

Ethosuximide—Amphetamines may delay intestinal absorption of ethosuximide.

Haloperidol—Haloperidol blocks dopamine and norepinephrine reuptake, thus inhibiting the central stimulant effects of amphetamines.

Lithium carbonate—The antiobesity and stimulatory effects of amphetamines may be inhibited by lithium carbonate.

Meperidine—Amphetamines potentiate the analgesic effect of meperidine.

Methenamine therapy—Urinary excretion of amphetamines is increased, and efficacy is reduced, by acidifying agents used in methenamine therapy.

Norepinephrine—Amphetamines enhance the adrenergic effect of norepinephrine.

Phenobarbital—Amphetamines may delay intestinal absorption of phenobarbital; co-administration of phenobarbital may produce a synergistic anticonvulsant action.

Phenytoin—Amphetamines may delay intestinal absorption of phenytoin; co-administration of phenytoin may produce a synergistic anticonvulsant action.

Propoxyphene—In cases of propoxyphene overdosage, amphetamine CNS stimulation is potentiated and fatal convulsions can occur.

Veratrum alkaloids—Amphetamines inhibit the hypotensive effect of veratrum alkaloids.

DRUG/LABORATORY TEST INTERACTIONS
■ Amphetamines can cause a significant elevation in plasma corticosteroid levels. This increase is greatest in the evening.

■ Amphetamines may interfere with urinary steroid determinations.

Carcinogenesis/Mutagenesis: Mutagenicity studies and long-term studies in animals to determine the carcinogenic potential of Dextroamphetamine Sulfate have not been performed.

Pregnancy—Teratogenic Effects: Pregnancy Category C. Dextroamphetamine Sulfate has been shown to have embryotoxic and teratogenic effects when administered to A/Jax mice and C57BL mice in doses approximately 41 times the maximum human dose. Embryotoxic effects were not seen in New Zealand white rabbits given the drug in doses 7 times the human dose nor in rats given 12.5 times the maximum human dose. There are no adequate and well-controlled studies in pregnant women. Dextroamphetamine Sulfate should be used during pregnancy only if the potential benefit justifies the potential risk to the fetus.

Nonteratogenic Effects: Infants born to mothers dependent on amphetamines have an increased risk of premature delivery and low birth weight. Also, these infants may experience symptoms of withdrawal as demonstrated by dysphoria, including agitation, and significant lassitude.

Nursing Mothers: Amphetamines are excreted in human milk. Mothers taking amphetamines should be advised to refrain from nursing.

Pediatric Use: Long-term effects of amphetamines in children have not been well established.

Amphetamines are not recommended for use as anorectic agents in children under 12 years of age, or in children under 3 years of age with Attention Deficit Disorder with Hyperactivity described under *"Indications and Usage".*

Clinical experience suggests that in psychotic children, administration of amphetamines may exacerbate symptoms of behavior disturbance and thought disorder.

Amphetamines have been reported to exacerbate motor and phonic tics and Tourette's syndrome. Therefore, clinical evaluation for tics and Tourette's syndrome in children and their families should precede use of stimulant medications.

Data are inadequate to determine whether chronic administration of amphetamines may be associated with growth inhibition: therefore, growth should be monitored during treatment.

Drug treatment is not indicated in all cases of Attention Deficit Disorder with Hyperactivity and should be considered only in light of the complete history and evaluation of the child. The decision to prescribe amphetamines should depend on the physician's assessment of the chronicity and severity of the child's symptoms and their appropriateness for his/her age. Prescription should not depend solely on the presence of one or more of the behavioral characteristics.

When these symptoms are associated with acute stress reactions, treatment with amphetamines is usually not indicated.

ADVERSE REACTIONS
Cardiovascular: Palpitations, tachycardia, elevation of blood pressure. There have been isolated reports of cardiomyopathy associated with chronic amphetamine use.

Central Nervous System: Psychotic episodes at recommended doses (rare), overstimulation, restlessness, dizziness, insomnia, euphoria, dyskinesia, dysphoria, tremor, headache, exacerbation of motor and phonic tics and Tourette's syndrome.

Gastrointestinal: Dryness of the mouth, unpleasant taste, diarrhea, constipation, other gastrointestinal disturbances.

Anorexia and weight loss may occur as undesirable effects when amphetamines are used for other than the anorectic effect.

Allergic: Urticaria.

Endocrine: Impotence, changes in libido.

DRUG ABUSE AND DEPENDENCE
Dextroamphetamine Sulfate is a Schedule II controlled substance.

Amphetamines have been extensively abused. Tolerance, extreme psychological dependence and severe social disability have occurred. There are reports of patients who have increased the dosage to many times that recommended.

Abrupt cessation following prolonged high dosage administration results in extreme fatigue and mental depression; changes are also noted on the sleep EEG.

Manifestations of chronic intoxication with amphetamines include severe dermatoses, marked insomnia, irritability, hyperactivity and personality changes.

The most severe manifestation of chronic intoxication is psychosis, often clinically indistinguishable from schizophrenia. This is rare with oral amphetamines.

OVERDOSAGE

Individual patient response to amphetamines varies widely. While toxic symptoms occasionally occur as an idiosyncrasy at doses as low as 2 mg, they are rare with doses of less than 15 mg; 30 mg can produce severe reactions, yet doses of 400 to 500 mg are not necessarily fatal.

In rats, the oral LD_{50} of Dextroamphetamine Sulfate is 96.8 mg/kg.

Manifestations of acute overdosage with amphetamines include restlessness, tremor, hyperreflexia, rhabdomyolysis, rapid respiration, hyperpyrexia, confusion, assaultiveness, hallucinations, panic states.

Fatigue and depression usually follow the central stimulation.

Cardiovascular effects include arrhythmias, hypertension or hypotension and circulatory collapse. Gastrointestinal symptoms include nausea, vomiting, diarrhea and abdominal cramps. Fatal poisoning is usually preceded by convulsions and coma.

Treatment —Management of acute amphetamine intoxication is largely symptomatic and includes gastric lavage and sedation with a barbiturate. Experience with hemodialysis or peritoneal dialysis is inadequate to permit recommendation in this regard. Acidification of the urine increases amphetamine excretion. If acute, severe hypertension complicates amphetamine overdosage, administration of intravenous phentolamine has been suggested. However, a gradual drop in blood pressure will usually result when sufficient sedation has been achieved.

Chlorpromazine antagonizes the central stimulant effects of amphetamines and can be used to treat amphetamine intoxication.

Since much of the capsule medication is coated for gradual release, therapy directed at reversing the effects of the ingested drug and at supporting the patient should be continued for as long as overdosage symptoms remain. Saline cathartics are useful for hastening the evacuation of pellets that have not already released medication.

DOSAGE AND ADMINISTRATION

Regardless of indication, amphetamines should be administered at the lowest effective dosage and dosage should be individually adjusted. Late evening doses—particulary with the capsule form—should be avoided because of the resulting insomnia.

Narcolepsy: Usual dose 5 to 60 mg per day in divided doses, depending on the individual patient response.

Narcolepsy seldom occurs in children under 12 years of age; however, when it does, Dextroamphetamine Sulfate may be used. The suggested initial dose for patients aged 6-12 is 5 mg daily; daily dose may be raised in increments of 5 mg at weekly intervals until optimal response is obtained. In patients 12 years of age and older, start with 10 mg daily; daily dosage may be raised in increments of 10 mg at weekly intervals until optimal response is obtained. If bothersome adverse reactions appear (e.g., insomnia or anorexia), dosage should be reduced. The capsules may be used for once-a-day dosage wherever appropriate. With tablets, give first dose on awakening; additional doses (1 or 2) at intervals of 4 to 6 hours.

Attention Deficit Disorder with Hyperactivity: Not recommended for children under 3 years of age.

In children from 3 to 5 years of age, start with 2.5 mg daily, by tablet; daily dosage may be raised in increments of 2.5 mg at weekly intervals until optimal response is obtained.

In children 6 years of age and older, start with 5 mg once or twice daily; daily dosage may be raised in increments of 5 mg at weekly intervals until optimal response is obtained. Only in rare cases will it be necessary to exceed a total of 40 mg per day.

The capsules may be used for once-a-day dosage wherever appropriate.

With tablets, give first dose on awakening; additional doses (1 or 2) at intervals of 4 to 6 hours.

Where possible, drug administration should be interrupted occasionally to determine if there is a recurrence of behavioral symptoms sufficient to require continued therapy.

Storage: Store at controlled room temperature (15° to 30°C; 59° to 86°F). Dispense in a tight, light-resistant container.

HOW SUPPLIED
CAPSULE, EXTENDED RELEASE (C-II): 5 MG

BRAND/MANUFACTURER	NDC	SIZE	AWP
○ **BRAND**			
DEXEDRINE: SK Beecham Pharm	00007-3512-15	50s	$20.30

CAPSULE, EXTENDED RELEASE (C-II): 10 MG

BRAND/MANUFACTURER	NDC	SIZE	AWP
○ **BRAND**			
DEXEDRINE: SK Beecham Pharm	00007-3513-15	50s	$25.30

CAPSULE, EXTENDED RELEASE (C-II): 15 MG

BRAND/MANUFACTURER	NDC	SIZE	AWP
○ **BRAND**			
DEXEDRINE: SK Beecham Pharm	00007-3514-15	50s	$32.30

TABLETS (C-II): 5 MG

AVERAGE UNIT PRICE (AVAILABLE SIZES)		GENERIC A-RATED AVERAGE PRICE (GAAP)	
BRAND	$0.19	100s	$19.60
GENERIC	$0.21	500s	$121.12

BRAND/MANUFACTURER	NDC	SIZE	AWP
◆ **BRAND**			
DEXEDRINE: SK Beecham Pharm	00007-3519-20	100s	$18.75
◆ **GENERICS**			
Rexar	00478-5451-01	100s	$19.33
DEXTROSTAT: Richwood	58521-0451-01	100s	$19.86
Rexar	00478-5451-05	500s	$95.00
Rugby	00536-3598-05	500s	$147.23
Rexar	00478-5451-10	1000s	$165.00

TABLETS (C-II): 10 MG

AVERAGE UNIT PRICE (AVAILABLE SIZES)	
GENERIC	$0.30

BRAND/MANUFACTURER	NDC	SIZE	AWP
◆ **GENERICS**			
Rexar	00478-5452-01	100s	$33.60
Rexar	00478-5452-05	500s	$155.16
Rexar	00478-5452-10	1000s	$257.58

Dextromethorphan Hydrobromide and Guaifenesin

DESCRIPTION

Each scored, sustained-release tablet provides 600 mg Guaifenesin and 30 mg Dextromethorphan Hydrobromide. Chemically, Guaifenesin is 3-(2-methoxyphenoxy)-1,2-propanediol. Its molecular formula is $C_{10}H_{14}O_4$ and molecular weight is 198.22.

Dextromethorphan Hydrobromide is a salt of the methyl either of the dextrorotatory isomer of lavorphanol, a narcotic analgesic. Chemically, it is 3-methoxy-17-methyl-9 +1a, 13 α, 14 α-morphinan hydrobromide monohydrate. Its molecular formula is $C_{18}H_{25}NO \cdot HBr \cdot H_2O$ and molecular weight in 370.33.

CLINICAL PHARMACOLOGY

Guaifenesin is an expectorant which increases respiratory tract fluid secretions and helps to loosen phlegm and bronchial secretions. By reducing the viscosity of secretions, Guaifenesin increases the efficiency of the mucociliary mechanism in removing accumulated secretions from the upper and lower airway. Guaifenesin is readily absorbed from the gastrointestinal tract and is rapidly metabolized and excreted in the urine. Guaifenesin has a plasma half-life of one hour. The major urinary metabolite is β-(2-methoxyphenoxy) lactic acid.

Dextromethorphan is an antitussive agent which, unlike the isometric levorphanol, has no analgesic or addictive properties. The drug acts centrally and elevates the threshold for coughing. It is about equal to codeine in depressing the cough reflex. In therapeutic dosage, Dextromethorphan does not inhibit ciliary activity. Dextromethorphan is rapidly absorbed from the gastrointestinal tract, metabolized by the liver and excreted primarily in the urine.

INDICATIONS AND USAGE

Dextromethorphan Hydrobromide/Guaifenesin tablets are indicated for the temporary relief of coughs associated with upper respiratory tract infections and related conditions such as sinusitis, pharyngitis, and bronchitis, particularly when these conditions are complicated by tenacious mucus and/or mucus plugs and congestion. The product is effective in productive as well as non-productive cough, but is of particular value in dry, non-productive cough which tends to injure the mucous membrane of the air passages.

CONTRAINDICATIONS

This drug is contraindicated in patients with hypersensitivity to Guaifenesin or Dextromethorphan and in patients receiving Monoamine Oxidase Inhibitor (MAOI) therapy and for 14 days after stopping MACI therapy. (See *"Drug Interactions"* section).

PRECAUTIONS

General: Before prescribing medication to suppress or modify cough, it is important that the underlying cause of cough is identified, that modification of cough does not increase the risk of clinical or physiological complications, and that appropriate therapy for the primary disease is instituted.

Dextromethorphan should be used with caution in sedated or debilitated patients, and in patients confined to the supine position.

Drug Interactions: Do not prescribe this product for use in patients that are now taking a prescription MAOI (certain drugs for depression, psychiatric or emotional conditions, or Parkinson's disease), or for 14 days after stopping the MAOI drug therapy.

Drug/Laboratory Test Interactions: Guaifenesin may increase renal clearance for urate and thereby lower serum uric acid levels. Guaifenesin may produce an increase in urinary 5-hydroxyindoleacetic acid and may therefore interfere with the interpretation of this test for the diagnosis of carcinoid syndrome. It may also

► SHOWN IN PRODUCT IDENTIFICATION GUIDE

falsely elevate the VMA test for catechols. Administration of this product should be discontinued 48 hours prior to the collection of urine specimens for such tests.

Carcinogenesis, Mutagenesis, Impairment of Fertility: No data are available on the long-term potential of Guaifenesin or of Dextromethorphan for carcinogenesis, mutagenesis, or impairment of fertility in animals or humans.

Pregnancy: Category C: Animal reproduction studies have not been conducted with Dextromethorphan Hydrobromide/Guaifenesin tablets. It is also not known whether tablets can cause fetal harm when administered to a pregnant woman or can affect reproduction capacity. Therefore, this product should be given to a pregnant woman only if clearly needed.

Nursing Mothers: It is not known whether Guaifenesin or Dextromethorphan is excreted in human milk. Because many drugs are excreted in human milk, caution should be exercised when this product is administered to a nursing woman and a decision should be made whether to discontinue nursing or to discontinue the drug, taking into account the importance of the drug to the mother.

ADVERSE REACTIONS
No serious side effects from Guaifenesin or Dextromethorphan have been reported.

OVERDOSAGE
Overdosage with Guaifenesin is unlikely to produce toxic effects since its toxicity is low. Guaifenesin, when administered by stomach tube to test animals in doses up to 5 grams/kg, produced no signs of toxicity. In severe cases of overdosage, treatment should be aimed at reducing further absorption of the drug. Gastric emptying (Syrup of Ipecac) and/or lavage is recommended as soon as possible after ingestions.

Overdosage with Dextromethorphan may produce central excitement and mental confusion. Very high doses may produce respiratory depression. One case of toxic psychosis (hyperactivity, marked visual and auditory hallucinations) after ingestion of a single 300 mg dose of Dextromethorphan has been reported.

DOSAGE AND ADMINISTRATION
Adults and children over 12 years of age: One or two tablets every 12 hours not to exceed 4 tablets in 24 hours.

Children 6 to 12 years: One tablet every 12 hours not to exceed 2 tablets in 24 hours.

Children 2 to 6 years: ½ tablet every 12 hours not to exceed 1 tablet in 24 hours.

Storage: Store at controlled room temperature between 15°C and 30°C (59°F and 86°F). Dispense in tight containers.

HOW SUPPLIED
CAPSULE, EXTENDED RELEASE: 15 MG-300 MG

BRAND/MANUFACTURER	NDC	SIZE	AWP
○ BRAND			
HUMIBID DM SPRINKLE: Adams	53014-0034-10	100s	$54.51

LIQUID (C-IV): 10 MG-100 MG/5 ML

BRAND/MANUFACTURER	NDC	SIZE	AWP
○ GENERICS			
HALOTUSSIN DM: Halsey Pharm	00879-0670-28	3840 ml	$43.65

SYRUP: 10 MG-100 MG/5 ML

BRAND/MANUFACTURER	NDC	SIZE	AWP
○ GENERICS			
Rugby	00536-0970-90	3840 ml	$33.75

TABLET, EXTENDED RELEASE:

BRAND/MANUFACTURER	NDC	SIZE	AWP
○ GENERICS			
Q-BID DM: Qualitest	00603-5542-21	100s	$42.30
GUIADRINE DM: Moore,H.L.	00839-7897-06	100s	$44.54
Q-BID DM: Qualitest	00603-5542-24	250s	$99.88
Q-BID DM: Qualitest	00603-5542-28	500s	$190.76

TABLET, EXTENDED RELEASE: 30 MG-600 MG

BRAND/MANUFACTURER	NDC	SIZE	AWP
○ BRAND			
► HUMIBID DM: Adams	53014-0030-10	100s	$58.81
	53014-0030-50	500s	$258.68
○ GENERICS			
GUAIFENEX DM: Ethex	58177-0213-04	100s	$39.14
FENESIN DM: Dura	51479-0014-01	100s	$41.50
MUCOBID DM: Econolab	55053-0090-01	100s	$41.50
Vintage	00254-5311-28	100s	$42.30
Rugby	00536-5591-01	100s	$44.03
Vintage	00254-5311-33	250s	$99.88
Vintage	00254-5311-35	500s	$190.76

TABLET, EXTENDED RELEASE: 600 MG-30 MG

BRAND/MANUFACTURER	NDC	SIZE	AWP
○ GENERICS			
FENEX-DM: TMK	59582-0917-01	100s	$41.50
Aligen	00405-4458-01	100s	$41.50
Goldline	00182-1042-01	100s	$50.40

TABLETS:

BRAND/MANUFACTURER	NDC	SIZE	AWP
○ GENERICS			
GUIADRINE DM: Pharmacist's Choice	54979-0150-01	100s	$41.50

TABLETS: 30 MG-600 MG

BRAND/MANUFACTURER	NDC	SIZE	AWP
○ GENERICS			
URL	00677-1486-01	100s	$46.35

TABLETS: 600 MG-30 MG

BRAND/MANUFACTURER	NDC	SIZE	AWP
○ GENERICS			
RESPA-DM: Respa Pharm	60575-0123-19	100s	$46.00

Dextromethorphan Hydrobromide and Promethazine Hydrochloride

DESCRIPTION
Each teaspoon (5 mL) contains 6.25 mg Promethazine Hydrochloride and 15 mg Dextromethorphan Hydrobromide in a flavored syrup base with a pH between 4.7 and 5.2 Alcohol 7%.

Promethazine Hydrochloride is a racemic compound; the empirical formula is $C_{17}H_{20}N_2S \cdot HCl$ and its molecular weight is 320.88.

Promethazine Hydrochloride, a phenothiazine derivative, is designated chemically as N,N,α-trimethyl-10*H*-phenothiazine-10-ethanamine monohydrochloride.

Promethazine Hydrochloride occurs as a white to faint yellow, practically odorless, crystalline powder which slowly oxidizes and turns blue on prolonged exposure to air. It is soluble in water and freely soluble in alcohol.

Dextromethorphan Hydrobromide is a salt of the methyl ether of the dextrorotatory isomer of levorphanol, a narcotic analgesic. It is chemically named as 3-methoxy-17-methyl-9α, 13α, 14α-morphinan hydrobromide monohydrate.

Dextromethorphan Hydrobromide monohydrate occurs as white crystals, is sparingly soluble in water, and is freely soluble in alcohol. The empirical formula is $C_{18}H_{25}NO \cdot HBr \cdot H_2O$, and the molecular weight of the monohydrate is is 370.33. Dextromethorphan HBr monohydrate is dextrorotatory with a specific rotation of + 27.6 degrees in water (20 degrees C, sodium D-line).

CLINICAL PHARMACOLOGY
PROMETHAZINE
Promethazine is a phenothiazine derivative which differs structurally from the antipsychotic phenothiazines by the presence of a branched side chain and no ring substitution. It is thought that this configuration is responsible for its relative lack (1/10 that of chlorpromazine) of dopaminergic (CNS) action.

Promethazine is an H_1 receptor blocking agent. In addition to its antihistaminic action, it provides clinically useful sedative and antiemetic effects. In therapeutic dosages, Promethazine produces no significant effects on the cardiovascular system.

Promethazine is well absorbed from the gastrointestinal tract. Clinical effects are apparent within 20 minutes after oral administration and generally last four to six hours, although they may persist as long as 12 hours. Promethazine is metabolized by the liver to a variety of compounds; the sulfoxides of Promethazine and N-demethylPromethazine are the predominant metabolites appearing in the urine.

DEXTROMETHORPHAN
Dextromethorphan is an antitussive agent and, unlike the isomeric levorphanol, it has no analgesic or addictive properties.

The drug acts centrally and elevates the threshold for coughing. It is about equal to codeine in depressing the cough reflex. In therapeutic dosage Dextromethorphan does not inhibit ciliary activity.

Dextromethorphan is rapidly absorbed from the gastrointestinal tract and exerts its effect in 15 to 30 minutes. The duration of action after oral administration is approximately three to six hours. Dextromethorphan is metabolized primarily by liver enzymes undergoing O-demethylation, N-demethylation, and partial conjugation with glucuronic acid and sulfate. In humans, (+)-3-hydroxy-N-methylmorphinan, (+)-3-hydroxymorphinan, and traces of unmetabolized drug were found in urine after oral administration.

INDICATIONS AND USAGE
Promethazine Hydrochloride with Dextromethorphan is indicated for the temporary relief of coughs and upper respiratory symptoms associated with allergy or the common cold.

◆ RATED THERAPEUTICALLY EQUIVALENT; ◇ THERAPEUTIC EQUIVALENCE UNCONFIRMED; ○ UNRATED

CONTRAINDICATIONS

Promethazine is contraindicted in individuals known to be hypersensitive or to have had an idiosyncratic reaction to Promethazine or to other phenothiazines.

Anthihistamines are contraindicated for use in the treatment of lower respiratory tract symptoms, including asthma. Dextromethorphan should not be used in patients receiving a monoamine oxidase inhibitor (MAOI).

WARNINGS

PROMETHAZINE

Promethazine may cause marked drowsiness. Ambulatory patients should be cautioned against such activities as driving or operating dangerous machinery until it is known that they do not become drowsy or dizzy from Promethazine therapy.

The sedative action of Promethazine Hydrochloride is additive to the sedative effects of central nervous system depressants; therefore, agents such as alcohol, narcotic analgesics, sedatives, hypnotics, and tranquilizers should either be eliminated or given in reduced dosage in the presence of Promethazine Hydrochloride. When given concomitantly with Promethazine Hydrochloride, the dose of barbiturates should be reduced by at least one-half, and the dose of analgesic depressants, such as morphine or meperidine, should be reduced by one-quarter to one-half.

Promethazine may lower seizure threshold. This should be taken into consideration when administering to persons with known seizure disorders or when giving in combination with narcotics or local anethetics which may also affect seizure threshold.

Sedative drugs or CNS depressants should be avoided in patients with a history of sleep apnea.

Antihistamines should be used with caution in patients with narrow-angle glaucoma, stenosing peptic ulcer, pyloroduodenal obstruction, and urinary bladder obstruction due to symptomatic prostatic hypertrophy and narrowing of the bladder neck.

Administration of Promethazine has been associated with reported cholestatic jaundice.

DEXTROMETHORPHAN

Administration of Dextromethorphan may be accompanied by histamine release and should be used with caution in atopic children.

PRECAUTIONS

Animal reproduction studies have not been conducted with the drug combination—Promethazine and Dextromethorphan. It is known whether this drug combination can cause fetal harm when administered to a pregnant woman or can affect reproduction capacity. Promethazine Hydrochloride with Dextromethorphan should be given to a pregnant woman only if clearly needed.

GENERAL

Promethazine should be used cautiously in persons with cardiovascular disease or with impairment of liver function. Dextromethorphan should be used with caution in sedated patients, in the debilitated, and in patients confined to the supine position.

INFORMATION FOR PATIENTS

Promethazine Hydrochloride with Dextromethorphan may cause marked drowsiness or impair the mental and/or physical abilities required for the performance of potentially harzardous tasks, such as driving a vehicle or operating machinery. Ambulatory patients should be told to avoid engaging in such activities until it is known that they do not become drowsy or dizzy from Promethazine Hydrochloride with Dextromethorphan therapy. Children should be supervised to avoid potential harm in bike riding or in other hazardous activities.

The concomitant use of alcohol or other central nervous system depressants, including narcotic analgesics, sedatives, hypnotics, and tranquilizers, may have an additive effect and should be avoided or their dosage reduced.

Patients should be advised to report any involuntary muscle movements or unusual sensitivity to sunlight.

DRUG INTERACTIONS

The sedative action of Promethazine is additive to the sedative effects of other central nervous system depressants, including alcohol, narcotic analgesics, sedatives, hypnotics, tricyclic antidepressants, and tranquilizers; therefore, these agents should be avoided or administered in reduced dosage to patients receiving Promethazine.

DRUG/LABORATORY TEST INTERACTIONS

The following laboratory tests may be affected in patients who are receiving therapy with Promethazine Hydrochloride:

Pregnancy Tests: Diagnostic pregnancy tests based on immunological reactions between HCG and anti-HCG may result in false-negative or false-positive interpretations.

Glucose Tolerance Test: An increase in blood glucose has been reported in patients receiving Promethazine.

CARCINOGENESIS, MUTAGENESIS, IMPAIRMENT OF FERTILITY

Long-term animal studies have not been performed to assess the carcinogenic potential of Promethazine or of Dextromethorphan. There are no animal or human data concerning the carcinogenicity, mutagenicity, or impairment of fertility with these drugs. Promethazine was nonmutagenic in the *Salmonella* test system of Ames.

PREGNANCY

Teratogenic Effects—Pregnancy Category C: Teratogenic effects have not been demonstrated in rat-feeding studies at doses of 6.25 and 12.5 mg/kg of Promethazine. These doses are 8.3 and 16.7 times the maximum recommended total daily dose for a 50-kg subject. Specific studies to test the action of the drug on parturition, lactation, and development of the animal neonate were not done, but a general preliminary study in rats indicated no effect on these parameters. Although antihistamines, including Promethazine, have been found to produce fetal mortality in rodents, the pharmacological effects of histamine in the rodent do not parallel those in man. There are no adequate and well-controlled studies of Promethazine in pregnant women.

Promethazine Hydrochloride with Dextromethorphan should be used during pregnancy only if the potential benefit justifies the potential risk to the fetus.

Nonteratogenic Effects: Promethazine taken within two weeks of delivery may inhibit platelet aggregation in the newborn.

LABOR AND DELIVERY

See *"Nonteratogenic Effects."*

NURSING MOTHERS

It is not known whether Promethazine or Dextromethorphan is excreted in human milk. Caution should be exercised when Promethazine Hydrochloride with Dextromethorphan is administered to a nursing woman.

PEDIATRIC USE

This product should not be used in children under 2 years of age because safety for that use has not been established.

ADVERSE REACTIONS

PROMETHAZINE

Nervous System: Sedation, sleepiness, occasional blurred vision, dryness of mouth, dizziness; rarely confusion, disorientation, and extrapyramidal symptoms such as oculogyric crisis, torticollis, and tongue protrusion (usually in association with parenteral injection or excessive dosage).

Cardiovascular: Increased or decreased blood pressure.

Dermatologic: Rash, rarely photosensitivity.

Hematologic: Rarely leukopenia, thrombocytopenia; agranulocytosis (1 case).

Gastrointestinal: Nausea and vomiting.

DEXTROMETHORPHAN

Dextromethorphan Hydrobromide occasionally causes slight drowsiness, dizziness, and gastrointestinal disturbances.

DRUG ABUSE AND DEPENDENCE

According to the WHO Expert Committee on Drug Dependence. Dextromethorphan could produce very slight psychic dependence but no physical dependence.

OVERDOSAGE

PROMETHAZINE

Signs and symptoms of overdosage with Promethazine range from mild depression of the central nervous system and cardiovascular system to profound hypotension, respiratory depression, and unconsciousness.

Stimulation may be evident, especially in children and geriatric patients. Convulsions may rarely occur. A paradoxical reaction has been reported in children receiving single doses of 75 mg to 125 mg orally, characterized by hyperexcitability and nightmares.

Atropine-like signs and symptoms—dry mouth, fixed, dilated pupils, flushing, as well as gastrointestinal symptoms, may occur.

DEXTROMETHORPHAN

Dextromethorphan may produce central excitement and mental confusion. Very high doses may produce respiratory depression. One case of toxic psychosis (hyperactivity, marked visual and auditory hallucinations) after ingestion of a single dose of 20 tablets (300 mg) of Dextromethorphan has been reported.

TREATMENT

Treatment of overdosage with Phenergan with Dextromethorphan is essentially symptomatic and supportive. Only in cases of extreme overdosage or individual sensitivity do vital signs including respiration, pulse, blood pressure, temperature, and EKG need to be monitored. Activated charcoal orally or by lavage may be given, or sodium or magnesium sulfate orally as a cathartic. Attention should be given to the reestablishment of adequate respiratory exchange through provision of a patent airway and institution of assisted or controlled ventilation. Diazepam may be used to control convulsions. Acidosis and electrolyte losses should be corrected. The antidotal efficacy of narcotic antagonists to Dextromethorphan has not been established; note that any of the depressant effects of Promethazine are not reversed by naloxone. Avoid analeptics, which may cause convulsions.

Severe hypotension usually responds to the administration of norepinephrine or phenylephrine. EPINEPHRINE SHOULD NOT BE USED, since its use in a patient with partial adrenergic blockade may further lower the blood pressure.

Limited experience with dialysis indicates that it is not helpful.

DOSAGE AND ADMINISTRATION

The average effective dose for adults is one teaspoon (5 mL) every 4 to 6 hours, not to exceed 30.0 mL in 24 hours. For children 6 years to under 12 years of age, the dose is one-half to one teaspoon (2.5 to 5.0 mL) every 4 to 6 hours, not to exceed 20.0 mL in 24 hours. For children 2 years to under 6 years of age, the dose is one-quarter to one half teaspoon (1.25 to 2.5 mL) every 4 to 6 hours, not to exceed 10.0 mL in 24 hours.

Promethazine Hydrochloride with Dextromethorphan is not recommended for children under 2 years of age.

Keep bottles tightly closed and store at room temperature between 15° and 25°C (59° and 77°F).

Protect from light.

Dispense in light-resistant, glass, tight containers.

HOW SUPPLIED
SYRUP:

BRAND/MANUFACTURER	NDC	SIZE	AWP
◆ GENERICS			
Barre	00472-1630-04	120 ml	$2.20

SYRUP: 15 MG-6.25 MG/5 ML

AVERAGE UNIT PRICE (AVAILABLE SIZES)		GENERIC A-RATED AVERAGE PRICE (GAAP)	
BRAND	$0.05	480 ml	$21.19
GENERIC	$0.01	3840 ml	$21.19
HCFA FUL (480 ml)	$0.01	120 ml	$2.38
		120 ml	$2.19
		480 ml	$6.29
		3840 ml	$41.84

BRAND/MANUFACTURER	NDC	SIZE	AWP
◆ BRAND			
PHENERGAN W/DM: Wyeth-Ayerst	00008-0548-03	480 ml	$20.95
	00008-0548-02	120 ml 24s	$138.49
◆ GENERICS			
Major	00904-1516-00	120 ml	$1.85
Rugby	00536-1765-97	120 ml	$2.25
Mason Dist	11845-0440-04	120 ml	$2.32
Halsey Pharm	00879-0516-04	120 ml	$2.40
Moore, H.L.	00839-7062-65	120 ml	$2.50
Rugby	00536-1765-85	480 ml	$4.94
Major	00904-1516-16	480 ml	$5.70
Moore, H.L.	00839-7062-69	480 ml	$5.79
Qualitest	00603-1579-58	480 ml	$5.84
Schein	00364-0734-16	480 ml	$5.85
URL	00677-0966-33	480 ml	$5.90
Barre	00472-1630-16	480 ml	$6.20
Aligen	00405-3650-16	480 ml	$6.50
Halsey Pharm	00879-0516-16	480 ml	$6.50
Mason Dist	11845-0440-13	480 ml	$6.52
Goldline	00182-1730-40	480 ml	$6.70
Geneva	00781-6030-16	480 ml	$7.71
Major	00904-1516-28	3840 ml	$34.35
Rugby	00536-1765-90	3840 ml	$37.43
Goldline	00182-1730-41	3840 ml	$41.70
Barre	00472-1630-28	3840 ml	$45.60
Halsey Pharm	00879-0516-28	3840 ml	$45.70

Dextrose

DESCRIPTION
Dextrose Injection, USP solutions are sterile and nonpyrogenic. They are parenteral solutions containing various concentrations of dextrose in water for injection intended for intravenous administration.

Each 100 mL of 5% Dextrose Injection, USP, contains Dextrose, hydrous 5 g in water for injection. The caloric value is 170 kcal/L. The osmolarity is 253 mOsmol/L (calc.), which is slightly hypotonic.

Each 100 mL of 10% Dextrose Injection, USP, contains dextrose, hydrous 10 g in water for injection. The caloric value is 340 kcal/L. The osmolarity is 505 mOsmol/L (calc.), which is hypertonic.

The pH for both concentrations is 4.3 (3.2 to 6.5).

The solutions contain no bacteriostat, antimicrobial agent or added buffer and each is intended only as a single-dose injection. When smaller doses are required the unused portion should be discarded.

The solutions are parenteral fluid and nutrient replenishers.

Dextrose, USP is chemically designated D-glucose monohydrate $(C_6H_{12}O_5 \cdot H_2O)$, a hexose sugar freely soluble in water.

Water for Injection, USP is chemically designated H_2O.

CLINICAL PHARMACOLOGY
When administered intravenously, these solutions provide a source of water and carbohydrate.

Isotonic and hypertonic concentrations of dextrose are suitable for parenteral maintenance of water requirements when salt is not needed or should be avoided.

Solutions containing carbohydrate in the form of Dextrose restore blood glucose levels and provide calories. Carbohydrate in the form of Dextrose may aid in minimizing liver glycogen depletion and exerts a protein-sparing action. Dextrose injected parenterally undergoes oxidation to carbon dioxide and water.

Water is an essential constituent of all body tissues and accounts for approximately 70% of total body weight. Average normal adult daily requirements range from two to three liters (1.0 to 1.5 liters each for insensible water loss by perspiration and urine production).

Water balance is maintained by various regulatory mechanisms. Water distribution depends primarily on the concentration of electrolytes in the body compartments and sodium (Na^+) plays a major role in maintaining physiologic equilibrium.

INDICATIONS AND USAGE
Intravenous solutions containing Dextrose are indicated for parenteral replenishment of fluid and minimal carbohydrate calories as required by the clinical condition of the patient.

CONTRAINDICATIONS
Dextrose Injection without electrolytes should not be administered simultaneously with blood through the same infusion set because of the possibility that pseudoagglutination of red cells may occur.

WARNINGS
Excessive administration of potassium-free solutions may result in significant hypokalemia.

The intravenous administration of these solutions can cause fluid and/or solute overloading resulting in dilution of serum electrolyte concentrations, overhydration, congested states or pulmonary edema.

The risk of dilutional states is inversely proportional to the electrolyte concentrations of administered parenteral solutions. The risk of solute overload causing congested states with peripheral and pulmonary edema is directly proportional to the electrolyte concentrations of such solutions.

PRECAUTIONS
Clinical evaluation and periodic laboratory determinations are necessary to monitor changes in fluid balance, electrolyte concentrations and acid-base balance during prolonged parenteral therapy or whenever the condition of the patient warrants such evaluation.

Solutions containing Dextrose should be used with caution in patients with known subclinical or overt diabetes mellitus.

Do not administer unless solution is clear and container is undamaged. Discard unused portion.

Carcinogenesis, Mutagenesis, Impairment of Fertility: Studies with Dextrose Injection, USP have not been performed to evaluate carcinogenic potential, mutagenic potential or effects on fertility.

Pregnancy: Teratogenic effects: Pregnancy Category C: Animal reproduction studies have not been conducted with Dextrose. It is also not known whether Dextrose can cause fetal harm when administered to a pregnant woman or can affect reproduction capacity. Dextrose should be given to a pregnant woman only if clearly needed.

Nursing Mothers: Caution should be exercised when Dextrose Injection, USP is administered to a nursing mother.

Pediatric Use: Safety and effectiveness in children have not been established.

ADVERSE REACTIONS
Reactions which may occur because of the solution or the technique of administration include febrile response, infection at the site of injection, venous thrombosis or phlebitis extending from the site of injection, extravasation and hypervolemia.

If an adverse reaction does occur, discontinue the infusion, evaluate the patient, institute appropriate therapeutic countermeasures and save the remainder of the fluid for examination if deemed necessary.

OVERDOSAGE
In the event of overhydration or solute overload, re-evaluate the patient and institute appropriate corrective measures. See *"Warnings"*, *"Precautions"*, and *"Adverse Reactions"*.

DOSAGE AND ADMINISTRATION
The dose is dependent upon the age, weight and clinical condition of the patient.

Drug Interactions: Additives may be incompatible. Consult with pharmacist, if available. When introducing additives, use aseptic technique, mix thoroughly and do not store.

Parenteral drug products should be inspected visually for particulate matter and discoloration prior to administration, whenever solution and container permit. See *"Precautions"*.

INSTRUCTIONS FOR USE
To Add Medications:
1. Prepare additive port.
2. Using aseptic technique and an additive delivery needle of appropriate length, puncture resealable additive port at target area, inner diaphragm and inject. Withdraw needle after injecting medication.
3. The additive port may be protected by covering with an additive cap.
4. Mix container contents thoroughly.

Preparation for Administration (Use aseptic technique):
1. Close flow control clamp of administration set.
2. Remove cover from outlet port at bottom of container.
3. Insert piercing pin of administration set into port with a twisting motion until the set is firmly seated. NOTE: When using a vented administration set, replace bacterial retentive air filter with piercing pin cover. Insert piercing pin with twisting motion until shoulder of air filter housing rests against the outlet port flange.

◆ RATED THERAPEUTICALLY EQUIVALENT; ◇ THERAPEUTIC EQUIVALENCE UNCONFIRMED; ○ UNRATED

4. Suspend container from hanger.
5. Squeeze and release drip chamber to establish proper fluid level in chamber.
6. Attach venipuncture device to set.
7. Open clamp to expel air from set and venipuncture device. Close clamp.
8. Perform venipuncture.
9. Regulate rate of administration with flow control clamp.

Warning: Do not use flexible container in series connections.

STORAGE
Exposure of pharmaceutical products to heat should be minimized. Avoid excessive heat. Protect from freezing. It is recommended that the product be stored at room temperature (25° C).

J CODES
500 ml = 1 unit IV—J7060

HOW SUPPLIED
INJECTION: 5%-0.3%-0.2%

BRAND/MANUFACTURER	NDC	SIZE	AWP
◆ GENERICS			
Abbott Hosp	00074-7922-09	1000 ml 12s	$132.24

INJECTION: 2.5%

BRAND/MANUFACTURER	NDC	SIZE	AWP
◆ GENERICS			
Abbott Hosp	00074-1508-05	1000 ml 6s	$76.17

INJECTION: 2.5%

BRAND/MANUFACTURER	NDC	SIZE	AWP
○ GENERICS			
Baxter	00338-0012-04	1000 ml 6s	$74.74

INJECTION: 5%

AVERAGE UNIT PRICE (AVAILABLE SIZES)		GENERIC A-RATED AVERAGE PRICE (GAAP)	
GENERIC	$0.11	500 ml	$9.70
		1000 ml	$10.69
		150 ml 12s	$90.15
		250 ml 12s	$118.60
		500 ml 12s	$118.60
		250 ml 24s	$258.02
		500 ml 24s	$224.17
		25 ml 48s	$634.25
		50 ml 80s	$974.25
		100 ml 80s	$974.25
		50 ml 96s	$928.51
		100 ml 96s	$928.51

BRAND/MANUFACTURER	NDC	SIZE	AWP
◆ GENERICS			
McGaw	00264-1510-36	50 ml	$14.63
McGaw	00264-1110-23	150 ml	$9.86
McGaw	00264-7510-20	250 ml	$9.12
McGaw	00264-1110-10	500 ml	$9.50
McGaw	00264-7510-10	500 ml	$9.90
McGaw	00264-1110-00	1000 ml	$10.69
McGaw	00264-7510-00	1000 ml	$10.69
Abbott Hosp	00074-1500-05	1000 ml 6s	$101.25
Abbott Hosp	00074-1523-01	50 ml 12s	$189.95
Abbott Hosp	00074-1523-11	100 ml 12s	$189.95
Baxter	00338-0015-01	150 ml 12s	$60.60
Abbott Hosp	00074-1522-01	150 ml 12s	$119.70
Baxter	00338-0016-02	250 ml 12s	$117.50
Abbott Hosp	00074-1522-02	250 ml 12s	$119.70
Baxter	00338-0016-03	500 ml 12s	$117.50
Abbott Hosp	00074-1522-03	500 ml 12s	$119.70
Baxter	00338-0017-04	1000 ml 12s	$129.73
Abbott Hosp	00074-7922-02	250 ml 24s	$226.29
Abbott Hosp	00074-7922-53	250 ml 24s	$226.29
Abbott Hosp	00074-7100-02	250 ml 24s	$321.48
Baxter	00338-0017-03	500 ml 24s	$222.05
Abbott Hosp	00074-7922-03	500 ml 24s	$226.29
Abbott Hosp	00074-1495-01	50 ml 25s	$95.89
Abbott Hosp	00074-1494-01	100 ml 25s	$99.75
Abbott Hosp	00074-7922-61	150 ml 32s	$301.72
Baxter	00338-0017-01	150 ml 36s	$333.08
Baxter	00338-0017-02	250 ml 36s	$333.08
Baxter	00338-0017-10	25 ml 48s	$542.88
Abbott Hosp	00074-7923-20	25 ml 48s	$725.61
Abbott Hosp	00074-7100-13	50 ml 48s	$531.24
Abbott Hosp	00074-7100-23	100 ml 48s	$531.24
McGaw	00264-1510-32	100 ml 64s	$614.40
Abbott Hosp	00074-7923-36	50 ml 80s	$788.50

BRAND/MANUFACTURER	NDC	SIZE	AWP
Baxter	00338-0551-11	50 ml 80s	$1160.00
Abbott Hosp	00074-7923-37	100 ml 80s	$788.50
Baxter	00338-0551-18	100 ml 80s	$1160.00
McGaw	00264-1510-31	50 ml 84s	$806.40
Baxter	00338-0017-11	50 ml 96s	$928.51
Baxter	00338-0017-31	50 ml 96s	$928.51
Baxter	00338-0017-41	50 ml 96s	$928.51
Baxter	00338-0017-18	100 ml 96s	$928.51
Baxter	00338-0017-38	100 ml 96s	$928.51
Baxter	00338-0017-48	100 ml 96s	$928.51

INJECTION: 5%

BRAND/MANUFACTURER	NDC	SIZE	AWP
○ GENERICS			
Intl Med Sys	00548-1181-00	10 ml 25s	$171.75

INJECTION: 10%

AVERAGE UNIT PRICE (AVAILABLE SIZES)		GENERIC A-RATED AVERAGE PRICE (GAAP)	
GENERIC	$0.06	500 ml	$15.15
		500 ml 12s	$207.75
		1000 ml 12s	$150.33
		500 ml 24s	$257.69

BRAND/MANUFACTURER	NDC	SIZE	AWP
◆ GENERICS			
McGaw	00264-1120-10	500 ml	$10.94
McGaw	00264-1120-01	500 ml	$19.36
McGaw	00264-1120-00	1000 ml	$14.48
Abbott Hosp	00074-5641-25	500 ml 6s	$120.34
Clintec	00338-0023-34	1000 ml 10s	$476.64
Abbott Hosp	00074-1530-02	250 ml 12s	$137.94
Baxter	00338-0023-12	500 ml 12s	$124.08
Abbott Hosp	00074-7938-19	500 ml 12s	$291.41
Baxter	00338-0023-04	1000 ml 12s	$148.90
Abbott Hosp	00074-7930-09	1000 ml 12s	$151.76
Clintec	00338-0023-13	500 ml 16s	$381.12
Baxter	00338-0023-03	500 ml 24s	$255.17
Abbott Hosp	00074-7930-03	500 ml 24s	$260.21
Abbott Hosp	00074-4089-02	5 ml 25s	$66.80
Solo Pak	39769-0158-17	17 ml 25s	$25.00
Baxter	00338-0023-02	250 ml 36s	$382.76

INJECTION: 10%

BRAND/MANUFACTURER	NDC	SIZE	AWP
○ GENERICS			
McGaw	00264-7520-20	250 ml	$10.97
McGaw	00264-7520-10	500 ml	$10.55
McGaw	00264-7520-00	1000 ml	$12.25
Abbott Hosp	00074-7930-02	250 ml 24s	$275.88
Sanofi Winthrop	00024-0341-06	3 ml 100s	$477.76

INJECTION: 20%

AVERAGE UNIT PRICE (AVAILABLE SIZES)		GENERIC A-RATED AVERAGE PRICE (GAAP)	
GENERIC	$0.04	500 ml	$18.73
		500 ml 6s	$102.53
		500 ml 12s	$235.76

BRAND/MANUFACTURER	NDC	SIZE	AWP
◆ GENERICS			
McGaw	00264-1125-10	500 ml	$15.06
McGaw	00264-1125-01	500 ml	$22.40
Baxter	00338-0030-13	500 ml 6s	$66.06
Abbott Hosp	00074-5642-25	500 ml 6s	$139.01
Clintec	00338-0711-34	1000 ml 10s	$550.40
Clintec	00338-0030-03	500 ml 10s	$183.60
Abbott Hosp	00074-1535-03	500 ml 12s	$187.10
Abbott Hosp	00074-7935-19	500 ml 12s	$336.59
Clintec	00338-0711-13	500 ml 16s	$440.25

INJECTION: 25%

BRAND/MANUFACTURER	NDC	SIZE	AWP
◆ GENERICS			
Abbott Hosp	00074-7898-01	10 ml 10s	$121.01

INJECTION: 25%

BRAND/MANUFACTURER	NDC	SIZE	AWP
○ GENERICS			
Intl Med Sys	00548-1015-00	10 ml 25s	$202.50

For additional alternatives, turn to the section beginning on page 2859.

➤ SHOWN IN PRODUCT IDENTIFICATION GUIDE

Dextrose and Electrolytes

DESCRIPTION
Dextrose/Electrolytes is a sterile, nonpyrogenic isotonic solution of balanced Electrolytes in water for injection. The solution is administered by intravenous infusion for parenteral replacement of acute losses of extracellular fluid.

Each 100 mL of Dextrose/Electrolytes contains sodium chloride, 526 mg; sodium acetate, 222 mg; sodium gluconate, 502 mg; potassium chloride, 37 mg; magnesium chloride hexahydrate, 30 mg. May contain HCl and/or NaOH for pH adjustment. pH 6.6 (5.5 - 8.0); 294 mOsm/liter (calc.).

Electrolytes per 1,000 mL (not including pH adjustment): Sodium 140 mEq; potassium 5 mEq; magnesium 3 mEq; chloride 98 mEq; acetate 27 mEq; gluconate 23 mEq.

The solution contains no bacteriostat, antimicrobial agent or added buffer (except for pH adjustment) and is intended only for use as a single-dose injection. When smaller doses are required, the unused portion should be discarded.

Dextrose/Electrolytes is a parenteral fluid and Electrolyte replenisher.

Sodium Chloride, USP, is chemically designated NaCl, a white crystalline powder freely soluble in water.

Potassium Chloride, USP, is chemically designated KCl, a white granular powder freely soluble in water.

Magnesium Chloride, USP, is chemically designated magnesium chloride hexahydrate ($MgCl_2$·$6H_2O$) deliquescent crystals very soluble in water.

Sodium acetate, USP, is chemically designated sodium acetate anhydrous ($C_2H_3NaO_2$), a hygroscopic powder soluble in water.

Sodium gluconate is chemically designated $C_6H_{11}NaO_7$, the normal sodium salt of gluconic acid soluble in water.

Water for Injection, USP, is chemically designated H_2O.

CLINICAL PHARMACOLOGY
When administered intravenously, Dextrose/Electrolytes provides water and electrolytes for replacement of acute extracellular fluid losses without disturbing normal electrolyte relationships. The electrolyte composition approaches that of the principal ions of normal plasma (extracellular fluid). The electrolyte concentration is approximately isotonic in relation to the extracellular fluid (approx. 280 mOsm/liter) and provides a physiologic sodium to chloride ratio, normal plasma concentrations of potassium and magnesium and two bicarbonate alternates, acetate and gluconate.

Solutions containing carbohydrate in the form of Dextrose restore blood glucose levels and supply calories. Carbohydrate in the form of dextrose may aid in minimizing liver glycogen depletion and exerts a protein-sparing action. Dextrose injected parenterally undergoes oxidation to carbon dioxide and water.

Sodium chloride in water dissociates to provide sodium (Na^+) and chloride (Cl^-) ions. Sodium (Na^+) is the principal cation of the extracellular fluid and plays a large part in the therapy of fluid and electrolyte disturbances. Chloride (Cl^-) has an integral role in buffering action when oxygen and carbon dioxide exchange occurs in the red blood cells. The distribution and excretion of sodium (Na^+) and chloride (Cl^-) are largely under the control of the kidney which maintains a balance between intake and output.

Potassium chloride in water dissociates to provide potassium (K^+) and chloride (Cl^-) ions. Potassium is the chief cation of body cells (160 mEq/liter of intracellular water). It is found in low concentration in plasma and extracellular fluids (3.5 to 5.0 mEq/liter in a healthy adult). Potassium plays an important role in electrolyte balance.

Potassium acetate in water dissociates to provide potassium (K^+) and acetate (CH_3COO^-) ions. Potassium is the chief cation of body cells (160 mEq/liter of intracellular water). It is found in low concentration in plasma and extracellular fluids (3.5 to 5.0 mEq/liter) in a healthy adult. Potassium plays an important role in electrolyte balance. Normally about 80% to 90% of the potassium intake is excreted in the urine; the remainder in the stools and to a small extent, in the perspiration. The kidney does not conserve potassium well, so that during fasting or in patients on a potassium-free diet, potassium loss from the body continues resulting in potassium depletion.

Magnesium acetate in water dissociates to provide magnesium (Mg^{++}) and acetate (CH_3COO^-) ions. Magnesium is the second most plentiful cation of the intracellular fluids. It is an important cofactor for enzymatic reactions and plays an important role in neurochemical transmission and muscular excitability. Normal plasma concentration ranges from 1.5 to 2.5 or 3.0 mEq per liter. Magnesium is excreted solely by the kidney at a rate proportional to the plasma concentration and glomerular filtration.

Normally about 80 to 90% of the potassium intake is excreted in the urine; the remainder in the stools and to a small extent, in the perspiration. The kidney does not conserve potassium well so that during fasting or in patients on a potassium-free diet, potassium loss from the body continues resulting in potassium depletion.

Magnesium chloride in water dissociates to provide magnesium (Mg^{++}) and chloride (Cl^-) ions. Magnesium is the second most plentiful cation of the intracellular fluids. It is an important cofactor for enzymatic reactions and plays an important role in neurochemical transmission and muscular excitability. Normal plasma concentration ranges from 1.5 to 2.5 or 3.0 mEq/liter. Magnesium is excreted solely by the kidney at a rate proportional to the plasma concentration and glomerular filtration.

Sodium acetate provides sodium (Na^+) and acetate (CH_3COO^-) ions, the latter anion (a source of hydrogen ion acceptors) serving as an alternate source of bicarbonate (HCO_3^-) by metabolic conversion in the liver. This has been shown to proceed readily even in the presence of severe liver disease. Thus, acetate anion exerts a mild systemic antiacidotic action that may be advantageous during fluid and electrolyte replacement therapy.

Sodium gluconate provides sodium (Na^+) and gluconate ($C_6H_{11}O_7^-$) ions. Although gluconate is a theoretical alternate metabolic source of bicarbonate (HCO_3^-) anion, a significant antiacidotic action has not been established. Thus, the gluconate anion serves primarily to complete the cation-anion balance of the solutions.

Water is an essential constituent of all body tissues and accounts for approximately 70% of total body weight. Average normal adult daily requirement ranges from two to three liters (1.0 to 1.5 liters each for insensible water loss by perspiration and urine production).

Water balance is maintained by various regulatory mechanisms. Water distribution depends primarily on the concentration of electrolytes in the body compartments and sodium (Na^+) plays a major role in maintaining physiologic equilibrium.

INDICATIONS AND USAGE
Dextrose/Electrolytes is indicated for *replacement* of acute extracellular fluid volume losses in surgery, trauma, burns or shock. Dextrose/Electrolytes also can be used as an adjunct to restore a decrease in circulatory volume in patients with moderate blood loss. Dextrose/Electrolytes is not intended to supplant transfusion of whole blood or packed red cells in the presence of uncontrolled hemorrhage or severe reductions of red cell volume.

Dextrose/Electrolytes is indicated for parenteral maintenance of routine daily fluid and Electrolyte requirements with minimal calories from Dextrose. Magnesium in the formula may help to prevent iatrogenic magnesium deficiency in patients receiving prolonged parenteral fluid therapy.

CONTRAINDICATIONS
None known.

WARNINGS
Solutions containing sodium ions should be used with great care, if at all, in patients with congestive heart failure, severe renal insufficiency and in clinical states in which there exists edema with sodium retention.

Solutions which contain potassium should be used with great care, if at all, in patients with hyperkalemia, severe renal failure and in conditions in which potassium retention is present.

In patients with diminished renal function, administration of solutions containing sodium or potassium ions may result in sodium or potassium retention.

Solutions containing acetate or gluconate ions should be used with great care in patients with metabolic or respiratory alkalosis. Acetate or gluconate should be administered with great care in those conditions in which there is an increased level or an impaired utilization of these ions, such as severe hepatic insufficiency.

The intravenous administration of this solution can cause fluid and/or solute overloading resulting in dilution of serum Electrolyte concentrations, overhydration, congested states or pulmonary edema.

The risk of dilutional states is inversely proportional to the Electrolyte concentrations of administered parenteral solutions. The risk of solute overload causing congested states with peripheral and pulmonary edema is directly proportional to the Electrolyte concentrations of such solutions.

PRECAUTIONS
Dextrose/Electrolytes should be used with caution in severe renal impairment because of the danger of hyperkalemia. As with all intravenous solutions, care be taken to avoid circulatory overload, especially in patients with cardiac or pulmonary disorders. Dextrose/Electrolytes is not intended to correct acidosis or large deficits of individual Electrolytes, nor to replace blood or plasma expanders when these are indicated.

Clinical evaluation and periodic laboratory determinations are necessary to monitor changes in fluid balance, Electrolyte concentrations and acid-base balance during prolonged parenteral therapy or whenever the condition of the patient warrants such evaluation.

Caution must be exercised in the administration of parenteral fluids, especially those containing sodium ions, to patients receiving corticosteroids or corticotropin.

Solutions containing acetate or gluconate ions should be used with caution, as excess administration may result in metabolic alkalosis.

Do not administer unless solution is clear and container is undamaged. Discard unused portion.

Pregnancy Category C: Animal reproduction studies have not been conducted with Dextrose/Electrolytes. It is also not known whether this solution can cause fetal harm when administered to a pregnant woman or can affect reproduction capacity. This solution should be given to a pregnant woman only if clearly needed.

ADVERSE REACTIONS
Reactions which may occur because of the solution or the technique of administration include febrile response, infection at the site of injection, venous thrombosis or phlebitis extending from the site of injection, extravasation and hypervolemia.

◆ RATED THERAPEUTICALLY EQUIVALENT; ◇ THERAPEUTIC EQUIVALENCE UNCONFIRMED; ○ UNRATED

If an adverse reaction does occur, discontinue the infusion, evaluate the patient, institute appropriate therapeutic countermeasures and save the remainder of the fluid for examination if deemed necessary.

OVERDOSAGE

In the event of overhydration or solute overload, re-evaluate the patient and institute appropriate corrective measures. See *"Warnings"*, *"Precautions"* and *"Adverse Reactions"*.

DOSAGE AND ADMINISTRATION

Dextrose/Electrolytes is administered by intravenous infusion. It may also be administered subcutaneously. The amount to be infused is based on replacement of losses of extracellular fluid volume in the individual patient. Up to 3 times the volume of estimated blood loss during and after surgery can be given to correct circulatory volume when there is only a moderate loss of blood.

DRUG INTERACTIONS

Additives may be incompatible. Consult with pharmacist, if available. When introducing additives, use aseptic technique, mix thoroughly and do not store.

Parenteral drug products should be inspected visually for particulate matter or discoloration prior to administration, whenever solution and container permit. See *"Precautions"*.

Dextrose/Electrolytes does not contain calcium to avoid precipitation of calcium salts that may occur when certain drugs are added. Solutions which contain calcium in amounts exceeding the normal plasma concentration may enhance clotting on contact with citrated blood. Hence, Dextrose/Electrolytes can be used for starting blood transfusion.

Electrolytes and 5% Dextrose Injection is administered by intravenous infusion. The dose is dependent upon the age, weight and clinical condition of the patient. A daily total amount of 1500 mL/M^2 of body surface will meet the usual adult daily requirements for water and principal electrolytes in patients unable to take anything by mouth. The usual daily maintenance amount for an average adult (70 kg and 1.8 square meters of body surface) is approximately three liters.

Pediatric patients may receive a total amount based on 1600 mL (under age 2 yrs.) to 2500 mL (under age 12 yrs.) per M^2 of body surface.

Parenteral drug products should be inspected visually for particulate matter or discoloration prior to administration, whenever solution and container permit. See *"Precautions."*

INSTRUCTIONS FOR USE

To Open: Tear outer wrap at notch and remove solution container. If supplemental medication is desired, follow directions below before preparing for administration. Some opacity of the plastic due to moisture absorption during the sterilization process may be observed. This is normal and does not affect the solution quality or safety. The opacity will diminish gradually.

To Add Medication:
1. Prepare additive port.
2. Using aseptic technique and an additive delivery needle of appropriate length, puncture resealable additive port at target area, inner diaphragm and inject. Withdraw needle after injecting medication.
3. The additive port may be protected by covering with an additive cap.
4. Mix container contents thoroughly.

Preparation for Administration (Use aseptic technique):
1. Close flow control clamp of administration set.
2. Remove cover from outlet port at bottom of container.
3. Insert piercing pin of administration set into port with a twisting motion until the set is firmly seated. *Note:* See full directions on administration set carton.
4. Suspend container from hanger.
5. Squeeze and release drip chamber to establish proper fluid level in chamber.
6. Open flow control clamp and clear air from set. Close clamp.
7. Attach set to venipuncture device. If device is not indwelling, prime and make venipuncture.
8. Regulate rate of administration with flow control clamp.

STORAGE

Exposure of pharmaceutical products to heat should be minimized. Avoid excessive heat. Protect from freezing. It is recommended that the product be stored at room temperature (25° C); however, brief exposure up to 40° C does not adversely affect the product.

HOW SUPPLIED

DEXTROSE/ELECTROLYTES

INJECTION:

AVERAGE UNIT PRICE (AVAILABLE SIZES)		GENERIC A-RATED AVERAGE PRICE (GAAP)	
BRAND	$0.03	1000 ml 12s	$166.56
GENERIC	$0.04	500 ml 24s	$295.68
		250 ml 36s	$443.52

BRAND/MANUFACTURER	NDC	SIZE	AWP
◆ **BRAND**			
PLASMA-LYTE: Baxter	00338-0156-04	1000 ml 6s	$89.94
	00338-0145-04	1000 ml 12s	$186.96
	00338-0149-04	1000 ml 12s	$231.70

BRAND/MANUFACTURER	NDC	SIZE	AWP
	00338-0147-04	1000 ml 12s	$232.13
NORMOSOL-R W/5% DEXTROSE: Abbott Hosp	00074-7968-09	1000 ml 12s	$236.12
NORMOSOL-M W/5% DEXTROSE: Abbott Hosp	00074-7965-09	1000 ml 12s	$236.55
PLASMA-LYTE: Baxter	00338-0149-03	500 ml 24s	$389.38
	00338-0145-03	500 ml 24s	$395.76
NORMOSOL-R W/5% DEXTROSE: Abbott Hosp	00074-7968-03	500 ml 24s	$397.01
PLASMA-LYTE: Baxter	00338-0147-03	500 ml 24s	$398.88
NORMOSOL-M W/5% DEXTROSE: Abbott Hosp	00074-7965-03	500 ml 24s	$406.70
◆ **GENERICS**			
Abbott Hosp	00074-4846-25	500 ml 6s	$237.83
Baxter	00338-0141-04	1000 ml 12s	$165.72
Baxter	00338-0143-04	1000 ml 12s	$167.40
Baxter	00338-0143-03	500 ml 24s	$264.24
Baxter	00338-0141-03	500 ml 24s	$327.12
Baxter	00338-0143-02	250 ml 36s	$396.36
Baxter	00338-0141-02	250 ml 36s	$490.68

INJECTION:

BRAND/MANUFACTURER	NDC	SIZE	AWP
○ **BRAND**			
ISOLYTE P W/DEXTROSE: McGaw	00264-1330-20	250 ml	$13.07
ISOLYTE M W/DEXTROSE: McGaw	00264-7720-20	250 ml	$20.72
ISOLYTE P W/DEXTROSE: McGaw	00264-7730-20	250 ml	$20.72
ISOLYTE M W/DEXTROSE: McGaw	00264-1320-10	500 ml	$16.75
ISOLYTE H W/DEXTROSE: McGaw	00264-7719-10	500 ml	$20.72
ISOLYTE M W/DEXTROSE: McGaw	00264-7720-10	500 ml	$20.72
ISOLYTE S W/DEXTROSE: McGaw	00264-7704-10	500 ml	$20.72
ISOLYTE P W/DEXTROSE: McGaw	00264-7730-10	500 ml	$20.77
ISOLYTE P W/DEXTROSE: McGaw	00264-1341-00	1000 ml	$17.71
ISOLYTE S W/DEXTROSE: McGaw	00264-7704-00	1000 ml	$18.46
ISOLYTE H W/DEXTROSE: McGaw	00264-1319-00	1000 ml	$19.14
ISOLYTE M W/DEXTROSE: McGaw	00264-7720-00	1000 ml	$23.52
ISOLYTE H W/DEXTROSE: McGaw	00264-7719-00	1000 ml	$23.57
ISOLYTE P W/DEXTROSE: McGaw	00264-7730-00	1000 ml	$23.57
ISOLYTE R W/DEXTROSE: McGaw	00264-7741-00	1000 ml	$23.57

SOLUTION:

AVERAGE UNIT PRICE (AVAILABLE SIZES)	
BRAND	$0.008

BRAND/MANUFACTURER	NDC	SIZE	AWP
◆ **BRAND**			
INPERSOL: Abbott Hosp	00074-7944-08	3000 ml 4s	$51.77
	00074-7943-08	3000 ml 4s	$52.96
	00074-7945-08	3000 ml 4s	$54.38
INPERSOL-LM: Abbott Hosp	00074-7892-07	1000 ml 6s	$67.33
INPERSOL-LM: Abbott Hosp	00074-7892-27	2000 ml 6s	$67.33
INPERSOL-LM: Abbott Hosp	00074-7893-07	2000 ml 6s	$67.33
INPERSOL: Abbott Hosp	00074-7943-07	2000 ml 6s	$69.11
	00074-7943-27	2000 ml 6s	$69.11
INPERSOL-LM: Abbott Hosp	00074-7893-07	2000 ml 6s	$69.11
	00074-7893-27	2000 ml 6s	$69.11
INPERSOL: Abbott Hosp	00074-7945-27	2000 ml 6s	$70.53
INPERSOL-LM: Abbott Hosp	00074-7894-07	2000 ml 6s	$70.53
	00074-7894-27	2000 ml 6s	$70.53
INPERSOL: Abbott Hosp	00074-7944-07	2000 ml 6s	$106.16
	00074-7945-07	2000 ml 6s	$111.79
	00074-7943-18	3000 ml 6s	$69.11
INPERSOL-LM: Abbott Hosp	00074-7893-18	3000 ml 6s	$69.11
	00074-7894-18	3000 ml 6s	$70.53
INPERSOL: Abbott Hosp	00074-7945-18	3000 ml 6s	$70.54
	00074-7944-15	1000 ml 12s	$96.18
INPERSOL-LM: Abbott Hosp	00074-7892-05	1000 ml 12s	$96.18
INPERSOL: Abbott Hosp	00074-7943-05	1000 ml 12s	$98.32
	00074-7943-15	1000 ml 12s	$98.32
INPERSOL-LM: Abbott Hosp	00074-7893-05	1000 ml 12s	$98.32
INPERSOL: Abbott Hosp	00074-7945-15	1000 ml 12s	$99.75
	00074-7944-05	1000 ml 12s	$243.11
	00074-7943-17	2000 ml 12s	$138.22
	00074-7945-17	2000 ml 12s	$141.07
	00074-7944-13	500 ml 24s	$192.37
	00074-7943-13	500 ml 24s	$196.65
	00074-7945-13	500 ml 24s	$199.50

SOLUTION:

BRAND/MANUFACTURER	NDC	SIZE	AWP
○ **BRAND**			
DIALYTE: McGaw	00264-2721-00	1000 ml	$12.08
	00264-2723-00	1000 ml	$12.08
	00264-2726-00	1000 ml	$12.08
	00264-2721-50	2000 ml	$19.60
	00264-2723-50	2000 ml	$19.60
	00264-2726-50	2000 ml	$19.63
	00264-2723-70	4000 ml	$23.09
	00264-2721-70	4000 ml	$23.14
	00264-2726-70	4000 ml	$23.14

ELECTROLYTES/MINERALS, MULTI

INJECTION:

AVERAGE UNIT PRICE (AVAILABLE SIZES)

BRAND	$0.22
GENERIC	$0.31

BRAND/MANUFACTURER	NDC	SIZE	AWP
◆ **BRAND**			
LYPHOLYTE II: Fujisawa	00469-1460-40	20 ml	$5.51
LYPHOLYTE: Fujisawa	00469-0900-40	20 ml	$6.60
TRACELYTE: Fujisawa	00469-0800-40	20 ml	$11.57
TRACELYTE II: Fujisawa	00469-1470-40	20 ml	$12.24
LYPHOLYTE II: Fujisawa	00469-1460-60	40 ml	$11.17
TRACELYTE DOUBLE ELECTROLYTES: Fujisawa	00469-1550-60	40 ml	$11.57
TRACELYTE II DOUBLE ELECTROLYTES: Fujisawa	00469-1570-60	40 ml	$11.57
LYPHOLYTE: Fujisawa	00469-0900-60	40 ml	$12.70
LYPHOLYTE II: Fujisawa	00469-1461-00	100 ml	$24.41
LYPHOLYTE: Fujisawa	00469-0901-00	100 ml	$29.86
LYPHOLYTE II: Fujisawa	00469-1462-00	200 ml	$41.83
LYPHOLYTE: Fujisawa	00469-0902-00	200 ml	$53.13
NORMOSOL-R PH 7.4: Abbott Hosp	00074-1570-05	1000 ml 6s	$163.31
PLASMA-LYTE 56: Baxter	00338-0167-04	1000 ml 12s	$121.68
	00338-0168-04	1000 ml 12s	$195.96
PLASMA-LYTE: Baxter	00338-0177-04	1000 ml 12s	$199.44
PLASMA-LYTE 148: Baxter	00338-0179-04	1000 ml 12s	$221.76

Dextrose and Electrolytes, Intraperitoneal

DESCRIPTION

Dextrose/Electrolytes (a peritoneal dialysis solution) is a sterile, nonpyrogenic formulation of electrolytes with three different concentrations of Dextrose in water for injection, each intended only as a dialyzing fluid for intraperitoneal administration. Each is administered by instillation into the peritoneal cavity followed by drainage as a means for removing body wastes, excessive body fluid, serum electrolytes and ingested dialyzable toxic substances. This product is also available with low magnesium content, with four dextrose concentrations.

Dextrose/Electrolytes with one of three dextrose concentrations is designated as follows: Dextrose/Electrolytes with 1.5% Dextrose; Dextrose/Electrolytes with 2.5% Dextrose; or Dextrose/Electrolytes with 4.25% Dextrose. Each 100 ml contains dextrose, hydrous 1.5 g, 2.5 g or 4.25 g respectively; sodium lactate, anhydrous 392 mg; sodium chloride, 567 mg; calcium chloride, dihydrate 25.7 mg and magnesium chloride, hexahydrate 15.2 mg. May contain hydrochloric acid or sodium hydroxide for pH adjustment; pH is 5.2 (approx.).

Electrolytes per 1000 ml (not including ions for pH adjustment): Na^+ 132 mEq; Ca^{++} 3.5 mEq; Mg^{++} 1.5 mEq; Cl^- 102 mEq; lactate $(CH_3CH(OH)COO^-)$ 35 mEq.

Dextrose/Electrolytes osmolar concentrations are as follows: Dextrose/Electrolytes with 1.5% Dextrose, 347 mOsm/liter (calc.); Dextrose/Electrolytes with 2.5% Dextrose, 398 mOsm/liter (calc.); Dextrose/Electrolytes with 4.25% Dextrose, 486 mOsm/liter (calc.).

Low Magnesium Dextrose/Electrolytes with one of four dextrose concentrations is designated as follows: Low Magnesium Dextrose/Electrolytes with 1.5% Dextrose; Low Magnesium Dextrose/Electrolytes with 2.5% Dextrose; Low Magnesium Dextrose/Electrolytes with 3.5% Dextrose; or Low Magnesium Dextrose/Electrolytes with 4.25% Dextrose. Each 100 mL contains dextrose, hydrous 1.5 g, 2.5 g, 3.5 g or 4.25 g respectively; sodium lactate, anhydrous 448 mg; sodium chloride, 538 mg; calcium chloride, dihydrate 25.7 mg; and magnesium chloride, hexahydrate 5.08 mg.

Electrolytes per 1000 mL (not including ions for pH adjustment): Na^+ 132 mEq; Ca^{++} 3.5 mEq; Mg^{++} 0.5 mEq; Cl^- 96 mEq; lactate $(CH_3CH(OH)COO^-)$ 40 mEq.

Low Magnesium Dextrose/Electrolytes osmolar concentrations are as follows: Low Magnesium Dextrose/Electrolytes with 1.5% Dextrose, 346 mOsmol/liter (calc.); Low Magnesium Dextrose/Electrolytes with 2.5% Dextrose, 396 mOsmol/liter (calc.); Low Magnesium Dextrose/Electrolytes with 3.5% Dextrose, 447 mOsmol/liter (calc.); Low Magnesium Dextrose/Electrolytes with 4.25% Dextrose, 485 mOsmol/liter (calc.).

The solutions contain no bacteriostat, antimicrobial agent or added buffer (except for pH adjustment) and each is intended only for use as a single-dose intraperitoneal injection. When smaller doses are required the unused portion should be discarded.

Dextrose/Electrolytes is classified as a peritoneal dialysis solution. Dextrose, USP is chemically designated D-glucose, monohydrate $(C_8H_{12}O_6 \cdot H_2O)$ a hexose sugar freely soluble in water.

Calcium Chloride, USP, is chemically designated calcium chloride, dihydrate $(CaCl_2 \cdot 2H_2O)$ white fragments or granules freely soluble in water.

Magnesium Chloride, USP is chemically designated magnesium chloride, hexahydrate $(MgCl_2 \cdot 6H_2O)$ colorless flakes or crystals very soluble in water.

Sodium Lactate, USP is chemically designated $(CH_3CH(OH)COONa)$, a 60% aqueous solution miscible in water.

Sodium Chloride, USP is chemically designated NaCl, a white, crystalline compound freely soluble in water.

Water for Injection, USP is chemically designated H_2O.

CLINICAL PHARMACOLOGY

Instillation of an appropriate peritoneal dialysis solution into the peritoneal cavity, followed by drainage after a suitable interval, allows exchange of fluid, Electrolytes and body wastes or toxins, according to the concentration gradient between the solution and blood constituents. It represents a simple but safe method of supplementing or bypassing the failing kidney or even the normal kidney when dialyzable substances not normally excreted in the urine, or potentially harmful to the kidney, must be removed.

Dextrose/Electrolytes with 1.5% Dextrose instilled into the peritoneal cavity removes abnormal solutes or abnormal amounts of solutes from the general circulation. Dextrose/Electrolytes with 2.5% Dextrose and 3.5% Dextrose, which have a higher osmotic concentration, provide an intermediate osmolar strength between the 1.5% and 4.25% concentrations. Instillation of Dextrose/Electrolytes with 4.25% Dextrose which is most highly osmotic, is effective for removing excess body water to correct fluid retention. Dextrose/Electrolytes is available without potassium so that hyperkalemia may be corrected.

The osmolar concentration of Dextrose/Electrolytes with 1.5% Dextrose has a calculated value of 347 mOsm/liter, that of Low Magnesium Dextrose/Electrolytes 346 mOsm/liter. The slight excess over the osmolar concentration of plasma is small and simply helps to assure that the amount of fluid returned will equal that instilled in patients having normal fluid balance. The reason for this difference is that in uremic states, the plasma is somewhat hypertonic because of the accumulation of products normally excreted by the kidney. The slight osmolar excess of Dextrose/Electrolytes with 1.5% Dextrose will help to prevent absorption of fluid instilled into the peritoneal cavity, thereby preventing overhydration of the patient.

The higher osmolarity (398 mOsm/liter, calc.) of Dextrose/Electrolytes with 2.5% Dextrose and of Low Magnesium Dextrose/Electrolytes with 2.5% and 3.5% Dextrose (396 and 447 mOsm/liter, calc.) may be more efficient than the 1.5% for removing excess body water and to a lesser extent waste products.

In patients with excessive fluid retention the use of Dextrose/Electrolytes with 4.25% Dextrose which has a calculated value of 486 mOsm/liter (Low Magnesium: 485 mOsm/liter) should be considered. By a solvent drag effect, the enhanced fluid removal may augment solute removal.

INDICATIONS AND USAGE

Dextrose/Electrolytes solutions are indicated for use in peritoneal dialysis. Peritoneal dialysis allows for removing excessive body wastes, excessive body fluid, excessive serum electrolytes and toxic ingestions. Indications include acute or chronic renal failure from any cause, poisoning with barbiturates or other systemic agents which are dialyzable or which cause acute renal insufficiency or failure, intractable edema, hepatic coma, hypercalcemia, hyperkalemia, azotemia and uremia. Peritoneal dialysis with Dextrose/Electrolytes solutions is not suggested as total therapy but as an aid to the management of patients for whom its use is indicated. In some instances, peritoneal dialysis may supplement hemodialysis.

Proper aseptic technique must be used throughout the procedure and at its termination in order to reduce the possibility of infection.

Heating the dialysis solution to 37° C by using a dry-heat cabinet or heating pad may decrease patient discomfort. The use of a water bath to heat the dialysis solution is not recommended.

Low Magnesium Dextrose/Electrolytes solutions are indicated for special peritoneal dialysis requirements. The magnesium concentrations of this formulation have been reduced to 0.5 mEq/L because average plasma magnesium levels in chronic CAPD patients have been observed to be elevated. The formulation may be used where hypermagnesemia is a problem, or where it is desired to increase oral magnesium intake. Furthermore, average serum bicarbonate levels in these patients have been observed to be somewhat lower than normal values; the bicarbonate precursor (lactate) concentration of this formulation has been raised to 40 mEq/L, to help prevent this biochemical condition.

CONTRAINDICATIONS

NOT FOR INJECTION.

The presence of multiple abdominal adhesions may be a mechanical impediment to the use of peritoneal dialysis by interfering with proper insertion of the catheter and by impairing both the instillation and removal of dialyzing fluid.

Peritonitis is no longer considered to be an absolute contraindication. It is treated by adding antibiotics to the dialysis solution and by systemic administration of antibiotics.

WARNINGS

FOR INTRAPERITONEAL ADMINISTRATION ONLY.

Solutions containing lactate ion should be used with great care in patients with metabolic or respiratory alkalosis. Lactate should be administered with great care in those conditions in which there is an increased level or an impaired utilization of this ion, such as severe hepatic insufficiency.

Do not heat container over 66° C (150° F) or administer solution above 37° C (98.6° F).

◆ RATED THERAPEUTICALLY EQUIVALENT; ◇ THERAPEUTIC EQUIVALENCE UNCONFIRMED; ○ UNRATED

PRECAUTIONS

Repeated instillation of potassium free peritoneal dialysis solutions may result in hypokalemia. Serum potassium as well as other serum electrolytes should be monitored, especially in patients receiving concomitant cardiac glycoside therapy (e.g., digitalis). When necessary, potassium may be added to the dialysis solution or given by mouth to maintain or restore normokalemic levels.

Recent or extensive abdominal surgery is a relative contraindication. The decision to use or withhold peritoneal dialysis in these cases lies with the physician. As a matter of record, peritoneal dialysis has been safely employed within three to ten days after numerous and varied intra-abdominal procedures.

Local edema from subcutaneous infiltration of the dialyzing solution may result if the catheter is incompletely inserted or if leakage from around the catheter is not controlled. Significant leakage may result in inaccurate determinations of fluid balance. The catheter may be readjusted if necessary.

Paralytic or adynamic ileus may occur, thus indicating the need for Wangensteen suction of the bowel as dialysis continues. However, this complication has occurred mainly during continuous irrigation and has rarely been seen during intermittent dialysis.

LABORATORY TESTS

When peritoneal dialysis is employed, careful attention must be given to maintaining fluid and electrolyte requirements, and controlling blood urea nitrogen (BUN) and serum creatinine concentrations.

Plasma electrolyte concentrations should be determined at regular intervals. Since protein depletion may occur during prolonged peritoneal dialysis, repeated determination of plasma protein concentration may be indicated. When necessary, protein replacement therapy should be instituted. Care should also be taken to avoid hyperglycemia during dialysis. If hyperglycemia does occur, appropriate insulin therapy should be instituted.

An accurate fluid balance record should be maintained and the weight of the patient carefully monitored.

Just as overhydration should be avoided, so should the two vigorous treatment of edema. Too rapid loss of fluid may result in a reduction of the effective circulating blood volume with consequent precipitation of shock and/or aggravation of renal impairment. Cardiac and central venous pressure status should be ascertained and appropriate measures to restore blood volume to normal or cardiogenic therapy should be instituted. Similarly, the overly rapid biochemical correction of severe uremia, due to the removal of urea more rapidly from the extracellular than from the intracellular water, may result in cellular and in particular, cerebral edema. Although such a complication occurs more commonly with hemodialysis, it has been seen occasionally in patients undergoing peritoneal lavage.

Hypernatremia should be avoided.

Solutions containing lactate ion should be used with caution as excess administration may result in metabolic alkalosis.

Do not administer unless solution is clear and container is undamaged. Discard unused portion.

When using Low Magnesium Dextrose/Electrolytes, plasma electrolyte concentrations should be determined at regular intervals. Serum magnesium levels should be monitored and if low, oral magnesium supplements or peritoneal dialysis solutions containing higher magnesium concentrations may be used.

Pregnancy Category C. Animal reproduction studies have not been conducted with Dextrose/Electrolytes solutions. It is also not known whether Dextrose/Electrolytes solutions can cause fetal harm when administered to a pregnant woman or can affect reproduction capacity. Dextrose/Electrolytes solutions should be given to a pregnant woman only if clearly needed.

ADVERSE REACTIONS

Adverse reactions in peritoneal dialysis include mechanical and solution related problems, as well as the results of contamination of equipment or improper technique in catheter placement.

Reactions to peritoneal dialysis in approximate decreasing order of severity are: uncontrolled infection (peritonitis, abdominal abscess, bowel perforation or necrosis, septicemia); ileus; abdominal pain; intra-abdominal hemorrhage or adhesions; hyperglycemia leading to hyperosmolar coma; hypoglycemia; electrolyte and fluid imbalance (edema, hypo- or hypervolemia, hypo- or hypertension, hypo- or hypernatremia, hypo- or hyperkalemia, metabolic alkalosis, disequilibrium syndrome, muscle cramps). The most frequent reactions to peritoneal dialysis are moderate abdominal pain and metabolic disturbances. These occur in about one-half of patients. Less frequent adverse reactions are: inadequate drainage (catheter obstruction, etc.), fluid leakage (around catheter site) and minimal to severe intra-abdominal hemorrhage which occur in about one-third of patients (approximately 35 in 100); occurrence of hyperglycemia, hypernatremia, hypo- and hyperkalemia, pulmonary atelectasis, pneumonia, and metabolic alkalosis ranges approximately 5 to 10 in 100 patients; other complications (including peritonitis) occur in a range of approximately less than 1 to 5 in 100 patients. The severity and incidence of adverse reactions during peritoneal dialysis is dependent upon the conduct of the procedure to prevent or control infection, to insure proper mechanical techniques, and to alter the dialyzing fluid as required to avoid complications.

If an adverse reaction does occur, discontinue dialysis, evaluate the patient, institute appropriate therapeutic measures and save the remainder of the fluid for examination if deemed necessary.

OVERDOSAGE

In the event of overhydration or solute overload, re-evaluate the patient and institute appropriate corrective measures. See *"Warnings," "Precautions"* and *"Adverse Reactions".*

DOSAGE AND ADMINISTRATION

Dextrose/Electrolytes solution is intended for intraperitoneal administration only. The mode of therapy, frequency, formulation, exchange volume, dwell time and length of dialysis should be selected by the physician who is responsible for treating each individual patient.

Heating the dialysis solution to 37° C by using a dry-heat cabinet or heating pad may decrease patient discomfort. The use of a water bath to heat the dialysis solution is not recommended.

The addition of heparin to the dialysis solution may be indicated to aid in prevention of catheter blockage when the solution drainage contains fibrinous or proteinaceous material.

To avoid the risk of severe dehydration and hypovolemia and to minimize the loss of protein, it is advisable to select the peritoneal dialysis solution with lowest level of osmolarity consistent with the fluid removal requirements for each exchange.

DRUG INTERACTIONS

Additives may be incompatible. Consult with pharmacist, if available. When introducing additives, use aseptic technique, mix thoroughly and do not store.

Parenteral drug products should be inspected visually for particulate matter and discoloration prior to administration, whenever solution and container permit. See *"Precautions".*

HOW SUPPLIED
INJECTION:

AVERAGE UNIT PRICE (AVAILABLE SIZES)		GENERIC A-RATED AVERAGE PRICE (GAAP)	
BRAND	$0.03	1000 ml 12s	$166.56
GENERIC	$0.04	500 ml 24s	$295.68
		250 ml 36s	$443.52

BRAND/MANUFACTURER	NDC	SIZE	AWP
◆ **BRAND**			
PLASMA-LYTE: Baxter	00338-0156-04	1000 ml 6s	$89.94
	00338-0145-04	1000 ml 12s	$186.96
	00338-0149-04	1000 ml 12s	$231.70
	00338-0147-04	1000 ml 12s	$232.13
NORMOSOL-R W/5% DEXTROSE: Abbott Hosp	00074-7968-09	1000 ml 12s	$236.12
NORMOSOL-M W/5% DEXTROSE: Abbott Hosp	00074-7965-09	1000 ml 12s	$236.55
PLASMA-LYTE: Baxter	00338-0149-03	500 ml 24s	$389.38
	00338-0145-03	500 ml 24s	$395.76
NORMOSOL-R W/5% DEXTROSE: Abbott Hosp	00074-7968-03	500 ml 24s	$397.01
PLASMA-LYTE: Baxter	00338-0147-03	500 ml 24s	$398.88
NORMOSOL-M W/5% DEXTROSE: Abbott Hosp	00074-7965-03	500 ml 24s	$406.70
◆ **GENERICS**			
Abbott Hosp	00074-4846-25	500 ml 6s	$237.83
Baxter	00338-0141-04	1000 ml 12s	$165.72
Baxter	00338-0143-04	1000 ml 12s	$167.40
Baxter	00338-0143-03	500 ml 24s	$264.24
Baxter	00338-0141-03	500 ml 24s	$327.12
Baxter	00338-0143-02	250 ml 36s	$396.36
Baxter	00338-0141-02	250 ml 36s	$490.68

INJECTION:

BRAND/MANUFACTURER	NDC	SIZE	AWP
○ **BRAND**			
ISOLYTE P W/DEXTROSE: McGaw	00264-1330-20	250 ml	$13.07
ISOLYTE M W/DEXTROSE: McGaw	00264-7720-20	250 ml	$20.72
ISOLYTE P W/DEXTROSE: McGaw	00264-7730-20	250 ml	$20.72
ISOLYTE M W/DEXTROSE: McGaw	00264-1320-10	500 ml	$16.75
ISOLYTE M W/DEXTROSE: McGaw	00264-7719-10	500 ml	$20.72
ISOLYTE M W/DEXTROSE: McGaw	00264-7720-10	500 ml	$20.72
ISOLYTE S W/DEXTROSE: McGaw	00264-7704-10	500 ml	$20.72
ISOLYTE P W/DEXTROSE: McGaw	00264-7730-10	500 ml	$20.77
ISOLYTE M W/DEXTROSE: McGaw	00264-1341-00	1000 ml	$17.71
ISOLYTE S W/DEXTROSE: McGaw	00264-7704-00	1000 ml	$18.46
ISOLYTE H W/DEXTROSE: McGaw	00264-1319-00	1000 ml	$19.14
ISOLYTE M W/DEXTROSE: McGaw	00264-7720-00	1000 ml	$23.52
ISOLYTE H W/DEXTROSE: McGaw	00264-7719-00	1000 ml	$23.57
ISOLYTE P W/DEXTROSE: McGaw	00264-7730-00	1000 ml	$23.57
ISOLYTE R W/DEXTROSE: McGaw	00264-7741-00	1000 ml	$23.57

SOLUTION:

AVERAGE UNIT PRICE (AVAILABLE SIZES)	
BRAND	$0.008

BRAND/MANUFACTURER	NDC	SIZE	AWP
◆ **BRAND**			
INPERSOL: Abbott Hosp	00074-7944-08	3000 ml 4s	$51.77
	00074-7943-08	3000 ml 4s	$52.96
	00074-7945-08	3000 ml 4s	$54.38
INPERSOL-LM: Abbott Hosp	00074-7892-07	1000 ml 6s	$67.33
INPERSOL: Abbott Hosp	00074-7944-27	2000 ml 6s	$67.33
INPERSOL-LM: Abbott Hosp	00074-7892-27	2000 ml 6s	$67.33
INPERSOL: Abbott Hosp	00074-7943-07	2000 ml 6s	$69.11

➤ **SHOWN IN PRODUCT IDENTIFICATION GUIDE**

BRAND/MANUFACTURER	NDC	SIZE	AWP
	00074-7943-27	2000 ml 6s	$69.11
INPERSOL-LM: Abbott Hosp	00074-7893-07	2000 ml 6s	$69.11
	00074-7893-27	2000 ml 6s	$69.11
INPERSOL: Abbott Hosp	00074-7945-27	2000 ml 6s	$70.53
INPERSOL-LM: Abbott Hosp	00074-7894-07	2000 ml 6s	$70.53
	00074-7894-27	2000 ml 6s	$70.53
INPERSOL: Abbott Hosp	00074-7944-07	2000 ml 6s	$106.16
	00074-7945-07	2000 ml 6s	$111.79
	00074-7943-18	3000 ml 6s	$69.11
INPERSOL-LM: Abbott Hosp	00074-7893-18	3000 ml 6s	$69.11
	00074-7894-18	3000 ml 6s	$70.53
INPERSOL: Abbott Hosp	00074-7945-18	3000 ml 6s	$70.54
INPERSOL-LM: Abbott Hosp	00074-7944-15	1000 ml 12s	$96.18
INPERSOL: Abbott Hosp	00074-7892-05	1000 ml 12s	$96.18
	00074-7943-05	1000 ml 12s	$98.32
	00074-7943-15	1000 ml 12s	$98.32
INPERSOL-LM: Abbott Hosp	00074-7893-05	1000 ml 12s	$98.32
INPERSOL: Abbott Hosp	00074-7945-15	1000 ml 12s	$99.75
	00074-7944-05	1000 ml 12s	$243.11
	00074-7943-17	2000 ml 12s	$138.22
	00074-7945-17	2000 ml 12s	$141.07
	00074-7944-13	500 ml 24s	$192.37
	00074-7943-13	500 ml 24s	$196.65
	00074-7945-13	500 ml 24s	$199.50

SOLUTION:

BRAND/MANUFACTURER	NDC	SIZE	AWP
○ BRAND			
DIALYTE: McGaw	00264-2721-00	1000 ml	$12.08
	00264-2723-00	1000 ml	$12.08
	00264-2726-00	1000 ml	$12.08
	00264-2721-50	2000 ml	$19.60
	00264-2723-50	2000 ml	$19.60
	00264-2726-50	2000 ml	$19.63
	00264-2723-70	4000 ml	$23.09
	00264-2721-70	4000 ml	$23.14
	00264-2726-70	4000 ml	$23.14

Dextrose and Potassium Chloride

DESCRIPTION
Dextrose/Potassium Chloride Injection, USP, is a sterile and nonpyrogenic solution in water for injection. It is for administration by intravenous infusion only and is available as 20, 30, or 40 mEq/liter Potassium Chloride in 5% Dextrose.

The solutions contain no bacteriostat, antimicrobial agent or added buffer and each is intended only for use as a single-dose injection. When smaller doses are required, the unused portion should be discarded.

These solutions are parenteral fluid, nutrient and electrolyte replenishers.

Dextrose, USP is chemically designated D-glucose monohydrate ($C_6H_{12}O_6 \cdot H_2O$), a hexose sugar freely soluble in water.

Potassium Chloride, USP, is chemically designated KCl, a white granular powder freely soluble in water.

Water for Injection, USP, is chemically designated H_2O.

CLINICAL PHARMACOLOGY
When administered intravenously, these solutions provide a source of water and Potassium Chloride with carbohydrate.

Solutions containing carbohydrate in the form of Dextrose restore blood glucose levels and provide calories. Carbohydrate in the form of Dextrose may aid in minimizing liver glycogen depletion and exerts a protein-sparing action. Dextrose injected parenterally undergoes oxidation to carbon dioxide and water.

Intravenous solutions containing Potassium Chloride are particularly intended to provide needed Potassium cation (K^+). Potassium is the chief cation of body cells (160 mEq/liter of intracellular water). It is found in low concentration in plasma and extracellular fluids (3.5 to 5.0 mEq/liter in a healthy adult). Potassium plays an important role in electrolyte balance. Normally about 80 to 90% of the Potassium intake is excreted in the urine; the remainder in the stools and to a small extent, in the perspiration. The kidney does not conserve Potassium well so that during fasting or in patients on a Potassium-free diet, Potassium loss from the body continues resulting in Potassium depletion. A deficiency of either Potassium or Chloride will lead to a deficit of the other.

Water is an essential constituent of all body tissues and accounts for approximately 70% of total body weight. Average normal adult daily requirement ranges from two three liters (1.0 to 1.5 liters each for insensible water loss by perspiration and urine production).

Water balance is maintained by various regulatory mechanisms. Water distribution depends primarily on the concentration of electrolytes in the body compartments and sodium (Na^+) plays a major role in maintaining physiologic equilibrium.

INDICATIONS AND USAGE
These solutions are indicated in patients requiring parenteral administration of Potassium Chloride with minimal carbohydrate calories.

CONTRAINDICATIONS
Solutions containing Potassium Chloride are contraindicated in diseases where high Potassium levels may be encountered.

WARNINGS
Solutions which contain Potassium ions should be used with great care, if at all, in patients with hyperkalemia, severe renal failure and in conditions in which Potassium retention is present.

To avoid Potassium intoxication, do not infuse these solutions rapidly. In patients with severe renal insufficiency or adrenal insufficiency, administration of Potassium Chloride may cause Potassium intoxication.

In patients with diminished renal function, administration of solutions containing Potassium ions may result in Potassium retention.

The intravenous administration of these solutions can cause fluid and/or solute overloading resulting in dilution of serum electrolyte concentrations, overhydration, congested states or pulmonary edema.

The risk of dilutional states is inversely proportional to the electrolyte concentration of administered parenteral solutions. The risk of solute overload causing congested states with peripheral and pulmonary edema is directly proportional to the electrolyte concentrations of such solutions.

PRECAUTIONS
Clinical evaluation and periodic laboratory determinations are necessary to monitor changes in fluid balance, electrolyte concentrations and acid-base balance during prolonged parenteral therapy or whenever the condition of the patient warrants such evaluation.

Solutions containing Dextrose should be used with caution in patients with known subclinical or overt diabetes mellitus.

Potassium replacement therapy should be guided primarily by serial electrocardiograms. Plasma Potassium levels are not necessarily indicative of tissue Potassium levels.

High plasma concentrations of Potassium may cause death through cardiac depression, arrhythmias or arrest.

Potassium-containing solutions should be used with caution in the presence of cardiac disease, particularly in digitalized patients or in the presence of renal disease.

Care should be exercised to insure that the needle (or catheter) is well within the lumen of the vein and that extravasation does not occur.

Do not administer unless solution is clear and container is undamaged. Discard unused portion.

Pregnancy Category C: Animal reproduction studies have not been conducted with Dextrose or Potassium Chloride. It is also not known whether Dextrose or Potassium Chloride can cause fetal harm when administered to a pregnant woman or can affect reproduction capacity. Dextrose or Potassium Chloride should be given to a pregnant woman only if clearly needed.

ADVERSE REACTIONS
Reactions which may occur because of the solution or technique of administration include febrile response, infection at the site of injection, venous thrombosis or phlebitis extending from the site of injection, extravasation and hypervolemia.

If an adverse reaction does occur, discontinue the infusion, evaluate the patient, institute appropriate therapeutic countermeasures and save the remainder of the fluid for examination if deemed necessary.

Nausea, vomiting, abdominal pain and diarrhea have been reported with Potassium therapy. The signs and symptoms of Potassium intoxication include paresthesias of the extremities, flaccid paralysis, listlessness, mental confusion, weakness and heaviness of the legs, hypotension, cardiac arrhythmias, heart block, electrocardiographic abnormalities such as disappearance of P waves, spreading and slurring of the QRS complex with development of a biphasic curve and cardiac arrest.

Potassium-containing solutions are intrinsically irritating to tissues. Therefore, extreme care should be taken to avoid perivascular infiltration. Local tissue necrosis and subsequent sloughing may result if extravasation occurs. Chemical phlebitis and venospasm have also been reported.

Should perivascular infiltration occur, I.V. administration at that site should be discontinued at once. Local infiltration of the affected area with procaine hydrochloride, 1%, to which hyaluronidase may be added, will often reduce venospasm and dilute the Potassium remaining in the tissues locally. Local application of heat may also be helpful.

OVERDOSAGE
In the event of Potassium overdosage, discontinue the infusion immediately and institute intensive corrective therapy to reduce serum Potassium levels. See *"Warnings"* and *"Precautions"*.

DOSAGE AND ADMINISTRATION
These solutions should be administered only by intravenous infusion and as directed by the physician. The dose and rate of injection are dependent upon the age, weight and clinical condition of the patient. If the serum Potassium level is greater than 2.5 mEq/liter, Potassium should be given at a rate not to exceed 10 mEq/hour in a concentration less than 30 mEq/liter. Somewhat faster rates and greater concentrations (usually up to 40 mEq/liter) of Potassium may be indicated in patients with more severe Potassium deficiency. The total 24-hour dose should not generally exceed 200 mEq of Potassium.

Parenteral drug products should be inspected visually for particulate matter and discoloration prior to administration, whenever solution and container permit. See *"Precautions"*.

◆ RATED THERAPEUTICALLY EQUIVALENT; ◇ THERAPEUTIC EQUIVALENCE UNCONFIRMED; ○ UNRATED

DRUG INTERACTIONS

Additives may be incompatible. Consult with pharmacist, if available. When introducing additives, use aseptic technique, mix thoroughly and do not store.

INSTRUCTIONS FOR USE

To Open: Tear outer wrap at notch and remove solution container. If supplemental medication is desired, follow directions below before preparing for administration.

To Add Medication:
1. Prepare additive port.
2. Using aseptic technique and an additive delivery needle of appropriate length, puncture resealable additive port at target area, inner diaphragm and inject. Withdraw needle after injecting medication.
3. The additive port may be protected by covering with an additive cap.
4. Mix container contents thoroughly.

Preparation for Administration (Use aseptic technique):
1. Close flow control clamp of administration set.
2. Remove cover from outlet port at bottom of container.
3. Insert piercing pin of administration set into port with a twisting motion until the set is firmly seated. *Note*: When using a vented administration set, replace bacterial retentive air filter with piercing pin cover. Insert piercing pin with twisting motion until shoulder of air filter housing rests against the outlet port flange.
4. Suspend container from hanger.
5. Squeeze and release drip chamber to establish proper fluid level in chamber.
6. Attach venipuncture device to set.
7. Open clamp to expel air from set and venipuncture device. Close clamp.
8. Perform venipuncture.
9. Regulate rate of administration with flow control clamp.
   WARNING: Do not use flexible container in series connections.

STORAGE

Exposure of pharmaceutical products to heat should be minimized. Avoid excessive heat. Protect from freezing. It is recommended that the product be stored at room temperature (25°C); however, brief exposure up to 40°C does not adversely affect the product.

HOW SUPPLIED
INJECTION: 5%-0.224%

AVERAGE UNIT PRICE (AVAILABLE SIZES)		GENERIC A-RATED AVERAGE PRICE (GAAP)	
GENERIC	$0.02	1000 ml 12s	$203.40

BRAND/MANUFACTURER	NDC	SIZE	AWP
◆ GENERICS			
Baxter	00338-0685-04	1000 ml 12s	$201.46
Abbott Hosp	00074-7996-09	1000 ml 12s	$205.34

INJECTION: 5%-0.075%

BRAND/MANUFACTURER	NDC	SIZE	AWP
◆ GENERICS			
Baxter	00338-0681-04	1000 ml 12s	$201.46

INJECTION: 5%-0.15%

AVERAGE UNIT PRICE (AVAILABLE SIZES)		GENERIC A-RATED AVERAGE PRICE (GAAP)	
GENERIC	$0.02	1000 ml 12s	$203.40

BRAND/MANUFACTURER	NDC	SIZE	AWP
◆ GENERICS			
Baxter	00338-0683-03	500 ml 12s	$79.92
Baxter	00338-0683-04	1000 ml 12s	$201.46
Abbott Hosp	00074-7905-09	1000 ml 12s	$205.34

INJECTION: 5%-0.3%

AVERAGE UNIT PRICE (AVAILABLE SIZES)		GENERIC A-RATED AVERAGE PRICE (GAAP)	
GENERIC	$0.03	1000 ml 12s	$203.40

BRAND/MANUFACTURER	NDC	SIZE	AWP
◆ GENERICS			
Baxter	00338-0687-03	500 ml 12s	$273.36
Baxter	00338-0687-04	1000 ml 12s	$201.46
Abbott Hosp	00074-7906-09	1000 ml 12s	$205.34
Abbott Hosp	00074-7906-03	500 ml 24s	$410.69

Dextrose and Ringer's

DESCRIPTION

These products are sterile, nonpyrogenic solutions each containing isotonic concentrations of electrolytes (with or without Dextrose) in water for injection. The solutions containing dextrose and electrolytes are hypertonic; those containing only electrolytes are isotonic. They are administered by intravenous infusion for parenteral replacement of extracellular losses of fluid and electrolytes, with or without minimal carbohydrate calories.

Each 100 mL of Ringer's Injection, USP contains sodium chloride 860 mg, potassium chloride 30 mg and calcium chloride, dihydrate 33 mg. May contain hydrochloric acid and/or sodium hydroxide for pH adjustment. A liter provides 147 mEq sodium (Na^+), 4 mEq potassium (K^+), 4 mEq calcium (Ca^{++}) and 155 mEq chloride (Cl^-). The electrolyte content is isotonic (309 mOsmol/liter, calc.) in relation to the extracellular fluid (approx. 280 mOsmol/liter). The pH of the solution is 5.4 (5.0-7.5).

Each 100 mL of 5% Dextrose and Ringer's Injection contains dextrose, hydrous 5 g plus the same ingredients and mEq values as Ringer's Injection, USP. A liter provides 170 calories (from dextrose) and has a hypertonic osmolar concentration of 561 mOsmol (calc.). The pH is 4.3 (3.5-6.5).

Each 100 mL of Lactated Ringer's Injection, USP contains sodium chloride 600 mg, sodium lactate, anhydrous 310 mg, potassium chloride 30 mg and calcium chloride, dihydrate 20 mg. May contain hydrochloric acid and/or sodium hydroxide for pH adjustment. A liter provides 9 calories (from lactate), sodium (Na^+), 130 mEq, potassium (K^+) 4 mEq, calcium (Ca^{++}) 3 mEq, chloride (Cl^-) 109 mEq and lactate [$CH_3CH(OH) COO^-$] 28 mEq. The electrolyte content is isotonic (273 mOsmol/liter, calc.) in relation to the extracellular fluid (approx. 280 mOsmol/liter). The pH of the solution is 6.6 (6.0-7.5).

Each 100 mL of 5% Dextrose and Lactated Ringer's Injection contains Dextrose, hydrous 5 g plus the same ingredients and mEq values as Lactated Ringer's Injection, USP (contains only hydrochloric acid for pH adjustment). A liter provides 179 calories (from dextrose and lactate) and has a hypertonic osmolar concentration of 525 mOsmol (calc.). The pH is 4.9 (4.5-5.2).

The solutions contain no bacteriostat, antimicrobial agent or added buffer (except for pH adjustment) and each is intended only for use as a single-dose injection. When smaller doses are required the unused portion should be discarded.

The solutions are parenteral fluid, nutrient and/or electrolyte replenishers.

Dextrose, USP, is chemically designated D-glucose, monohydrate ($C_6H_{12}O_6 \cdot H_2O$), a hexose sugar freely soluble in water.

Calcium Chloride, USP is chemically designated calcium chloride, dihydrate ($CaCl_2 \cdot 2 H_2O$), white fragments or granultes freely soluble in water.

Potassium Chloride, USP is chemically designated KCl, a white granular powder freely soluble in water.

Sodium Chloride, USP is chemically designated NaCl, a white crystalline powder freely soluble in water.

Sodium Lactate, USP is chemically designated monosodium lactate [$CH_3CH(OH)COONa$], a 60% aqueous solution miscible in water.

Water for Injection, USP is chemically designated H_2O.

CLINICAL PHARMACOLOGY

When administered intravenously, these solutions provide sources of water and electrolytes with or without minimal carbohydrate calories. Their electrolyte content resembles that of the principal ionic constituents of normal plasma and the solutions therefore are suitable for parenteral replacement of extracellular losses of fluid and electrolytes, with or without carbohydrate calories.

Solutions containing carbohydrate in the form of dextrose restore blood glucose levels and provide calories.

Carbohydrate in the form of dextrose may aid in minimizing liver glycogen depletion and exerts a protein-sparing action. Dextrose injected parenterally undergoes oxidation to carbon dioxide and water.

Calcium chloride in water dissociates to provide calcium (Ca^{++}) and chloride (Cl^-) ions. They are normal constituents of the body fluids and are dependent on various physiologic mechanisms for maintenance of balance between intake and output. Approximately 80% of body calcium is excreted in the feces as insoluble salts; urinary excretion accounts for the remaining 20%.

Potassium chloride in water dissociates to provide potassium (K^+) and chloride (Cl^-) ions. Potassium is found in low concentration in plasma and extracellular fluids (3.5 to 5.0 mEq/liter in a healthy adult). It is the chief cation of body cells (160 mEq/liter of intracellular water). Potassium plays an important role in electrolyte balance. Normally about 80 to 90% of the potassium intake is excreted in the urine; the remainder in the stools and to a small extent, in the perspiration. The kidney does not conserve potassium well so that during fasting or in patients on a potassium-free diet, potassium loss from the body continues resulting in potassium depletion.

Sodium chloride in water dissociates to provide sodium (Na^+) and chloride (Cl^-) ions. Sodium (Na^+) is the principal cation of the extracellular fluid and plays a large part in the therapy of fluid and electrolyte disturbances. Chloride (Cl^-) has an integral role in buffering action when oxygen and carbon dioxide exchange occurs in the red blood cells. The distribution and excretion of sodium (Na^+) and chloride (Cl^-) are largely under the control of the kidney which maintains a balance between intake and output.

Sodium lactate provides sodium (Na^+) and lactate ($C_3H_5O_3^-$) ions. The lactate anion is in equilibrium with pyruvate and has an alkalizing effect resulting from simultaneous removal by the liver of lactate and hydrogen ions. In the liver, lactate is metabolized to glycogen which is ultimately converted to carbon dioxide and water by oxidative metabolism. The sodium (Na^+) ion combines with bicarbonate ion produced from carbon dioxide of the body and thus retains bicarbonate to combat metabolic acidosis (bicarbonate deficiency). The normal plasma level of lactate ranges from 0.9 to 1.9 mEq/liter.

Water is an essential constituent of all body tissues and accounts for approximately 70% of total body weight. Average normal adult daily requirement ranges from two to three liters (1.0 to 1.5 liters each for insensible water loss by perspiration and urine production).

Water balance is maintained by various regulatory mechanisms. Water distribution depends primarily on the concentration of electrolytes in the body compartments and sodium (Na^+) plays a major role in maintaining physiologic equilibrium.

INDICATIONS AND USAGE

These solutions are indicated for parenteral replacement of extracellular losses of fluid and electrolytes, with or without minimal carbohydrate calories, as required by the clinical condition of the patient.

CONTRAINDICATIONS

Solutions containing lactate are NOT FOR USE IN THE TREATMENT OF LACTIC ACIDOSIS.

WARNINGS

Solutions containing calcium ions should not be administered simultaneously through the same administration set as blood because of the likelihood of coagulation.

Solutions which contain potassium should be used with great care, if at all, in patients with hyperkalemia, severe renal failure and in conditions in which potassium retention is present.

Solutions containing sodium ions should be used with great care, if at all, in patients with congestive heart failure, severe renal insufficiency and in clinical states in which there exists edema with sodium retention.

In patients with diminished renal function, administration of solutions containing sodium or potassium ions may result in sodium or potassium retention.

Solutions containing lactate ions should be used with great care in patients with metabolic or respiratory alkalosis. The administration of lactate ions should be done with great care where there is an increased level or an impaired utilization of lactate ions, as in severe hepatic insufficiency.

The intravenous administration of these solutions can cause fluid and/or solute overloading resulting in dilution of serum electrolyte concentrations, overhydration, congested states or pulmonary edema. The risk of dilutional states is inversely proportional to the electrolyte concentrations of administered parenteral solutions.

The risk of solute overload causing congested states with peripheral and pulmonary edema is directly proportional to the electrolyte concentrations of such solutions.

PRECAUTIONS

Clinical evaluation and periodic laboratory determinations are necessary to monitor changes in fluid balance, electrolyte concentrations and acid-base balance during prolonged parenteral therapy or whenever the condition of the patient warrants such evaluation.

Solutions containing dextrose should be used with caution in patients with known subclinical or overt diabetes mellitus.

Caution must be exercised in the administration of parenteral fluids, especially those containing sodium ions, to patients receiving corticosteroids or corticotropin.

Potassium containing solutions should be used with caution in the presence of cardiac disease, particularly in digitalized patients or in the presence of renal disease.

Solutions containing lactate ions should be used with caution as excess administration may result in metabolic alkalosis.

Do not administer unless solution is clear and container is undamaged. Discard unused portion.

Pregnancy Category C: Animal reproduction studies have not been conducted with Ringer's Injection, USP, Dextrose and Ringer's Injection, Lactated Ringer's Injection, USP or Dextrose and Lactated Ringer's Injection. It is also not known whether these injections can cause fetal harm when administered to a pregnant woman or can affect reproduction capacity. These injections should be given to a pregnant woman only if clearly needed.

ADVERSE REACTIONS

Reactions which may occur because of the solution or the technique of administration include febrile response, infection at the site of injection, venous thrombosis or phlebitis extending from the site of injection, extravasation and hypervolemia.

If an adverse reaction does occur, discontinue the infusion, evaluate the patient, institute appropriate therapeutic countermeasures and save the remainder of the fluid for examination if deemed necessary.

OVERDOSAGE

In the event of overhydration or solute overload, re-evaluate the patient and institute appropriate corrective measures. See *"Warnings," "Precautions,"* and *"Adverse Reactions"*.

DOSAGE AND ADMINISTRATION

The dose is dependent upon the age, weight and clinical condition of the patient.

DRUG INTERACTIONS

Additives may be incompatible. Consult with pharmacist, if available. When introducing additives, use aseptic technique, mix thoroughly and do not store.

The presence of calcium limits their compatibility with certain drugs that form precipitates of calcium salts, and also prohibits their simultaneous infusion through the same administration set as blood because of the likelihood of coagulation.

Parenteral drug products should be inspected visually for particulate matter and discoloration prior to administration, whenever solution and container permit. See *"Precautions"*.

To Add Medication:
1. Prepare additive port.
2. Using aseptic technique and an additive delivery needle of appropriate length, puncture resealable additive port at target area, inner diaphragm and inject. Withdraw needle after injecting medication.
3. The additive port may be protected by covering with an additive cap.
4. Mix container contents thoroughly.

Preparation for Administration (Use aseptic technique):
1. Close flow control clamp of administration set.
2. Remove cover from outlet port at bottom of container.
3. Insert piercing pin of administration set into port with a twisting motion until the set is firmly seated. *Note*: See full directions on administration set carton.
4. Suspend container from hanger.
5. Squeeze and release drip chamber to establish proper fluid level in chamber.
6. Open flow control clamp and clear air from set. Close clamp.
7. Attach set to venipuncture device. If device is not indwelling, prime and make venipuncture.
8. Regulate rate of administration with flow control clamp.

Storage: Exposure of pharmaceutical products to heat should be minimized. Avoid excessive heat. Protect from freezing. It is recommended that the product be stored at room temperature (25°C); however, brief exposure up to 40°C does not adversely affect the product.

WARNING: DO NOT USE FLEXIBLE CONTAINER IN SERIES CONNECTIONS.

HOW SUPPLIED
INJECTION: 2.5%

BRAND/MANUFACTURER	NDC	SIZE	AWP
◆ GENERICS			
Abbott Hosp	00074-1521-05	1000 ml 6s	$99.11

INJECTION: 5%

AVERAGE UNIT PRICE (AVAILABLE SIZES)		GENERIC A-RATED AVERAGE PRICE (GAAP)	
GENERIC	$0.02	1000 ml 12s	$175.42
		500 ml 24s	$275.98

BRAND/MANUFACTURER	NDC	SIZE	AWP
◆ GENERICS			
McGaw	00264-1351-10	500 ml	$11.06
McGaw	00264-1351-00	1000 ml	$13.31
Abbott Hosp	00074-7929-09	1000 ml 12s	$164.59
Baxter	00338-0111-04	1000 ml 12s	$179.14
Abbott Hosp	00074-7933-09	1000 ml 12s	$182.54
Abbott Hosp	00074-7929-03	500 ml 24s	$273.03
Baxter	00338-0111-03	500 ml 24s	$274.75
Abbott Hosp	00074-7933-03	500 ml 24s	$280.16

Dextrose and Sodium Chloride

DESCRIPTION

Dextrose and Sodium Chloride solutions are sterile and nonpyrogenic. They are large volume parenteral solutions containing various concentrations and combinations of these drugs in water for injection intended for intravenous administration.

See table for summary of content and characteristics of these solutions. (See related table).

The solutions contain no bacteriostat, antimicrobial agent or added buffer and each is intended only as a single-dose injection. When smaller doses are required the unused portion should be discarded.

The solutions are parenteral fluid, nutrient and electrolyte replenishers.

Dextrose, USP is chemically designated D-glucose monohydrate ($C_6H_{12}O_6 \cdot H_2O$), a hexose sugar freely soluble in water.

Sodium Chloride, USP is chemically designated NaCl, a white crystalline powder freely soluble in water.

Water for Injection, USP is chemically designated H_2O.

CLINICAL PHARMACOLOGY

When administered intravenously, these solutions provide a source of water, carbohydrate and electrolytes.

Solutions which provide combinations of hypotonic or isotonic concentrations of Dextrose and of Sodium Chloride are suitable for parenteral maintenance or replacement of water and electrolyte requirements with minimal carbohydrate calories.

Solutions containing carbohydrate in the form of Dextrose restore blood glucose levels and provide calories. Carbohydrate in the form of Dextrose may aid in minimizing liver glycogen depletion and exerts a protein-sparing action. Dextrose injected parenterally undergoes oxidation to carbon dioxide and water.

Sodium Chloride in water dissociates to provide sodium (N^+) and Chloride (Cl^-) ions. Sodium (Na^+) is the principal cation of the extracellular fluid and plays a large part in the therapy of fluid and electrolyte disturbances. Chloride

---

◆ RATED THERAPEUTICALLY EQUIVALENT; ◇ THERAPEUTIC EQUIVALENCE UNCONFIRMED; ○ UNRATED

(Cl^-) has an integral role in buffering action when oxygen and carbon dioxide exchange occurs in the red blood cells. The distribution and excretion of Sodium (Na^+) and Chloride (Cl^-) are largely under the control of the kidney which maintains a balance between intake and output.

Water is an essential constituent of all body tissues and accounts for approximately 70% of total body weight. Average normal adult daily requirements range from two to three liters (1.0 to 1.5 liters each for insensible water loss by perspiration and urine production).

Water balance is maintained by various regulatory mechanisms. Water distribution depends primarily on the concentration of electrolytes in the body compartments and Sodium (Na^+) plays a major role in maintaining physiologic equilibrium.

INDICATIONS AND USAGE
Intravenous solutions containing Dextrose and Sodium Chloride are indicated for parenteral replenishment of fluid, minimal carbohydrate calories, and Sodium Chloride as required by the clinical condition of the patient.

CONTRAINDICATIONS
None known.

WARNINGS
Solutions containing sodium ions should be used with great care, if at all, in patients with congestive heart failure, severe renal insufficiency and in clinical states in which there exists edema with Sodium retention.

Excessive administration of potassium-free solutions may result in significant hypokalemia.

In patients with diminished renal function, administration of solutions containing sodium ions may result in Sodium retention.

The intravenous administration of these solutions can cause fluid and/or solute overloading resulting in dilution of serum electrolyte concentrations, overhydration, congested states or pulmonary edema.

The risk of dilutional states is inversely proportional to the electrolyte concentrations of administered parenteral solutions. The risk of solute overload causing congested states with peripheral and pulmonary edema is directly proportional to the electrolyte concentrations of such solutions.

PRECAUTIONS
Clinical evaluation and periodic laboratory determinations are necessary to monitor changes in fluid balance, electrolyte concentrations and acid-base balance during prolonged parenteral therapy or whenever the condition of the patient warrants such evaluation.

Solutions containing Dextrose should be used with caution in patients with known subclinical or overt diabetes mellitus.

Caution must be exercised in the administration of parenteral fluids, especially those containing sodium ions to patients receiving corticosteroids or corticotropin.

Do not administer unless solution is clear and container is undamaged. Discard unused portion.

Pregnancy Category C: Animal reproduction studies have not been conducted with dextrose or sodium chloride. It is also not known whether dextrose or sodium chloride can cause fetal harm when administered to a pregnant woman or can affect reproduction capacity. Dextrose or Sodium Chloride should be given to a pregnant woman only if clearly needed.

ADVERSE REACTIONS
Reactions which may occur because of the solution or the technique of administration include febrile response, infection at the site of injection, venous thrombosis or phlebitis extending from the site of injection, extravasation and hypervolemia.

If an adverse reaction does occur, discontinue the infusion, evaluate the patient, institute appropriate therapeutic countermeasures and save the remainder of the fluid for examination if deemed necessary.

OVERDOSAGE
In the event of overhydration or solute overload, re-evaluate the patient and institute appropriate corrective measures. See *"Warnings," "Precautions"*, and *"Adverse Reactions"*.

DOSAGE AND ADMINISTRATION
The dose is dependent upon the age, weight and clinical condition of the patient.

Parenteral drug products should be inspected visually for particulate matter and discoloration prior to administration, whenever solution and container permit. See *"Precautions"*.

Drug Interactions: Additives may be incompatible. Consult with pharmacist, if available. When introducing additives, use aseptic technique, mix thoroughly and do not store.

INSTRUCTIONS FOR USE
To Add Medication:
1. Prepare additive port.
2. Using aseptic technique and an additive delivery needle of appropriate length, puncture resealable additive port at target area, inner diaphragm and inject. Withdraw needle after injecting medication.
3. The additive port may be protected by covering with an additive cap.
4. Mix container contents thoroughly.

Preparation for Administration (Use aseptic technique):
1. Close flow control clamp of administration set.
2. Remove cover from outlet port at bottom of container.
3. Insert piercing pin of administration set into port with a twisting motion until the set is firmly seated. *Note*: When using a vented administration set, replace bacterial retentive air filter with piercing pin cover. Insert piercing pin with twisting motion until shoulder of air filter housing rests against the outlet port flange.
4. Suspend container from hanger.
5. Squeeze and release drip chamber to establish proper fluid level in chamber.
6. Attach venipuncture device to set.
7. Open clamp to expel air from set and venipuncture device. Close clamp.
8. Perform venipuncture.
9. Regulate rate of administration with flow control clamp.

WARNING: Do not use flexible container in series connections.

STORAGE
Exposure of pharmaceutical products to heat should be minimized. Avoid excessive heat. Protect from freezing. It is recommended that the product be stored at room temperature (25°C); however, brief exposure up to 40°C does not adversely affect the product.

J CODES
500 ml = 1 unit IV—J7042

HOW SUPPLIED
INJECTION: 10%-0.9%

AVERAGE UNIT PRICE (AVAILABLE SIZES)			
GENERIC	$0.02		
BRAND/MANUFACTURER	NDC	SIZE	AWP
◆ GENERICS			
Abbott Hosp	00074-1534-05	1000 ml 6s	$91.84
Baxter	00338-0095-04	1000 ml 12s	$176.88
Baxter	00338-0095-03	500 ml 24s	$316.05

CONTENT AND CHARACTERISTICS

Product	Grams/100 mL		Per 1000 mL				Osmolarity	
	Dextrose (hydrous)	Sodium Chloride	Sodium Na^+	Chloride Cl^-	Caloric Value	Tonicity	mOsmol/L (calc)	pH
2.5% Dextrose and 0.45% Sodium Chloride Inj., USP	2.5	0.45	77 mEq	77 mEq	85	Isotonic	280	4.3 (3.5 to 6.5)
5% Dextrose and 0.225% Sodium Chloride Inj., USP	5	0.225	38.5 mEq	38.5 mEq	170	Hypertonic	329	4.3 (3.5 to 6.5)
5% Dextrose and 0.3% Sodium Chloride Inj., USP	5	0.3	51 mEq	51 mEq	170	Hypertonic	355	4.3 (3.5 to 6.5)
5% Dextrose and 0.45% Sodium Chloride Inj., USP	5	0.45	77 mEq	77 mEq	170	Hypertonic	406	4.3 (3.5 to 6.5)
5% Dextrose and 0.9% Sodium Chloride Inj., USP	5	0.9	154 mEq	154 mEq	170	Hypertonic	560	4.3 (3.5 to 6.5)

▶ SHOWN IN PRODUCT IDENTIFICATION GUIDE

INJECTION: 5%-0.2%

AVERAGE UNIT PRICE (AVAILABLE SIZES)

GENERIC	$0.02

BRAND/MANUFACTURER	NDC	SIZE	AWP
◆ GENERICS			
Baxter	00338-0077-04	1000 ml 12s	$141.70
Baxter	00338-0077-03	500 ml 24s	$238.46
Baxter	00338-0077-02	250 ml 36s	$357.69

INJECTION: 5%-0.3%

AVERAGE UNIT PRICE (AVAILABLE SIZES)

GENERIC	$0.02

BRAND/MANUFACTURER	NDC	SIZE	AWP
◆ GENERICS			
Abbott Hosp	00074-7925-09	1000 ml 12s	$144.50
Abbott Hosp	00074-7925-02	250 ml 24s	$243.11
Abbott Hosp	00074-7925-03	500 ml 24s	$243.11

INJECTION: 5%-0.9%

AVERAGE UNIT PRICE (AVAILABLE SIZES)

GENERIC	$0.02	GENERIC A-RATED AVERAGE PRICE (GAAP)	
		1000 ml 12s	$143.10
		500 ml 24s	$240.79

BRAND/MANUFACTURER	NDC	SIZE	AWP
◆ GENERICS			
Baxter	00338-0089-04	1000 ml 12s	$141.70
Abbott Hosp	00074-7941-09	1000 ml 12s	$144.50
Abbott Hosp	00074-7941-02	250 ml 24s	$243.11
Baxter	00338-0089-03	500 ml 24s	$238.46
Abbott Hosp	00074-7941-03	500 ml 24s	$243.11
Baxter	00338-0089-02	250 ml 36s	$357.69

INJECTION: 5%-0.33%

AVERAGE UNIT PRICE (AVAILABLE SIZES)

GENERIC	$0.02

BRAND/MANUFACTURER	NDC	SIZE	AWP
◆ GENERICS			
Baxter	00338-0081-04	1000 ml 12s	$141.70
Baxter	00338-0081-03	500 ml 24s	$238.46
Baxter	00338-0081-02	250 ml 36s	$357.69

INJECTION: 5%-0.45%

AVERAGE UNIT PRICE (AVAILABLE SIZES)

GENERIC	$0.02	GENERIC A-RATED AVERAGE PRICE (GAAP)	
		1000 ml 12s	$143.10
		500 ml 24s	$240.79

BRAND/MANUFACTURER	NDC	SIZE	AWP
◆ GENERICS			
Baxter	00338-0085-04	1000 ml 12s	$141.70
Abbott Hosp	00074-7926-09	1000 ml 12s	$144.50
Abbott Hosp	00074-7926-02	250 ml 24s	$243.11
Baxter	00338-0085-03	500 ml 24s	$238.46
Abbott Hosp	00074-7926-03	500 ml 24s	$243.11
Baxter	00338-0085-02	250 ml 36s	$357.69

INJECTION: 2.5%-0.45%

AVERAGE UNIT PRICE (AVAILABLE SIZES)

GENERIC	$0.02	GENERIC A-RATED AVERAGE PRICE (GAAP)	
		1000 ml 12s	$136.79
		500 ml 24s	$233.20

BRAND/MANUFACTURER	NDC	SIZE	AWP
◆ GENERICS			
Baxter	00338-0073-04	1000 ml 12s	$135.50
Abbott Hosp	00074-7940-09	1000 ml 12s	$138.08
Baxter	00338-0073-03	500 ml 24s	$230.98
Abbott Hosp	00074-7940-03	500 ml 24s	$235.41

INJECTION: 10%-0.2%

BRAND/MANUFACTURER	NDC	SIZE	AWP
◆ GENERICS			
Baxter	00338-0640-02	250 ml 12s	$73.06

INJECTION: 5%-0.225%

AVERAGE UNIT PRICE (AVAILABLE SIZES)

GENERIC	$0.02

BRAND/MANUFACTURER	NDC	SIZE	AWP
◆ GENERICS			
Abbott Hosp	00074-7924-09	1000 ml 12s	$144.50
Abbott Hosp	00074-7924-02	250 ml 24s	$243.11
Abbott Hosp	00074-7924-03	500 ml 24s	$243.11

For additional alternatives, turn to the section beginning on page 2859.

Dextrose/Electrolytes/Fructose/ Invert Sugar

DESCRIPTION

Dextrose/Electrolytes/Fructose/Invert Sugar Injections are sterile, nonpyrogenic hypertonic solutions for fluid and electrolyte replenishment and caloric supply in single dose glass containers for intravenous administration. They contain no antimicrobial agents. Sodium bisulfite is added as a stabilizer. Inverted and pH adjusted with hydrochloric acid. Composition, osmolarity, pH, ionic concentration and caloric content are shown in Table 1.

CLINICAL PHARMACOLOGY

Dextrose/Electrolytes/Fructose/Invert Sugar Injections have value as a source of water, electrolytes and calories. They are capable of inducing diuresis depending on the clinical condition of the patient.

Dextrose/Electrolytes/Fructose/Invert Sugar Injections produce a metabolic alkalinizing effect. Lactate ions are metabolized in the liver to glycogen, and ultimately to carbon dioxide and water, which requires the consumption of hydrogen cations.

INDICATIONS AND USAGE

Dextrose/Electrolytes/Fructose/Invert Sugar Injections are indicated as a source of water, electrolytes, and calories or as alkalinizing agents where hereditary Fructose intolerance can be ruled out.

CONTRAINDICATIONS

Dextrose/Electrolytes/Fructose/Invert Sugar Injections are contraindicated in patients with hereditary Fructose intolerance. It is imperative that a careful history be taken to detect any intolerance to sweets, sugar, fruits, or sorbitol sweeteners.

WARNINGS

Dextrose/Electrolytes/Fructose/Invert Sugar Injections should be used with great care, if at all, in patients with congestive heart failure, severe renal insufficiency, and in clinical states in which there exists edema with sodium retention.

Dextrose/Electrolytes/Fructose/Invert Sugar Injections should be used with great care, if at all, in patients with hyperkalemia, severe renal failure, and in conditions in which potassium retention is present.

Dextrose/Electrolytes/Fructose/Invert Sugar Injection should be used with great care in patients with metabolic or respiratory alkalosis. The administration of lactate ions should be done with great care in those conditions in which there is an increased level or an impaired utilization of these ions, such as severe hepatic insufficiency.

The intravenous administration of this injection can cause fluid and/or solute overloading resulting in dilution of serum electrolyte concentrations, overhydration, congested states, or pulmonary edema. The risk of dilutional states is inversely proportional to the electrolyte concentrations of the injection. The risk of solute overload causing congested states with peripheral and pulmonary edema is directly proportional to the electrolyte concentrations of the injection.

In patients with diminished renal function, administration of these injections may result in sodium or potassium retention.

These injections are not for use in the treatment of lactic acidosis.

Contains sodium bisulfite, a sulfite that may cause allergic-type reactions including anaphylactic symptoms and life-threatening or less severe asthmatic episodes in certain susceptible people. The overall prevalence of sulfite sensitivity in the general population is unknown and probably low.

Sulfite sensitivity is seen more frequently in asthmatic than in nonasthmatic people.

The safety and efficacy of this solution has not been demonstrated in pediatric patients (ages 0 to 12 years).

PRECAUTIONS

Clinical evaluation and periodic laboratory determinations are necessary to monitor changes in fluid balance, electrolyte concentrations, and acid base balance during prolonged parenteral therapy or whenever the condition of the patient warrants such evaluation.

Dextrose/Electrolytes/Fructose/Invert Sugar Injection should be used with caution. Excess administration may result in metabolic alkalosis.

Caution must be exercised in the administration of this injection to patients receiving corticosteroids or corticotropin.

Dextrose/Electrolytes/Fructose/Invert Sugar Injection should be used with caution in patients with overt or subclinical diabetes mellitus.

Rapid infusion of large quantities of this injection may raise serum uric acid levels. Unusually rapid infusion, approaching 500 mL/hr, has been associated with epigastric or substernal pain or discomfort, as well as cramping abdominal pain. Caution should be observed to prevent overhydration and serum electrolyte abnormalities.

PREGNANCY: TERATOGENIC EFFECTS

Pregnancy Category C. Animal reproduction studies have not been conducted with Dextrose/Electrolytes/Fructose/Invert Sugar and Electrolyte Injections. It is

◆ RATED THERAPEUTICALLY EQUIVALENT; ◇ THERAPEUTIC EQUIVALENCE UNCONFIRMED; ○ UNRATED

also not known whether Dextrose/Electrolytes/Fructose/Invert Sugar Injection can cause fetal harm when administered to a pregnant woman or can affect reproduction capacity. Dextrose/Electrolytes/Fructose/Invert Sugar Injection should be given to a pregnant woman only if clearly needed.

Do not administer unless vacuum is present and solution is clear, Unit must be used with a vented set or a nonvented set with a vented spike adapter.

ADVERSE REACTIONS

Reactions which may occur because of the solution or the technique of administration include febrile response, infection at the site of injection, venous thrombosis or phlebitis extending from the site of injection, extravasation, and hypervolemia.

Infusions of solutions containing Fructose to a patient with hereditary intolerance to Fructose may be fetal.

Lactic acidosis has been reported following injection of Fructose in patients with hepatic disease.

If an adverse reaction does occur, discontinue the infusion, evaluate the patient, institute appropriate therapeutic countermeasures, and save the remainder of the fluid for examination if deemed necessary.

DOSAGE AND ADMINISTRATION

As directed by a physician. Dosage is dependent upon the age, weight and clinical condition of the patient as well as laboratory determinations.

Parenteral drug products should be inspected visually for particulate matter and discoloration prior to administration whenever solution and container permit.

HOW SUPPLIED
INJECTION:

AVERAGE UNIT PRICE (AVAILABLE SIZES)		GENERIC A-RATED AVERAGE PRICE (GAAP)		
GENERIC	$0.02	**1000 ml 6s**		$109.68
BRAND/MANUFACTURER		NDC	SIZE	AWP
◆ **GENERICS**				
Baxter		00338-0236-04	1000 ml 6s	$98.34
Baxter		00338-0250-04	1000 ml 6s	$121.02

Dextrose/Lactated Ringer's/ Potassium Chloride

DESCRIPTION

Dextrose 5%/Lactated Ringer's/Potassium Chloride injection is a sterile, nonpyrogenic solution for fluid and electrolyte replenishment and caloric supply in a single dose container for intravenous administration. It contains no antimicrobial agents. Composition, osmolarity, pH, ionic concentration and caloric content are shown in Table 1.

CLINICAL PHARMACOLOGY

Dextrose/Lactated Ringer's/Potassium Chloride injection has value as a source of water, electrolytes, and calories. It is capable of inducing diuresis depending on the clinical condition of the patient.

Dextrose/Lactated Ringer's/Potassium Chloride Injection produces a metabolic alkalinizing effect. Lactate ions are metabolized ultimately to carbon dioxide and water, which requires the consumption of hydrogen cations.

INDICATIONS AND USAGE

Dextrose/Lactated Ringer's/Potassium Chloride injection is indicated as a source of water, electrolytes, and calories or as alkalinizing agents.

CONTRAINDICATIONS

None known.

WARNINGS

Dextrose/Lactated Ringer's/Potassium Chloride injection should be used with great care, if at all, in patients with congestive heart failure, severe renal insufficiency, and in clinical states in which there exists edema with sodium retention.

Dextrose/Lactated Ringer's/Potassium Chloride injection should be used with great care, if at all, in patients with hyperkalemia, severe renal failure, and in conditions in which potassium retention is present.

Dextrose/Lactated Ringer's/Potassium Chloride injection should be used with great care in patients with metabolic or respiratory alkalosis. The administration of lactate ions should be done with great care in those conditions in which there is an increased level or an impaired utilization of these ions, such as severe hepatic insufficiency.

Dextrose/Lactated Ringer's/Potassium Chloride injection should not be administered simultaneously with blood through the same administration set because of the likelihood of coagulation.

The intravenous administration of Dextrose/Lactated Ringer's/Potassium Chloride injection can cause fluid and/or solute overloading resulting in dilution of serum electrolyte concentrations, overhydration, congested states, or pulmonary edema. The risk of dilutional states is inversely proportional to the electrolyte concentrations of the injection.

The risk of solute overload causing congested states with peripheral and pulmonary edema is directly proportional to the electrolyte concentrations of the injection.

In patients with diminished renal function, administration of Dextrose/Lactated Ringer's/Potassium Chloride injection may result in sodium or potassium retention.

Dextrose/Lactated Ringer's/Potassium Chloride injection is not for use in the treatment of lactic acidosis.

PRECAUTIONS

Clinical evaluation and periodic laboratory determinations are necessary to monitor changes in fluid balance, electrolyte concentrations, and acid base balance during prolonged parenteral therapy or whenever the condition of the patient warrants such evaluation.

Dextrose/Lactated Ringer's/Potassium Chloride injection should be used with caution. Excess administration may result in metabolic alkalosis.

Caution must be exercised in the administration of Dextrose/Lactated Ringer's/Potassium Chloride injection to patients receiving corticosteroids or corticotropin.

Dextrose/Lactated Ringer's/Potassium Chloride injection should be used with caution in patients with overt or subclinical diabetes mellitus.

PREGNANCY, TERATOGENIC EFFECTS

Pregnancy Category C: Animal reproduction studies have not been conducted with Dextrose/Lactated Ringer's/Potassium Chloride injection. It is also not known whether Dextrose/Lactated Ringer's/Potassium Chloride injection can cause fetal harm when administered to a pregnant woman or can affect reproduction capacity. Dextrose/Lactated Ringer's /Potassium Chloride injection should be given to a pregnant woman only if clearly needed.

Do not administer unless solution is clear and seal is intact.

ADVERSE REACTIONS

Reactions which may occur because of the solution or the technique of administration include febrile response, infection at the site of injection, venous thrombosis or phlebitis extending from the site of injection, extravasation, and hypervolemia.

If an adverse reaction does occur, discontinue the infusion, evaluate the patient, institute appropriate therapeutic countermeasures, and save the remainder of the fluid for examination if deemed necessary.

DOSAGE AND ADMINISTRATION

As directed by a physician. Dosage is dependent upon the age, weight and clinical condition of the patient as well as laboratory determinations.

Parenteral drug products should be inspected visually for particulate matter and discoloration prior to administration whenever solution and container permit. Use of a final filter is recommended during administration of all parenteral solution, where possible.

Additives may be incompatible. Complete information is not available. Those additives known to be incompatible should not be used. Consult with pharmacist, if available. If, in the informed judgment of the physician, it is deemed advisable to introduce additives, use aseptic technique. Mix thoroughly when additives have been introduced. Do not store solutions containing additives.

Exposure of pharmaceutical products to heat should be minimized. Avoid excessive heat. It is recommended the product be stored at room temperature (25°C); brief exposure up to 40°C does not adversely affect the product.

Table 1
DEXTROSE/LACTATED RINGER'S/POTASSIUM CHLORIDE
mEq Potassium added

	20 mEq	40 mEq
Composition (g/L)		
Size (mL)	1000	1000
*Dextrose, Hydrous, USP	50	50
Sodium Chloride, USP (NaCl)	6.0	6.0
Sodium Lactate, ($C_3H_5NaO_3$)	3.1	3.1
Calcium Chloride, USP ($CaCl_2 \cdot 2H_2O$)	0.2	0.2
Potassium Chloride, USP (KCl)	1.79	3.25
**Osmolarity (mOsmol/L) (calc.)	565	605
pH	5.0	5.0
	(4.0 to 6.5)	(4.0 to 6.5)
Ionic Concentration (mEq/L)		
Sodium	130	130
Potassium	24	44
Calcium	3	3
Chloride	129	149
Lactate	28	28
Caloric Content (Kcal/L)	170	170

** *Normal physiologic osmolarity range is approximately 280 to 310 mOsmol/L. Administration of substantially hypertonic solutions (≥ 600 mOsmol/L) may cause vein damage.*

➤ SHOWN IN PRODUCT IDENTIFICATION GUIDE

HOW SUPPLIED
INJECTION:

AVERAGE UNIT PRICE (AVAILABLE SIZES)		GENERIC A-RATED AVERAGE PRICE (GAAP)	
GENERIC	$0.02	**1000 ml 12s**	**$232.22**

BRAND/MANUFACTURER	NDC	SIZE	AWP
◆ GENERICS			
Baxter	00338-0811-04	1000 ml 12s	$232.22
Baxter	00338-0815-04	1000 ml 12s	$232.22

Dextrose/Potassium Chloride/ Sodium Chloride

DESCRIPTION

Intravenous solutions with Potassium Chloride are sterile and nonpyrogenic solutions in water for injection. They are for administration by intravenous infusion only.

See tables for summary of content and characteristics of these solutions. The solutions contain no bacteriostat, antimicrobial agent or added buffer and each is intended only for use as a single-dose injection. When smaller doses are required, the unused portion should be discarded.

These solutions are parenteral fluid, nutrient and/or electrolyte replenishers. Dextrose, USP is chemically designated D-glucose, monohydrate ($C_6H_{12}O_6 \cdot H_2O$), a hexose sugar freely soluble in water.

Potassium Chloride, USP is chemically designated KCl, a white granular powder freely soluble in water.

Sodium Chloride, USP is chemically designated NaCl, a white crystalline powder freely soluble in water.

Water for Injection, USP is chemically designated H_2O.

CLINICAL PHARMACOLOGY

When administered intravenously, these solutions provide a source of water and Potassium Chloride with carbohydrate (Dextrose) and Sodium Chloride. See "How Supplied" section for specific concentrations of these various solutions.

Solutions containing carbohydrate in the form of Dextrose restore blood glucose levels and provide calories. Carbohydrate in the form of Dextrose may aid in minimizing liver glycogen depletion and exerts a protein-sparing action. Dextrose injected parenterally undergoes oxidation to carbon dioxide and water.

Intravenous solutions containing Potassium Chloride are particularly intended to provide needed potassium cation (K^+). Potassium is the chief cation of body cells (160 mEq/liter of intracellular water). It is found in low concentration in plasma and extracellular fluids (3.5 to 5.0 mEq/liter in a healthy adult). Potassium plays an important role in electrolyte balance. Normally about 80 to 90% of the potassium intake is excreted in the urine; the remainder in the stools and to a

Table 1

Potassium Chloride in 5% Dextrose and 0.225% Sodium Chloride Inj.

mEq Potassium	Size (mL)	Composition (g/L)			Calculated Osmolarity (mOsmol/L)	pH	Approx. Ionic Concentrations (mEq/L)			Approximate kcal/L
		Dextrose, Hydrous	Sodium Chloride	Potassium Chloride			Sodium (Na⁺)	Potassium (K⁺)	Chloride (Cl⁻)	
10 mEq	1000	50	2.25	0.745	349	4.2 (3.5 - 6.5)	38.5	10	48.5	170
10 mEq	500	50	2.25	1.49	370	4.2 (3.5 - 6.5)	38.5	20	58.5	170
20 mEq	1000	50	2.25	1.49	370	4.2 (3.5 - 6.5)	38.5	20	58.5	170
30 mEq	1000	50	2.25	2.24	389	4.2 (3.5 - 6.5)	38.5	30	68.5	170
40 mEq	1000	50	2.25	2.98	409	4.2 (3.5 - 6.5)	38.5	40	78.5	170

Table 2

Potassium Chloride in 5% Dextrose and 0.3% Sodium Chloride Inj.

mEq Potassium	Size (mL)	COMPOSITION (g/L)			Calculated Osmolarity (mOsmol/L)	pH	Approx. Ionic Concentrations (mEq/L)			Approximate kcal/L
		Dextrose, Hydrous	Sodium Chloride	Potassium Chloride			Sodium (Na⁺)	Potassium (K⁺)	Chloride (Cl⁻)	
10 mEq	500	50	3.0	1.49	395	4.2 (3.5 - 6.5)	51	20	71	170
20 mEq	1000	50	3.0	1.49	395	4.2 (3.5 - 6.5)	51	20	71	170
30 mEq	1000	50	3.0	2.24	415	4.2 (3.5 - 6.5)	51	30	81	170
40 mEq	1000	50	3.0	2.98	434	4.2 (3.5 - 6.5)	51	40	91	170

Table 3

Potassium Chloride in 5% Dextrose and 0.45% Sodium Chloride Inj.

mEq Potassium	Size (mL)	Composition (g/L)			Calculated Osmolarity (mOsmol/L)	pH	Approx. Ionic Concentrations (mEq/L)			Approximate kcal/L
		Dextrose, Hydrous	Sodium Chloride	Potassium Chloride			Sodium (Na⁺)	Potassium (K⁺)	Chloride (Cl⁻)	
10 mEq	1000	50	4.5	0.745	426	4.2 (3.5 - 6.8)	77	10	87	170
10 mEq	500	50	4.5	1.49	447	4.2 (3.5 - 6.5)	77	97	97	170
20 mEq	1000	50	4.5	1.49	447	4.2 (3.5 - 6.5)	77	20	97	170
30 mEq	1000	50	4.5	2.24	467	4.2 (3.5 - 6.5)	77	30	107	170
40 mEq	1000	50	4.5	2.98	487	4.2 (3.5 - 6.5)	77	40	117	170

Table 4

Potassium Chloride in 5% Dextrose and 0.9% Sodium Chloride Inj.

mEq Potassium	Size (mL)	Composition (g/L)			Calculated Osmolarity (mOsmol/L)	pH	Approx. Ionic Concentrations (mEq/L)			Approximate kcal/L
		Dextrose, Hydrous	Sodium Chloride	Potassium Chloride			Sodium (Na⁺)	Potassium (K⁺)	Chloride (Cl⁻)	
10 mEq	500	50	9	1.49	600	4.2 (3.5 - 6.5)	154	20	174	170
20 mEq	1000	50	9	1.49	600	4.2 (3.5 - 6.5)	154	20	174	170
40 mEq	1000	50	9	2.98	640	4.2 (3.5 - 6.5)	154	40	194	170

◆ RATED THERAPEUTICALLY EQUIVALENT; ◇ THERAPEUTIC EQUIVALENCE UNCONFIRMED; ○ UNRATED

small extent, in the perspiration. The kidney does not conserve potassium well so that during fasting or in patients on a Potassium-free diet, Potassium loss from the body continues resulting in Potassium depletion. A deficiency of either Potassium or Chloride will lead to a deficit of the other.

Sodium Chloride in water dissociates to provide Sodium (Na$^+$) and Chloride (Cl$^-$) ions. Sodium (Na$^+$) is the principal cation of the extracellular fluid and plays a large part in the therapy of fluid and electrolyte disturbances. Chloride (Cl$^-$) has an integral role in action when oxygen and carbon dioxide exchange occurs in the red blood cells. The distribution and excretion of Sodium (Na$^+$) and Chloride (Cl$^-$) are largely under the control of the kidney which maintains a balance between intake and output.

Water is an essential constituent of all body tissues and accounts for approximately 70% of total body weight. Average normal adult daily requirement ranges from two to three liters (1.0 to 1.5 liters each for insensible water loss by perspiration and urine production).

Water balance is maintained by various regulatory mechanisms. Water distribution depends primarily on the concentration of electrolytes in the body compartments and Sodium (Na$^+$) plays a major role in maintaining physiologic equilibrium.

INDICATIONS AND USAGE
These solutions are indicated in patients requiring parenteral administration of Potassium Chloride with minimal carbohydrate calories and Sodium Chloride.

CONTRAINDICATIONS
Solutions containing Potassium Chloride are contraindicated in diseases where high potassium levels may be encountered.

WARNINGS
Solutions which contain Potassium ions should be used with great care, if at all, in patients with hyperkalemia, severe renal failure and in conditions in which Potassium retention is present.

To avoid Potassium intoxication, do not infuse these solutions rapidly. In patients with severe renal insufficiency or adrenal insufficiency, administration of Potassium Chloride may cause Potassium intoxication.

Solutions containing sodium ions should be used with great care, if at all, in patients with congestive heart failure, severe renal insufficiency and in clinical states in which there exists edema with sodium retention.

In patients with diminished renal function, administration of solutions containing sodium or potassium ions may result in sodium or potassium retention.

The intravenous administration of these solutions can cause fluid and/or solute overloading resulting in dilution of serum electrolyte concentrations, overhydration, congested states or pulmonary edema.

The risk of dilutional states is inversely proportional to the electrolyte concentration of administered parenteral solutions. The risk of solute overload causing congested states with peripheral and pulmonary edema is directly proportional to the electrolyte concentrations of such solutions.

PRECAUTIONS
Clinical evaluation and periodic laboratory determinations are necessary to monitor changes in fluid balance, electrolyte concentrations and acid-base balance during prolonged parenteral therapy or whenever the condition of the patient warrants such evaluation.

Solutions containing Dextrose should be used with caution in patients with known subclinical or overt diabetes mellitus.

Caution must be exercised in the administration of parenteral fluids, especially those containing Sodium ions, to patients receiving corticosteroids or corticotropin.

Potassium replacement therapy should be guided primarily by serial electrocardiograms. Plasma potassium levels are not necessarily indicative of tissue potassium levels.

High plasma concentrations of Potassium may cause death through cardiac depression, arrhythmias or arrest.

Potassium-containing solutions should be used with caution in the presence of cardiac disease, particularly in digitalized patients or in the presence of renal disease.

Care should be exercised to insure that the needle (or catheter) is well within the lumen of the vein and that extravasation does not occur.

Do not administer unless solution is clear and container is undamaged. Discard unused portion.

Pregnancy Category C. Animal reproduction studies have not been conducted with Dextrose, Potassium Chloride or Sodium Chloride. It is also not known whether Dextrose, Potassium Chloride or Sodium Chloride can cause fetal harm when administered to a pregnant woman or can affect reproduction capacity. Dextrose, Potassium Chloride or Sodium Chloride should be given to a pregnant woman only if clearly needed.

ADVERSE REACTIONS
Reactions which may occur because of the solutions or technique of administration include febrile response, infection at the site of injection, venous thrombosis or phlebitis extending from the site of injection, extravasation and hypervolemia.

If an adverse reaction does occur, discontinue the infusion, evaluate the patient, institute appropriate therapeutic countermeasures and save the remainder of the fluid for examination if deemed necessary.

Nausea, vomiting, abdominal pain and diarrhea have been reported with Potassium therapy. The signs and symptoms of potassium intoxication include paresthesias of the extremities, flaccid paralysis, listlessness, mental confusion,

weakness and heaviness of the legs, hypotension, cardiac arrhythmias, heart block, electrocardiographic abnormalities such as disappearance of P waves, spreading and slurring of the QRS complex with development of a biphasic curve and cardiac arrest.

Potassium-containing solutions are intrinsically irritating to tissues. Therefore, extreme care should be taken to avoid perivascular infiltration. Local tissue necrosis and subsequent sloughing may result if extravasation occurs. Chemical phlebitis and venospasm have also been reported.

Should perivascular infiltration occur, I.V. administration at that site should be discontinued at once. Local infiltration of the affected area with procaine hydrochloride, 1%, to which hyaluronidase may be added, will often reduce venospasm and dilute the potassium remaining in the tissues locally. Local application of heat may also be helpful.

OVERDOSAGE
In the event of Potassium overdosage, discontinue the infusion immediately and institute intensive corrective therapy to reduce serum potassium levels. See *"Warnings"* and *"Precautions"*.

DOSAGE AND ADMINISTRATION
These solutions should be administered only by intravenous infusion and as directed by the physician. The dose and rate of injection are dependent upon the age, weight and clinical condition of the patient. If the serum potassium level is greater than 2.5 mEq/liter, potassium should be given at a rate not to exceed 10 mEq/hour in a concentration less than 30 mEq/liter. Somewhat faster rates and greater concentrations (usually up to 40 mEq/liter) of potassium may be indicated in patients with more severe potassium deficiency. The total 24-hour dose should not generally exceed 200 mEq of potassium.

DRUG INTERACTIONS
Additives may be incompatible. Consult with pharmacist, if available. When introducing additives, use aseptic technique, mix thoroughly and do not store.

Parenteral drug products should be inspected visually for particulate matter and discoloration prior to administration, whenever solution and container permit. See *"Precautions"*.

INSTRUCTIONS FOR USE
TO OPEN
Tear outer wrap at notch and remove solution container. If supplemental medication is desired, follow directions below before preparing for administration. Some opacity of the plastic due to moisture absorption during the sterilization process may be observed. This is normal and does not affect the solution quality or safety. The opacity will diminish gradually.

TO ADD MEDICATION
1. Prepare additive port.
2. Using aseptic technique and an additive delivery needle of appropriate length, puncture resealable additive port at target area, inner diaphragm and inject. Withdraw needle after injecting medication.
3. The additive port may be protected by covering with an additive cap.
4. Mix container contents thoroughly.

PREPARATION FOR ADMINISTRATION
(Use aseptic technique):

1. Close flow control clamp of administration set.
2. Remove cover from outlet port at bottom of container.
3. Insert piercing pin of administration set into port with a twisting motion until the set is firmly seated. *Note*: See full directions on administration set carton.
4. Suspend container from hanger.
5. Squeeze and release drip chamber to establish proper fluid level in chamber.
6. Open flow control clamp and clear air from set. Close clamp.
7. Attach set to venipuncture device. If device is not indwelling, prime and make venipuncture.
8. Regulate rate of administration with flow control clamp.

May contain HCl for pH adjustment.

STORAGE
Exposure of pharmaceutical products to heat should be minimized. Avoid excessive heat. Protect from freezing. It is recommended that the product be stored at room temperature (25° C); however, brief exposure up to 40° C does not adversely affect the product.

WARNINGS
Do not use flexible container in series connections.

HOW SUPPLIED
INJECTION: 5%-0.22%-0.3%

AVERAGE UNIT PRICE (AVAILABLE SIZES)		GENERIC A-RATED AVERAGE PRICE (GAAP)		
GENERIC	$0.02	1000 ml 12s		$203.40
BRAND/MANUFACTURER		NDC	SIZE	AWP
◆ GENERICS				
Baxter		00338-0605-04	1000 ml 12s	$201.46
Abbott Hosp		00074-7806-09	1000 ml 12s	$205.34

➤ SHOWN IN PRODUCT IDENTIFICATION GUIDE

INJECTION: 5%-0.15%-0.2%

AVERAGE UNIT PRICE (AVAILABLE SIZES)		GENERIC A-RATED AVERAGE PRICE (GAAP)		
GENERIC	$0.03	1000 ml 12s		$203.40
BRAND/MANUFACTURER		NDC	SIZE	AWP
◆ GENERICS				
Baxter		00338-0663-04	1000 ml 12s	$201.46
Abbott Hosp		00074-7901-09	1000 ml 12s	$205.34
Baxter		00338-0663-03	500 ml 18s	$273.36
Abbott Hosp		00074-7901-03	500 ml 24s	$631.56

INJECTION: 5%-0.15%-0.9%

AVERAGE UNIT PRICE (AVAILABLE SIZES)		GENERIC A-RATED AVERAGE PRICE (GAAP)		
GENERIC	$0.02	1000 ml 12s		$241.52
BRAND/MANUFACTURER		NDC	SIZE	AWP
◆ GENERICS				
Baxter		00338-0803-04	1000 ml 12s	$201.46
Abbott Hosp		00074-7107-09	1000 ml 12s	$281.58

INJECTION: 5%-0.15%-0.45%

AVERAGE UNIT PRICE (AVAILABLE SIZES)		GENERIC A-RATED AVERAGE PRICE (GAAP)		
GENERIC	$0.03	1000 ml 12s		$203.40
BRAND/MANUFACTURER		NDC	SIZE	AWP
◆ GENERICS				
Baxter		00338-0671-04	1000 ml 12s	$201.46
Abbott Hosp		00074-7902-09	1000 ml 12s	$205.34
Baxter		00338-0671-03	500 ml 18s	$273.36
Abbott Hosp		00074-7902-03	500 ml 24s	$631.56

INJECTION: 5%-0.22%-0.2%

AVERAGE UNIT PRICE (AVAILABLE SIZES)		GENERIC A-RATED AVERAGE PRICE (GAAP)		
GENERIC	$0.02	1000 ml 12s		$203.40
BRAND/MANUFACTURER		NDC	SIZE	AWP
◆ GENERICS				
Baxter		00338-0665-03	500 ml 12s	$170.78
Baxter		00338-0665-04	1000 ml 12s	$201.46
Abbott Hosp		00074-7991-09	1000 ml 12s	$205.34

INJECTION: 5%-0.22%-0.45%

AVERAGE UNIT PRICE (AVAILABLE SIZES)		GENERIC A-RATED AVERAGE PRICE (GAAP)		
GENERIC	$0.02	1000 ml 12s		$203.40
BRAND/MANUFACTURER		NDC	SIZE	AWP
◆ GENERICS				
Baxter		00338-0673-04	1000 ml 12s	$201.46
Abbott Hosp		00074-7903-09	1000 ml 12s	$205.34

INJECTION: 5%-0.3%-0.2%

AVERAGE UNIT PRICE (AVAILABLE SIZES)		GENERIC A-RATED AVERAGE PRICE (GAAP)		
GENERIC	$0.02	1000 ml 12s		$203.40
BRAND/MANUFACTURER		NDC	SIZE	AWP
◆ GENERICS				
Baxter		00338-0667-04	1000 ml 12s	$201.46
Abbott Hosp		00074-7992-09	1000 ml 12s	$205.34

INJECTION: 5%-0.3%-0.45%

AVERAGE UNIT PRICE (AVAILABLE SIZES)		GENERIC A-RATED AVERAGE PRICE (GAAP)		
GENERIC	$0.02	1000 ml 12s		$203.40
BRAND/MANUFACTURER		NDC	SIZE	AWP
◆ GENERICS				
Baxter		00338-0675-04	1000 ml 12s	$201.46
Abbott Hosp		00074-7904-09	1000 ml 12s	$205.34

INJECTION: 5%-0.3%-0.3%

AVERAGE UNIT PRICE (AVAILABLE SIZES)		GENERIC A-RATED AVERAGE PRICE (GAAP)		
GENERIC	$0.02	1000 ml 12s		$241.52
BRAND/MANUFACTURER		NDC	SIZE	AWP
◆ GENERICS				
Baxter		00338-0607-04	1000 ml 12s	$201.46
Abbott Hosp		00074-7105-09	1000 ml 12s	$281.58

INJECTION: 5%-0.075%-0.45%

AVERAGE UNIT PRICE (AVAILABLE SIZES)		GENERIC A-RATED AVERAGE PRICE (GAAP)		
GENERIC	$0.02	1000 ml 12s		$203.40
BRAND/MANUFACTURER		NDC	SIZE	AWP
◆ GENERICS				
Baxter		00338-0669-04	1000 ml 12s	$201.46
Abbott Hosp		00074-7993-09	1000 ml 12s	$205.34

For additional alternatives, turn to the section beginning on page 2859.

Dextrothyroxine Sodium

DESCRIPTION
Dextrothyroxine Sodium is the Sodium salt of the dextrorotatory isomer of thyroxine useful in the treatment of hyperlipidemia. It is chemically described as D-3,5,3',5'-tetraiodothyronine sodium salt.

Dextrothyroxine Sodium Tablets are available for oral use containing 1, 2 or 4 mg of Dextrothyroxine Sodium.

Following is its chemical structure:

CLINICAL PHARMACOLOGY
The predominant effect of Dextrothyroxine Sodium is the reduction of elevated serum cholesterol levels. Beta lipoprotein and triglyceride fractions may also be reduced from previously elevated levels.

Available evidence indicates that Dextrothyroxine Sodium stimulates the liver to increase catabolism and excretion of cholesterol and its degradation products via the biliary route into the feces. Cholesterol synthesis is not inhibited and abnormal metabolic end products do not accumulate in the blood.

INDICATION AND USAGE
Dextrothyroxine Sodium may be indicated as an adjunct to diet for the reduction of elevated low density lipoprotein (LDL) cholesterol in patients with primary hypercholesterolemia (Types IIa and IIb) with no known or suspected heart disease, whose response to diet and other nonpharmacologic measures has been inadequate

This is not an innocuous drug. Strict attention should be paid to the indications and contraindications.

After establishing that the elevation in serum cholesterol represents a primary disorder not due to secondary conditions such as poorly controlled diabetes mellitus, hypothyroidism, the nephrotic syndrome, liver disease, or dysproteinemias, it should be determined that a patient for whom treatment with Dextrothyroxine Sodium is being considered has a persistently elevated LDL cholesterol as the cause of an elevated total serum cholesterol. This may be particularly relevant for patients with elevated total triglycerides or with markedly elevated HDL-C values, where non-LDL lipoprotein fractions may contribute significantly to total cholesterol levels without apparent increase in cardiovascular risk. In most patients, LDL-C may be estimated according to the following equation LDL-C = Total cholesterol. $[(0.16 \times triglycerides) + HDL\text{-}C]$.

When total triglycerides are greater than 400 mg/dL this equation is less accurate. In such patients, LDL-Cholesterol may be obtained by ultracentrifugation.

It has not been clearly established whether Dextrothyroxine induced lowering of serum cholesterol or lipid levels has a detrimental, beneficial, or no effect on the morbidity or mortality due to atherosclerosis or coronary heart disease. Dextrothyroxine Sodium may have a detrimental effect on morbidity and mortality in patients with established coronary heart disease (see "Contraindications").

UNLABELED USES
Dextrothyroxine Sodium is used alone or as an adjunct in the treatment of hypothyroidism and scleroderma.

CONTRAINDICATIONS
The administration of Dextrothyroxine Sodium to euthyroid patients with one or more of the following conditions is contraindicated:

1. Known or suspected organic heart disease, especially coronary artery disease, including angina pectoris, history of myocardial infarction, cardiac arrhythmia or tachycardia, either active or in patients with demonstrated propensity for arrhythmias, rheumatic heart disease, history of congestive heart failure, and decompensated or borderline compensated cardiac status. In a large study, involving men who had had a myocardial infarction, use of the drug was discontinued because of a trend to increased mortality in Dextrothyroxine-treated subjects compared with placebo treated patients.
2. Hypertension (other than mild, labile systolic hypertension).
3. Pregnancy.
4. Nursing mothers.
5. History of iodism.
6. Safety and effectiveness in children have not been established.
7. In patients with advanced liver or kidney diseases.

◆ RATED THERAPEUTICALLY EQUIVALENT; ◇ THERAPEUTIC EQUIVALENCE UNCONFIRMED; ○ UNRATED

WARNINGS:

DRUGS WITH THYROID HORMONE ACTIVITY, ALONE OR TOGETHER WITH OTHER THERAPEUTIC AGENTS, HAVE BEEN USED FOR THE TREATMENT OF OBESITY. IN EUTHYROID PATIENTS, DOSES WITHIN THE RANGE OF DAILY HORMONAL REQUIREMENTS ARE INEFFECTIVE FOR WEIGHT REDUCTION. LARGER DOSES MAY PRODUCE SERIOUS OR EVEN LIFE THREATENING MANIFESTATIONS OF TOXICITY, PARTICULARLY WHEN GIVEN IN ASSOCIATION WITH SYMPATHOMIMETIC AMINES SUCH AS THOSE USED FOR THEIR ANORECTIC EFFECTS.

IN A LARGE STUDY, INVOLVING MEN WHO HAD HAD A MYOCARDIAL INFARCTION, USE OF THE DRUG WAS DISCONTINUED BECAUSE OF A TREND TO INCREASED MORTALITY IN DEXTROTHYROXINE-TREATED SUBJECTS COMPARED WITH PLACEBO-TREATED PATIENTS. EVEN IN SUBJECTS WITHOUT KNOWN OR SUSPECTED CORONARY DISEASE, THE POTENTIAL BENEFITS AND RISKS OF USING DEXTROTHYROXINE SODIUM SHOULD BE CAREFULLY CONSIDERED IN PATIENTS PRESENTING INCREASED RISK OF CORONARY DISEASE BECAUSE OF AGE, SEX, OBESITY, HISTORY OF SMOKING, HYPERTENSION AND/OR OTHER FACTORS INCREASING THE RISK OF CORONARY ARTERY DISEASE, SUCH AS A POSITIVE FAMILY HISTORY OF PREMATURE CORONARY DISEASE.

Dextrothyroxine Sodium may potentiate the effects of anticoagulants on prothrombin time.

Reductions of anticoagulant dosage by as much as 30% have been required in some patients.

Consequently, the dosage of anticoagulants should be reduced by one third upon initiation of Dextrothyroxine Sodium therapy and the dosage subsequently readjusted on the basis of prothrombin time. The prothrombin time of patients receiving anticoagulant therapy concomitantly with Dextrothyroxine Sodium therapy should be observed as frequently as necessary, at least weekly during the first few weeks of treatment.

In the surgical patient, it is wise to consider withdrawal of the drug two weeks prior to surgery if the use of anticoagulants during surgery is contemplated.

Dextrothyroxine Sodium should not be used with thyroid replacement drugs.

Since the possibility of precipitating cardiac arrhythmias during surgery may be greater in patients treated with thyroid harmones, it may be wise to discontinue Dextrothyroxine Sodium in euthyroid patients at least two weeks prior to an elective operation. Thus during emergency surgery in euthyroid patients, the patients should be carefully observed.

There are reports that Dextrothyroxine Sodium in diabetic patients is capable of increasing blood sugar levels with a resultant increase in requirements of insulin or oral hypoglycemic agents. Special attention should be paid to parameters necessary for good control of the diabetic state in dextrothyroxine sodium-treated subjects and to dosage requirements of insulin or other antidiabetic drugs if Dextrothyroxine Sodium is later withdrawn from patients who had required a dosage increase of insulin or oral hypoglycemic agents during its administration, the dosage of antidiabetic drugs should be reduced and adjusted to maintain good control of the diabetic state.

When impaired liver and/or kidney function are present, the advantages of Dextrothyroxine Sodium therapy must be weighed against the possibility of deleterious results (see "Contraindications").

PRECAUTIONS

General: It is expected that patients on Dextrothyroxine Sodium therapy will show increased serum thyroxine levels. These increased serum thyroxine values are evidence of absorption and transport of the drug, and should NOT be interpreted as evidence of hypermetabolism, therefore, they may not be used to determine the effective dose of Dextrothyroxine Sodium. Thyroxine values in the range of 10 to 25 mcg% in Dextrothyroxine Sodium-treated patients are common.

If signs or symptoms of iodism develop during Dextrothyroxine Sodium therapy, the drug should be discontinued.

The 2 mg Dextrothyroxine Sodium tablets contain FD&C Yellow No. 5 (tartrazine) which may cause allergic type reactions (including bronchial asthma) in certain susceptible individuals. Although the overall incidence of FD&C Yellow No. 5 (tartrazine) sensitivity in the general population is low, it is frequently seen in patients who also have aspirin hypersensitivity.

Information for Patients: Patients should receive instruction in appropriate dietary and nonpharmacologic measures designed to reduce serum cholesterol levels. These include restriction of intake of cholesterol, total calories, and saturated fatty acids, and increasing the ratio of polyunsaturated to saturated fats.

Patients should be instructed to notify physician if any of the following occur: palpitations, chest pain, diarrhea, excessive sweating, rash or acne, insomnia, headache, increasing nervousness, or visual disturbances.

Drug Interactions: Dextrothyroxine Sodium potentiates the effect of anticoagulants on prothrombin time, thus indicating a decrease in the dosage requirements of the anticoagulants. On the other hand, dosage requirements of antidiabetic drugs have been reported to be increased during Dextrothyroxine Sodium therapy (see "Warnings").

Carcinogenesis, Mutagenesis, Impairment of Fertility: Long term studies in animals to evaluate carcinogenic potential have not been performed.

Pregnancy: Pregnancy Category B: Reproduction studies have been performed in rabbits and rats at doses up to 100 times (mg/kg) the expected maximum daily dose for humans and have revealed no evidence of impaired fertility or harm to the fetus due to Dextrothyroxine Sodium. There are, however, no adequate and well-controlled studies in pregnant women. Because animal reproduction studies are not always predictive of human response, this drug should be used during pregnancy only if clearly needed.

Women of childbearing age who require drug therapy for hypercholesterolemia should consider use of a bile acid sequestering resin. Since pregnancy may occur despite the use of birth control procedures, administration of Dextrothyroxine Sodium to women of this age group should be undertaken only after weighing the possible risk to the fetus against the possible benefits to the mother.

Nursing Mothers: It is not known whether Dextrothyroxine Sodium is excreted in human milk. Because many drugs are excreted in human milk, caution should be exercised when Dextrothyroxine Sodium is administered to a nursing woman (see "Contraindications").

Pediatric Use: Safety and effectiveness in children have not been established (see "Contraindications").

ADVERSE REACTIONS

The side effects attributed to Dextrothyroxine Sodium therapy are, for the most part due to increased metabolism, and may be minimized by following the recommended dosage schedule. Adverse effects are least commonly seen in euthyroid patients with no signs or symptoms of organic heart disease.

In the absence of known organic heart disease, some cardiac changes may be precipitated during Dextrothyroxine Sodium therapy. Angina pectoris, extrasystoles, ectopic beats, supraventricular tachycardia, ECG evidence of ischemic myocardial changes and increase in heart size have all been observed. Myocardial infarctions, both fatal and nonfatal, have occurred, but these are not unexpected in untreated patients in the age groups studied. It is not known whether any of these infarcts were drug related. However, should any of these signs or symptoms develop, or other evidence of cardiac disease appear, Dextrothyroxine Sodium is contraindicated and should be discontinued.

Changes in clinical status that may be related to the metabolic action of the drug include the development of insomnia, nervousness, palpitations, tremors, loss of weight, lid lag, sweating, flushing, hyperthermia, hair loss, diuresis, and menstrual irregularities. Gastrointestinal complaints during therapy have included dyspepsia, nausea and vomiting, constipation, diarrhea, and decrease in appetite.

Other side effects reported to be associated with Dextrothyroxine Sodium therapy include the development of headache, changes in libido (increase or decrease), hoarseness, tinnitus, dizziness, peripheral edema, malaise, tiredness, visual disturbances, psychological changes, paresthesia, muscle pain, and various bizarre subjective complaints. Skin rashes, including a few which appeared to be due to iodism, and itching have been attributed to Dextrothyroxine Sodium by some investigators. Gallstones have been discovered in occasional Dextrothyroxine Sodium treated patients and cholestatic jaundice has occurred in one patient although its relationship to Dextrothyroxine Sodium therapy was not established.

In several instances, the previously existing conditions of the patient appeared to continue or progress during the administration of Dextrothyroxine Sodium. A worsening of peripheral vascular disease, altered sensorium, exophthalmos and retinopathy have been reported.

OVERDOSAGE

Overdosage with Dextrothyroxine Sodium may result in signs and symptoms of thyrotoxicosis. The dosage at which such symptoms may appear will depend on the previous thyroid status of the patient and their individual sensitivity to the drug Dextrothyroxine Sodium is somewhat protein-bound and would not be expected to be appreciably dialyzable. Treatment of overdosage is similar to that of thyrotoxic storm and may include hydration sedation and use of beta-adrenergic blocking agents.

DOSAGE AND ADMINISTRATION

For adult euthroid hypercholesterolemic patients, the recommended maintenance dose of Dextrothyroxine Sodium is 4 to 8 mg per day. The initial dose should be 1 to 2 mg daily, to be increased in 1 to 2 mg increments at intervals of not less than one month to a maximal level of 4 to 8 mg daily.

If signs or symptoms of cardiac disease develop during the treatment period, the drug should be withdrawn.

Store at controlled room temperature, 15°-30°C (59°-86°F).

HOW SUPPLIED
TABLETS: 1 MG

BRAND/MANUFACTURER	NDC	SIZE	AWP
○ BRAND CHOLOXIN: Boots Pharm	00048-1230-03	100s	$131.30

TABLETS: 2 MG

BRAND/MANUFACTURER	NDC	SIZE	AWP
○ BRAND CHOLOXIN: Boots Pharm	00048-1250-03	100s	$136.95

➤ SHOWN IN PRODUCT IDENTIFICATION GUIDE

TABLETS: 4 MG

BRAND/MANUFACTURER	NDC	SIZE	AWP
○ BRAND CHOLOXIN: Boots Pharm	00048-1270-03	100s	$168.20

Dezocine

DESCRIPTION

Dezocine is a synthetic opioid agonist-antagonist parenteral analgesic of the amino-tetralin series. The chemical name is (-)-[5R-(5α,11α,13S*)]-13-amino 5,6,7, 8,9,10,11,12-octahydro-5-methyl-5,11 -methanobenzocyclodecen-3-ol.

The molecular weight of the base is 245.4, and the molecular formula is $C_{16}H_{23}NO$. The n-octanol: water partition coefficient of Dezocine is 1.7.

Dezocine is available in three concentrations: 5, 10, and 15 mg of Dezocine per mL for intravenous or intramuscular administration. Each mL of the 5 mg strength contains 0.15 mg sodium metabisulfite and 7.236 mg lactic acid. Each mL of the 10 mg strength contains 0.15 mg sodium metabisulfite and 9.406 mg lactic acid. Each mL of the 15 mg strength contains 0.075 mg sodium metabisulfite and 11.578 mg lactic acid. Each mL of all three strengths contains 0.3 mL propylene glycol as a preservative and Water for Injection. The pH of Dezocine solutions is adjusted to 4.0 with sodium hydroxide.

Following is its chemical structure:

CLINICAL PHARMACOLOGY

PHARMACODYNAMICS

Dezocine is a strong opioid analgesic. Its analgesic potency, onset, and duration of action in the relief of postoperative pain are comparable to morphine. Pain relief in patients with postoperative pain is clinically evident when steady-state serum levels exceed 5 to 9 ng/mL. The side effects listed under **Adverse Reactions** were observed in patients whose average peak levels were less than 45 ng/mL. Peak analgesic effect lags peak serum levels by 20 to 60 minutes.

Table of Estimated Pharmacodynamic Parameters Following Intramuscular Doses of Dezocine

C(50)est1	5 to 9 ng/mL
C(toxic)est2	45 ng/mL

1. Estimated concentration required to obtain 50% decreases in pain intensity scores in post-operative pain.
2. Estimated concentration above which side effects may be more frequent.

PHARMACOKINETICS (SEE TABLE AND GRAPH)

Dezocine is completely and rapidly absorbed following intramuscular injection in normal volunteers with an average peak serum concentration of 19 ng/mL (range 10 to 38 ng/mL) occurring between 10 and 90 minutes after a 10 mg intramuscular injection. Following a 10 mg intravenous infusion over 5 minutes, the average terminal half-life of Dezocine is 2.4 hr (range 1.2 to 7.4 hr). The average volume of distribution (Vss) is 10.1 L/kg (range 4.7 to 20.1 L/kg), and the average total body clearance is 3.3 L/hr/kg (range 1.7 to 7.2 L/hr/kg). There is evidence of nonlinear (dose-dependent) pharmacokinetics at doses above 10 mg; in a study where 5, 10, and 20 mg intravenous doses of Dezocine were given (N = 12), dose-proportional serum levels were observed after 5 and 10 mg in injections, but the area under the serum concentration-time curve for the 20 mg dose was about 25% greater, and the total body clearance was about 20% lower, when compared to the 5 and 10 mg doses. The pharmacokinetics of Dezocine following chronic administration (steady-state pharmacokinetics) have not been experimentally determined, but predicted serum levels for 5 and 15 mg intramuscular doses given every 4 hr are presented in the graph.

Approximately two-thirds of a Dezocine dose is recovered in the urine with about 1% being excreted as unchanged Dezocine and the remainder as the glucuronide conjugate. Protein binding to Dezocine has not been studied.

MEAN (RANGE) PHARMACOKINETIC PARAMETERS OF DEZOCINE IN NORMAL VOLUNTEERS

	Dose		
IV	5 mg (N = 12)	10 mg (N = 36)	20 mg (N = 12)
Clearance (L/hr/kg)	3.52 (2.1-6.2)	3.33 (1.7-7.2)	2.76 (1.7-4.1)
Vss (L/kg)	10.7 (6.4-15.5)	10.1 (4.7-20.1)	8.8 (5.8-13.5)
t1/2 (hr)	1.7 (0.6-4.4)	2.4 (1.2-7.4)	2.4 (1.4-5.2)

(IM)	(N = 24)
Bioavailability	100%
Cmax1 (ng/mL)	10-38
tmax2 (min)	10-90

1. Peak plasma concentration.
2. Time-to-peak plasma concentration.

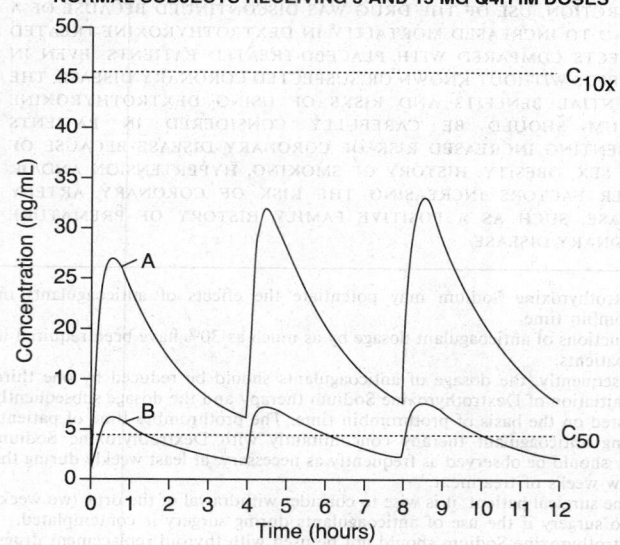

SIMULATED MEAN SERUM CONCENTRATIONS OF DEZOCINE IN NORMAL SUBJECTS RECEIVING 5 AND 15 MG Q4H IM DOSES

A — Dezocine 15 mg q4h
B — Dezocine 5 mg q4h
C_{tox} — Estimated concentration above which side effects may be more frequent
C_{50} — Estimated concentration required to obtain 50% decreases in pain intensity scores in postoperative pain

Hepatic insufficiency did not alter total body clearance in one study of 7 patients with cirrhosis. The volume of distribution and consequently the half-life, however, were increased by 30-50% relative to normal volunteers following a 10 mg intravenous dose. It is not known whether the free concentration of Dezocine is altered in cirrhotic patients.

The effect of renal insufficiency on Dezocine kinetics (urinary elimination) has not been studied. Because the primary elimination of Dezocine is through the urine as a glucuronide, however, use in patients with renal dysfunction should be done cautiously with reduced doses.

NARCOTIC ANTAGONIST ACTIVITY

Dezocine is a mixed opioid agonist-antagonist analgesic. Its opioid antagonist activity is less than that of nalorphine but greater than that of pentazocine when measured by antagonism of morphine-induced narcosis in rats.

EFFECT ON RESPIRATION

Dezocine and morphine produce a similar degree of respiratory depression when given in the usual analgesic doses. The effect is dose dependent and may be reversed by naloxone. As the dose of Dezocine is increased, there appears to be an upper limit to the magnitude of the respiratory depression produced by the drug in both animals and healthy human volunteers. Dezocine, like other mixed agonist-antagonist analgesics, may offer increased safety over pure agonist drugs such as morphine.

CARDIOVASCULAR EFFECTS

Dezocine has not been found to be associated with clinically important adverse effects on cardiac performance. Dezocine has been administered to patients as a 4-minute intravenous infusion at approximately 10 times the usual recommended intravenous dose without causing significant changes in mean systemic artery pressure, mean pulmonary artery pressure, pulmonary capillary wedge pressure, cardiac output, stroke index, and left ventricular stroke work index.

CLINICAL TRIALS

POSTOPERATIVE ANALGESIA

The analgesic efficacy of Dezocine was investigated in randomized controlled clinical trials in postoperative general surgical pain (orthopedic, gynecologic, and abdominal). The studies were primarily double-blind, single-dose, parallel trials in which Dezocine in intravenous (IV) doses of 2.5 to 10 mg (85 to 160 patients per treatment group) or intramuscular (IM) doses of 5 to 20 mg (39 to 221 patients per treatment group) was compared to 5 to 10 mg of morphine or 1 mg of IV butorphanol in patients with moderate-to-severe pain at baseline. The onset of analgesic action was similar to Dezocine morphine, and butorphanol, occurring

---

◆ RATED THERAPEUTICALLY EQUIVALENT; ◇ THERAPEUTIC EQUIVALENCE UNCONFIRMED; ○ UNRATED

within 15 minutes of IV and 30 minutes of IM administration of the drug Dezocine in 10 mg IM doses produced analgesia similar to that produced by 10 mg of IM morphine, while 5 mg of Dezocine IV was equivalent to 1 mg of IV butorphanol.

The peak analgesic effect and duration of analgesia were comparable for both routes of administration. The time by which approximately half of the patients remedicated was dose related and independent of the route of administration. Half of the patients remedicated within 2 hours after 5 mg of Dezocine or 1 mg of butorphanol IV, 3 hours after 10 mg of Dezocine or morphine IM, and 4 hours after 15 mg of Dezocine IM.

Another measure of the effect of Dezocine was the number of patients who did not require remedication during the six hours of the trial. The percentage of patients who did not request additional medication during the trial was 21% after a single dose of 15 mg of Dezocine 15% after 10 mg of Dezocine or morphine, and 4% after placebo.

Pain relief was proportional to the dose of Dezocine for single doses less than 20 mg. In one study with 39 to 42 patients per treatment group, comparing single doses of 20 or 10 mg of IM Dezocine with 10 mg of IM morphine, the patients receiving 20 mg of Dezocine did not obtain as much pain relief as that provided by 15 mg of the drug in other studies (the patients who received 10 mg of Dezocine or morphine in this study did obtain analgesia comparable to that seen in other trials). These results suggest that the maximally effective dose of Dezocine in postoperative pain may be 15 mg due to Dezocine's mixed agonist-antagonist pharmacology.

USE IN CHRONIC PAIN STATES
Data on the use of Dezocine in chronic pain has been gathered in trials of burn patients (n = 16) and cancer pain (n = 88). The daily dose of Dezocine for most patients with chronic pain has ranged between 20 and 60 mg per day, although doses as large as 90 to 140 mg per day have been used in 15 patients. Dezocine has not been adequately studied in the management of chronic pain. It is not recommended for use in patients who may have developed significant tolerance to opioid drugs from long-term use because of the risk of precipitating acute withdrawal symptoms.

INDICATIONS
Dezocine is indicated for the management of pain when the use of an opioid analgesic is appropriate (see "Clinical Trials").

CONTRAINDICATIONS
Dezocine should not be administered to patients who have been shown to be hypersensitive to it.

WARNINGS
Certain brands of Dezocine contain sodium metabisulfite, a sulfite that may cause allergic-type reactions including anaphylactic symptoms and life-threatening or less severe asthmatic episodes in certain susceptible people. The overall prevalence of sulfite sensitivity in the general population is unknown and probably low. Sulfite sensitivity is seen more frequently in asthmatic than in nonasthmatic people.

PATIENTS PHYSICALLY DEPENDENT ON NARCOTICS
Because of its opioid antagonist properties, Dezocine is not recommended for patients who are physically dependent on narcotics. Patients who have recently taken substantial amounts of narcotics may experience withdrawal symptoms. Because of the difficulty in assessing dependence in patients who have previously received substantial amounts of narcotic medication, caution should be used in the administration of Dezocine to such patients. To avoid precipitating an acute narcotic abstinence reaction, a sufficient period of withdrawal from opioids should be allowed before Dezocine is administered.

PRECAUTIONS
DEZOCINE IS A STRONG OPIOID ANALGESIC AND, LIKE ALL SUCH DRUGS, IT SHOULD BE ADMINISTERED IN CLINICAL SETTINGS WHERE RESPIRATORY DEPRESSION WILL BE PROMPTLY RECOGNIZED AND APPROPRIATELY MANAGED.

RESPIRATORY DEPRESSION INDUCED BY DEZOCINE CAN BE REVERSED WITH NALOXONE.

HEAD INJURY AND INCREASED INTRACRANIAL PRESSURE
Although there is no clinical experience in patients with head injury, the possible respiratory-depressant effect and the potential of strong analgesics to elevate cerebrospinal-fluid pressure (resulting from vasodilatation following CO_2 retention) may be markedly exaggerated in the presence of head injury, intracranial lesions, or a preexisting increase in intracranial pressure. Furthermore, strong analgesics can produce effects that may obscure the clinical course of patients with head injuries. In such patients, Dezocine should be used only when essential and with extreme caution.

USE IN CHRONIC OBSTRUCTIVE PULMONARY DISEASE
Because strong opioids cause some respiratory depression, they should be administered only with caution and in low doses to patients with preexisting respiratory depression (e.g., from other medication, uremia, or severe infection), severely limited respiratory reserve, bronchial asthma, obstructive respiratory conditions, or cyanosis. Respiratory depression induced by Dezocine can be reversed by naloxone.

USE IN HEPATIC OR RENAL DISEASE
Dezocine undergoes extensive hepatic metabolism and renal excretion of the glucuronide metabolite (see "Clinical Pharmacology"). Administration to patients with hepatic or renal dysfunction should be cautious using reduced doses.

USE IN BILIARY SURGERY
Although there is no evidence that Dezocine alters the tonic pressure within the common bile duct, therapeutic doses of other opioid analgesics can significantly increase pressure within the common bile duct. Therefore, Dezocine should be used with caution in such settings.

USE WITH OTHER CENTRAL NERVOUS SYSTEM DEPRESSANTS
Opioid analgesics, general anesthetics, sedatives, tranquilizers, hypnotics, or other CNS depressants (including alcohol) administered concomitantly with Dezocine may have an additive effect. When such combined therapy is contemplated, the dose of one or both agents should be reduced.

USE IN DRUG OR ALCOHOL DEPENDENCE
Use of Dezocine in combination with alcohol and/or other CNS depressant drugs will result in increased risk to the patient. Dezocine should be used with caution in individuals with active drug or alcohol addiction who are not in a medically controlled environment. Self-administration of any strong opioid may increase the relapse rate in populations recovering from addiction in abstinence-based recovery programs.

USE IN AMBULATORY PATIENTS
Strong opioid analgesics impair the mental or physical abilities required for the performance of potentially dangerous tasks such as driving a car or operating machinery. Patients who have been given Dezocine should not drive or operate dangerous machinery until the effects of the drug are no longer present.

PREGNANCY CATEGORY C
In reproductive studies Dezocine was shown to cause a dose-related suppression of body weight and food consumption of the parenteral generation in rats receiving either intravenous or intramuscular doses. Pup body weight was suppressed in a dose-related fashion. Teratology studies conducted in mice, rats, and rabbits revealed no evidence of teratogenic effects. There are no adequate and well-controlled studies in pregnant women. Dezocine should be used during pregnancy only if the potential benefit justifies the potential risk to the fetus.

LABOR AND DELIVERY
Safety to the mother and fetus after Dezocine administration during labor is unknown. The drug should be used in labor and delivery only when the physician deems its use essential to the welfare of the mother and infant.

NURSING MOTHERS
The use of Dezocine in mothers nursing infants is not recommended, since it is not known whether this drug is excreted in breast milk.

PEDIATRIC USE
Safety and efficacy in patients under the age of 18 years have not been established.

USE IN THE AGED
Like all strong, mixed opioid agonist-antagonist analgesics, Dezocine has the ability to depress respiration and reduce ventilatory drive to a clinically significant extent. It also has the potential to alter mental status or induce delirium in elderly patients. Dezocine has not undergone sufficient clinical testing in the geriatric population to assess its relative risk compared to other opioid analgesics, but the initial dose of all drugs of this class should be reduced in the geriatric patient and subsequent doses individualized.

ADVERSE REACTIONS
A total of 2192 patients have received Dezocine on an acute or chronic basis in the initial clinical trials of the drug. In nearly all cases, the type of incidence of side effects were those expected of a strong analgesic, and no unforeseen or unusual toxicity was reported. There is, as yet, limited information on the use of Dezocine for periods longer than 48 to 72 hours, but there was no evidence of hepatic, hematologic, or renal toxicity in 73 patients who received the drug for periods of time longer than 7 days.

The occurrence of adverse effects with Dezocine is based on data obtained from patients treated in both controlled and uncontrolled clinical trials. The adverse effects are listed below by frequency of occurrence within the body system affected.

The frequencies shown reflect the actual frequency of each adverse effect in patients who received Dezocine. There has been no attempt to correct for a placebo effect or to subtract the frequencies reported by placebo-treated patients in controlled trials.

The following adverse reactions were reported at a frequency of 1% or greater:

REACTIONS
Gastrointestinal System: Nausea* vomiting*.

Nervous System: Sedation*, dizziness/vertigo.

Skin: Injection-site reaction*.

(Reactions occurring with a frequency of 1 to < 3% are unmarked, while reactions occurring with a frequency of 3 to 9% are marked with an asterisk.*)

The following adverse reactions were reported with a frequency of less than 1% and are probably causally related to the administration of Dezocine:

Body as a Whole: Sweating, chills, flushing, low hemoglobin, edema.

Cardiovascular System: Hypotension, heart or pulse irregularity, hypertension, chest pain, pallor, thrombophlebitis.

Gastrointestinal System: Dry mouth, constipation, diarrhea, abdominal pain/distress/disorder.

Musculoskeletal System: Cramps/aching/pain.

Nervous System: Anxiety, confusion, crying, delusions, sleep disturbance, headache, delirium, depression.

Respiratory System: Respiratory depression, respiratory symptoms, atelectasis.

Skin: Pruritus, rash, erythema.

Special Senses: Diplopia, slurred speech, blurred vision.

Urogenital System: Urinary frequency, hesitancy, and retention.

The following adverse effects have been reported in less than 1% of the 2192 patients studied, and the association between these events and Dezocine administration is unknown. They are being listed to serve as alerting information for the physician.

Gastrointestinal: Increased alkaline phosphatase and SGOT.

Respiratory system: Hiccups.

Special senses: Congestion in ears, tinnitus.

There is no information available from postmarketing experience with the drug.

DRUG ABUSE AND DEPENDENCE

Dezocine has substituted for morphine in abuse-liability testing in animals. It has been identified as a narcotic in abuse-liability testing in experienced drug abusers, but has shown to evidence of abuse in clinical use during drug development. Mixed opioid agonist-antagonists of this type are generally recognized as having less potential for abuse than pure agonists such as morphine or meperidine, but all such drugs have abuse potential in certain individuals, especially those individuals with a prior history of opioid drug abuse or dependence.

Dezocine has a limited capacity to induce physical dependence in animal testing. Increasing tolerance to Dezocine or physical dependence on the drug were not seen in clinical trials.

OVERDOSAGE

CLINICAL PRESENTATION

Although there have been no incidents of overdosage with Dezocine during clinical trials, and thus no human experience with the drug, overdosage with Dezocine is possible. Based on the preclinical pharmacology of Dezocine, overdosage will produce acute respiratory depression, cardiovascular compromise, and delirium. The largest dose of Dezocine which has been given to nontolerant healthy volunteers without toxicity has been 30 mg/70 kg.

TREATMENT

The pharmacologic treatment of suspected Dezocine overdosage is intravenously administered naloxone. The respiratory and cardiac status of the patient should be evaluated constantly and appropriate supportive measures instituted, such as oxygen, intravenous fluids, vasopressors, and assisted or controlled respiration.

DOSAGE AND ADMINISTRATION

INTRAMUSCULAR

Although the recommended single dose for an adult is 5 to 20 mg, the majority of patients in clinical trials received an initial dose of 10 mg. Dosage should be adjusted according to the patient's weight, age, severity of pain, physical status, and other medications that the patient may be receiving. Dezocine may be repeated every 3 to 6 hours as necessary. The recommended maximum single dose is 20 mg, with a probable upper limit of 120 mg a day based on preclinical pharmacology of the drug. There is insufficient information regarding the risk of chronic use of Dezocine to establish limits for the maximum recommended duration of treatment with the drug.

INTRAVENOUS

The recommended range for intravenous administration of Dezocine is 2.5 to 10 mg repeated every 2 to 4 hours, with most patients in clinical trials receiving an initial intravenous dose of 5 mg.

SUBCUTANEOUS

Dezocine is not recommended for subcutaneous administration. Repeated injection of Dezocine at a single site has been associated with subcutaneous inflammation, vascular irritation, and venous thrombosis in animals. The significance of this finding for patients is unknown, although injection-site reactions occurred in 4% of patients treated with Dezocine in clinical trials.

CHILDREN AND ADOLESCENTS

Dezocine is not recommended for patients under 18 years of age.

SAFETY AND HANDLING INSTRUCTIONS

Dezocine is supplied in sealed dosage forms and at low concentrations which pose no known risk to health-care workers. Accidental dermal exposure to Dezocine should be treated by rinsing the affected area with fresh water.

Dezocine should be stored at room temperature and protected from light. As with all parenteral products, Dezocine should be inspected visually for particulate matter and discoloration prior to administration, whenever solution and container permit. Do not use if the solution contains a precipitate.

Dezocine, like other mixed agonist-antagonist opioid analgesics, has low abuse potential in patient populations. However, strong mixed agonist-antagonist drugs have reportedly been associated with abuse and dependence in health-care providers and others with ready access to such drugs. Dezocine should be handled accordingly.

HOW SUPPLIED
INJECTION: 5 MG/ML

BRAND/MANUFACTURER	NDC	SIZE	AWP
○ BRAND			
DALGAN: Astra	00186-1529-23	1 ml 10s	$68.49
	00186-1520-13	1 ml 25s	$166.75

INJECTION: 10 MG/ML

BRAND/MANUFACTURER	NDC	SIZE	AWP
○ BRAND			
DALGAN: Astra	00186-1522-12	10 ml 5s	$282.45
	00186-1524-23	1 ml 10s	$71.10
	00186-1521-13	1 ml 25s	$172.10

INJECTION: 15 MG/ML

BRAND/MANUFACTURER	NDC	SIZE	AWP
○ BRAND			
DALGAN: Astra	00186-1525-23	1 ml 10s	$72.76
	00186-1523-13	1 ml 25s	$177.43

DHC Plus SEE ACETAMINOPHEN/CAFFEINE/
DIHYDROCODEINE BITARTRATE

D.H.E. 45 SEE DIHYDROERGOTAMINE MESYLATE

DHT SEE DIHYDROTACHYSTEROL

DiaBeta SEE GLYBURIDE

Diabinese SEE CHLORPROPAMIDE

Dialyte SEE DEXTROSE AND ELECTROLYTES AND DEXTROSE
AND ELECTROLYTES, INTRAPERITONEAL

Diamox SEE ACETAZOLAMIDE

Diaphragm

DESCRIPTION

Diaphragms are available in three different types in a variety of sizes.

1. The Arcing spring diaphragm is a molded, buff-colored, natural rubber vaginal diaphragm containing a distortion-free, dual spring-within-a-spring which provides unique arcing action no matter where the rim is compressed. It is appropriate not only where ordinary diaphragms are indicated, but also in patients with mild cystocele, rectocele or retroversion. Arcing spring diaphragms are available in sizes 55mm through 95mm in 5mm increments. The contouring spring is actually 5 (five) springs in one.

2. The Coil spring diaphragm is a molded natural rubber vaginal diaphragm. The rim encases a tension-adjusted, cadmium-plated coil spring. Coil spring diaphragms are available in sizes 50mm through 105mm in 5mm increments.

3. The flat spring diaphragm is a molded, pure white, natural rubber vaginal diaphragm containing a flat, watch-type spring which allows compressibility in one plane only, thus facilitating insertion. Flat spring diaphragms are available in sizes 55mm through 95mm in 5mm increments.

Diaphragms are used in conjunction with spermicides, contraceptive jelly or contraceptive cream.

ACTION

These diaphragms when properly fitted serve two purposes:
   a. To stop the sperm from entering the cervical canal;
   b. To hold the spermicide.

◆ RATED THERAPEUTICALLY EQUIVALENT; ◇ THERAPEUTIC EQUIVALENCE UNCONFIRMED; ○ UNRATED

INDICATIONS

Diaphragms, in conjunction with an appropriate spermicide, are indicated for the prevention of pregnancy in women who elect to use diaphragms as a method of contraception.

CONTRAINDICATIONS

Known hypersensitivity to natural rubber products and prior history of Toxic Shock Syndrome (TSS).

WARNINGS

An association has been reported between diaphragm use and toxic shock syndrome (TSS), a serious condition which can be fatal.

For contraceptive effectiveness, the diaphragm should remain in place for six hours after intercourse and *should be removed as soon as possible thereafter.*

Continuous wearing of a contraceptive diaphragm for more than twenty-four hours is not recommended. Removal of the diaphragm before six hours may increase the risk of becoming pregnant. Retention of the diaphragm for any period of time may encourage the growth of certain bacteria in the vaginal tract. It has been suggested that under certain as yet unestablished conditions, overgrowth of these bacteria may lead to symptoms of toxic shock syndrome. Primary symptoms of TSS are sudden high fever (usually 102° or more), and vomiting, diarrhea, fainting or near fainting when standing up, dizziness or a rash that looks like sunburn. There may also be other signs of TSS such as aching of muscles and joints, redness of the eyes, sore throat and weakness. Patients should be instructed that if they experience sudden high fever and one or more of the other symptoms, they should remove the diaphragm and consult their physician immediately.

PRECAUTIONS

Diaphragm users should be instructed to consult their physician:
1. If they are not sure about the insertion and placement of the diaphragm.
2. If they or their partner feel or are made uncomfortable by the presence of the diaphragm.
3. If the diaphragm slips out of place when walking, coughing, or straining.
4. If the diaphragm no longer fits snugly above the public bone.
5. If at times other than menstruation there is blood on the diaphragm when it is removed.
6. If there are any holes, tears or other deterioration of the diaphragm.
7. If unable to remove the diaphragm.
8. *Important*—For contraceptive effectiveness, the diaphragm should remain in place for six hours after intercourse and *should be removed as soon as possible thereafter.* Continuous wearing of a contraceptive diaphragm for more than twenty-four hours is not recommended. Removal of the diaphragm before six hours may increase the risk of becoming pregnant. Retention of the diaphragm for any period of time may encourage the growth of certain bacteria in the vaginal tract. It has been suggested that under certain as yet unestablished conditions, overgrowth of these bacteria may lead to symptoms of toxic shock syndrome. Primary symptoms of TSS are sudden high fever (usually 102° or more), and vomiting, diarrhea, fainting or near fainting when standing up, dizziness or a rash that looks like a sunburn. There may also be other signs of TSS such as aching of muscles, redness of the eyes, sore throat and weakness. If the patient has a sudden high fever and one or more of the other symptoms, the diaphragm should be removed immediately and TSS should be considered.
9. Diaphragm users should have another diaphragm fitting if they have lost or gained more than ten pounds, have had the diaphragm for more than a year, or have had a baby or an abortion. As a matter of routine, each time a pelvic examination is performed, refitting should be done. The size and shape of the vagina changes and this may require a new size diaphragm. Even if the diaphragm size does not change, it is advisable to replace the diaphragm every two years or sooner.
10. Diaphragms may increase the risk of urinary tract infections especially if not properly fitted. Patients should be instructed to consult their physician if they experience any of the signs or symptoms of this type of infection which include pain on urination, blood in the urine, elevated temperature, frequent urination, or a sensation of obstruction while urinating.
11. Persons sensitive to natural rubber may have an allergic reaction to diaphragm use.

INSTRUCTIONS

1. Proper placement of the diaphragm is vital for effectiveness.
2. To be fully effective the diaphragm should never be used without contraceptive cream or jelly. The contraceptive cream or jelly must be spread around the inner surface of the diaphragm as well as around the rim.
3. To avoid pregnancy the diaphragm must be used every time there is intercourse.
4. The diaphragm may be inserted up to six hours before intercourse. If more than six hours has elapsed between insertion of the diaphragm and intercourse, additional contraceptive jelly or cream must be inserted. The diaphragm should not be removed to insert this additional cream or jelly.
The following Patient Instructions for insertion and removal are contained in the booklet.

PREPARING FOR INSERTION

1. It is recommended that you urinate and wash your hands before inserting the diaphragm.
2. Prior to inserting your diaphragm, put an applicatorful (about a teaspoon) of contraceptive jelly into the cup of the dome of the diaphragm. You may elect to simply squeeze the tube or use the applicator provided with the starter kit of contraceptive cream or jelly.
3. Spread a small amount around the edge with your fingertip, (if the amount applied to the rim is excessive, it will be difficult to control the diaphragm during insertion) then insert.
4. You can insert the diaphragm while you are standing with one leg up, squatting, or lying down. The position of the cervix and the walls of the vagina will be different depending on your position. If you are used to one position and then change to another, take extra care in positioning the diaphragm to be sure the cervix is covered.

INSERTING THE DIAPHRAGM

1. Hold the diaphragm with the dome down (spermicide up) and press the opposite sides of the rim together between your thumb and third finger. The diaphragm can be held from above or below.
2. Spread the lips of your vagina with your free hand. Hold the compressed diaphragm dome down (spermicide up) and push it gently inward along the rear wall of the vagina as far as it can go. Your index finger, kept on the outer rim of the diaphragm, helps you guide the diaphragm into place.
3. With your index finger, push the front rim of the diaphragm up until it is locked in place just above the pubic bone.
4. Check with your index finger to be sure the diaphragm is in place and is holding the contraceptive jelly or cream over the cervix. It is important that the cervix be covered by the diaphragm and spermicide and that the diaphragm be locked in place between the upper edge of the pubic bone and the rear wall of the vagina. You should be able to feel your cervix through the rubber shield. You can feel the front rim of the diaphragm above the pubic bone, but you may not be able to follow the rim all the way around since your fingers may not be long enough.
5. If, after some practice, you still find insertion awkward or difficult, vary your body and hand positions slightly until you can insert the diaphragm comfortably.

REMOVING THE DIAPHRAGM

To remove the diaphragm, put your index finger behind the front rim and pull the diaphragm down and out.

HOW TO FIT DIAPHRAGMS

1. To measure for diaphragm size:
Hold index and middle fingers together and insert into vagina up to the posterior fornix. Raise hand to bring surface of index finger to contact with pubic arch. Use tip of thumb to mark the point directly beneath the inferior margin of the pubic bone and withdraw finger in this position.
2. To determine diaphragm size:
Place one end of rim of fitting diaphragm or ring on tip of middle finger. The opposite end should lie just in front of the thumb tip. This is the approximate diameter of the diaphragm needed.
Insert a fitting diaphragm or ring of the appropriate size into the vagina.
Try both a larger and a smaller size before making a decision.
3. The proper size will fit snugly in the posterior fornix and behind the pubic arch without undue pressure.

HOW SUPPLIED
DIAPHRAGM:

BRAND/MANUFACTURER	NDC	SIZE	AWP
○ **BRAND**			
ORTHO ALL-FLEX: Ortho Pharm	00062-3301-00	1s	$18.30
	00062-3302-00	1s	$18.30
	00062-3303-00	1s	$18.30
	00062-3304-00	1s	$18.30
	00062-3305-00	1s	$18.30
	00062-3306-00	1s	$18.30
	00062-3307-00	1s	$18.30
	00062-3308-00	1s	$18.30
	00062-3309-00	1s	$18.30
○ **GENERICS**			
Milex	00396-9907-00	1s	$24.00

KIT:

BRAND/MANUFACTURER	NDC	SIZE	AWP
○ **BRAND**			
ORTHO COIL SPRING DIAPHRAGM KIT: Ortho Pharm	00062-3341-00	1s	$18.30
	00062-3342-00	1s	$18.30
	00062-3343-00	1s	$18.30
	00062-3344-00	1s	$18.30
	00062-3345-00	1s	$18.30
	00062-3346-00	1s	$18.30
	00062-3347-00	1s	$18.30
	00062-3348-00	1s	$18.30
	00062-3349-00	1s	$18.30
	00062-3350-00	1s	$18.30
	00062-3351-00	1s	$18.30
	00062-3352-00	1s	$18.30
ORTHO FLAT SPRING DIAPHRAGM KIT: Ortho Pharm	00062-3381-00	1s	$18.30
	00062-3382-00	1s	$18.30
	00062-3383-00	1s	$18.30

➤ SHOWN IN PRODUCT IDENTIFICATION GUIDE

BRAND/MANUFACTURER	NDC	SIZE	AWP
	00062-3384-00	1s	$18.30
	00062-3385-00	1s	$18.30
	00062-3386-00	1s	$18.30
	00062-3387-00	1s	$18.30
	00062-3388-00	1s	$18.30
	00062-3389-00	1s	$18.30

Diapid *SEE* LYPRESSIN

Diatrizoate Meglumine

DESCRIPTION

Diatrizoate Meglumine is a water-soluble, radiopaque diagnostic medium. It is a triiodinated benzoic acid derivative containing 47.06% or 141 mg/ml organically bound iodine. It is constituted as an iodinated anion (Diatrizoate) and a radiolucent cation (Meglumine).

Diatrizoate Meglumine is a sterile aqueous solution containing 30 or 60 gm of the meglumine salt of diatrizoic acid per 100 ml of solution. The solution is a clear, colorless to pale yellow liquid, and the pH is adjusted between 6.5 and 7.7. It is a relatively thermostable solution and may be autoclaved without harmful effects, although it should be protected from strong light.

Each 1 mL contains approximately 141 or 282 mg of organically bound iodine. The viscosity of the solution is 1.94 or 6.17 cp at 25°C and 1.42 or 4.12 cp at 37°C.

It is hypertonic to blood with an osmolality of 633 or 1415 mosm/kg (determined by VPO).

A 13% solution (w/v) is isotonic.

It is a colorless, microcrystalline solid which is readily soluble in water.

It is meglumine 3,5-diacetamido-2,4,6-triiodobenzoatel or 1-Deoxy-1-(methylamino)-D-glucitol 3,5-diacetamido-2,4,6-triiodobenzoate. The empirical formula is $(C_{11}H_9I_3N_2O_4 \cdot C_7H_{17}NO_5)$ and the molecular weight 809.13.

Following is its chemical structure:

CLINICAL PHARMACOLOGY

Intravascular injection of a radiopaque diagnostic agent opacifies those vessels in the path of the flow of the contrast medium, permitting radiographic visualization of the internal structures of the human body until significant hemodilution occurs.

Retrograde introduction of Diatrizoate Meglumine solution provides radiopacity of the contents of the urinary bladder. When used during micturation as a function test, it also opacifies the bladder neck and lower urinary tract. Continuous fluoroscopic and monitoring of urinary bladder contractions will demonstrate cystoureteric reflux and its extent, if present.

Diatrizoate Meglumine is not absorbed from the urinary tract to any extent (< 2%); therefore, systemic effects are rare. However, pyelorenal intravasation (especially in patients with ureteric reflux) can occur. Therefore, the potential for adverse effects, such as occur with intravascular use, are possible.

At physiologic pH, the water soluble contrast media are completely dissociated into a radiopaque anion and a solubilizing cation. While circulating in tissue fluids, the compound remains ionized. However, it is not metabolized but excreted unchanged in the urine, each Diatrizoate molecule remaining "obligated" to its Meglumine moiety.

Following intravenous injection, the radiopaque diagnostic agents are immediately diluted in the circulating plasma. Equilibrium is reached with the extracellular compartment at about 10 minutes. Hence, the plasma concentration at 10 minutes is closely related to the dose corrected to body size.

The pharmacokinetics of the intravenously administered radiopaque contrast media are usually best described by a two-compartment model with a rapid alpha phase for drug distribution and a slow beta phase for drug elimination. In patients with normal renal function, the alpha and beta half-lives were respectively 30 minutes and 120 minutes for Diatrizoate. But in patients with renal functional impairment, the elimination half-life for the beta phase can be prolonged up to several days.

Injectable radiopaque diagnostic agents are excreted either through the liver or through the kidneys. The two excretory pathways are not mutually exclusive, but the main route of excretion seems to be governed by the affinity of the contrast medium for serum albumin. From 0% to 10% of Diatrizoate sodium or Diatrizoate Meglumine is bound to serum protein.

Diatrizoate salts are excreted unchanged predominantly through the kidneys by glomerular filtration. The amount excreted by the kidney during any period of time is determined by the filtered load; ie, the product of plasma contrast media concentration and glomerular filtration rate. The plasma concentration is dependent upon the dose administered and the body size. The glomerular filtration rate varies with the body size, sex, age, circulatory dynamics, diuretic effect of the drug, and renal function. In patients with normal renal function the

maximum urinary concentration of Diatrizoate Meglumine occurs within 10 minutes with 12% of the administered dose being excreted. The mean values of cumulative urinary excretion for Diatrizoate Meglumine expressed as percentage of administered dose are 38% at 60 minutes, 45% at 3 hours, and 94 to 100% at 24 hours.

Urinary excretion of contrast media is delayed in infants younger than 1 month and in patients with urinary tract obstruction. The urinary iodine concentration is higher with the sodium salt of diatrizoic acid than with the meglumine salt.

The liver and small intestine provide the major alternate route of excretion for Diatrizoate. In patients free of severe renal disease, the fecal recovery is less than 2% of the administered dose. In patients with severe renal impairment the excretion of these contrast media through the gallbladder and into the small intestine sharply increases; up to 20% of the administered dose has been recovered in the feces in 48 hours.

Saliva is a minor secretory pathway for injectable radiopaque diagnostic agents. In patients with normal renal function, minimal amounts of contrast media are secreted unchanged. However, in uremic patients small amounts of free iodides resulting from deiodination prior to administration or *in vivo*, have been detected in the saliva.

Diatrizoate salts cross the placental barrier in humans by simple diffusion and appear to enter fetal tissue passively. No apparent harm to the fetus was observed when Diatrizoate sodium and Diatrizoate Meglumine were injected intravenously 24 hours prior to delivery. However, abnormal neonatal opacification of the small intestine and colon were detected 4 to 6 days after delivery. Procedures including radiation involve a certain risk related to the exposure of the fetus. (See "Precautions—General, Pregnancy Category C".)

Injectable radiopaque diagnostic agents are excreted unchanged in human milk. (See "Precautions—General, Nursing Mothers".)

Computerized Tomography: Diatrizoate Meglumine can be administered as an intravenous bolus for brain tissue enhancement using computerized tomography. Increased tissue contrast differential for the scan is achieved either because of increased vascular (arterial, venous, or capillary bed) contrast or by blood brain barrier penetration of the medium (or its absence) in certain localized areas of disrupted vascular permeability. The degree of tissue enhancement caused by increased blood contrast is directly related to blood iodine content. However, the degree of enhancement due to extravascular accumulation of iodine resulting from blood brain barrier disruption will depend on the extent of disruption, the blood level of iodine, and the time delay prior to scanning. The nature of the pathology will determine whether an immediate or delayed scan is optimal.

Effects of Steroid Therapy: The anti-inflammatory and antiedema effects in patients receiving steroid therapy have interfered with the expected distribution of CT tissue enhancement on the scan in certain diseases.

INDICATIONS AND USAGE

Diatrizoate Meglumine is indicated for excretory urography; cerebral angiography; peripheral arteriography; venography; operative, T-tube, or percutaneous transhepatic cholangiography; splenoportography; arthrography; discography; and contrast enhancement of computed tomographic head imaging. Some formulations are indicated for retrograde cystourethrography in adult and pediatric patients.

UROGRAPHY

Diatrizoate salts are used in small, medium, and large dose urography (see *"Dosage and Administration—Excretory Urography"*). Visualization of the urinary tract can be achieved by either direct intravenous bolus injection, intravenous drip infusion, or incidentally following intra-arterial procedures. Visualization of the urinary tract is delayed in infants less than 1 month old, and in patients with urinary tract obstruction (see *"Clinical Pharmacology"*).

CONTRAST ENHANCEMENT OF COMPUTED TOMOGRAPHIC HEAD IMAGING

Injectable radiopaque contrast media may be used to refine diagnostic precision in areas of the brain which may not otherwise have been satisfactorily visualized.

Tumors: Radiopaque diagnostic agents may be useful to investigate the presence and extent of certain malignancies such as: gliomas including malignant gliomas, glioblastomas, astrocytomas, oligodendrogliomas and gangliomas, ependymomas, medulloblastomas, meningiomas, neuromas, pinealomas, pituitary adenomas, craniopharyngiomas, germinomas, and metastatic lesions.

The usefulness of contrast enhancement for the investigation of the retrobulbar space and in cases of low grade or infiltrative glioma has not been demonstrated.

In calcified lesions, there is less likelihood of enhancement. Following therapy, tumors may show decreased or no enhancement.

The opacification of the inferior vermis following contrast media administration has resulted in false-positive diagnosis in a number of normal studies.

Nonneoplastic Conditions: The use of injectable radiopaque diagnostic agents may be beneficial in the image enhancement of nonneoplastic lesions. Cerebral infarctions of recent onset may be better visualized with contrast enhancement, while some infarctions are obscured if contrast media are used. The use of iodinated contrast media results in contrast enhancement in about 60% of cerebral infarctions studied from one to four weeks from the onset of symptoms.

Sites of active infection may also be enhanced following contrast media administration.

Arteriovenous malformations and aneurysms will show contrast enhancement. For these vascular lesions, the enhancement is probably dependent on the iodine content of the circulating blood pool.

◆ RATED THERAPEUTICALLY EQUIVALENT; ◇ THERAPEUTIC EQUIVALENCE UNCONFIRMED; ○ UNRATED

Hematomas and intraparenchymal bleeders seldom demonstrate any contrast enhancement. However, in cases of intraparenchymal clot, for which there is no obvious clinical explanation, contrast media administration may be helpful in ruling out the possibility of associated arteriovenous malformation.

ANGIOGRAPHY

Diatrizoate salts are used for radiographic studies throughout the cardiovascular system.

Intravascular radiopaque diagnostic agents of high concentration are not recommended for cerebral or spinal angiography (see *"Contraindications—General"*), and contrast agents with the lowest compatible viscosity and higher concentration of iodine (310 mg/ml to 480 mg/ml of bound iodine) must be used for angiocardiography. Contrast media approaching serum ionic content and osmolality have less potential for deleterious effects on the myocardium (see *"Precautions—General, Drug Interactions"*).

Addition of chelating agents may contribute to toxicity in coronary angiography, and the sodium content of angiographic agents used in coronary arteriography is of crucial importance.

In addition to the following general *"Contraindications"*, *"Warnings"*, *"Precautions"*, and *"Adverse Reactions"*, there are additional listings in these categories under the particular procedures.

CONTRAINDICATIONS
GENERAL

Diatrizoate Meglumine has no absolute contraindications in its recommended uses (see general *"Warnings"* and *"Precautions"*).

Do not use Diatrizoate Meglumine solution for myelography or for examination of dorsal cysts or sinuses which might communicate with the subarachnoid space. Even a small amount in the subarachnoid space may produce convulsions and result in fatality. Epidural injection is also contraindicated.

Urography and large dose vascular procedures are contraindicated in *dehydrated* azotemic patients. (See also *"Precautions, General"*.)

WARNINGS
GENERAL

Ionic iodinated contrast media inhibit blood coagulation, *in vitro*, more than nonionic contrast media. Nonetheless, it is prudent to avoid prolonged contact of blood with syringes containing ionic contrast media.

Serious, rarely fatal, thromboembolic events causing myocardial infarction and stroke have been reported during angiographic procedures with both ionic and nonionic contrast media. Therefore, meticulous intravascular administration technique is necessary, particularly during angiographic procedures, to minimize thromboembolic events. Numerous factors, including length of procedure, catheter and syringe material, underlying disease state and concomitant medications may contribute to the development of thromboembolic events. For these reasons, meticulous angiographic techniques are recommended including close attention to guidewire and catheter manipulation, use of manifold systems and/or three-way stopcocks, frequent catheter flushing with heparinized saline solutions and minimizing the length of the procedure. The use of plastic syringes in place of glass syringes has been reported to decrease but not eliminate the likelihood of *in vitro* clotting.

Serious or fatal reactions have been associated with the vascular entry of radiopaque media. It is important that a course of action be carefully planned in advance for the treatment of possible serious reactions.

Excretory urography is potentially hazardous in patients with multiple myeloma. In some of those patients, therapeutically resistant anuria resulting in progressive uremia, renal failure and eventually death has followed this procedure. Although neither the contrast agent nor dehydration has been proved separately to be the cause of anuria in myelomatous patients, it has been speculated that the combination of both may be causative. The risk of excretory urography in myelomatous patients is not a contraindication to the procedure; however, they require special precautions. Partial dehydration in the preparation of these patients for the examination is not recommended since this may predispose to the precipitation of myeloma protein in the renal tubules. Myeloma, which occurs most commonly in persons over age 40, should be considered before instituting urographic procedures.

Contrast media may promote sickling in individuals who are homozygous for sickle cell disease when the material is injected intravenously or intra-arterially.

Administration of radiopaque materials to patients known or suspected of having pheochromocytoma should be performed with extreme caution. If, in the opinion of the physician, the possible benefits of such procedures outweigh the considered risks, the procedures may be performed; however, the amount of radiopaque medium injected should be kept to an absolute minimum. The blood pressure should be assessed throughout the procedure and measures for treatment of a hypertensive crisis should be available.

Recent reports of thyroid storm occurring following the intravascular use of iodinated radiopaque diagnostic agents in patients with hyperthyroidism or with an autonomously functioning thyroid nodule suggest that this additional risk be evaluated in such patients before use of Diatrizoate Meglumine.

Contrast media administered for cardiac catheterization and angiocardiography may cause cellular injury to circulating lymphocytes. Chromosomal damage in humans includes inhibition of mitosis, increases in the number of micronuclei, and chromosome aberrations. The damages appear to be related to the contrast medium itself rather than to the x-ray radiation. It is to be noted that those agents have not been adequately tested in animal or laboratory systems.

Urography should be performed with caution in patients with severely impaired renal function and patients with combined renal and hepatic disease.

Subcutaneous extravasation, chiefly because of hypertonic cellulitis, causes transitory stinging. If the volume extravasated is small, ill effects are very unlikely. However, if the extravasation is extensive especially in poorly vascularized areas (eg, dorsum of the foot or hand), and especially in the presence of vascular disease, skin slough may occur. Injection of sterile water to dilute or addition of spreading agents to speed absorption have not been successful and may aggravate the condition.

Selective spinal arteriography or arteriography of trunks providing spinal branches can cause mild to severe muscle spasm. However, serious neurologic sequelae, including permanent paralysis, have occasionally been reported. (See also *"Angiography, Precaution"*.)

In patients with subarachnoid hemorrhage, a rare association between contrast administration and clinical deterioration, including convulsions and death, has been reported. Therefore, administration of intravascular iodinated ionic contrast media in these patients should be undertaken with caution.

PRECAUTIONS
GENERAL

Diagnostic procedures which involve the use of radiopaque diagnostic agents should be carried out only under the direction of personnel with the prerequisite training and with a thorough knowledge of the particular procedure to be performed. Appropriate facilities should be available for the management of any complication of the procedure, as well as for emergency treatment of severe reactions to the contrast agent itself. After parenteral administration of a radiopaque agent, competent personnel and emergency facilities should be available for at least 30 to 60 minutes since severe delayed reactions have occurred (see *"Adverse Reactions, General"*).

The possibility of a reaction, including serious, life-threatening, fatal, anaphylactic or cardiovascular reactions should always be considered (see *"Adverse Reactions"*). It is of utmost importance that a course of action be carefully planned in advance for immediate treatment of serious reactions, and that adequate and appropriate personnel be readily available in case of any reaction.

Preparatory dehydration for angiography and CT procedures is unnecessary and may be dangerous, contributing to acute renal failure in infants, young children, the elderly, patients with preexisting renal insufficiency, patients with advanced vascular disease, and diabetic patients. Dehydration in these patients seems to be enhanced by the osmotic diuretic action of urographic agents. Overnight fluid retention for urography may be undesirable and is considered unnecessary when using a relatively high (60%) concentration.

Although azotemia is not a contraindication, the medium should be used with great care in patients with advanced renal destruction associated with severe uremia. (See also *"Excretory Urography, Precautions"*.)

Acute renal failure has been reported in diabetic patients with diabetic nephropathy and in susceptible nondiabetic patients (often elderly with preexisting renal disease) following excretory urography. Therefore, careful consideration of the potential risks should be given before performing this radiographic procedure in these patients. (See also *"Excretory Urography, Precautions, Preparatory Dehydration"*.)

Immediately following surgery, excretory urography should be used with caution in renal transplant recipients.

The possibility of an idiosyncratic reaction in susceptible patients should always be considered (see *"Adverse Reactions, General"*). The susceptible population includes patients with a history of a previous reaction to a contrast medium, patients with a known sensitivity to iodine per se, and patients with a known clinical hypersensitivity: bronchial asthma, hay fever, and food allergies.

The occurrence of severe idiosyncratic reactions has prompted the use of several pretesting methods. However, pretesting cannot be relied upon to predict severe reactions and may itself be hazardous for the patient. It is suggested that a thorough medical history with emphasis on allergy and hypersensitivity, prior to injection of any contrast media, may be more accurate than pretesting in predicting potential adverse reactions.

Before injecting a contrast medium, the patient should be questioned for a history of allergy. A positive history of allergies or hypersensitivity does not arbitrarily contraindicate the use of a contrast agent, where a diagnostic procedure is thought essential, but caution should be exercised (see *"Adverse Reactions, General"*). Premedication with antihistamines or corticosteroids to avoid or minimize possible allergic reactions in such patients should be considered. Recent reports indicate that such pretreatment does not prevent serious life-threatening reactions, but may reduce both their incidence and severity.

Due to the transitory increase in the circulatory osmotic load, injections of urographic agents should be used with caution in patients with congestive heart failure. Such patients should be observed for several hours following the procedure to detect delayed hemodynamic disturbances.

General anesthesia may be indicated in the performance of some procedures in young or uncooperative children and in selected adult patients; however, a higher incidence of adverse reactions has been reported in these patients, and may be attributable to the inability of the patient to identify untoward symptoms, or to the hypotensive effect of anesthesia which can reduce cardiac output and increase the duration of exposure to the contrast agent.

Seizure activity is rare (about 0.01%) on intravenous injection of ionic contrast media. However, in the higher doses used for CT in patients with brain metastases the incidence can be much higher (1% to 10%). In these patients prophylactic use of a small parenteral dose of diazepam is suggested immediately before injection when extra high-dose CT regimens are employed.

In addition to the general precautions already described, excretory urography, cholangiography, and other uses also have hazards associated with the particular techniques employed. (see *"Individual Indications and Usage"* section.)

INFORMATION FOR PATIENTS
Patients receiving injectable radiopaque diagnostic agents should be instructed to:

1. Inform the physician if they are pregnant (see *"Clinical Pharmacology"*).

2. Inform the physician if they are diabetic or if they have multiple myeloma, pheochromocytoma, homozygous sickle cell disease or known thyroid disorder (see *"Warnings, General"*).

3. Inform the physician if they are allergic to any drugs, food, or if they have had any reactions to previous injections of dyes used for x-ray procedures (see *"Precautions, General"*).

4. Inform the physician about any other medications they are currently taking, including nonprescription drugs, before they are administered this drug.

DRUG INTERACTIONS
Renal toxicity has been reported in a few patients with liver dysfunction who were given oral cholecystographic agents followed by urographic agents. Administration of intravascular urographic agents should therefore be postponed in any patient with a known or suspected hepatic or biliary disorder who has recently received a cholecystographic contrast agent.

Addition of an inotropic agent to contrast agents may produce a paradoxical depressant response which can be deleterious to the ischemic myocardium.

Diphenhydramine hydrochloride may cause precipitation when mixed in the same syringe with Diatrizoate Meglumine.

Under certain circumstances (pH, temperature, concentrations, time), Diatrizoate solutions are incompatible with promethazine hydrochloride, diphenhydramine hydrochloride, brompheniramine maleate, or papaverine hydrochloride solutions. Diphenhydramine hydrochloride may cause precipitation when mixed in the same syringe with Diatrizoate Meglumine.

Do not prefill plastic syringes with Diatrizoate Meglumine for prolonged periods (ie, for several hours or longer) before use.

DRUG/LABORATORY TEST INTERACTIONS
Although interference with these laboratory tests have not been reported following cystography absorption (from the bladder or by pyelorenal back flow), they have occurred following direct *intravenous* injection.

If any of these studies, which might be affected by contrast media are indicated, it is recommended that they be performed prior to administration of the contrast medium or two or more days afterwards.

Diatrizoate salts interfere with several laboratory urine and blood tests.

BLOOD TESTS
Coagulation: Diatrizoate salts significantly inhibit all stages of coagulation. The fibrinogen concentration, Factors V, VII, and VIII are decreased. Prothrombin time and thromboplastin time are increased.

Platelet Aggregation: High levels of plasma diatrizoates inhibit platelet aggregation.

Serum Calcium: Diatrizoate salts may decrease serum calcium levels. However, this depletion of serum calcium may also be the result of the addition of chelating agents (edetate disodium) in the preparation of certain contrast media.

Red Cell Counts: Transitory decreases in red cell counts. Technetium-99m — RBC labeling interference.

Leukocyte Counts: Decrease.

Urea Nitrogen (BUN): Transitory increase (see *"Clinical Pharmacology"*).

Serum Creatinine: Transitory increase.

URINE TESTS
Contrast media which are excreted in the urine, may interfere with some laboratory determinations eg, proteinuria, specific gravity, osmolality, or bacterial cultures. Urine osmolarity and specific gravity are decreased due to induced diuresis. Diatrizoate in urine cultures may inhibit bacterial growth.

THYROID FUNCTION TESTS
Protein-bound Iodine (PBI) and Total Serum Organic Iodine: Transient increase of both tests following urography or cystography and retrograde pyelography have been noticed. The results of PBI and radioactive iodine uptake studies which depend on iodine estimations will not accurately reflect thyroid function for up to 16 days following administration of iodinated urographic media. However, thyroid function tests not depending on iodine estimations, eg, T_3 resin uptake or free thyroxine assays, are not affected.

CARCINOGENESIS, MUTAGENESIS, IMPAIRMENT OF FERTILITY
Long-term studies in animals have not been performed in order to evaluate carcinogenic potential, mutagenesis, or whether Diatrizoate Meglumine can affect fertility in males or females.

PREGNANCY CATEGORY C
Animal reproduction studies have not been conducted with Diatrizoate Meglumine. It is also not known whether Diatrizoate Meglumine can cause fetal harm when administered to a pregnant woman or can affect reproduction capacity. Diatrizoate Meglumine should be given to a pregnant woman only if clearly needed. Doses up to 2,500 mg/kg in rats, given IV daily, administered during gestation days 6 to 15 revealed no teratogenic abnormalities.

LABOR AND DELIVERY
It is not known whether use of these contrast agents during labor or delivery has immediate or delayed adverse effects on the fetus, prolongs the duration of labor or increases the likelihood that forceps delivery or other obstetrical intervention or resuscitation of the newborn will be necessary.

NURSING MOTHERS
Diatrizoate salts are excreted unchanged in human milk. Because of the potential adverse reactions, although it has not been established that serious adverse reactions occur in nursing infants, caution should be exercised when these intravascular contrast media are administered to a nursing woman.

PEDIATRIC USE
Infants and small children should not have any fluid restriction prior to excretory urography or any other procedures (see *"Precautions—General"*). Guidelines for pediatric dosages are presented in *"Dosage and Administration—General"*.

ADVERSE REACTIONS
GENERAL
Because inadvertent intravascular entry of Diatrizoate Meglumine is possible during urethrocystography (bladder absorption or pyelorenal back flow), the occurrence of systemic adverse effects is possible. However, the relative incidence and severity of the following reactions refer only to experience with direct *intravascular* injection.

Approximately 95% of adverse reactions accompanying the intravascular use of Diatrizoate salts are of mild to moderate severity. However, life-threatening reactions and fatalities, mostly of cardiovascular origin, have occurred.

Adverse reactions to injectable contrast media fall into two categories: chemotoxic reactions and idiosyncratic reactions.

Chemotoxic reactions results from the physicochemical properties of the contrast media, the dose, and the speed of injection. All hemodynamic disturbances and injuries to organs or vessels perfused by the contrast medium are included in this category.

Idiosyncratic reactions include all other reactions. They occur more frequently in patients 20 to 40 years old. Idiosyncratic reactions may or may not be dependent on the amount of dose injected, the speed of injection, the mode of injection, and the radiographic procedure. Idiosyncratic reactions are subdivided into minor, intermediate, and severe. The minor reactions are self-limited and of short duration; the severe reactions are life-threatening and treatment is urgent and mandatory.

The reported incidence of adverse reactions to contrast media in patients with a history of allergy are twice that of the general population. Patients with a history of previous reactions to a contrast medium are three times more susceptible than other patients. However, sensitivity to contrast media does not appear to increase with repeated examinations.

Most adverse reactions to injectable contrast media appear within one to three minutes after the start of injection, but delayed reactions may occur.

Adverse reactions are grouped by organ system and listed below by decreasing order of occurrence and with an approximate incidence of occurrence. Significantly more severe reactions are listed before the other reactions regardless of frequency.

GREATER THAN 1 IN 100 PATIENTS
Body as a Whole: Reported incidences of death range from 6.6 per 1 million (0.00066%) to 1 in 10,000 patients (0.01%). Most deaths occur during injection or 5 to 10 minutes later, the main feature being cardiac arrest with cardiovascular disease as the main aggravating factor.

Isolated reports of hypotensive collapse and shock following urography are found in the literature. The incidence of shock is estimated to occur in 1 out of 20,000 (0.005%) patients.

Cardiovascular System: The most frequent adverse reaction to Diatrizoate salts is vasodilation (feeling of warmth). The estimated incidence is 49%.

Digestive System: Nausea 6%, vomiting 3%.

Nervous System: Paresthesia 6%, dizziness 5%.

Respiratory System: Rhinitis 1%, increased cough 2%.

Skin and Appendages: Urticaria 1%.

Pain at the injection site is estimated to occur in about 12% of the patients undergoing urography. Pain is usually due to extravasation.

Painful hot erythematous swelling above the venipuncture site was estimated to occur in more than 1% of the patients undergoing phlebography.

Special Senses: Perversion of taste 11%.

Urogenital System: Osmotic nephrosis of the proximal tubular cells is estimated to occur in 23% of patients following excretory urography.

LESS THAN 1 IN 100 PATIENTS
Other infrequently reported reactions without accompanying incidence rates are listed below, grouped by organ system.

Body as a Whole: Malaria relapse, uremia, high creatinine and BUN (see *"Precautions, General Drug/Laboratory Test Interactions"*), thrombocytopenia, leukopenia and anemia.

Cardiovascular System: Cerebral hematomas, hemodynamic disturbances, sinus bradycardia, transient electrocardiographic abnormalities, ventricular fibrillation, petechiae, chest pain, cardiac arrest, tachycardia, and cardiorespiratory arrest.

◆ RATED THERAPEUTICALLY EQUIVALENT; ◇ THERAPEUTIC EQUIVALENCE UNCONFIRMED; ○ UNRATED

Digestive System: Severe unilateral or bilateral swelling of the parotid and submaxillary glands.

Nervous System: Convulsions, paralysis, coma, speech impairment and severe confusion (see *"Precautions, General"*).

Respiratory System: Asthma, dyspnea, laryngeal edema, pulmonary edema, bronchospasm, pulmonary embolus and respiratory arrest.

Skin and Appendages: Extravasation necrosis, urticaria with or without pruritus, mucocutaneous edema, and angioneurotic edema.

Special Senses: Bilateral ocular irritation, lacrimation, itching, conjunctival chemosis, infection, conjunctivitis, and unilateral blindness.

Urogenital: Renal failure, pain.

OVERDOSAGE

At dosage levels of 1 mL/lb, the incidence of unpleasant side effects increases. At total dosage of 2 mL/lb, administered over a short period of time (eg, 30 minutes), clinical signs of systemic intolerance appear (mostly related to hyperosmolar effects) and are manifest as tremors, irritability, and tachycardia. Above these maximal tolerated dosage levels in otherwise healthy adults, an increasing incidence and severity of dyspnea and pulmonary edema should be expected.

Four cases of overdosage in infants, during urography, are reported. Three of the infants died within 19 hours of the injection. The overdose ranged from slightly above the recommended pediatric dosage to a dose exceeding 19 gm/kg. The symptoms of overdosage appeared between 10 minutes to several hours after injection of the contrast medium. Adverse effects were life-threatening, affecting mainly the pulmonary and cardiovascular systems. The symptoms included: cyanosis, bradycardia, acidosis, pulmonary hemorrhage, convulsions, coma, and cardiac arrest. All infants showed a poor visualization of the kidneys and a diffuse opacification of all the tissues and vasculature. Autopsy findings showed acute pulmonary damage and/or edema of subcutaneous tissues. Treatment of an overdose of injectable radiopaque contrast media is directed toward the support of all vital functions, and prompt institution of symptomatic therapy.

The acute intravenous LD$_{50}$ of Diatrizoate Meglumine in mice is equivalent in iodine content of 5.3 gmI/kg to 8.0 gmI/kg and seems to be directly proportional to the rate of injection.

Diatrizoate Meglumine is dialyzable.

DOSAGE AND ADMINISTRATION

GENERAL

Preparation of the patient will vary with preference of the radiologist and the type of radiological procedure performed. Specific radiographic procedures used will depend on the state of the patient and the diagnostic indications. Individual dose should be tailored according to age, body size, and indication for examination. (See *"Individual Indications and Usage"* section for specific *"Dosage and Administration"*.)

Solutions of radiopaque diagnostic agents for intravascular use should be at body temperature when injected and may need to be warmed before use. In the event that crystallization occurs, the solution may be clarified by placing the vial in a water bath at 40°C to 50°C and shaking it gently for two to three minutes or until the solids redissolve. If the particles still persist, do not use this vial but discard it. The solution should be protected from light and any unused portion remaining in the container should be discarded.

Dilution and withdrawal of the contrast agents should be accomplished under aseptic conditions with sterile syringes.

Parenteral drug products should be inspected visually for particulate matter and discoloration prior to administration. Avoid contaminating catheters, syringes, needles, and contrast media with glove powder or cotton fibers.

PEDIATRIC DOSAGE

Pediatric doses of injectable radiopaque diagnostic agents are generally determined on a weight basis and should be calculated for each patient individually. (See *"Individual Indications and Usage"* section.)

DRUG INCOMPATIBILITIES

Diatrizoate salts are incompatible *in vitro* with some antihistamines and many other drugs. It is believed that one of the chief causes of *in vitro* incompatibility is an alteration of pH. Turbidity of solutions of intravascular contrast medium occurs between pH 2.5 and 4.1. Another cause is chemical interaction; therefore, other pharmaceuticals should not be mixed with contrast agents in the same syringe.

INDIVIDUAL INDICATIONS AND USAGE

The following sections for individual *"Indications and Usage"* contain *"Contraindications"*, *"Warnings,"* *"Precautions"*, *"Adverse Reactions"*, and *"Dosage and Administration"* sections related to the *specific procedures*. However, it should be understood that the information in the *general* sections is also likely to apply to all of these specific uses.

Hydration: With the possible exception of urography, patients should be fully hydrated prior to the following procedures.

EXCRETORY UROGRAPHY

Diatrizoate salts are used in small, medium, and large dose urography (see *"Dosage and Administration, Excretory Urography"*). Visualization of the urinary tract can be achieved by either direct intravenous injection, intravenous drip infusion, or sometimes by intramuscular or subcutaneous injections, or incidentally following intra-arterial procedure. Visualization of the urinary tract is delayed in infants less than 1 month old, and in patients with urinary tract obstruction (see *"Clinical Pharmacology"*).

Contraindication: Urography is contraindicated in patients with anuria.

Precautions: See *"Precautions, General"*. Some clinicians consider multiple myeloma a contraindication to excretory urography because of the great possibility of producing transient or fatal renal failure. Others believe that the risk of causing anuria is definite but small. If excretory urography is performed in the presence of multiple myeloma, dehydration should be avoided since it favors protein precipitation in renal tubules.

Although azotemia is not considered a contraindication, care is required in patients with advanced renal failure. The usual preparatory dehydration should be omitted, and urinary output should be observed for one to two days in these patients. Adequate visualization may be difficult or impossible to attain in patients with severely impaired renal and/or hepatic function. Use with extreme caution in patients with concomitant hepatorenal disease.

Because of the possibility of temporary suppression of urine, it is wise to allow an interval of at least 48 hours before excretory urography is repeated in patients with unilateral or bilateral reduction of normal renal function.

Preparatory Dehydration: Preparatory dehydration is dangerous in infants, young children, the elderly, and azotemic patients (especially those with polyuria, oliguria, diabetes, advanced vascular disease, or preexisting dehydration). The undesirable dehydration in these patients may be accentuated by the osmotic diuretic action of the medium.

Dehydration may improve image quality in patients with adequate renal function particularly if a low dose is used. Dehydration, however, *will not* improve contrast quality in patients with substantial renal insufficiencies and will increase risk of contrast induced renal damage. Dehydration in these patients is therefore contraindicated.

Adverse Reactions: See *"Adverse Reactions, General"*.

Dosage and Administration:

Intravenous Dosage:

Adults: A dose of 30 ml to 60 ml produces excellent shadows in the majority of adults subjected to partial dehydration and effective purgation. In persons of slight build, 20 ml produces adequate shadows. For best results and minimal reactions, the total 30 ml to 60 ml should be injected in one to three minutes and compression may be used. A small intravenous test dose may be administered as a possible aid in determining sensitivity to the medium. (See *"Precautions, General"*.)

Children: The suggested dosage for children up to 12 years old is presented in the table below. Children older than 12 years may be given an adult dose.

PEDIATRIC DOSAGE FOR EXCRETORY UROGRAPHY

Age	Body Weight	Dosage
Under 2 years	up to 10 lb	5 ml to 10 ml
	10 to 30 lb	10 ml to 15 ml
2 to 12 years	30 to 60 lb	15 ml to 30 ml
	over 60 lb	30 ml

Preliminary Preparation of Patient: Although clear shadows are often seen in patients who have had no preliminary preparation for urography, the largest percentage of satisfactory films is obtained in patients who abstain from fluids for 12 to 15 hours before the intravenous injection so that partial dehydration results. (See *"Precautions, General"* concerning dehydration.) Unless contraindicated, a laxative may be taken at bedtime to eliminate gas from the intestine.

Roentgenographic Technique: A preliminary scout film may be obtained before the intravenous injection. Excellent shadows can often be obtained immediately after administration of the radiopaque medium (within a five-minute period). If preliminary preparation has been carried out, the urinary organs are usually best visualized on films exposed 5, 10, or 15 minutes after intravenous injection. If a film of the bladder is required, it is generally taken 25 or 35 minutes after injection.

In patients with impaired renal function, the best shadows may not be obtainable until later (30 minutes or more) because of delayed excretion, and additional film may have to be exposed.

Most urologists and roentgenologists believe that compression immediately above the symphysis (obtained by application of a small hollow rubber ball about the size of a grapefruit or by the rolled bed sheet technique) assures adequate filling of the pelves and ureters, and hence is of great value. Although compression undoubtedly improves the urogram, it also seems to increase the possibility of pyelorenal backflow or reflux by raising the pressure within the urinary tract.

ANGIOGRAPHY

Precautions: Since serious neurologic complications, including quadriplegia, have occasionally been reported following spinal arteriography or selective injection of arterial trunks providing spinal artery branches (usually the thyrocervical, costocervical, subclavian, vertebral, bronchial, intercostal), great care is necessary to avoid entry of a large concentrated bolus of the medium. Thus, a "pilot" dose may establish correct position of the catheter tip. The concentration of the medium should not be over 60%. The carefully individualized dose is usually under 5 ml but preferably 3 ml to 4 ml and the number of repeat injections held to a minimum with appropriate intervals between injections. Pain or muscle spasm during the injection may require reevaluation of the procedure.

Angiography should be avoided whenever possible in patients with homocystinuria, because of the risk of inducing thrombosis and embolism.

CEREBRAL ANGIOGRAPHY
Indication: Diatrizoate Meglumine may be administered for visualization of the cerebral vessels. Inasmuch as cerebral angiography is a highly specialized procedure requiring the use of special techniques, it is recommended that Diatrizoate Meglumine be used for this purpose only by persons skilled and experienced in carrying out the procedure.

Contraindication: Carotid angiography during the progressive period of a stroke should be avoided, particularly on the left side because of the increased risk of cerebral complications.

Precautions: See "Precautions, General". Patients in whom cerebral angiography is to be performed should be selected with care.

Although cerebral angiography has been considered contraindicated in patients who have recently experienced cerebral embolism or thrombosis (stroke syndrome), many experts now believe that the diagnostic value of the procedure, when employed early as an aid in locating lesions amenable to operation, outweighs any added risk to the patient. Furthermore, a small number of postangiographic fatalities have been reported, including progressive thrombosis already clinically evident before angiography, in which the procedure did not appear to play any direct role. Patients with severe cerebrovascular disease should be examined primarily by indirect methods of angiography.

In cerebral angiography, every precaution must be taken to prevent untoward reactions. Reactions may vary directly with the concentration of the substance, the amount used, the speed and frequency of injections, and the interval between injections.

In subarachnoid hemorrhage, angiography is expected to be hazardous. In migraine, the procedure can be hazardous because of ischemic complications, particularly if performed during or soon after an attack.

Adverse Reactions: See "Adverse Reactions, General". With any contrast medium introduced into the cerebral vasculature, neurologic complications, including neuromuscular disorders, seizures, loss of consciousness, hemiplegia, unilateral dysesthesias, visual field defect, language disorders (aphasia), amnesia, and respiratory difficulties may occur, particularly when the extent of the intrinsic lesion is unknown. Such untoward reactions are for the most part temporary, although permanent visual field defects have been reported. Some investigators who are experienced in angiographic procedure emphasize the fact that they tend to occur after repeated injections or higher doses of the contrast medium. Other clinicians find that they occur most frequently in elderly patients. Inasmuch as the procedure itself is attended by technical difficulties regardless of the risk the patient presents (eg, mechanical catheter obstruction of the vertebral artery can cause transient blindness), the more experienced the radiologic team, the fewer the complications of any degree that are apt to arise.

Amaurosis can occur following carotid or especially selective vertebral arteriography. It is almost always transitory (4 to 48 hours).

Dosage and Administration: A dose of 8 ml to 12 ml injected at a rate not exceeding the normal flow in the carotid artery (about 5 ml per second) is suggested. The dose may be repeated as indicated; however, an increased risk attends each repeat injection. Children require a smaller dose in proportion to weight. Light anesthesia may be required in these procedures.

PERIPHERAL ARTERIOGRAPHY AND VENOGRAPHY
Indications: Diatrizoate Meglumine may be administered for peripheral arteriography and for venography.

Precautions: See "Precautions General". Extreme caution is advised in considering peripheral arteriography in patients suspected of having thromboangiitis obliterans (Buerger's disease) since any procedure (even insertion of a needle or catheter) may induce a severe arterial or venous spasm. Caution is also advisable in patients with severe ischemia associated with ascending infection.

Adverse Reactions: See "Adverse Reactions, General". Soreness in extremities has also been reported.

Adverse reactions observed during peripheral arteriography may sometimes be due to arterial trauma during the procedure (ie, insertion of needle or catheter, subintimal injection, perforation) as well as to the hypertonicity or effect of the medium. Reported adverse reactions include transient arterial spasm, extravasation, hemorrhage, hematoma formation with tamponade, injury to nerves in close proximity to artery, thrombosis, dissecting aneurysm, arteriovenous fistula (eg, with accidental perforation of femoral artery and vein during the needling), and transient leg pain from contraction of calf muscles in femoral arteriography. Transient hypotension has been reported after intra-arterial (brachial) injection of the medium. Also, brachial plexus injury has been reported with axillary artery injections.

During venography in the presence of venous stasis, inflammatory changes and thrombosis may occur. Thrombosis is rare if the vein is irrigated following the injection.

Dosage and Administration: Diagnostic arteriograms may be obtained with 20 ml to 40 ml Diatrizoate Meglumine introduced into the larger peripheral arteries by percutaneous or operative methods. Visualization of veins in the extremities may be accomplished with 10 ml to 20 ml.

DIRECT CHOLANGIOGRAPHY
Contraindication: Percutaneous transhepatic cholangiography is contraindicated in patients with coagulation defects and prolonged prothrombin times until normal, or near normal, coagulation is achieved (e.g., with vitamin K).

Precautions: In the presence of acute pancreatitis, direct cholangiography, if necessary, should be employed with caution, injecting no more than 5 ml to 10 ml without undue pressure.

Percutaneous transhepatic cholangiography should only be attempted when compatible blood for potential transfusions is in readiness and emergency surgical measures are available. The patient should be carefully monitored for at least 24 hours to insure prompt detection of bile leakage and hemorrhage. Cholespastic premedication, as with morphine, should be avoided. Respiratory movements should be controlled during introduction of the needle.

Adverse Reactions: Adverse reactions may often be attributed to injection pressure or excessive volume of the medium, resulting in overdistention. Such pressure may produce a sensation of epigastric fullness, followed by moderate pain in the back or right upper abdominal quadrant, which will subside when injection is stopped.

Hepatobiliary reflux of the medium may cause a pancholangitis or hepatitis which is usually transitory. Retrograde spread of the infection may produce liver abscess or septicemia. Pancreatic duct reflux may cause a transitory increase in serum amylase for a period of 6 to 18 hours without ill effects. Rarely it may cause pancreatitis.

In percutaneous transhepatic cholangiography, some discomfort is common, but severe pain is unusual. Complications of the procedure are often serious and have been reported in 4% to 6% of patients. These reactions have included bile leakage and peritonitis, which are more likely to occur in patients with obstructions that cause unrelieved high biliary pressure. Bleeding (sometimes massive with exsanguination) may occur, especially in patients with clotting abnormalities. Blood-bile fistula, manifested by an early urogram (within 2 minutes) has been reported. Hypotension with fever and chills, as manifestations of septicemia, have occurred. Tension pneumothorax, cholangitis, and bacteremia have been reported.

Dosage and Administration: The solution should be warmed to body temperature before administration. The injection is made slowly without undue pressure, taking great care to avoid introducing bubbles.

Operative: If no resistance is encountered, from 10 ml to 15 ml (sometimes up to 25 ml) of a 30% to 60% solution is injected or instilled into the cystic duct or common bile duct, as indicated. In patients with obstructive jaundice, 40 ml to 50 ml of the medium may be injected indirectly into the gallbladder after aspiration of its contents.

Postexploratory or Completion T Tube: Cholangiography may also be performed after exploration of the common bile duct.

Postoperative: Delayed cholangiograms are usually made from the fifth to the tenth postoperative day prior to removal of the T tube.

Percutaneous Transhepatic Cholangiography is recommended for carefully selected patients for the differential diagnosis of jaundice due to extrahepatic biliary obstruction or parenchymal disease. The procedure is only employed where oral or intravenous cholangiography and other procedures have failed to provide the necessary information. In obstructive cases, percutaneous transhepatic cholangiography is used to determine the cause and site of the obstruction to help plan surgery. The technique may also be of value in avoiding laparotomy in poor-risk jaundice patients since failure to enter a duct suggests hepatocellular disease. Careful attention to technique is essential for the success and safety of the procedure. The procedure is usually performed under local anesthesia following analgesic premedication (eg, 100 mg meperidine intramuscularly).

As the needle is advanced or withdrawn, a bile duct may be located by frequent aspiration for bile or mucus into a syringe filled with normal saline. As much bile as possible is aspirated. The usual dose of Diatrizoate Meglumine is 20 ml to 40 ml but the range can be from 10 ml to 60 ml depending on degree of biliary dilatation present. The injection may be repeated for exposures in different planes. If a duct is not readily located by aspiration, entry may be established by the injection of successive small doses of 1 ml or 2 ml of the medium under x-ray observation as the needle is withdrawn. If a duct is not located after three or four attempts, the procedure should be abandoned. Inability to enter a duct strongly suggests hepatocellular disease.

SPLENOPORTOGRAPHY
Indication: Splenoportography is usually performed under mild preoperative sedation and under local anesthesia.

Contraindications: Splenoportography should not be performed on any patient for whom splenectomy is contraindicated, since complications of the procedure at times make splenectomy necessary. Other contraindications include prolonged prothrombin time or other coagulation defects, significant thrombocytopenia, and any condition which may increase the possibility of rupture of the spleen.

Precautions: Prior gastrointestinal x-ray examination should include particular attention to the lower esophageal area. A hematologic survey, including prothrombin time and platelet count, should be performed. To minimize risk of bleeding, manipulation during or after entry of the needle should be avoided. Caution is advised in patients whose spleen has recently become tender and palpable.

Following splenoportography, the patient should lie on his left side for several hours and should be closely observed for 24 hours for signs of internal bleeding.

Adverse Reactions: Internal bleeding is the most common serious complication of splenoportography. Although leakage of up to 300 ml of blood is apparently not uncommon, sometimes blood transfusions and, rarely, splenectomy, may be required to control hemorrhage. Peritoneal extravasation may cause transient diaphragmatic irritation or mild to moderate transient pain which may sometimes be referred to the shoulder, the periumbilical region, or other areas. Because of the proximity of the pleural cavity, accidental pneumothorax has been known to occur. Inadvertent injection of the medium into other nearby structures is not likely to cause untoward consequences.

Dosage and Administration: A preliminary small "pilot" dose is injected to confirm splenic entry, followed usually by rapid injection of 20 ml to 25 ml of Diatrizoate Meglumine. Rapid serial exposures are started with the injection of the dose and continued until contrast is observed in the entire portal system.

ARTHROGRAPHY

Indications: Arthrography may be helpful in the diagnosis of posttraumatic or degenerative joint diseases, synovial rupture, the visualization of communicating bursae or cysts, and in meniscography. However, the technique is of little value unless the arthrograms are interpreted by well-trained personnel.

Contraindication: Arthrography is contraindicated when there is infection in or near the joint.

Precautions: See *"Precautions, General"*. A strict, aseptic technique is required to avoid introducing infection.

Adverse Reactions: See *"Adverse Reactions, General"*. Injection of Diatrizoate Meglumine into the joint usually causes immediate but transient discomfort. However, delayed, severe, or persistent pain may occur occasionally. Severe pain often results from undue use of pressure or the injection of large volumes. Joint swelling after injection is rare. Effusion, occasionally requiring aspiration, can occur in patients with rheumatoid arthritis.

Dosage and Administration: The procedure is usually performed with analgesic premedication and under local anesthesia. The amount of Diatrizoate Meglumine injected depends solely on the capacity of the joint. The damaged joint may require doses greatly exceeding those for normal joints. As much fluid as possible should first be aspirated from the joint; then, the medium should be injected gently to avoid overdistention of the joint capsule. Passive manipulation is sometimes used to disperse the medium in the joint. Sometimes, a 1 ml or 2 ml test dose in injected; immediate pain may indicate extravasation or extracapsular injection which, if confirmed by x-ray, requires relocation of the needle.

A single injection is usually adequate for multiple exposures. Contrast is good during the first 10 minutes after injection, adequate at 10 to 15 minutes, and begins to fade at 15 to 25 minutes.

The following approximate volumes have been used in normal adult joints:

Knee, shoulder, hip: 5 ml to 15 ml

Temporomandibular: 0.5 ml

Other: 1 ml to 4 ml

"Double contrast arthrography," using a mixture of the medium and air or a dilution of Diatrizoate Meglumine, has been employed.

DISCOGRAPHY

Indications: Cervical discography is a more hazardous procedure than lumbar discography, and the interpretation of the cervical discograms is more difficult.

The injected medium gradually diffuses throughout the disc and is absorbed rapidly. In a normal disc, good contrast is evident for 10 to 15 minutes. In a ruptured disc, the medium is absorbed more rapidly. Aspiration of the medium on completion of discography is considered unnecessary.

Contraindication: Discography is contraindicated when there is infection or open injury near the region to be examined.

Warning: Inadvertent subarachnoid injection must be avoided since even the small dose of the medium used in discography might result in convulsions and death. The onset of signs of pain, cramps, or convulsions (requiring anesthesia) may occur within minutes to an hour.

Precautions: A strict, aseptic technique is required to avoid introducing infection. The examination should be postponed if local or systemic infection is present. In cervical discography, care should be taken to avoid contamination of the disc by inadvertent puncture of the esophagus. Laceration of the disc by use of a needle that has become barbed by forceful impingement on a vertebra, should be avoided. The patient should be cautioned not to move during introduction of the needle.

Adverse Reactions: In the normal disc, only minor discomfort will occur during injection. More discomfort will result if excessive pressure or volume is used. Pain is unusual and may indicate extravasation.

In the damaged disc, however, the injection can cause pain, sometimes severe which mimics the symptoms. Transient backache or headache, as in lumbar puncture, often occurs. Extravasation from the disc into the lateral recesses and extradurally into the spinal canal or local soft tissue does not usually cause adverse effects.

During discography extreme care is advised to avoid inadvertent intrathecal injection since the injection of even small amounts of the contrast medium may cause convulsions, permanent sequelae, or fatality. Should the accident occur, the patient should be placed upright to confine the hyperbaric solution to a low level, anesthesia may be required to control convulsions, and if there is evidence of a large dose having been administered, a careful cerebrospinal fluid exchange-washout should be considered.

Dosage and Administration: Discography is usually performed with parenteral analgesia or sedation, and under local anesthesia. To minimize disc and tissue trauma, a two-needle technique is usually employed. An 18 to 20 gauge needle is used to penetrate to the disc and then a very fine (25 or 26 gauge) lumbar puncture-type needle is inserted through the needle to penetrate the disc.

Because of the resistance encountered, it is difficult to inject more than 0.2 ml to 0.3 ml of Diatrizoate Meglumine into a normal disc. Occasionally, however, a cervical disc can accept up to 0.5 ml and a lumbar disc, 1 ml (rarely, 2 ml) before resistance is encountered. Mild discomfort with little or no frank pain may indicate a normal disc.

In ruptured and some abnormal discs, 1 ml to 2 ml or more can be introduced without resistance; and, particularly if only one disc has pathology, the patient usually experiences pain, sometimes severe, with distribution characteristic of his symptoms. To minimize the amount of Diatrizoate Meglumine extravasated, no more than 2 ml is injected in any one disc.

The procedure should be planned so that the duration of the discogram allows multiple exposures with a single dose. It has been recommended that for diagnostic reasons that the procedure (injection and discogram) be performed on one disc at a time. Injection of a number of discs under suspicion, however, may be performed as part of one procedure.

CONTRAST ENHANCEMENT OF COMPUTED TOMOGRAPHIC HEAD IMAGING

Precautions: Metastatic Brain Lesions: Large doses of contrast media should be avoided in patients with suspected metastatic brain lesions. Intravenous administration of large doses to these patients is more likely to result in convulsions; however, these occurrences are rare. This has been attributed to tissue accumulation of the medium in the presence of blood brain barrier disruption caused by disease. Appropriate measures for seizure management should be immediately available.

Convulsion. (See *"Precautions—General".*)

Dosage and Administration: Bolus intravenous injection of 50 ml to 100 ml, or up to 150 ml by infusion. The rate of injection and the timing of scans will depend principally on the expected nature of the pathology. Dosage in children is proportional to adults, based on weight.

RETROGRADE CYSTOURETHROGRAPHY

After the bladder is emptied, Diatrizoate Meglumine is gently instilled without force, often beyond the first desire to micturate, but not beyond the point of urgency or mild discomfort. The volume required to fill the bladder to slightly less than capacity may vary from patient to patient.

Bladder capacity in normal adults is generally 200 ml to 300 ml, and rarely, up to 600 ml. Capacity at birth is 20 ml to 50 ml, and increases about 400% in the first year. In children 3 to 5 years old, bladder capacity is 150 ml to 180 ml. In children older than 8 years, it is in the low adult range.

In disease, bladder capacity in adults may vary from 50 ml in a hypertonic reflex bladder to over 1000 ml in an atonic or sensory paralytic bladder or chronic lower urinary tract obstruction.

Repeat examination may be required to detect reflux, or in function studies.

The concentration varies with technique and equipment used. Diatrizoate Meglumine may be diluted with sterile water or 5% dextrose solution, as indicated in the following tables. A 10% solution is isotonic.

250 ML OF DIATRIZOATE MEGLUMINE

	To Make		Add	Final Solution Contains
Final conc.	Final volume		Sterile water or 5% dextrose solution	Iodine
30%	250 ml		—	141 mg/ml
25%	300 ml		50 ml	118 mg/ml
21.4%	350 ml		100 ml	101 mg/ml
20%	375 ml		125 ml	94 mg/ml
18.8%	400 ml		150 ml	88 mg/ml
16.7%	450 ml		200 ml	78 mg/ml
15%	500 ml		250 ml	71 mg/ml

100 ML OF DIATRIZOATE MEGLUMINE (PEDIATRIC)

	To Make		Add	Final Solution Contains
Final conc.	Final volume		Sterile water or 5% dextrose solution	Iodine
30%	100 ml		—	141 mg/ml
24%	125 ml		25 ml	113 mg/ml
20%	150 ml		50 ml	94 mg/ml
15%	200 ml		100 ml	71 mg/ml
12%	250 ml		150 ml	56 mg/ml
10%	300 ml		200 ml	47 mg/ml

Dilution and withdrawal of the contrast agents should be accomplished under aseptic conditions with sterile syringes. The solution should be inspected visually for particulate matter and discoloration prior to administration.

STORAGE
Protect from strong light.

HOW SUPPLIED
INJECTION:

BRAND/MANUFACTURER	NDC	SIZE	AWP
◆ **BRAND**			
RENO-M-30: Bracco Diag	00003-0804-50	100 ml 25s	$450.63

INJECTION: 18%

BRAND/MANUFACTURER	NDC	SIZE	AWP
○ **BRAND**			
CYSTOGRAFIN-DILUTE: Bracco Diag	00003-1410-40	500 ml 6s	$196.85
	00003-1410-45	500 ml 6s	$214.99
	00003-1410-30	300 ml 10s	$243.71
	00003-1410-35	300 ml 10s	$273.01

INJECTION: 30%

AVERAGE UNIT PRICE (AVAILABLE SIZES)			
BRAND	$0.13		

BRAND/MANUFACTURER	NDC	SIZE	AWP
◆ **BRAND**			
CYSTOGRAFIN: Bracco Diag	00003-0149-55	300 ml 6s	$250.19
HYPAQUE MEGLUMINE: Sanofi Winthrop	00024-0740-20	100 ml 10s	$55.22
CYSTOGRAFIN: Bracco Diag	00003-0149-60	100 ml 10s	$231.61
HYPAQUE MEGLUMINE: Sanofi Winthrop	00024-0739-10	300 ml 10s	$174.41
RENO-M-DIP: Bracco Diag	00003-0809-75	300 ml 10s	$348.61
	00003-0809-76	300 ml 10s	$375.85
RENO-M-30: Bracco Diag	00003-0804-45	50 ml 25s	$251.40

INJECTION: 30%

BRAND/MANUFACTURER	NDC	SIZE	AWP
○ **BRAND**			
HYPAQUE-CYSTO: Sanofi Winthrop	00024-0735-10	300 ml 10s	$130.68
	00024-0734-10	500 ml 10s	$157.42

INJECTION: 60%

AVERAGE UNIT PRICE (AVAILABLE SIZES)			
BRAND	$0.21		

BRAND/MANUFACTURER	NDC	SIZE	AWP
◆ **BRAND**			
RENO-M-60: Bracco Diag	00003-0696-17	10 ml 10s	$50.71
HYPAQUE MEGLUMINE: Sanofi Winthrop	00024-0747-02	100 ml 10s	$120.36
RENO-M-60: Bracco Diag	00003-0696-55	100 ml 10s	$230.44
	00003-0696-65	150 ml 10s	$298.03
	00003-0696-70	150 ml 10s	$319.31
HYPAQUE MEGLUMINE: Sanofi Winthrop	00024-0749-20	200 ml 10s	$193.47
	00024-0750-10	200 ml 10s	$252.13
	00024-0744-04	20 ml 25s	$79.33
RENO-M-60: Bracco Diag	00003-0696-25	30 ml 25s	$191.95
HYPAQUE MEGLUMINE: Sanofi Winthrop	00024-0746-04	50 ml 25s	$151.40
RENO-M-60: Bracco Diag	00003-0696-50	50 ml 25s	$288.05
	00003-0696-60	100 ml 25s	$576.11

Diatrizoate Meglumine and Iodipamide Meglumine

DESCRIPTION
Diatrizoate Meglumine/Iodipamide Meglumine Injection is a sterile, nonpyrogenic, essentially colorless to pale yellow, aqueous radiopaque contrast medium for intrauterine instillation. Each mL provides 527 mg Diatrizoate Meglumine and 268 mg Iodipamide Meglumine.

Each mL contains approximately 380 mg organically bound iodine.

Diatrizoate Meglumine is designated chemically as 1-deoxy-1-(methylamino)-D-glucitol 3,5-diacetamido-2,4,6-triiodobenzoate (salt); Iodipamide Meglumine is 1-deoxy-1-(methylamino)-D-glucitol 3,3'-(adipoyldiimino)bis[2,4,6-triiodobenzoate] (2:1) (salt).

The molecular formula of Diatrizoate Meglumine is $C_{11}H_9I_3N_2O_4 \cdot C_7H_{17}NO_5$ its molecular weight is 809.13, originally bound iodine is 47.1% and its CAS number is 131-49-7.

The molecular formula of Iodipamide Meglumine is $C_{20}H_{14}I_6N_2O_6 \cdot 2C_7H_{17}NO_5$, its molecular weight is 1530.20, organically bound iodine is 49.8%, and its CAS number is 3521-84-4.

CLINICAL PHARMACOLOGY
The most important characteristic of contrast media is the iodine content. The relatively high atomic weight of iodine contributes sufficient radiodensity for radiographic contrast of the uterus and uterine tubes with surrounding tissues.

Diagnostic intrauterine radiopaque agents have few known pharmacological effects. Most of the medium within the uterine cavity is discharged immediately upon termination of the procedure. Any medium retained in the uterine cavity is completely absorbed within one hour, unless there is an obstruction and large hydrosalpinx, in which case absorption is generally complete within 24 hours. Any medium spilled into the peritoneal cavity is absorbed within 20 to 60 minutes and excreted by both the hepatic and renal systems.

INDICATIONS AND USAGE
Diatrizoate Meglumine/Iodipamide Maglumine Injection is indicated for use in hysterosalpingography.

CONTRAINDICATIONS
Hysterosalpingographic agents are contraindicated in pregnant women and those suspected of being pregnant. Hysterosalpingography should not be performed during the menstrual period or when infection of the external genitalia or genital tract is present. The procedure should not be attempted within 30 days following curettage or conization or within six months following the termination of pregnancy.

PRECAUTIONS
GENERAL
Diagnostic procedures which involve the use of radiopaque diagnostic agents should be carried out under the direction of personnel with the prerequisite training and with a thorough knowledge of the particular procedure to be performed.

In patients having or suspected of having carcinoma of the uterus and/or uterine tubes, the possible dispersion of carcinogenic cells during hysterosalpingography should be borne in mind.

The possibility of a reaction should always be considered. Patients at increased risk include those with a history of a previous reaction to a contrast medium, patients with a known sensitivity to iodine *per se*, and patients with a known clinical hypersensitivity: bronchial asthma, hay fever, and food allergies. A positive history of allergies or hypersensitivity does not arbitrarily contraindicate the use of a contrast agent where a diagnostic procedure is thought essential, but caution should be exercised (see *"Adverse Reactions"*, and *"Precautions, Information for the Patient"*).

INFORMATION FOR THE PATIENT
Patients receiving diagnostic agents for intrauterine radiography should be given the following information:

1. This drug has been prescribed to perform an x-ray study of the uterus and uterine tubes
2. Patients should be questioned regarding a recent history (within 30 days) of curettage or conization, pregnancy or a recent history (within six months) of termination of pregnancy, and a history of allergy to iodine, any foods, or x-ray dyes.
3. Patients should consult the physician if, at some future date, any thyroid tests are planned. The iodine in this agent may interfere with some thyroid tests.
4. This drug may cause adverse reactions (see *"Adverse Reactions"*) in some patients, but most reactions are mild and pass quickly.

DRUG/LABORATORY TEST INTERACTIONS
Thyroid Function Tests: Because a small amount of this medium may be absorbed, thyroid function tests such as protein bound iodine (PBI) and radioactive iodine uptake, if indicated, generally should be performed prior to instillation. However, thyroid function can be evaluated after use of any iodinated contrast agents by using T_3 resin uptake or free thyroxine assays.

PREGNANCY
See *"Contraindications"*.

NURSING MOTHERS
Diatrizoate Meglumine/Iodipamide Meglumine administered intravascularly has been found to be excreted in breast milk.

Because small amounts of these agents may be absorbed following intrauterine instillation, caution should be exercised when any diagnostic intrauterine radiopaque agent is administered to a nursing woman.

PEDIATRIC USE
Safety and effectiveness of hysterosalpingography has not been established in pediatric patients.

ADVERSE REACTIONS
Hypersensitivity reactions, which include sweating, flushing, pruritus, urticaria, skin rashes, arthralgia, respiratory distress, and circulatory collapse have occurred. Chills, fever, nausea, vomiting, and abdominal pain and tenderness are occasionally seen following instillation of the contrast medium.

It should be kept in mind that the serious or anaphylactoid reactions that may occur with intravascular administration of radiopaque contrast agents are theoretically possible following administration by other routes.

◆ RATED THERAPEUTICALLY EQUIVALENT; ◇ THERAPEUTIC EQUIVALENCE UNCONFIRMED; ○ UNRATED

DOSAGE AND ADMINISTRATION

As a convenience to the physician, the following guidelines which have proven satisfactory are provided (see *"Precautions, General"*). Patients should be counseled prior to radiographic examination (see *"Precautions, Information for the Patient"*).

Preparation of the Patient: Hysterosalpingography should be performed three to five days after the cessation of the patient's menstrual period as a precautionary measure. An enema and vaginal douche one hour before the examination are helpful, but not essential. The patient should empty her bladder before the examination. Since the procedure is remarkably free of pain when Diatrizoate Meglumine/Iodipamide Meglumine Injection is used, the use of a narcotic or anesthesia is unnecessary.

Dosage: 3 to 4 mL of Diatrizoate Meglumine/Iodipamide Meglumine, administered in fractional doses of approximately 1 mL, are usually adequate to visualize the uterus; an additional 3 to 4 mL will demonstrate the tubes. Total doses varying from 1.5 to 10 mL have been employed with satisfactory results.

Administration: The patient is placed in the lithotomy position and the vulva is cleansed with a suitable antiseptic solution. A Graves-type vaginal speculum is introduced, the cervix is exposed, and the vaginal vault is sponged with antiseptic solution.

A tenaculum is placed on the cervical lip, usually the anterior lip. A sterile sound may be passed to determine the position of the uterus and the direction of the cervical canal, and, when necessary, the cervical canal may be dilated. (Sounding the uterine cavity and dilatation of the canal are not usually required when a flexible cannula tip is used.)

A sterile syringe containing the Diatrizoate Meglumine/Iodipamide Meglumine Injection is attached by Luer-Lok to a uterine cannula. The two-way cannula valve is opened and all air bubbles in the cannula and syringe are expressed. About 1.5 to 2 mL of Diatrizoate Meglumine/Iodipamide Meglumine Injection are required to fill the cannula. (If preferred, a tubal insufflator under controlled pressure with a salpingogram attachment may be used instead of the syringe.)

The cannula tip is inserted into the cervical canal so that the adjustable rubber acorn obturator fits snugly at the external os. Careful placement of the cannula is important to avoid trauma and pain. Squeezing the trigger of the cannula to provide simultaneous traction on the tenaculum and forward pressure on the cannula should give a nonleaking cervical seal. Diatrizoate Meglumine/Iodipamide Meglumine Injection flows freely so that only gentle pressure on the plunger is necessary; however, the medium should be used as promptly as possible following withdrawal into the syringe. The syringe should be rinsed as soon after the procedure as possible to prevent freezing of the plunger.

The connection at the external os is checked for leakage. If the acorn obturator is inadequate, an inflatable balloon-obturator may be used to seal the cervical canal. When the equipment has been positioned satisfactorily, the tenaculum and cannula may be fixed in position until the procedure is terminated.

Radiography: A scout film may be made before the medium is administered. After the initial fractional injection, a film should be made using a Bucky diaphragm. After each successive injection of 1 mL, a film is taken, developed immediately, and inspected in the dark room before the next fractional dose of Diatrizoate Meglumine/Iodipamide Meglumine Injection is given, until the procedure is completed. Further injection and subsequent films can be made as required using posterior-anterior or oblique angles.

Clinical experience indicates that tubal patency, if present, will be demonstrable at the time of the injection and delayed films have not been required.

GENERAL

Diatrizoate Meglumine/Iodipamide Meglumine Injection should be inspected visually for particulate matter and discoloration prior to instillation whenever solution and container permit. The solution may vary in color from essentially colorless to pale yellow. Solutions which may have become substantially darker should not be used.

In the event that crystallization occurs, the solution may be clarified by placing the vial in hot water and shaking gently for several minutes or until the solution is clear. If cloudiness persists, the preparation should not be used. Allow the solution to cool to body temperature before administering.

STORAGE

Store at room temperature (20°-25°C). Protect from light.

HOW SUPPLIED
INJECTION: 52.7%-26.8%

BRAND/MANUFACTURER	NDC	SIZE	AWP
○ **BRAND**			
SINOGRAFIN: Bracco Diag	00003-0523-30	10 ml 10s	$361.16

Diatrizoate Sodium

DESCRIPTION

Diatrizoate Sodium is a radiopaque diagnostic agent, water-soluble organic iodide contrast medium. In pure form, it contains 59.87% organically bound iodine.

The 25% solution (w/v) contains 150 mg iodine per mL and 0.4 mEq (9.05 mg) sodium per mL. It has an osmolality of 696 mosm/kg (determined by VPO), at 25°C and is, therefore, hypertonic to blood. The viscosity (cp) is about 1.59 at 25°C and 1.19 at 37°C. The pKa is 3.4 for diatrizoic acid. The sterile aqueous solution is clear, colorless to pale yellow. It is relatively thermostable and may be autoclaved once.

Diatrizoate Sodium is a triiodinated benzoic acid derivative, the sodium salt of 3,5-diacetamido-2,4,6-triiodobenzoate. Its molecular weight is 635.90.

Following is its chemical structure:

CLINICAL PHARMACOLOGY
DISTRIBUTION

Intravascular injection of a radiopaque diagnostic agent opacifies those vessels in the path of the flow of the contrast medium, permitting radiographic visualization of the internal structures of the human body until significant hemodilution occurs. During use of Diatrizoate Sodium for infusion urography high serum levels of Diatrizoate Sodium are achieved and maintained.

At physiologic pH, the water-soluble contrast media are completely dissociated into a radiopaque anion and a solubilizing cation.

Following intravenous injection, Diatrizoate Sodium is immediately diluted in the circulating plasma. Equilibrium is reached with the extracellular compartment at about 10 minutes. Hence, the plasma concentration at 10 minutes is closely related to the dose corrected to body size.

The pharmacokinetics of the intravenously administered radiopaque contrast media are usually best described by a two compartment model with a rapid alpha phase for drug distribution and a slow beta phase for drug elimination. In patients with normal renal function, the alpha and beta half-lives were respectively 30 and 120 minutes for Diatrizoate Sodium. However, in patients with renal functional impairment, the elimination half-life for the beta phase can be prolonged up to several days.

EXCRETION

Diatrizoate Sodium is not metabolized but excreted unchanged in the urine, each Diatrizoate molecule remaining "obligated" to its sodium moiety. Excretion is accompanied by a dose-related osmotic diuresis which is less with the sodium than with the meglumine salt. Fluid deprivation may increase urinary iodine concentration; however, fluid restriction is usually not considered necessary with the higher dose infusion technique.

Diatrizoate solutions may be excreted either through the kidneys or the liver. These two excretory pathways are not mutually exclusive, but the main route of excretion seems to be governed by the affinity of the contrast medium for serum albumin. From 0% to 10% of Diatrizoate Sodium is bound to serum protein.

Diatrizoate salts are excreted predominantly unchanged through the kidneys by glomerular filtration. The amount excreted during any period of time is determined by the filtered load; ie, the product of plasma contrast media concentration and glomerular filtration rate. The plasma concentration is dependent upon the dose administered and the body size. The glomerular filtration rate varies with the body size, sex, age, circulatory dynamics, diuretic effect of the drug, and renal function. In patients with normal renal function the maximum urinary concentration of Diatrizoate Sodium occurs within 10 minutes with 12% of the administered dose being excreted. The mean values of cumulative urinary excretion for Diatrizoate Sodium expressed as percentage of administered doses are 38% at 60 minutes, 45% at 3 hours, and 94% to 100% at 24 hours.

Urinary excretion of contrast media is delayed in infants younger than 1 month and in patients with urinary tract obstruction. The urinary iodine concentration is higher with the sodium salt of diatrizoic acid than with the meglumine salt.

The liver and small intestine provide the major alternate route of excretion for Diatrizoate. In patients free of severe renal disease, the fecal recovery is less than 2% of the administered dose. In patients with severe renal impairment the excretion of these contrast media through the gallbladder and into the small intestine sharply increases; up to 20% of the administered dose has been recovered in the feces in 48 hours.

Saliva is a minor secretory pathway for injectable radiopaque diagnostic agents. In patients with normal renal function, minimal amounts of contrast media are secreted unchanged. However, in uremic patients small amounts of free iodides resulting from deiodination prior to administration or *in vivo*, have been detected in the saliva.

PREGNANCY AND LACTATION

Injectable radiopaque diagnostic agents cross the human placental barrier by simple diffusion and appear to enter fetal tissues passively. No apparent harm to the fetus was observed when Diatrizoate Sodium and Diatrizoate meglumine were injected intravenously 24 hours prior to delivery. However, abnormal neonatal opacification of the small intestine and colon were detected 4 to 6 days after delivery. Procedures including radiation involve a certain risk related to the exposure of the fetus.

Diatrizoate solutions are excreted unchanged in human milk.

CT ENHANCEMENT

Intravenous injection of Diatrizoate Sodium results in increased brain tissue contrast differentials. Initially, this may represent increased local vascular density. Later, however, in certain brain lesions which disrupt the function of the blood-brain barrier, tissue contrast distribution represents accumulated extravascular penetration of the medium.

INDICATIONS AND USAGE

UROGRAPHY

Diatrizoate salts are used in small, medium, and large dose urography (see *"Dosage and Administration"*). Visualization of the urinary tract can be achieved by either direct intravenous bolus injection or intravenous drip infusion. Visualization of the urinary tract is delayed in infants less than 1 month old, and in patients with urinary tract obstruction (see *"Clinical Pharmacology"*).

CONTRAST ENHANCEMENT OF COMPUTED TOMOGRAPHIC HEAD IMAGING

Injectable radiopaque contrast media may be used to refine diagnostic precision in areas of the brain which may not otherwise have been satisfactorily visualized.

Tumors: Radiopaque diagnostic agents may be useful to investigate the presence and extent of certain malignancies such as: gliomas including malignant gliomas, glioblastomas, astrocytomas, oligodendrogliomas and gangliomas, ependymomas, medulloblastomas, meningiomas, neuromas, pinealomas, pituitary adenomas, craniopharyngiomas, germinomas, and metastatic lesions.

The usefulness of contrast enhancement for the investigation of the retrobulbar space and in cases of low grade or infiltrative glioma has not been demonstrated.

In calcified lesions or cysts, there is less likelihood of enhancement. Following therapy, tumors may show decreased or no enhancement.

The opacification of the inferior vermis following contrast media administration has resulted in false-positive diagnosis in a number of normal studies.

Nonneoplastic Conditions: The use of injectable radiopaque diagnostic agents may be beneficial in the image enhancement of nonneoplastic lesions. Cerebral infarctions of recent onset may be better visualized with contrast enhancement in about 60% of cerebral infarctions studied from one to four weeks from the onset of symptoms.

Sites of active infection may also be enhanced following contrast media administration.

Arteriovenous malformations and aneurysms will show contrast enhancement. For these vascular lesions, the enhancement is probably dependent on the iodine content of the circulating blood pool.

Hematomas and intraparenchymal bleeders seldom demonstrate any contrast enhancement. However, in cases of intraparenchymal clot, for which there is no obvious clinical explanation, contrast media administration may be helpful in ruling out the possibility of associated arteriovenous malformation.

CONTRAINDICATIONS

Diatrizoate Sodium has no absolute contraindications in its recommended use (see *"Warnings"* and *"Precautions"*).

WARNINGS

Ionic iodinated contrast media inhibit blood coagulation, *in vitro*, more than nonionic contrast media. Nonetheless, it is prudent to avoid prolonged contact of blood with syringes containing ionic contrast media.

Serious, rarely fatal, thromboembolic events causing myocardial infarction and stroke have been reported during angiographic procedures with both ionic and nonionic contrast media. Therefore, meticulous intravascular administration technique is necessary, particularly during angiographic procedures, to minimize thromboembolic events. Numerous factors, including length of procedure, catheter and syringe material, underlying disease state and concomitant medications may contribute to the development of thromboembolic events. For these reasons, meticulous angiographic techniques are recommended including close attention to guidewire and catheter manipulation, use of manifold systems and/or three-way stopcocks, frequent catheter flushing with heparinized saline solutions and minimizing the length of the procedure. The use of plastic syringes in place of glass syringes has been reported to decrease but not eliminate the likelihood of *in vitro* clotting.

MYELOMATOSIS

Excretory urography is potentially hazardous in patients with multiple myeloma. In some of those patients, therapeutically resistant anuria resulting in progressive uremia, renal failure and eventually death has followed this procedure. Although neither the contrast agent nor dehydration has been proved separately to be the cause of anuria in myelomatous patients, it has been speculated that the combination of both may be causative. The risk of excretory urography in myelomatous patients is not a contraindication to the procedure; however, they require special precautions. Partial dehydration in the preparation of these patients for the examination is not recommended since this may predispose to the precipitation of myeloma protein in the renal tubules. Myeloma, which occurs most commonly in persons over age 40, should be considered before instituting urographic procedures.

SICKLE CELL

Contrast media may promote sickling in individuals who are homozygous for sickle cell disease when the material is injected intravenously or intra-arterially.

PHEOCHROMOCYTOMA

Administration of radiopaque materials to patients known or suspected of having pheochromocytoma should be performed with extreme caution. If, in the opinion of the physician, the possible benefits of such procedures outweigh the considered risks, the procedures may be performed; however, the amount of radiopaque medium injected should be kept to an absolute minimum. The blood pressure should be assessed throughout the procedure and measures for treatment of a hypertensive crisis should be available.

HYPERTHYROIDISM

Recent reports of thyroid storm occurring following the intravascular use of iodinated radiopaque diagnostic agents in patients with hyperthyroidism or with an autonomously functioning thyroid nodule suggest that this additional risk be evaluated in such patients before use of Diatrizoate Sodium.

RENAL AND HEPATIC DISEASE

Urography should be performed with caution in patients with severely impaired renal function and patients with combined renal and hepatic disease.

SUBARACHNOID HEMORRHAGE

In patients with subarachnoid hemorrhage, a rare association between contrast administration and clinical deterioration, including convulsions and death, has been reported. Therefore, administration of intravascular iodinated ionic contrast media in these patients should be undertaken with caution.

PRECAUTIONS

GENERAL

Diagnostic procedures which involve the use of radiopaque diagnostic agents should be carried out under the direction of personnel with the prerequisite training and with a thorough knowledge of the particular procedure to be performed. Appropriate facilities should be available for the management of any complication of the procedure, as well as for emergency treatment of severe reactions to the contrast agent itself. Competent personnel and emergency facilities should be available for at least 30 to 60 minutes since severe delayed reactions have occurred (see *"Adverse Reactions"*).

The possibility of a reaction, including serious, life-threatening, fatal, anaphylactic or cardiovascular reactions should always be considered (see *"Adverse Reactions"*). It is of utmost importance that a course of action be carefully planned in advance for immediate treatment of serious reactions, and that adequate and appropriate personnel be readily available in case of any reaction.

ALLERGIC HISTORY

Before injecting a contrast medium, the patient should be questioned for a history of allergy. A positive history does not arbitrarily contraindicate the use of a contrast agent where a diagnostic procedure is considered essential, but caution should be exercised (see *"Adverse Reactions"*).

The possibility of an idiosyncratic reaction in susceptible patients should always be considered (see *"Adverse Reactions"*). The susceptible population includes patients with a history of a previous reaction to a contrast media, patients with a known sensitivity to iodine per se, and patients with known clinical hypersensitivity (ie, bronchial asthma, hay fever, and food allergies).

Premedication with antihistamines or corticosteroids to avoid or minimize possible allergic reactions in such patients should be considered. Recent reports indicate that such pretreatment does not prevent serious life-threatening reactions, but may reduce both their incidence and severity.

TEST DOSE

The occurrence of severe idiosyncratic reactions has prompted the use of several pretesting methods. However, pretesting cannot be relied upon to predict severe reactions and may itself be hazardous for the patient. It is suggested that a thorough medical history with emphasis on allergy and hypersensitivity, prior to the injection of any contrast media, may be more accurate than pretesting in predicting potential adverse reactions.

PREPARATORY DEHYDRATION

Preparatory dehydration is dangerous and may contribute to acute renal failure in infants, young children, the elderly, patients with preexisting renal insufficiency, patients with advanced vascular disease especially in diabetic patients. Dehydration in these patients seems to be enhanced by the osmotic diuretic action of urographic agents. Routine overnight fluid restriction may be undesirable and is considered unnecessary when using the relatively large dose infusion urography technique. In CT enhancement studies, fluid restriction is unnecessary and undesirable.

DIABETES AND NEPHROPATHIES

Acute renal failure has been reported in diabetic patients with diabetic nephropathy and in susceptible nondiabetic patients (often elderly with preexisting renal disease) following excretory urography. Therefore, careful consideration of the potential risks should be given before performing this radiographic procedure in these patients.

RENAL TRANSPLANT

Immediately following surgery, excretory urography should be used with caution in renal transplant recipients.

EFFECTS OF OSMOTIC LOAD

Immediate adverse reactions to infusion urography have not been reported to occur at a higher frequency or greater severity than with routine excretory urography. However, sequelae of this procedure are possible some hours after the examination. The infusion imposes not only a sudden osmotic load, but may also present as much as 160 mEq of sodium (3.7 g) to patients with established, decreased glomerular filtration and renal tubular damage. In addition, these patients may also have coexisting or associated cardiovascular disease. Therefore, the possibility of the development of congestive heart failure hours after the procedure should be considered. Such patients should be observed for several hours following the procedure to detect delayed hemodynamic disturbances.

◆ RATED THERAPEUTICALLY EQUIVALENT; ◇ THERAPEUTIC EQUIVALENCE UNCONFIRMED; ○ UNRATED

Seizure activity is rare (about 0.01%) on intravenous injection of ionic contrast media. However, in the higher doses used for CT in patients with brain metastases the incidence can be much higher (1% to 10%). In these patients prophylactic use of a small parenteral dose of diazepam is suggested immediately before injection when extra high dose CT regimens are employed.

INFORMATION FOR PATIENTS
Patients receiving injectable radiopaque diagnostic agents should be instructed to:
1. Inform the physician if they are pregnant (see "Clinical Pharmacology").
2. Inform the physician if they are diabetic or if they have multiple myeloma, pheochromocytoma, homozygous sickle cell disease or known thyroid disorder (see "Warnings").
3. Inform the physician if they are allergic to any drugs, food, or if they have had any reactions to previous injections of dyes used for x-ray procedures (see "Precautions").
4. Inform the physician about any other medications they are currently taking, including nonprescription drugs, before they are administered this drug.

DRUG INTERACTIONS
Renal toxicity has been reported in a few patients with liver dysfunction who were given oral cholecystographic agents followed by urographic agents. Administration of intravascular urographic agents should therefore be postponed in any patient with a known or suspected hepatic or biliary disorder who has recently received a cholecystographic contrast agent.

Diphenhydramine hydrochloride may cause precipitation when mixed in the same syringe with Diatrizoate Sodium.

Under certain circumstances (pH, temperature, concentrations, time), Diatrizoate solutions are incompatible with promethazine hydrochloride, diphenhydramine hydrochloride, brompheniramine maleate, or papaverine hydrochloride solutions.

DRUG/LABORATORY TEST INTERACTIONS
If any of these studies, which might be affected by contrast media, are indicated, it is recommended that they be performed prior to administration of the contrast medium or two or more days afterwards.

Diatrizoate salts interfere with several laboratory urine and blood tests.

Blood Tests:

Coagulation: Diatrizoate salts significantly inhibit all stages of coagulation. The fibrinogen concentration, Factors V, VII, and VIII are decreased. Prothrombin time and thromboplastin time are increased.

Platelet Aggregation: High levels of plasma Diatrizoates inhibit platelet aggregation.

Serum Calcium: Diatrizoate salts may decrease serum calcium levels. However, this depletion of serum calcium may also be the result of the addition of chelating agents (edetate disodium) in the preparation of certain contrast media.

Red Cell Counts: Transitory decreases in red cell counts. Technetium-99m-RBC labeling interference.

Leukocyte Counts: Decrease following injection.

Urea Nitrogen (BUN): Transitory increase (see "Clinical Pharmacology").

Serum Creatinine: Transitory increase.

Urine Tests: Urine osmolality and specific gravity. Decreased due to induced diuresis.
Urine cultures. Diatrizoate in urine cultures may inhibit bacterial growth.

Thyroid Function Tests: Protein-bound Iodine (PBI) and Total Serum Organic Iodine: Transient increase of both tests following urography have been noticed. The results of PBI and radioactive iodine uptake studies which depend on iodine estimations will not accurately reflect thyroid function for up to 16 days following administration of iodinated urographic media. However, thyroid function tests not depending on iodine estimations, eg, T_3 resin uptake or free thyroxine assays are not affected.

CARCINOGENESIS, MUTAGENESIS, IMPAIRMENT OF FERTILITY
Long-term studies in animals have not been performed in order to evaluate carcinogenic potential, mutagenesis, or whether Diatrizoate Sodium can affect fertility in males or females.

PREGNANCY CATEGORY C
Animal reproduction studies have not been conducted with Diatrizoate Sodium. It is also not known whether Diatrizoate Sodium can cause fetal harm when administered to a pregnant woman or can affect reproduction capacity. Diatrizoate Sodium should be given to a pregnant woman only if clearly needed.

LABOR AND DELIVERY
It is not known whether use of these contrast agents during labor or delivery has immediate or delayed adverse effects on the fetus, prolongs the duration of labor or increases the likelihood that forceps delivery or other obstetrical intervention or resuscitation of the newborn will be necessary.

NURSING MOTHERS
Diatrizoate salts are excreted unchanged in human milk. Because of the potential adverse reactions, although it has not been established that serious adverse reactions occur in nursing infants, caution should be exercised when these intravascular contrast media are administered to a nursing woman.

PEDIATRIC USE
Infants and small children should not have fluid restriction prior to injection. Full hydration should be assured. (See "Precautions".)

ADVERSE REACTIONS
Approximately 95% of adverse reactions accompanying the intravascular use of Diatrizoate salts are of mild to moderate severity. However, life-threatening reactions and fatalities, mostly of cardiovascular origin, have occurred.

Adverse reactions to injectable contrast media fall into two categories: chemotoxic reactions and idiosyncratic reactions.

Chemotoxic reactions result from the physicochemical properties of the contrast media, the dose, and the speed of injection. All hemodynamic disturbances and injuries to organs or vessels perfused by the contrast medium are included in this category.

Idiosyncratic reactions include all other reactions. They occur more frequently in patients 20 to 40 years old. Idiosyncratic reactions may or may not be dependent on the amount of dose injected, the speed of injection, the mode of injection, and the radiographic procedure. Idiosyncratic reactions are subdivided into minor, intermediate, and severe. The minor reactions are self-limited and of short duration; the severe reactions are life-threatening and treatment is urgent and mandatory.

The reported incidence of adverse reactions to contrast media in patients with a history of allergy are twice that of the general population. Patients with a history of previous reactions to a contrast medium are three times more susceptible than other patients. However, sensitivity to contrast media does not appear to increase with repeated examinations.

Most adverse reactions to injectable contrast media appear within one to three minutes after the start of injection, but delayed reactions may occur.

Adverse reactions are grouped by organ system and listed below by decreasing order of occurrence and with an approximate incidence of occurrence. Significantly more severe reactions are listed before the other reactions regardless of frequency.

GREATER THAN 1 IN 100 PATIENTS
Body as a Whole: Reported incidences of death range from 6.6 per 1 million (0.00066%) to 1 in 10,000 patients (0.01%). Most deaths occur during injection or 5 to 10 minutes later, the main feature being cardiac arrest with cardiovascular disease as the main aggravating factor.

Isolated reports of hypotensive collapse and shock following urography are found in the literature. The incidence of shock is estimated to occur in 1 out of 20,000 (0.005%) patients.

Cardiovascular System: The most frequent adverse reaction to Diatrizoate salts is vasodilation (feeling of warmth). The estimated incidence is 49%.

Digestive System: Nausea 6%, vomiting 3%.

Nervous System: Paresthesia 6%, dizziness 5%.

Respiratory System: Rhinitis 1%, increased cough 2%.

Skin and Appendages: Urticaria 1%.

Pain at the injection site is estimated to occur in about 12% of the patients undergoing urography. Pain is usually due to extravasation.

Painful hot erythematous swelling above the venipuncture site was estimated to occur in more than 1% of the patients undergoing phlebography.

Special Senses: Perversion of taste 11%, and numbness.

Urogenital System: Osmotic nephrosis of the proximal tubular cells is estimated to occur in 23% of patients following excretory urography.

LESS THAN 1 IN 100 PATIENTS
Other infrequently reported reactions without accompanying incidence rates are listed below, grouped by organ system.

Body as a Whole: Malaria relapse, uremia, high creatinine and BUN (see "Precautions, Drug/Laboratory Test Interactions"), thrombocytopenia, leukopenia and anemia.

Cardiovascular System: Cerebral hematomas, hemodynamic disturbances, sinus bradycardia, transient electrocardiographic abnormalities, ventricular fibrillation, petechiae, chest pain, and cardiac arrest.

Digestive System: Severe unilateral or bilateral swelling of the parotid and submaxillary glands.

Nervous System: Convulsions, paralysis, coma, and agitation.

Respiratory System: Asthma, dyspnea, laryngeal edema, pulmonary edema, bronchospasm, and respiratory arrest.

Skin and Appendages: Extravasation necrosis, urticaria with or without pruritus, mucocutaneous edema, and angioneurotic edema.

Special Senses: Bilateral ocular irritation, lacrimation, itching, conjunctival chemosis, infection, and conjunctivitis.

Urogenital: Renal failure, pain.

OVERDOSAGE
At dosage levels of Diatrizoate Sodium above a level containing 45 g of iodine, the incidence of unpleasant side effects increases. At total dosage equivalent to 80 gI or 90 gI administered over a short period of time (eg, 30 minutes), clinical signs of systemic intolerance appear (mostly related to hyperosmolar effects) and are manifest as tremors, irritability, and tachycardia. Above these maximal tolerated

dosage levels in otherwise healthy adults, an increasing incidence and severity of dyspnea and pulmonary edemas should be expected.

The acute intravenous LD_{50} of Diatrizoate Sodium in mice is equivalent in iodine content of 5.3 gI/kg to 8.0 gI/kg and seem to be directly proportional to the rate of injection.

Diatrizoate Sodium is dialyzable.

DOSAGE AND ADMINISTRATION

Preparation of the patient will vary with preference of the radiologist and the type of radiological procedure performed. Specific radiographic procedures used will depend on the state of the patient and the diagnostic indications. Therefore, individual doses should be tailored according to age, conditions, body size, and indication for the examination.

Solutions of radiopaque diagnostic agents for intravascular use should be at body temperature when injected and may need to be warmed before use. In the event that crystallization occurs, the solution may be clarified by placing the vial in a water bath at 40°C to 50°C and shaking gently for two to three minutes or until the solids redissolve. If particles still persist, do not use this vial but discard it. The solution should be protected from strong light and any unused portion remaining in the container should be discarded.

Dilution and withdrawal of the contrast agents should be accomplished under aseptic conditions with sterile syringes.

Parenteral drug products should be inspected visually for particulate matter and discoloration prior to administration, whenever solution and container permit.

INFUSION UROGRAPHY

The recommended dose is calculated on the basis of 2 mL of Diatrizoate Sodium 25% per lb. of body weight. The average dose of the solution for adults is 300 mL; for optimum results, a minimum dose of 250 mL should be used. A maximum dose of 400 mL is generally sufficient for the largest of subjects.

The solution is administered intravenously through an 18-gauge needle over a period of three to ten minutes. Pyelographic films are taken at 10, 20, and 30 minutes from the beginning of the infusion. Early 2, 3, 4, and 5 minute films are obtained when indicated for the evaluation of hypertension. Nephrotomographic sections are best taken just at the end of the infusion, and voiding cystourethrograms when desired are usually made at 30 minutes.

CONTRAST ENHANCEMENT OF COMPUTED TOMOGRAPHIC HEAD IMAGING

The dose and administration will depend on the technique and equipment used. The usual dose in adults is 300 mL of Diatrizoate Sodium, infused over 10 to 20 minutes.

DRUG INCOMPATIBILITIES

Diatrizoate salts are incompatible *in vitro* with some antihistamines and many other drugs. It is believed that one of the chief causes of *in vitro* incompatibility is an alteration of pH. Turbidity of solutions of intravascular contrast medium occurs between pH 2.5 and 4.1. Another cause is chemical interaction; therefore, other pharmaceuticals should not be mixed with contrast agents in the same syringe.

STORAGE

The solution should be protected from strong light. Discard any unused portion remaining in the container.

HOW SUPPLIED
INJECTION: 20%

BRAND/MANUFACTURER	NDC	SIZE	AWP
○ BRAND			
HYPAQUE SODIUM: Sanofi Winthrop	00024-0754-10	100 ml 10s	$96.53

INJECTION: 25%

BRAND/MANUFACTURER	NDC	SIZE	AWP
○ BRAND			
HYPAQUE SODIUM: Sanofi Winthrop	00024-0758-10	300 ml 10s	$183.36

INJECTION: 50 GM/120 ML

BRAND/MANUFACTURER	NDC	SIZE	AWP
○ BRAND			
HYPAQUE SODIUM: Sanofi Winthrop	00024-0768-01	120 ml	$14.69

INJECTION: 50%

AVERAGE UNIT PRICE (AVAILABLE SIZES)	
BRAND	$0.12

BRAND/MANUFACTURER	NDC	SIZE	AWP
◆ BRAND			
HYPAQUE SODIUM: Sanofi Winthrop	00024-0770-15	200 ml 10s	$231.67
	00024-0766-04	50 ml 25s	$159.00

POWDER FOR RECONSTITUTION:

BRAND/MANUFACTURER	NDC	SIZE	AWP
○ BRAND			
HYPAQUE SODIUM: Sanofi Winthrop	00024-0769-01	250 gm	$52.02
	00024-0769-10	10 gm 10s	$27.24

Diazepam

DESCRIPTION

Diazepam is a benzodiazepine derivative. Chemically, Diazepam is 7- chloro - 1,3 - dihydro - 1 - methyl - 5 - phenyl - 2H- 1,4-benzodiazepin-2-one. It is a colorless crystalline compound, insoluble in water and has a molecular weight of 284.74.

Diazepam comes in tablets slow-release capsules, and an injectable form.

Following is its chemical structure:

PHARMACOLOGY

In animals, Diazepam appears to act on parts of the limbic system, the thalamus and hypothalamus, and induces calming effects. Diazepam, unlike chlorpromazine and reserpine, has no demonstrable peripheral autonomic blocking action, nor does it produce extrapyramidal side effects; however, animals treated with Diazepam do have a transient ataxia at higher doses. Diazepam was found to have transient cardiovascular depressor effects in dogs. Long-term experiments in rats revealed no disturbances of endocrine function. Injections into animals have produced localized irritation of tissue surrounding injection sites and some thickening of veins after intravenous use.

Oral LD_{50} of Diazepam is 720 mg/kg in mice and 1240 mg/kg in rats. Intraperitoneal administration of 400 mg/kg to a monkey resulted in death on the sixth day.

Reproduction Studies: A series of rat reproduction studies was performed with Diazepam in oral doses of 1, 10, 80 and 100 mg/kg. At 100 mg/kg there was a decrease in the number of pregnancies and surviving offspring in these rats. Neonatal survival of rats at doses lower than 100 mg/kg was within normal limits. Several neonates in these rat reproduction studies showed skeletal or other defects. Further studies in rats at doses up to and including 80 mg/kg/day did not reveal teratological effects on the offspring.

In humans, measurable blood levels of Diazepam were obtained in maternal and cord blood, indicating placental transfer of the drug.

The administration of one 15-mg Diazepam slow-release capsule results in blood levels of Diazepam over a 24-hour period which are comparable to those of 5-mg Diazepam tablets given three times daily.

The mean time to maximum plasma Diazepam concentrations after administration of 15-mg Diazepam slow-release capsules to eleven fasted subjects was 5.3 hours. The harmonic mean half-life of Diazepam was 36 hours. The range of average minimum steady-state plasma Diazepam concentrations during once daily administration of 15-mg Diazepam slow-release capsules to eleven normal subjects was 196 to 341 ng/mL.

INDICATIONS

Diazepam is indicated for the management of anxiety disorders or for the short-term relief of the symptoms of anxiety. Anxiety or tension associated with the stress of everyday life usually does not require treatment with an anxiolytic.

In acute alcohol withdrawal, Diazepam may be useful in the symptomatic relief of acute agitation, tremor, impending or acute delirium tremens and hallucinosis.

Injectable Diazepam is useful its an adjunct prior to endoscopic procedures if apprehension, anxiety or acute stress reactions are present, and to diminish the patient's recall of the procedures. (See *"Warnings".*)

Diazepam is a useful adjunct for the relief of skeletal muscle spasm due to reflex spasm to local pathology (such as inflammation of the muscles or joints, or secondary to trauma); spasticity caused by upper motor neuron disorders (such as cerebral palsy and paraplegia); athetosis; stiff-man syndrome; and tetanus.

Injectable Diazepam is a useful adjunct in status epilepticus and severe recurrent convulsive seizures. Injectable Diazepam is a useful premedication (the IM route is preferred) for relief of anxiety and tension in patients who are to undergo surgical procedures. Intravenously, prior to cardioversion for the relief of anxiety and tension and to diminish the patient's recall of the procedure.

Oral Diazepam may be used adjunctively in convulsive disorders, although it has not proved useful as the sole therapy. The effectiveness of Diazepam in long-term use, that is, more than 4 months, has not been assessed by systematic clinical studies. The physician should periodically reassess the usefulness of the drug for the individual patient.

UNLABELED USES

Diazepam is used alone or as an adjunct in the treatment of agoraphobia, chloroquine poisoning, LSD-induced flashback, Ménière's disease, panic disorder with or without agoraphobia, and tardive dyskinesia.

◆ RATED THERAPEUTICALLY EQUIVALENT; ◇ THERAPEUTIC EQUIVALENCE UNCONFIRMED; ○ UNRATED

CONTRAINDICATIONS

Diazepam is contraindicated in patients with a known hypersensitivity to this drug and, because of lack of sufficient clinical experience, in children under 6 months of age. It may be used in patients with open angle glaucoma who are receiving appropriate therapy, but is contraindicated in acute narrow angle glaucoma.

WARNINGS

Diazepam is not of value in the treatment of psychotic patients and should not be employed in lieu of appropriate treatment. As is true of most preparations containing CNS-acting drugs, patients receiving Diazepam should be cautioned against engaging in hazardous occupations requiring complete mental alertness such as operating machinery or driving a motor vehicle.

As with other agents which have anticonvulsant activity, when Diazepam is used as an adjunct in treating convulsive disorders, the possibility of an increase in the frequency and/or severity of grand mal seizures may require an increase in the dosage of standard anticonvulsant medication. Abrupt withdrawal of Diazepam in such cases may also be associated with a temporary increase in the frequency and/or severity of seizures. Tonic status epilepticus has been precipitated in patients treated with IV Diazepam for petit mal status or petit mal variant status.

Since Diazepam has a central nervous system depressant effect, patients should be advised against the simultaneous ingestion of alcohol and other CNS-depressant drugs during Diazepam therapy.

When used intravenously, the following procedures should be undertaken to reduce the possibility of venous thrombosis, phlebitis, local irritation, swelling, and rarely, vascular impairment: the solution should be injected slowly, taking at least 1 minute for each 5 mg (1 mL) given; do not use small veins, such as those on the dorsum of the hand or wrist; extreme care should be taken to avoid intra-arterial administration or extravasation.

Do not mix or dilute Diazepam with other solutions or drugs in syringe or infusion flask. If it is not feasible to administer Diazepam directly IV, it may be injected slowly through the infusion tubing as close as possible to the vein insertion.

Extreme care must be used in administering Injectable Diazepam, particularly by the IV route, to the elderly, to very ill patients and to those with limited pulmonary reserve because of the possibility that apnea and/or cardiac arrest may occur. Concomitant use of barbiturates, alcohol or other central nervous system depressants increases depression with increased risk of apnea. Resuscitative equipment including that necessary to support respiration should be readily available.

When Diazepam is used with a narcotic analgesic, the dosage of the narcotic should be reduced by at least one-third and administered in small increments. In some cases the use of a narcotic may not be necessary.

Injectable Diazepam should not be administered to patients in shock, coma or in acute alcoholic intoxication with depression of vital signs.

Usage in Pregnancy: **An increased risk of congenital malformations associated with the use of minor tranquilizers (Diazepam, meprobamate and chlordiazepoxide) during the first trimester of pregnancy has been suggested in several studies. Because use of these drugs is rarely a matter of urgency, their use during this period should almost always be avoided. The possibility that a woman of childbearing potential may be pregnant at the time of institution of therapy should be considered. Patients should be advised that if they become pregnant during therapy or intend to become pregnant they should communicate with their physicians about the desirability of discontinuing the drug.**

In humans, measurable amounts of Diazepam were found in maternal and cord blood, indicating placental transfer of the drug. Until additional information is available, injectable Diazepam is not recommended for obstetrical use.

Use in Children: Efficacy and safety of parenteral Diazepam has not been established in the neonate (30 days or less of age).

Prolonged central nervous system depression has been observed in neonates, apparently due to inability to biotransform Diazepam into inactive metabolites.

In pediatric use, in order to obtain maximal clinical effect with the minimum amount of drug and thus to reduce the risk of hazardous side effects, such as apnea or prolonged periods of somnolence, it is recommended that the drug be given slowly over a 3-minute period in a dosage not to exceed 0.26 mg/kg. After an interval of 15 to 30 minutes the initial dosage can be safely repeated. If, however, relief of symptoms is not obtained after a third administration, adjunctive therapy appropriate to the condition being treated is recommended.

Management of Overdosage: Manifestations of Diazepam overdosage include somnolence, confusion, coma and diminished reflexes. Respiration, pulse and blood pressure should be monitored, as in all cases of drug overdosage, although, in general, these effects have been minimal following overdosage. General supportive measures should be employed, along with immediate gastric lavage. Intravenous fluids should be administered and an adequate airway maintained. Hypotension may be combated by the use of levarterenol or metaraminol. Dialysis is of limited value. As with the management of intentional overdosage with any drug, it should be borne in mind that multiple agents may have been ingested.

Flumazenil, a specific benzodiazepine-receptor antagonist, is indicated for the complete or partial reversal of the sedative effects of benzodiazepines and may be used in situations when an overdose with a benzodiazepine is known or suspected. Prior to the administration of flumazenil, necessary measures should be instituted to secure airway, ventilation, and intravenous access. Flumazenil is intended as an adjunct to, not as a substitute for, proper management of benzodiazepine overdose. Patients treated with flumazenil should be monitored for resedation, respiratory depression and other residual benzodiazepine effects for an appropriate period after treatment. **The prescriber should be aware of a risk of seizure in association with flumazenil treatment, particularly in long-term benzodiazepine users and in cyclic antidepressant overdose.** The complete flumazenil package insert, including *"Contraindications," "Warnings"* and *"Precautions,"* should be consulted prior to use.

Withdrawal symptoms of the barbiturate type have occurred after the discontinuation of benzodiazepines. (See *"Drug Abuse and Dependence"* section.)

PRECAUTIONS

Although seizures may be brought under control promptly, a significant proportion of patients experience a return to seizure activity, presumably due to the short-lived effect of Diazepam after IV administration. The physician should be prepared to readminister the drug. However, Diazepam is not recommended for maintenance, and once seizures are brought under control, consideration should be given to the administration of agents useful in longer term control of seizures.

If Diazepam is to be combined with other psychotropic agents or anticonvulsant drugs, careful consideration should be given to the pharmacology of the agents to be employed—particularly with known compounds which may potentiate the action of Diazepam, such as phenothiazines, narcotics, barbiturates. MAO inhibitors and other antidepressants. The usual precautions are indicated for severely depressed patients or those in whom there is any evidence of latent depression; particularly the recognition that suicidal tendencies may be present and protective measures may be necessary. The usual precautions in treating patients with impaired renal or hepatic function should be observed.

Since an increase in cough reflex and laryngospasm may occur with peroral endoscopic procedures, the use of a topical anesthetic agent and the availability of necessary countermeasures are recommended.

Until additional information is available, Injectable Diazepam is not recommended for obstetrical use.

Injectable Diazepam has produced hypotension or muscular weakness in some patients particularly when used with narcotics, barbiturates or alcohol.

In elderly and debilitated patients, it is recommended that the dosage be limited to the smallest effective amount to preclude the development of ataxia or oversedation (2 mg to 2 1/2 mg once or twice daily, initially, to be increased gradually as needed and tolerated, or 2 mg to 5 mg Injectable Diazepam).

The clearance of Diazepam and certain other benzodiazepines can be delayed in association with cimetidine administration. The clinical significance of this is unclear.

Information for Patients: To assure the safe and effective use of benzodiazepines, patients should be informed that, since benzodiazepines may produce psychological and physical dependence, it is advisable that they consult with their physician before either increasing the dose or abruptly discontinuing this drug.

ADVERSE REACTIONS

Side effects most commonly reported were drowsiness, fatigue and ataxia; venous thrombosis and phlebitis at the site of injection with Injectable Diazepam. Infrequently encountered were confusion, constipation, depression, diplopia, dysarthria, headache, hypotension, incontinence, jaundice, changes in libido, nausea, changes in salivation, skin rash, slurred speech, tremor, urinary retention, vertigo and blurred vision; also, with Injectable Diazepam, hypoactivity, bradycardia, cardiovascular collapse, nystagmus, urticaria, hiccups. Paradoxical reactions such as acute hyperexcited states, anxiety, hallucinations, increased muscle spasticity, insomnia, rage, sleep disturbances and stimulation have been reported; should these occur, use of the drug should be discontinued.

In peroral endoscopic procedures, coughing, depressed respiration, dyspnea, hyperventilation, laryngospasm and pain in throat or chest have been reported.

Because of isolated reports of neutropenia and jaundice, periodic blood counts and liver function tests are advisable during long-term therapy. Minor changes in EEG patterns, usually low-voltage fast activity, have been observed in patients during and after Diazepam therapy and are of no known significance.

DRUG ABUSE AND DEPENDENCE

Withdrawal symptoms, similar in character to those noted with barbiturates and alcohol (convulsions, tremor, abdominal and muscle cramps, vomiting and sweating), have occurred following abrupt discontinuance of Diazepam. The more severe withdrawal symptoms have usually been limited to those patients who had received excessive doses over an extended period of time. Generally milder withdrawal symptoms (eg, dysphoria and insomnia) have been reported following abrupt discontinuation of benzodiazepines taken continuously at therapeutic levels for several months. Consequently, after extended therapy, abrupt discontinuation should generally be avoided and a gradual dosage tapering schedule followed. Addiction-prone individuals (such as drug addicts or alcoholics) should be under careful surveillance when receiving Diazepam or other psychotropic agents because of the predisposition of such patients to habituation and dependence.

DOSAGE AND ADMINISTRATION

Dosage should be individualized for maximum beneficial effect. While the usual daily dosages given below will meet the needs of most patients, there will be some who may require higher doses. In such cases dosage should be increased cautiously to avoid adverse effects.

Whenever oral Diazepam Tablets, 5 mg t.i.d. would be considered the appropriate dosage, one 15-mg, Slow-Release Diazepam capsule daily may be used.

➤ SHOWN IN PRODUCT IDENTIFICATION GUIDE

Slow-Release Diazepam 15-mg capsules are recommended for elderly or debilitated patients and children only when it has been determined that 5 mg oral Diazepam Tablets t.i.d. is the optimal daily dose. Oral Diazepam is not recommended for children under 6 months of age.

Adults:	Usual Daily Dose
Management of Anxiety Disorders and Relief of Symptoms of Anxiety.	Depending upon severity of symptoms—2 mg to 10 mg, 2 to 4 times daily; 1 or 2 (15 to 30 mg) Slow-Release capsules once daily
Symptomatic Relief in Acute Alcohol Withdrawal.	10 mg, 3 or 4 times during the first 24 hours reducing to 5 mg, 3 or 4 times daily as needed
Adjunctively for Relief of Skeletal Muscle Spasm.	2 mg to 10 mg, 3 or 4 times daily; 1 or 2 Slow-Release capsules (15 to 30 mg) once daily
Adjunctively in Convulsive Disorders.	2 mg to 10 mg, 2 to 4 times daily
Geriatric Patients, or in the presence of debilitating disease.	2 mg to 2 1/2 mg, 1 or 2 times daily initially; increase gradually as needed and tolerated

Children:	
Because of varied responses to CNS-acting drugs, initiate therapy with lowest dose and increase as required. Not for use in children under 6 months.	1 mg to 2 1/2 mg, 3 or 4 times daily initially; increase gradually as needed and tolerated

Injectable Diazepam: Dosage should be individualized for maximum beneficial effect. The usual recommended dose in older children and adults ranges from 2 mg to 20 mg IM or IV, depending on the indication and its severity. In some conditions, eg, tetanus, larger doses may be required. (See *"Dosage and Administration"* for specific indications.) In acute conditions the injection may be repeated within 1 hour although an interval of 3 to 4 hours is usually satisfactory. Lower doses (usually 2 mg to 5 mg) and slow increase in dosage should be used for elderly or debilitated patients and when other sedative drugs are administered. (See *"Warnings"* and *"Adverse Reactions"*.)

For dosage in infants above the age of 30 days and children, see the specific indications below. When intravenous use is indicated, facilities for respiratory assistance should be readily available.

Intramuscular: Injectable Diazepam should be injected deeply into the muscle.

Intravenous Use: (See *"Warnings"*, particularly for use in children.) The solution should be injected slowly, taking at least 1 minute for each 5 mg (1 mL) given. Do not use small veins, such as those on the dorsum of the hand or wrist. Extreme care should be taken to avoid intra-arterial administration or extravasation.

Do not mix or dilute Diazepam with other solutions or drugs in syringe or infusion flask. If it is not feasible to administer Diazepam directly IV, it may be injected slowly through the infusion tubing as close as possible to the vein insertion. (See related table).

Once the acute symptomatology has been properly controlled with Injectable Diazepam, the patient may be placed on oral therapy with Diazepam if further treatment is required.

ANIMAL PHARMACOLOGY

Oral LD_{50} of Diazepam is 720 mg/kg in mice and 1240 mg/kg in rats. Intraperitoneal administration of 400 mg/kg to a monkey resulted in death on the sixth day.

Reproduction Studies: A series of rat reproduction studies was performed with Diazepam in oral doses of 1, 10, 80 and 100 mg/kg given for periods ranging from 60 to 228 days prior to mating. At 100 mg/kg there was a decrease in the number of pregnancies and surviving offspring in these rats. These effects may be attributable to prolonged sedative activity, resulting in lack of interest in mating and lessened maternal nursing and care of the young. Neonatal survival of rats at doses lower than 100 mg/kg was within normal limits. Several neonates, both controls and experimentals, in these rat reproduction studies showed skeletal or other defects. Further studies in rats at doses up to and including 80 mg/kg/day did not reveal significant teratological effects on the offspring. Rabbits were maintained on doses of 1, 2, 5 and 8 mg/kg from day 6 through day 18 of gestation. No adverse effects on reproduction and no teratological changes were noted.

HOW SUPPLIED
CAPSULE, EXTENDED RELEASE (C-IV): 15 MG

BRAND/MANUFACTURER	NDC	SIZE	AWP
○ BRAND			
➤ VALRELEASE: Roche Labs	00004-0140-64	30s	$50.25
	00004-0140-01	100s	$166.76

INJECTION (C-IV): 5 MG/ML

AVERAGE UNIT PRICE (AVAILABLE SIZES)		GENERIC A-RATED AVERAGE PRICE (GAAP)	
BRAND	$2.05	10 ml	$11.28
GENERIC	$1.67	1 ml 10s	$29.84
		2 ml 10s	$29.53
		1 ml 25s	$73.85
		2 ml 25s	$78.82

BRAND/MANUFACTURER	NDC	SIZE	AWP
◆ BRAND			
VALIUM: Roche Prod	00140-1932-06	10 ml	$17.44
	00140-1931-06	2 ml 10s	$37.95
	00140-1933-06	2 ml 10s	$50.18
◆ GENERICS			
Moore,H.L.	00839-7190-30	10 ml	$8.09
Rugby	00536-4200-70	10 ml	$10.05
Major	00904-3904-10	10 ml	$11.05
URL	00677-1088-21	10 ml	$11.25
Goldline	00182-0094-63	10 ml	$11.25
Elkins-Sinn	00641-2289-41	10 ml	$11.88
Schein	00364-0825-54	10 ml	$13.35
Steris	00402-0445-10	10 ml	$13.35
Abbott Hosp	00074-3213-01	10 ml 5s	$31.83
Elkins-Sinn	00641-0369-23	1 ml 10s	$24.63
Elkins-Sinn	00641-3200-03	1 ml 10s	$30.63
Elkins-Sinn	00641-6288-11	1 ml 10s	$34.26
Abbott Hosp	00074-3210-01	2 ml 10s	$15.91
Elkins-Sinn	00641-1408-33	2 ml 10s	$25.88
Sanofi Winthrop	00024-0376-02	2 ml 10s	$30.00
Lederle Std Prod	00205-2810-46	2 ml 10s	$37.69
Elkins-Sinn	00641-6287-11	2 ml 10s	$38.18
Elkins-Sinn	00641-0369-25	1 ml 25s	$60.94
Schein	00364-0825-46	1 ml 25s	$86.76
Elkins-Sinn	00641-1408-35	2 ml 25s	$64.06
Elkins-Sinn	00641-0371-25	2 ml 25s	$70.31
Schein	00364-0825-48	2 ml 25s	$102.08

INJECTION (C-IV): 10 MG/2 ML

BRAND/MANUFACTURER	NDC	SIZE	AWP
◆ GENERICS			
Elkins-Sinn	00641-3201-03	2 ml 10s	$34.38

TABLETS (C-IV): 2 MG

AVERAGE UNIT PRICE (AVAILABLE SIZES)		GENERIC A-RATED AVERAGE PRICE (GAAP)	
BRAND	$0.39	100s	$11.84
GENERIC	$0.09	500s	$30.03
HCFA FUL (100s ea)	$0.02	1000s	$43.02

BRAND/MANUFACTURER	NDC	SIZE	AWP
◆ BRAND			
➤ VALIUM: Roche Prod	00140-0004-01	100s	$37.95
	00140-0004-49	100s ud	$40.04
	00140-0004-50	100s ud	$40.55
	00140-0004-14	500s	$188.67
◆ GENERICS			
Medirex	57480-0515-06	30s	$7.42
➤ Rugby	00536-3591-01	100s	$4.75
➤ Goldline	00182-1755-01	100s	$4.80
Geneva	00781-1482-01	100s	$4.85
➤ Mylan	00378-0271-01	100s	$4.89
Major	00904-3903-60	100s	$4.95
➤ Zenith	00172-3925-60	100s	$5.25
Barr	00555-0163-02	100s	$5.66
Schein	00364-0774-01	100s	$5.70
URL	00677-1048-01	100s	$5.75
Moore,H.L.	00839-7131-06	100s	$5.79
Purepac	00228-2051-10	100s	$7.50
Aligen	00405-0068-01	100s	$10.03
Lederle Std Prod	00005-3128-23	100s	$10.03
Parmed	00349-8448-01	100s	$13.89
Auro	55829-0831-10	100s ud	$14.70
Goldline	00182-1755-89	100s ud	$15.40
Vangard	00615-1532-13	100s ud	$17.96
Vangard	00615-1532-47	100s ud	$17.96
Geneva	00781-1482-13	100s ud	$18.10
Major	00904-3903-61	100s ud	$21.30
UDL	51079-0284-20	100s ud	$24.21
UDL	51079-0284-21	100s ud	$24.21
Medirex	57480-0515-01	100s ud	$24.75
Major	00904-3903-40	500s	$17.35
Schein	00364-0774-05	500s	$21.00
➤ Rugby	00536-3591-05	500s	$21.20
Goldline	00182-1755-05	500s	$21.30
Geneva	00781-1482-05	500s	$22.25
➤ Zenith	00172-3925-70	500s	$23.80
Qualitest	00603-3216-28	500s	$23.80
Martec	52555-0435-05	500s	$24.28
➤ Mylan	00378-0271-05	500s	$26.80
URL	00677-1048-05	500s	$37.45
Purepac	00228-2051-50	500s	$37.50
Aligen	00405-0068-02	500s	$40.41

◆ RATED THERAPEUTICALLY EQUIVALENT; ◇ THERAPEUTIC EQUIVALENCE UNCONFIRMED; ○ UNRATED

BRAND/MANUFACTURER	NDC	SIZE	AWP
Lederle Std Prod	00005-3128-31	500s	$46.40
Parmed	00349-8448-05	500s	$56.89
Barr	00555-0163-05	1000s	$31.01
Moore,H.L.	00839-7131-16	1000s	$31.12
Schein	00364-0774-02	1000s	$32.10
➤ Zenith	00172-3925-80	1000s	$34.75
➤ Rugby	00536-3591-10	1000s	$39.50
Aligen	00405-0068-03	1000s	$39.80
Major	00904-3903-80	1000s	$39.90
Parmed	00349-8448-10	1000s	$95.99
Parmed	00349-8448-52	2500s	$152.67

TABLETS (C-IV): 5 MG

AVERAGE UNIT PRICE (AVAILABLE SIZES)		GENERIC A-RATED AVERAGE PRICE (GAAP)	
BRAND	$0.60	100s	$17.65
GENERIC	$0.15	500s	$38.02
HCFA FUL (100s ea)	$0.03	1000s	$69.71

BRAND/MANUFACTURER	NDC	SIZE	AWP
◆ BRAND			
➤ VALIUM: Roche Prod	00140-0005-01	100s	$59.03
	00140-0005-49	100s ud	$61.10
	00140-0005-50	100s ud	$61.62
	00140-0005-14	500s	$294.02
◆ GENERICS			
Medirex	57480-0516-06	30s	$9.75
UDL	51079-0285-98	60s ud	$60.00
Major	00904-3901-60	100s	$6.85
➤ Schein	00364-0775-01	100s	$6.85
➤ Mylan	00378-0345-01	100s	$6.90
➤ Rugby	00536-3592-01	100s	$6.90

BRAND/MANUFACTURER	NDC	SIZE	AWP
Geneva	00781-1483-01	100s	$6.90
Goldline	00182-1756-01	100s	$6.95
➤ Zenith	00172-3926-60	100s	$7.45
Barr	00555-0363-02	100s	$7.92
Moore,H.L.	00839-7132-06	100s	$8.30
URL	00677-1049-01	100s	$10.70
Purepac	00228-2052-10	100s	$10.76
➤ Lederle Std Prod	00005-3129-23	100s	$15.96
Aligen	00405-0069-01	100s	$16.72
Parmed	00349-8449-01	100s	$22.89
Auro	55829-0832-10	100s ud	$21.73
Major	00904-3901-61	100s ud	$22.87
Goldline	00182-1756-89	100s ud	$23.20
Vangard	00615-1533-13	100s ud	$31.95
Vangard	00615-1533-47	100s ud	$31.95
UDL	51079-0285-20	100s ud	$32.14
UDL	51079-0285-21	100s ud	$32.14
Geneva	00781-1483-13	100s ud	$32.40
Medirex	57480-0516-01	100s ud	$35.50
Parmed	00349-8449-05	500s	$14.75
Geneva	00781-1483-05	500s	$22.50
Major	00904-3901-40	500s	$24.00
➤ Mylan	00378-0345-05	500s	$26.49
➤ Schein	00364-0775-05	500s	$27.83
➤ Zenith	00172-3926-70	500s	$30.55
Martec	52555-0436-05	500s	$31.15
➤ Rugby	00536-3592-05	500s	$31.75
Goldline	00182-1756-05	500s	$31.80
Qualitest	00603-3217-28	500s	$34.48
URL	00677-1049-05	500s	$53.75
Purepac	00228-2052-50	500s	$53.80
Lederle Std Prod	00005-3129-31	500s	$73.16
Aligen	00405-0069-02	500s	$76.20

RECOMMENDED DOSAGE FOR INJECTABLE DIAZEPAM

	Usual Adult Dosage	Dosage Range in Children (IV administration should be made slowly)
Moderate Anxiety Disorders and Symptoms of Anxiety.	2 mg to 5 mg, IM or IV. Repeat in 3 to 4 hours, if necessary.	
Severe Anxiety Disorders and Symptoms of Anxiety.	5 mg to 10 mg, IM or IV. Repeat in 3 to 4 hours, if necessary.	
Acute Alcohol Withdrawal: As an aid in symptomatic relief of acute agitation, tremor, impending or acute delirium tremens and hallucinosis.	10 mg, IM or IV initially, then 5 mg to 10 mg in 3 to 4 hours, if necessary.	
Endoscopic Procedures: Adjunctively, if apprehension, anxiety or acute stress reactions are present prior to endoscopic procedures. Dosage of narcotics should be reduced by at least a third and in some cases may be omitted. See "Precautions" for peroral procedures.	Titrate IV dosage to desired sedative response, such as slurring of speech, with slow administration immediately prior to the procedure. Generally 10 mg or less is adequate, but up to 20 mg IV may be given, particularly when concomitant narcotics are omitted. If IV cannot be used, 5 mg to 10 mg IM approximately 30 minutes prior to the procedure.	
Muscle Spasm: Associated with local pathology, cerebral palsy, athetosis, stiff-man syndrome or tetanus.	5 mg to 10 mg, IM or IV initially, then 5 mg to 10 mg in 3 to 4 hours, if necessary. For tetanus, larger doses may be required.	For tetanus in infants over 30 days of age, 1 mg to 2 mg IM or IV, slowly, repeated every 3 to 4 hours as necessary. In children 5 years or older, 5 mg to 10 mg repeated every 3 to 4 hours may be required to control tetanus spasms. Respiratory assistance should be available.
Status Epilepticus and Severe Recurrent Convulsive Seizures: In the convulsing patient, the IV route is by far preferred. This injection should be administered slowly. However, if IV administration is impossible, the IM route may be used.	5 mg to 10 mg initially (IV preferred). This injection may be repeated if necessary at 10 to 15 minute intervals up to a maximum dose of 30 mg. If necessary, therapy with Diazepam may be repeated in 2 to 4 hours; however, residual active metabolites may persist, and readministration should be made with this consideration. Extreme caution must be exercised with individuals with chronic lung disease or unstable cardiovascular status.	Infants over 30 days of age and children under 5 years, 0.2 mg to 0.5 mg slowly every 2 to 5 minutes up to a maximum of 5 mg (IV preferred). Children 5 years or older, 1 mg every 2 to 5 minutes up to a maximum of 10 mg (slow IV administration preferred). Repeat in 2 to 4 hours if necessary. EEG monitoring of the seizure may be helpful.
Preoperative Medication: To relieve anxiety and tension. (If atropine, scopolamine or other premedications are desired, they must be administered in separate syringes.)	10 mg, IM (preferred route), before surgery	
Cardioversion: To relieve anxiety and tension and to reduce recall of procedure.	5 mg to 15 mg, IV, within 5 to 10 minutes prior to the procedure.	

➤ SHOWN IN PRODUCT IDENTIFICATION GUIDE

BRAND/MANUFACTURER	NDC	SIZE	AWP
Moore,H.L.	00839-7132-16	1000s	$38.81
➤ Schein	00364-0775-02	1000s	$39.60
Barr	00555-0363-05	1000s	$46.78
➤ Zenith	00172-3926-80	1000s	$47.50
➤ Rugby	00536-3592-10	1000s	$60.00
Major	00904-3901-80	1000s	$60.10
Goldline	00182-1756-10	1000s	$60.10
Purepac	00228-2052-96	1000s	$107.60
Aligen	00405-0069-03	1000s	$108.35
Parmed	00349-8449-10	1000s	$128.25
Parmed	00349-8449-52	2500s	$232.35

TABLETS (C-IV): 10 MG

AVERAGE UNIT PRICE (AVAILABLE SIZES)		GENERIC A-RATED AVERAGE PRICE (GAAP)	
BRAND	$1.006	100s	$24.69
GENERIC	$0.18	500s	$55.41
HCFA FUL (100s ea)	$0.03	1000s	$88.97

BRAND/MANUFACTURER	NDC	SIZE	AWP
◆ BRAND			
➤ VALIUM: Roche Prod	00140-0006-01	100s	$99.45
	00140-0006-49	100s ud	$101.52
	00140-0006-50	100s ud	$102.05
	00140-0006-14	500s	$496.13
◆ GENERICS			
Medirex	57480-0517-06	30s	$11.70
Schein	00364-0776-01	100s	$10.67
➤ Zenith	00172-3927-60	100s	$11.30
➤ Mylan	00378-0477-01	100s	$11.50
➤ Rugby	00536-3593-01	100s	$11.50
Major	00904-3902-60	100s	$11.50
Geneva	00781-1484-01	100s	$11.50
Goldline	00182-1757-01	100s	$11.55
Barr	00555-0164-02	100s	$11.61
Moore,H.L.	00839-7133-06	100s	$12.76
URL	00677-1050-01	100s	$17.25
Purepac	00228-2053-10	100s	$17.29
Aligen	00405-0070-01	100s	$17.62
Lederle Std Prod	00005-3130-23	100s	$25.25
Parmed	00349-8450-01	100s	$39.49
Medirex	57480-0517-01	100s	$42.95
Major	00904-3902-61	100s ud	$25.41
Goldline	00182-1757-89	100s ud	$35.50
Auro	55829-0833-10	100s ud	$35.61
UDL	51079-0286-21	100s ud	$38.03
Vangard	00615-1534-13	100s ud	$42.22
Vangard	00615-1534-47	100s ud	$42.22
UDL	51079-0286-20	100s ud	$42.50
Geneva	00781-1484-13	100s ud	$42.75
Parmed	00349-8450-05	500s	$25.20
Moore,H.L.	00839-7133-12	500s	$29.11
Schein	00364-0776-05	500s	$29.32
➤ Zenith	00172-3927-70	500s	$32.80
Martec	52555-0437-05	500s	$33.80
Major	00904-3902-40	500s	$40.25
➤ Mylan	00378-0477-05	500s	$48.00
Geneva	00781-1484-05	500s	$48.00
➤ Rugby	00536-3593-05	500s	$54.80
Goldline	00182-1757-05	500s	$54.90
Qualitest	00603-3218-28	500s	$58.10
Aligen	00405-0070-02	500s	$80.22
URL	00677-1050-05	500s	$86.40
Purepac	00228-2053-50	500s	$86.45
Lederle Std Prod	00005-3130-31	500s	$123.84
Schein	00364-0776-10	1000s	$42.81
➤ Zenith	00172-3927-80	1000s	$69.50
Barr	00555-0164-05	1000s	$70.89
Moore,H.L.	00839-7133-16	1000s	$79.18
➤ Rugby	00536-3593-10	1000s	$102.40
Goldline	00182-1757-10	1000s	$102.50
Major	00904-3902-80	1000s	$102.70
Parmed	00349-8450-10	1000s	$141.75
Parmed	00349-8450-52	2500s	$370.75

Diazoxide

DESCRIPTION

Diazoxide is a nondiuretic benzothiadiazine derivative taken orally for the management of symptomatic hypoglycemia. The capsules contain 50 mg Diazoxide, USP. The suspension contains 50 mg of Diazoxide, USP in each milliliter; alcohol content is approximately 7.25%.

Diazoxide is 7-chloro-3-methyl-$2H$-1,2,4-benzothiadiazine 1,1-dioxide with the empirical formula $C_8H_7ClN_2O_2S$ and the molecular weight 230.7. It is a white powder practically insoluble to sparingly soluble in water.

Following is its chemical structure:

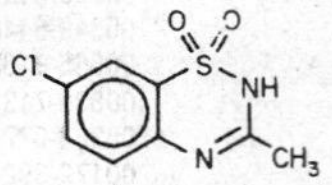

CLINICAL PHARMACOLOGY

Diazoxide administered orally produces a prompt dose-related increase in blood glucose level, due primarily to an inhibition of insulin release from the pancreas, and also to an extrapancreatic effect.

The hyperglycemic effect begins within an hour and generally lasts no more than eight hours in the presence of normal renal function.

Diazoxide decreases the excretion of sodium and water, resulting in fluid retention which may be clinically significant.

The hypotensive effect of Diazoxide on blood pressure is usually not marked with the oral preparation. This contrasts with the intravenous preparation of Diazoxide (see "Adverse Reactions").

Other pharmacologic actions of Diazoxide include increased pulse rate; increased serum uric acid levels due to decreased excretion; increased serum levels of free fatty acids' decreased chloride excretion; decreased para-amino-hippuric acid; (PAH) clearance with no appreciable effect on glomerular filtration rate.

The concomitant administration of a benzothiazide diuretic may intensify the hyperglycemic and hyperuricemic effects of Diazoxide. In the presence of hypokalemia, hyperglycemic effects are also potentiated.

Diazoxide-induced hyperglycemia is reversed by the administration of insulin or tolbutamide.

The inhibition of insulin release by Diazoxide is antagonized by alpha-adrenergic blocking agents.

Diazoxide is extensively bound (more than 90%) to serum proteins, and is excreted in the kidneys. The plasma half-life following I.V. administration is 28 + 8.3 hours. Limited data on oral administration revealed a half-life of 24 and 36 hours in two adults. In four children aged four months to six years, the plasma half-life varied from 9.5 to 24 hours on long-term oral administration. The half-life may be prolonged following overdosage, and in patients with impaired renal function.

INDICATIONS AND USAGE

Diazoxide is useful in the management of hypoglycemia due to hyperinsulinism associated with the following conditions:

Adults: Inoperable islet cell adenoma or carcinoma, or extrapancreatic malignancy.

Infants and Children: Leucine sensitivity, islet cell hyperplasia, nesidioblastosis, extrapancreatic malignancy, islet cell adenoma, or adenomatosis. Diazoxide may be used preoperatively as a temporary measure, and postoperatively, if hypoglycemia persists.

Diazoxide should be used only after a diagnosis of hypoglycemia due to one of the above conditions has been definitely established. When other specific medical therapy or surgical management either has been unsuccessful or is not feasible, treatment with Diazoxide should be considered.

CONTRAINDICATIONS

The use of Diazoxide for functional hypoglycemia is contraindicated. The drug should not be used in patients hypersensitive to Diazoxide or to other thiazides unless the potential benefits outweigh the possible risks.

WARNINGS

The antidiuretic property of Diazoxide may lead to significant fluid retention, which in patients with a compromised cardiac reserve, may precipitate congestive heart failure. The fluid retention will respond to conventional therapy with diuretics.

It should be noted that concomitantly administered thiazides may potentiate the hyperglycemic and hyperuricemic actions of Diazoxide (see "Drug Interactions" and "Animal Pharmacology and/or Toxicology"). Ketoacidosis and nonketoic hyperosmolar coma have been reported in patients treated with recommended doses of Diazoxide usually during intercurrent illness. Prompt recognition and treatment are essential (see "Overdosage"), and prolonged surveillance following the acute episode is necessary because of the long drug half-life of approximately 30 hours. The occurrence of these serious events may be reduced by careful education of patients regarding the need for monitoring the urine for sugar and ketones and for prompt reporting of abnormal findings and unusual symptoms to the physician.

Transient cataracts occur in association with hyperosmolar coma in an infant, and subsided on correction of the hyperosmolarity. Cataracts have been observed in several animals receiving daily doses of intravenous or oral Diazoxide.

The development of abnormal facial features in four children treated chronically (> 4 years) with Diazoxide for hypoglycemia hyperinsulinism in the same clinic has been reported.

PRECAUTIONS

General: Treatment with Diazoxide should be initiated under close clinical supervision, with careful monitoring of blood glucose and clinical response until the patient's condition has stabilized. This usually requires several days. If not effective in two to three weeks, the drug should be discontinued.

◆ RATED THERAPEUTICALLY EQUIVALENT; ◇ THERAPEUTIC EQUIVALENCE UNCONFIRMED; ○ UNRATED

Prolonged treatment requires regular monitoring of the urine for sugar and ketones, especially under stress conditions, with prompt reporting of any abnormalities to the physician. Additionally, blood sugar levels should be monitored periodically by the physician to determine the need for dose adjustment.

The effects of Diazoxide on the hematopoietic system and the level of serum uric acid should be kept in mind; the latter should be considered particularly in patients with hyperuricemia or a history of gout.

In some patients, higher blood levels have been observed with the oral suspension than with the capsule formulation of Diazoxide. Dosage should be adjusted as necessary in individual patients if changed from one formulation to the other.

Since the plasma half-life of Diazoxide is prolonged in patients with impaired renal function, a reduced dosage should be considered. Serum electrolyte levels should also be evaluated for such patients.

The antihypertensive effect of other drugs may be enhanced by Diazoxide, and this should be kept in mind when administering it concomitantly with antihypertensive agents.

Because of the protein binding, administration of Diazoxide with coumarin or its derivatives may require reduction in the dosage of the anticoagulant, although there has been no reported evidence of excessive anticoagulant effect. In addition, Diazoxide may possibly displace bilirubin from albumin; this should be kept in mind particularly when treating newborns with increased bilirubinemia.

Information for Patients: During treatment with Diazoxide the patient should be advised to consult regularly with the physician and to cooperate in the periodic monitoring of his condition by laboratory tests. In addition, the patient should be advised:

—to take the drug on a regular schedule as prescribed, not to skip doses, not to take extra doses;

—not to use this drug with other medications unless this is done with the physician's advice;

—not to allow anyone else to take this medication;

—to follow dietary instructions;

—to report promptly any adverse effects (i.e., increased urinary frequency, increased thirst, fruity breath odor);

—to report pregnancy or to discuss plans for pregnancy.

Laboratory Tests: The following procedures may be especially important in patient monitoring (not necessarily inclusive); blood glucose determinations (recommended at periodic intervals in patients taking Diazoxide orally for treatment of hypoglycemia, until stabilized); blood urea nitrogen (BUN) determinations and creatinine clearance determinations; hematocrit determinations; platelet count determinations; total and differential leukocyte counts; serum aspartate aminotransferase (AST) level determinations; serum uric acid level determinations; and urine testing for glucose and ketones (in patients being treated with Diazoxide for hypoglycemia, semi-quantitative estimation of sugar and ketones in serum performed by the patient and reported to the physician provides frequent and relatively inexpensive monitoring of the condition).

Drug Interactions: Since Diazoxide is highly bound to serum proteins, it may displace other substances which are also bound to protein, such as bilirubin or coumarin and its derivatives, resulting in higher blood levels of these substances. Concomitant administration of oral Diazoxide and diphenylhydantoin may result in a loss of seizure control. These potential interactions must be considered when administering Diazoxide *Capsules* or *Suspension.* The concomitant administration of thiazides or other commonly used diuretics may potentiate the hyperglycemic and hyperuricemic effects of Diazoxide.

Drug/Laboratory Test Interactions: The hyperglycemic and hyperuricemic effects of Diazoxide preclude proper assessment of these metabolic states. Increased renin secretion, IgG concentrations and decreased cortisol secretions have also been noted. Diazoxide inhibits glucagon-stimulated insulin release and causes a false-negative insulin response to glucagon.

Carcinogenesis, Mutagenesis, Impairment of Fertility: No long-term animal dosing study has been done to evaluate the carcinogenic potential of Diazoxide. No laboratory study of mutagenic potential or animal study of effects on fertility has been done.

Pregnancy Category C: Reproduction studies using the oral preparation in rats have revealed increased fetal resorptions and delayed parturition, as well as fetal skeletal anomalies; evidence of skeletal and cardiac teratogenic effects in rabbits has been noted with intravenous administration. The drug has also been demonstrated to cross the placental barrier in animals and to cause degeneration of the fetal pancreatic beta cells (see *"Animal Pharmacology and/or Toxicology"*). Since there are no adequate data on fetal effects of this drug when given to pregnant women, safety in pregnancy has not been established. When the use of Diazoxide is considered, the indications should be limited to those specified above for adults (see *"Indications and Usage"*), and the potential benefits to the mother must be weighed against possible harmful effects to the fetus.

Nonteratogenic Effects: Diazoxide crosses the placental barrier and appears in cord blood. When given to the mother prior to delivery of the infant, the drug may produce fetal or neonatal hyperbilirubinemia, thrombocytopenia, altered carbohydrate metabolism, and possibly other side effects that have occurred in adults.

Alopecia and hypertrichosis lanuginosa have occurred in infants whose mothers received oral Diazoxide during the last 19 to 60 days of pregnancy.

Labor and Delivery: Since intravenous administration of the drug during labor may cause cessation of uterine contractions, and administration of oxytocic agents may be required to reinstate labor, caution is advised in administering Diazoxide at that time.

Nursing Mothers: Information is not available concerning the passage of Diazoxide in breast milk. Because many drugs are excreted in human milk and because of the potential for adverse reactions from Diazoxide in nursing infants, a decision should be made whether to discontinue nursing or to discontinue the drug, taking into account the importance of the drug to the mother.

Pediatric Use: (See *"Indications and Usage"*.)

ADVERSE REACTIONS

Frequent and Serious: Sodium and fluid retention is most common in young infants and in adults and may precipitate congestive heart failure in patients with compromised cardiac reserve. It usually responds to diuretic therapy (see *"Drug Interactions"*).

Infrequent but Serious: Diabetic ketoacidosis and hyperosmolar nonketotic coma may develop very rapidly. Conventional therapy with insulin and restoration of fluid and electrolyte balance is usually effective if instituted promptly. Prolonged surveillance is essential in view of the long half life of Diazoxide (see *"Overdosage"*).

Other Frequent Adverse Reactions: Hirsutism of the lanugo type, mainly on the forehead, back and limbs, occurs most commonly in children and women and may be cosmetically unacceptable. It subsides on discontinuation of the drug.

Hyperglycemia or glycosuria may require reduction in dosage in order to avoid progression towards ketoacidosis or hyperosmolar coma.

Gastrointestinal intolerance may include anorexia, nausea, vomiting, abdominal pain, ileus, diarrhea, transient loss of taste. Tachycardia, palpitations, increased levels of serum uric acid are common.

Thrombocytopenia with or without purpura may require discontinuation of the drug. Neutropenia is transient, is not associated with increased susceptibility to infection, and ordinarily does not require discontinuation of the drug. Skin rash, headache, weakness, and malaise may also occur.

Other adverse reactions which have been observed are:

Cardiovascular: hypotension occurs occasionally, which may be augmented by thiazide diuretics given concurrently. A few cases of transient hypertension, for which no explanation is apparent, have been noted. Chest pain has been reported rarely.

Hematologic: eosinophilia; decreased hemoglobin/hematocrit; excessive bleeding, decreased IgG.

Hepato-renal: increased AST, alkaline phosphatase: azotemia, decreased creatinine clearance, reversible nephrotic syndrome, decreased urinary output, hematuria, albuminuria. Neurologic anxiety, dizziness, insomnia, polyneuritis, paresthesia, pruritus, extrapyramidal signs.

Ophthalmologic: transient cataracts, subconjunctival hemorrhage, ring scotoma, blurred vision, diplopia, lacrimation.

Skeletal, integumentary: monilial dermatitis, herpes, advance in bone-age; loss of scalp hair.

Systemic: fever, lymphadenopathy.

Other: gout, acute pancreatitis/pancreatic necrosis, galactorrhea, enlargement of lump in breast.

OVERDOSAGE

An overdosage of Diazoxide causes marked hyperglycemia which may be associated with ketoacidosis. It will respond to prompt insulin administration and restoration of fluid and electrolyte balance. Because of the drug's long half-life (approximately 30 hours), the symptoms of overdosage require prolonged surveillance for periods up to seven days until the blood sugar level stabilizes within the normal range. One investigator reported successful lowering of Diazoxide blood levels by peritoneal dialysis in one patient and by hemodialysis in another.

DOSAGE AND ADMINISTRATION

Patients should be under close clinical observation when treatment with Diazoxide is initiated. The clinical response and blood glucose level should be carefully monitored until the patient's condition has stabilized satisfactory; in most instances, this may be accomplished in several days. If administration of Diazoxide is not effective after two or three weeks, the drug should be discontinued.

The dosage of Diazoxide must be individualized based on the severity of the hypoglycemic condition and the blood glucose level and clinical response of the patient. The dosage should be adjusted until the desired clinical and laboratory effects are produced with the least amount of the drug. Special care should be taken to assure accuracy of dosage in infants and young children.

Adults and Children: The usual daily dosage is 3 to 8 mg/kg, divided into two or three equal doses every 8 to 12 hours. In certain instances, patients with refractory hypoglycemia may require higher dosages. Ordinarily, an appropriate starting dosage is 3 mg/kg/day, divided into three equal doses every 8 hours. Thus an average adult would receive a starting dosage of approximately 200 mg daily.

Infants and Newborns: The usual daily dosage is 8 to 15 mg/kg divided into two or three equal doses every 8 to 12 hours. An appropriate starting dosage is 10 mg/kg/day, divided into three equal doses every 8 hours.

Storage: Store between 2° and 30°C (36° and 86°F). Shake the suspension well before each use. Protect from light. Store in carton until contents are used.

ANIMAL PHARMACOLOGY AND/OR TOXICOLOGY

Oral Diazoxide in the mouse, rat, rabbit, dog, pig, and monkey produces a rapid and transient rise in blood glucose levels. In dogs, increased blood glucose is accompanied by increased free fatty acids, lactate, and pyruvate in the serum. In mice, a marked decrease in liver glycogen and an increase in the blood urea nitrogen level occur.

In acute toxicity studies the LD$_{50}$ for oral Diazoxide suspension is >5000 mg/kg in the rat, > 522 mg/kg in the neonatal rat, between 1900 and 2572 mg/kg in the mouse, and 219 mg/kg in the guinea pig. Although the oral LD$_{50}$ was not determined in the dog, a dosage of up to 500 mg/kg was well tolerated.

In subacute oral toxicity studies, Diazoxide at 400 mg/kg in the rat produced growth retardation, edema, increases in liver and kidney weights, and adrenal hypertrophy. Daily dosages up to 1080 mg/kg for three months produced hyperglycemia, an increase in liver weight and an increase in mortality. In dogs given oral Diazoxide at approximately 40 mg/kg/day for one month, no biologically significant gross or microscopic abnormalities were observed. Cataracts, attributed to markedly disturbed carbohydrate metabolism, have been observed in a few dogs given repeated daily doses of oral or intravenous Diazoxide. The lenticular changes resembled those which occur experimentally in animals with increased blood glucose levels. In chronic toxicity studies, rats given a daily dose of 200 mg/kg Diazoxide for 52 weeks had a decrease in weight gain and an increase in heart, liver, adrenal and thyroid weights. Mortality in drug-treated and control groups was not different. Dogs treated with Diazoxide at dosages of 50, 100, and 200 mg/kg/day for 82 weeks had higher blood glucose levels than controls. Mild bone marrow stimulation and increased pancreas weights were evident in the drug-treated dogs; several developed inguinal hernias, one had a testicular seminoma, and another had a mass near the penis. Two females had inguinal mammary swellings. The etiology of these changes was not established. There was no difference in mortality between drug-treated and control groups. In a second chronic oral toxicity study, dogs given milled Diazoxide at 50, 100, and 200 mg/kg/day had anorexia and severe weight loss, causing death in a few. Hematologic, biochemical, and histologic examination did not indicate any cause of death other than inanition. After one year of treatment, there is no evidence of herniation or tissue swelling in any of the dogs.

When Diazoxide was administered at high dosages concomitantly with either chlorothiazide to rats or trichlormethiazide to dogs, increased toxicity was observed. In rats, the combination was nephrotoxic; epithelial hyperplasia was observed in the collecting tubules. In dogs, a diabetic syndrome was produced which resulted in ketosis and death. Neither of the drugs given alone produced these effects.

Although the data are inconclusive, reproduction and teratology studies in several species of animals indicate that Diazoxide, when administered during the critical period of embryo formation, may interfere with normal fetal development, possibly through altered glucose metabolism. Parturition was occasionally prolonged in animals treated at term. Intravenous administration of Diazoxide to pregnant sheep, goats, and swine produced in the fetus an appreciable increase in blood glucose level and degeneration of the beta cells of the Islets of Langerhans. The reversibility of these effects was not studied.

HOW SUPPLIED
CAPSULE: 50 MG

BRAND/MANUFACTURER	NDC	SIZE	AWP
○ BRAND PROGLYCEM: Baker Norton	00575-6000-01	100s	$152.69

SUSPENSION: 50 MG/ML

BRAND/MANUFACTURER	NDC	SIZE	AWP
○ BRAND PROGLYCEM: Baker Norton	00575-6200-30	30 ml	$105.88

Diazoxide, Injectable

DESCRIPTION

Diazoxide, Injectable is a nondiuretic benzothiadiazine antihypertensive agent. Each ampule (20 ml) contains 300 mg Diazoxide, USP, in a clear, sterile, colorless aqueous solution; the pH is adjusted to approximately 11.6 with sodium hydroxide.

Diazoxide is 7-chloro-3-methyl-2*H*-1,2,4-benzothiadiazine 1,1-dioxide, with the empirical formula $C_8H_7ClN_2O_2S$, and the molecular weight 230.7. It is a white crystalline powder practically insoluble to sparingly soluble in water.

Following is its chemical structure:

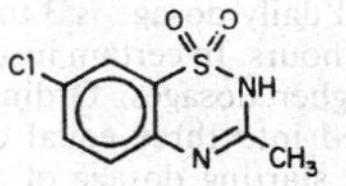

CLINICAL PHARMACOLOGY

Diazoxide, Injectable produces a prompt reduction of blood pressure in man by relaxing smooth muscle in the peripheral arterioles. Cardiac output is increased as blood pressure is reduced. Studies in animals demonstrate that coronary blood flow is maintained, while renal blood flow is increased after an initial decrease.

Transient hyperglycemia occurs in the majority of patients treated with Diazoxide, but usually requires treatment only in patients with diabetes mellitus. It will respond to the usual management measures, including insulin.

Blood glucose levels should be monitored especially in patients with diabetes and in those requiring multiple injections of Diazoxide. Cataracts have been observed in a few animals receiving repeated daily doses of intravenous Diazoxide.

Since Diazoxide causes sodium retention, repeated injections may precipitate edema and congestive heart failure. Increased volume of extracellular fluid may be a cause of treatment failure in nonresponsive patients. The increase in fluid volume characteristically responds to diuretic agents if adequate renal function exists. Concurrently administered thiazide diuretics may be expected to potentiate the antihypertensive and hyperuricemic actions of Diazoxide. (See *"Drug Interactions".*)

Diazoxide is extensively bound to serum protein (> 90%).

The plasma half-life is 28 ± 8.3 hours; however, the duration of its antihypertensive effect is variable, generally lasting less than 12 hours.

INDICATIONS AND USAGE

Diazoxide, Injectable is indicated for short-term use in the emergency reduction of blood pressure in severe, non-malignant and malignant hypertension in hospitalized adults; and in acute severe hypertension in hospitalized children, when prompt and urgent decrease of diastolic pressure is required. Treatment with orally effective antihypertensive agents should not be instituted until blood pressure has stabilized. The use of Diazoxide, Injectable for longer than 10 days is not recommended.

Diazoxide, Injectable is ineffective against hypertension due to pheochromocytoma.

CONTRAINDICATIONS

Diazoxide, Injectable should not be used in the treatment of compensatory hypertension, such as that associated with aortic coarctation or arteriovenous shunt, and should not be used in patients hypersensitive to Diazoxide, other thiazides, or other sulfonamide-derived drugs.

WARNINGS

Rapid Decrease of Blood Pressure: Caution must be observed when reducing severely elevated blood pressure. Diazoxide should only be administered utilizing the new 150 mg minibolus dosage. The use of a 300 mg intravenous dose of Diazoxide has been associated with angina and with myocardial and cerebral infarction. One instance of optic nerve infarction was reported when a 100 mmHg reduction in diastolic pressure occurred over ten minutes following a single 300 mg bolus. In one prospective trial conducted in patients with severe hypertension and coexistent coronary artery disease, a 50% incidence of ischemic changes in the electrocardiogram was observed following single 300 mg bolus injections of Diazoxide. The desired blood pressure lowering should therefore be achieved over as long a period of time as is compatible with the patient's status. At least several hours and preferably one or two days is tentatively recommended. Improved safety with equal efficacy can be achieved by administering Diazoxide, Injectable as a minibolus dose (1 to 3 mg/kg every 5 to 15 minutes up to a maximum of 150 mg in a single injection) until a diastolic blood pressure below 100 mmHg is achieved. Diazoxide, Injectable should not be administered in a bolus dose of 300 mg since this mode of administrated is less predictable and less controllable than the minibolus dosage. If hypotension severe enough to require therapy results from the reduction in blood pressure, it will usually respond to the Trendelenberg maneuver. If necessary, sympathomimetic agents such as dopamine or norepinephrine may be administered.

Special attention is required for patients with diabetes mellitus and those in whom retention of salt and water may present serious problems.

Myocardial Lesions in Animals: Intravenous administration of Diazoxide in dogs has induced subendocardial necrosis and necrosis of papillary muscles. These lesions, which are also produced by other vasodilator drugs (i.e., hydralazine, minoxidil) and by catecholamines, are presumed to be related to anoxia resulting from a combination of reflex tachycardia and decreased perfusion.

PRECAUTIONS

General: Diazoxide, Injectable is an effective antihypertensive agent requiring close monitoring of the patient's blood pressure at frequent intervals. Its administration may occasionally cause hypotension requiring treatment with sympathomimetic drugs. Therefore, Diazoxide, Injectable should be used primarily in the hospital or where adequate facilities exist to treat such untoward responses.

Diazoxide, Injectable should be administered only into a peripheral vein. Because the alkalinity of the solution is irritating to tissue, avoid extravascular injection or leakage. Subcutaneous administration has produced inflammation and pain without subsequent necrosis. If leakage into subcutaneous tissue occurs, the area should be treated with warm compresses and rest.

Diazoxide, Injectable should be used with care in patients who have impaired cerebral or cardiac circulation, that is, patients in whom abrupt reduction in blood pressure might be detrimental or those in whom mild tachycardia or decreased blood perfusion may be deleterious (see *"Warnings"*). Prolonged hypotension should be avoided so as not to aggravate preexisting renal failure.

Information for Patients: During and immediately following intravenous injection of Diazoxide, Injectable, the patient should remain supine.

Laboratory Tests: Diagnostic laboratory tests necessary to establish the patient's condition and status should be carried out prior to treatment with Diazoxide, Injectable. During and following treatment with Diazoxide, Injectable, laboratory tests to monitor the effects of treatment with this drug and the patient's condition should be done. Among the tests (not necessarily inclusive) are; hematologic (hematocrit, hemoglobin, white blood cell and platelet counts); metabolic (glucose, uric acid, total protein, albumin); electrolyte (sodium, potassium) and osmolality; renal function (creatinine, urine-protein); electrocardiogram.

Drug Interactions: Diazoxide is highly bound to serum protein. It can be expected to displace other substances which are also bound to protein, such as bilirubin or coumarin and its derivatives, resulting in higher blood levels of these substances.

An undesirable hypotension may result when Diazoxide is administered to patients who have received other antihypertensive medication within six hours.

One patient in a clinical study exhibited excessive hypotension after concomitant administration of Diazoxide with hydralazine and methyldopa. An episode of maternal hypotension and fetal bradycardia occurred in a patient in labor who received both reserpine and hydralazine prior to administration of Diazoxide. Neonatal hyperglycemia following intrapartum administration of Diazoxide, Injectable has also been reported.

Diazoxide, Injectable should not be administered within six hours of the administration of: hydralazine, reserpine, alphaprodine, methyldopa, beta-blockers, prazosin, minoxidil, the nitrites and other papaverine-like compounds. Concomitant administration with thiazides or other commonly used diuretics may be expected to potentiate the hyperuricemic and antihypertensive effects of Diazoxide.

Drug/Laboratory Test Interactions: The hyperglycemic and hyperuricemic effects of Diazoxide preclude proper assessment of these metabolic states. Increased renin secretion, IgG concentrations and decreased cortisol secretion have also been noted. Diazoxide inhibits glucagon-stimulated insulin release and will cause a false-negative insulin response to glucagon. In the rat, dog and monkey, Diazoxide increased serum free fatty acids and decreased plasma insulin levels.

Carcinogenesis, Mutagenesis, Impairment of Fertility: No long-term animal dosing study has been done to evaluate the carcinogenic potential of Diazoxide. No laboratory studies of mutagenic potential or animal studies of effects on fertility have been done.

Pregnancy Category C: Diazoxide has been shown to reduce fetal and/or pup survival: and to reduce fetal growth in rats, rabbits, and dogs at daily doses of 30.21, or 10 mg/kg, respectively. In rats treated at term, Diazoxide, at doses of 10 mg/kg and above, prolonged parturition.

The safety of Diazoxide, Injectable in pregnancy has not been established.

Nonteratogenic Effects: Diazoxide crosses the placental barrier and appears in cord blood. When given to the mother prior to delivery the drug may produce fetal or neonatal hyperbilirubinemia, thrombocytopenia, altered carbohydrate metabolism, and possibly other side effects that have occurred in adults.

Labor and Delivery: Diazoxide, Injectable is not indicated for use in pregnancy. Intravenous administration of the drug during labor may cause cessation of uterine contractions, requiring administration of an oxytocic agent.

Nursing Mothers: Information is not available concerning the passage of Diazoxide in breast milk. Because many drugs are excreted in human milk and because of the potential for adverse reactions in nursing infants from Diazoxide, a decision should be made whether to discontinue nursing or to discontinue the drug, taking into account the importance of the drug to the mother.

Pediatric Use: (See *"Indications and Usage"*.)

ADVERSE REACTIONS

It is reasonable to speculate that the currently recommended minibolus dosing regimen, which has replaced the 300 mg bolus dose in clinical practice, will result in adverse effects which are of similar character but of lesser frequency and severity.

In clinical experience with the rapid bolus administration of 300 mg, the most common adverse reactions reported were: hypotension (7%); nausea and vomiting (4%); dizziness and weakness (2%). Additional adverse reactions reported with bolus administration of 300 mg were as follows:

Cardiovascular: sodium and water retention after repeated injections, especially important in patients with impaired cardiac reserve; hypotension to shock levels; myocardial ischemia, usually transient and manifested by angina, atrial and ventricular arrhythmias, and marked electrocardiographic changes, but occasionally leading to myocardial infarction; optic nerve infarction following too rapid decrease in severely elevated blood pressure; supraventricular tachycardia and palpitation; bradycardia; chest discomfort or nonanginal "tightness in the chest."

Central Nervous System: cerebral ischemia, usually transient but occasionally leading to infarction and manifested by unconsciousness, convulsions, paralysis, confusion, or focal neurological deficit such as numbness of the hands; vasodilative phenomena, such as orthostatic hypotension, sweating, flushing, and generalized or localized sensations of warmth; various transient neurological findings secondary to alteration in regional blood flow to brain, such as headache (sometimes throbbing), dizziness, light-headedness, sleepiness (also reported as lethargy, somnolence or drowsiness), euphoria or "funny feeling," ringing in the ears and momentary hearing loss, and weakness of short duration; apprehension or anxiety.

Gastrointestinal: rarely, acute pancreatitis; nausea, vomiting and/or abdominal discomfort; anorexia; alteration in taste; parotid swelling; salivation; dry mouth; lacrimation; ileus; constipation and diarrhea.

Other: hyperglycemia in diabetic patients, especially after repeated injections; hyperosmolar coma in an infant; transient hyperglycemia in nondiabetic patients; transient retention of nitrogenous wastes; various respiratory findings secondary to the relaxation of smooth muscle, such as dyspnea, cough and choking sensation; warmth or pain along the injected vein; cellulitis without sloughing and/or phlebitis at the injection site of extravasation; back pain and increased nocturia; hypersensitivity reactions, such as rash, leukopenia and fever; papilledema induced by plasma volume expansion secondary to the administration of Diazoxide reported in a patient who had received eleven injections (300 mg/dose) over a 22-day period; malaise and blurred vision; transient cataract in an infant; hirsutism, and decreased libido.

OVERDOSAGE

Overdosage of Diazoxide, Injectable may cause an undesirable hypotension. Usually, this can be controlled with the Trendelenberg maneuver. If necessary, sympathomimetic agents, such as dopamine or norepinephrine, may be administered. Failure of blood pressure to rise in response to such agents suggests that the hypotension may have been caused by something other than Diazoxide. Excessive hyperglycemia resulting from overdosage will respond to conventional therapy of hyperglycemia.

DOSAGE AND ADMINISTRATION

Diazoxide, Injectable was originally recommended for use by bolus administration of 300 mg. Recent studies have shown that minibolus administration of Diazoxide, Injectable i.e., doses of 1 to 3 mg/kg repeated at intervals of 5 to 15 minutes is as effective in reducing blood pressure. Minibolus administration usually provides a more gradual reduction in blood pressure and thus may be expected to reduce the circulatory and neurological risks associated with acute hypotension.

Diazoxide, Injectable is administered undiluted and rapidly by intravenous injections of 1 to 3 mg/kg up to a maximum of 150 mg in a single injection. This dose may be repeated at intervals of 5 to 15 minutes until a satisfactory reduction in blood pressure (diastolic pressure below 100 mmHg) has been achieved.

With the patient recumbent, the calculated dose of Diazoxide , Injectable is administered intravenously in 30 seconds or less.

Diazoxide, Injectable should only be given into a peripheral vein. Do not administer it intramuscularly, subcutaneously, or into body cavities. Avoid extravasation of the drug into subcutaneous tissues.

Following the use of Diazoxide, Injectable, the blood pressure should be monitored closely until it has stabilized. Thereafter, measurements taken hourly during the balance of the effect should indicate any unusual response. A further decrease in blood pressure 30 minutes or more after injection should be investigated for causes other than the action of Diazoxide, Injectable. It is preferable that the patient remain supine for at least one hour after injection. In ambulatory patients, the blood pressure should also be measured with the patient standing before surveillance is ended. Repeated administration of Diazoxide, Injectable at intervals of 4 to 24 hours usually will maintain the blood pressure below pretreatment levels until a regimen of oral antihypertensive medication can be instituted. The interval between injections may be adjusted by the duration of the response to each injection. It is usually unnecessary to continue treatment with Diazoxide, Injectable for more than four to five days.

Since repeated administration of Diazoxide, Injectable can lead to sodium and water retention, administration of a diuretic may be necessary both for maximal blood pressure reduction and to avoid congestive heart failure. (See *"Clinical Pharmacology"*.)

Parenteral drug products should be inspected visually for particulate matter and discoloration prior to administration whenever solution and container permit.

Protect from light and freezing. Store between 2° and 30°C (36° and 86°F).

J CODES
Up to 300 mg IV—J1730

HOW SUPPLIED
INJECTION: 15 MG/ML

BRAND/MANUFACTURER	NDC	SIZE	AWP
◆ BRAND			
HYPERSTAT: Schering	00085-0201-05	20 ml	$83.86

Dibenzyline *SEE* PHENOXYBENZAMINE
HYDROCHLORIDE

Dichloroacetic Acid

DESCRIPTION
Dichloroacetic Acid (CHCl$_2$COOH) is a clear, colorless liquid (sp. gr. 1.56) supplied full strength ready to use. It does not contain or require a solvent or diluent, is always uniform in potency. Dichloroacetic Acid remains colorless and

retains its potency if kept in a tightly closed bottle and not contaminated with dissolved keratin or wooden applicators.

ACTIONS
Dichloroacetic Acid rapidly penetrates and cauterizes skin, keratin and other tissues. Its cauterizing effect is comparable to that obtained with such methods as electrocautery or freezing.

INDICATIONS
The lesions for which therapy with Dichloroacetic Acid is indicated are: calluses; hard and soft corns; xanthoma palpebrarum; seborrheic keratoses; ingrown nails; cysts and benign erosion of the cervix including endocervicitis and epistaxis.

CONTRAINDICATION
Topically applied chemical cauterant-keratolytics should not be used for the treatment of malignant or premalignant lesions.

WARNING
Dichloroacetic Acid is an extremely powerful keratolytic and cauterant. It should be restricted to those areas where these effects are desired.

DOSAGE AND ADMINISTRATION
The amount of Dichloroacetic Acid which should be applied varies with the nature of the lesion. Dense horny lesions such as corns and calluses require repeated extensive treatment. Lesions of light density such as xanthoma palpebrarum, soft corns, and seborrheic keratoses, should receive lighter applications.

Similarly, the number of treatments necessary will vary depending on the particular lesion being treated.

The treatment kit provides 10 mL Dichloroacetic Acid, 16 grams of petrolatum in a bottle, approximately 100 applicators, and a product insert with directions. Also included are a microdropper and holder and two sealed-stem acid receptacles of differing capacity.

HOW SUPPLIED
DEVICE:

BRAND/MANUFACTURER	NDC	SIZE	AWP
○ BRAND BICHLORACETIC ACID KAHLENBERG: Glenwood	00516-1009-00	100s	$5.24

GEL:

BRAND/MANUFACTURER	NDC	SIZE	AWP
○ BRAND BICHLORACETIC ACID KAHLENBERG: Glenwood	00516-1008-00	16 gm	$5.24

KIT:

BRAND/MANUFACTURER	NDC	SIZE	AWP
○ BRAND BICHLORACETIC ACID KAHLENBERG: Glenwood	00516-1004-11	1s	$76.51
	00516-1010-05	12s	$35.42

LIQUID:

BRAND/MANUFACTURER	NDC	SIZE	AWP
○ BRAND BICHLORACETIC ACID KAHLENBERG: Glenwood	00516-1007-11	10 ml	$43.28
	00516-1006-77	75 ml	$107.00

SOLUTION: 80%

BRAND/MANUFACTURER	NDC	SIZE	AWP
○ BRAND BICHLORACETIC ACID KAHLENBERG: Glenwood	00516-0080-15	15 ml	$37.56

Dichlorodifluoromethane and Trichloromonofluoromethane

INDICATIONS AND USAGE
Dichlorodifluoromethane/Trichloromonofluromethane spray is a vapocoolant intended for topical application in the management of myofascial pain, restricted motion, and muscle spasm, and for the control of pain associated with injections.

Clinical conditions that may respond to Spray and Stretch include low back pain (due to muscle spasm), acute stiff neck, torticollis, muscle spasm associated with osteoarthritis, ankle sprain, tight hamstring, masseter muscle spasm, certain types of headache, and referred pain due to trigger points. Relief of pain facilitates early mobilization in restoration of muscle function.

PRECAUTIONS
Care should be taken to minimize inhalation of vapors, especially with application around head or neck. Avoid contact with eyes. Dichlorodifluoromethane/Trichloromonofluoromethane should not be applied to the point of frost formation.

ADVERSE REACTIONS
Cutaneous sensitization may occur, but appears to be extremely rare. Freezing can occasionally alter pigmentation.

CONTRAINDICATIONS
Dichlorodifluoromethane/Trichloromonofluoromethane is contraindicated in individuals with a history of hypersensitivity to either agent. This product should not be used on patients having vascular impairment of the extremities.

WARNINGS
For external use only.

Dichlorodifluoromethane and Trichloromonofluoromethane are not classified as carcinogens. Based on animal studies and human experience, these fluorocarbons pose no hazard to man relative to systemic toxicity, carcinogenicity, mutagenicity, or teratogenicity when occupational exposure are below 1000 p.p.m. over an 8 hour time weighted average.

Contents under pressure. Store in a cool place. Do not store above 120°F. Do not store on or near high frequency ultrasound equipment.

DOSAGE AND ADMINISTRATION
To apply Dichlorodifluoromethane/Trichloromonofluoromethane invert the bottle over the treatment area approximately 12 inches (30 cm.) away from site of application. Open dispenseal spring valve completely, allowing the liquid to flow in a stream from the bottle.

1. Spray and Stretch Technique for Myofascial Pain
Spray and Stretch technique is a therapeutic system which involves three stages: EVALUATION, SPRAYING, and STRETCHING.

The therapeutic value of Spray and Stretch becomes most effective when the practitioner has mastered all stages and applies them in proper sequence.

I. Evaluation
During the evaluation phase the cause of pain is determined as local spasm or an irritated trigger point. The method of applying the spray to a muscle spasm differs slightly from application to a trigger point. A trigger point is a deep hypersensitive localized spot in a muscle which causes a referred pain pattern. With trigger points the source of pain is seldom the site of the pain. A trigger point may be detected by a snapping palpation over the muscle, causing the muscle in which the irritated trigger point is situated to "jump."

II. Spraying

A. Patient should assume a comfortable position.
B. Take precautions to cover the patient's eyes, nose, mouth, if spraying near face.
C. Hold bottle in an upside down position 12 to 18 inches (30 to 45 cm.) away from the treatment surface allowing the jet stream of vapocoolant to meet the skin at an acute angle to lessen the shock of impact.
D. The spray is directed in parallel sweeps 1.5 to 2 cm. apart. The rate of spraying is approximately 10 cm/sec. and is continued until the entire muscle has been covered. The number of sweeps is determined by the size of the muscle. In the case of a trigger point, the spray should be applied over the trigger point, through and over the reference zone. In the case of muscle spasm, the spray should be applied from origin to insertion.

III. Stretching
During application of the spray, the muscle is passively stretched. Force is gradually increased with successive sweeps, and the slack is smoothly taken up as the muscle relaxes, establishing a new stretch length.

Reaching the full normal length of the muscle is necessary to completely inactive trigger points and relieve pain.

After rewarming, the procedure may be repeated as necessary. Moist heat should be applied for 10 to 15 minutes following treatment.

For lasting benefit, any factors that perpetuate the trigger mechanism must be eliminated.

2. Pre-Injection Anesthesia
Prepare syringe and have it ready. Spray skin with Dichlorodifluoromethane/Trichloromonofluoromethane from a distance of about 12 inches (30 cm.) continuously for 3 to 5 seconds; do not frost the skin. Swab skin with alcohol and quickly introduce needle with skin taut.

HOW SUPPLIED
SPRAY:

BRAND/MANUFACTURER	NDC	SIZE	AWP
○ GENERICS Gebauer	00386-0003-04	120 ml	$14.73
Gebauer	00386-0003-05	120 ml	$14.73

Dichlorotetrafluoroethane and Ethyl Chloride

INDICATIONS AND USAGE
Dichlorotetrafluoroethane/Ethyl Chloride is a topical refrigerant anesthetic intended to control the pain associated with minor surgical procedures, dermabrasion, injections, contusions and minor strains.

◆ RATED THERAPEUTICALLY EQUIVALENT; ◇ THERAPEUTIC EQUIVALENCE UNCONFIRMED; ○ UNRATED

PRECAUTIONS
Inhalation of Dichlorotetrafluoroethane/Ethyl Chloride should be avoided as it may produce narcotic and general anesthetic effects, and may produce deep anesthesia, or fatal coma with respiratory or cardiac arrest. When used to produce local freezing of tissues, adjacent skin areas should be protected by application of petrolatum. The thawing process may be painful, and freezing may lower local resistance to infection and delay healing.

ADVERSE REACTIONS
Cutaneous sensitization may occur, but appears to be extremely rare. Freezing can occasionally alter pigmentation. Frostbite may occur.

CONTRAINDICATIONS
Dichlorotetrafluoroethane/Ethyl Chloride is contraindicated in individuals with a history of hypersensitivity to Ethyl Chloride or Dichlorotetrafluoroethane. Dichlorotetrafluoroethane/Ethyl Chloride should not be used on patients having vascular impairment of the extremities.

WARNINGS
For external use only.

The components of Dichlorotetrafluoroethane/Ethyl Chloride are not listed as carcinogens by IARC, NTP or OSHA. Based on animal studies and human experiences this mixture poses no hazard to man relative to systemic toxicity, carcinogenicity, mutagenicity, or teratogenicity when occupational exposures are below its recommended exposure limits.

Skin absorption of Ethyl Chloride can occur; no cases of chronic poisoning have been reported. Ethyl Chloride is known as a liver and kidney toxin; long term exposure may cause liver or kidney damage.

Dichlorotetrafluoroethane/Ethyl Chloride can cause frostbite.

Contents under pressure. Store in a cool place, do not store above 120°F.

DOSAGE AND ADMINISTRATION
To apply Dichlorotetrafluoroethane/Ethyl Chloride invert the container over the treatment area approximately 2 to 4 inches (5-10cm) from the site of application. Press gently on side of the spray valve allowing the liquid to emerge as a fine mist spray.

1. TOPICAL ANESTHESIA IN MINOR SURGERY
The operative site should be cleansed with a suitable antiseptic. Apply petrolatum to protect the adjacent area. Spray Dichlorotetrafluoroethane/Ethyl Chloride for a few seconds to the point of frost formation, when the tissue becomes white. Avoid prolonged spraying of skin beyond this state. The anesthetic action of Dichlorotetrafluoroethane/Ethyl Chloride rarely lasts more than a few seconds to a minute. Quickly swab operative site with antiseptic and promptly make incision. Reapply as needed.

2. DERMABRASION
The operative site should be cleansed with a suitable antiseptic. Apply petrolatum to protect adjacent areas. Take precautions to cover the patient's eyes, nose, mouth, if spraying near the face. To firm the skin and numb the dermabrasion site, spray treatment area for 20 to 30 seconds prior to starting the dermabrasion procedure. Reapply as necessary during the procedure to maintain desired skin firmness.

3. FOR PRE-INJECTION ANESTHESIA
Prepare syringe and have it ready. Spray skin with Dichlorotetrafluoroethane/Ethyl Chloride from a distance of about 4 inches (10 cm) continuously for 2 to 3 seconds; do not frost skin. Swab skin with alcohol and quickly introduce needle with skin taut.

4. CONTUSIONS AND MINOR STRAINS
The pain of bruises, contusions, and minor sprains may be controlled with Dichlorotetrafluoroethane/Ethyl Chloride.

Spray affected area from a distance of 6 to 12 inches (15 to 30 cm) for a few seconds until the tissue begins to frost and turn white. Avoid spraying of skin beyond this state. Use as you would ice. The amount of cooling depends on the dosage. The smallest dose needed to produce the desired effect should be used.

Determine the extent of injury (fracture, sprain, etc.). The anesthetic effect of Dichlorotetrafluoroethane/Ethyl Chloride rarely lasts more than a few seconds to a minute. This time interval is usually sufficient to help reduce or relieve the initial trauma of the injury.

HOW SUPPLIED
SPRAY:

BRAND/MANUFACTURER	NDC	SIZE	AWP
○ BRAND FLURO-ETHYL: Gebauer	00386-0002-09	270 ml	$16.61

Dichlorphenamide

DESCRIPTION
Dichlorphenamide is an oral carbonic anhydrase inhibitor. Dichlorphenamide, a dichlorinated benzenedisulfonamide, is known chemically as 4,5-dichloro-1,3-benzenedisulfonamide. Its empirical formula is $C_6H_6Cl_2N_2O_4S_2$.

Dichlorphenamide is a white or practically white, crystalline compound with a molecular weight of 305.16. It is very slightly soluble in water but soluble in dilute solutions of sodium carbonate and sodium hydroxide. Dilute alkaline solutions of Dichlorphenamide are stable at room temperature.

Dichlorphenamide is supplied as tablets, for oral administration, each containing 50 mg.

Following is its chemical structure:

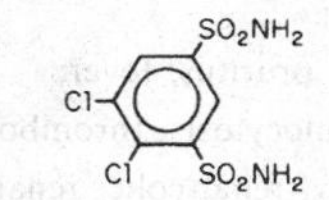

CLINICAL PHARMACOLOGY
Carbonic anhydrase inhibitors reduce intraocular pressure by partially suppressing the secretion of aqueous humor (inflow), although the mechanism by which they do this is not fully understood. Evidence suggests that HCO_3^- ions are produced in the ciliary body by hydration of carbon dioxide under the influence of carbonic anhydrase and diffuse into the posterior chamber with Na^+ ions. The aqueous fluid contains more Na^+ and HCO_3^- ions than dose plasma and consequently is hypertonic. Water is attracted to the posterior chamber by osmosis. Systemic administration of a carbonic anhydrase inhibitor has been shown to inactivate carbonic anhydrase in the ciliary body of the rabbit's eye and to reduce the high concentration of HCO_3^- ions in ocular fluids. As is the case with all carbonic anhydrase inhibitors, Dichlorphenamide in high doses causes some decrease in renal blood flow and glomerular filtration rate.

In man, Dichlorphenamide begins to act within an hour and maximal effect is observed in two to four hours. The lowered intraocular tension may be maintained for approximately 6 to 12 hours.

INDICATIONS AND USAGE
For adjunctive treatment of: chronic simple (open-angle) glaucoma, secondary glaucoma, and preoperatively in acute angle-closure glaucoma where delay of surgery is desired in order to lower intraocular pressure.

CONTRAINDICATIONS
Dichlorphenamide is contraindicated in hepatic insufficiency, renal failure, adrenocortical insufficiency, hyperchloremic acidosis, or in conditions in which serum levels of sodium or potassium are depressed. Dichlorphenamide should not be used in patients with severe pulmonary obstruction who are unable to increase their alveolar ventilation since their acidosis may be increased.

Dichlorphenamide is contraindicated in patients who are hypersensitive to this product.

PRECAUTIONS
GENERAL
Potassium excretion is increased by Dichlorphenamide and hypokalemia may develop with brisk diuresis, when severe cirrhosis is present, or during concomitant use of steroids or ACTH.

Interference with adequate oral electrolyte intake will also contribute to hypokalemia. Hypokalemia can sensitize or exaggerate the response of the heart to the toxic effects of digitalis (e.g., increased ventricular irritability). Hypokalemia may be avoided or treated by use of potassium supplements such as foods with a high potassium content. Dichlorphenamide should be used with caution in patients with respiratory acidosis.

DRUG INTERACTIONS
Caution is advised in patients receiving concomitant high-dose aspirin and carbonic anhydrase inhibitors, as anorexia, tachypnea, lethargy and coma have been rarely reported due to a possible drug interaction.

CARCINOGENESIS, MUTAGENESIS, IMPAIRMENT OF FERTILITY
Long-term studies in animals have not been performed to evaluate the effects upon fertility or carcinogenic potential of Dichlorphenamide.

PREGNANCY
Pregnancy Category C. Dichlorphenamide has been shown to be teratogenic in the rat (skeletal anomalies) when given in doses 100 times the human dose. There are no adequate and well-controlled studies in pregnant women. Dichlorphenamide should not be used in women of childbearing age or in pregnancy, especially during the first trimester, unless the potential benefits outweigh the potential risks.

NURSING MOTHERS
It is not known whether Dichlorphenamide is excreted in human milk. Because many drugs are excreted in human milk, caution should be exercised when Dichlorphenamide is administered to a nursing woman.

PEDIATRIC USE
Safety and effectiveness in children have not been established.

ADVERSE REACTIONS
Certain side effects characteristics of carbonic anhydrase inhibitors may occur with Dichlorphenamide, particularly with increasing doses. The most common effects include gastrointestinal disturbances (anorexia, nausea, and vomiting), drowsiness and paresthesias.

Included in the listing which follows are some adverse reactions which have not been reported with Dichlorphenamide. However, pharmacological similarities among the carbonic anhydrase inhibitors make it advisable to consider the following reactions when Dichlorphenamide is administered.

Central Nervous System/Psychiatric: ataxia, tremor, tinnitus, headache, weakness, nervousness, globus hystericus, lassitude, depression, confusion, disorientation, dizziness;

Gastrointestinal: constipation, hepatic insufficiency;

Metabolic: loss of weight, metabolic acidosis, electrolyte imbalance (hypokalemia, hyperchloremia), hyperuricemia;

Hypersensitivity: skin eruptions, pruritus, fever;

Hematologic: leukopenia, agranulocytosis, thrombocytopenia;

Genitourinary: urinary frequency, renal colic, renal calculi, phosphaturia.

OVERDOSAGE

The oral LD_{50} of Dichlorphenamide is 1710 and 2600 mg/kg in the mouse and rat respectively.

Symptoms of overdosage or toxicity may include drowsiness, anorexia, nausea, vomiting, dizziness, paresthesias, ataxia, tremor and tinnitus.

In the event of overdosage, induce emesis or perform gastric lavage. The electrolyte disturbance most likely to be encountered from overdosage is hyperchloremic acidosis that may respond to bicarbonate administration. Potassium supplementation may be required. The patient should be carefully observed and given supportive treatment.

DOSAGE AND ADMINISTRATION

Dichlorphenamide is usually given in conjunction with topical ocular hypotensive agents. In acute angle-closure glaucoma, it may be used together with miotics and osmotic agents in an attempt to reduce intraocular tension rapidly. If this is not quickly relieved, surgery may be mandatory.

Dosage must be adjusted carefully to meet the requirements of the individual patient. A priming dose of 100 to 200 mg of Dichlorphenamide (2 to 4 tablets) is suggested for adults, followed by 100 mg (2 tablets) every 12 hours until the desired response has been obtained. The recommended maintenance dosage for adults is 25 to 50 mg (½ to 1 tablet) once to three times daily.

HOW SUPPLIED
TABLETS: 50 MG

BRAND/MANUFACTURER	NDC	SIZE	AWP
○ BRAND			
DARANIDE: Merck	00006-0049-68	100s	$48.56

Diclofenac, Ophthalmic

DESCRIPTION

Diclofenac, Ophthalmic (Diclofenac Sodium) solution is a sterile, topical, nonsteroidal, anti-inflammatory product for ophthalmic use. Diclofenac Sodium is designated chemically as 2-[(2,6-dichlorophenyl) amino] benzeneacetic acid, monosodium salt, with an empirical formula of $C_{14}H_{10}CL_2NO_2Na$.

Diclofenac, Ophthalmic is available as a sterile solution. Each ml of solution contains: Diclofenac Sodium 1 mg Diclofenac Sodium is a faintly yellow-white to light-beige, slightly hygroscopic crystalline powder. It is freely soluble in methanol, sparingly soluble in water, very slightly soluble in acetonitrile, and insoluble in chloroform and in 0.1 N hydrochloric acid. Its molecular weight is 318.14. Diclofenac, Ophthalmic is an iso-osmotic physiologically compatible solution with an osmolality of about 300 mOsmol/1000 g, buffered at approximately pH 7.2.

Following is its chemical structure:

CLINICAL PHARMACOLOGY

Diclofenac Sodium is one of a series of phenylacetic acids that have demonstrated anti-inflammatory and analgesic properties in pharmacological studies. It is thought to inhibit the enzyme cyclooxygenase, which is essential in the biosynthesis of prostaglandins.

Prostaglandins have been shown in many animal models to be mediators of certain kinds of intraocular inflammation. In studies performed in animal eyes, prostaglandins have been shown to produce disruption of the blood-aqueous humor barrier, vasodilation, increased vascular permeability, leukocytosis, and increased intraocular pressure. Prostaglandins also appear to play a role in the mitotic response produced during ocular surgery by constricting the iris sphincter independently of cholinergic mechanisms. In clinical studies, Diclofenac, Ophthalmic has been shown to decrease the signs and symptoms of inflammation resulting from cataract surgery.

Results from clinical studies indicate that Diclofenac, Ophthalmic has no significant effect upon intraocular pressure; however, elevations in intraocular pressure may occur following cataract surgery.

Results from a bioavailability study established that plasma levels of Diclofenac following ocular instillation of two drops of Diclofenac, Ophthalmic to each eye were below the limit of quantitation (10 ng/mL) over a 4-hour period. This study suggests that limited, if any, systemic absorption occurs with Diclofenac, Ophthalmic.

In two doubled-masked, controlled, efficacy studies of postoperative inflammation, a total of 206 cataract patients were treated with Diclofenac, Ophthalmic and 103 patients were treated with vehicle placebo. Diclofenac, Ophthalmic was statistically favored over vehicle placebo at all three visits over a 2-week period for the clinical assessments of inflammation (anterior chamber cells and flare, conjunctival erythema and ciliary flush). Patients who participated in two other trials were safely continued on Diclofenac, Ophthalmic for a period of up to 6 weeks.

In two separate, double-masked, comparative studies the effects of Diclofenac, Ophthalmic and prednisolone sodium phosphate 1% on the blood-aqueous humor barrier were examined by anterior chamber fluorophotometry at 1 week post surgery. One study compared 27 patients in the Diclofenac, Ophthalmic group with 32 patients in the prednisolone group, and the other compared 32 patients in the Diclofenac, Ophthalmic group with 35 patients in the prednisolone group. Diclofenac, Ophthalmic was statistically more effective than prednisolone in expediting reestablishment of the blood-aqueous humor barrier disrupted by cataract extraction. However, the clinical benefit or harm in the reestablishment of the blood-aqueous barrier is unknown.

Diclofenac, Ophthalmic has been safely administered in conjunction with other ophthalmic medications such as antibiotics, beta blockers, carbonic anhydrase inhibitors, cycloplegics, and mydriatics.

INDICATIONS AND USAGE

Diclofenac, Ophthalmic is indicated for the treatment of postoperative inflammation in patients who have undergone cataract extraction.

CONTRAINDICATIONS

Diclofenac, Ophthalmic is contraindicated in patients concurrently wearing soft contact lenses and in patients who are hypersensitive to any component of the medication. Patients wearing hydrogel soft contact lenses who have used Diclofenac, Ophthalmic concurrently have experienced ocular irritation manifested by redness and burning.

WARNING

There is the potential for cross-sensitivity to acetylsalicylic acid, phenylacetic acid derivatives, and other nonsteroidal anti-inflammatory agents. Therefore, caution should be used when treating individuals who have previously exhibited sensitivities to these drugs.

With some nonsteroidal anti-inflammatory drugs, there exists the potential for increased bleeding time due to interference with thrombocyte aggregation. There have been reports that ocularly applied nonsteroidal anti-inflammatory drugs may cause increased bleeding of ocular tissues (including hyphemas) in conjunction with ocular surgery.

PRECAUTION

General: It is recommended that Diclofenac, Ophthalmic be used with caution in surgical patients with known bleeding tendencies or who are receiving other medications that may prolong bleeding time.

Diclofenac Sodium may slow or delay healing.

Carcinogenesis, Mutagenesis, Impairment of Fertility: Long-term carcinogenicity studies in rats given oral Diclofenac Sodium up to 2 mg/kg/day (approximately the human oral dose) have revealed no significant increases in tumor incidence. There was a slight increase in benign rat mammary fibroadenomas in mid-dose females (high-dose females had excessive mortality) but the increase was not significant for this common rat tumor. A 2-year carcinogenicity study conducted in mice employing oral Diclofenac Sodium up to 2 mg/kg/day did not reveal any oncogenic potential. Diclofenac Sodium did not show mutagenic potential in various mutagenicity studies including the Ames test. Diclofenac Sodium administered to male and female rats at 4 mg/kg/day did not affect fertility.

Pregnancy: Teratogenic Effects: Pregnancy Category B: Reproduction studies performed in mice at oral doses up to 5,000 times (20 mg/kg/day) and in rats and rabbits at oral doses up to 2,500 times (10 mg/kg/day) the human topical dose have revealed no evidence of teratogenicity due to Diclofenac Sodium, despite the induction of maternal toxicity and fetal toxicity. In rats, maternally toxic doses were associated with dystocia, prolonged gestation, reduced fetal weights and growth, and reduced fetal survival. Diclofenac Sodium has been shown to cross the placental barrier in mice and rats.

There are, however, no adequate and well-controlled studies in pregnant women. Because animal reproduction studies are not always predictive of human response, this drug should be used during pregnancy only if clearly needed.

Nonteratogenic Effects: Because of the known effects of prostaglandin-inhibiting drugs on the fetal cardiovascular system (closure of the ductus arteriosus), the use of Diclofenac, Ophthalmic during late pregnancy should be avoided.

Pediatric Use: Safety and effectiveness in children have not been established.

ADVERSE REACTIONS

Ocular: Transient burning and stinging was reported in 15% of patients across all studies with the use of topical Diclofenac, Ophthalmic. In cataract studies, keratitis occurred in 28% of patients receiving Diclofenac, Ophthalmic; most of the cases of keratitis occurred prior to drug therapy. Elevated intraocular pressure was reported in 15% of patients receiving Diclofenac, Ophthalmic, most of these cases occurred post surgery and prior to drug administration.

Other ocular medical problems included anterior chamber reaction and ocular allergy.

◆ RATED THERAPEUTICALLY EQUIVALENT; ◇ THERAPEUTIC EQUIVALENCE UNCONFIRMED; ○ UNRATED

Systemic: Nausea and vomiting occurred in 1% of patients receiving Diclofenac, Ophthalmic and in 0.5% of patients receiving vehicle alone. Viral infections occurred in ≤ 1% of each of the Diclofenac, Ophthalmic and vehicle groups.

OVERDOSAGE
Overdosage will not ordinarily cause acute problems. If accidentally ingested, fluids should be taken to dilute the medication.

DOSAGE AND ADMINISTRATION
One drop of Diclofenac, Ophthalmic should be applied to the affected eye four times daily beginning 24 hours after cataract surgery and continuing throughout the first 2 weeks of the postoperative period.

Store between 59°-86° F (15°-30° C). Protect from light.

Dispense in original, unopened container only.

HOW SUPPLIED
DROP: 0.1%

BRAND/MANUFACTURER	NDC	SIZE	AWP
○ **BRAND**			
VOLTAREN: Ciba Ophth	58768-0100-02	2.5 ml	$17.59
	58768-0100-05	5 ml	$27.44

Diclofenac, Oral

DESCRIPTION
Diclofenac, as the sodium or potassium salt, is a benzeneacetic acid derivative, designated chemically as 2-[(2,6-dichlorophenyl)amino] benzeneacetic acid, monosodium or monopotassium salt.

Diclofenac, as the sodium or potassium salt, is a faintly yellowish white to light beige, virtually odorless, slightly hygroscopic crystalline powder. Molecular weights of the sodium and potassium salts are 318.14 and 334.25, respectively. It is freely soluble in methanol, soluble in ethanol, and practically insoluble in chloroform and in dilute acid. Diclofenac sodium is sparingly soluble in water while Diclofenac potassium is soluble in water. The n-octanol/water partition coefficient is, for both Diclofenac salts, 13.4 at pH 7.4 and 1545 at pH 5.2. Both salts have a single dissociation constant (pKa) of 4.0 ± 0.2 at 25°C in water.

Diclofenac sodium is available as Diclofenac Delayed-Release (enteric-coated) Tablets of 25 mg, 50 mg, and 75 mg for oral administration.

Diclofenac potassium is available as Diclofenac Immediate-Release Tablets of 50 mg for oral administration.

CLINICAL PHARMACOLOGY
PHARMACODYNAMICS
Diclofenac, the anion, is a nonsteroidal anti-inflammatory drug (NSAID). In pharmacologic studies, Diclofenac has shown anti-inflammatory, analgesic, and antipyretic activity. As with other NSAIDs, its mode of action is not known; its ability to inhibit prostaglandin synthesis, however, may be involved in its anti-inflammatory activity, as well as contribute to its efficacy in relieving pain related to inflammation and primary dysmenorrhea. With regard to its analgesic effect, Diclofenac is not a narcotic.

PHARMACOKINETICS
Diclofenac Delayed-Release Tablets and Immediate-Release Tablets both contain the same therapeutic moiety, Diclofenac. They differ in the cationic portion of the salt (see *"Description"*) as well as in their release characteristics. Diclofenac Delayed-Release (enteric-coated) Tablets are in a pharmaceutical formulation that resists dissolution in the low pH of gastric fluid but allows a rapid release of drug in the higher pH-environment in the duodenum. Conversely, Diclofenac Immediate-Release Tablets are formulated to release Diclofenac in the stomach. The primary pharmacokinetic difference between the two products is in the pattern of drug release and absorption, as illustrated.

± 1 SD Plasma Diclofenac Sodium Concentration after a Single Dose of a Diclofenac Sodium Tablet 50 mg (N=38) and a Diclofenac Potassium Tablet 50 mg (N=48).

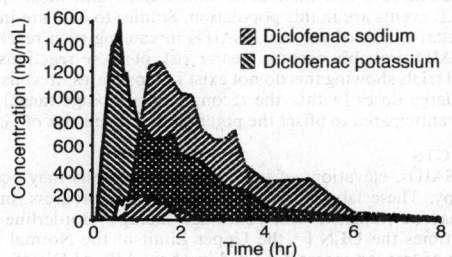

For this reason, separate sections are provided below to describe the different absorption profiles of Diclofenac Sodium Delayed-Release Tablets and Diclofenac Potassium Immediate-Release Tablets.

ABSORPTION
Diclofenac Sodium Delayed-Release Tablets: Diclofenac is completely absorbed from the gastrointestinal tract after fasting oral administration of Diclofenac. Of this, only 50% of the absorbed, dose of Diclofenac from Diclofenac Sodium is systemically available, due to first pass metabolism. Peak plasma levels are achieved in 2 hours in fasting normal volunteers, with a range from 1 to 4 hours. The area-under-the-plasma-concentration curve (AUC) is dose-proportional within the range of 25 mg to 150 mg. Peak plasma levels are less than dose-proportional and are approximately 1.0, 1.5, and 2.0 µg/mL for 25-mg, 50-mg, and 75-mg doses, respectively. It should be noted that the administration of several individual Diclofenac Sodium tablets may not yield equivalent results in peak concentration as the administration of one tablet of a higher strength. This is probably due to the staggered gastric emptying of tablets into the duodenum. After repeated oral administration of Diclofenac Sodium 50 mg b.i.d., Diclofenac did not accumulate in plasma.

When Diclofenac Sodium is taken with food, there is usually a delay in the onset of absorption of 1 to 4.5 hours, with delays as long as 10 hours in some patients, and a reduction in peak plasma levels of approximately 40%. The extent of absorption of Diclofenac Sodium however, is not significantly affected by food intake.

Diclofenac Potassium Immediate-Release Tablets: Diclofenac is rapidly and completely absorbed from the gastrointestinal tract, with measurable plasma levels being observed, in some fasting volunteers, within 10 minutes of dosing with Diclofenac Potassium. Peak plasma levels are achieved in approximately 1 hour in fasting normal volunteers, with a range from 0.33 to 2 hours. Only 50% of the absorbed dose of Diclofenac from Diclofenac Potassium systemically available, due to first pass metabolism.

The extent of absorption of Diclofenac from Diclofenac Potassium tablets is comparable to that from a buffered solution of Diclofenac Potassium. After repeated oral administration of Diclofenac Potassium 50 mg t.i.d., no accumulation of Diclofenac in plasma occurred.

The extent of Diclofenac absorption is not significantly affected when Diclofenac Potassium is taken with food. However, the rate of absorption is reduced by food, as indicated by a delay in T_{max} and decrease in C_{max} values by approximately 30%.

DISTRIBUTION
Plasma concentrations of Diclofenac decline from peak levels in a biexponential fashion, with the terminal phase having a half-life of approximately 2 hours. Clearance and volume of distribution are about 350 mL/min and 550 mL/kg, respectively. More than 99% of Diclofenac is reversibly bound to human plasma albumin.

A 4-week study, comparing plasma level profiles of Diclofenac Sodium 50 mg b.i.d., in younger (26-46 years) versus older (66-81 years) adults, did not show differences between age groups (10 patients per age group).

As with other NSAIDs, Diclofenac diffuses into and out of the synovial fluid. Diffusion into the joint occurs when plasma levels are higher than those in the synovial fluid, after which the process reverses and synovial fluid levels are higher than plasma levels. It is not known whether diffusion into the joint plays a role in the effectiveness of Diclofenac.

METABOLISM AND ELIMINATION
Diclofenac is eliminated through metabolism and subsequent urinary and biliary excretion of the glucuronide and the sulfate conjugates of the metabolites. Approximately 65% of the dose is excreted in the urine, and approximately 35% in the bile.

Conjugates of unchanged Diclofenac account for 5%-10% of the dose excreted in the urine and for less than 5% excreted in the bile. Little or no unchanged unconjugated drug is excreted. Conjugates of the principal metabolite account for 20%-30% of the dose excreted in the urine and for 10%-20% of the dose excreted in the bile. Conjugates of three other metabolites together account for 10%-20% of the dose excreted in the urine and for small amounts excreted in the bile. The elimination half-life values for these metabolites are shorter than those for the parent drug. Urinary excretion of an additional metabolite (half-life 80 hours) accounts for only 1.4% of the oral dose. The degree of accumulation of Diclofenac metabolites is unknown. Some of the metabolites may have activity.

PATIENTS WITH RENAL AND/OR HEPATIC IMPAIRMENT
To date, no differences in the pharmacokinetics of Diclofenac have been detected in studies of patients with renal (50 mg intravenously) or hepatic impairment (100 mg oral solution). In patients with renal impairment (N = 5, creatinine clearance 3 to 42 mL/min), AUC values and elimination rates were comparable to those in healthy subjects. In patients with biopsy-confirmed cirrhosis or chronic active hepatitis (variably elevated transaminases and mildly elevated bilirubins, N = 10), Diclofenac concentrations and urinary elimination values were comparable to those in healthy subjects.

CLINICAL STUDIES
Diclofenac Sodium Delayed-Release Tablets in Osteoarthritis: Diclofenac Sodium was evaluated for the management of the signs and symptoms of osteoarthritis of the hip or knee in a total of 633 patients treated for up to 3 months in placebo- and active-controlled clinical trials against aspirin (N = 449), and naproxen (N = 92). Diclofenac Sodium was given both in variable (100-150 mg/day) and fixed (150 mg/day) dosing schedules in either b.i.d. or t.i.d dosing regimens. In these trials, Diclofenac Sodium was found to be comparable to 2400 to 3600 mg/day of aspirin or 500 mg/day of naproxen. Diclofenac Sodium was effective when administered as either b.i.d. or t.i.d. dosing regimens.

Diclofenac Sodium Delayed-Release Tablets in Rheumatoid Arthritis: Diclofenac Sodium was evaluated for managing the signs and symptoms of rheumatoid arthritis in a total of 468 patients treated for up to 3 months in placebo- and active-controlled clinical trials against aspirin (N = 290), and ibuprofen (N = 74). Diclofenac Sodium was given in a fixed (150 or 200 mg/day) dosing schedule as either b.i.d. or t.i.d. dosing regimens. Diclofenac Sodium was found to be comparable to 3600 to 4800 mg/day of aspirin, and 2400 mg/day of ibuprofen. Diclofenac Sodium was used b.i.d. or t.i.d., administering 150 mg/day in most trials, but 50 mg q.i.d. (200 mg/day) was also studied.

Diclofenac Sodium Delayed-Release Tablets in Ankylosing Spondylitis: Diclofenac Sodium was evaluated for the management of the signs and symptoms of ankylosing spondylitis in a total of 132 patients in one active-controlled clinical trial against indomethacin (N = 130). Both Diclofenac Sodium and indomethacin patients were started on 25 mg t.i.d. and were permitted to increase the dose 25 mg/day each week to a maximum dose of 125 mg/day. Diclofenac Sodium 75-125 mg/day was found to be comparable to indomethacin 75-125 mg/day.

Diclofenac Potassium Immediate-Release Tablets in Analgesia/Primary Dysmenorrhea: The analgesic efficacy of Diclofenac Potassium was demonstrated in trials of patients with postoperative pain (following gynecologic, oral, and orthopedic surgery), osteoarthritis of the knee, and primary dysmenorrhea. The effectiveness of Diclofenac Potassium in studies of pain or primary dysmenorrhea showed that onset of analgesia began, in some patients, as soon as 30 minutes, and relief of pain lasted as long as 8 hours, following single 50-mg or 100-mg doses. Duration of pain relief was judged by the time at which approximately half of the patients needed remedication. The onset and duration of pain relief for either the 50-mg or 100-mg dose was essentially the same, whether patients had moderate or severe pain at baseline.

Diclofenac Potassium was studied in single-dose and multiple-dose pain trials. The pain models in single-dose studies were post-dental extraction and post-gynecologic surgery: the efficacy of the 50-mg dose (N = 258) and the 100-mg dose (N = 255) was comparable to aspirin 650 mg in onset of pain relief, but generally provided a longer duration of analgesia than aspirin. The pain models for multiple-dose trials were post-orthopedic surgery pain as well as pain associated with primary dysmenorrhea: the efficacy of the 50-mg dose (N = 101) and the 100-mg dose (N = 442), followed by 50 mg every 8 hours, was comparable to naproxen sodium 550 mg followed by 275 mg every 8 hours. In one study of chronic pain, in patients with osteoarthritis (N = 196), Diclofenac Potassium 50 mg t.i.d. was comparable in efficacy to ibuprofen 800 mg t.i.d. and Diclofenac Sodium Delayed-Release Tablets 50 mg t.i.d.

G.I. Blood Loss/Endoscopy Data: G.I. blood loss and endoscopy studies were performed with Diclofenac Sodium Delayed-Release (enteric-coated) Tablets that, unlike Immediate-Release Tablets, do not dissolve in the stomach where the endoscopic lesions are primarily seen; Diclofenac Potassium Immediate-Release Tablets have not been similarly studied. A repeat-dose endoscopy study, in patients with rheumatoid arthritis or osteoarthritis treated with Diclofenac Sodium Delayed-Release Tablets 75 mg b.i.d. (N = 101), or naproxen (immediate-release tablets) 500 mg b.i.d. (N = 103) for 3 months, resulted in a significantly smaller number of patients with an increase in endoscopy score from baseline and a significantly lower mean endoscopy score after treatment in the Diclofenac Sodium-treated patients. Two repeat-dose endoscopic studies, in normal volunteers showed that daily doses of Diclofenac Sodium Delayed-Release Tablets 75 or 100 mg (N = 6 and N = 14, respectively) for 1 week caused fewer gastric lesions, and those that did occur had lower scores than those observed following daily 500-mg doses of naproxen (immediate-release tablets). In healthy subjects, the daily administration of 150 mg of Diclofenac Sodium (N = 8) for 3 weeks resulted in a mean fecal blood loss less than that observed with 3.0 g of aspirin daily (N = 8). In four repeat-dose studies, mean fecal blood loss with 150 mg of Diclofenac Sodium was also less than that observed with 750 mg of naproxen (N = 8 and N = 6) or 150 mg of indomethacin (N = 8 and N = 6). *The clinical significance of these findings is unknown since there is no evidence available to indicate that Diclofenac Sodium is less likely than other drugs of its class to cause serious gastrointestinal lesions when used in chronic therapy.*

INDIVIDUALIZATION OF DOSAGE

Diclofenac, like other NSAIDs, shows interindividual differences in both pharmacokinetics and clinical response (pharmacodynamics). Consequently, the recommended strategy for initiating therapy is to use a starting dose likely to be effective for the majority of patients and to adjust dosage thereafter based on observation of Diclofenac's beneficial and adverse effects.

In patients weighing less than 60 kg (132 lb), or where the severity of the disease, concomitant medication, or other diseases warrant, the maximum recommended total daily dose of Diclofenac should be reduced. Experience with other NSAIDs has shown that starting therapy with maximum doses in patients at increased risk due to renal or hepatic disease, low body weight (< 60 kg), advanced age, a known ulcer diathesis, or known sensitivity to NSAID effects, is likely to increase frequency of adverse reactions and is not recommended (see *"Precautions"*).

Osteoarthritis/Rheumatoid Arthritis/Ankylosing Spondylitis: The usual starting dose of Diclofenac Delayed-Release or Immediate-Release Tablets for patients with osteoarthritis, is 100 to 150 mg/day, using a b.i.d. or t.i.d. dosing regimen. In two variable-dose clinical trials in osteoarthritis, of 266 patients started on 100 mg/day, 176 chose to increase the dose to 150 mg/day. Dosages above 150 mg/day have not been studied in patients with osteoarthritis.

The usual starting dose of Diclofenac Sodium Delayed-Release or Diclofenac Potassium Immediate-Release Tablets for most patients with rheumatoid arthritis is 150 mg/day, using a b.i.d. or t.i.d. dosing regimen. Patients requiring more relief of pain and inflammation may increase the dose to 200 mg/day. In clinical

trials, patients receiving 200 mg/day were less likely to drop from the trial due to lack of efficacy than patients receiving 150 mg/day. Dosages above 225 mg/day are not recommended in patients with rheumatoid arthritis because of increased risk of adverse events.

The recommended dose of Diclofenac Sodium Delayed-Release Tablets for patients with ankylosing spondylitis is 100 to 125 mg/day, using a q.i.d. dosing regimen (see *"Dosage and Administration"*) regarding the 125 mg/day dosing regimen). In a variable-dose clinical trial, of 132 patients started on 75 mg/day, 122 chose to increase the dose to 125 mg/day. Dosages above 125 mg/day have not been studied in patients with ankylosing spondylitis.

Analgesia/Primary Dysmenorrhea: Because of earlier absorption of Diclofenac from Diclofenac Potassium Immediate-Release Tablets, it is the formulation indicated for management of pain and primary dysmenorrhea when prompt onset of pain relief is desired. The results of clinical trials suggest an initial Diclofenac Potassium dose of 50 mg for pain or for primary dysmenorrhea, followed by doses of 50 mg every 8 hours, as needed. With experience, some patients with recurring pain, such as dysmenorrhea, may find that an initial dose of 100 mg of Diclofenac Potassium, followed by 50 mg doses, will provide better relief. After the first day, when the maximum recommended dose may be 200 mg, the total daily dose should generally not exceed 150 mg.

INDICATIONS AND USAGE

Diclofenac Delayed-Release or Immediate-Release Tablets are indicated for the acute and chronic treatment of signs and symptoms of rheumatoid arthritis, osteoarthritis, and ankylosing spondylitis. Only Diclofenac Potassium is indicated for the management of pain and primary dysmenorrhea, when prompt pain relief is desired, because it is formulated to provide earlier plasma concentrations of Diclofenac (see *"Clinical Pharmacology, Pharmacokinetics and Clinical Studies"*).

UNLABELED USES

Diclofenac is used alone or as an adjunct in the treatment of biliary colic, fever, and episiotomy pain. It is also used in the treatment of gout, migraine headache, and renal colic.

CONTRAINDICATIONS

Diclofenac in either formulation, Sodium or Potassium, is contraindicated in patients with hypersensitivity to Diclofenac. Diclofenac should not be given to patients who have experienced asthma, urticaria, or other allergic-type reactions after taking aspirin or other NSAIDs. Severe, rarely fatal, anaphylactic-like reactions to Diclofenac have been reported in such patients.

WARNINGS

GASTROINTESTINAL EFFECTS

Peptic ulceration and gastrointestinal bleeding have been reported in patients receiving Diclofenac. Physicians and patients should therefore remain alert for ulceration and bleeding in patients treated chronically with Diclofenac even in the absence of previous G.I. tract symptoms. It is recommended that patients be maintained on the lowest dose of Diclofenac possible, consistent with achieving a satisfactory therapeutic response.

Risk of G.I. Ulcerations, Bleeding, and Perforation with NSAID Therapy. Serious gastrointestinal toxicity such as bleeding, ulceration, and perforation can occur at any time, with or without warning symptoms, in patients treated chronically with NSAID therapy. Although minor upper gastrointestinal problems, such as dyspepsia, are common, usually developing early in therapy, physicians should remain alert for ulceration and bleeding in patients treated chronically with NSAIDs even in the absence of previous G.I. tract symptoms. In patients observed in clinical trials of several months to 2 years' duration, symptomatic upper G.I. ulcers, gross bleeding, or perforation appear to occur in approximately 1% of patients for 3-6 months, and in about 2%-4% of patients treated for 1 year. Physicians should inform patients about the signs and/or symptoms of serious G.I. toxicity and what steps to take if they occur.

Studies to date have not identified any subset of patients not at risk of developing peptic ulceration and bleeding. Except for a prior history of serious G.I. events and other risk factors known to be associated with peptic ulcer disease, such as alcoholism, smoking, etc., no risk factors (e.g., age, sex) have been associated with increased risk. Elderly or debilitated patients seem to tolerate ulceration or bleeding less well than other individuals, and most spontaneous reports of fatal G.I. events are in this population. Studies to date are inconclusive concerning the relative risk of various NSAIDs in causing such reactions. High doses of any NSAID probably carry a greater risk of these reactions, although controlled clinical trials showing this do not exist in most cases. In considering the use of relatively large doses (within the recommended dosage range), sufficient benefit should be anticipated to offset the potential increased risk of G.I. toxicity.

HEPATIC EFFECTS

As with other NSAIDs, elevations of one or more liver tests may occur during Diclofenac therapy. These laboratory abnormalities may progress, may remain unchanged, or may be transient with continued therapy. Borderline elevations (i.e., less than 3 times the ULN [= the Upper Limit of the Normal range]), or greater elevations of transaminases occurred in about 15% of Diclofenac-treated patients. Of the hepatic enzymes, ALT (SGPT) is the one recommended for the monitoring of liver injury.

In clinical trials, meaningful elevations (i.e., more than 3 times the ULN) of AST (SGOT) (ALT was not measured in all studies) occurred in about 2% of approximately 5700 patients at some time during Diclofenac Sodium treatment. In a large, open, controlled trial, meaningful elevations of ALT and/or AST occurred in about 4% of 3700 patients treated for 2-6 months, including marked elevations (i.e., more than 8 times the ULN) in about 1% of the 3700 patients. In that open-label study, a higher incidence of borderline (less than 3 times the ULN), moderate (3-8 times the ULN), and marked (> 8 times the ULN) elevations of ALT or AST was observed in patients receiving Diclofenac when compared to other NSAIDs. Transaminase elevations were seen more frequently in patients with osteoarthritis than in those with rheumatoid arthritis (see *"Adverse Reactions"*).

In addition to the enzyme elevations seen in clinical trials, rare cases of severe hepatic reactions, including jaundice and fatal fulminant hepatitis, have been reported.

Physicians should measure transminases periodically in patients receiving long-term therapy with Diclofenac because severe hepatotoxicity may develop without a prodrome of distinguishing symptoms. The optimum times for making the first and subsequent transaminase measurements are not known. In the largest U.S. trial (open-label) that involved 3700 patients monitored first at 8 weeks and 1200 patients monitored again at 24 weeks, almost all meaningful elevations in transaminases were detected before patients became symptomatic. In 42 of the 51 patients in all trials who developed marked transaminase elevations, abnormal tests occurred during the first 2 months of therapy with Diclofenac. Based on this experience, if Diclofenac is used chronically, the first transaminase measurement should be made no later than 8 weeks after the start of Diclofenac treatment. As with other NSAIDs, if abnormal liver tests persist or worsen, if clinical signs and/or symptoms consistent with liver disease develop, or if systemic manifestations occur (e.g., eosinophilia, rash, etc.), Diclofenac should be discontinued.

To minimize the possibility that hepatic injury will become severe between transaminase measurements, physicians should inform patients of the warning signs and symptoms of hepatotoxicity (e.g., nausea, fatigue, lethargy, pruritus, jaundice, right upper quadrant tenderness, and 'flu-like' symptoms), and the appropriate action patients should take if these signs and symptoms appear.

PRECAUTIONS
GENERAL
Allergic Reactions: As with other NSAIDs, allergic reactions including anaphylaxis have been reported with Diclofenac. Specific allergic manifestations consisting of swelling of eyelids, lips, pharynx, and larynx; urticaria; asthma; and broncho-spasm, sometimes with a concomitant fall in blood pressure (severe at times) have been observed in clinical trials and/or the marketing experience with Diclofenac. Anaphylaxis has rarely been reported from foreign sources; in U.S. clinical trials with Diclofenac in over 6000 patients, 1 case of anaphylaxis was reported. In controlled clinical trials, allergic reactions have been observed at an incidence of 0.5%. These reactions can occur without prior exposure to the drug.

Fluid Retention and Edema: Fluid retention and edema have been observed in some patients taking Diclofenac. Therefore, as with other NSAIDs, Diclofenac should be used with caution in patients with a history of cardiac decompensation, hypertension, or other conditions predisposing to fluid retention.

Renal Effects: As a class, NSAIDs have been associated with renal papillary necrosis and other abnormal renal pathology in long-term administration to animals. In oral Diclofenac studies in animals, some evidence of renal toxicity was noted. Isolated incidents of papillary necrosis were observed in a few animals at high doses (20-120 mg/kg) in several baboon subacute studies. In patients treated with Diclofenac, rare cases of interstitial nephritis and papillary necrosis have been reported (see *"Adverse Reactions"*). A second form of renal toxicity, generally associated with NSAIDs, is seen in patients with conditions leading to a reduction in renal blood flow or blood volume, where renal prostaglandins have a supportive role in the maintenance of renal perfusion. In these patients, administration of an NSAID results in a dose-dependent decrease in prostaglandin synthesis and, secondarily, in a reduction of renal blood flow, which may precipitate overt renal failure. Patients at greatest risk of this reaction are those with impaired renal function, heart failure, liver dysfunction, those taking diuretics, and the elderly. Discontinuation of NSAID therapy is typically followed by recovery to the pretreatment state Cases of significant renal failure in patients receiving Diclofenac have been reported from marketing experience, but were not observed in over 4000 patients in clinical trials during which serum creatinine and BUN values were followed serially. There were only 11 patients (0.3%) whose serum creatinine and concurrent serum BUN values were greater than 20 mg/dL and 40 mg/dL, respectively, while on Diclofenac (mean rise in the 11 patients: creatinine 2.3 mg/dL and BUN 28.4 mg/dL).

Since Diclofenac metabolites are eliminated primarily by the kidneys, patients with significantly impaired renal function should be more closely monitored than subjects with normal renal function.

Porphyria: The use of Diclofenac in patients with hepatic porphyria should be avoided. To date, 1 patient has been described in whom Diclofenac probably triggered a clinical attack of porphyria. The postulated mechanism, demonstrated in rats, for causing such attacks by Diclofenac, as well as some other NSAIDs, is through stimulation of the porphyrin precursor delta-aminolevulinic acid (ALA.)

INFORMATION FOR PATIENTS
Diclofenac, like other drugs of its class, is not free of side effects. The side effects of these drugs can cause discomfort and, rarely, there are more serious side effects, such as gastrointestinal bleeding, and more rarely, liver toxicity (see *"Warnings, Hepatic Effects"*), which may result in hospitalization and even fatal outcomes.

NSAIDs are often essential agents in the management of arthritis and have a major role in the management of pain, but they also may be commonly employed for conditions that are less serious.

Physicians may wish to discuss with their patients the potential risks (See *"Warnings"*, *"Precautions"*, and *"Adverse Reactions"*) and likely benefits of NSAID treatment, particularly when the drugs are used for less serious conditions where treatment without NSAIDs may represent an acceptable alternative to both the patient and physician.

LABORATORY TESTS
Because serious G.I. tract ulceration and bleeding can occur without warning symptoms, physicians should follow chronically treated patients for the signs and symptoms of ulceration and bleeding and should inform them of the importance of this follow-up (see *"Warnings, Risk of G.I. Ulcerations, Bleeding, and Perforation with NSAID Therapy"*). If Diclofenac is used chronically, patients should also be instructed to report any signs and symptoms that might be due to hepatotoxicity of Diclofenac; these symptoms may become evident between visits when periodic liver laboratory tests are performed (See *"Warnings, Hepatic Effects"*).

DRUG INTERACTIONS
Aspirin: Concomitant administration of Diclofenac and aspirin is not recommended because Diclofenac is displaced from its binding sites during the concomitant administration of aspirin, resulting in lower plasma concentrations, peak plasma levels, and AUC values.

Anticoagulants: While studies have not shown Diclofenac to interact with anticoagulants of the warfarin type, caution should be exercised, nonetheless, since interactions have been seen with other NSAIDs. Because prostaglandins play an important role in hemostatis, and NSAIDs affect platelet function as well, concurrent therapy with all NSAIDs, including Diclofenac and warfarin requires close monitoring of patients to be certain that no change in their anticoagulant dosage is required.

Digoxin, Methotrexate, Cyclosporine: Dicolfenac, like other NSAIDs, may affect renal prostaglandins and increase the toxicity of certain drugs. Ingestion of Diclofenac may increase serum concentrations of digoxin and methotrexate and increase cyclosporine's nephrotoxicity. Patients who begin taking Diclofenac or who increase their Diclofenac dose or any other NSAID while taking digoxin, methotrexate, or cyclosporine may develop toxicity characteristics for these drugs. They should be observed closely, particularly if renal function is impaired. In the case of digoxin, serum levels should be monitored.

Lithium: Diclofenac decreases lithium renal clearance and increases lithium plasma levels. In patients taking Diclofenac and lithium concomitantly, lithium toxicity may develop.

Oral Hypoglycemics: Diclofenac does not alter glucose metabolism in normal subjects nor does it alter the effects of oral hypoglycemic agents. There are rare reports, however, from marketing experiences of changes in effects of insulin or oral hypoglycemic agents in the presence of Diclofenac that necessitated changes in the doses of such agents. Both hypo- and hyperglycemic effects have been reported. A direct causal relationship has not been established, but physicians should consider the possibility that Diclofenac may alter a diabetic patient's response to insulin or oral hypoglycemic agents.

Diuretics: Diclofenac and other NSAIDs can inhibit the activity of diuretics. Concomitant treatment with potassium-sparing diuretics may be associated with increased serum potassium levels.

Other Drugs: In small groups of patients (7-10/interaction study), the concomitant administration of azathioprine, gold, chloroquine, D-penicillamine, prednisolone, doxycycline, or digitoxin did not significantly affect the peak levels and AUC values of Diclofenac.

PROTEIN BINDING
In vitro, Diclofenac interferes minimally or not at all with the protein binding of salicylic acid (20% decrease in binding), tolbutamide, prednisolone (10% decrease in binding), or warfarin. Benzylpenicillin, ampicillin, oxacillin, chlortetracycline, doxycycline, cephalothin, erythromycin, and sulfamethoxazole have no influence in vitro on the protein binding of Diclofenac in human serum.

DRUG/LABORATORY TEST INTERACTIONS
Effect on Blood Coagulation: Diclofenac increases platelet aggregation time but does not affect bleeding time, plasma thrombin clotting time, plasma fibrinogen, or factors V and VII to XII. Statistically significant changes in prothrombin and partial thromboplastin times have been reported in normal volunteers. The mean changes were observed to be less than 1 second in both instances, however, and are unlikely to be clinically important. Diclofenac is a prostaglandin synthetase inhibitor, however, and all drugs that inhibit prostaglandin synthesis interfere with platelet function to some degree; therefore, patients who may adversely affected by such an action should be carefully observed.

CARCINOGENESIS, MUTAGENESIS, IMPAIRMENT OF FERTILITY
Long-term carcinogenicity studies in rats given Diclofenac sodium up to 2 mg/kg/day or (12 mg/m²/day approximately the human dose) have revealed no significant increases in tumor incidence. There was a slight increase in benign mammary fibroadenomas in mid-dose-treated (0.5 mg/kg/day or 3 mg/m²/day) female rats (high-dose females had excessive mortality), but the increase was not significant for this common rat tumor. A 2-year carcinogenicity study conducted in mice employing Diclofenac Sodium at doses up to 0.3 mg/kg/day (0.9 mg/m²/day) in males and 1 mg/kg/day (3 mg/m²/day) in females did not reveal any oncogenic potential. Diclofenac Sodium did not show mutagenic activity in vitro point mutation assays in mammalian (mouse lymphoma) and microbial (yeast,

Ames) test systems and was nonmutagenic in several mammalian in vitro and in vivo tests, including dominant lethal and male germinal epithelial chromosomal studies in mice, and nucleus anomaly and chromosomal aberration studies in Chinese hamsters. Diclofenac Sodium administered to male and female rats at 4 mg/kg/day (24 mg/m^2/day) did not affect fertility.

TERATOGENIC EFFECTS

There are no adequate and well-controlled studies in pregnant women. Diclofenac should be used during pregnancy only if the benefits to the mother justify the potential risk to the fetus.

Pregnancy Category B: Reproduction studies have been performed in mice given Diclofenac Sodium (up to 20 mg/kg/day or 60 mg/m^2/day) and in rats and rabbits given Diclofenac Sodium (up to 10 mg/kg/day or 60 mg/m^2/day for rats, and 80 mg/m^2/day for rabbits), and have revealed no evidence of teratogenicity despite the induction of maternal toxicity and fetal toxicity. In rats, maternally toxic doses were associated with dystocia, prolonged gestation, reduced fetal weights and growth, and reduced fetal survival. Diclofenac has been shown to cross the placental barrier in mice and rats.

LABOR AND DELIVERY

The effects of Diclofenac on labor and delivery in pregnant women are unknown. Because the known effects of prostaglandin-inhibiting drugs on the fetal cardiovascular system (closure of ductus arteriosus), use of Diclofenac during late pregnancy should be avoided and, as with other nonsteriodal anti-inflammatory drugs, it is possible that Diclofenac may inhibit uterine contraction.

NURSING MOTHERS

Diclofenac has been found in the milk of nursing mothers. As with other drugs that are excreted in milk, Diclofenac is not recommended for use in nursing women.

PEDIATRIC USE

Safety and effectiveness of Diclofenac in children have not been established.

GERIATRIC USE

Of the more than 6000 patients treated with Diclofenac in U.S. trials, 31% were older than 65 years of age. No overall difference was observed between efficacy, adverse event or pharmacokinetic profiles of older and younger patients. As with any NSAID, the elderly are likely to tolerate adverse reactions less well than younger patients.

ADVERSE REACTIONS

Adverse reaction information is derived from blinded, controlled and open-label clinical trials, as well as worldwide marketing experience. In the description below, rates of more common events represent clinical study results; rarer events are derived principally from marketing experience and publications, and accurate rate estimates are generally not possible.

In a 6-month, double-blind trial comparing Diclofenac Sodium Delayed-Release Tablets (N = 197) vs. Diclofenac Potassium Immediate-Release Tablets (N = 196) vs. ibuprofen (N = 197), adverse reactions were similar in nature and frequency. In 718 patients treated for shorter periods, i.e., 2 weeks or less, with *Diclofenac Potassium Immediate-Release Tablets,* adverse reactions were reported one-half to one-tenth as frequently as by patients treated for longer periods.

The incidence of common adverse reactions (greater than 1%) is based upon controlled clinical trials in 1543 patients treated up to 13 weeks with *Diclofenac Sodium Delayed-Release Tablets.* By far the most common adverse effects were gastrointestinal symptoms, most of them minor, occuring in about 20%, and leading to discontinuation in about 3%, of patients. Peptic ulcer or G.I. bleeding occurred in clinical trials in 0.6% (95% confidence interval: 0.2% to 1%) of approximately 1800 patients during their first 3 months of Diclofenac treatment and in 1.6% (95% confidence interval: 0.8% to 2.4%) of approximately 800 patients followed for 1 year.

Gastrointestinal symptoms were followed in frequency by central nervous system side effects such as headache (7%) and dizziness (3%).

Meaningful (exceeding 3 times the Upper Limit of Normal) elevations of ALT (SGPT) or AST (SGOT) occurred at an overall rate of approximately 2% during the first 2 months of Diclofenac Sodium treatment. Unlike aspirin-related elevations, which occur more frequently in patients with rheumatoid arthritis, these elevations were more frequently observed in patients with osteoarthritis (2.6%) than in patients with rheumatoid arthritis (0.7%). Marked elevations (exceeding 8 times the ULN) were seen in 1% of patients treated for 2-6 months (See *"Warnings, Hepatic Effects"*).

The following adverse reactions were reported in patients treated with Diclofenac:

Incidence Greater Than 1%—Causal Relationship Probable: (All derived from clinical trials.)

Body as a Whole: Abdominal pain or cramps,* headache,* fluid retention, abdominal distention.

Digestive: Diarrhea,* indigestion,* nausea,* constipation,* flatulence, liver test abnormalities,* PUB, i.e., peptic ulcer, with or without bleeding and/or perforation, or bleeding without ulcer (see above and also *"Warnings"*).

*Incidence, 3% to 9% (incidence of unmarked reactions is 1%-3%).

Nervous System: Dizziness.

Skin and Appendages: Rash, pruritus.

Special Senses: Tinnitus.

Incidence Less Than 1%—Causal Relationship Probable: (The following reactions have been reported in patients taking Diclofenac under circumstances that do not permit a clear attribution of the reaction to Diclofenac. These reactions are being included as alerting information to physicians. Adverse reactions reported only in *worldwide marketing experience* or in the literature, not seen in clinical trials, are considered rare and are italicized.)

Body as a Whole: Malaise, swelling of lips and tongue, photosensitivity, *anaphylaxis,* anaphylactoid reactions.

Cardiovascular: Hypertension, congestive heart failure.

Digestive: Vomiting, jaundice, melena, aphthous stomatitis, dry mouth and mucous membranes, bloody diarrhea, hepatitis, *hepatic necrosis,* appetite change, pancreatitis with or without concomitant hepatitis, *colitis.*

Hemic and Lymphatic: Hemoglobin decrease, leukopenia, thrombocytopenia, *hemolytic anemia, aplastic anemia, agranulocytosis,* purpura, *allergic purpura.*

Metabolic and Nutritional Disorders: Azotemia.

Nervous System: Insomnia, drowsiness, depression, diplopia, anxiety, irritability, *aseptic meningitis.*

Respiratory: Epistaxis, asthma, laryngeal edema.

Skin and Appendages: Alopecia, urticaria, eczema, dermatitis, *bullous eruption erythema multiforme major,* angioedema, *Stevens-Johnson syndrome.*

Special Senses: Blurred vision, taste disorder, reversible hearing loss, scotoma.

Urogenital: Nephrotic syndrome, proteinuria, *oliguria, interstitial, nephritis, papillary necrosis,* acute renal failure.

Incidence Less Than 1%—Causal Relationship Unknown: (Adverse reactions reported only in worldwide marketing experience or in the literature, not seen in clinical trials, are considered rare and are italicized.)

Body as a Whole: Chest pain.

Cardiovascular: Palpitations, *flushing,* tachycardia, premature ventricular contractions, myocardial infarction.

Digestive: Esophageal lesions.

Hemic and Lymphatic: Bruising.

Metabolic and Nutritional Disorders: Hypoglycemia, *weight loss.*

Nervous System: Paresthesia, memory disturbance, nightmares, tremor, tic, *abnormal coordination,* convulsions, *disorientation, psychotic reaction.*

Respiratory: Dyspnea, hyperventilation, edema of pharynx.

Skin and Appendages: Excess perspiration, *exfoliative dermatitis.*

Special Senses: Vitreous floaters, night blindness, amblyopia.

Urogenital: Urinary frequency, nocturia, hematuria, impotence, vaginal bleeding.

OVERDOSAGE

Worldwide reports of overdosage with Diclofenac cover 66 cases. In approximately one-half of these reports of overdosage, concomitant medications were also taken. The highest dose of Diclofenac was 5.0 g in a 17-year-old male who suffered loss of consciousness, increased intracranial pressure, aspiration pneumonitis, and died 2 days after overdose. The next highest doses of Diclofenac were 4.0 g and 3.75 g. The 24-year-old female who took 4.0 g and the 28- and 42-year-old females, each of whom took 3.75 g, did not develop any clinically significant signs or symptoms. However, there was a report of a 17-year-old female who experienced vomiting and drowsiness after an overdose of 2.37 g of Diclofenac.

Animal LD$_{50}$ values show a wide range of susceptibilities to acute overdosage, with primates being more resistant to acute toxicity than rodents (LD$_{50}$ in mg/kg—rats, 55; dogs, 500; monkeys, 3200).

In case of acute overdosage, it is recommended that the stomach be emptied by vomiting or lavage. Forced diuresis may theoretically be beneficial because the drug is excreted in the urine. The effect of dialysis or hemoperfusion in the elimination of Diclofenac (99% protein-bound: see *"Clinical Pharmacology"*) remains unproven. In addition to supportive measures, the use of oral activated charcoal may help to reduce the absorption of Diclofenac.

DOSAGE AND ADMINISTRATION

Diclofenac may be administered as 25-mg, 50-mg, and 75-mg Diclofenac Sodium Delayed-Release Tablets or as 50-mg Diclofenac Potassium Immediate-Release Tablets. Regardless of the indication, the dosage of Diclofenac should be individualized to the lowest effective dose of Diclofenac Sodium or Diclofenac Potassium to minimize adverse effects (see *"Individualization of Dosage"*).

Osteoarthritis: The recommended dosage is 100 to 150 mg/day in divided doses, 50 mg b.i.d. or t.i.d. Diclofenac Sodium or Potassium or 75 mg b.i.d. (Diclofenac Sodium only). Dosages above 150 mg/day have not been studied in patients with osteoarthritis.

Rheumatoid Arthritis: The recommended dosage is 150-200 mg/day in divided doses, 50 mg t.i.d. or q.i.d. (Diclofenac Sodium or Potassium) or 75 mg b.i.d. (Diclofenac Sodium only). Dosages above 225 mg/day are not recommended in patients with rheumatoid arthritis.

Ankylosing Spondylitis: The recommended dosage is 100-125 mg/day administered as 25 mg q.i.d. with an extra 25-mg dose at bedtime if necessary. Dosages above 125 mg/day have not been studied in patients with ankylosing spondylitis.

◆ RATED THERAPEUTICALLY EQUIVALENT; ◇ THERAPEUTIC EQUIVALENCE UNCONFIRMED; ○ UNRATED

Analgesia and Primary Dysmenorrhea: The recommended starting dose of Diclofenac Potassium Immediate-Release Tablets is 50 mg t.i.d. With experience, physicians may find that in some patients an initial dose of 100 mg of Diclofenac Potassium, follow by 50-mg doses, will provide better relief. After the first day, when the maximum recommended dose may be 200 mg, the total daily dose should generally not exceed 150 mg.

Do not store above 86 ° F (30 ° C). Dispense in tight container (USP).

HOW SUPPLIED

DICLOFENAC SODIUM
ENTERIC COATED TABLETS: 25 MG

BRAND/MANUFACTURER	NDC	SIZE	AWP
○ **BRAND**			
➤ VOLTAREN: Geigy	00028-0258-60	60s	$28.13
	00028-0258-01	100s	$46.89
	00028-0258-61	100s ud	$50.16

ENTERIC COATED TABLETS: 50 MG

BRAND/MANUFACTURER	NDC	SIZE	AWP
○ **BRAND**			
➤ VOLTAREN: Geigy	00028-0262-60	60s	$54.67
	00028-0262-01	100s	$91.14
	00028-0262-61	100s ud	$97.53
	00028-0262-10	1000s	$895.79

ENTERIC COATED TABLETS: 75 MG

BRAND/MANUFACTURER	NDC	SIZE	AWP
○ **BRAND**			
➤ VOLTAREN: Geigy	00028-0264-60	60s	$66.23
	00028-0264-01	100s	$110.38
	00028-0264-61	100s ud	$118.12
	00028-0264-10	1000s	$1084.92

DICLOFENAC POTASSIUM
TABLETS: 50 MG

BRAND/MANUFACTURER	NDC	SIZE	AWP
○ **BRAND**			
➤ CATAFLAM: Geigy	00028-0151-01	100s	$130.00
	00028-0151-61	100s ud	$139.10

Dicloxacillin Sodium

DESCRIPTION
Dicloxacillin Sodium Monohydrate is an isoxazolyl penicillin which resists destruction by the enzyme penicillinase (beta-lactamase). It is the Monohydrate Sodium salt of 6-[3-(2, 6-Dichlorophenyl)-5-methyl-4-isoxazolecarboxamido]-3,3-dimethyl-7-oxo-4-thia-1-azabicyclo-[3.2.0] heptane-2-carboxylic acid.

Dicloxacillin Sodium Monohydrate capsules contain 250 mg or 500 mg Dicloxacillin.

Dicloxacillin Sodium Monohydrate oral suspension is a powder which when reconstituted as directed yields a suspension equivalent to 62.5 mg Dicloxacillin per 5 mL.

Following is its chemical structure:

ACTIONS
PHARMACOLOGY
Dicloxacillin Sodium Monohydrate is resistant to destruction by acid and is exceptionally well absorbed from the gastrointestinal tract. Oral administration of Dicloxacillin Sodium Monohydrate gives blood levels considerably higher than those obtained with equivalent doses of any other presently available oral penicillin.

MICROBIOLOGY
In vitro Dicloxacillin Sodium Monohydrate is active against certain gram-positive cocci, including most strains of beta-hemolytic streptococci, pneumococci, penicillin-G-sensitive staphylococci and, because of its resistance to penicillinase, penicillin-G-resistant staphylococci. Dicloxacillin Sodium Monohydrate has less intrinsic antibacterial activity and a narrower spectrum than penicillin G.

DISC SUSCEPTIBILITY TESTS
Quantitative methods that require measurement of zone diameters give the most precise estimates of antibiotic susceptibility. One such procedure[*] has been

---

* Bauer, A.W., Kirby, W.M.M., Sherris, J.C., and Turck, M.: Antibiotic Testing by a Standardized Single Discs Method. *Am. J. Clin. Pathol.*, 45:493, 1966: Standardized Disc Susceptibility Test. *FEDERAL REGISTER*37:20527-29, 1972.

recommended for use with discs for testing susceptibility to penicillinase-resistant penicillin-class antibiotics. Interpretations correlate diameters on the disc test with MIC values for penicillinase-resistant penicillins. With this procedure, a report from the laboratory of "susceptible" indicates that the infecting organism is likely to respond to therapy. A report of "resistant" indicates that the infecting organism is not likely to respond to therapy. A report of "intermediate susceptibility" suggests that the organism would be susceptible if high dosage is used, or if the infection is confined to tissues and fluids (e.g., urine), in which high antibiotic levels are attained.

INDICATIONS
Although the principal indications for Dicloxacillin Sodium Monohydrate is in the treatment of infections due to penicillinase-producing staphylococci, it may be used to initiate therapy in such patients in whom a staphylococcal infection is suspected. (See *"Important Note."*)

Bacteriologic studies to determine the causative organisms and their sensitivity to Dicloxacillin Sodium Monohydrate should be performed. In serious, life-threatening infections, oral preparations of the penicillinase-resistant penicillins should not be relied on for initial therapy.

Important Note: When it is judged necessary that treatment be initiated before definitive culture and sensitivity results are known, the choice of Dicloxacillin Sodium Monohydrate, should take into consideration the fact that it has been shown to be effective only in the treatment of infections caused by pneumococci, Group A beta-hemolytic streptococci, and penicillin-G-resistant and penicillin-G-sensitive staphylococci. If the bacteriology report later indicates the infection is due to an organism other than a penicillin-G-resistant staphylococcus sensitive to Dicloxacillin Sodium Monohydrate, the physician is advised to continue therapy with a drug other than Dicloxacillin Sodium Monohydrate or any other penicillinase-resistant penicillin.

Recent studies have reported that the percentage of staphylococcal isolates resistant to penicillin G outside the hospital is increasing, approximating the high percentage of resistant staphylococcal isolates found in the hospital. For this reason it is recommended that a penicillinase-resistant penicillin be used as initial therapy for any suspected staphylococcal infection until culture and sensitivity results are known.

Dicloxacillin Sodium Monohydrate acts through a mechanism similar to that of methicillin against penicillin-G-resistant staphylococci. Strains of staphylococci resistant to methicillin have existed in nature, and it is known that the number of these strains reported has been increasing. Such strains of staphylococci have been capable of producing serious disease, in some instances resulting in fatality. Because of this, there is concern that widespread use of the penicillinase-resistant penicillins may result in the appearance of an increasing number of staphylococcal strains which are resistant to these penicillins.

Methicillin-resistant strains are almost always resistant to all other penicillmase-resistant penicillins (cross-resistance with cephalosporin derivatives also occurs frequently). Resistance to any penicillinase-resistant penicillin should be interpreted as evidence of clinical resistance to all, in spite of the fact that minor variations in *in vitro* sensitivity may be encountered when more than one penicillinase-resistant penicillin is tested against the same strain of staphylococcus.

CONTRAINDICATIONS
A history of a previous hypersensitivity reaction to any of the penicillins is a contraindication.

WARNINGS
Serious and occasionally fatal hypersensitivity (anaphylactoid) reactions have been reported in patients on penicillin therapy. Although anaphylaxis is more frequent following parenteral therapy, it has occurred in patients on oral penicillins. These reactions are more apt to occur in individuals with a history of sensitivity to multiple allergens.

There have been reports of individuals with a history of penicillin hypersensitivity reactions who experienced severe hypersensitivity reactions when treated with cephalosporins. Before therapy with a penicillin, careful inquiry should be made concerning previous hypersensitivity reactions to penicillins, cephalosporins, and other allergens. If an allergic reaction occurs, appropriate therapy should be instituted and discontinuance of Dicloxacillin Sodium Monohydrate therapy considered. The usual agents (antihistamines, pressor amines, corticosteroids) should be readily available.

USAGE IN PREGNANCY
Safety for use in pregnancy has not been established.

PRECAUTIONS
As with any potent drug, periodic assessment of organ-system function, including renal, hepatic, and hematopoietic, should be made during prolonged therapy.

The possibility of bacterial and fungal superinfection should be kept in mind during long-term therapy. If overgrowth of resistant organisms occurs, appropriate measures should be taken.

This oral preparation should not be relied upon in patients with severe illness or with nausea, vomiting, gastric dilatation, cardiospasm, or intestinal hypermotility.

Since experience in neonates is limited, a dose for the newborn is not recommended at this time.

➤ **SHOWN IN PRODUCT IDENTIFICATION GUIDE**

ADVERSE REACTIONS

Gastrointestinal disturbances, such as nausea, vomiting, epigastric discomfort, flatulence, and loose stools, have been noted in some patients receiving Dicloxacillin Sodium Monohydrate. As with other penicillins, pruritus, urticaria, skin rashes, eosinophilia, anaphylactic reactions, and other allergic symptoms have been occasionally encountered.

Minor changes in the results of liver function tests such as transient elevation of SGOT and changes in cephalin flocculation tests have been reported. The clinical significance of these changes is unknown.

DOSAGE AND ADMINISTRATION

For mild-to-moderate upper-respiratory and localized skin and soft-tissue infections due to sensitive organisms:

Adults and children weighing 40 kg (88 lbs.) or more: 125 mg q. 6h.
Children weighing less than 40 kg (88 lbs.): 12.5 mg/kg/day in equally divided doses q. 6h.

For more severe infections such as those of the lower-respiratory tract or disseminated infections.

Adults and children weighing 40 kg (88 lbs.) or more: 250 mg q. 6h. or higher.
Children weighing less than 40 kg (88 lbs.): 25 mg/kg/day or higher in equally divided doses q. 6h.

Since experience in neonates is limited, a dose for the newborn is not recommended at this time.

Dicloxacillin Sodium Monohydrate is best absorbed when taken on an empty stomach, preferably one to two hours before meals.

N.B.: INFECTIONS CAUSED BY GROUP A BETA-HEMOLYTIC STREPTO-COCCI SHOULD BE TREATED FOR AT LEAST 10 DAYS TO HELP PREVENT THE OCCURRENCE OF ACUTE RHEUMATIC FEVER OR ACUTE GLOMERULONEPHRITIS.

Store capsules at room temperature, approximately 25° C (77°F). Keep tightly closed.

Dispense in tight container.

Store oval suspension at room temperature, approximately 25°C (77°F), before reconstitution.

Shake well before using.

Keep tightly closed.

After reconstitution store in refrigerator. Discard any unused portion after two weeks.

HOW SUPPLIED
CAPSULE: 125 MG

BRAND/MANUFACTURER	NDC	SIZE	AWP
◆ BRAND			
DYNAPEN: Apothecon	00015-7892-30	24s	$12.91

CAPSULE: 250 MG

AVERAGE UNIT PRICE (AVAILABLE SIZES)		GENERIC A-RATED AVERAGE PRICE (GAAP)	
BRAND	$0.94	100s	$38.67
GENERIC	$0.39		
HCFA FUL (100s ea)	$0.24		

BRAND/MANUFACTURER	NDC	SIZE	AWP
◆ BRAND			
DYNAPEN: Apothecon	00015-7893-60	100s	$93.95
◆ GENERICS			
Rugby	00536-1180-01	100s	$31.19
Qualitest	00603-3241-21	100s	$35.82
Warner Chilcott	00047-0945-24	100s	$36.78
Schein	00364-0856-01	100s	$37.50
Apothecon	57783-6058-01	100s	$37.57
Moore,H.L.	00839-6178-06	100s	$38.07
URL	00677-0930-01	100s	$39.50
Major	00904-2647-60	100s	$39.75
Geneva	00781-2220-01	100s	$39.75
Goldline	00182-1506-01	100s	$39.75
Lederle Std Prod	00005-3135-23	100s	$41.60
Biocraft	00332-3123-09	100s	$42.02
Aligen	00405-4322-01	100s	$42.20
DYCILL: SK Beecham Pharm	00029-6351-30	100s	$43.05
PATHOCIL: Wyeth-Ayerst	00008-0360-02	100s	$52.39
Raway	00686-0610-20	100s ud	$19.00
UDL	51079-0610-20	100s ud	$41.40

CAPSULE: 500 MG

AVERAGE UNIT PRICE (AVAILABLE SIZES)		GENERIC A-RATED AVERAGE PRICE (GAAP)	
BRAND	$1.76	100s	$66.43
GENERIC	$0.68		
HCFA FUL (100s ea)	$0.44		

BRAND/MANUFACTURER	NDC	SIZE	AWP
◆ BRAND			
DYNAPEN: Apothecon	00015-7658-50	50s	$87.77

BRAND/MANUFACTURER	NDC	SIZE	AWP
◆ GENERICS			
PATHOCIL: Wyeth-Ayerst	00008-0593-01	50s	$48.95
Rugby	00536-1190-01	100s	$54.88
Qualitest	00603-3242-21	100s	$60.50
Warner Chilcott	00047-0946-24	100s	$64.51
Moore,H.L.	00839-6614-06	100s	$66.35
Schein	00364-2071-01	100s	$66.75
Major	00904-2648-60	100s	$66.95
URL	00677-0931-01	100s	$67.35
Geneva	00781-2225-01	100s	$67.45
Goldline	00182-1507-01	100s	$67.45
Apothecon	57783-6058-01	100s	$67.62
Lederle Std Prod	00005-3136-23	100s	$74.11
Biocraft	00332-3125-09	100s	$75.63
Aligen	00405-4323-01	100s	$75.82
DYCILL: SK Beecham Pharm	00029-6352-30	100s	$76.85
Raway	00686-0611-20	100s ud	$36.00
UDL	51079-0611-20	100s ud	$74.60

SUSPENSION: 62.5 MG/5 ML

AVERAGE UNIT PRICE (AVAILABLE SIZES)	
BRAND	$0.08

BRAND/MANUFACTURER	NDC	SIZE	AWP
◆ BRAND			
DYNAPEN: Apothecon	00015-7856-40	100 ml	$8.77
	00015-7856-64	200 ml	$15.53

Dicumarol

DESCRIPTION

Dicumarol is a coumarin anticoagulant, chemically designated as 3,3'-methylene-bis [4-hydroxycoumarin].

Following is its chemical structure:

ACTIONS

Dicumarol and other coumarin anticoagulants act by depressing synthesis in the liver of several factors which are known to be active in the coagulation mechanisms in a variety of diseases characterized by thromboembolic phenomena. The resultant *in vivo* effect is a sequential depression of Factors VII, IX, X and II. The degree of depression is dependent upon the dosage administered. Anticoagulants have no direct effect on an established thrombus, nor do they reverse ischemic tissue damage. However, once a thrombosis has occurred, anticoagulant treatment aims to prevent further extension of the formed clot and prevents secondary thromboembolic complications which may result in serious and possible fatal sequelae.

Maximal plasma concentrations are reached in 1 to 9 hours. Approximately 97% is bound to albumin within the plasma. Dicumarol usually induces hypoprothrombinemia in 36 to 48 hours, and its duration of action may persist for 5 to 6 days, thus producing a smooth, long lasting response curve. Little is known of the metabolic pathways involved in the biotransformation of oral anticoagulants in man. However, their metabolites appear to be eliminated principally in the urine.

INDICATIONS

Dicumarol is indicated for the prophylaxis and treatment of venous thrombosis and its extension, the treatment of atrial fibrillation with embolization, the prophylaxis and treatment of pulmonary embolism, and as an adjunct in the treatment of coronary occlusion.

CONTRAINDICATIONS

Anticoagulation is contraindicated in any localized or general physical condition or personal circumstance in which the hazard of hemorrhage might be greater than its potential clinical benefits, such as:

Pregnancy: Dicumarol is contraindicated in pregnancy because the drug passes through the placental barrier and may cause fatal hemorrhage to the fetus in utero. Furthermore, there have been reports of birth malformations in children born to mothers who have been treated with dicumarol during pregnancy. Women of childbearing potential who are candidates for anticoagulant therapy should be carefully evaluated and the indications critically reviewed with the patient. If the patient becomes pregnant while taking this drug, she should be apprised of the potential risks to the fetus, and the possibility of termination of the pregnancy should be discussed in light of those risks.

Hemorrhagic tendencies or blood dyscrasias. Recent or comtemplated surgery of: (1) central nervous system; (2) eye; (3) traumatic surgery resulting in large open surfaces.

Bleeding tendencies associated with active ulceration or overt bleeding of: (1) gastrointestinal, genitourinary or respiratory tracts; (2) cerebrovascular hemor-

◆ RATED THERAPEUTICALLY EQUIVALENT; ◇ THERAPEUTIC EQUIVALENCE UNCONFIRMED; ○ UNRATED

rhage; (3) aneurysms—cerebral, dissecting aorta; (4) pericarditis and pericardial effusions.

Threatened abortion, eclampsia and preeclampsia.

Inadequate laboratory facilities or unsupervised senility, alcoholism, psychosis; or lack of patient cooperation.

Spinal puncture and other diagnostic or therapeutic procedures with potential for uncontrollable bleeding.

Miscellaneous: Major regional, lumbar block anesthesia, severe uncontrolled and/ or malignant hypertension, subacute bacterial endocarditis, open wounds, visceral carcinoma, vitamin K deficiency, and severe liver or kidney disease.

WARNINGS
The most serious risks associated with anticoagulant therapy with Dicumarol are hemorrhage in any tissue or organ and, less frequently, necrosis and/or gangrene of skin and other tissues. The risk of hemorrhage is related to the level of intensity and the duration of anticoagulant therapy. Hemorrhage and necrosis have in some cases been reported to result in death or permanent disability. Necrosis appears to be associated with local thrombosis and usually appears within a few days of the start of anticoagulant therapy. In severe cases of necrosis, treatment through debridement or amputation of the affected tissue, limb, breast or penis has been reported. Careful diagnosis is required to determine whether necrosis is caused by an underlying disease. Dicumarol therapy should be discontinued when Dicumarol is suspected to be the cause of developing necrosis and heparin therapy may be considered for anticoagulation. Although various treatments have been attempted, no treatment for necrosis has been considered uniformly effective. See below for information on predisposing conditions. These and other risks associated with anticoagulant therapy must be weighed against the risk of thrombosis or embolization in untreated cases.

Dicumarol is a potent drug with a half-life of 1 to 2 days; therefore its effects may become more pronounced as daily maintenance doses overlap. It cannot be emphasized too strongly that treatment of each patient is a highly individualized matter. Dosage should be controlled by periodic determinations of prothrombin time or other suitable coagulation tests. Determinations of whole blood clotting and bleeding times are not effective measures for control of therapy. Heparin prolongs the one-stage prothrombin time. Therefore, to obtain a valid prothrombin time when heparin and dicumarol are given together, a period of at least 5 hours should elapse after the last intravenous dose and 24 hours after the last subcutaneous dose of heparin, before blood is drawn.

Caution should be observed when Dicumarol is administered in any situation or in the presence of any predisposing condition where added risk of hemorrhage or necrosis is present.

Administration of anticoagulants in the following conditions will be based upon clinical judgment in which the risks of anticoagulant therapy are weighed against the risk of thrombosis or embolization in untreated cases. The following may be associated with these increased risks:

Lactation: Coumarins may pass into the milk of mothers and cause a prothrombinopenic state in the nursing infant.

Mild to moderate hepatic or renal insufficiency.

Infectious diseases or disturbances of intestinal flora: sprue, antibiotic therapy.

Trauma which may result in internal bleeding.

Surgery or trauma resulting in large exposed raw surfaces.

Indwelling catheters and/or drainage tubes in any orifice.

Mild to moderate hypertension.

Known or suspected hereditary, familial or clinical deficiency in protein C: This condition, which should be suspected if there is a history of recurrent episodes of thromboembolic disorders in the patient or in the family, has been associated with an increased risk of developing necrosis following Dicumarol administration. Skin necrosis may occur in the absence of protein C deficiency. It has been reported that initiation of anticoagulation therapy with heparin for 4 to 5 days before initiation of therapy with Dicumarol may minimize the incidence of this reaction. Dicumarol therapy should be discontinued when Dicumarol is suspected to be the cause of developing necrosis and heparin therapy may be considered for anticoagulation.

Miscellaneous: polycythemia vera, vasculitis, severe diabetes, severe allergic and anaphylactic disorders, active tuberculosis, history of ulcerative disease of the gastrointestinal tract and during the postpartum period.

Patients with congestive heart failure may become more sensitive to Dicumarol, thereby requiring more frequent laboratory monitoring, and reduced doses of dicumarol.

Use of anticoagulants with streptokinase or urokinase may be hazardous and caution should be exercised when used concomitantly. (Please note recommendations accompanying these preparations.)

Abrupt cessation of anticoagulant therapy is not generally recommended; taper dose gradually over 3 to 4 weeks.

PRECAUTIONS
Periodic determination of prothrombin time or other suitable coagulation test is essential.

Numerous factors, alone or in combination, including travel, changes in diet, environment, physical state and medication may influence response of the patient to anticoagulants. It is generally good practice to monitor the patient's response with additional prothrombin time determinations in the period immediately after discharge from the hospital, and whenever other medications are initiated, discontinued or taken haphazardly. The following factors are listed for your reference; however, other factors may also affect the prothrombin response.

The following factors, alone or in combination, may be responsible for increased prothrombin time response:

ENDOGENOUS FACTORS
Carcinoma; collagen disease; congestive heart failure; diarrhea; elevated temperature; hepatic disorders—infectious hepatitis, hyperthyroidism, jaundice; poor nutritional state; vitamin K deficiency—steatorrhea.

EXOGENOUS FACTORS
Alcohol†; allopurinol; aminosalicyclic acid; amiodarone; anabolic steroids; antibiotics; bromelains; chloral hydrate†; chloramphenicol; chlorpropamide; chymotrypsin; cimetidine; cinchophen; clofibrate; dicumarol overdosage; dextran; dextrothyroxine; diazoxide; dietary deficiencies; diflunisal; diuretics†; disulfiram; drugs affecting blood elements; ethacrynic acid; fenoprofen; glucagon; hepatotoxic drugs; ibuprofen; indomethacin; influenza virus vaccine; inhalation anesthetics; mefenamic acid; methyldopa; methylphenidate; methylthiouracil; metronidazole; miconazole; monoamine oxidase inhibitors; nalidixic acid; naproxen; nortriptyline; oxolinic acid; oxyphenbutazone; pentoxifylline; phenylbutazone; phenyramidol; phenytoin; prolonged hot weather; prolonged narcotics; propylthiouracil; pyrazolones; quinidine; quinine; ranitidine†; salicylates; sulfinpyrazone; sulfonamides, long acting; sulindac; thyroid drugs; tolbutamide; triclofos sodium; trimethoprim/sulfamethoxazole; unreliable prothrombin time determinations.

The following factors, alone or in combination, may be responsible for decreased prothrombin time response:

ENDOGENOUS FACTORS
Edema; hereditary resistance to coumarin therapy; hyperlipemia; hypothyroidism.

EXOGENOUS FACTORS
ACTH steroids; alcohol†; antacids; antihistamines; phenobarbital and other barbiturates; carbamazepine; chloral hydrate†; chlordiazepoxide; cholestyramine; Dicumarol underdosage; diet high in vitamin K; diuretics†; ethchlorvynol; glutethimide; griseofulvin; haloperidol; meprobamate; oral contraceptives; paraldehyde; primidone; ranitidine†; rifampin; unreliable prothrombin time determinations; vitamin C.

A patient may be exposed to a combination of the above factors, some of which may increase and some decrease his sensitivity to Dicumarol. Because the net effect on his prothrombin time response may be unpredictable under these circumstances, more frequent laboratory monitoring is advisable.

Drugs not yet shown to interact or not to interact with coumarins are best regarded with suspicion, and when their administration is started or stopped, the prothrombin time should be determined more often than usual.

Coumarins also affect the action of other drugs. Hypoglycemic agents (chlorpropamide and tolbutamide) and anticonvulsants (phenytoin and phenobarbital) may accumulate in the body as a result of interference with either their metabolism or excretion.

ADVERSE REACTIONS
Potential adverse reactions to Dicumarol may include:

Hemorrhage from any tissue or organ. This is a consequence of the anticoagulant effect. The signs and symptoms will vary according to the location and degree or extent of the bleeding. Therefore, the possibility of hemorrhage should be considered in evaluating the condition of any anticoagulated patient with complaints which do not indicate an obvious diagnosis. Bleeding during anticoagulant therapy does not always correlate with prothrombin activity. (See *"Treatment for Overdosage".*)

Adrenal hemorrhage with resultant acute adrenal insufficiency has occurred during anticoagulant therapy. Anticoagulant therapy should be discontinued in patients who develop signs and symptoms compatible with acute adrenal hemorrhage or insufficiency. Plasma cortisol levels should be measured immediately, and vigorous therapy with intravenous corticosteroids should be instituted promptly. Initiation of therapy should not depend upon laboratory confirmation of the diagnosis, since any delay in an acute situation may result in the patient's death.

Ovarian hemorrhage: Reports indicate that a woman receiving short- or long-term therapy with heparin or warfarin sodium may be at risk of developing ovarian hemorrhage at the time of ovulation. Caution should be observed when Dicumarol is administered since these compounds have similar actions.

Paralytic ileus and intestinal obstruction have been reported from submucosal or intramural hemorrhage.

Excessive uterine bleeding has occurred but menstrual flow is usually normal.

Bleeding which occurs when the prothrombin time is within the therapeutic range warrants diagnostic investigation since it may unmask a previously unsuspected lesion, e.g. tumor, ulcer, etc.

Necrosis of skin and other tissues. (See *"Warnings".*)

Other adverse reactions are infrequent and consist of alopecia, urticaria, dermatitis, fever, nausea, diarrhea, abdominal cramping, a syndrome called "purple toes", hypersensitivity reactions, leukopenia, and vomiting.

Priapism has been associated with anticoagulant administration, however, a causal relationship has not been established.

---

† Increased and decreased prothrombin time responses have been reported.

► SHOWN IN PRODUCT IDENTIFICATION GUIDE

OVERDOSAGE

Excessive prothrombinopenia, with or without bleeding, is readily controlled by discontinuing Dicumarol, and if necessary, the oral or parenteral administration of vitamin K$_1$. The appearance of microscopic hematuria, excessive menstrual bleeding, melena, petechiae or oozing from nicks made while shaving are early manifestations of hypoprothrombinemia beyond a safe and satisfactory level.

In excessive prothrombinopenia with mild or no bleeding, omission of one or more doses of Dicumarol may suffice; and if necessary, small doses of vitamin K$_1$ orally, 2 ½ to 10 mg, will usually correct the problem.

If minor bleeding persists, or progresses to frank bleeding, vitamin K$_1$ doses of 5 to 25 mg may be given parenterally. (Please note recommendations accompanying vitamin K preparations prior to use.)

Fresh whole blood transfusions should be considered in cases of severe bleeding or prothrombinopenic states unresponsive to vitamin K$_1$.

Resumption of Dicumarol administration reverses the effect of vitamin K$_1$, and a therapeutic hypoprothrombinemia level can again be obtained. A hypercoagulable state has been reported to occur following rapid reversal of a prolonged prothrombin time, therefore, caution must be used in determining the need for this vitamin.

DOSAGE AND LABORATORY CONTROL

The aim of anticoagulant therapy is to impede the coagulation or clotting mechanism to such an extent that thrombosis will not occur, but at the same time avoiding such extensive impairment as might produce spontaneous bleeding. Effective therapeutic levels with minimal complications can best be achieved in cooperative and well-instructed patients, who keep the doctor informed of their status between visits.

The administration and dosage of Dicumarol must be individualized for each patient according to the particular patient's sensitivity to the drug as indicated by the prothrombin time. The prothrombin time reflects the depression of vitamin K dependent Factors VII, X and II. These factors, in addition to Factor IX, are affected by coumarin anticoagulants. There are several modifications of the Quick one-stage prothrombin time and the physician should become familiar with the specific method used in his laboratory.

Administration of Dicumarol should be gauged according to prothrombin time determinations by a suitable method. The blood prothrombin time should usually be determined daily after the administration of the initial dose until prothrombin time results stabilize in the therapeutic range. Intervals between subsequent prothrombin time determinations should be based upon the physician's judgment of the patient's reliability and response to Dicumarol in order to maintain the individual within the therapeutic range. Acceptable intervals for prothrombin time determinations have usually fallen within the range of 1 to 4 weeks. Satisfactory levels for maintenance of therapeutic anticoagulation are 1 ½ to 2 ½ times the normal prothrombin time (e.g. 18 to 30 seconds, with a control of 12 seconds).

Induction: The dosage range for the average adult with normal prothrombin activity ranges from 200 to 300 mg the first day.

Maintenance: On subsequent days the dosage ranges from 25 to 200 mg. It is essential that prothrombin time be measured daily while establishing the correct maintenance dose. Once this has been determined, prothrombin times can be checked less frequently. Dicumarol tablets may not be interchangeable with Dicumarol capsules. Retitration of the dosage should be considered if the dosage form prescribed is changed.

Duration of Therapy: The duration of therapy in each patient should be individualized. In general, anticoagulant therapy should be continued until the danger of thrombosis and embolism has passed.

Treatment during Dentistry and Surgery: The management of patients who undergo dental and surgical procedures requires close liaison between attending physicians, surgeons and dentists. Interruption of anticoagulant therapy may precipitate thromboembolism, and conversely, if anticoagulants are maintained at full doses, some patients may hemorrhage excessively. If it is elected to administer anticoagulants prior to, during, or immediately following dental or surgical procedures, it is recommended that the dosage of Dicumarol be adjusted to maintain the prothrombin time at approximately 1 ½ to 2 ½ times the control level. The operative site should be sufficiently limited to permit the effective use of local procedures for hemostasis including absorbable hemostatic agents, sutures, and pressure dressings if necessary. Under these conditions dental and surgical procedures may be performed without undue risk of hemorrhage.

Dicumarol with Heparin: Since a delay intervenes between the administration of the initial dose and the therapeutic prolongation of prothrombin time, it may be advisable in emergency situations to administer sodium heparin initially along with Dicumarol.

It should be noted that heparin may affect the prothrombin time, and therefore, when patients are receiving both heparin and Dicumarol, the blood sample for prothrombin time determination should be drawn just prior to the next heparin dosage, at least 5 hours after the last intravenous injection or 24 hours after the last subcutaneous injection.

Recommended storage: Store below 77°F (25°C).

HOW SUPPLIED
TABLETS: 25 MG

BRAND/MANUFACTURER	NDC	SIZE	AWP
○ GENERICS			
Abbott Pharm	00074-3794-01	100s	$9.58

Dicyclomine Hydrochloride

DESCRIPTION

Dicyclomine Hydrochloride is an antispasmodic and anticholinergic (antimuscarinic) agent available in the following forms:

1. Dicyclomine Hydrochloride capsules for oral use 10 mg, hydrochloride USP.
2. Dicyclomine Hydrochloride tablets for oral use 20 mg.
3. Dicyclomine Hydrochloride syrup for oral use 10 mg in each 5 mL (1 teaspoonful).
4. Dicyclomine Hydrochloride injection is a sterile, pyrogen free, aqueous solution for intramuscular injection (NOT FOR INTRAVENOUS USE).

Ampul—2 mL—Each mL contains 10 mg Dicyclomine Hydrochloride in sterile water for injection, made isotonic with sodium chloride.

Vial—10 mL—Each mL contains 10 mg Dicyclomine Hydrochloride in sterile water for injection, made isotonic with sodium chloride. A preservative containing 0.5% chlorobutanol hydrous (chloral derivative) has been added.

Chemically, Dicyclomine Hydrochloride is [bicycloxyl]-1-carboxylic acid, 2-(diethylamino)ethyl ester, hydrochloride.

Dicyclomine Hydrochloride occurs as a fine, white, crystalline, practically odorless powder with a bitter taste. It is soluble in water, freely soluble in alcohol and chloroform, and very slightly soluble in ether.

Following is its chemical structure:

$$\text{COOCH}_2\text{CH}_2\text{N}(\text{C}_2\text{H}_5)_2 \cdot \text{HCl}$$

CLINICAL PHARMACOLOGY

Dicyclomine Hydrochloride relieves smooth muscle spasm of the gastrointestinal tract. Animal studies indicate that this action is achieved via a dual mechanism: (1) a specific anticholinergic effect (antimuscarinic) at the acetylcholine-receptor sites with approximately ⅛ the milligram potency of atropine (*in vitro*, guinea pig ileum); and (2) a direct effect upon smooth muscle (musculotropic) as evidenced by Dicyclomine Hydrochloride antagonism of bradykinin- and histamine-induced spasms of the isolated guinea pig ileum. Atropine did not affect responses to these two agonists. *In vitro* studies in cats and dogs showed Dicyclomine Hydrochloride to be equally potent against acetylcholine (ACh)- or barium chloride (BaCl$_2$)-induced intestinal spasm while atropine was at least 200 times more potent against effects of ACh than BaCl$_2$. Tests for mydriatic effects in mice showed that Dicyclomine Hydrochloride was approximately 1/500 as potent as atropine: antisialogogue tests in rabbits showed Dicyclomine Hydrochloride to be 1/300 as potent as atropine.

In man, Dicyclomine Hydrochloride is rapidly absorbed after oral administration, reaching peak values within 60-90 minutes. The principal route of elimination is via the urine (79.5% of the dose). Excretion also occurs in the feces, but to a lesser extent (8.4%). Mean half-life of plasma elimination in one study was determined to be approximately 1.8 hours when plasma concentrations were measured for 9 hours after a single dose. In subsequent studies, plasma concentrations were followed for up to 24 hours after a single dose, showing a secondary phase of elimination with a somewhat longer half-life. Mean volume of distribution for a 20 mg oral dose is approximately 3.65 L/kg suggesting extensive distribution in tissues.

In controlled clinical trials involving over 100 patients who received drug, 82% of patients treated for functional bowel/irritable bowel syndrome with Dicyclomine Hydrochloride at initial doses of 160 mg daily (40 mg q.i.d.) demonstrated a favorable clinical response compared with 55% treated with placebo. (P < .05). In these trials, most of the side effects were typically anticholinergic in nature (see table) and were reported by 61% of the patients.

Side Effect	Dicyclomine Hydrochloride (40 mg q.i.d.) %	Placebo %
Dry Mouth	33	5
Dizziness	29	2
Blurred Vision	27	2
Nausea	14	6
Light-headedness	11	3
Drowsiness	9	1
Weakness	7	1
Nervousness	6	2

Nine percent (9%) of patients were discontinued from the drug because of one or more of these side effects (compared with 2% in the placebo group). In 41% of the

---

◆ RATED THERAPEUTICALLY EQUIVALENT; ◇ THERAPEUTIC EQUIVALENCE UNCONFIRMED; ○ UNRATED

patients with side effects, side effects disappeared or were tolerated at the 160 mg daily dose without reduction. A dose reduction from 160 mg daily to an average daily dose of 90 mg was required in 46% of the patients with side effects who then continued to experience a favorable clinical response: their side effects either disappeared or were tolerated. (See *"Adverse Reactions"*).

INDICATIONS AND USAGE
For the treatment of functional bowel/irritable bowel syndrome.

CONTRAINDICATIONS
1. Obstructive uropathy
2. Obstructive disease of the gastrointestinal tract
3. Severe ulcerative colitis (see *"Precautions"*)
4. Reflux esophagitis
5. Unstable cardiovascular status in acute hemorrhage
6. Glaucoma
7. Myasthenia gravis
8. Evidence of prior hypersensitivity to Dicyclomine Hydrochloride or other ingredients of these formulations
9. Infants less than 6 months of age (see *"Warnings"* and *"Precautions: Information for Patients"*.)
10. Nursing Mothers (See *"Warnings"* and *"Precautions: Information for Patients"*.)

WARNINGS
In the presence of a high environmental temperature, heat prostration can occur with drug use (fever and heat stroke due to decreased sweating). If symptoms occur, the drug should be discontinued and supportive measures instituted. Diarrhea may be an early symptom of incomplete intestinal obstruction, especially in patients with ileostomy or colostomy. In this instance, treatment with this drug would be inappropriate and possibly harmful.

Dicyclomine Hydrochloride may produce drowsiness or blurred vision. The patient should be warned not to engage in activities requiring mental alertness, such as operating a motor vehicle or other machinery or performing hazardous work while taking this drug.

Psychosis has been reported in sensitive individuals given anticholinergic drugs. CNS signs and symptoms include confusion, disorientation, short-term memory loss, hallucinations, dysarthria, ataxia, coma, euphoria, decreased anxiety, fatigue, insomnia, agitation and mannerisms, and inappropriate affect. These CNS signs and symptoms usually resolve within 12 to 24 hours after discontinuation of the drug.

There are reports that administration of Dicyclomine Hydrochloride syrup to infants has been followed by serious respiratory symptoms (dyspnea, shortness of breath, breathlessness, respiratory collapse, apnea, asphyxia), seizures, syncope, pulse rate fluctuations, muscular hypotonia, and coma. Death has been reported. No causal relationship between these effects observed in infants and Dicyclomine Hydrochloride administration has been established. DICYCLOMINE HYDROCHLORIDE IS CONTRAINDICATED IN INFANTS LESS THAN 6 MONTHS OF AGE AND IN NURSING MOTHERS. (See *"Contraindications"* and *"Precautions: Nursing Mothers"* and *"Pediatric Use"*.)

Safety and efficacy of Dicyclomine Hydrochloride in children have not been established.

PRECAUTIONS
GENERAL
Use with caution in patients with:

1. Autonomic neuropathy
2. Hepatic or renal disease
3. Ulcerative colitis—large doses may suppress intestinal motility to the point of producing a paralytic ileus and the use of this drug may precipitate or aggravate the serious complication of toxic megacolon (see *"Contraindications"*)
4. Hyperthyroidism
5. Hypertension
6. Coronary heart disease
7. Congestive heart failure
8. Cardiac tachyarrhythmia
9. Hiatal hernia (see *"Contraindications: Reflux Esophagitis"*)
10. Known or suspected prostatic hypertrophy.

Investigate any tachycardia before administration of Dicyclomine Hydrochloride, since it may increase the heart rate. With overdosage, a curare-like action may occur (i.e., neuromuscular blockade leading to muscular weakness and possible paralysis).

INFORMATION FOR PATIENTS
Dicyclomine Hydrochloride may produce drowsiness or blurred vision. The patient should be warned not to engage in activities requiring mental alertness, such as operating a motor vehicle or other machinery or to perform hazardous work while taking this drug.

Dicyclomine Hydrochloride is contraindicated in infants less than 6 months of age and in nursing mothers. (See *"Contraindications,"* *"Warnings,"* and *"Precautions: Nursing Mothers"* and *"Pediatric Use"*.)

In the presence of a high environmental temperature, heat prostration can occur with drug use (fever and heat stroke due to decreased sweating). If symptoms occur, the drug should be discontinued and a physician contacted.

DRUG INTERACTIONS
The following agents may increase certain actions or side effects of anticholinergic drugs: amantadine, antiarrhythmic agents of class 1 (e.g., quinidine), antihistamines, antipsychotic agents (e.g., phenothiazines), benzodiazepines, MAO inhibitors, narcotic analgesics (e.g., meperidine), nitrates and nitrites, sympathomimetic agents, tricyclic antidepressants, and other drugs having anticholinergic activity. Anticholinergics antagonize the effects of antiglaucoma agents. Anticholinergic drugs in the presence of increased intraocular pressure may be hazardous when taken concurrently with agents such as corticosteroids. (See also *"Contraindications"*.)

Anticholinergic agents may affect gastrointestinal absorption of various drugs, such as slowly dissolving dosage forms of digoxin: increased serum digoxin concentrations may result. Anticholinergic drugs may antagonize the effects of drugs that alter gastrointestinal motility, such as metoclopramide. Because antacids may interfere with the absorption of anticholinergic agents, simultaneous use of these drugs should be avoided.

The inhibiting effects of anticholinergic drugs on gastric hydrochloric acid secretion are antagonized by agents used to treat achlorhydria and those used to test gastric secretion.

CARCINOGENESIS, MUTAGENESIS, INPAIRMENT OF FERTILITY
There are no known human data on long-term potential for carcinogenicity or mutagenicity.

Long-term studies in animals to determine carcinogenic potential are not known to have been conducted.

In studies in rats at doses of up to 100 mg/kg/day, Dicyclomine Hydrochloride produced no deleterious effects on breeding, conception, or parturition.

PREGNANCY
TERATOGENIC EFFECTS
Pregnancy Category B

Reproduction studies have been performed in rats and rabbits at doses up to 33 times the maximum recommended human dose based on 160 mg/day (3 mg/kg) and have revealed no evidence of impaired fertility or harm to the fetus due to Dicyclomine Hydrochloride. Epidemiologic studies in pregnant women with products containing Dicyclomine Hydrochloride (at doses up to 40 mg/day) have not shown that Dicyclomine Hydrochloride increases the risk of fetal abnormalities if administered during the first trimester of pregnancy. There are, however, no adequate and well-controlled studies in pregnant women at the recommended doses (80-160 mg/day). Because animal reproduction studies are not always predictive of human response, Dicyclomine Hydrochloride as indicated for functional bowel/irritable bowel syndrome should be used during pregnancy only if clearly needed.

NURSING MOTHERS
Since Dicyclomine Hydrochloride has been reported to be excreted in human milk, DICYCLOMINE HYDROCHLORIDE IS CONTRAINDICATED IN NURSING MOTHERS. (See *"Contraindications,"* *"Warnings,"* *"Precautions: Pediatric Use"* and *"Adverse Reactions."*)

PEDIATRIC USE:
(See *"Contraindications,"* *"Warnings,"* and *"Precautions: Nursing Mothers"*). DICYCLOMINE HYDROCHLORIDE IS CONTRAINDICATED IN INFANTS LESS THAN 6 MONTHS OF AGE.

Safety and effectiveness in children have not been established.

ADVERSE REACTIONS
Controlled clinical trials have provided frequency information for reported adverse effects of Dicyclomine Hydrochloride listed in a decreasing order of frequency. (See *"Clinical Pharmacology"*.)

Not all of the following adverse reactions have been reported with Dicyclomine Hydrochloride. Adverse reactions are included here that have been reported for pharmacologically similar drugs with anticholinergic/antispasmodic action.

Gastrointestinal: dry mouth, nausea, vomiting, constipation, bloated feeling, abdominal pain, taste loss, anorexia

Central Nervous System: dizziness, light-headedness, tingling, headache, drowsiness, weakness, nervousness, numbness, mental confusion and/or excitement (especially in elderly persons), dyskinesia, lethargy, syncope, speech disturbance, insomnia

Ophthalmologic: blurred vision, diplopia, mydriasis, cycloplegia, increased ocular tension

Dermatologic/Allergic: rash, urticaria, itching, and other dermal manifestations; severe allergic reaction or drug idiosyncrases including anaphylaxis

Genitourinary: urinary hesitancy urinary retention

Cardiovascular: tachycardia, palpitations

Respiratory: Dyspnea, apnea, asphyxia (see *"Warnings"*)

Other: decreased sweating, nasal stuffiness or congestion, sneezing, throat congestion, impotence, suppression of lactation (see *"Precautions: Nursing Mothers"*)

With the injectable form, there may be a temporary sensation of light-headedness. Some local irritation and focal coagulation necrosis may occur following the I.M. injection of the drug.

DRUG ABUSE AND DEPENDENCE

Tolerance, abuse, or dependence with Dicyclomine Hydrochloride has not been reported.

OVERDOSAGE

SIGNS AND SYMPTOMS

The signs and symptoms of overdosage are headache; nausea; vomiting; blurred vision; dilated pupils; hot, dry skin; dizziness; dryness of the mouth; difficulty in swallowing; and CNS stimulation. A curare-like action may occur (i.e., neuromuscular blockade leading to muscular weakness and possible paralysis).

ORAL LD$_{50}$

The acute oral LD$_{50}$ of the drug is 625 mg/kg in mice.

MINIMUM HUMAN LETHAL DOSE/MAXIMUM HUMAN DOSE RECORDED

The amount of drug in a single dose that is ordinarily associated with symptoms of overdosage or that is likely to be life threatening, has not been defined. The maximum human oral dose recorded was 600 mg by mouth in a 10-month-old child and approximately 1500 mg in an adult, each of whom survived.

In three of the infants who died following administration of Dicyclomine Hydrochloride (see "Warnings"), the blood concentrations of drug were 200, 220, and 505 ng/mL, respectively.

DIALYSIS

It is not known if Dicyclomine Hydrochloride is dialyzable.

TREATMENT

Treatment should consist of gastric lavage, emetics, and activated charcoal. Sedatives (e.g., short-acting barbiturates, benzodiazepines) may be used for management of overt signs of excitement. If indicated, an appropriate parenteral cholinergic agent may be used as an antidote.

DOSAGE AND ADMINISTRATION

DOSAGE MUST BE ADJUSTED TO INDIVIDUAL PATIENT NEEDS. (See "Clinical Pharmacology".)

Adults—Oral: The only oral dose clearly shown to be effective is 160 mg per day (in 4 equally divided doses). Since this dose is associated with a significant incidence of side effects, it is prudent to begin with 80 mg per day (in 4 equally divided doses). Depending upon the patient's response during the first week of therapy, the dose should be increased to 160 mg per day unless side effects limit dosage escalation.

If efficacy is not achieved within 2 weeks or side effects require doses below 80 mg per day, the drug should be discontinued. Documented safety data are not available for doses above 80 mg daily for periods longer than 2 weeks.

Adults—Intramuscular Injection: NOT FOR INTRAVENOUS USE.

The intramuscular dosage form is to be used temporarily when the patient cannot take oral medication. Intramuscular injection is about twice as bioavailable as oral dosage forms; consequently, the recommended intramuscular dose is 80 mg daily (in 4 equally divided doses).

Oral Dicyclomine Hydrochloride should be started as soon as possible and the intramuscular form should not be used for periods longer than 1 or 2 days.

ASPIRATE THE SYRINGE BEFORE INJECTING TO AVOID INTRAVASCULAR INJECTION, SINCE THROMBOSIS MAY OCCUR IF THE DRUG IS INADVERTENTLY INJECTED INTRAVASCULARLY. Parenteral drug products should be inspected visually for particulate matter and discoloration prior to administration, whenever solution and container permit.

Store capsules at room temperature, preferably below 86°F (30°C).

To prevent fading of tablets, avoid exposure to direct sunlight. Store tablets at room temperature, preferably below 86°F (30°C).

Store syrup at room temperature, preferably below 86°F (30°C).

Protect from excessive heat.

Store injection at room temperature, preferably below 86°F (30°C).

Protect from freezing.

J CODES

Up to 20 mg IM—J0500

HOW SUPPLIED

CAPSULE: 10 MG

AVERAGE UNIT PRICE (AVAILABLE SIZES)		GENERIC A-RATED AVERAGE PRICE (GAAP)	
BRAND	$0.24	100s	$21.97
GENERIC	$0.21	1000s	$197.58

BRAND/MANUFACTURER	NDC	SIZE	AWP
◆ BRAND			
➤ BENTYL: Marion Merrell Dow	00068-0120-61	100s	$24.36
◆ GENERICS			
Qualitest	00603-3265-21	100s	$19.94
Rugby	00536-3367-01	100s	$20.41
Huffman Labs.	54252-0110-01	100s	$22.05
URL	00677-0341-01	100s	$25.46
Aligen	00405-4328-03	1000s	$186.20
Qualitest	00603-3265-32	1000s	$186.70
Rugby	00536-3367-10	1000s	$185.00
URL	00677-0341-10	1000s	$232.41

INJECTION: 10 MG/ML

AVERAGE UNIT PRICE (AVAILABLE SIZES)	
BRAND	$5.12

BRAND/MANUFACTURER	NDC	SIZE	AWP
◆ BRAND			
BENTYL: Marion Merrell Dow	00068-0810-61	10 ml	$39.90
	00068-0809-23	2 ml 5s	$62.46
◆ GENERICS			
Goldline	00182-0708-63	10 ml	$14.10

SYRUP: 10 MG/5 ML

BRAND/MANUFACTURER	NDC	SIZE	AWP
◆ BRAND			
BENTYL: Marion Merrell Dow	00068-0125-16	480 ml	$27.12

TABLETS: 20 MG

AVERAGE UNIT PRICE (AVAILABLE SIZES)		GENERIC A-RATED AVERAGE PRICE (GAAP)	
BRAND	$0.35	100s	$30.03
GENERIC	$0.26		

BRAND/MANUFACTURER	NDC	SIZE	AWP
◆ BRAND			
➤ BENTYL: Marion Merrell Dow	00068-0123-61	100s	$34.80
◆ GENERICS			
➤ Rugby	00536-3377-01	100s	$29.11
Huffman Labs.	54252-0111-01	100s	$30.94
➤ Rugby	00536-3377-10	1000s	$190.62

Didanosine

WARNING

PANCREATITIS, WHICH HAS BEEN FATAL IN SOME CASES, IS THE MAJOR CLINICAL TOXICITY ASSOCIATED WITH DIDANOSINE THERAPY. PANCREATITIS MUST BE CONSIDERED WHENEVER A PATIENT RECEIVING DIDANOSINE DEVELOPS ABDOMINAL PAIN AND NAUSEA, VOMITING, OR ELEVATED BIOCHEMICAL MARKERS. UNDER THESE CIRCUMSTANCES, DIDANOSINE USE SHOULD BE SUSPENDED UNTIL THE DIAGNOSIS OF PANCREATITIS IS EXCLUDED (SEE "WARNINGS"). PATIENTS RECEIVING DIDANOSINE OR ANY ANTIRETROVIRAL THERAPY MAY CONTINUE TO DEVELOP OPPORTUNISTIC INFECTIONS AND OTHER COMPLICATIONS OF HIV INFECTION, AND THEREFORE SHOULD REMAIN UNDER CLOSE CLINICAL OBSERVATION BY PHYSICIANS EXPERIENCED IN THE TREATMENT OF PATIENTS WITH HIV ASSOCIATED DISEASES.

DESCRIPTION

Didanosine (formerly called dideoxyinosine [ddI]), a synthetic purine nucleoside analogue active against the Human Immunodeficiency Virus (HIV). Didanosine Chewable Dispersible Buffered Tablets are available for oral administration in strengths of 25, 50, 100 or 150 mg. Each tablet is buffered with dihydroxyaluminum sodium carbonate, magnesium hydroxide, and sodium citrate.

Didanosine Buffered Powder for Oral Solution is supplied for oral administration in single-dose packets containing 100, 167, 250, or 375 mg. Packets of each product strength also contain a citrate-phosphate buffer (composed of dibasic sodium phosphate, sodium, citrate, and citric acid) and sucrose.

Didanosine Pediatric Powder for Oral Solution is supplied for oral administration in 4- or 8-ounce glass bottles containing 2 or 4 grams respectively.

The chemical name for Didanosine is 2',3'-dideoxyinosine.

Didanosine is a white crystalline powder with the molecular formula $C_{10}H_{12}N_4O_3$ and a molecular weight of 236.2. The aqueous solubility of Didanosine at 25°C and pH of approximately 6 is 27.3 mg/mL. Didanosine is unstable in acidic solutions. For example, at pH <3 and 37°C, 10 percent of Didanosine decomposes to hypoxanthine in less than 2 minutes.

Following is its chemical structure:

◆ RATED THERAPEUTICALLY EQUIVALENT; ◇ THERAPEUTIC EQUIVALENCE UNCONFIRMED; ○ UNRATED

CLINICAL PHARMACOLOGY

MECHANISM OF ACTION

Didanosine, a nucleoside analogue of deoxyadenosine, inhibits the *in vitro* replication of HIV in human primary cell cultures and in established cell lines. After Didanosine enters the cell, it is converted by cellular enzymes to the active antiviral metabolite, dideoxyadenosine triphosphate (ddATP). The intracellular half-life of ddATP, calculated from results obtained from *in vitro* cell culture studies, varied from 8 to 24 hours.

A common feature of dideoxynucleosides (the class of compounds to which Didanosine belongs) is the lack of a free 3'-hydroxyl group. In nucleic acid replication, the 3'-hydroxyl of a naturally occurring nucleoside is the acceptor for covalent attachment of subsequent nucleoside 5'-monophosphates; its presence is therefore requisite for continued DNA chain extension. Because ddATP lacks a 3'-hydroxyl group, incorporation of ddATP into viral DNA leads to chain termination and, thus, inhibition of viral replication. In addition, ddATP further contributes to inhibition of viral replication through interference with the HIV-RNA dependent DNA polymerase (reverse transcriptase) by competing with the natural nucleoside triphosphate, dATP, for binding to the active site of the enzyme.

MICROBIOLOGY

The relationship between *in vitro* susceptibility of HIV to Didanosine and the inhibition of HIV replication in man or clinical response to therapy has not been established. *In vitro* sensitivity results vary greatly depending upon the time between virus infection and Didanosine treatment, the particular assay used, the cell type employed, the size of the virus inoculum and the laboratory performing the test. In addition, the reliability of methods currently available to measure virologic responses in clinical trials has not been established.

Didanosine has shown *in vitro* antiviral activity in a variety of HIV-infected T cell and monocyte/macrophage cell cultures. The concentration of drug necessary to inhibit viral replication 50 percent (ID_{50}) has been reported to range from 2.5 to 10μM (1 μM = 0.24 mg/mL) in T cells and from 0.01 to 0.1μM in monocyte/macrophage cell cultures. In H9 cells infected with HIV-1, expression of HIV-p24 gag protein was blocked with 10μM Didanosine while ATH8 cells infected with HIV-1 (strain HTLV-11IB) required > 10 μM for complete protection from cytopathic effects.

In a quantitative plaque (syncytium) reduction assay using HT4-6C cells, Didanosine ID_{50} values of 2.1 μM for HIV-1 and 5.6 μM for HIV-2 have been reported. The ID_{50} values of zidovudine determined using this assay system were 0.05 and 0.08 μM for HIV-1 and HIV-2, respectively. However, in infected human MT-2 cells in culture, Didanosine ID_{50} values reported for HIV-1 and HIV-2 were 1 and 10 μM, while ID_{50} values for zidovudine were 0.3 and > 100 μM, respectively.

The development of clinically significant Didanosine resistance in patients with HIV infection after receiving Didanosine therapy has not been studied adequately and the frequency of Didanosine-resistant isolates in the general population remains unknown. Pre- and posttherapy clinical isolates of HIV obtained from 14 patients on long-term Didanosine therapy have been evaluated *in vitro* for sensitivity to Didanosine. Results obtained showed that 12 of 14 pretherapy isolates had ID_{50} values of ≤ 5 μM, whereas, 2 of the 14 pretherapy isolates had ID_{50} values of 30 and 50 μM, respectively. Comparisons of posttherapy to pretherapy ID_{50} values, determined in isolates taken from the same patient, revealed that *in vitro* sensitivity to Didanosine decreased 15-fold in 1 patient, decreased 6-fold in 3 patients, and was not significantly altered in the remaining 10 patients evaluated. The clinical significance of these findings has not been established. In a quantitative plaque reduction assay using HT4-6C cells, Didanosine has shown activity *in vitro* (ID_{50} 0.7 μM) against one zidovudine-resistant HIV-1 strain isolated from a patient who had received long-term therapy with zidovudine.

The results of cytotoxicity studies in various cell lines have shown little cytotoxic action with Didanosine in cultured human bone marrow progenitor cells the concentration of drug necessary to inhibit cell growth 50 percent (IC_{50}) was > 100 μM for Didanosine. For zidovudine, IC_{50} values under similar assay conditions ranged from 0.13 to 5 μM.

Didanosine has shown antiviral activity in one mouse animal model. Mice with severe combined immunodeficiency, (SCID) of genetic origin have been shown to develop an immune system of human origin (SCID-hu) when transplanted with human fetal hematolymphoid organs. These SCID-hu mice, when innoculated with primary isolates of HIV become infected with HIV and subsequently develop viremia.

It has been shown that antiretroviral agents can prevent development of HIV viremia in this animal model system. In an assay in which Didanosine was administered to SCID-hu mice by intraperitoneal injection twice daily for 4 days commencing 24 hours prior to HIV infection and once daily for days 4 to 14 postinfection, the dose that protected 50 percent of the animals from developing viremia (PD_{50}) was reported to be 13.7 mg/kg/day. In a similar assay, the PD_{50} value for zidovudine administered orally in drinking water was determined to be 40.4 mg/kg/day.

ANIMAL TOXICOLOGY

Evidence of a dose-limiting skeletal muscle toxicity has been observed in mice and rats (but not in dogs) following long-term (greater than 90 days) dosing with Didanosine at doses that were approximately 1.2 to 12 times the estimated human exposure. The relationship of this finding to the potential of Didanosine to cause myopathy in humans is unclear. However, human myopathy has been associated with administration of other nucleoside analogues.

PHARMACOKINETICS

Didanosine is rapidly degraded at acidic pH. Therefore, all oral formulations contain buffering agents designed to increase the pH of the gastric environment. When Didanosine Chewable/Dispersible Buffered Tablets are administered each adult and pediatric dose must consist of 2 tablets in order to achieve adequate acid-neutralizing capacity for maximal absorption of Didanosine. The only exception is for pediatric patients who are less than 1 year of age; for these patients only 1 tablet is necessary to provide adequate acid neutralizing capacity.

Bioequivalence of Dosage Formulations: Results of a study in 18 asymptomatic HIV seropositive patients comparing a 375-mg dose of Didanosine Powder for Oral Solution and Didanosine Chewable/Dispersible Buffered Tablets indicate that Didanosine is 20 percent to 25 percent more bioavailable from the tablet compared to the solution. A separate study in 24 asymptomatic HIV seropositive patients demonstrated that a 375-mg dose of the Didanosine Buffered Powder for Oral Solution produced similar plasma concentrations to a 300-mg (2 × 150 mg tablets) dose of the Didanosine Chewable/Dispersible Buffered Tablets. Mean (±1 SD) peak plasma concentrations (C_{max}) were 1.6 (±0.6) μg/mL, range: 0.4 to 2.9 μg/mL, for the buffered solution and 1.6 (±0.5) μg/mL, range: 0.5 to 2.6 μg/mL, for the chewable tablet. Mean area under the plasma concentration versus time curve (AUC) values were 3.0 (±0.8) μg • hr/mL, range: 1.6 to 5.1 μg • hr/mL, for the buffered solution and 2.6 (0.7) μg • hr/mL, range: 1.1 to 3.9 μg • hr/mL, for the chewable tablet.

Effect of Food on Oral Absorption: All Didanosine formulations should be administered on an empty stomach: In a study which included 8 asymptomatic HIV seropositive patients, the administration of Didanosine Chewable/Dispersible Buffered Tablets within 5 minutes of a meal resulted in a 50 percent decrease in mean C_{max} and AUC values. The mean C_{max} was 2.8 μg/mL (range: 1.1 to 4.2 μg/mL) in the fasting state, versus 1.3 μg/mL (range: 0.7 to 2.2 μg/mL) in the fed state. The AUC values averaged 3.9 μg • hr/mL (range: 2.8 to 6.7 μg • hr/mL) under fasting conditions, versus 2.1 μg • hr/mL (range: 1.2 to 4.0 μg • hr/mL) following a meal.

Study Design in Adults: The pharmacokinetics of Didanosine were evaluated in 69 adult patients with AIDS or severe AIDS-Related Complex. These patients had creatinine clearance values of > 60 mL/min and no evidence of hepatic dysfunction. Patients received a 60-minute IV infusion of Didanosine administered once or twice a day for 2 weeks, at total daily doses ranging from 0.8 mg/kg to 33 mg/kg. Oral doses equivalent to twice the IV dose were administered for an additional 4 weeks. The oral doses were administered as a lyophilized formulation which was similar in composition to Didanosine Pediatric Powder for Oral Solution. Plasma Didanosine concentrations were obtained on the first day of dosing and at steady state after intravenous and oral dosing.

Absorption and Dose Linearity in Adults: Although there was significant variability between patients, the C_{max} and AUC values increased in proportion to dose over the range of doses administered in clinical practice. At doses of 7 mg/kg or less, the average absolute bioavailability was 33 (±14) percent after a single dose and 37 (±14) percent after 4 weeks of Didanosine dosing. Pharmacokinetic parameters at steady state were not significantly different from values obtained after the initial IV or oral dose.

Distribution in Adults: The steady state volume of distribution after IV administration averaged 54 L (range: 22 to 103 L). In a study of 5 adults, the concentration of Didanosine in the cerebrospinal fluid 1 hour after infusion of Didanosine averaged 21 percent of the simultaneous plasma concentration.[1]

Elimination in Adults: After oral administration of Didanosine, the average elimination half-life was 1.6 hours (range: 0.52 to 4.64 hours). Total body clearance averaged 800 mL/min (range: 412 to 1505 mL/min). Renal clearance represented approximately 50 percent of the total body clearance (average: 400, range: 95 to 860 mL/min), when Didanosine was administered either intravenously or orally. This indicates that active tubular secretion, in addition to glomerular filtration, is responsible for the renal elimination of Didanosine. Urinary recovery of Didanosine after a single dose was approximately 55 percent (range: 27 to 98 percent), and 20 percent (range: 3 to 31 percent) of the dose after IV and oral administration, respectively. There was no evidence of accumulation of Didanosine after either IV or oral dosing.

Study Design in Children: The pharmacokinetics of Didanosine have been evaluated in two pediatric studies. In one study (ACTG/St. Jude), 16 children and 4 adolescents received a single IV dose ranging from 40 to 90 mg/m² and multiple, twice daily oral doses of 80 to 180 mg/m² of Didanosine. In another study (NCl), 48 pediatric patients received a single IV dose and then multiple, three times daily oral doses ranging from 20 to 180 mg/m².[2] In both studies, oral doses were administered as a lyophilized formulation which was similar in composition to Didanosine Pediatric Powder for Oral Solution.

Absorption and Dose Linearity in Children: Although there was significant variability between patients, the C_{max} and AUC values increased in proportion to dose in both studies. These findings were similar to those in adult patients. The absolute bioavailability varied between patients in the ACTG/St. Jude study had averaged 32 (±12) percent, range: 13 to 53 percent, and 42 (±18) percent, range: 21 to 78 percent, after the first oral dose and at steady state, respectively. The NCl study also demonstrated significant variability in the oral absorption of Didanosine with an average absolute bioavailability of 19 (±17) percent, range: 2 to 89 percent in the ACTG/St. Jude study, the average steady state AUC was 1.4 (±0.4), 1.6 (±0.9) and 2.3 (±0.9) μg • hr/mL after the administration of oral doses of 80, 120, and 180 mg/m², respectively. The average corresponding steady state C_{max} values were 0.8 (±0.4), 1.4 (±0.7), and 1.7 (±0.9) μg/mL, respectively.

Distribution in Children: In the ACTG/St. Jude study, the volume of distribution after IV administration averaged 35.6 LM^2 (range, 18.4 to 60.7 Lm^2). In this study, the concentration of Didanosine ranged from 0.04 to 0.12 μg/mL in cerebrospinal fluid (CSF) samples collected from seven patients at times ranging from 1.5 to 3.5 hr after a single intravenous or oral dose. These CSF concentrations corresponded to 12 to 85 percent (mean: 46 percent) of the concentration in a simultaneous plasma sample.

Elimination in Children: In the ACTG/St. Jude study, the elimination half-life following oral administration averaged 0.8 hours (range: 0.51 to 1.2 hours). Total body clearance following IV administration averaged 532 mL min/m² (range 294 to 920 mL/min/m²). Mean renal clearance ranged from 190 to 319 mL/min/m² after the first oral dose and from 231 to 265 mL/min/m² at steady state. Urinary recovery averaged 21 percent (range 4 to 41 percent) at steady state. There was no evidence of accumulation of Didanosine after the administration of oral doses for an average of 26 days.

Metabolism: The metabolism of Didanosine has not been evaluated in man. When ^{14}C-radiolabeled Didanosine was administered to dogs as a single IV or oral dose, extensive metabolism occurred. The major metabolite identified in the urine, allantoin, represented approximately 61 percent of the administered radiolabel after oral administration. Three putative metabolites tentatively identified in the urine were hypoxanthine, xanthine, and uric acid. A similar metabolic profile was obtained using an isolated perfused rat liver preparation. The metabolic fate of the dideoxyribose moiety, released subsequent to enzymatic or chemical hydrolysis of the glycosidic bond, has not been determined. Based upon data from animal studies, it is presumed that the metabolism of Didanosine in man will occur by the same pathways responsible for the elimination of endogenous purines.

The intracellular half-life of ddATP, the metabolite presumed to be responsible for the antiretroviral activity of Didanosine, is reported to be 8 to 24 hours *in vitro*. The half-life of intracellular ddATP *in vivo* has not been measured. There are currently incomplete data concerning the effect of impaired renal or hepatic function on the pharmacokinetics of Didanosine. (See *"Precautions".*)

Because *in vitro* human plasma protein binding is less than 5 percent with Didanosine, drug interactions involving binding site displacement are not anticipated.

INDICATIONS AND USAGE

Didanosine is indicated for the treatment of adult patients with advanced HIV infection who have received prolonged prior zidovudine therapy. This indication is based on the results of a randomized, double-blind controlled clinical trial comparing two doses of Didanosine Buffered Powder for Oral Solution and zidovudine in patients with a median CD4 cell count of 95 cells/μL who were previously treated with zidovudine for a median duration of 13.7 months (range: 3-61 months).

Didanosine is also indicated for the treatment of adult and pediatric patients (over 6 months of age) with advanced HIV infections who have demonstrated intolerance or significant clinical or immunologic deterioration during zidovudine therapy. This indication is based primarily on the results of nonrandomized, Phase 1 studies in which an increase in CD4 cell counts was observed for many patients during Didanosine therapy (see "Description of Clinical Data").

Because initial therapy with zidovudine has been shown to prolong survival and decrease the incidence of opportunistic infections in patients with advanced HIV disease and because data are not yet available which evaluate the effect of initial therapy with Didanosine, zidovudine should be considered initial therapy for treatment of advanced HIV infection, unless contraindicated.

DESCRIPTION OF CLINICAL DATA

ADULTS

RESULTS FROM A CONTROLLED CLINICAL TRIAL[3]

A randomized, double-blind controlled clinical trial compared two weight-adjusted doses of Didanosine to zidovudine in patients who had tolerated four months or greater of prior zidovudine therapy. Doses of Didanosine Buffered Powder for Oral Solution were as follows:

Patient Weight	High Dose	Low (Recommended) Dose
≥ 60 kg	375 mg BID	250 mg BID
< 60 kg	250 mg BID	167 mg BID

Analyses were conducted on data from 913 patients who were accrued to the study from October 1989 to April 1991. Median duration of prior zidovudine was 13.7 months. The median entry CD4 cell count was 95 cells/μL (range: 0-627). Sixty percent of patients had ARC, 30 percent had AIDS and 10 percent had asymptomatic HIV disease. Median treatment duration during the study was 11.4 months.

Overall, participants randomized to Didanosine at the recommended dose had a statistically significant delay in time to first new AIDS-defining event or death compared to those randomized to zidovudine, (p = 0.015). There was no statistically significant difference between the high dose Didanosine and zidovudine arms in time to first new AIDS-defining event or death, (p = 0.46).

At one year the proportion of patients who developed a new AIDS-defining event or death was 40 percent in the zidovudine arm as compared to 28 percent and 34 percent for Didanosine at the recommended dose and Didanosine high dose, respectively.

There were no survival differences observed among the treatment arms, (high dose Didanosine versus zidovudine, p = 0.64 and Didanosine at the recommended dose versus zidovudine, p = 0.81).

The mean change in CD4 cell counts (cells/μL) by week 12 was +13 for high dose Didanosine and +11 for Didanosine at the recommended dose, compared to -9 for zidovudine. At week 24, the mean change was -9, -7 and -27, respectively. The 50:50 response (see *"Definitions of Outcome"*, below) was 10 percent for high dose Didanosine, 8 percent for Didanosine at the recommended dose, and 3 percent for zidovudine. The 10:10 response was 37 percent, 34 percent and 17 percent, respectively.

The major clinical adverse events associated with Didanosine during the course of study were pancreatitis and neuropathy. The one-year rates for pancreatitis were 13 percent for Didanosine high dose and 7 percent for Didanosine at the recommended dose as compared to 3 percent for zidovudine (p = 0.002 and p = 0.09, respectively). There were two episodes of fatal pancreatitis in the Didanosine high dose arm.

The one-year rates of grades 2, 3 or 4 peripheral neuropathy were 14 percent, 13 percent and 14 percent (high dose Didanosine versus zidovudine, p = 0.74 and Didanosine at the recommended dose versus zidovudine, p = 0.98).

The most commonly reported laboratory abnormalities in the controlled study were leukopenia and elevated amylase.

The one-year rates of leukopenia were 14 percent, 22 percent, and 26 percent for Didanosine high dose. Didanosine at the recommended dose and zidovudine respectively (high dose of Didanosine versus zidovudine, p < 0.001 and low dose of Didanosine versus zidovudine p < 0.001). The one-year rates for elevated amylase were 30 percent and 20 percent for patients receiving high and low dose Didanosine and compared to 6 percent for patients receiving zidovudine (p < 0.001 and p < 0.001). The one-year rates of grades 3,4 liver function test abnormalities were 21 percent and 43 percent for Didanosine high dose and low dose as compared to 23 percent zidovudine (p = 0.047 and p = 0.423).

PHASE 1 STUDIES

Four phase 1 trials, three of which were dose escalation studies, were conducted at five institutions (see Table 1). One-hundred seventy patients were enrolled, 75% of whom had previously received zidovudine therapy. Patients were primarily male and caucasian, and most had a history of homosexual or bisexual contact as their HIV risk factor. Median CD4 count at entry was 62 cells/μL. Dosages in these studies ranged from 0.8 to 66 mg/kg/day, and were given using several schedules and by two routes of administration (IV and PO) for a median duration of 38 weeks (range: 0 to 99 weeks). The median average daily dose was 10.3 mg/kg/day.

Table 1

DIDANOSINE ADULT PHASE 1 PROTOCOLS

Study	Deaconess	ACTG 064	Boston City	NCI
N	30	44	39	57
Accrual Dates	6/89 to 10/89	10/88 to 9/89	10/88 to 10/89	7/88 to 3/90
Median CD4	22	27	69	44
Range	0-270	4-415	2-540	0-496
% Caucasian	97	89	67	88
% Homosexual	77	82	64	88
% IVDU	10	2	18	2
% Prior ZDV	100*	81	53	71
% AIDS	73	36	46	44
Dose range (mg/kg/day) and schedule	6 PO & 750/ 1500 mg/ day PO BID	0.8 IV-66 PO BID	0.8 IV-30.4 PO QD	0.8 IV-51.2 PO BID or TID

* *All patients had documented hematologic intolerance to ZDV.*

In the phase 1 studies activity was assessed using CD4 cell counts which were obtained and analyzed at various time intervals. For comparison, an historical control database consisted of patients from the placebo groups of three randomized, blinded trials that compared zidovudine therapy to placebo, and patients from one open trial of dextran sulfate (now known not to be orally absorbed and therefore considered a placebo).

Additional safety data was derived from 7806 of the participants in the Didanosine U.S. Expanded Access Program who received weight-adjusted doses which approximated 6 to 10 mg/kg/day.

Definitions of outcome, which were applied *post hoc* to data from the patients receiving Didanosine in the phase 1 studies, included the following:

a) Presence of a "response", where response was defined as i) the greater of a 50-cell or 50 percent increase over baseline CD4 cell count maintained for a minimum of any consecutive 4 weeks during therapy (50:50); ii) the greater of a 10-cell or 10 percent increase defined similarly (10:10);

b) Percent change from baseline in CD4 cell count at various time points on therapy;

c) Longitudinal changes during study weeks 0 to 12: time weighted average of serial CD4 cell counts corrected for (normalized by) baseline CD4 cell count (NAUC). [Normalized area under the curve (NAUC) = (Cumulative AUC of CD4 cell count up to time t)/(baseline CD4 count × t).] NAUCs that exceed a value of 1 indicate that the average CD4 level during therapy is increased over the baseline CD4 cell count.

RESULTS FROM PHASE 1 STUDIES

Comparisons of CD4 cell counts between patients receiving Didanosine and historical controls must be considered with caution in light of differences in their

◆ RATED THERAPEUTICALLY EQUIVALENT; ◇ THERAPEUTIC EQUIVALENCE UNCONFIRMED; ○ UNRATED

comparability (e.g., entry CD4 cell counts, history of prior zidovudine therapy and secular changes in standards of care for HIV infected patients [Tables 1 and 2]).

Table 2
PRETREATMENT PATIENT COMPARISONS

	Historical Control Groups				
Study	All Phase 1	BWO2	ACTG 001	ACTG 016	ACTG 060
Population	ARC & AIDS	ARC & AIDS	Kaposi's Sarcoma	Early ARC	HIV Infection
N: Placebo	170	137	89	344	60
Accrual Dates	7/88 to 3/90	2/86 to 7/86	1/87 to 11/87	8/87 to 5/89	8/88 to 3/89
Median CD4 cell/mL	62	68	277	397	204
Range	0-540	0-1069	14-1316	151-862	4-621
% Caucasian	85	NA*	87	83	74
% Prior ZDV	75	0	0	0	25
% AIDS	48	55	100	0	25

* *NA = not available*

a) *Response:* 22 percent of patients receiving Didanosine had a 50:50 response in CD4 counts and 50 percent had a 10:10 response. In comparison, 2-12 percent of the historical control patients had a 50:50 response and 17-31 percent had a 10:10 response.

b) *Percent change from baseline:* In patients receiving Didanosine the percent increase from baseline CD4 cell counts was 29 percent at 4 weeks, 27 percent at 8 weeks, and 14 percent at 12 weeks. In comparison, historical control groups had progressive declines in CD4 cell counts.

c) *Longitudinal changes during study weeks 0 to 12:* 70 percent of patients receiving Didanosine had NAUC values exceeding 1, compared to 34 percent to 46 percent of the historical control patients. The mean NAUC in patients receiving Didanosine was 1.38 versus 0.99 to 1.04 in the historical control groups.

CHILDREN
RESULTS FROM PHASE 1 STUDIES
Two pediatric phase 1 does escalation clinical trials evaluated Didanosine in symptomatic patients with HIV disease (CDC P2 classification); both were open label studies without control patients. The larger study was conducted at the National Cancer Institute (NCI). Pediatric Branch, and the smaller study conducted under the auspices of the AIDS Clinical Trials Group (ACTG) and St. Jude Children's Research Hospital. The pediatric data included a total of 98 patients, 89 of whom met the criteria for symptomatic HIV-disease (CDC Class P2 [see Table 3]).

Table 3
BASELINE CHARACTERISTICS OF PEDIATRIC PHASE 1 PATIENTS

	NCI	ACTG/St. Jude
Total patients	78	20
Male:Female	48:30	12:8
Age (years)		
Median (Range)	6.9 (0.6-19)	6.3 (0.7-18)
Race		
Caucasian	52 (67)*	7 (35)
Black	17 (22)	11 (55)
Hispanic	4 (5)	2 (10)
Other	5 (6)	—
Prior ZDV	41 (52)	2 (10)
Mode of transmission		
Perinatal	39 (50)	10 (50)
Transfusion	21 (27)	4 (20)
Hemophiliac	18 (23)	6 (30)
Stage		
AIDS†	55 (70)	10 (50)
SHIV†	14 (18)	10 (50)
P1	9 (12)	—
Baseline CD4 cells/μL‡		
< 50	34 (45)	7 (35)
50-99	7 (9)	2 (10)
≥ 100	35 (46)	11 (55)
Median	70	205

* *Percentage of patients in this category for each study*
† *CDC class P2.*
‡ *Two patients did not have baseline CD4 counts*

Patients in these two studies received Didanosine at doses from 60 to 540 mg/m²/day. Based on an increased incidence of pancreatitis observed at the higher doses administered, all patients treated at doses > 360 mg/m²/day were dose reduced to this level or lower. Due to multiple dose adjustments, 77 percent of patients received average daily doses ≤ 300 mg/m²/day (see Table 4)

CD4 cell count, p24 antigenemia, and weight were each used to assess biologic activity of Didanosine. Although these definitions have not been definitively

correlated with clinical outcome for the purpose of describing the results of these studies, changes in these measures were analyzed by classifying patients by retrospectively applied definitions of "response." CD4 response definitions are as described for adult patients (see *"Definitions of outcome"* above). A response for p24 antigen was defined as a 50 percent reduction from baseline, or a decrease from between 32 to 64 pg/mL to < 32 pg/mL (assay sensitivity), occurring at any time during therapy and maintained for at least 4 weeks. Weight gain in children was also analyzed as either a 10 percent increase in weight (for smaller children) or a 2.5 increase (for children > 25 kg), also occurring at any time during therapy and maintained for at least 4 weeks.

Table 4
DOSING AND DURATION OF DIDANOSINE THERAPY IN CHILDREN

	NCI N = 78	ACTG/St. Jude N = 20
Total Daily Dose		
Range (mg/m²/day)	60-540	160-360
Regimen	TID	BID
Study Duration		
Median	35 weeks	37 weeks
Range	4-77 weeks	1-56 weeks
Cumulative Dose (mg/kg):		
Median (range)	2689 (3-7452)	2387 (29-3828)

Separate analyses with patients pooled from both studies were performed for CD4, p24, and weight responses for the 89 patients with symptomatic HIV disease (CDC class P2) and for the subset of 40 children previously exposed to zidovudine (see Table 5). The effect of Didanosine on survival and the incidence of opportunistic infections in children could not be assessed; therefore, zidovudine should be considered as initial therapy for the treatment of advanced HIV infection, unless contraindicated.

Table 5
RESPONSES POOLED PEDIATRIC DATA (CDC P2) N = 89

	Prior zidovudine Pts (N = 40)*	All Pts (N = 89)
Baseline CD4 (cells/μL), Median (range)	8 0-3140	60 0-3140
CD4 Response, 10:10 (%)	8/36 (22)	31/83 (37)
CD4 Response, 50:50 (%)	5/36 (14)	19/83 (23)
% CD4 Change at Week 8	+21	+27
p24 Response (%)†	10/18 (56)	36/49 (73)
CD4 (50:50) + weight (%)‡	1 (3)	4 (5)
p24 + weight (%)	4 (10)	9 (10)
CD4 (50:50) + p24 + weight (%)	1 (3)	9 (10)
Weight Response (%)	12/36 (33)	32/83 (39)
Neuropsychometric Response, NCI (%)§	7/21 (33)	12/43 (28)

* *Patients for whom the drug is currently recommended.*
† *p24 response was assessable only in patients with detectable p24 antigen at entry; 5 of 34 patients with undetectable antigen at entry became antigenemic during study.*
‡ *Patients who had both a 50:50 CD4 response and a weight response; subsequent categories are defined similarly.*
§ *The denominator reflects those patients with a baseline IQ score < 115; for the entire group, there was not a statistically significant change between entry and followup neuropsychometric scores.*

In general, hematologic parameters were stable during treatment with Didanosine. In addition, improvement in platelet counts were seen in 3 of 6 patients with idiopathic thrombocytopenic purpura (ITP) who entered the pediatric studies with this diagnosis. Patients enrolled in the NCI trial underwent detailed neuropsychometric testing at entry and at 6 months on study. An increment in an individual's IQ score of 10 percent and a minimum of 8 points relative to baseline was considered a response. Improvement was seen in 12 of 43 evaluable patients with a baseline IQ < 115. In the absence of a control group the contribution of drug to this increase is uncertain.

CONTRAINDICATION
Didanosine is contraindicated in patients with previously demonstrated clinically significant hypersensitivity to any of the components of the formulations.

WARNINGS
1. PANCREATITIS
PANCREATITIS, WHICH HAS BEEN FATAL IN SOME CASES, IS THE MAJOR CLINICAL TOXICITY ASSOCIATED WITH DIDANOSINE THERAPY. PANCREATITIS MUST BE CONSIDERED WHENEVER A PATIENT RECEIVING DIDANOSINE DEVELOPS ABDOMINAL PAIN AND NAUSEA,

VOMITING OR ELEVATED BIOCHEMICAL MARKERS. UNDER THESE CIRCUMSTANCES, DIDANOSINE USE SHOULD BE SUSPENDED UNTIL THE DIAGNOSIS OF PANCREATITIS IS EXCLUDED. When treatment with other drugs known to cause pancreatic toxicity is required (for example, IV centamidine), suspension of Didanosine should be considered.

In the controlled clinical trial comparing two doses of Didanosine to zidovudine the one-year rates of pancreatitis based on Kaplan-Meier estimates were 13 percent and 7 percent for Didanosine high dose and Didanosine at the recommended dose as compared to 3 percent for zidovudine (p = .001 and p = .09 respectively). Other symptoms suggestive of pancreatitis were also observed and are described in Table 6.

Table 6
PERCENTAGE OF PATIENTS WITH PANCREATITIS (CONTROLLED STUDY DATA)

	High Dose Didanosine	Recommended Dose Didanosine	Zidovudine
N	311	298	304
Pancreatitis	31 (10%)*	17 (6%)	6 (2%)
Abdominal pain/ Nausea and elevated amylase	1 (0.3%)	2 (0.6%)	3 (0.9%)
Elevated amylase	44 (14%)	30 (10%)	9 (3%)
Abdominal pain/ Nausea	4 (1%)	5 (2%)	13 (4%)

* *Two fatalities occurred in this group.*

The incidence of pancreatitis and potential manifestations of pancreatitis in the adult phase 1 studies are described in the table below.

Table 7
PERCENTAGE OF PATIENTS WITH PANCREATITIS (PHASE 1 STUDIES)

	Phase 1 ≤ 12.5 mg/kg/day	Phase 1 > 12.5 mg/kg/day
N	91	79
Pancreatitis	8 (9%)	21(27%)
Abdominal pain	9 (10%)	5 (6%)
Increased Amylase	16 (18%)	12 (15%)
Abdominal pain and increased amylase†	6 (7%)	5 (6%)

† *Some case reports recorded abdominal pain with elevated serum amylase, without reporting fully characterized pancreatitis.*

In the Expanded Access Program for Didanosine, 8 of 27 (30 percent) subjects with a history of pancreatitis who were treated with Didanosine developed pancreatitis. DIDANOSINE THERAPY SHOULD BE USED ONLY WITH EXTREME CAUTION IN THIS POPULATION.

Patients with a heightened risk of pancreatitis, such as those with a history of pancreatitis, alcohol consumption, elevated triglycerides, or evidence of advanced HIV infection, should be followed closely. Patients with renal impairment may be at greater risk for pancreatitis if treated without dose adjustment.

In pediatric studies, pancreatitis occurred in 2 of 60 (3 percent) patients treated at entry doses below 300 mg/m^2/day and in 5 of 38 (13 percent) patients treated at higher doses. In pediatric patients with symptoms similar to those described above, Didanosine use should be suspended until the diagnosis of pancreatitis is excluded.

2. PERIPHERAL NEUROPATHY
PERIPHERAL NEUROPATHY OCCURS IN PATIENTS TREATED WITH DIDANOSINE AND THE FREQUENCY APPEARS TO BE DOSE RELATED. PATIENTS SHOULD BE MONITORED FOR THE DEVELOPMENT OF A NEUROPATHY THAT IS USUALLY CHARACTERIZED BY DISTAL NUMBNESS, TINGLING, OR PAIN IN THE FEET OR HANDS. In the controlled trial comparing two doses of Didanosine to zidovudine, the one-year rates, based on Kaplan-Meier estimates, of grades 2, 3 or 4 peripheral neuropathy were 14 percent, 13 percent and 14 percent for high dose Didanosine, Didanosine at the recommended dose, and zidovudine, respectively, (high dose Didanosine versus zidovudine, p = 0.790 and Didanosine at the recommended dose versus zidovudine, p = 0.946).

Among the 91 adult phase 1 patients who received an average oral daily dose of Didanosine approximating 750 mg/day or less, 12 percent had neuropathy severe enough to require dose modification. Thirty-four percent of patients in these studies treated with Didanosine doses at or below 12.5 mg/kg/day developed neuropathy (see Table 8).

Table 8
INCIDENCE OF NEUROPATHY

	Phase 1 ≤ 12.5 mg/kg/day	Phase 1 > 12.5 mg/kg/day
N	91	79
Neuropathy	31 (34 %)	40 (51%)
Neuropathy requiring dose modification*	11 (12%)	27 (34%)

* *Twenty-one of 38 subjects were rechallenged following dose modification and tolerated ddI for periods ranging from 3 days to 45 weeks.*

Neuropathy occurred more frequently in patients with a history of neuropathy or neurotoxic drug therapy. These patients may be at increased risk of neuropathy during Didanosine therapy.

Neuropathy has been reported rarely in children treated with Didanosine. However, because signs and symptoms of neuropathy are difficult to assess in children, physicians should be alerted to the possibility of this event.

3. LIVER FAILURE
In the controlled clinical trial comparing two doses of Didanosine to zidovudine the one-year rates of grade 3-4 liver function test (LFT) alteration was 21 percent for high dose Didanosine, 13 percent for Didanosine at the recommended dose, and 14 percent for zidovudine (high dose Didanosine versus zidovudine, p = 0.047 and Didanosine at the recommended dose versus zidovudine, p = 0.423). Fatal liver failure of unknown etiology occurred during Didanosine therapy in 1/170 patients in the phase 1 studies and 14/7806 in the U.S. Expanded Access program but was not reported in the controlled trial.

4. RETINAL DEPIGMENTATION AND VISION
Four pediatric patients demonstrated retinal depigmentation at doses of Didanosine above 300 mg/m^2/day. Until further information is avaiable from ongoing clinical trials with children treated at currently recommended lower doses of Didanosine it has been proposed that children receiving Didanosine should undergo dilated retinal examination every 6 months or if a change in vision occurs. (See "Adverse Reactions").

PRECAUTIONS
GENERAL
Patients receiving Didanosine or any other antiretroviral therapy may continue to develop opportunistic infections and other complications of HIV infection, and therefore should remain under close clinical observation by physicians experienced in the treatment of patients with associated HIV diseases.

Ingestion of Didanosine with food reduces the absorption of Didanosine by as much as 50 percent. Therefore, Didanosine should be administered on an empty stomach.

Patients with Phenylketonuria: Didanosine Chewable/Dispersible Buffered Tablets contain the following quantities of phenylalanine:

Table 9

	150-mg Strength	All Other Strengths
Phenylalanine per 2-tablet dose	67.4 mg	45 mg
Phenylalanine per tablet	33.7 mg	22.6 mg

Patients on Sodium-Restricted Diets: Didanosine Chewable Dispersible Buffered Tablets: Each Didanosine buffered tablet contains 264.5 mg sodium. A 2-tablet dose of Didanosine buffered tablets contains 529 mg sodium. Didanosine Buffered Powder for Oral Solution. Each single-dose packet of Didanosine. Buffered Powder for Oral Solution contains 1380 mg sodium.

Patients With Renal Impairment: Patients with renal impairment (serum creatinine) > 1.5 mg/dL or creatinine clearance <60 mL/min may be at greater risk of toxicity from Didanosine due to decreased drug clearance; a dose reduction should be considered. The magnesium hydroxide content of each Didanosine tablet is 15.7 mEq which may present an excessive load of magnesium to patients with significant renal impairment, particularly after prolonged dosing.

Patients With Hepatic impairment: Patients with hepatic impairment may be at greater risk for toxicity related to Didanosine treatment due to altered metabolism: a dose reduction may be necessary.

Hyperuricemia: Didanosine has been associated with asymptomatic hyperuricemia: treatment suspension may be necessary if clinical measures aimed at reducing uric acids levels fail.

Diarrhea: Didanosine Buffered Powder for Oral Solution was associated with diarrhea in 34 percent of patients in the phase 1 adult studies (see "Adverse Reactions"). No data are available to demonstrate whether other formulations are associated with lower rates of diarrhea. However, if diarrhea develops in a patient receiving Didanosine Buffered Powder for Oral Solution, a trial of Didanosine Chewable/Dispersible Buffered Tablets should be considered.

INFORMATION FOR PATIENTS
Didanosine is not a cure for HIV infection, and patients may continue to develop HIV-associated illness, including opportunistic infection. Therefore, patients should remain under the care of a physician when using Didanosine.

Patients should be informed that the major toxicities of Didanosine are pancreatitis, which has been fatal in some patients and peripheral neuropathy. Symptoms of pancreatitis include abdominal pain, and nausea and vomiting.

◆ RATED THERAPEUTICALLY EQUIVALENT; ◇ THERAPEUTIC EQUIVALENCE UNCONFIRMED; ○ UNRATED

Symptoms of peripheral neuropathy include tingling, burning, pain or numbness in the hands or feet. Patients should be advised that these symptoms should be reported to their physicians. They should be counseled that these toxicities occur with greatest frequency in patients with a history of these events, and that dose modification and/or discontinuation of Didanosine may be required if toxicity develops. They should be cautioned about the use of other medications that may exacerbate the Didanosine, including alcohol.

Patients should be told that the long-term effects of Didanosine are unknown at this time. Patients should be advised that therapy has not been shown to reduce the risk of transmission of HIV to others through sexual contact or blood contamination.

DRUG INTERACTIONS
Coadministration of Didanosine with drugs that are known to cause peripheral neuropathy or pancreatitis may increase the risk of these toxicities (see "Warnings") and should be done only with extreme caution.

Drug interaction studies have demonstrated that there are no clinically significant interactions with Didanosine and ketoconazole or ranitidine. Drugs whose absorption can be affected by the level of acidity in the stomach (e.g., ketoconazole, dapsone), should be administered at least 2 hours prior to dosing with Didanosine. A study in 4 patients revealed that concomitant administration of ganciclovir does not significantly affect the pharmacokinetics of Didanosine. There is no evidence that Didanosine potentiates the myelosuppressive effects of ganciclovir.

As with other products containing magnesium and/or aluminum antacid components, Didanosine Chewable/Dispersible Buffered Tablets or Didanosine Pediatric Powder for Oral Solution should not be administered with a prescription antibiotic containing any form of tetracycline.

Plasma concentrations of some quinolone antibiotics are decreased when administered with antacids containing magnesium or aluminum. Therefore, doses of quinolone antibiotics should not be administered within 2 hours of taking Didanosine Chewable/Dispersible Buffered Tablets or Pediatric Powder for Oral Solution. Concomitant administration of antacids containing magnesium or aluminum with Didanosine Chewable/Dispersible Buffered Tablets or Pediatric Powder for Oral Solution may potentiate adverse effects associated with the antacid components.

CARCINOGENESIS AND MUTAGENESIS
Long-term carcinogenicity studies of Didanosine in animals have not been completed. No evidence of mutagenicity (with or without metabolic activation) was observed in Ames *Salmonella* mutagenicity assays or in a mutagenicity assay conducted with *Escherichia coli* tester strain WP2 uvrA where only a slight increase in revertants was observed with Didanosine. In a mammalian cell gene mutation assay conducted in L5178Y/TK ± mouse lymphoma cells, Didanosine was weakly positive both in the absence and presence of metabolic activation at concentrations of approximately 2000 µg/mL and above. In an *in vitro* cytogenic study performed in cultured human peripheral lymphocytes, high concentrations of Didanosine ($\geq$ 500 µg/mL) elevated the frequency of cells bearing chromosome aberrations. Another *in vitro* mammalian cell chromosome aberration study using Chinese Hamster Lung cells revealed that Didanosine produces chromosome aberrations at $\geq$ 500 µg/mL after 48 hours of exposure. However, no significant elevations in the frequency of cells with chromosome aberrations were seen at Didanosine concentrations up to 250 µg/mL. In a BALB/c 3T3 *in vitro* transformation assay, Didanosine was considered positive only at concentrations of 3000 µg/mL and above. No evidence of genotoxicity was observed in rat and mouse micronucleus assays.

The results from the genotoxicity studies suggest that Didanosine is not mutagenic at biologically and pharmacologically relevant doses. At significantly elevated doses *in vitro*, the genotoxic effects of Didanosine are similar in magnitude to those seen with natural DNA nucleosides.

PREGNANCY, REPRODUCTION AND FERTILITY
Pregnancy Category B. Reproduction studies have been performed in rats and rabbits at doses up to 12 and 14.2 times the estimated human exposure (based upon plasma levels), respectively and have revealed no evidence of impaired fertility or harm to the fetus due to Didanosine. At approximately 12 times the estimated human exposure, Didanosine was slightly toxic to female rats and their pups during mid and late lactation. These rats showed reduced food intake and body weight gains but the physical and functional development of the offspring was not impaired and there were no major changes in the F2 generation A study in rats showed that Didanosine and/or its metabolites are transferred to the fetus through the placenta. There are no adequate and well-controlled studies in pregnant women. Because animal reproduction studies are not always predictive of human response, this drug should be used during pregnancy only if clearly needed.

NURSING MOTHERS
It is not known whether Didanosine is excreted in human milk. A study in rats showed that, following oral administration, Didanosine and/or its metabolites were excreted into the milk of lactating rats. Because many drugs are excreted in human milk and because of the potential for serious adverse reactions from Didanosine in nursing infants, mothers should be instructed to discontinue nursing when taking Didanosine.

PEDIATRIC USE
See "Indications," "Warnings," and "Dosage and Administration" sections.

ADVERSE REACTIONS
THE MAJOR TOXICITIES OF DIDANOSINE ARE PANCREATITIS AND PERIPHERAL NEUROPATHY (see "Warnings").

Adults: Adverse events which occurred in at least 5 percent of adult patients in the controlled clinical trial comparing two doses of Didanosine to zidovudine are provided in Table 10.

Table 10
CLINICAL ADVERSE EVENTS/CUMULATIVE INCIDENCE $\geq$ 5 % AT DIDANOSINE RECOMMENDED DOSE (CONTROLLED STUDY DATA)

Adverse Events	High Dose Didanosine N = 311	Recommended Didanosine Dose N = 298	Zidovudine N = 304
Diarrhea	20	28	21
Neuropathy (all grades)	17	20	12
Chills/Fever	9	12	11
Rash/Pruritus	7	9	5
Abdominal pain	10	7	8
Asthenia	5	7	9
Headache	10	7	7
Pain	7	7	3
Nausea & Vomiting	6	7	6
Infection	5	6	5
Pancreatitis	10	6	2
Pneumonia	6	5	5

In the controlled clinical trial comparing two doses of Didanosine to zidovudine, the cumulative incidences of serious laboratory abnormalities in the 913 patients treated are listed in Table 11.

Table 11
CONTROLLED CLINICAL TRIAL/CUMULATIVE INCIDENCES OF ADULT LABORATORY ABNORMALITIES

Lab tests (Seriously Abnormal Level)	High Dose Didanosine N = 311	Recommended Didanosine Dose N = 298	Zidovudine N = 304
Leukopenia (< 2000/µL)	13	16	22
Amylase ($\geq$ 5 × ULN)	22	15	5
Granulocytopenia (< 750/µL)	8	8	15
Thrombocytopenia (< 50,000/µL)	2	2	3
SGPT (> 5 × ULN)	8	6	6
SGOT (> 5 × ULN)	8	7	6
Alkaline phosphate (> 5 × ULN)	4	1	1
Hemoglobin (< 8.0 g/dL)	2	3	5
Bilirubin (> 5 × ULN)	2	1	1
Uric Acid (> 5 × ULN)	1	2	1

Clinical adverse events which occurred in greater than one percent and up to 5 percent of patients enrolled in the controlled clinical trial are provided in Table 12.

Table 12
CLINICAL ADVERSE EVENTS/CUMULATIVE INCIDENCE $\geq$ 1% and < 5% AT DIDANOSINE RECOMMENDED DOSE (CONTROLLED STUDY DATA)

Adverse Events	High Dose Didanosine N = 311	Recommended Didanosine Dose N = 298	Zidovudine N = 304
Body as a Whole			
Allergic Reaction	2	1	1
Chest Pain	0	1	1
Malaise	1	1	3
Sarcoma	3	3	4
Cardiovascular			
Hemorrhage	0	1	0
Hypotension	0	1	0

Table 12

	%		
	High Dose Didanosine	Recommended Didanosine Dose	Zidovudine
Adverse Events	N = 311	N = 298	N = 304
Digestive			
Anorexia	1	2	2
Dry Mouth	3	2	0
Constipation	1	1	0
Oral Moniliasis	0	1	0
Metabolic/Nutritional			
Dehydration	1	1	1
Musculoskeletal			
Myopathy	2	3	6
Nervous			
Convulsion	2	2	2
Thinking			
Abnormal	1	2	1
Amnesia	1	1	0
Anxiety/Nervous/			
Twitch	2	1	2
Aphasia	0	1	0
Confusion	2	1	0
Depression	2	1	3
Dizziness	1	1	1
Hypertension	1	1	0
Respiratory			
Dyspnea	3	2	3
Bronchitis	1	1	1
Cough Increased	1	1	1
Skin and			
Appendages			
Herpes Zoster	0	1	0
Pruritus	0	1	1
Sweating	1	1	1
Special Senses			
Blurred Vision	0	1	1
Otitis Media	0	1	0
Retinitis	0	1	1

Events which occurred with a cumulative incidence of < 1 percent of patients enrolled in the controlled study who received the recommended dose are listed below:

Body as a Whole	Hypertonia
Abscess	Ileus
Cellulitis	Incoordination
Cyst	Intracranial Hemorrhage
Flu Syndrome	Paralysis
Hernia	Paranoid Reaction
Neck Rigidity	Psychosis
Numbness, Hands and Feet	Sleep Disorder
Cardiovascular	Speech Disorder
Migraine	Tremor
Palpitation	**Respiratory**
Peripheral Vascular Disorder	Asthma
Syncope	Epistaxis
Digestive	Laryngitis
Colitis	Lung Function Decreased
Eructation	Pharyngitis
Flatulence	Pneumonia Interstitial
Gastroenteritis	Respiratory Disorder
Gastrointestinal Hemorrhage	**Skin and Appendages**
Sialadenitis	Herpes Simplex
Stomach Ulcer Hemorrhage	Skin Disorder
Hemic/Lymphatic	**Special Senses**
Lymphoma Like Reaction	Conjunctivitis
Metabolic/Nutritional	Diplopia
Edema Peripheral	Dry Eye
Musculoskeletal	Ear Disorder
Arthralgia	Glaucoma
Arthritis	Otitis Externa
Hemiparesis	**Urogenital System**
Joint Disorder	Impotence
Leg Cramps	Kidney Calculus
Nervous	Kidney Failure
Acute Brain Syndrome	Kidney Function Abnormal
Ataxia	Nocturia
Grand Mal Convulsion	Urinary Frequency
Hyperesthesia	Vaginal Hemorrhage

Events which occurred with a cumulative incidence of < 1 percent in patients enrolled in the controlled study who received the high dose are listed above:

Body as a Whole	Drug Dependence
Abscess	Emotional Lability
Anaphylactoid Reaction	Encephalitis
Dementia	Foot Drop
Cardiovascular	Grand Mal Convulsion
Aortic Stenosis	Hyperesthesia
Cardiovascular Disorder	Insomnia
Heart Arrest	Manic Reaction
Heart Failure Right	Neuralgia
Hypotension	Reflexes Decreased
Intracranial Aneurysm	Reflexes Increased
Migraine	Speech Disorder
Myocardial Infarct	Withdrawal Syndrome
Digestive	**Respiratory**
Abnormal Stools	Epistaxis
Duodenitis	Hemoptysis
Esophagitis	Pharyngitis
Gastritis	**Skin and Appendages**
Gastrointestinal Carcinoma	Fungal Dermatitis
Gingivitis	Herpes Zoster
Hemorrhagic Pancreatitis	Pruritus
Hepatomegaly	Skin Discoloration
Oral Moniliasis	Urticaria
Pseudomembranous Enterocolitis	Vesiculobullous Rash
Rectal Hemorrhage	**Special Senses**
Tongue Disorder	Blurred Vision
Metabolic/Nutritional	Conjunctivitis
Acidosis	Eye Disorder
Generalized Edema	Photophobia
Thirst	Retinal Detachment
Musculoskeletal	Retinitis
Bone Disorder	Taste Perversion
Myositis	**Urogenital**
Pyogenic Arthritis	Acute Kidney Failure
Nervous	Kidney Function Abnormal
Abnormal Gait	Polyuria
CNS Depression	Urinary Frequency
	Vaginal Hemorrhage

Children: Adverse events reported in more than 5 percent of patients in the pediatric phase 1 trials (which includes all signs and symptoms on study) are listed in Table 13. There are no comparative controlled data to assess the incidence of adverse effects from Didanosine in children at this time; therefore, the adverse events reported in these pediatric studies should be considered as potential hazards of Didanosine treatment.

In pediatric studies, pancreatitis occurred in 2 of 60 (3 percent) patients treated at entry doses below 300 mg/m^2/day and in 5 of 38 (13 percent) patients treated at higher doses.

Table 13
PEDIATRIC CLINICAL ADVERSE EVENTS (CUMULATIVE INCIDENCES)

	%	
Adverse Events	Patients < 300 mg/m^2/day (n = 60)	Receiving All Patients (n = 98)
Body as a Whole		
Flu Syndrome	7	7
Malaise	38	29
Alopecia	7	5
Anorexia	52	51
Asthenia	42	41
Chills/Fever	82	82
Dehydration	7	5
Pain	27	31
Weight Loss	10	8
Increased Appetite	5	2
Change in Appetite	10	6
Failure to Thrive	13	9
GI System		
Liver Abnormalities	32	38
Melena	7	7
Oral Thrush	13	9
Abdominal Pain		
(see *"Warnings"*)	32	35
Constipation	10	12
Diarrhea (see *"Precautions"*)	82	81
Dry Mouth	7	4
Nausea/Vomiting (see *"Warnings"*)	57	58
Stomatitis/Mouth Sores	17	16
Pancreatitis (see *"Warnings"*)	3	7
Lympho-Hematologic		
Ecchymosis	15	15
Hemorrhage	10	10
Petechiae	3	7

◆ RATED THERAPEUTICALLY EQUIVALENT; ◇ THERAPEUTIC EQUIVALENCE UNCONFIRMED; ○ UNRATED

Musculoskeletal		
Muscle Atrophy	12	8
Myalgia	12	9
Arthritis	12	11
Decreased Strength	3	6
Cardiovascular		
Vasodilation	22	22
Arrhythmia	10	6
Nervous System		
Dizziness	5	7
Lethargy	7	4
Nervousness	33	27
Headache	58	55
Insomnia	10	8
Poor Coordination	8	6
Respiratory System		
Asthma	28	21
Cough	87	85
Dyspnea	27	23
Epistaxis	13	14
Hypoventilation	10	8
Pharyngitis	17	14
Rhinitis	48	48
Rhinorrhea	20	21
Rhonchi/Rales	8	6
Sinusitis	8	7
Congestion	5	3
Skin and Appendages		
Impetigo	5	6
Eczema	13	12
Excoriation	7	4
Skin Disorder	12	13
Sweating	8	7
Rash/Pruritus	72	70
Erythema	5	4
Special Senses		
Ear Pain/Otitis	13	11
Photophobia	8	5
Strabismus	8	5
Visual Impairment	5	5
Urogenital System		
Urinary Frequency	5	4

Serious adverse events reported from less than 5 percent of patients in the pediatric phase 1 trials are listed in Table 14.

Table 14
SERIOUS PEDIATRIC CLINICAL ADVERSE EVENTS (CUMULATIVE INCIDENCES IN <5 PERCENT OF PATIENTS)

Event	*%*
Seizure	1
Neurologic	2
Pneumonia	1
Diabetes Mellitus	1
Diabetes Insipidus	1

Four pediatric patients developed depigmentation of the retina while being treated with Didanosine at doses above 300 mg/m²/day. Two of the patients, treated at doses of 540 mg/m²/day, had progression of disease when treated with lower doses. One patient treated at lower doses has continued therapy without progression of disease. Until further information is available from ongoing clinical trials with children treated at currently recommended lower doses of Didanosine, it has been proposed that children receiving Didanosine should undergo dilated retinal examination every 6 months or if any change in vision occurs.

Serious laboratory abnormalities experienced by the pediatric patients are listed in Table 15. Laboratory abnormalities of grade 3 or 4 were observed more frequently among patients who began Didanosine therapy with abnormal values.

Table 15
PEDIATRIC PATIENT SERIOUS LABORATORY ABNORMALITIES (CUMULATIVE INCIDENCES)

	(Doses ≤ 300 mg/m²/day) N = 60	
Laboratory Test (Seriously Abnormal Level)	*Normal Baseline*	*Abnormal Baseline*
Leukopenia (< 2000 µL)	3%	36%
Granulocytopenia (< 1000 µL)	24%	62%
Thrombocytopenia (< 50,000 µL)	2%	67%
Anemia (Hb < 8.0 g/dL)	4%	27%

	(Doses ≤ 300 mg/m²/day) N = 60	
Laboratory Test (Seriously Abnormal Level)	*Normal Baseline*	*Abnormal Baseline*
SGPT (> 5 × ULN)	3%	25%
SGOT (> 5 × ULN)	0%	36%
Alkaline Phosphatase (> 5 × ULN)	0%	0%
Bilirubin (> 5 × ULN)	2%	0%
Uric Acid (> 1.25 × ULN)	0%	0%
Amylase (> 5 × ULN)	0%	0%

OVERDOSAGE

There is no known antidote for Didanosine overdosage. Experience in the phase 1 studies in which Didanosine was initially administered at doses ten times the currently recommended dose indicates that the complications of chronic overdosage would include pancreatitis, peripheral neuropathy, diarrhea, hyperuricemia or, possibly, hepatic dysfunction. It is not known whether Didanosine is dialyzable by peritoneal or hemodialysis.

DOSAGE AND ADMINISTRATION

DOSAGE

Adults: The dosing interval should be 12 hours. All Didanosine formulations should be administered on an empty stomach. Adult patients should take 2 tablets at each dose so that adequate buffering is provided to prevent gastric acid degradation of Didanosine. The recommended starting dose in adults is dependent on weight as outlined in the table below:

Table 16
ADULT DOSING

Patient Weight	*Didanosine Tablets*	*Didanosine Buffered Powder*
≥ 60 kg	200 mg BID	250 mg BID
< 60 kg	125 mg BID	167 mg BID

Children: The recommended dosing interval is 12 hours. All Didanosine formulations should be administered on an empty stomach. To prevent gastric acid degradation, children older than 1 year of age should receive a 2-tablet dose; children under 1 year should receive a 1-tablet dose. The recommended dose in children is dependent on body surface area as outlined in the table below (see Table 17). Doses equivalent to 100 mg/m²/day to 300 mg/m²/day of the Didanosine pediatric powder are currently being further evaluated in controlled clinical trials. The optimal dose of Didanosine for children has not been established and some investigators recommend doses of up to 300 mg/m²/day divided into three daily doses.

Table 17
PEDIATRIC DOSING (BASED ON 200 MG/M²/DAY AVERAGE RECOMMENDED DOSE)*

Body Surface Area (m²)	*Didanosine Tablets*	Didanosine Pediatric Powder	
		Dose	*Vol/10 mg/mL Admixture*
1.1-1.4	100 mg BID	125 mg BID	12.5 mL BID
0.8-1.0	75 mg BID	94 mg BID	9.5 mL BID
0.5-0.7	50 mg BID	62 mg BID	6 mL BID
≤ 0.4	25 mg BID	31 mg BID	3 mL BID

* *Based on Didanosine pediatric powder.*

DOSE ADJUSTMENT

Clinical signs suggestive of pancreatitis should prompt dose suspension and careful evaluation of the possibility of pancreatitis. Only after pancreatitis has been ruled out should dosing be resumed.

Patients who have presented symptoms of neuropathy may tolerate a reduced dose of Didanosine after resolution of these symptoms upon drug discontinuation.

There are insufficient data to recommend a specific dose adjustment of Didanosine in patients with impaired renal or hepatic function.

METHOD OF PREPARATION:

DIDANOSINE CHEWABLE/DISPERSIBLE BUFFERED TABLETS
Adult Dosing: Two tablets should be thoroughly chewed, manually crushed, or dispersed in at least 1 ounce of water prior to consumption. To disperse tablets, add 2 tablets to at least 1 ounce of drinking water. Stir until a uniform dispersion forms, and drink the entire dispersion immediately.

Pediatric Dosing: One or 2 tablets should be chewed, crushed, or dispersed in water prior to consumption, as described in the preceding *Adult-Dosing Method of Preparation.*

➤ SHOWN IN PRODUCT IDENTIFICATION GUIDE

DIDANOSINE BUFFERED POWDER FOR ORAL SOLUTION

1. Open packet carefully and pour contents into a container with approximately 4 ounces of drinking water. Do not mix with fruit juice or other acid-containing liquid.

2. Stir until the powder completely dissolves (approximately 2 to 3 minutes).

3. Drink the entire solution immediately.

DIDANOSINE PEDIATRIC POWDER FOR ORAL SOLUTION

Prior to dispensing, the pharmacist must constitute dry powder with Purified Water, USP, to an initial concentration of 20 mg/mL and immediately mix the resulting solution with antacid to a final concentration of 10 mg/mL as follows:

20 mg/mL Initial Solution: Constitute the product to 20 mg/mL by adding 100 mL or 200 mL of Purified Water, USP, to the 2 g or 4 g of Didanosine powder, respectively, in the product bottle.

10 mg/mL Final Admixture: 1. Immediately mix one part of the 20 mg/mL initial solution with one part of either Aluminum Hydroxide/Magnesium Hydroxide/ Simethicone Double Strength Liquid or Extra Strength Suspension for a final dispensing concentration of 10 mg Didanosine per mL. For patient home use, the admixture should be dispensed in appropriately sized, flint-glass bottles with child-resistant closures. This admixture is stable for 30 days under refrigeration 36° to 46°F (2° to 8°C).

2. Instruct the patient to shake the admixture thoroughly prior to use and to store the tightly closed container in the refrigerator, 36° to 46°F (2° to 8°C) up to 30 days.

The tablets should be stored in tightly closed bottles at 59° to 86°F (15° to 30°C). If dispersed in water, the dose may be held for up to 1 hour at ambient temperature.

The packets should be stored at 59° to 86°F (15° to to 30°C). After dissolving in water, the solution may be stored at ambient room temperature for up to 4 hours.

The bottles of powder should be stored at 59° to 86°F (15° to 30°C).

The Didanosine admixture may be stored up to 30 days in a refrigerator, 36° to 46°F (2° to 8°C). Discard any unused portion after 30 days.

HANDLING AND DISPOSAL

SPILL, LEAK AND DISPOSAL PROCEDURE

Avoid generating dust during clean-up of powdered products; use wet mop or damp sponge. Clean surface with soap and water as necessary. Containerize larger spills.

There is no single preferred method of disposal of containerized waste. Disposal options include incineration, landfill, or sewer as dictated by specific circumstances and relevant national, state, and local regulations.

REFERENCES

1. Hartman NR, et al. Pharmacokinetics of 2',3'-dideoxyadenosine and 2',3'-dideoxyinosine in patients with severe human immunodeficiency virus infection. *Clin Pharmacol Ther.* 1990;47:647-654. 2. Butler KM, et al. Dideoxyinosine in children with symptomatic human immunodeficiency virus infection. *New Eng. J Med.* 1991;324:137-144. 3. Kahn JK, et al. A controlled trial comparing continued Zidovudine with Didanosine in human immunodeficiency virus infection. *New Eng J Med.* 1992;327:581-587.

HOW SUPPLIED

CHEW TABLET: 25 MG

BRAND/MANUFACTURER	NDC	SIZE	AWP
○ BRAND			
VIDEX: Bristol-Myer Onc/Hiv	00087-6628-43	60s	$21.61

CHEW TABLET: 50 MG

BRAND/MANUFACTURER	NDC	SIZE	AWP
○ BRAND			
VIDEX: Bristol-Myer Onc/Hiv	00087-6624-43	60s	$43.21

CHEW TABLET: 100 MG

BRAND/MANUFACTURER	NDC	SIZE	AWP
○ BRAND			
▸ VIDEX: Bristol-Myer Onc/Hiv	00087-6627-43	60s	$86.42

CHEW TABLET: 150 MG

BRAND/MANUFACTURER	NDC	SIZE	AWP
○ BRAND			
VIDEX: Bristol-Myer Onc/Hiv	00087-6626-43	60s	$129.63

POWDER FOR RECONSTITUTION:

BRAND/MANUFACTURER	NDC	SIZE	AWP
○ BRAND			
VIDEX PEDIATRIC: Bristol-Myer Onc/Hiv	00087-6632-41	2 gm	$28.80
	00087-6633-41	4 gm	$57.60

POWDER FOR RECONSTITUTION: 100 MG

BRAND/MANUFACTURER	NDC	SIZE	AWP
○ BRAND			
VIDEX: Bristol-Myer Onc/Hiv	00087-6614-43	30s	$43.21

POWDER FOR RECONSTITUTION: 167 MG

BRAND/MANUFACTURER	NDC	SIZE	AWP
○ BRAND			
VIDEX: Bristol-Myer Onc/Hiv	00087-6615-43	30s	$72.17

POWDER FOR RECONSTITUTION: 250 MG

BRAND/MANUFACTURER	NDC	SIZE	AWP
○ BRAND			
VIDEX: Bristol-Myer Onc/Hiv	00087-6616-43	30s	$108.03

POWDER FOR RECONSTITUTION: 375 MG

BRAND/MANUFACTURER	NDC	SIZE	AWP
○ BRAND			
VIDEX: Bristol-Myer Onc/Hiv	00087-6617-43	30s	$162.05

Didrex *SEE* BENZPHETAMINE HYDROCHLORIDE

Didronel *SEE* ETIDRONATE DISODIUM, ORAL

Didronel I.V. *SEE* ETIDRONATE DISODIUM, INJECTABLE

Dienestrol Cream

1. ESTROGENS HAVE BEEN REPORTED TO INCREASE THE RISK OF ENDOMETRIAL CARCINOMA.

THREE INDEPENDENT CASE CONTROL STUDIES HAVE SHOWN AN INCREASED RISK OF ENDOMETRIAL CANCER IN POSTMENOPAUSAL WOMEN EXPOSED TO EXOGENOUS ESTROGENS FOR PROLONGED PERIODS.[1-3] THIS RISK WAS INDEPENDENT OF THE OTHER KNOWN RISK FACTORS FOR ENDOMETRIAL CANCER. THESE STUDIES ARE FURTHER SUPPORTED BY THE FINDING THAT INCIDENCE RATES OF ENDOMETRIAL CANCER HAVE INCREASED SHARPLY SINCE 1969 IN EIGHT DIFFERENT AREAS OF THE UNITED STATES WITH POPULATION-BASED CANCER REPORTING SYSTEMS, AN INCREASE WHICH MAY BE RELATED TO THE RAPIDLY EXPANDING USE OF ESTROGENS DURING THE LAST DECADE.[4]

THE THREE CASE CONTROL STUDIES REPORTED THAT THE RISK OF ENDOMETRIAL CANCER IN ESTROGEN USERS WAS ABOUT 4.5 TO 13.9 TIMES GREATER THAN IN NONUSERS. THE RISK APPEARS TO DEPEND ON BOTH DURATION OF TREATMENT[1] AND ON ESTROGEN DOSE.[3] IN VIEW OF THESE FINDINGS, WHEN ESTROGENS ARE USED FOR THE TREATMENT OF MENOPAUSAL SYMPTOMS, THE LOWEST DOSE THAT WILL CONTROL SYMPTOMS SHOULD BE UTILIZED AND MEDICATION SHOULD BE DISCONTINUED AS SOON AS POSSIBLE. WHEN PROLONGED TREATMENT IS MEDICALLY INDICATED, THE PATIENT SHOULD BE REASSESSED ON AT LEAST A SEMIANNUAL BASIS TO DETERMINE THE NEED FOR CONTINUED THERAPY. ALTHOUGH THE EVIDENCE MUST BE CONSIDERED PRELIMINARY, ONE STUDY SUGGESTS THAT CYCLIC ADMINISTRATION OF LOW DOSES OF ESTROGEN MAY CARRY LESS RISK THAN CONTINUOUS ADMINISTRATION;[3] IT THEREFORE APPEARS PRUDENT TO UTILIZE SUCH A REGIMEN.

CLOSE CLINICAL SURVEILLANCE OF ALL WOMEN TAKING ESTROGENS IS IMPORTANT. IN ALL CASES OF UNDIAGNOSED PERSISTENT OR RECURRING ABNORMAL VAGINAL BLEEDING, ADEQUATE DIAGNOSTIC MEASURES SHOULD BE UNDERTAKEN TO RULE OUT MALIGNANCY.

THERE IS NO EVIDENCE AT PRESENT THAT "NATURAL" ESTROGENS ARE MORE OR LESS HAZARDOUS THAN "SYNTHETIC" ESTROGENS AT EQUIESTROGENIC DOSES.

2. ESTROGENS SHOULD NOT BE USED DURING PREGNANCY

THE USE OF FEMALE SEX HORMONES, BOTH ESTROGENS AND PROGESTOGENS, DURING EARLY PREGNANCY MAY SERIOUSLY DAMAGE THE OFFSPRING. IT HAS BEEN SHOWN THAT FEMALES EXPOSED *IN UTERO* TO DIETHYLSTILBESTROL, A NON-STEROIDAL ESTROGEN, HAVE AN INCREASED RISK OF DEVELOPING IN LATER LIFE A FORM OF VAGINAL OR CERVICAL CANCER THAT ORDINARILY IS EXTREMELY RARE.[5,6] THIS RISK HAS BEEN ESTIMATED AS NOT GREATER THAN 4 PER 1000 EXPOSURES.[7] FURTHERMORE, A HIGH PERCENTAGE OF SUCH EXPOSED WOMEN (FROM 30 TO 90 PERCENT) HAVE BEEN FOUND TO HAVE VAGINAL ADENOSIS,[8-12] EPITHELIAL CHANGES OF THE VAGINA AND CERVIX. ALTHOUGH THESE CHANGES

◆ RATED THERAPEUTICALLY EQUIVALENT; ◇ THERAPEUTIC EQUIVALENCE UNCONFIRMED; ○ UNRATED

ARE HISTOLOGICALLY BENIGN, IT IS NOT KNOWN WHETHER THEY ARE PRECURSORS OF MALIGNANCY. ALTHOUGH SIMILAR DATA ARE NOT AVAILABLE WITH THE USE OF OTHER ESTROGENS, IT CANNOT BE PRESUMED THEY WOULD NOT INDUCE SIMILAR CHANGES.

SEVERAL REPORTS SUGGEST AN ASSOCIATION BETWEEN INTRAUTERINE EXPOSURE TO FEMALE SEX HORMONES AND CONGENITAL ANOMALIES, INCLUDING CONGENITAL HEART DEFECTS AND LIMB REDUCTION DEFECTS.[13-16] ONE CASE CONTROL STUDY[16] ESTIMATED A 4.7 FOLD INCREASED RISK OF LIMB REDUCTION DEFECTS IN INFANTS EXPOSED *IN UTERO* TO SEX HORMONES (ORAL CONTRACEPTIVES, HORMONE WITHDRAWAL TESTS FOR PREGNANCY, OR ATTEMPTED TREATMENT FOR THREATENED ABORTION). SOME OF THESE EXPOSURES WERE VERY SHORT AND INVOLVED ONLY A FEW DAYS OF TREATMENT. THE DATA SUGGEST THAT THE RISK OF LIMB REDUCTION DEFECTS IN EXPOSED FETUSES IS SOMEWHAT LESS THAN 1 PER 1000.

IN THE PAST, FEMALE SEX HORMONES HAVE BEEN USED DURING PREGNANCY IN AN ATTEMPT TO TREAT THREATENED OR HABITUAL ABORTION. THERE IS CONSIDERABLE EVIDENCE THAT ESTROGENS ARE INEFFECTIVE FOR THESE INDICATIONS, AND THERE IS NO EVIDENCE FROM WELL CONTROLLED STUDIES THAT PROGESTOGENS ARE EFFECTIVE FOR THESE USES.

IF DIENESTROL CREAM IS USED DURING PREGNANCY, OR IF THE PATIENT BECOMES PREGNANT WHILE USING THIS DRUG, SHE SHOULD BE APPRISED OF THE POTENTIAL RISKS TO THE FETUS, AND THE ADVISABILITY OF PREGNANCY CONTINUATION.

DESCRIPTION

Active ingredient: Dienestrol 0.01%.

Dienestrol is a synthetic, nonsteroidal estrogen. It is compounded in a cream base suitable for intravaginal use only. The cream base is composed of glyceryl monostearate, peanut oil, glycerin, benzoic acid, glutamic acid, butylated hydroxyanisole, citric acid, sodium hydroxide and water. The pH is approximately 4.3.

4.4'-(Diethylideneethylene)diphenol

Following is its chemical structure:

CLINICAL PHARMACOLOGY

Systemic absorption and mode of action of Dienestrol are undetermined.

INDICATIONS AND USAGE

Dienestrol Cream is indicated in the treatment of atrophic vaginitis and kraurosis vulvae.

DIENESTROL CREAM HAS NOT BEEN SHOWN TO BE EFFECTIVE FOR ANY PURPOSE DURING PREGNANCY AND ITS USE MAY CAUSE SEVERE HARM TO THE FETUS (see Boxed *"Warning"*).

UNLABELED USES
Dienestrol is used alone or as an adjunct in the treatment of labial adhesions.

CONTRAINDICATIONS

Estrogens may cause fetal harm when administered to a pregnant woman (see Boxed *"Warning"*). Estrogens are contraindicated in women who are or may become pregnant. If this drug is used during pregnancy, or if the patient becomes pregnant while using this drug, the patient should be apprised of the potential hazard to the fetus.

Estrogens should also not be used in women with any of the following conditions:
1. Known or suspected cancer of the breast.
2. Known or suspected estrogen-dependent neoplasia.
3. Undiagnosed abnormal genital bleeding.
4. Active thrombophlebitis or thromboembolic disorders.
5. A past history of thrombophlebitis, thrombosis, or thromboembolic disorders associated with previous estrogen use.

WARNINGS

1. Induction of Malignant Neoplasms: Long-term continuous administration of natural and synthetic estrogens in certain animal species increases the frequency of carcinomas of the breast, cervix, vagina, and liver. There is now evidence that estrogens increase the risk of carcinoma of the endometrium in humans. (See Boxed *"Warning"*.)

At the present time there is no satisfactory evidence that estrogens given to postmenopausal women increase the risk of cancer of the breast,[18] although a recent long-term followup of a single physician's practice has raised this possibility.[18a] Because of the animal data, there is a need for caution in prescribing estrogens for women with a strong family history of breast cancer or who have breast nodules, fibrocystic disease, or abnormal mammograms.

2. Gallbladder Disease: A recent study has reported a 2- to 3-fold increase in the risk of surgically confirmed gall bladder disease in women receiving postmenopausal estrogens,[18] similar to the 2-fold increase previously noted in users of oral contraceptives.[19,24] In the case of oral contraceptives the increased risk appeared after two years of use.[24]

3. Effects Similar to Those Caused by Estrogen-Progestogen Oral Contraceptives: There are several serious adverse effects of oral contraceptives, most of which have not, up to now, been documented as consequences of postmenopausal estrogen therapy. This may reflect the comparatively low doses of estrogen used in postmenopausal women. It would be expected that the larger doses of estrogen used to treat prostatic or breast cancer or postpartum breast engorgement are more likely to result in these adverse effects, and, in fact, it has been shown that there is an increased risk of thrombosis in men receiving estrogens for prostatic cancer and women for postpartum breast engorgement.[20-23]

a. Thromboembolic Disease: It is now well established that users of oral contraceptives have an increased risk of various thromboembolic and thrombotic vascular diseases, such as thrombophlebitis, pulmonary embolism, stroke, and myocardial infarction.[24-31] Cases of retinal thrombosis, mesenteric thrombosis, and optic neuritis have been reported in oral contraceptive users. There is evidence that the risk of several of these adverse reactions is related to the dose of the drug.[32,33] An increased risk of postsurgery thromboembolic complications has also been reported in users of oral contraceptives.[34,35] If feasible, estrogen should be discontinued at least 4 weeks before surgery of the type associated with an increased risk of thromboembolism, or during periods of prolonged immobilization.

While an increased rate of thromboembolic and thrombotic disease in postmenopausal users of estrogens has not been found,[18,36] this does not rule out the possibility that such an increase may be present or that subgroups of women who have underlying risk factors or who are receiving relatively large doses of estrogens may have increased risk. Therefore estrogens should not be used in persons with active thrombophlebitis or thromboembolic disorders, and they should not be used (except in treatment of malignancy) in persons with a history of such disorders in association with estrogen use. They should be used with caution in patients with cerebral vascular or coronary artery disease and only for those in whom estrogens are clearly needed.

Large doses of estrogen (5 mg conjugated estrogens per day), comparable to those used to treat cancer of the prostate and breast, have been shown in a large prospective clinical trial in men to increase the risk of nonfatal myocardial infarction, pulmonary embolism and thrombophlebitis. When estrogen doses of this size are used, any of the thromboembolic and thrombotic adverse effects associated with oral contraceptive use should be considered a clear risk.

b. Hepatic adenoma: Benign hepatic adenomas appear to be associated with the use of oral contraceptives,[38-40] Although benign, and rare, these may rupture and may cause death through intra-abdominal hemorrhage. Such lesions have not yet been reported in association with other estrogen or progestogen preparations but should be considered in estrogen users having abdominal pain and tenderness, abdominal mass, or hypovolemic shock. Hepatocellular carcinoma has also been reported in women taking estrogen-containing oral contraceptives.[39] The relationship of this malignancy to these drugs is not known at this time.

c. Elevated blood pressure: Increased blood pressure is not uncommon in women using oral contraceptives. There is now a report that this may occur with use of estrogens during menopause.[41] Blood pressure should be monitored with estrogen use, especially if high doses are used.

d. Glucose tolerance: A worsening of glucose tolerance has been observed in a significant percentage of patients on estrogen-containing oral contraceptives. For this reason, diabetic patients should be carefully observed while receiving estrogen.

4. Hypercalcemia: Administration of estrogens may lead to severe hypercalcemia in patients with breast cancer and bone metastases. If this occurs, the drug should be stopped and appropriate measures taken to reduce the serum calcium level.

PRECAUTIONS

A. GENERAL

1. A complete medical and family history should be taken prior to the initiation of any estrogen therapy. The pretreatment and periodic physical examinations should include special reference to blood pressure, breasts, abdomen, and pelvic organs, and should include a Papanicolaou smear. As a general rule, estrogen should not be prescribed for longer than one year without another physical examination being performed.

2. Fluid retention—Because estrogens may cause some degree of fluid retention, conditions which might be influenced by this factor such as epilepsy, migraine, and cardiac or renal dysfunction, require careful observation.

3. Certain patients may develop undesirable manifestations of excessive estrogenic stimulation, such as abnormal or excessive uterine bleeding, mastodynia, etc.

4. Oral contraceptives appear to be associated with an increased incidence of mental depression.[24] Although it is not clear whether this is due to the estrogenic or progestogenic component of the contraceptive, patients with a history of depression should be carefully observed.

5. Preexisting uterine leiomyomata may increase in size during estrogen use.

6. The pathologist should be advised of estrogen therapy when relevant specimens are submitted.

7. Patients with a past history of jaundice during pregnancy have an increased risk of recurrence of jaundice while receiving estrogen-containing oral contracep-

tive therapy. If jaundice develops in any patient receiving estrogen, the medication should be discontinued while the cause is investigated.

8. Estrogens may be poorly metabolized in patients with impaired liver function and they should be administered with caution in such patients.

9. Because estrogens influence the metabolism of calcium and phosphorus, they should be used with caution in patients with metabolic bone diseases that are associated with hypercalcemia or in patients with renal insufficiency.

10. Because of the effects of estrogens on epiphyseal closure, they should be used judiciously in young patients in whom bone growth is not complete.

11. The lowest effective dose appropriate for the specific indication should be utilized. Studies of the addition of a progestin for seven or more days of a cycle of estrogen administration have reported a lowered incidence of endometrial hyperplasia. Morphological and biochemical studies of endometrium suggest that 10 to 13 days of progestin are needed to provide maximal maturation of the endometrium and to eliminate any hyperplastic changes. Whether this will provide protection from endometrial carcinoma has not been clearly established. There are possible additional risks which may be associated with the inclusion of progestin in estrogen replacement regimens. The potential risks include adverse effects on carbohydrate and lipid metabolism. The choice of progestin and dosage may be important in minimizing these adverse effects.

B. INFORMATION FOR PATIENTS:
See text of patient package information which is reproduced below.

C. DRUG/LABORATORY TEST INTERACTIONS
Certain endocrine and liver function tests may be affected by estrogen-containing oral contraceptives. The following similar changes may be expected with larger doses of estrogen:

1. Increased sulfobromophthalein retention.

2. Increased prothrombin and factors VII, VIII, IX and X; decreased antithrombin 3; increased norepinephrine-induced platelet aggregability.

3. Increased thyroid-binding globulin (TBG) leading to increased circulating total thyroid hormone, as measured by PBI, T4 by column, or T4 by radioimmunoassay. Free T3 resin uptake is decreased, reflecting the elevated TBG; free T4 concentration is unaltered.

4. Impaired glucose tolerance.

5. Decreased pregnanediol excretion.

6. Reduced response to metyrapone test.

7. Reduced serum folate concentration.

8. Increased serum triglyceride and phospholipid concentration.

D. CARCINOGENESIS, MUTAGENESIS, IMPAIRMENT OF FERTILITY
See "Warnings" section for information on carcinogenesis, mutagenesis and impairment of fertility.

E. PREGNANCY
Teratogenic Effects.
Pregnancy Category X.
See "Contraindications" section.

F. NURSING MOTHERS
It is not known whether this drug is excreted in human milk. Because many drugs are excreted in human milk, caution should be exercised when estrogens are administered to a nursing woman.

ADVERSE REACTIONS

(See "Warnings" regarding induction of neoplasia, adverse effects on the fetus, increased incidence of gall bladder disease, and adverse effects similar to those of oral contraceptives, including thromboembolism.) The following additional adverse reactions have been reported with estrogenic therapy, including oral contraceptives:

1. *Genitourinary system:*
Increase in size of uterine fibromyomata.
Vaginal candidiasis.
Breakthrough bleeding, spotting, change in menstrual flow.
Dysmenorrhea.
Premenstrual-like syndrome.
Amenorrhea during and after treatment.
Change in cervical eversion and in degree of cervical secretion.
Cystitis-like syndrome.

2. *Breasts:*
Tenderness, enlargement, secretion.

3. *Gastrointestinal:*
Cholestatic jaundice.
Nausea, vomiting.
Abdominal cramps, bloating.

4. *Skin:*
Erythema multiforme.
Erythema nodosum.
Hemorrhagic eruption.
Loss of scalp hair.
Hirsutism.
Chloasma or melasma which may persist when drug is discontinued.

5. *Eyes:*
Steepening of corneal curvature.
Intolerance to contact lenses.

6. *CNS:*
Mental depression.
Headache, migraine, dizziness.
Chorea.

7. *Miscellaneous:*
Reduced carbohydrate tolerance.
Aggravation of porphyria.
Edema.
Changes in libido.
Increase or decrease in weight.

OVERDOSAGE

Numerous reports of ingestion of large doses of estrogen-containing oral contraceptives by young children indicate that serious ill effects do not occur. Overdosage of estrogen may cause nausea, and withdrawal bleeding may occur in females.

DOSAGE AND ADMINISTRATION

GIVEN CYCLICALLY FOR SHORT-TERM USE ONLY
For treatment of atrophic vaginitis, or kraurosis vulvae associated with the menopause.

The lowest dose that will control symptoms should be chosen and medication should be discontinued as promptly as possible.

Attempts to discontinue or taper medication should be made at 3 to 6 month intervals.

The usual dosage range is one or two applicatorsful per day for one or two weeks, then gradually reduced to one half initial dosage for a similar period. A maintenance dosage of one applicatorful, one to three times a week, may be used after restoration of the vaginal mucosa has been achieved.

Treated patients with an intact uterus should be monitored closely for signs of endometrial cancer and appropriate diagnostic measures should be taken to rule out malignancy in the event of persistent or recurring abnormal vaginal bleeding.

STORAGE
Store at controlled room temperature.

REFERENCES

1. Ziel, H.K. and W.D. Finkle, "Increased Risk of Endometrial Carcinoma Among Users of Conjugated Estrogens," *New England Journal of Medicine,* 293:1167-1170, 1975. 2. Smith, D.C., R. Prentice, D.J. Thompson, and W.L. Hermann, "Association of Exogenous Estrogen and Endometrial Carcinoma," *New England Journal of Medicine,* 293:1164-1167, 1975. 3. Mack, T.M., M.C. Pike, B.E. Henderson, R.I. Pfeffer, V.R. Gerkins, M. Arthur, and S.E. Brown, "Estrogens and Endometrial Cancer in a Retirement Community," *New England Journal of Medicine,* 294:1267-1287, 1976. 4. Weiss, N.S., D.R. Szekely and D.F. Austin, "Increasing Incidence of Endometrial Cancer in the United States," *New England Journal of Medicine,* 294:1259-1262, 1976. 5. Herbst, A.L., H. Ulfelder and D.C. Poskanzer, "Adenocarcinoma of Vagina," *New England Journal of Medicine,* 284:878-881, 1971. 6. Greenwald, P., J. Barlow, P. Nasca, and W. Burnett, "Vaginal Cancer after Maternal Treatment with Synthetic Estrogens," *New England Journal of Medicine,* 285:390-392, 1971. 7. Lanier, A., K. Noller, D. Decker, L. Elveback, and L. Kurland, "Cancer and Stilbestrol. A Follow-up of 1719 Persons Exposed to Estrogens in Utero and Born 1943-1959," *Mayo Clinic Proceedings,* 48:793-799, 1973. 8. Herbst, A., R. Kurman, and R. Scully, "Vaginal and Cervical Abnormalities After Exposure to Stilbestrol In Utero," *Obstetrics and Gynecology,* 40:287-298, 1972. 9. Herbst, A., S. Robboy, G. Macdonald, and R. Scully, "The Effects of Local Progesterone on Stilbestrol-Associated Vaginal Adenosis," *American Journal of Obstetrics and Gynecology* 118:607-615, 1974. 10. Herbst, A., D. Poskanzer, S. Robboy, L. Friedlander, and R. Scully, "Prenatal Exposure to Stilbestrol, A Prospective Comparison of Exposed Female Offspring with Unexposed Controls," *New England Journal of Medicine,* 292:334-339, 1975. 11. Staffi, A., R. Mattingly, D. Foley, and W. Fetherston, "Clinical Diagnosis of Vaginal Adenosis," *Obstetrics and Gynecology,* 43:118-128, 1974. 12. Sherman, A.I., M. Goldrath, A. Berlin, V. Vakhariya, F. Banooni, W. Michaels, P. Goodman, S. Brown, "Cervical-Vaginal Adenosis After *In Utero* Exposure to Synthetic Estrogens," *Obstetrics and Gynecology,* 44:531-545, 1974. 13. Gal, I., B. Kirman, and J. Stern, "Hormone Pregnancy Tests and Congenital Malformation," *Nature,* 216:83, 1967. 14. Levy, E.P., A. Cohen, and F.C. Fraser, "Hormone Treatment During Pregnancy and Congenital Heart Defects," *Lancet,* 1:611, 1973. 15. Nora, J. and A. Nora, "Birth Defects and Oral Contraceptives," *Lancet,* 1:941-942, 1973. 16. Janerich, D.T., J.M. Piper, and D.M. Glebatis, "Oral Contraceptives and Congenital Limb-Reduction Defects," *New England Journal of Medicine,* 291:697-700, 1974. 17. "Estrogens for Oral or Parenteral Use," *Federal Register,* 40:8212, 1975. 18. Boston Collaborative Drug Surveillance Program, "Surgically Confirmed Gall Bladder Disease, Venous Thromboembolism and Breast Tumors in Relation to Post-Menopausal Estrogen Therapy," *New England Journal of Medicine,* 290:15-19, 1974. 18a. Hoover, R., L.A. Gray, Sr., P. Cole, and B. MacMahon, "Menopausal Estrogens and Breast Cancer," *New England Journal of Medicine,* 295:401-405, 1976. 19. Boston Collaborative Drug Surveillance Program, "Oral Contraceptives and Venous Thromboembolic Disease, Surgically Confirmed Gall Bladder Disease, and Breast Tumors," *Lancet* 1:1399-1404, 1973. 20. Daniel, D.G., H. Campbell, and A.C. Turnbull, "Puerperal Thromboembolism and Suppression of Lactation," *Lancet,* 2:287-289, 1967. 21. The Veterans Administration Cooperative Urological Research Group, "Carcinoma of the Prostate: Treatment Comparisons," *Journal of Urology,* 98:516-522, 1967. 22. Bailer, J.C., "Thromboembolism and Oestrogen Therapy," *Lancet,* 2:560, 1967. 23. Blackard, C., R. Doe, G. Mellinger, and D. Byar, "Incidence of Cardiovascular Disease and Death In Patients Receiving Diethylstilbestrol for Carcinoma of the Prostate," *Cancer,* 26:249-256, 1970. 24. Royal College of General Practitioners, "Oral Contraception and Thromboembolic Disease," *Journal of the Royal College of General Practitioners,* 13:267-279, 1967. 25. Inman, W.H.W. and M.P. Vessey, "Investigation of Deaths from Pulmonary, Coronary, and Cerebral Thrombosis and Embolism in Women of Child-Bearing Age," *British Medical Journal,* 2:193-199, 1968. 26. Vessey, M.P. and R. Doll, "Investigation of Relation Between Use of Oral Contraceptives and Thromboembolic Disease, A Further Report," *British Medical Journal,* 2:651-657, 1969. 27. Sartwell, P.E., A.T. Masi, F.G. Arthes, G.R. Greene, and H.E. Smith, "Thromboembolism and Oral Contraceptives: An

Epidemiological Case Control Study," *American Journal of Epidemiology,* 90:365-380, 1969. 28. Collaborative Group for the Study of Stroke In Young Women, "Oral Contraception and Increased Risk of Cerebral Ischemia or Thrombosis," *New England Journal of Medicine,* 288:871-878, 1973. 29. Collaborative Group for the Study of Stroke in Young Women, "Oral Contraceptives and Stroke in Young Women: Associated Risk Factors," *Journal of the American Medical Association,* 231:718-722, 1975. 30. Mann, J.I. and W.H.W Inman, "Oral Contraceptives and Death from Myocardial Infarction," *British Medical Journal,* 2:245-248, 1975. 31. Mann, J.I., M.P. Vessey, M. Thorogood, and R. Doll., "Myocardial Infarction in Young Women with Special Reference to Oral Contraceptive Practice," *British Medical Journal,* 2:241-245, 1975. 32. Inman, W.H.W., V.P. Vessey, B. Westerholm, and A. Engelund, "Thromboembolic Disease and the Steroidal Content of Oral Contraceptives," *British Medical Journal,* 2:203-209, 1970. 33. Stolley, P.D., J.A. Tonascia, M.S. Tockman, P.E. Sartwell, A.H. Rutledge, and M.P. Jacobs, "Thrombosis with Low-Estrogen Oral Contraceptives," *American Journal of Epidemiology,* 102:197-208, 1975. 34. Vessey, M.P., R. Doll, A.S. Fairbairn, and G. Glober, "Post-Operative Thromboembolism and the Use of the Oral Contraceptives," *British Medical Journal,* 3:123-126, 1970. 35. Greene, G.R. and P.E. Sartwell, "Oral Contraceptive Use in Patients with Thromboembolism Following Surgery, Trauma or Infection," *American Journal of Public Health,* 62:680-685, 1972. 36. Rosenberg, L., M.B. Armstrong and H. Jick, "Myocardial Infarction and Estrogen Therapy in Postmenopausal Women," *New England Journal of Medicine,* 294:1256-1259, 1976. 37. Coronary Drug Project Research Group, "The Coronary Drug Project: Initial Findings Leading to Modifications of Its Research Protocol," *Journal of the American Medical Association,* 214:1303-1313, 1970. 38. Baum, J., F. Holtz, J.J. Bookstein, and E.W. Klein, "Possible Association between Benign Hepatomas and Oral Contraceptives," *Lancet,* 2:926-928, 1973. 39. Mays, E.T., W.M. Christopherson, M.M. Mahr, and H.C. Williams, "Hepatic Changes in Young Women Ingesting Contraceptive Steroids, Hepatic Hemorrhage and Primary Hepatic Tumors." *Journal of the American Medical Association,* 235:730-782, 1976. 40. Edmondson, H.A., B. Henderson, and B. Benton, "Liver Cell Adenomas Associated with the Use of Oral Contraceptives," *New England Journal of Medicine,* 294:470-472, 1976. 41. Pfeffer, R.I. and S. Van Den Noore, "Estrogen Use and Stroke Risk in Postmenopausal Women," *American Journal of Epidemiology,* 103:445-456, 1976.

PATIENT INFORMATION ABOUT ESTROGENS

Estrogens are female hormones produced by the ovaries. The ovaries make several different kinds of estrogens. In addition, scientists have been able to make a variety of synthetic estrogens. As far as we know, all these synthetic estrogens have similar properties and therefore much the same usefulness, side effects, and risks. This leaflet is intended to help you understand what estrogens are used for, some of the risks involved in their use, and to help minimize these risks. This leaflet includes important information about estrogens, but not all the information. If you want to know more, you can ask your doctor or pharmacist to let you read the package insert prepared for the doctor.

USES OF ESTROGEN

There is no proper use of estrogens in a pregnant woman

Estrogens are prescribed by doctors for a number of purposes, including:

1. To provide estrogen during a period of adjustment when a woman's ovaries no longer produce it, in order to prevent certain uncomfortable symptoms of estrogen deficiency. (All women normally decrease the production of estrogens, generally between the ages of 45 and 55; this is called the menopause.)

2. To prevent symptoms of estrogen deficiency when a woman's ovaries have been removed surgically before the natural menopause.

3. To prevent pregnancy. (Estrogens are given along with a progestogen, another female hormone; these combinations are called oral contraceptives or birth control pills. Patient labeling is available to women taking oral contraceptives and they will not be discussed in this leaflet.)

4. To treat certain cancers in women and men.

5. To prevent painful swelling of the breast after pregnancy in women who choose not to nurse their babies.

ESTROGENS IN THE MENOPAUSE

In the natural course of their lives, all women eventually experience a decrease in estrogen production. This usually occurs between ages 45 and 55 but may occur earlier or later. Sometimes the ovaries may need to be removed by an operation before natural menopause, producing a "surgical menopause."

When the amount of estrogen in the blood begins to decrease, many women may develop typical symptoms: Feelings of warmth in the face, neck, and chest or sudden intense episodes of heat and sweating throughout the body (called "hot flashes" or "hot flushes"). These symptoms are sometimes very uncomfortable. A few women eventually develop changes in the vagina (called "atrophic vaginitis") which cause discomfort, especially during and after intercourse.

Estrogens can be prescribed to treat these symptoms of the menopause. It is estimated that considerably more than half of all women undergoing the menopause have only mild symptoms or no symptoms at all and therefore do not need estrogens. Other women may need estrogens for a few months, while their bodies adjust to lower estrogen levels.

Sometimes the need will be for periods longer than six months. In an attempt to avoid over-stimulation of the uterus (womb), estrogens are usually given cyclically during each month of use, that is three weeks of pills followed by one week without pills.

Sometimes women experience nervous symptoms or depression during menopause. There is no evidence that estrogens are effective for such symptoms and they should not be used to treat them, although other treatment may be needed.

You may have heard that taking estrogens for long periods (years) after the menopause will keep your skin soft and supple and keep you feeling young. There is no evidence that this is so, however, and such long-term treatment carries important risks.

ESTROGENS TO PREVENT SWELLING OF THE BREASTS AFTER PREGNANCY

If you do not brest-feed your baby after delivery, your breasts may fill up with milk and become painful and engorged. This usually begins about three to four days after delivery and may last for a few days to up to a week or more. Sometimes the discomfort is severe, but usually it is not and can be controlled by pain-relieving drugs such as aspirin and by binding the breasts up tightly. Estrogens can be used to try to prevent the breasts from filling up. While this treatment is sometimes successful, in many cases the breasts fill up to some degree in spite of treatment. The dose of estrogens needed to prevent pain and swelling of the breasts is much larger than the dose needed to treat symptoms of the menopause and this may increase your chances of developing blood clots in the legs or lungs (see below). Therefore, it is important that you discuss the benefits and the risks of estrogen use with your doctor if you have decided not to breastfeed your baby.

SOME OF THE DANGERS OF ESTROGEN

1. Cancer of the Uterus: If estrogens are used in the postmenopausal period for more than a year, there is an increased risk of *endometrial cancer* (cancer of the uterus). Women taking estrogens have roughly five to ten times as great a chance of getting this cancer as women who take no estrogens. To put this another way, while a postmenopausal woman not taking estrogens has one chance in 1,000 each year of getting cancer of the uterus, a woman taking estrogens has five to ten chances in 1,000 each year. For this reason *it is important to take estrogens only when you really need them.*

The risk of this cancer is greater the longer estrogens are used and also seems to be greater when larger doses are taken. For this reason *it is important to take the lowest dose of estrogen that will control symptoms and to take it only as long as it is needed.* If estrogens are needed for longer periods of time, your doctor will want to reevaluate your need for estrogens at least every six months.

Women using estrogens should report any irregular vaginal bleeding to their doctors; such bleeding may be of no importance, but it can be an early warning of cancer of the uterus. If you have undiagnosed vaginal bleeding, you should not use estrogens until a diagnosis is made and you are certain there is no cancer of the uterus.

If you have had your uterus completely removed (total hysterectomy), there is no danger of developing cancer of the uterus.

2. Other Possible Cancers: Estrogens can cause development of other tumors in animals, such as tumors of the breast, cervix, vagina, or liver, when given for a long time. At present there is no good evidence that women using estrogen in the menopause have an increased risk of such tumors, but there is no way yet to be sure they do not; and one study raises the possibility that use of estrogens in the menopause may increase the risk of breast cancer many years later. This is a further reason to use estrogens only when clearly needed. While you are taking estrogens, it is important that you go to your doctor at least once a year for a physical examination. Also, if members of your family have had breast cancer or if you have breast nodules or abnormal mammograms (breast x-rays), your doctor may wish to carry out more frequent examinations of your breasts.

3. Gall Bladder Disease: Women who use estrogens after menopause are more likely to develop gall bladder disease needing surgery than women who do not use estrogens. Birth control pills have a similar effect.

4. Abnormal Blood Clotting: Oral contraceptives, some of which contain estrogens, increase the risk of blood clotting in various parts of the body. This can result in a stroke (if the clot is in the brain), a heart attack (clot in a blood vessel of the heart), or a pulmonary embolus (a clot which forms in the legs or pelvis, then breaks off and travels to the lungs). Any of these can be fatal. Blood clots may result in the loss of a limb, paralysis or loss of sight, depending on where the blood clot is formed or lodges if it breaks loose.

The larger doses of estrogen used to prevent swelling of the breasts after pregnancy have been reported to cause clotting in the legs and lungs.

It is recommended that if you have had any blood clotting disorders including clotting in the legs or lungs, or a heart attack or stroke, you should not use estrogens.

SPECIAL WARNING ABOUT PREGNANCY

You should not receive estrogen if you are pregnant. If this should occur, there is a greater than usual chance that the developing child will be born with a birth defect, although the possibility remains fairly small. A female child may have an increased risk of developing cancer of the vagina or cervix later in life (in the teens or twenties). Every possible effort should be made to avoid exposure to estrogens during pregnancy. If exposure occurs, see your doctor.

SOME OTHER EFFECTS OF ESTROGENS

In addition to the serious known risks of estrogens described above, estrogens have the following side effects and potential risks:

1. Nausea and Vomiting: The most common side effect of estrogen therapy is nausea. Vomiting is less common.

2. Effects on Breasts: Estrogens may cause breast tenderness or enlargement and may cause the breasts to secrete a liquid.

3. Effects on the Uterus: Estrogens may cause benign fibroid tumors of the uterus to get larger.

Some women will have menstrual bleeding when estrogens are stopped. But if the bleeding occurs on days you are still taking estrogens you should report this to your doctor.

4. Effects on Liver: Women taking estrogens develop on rare occasions a tumor of the liver which can rupture and bleed into the abdomen. You should report any swelling or unusual pain or tenderness in the abdomen to your doctor immediately.

Women with a past history of jaundice (yellowing of the skin and white parts of the eyes) may get jaundice again during estrogen use.

5. Other Effects: Estrogens may cause excess fluid to be retained in the body. This may make some conditions worse, such as epilepsy, migraine, heart disease, or kidney disease. If any of the above occur, stop taking estrogens and call your doctor.

SUMMARY

Estrogens have important uses, but they have serious risks as well. You must decide, with your doctor, whether the risks are acceptable to you in view of the benefits of treatment. Except where your doctor has prescribed estrogen for use in special cases of cancer of the breast or prostate, you should not use estrogens if you have cancer of the breast or uterus, are pregnant, have undiagnosed abnormal vaginal bleeding, blood clotting disorders including clotting in the legs or lungs, or have had a stroke, heart attack or angina.

You must understand that your doctor will require regular physical examinations while you are taking them and will try to discontinue the drug as soon as possible and use the smallest dose possible. You can help minimize the risk by being alert for signs of trouble including:

1. Abnormal bleeding from the vagina.
2. Pains in the calves or chest or sudden shortness of breath, or coughing blood (indicating possible clots in the legs, heart or lungs).
3. Severe headache, dizziness, faintness, or changes in vision (indicating possible developing clots in the brain or eye).
4. Breast lumps (you should ask your doctor how to examine your own breasts).
5. Jaundice (yellowing of the skin).
6. Mental depression.
7. *Any* other unusual condition or problem.

Based on his or her assessment of your medical needs, your doctor has prescribed this drug for you. Do not give the drug to anyone else.

HOW SUPPLIED
CREAM: 0.01%

AVERAGE UNIT PRICE (AVAILABLE SIZES)

BRAND			$0.29

BRAND/MANUFACTURER	NDC	SIZE	AWP
◆ BRAND			
ORTHO DIENESTROL: Ortho Pharm	00062-5450-00	78 gm	$21.90
	00062-5450-77	78 gm	$23.34

Diethylpropion Hydrochloride

DESCRIPTION

Diethylpropion Hydrochloride is available for oral administration in immediate-release tablets containing 25 mg and in controlled-release tablets containing 75 mg. Diethylpropion Hydrochloride is a sympathomimetic agent. The chemical name for Diethylpropion Hydrochloride is 1-phenyl-2-diethylamino-1-propanone hydrochloride.

In the controlled-release tablets, Diethylpropion Hydrochloride is dispersed in a hydrophilic matrix. On exposure to water, the Diethylpropion Hydrochloride is released at a relatively uniform rate as a result of slow hydration of the matrix. The result is controlled release of the anorectic agent.

Following is its chemical structure:

CLINICAL PHARMACOLOGY

Diethylpropion Hydrochloride is a sympathomimetic amine with some pharmacologic activity similar to that of the prototype drugs of this class used in obesity, the amphetamines. Actions include some central nervous system stimulation and elevation of blood pressure. Tolerance has been demonstrated with all drugs of this class in which these phenomena have been looked for.

Drugs of this class used in obesity are commonly known as "anorectics" or "anorexigenics." It has not been established, however, that the action of such drugs in treating obesity is primarily one of appetite suppression. For example, other central nervous system actions or metabolic effects may be involved.

Adult obese subjects instructed in dietary management and treated with "anorectic" drugs lose more weight on the average than those treated with placebo and diet, as determined in relatively short-term clinical trials.

The magnitude of increased weight loss of drug-treated patients over placebo-treated patients averages some fraction of a pound a week. However, individual weight loss may vary substantially from patient to patient. The rate of weight loss is greatest in the first weeks of therapy for both drug and placebo subjects and tends to decrease in succeeding weeks. The possible origins of the increased weight loss due to the various drug effects are not established. The amount of weight loss associated with the use of an "anorectic" drug varies from trial to trial,

and the increased weight loss appears to be related in part to variables other than the drug prescribed, such as the physician/investigator relationship, the population treated, and the diet prescribed. Studies do not permit conclusions as to the relative importance of the drug and non-drug factors on weight loss.

The natural history of obesity is measured in years, whereas most studies cited are restricted to a few weeks duration; thus, the total impact of drug-induced weight loss over that of diet alone is unknown.

Diethylpropion is rapidly absorbed from the GI tract after oral administration and is extensively metabolized through a complex pathway of biotransformation involving N-dealkylation and reduction. Many of these metabolites are biologically active and may participate in the therapeutic action of Diethylpropion Hydrochloride immediate-release or controlled-release tablets. Due to the varying lipid solubilities of these metabolites, their circulating levels are affected by urinary pH. Diethylpropion and/or its active metabolites are believed to cross the blood-brain barrier and the placenta.

Diethylpropion and its metabolites are excreted mainly by the kidney. It has been reported that between 75-106% of the dose is recovered in the urine within 48 hours after dosing. Using a phosphorescence assay that is specific for basic compounds containing a benzoyl group, the plasma half-life of the aminoketone metabolites is estimated to be between 4 to 6 hours.

The controlled-release characteristics of Diethylpropion Hydrochloride have been demonstrated by studies in humans in which plasma levels of Diethylpropion-related materials were measured by phosphorescence analysis. Plasma levels obtained with the 75 mg controlled-release formulation administered once daily indicated a more gradual release than the immediate-release formulation (three 25 mg tablets given in a single dose).

Diethylpropion Hydrochloride controlled-release tablets have not been shown superior in effectiveness to the same dosage of the immediate-release formulation (one 25 mg tablet three times daily). After administration of a single dose of Diethylpropion Hydrochloride (one 75 mg controlled-release tablet) or Diethylpropion Hydrochloride solution (75 mg dose) in a crossover study using normal human subjects, the amount of parent compound and its active metabolites recovered in the urine within 48 hours for the two dosage forms were not statistically different.

INDICATIONS AND USAGE

Diethylpropion Hydrochlorideis indicated in the management of exogenous obesity as a short-term adjunct (a few weeks) in a regimen of weight reduction based on caloric restriction. The usefulness of agents of this class (see *"Clinical Pharmacology"*) should be measured against possible risk factors inherent in their use such as those described below.

CONTRAINDICATIONS

Advanced arteriosclerosis, hyperthyroidism, known hypersensitivity, or idiosyncrasy to the sympathomimetic amines, glaucoma, severe hypertension (see *"Precautions."*)

Agitated states.

Patients with a history of drug abuse.

During or within 14 days following the administration of monoamine oxidase inhibitors, hypertensive crises may result.

WARNINGS

If tolerance develops, the recommended dose should not be exceeded in an attempt to increase the effect; rather, the drug should be discontinued. Diethylpropion Hydrochloride may impair the ability of the patient to engage in potentially hazardous activities such as operating machinery or driving a motor vehicle; the patient should therefore be cautioned accordingly.

When central nervous system active agents are used, consideration must always be given to the possibility of adverse interactions with alcohol.

PRECAUTIONS
GENERAL

Caution is to be exercised in prescribing Diethylpropion Hydrochloride for patients with hypertension or with symptomatic cardiovascular disease, including arrhythmias. Diethylpropion Hydrochloride should not be administered to patients with severe hypertension.

Reports suggest that Diethylpropion Hydrochloride may increase convulsions in some epileptics. Therefore, epileptics receiving Diethylpropion Hydrochloride should be carefully monitored. Titration of dose or discontinuance of Diethylpropion Hydrochloride may be necessary.

The least amount feasible should be prescribed or dispensed at one time in order to minimize the possibility of overdosage.

INFORMATION FOR PATIENT

The patient should be cautioned about concomitant use of alcohol or other CNS active drugs and Diethylpropion Hydrochloride. (See *"Warnings."*) The patient should be advised to observe caution when driving or engaging in any potentially hazardous activity.

LABORATORY TESTS
None

DRUG INTERACTIONS

Antidiabetic drug requirements (i.e., insulin) may be altered. Concurrent use with general anesthetics may result in arrhythmias. The pressor effects of Diethylpropion Hydrochloride and those of other drugs may be additive when the drugs are used concomitantly; conversely, Diethylpropion Hydrochloride may interfere with antihypertensive drugs (i.e., guanethidine, α-methyldopa). Concurrent use of

---

◆ RATED THERAPEUTICALLY EQUIVALENT; ◇ THERAPEUTIC EQUIVALENCE UNCONFIRMED; ○ UNRATED

phenothiazines may antagonize the anorectic effect of Diethylpropion Hydrochloride.

CARCINOGENESIS, MUTAGENESIS, AND IMPAIRMENT OF FERTILITY
No long-term studies have been done to evaluate Diethylpropion Hydrochloride for carcinogenicity. Mutagenicity studies have not been conducted. Animal reproduction studies revealed no evidence of impairment of fertility (see "Pregnancy").

PREGNANCY
Teratogenic Effects: Pregnancy Category B: Reproduction studies have been performed in rats at doses up to 9 times the human dose and have revealed no evidence of impaired fertility or harm to the fetus due to Diethylpropion Hydrochloride. There are, however, no adequate and well-controlled studies in pregnant women. Because animal reproduction studies are not always predictive of human response, this drug should be used during pregnancy only if clearly needed.

Nonteratogenic Effects: Abuse with Diethylpropion Hydrochloride during pregnancy may result in withdrawal symptoms in the human neonate.

Nursing Mothers: Since Diethylpropion Hydrochloride and/or its metabolites have been shown to be excreted in human milk, caution should be exercised when Diethylpropion Hydrochloride is administered to a nursing woman.

Pediatric Use: Since safety and effectiveness in children below the age of 12 have not been established, Diethylpropion Hydrochloride is *not* recommended for use in children under 12 years of age.

ADVERSE REACTIONS
Cardiovascular: Precordial pain, arrhythmia, ECG changes, tachycardia, elevation of blood pressure, palpitation.

Central Nervous System: In a few epileptics an increase in convulsive episodes has been reported; rarely psychotic episodes at recommended doses; dyskinesia, blurred vision, overstimulation, nervousness, restlessness, dizziness, jitteriness, insomnia, anxiety, euphoria, depression, dysphoria, tremor, mydriasis, drowsiness, malaise, headache.

Gastrointestinal: Vomiting, diarrhea, abdominal discomfort, dryness of the mouth, unpleasant taste, nausea, constipation, other gastrointestinal disturbances.

Allergic: Urticaria, rash, ecchymosis, erythema.

Endocrine: Impotence, changes in libido, gynecomastia, menstrual upset.

Hematopoietic System: Bone marrow depression, agranulocytosis, leukopenia.

Miscellaneous: A variety of miscellaneous adverse reactions has been reported by physicians. These include complaints such as dysuria, dyspnea, hair loss, muscle pain, increased sweating, and polyuria.

DRUG ABUSE AND DEPENDENCE
Diethylpropion Hydrochloride is a schedule IV controlled substance. Diethylpropion Hydrochloride has some chemical and pharmacologic similarities to the amphetamines and other related stimulant drugs that have been extensively abused. There have been reports of subjects becoming psychologically dependent on Diethylpropion Hydrochloride. The possibility of abuse should be kept in mind when evaluating the desirability of including a drug as part of a weight reduction program. Abuse of amphetamines and related drugs may be associated with varying degrees of psychologic dependence and social dysfunction which, in the case of certain drugs, may be severe. There are reports of patients who have increased the dosage to many times that recommended. Abrupt cessation following prolonged high dosage administration results in extreme fatigue and mental depression; changes are also noted on the sleep EEG. Manifestations of chronic intoxication with anorectic drugs include severe dermatoses, marked insomnia, irritability, hyperactivity, and personality changes. The most severe manifestation of chronic intoxication is psychosis, often clinically indistinguishable from schizophrenia.

OVERDOSAGE
Manifestations of acute overdosage include restlessness, tremor, hyperreflexia, rapid respiration, confusion, assaultiveness, hallucinations, panic states.

Fatigue and depression usually follow the central stimulation.

Cardiovascular effects include arrhythmias, hypertension or hypotension and circulatory collapse. Gastrointestinal symptoms include nausea, vomiting, diarrhea, and abdominal cramps. Overdosage of pharmacologically similar compounds has resulted in convulsions, coma and death.

The reported oral LD_{50} for mice is 600 mg/kg, for rats is 250 mg/kg and for dogs is 225 mg/kg.

Management of acute Diethylpropion Hydrochloride intoxication is largely symptomatic and includes lavage and sedation with a barbiturate. Experience with hemodialysis or peritoneal dialysis is inadequate to permit recommendation in this regard. Intravenous phentolamine has been suggested on pharmacologic grounds for possible acute, severe hypertension, if this complicates Diethylpropion Hydrochloride or overdosage.

DOSAGE AND ADMINISTRATION
Diethylpropion Hydrochloride immediate-release:
One immediate-release 25 mg tablet three times daily, one hour before meals, and in midevening if desired to overcome night hunger.
Diethylpropion Hydrochloride controlled-release:

One controlled-release 75 mg tablet daily, swallowed whole, in midmorning.
Keep tightly closed, store at room temperature, preferably below 86°F. Protect from excessive heat.

HOW SUPPLIED
TABLET (C-IV): 25 MG

AVERAGE UNIT PRICE (AVAILABLE SIZES)		GENERIC A-RATED AVERAGE PRICE (GAAP)	
BRAND	$0.38	100s	$5.61
GENERIC	$0.05	1000s	$34.74
HCFA FUL (100s ea)	$0.05		

BRAND/MANUFACTURER	NDC	SIZE	AWP
◆ **BRAND**			
TENUATE: Marion Merrell Dow	00068-0697-61	100s	$37.86
◆ **GENERICS**			
Moore,H.L.	00839-5109-06	100s	$5.20
Rugby	00536-3702-01	100s	$5.37
Camall	00147-0237-10	100s	$5.40
Goldline	00182-1436-01	100s	$6.45
Camall	00147-0237-20	1000s	$31.97
Rugby	00536-3702-10	1000s	$37.50

TABLET, EXTENDED RELEASE (C-IV): 75 MG

BRAND/MANUFACTURER	NDC	SIZE	AWP
◇ **BRAND**			
TENUATE DOSPAN: Marion Merrell Dow	00068-0698-61	100s	$94.92
	00068-0698-62	250s	$230.58
◇ **GENERICS**			
MD Pharm	43567-0450-07	100s	$45.88
Geneva	00781-1605-01	100s	$48.69
Qualitest	00603-3290-21	100s	$49.50
URL	00677-0436-01	100s	$61.00
Major	00904-0618-60	100s	$61.20
Goldline	00182-0870-01	100s	$63.00
Parmed	00349-2049-01	100s	$72.50
Rugby	00536-5673-01	100s	$79.90
Major	00904-0618-70	250s	$107.65
MD Pharm	43567-0450-10	250s	$112.32
Qualitest	00603-3290-24	250s	$118.60
Parmed	00349-2049-25	250s	$134.95
Goldline	00182-0870-02	250s	$156.00
Parmed	00349-2049-05	500s	$166.08

Diethylstilbestrol

1. USE OF ESTROGENS HAS BEEN REPORTED TO INCREASE THE RISK OF ENDOMETRIAL CARCINOMA: THREE INDEPENDENT CASE-CONTROL STUDIES HAVE REPORTED AN INCREASED RISK OF ENDOMETRIAL CANCER IN POSTMENOPAUSAL WOMEN EXPOSED TO EXOGENOUS ESTROGENS FOR MORE THAN 1 YEAR. THIS RISK WAS INDEPENDENT OF OTHER KNOWN RISK FACTORS FOR ENDOMETRIAL CANCER. THESE STUDIES ARE FURTHER SUPPORTED BY THE FINDING THAT, SINCE 1969, THE INCIDENCE RATE OF ENDOMETRIAL CANCER HAS INCREASED SHARPLY IN 8 DIFFERENT AREAS OF THE UNITED STATES WHICH HAVE POPULATION-BASED CANCER REPORTING SYSTEMS.

THE 3 CASE-CONTROL STUDIES REPORTED THAT THE RISK OF ENDOMETRIAL CANCER IN ESTROGEN USERS WAS ABOUT 4.5 TO 13.9 TIMES GREATER THAN IN NONUSERS. THE RISK APPEARS TO DEPEND ON BOTH THE DURATION OF TREATMENT AND THE DOSE OF ESTROGEN. IN VIEW OF THESE FINDINGS, THE LOWEST DOSE THAT WILL CONTROL SYMPTOMS SHOULD BE UTILIZED WHEN ESTROGENS ARE USED FOR THE TREATMENT OF MENOPAUSAL SYMPTOMS, AND MEDICATION SHOULD BE DISCONTINUED AS SOON AS POSSIBLE. WHEN PROLONGED TREATMENT IS MEDICALLY INDICATED, A REASSESSMENT SHOULD BE MADE ON AT LEAST A SEMI-ANNUAL BASIS TO DETERMINE THE NEED FOR CONTINUED THERAPY. ALTHOUGH THE EVIDENCE MUST BE CONSIDERED PRELIMINARY, 1 STUDY SUGGESTS THAT CYCLIC

► SHOWN IN PRODUCT IDENTIFICATION GUIDE

ADMINISTRATION OF LOW DOSES OF ESTROGEN MAY CARRY LESS RISK THAN DOES CONTINUOUS ADMINISTRATION; IT THEREFORE APPEARS PRUDENT TO UTILIZE SUCH A REGIMEN.

CLOSE CLINICAL SURVEILLANCE OF ALL WOMEN TAKING ESTROGENS IS IMPORTANT. IN ALL CASES OF UNDIAGNOSED PERSISTENT OR RECURRING ABNORMAL VAGINAL BLEEDING, ADEQUATE DIAGNOSTIC MEASURES SHOULD BE UNDERTAKEN TO RULE OUT MALIGNANCY.

AT PRESENT, THERE IS NO EVIDENCE THAT "NATURAL" ESTROGENS ARE MORE OR LESS HAZARDOUS THAN "SYNTHETIC" ESTROGENS AT EQUIVALENT ESTROGENIC DOSES.

2. ESTROGENS SHOULD NOT BE USED DURING PREGNANCY: THE USE OF FEMALE SEX HORMONES, BOTH ESTROGENS AND PROGESTOGENS, DURING EARLY PREGNANCY MAY AFFECT THE OFFSPRING. IT HAS BEEN REPORTED THAT FEMALES EXPOSED *IN UTERO* TO DIETHYLSTILBESTROL, A NONSTEROIDAL ESTROGEN, MAY HAVE AN INCREASED RISK OF DEVELOPING LATER IN LIFE A RARE FORM OF VAGINAL OR CERVICAL CANCER. THIS RISK HAS BEEN ESTIMATED TO BE 0.14 TO 1.4 PER 1,000 EXPOSURES. FURTHERMORE, FROM 30% TO 90% OF SUCH EXPOSED WOMEN HAVE BEEN FOUND TO HAVE VAGINAL ADENOSIS AND EPITHELIAL CHANGES OF THE VAGINA AND CERVIX. ALTHOUGH THESE CHANGES ARE HISTOLOGICALLY BENIGN, IT IS NOT KNOWN WHETHER THEY ARE PRECURSORS OF MALIGNANCY. EVEN THOUGH SIMILAR DATA ARE NOT AVAILABLE WITH THE USE OF OTHER ESTROGENS, IT CANNOT BE PRESUMED THAT THEY WOULD NOT INDUCE SIMILAR CHANGES.

SEVERAL REPORTS SUGGEST THAT THERE IS AN ASSOCIATION BETWEEN INTRAUTERINE EXPOSURE TO FEMALE SEX HORMONES AND CONGENITAL ANOMALIES, INCLUDING CONGENITAL HEART DEFECTS AND LIMB-REDUCTION DEFECTS. ONE CASE-CONTROL STUDY ESTIMATED A 4.7-FOLD INCREASED RISK OF LIMB-REDUCTION DEFECTS IN INFANTS EXPOSED *IN UTERO* TO SEX HORMONES (ORAL CONTRACEPTIVES, HORMONE WITHDRAWAL TESTS FOR PREGNANCY, OR ATTEMPTED TREATMENT FOR THREATENED ABORTION). SOME OF THESE EXPOSURES WERE VERY SHORT AND INVOLVED ONLY A FEW DAYS OF TREATMENT. THE DATA SUGGEST THAT THE RISK OF LIMB-REDUCTION DEFECTS IN EXPOSED FETUSES IS SOMEWHAT LESS THAN 1 PER 1,000.

IN THE PAST, FEMALE SEX HORMONES HAVE BEEN USED DURING PREGNANCY IN AN ATTEMPT TO TREAT THREATENED OR HABITUAL ABORTION; HOWEVER, THEIR EFFICACY WAS NEVER CONCLUSIVELY PROVED OR DISPROVED.

IF DIETHYLSTILBESTROL IS ADMINISTERED DURING PREGNANCY, OR IF THE PATIENT BECOMES PREGNANT WHILE TAKING THIS DRUG, SHE SHOULD BE APPRISED OF THE POTENTIAL RISKS TO THE FETUS AND OF THE ADVISABILITY OF PREGNANCY CONTINUATION.

This drug product should not be used as a postcoital contraceptive.

DESCRIPTION
Diethylstilbestrol is a crystalline synthetic estrogenic substance capable of producing all the pharmacologic and therapeutic responses attributed to natural estrogens. Diethylstilbestrol may be administered orally in the form of tablets, or intravenously in the form of a sterile solution. The injection is available as the diphosphate salt. Chemically, diethylstilbestrol is α,α'-diethyl-4,4'-stilbenediol.

CLINICAL PHARMACOLOGY
Putative receptor proteins for estrogens have been detected in estrogen-responsive tissues. Estrogens are first bound to a cytoplasmic receptor protein. Following modification, the estrogen-protein complex is translocated to the nucleus where ultimate binding of the estrogen containing complex occurs. As a result of such binding characteristic metabolic alterations ensue.

In the male patient with androgenic hormone dependent conditions such as metastatic carcinoma of the prostate gland, estrogens counter the androgenic influence by competing for the receptor sites. As a result of treatment with estrogens, metastatic lesions in the bone may also show improvement.

It has been demonstrated in animal studies that Diethylstilbestrol Diphosphate is rapidly hydrolysed to Diethylstilbesterol through phosphatase activity in the blood and tissues. When Diethylstilbestrol diphosphate (92 mg/kg body wt.) was injected intravenously into rabbits over a period of 2 to 3 minutes, free Diethylstilbestrol appeared in the blood stream as early as 5 minutes after termination of injection and within 15 minutes had reached a concentration of 16.3 ug/mL of plasma. This was followed by a rapid decline in concentration, only 1.2 ug/mL remaining after 2 hours. It is therefore expected that the high concentration of serum acid phosphatase in patients with prostatic carcinoma will hydrolyse Diethylstilbestrol diphosphate to free, active Diethylstilbestrol.

Diethylstilbestrol is metabolized by the body in much the same manner as the endogenous hormones. Inactivation of estrogen is carried out mainly in the liver. A certain proportion of the estrogen reaching that organ is excreted into the bile, only to be reabsorbed from the intestine. During this enterohepatic circulation, degradation of estrogen occurs through conversion to less active products, through oxidation to nonestrogenic substances, and through conjugation with sulfuric and glucuronic acids. These water-soluble conjugates are strong acids and are thus fully ionized in the body fluids; penetration into cells is therefore limited, and excretion by the kidney is favored because little tubular reabsorption is possible.

INDICATIONS AND USAGE
Diethylstilbestrol is indicated in the treatment of:

1. Breast cancer (for palliation only) in appropriately selected women and men with metastatic disease
2. Prostatic carcinoma—palliative therapy of advanced disease (only indication for the Diphosphate salt)

Diethylstilbestrol should not be used for any purpose during pregnancy. Its use may cause severe harm to the fetus (see boxed "Warning").

UNLABELED USES
Diethylstilbestrol is used alone or as an adjunct in the treatment of symptoms associated with menopause and in the prevention of stuttering attacks of priapism in sickle-cell disease. It is also used as a birth control for postcoital conception, suppression of postpartum lactation, and transsexual hormonal feminization.

CONTRAINDICATIONS
Estrogens should not be used in women or men with any of the following conditions:

1. Known or suspected cancer of the breast, except in appropriately selected patients being treated for metastatic disease
2. Known or suspected estrogen-dependent neoplasia
3. Known or suspected pregnancy (see boxed *"Warning"*)
4. Undiagnosed abnormal genital bleeding
5. Active thrombophlebitis or thromboembolic disorders
6. A past history of thrombophlebitis, thrombosis, or thromboembolic disorders associated with previous use of estrogen (except when used in treatment of breast or prostatic malignancy).

Diethylstilbestrol Diphosphate is not indicated in the treatment of any disorder in women.

WARNINGS
1. Induction of Malignant Neoplasms: In certain animal species, long-term continuous administration of natural and synthetic estrogens increases the frequency of carcinomas of the breast, cervix, vagina, kidney, and liver. There are now reports that prolonged use of estrogens increases the risk of carcinoma of the endometrium in humans (see boxed *"Warning"*).

At the present time, there is no satisfactory evidence that administration of estrogens to postmenopausal women increases the risk of cancer of the breast. This possibility, however, has been raised by a recent long-term follow-up of 1 physician's practice. Because of the animal data, there is a need for caution in prescribing estrogens for women with a family history of breast cancer or for women who have breast nodules, fibrocystic disease, or abnormal mammograms.

2. Gallbladder Disease: A recent study reported a 2-to-3-fold increase in the risk of gallbladder disease occurring in women receiving postmenopausal estrogen therapy, similar to the 2-fold increased risk previously noted in women using oral contraceptives. In the case of oral contraceptives, this increased risk appeared after 2 years of use.

3. Effects Similar to Those Caused by Estrogen-Progestogen Oral Contraceptives: There are several serious adverse effects associated with the use of oral contraceptives; however, most of these adverse effects have not as yet been documented as consequences of postmenopausal estrogen therapy. This may reflect the comparatively low doses of estrogen used in postmenopausal women. It would be expected that these adverse effects are more likely to occur following administration of the larger doses of estrogen used for treating prostatic or breast cancer. It has, in fact, been shown that there is an increased risk of thrombosis with the administration of estrogens for prostatic cancer in men and for postpartum breast engorgement in women.

a. Thromboembolic Disease: It is now well established that women taking oral contraceptives run an increased risk of various thromboembolic and thrombotic vascular diseases, such as thrombophlebitis, pulmonary embolism, stroke, and myocardial infarction. Cases of retinal thrombosis, mesenteric thrombosis, and optic neuritis have been reported in users of oral contraceptives. There is evidence that the risk of several of these adverse reactions is related to the dose of the drug. An increased risk of postsurgical thromboembolic complications has also been reported in users of oral contraceptives. If feasible, estrogen therapy should be discontinued at least 4 weeks before surgery such as that associated with an increased risk of thromboembolism, or that requiring periods of prolonged immobilization.

Although an increased rate of thromboembolic and thrombotic disease has not been noted in postmenopausal users of estrogen, this does not rule out the possibility that such an increase may be present or that it exists in subgroups of women who have underlying risk factors or who are receiving relatively large doses of estrogens. Therefore, estrogens should not be used in persons with active thrombophlebitis or thromboembolic disorders, nor should they be used (except in treatment of malignancy) in persons with a history of such disorders associated with estrogen therapy. Estrogens should be administered cautiously to patients with cerebral vascular or coronary artery disease and only when such therapy is clearly needed.

In a large prospective clinical trial in men, large doses of estrogen (5 mg of conjugated estrogens per day), comparable to those used to treat cancer of the prostate and breast, have been shown to increase the risk of nonfatal myocardial infarction, pulmonary embolism, and thrombophlebitis. When such large doses of estrogen are used, any of the thromboembolic and thrombotic adverse effects associated with the use of oral contraceptives should be considered a clear risk.

b. Hepatic Adenoma: Benign hepatic adenomas appear to be associated with the use of oral contraceptives. Although these adenomas are benign and rare, they may rupture and may cause death by intra-abdominal hemorrhage. Such lesions have not yet been reported in association with the administration of other estrogen or progestogen preparations, but they should be considered when abdominal pain and tenderness, abdominal mass, or hypovolemic shock occurs in persons receiving estrogen therapy. Hepatocellular carcinoma has also been reported in women taking estrogen-containing oral contraceptives. The relationship of this malignancy to these drugs is not known at this time.

c. Elevated Blood Pressure: Increased blood pressure is not uncommon in women taking oral contraceptives; in most cases, blood pressure returns to normal on discontinuing the drug. There is now 1 report that this may occur with use of estrogens in the menopause, and blood pressure should be monitored during estrogen therapy, especially if high doses are used.

d. Glucose Tolerance: A decrease in glucose tolerance has been observed in a significant percentage of patients on estrogen-containing oral contraceptives. For this reason, diabetic patients should be carefully observed while receiving estrogen.

4. Hypercalcemia: Administration of estrogens may lead to severe hypercalcemia in patients with breast cancer and bone metastases. If this occurs, the drug should be stopped and appropriate measures taken to reduce the serum calcium level.

PRECAUTIONS
GENERAL
1. A complete medical and family history should be taken prior to initiation of any estrogen therapy. In the pretreatment and periodic physical examinations, special consideration should be given to blood pressure, breasts, abdomen, and pelvic organs, and a Papanicolaou smear should be performed. As a general rule, estrogen should not be prescribed for longer than one year without another physical examination.

2. Fluid retention: Because estrogens may cause some degree of fluid retention, conditions which might be influenced by this factor, such as asthma, epilepsy, migraine, and cardiac or renal dysfunction, require careful observation.

3. Certain patients may develop undesirable manifestations of excessive estrogenic stimulation, such as abnormal or excessive uterine bleeding, mastodynia gynecomastia, etc.

4. Oral contraceptives appear to be associated with an increased incidence of mental depression. Although it is not clear whether this is due to the estrogenic or progestogenic component of the contraceptive agent, patients with a history of depression should be carefully observed.

5. Preexisting uterine leiomyomata may increase in size with administration of estrogens.

6. The pathologist should be advised of estrogen therapy when relevant specimens are submitted.

7. Patients with a past history of jaundice during pregnancy run an increased risk of recurrence of jaundice while receiving estrogen-containing oral contraceptive therapy. If jaundice develops in any patient receiving estrogen, the medication should be discontinued while the cause is investigated.

8. Estrogens may be poorly metabolized in patients with impaired liver function, and they should therefore be administered with caution in such patients.

9. Because estrogens influence the metabolism of calcium and phosphorus, they should be used with caution in patients with metabolic bone diseases associated with hypercalcemia or in patients with renal insufficiency.

10. Because of the effects of estrogens on epiphyseal closure, they should be used judiciously in young patients in whom bone growth is not complete.

11. Certain endocrine and liver function tests may be affected by estrogen-containing oral contraceptives. The following similar changes may be expected with larger doses of estrogen:

    a. Increased sulfobromophthalein retention

    b. Increased prothrombin and factors VII, VIII, IX, and X; decreased antithrombin 3; increased norepinephrine-induced platelet aggregability

    c. Increased thyroid-binding globulin (TBG) leading to increased circulating total thyroid hormone, as measured by PBI, T4 by column, or T4 by radioimmunoassay. Free T3 resin uptake is decreased, reflecting the elevated TBG; free T4 concentration is unaltered

    d. Impaired glucose tolerance

    e. Decreased pregnanediol excretion

    f. Reduced response to metyrapone test

    g. Reduced serum folate concentration

    h. Increased serum triglyceride and phospholipid concentration

INFORMATION FOR PATIENT:
1. The diphosphate salt only should not be used by women.
2. The following side effects have been reported in patients being treated with the diphosphate salt. If they occur they should be reported promptly to your physician:
- Mood changes, depression
- Nervousness, dizziness
- Loss of appetite, nausea, vomiting, abdominal cramps, bloating
- Skin rash

- Chest pain and shortness of breath
- Numbness or tingling about the nose or mouth
- Fluid accumulation
- Swelling tenderness of breasts
- Disturbances of vision
- Frequent or uncomfortable urination
- Painful swelling of extremities

3. The patient should consult a physician regularly for evaluation of blood pressure and heart rate.
4. Diabetic patients should monitor urines very carefully. Test of blood sugar may be necessary as well.
5. The following clinical problems are associated with the use of the diphosphate salt only:
- Hepatic cutaneous prophyria
- Erythema nodosum
- Erythema multiforme

A significant association has been shown between the use of estrogen containing drugs and the following serious reactions:
1. Thrombophlebitis
2. Pulmonary embolism
3. Cerebal thrombosis
4. There is suggestive evidence that there may be a relationship with coronary thrombosis.

The following adverse reactions are known to have occurred in patients receiving estrogens:

- Change in body weight
- Headache
- Loss of sex drive
- Post injection flare
- Aggravation of migraine headaches
- Loss of scalp hair
- Hemorrhagic eruption
- Fatigue
- Backache

CARCINOGENESIS, MUTAGENESIS, IMPAIRMENT OF FERTILITY
See *"Warnings"* regarding induction of neoplasia.

PREGNANCY CATEGORY X
See *"Contraindications"* and boxed *"Warning."*

The diphosphate salt is not indicated in the treatment of any disorder in women.

NURSING MOTHERS
As a general principle, the administration of any drug to nursing mothers should be done only when clearly necessary, since many drugs are excreted in human milk.

PEDIATRIC USE
Because of the effects of estrogens on epiphyseal closure, they should be used judiciously in young patients in whom bone growth is not complete.

ADVERSE REACTIONS
(See *"Warnings"* regarding induction of neoplasia, adverse effects on the fetus, increased incidence of gallbladder disease, and adverse effects similar to those of oral contraceptives, including thromboembolism.) The following additional adverse reactions have been reported with estrogenic therapy, including oral contraceptives:

1. Genitourinary System:
Breakthrough bleeding, spotting, change in menstrual flow
Dysmenorrhea
Premenstrual-like syndrome
Amenorrhea during and after treatment
Increase in size of uterine fibromyomata
Vaginal candidiasis
Change in cervical eversion and in degree of cervical secretion
Cystitis-like syndrome

2. Breasts:
Tenderness, enlargement, secretion

3. Gastrointestinal:
Nausea, vomiting
Abdominal cramps, bloating
Cholestatic jaundice

4. Skin:
Chloasma or melasma, which may persist when drug is discontinued
Erythema multiforme
Erythema nodosum
Hemorrhagic eruption
Loss of scalp hair
Hirsutism

5. Eyes:
Steepening of corneal curvature
Intolerance to contact lenses

6. CNS:
Headache, migraine, dizziness
Mental depression
Chorea

7. Miscellaneous:
Increase or decrease in weight
Reduced carbohydrate tolerance
Aggravation of porphyria
Edema
Changes in libido
Transient itching and burning sensation in the perineal region

OVERDOSAGE

Signs and Symptoms: Symptoms of acute overdose include anorexia, nausea, vomiting, abdominal cramps, and diarrhea. Withdrawal vaginal bleeding may follow large doses. Chronic toxicity may include salt and water retention, edema, headache, vertigo, leg cramps, gynecomastia, chloasma, and porphyria cutanea tarda. Polydipsia, polyuria, fatigue, and an abnormal glucose tolerance may occur in some patients with preclinical diabetes mellitus.

No information is available on the following: LD_{50}, concentration of Diethylstilbestrol in biologic fluids associated with toxicity and/or death, the amount of drug in a single dose usually associated with symptoms of overdosage, or the amount of Diethylstilbestrol in a single dose likely to be life threatening.

Numerous reports of ingestion of large doses of estrogen-containing oral contraceptives by young children indicate that acute serious ill effects do not occur.

Treatment: Chronic Diethylstilbestrol toxicity should be treated by discontinuing all estrogenic medications and providing supportive care for any symptoms that may be present.

To obtain up-to-date information about the treatment of overdose, a good resource is your certified Regional Poison Control Center. Telephone numbers of certified poison control centers are listed in the *Physicians' Desk Reference (PDR)*. In managing overdosage, consider the possibility of multiple drug overdoses, interaction among drugs, and unusual drug kinetics in your patient.

In treating acute overdose, protect the patient's airway and support ventilation and perfusion. Meticulously monitor and maintain, within acceptable limits, the patient's vital signs, blood gases, serum electrolytes, etc. Absorption of drugs from the gastrointestinal tract may be decreased by giving activated charcoal, which, in many cases, is more effective than emesis or lavage; consider charcoal instead of or in addition to gastric emptying. Repeated doses of charcoal over time may hasten elimination of some drugs that have been absorbed. Safeguard the patient's airway when employing gastric emptying or charcoal.

Forced diuresis, peritoneal dialysis, hemodialysis, or charcoal hemoperfusion have not been established as beneficial for an overdose of Diethylstilbestrol.

DOSAGE AND ADMINISTRATION

Given Chronically:

Inoperable progressing prostatic cancer
Diethylstilbestrol 1- and 5-mg tablets: 1 to 3 mg daily initially, increased in advanced cases; the dosage may later be reduced to an average of 1 mg daily.

Diethylstilbestrol phosphate 50-mg tablets: Start with one tablet three times a day and increase this dose level to four or more tablets three times a day, depending on the tolerance of the patient. Maximum daily dose not to exceed one gram.

Alternatively, if relief is not obtained with high oral dosages. Diethylstilbestrol Diphosphate may be administered intravenously. Diethylstilbestrol Diphosphate solution must be diluted before intravenous infusion.

Diethylstilbestrol Diphosphate Ampules 0.25 gram: It is recommended that 0.5 gram (2 ampules) dissolved in approximately 250 mL of normal saline for injection USP, or 5% dextrose for injection USP, be given intravenously the first day, and that each day thereafter one gram (4 ampules) be similarly administered in approximately 250 to 500 mL of normal saline for injection USP, or 5% dextrose for injection USP.

The infusion should be administered slowly (20-30) drops per minute) during the first 10-15 minutes and then the rate of flow adjusted so that the entire amount is given in a period of about one hour. This procedure should be followed for five days or more depending on the response of the patient. Following the first intensive course of therapy, 0.25-0.5 gram (1 or 2 ampules) may be administered in a similar manner once or twice weekly or maintenance obtained with Diethylstilbestrol Diphosphate tablets.

Stability of Solution: After reconstitution, if storage is desired, the solution should be kept at room temperature and away from direct light. Under these conditions the solution is stable for about 5 days, so long as cloudiness or evidence of a precipitate has not occurred.

Inoperable progressing breast cancer in appropriately selected men and postmenopausal women (see *"Indications"*): 15 mg daily.

Patients with an intact uterus should be closely monitored for signs of endometrial cancer, and appropriate diagnostic measures should be taken to rule out malignancy in the event of persistent or recurring abnormal vaginal bleeding.

Storage: Store Diethylstilbestrol Diphosphate at controlled room temperature (59°-86°F); protect from light.

J CODES
250 mg IV—J9165

HOW SUPPLIED

DIETHYLSTILBESTEROL DIPHOSPHATE
INJECTION: 0.25 GM/5 ML

BRAND/MANUFACTURER	NDC	SIZE	AWP
○ BRAND STILPHOSTROL: Miles Pharm	00026-8131-20	5 ml 20s	$250.37

TABLETS: 50 MG

BRAND/MANUFACTURER	NDC	SIZE	AWP
○ BRAND STILPHOSTROL: Miles Pharm	00026-8132-50	50s	$87.61

DIETHYLSTILBESTROL
TABLETS: 1 MG

BRAND/MANUFACTURER	NDC	SIZE	AWP
◇ GENERICS Lilly	00002-1052-02	100s	$9.14

TABLETS: 5 MG

BRAND/MANUFACTURER	NDC	SIZE	AWP
◇ GENERICS Lilly	00002-1054-02	100s	$24.35

Difil G *SEE* DYPHYLLINE AND GUAIFENESIN

Diflorasone Diacetate

DESCRIPTION
Diflorasone Diacetate is a synthetic corticosteroid for topical dermatological use. It is not for ophthalmic use.

Each gram of Diflorasone Diacetate Cream and Diflorasone Diacetate Ointment contains 0.5 mg Diflorasone Diacetate in a cream or ointment base respectively. Each gram of Diflorasone Diacetate Emollient Cream contains 0.5 mg Diflorasone Diacetate in an emollient cream base.

Chemically, Diflorasone Diacetate is: 6α, 9α-difluoro-11β, 17,21-trihydroxy-16β-methylpregna-1,4-diene-3,20-dione 17,21 diacetate.

Following is its chemical structure:

CLINICAL PHARMACOLOGY
Topical corticosteroids share anti-inflammatory, antipruritic and vasoconstrictive actions.

The mechanism of anti-inflammatory activity of the topical corticosteroids is unclear. However, corticosteroids are thought to act by the induction of phospholipase A_2 inhibitory proteins collectively called lipocortins. It is postulated that these proteins control the biosynthesis of potent mediators of inflammation such as prostaglandins and leukotrienes by inhibiting the release of their common precursor, arachidonic acid. Arachidonic acid is released from membrane phospholipids A_2. Various laboratory methods, including vasoconstrictor assays, are used to compare and predict potencies and/or clinical efficacies of the topical corticosteroids. There is some evidence to suggest that a recognizable correlation exists between vasoconstrictor potency and therapeutic efficacy in man.

Pharmacokinetics: The extent of percutaneous absorption of topical corticosteroids is determined by many factors including the vehicle, the integrity of the epidermal barrier and the use of occlusive dressings. Occlusive dressings with hydrocortisone for up to 24 hours have not been demonstrated to increase penetration; however, occlusion of hydrocortisone for 96 hours markedly enhances penetration.

Topical corticosteroids can be absorbed from normal intact skin. Inflammation and/or other disease processes in the skin increase percutaneous absorption. Occlusive dressings substantially increase the percutaneous absorption of topical corticosteroids. Thus, occlusive dressings may be a valuable therapeutic adjunct for treatment of resistant dermatoses. (See *"Dosage and Administration"*.)

Once absorbed through the skin, topical corticosteroids are handled through pharmacokinetic pathways similar to systemically administered corticosteroids.

◆ RATED THERAPEUTICALLY EQUIVALENT; ◇ THERAPEUTIC EQUIVALENCE UNCONFIRMED; ○ UNRATED

Corticosteroids are bound to plasma proteins in varying degrees. They are metabolized primarily in the liver and are then excreted by the kidneys. Some of the topical corticosteroids and their metabolites are also excreted into the bile.

INDICATIONS AND USAGE
Topical corticosteroids are indicated for relief of the inflammatory and pruritic manifestations of corticosteroids-responsive dermatoses.

CONTRAINDICATIONS
Topical steroids are contraindicated in those patients with a history of hypersensitivity to any of the components of the preparation.

PRECAUTIONS
GENERAL
Systemic absorption of topical corticosteroids has produced reversible hypothalamic-pituitary-adrenal (HPA) axis suppression with the potential for glucocorticoid insufficiency after withdrawal of treatment, manifestations of Cushing's syndrome, hyperglycemia, and glucosuria in some patients.

Conditions which augment systemic absorption include the application of the more potent steroids, use over large surface areas, prolonged use, and the addition of occlusive dressings.

Therefore, patients receiving a large dose of a potent topical steroid applied to a large surface area or under an occlusive dressing should be evaluated periodically for evidence of HPA axis suppression by using the urinary free-cortisol and ACTH stimulation tests, and, with some brands, A.M. plasma cortisol. Some brands of Diflorasone Diacetate Cream have a greater ability to produce adrenal suppression than does Diflorasone Diacetate Ointment, 0.05%. At 30 g per day (applied as 15 g twice daily) Diflorasone Diacetate Cream, 0.05% was shown to cause inhibition of the HPA axis in one of two patients following application for one week to psoriatic skin. At 15 g per day (applied as 7.5 g twice daily) Diflorasone Diacetate Cream was shown to cause mild inhibition of the HPA axis in one of five patients following application for one week to diseased skin (psoriasis or atopic dermatitis). These effects were reversible upon discontinuation of treatment. By comparison, Diflorasone Diacetate Ointment, 0.05% did not produce significant HPA axis suppression when used in divided doses at 30 g per day for one week in patients with psoriasis or atopic dermatitis. If HPA axis suppression is noted, an attempt should be made to withdraw the drug, to reduce the frequency of application, or to substitute a less potent steroid.

Recovery of HPA axis function is generally prompt and complete upon discontinuation of the drug. Infrequently, signs and symptoms of steroid withdrawal may occur, requiring supplemental systemic corticosteroids.

Children may absorb proportionally larger amounts of topical corticosteroids due to their larger skin surface to body mass ratios and thus are more susceptible to systemic toxicity. (See "Precautions—Pediatric Use").

If irritation develops, topical corticosteroids should be discontinued and appropriate therapy instituted. Allergic contact dermatitis with corticosteroids is usually diagnosed by observing failure to heal rather than noting a clinical exacerbation as with most topical products not containing corticosteroids. Such an observation should be corroborated with appropriate diagnostic patch testing.

In the presence of dermatological infections, the use of an appropriate antifungal or antibacterial agent should be instituted. If a favorable response does not occur promptly, the corticosteroid should be discontinued until the infection has been adequately controlled.

Diflorasone Diacetate Cream should not be used in the treatment of rosacea or perioral dermatitis, and it should not be used on the face, groin, or axillae.

Information for the Patient: Patients using topical corticosteroids should receive the following information and instructions:

1. This medication is to be used as directed by the physician. It is for external use only. Avoid contact with the eyes.
2. Patients should be advised not to use this medication for any disorder other than for which it was prescribed.
3. The treated skin area should not be bandaged or otherwise covered or wrapped as to be occlusive unless directed by the physician.
4. Patients should report any signs of local adverse reactions especially under occlusive dressing.
5. Parents of pediatric patients should be advised not to use tight-fitting diapers or plastic pants on a child being treated in the diaper area, as these garments may constitute occlusive dressings.

Laboratory Tests: The following tests may be helpful in evaluating the HPA axis suppression:
Urinary free cortisol test
ACTH stimulation test
A.M. plasma-cortisol test for some brands

Carcinogenesis, Mutagenesis, and Impairment of Fertility: Long-term animal studies have not been performed to evaluate the carcinogenic potential or the effect on fertility of topical corticosteroids.

Studies to determine mutagenicity with prednisolone and hydrocortisone have revealed negative results.

Diflorasone Diacetate was not found to be mutagenic in a micronucleus test in rats at dosage of 2400 mg/kg.

Studies in the rat following topical administration at doses up to 0.5 mg/kg revealed no effects on fertility.

Pregnancy Category C: Corticosteroids are generally teratogenic in laboratory animals when administered systemically at relatively low dosage levels. The more potent corticosteroids have been shown to be teratogenic after dermal application in laboratory animals. Diflorasone Diacetate has been shown to be teratogenic (cleft palate) in rats when applied topically at a dose of approximately 0.001 mg/kg/day to the shaven thorax of pregnant animals. This is approximately 0.3 times the human topical dose of Diflorasone Diacetate Cream. When pregnant rats were treated topically with approximately 0.5 mg/kg/day, uterine deaths were higher in the treated animals than in control animals.

In rabbits, cleft palate was seen when Diflorasone Diacetate was applied in topical doses as low as 20 mg/kg/day. In addition, fetal weight was depressed and litter sizes were smaller. There are no adequate and well-controlled studies in pregnant women on teratogenic effects from topically applied corticosteroids. Therefore, topical corticosteroids should be used during pregnancy only if the potential benefit justifies the potential risk to the fetus. Drugs of this class should not be used extensively on pregnant patients, in large amounts, or for prolonged periods of time.

Nursing Mothers: It is not known whether topical administration of corticosteroids could result in sufficient systemic absorption to produce detectable quantities in breast milk. Systemically administered corticosteroids are secreted into breast milk in quantities *not* likely to have a deleterious effect on the infant, although they could suppress growth, interfere with endogenous corticosteroid production, or cause other untoward effects. Nevertheless, caution should be exercised when topical corticosteroids are administered to a nursing woman.

Pediatric Use: Safety and effectiveness of Diflorasone Diacetate in children have not been established. *Pediatric patients may demonstrate greater susceptibility to topical corticosteroid-induced HPA axis suppression and Cushing's syndrome than mature patients because of a larger skin surface area to body weight ratio.* They are, therefore, also a greater risk of glucocorticosteroid insufficiency after withdrawal of treatment and of Cushing's syndrome while on treatment. Adverse effects including striae have been reported with inappropriate use of topical corticosteroids in infants and children.

Hypothalamic-pituitary-adrenal (HPA) axis suppression, Cushing's syndrome, and intracranial hypertension have been reported in children receiving topical corticosteroids. Manifestations of adrenal suppression in children include linear growth retardation, delayed weight gain, low plasma cortisol levels, and absence of response to ACTH stimulation. Manifestations of intracranial hypertension include bulging fontanelles, headaches, and bilateral papilledema.

Administration of topical corticosteroids to children should be limited to the least amount compatible with an effective therapeutic regimen. Chronic corticosteroid therapy may interfere with the growth and development of children.

ADVERSE REACTIONS
The following local adverse reactions have been reported with topical corticosteroids, but may occur more frequently with the use of occlusive dressings. These reactions are listed in an approximate decreasing order of occurrence:

1. Burning
2. Itching
3. Irritation
4. Dryness
5. Folliculitis
6. Hypertrichosis
7. Acneiform eruptions
8. Hypopigmentation
9. Perioral dermatitis
10. Allergic contact dermatitis
11. Maceration of the skin
12. Secondary infection
13. Skin atrophy
14. Striae
15. Miliaria

OVERDOSAGE
Topically applied corticosteroids can be absorbed in sufficient amounts to produce systemic effects (see "Precautions").

DOSAGE AND ADMINISTRATION
Diflorasone Diacetate is generally applied to the affected areas as a thin film from one to four times daily depending on the brand and the severity of the condition.

Diflorasone Diacetate Emollient should be applied to the affected areas as a thin film from one to three times daily depending on the severity or resistant nature of the condition.

Occlusive dressings may be used for the management of psoriasis or recalcitrant conditions.

If an infection develops, the use of occlusive dressings should be discontinued and appropriate antimicrobial therapy instituted.

Store some brands at controlled room temperature 15°-30°C (59°-86°F), others at or below 25°C (77°F).

HOW SUPPLIED
CREAM:

BRAND/MANUFACTURER	NDC	SIZE	AWP
○ **BRAND**			
PSORCON: Dermik	00066-0069-17	15 gm	$20.74
	00066-0069-31	30 gm	$28.49
	00066-0069-60	60 gm	$52.76

▶ SHOWN IN PRODUCT IDENTIFICATION GUIDE

CREAM: 0.05%

BRAND/MANUFACTURER	NDC	SIZE	AWP
○ **BRAND**			
FLORONE: Dermik	00066-0074-17	15 gm	$21.41
FLORONE E: Dermik	00066-0072-17	15 gm	$21.41
MAXIFLOR: Allergan Herbert	00023-0766-30	30 gm	$24.71
FLORONE: Dermik	00066-0074-31	30 gm	$30.56
FLORONE E: Dermik	00066-0072-31	30 gm	$30.56
MAXIFLOR: Allergan Herbert	00023-0766-60	60 gm	$40.11
FLORONE: Dermik	00066-0074-60	60 gm	$51.73
FLORONE E: Dermik	00066-0072-60	60 gm	$51.73

OINTMENT:

BRAND/MANUFACTURER	NDC	SIZE	AWP
○ **BRAND**			
PSORCON: Dermik	00066-0071-17	15 gm	$22.70
	00066-0071-31	30 gm	$31.20
	00066-0071-60	60 gm	$57.74

OINTMENT: 0.05%

BRAND/MANUFACTURER	NDC	SIZE	AWP
○ **BRAND**			
MAXIFLOR: Allergan Herbert	00023-0770-15	15 gm	$17.53
FLORONE: Dermik	00066-0075-17	15 gm	$21.41
MAXIFLOR: Allergan Herbert	00023-0770-30	30 gm	$24.71
FLORONE: Dermik	00066-0075-31	30 gm	$30.56
MAXIFLOR: Allergan Herbert	00023-0770-60	60 gm	$40.11
FLORONE: Dermik	00066-0075-60	60 gm	$51.73

Diflucan *SEE* FLUCONAZOLE

Diflunisal

DESCRIPTION

Diflunisal is 2′, 4′-difluoro-4-hydroxy-3-biphenylcarboxylic acid. Its empirical formula is $C_{13}H_8F_2O_3$.

Diflunisal has a molecular weight of 250.20. It is a stable, white, crystalline compound with a melting point of 211-213°C. It is practically insoluble in water at neutral or acidic pH. Because it is an organic acid, it dissolves readily in dilute alkali to give a moderately stable solution at room temperature. It is soluble in most organic solvents including ethanol, methanol, and acetone.

Diflunisal is available in 250 and 500 mg tablets for oral administration.

Following is its chemical structure:

CLINICAL PHARMACOLOGY

ACTION

Diflunisal is a nonsteroidal drug with analgesic, anti-inflammatory and antipyretic properties. It is a peripherally-acting non-narcotic analgesic drug. Habituation, tolerance and addiction have not been reported.

Diflunisal is a difluorophenyl derivative of salicyclic acid. Chemically, Diflunisal differs from aspirin (acetylsalicylic acid) in two respects. The first of these two is the presence of a difluorophenyl substituent at carbon 1. The second difference is the removal of the 0-acetyl group from the carbon 4 position. Diflunisal is not metabolized to salicylic acid, and the fluorine atoms are not displaced from the difluorophenyl ring structure.

The precise mechanism of the analgesic and anti-inflammatory actions of Diflunisal is not known. Diflunisal is a prostaglandin synthetase inhibitor. In animals, prostaglandins sensitize afferent nerves and potentiate the action of bradykinin in inducing pain. Since prostaglandins are known to be among the mediators of pain and inflammation, the mode of action of Diflunisal may be due to a decrease of prostaglandins in peripheral tissues.

PHARMACOKINETICS AND METABOLISM

Diflunisal is rapidly and completely absorbed following oral administration with peak plasma concentrations occurring between 2 to 3 hours. The drug is excreted in the urine as two soluble glucuronide conjugates accounting for about 90% of the administered dose. Little or no Diflunisal is excreted in the feces. Diflunisal appears in human milk in concentrations of 2-7% of those in plasma. More than 99% of Diflunisal in plasma is bound to proteins.

As is the case with salicylic acid, concentration-dependent pharmacokinetics prevail when Diflunisal is administered; a doubling of dosage produces a greater than doubling of drug accumulation. The effect becomes more apparent with repetitive doses. Following single doses, peak plasma concentrations of 41 ± 11 µg/mL (mean ± S.D.) were observed following 250 mg doses, 87 ± 17 µg/mL were observed following 500 mg and 124 ± 11 µg/mL following single 1000 mg doses. However, following administration of 250 mg b.i.d., a mean peak level of 56 ± 14 µg/mL was observed on day 8, while the mean peak level after 500 mg b.i.d. for 11 days was 190 ± 33 µg/mL. In contrast to salicylic acid which has a plasma half-life of 2 1/2 hours, the plasma half-life of Diflunisal is 3 to 4 times longer (8 to 12 hours), because of a difluorophenyl substituent at carbon 1. Because of its long half-life and nonlinear pharmacokinetics, several days are required for Diflunisal plasma levels to reach steady state following multiple doses. For this reason, an initial loading dose is necessary to shorten the time to reach steady state levels, and 2 to 3 days of observation are necessary for evaluating changes in treatment regimens if a loading dose is not used.

Studies in baboons to determine passage across the blood-brain barrier have shown that only small quantities of Diflunisal under normal or acidotic conditions are transported into the cerebrospinal fluid (CSF). The ratio of blood/CSF concentrations after intravenous doses of 50 mg/kg or oral doses of 100 mg/kg of Diflunisal was 100:1. In contrast, oral doses of 500 mg/kg of aspirin resulted in a blood/CSF ratio of 5:1.

MILD TO MODERATE PAIN

Diflunisal is a peripherally-acting analgesic agent with a long duration of action. Diflunisal produces significant analgesia within 1 hour and maximum analgesia within 2 to 3 hours.

Consistent with its long half-life, clinical effects of Diflunisal mirror its pharmacokinetic behavior, which is the basis for recommending a loading dose when instituting therapy. Patients treated with Diflunisal, on the first dose, tend to have a slower onset of pain relief when compared with drugs achieving comparable peak effects. However, Diflunisal produces longer-lasting responses than the comparative agents.

Comparative single dose clinical studies have established the analgesic efficacy of Diflunisal at various dose levels relative to other analgesics. Analgesic effect measurements were derived from hourly evaluations by patients during eight and twelve-hour postdosing observation periods. The following information may serve as a guide for prescribing Diflunisal.

Diflunisal 500 mg was comparable in analgesic efficacy to aspirin 650 mg, acetaminophen 600 mg or 650 mg, and acetaminophen 650 mg with propoxyphene napsylate 100 mg. Patients treated with Diflunisal had longer lasting responses than the patients treated with the comparative analgesics.

Diflunisal 1000 mg was comparable in analgesic efficacy to acetaminophen 600 mg with codeine 60 mg. Patients treated with Diflunisal had longer lasting responses than the patients who received acetaminophen with codeine.

A loading dose of 1000 mg provides faster onset of pain relief, shorter time to peak analgesic effect, and greater peak analgesic effect than an initial 500 mg dose.

In contrast to the comparative analgesics, a significantly greater proportion of patients treated with Diflunisal did not remedicate and continued to have a good analgesic effect eight to twelve hours after dosing. Seventy-five percent (75%) of patients treated with Diflunisal continued to have a good analgesic response at four hours. When patients having a good analgesic response to four hours were followed, 78% of these patients continued to have a good analgesic response at eight hours and 64% at twelve hours.

CHRONIC ANTI-INFLAMMATORY THERAPY IN OSTEOARTHRITIS AND RHEUMATOID ARTHRITIS

In the controlled, double-blind clinical trials in which Diflunisal (500 mg to 1000 mg a day) was compared with anti-inflammatory doses of aspirin (2-4 grams a day), patients treated with Diflunisal had a significantly lower incidence of tinnitus and of adverse effects involving the gastrointestinal system than patients treated with aspirin. (See also "Effect on Fecal Blood Loss").

OSTEOARTHRITIS

The effectiveness of Diflunisal for the treatment of osteoarthritis was studied in patients with osteoarthritis of the hip and/or knee. The activity of Diflunisal was demonstrated by clinical improvement in the signs and symptoms of disease activity.

In a double-blind multicenter study of 12 weeks' duration in which dosages were adjusted according to patient response, Diflunisal, 500 or 750 mg daily, was shown to be comparable in effectiveness of aspirin, 2000 or 3000 mg daily. In open-lable extensions of this study to 24 or 48 weeks, Diflunisal continued to show similar effectiveness and generally was well tolerated.

RHEUMUTOID ARTHRITIS

In controlled clinical trials, the effectiveness of Diflunisal was established for both acute exacerbations and long-term management of rheumatoid arthritis. The activity of Diflunisal was demonstrated by clinical improvement in the signs and symptoms of disease activity.

In a double-blind multicenter study of 12 weeks' duration in which dosages were adjusted according to patient response, Diflunisal 500 or 750 mg daily was comparable in effectiveness to aspirin 2,600 or 3,900 mg daily. In open-label extensions of this study to 52 weeks, Diflunisal continued to be effective and was generally well tolerated.

Diflunisal 500, 750, or 1000 mg daily was compared with aspirin 2000, 3000, or 4000 mg daily in a multicenter study of 8 weeks' duration in which dosages were adjusted according to patient response. In this study, Diflunisal was comparable in efficacy to aspirin.

In a double-blind multicenter study of 12 weeks' duration in which dosages were adjusted according to patient needs, Diflunisal 500 or 750 mg daily and ibuprofen 1600 or 2400 mg daily were comparable in effectiveness and tolerability. In a double-blind multicenter study of 12 weeks' duration, Diflunisal 750 mg daily was comparable in efficacy to naproxen 750 mg daily. The incidence of gastrointestinal adverse effects and tinnitus was comparable for both drugs.

◆ RATED THERAPEUTICALLY EQUIVALENT; ◇ THERAPEUTIC EQUIVALENCE UNCONFIRMED; ○ UNRATED

This study was extended to 48 weeks on an open-label basis. Diflunisal continued to be effective and generally well tolerated.

In patients with rheumatoid arthritis, Diflunisal and gold salts may be used in combination at their usual dosage levels. In clinical studies, Diflunisal added to the regimen of gold salts usually resulted in additional symptomatic relief but did not alter the course of the underlying disease.

ANTIPYRETIC ACTIVITY
Diflunisal is not recommended for use as an antipyretic agent. In single 250 mg, 500 mg, or 750 mg doses, Diflunisal produced measurable but not clinically useful decreases in temperature in patients with fever; however, the possibility that it may mask fever in some patients, particularly with chronic or high doses, should be considered.

URICOSURIC EFFECT
In normal volunteers, an increase in the renal clearance of uric acid and a decrease in serum uric acid was observed when Diflunisal was administered at 500 mg or 750 mg daily in divided doses. Patients on long-term therapy taking Diflunisal at 500 mg to 1000 mg daily in divided doses showed a prompt and consistent reduction across studies in mean serum uric acid levels, which were lowered as much as 1.4 mg%. It is not known whether Diflunisal interferes with the activity of other uricosuric agents.

EFFECT ON PLATELET FUNCTION
As an inhibitor of prostaglandin synthetase, Diflunisal has a dose-related effect on platelet function and bleeding time. In normal volunteers, 250 mg b.i.d. for 8 days had no effect on platelet function, and 500 mg b.i.d., the usual recommended dose, had a slight effect. At 1000 mg b.i.d., which exceeds the maximum recommended dosage, however, Diflunisal inhibited platelet function. In contrast to aspirin, these effects of Diflunisal were reversible, because of the absence of the chemically labile and biologically reactive O-acetyl group at the carbon 4 position. Bleeding time was not altered by a dose of 250 mg b.i.d., and was only slightly increased at 500 mg b.i.d. At 1000 mg b.i.d., a greater increase occurred, but was not statistically significantly different from the change in the placebo group.

EFFECT ON FECAL BLOOD LOSS
When Diflunisal was given to normal volunteers at the usual recommended dose of 500 mg twice daily, fecal blood loss was not significantly different from placebo. Aspirin at 1000 mg four times daily produced the expected increase in fecal blood loss. Diflunisal at 1000 mg twice daily (*Note:* exceeds the recommended dosage) caused a statistically significant increase in fecal blood loss, but this increase was only one-half as large as that associated with aspirin 1300 mg twice daily.

EFFECT ON BLOOD GLUCOSE
Diflunisal did not affect fasting blood sugar in diabetic patients who were receiving tolbutamide or placebo.

INDICATIONS AND USAGE
Diflunisal is indicated for acute or long-term use for symptomatic treatment of the following:

1. Mild to moderate pain
2. Osteoarthritis
3. Rheumatoid arthritis

UNLABELED USES
Diflunisal is used alone or as an adjunct in the treatment of dysmenorrhea and gout.

CONTRAINDICATIONS
Patients who are hypersensitive to this product.

Patients in whom acute asthmatic attacks, urticaria, or rhinitis are precipitated by aspirin or other nonsteroidal anti-inflammatory drugs.

WARNINGS
Peptic ulceration and gastrointestinal bleeding have been reported in patients receiving Diflunisal. Fatalities have occurred rarely. Gastrointestinal bleeding is associated with higher morbidity and mortality in patients acutely ill with other conditions, the elderly and patients with hemorrhagic disorders. In patients with active gastrointestinal bleeding or an active peptie ulcer the physician must weigh the benefits of therapy with Diflunisal against possible hazards, institute an appropriate ulcer regimen and carefully monitor the patient's progress. When Diflunisal is given to patients with a history of either upper or lower gastrointestinal tract disease, it should be given only after consulting the *"Adverse Reactions"* section and under close supervision.

RISK OF GI ULCERATIONS BLEEDING AND PERFORATION WITH NSAID THERAPY
Serious gastrointestinal toxicity such as bleeding, ulceration, and perforation, can occur at any time, with or without warning symptoms, in patients treated chronically with NSAID therapy. Although minor upper gastrointestinal problems, such as dyspepsia, are common, usually developing early in therapy, physicians should remain alert for ulceration and bleeding in patients treated chronically with NSAIDs even in the absence of previous GI tract symptoms. In patients observed in clinical trials of several months to two years duration, symptomatic upper GI ulcers, gross bleeding or perforation appear to occur in approximately 1% of patients treated for 3-6 months, and in about 2-4% of patients treated for one year. Physicians should inform patients about the signs and/or symptoms of serious GI toxicity and what steps to take if they occur.

Studies to date have not identified any subset of patients not at risk of developing peptic ulceration and bleeding. Except for a prior history of serious GI events and other risk factors known to be associated with peptic ulcer disease, such as alcoholism, smoking, etc., no risk factors (e.g., age, sex) have been associated with increased risk. Elderly or debilitated patients seem to tolerate ulceration or bleeding less well than other individuals and most spontaneous reports of fatal GI events are in this population. Studies to date are inconclusive concerning the relative risk of various NSAIDs in causing such reactions. High doses of any NSAID probably carry a greater risk of these reactions, although controlled clinical trials showing this do not exist in most cases. In considering the use of relatively large doses (within the recommended dosage range), sufficient benefit should be anticipated to offset the potential increased risk of GI toxicity.

PRECAUTIONS
GENERAL
Nonsteroidal anti-inflammatory drugs, including Diflunisal, may mask the usual signs and symptoms of infection. Therefore, the physician must be continually on the alert for this and should use the drug with extra care in the presence of existing infection.

Although Diflunisal has less effect on platelet function and bleeding time than aspirin, at higher doses it is an inhibitor of platelet function; therefore, patients who may be adversely affected should be carefully observed when Diflunisal is administered (see *"Clinical Pharmacology"*).

Because of reports of adverse eye findings with agents of this class, it is recommended that patients who develop eye complaints during treatment with Diflunisal have ophthalmologic studies.

Peripheral edema has been observed in some patients taking Diflunisal. Therefore, as with other drugs in this class, Diflunisal should be used with caution in patients with compromised cardiac function, hypertension, or other conditions predisposing to fluid retention.

Acetylsalicylic acid has been associated with Reye syndrome. Because Diflunisal is a derivative of salicylic acid, the possibility of its association with Reye syndrome cannot be excluded.

HYPERSENSITIVITY SYNDROME
A potentially life-threatening, apparent hypersensitivity syndrome has been reported. This multisystem syndrome includes constitutional symptoms (fever, chills), and cutaneous findings (see *"Adverse Reactions, Dermatologic"*). It may also include involvement of major organs (changes in liver function, jaundice, leukopenia, thrombocytopenia, eosinophilia, disseminated intravascular coagulation, renal impairment, including renal failure), and less specific findings (adenitis, arthralgia, myalgia, arthritis, malaise, anorexia, disorientation). If evidence of hypersensitivity occurs, therapy with Diflunisal should be discontinued.

RENAL EFFECTS
As with other nonsteroidal anti-inflammatory drugs, long term administration of Diflunisal to animals has resulted in renal papillary necrosis and other abnormal renal pathology. In humans, there have been reports of renal interstitial nephritis with hematuria and proteinuria and occasionally nephrotic syndrome.

A second form of renal toxicity has been seen in patients with prerenal and renal conditions leading to a reduction in renal blood flow or blood volume, where the renal prostaglandins have a supportive role in the maintenance of renal perfusion. In these patients administration of an NSAID may cause a dose dependent reduction in prostaglandin formation and may precipitate overt renal decompensation. Patients at greatest risk of this reaction are those with conditions such as renal or hepatic dysfunction, diabetes mellitus, advanced age, extracellular volume depletion from any cause, congestive heart failure, septicemia, pyelonephritis, or concomitant use of any nephrotoxic drug. Diflunisal or other NSAIDs should be given with caution and renal function should be monitored in any patient who may have reduced renal reserve. Discontinuation of NSAID therapy is typically followed by recovery to the pretreatment state.

Since Diflunisal is eliminated primarily by the kidneys, patients with significantly impaired renal function should be closely monitored; a lower daily dosage should be anticipated to avoid excessive drug accumulation.

INFORMATION FOR PATIENTS
Diflunisal, like other drugs of its class, is not free of side effects. The side effects of these drugs can cause discomfort and, rarely, there are more serious side effects such as gastrointestinal bleeding, which may result in hospitalization and even fatal outcomes.

NSAIDs (Nonsteroidal Anti-inflammatory Drugs) are often essential agents in the management of arthritis and have a major role in the treatment of pain, but they also may be commonly employed for conditions which are less serious. Physicians may wish to discuss with their patients the potential risks (see *"Warnings," "Precautions"* and *"Adverse Reactions"*) and likely benefits of NSAID treatment, particularly when the drugs are used for less serious conditions where treatment without NSAIDs may represent an acceptable alternative to both the patient and physician.

LABORATORY TESTS
Liver Function Tests: As with other non-steroidal anti-inflammatory drugs, borderline elevations of one or more liver tests may occur in up to 15% of patients. These abnormalities may progress, may remain essentially unchanged, or may be transient with continued therapy. The SGPT (ALT) test is probably the most sensitive indicator of liver dysfunction. Meaningful (3 times the upper limit of normal) elevations of SGPT or SGOT (AST) occurred in controlled clinical

trials in less than 1% of patients. A patient with symptoms and/or signs suggesting liver dysfunction, or in whom an abnormal liver test has occurred, should be evaluated for evidence of the development of more severe hepatic reactions while on therapy with Diflunisal, Severe hepatic reactions, including jaundice, have been reported with Diflunisal as well as with other non-steroidal anti-inflammatory drugs. Although such reactions are rare, if abnormal liver tests persist or worsen, if clinical signs and symptoms consistent with liver disease develop, or if systemic manifestations occur (e.g., eosinophilia, rash, etc.), Diflunisal should be discontinued, since liver reactions can be fatal.

Gastrointestinal: Because serious GI tract ulceration and bleeding can occur without warning symptoms, physicians should follow chronically treated patients for the signs and symptoms of ulceration and bleeding and should inform them of the importance of this follow-up (see *"Warnings, Risk of GI Ulcerations, Bleeding and Perforation with NSAID Therapy"*).

DRUG INTERACTIONS

Oral Anticoagulants: In some normal volunteers, the concomitant administration of Diflunisal and warfarin, acenocoumarol, or phenprocoumon resulted in prolongation of prothrombin time. This may occur because Diflunisal competitively displaces coumarins from protein binding sites. Accordingly, when Diflunisal is administered with oral anticoagulants, the prothrombin time should be closely monitored during and for several days after concomitant drug administration. Adjustment of dosage of oral anticoagulants may be required.

Tolbutamide: In diabetic patients receiving Diflunisal and tolbutamide, no significant effects were seen on tolbutamide plasma levels or fasting blood glucose.

Hydrochlorothiazide: In normal volunteers, concomitant administration of Diflunisal and hydrochlorothiazide resulted in significantly increased plasma levels of hydrochlorothiazide. Diflunisal decreased the hyperuricemic effect of hydrochlorothiazide.

Furosemide: In normal volunteers, the concomitant administration of Diflunisal and furosemide had no effect on the diuretic activity of furosemide. Diflunisal decreased the hyperuricemic effect of furosemide.

Antacids: Concomitant administration of antacids may reduce plasma levels of Diflunisal. This effect is small with occasional doses of antacids, but may be clinically significant when antacids are used on a continuous schedule.

Acetaminophen: In normal volunteers, concomitant administration of Diflunisal and acetaminophen resulted in an approximate 50% increase in plasma levels of acetaminophen. Acetaminophen had no effect on plasma levels of Diflunisal. Since acetaminophen in high doses has been associated with hepatotoxicity, concomitant administration of Diflunisal and acetaminophen should be used cautiously, with careful monitoring of patients.

Concomitant administration of Diflunisal and acetaminophen in dogs, but not in rats, at approximately 2 times the recommended maximum human therapeutic dose of each (40-52 mg/kg/day of Diflunisal acetaminophen), resulted in greater gastrointestinal toxicity than when either drug was administered alone. The clinical significance of these findings has not been established.

Methotrexate: Caution should be used if Diflunisal is administered concomitantly with methotrexate. Nonsteroidal anti-inflammatory drugs have been reported to decrease the tubular secretion of methotrexate and to potentiate its toxicity.

Cyclosporine: Administration of nonsteroidal anti-inflammatory drugs concomitantly with cyclosporine has been associated with an increase in cyclosporine-induced toxicity, possibly due to decreased synthesis of renal prostacyclin. NSAIDs should be used with caution in patients taking cyclosporine, and renal function should be carefully monitored.

Drug Interactions: Nonsteroidal Anti-inflammatory Drugs: The administration of Diflunisal to normal volunteers receiving indomethacin decreased the renal clearance and significantly increased the plasma levels of indomethacin. In some patients the combined use of indomethacin and Diflunisal has been associated with fatal gastrointestinal hemorrhage. Therefore, indomethacin and Diflunisal should not be used concomitantly.

Since no further clinical data are available about the safety and effectiveness of Diflunisal when used in combination with other non-steroidal anti-inflammatory drugs, no recommendation for their concomitant use can be made. The following information was obtained from studies in normal volunteers.

Aspirin: In normal volunteers, a small decrease in Diflunisal levels was observed when multiple doses of Diflunisal and aspirin were administered concomitantly.

Sulindac: The concomitant administration of Diflunisal and sulindac in normal volunteers resulted in lowering of the plasma levels of the active sulindac sulfide metabolite by approximately one-third.

Naproxen: The concomitant administration of Diflunisal and naproxen in normal volunteers had no effect on the plasma levels of naproxen, but significantly decreased the urinary excretion of naproxen and its glucuronide metabolite. Naproxen had no effect on plasma levels of Diflunisal.

DRUG/LABORATORY TEST INTERACTIONS

Serum Salicylate Assays: Caution should be used in interpreting the results of serum salicylate assays when Diflunisal is present. Salicylate levels have been found to be falsely elevated with some assay methods.

CARCINOGENESIS, MUTAGENESIS, IMPAIRMENT OF FERTILITY

Diflunisal did not affect the type or incidence of neoplasia in a 105-week study in the rat given doses up to 40 mg/kg/day (equivalent to approximately 1.3 times the maximum recommended human dose), or in long-term carcinogenic studies in mice given Diflunisal at doses up to 80 mg/kg/day (equivalent to approximately 2.7 times the maximum recommended human dose). It was concluded that there was no carcinogenic potential for Diflunisal.

Diflunisal passes the placental barrier to a minor degree in the rat. Diflunisal had no mutagenic activity after oral administration in the dominant lethal assay, in the Ames microbial mutagen test or in the V-79 Chinese hamster lung cell assay.

No evidence of impaired fertility was found in reproduction studies in rats at doses up to 50 mg/kg/day.

PREGNANCY

Pregnancy Category C: A dose of 60 mg/kg/day of Diflunisal (equivalent to two times the maximum human dose) was maternotoxic, embryotoxic, and teratogenic in rabbits. In three of six studies in rabbits, evidence of teratogenicity was observed at doses ranging from 40 to 50 mg/kg/day. Teratology studies in mice, at doses up to 45 mg/kg/day, and in rats at doses up to 100 mg/kg/day, revealed no harm to the fetus due to Diflunisal. Aspirin and other salicylates have been shown to be teratogenic in a wide variety of species, including the rat and rabbit, at doses ranging from 50 to 400 mg/kg/day (approximately one to eight times the human dose). There are no adequate and well controlled studies with Diflunisal in pregnant women. Diflunisal should be used during the first two trimesters of pregnancy only if the potential benefit justifies the potential risk to the fetus. Because of the known effect of drugs of this class on the human fetus (closure of the ductus arteriosus, platelet dysfunction with resultant bleeding, renal dysfunction or failure with oligohydramnios, gastrointestinal bleeding or perforation, and myocardial degenerative changes), use during the third trimester of pregnancy is not recommended.

In rats at a dose of one and one-half times the maximum human dose, there was an increase in the average length of gestation. Similar increases in the length of gestation have been observed with aspirin, indomethacin, and phenylbutazone, and may be related to inhibition of prostaglandin synthetase. Drugs of this class may cause dystocia and delayed parturition in pregnant animals.

NURSING MOTHERS

Diflunisal is excreted in human milk in concentrations of 2-7% of those in plasma. Because of the potential for serious adverse reactions in nursing infants from Diflunisal, a decision should be made whether to discontinue nursing or to discontinue the drug, taking into account the importance of the drug to the mother.

PEDIATRIC USE

The adverse effects observed following Diflunisal administration to neonatal animals appear to be species, age, and dose-dependent. At dose levels approximately 3 times the usual human therapeutic dose, both aspirin (200 to 400 mg/kg/day) and Diflunisal (80 mg/kg/day) resulted in death, leukocytosis, weight loss, and bilateral cataracts in neonatal (4 to 5-day-old) beagle puppies after 2 to 10 doses. Administration of an 80 mg/kg/day dose of Diflunisal to 25-day-old puppies resulted in lower mortality, and did not produce cataracts. In newborn rats, a 400 mg/kg/day dose of aspirin resulted in increased mortality and some cataracts, whereas the effects of Diflunisal administration at doses up to 140 mg/kg/day were limited to a decrease in average body weight gain.

Safety and effectiveness in infants and children have not been established, and use of the drug in children below the age of 12 years is not recommended.

ADVERSE REACTIONS

The adverse reactions observed in controlled clinical trials encompass observations in 2,427 patients.

Listed below are the adverse reactions reported in the 1,314 of these patients who received treatment in studies of two weeks or longer. Five hundred thirteen patients were treated for at least 24 weeks, 255 patients were treated for at least 48 weeks, and 46 patients were treated for 96 weeks. In general, the adverse reactions listed below were 2 to 14 times less frequent in the 1,113 patients who received short-term treatment for mild to moderate pain.

INCIDENCE GREATER THAN 1%

Gastrointestinal

The most frequent types of adverse reactions occurring with Diflunisal are gastrointestinal: these include nausea,* vomiting, dyspepsia*, gastrointestinal pain*, diarrhea*, constipation, and flatulence.

Psychiatric

Somnolence, insomnia.

Central Nervous System

Dizziness.

Special Senses

Tinnitus.

Dermatologic

Rash*

Miscellaneous

Headache*, fatigue/tiredness.

* Incidence between 3% and 9%. Those reactions occurring in 1% to 3% are not marked with an asterisk.

◆ RATED THERAPEUTICALLY EQUIVALENT; ◇ THERAPEUTIC EQUIVALENCE UNCONFIRMED; ○ UNRATED

INCIDENCE LESS THAN 1 IN 100

The following adverse reactions, occurring less frequently than 1 in 100, were reported in clinical trials or since the drug was marketed. The probability exists of a causal relationship between Diflunisal and these adverse reactions.

Dermatologic

Erythema multiforme, exfoliative dermatitis, Stevens-Johnson syndrome, toxic epidermal necrolysis, urticaria, pruritus, sweating, dry mucous membranes, stomatitis, photosensitivity.

Gastrointestinal

Peptic ulcer, gastrointestinal bleeding, anorexia, eructation, gastrointestinal perforation, gastritis.

Liver function abnormalities; jaundice, sometimes with fever; cholestasis; hepatitis.

Hematologic

Thrombocytopenia; agranulocytosis; hemolytic anemia.

Genitourinary

Dysuria; renal impairment, including renal failure; interstitial nephritis; hematuria; proteinuria.

Psychiatric

Nervousness, depression, hallucinations, confusion, disorientation.

Central Nervous System

Vertigo; light-headedness; paresthesias.

Special Senses

Transient visual disturbances including blurred vision.

Hypersensitivity Reactions

Acute anaphylactic reaction with bronchospasm; angioedema; flushing.

Hypersensitivity vasculitis.

Hypersensitivity syndrome (see *"Precautions"*).

Miscellaneous

Asthenia, edema.

CAUSAL RELATIONSHIP UNKNOWN

Other reactions have been reported in clinical trials or since the drug was marketed, but occurred under circumstances where a causal relationship could not be established. However, in these rarely reported events, that possibility cannot be excluded. Therefore, these observations are listed to serve as alerting information to physicians.

Respiratory

Dyspnea.

Cardiovascular

Palpitation, syncope.

Musculoskeletal

Muscle cramps.

Genitourinary

Nephrotic syndrome.

Miscellaneous

Chest pain.

A rare occurrence of fulminant necrotizing fasciitis, particularly in association with Group A β-hemolytic streptococcus, has been described in persons treated with non-steroidal anti-inflammatory agents, including Diflunisal, sometimes with fatal outcome (see also *"Precautions, General"*).

POTENTIAL ADVERSE EFFECTS

In addition, a variety of adverse effects not observed with Diflunisal in clinical trials or in marketing experience, but reported with other non-steroidal analgesic/anti-inflammatory agents should be considered potential adverse effects of Diflunisal.

OVERDOSAGE

Cases of overdosage have occurred and deaths have been reported. Most patients recovered without evidence of permanent sequelae. The most common signs and symptoms observed with overdosage were drowsiness, vomiting, nausea, diarrhea, hyperventilation, tachycardia, sweating, tinnitus, disorientation, stupor and coma. Diminished urine output and cardiorespiratory arrest have also been reported. The lowest dosage of Diflunisal at which a death has been reported was 15 grams without the presence of other drugs. In a mixed drug overdose, ingestion of 7.5 grams of Diflunisal resulted in death.

In the event of overdosage, the stomach should be emptied by inducing vomiting or by gastric lavage, and the patient carefully observed and given symptomatic and supportive treatment. Because of the high degree of protein binding, hemodialysis may not be effective.

The oral LD$_{50}$ of the drug is 500 mg/kg and 826 mg/kg in female mice and female rats respectively.

DOSAGE AND ADMINISTRATION

Concentration-dependent pharmacokinetics prevail when Diflunisal is administered; a doubling of dosage produces a greater than doubling of drug accumulation. The effect becomes more apparent with repetitive doses.

For mild to moderate pain, an initial dose of 1000 mg followed by 500 mg every 12 hours is recommended for most patients. Following the initial dose, some patients may require 500 mg every 8 hours.

A lower dosage may be appropriate depending on such factors as pain severity, patient response, weight, or advanced age; for example, 500 mg initially, followed by 250 mg every 8-12 hours.

For osteoarthritis and rheumatoid arthritis, the suggested dosage range is 500 mg to 1000 mg daily in two divided doses. The dosage of Diflunisal may be increased or decreased according to patient response.

Maintenance doses higher than 1500 mg a day are not recommended.

Diflunisal may be administered with water, milk or meals. Tablets should be swallowed whole, not crushed or chewed.

HOW SUPPLIED

TABLETS: 250 MG

AVERAGE UNIT PRICE (AVAILABLE SIZES)		GENERIC A-RATED AVERAGE PRICE (GAAP)	
BRAND	$0.94	60s	$47.26
GENERIC	$0.83	100s	$92.95

BRAND/MANUFACTURER	NDC	SIZE	AWP
◆ **BRAND**			
DOLOBID: Merck	00006-0675-61	60s	$55.30
	00006-0675-28	100s ud	$96.69
◆ **GENERICS**			
West Point	59591-0195-61	60s	$46.66
Roxane	00054-4210-21	60s	$47.85
Roxane	00054-8210-25	100s ud	$87.25
Major	00904-7763-61	100s ud	$98.65
West Point	59591-0195-74	500s	$349.94

TABLETS: 500 MG

AVERAGE UNIT PRICE (AVAILABLE SIZES)		GENERIC A-RATED AVERAGE PRICE (GAAP)	
BRAND	$1.17	60s	$57.75
GENERIC	$0.97	100s	$102.64
		500s	$430.48

BRAND/MANUFACTURER	NDC	SIZE	AWP
◆ **BRAND**			
DOLOBID: Merck	00006-0697-61	60s	$69.14
	00006-0697-28	100s ud	$119.65
◆ **GENERICS**			
Medirex	57480-0479-06	30s	$25.20
Schein	00364-2537-06	60s	$46.65
Lemmon	00093-0755-06	60s	$58.25
Aligen	00405-4330-31	60s	$58.25
Moore,H.L.	00839-7764-05	60s	$58.25
Goldline	00182-1954-26	60s	$58.30
West Point	59591-0196-61	60s	$58.33
Major	00904-7808-52	60s	$58.35
Roxane	00054-4220-21	60s	$59.90
Du Pont Multi	00056-0196-60	60s	$60.25
Rugby	00536-5563-08	60s	$60.92
URL	00677-1460-06	100s	$58.33
Lemmon	00093-0755-01	100s	$90.29
Roxane	00054-8220-25	100s ud	$104.28
UDL	51079-0754-20	100s ud	$104.50
Goldline	00182-1954-89	100s ud	$116.25
Major	00904-7764-61	100s ud	$119.85
Medirex	57480-0479-01	100s ud	$125.00
Lemmon	00093-0755-05	500s	$423.48
West Point	59591-0196-74	500s	$437.47

Digestive Enzymes/Hyoscyamine Sulfate/Phenyltloxamine Citrate

DESCRIPTION

Each capsule contains four standardized digestive enzymes: lipase, amylase, protease, cellulase, and Hyoscyamine Sulfate USP and Phenyltloxamine Citrate. Lipase, amylase, protease and cellulase are derived from fungal, plant and animal sources and are oral digestive enzyme supplements. Hyoscyamine Sulfate USP is one of the principal anticholinergic/antispasmodic components of belladonna alkaloids. Phenyltloxamine Citrate is a non-barbiturate sedative.

Each capsule contains:

lipase	.75 mg
amylase	.30 mg
protease	.6 mg
cellulase	.2 mg
Hyoscyamine Sulfate USP	0.0625 mg
Phenyltloxamine Citrate	.15 mg

CLINICAL PHARMACOLOGY

Diminution of secretions from exocrine glands is often a result of the normal aging process. This product provides a balanced combination of natural proteolytic, amylolytic cellulolytic and lipolytic enzymes to enhance digestion of proteins, starch and fat in the gastrointestinal tract. These enzymes do not exert any systemic pharmacologic effects. This product should be considered an enzyme supplement and not an enzyme replacement therapy. Enzymes in this product are basically derived from fungal and plant sources and possess a broad spectrum of pH activity. Enzymes are promptly released from the capsule and are bioavailable for digestion of food in the stomach and intestines. Hyoscyamine Sulfate provides a potent spasmolytic effect in reducing gastrointestinal hypermotility and intestinal spasm. A mild sedative effect is provided by Phenyltoloxamine Citrate.

INDICATIONS AND USAGE
This product is indicated for the relief of the symptoms of functional indigestion devoid of organic pathology commonly referred to as nervous indigestion and colloquially as "butterflies". The symptoms are bloating, gas, and fullness.

CONTRAINDICATIONS
Glaucoma, obstructive uropathy, obstructive disease of the gastrointestinal tract (as in achalasia, pyloroduodenal stenosis); paralytic ileus, intestinal atony of the elderly or debilitated patients; unstable cardiovascular status in acute hemorrhage; severe ulcerative colitis; toxic megacolon complicating ulcerative colitis; myasthenia gravis, or a hypersensitivity to any of the ingredients.

WARNINGS
Do not administer to patients who are allergic to pork products. In the presence of high environmental temperature, heat prostration can occur with drug use (fever and heat stroke due to decreased sweating). Diarrhea may be an early symptom of incomplete intestinal obstruction, especially in patients with ileostomy or colostomy. In this instance, treatment with this drug would be inappropriate This product may produce drowsiness or blurred vision. In this event, the patient should be warned not to engage in activities requiring mental alertness such as operating a motor vehicle or other machinery or to perform hazardous work while taking this drug.

PRECAUTIONS
GENERAL
Use with caution in patients with autonomic neuropathy, hyperthyroidism, coronary heart disease, congestive heart failure, cardiac arrhythmias, and hypertension. Investigate any tachycardia before giving any anticholinergic drug since they may increase the heart rate. Use with caution in patients with hiatal hernia associated with reflux esophagitis.

INFORMATION FOR PATIENTS
If capsules are opened, avoid inhalation of the powder. Sensitive individuals may experience allergic reactions.

CARCINOGENESIS, MUTAGENESIS, IMPAIRMENT OF FERTILITY
Long-term studies in animals have not been performed to evaluate the carcinogenic, mutagenic or impairment of fertility potential of this product.

PREGNANCY
Pregnancy Category C. Animal reproduction studies have not been conducted. It is also not known whether this product can cause fetal harm when administered to a pregnant woman or can affect reproduction capacity. It should be given to a pregnant woman only if clearly needed.

NURSING MOTHERS
Hyoscyamine Sulfate is excreted in human milk. It is not known whether the Enzymes or Phenyltoloxamine Citrate are excreted in human milk. Caution should be exercised when Enzymes/Hyoscyamine/Phenyltoloxamine is administered to a nursing woman.

ADVERSE REACTIONS
Occasionally a slight looseness of the stools may be noticed. If so, dosage should be reduced. Finely powdered pancreatic enzyme may be irritating to the mucous membranes and respiratory tract. Inhalation of the airborne powder may precipitate an asthma attack in sensitive individuals. Other adverse reactions may include dryness of the mouth; urinary hesitancy and retention; blurred vision; tachycardia; palpitations; mydriasis; cycloplegia; increased ocular tension; headache; nervousness; drowsiness; weakness; suppression of lactation; allergic reactions or drug idiosyncrasies; urticaria and other dermal manifestations and decreased sweating.

OVERDOSAGE
The signs and symptoms of overdose are headache, nausea, vomiting, blurred vision, dilated pupils, hot skin, dizziness, dryness of the mouth, difficulty in swallowing. Measures to be taken are immediate lavage of the stomach and injection of physostigmine 0.5 to 2 mg intravenously and repeated as necessary up to a total of 5 mg. Fever may be treated symptomatically. Excitement to a degree which demands attention may be managed with sodium thiopental 2% solution given slowly intravenously. In the event of paralysis of the respiratory muscles, artificial respiration should be instituted.

DOSAGE AND ADMINISTRATION
1 or 2 capsules taken with each meal or snack. Dosage may be adjusted according to the conditions and severity of symptoms to assure symptomatic control with a minimum of adverse effects.

Store at controlled room temperature 15°-30°C (59°-86°F).

HOW SUPPLIED
CAPSULE:

BRAND/MANUFACTURER	NDC	SIZE	AWP
○ BRAND			
KUTRASE: Schwarz	00091-3475-01	100s	$44.60

Digibind *SEE* DIGOXIN IMMUNE FAB (OVINE)

Digitoxin

DESCRIPTION
Digitoxin is a crystalline-pure single cardiac glycoside obtained from *Digitalis purpurea* and is identical in pharmacologic action with whole-leaf digitalis.

Digitoxin is the most slowly excreted of all digitalis compounds (excretion time is 14 to 21 days). It is most useful in patients with impaired renal function, since excretion and metabolism are independent of renal function.

Digitoxin is noted for its uniform potency, complete absorption, and lack of gastrointestinal irritation. It permits accurate dosage adjustments to produce maximum therapeutic effect smoothly and dependably.

Digitoxin for oral administration, is available in tablets containing 0.05 mg (0.07 μmol) or 0.1 mg (0.13 μmol) crystalline Digitoxin.

Digitoxin is a cardiotonic glycoside. The chemical name is card-20 (22)-enolide,3-[(O-2,6-dideoxy-β-D-ribo-hexopyranosyl-(1 → 4)-O-2,6 - dideoxy-β- D-ribo-hexopyranosyl (1 → 4)- 2,6-dideoxy- β-D- ribo- hexopyranosyl) oxy]-14-hydroxy, (3β,5β)-. The empirical formula of Digitoxin is $C_{41}H_{64}O_{13}$.

Following is its chemical structure:

CLINICAL PHARMACOLOGY
The cellular basis for the inotropic effects of digitalis is probably enhancement of excitation-contraction coupling, that process by which chemical energy is converted into mechanical energy when triggered by membrane depolarization. Most evidence relates this process to the entry of calcium ions into the cell during depolarization of the membrane and/or to the release of calcium from intracellular binding sites on the sarcoplasmic reticulum. The free calcium ion mediates the interaction of actin and myosin, resulting in contraction.

The amount of glycoside absorbed depends largely on its polarity, which is a function of the net electronic charge on the molecule. The more nonpolar or lipid soluble, the better is the absorption, because of the greater permeability of lipid membrane of the intestinal mucosa for lipid-soluble substances. The nonpolar, lipophilic Digitoxin is completely absorbed. Other glycosides are not as well absorbed.

Nonpolar Digitoxin is over 90% bound to tissue proteins. The firm binding of Digitoxin to protein is responsible for its long half-life (7 to 9 days).

Digitoxin differs from other commonly used glycosides not only in its firm binding to protein but also because it is metabolized in the liver, with the only active metabolite being digoxin, which represents only a small fraction of the total metabolites. All other metabolites are inert and are probably excreted as such in the urine. The portion of Digitoxin that is not metabolized is excreted in the bile to the intestines and recycled to the liver until it is completely metabolized. The portion of Digitoxin that is bound to protein is in equilibrium with free Digitoxin in the serum. Thus, as more and more of the free Digitoxin is metabolized after a single dose, there is proportionately less bound Digitoxin.

INDICATIONS AND USAGE
Digitoxin is indicated in the treatment of heart failure, atrial flutter, atrial fibrillation, and supraventricular tachycardia.

CONTRAINDICATIONS
If the indications are carefully observed, there are few contraindications to digitalis therapy except toxic response or idiosyncrasy to digitalis, ventricular tachycardia, beriberi, heart disease, and some instances of the hypersensitive carotid sinus syndrome.

Patients already taking Digitalis preparations must not be given the rapid digitalizing dose of Digitoxin or parenteral calcium.

◆ RATED THERAPEUTICALLY EQUIVALENT; ◇ THERAPEUTIC EQUIVALENCE UNCONFIRMED; ○ UNRATED

WARNINGS

Many of the arrhythmias for which digitalis is advised are identical with those reflecting digitalis intoxication. When the possibility of digitalis intoxication cannot be excluded, cardiac glycosides should be withheld temporarily if the clinical situation permits.

The patient with congestive heart failure may complain of nausea and vomiting. Since these symptoms may also be associated with digitalis intoxication, a clinical determination of their cause must be attempted before further administration of the drug.

Cases of idiopathic hypertrophic subaortic stenosis must be managed with extreme care. Unless cardiac failure is severe, it is doubtful whether digitalis should be employed.

Note: Digitalis glycosides are an important cause of accidental poisoning in children.

PRECAUTIONS

General: When the risk of digitalis intoxication is great, the use of a short-acting, rapidly eliminated glycoside, such as digoxin, is advisable. Although intoxication cannot always be prevented by the selection of one glycoside over another, certain glycosides may be preferred in patients who have fixed disabilities (eg, liver impairment, drug intolerance). However, Digitoxin can be used in patients with impaired renal function.

Special care must be exercised in elderly patients receiving digitalis, because their body mass tends to be small and renal clearance is likely to be reduced. Frequent electrocardiographic monitoring is important in these patients. In addition, digitalis must be used cautiously in the presence of active heart disease, such as acute myocardial infarction or acute myocarditis. In patients with acute or unstable chronic atrial fibrillation, digitalis may not normalize the ventricular rate even when the serum concentration exceeds the usual therapeutic level. Although these patients may be less sensitive to the toxic effects of digitalis than are patients with normal sinus rhythm, dosage should not be increased to potentially toxic levels.

Hypokalemia predisposes to digitalis toxicity, and even a moderate decrease in the concentration of serum potassium can precipitate serious arrhythmias.

Impaired liver function may necessitate reduction in dosage of any digitalis preparation, including Digitoxin.

Sensitive radioimmunoassay techniques have been developed for measuring serum levels of Digitoxin, and these procedures can be instituted in almost any hospital. Serum levels must, however, be evaluated in conjunction with clinical history and the results of the electrocardiogram and other laboratory tests. A therapeutic serum level for one patient may be excessive or inadequate for another patient.

Drug Interactions: The synthesis of microsomal enzymes that metabolize Digitoxin in the liver is subject to stimulation by a number of drugs, such as antihistamines, anti-convulsants, barbiturates, oral hypoglycemic agents, and others.

When Digitoxin is the glycoside used for digitalis maintenance, drugs that are liver-microsomal-enzyme inducers should not be used at the same time. Phenobarbital, phenylbutazone, and diphenylhydantoin will increase the rate of metabolism of Digitoxin. In patients receiving 60 mg of phenobarbital 3 times a day for 12 weeks, the steady-state concentration of Digitoxin in plasma fell approximately 50% when the drugs were administered concurrently and returned to previous levels when phenobarbital was discontinued.

When drugs that increase the rate of metabolism of Digitoxin in the liver are discontinued, toxicity may occur.

Hypokalemia is most frequently encountered in patients receiving concomitant diuretic therapy, because the most widely used and most effective diuretics (ie, thiazides and furosemide) increase the urinary loss of potassium. Prescribing a potassium-sparing agent (spironolactone or triamterene) together with the potassium-wasting diuretic is a reliable means for maintaining the serum potassium level. Alternatively, potassium chloride supplements may be prescribed.

Mineralocorticoids (eg, prednisone) and, rarely, certain antibiotics (eg, amphotericin B) may also cause increased excretion of potassium.

Usage in Pregnancy: Pregnancy Category C: Animal reproduction studies have not been conducted with Digitoxin. It is also not known whether this drug can cause fetal harm when administered to a pregnant woman or can affect reproduction capacity. Digitoxin should be given to a pregnant woman only if clearly needed.

Labor and Delivery: No information is available concerning the use of Digitoxin in labor and delivery.

Nursing Mothers: It is not known whether this drug is excreted in human breast milk. Because many drugs are excreted in human breast milk, caution should be exercised when Digitoxin is administered to a nursing woman.

ADVERSE REACTIONS

Anorexia, nausea, and vomiting have been reported. These effects are central in origin, but following large oral doses, there is also a local emetic action. Abdominal discomfort or pain and diarrhea may also occur.

OVERDOSAGE

Signs and Symptoms: Symptoms may include alterations in mental status, nausea, vomiting, bradycardia, visual disturbances, heart block, and all known cardiac arrhythmias. Hyperkalemia may be present following acute overdose, whereas hypokalemia is associated with chronic overdose. Peak toxic effects following acute overdose may be delayed up to 12 hours.

Older patients, particularly those with coronary insufficiency, are more susceptible to dysrhythmias. Ventricular fibrillation is the most common cause of death from digitalis poisoning. There is insufficient information to accurately determine the minimum toxic or lethal dose in humans. Death from ventricular fibrillation was reported 24 hours after admission in a patient with a plasma concentration of 124 ng/mL shortly before death.

Treatment: To obtain up-to-date information about the treatment of overdose, a good resource is your certified Regional Poison Control Center. Telephone numbers of certified poison control centers are listed in the *Physicians' Desk Reference (PDR)*. In managing overdosage, consider the possibility of multiple drug overdoses, interaction among drugs, and unusual drug kinetics in your patient.

Continuous ECG monitoring is necessary. For any suspected Digitoxin-induced dysrhythmia, discontinue the drug. Monitor potassium and Digitoxin concentrations. Severe hyperkalemia may require administration of sodium bicarbonate, glucose, and regular insulin.

Protect the patient's airway and support ventilation and perfusion. Meticulously monitor and maintain, within acceptable limits, the patient's vital signs, blood gases, serum electrolytes, etc. Absorption of drugs from the gastrointestinal tract may be decreased by giving activated charcoal, which, in many cases, is more effective than emesis or lavage; consider charcoal instead of or in addition to gastric emptying. Repeated doses of charcoal over time may hasten elimination of some drugs that have been absorbed. Safeguard the patient's airway when employing gastric emptying or charcoal.

Atropine or a pacemaker may be used for bradycardia and heart block. Phenytoin (15 mg/kg), at a rate not to exceed 50 mg/min, may be useful for treating ventricular dysrhythmias and to improve atrioventricular conduction. Lidocaine may also be used, but impaired AV conduction may require a pacemaker. Consider use of digitalis-specific Fab fragments.

Forced diuresis, peritoneal dialysis, hemodialysis, or charcoal hemoperfusion have not been established as beneficial for an overdose of Digitoxin.

Protect from light. Store at controlled room temperature, 59° to 86°F (15° to 30°C).

DOSAGE AND ADMINISTRATION

ADULTS:

Slow Digitalization: 0.2 mg twice daily for a period of 4 days, followed by maintenance dosage.

Rapid Digitalization: Preferably 0.6 mg initially, followed by 0.4 mg and then 0.2 mg at intervals of 4 to 6 hours.

Maintenance Dosage: Ranges from 0.05 to 0.3 mg daily, the most common dose being 0.15 mg daily.

HOW SUPPLIED

J CODES

J1155

HOW SUPPLIED

TABLETS: 0.1 MG

BRAND/MANUFACTURER	NDC	SIZE	AWP
○ **BRAND**			
CRYSTODIGIN: Lilly	00002-1060-02	100s	$5.14

Digoxin

DESCRIPTION

Digoxin is one of the cardiac (or digitalis) glycosides, a closely related group of drugs having in common specific effects on the myocardium. These drugs are found in a number of plants. Digoxin is extracted from the leaves of *Digitalis lanata*. The term "digitalis" is used to designate the whole group. The glycosides are composed of two portions: a sugar and a cardenolide (hence "glycosides").

Digoxin has the molecular formula $C_{41}H_{64}O_{14}$, a molecular weight of 780.95 and melting and decomposition points above 235°C. The drug is practically insoluble in water and in ether; slightly soluble in diluted (50%) alcohol and in chloroform; and freely soluble in pyridine. Digoxin powder is composed of odorless white crystals.

Digoxin has the chemical name: 3β-[(*O*-2,6-dideoxy-β-*D-ribo*-hexopyranosyl-(1→4)-*O*-2, 6-dideoxy-β-*D-ribo*-hexopyranosyl-(1→4)-2,6-dideoxy-β-*D-ribo*-hexopyranosyl) oxy]-12β, 14-dihydroxy-5β-card-20(22)-enolide.

Digoxin Tablets with 125 μg (0.125 mg), 250 μg (0.25 mg) or 500 μg (0.5 mg) Digoxin USP are intended for oral use.

Digoxin Solution in Capsules is a stable solution of Digoxin enclosed within a soft gelatin capsule for oral use available in 50 mcg, 100 mcg and 200 mcg. Each capsule contains the labeled amount of Digoxin USP dissolved in a solvent comprised of polyethylene glycol 400 USP, 8 percent ethyl alcohol, propylene glycol USP and purified water USP. Certain brands of Digoxin Solution in Capsules contain the inactive ingredients FD&C Red No. 40 (0.05 mg Capsule), D&C Yellow No. 10 (0.1 mg and 0.2 mg Capsules), FD&C Blue No. 1 (0.2 mg Capsule), gelatin, glycerin, methylparaben and propylparaben (added as preservatives), purified water, and sorbitol within the capsule shell.

Digoxin Pediatric Elixir is a stable solution of Digoxin specially formulated for oral use in infants and children. Each mL contains 50 μg (0.05 mg) Digoxin USP. Certain brands of elixir are lime-flavored and contain the inactive ingredients

➤ SHOWN IN PRODUCT IDENTIFICATION GUIDE

alcohol 10%, methylparaben 0.1% (added as a preservative), citric acid, D&C Green No. 5 and Yellow No. 10, flavor, propylene glycol, sodium phosphate, and sucrose. Each package is supplied with a specially calibrated dropper to facilitate the administration of accurate dosage even in premature infants. Starting at 0.2 mL, this 1 mL dropper is marked in divisions of 0.1 mL, each corresponding to 5 µg (0.005 mg) Digoxin.

Digoxin Injection is a sterile solution for intravenous or intramuscular injection. Certain brands of Digoxin Injection contain 40% propylene glycol and 10% alcohol and are buffered to a pH of 6.8 to 7.2 with 0.17% sodium phosphate and 0.08% anhydrous citric acid. Each 2 mL contains 500 µg (0.5 mg) Digoxin (250 µg [0.25 mg] per mL). Dilution is not required.

Digoxin Pediatric Injection is a sterile solution for intravenous or intramuscular injection. Certain brands of Digoxin Pediatric Injection contain 40% propylene glycol and 10% alcohol, and are buffered to a pH of 6.8 to 7.2 with 0.17% sodium phosphate and 0.08% anhydrous citric acid. Each 1 mL ampul contains 100 µg (0.1 mg) Digoxin. Dilution is not required.

Following is its chemical structure:

CLINICAL PHARMACOLOGY

Mechanism of Action: The influence of digitalis glycosides on the myocardium is dose-related, and involves both a direct action on cardiac muscle and the specialized conduction system, and indirect actions on the cardiovascular system mediated by the autonomic nervous system. The indirect actions mediated by the autonomic nervous system involve a vagomimetic action, which is responsible for the effects of digitalis on the sino-atrial (SA) and atrioventricular (AV) nodes; and also a baroreceptor sensitization which results in increased carotid sinus nerve activity and enhanced sympathetic withdrawal for any given increment in mean arterial pressure. The pharmacologic consequences of these direct and indirect effects are: 1) an increase in the force and velocity of myocardial systolic contraction (positive inotropic action); 2) a slowing of heart rate (negative chronotropic effect); and 3) decreased conduction velocity through the AV node. In higher doses, digitalis increases sympathetic outflow from the central nervous system (CNS) to both cardiac and peripheral sympathetic nerves. This increase in sympathetic activity may be an important factor in digitalis cardiac toxicity. Most of the extracardiac manifestations of digitalis toxicity are also mediated by the CNS.

PHARMACOKINETICS

Absorption: Gastrointestinal absorption of Digoxin is a passive process. Absorption of Digoxin from the tablet formulation has been demonstrated to be 60 to 80% complete compared to an identical intravenous dose of Digoxin (absolute bioavailability). When Digoxin tablets or capsules are taken after meals, the rate of absorption is slowed, but the total amount of Digoxin absorbed is usually unchanged. When the elixir is taken after meals, the rate of absorption is slowed, but the total amount of Digoxin absorbed is usually unchanged. When taken with meals high in bran fiber, however, the amount absorbed from an oral dose may be reduced. Absorption of Digoxin from Digoxin capsules has been demonstrated to be 90 to 100% complete compared to an identical intravenous dose of Digoxin. The enhanced absorption from Digoxin capsules compared to Digoxin tablets and elixir is associated with reduced between-patient and within-patient variability in steady-state serum concentrations. The peak serum concentrations are higher than those observed after tablets. Comparison of the systemic availability and equivalent doses for Digoxin preparations are shown in the following table:

Product	Absolute Bioavailability	Equivalent Doses (in mg*)		
Digoxin Tablet	60-80%	0.125	0.25	0.5
Digoxin Elixir	70-85%	0.125	0.25	0.5
Digoxin Injection/ I.M.	70-85%	0.125	0.25	0.5
Digoxin Injection/ I.V.	100%	0.1	0.2	0.4
Digoxin Capsules	90-100%	0.1	0.2	0.4

*1 mg = 1000 µg

In some patients, orally administered digoxin is converted to cardioinactive reduction products (e.g., dihydrodigoxin) by colonic bacteria in the gut. Data suggest that one in ten patients treated with Digoxin tablets will degrade 40% or more of the ingested dose. This phenomenon is minimized with Digoxin capsules because they are rapidly absorbed in the upper gastrointestinal tract.

Distribution: Following drug administration, a 6 to 8 hour distribution phase is observed. This is followed by a much more gradual serum concentration decline, which is dependent on Digoxin elimination from the body. The peak height and slope of the early portion (absorption/distribution phases) of the serum concentration-time curve are dependent upon the route of administration and the absorption characteristics of the formulation. Clinical evidence indicates that the early high serum concentrations (particularly high for Digoxin capsules) do not reflect the concentration of Digoxin at its site of action, but that with chronic use, the steady-state post-distribution serum levels are in equilibrium with tissue levels and correlate with pharmacologic effects. In individual patients, these post-distribution serum concentrations are linearly related to maintenance dosage and may be useful in evaluating therapeutic and toxic effects (see *"Serum Digoxin Concentrations"* in *"Dosage and Administration"* section).

Digoxin is concentrated in tissues and therefore has a large apparent volume of distribution. Digoxin crosses both the blood-brain barrier and the placenta. At delivery, serum Digoxin concentration in the newborn is similar to the serum level in the mother. Approximately 20 to 25% of plasma Digoxin is bound to protein. Serum Digoxin concentrations are not significantly altered by large changes in fat tissue weight, so that its distribution space correlates best with lean (ideal) body weight, not total body weight.

Pharmacologic Response: The approximate times to onset of effect and to peak effect of all the Digoxin preparations are given in the following table:

Product	Time to Onset of Effect*	Time to Peak Effect*
Digoxin Tablet	0.5-2 hours	2-6 hours
Digoxin Elixir	0.5-2 hours	2-6 hours
Digoxin Injection/I.M.	0.5-2 hours	2-6 hours
Digoxin Injection/I.V.	5-30 minutes†	1-4 hours
Digoxin Capsules	0.5-2 hours	2-6 hours

*Documented for ventricular response rate in atrial fibrillation, inotropic effect and electrocardiographic changes.
†Depending upon rate of infusion.

Excretion: Elimination of Digoxin follows first-order kinetics (that is, the quantity of digoxin eliminated at any time is proportional to the total body content). Following intravenous administration to normal subjects, 50 to 70% of a Digoxin dose is excreted unchanged in the urine. Renal excretion of Digoxin is proportional to glomerular filtration rate and is largely independent of urine flow. In subjects with normal renal function, Digoxin has a half-life of 1.5 to 2.0 days. The half-life in anuric patients is prolonged to 4 to 6 days. Digoxin is not effectively removed from the body by dialysis, exchange transfusion or during cardiopulmonary by-pass because most of the drug is in tissue rather than circulating in the blood.

INDICATIONS AND USAGE

Heart Failure: The increased cardiac output resulting from the inotropic action of Digoxin ameliorates the disturbances characteristic of heart failure (venous congestion, edema, dyspnea, orthopnea and cardiac asthma).

Digoxin is more effective in "low output" (pump) failure than in "high output" heart failure secondary to arteriovenous fistula, anemia, infection or hyperthyroidism.

Digoxin is usually continued after failure is controlled, unless some known precipitating factor is corrected. Studies have shown, however, that even though hemodynamic effects can be demonstrated in almost all patients, corresponding improvement in the signs and symptoms of heart failure is not necessarily apparent. Therefore, in patients in whom Digoxin may be difficult to regulate, or in whom the risk of toxicity may be great (e.g., patients with unstable renal function or whose potassium levels tend to fluctuate) a cautious withdrawal of Digoxin may be considered. If Digoxin is discontinued, the patient should be regularly monitored for clinical evidence of recurrent heart failure.

Atrial Fibrillation: Digoxin reduces ventricular rate and thereby improves hemodynamics. Palpitation, precordial distress or weakness are relieved and concomitant congestive failure ameliorated. Digoxin should be continued in doses necessary to maintain the desired ventricular rate.

Atrial Flutter: Digoxin slows the heart and regular sinus rhythm may appear. Frequently the flutter is converted to atrial fibrillation with a controlled ventricular response. Digoxin treatment should be maintained if atrial fibrillation persists. (Electrical cardioversion is often the treatment of choice for atrial flutter. See discussion of cardioversion in *"Precautions"* section.)

Paroxysmal Atrial Tachycardia (PAT): Digoxin may convert PAT to sinus rhythm by slowing conduction through the AV node. If heart failure has ensued or paroxysms recur frequently, Digoxin should be continued. In infants, Digoxin is usually continued for 3 to 6 months after a single episode of PAT to prevent recurrence.

UNLABELED USES

Digoxin is used as an adjunct in the treatment of myocardial infarction and congested circulatory states secondary to ventricular septal defects in infants.

◆ RATED THERAPEUTICALLY EQUIVALENT; ◇ THERAPEUTIC EQUIVALENCE UNCONFIRMED; ○ UNRATED

CONTRAINDICATIONS

Digitalis glycosides are contraindicated in ventricular fibrillation.

In a given patient, an untoward effect requiring permanent discontinuation of other digitalis preparations usually constitutes a contraindication to Digoxin. Hypersensitivity to Digoxin itself is a contraindication to its use. Allergy to Digoxin, though rare, does occur. It may not extend to all such preparations, and another digitalis glycoside may be tried with caution.

WARNINGS

Digitalis alone or with other drugs has been used in the treatment of obesity. This use of Digoxin or other digitalis glycosides is unwarranted. Moreover, since they may cause potentially fatal arrhythmias or other adverse effects, the use of these drugs solely for the treatment of obesity is dangerous.

It is recommended that Digoxin in soft capsules be administered in divided daily doses to minimize any potential adverse reactions, since peak serum Digoxin concentrations resulting from the capsules are approximately twice those after bioequivalent tablet doses (400 μg of Digoxin capsules are bioequivalent to 500 μg of tablets). Studies are underway to determine if there are any increased risks associated with the higher peaks that occur with single daily dosing of soft gelatin capsules.

Anorexia, nausea, vomiting and arrhythmias may accompany heart failure or may be indications of digitalis intoxication. Clinical evaluation of the cause of these symptoms should be attempted before further digitalis administration. In such circumstances determination of the serum Digoxin concentration may be an aid in deciding whether or not digitalis toxicity is likely to be present. If the possibility of digitalis intoxication cannot be excluded, cardiac glycosides should be temporarily withheld, if permitted by the clinical situation.

Patients with renal insufficiency require smaller than usual maintenance doses of Digoxin (see *"Dosage and Administration"* section).

Heart failure accompanying acute glomerulonephritis requires extreme care in digitalization. Relatively low loading and maintenance doses and concomitant use of antihypertensive drugs may be necessary and careful monitoring is essential. Digoxin should be discontinued as soon as possible. Patients with severe carditis, such as carditis associated with rheumatic fever or viral myocarditis, are especially sensitive to digoxin-induced disturbances of rhythm.

Newborn infants display considerable variability in their tolerance to Digoxin. Premature and immature infants are particularly sensitive, and dosage must not only be reduced but must be individualized according to their degree of maturity.

Note: Digitalis glycosides are an important cause of accidental poisoning in children.

PRECAUTIONS

General: Digoxin toxicity develops more frequently and lasts longer in patients with renal impairment because of the decreased excretion of Digoxin. Therefore, it should be anticipated that dosage requirements will be decreased in patients with moderate to severe renal disease (see *"Dosage and Administration"* section). Because of the prolonged half-life, a longer period of time is required to achieve an initial or new steady-state concentration in patients with renal impairment than in patients with normal renal function. In patients with hypokalemia, toxicity may occur despite serum Digoxin concentrations within the "normal range," because potassium depletion sensitizes the myocardium to Digoxin. Therefore, it is desirable to maintain normal serum potassium levels in patients being treated with Digoxin. Hypokalemia may result from diuretic, amphotericin B or corticosteroid therapy, and from dialysis or mechanical suction of gastrointestinal secretions. It may also accompany malnutrition, diarrhea, prolonged vomiting, old age and long-standing heart failure. In general, rapid changes in serum potassium or other electrolytes should be avoided, and intravenous treatment with potassium should be reserved for special circumstances as described below (see *"Treatment of Arrhythmias Produced by Overdosage"* section).

Calcium, particularly when administered rapidly by the intravenous route, may produce serious arrhythmias in digitalized patients. Hypercalcemia from any cause predisposes the patient to digitalis toxicity. On the other hand, hypocalcemia can nullify the effects of Digoxin in man; thus, Digoxin may be ineffective until serum calcium is restored to normal. These interactions are related to the fact that calcium affects contractility and excitability of the heart in a manner similar to Digoxin.

Hypomagnesemia may predispose to digitalis toxicity. If low magnesium levels are detected in a patient on Digoxin, replacement therapy should be instituted.

Quinidine, verapamil, amiodarone, propafenone, indomethacin and itraconazole cause a rise in serum Digoxin concentration, with the implication that digitalis intoxication may result. This rise appears to be proportional to the dose. The effect is mediated by a reduction in the Digoxin clearance and, in the case of quinidine, decreased volume of distribution as well.

Certain antibiotics may increase Digoxin absorption in patients who convert Digoxin to inactive metabolites in the gut (see *"Pharmacokinetics"* portion of the *"Clinical Pharmacology"* section). Recent studies have shown that specific colonic bacteria in the lower gastrointestinal tract convert Digoxin to cardioinactive reduction products, thereby reducing its bioavailability. Although inactivation of these bacteria by antibiotics is rapid, the serum Digoxin concentration will rise at a rate consistent with the elimination half-life of Digoxin. The magnitude of rise in serum Digoxin concentration relates to the extent of bacterial inactivation, and may be as much as two-fold in some cases. This interaction is significantly reduced if Digoxin is given as capsules. Patients with acute myocardial infarction or severe pulmonary disease may be unusually sensitive to Digoxin-induced disturbances of rhythm.

Atrial arrhythmias associated with hypermetabolic states (e.g. hyperthyroidism) are particularly resistant to Digoxin treatment. Large doses of Digoxin are not recommended as the only treatment of these arrhythmias and care must be taken to avoid toxicity if large doses of Digoxin are required. In hypothyroidism, the Digoxin requirements are reduced. Digoxin responses in patients with compensated thyroid disease are normal.

Reduction of Digoxin dosage may be desirable prior to electrical cardioversion to avoid induction of ventricular arrhythmias, but the physician must consider the consequences of rapid increase in ventricular response to atrial fibrillation if Digoxin is withheld 1 to 2 days prior to cardioversion. If there is a suspicion that digitalis toxicity exists, elective cardioversion should be delayed. If it is not prudent to delay cardioversion, the energy level selected should be minimal at first and carefully increased in an attempt to avoid precipitating ventricular arrhythmias.

Incomplete AV block, especially in patients with Stokes-Adams attacks, may progress to advanced or complete heart block if Digoxin is given.

In some patients with sinus node disease (i.e., Sick Sinus Syndrome), Digoxin may worsen sinus bradycardia or sino-atrial block.

In patients with Wolff-Parkinson-White Syndrome and atrial fibrillation, Digoxin can enhance transmission of impulses through the accessory pathway. This effect may result in extremely rapid ventricular rates and even ventricular fibrillation.

Digoxin may worsen the outflow obstruction in patients with idiopathic hypertrophic subaortic stenosis (IHSS). Unless cardiac failure is severe, it is doubtful whether Digoxin should be employed.

Patients with chronic constrictive pericarditis may fail to respond to Digoxin. In addition, slowing of the heart rate by Digoxin in some patients may further decrease cardiac output.

Patients with heart failure from amyloid heart disease or constrictive cardiomyopathies respond poorly to treatment with Digoxin.

Digoxin is not indicated for the treatment of sinus tachycardia unless it is associated with heart failure.

Digoxin may produce false positive ST-T changes in the electrocardiogram during exercise testing.

Intramuscular injection of Digoxin is extremely painful and offers no advantages unless other routes of administration are contraindicated.

Laboratory Tests: Patients receiving Digoxin should have their serum electrolytes and renal function (BUN and/or serum creatinine) assessed periodically; the frequency of assessments will depend on the clinical setting. For discussion of serum Digoxin concentrations, see *"Dosage and Administration"* section.

Drug Interactions: Potassium-depleting *corticosteroids* and *diuretics* may be major contributing factors to digitalis toxicity. *Calcium*, particularly if administered rapidly by the intravenous route, may produce serious arrhythmias in digitalized patients. *Quinidine, verapamil, amiodarone, propafenone, indomethacin and itraconazole* cause a rise in serum Digoxin concentration, with the implication that digitalis intoxication may result. Certain *antibiotics* increase Digoxin absorption in patients who inactivate Digoxin by bacterial metabolism in the lower intestine, so that digitalis intoxication may result. *Propantheline* and *diphenoxylate,* by decreasing gut motility, may increase Digoxin absorption. *Antacids, kaolin-pectin, sulfasalazine, neomycin, cholestyramine,* certain *anticancer drugs,* and *metoclopramide* may reduce intestinal Digoxin absorption, resulting in unexpectedly low serum concentrations. There have been inconsistent reports regarding the effects of other drugs on the serum Digoxin concentration. *Thyroid* administration to a digitalized, hypothyroid patient may increase the dose requirement of Digoxin. Concomitant use of Digoxin and *sympathomimetics* increases the risk of cardiac arrhythmias because both enhance ectopic pacemaker activity. *Succinylcholine* may cause a sudden extrusion of potassium from muscle cells, and may thereby cause arrhythmias in digitalized patients. Although β adrenergic blockers or calcium channel blockers and Digoxin may be useful in combination to control atrial fibrillation, their additive effects on AV node conduction can result in complete heart block.

Due to the considerable variability of these interactions, Digoxin dosage should be carefully individualized when patients receive coadministered medications. Furthermore, caution should be exercised when combining Digoxin with any drug that may cause a significant deterioration in renal function, since this may impair the excretion of Digoxin.

Carcinogenesis, Mutagenesis, Impairment of Fertility: There have been no long-term studies performed in animals to evaluate carcinogenic potential.

Pregnancy: Teratogenic Effects: Pregnancy Category C. Animal reproduction studies have not been conducted with Digoxin. It is also not known whether Digoxin can cause fetal harm when administered to a pregnant woman or can affect reproduction capacity. Digoxin should be given to a pregnant woman only if clearly needed.

Nursing Mothers: Studies have shown that Digoxin concentrations in the mother's serum and milk are similar. However, the estimated daily dose to a nursing infant will be far below the usual infant maintenance dose. Therefore, this amount should have no pharmacologic effect upon the infant. Nevertheless, caution should be exercised when Digoxin is administered to a nursing woman.

ADVERSE REACTIONS

The frequency and severity of adverse reactions to Digoxin depend on the dose and route of administration, as well as on the patient's underlying disease or concomitant therapies (see *"Precautions"* section and *"Serum Digoxin Concentrations"* subsection of *"Dosage and Administration"*). The overall incidence of adverse reactions has been reported as 5 to 20%, with 15 to 20% of them being considered serious (one to four percent of patients receiving Digoxin). Evidence suggests that the incidence of toxicity has decreased since the introduction of the serum Digoxin assay and improved standardization of Digoxin tablets. Cardiac toxicity accounts for about one-half, gastrointestinal disturbances for about one-fourth, and CNS and other toxicity for about one-fourth of these adverse reactions.

ADULTS
Cardiac: Unifocal or multiform ventricular premature contractions, especially in bigeminal or trigeminal patterns are the most common arrhythmias associated with Digoxin toxicity in adults with heart disease.

Ventricular tachycardia may result from digitalis toxicity. Atrioventricular (AV) dissociation, accelerated junctional (nodal) rhythm and atrial tachycardia with block are also common arrhythmias caused by Digoxin overdosage.

Excessive slowing of the pulse is a clinical sign of Digoxin overdosage. AV block (Wenckebach) of increasing degree may proceed to complete heart block.

Note: The electrocardiogram is fundamental in determining the presence and nature of these cardiac disturbances. Digoxin may also induce other changes in the ECG (e.g., PR prolongation, ST depression), which represent Digoxin effect and may or may not be associated with digitalis toxicity.

Gastrointestinal: Anorexia, nausea, vomiting and less commonly diarrhea are common early symptoms of overdosage. However, uncontrolled heart failure may also produce such symptoms. Digitalis toxicity very rarely may cause abdominal pain and hemorrhagic necrosis of the intestines.

CNS: Visual disturbances (blurred or yellow vision), headache, weakness, dizziness, apathy and psychosis can occur.

Other: Gynecomastia is occasionally observed. Maculopapular rash or other skin reactions are rarely observed.

INFANTS AND CHILDREN
Toxicity differs from the adult in a number of respects. Anorexia, nausea, vomiting, diarrhea and CNS disturbances may be present but are rare as initial symptoms in infants. Cardiac arrhythmias are more reliable signs of toxicity. Digoxin in children may produce any arrhythmia. The most commonly encountered are conduction disturbances or supraventricular tachyarrhythmias, such as atrial tachycardia with or without block and junctional (nodal) tachycardia. Ventricular arrhythmias are less common. Sinus bradycardia may also be a sign of impending Digoxin intoxication, especially in infants, even in the absence of first degree heart block. Any arrhythmia or alteration in cardiac conduction that develops in a child taking Digoxin should initially be assumed to be a consequence of Digoxin intoxication.

OVERDOSAGE
TREATMENT OF ARRHYTHMIAS PRODUCED BY OVERDOSAGE
Adults: Digoxin should be discontinued until all signs of toxicity are gone. Discontinuation may be all that is necessary if toxic manifestations are not severe and appear only near the expected time for maximum effect of the drug.

Correction of factors that may contribute to toxicity such as electrolyte disturbances, hypoxia, acid-base disturbances and removal of aggravating agents such as catecholamines, should also be considered. Potassium salts may be indicated, particularly if hypokalemia is present. Potassium administration may be dangerous in the setting of massive digitalis overdosage (see *"Massive Digitalis Overdosage"* subsection below). Potassium chloride in divided oral doses totaling 3 to 6 grams of the salt (40 to 80 mEq K+) for adults may be given provided renal function is adequate (see below for potassium recommendations in Infants and Children).

When correction of the arrhythmia is urgent and the serum potassium concentration is low or normal, potassium should be administered intravenously in 5% dextrose injection. For adults, a total of 40 to 80 mEq (diluted to a concentration of 40 mEq per 500 mL) may be given at a rate not exceeding 20 mEq per hour, or slower if limited by pain due to local irritation. Additional amounts may be given if the arrhythmia is uncontrolled and potassium well-tolerated. ECG monitoring should be performed to watch for any evidence of potassium toxicity (e.g., peaking of T waves) and to observe the effect on the arrhythmia. The infusion may be stopped when the desired effect is achieved.

Note: Potassium should not be used and may be dangerous in heart block due to Digoxin, unless primarily related to supraventricular tachycardia.

Other agents that have been used for the treatment of Digoxin intoxication include lidocaine, procainamide, propranolol and phenytoin, although use of the latter must be considered experimental. In advanced heart block, atropine and/or temporary ventricular pacing may be beneficial. Digoxin Immune Fab (Ovine) can be used to reverse potentially life-threatening Digoxin (or digitoxin) intoxication. Improvement in signs and symptoms of digitalis toxicity usually begins within ½ hour of Digoxin Immune Fab (Ovine) administration. Each 40 mg vial of Digoxin Immune Fab (Ovine) will neutralize 0.6 mg of Digoxin (which is a usual body store of an adequately digitalized 70 kg patient).

Infants and Children: See *"Adult"* section for general recommendations for the treatment of arrhythmias produced by overdosage and for cautions regarding the use of potassium. If a potassium preparation is used to treat toxicity, it may be given orally in divided doses totaling 1 to 1.5 mEq K+ per kilogram (kg) body weight (1 gram of potassium chloride contains 13.4 mEq K+).

When correction of the arrhythmia with potassium is urgent, approximately 0.5 mEq/kg of potassium per hour may be given intravenously, with careful ECG

monitoring. The intravenous solution of potassium should be dilute enough to avoid local irritation; however, especially in infants, care must be taken to avoid intravenous fluid overload.

MASSIVE DIGITALIS OVERDOSAGE
Manifestations of life-threatening toxicity include severe ventricular arrhythmias such as ventricular tachycardia or ventricular fibrillation, or progressive bradyarrhythmias such as severe sinus bradycardia or second or third degree heart block not responsive to atropine. An overdosage of more than 10 mg of Digoxin in previously healthy adults or 4 mg in previously healthy children or overdosage resulting in steady-state serum concentrations greater than 10 mg/mL, often results in cardiac arrest.

Severe digitalis intoxication can cause life-threatening elevation in serum potassium concentration by shifting potassium from inside to outside the cell resulting in hyperkalemia. Administration of potassium supplements in the setting of massive intoxication may be hazardous.

Digoxin Immune Fab (Ovine) may be used at a dose equimolar to Digoxin in the body to reverse the effects of ingestion of a massive overdose. The decision to administer Digoxin Immune Fab (Ovine) before the onset of toxic manifestations will depend on the likelihood that life-threatening toxicity will occur (see above).

Patients with massive digitalis ingestion should receive large doses of activated charcoal to prevent absorption and bind Digoxin in the gut during enteroenteric recirculation. Emesis of gastric lavage may be indicated especially if ingestion has occurred within 30 minutes of the patient's presentation at the hospital. Emesis should not be induced in patients who are obtunded. If a patient presents more than 2 hours after ingestion or already has toxic manifestations, it may be unsafe to induce vomiting or attempt passage of a gastric tube, because such maneuvers may induce an acute vagal episode that can worsen digitalis-toxic arrhythmias.

DOSAGE AND ADMINISTRATION
Recommended dosages are average values that may require considerable modification because of individual sensitivity or associated conditions. Diminished renal function is the most important factor requiring modification of recommended doses.

Due to the more complete absorption of Digoxin from soft capsules, recommended oral doses are only 80 percent of those for tablets, elixir and injection.

Because the significance of the higher peak serum concentrations associated with once daily capsules is not established, divided daily dosing is presently recommended for:

1. Infants and children under 10 years of age;
2. Patients requiring a daily dose of 300 µg (0.3 mg) or greater;
3. Patients with a previous history of digitalis toxicity;
4. Patients considered likely to become toxic;
5. Patients in whom compliance is not a problem.

Where compliance is considered a problem, single daily dosing may be appropriate.

Parenteral administration of Digoxin should be used only when the need for rapid digitalization is urgent or when the drug cannot be taken orally. Intramuscular injection can lead to severe pain at the injection site, thus intravenous administration is preferred. If the drug must be administered by the intramuscular route, it should be injected deep into the muscle followed by massage. No more than 500 µg (2 mL) should be injected into a single site.

Digoxin Injection can be administered undiluted or diluted with a 4-fold or greater volume of Sterile Water for Injection, 0.9% Sodium Chloride Injection or 5% Dextrose Injection. The use of less than a 4-fold volume of diluent could lead to precipitation of the Digoxin. Immediate use of the diluted product is recommended.

If tuberculin syringes are used to measure very small doses, one must be aware of the problem of inadvertent overadministration of Digoxin. The syringe should *not* be flushed with the parenteral solution after its contents are expelled into an indwelling vascular catheter.

Slow infusion of Digoxin Injection is preferable to bolus administration. Rapid infusion of digitalis glycosides has been shown to cause systemic and coronary arteriolar constriction, which may be clinically undesirable. Caution is thus advised and Digoxin Injection should probably be administered over a period of 5 minutes or longer. Mixing of Digoxin Injection with other drugs in the same container or simultaneous administration in the same intravenous line is not recommended.

In deciding the dose of Digoxin, several factors must be considered:

1. The disease being treated. Atrial arrhythmias may require larger doses than heart failure.
2. The body weight of the patient. Doses should be calculated based upon lean or ideal body weight.
3. The patient's renal function, preferably evaluated on the basis of creatinine clearance.
4. Age is an important factor in infants and children.
5. Concomitant disease states, drugs or other factors likely to alter the expected clinical response to Digoxin (see *"Precautions"* and *"Drug Interactions"* sections).

Digitalization may be accomplished by either of two general approaches that vary in dosage and frequency of administration, but reach the same endpoint in terms of total amount of Digoxin accumulated in the body.

1. Rapid digitalization may be achieved by administering a loading dose based upon projected peak body Digoxin stores, then calculating the maintenance dose as a percentage of the loading dose.

---

2. More gradual digitalization may be obtained by beginning an appropriate maintenance dose, thus allowing Digoxin body stores to accumulate slowly. Steady-state serum Digoxin concentrations will be achieved in approximately 5 half-lives of the drug for the individual patient. Depending upon the patient's renal function, this will take between one and three weeks.

ADULTS

Adults—Rapid Digitalization with a Loading Dose. Peak body Digoxin stores of 8 to 12 µg/kg should provide therapeutic effect with minimum risk of toxicity in most patients with heart failure and normal sinus rhythm. Larger stores (10 to 15 µg/kg) are often required for adequate control of ventricular rate in patients with atrial flutter or fibrillation. Because of altered Digoxin distribution and elimination, projected peak body stores for patients with renal insufficiency should be conservative (i.e., 6 to 10 µg/kg) [see "Precautions" section].

The loading dose should be based on the projected peak body stores and administered in several portions, with roughly half the total given as the first dose. Additional fractions of this planned total dose may be given at 6 to 8 hour intervals, *with careful assessment of clinical response before each additional dose.*

If the patient's clinical response necessitates a change from the calculated dose of Digoxin, then calculation of the maintenance dose should be based upon the amount actually given.

In previously undigitalized patients, a single initial Digoxin Tablet dose of 500 to 750 µg (0.5 to 0.75 mg) or Digoxin capsule dose of 400 to 600 mcg (0.4 to 0.6 mg) usually produces a detectable effect in 0.5 to 2 hours that becomes maximal in 2 to 6 hours. Additional doses of 125 to 375 µg (0.125 to 0.375) mg of the tablets and 100 to 300 mcg (0.1 to 0.3 mg) of the capsules may be given cautiously at 6 to 8 hour intervals until clinical evidence of an adequate effect is noted. The usual amount of Digoxin tablets that a 70 kg patient requires to achieve 8 to 15 µg/kg peak body stores is 750 to 1250 µg (0.75 to 1.25 mg). The usual amount of Digoxin capsules that a 70 kg patient requires to achieve 8 to 15 µg/kg peak body stores is 600 to 1000 µg (0.6 to 1.0 mg).

In previously undigitalized patients, a single initial intravenous Digoxin Injection dose of 400 to 600 µg (0.4 to 0.6 mg) usually produces a detectable effect in 5 to 30 minutes that becomes maximal in 1 to 4 hours. Additional doses of 100 to 300 µg (0.1 to 0.3 mg) may be given cautiously at 4 to 8 hour intervals until clinical evidence of an adequate effect is noted. The usual amount of Digoxin Injection that a 70 kg patient requires to achieve 8 to 15 µg/kg peak body stores is 600 to 1000 µg (0.6 to 1.0 mg).

Although peak body stores are mathematically related to loading doses and are utilized to calculate maintenance doses, they do not correlate with measured serum concentrations. This discrepancy is caused by Digoxin distribution within the body during the first 6 to 8 hours following a dose. Serum concentrations drawn during this time are usually not interpretable.

The maintenance dose should be based upon the percentage of the peak body stores lost each day through elimination. The following formula has had wide clinical use:

$$\text{Maintenance Dose} = \text{Peak Body Stores} \times \frac{\% \text{ Daily Loss}}{100}$$
$$(\text{i.e., Loading Dose})$$

Where: % Daily Loss = 14 + Ccr/5

Ccr is creatinine clearance, corrected to 70 kg body weight or 1.73 m² body surface area. *For adults,* if only serum creatinine concentrations (Scr) are available, a Ccr (corrected to 70 kg body weight) may be estimated in men as (140 − Age)/Scr. For women, this result should be multiplied by 0.85.

Note: This equation cannot be used for estimating creatinine clearance in infants or children.

A common practice involves the use of Digoxin Injection to achieve rapid digitalization, with conversion to Digoxin Tablets or Capsules for maintenance therapy. If patients are switched from intravenous to oral Digoxin formulations, allowances must be made for differences in bioavailability when calculating maintenance dosages (see table, "Clinical Pharmacology" section).

Adults—Gradual Digitalization with a Maintenance Dose: The following tables provide respective average Digoxin Tablet daily maintenance dose requirements for patients with heart failure based upon lean body weight and renal function:
(See related table).
(See related table).

Example: based on the above tables, a patient in heart failure with an estimated lean body weight of 70 kg and a Ccr of 60 mL/min, should be given a 250 µg (0.25 mg) Digoxin Tablet or 200 mcg (0.2 mg) Digoxin Capsules each day. The tablets are usually taken after the morning meal whereas the capsules are taken as a 100 µg (0.1 mg) capsule after the morning and evening meals. Steady-state serum concentrations should not be anticipated before 11 days.

INFANTS AND CHILDREN

Digitalization must be individualized. Divided daily dosing is recommended for infants and young children. In these patients, where dosage adjustment is frequent and outside the fixed dosages available, Digoxin Capsules may not be the formulation of choice. Children over 10 years of age require adult dosages in proportion to their body weight.

In the newborn period, renal clearance of Digoxin is diminished and suitable dosage adjustments must be observed. This is especially pronounced in the premature infant. Beyond the immediate newborn period, children generally require proportionally larger doses than adults on the basis of body weight or body surface area.

Digoxin Injection Pediatric can be used to achieve rapid digitalization, with conversion to an oral Digoxin formulation for maintenance therapy. If patients are switched from intravenous to oral Digoxin Tablets or Elixir, allowances must be made for differences in bioavailability when calculating maintenance dosages (see bioavailability table in "Clinical Pharmacology" section and dosing table below).

Intramuscular injection of Digoxin is extremely painful and offers no advantages unless other routes of administration are contraindicated.

Digitalizing and daily maintenance doses for each age group are given below and should provide therapeutic effect with minimum risk of toxicity in most patients with heart failure and normal sinus rhythm. Larger doses are often required for adequate control of ventricular rate in patients with atrial flutter or fibrillation.

The loading dose should be administered in several portions, with roughly half the total given as the first dose. Additional fractions of this planned total dose may be given at 6 to 8 hour intervals, *with careful assessment of clinical response before each additional dose.* If the patient's clinical response necessitates a change from the calculated dose of Digoxin, then calculation of the maintenance dose should be based upon the amount actually given.

USUAL DIGITALIZING AND MAINTENANCE DOSAGES FOR DIGOXIN TABLETS IN CHILDREN WITH NORMAL RENAL FUNCTION BASED ON LEAN BODY WEIGHT

Age	Digitalizing* Dose (µg/kg)	Daily† Maintenance Dose (µg/kg)
2 to 5 Years	30 to 40	
5 to 10 Years	20 to 35	25 to 35% of *oral* loading dose‡
Over 10 Years	10 to 15	

* *I.V. digitalizing doses are 80% of oral digitalizing doses.*
† *Divided daily dosing is recommended for children under 10 years of age.*
‡ *Projected or actual digitalizing dose providing clinical response.*

USUAL DIGITALIZING AND MAINTENANCE DOSAGES FOR DIGOXIN CAPSULES IN CHILDREN WITH NORMAL RENAL FUNCTION BASED ON LEAN BODY WEIGHT

Age	Digitalizing* Dose (µg/kg)	Daily† Maintenance Dose (µg/kg)
2 to 5 Years	25—35	25 to 35% of the oral or I.V. loading dose‡
5 to 10 Years	15—30	
Over 10 Years	8—12	

* *I.V. digitalizing doses are the same as Digoxin capsule digitalizing doses.*
† *Divided daily dosing is recommended for children under 10 years of age.*
‡ *Projected or actual digitalizing dose providing desired clinical response.*

USUAL DIGITALIZING AND MAINTENANCE DOSAGES FOR DIGOXIN ELIXIR PEDIATRIC IN CHILDREN WITH NORMAL RENAL FUNCTION BASED ON LEAN BODY WEIGHT

Age	Digitalizing* Dose (µg/kg)	Daily† Maintenance Dose (µg/kg)
Premature	20—30	20—30% of *oral* loading dose‡
Full Term	25—35	
1—24 Months	35—60	
2—5 Years	30—40	25—35% of *oral* loading dose‡
5—10 Years	20—35	
Over 10 Years	10—15	

* *I.V. digitalizing doses are 80% of oral digitalizing doses.*
† *Divided daily dosing is recommended for children under 10 years of age.*
‡ *Projected or actual digitalizing dose providing clinical response.*

USUAL DIGITALIZING AND MAINTENANCE DOSAGES FOR DIGOXIN INJECTION IN CHILDREN WITH NORMAL RENAL FUNCTION BASED ON LEAN BODY WEIGHT

Age	Digitalizing* Dose (µg/kg)	Daily† I.V. Maintenance Dose (µg/kg)
2 to 5 Years	25 to 35	
5 to 10 Years	15 to 30	25 to 35% of the I.V. loading dose‡
Over 10 Years	8 to 12	

* *I.V. digitalizing doses are 80% of oral digitalizing doses.*
† *Divided daily dosing is recommended for children under 10 years of age.*
‡ *Projected or actual digitalizing dose providing clinical response.*

USUAL DIGITALIZING AND MAINTENANCE DOSAGES FOR DIGOXIN INJECTION PEDIATRIC IN CHILDREN WITH NORMAL RENAL FUNCTION BASED ON LEAN BODY WEIGHT

Age	Digitalizing* Dose (µg/kg)	Daily† I.V. Maintenance Dose (µg/kg)
Premature	15 to 25	20 to 30% of the I.V. loading dose‡

Age	Digitalizing* Dose (µg/kg)	Daily† I.V. Maintenance Dose (µg/kg)
Full-Term	20 to 30	
1 to 24 Months	30 to 50	
2 to 5 Years	25 to 35	25 to 35% of the I.V. loading dose‡
	15 to 30	
5 to 10 Years		
Over 10 Years	8 to 12	

* *I.V. digitalizing doses are 80% of oral digitalizing doses.*
† *Divided daily dosing is recommended for children under 10 years of age.*
‡ *Projected or actual digitalizing dose providing clinical response.*

More gradual digitalization can also be accomplished by beginning an appropriate maintenance dose. The range of percentages provided above can be used in calculating this dose for patients with normal renal function. In children with renal disease, Digoxin dosing must be carefully titrated based upon clinical response.

Long-term use of Digoxin is indicated in many children who have been digitalized for acute heart failure, unless the cause is transient. Children with severe congenital heart disease, even after surgery, may require Digoxin for prolonged periods.

It cannot be overemphasized that both the adult and pediatric dosage guidelines provided are based upon average patient response and substantial individual variation can be expected. Accordingly, ultimate dosage selection must be based upon clinical assessment of the patient.

Serum Digoxin Concentrations: Measurement of serum Digoxin concentrations can be helpful to the clinician in determining the state of digitalization and in assigning certain probabilities to the likelihood of Digoxin intoxication. Studies in adults considered adequately digitalized (without evidence of toxicity) show that about two-thirds of such patients have serum Digoxin levels ranging from 0.8 to 2.0 ng/mL. Patients with atrial fibrillation or atrial flutter require and appear to tolerate higher levels than do patients with other indications. On the other hand, in adult patients with clinical evidence of Digoxin toxicity, about two-thirds will have serum Digoxin levels greater than 2.0 ng/mL. Thus, whereas levels less than 0.8 ng/mL are infrequently associated with toxicity, levels greater than 2.0 ng/mL are often associated with toxicity. Values in between are not very helpful in deciding whether a certain sign or symptom is more likely caused by Digoxin toxicity or by something else. There are rare patients who are unable to tolerate Digoxin even at serum concentrations below 0.8 ng/mL. Some researchers suggest that infants and young children tolerate slightly higher serum concentrations than do adults.

To allow adequate time for equilibration of Digoxin between serum and tissue, *sampling of serum concentrations for clinical use should be at least 6 to 8 hours after the last dose,* regardless of the route of administration or formulation used. On a twice daily dosing schedule, there will be only minor differences in serum Digoxin concentrations whether sampling is done at 8 or 12 hours after a dose.

After a single daily dose, the concentration will be 10 to 25% lower when sampled at 24 versus 8 hours, depending upon the patient's renal function. Ideally, sampling for assessment of steady-state concentrations should be done just before the next dose.

If a discrepancy exists between the reported serum concentration and the observed clinical response, the clinician should consider the following possibilities:

1. Analytical problems in the assay procedure.
2. Inappropriate serum sampling time.
3. Administration of a digitalis glycoside other than Digoxin.
4. Conditions (described in *"Warnings"* and *"Precautions"* sections) causing an alteration in the sensitivity of the patient to Digoxin.
5. The patient falls outside the norm in his response to or handling of Digoxin. This decision should only be reached after exclusion of the other possibilities and generally should be confirmed by additional correlations of clinical observations with serum Digoxin concentrations.

The serum concentration data should always be interpreted in the overall clinical context and an isolated serum concentration value should not be used alone as a basis for increasing or decreasing Digoxin dosage.

Adjustment of Maintenance Dose in Previously Digitalized Patients:
Digoxin Tablet maintenance doses in individual patients on steady-state digoxin can be adjusted upward or downward in proportion to the ratio of the desired versus the measured serum concentration. For example, a patient at steady-state on 125 µg (0.125 mg) of Digoxin tablets or 100 mcg (0.1 mg) Digoxin Injection per day with a measured serum concentration of 0.7 ng/mL, should have the dose increased to 250 µg (0.25 mg) or 200 mcg (0.2 mg) respectively, per day to achieve a steady-state serum concentration of 1.4 ng/mL, *assuming the serum Digoxin concentration measurement is correct, renal function remains stable during this time and the needed adjustment is not the result of a problem with compliance.*

Another example is a patient at steady-state on 100 µg (0.1 mg) of Digoxin Capsules per day with a measured serum concentration of 0.7 ng/mL, should have the dose increased to 200 µg (0.2 mg) per day to achieve a steady-state serum concentration of 1.4 ng/mL, *assuming the serum Digoxin concentration measurement is correct, renal function remains stable during this time and the needed adjustment is not the result of a problem with compliance.*

Dosage Adjustment When Changing Preparations: The difference in bioavailability between injectable Digoxin or Digoxin Capsules and Digoxin Elixir Pediatric or Digoxin Tablets must be considered when changing patients from one dosage form to another. The absolute bioavailability of the capsule formulation is greater than that of the standard tablets and very near that of the intravenous dosage form. As a result the doses recommended for Digoxin capsules are the same as those for Digoxin Injection (see *"Clinical Pharmacology"* section).

Digoxin Injection and Digoxin Capsule doses of 100 µg (0.1 mg) and 200 µg (0.2 mg) are approximately equivalent to 125 µg (0.125 mg) and 250 µg (0.25 mg)

USUAL DIGOXIN TABLET DAILY MAINTENANCE DOSE REQUIREMENTS (µg)
FOR ESTIMATED PEAK BODY STORES OF 10 µg/kg

		Lean Body Weight (kg/lbs)							
		50/110	60/132	70/154	80/176	90/198	100/220		
	0	63*†	125	125	125	188††	188	22	
	10	125	125	125	188	188	188	19	
	20	125	125	188	188	188	250	16	
Corrected	30	125	188	188	188	250	250	14	Number of
Ccr	40	125	188	188	250	250	250	13	Days
(mL/min	50	188	188	250	250	250	250	12	Before
per 70 kg)	60	188	188	250	250	250	375	11	Steady-State
	70	188	250	250	250	250	375	10	Achieved
	80	188	250	250	250	375	375	9	
	90	188	250	250	250	375	500	8	
	100	250	250	250	375	375	500	7	

* *63 µg = 0.063 mg*
† *½ of 125 µg tablet or 125 µg every other day*
†† *1½ of 125 µg tablet.*

USUAL DIGOXIN CAPSULE DAILY MAINTENANCE DOSE REQUIREMENTS (µg)
FOR ESTIMATED PEAK BODY STORES OF 10 µg/kg

		Lean Body Weight (kg/lbs)							
		50/110	60/132	70/154	80/176	90/198	100/220		
	0	50	100	100	100	150	150	22	
	10	100	100	100	150	150	150	19	
	20	100	100	150	150	150	200	16	
Corrected	30	100	150	150	150	200	200	14	Number of
Ccr	40	100	150	150	200	200	250	13	Days
(mL/min	50	150	150	200	200	250	250	12	Before
per 70 kg)	60	150	150	200	200	250	300	11	Steady-State
	70	150	200	200	250	250	300	10	Achieved
	80	150	200	200	250	300	300	9	
	90	150	200	250	250	300	350	8	
	100	200	200	250	300	300	350	7	

◆ RATED THERAPEUTICALLY EQUIVALENT; ◇ THERAPEUTIC EQUIVALENCE UNCONFIRMED; ○ UNRATED

doses of Digoxin Tablets and Elixir Pediatric (see table of *"Clinical Pharmacology"* section).

Adjustments in dosage will seldom be necessary when converting a patient from intravenous to Digoxin Capsule formulation. The differences in bioavailability between injectable Digoxin or Digoxin Capsules, and Digoxin Elixir Pediatric or Digoxin Tablets must be considered when changing patients from one dosage form to another. Intramuscular injection of Digoxin is extremely painful and offers no advantages unless other routes of administration are contraindicated.

Storage: Store at 15° to 25°C (59° to 77°F) in a dry place and protect from light.

J CODES
Up to 0.5 mg IM,IV—J1160

HOW SUPPLIED
CAPSULE: 0.05 MG

BRAND/MANUFACTURER	NDC	SIZE	AWP
○ **BRAND**			
➤ LANOXICAPS: Burr Wellcome	00081-0270-55	100s	$13.67

CAPSULE: 0.1 MG

BRAND/MANUFACTURER	NDC	SIZE	AWP
○ **BRAND**			
➤ LANOXICAPS: Burr Wellcome	00081-0272-30	30s	$6.50
	00081-0272-55	100s	$14.93

CAPSULE: 0.2 MG

BRAND/MANUFACTURER	NDC	SIZE	AWP
○ **BRAND**			
➤ LANOXICAPS: Burr Wellcome	00081-0274-30	30s	$7.97
	00081-0274-55	100s	$17.36

ELIXIR: 0.05 MG/ML

BRAND/MANUFACTURER	NDC	SIZE	AWP
○ **BRAND**			
LANOXIN: Burr Wellcome	00081-0264-27	60 ml	$17.06
○ **GENERICS**			
Liquipharm	54198-0148-02	60 ml	$9.25
Bausch&Lomb Pharm	24208-0360-67	60 ml	$9.63
Roxane	00054-3192-46	60 ml	$10.40
Roxane	00054-8192-16	2.5 ml 40s ud	$41.93
Roxane	00054-8193-16	5 ml 40s ud	$62.30

INJECTION: 0.1 MG/ML

BRAND/MANUFACTURER	NDC	SIZE	AWP
◆ **BRAND**			
LANOXIN: Burr Wellcome	00081-0262-10	1 ml 10s	$51.66

INJECTION: 0.25 MG/ML

AVERAGE UNIT PRICE (AVAILABLE SIZES)	
BRAND	$0.98
GENERIC	$1.33

BRAND/MANUFACTURER	NDC	SIZE	AWP
◆ **BRAND**			
LANOXIN: Burr Wellcome	00081-0260-10	2 ml 10s	$21.50
	00081-0260-35	2 ml 50s	$87.84
◆ **GENERICS**			
Wyeth-Ayerst	00008-0480-02	1 ml 10s	$22.94
Wyeth-Ayerst	00008-0480-01	2 ml 10s	$23.29
Elkins-Sinn	00641-1410-36	2 ml 100s	$103.95

INJECTION: 0.25 MG/ML

BRAND/MANUFACTURER	NDC	SIZE	AWP
○ **GENERICS**			
Allscrips	54569-2217-00	1 ml 10s	$22.94

TABLET: 0.125 MG

BRAND/MANUFACTURER	NDC	SIZE	AWP
○ **BRAND**			
➤ LANOXIN: Burr Wellcome	00081-0242-30	30s	$5.76
	00081-0242-55	100s	$11.26
	00081-0242-56	100s ud	$15.72
	00081-0242-75	1000s	$86.52
○ **GENERICS**			
Phys Total Care	54868-2134-03	30s	$2.11
Medirex	57480-0343-06	30s	$4.50
Southwood	58016-0354-30	30s	$5.07
Southwood	58016-0354-60	60s	$6.53
Phys Total Care	54868-2134-01	100s	$4.44
Moore,H.L.	00839-7641-06	100s	$9.52

BRAND/MANUFACTURER	NDC	SIZE	AWP
Southwood	58016-0354-00	100s	$9.63
Vangard	00615-0547-13	100s ud	$14.75
Raway	00686-0547-13	100s ud	$15.50
Moore,H.L.	00839-7641-16	1000s	$74.86
Moore,H.L.	00839-7641-20	5000s	$353.30

For additional alternatives, turn to the section beginning on page 2859.

Digoxin Immune Fab (Ovine)

DESCRIPTION
Digoxin Immune Fab (Ovine), is a sterile lyophilized powder of antigen binding fragments (Fab) derived from specific antidigoxin antibodies raised in sheep. Production of antibodies specific for Digoxin involves conjugation of Digoxin as a hapten to human albumin. Sheep are immunized with this material to produce antibodies specific for the antigenic determinants of the digoxin molecule. The antibody is then papain digested and Digoxin-specific Fab fragments of the antibody are isolated and purified by affinity chromatography. These antibody fragments have a molecular weight of approximately 50,000.

Each vial, which will bind approximately 0.6 mg of Digoxin (or digitoxin), contains 40 mg of Digoxin-specific Fab fragments derived from sheep.

Digoxin Immune Fab (Ovine) is administered by intravenous injection after reconstitution with Sterile Water for Injection (4 mL per vial).

CLINICAL PHARMACOLOGY
After intravenous injection of Digoxin Immune Fab (Ovine) in the baboon, Digoxin-specific Fab fragments are excreted in the urine with a biological half-life of about 9 to 13 hours.[1] In humans with normal renal function the half-life appears to be 15 to 20 hours.[2] Experimental studies in animals indicate that these antibody fragments have a large volume of distribution in the extracellular space, unlike whole antibody which distributes in a space only about twice the plasma volume.[1] Ordinarily, following administration of Digoxin Immune Fab (Ovine), improvement in signs and symptoms of digitalis intoxication begins within one-half hour or less.[2,3,4,5]

The affinity of Digoxin Immune Fab (Ovine) for Digoxin is in the range of 10^9 to 10^{10} M^{-1}, which is greater than the affinity of Digoxin for (sodium, potassium) ATPase, the presumed receptor for its toxic effects. The affinity of Digoxin Immune Fab (Ovine) for digitoxin is about 10^8 to 10^9 M^{-1}.[6]

Digoxin Immune Fab (Ovine) binds molecules of Digoxin, making them unavailable for binding at their site of action on cells in the body. The Fab fragment-Digoxin complex accumulates in the blood, from which it is excreted by the kidney. The net effect is to shift the equilibrium away from binding of Digoxin to its receptors in the body, thereby reversing its effects.

INDICATIONS AND USAGE
Digoxin Immune Fab (Ovine) is indicated for treatment of potentially life-threatening Digoxin intoxication.[3] Although designed specifically to treat life-threatening Digoxin overdose, it has also been used successfully to treat life-threatening digitoxin overdose.[3] Since human experience is limited and the consequences of repeated exposures are unknown, Digoxin Immune Fab (Ovine) is not indicated for milder cases of digitalis toxicity.

Manifestations of life-threatening toxicity include severe ventricular arrhythmias such as ventricular tachycardia or ventricular fibrillation, or progressive bradyarrhythmias such as severe sinus bradycardia or second or third degree heart block not responsive to atropine.

Ingestion of more than 10 mg of Digoxin in previously healthy adults or 4 mg of Digoxin in previously healthy children, or ingestion causing steady-state serum concentrations greater than 10 ng/ml, often results in cardiac arrest. Digitalis-induced progressive elevation of the serum potassium concentration also suggests imminent cardiac arrest. If the potassium concentration exceeds 5 mEq/L in the setting of severe digitalis intoxication, Digoxin Immune Fab (Ovine) therapy is indicated.

CONTRAINDICATIONS
There are no known contraindications to the use of Digoxin Immune Fab (Ovine).

WARNINGS
Suicidal ingestion often involves more than one drug; thus toxicity from other drugs should not be overlooked.

One should consider the possibility of anaphylactic, hypersensitivity or febrile reactions. If an anaphylactoid reaction occurs, the drug infusion should be discontinued and appropriate therapy initiated using aminophylline, oxygen, volume expansion, diphenydramine, corticosteroids and airway management as indicated. The need for epinephrine should be balanced against its potential risk in the setting of digitalis toxicity.

Since the Fab fragment of the antibody lacks the antigenic determinants of the Fc fragment, it should pose less of an immunogenic threat to patients than does an intact immunoglobulin molecule. Patients with known allergies would be particularly at risk, as would individuals who have previously received antibodies or Fab fragments raised in sheep. Papain is used to cleave the whole antibody into Fab and Fc fragments, and traces of papain or inactivated papain residues may be present in Digoxin Immune Fab (Ovine). Patients with allergies to papain, chymopapain, or other papaya extracts also may be particularly at risk.

Skin testing for allergy was performed during the clinical investigation of Digoxin Immune Fab (Ovine). Only one patient developed erythema at the site of skin testing, with no accompanying wheal reaction; this individual had no adverse reaction to systemic treatment with Digoxin Immune Fab (Ovine). Since allergy testing can delay urgently needed therapy, it is not routinely required before treatment of life-threatening digitals toxicity with Digoxin Immune Fab (Ovine).

Skin testing may be appropriate for high risk individuals, especially patients with known allergies or those previously treated with Digoxin Immune Fab (Ovine). The intradermal skin test can be performed by: 1. Diluting 0.1 mL of reconstituted Digoxin Immune Fab (Ovine) (10 mg/mL) in 9.9 mL sterile isotonic saline (1:100 dilution, 100 μg/mL). 2. Injecting 0.1 mL of the 1:100 dilution (10 μg) intradermally and observing for an urticarial wheal surrounded by a zone of erythema. The test should be read at 20 minutes.

The scratch test procedure is performed by placing one drop of a 1:100 dilution of Digoxin Immune Fab (Ovine) on the skin and then making a 1/4-inch scratch through the drop with a sterile needle. The scratch site is inspected at 20 minutes for an urticarial wheal surrounded by erythema.

If skin testing causes a systemic reaction, a tourniquet should be applied above the site of testing and measures to treat anaphylaxis should be instituted. Further administration of Digoxin Immune Fab (Ovine) should be avoided unless its use is absolutely essential, in which case the patient should be pretreated with corticosteroids and diphenhydramine. The physician should be prepared to treat anaphylaxis.

PRECAUTIONS
GENERAL

Standard therapy for digitalis intoxication includes withdrawal of the drug and correction of factors that may contribute to toxicity, such as electrolyte disturbances, hypoxia, acid-base disturbances and agents such as catecholamines. Also, treatment of arrhythmias may include judicious potassium supplements, lidocaine, phenytoin, procainamide and/or propranolol; treatment of sinus bradycardia or atrioventricular block may involve atropine or pacemaker insertion. Massive digitalis intoxication can cause hyperkalemia; administration of potassium supplements in the setting of massive intoxication may be hazardous (see "Laboratory Tests"). After treatment with Digoxin Immune Fab (Ovine), the serum potassium concentration may drop rapidly[2] and must be monitored frequently, especially over the first several hours after Digoxin Immune Fab (Ovine) is given (see "Laboratory Tests").

The elimination half-life in the setting of renal failure has not been clearly defined. Patients with renal dysfunction have been successfully treated with Digoxin Immune Fab (Ovine).[4] There is no evidence to suggest the time-course of therapeutic effect is any different in these patients than in patients with normal renal function, but excretion of the Fab fragment-Digoxin complex from the body is probably delayed. In patients who are functionally anephric, one would anticipate failure to clear the Fab fragment-Digoxin complex from the blood by glomerular filtration and renal excretion. Whether failure to eliminate the Fab fragment-Digoxin complex in severe renal failure can lead to reintoxication following release of newly unbound Digoxin into the blood is uncertain. Such patients should be monitored for a prolonged period for possible recurrence of digitalis toxicity.

Patients with intrinsically poor cardiac function may deteriorate from withdrawal of the inotropic action of Digoxin. Studies in animals have shown that the reversal of inotropic effect is relatively gradual, occurring over hours. When needed, additional support can be provided by use of intravenous inotropes, such as dopamine or dobutamine, or vasodilators. One must be careful in using catecholamines not to aggravate digitalis toxic rhythm disturbances. Clearly, other types of digitalis glycosides should not be used in this setting. Redigitalization should be postponed, if possible, until the Fab fragments have been eliminated from the body, which may require several days. Patients with impaired renal function may require a week or longer.

Laboratory Tests: **Digoxin Immune Fab (Ovine) will interfere with digitalis immunoassay measurements.[7] Thus, the standard serum Digoxin concentration measurement can be clinically misleading until the Fab Fragment is eliminated from the body.**

Serum Digoxin or digitoxin concentration should be obtained before Digoxin Immune Fab (Ovine) administration if at all possible. These measurements may be difficult to interpret if drawn soon after the last digitalis dose, since at least 6 to 8 hours are required for equilibration of Digoxin between serum and tissue. Patients should be closely monitored, including temperature, blood pressure, electrocardiogram and potassium concentration, during and after administration of Digoxin Immune Fab (Ovine). The total serum Digoxin concentration may rise precipitously following administration of Digoxin Immune Fab (Ovine) but this will be almost entirely bound to the Fab fragment and therefore not able to react with receptors in the body.

Potassium concentrations should be followed carefully. Severe digitalis intoxication can cause life-threatening elevation in serum potassium concentration by shifting potassium from inside to outside the cell. The elevation in serum potassium concentration can lead to increased renal excretion of potassium. Thus, these patients may have hyperkalemia with a total body deficit of potassium. When the effect of digitalis is reversed by Digoxin Immune Fab (Ovine), potassium shifts back inside the cell, with a resulting decline in serum potassium concentration.[4] Hypokalemia may thus develop rapidly. For these reasons, serum potassium concentration should be monitored repeatedly, especially over the first several hours after Digoxin Immune Fab (Ovine) is given, and cautiously treated when necessary.

Carcinogenesis, Mutagenesis, Impairment of Fertility: There have been no long-term studies performed in animals to evaluate carcinogenic potential.

Pregnancy: Pregnancy Category C. Animal reproduction studies have not been conducted with Digoxin Immune Fab (Ovine). It is also not known whether Digoxin Immune Fab (Ovine) can cause fetal harm when administered to a pregnant woman or can affect reproduction capacity. Digoxin Immune Fab (Ovine) should be given to a pregnant woman only if clearly needed.

Nursing Mothers: It is not known whether this drug is excreted in human milk. Because many drugs are excreted in human milk, caution should be exercised when Digoxin Immune Fab (Ovine) is administered to a nursing woman.

Pediatric Use: Digoxin Immune Fab (Ovine) has been successfully used in infants with no apparent adverse sequelae. As in all other circumstances, use of this drug in infants should be based on careful consideration of the benefits of the drug balanced against the potential risk involved.

ADVERSE REACTIONS

Allergic reactions to Digoxin Immune Fab (Ovine) have been reported rarely. Patients with a history of allergy, especially to antibiotics, appear to be at particular risk (see "Warnings"). In a few instances, low cardiac output states and congestive heart failure could have been exacerbated by withdrawal of the inotropic effects of digitalis. Hypokalemia may occur from re-activation of (sodium, potassium) ATPase (see "Laboratory Tests"). Patients with atrial fibrillation may develop a rapid ventricular response from withdrawal of the effects of digitalis on the atrioventricular node.[4]

DOSAGE AND ADMINISTRATION
GENERAL GUIDELINES

The dosage of Digoxin Immune Fab (Ovine) varies according to the amount of Digoxin (or digitoxin) to be neutralized. The average dose used during clinical testing was 10 vials.

Dosage for Acute Ingestion of Unknown Amount: Twenty (20) vials (800 mg) of Digoxin Immune Fab (Ovine) is adequate to treat most life-threatening ingestions in both *adults and children.* However, in children it is important to monitor for volume overload. In general, a large Digoxin Immune Fab (Ovine) dose has a faster onset of effect but may enhance the possibility of a febrile reaction. The physician may consider administering 10 vials, observing the patients response, and following with an additional 10 vials if clinically indicated.

Dosage for Toxicity During Chronic Therapy: For adults, 6 vials (240 mg) usually is adequate to reverse most cases of toxicity. This dose can be used in patients who are in acute distress or for whom a serum Digoxin or digitoxin concentration is not available. In infants and small children ($\leq$ 20 kg) a single vial usually should suffice.

Methods for calculating the dose of Digoxin Immune Fab (Ovine) required to neutralize the known or estimated amount of Digoxin or digitoxin in the body are given below (see "Dosage Calculation" section).

When determining the dose for Digoxin Immune Fab (ovine), the following guidelines should be considered:

—Erroneous calculations may result from inaccurate estimates of the amount of digitalis ingested or absorbed or from nonsteady-state serum digitalis concentrations. Inaccurate serum digitalis concentration measurements are a possible source of error. Most serum Digoxin assay kits are designed to measure values less than 5 ng/mL. Dilution of samples is required to obtain accurate measures above 5 ng/mL.

—Dosage calculations are based on a steady-state volume of distribution of approximately 6 L/kg for Digoxin (0.6 L/kg for digitoxin) to convert serum digitalis concentration to the amount of digitalis in the body. The conversion is based on the principle that body load equals drug steady-state serum concentration multiplied by volume of distribution. These volumes are population averages and vary widely among individuals. Many patients may require higher doses for complete neutralization. Doses should ordinarily be rounded up to the next whole vial.

—If toxicity has not adequately reversed after several hours or appears to recur, readministration of Digoxin Immune Fab (Ovine) at a dose guided by clinical judgment may be required.

—Failure to respond to Digoxin Immune Fab (Ovine) raises the possibility that the clinical problem is not caused by digitalis intoxication. If there is no response to an adequate dose of Digoxin Immune Fab (Ovine), the diagnosis of digitalis toxicity should be questioned.

DOSAGE CALCULATION

Acute Ingestion of Known Amount: Each vial of Digoxin Immune Fab (Ovine) contains 40 mg of purified Digoxin-specific Fab fragments which will bind approximately 0.6 mg of Digoxin (or digitoxin). Thus one can calculate the total number of vials required by dividing the total digitalis body load in mg by 0.6 mg/vial (see Formula 1).

For toxicity from an acute ingestion, total body load in milligrams will be approximately equal to the amount ingested in milligrams for Digoxin capsules and digitoxin, or the amount ingested in milligrams multiplied by 0.80 (to account for incomplete absorption) for Digoxin tablets.

Table 1 gives dosage estimates in number of vials for *adults and children* who have ingested a single large dose of Digoxin and for whom the approximate number of tablets or capsules is known. The Digoxin Immune Fab (Ovine) dose (in number of vials) represented in Table 1 can be approximated using the following formula:

Formula 1

$$\text{Dose (in \# of vials)} = \frac{\text{Total digitalis body load in mg}}{0.6 \text{ mg of digitalis bound/vial}}$$

◆ RATED THERAPEUTICALLY EQUIVALENT; ◇ THERAPEUTIC EQUIVALENCE UNCONFIRMED; ○ UNRATED

Table 1
APPROXIMATE DIGOXIN IMMUNE FAB (OVINE) DOSE FOR REVERSAL OF A SINGLE LARGE DIGOXIN OVERDOSE

Number of Digoxin Tablets Capsules Ingested*	Digoxin Immune Fab (Ovine) Dose # of Vials
25	9
50	17
75	25
100	34
150	50
200	67

* *0.25 mg tablets with 80% bioavailability or 0.2 mg Digoxin capsules with 100% biovailability.*

Calculations Based on Steady-State Serum Digoxin Concentration: Table 2 gives dosage estimates in number of vials for *adults patients* for whom a steady-state serum Digoxin concentration is known. The Digoxin Immune Fab (Ovine) dose (in number of vials) represented in Table 2 can be approximated using the following formula:

Formula 2

$$\text{Dose (in \# of vials)} = \frac{(\text{Serum Digoxin concentration}) \text{ in ng/mL}) (\text{weight in kg})}{100}$$

Table 2
ADULT DOSE ESTIMATE OF DIGOXIN IMMUNE FAB (OVINE) (IN # OF VIALS) FROM STEADY-STATE SERUM DIGOXIN CONCENTRATION

Patient Weight (kg)	Serum Digoxin Concentration (ng/mL)						
	1	2	4	8	12	16	20
40	0.5 v	1 v	2 v	3 v	5 v	7 v	8 v
60	0.5 v	1 v	3 v	5 v	7 v	10 v	12 v
70	1 v	2 v	3 v	6 v	9 v	11 v	14 v
80	1 v	2 v	3 v	7 v	10 v	13 v	16 v
100	1 v	2 v	4 v	8 v	12 v	16 v	20 v

v = vials

Table 3 gives dosage estimates in milligrams *for infants and small children* based on the steady-state serum Digoxin concentration. The Digoxin Immune Fab (Ovine) dose represented in Table 3 can be estimated by multiplying the dose (in number of vials) calculated from Formula 2 by the amount of Digoxin Immune Fab (Ovine) contained in a vial (40 mg/vial) (see Formula 3). Since infants and small children can have much smaller dosage requirements, it is recommended that the 40 mg vial be reconstituted as directed and administered with a tuberculin syringe. For very small doses, a reconstituted vial can be diluted with 36 mL of sterile isotonic saline to achieve a concentration of 1 mg/mL.

Formula 3
Dose (in mg) = (Dose [in # of vials]) (40 mg/vial)

Table 3
INFANTS AND SMALL CHILDREN DOSE ESTIMATES OF DIGOXIN IMMUNE FAB (OVINE) (IN MG) FROM STEADY-STATE SERUM DIGOXIN CONCENTRATION

Patient Weight (kg)	Serum Digoxin Concentration (ng/mL)						
	1	2	4	8	12	16	20
1	0.4* mg	1* mg	1.5* mg	3* mg	5 mg	7 mg	8 mg
3	1* mg	3* mg	5 mg	10 mg	15 mg	19 mg	24 mg
5	2* mg	4 mg	8 mg	16 mg	24 mg	32 mg	40 mg
10	4 mg	8 mg	16 mg	32 mg	48 mg	64 mg	80 mg
20	8 mg	16 mg	32 mg	64 mg	96 mg	128 mg	160 mg

*Dilution of reconstituted vial of 1 mg/mL may be desirable

Calculation Based on Steady-State Digitoxin Concentration: The Digoxin Immune Fab (Ovine) dose for digitoxin toxicity can be approximated using the following formula:

Formula 4

$$\text{Dose (in \# of vials)} = \frac{(\text{Serum digitoxin concentration in ng/mL}) (\text{weight in kg})}{1000}$$

If the dose based on ingested amount differs substantially from that calculated from the serum Digoxin or digitoxin concentration, it may be preferable to use the higher dose.

ADMINISTRATION

The contents in each vial to be used should be dissolved with 4 mL of Sterile Water for Injection, by gentle mixing, to give a clear, colorless, approximately isosmotic solution with a protein concentration of 10 mg/mL. Reconstituted product should be used promptly. If it is not used immediately, it may be stored under refrigeration at 2 to 8°C (36 to 46°F) for up to 4 hours. The reconstituted product may be diluted with sterile isotonic saline to a convenient volume. Parenteral drug products should be inspected visually for particulate matter and discoloration prior to administration, whenever solution and container permit.

Digoxin Immune Fab (Ovine) is administered by the intravenous route over 30 minutes. It is recommended that it be infused through a 0.22 micron membrane filter to ensure no undissolved particulate matter is administered. If cardiac arrest is imminent, it can be given as a bolus injection.

Refrigerate at 2 to 8°C (36 to 46°F). Unreconstituted vials can be stored at up to 30°C (86°F) for a total of 30 days.

REFERENCES

1. Smith TW, Lloyd BL, Spicer N, Haber E. Immunogenicity and kinetics of distribution and elimination of sheep Digoxin-specific IgG and Fab fragments in the rabbit and baboon. *Clin Exp Immunol* 1979; 36:384-396.   2. Smith TW, Haber E, Yeatman L, Butler VP Jr. Reversal of advanced Digoxin intoxication with Fab fragments of Digoxin-specific antibodies. *N Engl J Med* 1976; 294:797-800.   3. Smith TW, Butler VP Jr, Haber E, Fozzard H, Marcus Fl, Bremner WF, Schulman IC, Phillips A. Treatment of life-threatening digitalis intoxication with Digoxin-specific Fab antibody fragments: Experience in 26 cases. *N Engl J Med* 1982; 307:1357-1362.   4. Wenger TL, Butler VP Jr, Haber E, Smith TW. Treatment of 63 severely digitalis-toxic patients with Digoxin-specific antibody fragments. *J Am Coll Cardiol* 1985; 5:118A-123A.   5. Spiegel A, Marchlinski FE. Time course for reversal of Digoxin toxicity with Digoxin-specific antibody fragments. *Am Heart J* 1985; 109:1397-1399.   6. Smith TW, Butler VP, Haber E. Characterization of antibodies of high affinity and specificity for the digitalis glycoside Digoxin. *Biochemistry* 1970; 9:331-337.   7. Gibb I, Adams PC, Parnham AJ, Jennings K. Plasma Digoxin: Assay anomalies in Fab-treated patients. *Br J Clin Pharmacol* 1983; 16:445-447.

HOW SUPPLIED
INJECTION: 10 MG/ML

BRAND/MANUFACTURER	NDC	SIZE	AWP
○ BRAND			
DIGIBIND: Burr Wellcome	00081-0230-44	4 ml	$386.53

Dihydroergotamine Mesylate

DESCRIPTION

Dihydroergotamine Mesylate is ergotamine hydrogenated in the 9, 10 position as the mesylate salt. Dihydroergotamine Mesylate is known chemically as ergotaman-3',6',18-trione,9,10-dihydro-12'-hydroxy-2'-methyl-5'- (phenylmethyl)-,(5'α,10α)-, monomethanesulfonate (salt).

The empirical formula is $C_{33}H_{37}N_5O_5.CH_4O_3S$ and the molecular weight is 679.79. Dihydroergotamine Mesylate is a clear, colorless solution supplied in sterile ampuls for Intravenous or Intramuscular administration. Each ml contains: Dihydroergotamine Mesylate 1 mg.

Following is its chemical structure:

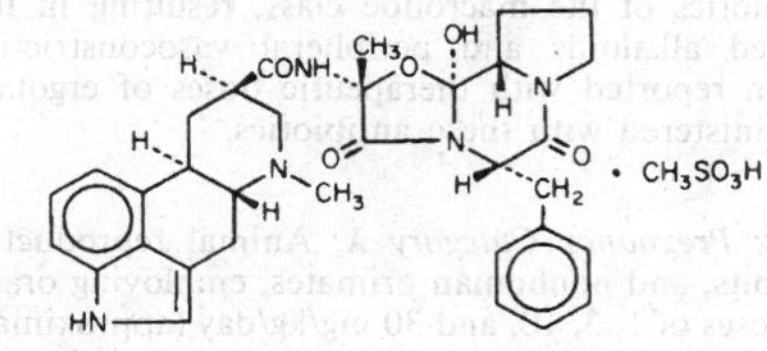

ACTIONS

Dihydroergotamine is an alpha adrenergic blocking agent with a direct stimulating effect on the smooth muscle of peripheral and cranial blood vessels, and produces depression of central vasomotor centers. The compound also has the properties of serotonin antagonism. In comparison to ergotamine, the adrenergic blocking actions are more pronounced, the vasoconstrictive actions somewhat less pronounced, and there is reduced incidence and degree of nausea and vomiting.

Onset of action occurs in 15-30 minutes following intramuscular administration and persists for 3-4 hours.

Repeated dosage at 1 hour intervals up to 3 hours may be required to obtain maximal effect.

INDICATIONS

Dihydroergotamine Mesylate injection therapy is indicated to abort or prevent vascular headache, e.g., migraine, migraine variants, or so-called "histaminic cephalalgia" when rapid control is desired or when other routes of administration are not feasible.

For best results, treatment should commence at the first symptom or sign of a migraine headache attack.

UNLABELED USES

Dihydroergotamine is used alone or as an adjunct in the treatment of antidepressant-induced xerostomia, cyclic idiopathic edema in women, and acute and chronic diarrhea. It is also used as a prophylactic adjunct for the prophylaxis of deep vein thrombosis in total hip replacement, in orthostatic hypotension, pelvic congestion with pain, and intracranial hypertension in patients with cerebral edema.

CONTRAINDICATIONS

Dihydroergotamine Mesylate is contraindicated in patients who have previously shown hypersensitivity to ergot alkaloids.

The drug is also contraindicated in patients having conditions predisposing to vasospastic reactions such as known peripheral arterial disease, coronary artery disease (in particular, unstable or vasospastic angina), sepsis, vascular surgery, uncontrolled hypertension, and severely impaired hepatic or renal function.

Dihydroergotamine possesses oxytocic properties and, therefore, should not be administered during pregnancy.

Dihydroergotamine should not be used in nursing mothers (see *"Precautions"*).

Dihydroergotamine should not be used with vasoconstrictors because the combination may result in extreme elevation of blood pressure.

WARNINGS

VASOSPASM

Dihydroergotamine, like other ergot alkaloids, can cause vasospastic reactions, including angina, although it seems to do so less frequently than other ergots. This action appears to be dose related; however, some patients may demonstrate individual sensitivity to the agent.

Vasospastic reactions are manifested by intense arterial vasoconstriction, producing signs and symptoms of peripheral vascular ischemia (e.g., muscle pains, numbness, coldness, and pallor or cyanosis of the digits), angina or unusual syndromes, such as mesenteric ischemia. Because persistent vasospasm can result in gangrene or death, Dihydroergotamine Mesylate injection should be discontinued immediately if signs or symptoms of vasoconstriction develop.

PRECAUTIONS

INFORMATION FOR PATIENTS

No more than 3 mL intramuscularly or 2 mL intravenously should be injected for any single migraine attack. No more than 6 mL should be injected during any 7-day period.

Dihydroergotamine Mesylate injection should be used only for vascular headaches of the migraine type. It is not effective for other types of headaches and it lacks analgesic properties. Patients should be advised to report to the physician immediately any of the following: numbness or tingling in the fingers and toes, muscle pain in the arms and legs, weakness in the legs, pain in the chest, or temporary speeding or slowing of the heart rate, swelling, or itching.

DRUG INTERACTIONS

Vasoconstrictors: Dihydroergotamine Mesylate injection should not be administered with vasoconstrictors or sympathomimetics (pressor agents) because the combination may cause extreme elevation of blood pressure.

Beta Blockers: There have been reports that propranolol may potentiate the vasoconstrictive action of ergotamine by blocking the vasodilating property of epinephrine.

Nicotine: Nicotine may provoke vasoconstriction in some patients, predisposing to a greater ischemic response to ergot therapy.

Macrolide Antibiotics (e.g. Erythromycin): Agents of the ergot alkaloid class, of which Dihydroergotamine Mesylate injection is a member, have been shown to interact with antibiotics of the macrolide class, resulting in increased plasma levels of unchanged alkaloids and peripheral vasoconstriction. Vasospastic reactions have been reported with therapeutic doses of ergotamine-containing drugs when coadministered with these antibiotics.

PREGNANCY

Teratogenic Effects: Pregnancy Category X: Animal reproductive (teratogenic) studies in rats, rabbits, and nonhuman primates, employing oral Dihydroergotamine Mesylate at doses of 1, 3, 10, and 30 mg/kg/day (approximately 12, 36, 120, and 360 times the maximum recommended daily dose based on a 50 kg man) did not produce any evidence of adverse reproductive effects. There are no studies on the placental transfer or teratogenicity of Dihydroergotamine Mesylate. Ergotamine crosses the placenta in small amounts, although it does not appear to be embryotoxic. However, prolonged vasoconstriction of the uterine vessels and/or increased myometrial tone leading to reduced myometrial and placenta blood flow may contribute to fetal growth retardation in animals. (See *"Contraindications."*)

NURSING MOTHERS

Ergot drugs are known to inhibit prolactin. It is likely that Dihydroergotamine Mesylate is excreted in human milk. However, there are no data on the concentration of Dihydroergotamine in human milk. It is known that ergotamine is excreted in breast milk and may cause vomiting, diarrhea, weak pulse and unstable blood pressure in nursing infants. Because of the potential for these serious adverse reactions in nursing infants from Dihydroergotamine Mesylate, nursing should not be undertaken during the use of Dihydroergotamine Mesylate.

PEDIATRIC USE

Safety and effectiveness of Dihydroergotamine Mesylate in children have not been established.

ADVERSE REACTIONS

Numbness and tingling of fingers and toes, muscle pains in the extremities, weakness in the legs, precordial distress and pain, transient tachycardia or bradycardia, nausea, vomiting, localized edema, itching, and injection site reactions.

In studies with normal volunteers, doses of Dihydroergotamine Mesylate injection of 2-3 mg resulted in an increased frequency of headache, leg cramps and soreness, nausea, and vomiting.

There have been reports of pleural and retroperitoneal fibrosis in patients following prolonged use of Dihydroergotamine.

DRUG ABUSE AND DEPENDENCE

ABUSE AND DEPENDENCE

Currently available data have not demonstrated drug abuse and psychological dependence with Dihydroergotamine. However, cases of drug abuse and psychological dependence in patients on other forms of ergot therapy have been reported. Thus, due to the chronicity of vascular headaches, it is imperative that patients be advised not to exceed recommended dosages.

OVERDOSAGE

To date, there have been no reports of acute overdosage with this drug. Due to the risk of vascular spasm, exceeding the recommended dosages of Dihydroergotamine Mesylate injection is to be avoided. Excessive doses of Dihydroergotamine may result in peripheral signs and symptoms of *ergotism*. Treatment includes discontinuance of the drug, local application of warmth to the affected area, the administration of vasodilators, and nursing care to prevent tissue damage.

In general, the symptoms of an acute Dihydroergotamine Mesylate overdose are similar to those of an ergotamine overdose, although there is less pronounced nausea and vomiting with Dihydroergotamine Mesylate. The symptoms of an ergotamine overdose include the following: numbness, tingling, pain, and cyanosis of the extremities associated with diminished or absent peripheral pulses; respiratory depression; an increase and/or decrease in blood pressure, usually in that order; confusion, delirium, convulsions, and coma; and/or some degree of nausea; vomiting; and abdominal pain.

DOSAGE AND ADMINISTRATION

Dihydroergotamine Mesylate should be administered in a dose of 1 mL intramuscularly at the first warning sign of headache, and repeated at 1 hour intervals to a total dose of 3 mL. Optimal results are obtained by titrating the dose over the course of several headaches to find the minimal effective dose for each patient; this dose should then be employed at onset of subsequent attacks. Where more rapid effect is desired, the intravenous route may be employed to a maximum of 2 mL. Total weekly dosage should not exceed 6 mL.

To assure constant potency, protect the ampuls from light and heat. Store and dispense below 77°F (25°C), in light-resistant containers. Administer only if clear and colorless.

J CODES

Up to 1 mg IM,IV—J1110

HOW SUPPLIED

INJECTION: 1 MG/ML

BRAND/MANUFACTURER	NDC	SIZE	AWP
○ **BRAND**			
D.H.E. 45: Sandoz Pharm	00078-0041-03	1 ml 20s	$193.80

Dihydrotachysterol

DESCRIPTION

Each tablet contains:

Dihydrotachysterol ....0.125 mg, 0.2 mg, or 0.4 mg

Each mL of oral solution contains:

Dihydrotachysterol ....0.2 mg

Dihydrotachysterol is a synthetic reduction product of tachysterol, a close isomer of vitamin D. Chemically Dihydrotachysterol is *9,10-Secoergosta-5,7,22-tri-en-3β-ol.*

Dihydrotachysterol acts as a blood calcium regulator.

Following is its chemical structure:

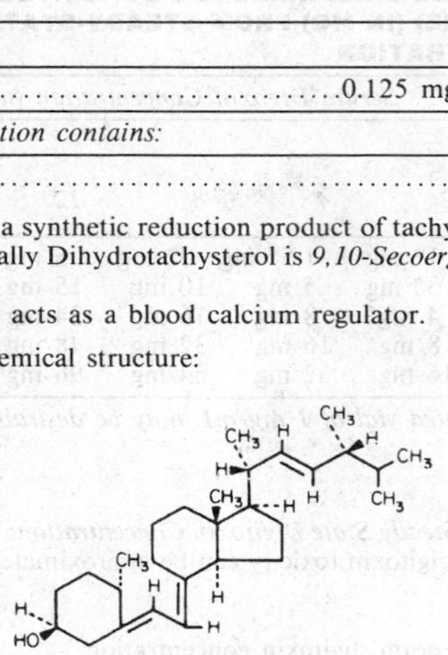

CLINICAL PHARMACOLOGY

Dihydrotachysterol is hydroxylated in the liver to 25-hydroxydihydrotachysterol, which is the major circulating active form of the drug. It does not undergo further hydroxylation by the kidney and therefore is the analogue of 1,25-dihydroxyvitamin D. Dihydrotachysterol is effective in the elevation of serum calcium by stimulating intestinal calcium absorption and mobilizing bone calcium in the absence of parathyroid hormone and of functioning renal tissue. Dihydrotachysterol also increases renal phosphate excretion. In contrast to parathyroid extract, Dihydrotachysterol is active when taken orally, exerts a slow but persistent effect, and may be used for long periods without increasing the dosage or causing tolerance. Dihydrotachysterol is faster-acting than pharmacologic doses of vitamin D and is less persistent after cessation of treatment, thus decreasing the risk of accumulation and of hypercalcemia.

INDICATIONS AND USAGE

Dihydrotachysterol is indicated for the treatment of acute, chronic, and latent forms of postoperative tetany, idiopathic tetany, and hypoparathyroidism.

UNLABELED USES
Dihydrotachysterol is used alone or as an adjunct in the treatment of renal osteodystrophy.

CONTRAINDICATIONS

Contraindicated in patiens with hypercalcemia, abnormal sensitivity to the effects of vitamin D, and hypervitaminosis D.

PRECAUTIONS

General: The difference between therapeutic dose and intoxicating dose may be small in any patient and therefore dosage must be individualized and periodically revaluated. In patients with renal osteodystrophy accompanied by hyperphosphatemia, maintenance of a normal serum phosphorus level by dietary phosphate restriction and/or administration of aluminum gels as intestinal phosphate binders is essential to prevent metastatic calcification.

Because of its effect on serum calcium, Dihydrotachysterol should be administered to pregnant patients or to patients with renal stones only when, in the judgment of the physician, the potential benefits outweigh the possible hazards.

Laboratory Tests: To prevent hypercalcemia, treatment should always be controlled by regular determination of blood calcium level, which should be maintained within the normal range.

Drug Interactions: Administration of thiazide diuretics to hypoparathyroid patients who are concurrently being treated with Dihydrotach- ysterol may cause hypercalcemia.

Pregnancy Teratogenic Effects—Pregnancy Category C: Animal reproduction studies have shown fetal abnormalities in several species associated with hypervitaminosis D. These are similar to the supravalvular aortic stenosis syndrome described in infants by Black in England (1963). This syndrome was characterized by supravalvular aortic stenosis, elfin facies, and mental retardation.

There are no adequate and well-controlled studies in pregnant women. Dihydrotachysterol should be used during pregnancy only if the potential benefit justifies the potential risk to the fetus.

Nursing Mothers: It is not known whether this drug is excreted in human milk. Because many drugs are excreted in human milk, caution should be exercised when Dihydrotachysterol is administered to a nursing woman.

OVERDOSAGE

The effect of Dihydrotachysterol can persist for up to one month after cessation of treatment.

Manifestations: Toxicity associated with Dihydrotachysterol is similar to that seen with large doses of vitamin D. Overdosage is manifested by symptoms of hypercalcemia, i.e., weakness, headache, anorexia, nausea, vomiting, abdominal cramps, diarrhea, constipation, vertigo, tinnitus, ataxia, hypotonia, lethargy, depression, amnesia, diaorientation, hallucinations, syncope, and coma. Impairment of renal function may result in polyuria, polydipsia, and albuminuria. Widespread calcification of soft tissues, including heart, blood vessels, kidneys, and lungs, can occur. Death can result from cardiovascular or renal failure.

Treatment: Treatment of overdosage consists of withdrawal of Dihydrotachysterol, bed rest, liberal intake of fluids, a low-calcium diet, and administration of a laxative. Hypercalcemic crisis with dehydration, stupor, coma, and azotemia requires more vigorous treatment. The first step should be hydration of the patient. Intravenous saline may quickly and significantly increase urinary calcium excretion. A loop diuretic (furosemide or ethacrymic acid) may be given with the saline infusion to further increase renal calcium excretion.

Other reported therapeutic measures include dialysis or the administration of citrates, sulfates, phosphates, corticosteroids, EDTA (ethylenediaminetetraacetic acids), and mithramycin via appropriate regimens.

DOSAGE AND ADMINISTRATION

The dosage depends on the nature and seriousness of the disorder and should be adapted to each individual patient. Serum calcium levels should be maintained between 9 to 10 mg per 100 mL.

The following dosage schedule will serve as a guide:

Initial Dose: 0.8 mg to 2.4 mg daily for several days.

Maintenance Dose: 0.2 mg to 1.0 mg daily as required for normal serum calcium levels. The average maintenance dose is 0.6 mg daily. This dose may be supplemented with 10 to 15 grams of calcium lactate or gluconate by mouth daily.

HOW SUPPLIED
CAPSULE: 0.125 MG

BRAND/MANUFACTURER	NDC	SIZE	AWP
○ **BRAND**			
HYTAKEROL: Sanofi Winthrop	00024-0792-02	50s	$109.41

LIQUID: 0.2 MG/ML

BRAND/MANUFACTURER	NDC	SIZE	AWP
○ **BRAND**			
DHT: Roxane	00054-3170-44	30 ml	$32.75

TABLETS: 0.125 MG

BRAND/MANUFACTURER	NDC	SIZE	AWP
○ **BRAND**			
DHT: Roxane	00054-4190-19	50s	$43.88
	00054-8172-25	100s ud	$92.86

TABLETS: 0.2 MG

BRAND/MANUFACTURER	NDC	SIZE	AWP
○ **BRAND**			
DHT: Roxane	00054-4189-25	100s	$88.64
	00054-8182-25	100s ud	$101.87

TABLETS: 0.4 MG

BRAND/MANUFACTURER	NDC	SIZE	AWP
○ **BRAND**			
DHT: Roxane	00054-4191-19	50s	$78.65

Dilacor XR *SEE* DILTIAZEM HYDROCHLORIDE

Dilantin *SEE* PHENYTOIN

Dilaudid *SEE* HYDROMORPHONE HYDROCHLORIDE

Dilaudid Cough Syrup *SEE* GUAIFENESIN AND HYDROMORPHONE HYDROCHLORIDE

Diltiazem Hydrochloride

DESCRIPTION

Diltiazem Hydrochloride is a calcium ion influx inhibitor (slow channel blocker or calcium antagonist). It is available as extended-release and sustained-release capsules, tablets, and a solution for intravenous injection or infusion.

Each extended-release capsule contains:
Diltiazem Hydrochloride ....120, 180, 240, or 300 mg

Each sustained-release capsule contains:
Diltiazem Hydrochloride ....60, 90, or 120 mg

Each tablet contains:
Diltiazem Hydrochloride ....30, 60, 90, or 120 mg

Each ml of solution for injection contains:
Diltiazem Hydrochloride ....5 mg

Chemically, Diltiazem Hydrochloride is 1,5-Benzothiazepin-4(5H)one,3-(acetyloxy)-5-[2-(dimethylamino)ethyl]-2,3-dihydro-2-4-methoxyphenyl)-, monohydrochloride, (+)-cis-.

Diltiazem Hydrochloride is a white to off-white crystalline powder with a bitter taste. It is soluble in water, methanol, and chloroform. Its molecular formula is $C_{22}H_{26}N_2O_4S\cdot HCl$ and it has a molecular weight of 450.98.

Following is its chemical structure:

CLINICAL PHARMACOLOGY

The therapeutic effects of Diltiazem HCl are believed to be related to its ability to inhibit the influx of calcium ions during membrane depolarization of cardiac and vascular smooth muscle.

MECHANISMS OF ACTION

Hypertension: Diltiazem HCl produces its antihypertensive effect primarily by relaxation of vascular smooth muscle and the resultant decrease in peripheral vascular resistance. The magnitude of blood pressure reduction is related to the degree of hypertension, thus hypertensive individuals experience an antihypertensive effect, whereas there is only a modest fall in blood pressure in normotensives.

Angina: Although precise mechanisms of its antianginal actions are still being delineated. Diltiazem HCl is believed to act in the following ways: Diltiazem HCl has been shown to produce increases in exercise tolerance, probably due to its ability to reduce myocardial oxygen demand. This is accomplished via reductions in heart rate and systemic blood pressure at submaximal and maximal work loads. Diltiazem has been shown to be a potent dilator of coronary arteries, both epicardial and subendocardial. Spontaneous and ergonovine-induced coronary artery spasm are inhibited by Diltiazem. In animal models, Diltiazem interferes with the slow inward (depolarizing) current in excitable tissue. It causes excitation-contraction uncoupling in various myocardial tissues without changes in the configuration of the action potential. Diltiazem produces relaxation of coronary vascular smooth muscle and dilation of both large and small coronary arteries at drug levels which cause little or no negative inotropic effect The resultant increases in coronary blood flow (epicardial and subendocardial) occur in ischemic and nonischemic models and are accompanied by dose-dependent decreases in systemic blood pressure and decreases in peripheral resistance.

Supraventricular Tachycardias: The therapeutic benefits of Diltiazem HCl intravenous (IV) in supraventricular tachycardias are related to its ability to slow AV nodal conduction time and prolong AV nodal refractoriness. Diltiazem HCl IV exhibits frequency (use) dependent effects on AV nodal conduction such that it may selectively reduce the heart rate during tachycardias involving the AV node with little or no effect on normal AV nodal conduction at normal heart rates.

Diltiazem HCl IV slows the ventricular rate in patients with a rapid ventricular response during atrial fibrillation or atrial flutter. Diltiazem HCl IV converts paroxysmal supraventricular tachycardia (PSVT) to normal sinus rhythm by interrupting the reentry circuit in AV nodal reentrant tachycardias and reciprocating tachycardias, eg. Wolff-Parkinson-White syndrome (WPW).

Diltiazem HCl IV prolongs the sinus cycle length. It has no effects on the sinus node recovery time or on the sinoatrial conduction time in patients without SA nodal dysfunction. Diltiazem HCl IV has no significant electrophysiologic effect on tissues in the heart that are fast sodium channel dependent, eg. His-Purkinje tissue, atrial and ventricular muscle, and extranodal accessory pathways.

HEMODYNAMIC AND ELECTROPHYSIOLOGIC EFFECTS

Like other calcium channel antagonists, Diltiazem decreases sinoatrial and atrioventricular conduction in isolated tissues and has a negative inotropic effect in isolated preparations. In the intact animal, prolongation of the AH interval can be seen at higher doses.

In man, Diltiazem prevents spontaneous and ergonovine-provoked coronary artery spasm. It causes a decrease in peripheral vascular resistance and a modest fall in blood pressure in normotensive individuals and in exercise tolerance studies in patients with ischemic heart disease, reduces the heart rate-blood pressure product for any given work load. Studies to date, primarily in patients with good ventricular function, have not revealed evidence of a negative inotropic effect; cardiac output ejection fraction, and left ventricular end diastolic pressure have not been affected. Such data have no predictive value with respect to effects in patients with poor ventricular function, and increased heart failure has been reported in patients with preexisting impairment of ventricular function. There are as yet few data on the interaction of Diltiazem and beta-blockers in patients with poor ventricular function. Resting heart rate is usually unchanged or slightly reduced by Diltiazem.

In hypertensive patients, Diltiazem HCl produces antihypertensive effects both in the supine and standing positions. In a double-blind, parallel, dose-response study utilizing doses ranging from 90 to 540 mg once daily, extended-release Diltiazem HCl lowered supine diastolic blood pressure in an apparent linear manner over the entire dose range studied. The changes in diastolic blood pressure, measured at trough, for placebo, 90 mg, 180 mg, 360 mg, and 540 mg were -2.9, -4.5. -6.1, -9.5, and -10.5 mm Hg, respectively. In two short-term, double-blind, placebo-controlled studies, 303 hypertensive patients were treated with once-daily extended-release Diltazem HCl in doses of up to 540 mg. There were no instances of greater than first-degree atrioventricular block, and the maximum increase in the PR interval was .08 seconds. No patients were prematurely discontinued from the medication due to symptoms related to prolongation of the PR interval. Postural hypotension is infrequently noted upon suddenly assuming an upright position. No reflex tachycardia is associated with the chronic antihypertensive effects. Diltiazem HCl decreases vascular resistance, increases cardiac output by increasing stroke volume, and produces a slight decrease or no change in heart rate. During dynamic exercise increases in diastolic pressure are inhibited while maximum achievable systolic pressure is usually reduced. Heart rate at maximum exercise does not change or is slightly reduced. Chronic therapy with Diltiazem HCl produces no change or an increase in plasma catecholamines. No increased activity of the renin-angiotensin-aldosterone axis has been observed. Diltiazem HCl reduces or antagonizes the renal and peripheral effects of angiotension II. Hypertensive animal models respond to Diltiazem with reductions in blood pressure and increased urinary output and natriuresis without a change in urinary sodium/potassium ratio. In man, transient natriuresis and kaliuresis have been reported, but only in high intravenous doses of 0.5 mg/kg of body weight.

In a double-blind, parallel dose response study of doses from 60 mg to 480 mg once daily, extended release Diltiazem HCl increased time to termination of exercise in a linear manner over the entire dose range studied. The improvement in time to termination of exercise utilizing a Bruce exercise protocol, measured at trough, for placebo, 60 mg, 120 mg, 240 mg, 360 mg, and 480 mg was 29, 40, 56, 51, 69 and 68 seconds, respectively. As doses of extended-release Diltiazem HCl were increased overall angina frequency was decreased, extended-release Diltiazem HCl, 180 mg once daily, or placebo was administered in a double-blind study to patients receiving concomitant treatment with long-acting nitrates and or beta-blockers. A significant increase in time to termination of exercise and a significant decrease in overall angina frequency was observed. In this trial the overall frequency of adverse events in the extended-release Diltiazem HCl treatment group was the same as the placebo group.

Intravenous Diltiazem in doses of 20 mg prolongs AH conduction time and AV node functional and effective refractory periods by approximately 20%. In a study involving single oral doses of 300 mg of Diltiazem HCL in six normal volunteers, the average maximum PR prolongation was 14% with no instances of greater than first-degree AV block. Diltiazem-associated prolongation of the AH interval is not more pronounced in patients with first-degree heart block. In patients with sick sinus syndrome, Diltiazem significantly prolongs sinus cycle length (up to 50% in some cases).

Chronic oral administration of Diltiazem HCl to patients in doses of up to 240 (tablets), 360 (sustained-release), or 540 (extended-release) mg/day has resulted in small increases in PR interval, and on occasion produces abnormal prolongation. (See *"Warnings"*).

In patients with cardiovascular disease, Diltiazem HCl injection administered intravenously in single bolus doses, followed in some cases by a continuous infusion, reduced blood pressure, systemic vascular resistance, the rate-pressure product, and coronary vascular resistance and increased coronary blood flow. In a limited number of studies of patients with compromised myocardium (severe congestive heart failure, acute myocardial infarction, hypertrophic cardiomyopathy), administration of intravenous Diltiazem produced no significant effect on contractility, left ventricular end diastolic pressure or pulmonary capillary wedge pressure. The mean ejection fraction and cardiac output/index remained unchanged or increased. Maximal hemodynamic effects usually occurred within 2 to 5 minutes of an injection. However, in rare instances, worsening of congestive heart failure has been reported in patients with preexisting impaired ventricular function.

PHARMACODYNAMICS

In one short-term, double-blind, placebo-controlled study, extended-release Diltiazem HCl 120, 240, 360 and 480 mg/day demonstrated a dose-related antihypertensive response among patients with mild to moderate hypertension. Statistically significant decreases in trough mean supine diastolic blood pressure were seen through four weeks of treatment: 120 mg/day (-5.1 mmHg); 240 mg/day (-6.9 mmHg); 360 mg/day (-6.9 mmHg); and 480 mg/day (-10.6 mmHg). Statistically significant decreases in trough mean supine systolic blood pressure were also seen through four weeks of treatment; 120 mg/day (-2.6 mmHg); 240 mg/day (-6.5 mmHg); 360 mg/day (-4.8 mmHg); and 480 mg/day (-10.6 mmHg). The proportion of evaluable patients exhibiting a therapeutic response (supine diastolic blood pressure < 90 mmHg or decrease > 10 mmHg) was greater as the dose increased: 31%, 42%, 48%, and 69% with the 120, 240, 360 and 480 mg/day Diltiazem groups, respectively. Similar findings were observed for standing systolic and diastolic blood pressures. The trough (24 hours after a dose) antihypertensive effect of extended-release Diltiazem HCl retained more than one-half of the response seen at peak (3-6 hours after administration).

Significant reductions of mean supine blood pressure (at trough) in patients with mild to moderate hypertension were also seen in a short-term, double-blind, dose-escalation, placebo-controlled study after 2 weeks of once-daily extended-release Diltiazem HCl 180 mg/day (diastolic: -6.1 mmHg; systolic: -4.7 mmHg) and again, 2 weeks after escalation to 360 mg/day (diastolic: -9.3 mmHg; systolic: -7.2 mmHg). However, a further increase in dose to 540 mg/day for 2 weeks provided only a minimal further increase in the antihypertensive effect (diastolic: -10.2 mmHg; systolic: -6.7 mmHg).

With IV administration, the prolongation of PR interval correlated significantly with plasma Diltiazem concentration in normal volunteers using the Sigmoidal E_{max} model. Changes in heart rate, systolic blood pressure, and diastolic blood pressure did not correlate with Diltiazem plasma concentrations in normal volunteers. Reduction in mean arterial pressure correlated linearly with Diltiazem plasma concentration in a group of hypertensive patients.

In patients with atrial fibrillation and atrial flutter, a significant correlation was observed between the percent reduction in HR and plasma Diltiazem concentration using the Sigmoidal E_{max} model. Based on this relationship the mean plasma Diltiazem concentration required to produce a 20% decrease in heart rate was determined to be 80 ng mL. Mean plasma Diltiazem concentrations of 130 ng mL and 300 ng mL were determined to produce reductions in heart rate of 30% and 40%.

PHARMACOKINETICS AND METABOLISM

Diltiazem is well absorbed from the gastrointestinal tract (to about 80% of a reference capsule from the tablet formulation) and is subject to an extensive first-pass effect. When given as an immediate-release oral formulation, the absolute bioavailability (compared to intravenous administration) is about 40%. After oral administration, Diltiazem HCl undergoes extensive metabolism in man by deacetylation. N-demethylation, and O-demethylation via cytochrome P-450 (oxidative metabolism) in addition to conjugation. Metabolites N-monodesmethyldiltiazem, desacetyldiltiazem, desacetyl-N-monodesmethyl- diltiazem, desacetyl-O-desmethyldiltiazem, and desacetyl-N, O-desmethyldiltiazem have been identified in human urine. Following oral administration, 2% to 4% of the unchanged Diltiazem HCl appears in the urine.

Drugs which induce or inhibit hepatic microsomal enzymes may alter Diltiazem disposition.

Following single intravenous injection of Diltiazem HCl, however, plasma concentrations of N-monodesmethyldiltiazem and desacetyldiltiazem, two principal metabolites found in plasma after oral administration, are typically not detected. These metabolites are observed, however, following 24-hour constant rate intravenous infusion.

Total radioactivity measurement following short IV administration in healthy volunteers suggests the presence of other unidentified metabolites which attain higher concentrations than those of Diltiazem and are more slowly eliminated: half-life of total radioactivity is about 20 hours compared to 2 to 5 hours for Diltiazem.

In vitro binding studies show Diltiazem HCl is 70% to 80% bound to plasma proteins. *In vitro* studies suggest alpha-acid glycoprotein binds approximately 40% of the drug at clinically significant concentrations. Albumin appears to bind approximately 30% of the drug, while other constituents bind the remaining bound fraction. Competitive *in vitro* ligand binding studies have also shown Diltiazem HCl binding is not altered by therapeutic concentrations of digoxin, hydrochlorothiazide, indomethacin, phenylbutazone, propranolol, salicylic acid tolbutamide, or warfarin. Single oral doses of 30 to 120 mg of Diltiazem Hydrochloride result in detectable plasma levels within 30 to 60 minutes and peak plasma levels two to three hours after drug administration. The plasma elimination half-life following single or multiple drug administration is approximately 3.0 to 4.5 hours. Desacetyl Diltiazem is also present in the plasma at levels of 10% to 20% of the parent drug and is 25% to 50% as potent a coronary vasodilator as Diltiazem. Minimum therapeutic plasma Diltiazem concentrations appear to be in the range of 40 or 50 to 200 ng/mL. There is a departure from linearity when dose strengths are increased: the half-life is slightly increased with dose. When single doses above 60 mg are given, a 120-mg dose gave blood levels three times that of the 60-mg dose. A study that compared patients with normal hepatic function to patients with cirrhosis found an increase in half-life and a 69% increase in bioavailability in the hepatically impaired patients. A single study in patients with severely impaired renal function showed no difference in the pharmacokinetic profile of Diltiazem compared to patients with normal renal function.

DILTIAZEM HCL EXTENDED-RELEASE CAPSULES
When compared to a regimen of Diltiazem HCl tablets at steady-state, more than 95% of drug is absorbed from the extended-release Diltiazem HCl formulation. Controlled absorption of Diltiazem begins within 1 hour, with maximum plasma concentrations being achieved 4 to 6 hours after administration. A single 360-mg dose of the capsule results in detectable plasma levels within 2 hours and peak plasma levels between 10 and 14 hours: absorption occurs throughout the dosing interval.

In-vivo release of Diltiazem occurs throughout the gastrointestinal tract, with controlled release still occurring for up to 24 hours after administration, as determined by radiolabelled methods.

The presence of food did not affect the ability of Diltiazem HCl extended-release to maintain a continuous release of drug for up to 24 hours after administration.

When extended-release Diltiazem HCl was coadministered with a high fat content breakfast, the extent of Diltiazem absorption was not affected; there was a modest effect on Diltiazem bioavailability with AUC increasing by 13% and C_{max} by 37%. Dose-dumping does not occur. The apparent elimination half-life after single or multiple dosing is 5 to 8 hours. The apparent stead-state half-life of Diltiazem following once-daily administration of Diltiazem HCl extended-release ranges from 5 to 10 hours. This prolongation of half-life is attributed to continued absorption of Diltiazem rather than to alterations in its elimination.

Neither the absolute bioavailability of Diltiazem HCl extended-release capsules nor its relative bioavailability compared to immediate release products has been definitively determined. No information is currently available as to the relative bioavailability of Diltiazem HCl extended-release capsules compared to other approved controlled-release Diltiazem products.

A departure from linearity similar to that seen with Diltiazem HCl tablets and Diltiazem HCl sustained-release capsules is observed. As the dose of Diltiazem HCl extended-release capsules is increased from a daily dose of 120 mg to 240 mg, there is an increase in the area-under-the-curve of 2.3 to 2.7 times. When the dose is increased from 240 mg to 360 mg there is an increase in the area-under-the-curve of 1.6 times and when the dose is increased from 240 mg to 480 mg, AUC increases 2.4-fold.

DILTIAZEM HCL SUSTAINED-RELEASE CAPSULES
Diltiazem is absorbed from the capsule formulation to about 92% of a reference solution at steady-state. A single 120-mg dose of the capsule results in detectable plasma levels within two to three hours and peak plasma levels at six to 11 hours. The apparent elimination half-life after single or multiple dosing is five to seven hours. A departure from linearity similar to that observed with the Diltiazem HCl tablet is observed. As the dose of Diltiazem HCl sustained-release capsules is increased from a daily dose of 120 mg (60 mg bid) to 240 mg (120 mg bid) daily,

there is an increase in area-under-the-curve of 2.6 times. When the dose is increased from 240 mg to 360 mg daily, there is an increase in the area-under-the-curve of 1.8 times. The average plasma levels of the capsule dosed twice daily at steady-state are equivalent to the tablet dosed four times daily when the same total daily dose is administered.

INTRAVENOUS DILTIAZEM HCL
Following a single intravenous injection in healthy male volunteers Diltiazem HCl appears to obey linear pharmacokinetics over a dose range of 10.5 to 21.0 mg. The plasma elimination half-life is approximately 3.4 hours. The apparent volume of distribution of Diltiazem HCl is approximately 305 L Diltiazem HCl is extensively metabolized in the liver with a systemic clearance of approximately 65 L/h.

After constant rate intravenous infusion to healthy male volunteers, Diltiazem exhibits nonlinear pharmacokinetics over an infusion range of 4.8 to 13.2 mg h for 24 hours. Over this infusion range, as the dose is increased systemic clearance decreases from 64 to 48 L/h while the plasma elimination half-life increases from 4.1 to 4.9 hours. The apparent volume of distribution remains unchanged (360 to 391 L). In patients with atrial fibrillation or atrial flutter, Diltiazem systemic clearance has been found to be decreased compared to healthy volunteers. In patients administered bolus doses ranging from 2.5 mg to 38.5 mg, systemic clearance averaged 36 L/h. In patients administered continuous infusions at 10 mg/h or 15 mg/h for 24 hours, Diltiazem systemic clearance averaged 42 L/h and 31 L/h, respectively.

Based on the results of pharmacokinetic studies in healthy volunteers administered different *oral* Diltiazem HCl formulations, constant rate intravenous infusions of Diltiazem HCl at 3, 5, 7, and 11 mg/h are predicted to produce steady-state plasma Diltiazem concentrations equivalent to 120-, 180-, 240-, and 360-mg total daily oral doses of Diltiazem HCl tablets or Diltiazem HCl sustained-release capsules.

INDICATIONS AND USAGE
Diltiazem HCl extended-release and sustained-release capsules are indicated for the treatment of hypertension. They may be used alone or in combination with other antihypertensive medications, such as diuretics.

Diltiazem HCl tablets and extended-release capsules are indicated for the management of chronic stable angina and angina due to coronary artery spasm.

Diltiazem HCl IV is indicated for the following:

1. Atrial Fibrillation or Atrial Flutter: Temporary control of rapid ventricular rate in atrial fibrillation or atrial flutter. It should not be used in patients with atrial fibrillation or atrial flutter associated with an accessory bypass tract such as in Wolff-Parkinson-White (WPW) syndrome or short PR syndrome.

2. Paroxysmal Supraventricular Tachycardia: Rapid conversion of paroxysmal supraventricular tachycardias (PSVT) to sinus rhythm. This includes AV nodal reentrant tachycardias and reciprocating tachycardias associated with an extranodal accessory pathway such as the WPW syndrome or short PR syndrome. Unless otherwise contraindicated, appropriate vagal maneuvers should be attempted prior to administration of Diltiazem HCl IV.

The use of Diltiazem HCl IV for control of ventricular response in patients with atrial fibrillation or atrial flutter or conversion to sinus rhythm in patients with PSVT should be undertaken with caution when the patient is compromised hemodynamically or is taking other drugs that decrease any or all of the following: peripheral resistance, myocardial filling, myocardial contractility, or electrical impulse propagation in the myocardium.

For either indication and particularly when employing continuous intravenous infusion, the setting should include continuous monitoring of the ECG and frequent measurement of blood pressure. A defibrillator and emergency equipment should be readily available.

In domestic controlled trials in patients with atrial fibrillation or atrial flutter, bolus administration of Diltiazem HCl IV was effective in reducing heart rate by at least 20% in 95% of patients. Diltiazem HCl IV rarely converts atrial fibrillation or atrial flutter to normal sinus rhythm. Following administration of one or two intravenous bolus doses of Diltiazem HCl IV, response usually occurs within 3 minutes and maximal heart rate reduction generally occurs in 2 to 7 minutes. Heart rate reduction may last from 1 to 3 hours. If hypotension occurs, it is generally short-lived, but may last from 1 to 3 hours.

A 24-hour continuous infusion of Diltiazem HCl IV in the treatment of atrial fibrillation or atrial flutter maintained at least a 20% heart rate reduction during the infusion in 83% of patients. Upon discontinuation of infusion, heart rate reduction may last from 0.5 hours to more than 10 hours (median duration, 7 hours). Hypotension, if it occurs, may be similarly persistent.

In the controlled clinical trials 3.2% of patients required some form of intervention (typically, use of intravenous fluids or the Trendelenburg position) for blood pressure support following Diltiazem HCl IV.

In domestic controlled trials, bolus administration of Diltiazem HCl IV was effective in converting PSVT to normal sinus rhythm in 88% of patients within 3 minutes of the first or second bolus dose.

Symptoms associated with the arrhythmia were improved in conjunction with decreased heart rate or conversion to normal sinus rhythm following administration of Diltiazem HCl IV.

UNLABELED USES
Diltiazem Hydrochloride is used alone or as an adjunct in the treatment of unstable angina, in patients with Wolff-Parkinson-White syndrome to treat reentrant arrhythmias, congestive heart failure, and hypertensive crisis. It is also used in pulmonary hypertension, hypertrophic cardiomyopathy, silent ischemia,

to prevent early reinfarction and severe angina following a non-Q-wave myocardial infarction, and in the prophylaxis of refractory migraine headache. In addition, Diltiazem Hydrochloride is also prescribed in proctalgia fugax, to reduce the frequency of involuntary movements in patients with tardive dyskinesia, to improve symptoms of chest pain and dysphagia in patients with nutcracker esophagus, and other esophageal disorders. It is also used to treat proteinuria in diabetic, hypertensive patients, in thyrotoxicosis, to overcome resistance to vincristine therapy in patients with acute lymphocytic leukemia, Raynaud's phenomenon, and to reduce acute renal failure in renal transplantation.

CONTRAINDICATIONS

Diltiazem HCl is contraindicated in:

(1) patients with sick sinus syndrome except in the presence of a functioning ventricular pacemaker.

(2) patients with second- or third-degree AV block except in the presence of a functioning ventricular pacemaker.

(3) patients with hypotension (less than 90 mm Hg systolic) or cardiogenic shock,

(4) patients who have demonstrated hypersensitivity to the drug, and

(5) patients with acute myocardial infarction and pulmonary congestion documented by x-ray on admission.

Intravenous Diltiazem and intravenous beta-blockers should not be administered together or in close proximity within a few hours.

Diltiazem HCl IV is also contraindicated in:

(6) Patients with atrial fibrillation or atrial flutter associated with an accessory bypass tract such as in WPW syndrome or short PR syndrome.

As with other agents which slow AV nodal conduction and do not prolong the refractoriness of the accessory pathway (eg, verapamil, digoxin), in rare instances patients in atrial fibrillation or atrial flutter associated with an accessory bypass tract may experience a potentially life-threatening increase in heart rate accompanied by hypotension when treated with Diltiazem HCl IV. As such, the initial use of Diltiazem HCl IV should be, if possible, in a setting where monitoring and resuscitation capabilities, including DC cardioversion/defibrillation, are present (see "Overdosage"). Once familiarity of the patient's response is established, use in an office setting may be acceptable.

(7) Patients with ventricular tachycardia. Administration of other calcium channel blockers to patients with wide complex tachycardia (QRS ≥ 0.12 seconds) has resulted in hemodynamic deterioration and ventricular fibrillation. It is important that an accurate pretreatment diagnosis distinguish wide complex QRS tachycardia of supraventricular origin from that of ventricular origin prior to administration of Diltiazem HCl IV.

WARNINGS

1. Cardiac Conduction: Diltiazem HCl prolongs AV node conduction and refractory periods that may rarely result in second- or third-degree AV block in sinus rhythm without significantly prolonging sinus node recovery time, except in patients with sick sinus syndrome. The effect may rarely result in abnormally slow heart rates particularly in patients with sick sinus syndrome or second- or third-degree AV block. Concomitant use of Diltiazem with agents known to affect cardiac conduction, e.g., beta-blockers or digitalis, may result in additive effects on cardiac conduction. A patient with Prinzmetal's angina developed periods of asystole (2 to 5 seconds) after a single dose of 60 mg of Diltiazem.

If high-degree AV block occurs in sinus rhythm, intravenous Diltiazem should be discontinued and appropriate supportive measures instituted (see "Overdosage").

2. Congestive Heart Failure: Although Diltiazem has a negative inotropic effect in isolated animal tissue preparations, hemodynamic studies in humans with normal ventricular function and in patients with a compromised myocardium, such as severe CHF acute MI and hypertrophic cardiomyopathy, have not shown a reduction in cardiac index nor consistent negative effects on contractility (dp/dt). An acute study of oral Diltiazem in patients with impaired ventricular function rejection fraction 24% ± 6% showed improvement in indices of ventricular function without significant decrease in contractile function (dp/dt). Worsening of congestive heart failure has been reported in patients with preexisting impairment of ventricular function. Experience with the use of Diltiazem HCl alone or in combination with beta-blockers or Diltiazem HCl IV in patients with impaired ventricular function is limited. Caution should be exercised when using the drug in such patients or when using this combination.

3. Hypotension: Decreases in blood pressure associated with Diltiazem HCl therapy may occasionally result in symptomatic hypotension. The use of intravenous Diltiazem for control of ventricular response in patients with supraventricular arrhythmias should be undertaken with caution when the patient is compromised hemodynamically. In addition, caution should be used in patients taking other drugs that decrease peripheral resistance, intravascular volume, myocardial contractility or conduction.

4. Acute Hepatic Injury: Mild elevations of transaminases with and without concomitant elevation in alkaline phosphatase and bilirubin have been observed in clinical studies. Such elevations were usually transient and frequently resolved even with continued Diltiazem treatment. In rare instances, significant elevations in enzymes such as alkaline phosphatase. LDH, SGOT, SGPT, and other phenomena consistent with acute hepatic injury have been noted following oral Diltiazem HCl. Therefore, the potential for acute hepatic injury exists following administration of intravenous Diltiazem. These reactions tended to occur early after therapy initiation (1 to 6 or 8 weeks) and have been reversible upon

discontinuation of drug therapy. The relationship to Diltiazem HCl is uncertain in some cases, but probable in some. (See "Precautions".)

5. Ventricular Premature Beats (VPBs): VPBs may be present on conversion of PSVT to sinus rhythm with Diltiazem HCl IV. These VPBs are transient, are typically considered to be benign, and appear to have no clinical significance. Similar ventricular complexes have been noted during cardioversion, other pharmacologic therapy, and during spontaneous conversion of PSVT to sinus rhythm.

PRECAUTIONS

GENERAL

Diltiazem HCl is extensively metabolized by the liver and excreted by the kidneys and in bile. As with any drug given over prolonged periods, laboratory parameters of renal and hepatic function should be monitored at regular intervals. The drug should be used with caution in patients with impaired renal or hepatic function. In subacute and chronic dog and rat studies designed to produce toxicity, high oral doses of Diltiazem were associated with hepatic damage. In special subacute hepatic studies, oral doses of 125 mg/kg and higher in rats were associated with histological changes in the liver which were reversible when the drug was discontinued. In dogs, doses of 20 mg/kg were also associated with hepatic changes; however, these changes were reversible with continued dosing. High intravenous dosages (4.5 mg/kg tid) administered to dogs resulted in significant bradycardia and alterations in AV conduction.

Dermatological events (see "Adverse Reactions" section) may be transient and may disappear despite continued use of Diltiazem HCl. However, skin eruptions progressing to erythema multiforme and/or exfoliative dermatitis have also been infrequently reported following oral Diltiazem. Therefore, the potential for these dermatologic reactions exists following exposure to intravenous Diltiazem. Should a dermatologic reaction persist, the drug should be discontinued.

Information for Patients: Diltiazem HCl extended-release capsules should be taken on an empty stomach. Patients should be cautioned that Diltiazem HCl extended-release capsules should not be opened, chewed or crushed, and should be swallowed whole.

DRUG INTERACTIONS

Due to the potential for additive effects, caution and careful titration are warranted in patients receiving Diltiazem HCl concomitantly with other agents known to affect cardiac contractility and or conduction. (See "Warnings".) Pharmacologic studies indicate that there may be additive effects in prolonging AV conduction when using beta-blockers or digitalis concomitantly with Diltiazem HCl. (See "Warnings".)

As with all drugs, care should be exercised when treating patients with multiple medications. Diltiazem HCl undergoes biotransformation by cytochrome P-450 mixed function oxidase. Coadministration of Diltiazem HCl with other agents which follow the same route of biotransformation may result in the competitive inhibition of metabolism.

Especially in patients with renal and/or hepatic impairment, dosages of similarly metabolized drugs, particularly those of low therapeutic ratio, may require adjustment when starting or stopping concomitantly administered Diltiazem HCl to maintain optimum therapeutic blood levels. stopping concomitantly administered diltiazem to maintain optimum therapeutic blood levels.

Beta-blockers: Controlled and uncontrolled domestic studies suggest that concomitant use of Diltiazem HCl and beta-blockers is usually well tolerated, but available data are not sufficient to predict the effects of concomitant treatment in patients with left ventricular dysfunction or cardiac conduction abnormalities.

Administration of oral Diltiazem HCl concomitantly with propranolol in five normal volunteers resulted in increased propranolol levels in all subjects and bioavailability of propranolol was increased approximately 50%. *In vitro,* propranolol appears to be displaced from its binding sites by Diltiazem. If combination therapy is initiated or withdrawn in conjunction with propranolol, an adjustment in the propranolol dose may be warranted (See "Warnings").

Intravenous Diltiazem has been administered to patients on chronic oral beta-blocker therapy. The combination of the two drugs was generally well tolerated without serious adverse effects. If intravenous Diltiazem is administered to patients receiving chronic oral beta-blocker therapy, the possibility for bradycardia. AV block and/or depression of contractility should be considered (see "Contraindications").

Cimetidine: A study in six healthy volunteers has shown a significant increase in peak Diltiazem plasma levels (58%) and area-under-the-curve (53%) after a 1-week course of cimetidine at 1200 mg per day and a single dose of Diltiazem 60 mg. Ranitidine produced smaller, nonsignificant increases. The effect may be mediated by cimetidine's known inhibition of hepatic cytochrome P-450, the enzyme system responsible for the first-pass metabolism of Diltiazem. Patients currently receiving Diltiazem therapy should be carefully monitored for a change in pharmacological effect when initiating and discontinuing therapy with cimetidine. An adjustment in the Diltiazem dose may be warranted.

Digitalis: Administration of Diltiazem HCl with digoxin in 24 healthy male subjects increased plasma digoxin concentrations approximately 20%. Another investigator found no increase in digoxin levels in 12 patients with coronary artery disease. Since there have been conflicting results regarding the effect of digoxin levels, it is recommended that digoxin levels be monitored when initiating, adjusting, and discontinuing Diltiazme HCl therapy to avoid possible over or under-digitalization. (See "Warnings").

Intravenous Diltiazem has been administered to patients receiving either intravenous or oral Digitalis therapy. The combination of the two drugs was well tolerated without serious adverse effects. However, since both drugs affect AV nodal conduction, patients should be monitored for excessive slowing of the heart rate and or AV block.

Anesthetics: The depression of cardiac contractility, conductivity, and automaticity as well as the vascular dilation associated with anesthetics may be potentiated by calcium channel blockers. When used concomitantly, anesthetics and calcium blockers should be titrated carefully.

Cyclosporine: A pharmacokinetic interaction between Diltiazem and cyclosporine has been observed during studies involving renal and cardic transplant patients. In renal and cardiac transplant recipients, a reduction of cyclosporine dose ranging from 15% to 48% was necessary to maintain cyclosporine trough concentrations similar to those seen prior to the addition of Diltiazem. If these agents are to be administered concurrently, cyclosporine concentrations should be monitored, especially when Diltiazem therapy is initiated, adjusted, or discontinued.

The effect of cyclosporine on Diltiazem plasma concentrations has not been evaluated.

Carbamazepine: Concomitant administration of Diltiazem with carbamazepine has been reported to result in elevated serum levels of carbamazepine (40% to 72% increase) resulting in toxicity in some cases. Patients receiving these drugs concurrently should be monitored for a potential drug interaction.

CARCINOGENESIS, MUTAGENESIS, IMPAIRMENT OF FERTILITY
A 24-month study in rats at oral dosage levels of up to 100 mg/kg/day and a 21-month study in mice at oral dosage levels of up to 30 mg/kg/day showed no evidence of carcinogenicity. There was no mutagenic response *in vitro* or *in vivo* in mammalian cell assays or *in vitro* in bacteria. No evidence of impaired fertility was observed in a study performed in male and female rats at oral dosages of up to 100 mg/kg/day.

PREGNANCY
Category C: Reproduction studies have been conducted in mice, rats, and rabbits. Administration of oral doses ranging from four to ten times greater (on a mg/kg basis) than the daily recommended oral antianginal therapeutic dose has resulted in embryo and fetal lethality. These doses, in some studies, have been reported to cause skeletal abnormalities and abnormalities of the heart, retina, and tongue. In the perinatal/postnatal studies, there was some reduction in early individual pup weights and survival rates. There was an increase incidence of stillbirths at doses of 20 times the human oral antianginal dose or greater. There are no well-controlled studies in pregnant women: therefore, use Diltiazem HCl in pregnant women only if the potential benefit justifies the potential risk to the fetus.

NURSING MOTHERS
Diltiazem is excreted in human milk. One report with oral Diltiazem suggests that concentrations in breast milk may approximate serum levels. If use of Diltiazem HCl is deemed essential, an alternative method of infant feeding should be instituted.

PEDIATRIC USE
Safety and effectiveness in children have not been established.

ADVERSE REACTIONS
Serious adverse reactions have been rare in studies carried out to date, but it should be recognized that patients with impaired ventricular function and cardiac conduction abnormalities have usually been excluded from these studies.

In domestic placebo-controlled angina trials, the incidence of adverse reactions reported during Diltiazem HCl therapy was not greater than that reported during placebo therapy.

The following table presents the most common adverse reactions reported in placebo-controlled angina and hypertension trials in patients receiving extended-release Diltiazem HCl up to 360 mg with rates in placebo patients shown for comparison.

DILTIAZEM HCL EXTENDED-RELEASE CAPSULE PLACEBO-CONTROLLED ANGINA AND HYPERTENSION TRIALS COMBINED

Adverse Reaction	Extended-release Diltiazem HCl N = 607	Placebo N = 301
Headache	5.4%	5.0%
Dizziness	3.0%	3.0%
Bradycardia	3.3%	1.3%
AV Block First Degree	3.3%	0.0%
Edema	2.6%	1.3%
ECG Abnormality	1.6%	2.3%
Asthenia	1.8%	1.7%

The most common adverse events (frequency ≥ 1%) in placebo-controlled clinical hypertension studies with extended-release Diltiazem HCl using daily doses up to 540 mg are listed in the table below with placebo-treated patients included for comparison.

MOST COMMON ADVERSE EVENTS IN DOUBLE-BLIND, PLACEBO-CONTROLLED HYPERTENSION TRIALS

Adverse Events (COSTART Term)	Extended-release Diltiazem HCl N = 303 - pts (%)	Placebo N = 87 - pts (%)
rhinitis	29 (9.6)	7 (8.0)
headache	27 (8.9)	12 (13.8)
pharyngitis	17 (5.6)	4 (4.6)
constipation	11 (3.6)	2 (2.3)
cough increase	9 (3.0)	2 (2.3)
flu syndrome	7 (2.3)	1 (1.1)
edema peripheral	7 (2.3)	0 (0.0)
myalgia	7 (2.3)	0 (0.0)
diarrhea	6 (2.0)	0 (0.0)
vomiting	6 (2.0)	0 (0.0)
sinusitis	6 (2.0)	1 (1.1)
asthenia	5 (1.7)	0 (0.0)
pain, back	5 (1.7)	2 (2.3)
nausea	5 (1.7)	1 (1.1)
dyspepsia	4 (1.3)	0 (0.0)
vasodilatation	4 (1.3)	0 (0.0)
injury, accident	4 (1.3)	0 (0.0)
pain, abdominal	3 (1.0)	0 (0.0)
arthrosis	3 (1.0)	0 (0.0)
insomnia	3 (1.0)	0 (0.0)
dyspnea	3 (1.0)	0 (0.0)
rash	3 (1.0)	1 (1.1)
tinnitus	3 (1.0)	0 (0.0)

* Adverse events occurring in 1% or more of patients receiving extended-release Diltiazem HCl.

The adverse events described below represent events observed in clinical studies of hypertensive patients receiving either Diltiazem HCl tablets or Diltiazem HCl sustained-release capsules as well as experiences observed in studies of angina and during marketing. The most common events in hypertension studies are shown in a table with rates in placebo patients shown for comparison. Less common events are listed by body system; these include any adverse reactions seen in angina studies that were not observed in hypertension studies in all hypertensive patients studied (over 900), the most common adverse events were edema (9%), headache (8%), dizziness (6%), asthenia (5%), sinus bradycardia (3%), flushing (3%), and first degree AV block (3%). Only edema and perhaps bradycardia and dizziness were dose related. The most common events observed in clinical studies (over 2,100 patients) of angina patients and hypertensive patients receiving Diltiazem HCl tablets or Diltiazem HCl sustained-release capsules were (ie. greater than 1% edema (5.4%), headache (4.5%), dizziness (3.4%) asthenia (2.8%), first degree AV block (1.8%), flushing (1.7%), nausea (1.6%), bradycardia (1.5%), and rash (1.5%).

DOUBLE BLIND PLACEBO CONTROLLED HYPERTENSION TRIALS

Adverse Events	Diltiazem N = 315 - pts (%)	Placebo N = 211 - pts (%)
Headache	38 (12%)	17 (8%)
AV block first degree	24 (7.6%)	4 (1.9%)
Dizziness	22 (7%)	6 (2.8%)
Edema	19 (6%)	2 (0.9%)
Bradycardia	19 (6%)	3 (1.4%)
ECG abnormality	13 (4.1%)	3 (1.4%)
Asthenia	10 (3.2%)	1 (0.5%)
Constipation	5 (1.6%)	2 (0.9%)
Dyspepsia	4 (1.3%)	1 (0.5%)
Nausea	4 (1.3%)	2 (0.9%)
Palpitations	4 (1.3%)	2 (0.9%)
Polyuria	4 (1.3%)	2 (0.9%)
Somnolence	4 (1.3%)	—
Alk phos increase	3 (1%)	1 (0.5%)
Hypotension	3 (1%)	1 (0.5%)
Insomnia	3 (1%)	1 (0.5%)
Rash	3 (1%)	1 (0.5%)
AV block second degree	2 (0.6%)	—

In clinical trials of Diltiazem HCl extended-release capsules, Diltiazem HCl tablets, and Diltiazem HCl sustained-release capsules involving over 3200 patients, the most common events (ie, greater than 1% were edema (4.6%), headache (4.6%), dizziness (3.5%), asthenia (2.6%), first degree AV block (2.4%), bradycardia (1.7%), flushing (1.4%), nausea (1.4%), and rash (1.2%). Percentages vary in other studies.

In addition, the following events were reported infrequently (less than 1%) in angina or hypertension trials.

Cardiovascular: Angina, arrhythmia AV block (first, second-or third-degree), bradycardia bundle branch block, congestive heart failure, ECG abnormalities, flushing, hypotension, postural hypotension, pallor, palpitations, phlebitis, ST elevation, syncope, tachycardia, ventricular extrasystoles.

Nervous System: Abnormal dreams, amnesia, depression, dizziness, gait abnormality, hallucinations, hypertonia, insomnia, nervousness, paresthesia, personality change, somnolence, tinnitus, tremor vertigo.

Gastrointestinal: Anorexia, constipation, diarrhea, dry mouth, dysgeusia, dyspepsia, eructation, mild elevations of SGOT, SGPT, LDH, and alkaline phosphatase (see *"Hepatic Warnings"*), thirst, tooth disorder, vomiting, weight increase.

Dermatological: Petechiae, photosensitivity, pruritus, skin hypertrophy (nevus), sweating, urticaria.

Respiratory System: Epistaxis, bronchitis, respiratory disorder.

Urogenital System: Cystitis, kidney calculus, impotence, dysmenorrhea, vaginitis, prostate disease.

Metabolic and Nutritional Disorders: Gout, edema.

Musculoskeletal System: Arthralgia, bursitis, bone pain.

Hemic and Lymphatic System: Lymphadenopathy.

Body as a Whole: Pain, unevaluable reaction, neck pain, neck rigidity, fever, chest pain, malaise.

Other: Amblyopia, CPK increase, dyspnea, ear pain, epistaxis, eye irritation, hyperglycemia, hyperuricemia, impotence, muscle cramps, nasal congestion, nocturia, osteoarticular pain, polyuria, sexual difficulties.

The following postmarketing events have been reported infrequently in patients receiving Diltiazem HCl: alopecia, erythema multiforme, exfoliative dermatitis, extrapyramidal symptoms, gingival hyperplasia, hemolytic anemia, increased bleeding time, leukopenia, purpura, retinopathy, and thrombocytopenia. In addition, events such as myocardial infarction have been observed which are not readily distinguishable from the natural history of the disease in these patients. A number of well-documented cases of generalized rash, characterized as leukocyloclastic vasculitis, have been reported. However, a definitive cause and effect relationship between these events and Diltiazem HCl therapy is yet to be established.

The following adverse reaction rates are based on the use of Diltiazem HCl IV in over 400 domestic clinical trial patients with atrial fibrillation/flutter or PSVT under double-blind or open-label conditions. Worldwide experience in over 1,300 patients was similar.

Adverse events reported in controlled and uncontrolled clinical trials were generally mild and transient. Hypotension was the most commonly reported adverse event during clinical trials. Asymptomatic hypotension occurred in 4.3% of patients. Symptomatic hypotension occurred in 3.2% of patients. When treatment for hypotension was required, it generally consisted of administration of saline or placing the patient in the Trendelenburg position. Other events reported in at least 1% of the Diltiazem-treated patients were injection site reactions (eg. itching, burning—3.9%, vasodilation (flushing)—1.7%, and arrhythmia (junctional rhythm or isorhythmic dissociation)—1.0%.

In addition, the following events were reported infrequently (less than 1%):

Cardiovascular: Atrial flutter, AV block first degree, AV block second degree, bradycardia, chest pain, congestive heart failure, sinus pause, sinus node dysfunction, syncope, ventricular arrhythmia, ventricular fibrillation, ventricular tachycardia.

Dermatologic: Pruritus, sweating.

Gastrointestinal: Constipation, elevated SGOT or alkaline phosphatase, nausea, vomiting.

Nervous System: Dizziness, paresthesia.

Other: Amblyopia, asthenia, dry mouth, dyspnea, edema, headache, hyperuricemia.

Although not observed in clinical trials with Diltiazem HCl IV other reactions associated with oral Diltiazem may occur.

OVERDOSAGE

The oral LD$_{50}$'s in mice and rats range from 415 to 740 mg/kg and from 560 to 810 mg kg respectively. The intravenous LD$_{50}$'s is these species were 60 and 38 mg kg, respectively. The oral LD$_{50}$ in dogs is considered to be in excess of 50 mg kg, while lethality was seen in monkeys at 360 mg/kg. The toxic dose in man not known. Due to extensive metabolism, blood levels after a standard dose of Diltiazem can vary over tenfold, limiting the usefulness of blood levels in overdose cases.

There have been 29 reports of Diltiazem overdose in doses ranging from less than 1 gm to 10.8 gm. Sixteen of these reports involved multiple drug ingestions.

Twenty-two reports indicated patients had recovered from Dilitiazem overdose ranging from less than 1 gm to 10.8 gm. There were seven reports with a fatal outcome: although the amount of Diltiazem ingested was unknown, multiple drug ingestions were confirmed in six of the seven reports.

Events observed following Diltiazem overdose included bradycardia, hypotension, heart block, and cardiac failure. Most reports of overdose described some supportive medical measure and/or drug treatment. The administration of ipecac to induce vomiting and activated charcoal to reduce drug absorption have been advocated as initial means of intervention. Bradycardia frequently responded favorably to atropine as did heart block, although cardiac pacing was also frequently utilized to treat heart block. Fluids and vasopressors were used to maintain blood pressure, and in cases of cardiac failure, inotropic agents were administered. In addition, some patients received treatment with ventilatory support, gastric lavage, and/or intravenous calcium. Evidence of the effectiveness of intravneous calcium administration to reverse the pharmacological effects of Diltiazem overdose was conflicting.

Charcoal hemoperfusion has been used successfully as an adjunct therapy to hasten drug elimination. Overdoses with as much of 10.8 gm of oral Diltiazem have been successfully treated using appropriate supportive care.

In the event of overdose or exaggerated response, appropriate supportive measures should be employed in addition to gastrointestinal decontamination. Diltiazem does not appear to be removed by peritoneal or hemodialysis. Based on the known pharmacological effects of Diltiazem and/or reported clinical experiences, the following measures may be considered.

Bradycardia: Administer atropine (0.60 to 1.0 mg). If there is no response to vagal blockade, administer isoproterenol cautiously.

High-degree AV Block: Treat as for bradycardia above Fixed high-degree AV block should be treated with cardiac pacing.

Cardiac Failure: Administer inotropic agents (isoproterenol, dopamine, or dobutamine) and diuretics.

Hypotension: Vasopressors (eg., dopamine or levarterenol bitartrate).

Actual treatment and dosage should depend on the severity of the clinical situation and the judgement and experience of the treating physician.

DOSAGE AND ADMINISTRATION

Extended-release capsules patients controlled on Diltiazem alone or in combination with other medications may be switched to Diltiazem HCl extended-release capsules at the nearest equivalent total daily dose. Higher doses of extended-release Diltiazem HCl may be needed in some patients. Patients should be closely monitored. Subsequent titration to higher or lower doses may be necessary and should be intiated as clinically warranted. There is limited general clinical experience with doses above 360 mg, but doses to 540 mg have been studied in clinical trials. The incidence of side effects increases as the dose increases with first-degree AV block, dizziness, and sinus bradycardia bearing the strongest relationship to dose.

Hypotension: Dosage needs to be adjusted by titration to individual patient needs. When used as monotherapy reasonable starting doses are 180 to 240 mg once daily, although individual patients, particularly ≥ 60 years of age, may respond to a lower dose of 120 mg. Maximum hypertensive effect is usually observed by 14 days of chronic therapy, therefore, dosage adjustments should be scheduled accordingly the usual dosage range studied in clinical trials was 180 mg to 480 mg once daily. Although current clinical experience with the 540 mg dose is limited, the dose may be increased to 540 mg with little or no increased risk of adverse reactions.

While a dose of extended-release Diltiazem HCl given once-daily may produce an antihypertensive effect similar to the same total daily dose given in divided doses, individual dose adjustment may be needed.

Administration: Studies have shown a slight increase in the rate of absorption of extended-release Diltiazem HCl when ingested with a high-fat breakfast: therefore, administration in the morning on an empty stomach is recommended.

Patients should be cautioned that the extended-release Diltiazem HCl capsules should not be opened, chewed or crushed, and should be swallowed whole.

Angina: Dosages for the treatment of angina should be adjusted to each patient's needs, starting with a dose of 120 or 180 mg once daily. Individual patients may respond to higher doses of up to 480 mg once daily. When necessary, titration may be carried out over a 7 to 14 day period.

CONCOMITANT USE WITH OTHER CARDIOVASCULAR AGENTS

1. Sublingual NTG: may be taken as required to abort acute anginal attacks during Diltiazem HCl therapy.

2. Prophylactic Nitrate Therapy: Diltiazem HCl may be safely coadministered with short- and long-acting nitrates.

3. Beta-blockers: (see *"Warnings"* and *"Precautions"*)

4. Antihypertensives: Diltiazem HCl has an additive antihypertensive effect when used with other antihypertensive agents. Therefore, the dosage of Diltiazem HCl or the concomitant antihypertensives may need to be adjusted when adding one to the other.

SUSTAINED-RELEASE CAPSULES

Dosages must be adjusted to each patient's needs, starting with 60 to 120 mg twice daily. Maximum antihypertensive effect is usually observed by 14 days of chronic therapy: therefore, dosage adjustments should be scheduled accordingly. Although individual patients may respond to lower doses, the usual optimum dosage range in clinical trials was 240 to 360 mg/day.

Diltiazem HCl has an additive antihypertensive effect when used with other antihypertensive agents. Therefore, the dosage of Diltiazem HCl or the concomitant antihypertensives may need to be adjusted when adding one to the other. (See *"Warnings"* and *"Precautions"*) regarding use with beta-blockers.

Exertional Angina Pectoris Due to Atherosclerotic Coronary Artery Disease or Angina Pectoris at Rest Due to Coronary Artery Spasm: Dosage must be adjusted to each patient's needs. Starting with 30 mg four times daily, before meals and at bedtime, dosage should be increased gradually (given in divided doses three or four times daily) at one- to two-day intervals until optimum response is obtained. Although individual patients may respond to any dosage level, the average optimum dosage range appears to be 180 to 360 mg/day. There are no available data concerning dosage requirements in patients with impaired renal or hepatic function. If the drug must be used in such patients, titration should be carried out with particular caution.

CONCOMITANT USE WITH OTHER CARDIOVASCULAR AGENTS

1. Sublingual NTG: may be taken as required to abort acute anginal attacks during Diltiazem HCl therapy.

2. Prophylactic Nitrate Therapy: Diltiazem HCl may be safely coadministered with short- and long-acting nitrates, but there have been no controlled studies to evaluate the antianginal effectiveness of this combination.

3. Beta-blockers: (see *"Warnings"* and *"Precautions"*)

IV INJECTION

Direct Intravenous Single Injections (Bolus): The initial dose of Diltiazem HCl IV should be 0.25 mg kg actual body weight as a bolus administered over 2 minutes (20 mg is a reasonable dose for the average patient). If response is inadequate, a second dose may be administered after 15 minutes. The second bolus dose of Diltiazem HCl IV should be 0.35 mg/kg actual body weight administered over 2 minutes (25 mg is a reasonable dose for the average patient). Subsequent intravenous bolus doses should be individualized for each patient. Patients with low body weights should be dosed on a mg/kg basis. Some patients may respond to an initial dose of 0.15 mg/kg, although duration of action may be shorter. Experience with this dose is limited.

Continuous Intravenous Infusion: For continued reduction of the heart rate up to 24 hours) in patients with atrial fibrillation or atrial flutter, an intravenous infusion of Diltiazem HCl IV may be administered. Immediately following bolus administration of 20 mg (0.25 mg/kg) or 25 mg (0.35 mg/kg) Diltiazem HCl IV and reduction of heart rate, begin an intravenous infusion of Diltiazem HCl IV. The recommended initial infusion rate of Diltiazem HCl IV is 10 mg/h. Some patients may maintain response to an initial rate of 5 mg/h. The infusion rate may be increased in 5 mg/h increments up to 15 mg/h as needed, if further reduction in heart rate is required. The infusion may be maintained for up to 24 hours. Diltiazem shows dose-dependent, non-linear pharmacokinetics. Duration of infusion longer than 24 hours and infusion rates greater than 15 mg/h have not been studied. Therefore, infusion duration exceeding 24 hours and infusion rates exceeding 15 mg/h are not recommended.

Dilution: To prepare Diltiazem HCl IV for continuous intravenous infusion aseptically transfer the appropriate quantity (see chart) of Diltiazem HCl IV to the desired volume of either normal saline. DSW, or D5W/0.45% NaCl. Mix thoroughly. Use within 24 hours. Keep refrigerated until use.

Diluent Volume	Quantity of Diltiazem HCl Injection	Final Concentration	Administration Dose*	Infusion Rate
100 mL	125 mg (25 mL)	1.0 mg/mL	10 mg/h 15 mg/h	10 mL/h 15 mL/h
250 mL	250 mg (50 mL)	0.83 mg/mL	10 mg/h 15 mg/h	12 mL/h 18 mL/h
500 mL	250 mg/ 50 mL	0.45 mg/mL	10 mg/h 15 mg/h	22 mL/h 33 mL/h

* 5 mg/h may be appropriate for some patients

Diltiazem HCl IV was tested for compatibility with three commonly used intravenous fluids at a maximal concentration of 1 mg Diltiazem HCl per ml Diltiazem HCl IV was found to be physically compatible and chemically stable in the following parenteral solutions for at least 24 hours when stored in glass or polyvinyl-chloride (PVC) bags at controlled room temperature 15-30°C (59-86°F) or under refrigeration 2-8°C (36-46°F).

- dextrose (5%) injection USP
- sodium chloride (0.9%) injection USP
- dextrose (5%) and sodium chloride (0.45%) injection USP

Because of potential physical incompatibilities, it is recommended that Diltiazem HCl IV not be mixed with any other drugs in the same container.

If possible, it is recommended that Diltiazem HCl IV not be co-infused in the same intravenous line.

Physical incompatibilities (precipitate formation or cloudiness) were observed when Diltiazem HCl IV was infused in the same intravenous line with the following drugs: acetazolamide, acyclovir, aminophylline, ampicillin, ampicillin sodium, sulbactam sodium, cefamandole, cefoperazone, diazepam, furosemide, hydrocortisone sodium succinate, insulin, (regular: 100 units/mL), methylprednisolone, sodium succinate, mezlocillin, nafcillin, phenytoin, rifampin, and sodium bicarbonate.

Parenteral drug products should be inspected visually for particulate matter and discoloration prior to administration whenever solution and container permit.

Translation to Further Antiarrhythmic Therapy: Transition to other antiarrhythmic agents following administration of Diltiazem HCl IV is generally safe. However, reference should be made to the respective agent manufacturer's package insert for information relative to dosage and administration.

In controlled clinical trials, therapy with antiarrhythmic agents to maintain reduced heart rate in atrial fibrillation or atrial flutter or for prophylaxis of PSVT was generally started within 3 hours after bolus administration of Diltiazem HCl IV. These antiarrhythmic agents were intravenous or oral digoxin, Class I

antiarrhythmics (eg. quinidine, procainamide), calcium channel blockers, and oral beta-blockers.

Experience in the use of antiarrhythmic agents following maintenance infusion of Diltiazem HCl IV is limited. Patients should be dosed on an individual basis and reference should be made to the respective manufacturer's package insert for information relative to dosage and administration.

STORAGE CONDITIONS

Store at controlled room temperature 58-86°F 15-80°C.

Store injection under refrigeration 2-8°C (36-46°F). Do not freeze; may be stored at room temperature for up to 1 month. Destroy after 1 month at room temperature.

HOW SUPPLIED

CAPSULE, EXTENDED RELEASE: 60 MG

AVERAGE UNIT PRICE (AVAILABLE SIZES)		GENERIC A-RATED AVERAGE PRICE (GAAP)	
BRAND	$0.85	100s	$74.92
GENERIC	$0.78		
HCFA FUL (100s ea)	$0.71		

BRAND/MANUFACTURER	NDC	SIZE	AWP
◆ BRAND			
➤ CARDIZEM SR: Marion Merrell Dow	00088-1777-47	100s	$80.00
	00088-1777-49	100s ud	$89.75
◆ GENERICS			
Medirex	57480-0804-06	30s	$25.78
Major	00904-7840-60	100s	$69.20
Lemmon	00093-0021-01	100s	$69.60
Medirex	57480-0804-01	100s	$85.95

CAPSULE, EXTENDED RELEASE: 90 MG

AVERAGE UNIT PRICE (AVAILABLE SIZES)		GENERIC A-RATED AVERAGE PRICE (GAAP)	
BRAND	$0.97	100s	$85.45
GENERIC	$0.88		
HCFA FUL (100s ea)	$0.81		

BRAND/MANUFACTURER	NDC	SIZE	AWP
◆ BRAND			
➤ CARDIZEM SR: Marion Merrell Dow	00088-1778-47	100s	$91.50
	00088-1778-49	100s ud	$102.81
◆ GENERICS			
Medirex	57480-0805-06	30s	$29.08
Major	00904-7841-60	100s	$79.20
Lemmon	00093-0022-01	100s	$80.20
Medirex	57480-0805-01	100s ud	$96.95

CAPSULE, EXTENDED RELEASE: 120 MG

AVERAGE UNIT PRICE (AVAILABLE SIZES)		GENERIC A-RATED AVERAGE PRICE (GAAP)	
BRAND	$1.27	100s	$103.70
GENERIC	$1.04		

BRAND/MANUFACTURER	NDC	SIZE	AWP
◆ BRAND			
➤ CARDIZEM SR: Marion Merrell Dow	00088-1779-47	100s	$119.19
	00088-1779-49	100s ud	$133.81
◆ GENERICS			
Major	00904-7842-60	100s	$103.15
Lemmon	00093-0023-01	100s	$104.25

CAPSULE, EXTENDED RELEASE: 120 MG

BRAND/MANUFACTURER	NDC	SIZE	AWP
◇ BRAND			
➤ CARDIZEM CD: Marion Merrell Dow	00088-1795-30	30s	$31.32
	00088-1795-42	90s	$89.34
➤ DILACOR XR: RPR	00075-0250-00	100s	$92.62
➤ CARDIZEM CD: Marion Merrell Dow	00088-1795-49	100s ud	$99.06
	00088-1795-90	5000s	$4963.74

CAPSULE, EXTENDED RELEASE: 120 MG

BRAND/MANUFACTURER	NDC	SIZE	AWP
○ BRAND			
➤ DILACOR XR: RPR	00075-0250-99	1000s	$852.00
○ GENERICS			
Allscrips	54569-3786-00	30s	$31.28
Aligen	00405-4349-01	100s	$104.21

CAPSULE, EXTENDED RELEASE: 180 MG

BRAND/MANUFACTURER	NDC	SIZE	AWP
◇ BRAND			
➤ CARDIZEM CD: Marion Merrell Dow	00088-1796-30	30s	$38.82
➤ CARDIZEM CD: Marion Merrell Dow	00088-1796-42	90s	$107.82
➤ DILACOR XR: RPR	00075-0251-00	100s	$103.86
	00075-0251-62	100s ud	$109.08
➤ CARDIZEM CD: Marion Merrell Dow	00088-1796-49	100s ud	$119.10
	00088-1796-90	5000s	$5991.24

➤ SHOWN IN PRODUCT IDENTIFICATION GUIDE

CAPSULE, EXTENDED RELEASE: 180 MG

BRAND/MANUFACTURER	NDC	SIZE	AWP
○ BRAND			
➤ DILACOR XR: RPR	00075-0251-99	1000s	$955.54

CAPSULE, EXTENDED RELEASE: 240 MG

BRAND/MANUFACTURER	NDC	SIZE	AWP
◇ BRAND			
➤ CARDIZEM CD: Marion Merrell Dow	00088-1797-30	30s	$52.62
	00088-1797-42	90s	$152.94
➤ DILACOR XR: RPR	00075-0252-00	100s	$103.86
	00075-0252-62	100s	$109.08
➤ CARDIZEM CD: Marion Merrell Dow	00088-1797-49	100s ud	$169.26
	00088-1797-90	5000s	$8499.24

CAPSULE, EXTENDED RELEASE: 240 MG

BRAND/MANUFACTURER	NDC	SIZE	AWP
○ BRAND			
➤ DILACOR XR: RPR	00075-0252-99	1000s	$955.54

CAPSULE, EXTENDED RELEASE: 300 MG

BRAND/MANUFACTURER	NDC	SIZE	AWP
○ BRAND			
➤ CARDIZEM CD: Marion Merrell Dow	00088-1798-30	30s	$68.94
	00088-1798-42	90s	$198.12
	00088-1798-49	100s ud	$218.16
	00088-1798-90	5000s	$11007.24

INJECTION: 5 MG/ML

BRAND/MANUFACTURER	NDC	SIZE	AWP
○ BRAND			
CARDIZEM: Marion Merrell Dow	00088-1790-32	5 ml 6s	$77.82
	00088-1790-33	10 ml 6s	$144.00

TABLET: 30 MG

AVERAGE UNIT PRICE (AVAILABLE SIZES)		GENERIC A-RATED AVERAGE PRICE (GAAP)	
BRAND	$0.45	100s	$37.68
GENERIC	$0.37	500s	$178.53
HCFA FUL (100s ea)	$0.12	1000s	$318.42

BRAND/MANUFACTURER	NDC	SIZE	AWP
◆ BRAND			
➤ CARDIZEM: Marion Merrell Dow	00088-1771-47	100s	$43.50
	00088-1771-49	100s ud	$49.19
	00088-1771-55	500s	$213.56
	00088-1771-90	5000s	$2135.88
◆ GENERICS			
Aligen	00405-4340-01	100s	$34.37
➤ Rugby	00536-3101-01	100s	$34.37
Copley	38245-0631-10	100s	$34.37
West Point	59591-0071-68	100s	$34.37
Major	00904-7714-60	100s	$34.90
Martec	52555-0465-01	100s	$34.90
Schein	00364-2541-01	100s	$35.39
Lederle Std Prod	00005-3333-43	100s	$35.45
Qualitest	00603-3319-21	100s	$35.96
Geneva	00781-1158-01	100s	$36.23
URL	00677-1451-01	100s	$36.25
Mylan	00378-0023-01	100s	$37.70
Goldline	00182-1937-01	100s	$37.70
Moore,H.L.	00839-7748-06	100s	$39.95
Major	00904-7714-61	100s ud	$40.40
➤ Rugby	00536-3101-21	100s ud	$41.00
Goldline	00182-1937-89	100s ud	$42.50
UDL	51079-0745-20	100s ud	$44.94
Vangard	00615-3548-13	100s ud	$45.15
Martec	52555-0465-05	500s	$173.40
Major	00904-7714-40	500s	$173.95
Qualitest	00603-3319-28	500s	$177.45
Moore,H.L.	00839-7748-12	500s	$179.48
➤ Rugby	00536-3101-05	500s	$182.01
Mylan	00378-0023-05	500s	$184.90
Goldline	00182-1937-10	1000s	$300.00
Lederle Std Prod	00005-3333-34	1000s	$336.83

For additional alternatives, turn to the section beginning on page 2859.

Dimenhydrinate, Injectable

DESCRIPTION

Dimenhydrinate, an antinauseant/antiemetic, is the 8-chloro-theophylline salt of diphenhydramine. It contains not less than 53% and not more than 55.5% of diphenhydramine and not less than 44% and not more than 47% of 8-chlorotheophylline, calculated on the dried basis. Chemically it is 8-chlorotheophylline, compound with 2-(diphenylmethoxy)-N,N-dimethylethylamine (1:1). $C_{17}H_{21}NO\text{-}C_7H_7ClN_4O_2$

Dimenhydrinate Injection ampules and vials contain a sterile solution. Each mL contains: Dimenhydrinate 50 mg.

Following is its chemical structure:

CLINICAL PHARMACOLOGY

While the precise mode of action of Dimenhydrinate is not known, it has a depressant action on hyperstimulated labyrinthine function.

INDICATIONS AND USAGE

Dimenhydrinate Injection is indicated for the prevention and treatment of the nausea, vomiting, or vertigo of motion sickness.

CONTRAINDICATIONS

Neonates and patients with a history of hypersensitivity to Dimenhydrinate or its components (diphenhydramine or 8-chlorotheophylline) should not be treated with Dimenhydrinate.

Note: This product contains benzyl alcohol. Benzyl alcohol has been associated with a fatal "Gasping Syndrome" in premature infants and infants of low birth weight.

WARNINGS

Caution should be used when Dimenhydrinate is given in conjunction with certain antibiotics that may cause ototoxicity, since Dimenhydrinate is capable of masking ototoxic symptoms and an irreversible state may be reached.

This drug may impair the mental and/or physical abilities required for the performance of potentially hazardous tasks, such as driving a vehicle or operating machinery. The concomitant use of alcohol or other central nervous system depressants may have an additive effect. Therefore, patients should be warned accordingly.

Dimenhydrinate should be used with caution in patients having conditions which might be aggravated by anticholinergic therapy (i.e., prostatic hypertrophy, stenosing peptic ulcer, pyloroduodenal obstruction, bladder neck obstruction, narrow-angle glaucoma, bronchial asthma, or cardiac arrhythmias).

The preparation should not be injected intra-arterially.

Usage in Children: For infants and children especially, antihistamines in overdosage may cause hallucinations, convulsions, or death.

As in adults, antihistamines may diminish mental alertness in children, in the young child, particularly, they may produce excitation. (See "Contraindications" section).

PRECAUTIONS

General: Drowsiness may be experienced by some patients, especially with high dosage. This effect frequently is not undesirable in conditions for which the drug is used.

Information for Patients: Because of the potential for drowsiness, patients taking Dimenhydrinate should be cautioned against operating automobiles or dangerous machinery. (See "Warnings" section.)

Carcinogenesis, Mutagenesis, Impairment of Fertility: Mutagenicity screening tests performed with Dimenhydrinate, diphenhydramine, and 8-chlorotheophylline produced positive results in the bacterial systems and negative results in the mammalian systems. There are no human data that indicate Dimenhydrinate is a carcinogen or mutagen or that it impairs fertility.

Pregnancy: Pregnancy Category B: Reproduction studies have been performed in rats at doses up to 20 times the human dose, and in rabbits at doses up to 25 times the human dose (on a mg/kg basis), and have revealed no evidence of impaired fertility or harm to the fetus due to Dimenhydrinate. There are no adequate and well-controlled studies in pregnant women. However, clinical studies in pregnant women have not indicated that Dimenhydrinate increases the risk of abnormalities when administered in any trimester of pregnancy. It would appear that the possibility of fetal harm is remote when the drug is used during pregnancy. Nevertheless, because the studies in humans cannot rule out the possibility of harm, Dimenhydrinate should be used during pregnancy only if clearly needed.

Labor and Delivery: The safety of Dimenhydrinate Injection given during labor and delivery has not been established. Reports have indicated Dimenhydrinate may have an oxytocic effect. Caution is advised when this effect is unwanted or in situations where it may prove detrimental.

Nursing Mothers: Small amounts of Dimenhydrinate are excreted in breast milk. Because of the potential for adverse reactions in nursing infants from Dimenhydrinate, a decision should be made whether to discontinue nursing or to discontinue the drug, taking into account the importance of the drug to the mother.

ADVERSE REACTIONS

The most frequent adverse reaction to Dimenhydrinate is drowsiness. Dizziness may also occur. Symptoms of dry mouth, nose and throat, blurred vision, difficult or painful urination, headache, anorexia, nervousness, restlessness or insomnia (especially in children), skin rash, thickening of bronchial secretions, tachycardia, epigastric distress, lassitude, excitation, and nausea have been reported.

◆ RATED THERAPEUTICALLY EQUIVALENT; ◇ THERAPEUTIC EQUIVALENCE UNCONFIRMED; ○ UNRATED

OVERDOSAGE

Drowsiness is the usual clinical side effect. Convulsions, coma, and respiratory depression may occur with massive overdosage. No specific antidote is known. If respiratory depression occurs, mechanically assisted respiration should be initiated and oxygen administered. Convulsions should be treated with appropriate doses of diazepam. Phenobarbital (5 to 6 mg/kg) may be given to control convulsions in children.

The oral LD_{50} in mice and rats is 203 mg/kg and 1320 mg/kg, respectively. The intraperitoneal LD_{50} in mice is 149 mg/kg.

DOSAGE AND ADMINISTRATION

Dimenhydrinate in the injectable form is indicated when the oral form is impractical.

Adults: Nausea or vomiting may be expected to be controlled for approximately 4 hours with 50 mg, and prevented by a similar dose every 4 hours. Its administration may be attended by some degree of drowsiness in some patients, and 100 mg every 4 hours may be given in conditions in which drowsiness is not objectionable or is even desirable.

For intramuscular administration, each milliliter (50 mg) of solution is injected as needed, but for intravenous administration, each milliliter (50 mg) of solution must be diluted in 10 mL of 0.9% Sodium Chloride Injection USP and injected over a period of 2 minutes.

Pediatric: For intramuscular administration, 1.25 mg/kg of body weight or 37.5 mg/m^2 of body surface area is administered four times daily. The maximum dose should not exceed 300 mg daily (see *"Contraindications"* section.)

Parenteral drug products should be inspected visually for particulate matter and discoloration prior to administration, whenever solution and container permit.

Store at 15° - 30° C (59° - 86° F).

J CODES

Up to 50 mg IM,IV—J1240

HOW SUPPLIED

INJECTION: 50 MG/ML

AVERAGE UNIT PRICE (AVAILABLE SIZES)		GENERIC A-RATED AVERAGE PRICE (GAAP)		
GENERIC	$1.17	10 ml		$6.92
BRAND/MANUFACTURER		NDC	SIZE	AWP
◆ GENERICS				
Steris		00402-0241-81	1 ml	$1.73
Schein		00364-6529-54	10 ml	$5.17
Steris		00402-0241-10	10 ml	$5.17
HYDRATE: Hyrex		00314-0661-70	10 ml	$6.90
URL		00677-0599-21	10 ml	$7.10
Rugby		00536-4430-70	10 ml	$7.12
Goldline		00182-0938-63	10 ml	$10.05
Wyeth-Ayerst		00008-0485-01	1 ml 10s	$28.70
Schein		00364-6529-46	1 ml 25s	$43.35

INJECTION: 50 MG/ML

BRAND/MANUFACTURER	NDC	SIZE	AWP
○ GENERICS			
DYMENATE: Keene	00588-5131-70	10 ml	$3.25
Truxton	00463-1086-10	10 ml	$4.05
WEHAMINE: Roberts/Hauck	59441-0630-10	10 ml	$4.22
CMC-Cons	00223-7475-10	10 ml	$4.25
Allscrips	54569-2706-00	10 ml	$6.07
Veratex	17022-1358-03	10 ml 10s	$3.60

Dimercaprol

DESCRIPTION

Dimercaprol (2,3-dimercapto-1-propanol) is a colorless or almost colorless liquid, having a disagreeable, mercaptan-like odor. Each 1 ml sterile Dimercaprol ampule contains 100 mg in 200 mg benzyl benzoate and 700 mg peanut oil.

Following is its chemical structure:

$$\underset{\underset{SH}{|}}{CH_2} \underset{\underset{SH}{|}}{CH} CH_2OH$$

ACTION

Dimercaprol promotes the excretion of arsenic, gold and mercury in cases of poisoning. It is also used in combination with edetate calcium disodium injection, USP to promote the excretion of lead.

INDICATIONS

Dimercaprol Injection is indicated in the treatment of arsenic, gold and mercury poisoning. It is indicated in acute lead poisoning when used concomitantly with edetate calcium disodium injection, USP.

Dimercaprol Injection, USP is effective for use in acute poisoning by mercury salts if therapy is begun within one or two hours following ingestion. It is not very effective for chronic mercury poisoning.

Dimercaprol Injection, USP is of questionable value in poisoning caused by other heavy metals such as antimony and bismuth. It should not be used in iron, cadmium, or selenium poisoning because the resulting Dimercaprol-metal complexes are more toxic than the metal alone, especially to the kidneys.

CONTRAINDICATIONS

Dimercaprol is contraindicated in most instances of hepatic insufficiency with the exception of postarsenical jaundice. The drug should be discontinued or used only with extreme caution if acute renal insufficiency develops during therapy.

WARNINGS

There may be local pain at the site of the injection. A reaction apparently peculiar to children is fever which may persist during therapy. It occurs in approximately 30% of children. A transient reduction of the percentage of polymorphonuclear leukocytes may also be observed.

PRECAUTIONS

Because the Dimercaprol-metal complex breaks down easily in an acid medium, production of an alkaline urine affords protection to the kidney during therapy. Medicinal iron should not be administered to patients under therapy with Dimercaprol. Data is not available regarding the use of Dimercaprol during pregnancy and it should not be used unless judged by the physician to be necessary in the treatment of life threatening acute poisoning.

ADVERSE REACTIONS

One of the most consistent responses to Dimercaprol Injection, USP is a rise in blood pressure accompanied by tachycardia. This rise is roughly proportional to the dose administered. Doses larger than those recommended may cause other transitory signs and symptoms in approximate order of frequency as follows: (1) nausea and, in some instances, vomiting; (2) headache; (3) a burning sensation in the lips, mouth and throat; (4) a feeling of constriction, even pain, in the throat, chest, or hands; (5) conjunctivitis, lacrimation, blepharal spasm, rhinorrhea, and salivation; (6) tingling of the hands; (7) a burning sensation in the penis; (8) sweating of the forehead, hands and other areas; (9) abdominal pain; and (10) occasional appearance of painful sterile abscesses. Many of the above symptoms are accompanied by a feeling of anxiety, weakness, and unrest and often are relieved by administration of an antihistamine.

DOSAGE AND ADMINISTRATION

By deep intramuscular injection only. For mild arsenic or gold poisoning, 2.5 mg/kg of body weight four times daily for two days, two times on the third day, and once daily thereafter for ten days; for severe arsenic or gold poisoning, 3 mg/kg every four hours for two days, four times on the third day, then twice daily thereafter for ten days. For mercury poisoning, 5 mg/kg initially, followed by 2.5 mg/kg one or two times daily for ten days. For acute lead encephalopathy 4 mg/kg body weight is given alone in the first dose and thereafter at four hour intervals in combination with edetate calcium disodium injection, USP administered at a separate site. For less severe poisoning the dose can be reduced to 3 mg/kg after the first dose. Treatment is maintained for two to seven days depending on clinical response. Successful treatment depends on beginning injections at the earliest possible moment and on the use of adequate amounts at frequent intervals. Other supportive measures should always be used in conjunction with Dimercaprol therapy.

Dimercaprol should be inspected visually for particulate matter and discoloration prior to administration.

Store at 15° to 30°C (59° to 85°F).

J CODES

Up to 100 mg IM—J0470

HOW SUPPLIED

INJECTION: 10%

BRAND/MANUFACTURER	NDC	SIZE	AWP
○ BRAND			
BAL IN OIL: BD Microbiology	00011-8341-09	3 ml 10s	$330.00

Dimetane *SEE* BROMPHENIRAMINE MALEATE/CODEINE PHOSPHATE/PHENYLPROPANOLAMINE HYDROCHLORIDE *AND* BROMPHENIRAMINE/DEXTROMETHORPHAN/PSEUDOEPHEDRINE

Dimethyl Sulfoxide

DESCRIPTION

Each ml of Dimethyl Sulfoxide 50% w/w Aqueous Solution for intravesical instillation contains 0.54 gm Dimethyl Sulfoxide. It is a sterile and nonpyrogenic intravesical installation for the treatment of interstitial cystitis.

NOT FOR I.M. OR I.V. INJECTION; DO NOT AUTOCLAVE.

The active component Dimethyl Sulfoxide has the empirical formula C_2H_6OS.

Dimethyl Sulfoxide is a clear, colorless and essentially odorless liquid which is miscible with water and most organic solvents. Other physical characteristics include molecular weight 78.13, melting point 18.3° to 18.4° C, and a specific gravity of 1.096.

➤ SHOWN IN PRODUCT IDENTIFICATION GUIDE

Following is its chemical structure:

$$CH_3{-}S{=}O$$
$$CH_3$$

CLINICAL PHARMACOLOGY

Dimethyl Sulfoxide is metabolized in man by oxidation to Dimethyl sulfone or by reduction to dimethyl sulfide. Dimethyl Sulfoxide and dimethyl sulfone are excreted in the urine and feces. Dimethyl sulfide is eliminated through the breath and skin and is responsible for the characteristic odor from patients on Dimethyl Sulfoxide medication. Dimethyl sulfone can persist in serum for longer than two weeks after a single intravesical instillation. No residual accumulation of Dimethyl Sulfoxide has occurred in man or lower animals who have received treatment for protracted periods of time. Following topical application, Dimethyl Sulfoxide is absorbed and generally distributed in the tissues and body fluids.

INDICATIONS AND USAGE

Dimethyl Sulfoxide is indicated for the symptomatic relief of patients with interstitial cystitis. Dimethyl Sulfoxide has not been approved as being safe and effective for any other indication. There is no clinical evidence of effectiveness of Dimethyl Sulfoxide in the treatment of bacterial infections of the urinary tract.

UNLABELED USES

Dimethyl Sulfoxide is used alone or as an adjunct in the treatment of renal amyloidosis and cytotoxic drug extravasation, and in the topical relief of pain. Dimethyl Sulfoxide is also used for topical relief of neurogenic pain following herpes zoster infections.

CONTRAINDICATIONS

None known.

WARNINGS

Dimethyl Sulfoxide can initiate the liberation of histamine and there has been an occasional hypersensitivity reaction with topical administration of Dimethyl Sulfoxide. This hypersensitivity has been reported in one patient receiving intravesical Dimethyl Sulfoxide. The physician should be cognizant of this possibility in prescribing Dimethyl Sulfoxide. If anaphylactoid symptoms develop, appropriate therapy should be instituted.

PRECAUTIONS

Changes in the refractive index and lens opacities have been seen in monkeys, dogs and rabbits given high doses of Dimethyl Sulfoxide chronically. Since lens changes were noted in animals, full eye evaluations, including slit lamp examinations, are recommended prior to and periodically during treatment.

Approximately every six months patients receiving Dimethyl Sulfoxide should have a biochemical screening, particularly liver and renal function tests, and complete blood count.

Intravesical instillation of Dimethyl Sulfoxide may be harmful to patients with urinary tract malignancy because of Dimethyl Sulfoxide-induced vasodilation.

Some data indicate that Dimethyl Sulfoxide potentiates other concomitantly administered medications.

Pregnancy Category C: Dimethyl Sulfoxide caused teratogenic responses in hamsters, rats and mice when administered intraperitoneally at high doses (2.5-12 gm/kg). Oral or topical doses of Dimethyl Sulfoxide did not cause problems of reproduction in rats, mice and hamsters. Topical doses (5 gm/kg first two days, then 2.5 gm/kg - last eight days) produced terata in rabbits, but in another study, topical doses of 1.1 gm/kg days 3 through 16 of gestation failed to produce any abnormalities. There are no adequate and well controlled studies in pregnant women. Dimethyl Sulfoxide should be used during pregnancy only if the potential benefit justifies the potential risk to the fetus.

It is not known whether this drug is excreted in human milk. Because many drugs are excreted in human milk, caution should be exercised when Dimethyl Sulfoxide is administered to a nursing woman.

Safety and effectiveness in children have not been established.

Information available to be given to the patient is reprinted at the end of this text.

ADVERSE REACTIONS

A garlic-like taste may be noted by the patient within a few minutes after instillation of Dimethyl Sulfoxide. This taste may last several hours and because of the presence of metabolites, an odor on the breath and skin may remain for 72 hours.

Transient chemical cystitis has been noted following instillation of Dimethyl Sulfoxide.

The patient may experience moderately severe discomfort on administration. Usually this becomes less prominent with repeated administration.

DRUG ABUSE AND DEPENDENCE

None known.

OVERDOSAGE

The oral LD$_{50}$ of Dimethyl Sulfoxide in the dog is greater than 10 gm/kg. It is improbable that this dosage level could be obtained with intravesical instillation of Dimethyl/Sulfoxide in the patient.

In case of accidental oral ingestion, specific measures should be taken to induce emesis. Additional measures which may be considered are gastric lavage, activated charcoal and forced diuresis.

DOSAGE AND ADMINISTRATION

Instillation of 50 ml of Dimethyl Sulfoxide directly into the bladder may be accomplished by catheter or asepto syringe and allowed to remain for 15 minutes. Application of an analgesic lubricant gel such as lidocaine jelly to the urethra is suggested prior to insertion of the catheter to avoid spasm. The medication is expelled by spontaneous voiding. It is recommended that the treatment be repeated every two weeks until maximum symptomatic relief is obtained. Thereafter, time intervals between therapy may be increased appropriately.

Administration of oral analgesic medication or suppositories containing belladonna and opium prior to the instillation of Dimethyl Sulfoxide can reduce bladder spasm.

In patients with severe interstitial cystitis with very sensitive bladders, the initial treatment, and possibly the second and third (depending on patient response) should be done under anesthesia. (Saddle block has been suggested).

Protect from strong light.

Store at room temperature (59° to 86°F; 15° to 30° C).

Do not autoclave.

INFORMATION FOR PATIENTS

(Physician Copy)

Dimethyl Sulfoxide is a sterile solution of 50% Dimethyl Sulfoxide (DMSO) and 50% water that has been approved by the U.S. Food and Drug Administration for use in the symptomatic relief of patients with interstitial cystitis.

DMSO will be instilled in the bladder on an inpatient or outpatient basis, which will be determined by your physician.

Some data indicate that DMSO could change the effectiveness of any medication(s) that you may be presently receiving. Be sure to mention the name and dosage of all medications you are taking to your physician before a DMSO instillation. A garlic-like taste may be noted by the patient within a few minutes after instillation of DMSO. This taste may last several hours. An odor on the breath and skin may be present and remain for up to 72 hours.

Some patients may experience discomfort on administration of the drug. Usually this becomes less prominent with repeated administration.

If you are pregnant or nursing, ask your physician about the advisability of using DMSO.

Some eye changes have been observed in animals treated with DMSO in large doses for prolonged periods. Therefore your doctor may want you to have eye evaluations, including slit lamp examinations, prior to and periodically during treatment.

INFORMATION FOR PATIENTS

(Patient Copy)

Dimethyl/Sulfoxide is a sterile solution of 50% Dimethyl Sulfoxide (DMSO) and 50% water that has been approved by the U.S. Food and Drug Administration for use in the symptomatic relief of patients with interstitial cystitis.

DMSO will be instilled in the bladder on an inpatient or outpatient basis, which will be determined by your physician.

Some data indicate that DMSO could change the effectiveness of any medication(s) that you may be presently receiving. Be sure to mention the name and dosage of all medications you are taking to your physician before a DMSO instillation.

A garlic-like taste may be noted by the patient within a few minutes after instillation of DMSO. This taste may last several hours. An odor on the breath and skin may be present and remain for up to 72 hours.

Some patients may experience discomfort on administration of the drug. Usually this becomes less prominent with repeated administration.

If you are pregnant or nursing, ask your physician about the advisability of using DMSO.

Some eye changes have been observed in animals treated with DMSO in large doses for prolonged periods. Therefore your doctor may want you to have eye evaluations, including slit lamp examinations, prior to and periodically during treatment.

J CODES
OTH—J1212

HOW SUPPLIED
INJECTION: 50%

BRAND/MANUFACTURER	NDC	SIZE	AWP
○ GENERICS			
McGuff	49072-0433-05	50 ml	$34.50

INJECTION: 100%

BRAND/MANUFACTURER	NDC	SIZE	AWP
○ GENERICS			
McGuff	49072-0840-88	70 ml	$27.95

SOLUTION: 50%

BRAND/MANUFACTURER	NDC	SIZE	AWP
○ BRAND			
RIMSO-50: Research Ind	00433-0433-05	50 ml doz	$564.00

◆ RATED THERAPEUTICALLY EQUIVALENT; ◇ THERAPEUTIC EQUIVALENCE UNCONFIRMED; ○ UNRATED

Dinoprostone, Cervical

DESCRIPTION

Dinoprostone Gel contains Dinoprostone as the naturally occurring form of prostaglandin E_2 (PGE_2) and is designated chemically as (5Z, 11α, 13E, 15S)-11,15-Dihydroxy-9-oxoprosta-5, 13-dien-1-oic acid. The molecular formula is $C_{20}H_{32}O_5$ and the molecular weight is 352.5. Dinoprostone occurs as a white to off-white crystalline powder with a melting point within the range of 65° to 69°C. It is soluble in ethanol, in 25% ethanol in water, and in water to the extent of 130 mg/100 mL. The active constituent is Dinoprostone 0.5 mg/3g (2.5 mL gel); other constituents are colloidal silicon dioxide NF (240 mg/3 g) and triacetin USP (2760 mg/3 g).

Following is its chemical structure:

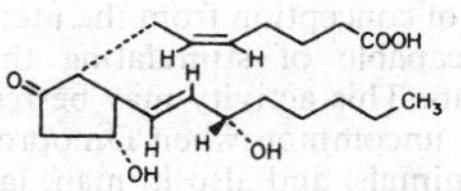

CLINICAL PHARMACOLOGY

Dinoprostone Gel administered endocervically may stimulate the myometrium of the gravid uterus to contract in a manner similar to contractions seen in the term uterus during labor. Whether or not this action results from a direct effect of Dinoprostone on the myometrium has not been determined. Dinoprostone is also capable of stimulating smooth muscle of the gastrointestinal tract in humans. This activity may be responsible for the vomiting and/or diarrhea that is occasionally seen when Dinoprostone is used for preinduction cervical ripening.

In laboratory animals, and also in humans, large doses of Dinoprostone can lower blood pressure, probably as a result of its effect on smooth muscle of the vascular system. With the doses of Dinoprostone used for cervical ripening this effect has not been seen. In laboratory animals, and also in humans, Dinoprostone can elevate body temperature; however, with the dosing used for cervical ripening this effect has not been seen.

In addition to an oxytocic effect, there is evidence suggesting that this agent has a local cervical effect in initiating softening, effacement, and dilation. These changes, referred to as cervical ripening, occur spontaneously as the normal pregnancy progresses toward term and allow evacuation of uterine contents by decreasing cervical resistance at the same time that myometrial activity increases. While not completely understood, biochemical changes within the cervix during natural cervical ripening are similar to those following PGE_2-induced ripening. Further, it has been shown that these changes can take place independent of myometrial activity; however, it is quite likely that PGE_2 administered endocervically produces effacement and softening by combined contraction-inducing and cervical-ripening properties. There is evidence to suggest that the changes that take place within the cervix are due to collagen degradation resulting from collagenase secretion as a response, at least in part, to PGE_2.

Using an unvalidated assay, the following information was determined. When Dinoprostone Gel was administered endocervically to women undergoing preinduction ripening, results from measurement of plasma levels of the metabolite 13, 14-dihydro-15-keto-PGE_2 (DHK-PGE_2) showed that PGE_2 was relatively rapidly absorbed and the T_{max} was 0.5 to 0.75 hours. Plasma mean C_{max} for gel-treated subjects was 433 ± 51 pg/mL versus 137 ± 24 pg/mL for untreated controls. In those subjects in which a clinical response was observed, mean C_{max} was 484 ± 54 pg/mL versus 213 ± 69 pg/mL in nonresponders and 219 ± 92 pg/mL in control subjects who had positive clinical progression toward normal labor. These elevated levels in gel-treated subjects appear to be largely a result of absorption of PGE_2 from the gel rather than from endogenous sources. PGE_2 is completely metabolized in humans. PGE_2 is extensively metabolized in the lungs, and the resulting metabolites are further metabolized in the liver and kidney. The major route of elimination of the products of PGE_2 metabolism is the kidneys.

INDICATIONS AND USAGE

Dinoprostone Gel is indicated for ripening an unfavorable cervix in pregnant women at or near term with a medical or obstetrical need for labor induction.

CONTRAINDICATIONS

Endocervically administered Dinoprostone Gel is not recommended for the following:

a. Patients in whom oxytocic drugs are generally contraindicated or where prolonged contractions of the uterus are considered inappropriate, such as:
- cases with a history of cesarean section or major uterine surgery
- cases in which cephalopelvic disproportion is present
- cases in which there is a history of difficult labor and/or traumatic delivery
- grand multiparae with six or more previous term pregnancies
- cases with non-vertex presentation
- cases with hyperactive or hypertonic uterine patterns
- cases of fetal distress where delivery is not imminent
- in obstetric emergencies where the benefit-to-risk ratio for either the fetus or the mother favors surgical intervention.

b. Patients with ruptured membranes.
c. Patients with hypersensitivity to prostaglandins or constituents of the gel.
d. Patients with placenta previa or unexplained vaginal bleeding during this pregnancy.
e. Patients for whom vaginal delivery is not indicated, such as vasa previa or active herpes genitalia.

WARNINGS

FOR HOSPITAL USE ONLY

Dinoprostone, as with other potent oxytocic agents, should be used only with strict adherence to recommended dosages. Dinoprostone should be administered by physicians in a hospital that can provide immediate intensive care and acute surgical facilities.

PRECAUTIONS

1. GENERAL PRECAUTIONS

During use, uterine activity, fetal status, and character of the cervix (dilation and effacement) should be carefully monitored either by auscultation or electronic fetal monitoring to detect possible evidence of undesired responses, eg, hypertonus, sustained uterine contractility, or fetal distress. In cases where there is a history of hypertonic uterine contractility or tetanic uterine contractions, it is recommended that uterine activity and the state of the fetus should be continuously monitored. The possibility of uterine rupture should be borne in mind when high-tone myometrial contractions are sustained.

Feto-pelvic relationships should be carefully evaluated before use of Dinoprostone Gel (see "Contraindications").

Caution should be exercised in administration of Dinoprostone Gel in patients with:

- asthma or history of asthma
- glaucoma or raised intraocular pressure

Caution should be taken so as not to administer Dinoprostone Gel above the level of the internal os. Careful vaginal examination will reveal the degree of effacement which will regulate the size of the shielded endocervical catheter to be used. That is, the 20 mm endocervical catheter should be used if no effacement is present, and the 10 mm catheter should be used if the cervix is 50% effaced. Placement of Dinoprostone Gel into the extra-amniotic space has been associated with uterine hyperstimulation.

As Dinoprostone Gel is extensively metabolized in the lung, liver, and kidney, and the major route of elimination is the kidney, Dinoprostone Gel should be used with caution in patients with renal and hepatic dysfunction.

2. DRUG INTERACTIONS

Dinoprostone Gel may augment the activity of other oxytocic agents and their concomitant use is not recommended. For the sequential use of oxytocin following Dinoprostone Gel administration, a dosing interval of 6-12 hours is recommended.

3. CARCINOGENESIS, MUTAGENESIS, IMPAIRMENT OF FERTILITY

Carcinogenic bioassay studies have not been conducted in animals with Dinoprostone Gel due to the limited indications for use and short duration of administration. No evidence of mutagenicity was observed in the Micronucleus Test or Ames Assay.

PREGNANCY, TERATOGENIC EFFECTS

Pregnancy Category C: Prostaglandin E_2 produced an increase in skeletal anomalies in rats and rabbits. No effect would be expected clinically, when used as indicated, since Dinoprostone Gel is administered after the period of organogenesis. Dinoprostone Gel has been shown to be embryotoxic in rats and rabbits, and any dose that produces sustained increased uterine tone could put the embryo or fetus at risk. See statements under "General Precautions."

ADVERSE REACTIONS

Dinoprostone Gel is generally well-tolerated. In controlled trials, in which 1731 women were entered, the following events were reported at an occurrence of ≥ 1%:

Adverse Reaction	PGE_2 (N = 884)	Control* (N = 847)
	N (%)	N (%)
Maternal		
Uterine contractile abnormality	58 (6.6)	34 (4.0)
Any gastrointestinal effect	50 (5.7)	22 (2.6)
Back pain	27 (3.1)	0 (0)
Warm feeling in vagina	13 (1.5)	0 (0)
Fever	12 (1.4)	10 (1.2)
Fetal		
Any fetal heart rate abnormality	150 (17.0)	123 (14.5)
Bradycardia	36 (4.1)	26 (3.1)
Deceleration		
Late	25 (2.8)	18 (2.1)
Variable	38 (4.3)	29 (3.4)
Unspecified	19 (2.1)	19 (2.2)

*placebo gel or no treatment

In addition, in other trials amnionitis and intrauterine fetal sepsis have been associated with extra-amniotic intrauterine administration of PGE_2. Uterine rupture has been reported in association with the use of Dinoprostone Gel intracervically. Additional events reported in the literature, associated by the authors with the use of Dinoprostone Gel, included premature rupture of membranes, fetal depression (1 min Apgar <7), and fetal acidosis (umbilical artery pH <7.15).

DRUG ABUSE AND DEPENDENCE

No drug abuse or drug dependence has been seen with the use of Dinoprostone Gel.

OVERDOSAGE

Overdosage with Dinoprostone Gel may be expressed by uterine hypercontractility and uterine hypertonus. Because of the transient nature of PGE_2-induced myometrial hyperstimulation, nonspecific, conservative management was found to be effective in the vast majority of the cases: ie, maternal position change and administration of oxygen to the mother. β-adrenergic drugs may be used as a treatment of hyperstimulation following the administration of PGE_2 for cervical ripening.

DOSAGE AND ADMINISTRATION

Note: USE CAUTION IN HANDLING THIS PRODUCT TO PREVENT CONTACT WITH SKIN. WASH HANDS THOROUGHLY WITH SOAP AND WATER AFTER ADMINISTRATION.

Dinoprostone Gel should be brought to room temperature (59° to 86°F; 15° to 30°C) just prior to administration. Do not force the warming process by using a water bath or other source of external heat (eg, microwave oven).

To prepare the product for use, remove the peel-off seal from the end of the syringe. Then remove the protective end cap (to serve as plunger extension) and insert the protective end cap into the plunger stopper assembly in the barrel of syringe. Choose the appropriate length shielded catheter (10 mm or 20 mm) and aseptically remove the sterile shielded catheter from the package. Careful vaginal examination will reveal the degree of effacement which will regulate the size of the shielded endocervical catheter to be used. That is, the 20 mm endocervical catheter should be used if no effacement is present, and the 10 mm catheter should be used if the cervix is 50% effaced. Firmly attach the catheter hub to the syringe tip as evidenced by a distinct click. Fill the catheter with sterile gel by pushing the plunger assembly to expel air from the catheter prior to administration to the patient.

To administer the product properly, the patient should be in a dorsal position with the cervix visualized using a speculum. Using sterile technique, introduce the gel with the catheter provided into the cervical canal just below the level of the internal os. Administer the contents of the syringe by gentle expulsion and then remove the catheter. The gel is easily extrudable from the syringe. Use the contents of one syringe for one patient only. No attempt should be made to administer the small amount of gel remaining in the catheter. The syringe, catheter, and any unused package contents should be discarded after use. Following Dinoprostone Gel administration, the patient should remain in the supine position for at least 15-30 minutes to minimize leakage from the cervical canal. If the desired response is obtained from the starting dose of Dinoprostone Gel, the recommended interval before giving intravenous oxytocin is 6-12 hours. If there is no cervical/uterine response to the initial dose of Dinoprostone Gel, repeat dosing may be given. The recommended repeat dose is 0.5 mg Dinoprostone with a dosing interval of 6 hours. The need for additional dosing and the interval must be determined by the attending physician based on the course of clinical events. The maximum recommended cumulative dose for a 24-hour period is 1.5 mg of Dinoprostone (7.5 mL Dinoprostone Gel).

Dinoprostone Gel has a shelf life of 24 months when stored under continuous refrigeration (36° to 46°F; 2° to 8°C).

HOW SUPPLIED
GEL: 0.5 MG

BRAND/MANUFACTURER	NDC	SIZE	AWP
○ **BRAND** PREPIDIL: Upjohn	00009-3359-01	3 gm	$93.75

SUPPOSITORY: 20 MG

BRAND/MANUFACTURER	NDC	SIZE	AWP
○ **BRAND** PROSTIN E2: Upjohn	00009-0827-01	1s	$111.83

Dinoprostone, Vaginal

DESCRIPTION

Dinoprostone Vaginal Suppository, an oxytocic, contains the naturally occurring prostaglandin E2 (PGE2).

Its chemical name is (5Z,11α,13E,15S)-11,15-Dihydroxy-9-oxo-prosta-5,13-dien-1-oic acid.

The molecular formula is $C_{20}H_{32}O_5$. The molecular weight of Dinoprostone is 352.5. Dinoprostone occurs as a white crystalline powder. It has a melting point within the range of 64° to 71° C. Dinoprostone is soluble in ethanol and in 25% ethanol in water. It is soluble in water to the extent of 130 mg/100 mL.

Each suppository contains 20 mg of Dinoprostone in a mixture of glycerides of fatty acids.

Following is its chemical structure:

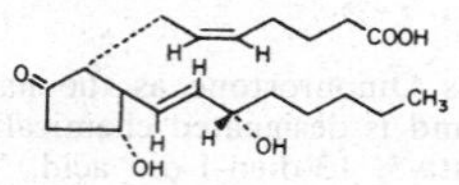

CLINICAL PHARMACOLOGY

Dinoprostone Vaginal Suppository administered intravaginally stimulates the myometrium of the gravid uterus to contract in a manner that is similar to the contractions seen in the term uterus during labor. Whether or not this action results from a direct effect of Dinoprostone on the myometrium has not been determined with certainty at this time. Nonetheless, the myometrial contractions induced by the vaginal administration of Dinoprostone are sufficient to produce evacuation of the products of conception from the uterus in the majority of cases.

Dinoprostone is also capable of stimulating the smooth muscle of the gastrointestinal tract of man. This activity may be responsible for the vomiting and/or diarrhea that is not uncommon when Dinoprostone is used to terminate pregnancy. In laboratory animals, and also in man, large doses of Dinoprostone can lower blood pressure, probably as a consequence of its effect on the smooth muscle of the vascular system. With the doses of Dinoprostone used for terminating pregnancy this effect has not been clinically significant. In laboratory animals, and also in man, Dinoprostone can elevate body temperature. With the clinical doses of Dinoprostone used for the termination of pregnancy some patients do exhibit temperature increases.

INDICATIONS AND USAGE

1. Dinoprostone Vaginal Suppository is indicated for the termination of pregnancy from the 12th through the 20th gestational week as calculated from the first day of the last normal menstrual period.
2. Dinoprostone is also indicated for evacuation of the uterine contents in the management of missed abortion or intrauterine fetal death up to 28 weeks of gestational age as calculated from the first day of the last normal menstrual period.
3. Dinoprostone is indicated in the management of nonmetastatic gestational trophoblastic disease (benign hydatidiform mole).

CONTRAINDICATIONS

1. Hypersensitivity to Dinoprostone
2. Acute pelvic inflammatory disease
3. Patients with active cardiac, pulmonary, renal, or hepatic disease

> ### WARNINGS
> DINOPROSTONE, AS WITH OTHER POTENT OXYTOCIC AGENTS, SHOULD BE USED ONLY WITH STRICT ADHERENCE TO RECOMMENDED DOSAGES. DINOPROSTONE SHOULD BE USED BY MEDICALLY TRAINED PERSONNEL IN A HOSPITAL WHICH CAN PROVIDE IMMEDIATE INTENSIVE CARE AND ACUTE SURGICAL FACILITIES.

Dinoprostone does not appear to directly affect the fetoplacental unit. Therefore, the possibility does exist that the previable fetus aborted by Dinoprostone could exhibit transient life signs. Dinoprostone is not indicated if the fetus in utero has reached the stage of viability. Dinoprostone should not be considered a feticidal agent.

Evidence from animal studies has suggested that certain prostaglandins may have some teratogenic potential. Therefore, any failed pregnancy termination with Dinoprostone should be completed by some other means.

Dinoprostone Vaginal Suppository should not be used for extemporaneous preparation of any other dosage form.

Neither the Dinoprostone Vaginal Suppository, as dispensed nor any extemporaneous formulation made from the Dinoprostone Vaginal Suppository should be used for cervical ripening or other indication in the patient with term pregnancy.

PRECAUTIONS

1. GENERAL PRECAUTIONS
Animal studies lasting several weeks at high doses have shown that prostaglandins of the E and F series can induce proliferation of bone. Such effects have also been noted in newborn infants who have received prostaglandin E1 during prolonged treatment. There is no evidence that short term administration of Dinoprostone Vaginal Suppository can cause similar bone effects.

As in spontaneous abortion, where the process is sometimes incomplete, abortion induced by Dinoprostone may sometimes be incomplete. In such cases, other measures should be taken to assure complete abortion.

In patients with a history of asthma, hypo- or hypertension, cardiovascular disease, renal disease, hepatic disease, anemia, jaundice, diabetes or history of epilepsy, Dinoprostone should be used with caution.

Dinoprostone administered by the vaginal route should be used with caution in the presence of cervicitis, infected endocervical lesions, or acute vaginitis.

As with any oxytocic agent, Dinoprostone should be used with caution in patients with compromised (scarred) uteri. Dinoprostone vaginal therapy is associated with transient pyrexia that may be due to its effect on hypothalamic thermoregulation. In the patients studied, temperature elevations in excess of 2°F

◆ RATED THERAPEUTICALLY EQUIVALENT; ◇ THERAPEUTIC EQUIVALENCE UNCONFIRMED; ○ UNRATED

Endometritis pyrexia

1. Time of onset: Typically, on third post-abortional day (38°C or higher).
2. Duration: Untreated pyrexia and infection continue and may give rise to other infective pelvic pathology.
3. Retention: Products of conception are often retained in the cervical os or uterine cavity.
4. Histology: Endometrium shows evidence of inflammatory lymphocytic infiltration with areas of necrotic hemorrhagic tissue.
5. The uterus: Often remains boggy and soft with tenderness over the fundus, and pain on moving the cervix, on bimanual examination.
6. Discharge: Often associated foul-smelling lochia and leukorrhea.
7. Cervical culture
   The culture of pathological organisms from the cervix or uterine cavity after abortion does not, of itself, warrant the diagnosis of septic abortion in the absence of clinical evidence of sepsis. It is not uncommon to culture pathogens from cases of recent abortion *not* clinically infected. Persistent positive culture with clear clinical signs of infection are significant in the differential diagnosis.
8. Blood count
   Leukocytosis and differential white cell counts are not of major clinical importance in distinguishing between the two conditions, since total WBC's may be increased as a result of infection and transient leukocytosis may also be drug induced.
In the absence of clinical or bacteriological evidence of intrauterine infection, supportive therapy for drug induced fevers includes the forcing of fluids. As all PGE2-induced fevers have been found to be transient or self-limiting, it is doubtful if any simple empirical measures for temperature reduction are indicated.

PGE2 Induced pyrexia

Within 15-45 minutes of suppository administration.

Elevations revert to pretreatment levels within 2-6 hours after discontinuation of therapy or removal of suppository from vagina without any other treatment.
Elevation occurs irrespective of any retained tissue.

Although the endometrial stroma may be edematous and vascular, there relative absence of inflammatory reaction.
Normal uterine involution not tender.

Lochia normal.

(1.1°C) were observed in approximately one-half of the patients on the recommended dosage regimen. In all cases, temperature returned to normal on discontinuation of therapy. Differentiation of post-abortion endometritis from drug-induced temperature elevations is difficult, but with increasing clinical exposure and experience with PGE2 vaginal therapy the distinctions become more obviously apparent and are summarized below: (See related table).

2. LABORATORY TESTS
When a pregnancy diagnosed as missed abortion is electively interrupted with intravaginal administration of Dinoprostone, confirmation of intrauterine fetal death should be obtained in respect to a *negative pregnancy test* for chorionic gonadotropic activity (U.C.G. test or equivalent). When a pregnancy with late fetal intrauterine death is interrupted with intravaginal administration of Dinoprostone, confirmation of intrauterine fetal death should be obtained prior to treatment.

3. DRUG INTERACTIONS
Dinoprostone may augment the activity of other oxytocic drugs. Concomitant use with other oxytocic agents is not recommended.

4. CARCINOGENESIS, MUTAGENESIS, IMPAIRMENT OF FERTILITY
Carcinogenic bioassay studies have not been conducted in animals with Dinoprostone due to the limited indications for use and short duration of administration. No evidence of mutagenicity was observed in the Micronucleus Test or Ames Assay.

5. PREGNANCY:
Teratogenic Effects: Pregnancy Category C. Animal studies do not indicate that Dinoprostone is teratogenic, however, it has been shown to be embryotoxic in rats and rabbits and any dose which produces increased uterine tone could put the embryo or fetus at risk. See *"Warnings"* section.

ADVERSE REACTIONS
The most frequent adverse reactions observed with the use of Dinoprostone for abortion are related to its contractile effect on smooth muscle.
   In the patients studied, approximately two-thirds experienced vomiting, one-half temperature elevations, two-fifths diarrhea, one-third some nausea, one-tenth headache, and one-tenth shivering and chills.
   In addition, approximately one-tenth of the patients studied exhibited transient diastolic blood pressure decreases of greater than 20 mmHg.
   Two cases of myocardial infarction following the use of Dinoprostone have been reported in patients with a history of cardiovascular disease.
   It is not known whether these events were related to the administration of Dinoprostone.
   Adverse effects in decreasing order of their frequency, observed with the use of Dinoprostone, not all of which are clearly drug related include:
Vomiting
Diarrhea
Nausea
Fever
Headache
Chills or shivering
Backache
Joint inflammation or pain new or exacerbated
Flushing or hot flashes
Dizziness
Arthralgia
Vaginal pain
Chest pain
Dyspnea
Endometritis
Syncope or fainting sensation

Vaginitis or vulvitis
Weakness
Muscular cramp or pain
Tightness in chest
Nocturnal leg cramps
Uterine rupture
Breast tenderness
Blurred vision
Coughing
Rash
Myalgia
Stiff neck
Dehydration
Tremor
Paresthesia
Hearing impairment
Urine retention
Pharyngitis
Laryngitis
Diaphoresis
Eye pain
Wheezing
Cardiac arrhythmia
Skin discoloration
Vaginismus
Tension

DOSAGE AND ADMINISTRATION
STORE IN A FREEZER NOT ABOVE -20°C (-4°F) BUT BRING TO ROOM TEMPERATURE JUST PRIOR TO USE. REMOVE FOIL BEFORE USE.
   A suppository containing 20 mg of Dinoprostone should be inserted high into the vagina. The patient should remain in the supine position for ten minutes following insertion.
   Additional intravaginal administration of each subsequent suppository should be at 3- to 5-hour intervals until abortion occurs. Within the above recommended intervals administration time should be determined by abortifacient progress, uterine contractility response, and by patient tolerance. Continuous administration of the drug for more than 2 days is not recommended.

HOW SUPPLIED
SUPPOSITORY: 20 MG

BRAND/MANUFACTURER	NDC	SIZE	AWP
○ BRAND			
PROSTIN E2: Upjohn	00009-0827-01	1s	$111.83

Dipentum *SEE* OLSALAZINE SODIUM

Diphenhydramine Hydrochloride

DESCRIPTION
Diphenhydramine Hydrochloride/(HCl) is an antihistamine drug having the chemical name 2-(Diphenylmethoxy)-N, N-dimethylethylamine hydrochloride. It occurs as a white crystalline powder, is freely soluble in water and alcohol and has a molecular weight of 291.82. The molecular formula is $C_{17}H_{21}NO \cdot HCl$.
   Diphenhydramine is available as:

Capsules containing:

25 mg Diphenhydramine HCl
50 mg Diphenhydramine HCl

► SHOWN IN PRODUCT IDENTIFICATION GUIDE

Injection containing:
10 mg/ml Diphenhydramine HCl
50 mg/ml Diphenhydramine HCl

Following is its chemical structure:

CLINICAL PHARMACOLOGY

Diphenhydramine HCl is an antihistamine with anticholinergic (drying) and sedative side effects. Antihistamines appear to compete with histamine for cell receptor sites on effector cells.

A single oral dose of Diphenhydramine HCl is quickly absorbed with maximum activity occurring in approximately one hour. The duration of activity following an average dose of Diphenhydramine HCl is from four to six hours. Diphenhydramine is widely distributed throughout the body, including the CNS. Little, if any, of the oral dose is excreted unchanged in the urine; most appears as the degradation products of metabolic transformation in the liver, which are almost completely excreted within 24 hours.

Diphenhydramine HCl in the injectable form has a rapid onset of action. Diphenhydramine HCl is widely distributed throughout the body, including the CNS. A portion of the injected drug is excreted unchanged in the urine, while the rest is metabolized via the liver. Detailed information on the pharmacokinetics of Diphenhydramine HCl injection is not available.

INDICATIONS AND USAGE

Diphenhydramine HCl in the oral form is effective for the following indications:

Antihistaminic: For allergic conjunctivitis due to foods; mild, uncomplicated allergic skin manifestations of urticaria and angioedema; amelioration of allergic reactions to blood or plasma; dermatographism; as therapy for anaphylactic reactions *adjunctive* to epinephrine and other standard measures after the acute manifestations have been controlled.

Motion sickness: For active and prophylactic treatment of motion sickness.

Antiparkinsonism: For parkinsonism (including drug-induced) in the elderly unable to tolerate more potent agents; mild cases of parkinsonism (including drug-induced) in other age groups; in other cases of parkinsonism (including drug-induced) in combination with centrally acting anticholinergic agents.

Diphenhydramine HCl in the injectable form is effective for the following conditions when Diphenhydramine HCl in the oral form is impractical. Antihistaminic: For amelioration of allergic reactions to blood or plasma, in anaphylaxis as an adjunct to epinephrine and other standard measures after the acute symptoms have been controlled, and for other uncomplicated allergic conditions of the immediate type when oral therapy is impossible or contraindicated.

Motion Sickness: For active treatment of motion sickness.

Antiparkinsonism: For use in parkinsonism, when oral therapy is impossible or contraindicated, as follows: parkinsonism in the elderly who are unable to tolerate more potent agents, mild cases of parkinsonism in other age groups, and in other cases of parkinsonism in combination with centrally acting anticholinergic agents.

UNLABELED USES
Diphenhydramine HCl is used alone or as an adjunct in patients with a prior history of allergic reactions to contrast media, and to provide local anesthesia.

CONTRAINDICATIONS

Use in Newborn or Premature Infants: This drug should *not* be used in newborn or premature infants.

Use in Nursing Mothers: Because of the higher risk of antihistamines for infants generally, and for newborns and prematures in particular, antihistamine therapy is contraindicated in nursing mothers.

Use as a Local Anesthetic: Because of the risk of local necrosis, this drug should not be used as a local anesthesia.

Antihistamines are Also Contraindicated in the Following Conditions: Hypersensitivity to Diphenhydramine HCl and other antihistamines of similar chemical structure.

WARNINGS

Antihistamines should be used with considerable caution in patients with narrow-angle glaucoma, stenosing peptic ulcer, pyloroduodenal obstruction, symptomatic prostatic hypertrophy, or bladder-neck obstruction.

USE IN CHILDREN
In infants and children, especially, antihistamines in *overdosage* may cause hallucinations, convulsions, or death. As in adults, antihistamines may diminish mental alertness in children. In the young child, particularly, they may produce excitation.

USE IN THE ELDERLY (APPROXIMATELY 60 YEARS OR OLDER)
Antihistamines are more likely to cause dizziness, sedation, and hypotension in elderly patients.

PRECAUTIONS

General: Diphenhydramine HCl has an atropine-like action and therefore should be used with caution in patients with a history of bronchial asthma, increased intraocular pressure, hyperthyroidism, cardiovascular disease or hypertension. Use with caution in patients with lower respiratory disease, including asthma.

Information for Patients: Patients taking Diphenhydramine HCl should be advised that this drug may cause drowsiness and has an additive effect with alcohol. Patients should be warned about engaging in activities requiring mental alertness such as driving a car or operating appliances, machinery, etc.

Drug Interactions: Diphenhydramine HCl has additive effects with alcohol and other CNS depressants (hypnotics, sedatives, tranquilizers, etc).

Caution: Patients taking monoamine oxidase inhibitors should not receive antihistamine therapy concurrently.

MAO inhibitors prolong and intensify the anticholinergic (drying) effects of antihistamines.

Carcinogenesis, Mutagenesis, Impairment of Fertility: Long-term studies in animals to determine mutagenic and carcinogenic potential have not been performed.

Pregnancy: Pregnancy Category B. Reproduction studies have been performed in rats and rabbits at doses up to 5 times the human dose and have revealed no evidence of impaired fertility or harm to the fetus due to Diphenhydramine HCl. There are, however, no adequate and well-controlled studies in pregnant women. Because animal reproduction studies are not always predictive of human response, this drug should be used during pregnancy only if clearly needed.

ADVERSE REACTIONS

THE MOST FREQUENT ADVERSE REACTIONS ARE ITALICIZED
1. *General:* Urticaria, drug rash, anaphylactic shock, photosensitivity, excessive perspiration, chills, dryness of mouth, nose, and throat.

2. *Cardiovascular System:* Hypotension, headache, palpitations, tachycardia, extrasystoles

3. *Hematologic System:* Hemolytic anemia, thrombocytopenia, agranulocytosis

4. *Nervous System: Sedation, sleepiness, dizziness, disturbed coordination*, fatigue, confusion, restlessness, excitation, nervousness, tremor, irritability, insomnia, euphoria, paresthesia, blurred vision, diplopia, vertigo, tinnitus, acute labyrinthitis, neuritis, convulsions

5. *GI System: Epigastric distress*, anorexia, nausea, vomiting, diarrhea, constipation

6. *GU System:* Urinary frequency, difficult urination, urinary retention, early menses

7. *Respiratory System: Thickening of bronchial secretions*, tightness of chest and wheezing, nasal stuffiness

OVERDOSAGE

Antihistamine overdosage reactions may vary from central nervous system depression to stimulation. Stimulation is particularly likely in children. Atropine-like signs and symptoms, dry mouth: fixed, dilated pupils; flushing, and gastrointestinal symptoms may also occur.

If vomiting has not occurred spontaneously: the patient should be induced to vomit. This is best done by having him drink a glass of water or milk after which he should be made to gag. Precautions against aspiration must be taken, especially in infants and children.

If vomiting is unsuccessful: gastric lavage is indicated within 3 hours after ingestion and even later if large amounts of milk or cream were given beforehand. Isotonic or ½ isotonic saline is the lavage solution of choice.

Saline cathartics: as milk of magnesia, by osmosis draw water into the bowel and therefore are valuable for their action in rapid dilution of food content.

Stimulants: should not be used.

Vasopressors may be used to treat hypotension.

DOSAGE AND ADMINISTRATION

A single oral dose of Diphenhydramine HCl is quickly absorbed with maximum activity occurring in approximately one hour. The duration of activity following an average dose of Diphenhydramine HCl is from four to six hours.

Adults: 25 to 50 mg three or four times daily. The night-time sleep-aid dosage is 50 mg at bedtime.

Children: (over 20 lb): 12.5 to 25 mg three to four times daily. Maximum daily dosage not to exceed 300 mg. For physicians who wish to calculate the dose on the basis of body weight or surface area, the recommended dosage is 5 mg/kg/24 hours or 150 mg/m^2/24 hours.

Data are not available on the use of Diphenhydramine HCl as a nighttime sleep-aid in children under 12 years. The basis for determining the most effective dosage regimen will be the response of the patient to medication and the condition under treatment.

◆ RATED THERAPEUTICALLY EQUIVALENT; ◇ THERAPEUTIC EQUIVALENCE UNCONFIRMED; ○ UNRATED

In motion sickness, full dosage is recommended for prophylactic use, the first dose to be given 30 minutes before exposure to motion and similar doses before meals and upon retiring for the duration of exposure.

Diphenhydramine in the injectable form is indicated when the oral form is impractical.

Parenteral drug products should be inspected visually for particulate matter and discoloration prior to administration, whenever solution and container permit.

Children: 5 mg/kg/24 hr or 150 mg/m^2/24 hr. Maximum daily dosage is 300 mg. Divide into four doses, administered intravenously or deeply intramuscularly.

Adults: 10 to 50 mg intravenously or deeply intramuscularly; 100 mg if required; maximum daily dosage is 400 mg.

Storage: Store at controlled room temperature, 15°-30°C (59°-86°F).
Protect injection from freezing light; protect tablets from moisture.

J CODES
Up to 50 mg IV,IM—J1200

HOW SUPPLIED
CAPSULE: 25 MG

AVERAGE UNIT PRICE (AVAILABLE SIZES)		GENERIC A-RATED AVERAGE PRICE (GAAP)	
BRAND	$0.22	30s	$2.68
GENERIC	$0.05	100s	$6.37
HCFA FUL (100s ea)	$0.02	1000s	$21.90

BRAND/MANUFACTURER	NDC	SIZE	AWP
◆ BRAND			
BENADRYL: Parke-Davis	00071-0471-24	100s	$21.69
◆ GENERICS			
Major	00904-2055-46	30s	$1.90
Medirex	57480-0321-06	30s	$3.46
Richlyn	00115-1110-01	100s	$2.83
Rugby	00536-3758-01	100s	$2.88
Major	00904-2055-60	100s	$3.75
Geneva	00781-2458-01	100s	$4.25
Moore,H.L.	00839-1278-06	100s	$4.85
Purepac	00228-2191-10	100s	$6.19
Mutual	53489-0113-01	100s	$6.30
Aligen	00405-4344-01	100s	$6.32
URL	00677-0063-01	100s	$6.35
Parmed	00349-8871-01	100s	$9.70
Major	00904-2055-61	100s ud	$6.85
Auro	55829-0627-10	100s ud	$8.02
Vangard	00615-0368-13	100s ud	$9.73
Medirex	57480-0321-01	100s ud	$11.20
Rugby	00536-3758-10	1000s	$16.75
Raway	00686-3136-10	1000s	$17.00
Goldline	00182-0492-10	1000s	$18.00
Major	00904-2055-80	1000s	$18.50
Qualitest	00603-3337-32	1000s	$19.95
Geneva	00781-2458-10	1000s	$20.25
Moore,H.L.	00839-1278-16	1000s	$21.45
Richlyn	00115-1110-03	1000s	$21.75
URL	00677-0063-10	1000s	$23.00
Schein	00364-0116-02	1000s	$23.00
Mutual	53489-0113-10	1000s	$23.00
Aligen	00405-4344-03	1000s	$23.12
Parmed	00349-8871-10	1000s	$24.50
Purepac	00228-2191-96	1000s	$36.34

CAPSULE: 50 MG

AVERAGE UNIT PRICE (AVAILABLE SIZES)		GENERIC A-RATED AVERAGE PRICE (GAAP)	
BRAND	$0.31	30s	$3.09
GENERIC	$0.08	100s	$7.32
HCFA FUL (100s ea)	$0.02	1000s	$26.31

BRAND/MANUFACTURER	NDC	SIZE	AWP
◆ BRAND			
BENADRYL: Parke-Davis	00071-0373-24	100s	$29.25
	00071-0373-40	100s ud	$32.13
◆ GENERICS			
Major	00904-2056-46	30s	$1.95
Medirex	57480-0322-06	30s	$4.22
UDL	51079-0066-98	60s	$60.00
Richlyn	00115-1111-01	100s	$3.16
Rugby	00536-3762-01	100s	$3.69
Major	00904-2056-60	100s	$3.95
Schein	00364-0117-01	100s	$4.32
Geneva	00781-2498-01	100s	$4.75
Moore,H.L.	00839-1280-06	100s	$4.85
Barr	00555-0059-02	100s	$4.88
URL	00677-0064-01	100s	$4.90
Mutual	53489-0114-01	100s	$4.90
Purepac	00228-2192-10	100s	$6.80
Aligen	00405-4345-01	100s	$6.98
Parmed	00349-8872-01	100s	$18.18
Raway	00686-0369-13	100s ud	$6.50
Schein	00364-0117-90	100s ud	$6.95
Major	00904-2056-61	100s ud	$7.09

BRAND/MANUFACTURER	NDC	SIZE	AWP
Auro	55829-0628-10	100s ud	$9.69
Vangard	00615-0369-13	100s ud	$10.66
UDL	51079-0066-20	100s ud	$13.45
Medirex	57480-0322-01	100s ud	$13.45
Goldline	00182-0135-10	1000s	$19.50
Rugby	00536-3762-10	1000s	$20.38
Major	00904-2056-80	1000s	$21.05
Moore,H.L.	00839-1280-16	1000s	$21.45
Geneva	00781-2498-10	1000s	$23.25
Richlyn	00115-1111-03	1000s	$24.30
Qualitest	00603-3338-32	1000s	$24.31
Dixon-Shane	17236-0518-10	1000s	$24.50
Barr	00555-0059-05	1000s	$24.55
Mutual	53489-0114-10	1000s	$26.60
URL	00677-0064-10	1000s	$26.78
Schein	00364-0117-02	1000s	$26.80
Parmed	00349-8872-10	1000s	$27.90
Aligen	00405-4345-03	1000s	$41.62
Purepac	00228-2192-96	1000s	$41.65

ELIXIR:

BRAND/MANUFACTURER	NDC	SIZE	AWP
◆ GENERICS			
URL	00677-1524-33	480 ml	$4.45

ELIXIR: 12.5 MG/5 ML

AVERAGE UNIT PRICE (AVAILABLE SIZES)		GENERIC A-RATED AVERAGE PRICE (GAAP)	
GENERIC	$0.02	120 ml	$2.06
HCFA FUL (480 ml)	$0.01	480 ml	$4.83
		3840 ml	$21.58

BRAND/MANUFACTURER	NDC	SIZE	AWP
◆ GENERICS			
HYDRAMINE: Moore,H.L.	00839-5162-65	120 ml	$1.96
Cenci,H.R.	00556-0061-04	120 ml	$2.16
HYDRAMINE: Moore,H.L.	00839-5162-69	480 ml	$3.71
Cenci,H.R.	00556-0061-16	480 ml	$3.90
Qualitest	00603-1175-58	480 ml	$4.66
Purepac	00228-2188-16	480 ml	$5.67
Major	00904-1227-16	480 ml	$6.20
HYDRAMINE: Moore,H.L.	00839-5162-70	3840 ml	$20.78
Major	00904-1227-28	3840 ml	$21.85
Cenci,H.R.	00556-0061-28	3840 ml	$22.10
Pharm Assoc	00121-0489-05	5 ml 100s ud	$43.83
Pharm Assoc	00121-0489-10	10 ml 100s ud	$48.18
Pharm Assoc	00121-0489-20	20 ml 100s ud	$61.25

ELIXIR: 25 MG/10 ML

BRAND/MANUFACTURER	NDC	SIZE	AWP
◆ GENERICS			
Roxane	00054-8190-04	10 ml 100s ud	$51.89

INJECTION: 10 MG/ML

AVERAGE UNIT PRICE (AVAILABLE SIZES)		GENERIC A-RATED AVERAGE PRICE (GAAP)	
GENERIC	$0.22	30 ml	$6.65

BRAND/MANUFACTURER	NDC	SIZE	AWP
◆ GENERICS			
Schein	00364-6530-56	30 ml	$4.75
Steris	00402-0826-30	30 ml	$4.75
Moore,H.L.	00839-5569-36	30 ml	$6.74
Rugby	00536-4451-75	30 ml	$10.35

INJECTION: 50 MG/ML

AVERAGE UNIT PRICE (AVAILABLE SIZES)		GENERIC A-RATED AVERAGE PRICE (GAAP)	
BRAND	$1.39	10 ml	$7.15
GENERIC	$1.18	1 ml 25s	$59.65

BRAND/MANUFACTURER	NDC	SIZE	AWP
◆ BRAND			
BENADRYL: Parke-Davis	00071-4402-10	10 ml	$9.47
	00071-4259-03	1 ml 10s	$15.24
	00071-4259-40	1 ml 10s	$16.84
◆ GENERICS			
Schein	00364-6531-54	10 ml	$5.40
Steris	00402-0827-10	10 ml	$5.40
Insource	58441-1117-01	10 ml	$5.89
Genl Inject	52584-0117-10	10 ml	$5.89
Major	00904-0835-10	10 ml	$6.40
HYREXIN: Hyrex	00314-0673-70	10 ml	$6.90
Moore,H.L.	00839-6305-30	10 ml	$7.28
Rugby	00536-4460-70	10 ml	$12.75
Wyeth-Ayerst	00008-0384-01	1 ml 10s	$25.91
Elkins-Sinn	00641-0376-25	1 ml 25s	$14.89
Intl Med Sys	00548-1390-00	1 ml 25s	$104.40

▶ SHOWN IN PRODUCT IDENTIFICATION GUIDE

INJECTION: 50 MG

BRAND/MANUFACTURER		NDC	SIZE	AWP
◆ GENERICS				
Goldline		00182-3024-63	10 ml	$9.90

SYRUP: 12.5 MG/5 ML

AVERAGE UNIT PRICE (AVAILABLE SIZES)				
GENERIC	$0.01			

BRAND/MANUFACTURER		NDC	SIZE	AWP
◆ GENERICS				
HYDRAMINE: Moore,H.L.		00839-6122-65	120 ml	$2.01
HYDRAMINE: Moore,H.L.		00839-6122-69	480 ml	$4.44

TABLETS: 25 MG

BRAND/MANUFACTURER	NDC	SIZE	AWP
◆ GENERICS			
Geneva	00781-2458-13	100s ud	$9.95

TABLETS: 50 MG

BRAND/MANUFACTURER	NDC	SIZE	AWP
◆ GENERICS			
Geneva	00781-2498-13	100s ud	$11.25

Diphenidol

Diphenidol may cause hallucinations, disorientation, or confusion. For this reason, its use is limited to patients who are hospitalized or under comparable, continuous, close, professional supervision. Even then, the physician should carefully weigh the benefits against the possible risks and give due consideration to alternate therapeutic measures.

DESCRIPTION

Diphenidol, α, α-diphenyl-1-piperidinebutanol, is a compound not related to the antihistamines, phenothiazines, barbiturates, or other agents with antivertigo or antiemetic action.

Each tablet contains Diphenidol hydrochloride, equivalent to Diphenidol 25 mg.

Following is its chemical structure:

ACTIONS

Diphenidol apparently exerts a specific antivertigo effect on the vestibular apparatus to control vertigo and inhibits the chemoreceptor trigger zone to control nausea and vomiting.

INDICATIONS (SEE "WARNINGS").

1) Vertigo: Diphenidol is indicated in peripheral (labyrinthine) vertigo and associated nausea and vomiting, as seen in such conditions as: Meniere's disease, middle- and inner-ear surgery (labyrinthitis).

2) Nausea and vomiting: Diphenidol is indicated in the control of nausea and vomiting, as seen in such conditions as: postoperative states, malignant neoplasms and labyrinthine disturbances.

CONTRAINDICATIONS

Known hypersensitivity to the drug is a contraindication. Anuria is a contraindication. (Since approximately 90% of the drug is excreted in the urine, renal shutdown could cause systemic accumulation.)

WARNINGS

Diphenidol may cause hallucinations, disorientation or confusion. For this reason, its use is limited to patients who are hospitalized or under comparable, continuous, close, professional supervision. Even then, the physician should carefully weigh the benefits against the possible risks and give due consideration to alternate therapeutic measures.

The incidence of auditory and visual hallucinations, disorientation and confusion appears to be less than 1/2% or approximately one in 350 patients. The reaction has usually occurred within three days of starting the drug in recommended dosage and has subsided spontaneously usually within three days after discontinuation of the drug. Patients on Diphenidol should be observed closely and in the event of such a reaction the drug should be stopped.

Usage in Pregnancy: Use of any drug in pregnancy, lactation or in women of childbearing age requires that the potential benefits of the drug be weighed against its possible hazards to the mother and child.

In animal teratogenesis and reproduction studies of Diphenidol, there were no significant differences between drug-treated groups and untreated control groups, except as noted under animal Reproduction Studies (see "Animal Pharmacology").

In 936 patients who received Diphenidol during pregnancy, the incidences of normal and abnormal birth were comparable to those reported in the literature for the average population of pregnant patients. And in no instance was there any evidence that Diphenidol played a part in birth abnormality (see "In Pregnancy").

Diphenidol is not indicated for use in nausea and vomiting of pregnancy, since the therapeutic value and safety in this indication have not yet been determined.

PRECAUTIONS

The antiemetic action of Diphenidol may mask signs of overdose of drugs (e.g., digitalis) or may obscure diagnosis of conditions such as intestinal obstruction and brain tumor.

Although there have been no reports of blood dyscrasias with Diphenidol, patients should be observed regularly for any idiosyncratic reactions.

Diphenidol, has a weak peripheral anticholinergic effect and should be used with care in patients with glaucoma, obstructive lesions of the gastrointestinal and genitourinary tracts, such as stenosing peptic ulcer, prostatic hypertrophy, pyloric and duodenal obstruction, and organic cardiospasm.

Certain brands of Diphenidol contain FD&C Yellow No. 5 (tartrazine) which may cause allergic-type reactions (including bronchial asthma) in certain susceptible individuals. Although the overall incidence of FD&C Yellow No. 5 (tartrazine) sensitivity in the general population is low, it is frequently seen in patients who also have aspirin hypersensitivity.

Usage in Children: Diphenidol is not recommended for use in children under 50 pounds. (see "Dosage and Administration—Children").

ADVERSE REACTIONS

Auditory and visual hallucinations, disorientation and confusion have been reported. Drowsiness, overstimulation, depression, sleep disturbance, dry mouth, G.I. irritation (nausea and indigestion), or blurred vision may occur.

Rarely, slight dizziness, skin rash, malaise, headache, or heartburn may occur. Mild jaundice of questionable relationship to the use of Diphenidol has been reported. Slight, transient lowering of blood pressure has been reported in a few patients.

(See laboratory studies under "Human Pharmacology".)

DOSAGE AND ADMINISTRATION (SEE "WARNINGS").

ADULTS
For Vertigo or Nausea and Vomiting: The usual dose is one tablet (25 mg) every four hours as needed. Some patients may require two tablets (50 mg).

CHILDREN
For Nausea and Vomiting: These recommendations are for nausea and vomiting only. There has been no experience with Diphenidol in vertigo in children. Unit doses in children are best calculated by body weight: usually 0.4 mg./lb.

Children's doses usually should not be given more often than every four hours. However, if symptoms persist after the first dose, administration may be repeated after one hour. Thereafter, doses may be given every four hours as needed. The total dose in 24 hours should not exceed 2.5 mg./lb.

Note: The drug is not recommended for use in children under 50 pounds. The dosage for children 50 to 100 pounds is one tablet (25 mg).

OVERDOSAGE

In the event of overdosage, the patient should be managed according to his symptoms. Treatment is essentially supportive, with maintenance of blood pressure and respiration, plus careful observation. Early gastric lavage may be indicated depending on the amount of overdose and nature of symptoms.

ANIMAL PHARMACOLOGY

Diphenidol, exerts its antiemetic effect primarily by inhibiting the chemoreceptor trigger zone, as evidenced by its activity in blocking emesis induced by apomorphine in dogs. In this regard Diphenidol, as the hydrochloride salt, has a potency equal to the potent phenothiazine antiemetic, chlorpomazine hydrochloride. In animals Diphenidol has only weak parasympatholytic activity and no significant sedative, tranquilizing or antihistaminic action or effects on blood pressure, heart rate, respiration or the electrocardiogram.

Subacute and chronic toxicity studies in rats and dogs, in which large doses of Diphenidol, as the hydrochloride salt, were administered orally and intramuscularly for periods up to one year, revealed no significant effects on hematology, liver function, kidney function or blood glucose determinations. Histological examination of the animals' tissues did not reveal any significant lesions attributable to administration of Diphenidol.

Reproduction Studies: Teratogenesis and reproduction studies were carried out in rats and rabbits. In rats, Diphenidol, as the hydrochloride salt, was fed daily to male and female animals in doses of 20 mg./kg. and 40 mg./kg. (approximately three and six times the maximum recommended daily dose in adult humans) for 60 days before mating, and during mating, gestation and lactation for each of two litters. There were no significant differences between drug-treated and untreated control groups with regard to conception rate, litter size, live birth or viability in either of the two litters. There was no congenital anomaly among the offspring. In rabbits, Diphenidol, as the hydrochloride salt, was fed in the diets in doses of 5 mg./kg. or 75 mg./kg. (approximately equal to, and 12 times as much as, the maximum recommended daily dose in adult humans) from the first day of gestation through the 26th or 27th day of gestation, when the young were delivered by Cesarean section. There were no significant differences between drug-treated and control groups with regard to number and weight of fetuses, numbers of resorption sites or viable fetuses. There was also no statistically significant difference between drug-treated and control groups with regard to the total percentage of under-developed fetuses. However, when data were calculated on the basis of a ratio between underdeveloped fetuses and number of pregnant does, an adverse dose-related effect was observed in the high-dose test group.

HUMAN PHARMACOLOGY

Three double-blind controlled studies comparing Diphenidol to placebo were carried out: one in 32 male volunteers over a four-week period; one in 45 volunteers of whom 15 were studied for 12 weeks and 17 for 24 weeks; and one in 48 volunteers of whom 36 were studied for 12 weeks.

In the first study Diphenidol, as the hydrochloride salt, was given orally in daily doses that were started at 75 mg. during the first week and graduated up to 200 mg. by the fourth week. In the second study, one group received Diphenidol orally, as the hydrochloride salt, titrated up to 500 mg. daily, then down to 200 mg. daily; another group received a maximum of 200 mg. daily. In the third study, patients received oral doses of 200 mg. to 300 mg. of Diphenidol daily, as the hydrochloride or pamoate salts.

The studies included these laboratory determinations: complete blood counts (including hemoglobin and hematocrit determinations), urinalyses (including microscopic examination), serum alkaline phosphatase, serum bilirubin, and bromsulphalein retention. The studies also included records of weight and blood pressure and, in one, electrocardiograms.

In two of these studies, clinical laboratory changes were seen among volunteers in both treated and control groups. The changes included: extrasystoles, white cells in the urine, increase in prothrombin time, rise in hematocrit, rise in leucocytes, rise in eosinophils, and rise or reduction in neutrophils. At no time in any study did changes in the treated group differ significantly from those in the control group. Diphenidol, as the hydrochloride salt, was given orally to 17 children (aged five to 15). Total daily doses ranged from 90 to 240 mg. Complete blood counts and, in some patients, urinalyses were done before treatment and after approximately four days of treatment. There was no significant difference between pre- and post-treatment laboratory determinations in any child. No side effects were seen.

Excretion: Following oral administration of Diphenidol to dogs, as the hydrochloride or pamoate salts, and to humans, as the hydrochloride salt, peak blood concentration of the drug generally occurs in one and a half to three hours. In dogs and rats, virtually all of an oral dose of C^{14}-labeled Diphenidol is excreted in the urine and feces within three to four days, as determined by radioactivity counts. Approximately the same percentage of an administered dose appeared in the urine of dogs following either oral administration of the hydrochloride salt or rectal administration of the free base.

In Pregnancy: Investigators kept follow-up records on 936 patients who had received Diphenidol at some time during pregnancy, primarily during the first trimester.

Of the 936 women, 864 (92%) had normal births of normal infants.

Seventy-two (8%) of the women experienced some birth abnormality. Of the 72, six patients had premature but otherwise normal infants, 40 patients aborted, 10 had stillbirths, and 16 had infants with miscellaneous defects. These included hernias, congenital heart defects, hydrocephalus, internal strabismus, anencephalus, enlarged thyroid, and hypospadia.

These incidences of abnormal birth are lower than those generally reported in the literature for the average population of pregnant patients. And in no instance was there any evidence that the administration of Diphenidol played a part in birth abnormality.

HOW SUPPLIED

Current prices are unavailable. Check wholesaler for further information.

Diphtheria Antitoxin

DESCRIPTION

Diphtheria Antitoxin is a sterile solution of pepsin treated antitoxic substances obtained from the sera of horses immunized against diphtheria toxin with diphtheria toxoid alone or in conjunction with diphtheria toxin.

INDICATIONS AND USAGE

For prevention or treatment of diphtheria.

Diphtheria Antitoxin neutralizes the toxins produced by *Corynebacterium diphtheriae.*

CONTRAINDICATIONS

None known. If diphtheria is present, antitoxin must be given.

PRECAUTIONS

SENSITIVITY TESTING

Before giving Diphtheria Antitoxin to *anyone*, make a complete record of:

Previous injections of "serum" of any type.
Any allergic manifestations the patient has ever had.
Then, test for sensitivity to horse serum, and *record the results.*
Regardless of the history, a sensitivity test with suitable controls must be performed before the administration of antitoxin. Whenever possible, both the Conjunctival Test and the Intracutaneous or the Scratch Test should be performed.

Epinephrine Injection (1:1,000), a tourniquet and a hypodermic syringe with needle always should be at hand while performing sensitivity tests or administering antitoxin.

CONJUNCTIVAL TEST
Place one drop of a 1:10 dilution of Diphtheria Antitoxin in the lower conjunctival sac of one eye, and a drop of normal saline in the other eye to serve as a control.[1]

A positive (sensitivity) reaction consists of itching, burning, redness and lacrimation appearing within 15 minutes; these symptoms can be relieved by instilling a drop of epinephrine solution. The control eye should remain normal. If BOTH eyes remain normal, the conjunctival test is negative.

INTRACUTANEOUS TEST (MOST SENSITIVE)
Inject Intracutaneously 0.1 mL of a 1:100 dilution of Diphtheria Antitoxin. A separate but comparable skin site is injected intracutaneously with 0.1 mL of normal saline to serve as a control.[1] The results of the intracutaneous tests are read after an interval of 20 minutes by comparing the two injection sites. A positive sensitivity test to Diphtheria Antitoxin consists of an urticarial wheal, with or without pseudopods, surrounded by a halo of erythema. This is in contradistinction to a negative or minimal reaction, with no wheal or pseudopods, at the saline injection site.

Note: For allergic individuals, a preliminary test with 0.05 mL of a 1:1,000 dilution, intradermally, is advisable.[1]

SCRATCH TEST
A 1/4" skin scratch is made through a drop of 1:100 dilution of Diphtheria Antitoxin. To serve as a control, a similar scratch is made through a drop of normal saline placed on a different but comparable skin site. The results of the scratch test are read after an interval of 20 minutes by comparing the two sites. A positive sensitivity test to Diphtheria Antitoxin consists of an urticarial wheal, with or without pseudopods, surrounded by a halo of erythema. This is in contradistinction to a negative or minimal reaction, with no wheal or pseudopods, at the saline scratch site.

Note: Whenever possible, both the conjunctival test *and* the intracutaneous or scratch test should be performed.

Caution: A negative intracutaneous, scratch or conjunctival sensitivity test is usually considered reliable but does not completely rule out systemic sensitivity.

DESENSITIZATION[1]
In the event of a positive sensitivity test or a doubtful reaction, careful desensitization of the patient should be carried out. Serial injections of diluted Diphtheria Antitoxin as indicated below may be made at intervals of 15 minutes provided no reaction occurs. If a reaction occurs after an injection one should wait an hour and then repeat the last dose which failed to cause a reaction.

1. 0.05 mL of 1:20 dilution, subcutaneously;
2. 0.1 mL of 1:10 dilution, subcutaneously;
3. 0.3 mL of 1:10 dilution, subcutaneously;
4. 0.1 mL undiluted serum, subcutaneously;
5. 0.2 mL undiluted serum, subcutaneously;
6. 0.5 mL undiluted serum, intramuscularly;
7. Inject remaining therapeutic dose intramuscularly.

Note: For passive immunization, step 7 may be omitted, and the remaining amount of antitoxin may be administered intravenously with caution (not to exceed 1.0 mL per min.) in the proportion of 0.5 mL of antitoxin to 10 mL of sodium chloride injection USP or 5% dextrose injection. In severe diseases the preferred route of administration is intravenous to neutralize toxin as rapidly as possible.

EPINEPHRINE INJECTION (1:1000) must be immediately available.

ADVERSE REACTIONS

The incidence of acute anaphylaxis characterized by sudden onset of urticaria, respiratory distress and vascular collapse, or serum sickness (usually appearing 7-12 days after administration) characterized by fever, arthralgias, skin rash and lymphadenopathy is largely related to the amount of horse serum administered, the hypersensitivity of the patient and the history of previous serum injection.

Caution: A separate, sterile syringe and needle should be used for each individual patient to prevent transmission of hepatitis or other infectious agents from one person to another.

ADMINISTRATION

Intramuscularly or by slow intravenous infusion.
Antitoxin should be warmed to 32°—34°C (90°—95°F) before injection.
Do not warm above recommended temperature.

DOSAGE[1]

With prophylactic doses the incidence of serum sickness is generally below 10%; with therapeutic dosage a higher incidence should be anticipated, depending upon the amount administered. The incubation period varies from 7 to 12 days. A short incubation period (accelerated serum sickness) occurs in individuals who have been sensitized by previous serum therapy.

THERAPEUTIC REGIMEN
1. Perform sensitivity tests.

2. Give all of the required antitoxin, intramuscularly or intravenously, at once. Each hour's delay increases the dosage requirements and decreases the beneficial effects.

3. Suggested ranges are: pharyngeal or laryngeal disease of 48 hours' duration, 20,000 to 40,000 units; nasopharyngeal lesions, 40,000 to 60,000 units; extensive disease of 3 or more days' duration or any patient with brawny swelling of the neck, 80,000 to 120,000 units.

4. Give children the same dose as adults.

5. *In addition*, appropriate antimicrobial agents in full therapeutic dosage should be started.

Any person with clinical symptoms of diphtheria should receive Diphtheria Antitoxin at once without waiting for bacteriologic confirmation of the diagnosis. Observation and supportive treatment should be continued until all local and general symptoms are controlled, or until some other etiologic agent has been identified.

PROPHYLACTIC REGIMEN

All asymptomatic, unimmunized contacts of patients with diphtheria should receive prompt prophylaxis with appropriate antimicrobial therapy with cultures before and after treatment, immunization with Diphtheria toxoid, and continued surveillance for seven days.

Close contacts not under surveillance should receive appropriate antimicrobial therapy, immunization with Diphtheria toxoid and Diphtheria Antitoxin.[2] Prior to administering Diphtheria Antitoxin:

1. Perform appropriate sensitivity tests.

2. If sensitivity testing is negative, give 10,000 units intramuscularly.[3] The dose is dependent upon length of time since exposure, the extent of the exposure and the medical condition of the individual.

3. If sensitivity testing is positive, proceed with desensitization schedule outlined above.

STORAGE

Store between 2°—8°C (35°—46°F). Potency not affected by freezing.

REFERENCES

1. Report of the Committee on Infectious Diseases, American Academy of Pediatrics, Evanston, Illinois, p. 20,21, and 62, 1977 2. Diphtheria Antitoxin for case contacts. MMWR 26: 402, 1977 3. Report of the Committee on Infectious Diseases, American Academy of Pediatrics, Evanston, Illinois, p. 47, 1970

HOW SUPPLIED

INJECTION: 20,000 U

BRAND/MANUFACTURER	NDC	SIZE	AWP
○ GENERICS Connaught	49281-0230-89	1 ml	$331.25

Diphtheria and Tetanus Toxoids

DESCRIPTION

Diphtheria and Tetanus Toxoids is a sterile combination of refined Diphtheria and Tetanus Toxoids for intramuscular use only. After shaking, the vaccine is a homogeneous white suspension.

The Diphtheria and Tetanus Toxins are produced according to the method of Mueller and Miller[1,2] and are refined by the Pillemer alcohol fractionation method[3].

Each 0.5 mL dose is formulated to contain 2 (adult) or 12.5 (pediatric) Lf units of diphtheria toxoid, and 5 Lf units of tetanus toxoid.

CLINICAL PHARMACOLOGY

Diphtheria is primarily a localized and generalized intoxication caused by diphtheria toxin, an extracellular protein metabolite of toxinogenic strains of *Corynebacterium diphtheriae*. While the incidence of diphtheria in the U.S. has decreased from over 200,000 cases reported in 1921 before the general use of diphtheria toxoid, to only 15 cases reported from 1980 through 1983, the ratio of fatalities to attack rate has remained constant at about 5% to 10%[4]. The highest case fatality rates are in the very young and the elderly.

Following adequate immunization with diphtheria toxoid, which induces antitoxin, it is thought that protection lasts for at least 10 years.[4] This significantly reduces both the risk of developing diphtheria and the severity of clinical illness. It does not, however, eliminate carriage of *C diphtheriae* in the pharynx or on the skin.[4]

Tetanus is an intoxication manifested primarily by neuromuscular dysfunction, caused by a potent exotoxin elaborated by *Clostridium tetani*. The incidence of tetanus in the U.S. has dropped dramatically with the routine use of tetanus toxoid, remaining relatively constant over the last decade at about 90 cases reported annually.[4] Spores of *C tetani* are ubiquitous, and there is essentially no natural immunity to tetanus toxin. Thus, universal primary immunization with tetanus toxoid, and subsequent maintenance of adequate antitoxin levels by means of timed boosters, is necessary to protect all age groups.[4] Tetanus toxoid is a highly effective antigen, and a completed primary series generally induces protective levels of serum antitoxin that persist for at least 10 years.[4]

INDICATIONS AND USAGE

Diphtheria and Tetanus Toxoids (pediatric) is indicated for active immunization of infants and children from 2 months of age up to their seventh birthday both for routine protection and as a preventive measure against diphtheria and tetanus, in circumstances in which the use of a combined triple vaccine containing pertussis antigen is contraindicated.[4,5]

Diphtheria and Tetanus Toxoids (adult) is indicated for active immunization against tetanus and diphtheria in adults and children 7 years of age and older.[4,6]

The Immunization Practices Advisory Committee (ACIP) of the U.S. Public Health Service recommends the use of the combined toxoids vaccine rather than single component vaccines for both primary and booster injections, including active tetanus immunization in wound management.[4]

Tetanus or diphtheria infection may not confer immunity; therefore, initiation or completion of active immunization is indicated at the time of recovery from these infections.[4]

There is no evidence that Diphtheria and Tetanus Toxoids are teratogenic. A previously unimmunized pregnant woman, who may deliver her child under nonhygienic circumstances and/or surroundings, should receive two properly spaced doses of Diphtheria and Tetanus Toxoids before delivery, preferably during the last two trimesters. Incompletely immunized pregnant women should complete the three-dose series. Those immunized more than 10 years previously should have a booster dose.[4] (See also pregnancy information under *"Precautions."*)

CONTRAINDICATIONS

Hypersensitivity to any component of the vaccine including thimerosal (a mercury derivative contained in some brands) is a contraindication.

The occurrence of any neurological symptoms or signs following administration of this product is a contraindication to further use.

Immunization should be deferred during the course of any febrile illness or acute infection. A minor afebrile illness such as a mild upper respiratory infection is not usually reason to defer immunization.[4,5]

The clinical judgment of the attending physician should prevail at all times.

Routine immunization should be deferred during an outbreak of poliomyelitis, providing the patient has not sustained an injury that increases the risk of tetanus and providing an outbreak of diphtheria does not occur simultaneously.

WARNINGS

THE PEDIATRIC FORMULATION IS NOT RECOMMENDED FOR IMMUNIZING PERSONS ON OR AFTER THEIR SEVENTH BIRTHDAY; THE ADULT FORMULATION IS NOT RECOMMENDED FOR IMMUNIZING PERSONS LESS THAN 7 YEARS OF AGE.

The concentration of diphtheria toxoid in preparations intended for use in persons 7 years of age or older is lower than that of the pediatric formulation; a lower dosage of diphtheria toxoid is recommended for persons 7 years of age or older because adverse reactions to the diphtheria component are thought to be related to both dose and age.[4]

THE OCCURRENCE OF A NEUROLOGICAL OR SEVERE HYPERSENSITIVITY REACTION FOLLOWING A PREVIOUS DOSE IS A CONTRAINDICATION TO FURTHER USE OF THIS PRODUCT.[4]

THE ADMINISTRATION OF BOOSTER DOSES MORE FREQUENTLY THAN RECOMMENDED (see *"Dosage and Administration"*) MAY BE ASSOCIATED WITH INCREASED INCIDENCE AND SEVERITY OF REACTIONS.[4]

Persons who experience Arthus-type hypersensitivity reactions or temperature greater than 39.4°C (103°F), after a previous dose of tetanus toxoid usually have very high serum tetanus antitoxin levels and should not be given even emergency doses of Diphtheria and Tetanus Toxoids more frequently than every 10 years, even if they have a wound that is neither clean nor minor.[4]

If a contraindication to using tetanus toxoid-containing preparations exists in a person who has not completed a primary immunizing course of tetanus toxoid, and other than a clean, minor wound is sustained, only passive immunization should be given using human Tetanus, Immune Globulin (TIG).[4]

DT should not be given to individuals with thrombocytopenia or any coagulation disorder that would contraindicate intramuscular injection unless the potential benefits clearly outweigh the risk of administration.

Patients with impaired immune responsiveness, whether due to the use of immunosuppressive therapy (including irradiation, corticosteroids, antimetabolites, alkylating agents, and cytotoxic agents), a genetic defect, human immunodeficiency virus (HIV) infection, or other causes, may have a reduced antibody response to active immunization procedures.[4,5,6,7] Deferral of administration of vaccine may be considered in individuals receiving immunosuppressive therapy.[4,5,6] Other groups should generally receive this vaccine according to the usual recommended schedule.[4,5,7,8]

Special care should be taken to prevent injection into a blood vessel.

PRECAUTIONS

GENERAL

1. THE PEDIATRIC FORMULATION SHOULD BE USED FOR THE AGE GROUP BETWEEN 2 MONTHS AND THE SEVENTH BIRTHDAY; THE ADULT FORMULATION SHOULD BE USED FOR INDIVIDUALS 7 YEARS OF AGE OR OLDER.

2. PRIOR TO ADMINISTRATION OF ANY DOSE OF DIPHTHERIA AND TETANUS TOXOIDS, THE PARENT, GUARDIAN OR ADULT PATIENT SHOULD BE ASKED ABOUT THE RECENT HEALTH STATUS AND IMMUNIZATION STATUS OF THE PATIENT TO BE IMMUNIZED IN ORDER TO DETERMINE THE EXISTENCE OF ANY CONTRAINDICATION TO IMMUNIZATION WITH DIPHTHERIA AND TETANUS TOXOIDS. (SEE *"CONTRAINDICATIONS, WARNINGS"*).

3. WHEN THE PATIENT RETURNS FOR THE NEXT DOSE IN A SERIES, THE PARENT, GUARDIAN, OR ADULT PATIENT SHOULD BE QUES-

TIONED CONCERNING OCCURRENCE OF ANY SYMPTOM AND/OR SIGN OF AN ADVERSE REACTION AFTER THE PREVIOUS DOSE. (SEE "CONTRAINDICATIONS, ADVERSE REACTIONS").

4. BEFORE THE INJECTION OF ANY BIOLOGICAL, THE PHYSICIAN SHOULD TAKE ALL PRECAUTIONS KNOWN FOR PREVENTION OF ALLERGIC OR ANY OTHER SIDE REACTIONS. This should include: a review of the patient's history regarding possible sensitivity; the ready availability of epinephrine 1:1,000 and other appropriate agents used for control of immediate allergic reactions; and a knowledge of the recent literature pertaining to use of the biological concerned, including the nature of side effects and adverse reactions that may follow its use.

5. A separate sterile syringe and needle or a sterile disposable unit should be used for each individual patient to prevent transmission of hepatitis or other infectious agents from one person to another.

6. *Shake vigorously before withdrawing each dose to resuspend the contents of the container.*

7. NATIONAL CHILDHOOD VACCINE INJURY ACT OF 1986 (AS AMENDED IN 1987)

This Act requires that the manufacturer and lot number of the vaccine administered be recorded by the health care provider in the vaccine recipient's permanent medical record, along with the date of administration of the vaccine and the name, address and title of the person administering the vaccine.

The Act further requires the health care provider to report to a health department or to the FDA the occurrence following immunization of any event set forth in the Vaccine Injury Table including: anaphylaxis or anaphylactic shock within 24 hours, encephalopathy or encephalitis within 7 days, residual seizure disorder, any acute complication or sequelae (including death) of above events, or any event that would contraindicate further doses of vaccine, according to this package insert.[9]

INFORMATION FOR THE PATIENT
PRIOR TO THE ADMINISTRATION OF THIS VACCINE, HEALTH CARE PERSONNEL SHOULD INFORM THE PARENT, GUARDIAN OR OTHER RESPONSIBLE ADULT, OR ADULT PATIENT OF THE BENEFITS AND RISKS OF VACCINATION AGAINST DIPHTHERIA AND TETANUS.

USE IN PREGNANCY
The pediatric formulation is not recommended for administration to females of child-bearing age.

Pregnancy Category C: Animal reproductive studies have not been conducted with Diphtheria and Tetanus Toxoids (adult). There is no evidence that Diphtheria and Tetanus Toxoids (adult) are teratogenic. Diphtheria and Tetanus Toxoids (adult) should be given to inadequately immunized pregnant women because it affords protection against neonatal tetanus.[10] Waiting until the second trimester is a reasonable precaution to minimize any theoretical concern.[4] Maintenance of adequate immunization by routine boosters in nonpregnant women of childbearing age (see *"Dosage and Administration"*) can obviate the need to vaccinate women during pregnancy.

ADVERSE REACTIONS
Local reactions, manifested by varying degrees of erythema, induration, and tenderness, may occur after administration of Diphtheria and Tetanus Toxoids.[11-16] Such local reactions are usually self-limited and require no therapy. Nodule,[17] sterile abscess formation, or subcutaneous atrophy may occur at the site of injection.

Systemic symptoms, including drowsiness, fretfulness, vomiting, anorexia, and persistent crying have been described following Diphtheria and Tetanus Toxoid (pediatric) immunization.[11,12]

In one study, fever $\geq38°C$ (100.4°F) was reported in 9.3% of Diphtheria and Tetanus Toxoid (pediatric) recipients, and fever $\geq39°C$ (102.2°F) was reported in 0.7% of recipients.[11]

Pallor, coldness, and hyporesponsiveness have been reported in a child receiving a Diphtheria and Tetanus Toxoid (pediatric) vaccine.[12]

Systemic reactions, such as fever, chills, myalgias, and headaches, also may occur[13-16] with Diphtheria and Tetanus Toxoids (adult).

Arthus-type hypersensitivity reactions, or high fever, may occur in persons who have very high serum antitoxin antibodies due to overly frequent injections of toxoid (see *"Warnings"*).

NEUROLOGICAL COMPLICATIONS[18] SUCH AS CONVULSIONS,[13] ENCEPHALOPATHY,[19,20] AND VARIOUS MONO- AND POLYNEUROPATHIES,[20-26] INCLUDING GUILLIAN-BARRE SYNDROME,[27,28] HAVE BEEN REPORTED FOLLOWING ADMINISTRATION OF PREPARATIONS CONTAINING DIPHTHERIA AND/OR TETANUS ANTIGENS.

URTICARIA, ERYTHEMA MULTIFORME OR OTHER RASH. ARTHRALGIAS[19] AND, MORE RARELY, A SEVERE ANAPHYLACTIC REACTION (IE. URTICARIA WITH SWELLING OF THE MOUTH, DIFFICULTY BREATHING, HYPOTENSION, OR SHOCK) HAVE BEEN REPORTED FOLLOWING ADMINISTRATION OF PREPARATIONS CONTAINING DIPHTHERIA AND/OR TETANUS ANTIGENS.

DOSAGE AND ADMINISTRATION
For Intramuscular Use Only: Shake vigorously before withdrawing each dose to resuspend the contents of the container.

Parenteral drug products should be inspected visually for particulate matter and discoloration prior to administration. (See *"Description"*).

The vaccine should be injected intramuscularly, preferably into the midlateral muscles of the thigh (pediatric) or deltoid (pediatric and adult), with care to avoid major peripheral nerve trunks.

Before injection, the skin at the injection site should be cleansed and prepared with a suitable germicide.

After insertion of the needle, aspirate to help avoid inadvertent injection into a blood vessel.

Pediatric Formulation: This combined preparation against both diphtheria and tetanus is designed particularly to meet the need of children less than 7 years of age for whom the use of a combined triple vaccine containing pertussis antigen is contraindicated.

It is recommended that active immunization against diphtheria and tetanus be started at 2 months of age.

Unimmunized infants and children less than 1 year of age for whom vaccine containing pertussis antigen is contraindicated should receive three doses of 0.5 mL each of Diphtheria and Tetanus Toxoids at 4 to 8 week intervals, followed by a fourth (reinforcing) dose of 0.5 mL 6 to 12 months after the third dose, for the primary series.

Unimmunized children 1 year of age or older for whom vaccine containing pertussis antigen is contraindicated should receive two doses of 0.5 mL each of Diphtheria and Tetanus Toxoids, 4 to 8 weeks apart, followed by a third (reinforcing) dose 6 to 12 months later, for the primary series.

If after beginning a Diphtheria/Tetanus/Pertussis series, further doses of vaccine containing pertussis antigen become contraindicated, Diphtheria and Tetanus Toxoids should be substituted for each of the remaining doses[4,5].

The reinforcing dose is an integral part of the primary immunizing series.

Interruption of the recommended schedule with a delay between doses does not interfere with the final immunity achieved, nor does it necessitate starting the series over again, regardless of the length of time elapsed between doses.[4,5]

A booster dose of 0.5 mL is indicated at age 4 to 6 years, preferably prior to entrance into kindergarten or elementary school. However, if the last dose of the primary immunizing series was administered after the fourth birthday, a booster prior to school entry is not considered necessary.[4,5]

Adult Formulation: The primary immunizing course for unimmunized individuals 7 years of age or older consists of two doses of 0.5 mL each, 4 to 8 weeks apart, followed by a third (reinforcing) dose of 0.5 mL 6 to 12 months after the second dose. The reinforcing dose is an integral part of the primary immunizing course.[4] Interruption of the recommended schedule with a delay between doses does not interfere with the final immunity achieved, nor does it necessitate starting the series over again, regardless of the length of time elapsed between doses.[4]

A booster dose of 0.5 mL of Diphtheria and Tetanus Toxoids is given 10 years after completion of primary immunization and every 10 years thereafter. If a dose is given sooner than 10 years, as part of wound management or on exposure to diphtheria, the next booster is not needed for 10 years thereafter. (See *"Warnings"*.) MORE FREQUENT BOOSTER DOSES ARE NOT INDICATED AND MAY BE ASSOCIATED WITH INCREASED INCIDENCE AND SEVERITY OF REACTIONS.[4] (See *"Warnings"*.)

Diphtheria Prophylaxis for Case Contacts: All case contacts, household and others, who have previously received fewer than three doses of diphtheria toxoid should receive an immediate dose of an appropriate diphtheria toxoid-containing preparation and should complete the series according to schedule. Case contacts who previously received three or more doses, but who have not received a dose of a preparation containing diphtheria toxoid within the previous 5 years, should receive a dose of a diphtheria toxoid-containing preparation appropriate for their age.

TETANUS PROPHYLAXIS IN WOUND MANAGEMENT
Pediatric: For routine wound management of children under 7 years of age who are not completely immunized, Diphtheria and Tetanus Toxoids (pediatric) should be used instead of single-antigen tetanus toxoid (if pertussis antigen is contraindicated or individual circumstances are such that potential febrile reactions following Diphtheria/Tetanus/Pertussis might confound the management of the patient).[4] Completion of primary vaccination thereafter should be ensured.

For tetanus-prone wounds in children who have had fewer than three, or an unknown number of immunizations with a tetanus-toxoid containing product, passive immunization with human Tetanus- Immune Globulin (TIG) is also recommended.[4] A separate syringe and site of injection should be used.

Adult: The need for active immunization with a tetanus toxoid-containing preparation, with or without passive immunization with human Tetanus Immune Globulin (TIG) depends on both the condition of the wound and the patient's immunization history. Tetanus has rarely occurred among persons with a documented primary series of tetanus toxoid injections. A thorough attempt must be made to determine whether a patient has completed primary immunization.[4]

Individuals who have completed primary immunization against tetanus, and who sustain wounds which are minor and uncontaminated, should receive a booster dose of a tetanus-toxoid preparation only if they have not received tetanus toxoid within the preceding 10 years. For other wounds, a booster is appropriate if the patient has not received tetanus toxoid within the preceding 5 years. Antitoxin antibodies develop rapidly in persons who have previously received at least two doses of tetanus toxoid.[4]

Individuals who have not completed primary immunization against tetanus, or whose immunization history is unknown or uncertain, should be immunized with a tetanus toxoid-containing product. Completion of primary immunization thereafter should be ensured. In addition, if these individuals have sustained a tetanus-prone wound, the use of human TIG is recommended. A separate syringe and site of administration should be used.[4]

SUMMARY GUIDE TO TETANUS PROPHYLAXIS IN ROUTINE WOUND MANAGEMENT[4]*

History of Tetanus toxoid (doses)	Clean, minor wounds		All other wounds†	
	Diphtheria and Tetanus Toxoids	TIG	Diphtheria and Tetanus Toxoids	TIG
Unknown < three	Yes	No	Yes	Yes
≥ three ‡	No§	No	No"	No

*Important details are in the text.

†Such as, but not limited to, wounds contaminated with dirt, feces, soil, saliva, etc.; puncture wounds; avulsions; and wounds resulting from missiles, crushing, burns, and frost-bite.

‡If only three doses of fluid toxoid have been received, a fourth dose of toxoid, preferably an adsorbed toxoid, should be given.

§Yes, if more than 10 years since last dose.

"Yes, if more than 5 years since last dose. (More frequent boosters are not needed and can accentuate side effects.)

Diphtheria and Tetanus Toxoids (adult) is the preferred preparation for active tetanus immunization in wound management of patients 7 years of age or older. This is to enhance diphtheria protection, since a large proportion of adults are susceptible. Thus, by taking advantage of acute health care visits for wound management, some patients can be protected who otherwise would remain susceptible.[4]

STORAGE

Do not freeze. Store refrigerated, away from freezer compartment, at 2°C to 8°C (36°F to 46°F).

REFERENCES

1. Mueler JH, Miller PA: Production of diphtheria toxin of high potency (100Lf) on a reproducible medium. J Immunol 1941:40:21-32. 2. Mueller JH, Miller PA: Factors influencing the production of tetanal toxin. J Immunol 1947:56:143-147. 3. Pillemer L. Grossberg DB, Wittler RG: The immunochemistry of toxins and toxoids. II. The preparation and immunological evaluation of purified tetanal toxoid. J Immunol 1946:54:213-224. 4. Recommendation of the Immunization Practices Advisory Committee (ACIP): Diphtheria, tetanus and pertussis: Guidelines for vaccine prophylaxis and other preventive measures. MMWR 1985:34:405-426. 5. American Academy of Pediatrics: Report of the Committee on Infectious Diseases, ed 20. Elk Grove Village, IL, American Academy of Pediatrics, 1986. 6. Committee on Immunization, Council of Medical Societies American College of Physicians: Guide for Adult Immunization, 1st Edition 1985: Philadelphia, PA. 7. Recommendation of the ACIP: Immunization of children infected with Human T-Lymphotrophic Virus Type III/Lymphadenopathy associated virus. MMWR 1986; 35(38):595-606. 8. Immunization of children infected with Human Immunodeficiency Virus-Supplementary ACIP statement. MMWR 1988:37(12):181-183. 9. National Childhood Vaccine Injury Act: Requirements for permanent vaccination records and for reporting of selected events after vaccination. MMWR 1988:37(13):197-200. 10. Recommendations of the ACIP: General recommendations on immunization. MMWR 1983:32(1):1-17. 11. Cody C, et al: Nature and rates of adverse reactions associated with DTP and DT immunizations in infants and children. Pediatrics 1981:68:650-660. 12. Feery BJ: Incidence and type of reactions to triple antigen (DTP) and DT (CDT) vaccines. Med Jour of Australia 1982:2:511-515. 13. Deacon SP, et al: A comparative clinical study of adsorbed tetanus vaccine and adult-type tetanus-diphtheria vaccine. J Hyg (Cambridge) 1982:89:513-519. 14. Macko MB, Powell CE: Comparison of the morbidity of tetanus toxoid boosters with tetanus-diphtheria toxoid boosters. Ann Emerg Med 1985:14(1):33-35. 15. Myers MG, et al: Primary immunization with tetanus and diphtheria toxoids. JAMA 1982:248(19):2478-2480. 16. Sisk CW, et al: Reactions to tetanus-diphtheria toxoid (adult). Arch Environ Health 1965:11:34-36. 17. Fawcett HA, Smith NP: Injection-site granuloma due to aluminum. Arch Dermatol 1984:120:1318-1322. 18. Rutledge SL, Snead OC: Neurological complications of immunizations. J Pediatr 1986:109:917-924. 19. Adverse Events Following Immunization. MMWR 1985:34(3):43-47. 20. Schlenska GK: Unusual neurological complications following tetanus toxoid administration. J Neurol 1977:215:299-302. 21. Blumstein GI, Kreithen H: Peripheral neuropathy following tetanus toxoid administration. JAMA 1966:198:1030-1031. 22. Reinstein L. Pargament JM. Goodman JS: Peripheral neuropathy after multiple tetanus toxoid injections. Arch Phys Med Rehabil 1982:63:332-334. 23. Tsairis P, Duck PJ, Mulder DW: Natural history of brachial plexus neuropathy. Arch Neurol 1972:27:109-117. 24. Quast U, Hennessen W, Widmark RM: Mono- and polyneuritis after tetanus vaccination. Devel Bio Stand 1979:43:25-32. 25. Holliday PL, Bauer RB: Polyradiculoneuritis secondary to immunization with tetanus and diphtheria toxoids. Arch Neurol 1983:40:56-57. 26. Fenichel GM: Neurological complications of tetanus toxoid. Arch Neurol 1983:40:390. 27. Pollard JD, Selby G: Relapsing neuropathy due to tetanus toxoid. J Neurol Sci 1978:37:113-125. 28. Newton N, Janati A: Guillain-Barre syndrome after vaccination with purified tetanus toxoid. S Med J 1987:80:1053-1054.

HOW SUPPLIED
INJECTION:

BRAND/MANUFACTURER	NDC	SIZE	AWP
○ GENERICS			
Sclavo	42021-0210-11	5 ml	$7.50
Sclavo	42021-0211-09	5 ml	$7.50
Lederle Labs	00005-1858-31	5 ml	$13.24

BRAND/MANUFACTURER	NDC	SIZE	AWP
Lederle Labs	00005-1875-31	5 ml	$13.24
Wyeth-Ayerst	00008-0338-02	5 ml	$13.64
Wyeth-Ayerst	00008-0341-02	5 ml	$13.64
Connaught	49281-0275-10	5 ml	$13.75
Connaught	49281-0271-83	5 ml	$13.75
Lederle Labs	00005-1875-47	0.5 ml 10s ud	$36.48
Wyeth-Ayerst	00008-0338-01	1 ml 10s	$25.31
Wyeth-Ayerst	00008-0341-01	1 ml 10s	$25.31

Diphtheria/Haemophilus b/ Pertussis/Tetanus Vaccine

DESCRIPTION

Diphtheria/Haemophilus b/Pertussis/Tetanus is a sterile combination of vaccines. Diphtheria/Haemophilus b/Pertussis/Tetanus is for intramuscular use only. After shaking, the vaccine is a homogeneous white suspension.

The Diphtheria and Tetanus toxoids are derived from Corynebacterium diphtheriae and Clostridium tetani, respectively, which are grown in media according to the method of Mueller and Miller.[1,2] C. diphtheriae is grown in a defined medium containing casamino acids and C. tetani in a medium containing beef heart infusion. They are detoxified by use of formaldehyde. The toxoids are refined by the Pillemer alcohol fractionation method[3] and are diluted with a solution containing sodium phosphate monobasic, sodium phosphate dibasic, glycine, and thimerosal (mercury derivative) as a preservative.

Pertussis Vaccine is prepared by growing Phase I Bordetella pertussis in a modified Cohen-Wheeler broth containing acid hydrolysate of casein. The B. pertussis is inactivated with thimerosal, harvested, and then suspended in a solution containing potassium phosphate monobasic, sodium phosphate dibasic, sodium chloride, and thimerosal (mercury derivative) as a preservative.

The oligosaccharides for the Haemophilus b conjugate component are derived from highly purified capsular polysaccharide, polyribosylribitol phosphate, isolated from Haemophilus influenzae type b (Haemophilus b) grown in a chemically defined medium (a mixture of mineral salts, amino acids, and cofactors). The oligosaccharides are purified and sized by diafiltrations through a series of ultrafiltration membranes, and coupled by reductive amination directly to highly purified CRM_{197}.[4,5] CRM_{197} is a nontoxic variant of diphtheria toxin isolated from cultures of C. diphtheriae C7 (β 197) grown in a casamino acids and yeast extract-based medium. The conjugate is purified through ultrafiltration, ammonium sulfate precipitation, and ion-exchange chromatography to high purity.

The Haemophilus b conjugate component is combined with the diphtheria and tetanus toxoids and pertussis vaccine adsorbed to produce the final vaccine. As a preservative, thimerosal (mercury derivative) is added to the combination vaccine to a final concentration of 1:10,000. The aluminum content (from aluminum phosphate adjuvant) of the final product does not exceed 0.85 mg per 0.5 mL dose as determined by assay. The residual-free formaldehyde content by assay is ≤ 0.02%.

Each single dose of 0.5 mL of Diphtheria/Haemophilus b/Pertussis/Tetanus Vaccine is formulated to contain 12.5 Lf of diphtheria toxoid, 5 Lf of tetanus toxoid (both toxoids induce not less than 2 units of antitoxin per mL in the guinea pig potency test), 10 µg of purified Haemophilus b saccharide, and approximately 25 µg of CRM_{197} protein. Each 0.5 mL dose of vaccine is formulated to contain less than 16 OPUs of inactivated pertussis cells. The total human immunizing dose (the first three 0.5 mL doses given) contains an estimate of 12 units of Pertussis Vaccine with an estimate of 4 protective units per single human dose, as determined by the mouse pertussis potency test. The potency for the Haemophilus b conjugate component of Diphtheria/Haemophilus b/Pertussis/Tetanus Vaccine (Diphtheria CRM_{197} Protein Conjugate) is determined by gas chromatography assay for total saccharide. Each component of the vaccine—Diphtheria, Haemophilus b, Pertussis, and Tetanus meets the required potency standards, and contains no other active ingredients.

CLINICAL PHARMACOLOGY

Simultaneous immunization against diphtheria, pertussis, and tetanus during infancy and childhood has been a routine practice in the United States since the late 1940s, and immunization against Haemophilus b has been a routine practice since 1985. These immunizations have played a major role in markedly reducing the incidence of cases and deaths from each of these diseases.

Diphtheria is primarily a localized and generalized intoxication caused by Diphtheria toxin, an extracellular protein metabolite of toxinogenic strains of C. diphtheriae. While the incidence of Diphtheria in the US has decreased from over 200,000 cases reported in 1921, before the general use of Diphtheria toxoid, to only 15 cases reported from 1980 to 1983,[6] the case fatality rate has remained constant at about 5% to 10%. The highest case fatality rates are in the very young and in the elderly.

Following adequate immunization with Diphtheria toxoid, it is thought that protection lasts for at least 10 years.[6]

Antitoxin levels of at least 0.01 antitoxin units/mL are generally regarded as protective.[7] This significantly reduces both the risk of developing diphtheria and the severity of clinical illness. It does not, however, eliminate carriage of C. diphtheriae in the pharynx or on the skin.[6]

Tetanus is an intoxication manifested primarily by neuromuscular dysfunction caused by a potent exotoxin elaborated by C. tetani. The incidence of tetanus in the US has dropped dramatically with the routine use of Tetanus toxoid, remaining relatively constant over the last decade at about 90 cases reported annually. Spores of *C. tetani* are ubiquitous, and there is essentially no natural immunity to tetanus toxin.

Thus, universal primary immunization with Tetanus toxoid with subsequent maintenance of adequate antitoxin levels, by means of timed boosters, is recommended to protect all age groups.[6] Tetanus toxoid is a highly effective antigen and a completed primary series generally induces serum antitoxin levels of at least 0.01 antitoxin units, a level that has been reported to be protective.[8] It is thought that protection persists for at least 10 years.[6]

The toxoids of Tetanus and Diphtheria induce neutralizing antibodies to the toxins produced by the infecting organism. In clinical studies with Diphtheria and Tetanus toxoids, administered in combination with Pertussis vaccine, serum antitoxin levels have been shown to be greater than 0.01 antitoxin units/mL in 97% to 100% of 372 infants following three doses.[9,10] These levels are generally regarded to be protective.[7,8]

Pertussis (whooping cough) is a disease of the respiratory tract caused by *B. pertussis*. This gram-negative cocobacillus produces a variety of active components including endotoxin and a number of other substances that have been defined primarily on the basis of their biological activity in animals. These active components have been associated with a number of effects, such as lymphocytosis, leukocytosis, sensitivity to histamine, changes in glucose and/or insulin levels, possible neurological effects and adjuvant activity.[11] The roles of each of the different components in either the pathogenesis of, or immunity to, pertussis is not well understood.

Pertussis (whooping cough) is a highly communicable disease of the respiratory tract. Attack rates of over 90% have been reported in unimmunized household contacts.[12] Since immunization against pertussis (whooping cough) became widespread, the number of reported cases and associated mortality in the US has declined from about 120,000 cases and 1,100 deaths in 1950,[13] to an annual average of about 3,500 cases and 10 fatalities in recent years.[6,14] Precise data do not exist since bacteriological confirmation of pertussis can be obtained in less than half of the suspected cases. Most reported illness from *B. pertussis* occurs in infants and young children; two-thirds of reported deaths occur in children less than 1 year old. Older children and adults, in whom classic signs are often absent, may go undiagnosed and serve as reservoirs of disease.[6,15]

The potency of the Pertussis component of the vaccine is measured and shown to be acceptable in the mouse potency test. Previously, serum agglutinin titers of Pertussis vaccines have been correlated with clinical protection in the Medical Research Council trials.[8] The Pertussis component induces immunity against pertussis disease in humans.

Haemophilus influenzae type b was the most common cause of invasive bacterial disease, including meningitis, in young children in the US prior to licensure of vaccines for this disease. Although nonencapsulated *H. influenzae* are common and six capsular polysaccharide types are known, strains with the type b capsule caused most of the invasive Haemophilus diseases prior to the introduction of Haemophilus b conjugate vaccines.[16]

Prior to routine immunization, Haemophilus b disease occurred primarily in children under 5 years of age. In the US, the incidence of invasive Haemophilus b disease peaked between 6 months and 1 year of age, and approximately 55% of disease occurred between 6 and 18 months of age.[16] The cumulative risk of developing invasive Haemophilus b disease during the first 5 years of life was about 1 in 200 prior to the introduction of Haemophilus b conjugate vaccines. Approximately 60% of cases were meningitis. Cellulitis, epiglottitis, pericarditis, pneumonia, sepsis, or septic arthritis made up the remaining 40%. An estimated 12,000 cases of Haemophilus b meningitis occurred annually prior to the routine use of conjugate vaccines in infants and toddlers.[16,17] The mortality rate can be 5%, and neurologic sequelae have been observed in up to 38% of survivors.[18]

The incidence of invasive Haemophilus b disease is increased in certain children, such as those who are native Americans, black, or from lower socioeconomic status and those with medical conditions such as asplenia, sickle cell disease, malignancies associated with immunosuppression, and antibody deficiency syndromes.[16,17,19]

The protective activity of antibody to Haemophilus b polysaccharide was demonstrated by the efficacy study of Haemophilus b polysaccharide (HbPs) vaccine.[20] Data from passive antibody studies indicate that a preexisting titer of antibody to HbPs of 0.15 µg/mL correlates with protection.[21] Data from a Finnish field trial in children 18 to 71 months of age indicate that a titer of $\geq$ 1.0 µg/mL 3 weeks after vaccination is associated with long-term protection.[22]

Linkage of Haemophilus b saccharides to a protein such as CRM_{197} converts the saccharide (HbO) to a T-dependent (HbOC) antigen, and results in an enhanced antibody response to the saccharide in young infants that primes for an anamnestic response and is predominantly of the IgG class.[23] Laboratory evidence indicates that the native state of the CRM_{197} protein and the use of oligosaccharides in the formulation of, Haemophilus b Conjugate Vaccine (Diphtheria CRM_{197} Protein Conjugate) (HbOC), enhances its immunogenicity.[24-26] NO PUBLISHED DATA ARE AVAILABLE TO SUPPORT THE INTERCHANGEABILITY OF HbOC AND OTHER HAEMOPHILUS b CONJUGATE VACCINES WITH ONE ANOTHER FOR PRIMARY IMMUNIZATION.

HbOC was shown to be effective in a large-scale controlled clinical trial in a multiethnic population in northern California carried out between February 1988 and June 1990.[27,28] It should be noted that DTP was administered simultaneously with HbOC but at a separate site. There were no (0) vaccine failures in infants who received three doses of HbOC and 12 cases of Haemophilus b disease (6 cases of meningitis) in the control group. The estimate of efficacy is 100% (P = .0002)

with 95% Confidence Intervals of 68% to 100%. Through the end of 1991, with an additional 49,000 person-years of follow-up, there were still no cases of Haemophilus b disease in fully vaccinated infants less than 2 years of age.[10,29] Person-years may be defined as the number of individuals receiving the appropriate number of doses times the average number of years of follow-up for all of the individuals. One case of disease has been reported in a 3 1/2-year-old child who did not receive the recommended booster dose.

Evidence of efficacy postlicensure of Haemophilus b conjugate vaccines in the US is indicated by reports of significant reductions (71% to 94%) in Haemophilus b disease that are closely associated with increases in the net doses of Haemophilus b conjugate vaccines distributed.[29,30] Occasional cases of vaccine failures have, however, been reported to the US Department of Health and Human Services through the Vaccine Adverse Event Reporting System (VAERS) since licensure of Haemophilus b conjugate vaccines.

Diphtheria/Haemophilus b/Pertussis/Tetanus Vaccine has been given to 6,793 children as part of a series of studies to test the safety and immunogenicity of this combined product when compared to separate administration of DTP and HbOC. The vaccines were given at 2, 4, and 6 months of age or at 15 to 18 months of age. Local reactions and systemic events after vaccination were generally comparable between the groups which received the combination product or separate injections. (It should be noted that comparison of local reactions was done by comparing the combined product to the separate injection site that gave the largest reactions or to the DTP injection site.) Scattered reactions occurred more frequently (P < 0.05) in the combination group for some doses (swelling and drowsiness after the first dose; irritability and restless sleep after the second dose; injection site warmth and irritability after the third dose; injection site swelling, warmth, tenderness, irritability after the toddler dose). Rash was seen more commonly in the separate group. There was no consistent or identifiable pattern to these group differences across studies or doses. The large trial with 6,497 infants receiving Diphtheria/Haemophilus b/Pertussis/Tetanus Vaccine allowed analysis of rare adverse events, including SIDS (sudden infant death syndrome), hospitalizations, and emergency room visits, following vaccination. No differences were found between the cohorts (see *"Adverse Reactions"*).[10] Taken together the safety studies conducted in infants and in toddlers indicate that this vaccine is safe and that there was no consistent pattern of enhanced adverse events following combined Diphtheria/Haemophilus b/Pertussis/Tetanus Vaccine as compared to separate injections.

The antibody response to each of the components of Diphtheria/Haemophilus b/Pertussis/Tetanus Vaccine was measured (n = 189) and compared to separate administration of the DTP and HbOC vaccines (n = 189). After three doses, the antibody response to Diphtheria/Haemophilus b/Pertussis/Tetanus Vaccine was equal to or higher for all four components: tetanus (IU/mL), diphtheria (IU/mL), pertussis (microagglutination), and *H. influenzae* b polysaccharide (µg IgG/mL as per ELISA). In addition, responses to specific pertussis antigens (ie, pertussis toxin, FHA, and 69K protein) were found to be as high or higher in the Diphtheria/Haemophilus b/Pertussis/Tetanus Vaccine product compared to separate administration of DTP. Therefore, the immunogenicity of the combined vaccine is at least as good as the two vaccines given separately.[10]

INDICATIONS AND USAGE

Diphtheria/Haemophilus b/Pertussis/Tetanus Vaccine is indicated for the active immunization of children 2 months of age to 5 years of age for protection against diphtheria, Haemophilus b, Pertussis, and Tetanus disease when indications for immunization with DTP vaccine and Haemophilus b Conjugate Vaccine coincide. Typically, this is at 2, 4, 6, and 15 months of age.

Children who have recovered from culture-confirmed pertussis need not receive further doses of a vaccine containing Pertussis.[6] However, these children should receive additional doses of Diphtheria and Tetanus Toxoids Adsorbed, for Pediatric Use (DT) as well as Haemophilus b Conjugate Vaccine as appropriate to complete the series.

The American Academy of Pediatrics has recommended that children who have experienced invasive Haemophilus b disease when < 24 months of age should continue immunization against Haemophilus b, but that children whose disease occurred at $\geq$ 24 months need not receive further doses of Haemophilus b Conjugate Vaccine.[31] However, these children should receive additional doses of DTP (or if pertussis is contraindicated, DT should be used) as appropriate to complete the series.

Diphtheria/Haemophilus b/Pertussis/Tetanus Vaccine is intended for active immunization against diphtheria, Haemophilus type b, pertussis, and tetanus diseases and is not to be used for treatment of actual infection. Diphtheria/Haemophilus b/Pertussis/Tetanus Vaccine is not routinely recommended for immunization of persons older than 5 years of age. Under certain circumstances, Diphtheria/Haemophilus b/Pertussis/Tetanus Vaccine may be used beyond age 5 years. Because Diphtheria/Haemophilus b/Pertussis/Tetanus Vaccine contains pediatric DTP vaccine, it is not recommended for use beyond the seventh birthday.

As with any vaccine, Diphtheria/Haemophilus b/Pertussis/Tetanus Vaccine may not protect 100% of individuals receiving the vaccine.

If passive immunization is needed, Tetanus Immune Globulin (human TIG) and/or Diphtheria Antitoxin are recommended for tetanus and diphtheria, respectively (see *"Dosage and Administration"*).[6]

CONTRAINDICATIONS

HYPERSENSIVITY TO ANY COMPONENT OF THE VACCINE, INCLUDING THIMEROSAL, A MERCURY DERIVATIVE, IS A CONTRAINDICATION.

bility and death have also been reported rarely in temporal relation to immunization although a causal relationship has not been established.

DOSAGE AND ADMINISTRATION

FOR INTRAMUSCULAR USE ONLY

For infants beginning at 2 months of age, the immunization series for Diphtheria/Haemophilus b/Pertussis/Tetanus Vaccine consists of three doses of 0.5 mL each at approximately 2-month intervals, followed by a fourth dose of 0.5 mL at approximately 15 months of age. Diphtheria/Haemophilus b/Pertussis/Tetanus Vaccine may be substituted for DTP and Haemophilus b conjugate vaccine administered separately, whenever the recommended schedules for use of these two vaccines coincide (see DTP and Haemophilus b conjugate vaccine recommended dosage schedules).[6,31,32,69] However, no published data are available to support the interchangeability of the Haemophilus b conjugate vaccin in the Diphtheria/Haemophilus b/ Pertussis/ Tetanus vaccine and Haemophilus b conjugate vaccine with other Haemophilus b conjugate vaccines for the primary series. Therefore, it is recommended that the same conjugate vaccine be used throughout the primary series, consistent with the data supporting licensure of the vaccine.[31]

RECOMMENDED IMMUNIZATION SCHEDULES

For Previously Unvaccinated Younger Children

Dose	*Age*	*Immunization*
1	2 months	Diphtheria/Haemophilus b/Pertussis/Tetanus Vaccine
2	4 months	Diphtheria/Haemophilus b/Pertussis/Tetanus Vaccine
3	6 months	Diphtheria/Haemophilus b/Pertussis/Tetanus Vaccine
4	15-18 months	Diphtheria/Haemophilus b/Pertussis/Tetanus Vaccine*
5	4-6 years	DTP or DTaP

* *Children 15-18 months of age may receive DTaP plus a Haemophilus b conjugate vaccine as separate injections.*

FOR PREVIOUSLY UNVACCINATED *OLDER* CHILDREN[32]

Immunization schedules should be considered on an individual basis for children not vaccinated according to the recommended schedule. Three doses of a product containing DTP, given at approximately 2 month intervals, are required followed by a fourth dose of a product containing DTP or DTaP approximately 12 months later and a fifth dose of a product containing DTP or DTaP at 4-6 years of age. If the fourth dose of a Pertussis-containing vaccine is not given until after the fourth birthday, no further doses of a Pertussis-containing vaccine are necessary.

The number of doses of an HbOC-containing product indicated depends on the age that immunization is begun. A child 7-11 months of age should receive 3 doses of a product containing HbOC. A child 12-14 months of age should receive 2 doses of a product containing HbOC. A child 15-59 months of age should receive 1 dose of a product containing HbOC.

As indicated previously, Diphtheria/Haemophilus b/Pertussis/Tetanus Vaccine may be substituted for DTP and Haemophilus b conjugate vaccine administered separately, whenever the recommended schedule for use of these two vaccines coincides.

Preterm infants should be vaccinated with Diphtheria/Haemophilus b/Pertussis/Tetanus Vaccine according to their chronological age, from birth.[6]

Interruption of the recommended schedules with a delay between doses does not interfere with the final immunity achieved; nor does it necessitate starting the series over again, regardless of the length of time elapsed between doses.[6,32]

If a contraindication to the Pertussis vaccine component occurs, Diphtheria and Tetanus Toxoids Adsorbed, for Pediatric Use (DT) and Haemophilus b Conjugate Vaccine, as separate injections, should be substituted for each of the remaining doses.

The use of reduced volume (fractional doses) is not recommended. The effect of such practices on the frequency of serious adverse events and on protection against disease has not been determined.

Shake vigorously to obtain a uniform suspensin prior to withdrawing each dose from the multiple dose vial. The vaccine should not be used if it cannot be resuspended.

Parenteral drug products should be inspected visually for particulate matter and discoloration prior to administration whenever solution and container permit. (See *"Description."*)

The vaccine should be injected intramuscularly. The preferred sites are the anterolateral aspect of the thigh or the deltoid muscle of the upper arm. The vaccine should not be injected in the gluteal area or areas where there may be a major nerve trunk. Before injection, the skin at the injection site should be cleansed and prepared with a suitable germicide.

After insertion of the needle, aspirate to help avoid inadvertent injection into a blood vessel.

For either primary or booster immunization against tetanus and diphtheria of individuals 7 years of age and older, the use of Tetanus and Diphtheria Toxoids Adsorbed for Adult Use (Td) is recommended.[6,32]

For passive immunization against tetanus and diphtheria, human TIG, and/or Diphtheria Antitoxin are recommended.[6] A separate syringe and site of injection should be used.

STORAGE

Do not freeze. Store refrigerated, away from freezer compartment, AT 2°C TO 8°C (36°F TO 46°F).

REFERENCES

1. Mueller JH, Miller PA. Production of diphtheria toxin of high potency (100 Lf) on a reproducible medium. *J Immunol.* 1941; 40:21-32. 2. Mueller JH, Miller PA. Factors influencing the production of tetanal toxin. *J Immunol.* 1947; 56: 143-147. 3. Pillemer L, Grossberg DB, Wittler RG. The immuno-chemistry of toxins and toxoids, II. The preparation and immunologic evaluation of purified tetanal toxoid. *J Immunol.* 1946; 54:213-224. 4. United States Patent Number 4,902,506 by Anderson PW, Eby RJ filed May 5, 1986 issued February 20, 1990. 5. Seid RC Jr, Boykins RA, Liu DF, et al. Chemical evidence for covalent linkage of a semi-synthetic glycoconjugate vaccine for *Haemophilus influenzae* type b disease. *Glycoconjugate J.* 1989; 6:489-498. 6. Diphtheria, tetanus and pertussis: Recommendations for vaccine use and other preventive measures—recommendations of the Immunization Practices Advisory Committee (ACIP). *MMWR.* 1991: 40/No. RR-10. 7. Pappenheimer AM Jr. Diphtheria. In: ermanier R, ed. *Bacterial Vaccines.* New York, NY: Academic Press Inc; 1984: 1-36. 8. *Federal Register Notice*, Friday, December 13, 1985, Vol. 50, No. 240. 9. Blumberg DA, Mink CM, Cherry JD, et al. Comparison of acellular and whole-cell pertussis-component diphtheria-tetanus-pertussis vaccines in infants. *J Pediatr.* 1991; 119:194-204. 10. Unpublished data available from Praxis Biologics, Inc. and Lederle Laboratories. 11. Manclark CR, Cowell JL. Pertussis Vaccine. In: Germanier R, ed. *Bacterial Vaccines.* New York, NY: Academic Press Inc: 1984: 69-106. 12. Kendrick PL. Secondary familial attack rates from pertussis in vaccinated and unvaccinated children. *Am J Hygiene.* 1940; 32:89-91. 13. Reported incidence of notifiable diseases in the United States. *MMWR.* 1970; 19(53):44. 14. Pertussis surveillance—United States, 1986-1988, *MMWR.* 1990; 39(4):57-66. 15. Mortimer EA Jr. Pertussis and its prevention: a family affair. *J Infect Dis.* 161:437-479. 16. Wenger JD, Ward JL, Broome CV. Prevention of *Haemophilus influenzae* type b disease: vaccines and passive prophylaxis. InRE,MINGTON JS, Swartz MS, eds. *Current Clinical Topics in Infectious Diseases.* New York, NY: McGraw-Hill Inc; 1989; 10:306-339. 17. Recommendation of the Immunization Practices Advisory Committee (ACIP). Polysaccharide vaccine for prevention of *Haemophilus influenzae* type b disease. *MMWR.* 1985; 34:201-205. 18. Sell SH. Long term sequelae of bacterial meningitis in children. *Pediatr Infect Dis J.* 1983; 2:90-93. 19. Broome CV. Epidemiology of *Haemophilus influenzae* type b infections in the United States. *Pediatr Infect Dis J.* 1987; 6:779-782. 20. Peltola H, Kayhty H, Sivonen A. *Haemophilus influenzae* type b capsular polysaccharide vaccine in children: a double-blind field study of 100,000 vaccines 3 months to 5 years of age in Finland. *Pediatrics.* 1977; 60:730-737. 21. Robbins JB, Parke JC, Schneerson R. Quantitative measurement of "natural" and immunization-induced *Haemophilus influenzae* type b capsular polysaccharide antibodies. *Pediatr Res.* 1973; 7:103-110. 22. Kayhty H, Peltola H, Karanko V, et al. The protective level of serum antibodies to the capsular polysaccharide of *Haemophilus influenzae* type b. *J Infect Dis.* 1983; 147:1100. 23. Weinberg GA, Granoff DM. Polysaccharide-protein conjugate vaccines for the prevention of *Haemophilus influenzae* type b disease. *J Pediatr.* 1988; 113:621-631. 24. Makela O, Peterfy F, Outshoorn IG, et al. Immunogenic properties of a (1-6) dextran, its protein conjugates, and conjugates of its breakdown products in mice. *Scand J Immunol.* 1984; 19:541-550. 25. Anderson P, Pichichero ME, Insel RA. Immunogens consisting of oligosaccharides from *Haemophilus influenzae* type b coupled to diphtheria toxoid or the toxin protein CRM_{197} *J Clin Invest.* 1985; 76:52-59. 26. Madore DV, Phipps DC, Eby R, et al. Immune response of young children vaccinated with *Haemophilus influenzae* type b conjugate vaccines. In: Cruse JM, Lewis RE, eds. *Contributions to Microbiology and Immunology: Conjugate Vaccines.* New York, NY: Karger Medical and Scientific Publishers; 1989; 10:125-150. 27. Black SB, Shinefield HR, Lampert D, et al. Safety and immunogenicity of oligosaccharide conjugate *Haemophilus influenzae* type b. (HbOC) vaccine in infancy. *Pediatr Infect Dis J.* 1991; 10:92-96. 28. Black SB, Shinefield HR, Fireman B, et al. Efficacy in infancy of oligosaccharide conjugate *Haemophilus influenzae* type b (HbOC) vaccine in a United States population of 61,080 children. *Pediatr Infect Dis J.* 1991; 10:97-104. 29. Black SB, Shinefield HR, The Kaiser Permanente Pediatric Vaccine Study Group. Immunization with oligosaccharide conjugate *Haemophilus influenzae* type b (HbOC) vaccine on a large health maintenance organization population: extended follow-up and impact on *Haemophilus influenzae* disease epidemiology. *Pediatr Infect Dis J.* 1992; 11:610-613. 30. Adams WG, Deaver KA, Cochi SL, et al. Decline of childhood *Haemophilus influenzae* type b (Hib) disease in the Hib vaccine era. *JAMA.* 1993; 269:221-226. 31. Recommendations of the AAP. *Haemophilus influenzae* type b conjugate vaccine: recommendations for immunization of infants and children 2 months of age and older: update. *Pediatrics.* 1991: 88:169-172. 32. American Academy of Pediatrics: Report of the Committee on Infectious Diseases. 22nd ed. Elk Grove Village, Ill: American Academy of Pediatrics; 1991. 33. Pertussis immunization: family history of convulsions and use of antipyretics—supplementary ACIP statement. *MMWR.* 1987; 36(18):281-282. 34. Stetler HC, Orenstein WA, Bart KJ, et al. History of convulsions and use of pertussis vaccine. *J Pediatr.* 1985; 107(2):175-179. 35. Hirtz DG, Nelson KB, Ellenberg JH. Seizures following childhood immunizations. *J Pediatr.* 1983; 102(1):14-18. 36. Ipp MM, Gold R, Greenberg S, et al. Acetaminophen prophylaxis of adverse reactions following vaccination of infants with diphtheria-pertussis-tetanus toxoids-polio vaccine. *Pediatr Infect Dis J.* 1987; 6:721-725. 37. Sutter RW, Patriarca PA, Suleiman AJM, et al. Attributable risk of DTP (Diphtheria and Tetanus Toxoids and Pertussis Vaccine) injection in provoking paralytic poliomyelitis during a large outbreak in Oman. *J Infect Dis.* 1992; 165:444-449. 38. Bernier R, Frank JA, Dondero TJ, et al. Diphtheria-tetanus toxoids, pertussis vaccination and sudden infant deaths in Tennessee. *J Pediatr.* 1982; 101:419-421. 39. Baraff L, Ablon WJ, Weiss RC. Possible temporal association between diptheria-tetanus toxoid, pertussis vaccination and sudden infant death syndrome. *Pediatr Inf Dis.* 1983; 2:7-11. 40. Walker AM, Jick H, Perera DR, et al. Diphtheria-Tetanus-pertussis immunization and sudden infant death. *AJPH.* 1987; 77(8):945-951. 41. Hoffman HJ, Hunter JC, Damus K, et al. Diphtheria-tetanus-pertussis immunization and sudden infant death: results of the National Institute of Child Health and Human Development cooperative study of sudden infant death syndrome risk factors. *Pediatrics.* 1987; 79(4):598-611. 42. Mortimer EA. Efficacy of Haemophilus b polysaccharide vaccine: an enigma. *JAMA.* 1988; 260:1454-1455. 43. Scheifele D, Bjornsen

GLG, Arcand T, et al. Antigenuria after receipt of Haemophilus b Diphtheria Toxoid Conjugate Vaccine. *Pediatr Infect Dis J.* 1989; 8:887-888. 44. Recommendation of the ACIP—Immunization of children infected with human T-lymphotrophic virus type III/lymphadenopathy-associated virus. *MMWR.* 1986; 35(38):595-606. 45. Immunization of children infected with human immunodeficiency virus—supplementary ACIP statement. *MMWR.* 1988; 37(12):181-183. 46. General Recommendations on Immunization—Recommendations of the Immunization Practices Advisory Committee (ACIP). *MMWR.* 1989; 38(13):221. 47. CDC. Vaccine Adverse Event Reporting System—United States. *MMWR.* 1990; 39:730-733. 48. Fawcett HA, Smith NP. Injection-site granuloma due to aluminum. *Arch Dermatol.* 1984; 120:1318-1322. 49. Bellman MH, Ross EM, Miller DL. Infantile spasms and pertussis immunization. *Lancet.* 1983; 1:1031-1034. 50. Mathur R, Kumari S. Bulging fontanel following triple vaccine (letter). *Indian Pediatrics.* 1981; 18(6):417-418. 51. Shendurnikar N, Gandhi DJ, Patel J, et al. Bulging fontanel following DTP vaccine (letter). *Indian Pediatrics.* 1986; 23(11):960. 52. Jacob J, Mannino F. Increased intracranial pressure after diphtheria, tetanus, and pertussis immunization. *Am J Dis Child.* 1979; 133:217-218. 53. Leung A. Congenital heart disease and DTP vaccination. *Can Med Assoc J.* 1984; 131:541. 54. Park JM, Ledbetter EO, South MA, et al. Paroxysmal supraventricular tachycardia precipitated by pertussis vaccine. *Pediatrics.* 1983; 102(6):883-885. 55. Amsel SG, Hanukoglu A, Fried D, et al. Myocarditis after triple immunization. *Arch Dis Child.* 1986; 61:403-404. 56. CDC. Adverse events following immunization. *MMWR.* 1985; 34:43-47. 57. Rutledge SL, Snead OC. Neurologic complications of immunizations. *J Pediatr.* 1986; 109:917-924. 58. Milstein JB, Gross TP, Kuritsky JN. Adverse reactions reported following receipt of *Haemophilus influenzae* type b vaccine: an analysis after one year of marketing *Pediatrics.* 1987; 80:270-274. 59. Schlenska GK. Unusual neurological complications following tetanus toxoid administration. *J Neurol.* 1977; 215:299-302. 60. Blumstein GI, Kreithen H. Peripheral neuropathy following tetanus toxoid administration. *JAMA.* 1966; 198:1030-1031. 61. Reinstein L. Pargament JM, Goodman JS. Peripheral neuropathy after multiple tetanus toxoid injections. *Arch Phys Med Rehabil.* 63:332-334. 62. Tsairis P, Dyck PJ, Mulder DW. Natural history of brachial plexus neuropathy. *Arch Neurol.* 1972; 27:109-117. 63. Quast U, Hennessen W, Widmark RM. Mono- and polyneuritis after tetanus vaccination. *Devel Bio Stand.* 1979; 43:25-32. 64. Holliday PL, Bauer RB. Polyradiculoneuritis secondary to immunization with tetanus and diphtheria toxoids. *Arch Neurol.* 1983; 40:56-57. 65. Fenichel GM. Neurological complications of tetanus toxoid. *Arch Neurol.* 1983; 40-390. 66. Pollard JD, Selby G. Relapsing neuropathy due to tetanus toxoid. *J Neurol Sci.* 1978; 37:113-125. 67. Newton N, Janati A. Guillain-Barre syndrome after vaccination with purified tetanus toxoid. *S Med J.* 1987; 80:1053-1054. 68. D'Cruz DF, Sharpiro ED, Spiegelman KN, et al. Acute inflammatory demyelinating polyradiculoneuropathy (Guillian-Barre syndrome) after immunization with *Haemophilus influenzae* type b conjugate vaccine. *J Pediatr.* 1989; 115:743-746. 69. Recommendation of the ACIP: Haemophilus B conjugate vaccines for prevention of *Haemophilus influenzae* type b disease among infants and children two months of age and older. *MMWR.* 1991; 40:1-7.

HOW SUPPLIED

INJECTION:

BRAND/MANUFACTURER	NDC	SIZE	AWP
○ BRAND			
TETRAMUNE: Lederle Labs	00005-1960-31	5 ml	$323.31

Diphtheria/Pertussis/Tetanus

DESCRIPTION

Diphtheria/Pertussis/Tetanus, whole-cell and acellular, combines diphtheria and tetanus toxoids, adsorbed with pertussis vaccine, for intramuscular use, in a sterile isotonic solution.

Corynebacterium diptheriae cultures are grown in a modified Mueller and Miller medium.[1] *Clostridium tetani* cultures are grown in a peptone-based medium. Both toxins are detoxified with formaldehyde.

The pertussis vaccine component is derived from *Bordetalla pertussis* cultures.

The toxoids are absorbed to aluminum as aluminum potassium sulfate talum: or aluminum hydroxide and aluminum phosphate. The adsorbed diptheria and tetanus toxoids are combined with pertussis vaccine concentrate, and diluted to a final volume using sterile phosphate-buffered physiological saline. Each 0.5 mL dose contains, by assay, not more than 0.17 to 0.85 mg of aluminum and not more than 0.001% to 0.02% of residual formaldehyde.

Each 0.5 mL dose is formulated to contain 6.5, 6.7, 7.5, or 12.5 Lf of diphtheria toxoid and 5 or 5.5 Lf of tetanus toxoid (both toxoids induce at least 2 units of antitoxin per mL in the guinea pig potency test) and 46.8 µg of pertussis antigens.

The total human immunizing dose (the first three 0.5 mL doses administered) contains an estimate of 12 units of pertussis vaccine (4 protective units per single dose).[2]

CLINICAL PHARMACOLOGY

Simultaneous immunization against diphtheria, tetanus, and pertussis, using a conventional "whole-cell" Diphtheria/Pertussis/Tetanus Vaccine, has been a routine practice during infancy and childhood in the United States since the late 1940s. This practice has played a major role in markedly reducing the incidence rates of cases and deaths from each of these diseases.[2]

DIPHTHERIA

Corynebacterium diphtheriae may cause both a localized and generalized disease. Systemic intoxication is caused by diphtheria exotoxin, an extracellular protein metabolite of toxigenic strains of *C. diphtheriae.* Protection against disease is due to the development of neutralizing antibodies to diphtheria toxin.

At one time, diphtheria was common in the United States. More than 200,000 cases, primarily among young children. were reported in 1921. Approximately 5% to 10% of cases were fatal; the highest case-fatality ratios were recorded for the very young and the elderly. Reported cases of diphtheria of all types declined from 306 in 1975 to 59 in 1979; most were cutaneous diphtheria reported from a single state. After 1979, cutaneous diphtheria was no longer a notifiable disease. From 1980 to 1989, only 24 cases of respiratory diphtheria were reported; two cases were fatal, and 18 (75%) occurred among persons 20 years of age or older.[2]

Diphtheria is currently a rare disease in the United States primarily because of the high level of appropriate vaccination among children (97% of children entering school have received ≥ three doses of Diphtheria/Pertussis/Tetanus) and because of an apparent reduction in the prevalence of toxigenic strains of *C. diptheria.* Most cases occur among unvaccinated or inadequately immunized persons.[2]

Both toxigenic and nontoxigenic strains of *C. diphtheriae* can cause disease, but only strains that produce diphtheria toxin cause severe manifestations such as myocarditis and neutritis. Toxigenic strains are more often associated with severe or fatal illness in noncutaneous (respiratory or other mucosal surface) infections and are more commonly recovered in association with respiratory than from cutaneous infections.[2] Diptheria remains a serious disease, with the highest case-fatality rates among infants and the elderly.[2]

There is essentially no natural immunity to diphtheria toxin. Thus, universal primary immunization with diphtheria toxoid, with subsequent maintenance of adequate antitoxin levels by means of timed boosters, is necessary to protect all age groups. Following adequate immunization with diphtheria toxoid, which induces antitoxin and neutralizing antibodies, it is thought that protection lasts for at least 10 years.[1] Serologic data demonstrate the ability of Diphtheria/Pertussis/Tetanus vaccine to stimulate neutralizing antibody against diphtheria antigen in humans—the protective level is ≥ 0.01 units/mL. Following administration of three doses of diphtheria vaccine (having a potency of 2 to 4 antitoxin-inducing units per mL) geometric mean titers (GMTs) were 3.7 to 9.3 antitoxin units.[3,4] This significantly reduces both the risk of developing diphtheria and the severity of clinical illness.

Vaccination does not however, eliminate carriage of *C. diphtheriae* in the pharynx or nose or on the skin.[2]

TETANUS

Tetanus is an intoxication manifested primarily by neuromuscular dysfunction caused by a potent exotoxin elaborated by *Clostridium tetani.*

The occurrence of tetanus in the United States has decreased dramatically from 560 reported cases in 1947 to a record low of 48 reported cases in 1987. Tetanus in the United States is primarily a disease of older adults. Of 99 tetanus patients with complete information reported to the Centers for Disease Control and Prevention (CDC) during 1987 and 1988, 68% were ≥ 50 years of age, while only six were < 20 years of age. Overall, the case-fatality rate was 21%. In 1992, 45 cases were reported of which 82% were ≥ 50 years of age.[5] The disease continues to occur almost exclusively among persons who are unvaccinated or inadequately vaccinated or whose vaccination histories are unknown or uncertain.[2]

In 4% of tetanus cases reported during 1987 and 1988, no wound or other condition could be implicated. Non-acute skin lesions, such as ulcers, or medical conditions, such as abscesses, were reported in 14% of cases.[2]

Spores of *C. tetani* are ubiquitous. Serologic tests indicate that naturally acquired immunity to tetanus toxin does not occur in the United States.[2] Thus, universal primary vaccination, with subsequent maintenance of adequate antitoxin levels by means of appropriately timed boosters, is necessary to protect persons among all age-groups. Tetanus toxoid is a highly effective antigen, and a completed primary series generally induces protective levels of neutralizing antibodies to tetanus toxin that persist for ≤ 10 years.[2]

Serologic data demonstrate the ability of vaccine to stimulate neutralizing antibody against tetanus antigen in humans. Following administration of three doses of tetanus vaccine (having a potency of 2 to 4 antitoxin-inducing units per mL) GMTs were 13.5 units to 29.1 antitoxin units.[3,4]

The potency of diphtheria and tetanus toxoids was determined on the basis of immunogenicity studies with a comparison to a serological correlate of protection (0.01 I.U./mL) established by the Panel of Review of Bacterial Vaccines & Toxoids.[6]

EFFICACY OF DIPHTHERIA AND TETANUS TOXOID VACCINES

Circulating protective levels of neutralizing antibodies to diphtheria and tetanus toxins can be induced by the administration of diphtheria and tetanus toxoids adsorbed or Diphtheria/Pertussis/Tetanus.

A clinical study was performed in 20 children under one year of age to determine the serological responses and the adverse reactions when diphtheria and tetanus toxoids was administered as a primary series of three doses. Protective levels of diphtheria and tetanus antitoxins that were equal to or greater than 0.01 I.U./mL were detected in 100% of the children following two doses of the vaccine. However, maternal antibody may have contributed to the total neutralizing antibody in some of these infants. Protective levels of antitoxin were observed in 100% of these infants following three doses of diphtheria and tetanus toxoids. No local or systemic reactions were observed in approximately half of the infants and only mild or moderate reactions were observed in the remainder of the diphtheria and tetanus toxoids study group.[7]

Another clinical study to evaluate serological responses and adverse reactions of diphtheria and tetanus toxoids was performed in 40 children under one year of age. One group of 20 children received 0.5 mL doses of diphtheria and tetanus toxoids at two, four and six months of age, respectively. The second group of 20 children received 0.5 mL doses of Diphtheria/Pertussis/Tetanus and diphtheria and tetanus toxoids respectively, at the same ages. The immunologic protection against diphtheria and tetanus as measured by toxin neutralizing antibodies induced by diphtheria and tetanus toxoids was comparable when administered as either a second or third dose.[8]

The incidence of adverse reactions was significantly lower following diphtheria and tetanus toxoids administration (p < 0.05). Although the number of vaccinees was small, no persistent screaming episodes or severe neurological reactions such as seizures or encephalopathy were observed with either vaccine in this study.[8]

PERTUSSIS

Pertussis (whooping cough) is a highly communicable disease of the respiratory tract caused by *Bordetella pertussis* that has an attack rate in unimmunized houshold contacts of over 90%. This gram-negative coccobacillus produces a variety of biologically active components. One of these components, pertussis toxin, a 69-kd outer membrane protein, has been associated with a number of effects such as lymphocytosis, leukocytosis, sensitivity to histamine, changes in glucose and/or insulin levels, neurological effects, and adjuvant activity.[9] The role of the different components produced by *B. pertussis* in either the pathogenesis of, or the immunity to, pertussis is not well understood. Immunization with vaccines containing inactivated pertussis toxin and filamentous hemagglutinin, have been associated with protection in clinical studies. Another biologically active component, endotoxin, may contribute to reactogenicity of pertussis vaccines.[13]

Pertussis is highly communicable (attack rates of ≤ 90% have been reported among unvaccinated household contacts)[10] and can cause severe disease particularly among very young children.

Pertussis was once a major cause of infant and childhood morbidity and mortality in the United States. Pertussis became a nationally notifiable disease in 1922, and reports received a peak of 265,269 cases and 7,518 deaths in 1934. The highest number of reported pertussis deaths (9,269) occurred in 1923. The introduction and widespread use of standardized whole-cell pertussis vaccines combined with diphtheria and tetanus toxoids in the late 1940s resulted in a substantial decline in pertussis disease, a decline which continued without interruption for nearly 30 years.[2]

By 1970, the annual reported incidence of pertussis had been reduced by 99%. During the 1970s the annual numbers of reported cases stabilized at an average of approximately 2,300 cases each year. During the 1980s, however, the annual numbers of reported cases gradually increased from 1,730 cases in 1980 to 4,517 cases in 1989. An average of eight pertussis-associated fatalities was reported each year throughout the 1980s.[2]

From 1989 to 1991, 11,446 cases of pertussis were reported for an unadjusted incidence per 100,000 population of 1.7 in 1989, 1.8 in 1990 and 1.1 in 1991. The incidence for 1992 was 1.6 per 100,000. Age specific incidence and hospitalization rates were highest in the first year of life, decreasing with increasing age. Trends of the past years suggest an increase in reported pertussis since 1976, with the peak year being 1990.[11]

Accurate data do not exist, as bacteriological confirmation of pertussis can be obtained in less than half of the suspected cases.

Of 10,749 patients < 1 year of age reported nationally as having pertussis during the period 1980 to 1989, 69% were hospitalized, 22% had pneumonia, 3.0% had ≥ one seizure, 0.9% had encephalopathy, and 0.6% died.[12]

During the period 1989 to 1991, of 3,900 reports of hospitalization, 1,115 had developed pneumonia, seizures occurred in 157 cases, encephalopathy was reported for 12, and there were 20 pertussis attributed deaths. These events were more frequently reported in children less than 6 months of age and were generally less frequent with increasing age.[13] Of patients 3 months through 4 years of age, where vaccination status was known, 65% of 4,471 patients had not received the recommended schedule of immunization and 39% had not received any pertussis containing vaccine.[5]

Among older children and adults, including those previously vaccinated, *B. pertussis* infection may result in symptoms of bronchitis or an upper-respiratory-tract infection. Pertussis may not be diagnosed because classic signs, especially the inspiratory whoop, may be absent. Older preschool children and school-age siblings who are not fully vaccinated and who develop pertussis can be important sources of infection for infants < 1 year of age, the group at highest risk of disease and disease severity.[2] Adults also play an important role in the transmission of pertussis to unvaccinated or incompletely vaccinated infants and young children.[2]

Because the severity of pertussis decreases with age, and the vaccine may cause side effects and adverse reactions, routine pertussis immunization is not recommended for persons 7 years of age or older.[14]

EFFICACY OF PERTUSSIS VACCINE

Although Diphtheria/Pertussis/Tetanus has been evaluated as a control vaccine in a number of clinical trials of acellular pertussis vaccines, no formal efficacy trial was performed prior to approval. Approval was based on historical and continuing evidence of protection (surveillance) in the population at risk. It was also shown that vaccines with acceptable mouse protection potencies induced protective serum agglutinin antibody titers.[6]

Potency of the pertussis component of the vaccine is measured and shown to be acceptable in the mouse potency test. Serum agglutinin titers of vaccinees were correlated with clinical protection in the Medical Research Council trials. In the second Medical Research Council Field Trial, which compared five pertussis vaccines (including the nonadsorbed component of the present vaccine) and involved more than 30,000 children aged 6 months to 3 years, attack rates in exposed vaccinated children ranged from 4% to 29%. In an earlier trial, the attack

rate in unvaccinated exposed children was 87%. Efficacy of the present vaccine has been estimated at 80% to 85%.[15,16] All five vaccines were found to be efficacious. In this trial, protection was found to correlate with protection of mice against intracerebral infection, production of specific agglutinin in mice, and production of specific agglutinin in children.[15,16]

General use of whole-cell pertussis Diphtheria/Pertussis/Tetanus vaccines has resulted in a substantial reduction in cases and deaths from pertussis disease.[17,18] The use of acellular Diphtheria/Pertussis/Tetanus as the fourth or fifth dose evokes an antibody response at least as great as whole-cell pertussis Diphtheria/Pertussis/Tetanus vaccine following a primary series with commercially available U.S. whole-cell pertussis DTP with respect to pertussis toxin and filamentous hemagglutinin antibodies.[19,20]

Acellular pertussis vaccines have been used in Japan since 1981, mostly in 2-year-old children. Evidence for the efficacy of these vaccines, as a group, is demonstrated by the decline in pertussis disease with their routine use in that country.[17,21] In addition, a review of epidemiological studies of the Japanese acellular pertussis vaccines estimated that these vaccines, as a group, were 88% efficacious in protecting against clinical pertussis on household exposure, with a 95% confidence interval of 79% to 93%.[22]

In three Japanese household contact studies which employed retrospective case ascertainment and nonstandard case definitions, the vaccine-specific efficacy of the vaccine ranged between 89% and 94% but confidence intervals were wide, due to the small number of children in each study.[23-26] Although there were differences in study methods, these estimates of efficacy are quite comparable to that for whole-cell pertussis vaccine in the United States.[27]

Efficacy of the Diphtheria/Pertussis/Tetanus vaccine containing the acellular pertussis vaccine component was examined, in particular, in a nonblinded household contact study that included both retrospective and prospective case evaluation.[28] As a consequence of the immunization schedule in Japan at the time of study, none of the vaccinated contacts were less than 2 years of age while some of the unvaccinated contacts were less than 2 years of age. When analysis of results was limited to vaccinated and unvaccinated household contacts 2 years of age and over, efficacy was estimated to be 79% (95% confidence interval, 60% to 89%) for physician-diagnosed pertussis disease. This included respiratory illness that may have been mild pertussis. When cases were restricted to disease diagnosed as typical pertussis, omitting mild suspect cases, efficacy was estimated to be 97% (95% confidence interval, 82% to 99%).

When unvaccinated household contacts under 2 years of age are also included in the analysis, efficacy was estimated to be 81% (95% confidence interval, 64% to 90%) against pertussis disease (including mild suspect cases) and 98% (95% confidence interval, 84% to 99%) against typical pertussis.

A large placebo-controlled efficacy trial of two acellular pertussis vaccines was carried out in Sweden in 1986-1987. One of the vaccines contained a two-component acellular pertussis vaccine. In its first phase, the trial in Sweden was a randomized, blinded prospective trial using a standardized case definition and active case ascertainment. In this phase, 1,389 children, 5 to 11 months of age, received two doses of the inactivated acellular pertussis vaccine 7 to 13 weeks apart and 954 received a placebo control. During the 15 months of follow-up from 30 days after the second dose, culture-confirmed whooping cough (cough and a positive culture of *Bordetella pertussis*) occurred in 40 placebo and 18 acellular pertussis vaccine recipients. The point estimate of protective efficacy for the vaccine was 69% (95% confidence interval: 47% to 82%) for all cases of culture-confirmed pertussis and 80% (95% confidence interval: 59% to 91%) for culture confirmed cases with cough of over 30 days duration.[29]

A three-year unblinded passive follow-up of vaccine and placebo recipients from the above Swedish study has shown a post-trial efficacy of 77% (95% confidence interval; 65% to 85%) for all culture-proven cases of pertussis, and an efficacy of 92% (95% confidence interval; 84% to 96%) for culture-proven cases with a cough of over 30 days duration.[30]

Anti-pertussis toxin and anti-filamentous hemagglutinin antibody responses in children enrolled in the trial in Sweden were subsequently compared to responses observed in clinical trials of acellular Diphtheria/Pertussis/Tetanus conducted in the U.S. In the U.S. trials, children 15 to 20 months of age who had previously received three doses of licensed whole-cell pertussis Diphtheria/Pertussis/Tetanus and children 4 to 6 years of age who had previously received four doses of licensed whole-cell pertussis Diphtheria/Pertussis/Tetanus were immunized with a single dose of acellular Diphtheria/Pertussis/Tetanus. The anti-pertussis toxin and anti-filamentous hemagglutinin antibody responses to acellular Diphtheria/Pertussis/Tetanus in the U.S. trials were found to be similar to the responses observed in children enrolled in the trial in Sweden. Although the Swedish efficacy trial immunization with an inactivated pertussis toxin/filamentous hemagglutinin vaccine was shown to protect against pertussis, no specific serological correlate or measure of protective immune response was found.[29] The role in clinical protection of specific serum antibodies is, therefore, not known at this time.

Additionally, the antibody responses in children immunized with acellular Diphtheria/Pertussis/Tetanus were compared to those in children immunized with whole-cell pertussis Diphtheria/Pertussis/Tetanus vaccine. Immunogenicity data from the clinical trials in the U.S. are summarized in Table 1. Anti-pertussis toxin and anti-filamentous hemagglutinin responses to acellular Diphtheria/Pertussis/Tetanus were significantly higher than those to whole-cell pertussis Dipherthia/Pertussis/Tetanus vaccine. Serological responses to diphtheria and tetanus antigens, not shown in Table 1, were equal to or greater than those produced by whole-cell pertussis Diphtheria/Pertussis/Tetanus vaccine.[19,20]

Clinical experience (immunogenicity) in the United States is summarized in Table 1.[19,20] (See related table).

A total of 3,700 doses of Acellular Diphtheria/Pertussis/Tetanus have been administered in U.S. clinical trials, in children 15-20 months of age and 4-6 years of age. When compared to whole-cell pertussis Diphtheria/Pertussis/Tetanus vaccine, acellular Diphtheria/Pertussis/Tetanus produced fewer and milder local reactions such as erythema, swelling, and tenderness at the injection site; as well as fewer and milder systemic reactions such as fever, irritability, drowsiness, vomiting, anorexia and high-pitched unusual cry. Rates of more serious and infrequent adverse experiences for acellular Diphtheria/Pertussis/Tetanus are not known at this time.

INDICATIONS AND USAGE

Diphtheria/Pertussis/Tetanus whole-cell vaccine is recommended for active immunization of children up to 7 years against diphtheria, tetanus and pertussis (whooping cough) simultaneously. However, in instances where the pertussis vaccine component is contraindicated, or where the physician decies that pertussis vaccine is not to be administered, diphteria and tetanus toxoids should be used. When confirmation is lacking, Diphtheria/Pertussis/Tetanus vaccination should be completed.[2] Diphtheria/Pertussis/Tetanus may be used concomitantly with tetanus immune globulin and diphtheria antitoxin (see *"Dosage and Administration"*). Immunization should be started at 6 weeks to 2 months of age and be completed before the seventh birthday.[2,34] Diphtheria/Pertussis/Tetanus acellular vaccine is indicated as a fourth and/or fifth dose for immunization of children 15 months to 7 years of age (prior to seventh birthday) who have previously been immunized against diphtheria, tetanus and pertussis with three or four doses of whole-cell pertussis Diphtheria/Pertussis/Tetanus vaccine. However, in instances where the pertussis vaccine component is contraindicated, diphtheria and tetanus toxoids should be used for each of the remaining doses.

Persons recovering from confirmed pertussis do not need additional doses of Diphtheria/Pertussis/Tetanus but should receive additional doses of diphtheria and tetanus toxoids to complete the series.[2]

Available data indicate that the appropriate age for institution of immunizations in prematurely born infants is the usual chronological age of 2 months. Vaccine doses should not be reduced for preterm infants.[2,34] Diphtheria/Pertussis/Tetanus may be used concomitantly with tetanus immune globulin and diphtheria antitoxin (see *"Dosage and Administration"*).

If passive immunization is required, tetanus immune globulin (human) and/or equine diphtheria antitoxin are the products of choice for tetanus and diphtheria, respectively (see *"Dosage and Administration section"*).

When Diphtheria/Pertussis/Tetanus whole-cell vaccine is used to reconstitute Haemophilus b conjugate vaccine, the combined vaccines are indicated for the active immunization of infants and children 2 months through 5 years of age for the prevention of invasive diseases caused by diphtheria, tetanus, pertussis and *H influenzae* type b.[35,36]

A single injection containing diphtheria, tetanus, pertussis and Haemophilus b conjugate antigens may be more acceptable to parents and may increase compliance with vaccination programs. Therefore, in those situations where, in the judgment of the physician, it is of benefit to administer a single injection of whole-cell Diphtheria/Pertussis/Tetanus vaccine and Haemophilus b conjugate vaccine concomitantly; *only whole-cell Diphtheria/Pertussis/Tetanus vaccine may be used for reconstitution of lyophilized Haemophilus b conjugate vaccine*. Antibody levels associated with protection may not be achieved earlier than two weeks following the last recommended dose. (See *"Dosage and Administration"* section.)

As with any vaccine, vaccination with Diptheria/Pertussis/Tetanus or combined vaccines Diphtheria/Pertussis/Tetanus and Haemophilus b conjugate vaccine may not protect 100% of susceptible individuals.

This vaccine is NOT to be used for the treatment of diphtheria, tetanus, pertussis or H influenzae type b infection. This vaccine should NOT be used for immunizing persons 7 years of age and older. In children 7 years of age and older and in adults, tetanus and diphtheria toxoids adsorbed for adult use is preferable to use of either tetanus or diphtheria vaccines alone.

The administration of acellular Diphtheria/Pertussis/Tetanus may be considered for children as young as 15 months of age when it is expected that the child will not return at 18 months to receive the fourth dose in this immunization series although studies in this age group have not been completed. *Diphtheria/Pertussis/Tetanus Acellular Vaccine is not recommended for use in children below the age of 15 months. This vaccine is not recommended for use as a primary series in children of any age.*

CONTRAINDICATIONS

Hypersensitivity to any component of the vaccine is a contraindication for further use of this vaccine.

It is a contraindication to use this or any other related vaccine after an immediate anaphylactic reaction or other serious adverse reaction associated with a previous dose. Immunization with acellular Diphtheria/Pertussis/Tetanus is contraindicated if the child has experienced any event following previous immunization with pertussis vaccine (whole-cell) Diphtheria/Pertussis/Tetanus or acellular pertussis-containing Diphtheria/Pertussis/Tetanus vaccine), which is considered by the ACIP or AAP to be a contraindication to further doses of pertussis vaccine.

It is a contraindication to administer this vaccine in the presence of any evolving neurological condition.

Encephalopathy not due to an identifiable cause, occurring within 7 days of a prior whole-cell Diphtheria/Pertussis/Tetanus or acellular Diphtheria/Pertussis/Tetanus immunization and consisting of major alterations of consciousness, unresponsiveness, generalized or focal seizures that persist for more than a few hours and failure to recover within 24 hours should be considered a contraindication to further use; this includes severe alterations in consciousness with generalized or focal neurologic signs. Even though causation cannot be established, no subsequent doses should be given.[2]

The presence of any evolving or changing disorder affecting the central nervous system is a contraindication to administration of Diphtheria/Pertussis/Tetanus regardless of whether the suspected neurological disorder is associated with occurrence of seizure activity of any type.

Studies have indicated that a personal or family history of seizures is associated with increased frequency of seizures following pertussis immunization.[10]

Personal History: The Immunization Practices Advisory Committee (ACIP) of the U.S. Public Health Service states: "The presence of a neurologic condition characterized by changing developmental or neurologic findings. Regardless of whether a definitive diagnosis has been made is... considered a contraindication to receipt of Pertussis vaccine. Because administration of 'DTP' may coincide with or possibly even aggravate manifestations of the disease. Such disorders include uncontrolled epilepsy, infantile spasms, and progressive encephalopathy."[14]

The Immunization Practices Advisory Committee (ACIP) and the American Academy of Pediatrics (AAP) recognize certain circumstances in which children with stable central nervous system disorders, including well-controlled seizures or statisfactorily explained single seizures, may receive pertussis vaccine. The decision to administer vaccine to such children must be made by the physician on an individual basis with consideration of all relevant factors. To allow an accurate assessment of risks and benefits for that individual, the physician should review

Table 1.[19,20]

COMPARISON OF IgG ANTIBODY TO PERTUSSIS TOXIN (PT) AND FILAMENTOUS HEMAGGLUTININ (FHA) IN ELISA UNITS (EU) AND CHO-CELL NEUTRALIZATION TITERS (CHO) INDUCED BY A SINGLE DOSE OF EITHER ACELLULAR DIPHTHERIA/PERTUSSIS/TETANUS PERTUSSIS WHOLE-CELL OR DIPHTHERIA/PERTUSSIS/TETANUS VACCINE IN CHILDREN 15 TO 20 MONTHS OF AGE* AND 4 TO 6 YEARS OF AGE**

Vaccine	Age Group (n =)	PT/GMT† (EU)		FHA/GMT† (EU)		CHO	
		Pre-Vaccination	Post-Vaccination‡	Pre-Vaccination	Post-Vaccination‡	Pre-Vaccination	Post-Vaccination†
Acellular Diphtheria/Pertussis/Tetanus	15-20 Months (354)	14.5	443.0††	7.0	65.0††	25.3	300††
Whole-Cell Diphtheria/Pertussis/Tetanus	15-20 Months (175)	14.5	67.0	6.0	19.0	24.8	119
Acellular Diphtheria/Pertussis/Tetanus	4-6 Years (211)	14.5	408.0††	18.9	36.0††	23.6	210††
Whole-Cell Diphteria/Pertussis/Tetanus	4-6 Years (65)	15.2	81.0	19.2	104.0	27.9	107

* All children in the 15-to 20-month group received U.S. licensed whole-cell pertussis Diphtheria/Pertussis/Tetanus vaccine for the first three doses of their primary series.

** All children in the 4- to 6-year group received U.S. licensed whole-cell pertussis Diphtheria/Pertussis/Tetanus vaccine for the first four doses in their primary series.

‡ Geometric mean titer.

† Post-vaccination 4 to 6 weeks.

£ Post-vaccination GMT for the Acellular Diphtheria/Pertussis/Tetanus group, (4 to 6 years olds), is significantly higher than that of the whole-cell pertussis Diphtheria/Pertussis/Tetanus vaccine group (P < 0.05).

†† Post-vaccination GMT's for the Acellular Diphtheria/Pertussis/Tetanus group, at 15 to 20 months and at 4 to 6 years, are significantly higher than those of the matching whole-cell Diphtheria/Pertussis/Tetanus group, (P < 0.001 in each case).

➤ SHOWN IN PRODUCT IDENTIFICATION GUIDE

the full text of the ACIP and AAP guidelines prior to considering vaccination for such children.[14,33,37] The parent or guardian should be advised of the increased risk involved.

Immunization should be deferred during the course of an acute illness. Vaccination of infants and children with severe, febrile illness should generally be deferred until these persons have recovered. However, the presence of minor illnesses such as mild upper respiratory infections with or without low-grade fever are not contraindications to further use.[2]

Elective immunization procedures should be deferred during an outbreak of poliomyelitis, providing the patient has not sustained an injury that increases the risk of tetanus and providing an outbreak of diphtheria or pertussis does not occur simultaneously.[40]

Data on the use of acellular Diphtheria/Pertussis/Tetanus in children for whom whole-cell pertussis Diphtheria/Pertussis/Tetanus vaccine is contraindicated are not available. Until such data are available, it would be prudent to consider the Immunization Practices Advisory Committee (ACIP) and American Academy of Pediatrics (AAP) contraindications to whole-cell pertussis Diphtheria/Pertussis/Tetanus vaccine to be contraindications to Diphtheria/Pertussis/Tetanus.

WARNINGS

If any of the following events occur in temporal relation to receipt of Diphtheria/Pertussis/Tetanus, the decision to give subsequent doses of vaccine containing the Pertussis component should be carefully considered. There may be circumstances, such as a high incidence of pertussis, when the potential benefits outweigh possible risks, particularly since these events are not associated with permanent sequelae.[2]

THE FOLLOWING EVENTS WERE PREVIOUSLY CONSIDERED CONTRAINDICATIONS AND ARE NOW CONSIDERED WARNINGS.[2]

Temperature of ≥ 40.5°C (105°F) within 48 hours not due to another identifiable cause: Such a temperature is considered a warning because of the likelihood that fever following a subsequent dose of Diphtheria/Pertussis/Tetanus Vaccine also will be high. Because such febrile reactions are usually attributed to the pertussis component, vaccination with diphtheria and tetanus toxoids should not be discontinued.[2]

Collapse or shock-like state (hypotonic-hyporesponsive episode) within 48 hours: Although these uncommon events have not been recognized to cause death nor to induce permanent neurological sequelae, it is prudent to continue vaccination with diphtheria and tetanus toxoids, omitting the pertussis component.[2]

Persistent, inconsolable crying lasting ≥ 3 hours, occurring within 48 hours: Follow-up of infants who have cried inconsolably following Diphtheria/Pertussis/Tetanus vaccination has indicated that this reaction, though unpleasant, is without long-term sequelae and not associated with other reactions of greater significance.[2] Evidence is insufficient to indicate whether pertussis vaccine-associated protracted, inconsolable, or high-pitched crying or screaming does, or does not, lead to chronic neurologic damage.[41] Inconsolable crying occurs most frequently following the first dose and is less frequently reported following subsequent doses of Diphtheria/Pertussis/Tetanus vaccine. However, crying for > 30 minutes following Diphtheria/Pertussis/Tetanus vaccination can be a predictor of increased likelihood of recurrence of persistent crying following subsequent doses. Children with persistent crying have had a higher rate of local reactions than children who had other Diphtheria/Pertussis/Tetanus associated reactions (including high fever, seizures, and hypotonic-hyporesponsive episodes), suggesting that prolonged crying was really a pain reaction.[2]

Convulsions with or without fever occurring within three days: Short-lived convulsions, with or without fever, have not been shown to cause permanent sequelae. Furthermore, the occurrence of prolonged febrile seizures (i.e., status epilepticus — any seizure lasting > 30 minutes or recurrent seizures lasting a total of 30 minutes without the child fully regaining consciousness), irrespective of their cause, involving an otherwise normal child does not substantially increase the risk for subsequent febrile (brief or prolonged) or afebrile seizures. The risk is significantly increased (p = 0.018) only among those children who are neurologically abnormal before their episode of status epilepticus.[2] Accordingly, although a convulsion following Diphtheria/Pertussis/Tetanus vaccination has previously been considered a contraindication to further doses, under certain circumstances subsequent doses may be indicated, particularly if the risk of pertussis in the community is high. If a child has a seizure following the first or second dose of Diphtheria/Pertussis/Tetanus, it is desirable to delay subsequent doses until the child's neurologic status is better defined. By the end of the first year of life, the presence of an underlying neurologic disorder has usually been determined, and appropriate treatment instituted. Diphtheria and tetanus toxoids vaccine should not be administered before a decision has been made about whether to continue the Diphtheria/Pertussis/Tetanus series. Regardless of which vaccine is given, it is prudent also to administer acetaminophen[2], 15 mg/kg of body weight, at the time of vaccination and every 4 hours subsequently for 24 hours, to reduce the possibility of post-vaccination fever.

The clinical judgment of the attending physician should prevail at all times.

Persons who experienced Arthus-type hypersensitivity reactions or a temperature of > 103°F (39.4°C) following prior dose of tetanus toxoid usually have high serum tetanus antitoxin levels and should not be given even emergency doses of diphtheria and tetanus toxoids more frequently than every 10 years, even if they have a wound that is neither clean nor minor.[2]

Diphtheria/Pertussis/Tetanus should not be given to children with any coagulation disorder, including thrombocytopenia, that would contraindicate intramuscular injection unless the potential benefit clearly outweighs the risk of administration.

Recent studies suggest that infants and children with a history of convulsions in first-degree family members (i.e., siblings and parents) have a 3.2-fold increased risk for neurologic events compared with those without such histories.[37] *However, the ACIP has concluded that a family history of convulsions in parents and siblings is not a contraindication to pertussis vaccination and that children with such family histories should receive Pertussis vaccine according to the recommended schedule.*[2]

A recent review of all available data by the IOM found evidence is consistent with a causal relation between Diphtheria/Pertussis/Tetanus vaccine and acute encephalopathy, but that there is insufficient evidence to indicate a causal relation between Diphtheria/Pertussis/Tetanus vaccine and serious acute neurologic illness or permanent neurologic damage.[41]

Infants and children with recognized possible or potential underlying neurologic conditions seem to be at enhanced risk for the appearance of manifestations of the underlying neurologic disorder within two or three days following vaccination.[2] Whether to administer Diphtheria/Pertussis/Tetanus to children with proven or suspected underlying neurologic disorders must be decided on an individual basis. Important considerations include the current local incidence of pertussis, the near absence of diptheria in the United States and the low risk of infection with *C. tetani*.[2]

Although these events were considered absolute contraindications in previous ACIP recommendations, there may be circumstances, such as a high incidence of pertussis, in which the potential benefits outweigh possible risks, particularly because these events are not associated with permanent sequelae.[2]

The administration of Diphtheria/Pertussis/Tetanus to children with proven or suspected underlying neurologic disorders that are not actively evolving must be decided on an individual basis.

Only full doses (0.5 mL) of Diphtheria/Pertussis/Tetanus vaccine should be given; if a specific contraindication to Diphtheria/Pertussis/Tetanus exists, the vaccine should not be given.[2]

Controversy regarding the safety of pertussis vaccine during the 1970s led to several studies of the benefits and risks of this vaccination during the 1980s. These epidemiologic analyses clearly indicate that the benefits of pertussis vaccination outweigh any risks and have not shown a cause and effect with neurologic illness.[2,34]

The occurrence of sudden infant death syndrome (SIDS) has been reported following administration of Diphtheria/Pertussis/Tetanus.[42-44] However, a large case-control study in the U.S. revealed no causal relationship between receipt of Diphtheria/Pertussis/Tetanus vaccine and SIDS.[45]

Onset of infantile spasms has occurred in infants who have recently received Diphtheria/Pertussis/Tetanus or diphtheria and tetanus toxoids. Analysis of data from the National Childhood Encephalopathy Study on children with infantile spasms showed that receipt of Diphtheria/Pertussis/Tetanus or diphtheria and tetanus toxoids was not causally related to infantile spasms.[46] The incidence of onset of infantile spasms increases at 3 to 9 months of age, the time period in which the second and third doses of Diphtheria/Pertussis/Tetanus are generally given. Therefore, some cases of infantile spasms can be expected to be related by chance alone to recent receipt of Diphtheria/Pertussis/Tetanus.[14]

Patients with impaired immune responsiveness, whether due to the use of immunosuppressive therapy (including irradiation, corticosteroids, antimetabolites, alkylating agents, and cytotoxic agents), a genetic defect, human immunodeficiency virus (HIV) infection, or other causes, may have a reduced antibody response to active immunization procedures.[14,33,47] Deferral of administration of vaccine may be considered in individuals receiving immunosuppressive therapy.[14,33] Other groups should receive this vaccine according to the usual recommended schedule.[14,33,47,48]

Special care should be taken to prevent injection into a blood vessel.

Deaths have been reported in temporal association with the administration of Diphtheria/Pertussis/Tetanus vaccine (see "*Adverse Reactions*" section).

When Diphtheria/Pertussis/Tetanus vaccine is used alone or to reconstitute Haemophilus b conjugate vaccine and administered to immunosuppressed persons or persons receiving immunosuppressive therapy, the expected antibody responses may not be obtained. This includes patients with severe combined immunodeficiency, hypogammaglobulinemia, or agammaglobulinemia; altered immune states due to diseases such as leukemia, lymphoma, or generalized malignancy, or an immune system compromised by treatment with corticosteroids, alkylating drugs, antimetabolites or radiation.[49]

Administration of Diphtheria/Pertussis/Tetanus and/or Haemophilus b conjugate vaccine is not contraindicated in individuals with HIV infection.

Diphtheria/Pertussis/Tetanus acellular vaccine is not recommended for use in children below the age of 15 months. Studies in children 15 to 17 months of age have not been completed.

No determination of efficacy in infants has been made to date. Studies designed to evaluate efficacy in infants are ongoing but are not yet complete. Although antibody responses to diphtheria, tetanus, and pertussis toxin, and filamentous hemagglutinin in infants immunized with Diphtheria/Pertussis/Tetanus acellular vaccine were at least equivalent to those for whole-cell pertussis Diphtheria/Pertussis/Tetanus vaccine, the role of serum antibodies in protection against pertussis is unknown.

Diphtheria/Pertussis/Tetanus is not recommended for immunization on or after the seventh birthday.

PRECAUTIONS
GENERAL
Care is to be taken by the health-care provider for the safe and effective use of DTP.

Epinephrine Injection (1:1000) must be immediately available should an acute anaphylactic reaction occur due to any component of the vaccine.

Prior to an injection of any vaccine, all known precautions should be taken to prevent adverse reactions. This includes a review of the patient's history with respect to possible sensitivity and any previous adverse reactions to the vaccine or similar vaccines, previous immunization history, current health status (see "Contraindications," "Warnings" sections), and a current knowledge of the literature concerning the use of the vaccine under consideration.

Children with impaired immune responsiveness, whether due to the use of immunosuppressive therapy (including irradiation, corticosteroids, antimetabolites, alkylating agents, and cytotoxic agents), a genetic defect, human immunodeficiency virus (HIV) infection, or other causes, may have reduced antibody response to active immunization procedures.[2,34,50] Deferral of administration of vaccine may be considered in individuals receiving immunosuppressive therapy.[2,34] Other groups should receive this vaccine according to the usual recommended schedule.[2,34,50,51] (See "Drug Interactions".)

This product is not contraindicated for use in individuals with HIV.

Prior to administration of Diphtheria/Pertussis/Tetanus, health-care personnel should inform the parent or guardian of the patient the benefits and risks of immunization, and also inquire about the recent health status of the patient to be injected.

Special care should be taken to ensure that the injection does not enter a blood vessel.

If the product is a suspension containing an adjuvant, shake vigorously to obtain a uniform suspension prior to withdrawing each dose from the multiple dose vial.

A separate, sterile syringe and needle or a sterile disposable unit should be used for each patient to prevent transmission of hepatitis or other infectious agents from person to person. Needles should not be recapped and should be disposed of properly.

Previous immunization history should be ascertained to confirm that at least three doses of whole-cell pertussis Diphtheria/Pertussis/Tetanus vaccine have been given before administering acellular Diphtheria/Pertussis/Tetanus.

INFORMATION FOR PATIENTS
As part of the child's immunization record, the date, lot number and manufacturer of the vaccine administered *must* be recorded.[52,53,54]

Parents should be fully informed of the benefits and risks of immunization with Diphtheria/Pertussis/Tetanus. The health-care provider should inform the parent or guardian of the patient about the recommended immunization schedule, the benefits and risks of the vaccine, and the potential for adverse reactions that have been temporally associated with administration and obtain informed consent. Parents or guardians should be instructed to report any serious adverse reactions to their health-care provider. Guidance should be provided on other measures to be taken should adverse events occur, e.g., antipyretic measures for elevated temperatures.

It is extremely important when the children returns for the next dose in the series that the parent or guardian of the patient should be questioned concerning occurrence of any symptoms and/or signs of an adverse reaction after the previous dose (See "Contraindications," "Adverse Reactions" sections).

The health-care provider should inform the parent or guardian of the patient the importance of completing the immunization series.

The health-care provider should provide the vaccine information materials or pamphlets which are required to be given with each immunization.

The U.S. Department of Health and Human Services has established a Vaccine Adverse Event Reporting System (VAERS) to accept all reports of suspected adverse events after the administration of any vaccine, including but not limited to the reporting of events required by the National Childhood Vaccine Injury Act of 1986.[52] The toll-free number for VAERS forms and information is 1-800-822-7967.

The National Vaccine Injury Compensation Program, established by the National Childhood Vaccine Injury Act of 1986. requires that the manufacturer and lot number of the vaccine administered be recorded by the health care provider in the vaccine recipient's permanent medical record, along with the date of administration of the vaccine and the name, address, and title of the person administering the vaccine.

The Act further requires the health care provider to report to a health department or to the FDA the occurrence following immunization of any event set forth in the Vaccine Injury Table including: anaphylaxis or anaphylactic shock within 24 hours, encephalopathy or encephalitis within 7 days, shock-collapse or hypotonic-hyporesponsive collapse within 7 days, residual seizure disorder, any acute complication or sequelae (including death) of above events, or any event that would contraindicate further doses of vaccine.[53,54]

DRUG INTERACTIONS
If Diphtheria/Pertussis/Tetanus and tetanus immune globulin or diphtheria antitoxin are administered concurrently, separate syringes and separate sites should be used.

As with other intramuscular injections, use with caution in patients on anticoagulant therapy.

Immunosuppressive therapies, including irradiation, antimetabolites, alkylating agents, cytotoxic drugs, and corticosteroids (used in greater than physiologic

doses), may reduce the immune response to vaccines. Short-term (< 2 weeks) corticosteroid therapy or intra-articular, bursal, or tendon injections with corticosteroids should not be immunosuppressive. Although no specific studies with pertussis vaccine are available, if immunosuppressive therapy will be discontinued shortly, it is reasonable to defer vaccination until the patient has been off therapy for one month: otherwise, the patient should be vaccinated while still on therapy.[2]

If Diphtheria/Pertussis/Tetanus has been administered to persons receiving immunosuppressive therapy, a recent injection of immunoglobulin or having an immunodeficiency disorder, an adequate immunologic response may not be obtained.

Influenza virus vaccine should not be given within three days of the administration of Diphtheria/Pertussis/Tetanus.[34]

CARCINOGENESIS, MUTAGENESIS, IMPAIRMENT OF FERTILITY
No studies have been performed to evaluate carcinogenicity, mutagenic potential, or impact on fertility.

PREGNANCY
Pregnancy Category C: This vaccine is not recommended for persons 7 years of age and older. Animal reproduction studies have not been conducted with Diphtheria/Pertussis/Tetanus. It is also not known whether Diphtheria/Pertussis/Tetanus can cause fetal harm when administered to a pregnant woman or can affect reproductive capacity.

PEDIATRIC USE
Safety and effectiveness of Diphtheria/Pertussis/Tetanus whole-cell vaccine or at the time when Diphtheria/Pertussis/Tetanus whole-cell vaccine is used to reconstitute Haemophilus B conjugate vaccine in infants below the age of six weeks have not been established. (See "Dosage and Administration" section.)

Diphtheria/Pertussis/Tetanus whole-cell vaccine is recommended for immunizing children 6 weeks of age through 6 years of age (up to the seventh birthday). Diphtheria/Pertussis/Tetanus whole-cell vaccine is the preferred vaccine in this age group, but in those situations where an *absolute contraindication* to pertussis vaccination exists, or where in the opinion of the physician the pertussis vaccine should not be administered. diphtheria and tetanus toxoids is the appropriate alternative.

Full protection is achieved upon completion of primary immunization with either four doses of Diphtheria/Pertussis/Tetanus whole-cell vaccine, or three doses of Diphtheria/Pertussis/Tetanus whole-cell vaccine followed by a dose of an approved acellular Diphtheria/Pertussis/Tetanus whole-cell vaccine. A fifth dose of Diphtheria/Pertussis/Tetanus whole-cell vaccine or an approved acellular Diphtheria/Pertussis/Tetanus whole-cell vaccine is required.

This vaccine is not recommended for persons 7 years of age and older. For persons 7 years of age and older, the recommended vaccine is diphtheria and tetanus toxoids for adult use, in preference to either diphtheria or tetanus vaccine alone.

Efficacy data for Diphtheria/Pertussis/Tetanus acellular vaccine in infants is not available. Although antibody responses to diphtheria, tetanus, and pertussis toxin and filamentous hemagglutinin in infants immunized with Diphtheria/Pertussis/Tetanus acellular vaccine were at least equivalent to those for whole-cell pertussis Diphtheria/Pertussis/Tetanus vaccine, the role of serum antibodies in protection against pertussis is unknown at this time.

Diphtheria/Pertussis/Tetanus acellular vaccine is not recommended for use in children below 15 months of age. This vaccine is not recommended for use as a primary series in children of any age.

ADVERSE REACTIONS
Adverse reactions associated with the use of Diphtheria/Pertussis/Tetanus include local redness, warmth, edema, induration with or without tenderness, as well as arthralgias, urticaria and rash. Some data suggest that febrile reactions are more likely to occur in those who have experienced such responses after prior doses.[8]

The frequency of local reactions following Diphtheria/Pertussis/Tetanus vaccination is significantly higher with increasing numbers of doses of Diphtheria/Pertussis/Tetanus, while other mild to moderate systemic reactions (e.g., fretfulness, vomiting) are significantly less frequent.[55] Approximately 50% of Diphtheria/Pertussis/Tetanus recipients will develop temperature elevations > 38°C (100.4°F) after one or more doses of the series; approximately 6% > 39°C (102.2°F);[56] and approximately 0.3% ≥ 40.5°C (105°F).[14] Some data suggest that febrile reactions are more likely to occur in those who have experienced such responses after prior doses.[13] If local redness 2.5 cm occurs, the likelihood of recurrence after another Diphtheria/Pertussis/Tetanus dose increases significantly.[8] Evidence does not indicate a causal relation between Diphtheria/Pertussis/Tetanus vaccine and SIDS. Studies showing a temporal relation between these events are consistent with the expected occurrence of SIDS over the age range in which Diphtheria/Pertussis/Tetanus immunization typically occurs.[41]

Deaths due to causes other than SIDS, including deaths due to serious infections, have occurred in infants following the administration of Diphtheria/Pertussis/Tetanus. No association has been shown for hospitalizations due to infectious disease and receipt of Diphtheria/Pertussis/Tetanus.[57]

Approximate rates for adverse events following receipt of Diphtheria/Pertussis/Tetanus vaccine (regardless of dose number in the series) are indicated in Table 2.[2]

Table 2[2]

ADVERSE EVENTS OCCURRING WITHIN 48 HOURS OF DIPHTHERIA/PERTUSSIS/TETANUS VACCINATIONS

Event	Frequency*
Local	
Redness	1 in 3 doses
Swelling	2 in 5 doses
Pain	1 in 2 doses
Systemic	
Fever ≥ 38°C (100 4°F)	1 in 2 doses
Drowsiness	1 in 3 doses
Fretfulness	1 in 3 doses
Vomiting	1 in 2 doses
Anorexia	1 in 15 doses
Persistent, inconsolable crying (duration ≥ 3 hours)	1 in 100 doses
Fever ≥ 40.5°C (≥ 105°F)	1 in 330 doses
Nervous System	
Collapse (hypotonic-hyporesponsive (episode)	1 in 1,750 doses
Convulsions (with or without fever)	1 in 1,750 doses

* *Rate per total number of doses regardless of dose number in Diphtheria/Pertussis/Tetanus series.*

In a prospective study of serious reactions to Michigan Department of Public Health's Diphtheria/Pertussis/Tetanus vaccine within 48 hours of vaccination, the following rates of adverse events were reported via mail-in questionnaires completed by parents followed by telephone contacts of positive responses: prolonged crying > 3 hours 1:442; unusual crying 1:1,457; fever > 40.5°C 1:1,770; hypotension/hyporesponsiveness 1:3,539 and seizure 1:24,776.[58]

Table 3 lists the frequency of adverse reactions in 372 children who received acellular Diphtheria/Pertussis/Tetanus at 15 to 20 months and 239 children who received acellular Diphtheria/Pertussis/Tetanus at 4 to 6 years of age. These children had previously received three or four doses of whole-cell pertussis Diphtheria/Pertussis/Tetanus vaccine at approximately 2, 4, 6 and 18 months of age. (See related table).

Adverse reactions associated with acellular Diphtheria/Pertussis/Tetanus have been evaluated in 911 children receiving this vaccine as the fourth or fifth dose in the Diphtheria/Petussis/Tetanus series. The percent of children experiencing common symptoms at any time within 72 hours following immunization is summarized below.[32]

Symptom	% of children* reporting symptoms within 72 hours of immunization (n = 911)
Tenderness	26
Erythema (> 2 cm)	10
Induration (> 2 cm)	7
Injection site temp	17
Fever ≥ 38°C (100.4°F)	19
> 39°C (102.2°F)	1.5

Table 3[1]

Symptom	% of children* reporting symptoms within 72 hours of immunization (n = 911)
Drowsiness	6
Fretfulness	17
Vomiting	2

* *Children age groups 17 to 24 months and 4 to 6 years of age (fourth and fifth doses) are included.*

During a 72-hour period following immunization, the most frequently reported adverse events, excluding those listed frequently reported adverse events, including those listed above, in decreasing order of frequency were: upper respiratory infection/rhinitis (6%), diarrhea/loose stools (3.5%), rash (1.2%). One child experienced a febrile seizure 78 hours after immunization.[32] A cause and effort relationship between these latter events and vaccination has not been established.

In investigational studies in 2,041 infants administered a total of 5,719 doses of acellular Diphtheria/Pertussis/Tetanus the combined frequency of common symptoms, at any time within 72 hours following any dose was as follows: erythema > 2 cm, 4%; induration > cm, 1.5%; fever 38°C (100.4°F), 7%; drowsiness, 12%; fretfulness, 20%; vomiting, 3%. During this period, events judged by the investigators to contraindicate further doses of vaccine occurred in the indicated number of children, persistent or unusual cry (11); fever 40.5°C (104.9°F) (1); possible seizure (1); hypotonic-hyporesponsive episode (1); lethargy (1); injection site rash (1). One child died suddenly 6 weeks after immunization following apparent recovery from an enteroviral meningitis;[32] however, a causal relationship with acellular Diphtheria/Pertussis/Tetanus has not been established.

BODY SYSTEM AS A WHOLE

Mild systemic reactions such as fever, drowsiness, fretfulness, and anorexia, occur quite frequently. These reactions are significantly more common following administration of Diphtheria/Pertussis/Tetanus than following diphtheria and tetanus toxoids, are usually self-limited, and need no therapy other than symptomatic treatment such as acetaminophen.[2]

Rarely, an anphylactic reaction (i.e., hives, swelling of the mouth, difficulty breathing, hypotension, or shock) and death have been reported after receiving preparations containing diphtheria, tetanus, and/or pertussis antigens.[2]

Arthus-type hypersensitivity reactions, characterized by severe local reactions (generally starting 2 to 8 hours after an injection), may follow receipt of tetanus toxoid.[2] A few cases of peripheral neuropathy have been reported following tetanus toxoid administration, although a causal relationship has not been established.[2]

Significant reactions attributed to the pertussis vaccine component have been: high fever of 40.5°C (105°F), a transient shock-like episode, excessive screaming (persistent crying or screaming for 3 or more hours duration), an unusual high-pitched cry, and convulsions. These events occur infrequently and appear to be without sequelae.[2]

Occasionally, a nodule may be palpable at the injection site of adsorbed products for several weeks. Sterile abscesses at the site of injection have been reported (6 to 10 per million doses)[2] subcutaneous atrophy may occur. Cervical lymphadenopathy has been reported following Diphtheria/Pertussis/Tetanus injections into the arm.[59]

NERVOUS SYSTEM

Pertussis vaccine has been associated with a greater proportion of adverse reactions than many other childhood immunizations.[60] Should symptomatology

Table 3[1]

ADVERSE EVENTS OCCURRING 24, 48 AND 72 HOURS FOLLOWING DIPHTHERIA AND TETANUS TOXOIDS AND ACELLULAR PERTUSSIS VACCINE ADSORBED IMMUNIZATIONS GIVEN AT 15 TO 20 MONTHS AND 4 TO 6 YEARS OF AGE.

Event	Frequency					
	15 to 20 Months Reaction % (n = 372)			4 to 6 Years Reactions % (n = 239)		
	24 hr	48 hr	72 hr	24 hr	48 hr	72 hr
Local						
Erythema*	13%	7%	3%	25%	23%	14%
Swelling*	6%	2%	1%	21%	20%	14%
Tenderness	6%	4%	2%	35%	20%	8
Mild/Moderate Systemic						
Fever > 101°F (rectal)	4%	1%	1%	3%	2%	1%
Gastrointestinal						
Diarrhea	3%	3%	2%	0%	0%	0%
Vomiting	2%	1%	0%	1%	1%	0%%
Anorexia	6%	4%	3%	5%	3%	1%
Neurological						
Drowsiness	11%	4%	1%	13%	3%	2%
Irritability	15%	9%	5%	10%	7%	5%
High-pitched unusual cry	1%	1%	0%	0%	0%	0%

* *Includes all occurrences of erythema.*
** *Includes all occurrences of swelling.*

◆ RATED THERAPEUTICALLY EQUIVALENT; ◇ THERAPEUTIC EQUIVALENCE UNCONFIRMED; ○ UNRATED

referable to the central nervous system develop within 7 days following administration, further immunization with this product is contraindicated (see *"Contraindications"*).

The following neurologic illness have been reported as temporally associated with vaccine containing tetanus toxoid: neurological complications[61,62] including cochlear lesion,[63] brachial plexus neuropathies,[63,64] paralysis of the radial nerve,[65] paralysis of the recurrent nerve[63] accommodation paresis, and EEG disturbances with encephalopathy.[55] The report from the IOM suggests that there is a causal relation between Guillain-Barre syndrome (GBS) and vaccines containing tetanus toxoid.[66] In the differential diagnosis of polyradiculoneuropathies following administration of a vaccine containing tetanus toxoid should be considered as a possible etiology.[55,67]

Short-lived convulsions (usually febrile), or collapse (hypotonic-hyporesponsive episode) occur infrequently and appear to be without sequelae.[2]

More severe neurologic events, such as a prolonged convulsion, or encephalopathy, although rare, have been reported in temporal association with Diphtheria/Pertussis/Tetanus administration. An analysis of these data failed to show any cause and effect association.[2] One study suggests the incidence of encephalopathy occurring within 7 days of vaccination may be 1 per 140,000 doses, with encephalopathy resulting in death or permanent damage to the central nervous system estimated to occur in 1 per 330,000 doses.[67] (See *"Contraindications"* and *"Warnings"* .)

The incidence of convulsion or transient shock-like episode occurring within 48 hours of vaccination has been estimated to be 1 per 1,750 doses.[55]

Permanent neurological disability and death have been reported rarely in temporal relation to immunization with vaccines containing pertussis antigens.

In the National Childhood Encephalopathy Study (NCES), a large, case-control study in England, children 2 to 35 months of age with serious, acute neurologic disorders, such as encephalopathy or complicated convulsion(s), were more likely to have received Diphtheria/Pertussis/Tetanus in the 7 days preceding onset than their age-, sex-, and neighborhood-matched controls. Among children known to be neurologically normal before entering the study, the relative risk (estimated by odds ratio) of a neurologic illness occurring within the 7-day period following receipt of Diphtheria/Pertussis/Tetanus dose, compared to children not receiving Diphtheria/Pertussis/Tetanus in the 7-day period before onset of their illness, was 3.3 (p < 0.001).[2]

Within this 7-day period, the risk was significantly increased for immunized children only within 3 days of vaccination (relative risk 4.2, p < 0.001). The relative risk for illness occurring 4-7 days after vaccination was 2.1 (p < 0.1). Serious neurologic illnesses requiring hospitalization attributable to pertussis vaccine are rare. Final analysis of a comprehensive case-control study has estimated that the attributable risk of such illnesses is 1 in 140,000 doses administered. An earlier analysis had estimated this risk at 1/110,000 doses. In contrast, final analysis of the case-control study found that the risk of serious neurologic illness following pertussis disease was 1/11,000 pertussis cases. The estimated risk for a permanent neurologic deficit was one in 330,000 doses with a wide confidence interval.[2] No specific clinical syndrome was identified. Overall, Diphtheria/Pertussis/Tetanus vaccine accounted for only a small proportion of cases of serious neurologic disorders reported in the population studied. Repeated evaluations have shown that the benefits of vaccine outweigh the risks[2,34]; therefore, both the ACIP and the American Academy of Pediatrics continue to recommend the use of Diphtheria/Pertussis/Tetanus vaccine.[2,34] The methods and results of the NCES have been thoroughly scrutinized since publication of the study. This reassessment by multiple groups has determined that the number of patients was too small and their classification subject to enough uncertainty to preclude drawing valid conclusions about whether a causal relation exists between pertussis vaccine and permanent neurologic damage. Preliminary data from a 10-year follow-up study of some of the children studied in the original NCES study also suggested a relation between symptoms following Diphtheria/Pertussis/Tetanus vaccination and permanent neurologic disability. However, details are not available to evaluate this study adequately, and the same concerns remain about Diphtheria/Pertussis/Tetanus precipitating initial manifestations of pre-existing neurologic disorders.[2]

An IOM report by the Committee to review the adverse consequences of pertussis and rubella vaccines concluded that evidence is consistent with a causal relation between Diphtheria/Pertussis/Tetanus vaccine and acute encephalopathy, defined in the controlled studies reviewed as encephalopathy, encephalitis, or encepohalomyelitis. On the basis of review of the evidence bearing on this relation, the Committee concludes that the range of excess risk of acute encephalopathy following Diphtheria/Pertussis/Tetanus immunization is consistent with that estimated for the NCES: 0.0 to 10.5 per million immunizations. The report also states that there is insufficient evidence to indicate a causal relation between Diphtheria/Pertussis/Tetanus vaccine and permanent neurologic damage.[41]

Onset of infantile spasms has occurred in infants who have recently received Diphtheria/Pertussis/Tetanus or diphtheria and tetanus toxoids. Analysis of data from the NCES on children with infantile spasms showed that receipt of diphtheria and tetanus toxoids or Diphtheria/Pertussis/Tetanus was not causally related to infantile spasms.[46] The incidence of onset of infantile spasms increases at 3-9 months of age, the time period in which the second and third doses of Diphtheria/Pertussis/Tetanus are generally given. Therefore, some cases of infantile spasms can be expected to be related by chance alone to recent receipt of Diphtheria/Pertussis/Tetanus.[2]

A bulging fontanelle associated with increased intracranial pressure which occurred within 24 hours following Diphtheria/Pertussis/Tetanus immunization has been reported. A causal relationship has not been established.[68,69,70]

CARDIOVASCULAR SYSTEM

An infant who developed myocarditis several hours after immunization has been reported.[71] Hypotension may occur.

RESPIRATORY SYSTEM

Respiratory difficulties, including apnea, have been observed.

LOCAL

Rash and allergic reactions have been observed.

Sudden infant death syndrome (SIDS) has temporally occurred in infants following administration of Diphtheria/Pertussis/Tetanus. A large case-control study of SIDS in the United States showed that receipt of Diphtheria/Pertussis/Tetanus was not causally related to SIDS.[44,45,72] It should be recognized that the first three primary immunizing doses of Diphtheria/Pertussis/Tetanus are usually administered to infants 2 to 6 months of age and that approximately 85% of SIDS cases occur at ages 1-6 months, with the peak incidence occurring at 6 weeks to 4 months of age. By chance alone, some SIDS victims can be expected to have recently received Diphtheria/Pertussis/Tetanus.[44,45,72]

When whole-cell Diphtheria/Pertussis/Tetanus was administered concomitantly (at separate sites with separate syringes) with Haemophilus b conjugate vaccine the systemic adverse experience profile was not different from that seen when whole-cell Diphtheria/Pertussis/Tetanus vaccine was administered alone.[35,36]

In general, the rates of minor systemic reactions after Diphtheria/Pertussis/Tetanus was used to reconstitute Haemophilus b conjugate vaccine were comparable to those usually reported after Diphtheria/Pertussis/Tetanus vaccine alone.[8,55,73]

When whole-cell Diphtheria/Pertussis/Tetanus was used to reconstitute Haemophilus b conjugate vaccine and administered to infants at 2, 4 and 6 months of age, the systemic adverse experience profile was comparable to that observed when the two vaccines were given separately. An increase in the rate of local reactions was observed in some instances within the 24-hour period after immunization.[35,36]

REPORTING OF ADVERSE EVENTS

Reporting by parents or guardians of all adverse events occurring after vaccine administration should be encouraged. Adverse events following immunization with vaccine should be reported by health-care providers to the U.S. Department of Health and Human Services (DHHS) Vaccine Adverse Event Reporting System (VAERS). Reporting forms and information about reporting requirements or completion of the form can be obtained from VAERS through a toll-free number 1-800-822-7967.[52,53,54]

DOSAGE AND ADMINISTRATION

Parenteral drug products should be inspected visually for extraneous particulate matter and/or discoloration prior to administration whenever solution and container permit. If these conditions exist, vaccine should not be administered.

Shake vial well before withdrawing each dose.

Vigorous agitation is required to resuspend the contents of the vial. Discard if vaccine cannot be resuspended.

FOR ADMINISTRATION OF DIPHTHERIA/PERTUSSIS/TETANUS WHOLE-CELL OR ACELLULAR VACCINE

The primary series of whole-cell vaccine for children less than 7 years of age is four doses of 0.5 mL each given intramuscularly. The customary age for the first dose is 2 months of age but may be given as young as 6 weeks of age and up to the seventh birthday. The acellular vaccine is indicated for the fourth and fifth doses of the series. The customary age is 15 months and up.

Inject 0.5 ml intramuscularly only. The preferred injection sites are the anterolateral aspect of the thigh and the deltoid muscle of the upper arm. The vaccine should not be injected into the gluteal area or areas where there may be a major nerve trunk. During the course of primary immunizations, injections should not be made more than once at the same site.

The use of reduced volume (fractional dose) is not recommended. The effect of such practices on the frequency of serious adverse events and on protection against disease has not been determined.

Do NOT administer this product subcutaneously.

Special care (aspiration) should be taken to ensure that the injection does not enter a blood vessel.

Primary Immunization: The whole-cell vaccine is recommended for children 6 weeks through 6 years of age (up to seventh birthday) ideally beginning when the infant is 6 weeks to 2 months of age.

The primary series consists of four doses. For infants 6 weeks through 12 months of age, administer three 0.5 mL doses intramuscularly at least 4 to 8 weeks apart. The fourth dose is administered 6 to 12 months after the third injection.

The acellular vaccine is indicated for the fourth dose (0.5 mL) of the diphtheria, tetanus and pertussis immunization series. The acellular vaccine may be given 6 to 12 months after the third dose of whole-cell pertussis Diphtheria/Pertussis/Tetanus to maintain adequate immunity during the preschool years. This dose is an integral part of the primary vaccinating course.

Acellular Diphtheria/Pertussis/Tetanus is indicated for the fifth dose (0.5 mL) of the Diphtheria, Tetanus and Pertussis immunization series. Prior immunizations may consist of three doses of whole-cell pertussis Diphtheria/Pertussis/Tetanus and one dose of acellular pertussis Diphtheria/Pertussis/Tetanus or four doses of whole-cell pertussis Diphtheria/Pertussis/Tetanus. Acellular Diphtheria/Pertussis/Tetanus may be given to children 4 to 6 years of age, before entering kindergarten or elementary school (not considered necessary if fourth primary vaccinating dose administered after four birthday).

▶ SHOWN IN PRODUCT IDENTIFICATION GUIDE

Booster Immunization: For children between 4 and 6 years of age (preferably at time of kindergarten or elementary school entrance), a booster of 0.5 mL should be administered intramuscularly. Those who receive all four primary immunizing doses before their fourth birthday should receive a single dose of Diphtheria/Pertussis/Tetanus just before entering kindergarten or elementary school. This booster dose is not necessary if the fourth dose in the primary series was administered after the fourth birthday. Thereafter, routine booster immunizations should be with diphtheria and tetanus toxoids (adult) at intervals of 10 years. Persons 7 years of age and older should not be immunized with Diphtheria/Pertussis/Tetanus.

Table 4[2]
ROUTINE DIPHTHERIA/PERTUSSIS/TETANUS VACCINATION SCHEDULES SUMMARY FOR CHILDREN < 7 YEARS OLD —UNITED STATES, 1991

Dose	Customary Age	Age/Interval[†]	Product
Primary 1	2 Months	6 weeks old or older	Diphtheria/Pertussis/Tetanus
Primary 2	4 Months	4-8 weeks after first dose*	Diphtheria/Pertussis/Tetanus
Primary 3	6 Months	4-8 weeks after second dose*	Diphtheria/Pertussis/Tetanus
Primary 4	15 Months	6-12 months after third dose*	Diphtheria/Pertussis/Tetanus
Booster	4-6 years old, before entering kindergarten or elementary school (not necessary if fourth primary vaccinating dose administered on or after fourth birthday)		Diphtheria/Pertussis/Tetanus
Additional boosters		Every 10 years after last dose	Diphtheria and tetanus toxoids

* *Use Diphtheria and tetanus toxoids if pertussis vaccine is contraindicated. If the child is ≥ 1 year of age at the time that primary dose three is due, a third dose 6 to 12 months after the second dose completes primary vaccination with Diphtheria and tetanus toxoids.*
† *Prolonging the interval dose does not require restarting series.*

Preterm infants should be vaccinated according to their chronological age from birth.[2,34]

Interruption of the recommended schedule with a delay between doses does not interfere with the final immunity achieved with Diptheria/Pertussis/Tetanus. There is no need to start the series over again, regardless of the time elapsed between doses.

Acellular Diphtheria/Pertussis/Tetanus can be interchangeably used with whole-cell Diphtheria/Pertussis/Tetanus for the fourth and fifth doses. However, Haemophilus b conjugate vaccine cannot be reconstituted with Acellular Diphtheria/Pertussis/Tetanus.

The simultaneous administration of whole-cell Diphtheria/Pertussis/Tetanus, oral poliovirus vaccine (OPV), and measles-mumps-rubella vaccine (MMR) has resulted in seroconversion rates and rates of side effects similar to those observed when the vaccines are administered separately. The simultaneous administration of Diphtheria/Pertussis/Tetanus and Haemophilus b conjugate vaccine has resulted in antibody responses to the individual antigens and rates of side effects similar to those observed when the vaccines are administered separately.[74] Simultaneous vaccination (at separate sites with separate syringes) with whole-cell Diphtheria/Pertussis/Tetanus, MMR, OPV, or inactivated poliovirus vaccine (IPV), and Haemophilus b conjugate vaccine (HbCV) is also acceptable.[2] The simultaneous administration of acellular Diphtheria/Pertussis/Tetanus, OPV, and MMR has not been evaluated. However, on the basis of studies using whole-cell, Diphtheria/Pertussis/Tetanus, the ACIP does not anticipate any differences in seroconversion rates and rates of side effects from those observed when the vaccines are administered separately. The ACIP recommends the simultaneous administration, at separate sites with separate syringes, of all vaccines appropriate to the age and previous vaccination status of the recipients including the special circumstance of simultaneous administration of whole-cell and acellular Diphtheria/Pertussis/Tetanus, OPV, HbCV, and MMR at ≥ 15 months of age.[2]

If passive immunization is needed for tetanus, tetanus immune globulin (human) is the product of choice. It provides longer protection than antitoxin of animal origin and causes few adverse reactions. The currently recommended prophylactic dose of tetanus immune globulin (human) for wounds of average severity is 250 units intramuscularly. When tetanus toxoid and tetanus immune globulin (human) are administered concurrently, separate syringes and separate sites should be used. The ACIP recommends the use of only adsorbed toxoid in this situation.[2]

The American Academy of Pediatrics recommends that influenza virus vaccine should not be administered within 3 days of immunization with a pertussis-containing vaccine.[5]

WHEN RECONSTITUTING HAEMOPHILUS B CONJUGATE VACCINE
Whole-cell Diphtheria/Pertussis/Tetanus vaccine also can be used for reconstitution of Haemophilus b conjugate vaccine. Cleanse both the Diphtheria/Pertussis/

Tetanus and vaccine vial rubber barriers with a suitable germicide prior to reconstitution. Thoroughly agitate the vial of whole-cell Diphtheria/Pertussis/Tetanus vaccine, then withdraw 0.6 mL dose and inject into the vial of lyophilized Haemophilus b conjugate vaccine. Withdraw and administer 0.5 mL dose of Diphtheria/Pertussis/Tetanus Haemophilus b conjugate vaccine vaccines.

When whole-cell Diphtheria/Pertussis/Tetanus vaccine is used to reconstitute Haemophilus b conjugate vaccine, administer *intramuscularly only. Vaccine should be used immediately (i.e. within 30 minutes) after reconstitution.*

Before injection, the skin over the site to be injected should be cleansed with a suitable germicide. After insertion of the needle, aspirate to ensure that the needle has not entered a blood vessel.

Each dose of Diphtheria/Pertussis/Tetanus or Haemophilus b conjugate vaccines is administered intramuscularly in the outer aspect of the vastus lateralis (mid-thigh) or deltoid. The vaccine should not be injected into the gluteal area or areas where there may be a nerve trunk. During the course of primary immunizations, injections should not be made more than once at the same site.

When Diphtheria/Pertussis/Tetanus vaccine is used to reconstitute Haemophilus b conjugate vaccine, the combined vaccines are indicated for infants and children 2 months through 5 years of age for intramuscular administration in accordance with the schedule indicated in Table 5.[5,35]

Table 5[35]
RECOMMENDED IMMUNIZATION SCHEDULE FOR PREVIOUSLY UNVACCINATED CHILDREN

Dose	Age	Immunization
First, Second and Third	At 2, 4 and 6 months	Diphtheria/Pertussis/Tetanus alone or with Haemophilus b conjugate
Fourth	At 15 to 18 months	Diphtheria/Pertussis/Tetanus alone or with Haemophilus b conjugate
Fifth	At 4 to 6 years	Diphtheria/Pertussis/Tetanus or Acellular Diphtheria/Pertussis/Tetanus

* *Acellular Pertussis (DTaP) should NOT be used to reconstitute Haemophilus b conjugate vaccine. When administering DTaP for the fourth dose. Haemophilus influenzae type b vaccine also should be administered at this time in a separate syringe at a different site.*

FOR PREVIOUSLY UNVACCINATED CHILDREN
Immunization schedules should be considered on an individual basis for children not vaccinated according to the recommended schedule. Three doses of a product containing Diphtheria/Pertussis/Tetanus whole-cell or acellular, given at approximately 2-month intervals are required followed by a fourth dose of a product containing Diphtheria/Pertussis/Tetanus whole-cell or acellular approximately 12 months later and a fifth dose of a product containing whole-cell or acellular, Diphtheria/Pertussis/Tetanus at 4 to 6 years of age. If the fourth dose of a pertussis-containing vaccine is not given until after the fourth birthday, no further doses of a pertussis-containing vaccine are necessary.

The number of doses of a product containing *H influenzae* type b conjugate vaccine indicated depends on the age that immunization is begun. A child 7 to 11 months of age should receive 3 doses of a product containing *H influenzae* type b conjugate vaccine. A child 12 to 14 months of age should receive 2 doses of a product containing *H influenzae* type b conjugate vaccine. A child 15 to 59 months of age should receive 1 dose of a product containing *H influenzae* type b conjugate vaccine.

Preterm infants should be vaccinated according to their chronological age from birth.[34]

Interruption of the recommended schedule with a delay between doses should not interfere with the final immunity achieved with whole-cell Diphtheria/Pertussis/Tetanus vaccine is used to reconstitute Haemophilus b conjugate vaccine. There is no need to start the series over again, regardless of the time elapsed between doses.

It is recommended that the same conjugate vaccine be used throughout each immunization schedule, consistent with the data supporting approval and insure of the vaccine.

STORAGE
Store between 2°-8°C (35°-46°F) *Do not freeze.* Temperature extremes may adversely affect resuspendability of this vaccine.

REFERENCES
1. Mueller JH, et al. Production of diphtheria toxin of high potency (100 Lf) on a reproducible medium. J Immunol 40:21-32. 1941. 2. Recommendations of the Immunization Practices Advisory Committee (ACIP), Diphtheria, Tetanus, and Pertussis: Recommendations for vaccine use and other preventive measures. MMWR 40: No. RR-10, 1991 (NOTE: Articles relevant to reference cited are listed in the MMWR publication.) 3. Brown GC, Volk VK, Gottshall RY, et al: Responses of infants to DTP-P vaccine used in nine injection schedules. *Public Health Reports.* 1964;79:585-601. 4. Volk VK, Gottshall RY, Anderson HD, et al: Antibody response to booster dose of diphtheria and tetanus toxoids and pertussis vaccine. *Public Health Reports.* 1964;79:424-434. 5. CDC. Summary of Notifiable Disease, United States 1992. MMWR 41:No. 55, 1993. 6. Department of Health and Human Services, Food and Drug Administration. Biological Products: Bacterial Vaccines and Toxoids: Implemen-

tation of Efficacy Review; view; Proposed Rule, Federal Register Vol 50 No. 240, pp 51002-51117, 1985 7. Pichichero ME, et al. Pediatric diphtheria and tetanus toxoids-adsorbed vaccine: Immune response to the first booster following the diphtheria and tetanus toxoids vaccine primary series. Pediatr Infect Dis 5:428-430, 1986 8. Barkin RM, et al. Pediatric diphtheria and tetanus toxoids (DT) vaccine: Clinical and immunologic response when administered as theprimary series. J Pediatr 106:779-781, 1985 9. Manclark CR, et al. Pertussis. In: R. Germainier (ed), Bacterial Vaccines Academic Press INc., NY 69-106, 1984 10. Report of the Committee on Infectious Diseases. Elk Grove Village, IL, American Academy of Pediatrics, 358-369, 1991 11. Centers for Disease Control and Prevention (CDC). Tetanus surveillance—United States. 1989-1991. MMWR 41:No. SS-8, 1992 12. farizo KM, et al. Epidemiologic features of pertussis in the United States, 1980-1989. Rev Infect Dis (IN PRESS) 13. Baraff L, et al. DTP—associated reactions: An analysis by injection site, manufacturer, prior reactions and dose, Pediatr 73;31, 1984 14 Diphtheria, tetanus and pertussis: Cuidelines for vaccine prophylaxis and other preventive measures—recommendation of the Immunization Practices Advisory Committee (ACIP). *MMWR.* 1985:35(27r405-426. 15 *Feeral Register.* December 13, 1985;50)240). 16 Whooping Cough Immunization Committee of the Medical Research Council: Vaccination against whooping cough. *Br Med J.* Aug 25, 1956;ii:454-462. 17. Pertussis. Report of the Committee on INfectious Diseases. American Academy of Pediatrics, Evanston, Illinois. Twenty-second Edition, 1991 18. CDC. Pertussis Surveillance—United States, 1986 and 1998. MMWR 39: 57-66, 1990 19. Bernstein H, et al. Clinical reactions and immunogenicity of the BIKEN Acellular Diphtheria and Tetanus Toxoids and Pertussis Vaccine in 4-through 6-year-old US childrren. AJDC 146: 556-559, 1992 20. Feldman S, et al. Comparison of acellular (B-Type) and whole-cell pertussis-component diphtheria-tetanus-pertussis vaccines as the first booster immunization in 15- to 24-month-old children. J Pediatr, IN PRESS 21. Kimura M, et al. Developments in pertussis immunisation in Japan. The Lancet: 30-32, 1990 22. Noble GR, et al. Acellular and whole-cell pertussis vaccines in Japan. JAMA 257:1351-1356, 1987 23. Noble GR, Bernier RH, Esber EC, et al. Acellular and whole-cell pertussis vaccine in Japan. *JAMA* 1987; 257:1351-1356. 24. Pertussis—United States, 1982 and 1983. *MMWR* 1984; 33(40):573-575. 25. Isomura S, Suzuki S, Sato Y. Clinical efficacy of the Japanese acellular pertussis vaccine after intrafamiliar exposure to pertussis patients. Proceedings of the Fourth International Symposium on Pertussis, Joint IABS/WHO Meeting, Geneva, Switzerland, 1984. *Dev. Biol. Standard.* Vol. 61:531-537 (s. Karger, Basel, 1985). 26. Aoyama T, Murase Y, Gonda T, Iwata T. Type-specific efficacy of acellular pertussis vaccine. *AJDC* 1988; 142:40-42. 27. Kato T, Goshima t, Nakajima N, Kaku H, Arimoto Y, Hayashi F. Protection against pertussis by acellular pertussis vaccines (Takeda, Japan): Household contact studies in Kawasaki City, Japan. *Acta paediatr Jpn* 1989; 31:698-701. 28. Mortimer EA, Kimura M, Cherry JD, et al. Protective efficacy of the Takeda Acellular Pertussis Vaccine combined with diphtheria and tetanus toxoids following household exposure of Japanese children. *AJDC* 1990; 144:899-904. 29. Blumberg DA, Mink CM, Cherry JD, et al. Comparison of Acellular and whole-cell pertussis-component diphtheria-tetanus-pertussis vaccines in infants. *J. Pediatr.* 1991;119:1948204. 30. Morgan CM, Blumberg DA, Cherry JD, et al. Comparison of acellular and whole-cell pertussis-component DTP vaccines. *ADJC.* 1990;144:41-45. 31. Blumaberg DA, Mink CM, Cherry JD et al. Comparison of an acellular pertussis-component DTP vaccine with a whole-cell pertussis-component DTP vaccine in 17- to 24- month-old children, with measurement of 69-kilodalton outer membrane protein antibody. *J Pediatr.* 1990;117:46-51. 32. Data on file, Lederle Laboratories, Pearl River, NY. 33. American Academy of Pediatrics: Report of the Committee on Infectious Diseases, ed 21. Elk Grove Village, IL: American Academy of Pediatrics, 1988. 34. Report of the Committee on Infectious Disease. American Academy of Pediatrics, Elk Grove Village, IL, 1991 35. Data on file. Pasteur Merieux Serums * Vaccins S.A. 36. Data on file. Connaught Laboratories, Inc. 37. Pertussis immunization: family history of convulsions and use of antipyretics—supplementary ACIP statement. *MMWR.* 1987:36(18):281-282. 38. Stetler HC, et al: History of convulsions and use of pertussis vaccine. *J Pediatr.* 1985:107)2):175-179. 39. Hirtz DG, et al: Seizures following childhood immunizations. *J. Pediatr.* 1983;102(1):14-18. 41. Howson CP, et al. *Adverse Effects of Pertussis and Rubella Vaccines.* National Academy Press, Washington, DC, 1991 42. Bernier R, et al: Diphtheria-tetanus toxoids, pertussis vaccination and sudden infant deaths in Tennessee. *J Pediatr.* 1982;101:419-421. 43. Baraff L. et al: Possible temporal association between diphtheria-tetanus toxoid, pertussis vaccination and sudden infant death syndrome. *Pediatr Inf Dis.* 1983;2:7-11. 44. Walker AM. et al: Diphtheria-tetanus-pertussis immunization and sudden infant death syndrome. *AJPH.* 1987;77(8):945-951. 45. Hoffman HJ, et al: Diphtheria-tetanus-pertussis immunization and sudden infant death: results of the national Institute of Child Health and Human Development cooperative study of sudden infant death syndrome risk factors. *Pediatrics.* 1987;79(4):598-611. 46. Bellman MH, et al: Infantile spasms and pertussis immunization. *Lancet.* 1983;1:1031-1034. 47. Recommendation of the ACIP: Immunization of children infected with Human T-Lymphotrophic Virus Type III/Lymphadenopathy-associated virus *MMWR.* 1986; 35(38):595-606. 48. Immunization of children infected with Human Immunodeficiency Virus—Supplementary ACIP statement. *MMWR.* 1988:37(12):181-183. 49. ACIP. General recommendations on immunization. *MMWR* 38:205-227, 1989. 50. Recommendation of the ACIP: immunization of children infected with human T-lymphotropic virus type III/lymphadenopathy-associated virus. *MMWR.* 1986; 35((38):595-606. 51. Immunization of children infected with human immunodeficiency virus—supplementary ACIP statement. *MMWR.* 1988;37(12):181-183. 52. CDC. Vaccine Adverse Event Reporting System—United States. *MMWR* 39:730-733, 1990. 53. CDC. National Childhood Vaccine Injury Act: requirements for permanent vaccination records and for reporting of selected events after vaccination. *MMWR* 37:197-200, 1988. 54. Food and Drug Administration. New reporting requirements for vaccine adverse events. FDA Drug Bull 18 (2), 16-18, 1988. 55. Cody CL, et al. Nature and rates of adverse reactions associated with DTP adn DT immunizations in infants and children. *Pediatr* 68: 650-660, 1981. 56. Bernier R, et al: Abscesses complicating DTP vaccination. *Am J Dis Child.* 1981;135:826-828. 57. Joffe LS, et al. Diphtheria-tetanus toxoids-pertussis vaccination does not increase the risk of hospitalization with an infectious illness. *Pediatr Infect Dis J* 11:730-735, 1992. 58. Murray d,Wilcok K, Berlin B and the Michigan DTP Study Group: Serious reactions to DTP vaccine: a Michigan survey. *Pediatr Res.* 1988;42(4 part 2) Abst. No. 1054. 59. Omokoku B, Castells S: Post-DPT inoculation-caused lymphadenitis in children. *NY State J Med.* 1981;81:1667-1668. 60. Adverse events following immunization. *MMWR.* 1985;34:43-47. 61. Rutledge SL, et al. Neurological complications of immunization. *J Pediatr* 109:917-924, 1986. 62. Walker AM, et al. Neurologic events following Diphtheria-Tetanus-Pertussis immunization. *Pediatr* 81:345-349, 1988. 63. Wilson GS. The Hazards of Immunization. Allergic manifestations: Post-vaccinal neuritis, pp 153-156, 1967. 64. Tsairis P, et al. Natural history of brachial plexus neuropathy. *Arch Neurol* 27: 109-117, 1972. 65. Blumstein GI. et al. Peripheral neuropathy following tetanus toxoid administration. *JAMA* 198:1030-1031, 1966. 66 Stratton KB, et al. *Adverse Evants Associated with Childhood Vaccines: Evidence Bearing on Causality. National Academy Press, Washington, DC, 1993.* 67. Schlenska GK. Unusual neurological complications following tetanus toxoid administration. *J Neurol* 215:299-302, 1997. 68. Jacob J, et al. Increased intracranial pressure after diphtheria, tetanus and pertussis immunization. Am J Dis Child Vol 133:217-218, 1979 69. Mathur R. et al. Bulging fontanel following triple vaccine. *Indian Pediatr* 18 (6): 417-418, 1981 70. Shendurnikar N, et al. Bulging fontanel following DTP vaccine. *Indian Pediatr* 23 (11):960, 1966. 71. CDC. *Adverse events following immunization.* Surveillance Report No. 3, 1985-1986. Issued February 1989. 72. Griffin MR, et al. Risk of sudden infant death syndrome after immunization with the Diphtheria-Tetanus-Pertussis Vaccine. *N Engl J Med* 618-623, 1988. 73. Long SS, et al. Longitudinal study of adverse reactions following diphtheria-tetanus-pertussis vaccine in infancy. *Pediatr* 85:294-302, 1990.

HOW SUPPLIED

INJECTION:

BRAND/MANUFACTURER	NDC	SIZE	AWP
○ **BRAND**			
TRI-IMMUNOL: Lederle Labs	00005-1948-33	7.5 ml	$172.98
TRIPEDIA: Connaught	49281-0282-15	7.5 ml	$315.44
ACEL-IMUNE: Lederle Labs	00005-1950-31	5 ml	$198.63
WHOLE CELL DTP VACCINE: SK Beecham Pharm	00007-3555-01	5 ml 10s	$65.60
○ **GENERICS**			
DTP VACCINE: Connaught	49281-0280-84	7.5 ml	$193.81

Dipivefrin Hydrochloride

DESCRIPTION

Dipivefrin Hydrochloride is supplied in a sterile, isotonic solution. Dipivefrin Hydrochloride is a white, crystalline powder, freely soluble in water.

Empirical Formula: $C_{19}H_{29}O_5N \cdot HCl$

Chemical Name: (±)-3,4-Dihydroxy-α-[(methylamino)methyl]benzyl alcohol 3,4-dipivalate hydrochloride.

Contains:

Dipivefrin Hydrochloride 0.1%

Following is its chemical structure:

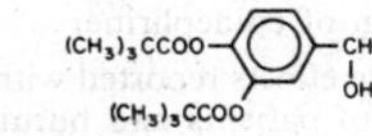

CLINICAL PHARMACOLOGY

Dipivefrin Hydrochloride is a member of a class of drugs known as prodrugs. Prodrugs are usually not active in themselves and require biotransformation to the parent compound before therapeutic activity is seen. These modifications are undertaken to enhance absorption, decrease side effects and enhance stability and comfort, thus making the parent compound a more useful drug. Enhanced absorption makes the prodrug a more efficient delivery system for the parent drug because less drug will be needed to produce the desired therapeutic response.

Dipivefrin Hydrochloride is a prodrug of epinephrine formed by the diesterification of epinephrine and pivalic acid. The addition of pivaloyl groups to the epinephrine molecule enhances its lipophilic character and, as a consequence, its penetration into the anterior chamber.

Dipivefrin Hydrochloride is converted to epinephrine inside the human eye by enzyme hydrolysis. The liberated epinephrine, an adrenergic agonist, appears to exert its action by decreasing aqueous production and by enhancing outflow facility. The Dipivefrin Hydrochloride prodrug delivery system is a more efficient way of delivering the therapeutic effects of epinephrine, with fewer side effects than are associated with conventional epinephrine therapy.

The onset of action with one drop of Dipivefrin Hydrochloride occurs about 30 minutes after treatment, with maximum effect seen at about one hour.

Using a prodrug means that less drug is needed for therapeutic effect since absorption is enhanced with the prodrug. Dipivefrin Hydrochloride at 0.1% Dipivefrin was judged less irritating than a 1% solution of epinephrine hydrochloride or bitartrate. In addition only 8 of 455 patients (1.8%) treated with Dipivefrin Hydrochloride reported discomfort due to photophobia, glare or light sensitivity.

INDICATIONS

Dipivefrin Hydrochloride is indicated as initial therapy for the control of intraocular pressure in chronic open-angle glaucoma. Patients responding inadequately to other antiglaucoma therapy may respond to addition of Dipivefrin Hydrochloride.

In controlled and open-label studies of glaucoma, Dipivefrin Hydrochloride demonstrated a statistically significant intraocular pressure-lowering effect. Patients using Dipivefrin Hydrochloride twice daily in studies with mean durations of 76-146 days experienced mean pressure reductions ranging from 20-24%.

Therapeutic response to Dipivefrin Hydrochloride twice daily is somewhat less than 2% epinephrine twice daily. Controlled studies showed statistically significant differences in lowering of intraocular pressure between Dipivefrin Hydrochloride and 2% epinephrine. In controlled studies in patients with a history of epinephrine intolerance, only 3% of patients treated with Dipivefrin Hydrochloride exhibited intolerance, while 55% of those treated with epinephrine again developed an intolerance.

Therapeutic response to Dipivefrin Hydrochloride twice daily therapy is comparable to 2% pilocarpine 4 times daily. In controlled clinical studies comparing Dipivefrin Hydrochloride and 2% pilocarpine, there were no statistically significant differences in the maintenance of IOP levels for the two medications, Dipivefrin Hydrochloride does not produce miosis or accommodative spasm which cholinergic agents are known to produce. The blurred vision and night blindness often associated with miotic agents are not present with Dipivefrin Hydrochloride therapy. Patients with cataracts avoid the inability to see around lenticular opacities caused by constricted pupil.

CONTRAINDICATIONS

Dipivefrin Hydrochloride should not be used in patients with narrow angles since any dilation of the pupil may predispose the patient to an attack of angle-closure glaucoma. This product is contraindicated in patients who are hypersensitive to any of its components.

PRECAUTIONS

Aphakic Patients: Macular edema has been shown to occur in up to 30% of aphakic patients treated with epinephrine. Discontinuation of epinephrine generally results in reversal of the maculopathy.

Pregnancy: Pregnancy Category B: Reproduction studies have been performed in rats and rabbits at daily oral doses up to 10 mg/kg body weight (5 mg/kg in teratogenicity studies), and have revealed no evidence of impaired fertility or harm to the fetus due to Dipivefrin Hydrichloride. There are, however, no adequate and well-controlled studies in pregnant women. Because animal reproduction studies are not always predictive of human response, this drug should be used during pregnancy only if clearly needed.

Nursing Mothers: It is known whether this drug is excreted in human milk. Because many drugs are excreted in human milk, caution should be exercised when Dipivefrin Hydrochloride is administered to a nursing woman.

Usage in Children: Clinical studies for safety and efficacy in children have not been done.

Animal Studies: Rabbit studies indicated a dose-related incidence of meibomian gland retention cysts following topical administration of both Dipivefrin Hydrochloride and epinephrine.

ADVERSE REACTIONS

Cardiovascular Effects: Tachycardia, arrhythmias and hypertension have been reported with ocular administration of epinephrine.

Local Effects: The most frequent side effects reported with Dipivefrin Hydrochloride alone were injection in 6.5% of patients and burning and stinging in 6%. Follicular conjunctivitis, mydriasis and allergic reactions to Dipivefrin Hydrochloride have been reported infrequently. Epinephrine therapy can lead to adrenochrome deposits in the conjunctiva and cornea.

DOSAGE AND ADMINISTRATION

Initial Glaucoma Therapy: The usual dosage of Dipivefrin Hydrochloride is one drop in the eye(s) every 12 hours.

Replacement with Dipivefrin Hydrochloride: When patients are being transferred to Dipivefrin Hydrochloride from antiglaucoma agents other than epinephrine, on the first day continue the previous medication and add one drop of Dipivefrin Hydrochloride in each eye every 12 hours. On the following day, discontinue the previously used antiglaucoma agent and continue with Dipivefrin Hydrochloride.

In transferring patients from conventional epinephrine therapy to Dipivefrin Hydrochloride, simply discontinue the epinephrine medication and institute the Dipivefrin Hydrochloride regimen.

Addition of Dipivefrin Hydrochloride: When patients on other antiglaucoma agents require additional therapy, add one drop of Dipivefrin Hydrochloride every 12 hours.

Concomitant Therapy: For difficult to control patients, the addition of Dipivefrin Hydrochloride to other agents such as pilocarpine, carbachol, echothiophate iodide or acetazolamide has been shown to be effective.

Note: Not for injection.

Note: Store in tight, light-resistant containers.

HOW SUPPLIED
DROP: 0.1%

AVERAGE UNIT PRICE (AVAILABLE SIZES)

| BRAND | $2.82 |
| GENERIC | $2.28 |

BRAND/MANUFACTURER	NDC	SIZE	AWP
◆ **BRAND**			
PROPINE: Allergan Inc	11980-0260-25	5 ml	$15.14
	11980-0260-20	10 ml	$27.48
	11980-0260-21	15 ml	$40.45
◆ **GENERICS**			
Alcon Ophthalmic	00065-0235-05	5 ml	$12.00
Alcon Ophthalmic	00065-0235-10	10 ml	$22.00
Alcon Ophthalmic	00065-0235-15	15 ml	$33.50

For additional alternatives, turn to the section beginning on page 2859.

Diprivan *SEE* PROPOFOL
Diprolene *SEE* BETAMETHASONE, TOPICAL
Diprosone *SEE* BETAMETHASONE, TOPICAL

Dipyridamole, Injectable

DESCRIPTION

Dipyridamole for intravenous injection is a coronary vasodilator described as 2.6 bis-(diethanolamino)-4,8-dipiparidino-pyrimido-(5,4-d)pyrimidine.

Dipyridamole in solution is an odorless, pale yellow liquid which can be diluted in normal saline and dextrose and water for intravenous administration.

Dipyridamole, Injectable, as a sterile solution for intravenous administration contains:

Active ingredient: AMPULES 2 ml: Dipyridamole USP 10 mg. AMPULES 10 ml: Dipyridamole USP 50 mg.

Following is its chemical structure:

CLINICAL PHARMACOLOGY

In a study of 10 patients with angiographically normal or minimally (less than 25% luminal diameter narrowing) coronary vessels, IV Dipyridamole in a dose of 0.58 mg/kg infused over 4 minutes resulted in an average fivefold increase in coronary blood flow velocity compared to resting coronary flow velocity (range 3.8 to 7 times resting velocity). The mean time to peak flow velocity was 6.5 minutes from the start of the 4-minute infusion (range 2.5 to 8.7 minutes). Cardiovascular responses to the intravenous administration of Dipyridamole when given to patients in the supine position, include a mild but significant increase in heart rate of approximately 20% and mild but significant decreases in both systolic and diastolic blood pressure of approximately 2-8%, with vital signs returning to baseline values in approximately 30 minutes.

Mechanism of Action: Dipyridamole is a coronary vasodilator in man. The mechanism of vasodilation has not been fully elucidated, but may result from inhibition of uptake of adenosine, an important mediator of coronary vasodilation. The vasodilatory effects of Persantine are abolished by administration of the adenosine receptor antagonist theophylline.

How Dipyridamole induced vasodilation leads to abnormalities in thallium distribution and ventricular function is also uncertain but presumably represents a "steal" phenomenon in which relatively intact vessels dilate, and sustain enhanced flow, leaving reduced pressure and flow across areas of hemodynamically important coronary vascular constriction.

Pharmacokinetics and Metabolism: Plasma Dipyridamole concentrations decline in a inexponential fashion following intravenous infusion of Dipyridamole, with half-lives averaging 3-12 minutes, 33-62 minutes, and 11.6-15 hours. Two minutes following a 0.568 mg/kg dose of IV Dipyridamole administered as a 4-minute infusion, the mean dipyridamole serum concentration was 4.6 ± 1.3 mog/ml. The average plasma protein binding of Dipyridamole is approximately 99%, primarily to α_1-glycoprotein. Dipyridamole is metabolized in the liver to the glucuronic acid conjugate and excreted with the bile. The average total body clearance is 2.3-3.5 ml/min/kg, with an apparent volume of distribution at steady state of 1-2.5 l/kg and a central apparent volume of 3-5 liters.

INDICATIONS AND USAGE

IV Dipyridamole is indicated as an alternative to exercise in thallium myocardial perfusion imaging for the evaluation of coronary artery disease in patients who cannot exercise adequately.

In a study of about 100 patients who underwent coronary arteriography and IV Dipyridamole assisted thallium imaging, the results of both tests were interpreted blindly and the sensitivity and specificity of the Dipyridamole thallium study in predicting the angiographic outcome were calculated. The sensitivity of the Dipyridamole test (true positive Dipyridamole divided by the total number of patients with positive angiography) was about 85%. The specificity (true negative divided by the number of patients with negative angiograms) was about 50%.

In a subset of patients who had exercise thallium imaging as well as Dipyridamole thallium imaging, sensitivity and specificity of the two tests was almost identical.

UNLABELED USES

Dipyridamole Intravenous Injection is used as an adjunct in the treatment of congestive heart failure.

◆ RATED THERAPEUTICALLY EQUIVALENT; ◇ THERAPEUTIC EQUIVALENCE UNCONFIRMED; ○ UNRATED

CONTRAINDICATIONS
Hypersensitivity to Dipyridamole.

WARNINGS
Serious adverse reactions associated with the administration of intravenous Dipyridamole have included fatal and non-fatal myocardial infarction, ventricular fibrilation, symptomatic ventricular tachycardia, stroke, transient cerebral ischemia, and bronchospasm.

In a study of 3911 patients given intravenous Dipyridamole as an adjunct to thallium myocardial perfusion imaging, two types of serious adverse events were reported: 1) four cases of myocardial infarction (0.1%), two fatal (0.05%); and two non-fatal (0.05%); and 2) six cases of severe bronchospasm (0.2%). Although the incidence of these serious adverse events was small (0.3%, 10 of 3911), the potential clinical information to be gained through use of intravenous Dipyridamole thallium imaging (see *"Indications and Usage"* noting the rate of false positive and false negative results) must be weighed against the risk to the patient. Patients with a history of unstable angina may be at a greater risk for severe myocardial ischemia. Patients with a history of asthma may be at a greater risk for bronchospasm during IV Dipyridamole use.

When thallium, myocardial perfusion imaging is performed with intravenous Dipyridamole, parenteral aminophylline should be readily available for relieving adverse events such as bronchospasm or chest pain. Vital signs should be monitored during, and for 10-15 minutes following, the intravenous infusion of Dipyridamole and an electrocardiographic tracing should be obtained using at least one chest lead. Should severe chest pain or bronchospasm occur, parenteral aminophylline may be administered by slow intravenous injection (50-100 mg over 30-60 seconds) in doses ranging from 50 to 250 mg. In the case of severe hypotension, the patient should be placed in a supine position with the head tilted down if necessary, before administration of parenteral aminophylline. If 250 mg of aminophylline does not relieve chest pain symptoms within a few minutes, sublingual nitroglycerin may be administered. If chest pain continues despite use of aminophylline and nitroglycerin, the possibility of myocardial infarction should be considered. If the clinical condition of a patient with an adverse event permits a one minute delay in the administration of parenteral aminophylline, thallium-20 may be injected and allowed to circulate for one minute before the injection of aminophylline. This will allow initial thallium perfusion imaging to be performed before reversal of the pharmacologic effects of Dipyridamole on the coronary circulation.

PRECAUTIONS
See *"Warnings"*.

Drug Interaction: Oral maintenance theophylline may abolish the coronary vasodilation induced by intravenous Dipyridamole administration. This could lead to a false negative thallium imaging result (see *"Mechanism of Action"*).

Carcinogenesis, Mutagenesis, Impairment of Fertility: In studies in which Dipyridamole was administered in the feed at doses of up to 75 mg/kg/day (9.4 times the maximum recommended daily human oral dose) in mice (up to 128 weeks in males and up to 142 weeks in females) and rats (up to 111 weeks in males and females), there was no evidence of drug related carcinogenesis. Mutagenicity tests of Dipyridamole with bacterial and mammalian cell systems were negative. There was no evidence of impaired fertility when Dipyridamole was administered to male and female rats at oral doses up to 50 mg/kg/day (63 times the maximum recommended daily human oral dose). A significant reduction in number of corpora lutea with consequent reduction in implantations and live fetuses was, however, observed at 1250 mg/kg/day.

Pregnancy Category B: Reproduction studies performed in mice and rats at daily oral doses of up to 125 mg/kg (15.8 times* the maximum recommended daily human oral dose) have revealed no evidence of impaired embryonic development due to Dipyridamole. There are, however, no adequate and well controlled studies in pregnant women. Because animal reproduction studies are not always predictive of human responses, this drug should be used during pregnancy only if clearly needed.

Nursing Mothers: Dipyridamole is excreted in human milk.

Pediatric Use: Safety and effectiveness in children have not been established.

ADVERSE REACTIONS
Adverse reaction information concerning intravenous Dipyridamole is derived from a study of 3911 patients in which intravenous Dipyridamole as an adjunct to thallium myocardial perfusion imaging and from spontaneous reports of adverse reactions and the published literature.

Serious adverse events (fatal and nonfatal myocardial infarction, severe ventricular arrhythmias, and serious CNS abnormalities) are described above (see *"Warnings"*).

In the study of 3911 patients, the most frequent adverse reactions were: chest pain/angina pectoris (19.7%), electrocardiographic changes (most commonly ST-T changes) (15.9%), headache (12.2%), and dizziness (11.8%).

ADVERSE REACTIONS OCCURRING IN GREATER THAN 1% OF THE PATIENTS IN THE STUDY ARE SHOWN IN THE FOLLOWING TABLES:

	Incidence (%) of Drug-Related Adverse Events
Chest pain/angina pectoris	19.7
Headache	12.8
Dizziness	11.5
Electrocardiographic Abnormalities/ BT-T changes	7.5
Electrocardiographic Abnormalities/ Extrasystoles	3.2
Hypotention	4.6
Nausea	4.6
Flushing	3.4
Electrocardiographic Abnormalities/ Tachycardia	3.2
Dyspnea	2.6
Pain Unspecified	2.6
Blood Pressure Liability	1.6
Hypertension	1.5
Paresthesia	1.3
Fatigue	1.2

* Calculation based on assumed body weight of 50 kg.

Less common adverse reactions occurring in 1% or less of the patients within the study included:

Cardiovascular System: Electrocardiographic abnormalities unspecified (0.8%), arrhythmia unspecified (0.6%), palpitation (0.3%), ventricular tachycardia (0.2%, see *"Warnings"*), bradycardia (0.2%), myocardial infarction (0.1%, see *"Warnings"*), AV block (0.1%), syncope (0.1%), orthostatic hypotension (0.1%), atrial fibrillation (0.1%), supraventricular tachycardia (0.1%), ventricular arrhythmia unspecified (0.09%, see *"Warnings"*), heart block unspecified (0.03%), cardiomyopathy (0.03%), edema (0.03%).

Central and Peripheral Nervous System: Hypothesia (0.5%), hypertonia (0.3%), nervousness/anxiety (0.2%), tremor (0.1%), abnormal coordination (0.03%), somnolence (0.09%), dysphonia (0.03%), migraine (0.03%), vertigo (0.03%).

Gastrointestinal System: Dyspepsia (1.0%), dry mouth (0.8%), abdominal pain (0.7%), flatulence (0.6%), vomiting (0.4%), eruciation (0.1%), dysphagia (0.03%), tenesmus (0.03%), appetite increased (0.03%).

Respiratory System: Pharyngitis (0.3%), bronchospasm (0.2%, see *"Warnings"*), hyperventilation (0.1%), rhinitis (0.1%), coughing (0.03%), pleural pain (0.03%).

Other: Myalgia (0.9%), back pain (0.8%), injection site reaction unspecified (0.4%), diaphoresis (0.4%), asthenia (0.3%), malaise (0.3%), antralgia (0.3%), injection site pain (0.1%), rigor (0.1%), sarache (0.1%), tinnitus (0.03%), eye pain (0.03%), renal pain (0.03%), perineal pain (0.03%), breast pain (0.03%), intermittent claudication (0.03%), leg cramping (0.03%).

OVERDOSAGE
No cases of overdosage in humans have been reported. It is unlikely that overdosage will occur because of the nature of use (i.e., single intravenous administration in controlled settings). See *"Warnings."*

DOSAGE AND ADMINISTRATION
The dose of intravenous Dipyridamole as an adjunct to thallium myocardial perfusion imaging should be adjusted to the weight of the patient. The recommended dose is 0.142 mg/kg/minute (0.57 mg/kg total) infused over 4 minutes. Although the maximum tolerated dose has not been determined, clinical experience suggests that a total dose beyond 50 mg is not needed for any patient.

Prior to intravenous administration, IV Dipyridamole should be diluted in at least 1:2 ratio with 0.45% sodium chloride injection, 0.9% sodium chloride injection, or 5% dextrose injection for a total volume of approximately 20 to 50 ml. Infusion of undiluted Dipyridamole may cause local irritation.

Thallium-201 should be injected within 5 minutes following the 4-minute infusion of Dipyridamole.

Do not mix IV Dipyridamole with other drugs in the same syringe or infusion container.

Parenteral drug product should be inspected visually for particulate matter and discoloration prior to admiration, whenever solution and container permit.

Store between 15° C (59° F) - 25° C (77° F). Protect from direct light. Avoid freezing.

J CODES
Per 10 mg IV—J1245

HOW SUPPLIED
INJECTION: 5 MG/ML

BRAND/MANUFACTURER	*NDC*	*SIZE*	*AWP*
○ **BRAND**			
PERSANTINE: Du Pont Pharma	00590-0302-21	2 ml 5s	$150.00

Dipyridamole, Oral

DESCRIPTION
Dipyridamole is a platelet inhibitor chemically described as 2,6-bis-(diethanolamino)-4,8-dipiperidino-pyrimido-(5,4-d) pyrimidine. Its molecular formula is $C_{24}H_{40}N_8O_4$ and its molecular weight is 504.63.

Dipyridamole is an odorless yellow crystalline powder, having a bitter taste. It is soluble in dilute acids, methanol and chloroform, and practically insoluble in water.

Dipyridamole tablets for oral administration contain:

Active Ingredient: Tablets 25, 50 and 75 mg: Dipyridamole USP 25, 50 and 75 mg respectively.

Following is its chemical structure:

$$(HOCH_2CH_2)_2N \quad N(CH_2CH_2OH)_2$$

CLINICAL PHARMACOLOGY

It is believed that platelet reactivity and interaction with prosthetic cardiac valve surfaces, resulting in abnormally shortened platelet survival time, is a significant factor in thromboembolic complications occurring in connection with prosthetic heart valve replacement.

Dipyridamole has been found to lengthen abnormally shortened platelet survival time in a dose-dependent manner.

In three randomized controlled clinical trials involving 854 patients who had undergone surgical placement of a prosthetic heart valve, Dipyridamole in combination with warfarin, decreased the incidence of postoperative thromboembolic events by 62% to 91% compared to warfarin treatment alone. The incidence of thromboembolic events in patients receiving the combination of Dipyridamole and warfarin ranged from 1.2% to 1.8%. In three additional studies involving 392 patients taking Dipyridamole and coumarin-like anticoagulants, the incidence of thromboembolic events ranged from 2.3% to 6.9%.

In these trials, the coumarin anticoagulant was begun between 24 hours and 4 days postoperatively, and the Dipyridamole was begun between 24 hours and 10 days postoperatively. The length of follow-up in these trials varied from 1 to 2 years.

Dipyridamole does not influence prothrombin time or activity measurements when administered with warfarin.

Mechanism of Action: Dipyridamole is a platelet adhesion inhibitor, although the mechanism of action has not been fully elucidated. The mechanism may relate to inhibition of red blood cell uptake of adenosine, itself an inhibitor of platelet reactivity, phosphodiesterase inhibition leading to increased cyclic-3',5'-adenosine monophosphate within platelets, and inhibition of thromboxane A_2 formation, which is a potent stimulator of platelet activation.

Hemodynamics: In dogs intraduodenal doses of Dipyridamole of 0.5 to 4.0 mg/kg produced dose-related decreases in systemic and coronary vascular resistance leading to decreases in systemic blood pressure and increases in coronary blood flow. Onset of action was in about 24 minutes and effects persisted for about 3 hours.

Similar effects were observed following IV Dipyridamole in doses ranging from 0.025 to 2.0 mg/kg.

In man the same qualitative hemodynamic effects have been observed. However, acute intravenous administration of Dipyridamole may worsen regional myocardial perfusion distal to partial occlusion of coronary arteries.

Pharmacokinetics and Metabolism: Following an oral dose of Dipyridamole, the average time to peak concentration is about 75 minutes. The decline in plasma concentration following a dose of Dipyridamole fits a two-compartment model. The alpha half-life (the initial decline following peak concentration) is approximately 40 minutes. The beta half-life (the terminal decline in plasma concentration) is approximately 10 hours. Dipyridamole is highly bound to plasma proteins. It is metabolized in the liver where it is conjugated as a glucuronide and excreted with the bile.

INDICATIONS AND USAGE

Dipyridamole is indicated as an adjunct to coumarin anticoagulants in the prevention of post-operative thromboembolic complications of cardiac valve replacement.

UNLABELED USES

Dipyridamole is used alone or as an adjunct in the treatment of angina, to prevent graft occlusion in patients undergoing arterial reconstructive bypass surgery, intralingual bypass grafts, and to prevent deterioration of coronary vessel patency after percutaneous transluminal angioplasty. It is also used to slow the progression of microaneurysm in patients with early diabetic retinopathy, in high-risk patients with a history of idiopathic fetal growth retardation and placental infarction, hypertrophic cardiomyopathy, and membranoproliferative glomerulonephritis. Dipyridamole is also prescribed with aspirin for the prophylaxis of migraine headache, myocardial reinfarction, in diabetic necrobiosis lesions, to reduce platelet aggregation at the carotid endarterectomy, to slow progression of peripheral occlusive arterial disease, to increase inulin clearance in peritoneal dialysis, to reduce proteinuria due to chronic renal failure, to reduce the incidence of deep venous thrombosis, to reduce the number of platelets deposited on dacron aortofemoral artery grafts, and transient ischemic attacks.

CONTRAINDICATIONS
None known.

PRECAUTIONS

General: Dipyridamole should be used with caution in patients with hypotension since it can produce peripheral vasodilation.

Carcinogenesis, Mutagenesis, Impairment of Fertility: In a 111 week oral study in mice and in a 128-142 week oral study in rats, Dipyridamole produced no significant carcinogenic effects at doses of 8, 25 and 75 mg/kg (1, 3.1 and 9.4 times the maximum recommended daily human dose). Mutagenicity testing with Dipyridamole was negative. Reproduction studies with Dipyridamole revealed no evidence of impaired fertility in rats at dosages up to 60 times the maximum recommended human dose. A significant reduction in number of corpora lutea with consequent reduction in implantations and live fetuses was, however, observed at 155 times the maximum recommended human dose.

Teratogenic Effects: Pregnancy Category B: Reproduction studies have been performed in mice and rats at doses up to 125 mg/kg (15.6 times the maximum recommended daily human dose) and rabbits at doses up to 20 mg/kg and have revealed no evidence of harm to the fetus due to Dipyridamole. There are, however, no adequate and well-controlled studies in pregnant women. Because animal reproduction studies are not always predictive of human response, this drug should be used during pregnancy only if clearly needed.

Nursing Mothers: As Dipyridamole is excreted in human milk, caution should be exercised when Dipyridamole is administered to a nursing woman.

Pediatric Use: Safety and effectiveness in children below the age of 12 years have not been established.

ADVERSE REACTIONS

Adverse reactions at therapeutic doses are usually minimal and transient. On long-term use of Dipyridamole initial side effects usually disappear. The following reactions were reported in two heart valve replacement trials comparing Dipyridamole and warfarin therapy to either warfarin alone or warfarin and placebo:

	Dipyridamole Warfarin (N = 147)	Placebo/Warfarin (N = 170)
Dizziness	13.6%	8.2%
Abdominal distress	6.1%	3.5%
Headache	2.3%	0.0
Rash	2.3%	1.1%

Other reactions from uncontrolled studies include diarrhea, vomiting, flushing and pruritus. In addition, angina pectoris has been reported rarely and there have been rare reports of liver dysfunction. On those uncommon occasions when adverse reactions have been persistent or intolerable, they have ceased on withdrawal of the medication.

When Dipyridamole was administered concomitantly with warfarin, bleeding was no greater in frequency or severity than that observed when warfarin was administered alone.

OVERDOSAGE

Hypotension, if it occurs, is likely to be of short duration, but a vasopressor drug may be used if necessary. The oral LD_{50} in rats is greater than 6,000 mg/kg, while in the dogs, the oral LD_{50} is approximately 400 mg/kg. Since Dipyridamole is highly protein bound, dialysis is not likely to be of benefit.

DOSAGE AND ADMINISTRATION

Adjunctive Use in Prophylaxis of Thromboembolism after Cardiac Valve Replacement: The recommended dose is 75-100 mg four times daily as an adjunct to the usual warfarin therapy. Please note that aspirin is not to be administered concomitantly with coumarin anticoagulants.

Store below 86°F (30°C).

HOW SUPPLIED
TABLETS: 25 MG

AVERAGE UNIT PRICE (AVAILABLE SIZES)		GENERIC A-RATED AVERAGE PRICE (GAAP)	
BRAND	$0.32	100s	$8.40
GENERIC	$0.07	500s	$33.30
HCFA FUL (100s ea)	$0.02	1000s	$40.87

BRAND/MANUFACTURER	NDC	SIZE	AWP
◆ BRAND			
➤ PERSANTINE: Boehr Ingelheim	00597-0017-01	100s	$31.85
	00597-0017-61	100s ud	$33.46
	00597-0017-10	1000s	$302.03
◆ GENERICS			
Rugby	00536-3570-01	100s	$4.13
Moore,H.L.	00839-6327-06	100s	$4.79
Qualitest	00603-3383-21	100s	$4.84
Major	00904-1083-60	100s	$5.20
Major	00904-1086-60	100s	$5.20
Goldline	00182-1568-01	100s	$6.00

◆ RATED THERAPEUTICALLY EQUIVALENT; ◇ THERAPEUTIC EQUIVALENCE UNCONFIRMED; ○ UNRATED

BRAND/MANUFACTURER	NDC	SIZE	AWP
Purepac	00228-2193-10	100s	$6.27
Aligen	00405-5350-01	100s	$6.28
Schein	00364-2491-01	100s	$6.50
➤ Geneva	00781-1890-01	100s	$6.75
Barr	00555-0252-02	100s	$8.10
Aligen	00405-4350-01	100s	$8.15
Lederle Std Prod	00005-3743-23	100s	$8.56
Parmed	00349-2344-01	100s	$8.83
Parmed	00349-8908-01	100s	$8.83
Major	00904-1083-61	100s ud	$6.39
Raway	00686-0068-20	100s ud	$6.50
Goldline	00182-1568-89	100s ud	$6.90
Goldline	00182-1156-89	100s ud	$9.80
Vangard	00615-1543-13	100s ud	$13.58
Auro	55829-0235-10	100s ud	$13.97
➤ Geneva	00781-1890-13	100s ud	$14.00
Major	00904-1086-61	100s ud	$14.69
UDL	51079-0068-20	100s ud	$17.30
Barr	00555-0252-04	500s	$32.75
Lederle Std Prod	00005-3743-31	500s	$33.85
Goldline	00182-1156-10	1000s	$19.25
Rugby	00536-3570-10	1000s	$25.73
Moore,H.L.	00839-6327-16	1000s	$29.01
Major	00904-1083-80	1000s	$29.20
Major	00904-1086-80	1000s	$29.20
Goldline	00182-1568-10	1000s	$30.00
➤ Geneva	00781-1890-10	1000s	$37.10
Qualitest	00603-3383-32	1000s	$37.48
Schein	00364-2491-02	1000s	$39.54
Barr	00555-0252-05	1000s	$40.05
Aligen	00405-4350-03	1000s	$40.19
Aligen	00405-5350-03	1000s	$41.22
Purepac	00228-2193-96	1000s	$41.91
Parmed	00349-2344-10	1000s	$86.62
Parmed	00349-8908-10	1000s	$86.62
Parmed	00349-2344-52	2500s	$180.00

TABLETS: 50 MG

AVERAGE UNIT PRICE (AVAILABLE SIZES)		GENERIC A-RATED AVERAGE PRICE (GAAP)	
BRAND	$0.51	100s	$13.17
GENERIC	$0.11	500s	$45.11
HCFA FUL (100s ea)	$0.04	1000s	$63.40

BRAND/MANUFACTURER	NDC	SIZE	AWP
◆ BRAND			
➤ PERSANTINE: Boehr Ingelheim	00597-0018-01	100s	$51.31
	00597-0018-61	100s ud	$53.88
	00597-0018-10	1000s	$487.50
◆ GENERICS			
Rugby	00536-3619-01	100s	$6.80
Goldline	00182-1405-01	100s	$6.85
Moore,H.L.	00839-6494-06	100s	$7.90
Major	00904-1085-60	100s	$8.50
Qualitest	00603-3384-21	100s	$9.11
Goldline	00182-1569-01	100s	$9.50
➤ Geneva	00781-1678-01	100s	$10.20
Purepac	00228-2183-10	100s	$10.34
Aligen	00405-5351-01	100s	$10.38
➤ Barr	00555-0285-02	100s	$10.78
Aligen	00405-4351-01	100s	$10.82
➤ Lederle Std Prod	00005-3790-23	100s	$11.25
Schein	00364-2492-01	100s	$11.76
Raway	00686-0069-20	100s ud	$7.00
Major	00904-1085-61	100s ud	$9.59
Goldline	00182-1569-89	100s ud	$9.90
Goldline	00182-1405-89	100s ud	$15.00
Auro	55829-0236-10	100s ud	$16.62
Major	00904-1087-61	100s ud	$25.75
Vangard	00615-1573-13	100s ud	$25.88
➤ Geneva	00781-1678-13	100s ud	$26.00
UDL	51079-0069-20	100s ud	$29.75
Rugby	00536-3619-05	500s	$31.80
➤ Barr	00555-0285-04	500s	$50.94
➤ Lederle Std Prod	00005-3790-31	500s	$52.60
Rugby	00536-3619-10	1000s	$46.70
Goldline	00182-1405-10	1000s	$46.75
Major	00904-1085-80	1000s	$49.85
Major	00904-1087-80	1000s	$49.85
Moore,H.L.	00839-6494-16	1000s	$60.08
➤ Geneva	00781-1678-10	1000s	$64.10
Goldline	00182-1569-10	1000s	$65.00
Qualitest	00603-3384-32	1000s	$68.88
Schein	00364-2492-02	1000s	$70.16
➤ Barr	00555-0285-05	1000s	$75.11
Aligen	00405-4351-03	1000s	$75.22
Purepac	00228-2183-96	1000s	$76.16
Aligen	00405-5351-03	1000s	$76.34

TABLETS: 75 MG

AVERAGE UNIT PRICE (AVAILABLE SIZES)		GENERIC A-RATED AVERAGE PRICE (GAAP)	
BRAND	$0.69	100s	$20.45
GENERIC	$0.16	500s	$69.89
HCFA FUL (100s ea)	$0.04	1000s	$101.23

BRAND/MANUFACTURER	NDC	SIZE	AWP
◆ BRAND			
➤ PERSANTINE: Boehr Ingelheim	00597-0019-01	100s	$68.64
	00597-0019-61	100s ud	$72.06
	00597-0019-05	500s	$332.96
◆ GENERICS			
Rugby	00536-3620-01	100s	$9.80
Goldline	00182-1354-01	100s	$9.90
Moore,H.L.	00839-6429-06	100s	$11.19
Major	00904-1084-60	100s	$11.25
Goldline	00182-1570-01	100s	$14.00
Purepac	00228-2185-10	100s	$15.02
Aligen	00405-5352-01	100s	$15.10
Geneva	00781-1478-01	100s	$15.75
Qualitest	00603-3385-21	100s	$18.10
Barr	00555-0286-02	100s	$18.78
Aligen	00405-4352-01	100s	$18.82
Parmed	00349-8378-01	100s	$19.25
Lederle Std Prod	00005-3791-23	100s	$19.88

Disalcid SEE SALSALATE

Disopyramide Phosphate

DESCRIPTION

Disopyramide Phosphate is an antiarrhythmic drug available for oral administration in immediate-release and controlled-release capsules containing 100 mg or 150 mg of disopyramide base, present as the phosphate. The base content of the phosphate salt is 77.6%.

Disopyramide Phosphate is α-[2-(diisopropylamino) ethyl]-α-phenyl-2-pyridine-acetamide phosphate

Disopyramide Phosphate is freely soluble in water, and the free base (pKa 10.4) has an aqueous solubility of 1 mg/ml. The chloroform: water partition coefficient of the base is 3.1 at pH 7.2.

Norpace is a racemic mixture of d- and l-isomers. This drug is not chemically related to other antiarrhythmic drugs.

Disopyramide Phosphate controlled-release capsules are designed to afford a gradual and consistent release of Disopyramide. Thus, for maintenance therapy, Disopyramide Phosphate Controlled Release provides the benefit of less-frequent dosing (every 12 hours) as compared with the every-6-hour dosage schedule of immediate-release Disopyramide Phosphate capsules.

Following is its chemical structure:

$$(CH_3)_2CH-NCH_2CH_2-\overset{\displaystyle C_6H_5}{\underset{(CH_3)_2CH}{C}}-CONH_2$$

CLINICAL PHARMACOLOGY

MECHANISMS OF ACTION

Disopyramide Phosphate is a Type 1 antiarrhythmic drug (ie, similar to procainamide and quinidine). *In animal studies* Disopyramide Phosphate decreases the rate of diastolic depolarization (phase 4) in cells with augmented automaticity, decreases the upstroke velocity (phase 0) and increases the action potential duration of normal cardiac cells, decreases the disparity in refractoriness between infarcted and adjacent normally perfused myocardium, and has no effect on alpha- or beta-adrenergic receptors.

ELECTROPHYSIOLOGY

In man, Disopyramide Phosphate at therapeutic plasma levels shortens the sinus node recovery time, lengthens the effective refractory period of the atrium, and has a minimal effect on the effective refractory period of the AV node. Little effect has been shown on AV-nodal and His-Purkinje conduction times or QRS duration. However, prolongation of conduction in accessory pathways occurs.

HEMODYNAMICS

At recommended oral doses, Disopyramide Phosphate rarely produces significant alterations of blood pressure in patients without congestive heart failure (see "Warnings"). With intravenous Disopyramide Phosphate, either increases in systolic/diastolic or decreases in systolic blood pressure have been reported, depending on the infusion rate and the patient population. Intravenous Disopyramide Phosphate may cause cardiac depression with an approximate mean 10% reduction of cardiac output, which is more pronounced in patients with cardiac dysfunction.

➤ SHOWN IN PRODUCT IDENTIFICATION GUIDE

ANTICHOLINERGIC ACTIVITY

The *in vitro* anticholinergic activity of Disopyramide Phosphate is approximately 0.06% that of atropine; however, the usual dose for Disopyramide Phosphate is 150 mg every 6 hours and for Disopyramide Phosphate Controlled Release 300 mg every 12 hours, compared to 0.4 to 0.6 mg for atropine (see *"Warnings"* and *"Adverse Reactions"* for anticholinergic side effects).

PHARMACOKINETICS

Following oral administration of immediate-release Disopyramide Phosphate, the drug is rapidly and almost completely absorbed, and peak plasma levels are usually attained within 2 hours. The usual therapeutic plasma levels of Disopyramide base are 2 to 4 mcg/ml, and at these concentrations protein binding varies from 50% to 65%. Because of concentration-dependent protein binding, it is difficult to predict the concentration of the free drug when total drug is measured.

The mean plasma half-life of Disopyramide in healthy humans is 6.7 hours (range of 4 to 10 hours). In six patients with impaired renal function (creatinine clearance less than 40 ml/min), Disopyramide half-life values were 8 to 18 hours. After the oral administration of 200 mg of Disopyramide to 10 cardiac patients with borderline to moderate heart failure, the time to peak serum concentration of 2.3 ± 1.5 hours (mean $\pm$ SD) was increased, and the mean peak serum concentration of 4.8 ± 1.6 mcg/ml was higher than in healthy volunteers. After intravenous administration in these same patients, the mean elimination half-life was 9.7 ± 4.2 hours (range in healthy volunteers of 4.4 to 7.8 hours). In a second study of the oral administration of Disopyramide to 7 patients with heart disease, including left ventricular dysfunction, the mean plasma half-life was slightly prolonged to 7.8 ± 1.9 hours (range of 5 to 9.5 hours).

In healthy men, about 50% of a given dose of Disopyramide is excreted in the urine as the unchanged drug, about 20% as the mono-N-dealkylated metabolite, and 10% as the other metabolites. The plasma concentration of the major metabolite is approximately one tenth that of Disopyramide. Altering the urinary pH in man does not affect the plasma half-life of Disopyramide.

In a crossover study in healthy subjects, the bioavailability of Disopyramide from Disopyramide Phosphate Controlled Release capsules was similar to that from the immediate-release capsules. With a single 300-mg oral dose, peak Disopyramide plasma concentrations of 3.23 ± 0.75 mcg/ml (mean $\pm$ SD) at 2.5 ± 2.3 hours were obtained with two 150-mg immediate-release capsules and 2.22 ± 0.47 mcg/ml at 4.9 ± 1.4 hours with two 150-mg Disopyramide Phosphate Controlled Release capsules. The elimination half-life of Disopyramide was 8.31 ± 1.83 hours with the immediate-release capsules and 11.65 ± 4.72 hours with Disopyramide Phosphate Controlled Release capsules. The amount of Disopyramide and mono-N-dealkylated metabolite excreted in the urine in 48 hours was 128 and 48 mg, respectively, with the immediate-release capsules, and 112 and 33 mg, respectively, with Disopyramide Phosphate Controlled Release capsules. The differences in the urinary excretion of either constituent were not statistically significant.

Following multiple doses, steady-state plasma levels of between 2 and 4 mcg/ml were attained following either 150 mg every-6-hour dosing with immediate-release capsules or 300 mg every-12-hour dosing with Disopyramide Phosphate Controlled Release capsules.

INDICATIONS AND USAGE

Disopyramide Phosphate and Disopyramide Phosphate Controlled Release are indicated for the treatment of documented ventricular arrhythmias, such as sustained ventricular tachycardia, that, in the judgment of the physician, are life-threatening. Because of the proarrhythmic effects of Disopyramide Phosphate and Disopyramide Phosphate Controlled Release, their use with lesser arrhythmias is generally not recommended. Treatment of patients with asymptomatic ventricular premature contractions should be avoided.

Initiation of Disopyramide Phosphate and Disopyramide Phosphate Controlled Release treatment, as with other antiarrhythmic agents used to treat life-threatening arrhythmias, should be carried out in the hospital. Disopyramide Phosphate Controlled Release should not be used initially if rapid establishment or Disopyramide plasma levels is desired.

Antiarrhythmic drugs have not been shown to enhance survival in patients with ventricular arrhythmias.

UNLABELED USES

Disopyramide Phosphate is used alone or as an adjunct in the treatment of supraventricular arrhythmias.

CONTRAINDICATIONS

Disopyramide Phosphate and Disopyramide Phosphate Controlled Release are contraindicated in the presence of cardiogenic shock, preexisting second- or third-degree AV block (if no pacemaker is present), congenital Q-T prolongation, or known hypersensitivity to the drug.

WARNINGS

MORTALITY:

In the National Heart, Lung and Blood Institute's Cardiac Arrhythmia Suppression Trial (CAST), a long-term, multicentered, randomized, double-blind study in patients with asymptomatic non-life-threatening ventricular arrhythmias who had had myocardial infarctions more than 6 days but less than 2 years previously, an excessive mortality or non-fatal cardiac arrest rate was seen in patients treated with encainide or flecainide (56/730) compared with that seen in patients assigned to matched placebo-treated groups (22/725). The average duration of treatment with encainide or flecainide in this study was 10 months.

The applicability of these results to other populations (eg, those without recent myocardial infarctions) or to other antiarrhythmic drugs is uncertain, but at present it is prudent to consider any antiarrhythmic agent to have a significant risk in patients with structural heart disease.

NEGATIVE INOTROPIC PROPERTIES

HEART FAILURE/HYPOTENSION

Disopyramide Phosphate or Disopyramide Phosphate Controlled Release may cause or worsen congestive heart failure or produce severe hypotension as a consequence of its negative inotropic properties. Hypotension has been observed primarily in patients with primary cardiomyopathy or inadequately compensated congestive heart failure. Disopyramide Phosphate or Disopyramide Phosphate Controlled Release should not be used in patients with uncompensated or marginally compensated congestive heart failure or hypotension unless the congestive heart failure or hypotension is secondary to cardiac arrhythmia. Patients with a history of heart failure may be treated with Disopyramide Phosphate or Disopyramide Phosphate Controlled Release, but careful attention must be given to the maintenance of cardiac function, including optimal digitalization. If hypotension occurs or congestive heart failure worsens, Disopyramide Phosphate or Disopyramide Phosphate Controlled Release should be discontinued and, if necessary, restarted at a lower dosage only after adequate cardiac compensation has been established.

QRS WIDENING

Although it is unusual, significant widening (greater than 25%) of the QRS complex may occur during Disopyramide Phosphate or Disopyramide Phosphate Controlled Release administration: in such cases Disopyramide Phosphate or Disopyramide Phosphate Controlled Release should be discontinued.

Q-T PROLONGATION

As with other Type 1 antiarrhythmic drugs, prolongation of the Q-T interval (corrected) and worsening of the arrhythmia, including ventricular tachycardia and ventricular fibrillation, may occur. Patients who have evidenced prolongation of the Q-T interval in response to quinidine may be at particular risk. As with other Type 1A antiarrhythmics, Disopyramide Phosphate has been associated with torsade de pointes.

If a Q-T prolongation of greater than 25% is observed and if ectopy continues, the patient should be monitored closely, and consideration be given to discontinuing Disopyramide Phosphate or Disopyramide Phosphate Controlled Release.

HYPOGLYCEMIA

In rare instances significant lowering of blood glucose values has been reported during Disopyramide Phosphate administration. The physician should be alert to this possibility, especially in patients with congestive heart failure, chronic malnutrition, hepatic, renal, or other diseases, or drugs (eg, beta adrenoceptor blockers, alcohol) which could compromise preservation of the normal glucoregulatory mechanisms in the absence of food. In these patients the blood glucose levels should be carefully followed.

CONCOMITANT ANTIARRHYTHMIC THERAPY

The concomitant use of Disopyramide Phosphate or Disopyramide Phosphate Controlled Release with other Type 1A antiarrhythmic agents (such as quinidine or procainamide), Type 1C antiarrhythmics (such as encainide, flecainide or propafenone), and/or propranolol be reserved for patients with life-threatening arrhythmias who are demonstrably unresponsive to single-agent antiarrhythmic therapy. Such use may produce serious negative inotropic effects, or may excessively prolong conduction. This should be considered particularly in patients with any degree of cardiac decompensation or those with a prior history thereof. Patients receiving more than one antiarrhythmic drug must be carefully monitored.

HEART BLOCK

If first-degree heart block develops in a patient receiving Disopyramide Phosphate or Disopyramide Phosphate Controlled Release the dosage should be reduced. If the block persists despite reduction of dosage, continuation of the drug must depend upon weighing the benefit being obtained against the risk of higher degrees of heart block. Development of second- or third-degree AV block or unifascicular, bifascicular, or trifascicular block requires discontinuation of Disopyramide Phosphate or Disopyramide Phosphate Controlled Release therapy, unless the ventricular rate is adequately controlled by a temporary or implanted ventricular pacemaker.

ANTICHOLINERGIC ACTIVITY

Because of its anticholinergic activity, Disopyramide Phosphate should not be used in patients with glaucoma, myasthenia gravis, or urinary retention unless adequate overriding measures are taken; these consist of the topical application of potent miotics (eg, pilocarpine) for patients with glaucoma, and catheter drainage or operative relief for patients with urinary retention. Urinary retention may occur in patients of either sex as a consequence of Disopyramide Phosphate or Disopyramide Phosphate Controlled Release administration, but males with benign prostatic hypertrophy are at particular risk. In patients with a family history of glaucoma, intraocular pressure should be measured before initiating Disopyramide Phosphate or Disopyramide Phosphate Controlled Release therapy. Disopyramide Phosphate should be used with special care in patients with myasthenia gravis since its anticholinergic properties could precipitate a myasthenic crisis in such patients.

PRECAUTIONS

GENERAL

Atrial Tachyarrhythmias: Patients with atrial flutter or fibrillation should be digitalized prior to Disopyramide Phosphate or Disopyramide Phosphate Controlled Release administration to ensure that drug-induced enhancement of AV conduction does not result in an increase of ventricular rate beyond physiologically acceptable limits.

Conduction Abnormalities: Care should be taken when prescribing Disopyramide Phosphate or Disopyramide Phosphate Controlled Release for patients with sick sinus syndrome (bradycardiatachycardia syndrome), Wolff-Parkinson-White syndrome (WPW), or bundle branch block. The effect of Disopyramide Phosphate in these conditions is uncertain at present.

Cardiomyopathy: Patients with myocarditis or other cardiomyopathy may develop significant hypotension in response to the usual dosage of Disopyramide Phosphate, probably due to cardiodepressant mechanisms. Therefore, a loading dose of Disopyramide Phosphate should not be given to such patients, and initial dosage and subsequent dosage adjustments should be made under close supervision (see *"Dosage and Administration"*).

Renal Impairment: More than 50% of Disopyramide is excreted in the urine unchanged. Therefore, Disopyramide Phosphate dosage should be reduced in patients with impaired renal function (see *"Dosage and Administration"*). The electrocardiogram should be carefully monitored for prolongation of PR interval, evidence of QRS widening, or other signs of overdosage (see *"Overdosage"*).

Disopyramide Phosphate Controlled Release is not recommended for patients with severe renal insufficiency (creatinine clearance 40 ml/min or less).

Hepatic Impairment: Hepatic impairment also causes an increase in the plasma half-life of Disopyramide. Dosage should be reduced for patients with such impairment. The electrocardiogram should be carefully monitored for signs of overdosage (see *"Overdosage"*).

Patients with cardiac dysfunction have a higher potential for hepatic impairment; this should be considered when administering Disopyramide Phosphate or Disopyramide Phosphate Controlled Release.

Potassium Imbalance: Antiarrhythmic drugs may be ineffective in patients with hypokalemia, and their toxic effects may be enhanced in patients with hyperkalemia. Therefore, potassium abnormalities should be corrected before starting Disopyramide Phosphate or Disopyramide Phosphate Controlled Release therapy.

DRUG INTERACTIONS

If phenytoin or other hepatic enzyme inducers are taken concurrently with Disopyramide Phosphate or Disopyramide Phosphate Controlled Release, lower plasma levels of Disopyramide may occur. Monitoring of Disopyramide plasma levels is recommended in such concurrent use to avoid ineffective therapy. Other antiarrhythmic drugs (eg, quinidine, procainamide, lidocaine, propranolol) have occasionally been used concurrently with Disopyramide Phosphate. Excessive widening of the QRS complex and/or prolongation of the Q-T interval may occur in these situations (see *"Warnings"*). In healthy subjects, no significant drug-drug interaction was observed when Disopyramide Phosphate was coadministered with either propranolol or diazepam. Concomitant administration of Disopyramide Phosphate and quinidine resulted in slight increases in plasma Disopyramide levels and slight decreases in plasma quinidine levels. Disopyramide Phosphate does not increase serum digoxin levels.

Until data on possible interactions between verapamil and Disopyramide Phosphate are obtained, Disopyramide should not be administered within 48 hours before or 24 hours after verapamil administration.

CARCINOGENESIS, MUTAGENESIS, IMPAIRMENT OF FERTILITY

Eighteen months of Disopyramide Phosphate administration to rats, at oral doses up to 400 mg/kg/day (about 30 times the usual daily human dose of 600 mg/day, assuming a patient weight of at least 50 kg), revealed no evidence of carcinogenic potential. An evaluation of mutagenic potential by Ames test was negative. Disopyramide Phosphate, at doses up to 250 mg/kg/day, did not adversely affect fertility of rats.

PREGNANCY

Teratogenic Effects: Pregnancy Category C. Disopyramide Phosphate was associated with decreased numbers of implantation sites and decreased growth and survival of pups when administered to pregnant rats at 250 mg/kg/day (20 or more times the usual daily human dose of 12 mg/kg, assuming a patient weight of at least 50 kg), a level at which weight gain and food consumption of dams were also reduced. Increased resorption rates were reported in rabbits at 60 mg/kg/day (5 or more times the usual daily human dose). Effects on implantation, pup growth, and survival were not evaluated in rabbits. There are no adequate and well-controlled studies in pregnant women. Disopyramide Phosphate or Disopyramide Phosphate Controlled Release should be used during pregnancy only if the potential benefit justifies the potential risk to the fetus.

Nonteratogenic Effects: **Disopyramide Phosphate has been reported to stimulate contractions of the pregnant uterus.** Disopyramide has been found in human fetal blood.

LABOR AND DELIVERY

It is not known whether the use of Disopyramide Phosphate or Disopyramide Phosphate Controlled Release during labor or delivery has immediate or delayed adverse effects on the fetus, or whether it prolongs the duration of labor or increases the need for forceps delivery or other obstetric intervention.

NURSING MOTHERS

Studies in rats have shown that the concentration of Disopyramide and its metabolites is between one and three times greater in milk than it is in plasma. Following oral administration, Disopyramide has been detected in human milk at a concentration not exceeding that in plasma. Because of the potential for serious adverse reactions in nursing infants from Disopyramide Phosphate or Disopyramide Phosphate Controlled Release a decision should be made whether to discontinue nursing or to discontinue the drug, taking into account the importance of the drug to the mother.

ADVERSE REACTIONS

The adverse reactions which were reported in Disopyramide Phosphate clinical trials encompass observations in 1,500 patients, including 90 patients studied for at least 4 years. The most serious adverse reactions are hypotension and congestive heart failure. The most common adverse reactions, which are dose dependent, are associated with the anticholinergic properties of the drug. These may be transitory, but may be persistent or can be severe. Urinary retention is the most serious anticholinergic effect.

The following reactions were reported in 10% to 40% of patients:
Anticholinergic: dry mouth (32%), urinary hesitancy (14%), constipation (11%)

The following reactions were reported in 3% to 9% of patients:
Anticholinergic: blurred vision, dry nose/eyes/throat
Genitourinary: urinary retention, urinary frequency and urgency
Gastrointestinal: nausea, pain/bloating/gas
General: dizziness, general fatigue/muscle weakness, headache, malaise, aches/pains

The following reactions were reported in 1% to 3% of patients:
Genitourinary: impotence
Cardiovascular: hypotension with or without congestive heart failure, increased congestive heart failure (see *"Warnings"*), cardiac conduction disturbances (see *"Warnings"*), edema/weight gain, shortness of breath, syncope, chest pain
Gastrointestinal: anorexia, diarrhea, vomiting
Dermatologic: generalized rash/dermatoses, itching Central nervous system: nervousness
Other: hypokalemia, elevated cholesterol/triglycerides

The following reactions were reported in less than 1%:
Depression, insomnia, dysuria, numbness/tingling, elevated liver enzymes, AV block, elevated BUN, elevated creatinine, decreased hemoglobin/hematocrit
Hypoglycemia has been reported in association with Disopyramide Phosphate administration (see *"Warnings"*).

Infrequent occurrences of reversible cholestatic jaundice, fever, and respiratory difficulty have been reported in association with Disopyramide therapy, as have rare instances of thrombocytopenia, reversible agranulocytosis, and gynecomastia. Some cases of LE (lupus erythematosus) symptoms have been reported; most cases occurred in patients who had been switched to Disopyramide from procainamide following the development of LE symptoms. Rarely, acute psychosis has been reported following Disopyramide Phosphate therapy, with prompt return to normal mental status when therapy was stopped. The physician should be aware of these possible reactions and should discontinue Disopyramide Phosphate or Disopyramide Phosphate Controlled Release therapy promptly if they occur.

OVERDOSAGE

SYMPTOMS

Deliberate or accidental overdosage of oral Disopyramide may be followed by apnea, loss of consciousness, cardiac arrhythmias, and loss of spontaneous respiration. Death has occurred following overdosage.

Toxic plasma levels of Disopyramide produce excessive widening of the QRS complex and Q-T interval, worsening of congestive heart failure, hypotension, varying kinds and degrees of conduction disturbance, bradycardia, and finally asystole. Obvious anticholinergic effects are also observed.

The approximate oral LD50 of Disopyramide Phosphate is 580 and 700 mg/kg for rats and mice, respectively.

TREATMENT

Experience indicates that prompt and vigorous treatment of overdosage is necessary, even in the absence of symptoms. Such treatment may be lifesaving. No specific antidote for Disopyramide Phosphate has been identified. Treatment should be symptomatic and may include induction of emesis or gastric lavage, administration of a cathartic followed by activated charcoal by mouth or stomach tube, intravenous administration of isoproterenol and dopamine, insertion of an intra-aortic balloon for counterpulsation, and mechanically assisted ventilation. Hemodialysis or, preferably, hemoperfusion with charcoal may be employed to lower serum concentration of the drug.

The electrocardiogram should be monitored, and supportive therapy with cardiac glycosides and diuretics should be given as required.

If progressive AV block should develop, endocardial pacing should be implemented. In case of any impaired renal function, measures to increase the glomerular filtration rate may reduce the toxicity (Disopyramide is excreted primarily by the kidney).

The anticholinergic effects can be reversed with neostigmine at the discretion of the physician.

Altering the urinary pH in humans does not affect the plasma half-life or the amount of Disopyramide excreted in the urine.

DOSAGE AND ADMINISTRATION

The dosage of Disopyramide Phosphate or Disopyramide Phosphate Controlled Release must be individualized for each patient on the basis of response and tolerance. The usual adult dosage of Disopyramide Phosphate or Disopyramide Phosphate Controlled Release is 400 to 800 mg per day given in divided doses.

The recommended dosage for most adults is 600 mg/day given in divided doses (either 150 mg every 6 hours for immediate-release Disopyramide Phosphate or 300 mg every 12 hours for Disopyramide Phosphate Controlled Release). For patients whose body weight is less than 110 pounds (50 kg), the recommended dosage is 400 mg/day given in divided doses (either 100 mg every 6 hours for immediate-release Disopyramide Phosphate or 200 mg every 12 hours for Disopyramide Phosphate Controlled Release).

For patients with cardiomyopathy or possible cardiac decompensation, a loading dose, as discussed below, should not be given, and initial dosage should be limited to 100 mg of immediate-release Disopyramide Phosphate every 6 to 8 hours. Subsequent dosage adjustments should be made gradually, with close monitoring for the possible development of hypotension and/or congestive heart failure (see "Warnings").

For patients with moderate renal insufficiency (creatinine clearance greater than 40 ml/min) or hepatic insufficiency, the recommended dosage is 400 mg/day given in divided doses (either 100 mg every 6 hours for immediate-release Disopyramide Phosphate or 200 mg every 12 hours for Disopyramide Phosphate Controlled Release).

For patients with severe renal insufficiency (C_{cr} 40 ml/min or less), the recommended dosage regimen of immediate-release Disopyramide Phosphate is 100 mg at intervals shown in the table below, with or without an initial loading dose of 150 mg.

IMMEDIATE-RELEASE DISOPYRAMIDE PHOSPHATE DOSAGE INTERVAL FOR PATIENTS WITH RENAL INSUFFICIENCY

Creatinine clearance (ml/min)	40-30	30-15	less than 15
Approximate maintenance-dosing interval	q 8 hr	q 12 hr	q 24 hr

The above dosing schedules are for Disopyramide Phosphate immediate-release capsules; Disopyramide Phosphate Controlled Release is not recommended for patients with severe renal insufficiency.

For patients in whom rapid control of ventricular arrhythmia is essential, an initial loading dose of 300 mg of immediate-release Disopyramide Phosphate (200 mg for patients whose body weight is less than 110 pounds) is recommended, followed by the appropriate maintenance dosage. Therapeutic effects are usually attained 30 minutes to 3 hours after administration of a 300-mg loading dose. If there is no response or evidence of toxicity within 6 hours of the loading dose, 200 mg of immediate-release Disopyramide Phosphate every 6 hours may be prescribed instead of the usual 150 mg. If there is no response to this dosage within 48 hours, either Disopyramide Phosphate should then be discontinued or the physician should consider hospitalizing the patient for careful monitoring while subsequent immediate-release Disopyramide Phosphate doses of 250 mg or 300 mg every 6 hours are given. A limited number of patients with severe refractory ventricular tachycardia have tolerated daily doses of Disopyramide Phosphate up to 1600 mg per day (400 mg every 6 hours), resulting in Disopyramide plasma levels up to 9 mcg/mL. If such treatment is warranted, it is essential that patients be hospitalized for close evaluation and continuous monitoring.

Disopyramide Phosphate Controlled Release should not be used initially if rapid establishment of Disopyramide plasma levels is desired.

TRANSFERRING TO DISOPYRAMIDE PHOSPHATE OR DISOPYRAMIDE PHOSPHATE CONTROLLED RELEASE

The following dosage schedule based on theoretical considerations rather than experimental data is suggested for transferring patients with normal renal function from either quinidine sulfate or procainamide therapy (Type 1 antiarrhythmic agents) to Disopyramide Phosphate or Disopyramide Phosphate Controlled Release therapy:

Disopyramide Phosphate or Disopyramide Phosphate Controlled Release should be started using the regular maintenance schedule **without a loading dose** 6 to 12 hours after the last dose of quinidine sulfate or 3 to 6 hours after the last dose of procainamide.

In patients in whom withdrawal of quinidine sulfate or procainamide is likely to produce life-threatening arrhythmias, the physician should consider hospitalization of the patient.

When transferring a patient from immediate-release Disopyramide Phosphate to Disopyramide Phosphate Controlled Release the maintenance schedule of Disopyramide Phosphate Controlled Release may be started 6 hours after the last dose of immediate-release Disopyramide Phosphate.

PEDIATRIC DOSAGE

Controlled clinical studies have not been conducted in pediatric patients; however, the following suggested dosage table is based on published clinical experience.

Total daily dosage should be divided and equal doses administered orally every 6 hours or at intervals according to individual patient needs. Disopyramide plasma levels and therapeutic response must be monitored closely. Patients should be hospitalized during the initial treatment period, and dose titration should start at the lower end of the ranges provided below.

SUGGESTED TOTAL DAILY DOSAGE*

Age (years)	Disopyramide (mg/kg body weight/day)
Under 1	10 to 30
1 to 4	10 to 20
4 to 12	10 to 15
12 to 18	6 to 15

* *Dosage is expressed in milligrams of Disopyramide base. Since Disopyramide Phosphate 100-mg capsules contain 100 mg of Disopyramide base, the pharmacist can readily prepare a 1-mg/mL to 10-mg/mL liquid suspension by adding the entire contents of Disopyramide Phosphate capsules to cherry syrup, NF. The resulting suspension, when refrigerated, is stable for one month and should be thoroughly shaken before the measurement of each dose. The suspension should be dispensed in an amber glass bottle with a child-resistant closure. Disopyramide Phosphate Controlled Release capsules should not be used to prepare the above suspension.*

Store below 86°F (30°C).

HOW SUPPLIED
CAPSULE: 100 MG

AVERAGE UNIT PRICE (AVAILABLE SIZES)

BRAND	$0.52	GENERIC A-RATED AVERAGE PRICE (GAAP)	
GENERIC	$0.24	100s	$24.10
HCFA FUL (100s ea)	$0.10	500s	$109.86

BRAND/MANUFACTURER	NDC	SIZE	AWP
◆ **BRAND**			
NORPACE: Searle	00025-2752-31	100s	$52.53
	00025-2752-34	100s ud	$54.99
	00025-2752-52	1000s	$484.31
◆ **GENERICS**			
Biocraft	00332-3127-09	100s	$20.18
Geneva	00781-2110-01	100s	$22.25
Aligen	00405-4357-01	100s	$22.30
Moore,H.L.	00839-7091-06	100s	$22.88
Schein	00364-0739-01	100s	$22.95
Goldline	00182-1743-01	100s	$22.95
Qualitest	00603-3408-21	100s	$22.96
Caremark	00339-5681-12	100s	$23.00
URL	00677-1020-01	100s	$23.90
Rugby	00536-3595-01	100s	$23.95
Major	00904-2482-60	100s	$23.95
U.S. Trading	56126-0330-11	100s ud	$12.38
Raway	00686-0296-20	100s ud	$19.00
Schein	00364-0739-90	100s ud	$33.75
UDL	51079-0296-20	100s ud	$34.53
Auro	55829-0631-10	100s ud	$34.60
Biocraft	00332-3127-13	500s	$95.90
Moore,H.L.	00839-7091-12	500s	$108.68
Schein	00364-0739-05	500s	$111.50
Rugby	00536-3595-05	500s	$116.50
Major	00904-2482-40	500s	$116.70

CAPSULE: 150 MG

AVERAGE UNIT PRICE (AVAILABLE SIZES)

BRAND	$0.61	GENERIC A-RATED AVERAGE PRICE (GAAP)	
GENERIC	$0.29	100s	$29.73
HCFA FUL (100s ea)	$0.12	500s	$128.64

BRAND/MANUFACTURER	NDC	SIZE	AWP
◆ **BRAND**			
NORPACE: Searle	00025-2762-31	100s	$62.04
	00025-2762-34	100s ud	$64.53
	00025-2762-52	1000s	$572.06
◆ **GENERICS**			
Biocraft	00332-3129-09	100s	$23.84
Aligen	00405-4358-01	100s	$26.35
Schein	00364-0740-01	100s	$26.75
Geneva	00781-2115-01	100s	$26.80
Caremark	00339-5683-12	100s	$27.58
Moore,H.L.	00839-7092-06	100s	$27.66
Qualitest	00603-3409-21	100s	$28.40
URL	00677-1021-01	100s	$28.50
Goldline	00182-1744-01	100s	$28.50
Rugby	00536-3596-01	100s	$28.69
Major	00904-2483-60	100s	$28.75
Raway	00686-0297-20	100s ud	$21.00
Major	00904-2483-61	100s ud	$32.93
Schein	00364-0740-90	100s ud	$39.75
UDL	51079-0297-20	100s ud	$39.80
Auro	55829-0632-10	100s ud	$40.44
Biocraft	00332-3129-13	500s	$113.29
Moore,H.L.	00839-7092-12	500s	$131.21
Major	00904-2483-40	500s	$131.25
Schein	00364-0740-05	500s	$131.25
Rugby	00536-3596-05	500s	$136.21

CAPSULE, EXTENDED RELEASE: 100 MG

AVERAGE UNIT PRICE (AVAILABLE SIZES)		GENERIC A-RATED AVERAGE PRICE (GAAP)		
BRAND	$0.63	100s		$49.61
GENERIC	$0.49			

BRAND/MANUFACTURER		NDC	SIZE	AWP
◆ BRAND				
NORPACE CR: Searle		00025-2732-31	100s	$63.25
		00025-2732-34	100s ud	$66.23
		00025-2732-51	500s	$300.62
◆ GENERICS				
Ethex		58177-0003-04	100s	$46.12
Major		00904-2488-60	100s	$53.10
Major		00904-2488-40	500s	$230.80

CAPSULE, EXTENDED RELEASE: 150 MG

AVERAGE UNIT PRICE (AVAILABLE SIZES)		GENERIC A-RATED AVERAGE PRICE (GAAP)		
BRAND	$0.75	100s		$53.94
GENERIC	$0.54			

BRAND/MANUFACTURER		NDC	SIZE	AWP
◆ BRAND				
NORPACE CR: Searle		00025-2742-31	100s	$74.76
		00025-2742-34	100s ud	$77.74
		00025-2742-51	500s	$355.17
◆ GENERICS				
Caremark		00339-5684-12	100s	$53.36
Ethex		58177-0002-04	100s	$54.51
Major		00904-2489-40	500s	$270.95

Disotate SEE EDETATE DISODIUM

Disulfiram

> **WARNING**
> DISULFIRAM SHOULD *NEVER* BE ADMINISTERED TO A PATIENT WHEN HE IS IN A STATE OF ALCOHOL INTOXICATION, OR WITHOUT HIS FULL KNOWLEDGE.
> THE PHYSICIAN SHOULD INSTRUCT RELATIVES ACCORDINGLY.

DESCRIPTION

Chemical Name: bis(diethylthiocarbamoyl) disulfide

Disulfiram occurs as a white to off-white, odorless, and almost tasteless powder, soluble in water to the extent of about 20 mg in 100 mL, and in alcohol to the extent of about 3.8 g in 100 mL.

Following is its chemical structure:

$$(C_2H_5)_2NC-S-S-CN(C_2H_5)_2$$

ACTION

Disulfiram produces a sensitivity to alcohol which results in a highly unpleasant reaction when the patient under treatment ingests even small amounts of alcohol.

Disulfiram blocks the oxidation of alcohol at the acetaldehyde stage. During alcohol metabolism following Disulfiram intake, the concentration of acetaldehyde occurring in the blood may be 5- to 10-times higher than that found during metabolism of the same amount of alcohol alone.

Accumulation of acetaldehyde in the blood produces a complex of highly unpleasant symptoms referred to hereinafter as the Disulfiram-alcohol reaction. This reaction, which is proportional to the dosage of both Disulfiram and alcohol, will persist as long as alcohol is being metabolized. Disulfiram does not appear to influence the rate of alcohol elimination from the body.

Disulfiram is absorbed slowly from the gastrointestinal tract and eliminated slowly from the body. One (or even two) weeks after a patient has taken his last dose of Disulfiram, ingestion of alcohol may produce unpleasant symptoms.

Prolonged administration of Disulfiram does not produce tolerance; the longer a patient remains on therapy, the more exquisitely sensitive he becomes to alcohol.

INDICATION

Disulfiram is an aid in the management of selected chronic alcoholic patients who *want* to remain in a state of enforced sobriety so that supportive and psychotherapeutic treatment may be applied to best advantage.

Disulfiram is not a cure for alcoholism. When used alone, without proper motivation and supportive therapy, it is unlikely that it will have any substantive effect on the drinking pattern of the chronic alcoholic.

CONTRAINDICATIONS

Patients who are receiving or have recently received metronidazole, paraldehyde, alcohol, or alcohol-containing preparations, e.g., cough syrups, tonics and the like, should not be given Disulfiram.

Disulfiram is contraindicated in the presence of severe myocardial disease or coronary occlusion, psychoses, and hypersensitivity to Disulfiram or to other thiuram derivatives used in pesticides and rubber vulcanization.

> **WARNINGS**
> DISULFIRAM SHOULD *NEVER* BE ADMINISTERED TO A PATIENT WHEN HE IS IN A STATE OF ALCOHOL INTOXICATION, OR WITHOUT HIS FULL KNOWLEDGE.
> THE PHYSICIAN SHOULD INSTRUCT RELATIVES ACCORDINGLY.

The patient must be fully informed of the Disulfiram-alcohol reaction. He must be strongly cautioned against surreptitious drinking while taking the drug, and he must be fully aware of possible consequences. He should be warned to avoid alcohol in disguised form, i.e., in sauces, vinegars, cough mixtures, and even aftershave lotions and back rubs. He should also be warned that reactions may occur with alcohol up to 14 days after ingesting Disulfiram.

THE DISULFIRAM-ALCOHOL REACTION

Disulfiram plus alcohol, even small amounts, produces flushing, throbbing in head and neck, throbbing headache, respiratory difficulty, nausea, copious vomiting, sweating, thirst, chest pain, palpitation, dyspnea, hyperventilation, tachycardia, hypotension, syncope, marked uneasiness, weakness, vertigo, blurred vision, and confusion. In severe reactions there may be respiratory depression, cardiovascular collapse, arrhythmias, myocardial infarction, acute congestive heart failure, unconsciousness, convulsions, and death.

The intensity of the reaction varies with each individual but is generally proportional to the amounts of Antabuse and alcohol ingested. Mild reactions may occur in the sensitive individual when the blood alcohol concentration is increased to as little as 5 to 10 mg per 100 mL. Symptoms are fully developed at 50 mg per 100 mL, and unconsciousness usually results when the blood alcohol level reaches 125 to 150 mg.

The duration of the reaction varies from 30 to 60 minutes, to several hours in the more severe cases, or as long as there is alcohol in the blood.

DRUG INTERACTIONS

Disulfiram appears to decrease the rate at which certain drugs are metabolized and therefore may increase the blood levels and the possibility of clinical toxicity of drugs given concomitantly.

DISULFIRAM SHOULD BE USED WITH CAUTION IN THOSE PATIENTS RECEIVING PHENYTOIN AND ITS CONGENERS, SINCE THE CONCOMITANT ADMINISTRATION OF THESE TWO DRUGS CAN LEAD TO PHENYTOIN INTOXICATION. PRIOR TO ADMINISTERING DISULFIRAM TO A PATIENT ON PHENYTOIN THERAPY, A BASELINE PHENYTOIN SERUM LEVEL SHOULD BE OBTAINED, SUBSEQUENT TO INITIATION OF DISULFIRAM THERAPY, SERUM LEVELS OF PHENYTOIN SHOULD BE DETERMINED ON DIFFERENT DAYS FOR EVIDENCE OF AN INCREASE OR FOR A CONTINUING RISE IN LEVELS. INCREASED PHENYTOIN LEVELS SHOULD BE TREATED WITH APPROPRIATE DOSAGE ADJUSTMENT.

It may be necessary to adjust the dosage of oral anticoagulants upon beginning or stopping Disulfiram, since Disulfiram may prolong prothrombin time.

Patients taking isoniazid when Disulfiram is given should be observed for the appearance of unsteady gait or marked changes in mental status; the Disulfiram should be discontinued if such signs appear.

In rats, simultaneous ingestion of Disulfiram and nitrite in the diet for 78 weeks has been reported to cause tumors, and it has been suggested that Disulfiram may react with nitrites in the rat stomach to form a nitrosamine, which is tumorigenic. Disulfiram alone in the rats' diet did not lead to such tumors. The relevance of this finding to humans is not known at this time.

CONCOMITANT CONDITIONS

Because of the possibility of an accidental Disulfiram-alcohol reaction Disulfiram should be used with extreme caution in patients with any of the following conditions: diabetes mellitus, hypothyroidism, epilepsy, cerebral damage, chronic and acute nephritis, hepatic cirrhosis or insufficiency.

USAGE IN PREGNANCY

The safe use of this drug in pregnancy has not been established. Therefore, Disulfiram should be used during pregnancy only when, in the judgment of the physician, the probable benefits outweigh the possible risks.

PRECAUTIONS

Patients with a history of rubber contact dermatitis should be evaluated for hypersensitivity to thiuram derivatives before receiving Disulfiram (see *"Contraindications"*).

It is suggested that every patient under treatment carry an *Identification Card*, stating that he is receiving Disulfiram and describing the symptoms most likely to occur as a result of the Disulfiram-alcohol reaction. In addition, this card should indicate the physician or institution to be contacted in an emergency.

Alcoholism may accompany or be followed by dependence on narcotics or sedatives. Barbiturates and Disulfiram have been administered concurrently

► SHOWN IN PRODUCT IDENTIFICATION GUIDE

without untoward effects; the possibility of initiating a new abuse should be considered. Baseline and follow-up transaminase tests (10 to 14 days) are suggested to detect any hepatic dysfunction that may result with Disulfiram therapy. In addition, a complete blood count and a sequential multiple analysis-12 (SMA-12) test should be made every six months.

Patients taking Disulfiram Tablets should not be exposed to ethylene dibromide or its vapors. This precaution is based on preliminary results of animal research currently in progress that suggest a toxic interaction between inhaled ethylene dibromide and ingested Disulfiram resulting in a higher incidence of tumors and mortality in rats. A correlation between this finding and humans, however, has not been demonstrated.

ADVERSE REACTIONS
(See *"Contraindications," "Warnings,"* and *"Precautions".*) OPTIC NEURITIS, PERIPHERAL NEURITIS, POLYNEURITIS, AND PERIPHERAL NEUROPATHY MAY OCCUR FOLLOWING ADMINISTRATION OF DISULFIRAM.

Multiple cases of hepatitis, including both cholestatic and fulminant hepatitis, have been reported to be associated with administration of Antabuse.

Occasional skin eruption are, as a rule, readily controlled by concomitant administration of an antihistaminic drug.

In a small number of patients, a transient mild drowsiness, fatigability, impotence, headache, acneform eruptions, allergic dermatitis, or a metallic or garlic-like aftertaste may be experienced during the first two weeks of therapy. These complaints usually disappear spontaneously with the continuation of therapy, or with reduced dosage.

Psychotic reactions have been noted, attributable in most cases to high dosage, combined toxicity (with metronidazole or isoniazid), or to the unmasking of underlying psychoses in patients stressed by the withdrawal of alcohol.

DOSAGE AND ADMINISTRATION
Disulfiram should never be administered until the patient has abstained from alcohol for at least 12 hours.

INITIAL DOSAGE SCHEDULE
In the first phase of treatment, a *maximum* of 500 mg daily is given in a single dose for one to two weeks. Although usually taken in the morning, Disulfiram may be taken on retiring by patients who experience a sedative effect. Alternatively, to minimize, or eliminate, the sedative effect, dosage may be adjusted downward.

MAINTENANCE REGIMEN
The average maintenance dose is 250 mg daily (range, 125 to 500 mg); it should not exceed 500 mg daily.

Note: Occasionally patients, while seemingly on adequate maintenance doses of Disulfiram, report that they are able to drink alcoholic beverages with impunity and without any symptomatology. All appearances to the contrary, such patients must be presumed to be disposing of their tablets in some manner without actually taking them. Until such patients have been observed reliably taking their daily Disulfiram tablets (preferably crushed and well mixed with liquid), it cannot be concluded that Disulfiram is ineffective.

DURATION OF THERAPY
The daily, uninterrupted administration of Disulfiram must be continued until the patient is fully recovered socially and a basis for permanent self-control is established. Depending on the individual patient, maintenance therapy may be required for months, or even years.

TRIAL WITH ALCOHOL
During early experience with Disulfiram, it was thought advisable for each patient to have at least one supervised alcohol-drug reaction. More recently, the test reaction has been largely abandoned. Furthermore, such a test reaction should never be administered to a patient over 50 years of age. A clear, detailed, and convincing description of the reaction is felt to be sufficient in most cases.

However, where a test reaction is deemed necessary, the suggested procedure is as follows:

After the first one to two weeks' therapy with 500 mg daily, a drink of 15 mL (½ oz) of 100 proof whiskey, or equivalent, is taken slowly. This test dose of alcoholic beverage may be repeated once only, so that the total dose does not exceed 30 mL (1 oz) of whiskey. Once a reaction develops, no more alcohol should be consumed. Such tests should be carried out only when the patient is hospitalized, or comparable supervision and facilities, including oxygen, are available.

MANAGEMENT OF DISULFIRAM-ALCOHOL REACTION
In severe reactions, whether caused by an excessive test dose or by the patient's unsupervised ingestion of alcohol, supportive measures to restore blood pressure and treat shock should be instituted. Other recommendations include: oxygen, carbogen (95% oxygen and 5% carbon dioxide), vitamin C intravenously in massive doses (1 g), and ephedrine sulfate. Antihistamines have also been used intravenously. Potassium levels should be monitored, particularly in patients on digitalis, since hypokalemia has been reported.

Store at room temperature, approx. 25°C.

HOW SUPPLIED
TABLETS: 250 MG

BRAND/MANUFACTURER	NDC	SIZE	AWP
◇ **BRAND**			
ANTABUSE: Wyeth-Ayerst	00046-0809-81	100s	$66.11
◇ **GENERICS**			
Rugby	00536-3767-01	100s	$7.43
Major	00904-1180-60	100s	$7.65
Schein	00364-0336-01	100s	$7.87
Geneva	00781-1060-01	100s	$7.90
Qualitest	00603-3431-21	100s	$7.91
Goldline	00182-0532-01	100s	$7.95
URL	00677-1001-01	100s	$8.05
Moore,H.L.	00839-1286-06	100s	$8.09
Sidmak	50111-0331-01	100s	$8.30
Major	00904-1180-61	100s ud	$16.10
Sidmak	50111-0331-03	1000s	$60.80

TABLETS: 500 MG

BRAND/MANUFACTURER	NDC	SIZE	AWP
◇ **BRAND**			
ANTABUSE: Wyeth-Ayerst	00046-0810-50	50s	$39.88
◇ **GENERICS**			
Schein	00364-0337-50	50s	$9.35
Major	00904-1181-60	100s	$11.95
Geneva	00781-1070-01	100s	$12.88
Qualitest	00603-3432-21	100s	$13.86
Goldline	00182-0533-01	100s	$15.00

Ditropan SEE OXYBUTYNIN CHLORIDE

Diucardin SEE HYDROFLUMETHIAZIDE

Diupres SEE CHLOROTHIAZIDE WITH RESERPINE

Diuril SEE CHLOROTHIAZIDE

Diutensen-R SEE METHYCLOTHIAZIDE WITH RESERPINE

Divalproex Sodium

> ## WARNING
> HEPATIC FAILURE RESULTING IN FATALITIES HAS OCCURRED IN PATIENTS RECEIVING VALPROIC ACID AND ITS DERIVATIVES. EXPERIENCE HAS INDICATED THAT CHILDREN UNDER THE AGE OF TWO YEARS ARE AT A CONSIDERABLY INCREASED RISK OF DEVELOPING FATAL HEPATOTOXICITY, ESPECIALLY THOSE ON MULTIPLE ANTICONVULSANTS, THOSE WITH CONGENITAL METABOLIC DISORDERS, THOSE WITH SEVERE SEIZURE DISORDERS ACCOMPANIED BY MENTAL RETARDATION, AND THOSE WITH ORGANIC BRAIN DISEASE. WHEN DIVALPROEX SODIUM IS USED IN THIS PATIENT GROUP, IT SHOULD BE USED WITH EXTREME CAUTION AND AS A SOLE AGENT. THE BENEFITS OF SEIZURE CONTROL SHOULD BE WEIGHED AGAINST THE RISKS. ABOVE THIS AGE GROUP, EXPERIENCE HAS INDICATED THAT THE INCIDENCE OF FATAL HEPATOTOXICITY DECREASES CONSIDERABLY IN PROGRESSIVELY OLDER PATIENT GROUPS.
>
> THESE INCIDENTS USUALLY HAVE OCCURRED DURING THE FIRST SIX MONTHS OF TREATMENT. SERIOUS OR FATAL HEPATOTOXICITY MAY BE PRECEDED BY NON-SPECIFIC SYMPTOMS SUCH AS LOSS OF SEIZURE CONTROL, MALAISE, WEAKNESS, LETHARGY, FACIAL EDEMA, ANOREXIA, AND VOMITING. PATIENTS SHOULD BE MONITORED CLOSELY FOR APPEARANCE OF THESE SYMPTOMS. LIVER FUNCTION TESTS SHOULD BE PERFORMED PRIOR TO THERAPY AND AT FREQUENT INTERVALS THEREAFTER, ESPECIALLY DURING THE FIRST SIX MONTHS.

DESCRIPTION
Divalproex Sodium is a stable co-ordination compound comprised of sodium valproate and valproic acid in a 1:1 molar relationship and formed during the partial neutralization of valproic acid with 0.5 equivalent of sodium hydroxide. Chemically it is designated as sodium hydrogen bis (2-propylpentanoate).

Divalproex Sodium occurs as a white powder with a characteristic odor.

Divalproex Sodium tablets and Sprinkle capsules are antiepileptics for oral administration. Divalproex Sodium Sprinkle capsules contain specially coated particles of Divalproex Sodium equivalent to 125 mg of valproic acid in a hard gelatin capsule. Divalproex Sodium tablets are supplied in three dosage strengths containing Divalproex Sodium equivalent to 125 mg, 250 mg, or 500 mg of valproic acid.

Following is its chemical structure:

$$CH_3CH_2CH_2 \quad CH{-}CH_2CH_2CH_3$$
$$HO{-}C{=}O$$
$$O{=}C{-}O^- \quad Na^+$$
$$CH_3CH_2CH_2{-}CH{-}CH_2CH_2CH_3$$

CLINICAL PHARMACOLOGY

Divalproex Sodium is an antiepileptic agent which dissociates to the valproate ion in the gastrointestinal tract. The mechanism by which valproate exerts its antiepileptic effects has not been established. It has been suggested that its activity is related to increased brain levels of gamma-aminobutyric acid (GABA).

Equivalent oral doses of Divalproex Sodium products and valproic acid capsules deliver equivalent quantities of valproate ion systemically. However, the rate of valproate ion absorption may vary with the conditions of use (e.g., fasting or postprandial) and the method of administration (e.g., whether the contents of the capsule are sprinkled on food or the capsule is taken intact).

When subjects are in a fasting state, peak plasma concentrations of valproate ion are observed approximately 3 to 4 hours following administration of all Divalproex Sodium products. Experiments indicate that feeding can influence the rate of systemic absorption of valproate. In studies in which the contents of Divalproex Sodium Sprinkle capsules were sprinkled on applesauce, feeding was found to delay the time to peak plasma concentration by approximately 1.5 hours.

Compared to Divalproex Sodium tablets, however, Divalproex Sodium Sprinkle capsules (in the fasting state) exhibit a slower rate of absorption, resulting in lower peak plasma concentrations (i.e., fluctuations between minimum and maximum plasma valproate concentrations are attenuated).

While absorption rate from the GI tract and fluctuation in valproate plasma concentrations vary with dosing regimen and formulation, the efficacy of valproate in chronic use is not affected. Experience employing dosing regimens from once-a-day to four-times-a-day, as well as studies in primate epilepsy models involving constant rate infusion, indicate that total daily systemic bioavailability (extent of absorption) is the primary determinant of seizure control and that differences in the ratios of plasma peak to trough concentrations between valproate formulations are inconsequential from a practical clinical standpoint.

Accordingly, coadministration of oral valproate products with food and substitution among the various Divalproex Sodium and valproic acid formulations should cause no clinical problems (see *"Dosage and Administration"*). Nonetheless, any changes in dosage administration, or the addition or discontinuance of concomitant drugs should ordinarily be accompanied by close monitoring of clinical status and valproate plasma concentrations.

The plasma half-life of valproate is typically in the range of 6 to 16 hours. Half-lives in the lower part of the range are usually found in patients taking other antiepileptic drugs capable of enzyme induction.

Valproate is primarily metabolized in the liver. The major metabolic routes are glucuronidation, mitochondrial beta oxidation, and microsomal oxidation. The major metabolites formed are the glucuronide conjugate, 2-propyl-3-keto-pentanoic acid, and 2-propylhydroxypentanoic acids. Other unsaturated metabolites have been reported. The major route of elimination of these metabolites is in the urine.

Patients on monotherapy will generally have longer half-lives and higher concentrations of valproate at a given dosage than patients receiving polytherapy. This is primarily due to enzyme induction caused by other antiepileptics, which results in enhanced clearance of valproate by glucuronidation and microsomal oxidation. Because of these changes in valproate clearance, monitoring of antiepileptic concentrations should be intensified whenever concomitant antiepileptics are introduced or withdrawn.

The therapeutic range is commonly considered to be 50 to 100 mcg/ml of total valproate, although some patients may be controlled with lower or higher plasma concentrations.[1] Valproate is highly bound (90%) to plasma proteins in the therapeutic range; however, protein binding is concentration-dependent and decreases at high valproate concentrations. The binding is variable among patients and may be affected by fatty acids or by highly bound drugs such as salicylate. Some clinicians favor monitoring free valproate concentrations, which may more accurately reflect CNS penetration of valproate. As yet, a consensus on the therapeutic range of free concentrations has not been established; however, monitoring total and free valproate may be informative when there are changes in clinical status, concomitant medication, or valproate dosage.

INDICATIONS AND USAGE

Divalproex Sodium is indicated for use as sole and adjunctive therapy in the treatment of simple and complex absence seizures, and adjunctively in patients with multiple seizure types that include absence seizures.

Simple absence is defined as very brief clouding of the sensorium or loss of consciousness accompanied by certain generalized epileptic discharges without other detectable clinical signs. Complex absence is the term used when other signs are also present.

SEE *"WARNINGS"* for STATEMENT REGARDING FATAL HEPATIC DYSFUNCTION.

➤ SHOWN IN PRODUCT IDENTIFICATION GUIDE

UNLABELED USES

Divalproex Sodium is used alone or as an adjunct in the treatment of incapacitating, intractable hiccups, prophylactic therapy against migraine headache, and Nelson's syndrome associated with Cushing's disease. It is also used in the treatment of psychotic disorder, febrile seizures, infantile seizures, and myoclonic seizures.

CONTRAINDICATIONS

DIVALPROEX SODIUM SHOULD NOT BE ADMINISTERED TO PATIENTS WITH HEPATIC DISEASE OR SIGNIFICANT DYSFUNCTION.

Divalproex Sodium is contraindicated in patients with known hypersensitivity to the drug.

WARNINGS

Hepatic failure resulting in fatalities has occurred in patients receiving valproic acid. These incidents usually have occurred during the first six months of treatment. Serious or fatal hepatotoxicity may be preceded by nonspecific symptoms such as loss of seizure control, malaise, weakness, lethargy, facial edema, anorexia, and vomiting. Patients should be monitored closely for appearance of these symptoms. Liver function tests should be performed prior to therapy and at frequent intervals thereafter, especially during the first six months. However, physicians should not rely totally on serum biochemistry since these tests may not be abnormal in all instances, but should also consider the results of careful interim medical history and physical examination. Caution should be observed when administering Divalproex Sodium products to patients with a prior history of hepatic disease. Patients on multiple anticonvulsants, children, those with congenital metabolic disorders, those with severe seizure disorders accompanied by mental retardation, and those with organic brain disease may be at particular risk. Experience has indicated that children under the age of two years are at considerably increased risk of developing fatal hepatotoxicity, especially those with the aforementioned conditions. When Divalproex Sodium is used in this patient group, it should be used with extreme caution and as a sole agent. The benefits of seizure control should be weighed against the risks. Above this age group, experience has indicated that the incidence of fatal hepatotoxicity decreases considerably in progressively older patient groups.

The drug should be discontinued immediately in the presence of significant hepatic dysfunction, suspected or apparent. In some cases, hepatic dysfunction has progressed in spite of discontinuation of drug.

The frequency of adverse effects (particularly elevated liver enzymes) may be dose-related. The benefit of improved seizure control which may accompany the higher doses should therefore be weighed against the possibility of a greater incidence of adverse effects.

Usage in Pregnancy: ACCORDING TO PUBLISHED AND UNPUBLISHED REPORTS, VALPROIC ACID MAY PRODUCE TERATOGENIC EFFECTS IN THE OFFSPRING OF HUMAN FEMALES RECEIVING THE DRUG DURING PREGNANCY.

THERE ARE MULTIPLE REPORTS IN THE CLINICAL LITERATURE WHICH INDICATE THAT THE USE OF ANTIEPILEPTIC DRUGS DURING PREGNANCY RESULTS IN AN INCREASED INCIDENCE OF BIRTH DEFECTS IN THE OFFSPRING. ALTHOUGH DATA ARE MORE EXTENSIVE WITH RESPECT TO TRIMETHADIONE, PARAMETHADIONE, PHENYTOIN, AND PHENOBARBITAL, REPORTS INDICATE A POSSIBLE SIMILAR ASSOCIATION WITH THE USE OF OTHER ANTIEPILEPTIC DRUGS. THEREFORE, ANTIEPILEPTIC DRUGS SHOULD BE ADMINISTERED TO WOMEN OF CHILDBEARING POTENTIAL ONLY IF THEY ARE CLEARLY SHOWN TO BE ESSENTIAL IN THE MANAGEMENT OF THEIR SEIZURES.

THE INCIDENCE OF NEURAL TUBE DEFECTS IN THE FETUS MAY BE INCREASED IN MOTHERS RECEIVING VALPROATE DURING THE FIRST TRIMESTER OF PREGNANCY. THE CENTERS FOR DISEASE CONTROL (CDC) HAS ESTIMATED THE RISK OF VALPROIC ACID EXPOSED WOMEN HAVING CHILDREN WITH SPINA BIFIDA TO BE APPROXIMATELY 1 TO 2%.[2]

OTHER CONGENITAL ANOMALIES (E.G., CRANIOFACIAL DEFECTS, CARDIOVASCULAR MALFORMATIONS AND ANOMALIES INVOLVING VARIOUS BODY SYSTEM), COMPATIBLE AND INCOMPATIBLE WITH LIFE, HAVE BEEN REPORTED, SUFFICIENT DATA TO DETERMINE THE INCIDENCE OF THESE CONGENITAL ANOMALIES IS NOT AVAILABLE.

THE HIGHER INCIDENCE OF CONGENITAL ANOMALIES IN ANTIEPILEPTIC DRUG-TREATED WOMEN WITH SEIZURE DISORDERS CANNOT BE REGARDED AS A CAUSE AND EFFECT RELATIONSHIP. THERE ARE INTRINSIC METHODOLOGIC PROBLEMS IN OBTAINING ADEQUATE DATA ON DRUG TERATOGENICITY IN HUMANS: GENETIC FACTORS OR THE EPILEPTIC CONDITION ITSELF MAY BE MORE IMPORTANT THAN DRUG THERAPY IN CONTRIBUTING TO CONGENITAL ANOMALIES.

PATIENTS TAKING VALPROATE MAY DEVELOP CLOTTING ABNORMALITIES. A PATIENT WHO HAD LOW FIBRINOGEN WHEN TAKING MULTIPLE ANTI-CONVULSANTS INCLUDING VALPROATE GAVE BIRTH TO AN INFANT WITH AFIBRINOGENEMIA WHO SUBSEQUENTLY DIED OF HEMORRHAGE. IF VALPROATE IS USED IN PREGNANCY, THE CLOTTING PARAMETERS SHOULD BE MONITORED CAREFULLY. HEPATIC FAILURE, RESULTING IN THE DEATH OF A NEWBORN AND OF AN INFANT, HAVE BEEN REPORTED FOLLOWING THE USE OF VALPROATE DURING PREGNANCY.

ANIMAL STUDIES ALSO HAVE DEMONSTRATED VALPROATE INDUCED TERATOGENICITY. Studies in rats and human females demonstrated placental transfer of the drug. Doses greater than 65 mg/kg/day given to pregnant rats and mice produced skeletal abnormalities in the off-spring primarily involving ribs and vertebrate; doses greater than 150 mg/kg/day given to pregnant rabbits produced fetal resorptions and (primarily) soft-tissue abnormalities in the offspring. In rats a dose-related delay in the onset of parturition was noted. Postnatal growth and survival of the progeny were adversely affected, particularly when drug administration spanned the entire gestation and early lactation period.

Antiepileptic drugs should not be discontinued in patients in whom the drug is administered to prevent major seizures because of the strong possibility of precipitating status epilepticus with attendant hypoxia and threat to life. In individual cases where the severity and frequency of the seizure disorder are such that the removal of medication does not pose a serious threat to the patient, discontinuation of the drug may be considered prior to and during pregnancy, although it cannot be said with any confidence that even minor seizures do not pose some hazard to the developing embryo or fetus.

The prescribing physician will wish to weigh these considerations in treating or counseling epileptic women of childbearing potential.

Tests to detect neural tube and other defects using current accepted procedures should be considered a part of routine prenatal care in childbearing women receiving valproate.

PRECAUTIONS

Hepatic Dysfunction: See boxed *"Warning"*, *"Contraindications"* and *"Warnings"*.

General: Based of reports of thrombocytopenia, inhibition of the second phase of platelet aggregation, and abnormal coagulation parameters (e.g., low fibrogen), platelet counts and coagulation tests are recommended before initiating therapy and at periodic intervals. It is recommended that patients receiving Divalproex Sodium be monitored for platelet count and coagulation parameters prior to planned surgery. Evidence of hemorrhage, bruising, or a disorder of hemostasis/ coagulation is an indication for reduction of the dosage or withdrawal of therapy.

Hyperammonemia with or without lethargy or coma has been reported and may be present in the absence of abnormal liver function tests. Asympatomatic elevations of ammonia are more common and when present require more frequent monitoring. If clinically significant symptoms occur, Divalproex Sodium therapy should be modified or discontinued.

Since valproate may interact with concurrently administered antiepileptic drugs, periodic plasma concentration determinations of concomitant antiepileptic drugs are recommended during the early course of therapy. (See *"Drug Interactions."*)

Valproate is partially eliminated in the urine as a keto-metabolite which may lead to a false interpretation of the urine ketone test.

There have been reports of altered thyroid function tests associated with valproate. The clinical significance of these is unknown.

Information for Patients: Since Divalproex Sodium products may produce CNS depression, especially when combined CNS depressants (e.g., alcohol), patients should be advised not to engage in hazardous activities, such as driving an automobile or operating dangerous machinery, until it is known that they do not become drowsy from the drug.

The specially coated particles in Divalproex Sodium Sprinkle capsules have been observed in the stool, but this occurrence has not been associated with clinically significant effects.

Drug Interactions: Valproate may potentiate the action of CNS depressants (i.e., alcohol, benzodiazepines, etc).

The concomitant administration of valproate with drugs that exhibit extensive protein binding (e.g., aspirin, carbamazepine, dicumarol, and phenytoin) may result in alteration of serum drug concentrations.

There is evidence that valproate can cause an increase in serum phenobarbital concentrations by impairment of nonreal clearance. This pnenomenon can result in severe CNS depression. The combination of valproate and phenobarbital has also been reported to produce CNS depression without significant elevations of barbiturate or valproate serum concentrations. All patients receiving concomitant barbiturate therapy should be closely monitored for neurological toxicity. Serum barbiturate levels should be obtained, if possible, and the barbiturate dosage decreased, if appropriate.

Primidone is metabolized to a barbiturate and, therefore, may also be involved in a similar or identical interaction. There have been reports of breakthrough seizures occurring with the combination of valproate and phenytoin. Most reports have noted a decrease in total plasma phenytoin serum concentration have been reported. An initial fall with subsequent increase in total phenytoin concentrations has also been reported. In addition, a decrease in total serum phenytoin with an increase in the free vs. protein bound phenytoin concentrations has been reported. The dosage of phenytoin should be adjusted as required by the clinical situation.

The concomitant use of valproic acid and clonazepam may induce absence status in patients with a history of absence type seizures.

There is inconclusive evidence regarding the effect of valproate on serum ethosuximide concentrations. Patients receiving valproate and ethosuximide, especially along with other anticonvulsants, should be monitored for alterations in serum concentrations of both drugs.

Caution is recommended when valproate is used with drugs affecting coagulation, (e.g., aspirin, warfarin). See *"Adverse Reactions"*.

Evidence suggests that there is an association between the use of certain antiepileptics and failure of oral contraceptives. One explanation for this interaction is that enzyme-inducing antiepileptics effectively lower plasma concentrations of the relevant steroid hormones, resulting in unimpaired ovulation. However, other mechanisms, not related to enzyme induction, may contribute to the failure of oral contraceptives. While valproate is not a significant enzyme inducer, and, therefore, would not be expected to decrease concentrations of steroid hormones, clinical data about the interaction of valproate with oral contraceptives is minimal.[3]

Carcinogenesis: Valproic acid was administered to Sprague Dawley rats and ICR (HA /ICR) mice at doses of 0, 80, and 170 mg/kg/day for two years. A variety of neoplasms were observed in both species. The chief findings were a statistically significant increase in the incidence of subcutaneous fibrosarcomas in high dose male rats receiving valproic acid and a statistically significant dose-related trend for benign pulmonary adenomas in male mice receiving valproic acid. The significance of these findings for humans is unknown.

Mutagenesis: Studies of valproate have been performed using bacterial and mammalian systems. These studies have provided no evidence of a mutagenic potential for valproate.

Fertility: Chronic toxicity studies in juvenile and adult rats and dogs demonstrated reduced spermatogenesis and testicular atrophy at doses greater than 200 mg/kg/day in rats and greater than 90 mg/kg/day in dogs. Segment I fertility studies in rats have shown doses up to 350 mg/kg/day for 60 days to have no effect on fertility. THE EFFECT OF VALPROATE ON TESTICULAR DEVELOPMENT AND ON SPERM PRODUCTION AND FERTILITY IN HUMANS IS UNKNOWN.

Pregnancy: Pregnancy Category D: see *"Warnings"*.

Nursing Mothers: Valproate is excreted in breast milk. Concentrations in breast milk have been reported to be 1-10% of serum concentrations. It is not known what effect this would have on a nursing infant. Caution should be exercised when Divalproex Sodium is administered to a nursing woman.

ADVERSE REACTIONS

Since Divalproex Sodium has usually been used with other antiepileptic drugs, it is not possible, in most cases, to determine whether the following adverse reactions can be ascribed to Divalproex Sodium alone, or the combination of drugs.

Gastrointestinal: The most commonly reported side effects at the initiation of therapy are nausea, vomiting and indigestion. These effects are usually transient and rarely require discontinuation of therapy. Diarrhea, abdominal cramps, and constipation have been reported. Both anorexia with some weight loss and increased appetite with weight gain have also been reported. The administration of delayed-release Divalproex Sodium may result in reduction of gastrointestinal side effects in some patients.[4]

CNS Effects: Sedative effects have occurred in patients receiving valproate alone but occur most often in patients receiving combination therapy. Sedation usually abates upon reduction of other antiepileptic medication. Tremor (may be dose-related), hallucinations, ataxia, headache, nystagmus, diplopia, asterixis, "spots before eyes", dysarthria, dizziness, and incoordination. Rare cases of coma have occurred in patients receiving valproate alone or in conjunction with phenobarbital. In rare instances encephalopathy with fever has developed shortly after the introduction of valproate monotherapy without evidence of hepatic dysfunction or inappropriate plasma levels; all patients recovered after the drug was withdrawn.

Dermatologic: Transient hair loss, skin rash, photosensitivity, generalized pruritus, erythema multiforme, and Stevens-Johnson syndrome. A case of fatal epidermal necrolysis has been reported in a 6 month old infant taking valproate and several other concomitant medications.

Psychiatric: Emotional upset, depression, psychosis, aggression, hyperactivity and behavioral deterioration.

Musculoskeletal: Weakness.

Hematologic: Thrombocytopenia and inhibition of the secondary phase of platelet aggregation may be reflected in altered bleeding time, petechiae, bruising, hematoma formation, and frank hermorrhage (see *"Precautions"—General and Drug Interactions*). Relative lymphocytosis, macrocytosis, hypofibrinogenemia, leukopenia, eosinophilia, anemia including macrocytic with or without folate deficiency, bone marrow suppression, and acute intermittent porphyria.

Hepatic: Minor elevations of transaminases (e.g., SGOT and SGPT) and LDH are frequent and appear to be dose-related. Occasionally, laboratory test results include increases in serum bilirubin and abnormal changes in other liver function tests. These results may reflect potentially serious hepatotoxicity (see *"Warnings"*).

Endocrine: Irregular menses and secondary amenorrhea, breast enlargement, galactorrhea and parotid gland swelling. Abnormal thyroid function tests (see *"Precautions"*).

Pancreatic: Acute pancreatitis including fatalities.

Metabolic: Hyperammonemia (see *"Precautions"*), hyponatremia, and inappropriate ADH secretion.

Decreased carnitine concentrations have been reported although the clinical relevance is undermined.

Hyperglycinemia has occurred and was associated with a fatal outcome in a patient with preexistent nonketotic hyperglycinemia.

Genitourinary: Enuresis.

Special Senses: Hearing loss, either reversible or irreversible, has been reported; however, a cause and effect relationship has not been established.

Other: Edema of the extremities, lupus erythematosus, and fever.

OVERDOSAGE

Overdosage with valproate may result in somnolence, heart block, and deep coma. Fatalities have been reported.

The benefit of gastric lavage or emesis will vary with the time since ingestion. General supportive measures should be applied with particular attention to the maintenance of adequate urinary output.

Naloxone has been reported to reverse the CNS depressant effects of valproate overdosage. Because naloxone could theoretically also reverse the antiepileptic effects of valproate, it should be used with caution.

DOSAGE AND ADMINISTRATION

Divalproex Sodium tablets and Sprinkle capsules are administered orally. The recommended initial dose is 15 mg/kg/day, increasing at one week intervals by 5 to 10 mg/kg/day until seizures are controlled or side effects preclude further increases. The maximum recommended dosage is 60 mg/kg/day. If the total daily dose exceeds 250 mg, it should be given in a divided regimen.

Administration of Sprinkle Capsule: Divalproex Sodium Sprinkle capsules may be swallowed whole or may be administered by carefully opening the capsule and sprinkling the entire contents on a small amount (teaspoonful) of soft food such as applesauce or pudding. The drug/food mixture should be swallowed immediately (avoid chewing) and not stored for future use. Each capsule is oversized to allow ease of opening.

Conversion from Divalproex Sodium to Divalproex Sodium: In patients previously receiving Divalproex Sodium (valproic acid) therapy, Divalproex Sodium products should be initiated at the same daily dose and dosing schedule. After the patient is stabilized on a Divalproex Sodium product, a dosing schedule of two or three times a day may be elected in selected patients.[5]

Divalproex Sodium products provide equal extents of absorption, although they may not produce identical trough and peak valproate concentrations. Divalproex Sodium tablets produce slightly higher peak concentrations than Divalproex Sodium Sprinkle capsules. Such differences in the maximum and minimum valproate plasma concentrations are unlikely to be of clinical significance; however, changes in dosage administration of valproate or concomitant medications should be accompanied by increased monitoring of plasma concentrations of valproate and other medications, as well as the patient's clinical status.

The frequency of adverse effects (particularly elevated liver enzymes) may be dose-related. The benefit of improved seizure control with higher doses should be weighed against the possibility of a greater incidence of adverse reactions.

A good correlation has not been established between daily dose, serum concentration and therapeutic effect. However, therapeutic valproate serum concentrations for most patients will range from 50 to 100 mcg/mL. Some patients may be controlled with lower or higher serum concentrations (see *"Clinical Pharmacology"*).

As the Divalproex Sodium dosage is titrated upward, blood concentrations of phenobarbital and/or phenytoin may be affected. (See *"Precautions".*)

Patients who experience G. I. irritation may benefit from administration of the drug with food or by slowly building up the dose from an initial low level.

Recommended Storage: Store capsules below 86°F(30°C).

REFERENCES
1. Hurst DL. Expanded therapeutic range of valproate. *Pediatr Neurol.* 1987, 3:342-344. 2. Centers for Disease Control, valproate: a new cause of birth defects—report from Italy and follow-up from France. *Morbidity and Mortality Weekly Report.* 1983; 32(33); 438-439. 3. Mattson RH, et al. Use of oral contraceptives by women with epilepsy. *JAMA.* 1986; 256(2): 238-240. 4. Wilder, BJ, et al. Gastrointestinal tolerance of divalproex sodium. *Neurology.* 1983; 33: 808-811. 5. Wilder BJ, et al. Twice-daily dosing of valproate with divalproex, *Clin Pharmacol Ther.* 1983; 34(4): 501-504.

HOW SUPPLIED
CAPSULE: 125 MG

BRAND/MANUFACTURER	NDC	SIZE	AWP
○ BRAND			
➤ DEPAKOTE SPRINKLES: Abbott Pharm	00074-6114-13	100s	$29.95
	00074-6114-11	100s ud	$33.40

ENTERIC COATED TABLETS: 125 MG

BRAND/MANUFACTURER	NDC	SIZE	AWP
○ BRAND			
➤ DEPAKOTE: Abbott Pharm	00074-6212-13	100s	$29.79
	00074-6212-11	100s ud	$33.23

ENTERIC COATED TABLETS: 250 MG

BRAND/MANUFACTURER	NDC	SIZE	AWP
○ BRAND			
➤ DEPAKOTE: Abbott Pharm	00074-6214-13	100s	$58.49
	00074-6214-11	100s ud	$63.44
	00074-6214-53	500s	$292.43

ENTERIC COATED TABLETS: 500 MG

BRAND/MANUFACTURER	NDC	SIZE	AWP
○ BRAND			
➤ DEPAKOTE: Abbott Pharm	00074-6215-13	100s	$107.88
	00074-6215-11	100s ud	$115.43
	00074-6215-53	500s	$539.36

Dobutamine Hydrochloride

DESCRIPTION

Dobutamine Hydrochloride Injection is 1,2-benzenediol, 4-[2-[[3-(4-hydroxyphenyl)-1-methyl- propyl]amino]ethyl]-, hydrochloride, (±)-. It is a synthetic catecholamine.

The clinical formulation is supplied in a sterile form for intravenous use only. Each mL contains 12.5 mg (41.5 μmol) dobutamine, 0.24 mg sodium bisulfite (added during manufacture), and water for injection, q.s. Hydrochloric acid and/or sodium hydroxide may have been added during manufacture to adjust the pH.

Following is its chemical structure:

$$ HO-\text{(ring)}-HO-(CH_2)_2NHCH\overset{CH_3}{|}CH(CH_2)_2-\text{(ring)}-OH $$

CLINICAL PHARMACOLOGY

Dobutamine Hydrochloride Injection is a direct-acting inotropic agent whose primary activity results from stimulation of the β receptors of the heart while producing comparatively mild chronotropic, hypertensive, arrhythmogenic, and vasodilative effects. It does not cause the release of endogenous norepinephrine, as does dopamine. In animal studies, Dobutamine produces less increase in heart rate and less decrease in peripheral vascular resistance for a given inotropic effect than does isoproterenol.

In patients with depressed cardiac function, both Dobutamine and isoproterenol increase the cardiac output to a similar degree. In the case of Dobutamine, this increase is usually not accompanied by marked increases in heart rate (although tachycardia is occasionally observed), and the cardiac stroke volume is usually increased. In contrast, isoproterenol increases the cardiac index primarily by increasing the heart rate while stroke volume changes little or declines. Facilitation of atrioventricular conduction has been observed in human electrophysiologic studies and in patients with atrial fibrillation.

Systemic vascular resistance is usually decreased with administration of Dobutamine. Occasionally, minimum vasoconstriction has been observed.

Most clinical experience with Dobutamine is short-term—not more than several hours in duration. In the limited number of patients who were studied for 24, 48, and 72 hours, a persistent increase in cardiac output occurred in some, whereas output returned toward baseline values in others.

The onset of action of Dobutamine Hydrochloride is within 1 to 2 minutes; however, as much as 10 minutes may be required to obtain the peak effect of a particular infusion rate.

The plasma half-life of Dobutamine in humans is 2 minutes.

The principal routes of metabolism are methylation of the catechol and conjugation. In human urine, the major excretion products are the conjugates of Dobutamine and 3-O-methyl Dobutamine. The 3-O-methyl derivative of Dobutamine is inactive.

Alteration of synaptic concentrations of catecholamines with either reserpine or tricyclic antidepressants does not alter the actions of Dobutamine in animals, which indicates that the actions of Dobutamine are not dependent on presynaptic mechanisms.

INDICATIONS AND USAGE

Dobutamine Hydrochloride Injection is indicated when parenteral therapy is necessary for inotropic support in the short-term treatment of adults with cardiac decompensation due to depressed contractility resulting either from organic heart disease or from cardiac surgical procedures.

In patients who have atrial fibrillation with rapid ventricular response, a digitalis preparation should be used prior to institution of therapy with Dobutamine Hydrochloride.

CONTRAINDICATIONS

Dobutamine Hydrochloride Injection is contraindicated in patients with idiopathic hypertrophic subaortic stenosis and in patients who have shown previous manifestations of hypersensitivity to Dobutamine Hydrochloride.

WARNINGS

1. Increase in Heart Rate or Blood Pressure: Dobutamine Hydrochloride Injection may cause a marked increase in heart rate or blood pressure, especially systolic pressure. Approximately 10% of patients in clinical studies have had rate increases of 30 beats/minute or more, and about 7.5% have had a 50 mm Hg or greater increase in systolic pressure. Usually, reduction of dosage promptly reverses these effects. Because Dobutamine facilitates atrioventricular conduction, patients with atrial fibrillation are at risk of developing rapid ventricular response. Patients with preexisting hypertension appear to face an increased risk of developing an exaggerated pressor response.

➤ SHOWN IN PRODUCT IDENTIFICATION GUIDE

2. *Ectopic Activity:* Dobutamine Hydrochloride may precipitate or exacerbate ventricular ectopic activity, but it rarely has caused ventricular tachycardia.

3. *Hypersensitivity:* Reactions suggestive of hypersensitivity associated with administration of Dobutamine Hydrochloride including skin rash, fever, eosinophilia, and bronchospasm, have been reported occasionally.

4. Dobutamine Hydrochloride contains sodium bisulfite, a sulfite that may cause allergic-type reactions, including anaphylactic symptoms and life-threatening or less severe asthmatic episodes, in certain susceptible people. The overall prevalence of sulfite sensitivity in the general population is unknown and probably low. Sulfite sensitivity is seen more frequently in asthmatic than in nonasthmatic people.

PRECAUTIONS

1. During the administration of Dobutamine Hydrochloride Injection, as with any adrenergic agent, ECG and blood pressure should be continuously monitored. In addition, pulmonary wedge pressure and cardiac output should be monitored whenever possible to aid in the safe and effective infusion of Dobutamine Hydrochloride.

2. Hypovolemia should be corrected with suitable volume expanders before treatment with Dobutamine Hydrochloride is instituted.

3. Animal studies indicate that Dobutamine may be ineffective if the patient has recently received a β-blocking drug. In such a case, the peripheral vascular resistance may increase.

4. No improvement may be observed in the presence of marked mechanical obstruction, such as severe valvular aortic stenosis.

5. Dobutamine, like other β_2-agonists, can produce a mild reduction in serum potassium concentration, rarely to hypokalemic levels. Accordingly, consideration should be given to monitoring serum potassium.

Usage Following Acute Myocardial Infarction: Clinical experience with Dobutamine Hydrochloride following myocardial infarction has been insufficient to establish the safety of the drug for this use. There is concern that any agent that increases contractile force and heart rate may increase the size of an infarction by intensifying ischemia, but it is not known whether Dobutamine does so.

Usage in Pregnancy: Reproduction studies performed in rats and rabbits have revealed no evidence of impaired fertility, harm to the fetus, or teratogenic effects due to Dobutamine. However, the drug has not been administered to pregnant women and should be used only when the expected benefits clearly outweigh the potential risks to the fetus.

Pediatric Use: The safety and effectiveness of Dobutamine Hydrochloride for use in children have not been studied.

Drug Interaction: There was no evidence of drug interactions in clinical studies in which Dobutamine Hydrochloride was administered concurrently with other drugs, including digitalis preparations, furosemide, spironolactone, lidocaine, glyceryl trinitrate, isosorbide dinitrate, morphine, atropine, heparin, protamine, potassium chloride, folic acid, and acetaminophen. Preliminary studies indicate that the concomitant use of Dobutamine and nitroprusside results in a higher cardiac output and, usually, a lower pulmonary wedge pressure than when either drug is used alone.

ADVERSE REACTIONS

Increased Heart Rate, Blood Pressure, and Ventricular Ectopic Activity: A 10- to 20-mm increase in systolic blood pressure and an increase in heart rate of 5 to 15 beats/minute have been noted in most patients (see Warnings regarding exaggerated chronotropic and pressor effects). Approximately 5% of patients have had increased premature ventricular beats during infusions. These effects are dose related.

Hypotension: Precipitous decreases in blood pressure have occasionally been described in association with Dobutamine therapy. Decreasing the dose or discontinuing the infusion typically results in rapid return of blood pressure to baseline values. In rare cases, however, intervention may be required and reversibility may not be immediate.

Reactions at Sites of Intravenous Infusion: Phlebitis has occasionally been reported. Local inflammatory changes have been described following inadvertent infiltration.

Miscellaneous Uncommon Effects: The following adverse effects have been reported in 1% to 3% of patients: nausea, headache, anginal pain, nonspecific chest pain, palpitations, and shortness of breath.

Administration of Dobutamine Hydrochloride Injection, like other catecholamines, can produce a mild reduction in serum potassium concentration, rarely to hypokalemic levels (see *"Precautions"*).

Longer-Term Safety: Infusions of up to 72 hours have revealed no adverse effects other than those seen with shorter infusions.

OVERDOSAGE

Overdoses of Dobutamine have been reported rarely. The following is provided to serve as a guide if such an overdose is encountered.

Signs and Symptoms: Toxicity from Dobutamine Hydrochloride is usually due to excessive cardiac β-receptor stimulation. The duration of action of Dobutamine Hydrochloride is generally short ($T_{1/2}$ = 2 minutes) because it is rapidly metabolized by catechol-O-methyltransferase. The symptoms of toxicity may include anorexia, nausea, vomiting, tremor, anxiety, palpitations, headache,

shortness of breath, and anginal and nonspecific chest pain. The positive inotropic and chronotropic effects of Dobutamine on the myocardium may cause hypertension, tachyarrhythmias, myocardial ischemia, and ventricular fibrillation. Hypotension may result from vasodilation.

If the product is ingested, unpredictable absorption may occur from the mouth and the gastrointestinal tract.

Treatment: To obtain up-to-date information about the treatment of overdose, a good resource is your certified Regional Poison Control Center. Telephone numbers of certified poison control centers are listed in the *Physicians' Desk Reference (PDR)*. In managing overdosage, consider the possibility of multiple drug overdoses, interaction among drugs, and unusual drug kinetics in your patient.

The initial actions to be taken in a Dobutamine Hydrochloride overdose are discontinuing administration, establishing an airway, and ensuring oxygenation and ventilation. Resuscitative measures should be initiated promptly. Severe ventricular tachyarrhythmias may be successfully treated with propranolol or lidocaine. Hypertension usually responds to a reduction in dose or discontinuation of therapy.

Protect the patient's airway and support ventilation and perfusion. If needed, meticulously monitor and maintain, within acceptable limits, the patient's vital signs, blood gases, serum electrolytes, etc. Absorption of drugs from the gastrointestinal tract may be decreased by giving activated charcoal, which, in many cases, is more effective than emesis or lavage; consider charcoal instead of or in addition to gastric emptying. Repeated doses of charcoal over time may hasten elimination of some drugs that have been absorbed. Safeguard the patient's airway when employing gastric emptying or charcoal.

Forced diuresis, peritoneal dialysis, hemodialysis, or charcoal hemoperfusion have not been established as beneficial for an overdose of Dobutamine Hydrochloride.

DOSAGE AND ADMINISTRATION

Note: Do not add Dobutamine Hydrochloride Injection to 5% Sodium Bicarbonate Injection or to any other strongly alkaline solution. Because of potential physical incompatibilities, it is recommended that Dobutamine Hydrochloride not be mixed with other drugs in the same solution. Dobutamine Hydrochloride should not be used in conjunction with other agents or diluents containing both sodium bisulfite and ethanol.

Reconstitution and Stability: At the time of administration, Dobutamine Hydrochloride must be further diluted in an IV container to at least a 50-mL solution using 1 of the following intravenous solutions as a diluent: 5% Dextrose Injection, 5% Dextrose and 0.45% Sodium Chloride Injection, 5% Dextrose and 0.9% Sodium Chloride Injection, 10% Dextrose Injection, Isolyte® M with 5% Dextrose Injection, Lactated Ringer's Injection, 5% Dextrose in Lactated Ringer's Injection, Normosol® M in D5-W, 20% Osmitrol® in Water for Injection, 0.9% Sodium Chloride Injection, or Sodium Lactate Injection. Intravenous solutions should be used within 24 hours.

Solutions containing Dobutamine Hydrochloride may exhibit a pink color that, if present, will increase with time. This color change is due to slight oxidation of the drug, but there is no significant loss of potency during the reconstitution time period stated above.

Recommended Dosage: The rate of infusion needed to increase cardiac output usually ranged from 2.5 to 10 µg/kg/min (see *"Table"*). On rare occasions, infusion rates up to 40 µg/kg/min have been required to obtain the desired effect.

DOBUTAMINE HYDROCHLORIDE INJECTION—RATES OF INFUSION FOR CONCENTRATIONS OF 250, 500, AND 1,000 µg/ML

Drug Delivery Rate (µg/kg/min)	Infusion Delivery Rate		
	250 µg/mL* (mL/kg/min)	500 µg/mL† (mL/kg/min)	1,000 µg/mL‡ (mL/kg/min)
2.5	0.01	0.005	0.0025
5	0.02	0.01	0.005
7.5	0.03	0.015	0.0075
10	0.04	0.02	0.01
12.5	0.05	0.025	0.0125
15	0.06	0.03	0.015

*   *250 µg/mL of diluent*
†   *500 µg/mL or 250 mg/500 mL of diluent*
‡   *1,000 µg/mL or 250 mg/250 mL of diluent*

The rate of administration and the duration of therapy should be adjusted according to the patient's response as determined by heart rate, presence of ectopic activity, blood pressure, urine flow, and, whenever possible, measurement of central venous or pulmonary wedge pressure and cardiac output.

Concentrations up to 5,000 µg/mL have been administered to humans (250 mg/50 mL). The final volume administered should be determined by the fluid requirements of the patient.

Store at controlled room temperature, 59° to 86°F (15° to 30°C).

◆ RATED THERAPEUTICALLY EQUIVALENT; ◇ THERAPEUTIC EQUIVALENCE UNCONFIRMED; ○ UNRATED

HOW SUPPLIED
INJECTION: 12.5 MG/ML

AVERAGE UNIT PRICE (AVAILABLE SIZES)

BRAND	$2.54
GENERIC	$2.32

BRAND/MANUFACTURER	NDC	SIZE	AWP
◆ BRAND			
DOBUTREX: Lilly	00002-7175-01	20 ml	$50.77
	00002-7175-10	20 ml 10s	$507.75
◆ GENERICS			
Schein	00364-3031-55	20 ml	$43.15
Gensia	00703-1815-03	20 ml 10s	$495.38

INJECTION: 125 MG

BRAND/MANUFACTURER	NDC	SIZE	AWP
◆ GENERICS			
Abbott Hosp	00074-2345-32	250 ml 12s	$696.40

INJECTION: 250 MG

AVERAGE UNIT PRICE (AVAILABLE SIZES)

GENERIC	$1.20

BRAND/MANUFACTURER	NDC	SIZE	AWP
◆ GENERICS			
Abbott Hosp	00074-2344-01	20 ml	$45.26
Abbott Hosp	00074-2344-02	20 ml 10s	$428.09
Abbott Hosp	00074-2346-32	250 ml 12s	$769.79
Abbott Hosp	00074-2345-34	500 ml 12s	$805.36

INJECTION: 500 MG

AVERAGE UNIT PRICE (AVAILABLE SIZES)

GENERIC	$0.36

BRAND/MANUFACTURER	NDC	SIZE	AWP
◆ GENERICS			
Abbott Hosp	00074-2347-32	250 ml 12s	$1423.72
Abbott Hosp	00074-2346-34	500 ml 12s	$1460.48

Dobutrex SEE DOBUTAMINE HYDROCHLORIDE

Dolobid SEE DIFLUNISAL

Dolophine HCl SEE METHADONE HYDROCHLORIDE

Domeboro SEE ACETIC ACID, OTIC

Donnatal SEE BELLADONNA AND PHENOBARBITAL

Donnazyme SEE PANCRELIPASE

Dopamine Hydrochloride

DESCRIPTION
Dopamine Hydrochloride (Dopamine HCl) injection, USP is a clear, practically colorless, aqueous, additive solution for intravenous infusion after dilution. Each mL contains either 40 mg, 80 mg, or 160 mg Dopamine HCl, USP (equivalent to 32.3 mg, 64.6 mg and 129.2 mg Dopamine base, respectively) in Water for Injection, USP containing 1% sodium metabisulfite, NF as an antioxidant. Hydrochloric acid or sodium hydroxide added to adjust pH when necessary. The solution is sterile and nonpyrogenic. The pH is 2.5-5. Dopamine HCl, a naturally occurring catecholamine, is an inotropic vasopressor agent. Its chemical name is 3,4-dihydroxyphenethylamine hydrochloride. The molecular weight is 189.65.

Dopamine HCl is sensitive to alkalis, iron salts and oxidizing agents **Dopamine HCl must be diluted in an appropriate, sterile parenteral solution (see "Dosage And Administration" section) before intravenous administration.**

Following is its chemical structure:

$$HO - \text{(benzene ring)} - CH_2CH_2NH_2 \cdot HCl$$

CLINICAL PHARMACOLOGY
Dopamine is a natural catecholamine formed by the decarboxylation of 3,4-dihydroxyphenylalanine (DOPA). It is a precursor to norepinephrine in noradrenergic nerves and is also a neurotransmitter in certain areas of the central nervous system, especially in the nigrostriatal tract, and in a few peripheral sympathetic nerves.

Dopamine produces positive chronotropic and inotropic effects on the myocardium, resulting in increased heart rate and cardiac contractility. This is accomplished directly by exerting an agonist action on beta-adrenoceptors and indirectly by causing release of norepinephrine from storage sites in sympathetic nerve endings.

Dopamine's onset of action occurs within five minutes of intravenous administration, and with Dopamine's plasma half-life of about two minutes, the duration of action is less than ten minutes. If monoamine oxidase (MAO) inhibitors are present, however, the duration may increase to one hour. The drug is widely distributed in the body but does not cross the blood-brain barrier to a significant extent. Dopamine is metabolized in the liver, kidney, and plasma by MAO and catechol-O-methyltransferase to the inactive compounds homovanillic acid (HVA) and 3,4-dihydroxyphenylacetic acid. About 25% of the dose is taken up into specialized neurosecretory vesicles (the adrenergic nerve terminals), where it is hydroxylated to form norepinephrine. It has been reported that about 80% of the drug is excreted in the urine within 24 hours, primarily as HVA and its sulfate and glucuronide conjugates and as 3,4-dihydroxyphenylacetic acid. A very small portion is excreted unchanged.

The predominant effects of Dopamine are dose-related, although actual response of an individual patient will largely depend on the clinical status of the patient at the time the drug is administered. At low rates of infusion (0.5-2 mcg/kg/min) Dopamine causes vasodilation that is presumed to be due to a specific agonist action on Dopamine receptors (distinct from alpha- and beta-adrenoceptors) in the renal, mesenteric, coronary, and intracerebral vascular beds. At these Dopamine receptors, haloperidol is an antagonist. The vasodilation in these vascular beds is accompanied by increased glomerular filtration rate, renal blood flow, sodium excretion, and urine flow. Hypotension sometimes occurs. An increase in urinary output produced by Dopamine is usually not associated with a decrease in osmolarity of the urine.

At intermediate rates of infusion (2-10 mcg/kg/min) Dopamine acts to stimulate the beta$_1$-adrenoceptors, resulting in improved myocardial contractility, increased SA rate and enhanced impulse conduction in the heart. There is little, if any, stimulation of the beta$_2$-adrenoceptors (peripheral vasodilation). Dopamine causes less increase in myocardial oxygen consumption than isoproterenol, and its use is not usually associated with a tachyarrhythmia. Clinical studies indicate that it usually increases systolic and pulse pressure with either no effect or a slight increase in diastolic pressure. Blood flow to the peripheral vascular beds may decrease while mesenteric flow increases due to increased cardiac output. At low and intermediate doses, total peripheral resistance (which would be raised by alpha activity) is usually unchanged.

At higher rates of infusion (10-20 mcg/kg/min) there is some effect on alpha-adrenoceptors, with consequent vasoconstrictor effects and a rise in blood pressure. The vasoconstrictor effects are first seen in the skeletal muscle vascular beds, but with increasing doses they are also evident in the renal and mesenteric vessels. At very high rates of infusion (above 20 mcg/kg/min), stimulation of alpha-adrenoceptors predominates and vasoconstriction may compromise the circulation of the limbs and override the Dopaminergic effects of Dopamine, reversing renal dilation and natriuresis.

INDICATIONS
Dopamine HCl injection, is indicated for the correction of hemodynamic imbalances present in the shock syndrome due to myocardial infarctions, trauma, endotoxic septicemia, open heart surgery, renal failure, and chronic cardiac decompensation as in congestive failure. Where appropriate, restoration of blood volume with a suitable plasma expander or whole blood should be instituted or completed prior to administration of Dopamine HCl.

Patients most likely to respond adequately to Dopamine HCl are those in whom physiological parameters, such as urine flow, myocardial function, and blood pressure, have not undergone profound deterioration. Multiclinic trials indicate that the shorter the time interval between onset of signs and symptoms and initiation of therapy with volume correction and Dopamine HCl, the better the prognosis.

Poor Perfusion of Vital Organs: Urine flow appears to be one of the better diagnostic signs by which adequacy of vital organ perfusion can be monitored. Nevertheless, the physician should also observe the patient for signs of reversal of confusion or comatose condition. Loss of pallor, increase in toe temperature, and/or adequacy of nail bed capillary filling may also be used as indices of adequate dosage. Clinical studies have shown that when Dopamine HCl is administered before urine flow has diminished to levels approximating 0.3 mL/minute, prognosis is more favorable. Nevertheless, in a number of oliguric or anuric patients, administration of Dopamine HCl has resulted in an increase in urine flow which in some cases reached normal levels Dopamine HCl may also increase urine flow in patients whose output is within normal limits and thus may be of value in reducing the degree of preexisting fluid accumulation. It should be noted that at doses above those optimal for the individual patient, urine flow may decrease, necessitating reduction of dosage. Concurrent administration of Dopamine HCl and diuretic agents may produce an additive or potentiating effect.

Low Cardiac Output: Increased cardiac output is related to the direct inotropic effect of Dopamine HCl on the myocardium. Increased cardiac output at low or moderate doses appears to be related to a favorable prognosis. Increase in cardiac output has been associated with either static or decreased systemic vascular resistance (SVR). Static or decreased SVR associated with low or moderate increments in cardiac output is believed to be a reflection of differential effects on specific vascular beds with increased resistance in peripheral beds (e.g., femoral) and concomitant decreases in mesenteric and renal vascular beds. Redistribution of blood flow parallels these changes so that an increase in cardiac output is accompanied by an increase in mesenteric and renal blood flow. In many instances the renal fraction of the total cardiac output has been found to increase. The increase in cardiac output produced by Dopamine HCl is not associated with substantial decreases in systemic vascular resistance as may occur with isoproterenol.

Hypotension: Hypotension due to inadequate cardiac output can be managed by administration of low to moderate doses of Dopamine HCl, which have little effect on SVR. At high therapeutic doses, the alpha adrenergic activity of Dopamine HCl becomes more prominent and thus may correct hypotension due to diminished SVR. As in the case of other circulatory decompensation states, prognosis is better in patients whose blood pressure and urine flow have not undergone profound deterioration. Therefore, it is suggested that the physician administer Dopamine HCl as soon as a definite trend toward decreased systolic and diastolic pressure becomes evident.

CONTRAINDICATIONS

Dopamine HCl should not be used in patients with pheochromocytoma.

WARNINGS

Dopamine HCl should not be administered in the presence of uncorrected tachyarrhythmias or ventricular fibrillation. Do *Not* add Dopamine HCl to any alkaline diluent solution, since the drug is inactivated in alkaline solution.

Patients who have been treated with monoamine oxidase (MAO) inhibitors prior to the administration of Dopamine HCl will require substantially reduced dosage. Dopamine is metabolized by MAO, and inhibition of this enzyme prolongs and potentiates the effect of Dopamine HCl. The starting dose in such patients should be reduced to at least one-tenth ($^1/_{10}$) of the usual dose.

Contains sodium metabisulfite, a sulfite that may cause allergic-type reactions including anaphylactic symptoms and life-threatening or less severe asthmatic episodes in certain susceptible people. The overall prevalence of sulfite sensitivity in the general population is unknown, and probably low. Sulfite sensitivity is seen more frequently in asthmatic than in nonasthmatic people.

PRECAUTIONS:

GENERAL

Careful Monitoring Required: Close monitoring of the following indices—urine flow, cardiac output and blood pressure during Dopamine HCl infusion is necessary as in the case of any adrenergic agent.

Avoid Hypovolemia: Prior to treatment with Dopamine HCl, hypovolemia should be fully corrected, if possible, with either whole blood or plasma as indicated.

Decreased Pulse Pressure: If a disproportionate rise in the diastolic pressure (i.e., a marked decrease in the pulse pressure) is observed in patients receiving Dopamine HCl injection, the infusion rate should be decreased and the patient observed carefully for further evidence of predominant vasoconstrictor activity, unless such an effect is desired.

Extravasation: Dopamine HCl should be infused into a large vein whenever possible to prevent the possibility of extravensation into tissue adjacent to the infusion site. Extravasation may cause necrosis and sloughing of surrounding tissue. Large veins of the antecubital fossa are preferred to veins in the dorsum of the hand or ankle. Less suitable infusion sites should be used only if the patient's condition requires immediate attention. The physician should switch to more suitable sites as rapidly as possible. The infusion site should be continuously monitored for free flow.

Occlusive Vascular Disease: Patients with a history of occlusive vascular disease (for example, atherosclerosis, arterial embolism, Raynaud's disease, cold injury, diabetic endarteritis, and Buerger's disease) should be closely monitored for any changes in color or temperature of the skin in the extremities. If a change in skin color or temperature occurs and is thought to be the result of compromised circulation to the extremities, the benefits of continued Dopamine HCl infusion should be weighed against the risk of possible necrosis. This condition may be reversed by either decreasing or discontinuing the rate of infusion.

IMPORTANT—ANTIDOTE FOR PERIPHERAL ISCHEMIA: TO PREVENT SLOUGHING AND NECROSIS IN ISCHEMIC AREAS, THE AREA SHOULD BE INFILTRATED AS SOON AS POSSIBLE WITH 10 TO 15 mL OF SALINE SOLUTION CONTAINING FROM 5 TO 10 mg OF REGITINE® (BRAND OF PHENTOLAMINE), AN ADRENERGIC BLOCKING AGENT. A SYRINGE WITH A FINE HYPODERMIC NEEDLE SHOULD BE USED, AND THE SOLUTION LIBERALLY INFILTRATED THROUGHOUT THE ISCHEMIC AREA. SYMPATHETIC BLOCKADE WITH PHENTOLAMINE CAUSES IMMEDIATE AND CONSPICUOUS LOCAL HYPEREMIC CHANGES IF THE AREA IS INFILTRATED WITHIN 12 HOURS. THEREFORE, PHENTOLAMINE SHOULD BE GIVEN AS SOON AS POSSIBLE AFTER THE EXTRAVASATION IS NOTED.

DRUG INTERACTIONS

Avoid cyclopropane or halogenated hydrocarbon anesthetics: Cyclopropane or halogenated hydrocarbon anesthetics increase cardiac autonomic irritability and therefore may sensitize the myocardium to the action of certain intravenously administered catecholamines. This interaction appears to be related both to pressor activity and to beta adrenergic stimulating properties of these catecholamines. Therefore, as with certain other catecholamines, and because of the theoretical arrhythmogenic potential, Dopamine HCl should be used with *EXTREME CAUTION* in patients inhaling cyclopropane or halogenated hydrocarbon anesthetics.

Carcinogenesis, Mutagenesis, Impairment of Fertility: Longterm studies in animals have not been performed to evaluate carcinogenic potential.

Pregnancy—Pregnancy Category C: Animal studies have revealed no evidence of teratogenic effects from Dopamine HCl. In one study, administration of Dopamine HCl to pregnant rats resulted in a decreased survival rate of the newborn and a potential for cataract formation in the survivors. There are no adequate and well-controlled studies in pregnant women. Dopamine HCl should be used during pregnancy only if the potential benefit justifies the potential risk to the fetus.

Labor and Delivery: Information on labor and delivery is unknown.

Nursing Mothers: It is not known whether this drug is excreted in human milk. Because many drugs are excreted in human milk, caution should be exercised when Dopamine HCl is administered to a nursing mother.

Pediatric Use: Safety and effectiveness in children have not been established. However, peripheral gangrene has been reported in neonates and children.

ADVERSE REACTIONS

The most frequent adverse reactions observed in clinical evaluation of Dopamine HCl included ectopic beats, nausea, vomiting, tachycardia, anginal pain, palpitation, dyspnea, headache, hypotension, and vasoconstriction. Other adverse reactions which have been reported infrequently were aberrant conduction, bradycardia, piloerection, widened QRS complex, azotemia, and elevated blood pressure.

OVERDOSAGE

In case of accidental overdosage, as evidenced by excessive blood pressure elevation, reduce rate of administration or temporarily discontinue Dopamine HCl until patient's condition stabilizes. Since the duration of action of Dopamine HCl is quite short, no additional remedial measures are usually necessary. If these measures fail to stabilize the patient's condition, use of the short-acting alpha adrenergic blocking agent, phentolamine, should be considered.

DOSAGE AND ADMINISTRATION

Warning: This is a potent drug: It must be diluted before administration to patient.

Suggested Dilution: Transfer contents of one or more ampuls or vials by aseptic technique to either a 250 mL or 500 mL bottle of one of the following sterile intravenous solutions:

1) Sodium Chloride Injection, USP
2) Dextrose (5%) Injection, USP
3) Dextrose (5%) and Sodium Chloride (0.9%) Injection, USP
4) 5% Dextrose in 0.45% Sodium Chloride Solution
5) Dextrose (5%) in Lactated Ringer's Solution
6) Sodium Lactate ($^1/_6$ Molar) Injection, USP
7) Lactated Ringer's Injection, USP

◆ RATED THERAPEUTICALLY EQUIVALENT; ◇ THERAPEUTIC EQUIVALENCE UNCONFIRMED; ○ UNRATED

Dopamine HCl injection, has been found to be stable for a minimum of 24 hours after dilution in the sterile intravenous solutions listed above. However, as with all intravenous admixtures, dilution should be made just prior to administration.

Do *Not* add Dopamine HCl Injection to Sodium Bicarbonate or other alkaline intravenous solutions, since the drug is inactivated in alkaline solution.

Rate of Administration: Dopamine HCl after dilution, is administered intravenously through a suitable intravenous catheter or needle. An IV drip chamber or other suitable metering device is essential for controlling the rate of flow in drops/minute. Each patient must be individually titrated to the desired hemodynamic and/or renal response with Dopamine HCl. In titrating to the desired increase in systolic blood pressure, the optimum dosage rate for renal response may be exceeded, thus necessitating a reduction in rate after the hemodynamic condition is stabilized.

Administration at rates greater than 50 mcg/kg/minute have safely been used in advanced circulatory decompensation states. If unnecessary fluid expansion is of concern, adjustment of drug concentration may be preferred over increasing the flow rate of a less concentrated dilution.

SUGGESTED REGIMEN

1. When appropriate, increase blood volume with whole blood or plasma until central venous pressure is 10 to 15 cm H_2O or pulmonary wedge pressure is 14-18 mm Hg.

2. Begin administration of diluted solution at doses of 2-5 mcg/kg/minute Dopamine HCl in patients who are likely to respond to modest increments of heart force and renal perfusion.

In more seriously ill patients, begin administration of diluted solution at doses of 5 mcg/kg/minute Dopamine HCl and increase gradually using 5 to 10 mcg/kg/minute increments, up to 20 to 50 mcg/kg/minute as needed. If doses of Dopamine HCl in excess of 50 mcg/kg/minute are required, it is suggested that urine output be checked frequently. Should urine flow begin to decrease in the absence of hypotension, reduction of Dopamine HCl dosage should be considered. Multiclinic trials have shown that more than 50% of the patients were satisfactorily maintained on doses of Dopamine HCl less than 20 mcg/kg/minute. In patients who do not respond to these doses with adequate arterial pressures or urine flow, additional increments of Dopamine HCl may be employed in an effort to produce an appropriate arterial pressure and central perfusion.

3. Treatment of all patients requires constant evaluation of therapy in terms of the blood volume, augmentation of myocardial contractility, and distribution of peripheral perfusion. Dosage of Dopamine HCl should be adjusted according to the patient's response, with particular attention to diminution of established urine flow rate, increasing tachycardia or development of new dysrhythmias as indices for decreasing or temporarily suspending the dosage.

4. As with all potent intravenously administered drugs, care should be taken to control the rate of administration so as to avoid inadvertent administration of a bolus of drug.

Store at controlled room temperature 15°-30°C (59°-86°F). WARNING: NOT FOR DIRECT INTRAVENOUS INJECTION. MUST BE DILUTED BEFORE USE.

HOW SUPPLIED
INJECTION: 40 MG/ML

AVERAGE UNIT PRICE (AVAILABLE SIZES)		GENERIC A-RATED AVERAGE PRICE (GAAP)	
GENERIC	$1.31	5 ml 20s	$60.63
		5 ml 25s	$96.72
		10 ml 25s	$479.78

BRAND/MANUFACTURER	NDC	SIZE	AWP
◆ GENERICS			
Abbott Hosp	00074-5819-01	5 ml 5s	$64.13
Abbott Hosp	00074-9105-01	10 ml 5s	$118.69
Astra	00186-0638-01	5 ml 10s	$75.00
Astra	00186-0639-01	10 ml 10s	$154.00
INTROPIN: Du Pont Multi	00590-0040-05	5 ml 20s	$60.00
INTROPIN: Du Pont Multi	00590-0040-06	5 ml 20s	$61.25
Elkins-Sinn	00641-1416-35	5 ml 25s	$37.50
Elkins-Sinn	00641-0112-25	5 ml 25s	$48.13
Amer Regent	00517-1805-25	5 ml 25s	$54.69
Solo Pak	39769-0009-05	5 ml 25s	$73.44
Abbott Hosp	00074-5820-10	5 ml 25s	$269.86
Intl Med Sys	00548-6137-00	10 ml 25s	$424.88
Abbott Hosp	00074-9104-20	10 ml 25s	$534.67
Intl Med Sys	00548-6135-00	20 ml 25s	$705.00

INJECTION: 80 MG/ML

AVERAGE UNIT PRICE (AVAILABLE SIZES)		GENERIC A-RATED AVERAGE PRICE (GAAP)	
GENERIC	$1.78	5 ml 25s	$103.52
		10 ml 25s	$906.36

BRAND/MANUFACTURER	NDC	SIZE	AWP
◆ GENERICS			
Astra	00186-0641-01	5 ml 10s	$125.00
INTROPIN: Du Pont Multi	00590-0046-06	5 ml 20s	$120.00
Elkins-Sinn	00641-1413-35	5 ml 25s	$75.00
Elkins-Sinn	00641-0114-25	5 ml 25s	$96.25
Amer Regent	00517-1905-25	5 ml 25s	$102.19
Solo Pak	39769-0010-05	5 ml 25s	$140.63
Abbott Hosp	00074-4265-01	10 ml 25s	$862.42
Abbott Hosp	00074-4266-01	10 ml 25s	$950.30

INJECTION: 160 MG/ML

AVERAGE UNIT PRICE (AVAILABLE SIZES)	
GENERIC	$2.40

BRAND/MANUFACTURER	NDC	SIZE	AWP
◆ GENERICS			
Astra	00186-0642-01	5 ml 10s	$165.38
INTROPIN: Du Pont Multi	00590-0047-06	5 ml 20s	$225.00
Amer Regent	00517-1305-25	5 ml 25s	$203.44

Dopar SEE LEVODOPA

Dopram SEE DOXAPRAM HYDROCHLORIDE

Doral SEE QUAZEPAM

Dornase Alfa

DESCRIPTION

Dornase Alfa inhalation solution is a sterile, clear, colorless, highly purified solution of recombinant human deoxyribonuclease I (rhDNase), an enzyme which selectively cleaves DNA. The protein is produced by genetically engineered Chinese Hamster Ovary (CHO) cells containing DNA encoding for the native human protein, deoxyribonuclease I (DNase). The product is purified by tangential flow filtration and column chromatography. The purified glycoprotein contains 260 amino acids with an approximate molecular weight of 37,000 daltons (1). The primary amino acid sequence is identical to that of the native human enzyme.

Dornase Alfa is administered by inhalation of an aerosol mist produced by a compressed air driven nebulizer system (see *"Clinical Experience;" "Dosage and Administration"*). Each Dornase Alfa single-use ampule will deliver 2.5 mL of the solution to the nebulizer bowl.

Each ml of aqueous solution contains:

Dornase Alfa ....1.0 mg

The nominal pH of the solution is 6.3.

CLINICAL PHARMACOLOGY

GENERAL

In cystic fibrosis (CF) patients, retention of viscous purulent secretions in the airways contributes both to reduced pulmonary function and to exacerbations of infection (2,3).

Purulent pulmonary secretions contain very high concentrations of extracellular DNA released by degenerating leukocytes that accumulate in response to infection (4). In vitro, Dornase Alfa hydrolyzes the DNA in sputum of CF patients and reduces sputum viscoelasticity (1).

PHARMACOKINETICS

When 2.5 mg Dornase Alfa was administered by inhalation to eighteen CF patients, mean sputum concentrations of 3 µ/mL DNase were measurable within 15 minutes. Mean sputum concentrations declined to an average of 0.6 µ/mL two hours following inhalation. Inhalation of up to 10 mg TID of Dornase Alfa by 4 CF patients for six consecutive days, did not result in a significant elevation of serum concentrations of DNase above normal endogenous levels (5,6). After administration of up to 2.5 mg of Dornase Alfa twice daily for six months to 321 CF patients, no accumulation of serum DNase was noted.

CLINICAL EXPERIENCE

Dornase Alfa has been evaluated in a large, randomized, placebo-controlled trial of clinically stable cystic fibrosis patients, 5 years of age and older, with baseline forced vital capacity (FVC) greater than or equal to 40% of predicted and receiving standard therapies for cystic fibrosis (7). Patients were treated with placebo (325 patients), 2.5 mg of Dornase Alfa once a day (321 patients), or 2.5 mg of Dornase Alfa twice a day (321 patients) for six months administered via a Hudson T Up-draft II nebulizer with a Pulmo-Aide compressor.

Both doses of Dornase Alfa resulted in significant reductions compared with the placebo group in the number of patients experiencing respiratory tract infections requiring use of parenteral antibiotics. Administration of Dornade Alfa reduced the relative risk of developing a respiratory tract infection by 27% and 29% for the 2.5 mg daily dose and the 2.5 mg twice daily dose, respectively (see Table 1). The data suggest that the effects of Dornase Alfa on respiratory tract infections in older patients (> 21 years) may be smaller than in younger patients, and that twice daily dosing may be required in the older patients. Patients with baseline FVC > 85% may also benefit from twice a day dosing (see Table 1). The reduced risk of respiratory infection observed in Dornase Alfa treated patients did not directly correlate with improvement in FEV_1 during the initial two weeks of therapy.

Within 8 days of the start of treatment with Dornase Alfa, mean FEV_1 increased 7.9% in those treated once a day and 9.0% in those treated twice a day compared to the baseline values. The mean FEV_1 observed during long-term therapy increased 5.8% from baseline at the 2.5 mg daily dose level and 5.6% from baseline at the 2.5 mg twice daily dose level. Placebo recipients did not show significant mean changes in pulmonary function testing (see Figure 1).

For patients 5 years of age or older, with baseline FVC greater than or equal to 40%, administration of Dornase Alfa decreased the incidence of occurrence of first respiratory tract infection requiring parenteral antibiotics, and improved mean FEV_1, regardless of age or baseline FVC.

Table 1

INCIDENCE OF FIRST RESPIRATORY TRACT INFECTION REQUIRING PARENTERAL ANTIBIOTICS IN A CONTROLLED TRIAL

	Placebo *N = 325*	*2.5 mg QD* *N = 322*	*2.5 mg BID* *N = 321*
Percent of Patients			
Infected	43%	34%	33%
Relative Risk (vs placebo)		0.73	0.71
p-value (vs placebo)		0.015	0.007
Subgroup by Age and *Baseline FVC*	*Placebo* *(N)*	*2.5 mg QD* *(N)*	*2.5 mg BID* *(N)*
Age			
5-20 years	42% (201)	25% (199)	28% (184)
21 years and older	44% (124)	48% (123)	39% (137)
Baseline FVC			
40-85% Predicted	54% (194)	41% (201)	44% (203)
> 85% Predicted	27% (131)	21% (121)	14% (118)

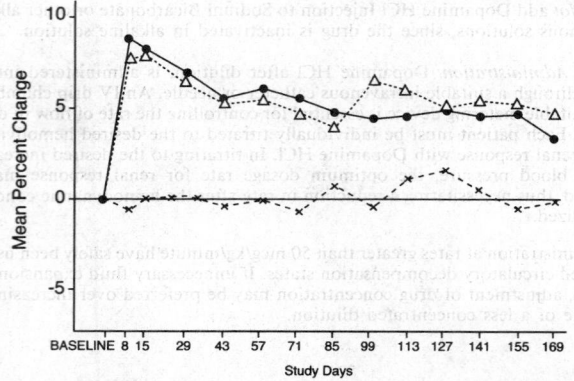

Figure 1

MEAN PERCENT CHANGE FROM BASELINE FEV₁ IN A CONTROLLED TRIAL

Treatment: x······· Placebo   △--- rhNDase 2.5 mg QD   ●— rhNDase 2.5 mg BID

OTHER STUDIES

Dornase Alfa did not produce a pulmonary function benefit in short-term usage in patients with FVC less than 40% of predicted. Studies are in progress to assess the impact of chronic use on pulmonary function and infection risk in this population.

Clinical trials have indicated that Dornase Alfa therapy can be continued or initiated during an acute respiratory exacerbation.

Short-term dose ranging studies demonstrated that doses in excess of 2.5 mg BID did not provide further improvement in FEV_1. Patients who have received drug on a cyclical regimen (ie, administration of Dornase Alfa 10 mg BID for 14 days, followed by a 14 day wash out period) showed rapid improvement in FEV_1 with the initiation of each cycle and a return to baseline with each Dornase Alfa withdrawal.

INDICATIONS AND USAGE

Daily administration of Dornase Alfa in conjunction with standard therapies is indicated in the management of cystic fibrosis patients to reduce the frequency of respiratory infections requiring parenteral antibiotics and to improve pulmonary function. Safety and efficacy of daily administration have not been demonstrated in patients under the age of 5 years, or with FVC < 40% of predicted, or for longer than twelve months.

CONTRAINDICATIONS

Dornase Alfa is contraindicated in patients with known hypersensitivity to it, to. Chinese Hamster Ovary cell products, or to any component of the product.

WARNINGS

None.

PRECAUTIONS

GENERAL

Dornase Alfa should be used in conjunction with standard therapies for CF.

INFORMATION FOR PATIENTS

Dornase Alfa must be stored in the refrigerator at 2-8 °C (36-46 °F) and protected from strong light. It should be kept refrigerated during transport and should not be exposed to room temperatures for a total time of 24 hours. The solution should be discarded if it is cloudy or discolored. Some brands contain no preservative and, once opened, the entire ampule must be used or discarded. Patients should be instructed in the proper use and maintenance of th enebulizer and compressor system used in its delivery.

Dornase Alfa should not be diluted or mixed with other drugs in the nebulizer. Mixing of Dornase Alfa with other drugs could lead to adverse physicochemical and/or functional changes in Dornase Alfa or the admixed compound.

DRUG INTERACTIONS

Clinical trials have indicated that Dornase Alfa can be effectively and safely used to in conjunction with standard cystic fibrosis therapies including oral, inhaled and parenteral antibiotics, bronchodilators, enzyme supplements, vitamins, oral and inhaled corticosteroids, and analgesics. No formal drug interaction studies have been performed.

CARCINOGENESIS, MUTAGENESIS, IMPAIRMENT OF FERTILITY

Carcinogenesis: A two year inhalation (head-only) toxicity study of Dornase Alfa in rats to assess oncogenic potential is in progress.

Mutagenesis: Ames tests using six different tester strains of bacteria (4 of S. typhimurium and 2 of E. coli) at concentrations up to 5000 µg/plate, a cytogenetic assay using human peripheral blood lymphocytes at concentrations up to 2000 µg/plate, and a mouse lymphocytes at concentrations up to 1000 µg/plate, with and without metabolic activation, revealed no evidence of mutagenesis potential. Dornase Alfa was tested in a micronucleus (in vivo) assay for its potential to produce chromosome damage in bone marrow cells of mice following a bolus intravenous dose of 10 mg/kg on two consecutive days. No evidence of chromosomal damage was noted.

Impairment of Fertility: In studies with rats receiving up to 10 mg/kg/day, a dose representing systemic exposures greater than 600 times that expected following the recommended human dose, fertility and reproductive performance of both males and females was not affected.

PREGNANCY (CATEGORY B)

Reproduction studies have been performed in rats and rabbits with intravenous doses up to 10 mg/kg/day, representing systemic exposures greater than 600 times that expected following the recommended human dose. These studies have revealed no evidence of impaired fertility, harm to the fetus or effects on development due to Dornase Alfa. There are, however, no adequate and well-controlled studies in pregnant women. Because animal reproductive studies are not always predictive of the human response, this drug should be used during pregnancy only if clearly needed.

NURSING MOTHERS

It is not known whether the drug is excreted in human milk. Because many drugs are excreted in human milk, caution should be exercised when Dornase Alfa is administered to a nursing woman.

PEDIATRIC USE

Safety and effectiveness of Dornase Alfa in children under the age of 5 years has not been studied.

ADVERSE REACTIONS

Patients have been exposed to Dornase Alfa for up to 12 months in clinical trials. In a large, randomized, placebo-controlled clinical trial, over 600 patients received once or twice daily for six months; most adverse events were not more common on Dornase Alfa than on placebo and probably reflected the sequelae of the underlying lung disease. In most cases events that were increased were mild, transient in nature, and did not require alterations in dosing. Few patients experienced adverse events resulting in permanent discontinuation from Dornase Alfa, and the discontinuation rate was similar for placebo (2%) and Dornase Alfa (3%).

Events that were more frequent in Dornase Alfa treated patients than in placebo treated patients are listed in Table 2.

Table 2
ADVERSE EVENTS REPORTED IN A CONTROLLED TRIAL

Adverse Event	Placebo n = 325	Dornase Alfa QD n = 322	Dornase Alfa BID n = 321
Voice alteration	7%	12%	16%
Pharyngitis	33%	36%	40%
Laryngitis	1%	3%	4%
Rash	7%	10%	12%
Chest pain	16%	18%	21%
Conjunctivitis	2%	4%	5%

EVENTS OBSERVED AT SIMILAR RATES IN DORNASE ALFA AND PLACEBO TREATED PATIENTS

Body as a Whole: Abdominal pain, Asthenia, Fever, Flu syndrome, Malaise, Sepsis.

Digestive System: Intestinal Obstruction, Gall Bladder disease, Liver disease, Pancreatic disease.

Metabolic Nutritional: Diabetes Mellitus, Hypoxia.

System: Weight Loss.

Respiratory System: Apnea, Bronchiectasia, Bronchitis, Change in Sputum, Cough Increase, Dyspnea, Hemoptysis, Lung Function Decrease, Nasal Polyps, Pneumonia, Pneumothorax, Rhinitis, Sinusitis, Sputum Increase, Wheeze

Mortality rates observed in a controlled trial were similar for the placebo (1%) and Dornase Alfa (1%). Causes of death were consistent with progression of cystic fibrosis and included apnea, cardiac arrest, cardiopulmonary arrest, cor pulmonale, heart failure, massive hemoptysis, pneumonia, pneumothorax, and respiratory failure.

ALLERGIC REACTIONS

There have been no reports of anaphylaxis attributed to the administration of Dornase Alfa date. Skin rash and urticaria have been observed, and were mild and transient in nature. Within all of the studies, a small percentage (average of 2-4%) of patients treated with Dornase Alfa developed serum antibodies to Dornase Alfa. None of these patients developed anaphylaxis, and the clinical significance of serum antibodies to Dornase Alfa is unknown.

OVERDOSAGE

Single-dose inhalation studies in rats and monkeys at doses up to 180-times higher than doses routinely used in clinical studies are well tolerated. Single dose oral administration of Dornase Alfa in doses up to 200 mg/kg are also well tolerated by rats.

Cystic fibrosis patients have received up to 20 mg BID for up to 6 days and 10 mg BID intermittently (2 weeks on/2 weeks off drug) for 168 days. These doses were well tolerated.

DOSAGE AND ADMINISTRATION

The recommended dose for use in most cystic fibrosis patients is one 2.5 mg single-use ampule inhaled once daily using a recommended nebulizer. Some patients may benefit from twice daily administration (see Clinical Experience, Table 1). Clinical trials have been performed with the following nebulizers and compressors the disposable jet nebulizer Hudson T Up-draft II and disposable jet nebulizer Marquest Acorn II in conjunction with a Pulmo-Aide compressor, and the reusable PARI LC Jet⁺ nebulizer, in conjunction with the PARI PRONEB compressor. Safety and efficacy have been demonstrated only with these recommended nebulizer systems. No clinical data are currently available that support the safety and efficacy of administration of Dornase Alfa with other nebulizer systems. The patient should follow the manufacturer's instructions on the use and maintenance of the equipment.

Dornase Alfa should not be diluted or mixed with other drugs in the nebulizer. Mixing of Dornase Alfa with other drugs could lead to adverse physicochemical and/or functional changes in Dornase Alfa or the admixed compound.

Dornase Alfa should be stored under refrigeration (2-8°C/36-46°F). Ampules should be protected from light. Do not use beyond the expiration date stamped on the ampule. Unused ampules should be stored in their protective foil pouch under refrigeration.

REFERENCES

1. Shak S, Capon DJ, Hellmiss R, Marsters SA, Baker CL. Recombinant human DNase 1 reduces the viscosity of cystic fibrosis sputum. Proc Natl Acad Sci USA 1990; 87:9188-92. 2. Boat TF. Cystic Fibrosis, In: Murray JF, Nadel JA, editors. Textbook of respiratory medicine, Philadelphia: Saunders WB, 1988;1:1126-52. 3. Collins FS. Cystic Fibrosis: molecular biology and therapeutic implications. Science 1992;256:774-9. 4. Potter JL, Spector S, Matthews LW, Lemm J. Studies of pulmonary secretions. Amer Rev of Respiratory Disease 1969;99;909-15. 5. Hubbard RC, McElvaney NG, Birrer P, Shak S, Robinson WW, Jolley C, et al. A preliminary study of aerosolized recombinant human deoxyribonuclease I in the treatment of cystic fibrosis New Eng J. Med 1992;326:812-5. 6. Aitken ML, Burke W, McDonald G, Shak S, Montgomery AB, Smith A. Recombinant human DNase inhalation in normal subjects and patients with cystic fibrosis. JAMA 1992;267(14):1947-51. 7. Fuchs HJ, Borowitz D, Christianson D, Morris E, Nash M, Ramsey B, et al. Aerosolized recombinant human DNase reduces pulmonary exacerbations and improves pulmonary function in patients with cystic fibrosis. Presented by Mary Ellen Wohl, M.D. at the 36th Annual Conference on Chest Disease, Intermountain Thoracic Society, January 26, 1993.

HOW SUPPLIED
SOLUTION: 2.5 MG/2.5 ML

BRAND/MANUFACTURER	NDC	SIZE	AWP
BRAND			
PULMOZYME: Genentech	50242-0100-38	2.5 ml 14s	$453.60
	50242-0100-40	2.5 ml 30s	$972.00

Doryx *SEE DOXYCYCLINE*

Dovonex *SEE CALCIPOTRIENE*

Doxacurium Chloride

This drug should be administered only by adequately trained individuals familiar with its actions, characteristics, and hazards.

DESCRIPTION

Doxacurium Chloride is a long-acting, nondepolarizing skeletal muscle relaxant for intravenous administration. Doxacurium Chloride is *trans, trans*-2,2'-[succinyl-bis(oxytrimethylene)]bis[1,2,3,4-tetrahydro-6, 7, 8-trimeth-oxy-2-methyl-1-(3,4,5-trimethoxybenzyl)isoquinolinium] dichloride. The molecular formula is $C_{56}H_{78}Cl_2N_2O_{16}$ and the molecular weight is 1106.14. The compound does not partition into the 1-octanol phase of a distilled water/1-octanol system, *i.e.*, the n-octanol:water partition coefficient is 0.

Doxacurium Chloride is a mixture of the three *trans, trans* stereoisomers, a *dl* pair [(1*R*, 1' *R*, 2*S*, 2' *S*) and (1*S*, 1' *S*, 2*R*, 2' *R*)] and a meso form (1*R*, 1' *S*, 2*S*, 2' *R*).

Doxacurium Chloride Injection is a sterile, non-pyrogenic aqueous solution (pH 3.9 to 5.0) containing 1 mg/mL Doxacurium in Water for Injection. Hydrochloric acid may have been added to adjust pH. Doxacurium Chloride Injection contains 0.9% w/v benzyl alcohol.

Following is its chemical structure:

CLINICAL PHARMACOLOGY

Doxacurium Chloride binds competitively to cholinergic receptors on the motor end-plate to antagonize the action of acetylcholine, resulting in a block of neuromuscular transmission. This action is antagonized by acetylcholinesterase inhibitors, such as neostigmine.

Pharmacodynamics: Doxacurium Chloride is approximately 2.5 to 3 times more potent than pancuronium and 10 to 12 times more potent than metocurine. Doxacurium Chloride in doses of 1.5 to $2 \times ED_{95}$ has a clinical duration of action (range and variability) similar to that of equipotent doses of pancuronium and metocurine (historic data and limited comparison). The average ED_{95} (dose required to produce 95% suppression of the adductor pollicis muscle twitch response to ulnar nerve stimulation) of Doxacurium Chloride is 0.025 mg/kg (range: 0.020 to 0.033) in adults receiving balanced anesthesia.

The onset and clinically effective duration (time from injection to 25% recovery) of Doxacurium Chloride administered alone or after succinylcholine during stable balanced anesthesia are shown in Table 1.

Table 1

PHARMACODYNAMIC DOSE RESPONSE* BALANCED ANESTHESIA

	Initial Doxacurium Chloride Dose (mg/kg)		
	0.025† (n=34)	0.05 (n=27)	0.08 (n=9)
Time to Maximum Block (min)	9.3 (5.4-16)	5.2 (2.5-13)	3.5 (2.4-5)
Clinical Duration (min) (Time to 25% Recovery)	55 (9-145)	100 (39-232)	160 (110-338)

* Values shown are means (range).
† Doxacurium Chloride administered after 10% to 100% recovery from an intubating dose of succinylcholine.

Initial doses of 0.05 mg/kg ($2 \times ED_{95}$) and 0.08 mg/kg ($3 \times ED_{95}$) Doxacurium Chloride administered during the induction of thiopental-narcotic anesthesia produced good-to-excellent conditions for tracheal intubation in 5 minutes (13 of 15 cases studied) and 4 minutes (8 of 9 cases studied)(which are before maximum block), respectively.

As with other long-acting agents, the clinical duration of neuromuscular block associated with Doxacurium Chloride shows considerable interpatient variability. An analysis of 390 cases in U.S. clinical trials utilizing a variety of premedications, varying lengths of surgery, and various anesthetic agents, indicates that approximately two-thirds of the patients had clinical durations within 30 minutes of the duration predicted by dose (based on mg/kg actual body weight). Patients ≥ 60 years old are approximately twice as likely to experience prolonged clinical duration (30 minutes longer than predicted) than patients < 60 years old; thus, care should be used in older patients when prolonged recovery is undesirable (see *"Geriatic Use"* subsection of *"Precautions"* and *"Individualization of Dosages"* subsection of *"Clinical Pharmacology"*). In addition, obese patients (patients weighing ≥ 30% more than ideal body weight for height) were almost twice as likely to experience prolonged clinical duration than nonobese patients; therefore, dosing should be based on ideal body weight (IBW) for obese patients (see *"Individualization of Dosages"* subsection of *"Clinical Pharmacology"*).

The mean time for spontaneous T_1 recovery from 25% to 50% of control following initial doses of Doxacurium Chloride is approximately 26 minutes (range: 7 to 104, n=253) during balanced anesthesia. The mean time for spontaneous T_1 recovery from 25% to 75% is 54 minutes (range: 14 to 184, n=184).

Most patients receiving Doxacurium Chloride in clinical trials required pharmacologic reversal prior to full spontaneous recovery from neuromuscular block (see *"Antagonism of Neuromuscular Block"* subsection of *"Overdosage"*); therefore, relatively few data are available on the time from injection to 95% spontaneous recovery of the twitch response. As with other long-acting neuromuscular blocking agents, Doxacurium Chloride may be associated with prolonged times to full spontaneous recovery. Following an initial dose of 0.025 mg/kg Doxacurium Chloride, some patients may require as long as 4 hours to exhibit full spontaneous recovery.

Cumulative neuromuscular blocking effects are not associated with repeated administration of maintenance doses of Doxacurium Chloride at 25% T_1 recovery. As with initial doses, however, the duration of action following maintenance doses of Doxacurium Chloride may vary considerably among patients.

The Doxacurium Chloride ED_{95} for children 2 to 12 years of age receiving halothane anesthesia is approximately 0.03 mg/kg. Children require higher Doxacurium Chloride doses on a mg/kg basis than adults to achieve comparable levels of block. The onset time and duration of block are shorter in children than adults. During halothane anesthesia, doses of 0.03 mg/kg and 0.05 mg/kg Doxacurium Chloride produce maximum block in approximately 7 and 4 minutes, respectively. The duration of clinically effective block is approximately 30 minutes after an initial dose of 0.03 mg/kg and approximately 45 minutes after 0.05 mg/kg. Doxacurium Chloride has not been studied in children below the age of 2 years.

The neuromuscular block produced by Doxacurium Chloride may be antagonized by anticholinesterase agents. As with other nondepolarizing neuromuscular blocking agents, the more profound the neuromuscular block at reversal, the longer the time and the greater the dose of anticholinesterase required for recovery of neuromuscular function.

Hemodynamics: Administration of Doxacurium Chloride doses up to and including 0.08 mg/kg ($\sim 3 \times ED_{95}$) over 5 to 15 seconds to healthy adult patients during stable state balanced anesthesia and to patients with serious cardiovascular disease undergoing coronary artery bypass grafting, cardiac valvular repair, or vascular repair produced no dose-related effects on mean arterial blood pressure (MAP) or heart rate (HR).

No dose-related changes in MAP and HR were observed following administration of up to 0.05 mg/kg Doxacurium Chloride over 5 to 15 seconds in 2 - to 12-year-old children receiving halothane anesthesia.

Doses of 0.03 to 0.08 mg/kg (1.2 to $3 \times ED_{95}$) were not associated with dose-dependent changes in mean plasma histamine concentration. Clinical experience with more than 1,000 patients indicates that adverse experiences typically associated with histamine release (*i.e.,* bronchospasm, hypotension, tachycardia, cutaneous flushing, urticaria, *etc.*) are very rare following the administration of Doxacurium Chloride (see *"Adverse Reactions"*).

Pharmacokinetics: Pharmacokinetic and pharmacodynamic results from a study of 24 healthy young adult patients and 8 healthy elderly patients are summarized in Table 2. The pharmacokinetics are linear over the dosage range tested (*i.e.,* plasma concentrations are approximately proportional to dose). The pharmacokinetics of Doxacurium Chloride are similar in healthy young adult and elderly patients. Some healthy elderly patients tend to be more sensitive to the neuromuscular blocking effects of Doxacurium Chloride than healthy young adult patients receiving the same dose. The time to maximum block is longer in elderly patients than in young adult patients (11.2 versus 7.7 minutes at 0.025 mg/kg Doxacurium Chloride). In addition, the clinically effective durations of block are more variable and tend to be longer in healthy elderly patients than in healthy young adult patients receiving the same dose. (See related table).

Table 3 summarizes the pharmacokinetic and pharmacodynamic results from a study of 9 healthy young adult patients, 8 patients with end-stage kidney disease undergoing kidney transplantation, and 7 patients with end-stage liver disease undergoing liver transplantation. The results suggest that a longer $t_{1/2}$ can be expected in patients with end-stage kidney disease; in addition, these patients may be more sensitive to the neuromuscular blocking effects of Doxacurium Chloride. The time to maximum block was slightly longer and the clinically effective duration of block was prolonged in patients with end-stage kidney disease.

Table 3

PHARMACOKINETIC AND PHARMACODYNAMIC PARAMETERS[1] OF DOXACURIUM CHLORIDE IN HEALTHY PATIENTS AND IN PATIENTS UNDERGOING KIDNEY OR LIVER TRANSPLANTATION (ISOFLURANE ANESTHESIA)

Parameter	Healthy Young Adult Patients 0.015 mg/kg (n=9)	Kidney Transplant Patients 0.015 mg/kg (n=8)	Liver Transplant Patients 0.015 mg/kg (n=7)
$t_{1/2}$ elimination (min)	99 (48-193)	221 (84-592)	115 (69-148)
Volume of Distribution at Steady State (L/kg)	0.22 (0.11-0.43)	0.27 (0.17-0.55)	0.29 (0.17-0.35)
Plasma Clearance (mL/min/kg)	2.66 (1.35-6.66)	1.23 (0.48-2.40)	2.30 (1.96-3.05)
Maximum Block (%)	86 (59-100)	98 (95-100)	70 (0-100)
Clinically Effective Duration of Block (min)	36 (19-80)	80 (29-133)	52 (20-91)

[1] Values shown are means (range).

No data are available from patients with liver disease not requiring transplantation. There are no significant alterations in the pharmacokinetics of Doxacurium Chloride in liver transplant patients. Sensitivity to the neuromuscular blocking effects of Doxacurium Chloride was highly variable in patients undergoing liver transplantation. Three of 7 patients developed ≤ 50% block, indicating that a reduced sensitivity to Doxacurium Chloride may occur in such patients. In those patients who developed > 50% neuromuscular block, the time to maximum block and the clinically effective duration tended to be longer than in healthy young adult patients (see *"Individualization of Dosages"* subsection of *"Clinical Pharmacology"*).

Consecutively administered maintenance doses of 0.005 mg/kg Doxacurium Chloride each given at 25% T_1 recovery following the preceding dose, do not result in a progressive increase in the plasma concentration of Doxacurium or a progressive increase in the depth or duration of block produced by each dose.

Doxacurium Chloride is not metabolized *in vitro* in fresh human plasma. Plasma protein binding of Doxacurium Chloride is approximately 30% in human plasma.

In vivo data from humans suggest that Doxacurium Chloride is not metabolized and that the major elimination pathway is excretion of unchanged drug in urine and bile. In studies of healthy adult patients, 24% to 38% of an administered dose was recovered as parent drug in urine over 6 to 12 hours after dosing. High bile concentrations of Doxacurium Chloride (relative to plasma) have been found 35 to 90 minutes after administration. The overall extent of biliary excretion is unknown. The data derived from analysis of human urine and bile are consistent with data from *in vivo* studies in the rat, cat, and dog, which indicate that all of an administered dose of Doxacurium Chloride is recovered as parent drug in the urine and bile of these species.

Individualization of Dosages: In elderly patients or patients who have impaired renal function, the potential for a prolongation of block may be reduced by decreasing the initial Doxacurium Chloride dose and by titrating the dose to achieve the desired depth of block. In obese patients (patients weighing ≥ 30% more than ideal body weight for height), the Doxacurium Chloride dose should be determined using the patient's ideal body weight (IBW), according to the following formulae:

Men: IBW in kg=[106 +(6 × inches in height above 5 feet)]/2.2
Women: IBW in kg = [100 + (5 × inches in height above 5 feet)]/2.2

Dosage requirements for patients with severe liver disease are variable; some patients may require a higher than normal initial Doxacurium Chloride dose to achieve clinically effective block. Once adequate block is established, the clinical duration of block may be prolonged in such patients relative to patients with normal liver function.

As with pancuronium, metocurine, and vecuronium, resistance to Doxacurium Chloride, manifested by a reduced intensity and/or shortened duration of block, must be considered when Doxacurium Chloride is selected for use in patients receiving phenytoin or carbamazepine (see *"Drug Interactions"* subsection of *"Precautions"*).

As with other nondepolarizing neuromuscular blocking agents, a reduction in dosage of Doxacurium Chloride must be considered in cachectic or debilitated patients, in patients with neuromuscular diseases, severe electrolyte abnormalities, or carcinomatosis, and in other patients in whom potentiation of neuromuscular block or difficulty with reversal is anticipated. Increased doses of Doxacurium Chloride may be required in burn patients (see *"Precautions"*).

INDICATIONS AND USAGE
Doxacurium Chloride is a long-acting neuromuscular blocking agent, indicated as an adjunct to general anesthesia, to provide skeletal muscle relaxation during surgery. Doxacurium Chloride can also be used to provide skeletal muscle relaxation for endotracheal intubation.

CONTRAINDICATIONS
Doxacurium Chloride is contraindicated in patients known to have hypersensitivity to it.

WARNINGS
DOXACURIUM CHLORIDE SHOULD BE ADMINISTERED IN CAREFULLY ADJUSTED DOSAGE BY OR UNDER THE SUPERVISION OF EXPERIENCED CLINICIANS WHO ARE FAMILIAR WITH THE DRUG'S ACTIONS AND THE POSSIBLE COMPLICATIONS OF ITS USE. THE DRUG SHOULD NOT BE ADMINISTERED UNLESS FACILITIES FOR INTUBATION, ARTIFICIAL RESPIRATION, OXYGEN THERAPY, AND AN ANTAGONIST ARE WITHIN IMMEDIATE REACH. IT IS RECOMMENDED THAT CLINICIANS ADMINISTERING LONG-ACTING NEUROMUSCULAR BLOCKING AGENTS SUCH AS DOXACURIUM CHLORIDE EMPLOY A PERIPHERAL NERVE STIMULATOR TO MONITOR DRUG RESPONSE, NEED FOR ADDITIONAL RELAXANTS, AND ADEQUACY OF SPONTANEOUS RECOVERY OR ANTAGONISM.

DOXACURIUM CHLORIDE HAS NO KNOWN EFFECT ON CONSCIOUSNESS, PAIN THRESHOLD, OR CEREBRATION. TO AVOID DISTRESS TO THE PATIENT, NEUROMUSCULAR BLOCK SHOULD NOT BE INDUCED BEFORE UNCON- SCIOUSNESS.

Doxacurium Chloride Injection is acidic (pH 3.9 to 5.0) and may not be compatible with alkaline solutions having a pH greater than 8.5 (*e.g.,* barbiturate solutions).

Doxacurium Chloride Injection contains benzyl alcohol. In newborn infants, benzyl alcohol has been associated with an increased incidence of neurological and other complications which are sometimes fatal. See *"Pediatric Use"* subsection of *"Precautions"*.

PRECAUTIONS
General: Doxacurium Chloride has no clinically significant effects on heart rate; therefore, Doxacurium Chloride will not counteract the bradycardia produced by many anesthetic agents or by vagal stimulation.

Neuromuscular blocking agents may have a profound effect in patients with neuromuscular diseases (*e.g.,* myasthenia gravis and the myasthenic syndrome). In these and other conditions in which prolonged neuromuscular block is a possibility (*e.g.,* carcinomatosis), the use of a peripheral nerve stimulator and a small test dose of Doxacurium Chloride is recommended to assess the level of neuromuscular block and to monitor dosage requirements. Shorter acting muscle relaxants than Doxacurium Chloride may be more suitable for these patients. Resistance to nondepolarizing neuromuscular blocking agents may develop in patients with burns depending upon the time elapsed since the injury and the size of the burn. Doxacurium Chloride has not been studied in patients with burns. Acid-base and/or serum electrolyte abnormalities may potentiate or antagonize the action of neuromuscular blocking agents. The action of neuromuscular blocking agents may be enhanced by magnesium salts administered for the management of toxemia of pregnancy.

Doxacurium Chloride has not been studied in patients with asthma.

No data are available to support the use of Doxacurium Chloride by intramuscular injection.

Renal and Hepatic Disease: Doxacurium Chloride has been studied in patients with end-stage kidney (n=8) or liver (n=7) disease undergoing transplantation procedures (see *"Clinical Pharmacology"*). The possibility of prolonged neuromuscular block in patients undergoing renal transplantation and the possibility of a variable onset and duration of neuromuscular block in patients undergoing liver transplantation must be considered when Doxacurium Chloride is used in such patients.

Obesity: Administration of Doxacurium Chloride on the basis of actual body weight is associated with a prolonged duration of action in obese patients (patients weighing ≥ 30% more than ideal body weight for height) (see *"Clinical Pharmacology"*). Therefore, the dose of Doxacurium Chloride should be based upon ideal body weight in obese patients (see *"Individualization of Dosages"* subsection of *"Clinical Pharmacology"*).

Malignant Hyperthermia (MH): In a study of MH-susceptible pigs, Doxacurium Chloride did not trigger MH. Doxacurium Chloride has not been studied in MH-susceptible patients. Since MH can develop in the absence of established triggering agents, the clinician should be prepared to recognize and treat MH in any patient scheduled for general anesthesia.

Long-Term Use in the Intensive Care Unit (ICU): No data are available on the long-term use of Doxacurium Chloride in patients undergoing mechanical ventilation in the ICU.

Drug Interactions: Prior administration of succinylcholine has no clinically important effect on the neuromuscular blocking action of Doxacurium Chloride.

Table 2
PHARMACOKINETIC AND PHARMACODYNAMIC PARAMETERS[1] OF DOXACURIUM CHLORIDE IN YOUNG ADULT AND ELDERLY PATIENTS (ISOFLURANE ANESTHESIA)

| Parameter | Healthy Young Adult Patients (22 to 49 yrs) | | | Healthy Elderly Patients (67 to 72 yrs) |
	0.025 mg/kg (n=8)	0.05 mg/kg (n=8)	0.08 mg/kg (n=8)	0.025 mg/kg (n=8)
t½ elimination (min)	86 (25-171)	123 (61-163)	98 (47-163)	96 (50-114)
Volume of Distribution at Steady State (L/kg)	0.15 (0.10-0.21)	0.24 (0.13-0.30)	0.22 (0.16-0.33)	0.22 (0.14-0.40)
Plasma Clearance (mL/min/kg)	2.22 (1.02-3.95)	2.62 (1.21-5.70)	2.53 (1.88-3.38)	2.47 (1.58-3.60)
Maximum Block (%)	97 (88-100)	100 (100-100)	100 (100-100)	96 (90-100)
Clinically Effective Duration of Block[2] (min)	68 (35-90)	91 (47-132)	177 (74-268)	97 (36-179)

[1] Values shown are means (range).
[2] Time from injection to 25% recovery of the control twitch height.

The use of Doxacurium Chloride before succinylcholine to attenuate some of the side effects of succinylcholine has not been studied.

There are no clinical data on concomitant use of Doxacurium Chloride and other nondepolarizing neuromuscular blocking agents. Isoflurane, enflurane and halothane decrease the ED_{50} of Doxacurium Chloride by 30% to 45%. These agents may also prolong the clinically effective duration of action by up to 25%.

Other drugs which may enhance the neuromuscular blocking action of nondepolarizing agents such as Doxacurium Chloride include certain antibiotics (e.g., aminoglycosides, tetracyclines, bacitracin, polymyxins, lincomycin, clindamycin, colistin, and sodium colistimethate), magnesium salts, lithium, local anesthetics, procainamide, and quinidine.

As with some other nondepolarizing neuromuscular blocking agents, the time of onset of neuromuscular block induced by Doxacurium Chloride is lengthened and the duration of block is shortened in patients receiving phenytoin or carbamazepine.

Carcinogenesis, Mutagenesis, Impairment of Fertility: Carcinogenesis and fertility studies have not been performed. Doxacurium Chloride was evaluated in a battery of four short-term mutagenicity tests. It was non-mutagenic in the Ames Salmonella assay, in the mouse lymphoma assay, and in the human lymphocyte assay. In the *in vivo* rat bone marrow cytogenetic assay, statistically significant increases in the incidence of structural abnormalities, relative to vehicle controls, were observed in male rats dosed with 0.1 mg/kg (0.625 mg/m^2 Doxacurium Chloride and sacrificed at 6 hours, but not at 24 or 48 hours, and in female rats dosed with 0.2 mg/kg (1.25 mg/m^2) Doxacurium Chloride and sacrificed at 24 hours, but not at 6 or 48 hours. There was no increase in structural abnormalities in either male or female rats given 0.3 mg/kg (1.875 mg/m^2) Doxacurium Chloride and sacrificed at 6, 24, or 48 hours. Thus, the incidence of abnormalities in the *in vivo* rat bone marrow cytogenetic assay was not dose-dependent and, therefore, the likelihood that the observed abnormalities were treatment-related or clinically significant is low.

Pregnancy: Teratogenic Effects: Pregnancy Category C. Teratology testing in nonventilated, pregnant rats and mice treated subcutaneously with maximum subparalyzing doses of Doxacurium Chloride revealed no maternal or fetal toxicity or teratogenic effects. There are no adequate and well-controlled studies of Doxacurium Chloride in pregnant women. Because animal studies are not always predictive of human response and the doses used were subparalyzing, Doxacurium Chloride should be used during pregnancy only if the potential benefit justifies the potential risk to the fetus.

Labor and Delivery: The use of Doxacurium Chloride during labor, vaginal delivery, or cesarean section has not been studied. It is not known whether Doxacurium Chloride administered to the mother has immediate or delayed effects on the fetus. The duration of action of Doxacurium Chloride exceeds the usual duration of operative obstetrics (cesarean section). Therefore, Doxacurium Chloride is not recommended for use in patients undergoing C-section.

Nursing Mothers: It is not known whether Doxacurium Chloride is excreted in human milk. Because many drugs are excreted in human milk, caution should be exercised following Doxacurium Chloride administration to a nursing woman.

Pediatric Use: Doxacurium Chloride has not been studied in children below the age of 2 years. See *"Clinical Pharmacology"* and *"Dosage and Administration"* for clinical experience and recommendations for use in children 2 to 12 years of age.

Geriatric Use: Doxacurium Chloride has been used in elderly patients, including patients with significant cardiovascular disease. In elderly patients the onset of maximum block is slower and the duration of neuromuscular block produced by Doxacurium Chloride is more variable and, in some cases, longer than in young adult patients (see *"Pharmacodynamics"* and *"Individualization of Dosages"* subsections of *"Clinical Pharmacology"*).

ADVERSE REACTIONS

The most frequent adverse effect of nondepolarizing blocking agents as a class consists of an extension of the pharmacological action beyond the time needed for surgery and anesthesia. This effect may vary from skeletal muscle weakness to profound and prolonged skeletal muscle paralysis resulting in respiratory insufficiency and apnea which require manual or mechanical ventilation until recovery is judged to be clinically adequate (see *"Overdosage"*). Inadequate reversal of neuromuscular block from Doxacurium Chloride is possible, as with all nondepolarizing agents. Prolonged neuromuscular block and inadequate reversal may lead to post-operative complications.

Observed in Clinical Trials: Adverse experiences were uncommon among the 1034 surgical patients and volunteers who received Doxacurium Chloride and other drugs in U.S. clinical studies in the course of a wide variety of procedures conducted during balanced or inhalational anesthesia. The following adverse experiences were reported in patients administered Doxacurium Chloride (all events judged by investigators during the clinical trials to have a possible causal relationship):

Incidence Greater than 1%: None

Incidence Less than 1%: Cardiovascular:* hypotension,† flushing,† ventricular fibrillation, myocardial infarction
  Respiratory: bronchospasm, wheezing

---

* Reports of ventricular fibrillation (n=1) and myocardial infarction (n=1) were limited to ASA Class 3-4 patients undergoing cardiac surgery (n=142).
† 0.3% incidence. All other reactions unmarked were ≤ 0.1%.

Dermatological: urticaria, injection site reaction
Special Senses: diplopia
  Nonspecific: difficult neuromuscular block reversal, prolonged drug effect, fever

OVERDOSAGE

Overdosage with neuromuscular blocking agents may result in neuromuscular block beyond the time needed for surgery and anesthesia. The primary treatment is maintenance of a patent airway and controlled ventilation until recovery of normal neuromuscular function is assured. Once evidence of recovery from neuromuscular block is observed, further recovery may be facilitated by administration of an anticholinesterase agent (e.g., neostigmine, edrophonium) in conjunction with an appropriate anticholinergic agent (see *"Antagonism of Neuromuscular Block"*).

Antagonism of Neuromuscular Block: ANTAGONISTS (SUCH AS NEOSTIGMINE) SHOULD NOT BE ADMINISTERED PRIOR TO THE DEMONSTRATION OF SOME SPONTANEOUS RECOVERY FROM NEUROMUSCULAR BLOCK. THE USE OF A NERVE STIMULATOR TO DOCUMENT RECOVERY AND ANTAGONISM OF NEUROMUSCULAR BLOCK IS RECOMMENDED. T_4/T_1 SHOULD BE > ZERO BEFORE ANTAGONISM IS ATTEMPTED.

In an analysis of patients in whom antagonism of neuromuscular block was evaluated following administration of single doses of neostigmine averaging 0.06 mg/kg (range: 0.05 to 0.075) administered at approximately 25% T_1 spontaneous recovery during balanced anesthesia, 71% of patients exhibited $T_4/T_1 \geq 0.7$ before monitoring was discontinued. For these patients, the mean time to $T_4/T_1 \geq 0.7$ was 19 minutes (range: 7 to 55). As with other long-acting nondepolarizing neuromuscular blocking agents, the time for recovery of neuromuscular function following administration of neostigmine is dependent upon the level of residual neuromuscular block at the time of attempted reversal; longer recovery times than those cited above may be anticipated when neostigmine is administered at more profound levels of block (i.e., at < 25% T_1 recovery).

Patients should be evaluated for adequate clinical evidence of antagonism, e.g., 5-second head lift, and grip strength. Ventilation must be supported until no longer required. As with other neuromuscular blocking agents, physicians should be alert to the possibility that the action of the drugs used to antagonize neuromuscular block may wear off before the effects of Doxacurium Chloride on the neuromuscular junction have declined sufficiently.

Antagonism may be delayed in the presence of debilitation, carcinomatosis, and the concomitant use of certain broad spectrum antibiotics, or anesthetic agents and other drugs which enhance neuromuscular block or separately cause respiratory depression (see *"Drug Interactions"* subsection of *"Precautions"*). Under such circumstances the management is the same as that of prolonged neuromuscular block. In clinical trials, a dose of 1 mg/kg edrophonium was not as effective as a dose of 0.06 mg/kg neostigmine in antagonizing moderate to deep levels of neuromuscular block (i.e., < 60% T_1 recovery). Therefore, the use of 1 mg/kg edrophonium is not recommended for reversal from moderate to deep levels of block. The use of pyridostigmine has not been studied.

DOSAGE AND ADMINISTRATION

DOXACURIUM CHLORIDE SHOULD ONLY BE ADMINISTERED INTRAVENOUSLY.

Doxacurium Chloride, like other long-acting neuromuscular blocking agents, displays variability in the duration of its effect. The potential for a prolonged clinical duration of neuromuscular block must be considered when Doxacurium Chloride is selected for administration. The dosage information provided below is intended as a guide only. Doses should be individualized (see *"Individualization of Dosages"* subsection of *"Clinical Pharmacology"*). Factors that may warrant dosage adjustment include: advancing age, the presence of kidney or liver disease, or obesity (patients weighing ≥ 30% more than ideal body weight for height). The use of a peripheral nerve stimulator will permit the most advantageous use of Doxacurium Chloride, minimize the possibility of overdosage or underdosage, and assist in the evaluation of recovery.

Parenteral drug products should be inspected visually for particulate matter and discoloration prior to administration whenever solution and container permit.

ADULTS

Initial Doses: When administered as a component of a thiopental/narcotic induction-intubation paradigm as well as for production of long-duration neuromuscular block during surgery, 0.05 mg/kg (2 × ED$_{95}$) Doxacurium Chloride produces good-to-excellent conditions for tracheal intubation in 5 minutes in approximately 90% of patients. Lower doses of Doxacurium Chloride may result in a longer time for development of satisfactory intubation conditions. Clinically effective neuromuscular block may be expected to last approximately 100 minutes on average (range: 39 to 232) following 0.05 mg/kg Doxacurium Chloride administered to patients receiving balanced anesthesia.

An initial Doxacurium Chloride dose of 0.08 mg/kg (3 × ED$_{95}$) should be reserved for instances in which a need for very prolonged neuromuscular block is anticipated. In approximately 90% of patients, good-to-excellent intubation conditions may be expected in 4 minutes after this dose; however, clinically effective block may be expected to persist for as long as 160 minutes or more (range: 110 to 338) (see *"Clinical Pharmacology"*).

If Doxacurium Chloride is administered during stead-state isoflurane, enflurane, or halothane anesthesia, reduction of the Doxacurium Chloride dose by one-third should be considered.

◆ RATED THERAPEUTICALLY EQUIVALENT; ◇ THERAPEUTIC EQUIVALENCE UNCONFIRMED; ○ UNRATED

When succinylcholine is administered to facilitate tracheal intubation in patients receiving balanced anesthesia, an initial dose of 0.025 mg/kg (ED$_{95}$) Doxacurium Chloride provides about 60 minutes (range: 9 to 145) of clinically effective neuromuscular block for surgery. For a longer duration of action, a larger initial dose may be administered.

Maintenance Doses: Maintenance dosing will generally be required about 60 minutes after an initial dose of 0.025 mg/kg Doxacurium Chloride or 100 minutes after an initial dose of 0.05 mg/kg Doxacurium Chloride during balanced anesthesia. Repeated maintenance doses administered at 25% T$_1$ recovery may be expected to be required at relatively regular intervals in each patient. The interval may vary considerably between patients. Maintenance doses of 0.005 and 0.01 mg/kg Doxacurium Chloride each provide an average 30 minutes (range: 9 to 57) and 45 minutes (range: 14 to 108), respectively, of additional clinically effective neuromuscular block. For shorter or longer desired durations, smaller or larger maintenance doses may be administered.

CHILDREN
When administered during halothane anesthesia, an initial dose of 0.03 mg/kg (ED$_{95}$) produces maximum neuromuscular block in about 7 minutes (range: 5 to 11) and clinically effective block for an average of 30 minutes (range: 12 to 54). Under halothane anesthesia, 0.05 mg/kg produces maximum block in about 4 minutes (range: 2 to 10) and clinically effective block for 45 minutes (range: 30 to 80). Maintenance doses are generally required more frequently in children than in adults. Because of the potentiating effect of halothane seen in adults, a higher dose of Doxacurium Chloride may be required in children receiving balanced anesthesia than in children receiving halothane anesthesia to achieve a comparable onset and duration of neuromuscular block. Doxacurium Chloride has not been studied in children below the age of 2 years.

COMPATIBILITY
Y-site Administration: Doxacurium Chloride Injection may not be compatible with alkaline solutions with a pH greater than 8.5 (*e.g.,* barbiturate solutions).
  Doxacurium Chloride is compatible with:

- 5% Dextrose Injection USP
- 0.9% Sodium Chloride Injection USP
- 5% Dextrose and 0.9% Sodium Chloride Injection USP
- Lactated Ringer's Injection USP
- 5% Dextrose and Lactated Ringer's Injection
- Sufentanil citrate Injection, diluted as directed
- Alfentanil hydrochloride Injection, diluted as directed
- Fentanyl citrate Injection, diluted as directed

Dilution Stability: Doxacurium Chloride diluted up to 1:10 in 5% Dextrose Injection USP or 0.9% sodium chloride injection USP have been shown to be physically and chemically stable when stored in polypropylene syringes at 5° to 25°C (41° to 77°F), for up to 24 hours. Since dilution diminishes the preservative effectiveness of benzyl alcohol, aseptic techniques should be used to prepare the diluted product. Immediate use of the diluted product is preferred, and any unused portion of diluted Doxacurium Chloride should be discarded after 8 hours.

STORAGE
Store Doxacurium Chloride Injection at room temperature of 15° to 25°C (59° to 77°F). DO NOT FREEZE.

HOW SUPPLIED
INJECTION: 1 MG/ML

BRAND/MANUFACTURER	NDC	SIZE	AWP
○ **BRAND** NUROMAX: Burr Wellcome	00081-0763-44	5 ml 10s	$345.18

Doxapram Hydrochloride

DESCRIPTION
Doxapram Hydrochloride Injection, is a clear, colorless, sterile, non-pyrogenic, aqueous solution with pH 3.5-5.0, for intravenous administration.

Each 1 mL contains:

Doxapram Hydrochloride . . . . .20 mg.

Certain brands of Doxapram Hydrochloride contain benzyl alcohol.
  Doxapram Hydrochloride Injectable is a respiratory stimulant.
  Doxapram Hydrochloride is a white to off-white, crystalline powder, sparingly soluble in water, alcohol and chloroform.
  It has the following chemical name: 1-ethyl-4-[2-(4-morpholinyl)ethyl]-3,3-diphenyl-2-pyrrolidinone monohydrochloride, monohydrate.

  Following is its chemical structure:

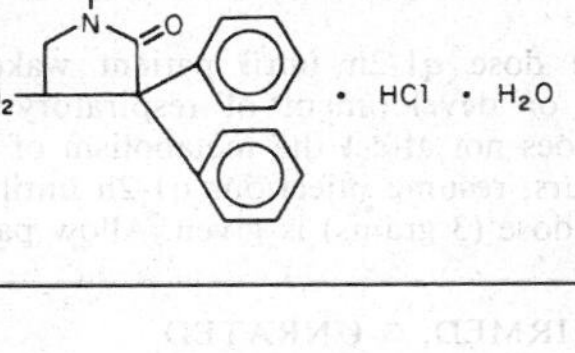

CLINICAL PHARMACOLOGY
Doxapram Hydrochloride produces respiratory stimulation mediated through the peripheral carotid chemoreceptors. As the dosage level is increased, the central respiratory centers in the medulla are stimulated with progressive stimulation of other parts of the brain and spinal cord.
  The onset of respiratory stimulation following the recommended single intravenous injection of Doxapram Hydrochloride usually occurs in 20-40 seconds with peak effect at 1-2 minutes. The duration of effect may vary from 5-12 minutes. The respiratory stimulant action is manifested by an increase in tidal volume associated with a slight increase in respiratory rate.
  A pressor response may result following Doxapram administration. Provided there is no impairment of cardiac function, the pressor effect is more marked in hypovolemic than in normovolemic states. The pressor response is due to the improved cardiac output rather than peripheral vasoconstriction. Following Doxapram administration an increased release of catecholamines has been noted.
  Although opiate induced respiratory depression is antagonized by Doxapram, the analgesic effect is not affected.

INDICATIONS
1. POSTANESTHESIA
a. When the possibility of airway obstruction and/or hypoxia have been eliminated, Doxapram may be used to stimulate respiration in patients with drug-induced postanesthesia respiratory depression or apnea other than that due to muscle relaxant drugs.
b. To pharmacologically stimulate deep breathing in the so-called "stir-up" regimen in the postoperative patient. (Simultaneous administration of oxygen is desirable.)

2. DRUG-INDUCED CENTRAL NERVOUS SYSTEM DEPRESSION
Exercising care to prevent vomiting and aspiration, Doxapram may be used to stimulate respiration, hasten arousal, and to encourage the return of laryngopharyngeal reflexes in patients with mild to moderate respiratory and CNS depression due to drug overdosage.

3. CHRONIC PULMONARY DISEASE ASSOCIATED WITH ACUTE HYPERCAPNIA
Doxapram is indicated as a temporary measure in hospitalized patients with acute respiratory insufficiency superimposed on chronic obstructive pulmonary disease. Its use should be for a short period of time (approximately 2 hours) as an aid in the prevention of elevation of arterial CO$_2$ tension during the administration of oxygen. It should not be used in conjunction with mechanical ventilation.

CONTRAINDICATIONS
Due to its benzyl alcohol content, Doxapram Hydrochloride Injectable should not be used in newborns.
  Doxapram should not be used in patients with epilepsy or other convulsive disorders.
  Doxapram is contraindicated in patients with mechanical disorders of ventilation such as mechanical obstruction, muscle paresis, flial chest, pneumothorax, acute bronchial asthma, pulmonary fibrosis or other conditions resulting in restriction of chest wall, muscles of respiration or alveolar expansion.
  Doxapram is contraindicated in patients with evidence of head injury or cerebral vascular accident and in those with significant cardiovascular impairment, severe hypertension, or known hypersensitivity to the drug.

WARNINGS
1. IN POSTANESTHETIC USE
a. Doxapram is neither an antagonist to muscle relaxant drugs nor a specific narcotic antagonist. Adequacy of airway and oxygenation must be assured prior to Doxapram administration.
b. Doxapram should be administered with great care and only under careful supervision to patients with hypermetabolic states such as hyperthyroidism or pheochromocytoma.
c. Since narcosis may recur after stimulation with Doxapram, care should be taken to maintain close observation until the patient has been fully alert for ½ to 1 hour.

2. IN DRUG-INDUCED CNS AND RESPIRATORY DEPRESSION
Doxapram alone may not stimulate adequate spontaneous breathing or provide sufficient arousal in patients who are *severely* depressed either due to respiratory failure or to CNS depressant drugs, but should be used as an adjunct to established supportive measures and resuscitative techniques.

3. IN CHRONIC OBSTRUCTIVE PULMONARY DISEASE
a. Because of the associated increased work of breathing, do not increase the rate of infusion of Doxapram in severely ill patients in an attempt to lower pCO$_2$.
b. Doxapram should not be used in conjunction with mechanical ventilation.

PRECAUTIONS
1. GENERAL
a. An adequate airway is essential.
b. Recommended dosages of Doxapram Hydrochloride should be employed and maximum total dosages should not be exceeded. In order to avoid side effects, it is advisable to use the minimum effective dosage.
c. Monitoring of the blood pressure and deep tendon reflexes is recommended to prevent overdosage.

➤ SHOWN IN PRODUCT IDENTIFICATION GUIDE

d. Vascular extravasation or use of a single injection site over an extended period should be avoided since either may lead to thrombophlebitis or local skin irritation.

e. Rapid infusion may result in hemolysis.

f. Lowered pCO_2 induced by hyperventilation produces cerebral vasoconstriction and slowing of the cerebral circulation. This should be taken into consideration on an individual basis.

g. Intravenous short-acting barbiturates, oxygen and resuscitative equipment should be readily available to manage overdosage manifested by excessive central nervous system stimulation. Slow administration of the drug, and careful observation of the patient during administration and for some time subsequently are advisable. These precautions are to assure that the protective reflexes have been restored and to prevent possible post-hyperventilation hypoventilation.

h. Doxapram should be administered cautiously to patients receiving sympathomimetic or monoamine oxidase inhibiting drugs, since and additive pressor effect may occur.

i. Blood pressure increases are generally modest but significant increases have been noted in some patients. Because of this Doxapram is not recommended for use in severe hypertension (see *"Contraindications"*).

j. If sudden hypotension or dyspnea develops, Doxapram should be stopped.

2. IN POSTANESTHETIC USE.

a. The same consideration to pre-existing disease states should be exercised as in non-anesthetized individuals. See *"Contraindications"* and *"Warning"* covering use in hypertension, asthma, disturbances of respiratory mechanics including airway obstruction, CNS disorders including increased cerebrospinal fluid pressure, convulsive disorders, acute agitation, and profound metabolic disorders.

b. See *"Drug Interactions"*.

3. IN CHRONIC OBSTRUCTIVE PULMONARY DISEASE

a. Arrhythmias seen in some patients in acute respiratory failure secondary to chronic obstructive pulmonary disease are probably the result of hypoxia. Doxapram should be used with caution in these patients.

b. Arterial blood gases should be drawn prior to the initiation of Doxapram infusion and oxygen administration, then at least every ½ hour. Doxapram administration does not diminish the need for careful monitoring of the patient or the need for supplemental oxygen in patients with acute respiratory failure. Doxapram should be stopped if the arterial blood gases deteriorate, and mechanical ventilation initiated.

Drug Interactions: Administration of Doxapram to patients who are receiving sympathomimetic or monoamine oxidase inhibiting drugs may result in an additive pressor effect. (See *"Precautions"*).

In patients who have received muscle relaxants, Doxapram may temporarily mask the residual effects of muscle relaxant drugs.

In patients who have received anesthetics known to sensitize the myocardium to catecholamines, such as halothane, cyclopropane and enflurane, initiation of Doxapram therapy should be delayed for at least 10 minutes following discontinuance of anesthesia, since an increase in epinephrine release has been noted with Doxapram.

Carcinogenesis, Mutagenesis, Impairment of Fertility: No carcinogenic or mutagenic studies have been performed using Doxapram. Doxapram did not adversely affect the breeding performance of rats.

Pregnancy Category B: Reproduction studies have been performed in rats at doses up to 1.6 times the human dose and have revealed no evidence of impaired fertility or harm to the fetus due to Doxapram. There are, however, no adequate and well-controlled studies in pregnant women. Since the animals in the reproduction studies were dosed by the IM and oral routes and animal reproduction studies, in general, are not always predictive of human response, this drug should be used during pregnancy only if clearly needed.

Nursing mothers: It is not known whether this drug is excreted in human milk. Because many drugs are excreted in human milk, caution should be exercised when Doxapram Hydrochloride is administered to a nursing mother.

Pediatric use: The use of the preservative benzyl alcohol in the newborn has been associated with metabolic, CNS, respiratory, circulatory, and renal dysfunction. Safety and effectiveness in children below the age of 12 years have not been established.

ADVERSE REACTIONS

The following adverse reactions have been reported:

1. CENTRAL AND AUTONOMIC NERVOUS SYSTEMS

Pyrexia, flushing, sweating: pruritus and paresthesia, such as a feeling of warmth, burning, or hot sensation, especially in the area of genitalia and perineum; apprehension, disorientation, pupillary dilatation, headache, dizziness, hyperactivity, involuntary movements, muscle spasticity, increased deep tendon reflexes, clonus, bilateral Babinski, and convulsion.

2. RESPIRATORY

Dyspnea, cough, tachypnea, laryngospasm, bronchospasm, hiccough, and rebound hypoventilation.

3. CARDIOVASCULAR

Phlebitis, variations in heart rate, lowered T-waves, arrhythmias, chest pain, tightness in chest. A mild to moderate increase in blood pressure is commonly noted and may be of concern in patients with severe cardiovascular diseases.

4. GASTROINTESTINAL

Nausea, vomiting, diarrhea, desire to defecate.

5. GENITOURINARY

Stimulation of urinary bladder with spontaneous voiding; urinary retention.

6. LABORATORY DETERMINATIONS

A decrease in hemoglobin, hematocrit, or red blood cell count has been observed in postoperative patients. In the presence of pre-existing leukopenia, a further decrease in WBC has been observed following anesthesia and treatment with Doxapram Hydrochloride. Elevation of BUN and albuminuria have also been observed. As some of the patients cited above had received multiple drugs concomitantly, a cause and effect relationship could not be determined.

OVERDOSAGE

Signs and Symptoms: Symptoms of overdosage are extensions of the pharmacologic effects of the drug. Excessive pressor effect, tachycardia, skeletal muscle hyperactivity, and enhanced deep tendon reflexes may be early signs of overdosage. Therefore, the blood pressure, pulse rate and deep tendon reflexes should be evaluated periodically and the dosage or infusion rate adjusted accordingly.

Convulsive seizures are unlikely at recommended dosages. In unanesthetized animals, the convulsant dose is 70 times greater than the respiratory stimulant dose. Intravenous LD_{50} values in the mouse and rat were approximately 75 mg/kg and in the cat and dog were 40-80 mg/kg.

Except for management of chronic obstructive pulmonary disease associated with acute hypercapnia, the maximum recommended dosage is 3 GRAMS/24 HOURS. (See *"Dosage and Administration"*.)

Management: There is no specific antidote for Doxapram. Management should be symptomatic. Short-acting intravenous barbiturates, oxygen and resuscitative equipment should be used as needed for supportive treatment.

There is no evidence that Doxapram is dialyzable; further, the half-life of Doxapram makes it unlikely that dialysis would be appropriate in managing overdose with this drug.

DOSAGE AND ADMINISTRATION

1. Doxapram Hydrochloride is compatible with 5% and 10% dextrose in water or normal saline. ADMIXTURE OF DOXAPRAM WITH ALKALINE SOLUTIONS SUCH AS 2.5% THIOPENTAL SODIUM, BICARBONATE, OR AMINOPHYLLINE WILL RESULT IN PRECIPITATION OR GAS FORMATION.

2. IN POSTANESTHETIC USE

a. By I.V. injection (see Table I. Dosage for postanesthetic use—I.V.). Slow administration of the drug and careful observation of the patient during administration and for some time subsequently are advisable. (See related table).

b. By infusion. The solution is prepared by adding 250 mg of Doxapram (12.5 mL) to 250 mL of dextrose or saline solution. The infusion is initiated at a rate of approximately 5 mg/minute until a satisfactory respiratory response is observed, and maintained at a rate of 1-3 mg/minute. The rate of infusion should be adjusted to sustain the desired level of respiratory stimulation with a minimum of side effects. The recommended total dosage by infusion is 4 mg/kg (2.0 mg/lb), or approximately 300 mg for the average adult.

3. IN THE MANAGEMENT OF DRUG INDUCED CNS DEPRESSION.
(See *Table 2. Dosage for drug-induced CNS depression*)

Table 2

DOXAPRAM HYDROCHLORIDE INJECTABLE DOSAGE FOR DRUG-INDUCED CNS DEPRESSION.

Level of Depression	Method One Priming dose single/repeat i.v. injection		Method Two Rate of intermittent i.v. infusion	
	mg/kg	mg/lb	mg/kg/hr	mg/lb/hr
Mild*	1.0	0.5	1.0-2.0	0.5-1.0
Moderate†	2.0	1.0	2.0-3.0	1.0-1.5

* *Mild Depression*
   Class 0: Asleep, but can be aroused and can answer questions.
   Class 1: Comatose, will withdraw from painful stimuli, reflexes intact.
† *Moderate Depression*
   Class 2: Comatose, will not withdraw from painful stimuli, reflexes intact.
   Class 3: Comatose, reflexes absent, no depression of circulation or respiration.

METHOD ONE

Using Single and/or Repeat Single I.V. *Injections.*

a. Give priming dose of 1.0 mg/lb (2.0 mg/kg) body weight and repeat in 5 minutes.

b. Repeat same dose q1-2h until patient wakens. Watch for relapse into unconsciousness or development of respiratory depression, since Doxapram Hydrochloride does not affect the metabolism of CNS-depressant drugs.

c. If relapse occurs, resume injections q1-2h until arousal is sustained, or total maximum daily dose (3 grams) is given. Allow patients to sleep until 24 hours

Table 1
DOXAPRAM HYDROCHLORIDE INJECTABLE DOSAGE FOR POSTANESTHETIC USE—I.V.

I.V. Administration	Recommended dosage			Maximum dose per single injection		Maximum total dose	
	mg/kg	mg/lb	mg/kg	mg/lb	mg/kg	mg/lb	
Single Injection	0.5-1.0	0.25-0.5	1.5	0.70	1.5	0.70	
Repeat Injection (5 min. intervals)	0.5-1.0	0.25-0.5	1.5	0.70	2.0	1.0	
Infusion	0.5-1.0	0.25-0.5	—	—	4.0	2.0	

have elapsed from first injection of Doxapram Hydrochloride using assisted or automatic respiration if necessary.

d. Repeat procedure the following day until patient breathes spontaneously and sustains desired level of consciousness, or until maximum dosage (3 grams) is given.

e. Repetitive doses should be administered only to patients who have shown response to the initial dose.

f. Failure to respond appropriately indicates the need for neurologic evaluation for a possible nervous system source of sustained coma.

METHOD TWO
By Intermittent I.V. *infusion.*

a. Give priming dose as in Method One.

b. If patient wakens, watch for relapse; if no response, continue general supportive treatment for 1-2 hours and repeat Doxapram Hydrochloride. If some respiratory stimulation occurs, prepare I.V. infusion by adding 250 mg of Doxapram Hydrochloride (12.5 mL) to 250 mL of saline or dextrose solution. Deliver at rate of 1-3 mg/min (60-180 mL/hr) according to size of patient and depth of coma. Discontinue Doxapram Hydrochloride if patient begins to waken or at end of 2 hours.

c. Continue supportive treatment for ½ to 2 hours and repeat Step b.

d. Do not exceed 3 grams/day.

4. CHRONIC OBSTRUCTIVE PULMONARY DISEASE ASSOCIATED WITH ACUTE HYPERCAPNIA

a. One vial of Doxapram (400 mg) should be mixed with 180 mL of dextrose or saline solution (concentration of 2.0 mg/mL). The infusion should be started at 1-2 mg/minute (½-1 mL/minute): if indicated, increase to a maximum of 3 mg/minute. Arterial blood gases should be determined prior to the onset of Doxapram's administration and at least every half hour during thg two hours of infusion to insure against the insidious development of CO_2-RETENTION AND ACIDOSIS. Alteration of oxygen concentration or flow rate may necessetate adjustment in the rate of Doxapram infusion.

b. Predictable blood gas patterns are more readily established with a continuous infusion of Doxapram. If the blood gases show evidence of deterioration, the infusion of Doxapram should be discontinued.

c. ADDITIONAL INFUSIONS BEYOND THE SINGLE MAXIMUM TWO HOUR ADMINISTRATION PERIOD ARE NOT RECOMMENDED.

Parenteral drug products should be inspected visually for particulate matter and discoloration prior to administration, whenever solution and container permit.

Store at controlled room temperature, between 15°C and 30°C (59°F and 86°F).

HOW SUPPLIED
INJECTION: 20 MG/ML

BRAND/MANUFACTURER	NDC	SIZE	AWP
◆ **BRAND**			
DOPRAM: Robins Pharm	00031-4849-83	20 ml	$42.75
◆ **GENERICS**			
Schein	00364-3021-55	20 ml	$40.85

Doxazosin Mesylate

DESCRIPTION
Doxazosin Mesylate is a quinazoline compound that is a selective inhibitor of the alpha$_1$ subtype of alpha adrenergic receptors. The chemical name of Doxazosin Mesylate is 1-(4-amino-6,7-dimethoxy-2-quinazolinyl)-4-(1,4-benzodioxan-2-yl-carbonyl) piperazine methanesulfonate.

The empirical formula for Doxazosin Mesylate is $C_{23}H_{25}$- $N_5O_5 \cdot CH_4O_3S$ and the molecular weight is 547.6.

Doxazosin Mesylate is freely soluble in dimethylsulfoxide, soluble in dimethylformamide, slightly soluble in methanol, ethanol, and water (0.8% at 25°C), and very slightly soluble in acetone and methylene chloride.

Following is its chemical structure:

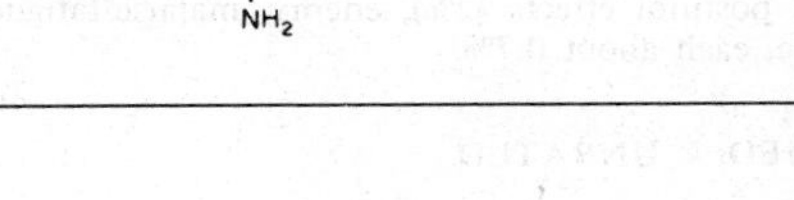

CLINICAL PHARMACOLOGY
MECHANISM OF ACTION
The mechanism of action of Doxazosin Mesylate is selective blockade of the alpha$_1$ (postjunctional) subtype of alpha adrenergic receptors. Studies in normal human subjects have shown that Doxazosin competitively antagonized the pressor effects of phenylephrine (an alpha$_1$ agonist) and the systolic pressor effect of norepinephrine. Doxazosin and prazosin have similar abilities to antagonize phenylephrine. The antihypertensive effect of Doxazosin Mesylate results from a decrease in systemic vascular resistance. The parent compound, Doxazosin, is primarily responsible for the antihypertensive activity. The low plasma concentrations of known active and inactive metabolites of Doxazosin (2-piperazinyl, 6'- and 7'-hydroxy and 6- and 7-O-desmethyl compounds) compared to parent drug indicate that the contribution of even the most potent compound (6'-hydroxy) to the antihypertensive effect of Doxazosin in man is probably small.

PHARMACOKINETICS
After oral administration of therapeutic doses, peak plasma levels of Doxazosin Mesylate occur at about 2-3 hours. Bioavailability is approximately 65%, reflecting first pass metabolism of Doxazosin by the liver. The effect of food on the bioavailability of Doxazosin has not been determined. Doxazosin Mesylate is extensively metabolized in the liver, mainly by O-demethylation of the quinazoline nucleus or hydroxylation of the benzodioxan moiety. In a study of two subjects administered radiolabelled Doxazosin 2 mg orally and 1 mg intravenous on two separate occasions, approximately 63% of the dose was eliminated in the feces and 9% of the dose was found in the urine. On average only 4.8% of the dose was excreted as unchanged drug in the feces and only a trace of the total radioactivity in the urine was attributed to unchanged drug. At the plasma concentrations achieved by therapeutic doses approximately 98% of the circulating drug is bound to plasma proteins.

Plasma elimination of Doxazosin is biphasic, with a terminal elimination half life of about 22 hours. Steady-state studies in hypertensive patients given Doxazosin doses of 2-16 mg once daily showed linear kinetics and dose proportionality. In two studies, following the administration of 2 mg orally once daily, the mean accumulation ratios (steady state AUC vs first dose AUC) were 1.2 and 1.7. Enterohepatic recycling is suggested by secondary peaking of plasma Doxazosin concentrations.

Although several active metabolites of Doxazosin have been identified, the pharmacokinetics of these metabolites have not been characterized.

Pharmacokinetic studies in elderly patients and patients with renal impairment have shown no significant alterations compared to younger patients with normal renal function. There have, however, been no studies of patients with liver impairment, and there are only limited data on the effects of drugs known to influence hepatic metabolism [e.g. cimetidine (See "Precautions")]. Use of Doxazosin in patients with altered liver function should be undertaken with particular caution, if at all, as excretion is almost wholly hepatic.

PHARMACODYNAMICS
Administration of Doxazosin Mesylate results in a reduction in systemic vascular resistance. In patients with hypertension there is little change in cardiac output. Maximum reductions in blood pressure usually occur 2-6 hours after dosing and are associated with a small increase in standing heart rate. Like other alpha$_1$-adrenergic blocking agents, Doxazosin has a greater effect on blood pressure and heart rate in the standing position.

In a pooled analysis of placebo controlled studies with about 300 patients per treatment group, Doxazosin, at doses of 1-16 mg given once daily, lowered blood pressure at 24 hours by about 10/8 mmHg compared to placebo in the standing position and about 9/5 mmHg in the supine position. Peak blood pressure effects (1-6 hours) were larger by about 50-75% (i.e., trough values were about 55-70% of peak effect), with the larger peak-trough differences seen in systolic pressures. There was no apparent difference in the blood pressure response of Caucasians and blacks or of patients above and below age 65. In these predominantly normocholesterolemic patients Doxazosin produced small reductions in total serum cholesterol (2-3%), LDL cholesterol (4%), and a similarly small increase in HDL/total cholesterol ratio (4%). The clinical significance of these findings is uncertain. In the same patient population, patients receiving Doxazosin Mesylate gained a mean of 0.6 kg compared to a mean loss of 0.1 kg for placebo patients.

INDICATIONS AND USAGE
Doxazosin Mesylate is indicated for the treatment of hypertension. Doxazosin Mesylate may be used alone or in combination with diuretics or beta-adrenergic blocking agents. There is limited experience with Doxazosin Mesylate in combination with angiotensin converting enzyme inhibitors or calcium channel blockers.

➤ SHOWN IN PRODUCT IDENTIFICATION GUIDE

UNLABELED USES

Doxazosin Mesylate is used alone or as an adjunct in the treatment of congestive heart failure, pheochromocytoma, and for symptomatic relief of benign prostatic hyperplasia.

CONTRAINDICATIONS

Doxazosin Mesylate is contraindicated in patients with a known sensitivity to quinazolines (e.g. prazosin, terazosin).

WARNINGS

Syncope and "First-dose" Effect:

Doxazosin, like other alpha-adrenergic blocking agents, can cause marked hypotension, especially in the upright position, with syncope and other postural symptoms such as dizziness. Marked orthostatic effects are most common with the first dose but can also occur when there is a dosage increase, or if therapy is interrupted for more than a few days. To decrease the likelihood of excessive hypotension and syncope, it is essential that treatment be initiated with the 1 mg dose. The 2, 4, and 8 mg tablets are not for initial therapy. Dosage should then be adjusted slowly (see *"Dosage and Administration"* section) with increases in dose every two weeks. Additional antihypertensive agents should be added with caution.

Patients being titrated with Doxazosin should be cautioned to avoid situations where injury could result should syncope occur.

In an early investigational study of the safety and tolerance of increasing daily doses of Doxazosin in normotensives beginning at 1 mg/day, only 2 of 6 subjects could tolerate more than 2 mg/day without experiencing symptomatic postural hypotension. In another study of 24 healthy normotensive male subjects receiving initial doses of 2 mg/day of Doxazosin, seven (29%) of the subjects experienced symptomatic postural hypotension between 0.5 and 6 hours after the first dose necessitating termination of the study. In this study 2 of the normotensive subjects experienced syncope. Subsequent trials in hypertensive patients always began Doxazosin dosing at 1 mg/day resulting in a 4% incidence of postural side effects at 1 mg/day with no cases of syncope.

In multiple dose clinical trials involving over 1500 patients with dose titration every one to two weeks, syncope was reported in 0.7% of patients. None of these events occurred at the starting dose of 1 mg and 1.2% (8/664) occurred at 16 mg/day.

If syncope occurs, the patient should be placed in a recumbent position and treated supportively as necessary.

PRECAUTIONS

GENERAL

1. Orthostatic Hypotension: While syncope is the most severe orthostatic effect of Doxazosin Mesylate, other symptoms of lowered blood pressure, such as dizziness, light-headedness, or vertigo, can occur, especially at initiation of therapy or at the time of dose increases. These were common in clinical trials, occurring in up to 23% of all patients treated and causing discontinuation of therapy in about 2%.

In placebo controlled titration trials orthostatic effects were minimized by beginning therapy at 1 mg per day and titrating every two weeks to 2, 4, or 8 mg per day. There was an increased frequency of orthostatic effects in patients given 8 mg or more, 10%, compared to 5% at 1-4 mg and 3% in the placebo group.

Patients in occupations in which orthostatic hypotension could be dangerous should be treated with particular caution.

If hypotension occurs, the patient should be placed in the supine position and, if this measure is inadequate, volume expansion with intravenous fluids or vasopressor therapy may be used. A transient hypotensive response is not a contraindication to further doses of Doxazosin Mesylate.

2. Impaired Liver Function: Doxazosin Mesylate should be administered with caution to patients with evidence of impaired hepatic function or to patients receiving drugs known to influence hepatic metabolism (see *"Clinical Pharmacology"*). There is no controlled clinical experience with Doxazosin Mesylate in patients with these conditions.

3. Leukopenia/Neutropenia: Analysis of hematologic data from patients receiving Doxazosin Mesylate in controlled clinical trials showed that the mean WBC (N = 474) and mean neutrophil counts (N = 419) were decreased by 2.4% and 1.0% respectively, compared to placebo, a phenomenon seen with other alpha blocking drugs. A search through a data base of 2400 patients revealed 4 in which drug-related neutropenia could not be ruled out. Two had a single low value on the last day of treatment. Two had stable, non-progressive neutrophil counts in the 1000/mm^3 range over periods of 20 and 40 weeks. In cases where follow-up was available the WBCs and neutrophil counts returned to normal after discontinuation of Doxazosin Mesylate. No patients became symptomatic as a result of the low WBC or neutrophil counts.

INFORMATION FOR PATIENTS

Patients should be made aware of the possibility of syncopal and orthostatic symptoms, especially at the initation of therapy, and urged to avoid driving or hazardous tasks for 24 hours after the first dose, after a dosage increase, and after interruption of therapy when treatment is resumed. They should be cautioned to avoid situations where injury could result should syncope occur during initiation of Doxazosin therapy. They should also be advised of the need to sit or lie down when symptoms of lowered blood pressure occur, although these symptoms are not always orthostatic, and to be careful when rising from a sitting or lying position. If dizziness, light-headedness, or palpitations are bothersome they should be reported to the physician, so that dose adjustment can be considered. Patients should also be told that drowsiness or somnolence can occur with Doxazosin, requiring caution in people who must drive or operate heavy machinery.

DRUG INTERACTIONS

Most (98%) of plasma Doxazosin is protein bound. *In vitro* data in human plasma indicate that Doxazosin Mesylate has no effect on protein binding of dioxin, warfarin, phenytoin or indomethacin. There is no information on the effect of other highly plasma protein bound drugs on Doxazosin binding. Doxazosin Mesylate has been administered without any evidence of an adverse drug interaction to patients receiving thiazide diuretics, beta-blocking agents, and nonsteroidal anti-inflammatory drugs.

CIMETIDINE

In a placebo-controlled trial in normal volunteers, the administration of a single 1 mg dose of Doxazosin on day 1 of a four-day regimen of oral cimetidine (400 mg twice daily) resulted in a 10% increase in mean AUC of Doxazosin (p=0.006), and a slight but not statistically significant increase in mean Cmax and mean half-life of Doxazosin. The clinical significance of this increase in Doxazosin AUC is unknown.

DRUG/LABORATORY TEST INTERACTIONS

None known.

CARDIAC TOXICITY IN ANIMALS

An increased incidence of myocardial necrosis or fibrosis was displayed by Sprague-Dawley rats after 6 months of dietary administration at concentrations calculated to provide 80 mg Doxazosin/kg/day and after 12 months of dietary administration at concentrations calculated to provide 40 mg Doxazosin/kg/day (150 times the maximum recommended human dose assuming a patient weight of 60 kg). Myocardial fibrosis was observed in both rats and mice treated in the same manner with 40 mg Doxazosin/kg/day for 18 months. No cardiotoxicity was observed at lower doses (up to 10 to 20 mg/kg/day, depending on the study) in either species. These lesions were not observed after 12 months of oral dosing in dogs and Wistar rats at maximum doses of 20 mg/kg/day and 100 mg/kg/day, respectively. There is no evidence that similar lesions occur in humans.

CARCINOGENESIS, MUTAGENESIS AND
IMPAIRMENT OF FERTILITY

Chronic dietary administration (up to 24 months) of Doxazosin Mesylate at maximally tolerated concentrations (highest dose 40 mg/kg: about 150 times the maximum recommended human dose of 16 mg/60 kg) revealed no evidence of carcinogenicity in rats. There was also no evidence of carcinogenicity in a similarly conducted study (up to 18 months of dietary administration) in mice. The mouse study, however, was compromised by the failure to use a maximally tolerated dose of Doxazosin.

Mutagenicity studies revealed no drug- or metabolite-related effects at either chromosomal or subchromosomal levels.

Studies in rats showed reduced fertility in males treated with Doxazosin at oral doses of 20 (but not 5 or 10) mg/kg/day, about 75 times the maximum recommended human dose. This effect was reversible within two weeks of drug withdrawal.

PREGNANCY

Teratogenic Effects, Pregnancy Category C: Studies in pregnant rabbits and rats at daily oral doses of up to 41 and 20 mg/kg, respectively (154 and 75 times the maximum recommended daily dose of 16 mg, assuming a patient weight of 60 kg), have revealed no evidence of harm to the fetus. A dosage regimen of 82 mg/kg/day in the rabbit was associated with reduced fetal survival. There are no adequate and well-controlled studies in pregnant women. Because animal reproduction studies are not always predictive of human response, Doxazosin Mesylate should be used during pregnancy if clearly needed.

Radioactivity was found to cross the placenta following oral administration of labelled Doxazosin to pregnant rats.

Nonteratogenic Effects: In peri-postnatal studies in rats, postnatal development at maternal doses of 40 or 50 mg/kg/day of Doxazosin was delayed as evidenced by slower body weight gain and a slightly later appearance of anatomical features and reflexes.

NURSING MOTHERS

Studies in lactating rats given a single oral dose of 1 mg/kg of [2-^{14}C]-Doxazosin indicate that Doxazosin accumulates in rat breast milk with a maximum concentration about 20 times greater than the maternal plasma concentration. It is not known whether this drug is excreted in human milk. Because many drugs are excreted in human milk, caution should be exercised when Doxazosin Mesylate is administered to a nursing mother.

PEDIATRIC USE

Safety and effectiveness in children have not been established.

ADVERSE REACTIONS

Doxazosin Mesylate has been administered to approximately 4000 patients, of whom 1679 were included in the clinical development program. In that program, minor adverse effects were frequent, but led to discontinuation of treatment in only 7% of patients. In placebo-controlled studies adverse effect occurred in 49% and 40% of patients in the Doxazosin and placebo groups, respectively, and to discontinuation in 2% of patients in each group. The major reasons for discontinuation were postural effects (2%), edema, malaise/fatigue, and some heart rate disturbance, each about 0.7%.

In controlled clinical trials directly comparing Doxazosin Mesylate to placebo there was no significant difference in the incidence of side effects, except for dizziness (including postural), weight gain, somnolence and fatigue/malaise. Postural effects and edema appeared to be dose related.

The prevalence rates presented below are based on combined data from placebo-controlled studies involving once daily administration of Doxazosin at doses ranging from 1-16 mg. Table 1 summarizes those adverse experiences (possibly/probably related) reported for patients in these studies where the prevalence rate in the Doxazosin group was at least 0.5% or where the reaction is of particular interest.

Table 1
ADVERSE REACTIONS DURING PLACEBO CONTROLLED STUDIES

	Doxazosin (N=339)	*Placebo* (N=336)
CARDIOVASCULAR		
Dizziness	19%	9%
Vertigo	2%	1%
Postural Hypotension	0.3%	0%
Edema	4%	3%
Palpitation	2%	3%
Arrhythmia	1%	0%
Hypotension	1%	0%
Tachycardia	0.3%	1%
Peripheral Ischemia	0.3%	0%
SKIN APPENDAGES		
Rash	1%	1%
Pruritus	1%	1%
MUSCULOSKELETAL		
Arthralgia/Arthritis	1%	0%
Muscle Weakness	1%	0%
Myalgia	1%	0%
CENTRAL & PERIPHERAL N.S.		
Headache	14%	16%
Paresthesia	1%	1%
Kinetic Disorders	1%	0%
Ataxia	1%	0%
Hypertonia	1%	0%
Muscle Cramps	1%	0%
AUTONOMIC		
Mouth Dry	2%	2%
Flushing	1%	0%
SPECIAL SENSES		
Vision Abnormal	2%	1%
Conjunctivitis/Eye Pain	1%	1%
Tinnitus	1%	0.3%
PSYCHIATRIC		
Somnolence	5%	1%
Nervousness	2%	2%
Depression	1%	1%
Insomnia	1%	1%
Sexual Dysfunction	2%	1%
GASTROINTESTINAL		
Nausea	3%	4%
Diarrhea	2%	3%
Constipation	1%	1%
Dyspepsia	1%	1%
Flatulence	1%	1%
Abdominal Pain	0%	2%
Vomiting	0%	1%
RESPIRATORY		
Rhinitis	3%	1%
Dyspnea	1%	1%
Epistaxis	1%	0%
URINARY		
Polyuria	2%	0%
Urinary Incontinence	1%	0%
Micturation Frequency	0%	2%
GENERAL		
Fatigue/Malaise	12%	6%
Chest Pain	2%	2%
Asthenia	1%	1%
Face Edema	1%	0%
Pain	2%	2%

Additional adverse reactions have been reported, but these are, in general, not distinguishable from symptoms that might have occurred in the absence of exposure to Doxazosin. The following adverse reactions occurred with a frequency of between 0.5% and 1%: syncope, hypoesthesia, increased sweating, agitation, increased weight. The following additional adverse reactions were reported by <0.5% of 3960 patients who received Doxazosin in controlled or open, short- or long-term clinical studies, including international studies.

Cardiovascular System: angina pectoris, myocardial infarction, cerebrovascular accident;

Autonomic Nervous System: pallor;

Metabolic: thirst, gout, hypokalemia;

Hematopoietic: lymphadenopathy, purpura;

Reproductive System: breast pain;

Skin Disorders: alopecia, dry skin, eczema;

Central Nervous System: paresis, tremor, twitching, confusion, migraine, impaired concentration;

Psychiatric: paroniria, amnesia, emotional lability, abnormal thinking, depersonalization;

Special Senses: parosmia, earache, taste perversion, photophobia, abnormal lacrimation;

Gastrointestinal System: increased appetite, anorexia, fecal incontinence, gastroenteritis;

Respiratory System: bronchospasm, sinusitis, coughing, pharyngitis;

Urinary System: renal calculus;

General Body System: hot flushes, back pain, infection, fever/rigors, decreased weight, influenza-like symptoms.

Doxazosin Mesylate has not been associated with any clinically significant changes in routine biochemical tests. No clinically relevant adverse effects were noted on serum potassium, serum glucose, uric acid, blood urea nitrogen, creatinine or liver function tests. Doxazosin Mesylate has been associated with decreases in white blood cell counts (See *"Precautions"*).

OVERDOSAGE
No data are available in regard to overdosage in humans. The oral LD_{50} of Doxazosin is greater than 1000 mg/kg in mice and rats. The most likely manifestation of overdosage would be hypotension, for which the usual treatment would be intravenous infusion of fluid. As Doxazosin is highly protein bound, dialysis would not be indicated.

DOSAGE AND ADMINISTRATION
Dosage Must Be Individualized: The initial dosage of Doxazosin Mesylate in hypertensive patients is 1 mg given once daily. This starting dose is intended to minimize the frequency of postural hypotension and first dose syncope associated with Doxazosin Mesylate. Postural effects are most likely to occur between 2 and 6 hours after a dose. Therefore blood pressure measurements should be taken during this time period after the first dose and with each increase in dose. Depending on the individual patient's standing blood pressure response (based on measurements taken at 2-6 hours postdose and 24 hours postdose), dosage may then be increased to 2 mg and thereafter if necessary to 4 mg, 8 mg and 16 mg to achieve the desired reduction in blood pressure. **Increases in dose beyond 4 mg increase the likelihood of excessive postural effects including syncope, postural dizziness/ vertigo, postural hypotension. At a titrated dose of 16 mg once daily the frequency of postural effects is about 12% compared to 3% for placebo.**

Store below 86°F (30°C).

HOW SUPPLIED
TABLETS: 1 MG

BRAND/MANUFACTURER	NDC	SIZE	AWP
○ BRAND			
➤ CARDURA: Roerig,J.B.	00049-2750-66	100s	$85.26
	00049-2750-41	100s ud	$87.81

TABLETS: 2 MG

BRAND/MANUFACTURER	NDC	SIZE	AWP
○ BRAND			
➤ CARDURA: Roerig,J.B.	00049-2760-66	100s	$85.26
	00049-2760-41	100s ud	$87.81

TABLETS: 4 MG

BRAND/MANUFACTURER	NDC	SIZE	AWP
○ BRAND			
➤ CARDURA: Roerig,J.B.	00049-2770-66	100s	$89.51
	00049-2770-41	100s ud	$92.20

➤ SHOWN IN PRODUCT IDENTIFICATION GUIDE

Doxepin Hydrochloride

DESCRIPTION

Doxepin Hydrochloride is one of a class of psychotherapeutic agents known as dibenzoxepin tricyclic compounds. The molecular formula of the compound is $C_{19}H_{21}NO \cdot HCl$ having a molecular weight of 316. It is a white crystalline solid readily soluble in water, lower alcohols and chloroform.

Chemically, Doxepin Hydrochloride is a dibenzoxepin derivative and is the first of a family of tricyclic psychotherapeutic agents. Specifically, it is an isomeric mixture of 1-Propanamine, 3-Dibenz[b,e] oxepin-11(6H)ylidene-N,N-dimethyl-hydrochloride.

All capsule and oral concentrate strengths for oral administration contain Doxepin base as the Hydrochloride.

Each capsule contains:

Doxepin ....10, 25, 50, 75, 100, or 150 mg.

Each ml of oral concentrate contains:

Doxepin ....10 mg.

Following is its chemical structure:

$$CHCH_2CH_2N(CH_3)_2$$

· HCl

CLINICAL PHARMACOLOGY

The mechanism of action of Doxepin HCl is not definitely known. It is not a central nervous system stimulant nor a monoamine oxidase inhibitor. The current hypothesis is that the clinical effects are due, at least in part, to influences on the adrenergic activity at the synapses so that deactivation of norepinephrine by reuptake into the nerve terminals is prevented. Animal studies suggest that Doxepin HCl does not appreciably antagonize the antihypertensive action of guanethidine. In animal studies anticholinergic, antiserotonin and antihistamine effects on smooth muscle have been demonstrated. At higher than usual clinical doses norepinephrine response was potentiated in animals. The effect was not demonstrated in humans.

At clinical dosages up to 150 mg per day, Doxepin HCl can be given to man concomitantly with guanethidine and related compounds without blocking the antihypertensive effect. At dosages above 150 mg per day blocking of the antihypertensive effect of these compounds has been reported.

Doxepin is virtually devoid of euphoria as a side effect. Characteristic of this type of compound, Doxepin has not been demonstrated to produce the physical tolerance or psychological dependence associated with addictive compounds.

INDICATIONS AND USAGE

Doxepin HCl is recommended for the treatment of:
1. Psychoneurotic patients with depression and/or anxiety.
2. Depression and/or anxiety associated with alcoholism (not to be taken concomitantly with alcohol).
3. Depression and/or anxiety associated with organic disease (the possibility of drug interaction should be considered if the patient is receiving other drugs concomitantly).
4. Psychotic depressive disorders associated with anxiety including involutional depression and manic-depressive disorders.

The target symptoms of psychoneurosis that respond particularly well to Doxepin HCl include anxiety, tension, depression, somatic symptoms and concerns, sleep disturbances, guilt, lack of energy, fear, apprehension and worry.

Clinical experience has shown that Doxepin HCl is safe and well-tolerated even in the elderly patient. Owing to a lack of clinical experience in the pediatric population, Doxepin HCl is not recommended for use in children under 12 years of age.

UNLABELED USES

Doxepin is used alone or as an adjunct in the treatment of anorexia nervosa, detrusor overactivity and associated symptoms in female cocaine dependence patients, and refractory depression. It is also used in patients with psychogenic headache, duodenal ulcer, night terrors, to reduce postprandial hypoglycemia, and posttraumatic stress disorder. Doxepin is also prescribed for premenstrual syndrome, pruritus, chronic cancer pain, tobacco smoking cessation, and idiopathic urticaria.

CONTRAINDICATIONS

Doxepin HCl is contraindicated in patients who have shown hypersensitivity to the drug. Possibility of cross sensitivity with other dibenzoxepines should be kept in mind.

Doxepin HCl is contraindicated in patients with glaucoma or a tendency to urinary retention. The disorders should be ruled out, particularly in older patients.

WARNINGS

The once-a-day dosage regimen of Doxepin HCl in patients with intercurrent illness or patients taking other medications should be carefully adjusted. This is especially important in patients receiving other medications with anticholinergic effects.

Usage in Geriatrics: The use of Doxepin HCl on a once-a-day dosage regimen in geriatric patients should be adjusted carefully based on the patient's condition.

Usage in Pregnancy: Reproduction studies have been performed in rats, rabbits, monkeys and dogs and there was no evidence of harm to the animal fetus. The relevance to humans is not known. Since there is no experience in pregnant women who have received this drug, safety in pregnancy has not been established. There has been a report of apnea and drowsiness occurring in a nursing infant whose mother was taking Doxepin.

Usage in Children: The use of Doxepin HCl in children under 12 years of age is not recommended, because safe conditions for its use have not been established.

DRUG INTERACTIONS

MAO Inhibitors: Serious side effects and even death have been reported following the concomitant use of certain drugs with MAO inhibitors. Therefore, MAO inhibitors should be discontinued at least two weeks prior to the cautious initiation of therapy with Doxepin HCl. The exact length of time may vary and is dependent upon the particular MAO inhibitor being used, the length of time it has been administered, and the dosage involved.

Cimetidine: Cimetidine has been reported to produce clinically significant fluctuations in steady-state serum concentrations of various tricyclic antidepressants. Serious anticholinergic symptoms (i.e., severe dry mouth, urinary retention and blurred vision) have been associated with elevations in the serum levels of tricyclic antidepressant when cimetidine therapy is initiated. Additionally, higher than expected tricyclic antidepressant levels have been observed when they are begun in patients already taking cimetidine. In patients who have been reported to be well controlled on tricyclic antidepressants receiving concurrent cimetidine therapy, discontinuation of cimetidine has been reported to decrease established steady-state serum tricyclic antidepressant levels and compromise their therapeutic effects.

Usage with Alcohol: It should be borne in mind that alcohol ingestion may increase the danger inherent in any intentional or unintentional Doxepin HCl overdosage. This is especially important in patients who may use alcohol excessively.

Tolazamide: A case of severe hypoglycemia has been reported in a type II diabetic patient maintained on tolazamide (1 gm/day) 11 days after the addition of Doxepin (75 mg/day).

PRECAUTIONS

Since drowsiness may occur with the use of this drug, patients should be warned of the possibility and cautioned against driving a car or operating hazardous machinery while taking the drug. Patients should also be cautioned that their response to alcohol may be potentiated.

Since suicide is an inherent risk in any depressed patient and may remain so until significant improvement has occurred, patients should be closely supervised during the early course of therapy. Prescriptions should be written for the smallest feasible amount.

Should increased symptoms of psychosis or shift to manic symptomatology occur, it may be necessary to reduce dosage or add a major tranquilizer to the dosage regimen.

ADVERSE REACTIONS

Note: Some of the adverse reactions noted below have not been specifically reported with Doxepin HCl use. However, due to the close pharmacological similarities among the tricyclics, the reactions should be considered when prescribing Doxepin HCl.

Anticholinergic Effects: Dry mouth, blurred vision, constipation and urinary retention have been reported. If they do not subside with continued therapy or become severe, it may be necessary to reduce the dosage.

Central Nervous System Effects: Drowsiness is the most commonly noticed side effect. This tends to disappear as therapy is continued. Other infrequently reported CNS side effects are confusion, disorientation, hallucinations, numbness, paresthesias, ataxia, extrapyramidal symptoms, seizures, tardive dyskinesia, and tremor.

Cardiovascular Effects: Cardiovascular effects including hypotension, hypertension, and tachycardia have been reported occasionally.

Allergic: Skin rash, edema, photosensitization, and pruritus have occasionally occurred.

Hematologic: Eosinophilia has been reported in a few patients. There have been occasional reports of bone marrow depression manifesting as agranulocytosis, leukopenia, thrombocytopenia, and purpura.

Gastrointestinal: Nausea, vomiting, indigestion, taste disturbances, diarrhea, anorexia, and aphthous stomatitis have been reported. (See *"Anticholinergic Effects"*.)

Endocrine: Raised or lowered libido, testicular swelling, gynecomastia in males, enlargement of breasts and galactorrhea in the female, raising or lowering of blood sugar levels and syndrome of inappropriate antidiuretic hormone secretion have been reported with tricyclic administration.

Other: Dizziness, tinnitus, weight gain, sweating, chills, fatigue, weakness, flushing, jaundice, alopecia, headache, exacerbation of asthma, and hyperpyrexia (in association with chlorpromazine) have been occasionally observed as adverse effects.

Withdrawal Symptoms: The possibility of development of withdrawal symptoms upon abrupt cessation of treatment after prolonged Doxepin HCl administration should be borne in mind. These are not indicative of addiction and gradual withdrawal of medication should not cause these symptoms.

OVERDOSAGE

A. SIGNS AND SYMPTOMS
1. *Mild:* Drowsiness, stupor, blurred vision, excessive dryness of mouth.
2. *Severe:* Respiratory depression, hypotension, coma, convulsions, cardiac arrhythmias and tachycardias.

Also: urinary retention (bladder atony), decreased gastrointestinal motility (paralytic ileus), hyperthemia (or hypothermia), hypertension, dilated pupils, hyperactive reflexes.

B. MANAGEMENT AND TREATMENT
1. *Mild* : Observation and supportive therapy is all that is usually necessary.
2. *Severe* : Medical management of severe Doxepin HCl overdosage consists of aggressive supportive therapy. If the patient is conscious, gastric lavage, with appropriate precautions to prevent pulmonary aspiration, should be performed even though Doxepin HCl is rapidly absorbed. The use of activated charcoal has been recommended, as has continuous gastric lavage with saline for 24 hours or more. An adequate airway should be established in comatose patients and assisted ventilation used if necessary. EKG monitoring may be required for several days, since relapse after apparent recovery has been reported. Arrhythmias should be treated with appropriate antiarrhythmic agents. It has been reported that many of the cardiovascular and CNS symptoms of tricyclic antidepressant poisoning in adults may be reversed by the slow intravenous administration of 1 mg to 3 mg of physostigmine salicylate. Because physostigmine is rapidly metabolized, the dosage should be repeated as required. Convulsions may respond to standard anticonvulsant therapy; however, barbiturates may potentiate any respiratory depression. Dialysis and forced diuresis generally are not of value in the management of overdosage due to high tissue and protein binding of Doxepin HCl.

DOSAGE AND ADMINISTRATION

For most patients with illness of mild to moderate severity, a starting daily dose of 75 mg is recommended. Dosage may subsequently be increased or decreased at appropriate intervals and according to individual response. The usual optimum dose range is 75 mg per day to 150 mg per day.

In more severely ill patients higher doses may be required with subsequent gradual increase to 300 mg per day, if necessary. Additional therapeutic effect is rarely to be obtained by exceeding a dose of 300 mg per day.

In patients with very mild symptomatology or emotional symptoms accompanying organic disease, lower doses may suffice. Some of these patients have been controlled on doses as low as 25-50 mg per day.

The total daily dosage of Doxepin may be given on a divided or once-a-day dosage schedule. If the once-a-day schedule is employed, the maximum recommended dose is 150 mg per day. This dose may be given at bedtime. **The 150 mg capsule strength is intended for maintenance therapy only and is not recommended for intiation of treatment.**

Antianxiety effect is apparent before the antidepressant effect. Optimal antidepressant effect may not be evident for two to three weeks.

Just prior to administration, Doxepin HCl oral concentrate should be diluted with approximately 120 ml of water, whole or skimmed milk, or orange, grapefruit, tomato, prune or pineapple juice. Doxepin HCl Oral Concentrate is not physically compatible with a number of carbonated beverages. For those patients requiring antidepressant therapy who are on methadone maintenance, Doxepin HCl Oral Concentrate and methadone syrup can be mixed together with lemonade, orange juice, sugar water, or water, but not with grape juice. Preparation and storage of bulk dilutions is not recommended.

STORAGE
Store at controlled room temperature, 15-30°C (59-86°F). Protect from light.
Dispense in a tight, light-resistant container using a child-resistant closure.

HOW SUPPLIED
CAPSULE: 10 MG

AVERAGE UNIT PRICE (AVAILABLE SIZES)		GENERIC A-RATED AVERAGE PRICE (GAAP)	
BRAND	$0.31	100s	$13.21
GENERIC	$0.12	1000s	$97.46
HCFA FUL (100s ea)	$0.05		

BRAND/MANUFACTURER	NDC	SIZE	AWP
◆ **BRAND**			
ADAPIN: Lotus Biochemical	59417-0356-71	100s	$28.31
➤ SINEQUAN: Roerig	00662-5340-66	100s	$32.56
	00662-5340-41	100s ud	$35.61
	00662-5340-82	1000s	$284.24

BRAND/MANUFACTURER	NDC	SIZE	AWP
◆ **GENERICS**			
Qualitest	00603-3455-21	100s	$9.05
Caraco	57664-0130-08	100s	$9.20
Schein	00364-2113-01	100s	$9.20
Goldline	00182-1325-01	100s	$10.00
Martec	52555-0294-01	100s	$10.05
Geneva	00781-2800-01	100s	$10.26
Major	00904-1260-60	100s	$10.50
Rugby	00536-4563-01	100s	$11.95
Aligen	00405-4369-01	100s	$12.20
URL	00677-1101-01	100s	$12.70
Mylan	00378-1049-01	100s	$12.76
Moore,H.L.	00839-7220-06	100s	$12.89
Royce	51875-0309-01	100s	$12.90
Par	49884-0217-01	100s	$12.95
Mason Dist	11845-0346-01	100s	$12.95
Moore,H.L.	00839-7892-06	100s	$13.56
Parmed	00349-8591-01	100s	$13.65
Raway	00686-0436-20	100s	$15.00
U.S. Trading	56126-0345-11	100s ud	$6.41
Goldline	00182-1325-89	100s ud	$14.99
Geneva	00781-2800-13	100s ud	$15.72
Schein	00364-2113-90	100s ud	$18.00
Major	00904-1260-61	100s ud	$19.40
Vangard	00615-0395-13	100s ud	$19.57
UDL	51079-0436-20	100s ud	$24.40
Par	49884-0217-05	500s	$64.50
Rugby	00536-4563-10	1000s	$49.50
Aligen	00405-4369-03	1000s	$54.45
Qualitest	00603-3455-32	1000s	$80.43
Major	00904-1260-80	1000s	$80.55
Mylan	00378-1049-10	1000s	$113.88
Royce	51875-0309-04	1000s	$115.20
Par	49884-0217-10	1000s	$125.62
Mason Dist	11845-0346-04	1000s	$125.62
Moore,H.L.	00839-7892-16	1000s	$131.89

CAPSULE: 25 MG

AVERAGE UNIT PRICE (AVAILABLE SIZES)		GENERIC A-RATED AVERAGE PRICE (GAAP)	
BRAND	$0.39	100s	$15.20
GENERIC	$0.14	1000s	$116.58
HCFA FUL (100s ea)	$0.05		

BRAND/MANUFACTURER	NDC	SIZE	AWP
◆ **BRAND**			
➤ ADAPIN: Lotus Biochemical	59417-0357-71	100s	$36.51
➤ SINEQUAN: Roerig	00662-5350-66	100s	$42.00
	00662-5350-41	100s ud	$44.75
	00662-5350-82	1000s	$366.29
	00662-5350-94	5000s	$1794.93
◆ **GENERICS**			
Qualitest	00603-3456-21	100s	$11.60
Caraco	57664-0131-08	100s	$11.75
Goldline	00182-1326-01	100s	$11.75
Schein	00364-2114-01	100s	$11.90
Martec	52555-0295-01	100s	$12.20
Rugby	00536-4564-01	100s	$12.75
➤ Geneva	00781-2801-01	100s	$12.87
Major	00904-1261-60	100s	$12.95
URL	00677-1102-01	100s	$13.08
➤ Mylan	00378-3125-01	100s	$13.12
Aligen	00405-4370-01	100s	$13.20
Par	49884-0218-01	100s	$13.25
Royce	51875-0310-01	100s	$13.25
Mason Dist	11845-0347-01	100s	$13.25
Moore,H.L.	00839-7221-06	100s	$13.49
Moore,H.L.	00839-7893-06	100s	$13.91
Parmed	00349-8592-01	100s	$14.04
Raway	00686-0437-20	100s	$15.50
U.S. Trading	56126-0346-11	100s ud	$7.77
Goldline	00182-1326-89	100s ud	$17.99
➤ Geneva	00781-2801-13	100s ud	$19.60
Schein	00364-2114-90	100s ud	$22.00
Vangard	00615-0396-13	100s ud	$23.83
Major	00904-1261-61	100s ud	$24.22
UDL	51079-0437-20	100s ud	$30.66
Par	49884-0218-05	500s	$66.25
Schein	00364-2114-02	1000s	$76.80
Major	00904-1261-80	1000s	$89.50
Caraco	57664-0131-18	1000s	$107.75
➤ Geneva	00781-2801-10	1000s	$110.50
Qualitest	00603-3456-32	1000s	$110.91
➤ Mylan	00378-3125-10	1000s	$115.62
Rugby	00536-4564-10	1000s	$115.75
Royce	51875-0310-04	1000s	$120.05
Par	49884-0218-10	1000s	$128.53
Mason Dist	11845-0347-04	1000s	$128.53
Aligen	00405-4370-03	1000s	$128.90
Moore,H.L.	00839-7221-16	1000s	$141.35
Moore,H.L.	00839-7893-16	1000s	$141.35

➤ SHOWN IN PRODUCT IDENTIFICATION GUIDE

CAPSULE: 50 MG

AVERAGE UNIT PRICE (AVAILABLE SIZES)		GENERIC A-RATED AVERAGE PRICE (GAAP)	
BRAND	$0.53	**100s**	$21.36
GENERIC	$0.20	**1000s**	$161.17
HCFA FUL (100s ea)	$0.07		

BRAND/MANUFACTURER	NDC	SIZE	AWP
◆ **BRAND**			
➤ ADAPIN: Lotus Biochemical	59417-0358-71	100s	$51.42
➤ SINEQUAN: Roerig	00662-5360-66	100s	$59.13
	00662-5360-82	1000s	$515.96
	00662-5360-94	5000s	$2528.03
◆ **GENERICS**			
Qualitest	00603-3457-21	100s	$16.61
Caraco	57664-0132-08	100s	$16.80
Schein	00364-2115-01	100s	$16.80
Martec	52555-0296-01	100s	$16.90
Goldline	00182-1327-01	100s	$18.00
Geneva	00781-2802-01	100s	$18.04
Major	00904-1262-60	100s	$18.25
URL	00677-1103-01	100s	$18.35
Mylan	00378-4250-01	100s	$18.38
Par	49884-0219-01	100s	$18.90
Mason Dist	11845-0348-01	100s	$18.90
Aligen	00405-4371-01	100s	$18.94
Royce	51875-0311-01	100s	$19.02
Moore,H.L.	00839-7222-06	100s	$19.24
Moore,H.L.	00839-7894-06	100s	$19.24
Rugby	00536-4565-01	100s	$19.25
Raway	00686-0438-20	100s	$19.50
Parmed	00349-8593-01	100s	$19.67
U.S. Trading	56126-0347-11	100s ud	$9.23
Goldline	00182-1327-89	100s ud	$25.99
Geneva	00781-2802-13	100s ud	$27.60
Schein	00364-2115-90	100s ud	$31.50
Vangard	00615-0397-13	100s ud	$32.64
Major	00904-1262-61	100s ud	$33.41
UDL	51079-0438-20	100s ud	$42.74
Par	49884-0219-05	500s	$94.50
Qualitest	00603-3457-32	1000s	$100.67
Schein	00364-2115-02	1000s	$110.00
Major	00904-1262-80	1000s	$138.50
Caraco	57664-0132-18	1000s	$138.90
Rugby	00536-4565-10	1000s	$146.75
Geneva	00781-2802-10	1000s	$158.60
Mylan	00378-4250-10	1000s	$169.38
Royce	51875-0311-04	1000s	$176.00
Par	49884-0219-10	1000s	$183.33
Mason Dist	11845-0348-04	1000s	$183.33
Aligen	00405-4371-03	1000s	$183.52
Moore,H.L.	00839-7894-16	1000s	$203.10
Moore,H.L.	00839-7222-16	1000s	$203.11

CAPSULE: 75 MG

AVERAGE UNIT PRICE (AVAILABLE SIZES)		GENERIC A-RATED AVERAGE PRICE (GAAP)	
BRAND	$0.91	**100s**	$36.66
GENERIC	$0.35	**500s**	$140.00
HCFA FUL (100s ea)	$0.10	**1000s**	$277.00

BRAND/MANUFACTURER	NDC	SIZE	AWP
◆ **BRAND**			
ADAPIN: Lotus Biochemical	59417-0361-71	100s	$85.27
➤ SINEQUAN: Roerig	00662-5390-66	100s	$98.05
	00662-5390-82	1000s	$891.80
◆ **GENERICS**			
Qualitest	00603-3458-21	100s	$19.12
Martec	52555-0331-01	100s	$28.25
Major	00904-1263-60	100s	$29.00
Goldline	00182-1328-01	100s	$29.00
Schein	00364-2116-01	100s	$29.10
Geneva	00781-2803-01	100s	$29.90
Rugby	00536-3737-01	100s	$30.75
URL	00677-1104-01	100s	$35.25
Mylan	00378-5375-01	100s	$35.50
Par	49884-0220-01	100s	$35.75
Mason Dist	11845-0349-01	100s	$35.75
Aligen	00405-4372-01	100s	$35.82
Moore,H.L.	00839-7223-06	100s	$36.38
Moore,H.L.	00839-7895-06	100s	$37.53
Parmed	00349-8594-01	100s	$37.99
U.S. Trading	56126-0348-11	100s ud	$11.85
Goldline	00182-1328-89	100s ud	$30.00
Geneva	00781-2803-13	100s ud	$44.10
Schein	00364-2116-90	100s ud	$50.00
Vangard	00615-0398-13	100s ud	$58.36
Major	00904-1263-61	100s ud	$58.61
UDL	51079-0645-20	100s ud	$68.43
Rugby	00536-3737-05	500s	$101.25
Par	49884-0220-05	500s	$178.75
Qualitest	00603-3458-32	1000s	$134.91
Mason Dist	11845-0349-04	1000s	$197.60
Mylan	00378-5375-10	1000s	$341.62

BRAND/MANUFACTURER	NDC	SIZE	AWP
Par	49884-0220-10	1000s	$346.78
Moore,H.L.	00839-7895-16	1000s	$364.10

CAPSULE: 100 MG

AVERAGE UNIT PRICE (AVAILABLE SIZES)		GENERIC A-RATED AVERAGE PRICE (GAAP)	
BRAND	$0.98	**100s**	$41.74
GENERIC	$0.41	**1000s**	$358.16
HCFA FUL (100s ea)	$0.12		

BRAND/MANUFACTURER	NDC	SIZE	AWP
◆ **BRAND**			
ADAPIN: Lotus Biochemical	59417-0359-71	100s	$92.96
➤ SINEQUAN: Roerig	00662-5380-66	100s	$106.90
	00662-5380-82	1000s	$944.36
◆ **GENERICS**			
Raway	00686-0465-20	100s	$27.50
Qualitest	00603-3459-21	100s	$29.96
Geneva	00781-2804-01	100s	$30.05
Schein	00364-2117-01	100s	$30.90
Goldline	00182-1329-01	100s	$32.00
Martec	52555-0332-01	100s	$32.40
Rugby	00536-4566-01	100s	$39.50
Major	00904-1264-60	100s	$39.50
URL	00677-1105-01	100s	$41.59
Mylan	00378-6410-01	100s	$41.62
Par	49884-0221-01	100s	$42.05
Mason Dist	11845-0350-01	100s	$42.05
Aligen	00405-4373-01	100s	$42.32
Moore,H.L.	00839-7224-06	100s	$42.65
Moore,H.L.	00839-7896-06	100s	$42.65
Parmed	00349-8595-01	100s	$44.89
U.S. Trading	56126-0349-11	100s ud	$14.42
Goldline	00182-1329-89	100s ud	$35.00
Geneva	00781-2804-13	100s ud	$48.99
Schein	00364-2117-90	100s ud	$52.00
Vangard	00615-0399-13	100s ud	$65.14
Major	00904-1264-61	100s ud	$66.25
UDL	51079-0651-20	100s ud	$76.64
Par	49884-0221-05	500s	$210.25
Rugby	00536-4566-10	1000s	$193.75
Mylan	00378-6410-10	1000s	$402.76
Par	49884-0221-10	1000s	$407.89
Moore,H.L.	00839-7896-16	1000s	$428.22

CAPSULE: 150 MG

AVERAGE UNIT PRICE (AVAILABLE SIZES)		GENERIC A-RATED AVERAGE PRICE (GAAP)	
BRAND	$1.65	**100s**	$50.85
GENERIC	$0.51		
HCFA FUL (100s ea)	$0.31		

BRAND/MANUFACTURER	NDC	SIZE	AWP
◆ **BRAND**			
ADAPIN: Lotus Biochemical	59417-0370-65	50s	$77.18
➤ SINEQUAN: Roerig	00662-5370-50	50s	$88.75
	00662-5370-73	500s	$807.65
◆ **GENERICS**			
Raway	00686-0301-13	100s	$34.00
Qualitest	00603-3460-21	100s	$48.10
Goldline	00182-1878-01	100s	$51.00
Major	00904-1265-60	100s	$52.45
Schein	00364-2525-01	100s	$52.96
Par	49884-0222-01	100s	$55.50
Moore,H.L.	00839-7509-06	100s	$58.25
Martec	52555-0322-01	100s	$59.85
Rugby	00536-3738-01	100s	$59.93
U.S. Trading	56126-0401-11	100s ud	$36.47
Par	49884-0222-05	500s	$277.50

CONCENTRATE: 10 MG/ML

AVERAGE UNIT PRICE (AVAILABLE SIZES)		GENERIC A-RATED AVERAGE PRICE (GAAP)	
BRAND	$0.21	**120 ml**	$15.33
GENERIC	$0.13		
HCFA FUL (120 ml)	$0.14		

BRAND/MANUFACTURER	NDC	SIZE	AWP
◆ **BRAND**			
SINEQUAN: Roerig	00662-5100-47	120 ml	$25.13
◆ **GENERICS**			
Copley	38245-0612-14	120 ml	$13.00
Warner Chilcott	00047-2623-35	120 ml	$14.00
Pennex	00426-8651-04	120 ml	$14.63
Pennex	00832-8651-04	120 ml	$14.63
Goldline	00182-6043-71	120 ml	$16.00
UDL	51079-0688-37	120 ml	$19.70

CREAM: 5%

BRAND/MANUFACTURER	NDC	SIZE	AWP
○ **BRAND**			
ZONALON: Genderm	52761-0523-30	30 gm	$19.80

◆ RATED THERAPEUTICALLY EQUIVALENT; ◇ THERAPEUTIC EQUIVALENCE UNCONFIRMED; ○ UNRATED

LIQUID: 10 MG/ML

AVERAGE UNIT PRICE (AVAILABLE SIZES)		GENERIC A-RATED AVERAGE PRICE (GAAP)	
GENERIC	$0.12	120 ml	$14.74

BRAND/MANUFACTURER		NDC	SIZE	AWP
◆ **GENERICS**				
Raway		00686-0612-14	120 ml	$13.00
Schein		00364-2278-77	120 ml	$14.70
Moore,H.L.		00839-7470-65	120 ml	$14.90
Rugby		00536-0685-97	120 ml	$16.35

SOLUTION: 10 MG/ML

BRAND/MANUFACTURER	NDC	SIZE	AWP
◆ **GENERICS**			
Aligen	00405-2680-76	120 ml	$15.20

TABLETS: 50 MG

AVERAGE UNIT PRICE (AVAILABLE SIZES)	
GENERIC	$0.44

BRAND/MANUFACTURER	NDC	SIZE	AWP
◆ **GENERICS**			
Medirex	57480-0464-06	30s	$13.20
Medirex	57480-0464-01	100s	$44.00

TABLETS: 150 MG

BRAND/MANUFACTURER	NDC	SIZE	AWP
◆ **GENERICS**			
Par	49884-0222-03	50s	$33.50

Doxorubicin Hydrochloride

WARNINGS

1. SEVERE LOCAL TISSUE NECROSIS WILL OCCUR IF THERE IS EXTRAVASATION DURING ADMINISTRATION (SEE *"DOSAGE AND ADMINISTRATION"*). DOXORUBICIN MUST NOT BE GIVEN BY THE INTRAMUSCULAR OR SUBCUTANEOUS ROUTE.

2. SERIOUS IRREVERSIBLE MYOCARDIAL TOXICITY WITH DELAYED CONGESTIVE HEART FAILURE OFTEN UNRESPONSIVE TO ANY CARDIAC SUPPORTIVE THERAPY MAY BE ENCOUNTERED AS TOTAL DOSAGE APPROACHES 550 MG/M^2. THIS TOXICITY MAY OCCUR AT LOWER CUMULATIVE DOSES IN PATIENTS WITH PRIOR MEDIASTINAL IRRADIATION OR ON CONCURRENT CYCLOPHOSPHAMIDE THERAPY.

3. DOSAGE SHOULD BE REDUCED IN PATIENTS WITH IMPAIRED HEPATIC FUNCTION.

4. SEVERE MYELOSUPPRESSION MAY OCCUR.

5. DOXORUBICIN SHOULD BE ADMINISTERED ONLY UNDER THE SUPERVISION OF A PHYSICIAN WHO IS EXPERIENCED IN THE USE OF CANCER CHEMOTHERAPEUTIC AGENTS.

DESCRIPTION

Doxorubicin is a cytotoxic anthracycline antibiotic isolated from cultures of *Streptomyces peucetius* var. *caesius*, with the chemical name of 8-Hydroxyacetyl (8S,10S)-10-((3-amino-2,3,6-trideoxy-alpha-L-lyxo-hexopyr anosylloxy)-6,8,11-trihydroxy-1 methoxy-7,8,9,10-tetra hydronaphthacene-5,12-dione hydrochloride. Doxorubicin consists of a naphthacenequinone nucleus linked through a glycosidic bond at ring atom 7 to an amino sugar, daunosamine.

The molecular formula of Doxorubicin is $C_{27}H_{29}NO_{11} \cdot HCl$. The molecular weight is 579.99.

Doxorubicin binds to nucleic acids, presumably by specific intercalation of the planar anthracycline nucleus with the DNA double helix. The anthracycline ring is lipophilic but the saturated end of the ring system contains abundant hydroxyl groups adjacent to the amino sugar, producing a hydrophilic center. The molecule is amphoteric, containing acidic functions in the ring phenolic groups and a basic function in the sugar amino group. It binds to cell membranes as well as plasma proteins.

Doxorubicin is available as sterile lypholized powder in vials containing 10 mg, 20 mg or 50 mg per vial, and as a parenteral isotonic or sterile aqueous solution in with a concentration of 2 mg/ml. Vial sizes of the solution are 5 ml, 10 ml, 25 ml, and 100 ml.

Following is its chemical structure:

CLINICAL PHARMACOLOGY

Though not completely elucidated, the mechanism of action of Doxorubicin is related to its ability to bind to DNA and inhibit nucleic acid synthesis. Cell culture studies have demonstrated rapid cell penetration and perinucleolar chromatin binding, rapid inhibition of mitotic activity and nucleic acid synthesis, mutagenesis and chromosomal aberrations. Animal studies have shown activity in a spectrum of experimental tumors, immunosuppression, carcinogenic properties in rodents, induction of a variety of toxic effects, including delayed and progressive cardiac toxicity, myelosuppression in all species and atrophy to testes in rats and dogs.

Pharmacokinetic studies show the intravenous administration of normal or radiolabeled Doxorubicin is followed by rapid plasma clearance and significant tissue binding. Urinary excretion, as determined by fluorimetric methods, accounts for approximately 4-5% of the administered dose in five days. Biliary excretion represents the major excretion route, 40-50% of the administered dose being recovered in the bile or the feces in seven days. Impairment of liver function results in slower excretion, and consequently, increased retention and accumulation in plasma and tissue. Doxorubicin does not cross the blood brain barrier.

INDICATIONS AND USAGE

Doxorubicin Hydrochloride for injection has been used successfully to produce regression in disseminated neoplastic conditions such as acute lymphoblastic leukemia, acute myeloblastic leukemia, Wilms' tumor, neuroblastoma, soft tissue and bone sarcomas, breast carcinoma, ovarian carcinoma, transitional cell bladder carcinoma, thyroid carcinoma, lymphomas of both Hodgkin and non-Hodgkin types, bronchogenic carcinoma in which the small cell histologic type is the most responsive compared to other cell types and gastric carcinoma.

A number of other solid tumors have also shown some responsiveness but in numbers too limited to justify specific recommendation. Studies to date have shown malignant melanoma, kidney carcinoma, large bowel carcinoma, brain tumors and metastases to the central nervous system not to be significantly responsive to Doxorubicin HCl therapy.

UNLABELED USES

Doxorubicin is used as an adjunct in the treatment of adenocarcinoma, apudomas, to treat recurrent or metastatic cervical carcinoma, chronic lymphocytic leukemia, advanced or recurrent endometrial carcinoma, and pancreatic islet cell carcinomas. It is also used in combination with other antineoplastic agents to treat AIDS-related Kaposi's sarcoma, advanced diffuse large-cell lymphomas, liver cancer including hepatoblastoma, multiple myeloma, advanced ovarian cancer, endocrine-unresponsive metastatic prostatic cancer, and basal cell carcinoma and squamous cell carcinoma.

CONTRAINDICATIONS

Doxorubicin HCl therapy should not be started in patients who have marked myelosuppression induced by previous treatment with other antitumor agents or by radiotherapy. Conclusive data are not available on pre-existing heart disease as a co-factor of increased risk of Doxorubicin HCl induced cardiac toxicity. Preliminary data suggest that in such cases cardiac toxicity may occur at doses lower than the recommended cumulative limit. It is therefore not recommended to start Doxorubicin HCl in such cases. Doxorubicin HCl treatment is contraindicated in patients who received previous treatment with complete cumulative doses of Doxorubicin HCl and/or daunorubicin.

WARNINGS

Special attention must be given to the cardiac toxicity exhibited by Doxorubicin HCl. Although uncommon, acute left ventricular failure has occurred, particularly in patients who have received total dosage of the drug exceeding the currently recommended limit of 550 mg/m^2. This limit appears to be lower (400 mg/m^2) in patients who received radiotherapy to the mediastinal area or concomitant therapy with other potentially cardiotoxic agents such as cyclophosphamide. The total dose of Doxorubicin HCl administered to the individual patient should also take into account a previous or concomitant therapy with related compounds such as daunorubicin. Congestive heart failure and/or cardiomyopathy may be encountered several weeks after discontinuation of Doxorubicin HCl therapy.

Cardiac failure is often not favorably affected by presently known medical or physical therapy for cardiac support. Early clinical diagnosis of drug-induced heart failure appears to be essential for successful treatment with digitalis, diuretics, low salt diet and bed rest. Severe cardiac toxicity may occur precipitously without antecedent EKG changes. A baseline EKG and EKGs performed prior to each dose or course after 300 mg/m^2 cumulative dose has been given is suggested. Transient EKG changes consisting of T-wave flattening, S-T depression and arrhythmias lasting for up to two weeks after a dose or course of Doxorubicin HCl are presently not considered indications for suspension of Doxorubicin HCl therapy. Doxorubicin HCl cardiomyopathy has been reported to be associated with a persistent reduction in the voltage of the QRS wave, a prolongation of the systolic time interval and a reduction of the ejection fraction as determined by echocardiography or radionuclide angiography. None of these tests have yet been confirmed to consistently identify those individual patients that are approaching their maximally tolerated cumulative dose of Doxorubicin HCl. If test results indicate change in cardiac function associated with Doxorubicin HCl the benefit of continued therapy must be carefully evaluated against the risk of producing irreversible cardiac damage.

Acute life-threatening arrhythmias have been reported to occur during or within a few hours after Doxorubicin HCl administration.

There is a high incidence of bone marrow depression, primarily of leukocytes, requiring careful hematologic monitoring. With the recommended dosage schedule, leukopenia is usually transient, reaching its nadir at 10-14 days after treatment with recovery usually occurring by the 21st day. White blood cell counts as low as 100/mm^3 are to be expected during treatment with appropriate doses of Doxorubicin HCl. Red blood cell and platelet levels should also be monitored since they may also be depressed. Hematologic toxicity may require dose reduction or suspension or delay of Doxorubicin HCl therapy. Persistent severe myelosuppression may result in superinfection and/or hemorrhage.

Doxorubicin HCl may potentiate the toxicity of other anticancer therapies. Exacerbation of cyclophosphamide induced hemorrhagic cystitis and enhancement of the hepatotoxicity of 6-mercaptopurine have been reported. Radiation-induced toxicity to the myocardium, mucosae, skin and liver have been reported to be increased by the administration of Doxorubicin HCl.

Toxicity to recommended doses of Doxorubicin HCl is enhanced by hepatic impairment; therefore, prior to the individual dosing, evaluation of hepatic function is recommended using conventional clinical laboratory tests such as SGOT, SGPT, alkaline phosphatase and bilirubin. (See "Dosage and Administration".)

Necrotizing colitis manifested by typhlitis (cecal inflammation), bloody stools and severe and sometimes fatal infections have been associated with a combination of Doxorubicin HCl given by IV push daily for 3 days and cytarabine given by continuous infusion daily for 7 or more days.

On intravenous administration of Doxorubicin HCl extravasation may occur with or without an accompanying stinging or burning sensation and even if blood returns well on aspiration of the infusion needle (see "Dosage and Administration"). If any signs or symptoms of extravasation have occurred the injection or infusion should be immediately terminated and restarted in another vein.

Doxorubicin HCl and related compounds have also been shown to have mutagenic and carcinogenic properties when tested in experimental models.

Usage in Pregnancy: Safe use of Doxorubicin HCl in pregnancy has not been established. Doxorubicin HCl is embryotoxic and teratogenic in rats and embryotoxic and abortifacient in rabbits. Therefore, the benefits to the pregnant patient should be carefully weighed against the potential toxicity to fetus and embryo. The possible adverse effects on fertility in males and females in humans or experimental animals have not been adequately evaluated.

PRECAUTIONS

Initial treatment with Doxorubicin HCl requires close observation of the patient and extensive laboratory monitoring. It is recommended, therefore, that patients be hospitalized at least during the first phase of the treatment.

Like other cytotoxic drugs, Doxorubicin HCl may induce hyperuricemia secondary to rapid lysis of neoplastic cells. The clinician should monitor the patient's blood uric acid level and be prepared to use such supportive and pharmacologic measures as might be necessary to control this problem.

Doxorubicin HCl imparts a red coloration to the urine for 1-2 days after administration and patients should be advised to expect this during active therapy.

Doxorubicin HCl is not an anti-microbial agent.

ADVERSE REACTIONS

Dose limiting toxicities of therapy are myelosuppression and cardiotoxicity (see "Warnings"). Other reactions reported are:

Cutaneous: Reversible complete alopecia occurs in most cases. Hyperpigmentation of nailbeds and dermal creases, primarily in children, and onycholysis have been reported in a few cases. Recall of skin reaction due to prior radiotherapy has occurred with Doxorubicin HCl administration.

Gastrointestinal: Acute nausea and vomiting occurs frequently and may be severe. This may be alleviated by antiemetic therapy. Mucositis (stomatitis and esophagitis) may occur 5-10 days after administration. The effect may be severe leading to ulceration and represents a site of origin for severe infections. The dose regimen consisting of administration of Doxorubicin HCl on three successive days results in the greater incidence and severity of mucositis. Ulceration and necrosis of the colon, especially the cecum, may occur leading to bleeding or severe infections which can be fatal. This reaction has been reported in patients with acute non-lymphocytic leukemia treated with a 3-day course of Doxorubicin HCl combined with cytarabine. Anorexia and diarrhea have been occasionally reported.

Vascular: Phlebosclerosis has been reported especially when small veins are used or a single vein is used for repeated administration. Facial flushing may occur if the injection is given too rapidly.

Local: Severe cellulitis, vesication and tissue necrosis will occur if Doxorubicin HCl is extravasated during administration. Erythematous streaking along the vein proximal to the site of the injection has been reported (see "Dosage and Administration").

Hypersensitivity: Fever, chills and urticaria have been reported occasionally. Anaphylaxis may occur. A case of apparent cross sensitivity to lincomycin has been reported.

Other: Conjunctivitis and lacrimation occur rarely.

OVERDOSAGE

Acute overdosage with Doxorubicin HCl enhances the toxic effects of mucositis, leukopenia and thrombopenia. Treatment of acute overdosage consists of treatment of the severely myelosuppressed patient with hospitalization, antibiotics, platelet and granulocyte transfusions and symptomatic treatment of mucositis.

Chronic overdosage with cumulative doses exceeding 550 mg/m^2 increases the risk of cardiomyopathy and resultant congestive heart failure. Treatment consists of vigorous management of congestive heart failure with digitalis preparations and diuretics. The use of peripheral vasodilators has been recommended.

DOSAGE AND ADMINISTRATION

Care in the administration of Doxorubicin HCl will reduce the chance of perivenous infiltration. It may also decrease the chance of local reactions such as urticaria and erythematous streaking. On intravenous administration of Doxorubicin HCl, extravasation may occur with or without an accompanying stinging or burning sensation and even if blood returns well on aspiration of the infusion needle. If any signs or symptoms of extravasation have occurred, the injection or infusion should be immediately terminated and restarted in another vein. If it is known or suspected that subcutaneous extravasation has occurred, local infiltration with an injectable corticosteroid and flooding the site with normal saline has been reported to lessen the local reaction. Because of the progressive nature of extravasation reactions, the area of injection should be frequently examined and plastic surgery consultation obtained. If ulceration begins, early wide excision of the involved area should be considered.[1]

The most commonly used dosage schedule is 60-75 mg/m^2 as a single intravenous injection administered at 21-day intervals. The lower dose should be given to patients with inadequate marrow reserves due to old age, or prior therapy, or neoplastic marrow infiltration. An alternative dose schedule is weekly doses of 20 mg/m^2 which has been reported to produce a lower incidence of congestive heart failure. Thirty mg/m^2 on each of three successive days repeated every 4 weeks has also been used. Doxorubicin HCl dosage must be reduced if the bilirubin is elevated as follows: serum bilirubin 1.2-3.0 mg/dL — give ½ normal dose, >3 mg/dL — give ¼ normal dose.

Preparation of Solution: Doxorubicin HCl 10 mg, 20 mg, 50 mg, and 150 mg vials should be reconstituted with 5 mL, 10 mL, 25 mL, and 75 mL respectively, of Sodium Chloride Injection, USP (0.9%) to give a final concentration of 2 mg/mL of Doxorubicin Hydrochloride. An appropriate volume of air should be withdrawn from the vial during reconstitution to avoid excessive pressure build-up. Bacteriostatic diluents are not recommended.

After adding the diluent, the vial should be shaken and the contents allowed to dissolve. The reconstituted solution is stable for 24 hours to 7 days at room temperature, depending on the brand, and under refrigeration (2°-8°C). It should be protected from exposure to sunlight. Discard any unused solution from the 10 mg, 20 mg and 50 mg single dose vials. Unused solutions of the multiple dose vial remaining beyond the recommended storage times should be discarded.

It is recommended that Doxorubicin HCl be slowly administered into the tubing of a freely running intravenous infusion of Sodium Chloride Injection USP or 5% Dextrose Injection USP. The tubing should be attached to a Butterfly® needle inserted preferably into a large vein. If possible, avoid veins over joints or in extremities with compromised venous or lymphatic drainage. The rate of administration is dependent on the size of the vein and the dosage. However, the dose should be administered in not less than 3 to 5 minutes. Local erythematous streaking along the vein as well as facial flushing may be indicative of too rapid an administration. A burning or stinging sensation may be indicative of perivenous infiltration and the infusion should be immediately terminated and restarted in another vein. Perivenous infiltration may occur painlessly.

Doxorubicin HCl should not be mixed with heparin or 5-fluorouracil since it has been reported that these drugs are incompatible to the extent that a precipitate may form. Until specific compatibility data are available, it is not recommended that Doxorubicin HCl be mixed with other drugs. Doxorubicin HCl has been used concurrently with other approved chemotherapeutic agents. Evidence is available that in some types of neoplastic disease combination chemotherapy is superior to single agents. The benefits and risks of such therapy continue to be elucidated.

Parenteral drug products should be inspected visually for particulate matter and discoloration prior to administration, whenever solution and container permit.

Handling and Disposal: Skin reactions associated with Doxorubicin HCl have been reported. Caution in the handling and preparation of the powder and of the solution must be exercised and the use of gloves is recommended. If Doxorubicin HCl powder or solution contacts the skin or mucosae, immediately wash thoroughly with soap and water.

Procedures for proper handling and disposal of anti-cancer drugs should be considered. Several guidelines on this subject have been published.[2-8] There is no general agreement that all of the procedures recommended in the guidelines are necessary or appropriate.

Storage: Store the solution under refrigeration 2°-8°C (36°-46°F), protect from light and retain in carton until time of use. Discard unused portion.

Store the lyopholized powder at controlled room temperature, 15°-30°C (59°-86°F). After reconstitution the solution is stable for 24 hours at room temperature and 48 hours under refrigeration, 2°-8°C (36°-46°F). Protect from exposure to light, including sunlight.

REFERENCES
1. Rudolph R et al: Skin Ulcers Due to Doxorubicin HCl. Cancer 38: 1087-1094, Sept. 1976.   2. Recommendations for the Safe Handling of Parenteral Antineoplastic Drugs. NIH Publication No. 83-2621. For sale by the Superintendent of Documents, U.S. Government Printing Office, Washington, D.C. 20402.   3. AMA Council Report, Guidelines for Handling Parenteral Antineoplastics. JAMA, March 15, 1985.   4. National Study Commission on Cytotoxic Exposure—Recommendations for Handling Cytotoxic Agents. Available from Louis P. Jeffrey, Sc. D., Director of Pharmacy Services, Rhode Island Hospital, 593 Eddy Street, Providence, Rhode Island 02902.   5. Clinical Oncological Society of Australia: Guidelines and recommendations for safe handling of antineoplastic agents. Med J. Australia 1:426-428, 1983.   6. Jones R., et al. Safe handling of chemotherapeutic agents: A report from the Mount Sinai Medical Center. Ca—A Cancer Journal for Clinicians Sept/Oct, 258-263, 1983.   7. American Society of Hospital Pharmacists technical assistance bulletin on handling cytotoxic drugs in hospitals. Am J Hosp Pharm 42:131-137, 1985.   8. OSHA Work-Practice Guidelines for Personnel Dealing with Cytotoxic (Antineoplastic) Drugs. *Am J Hosp Pharm.* 43:1193-1204, 1986.

J CODES
50 mg IV—J9010
10 mg IV—J9000

HOW SUPPLIED
INJECTION: 2 MG/ML

AVERAGE UNIT PRICE (AVAILABLE SIZES)			
BRAND	$9.61		
GENERIC	$9.47		

BRAND/MANUFACTURER	NDC	SIZE	AWP
◆ BRAND			
ADRIAMYCIN PFS: Pharmacia	00013-1136-91	5 ml	$48.31
	00013-1146-94	10 ml	$96.63
	00013-1156-79	25 ml	$241.56
	00013-1166-83	100 ml	$946.94
◆ GENERICS			
Chiron Therapeutics	53905-0237-01	25 ml	$236.74
Chiron Therapeutics	53905-0235-10	5 ml 10s	$473.50
Chiron Therapeutics	53905-0236-10	10 ml 10s	$947.00

INJECTION: 2 MG/ML

BRAND/MANUFACTURER	NDC	SIZE	AWP
○ BRAND			
ADRIAMYCIN PFS: Pharmacia	00013-1176-87	37.5 ml	$362.35

POWDER FOR INJECTION: 10 MG

AVERAGE UNIT PRICE (AVAILABLE SIZES)		GENERIC A-RATED AVERAGE PRICE (GAAP)	
BRAND	$44.91	10s	$395.56
GENERIC	$39.56		

BRAND/MANUFACTURER	NDC	SIZE	AWP
◆ BRAND			
RUBEX: Bristol-Myer Onc/Hiv	00015-3351-22	1s	$43.81
ADRIAMYCIN RDF: Pharmacia	00013-1086-91	1s	$46.00
◆ GENERICS			
Astra	00186-1530-13	10s	$207.25
VHA	00702-0231-10	10s	$450.75
Chiron Therapeutics	53905-0231-10	10s	$450.75
VHA	00702-0235-10	10s	$473.50

POWDER FOR INJECTION: 20 MG

AVERAGE UNIT PRICE (AVAILABLE SIZES)		GENERIC A-RATED AVERAGE PRICE (GAAP)	
BRAND	$92.000	6s	$554.59
GENERIC	$91.67		

BRAND/MANUFACTURER	NDC	SIZE	AWP
◆ BRAND			
ADRIAMYCIN RDF: Pharmacia	00013-1096-94	1s	$92.00
◆ GENERICS			
VHA	00702-0232-06	6s	$540.98
VHA	00702-0236-06	6s	$568.20
Chiron Therapeutics	53905-0232-10	10s	$901.60

POWDER FOR INJECTION: 50 MG

AVERAGE UNIT PRICE (AVAILABLE SIZES)		GENERIC A-RATED AVERAGE PRICE (GAAP)	
BRAND	$213.58	1s	$197.64
GENERIC	$197.64		

BRAND/MANUFACTURER	NDC	SIZE	AWP
◆ BRAND			
RUBEX: Bristol-Myer Onc/Hiv	00015-3352-22	1s	$197.15
ADRIAMYCIN RDF: Pharmacia	00013-1106-79	1s	$230.00
◆ GENERICS			
Astra	00186-1531-01	1s	$103.00
VHA	00702-0233-01	1s	$225.40
Chiron Therapeutics	53905-0233-01	1s	$225.40

BRAND/MANUFACTURER	NDC	SIZE	AWP
VHA	00702-0237-01	1s	$236.74

POWDER FOR INJECTION: 100 MG

BRAND/MANUFACTURER	NDC	SIZE	AWP
◆ BRAND			
RUBEX: Bristol-Myer Onc/Hiv	00015-3353-22	1s	$394.29

POWDER FOR INJECTION: 150 MG

BRAND/MANUFACTURER	NDC	SIZE	AWP
◆ BRAND			
ADRIAMYCIN RDF: Pharmacia	00013-1116-83	1s	$676.19

Doxycycline

DESCRIPTION
Doxycycline is a broad-spectrum antibiotic synthetically derived from oxytetracycline and is available as a syrup, capsules, oral suspension, and tablets for oral administration, and as an injection for intravenous use.

Each 5 ml (teaspoonful) of syrup contains:
Doxycycline Calcium equivalent to ....50 mg Doxycycline

Each capsule contains:
Doxycycline Hyclate equivalent to ....50 or 100 mg Doxycycline
Doxycycline Monohydrate equivalent to.. 50 or 100 mg Doxycycline

Each 5 ml (teaspoonful) of oral suspension contains:
Doxycycline Monohydrate equivalent to ....25 mg Doxycycline

Each tablet contains:
Doxycycline Hyclate equivalent to ....100 mg Doxycycline

Each unit of powder for injection contains:
Doxycycline Hyclate equivalent to ....100 mg Doxycycline

Each unit for injection contains:
Doxycycline Hyclate equivalent to ....200 mg Doxycycline

Doxycycline monohydrate has a molecular formula of $C_{22}H_{24}N_2O_8 \cdot H_2O$ and a molecular weight of 462.46. The chemical designation for Doxycycline is 4-(Dimethylamino)-1, 4, 4a, 5, 5a, 6, 11, 12a-octahydro-3, 5, 10, 12, 12a-pentahydroxy-6-methyl-1, 11-dioxo-2-naphthacenecarboxamide monohydrate. The molecular formula for Doxycycline hyclate (hydrochloride hemiethanolate hemihydrate) is $(C_{22}H_{24}N_2O_8 \cdot HCl)_2 \cdot C_2H_6O \cdot H_2O$ and the molecular weight is 1025.89. Doxycycline is a light-yellow crystalline powder. Doxycycline hyclate is soluble in water, while Doxycycline monohydrate is very slightly soluble in water. Doxycycline hyclate pelletized capsules contain specially coated pellets of Doxycycline hyclate for oral administration. The chemical designation is alpha-6-desoxy-5-oxytetracycline.

Doxycycline has a high degree of lipoid solubility and a low affinity for calcium binding. It is highly stable in normal human serum. Doxycycline will not degrade into an epianhydro form. Certain brands of Doxycycline calcium syrup contain sodium metabisulfite, a sulfite that may cause allergic type reactions including anaphylactic symptoms and life threatening or less severe asthmatic episodes in certain susceptible people.

CLINICAL PHARMACOLOGY
Tetracyclines are readily absorbed and are bound to plasma proteins in varying degree. They are concentrated by the liver in the bile, and excreted in the urine and feces at high concentrations and in a biologically active form. Doxycycline is virtually completely absorbed after oral administration.

Following a 200 mg dose, normal adult volunteers averaged peak serum levels of 2.6 mcg/mL of Doxycycline at 2 hours decreasing to 1.45 mcg/ml at 24 hours. Following a 200 mg dose of Doxycycline monohydrate, 24 normal adult volunteers averaged the following serum concentration values:

Time (hr):	0.5	1.0	1.5	2.0	3.0	4.0
Conc. (mcg/ml)	1.02	2.26	2.67	3.01	3.16	3.03

Time (hr):	8.0	12.0	24.0	48.0	72.0
Conc. (mcg/ml)	2.03	1.62	0.95	0.37	0.15

Average Observed Values

Maximum Concentration	3.61 mcg/mL (± 0.9 sd)
Time of Maximum Concentration	2.60 hr (± 1.10 sd)
Elimination Rate Constant	0.049 per hr (± 0.030 sd)
Half-Life	16.33 hr (± 4.53 sd)

Following a single 100 mg dose administered in a concentration of 0.4 mg/ml in a one-hour infusion, normal adult volunteers average a peak of 2.5 mcg/ml, while 200 mg of a concentration of 0.4 mg/ml administered over two hours averaged a peak of 3.6 mcg/ml.

► SHOWN IN PRODUCT IDENTIFICATION GUIDE

Excretion of Doxycycline by the kidney is about 40%/72 hours in individuals with normal function (creatinine clearance about 75 ml/min.). This percentage excretion may fall as low as 1-5%/72 hours in individuals with severe renal insufficiency (creatinine clearance below 10 ml/min.). Studies have shown no significant difference in serum half-life of Doxycycline (range 18-22 hours) in individuals with normal and severely impaired renal function.

Hemodialysis does not alter serum half-life.

Results of animal studies indicate that tetracyclines cross the placenta and are found in fetal tissues.

MICROBIOLOGY

The tetracyclines are primarily bacteriostatic and are thought to exert their antimicrobial effect by the inhibition of protein synthesis. The tetracyclines, including Doxycycline, have a similar antimicrobial spectrum of activity against a wide range of gram-positive and gram-negative organisms. Cross-resistance of these organisms to tetracyclines is common.

While *in vitro* studies have demonstrated the susceptibility of most strains of the following microorganisms, clinical efficacy for infections other than those included in the *"Indications and Usage"* section has not been documented.

GRAM-NEGATIVE BACTERIA
Neisseria gonorrhoeae
Calymmatobacterium granulomatis
Haemophilus ducreyi
Haemophilus influenzae
Yersinia pestis (formerly *Pasteurella pestis*)
Francisella tularensis (formerly *Pasteurella tularensis*)
Vibrio cholera (formerly *Vibrio comma*)
Vibrio fetus
Bartonella bacilliformis
Brucella species

Because many strains of the following groups of gram-negative microorganisms have been shown to be resistant to tetracyclines, culture and susceptibility testing are recommended:
Escherichia coli
Klebsiella species
Enterobacter aerogenes
Shigella species
Acinetobacter species (formerly *Mima* species and *Herellea* species)
Bacteroides species

GRAM-POSITIVE BACTERIA
Because many strains of the following groups of gram-positive microorganisms have been shown to be resistant to tetracyclines, culture and susceptibility testing are recommended. Up to 44 percent of strains of *Streptococcus pyogenes* and 74 percent of *Streptococcus faecalis* have been found to be resistant to tetracycline drugs. Therefore, tetracyclines should not be used for streptococcal disease unless the organism has been demonstrated to be susceptible.
Streptococcus pyogenes
Streptococcus pneumoniae
Enterococcus group (*Streptococcus faecalis* and *Streptococcus fae- cium*)
Alpha-hemolytic streptococci (viridans group)

OTHER MICROORGANISMS
Rickettsaie
Chlamydia psittaci
Chlamydia trachomatis
Mycoplasma pneumoniae
Ureaplasma urealyticum
Borrelia recurrentis
Treponema pallidum
Treponema pertenue
Clostridium species
Fusobacterium fusiforme
Actinomyces species
Bacillus anthracis
Propionbacterium acnes
Entamoeba species
Balantidium coli
Plasmodium falciparum

Doxycycline has been found to be active against the asexual erythrocytic forms of *Plasmodium falciparum* but not against the gametocytes of *P. falciparum*. The precise mechanism of action of the drug is not known.

SUSCEPTIBILITY TESTS:
Diffusion techniques: Quantitative methods that require measurement of zone diameters give the most precise estimate of the susceptibility of bacteria to antimicrobial agents. One such standard procedure[1] which has been recommended for use with disks to test susceptibility of organisms to Doxycycline uses the 30-mcg tetracycline-class disk or the 30-mcg Doxycycline disk. Interpretation involves the correlation of the diameter obtained in the disk test with the minimum inhibitory concentration (MIC) for tetracycline or Doxycycline, respectively.

Reports from the laboratory giving results of the standard single-disk susceptibility test with a 30-mcg tetracycline-class disk or the 30-mcg Doxycycline disk should be interpreted according to the following criteria:

| Zone Diameter (mm) | | Interpretation |
Tetracycline	Doxycycline	
≥19	≥16	Susceptible
15-18	13-15	Intermediate
≤14	≤12	Resistant

A report of "Susceptible" indicates that the pathogen is likely to be inhibited by generally achievable blood levels. A report of "Intermediate" suggests that the organism would be susceptible if a high dosage is used or if the infection is confined to tissues and fluids (e.g., urine) in which high antimicrobial levels are attained. A report of "Resistant" indicates that achievable concentrations are unlikely to be inhibitory, and other therapy should be selected.

Standardized procedures require the use of laboratory control organisms. The 30-mcg tetracycline-class disk or the 30-mcg Doxycyc- line disk should give the following zone diameters:

| Organism | Zone Diameter (mm) | |
	Tetracycline	Doxycycline
E. coli ATCC 25922	18-25	18-24
S. aureus ATCC 25923	19-28	23-29

Dilution techniques: Use a standardized dilution method[2] (broth, agar, microdilution) or equivalent with tetracycline powder. The MIC values obtained should be interpreted according to the following criteria:

MIC (mcg/mL)	Interpretation
≤4	Susceptible
8	Intermediate
≥16	Resistant

As with standard diffusion techniques, dilution methods require the use of laboratory control organisms. Standard tetracycline powder should provide the following MIC values:

Organism	MIC (mcg/mL)
E. coli ATCC 25922	1.0-4.0
S. aureus ATCC 29213	0.25-1.0
E. faecalis ATCC 29212	8-32
P. aeruginosa ATCC 27853	8-32

INDICATIONS AND USAGE
TREATMENT
Doxycycline is indicated for the treatment of the following infections:

Rocky mountain spotted fever, typhus fever and the typhus group, Q fever, rickettsialpox, and tick fevers caused by Rickettsiae.

Respiratory tract infections caused by *Mycoplasma pneumoniae*. (PPLO. Eaton's agent)

Lymphogranuloma venereum caused by *Chlamydia trachomatis*.

Psittacosis (ornithosis) caused by *Chlamydia psittaci*.

Trachoma caused by *Chlamydia trachomatis*, although the infectious agent is not always eliminated as judged by immunofluorescence.

Inclusion conjunctivitis caused by *Chlamydia trachomatis*. (May be treated with oral Doxycycline alone, or with a combination of topical agents.)

Uncomplicated urethral, endocervical or rectal infections in adults caused by *Chlamydia trachomatis*.

Nongonococcal urethritis caused by *Ureaplasma urealyticum* and *Chlamydia trachomatis*.

Acute epididymo-orchitis caused by *Chlamydia trachomatis*.[4]

Uncomplicated gonococcal infections in adults (except for anorectal infections in men), the gonococcal arthritis-dermatitis syndrome and acute epididymo-orchitis caused by *N. gonorrhoeae*.[4]

Relapsing fever due to *Borrelia recurrentis*.

Doxycycline is also indicated for the treatment of infections caused by the following gram-negative microorganisms:

Chancroid caused by *Haemophilus ducreyi*.

Plaque due to *Yersinia pestis* (formerly *Pasteurella pestis*).

Tuleremia due to *Francisella tulerensis* (formerly *Pasteurella tulerensis*).

Cholera caused by *Vibrio cholerae* (formerly *Vibrio comma*).

Campylobacter fetus infections caused by *Campylobacter fetus* (formerly *Vibrio fetus*).

Brucellosis due to *Brucella* species (in conjunction with streptomycin).

Bartonellosis due to *Bartonella bacilliformis*.

Granuloma inguinale caused by *Calymmatobacterium granulomatis*.

Infections due to *Bacteroides* species.

Because many strains of the following groups of microorganisms have been shown to be resistant to Doxycycline, culture and susceptibility testing are recommended.

◆ RATED THERAPEUTICALLY EQUIVALENT; ◇ THERAPEUTIC EQUIVALENCE UNCONFIRMED; ○ UNRATED

Doxycycline is indicated for treatment of infections caused by the following gram-negative microorganisms, when bacteriologic testing indicates appropriate susceptibility to the drug:

Escherichia coli.
Enterobacter aerogenes (formerly *Aerobacter aerogenes*).
Shigella species.
Acinetobacter species (formerly *Mima* species and *Herellea* species).
Respiratory tract infections caused by *Haemophilus influenzae.*
Respiratory tract and urinary tract infections caused by *Klebsiella* species.

Doxycycline is indicated for treatment of infections caused by the following gram-positive microorganisms when bacteriologic testing indicates appropriate susceptibility to the drug:

Upper respiratory infections caused by *Streptococcus pneumoniae* (formerly *Diplococcus pneumoniae*).

Streptococcus species: Up to 44 percent of strains of *Streptococcus pyogenes* and 74 percent of *Streptococcus faecalis* have been found to be resistant to tetracycline drugs. Therefore, tetracyclines should not to be used for streptococcal disease unless the organism has been demonstrated to be susceptible.

For upper respiratory infections due to group A beta-hemolytic streptococci, penicillin is the usual drug of choice, including prophylaxis of rheumatic fever.

Staphylococcus aureus, (respiratory, skin and soft-tissue infections). Tetracyclines are not the drug of choice in the treatment of any type of staphylococcal infection.

When penicillin is contraindicated, Doxycycline is an alternative drug in the treatment of the following infections:
Uncomplicated gonorrhea caused by *Neisseria gonorrhoeae.*
Infections due to *Neisseria meningitidis.*
Syphilis caused by *Treponema pallidum.*
Yaws caused by *Treponema pertenue.*
Listeriosis due to *Listeria monocytogenes.*
Anthrax due to *Bacillus anthracis.*
Vincent's infection caused by *Fusobacterium fusiforme.*
Actinomycosis caused by *Actinomyces israelii*, and other infections due to *Actinomyces* species.
Infections caused by *Clostridium* species.

In acute intestinal amebiasis, Doxycycline may be a useful adjunct to amebicides.

In severe acne, Doxycycline may be useful adjunctive therapy.

PROPHYLAXIS
Doxycycline is indicated for the prophylaxis of malaria due to *Plasmodium falciparum* in short-term travelers (<4 months) to areas with chloroquine and/or pyrimethamine-sulfadoxine resistant strains. See *"Dosage and Administration"* section and *"Information for Patients"* subsection of the *"Precautions"* section.

UNLABELED USES
Doxycycline is used alone or as an adjunct in the treatment of gynecologic infections including serious infections in patients with radical hysterectomy, infertility, anicteric leptospirosis, stage I Lyme disease, and pericarditis. It is also used in premenstrual syndrome, proctitis, proctocolitis, enteritis, and recurrent periodontitis. In addition, Doxycycline is also used in Sweet's syndrome, epididymitis, and as an prophylaxis in colonic surgery.

CONTRAINDICATIONS
This drug is contraindicated in persons who have shown hypersensi- tivity to any of the tetracyclines.

WARNINGS
THE USE OF DRUGS OF THE TETRACYCLINE CLASS DURING TOOTH DEVELOPMENT (LAST HALF OF PREGNANCY, INFANCY AND CHILDHOOD TO THE AGE OF 8 YEARS) MAY CAUSE PERMANENT DISCOLORATION OF THE TEETH (YELLOW-GRAY-BROWN).

This adverse reaction is more common during long-term use of the drugs, but has been observed following repeated short-term courses. Enamel hypoplasia has also been reported.

TETRACYCLINE DRUGS, THEREFORE, SHOULD NOT BE USED IN THIS AGE GROUP UNLESS OTHER DRUGS ARE NOT LIKELY TO BE EFFECTIVE OR ARE CONTRAINDICATED.

All tetracyclines form a stable calcium complex in any bone-forming tissue. A decrease in fibula growth rate has been observed in prematures given oral tetracycline in doses of 25 mg/kg every 6 hours. This reaction was shown to be reversible when the drug was discontinued.

Results of animal studies indicate that tetracyclines cross the placenta, are found in fetal tissues, and can have toxic effects on the developing fetus (often related to retardation of skeletal development). Evidence of embryotoxicity has also been noted in animals treated early in pregnancy. Doxycycline has not been studied in pregnant patients. It should not be used in pregnant women unless, in the judgment of the physician, it is essential for the welfare of the patient. If any tetracycline is used during pregnancy or if the patient becomes pregnant while taking this drug, the patient should be apprised of the potential hazard to the fetus.

The antianabolic action of the tetracyclines may cause an increase in BUN. Studies to date indicate that this does not occur with the use of Doxycycline in patients with impaired renal function.

Photosensitivity manifested by an exaggerated sunburn reaction has been observed in some individuals taking tetracyclines. Patients apt to be exposed to direct sunlight or ultraviolet light should be advised that this reaction can occur with tetracycline drugs, and treatment should be discontinued at the first evidence of skin erythema.

Some brands or formulations contain sodium metabisulfite, a sulfite that may cause allergic-type reactions including anaphylactic symptoms and life-threatening or less severe asthmatic episodes in certain susceptible people. The over-all prevalence of sulfite sensitivity in the general population is unknown and probably low. Sulfite sensitivity is seen more frequently in asthmatic than in nonasthmatic people.

PRECAUTIONS
GENERAL
As with other antibiotic preparations, use of this drug may result in overgrowth of nonsusceptible organisms, including fungi. If superinfection occurs, the antibiotic should be discontinued and appropriate therapy instituted.

Bulging fontanels in infants and benign intracranial hypertension in adults have been reported in individuals receiving tetracyclines. These conditions disappeared when the drug was discontinued.

Incision and drainage or other surgical procedures should be performed in conjunction with antibiotic therapy, when indicated.

Doxycycline offers substantial but not complete suppression of the asexual blood stages of *Plasmodium* strains.

Doxycycline does not suppress *P. falciparium's* sexual blood stage gametocytes. Subjects completing this prophylactic regimen may still transmit the infection to mosquitoes outside endemic areas.

All infections due to group A beta-hemolytic streptococci should be treated for at least 10 days.

INFORMATION FOR PATIENTS
Patients taking Doxycycline for malaria prophylaxis should be advised:
— that no present-day antimalarial agent, including Doxycycline, guarantees protection against malaria.
— to avoid being bitten by mosquitoes by using personal protective measures that help avoid contact with mosquitoes, especially from dusk to dawn (e.g., staying in well-screened areas, using mosquito nets, covering the body with clothing, and using an effective insect repellent.)
— that Doxycycline prophylaxis:
— should begin 1-2 days before travel to the malarious area,
— should be continued daily while in the malarious area and after the malarious area,
— should be continued for 4 further weeks to avoid development of malaria after returning from an endemic area,
— should not exceed 4 months.
All patients taking Doxycycline should be advised:
— to avoid excessive sunlight or artificial ultraviolet light while receiving Doxycycline and to discontinue therapy if phototoxicity (e.g., skin eruption, etc) occurs. Sunscreen or sunblock should be considered. (See *"Warnings".*)
— to drink fluids liberally along with Doxycycline to reduce the risk of esophegeal irritation and ulceration. (See *"Adverse Reactions".*)
— that the absorption of tetracyclines is reduced when taken with foods, especially those which contain calcium. However, the absorption of Doxycycline is not markedly influenced by simultaneous ingestion of food or milk. (See *"Drug Interactions".*)
— that the absorption of tetracyclines is reduced when taking bismuth subsalicylate. (See *"Drug Interactions".*)
— that the use of Doxycycline might increase the incidence of vaginal candidiasis.

LABORATORY TESTS
In venereal disease, when co-existent syphilis is suspected, dark field examination should be done before treatment is started and the blood serology repeated monthly for at least 4 months.

In long-term therapy, periodic laboratory evalution of organ systems, including hematopoietic, renal, and hepatic studies, should be performed.

DRUG INTERACTIONS
Because tetracyclines have been shown to depress plasma prothrombin activity, patients who are on anticoagulant therapy may require downward adjustment of their anticoagulant dosage.

Since bacteriostatic drugs may interfere with the bactericidal action of penicillin, it is advisable to avoid giving tetracyclines in conjunction with penicillin.

Absorption of tetracyclines is impaired by antacids containing aluminum, calcium, or magnesium, and iron-containing preparations.

Absorption of tetracyclines is impaired by bismuth subsalicylate.

Barbiturates, carbamazepine, and phenytoin decrease the half-life of Doxycycline.

The concurrent use of tetracycline and methoxyflurane has been reported to result in fatal renal toxicity.

Concurrent use of tetracycline may render oral contraceptives less effective.

DRUG/LABORATORY TEST INTERACTIONS
False elevations of urinary catecholamine levels may occur due to interference with the fluorescence test.

CARCINOGENESIS, MUTAGENESIS, IMPAIRMENT OF FERTILITY
Long-term studies in animals to evaluate carcinogenic potential of Doxycycline have not been conducted. However, there has been evidence of oncogenic activity

in rats in studies with the related antibiotics, oxytetracycline (adrenal and pituitary tumors), and minocycline (thyroid tumors). Long term studies are currently being conducted to determine whether tetracyclines have carcinogenic potential. Animal studies conducted in rats and mice have not provided conclusive evidence that tetracyclines may be carcinogenic or that they impair fertility.

Likewise, although mutagenicity studies of Doxycycline have not been conducted, positive results in *in vitro* mammalian cell assays have been reported for related antibiotics (tetracycline, oxytetracycline). In two mammalian cell assays (L51784 mouse lymphoma and Chinese hamster lung cells *in vitro*) positive responses for mutagenicity occurred at concentrations of 60 and 10 mcg/mL respectively. In humans no association between tetracyclines and these effects have been made.

Doxycycline administered orally at dosage levels as high as 250 mg/kg/day had no apparent effect on the fertility of female rats. Effect on male fertility has not been studied.

PREGNANCY CATEGORY
Teratogenic effects: Category "D" — (see *"Warnings"*).
Nonteratogenic effects: (see *"Warnings"*).

LABOR AND DELIVERY
The effect of tetracyclines on labor and delivery is unknown.

NURSING MOTHERS
Tetracyclines are excreted in human milk. Because of the potential for serious adverse reactions in nursing infants from Doxycycline, a decision should be made whether to discontinue nursing or to discontinue the drug, taking into account the importance of the drug to the mother. (See *"Warnings"*.)

PEDIATRIC USE
The use of Doxycycline in children under 8 years is not recommended because safe conditions for its use have not been established. (See *"Warnings"* and *"Dosage and Administration"*.)

ADVERSE REACTIONS
Due to oral Doxycycline's virtually complete absorption, side effects of the lower bowel, particularly diarrhea, have been infrequent. The following adverse reactions have been observed in patients receiving tetracyclines:

Gastrointestinal: anorexia, nausea, vomiting, diarrhea, glossitis, dysphagia, enterocolitis, and inflammatory lesions (with monilial overgrowth) in the anogenital region. Hepatotoxicity has been reported rarely. These reactions have been caused by both the oral and parenteral administration of tetracyclines. Rare instances of esophagitis and esophageal ulcerations have been reported in patients receiving capsule and tablet forms of the drugs in the tetracycline class. Most of these patients took medications immediately before going to bed. (See *"Dosage and Administration"*.)

Skin: malculopapular and erythematous rashes. Exfoliative dermatitis has been reported but is uncommon. Photosensitivity is discussed above. (See *"Warnings"*.)

Renal toxicity: Rise in BUN has been reported and is appearently dose related. (See *"Warnings"*.)

Hypersensitivity reactions: urticaria, angioneurotic edema, anaphylaxis, anaphylactoid purpura, serum sickness, pericarditis, and exacerbation of systemic lupus erythematosus.

Blood: Hemolytic anemia, thrombocytopenia, neutropenia, and eosinophilia have been reported.

Other: bulging fontanels in infants and intracranial hypertension in adults. (See *"Precautions—General"*.)

When given over prolonged periods, tetracyclines have been reported to produce brown-black microscopic discoloration of the thyroid gland. No abnormalities of thyroid function studies are known to occur.

OVERDOSAGE
In case of overdosage, discontinue medication, treat symptomatically and institute supportive measures. Dialysis does not alter serum half-life and thus would not be of benefit in treating cases of overdosage.

DOSAGE AND ADMINISTRATION
THE USUAL DOSAGE AND FREQUENCY OF ADMINISTRATION OF DOXYCYCLINE DIFFERES FROM THAT OF THE OTHER TETRACYCLINES. EXCEEDING THE RECOMMENDED DOSAGE MAY RESULT IN AN INCREASED INCIDENCE OF SIDE EFFECTS.

ORAL DOXYCYCLINE
Adults: The usual dose of oral Doxycycline is 200 mg on the first day of treatment (administered 100 mg every 12 hours or 50 mg every 6 hours) followed by a maintenance dose of 100 mg/day. The maintenance dose may be administered as a single dose or as 50 mg every 12 hours.

In the management of more severe infections (particularly chronic infections of the urinary tract), 100 mg every 12 hours is recommended.

For children above eight years of age: The recommended dosage schedule for children weighing 100 pounds or less is 2 mg/lb of body weight divided into two doses on the first day of treatment, followed by 1 mg/lb of body weight given as a single daily dose or divided into two doses, on subsequent days. For more severe

infections up to 2 mg/lb of body weight may be used. For children over 100 lb the usual adult dose should be used.

The therapeutic antibacterial serum activity will usually persist for 24 hours following recommended dosage.

When used in streptococcal infections, therapy should be continued for 10 days.

Administration of adequate amounts of fluid along with capsule and tablet forms of drugs in the tetracycline class is recommended to wash down the drugs and reduce the risk of esophageal irritation and ulceration. (See *"Adverse Reactions"*.)

If gastric irritation occurs, it is recommended that Doxycycline be given with food or milk. The absorption of Doxycycline is not markedly influenced by simultaneous ingestion of food or milk. Ingestion of a high fat meal has been shown to delay the time to peak plasma concentrations by an average of one hour and 20 minutes. However, in the same study, food enhanced the average peak concentration by 7.5% and the area under the curve by 5.7%.

Antacids containing aluminum, calcium or magnesium, sodium bicarbonate, and iron-containing preparations should not be given to patients taking oral tetracyclines.

Studies to date have indicated that administration of Doxycycline at the usual recommended doses does not lead to excessive accumulation of the antibiotic in patients with renal impairment.

Uncomplicated gonococcal infections in adults (except anorectal infections in men): 100 mg, by mouth, twice a day for 7 days. As an alternate single visit dose, administer 300 mg stat followed in one hour by a second 300 mg dose. The dose may be administered with food, including milk or carbonated beverage, as required.

Uncomplicated urethral, endocervical, or rectal infection in adults caused by Chlamydia trachomatis: 100 mg by mouth twice a day for at least 7 days.

Nongonococcal urethritis (NGU) caused by C. trachomatis or U. urealyticum: 100 mg by mouth twice a day for at least 7 days.

Syphilis, early: Patients who are allergic to penicillin should be treated with Doxycycline 100 mg by mouth twice a day for 2 weeks.

Syphilis of more than one year's duration: Patients who are allergic to penicillin should be treated with Doxycycline 100 mg by mouth twice a day for 4 weeks.

Alternatively, in primary and secondary syphilis: 300 mg a day in divided doses for at least 10 days.

Acute epididymo-orchitis caused by N. gonorrhoeae: 100 mg, by mouth, twice a day for at least 10 days.

Acute epididymo-orchitis caused by C. trachomatis: 100 mg, by mouth, twice a day for at least 10 days.

For prophylaxis of malaria: For adults, the recommended dose is 100 mg daily. For children over 8 years of age, the recommended dose is 2 mg/kg given once daily up to the adult dose. Prophylaxis should begin 1-2 days before travel to the malarious area. Prophylaxis should be continued daily during travel in the malarious area and for 4 weeks after the traveler leaves the malarious area.

INTRAVENOUS DOXYCYCLINE
Rapid administration of intravenous Doxycycline hyclate is to be avoided. Parenteral therapy is indicated only when oral therapy is not indicated. Oral therapy should be instituted as soon as possible. If intravenous therapy is given over prolonged periods of time, thrombophlebitis may result.

Adults: The usual dosage of Doxycycline Hyclate IV is 200 mg on the first day of treatment administered in one or two infusions.

Subsequent daily dosage is 100 to 200 mg depending upon the severity of infection, with 200 mg administered in one or two infusions.

In the treatment of primary and secondary syphilis, the recom- mended dosage is 300 mg daily for at least 10 days.

For children above eight years of age: The recommended dosage schedule for children weighing 100 lbs or less is 2 mg/lb. of body weight on the first day of treatment, administered in one or two infusions. Subsequent daily dosage is 1 to 2 mg/lb. of body weight given as one or two infusions, depending on the severity of the infection. For children over 100 lbs the usual adult dose should be used. (See *"Warnings"* section for *"Usage in Children"*.)

General: The duration of infusion may vary with the dose (100 to 200 mg per day), but is usually one to four hours. A recommended minimum infusion time for 100 mg of a 0.5 mg/ml solution is one hour. Therapy should be continued for at least 24-48 hours after symptoms and fever have subsided. The therapeutic antibacterial serum activity will usually persist for 24 hours following recommended dosage.

Intravenous solutions should not be injected intramuscularly or subcutaneously. Caution should be taken to avoid the inadvertent introduction of the intravenous solution into the adjacent soft tissue.

PREPARATION OF SOLUTION
To prepare a solution containing 10 mg/ml, reconstitute 100 mg or 200 mg powder with 10 ml or 20 ml of sterile water for injection or any of the ten intravenous infusion solutions listed below. Each 100 mg of Doxycycline hyclate is further diluted with 100 ml to 1000 ml of the intravenous solutions listed below. Each 200 mg of Doxycycline hyclate is further diluted with 200 ml to 2000 ml of the following intravenous solutions:
  1. Sodium Chloride Injection, USP
  2. 5% Dextrose Injection, USP

◆ RATED THERAPEUTICALLY EQUIVALENT; ◇ THERAPEUTIC EQUIVALENCE UNCONFIRMED; ○ UNRATED

3. Ringer's Injection, USP
4. Invert Sugar, 10% in Water
5. Lactated Ringer's Injection, USP
6. Dextrose 5% in Lactated Ringer's
7. Normosol-M® in D5-W (Abbott)
8. Normosol-R® in D5-W (Abbott)
9. Plasma-Lyte® 56 in 5% Dextrose (Travenol)
10. Plasma-Lyte® 148 in 5% Dextrose (Travenol)

This will result in desired concentrations of 0.1 to 1.0 mg/ml. Concentrations lower than 0.1 mg/ml or higher than 1.0 mg/ml are not recommended.

Stability: Doxycycline hyclate IV is stable for 48 hours in solution when diluted with sodium chloride injection or 5% dextrose injection, to concentrations between 1.0 mg/ml and 0.1 mg/ml and stored at 25°C. Doxycycline hyclate IV in these solutions is stable under fluorescent light for 48 hours, but must be protected from direct sunlight during storage and infusion. Reconstituted solutions (1.0 to 0.1 mg/ml) may be stored up to 72 hours prior to start of infusion if refrigerated and protected from sunlight and artificial light. Infusion must then be completed within 12 hours. Solutions must be used within these time periods or discarded.

Doxycycline hyclate IV, when diluted with Ringer's injection, USP, or invert sugar, 10% in Water, or Normosol-M® in D5-W (Abbott), or Normosol-R® in D5-W (Abbott), or Plasma-Lyte® 56 in 5% Dextrose (Travenol), or Plasma-Lyte® 148 in 5% Dextrose (Travenol) to a concentration between 1.0 mg/ml and 0.1 mg/ml, must be completely infused within 12 hours after reconstitution to ensure adequate stability. During infusion, the solution must be protected from direct sunlight. Reconstituted solutions (1.0 to 0.1 mg/ml) may be stored up to 72 hours prior to start of infusion if refrigerated and protected from sunlight and artifical light. Infusion must then be completed within 12 hours. Solutions must be used within these time periods or discarded.

When diluted with Lactated Ringer's Injection, USP, or Dextrose 5% in Lactated Ringer's, infusion of the solution (ca. 1.0 mg/ml) or lower concentrations (not less than 0.1 mg/ml) must be completed within six hours after reconstitution to ensure adequate stability. During infusion, the solution must be protected from direct sunlight. Solutions must be used within this time period or discarded.

Solutions of Doxycycline hyclate for injection at a concentration of 10 mg/ml in sterile water for injection, when frozen immediately after reconstitution are stable for 8 weeks when stored at −20°C. If the product is warmed, care should be taken to avoid heating it after the thawing is complete. Once thawed the solution should not be refrozen.

STORAGE
All products are to be stored at controlled room temperature, 59°-86°F (15°-30°C) and dispensed in tight, light-resistant containers (USP). The unit dose packs should also be stored in a dry place.

ANIMAL PHARMACOLOGY AND ANIMAL TOXICOLOGY
Hyperpigmentation of the thyroid has been produced by members of the tetracycline class in the following species: in rats by oxytetracycline, Doxycycline, tetracycline PO$_4$, and methacycline; in minipigs by Doxycycline, minocycline, tetracycline PO$_4$, and methacycline; in dogs by Doxycycline and minocycline; in monkeys by minocycline.

Minocycline, tetracycline PO$_4$, methacycline, Doxycycline, tetracycline base, oxytetracycline HCl, and tetracycline HCl were goitrogenic in rats fed a low iodine diet. This goitrogenic effect was accompanied by high radioactive iodine uptake. Administration of minocycline also produced a large goiter with high radioiodine uptake in rats fed a relatively high iodine diet.

Treatment of various animal species with this class of drugs has also resulted in the induction of thyroid hyperplasia in the following: in rats and dogs (minocycline); in chickens (chlortetracycline); and in rats and mice (oxytetracycline). Adrenal gland hyperplasia has been observed in goats and rats treated with oxytetracycline.

REFERENCES
1. National Committee for Clinical Laboratory Standards, *Performance Standards for Antimicrobial Disk Susceptibility Test,* Fourth Edition. Approved Standard NCCLS Document M2-A4, Vol. 10, No. 7 NCCLS, Villanova, PA, April 1990. 2. National Committee for Clinical Laboratory Standards, *Methods for Dilution Antimicrobial Susceptibility Tests for Bacteria that Grow Aerobically,* Second Edition. Approved Standard NCCLS Document M7-A2, Vol. 10, No. 8 NCCLS, Villanova, PA, April 1990. 3. NCCLS Approved Standard: M2-A3, Vol. 4, Performance Standards for Antimicrobial Disk Susceptibility Tests, Third Edition: available from the National Committee for Clinical Laboratory Standards, 771 East Lancaster Avenue, Villanova, Pa. 19085 4. CDC Sexually Transmitted Diseases Treatment Guidelines 1982

HOW SUPPLIED
CAPSULE: 50 MG

AVERAGE UNIT PRICE (AVAILABLE SIZES)		GENERIC A-RATED AVERAGE PRICE (GAAP)	
		50s	$11.54
BRAND	$1.89	100s	$48.73
GENERIC	$0.26	500s	$70.83

BRAND/MANUFACTURER	NDC	SIZE	AWP
◆ BRAND			
▶ VIBRAMYCIN HYCLATE: Pfizer Labs	00069-0940-50	50s	$94.48
◆ GENERICS			
Qualitest	00603-3480-19	50s	$7.45
Geneva	00781-2525-50	50s	$8.02
Caraco	57664-0111-05	50s	$8.15

BRAND/MANUFACTURER	NDC	SIZE	AWP
Rugby	00536-0280-06	50s	$8.25
Schein	00364-2032-50	50s	$8.26
West-Ward	00143-3141-50	50s	$9.00
DOXY-D: Dunhall	00217-0804-50	50s	$9.50
Moore, H.L.	00839-1288-04	50s	$9.65
Major	00904-0427-51	50s	$10.70
Lemmon	00093-0642-53	50s	$10.75
Halsey Pharm	00879-0525-50	50s	$11.03
Mylan	00378-0145-89	50s	$11.06
Zenith	00172-2984-48	50s	$11.10
Goldline	00182-1090-19	50s	$11.50
Martec	52555-0433-00	50s	$11.65
Warner Chilcott	00047-0829-19	50s	$11.74
URL	00677-0598-02	50s	$11.90
Mutual	53489-0118-02	50s	$11.90
Purepac	00228-2194-05	50s	$15.86
Aligen	00405-4378-50	50s	$15.93
Parmed	00349-1007-50	50s	$28.95
Raway	00686-0148-20	100s ud	$19.20
Major	00904-0427-61	100s ud	$32.20
Schein	00364-2032-90	100s ud	$34.35
Auro	55829-0661-10	100s ud	$78.61
UDL	51079-0148-20	100s ud	$79.27
West-Ward	00143-3141-05	500s	$52.50
Halsey Pharm	00879-0525-05	500s	$75.50
Zenith	00172-2984-70	500s	$76.70
Mutual	53489-0118-05	500s	$78.60

CAPSULE: 50 MG

BRAND/MANUFACTURER	NDC	SIZE	AWP
○ BRAND			
▶ MONODOX: Oclassen	55515-0260-06	100s	$94.80

CAPSULE: 100 MG

AVERAGE UNIT PRICE (AVAILABLE SIZES)		GENERIC A-RATED AVERAGE PRICE (GAAP)	
BRAND	$3.25	50s	$23.79
GENERIC	$0.43	100s	$66.46
HCFA FUL (50s ea)	$0.11	500s	$152.55

BRAND/MANUFACTURER	NDC	SIZE	AWP
◆ BRAND			
▶ VIBRAMYCIN HYCLATE: Pfizer Labs	00069-0950-50	50s	$169.86
	00069-0950-41	100s ud	$341.02
	00069-0950-73	500s	$1470.90
◆ GENERICS			
Major	00904-0428-95	20s	$4.40
Qualitest	00603-3481-19	50s	$8.35
▶ Rugby	00536-0230-06	50s	$8.55
Geneva	00781-2522-50	50s	$9.68
Caraco	57664-0115-05	50s	$11.95
▶ Schein	00364-2033-50	50s	$11.95
Moore, H.L.	00839-1289-04	50s	$12.83
Major	00904-0428-51	50s	$17.50
West-Ward	00143-3142-50	50s	$17.95
Warner Chilcott	00047-0830-19	50s	$18.40
▶ Mylan	00378-0148-89	50s	$18.45
Halsey Pharm	00879-0526-19	50s	$18.45
Goldline	00182-1035-19	50s	$18.50
▶ Zenith	00172-2985-48	50s	$18.70
URL	00677-0562-02	50s	$19.20
▶ Mutual	53489-0119-02	50s	$19.20
Martec	52555-0434-00	50s	$19.65
Lemmon	00093-0653-53	50s	$22.75
Aligen	00405-4377-50	50s	$24.82
Parmed	00349-1008-50	50s	$29.65
Lederle Std Prod	00005-3768-18	50s	$29.85
Apothecon	00003-0814-05	50s	$64.45
Major	00904-0429-51	50s	$102.50
U.S. Trading	56126-0019-11	100s ud	$12.02
Raway	00686-0522-20	100s ud	$21.00
Major	00904-0428-61	100s ud	$32.82
West-Ward	00143-3142-25	100s ud	$39.00
▶ Schein	00364-2033-90	100s ud	$46.43
Vangard	00615-0385-13	100s ud	$94.22
UDL	51079-0522-20	100s ud	$110.90
Auro	55829-0662-10	100s ud	$119.86
Goldline	00182-1035-89	100s ud	$121.90
▶ Rugby	00536-0230-32	200s	$31.95
▶ Schein	00364-2033-05	500s	$69.85
▶ Rugby	00536-0230-05	500s	$75.00
West-Ward	00143-3142-05	500s	$75.00
Caraco	57664-0115-13	500s	$76.00
Geneva	00781-2522-50	500s	$82.95
Major	00904-0428-40	500s	$94.25
Moore, H.L.	00839-1289-12	500s	$108.61
Goldline	00182-1035-05	500s	$115.00
Parmed	00349-1008-05	500s	$115.50
DOXY-D: Dunhall	00217-0805-03	500s	$135.00
Qualitest	00603-3481-28	500s	$140.11
Halsey Pharm	00879-0526-05	500s	$142.43

BRAND/MANUFACTURER	NDC	SIZE	AWP
➤ Mylan	00378-0148-05	500s	$142.50
➤ Zenith	00172-2985-70	500s	$147.80
URL	00677-0562-05	500s	$149.00
➤ Mutual	53489-0119-05	500s	$149.00
Martec	52555-0434-05	500s	$155.20
Aligen	00405-4377-02	500s	$198.00
Lemmon	00093-0653-05	500s	$204.50
Lederle Std Prod	00005-3768-31	500s	$269.48
Apothecon	00003-0814-01	500s	$558.38

CAPSULE: 100 MG

BRAND/MANUFACTURER	NDC	SIZE	AWP
○ BRAND			
➤ MONODOX: Oclassen	55515-0259-04	50s	$77.40
	55515-0259-07	250s	$372.00

CAPSULE, EXTENDED RELEASE: 100 MG

BRAND/MANUFACTURER	NDC	SIZE	AWP
◆ GENERICS			
Moore,H.L.	00839-7654-04	50s	$79.64

ENTERIC COATED CAPSULES: 100 MG

BRAND/MANUFACTURER	NDC	SIZE	AWP
◆ BRAND			
➤ DORYX: Parke-Davis	00071-0838-19	50s	$121.95
◆ GENERICS			
Sidmak	50111-0377-05	50s	$72.00
Warner Chilcott	00047-0091-19	50s	$86.32

POWDER FOR INJECTION: 100 MG

AVERAGE UNIT PRICE (AVAILABLE SIZES)		GENERIC A-RATED AVERAGE PRICE (GAAP)	
BRAND	$21.07	1s	$17.80
GENERIC	$17.80		

BRAND/MANUFACTURER	NDC	SIZE	AWP
◆ BRAND			
VIBRAMYCIN HYCLATE: Roerig	00049-0960-77	5s	$105.35
◆ GENERICS			
Elkins-Sinn	00641-2292-41	1s	$16.70
Fujisawa	00469-1300-30	1s	$18.89

POWDER FOR INJECTION: 200 MG

BRAND/MANUFACTURER	NDC	SIZE	AWP
◆ GENERICS			
Fujisawa	00469-1640-40	1s	$37.24

POWDER FOR RECONSTITUTION: 25 MG/5 ML

BRAND/MANUFACTURER	NDC	SIZE	AWP
◆ BRAND			
VIBRAMYCIN MONOHYDRATE: Pfizer Labs	00069-0970-65	60 ml	$10.35

SYRUP: 50 MG/5 ML

BRAND/MANUFACTURER	NDC	SIZE	AWP
○ BRAND			
VIBRAMYCIN CALCIUM: Pfizer Labs	00069-0971-51	30 ml	$10.35
	00069-0971-93	480 ml	$157.18

TABLETS: 100 MG

AVERAGE UNIT PRICE (AVAILABLE SIZES)		GENERIC A-RATED AVERAGE PRICE (GAAP)	
BRAND	$3.25	50s	$21.04
GENERIC	$0.44	100s	$60.87
HCFA FUL (50s ea)	$0.13	500s	$162.38

BRAND/MANUFACTURER	NDC	SIZE	AWP
◆ BRAND			
➤ VIBRA-TABS: Pfizer Labs	00069-0990-50	50s	$169.86
	00069-0990-41	100s ud	$341.02
	00069-0990-73	500s	$1470.90
◆ GENERICS			
Allscrips	54569-3074-06	2s	$0.83
UDL	51079-0522-90	30s ud	$60.00
Rugby	00536-0340-06	50s	$8.04
Schein	00364-2063-50	50s	$8.25
Moore,H.L.	00839-6641-04	50s	$12.83
Mylan	00378-0167-89	50s	$17.45
Halsey Pharm	00879-0725-50	50s	$17.45
Major	00904-0430-51	50s	$17.50
Zenith	00172-3626-48	50s	$17.70
Warner Chilcott	00047-0813-19	50s	$17.76
Geneva	00781-1075-50	50s	$17.85
Qualitest	00603-3482-19	50s	$18.45

BRAND/MANUFACTURER	NDC	SIZE	AWP
Goldline	00182-1535-19	50s	$18.50
Martec	52555-0229-00	50s	$18.60
URL	00677-0799-02	50s	$19.20
Mutual	53489-0120-02	50s	$19.20
Lemmon	00093-0750-53	50s	$22.75
Aligen	00405-4379-50	50s	$25.01
Parmed	00349-1100-50	50s	$28.95
Lederle Std Prod	00005-3116-18	50s	$29.85
Apothecon	00003-0812-40	50s	$64.45
DOXI FILM: Wakefield	59310-0106-10	100s	$35.91
Raway	00686-0554-20	100s ud	$19.00
Major	00904-0430-61	100s ud	$32.82
Schein	00364-2063-90	100s ud	$44.70
UDL	51079-0554-20	100s ud	$110.90
Goldline	00182-1535-89	100s ud	$121.90
Rugby	00536-0340-32	200s	$31.44
Major	00904-0430-40	500s	$63.75
Rugby	00536-0340-05	500s	$71.70
Schein	00364-2063-05	500s	$78.50
Moore,H.L.	00839-6641-12	500s	$108.61
Goldline	00182-1535-05	500s	$115.00
Parmed	00349-1100-05	500s	$115.50
Halsey Pharm	00879-0725-05	500s	$139.40
Mylan	00378-0167-05	500s	$139.50
Zenith	00172-3626-70	500s	$140.55
Qualitest	00603-3482-28	500s	$142.40
Martec	52555-0229-05	500s	$144.80
Geneva	00781-1075-05	500s	$148.60
URL	00677-0799-05	500s	$149.00
Mutual	53489-0120-05	500s	$149.00
Aligen	00405-4379-02	500s	$184.22
Lemmon	00093-0750-05	500s	$204.50
Lederle Std Prod	00005-3116-31	500s	$269.48
Apothecon	00003-0812-60	500s	$558.38

Drisdol SEE ERGOCALCIFEROL

Dritho-Scalp SEE ANTHRALIN

Drithocreme SEE ANTHRALIN

Dronabinol

DESCRIPTION

Dronabinol is a cannabinoid designated chemically as (6aR-trans)-6a,7,8,10a-tetrahydro-6,6,9-trimethyl-3-pentyl-6 H-dibenzo [b,d]pyran-1-ol. ($C_{21}H_{30}O_2$, molecular weight = 314.47)

Dronabinol, delta-9-tetrahydrocannabinol (delta-9-THC), is naturally-occurring and has been extracted from Cannabis sativa L. (marijuana).

Dronabinol is also chemically synthesized and is a light-yellow resinous oil that is sticky at room temperature and hardens upon refrigeration. Dronabinol is insoluble in water and is formulated in sesame oil. It has a pK_a of 10.6 and an octanol-water partition coefficient: 6,000:1 at pH7.

Capsules for oral administration: Dronabinol is supplied as round soft gelatin capsules containing either 2.5 mg, 5 mg, or 10 mg Dronabinol.

Following is its chemical structure:

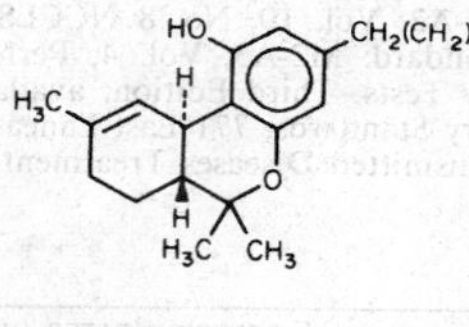

CLINICAL PHARMACOLOGY

Dronabinol is an orally active cannabinoid which, like other cannabinoids, has complex effects on the central nervous system (CNS), including central sympathomimetic activity. Cannabinoid receptors have been discovered in neural tissues. These receptors may play a role in mediating the effects of Dronabinol and other cannabinoids.

Pharmacodynamics: Dronabinol-induced sympathomimetic activity may result in tachycardia and/or conjunctival injection. Its effects on blood pressure are inconsistent, but occasional subjects have experienced orthostatic hyptotension and/or syncope upon abrupt standing.

◆ RATED THERAPEUTICALLY EQUIVALENT; ◇ THERAPEUTIC EQUIVALENCE UNCONFIRMED; ○ UNRATED

Dronabinol also demonstrates reversible effects on appetite, mood, cognition, memory, and perception. These phenomena appear to be dose-related, increasing in frequency with higher dosages, and subject to great interpatient variability After oral administration, Dronabinol has an onset of action of approximately 0.5 to 1 hours and peak effect at 2 to 4 hours. Duration of action for psychoactive effects is 4 to 6 hours, but the appetite stimulant effect of Dronabinol may continue for 24 hours or longer after administration. Tachyphylaxis and tolerance develop to some of the pharmacologic effects of Dronabinol and other cannabinoids with chronic use, suggesting an indirect effect on sympathetic neurons. In a study of the pharmacodynamics of chronic Dronabinol exposure, healthy male volunteers (N = 12) received 210 mg/day Dronabinol, administered orally in divided doses, for 16 days. An initial tachycardia induced by Dronabinol was replaced successively by normal sinus rhythm and then bradycardia. A decrease in supine blood pressure, made worse by standing, was also observed initially. These volunteers developed tolerance to the cardiovascular and subjective adverse CNS effects of Dronabinol within 12 days of treatment initiation.

Tachyphylaxis and tolerance do not, however, appear to develop to the appetite stimulant effect of Dronabinol. In studies involving patients with Acquired Immune Deficiency Syndrome (AIDS), the appetite stimulant effect of Dronabinol has been sustained for up to five months in clinical trials, at dosages ranging from 2.5 mg/day to 20 mg/day.

PHARMACOKINETICS

Absorption and Distribution. Dronabinol is almost completely absorbed (90 to 95%) after single oral doses. Due to the combined effects of first pass hepatic metabolism and high lipid solubility, only 10 to 20% of the administered dose reaches the systemic circulation. Dronabinol has a large apparent volume of distribution, approximately 10 L/kg, because of its liquid solubility. The plasma protein binding of Dronabinol and its metabolites is approximately 97%.

The elimination phase of Dronabinol can be described using a two compartment model with an initial (alpha) half-life of about 4 hours and a terminal (beta) half-life of 25 to 36 hours. Because of its large volume of distribution, Dronabinol and its metabolites may be excreted at low levels for prolonged periods of time.

Metabolism. Dronabinol undergoes extensive first-pass hepatic metabolism, primarily by microsomal hydroxylation, yielding both active and inactive metabolites. Dronabinol and its principal active metabolite, 11-OH-delta-9-THC, are present in approximately equal concentrations in plasma. Concentrations of both parent drug and metabolite peak at approximately 2 to 4 hours after oral dosing and decline over several days. Values for clearance average about 0.2 L/kg-hr, but are highly variable due to the complexity of cannabinoid distribution.

Elimination. Dronabinol and its biotransformation products are excreted in both feces and urine. Biliary excretion is the major route of elimination with about half of a radiolabeled oral dose being recovered from the feces within 72 hours as contrasted with 10 to 15% recovered from urine. Less than 5% of an oral dose is recovered unchanged in the feces.

Following single dose administration, low levels of Dronabinol metabolites have been detected for more than 5 weeks in the urine and feces.

In a study of Dronabinol involving AIDS patients, urinary cannabinoid/creatinine concentration ratios were studied biweekly over a six week period. The urinary cannabinoid/creatinine ratio was closely correlated with dose. No increase in the cannabinoid/creatinine ratio was observed after the first two weeks of treatment, indicating that steady-state cannabinoid levels had been reached. This conclusion is consistent with predictions based on the observed terminal half-life of Dronabinol.

Special Populations. The pharmacokinetic profile of Dronabinol has not been investigated in either pediatric or geriatric patients.

CLINICAL TRIALS

Appetite Stimulation. The appetite stimulant effect of Dronabinol in the treatment of AIDS-related anorexia associated with weight loss was studied in a randomized, double-blind, placebo-controlled study involving 139 patients. The initial dosage of Dronabinol in all patients was 5 mg/day, administered in doses of 2.5 mg one hour before lunch and one hour before supper. In pilot studies, early morning administration of Dronabinol appeared to have been associated with an increased frequency of adverse experiences, as compared to dosing later in the day. The effect of Dronabinol on appetite, weight, mood, and nausea was measured at scheduled intervals during the six-week treatment period. Side effects (feeling high, dizziness, confusion, somnolence) occurred in 13 to 72 patients (18%) at this dosage level and the dosage was reduced to 2.5 mg/day, administered as a single dose at supper or bedtime.

As compared to placebo, Dronabinol treatment resulted in a statistically significant improvement in appetite as measured by visual analog scale (see figure). Trends toward improved body weight and mood, and decreases in nausea were also seen.

After completing the 6-week study, patients were allowed to continue treatment with Dronabinol in an open-label study, in which there was a sustained improvement in appetite.

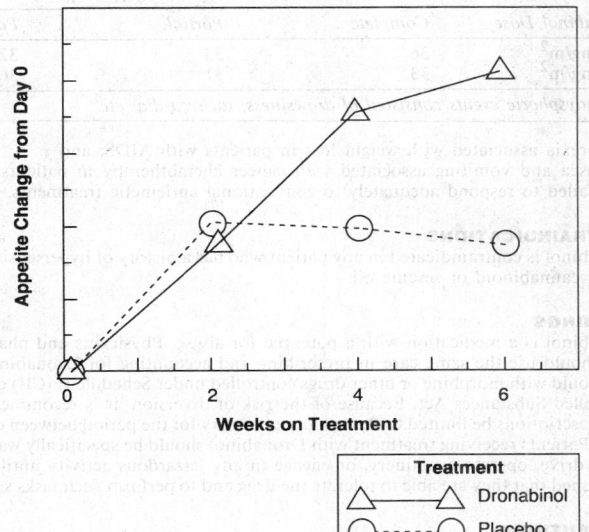

Appetite Change from Baseline

Antiemetic. Dronabinol treatment of chemotherapy-induced emesis was evaluated in 454 patients with cancer, who received a total of 750 courses of treatment of various malignancies. The antiemetic efficacy of Dronabinol was greatest in patients receiving cytotoxic therapy with MOPP for Hodgkin's and non-Hodgkin's lymphomas. Dronabinol dosages ranged from 2.5 mg/day to 40 mg/day, administered in equally divided doses every four to six hours (four times daily). As indicated in the following table, escalating the Dronabinol dose above 7 mg/m² increased the frequency of adverse experiences, with no additional antiemetic benefit. (See related table).

Combination antiemetic therapy with Dronabinol and a phenothiazine (prochlorperazine) may result in synergistic or additive antiemetic effects and attenuate the toxicities associated with each of the agents.

INDIVIDUALIZATION OF DOSAGES

The pharmacologic effects of Dronabinol are dose-related and subject to considerable interpatient variability. Therefore, dosage individualization is critical in achieving the maximum benefit of Dronabinol treatment.

Appetite Stimulation: In the clinical trials, the majority of patients were treated with 5 mg/day Dronabinol although the dosages ranged from 2.5 to 20 mg/day. For an adult:

1. Begin with 2.5 mg before lunch and 2.5 mg before supper. If CNS symptoms (feeling high, dizziness, confusion, somnolence) do occur, they usually resolve in 1 to 3 days with continued dosage.
2. If CNS symptoms are severe or persistent, reduce the dose to 2.5 mg before supper. If symptoms continue to be a problem, taking the single dose in the evening or at bedtime may reduce their severity.
3. When adverse effects are absent or minimal and further therapeutic effect is desired, increase the dose to 2.5 mg before lunch and 5 mg before supper or 5 and 5 mg. Although most patients respond to 2.5 mg twice daily, 10 mg twice daily has been tolerated in about half of the patients in appetite stimulation studies.

The pharmacologic effects of Dronabinol are reversible upon treatment cessation.

Antiemetic: Most patients respond to 5 mg three or four times daily. Dosage may be escalated during a chemotherapy cycle or at subsequent cycles, based upon initial results. Therapy should be initiated at the lowest recommended dosage and titrated to clinical response. Administration of Dronabinol with phenothiazines, such as prochlorperazine, has resulted in improved efficacy as compared to either drug alone, without additional toxicity.

Pediatrics: Dronabinol is not recommended for AIDS-related anorexia in pediatric patients because it has not been studied in this population. The pediatric dosage for the treatment of chemotherapy-induced emesis is the same as in adults. Caution is recommended in prescribing Dronabinol for children because of the psychoactive effects.

Geriatrics: Caution is advised in prescribing Dronabinol in elderly patients because they are generally more sensitive to the psychoactive effects of drugs. In antiemetic studies, no difference in tolerance or efficacy was apparent in patients > 55 years old.

INDICATIONS AND USAGE

Dronabinol is indicated for the treatment of:

➤ SHOWN IN PRODUCT IDENTIFICATION GUIDE

DRONABINOL DOSE: RESPONSE FREQUENCY AND ADVERSE EXPERIENCES*
N = 750 TREATMENT COURSES

Dronabinol Dose	Response Frequency (%)				Adverse Events Frequency (%)		
	Complete	Partial	Poor		None	Nondysphoric	Dysphoric
< 7 mg/m^2	36	32	32		23	65	12
> 7 mg/m^2	33	31	36		13	58	28

Nondysphoric events consisted of drowsiness, tachycardia, etc.

1. anorexia associated with weight loss in patients with AIDS; and
2. nausea and vomiting associated with cancer chemotherapy in patients who have failed to respond adequately to conventional antiemetic treatments.

CONTRAINDICATIONS

Dronabinol is contraindicated in any patient who has a history of hypersensitivity to any cannabinoid or sesame oil.

WARNINGS

Dronabinol is a medication with a potential for abuse. Physicians and pharmacists should use the same care in prescribing and accounting for Dronabinol as they would with morphine or other drugs controlled under Schedule II (CII) of the Controlled Substances Act. Because of the risk of diversion, it is recommended that prescriptions be limited to the amount necessary for the period between clinic visits. Patients receiving treatment with Dronabinol should be specifically warned not to drive, operate machinery, or engage in any hazardous activity until it is established that they are able to tolerate the drug and to perform such tasks safely.

PRECAUTIONS

General: The risk/benefit ratio of Dronabinol use should be carefully evaluated in patients with the following medical conditions because of individual variation in response and tolerance to the effects of Dronabinol.

Dronabinol should be used with caution in patients with cardiac disorders because of occasional hypotension, possible hypertension, syncope, or tachycardia (see "Clinical Pharmacology").

Dronabinol should be used with caution in patients with a history of substance abuse, including alcohol abuse or dependence, because they may be more prone to abuse Dronabinol as well. Multiple substance abuse is common and marijuana, which contains the same active compound, is a frequently abused substance.

Dronabinol should be used with caution and careful psychiatric monitoring in patients with mania, depression, or schizophrenia because Dronabinol may exacerbate these illnesses. Dronabinol should be used with caution in patients receiving concomitant therapy with sedatives, hypnotics or other psychoactive drugs because of the potential for additive or synergistic CNS effects.

Dronabinol should be used with caution in pregnant patients, nursing mothers, or pediatric patients because it has not been studied in these patient populations.

Dronabinol should be used with caution for treatment of anorexia and weight loss in elderly patients with AIDS because they may be more sensitive to the psychoactive effects and because its use in these patients has not been studied.

Information for Patients: Patients receiving treatment with Dronabinol should be alerted to the potential for additive central nervous system depression if Dronabinol is used concomitantly with alcohol or other CNS depressants such as benzodiazepines and barbiturates.

Patients receiving treatment with Dronabinol should be specifically warned not to drive, operate machinery, or engage in any hazardous activity until it is established that they are able to tolerate the drug and to perform such tasks safely. Patients using Dronabinol should be advised of possible changes in mood and other adverse behavioral effects of the drug so as to avoid panic in the event of such manifestations. Patients should remain under the supervision of a responsible adult during initial use of Dronabinol and following dosage adjustments.

Drug Interactions: In studies involving patients with AIDS and/or cancer, Dronabinol has been co-administered with a variety of medications (e.g., cytotoxic agents, anti-infective agents, sedatives, or opioid analgesics) without resulting in any clinically significant drug/drug interactions. Although no drug/drug interactions were discovered during the clinical trials of Dronabinol, cannabinoids may interact with other medications through both metabolic and pharmacodynamic mechanisms. Dronabinol is highly protein bound to plasma proteins, and therefore, might displace other protein-bound drugs. Although this displacement has not been confirmed *in vivo*, practitioners should monitor patients for a change in dosage requirements when administering Dronabinol to patients receiving other highly protein-bound drugs. Published reports of drug/drug interactions involving cannabinoids are summarized in the following table.

Concomitant Drug	Clinical Effects(s)
Amphetamines, cocaine, other sympathomimetic agents	Additive hypertension, tachycardia possibly cardiotoxicity
Atropine, scopolamine, antihistamines, other anticholinergic agents	Additive or super-additive tachycardia, drowsiness
Amitriptyline, amoxapine, desipramine, other tricyclic antidepressants	Additive tachycardia, hypertension, drowsiness

Concomitant Drug	Clinical Effects(s)
Barbiturates, benzodiazepines, ethanol, lithium, opioids, buspirone, antihistamines, muscle relaxants, other CNS depressants	Additive drowsiness and CNS depression
Disulfiram	A reversible hypomanic reaction was reported in a 28 y/o man who smoked marijuana; confirmed by dechallenge and rechallenge
Fluoxetine	A 21 y/o female with depression and bulimia receiving 20 mg/day fluoxetine × 4 wks became hypomanic after smoking marijuana; symptoms resolved after 4 days
Antipyrine, barbiturates	Decreased clearance of these agents, presumably via competitive inhibition of metabolism
Theophylline	Increased theophylline metabolism reported with smoking of marijuana; effect similar to that following smoking tobacco

Carcinogenesis, Mutagenesis, Impairment of Fertility: Carcinogenicity studies have not been performed with Dronabinol. Mutagenicity testing of Dronabinol was negative in an Ames test. In a long-term study (77 days) in rats, oral administration of Dronabinol at doses of 30 to 150 mg/m^2, equivalent to 0.3 to 1.5 times maximum recommended human dose (MRHD) of 90 mg/m^2/day in cancer patients or 2 to 10 times MRHD of 15 mg/m^2/day in AIDS patients, reduced ventral prostate, seminal vesicle and epididymal weights and caused a decrease in seminal fluid volume. Decreases in spermatogenesis, number of developing germ cells, and number of Leydig cells in the testis were also observed. However, sperm count, mating success and testosterone levels were not affected. The significance of these animal findings in humans is not known.

Pregnancy: Pregnancy Category C. Reproduction studies with Dronabinol have been performed in mice at 15 to 450 mg/m^2, equivalent to 0.2 to 5 times maximum recommended human dose (MRHD) of 90 mg/m^2/day in cancer patients or 1 to 30 times MRHD of 15 mg/m^2/day in AIDS patients, and in rats at 74 to 295 mg/m^2 (equivalent to 0.8 to 3 times MRHD of 90 mg/m^2 in cancer patients or 5 to 20 times MRHD of 15 mg/m^2/day in AIDS patients). These studies have revealed no evidence of teratogenicity due to Dronabinol. At these dosages in mice and rats, Dronabinol decreased maternal weight gain and number of viable pups and increased fetal mortality and early resorptions. Such effects were dose dependent and less apparent at lower doses which produced less maternal toxicity. There are no adequate and well-controlled studies in pregnant women. Dronabinol should be used only if the potential benefit justifies the potential risk to the fetus.

Nursing Mothers: Use of Dronabinol is not recommended in nursing mothers since, in addition to the secretion of HIV virus in breast milk, Dronabinol is concentrated in and secreted in human breast milk and is absorbed by the nursing baby.

ADVERSE REACTIONS

Adverse experiences information summarized in the tables below was derived from well-controlled clinical trials conducted in the US and US territories involving 474 patients exposed to Dronabinol. Studies of AIDS-related weight loss included 157 patients receiving Dronabinol at a dose of 2.5 mg twice daily and 67 receiving placebo. Studies of nausea and vomiting related to cancer chemotherapy included 317 patients receiving Dronabinol and 68 receiving placebo.

A cannabinoid dose-related "high" (easy laughing, elation and heightened awareness) has been reported by patients receiving Dronabinol in both the antiemetic (24%) and the lower dose appetite stimulant clinical trials (8%) (see "Clinical Trials").

The most frequently reported adverse experiences in patients with AIDS during placebo-controlled clinical trials involved the CNS and were reported by 33% of patients receiving Dronabinol. The frequency of adverse experiences did not correlate with the duration of therapy.

PROBABLY CAUSALLY RELATED: INCIDENCE GREATER THAN 1%
Rates derived from clinical trials in AIDS-related anorexia (N = 157) and chemotherapy-related nausea (N = 317). Rates were generally higher in the antiemetic use (given in parentheses).

Body as a Whole: Asthenia.

◆ RATED THERAPEUTICALLY EQUIVALENT; ◇ THERAPEUTIC EQUIVALENCE UNCONFIRMED; ○ UNRATED

Cardiovascular: Palpitations, tachycardia, vasodilation.

Digestive: Nausea*, vomiting*.

Nervous System: (Amnesia), (ataxia), confusion, depersonalization, dizziness*, euphoria* (24%), (hallucination), paranoid reaction*, somnolence*, thinking abnormal.

Special Senses: Vision difficulties.
* Incidence of events 3% to 10%

PROBABLY CAUSALLY RELATED: INCIDENCE LESS THAN 1%
Event rates derived from clinical trials in AIDS-related anorexia (N = 157) and chemotherapy-related nausea (N = 317).

Cardiovascular: Conjunctivitis*, hypotension*.

Digestive: Diarrhea*, fecal incontinence.

Musculoskeletal: Myalgias.

Nervous System: Depression, emotionallability, nightmares, speech difficulties, tinnitus.

Respiratory: Cough, rhinitis, sinusitis.

Skin and Appendages: Flushing*.
* Incidence of events 0.3% to 1%.

CAUSAL RELATIONSHIP UNKNOWN: INCIDENCE LESS THAN 1%
The clinical significance of the association of these events with Dronabinol treatment is unknown, but they are reported as alerting information for the clinician.

Body as a Whole: Headache.

Digestive: Anorexia, hepatic enzyme elevation.

Nervous System: Anxiety/nervousness, tremors.

Skin and Appendages: Sweating.

DRUG ABUSE AND DEPENDENCE
Dronabinol is one of the psychoactive compounds present in cannabis, and is abusable and controlled Schedule II (CII) under the Controlled Substances Act. Both psychological and physiological dependence have been noted in healthy individuals receiving Dronabinol, but addiction is uncommon and has only been seen after prolonged high dose administration.

Chronic abuse of cannabis has been associated with decrements in motivation, cognition, judgement, and perception. The etiology of these impairments is unknown, but may be associated with the complex process of addiction rather than an isolated effect of the drug. No such decrements in psychological, social or neurological status have been associated with the administration of Dronabinol for therapeutic purposes. In an open-label study in patients with AIDS who received Dronabinol for up to five months, no abuse, diversion or systematic change in personality or social functioning were observed despite the inclusion of a substantial number of patients with a past history of drug abuse.

An abstinence syndrome has been reported after the abrupt discontinuation of Dronabinol in volunteers receiving dosages of 210 mg/day for 12 to 16 consecutive days. Within 12 hours after discontinuation, these volunteers manifested symptoms such as irritability, insomnia, and restlessness. By approximately 24 hours post-Dronabinol discontinuation, withdrawal symptoms intensified to include "hot flashes", sweating, rhinorrhea, loose stools, hiccoughs and anorexia. These withdrawal symptoms gradually dissipated over the next 48 hours. Electroencephalographic changes consistent with the effects of drug withdrawal (hyperexcitation) were recorded in patients after abrupt dechallenge. Patients also complained of disturbed sleep for several weeks after discontinuing therapy with high dosages of Dronabinol.

OVERDOSAGE
Signs and symptoms following MILD Dronabinol intoxication include drowsiness, euphoria, heightened sensory awareness, altered time perception, reddened conjunctiva, dry mouth and tachycardia: following MODERATE intoxication include memory impairment, depersonalization, mood alteration, urinary retention, and reduced bowel motility; and following SEVERE intoxication include decreased motor coordination, lethargy, slurred speech, and postural hypotension. Apprehensive patients may experience panic reactions and seizures may occur in patients with existing seizure disorders.

The estimated lethal human dose of intravenous Dronabinol is 30 mg/kg (2100 mg/70kg). Significant CNS symptoms in antiemetic studies followed oral doses of 0.4 mg/kg (28 mg/70 kg) of Dronabinol.

Management: A potentially serious oral ingestion, if recent, should be managed with gut decontamination. In unconscious patients with a secure airway, instill activated charcoal (30 to 100 g in adults, 1 to 2 g/kg in infants) via a nasogastric tube. A saline cathartic or sorbitol may be added to the first dose of activated charcoal. Patients experiencing depressive, hallucinatory or psychotic reactions should be placed in a quiet area and offered reassurance. Benzodiazepines (5 to 10 mg diazepam *po*) may be used for treatment of extreme agitation. Hypotension usually responds to Trendelenburg position and IV fluids. Pressors are rarely required.

DOSAGE AND ADMINISTRATION
Appetite Stimulation: Initially, 2.5 mg Dronabinol should be administered orally twice daily (b.i.d.) before lunch and supper. For patients unable to tolerate this 5 mg/day dosage of Dronabinol the dosage can be reduced to 2.5 mg/day,

administered as a single dose in the evening or at bedtime. If clinically indicated and in the absence of significant adverse effects, the dosage may be gradually increased to a maximum of 20 mg/day Dronabinol administered in divided oral doses. Caution should be exercised in escalating the dosage of Dronabinol because of the increased frequency of dose-related adverse experiences at higher dosages (see *"Precautions"*).

Antiemetic: Dronabinol is best administered at an initial dose of 5 mg/m², given 1 to 3 hours prior to the administration of chemotherapy, then every 2 to 4 hours after chemotherapy is given, for a total of 4 to 6 doses/day. Should the 5 mg/m² dose prove to be ineffective, and in the absence of significant side effects, the dose may be escalated by 2.5 mg/m² increments to a maximum of 15 mg/m² per dose. Caution should be exercised in dose escalation, however, as the incidence of disturbing psychiatric symptoms increases significantly at maximum dose (See *"Precautions"*).

Safety and Handling: Dronabinol should be packaged in a well-closed container and stored in a cool environment between 8° and 15°C (46° and 59°F). Protect from freezing. No particular hazard to health care workers handling the capsules has been identified.

Access to abusable drugs such as Dronabinol presents an occupational hazard for addiction in the health care industry. Routine procedures for handling controlled substances developed to protect the public may not be adequate to protect health care workers. Implementation of more effective accounting procedures and measures to appropriately restrict access to drugs of this class may minimize the risk of self-administration by health care providers.

HOW SUPPLIED
CAPSULE (C-II): 2.5 MG

BRAND/MANUFACTURER	NDC	SIZE	AWP
○ **BRAND**			
MARINOL: Roxane	00054-2601-11	25s	$78.47
	00054-2601-21	60s	$179.40
	00054-2601-25	100s	$268.50

CAPSULE (C-II): 5 MG

BRAND/MANUFACTURER	NDC	SIZE	AWP
○ **BRAND**			
MARINOL: Roxane	00054-2602-11	25s	$154.70
	00054-2602-25	100s	$528.00

CAPSULE (C-II): 10 MG

BRAND/MANUFACTURER	NDC	SIZE	AWP
○ **BRAND**			
MARINOL: Roxane	00054-2603-11	25s	$309.40

Droperidol

DESCRIPTION
Droperidol is a neuroleptic (tranquilizer) agent available in ampuls and vials. Each milliliter contains 2.5 mg of Droperidol in an aqueous solution adjusted to pH 3.4 ± 0.4 with lactic acid. Droperidol in 10 mL multidose vials also contains 1.8 mg of methylparaben and 0.2 mg propylparaben. Droperidol is chemically identified as 1-(1-[3-(p-fluorobenzoyl) propyl]-1,2,3,6-tetrahydro-4-pyridyl)-2-benzimidazolinone with a molecular weight of 379.43.

Droperidol is a sterile, non-pyrogenic aqueous solution for intravenous or intramuscular injection.

Following is its chemical structure:

CLINICAL PHARMACOLOGY
Droperidol produces marked tranquilization and sedation. It allays apprehension and provides a state of mental detachment and indifference while maintaining a state of reflex alertness.

Droperidol produces an antiemetic effect as evidenced by the antagonism of apomorphine in dogs. It lowers the incidence of nausea and vomiting during surgical procedures and provides antiemetic protection in the postoperative period.

Droperidol potentiates other CNS depressants. It produces mild alpha-adrenergic blockade, peripheral vascular dilatation and reduction of the pressor effect of epinephrine. It can produce hypotension and decreased peripheral vascular resistance and may decrease pulmonary arterial pressure (particularly if it is abnormally high). It may reduce the incidence of epinephrine-induced arrhythmias, but it does not prevent other cardiac arrhythmias.

The onset of action of single intramuscular and intravenous doses is from three to ten minutes following administration, although the peak effect may not be apparent for up to thirty minutes. The duration of the tranquilizing and sedative effects generally is two to four hours, although alteration of alertness may persist for as long as twelve hours.

INDICATIONS AND USAGE

Droperidol is indicated:

■ to produce tranquilization and to reduce the incidence of nausea and vomiting in surgical and diagnostic procedures.

■ for premedication, induction, and as an adjunct in the maintenance of general and regional anesthesia.

■ in neuroleptanalgesia in which Droperidol is given concurrently with an opioid analgesic, such as fentanyl citrate, Injection, to aid in producing tranquility and decreasing anxiety and pain.

UNLABELED USES

Droperidol is used alone or as an adjunct in the treatment of hiccup and chemotherapy-induced nausea and vomiting. It is also used during endotracheal intubation and is prescribed to control agitation in severely agitated psychotic patients and patients with Ménière's disease.

CONTRAINDICATIONS

Droperidol is contraindicated in patients with known hypersensitivity to the drug.

WARNINGS

FLUIDS AND OTHER COUNTERMEASURES TO MANAGE HYPOTENSION SHOULD BE READILY AVAILABLE.

As with other CNS depressant drugs, patients who have received Droperidol should have appropriate surveillance.

It is recommended that opioids, when required, initially be used in reduced doses.

As with other neuroleptic agents, very rare reports of neuroleptic malignant syndrome (altered consciousness, muscle rigidity and autonomic instability) have occurred in patients who have received Droperidol.

Since it may be difficult to distinguish neuroleptic malignant syndrome from malignant hyperpyrexia in the perioperative period, prompt treatment with dantrolene should be considered if increases in temperature, heart rate or carbon dioxide production occur.

Cases of sudden death have been reported following use of Droperidol at high doses (generally 25 mg or greater) in patients at risk for cardiac dysrhythmia due to anoxia, hypercarbia, severe electrolyte disturbances, or alcohol withdrawal. While these reports do not establish the cause of such death, QT prolongation after Droperidol administration has been reported and there is at least one case of nonfatal torsade de pointes confirmed by rechallenge.

Because of these reports Droperidol is not recommended in the treatment of alcohol withdrawal or in other clinical situations where high doses are likely to be needed in patients at risk for dysrhythmia.

PRECAUTIONS

General: The initial dose of Droperidol should be appropriately reduced in elderly, debilitated and other poor-risk patients. The effect of the initial dose should be considered in determining incremental doses.

Certain forms of conduction anesthesia, such as spinal anesthesia and some peridural anesthetics, can alter respiration by blocking intercostal nerves and can cause peripheral vasodilatation and hypotension because of sympathetic blockade. Through other mechanisms (see *"Clinical Pharmacology"*), Droperidol can also alter circulation. Therefore, when Droperidol is used to supplement these forms of anesthesia, the anesthetist should be familiar with the physiological alterations involved, and be prepared to manage them in the patients elected for these forms of anesthesia.

If hypotension occurs, the possibility of hypovolemia should be considered and managed with appropriate parenteral fluid therapy. Repositioning the patient to improve venous return to the heart should be considered when operative conditions permit. It should be noted that in spinal and peridural anesthesia, tilting the patient into a head-down position may result in a higher level of anesthesia than is desirable, as well as impair venous return to the heart. Care should be exercised in moving and positioning of patients because of a possibility of orthostatic hypotension. If volume expansion with fluids plus these other countermeasures do not correct the hypotension, then the administration of pressor agents other than epinephrine should be considered. Epinephrine may paradoxically decrease the blood pressure in patients treated with Droperidol due to the alpha-adrenergic blocking action of Droperidol.

Since Droperidol may decrease pulmonary arterial pressure, this fact should be considered by those who conduct diagnostic or surgical procedures where interpretation of pulmonary arterial pressure measurements might determine final management of the patient.

Vital signs should be monitored routinely.

When the EEG is used for postoperative monitoring, it may be found that the EEG pattern returns to normal slowly.

Impaired Hepatic or Renal Function: Droperidol should be administered with caution to patients with liver and kidney dysfunction because of the importance of these organs in the metabolism and excretion of drugs.

Pheochromocytoma: In patients with diagnosed/suspected pheochromocytoma, severe hypertension and tachycardia have been observed after the administration of Droperidol.

Drug Interactions: Other CNS depressant drugs (e.g. barbiturates, tranquilizers, opioids and general anesthetics) have additive or potentiating effects with Droperidol. When patients have received such drugs, the dose of Droperidol

required will be less than usual. Following the administration of Droperidol the dose of other CNS depressant drugs should be reduced.

Carcinogenesis, Mutagenesis, Impairment of Fertility: No carcinogenicity studies have been carried out with Droperidol. The micronucleus test in female rats revealed no mutagenic effects in single oral doses as high as 160 mg/kg. An oral study in rats (Segment I) revealed no impairment of fertility in either male or females at 0.63, 2.5 and 10 mg/kg doses (approximately 2, 9 and 36 times maximum recommended human iv/im dosage).

Pregnancy—Category C: Droperidol administered intravenously has been shown to cause a slight increase in mortality of the newborn rat at 4.4 times the upper human dose. At 44 times the upper human dose, mortality rate was comparable to that for control animals. Following intramuscular administration, increased mortality of the offspring at 1.8 times the upper human dose is attributed to CNS depression in the dams who neglected to remove placentae from their offspring. Droperidol has not been shown to be teratogenic in animals. There are no adequate and well-controlled studies in pregnant women. Droperidol should be used during pregnancy only if the potential benefit justifies the potential risk to the fetus.

Labor and Delivery: There are insufficient data to support the use of Droperidol in labor and delivery. Therefore, such use is not recommended.

Nursing Mothers: It is not known whether Droperidol is excreted in human milk. Because many drugs are excreted in human milk, caution should be exercised when Droperidol is administered to a nursing mother.

Pediatric Use: The safety of Droperidol in children younger than two years of age has not been established.

ADVERSE REACTIONS

The most common somatic adverse reactions reported to occur with Droperidol are mild to moderate hypotension and tachycardia, but these effects usually subside without treatment. If hypotension occurs and is severe or persists, the possibility of hypovolemia should be considered and managed with appropriate parenteral fluid therapy.

The most common behavioral adverse effects of Droperidol include dysphoria, postoperative drowsiness, restlessness, hyperactivity and anxiety, which can either be the result of an inadequate dosage (lack of adequate treatment effect) or of an adverse drug reaction (part of the symptom complex of akathisia).

Care should be taken to search for extrapyramidal signs and symptoms (dystonia, akathisia, oculogyric crisis) to differentiate these different clinical conditions, when extrapyramidal symptoms are the cause, they can usually be controlled with anticholinergic agents.

Postoperative hallucinatory episodes (sometimes associated with transient periods of mental depression) have also been reported.

Other less common reported adverse reactions include anaphylaxis, dizziness, chills and/or shivering, laryngospasm, and bronchospasm.

Elevated blood pressure, with or without pre-existing hypertension, has been reported following administration of Droperidol combined with fentanyl citrate or other parenteral analgesics. This might be due to unexplained alterations in sympathetic activity following large doses; however, it is also frequently attributed to anesthetic or surgical stimulation during light anesthesia.

OVERDOSAGE

Manifestations: The manifestations of Droperidol overdosage are an extension of its pharmacologic actions.

Treatment: In the presence of hypoventilation or apnea, oxygen should be administered and respiration should be assisted or controlled as indicated. A patent airway must be maintained; an oropharyngeal airway or endotracheal tube might be indicated. The patient should be carefully observed for 24 hours; body warmth and adequate fluid intake should be maintained. If hypotension occurs and is severe or persists, the possibility of hypovolemia should be considered and managed with appropriate parenteral fluid therapy. (See *"Precautions"*.)

If significant extrapyramidal reactions occur in the context of an overdose, an anticholinergic should be administered. The intravenous LD_{50} of Droperidol is 20-43 mg/kg in mice; 30 mg/kg in rats; 25 mg/kg in dogs and 11-13 mg/kg in rabbits. The intramuscular LD_{50} of Droperidol is 195 mg/kg in mice; 104-110 mg/kg in rats; 97 mg/kg in rabbits and 200 mg/kg in guinea pigs.

DOSAGE AND ADMINISTRATION

Dosage should be individualized: Some of the factors to be considered in determining the dose are age, body weight, physical status, underlying pathological condition, use of other drugs, type of anesthesia to be used and the surgical procedure involved. Vital signs should be monitored routinely.

USUAL ADULT DOSAGE

I. Premedication: (to be appropriately modified in the elderly, debilitated and those who have received other depressant drugs) 2.5 to 10 mg (1 to 4 mL) may be administered intramuscularly 30 to 60 minutes preoperatively.

II. Adjunct to General Anesthesia:

Induction: 2.5 mg (1 mL) per 20 to 25 pounds may be administered (usually intravenously) along with an analgesic and/or general anesthetic. Smaller doses may be adequate. The total amount of Droperidol administered should be titrated to obtain the desired effect based on the individual patient's response.

Maintenance: 1.25 to 2.5 mg (0.5 to 1 mL) usually intravenously.

III. Use without a general anesthetic in diagnostic procedures: Administer the usual I.M. premedication 2.5 to 10 mg (1 to 4 mL) 30 to 60 minutes before the

---

procedure. Additional 1.25 to 2.5 mg (0.5 to 1 mL) amounts of Droperidol may be administered, usually intravenously.

Note: When Droperidol is used in certain procedures, such as bronchoscopy, appropriate topical anesthesia is still necessary.

IV. Adjunct to regional anesthesia: 2.5 to 5 mg (1 to 2 mL) may be administered intramuscularly or slowly intravenously when additional sedation is required.

USUAL CHILDREN'S DOSAGE

For children two to 12 years of age, a reduced dose as low as 1.0 to 1.5 mg (0.4 to 0.6 mL) per 20 to 25 pounds is recommended for premedication or for induction of anesthesia. See *"Warnings"* and *"Precautions"* for use of Droperidol with other CNS depressants and in patients with altered response.

Parenteral drug products should be inspected visually for particulate matter and discoloration prior to administration, whenever solution and container permit. If such abnormalities are observed, the drug should not be administered.

STORAGE

Protect from Light. Store at Room Temperature 15°C-30°C (59°F-86°F).

J CODES

Up to 5 mg IM,IV—J1790

HOW SUPPLIED
INJECTION: 2.5 MG/ML

AVERAGE UNIT PRICE (AVAILABLE SIZES)		GENERIC A-RATED AVERAGE PRICE (GAAP)	
BRAND	$3.45	2 ml 10s	$39.86
GENERIC	$1.56	5 ml 10s	$56.31

BRAND/MANUFACTURER	NDC	SIZE	AWP
◆ **BRAND**			
INAPSINE: Janssen	50458-0010-01	1 ml 10s	$42.50
	50458-0010-02	2 ml 10s	$53.06
◆ **GENERICS**			
Astra	00186-1224-12	10 ml 5s	$51.50
Du Pont Multi	00590-5981-53	2 ml 10s	$26.25
Astra	00186-1220-03	2 ml 10s	$31.56
Solo Pak	39769-0123-02	2 ml 10s	$34.38
Astra	00186-1226-13	2 ml 10s	$36.88
Amer Regent	00517-9702-10	2 ml 10s	$42.50
Abbott Hosp	00074-1187-01	2 ml 10s	$67.57
Du Pont Multi	00590-5981-61	5 ml 10s	$35.00
Astra	00186-1221-03	5 ml 10s	$54.00
Astra	00186-1227-13	5 ml 10s	$61.25
Amer Regent	00517-9705-10	5 ml 10s	$75.00
Amer Regent	00517-9710-10	10 ml 10s	$118.75

Droperidol and Fentanyl Citrate

THE TWO COMPONENTS OF THIS INJECTION, FENTANYL CITRATE AND DROPERIDOL, HAVE DIFFERENT PHARMACOLOGIC ACTIONS. BEFORE ADMINISTERING DROPERIDOL/FENTANYL CITRATE INJECTION, THE USER SHOULD BECOME FAMILIAR WITH THE SPECIAL PROPERTIES OF EACH DRUG, PARTICULARLY THE WIDELY DIFFERING DURATIONS OF ACTION.

DESCRIPTION

Droperidol/Fentanyl Citrate is a potent opioid analgesic (Fentanyl Citrate) and a neuroleptic (tranquilizer) agent (Droperidol). Each milliliter contains (in a 1:50 ratio) Fentanyl Citrate equivalent to 50 µg of fentanyl base and 2.5 mg of Droperidol in a solution.

The chemical name of Fentanyl Citrate is N- (1-phenethyl-4-piperidyl) propionanilide citrate (1:1). Molecular weight: 528.60

The chemical name of Droperidol is 1-[1-[3-(p-fluorobenzoyl)propyl]-1,2,3,6-tetrahydro-4-pyridyl] -2-benzimidazolinone. Molecular weight: 379.43

Droperidol/Fentanyl Citrate is a sterile, preservative free aqueous solution for intravenous or intramuscular injection.

CLINICAL PHARMACOLOGY

Droperidol/Fentanyl Citrate is a combination drug containing an opioid analgesic, Fentanyl Citrate, and a neuroleptic (major tranquilizer), Droperidol. The combined effect, sometimes referred to as neuroleptanalgesia, is characterized by general quiescence, reduced motor activity, and profound analgesia; complete loss of consciousness usually does not occur from use of Droperidol/Fentanyl Citrate Injection alone. The incidence of early postoperative pain and emesis may be reduced.

A. Fentanyl Citrate is an opioid analgesic. A dose of 100 µg (0.1 mg) (2.0 mL), is approximately equivalent in analgesic activity to 10 mg of morphine or 75 mg of meperidine. The principal actions of therapeutic value are analgesia and sedation. Alterations in respiratory rate and alveolar ventilation, associated with opioid analgesics, may last longer than the analgesic effect. As the dose of opioid is increased, the decrease in pulmonary exchange becomes greater. Large doses may produce apnea. Fentanyl Citrate appears to have less emetic activity than either morphine or meperidine. Histamine assays and skin wheal testing in man indicate that clinically significant histamine release rarely occurs with Fentanyl

Citrate. Assays in man show no clinically significant histamine release in dosages up to 50 µg/kg (0.05 mg/kg) (1 mL/kg). The pharmacokinetics of Fentanyl Citrate can be described as a three-compartment model, with a distribution time of 1.7 minutes, redistribution of 13 minutes and a terminal elimination half-life of 219 minutes. The volume of distribution for Fentanyl Citrate is 4 L/kg.

Fentanyl Citrate plasma protein binding capacity increases with increasing ionization of the drug. Alterations in pH may affect its distribution between plasma and the central nervous system. It accumulates in skeletal muscle and fat, and is released slowly into the blood. Fentanyl Citrate, which is primarily transformed in the liver, demonstrates a high first pass clearance and releases approximately 75% of an intravenous dose in urine, mostly as metabolites with less than 10% representing the unchanged drug. Approximately 9% of the dose is recovered in the feces, primarily as metabolites. The onset of action of Fentanyl Citrate is almost immediate when the drug is given intravenously; however, the maximal analgesic and respiratory depressant effect may not be noted for several minutes. The usual duration of action of the analgesic effect is 30 to 60 minutes after a single intravenous dose of up to 100 µg (0.1 mg) (2.0 mL). Following intramuscular administration, the onset of action is from seven to eight minutes, and the duration of action is one to two hours. As with longer acting opioid analgesics, the duration of the respiratory depressant effect of Fentanyl Citrate may be longer than the analgesic effect. The following observations have been reported concerning altered respiratory response to CO_2 stimulation following administration of Fentanyl Citrate to man:

1. DIMINISHED SENSITIVITY TO CO_2 STIMULATION MAY PERSIST LONGER THAN DEPRESSION OF RESPIRATORY RATE. [Altered sensitivity to CO_2 stimulation has been demonstrated for up to four hours following a single dose of 600 µg (0.6 mg) (12 mL) Fentanyl Citrate to healthy volunteers.] Fentanyl Citrate frequently slows the respiratory rate, duration and degree of respiratory depression being dose related.

2. The peak respiratory depressant effect of a single intravenous dose of Fentanyl Citrate is noted 5 to 15 minutes following injection. See also *"Warnings"* and *"Precautions"* concerning respiratory depression.

B. Droperidol produces marked tranquilization and sedation. Droperidol allays apprehension and provides a state of mental detachment and indifference while maintaining a state of reflex alertness.

Droperidol also produces an antiemetic effect as evidenced by the antagonism of apomorphine in dogs. It lowers the incidence of nausea and vomiting during surgical procedures and provides antiemetic protection in the postoperative period.

Droperidol potentiates other CNS depressants. It produces mild alpha-adrenergic blockade, peripheral vascular dilatation and reduction of the pressor effect of epinephrine. It can produce hypotension and decreased peripheral vascular resistance and may decrease pulmonary arterial pressure (particularly if it is abnormally high). It may reduce the incidence of epinephrine-induced arrhythmias, but does not prevent other cardiac arrhythmias.

The onset of action of single intramuscular and intravenous doses of droperidol is from three to ten minutes following administration, although the peak effect may not be apparent for up to thirty minutes. The duration of the tranquilizing and sedative effects generally is two to four hours, although alteration of consciousness may persist for as long as twelve hours. This is in contrast to the much shorter duration of Fentanyl Citrate.

INDICATIONS AND USAGE

Droperidol/Fentanyl Citrate is indicated to produce tranquilization and analgesia for surgical and diagnostic procedures. It may be used as an anesthetic premedication, as an adjunct to the induction of anesthesia, and as an adjunct in the maintenance of general and regional anesthesia. If the supplementation of analgesia is necessary, Fentanyl Citrate alone rather than the combination drug, Droperidol/Fentanyl Citrate, should usually be used, see *"Dosage and Administration"* section.

CONTRAINDICATIONS

Droperidol/Fentanyl Citrate is contraindicated in patients with known hypersensitivity to either component.

WARNINGS

DROPERIDOL/FENTANYL CITRATE SHOULD BE ADMINISTERED ONLY BY PERSONS SPECIFICALLY TRAINED IN THE USE OF INTRAVENOUS ANESTHETICS AND MANAGEMENT OF THE RESPIRATORY EFFECTS OF POTENT OPIOIDS.

AN OPIOID ANTAGONIST, RESUSCITATIVE AND INTUBATION EQUIPMENT AND OXYGEN SHOULD BE READILY AVAILABLE.

See also discussion of opioid antagonists in *"Precautions"* and *"Overdosage"* sections.

FLUIDS AND OTHER COUNTERMEASURES TO MANAGE HYPOTENSION SHOULD ALSO BE AVAILABLE.

The respiratory depressant effect of opioids persists longer than the measured analgesic effect. When used with Droperidol/Fentanyl Citrate the total dose of all opioid analgesics administered should be considered by the practitioner before ordering opioid analgesics during recovery from anesthesia. It is recommended that opioids, when required, be used in reduced doses initially, as low as 1/4 to 1/3 those usually recommended.

Droperidol/Fentanyl Citrate may cause muscle rigidity, particularly involving the muscles of respiration. This effect is due to the Fentanyl Citrate component and is related to the dose and speed of injection. Its incidence can be reduced by the use of slow intravenous injection. Once the effect occurs, it is managed by the use of assisted or controlled respiration and, if necessary, by a neuromuscular blocking agent compatible with the patient's condition.

Head Injuries and Increased Intracranial Pressure: Droperidol/Fentanyl Citrate should be used with caution in patients who may be particularly susceptible to respiratory depression such as comatose patients who may have a head injury or brain tumor. In addition, Droperidol/Fentanyl Citrate may obscure the clinical course of patients with head injury.

As with other neuroleptic agents, very rare reports of neuroleptic malignant syndrome (altered consciousness, muscle rigidity and autonomic instability) have occurred in patients who have received the Droperidol component of Droperidol/Fentanyl Citrate. Since it may be difficult to distinguish neuroleptic malignant syndrome from malignant hyperpyrexia in the peri-operative period, prompt treatment with dantrolene should be considered if increases in temperature, heart rate or carbon dioxide production occur.

Cases of sudden death have been reported following use of Droperidol at high doses (generally 25 mg or greater) in patients at risk for cardiac dysrhythmia due to anoxia, hypercarbia, severe electrolyte disturbances, or alcohol withdrawal. While these reports do not establish the cause of such death, QT prolongation after administration of the Droperidol component of Droperidol/Fentanyl Citrate has been reported and there is at least one case of non-fatal torsades de pointes confirmed by re-challenge.

Because of these reports, Droperidol/Fentanyl Citrate is not recommended in the treatment of alcohol withdrawal or in other clinical situations where high doses are likely to be needed in patients at risk for dysrhythmia.

PRECAUTIONS

General: The initial dose of Droperidol/Fentanyl Citrate should be appropriately reduced in elderly, debilitated and other poor-risk patients. The effect of the initial dose should be considered in determining incremental doses. Certain forms of conduction anesthesia, such as spinal anesthesia and some peridural anesthetics, can alter respiration by blocking intercostal nerves and can cause peripheral vasodilation and hypotension because of sympathetic blockade. Through other mechanisms (see *"Clinical Pharmacology"*) Fentanyl Citrate and Droperidol can also depress respiration and blood pressure. Therefore, when Droperidol/Fentanyl Citrate is used to supplement these forms of anesthesia, the anesthetist should be familiar with the physiological alterations involved, and be prepared to manage them in the patients selected for these forms of anesthesia.

The Droperidol component of Droperidol/Fentanyl Citrate may decrease pulmonary arterial pressure. This fact should be considered by those who conduct diagnostic or surgical procedures where interpretation of pulmonary arterial pressure measurements might determine final management of the patient.

Vital signs should be monitored routinely.

When the EEG is used for postoperative monitoring, it may be found that the EEG pattern returns to normal slowly.

Hypotension: If hypotension occurs, the possibility of hypovolemia should be considered and managed with appropriate parenteral fluid therapy. Repositioning the patient to improve venous return to the heart should be considered when operative conditions permit. It should be noted that in spinal and peridural anesthesia, tilting the patient into a head down position may result in a higher level of anesthesia than is desirable, as well as impair venous return to the heart. Care should be exercised in the moving and positioning of patients because of a possibility of orthostatic hypotension. If volume expansion with fluids plus these other countermeasures do not correct the hypotension, then the administration of pressor agents other than epinephrine should be considered. Epinephrine may paradoxically decrease the blood pressure in patients treated with Droperidol/Fentanyl Citrate due to the alpha-adrenergic blocking action of Droperidol.

Impaired Respiration: Droperidol/Fentanyl Citrate and Fentanyl Citrate should be used with caution in patients with chronic obstructive pulmonary disease, patients with decreased respiratory reserve and others with potentially compromised ventilation. In such patients opioids may additionally decrease respiratory drive and increase airway resistance. During anesthesia, this can be managed by assisted or controlled respiration. Respiratory depression caused by opioid analgesics can be reversed by opioid antagonists. Appropriate surveillance should be maintained because the duration of respiratory depression of doses of Fentanyl Citrate as Fentanyl Citrate or Droperidol/Fentanyl Citrate employed during anesthesia may be longer than the duration of the opioid antagonist action. Consult individual prescribing information (levallorphan, nalorphine and naloxone) before employing opioid antagonists.

Impaired Hepatic or Renal Function: Droperidol/Fentanyl Citrate should be administered with caution to patients with liver and kidney dysfunction because of the importance of these organs in the metabolism and excretion of drugs.

Pheochromocytoma: In patients with diagnosed/suspected pheochromocytoma, severe hypertension and tachycardia have been observed after the administration of the droperidol component of Droperidol/Fentanyl Citrate.

Cardiovascular Effects: The Droperidol/Fentanyl Citrate component may produce bradycardia, which may be treated with atropine. Droperidol/Fentanyl Citrate should be used with caution in patients with cardiac bradyarrhythmias.

Drug Interactions: Other CNS depressant drugs (e.g. barbiturates, tranquilizers, opioids and general anesthetics) have additive or potentiating effects with Droperidol/Fentanyl Citrate. When patients have received such drugs, the dose of Droperidol/Fentanyl Citrate required will be less than usual. Following the administration of Droperidol/Fentanyl Citrate, the dose of the other CNS depressant drugs should be reduced.

Carcinogenesis Mutagenesis, Impairment of Fertility: No carcinogenicity studies have been conducted with Droperidol/Fentanyl Citrate or its components. A subcutaneous study of Droperidol/Fentanyl Citrate in female rats revealed no impairment of fertility at doses 9 times the upper human dose. An intravenous study revealed no effects on fertility at 2 times the upper human dose (highest dosage level tested).

Pregnancy: Category C: Droperidol/Fentanyl Citrate had no embryotoxic effects in rats at intravenous doses approximately 2 times the upper human dose. A subcutaneous study of Droperidol/Fentanyl Citrate in female rats showed increased fetal resorptions at 18 times the upper human dose. No teratogenic effects were revealed at 36 times the upper human dose. In rabbits, increased resorptions and decreased litter size were found at intravenous doses approximately 2 times the upper human dose. Maternal mortality occurred at 7 times the upper human dose.

Droperidol/Fentanyl Citrate has not been shown to be teratogenic in animals. There are no adequate and well-controlled studies in pregnant women. Droperidol/Fentanyl Citrate should be used during pregnancy only if the potential benefit justifies the potential risk to the fetus.

Labor and Delivery: There are insufficient data to support the use of Droperidol/Fentanyl Citrate in labor and delivery. Therefore, such use is not recommended.

Nursing Mothers: It is not known whether Fentanyl Citrate or Droperidol are excreted in human milk. Because many drugs are excreted in human milk, caution should be exercised when Droperidol/Fentanyl Citrate is administered to a nursing woman.

Pediatric Use: The safety and efficacy of Droperidol/Fentanyl Citrate in children under two years of age has not been established.

ADVERSE REACTIONS

The most common serious adverse reactions reported to occur with (Droperidol/Fentanyl Citrate) are respiratory depression, apnea, and muscular rigidity; if these remain untreated, respiratory arrest, circulatory depression or cardiac arrest could occur. Mild to moderate hypotension and tachycardia also occur, but these effects usually subside without treatment. If hypotension occurs and is severe or persists, the possibility of hypovolemia should be considered and managed with appropriate parenteral fluid therapy.

The most common behavioral adverse effects of (Droperidol/Fentanyl Citrate) include dysphoria, postoperative drowsiness, restlessness, hyperactivity and anxiety, which can either be the result of an inadequate dosage (lack of adequate treatment effect) or of an adverse drug reaction (part of the symptom complex of akathisia).

Care should be taken to search for extrapyramidal signs and symptoms (dystonia, akathisia, oculogyric crisis) to differentiate these different clinical conditions. When extrapyramidal symptoms are the cause, they can usually be controlled with anticholinergic agents.

Postoperative hallucinatory episodes (sometimes associated with transient periods of mental depression) have also been reported.

Other less common reported adverse reactions include anaphylaxis, dizziness, chills and/or shivering, twitching, blurred vision, laryngospasm, bronchospasm, bradycardia, nausea and emesis, diaphoresis, and emergence delirium.

DRUG ABUSE AND DEPENDENCE

The Fentanyl Citrate component of Droperidol/Fentanyl Citrate is a Schedule II opioid that can produce drug dependence of the morphine type and, therefore, has the potential for being abused.

OVERDOSAGE

Manifestations: The manifestations of Droperidol/Fentanyl Citrate overdosage are an extension of its pharmacologic actions.

Treatment: In the presence of hypoventilation or apnea, oxygen should be administered and respiration should be assisted or controlled as indicated. A patent airway must be maintained; an oropharyngeal airway or endotracheal tube might be indicated. If depressed respiration is associated with muscular rigidity, an intravenous neuromuscular blocking agent might be required to facilitate assisted or controlled respiration. The patient should be carefully observed for 24 hours; body warmth and adequate fluid intake should be maintained. If hypotension occurs and is severe or persists, the possibility of hypovolemia should be considered and managed with appropriate parenteral fluid therapy (see *"Precautions"*). A specific opioid antagonist such as nalorphine, levallorphan or naloxone should be available for use as indicated to manage respiratory depression caused by the opioid component Fentanyl Citrate. This does not preclude the use of more immediate countermeasures. The duration of respiratory depression following overdose of Fentanyl Citrate may be longer than the duration of opioid antagonist action. Consult the package inserts of the individual opioid antagonists for details about use.

If significant extrapyramidal reactions occur in the context of an overdose, an anticholinergic should be administered. The LD_{50} values after intravenous administration were 4.1-5.27 mg/kg for the rat and the rabbit and 17 mg/kg or more for the mouse and the dog. After intramuscular administration LD_{50} determinations were 6.7-14.5 mg/kg for the rabbit and 75 mg/kg for the mouse.

DOSAGE AND ADMINISTRATION

Dosage should be individualized. Some of the factors to be considered in determining dose are age, body weight, physical status, underlying pathological condition, use of other drugs, the type of anesthesia to be used and the surgical procedure involved.

◆ RATED THERAPEUTICALLY EQUIVALENT; ◇ THERAPEUTIC EQUIVALENCE UNCONFIRMED; ○ UNRATED

Vital signs should be monitored routinely.

Most patients who have received Droperidol/Fentanyl Citrate do not require opioid analgesics during the immediate postoperative period.

It is recommended that opioid analgesics, when required, be used initially in reduced doses, as low as ¼ to ⅓ those usually recommended.

USUAL ADULT DOSAGE:

I. Premedication—(to be appropriately modified in the elderly, debilitated and those who have received other depressant drugs)—0.5 to 2.0 mL may be administered *intramuscularly* 45 to 60 minutes prior to surgery with or without atropine.

II. Adjunct to General Anesthesia—Induction: 1 mL per 20 to 25 pounds of body weight may be slowly administered intravenously. Smaller doses may be adequate.

The total amount of Droperidol/Fentanyl Citrate administered should be carefully titrated to obtain the desired effect based on the individual patient's response.

There are several methods of administration of Droperidol/Fentanyl Citrate Injection for induction of anesthesia.

A. Intravenous injection—To allow for the variable needs of patients Droperidol/Fentanyl Citrate may be administered intravenously in fractional parts of the calculated dose. With the onset of somnolence, the general anesthetic may be administered.

B. Intravenous drip—10 mL of Droperidol/Fentanyl Citrate are added to 250 mL of 5% dextrose in water and the drip given rapidly until the onset of somnolence. At that time, the drip may be either slowed or stopped and the general anesthetic administered.

Maintenance: Droperidol/Fentanyl Citrate is not indicated as the sole agent for the maintenance of surgical anesthesia. It is customarily used in combination with other measures such as nitrous oxide-oxygen, other inhalation anesthetics and/or topical or regional anesthesia.

To prevent the possibility of excessive accumulation of the relatively long-acting Droperidol component, Fentanyl Citrate alone should be used in increments of 25 to 50 µg (0.025 to 0.05 mg) (0.5 to 1.0 mL) for the maintenance of analgesia in patients initially given Droperidol/Fentanyl Citrate as an adjunct to general anesthesia. (See Fentanyl Citrate package insert for additional prescribing information.) However, in prolonged operations, additional 0.5 to 1.0 mL amounts of Droperidol/Fentanyl Citrate may be administered with caution intravenously if changes in the patient's condition indicate lightening of tranquilization and analgesia.

III. Use Without a General Anesthetic in Diagnostic Procedures: Administer the usual intramuscular premedication (0.5 to 2.0 mL) 45 to 60 minutes before the procedure. To prevent the possibility of excessive accumulation of the relatively long-acting Droperidol component, Fentanyl Citrate alone should be used in increments of 25 to 50 µg (0.025 to 0.05 mg) (0.5 to 1.0 mL) for the maintenance of analgesia in patients initially given Droperidol/Fentanyl Citrate Injection. See Fentanyl Citrate package insert for additional information. However, in prolonged operations, additional 0.5 to 1.0 mL amounts of Droperidol/Fentanyl Citrate may be administered with caution intravenously if changes in the patient's condition indicate lightening of tranquilization and analgesia. *Note:* When Droperidol/Fentanyl Citrate is used in certain procedures such as bronchoscopy, appropriate topical anesthesia is still necessary.

IV. Adjunct to Regional Anesthesia: 1 to 2 mL may be administered intramuscularly or slowly intravenously when additional sedation and analgesia are required.

USUAL CHILDREN'S DOSAGE:
For premedication and as an adjunct to general anesthesia in children over 2 years of age (see *"Precautions"*):

I. Premedication: 0.25 mL per 20 lbs, body weight administered *intramuscularly* 45 to 60 minutes prior to surgery with or without atropine.

II. Adjunct to General Anesthesia: The total combined dose for induction and maintenance averages 0.5 mL per 20 lbs. body weight. Following induction with Droperidol/Fentanyl Citrate Injection, Fentanyl Citrate alone in a dose of 1/4 to 1/3 that recommended in the adult dosage section should usually be used when indicated to avoid the possibility of excessive accumulation of droperidol. However, in prolonged operations, additional increments of Droperidol/Fentanyl Citrate may be administered with caution when changes in the patient's condition indicate lightening of tranquilization and analgesia.

See *"Warnings"* and *"Precautions"* for use of Droperidol/Fentanyl Citrate with other CNS depressants, and in patients with altered response.

Parenteral drug products should be inspected visually for particulate matter and discoloration prior to administration, whenever solution and container permit. If such abnormalities are observed, the drug should not be administered.

(FOR INTRAVENOUS USE BY HOSPITAL PERSONNEL SPECIFICALLY TRAINED IN THE USE OF OPIOID ANALGESICS.)

Protect From Light. Store at Room Temperature 15°-30°C (59°-86°F).

J CODES
Up to 2 ml ampule IM,IV—J1810

HOW SUPPLIED
INJECTION (C-II): 2.5 MG-0.05 MG/ML

AVERAGE UNIT PRICE (AVAILABLE SIZES)		GENERIC A-RATED AVERAGE PRICE (GAAP)	
BRAND	$6.77	2 ml 10s	$102.51
GENERIC	$4.90	5 ml 10s	$165.01

BRAND/MANUFACTURER	NDC	SIZE	AWP
◆ BRAND			
INNOVAR: Janssen	50458-0020-02	2 ml 10s	$135.29
◆ GENERICS			
Astra	00186-1230-03	2 ml 10s	$99.38
Astra	00186-1232-13	2 ml 10s	$105.63
Astra	00186-1233-13	5 ml 10s	$164.38
Astra	00186-1231-03	5 ml 10s	$165.63
Abbott Hosp	00074-1186-12	2 ml 100s	$1534.25

Drotic SEE HYDROCORTISONE/NEOMYCIN SULFATE/ POLYMYXIN B SULFATE

Drysol SEE ALUMINUM CHLORIDE (HEXAHYDRATE)

DTIC-Dome SEE DACARBAZINE

Duo-Medihaler SEE ISOPROTERENOL HYDROCHLORIDE WITH PHENYLEPHRINE BITARTRATE

Durabolin SEE NANDROLONE

Duragesic SEE FENTANYL

Duranest SEE ETIDOCAINE HYDROCHLORIDE

Duricef SEE CEFADROXIL MONOHYDRATE

Duvoid SEE BETHANECHOL CHLORIDE

Dyazide SEE HYDROCHLOROTHIAZIDE AND TRIAMTERENE

Dyclone SEE DYCLONINE HYDROCHLORIDE

Dyclonine Hydrochloride

DESCRIPTION
Dyclonine HCl 0.5% and 1% Topical Solutions contain a local anesthetic agent and are administered topically. See *"Indications"* for specific uses.

Dyclonine HCl 0.5% and 1% Topical Solutions contain Dyclonine HCl, which is chemically designated as 4'-butoxy-3-piperidinopropiophenone HCl. Dyclonine HCl is a white crystalline powder that is sparingly soluble in water.

Following is its chemical structure:

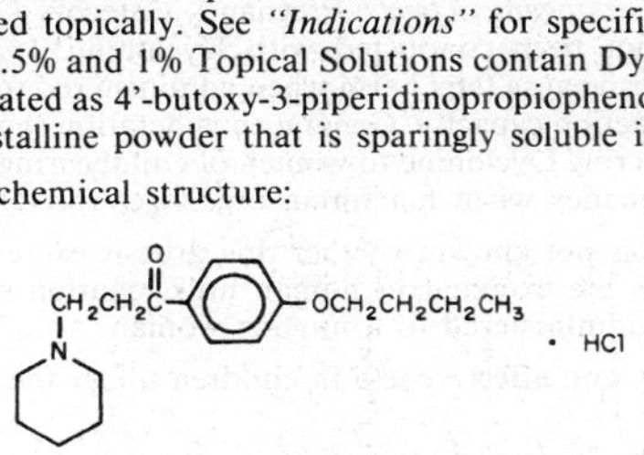

COMPOSITIONS OF DYCLONINE HCL 0.5% AND 1% TOPICAL SOLUTIONS
Each mL of Dyclonine HCl 0.5% Solution contains Dyclonine HCl, 5 mg.
Each mL of Dyclonine HCl 1% Solution contains Dyclonine HCl, 10 mg.

► SHOWN IN PRODUCT IDENTIFICATION GUIDE

Both solutions also contain chlorbutanol hydrous and sodium chloride, and the pH is adjusted to 3.0-5.0 by means of hydrochloric acid.

CLINICAL PHARMACOLOGY

Dyclonine HCl Topical Solutions effect surface anesthesia when applied topically to mucous membranes. Effective anesthesia varies with different patients, but usually occurs from 2 to 10 minutes after application and persists for approximately 30 minutes.

INDICATIONS AND USAGE

Dyclonine HCl Topical Solutions are indicated for anesthetizing accessible mucous membranes (e.g., the mouth, pharynx, larynx, trachea, esophagus, and urethra) prior to various endoscopic procedures.

Dyclonine HCl 0.5% Topical Solution may also be used to block the gag reflex, to relieve the pain of oral ulcers or stomatitis and to relieve pain associated with ano-genital lesions.

UNLABELED USES

Dyclonine HCl is used alone or as an adjunct in the symptomatic treatment of sore throat.

CONTRAINDICATIONS

Dyclonine is contraindicated in patients known to be hypersensitive (allergic) to the local anesthetic or to other components of Dyclonine HCl Topical Solutions.

WARNINGS

IN ORDER TO MANAGE POSSIBLE ADVERSE REACTIONS, RESUSCITATIVE EQUIPMENT, OXYGEN AND OTHER RESUSCITATIVE DRUGS SHOULD BE IMMEDIATELY AVAILABLE WHENEVER LOCAL ANESTHETIC AGENTS, SUCH AS DYCLONINE, ARE ADMINISTERED TO MUCOUS MEMBRANES.

Dyclonine HCl Topical Solutions should not be injected into tissue or used in the eyes because of highly irritant properties.

Dyclonine HCl Topical Solutions should be used with extreme caution in the presence of sepsis or severely traumatized mucosa in the area of application since under such conditions there is the potential for rapid systemic absorption.

PRECAUTIONS

General: The safety and effectiveness of Dyclonine depend on proper dosage, correct technique, adequate precautions, and readiness for emergencies (see *"Warnings"* and *"Adverse Reactions"*). The lowest dosage that results in effective anesthesia should be used to avoid high plasma levels and serious adverse effects. Repeated doses of Dyclonine HCl may cause significant increases in blood levels with each repeated dose because of slow accumulation of the drug or its metabolites. Tolerance to elevated blood levels varies with the status of the patient. Debilitated, elderly patients, acutely ill patients, and children should be given reduced doses commensurate with their age, weight and physical condition. Dyclonine should also be used with caution in patients with severe shock or heart block.

Dyclonine HCl Topical Solutions should be used with caution in persons with known drug sensitivities.

Information for Patients: When topical anesthetics are used in the mouth or throat, the patient should be aware that the production of topical anesthesia may impair swallowing and thus enhance the danger of aspiration. For this reason, food should not be ingested for 60 minutes following use of local anesthetic preparations in the mouth or throat area. This is particularly important in children because of their frequency of eating.

Numbness of the tongue or buccal mucosa may increase the danger of biting trauma. When Dyclonine HCl 0.5% Topical Solution is used to relieve the pain of oral ulcers or stomatitis which interferes with eating, patients should be warned about the risk of biting trauma before they accept this treatment; caution should be exercised in selecting food and eating. Following other uses in the mouth and throat area, food and/or chewing gum should not be used while the area is anesthetized.

Drug/Laboratory Test Interactions: Dyclonine HCl Topical Solutions should not be used in cystoscopic procedures following intravenous pyelography because an iodine precipitate occurs which interferes with visualization.

Carcinogenesis, mutagenesis, impairment of fertility: Studies of Dyclonine in animals to evaluate the carcinogenic and mutagenic potential or the effect on fertility have not been conducted.

Use in Pregnancy: Teratogenic Effects: Pregnancy Category C. Animal reproduction studies have not been conducted with Dyclonine. It is also not known whether Dyclonine can cause fetal harm when administered to a pregnant woman or can affect reproduction capacity. General consideration should be given to this fact before administering Dyclonine to women of childbearing potential, especially during early pregnancy when maximum organogenesis takes place.

Nursing Mothers: It is not known whether this drug is excreted in human milk. Because many drugs are excreted in human milk, caution should be exercised when Dyclonine is administered to a nursing woman.

Pediatric Use: Safety and effectiveness in children under the age of 12 have not been established.

ADVERSE REACTIONS

Adverse experiences following the administration of Dyclonine are similar in nature to those observed with other local anesthetic agents. These adverse experiences are, in general, dose-related and may result from high plasma levels caused by excessive dosage or rapid absorption, or may result from a hypersensi-

tivity, idiosyncrasy or diminished tolerance on the part of the patient. Serious adverse experiences are generally systemic in nature. The following types are those most commonly reported:

Central Nervous System: CNS manifestations are excitatory and/or depressant and may be characterized by light-headedness, nervousness, apprehension, euphoria, confusion, dizziness, drowsiness, tinnitus, blurred or double vision, vomiting, sensations of heat, cold or numbness, twitching, tremors, convulsions, unconsciousness, repiratory depression and arrest. The excitatory manifestations may be very brief or may not occur at all, in which case the first manifestation of toxicity may be drowsiness merging into unconsciousness and respiratory arrest.

Drowsiness following the administration of Dyclonine is usually an early sign of a high blood level of the drug and may occur as a consequence of rapid absorption.

Cardiovascular System: Cardiovascular manifestations are usually depressant and are characterized by bradycardia, hypotension, and cardiovascular collapse, which may lead to cardiac arrest.

Allergic: Allergic reactions are characterized by cutaneous lesions, urticaria, edema or anaphylactoid reactions. Allergic reactions may occur as a result of sensitivity either to the local anesthetic agent or to the other ingredients used in this formulation. Allergic reactions, if they occur, should be managed by conventional means. The detection of sensitivity by skin testing is of doubtful value. Local reactions include irritation, stinging, urethritis with and without bleeding.

OVERDOSAGE

Acute emergencies from local anesthetics are generally related to high plasma levels encountered during therapeutic use of local anesthetics. (See *"Adverse Reactions," "Warnings,"* and *"Precautions"*).

Management of Local Anesthetic Emergencies: The first consideration is prevention, best accomplished by careful and constant monitoring of cardiovascular and respiratory vital signs and the patient's state of consciousness after each local anesthetic administration.

The first step in the management of convulsions consists of immediate attention to the maintenance of a patent airway and assisted or controlled ventilation with oxygen and a delivery system capable of permitting immediate positive airway pressure by mask. Immediately after the institution of these ventilatory measures, the adequacy of the circulation should be evaluated, keeping in mind that drugs used to treat convulsions sometimes depress the circulation when administered intravenously. Should convulsions persist despite adequate respiratory support, and if the status of the circulation permits, small increments of an ultra-short acting barbiturate (such as thiopental or thiamylal) or a benzodiazepine (such as diazepam) may be administered intravenously. The clinician should be familiar, prior to use of local anesthetics, with these anticonvulsant drugs. Supportive treatment of circulatory depression may require administration of intravenous fluids and, when appropriate, a vasopressor as directed by the clinical situation (e.g., ephedrine).

If not treated immediately, both convulsions and cardiovascular depression can result in hypoxia, acidosis, bradycardia, arrhythmias and cardiac arrest. If cardiac arrest should occur, standard cardiopulmonary resuscitative measures should be instituted.

The mean lethal dose (LD_{50}) of Dyclonine HCl administered orally to female rats is 176 mg/kg and 90 mg/kg in female mice. Intraperitoneally the LD_{50} in female rats is 31 mg/kg and 43 mg/kg in female mice.

DOSAGE AND ADMINISTRATION

As with all local anesthetics, the dosage varies and depends upon the area to be anesthetized, vascularity of the tissues, individual tolerance and the technique of anesthesia. The lowest dosage needed to provide effective anesthesia should be administered.

A maximum dose of 30 mL of 1% Dyclonine HCl Topical Solution (300 mg of Dyclonine HCl) may be used, although satisfactory anesthesia is usually produced within the range of 4 to 20 mL. For specific techniques and procedures refer to standard textbooks.

Although as much as 300 mg of Dyclonine HCl (as a 1% solution) have been tolerated, this dosage as a 0.5% solution has not been administered primarily because satisfactory anesthesia in endoscopic procedures can usually be produced by lesser amounts. For specific techniques for endoscopic procedures refer to standard textbooks.

PROCTOLOGY

Apply pledgets of cotton or sponges moistened with the Dyclonine HCl 0.5% Solution to postoperative wounds for the relief of discomfort and pain.

GYNECOLOGY

Apply Dyclonine HCl 0.5% Solution as wet compresses or as a spray to relieve the discomfort of episiotomy or perineorrhaphy wounds.

ONCOLOGY-RADIOLOGY

Apply Dyclonine HCl 0.5% Solution as a rinse or swab to inflamed or ulcerated mucous membrane of the mouth caused by antineoplastic chemotherapy or radiation therapy. In lesions of the esophagus, 5-15 mL of the anesthetic may be swallowed to relieve pain and allow more comfortable deglutition.

OTORHINOLARYNGOLOGY

To suppress the gag reflex and to facilitate examination of the posterior pharynx or larynx, apply Dyclonine HCl 0.5% Solution as a spray or gargle.

Dyclonine HCl 0.5% Solution may be applied as a rinse or swab to relieve the discomfort of aphthous stomatitis, herpetic stomatitis, or other painful oral lesions.

DENTISTRY

Dyclonine HCl 0.5% Topical Solution is useful to suppress the gag reflex in the positioning of x-ray films, making prosthetic impressions, and doing surgical procedures in the molar areas. It is also useful as a preinjection mucous membrane anesthetic or applied to the gums prior to scaling (prophylaxis). The anesthetic can be applied as a mouthwash or gargle and the excess spit out.

Keep tightly closed. Store at controlled room temperature: 15°-30°C (59°-86°F). Avoid excessive heat (temperatures above 40°C (104°F). Subject to damage by freezing.

HOW SUPPLIED
SOLUTION: 0.5%

BRAND/MANUFACTURER	NDC	SIZE	AWP
◆ BRAND			
DYCLONE: Astra	00186-3001-67	30 ml	$26.29

SOLUTION: 1%

BRAND/MANUFACTURER	NDC	SIZE	AWP
◆ BRAND			
DYCLONE: Astra	00186-3002-67	30 ml	$35.41

Dymelor SEE ACETOHEXAMIDE

Dynacin SEE MINOCYCLINE HYDROCHLORIDE

DynaCirc SEE ISRADIPINE

Dynapen SEE DICLOXACILLIN SODIUM

Dyphylline

DESCRIPTION

Dyphylline, a xanthine derivative, is a bronchodilator available for oral administration as tablets of 200 mg and 400 mg.

Chemically, Dyphylline is 7-(2,3-dihydroxypropyl)-theophylline, a white, extremely bitter, amorphous powder that is freely soluble in water and soluble in alcohol to the extent of 2g/100 ml. Dyphylline forms a neutral solution that is stable in gastrointestinal fluids over a wide range of pH.

The molecular formula for Dyphylline is $C_{10}H_{14}N_4O_4$ with a molecular weight of 254.25.

Following is its chemical structure:

(chemical structure of Dyphylline)

CLINICAL PHARMACOLOGY

Dyphylline is a xanthine derivative with pharmacologic actions similar to theophylline and other members of this class of drugs. Its primary action is that of bronchodilation, but it also exhibits peripheral vasodilatory and other smooth muscle relaxant activity to a lesser degree. The bronchodilatory action of Dyphylline, as with other xanthines, is thought to be mediated through competitive inhibition of phosphodiesterase with a resulting increase in cyclic AMP producing relaxation of bronchial smooth muscle.

Dyphylline is well tolerated and produces less nausea than aminophylline and other alkaline theophylline compounds when administered orally. Unlike the hydrolyzable salts of theophylline, Dyphylline is not converted to free theophylline *in vivo*. It is absorbed rapidly in therapeutically active form and in healthy volunteers reaches a mean peak plasma concentration of 17.1 mcg/ml in approximately 45 minutes following a single oral dose of 1000 mg of Dyphylline.

Dyphylline exerts its bronchodilatory effects directly and, unlike theophylline, is excreted unchanged by the kidneys without being metabolized by the liver. Because of this, Dyphylline pharmacokinetics and plasma levels are not influenced by various factors that affect liver function and hepatic enzyme activity, such as smoking, age, congestive heart failure or concomitant use of drugs which affect liver function.

The elimination half-life of Dyphylline is approximately two hours (1.8-2.1 hr) and approximately 88% of a single oral dose can be recovered from the urine unchanged. The renal clearance would be correspondingly reduced in patients with impaired renal function. In anuric patients, the half-life may be increased 3 to 4 times normal.

Dyphylline plasma levels are dose-related and generally predictable. The range of plasma levels within which Dyphylline can be expected to produce effective bronchodilation has not been determined.

Dyphylline plasma concentrations can be accurately determined using high pressure liquid chromatography (HPLC)[*] or gas-liquid chromatography (GLC).

INDICATIONS AND USAGE

For relief of acute bronchial asthma and for reversible bronchospasm associated with chronic bronchitits and emphysema.

CONTRAINDICATIONS

Hypersensitivity to Dyphylline or related xanthine compounds.

WARNINGS

Dyphylline is not indicated in the management of status asthmaticus, which is a serious medical emergency.

Although the relationship between plasma levels of Dyphylline and appearance of toxicity is unknown, excessive doses may be expected to be associated with an increased risk of adverse effects.

PRECAUTIONS

General: Use Dyphylline with caution in patients with severe cardiac disease, hypertension, hyperthyroidism, acute myocardial injury or peptic ulcer.

Drug Interactions: Synergism between xanthine bronchodilators (e.g., theophylline), ephedrine and other sympathomimetic bronchodilators has been reported. This should be considered whenever these agents are prescribed concomitantly. Concurrent administration of Dyphylline and probenecid, which competes for tubular secretion, has been shown to increase the plasma half-life of Dyphylline (see *"Clinical Pharmacology"*).

Carinogenesis, Mutagenesis, Impairment of Fertility. No long-term animal studies have been performed with Dyphylline.

Pregnancy: Teratogenic effects—Pregnancy Category C. Animal reproduction studies have not been conducted with Dyphylline. It is also not known if Dyphylline can cause fetal harm when administered to a pregnant woman or can affect reproduction capacity. Dyphylline should be given to a pregnant woman only if clearly needed.

Nursing mothers: Dyphylline is present in human milk at approximately twice the maternal plasma concentration. Caution should be exercised when Dyphylline is administered to a nursing woman.

Pediatric use: Safety and effectiveness in children have not been established.

ADVERSE REACTIONS

Adverse reactions with the use of Dyphylline have been infrequent, relatively mild, and rarely required reduction in dosage or withdrawal of therapy.

The following adverse reactions which have been reported with other xanthine bronchodilators, and which have most often been related to excessive drug plasma levels, should be considered as potential adverse effects when Dyphylline is administered:

Gastrointestinal: nausea, vomiting, epigastric pain, hematemesis, diarrhea.

Central nervous system: headache, irritability, restlessness, insomnia, hyperexcitability, agitation, muscle twitching, generalized clonic and tonic convulsions.

Cardiovascular: palpitation, tachycardia, extrasystoles, flushing, hypotension, circulatory failure, ventricular arrhythmias.

Respiratory: tachypnea.

Renal: albuminuria, gross and microscopic hematuria, diuresis.

Other: hyperglycemia, inappropriate ADH syndrome.

OVERDOSAGE

There have been no reports, in the literature, of overdosage with Dyphylline. However, the following information based on reports of theophylline overdosage are considered typical of the xanthine class of drugs and should be kept in mind.

Signs and symptoms: Restlessness, anorexia, nausea, vomiting, diarrhea, insomnia, irritability, and headache. Marked overdosage with resulting severe toxicity has produced agitation, severe vomiting, dehydration, excessive thirst, tinnitus, cardiac arrhythmias, hyperthermia, diaphoresis, and generalized clonic and tonic convulsions. Cardiovascular collapse has also occurred, with some fatalities. Seizures have occurred in some cases associated with very high theophylline plasma concentrations, without any premonitory symptoms of toxicity.

Treatment: There is no specific antidote for overdosage with drugs of the xanthine class. Symptomatic treatment and general supportive measures should be instituted with careful monitoring and maintenance of vital signs, fluids and electrolytes. The stomach should be emptied by inducing emesis if the patient is conscious and responsive, or by gastric lavage, taking care to protect against aspiration, especially in stuporous or comatose patients. Maintenance of an adequate airway is essential in case oxygen or assisted respiration is needed. Sympathomimetic agents should be avoided but sedatives such as short-acting barbiturates may be useful.

[*] *See et al. J. Chromatogr.* **221**: 170 (1980)

➤ SHOWN IN PRODUCT IDENTIFICATION GUIDE

Dyphylline is dialyzable and, although not recommended as a routine procedure in overdosage cases, hemodialysis may be of some benefit when severe intoxication is present or when the patient has not responded to general supportive and symptomatic treatment.

DOSAGE AND ADMINISTRATION

Dosage should be individually titrated according to the severity of the condition and the response of the patient.

Usual Adult Dosage: Up to 15 mg/kg every six hours.

Appropriate dosage adjustments should be made in patients with impaired renal function (see *"Clinical Pharmacology"*).

Store at controlled room temperature 15°-30°C (59°-86°F).

Dispense in a tight container.

J CODES

Up to 500 mg IM—J1180

HOW SUPPLIED

ELIXIR: 100 MG/15 ML

BRAND/MANUFACTURER	NDC	SIZE	AWP
○ BRAND			
LUFYLLIN: Wallace	00037-0515-68	480 ml	$56.53
	00037-0515-69	3840 ml	$414.42

INJECTION: 250 MG/ML

BRAND/MANUFACTURER	NDC	SIZE	AWP
○ BRAND			
LUFYLLIN: Wallace	00037-0537-01	2 ml 25s	$368.76

TABLETS:

BRAND/MANUFACTURER	NDC	SIZE	AWP
◇ GENERICS			
DYFLEX: EconoMed	38130-0066-01	100s	$9.75
DYFLEX: EconoMed	38130-0066-10	1000s	$84.75

TABLETS: 200 MG

BRAND/MANUFACTURER	NDC	SIZE	AWP
○ BRAND			
LUFYLLIN: Wallace	00037-0521-92	100s	$90.25
	00037-0521-97	1000s	$840.00
	00037-0521-85	1000s ud	$1050.65
	00037-0521-98	5000s	$3940.79
◇ GENERICS			
NEOTHYLLINE: Major	00904-1556-60	100s	$11.95
NEOTHYLLINE: Lemmon	00093-0030-01	100s	$13.78
DILOR-200: Savage	00281-1115-53	100s	$24.12
DILOR-200: Savage	00281-1115-63	100s ud	$38.48
DILOR-200: Savage	00281-1115-57	1000s	$213.34

TABLETS: 400 MG

BRAND/MANUFACTURER	NDC	SIZE	AWP
○ BRAND			
LUFYLLIN-400: Wallace	00037-0731-92	100s	$132.55
	00037-0731-97	1000s	$1029.20
	00037-0731-99	2500s	$2573.03
◇ GENERICS			
NEOTHYLLINE: Major	00904-1557-60	100s	$13.30
NEOTHYLLINE: Lemmon	00093-0037-01	100s	$16.86
URL	00677-1036-01	100s	$16.95
DILOR-400: Savage	00281-1115-53	100s	$35.15
DILOR-400: Savage	00281-1116-63	100s ud	$55.49
DILOR-400: Savage	00281-1116-57	1000s	$262.18

Dyphylline and Guaifenesin

DESCRIPTION

Dyphylline/Guaifenesin is a bronchodilator/expectorant combination available for oral administration as *Tablets* and *Elixir*.

Each 15 mL (one tablespoonful) of elixir contains:

Dyphylline	100 mg
Guaifenesin	100 mg
Alcohol (by volume)	17%

Each tablet contains:

Dyphylline	200 mg
Guaifenesin	200 mg

Dyphylline is 7-(2,3-dihydroxypropyl)-theophylline, a white, extremely bitter, amorphous powder that is fully soluble in water and soluble in alcohol to the extent of 2 g/100 mL. Dyphylline forms a neutral solution that is stable in gastrointestinal fluids over a wide range of pH.

CLINICAL PHARMACOLOGY

Dyphylline is a xanthine derivative with pharmacologic actions similar to theophylline and other members of this class of drugs. Its primary action is that of bronchodilation, but it also exhibits peripheral vasodilatory and other smooth muscle relaxant activity to a lesser degree. The bronchodilatory action of Dyphylline, as with as other xanthines, is thought to be mediated through competitive inhibition of phosphodiesterase with a resulting increase in cyclic AMP producing relaxation of bronchial smooth muscle.

Dyphylline in Dyphylline/Guaifenesin is well tolerated and produces less nausea than aminophylline and other alkaline theophylline compounds when administered orally. Unlike the hydrolyzable salts of theophylline, Dyphylline is not converted to free theophylline, *in vivo*. It is absorbed rapidly in therapeutically active form and in healthy volunteers reaches a mean peak plasma concentration of 17.1 mcg/mL in approximately 45 minutes following a single oral dose of 1000 mg of Dyphylline.

Dyphylline exerts its bronchodilatory effects directly and, unlike theophylline, is excreted unchanged by the kidneys without being metabolized by the liver. Because of this, Dyphylline pharmacokinetics and plasma levels are not influenced by various factors that affect liver function and hepatic enzyme activity, such as smoking, age, or concomitant use of drugs which affect liver function.

The elimination half-life of Dyphylline is approximately two hours (1.8-2.1 hr) and approximately 88% of a single oral dose can be recovered from the urine unchanged. The renal clearance would be correspondingly reduced in patients with impaired renal function. In anuric patients, the half-life may be increased 3 to 4 times normal.

Dyphylline plasma levels are dose-related and generally predictable. The therapeutic range of plasma levels within which Dyphylline can be expected to produce effective bronchodilation has not been determined.

Dyphylline plasma concentrations can be accurately determined using high pressure liquid chromatography (HPLC)* or gas-liquid chromatography (GLC).

Guaifenesin is an expectorant whose action helps increase the output of thin respiratory tract fluid to facilitate mucociliary clearance and removal of inspissated mucus.

INDICATIONS AND USAGE

For relief of acute bronchial asthma and for reversible bronchospasm associated with chronic bronchitis and emphysema.

CONTRAINDICATIONS

Hypersensitivity to any of the ingredients or related compounds.

WARNINGS

Dyphylline/Guaifenesin is not indicated in the management of status asthmaticus, which is a serious medical emergency.

Although the relationship between plasma levels of Dyphylline and appearance of toxicity is unknown, excessive doses may be expected to be associated with an increased risk of adverse effects.

PRECAUTIONS

General: Use Dyphylline/Guaifenesin with caution in patients with severe cardiac disease, hypertension, hyperthyroidism, acute myocardial injury or peptic ulcer.

Drug Interactions: Synergism between xanthine bronchodilators (e.g., theophylline), ephedrine and other sympathomimetic bronchodilators has been reported. This should be considered whenever these agents are prescribed concomitantly. Concurrent administration of Dyphylline and probenecid, which competes for tubular secretion, has been shown to increase plasma half-life of Dyphylline (see *"Clinical Pharmacology"*).

Carcinogenesis, Mutagenesis, Impairment of Fertility: No long-term animal studies have been performed with Dyphylline/Guaifenesin.

Pregnancy: Teratogenic effects—Pregnancy Category C. Animal reproduction studies have not been conducted with Dyphylline/Guaifenesin. It is also not known whether this product can cause fetal harm when administered to a pregnant woman or can affect reproduction capacity. Dyphylline/Guaifenesin should be given to a pregnant woman only if clearly needed.

Nursing Mothers: Dyphylline is present in human milk at approximately twice the maternal plasma concentration. Caution should be exercised when Dyphylline/Guaifenesin is administered to a nursing woman.

Pediatric Use: Safety and effectiveness in children below the age of six have not been established. Use caution when administering to children six years of age or older.

ADVERSE REACTIONS

Dyphylline/Guaifenesin may cause nausea, headache, cardiac palpitation and CNS stimulation. Postprandial administration may help avoid gastric discomfort.

The following adverse reactions which have been reported with other xanthine bronchodilators, and which have most often been related to excessive drug plasma levels, should be considered as potential adverse effects when Dyphylline is administered:

Gastrointestinal: nausea, vomiting, epigastric pain, hematemesis, diarrhea.

Central nervous system: headache, irritability, restlessness, insomnia, hyperexcitability, agitation, muscle twitching, generalized clonic and tonic convulsions.

---

* See Valia, et al: *J. Chromatog.* 221:170 (1980).

Cardiovascular: palpitation, tachycardia, extrasystoles, flushing, hypotension, circulatory failure, ventricular arrhythmias.

Respiratory: tachypnea.

Renal: albuminuria, gross and microscopic hematuria, diuresis.

Other: hyperglycemia, inappropriate ADH syndrome.

OVERDOSAGE

There have been no reports, in the literature, of overdosage with Dyphylline/Guaifenesin. However, the following information based on reports of theophylline overdosage are considered typical of the xanthine class of drugs and should be kept in mind.

Signs and symptoms: Restlessness, anorexia, nausea, vomiting, diarrhea, insomnia, irritability, and headache. Marked overdosage with resulting severe toxicity has produced agitation, severe vomiting, dehydration, excessive thirst, tinnitus, cardiac arrhythmias, hyperthermia, diaphoresis, and generalized clonic and tonic convulsions. Cardiovascular collapse has also occurred, with some fatalities. Seizures have occurred in some cases associated with very high theophylline plasma concentrations, without any premonitory symptoms of toxicity.

Treatment: There is no specific antidote for overdosage with drugs of the xanthine class. Symptomatic treatment and general supportive measures should be instituted with careful monitoring and maintenance of vital signs, fluids and electrolytes: The stomach should be emptied by inducing emesis if the patient is conscious and responsive, or by gastric lavage, taking care to protect against aspiration, especially in stuporous or comatose patients. Maintenance of an adequate airway is essential in case oxygen or assisted respiration is needed. Sympathomimetic agents should be avoided but sedatives such as short-acting barbiturates may be useful.

Dyphylline is dialyzable and, although not recommended as a routine procedure in overdosage cases, hemodialysis may be of some benefit when severe intoxication is present or when the patient has not responded to general supportive and symptomatic treatment.

DOSAGE AND ADMINISTRATION

Dosage should be individually titrated according to the severity of the condition and the response of the patient.

Usual Adult Dosage: 1 tablet or 30 mL (2 tablespoonfuls) elixir, four times daily.

Children above Age Six: ½ to 1 tablet or 15 to 30 mL (1 to 2 tablespoonfuls) elixir, 3 or 4 times daily.

Not recommended for use in children below age six: (see "Precautions").
Tablets and Elixir: Store at controlled room temperature 15°-30°C (59°-86°F).
Dispense in a tight container.

HOW SUPPLIED
CAPSULE: 200 MG-100 MG

BRAND/MANUFACTURER	NDC	SIZE	AWP
○ GENERICS			
EMFASEEM: Saron	00834-4019-91	100s	$20.00

ELIXIR: 100 MG-100 MG/15 ML

BRAND/MANUFACTURER	NDC	SIZE	AWP
○ BRAND			
LUFYLLIN-GG: Wallace	00037-0545-68	480 ml	$78.77
	00037-0545-69	3840 ml	$585.31
○ GENERICS			
DYPHYL GG: Norton,HN	50732-0897-16	473 ml	$13.50
Hi-Tech	50383-0806-16	480 ml	$10.00
DYFILIN GG: Mikart	46672-0614-16	480 ml	$12.50
Silarx	54838-0513-08	480 ml	$12.60
Rugby	00536-0690-85	480 ml	$14.15
Goldline	00182-1375-40	480 ml	$14.40
Qualitest	00603-1190-58	480 ml	$15.30
Barre	00472-1238-16	480 ml	$15.75
DYPHYL GG: Norton,HN	50732-0897-28	3785 ml	$97.20

LIQUID: 100 MG-100 MG/15 ML

BRAND/MANUFACTURER	NDC	SIZE	AWP
○ BRAND			
DIFIL G: Stewart Jackson	45565-0306-17	480 ml	$12.00

For additional alternatives, turn to the section beginning on page 2859.

Dyrenium *SEE* TRIAMTERENE

Ear-Eze *SEE* HYDROCORTISONE/NEOMYCIN SULFATE/
POLYMYXIN B SULFATE

Easprin *SEE* ASPIRIN

Echothiophate Iodide

DESCRIPTION
Chemical name: (2-mercaptoethyl) trimethylammonium iodide O,O-diethyl phosphorothioate.

Echothiophate Iodide occurs as a white, crystalline, water-soluble, hygroscopic solid having a slight mercaptan-like odor. When freeze-dried in the presence of potassium acetate, the mixture appears as a white amorphous deposit on the walls of the bottle.

Each package contains materials for dispensing 5 mL of eyedrops: (1) bottle containing sterile Echothiophate Iodide in one of four potencies [1.5 mg (0.03%), 3 mg (0.06%), 6.25 mg (0.125%), or 12.5 mg (0.25%)] as indicated on the lable.

Following is its chemical structure:

$$\left[(CH_3)_3N^+CH_2CH_2 - S - \overset{\overset{O}{\|}}{P} \overset{OC_2H_5}{\underset{OC_2H_5}{\diagup}} \right] \; I^-$$

CLINICAL PHARMACOLOGY
Echothiophate Iodide is a long-acting cholinesterase inhibitor for topical use which enhances the effect of endogenously liberated acetylcholine in iris, ciliary muscle, and other parasympathetically innervated structures of the eye. It thereby causes miosis, increase in facility of outflow of aqueous humor, fall in intraocular pressure, and potentiation of accommodation.

Echothiophate Iodide will depress both plasma and erythrocyte cholinesterase levels in most patients after a few weeks of eyedrop therapy.

INDICATIONS AND USAGE
Glaucoma: Chronic open-angle glaucoma. Subacute or chronic angle-closure glaucoma after iridectomy or where surgery is refused or contraindicated. Certain non-uveitic secondary types of glaucoma, especially glaucoma following cataract surgery.

Accommodative Esotropia: Concomitant esotropias with a significant accommodative component.

CONTRAINDICATIONS
1. Active uveal inflammation.
2. Most cases of angle-closure glaucoma, due to the possibility of increasing angle block.
3. Hypersensitivity to the active or inactive ingredients.

WARNINGS
1. Succinylcholine should be administered only with great caution, if at all, prior to or during general anesthesia to patients receiving anticholinesterase medication because of possible respiratory or cardiovascular collapse.
2. Caution should be observed in treating glaucoma with Echothiophate Iodide in patients who are at the same time undergoing treatment with systemic anticholinesterase medications for myasthenia gravis, because of possible adverse additive effects.
(See "Precautions—Drug Interactions" for further information.)

PRECAUTIONS
GENERAL
1. Gonioscopy is recommended prior to initiation of therapy. Routine examination to detect lens opacity should accompany clinical use of Echothiophate Iodide.
2. Where there is a quiescent uveitis or a history of this condition, anticholinesterase therapy should be avoided or used cautiously because of the intense and persistent miosis and ciliary muscle contraction that may occur.
3. While systemic effects are infrequent, proper use of the drug requires digital compression of the nasolacrimal ducts for a minute or two following instillation to minimize drainage into the nasal chamber with its extensive absorption area. To prevent possible skin absorption, hands should be washed following instillation.
4. Temporary discontinuance of medication is necessary if cardiac irregularities occur.
5. Anticholinesterase drugs should be used with extreme caution, if at all, in patients with marked vagotonia, bronchial asthma, spastic gastrointestinal disturbances, peptic ulcer, pronounced bradycardia and hypotension, recent myocardial infarction, epilepsy, parkinsonism, and other disorders that may respond adversely to vagotonic effects.
6. Anticholinesterase drugs should be employed prior to ophthalmic surgery only as a considered risk because of the possible occurrence of hyphema.
7. Echothiophate Iodide should be used with great caution, if at all, where there is a prior history of retinal detachment.
8. Temporary discontinuance of medication is necessary if salivation, urinary incontinence, diarrhea, profuse sweating, muscle weakness, or respiratory difficulties occur.
9. Patients receiving Echothiophate Iodide who are exposed to carbamate- or organophosphate-type insecticides and pesticides (professional gardeners, farmers, workers in plants manufacturing or formulating such products, etc.) should be warned of the additive systemic effects possible from absorption of the pesticide through the respiratory tract or skin. During periods of exposure to such pesticides, the wearing of respiratory masks, and frequent washing and clothing changes may be advisable.

➤ SHOWN IN PRODUCT IDENTIFICATION GUIDE

Drug Interactions: Echothiophate Iodide potentiates other cholinesterase inhibitors such as succinylcholine or organophosphate and carbamate insecticides. Patients undergoing systemic anticholinesterase treatment should be warned of the possible additive effects of Echothiophate Iodide.

Carcinogenesis, Mutagenesis, Impairment of Fertility: No data is available regarding carcinogenesis, mutagenesis, and impairment of fertility.

Pregnancy: Teratogenic Effects—Pregnancy Category C: Animal reproduction studies have not been conducted with Echothiophate Iodide. It is also not known whether Echothiophate Iodide can cause fetal harm when administered to a pregnant woman or can affect reproduction capacity. Echothiophate Iodide should be given to a pregnant woman only if clearly needed.

Nursing Mothers: Because of the potential for serious adverse reactions in nursing infants from Echothiophate Iodide, a decision should be made whether to discontinue nursing or to discontinue the drug, taking into account the importance of the drug to the mother.

ADVERSE REACTIONS

1. Although the relationship, if any, of retinal detachment to the administration of Echothiophate Iodide has not been established, retinal detachment has been reported in a few cases during the use of Echothiophate Iodide in adult patients without a previous history of this disorder.

2. Stinging, burning, lacrimation, lid muscle twitching, conjunctival and ciliary redness, browache, induced myopia with visual blurring may occur.

3. Activation of latent iritis or uveitis may occur.

4. Iris cysts may form, and if treatment is continued, may enlarge and obscure vision. This occurrence is more frequent in children. The cysts usually shrink upon discontinuance of the medication, reduction in strength of the drops or frequency of instillation. Rarely, they may rupture or break free into the aqueous. Regular examinations are advisable when the drug is being prescribed for the treatment of accommodative esotropia.

5. Prolonged use may cause conjunctival thickening, obstruction of nasolacrimal canals.

6. Lens opacities occurring in patients under treatment for glaucoma with Echothiophate Iodide have been reported and similar changes have been produced experimentally in normal monkeys. Routine examinations should accompany clinical use of the drug.

7. Paradoxical increase in intraocular pressure may follow anticholinesterase instillation. This may be alleviated by prescribing a sympathomimetic mydriatic such as phenylephrine.

8. Cardiac irregularities.

DOSAGE AND ADMINISTRATION

DIRECTIONS FOR PREPARING EYEDROPS

1. USE ASEPTIC TECHNIQUE.

2. TEAR OFF ALUMINUM SEALS, AND REMOVE AND DISCARD RUBBER PLUGS FROM BOTH DRUG AND DILUENT CONTAINERS.

3. POUR DILUENT INTO DRUG CONTAINER.

4. REMOVE DROPPER ASSEMBLY FROM ITS STERILE WRAPPING. HOLDING DROPPER ASSEMBLY BY THE SCREW CAP AND, *WITHOUT COMPRESSING RUBBER BULB,* INSERT INTO DRUG CONTAINER AND SCREW DOWN TIGHTLY.

5. SHAKE FOR SEVERAL SECONDS TO ENSURE MIXING.

6. DO NOT COVER NOR OBLITERATE INSTRUCTIONS TO PATIENT REGARDING STORAGE OF EYEDROPS.

GLAUCOMA

Selection of Therapy: The *medication prescribed* should be that which will control the intraocular pressure around-the-clock with the least risk of side effects or adverse reactions. "Tonometric glaucoma" (ocular hypertension without other evidence of the disease) is frequently not treated with any medication, and Echothiophate Iodide is certainly not recommended for this condition. In early chronic simple glaucoma with field loss or disc changes, pilocarpine is generally used for initial therapy and can be recommended so long as control is thereby maintained over the 24 hours of the day.

When this is not the case, Echothiophate Iodide 0.03% may be effective and probably has no greater potential for side effects. If this dosage is inadequate, epinephrine and a carbonic anhydrase inhibitor may be added to the regimen. When still more effective medication is required, the higher strengths of Echothiophate Iodide may be prescribed with the recognition that the control of the intraocular pressure should have priority regardless of potential side effects. In secondary glaucoma following cataract surgery, the higher strengths of the drug are frequently needed and are ordinarily very well tolerated. The *dosage regimen* prescribed should call for the lowest concentration that will control the intraocular pressure around-the-clock. Where tonometry around-the-clock is not feasible, it is suggested that appointments for tension-taking be made at different times of the day so that inadequate control may be more readily detected. Two doses a day are preferred to one in order to maintain as smooth a diurnal tension curve as possible, although a single dose per day or every other day has been used with satisfactory results. Because of the long duration of action of the drug, it is never necessary or desirable to exceed a schedule of twice a day. The daily dose or one of the two daily doses should always be instilled just before retiring to avoid inconvenience due to the miosis.

Early Chronic Simple Glaucoma: Echothiophate Iodide 0.03% instilled twice a day, just before retiring and in the morning, may be prescribed advantageously for cases of early chronic simple glaucoma that are not controlled around-the-clock with other less potent agents. Because of prolonged action, control during the night and early morning hours may then sometimes be obtained. A change in therapy is indicated if, at any time, the tension fails to remain at an acceptable level on this regimen.

Advanced Chronic Simple Glaucoma and Glaucoma Secondary to Cataract Surgery: These cases may respond satisfactorily to Echothiophate Iodide 0.03% twice a day as above. When the patient is being transferred to Echothiophate Iodide because of unsatisfactory control with pilocarpine, carbachol, epinephrine, etc., one of the higher strengths, 0.06%, 0.125%, or 0.25% will usually be needed. In this case, a brief trial with the 0.03% eyedrops will be advantageous in that the higher strengths will then be more easily tolerated.

Concomitant Therapy: Echothiophate Iodide may be used concomitantly with epinephrine, a carbonic anhydrase inhibitor, or both.

Technique: Good technique in the administration of Echothiophate Iodide requires that finger pressure at the inner canthus should be exerted for a minute or two following instillation of the eyedrops, to minimize drainage into the nose and throat. Excess solution around the eye should be removed with tissue and any medication on the hands should be rinsed off.

ACCOMMODATIVE ESOTROPIA (PEDIATRIC USE)

In Diagnosis: One drop of 0.125% may be instilled once a day in both eyes on retiring, for a period of two or three weeks. If the esotropia is accommodative, a favorable response will usually be noted which may begin within a few hours.

In Treatment: Echothiophate Hydrochloride is prescribed at the lowest concentration and frequency which gives satisfactory results. After the initial period of treatment for diagnostic purposes, the schedule may be reduced to 0.125% every other day or 0.06% every day. These dosages can often be gradually lowered as treatment progresses. The 0.03% strength has proven to be effective in some cases. The maximum usually recommended dosage is 0.125% once a day, although more intensive therapy has been used for short periods.

Technique: (See *"Dosage and Administration—Glaucoma."*)

Duration of Treatment: In diagnosis, only a short period is required and little time will be lost in instituting other procedures if the esotropia proves to be unresponsive. In therapy, there is no definite limit so long as the drug is well tolerated. However, if the eyedrops, with or without eyeglasses, are gradually withdrawn after about a year or two and deviation recurs, surgery should be considered. As with other miotics, tolerance may occasionally develop after prolonged use. In such cases, a rest period will restore the original activity of the drug.

HANDLING AND STORAGE
Store at or below room temperature (approximately 25°C).

After reconstitution, keep eyedrops in refrigerator to obtain maximum useful life of 6 months. Room temperature is acceptable if drops will be used within a month.

HOW SUPPLIED
POWDER FOR RECONSTITUTION: 0.03%

BRAND/MANUFACTURER	NDC	SIZE	AWP
○ **BRAND** PHOSPHOLINE IODIDE: Wyeth-Ayerst	00046-1062-05	5 ml	$21.13

POWDER FOR RECONSTITUTION: 0.06%

BRAND/MANUFACTURER	NDC	SIZE	AWP
○ **BRAND** PHOSPHOLINE IODIDE: Wyeth-Ayerst	00046-1064-05	5 ml	$22.14

POWDER FOR RECONSTITUTION: 0.125%

BRAND/MANUFACTURER	NDC	SIZE	AWP
○ **BRAND** PHOSPHOLINE IODIDE: Wyeth-Ayerst	00046-1065-05	5 ml	$24.83

POWDER FOR RECONSTITUTION: 0.25%

BRAND/MANUFACTURER	NDC	SIZE	AWP
○ **BRAND** PHOSPHOLINE IODIDE: Wyeth-Ayerst	00046-1066-05	5 ml	$27.98

Econazole Nitrate

DESCRIPTION
Econazole Nitrate Cream contains the antifungal agent, Econazole Nitrate 1%, in a water-miscible base consisting of pegoxol 7 stearate, peglicol 5 oleate, mineral oil, benzoic acid, butylated hydroxyanisole, and purified water. The white to off-white soft cream is for topical use only.

Chemically, Econazole Nitrate is 1-[2-[(4-chlorophenyl) methoxy]-2-(2,4-dichlorophenyl)ethyl]-1H-imidazole mononitrate.

Following is its chemical structure:

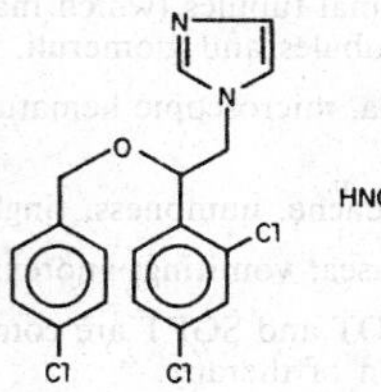

CLINICAL PHARMACOLOGY

After topical application to the skin of normal subjects, systemic absorption of Econazol Nitrate is extremely low. Although most of the applied drug remains on the skin surface, drug concentrations were found in the stratum corneum which, by far, exceeded the minimum inhibitory concentration for dermatophytes. Inhibitory concentrations were achieved in the epidermis and as deep as the middle region of the dermis. Less than 1% of the applied dose was recovered in the urine and feces.

Microbiology: In *vitro* studies, Econazole Nitrate exhibits broad-spectrum antifungal activity against the dermatophytes, *Trichophyton rubrum*, *Trichophyton mentagrophytes*, *Trichophyton tonsurans*, *Microsporum canis*, *Microsporum audouini*, *Microsporum gypseum*, and *Epidermophyton floccosum*, the yeast, *Candida albicans* and *Pityrosporum orbiculare* (the organism responsible for tinea versicolor), and certain gram positive bacteria.

INDICATIONS AND USAGE

Econazole Nitrate Cream is indicated for topical application in the treatment of tinea pedis, tinea cruris, and tinea corporis caused by *Trichophyton rubrum*, *Trichophyton mentagrophytes*, *Trichophyton tonsurans*, *Microsporum canis*, *Microsporum audouini*, *Microsporum gypseum*, and *Epidermophyton floccosum*, in the treatment of cutaneous candidiasis, and in the treatment of tinea versicolor.

CONTRAINDICATIONS

Econazole Nitrate Cream is contraindicated in individuals who have shown hypersensitivity to any of its ingredients.

WARNINGS

Econazole Nitrate is not for ophthalmic use.

PRECAUTIONS

General: If a reaction suggesting sensitivity or chemical irritation should occur, use of the medication should be discontinued.

For external use only. Avoid introduction of Econazole Nitrate Cream into the eyes.

Carcinogenicity Studies: Long-term animal studies to determine carcinogenic potential have not been performed.

Fertility (Reproduction): Oral administration of Econazole Nitrate in rats has been reported to produce prolonged gestation. Intravaginal administration in humans has not shown prolonged gestation or other adverse reproductive effects attributable to Econazole Nitrate therapy.

Pregnancy: Pregnancy Category C: Econazole Nitrate has not been shown to be teratogenic when administered orally to mice, rabbits or rats. Fetotoxic or embryotoxic effects were observed in Segment I oral studies with rats receiving 10 to 40 times the human dermal dose. Similar effects were observed in Segment II or Segment III studies with mice, rabbits and/or rats receiving oral doses 80 or 40 times the human dermal dose.

Econazole Nitrate should be used in the first trimester of pregnancy only when the physician considers it essential to the welfare of the patient. The drug should be used during the second and third trimesters of pregnancy only if clearly needed.

Nursing Mothers: It is not known whether Econazole Nitrate is excreted in human milk. Following oral administration of Econazole Nitrate to lactating rats, Econazole and/or metabolites were excreted in milk and were found in nursing pups. Also, in lactating rats receiving large oral doses (40 or 80 times the human dermal dose), there was a reduction in postpartum viability of pups and survival to weaning: however, at these high doses, maternal toxicity was present and may have been a contributing factor. Caution should be exercised when Econazole Nitrate is administered to a nursing woman.

ADVERSE REACTIONS

During clinical trials, approximately 3% of patients treated with Econazole Nitrate 1% cream reported side effects thought possibly to be due to the drug, consisting mainly of burning, itching, stinging and erythema. One case of pruritic rash has also been reported.

OVERDOSE

Overdosage of Econazole Nitrate in humans has not been reported to date. In mice, rats, guinea pigs and dogs, the oral LD 50 values were found to be 462, 668, 272, and > 160 mg/kg, respectively.

DOSAGE AND ADMINISTRATION

Sufficient Econazole Nitrate Cream should be applied to cover affected areas once daily in patients with tinea pedis, tinea cruris, tinea corporis, and tinea versicolor, and twice daily (morning and evening) in patients with cutaneous candidiasis.

Early relief of symptoms is experienced by the majority of patients and clinical improvement may be seen fairly soon after treatment is begun; however, candidal infections and tinea cruris and corporis should be treated for two weeks and tinea pedis for one month in order to reduce the possibility of recurrence. If a patient shows no clinical improvement after the treatment period, the diagnosis should be redetermined. Patients with tinea versicolor usually exhibit clinical and mycological clearing after two weeks of treatment.

Store Econazole Nitrate Cream below 86°F.

HOW SUPPLIED
CREAM: 1%

BRAND/MANUFACTURER	NDC	SIZE	AWP
○ BRAND			
SPECTAZOLE: Ortho Pharm	00062-5460-02	15 gm	$11.04
	00062-5460-01	30 gm	$18.72
	00062-5460-03	85 gm	$36.12

Econopred *SEE* PREDNISOLONE ACETATE, OPHTHALMIC *AND* PREDNISOLONE, SYSTEMIC

Edecrin *SEE* ETHACRYNIC ACID

Edetate Calcium Disodium

WARNINGS

EDETATE CALCIUM DISODIUM IS CAPABLE OF PRODUCING TOXIC EFFECTS WHICH CAN BE FATAL. LEAD ENCEPHALOPATHY IS RELATIVELY RARE IN ADULTS, BUT OCCURS MORE OFTEN IN CHILDREN IN WHOM IT MAY BE INCIPIENT AND THUS OVERLOOKED. THE MORTALITY RATE IN THESE CHILDREN HAS BEEN HIGH. PATIENTS WITH LEAD ENCEPHALOPATHY AND CEREBRAL EDEMA MAY EXPERIENCE A LETHAL INCREASE IN INTRACRANIAL PRESSURE FOLLOWING INTRAVENOUS INFUSION: THE INTRAMUSCULAR ROUTE IS PREFERRED FOR THESE PATIENTS AND FOR YOUNG CHILDREN. IN CASES WHERE THE INTRAVENOUS ROUTE IS NECESSARY, AVOID RAPID INFUSION. THE DOSAGE SCHEDULE SHOULD BE FOLLOWED AND AT NO TIME SHOULD THE RECOMMENDED DAILY DOSE BE EXCEEDED.

DESCRIPTION

Edetate Calcium Disodium is a sterile, injectable, chelating agent in concentrated solution for intravenous infusion or intramuscular injection. Each 5 ml ampul contains 1000 mg of Edetate Calcium Disodium [equivalent to 200 mg/ml] in water for injection. Chemically, this product is called [[N,N',-1,2-ethanediylbis[N-(carboxymethyl)-glycinato]](4)-N,N',O, O^N,O^N]-,disodium,hydrate, (OC-6-21)-Calciate(2-).

Following is its chemical structure:

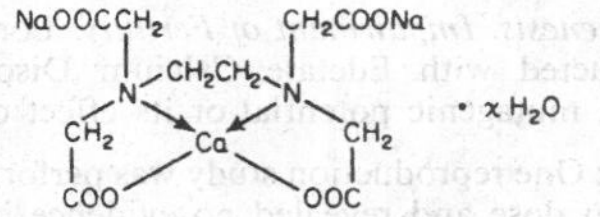

CLINICAL PHARMACOLOGY

The pharmacologic effects of Edetate Calcium Disodium are due to the formation of chelates with divalent and trivalent metals. A stable chelate will form with any metal that has the ability to displace calcium from the molecule, a feature shared by lead, zinc, cadmium, manganese, iron and mercury. The amounts of manganese and iron mobilized for chelation are not significant. Copper[1] is not mobilized and mercury is unavailable for chelation because it is too tightly bound to body ligands or it is stored in inaccessible body compartments. The excretion of calcium by the body is not increased following intravenous administration of Edetate Calcium Disodium, but the excretion of zinc is considerably increased.[1]

Edetate Calcium Disodium is poorly absorbed from the gastrointestinal tract. In blood, all the drug is found in the plasma. Edetate Calcium Disodium does not appear to penetrate cells; it is distributed primarily in the extracellular fluid with only about 5% of the plasma concentration found in spinal fluid.

The half life of Edetate Calcium Disodium is 20 to 60 minutes.

It is excreted primarily by the kidney, with about 50% excreted in one hour and over 95% within 24 hours.[2] Almost none of the compound is metabolized.

The primary source of lead chelated by Edetate Calcium Disodium is from bone; subsequently, soft-tissue lead is redistributed to bone when chelation is stopped.[3,4] There is also some reduction in kidney lead levels following chelation therapy.

It has been shown in animals that following a single dose of Edetate Calcium Disodium urinary lead output increases, blood lead concentration decreases, but brain lead is significantly increased due to internal redistribution of lead.[5] (See "Warnings".) These data are in agreement with the recent results of others in experimental animals showing that after a five day course of treatment there is no net reduction in brain lead.[6]

INDICATIONS AND USAGE

Edetate Calcium Disodium is indicated for the reduction of blood levels and depot stores of lead in lead poisoning (acute and chronic) and lead encephalopathy, in both children and adults.

Chelation therapy should not replace effective measures to eliminate or reduce further exposure to lead.

CONTRAINDICATIONS

Edetate Calcium Disodium should not be given during periods of anuria, nor to patients with active renal disease or hepatitis.

WARNINGS

See boxed "warning."

PRECAUTIONS

General Precautions: Edetate Calcium Disodium may produce the same renal damage as lead poisoning, such as proteinuria and microscopic hematuria. Treatment-induced nephrotoxicity is dose-dependent and may be reduced by assuring adequate diuresis before therapy begins. Urine flow must be monitored throughout therapy which must be stopped if anuria or severe olyguria develop. The proximal tubule hydropic degeneration usually recovers upon cessation of therapy. Edetate Calcium Disodium must be used in reduced doses in patients with pre-existing mild renal disease.

Patients should be monitored for cardiac rhythm irregularities and other ECG changes during intravenous therapy.

Information for Patients: Patients should be instructed to immediately inform their physician if urine output stops for a period of 12 hours.

Laboratory Tests: Urinarlysis and urine sediment, renal and hepatic function and serum electrolyte levels should be checked before each course of therapy and then be monitored daily during therapy in severe cases, and in less serious cases after the second and fifth day of therapy. Therapy must be discontinued at the first sign of renal toxicity. The presence of large renal epithelial cells or increasing number of red blood cells in urinary sediment or greater proteinuria call for immediate stopping of Edetate Calcium Disodium administration. Alkaline phosphatase values are frequently depressed (possibly due to decreased serum zinc levels), but return to normal within 48 hours after cessation of therapy. Elevated erythrocyte protoporphyrin levels (> 35 mcg/dl of whole blood) indicate the need to perform a venous blood lead determination. If the whole blood lead concentration is between 25-55 mcg/dl a mobilization test can be considered.[7,8] (See "Diagnostic Test".) An elevation of urinary coproporphyrin (adults: > 250 mcg/day; children under 80 lbs; > 75 mcg/day) and elevation of urinary delta aminolevulinic acid (ALA) (adults: > 4 mg/day; children: > 3 mg/m^2/day) are associated with blood lead levels > 40 mcg/dl. Urinary coproporphyrin may be falsely negative in terminal patients and in severely iron-depleted children who are not regenerating heme.[9] In growing children long bone x-rays showing lead lines and abdominal x-rays showing radio-opaque material in the abdomen may be of help in estimating the level of exposure to lead.

Drug Interactions: There is no known drug interference with standard clinical laboratory tests. Steroids enhance the renal toxicity of Edetate Calcium Disodium in animals.[7] (Edetate Calcium Disodium interferes with the action of zinc insulin preparations by chelating the zinc.[7]

Carcinogenesis, Mutagenesis, Impairment of Fertility: Long term animal studies have not been conducted with Edetate Calcium Disodium to evaluate its carcinogenic potential, mutagenic potential or its effect on fertility.

Pregnancy: Category B: One reproduction study was performed in rats at doses up to 13 times the human dose and revealed no evidence of impaired fertility or harm to the fetus due to Edetate Calcium Disodium.[10] Another reproduction study performed in rats at doses up to about 25 to 40 times the human dose revealed evidence of fetal malformations due to Edetate Calcium Disodium, which were prevented by simultaneous supplementation of dietary zinc.[11]

There are, however, no adequate and well-controlled studies in pregnant women. Because animal reproduction studies are not always predictive of human response, this drug should be used during pregnancy only if clearly needed.

Labor and Delivery: Edetate Calcium Disodium has no recognized use during labor and delivery, and its effects during these processes are unknown.

Nursing Mothers: It is not known whether this drug is excreted in human milk. Because many drugs are excreted in human milk, caution should be exercised when Edetate Calcium Disodium is administered to a nursing woman.

Pediatric Use: Since lead poisoning occurs in children and adults but is frequently more severe in children Edetate Calcium Disodium is used in patients of all ages.

ADVERSE REACTIONS

The following adverse effects have been associated with the use of Edetate Calcium Disodium:

Body as a Whole: pain at intramuscular injection site, fever, chills, malaise, fatigue, myalgia, arthralgia.

Cardiovascular: hypotension, cardiac rhythm irregularities.

Renal: acute necrosis of proximal tubules (which may result in fatal nephrosis), infrequent changes in distal tubules and glomeruli.

Urinary: glycosuria, proteinuria, microscopic hematuria and large epithelial cells in urinary sediment.

Nervous System: tremors, headache, numbness, tingling.

Gastrointestinal: cheilosis, nausea, vomiting, anorexia, excessive thirst.

Hepatic: mild increases in SGOT and SGPT are common, and return to normal within 48 hours after cessation of therapy.

Immunogenic: histamine-like reactions (sneezing, nasal congestion, lacrimation), rash.

Hematopoietic: transient bone marrow depression, anemia.

Metabolic: zinc deficiency, hypercalcemia.

OVERDOSAGE

Symptoms: Inadvertent administration of 5 times the recommended dose, infused intravenously over a 24 hour period, to an asymptomatic 16 month old patient with a blood lead content of 56 mcg/dl did not cause any ill effects Edetate Calcium Disodium can aggravate the symptoms of severe lead poisoning, therefore, most toxic effects (cerebral edema, renal tubular necrosis) appear to be associated with lead poisoning. Because of cerebral edema, a therapeutic dose may be lethal to an adult or a child with lead encephalopathy. Higher dosage of Edetate Calcium Disodium may produce a more severe zinc deficiency.

Treatment: Cerebral edema should be treated with repeated doses of mannitol. Steroids enhance the renal toxicity of Edetate Calcium Disodium in animals and, therefore, are no longer recommended.[7] Zinc levels must be monitored. Good urinary output must be maintained because diuresis will enhance drug elimination. It is not known if Edetate Calcium Disodium is dialyzable.

DOSAGE AND ADMINISTRATION

When a source for the lead intoxication has been identified, the patient should be removed from the source, if possible. The recommended dose of Edetate Calcium Disodium for asymptomatic adults and children whose blood lead level is < 70 mcg/dl but < 20 mcg/dl (World Health Organization recommended upper allowable level) is 1000 mg/m^2/day whether given intravenously or intramuscularly. (See Surface Area Nomogram.)

SURFACE AREA NOMOGRAM

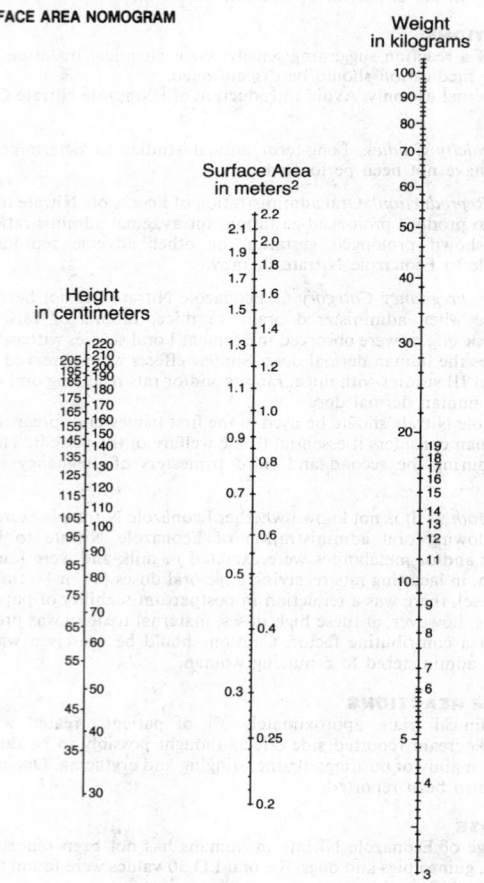

For adults with lead nephropathy, the following dosage regimen has been suggested: 500 mg/m^2 every 24 hours for 5 days for patients with serum creatinine levels of 2-3 mg/dl, every 48 hours for 3 doses for patients with creatinine levels of 3-4 mg/dl, and once weekly for patients with creatinine levels above 4 mg/dl. These regimens may be repeated at one month intervals.[12]

Edetate Calcium Disodium, used alone, may aggravate symptoms in patients with very high blood lead levels. When the blood lead level is $\geq$ 70 mcg/dl or clinical symptoms consistent with lead poisoning are present, it is recommended that Edetate Calcium Disodium be used in conjunction with dimercaprol. Please consult published protocols and specialized references for dosage recommendations of combination therapy.[14-18]

Therapy of lead poisoning in adults and children with Edetate Calcium Disodium is continued over a period of five days. Therapy is then interrupted for 2 to 4 days to allow redistribution of the lead and to prevent severe depletion of zinc and other essential metals. Two courses of treatment are usually employed; however, it depends on severity of the lead toxicity and the patient's tolerance of the drug.

Edetate Calcium Disodium is equally effective whether administered intravenously or intramuscularly. The intramuscular route is used for all patients with overt lead encephalopathy and this route is recommended for young children.

Acutely ill individuals may be dehydrated from vomiting. Since Edetate Calcium Disodium is excreted almost exclusively in the urine, it is very important to establish urine flow with intravenous fluid administration before the first dose of the chelating agent is given; however, excessive fluid must be avoided in patients with encephalopathy. Once urine flow is established, further intravenous fluid is restricted to basal water and electrolyte requirements. Administration of Edetate Calcium Disodium should be stopped whenever there is cessation of urine flow in order to avoid unduly high tissue levels of the drug. Edetate Calcium Disodium must be used in reduced doses in patients with pre-existing mild renal disease.

Intravenous Administration: Add the total daily dose of Edetate Calcium Disodium (1000 mg/m^2/day) to 250-500 ml of 5% dextrose or 0.9% sodium chloride injection. The total daily dose should be infused over a period of 8-12 hours. Edetate Calcium Disodium injection is incompatible with 10% dextrose, 10% invert sugar in 0.9% sodium chloride, lactate Ringer's, Ringer's, one-sixth molar sodium lactate injections, and with injectable amphotericin B and hydralazine hydrochloride.

Intramuscular Administration: The total daily dosage (1000 mg/m^2/day) should be divided into equal doses spaced 8-12 hours apart. Lidocaine or procaine should be added to the Edetate Calcium Disodium injection to minimize pain at the injection site. The final lidocaine or procaine concentration of 5 mg/ml (0.5%) can be obtained as follows: 0.25 ml of 10% lidocaine solution per 5 ml (entire content of ampul) concentrated Edetate Calcium Disodium; 1 ml of 1% lidocaine or procaine solution per ml of concentrated Edetate Calcium Disodium. When used alone, regardless of method of administration. Edetate Calcium Disodium should not be given at doses larger than those recommended.

Diagnostic Test: Several methods have been described for lead mobilization tests using Edetate Calcium Disodium to assess body stores.[7,9,12,13,18]

These procedures have advantages and disadvantages that should be reviewed in current references. Edetate Calcium Disodium mobilization test should not be performed in symptomatic patients and in patients with blood lead levels above 55 mcg/dl for whom appropriate therapy is indicated.

Parenteral drug should be inspected visually for particulate matter and discoloration prior to administration, whenever solution and container permit.

Store at controlled room temperature, 15-30°C (59-86°F).

REFERENCES

1. Thomas DJ, Chisolm JJ. Lead, zinc and copper decorporation during calcium disodium ethylenediamine tetra-acetate treatment of lead-poisoned children. J Pharmacol Exp Therapeu 1986; 239:829-835. 2. The Pharmacological Basis of Therapeutics, 7th edition, Goodman and Gilman, editors. Macmillan Publishing Company, New York, 1985, pp. 1619-1622. 3. Hammond PB, Aronson AL, Olson WC. The mechanism of mobilization of lead by ethylenediaminetetraacetate. J Pharmacol Exp Therapeu 1967; 157:196-206. 4. Van de Vyver FL, D'Haese PC, Visser WJ, et al. Bone lead in dialysis patients. Kidney Intl 1988; 33:601-607. 5. Cory-Slecta DA, Weiss B, Cox C. Mobilization and redistribution of lead over the course of calcium disodium ethylenediamine tetraacetate chelation therapy. J Pharmacol Exp Therapeu 1987; 243:804-813. 6. Chisolm JJ. Mobilization of lead by calcium disodium edetate. Am J Dis Child 1987; 141:1256-1257. 7. Drug Evaluations, 6th Edition, American Medical Association, Saunders, Philadelphia, 1986, pp. 1637-1639. 8. Centers for Disease Control: Preventing lead poisoning in young children. Atlanta, GA, Department of Health and Human Services, 1985 Jan. 9. Finberg L, Rajagopal V. Diagnosis and treatment of lead poisoning in children. J Family Med 1985 April: 3-12. 10. Schardein JL, Sakowski R, Petrere J, et al. Teratogenesis studies with EDTA and its salts in rats. Toxicol Appl Pharmacol 1981; 61:423-428. 11. Swenerton H, Hurley LS. Teratogenic effects of a chelating agent and their prevention by zinc. Science 1971; 173:62-64. 12. American Hospital Formulary Service, Drug Information, 1988, pp. 1695-1698. 13. Markowitz ME, Rosen JF. Assessment of lead stores in children: Validation of an 8-hour CaNa₂EDTA (Calcium Disodium Versenate) provocative test. J Pediatrics 1984; 104:337-341. 14. Piomelli S, Rosen JF, Chisolm JJ, et al. Management of childhood lead poisoning, J Pediatrics 1984; 105:523-532. 15. Sachs HK, Blanksma LA, Murray EF, et al. Ambulatory treatment of lead poisoning: Report of 1,155 cases. Pediatrics 1970; 46:389. 16. Chisolm JJ. The use of chelating agents in the treatment of acute and chronic lead intoxication in childhood. J Pediatrics 1968; 73:1. 17. Coffin R, Phillips JL, Staples WI, et al. Treatment of lead encephalopathy in children. J Pediatrics 1966; 69: 198-206. 18. Chisolm JJ. Increased lead absorption and acute lead poisoning. Current Pediatric Therapy 12, Gillis and Kagan, editors, WB Saunders, Philadelphia, 1986, pp. 667-671.

J CODES

Up to 200 mg IV,SC,IM—J0600

HOW SUPPLIED

INJECTION: 200 MG/ML

BRAND/MANUFACTURER	NDC	SIZE	AWP
○ **BRAND**			
CALCIUM DISODIUM VERSENATE: 3M Pharm	00089-0510-06	5 ml 6s	$189.78

Edetate Disodium

> **WARNING**
>
> THE USE OF THIS DRUG IN ANY PARTICULAR PATIENT IS RECOMMENDED ONLY WHEN THE SEVERITY OF THE CLINICAL CONDITION JUSTIFIES THE AGGRESSIVE MEASURES ASSOCIATED WITH THIS TYPE OF THERAPY.

DESCRIPTION

Edetate Disodium is a sterile, nonpyrogenic, concentrated solution of Edetate Disodium in water for injection which as a result of a pH adjustment with sodium hydroxide contains varying amounts of disodium and trisodium salts. After dilution, it is administered by intravenous infusion.

Each milliliter (mL) contains Edetate Disodium, anhydrous 150 mg. May contain sodium hydroxide for pH adjustment. pH is 7.0 (6.5 to 7.5).

Edetate Disodium is classified as a clinical chelating agent for emergency lowering of serum calcium in hypercalcemia.

The solution contains no bacteriostat, antimicrobial agent or buffer (except for pH adjustment) and is intended only for use (after dilution) as a single-dose infusion. When smaller doses are required, the unused portion should be discarded.

Edetate Disodium, USP is chemically designated disodium (ethylenedinitrilo) tetraacetate dihydrate, a white crystalline powder soluble in water. It is also described as the disodium salt of ethylenediamine tetraacetic acid (EDTA).

Following is its chemical structure:

$$\begin{array}{c} NaOOCCH_2 \\ \\ HOOCCH_2 \end{array} NCH_2CH_2N \begin{array}{c} CH_2COONa \\ \\ CH_2COOH \end{array} \cdot 2H_2O$$

CLINICAL PHARMACOLOGY

Edetate Disodium Injection, USP forms chelates with the cations of calcium and many divalent and trivalent metals. Because of its affinity for calcium, Edetate Disodium will produce a lowering of the serum calcium level during intravenous infusion. Slow infusion over a protracted period may cause mobilization of extracirculatory calcium stores. Edetate Disodium exerts a negative inotropic effect upon the heart.

After intravenous administration, the chelate formed is excreted in the urine with 50% appearing in 1 hour and over 95% in 24 hours.

Edetate Disodium likewise forms chelates with other polyvalent metals and produces increases in urinary excretion of magnesium, zinc and other trace elements. It does not form a chelate with potassium but may reduce the serum level and increase urinary loss of potassium.

INDICATIONS AND USAGE

Edetate Disodium is indicated in selected patients for the emergency treatment of hypercalcemia and for the control of ventricular arrhythmias associated with digitalis toxicity.

CONTRAINDICATIONS

Edetate Disodium is contraindicated in anuric patients. It is not indicated for the treatment of generalized arteriosclerosis associated with advancing age.

WARNINGS

See *"Warning"* statement.

Rapid intravenous infusion or attainment of high serum concentration of Edetate Disodium may cause a precipitous drop in the serum calcium level and may result in fatality. Toxicity appears to be dependent upon both total dosage and speed of administration. The rate of administration and dosage should not exceed that indicated in *"Dosage and Administration"*.

Because of its irritant effect on the tissues and because of the danger of serious side effects if administered in the undiluted form, Edetate Disodium should be diluted before infusion. See *"Dosage and Administration"*.

PRECAUTIONS

After the infusion of Edetate Disodium, the patient should remain in bed for a short time because of the possibility of postural hypotension.

The possibility of an adverse effect on myocardial contractility should be considered when administering the drug to patients with heart disease. Caution is dictated in the use of this drug in patients with limited cardiac reserve or incipient congestive failure.

Edetate Disodium Injection therapy should be used with caution in patients with clinical or subclinical potassium deficiency states. In such cases it is

► SHOWN IN PRODUCT IDENTIFICATION GUIDE

advisable to perform serum potassium blood levels for possible hypokalemia and to monitor ECG changes.

The possibility of hypomagnesemia should be kept in mind during prolonged therapy.

Treatment with Edetate Disodium has been shown to cause a lowering of blood sugar and insulin requirements in patients with diabetes who are treated with insulin.

Do not use unless solution is clear and container is intact.

Discard unused portion.

LABORATORY TEST

Renal excretory function should be assessed prior to treatment. Periodic BUN and creatinine determinations and daily urinalysis should be performed on patients receiving this drug.

Because of the possibility of inducing an electrolyte imbalance during treatment with Edetate Disodium, appropriate laboratory determinations and studies to evaluate the status of cardiac function should be performed. Repetition of these tests is recommended as often as clinically indicated, particularly in patients with ventricular arrhythmia and those with a history of seizure disorders or intracranial lesions. If clinical evidence suggests any disturbance of liver function during treatment, appropriate laboratory determinations should be performed and withdrawal of the drug may be required.

DRUG/LABORATORY TEST INTERACTIONS

The oxalate method of determining serum calcium tends to give low readings in the presence of Edetate Disodium; modification of this method, as by acidifying the sample or use of a different method may be required for accuracy. The least interference will be noted immediately before a subsequent dose is administered.

CARCINOGENESIS, MUTAGENESIS, IMPAIRMENT OF FERTILITY

Definitive statements cannot be made due to insufficient data and conflicting information.

Pregnancy Category C: Animal reproduction studies have not been conducted with Edetate Disodium Injection. It is also not known whether Edetate Disodium Injection can cause fetal harm when administered to a pregnant woman or can affect reproduction capacity. Edetate Disodium Injection should be given to a pregnant woman only if clearly needed.

Nursing Mothers: The safety of this product in nursing mothers has not been established.

ADVERSE REACTIONS

Gastrointestinal symptoms such as nausea, vomiting and diarrhea are fairly common following administration of this drug. Transient symptoms such as circumoral paresthesia, numbness and headache and a transient drop in systolic and diastolic blood pressure may occur. Thrombophlebitis, febrile reactions, hyperuricemia, anemia, exfoliative dermatitis and other toxic skin and mucous membrane reactions have been reported.

Nephrotoxicity and damage to the reticuloendothelial system with hemorrhagic tendencies have been reported with excessive dosages.

OVERDOSAGE

Because of the possibility that Edetate Disodium may produce a precipitous drop in the serum calcium level, a source of calcium replacement suitable for intravenous administration (such as calcium gluconate) should be instantly available at the bedside before Edetate Disodium is administered. Extreme caution is dictated in the use of intravenous calcium in the treatment of tetany, especially in digitalized patients because the action of the drug and the replacement of calcium ions may produce a reversal of the desired digitalis effect.

DOSAGE AND ADMINISTRATION

Edetate Disodium Injection, USP is administered by intravenous infusion only after dilution.

For Adults: The recommended daily dosage is 50 mg/kg of body weight to a maximum dose of 3 g in 24 hours. The dose, calculated by body weight, should be diluted in 500 mL of 5% Dextrose Injection, USP or 0.9% Sodium Chloride Injection, USP. The intravenous infusion should be regulated so that three or more hours are required for completion and the cardiac reserve of the patient is not exceeded. A suggested regimen includes five consecutive daily doses followed by two days without medication, with repeated courses as necessary to a total of 15 doses.

For Children: The recommended daily dosage is 40 mg/kg (1 g per 25 kg) of body weight. The dose, calculated by body weight, should be diluted in a sufficient volume of 5% Dextrose Injection, USP or 0.9% Sodium Chloride Injection, USP to bring the final concentration of Edetate Disodium to not more than 3%. The intravenous infusion should be regulated so that three or more hours are required for completion and the cardiac reserve of the patient is not exceeded. The maximum dose is 70 mg/kg per 24-hour period.

Parenteral drug products should be inspected visually for particulate matter and discoloration prior to administration, whenever solution and container permit. See *"Precautions"*.

DRUG INTERACTIONS

Additives may be incompatible with the reconstituted (diluted) solution required for intravenous infusion. Consult with pharmacist, if available. When introducing additives, use aseptic technique, mix thoroughly and do not store.

STORAGE

Store at controlled room temperature, 15°C to 30°C (59°F to 86°F).

J CODES

IV—J3520

HOW SUPPLIED
INJECTION: 150 MG/ML

AVERAGE UNIT PRICE (AVAILABLE SIZES)		GENERIC A-RATED AVERAGE PRICE (GAAP)	
BRAND	$1.28	20 ml	$14.25
GENERIC	$0.71		

BRAND/MANUFACTURER	NDC	SIZE	AWP
◆ **BRAND**			
ENDRATE: Abbott Hosp	00074-6940-03	20 ml 5s	$128.37
◆ **GENERICS**			
Schein	00364-2485-55	20 ml	$14.25
Steris	00402-0277-20	20 ml	$14.25

INJECTION: 150 MG/ML

BRAND/MANUFACTURER	NDC	SIZE	AWP
○ **BRAND**			
DISOTATE: Forest Pharm	00456-0724-17	20 ml	$4.00

Edrophonium Chloride

DESCRIPTION

Edrophonium Chloride is a short and rapid-acting cholinergic drug. Chemically, Edrophonium Chloride is ethyl (*m*-hydroxyphenyl)-dimethylammonium chloride.

10- or 15-ml vials: Each ml contains, in a sterile solution, 10 mg Edrophonium Chloride; pH is adjusted to approximately 5.4.

1-ml ampuls: Each ml contains, in a sterile solution, 10 mg Edrophonium Chloride; pH is adjusted to approximately 5.4.

Edrophonium Chloride is intended for IV and IM use.

Following is its chemical structure:

$$HO-\bigcirc-N^+(CH_3)_2 \quad C_2H_5 \quad Cl^-$$

ACTIONS

Edrophonium Chloride is an anticholinesterase drug. Its pharmacological action is due primarily to the inhibition or inactivation of acetylcholinesterase at sites of cholinergic transmission. Its effect is manifest within 30 to 60 seconds after injection and lasts an average of 10 minutes.

INDICATIONS

Edrophonium Chloride is recommended for the differential diagnosis of myasthenia gravis and as an adjunct in the evaluation of treatment requirements in this disease. It may also be used for evaluating emergency treatment in myasthenic crises. Because of its brief duration of action, it is not recommended for maintenance therapy in myasthenia gravis.

Edrophonium Chloride is also useful whenever a curare antagonist is needed to reverse the neuromuscular block produced by curare, tubocurarine, gallamine triethiodide or dimethyl-tubocurarine. It is *not* effective against decamethonium bromide and succinylcholine chloride. It may be used adjunctively in the treatment of respiratory depression caused by curare overdosage.

CONTRAINDICATIONS

Known hypersensitivity to anticholinesterase agents; intestinal and urinary obstructions of mechanical type.

WARNINGS

Whenever anticholinesterase drugs are used for testing, a syringe containing 1 mg of atropine sulfate should be immediately available to be given in aliquots intravenously to counteract severe cholinergic reactions which may occur in the hypersensitive individual, whether he is normal or myasthenic. Edrophonium Chloride should be used with caution in patients with bronchial asthma or cardiac dysrhythmias. The transient bradycardia which sometimes occurs can be relieved by atropine sulfate. Isolated instances of cardiac and respiratory arrest following administration of Edrophonium Chloride have been reported. It is postulated that these are vagotonic effects.

Certain brands of Edrophonium Chloride contain sodium sulfite, a sulfite that may cause allergic-type reactions, including anaphylactic symptoms and life-threatening or less severe asthmatic episodes in certain susceptible people. The overall prevalence of sulfite sensitivity in the general population is unknown and probably low. Sulfite sensitivity is seen more frequently in asthmatic than in nonasthmatic people.

Usage in Pregnancy: The safety of Edrophonium Chloride during pregnancy or lactation in humans has not been established. Therefore, use of Edrophonium Chloride in women who may become pregnant requires weighing the drug's potential benefits against its possible hazards to mother and child.

◆ RATED THERAPEUTICALLY EQUIVALENT; ◇ THERAPEUTIC EQUIVALENCE UNCONFIRMED; ○ UNRATED

PRECAUTIONS

Patients may develop "anticholinesterase insensitivity" for brief or prolonged periods. During these periods the patients should be carefully monitored and may need respiratory assistance. Dosages of anticholinesterase drugs should be reduced or withheld until patients again become sensitive to them.

ADVERSE REACTIONS

Careful observation should be made for severe cholinergic reactions in the hyperreactive individual. The myasthenic patient in crisis who is being tested with Edrophonium Chloride should be observed for bradycardia or cardiac standstill and cholinergic reactions if an overdose is given. The following reactions common to anticholinesterase agents may occur, although not all of these reactions have been reported with the administration of Edrophonium Chloride, probably because of its short duration of action and limited indications:

Eye: Increased lacrimation, pupillary constriction, spasm of accommodation, diplopia, conjunctival hyperemia.

CNS: Convulsions, dysarthria, dysphonia, dysphagia.

Respiratory: Increased tracheobronchial secretions, laryngospasm, bronchiolar constriction, paralysis of muscles of respiration, central respiratory paralysis.

Cardiac: Arrhythmias (especially bradycardia), fall in cardiac output leading to hypotension.

G.I.: Increased salivary, gastric and intestinal secretion, nausea, vomiting, increased peristalsis, diarrhea, abdominal cramps.

Skeletal Muscle: Weakness, fasciculations.

Miscellaneous: Increased urinary frequency and incontinence, diaphoresis.

Parenteral drug products should be inspected visually for particulate matter and discoloration prior to administration, whenever solution and container permit.

DRUG INTERACTIONS

Care should be given when administering this drug to patients with symptoms of myasthenic weakness who are also on anticholinesterase drugs. Since symptoms of anticholinesterase overdose (cholinergic crisis) may mimic underdosage (myasthenic weakness), their condition may be worsened by the use of this drug. (See "Overdosage" section for treatment.)

OVERDOSAGE

With drugs of this type, muscarine-like symptoms (nausea, vomiting, diarrhea, sweating, increased bronchial and salivary secretions and bradycardia) often appear with overdosage (cholinergic crisis). An important complication that can arise is obstruction of the airway by bronchial secretions. These may be managed with suction (especially if tracheostomy has been performed) and by the use of atropine. Many experts have advocated a wide range of dosages of atropine (*for Edrophonium Chloride see atropine dosage below*), but if there are copious secretions, up to 1.2 mg intravenously may be given initially and repeated every 20 minutes until secretions are controlled. Signs of atropine overdosage such as dry mouth, flush and tachycardia should be avoided as tenacious secretions and bronchial plugs may form. A total dose of atropine of 5 to 10 mg or even more may be required. The following steps should be taken in the management of overdosage of Edrophonium Chloride:

1. Adequate respiratory exchange should be maintained by assuring an open airway, and by the use of assisted respiration augmented by oxygen.
2. Cardiac function should be monitored until complete stabilization has been achieved.
3. Atropine sulfate in doses of 0.4 to 0.5 mg should be administered intravenously. This may be repeated every 3 to 10 minutes. Because of the short duration of action of Edrophonium Chloride the total dose required will seldom exceed 2 mg.
4. Pralidoxime chloride (a cholinesterase reactivator) may be given intravenously at the rate of 50 to 100 mg per minute; usually the total dose does not exceed 1000 mg. Extreme caution should be exercised in the use of pralidoxime chloride when the cholinergic symptoms are induced by double-bond phosphorous anticholinesterase drugs.[9]
5. If convulsions or shock is present, appropriate measures should be instituted.

DOSAGE AND ADMINISTRATION

EDROPHONIUM CHLORIDE TEST IN THE DIFFERENTIAL DIAGNOSIS OF MYASTHENIA GRAVIS:[1-8]

Intravenous Dosage (Adults): A tuberculin syringe containing 1 ml (10 mg) of Edrophonium Chloride is prepared with an intravenous needle, and 0.2 ml (2 mg) is injected intravenously within 15 to 30 seconds. The needle is left *in situ.* Only if no reaction occurs after 45 seconds is the remaining 0.8 ml (8 mg) injected. If a cholinergic reaction (muscarinic side effects, skeletal muscle fasciculations and increased muscle weakness) occurs after injection of 0.2 ml (2 mg), the test is discontinued and atropine sulfate 0.4 mg to 0.5 mg is administered intravenously. After one-half hour the test may be repeated.

Intramuscular Dosage (Adults): In adults with inaccessible veins, dosage for intramuscular injection is 1 ml (10 mg) of Edrophonium Chloride. Subjects who demonstrate hyperreactivity to this injection (cholinergic reaction), should be retested after one-half hour with 0.2 ml (2 mg) of Edrophonium Chloride intramuscularly to rule out false-negative reactions.

Dosage (Children): The intravenous testing dose of Edrophonium Chloride in children weighing up to 75 lbs is 0.1 ml (1 mg); above this weight, the dose is 0.2 ml (2 mg). If there is no response after 45 seconds, it may be titrated up to 0.5 ml (5 mg) in children under 75 lbs, given in increments of 0.1 ml (1 mg) every 30 to 45 seconds and up to 1 ml (10 mg) in heavier children. In infants, the recommended dose is 0.05 ml (0.5 mg). Because of technical difficulty with intravenous injection in children, the intramuscular route may be used. In children weighing up to 75 lbs, 0.2 ml (2 mg) is injected intramuscularly. In children weighing more than 75 lbs, 0.5 ml (5 mg) is injected intramuscularly. All signs which would appear with the intravenous test appear with the intramuscular test except that there is a delay of two to ten minutes before a reaction is noted.

Edrophonium Chloride Test for Evaluation of Treatment Requirements in Myasthenia Gravis: The recommended dose is 0.1 ml to 0.2 ml (1 mg to 2 mg) of Edrophonium Chloride, administered intravenously one hour after oral intake of the drug being used in treatment.[1-5] Response will be myasthenic in the undertreated patient, adequate in the controlled patient, and cholinergic in the overtreated patient. Responses to Edrophonium Chloride in myasthenic and nonmyasthenic individuals are summarized in the accompanying chart.[2]

	Myasthenic*	Adequate†	Cholinergic‡
Muscle Strength (ptosis, diplopia, dysphonia, dysphagia, dysarthria, respiration, limb strength)	Increased	No change	Decreased
Fasciculations (orbicularis oculi, facial muscles, limb muscles)	Absent	Present or absent	Present or absent
Side reactions (lacrimation, diaphoresis, salivation, abdominal cramps, nausea, vomiting, diarrhea)	Absent	Minimal	Severe

* *Myasthenic Response—occurs in untreated myasthenics and may serve to establish diagnosis; in patients under treatment, indicates that therapy is inadequate.*

† *Adequate Response—observed in treated patients when therapy is stabilized; a typical response in normal individuals. In addition to this response in nonmyasthenics, the phenomenon of forced lid closure is often observed in psychoneurotics.*

‡ *Cholinergic Response—seen in myasthenics who have been overtreated with anticholinesterase drugs.*

Edrophonium Chloride Test in Crisis: The term *crisis* is applied to the myasthenic whenever severe respiratory distress with objective ventilatory inadequacy occurs and the response to medication is not predictable. This state may be secondary to a sudden increase in severity of myasthenia gravis (myasthenic crisis), or to overtreatment with anticholinesterase drugs (cholinergic crisis).

When a patient is apneic, controlled ventilation must be secured immediately in order to avoid cardiac arrest and irreversible central nervous system damage. No attempt is made to test with Edrophonium Chloride until respiratory exchange is adequate. *Dosage used at this time is most important:* If the patient is cholinergic, Edrophonium Chloride will cause increased oropharyngeal secretions and further weakness in the muscles of respiration. If the crisis is myasthenic, the test clearly improves respiration and the patient can be treated with longer-acting intravenous anticholinesterase medication. When the test is performed, there should not be more than 0.2 ml (2 mg) Edrophonium Chloride in the syringe. An intravenous dose of 0.1 ml (1 mg) is given initially. The patient's heart action is carefully observed. If, after an interval of one minute, this dose does not further impair the patient, the remaining 0.1 ml (1 mg) can be injected. If no clear improvement of respiration occurs after 0.2 ml (2 mg) dose, it is usually wisest to discontinue all anticholinesterase drug therapy and secure controlled ventilation by tracheostomy with assisted respiration.[5]

For Use as a Curare Antagonist: Edrophonium Chloride should be administered by intravenous injection in 1 ml (10 mg) doses given slowly over a period of 30 to 45 seconds so that the onset of cholinergic reaction can be detected. This dosage may be repeated whenever necessary. The maximal dose for any one patient should be 4 ml (40 mg). Because of its brief effect, Edrophonium Chloride should not be given prior to the administration of curare, tubocurarine, gallamine triethiodide or dimethyl-tubocurarine; it should be used at the time when its effect is needed. When given to counteract curare overdosage, the effect of each dose on the respiration should be carefully observed before it is repeated, and assisted ventilation should always be employed.

Parental drug products should be inspected visually for particulate matter and discoloration prior to administration, whenever solution and container permit.

Storage: Edrophonium Chloride should be stored between 15°C and 30°C (59°F and 86°F).

REFERENCES

1. Osserman, K.E. and Kaplan, L.I., *J.A.M.A., 150: 265, 1952.* 2. Osserman, K.E., Kaplan, L.I. and Besson, G., *J. Mt. Sinai Hosp., 20:* 165, 1953. 3. Osserman, K.E. and Kaplan, L.I., *Arch. Neurol. & Psychiat., 70:* 385, 1953. 4. Osserman, K.E. and Teng, P., *J.A.M.A., 160:*153, 1956. 5. Osserman, K.E. and Genkins, G., *Ann. N.Y. Acad. Sci., 135:* 312, 1966. 6. Tether, J.E., Second International Symposium Proceedings, Myasthenia Gravis, 1961, p. 444. 7. Tether, J.E., in H.F. Conn: *Current Therapy 1960,* Philadelphia, W. B. Saunders Company, p. 551. 8. Tether, J.E., in H.F. Conn: *Current Therapy 1965,* Philadelphia, W. B. Saunders Company, p. 556. 9. Grob, D. and Johns, R.J., *J.A.M.A., 166:* 1855, 1958.

HOW SUPPLIED
INJECTION: 10 MG/ML

AVERAGE UNIT PRICE (AVAILABLE SIZES)

BRAND			$1.85

BRAND/MANUFACTURER	NDC	SIZE	AWP
◆ BRAND			
ENLON: Ohmeda	10019-0873-15	15 ml	$10.29
TENSILON: ICN	00187-3200-10	1 ml 10s	$40.80
	00187-3200-20	10 ml 10s	$184.62
REVERSOL: Organon	00052-0466-34	10 ml 25s	$198.00

E.E.S. *SEE* ERYTHROMYCIN, ORAL

Effexor *SEE* VENLAFAXINE HYDROCHLORIDE

Efudex *SEE* FLUOROURACIL, TOPICAL

Efudex *SEE* FLUOROURACIL, SYSTEMIC

Elase *SEE* CHLORAMPHENICOL/DESOXYRIBONUCLEASE/ FIBRINOLYSIN

Elavil *SEE* AMITRIPTYLINE HYDROCHLORIDE

Eldepryl *SEE* SELEGILINE HYDROCHLORIDE

Eldopaque Forte *SEE* HYDROQUINONE

Eldoquin Forte *SEE* HYDROQUINONE

Electrolytes and Polyethylene Glycol 3350

DESCRIPTION

Electrolytes/Polyethylene Glycol 3350 is available as a powder for reconstitution containing, under the trade name GOLYTELY:

Polyethylene Glycol 3350	236 g
Sodium Sulfate	22.74 g
Sodium Bicarbonate	6.74 g
Sodium Chloride	5.86 g
Potassium Chloride	2.97 g

OR, under the trade name NULYTELY:

Polyethylene Glycol 3350	420 g
Sodium Bicarbonate	5.72 g
Sodium Chloride	11.2 g
Potassium Chloride	1.48 g

OR, under the trade name COLYTE: (in solution)

Polyethylene Glycol 3350	60 g/L
Sodium Chloride	1.46 g/L
Potassium Chloride	0.745 g/L
Sodium Bicarbonate	1.68 g/L
Sodium Sulfate	5.68 g/L
Flavor ingredients (when present)	0.483 g/L

When dissolved in sufficient water to make 4 liters, the final solution contains 125 mEq/L sodium, 10 mEq/L potassium, 20 mEq/L bicarbonate, 80 mEq/L sulfate, 35 mEq/L chloride and 18 mEq/L Polyethylene Glycol 3350.

When dissolved in water to a volume of 4 liters, Electrolytes/Polyethylene Gylcol 3350 is an isosmotic solution. Electrolytes/Polyethylene Glycol 3350 is administered orally or via nasogastric tube.

CLINICAL PHARMACOLOGY
Electrolytes/Polyethylene Glycol 3350 induces a diarrhea which rapidly cleanses the bowel, usually within four hours. The osmotic activity of Polyethylene Glycol 3350 and the Electrolyte concentration result in virtually no net absorption or excretion of ions or water. Accordingly, large volumes may be administered without significant changes in fluid or electrolyte balance.

INDICATIONS AND USAGE
Electrolytes/Polyethylene Glycol 3350 is indicated for bowel cleansing prior to colonoscopy and barium enema x-ray examination.

CONTRAINDICATIONS
Electrolytes/Polyethylene Glycol 3350 is contraindicated in patients with gastrointestinal obstruction, gastric retention, bowel perforation, toxic colitis, toxic megacolon or ileus.

WARNINGS
No additional ingredients, e.g., flavorings, should be added to the solution. Electrolytes/Polyethylene Glycol 3350 should be used with caution in patients with severe ulcerative colitis.

PRECAUTIONS
General: Patients with impaired gag reflex, unconscious or semiconscious patients, and patients prone to regurgitation or aspiration should be observed during the administration of Electrolyte/Polyethylene Glycol 3350, especially if it is administered via nasogastric tube. If a patient experiences severe bloating, distention or abdominal pain, administration should be slowed or temporarily discontinued until the symptoms abate. If gastrointestinal obstruction or perforation is suspected, appropriate studies should be performed to rule out these conditions before administration of Electrolytes/Polyethylene Glycol 3350.

Information for Patients: Electrolytes/Polyethylene Glycol 3350 produces a watery stool which cleanses the bowel before examination. Prepare the solution according to the instructions on the bottle. It is more palatable if chilled. For best results, no solid food should be consumed during the 3 to 4 hour period before drinking the solution, but in no case should solid foods be eaten within 2 hours of taking Electrolytes/Polyethylene Glycol 3350.

Drink 240 ml (8 fl. oz.) every 10 minutes. Rapid drinking of each portion is better than drinking small amounts continuously. The first bowel movement should occur approximately one hour after the start of Electrolytes/Polyethylene Glycol 3350 admininstration. You may experience some abdominal bloating and distention before the bowels start to move. If severe discomfort or distention occurs, stop drinking temporarily or drink each portion at longer intervals until these symptoms disappear. Continue drinking until the watery stool is clear and free of solid matter. This usually requires at least 3 liters and it is best to drink all of the solution. Any unused portion should be discarded.

Drug Interactions: Oral medication administered within one hour of the start of administration of Electrolytes/Polyethylene Glycol 3350 may be flushed from the gastrointestinal tract and not absorbed.

Carcinogenesis, Mutagenesis, Impairment of Fertility: Carcinogenic and reproductive studies with animals have not been performed.

Pregnancy: Category C. Animal reproduction studies have not been conducted with Electrolytes/Polyethylene Glycol 3350. It is also not known whether Electrolytes/Polyethylene Glycol 3350 can cause fetal harm when administered to a pregnant woman or can affect reproductive capacity. Electrolytes/Polyethylene Glycol 3350 should be given to a pregnant woman only if clearly needed.

Pediatric Use: Safety and effectiveness in children have not been established.

ADVERSE REACTIONS
Nausea, abdominal fullness and bloating are the most common adverse reactions (occurring in up to 50% of patients) to administration of Electrolytes/Polyethylene Glycol 3350. Abdominal cramps, vomiting and anal irritation occur less frequently. These adverse reactions are transient and subside rapidly. Isolated cases of urticaria, rhinorrhea, dermatitis and (rarely) anaphylactic reaction have been reported which may represent allergic reactions.

DOSAGE AND ADMINISTRATION
The recommended dose for adults is 4 liters of Electrolytes/Polyethylene Glycol 3350 solution prior to gastrointestinal examination, as ingestion of this dose produces a satisfactory preparation in over 95% of patients. Ideally the patient should fast for approximately three or four hours prior to Electrolytes/Polyethylene Glycol 3350 administration, but in no case should solid food be given for at least two hours before the solution is given.

Electrolytes/Polyethylene Glycol 3350 is usually administered orally, but may be given via nasogastric tube to patients who are unwilling or unable to drink the solution. *Oral administration* is at a rate of 240 ml (8 fl. oz.) every 10 minutes, until 4 liters are consumed or the rectal effluent is clear. Rapid drinking of each portion is preferred to drinking small amounts continuously. *Nasogastric tube administration* is at the rate of 20-30 ml per minute (1.2-1.8 liters per hour). The first bowel movement should occur approximately one hour after the start of Electrolytes/Polyethylene Glycol 3350 administration.

Various regimens have been used. One method is to schedule patients for examination in midmorning or later, allowing the patients three hours for drinking and an additional one hour period for complete bowel evacuation. Another method is to administer Electrolytes/Polyethylene Glycol 3350 on the evening before the examination, particularly if the patient is to have a barium enema.

◆ RATED THERAPEUTICALLY EQUIVALENT; ◇ THERAPEUTIC EQUIVALENCE UNCONFIRMED; ○ UNRATED

Preparation of the Solution: Electrolytes/Polyethylene Glycol 3350 solution is prepared by filling the container to the 4 liter mark with water and shaking vigorously several times to insure that the ingredients are dissolved or dissolving the powder in a one-gallon food-grade container, in a sufficient quantity of water to produce the final volume according to package directions and mixing well. Dissolution is facilitated by using lukewarm water. The solution is more palatable if chilled before administration. The reconstituted solution should be refrigerated and used within 48 hours. Discard any unused portion.

Storage: Store in sealed container at controlled room temperature 59°-86°F (15°-30°C) or at 25°C for some brands. When reconstituted, keep solution refrigerated. Use within 48 hours. Discard unused portion.

HOW SUPPLIED
POWDER FOR RECONSTITUTION:

AVERAGE UNIT PRICE (AVAILABLE SIZES)		GENERIC A-RATED AVERAGE PRICE (GAAP)	
BRAND	$0.003	4000 gm	$12.17
GENERIC	$0.003	4000 ml	$12.17
		4000 gm	$12.13
		4000 ml	$12.13

BRAND/MANUFACTURER	NDC	SIZE	AWP
◆ BRAND			
GOLYTELY: Braintree	52268-0700-01	3840 gm	$7.80
	52268-0100-01	4000 gm	$14.46
COLOVAGE: Dynapharm	55516-0101-01	3800 ml	$13.36
COLYTE FL: Reed & Carnrick	00021-4403-13	3840 ml	$9.89
	00021-4401-49	3840 ml	$8.75
	00021-4401-23	4000 ml	$14.57
	00021-4403-05	4000 ml	$16.48
◆ GENERICS			
GO-EVAC: Rugby	00536-2776-90	4000 gm	$12.25
CO-LAV: Copley	38245-0688-18	4000 ml	$12.00
Goldline	00182-7026-86	4000 ml	$12.00
Stafford-Miller	55372-4460-01	4000 ml	$12.50
GO-EVAC: Copley	38245-0690-18	4000 ml	$12.00

POWDER FOR RECONSTITUTION:

BRAND/MANUFACTURER	NDC	SIZE	AWP
○ BRAND			
NULYTELY: Braintree	52268-0300-01	4000 ml	$15.06

Electrolytes, Injectable

DESCRIPTION
Electrolytes, Injectable, (multiple electrolyte additive) is a sterile, nonpyrogenic, *concentrated* solution of intra- and extracellular ions for intravenous infusion after dilution as a maintenance electrolyte replenisher only. The pH is 6.0 to 7.5. Osmolarity is 4.32 to 7.52 mOsmol/mL (calc.); specific gravity is 1.093 to 1.176.

Some brands are provided in a Pharmacy Bulk Package, a sterile dosage form which contains multiple single doses for use only in a pharmacy bulk admixture program.

The salts and ionic composition of a typical 20 mL dose are as follows:

Ingredient or Ion	mg/20 mL	mEq/20 mL
Sodium Acetate (trihydrate)	2700	
Sodium Gluconate	1100	
Potassium Chloride	2500	
Potassium Acetate	690	
Magnesium Acetate (tetrahydrate)	860	
Calcium Acetate (anhydrous)	395	
Sodium (Na^+)		25
Potassium (K^+)		40.6
Calcium (Ca^{++})		5
Magnesium (Mg^{++})		8
Acetate (CH_3COO^-)		40.6*
Chloride (Cl^-)		33.5
Gluconate ($C_6H_{11}O_7^-$)		5

* *May include ion for pH adjustment*

or

Ingredient or Ion	mg/20 mL	mEq/20 mL
Sodium Chloride	321	
Calcium Chloride (dihydrate)	331	
Potassium Chloride	1491	
Magnesium Chloride (hexahydrate)	508	
Sodium Acetate (anhydrous)	2420	
Sodium (Na^+)		35
Potassium (K^+)		20
Calcium (Ca^{++})		4.5
Magnesium (Mg^{++})		5
Chloride (Cl^-)		35
Acetate (CH_3COO^-)		29.5

or

Ingredient or Ion	mg/20 mL	mEq/20 mL
Sodium Chloride	438	
Sodium Acetate (anhydrous)	861	
Potassium Chloride	1342	
Magnesium Chloride (hexahydrate)	508	
Calcium Chloride (dihydrate)	331	
Sodium (Na^+)		18
Potassium (K^+)		18
Calcium (Ca^{++})		4.5
Magnesium (Mg^{++})		5
Chloride (Cl^-)		35
Acetate (CH_3COO^-)		10.5

Sodium Acetate, USP, (trihydrate) is chemically designated $CH_3COONa \cdot 3H_2O$, a white, granular powder very soluble in water. Sodium Acetate, USP, (anhydrous) is chemically designated $C_2H_3NaO_2$.

Sodium Gluconate, USP is chemically designated $C_6H_{11}NaO_7$, the normal sodium salt of gluconic acid soluble in water.

Sodium Chloride, USP is chemically designated NaCl, a white crystalline compound freely soluble in water.

Calcium Chloride, USP dihydrate is chemically designated $CaCl_2 \cdot 2H_2O$, white, odorless fragments or granules, freely soluble in water.

Potassium Chloride, USP is chemically designated KCl, a white granular powder freely soluble in water.

Potassium Acetate, USP is chemically designated CH_3COOK, colorless crystals or white crystalline powder very soluble in water.

Magnesium Acetate (tetrahydrate) is chemically designated $(CH_3COO)_2Mg \cdot 4H_2O$, colorless or white crystals very soluble in water.

Magnesium Chloride, USP hexahydrate is chemically designated $MgCl_2 \cdot 6H_2O$, deliquescent crystals very soluble in water.

Sodium Acetate, USP anhydrous is chemically designated $C_2H_3N_aO_2$, a hygroscopic powder very soluble in water.

Calcium Acetate (anhydrous) is chemically designated $(CH_3COO)_2Ca$, a crystalline hygroscopic powder soluble in water.

Water for Injection, USP is chemically designated H_2O.

The Pharmacy Bulk Package is designed for use with manual, gravity flow operations and automated compounding devices for preparing sterile parenteral nutrient admixtures. Multiple single doses may be dispensed during continual aliquoting operations. The entire contents should be dispensed within 24 hours.

CLINICAL PHARMACOLOGY
Electrolytes, Injectable, helps to maintain normal cellular metabolism during total parenteral nutrition (TPN). Providing Electrolytes in appropriate amounts prevents deficiency symptoms which otherwise would occur in their absence.

Cations: Sodium is the principal extracellular cation; it helps maintain motor nerve depolarization, proper fluid balance and normal renal metabolism. Potassium is the principal intracellular cation; it helps transport dextrose across the cell membrane and contributes to normal renal function. Magnesium is an important cofactor for enzymatic reactions and helps to maintain normal CNS (central nervous system) activity and amino acid utilization. Calcium participates in muscle contraction, blood coagulation and helps maintain normal neuromuscular function.

Anions: Chloride is the principal extracellular anion which, along with bicarbonate, is involved in maintaining proper anion balance. Acetate is an important metabolic intermediate in the tricarboxylic acid cycle and is a bicarbonate alternate. Gluconate is a theoretical metabolic alternate to bicarbonate, but its primary purpose is to complete the anion-cation balance of the solution.

The distribution and excretion of sodium (Na^+) and chloride (Cl^-) are largely under the control of the kidney which maintains a balance between intake and output.

Approximately 80% of body calcium (Ca^{++}) is excreted in the feces as insoluble salts; urinary excretion accounts for the remaining 20%.

Potassium (K^+) is found in low concentration in the plasma and extracellular fluids (3.5 to 5.0 mEq/liter in a healthy adult). Normally about 80% to 90% of the potassium intake is excreted in the urine, the remainder in the stools and to a small extent, in the perspiration. The kidney does not conserve potassium well so that during fasting or in patients on a potassium-free diet, potassium loss from the body continues resulting in potassium depletion.

Magnesium (Mg^{++}) is the second most plentiful intracellular cation. Normal plasma concentration ranges from 1.5 to 2.5 or 3 mEq/L. Magnesium is excreted solely by the kidney at a rate proportional to the plasma concentration and glomerular filtration.

Acetate (CH_3COO^-) provides bicarbonate (HCO_3^-) by metabolic conversion in the liver. This has been shown to proceed readily even in the presence of severe liver disease. Although gluconate is a theoretical alternate metabolic source of bicarbonate, a significant antiacidotic action has not been established. Gluconate serves primarily to complete the cation-anion balance of the solution.

INDICATIONS AND USAGE
Electrolytes, Injectable, is indicated for use as a supplement to nutritional solutions containing concentrated dextrose and amino acids delivered by central venous infusion, to help maintain Electrolyte homeostasis in adult patients.

TPN Electrolytes II (multiple electrolyte additive) is indicated for use with Potassium Phosphates Injection, USP as a supplement to nutritional solutions containing concentrated dextrose and amino acids (in particular, Aminosyn II) delivered by central venous infusion, to help maintain electrolyte homeostasis in adult patients.

CONTRAINDICATIONS

Electrolytes, Injectable, is contraindicated in pathological conditions where additives of potassium, sodium, calcium, magnesium or chloride could be clinically deleterious, e.g. anuria, hyperkalemia, heart block or myocardial damage and severe edema due to cardiovascular, renal or hepatic failure.

WARNINGS

Concentrated, Hypertonic, Additive Solution. **Must be diluted** in TPN solution and thoroughly mixed prior to administration.

Contains No Phosphate. Patients receiving TPN solutions containing concentrated dextrose require additive phosphate, in addition to Electrolytes, Injectable. Between 10 and 15 mM (310 to 465 mg) phosphorus are physically compatible with as much as 10 to 12 mEq calcium in the same 1000 mL admixture. A potassium phosphate additive will supply needed phosphorus as well as potassium for central vein TPN, or, as the concentration of sodium in some brands of Electrolytes, Injectable, is only 25 mEq/20 mL (target for TPN is 35 to 45 mEq/L), a sodium phosphate additive will supply needed phosphorus as well as sodium for central vein TPN. The phosphate supplement should first be added to the amino acid or dextrose container and diluted well to avoid precipitation with calcium.

The target concentration for sodium in TPN ranges from 35 to 45 mEq/L. If a sufficient amount of sodium is not present in the final admixture, consider adding more sodium.

The potassium content of other additives, such as potassium phosphate or potassium-containing antibiotics, must be considered in the context of total potassium delivered. TPN patients usually require 30 to 50 mEq of potassium per liter of TPN solution containing concentrated (20 to 25%) dextrose.

Not Intended For Pediatric Use.

Solutions containing sodium ions should be used with great care, if at all, in patients with congestive heart failure, severe renal insufficiency and in clinical states in which there exists edema with sodium retention.

Solutions which contain potassium ions should be used with great care, if at all, in patients with hyperkalemia, severe renal failure and in conditions in which potassium retention is present.

In patients with diminished renal function, administration of solutions containing sodium or potassium ions may result in sodium or potassium retention.

Solutions containing acetate ions should be used with great care in patients with metabolic or respiratory alkalosis. Acetate should be administered with great care in those conditions in which there is an increased level or an impaired utilization of this ion, such as severe hepatic insufficiency.

PRECAUTIONS

Do not administer unless solution is clear and seal is intact. Discard unused portion.

Blood levels of sodium, potassium, calcium, magnesium, phosphorus and chloride should be monitored frequently during TPN. Significant deviations from normal may justify further supplementation or substitution of individual Electrolyte additives (in place of Electrolytes, Injectable) to tailor the Electrolyte supplement to meet individual patient requirements.

In patients with renal dysfunction or cardiovascular insufficiency, especially in elderly or postsurgical patients, consider the potential effects of sodium and potassium present in each 20 mL volume of Electrolytes, Injectable.

Extraordinary Electrolyte losses are not necessarily corrected by Electrolytes, Injectables. In protracted vomiting or diarrhea or in patients with fistula drainage or nasogastric suction, separate replacement therapy may be necessary, based upon analysis of losses sustained.

Caution must be exercised in the administration of parenteral fluids, especially those containing sodium ions, to patients receiving corticosteroids or corticotropin.

Solutions containing acetate ions should be used with caution as excess administration may result in metabolic alkalosis.

Pregnancy Category C: Animal reproduction studies have not been conducted with Electrolytes, Injectable. It is also not known whether Electrolytes, Injectable, can cause fetal harm when administered to a pregnant woman or can affect reproduction capacity. Electrolytes, Injectable, should be given to a pregnant woman only if clearly needed.

ADVERSE REACTIONS

Symptoms may result from an excess or deficit of one or more of the ions present in Electrolytes, Injectable. Therefore, frequent monitoring of Electrolyte blood levels is recommended. Sodium excess can cause edema and exacerbation of congestive heart failure. Excess potassium can cause deviations from the normal ECG (electrocardiogram). Potassium deficits can impair neuromuscular function, causing muscle weakness or frank paralysis, intestinal dilatation and ileus. Calcium deficits can produce neuromuscular hyperexcitability, ranging from paresthesias, cramps and laryngospasm to tetany and grand mal seizures. Depressed calcium levels can accompany administration of parenteral phosphorus or large amounts of albumin. Magnesium deficiency can precipitate neuromuscular dysfunction, hyperirritability, psychotic behavior, tachycardia and hypertension. Magnesium excess can cause muscle weakness, ECG changes, sedation and mental confusion.

DRUG ABUSE AND DEPENDENCE

None known.

OVERDOSAGE

In the event of overhydration or solute overload, re-evaluate the patient and institute appropriate corrective measures. See *"Warnings"* and *"Precautions"*.

DOSAGE AND ADMINISTRATION

Electrolytes, Injectable, in the Pharmacy Bulk Package is designed for use with manual, gravity flow operations and automated compounding devices for preparing sterile nutrient admixtures.

One 20 mL volume of Electrolytes, Injectable, is added to each liter of amino acid/dextrose solution. Alternatively, the Electrolytes, Injectable, can be added to the container of amino acids or concentrated dextrose, to permit addition of the necessary phosphate additive to the remaining container. This latter technique helps avoid physical incompatibilities between calcium and phosphorus. A sodium or potassium phosphate additive is recommended for addition to nutritional solutions containing Electrolytes, Injectable. The final concentration of sodium or potassium for central vein TPN admixtures usually approximates 40 mEq/L (± 10 mEq/L).

Between two and three liters of TPN solution with added Electrolytes, Injectable, are usually administered daily to adults. Solutions are given continuously over the entire 24-hour period at a constant rate, ranging from 83 to 125 mL/hour. TPN solutions containing Electrolytes, Injectable, and concentrated dextrose are administered intravenously, through a central venous catheter.

Parenteral drug products should be inspected visually for particulate matter and discoloration prior to administration, whenever solution and container permit. See *"Precautions"*.

RECOMMENDED DIRECTIONS FOR USE OF THE PHARMACY BULK PACKAGE

Use Aseptic Technique:

1. During use, container must be stored, and all manipulations performed, in an appropriate laminar flow hood.

2. Remove fliptop from vial and cleanse stopper with antiseptic.

3. Pierce stopper with transfer device. Insertion of transfer device into stopper should be performed only once in a Pharmacy Bulk Package solution without antimicrobial preservative. The time frame permitted for container withdrawals should be as brief as possible, usually no longer than needed to systematically complete aliquoting operations without interruption. Discard container within 24 hours after penetration.

4. Sequentially dispense aliquots of Electrolytes, Injectable, into pooling containers using appropriate transfer device. During fluid transfer operations, the Pharmacy Bulk Package should be maintained under the recommended storage conditions.

STORAGE

Exposure of pharmaceutical products to heat should be minimized. Avoid excessive heat. Protect from freezing. It is recommended that the product be stored at room temperature (25° C); however, brief exposure up to 40°C does not adversely affect the product.

Store the Pharmacy Bulk Package at controlled room temperature 15° to 30°C (59° to 86°F).

HOW SUPPLIED
INJECTION:

AVERAGE UNIT PRICE (AVAILABLE SIZES)

BRAND	$0.22
GENERIC	$0.31

BRAND/MANUFACTURER	NDC	SIZE	AWP
◆ **BRAND**			
LYPHOLYTE II: Fujisawa	00469-1460-40	20 ml	$5.51
LYPHOLYTE: Fujisawa	00469-0900-40	20 ml	$6.60
TRACELYTE: Fujisawa	00469-0800-40	20 ml	$11.57
TRACELYTE II: Fujisawa	00469-1470-40	20 ml	$12.24
LYPHOLYTE: Fujisawa	00469-1460-60	40 ml	$11.11
TRACELYTE DOUBLE ELECTROLYTES: Fujisawa	00469-1550-60	40 ml	$11.57
TRACELYTE II DOUBLE ELECTROLYTES: Fujisawa	00469-1570-60	40 ml	$11.57
LYPHOLYTE: Fujisawa	00469-0900-60	40 ml	$12.70
LYPHOLYTE II: Fujisawa	00469-1461-00	100 ml	$24.41
LYPHOLYTE: Fujisawa	00469-0901-00	100 ml	$29.86
LYPHOLYTE II: Fujisawa	00469-1462-00	200 ml	$41.83
LYPHOLYTE: Fujisawa	00469-0902-00	200 ml	$53.13
NORMOSOL-R PH 7.4: Abbott Hosp	00074-1570-05	1000 ml 6s	$163.31
PLASMA-LYTE 56: Baxter	00338-0167-04	1000 ml 12s	$121.68
	00338-0168-04	1000 ml 12s	$195.96
PLASMA-LYTE: Baxter	00338-0177-04	1000 ml 12s	$199.44
PLASMA-LYTE 148: Baxter	00338-0179-04	1000 ml 12s	$221.76
NORMOSOL-R: Abbott Hosp	00074-7967-09	1000 ml 12s	$226.01
PLASMA-LYTE A PH-7.4: Baxter	00338-0221-04	1000 ml 12s	$301.10
NORMOSOL-R PH 7.4: Abbott Hosp	00074-7670-09	1000 ml 12s	$306.95
PLASMA-LYTE 148: Baxter	00338-0179-03	500 ml 24s	$387.65
NORMOSOL-R: Abbott Hosp	00074-7967-03	500 ml 24s	$395.01
PLASMA-LYTE A PH-7.4: Baxter	00338-0221-03	500 ml 24s	$498.82
NORMOSOL-R PH 7.4: Abbott Hosp	00074-7670-03	500 ml 24s	$508.44
TPN ELECTROLYTES: Abbott Hosp	00074-5779-01	20 ml 25s	$181.39
TPN ELECTROLYTES III: Abbott Hosp	00074-3844-01	20 ml 25s	$187.03
TPN ELECTROLYTES: Abbott Hosp	00074-5881-01	20 ml 25s	$231.56

◆ RATED THERAPEUTICALLY EQUIVALENT; ◇ THERAPEUTIC EQUIVALENCE UNCONFIRMED; ○ UNRATED

BRAND/MANUFACTURER	NDC	SIZE	AWP
	00074-5882-01	20 ml 25s	$297.17
	00074-3296-06	100 ml 25s	$598.80
TPN ELECTROLYTES III: Abbott Hosp	00074-3298-06	100 ml 25s	$617.80
◆ GENERICS			
Abbott Hosp	00074-3236-01	20 ml 25s	$187.03
Abbott Hosp	00074-3297-06	100 ml 25s	$617.80

INJECTION:

BRAND/MANUFACTURER	NDC	SIZE	AWP
○ BRAND			
HYPERLYTE: McGaw	00703-5300-04	25 ml	$7.19
HYPERLYTE R: McGaw	00703-5310-04	25 ml	$7.19
HYPERLYTE: McGaw	00264-1943-20	250 ml	$29.78
ISOLYTE S PH 7.4: McGaw	00264-7707-10	500 ml	$20.72
ISOLYTE S: McGaw	00264-7703-10	500 ml	$23.47
ISOLYTE E: McGaw	00264-7700-00	1000 ml	$18.49
ISOLYTE S: McGaw	00264-7703-00	1000 ml	$25.46
ISOLYTE S PH 7.4: McGaw	00264-7707-00	1000 ml	$25.50

Elimite SEE PERMETHRIN

Elixophyllin SEE GUAIFENESIN AND THEOPHYLLINE, THEOPHYLLINE AND POTASSIUM IODIDE AND THEOPHYLLINE

Elocon SEE MOMETASONE FUROATE

Elspar SEE ASPARAGINASE

Emcyt SEE ESTRAMUSTINE PHOSPHATE SODIUM

Emete-con SEE BENZQUINAMIDE HYDROCHLORIDE

Eminase SEE ANISTREPLASE

EMLA SEE LIDOCAINE WITH PRILOCAINE

Empirin with Codeine SEE ASPIRIN WITH CODEINE PHOSPHATE

E-Mycin SEE ERYTHROMYCIN, ORAL

Enalapril

USE IN PREGNANCY
WHEN USED IN PREGNANCY DURING THE SECOND AND THIRD TRIMESTERS, ACE INHIBITORS CAN CAUSE INJURY AND EVEN DEATH TO THE DEVELOPING FETUS. WHEN PREGNANCY IS DETECTED, ENALAPRIL SHOULD BE DISCONTINUED AS SOON AS POSSIBLE. SEE *"WARNINGS. FETAL/NEONATAL MORBIDITY AND MORTALITY."*

DESCRIPTION
Enalapril Maleate is the maleate salt of Enalapril, the ethyl ester of a long-acting angiotensin converting enzyme inhibitor, enalaprilat. Enalapril Maleate is chemically described as (S)-1-[N-[1-(ethoxycarbonyl)-3-phenylpropyl]-L-al anyl] -L-proline, (Z)-2-butenedioate salt (1:1). Its empirical formula is $C_{20}H_{28}N_2O_5 \cdot C_4H_4O_4$.

Enalapril Maleate is a white to off-white, crystalline powder with a molecular weight of 492.53. It is sparingly soluble in water, soluble in ethanol, and freely soluble in methanol. Enalapril is a pro-drug; following oral administration, it is bioactivated by hydrolysis of the ethyl ester to Enalaprilat, which is the active angiotensin converting enzyme inhibitor.

Enalaprilat is a sterile aqueous solution for intravenous administration. It is chemically described as (S)-1-[N-(1-carboxy-3-phenylpropyl)-L-alanyl]-L-proline dihydrate. Its empirical formula is $C_{18}H_{24}N_2O_5 \cdot 2H_2O$.

Enalaprilat is a white to off-white, crystalline powder with a molecular weight of 384.43. It is sparingly soluble in methanol and slightly soluble in water.

Each tablet contains:
Enalapril Maleate 2.5, 5, 10, or 20 mg

Each mL of intravenous solution contains:
Enalaprilat 1.25 mg

Following is its chemical structure:

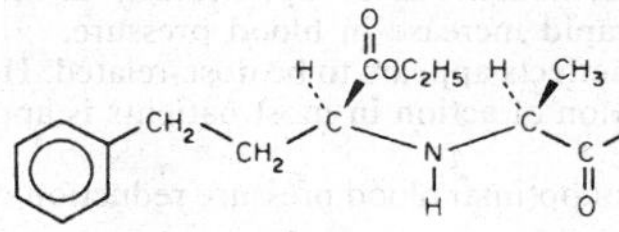

CLINICAL PHARMACOLOGY
Enalaprilat, an angiotensin-converting enzyme (ACE) inhibitor when administered intravenously, is the active metabolite of the orally administered pro-drug, Enalapril Maleate. Enalaprilat is poorly absorbed orally.

MECHANISM OF ACTION
Intravenous Enalaprilat, or oral Enalapril, after hydrolysis to enalaprilat, inhibits angiotensin-converting enzyme (ACE) in human subjects and animals. ACE is a peptidyl dipeptidase that catalyzes the conversion of angiotensin I to the vasoconstrictor substance, angiotensin II. Angiotensin II also stimulates aldosterone secretion by the adrenal cortex. The beneficial effects of Enalapril in hypertension and heart failure appear to result primarily from suppression of the renin-angiotensin-aldosterone system. Inhibition of ACE results in decreased plasma angiotensin II, which leads to decreased vasopressor activity and to decreased aldosterone secretion. Although the latter decrease is small, it results in small increases of serum potassium. In hypertensive patients treated with Enalapril alone for up to 48 weeks, mean increases in serum potassium of approximately 0.2 mEq/L were observed. In patients treated with Enalapril plus a thiazide diuretic, there was essentially no change in serum potassium. (See *"Precautions."*) Removal of angiotensin II negative feedback on renin secretion leads to increased plasma renin activity.

ACE is identical to kininase, an enzyme that degrades bradykinin. Whether increased levels of bradykinin, a potent vasodepressor peptide, play a role in the therapeutic effects of Enalapril remains to be elucidated.

While the mechanism through which Enalapril lowers blood pressure is believed to be primarily suppression of the renin-angiotensin-aldosterone system, Enalapril is antihypertensive even in patients with low-renin hypertension. Although Enalaprilat was antihypertensive in all races studied, black hypertensive patients (usually a low-renin hypertensive population) had a smaller average response to Enalapril or enalaprilat monotherapy than non-black patients.

PHARMACOKINETICS AND METABOLISM
Following oral administration of Enalapril, peak serum concentrations of Enalapril occur within about one hour. Based on urinary recovery, the extent of absorption of Enalapril is approximately 60 percent. Enalapril absorption is not influenced by the presence of food in the gastrointestinal tract. Following absorption, Enalapril is hydrolyzed to enalaprilat, which is a more potent angiotensin converting enzyme inhibitor than Enalapril; enalaprilat is poorly absorbed when administered orally. Peak serum concentrations of Enalaprilat occur three to four hours after an oral dose of Enalapril Maleate. Excretion of Enalapril/enalaprilat is primarily renal. Approximately 94 percent of the dose is recovered in the urine and feces as Enalaprilat or Enalapril within 24 hours. The principal components in urine are Enalaprilat, accounting for about 40 percent of the dose, and intact Enalapril. There is no evidence of metabolites of Enalapril, other than Enalaprilat.

Following intravenous administration of a single dose, the serum concentration profile of enalaprilat is polyexponential with a prolonged terminal phase, apparently representing a small fraction of the administered dose that has been bound to ACE. The amount bound does not increase with dose, indicating a saturable site of binding. The effective half-life for accumulation of Enalaprilat following multiple doses of Enalapril Maleate is 11 hours.

The disposition of Enalapril and enalaprilat in patients with renal insufficiency is similar to that in patients with normal renal function until the glomerular filtration rate is 30 mL/min or less. With glomerular filtration rate ≤ 30 mL/min, peak and trough Enalaprilat levels increase, time to peak concentration increases and time to steady state may be delayed. The effective half-life of Enalapril after intravenous administration of following multiple doses of Enalapril Maleate is prolonged at this level of renal insufficiency. (See *"Dosage and Administration."*) Enalaprilat is dialyzable at the rate of 62 mL/min. Studies in dogs indicate that Enalapril crosses the blood-brain barrier poorly, if at all; Enalaprilat does not enter the brain. Multiple doses of Enalapril Maleate in rats do not result in accumulation in any tissues. Milk of lactating rats contains radioactivity following administration of [14]C Enalapril Maleate. Radioactivity was found to cross the placenta following administration of labeled drug to pregnant hamsters.

► SHOWN IN PRODUCT IDENTIFICATION GUIDE

PHARMACODYNAMICS AND CLINICAL EFFECTS

Hypertension: Administration of Enalapril or enalaprilat to patients with hypertension of severity ranging from mild to severe results in a reduction of both supine and standing systolic and diastolic blood pressure usually with no orthostatic component. Symptomatic postural hypotension is therefore infrequent, although it might be anticipated in volume-depleted patients. (See *"Warnings."*)

In most patients studied, after oral administration of a single dose of Enalapril, onset of antihypertensive activity was seen at one hour with peak reduction of blood pressure achieved by four to six hours.

At recommended doses, antihypertensive effects have been maintained for at least 24 hours. In some patients the effects may diminish toward the end of the dosing interval (see *"Dosage and Administration."*) The onset of action usually occurs within fifteen minutes of administration of Enalaprilat with the maximum effect occurring within one to four hours. The abrupt withdrawal of Enalaprilat has not been associated with a rapid increase in blood pressure.

The duration of hemodynamic effects appears to be dose-related. However, for the recommended dose, the duration of action in most patients is approximately six hours.

In some patients achievement of optimal blood pressure reduction may require several weeks of therapy.

The antihypertensive effects of Enalapril have continued during long term therapy. Abrupt withdrawal of Enalapril has not been associated with a rapid increase in blood pressure.

In hemodynamic studies in patients with essential hypertension, blood pressure reduction was accompanied by a reduction in peripheral arterial resistance with an increase in cardiac output and little or no change in heart rate. Following administration of Enalapril or enalaprilat, there is an increase in renal blood flow; glomerular filtration rate is usually unchanged. The effects appear to be similar in patients with renovascular hypertension.

When given together with thiazide-type diuretics, the blood pressure lowering effects of Enalapril are approximately additive.

In a clinical pharmacology study, indomethacin or sulindac was administered to hypertensive patients receiving Enalapril. In this study there was no evidence of a blunting of the antihypertensive action of Enalapril.

Heart Failure: In trials in patients treated with digitalis and diuretics, treatment with Enalapril resulted in decreased systemic vascular resistance, blood pressure, pulmonary capillary wedge pressure and heart size, and increased cardiac output and exercise tolerance. Heart rate was unchanged or slightly reduced, and mean ejection fraction was unchanged or increased. There was a beneficial effect on severity of heart failure as measured by the New York Heart Association (NYHA) classification and on symptoms of dyspnea and fatigue. Hemodynamic effects were observed after the first dose, and appeared to be maintained in uncontrolled studies lasting as long as four months. Effects on exercise tolerance, heart size, and severity and symptoms of heart failure were observed in placebo-controlled studies lasting from eight weeks to over one year. From the results of one trial involving an ACE inhibitor other than Enalapril, it appears that the symptomatic benefit associated with that ACE inhibitor's use dose not depend upon digitalis being present.

Heart Failure, Mortality Trials: In a multicenter, placebo-controlled clinical trial, 2,569 patients with all degrees of symptomatic heart failure and ejection fraction ≤ 35 percent were randomized to placebo or Enalapril and followed for up to 55 months (SOLVD-Treatment). Use of Enalapril was associated with an 11 percent reduction in all cause mortality and a 30 percent reduction in hospitalization for heart failure. Disease that excluded patients from enrollment in the study included severe stable angina (> 2 attacks/day), hemodynamically significant valvular or outflow tract obstruction, renal failure (creatinine > 2.5 mg/dL), cerebral vascular disease (e.g., significant carotid artery disease), advanced pulmonary disease, malignancies, active myocarditis and constrictive pericarditis. The mortality benefit associated with Enalapril does not appear to depend upon digitalis being present.

A second multicenter trial used the SOLVD protocol for study of asymptomatic or minimally symptomatic patients. SOLVD-Prevention patients, who had left ventricular ejection fraction ≤ 35% and no history of symptomatic heart failure, were randomized to placebo (n = 2117) or Enalapril (n = 2111) and followed for up to 5 years. The majority of patients in the SOLVD-Prevention trial had a history of ischemic heart disease. A history of myocardial infarction was present in 80 percent of patients, current angina pectoris in 34 percent, and a history of hypertension in 37 percent. No statistically significant mortality effect was demonstrated in this population. Enalapril-treated subjects had 32% fewer first hospitalizations for heart failure, and 32% fewer total heart failure hospitalizations. Compared to placebo, 32 percent fewer patients receiving Enalapril developed symptoms of overt heart failure. Hospitalizations for cardiovascular reasons were also reduced. There was an insignificant reduction in hospitalizations for any cause in the Enalapril treatment group (for Enalapril vs. placebo, respectively, 1166 vs. 1201 first hospitalizations, 2649 vs. 2840 total hospitalizations), although the study was not powered to look for such an effect.

The SOLVD-Prevention trial was not designed to determine whether treatment of asymptomatic patients with low ejection fraction would be superior, with respect to preventing hospitalization, to closer follow-up and use of Enalapril at the earliest sign of heart failure. However, under the conditions of follow-up in the SOLVD-Prevention trial (every 4 months at the study clinic; personal physician as needed), 68% of patients on placebo who were hospitalized for heart failure had no prior symptoms recorded which would have signaled initiation of treatment.

The SOLVD-Prevention trial was also not designed to show whether Enalapril modified the progression of underlying heart disease.

In another multicenter, placebo-controlled trial (CONSENSUS) limited to patients with NYHA class IV congestive heart failure and radiographic evidence of cardiomegaly, use of Enalapril was associated with improved survival. The results are shown in the following table.

| | Survival (%) | |
	Six Months	One Year
Enalapril (n = 127)	74	64
Placebo (n = 126)	56	48

In both CONSENSUS and SOLVD-Treatment trials, patients were also usually receiving digitalis, diuretics or both.

INDICATIONS AND USAGE

Hypertension: Enalapril is indicated for the treatment of hypertension. Enalapril is effective alone or in combination with other antihypertensive agents, especially thiazide-type diuretics. The blood pressure lowering effects of Enalapril and thiazides are approximately additive.

Intravenous enalaprilat is indicated for the treatment of hypertension when oral therapy is not practical.

Intravenous enalaprilat has been studied with only one other antihypertensive agent, furosemide, which showed approximately additive effects on blood pressure. Enalapril, the pro-drug of Enalaprilat, has been used extensively with a variety of other antihypertensive agents, without apparent difficulty except for occasional hypotension.

Heart Failure: Enalapril is indicated for the treatment of symptomatic congestive heart failure, usually in combination with diuretics and digitalis. In these patients Enalapril improves symptoms, increases survival, and decreases the frequency of hospitalization (see *"Clinical Pharmacology, Heart Failure, Mortality Trials"* for details and limitations of survival trials).

In using Enalapril consideration should be given to the fact that another angiotensin converting enzyme inhibitor, captopril, has caused agranulocytosis, particularly in patients with renal impairment or collagen vascular disease and that available data are insufficient to show that Enalapril does not have a similar risk. (See *"Warnings."*)

Asymptomatic Left Ventricular Dysfunction: In clinically stable asymptomatic patients with left ventricular dysfunction (ejection fraction ≤ 35 percent), Enalapril decreases the rate of development of overt heart failure and decreases the incidence of hospitalization for heart failure. (See *"Clinical Pharmacology, Heart Failure, Mortality Trials"* for details and limitations of survival trials.)

UNLABELED USES

Enalapril is used alone or as an adjunct in the treatment of angina, diabetic nephropathy, and Raynaud's disease. It is also used in hypertension associated with scleroderma renal crisis.

CONTRAINDICATIONS

Enalapril and enalaprilat are contraindicated in patients who are hypersensitive to this product and in patients with a history of angioedema related to previous treatment with an angiotensin converting enzyme inhibitor.

WARNINGS

ANGIOEDEMA

Angioedema of the face, extremities, lips, tongue, glottis and/or larynx has been reported in patients treated with angiotensin converting enzyme inhibitors, including Enalapril and enalaprilat. This may occur at any time during treatment. In such cases Enalapril or enalaprilat should be promptly discontinued and appropriate therapy and monitoring should be provided until complete and sustained resolution of signs and symptoms has occurred. In instances where swelling has been confined to the face and lips the condition has generally resolved without treatment, although antihistamines have been useful in relieving symptoms. Angioedema associated with laryngeal edema may be fatal. **Where there is involvement of the tongue, glottis or larynx, likely to cause airway obstruction, appropriate therapy, e.g., subcutaneous epinephrine solution 1:1000 (0.3 mL to 0.5 mL) and/or measures necessary to ensure a patent airway, should be promptly provided.** (See *"Adverse Reactions."*)

Patients with a history of angioedema unrelated to ACE inhibitor therapy may be at increased risk of angioedema while receiving an ACE inhibitor (see also *"Contraindications"*).

Hypotension: Excessive hypotension is rare in uncomplicated hypertensive patients treated with Enalapril alone but is a possible consequence of the use of Enalaprilat especially in severely salt/volume depleted persons such as those treated vigorously with diuretics or patients on dialysis. Patients with heart failure given Enalapril commonly have some reduction in blood pressure, especially with the first dose, but discontinuation of therapy for continuing symptomatic hypotension usually is not necessary when dosing instructions are followed: caution should be observed when initiating therapy. (See *"Dosage and Administration."*) Patients at risk for excessive hypotension, sometimes associated with oliguria and/or progressive azotemia, and rarely with acute renal failure and/or death, include those with the following conditions or characteristics: heart failure, hyponatremia, high dose diuretic therapy, recent intensive diuresis or increase in diuretic dose, renal dialysis, or severe volume and/or salt depletion of any etiology. It may be advisable to eliminate the diuretic (except in patients with heart failure), reduce the diuretic dose or increase salt intake cautiously before initiating therapy with Enalapril or enalaprilat in patients at risk for excessive hypotension who are able to tolerate such adjustments. (See *"Precautions, Drug Interactions"* and *"Adverse Reactions."*) In patients at risk for excessive hypotension, therapy should be started under very close medical supervision and such patients should be followed closely for the first two weeks of treatment and whenever the dose of Enalapril and/or diuretic is increased. Similar considerations may apply to patients with ischemic heart or cerebrovascular disease, in whom an excessive fall in blood pressure could result in a myocardial infarction or cerebrovascular accident.

In patients with heart failure given intravenous Enalaprilat, with or without associated renal insufficiency, excessive hypotension has been observed and may be associated with oliguria and/or progressive azotemia, and rarely with acute renal failure and/or death. Because of the potential for an excessive fall in blood pressure especially in these patients, therapy should be followed closely whenever the dose of Enalaprilat is adjusted and/or diuretic is increased. Similar consideration may apply to patients with ischemic heart or cerebrovascular disease, in whom an excessive fall in blood pressure could result in a myocardial infarction or cerebrovascular accident.

If excessive hypotension occurs, the patient should be placed in the supine position and, if necessary, receive an intravenous infusion of normal saline. A transient hypotensive response is not a contraindication to further doses of Enalapril or enalaprilat, which usually can be given without difficulty once the blood pressure has stabilized. If symptomatic hypotension develops, a dose reduction or discontinuation of Enalapril or concomitant diuretic may be necessary.

Neutropenia/Agranulocytosis: Another angiotensin converting enzyme inhibitor, captopril, has been shown to cause agranulocytosis and bone marrow depression, rarely in uncomplicated patients but more frequently in patients with renal impairment especially if they also have a collagen vascular disease. Available data from clinical trials of Enalapril are insufficient to show that Enalapril does not cause agranulocytosis at similar rates. Marketing experience has revealed several cases of neutropenia or agranulocytosis in which a causal relationship to Enalapril cannot be excluded. Periodic monitoring of white blood cell counts in patients with collagen vascular disease and renal disease should be considered.

Fetal/Neonatal Morbidity and Mortality: ACE inhibitors can cause fetal and neonatal morbidity and death when administered to pregnant women. Several dozen cases have been reported in the world literature. When pregnancy is detected, ACE inhibitors should be discontinued as soon as possible.

The use of ACE inhibitors during the second and third trimesters of pregnancy has been associated with fetal and neonatal injury, including hypotension, neonatal skull hypoplasia, anuria, reversible or irreversible renal failure, and death. Oligohydramnios has also been reported, presumably resulting from decreased fetal renal function: oligohydramnios in this setting has been associated with fetal limb contractures, craniofacial deformation, and hypoplastic lung development. Prematurity, intrauterine growth retardation, and patent ductus arteriosus have also been reported, although it is not clear whether these occurrences were due to the ACE-inhibitor exposure.

These adverse effects do not appear to have resulted from intrauterine ACE-inhibitor exposure that has been limited to the first trimester. Mothers whose embryos and fetuses are exposed to ACE inhibitors only during the first trimester should be so informed. Nonetheless, when patients become pregnant, physicians should make every effort to discontinue the use of enalaprilat as soon as possible.

Rarely (probably less often than once in every thousand pregnancies), no alternative to ACE inhibitors will be found. In these rare cases, the mothers should be apprised of the potential hazards to their fetuses, and serial ultrasound examinations should be performed to assess the intraamniotic environment.

If oligohydramnios is observed, enalaprilat should be discontinued unless it is considered lifesaving for the mother. Contraction stress testing (CST), a non-stress test (NST), or biophysical profiling (BPP) may be appropriate, depending upon the week of pregnancy. Patients and physicians should be aware, however, that oligohydramnios may not appear until after the fetus has sustained irreversible injury.

Infants with histories of *in utero* exposure to ACE inhibitors should be closely observed for hypotension, oliguria, and hyperkalemia. If oliguria occurs, attention should be directed toward support of blood pressure and renal perfusion. Exchange transfusion or dialysis may be required as means of reversing hypotension and/or substituting for disordered renal function. Enalapril, which crosses the placenta, has been removed from neonatal circulation by peritoneal dialysis with some clinical benefit, and theoretically may be removed by exchange transfusion, although there is no experience with the latter procedure.

No teratogenic effects of oral Enalapril were seen in studies of pregnant rats and rabbits. On a mg/kg basis, the doses used were up to 333 times (in rats), and 50 times (in rabbits) the maximum recommended human dose.

PRECAUTIONS
GENERAL
Impaired Renal Function: As a consequence of inhibiting the renin-angiotensin-aldosterone system, changes in renal function may be anticipated in susceptible individuals. In patients with severe heart failure whose renal function may depend on the activity of the renin-angiotensin-aldosterone system, treatment with angiotensin converting enzyme inhibitors, including Enalapril or enalaprilat, may be associated with oliguria and/or progressive azotemia and rarely with acute renal failure and/or death.

In clinical studies in hypertensive patients with unilateral or bilateral renal artery stenosis, increases in blood urea nitrogen and serum creatinine were observed in 20 percent of patients receiving Enalapril. These increases were almost always reversible upon discontinuation of Enalapril or enalaprilat and/or diuretic therapy. In such patients renal function should be monitored during the first few weeks of therapy.

Some patients with hypertension or heart failure with no increases in blood urea and serum creatinine, usually minor and transient, especially when Enalapril, or, in the case of hypertension, Enalaprilat, has been given concomitantly with a diuretic. This is more likely to occur in patients with pre-existing renal impairment. Dosage reduction of Enalaprilat and/or discontinuation of the diuretic and/or Enalapril may be required.

Evaluation or patients with hypertension or heart failure should always include assessment of renal function. (See *"Dosage and Administration."*)

Hemodialysis Patients: Anaphylactoid reactions have been reported in patients dialyzed with high-flux membranes and treated concomitantly with an ACE inhibitor. In these patients consideration should be given to using a different type of dialysis membrane or a different class of antihypertensive agent.

Hyperkalemia: Elevated serum potassium (greater than 5.7 mEq/L) was observed in approximately one percent of hypertensive patients in clinical trials receiving Enalapril. In most cases these were isolated values which resolved despite continued therapy. Hyperkalemia was a cause of discontinuation of therapy in 0.28 percent of hypertensive patients. In clinical trials in heart failure, hyperkalemia was observed in 3.8 percent of patients but was not a cause for discontinuation.

Risk factors for the development of hyperkalemia include renal insufficiency, diabetes mellitus, and the concomitant use of potassium-sparing diuretics, potassium supplements and/or potassium-containing salt substitutes, which should be used cautiously, if at all, with Enalapril or enalaprilat. (See *"Drug Interactions."*)

Cough: Cough has been reported with the use of ACE inhibitors. Characteristically, the cough is nonproductive, persistent and resolves after discontinuation of therapy. ACE inhibitor-induced cough should be considered as part of the differential diagnosis of cough.

Surgery/Anesthesia: In patients undergoing major surgery or during anesthesia with agents that produce hypotension, Enalapril may block angiotensin II formation secondary to compensatory renin release. If hypotension occurs and is considered to be due to this mechanism, it can be corrected by volume expansion.

INFORMATION FOR PATIENTS
Angioedema: Angioedema, including laryngeal edema, may occur at any time during treatment with angiotensin converting enzyme inhibitors, including Enalapril. Patients should be so advised and told to report immediately any signs of symptoms suggesting angioedema (swelling of face, extremities, eyes, lips, tongue, difficulty in swallowing or breathing) and to take no more drug until they have consulted with the prescribing physician.

Hypotension: Patients should be cautioned to report light-headedness, especially during the first few days of therapy. If actual syncope occurs, the patients should be told to discontinue the drug until they have consulted with the prescribing physician.

All patients should be cautioned that excessive perspiration and dehydration may lead to an excessive fall in blood pressure because of reduction in fluid volume. Other causes of volume depletion such as vomiting or diarrhea may also lead to a fall in blood pressure; patients should be advised to consult with the physician.

Hyperkalemia: Patients should be told not to use salt substitutes containing potassium without consulting their physician.

Neutropenia: Patients should be told to report promptly any indication of infection (e.g., sore throat, fever) which may be a sign of neutropenia.

Pregnancy: Female patients of childbearing age should be told about the consequences of second- and third-trimester exposure to ACE inhibitors, and they should also be told that these consequences do not appear to have resulted from intrauterine ACE-inhibitor exposure that has been limited to the first trimester. These patients should be asked to report pregnancies to their physicians as soon as possible.

Note: As with many other drugs, certain advice to patients being treated with Enalapril is warranted. This information is intended to aid in the safe and effective use of this medication. It is not a disclosure of all possible adverse or intended effects.

DRUG INTERACTIONS
Hypotension-Patients on Diuretic Therapy: Patients on diuretics and especially those in whom diuretic therapy was recently instituted, may occasionally experience an excessive reduction of blood pressure after initiation of therapy with Enalapril or enalaprilat. The possibility of hypotensive effects with Enalapril can be minimized by either discontinuing the diuretic or increasing the salt intake prior to initiation of treatment with Enalapril; the possibility of hypotensive effects with enalaprilat can be minimized by administration of an intravenous infusion of normal saline, discontinuing the diuretic or increasing the salt intake prior to initiation of treatment with enalaprilat. If it is necessary to continue the diuretic, provide close medical supervision after the initial dose for at least two hours with Enalapril, one hour with Enalaprilat, and until blood pressure has

stabilized for at least an additional hour. (See "Warnings" and "Dosage and Administration.")

Agents Causing Renin Release: The antihypertensive effect of Enalapril and enalaprilat is augmented by antihypertensive agents that cause renin release (e.g., diuretics).

Other Cardiovascular Agents: Enalapril and enalaprilat have been used concomitantly with beta adrenergic-blocking agents, methyldopa, nitrates, calcium-blocking agents, hydralazine, prazosin and digoxin without evidence of clinically significant adverse interactions.

Agents Increasing Serum Potassium: Enalapril and enalaprilat attenuate potassium loss caused by thiazide-type diuretics. Potassium-sparing diuretics (e.g., spironolactone, triamterene, or amiloride), potassium supplements, or potassium-containing salt substitutes may lead to significant increases in serum potassium. Therefore, if concomitant use of these agents is indicated because of demonstrated hypokalemia, they should be used with caution and with frequent monitoring of serum potassium. Potassium sparing agents should generally not be used in patients with heart failure receiving Enalapril.

Lithium: Lithium toxicity has been reported in patients receiving lithium concomitantly with drugs which cause elimination of sodium, including ACE inhibitors. A few cases of lithium toxicity have been reported in patients receiving concomitant Enalapril and lithium and were reversible upon discontinuation of both drugs. It is recommended that serum lithium levels be monitored frequently if Enalapril is administered concomitantly with lithium.

Carcinogenesis, Mutagenesis, Impairment of Fertility: Carcinogenity studies have not been done with enalaprilat. Enalaprilat is the bioactive form of its ethyl ester, Enalapril Maleate. There was no evidence of a tumorigenic effect when Enalapril was administered for 106 weeks to rats at doses up to 90 mg/kg/day (150 times* the maximum daily human dose). Enalapril has also been administered for 94 weeks to male and female mice at oral doses up to 90 and 180 mg/kg/day, respectively (150 and 300 times* the maximum oral daily dose for humans) and showed no evidence of carcinogenicity.

Neither Enalapril Maleate nor the active diacid was mutagenic in the Ames microbial mutagen test with or without metabolic activation. Enalapril was also negative in the following genotoxicity studies: rec-assay, reverse mutation assay with *E. coli*, sister chromatid exchange with cultured mammalian cells, and the micronucleus test with mice, as well as in an *in vivo* cytogenic study using mouse bone marrow.

There were no adverse effects on reproductive performance in male and female rats treated with 10 to 90 mg/kg/day of Enalapril.

PREGNANCY
Pregnancy Categories C: (first trimester) and D (second and third trimesters). See *"Warnings, Fetal/Neonatal Morbidity and Mortality."*

NURSING MOTHERS
Enalapril and Enalaprilat are detected in human milk in trace amounts. Caution should be exercised when Enalapril or Enalaprilat is given to a nursing mother.

PEDIATRIC USE
Safety and effectiveness in children have not been established.

ADVERSE REACTIONS
Enalapril has been evaluated for safety in more than 10,000 patients, including over 1000 patients treated for one year or more. Enalapril has been found to be generally well tolerated in controlled clinical trials involving 2987 patients.

For the most part, adverse experiences were mild and transient in nature. In clinical trials, discontinuation of therapy due to clinical adverse experiences was required in 3.3 percent of patients with hypertension and in 5.7 percent of patients with heart failure. The frequency of adverse experiences was not related to total daily dosage within the usual dosage ranges. In patients with hypertension the overall percentage of patients treated with Enalapril reporting adverse experiences was comparable to placebo.

Enalaprilat has been found to be generally well tolerated in controlled clinical trials involving 349 patients (168 with hypertension, 153 with congestive heart failure and 28 with coronary artery disease). The most frequent clinically significant adverse experience was hypotension (3.4 percent), occurring in eight patients (5.2 percent) with congestive heart failure, three (1.8 percent) with hypertension and one with coronary artery disease. Other adverse experiences occurring in greater than one percent of patients were: headache (2.9 percent) and nausea (1.1 percent).

Hypertension: Adverse experiences occurring in greater than one percent of patients with hypertension treated with Enalapril in controlled clinical trials are shown below. In patients treated with Enalapril, the maximum duration of therapy was three years; in placebo treated patients the maximum duration of therapy was 12 weeks.

	Enalapril (n = 2314) Incidence (discontinuation)	Placebo (n = 230) Incidence
Body As A Whole		
Fatigue	3.0 (< 0.1)	2.6
Orthostatic Effects	1.2 (< 0.1)	0.0
Asthenia	1.1 (0.1)	0.9
Digestive		
Diarrhea	1.4 (< 0.1)	1.7
Nausea	1.4 (0.2)	1.7
Nervous/Psychiatric		
Headache	5.2 (0.3)	9.1
Dizziness	4.3 (0.4)	4.3
Respiratory		
Cough	1.3 (0.1)	0.9
Skin		
Rash	1.4 (0.4)	0.4

Heart Failure: Adverse experiences occurring in greater than one percent of patients with heart failure treated with Enalapril are shown below. The incidences represent the experiences from both controlled and uncontrolled clinical trials (maximum duration of therapy is approximately one year). In the placebo treated patients, the incidences reported are from the controlled trials (maximum duration of therapy is 12 weeks). The percentage of patients with severe heart failure (NYHA Class IV) was 29 percent and 43 percent for patients treated with Enalapril and placebo, respectively.

	Enalapril (n = 673) Incidence (discontinuation)	Placebo (n = 339) Incidence
Body As A Whole		
Orthostatic Effects	2.2 (0.1)	0.3
Syncope	2.2 (0.1)	0.9
Chest Pain	2.1 (0.0)	2.1
Fatigue	1.8 (0.0)	1.8
Abdominal Pain	1.6 (0.4)	2.1
Asthenia	1.6 (0.1)	0.3
Cardiovascular		
Hypotension	6.7 (1.9)	0.6
Orthostatic Hypotension	1.6 (0.1)	0.3
Angina Pectoris	1.5 (0.1)	1.8
Myocardial Infarction	1.2 (0.3)	1.8
Digestive		
Diarrhea	2.1 (0.1)	1.2
Nausea	1.3 (0.1)	0.6
Vomiting	1.3 (0.0)	0.9
Nervous/Psychiatric		
Dizziness	7.9 (0.6)	0.6
Headache	1.8 (0.1)	0.6
Vertigo	1.6 (0.1)	1.2
Respiratory		
Cough	2.2 (0.0)	0.6
Bronchitis	1.3 (0.0)	0.9
Dyspnea	1.3 (0.1)	0.4
Pneumonia	1.0 (0.0)	2.4
Skin		
Rash	1.3 (0.0)	2.4
Urogenital		
Urinary Tract Infection	1.3 (0.0)	2.4

Other serious clinical adverse experiences occurring since the drug was marketed or adverse experiences occurring in 0.5 to 1.0 percent of patients with hypertension or heart failure in clinical trials are listed below.

Body as a Whole: Anaphylactoid reactions syncope, orthostatic effects, chest pain, abdominal pain, asthenia (see "Precautions, Hemodialysis Patients").

Cardiovascular: Cardiac arrest; myocardial infarction or cerebrovascular accident, possibly secondary to excessive hypotension in high risk patients (see "Warnings, Hypotension"); pulmonary embolism and infarction; pulmonary edema; rhythm disturbances including atrial tachycardia and bradycardia; atrial fibrillation; palpitation, orthostatic hypotension, angina pectoris.

Digestive: Ileus, pancreatitis, hepatic failure, hepatitis (hepatocellular [proven on rechallenge] or cholestatic jaundice), melena, anorexia, dyspepsia, constipation, glossitis, stomatitis, dry mouth, diarrhea, vomiting

Hematologic: Rare cases of neutropenia, thrombocytopenia and bone marrow depression

Musculoskeletal: Muscle cramps.

Nervous/Psychiatric: Depression, confusion, ataxia, somnolence, insomnia, nervousness, peripheral neuropathy (e.g., paresthesia, dysesthesia), vertigo.

Respiratory: Bronchospasm, dyspnea, pneumonia, bronchitis, cough rhinorrhea, sore throat and hoarseness, asthma, upper respiratory infection, pulmonary infiltrates.

Skin: Exfoliative dermatitis, toxic epidermal necrolysis, Stevens-Johnson syndrome, pemphigus, herpes zoster, erythema multiforme, urticaria, pruritus, alopecia, flushing, diaphoresis, photosensitivity.

---

* Based on patient weight of 50 kg

◆ RATED THERAPEUTICALLY EQUIVALENT; ◇ THERAPEUTIC EQUIVALENCE UNCONFIRMED; ○ UNRATED

Special Senses: Blurred vision, taste alteration, anosmia, tinnitus, conjunctivitis, dry eyes, tearing.

Urogenital: Renal failure, oliguria, renal dysfunction (see *"Precautions"* and *"Dosage and Administration"*), urinary tract infection, flank pain, gynecomastia, impotence.

Miscellaneous: A symptom complex has been reported which may include a positive ANA, an elevated erythrocyte sedimentation rate, arthralgia/arthritis, myalgia/myositis, fever, serositis, vasculitis, leukocytosis, eosinophilia, photosensitivity, rash and other dermatologic manifestations.

Angioedema: Angioedema has been reported in patients receiving Enalapril/Enalaprilat. Angioedema associated with laryngeal edema may be fatal. If angioedema of the face, extremities, lips, tongue, glottis and/or larynx occurs, treatment with Enalapril/Enalaprilat should be discontinued and appropriate therapy instituted immediately. (See *"Warnings."*)

Hypotension: Combining the results of clinical trials in patients with hypertension or congestive heart failure, hypotension (including postural hypotension, and other orthostatic effects) was reported in 2.3 percent of patients following the initial dose of Enalapril or during extended therapy. In the hypertensive patients, hypotension occurred in 0.9 percent and syncope occurred in 0.5 percent of patients. Hypotension or syncope was a cause for discontinuation of therapy in 0.1 percent of hypertensive patients. (See *"Warnings."*)

Fetal/Neonatal Morbidity and Mortality: See *"Warnings, Fetal/Neonatal Morbidity and Mortality."*

Cough: See *"Precautions, Cough."*

CLINICAL LABORATORY TEST FINDINGS

Serum Electrolytes: Hyperkalemia (see *"Precautions"*), hyponatremia.

Creatinine, Blood Urea Nitrogen: In controlled clinical trials minor increases in blood urea nitrogen and serum creatinine, reversible upon discontinuation of therapy, were observed in about 0.2 percent of patients with essential hypertension treated with Enalapril alone. Increases are more likely to occur in patients receiving concomitant diuretics or in patients with renal artery stenosis. (See *"Precautions."*) In patients with heart failure who were also receiving diuretics with or without digitalis, increases in blood urea nitrogen or serum creatinine, usually reversible upon discontinuation of Enalapril and/or other concomitant diuretic therapy, were observed in about 11 percent of patients. Increases in blood urea nitrogen or creatinine were a cause for discontinuation in 1.2 percent of patients.

Hematology: Small decreases in hemoglobin and hematocrit (mean decreases of approximately 0.3 g percent and 1.0 vol percent, respectively) occur frequently in either hypertension or congestive heart failure patients treated with Enalapril but are rarely of clinical importance unless another cause of anemia coexists. In clinical trials, less than 0.1 percent of patients discontinued therapy due to anemia. Hemolytic anemia, including cases of hemolysis in patients with G-6-PD deficiency, has been reported; a causal relationship to Enalapril has not been established.

Liver Function Tests: Elevations of liver enzymes and/or serum bilirubin have occurred.

Adverse experiences occurring in 0.5 to 1.0 percent of patients in controlled clinical trials of enalaprilat included: myocardial infarction, fatigue, dizziness, fever, rash and constipation.

Since Enalapril is converted to enalaprilat, those adverse experiences associated with Enalapril might also be expected to occur with enalaprilat.

OVERDOSAGE

Limited data are available in regard to overdosage in humans.

In clinical studies, some hypertensive patients received a maximum dose of 80 mg of Enalaprilat intravenously over a fifteen minute period. At this high dose, no adverse effects beyond those as associated with the recommended dosages were observed.

The intravenous LD$_{50}$ of enalaprilat is 3740-5890 mg/kg in female mice.

The oral LD$_{50}$ of Enalapril is 2000 mg/kg in mice and rats. The most likely manifestation of overdosage would be hypotension, for which the usual treatment would be intravenous infusion of normal saline solution.

Enalaprilat may be removed from general circulation by hemodialysis and has been removed from neonatal circulation by peritoneal dialysis.

DOSAGE AND ADMINISTRATION

ENALAPRIL

Hypertension: In patients who are currently being treated with a diuretic, symptomatic hypotension occasionally may occur following the initial dose of Enalapril. The diuretic should, if possible, be discontinued for two to three days before beginning therapy with Enalapril to reduce the likelihood of hypotension. (See *"Warnings."*) If the patient's blood pressure is not controlled with Enalapril alone, diuretic therapy may be resumed.

If the diuretic cannot be discontinued an initial dose of 2.5 mg should be used under medical supervision for at least two hours and until blood pressure has stabilized for at least an additional hour. (See *"Warnings"* and *"Precautions, Drug Interactions."*)

The recommended initial dose in patients not on diuretics is 5 mg once a day. Dosage should be adjusted according to blood pressure response. The usual dosage range is 10 to 40 mg per day administered in a single dose or two divided doses. In some patients treated once daily, the antihypertensive effect may

diminish toward the end of the dosing interval. In such patients, an increase in dosage or twice daily administration should be considered. If blood pressure is not controlled with Enalapril alone, a diuretic may be added. Concomitant administration of Enalapril with potassium supplements, potassium salt substitutes, or potassium-sparing diuretics may lead to increases of serum potassium (see *"Precautions"*).

Dosage Adjustment in Hypertensive Patients with Renal Impairment: The usual dose of Enalapril is recommended for patients with a creatinine clearance > 30 mL/min (serum creatinine of up to approximately 3 mg/dL). For patients with creatinine clearance ≤ 30 mL/min (serum creatinine ≥ 3 mg/dL), the first dose is 2.5 mg once daily. The dosage may be titrated upward until blood pressure is controlled or to a maximum of 40 mg daily.

Renal Status	Creatinine-Clearance mL/min	Initial Dose mg/day
Normal Renal Function	> 80 mL/min	5 mg
Mild Impairment	≤ 80 > 30 mL/min	5 mg
Moderate to Severe impairment	≤ 30mL/min	2.5 mg
Dialysis Patients*		2.5 mg on dialysis days**

* *See "Precautions, Hemodialysis Patients"*
** *Dosage on nondialysis days should be adjusted depending on the blood pressure response.*

Heart Failure: Enalapril is indicated for the treatment of symptomatic congestive heart failure, usually in combination with diuretics and digitalis.

The recommended starting dose is 2.5 mg administered once or twice daily. The usual therapeutic dosing range is 5 to 20 mg daily, given as a single dose or two divided doses; the majority of patient experience in clinical studies has been with twice daily dosing. Dosage may be adjusted depending upon clinical response (see *"Warnings"*). In the placebo-controlled studies which demonstrated improved survival, the dose of Enalapril was titrated upward as tolerated by the patient. The maximum daily dose administered in clinical trials was 40 mg.

Asymptomatic Left Ventricular Dysfunction: In the trial that demonstrated efficacy, patients were started on 2.5 mg twice daily and were titrated as tolerated to the targeted daily dose of 20 mg (in divided doses).

After the initial dose of Enalapril, the patient should be observed under medical supervision for at least two hours and until blood pressure has stabilized for at least an additional hour. (see *"Warnings"* and *"Precautions, Drug Interactions."*) If possible, the dose of any concomitant diuretic should be reduced which may diminish the likelihood of hypotension. The appearance of hypotension after the initial dose of Enalapril does not preclude subsequent careful dose titration with the drug, following effective management of the hypotension.

Dosage Adjustment in Patients with Heart Failure and Renal Impairment or Hyponatremia: In patients with heart failure who have hyponatremia (serum sodium less than 130 mEq/L) or with serum creatinine greater than 1.6 mg/dL, therapy should be initiated at 2.5 mg daily under close medical supervision. (See *"Dosage and Administration, Heart Failure"*, *"Warnings"* and *"Precautions, Drug Interactions."*) The dose may be increased to 2.5 mg b.i.d., then 5 mg b.i.d. and higher as needed, usually at intervals of four days or more if at the time of dosage adjustment there is not excessive hypotension or significant deterioration of renal function. The maximum daily dose is 40 mg.

FOR INTRAVENOUS ADMINISTRATION ONLY

The dose in hypertension is 1.25 mg every six hours administered intravenously over a five minute period. A clinical response is usually seen within 15 minutes. Peak effects after the first dose may not occur for up to four hours after dosing. The peak effects of the second and subsequent doses may exceed those of the first.

No dosage regimen for enalaprilat has been clearly demonstrated to be more effective in treating hypertension than 1.25 mg every six hours. However, in controlled clinical studies in hypertension, doses as high as 5 mg every six hours were well tolerated for up to 36 hours. There has been inadequate experience with doses greater than 20 mg per day.

In studies of patients with hypertension, enalaprilat has not been administered for periods longer than 48 hours. In other studies, patients have received enalaprilat for as long as seven days.

The dose for patients being converted to Enalaprilat from oral therapy for hypertension with Enalapril Maleate is 1.25 mg every six hours. For conversion from intravenous to oral therapy, the recommended initial dose of Enalaprilat Maleate is 5 mg once a day with subsequent dosage adjustments as necessary.

Patients on Diuretic Therapy: For patients on diuretic therapy the recommended starting dose for hypertension is 0.625 mg administered intravenously over a five minute period. A clinical response is usually seen within 15 minutes. Peak effects after the first dose may not occur for up to four hours after dosing, although most of the effect is usually apparent within the first hour. If after one hour there is an inadequate clinical response, the 0.625 mg dose may be repeated. Additional doses of 1.25 mg may be administered at six hour intervals.

For conversion from intravenous to oral therapy, the recommended initial dose of Enalapril Maleate for patients who have responded to 0.625 mg of enalaprilat every six hours is 2.5 mg once a day with subsequent dosage adjustment as necessary.

Dosage Adjustment in Renal Impairment: The usual dose of 1.25 mg of Enalaprilat every six hours is recommended for patients with a creatinine clearance > 30 mL/min (serum creatinine of up to approximately 3 mg/dL). For patients with creatinine clearance ≤ 30 mL/min (serum creatinine ≥ 3 mg/dL), the initial dose is 0.625 mg. (See "Warnings.")

If after one hour there is an inadequate clinical response, the 0.625 mg dose may be repeated. Additional doses of 1.25 mg may be administered at six hour intervals.

For dialysis patients, see below, "Patients at Risk of Excessive Hypotension."

For conversion from intravenous to oral therapy, the recommended initial dose of Enalapril Maleate is 5 mg once a day for patients with creatinine clearance > 30 mL/min and 2.5 mg once daily for patients with creatinine clearance ≤ 30 mL/min. Dosage should then be adjusted according to blood pressure response.

Patients at Risk of Excessive Hypotension: Hypertensive patients at risk of excessive hypotension include those with the following concurrent conditions or characteristics: heart failure, hyponatremia, high dose diuretic therapy, recent intensive diuresis or increase in diuretic dose, renal dialysis, or severe volume and/or salt depletion of any etiology (see "Warnings"). Single doses of enalaprilat as low as 0.2 mg have produced excessive hypotension in normotensive patients with these diagnoses. Because of the potential for an extreme-hypotensive response in these patients, therapy should be started under very close medical supervision. The starting dose should be no greater than 0.625 mg administered intravenously over a period of no less than five minutes and preferably longer (up to one hour). Patients should be followed closely whenever the dose of enalaprilat is adjusted and/or diuretic is increased.

Administration: Enalaprilat should be administered as a slow intravenous infusion, as indicated above, over at least five minutes. It may be administered as provided or diluted with up 50 mL of a compatible diluent.

Parenteral drug products should be inspected visually for particulate matter and discoloration prior to use whenever solution and container permit.

Storage: Store tablets below 30°C (86°F) and avoid transient temperatures above 50°C (122°F). Keep container tightly closed. Protect moisture.

Dispense in a tight container, if product package is subdivided.

Store intravenous solution below 30°C (86°F).

HOW SUPPLIED

ENALAPRIL MALEATE
TABLETS: 2.5 MG

BRAND/MANUFACTURER	NDC	SIZE	AWP
○ **BRAND**			
▶ VASOTEC: Merck	00006-0014-68	100s	$71.76
	00006-0014-28	100s ud	$75.55
	00006-0014-82	1000s	$717.73
	00006-0014-94	1080s	$775.20
	00006-0014-98	2160s	$1550.41
	00006-0014-87	10000s	$7177.25

TABLETS: 5 MG

BRAND/MANUFACTURER	NDC	SIZE	AWP
○ **BRAND**			
▶ VASOTEC: Merck	00006-0712-68	100s	$91.18
	00006-0712-28	100s ud	$94.98
	00006-0712-82	1000s	$911.85
	00006-0712-94	1080s	$984.93
	00006-0712-98	2160s	$1969.88
	00006-0712-81	4000s	$3647.43
	00006-0712-87	10000s	$9118.59

TABLETS: 10 MG

BRAND/MANUFACTURER	NDC	SIZE	AWP
○ **BRAND**			
▶ VASOTEC: Merck	00006-0713-68	100s	$95.74
	00006-0713-28	100s ud	$99.53
	00006-0713-82	1000s	$957.48
	00006-0713-94	1080s	$1034.23
	00006-0713-98	2160s	$2068.46
	00006-0713-81	4000s	$3829.94
	00006-0713-87	10000s	$9574.84

TABLETS: 20 MG

BRAND/MANUFACTURER	NDC	SIZE	AWP
○ **BRAND**			
▶ VASOTEC: Merck	00006-0714-68	100s	$136.19
	00006-0714-28	100s ud.	$140.00
	00006-0714-82	1000s	$1361.91
	00006-0714-94	1080s	$1471.05
	00006-0714-87	10000s	$13619.08

ENALAPRILATE
INJECTION: 1.25 MG/ML

BRAND/MANUFACTURER	NDC	SIZE	AWP
○ **BRAND**			
VASOTEC I.V.: Merck	00006-3508-01	1 ml	$12.80
	00006-3508-04	2 ml	$25.63

Enalapril Maleate with Hydrochlorothiazide

> **USE IN PREGNANCY**
> WHEN USED IN PREGNANCY DURING THE SECOND AND THIRD TRIMESTERS, ACE INHIBITORS CAN CAUSE INJURY AND EVEN DEATH TO THE DEVELOPING FETUS. WHEN PREGNANCY IS DETECTED, ENALAPRIL MALEATE/HCTZ SHOULD BE DISCONTINUED AS SOON AS POSSIBLE. SEE "WARNINGS, PREGNANCY, ENALAPRIL MALEATE/HCTZ, FETAL/NEONATAL MORBIDITY AND MORTALITY".

DESCRIPTION
Enalapril Maleate/HCTZ combines an angiotensin converting enzyme inhibitor and a diuretic. Enalapril Maleate is the Maleate salt of Enalapril, the ethyl ester of a long-acting angiotensin converting enzyme inhibitor, Enalaprilat. Enalapril Maleate is chemically described as (S)-1-[N-[1-(ethoxycarbonyl)-3-phenylpropyl]-L-alanyl]-L- proline, (Z)-2-butenedioate salt (1:1). Its empirical formula is $C_{20}H_{28}N_2O_5.C_4H_4O_4$.

Enalapril Maleate is a white to off-white crystalline powder with a molecular weight of 492.53. It is sparingly soluble in water, soluble in ethanol, and freely soluble in methanol.

Enalapril is a pro-drug; following oral administration, it is bioactivated by hydrolysis of the ethyl ester to Enalaprilat, which is the active angiotensin converting enzyme inhibitor. Hydrochlorothiazide is 6-chloro-3,4-dihydro-2H-1,2,4-benzothiadiazine-7-sulfonamide 1,1-dioxide. Its empirical formula is $C_7H_8ClN_3O_4S_2$.

It is a white, or practically white, crystalline powder with a molecular weight of 297.72, which is slightly soluble in water, but freely soluble in sodium hydroxide solution.

Enalapril Maleate/HCTZ is available for oral use as tablets containing 10 mg of Enalapril Maleate, 25 mg of Hydrochlorothiazide.

CLINICAL PHARMACOLOGY
As a result of its diuretic effects, Hydrochlorothiazide increases plasma renin activity, increases aldosterone secretion, and decreases serum potassium. Administration of Enalapril Maleate blocks the renin-angiotensin-aldosterone axis and tends to reverse the potassium loss associated with the diuretic.

In clinical studies, the extent of blood pressure reduction seen with the combination of Enalapril Maleate and Hydrochlorothiazide was approximately additive. The antihypertensive effect of Enalapril Maleate/HCTZ was usually sustained for at least 24 hours.

Concomitant administration of Enalapril Maleate and Hydrochlorothiazide has little, or no effect on the bioavailability of either drug. The combination tablet is bioequivalent to concomitant administration of the separate entities.

ENALAPRIL MALEATE
Mechanism of Action: Enalapril, after hydrolysis to enalaprilat, inhibits angiotensin-converting enzyme (ACE) in human subjects and animals. ACE is a peptidyl dipeptidase that catalyzes the conversion of angiotensin I to the vasoconstrictor substance, angiotensin II. Angiotensin II also stimulates aldosterone secretion by the adrenal cortex. Inhibition of ACE results in decreased plasma angiotensin II, which leads to decreased vasopressor activity and to decreased aldosterone secretion. Although the latter decrease is small, it results in small increases of serum potassium. In hypertensive patients treated with Enalapril Maleate alone for up to 48 weeks, mean increases in serum potassium of approximately 0.2 mEq/L were observed. In patients treated with Enalapril Maleate plus a thiazide diuretic, there was essentially no change in serum potassium. (See "Precautions".) Removal of angiotensin II negative feedback on renin secretion leads to increased plasma renin activity.

ACE is identical to kininase, an enzyme that degrades bradykinin. Whether increased levels of bradykinin, a potent vasodepressor peptide, play a role in the therapeutic effects of Enalapril remains to be elucidated.

While the mechanism through which Enalapril lowers blood pressure is believed to be primarily suppression of the renin-angiotensin-aldosterone system, Enalapril is antihypertensive even in patients with low-renin hypertension. Although Enalapril was antihypertensive in all races studied, black hypertensive patients (usually a low-renin hypertensive population) had a smaller average

---

◆ RATED THERAPEUTICALLY EQUIVALENT; ◇ THERAPEUTIC EQUIVALENCE UNCONFIRMED; ○ UNRATED

response to Enalapril Maleate monotherapy than nonblack patients. In contrast, Hydrochlorothiazide was more effective in black patients than Enalapril. Concomitant administration of Enalapril Maleate and Hydrochlorothiazide was equally effective in black and nonblack patients.

Pharmacokinetics and Metabolism: Following oral administration of Enalapril Maleate, peak serum concentrations of Enalapril occur within about one hour. Based on urinary recovery, the extent of absorption of Enalapril is approximately 60 percent. Enalapril absorption is not influenced by the presence of food in the gastrointestinal tract. Following absorption, Enalapril is hydrolyzed to Enalaprilat, which is a more potent angiotensin converting enzyme inhibitor than Enalapril; Enalaprilat is poorly absorbed when administered orally. Peak serum concentrations of Enalaprilat occur three to four hours after an oral dose of Enalapril Maleate. Excretion of Enalaprilat and Enalapril is primarily renal. Approximately 94 percent of the dose is recovered in the urine and feces as Enalaprilat or Enalapril. The principal components in urine are enalaprilat, accounting for about 40 percent of the dose, and intact Enalapril. There is no evidence of metabolites of Enalapril, other than enalaprilat. The serum concentration profile of Enalaprilat exhibits a prolonged terminal phase, apparently representing a small fraction of the administered dose that has been bound to ACE. The amount bound does not increase with dose, indicating a saturable site of binding. The effective half-life for accumulation of Enalaprilat following multiple doses of Enalapril Maleate is 11 hours.

The disposition of Enalapril and Enalaprilat in patients with renal insufficiency is similar to that in patients with normal renal function until the glomerular filtration rate is 30 mL/min or less. With glomerular filtration rate $\leq$ 30 mL/min, peak and trough Enalaprilat levels increase, time to peak concentration increases and time to steady state may be delayed. The effective half-life of Enalaprilat following multiple doses of Enalapril Maleate is prolonged at this level of renal insufficiency. Enalaprilat is dialyzable at the rate of 62 mL/min.

Studies in dogs indicate that Enalapril crosses the blood-brain barrier poorly, if at all; Enalaprilat does not enter the brain. Multiple doses of Enalapril Maleate in rats do not result in accumulation in any tissues. Milk of lactating rats contains radioactivity following administration of ^{14}C Enalapril Maleate. Radioactivity was found to cross the placenta following administration of labeled drug to pregnant hamsters.

Pharmacodynamics: Administration of Enalapril Maleate to patients with hypertension of severity ranging from mild to severe results in a reduction of both supine and standing blood pressure usually with no orthostatic component. Symptomatic postural hypotension is infrequent with Enalapril alone but it can be anticipated in volume-depleted patients, such as patients treated with diuretics. In clinical trials with Enalapril and Hydrochlorothiazide administered concurrently, syncope occurred in 1.3 percent of patients. (See *"Warnings"* and *"Dosage"* and *"Administration"*.) In most patients studied, after oral administration of a single dose of Enalapril Maleate, onset of antihypertensive activity was seen at one hour with peak reduction of blood pressure achieved by four to six hours.

At recommended doses, antihypertensive effects of Enalapril Maleate monotherapy have been maintained for at least 24 hours. In some patients the effects may diminish toward the end of the dosing interval; this was less frequently observed with concomitant administration of Enalapril Maleate and Hydrochlorothiazide.

Achievement of optimal blood pressure reduction may require several weeks of Enalapril therapy in some patients. The antihypertensive effects of Enalapril have continued during long term therapy. Abrupt withdrawal of Enalapril has not been associated with a rapid increase in blood pressure.

In hemodynamic studies in patients with essential hypertension, blood pressure reduction produced by Enalapril was accompanied by a reduction in peripheral arterial resistance with an increase in cardiac output and little or no change in heart rate. Following administration of Enalapril Maleate, there is an increase in renal blood flow; glomerular filtration rate is usually unchanged. The effects appear to be similar in patients with renovascular hypertension.

In a clinical pharmacology study, indomethacin or sulindac was administered to hypertensive patients receiving Enalapril Maleate. In this study there was no evidence of a blunting of the antihypertensive action of Enalapril Maleate.

HYDROCHLOROTHIAZIDE

The mechanism of the antihypertensive effect of thiazides is unknown. Thiazides do not usually affect normal blood pressure. Hydrochlorothiazide is a diuretic and antihypertensive. It affects the distal renal tubular mechanism of electrolyte reabsorption. Hydrochlorothiazide increases excretion of sodium and chloride in approximately equivalent amounts. Natriuresis may be accompanied by some loss of potassium and bicarbonate. After oral use diuresis begins within two hours, peaks in about four hours and lasts about 6 to 12 hours. Hydrochlorothiazide is not metabolized but is eliminated rapidly by the kidney. When plasma levels have been followed for at least 24 hours, the plasma half-life has been observed to vary between 5.6 and 14.8 hours. At least 61 percent of the oral dose is eliminated unchanged within 24 hours. Hydrochlorothiazide crosses the placental but not the blood-brain barrier.

INDICATIONS AND USAGE

Enalapril Maleate/HCTZ is indicated for the treatment of hypertension in patients for whom combination therapy is appropriate. **This fixed dose combination is not indicated for initial therapy. Patients already receiving a diuretic when Enalapril is initiated, or given a diuretic and Enalapril simultaneously, can develop symptomatic hypotension. In the initial titration of the individual entities, it is important, if possible, to stop the diuretic for several days before starting Enalapril or, if this is not possible, begin Enalapril at a low initial dose (see** *"Dosage and Administration"*). **This fixed dose combination is not suitable for titration but may be**

substituted for the individual components if the titrated doses are the same as those in the combination.

In using Enalapril Maleate/HCTZ, consideration should be given to the fact that another angiotensin converting enzyme inhibitor, Captopril, has caused agranulocytosis, particularly in patients with renal impairment or collagen vascular disease, and that available data are insufficient to show that Enalapril does not have a similar risk. (See *"Warnings".*)

CONTRAINDICATIONS

Enalapril Maleate/HCTZ is contraindicated in patients who are hypersensitive to any component of this product and in patients with a history of angioedema related to previous treatment with an angiotensin converting enzyme inhibitor. Because of the Hydrochlorothiazide component, this product is contraindicated in patients with anuria or hypersensitivity to other sulfonamide-derived drugs.

WARNINGS
GENERAL
ENALAPRIL MALEATE

Hypotension: Excessive hypotension was rarely seen in uncomplicated hypertensive patients but is a possible consequence of Enalapril use in severely salt/volume depleted persons such as those treated vigorously with diuretics or patients on dialysis.

Syncope has been reported in 1.3 percent of patients receiving Enalapril Maleate/HCTZ. In patients receiving Enalapril alone, the incidence of syncope is 0.5 percent. The overall incidence of syncope may be reduced by proper titration of the individual components. (See *"Precautions: Drug Interactions"*, *"Adverse Reactions"* and *"Dosage and Administration"*.)

In patients with severe congestive heart failure, with or without associated renal insufficiency, excessive hypotension has been observed and may be associated with oliguria and/or progressive azotemia, and rarely with acute renal failure and/or death. Because of the potential fall in blood pressure in these patients, therapy should be started under very close medical supervision. Such patients should be followed closely for the first two weeks of treatment and whenever the dose of Enalapril and/or diuretic is increased. Similar considerations may apply to patients with ischemic heart or cerebrovascular disease, in whom an excessive fall in blood pressure could result in a myocardial infarction or cerebrovascular accident.

If hypotension occurs, the patient should be placed in the supine position and, if necessary, receive an intravenous infusion of normal saline. A transient hypotensive response is not a contraindication to further doses, which usually can be given without difficulty once the blood pressure has increased after volume expansion.

Angioedema: Angioedema of the face, extremities, lips, tongue, glottis and/or larynx has been reported in patients treated with angiotensin converting enzyme inhibitors, including Enalapril. This may occur at any time during treatments. In such cases Enalapril Maleate/HCTZ should be promptly discontinued and appropriate therapy and monitoring should be provided until complete and sustained resolution of signs and symptoms has occurred. In instances where swelling has been confined to the face and lips the condition has generally resolved without treatment, although antihistamines have been useful in relieving symptoms. Angioedema associated with laryngeal edema may be fatal. **Where there is involvement of the tongue, glottis or larynx, likely to cause airway obstruction, appropriate therapy, e.g., subcutaneous epinephrine solution 1:1000 (0.3 mL to 0.5 mL) and/or measures necessary to ensure a patent airway, should be promptly provided** (See *"Adverse Reactions".*)

Patients with a history of angioedema unrelated to ACE inhibitor therapy may be at increased risk of angioedema while receiving an ACE inhibitor (see also *"Contraindications"*).

Neutropenia/Agranulocytosis: Another angiotensin converting enzyme inhibitor, captopril, has been shown to cause agranulocytosis and bone marrow depression, rarely in uncomplicated patients but more frequently in patients with renal impairment especially if they also have a collagen vascular disease. Available data from clinical trials of Enalapril are insufficient to show that Enalapril does not cause agranulocytosis at similar rates. Marketing experience has revealed several cases of neutropenia or agranulocytosis in which a causal relationship to Enalapril cannot be excluded. Periodic monitoring of white blood cell counts in patients with collagen vascular disease and renal disease should be considered.

HYDROCHLOROTHIAZIDE

Thiazides should be used with caution in severe renal disease. In patients with renal disease, thiazides may precipitate azotemia. Cumulative effects of the drug may develop in patients with impaired renal function.

Thiazides should be used with caution in patients with impaired hepatic function or progressive liver disease, since minor alterations of fluid and electrolyte balance may precipitate hepatic coma.

Sensitivity reactions may occur in patients with or without a history of allergy or bronchial asthma.

The possibility of exacerbation or activation of systemic lupus erythematosus has been reported.

Lithium generally should not be given with thiazides (see *"Precautions: Drug Interactions, Enalapril Maleate and Hydrochlorothiazide"*).

PREGNANCY
ENALAPRIL-HYDROCHLOROTHIAZIDE

There was no teratogenicity in rats given up to 90 mg/kg/day of Enalapril (150 times the maximum human dose) in combination with 10 mg/kg/day of

Hydrochlorothiazide (2½ times the maximum human dose) or in mice given up to 30 mg/kg/day of Enalapril (50 times the maximum human dose) in combination with 10 mg/kg/day of Hydrochlorothiazide (2½ times the maximum human dose). At these doses, fetotoxicity expressed as a decrease in average fetal weight occurred in both species. No fetotoxicity occurred at lower doses; 30/10 mg/kg/day of Enalapril Hydrochlorothiazide in rats and 10/10 mg/kg/day of Enalapril Hydrochlorothiazide in mice.

When used in pregnancy during the second and third trimesters, ACE inhibitors can cause injury and even death to the developing fetus. When pregnancy is detected, Enalapril Maleate/HCTZ should be discontinued a soon as possible. (See *"Enalapril Maleate, Fetal/Neonatal Morbidity and Mortality"* below.)

ENALAPRIL MALEATE
Fetal/Neonatal Morbidity and Mortality: ACE inhibitors can cause fetal and neonatal morbidity and death when administered to pregnant women. Several dozen cases have been reported in the world literature. When pregnancy is detected, ACE inhibitors should be discontinued as soon as possible.

The use of ACE inhibitors during the second and third trimesters of pregnancy has been associated with fetal and neonatal injury, including hypotension, neonatal skull hypoplasia, anuria, reversible or irreversible renal failure, and death. Oligohydramnios has also been reported, presumably resulting from decreased fetal renal function; oligohydramnios in this setting has been associated with fetal limb contractures, craniofacial deformation, and hypoplastic lung development. Prematurity, intrauterine growth retardation, and patent ductus arteriosus have also been reported, although it is not clear whether these occurrences were due to the ACE-inhibitor exposure.

These adverse effects do not appear to have resulted from intrauterine ACE-inhibitor exposure that has been limited to the first trimester. Mothers whose embryos and fetuses are exposed to ACE inhibitors only during the first trimester should be so informed. Nonetheless, when patients become pregnant, physicians should make every effort to discontinue the use of Enalapril Maleate/HCTZ as soon as possible.

Rarely (probably less often than one in every thousand pregnancies), no alternative to ACE inhibitors will be found. In these rare cases, the mothers should be apprised of the potential hazards to their fetuses, and serial ultrasound examinations should be performed to assess the intraamniotic environment.

If oligohydramnios is observed, Enalapril Maleate/HCTZ should be discontinued unless it is considered lifesaving for the mother. Contraction stress testing (CST), a non-stress test (NST), or biophysical profiling (BPP) may be appropriate, depending upon the week of pregnancy. Patients and physicians should be aware, however, that oligohydramnios may not appear until after the fetus has sustained irreversible injury.

Infants with histories of *in utero* exposure to ACE inhibitors should be closely observed for hypotension, oliguria, and hyperkalemia. If oliguria occurs, attention should be directed toward support of blood pressure and renal perfusion. Exchange transfusion or dialysis may be required as means of reversing hypotension and/or substituting for disordered renal function. Enalapril, which crosses the placenta, has been removed from neonatal circulation by peritoneal dialysis with some clinical benefit, and theoretically may be removed by exchange transfusion, although there is no experience with the latter procedure.

No teratogenic effects of Enalapril were seen in studies of pregnant rats, and rabbits. On a mg/kg basis, the doses used were up to 333 times (in rats), and 50 times (in rabbits) the maximum recommended human dose.

HYDROCHLOROTHIAZIDE
Teratogenic Effects: Reproduction studies in the rabbit, the mouse and the rat at doses up to 100 mg/kg/day (50 times the human dose) showed no evidence of external abnormalities of the fetus due to Hydrochlorothiazide. Hydrochlorothiazide given in a two-litter study in rats at doses of 4-5.6 mg/kg/day (approximately 1-2 times the usual daily human dose) did not impair fertility or produce birth abnormalities in the offspring. Thiazides cross the placental barrier and appear in cord blood.

Nonteratogenic Effects: These may include fetal or neonatal jaundice, thrombocytopenia, and possibly other adverse reactions which have occurred in the adult.

PRECAUTIONS
GENERAL ENALAPRIL MALEATE
Impaired Renal Function: As a consequence of inhibiting the renin-angiotensin-aldosterone system, changes in renal function may be anticipated in susceptible individuals. In patients with severe congestive heart failure whose renal function may depend on the activity of the renin-angiotensin-aldosterone system, treatment with angiotensin converting enzyme inhibitors, including Enalapril, may be associated with oliguria and/or progressive azotemia and rarely with acute renal failure and/or death.

In clinical studies in hypertensive patients with unilateral or bilateral renal artery stenosis, increases in blood urea nitrogen and serum creatinine were observed in 20 percent of patients. These increases were almost always reversible upon discontinuation of Enalapril and/or diuretic therapy. In such patients renal function should be monitored during the first few weeks of therapy.

Some patients with hypertension or heart failure with no apparent pre-existing renal vascular disease have developed increases in blood urea and serum creatinine, usually minor and transient, especially when Enalapril has been given concomitantly with a diuretic. This is more likely to occur in patients with pre-existing renal impairment. Dosage reduction of Enalapril and/or discontinuation of the diuretic may be required.

Evaluation of the hypertensive patient should always include assessment of renal function.

Hemodialysis Patients: Anaphylactoid reactions have been reported in patients dialyzed with high-flux membranes (e.g., AN 69*) and treated concomitantly with an ACE inhibitor. In these patients consideration should be given to using a different type of dialysis membrane or a different class of antihypertensive agent.

Hyperkalemia: Elevated serum potassium (greater than 5.7 mEq/L) was observed in approximately one percent of hypertensive patients in clinical trials treated with Enalapril alone. In most cases these were isolated values which resolved despite continued therapy, although hyperkalemia was a cause of discontinuation of therapy in 0.28 percent of hypertensive patients. Hyperkalemia was less frequent (approximately 0.1 percent) in patients treated with Enalapril plus Hydrochlorothiazide. Risk factors for the development of hyperkalemia include renal insufficiency, diabetes mellitus, and the concomitant use of potassium-sparing diuretics, potassium supplements and/or potassium-containing salt substitutes, which should be used cautiously, if at all, with Enalapril. (See *"Drug Interactions"*.)

Cough: Cough has been reported with the use of ACE inhibitors. Characteristically, the cough is nonproductive, persistent and resolves after discontinuation of therapy. ACE inhibitor-induced cough should be considered as part of the differential diagnosis of cough.

Surgery/Anesthesia: In patients undergoing major surgery or during anesthesia with agents that produce hypotension, Enalapril may block angiotensin II formation secondary to compensatory renin release. If hypotension occurs and is considered to be due to this mechanism, it can be corrected by volume expansion.

HYDROCHLOROTHIAZIDE
Periodic determination of serum electrolytes to detect possible electrolyte imbalance should be performed at appropriate intervals. All patients receiving thiazide therapy should be observed for clinical signs of fluid or electrolyte imbalance: namely hyponatremia, hypochloremic alkalosis, and hypokalemia. Serum and urine electrolyte determinations are particularly important when the patient is vomiting excessively or receiving parenteral fluids. Warning signs or symptoms of fluid and electrolyte imbalance, irrespective of cause, include dryness of mouth, thirst, weakness, lethargy, drowsiness, restlessness, confusion, seizures, muscle pains or cramps, muscular fatigue, hypotension, oliguria, tachycardia, and gastrointestinal disturbances such as nausea and vomiting.

Hypokalemia may develop, especially with brisk diuresis, when severe cirrhosis is present, or after prolonged therapy. Interference with adequate oral electrolyte intake will also contribute to hypokalemia. Hypokalemia may cause cardiac arrhythmia and may also sensitize or exaggerate the response of the heart to the toxic effects of digitalis (e.g., increased ventricular irritability). Because Enalapril reduces the production of aldosterone, concomitant therapy with Enalapril attenuates the diuretic-induced potassium loss (see *"Drug Interactions, Agents Increasing Serum Potassium"*).

Although any chloride deficit is generally mild and usually does not require specific treatment except under extraordinary circumstances (as in liver disease or renal disease), chloride replacement may be required in the treatment of metabolic alkalosis.

Dilutional hyponatremia may occur in edematous patients in hot weather; appropriate therapy is water restriction, rather than administration of salt except in rare instances when the hyponatremia is life-threatening. In actual salt depletion, appropriate replacement is the therapy of choice. Hyperuricemia may occur or frank gout may be precipitated in certain patients receiving thiazide therapy.

In diabetic patients dosage adjustments of insulin or oral hypoglycemic agents may be required. Hyperglycemia may occur with thiazide diuretics. Thus latent diabetes mellitus may become manifest during thiazide therapy.

The antihypertensive effects of the drug may be enhanced in the postsympathectomy patient.

If progressive renal impairment becomes evident consider withholding or discontinuing diuretic therapy.

Thiazides have been shown to increase the urinary excretion of magnesium; this may result in hypomagnesemia.

Thiazides may decrease urinary calcium excretion.

Thiazides may cause intermittent and slight elevation of serum calcium in the absence of known disorders of calcium metabolism. Marked hypercalcemia may be evidence of hidden hyperparathyroidism. Thiazides should be discontinued before carrying out tests for parathyroid function.

Increases in cholesterol and triglyceride levels may be associated with thiazide diuretic therapy.

INFORMATION FOR PATIENTS
Angioedema: Angioedema, including laryngeal edema, may occur at any time during treatment with angiotensin converting enzyme inhibitors, including Enalapril. Patients should be so advised and told to report immediately any signs or symptoms suggesting angioedema (swelling of face, extremities, eyes, lips, tongue, difficulty in swallowing or breathing) and to take no more drug until they have consulted with the prescribing physician.

Hypotension: Patients should be cautioned to report light-headedness especially during the first few days of therapy. If actual syncope occurs the patients should be told to discontinue the drug until they have consulted with the prescribing physician.

---

* Registered trademark of Hospal Ltd.

All patients should be cautioned that excessive perspiration and dehydration may lead to an excessive fall in blood pressure because of reduction in fluid volume. Other causes of volume depletion such as vomiting or diarrhea may also lead to a fall in blood pressure; patients should be advised to consult with the physician.

Hyperkalemia: Patients should be told not to use salt substitutes containing potassium without consulting their physician.

Neutropenia: Patients should be told to report promptly any indication of infection (e.g., sore throat, fever) which may be a sign of neutropenia.

Pregnancy: Female patients of childbearing age should be told about the consequences of second- and third-trimester exposure to ACE inhibitors, and they should also be told that these consequences do not appear to have resulted from intrauterine ACE-inhibitor exposure that has been limited to the first trimester. These patients should be asked to report pregnancies to their physicians as soon as possible.

Note: As with many other drugs, certain advice to patients being treated with Enalapril Maleate/HCTZ is warranted. This information is intended to aid in the safe and effective use of this medication. It is not a disclosure of all possible adverse or intended effects.

DRUG INTERACTIONS
ENALAPRIL MALEATE
Hypotension — Patients on Diuretic Therapy: Patients on diuretics and especially those in whom diuretic therapy was recently instituted, may occasionally experience an excessive reduction of blood pressure after initiation of therapy with Enalapril. The possibility of hypotensive effects with Enalapril can be minimized by either discontinuing the diuretic or increasing the salt intake prior to initiation of treatment with Enalapril. If it is necessary to continue the diuretic, provide medical supervision for at least two hours and until blood pressure has stabilized for at least an additional hour. (See *"Warnings"* and *"Dosage and Administration"*.)

Agents Causing Renin Release: The antihypertensive effect of Enalapril is augmented by antihypertensive agents that cause renin release (e.g., diuretics).

Other Cardiovascular Agents: Enalapril has been used concomitantly with beta adrenergic-blocking agents, methyldopa, nitrates, calcium-blocking agents, hydralazine and prazosin without evidence of clinically significant adverse interactions.

Agents Increasing Serum Potassium: Enalapril attenuates diuretic-induced potassium loss. Potassium-sparing diuretics (e.g., spironolactone, triamterene, or amiloride), potassium supplements, or potassium-containing salt substitutes may lead to significant increases in serum potassium. Therefore, if concomitant use of these agents is indicated because of demonstrated hypokalemia they should be used with caution and with frequent monitoring of serum potassium.

Lithium: Lithium toxicity has been reported in patients receiving lithium concomitantly with drugs which cause elimination of sodium, including ACE inhibitors. A few cases of lithium toxicity have been reported in patients receiving concomitant Enalapril and lithium and were reversible upon discontinuation of both drugs. It is recommended that serum lithium levels be monitored frequently if Enalapril is administered concomitantly with lithium.

HYDROCHLOROTHIAZIDE
When administered concurrently the following drugs may interact with thiazide diuretics:

Alcohol, Barbiturates, or Narcotics: potentiation of orthostatic hypotension may occur.

Antidiabetic Drugs (Oral Agents and Insulin): dosage adjustment of the antidiabetic drug may be required.

Other Antihypertensive Drugs: additive effect or potentiation.

Cholestyramine and Colestipol Resins: Absorption of Hydrochlorothiazide is impaired in the presence of anionic exchange resins. Single doses of either cholestyramine or colestipol resins bind the Hydrochlorothiazide and reduce its absorption from the gastrointestinal tract by up to 85 and 43 percent, respectively.

Corticosteroids, ACTH: intensified electrolyte depletion, particularly hypokalemia.

Pressor Amines (e.g., norepinephrine): possible decreased response to pressor amines but not sufficient to preclude their use.

Skeletal Muscle Relaxants, Nondepolarizing (e.g., tubocurarine): possible increased responsiveness to the muscle relaxant.

Lithium: should not generally be given with diuretics. Diuretic agents reduce the renal clearance of lithium and add a high risk of lithium toxicity. Refer to the package insert for lithium preparations before use of such preparations with Enalapril Maleate/HCTZ.

Nonsteroidal Anti-inflammatory Drugs: In some patients, the administration of a non-steroidal anti-inflammatory agent can reduce the diuretic, natriuretic, and antihypertensive effects of loop, potassium-sparing and thiazide diuretics. Therefore, when Enalapril Maleate and non-steroidal anti-inflammatory agents are used concomitantly, the patient should be observed closely to determine if the desired effect of the diuretic is obtained.

CARCINOGENESIS, MUTAGENESIS, IMPAIRMENT OF FERTILITY
Enalapril in combination with Hydrochlorothiazide was not mutagenic in the Ames microbial mutagen test with or without metabolic activation. Enalapril

Hydrochlorothiazide did not produce DNA single strand breaks in an *in vitro* alkaline elution assay in rat hepatocytes or chromosomal aberrations in an *in vivo* mouse bone marrow assay.

ENALAPRIL MALEATE
There was no evidence of a tumorigenic effect when Enalapril was administered for 106 weeks to rats at doses up to 90 mg/kg/day (150 times[*] the maximum daily huamn dose). Enalapril has also been administered for 94 weeks to male and female mice at doses up to 90 and 180 mg/kg/day, respectively, (150 and 300 times[*] the maximum daily dose for humans) and showed no evidence of carcinogenicity.

Neither Enalapril Maleate nor the active diacid was mutagenic in the Ames microbial mutagen test with or without metabolic activation. Enalapril was also negative in the following genotoxicity studies: rec-assay, reverse mutation assay with *E. coli*, sister chromatid exchange with cultured mammalian cells, and the micronucleus test with mice, as well as in an *in vivo* cytogenic study using mouse bone marrow.

There were no adverse effects on reproductive performance in male and female rats treated with 10 to 90 mg/kg/day of Enalapril.

HYDROCHLOROTHIAZIDE
Two-year feeding studies in mice and rats conducted under the auspices of the National Toxicology Program (NTP) uncovered no evidence of a carcinogenic potential of Hydrochlorothiazide in female mice (at doses of up to approximately 600 mg/kg/day) or in male and female rats (at doses of up to approximately 100 mg/kg/day). The NTP, however, found equivocal evidence for hepatocarcinogenicity in male mice. Hydrochlorothiazide was not genotoxic *in vitro* in the Ames mutagenicity assay of *Salmonella typhimurium* strains TA 98, TA 100, TA 1535, TA 1537, and TA 1538 and in the Chinese Hamster Ovary (CHO) test for chromosomal aberrations, or *in vivo* in assays using mouse germinal cell chromosomes, Chinese hamster bone marrow chromosomes, and the *Drosophila* sex-linked recessive lethal trait gene. Positive test results were obtained only in the *in vitro* CHO Sister Chromatid Exchange (clastogenicity) and in the Mouse Lymphoma Cell (mutagenicity) assays, using concentrations of Hydrochlorothiazide from 43 to 1300 µg/mL, and in the *Aspergillus nidulans* nondisjunction assay at an unspecified concentration.

Hydrochlorothiazide had no adverse effects on the fertility of mice and rats of either sex in studies wherein these species were exposed, via their diet, to doses of up to 100 and 4 mg/kg, respectively, prior to conception and throughout gestation.

PREGNANCY
Pregnancy Categories C (first trimester) and D (second and third trimesters.) See *"Warnings, Pregnancy, Enalapril Maleate, Fetal/Neonatal Morbidity and Mortality".*

NURSING MOTHERS
Enalapril and Enalaprilat are detected in human milk in trace amounts. Thiazides do appear in human milk. Because of the potential for serious reactions in nursing infants from either drug, a decision should be made whether to discontinue nursing or to discontinue Enalapril Maleate/HCTZ taking into account the importance of the drug to the mother.

PEDIATRIC USE
Safety and effectiveness in children have not been established.

ADVERSE REACTIONS
Enalapril Maleate/HCTZ has, been evaluated for safety in more than 1500 patients, including over 300 patients treated for one year or more. In clinical trials with Enalapril Maleate/HCTZ no adverse experiences peculiar to this combination drug have been observed. Adverse experiences that have occurred, have been limited to those that have been previously reported with Enalapril or Hydrochlorothiazide.

The most frequent clinical adverse experiences in controlled trials were: dizziness (8.6 percent), headache (5.5 percent), fatigue (3.9 percent) and cough (3.5 percent). Generally, adverse experiences were mild and transient in nature. Adverse experiences occurring in greater than two percent of patients treated with Enalapril Maleate/HCTZ in controlled clinical trials are shown below.

	Percent of Patients in Controlled Studies	
	Enalapril Maleate/ HCTZ (n = 1580) Incidence (discontinuation)	*Placebo (n = 230) Incidence*
Dizziness	8.6 (0.7)	4.3
Headache	5.5 (0.4)	9.1
Fatigue	3.9 (0.8)	2.6
Cough	3.5 (0.4)	0.9
Muscle Cramps	2.7 (0.2)	0.9
Nausea	2.5 (0.4)	1.7
Asthenia	2.4 (0.3)	0.9
Orthostatic Effects	2.3 (< 0.1)	0.0
Impotence	2.2 (0.5)	0.5
Diarrhea	2.1 (< 0.1)	1.7

* Based on patient weight of 50 kg

► SHOWN IN PRODUCT IDENTIFICATION GUIDE

Clinical adverse experiences occurring in 0.5 to 2.0 percent of patients in controlled trials included.

Body As A Whole: Syncope, chest pain, abdominal pain;

Cardiovascular: Orthostatic hypotension, palpitation, tachycardia;

Digestive: Vomiting, dyspepsia, constipation, flatulence, dry mouth;

Nervous/Psychiatric: Insomnia, nervousness, paresthesia, somnolence, vertigo;

Skin: Pruritus, rash;

Other: Dyspnea, gout, back pain, arthralgia, diaphoresis, decreased libido, tinnitus, urinary tract infection.

Angioedema: Angioedema has been reported in patients receiving Enalapril Maleate/HCTZ (0.6 percent). Angioedema associated with laryngeal edema may be fatal. If angioedema of the face, extremities, lips, tongue, glottis and/or larynx occurs, treatment with Enalapril Maleate/HCTZ should be discontinued and appropriate therapy instituted immediately. (See *"Warnings".*)

Hypotension: In clinical trials, adverse effects relating to hypotension occurred as follows: hypotension (0.9 percent), orthostatic hypotension (1.5 percent), other orthostatic effects (2.3 percent). In addition syncope occurred in 1.3 percent of patients. (See *"Warnings".*)

Cough: See *"Precautions, Cough,".*

CLINICAL LABORATORY TEST FINDINGS
Serum Electrolytes: See *"Precautions".*

Creatinine, Blood Urea Nitrogen: In controlled clinical trials minor increases in blood urea nitrogen and serum creatine, reversible upon discontinuation of therapy, were observed in about 0.6 percent of patients with essential hypertension treated with Enalapril Maleate/HCTZ. More marked increases have been reported in other Enalapril experience. Increases are more likely to occur in patients with renal artery stenosis. (See *"Precautions".*)

Serum Uric Acid, Glucose, Magnesium, and Calcium: See *"Precautions".*

Hemoglobin and Hematocrit: Small decreases in hemoglobin and hematocrit (mean decreases of approximately 0.3 g percent and 1.0 vol percent, respectively) occur frequently in hypertensive patients treated with Enalapril Maleate/HCTZ but are rarely of clinical importance unless another cause of anemia coexists. In clinical trials, less than 0.1 percent of patients discontinued therapy due to anemia.

Liver Function Tests: Rarely, elevations of liver enzymes and/or serum bilirubin have occurred.

Other adverse reactions that have been reported with the individual components are listed below and, within each category, are in order of decreasing severity.

ENALAPRIL MALEATE
Enalapril has been evaluated for safety in more than 10,000 patients. In clinical trials adverse reactions which occurred with Enalapril were also seen with Enalapril Maleate/HCTZ. However, since Enalapril has been marketed, the following adverse reactions have been reported:

Body As A Whole: Anaphylactoid reactions (see *"Precautions Hemodialysis Patients"*)

Cardiovascular: Cardiac arrest; myocardial infarction or cerebrovascular accident, possibly secondary to excessive hypotension in high risk patients (see *"Warnings, Hypotension"*); pulmonary embolism and infarction; pulmonary edema; rhythm disturbances including atrial tachycardia and bradycardia, atrial fibrillation; hypotension; angina pectoris;

Digestive: Ileus, pancreatitis, hepatic failure, hepatitis (hepatocellular [proven on rechallenge] or cholestatic jaundice), melena, anorexia, glossitis, stomatitis, dry mouth;

Hematologic: Rare cases of neutropenia, thrombocytopenia and bone marrow depression. Hemolytic anemia, including cases of hemolysis in patients with G-6-PD deficiency, has been reported: a causal relationship to Enalapril has not been established;

Nervous System/Psychiatric: Depression, confusion, ataxia, peripheral neuropathy, (e.g., paresthesia, dysesthesia);

Urogenital: Renal failure, oliguria, renal dysfunction, (see *"Precautions"* and *"Dosage and Administration"*), flank pain, gynecomastia;

Respiratory: Pulmonary infiltrates, bronchospasm, pneumonia, bronchitis, rhinorrhea, sore throat and hoarseness, asthma, upper respiratory infection;

Skin: Exfoliative dermatitis, toxic epidermal necrolysis, Stevens-Johnson syndrome, herpes zoster, erythema multiforme, urticaria, pemphigus, alopecia, flushing, photosensitivity;

Special Senses: Blurred vision, taste alteration, anosmia, conjunctivitis dry eyes, tearing;

Miscellaneous: A symptom complex has been reported which may include a positive ANA, an elevated erythrocyte sedimentation rate, arthralgia/arthritis, myalgia/myositis, fever, serositis, vasculitis, leukocytosis, eosinophilia, photosensitivity, rash and other dermatologic manifestations.

Fetal/Neonatal Morbidity and Mortality: See *"Warnings, Pregnancy, Enalapril Maleate, Fetal/Neonatal Morbidiy and Mortality."*

HYDROCHLOROTHIAZIDE
Body as a Whole: Weakness;

Digestive: Pancreatitis, jaundice, (intrahepatic cholestatic jaundice), sialadenitis, cramping, gastric irritation, anorexia;

Hematologic: Aplastic anemia, agranulocytosis, leukopenia, hemolytic anemia, thrombocytopenia;

Hypersensitivity: Purpura, photosensitivity, urticaria, necrotizing angiitis (vasculitis and cutaneous vasculitis), fever, respiratory distress including pneumonitis and pulmonary edema, anaphylactic reactions;

Musculoskeletal: Muscle spasm;

Nervous system/Psychiatric: Restlesness;

Renal: Renal failure, renal dysfunction, interstitial nephritis (see *"Warnings"*);

Skin: Erythema multiforme including Stevens-Johnson syndrome, exfoliative dermatitis including toxic epidermal necrolysis, alopecia;

Special Senses: Transient blurred vision, xanthopsia.

OVERDOSAGE
No specific information is available on the treatment of overdosage with Enalapril Maleate/HCTZ. Treatment is symptomatic and supportive. Therapy with Enalapril Maleate/HCTZ should be discontinued and the patient observed closely. Suggested measures include induction of emesis and/or gastric lavage, and correction of dehydration, electrolyte imbalance and hypotension by established procedures.

Enalapril Maleate: The oral LD_{50} of Enalapril is 2000 mg/kg in mice and rats. The most likely manifestation of overdosage would be hypotension, for which the usual treatment would be intravenous infusion of normal saline solution. Enalaprilat may be removed from general circulation by hemodialysis and has been removed from neonatal circulation by peritoneal dialysis.

Hydrochlorothiazide: The oral LD_{50} of Hydrochlorothiazide is greater than 10.0 g/kg in both mice and rats. The most common signs and symptoms observed are those caused by electrolyte depletion (hypokalemia, hypochloremia, hyponatremia) and dehydration resulting from excessive diuresis. If digitalis has also been administered, hypokalemia may accentuate cardiac arrhythmias.

DOSAGE AND ADMINISTRATION
DOSAGE MUST BE INDIVIDUALIZED. THE FIXED COMBINATION IS NOT FOR INITIAL THERAPY. THE DOSE OF ENALAPRIL MALEATE/HCTZ SHOULD BE DETERMINED BY THE TITRATION OF THE INDIVIDUAL COMPONENTS.
Once the patient has been successfully titrated with the individual components as described below, Enalapril Maleate/HCTZ (one or two 10-25 tablets once daily) may be substituted if the titrated doses are the same as those in the fixed combination. (See *"Indications and Usage"* and *"Warnings"*). Patients usually do not require doses in excess of 50 mg of Hydrochlorothiazide daily when combined with other antihypertensive agents. Therefore, since each tablet of Enalapril Maleate/HCTZ includes 25 mg of Hydrochlorothiazide, the daily dosage of Enalapril Maleate/HCTZ should not exceed two tablets. If further blood pressure control is indicated, additional doses of Enalapril or other nondiuretic antihypertensive agents should be considered.
For Enalapril monotherapy the recommended initial dose in patients not on diuretics is 5 mg of Enalapril once a day. Dosae should be adjusted according to blood pressure response. The usual dosage range of Enalapril is 10 to 40 mg per day administered in a single dose or two divided doses. In some patients treated once daily, the antihypertensive effects may diminish toward the end of the dosing interval. In such patients, an increase in dosage or twice daily administration should be considered. If blood pressure is not controlled with Enalapril alone, a diuretic may be added.
In patients who are currently being treated with a diuretic, symptomatic hypotension occasionally may occur following the initial dose of Enalapril. The diuretic should, if possible, be discontinued for two to three days before beginning therapy with Enalapril to reduce the likelihood of hypotension. (See *"Warnings".*) If the patient's blood pressure is not controlled with Enalapril alone, diuretic therapy may be resumed.
If the diuretic cannot be discontinued an initial dose of 2.5 mg of Enalapril should be used under medical supervision for at least two hours and until blood pressure has stabilized for at least an additional hour. (See *"Warnings"* and *"Precautions: Drug Interactions".*)
Concomitant administration of Enalapril Maleate/HCTZ with potassium supplements, potassium salt substitutes, or potassium sparing agents may lead to increases of serum potassium. (See *"Precautions".*)

Dosage Adjustment in Renal Impairment: The usual dose of Enalapril Maleate/HCTZ is recommended for patients with a creatinine clearance > 30 mL/min (serum creatinine of up to approximately 3 mg/dL).
When concomitant diuretic therapy is required in patients with severe renal impairment, a loop diuretic, rather than a thiazide diuretic is preferred for use with Enalapril; therefore, for patients with severe renal dysfunction the Enalapril Maleate Hydrochlorothiazide combination tablet is not recommended.

Storage: Store below 30°C (86°F) and avoid transient temperatures above 50°C (122°F). Keep container tightly closed. Protect from moisture.
Dispense in a tight container, if product package is sub-divided.

◆ RATED THERAPEUTICALLY EQUIVALENT; ◇ THERAPEUTIC EQUIVALENCE UNCONFIRMED; ○ UNRATED

HOW SUPPLIED
TABLETS: 10 MG-25 MG

BRAND/MANUFACTURER	NDC	SIZE	AWP
○ **BRAND**			
▶ VASERETIC 10-25: Merck	00006-0720-68	100s	$106.60

Endafed *SEE* BROMPHENIRAMINE MALEATE AND PSEUDOEPHEDRINE HYDROCHLORIDE

Endrate *SEE* EDETATE DISODIUM

Enduron *SEE* METHYCLOTHIAZIDE

Enduronyl *SEE* DESERPIDINE AND METHYCLOTHIAZIDE

Enflurane

DESCRIPTION
Enflurane, a nonflammable liquid administered by vaporizing, is a general inhalation anesthetic drug. It is 2-chloro-1,1,2-trifluoroethyl difluoromethyl ether (CHF_2OCF_2CHFCl). The boiling point is 56.5° C at 760 mm Hg, and the vapor pressure (in mm Hg) is 175 at 20° C, 218 at 25° C, and 345 at 36° C. Vapor pressures can be calculated using the equation:

$$\log_{10}P_{vap} = A + \frac{B}{T}$$

$$A = 7.967$$
$$B = -1678.4$$
$$T = °C + 273.16 \text{ (Kelvin)}$$

The specific gravity (25°/25° C) is 1.517. The refractive index at 20° C is 1.3026-1.3030. The blood/gas coefficient is 1.91 at 37° C and the oil/gas coefficient is 98.5 at 37° C.

Enflurane is a clear, colorless, stable liquid whose purity exceeds 99.9% (area percent by gas chromatography). No stabilizers are added as these have been found, through controlled laboratory tests, to be unnecessary even in the presence of ultraviolet light. Enflurane is stable to strong base, does not decompose in contact with soda lime (at normal operating temperatures), and does not react with aluminium, tin, brass, iron or copper. The partition coefficients of Enflurane at 25° C are 74 in conductive rubber and 120 in polyvinyl chloride.

Following is its chemical structure:

```
    F   F F
    |   | |
H - C - O-C-C - H
    |   | |
    F   F Cl
```

CLINICAL PHARMACOLOGY
Enflurane is an inhalation anesthetic. The MAC (minimum alveolar concentration) in man is 1.68% in pure oxygen, 0.57 in 70% nitrous oxide-30% oxygen, and 1.17 in 30% nitrous oxide-70% oxygen.

Induction of and recovery from anesthesia with Enflurane are rapid. Enflurane has a mild, sweet odor. Enflurane may provide a mild stimulus to salivation or tracheobronchial secretions. Pharyngeal and laryngeal reflexes are readily obtunded. The level of anesthesia can be changed rapidly by changing the inspired Enflurane concentration. Enflurane reduces ventilation as depth of anesthesia increases. High $PaCO_2$ levels can be obtained at deeper levels of anesthesia if ventilation is not supported. Enflurane provokes a sigh response reminiscent of that seen with diethyl ether.

There is a decrease in blood pressure with induction of anesthesia, followed by a return to near normal with surgical stimulation. Progressive increases in depth of anesthesia produce corresponding increases in hypotension. Heart rate remains relatively constant without significant bradycardia. Electrocardiographic monitoring or recordings indicate that cardiac rhythm remains stable. Elevation of the carbon dioxide level in arterial blood does not alter cardiac rhythm.

Studies in man indicate a considerable margin of safety in the administration of epinephrine-containing solutions during Enflurane anesthesia. Enflurane anesthesia has been used in excision of pheochromocytoma in man without ventricular arrhythmias. On the basis of studies in patients anesthetized with Enflurane and injected with epinephrine-containing solutions to achieve hemostasis in a highly vascular area (transsphenoidal surgery), up to 2 micrograms per kilogram (2 µg/kg) of epinephrine may be injected subcutaneously over a 10 minute period in patients judged to have ordinary tolerance to epinephrine administration. This would represent up to 14 mL of 1:100,000 epinephrine-containing solution (10 µg/mL), or the equivalent quantity, in a 70 kilogram patient. This may be repeated up to 3 times per hour (total 42 mL per hour). The concomitant administration of lidocaine enhances the safety of the use of epinephrine during Enflurane anesthesia. This effect of lidocaine is dose related.

All customary precautions in the use of vasoconstrictor substances should be observed.

Muscle relaxation may be adequate for intra-abdominal operations at normal levels of anesthesia. Muscle relaxants may be used to achieve greater relaxation and all commonly used muscle relaxants are compatible with Enflurane. THE NONDEPOLARIZING MUSCLE RELAXANTS ARE POTENTIATED. In the normal 70 kg adult, 6 to 9 mg of d-tubocuraine or 1.0 to 1.5 mg of pancuronium will produce a 90% or greater depression of twitch height. Neostigmine does not reverse the direct effect of Enflurane.

Enflurane 0.25 to 1.0% (average 0.5%) provides analgesia equal to that produced by 30 to 60% (average 40%) nitrous oxide for vaginal delivery. With either agent, patients remain awake, cooperative and oriented. Maternal blood losses are comparable. These clinical approaches produce normal Apgar scores. Serial neurobehavioral testing of the newborn during the first 24 hours of life reveals that neither Enflurane nor nitrous oxide analgesia is associated with obvious neurobehavioral alterations. Neither Enflurane nor nitrous oxide when used for obstetrical analgesia alters BUN, creatinine, uric acid or osmolality. The only difference in the use of these two agents for obstetrical analgesia appears to be higher inspired oxygen concentration that may be used with Enflurane.

Analgetic doses of Enflurane, up to approximately 1.0%, do not significantly depress the rate or force of uterine contraction during labor and delivery. A slowing of the rate of uterine contraction and a diminution of the force of uterine contraction is noted between the administration of 1.0 to 2.0% delivered Enflurane; concentrations somewhere between 2.0 and 3.0% delivered Enflurane may abolish uterine contractions. Enflurane displaces the myometrial response curve to oxytocin so that at lower concentrations of Enflurane oxytocin will restore uterine contractions; however, as the dose of Enflurane progresses (somewhere between 1.5 and 3.0% delivered Enflurane) the response to oxytocin is diminished and then abolished. Uterine bleeding may be increased when Enflurane is used in higher concentrations for vaginal delivery or to facilitate delivery by Cesarean section; however, this has not been demonstrated within the recommended dosage range (see *"Dosage and Administration"* section). Mean estimated blood loss in patients anesthetized for therapeutic termination of pregnancy with 1.0% Enflurane in 70% nitrous oxide with oxygen is approximately twice that noted following therapeutic termination of pregnancy performed with the use of a local anesthetic technique (40 mL versus 20 mL).

Pharmacokinetics: Biotransformation of Enflurane in man results in low peak levels of serum fluoride averaging 15 µmol/L. These levels are well below the 50 µmol/L threshold level which can produce minimal renal damage in normal subjects. However, patients chronically ingesting isoniazid or other hydrazine-containing compounds may metabolize greater amounts of Enflurane. Although no significant renal dysfunction has been found thus far in such patients, peak serum fluoride levels can exceed 50 µmol/L, particularly when anesthesia goes beyond 2 MAC hours. Depression of lymphocyte transformation does not follow prolonged Enflurane anesthesia in man in the absence of surgery. Thus Enflurane does not depress this aspect of the immune response.

INDICATIONS AND USAGE
Enflurane may be used for induction and maintenance of general anesthesia. Enflurane may be used to provide analgesia for vaginal delivery. Low concentrations of Enflurane (see *"Dosage and Administration"*) may also be used to supplement other general anesthetic agents during delivery by Cesarean section. Higher concentrations of Enflurane may produce uterine relaxation and an increase in uterine bleeding.

CONTRAINDICATIONS
Seizure disorders (see *"Warnings"*).
　Known sensitivity to Enflurane or other halogenated anesthetics.
　Known or suspected genetic susceptibility to malignant hyperthermia.

WARNINGS
Increasing depth of anesthesia with Enflurane may produce a change in the electroencephalogram characterized by high voltage, fast frequency, progressing through spike-dome complexes alternating with periods of electrical silence to frank seizure activity. The latter may or may not be associated with motor movement. Motor activity, when encountered, generally consists of twitching or "jerks" of various muscle groups; it is self-limiting and can be terminated by lowering the anesthetic concentration. This electroencephalographic pattern associated with deep anesthesia is exacerbated by low arterial carbon dioxide tension. A reduction in ventilation and anesthetic concentrations usually suffices to eliminate seizure activity. Cerebral blood flow and metabolism studies in normal volunteers immediately following seizure activity show no evidence of cerebral hypoxia. Mental function testing does not reveal any impairment of performance following prolonged Enflurane anesthesia associated with or not associated with seizure activity.

Since levels of anesthesia may be altered easily and rapidly, only vaporizers producing predictable concentrations should be used. Hypotension and respiratory exchange can serve as a guide to depth of anesthesia. Deep levels of anesthesia may produce marked hypotension and respiratory depression.

When previous exposure to a halogenated anesthetic is known to have been followed by evidence of unexplained hepatic dysfunction, consideration should be given to use of an agent other than Enflurane.

PRECAUTIONS
General: Enflurane should be used with caution in patients who by virtue of medical or drug history could be considered more susceptible to cortical stimulation produced by the drug.

Information to Patients: Enflurane, as well as other general anesthetics, may cause a slight decrease in intellectual function for 2 to 3 days following anesthesia. As with other anesthetics, small changes in moods and symptoms may persist for several days following administration.

Laboratory Tests: Bromsulfalein (BSP) retention is mildly elevated postoperatively in some cases. This may relate to the effect of surgery since prolonged anesthesia (5 to 7 hours) in human volunteers does not result in BSP elevation. There is some elevation of glucose and white blood count intraoperatively. Glucose elevation should be considered in diabetic patients.

Drug Interactions: The action of nondepolarizing relaxants is augmented by Enflurane. Less than the usual amounts of these drugs should be used. If the usual amounts of nondepolarizing relaxants are given, the time for recovery from neuromuscular blockade will be longer in the presence of Enflurane than when halothane or nitrous oxide with a balanced technique are used.

Carcinogenesis/Mutagenesis: Swiss ICR mice were given Enflurane to determine whether such exposure might induce neoplasia. Enflurane was given at 1/2, 1/8 and 1/32 MAC for four in-utero exposures and for 24 exposures to the pups during the first nine weeks of life. The mice were killed at 15 months of age. The incidence of tumors in these mice was the same as in untreated control mice who were given the same background gases, but not the anesthetic.

Exposure of mice to 20 hours of 1.2% Enflurane causes a small (about 1/2 of 1.0%) but statistically significant increase in sperm abnormalities. In contrast to these results, in vitro approaches to the study of mutagenesis (Ames test, sister chromatid exchange test, and the 8-azaguanine system) have not shown a mutagenic effect of Enflurane.

Pregnancy Category B: Reproduction studies have been performed in rats and rabbits at doses up to four times the human dose and have revealed no evidence of impaired fertility or harm to the fetus due to Enflurane. There are, however, no adequate and well controlled studies in pregnant women. Because animal reproduction studies are not always predictive of human response, this drug should be used during pregnancy only if clearly needed.

Nursing Mothers: It is not known whether this drug is excreted in human milk. Because many drugs are excreted in human milk, caution should be exercised when Enflurane is administered to a nursing woman.

Malignant Hyperthermia: In susceptible individuals, Enflurane anesthesia may trigger a skeletal muscle hypermetabolic state leading to high oxygen demand and the clinical syndrome known as malignant hyperthermia. The syndrome includes nonspecific features such as muscle rigidity, tachycardia, tachypnea, cyanosis, arrhythmias and unstable blood pressure. (It should also be noted that many of these nonspecific signs may appear with light anesthesia, acute hypoxia, etc. The syndrome of malignant hyperthermia secondary to Enflurane appears to be rare; by March 1980, 35 cases had been reported in North America for an approximate incidence of 1:725,000 Enflurane anesthetics.) An increase in overall metabolism may be reflected in an elevated temperature (which may rise rapidly early or late in the case, but usually is not the first sign of augmented metabolism) and an increased usage of CO_2 absorption system (hot canister). PaO_2 and pH may decrease, and hyperkalemia and a base deficit may appear. Treatment includes discontinuance of triggering agents (e.g., Enflurane), administration of intravenous dantrolene sodium, and application of supportive therapy. Such therapy includes vigorous efforts to restore body temperature to normal, respiratory and circulatory support as indicated, and management of electrolyte-fluid-acid-base derangement. (Consult prescribing information for dantrolene sodium intravenous for additional information on patient management.) Renal failure may appear later, and urine flow should be sustained if possible.

ADVERSE REACTIONS

1. Malignant hyperthermia (see *"Precautions"*).
2. Motor activity exemplified by movements of various muscle groups and/or seizures may be encountered with deep levels of Enflurane anesthesia, or light levels with hypocapnia.
3. Hypotension and respiratory depression have been reported.
4. Arrhythmias, shivering, nausea and vomiting have been reported.
5. Elevation of the white blood count has been observed.
6. Unexplained mild, moderate and severe liver injury may rarely follow anesthesia with Enflurane. Serum transaminases may be increased and histologic evidence of injury may be found. The histologic changes are neither unique nor consistent. In several of these cases, it has not been possible to exclude Enflurane as the cause or as a contributing cause to liver injury. The incidence of unexplained hepatotoxicity following the administration of Enflurane is unknown, but it appears to be rare and not dose related.

OVERDOSAGE

In the event of overdosage, or what may appear to be overdosage, the following action should be taken:

Stop drug administration, establish a clear airway and initiate assisted or controlled ventilation with pure oxygen.

DOSAGE AND ADMINISTRATION

The concentration of Enflurane being delivered from a vaporizer during anesthesia should be known. This may be accomplished by using:

a) vaporizers calibrated specifically for Enflurane;
b) vaporizers from which delivered flows can easily and readily be calculated.

Preanesthetic Medication: Preanesthetic medication should be selected according to the need of the individual patient, taking into account that secretions are

weakly stimulated by Enflurane and that Enflurane does not alter heart rate. The use of anticholinergic drugs is a matter of choice.

Surgical Anesthesia: Induction may be achieved using Enflurane alone with oxygen or in combination with oxygen-nitrous oxide mixtures. Under these conditions some excitement may be encountered. If excitement is to be avoided, a hypnotic dose of a short-acting barbiturate should be used to induce unconsciousness, followed by the Enflurane mixture. In general, inspired concentrations of 2.0 to 4.5% Enflurane produce surgical anesthesia in 7 to 10 minutes.

Maintenance: Surgical levels of anesthesia may be maintained with 0.5 to 3.0% Enflurane. Maintenance concentrations should not exceed 3.0%. If added relaxation is required, supplemental doses of muscle relaxants may be used. Ventilation to maintain the tension of carbon dioxide in arterial blood in the 35 to 45 mm Hg range is preferred. Hyperventilation should be avoided in order to minimize possible CNS excitation.

The level of blood pressure during maintenance is an inverse function of Enflurane concentration in the absence of other complicating problems. Excessive decreases (unless related to hypovolemia) may be due to depth of anesthesia and in such instances should be corrected by lightening the level of anesthesia.

Analgesia: Enflurane 0.25 to 1.0% provides analgesia for vaginal delivery equal to that produced by 30 to 60% nitrous oxide. These concentrations normally do not produce amnesia. See also the information on the effects of Enflurane on uterine contraction contained in the *"Clinical Pharmacology"* section.

Cesarean Section: Enflurane should ordinarily be administered in the concentration range of 0.5 to 1.0% to supplement other general anesthetics. See also the information on the effects of Enflurane on uterine contraction contained in the *"Clinical Pharmacology"* section.

Storage: Store at room temperature 15° - 30° C (59° - 86° F). Enflurane contains no additives and has been demonstrated to be stable at room temperature for periods in excess of five years.

HOW SUPPLIED
SOLUTION:

BRAND/MANUFACTURER	NDC	SIZE	AWP
○ **BRAND**			
ETHRANE: Ohmeda	10019-0350-50	125 ml	$96.00
	10019-0350-60	250 ml	$162.00
○ **GENERICS**			
Abbott Hosp	00074-9406-01	125 ml	$123.29
Abbott Hosp	00074-9406-02	250 ml	$208.05

Engerix-B *SEE* HEPATITIS B VACCINE, RECOMBINANT

Enlon *SEE* ATROPINE SULFATE AND EDROPHONIUM CHLORIDE *AND* EDROPHONIUM CHLORIDE

Enoxacin

DESCRIPTION

Enoxacin is a broad-spectrum azafluoroquinolone antibacterial agent for oral administration. Enoxacin is 1-ethyl-6-fluoro-1,4-dihydro-4-oxo-7-(1-piperazinyl)-1,8-naphthyridine -3-carboxylic acid sesquihydrate.

Its empirical formula is $C_{15}H_{17}N_4O_3F \cdot \frac{1}{2}H_2O$, and its molecular weight is 320.32 (anhydrous). Enoxacin is an ivory-to-slightly yellow powder. In dilute aqueous solution, it is unstable in strong sunlight.

Enoxacin is available in 200-mg and 400-mg film-coated tablets. Each "200" and "400" tablet contains enoxacin sesquihydrate equivalent to 200 mg and 400 mg of anhydrous Enoxacin respectively.

Following is its chemical structure:

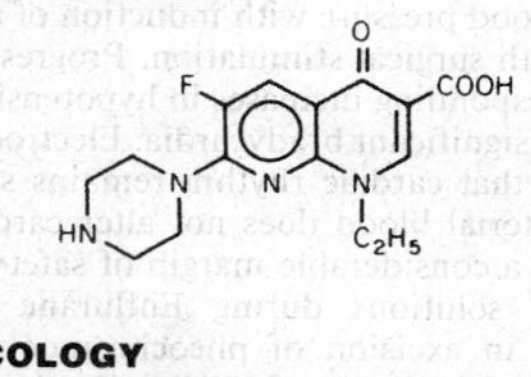

CLINICAL PHARMACOLOGY

Following oral administration to healthy subjects, peak plasma Enoxacin concentrations were achieved within 1 to 3 hours. Absolute oral bioavailability of Enoxacin is approximately 90%. Maximum plasma concentrations of Enoxacin average 0.93 mcg/mL and 2.0 mcg/mL after single 200-mg and 400-mg doses, respectively. Enoxacin plasma half-life is 3 to 6 hours. Enoxacin is excreted primarily via the kidney. After a single dose, greater than 40% was recovered in urine by 48 hours as unchanged drug. In elderly patients, the mean peak Enoxacin plasma concentration was 50% higher than that in young adult volunteers receiving comparable single doses of Enoxacin. This appears to correspond to age-associated reduction of renal function in the elderly population. Five metabolites of Enoxacin have been identified in human urine and account for 15% to 20% of the administered dose. Enoxacin diffuses into cervix, fallopian tube, and myometrium at levels approximately 1-2 times those achieved in plasma, and into kidney and prostate at levels approximately 2-4 times those achieved in plasma. Studies have not been conducted to assess the penetration of Enoxacin into human cerebrospinal fluid.

Enoxacin is approximately 40% bound to plasma proteins in healthy subjects and is approximately 14% bound to plasma proteins in patients with impaired renal function.

The effect of food on the absorption of Enoxacin from the tablet formulation has not been studied.

Some isozymes of the cytochrome P-450 hepatic microsomal enzyme system are inhibited by Enoxacin. This inhibition results in significant drug/drug interactions with theophylline and caffeine. Enoxacin interferes with the metabolism of theophylines, resulting in a dose related decrease in theophylline clearance. Elevated serum theophylline concentrations may increase the risk of theophylline-related adverse reactions. (See "Drug Interactions".)

Clearance of Enoxacin is reduced in patients with impaired renal function (creatinine clearance ≤ 30 mL/min/1.73 m^2), and dosage adjustment is necessary. (See "Dosage and Administration".)

MICROBIOLOGY

Enoxacin is an inhibitor of the bacterial enzyme DNA gyrase and is a bactericidal agent. Enoxacin may be active against pathogens resistant to drugs that act by different mechanisms.

Enoxacin has been shown to be active against most strains of the following organisms both in vitro and in clinical infections: (See "Indications and Usage".)

Gram-positive aerobes: Staphylococcus epidermidis, Staphyloccus saprophyticus.

Gram-negative aerobes: Enterobacter cloacae, Escherichia coli, Klebsiella pneumoniae, Neisseria gonorrhoeae, Proteus mirabilis, Pseudomonas aeruginosa.

The following in vitro data are available but their clinical significance is unknown.

In addition, Enoxacin exhibits in vitro minimum inhibitory concentrations (MICs) of 2.0 mcg/mL or less against most strains of the following organisms; however, the safety and effectiveness of Enoxacin in treating clinical infections due to these organisms have not been established in adequate and well-controlled trials.

Gram-negative aerobes: Aeromonas hydrophila, Citrobacter diversus, Citrobacter freundii, Citrobacter koseri, Enterobacter aerogenes, Haemophilus ducreyi, Klebsiella oxytoca, Klebsiella ozaenae, Morganella morganii, Proteus vulgaris, Providencia stuartii, Providencia alcalifaciens, Serratia marcescens, Serratia proteomaculans (formerly S. liquefaciens).

Many strains of Streptococcus species and anaerobes are usually resistant to Enoxacin.

The activity of Enoxacin against Treponema pallidum has not been evaluated; however, other quinolones are not active against T. pallidum. (See "Warnings".)

Cross-resistance with other quinolones has been demonstrated.

The addition of human serum has no effect on the in vitro MIC values; however, Enoxacin activity is decreased in acidic (pH 5.5) environments.

SUSCEPTIBILITY TESTING

Diffusion Techniques: Quantitative methods that require measurement of zone diameters give the most precise estimate of susceptibility of bacteria to antimicrobial agents. One such standardized procedure[1] that has been recommended for use with disks to test susceptibility of organisms to Enoxacin uses the 10-mcg Enoxacin disk.

Interpretation involves the correlation of the diameter obtained in the disk test with the minimum inhibitory concentration (MIC) for Enoxacin.

Reports from the laboratory giving results of the standard single-disk susceptibility test with a 10-mcg Enoxacin disk should be interpreted according to the following criteria:

Zone Diameter (mm)	Interpretation
≥ 18	(S) Susceptible
15-17	(MS) Moderately susceptible
≤ 14	(R) Resistant

A report of "susceptible" indicates that the pathogen is likely to be inhibited by generally achievable blood concentrations. A report of "moderately susceptible" suggests that the organism would be susceptible if high dosage is used or if the infection is confined to tissues or fluids in which high antimicrobial levels are attained. A report of "resistant" indicates that achievable drug concentrations are unlikely to be inhibitory, and other therapy should be selected.

Standardized susceptibility test procedures require the use of laboratory control organisms. The 10-mcg Enoxacin disk should give the following zone diameters:

Organism	Zone Diameter (mm)
Escherichia coli (ATCC 25922)	28-36
Neisseria Gonorrhoeae (ATCC 49226)	43-51
Pseudomonas aeruginosa (ATCC 27853)	22-28

Organism	Zone Diameter (mm)
Staphylococcus aureus (ATCC 25923)	22-28

Other quinolone antibacterial disks should not be substituted when performing susceptibility tests for Enoxacin because of spectrum differences. The 10-mcg Enoxacin disk should be used for all in vitro testing of isolates for Enoxacin susceptibility using diffusion techniques.

Dilution Techniques: Use a standardized dilution method[2] (broth, agar, or microdilution) or equivalent with Enoxacin powder. The MIC values obtained should be interpreted according to the following criteria:

MIC (mcg/mL)	Interpretation
≥ 2	(S) Susceptible
4	(MS) Moderately susceptible
≤ 8	(R) Resistant

As with standard diffusion methods, dilution procedures require the use of laboratory control organisms. Standard Enoxacin powder should give the following MIC values:

Organism	MIC (mcg/mL)
Enterococcus faecalis (ATCC 29212)	2-16
Escherichia coli (ATCC 25922)	0.06-0.25
Neisseria gonorrhoeae (ATCC 49226)	0.015-0.06
Pseudomonas aeruginosa (ATCC 27853)	2-8
Staphylococcus aureus (ATCC 29213)	0.5-2

INDICATIONS AND USAGE

Enoxacin is indicated for the treatment of adults (≥ 18 years of age) with the following infections caused by susceptible strains of the designated microorganisms:

Sexually Transmitted Diseases: (See "Warnings".) Uncomplicated urethral or cervical gonorrhea due to Neisseria gonorrhoeae.

Urinary Tract: Uncomplicated urinary tract infections (cystitis) due to Escherichia coli, Staphylococcus epidermidis,* or Staphylococcus saprophyticus.*

Complicated urinary tract infections: due to Escherichia coli, Klebsiella pneumoniae, Proteus mirabilis, Pseudomonas aeruginosa, Staphylococcus epidermidis, or Enterobacter cloacae.* The dosage regimens for complicated and uncomplicated urinary tract infections are different. (See "Dosage and Administration".)

Penicillinase production should have no effect on Enoxacin activity.

Appropriate culture and susceptibility tests should be performed before treatment in order to isolate and identify organisms causing the infection and to determine their susceptibility to Enoxacin. Therapy with Enoxacin may be initiated while awaiting the results of these studies; therapy should be adjusted if necessary once the results are known. Culture and susceptibility testing performed periodically during therapy will provide information not only on the therapeutic effect of the antimicrobial agent but also on the possible emergence of bacterial resistance.

CONTRAINDICATIONS

Enoxacin is contraindicated for individuals with a history of hypersensitivity to Enoxacin or to any of the other members of the quinolone class of antimicrobial agents.

WARNINGS

THE SAFETY AND EFFECTIVENESS OF ENOXACIN IN CHILDREN, ADOLESCENTS (UNDER THE AGE OF 18 YEARS), PREGNANT WOMEN, AND LACTATING WOMEN HAVE NOT BEEN ESTABLISHED. (See "Precautions"—Pregnancy, Nursing Mothers, and Pediatric Use). Enoxacin has been shown to cause arthropathy in immature rats and dogs when given in oral doses approximately 1.5 and 3.8 times, respectively, the highest human clinical dose based on a mg/m^2 basis after a four-week dosage regimen. Gross and histopathological examination of the weight-bearing joints of the dogs revealed lesions of the cartilage. Other quinolones also produce erosions of cartilage of weight-bearing joints and other signs of arthropathy in immature animals of various species. (See "Animal Pharmacology".)

Enoxacin has not been shown to be effective in the treatment of syphilis. Antimicrobial agents used in high doses for short periods of time to treat gonorrhea may mask or delay the symptoms of incubating syphilis. All patients with gonorrhea should have a serologic test for syphilis at the time of diagnosis. Patients treated with Enoxacin should have a follow-up serologic test for syphilis after 3 months.

Serious and occasionally fatal hypersensitivity (anaphylactoid or anaphylactic) reactions, some following the first dose, have been reported in patients receiving quinolone therapy. Some reactions were accompanied by cardiovascular collapse,

---

* Efficacy for this organism in this organ system at the recommended dose was studied in fewer than ten infections.

loss of consciousness, tingling, pharyngeal or facial edema, dyspnea, urticaria, or itching. Only a few patients had a history of previous hypersensitivity reactions. Serious hypersensitivity reactions have also been reported following treatment with Enoxacin. If an allergic reaction to Enoxacin occurs, discontinue the drug. Serious acute hypersensitivity reactions may require immediate treatment with epinephrine. Oxygen, intravenous fluids, antihistamines, corticosteroids, pressor amines, and airway management, including intubation, should be administered as indicated.

Convulsions and abnormal electroencephalograms have been reported in some patients receiving Enoxacin. Convulsions, increased intracranial pressure, and/or toxic psychoses have also been reported in patients receiving other drugs in this class. Quinolones may also cause central nervous system (CNS) stimulation which may lead to tremors, restlessness, lightheadedness, confusion, or hallucinations. If these reactions occur in patients receiving Enoxacin, the drug should be discontinued and appropriate measures instituted. Enoxacin, as well as other quinolones, should be used with caution in patients with known or suspected CNS disorders, such as severe cerebral arteriosclerosis, epilepsy, and other factors that predispose to seizures. (See "Adverse Reactions".)

Pseudomembranous colitis has been reported with nearly all antibacterial agents, including Enoxacin, and may range in severity from mild to life-threatening. Therefore, it is important to consider this diagnosis in patients who present with diarrhea subsequent to the administration of antibacterial agents.

Treatment with broad-spectrum antibacterial agents alters the normal flora of the colon and may permit overgrowth of clostridia. Studies indicate that a toxin produced by *Clostridium difficile* is a primary cause of "antibiotic-associated colitis."

After the diagnosis of pseudomembranous colitis has been established, therapeutic measures should be initiated.

Mild cases of pseudomembranous colitis usually respond to discontinuation of the drug alone. In moderate to severe cases, consideration should be given to management with fluids and electrolytes, protein supplementation, and treatment with an antibacterial drug clinically effective against *C. difficile* colitis.

Enoxacin is a potent inhibitor of the hepatic microsomal enzyme system, resulting in significant drug/drug interactions with theophylline and caffeine. (See "Drug Interactions".)

PRECAUTIONS

General: Alteration of the dosage regimen is necessary for patients with impaired renal function (creatinine clearance ≤ 30 mL/min/1.73 m^2). (See "Dosage and Administration".)

Moderate-to-severe phototoxicity reactions have been observed in patients exposed to direct sunlight while receiving Enoxacin or some other drugs in this class. Excessive sunlight should be avoided. Therapy should be discontinued if phototoxicity occurs.

Ophthalmologic abnormalities, including cataracts and multiple punctate lenticular opacities, have been noted in patients undergoing treatment with Enoxacin, as well as with some other quinolones, but have also been observed in patients receiving placebo in comparative trials. In clinical trials using multiple-dose therapy, ophthalmic tissue levels of Enoxacin and other quinolones were significantly higher than respective plasma concentrations. The causal relationship, if any, of quinolones to lenticular abnormalities has not been established.

Decreased spermatogenesis and subsequent decreased fertility were noted in rats and dogs treated with doses of Enoxacin that produced plasma levels in the animals three times higher than those produced in humans at the recommended therapeutic dosage. The potential for Enoxacin to affect spermatogenesis in male patients is unknown.

Information for Patients: Patients should be advised:

■ not to take magnesium-, aluminum-, or calcium-containing antacids, bismuth subsalicylate, products containing iron, or multivitamins containing zinc for 8 hours prior to Enoxacin or for 2 hours after Enoxacin administration (see "Precautions—Drug Interactions");
■ to drink fluids liberally;
■ to avoid consumption of caffeine-containing products (certain drugs, coffee, tea, chocolate, certain carbonated beverages) during Enoxacin therapy (see "Precautions—Drug Interactions");
■ that Enoxacin may cause dizziness and light-headedness and, therefore, patients should know how they react to Enoxacin before they operate an automobile or machinery or engage in activities requiring mental alertness and coordination;
■ that Enoxacin may be associated with hypersensitivity reaction, even following the first dose, and to discontinue the drug at the first sign of a skin rash or other allergic reaction;
■ to avoid undue exposure to excessive sunlight while receiving Enoxacin and to discontinue therapy if phototoxicity occurs.

DRUG INTERACTIONS

Bismuth: Bismuth subsalicylate, given concomitantly with Enoxacin or 60 minutes following Enoxacin administration, decreased Enoxacin bioavailability by approximately 25%. Thus, concomitant administration of Enoxacin and bismuth subsalicylate should be avoided.

Caffeine: Enoxacin is a potent inhibitor of the cytochrome P-450 isozymes responsible for the metabolism of methylxanthines. In a multiple-dose study, Enoxacin caused a dose-related increase in the mean elimination half-life of caffeine, thereby decreasing the clearance of caffeine by up to 80% and leading to a five-fold increase in the AUC and the half-life of caffeine. Trough plasma Enoxacin levels were also 20% higher when caffeine and Enoxacin were

administered concomitantly. Caffeine-related adverse effects have occurred in patients consuming caffeine while on therapy with Enoxacin. (See "Warnings".)

Cyclosporine: Elevated serum levels of cyclosporine have been reported with concomitant use of cyclosporine with other members of the quinolone class.

Digoxin: Enoxacin may raise serum digoxin levels in some individuals. If signs and symptoms suggestive of digoxin toxicity occur when Enoxacin and digoxin are given concomitantly, physicians are advised to obtain serum digoxin levels and adjust digoxin doses appropriately.

Nonsteroidal Anti-Inflammatory Agents: Seizures have been reported in patients taking Enoxacin concomitantly with the nonsteroidal anti-inflammatory drug fenbufen. Animal studies also suggest an increased potential for seizures when these two drugs are given concomitantly. Fenbufen is not approved in the United States at this time.

Sucralfate and Antacids: Quinolones form chelates with metal cations. Therefore, administration of quinolones with antacids containing calcium, magnesium, or aluminum; with sucralfate; with divalent or trivalent cations such as iron; or with multivitamins containing zinc may substantially interfere with drug absorption and result in insufficient plasma and tissue quinolone concentrations. Antacids containing aluminum hydroxide and magnesium hydroxide reduce the oral absorption of Enoxacin by 75%. The oral bio-availability of Enoxacin is reduced by 60% with coadministration of ranitidine. These agents should not be taken for 8 hours before or for 2 hours after Enoxacin administration.

Theophylline: Enoxacin is a potent inhibitor of the cytochrome P-450 isozymes responsible for the metabolism of methylxanthines. Enoxacin interferes with the metabolism of theophylline resulting in a 42% to 74% dose-related decrease in theophylline clearance and a subsequent 260% to 350% increase in serum theophylline levels. Theophylline-related adverse effects have occurred in patients when theophylline and Enoxacin were coadministered. (See "Warnings".)

Warfarin: Quinolones including Enoxacin, decrease the clearance of R-warfarin, the less active isomer of racemic warfarin. Enoxacin does not affect the clearance of the active S-isomer, and changes in clotting time have not been observed when Enoxacin and warfarin were coadministered. Nevertheless, the prothrombin time or other suitable coagulation test should be monitored when warfarin or its derivatives and Enoxacin are given concomitantly.

Carcinogenesis, Mutagenesis, Impairment of Fertility: Long-term studies in animals to determine the carcinogenic potential of Enoxacin have not been conducted.

Genetic toxicology tests included *in vitro* mutagenicity and cytogenetic assays and *in vivo* cytogenetic and micronucleus tests. Enoxacin did not induce point mutations in bacterial cells or mitotic gene conversion in yeast cells, with or without metabolic activation. Enoxacin did not induce sister chromatid exchanges or structural chromosomal aberrations in mammalian cells *in vitro*, with or without metabolic activation. In addition, Enoxacin did not induce chromosomal aberrations in mice.

There was a minimal, dose-related, statistically significant increase in micronuclei at high doses in mice. The significance of these findings, in the absence of effects in other test systems, is not established.

Enoxacin produced no consistent effects on fertility and reproductive parameters in female rats given oral doses of Enoxacin at levels up to 1000 mg/kg. Decreased spermatogenesis and subsequent impaired fertility was noted in male rats given oral doses of 1000 mg/kg. This dose is approximately 13-fold greater than the highest human clinical daily oral dose of 16 mg/kg, assuming a 50 kg person and based on a mg/m^2 basis.

Pregnancy: Teratogenic Effects. Pregnancy Category C. Studies with Enoxacin given orally to mice and rats have shown no evidence of teratogenic potential. The intravenous infusion of Enoxacin into pregnant rabbits at doses of 10 to 50 mg/kg caused dose-related maternal toxicity (venous irritation, body weight loss, and reduced food intake) and, at 50 mg/kg, fetal toxicity (increased post-implantation loss and stunted fetuses).

At 50 mg/kg, the incidence of fetal malformations was significantly increased in the presence of overt maternal and fetal toxicity. There are no adequate and well-controlled studies in pregnant women. Enoxacin should be used during pregnancy only if the potential benefit justifies the potential risk to the fetus. (See "Warnings".)

Nursing Mothers: It is not known whether Enoxacin is excreted in human milk. Enoxacin is excreted in the milk of lactating rats. Because drugs of this class are excreted in human milk and because of the potential for serious adverse reactions from Enoxacin in nursing infants, a decision should be made whether to discontinue nursing or to discontinue the drug, taking into account the importance of the drug to the mother.

Pediatric Use: Safety and effectiveness in children and adolescents below the age of 18 years have not been established. Enoxacin causes arthropathy in juvenile animals. (See "Warnings" and "Animal Pharmacology".)

Geriatric Use: In multiple-dose clinical trials of Enoxacin, elderly patients (≥ 65 years of age) experienced significantly more overall adverse events than patients under 65 years of age. However, the incidence of drug-related adverse reactions was comparable between age groups.

ADVERSE REACTIONS

Single-Dose Studies: During clinical trials, approximately 9% of patients treated with a single dose of 400 mg of Enoxacin for uncomplicated urethral or endocervical gonorrhea reported adverse events.

The most frequently reported events in single-dose trials, without regard to drug relationship, were nausea and vomiting (2%). Events that occurred in less than 1% of patients are listed below.

Central Nervous System: headache, dizziness, somnolence.

Gastrointestinal: abdominal pain.

Gynecologic: vaginal moniliasis.

Skin/Hypersensitivity: rash.

Laboratory Abnormalities: increased AST (SGOT), decreased hemoglobin, decreased hematocrit, eosinophilia, leukocytosis, leukopenia, thrombocytosis, increased urinary protein, increased alkaline phosphatase, increased ALT (SGPT), increased bilirubin, hyperkalemia.

Multiple-Dose Studies: The incidence of adverse events reported by patients in multiple-dose clinical trials, without regard to drug relationship, was 23%. The incidence of drug-related adverse reactions in multiple-dose clinical trials was 16%. Among patients receiving multiple-dose therapy Enoxacin was discontinued because of an adverse event in 3.8% of patients.

The following events were considered likely to be drug-related in patients receiving multiple doses of Enoxacin in clinical trials: nausea and/or vomiting 6%, dizziness 2%, headache 1%, abdominal pain 1%, diarrhea 1%, dyspepsia 1%. The most frequently reported events in all multiple-dose clinical trials, without regard to drug relationship, were as follows: nausea and/or vomiting 8%, dizziness and/or vertigo 3%, headache 2%, diarrhea 2%, abdominal pain 2%, insomnia 1%, dyspepsia 1%, rash 1%, nervousness and/or anxiety 1%, unusual taste 1%, pruritus 1%.

Additional events that occurred in less than 1% of patients but > 0.1% of patients are listed below.

Body as a Whole: asthenia, fatigue, fever, malaise, back pain, chest pain, edema, chills.

Gastrointestinal: flatulence, constipation, dry mouth/throat, stomatitis, anorexia, gastritis, bloody stools.

Central Nervous System: somnolence, tremor, convulsions, paresthesia, confusion, agitation, depression, syncope, myoclonus, depersonalization, hypertonia.

Skin/Hypersensitivity: photosensitivity reaction, urticaria, hyperhidrosis, mycotic infection, erythema multiforme, toxic epidermal necrolysis, Stevens-Johnson syndrome.

Special Senses: tinnitus, conjunctivitis, visual disturbances including amblyopia.

Musculoskeletal: myalgia, arthralgia.

Cardiovascular: palpitations, tachycardia, vasodilation.

Respiratory: dyspnea, cough, epistaxis.

Hemic and Lymphatic: purpura.

Urogenital: vaginal moniliasis, vaginitis, urinary incontinence, renal failure.

The following adverse events occurred in less than 0.1% of patients in multiple-dose clinical trials but were considered significant: pseudomembranous colitis, hyperkinesia, amnesia, ataxia, hypotonia, psychosis, emotional lability, hallucination, schizophrenic reaction.

Laboratory Changes: The following laboratory abnormalities appeared in ≥ 1.0% of patients receiving multiple doses of Enoxacin: elevated AST (SGOT), elevated ALT (SGPT). It is not known whether these abnormalities were caused by the drug or the underlying conditions.

Worldwide Postmarketing Experience: The most frequent spontaneously-reported adverse events in the worldwide post-marketing experience with multiple- and single-dose Enoxacin use have been rashes, seizures/convulsions, and photosensitivity reactions; however, there is no evidence that the incidences of these events were larger than those observed in the clinical trials population.

Quinolone-class Adverse Reactions: Although not reported in completed clinical studies with Enoxacin, a variety of adverse events have been reported with other quinolones.

Clinical Adverse Events Include: erythema nodosum, hepatic necrosis, possible exacerbation of myasthenia gravis, nystagmus, intestinal perforation, hyperpigmentation, interstitial nephritis, polyuria, urinary retention, renal calculi, cardiopulmonary arrest, cerebral thrombosis, and laryngeal or pulmonary edema.

Laboratory Adverse Events Include: agranulocytosis, elevation of serum triglycerides and/or serum cholesterol, prolongation of the prothrombin time, candiduria, and crystalluria.

OVERDOSAGE

In the event of acute overdosage, the stomach should be emptied by inducing vomiting or by gastric lavage and the patient carefully observed and given supportive treatment. Enoxacin is poorly removed (< 5% over 4 hours) by hemodialysis.

DOSAGE AND ADMINISTRATION

Enoxacin should be taken at least one hour before or at least two hours after a meal. See *"Indications and Usage"* for information on appropriate pathogens and patient populations.

SEXUALLY TRANSMITTED DISEASES

Uncomplicated urethral or cervical gonorrhea: 400 mg single dose.

URINARY TRACT INFECTIONS

Uncomplicated urinary tract infections: 200 mg q12h for 7 days.
Complicated urinary tract infections: 400 mg q12h for 14 days.

Dosage Adjustment for Renal Impairment: Dosage should be adjusted in patients with a creatinine clearance value of 30 mL/min/1.73 m² or less. After a normal initial dose, the dosing interval should be adjusted as follows:

Creatinine Clearance	Dosage Adjustment	Dose Interval
> 30 mL/min/1.73m²	None	12 hours
≤ 30 mL/min/1.73m²	½ recommended dose	12 hours

When only the serum creatinine is known, the following formula may be used to estimate creatinine clearance.

Men:

$$\text{creatinine clearance (mL/min)} = \frac{\text{Weight (kg)} \times (140\text{-age})}{72 \times \text{serum creatinine (mg/dL)}}$$

Women: 0.85 × the value calculated for men.

The serum creatinine should represent a steady state of renal function.

Dosage adjustment is not necessary in elderly patients with normal renal function, but dose should be adjusted according to the previous guidelines in elderly patients with compromised renal function.

Store at controlled room temperature, 15°C to 30°C (59°F to 86°F).

ANIMAL PHARMACOLOGY

Enoxacin and other members of the quinolone class have been shown to cause arthropathy in immature animals of most species tested. (See *"Warnings".*)

REFERENCES

1. National Committee for Clinical Laboratory Standards, Performance Standards for Antimicrobial Disk Susceptibility Tests—Fourth Edition. Approved Standard NCCLS Document M2-A4, Vol. 10, No. 7, NCCLS, Villanova, PA, 1990. 2. National Committee for Clinical Laboratory Standards, Methods for Dilution Antimicrobial Susceptibility Tests for Bacteria that Grow Aerobically—Second Edition. Approved Standard NCCLS Document M7-A2, Vol. 10, No. 8, NCCLS, Villanova, PA, 1990.

HOW SUPPLIED

TABLETS: 200 MG

BRAND/MANUFACTURER	NDC	SIZE	AWP
○ BRAND PENETREX: RPR	00075-5100-50	50s	$136.50

TABLETS: 400 MG

BRAND/MANUFACTURER	NDC	SIZE	AWP
○ BRAND PENETREX: RPR	00075-5140-50	50s	$136.50

Enoxaparin

DESCRIPTION

Enoxaparin is a sterile, low molecular weight heparin for injection. Each syringe contains 30 mg Enoxaparin in 0.3 mL Water for Injection. The approximate anti-Factor Xa activity per syringe is 3000 IU (with reference to the W.H.O. First International Low Molecular Weight Heparin Reference Standard). Nitrogen is used in the headspace to inhibit oxidation. The pH of the injection is 5.5-7.5. The solution is preservative-free and intended for use only as a single-dose injection.

Enoxaparin is obtained by alkaline degradation of heparin benzyl ester derived from porcine intestinal mucosa. Its structure is characterized by a 2-O-sulfo-4-enepyranosuronic acid group at the non-reducing end and a 2-N,6-O-disulfo-D-glucosamine at the reducing end of the chain. The substance is the sodium salt. The average molecular weight is about 4500. The molecular weight distribution is:

CLINICAL PHARMACOLOGY

Enoxaparin is a low molecular weight heparin which has antithrombotic properties. In man Enoxaparin is characterized by a higher ratio of anti-Factor Xa to anti-Factor IIa activity (3.35 ± 0.89) than unfractionated heparin (1.22 ± 0.13). Following the administration of a single subcutaneous dose of up to 90 mg Enoxaparin to healthy subjects, no appreciable change was observed in fibrinogen level and other parameters of fibrinolysis. At the recommended doses, single injections of Enoxaparin do not significantly influence platelet aggregation or affect global clotting tests (i.e. prothrombin time [PT] or activated partial thromboplastin time [APTT]).

PHARMACODYNAMICS

Maximum anti-Factor Xa and antithrombin (anti-Factor IIa) activities occur 3 to 5 hours after subcutaneous injection of Enoxaparin. Mean peak anti-Factor Xa activity was 0.16 IU/mL (1.58 µg/mL) and 0.38 IU/mL (3.83 µg/mL) after the 20 mg and the 40 mg clinically tested doses, respectively. Mean absolute bioavailability of Enoxaparin based on anti-Factor Xa activity is 92% in healthy volunteers. The volume of distribution of anti-Factor Xa activity is about 6 L. Following i.v. dosing, the total body clearance of Enoxaparin is 25 mL/min. Elimination half-life based on anti-Factor Xa activity was about 4.5 hours after subcutaneous administration. Following a 40 mg dose significant anti-Factor Xa activity persists in plasma for about 12 hours. There appears to be no appreciable increase in anti-Factor Xa activity after dosing for 3 days in young healthy subjects. Clearance, C_{max}, and AUC for anti-Factor Xa values following single and multiple s.c. dosing in elderly subjects and subjects with renal failure were close to those observed in normal subjects. An increase of 25% in the area under anti-Factor Xa activity versus time curve was observed following once daily dosing in healthy elderly subjects for 10 days. The kinetics of anti-Factor Xa activity in anuric patients undergoing dialysis are similar to those in normal subjects following i.v. dosing.

The decline of anti-Factor Xa activity with time was parallel to the decay curve of plasma total radioactivity (^{99m}TC) in healthy volunteers. Following intravenous dosing of Enoxaparin labeled with the gamma-emitter, ^{99m}Tc, 40% of radioactivity and 8-20% of anti-Factor Xa activity were recovered in urine in 24 hours.

CLINICAL TRIALS

Enoxaparin has been shown to prevent postoperative deep vein thrombosis (DVT) following hip replacement surgery. The data from two controlled clinical trials are summarized in the following tables. In all studies, efficacy is based on "all treated patients" analysis.

In a double-blind study Enoxaparin 30 mg q12h sc was compared to placebo. Treatment was initiated within 12-24 hours post-surgery and was continued for 10-14 days post-operatively.

Treatment Group	Treatment Group	
	Enoxaparin	Placebo
Dosing Regimen	30 mg q12h	q12h
	n (%)	n (%)
All Treated Patients	50 (100%)	50 (100%)
Treatment Failures		
Total DVT (%)	5 (10%)	23 (46%)*
Proximal DVT (%)	1 (2%)	11 (22%)**

* p value versus placebo = 0.0002
** p value versus placebo = 0.0134

A double-blind, multicenter study compared three dosing regimens of Enoxaparin. Treatment was initiated within two days post-surgery and was continued for up to 7 days postoperatively.

Dose	Treatment Group, Enoxaparin		
	10 mg QD n (%)	30 mg g 12h n (%)	40 mg QD n (%)
All Treated Patients	161 (100%)	208 (100%)	199 (100%)
Treatment Failures			
Total DVT (%)	40 (25%)	22 (11%)*	27 (14%)**
Proximal DVT (%)	17 (11%)	8 (4%)	9 (5%)

* p value versus Enoxaparin ® 10 mg QD = 0.0008
** p value versus Enoxaparin ® 10 mg QD = 0.0168

There was no significant difference between the 30 mg BID and 40 mg QD regimens.

INDICATION AND USAGE

Enoxaparin Injection is indicated for the prevention of deep vein thrombosis, which may lead to pulmonary embolism, following hip replacement surgery.

CONTRAINDICATIONS

Enoxaparin Injection is contraindicated in patients with active major bleeding, in patients with thrombocytopenia associated with a positive *in vitro* test for anti-platelet antibody in the presence of Enoxaparin Injection, or in patients with hypersensitivity to Enoxaparin Injection.

Patients with known hypersensitivity to heparin or pork products should not be treated with Enoxaparin.

WARNINGS

Enoxaparin Injection is not intended for intramuscular administration.

Enoxaparin cannot be used interchangeably (unit for unit) with unfractionated heparin or other low molecular weight heparins.

Enoxaparin should be used with extreme caution in patients with history of heparin-induced thrombocytopenia.

HEMORRHAGE:
Enoxaparin Injection like other anticoagulants, should be used with extreme caution in conditions with increased risk of hemorrhage, such as bacterial endocarditis, congenital or acquired bleeding disorders, active ulceration and angiodysplastic gastrointestinal disease, hemorrhagic stroke or shortly after brain, spinal or ophthalmological surgery.

Bleeding can occur at any site during therapy with Enoxaparin. An unexplained fall in hematocrit or blood pressure should lead to a search for a bleeding site.

THROMBOCYTOPENIA:
Moderate thrombocytopenia (platelet counts < 100,000/mm^3 and > 50,000/mm^3) occurred at a rate of about 2% in patients given Enoxaparin, 3% in patients given

heparin, and 0% in patients receiving placebo in clinical trials. Thrombocytopenia of any degree should be monitored closely.

PRECAUTIONS
GENERAL
Enoxaparin Injection should not be mixed with other injections or infusions. Enoxaparin Injection should be used with care in patients with a bleeding diathesis, uncontrolled arterial hypertension or a history of recent gastrointestinal ulceration and hemorrhage. Elderly patients and patients with renal insufficiency may show delayed elimination of Enoxaparin. Enoxaparin should be used with care in these patients.

If thromboembolic events occur despite Enoxaparin prophylaxis Enoxaparin should be discontinued and appropriate therapy initiated.

LABORATORY TESTS
Periodic complete blood counts, including platelet count, and stool occult blood tests are recommended during the course of treatment with Enoxaparin Injection.

DRUG INTERACTIONS
Enoxaparin Injection should be used with care in patients receiving oral anticoagulants, and/or platelet inhibitors.

DRUG/LABORATORY TEST INTERACTIONS
ELEVATIONS OF SERUM TRANSAMINASES
Asymptomatic increases in transaminase levels (SGOT [AST] and SGPT [ALT]) greater than three times the upper limit of normal of the laboratory reference range have been reported in 2 of 10 normal subjects and in up to 5% of patients during treatment with Enoxaparin Injection. Similar significant increases in transaminase levels have also been observed in patients and normal volunteers treated with heparin and other low molecular weight heparins. Such elevations are fully reversible and are rarely associated with increases in bilirubin. Since transaminase determinations are important in the differential diagnosis of myocardial infarction, liver disease and pulmonary emboli, elevations that might be caused by drugs like Enoxaparin should be interpreted with caution.

CARCINOGENESIS, MUTAGENESIS, IMPAIRMENT OF FERTILITY
No long-term studies in animals have been performed to evaluate carcinogenic potential of Enoxaparin. Enoxaparin was not mutagenic in *in vitro* tests, including the Ames test, mouse lymphoma cell forward mutation test, and human lymphocyte chromosomal aberration test and the *in vivo* rat bone marrow chromosomal aberration test. Enoxaparin was found to have no effect on fertility or reproductive performance of male and female rats at subcutaneous doses up to 20 mg/kg/day or 141 mg/m^2/day. The maximum received human dose in clinical trials was 1.5 mg/kg/day or 48.4 mg/m^2/day.

PREGNANCY: TERATOGENIC EFFECTS
Pregnancy category B: Teratology studies have been conducted in rats and rabbits at subcutaneous doses of Enoxaparin up to 30 mg/kg/day or 211 mg/m^2/day and 410 mg/m^2/day, respectively. The maximum received human dose in clinical trials was 1.5 mg/kg/day or 48.4 mg/m^2/day. There was no evidence of teratogenic effects or fetotoxicity due to Enoxaparin. There are, however, no adequate and well controlled studies in pregnant women. Because animal reproduction studies are not always predictive of human response, this drug should be used during pregnancy only if clearly needed.

NURSING MOTHERS:
It is not known whether this drug is excreted in human milk. Because many drugs are excreted in human milk, caution should be exercised when Enoxaparin is administered to nursing women.

PEDIATRIC USE
Safety and effectiveness of Enoxaparin in children has not been established.

ADVERSE REACTIONS
HEMORRHAGE
The incidence of hemorrhagic complications during Enoxaparin Injection treatment has been low.

The following rates of major bleeding events have been reported during clinical trials with Enoxaparin Injection and heparin and placebo in patients undergoing hip replacement surgery.

MAJOR BLEEDING EPISODE*

Enoxaparin	Heparin	Placebo
30 mg q12h	15000 U/24h	
n = 786	n = 541	n = 50
31[4%]	32[6%]	2[4%]

* Bleeding complication considered major if accompanied by a significant clinical event or if hemoglobin decreased by ≥ 2 g/dL or transfusion of 2 or more units of blood products was required.

THROMBOCYTOPENIA
During clinical trials with Enoxaparin Injection, moderate thrombocytopenia, defined as a platelet count less than 100,000/mm^3, was reported in 2% of patients given Enoxaparin 3% in patients given heparin and 0% in patients receiving placebo. (see "Warnings").

LOCAL IRRITATION
Mild local irritation, pain, hematoma and erythema may follow subcutaneous injection of Enoxaparin Injection.

OTHER
Other adverse effects that were thought to be possibly or probably related to treatment with Enoxaparin Injection, heparin or placebo in clinical trials, and that occurred at a rate of at least 2% in the Enoxaparin group, are shown below.

ADVERSE EVENTS OCCURRING AT ≥ 2% INCIDENCE IN ENOXAPARIN TREATED PATIENTS (EXCLUDING UNRELATED ADVERSE EVENTS)

Adverse Event	Enoxaparin 30 mg q12h n = 786 Severe	Total	Heparin 15000 U/24h n = 541 Severe	Total	Placebo n = 50 Severe	Total
Fever	< 1%	4%	< 1%	3%	0%	4%
Pain	< 1%	2%	1%	3%	0%	8%
Hemorrhage	< 1%	5%	< 1%	5%	0%	2%
Nausea	< 1%	3%	< 1%	2%	0%	2%
Ecchymosis	< 1%	2%	< 1%	2%	0%	2%
Hypochromic anemia	1%	3%	3%	7%	2%	16%
Edema	1%	3%	< 1%	2%	0%	4%
Peripheral edema	1%	3%	1%	5%	0%	0%
Confusion	< 1%	2%	< 1%	1%	0%	0%

OVERDOSAGE
SYMPTOMS/TREATMENT
Accidental overdosage following administration of Enoxaparin Injection may lead to hemorrhagic complications. This may be largely neutralized by the slow intravenous injection of protamine sulfate (1% solution). The dose of protamine sulfate should be equal to the dose of Enoxaparin Injection injected: 1 mg protamine sulfate should be administered to neutralize 1 mg Enoxaparin Injection. A second infusion of 0.5 mg/mg protamine sulfate may be administered if the APTT measured 2 to 4 hours after the first infusion remains prolonged. However, even with higher doses of protamine, the APTT may remain more prolonged than under normal conditions found following administration of conventional heparin. In all cases, the anti-Factor Xa activity is never completely neutralized (maximum about 60%). Particular care should be taken to avoid overdosage with protamine sulfate. Administration of protamine sulfate can cause severe hypotensive and anaphylactoid reactions. Because fatal reactions, often resembling anaphylaxis, have been reported with protamine sulfate, it should be given only when resuscitation techniques and treatment of anaphylactic shock are readily available. For additional information consult the labeling of Protamine Sulfate Injection, USP, products.

A single subcutaneous dose of 46.4 mg/kg Enoxaparin was lethal to rats. The symptoms of acute toxicity were ataxia, decreased motility, dyspnea, cyanosis and coma.

DOSAGE AND ADMINISTRATION
ADULT DOSAGE
In patients undergoing hip replacement, the recommended dose of Enoxaparin Injection is 30 mg twice daily administered by subcutaneous injection with the initial dose given as soon as possible after surgery, but not more than 24 hours post-operatively. Treatment should be continued throughout the period of post-operative care until the risk of deep vein thrombosis has diminished. Up to 14 days administration has been well tolerated in controlled clinical trials. The average duration of administration is 7 to 10 days.

All patients should be screened prior to prophylactic administration of Enoxaparin to rule out a bleeding disorder. There is usually no need for daily monitoring of the effect of Enoxaparin in patients with normal presurgical coagulation parameters.

ADMINISTRATION
Enoxaparin Injection is administered by subcutaneous injection. It must not be administered by intramuscular injection. Subcutaneous injection technique: Patients should be lying down and Enoxaparin Injection administered by deep subcutaneous injection. Administration should be alternated between the left and right anterolateral and left and right posterolateral abdominal wall. The whole length of the needle should be introduced into a skin fold held between the thumb and forefinger; the skin fold should be held throughout the injection.

Enoxaparin injection is a clear colorless to pale-yellow sterile solution and as with other parenteral drug products should be inspected visually for particulate matter and discoloration prior to administration.

Enoxaparin Injection should be stored at or below 25°C. Do not freeze.

HOW SUPPLIED
INJECTION: 30 MG

BRAND/MANUFACTURER	NDC	SIZE	AWP
○ **BRAND**			
LOVENOX: RPR	00075-0624-30	0.3 ml 10s	$150.09

Entex *SEE* **GUAIFENESIN AND PHENYLPROPANOLAMINE HYDROCHLORIDE, GUAIFENESIN AND PSEUDOEPHEDRINE HYDROCHLORIDE** *AND* **GUAIFENESIN/PHENYLEPHRINE HYDROCHLORIDE/PHENYLPROPANOLAMINE HYDROCHLORIDE**

Ephedrine Hydrochloride with Guaifenesin

DESCRIPTION
Each teaspoonful (5ml) contains:

Active ingredients:
Ephedrine HCl ....6.25 mg.
Guaifenesin ....100.00 mg.

INDICATIONS
For the temporary relief of shortness of breath, tightness of chest and wheezing due to bronchial asthma. For the symptomatic control of bronchial asthma. Eases breathing for asthma patients by reducing spasms of bronchial muscles. For the symptomatic relief of cough due to colds and minor upper respiratory infections.

CONTRAINDICATIONS
Sensitivity to any of the ingredients. Contraindicated in marked hypertension, hyperthyroidism or in patients who are receiving MAO inhibitors or antihypertensive medicine.

WARNINGS
Do not use this product unless a diagnosis of asthma has been made by a doctor. Do not use this product if you have heart disease, high blood pressure, thyroid disease, diabetes, or difficulty in urination due to enlargement of the prostrate gland unless directed by a doctor. Do not use this product if you have ever been hospitalized for asthma or if you are taking any prescription drug for asthma unless directed by a doctor.

PRECAUTIONS
Drug Interactions: Do not use this product if you are presently taking a prescription drug for high blood pressure or depression without first consulting your doctor.

Do not continue to use this product and seek medical assistance immediately if symptoms are not relieved within 1 hour or become worse.

Some users of this product may experience nervousness, tremor, sleeplessness, nausea and loss of appetite. If these symptoms persist or become worse, consult your doctor.

Diagnostic Interference: Urinary 5-hydroxyindoleacetic acid (5-HIAA) determinations. Urinary Vanillylmandelic Acid (VMA) determinations.

ADVERSE REACTIONS
Possible adverse reactions include diarrhea, drowsiness, nausea, vomiting and stomach pain.

Caution: As with any drug, if you are pregnant or nursing a baby, seek the advice of your physician before using this product.

DOSAGE
Adults: Two to four teaspoonfuls every 4 hours, not to exceed 24 teaspoonfuls in 24 hours, or as directed.

Children under 12 years of age: Consult a doctor.

PROFESSIONAL LABELING ONLY
Children 6-12: One teaspoonful every 4 hours, not to exceed 6 teaspoonfuls in 24 hours.

Children 2-6: ½ teaspoonful every 4 hours, not to exceed 3 teaspoonfuls in 24 hours.

STORAGE
Keep this and all drugs out of the reach of children.
Dispense in tight, light resistant containers as defined in the USP/NF.
Store between 59°-86° (15°-30°C)

HOW SUPPLIED
CAPSULE:

BRAND/MANUFACTURER	NDC	SIZE	AWP
○ **BRAND**			
BRONCHOLATE: Bock	00563-0276-01	100s	$14.13

➤ SHOWN IN PRODUCT IDENTIFICATION GUIDE

SYRUP:

BRAND/MANUFACTURER	NDC	SIZE	AWP
○ **BRAND**			
BRONCHOLATE SYRUP: Bock	00563-0280-16	480 ml	$10.74

Ephedrine Hydrochloride/ Phenobarbital/Potassium Iodide/ Theophylline

DESCRIPTION

Each Ephedrine Hydrochloride/Phenobarbital/Potassium Iodide/Theophylline tablet contains Ephedrine Hydrochloride 24 mg: Phenobarbital 24 mg [Warning: May be habit forming]; Potassium Iodide 320 mg Theophylline calcium salicylate 130 mg (equivalent to 65 mg anhydrous Theophylline).

This combination contains two bronchodilators, Theophylline and Ephedrine. Phenobarbital serves as a mild sedative to help counteract central nervous system stimulation which may be caused by Ephedrine. Wheezing and coughing are relieved by improved bronchodilation while the expectorant action of Potassium Iodide helps to remove secretions from the bronchial tree. Dyspnea is thus relieved or prevented and acute episodes of bronchospasm are often eliminated with consequent lessening of apprehension and distress.

CLINICAL PHARMACOLOGY

Theophylline directly relaxes the smooth muscle of the bronchial airways and pulmonary blood vessels, thus acting mainly as a bronchodilator, pulmonary vasodilator and smooth muscle relaxant. It also possesses other actions typical of the xanthine derivatives: coronary vasodilator, diuretic, and cardiac, cerebral, and skeletal muscle stimulant. The actions of Theophylline may be mediated through inhibition of phosphodiesterase and a resultant increase in intracellular cyclic AMP which could mediate smooth muscle relaxation.

In vitro, Theophylline has been shown to react synergistically with beta agonists (such as isoproterenol) that increase intracellular cyclic AMP through the stimulation of adenyl cyclase, but synergism has not been demonstrated in clinical studies and more data are needed to determine if Theophylline and beta agonists have clinically important additive effects *in vivo*.

Apparently, tolerance does not develop with chronic use of Theophylline.

The half-life is shortened with cigarette smoking. The half-life of Theophylline in smokers (1 to 2 packs/day) averaged 4 to 5 hours in various studies, much shorter than the 7 to 9 hour half-life in nonsmokers. The increase in Theophylline clearance caused by smoking is probably the result of induction of drug metabolizing enzymes that do not readily normalize after cessation of smoking. It appears that between 3 months and 2 years may be necessary for normalization of the effect of smoking on Theophylline pharmacokinetics.

The half-life is prolonged in alcoholism, reduced hepatic or renal function, congestive heart failure, and in patients receiving cimetidine or antibiotics such as troleandomycin (TAO, Cyclamycin), erythromycin, lincomycin and clindamycin. High fever for prolonged periods may decrease Theophylline elimination.

Newborn infants have extremely slow clearances with half-lives exceeding 24 hours. These approach those seen for older children after about 3-6 months.

Older adults with chronic obstructive pulmonary disease, patients with cor pulmonale or other causes of heart failure, and patients with liver pathology may have much lower clearances with half-lives that may exceed 24 hours.

THEOPHYLLINE ELIMINATION CHARACTERISTICS

	Theophylline Clearance Rates (mean ± S.D.)	Half-life Average (mean ± S.D.)
Children (over 6 months of age)	1.45 ± .58 mL/kg/min	3.7 ± 1.1 hours
Adult nonsmokers with uncomplicated asthma	0.65 ± .19 mL/kg/min	8.7 ± 2.2 hours

INDICATIONS

For chronic respiratory disease in which tenacious mucus and bronchospasm are dominant symptoms, such as bronchial asthma, chronic bronchitis and pulmonary emphysema.

CONTRAINDICATIONS

Use of this combination is contraindicated in patients with enlarged thyroid or goiter or with known sensitivity to Theophylline, Potassium Iodide, Ephedrine or sympathomimetics, or barbiturates.

The Iodide in this combination can cause fetal harm when administered to a pregnant woman. Development of goiter has been reported in infants whose mothers received Iodide-containing medications during pregnancy. A few neonatal deaths resulting from tracheal obstruction due to congenital goiters have been reported. Use of barbiturates during pregnancy may cause physical dependence with resulting withdrawal symptoms in the neonate; may cause birth defects; may be associated with neonatal hemorrhage due to reduction in levels of vitamin K-dependent clotting factors in the neonate; may cause respiratory depression in the neonate. This combination is contraindicated in women who are or may become pregnant. If this drug is used during pregnancy, or if the patient becomes pregnant while taking this drug, the patient should be apprised of the potential hazard to the fetus.

WARNINGS

This combination contains thiosulfate, a sulfite that may cause allergic-type reactions including anaphylactic symptoms and life-threatening or less severe asthmatic episodes in certain susceptible people. The overall prevalence of sulfite sensitivity in the general population is unknown and probably low. Sulfite sensitivity is seen more frequently in asthmatic than non-asthmatic people.

This combination contains Theophylline calcium salicylate. Salicylates have been reported to be associated with the development of Reye's syndrome in children and teenagers with chickenpox or flu.

Excessive Theophylline doses may be associated with toxicity; determination of serum Theophylline levels is recommended to assure maximal benefit without excessive risk. Incidence of toxicity increases at serum levels greater than 20 mcg/mL. Because of the Theophylline content of this combination, it is unlikely that toxic levels of Theophylline would be reached unless a serious overdosage occurs.

Morphine, curare, and stilbamidine should be used with caution in patients with airflow obstruction since they stimulate histamine release and can induce asthmatic attacks. They may also suppress respiration leading to respiratory failure. Alternative drugs should be chosen whenever possible.

There is an excellent correlation between clinical manifestations of toxicity and high blood levels of Theophylline resulting from conventional doses in patients with lowered body plasma clearances (due to transient cardiac decompensation), patients with liver dysfunction or chronic obstructive lung disease, and patients who are older than 55 years of age, particularly males. In about 50% of patients, nausea and restlessness precede more severe manifestations of toxicity. In other patients, ventricular arrhythmias or seizures may be the first signs of toxicity. These more serious side effects are more likely to occur after intravenous administration of Theophylline. Many patients who have high Theophylline serum levels exhibit a tachycardia, and Theophylline may worsen preexisting arrhythmias.

PRECAUTIONS

Mean half-life in smokers is shorter than in nonsmokers; therefore smokers may require larger doses of Theophylline. This combination, like all Theophylline products, should not be administered concurrently with other xanthine medications. Use with caution in patients with severe cardiac disease, severe hypoxemia, hypertension, hyperthyroidism, acute myocardial injury, cor pulmonale, congestive heart failure, liver disease, peptic ulcer and in the elderly (especially males) and in neonates. Great caution should be used especially in giving Theophylline to patients in congestive heart failure; such patients have shown markedly prolonged Theophylline blood level curves with Theophylline persisting in serum for long periods following discontinuation of the drug. Theophylline may occasionally act as a local irritant to the G.I. tract although gastrointestinal symptoms are more commonly central in origin and associated with serum concentrations over 20 mcg/mL.

Ephedrine-containing medications should be used with caution in patients with cardiovascular disease, diabetes mellitus, predisposition to glaucoma, hypertension, hyperthyroidism, or prostatic hypertrophy.

Potassium Iodide may aggravate acne in adolescents and adults.

Phenobarbital should be used with caution in patients with a history of drug abuse or dependence, impaired renal or hepatic function, hyperkinesis, uncontrolled pain, or history of porphyria.

Usage in Pregnancy: Pregnancy Category X. See *"Contraindications"* section.

Nursing Mothers: Because of the potential for serious adverse reactions in nursing infants from the Potassium Iodide, Ephedrine and Phenobarbital in this combination, a decision should be made whether to discontinue nursing or to discontinue the drug, taking into account the importance of the drug to the mother.

Pediatric Use: This combination is indicated for use in children on a short term basis. Chronic use should be reserved for patients in whom other expectorants have not been effective. If this combination is used chronically in children, the patient should be observed for signs of thyroid enlargement and worsening of acne.

Geriatric Patients: Geriatric patients may be more sensitive to the effects of Ephedrine.

ADVERSE REACTIONS

The most frequent adverse reactions to Theophylline are usually due to overdose (serum levels in excess of 20 mcg/mL) and are: nausea, vomiting, epigastric pain, hematemesis, diarrhea, headaches, irritability, restlessness, insomnia, reflex hyperexcitability, muscle twitching, clonic and tonic generalized convulsions, palpitations, tachycardia, extra systoles, flushing, hypotension, circulatory failure, ventricular arrhythmias, tachypnea, albuminuria, increased excretion of renal tubular cells and red blood cells, potentiation of diuresis, hyperglycemia and inappropriate ADH syndrome. Thyroid adenoma, goiter and myxedema are possible side effects of Potassium Iodide.

Hypersensitivity to Iodides may be manifested by angioneurotic edema, cutaneous and mucosal hemorrhages, and symptoms resembling serum sickness, such as fever, arthralgia, lymph node enlargement and eosinophilia.

Chronic ingestion of Iodides may result in chronic Iodide poisoning, or iodism. Initial symptoms include an unpleasant brassy taste, burning in the mouth and

---

◆ RATED THERAPEUTICALLY EQUIVALENT; ◇ THERAPEUTIC EQUIVALENCE UNCONFIRMED; ○ UNRATED

throat, soreness of the teeth and gums, increased salivation, coryza, sneezing, irritation of the eyes with swelling of the eyelids, headache, cough, skin lesions, diarrhea, gastric irritation, anorexia, fever and depression. The symptoms of iodism disappear spontaneously within a few days after stopping the administration of Iodide. Therefore, treatment consists of stopping therapy with this combination and providing supportive measures as indicated by the symptoms. Abundant fluid and sodium chloride intake may hasten Iodide elimination. In severe cases, the use of mannitol to establish an osmotic diuresis may be appropriate. Potassium Iodide may produce hyperkalemia and, if ingested chronically, may lead to goiter.

Adverse reactions to Ephedrine include nervousness, restlessness, trouble in sleeping, irregular heartbeat, difficult or painful urination, dizziness or light-headedness, headache, loss of appetite, nausea or vomiting, trembling, troubled breathing, unusual increase in sweating, unusual paleness, feeling of warmth, and weakness. Tolerance to Ephedrine may develop with prolonged or excessive use.

Adverse reactions to Phenobarbital include mental confusion or depression, shortness of breath or troubled breathing, skin rash, hives, swelling of eyelids, face or lips, wheezing or tightness in chest, sore throat and fever, unusual bleeding or bruising, unusual excitement, tiredness or weakness, unusually slow heartbeat, yellowing of eyes or skin.

DRUG INTERACTIONS

Toxic synergism of Theophylline with Ephedrine has been documented and may occur with some other sympathomimetic bronchodilators.

Drug	Effect
Aminophylline with lithium carbonate	Increased excretion of lithium carbonate
Potassium iodide with lithium	Increased hypothyroid and goiterogenic effects
Aminophylline with propranolol	Antagonism of propranolol effect
Theophylline with furosemide	Increased diuresis
Theophylline with hexamethonium	Decreased hexamethonium induced chronotropic effect
Theophylline with reserpine	Reserpine-induced tachycardia
Theophylline with chlordiazepoxide	Chlordiazepoxide-induced fatty acid mobilization
Theophylline with troleandomycin (TAO, Cyclamycin), erythromycin, lincomycin, clindamycin	Increased Theophylline plasma levels
Theophylline with phenytoin	Decreased phenytoin levels
Theophylline with cimetidine	Increased Theophylline blood levels
Ephedrine with digitalis glycosides or anesthetics	May cause cardiac arrhythmias
Ephedrine with ergonovine, methylergonovine or oxytocin	Hypertension
Ephedrine with guanethidine	Decreased hypotensive effect
Ephedrine with MAO inhibitors	Potentiation of pressor effect of ephedrine
Ephedrine with reserpine	Decreased pressor effect of ephedrine
Ephedrine with other sympathomimetics	Increased effects of either medication
Ephedrine with tricyclic antidepressants	May antagonize the pressor action of ephedrine
Phenobarbital with alcohol, general anesthetics, other CNS depressants, or MAO inhibitors	Increased effects of either medication
Phenobarbital with oral anticoagulants	Decreased anticoagulant effects
Phenobarbital with corticosteroids, digitalis, digitoxin, doxycycline, tricyclic antidepressants, griseofulvin or phenytoin	Decreased effects of these drugs

OVERDOSAGE

A. If potential overdose is established and seizure has not occurred and patient is conscious:

1) Induce vomiting.
2) Administer a cathartic.
3) Administer activated charcoal.

B. If patient is having a seizure:

1) Establish an airway.
2) Administer O$_2$.
3) Treat the seizure with intravenous diazepam, 0.1 to 0.3 mg/kg up to 10 mg.
4) Monitor vital signs, maintain blood pressure and provide adequate hydration.

C. Post-seizure coma:

1) Maintain airway and oxygenation.
2) Follow above recommendations to prevent absorption of drug, but intubation and lavage will have to be performed instead of inducing emesis, and introduce the cathartic and charcoal via a large bore gastric lavage tube.
3) Continue to provide full supportive care and adequate hydration while waiting for drug to be metabolized. In general, the drug is metabolized sufficiently rapidly so as not to require dialysis.

DOSAGE AND ADMINISTRATION

When rapidly absorbed products such as uncoated tablets with rapid dissolution are used, dosing to maintain "around the clock" blood levels generally requires administration every 6 hours in children; dosing intervals up to 8 hours may be satisfactory for adults because of their slower elimination rate.

Pulmonary function measurements before and after a period of treatment permit an objective assessment of response to this product.

USUAL DOSE:

Adults—One tablet 3 or 4 times daily; if needed, an additional one tablet upon retiring for nighttime relief. In severe attacks, the usual dose may be increased by one half.

Children 6 to 12 years—one half tablet three times daily.

Children under 6 years—dose is proportionately less.

STORAGE

Store at 59°-86°F (15°-30°C). Dispense in tight, light-resistant container as defined in USP.

HOW SUPPLIED
TABLETS:

BRAND/MANUFACTURER	NDC	SIZE	AWP
○ BRAND			
QUADRINAL: Knoll	00044-4520-02	100s	$37.82

Ephedrine Sulfate

DESCRIPTION

Ephedrine Sulfate is an alkaloid drug that produces sympathomimetic effects when administered orally, parenterally, or topically. It stimulates the central nervous system, increases blood pressure, stimulates heart muscle, constricts arterioles, relaxes smooth muscle of the bronchi and gastrointestinal tract, dilates the pupil, and increases the metabolic rate.

Ephedrine Sulfate is available in the following form: 25 mg (0.058 mmol) or 50 mg (0.117 mmol) in 1 mL ampoules for intravenous, subcutaneous, or intramuscular injection.

The chemical name for Ephedrine Sulfate is $(C_{10}H_{15}NO)_2 \cdot H_2SO_4$ benzenemethanol, α-[1-(methylamino)-ethyl]-, [R-(R*,S*)]-, sulfate (2:1) (salt). Its molecular weight is 428.54.

Ephedrine Sulfate occurs as fine, white odorless crystals or powder and darkens on exposure to light. It is freely soluble in water and slightly soluble in alcohol.

Following is its chemical structure:

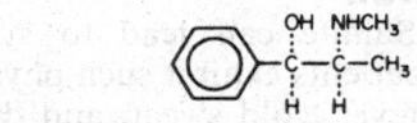

CLINICAL PHARMACOLOGY

Ephedrine is a potent sympathomimetic that stimulates both α and β receptors and has clinical uses related to both actions. Its peripheral actions, which it owes in part to the release of epinephrine, simulate responses that are obtained when adrenergic nerves are stimulated. These include an increase in blood pressure, stimulation of heart muscle, constriction of arterioles, relaxation of the smooth muscle of the bronchi and gastrointestinal tract, and dilation of the pupils. In the bladder, relaxation of the detrusor muscle is not prominent, but the tone of the trigone and vesicle sphincter is increased.

Ephedrine also has a potent effect on the central nervous system. It stimulates the cerebral cortex and subcortical centers, which accounts for its use in the treatment of narcolepsy.

The cardiovascular responses reported in man include moderate tachycardia, unchanged or augmented stroke volume, enhanced cardiac output, variable alterations in peripheral resistance, and, usually, a rise in blood pressure. The action of Ephedrine is more prominent on the heart than on the blood vessels. Ephedrine increases the flow of coronary, cerebral, and muscle blood.

In patients with myasthenia gravis, administration of Ephedrine produces a real but modest increase in motor power. The exact mechanism by which ephedrine affects skeletal muscle contraction is unknown.

INDICATIONS AND USAGE

Ephedrine Sulfate is indicated for parenteral treatment of allergic disorders, such as bronchial asthma. The drug has long been used as a pressor agent, particularly during spinal anesthesia when hypotension frequently occurs. In Stokes-Adams syndrome with complete heart block, ephedrine has a value similar to that of epinephrine. It is administered as a central nervous system stimulant in narcolepsy and depressive states.

UNLABELED USES

Ephedrine Sulfate is used alone or as an adjunct in the treatment of ejaculatory failure to produce an increase in volume of ejaculate and an increase in motility of sperm, in the prevention of postoperative nausea and vomiting, and diabetic neuropathy.

CONTRAINDICATIONS

Allergic reactions to ephedrine are rare. This hypersensitivity, if known, is a specific contraindication.

PRECAUTIONS

General: Special care should be used in administering Ephedrine Sulfate to patients with heart disease, angina pectoris, diabetes, hyperthyroidism, prostatic hypertrophy, or hypertension and to patients receiving digitalis. Prolonged use may produce a syndrome resembling an anxiety state. Tolerance to ephedrine may develop, but temporary cessation of the drug restores its original effectiveness.

Information for Patients: Many patients develop nervousness when taking therapeutic doses of Ephedrine, and the patient should be made aware of this and the fact that a sedative may be necessary to relieve symptoms. Occasionally, tolerance to the drug may develop; however, temporary discontinuation of the medication restores the patient's original response to the drug. Therapeutic doses of Ephedrine Sulfate can counteract the blood-pressure-lowering effect of some hypotensive drugs.

Drug Interactions: Therapeutic doses of Ephedrine Sulfate can inhibit the hypotensive action of guanethidine, bethanidine, and debrisoquin by displacing these adrenergic blockers from their site of action in the sympathetic neurons. The effects in man are seen as a relative or complete blockade of the antihypertensive drug by a sudden rise in blood pressure. Decongestants, medications for treating colds, and bronchodilators may contain ephedrine sulfate and should not be used concomitantly with antihypertensive therapy.

Usage in Pregnancy: Pregnancy Category C: Animal reproduction studies have not been conducted with Ephedrine Sulfate. Also, it is not known whether the drug can cause fetal harm when administered to a pregnant woman or can affect reproduction capacity. Ephedrine Sulfate should be given to a pregnant woman only if clearly needed.

It is not known what effect Ephedrine Sulfate may have on the newborn or on the child's later growth and development when the drug is administered to the mother just before or during labor.

Nursing Mothers: It is not known whether this drug is excreted in human milk. Because many drugs are excreted in human milk, caution should be exercised when Ephedrine Sulfate is administered to a nursing mother.

ADVERSE REACTIONS

With large doses of Ephedrine Sulfate, most patients will experience nervousness, insomnia, vertigo, headache, tachycardia, palpitation, and sweating. Some patients have nausea, vomiting, and anorexia. Vesical sphincter spasm may occur and result in difficult and painful urination. Urinary retention may develop in males with prostatism.

Precordial pain and cardiac arrhythmias may occur following administration of Ephedrine.

Contact dermatitis has been reported after topical application.

DRUG ABUSE AND DEPENDENCE

Prolonged abuse of Ephedrine Sulfate can lead to symptoms of paranoid schizophrenia. When this occurs, patients exhibit such physical signs as tachycardia, poor nutrition and hygiene, fever, cold sweat, and dilated pupils.

Some measure of tolerance to the actions of Ephedrine develops, but addiction does not occur. Temporary cessation of medication restores the patient's original response to the drug.

OVERDOSAGE

Signs and Symptoms: In acute poisoning following injection, ingestion, or absorption via mucous membranes the following may be noted: nausea, vomiting, chills, fever, irritability, nervousness, suicidal behavior, personality changes, dilated pupils, blurred vision, and tachycardia. More severe effects include opisthotonos, spasms, convulsions, pulmonary edema, gasping respirations, respiratory failure, cyanosis, and tachyarrhythmias. Initially there may be hypertension, followed later by hypotension accompanied by anuria. In chronic poisoning. prolonged exposure of the nasal mucosa to the drug leads to chronic nasal congestion. Large doses may lead to personality changes with a psychic craving for the drug. Chronic use of Ephedrine can also cause symptoms of tension and anxiety that may progress to psychosis. Laboratory findings in these instances are not useful in making a diagnosis.

In man, the probable lethal dose is 50 mg/kg. In children up to 2 years of age, the minimum oral lethal dose is approximately 200 mg. Information is not available on serum concentrations that may be toxic or lethal.

Treatment: To obtain up-to-date information about the treatment of overdose, a good resource is your certified Regional Poison Control Center. Telephone numbers of certified poison control centers are listed in the *Physicians' Desk Reference (PDR).* In managing overdosage, consider the possibility of multiple drug overdoses, interaction among drugs, and unusual drug kinetics in your patient.

Protect the patient's airway and support ventilation and perfusion. Meticulously monitor and maintain, within acceptable limits, the patient's vital signs, blood gases, serum electrolytes, etc. Absorption of drugs from the gastrointestinal tract may be decreased by giving activated charcoal which, in many cases, is more effective than emesis or lavage; consider charcoal instead of or in addition to gastric emptying. Repeated doses of charcoal over time may hasten elimination of some drugs that have been absorbed. Safeguard the patient's airway when employing gastric emptying or charcoal.

If marked hypertension is present, consider use of nitroprusside or phentolamine infusion. For hypotension, consider intravenous fluids, elevation of the legs, or inotropic vasopressors such as levarterenol.

Life-threatening supraventricular or ventricular tachycardias may be treated by slow intravenous administration of propranolol. Monitoring of the electrocardiogram and vital signs should be done continuously.

If the patient develops convulsions, diazepam, phenytoin, or phenobarbital may be considered. For refractory seizures, general anesthesia with thiopental or halothane and paralysis with a neuromuscular blocking agent may be necessary.

Forced diuresis, peritoneal dialysis, hemodialysis, or charcoal hemoperfusion have not been established as beneficial for an overdose of Ephedrine Sulfate.

DOSAGE AND ADMINISTRATION

Adults: The usual parenteral dose is 25 to 50 mg, given subcutaneously, intramuscularly, or infused *slowly* (over at least 15 minutes) intravenously.

Infants and Children: The usual subcutaneous or IV dose is 3 mg/kg/day, or 100 mg/m^2/day divided into 4 to 6 doses.

Parenteral drug products should be inspected visually for particulate matter and discoloration prior to administration, whenever solution or container permits.

Storage: Store at controlled room temperature, 59° to 86°F (15° to 30°C).

HOW SUPPLIED
INJECTION: 50 MG/ML

BRAND/MANUFACTURER	NDC	SIZE	AWP
◆ GENERICS			
Abbott Hosp	00074-3073-03	1 ml 10s	$14.73

Ephedrine Sulfate/Hydroxyzine Hydrochloride/Theophylline

DESCRIPTION
Ephedrine Sulfate/Hydroxyzine Hydrochloride/Theophylline is available in tablets and dye-free syrup.

Each tablet contains:

Ephedrine Sulfate	.25 mg
Theophylline	130 mg

Each teaspoon (5 mL) syrup contains:

Ephedrine Sulfate	6.25 mg
Hydroxyzine Hydrochloride	2.5 mg
Theophylline	32.50 mg
Alcohol (Ethyl Alcohol)	5% v/v.

ACTIONS
The action of Ephedrine as a vasoconstrictor is well known. It is therefore of significant benefit in symptomatic relief of the congestion occurring in bronchial asthma. As a bronchodilator, it has a slower onset but longer duration of action than does epinephrine, which, in contrast to Ephedrine, is not effective upon oral administration.

The diverse actions of Theophylline—bronchospasmolytic, cardiovascular, and diuretic—are well established, and make it a particularly useful drug in the treatment of bronchial asthma, both in the acute attack and in the prophylactic therapy of the disease.

Hydroxyzine Hydrochloride modifies the central stimulatory action of Ephedrine preventing excessive excitation in patients on Ephedrine Sulfate/Hydroxyzine Hydrochloride/Theophylline therapy.

Hydroxyzine Hydrochloride has demonstrated antiserotonin activity and antispasmodic potency of a nonspecific nature. Ephedrine Sulfate/Hydroxyzine Hydrochloride/Theophylline Syrup produces an expectorant action wherein the tenacity of the sputum is decreased and the ease of expectoration is increased.

INDICATIONS

BASED ON A REVIEW OF THIS DRUG BY THE NATIONAL ACADEMY OF SCIENCES-NATIONAL RESEARCH COUNCIL AND/OR OTHER INFORMATION, FDA HAS CLASSIFIED THE INDICATIONS AS FOLLOWS:
"POSSIBLY" EFFECTIVE: FOR CONTROLLING BRONCHOSPASTIC DISORDERS.
FINAL CLASSIFICATION OF THE LESS THAN EFFECTIVE INDICATION REQUIRES FURTHER INVESTIGATION.

CONTRAINDICATIONS
Because of the Ephedrine, Ephedrine Sulfate/Hydroxyzine Hydrochloride/Theophylline is contraindicated in cardiovascular disease, hyperthyroidism, and hypertension. This drug is contraindicated in individuals who have shown hypersensitivity to the drug or its components.

Hydroxyzine, when administered to the pregnant mouse, rat, and rabbit induced fetal abnormalities in the rat at doses substantially above the human therapeutic range. Clinical data in human beings are inadequate to establish safety in early pregnancy. Until such data are available, Hydroxyzine is contraindicated in early pregnancy.

◆ RATED THERAPEUTICALLY EQUIVALENT; ◇ THERAPEUTIC EQUIVALENCE UNCONFIRMED; ○ UNRATED

PRECAUTIONS

Because of the Ephedrine component this drug should be used with caution in elderly males or those with known prostatic hypertrophy.

The potentiating action of Hydroxyzine, although mild, must be taken into consideration when the drug is used in conjunction with central nervous system depressants; and when other central nervous system depressants are administered concomitantly with Hydroxyzine their dosage should be reduced. Patients should be cautioned that Hydroxyzine can increase the effect of alcohol.

Patients should be warned—because of the Hydroxyzine component—of the possibility of drowsiness occurring and cautioned against driving a car or operating dangerous machinery while taking this drug.

ADVERSE REACTIONS

With large doses of Ephedrine, excitation, tremulousness, insomnia, nervousness, palpitation, tachycardia, precordial pain, cardiac arrhythmias, vertigo, dryness of the nose and throat, headache, sweating, and warmth may occur. Because Ephedrine is a sympathomimetic agent some patients may develop vesical sphincter spasm and resultant urinary hesitation, and occasionally acute urinary retention. This should be borne in mind when administering preparations containing Ephedrine to elderly males or those with known prostatic hypertrophy. At the recommended dose for Ephedrine Sulfate/Hydroxyzine Hydrochloride/Theophylline, a side effect occasionally reported is palpitation, and this can be controlled with dosage adjustment, additional amounts of concurrently administered Hydroxyzine Hydrochloride, or discontinuation of the medication. When Ephedrine is given three or more times daily patients may develop tolerance after several weeks of therapy.

Theophylline when given on an empty stomach frequently causes gastric irritation accompanied by upper abdominal discomfort, nausea, and vomiting. Administration of the medication after meals will serve to minimize this side effect. Theophylline may cause diuresis and cardiac stimulation. The amount of Hydroxyzine Hydrochloride present in Ephedrine Sulfate/Hydroxyzine Hydrochloride/Theophylline has not resulted in disturbing side effects. When used alone specifically as a tranquilizer in the normal dosage range (25 to 50 mg, three or four times a day), side effects are infrequent; even at these higher doses, no serious side effects have been reported and confirmed to date. Those which do occasionally occur when Hydroxyzine Hydrochloride is used alone are drowsiness, xerostomia and, at extremely high doses, involuntary motor activity, unsteadiness of gait, neuromuscular weakness, all of which may be controlled by reduction of the dosage or discontinuation of the medication.

With the relatively low dose of Hydroxyzine Hydrochloride in Ephedrine Sulfate/Hydroxyzine Hydrochloride/Theophylline, these effects are not likely to occur. In addition, the ataractic action of Hydroxyzine Hydrochloride may modify the cardiac stimulatory action of Ephedrine, and concurrently, increasing the amount of Hydroxyzine Hydrochloride may control or abolish this undesirable effect of Ephedrine.

DOSAGE AND ADMINISTRATION

The dosage of Ephedrine Sulfate/Hydroxyzine Hydrochloride/Theophylline should be adjusted according to the severity of complaints, and the patient's individual toleration.

Tablets: In general, an adult dose of 1 tablet, 2 to 4 times daily, should be sufficient. Some patients are controlled adequately with ½ to 1 tablet at bedtime. The time interval between doses should not be shorter than four hours. The dosage for children over 5 years of age and for adults who are sensitive to Ephedrine, is one-half the usual adult dose. Clinical experience to date has been confined to ages above 5 years.

Syrup: The dose for children over 5 years of age is 1 teaspoon (5 ml.), 3 to 4 times daily. Dosage for children 2 to 5 years of age is ½ to 1 teaspoon (2.5-5 ml.), 3 to 4 times daily. Not recommended for children under 2 years of age.

Dispense syrup in tight light-resistant containers (USP).

HOW SUPPLIED
SYRUP: 18.75 MG-7.5 MG-97.5 MG

BRAND/MANUFACTURER	NDC	SIZE	AWP
○ **BRAND**			
MARAX DF: Roerig	00049-2550-93	480 ml	$38.25
○ **GENERICS**			
THEOMAX DF: Barre	00472-1552-16	480 ml	$11.55

For additional alternatives, turn to the section beginning on page 2859.

Epidural Single Shot W/Lidocaine
***SEE* LIDOCAINE HYDROCHLORIDE, INJECTABLE *AND* LIDOCAINE HYDROCHLORIDE, LOCAL ANESTHESIA**

Epifoam *SEE* **HYDROCORTISONE ACETATE AND PRAMOXINE HYDROCHLORIDE**

Epifrin *SEE* EPINEPHRINE, OPHTHALMIC

E-Pilo *SEE* EPINEPHRINE BITARTRATE AND PILOCARPINE HYDROCHLORIDE

Epinal *SEE* EPINEPHRINE, OPHTHALMIC

Epinephrine Bitartrate and Pilocarpine Hydrochloride

DESCRIPTION

Epinephrine Bitartrate/Pilocarpine Hydrochloride ophthalmic solution is a sterile solution for ophthalmic administration having the following composition:

Pilocarpine Hydrochloride	10 mg/mL
(cholinergic/parasympathomimetic)	
*Epinephrine Bitartrate	10 mg/mL
(sympathomimetic)	
Pilocarpine Hydrochloride	20 mg/mL
*Epinephrine Bitartrate	10 mg/mL
Pilocarpine Hydrochloride	30 mg/mL
*Epinephrine Bitartrate	10 mg/mL
Pilocarpine Hydrochloride	40 mg/mL
*Epinephrine Bitartrate	10 mg/mL
Pilocarpine Hydrochloride	60 mg/mL
*Epinephrine Bitartrate	10 mg/mL

* *Epinephrine Base 5.5 mg/mL*

The chemical name for Epinephrine Bitartrate is 1,2-Benzenediol,4-[1-hydroxy-2-(methylamino)ethyl]-,(R)-,[R-(R*, R*)]-2,3-dihydroxybutanedioate (1:1) salt.

The chemical name for Pilocarpine Hydrochloride is 2(3H)-Furanone,3-ethyl-dihydro-4-[(1-methyl-1H-imidazol-5-yl) methyl]-,monohydrochloride,(3S-cis)-.

CLINICAL PHARMACOLOGY

Epinephrine is an alpha and beta sympathetic receptor agonist (sympathomimetic), reduces aqueous flow, and increases the facility of outflow. Pilocarpine is a direct-acting cholinergic (parasympathomimetic) agent and increases the facility of outflow.

INDICATIONS AND USAGE

Epinephrine Bitartrate/Pilocarpine HCl ophthalmic solution is indicated for the treatment of chronic primary open-angle glaucoma. It may be used in combination with carbonic anhydrase inhibitors, hyperosmotic agents, or beta-adrenergic blocking agents.

CONTRAINDICATIONS

Narrow or shallow angle (angle closure) glaucoma. Miotics are contraindicated when constriction is undesirable such as in acute iritis and in persons hypersensitive to one or more of the components in this preparation.

WARNINGS

To avoid inducing angle closure glaucoma, an estimation of the depth of the angle of the anterior chamber should be made. Use with caution in individuals with a history of hyperthyroidism, hypertension, organic cardiac disease and long-standing bronchial asthma. Maculopathy with associated decrease in visual acuity may occur in the aphakic eye; in this event, administration should be discontinued promptly.

Some brands contain sodium bisulfite, a sulfite that may cause allergic-type reactions including anaphylactic symptoms and life-threatening or less severe asthmatic episodes in certain susceptible people. The overall prevalence of sulfite sensitivity in the general population is unknown and probably low. Sulfite sensitivity is seen more frequently in asthmatic than in nonasthmatic people.

PRECAUTIONS

Aphakic patients should be warned to consult their physicians immediately if they note any decrease in visual acuity because Epinephrine maculopathy may occur.

Topical use of Epinephrine in any form should be interrupted prior to general anesthesia with certain anesthetics such as cyclopropane, or halogenated hydrocarbon anesthetics such as halothane because the myocardium may be sensitized to sympathomimetics.

Tricyclic antidepressants, some antihistamines (diphenhydramine, tripelennamine, and dexchlorpheniramine) and thyroid hormones may potentiate the effects of Epinephrine, especially on heart rhythm and rate.

The Pilocarpine-induced miosis may cause difficulty in dark adaptation. The patient should exercise caution when involved in night driving or other hazardous activities in poor light.

This preparation should not be used in conjunction with the wearing of soft contact lenses.

For topical ophthalmic use only. Not for injection. To prevent contaminating the dropper tip and solution, care should be taken not to touch the eyelids or surrounding areas with the dropper tip of the bottle. Keep bottle tightly closed when not in use and protect from light. Do not use if color of solution is pinkish or darker than slightly yellow or if it contains a precipitate.

Carcinogenesis, Mutagenesis, Impairment of Fertility: There have been no long-term studies done using Pilocarpine and/or Epinephrine in animals to evaluate carcinogenic potential.

Pregnancy: Pregnancy Category C. Animal reproduction studies have not been conducted with Pilocarpine and/or Epinephrine. It is also not known whether Pilocarpine and/or Epinephrine can cause fetal harm when administered to a pregnant woman or can affect reproduction capacity. Pilocarpine and/or Epinephrine should be given to a pregnant woman only if clearly needed.

Nursing Mothers: It is not known whether these drugs are excreted in human milk. Because many drugs are excreted in human milk, caution should be exercised when Pilocarpine and/or Epinephrine is administered to a nursing woman.

Pediatric Use: Safety and effectiveness in children have not been established.

ADVERSE REACTIONS

Ocular: Prolonged use may be associated with conjunctival or corneal pigmentation. Following prolonged administration, ocular irritation (hypersensitivity) may develop in a significant number of patients. Maculopathy with associated decrease in visual acuity may occur in the aphakic eye. As with all miotics, ocular side effects such as slight ciliary spasm, conjunctival vascular congestion, temporal or supraorbital headache, lacrimation, and induced myopia may occur. This is especially true in younger individuals who have recently begun administration.

Systemic: Systemic side effects such as headache, palpitation, faintness, tachycardia, and extrasystoles may occur. Severe side effects such as hypertension and cardiac arrhythmia have been reported.

DOSAGE AND ADMINISTRATION

The initial dose is one or two drops in the affected eye(s) twice daily. The medication may be used more frequently if necessary. The frequency of instillation and the concentration of Epinephrine Bitartrate/Pilocarpine HCl ophthalmic solution are determined by the severity of the glaucoma and the response of the patient.

Concomitant use of this product and soft contact lens wear may lead to soft contact lens discoloration. Patients should be advised not to wear their soft contact lenses for the duration of use of this product.

Store at controlled room temperature 15°-30°C (59°-86°F). Keep tightly closed when not in use. Protect from light.

HOW SUPPLIED

DROP:

BRAND/MANUFACTURER	NDC	SIZE	AWP
○ **BRAND**			
E-PILO-1: Iolab	00058-2344-10	10 ml	$12.78
E-PILO-2: Iolab	00058-2345-10	10 ml	$13.02
E-PILO-4: Iolab	00058-2355-10	10 ml	$14.04
E-PILO-6: Iolab	00058-2357-10	10 ml	$14.52
P1E1: Alcon Labs	00998-0365-15	15 ml	$17.13
P2E1: Alcon Labs	00998-0366-15	15 ml	$17.13
P3E1: Alcon Labs	00998-0367-15	15 ml	$17.88
P4E1: Alcon Labs	00998-0368-15	15 ml	$18.75
P6E1: Alcon Labs	00998-0369-15	15 ml	$19.69

Epinephrine, Ophthalmic

DESCRIPTION

Epinephrine, Ophthalmic is a sterile topical ophthalmic solution.

The chemical name of Epinephrine is 1,2-Benzenediol, 4-[1-hydroxy-2-(methylamino)ethyl]-, (R)-; of Epinephrine Hydrochloride 1,2-Benzenediol, 4-[1-hydroxy-2-(methylamino)ethyl]-, (R)-, monohydro- chloride; and of Epinephryl Barate 1, 3, 2-Benzodioxaborole-5-methanol, 2-hydroxy-α-[(methylamino) methyl]-,(R)-, (—)-3, 4-Dihydroxy-α-[(methylamino) methyl] benzyl alcohol, cyclic 3, 4-ester with boric acid.

Each mL contains: Active: Epinephrine Hydrochloride equivalent to 1.0% or 2.0% Epinephrine base; or Epinephryl Borate equivalent to Epinephrine 0.5% or 1%.

CLINICAL PHARMACOLOGY

Lowers intraocular pressure by reducing the production of aqueous and increasing the facility of outflow.

Epinephrine is an adrenergic agonist that stimulates α- and β-adrenergic receptors. The capacity of Epinephrine, Ophthalmic to decrease the aqueous inflow in open-angle glaucoma has been well documented. Studies have also shown that prolonged topical Epinephrine therapy offers significant improvement in the coefficient of aqueous outflow.

Epinephrine, Ophthalmic is effective alone in reducing intraocular pressure and is particularly useful in combination with miotics or beta-adrenergic blocking agents for the difficult-to-control patients. The addition of Epinephrine, Ophthal-

mic to the patient's regimen often provides better control of intraocular pressure than the original agent alone.

INDICATIONS AND USAGE

For the control of simple (open angle) glaucoma. It may be used in combination with miotics, beta blockers, hyperosmotic agents, or carbonic anhydrase inhibitors when indicated.

CONTRAINDICATIONS

Do not use in narrow or shallow angle (angle closure) glaucoma.

Contraindicated in those persons who have shown hypersensitivity to any component of this preparation.

WARNINGS

For topical eye use only—not for injection or intraocular use. Epinephrine, Ophthalmic, should be used with caution in patients with a narrow angle, since dilation of the pupil may trigger an acute attack of narrow-angle glaucoma. To avoid inducing angle closure glaucoma, an estimation of the depth of the angle of the anterior chamber should be made. Maculopathy or reversible macular edema with associated decrease in visual acuity may occur in the aphakic eye; in this event, administration should be discontinued promptly. Systemic effects from ophthalmic instillation are uncommon; however, use with caution in the elderly and in patients with a history of cardiac disease, hypertensive cardiovascular disease, coronary artery disease, diabetes, cerebral arteriosclerosis, hyperthyroidism, hypertension and bronchial asthma. Interrupt use prior to general anesthesia with anesthetics which sensitize the myocardium to sympathomimetics (e.g., cyclopropane or halothane). Careful supervision and adjustment of dosages are required when administered simultaneously or up to 21 days after administration of MAO inhibitors, since exaggerated adrenergic effects may result. The pressor response of adrenergic agents may also be potentiated by concurrent use of tricyclic antidepressants. Do not use if solution is brown or contains a precipitate. Certain brands of Epinephrine Ophthalmic solution contain sodium metabisulfite, a sulfite that may cause allergic-type reactions including anaphylactic symptoms and life-threatening or less severe asthmatic episodes in certain susceptible people. The overall prevalence of sulfite sensitivity in the general population is unknown and probably low. Sulfite sensitivity is seen more frequently in asthmatic than in nonasthmatic people.

PRECAUTIONS

General: Do not use this preparation while wearing soft contact lenses. Epinephrine in any form is relatively uncomfortable upon instillation. However, discomfort lessens as the concentration of Epinephrine decreases. Epinephrine, Ophthalmic, is not for injection. If a general anesthetic is to be used, consult the anesthesiologist.

Information For Patients: Do not touch dropper tip to any surface, as this may contaminate the solution. Patient should immediately report any decrease in visual acuity.

Carcinogenesis, Mutagenesis, Impairment of Fertility: There have been no long-term studies done using Epinephryl Borate or Epinephrine, Ophthalmic, solution in animals or humans to evaluate carcinogenic potential.

Pregnancy: Pregnancy Category C Animal reproduction studies have not been conducted with Epinephryl Borate or Epinephrine. It is also not known whether Epinephryl Borate or Epinephrine can cause fetal harm when administered to a pregnant woman or can affect reproduction capacity. Epinephrine, Ophthalmic, solution should be given to a pregnant woman only if clearly needed.

Pediatric Use: Safety and effectiveness in children have not been established.

Nursing Mothers: It is not known whether these drugs are excreted in human milk. Because many drugs are excreted in human milk, caution should be exercised when Epinephryl Borate or Epinephrine is administered to a nursing woman.

ADVERSE REACTIONS

Transient symptoms of stinging and burning may occur. Prolonged use may be associated with conjunctival or corneal pigmentation. Following prolonged administration, ocular irritation (hypersensitivity) may develop. Systemic side effects such as headache, palpitation, faintness, tachycardia, and extrasystoles may occur. Severe side effects such as hypertension and cardiac arrhythmia have been reported. Other undesirable reactions to topical Epinephrine include eye pain or ache, browache, conjunctival hyperemia and allergic lid reactions. Topical Epinephrine has been reported to produce reversible macular edema or macolopathy in some aphakic patients.

OVERDOSAGE

Accidental ingestion will not cause problems because pharmacologically active concentrations of Epinephrine cannot be achieved orally in man. Should accidental overdosage in the eye(s) occur, flush eye(s) with water or normal saline.

DOSAGE AND ADMINISTRATION

Usual dosage is one drop topically in the eye(s) one or two times daily for the control of glaucoma. The dosage should be adjusted to meet the needs of the individual patient.

Storage: Store at 36° to 75°F (2° to 24° C).

Note: Protect from light and excessive heat. If the solution discolors or a precipitate forms, it should be discarded.

Epinephryl Borate: Store in upright position with the dropper tightly sealed.

◆ RATED THERAPEUTICALLY EQUIVALENT; ◇ THERAPEUTIC EQUIVALENCE UNCONFIRMED; ○ UNRATED

Protect from excessive heat and light. Store at 2°-24°C (36°-75°F) in a dark place. Do not freeze.

HOW SUPPLIED

EPINEPHRINE BORATE

DROP: 0.5%

BRAND/MANUFACTURER	NDC	SIZE	AWP
○ **BRAND**			
EPPY/N: Paragon	00077-0321-75	7.5 ml	$10.38
EPINAL: Alcon Ophthalmic	00065-0265-07	7.5 ml	$14.25

DROP: 1%

BRAND/MANUFACTURER	NDC	SIZE	AWP
○ **BRAND**			
EPPY/N: Akorn	00077-0322-75	7.5 ml	$12.19
EPINAL: Alcon Ophthalmic	00065-0264-07	7.5 ml	$14.88

DROP: 2%

BRAND/MANUFACTURER	NDC	SIZE	AWP
○ **BRAND**			
EPPY/N: Akorn	00077-0333-75	7.5 ml	$12.81

EPINEPHRINE HYDROCHLORIDE

DROP: 0.5%

BRAND/MANUFACTURER	NDC	SIZE	AWP
○ **BRAND**			
EPIFRIN: Allergan Inc	11980-0119-15	15 ml	$26.50

DROP: 1%

BRAND/MANUFACTURER	NDC	SIZE	AWP
○ **BRAND**			
GLAUCON: Alcon Ophthalmic	00998-0249-10	10 ml	$16.88
EPIFRIN: Allergan Inc	11980-0122-15	15 ml	$28.41

DROP: 2%

BRAND/MANUFACTURER	NDC	SIZE	AWP
○ **BRAND**			
GLAUCON: Alcon Ophthalmic	00998-0250-10	10 ml	$18.38
EPIFRIN: Allergan Inc	11980-0058-15	15 ml	$32.46

Epinephrine, Systemic

DESCRIPTION

Epinephrine, Systemic, is available as a solution for subcutaneous or intramuscular injection and a suspension for subcutaneous use. When diluted, the solution may also be administered intracardially or intravenously. Each ml of solution contains 1 mg Epinephrine as the hydrochloride dissolved in Water for Injection, USP. Each ml of Epinephrine Suspension for subcutaneous injection contains 5 mg Epinephrine in a sterile aqueous vehicle containing ascorbic acid 10 mg and thioglycolic acid 6.6 mg (as sodium salts) phenol 5 mg and glycerin (USP) 325 mg. Sodium hydroxide is added to adjust the pH. Approximately 80% of the total Epinephrine is in suspension.

Epinephrine Injection is also available in a pre-filled syringe containing 2 ml Epinephrine Injection for emergency intramuscular use. Each syringe delivers a single dose of either 0.3 mg (0.3 ml) Epinephrine (1:1000) for adults or 0.15 mg (0.3 ml) Epinephrine (1:2000) for pediatric patients.

Epinephrine is the active principle of the adrenal medulla, chemically described as (-)-3,4-Dihydroxy-α-[(methylamino) methyl] benzyl alcohol. Epinephrine is a white to off-white, odorless, microcrystalline powder or granules. It is affected by light. Its molecular formula is $C_9H_{13}NO_6$ and its molecular weight 183.21.

Following is its chemical structure:

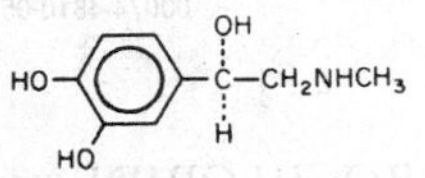

CLINICAL PHARMACOLOGY

Epinephrine is a sympathomimetic drug. It activates an adrenergic receptive mechanism on effector cells and imitates all actions of the sympathetic nervous system except those on the arteries of the face and sweat glands. It is the drug of choice for the emergency treatment of severe allergic reactions (Type I) to insect stings or bites, foods, drugs, and other allergens. It can also be used in the treatment of idiopathic or exercise-induced anaphylaxis. Epinephrine when given subcutaneously or intramuscularly has a rapid onset and short duration of action. Epinephrine acts on both alpha and beta receptors and is the most potent alpha receptor activator. Beta stimulation provides bronchodilator action by relaxing bronchial muscle. Alpha stimulation increases vital capacity by relieving congestion of the bronchial mucosa and by constricting pulmonary vessels.

Recent studies in laboratory animals (minipigs, rodents, and dogs) recorded the occurrence of cardiac arrhythmias and sudden death (with histologic evidence of myocardial necrosis) when beta agonists and methylxanthines were administered concurrently. The significance of these findings when applied to humans is currently unknown.

INDICATIONS AND USAGE

In general, the most common uses of the sterile solution of Epinephrine are to relieve respiratory distress due to bronchospasm, to provide rapid relief of hypersensitivity reactions to drugs and other allergens, and to prolong the action of infiltration anesthetics. Its cardiac effects may be of use in restoring cardiac rhythm in cardiac arrest due to various causes, but it is not used in cardiac failure or in hemorrhagic, traumatic, or cardiogenic shock.

Epinephrine is used as a hemostatic agent. It is also used in treating mucosal congestion of hay fever, rhinitis, and acute sinusitis; to relieve bronchial asthmatic paroxysms; in syncope due to complete heart block or carotid sinus hypersensitivity; for symptomatic relief of serum sickness, urticaria, angioneurotic edema; for resuscitation in cardiac arrest following anesthetic accidents; in simple (open angle) glaucoma; for relaxation of uterine musculature and to inhibit uterine contractions. Epinephrine Injection can be utilized to prolong the action of intraspinal and local anesthetics (see "Contraindications" section).

The suspension is specifically used for the symptomatic treatment of bronchial asthma, and reversible bronchospasm associated with chronic bronchitis and emphysema.

The pre-filled syringes of Epinephrine are indicated in the emergency treatment of allergic reactions (anaphylaxis) to insect stings or bites, foods, drugs and other allergens as well as idiopathic or exercise-induced anaphylaxis. They are intended for immediate self-administration by a person with a history of an anaphylactic reaction. Such reactions may occur within minutes after exposure and consist of flushing, apprehension, syncope, tachycardia, thready or unobtainable pulse associated with a fall in blood pressure, convulsions, vomiting, diarrhea and abdominal cramps, involuntary voiding, wheezing, dyspnea due to laryngeal spasm, pruritis, rashes, urticaria or angioedema. The Epinephrine pre-filled syringe is designed as emergency supportive therapy only and is not a replacement or substitute for immediate medical or hospital care.

CONTRAINDICATIONS

Epinephrine is contraindicated in narrow angle (congestive) glaucoma, shock, during general anesthesia with halogenated hydrocarbons or cyclopropane and in individuals with organic brain damage or organic heart disease. Epinephrine is also contraindicated with local anesthesia of certain areas, eg, fingers, toes, because of the danger of vasoconstriction producing sloughing of tissue; in labor because it may delay the second stage; in cardiac dilatation and coronary insufficiency.

Hypersensitivity to any of the components.

There are no absolute contraindications in a life-threatening situation.

WARNINGS

Administer with caution to elderly people; children; to those with cardiovascular disease, hypertension, diabetes or hyperthyroid in psychoneurotic individuals, and in pregnancy. Epinephrine is essential for the treatment of anaphylaxis. Therefore, patients with these conditions, and/or any other person who might be in a position to administer Epinephrine pre-filled syringe to a patient experiencing anaphylaxis should be carefully instructed in regard to the circumstances under which this lifesaving medication should be used.

Patients with long-standing bronchial asthma and emphysema who have developed degenerative heart disease should be administered the drug with extreme caution.

Cardiac arrhythmias may follow administration of Epinephrine. Overdosage or inadvertent intravenous injection of Epinephrine may cause cerebrovascular hemorrhage resulting from the sharp rise in blood pressure.

Fatalities may also result from pulmonary edema because of the peripheral constriction and cardiac stimulation produced. Rapidly acting vasodilators such as nitrites, or alpha blocking agents may counteract the marked pressor effects of Epinephrine.

Epinephrine is the preferred treatment for serious allergic or other emergency situations even though this product contains sodium bisulfite or sodium metabisulfite, a sulfites that may in other products cause allergic-type reactions including anaphylactic symptoms or life-threatening or less severe asthmatic episodes in certain susceptible persons. The alternatives to using Epinephrine in a life-threatening situation may not be satisfactory. The presence of a sulfite in this product should not deter administration of the drug for treatment of serious allergic or other emergency situations.

PRECAUTIONS

Do not remove ampules or vials from carton until ready to use. The solution should not be used if it is pinkish or darker than slightly yellow or if it contains a precipitate.

Epinephrine is readily destroyed by alkalies and oxidizing agents. In the latter category are oxygen, chlorine, bromine, iodine, permanganates, chromates, nitrites and salts of easily reducible metals, especially iron.

The suspension should not be employed to correct drug-induced hypotension.

Replace the syringe if the solution is discolored or contains a precipitate. Avoid possible inadvertent intravascular administration. Select an appropriate injection site such as the thigh. DO NOT INJECT INTO BUTTOCK. Large doses or accidental intravenous injection of Epinephrine may result in cerebral hemorrhage due to sharp rise in blood pressure. DO NOT INJECT INTRAVENOUSLY.

Patients should be instructed to contact a physician immediately if severe pain at the site of injection develops.

Drug Interactions: Use of Epinephrine with excessive doses of digitalis, mercurial diuretics, or other drugs that sensitize the heart to arrhythmias is not recommended. Anginal pain may be induced when coronary insufficiency is present.

Epinephrine should not be administered concomitantly with other sympathomimetic agents, since their combined effects on the cardiovascular system may be deleterious to the patient.

The effects of epinephrine may be potentiated by tricyclic antidepressants monoamine oxidose inhibitors; certain antihistamines, e.g., diphenhydramine, tripelennamine, d-chlorpheniramine; and sodium l-thyroxine.

Carcinogenesis, Mutagenesis, Impairment of Fertility: Studies of Epinephrine in animals to evaluate the carcinogenic and mutagenic potential or the effect on fertility have not been conducted.

Usage in Pregnancy: Pregnancy Category C. Epinephrine has been shown to be teratogenic in rats when given in doses about 25 times the human dose. There are no adequate and well controlled studies in pregnant women. Epinephrine should be used during pregnancy only if the potential benefit justifies the potential risk to the fetus.

Pediatric Use: Epinephrine may be given safely to children at a dosage appropriate to body weight (see *"Dosage and Administration"*).

ADVERSE REACTIONS

Transient and minor side effects of anxiety, headache, tachycardia, restlessness, sweating, nausea and vomiting, respiratory difficulty, pallor, dizziness, weakness, tremor, nervousness, fear and palpitations often occur with therapeutic doses, especially in hyperthyroid individuals. Repeated local injections can result in necrosis at sites of injection from vascular constriction. "Epinephrine-fastness" can occur with prolonged use. With the Suspension, occlusion of the central retinal artery, clostridial myonecrosis and shock have also been reported.

Also, urticaria, wheal and hemorrhage at the site of injection may occur. Repeated injections at the same site may result in necrosis from vascular constriction.

Tolerance to epinephrine may occur with prolonged use.

OVERDOSAGE

Overdosage or inadvertent intravenous injection may cause cerebrovascular hemorrhage resulting from the sharp rise in blood pressure. Fatalities may also result from pulmonary edema because of peripheral constriction and cardiac stimulation produced. Rapidly acting vasodilators such as nitrites, or alpha blocking agents may counteract the marked pressor effects. Cardiac arrhythmias may be countered by administering rapidly acting antiarrhythmic or beta blocking agents.

DOSAGE AND ADMINISTRATION

Parenteral drug products should be inspected visually for particulate matter and discoloration whenever solution and container permit.

Subcutaneously or intramuscularly: 0.2 to 1 ml (mg). Start with a small dose and increase if required.

Epinephrine solution 1:1000: Note: The subcutaneous is the preferred route of administration. If given intramuscularly, injection into the buttocks should be avoided.

For bronchial asthma and certain allergic, manifestations, eg. angioedema, urticaria, serum sickness, anaphylactic shock, use Epinephrine subcutaneously. For bronchial asthma in pediatric patients, administer 0.1 mg/kg or 0.3 mg/m^2 to a maximum of 0.5 mg subcutaneously, repeated every four hours if required.

For cardiac resuscitation, a dose of 0.5 ml (0.5 mg) diluted to 10 ml with sodium chloride injection can be administered intraveneously or intracardially to restore myocardial contractility. External cardiac massage should follow intracardial administration to permit the drug to enter coronary circulation. The drug should be used secondarily to unsuccessful attempt with physical or electromechanical methods.

In ophthalmologic use (for producing conjunctival decongestion, to control hemorrhage, produce mydriasis and reduce intraocular pressure), use a concentration of 1:10,000 (0.1 mg/ml) to 1:1,00 (1 mg/ml).

For Intraspinal use (Amp 88), usual dose is 0.2 to 0.4 ml (0.2 to 0.4 mg) added to anesthetic spinal fluid mixture (may prolong anesthetic action by limiting absorption). For use with local anesthetic, Epinephrine 1:100,000 (0.01 mg/ml) to 1:20,00 (0.05 mg/ml) is the usual concentration employed.

Note: Inject subcutaneously.

Epinephrine Suspension (1:200): As with all sterile products, failure to follow aseptic procedures may result in microbial contamination causing adverse consequences which could lead to life threatening illness.

It is suggested that Epinephrine be administered with a turberculin syringe and a 26 gauge, ½ inch needle.

A small initial test dose may be administered subcutaneously as a possible aid in determining patient sensitivity to epinephrine.

Site of injection should be varied to avoid necrosis at the site of injection.

Each time before withdrawing Epinephrine into syringe, *Shake vial or ampoule thoroughly* to disperse particles and obtain a uniform suspension. Inject promptly subcutaneously to avoid setting of suspension in the syringe.

Adults: Adult dosage range is 0.1 to 0.3 mL depending on patient response.

Subsequent doses should be administered only when necessary and not more frequently than every six hours.

Infants 1 month to 2 years and Children 2 to 12 years: Pediatric dose is 0.005 mL/kg (2.2 lb) body weight injected subcutaneously.

For children 30 kg or less maximum single dose is 0.5 mL: Subsequent doses should be administered only when necessary and not more frequently than every six hours.

Epinephrine pre-Filled Syringes: Useful epinephrine adult dose for allergic emergencies is 0.3 mg. For pediatric use, the appropriate dosage may be 0.15 or 0.30 mg depending upon the body weight of the patient. However, the prescribing physician has the option of prescribing more or less than these amounts, based on careful assessment of each individual patient and recognize the life-threatening nature of the reactions for which this drug is being prescribed. With severe persistent anaphylaxis, repeat injections with an additional syringe may be necessary.

Storage: Store Epinephrine solution (1:1000) between 59° and 77° F (15° and 25° C). Protect from light and freezing. Store suspension under refrigeration. Do not freeze.

Do not expose to temperature above 86° F (30° C).

Epinephrine is light sensitive and should be stored in the tube provided. Store at room temperature (15°-30° C/59°-86° F). Do not refrigerate. Before using, check to make sure solution is not discolored.

CLINICAL STUDIES

Controlled studies comparing the effectiveness of Epinephrine suspension 1:200 and an aqueous solution of Epinephrine 1:1000 were conducted in both pediatric and adult asthmatics. The studies demonstrated rapid bronchodilator activity following administration of either Epinephrine or Epinephrine Suspension administration. Improvement in Wright Peak Expiratory Flow Rate was greater for Epinephrine Suspension than Epinephrine 1:1000 3 to 8 hours following administration (10 hours study duration).

J CODES
Up to 1 ml ampule SC, IM—J0170

HOW SUPPLIED

EPINEPHRINE
INJECTION: 1 MG/ML

BRAND/MANUFACTURER	NDC	SIZE	AWP
○ **BRAND**			
ANA-GUARD: Miles Allergy	00118-9984-01	1 ml	$12.33
	00118-9984-06	1 ml 6s	$90.00

INJECTION: 5 MG/ML

BRAND/MANUFACTURER	NDC	SIZE	AWP
○ **GENERICS**			
SUS-PHRINE INJECTION: Forest Pharm	00456-0664-05	5 ml	$35.68
SUS-PHRINE INJECTION: Forest Pharm	00456-0664-39	0.3 ml 10s	$43.14
SUS-PHRINE INJECTION: Forest Pharm	00456-0664-34	0.3 ml 25s	$103.81

KIT: 0.5 MG/ML

BRAND/MANUFACTURER	NDC	SIZE	AWP
○ **GENERICS**			
EPI-PEN JR AUTO-INJECTOR: Center	00268-0302-01	1s	$30.84

KIT: 1 MG/ML

BRAND/MANUFACTURER	NDC	SIZE	AWP
○ **GENERICS**			
EPI-PEN AUTO-INJECTOR: Center	00268-0301-01	1s	$30.84

SET:

BRAND/MANUFACTURER	NDC	SIZE	AWP
○ **GENERICS**			
Abbott Hosp	00074-3096-05	10s	$478.44
Abbott Hosp	00074-4810-05	10s	$478.44

EPINEPHRINE HYDROCHLORIDE
INJECTION: 0.1 MG/ML

AVERAGE UNIT PRICE (AVAILABLE SIZES)		GENERIC A-RATED AVERAGE PRICE (GAAP)	
GENERIC	$1.28	10 ml 10s	$127.10

BRAND/MANUFACTURER	NDC	SIZE	AWP
◆ **GENERICS**			
Abbott Hosp	00074-4921-01	10 ml 10s	$118.04
Abbott Hosp	00074-4921-23	10 ml 10s	$130.86
Abbott Hosp	00074-4901-01	10 ml 10s	$132.41
Abbott Hosp	00074-4921-33	10 ml 25s	$327.16

◆ RATED THERAPEUTICALLY EQUIVALENT; ◇ THERAPEUTIC EQUIVALENCE UNCONFIRMED; ○ UNRATED

INJECTION: 1 MG/ML

BRAND/MANUFACTURER	NDC	SIZE	AWP
◆ GENERICS			
Abbott Hosp	00074-7241-01	1 ml 25s	$21.97

INJECTION: 1 MG/ML

BRAND/MANUFACTURER	NDC	SIZE	AWP
○ BRAND			
ADRENALIN: Parke-Davis	00071-4011-13	30 ml	$9.81
	00071-4188-03	1 ml 10s	$14.46
○ GENERICS			
Amer Regent	00517-1130-01	30 ml	$9.25
Allscrips	54569-1422-00	1 ml 10s	$23.40
Veratex	17022-1442-07	30 ml 10s	$1.20
Elkins-Sinn	00641-1420-35	1 ml 25s	$11.25
Amer Regent	00517-1061-25	1 ml 25s	$12.19
CMC-Cons	00223-7520-25	1 ml 25s	$22.50
Allscrips	54569-3075-00	1 ml 25s	$38.76
Amer Regent	00517-1071-25	1 ml 25s	$109.38
Raway	00686-1071-25	1 ml 25s	$110.00
Intl Med Sys	00548-1071-00	1 ml 25s	$130.50
Elkins-Sinn	00641-1420-36	1 ml 100s	$36.88

Epoetin Alfa

DESCRIPTION

Erythropoietin is a glycoprotein which stimulates red blood cell production. It is produced in the kidney and stimulates the division and differentiation of committed erythroid progenitors in the bone marrow. Epoetin Alfa has been selected as the proper name for recombinant human erythropoietin. Epoetin Alfa, a 165 amino acid glycoprotein manufactured by recombinant DNA technology, has the same biological effects as endogenous erythropoietin.[1] It has a molecular weight of 30,400 daltons and is produced by mammalian cells into which the human erythropoietin gene has been introduced. The product contains the identical amino acid sequence of isolated natural erythropoietin.

Epoetin Alfa is formulated as a sterile, colorless, preservative-free liquid for intravenous or subcutaneous administration. Each single use vial contains 2,000, 3,000, 4,000, or 10,000 units of Epoetin Alfa.

Following is its chemical structure:

CLINICAL PHARMACOLOGY

Chronic Renal Failure Patients: Erythropoietin is a glycoprotein which stimulates red blood cell production. Endogenous production of erythropoietin is normally regulated by the level of tissue oxygenation. Hypoxia and anemia generally increase the production of erythropoietin, which in turn stimulates erythropoiesis.[2] In normal subjects, plasma erythropoietin levels range from 0.01 to 0.03 Units/mL,[2,3] and increase up to 100- to 1000-fold during hypoxia or anemia.[2,3] In contrast, in patients with chronic renal failure (CRF), production of erythropoietin is impaired, and this erythropoietin deficiency is the primary cause of their anemia.[3,4]

Chronic renal failure is the clinical situation in which there is a progressive and usually irreversible decline in kidney function. Such patients may manifest the sequelae of renal dysfunction, including anemia, but do not necessarily require regular dialysis. Patients with end-stage renal disease (ESRD) are those patients with CRF who require regular dialysis or kidney transplantation for survival.

Epoetin Alfa has been shown to stimulate erythropoiesis in anemic patients with CRF, including both patients on dialysis and those who do not require regular dialysis.[4-13] The first evidence of a response to the three times weekly (T.I.W.) administration of Epoetin Alfa is an increase in the reticulocyte count within 10 days, followed by increases in the red cell count, hemoglobin, and hematocrit, usually within 2-6 weeks.[4,5] *Because of the length of time required for*

erythropoiesis—several days for erythroid progenitors to mature and be released into the circulation—a clinically significant increase in hematocrit is usually not observed in less than 2 weeks and may require up to 6 weeks in some patients. Once the hematocrit reaches the target range (30-33%), that level can be sustained by Epoetin Alfa therapy in the absence of iron deficiency and concurrent illnesses. The rate of hematocrit increase varies between patients and is dependent upon the dose of Epoetin Alfa, within a therapeutic range of approximately 50-300 Units/kg T.I.W.[4]; a greater biologic response is not observed at doses exceeding 300 Units/kg T.I.W.[6] Other factors affecting the rate and extent of response include availability of iron stores, the baseline hematocrit, and the presence of concurrent medical problems.

Zidovudine Treated HIV-Infected Patients: Responsiveness to Epoetin Alfa in HIV-infected patients is dependent upon the endogenous serum erythropoietin level prior to treatment. Patients with endogenous serum erythropoietin levels ≤ 500 mUnits/mL, and who are receiving a dose of zidovudine ≤ 4200 mg/week, may respond to Epoetin Alfa therapy. Patients with endogenous serum erythropoietin levels > 500 mUnits/mL do not appear to respond to Epoetin Alfa therapy. In a series of four clinical trials involving 255 patients, 60-80% of HIV-infected patients treated with zidovudine had endogenous serum erythropoietin levels ≤ 500 mUnits/mL.

Response to Epoetin Alfa in zidovudine-treated HIV-infected patients is manifested by reduced transfusion requirements and increased hematocrit.

Cancer Patients on Chemotherapy: Anemia in cancer patients may be related to the disease itself or the effect of concomitantly administered chemotherapeutic agents. Epoetin Alfa has been shown to increase hematocrit and decrease transfusion requirements after the first month of therapy, (Months 2 and 3 of therapy), in anemic cancer patients undergoing chemotherapy.

A series of clinical trials enrolled 131 anemic cancer patients who were receiving cyclic cisplatin- or non cisplatin-containing chemotherapy. Endogenous baseline serum erythropoietin levels varied among patients in these trials with approximately 75% (N=83/110) having endogenous serum erythropoietin levels ≤132 mUnits/mL, and approximately 4% (N=4/110) of patients having endogenous serum erythropoietin levels >500 mUnits/mL. In general, patients with lower baseline serum erythropoietin levels responded more vigorously to Epoetin Alfa than patients with higher baseline serum erythropoietin levels. Although no specific serum erythropoietin levels can be stipulated above which patients would be unlikely to respond to Epoetin Alfa therapy, treatment of patients with grossly elevated serum erythropoietin levels (e.g., >200 mUnits/mL) is not recommended.

Pharmacokinetics: Intravenously administered Epoetin Alfa is eliminated at a rate consistent with first order kinetics with a circulating half-life ranging from approximately 4 to 13 hours in patients with CRF. Within the therapeutic dose range, detectable levels of plasma erythropoietin are maintained for at least 24 hours.[7] After subcutaneous administration of Epoetin Alfa to patients with CRF, peak serum levels are achieved within 5-24 hours after administration and decline slowly thereafter. There is no apparent difference in half-life between patients not on dialysis whose serum creatinine levels were greater than 3, and patients maintained on dialysis.

In normal volunteers, the half-life of intravenously administered Epoetin Alfa is approximately 20% shorter than the half-life in CRF patients. The pharmacokinetics of Epoetin Alfa have not been studied in HIV-infected patients.

INDICATIONS AND USAGE

Treatment of Anemia of Chronic Renal Failure Patients: Epoetin Alfa is indicated in the treatment of anemia associated with chronic renal failure, including patients on dialysis (end stage renal disease) and patients not on dialysis. Epoetin Alfa is indicated to elevate or maintain the red blood cell level (as manifested by the hematocrit or hemoglobin determinations) and to decrease the need for transfusions in these patients.

Epoetin Alfa is not intended for patients who require immediate correction of severe anemia. Epoetin Alfa may obviate the need for maintenance transfusions but is not a substitute for emergency transfusion.

Prior to initiation of therapy, the patient's iron stores, including transferrin saturation and serum ferritin, should be evaluated. Transferrin saturation should be at least 20% and ferritin at least 100 ng/mL. Blood pressure should be adequately controlled prior to initiation of Epoetin Alfa therapy, and must be closely monitored and controlled during therapy. Non-dialysis patients with symptomatic anemia considered for therapy should have a hematocrit less than 30%. All patients on Epoetin Alfa therapy should be regularly monitored (see *"Laboratory Monitoring"* and *"Precautions"*).

Epoetin Alfa should be administered under the guidance of a qualified physician (see *"Dosage and Administration"*).

Treatment of Anemia in Zidovudine-Treated HIV-Infected Patients: Epoetin Alfa is indicated for the treatment of anemia related to therapy with zidovudine in HIV-infected patients. Epoetin Alfa is indicated to elevate or maintain the red blood cell level (as manifested by the hematocrit or hemoglobin determinations) and to decrease the need for transfusions in these patients Epoetin Alfa is not indicated for the treatment of anemia in HIV-infected patients due to other factors such as iron or folate deficiencies, hemolysis or gastrointestinal bleeding, which should be managed appropriately.

Epoetin Alfa, at a dose of 100 Units/kg three times per week, is effective in decreasing the transfusion requirement and increasing the red blood cell level of anemic, HIV-infected patients treated with zidovudine, when the endogenous serum erythropoietin level is ≤ 500 mUnits/mL and when patients are receiving a dose of zidovudine ≤ 4200 mg/week.

Treatment of Anemia in Cancer Patients on Chemotherapy: Epoetin Alfa is indicated for the treatment of anemia in patients with non-myeloid malignancies where anemia is due to the effect of concomitantly administered chemotherapy. Epoetin Alfa is indicated to decrease the need for transfusions in patients who will be receiving concomitant chemotherapy for a minimum of two months. Epoetin Alfa is not indicated for the treatment of anemia in cancer patients due to other factors such as iron or folate deficiencies, hemolysis or gastrointestinal bleeding which should be managed appropriately.

CLINICAL EXPERIENCE: RESPONSE TO EPOETIN ALFA
Chronic Renal Failure Patients: Response to Epoetin Alfa was consistent across all studies. In the presence of adequate iron stores (see *"Pre-Therapy Iron Evaluation"*), the time to reach the target hematocrit is a function of the baseline hematocrit and the rate of hematocrit rise.

The rate of increase in hematocrit is dependent upon the dose of Epoetin Alfa administered and individual patient variation. In clinical trials at starting doses of 50-150 Units/kg T.I.W., patients responded with an average rate of hematocrit rise of:

	Hematocrit Increase	
Starting Dose (T.I.W. IV)	Hematocrit Points/Day	Hematocrit Points/2 Weeks
50 Units/kg	0.11	1.5
100 Units/kg	0.18	2.5
150 Units/kg	0.25	3.5

Over this dose range, approximately 95% of all patients responded with a clinically significant increase in hematocrit, and by the end of approximately 2 months of therapy virtually all patients were transfusion-independent. Once the target hematocrit was achieved, the maintenance dose was individualized for each patient.

Patients on Dialysis: Thirteen clinical studies were conducted, involving intravenous administration to a total of 1,010 anemic patients on dialysis for 986 patient-years of Epoetin Alfa therapy. In the three largest of these clinical trials, the median maintenance dose necessary to maintain the hematocrit between 30-36% was approximately 75 Units/kg (T.I.W.). In the U.S. multicenter Phase III study, approximately 65% of the patients required doses of 100 Units/kg T.I.W., or less, to maintain their hematocrit at approximately 35%. Almost 10% of patients required a dose of 25 Units/kg, or less, and approximately 10% required a dose of more than 200 Units/kg T.I.W. to maintain their hematocrit at this level.

Patients with CRF Not Requiring Dialysis: Four clinical trials were conducted in patients with CRF not on dialysis involving 181 Epoetin Alfa-treated patients for approximately 67 patient-years of experience. These patients responded to Epoetin Alfa therapy in a manner similar to that observed in patients on dialysis. Patients with CRF not on dialysis demonstrated a dose-dependent and sustained increase in hematocrit when Epoetin Alfa was administered by either an intravenous (IV) or subcutaneous (SC) route, with similar rates of rise of hematocrit when Epoetin Alfa was administered by either route. Moreover, Epoetin Alfa doses of 75-150 Units/kg per week have been shown to maintain hematocrits of 36-38% for up to 6 months.

Zidovudine-Treated HIV-Infected Patients: Epoetin Alfa has been studied in four placebo-controlled trials enrolling 297 anemic (hematocrit < 30%) HIV-infected (AIDS) patients receiving concomitant therapy with zidovudine (all patients were treated with Epoetin Alfa manufactured by Amgen Inc.). In the subgroup of patients (89/125 Epoetin Alfa, and 88/130 placebo) with prestudy endogenous serum erythropoietin levels ≤ 500 mUnits/mL (normal endogenous serum erythropoietin levels are 4-26 mUnits/mL), Epoetin Alfa reduced the mean cumulative number of units of blood transfused per patient by approximately 40%, as compared to the placebo group.[14] Among those patients who required transfusions at baseline, 43% of Epoetin Alfa-treated patients versus 18% of placebo-treated patients were transfusion-independent during the second and third months of therapy. Epoetin Alfa therapy also resulted in significant increases in hematocrit in comparison to placebo. When examining the results according to the weekly dose of zidovudine received during Month 3 of therapy, there was a statistically significant (p < 0.003) reduction in transfusion requirements in Epoetin Alfa-treated patients (N=51) compared to placebo treated patients (N=54) whose mean weekly zidovudine dose was ≤ 4200 mg/week.[14] Approximately 17% of the patients with endogenous serum erythropoietin levels ≤ 500 mUnits/mL receiving Epoetin Alfa in doses from 100-200 Units/kg three times weekly (T.I.W.) achieved a hematocrit of 38% unrelated to transfusions or to a significant reduction in zidovudine dose. In the subgroup of patients whose prestudy endogenous serum erythropoietin levels were > 500 mUnits/mL Epoetin Alfa therapy did not reduce transfusion requirements or increase hematocrit, compared to the corresponding responses in placebo-treated patients.

Responsiveness to Epoetin Alfa therapy may be blunted by intercurrent infectious/inflammatory episodes and by an increase in zidovudine dosage. Consequently, the dose of Epoetin Alfa must be titrated based on these factors to maintain the desired erythropoietic response.

Cancer Patients on Chemotherapy: Epoetin Alfa has been studied in a series of placebo-controlled, double-blind trials in a total of 131 anemic cancer patients. Within this group, 72 patients were treated with concomitant non cisplatin-containing chemotherapy regimens and 59 patients were treated with concomitant

cisplatin-containing chemotherapy regimens. Patients were randomized to Epoetin Alfa 150 Units/kg or placebo subcutaneously T.I.W. for 12 weeks. Epoetin Alfa therapy was associated with a significantly (p < 0.008) greater hematocrit response than in the corresponding placebo-treated patients (see *"Table"*).

HEMATOCRIT (%): MEAN CHANGE FROM BASELINE TO FINAL VALUE*

Study	Epoetin Alfa	Placebo
Chemotherapy	7.6	1.3
Cisplatin	6.9	0.6

* *Significantly higher in Epoetin Alfa patients than in placebo patients (p > 0.008)*

In the two types of chemotherapy studies, (utilizing an Epoetin Alfa dose of 150 Units/kg T.I.W.), the mean number of units of blood transfused per patient after the first month of therapy was significantly (p < 0.02) lower in Epoetin Alfa treated patients (0.71 units in Months 2, 3) than in corresponding placebo-treated patients (1.84 units in Months 2, 3). Moreover, the proportion of patients transfused during Months 2 and 3 of therapy combined was significantly (p < 0.03) lower in the Epoetin Alfa-treated patients than in the corresponding placebo-treated patients (22% versus 43%).[14]

Comparable intensity of chemotherapy in the Epoetin Alfa and placebo groups in the chemotherapy trials was suggested by a similar area under the neutrophil time curve in Epoetin Alfa- and placebo-treated patients as well as by a similar proportion of patients in Epoetin Alfa- and placebo-treated groups whose absolute neutrophil counts fell below 1,000 cells/μL. Available evidence suggests that patients with lymphoid and solid cancers respond to Epoetin Alfa therapy, and that patients with or without tumor infiltration of the bone marrow respond to Epoetin Alfa therapy.

UNLABELED USES
Epoetin Alfa is used alone or as an adjunct in the treatment of anemia of prematurity, anemia associated with multiple myeloma, and sexual dysfunction in hemodialysis patients.

CONTRAINDICATIONS
Epoetin Alfa is contraindicated in patients with:
1. Uncontrolled hypertension.
2. Known hypersensitivity to mammalian cell-derived products.
3. Known hypersensitivity to Albumin (Human).

WARNINGS
CHRONIC RENAL FAILURE PATIENTS
Hypertension: Patients with uncontrolled hypertension should not be treated with Epoetin Alfa; blood pressure should be controlled adequately before initiation of therapy. Blood pressure may rise during Epoetin Alfa therapy, often during the early phase of treatment when the hematocrit is increasing.

For patients who respond to Epoetin Alfa with a rapid increase in hematocrit (e.g., more than 4 points in any 2-week period), the dose of Epoetin Alfa should be reduced because of the possible association of excessive rate of rise of hematocrit with an exacerbation of hypertension.

Seizures: Seizures have occurred in patients with CRF participating in Epoetin Alfa clinical trials.

In patients on dialysis, there was a higher incidence of seizures during the first 90 days of therapy (occurring in approximately 2.5% of patients), as compared with later timepoints.

Given the potential for an increased risk of seizures during the first 90 days of therapy, blood pressure and the presence of premonitory neurologic symptoms should be monitored closely. Patients should be cautioned to avoid potentially hazardous activities such as driving or operating heavy machinery during this period.

Thrombotic Events: During hemodialysis, patients treated with Epoetin Alfa may require increased anticoagulation with heparin to prevent clotting of the artificial kidney. Clotting of the vascular access (A-V shunt) has occurred at an annualized rate of about 0.25 events per patient-year on Epoetin Alfa therapy.

Overall, for patients with CRF (whether on dialysis or not), other thrombotic events (e.g., myocardial infarction, cerebrovascular accident, transient ischemic attack) have occurred at an annualized rate of less than 0.04 events per patient year of Epoetin Alfa therapy. Patients with pre-existing vascular disease should be monitored closely.

ZIDOVUDINE-TREATED HIV-INFECTED PATIENTS
In contrast to CRF patients, Epoetin Alfa therapy has not been linked to exacerbation of hypertension, seizures, and thrombotic events in HIV-infected patients.

PRECAUTIONS
CHRONIC RENAL FAILURE PATIENTS AND ZIDOVUDINE-TREATED HIV-INFECTED PATIENTS, AND CANCER PATIENTS ON CHEMOTHERAPY
General: The parenteral administration of any biologic product should be attended by appropriate precautions in case allergic or other untoward reactions occur (see *"Contraindications"*). While transient rashes have occasionally been observed concurrently with Epoetin Alfa therapy, no serious allergic or anaphylactic reactions have been reported.

The safety and efficacy of Epoetin Alfa therapy have not been established in patients with a known history of a seizure disorder or underlying hematologic disease (e.g., sickle cell anemia, myelodysplastic syndromes, or hypercoagulable disorders).

In some female patients, menses have resumed following Epoetin Alfa therapy; the possibility of potential pregnancy should be discussed and the need for contraception evaluated.

Hematology: Exacerbation of porphyria has been observed rarely in Epoetin Alfa-treated patients with CRF. However, Epoetin Alfa has not caused increased urinary excretion of porphyrin metabolites in normal volunteers, even in the presence of a rapid erythropoietic response. Nevertheless, Epoetin Alfa should be used with caution in patients with known porphyria.

In pre-clinical studies in dogs and rats, but not in monkeys, Epoetin Alfa therapy was associated with subclinical bone marrow fibrosis. Bone marrow fibrosis is a known complication of CRF in humans and may be related to secondary hyperparathyroidism or unknown factors. The incidence of bone marrow fibrosis was not increased in a study of patients on dialysis who were treated with Epoetin Alfa for 12-19 months, compared to the incidence of bone marrow fibrosis in a matched group of patients who had not been treated with Epoetin Alfa.

Hematocrit in CRF patients should be measured twice a week; zidovudine-treated HIV-infected, and cancer patients should have hematocrit measured once a week until hematocrit has been stabilized, and measured periodically thereafter.

Delayed or Diminished Response: If the patient fails to respond or to maintain a response, the following etiologies should be considered and evaluated:
1. Iron deficiency: functional iron deficiency may develop with normal ferritin levels but low transferrin saturation (less than 20%), presumably due to the inability to mobilize iron stores rapidly enough to support increased erythropoiesis. Virtually all patients will eventually require supplemental iron therapy.
2. Underlying infectious, inflammatory, or malignant processes.
3. Occult blood loss.
4. Underlying hematologic diseases (i.e., thalassemia, refractory anemia, or other myelodysplastic disorders).
5. Vitamin deficiencies: folic acid or vitamin B_{12}.
6. Hemolysis.
7. Aluminum intoxication.
8. Osteitis fibrosa cystica.

Iron Evaluation: Prior to and during Epoetin Alfa therapy, the patient's iron stores, including transferrin saturation (serum iron divided by iron binding capacity) and serum ferritin, should be evaluated. Transferrin saturation should be at least 20%, and ferritin should be at least 100 ng/mL. Supplemental iron may be required to increase and maintain transferrin saturation to levels that will adequately support Epoetin Alfa-stimulated erythropoiesis.

Drug Interaction: No evidence of interaction of Epoetin Alfa with other drugs was observed in the course of clinical trials.

Carcinogenesis, Mutagenesis, and Impairment of Fertility: Carcinogenic potential of Epoetin Alfa has not been evaluated. Epoetin Alfa does not induce bacterial gene mutation (Ames Test), chromosomal aberrations in mammalian cells, micronuclei in mice, or gene mutation at the HGPRT locus. In male and female rats treated intravenously with Epoetin Alfa, there was a trend for slightly increased fetal wastage at doses of 100 and 500 Units/kg.

Pregnancy Category C: Epoetin Alfa has been shown to have adverse effects in rats when given in doses five times the human dose. There are no adequate and well-controlled studies in pregnant women. Epoetin Alfa should be used during pregnancy only if potential benefit justifies the potential risk to the fetus.

In studies in female rats, there were decreases in body weight gain, delays in appearance of abdominal hair, delayed eyelid opening, delayed ossification, and decreases in the number of caudal vertebrae in the F1 fetuses of the 500 Units/kg group. In female rats treated intravenously, there was a trend for slightly increased fetal wastage at doses of 100 and 500 Units/kg. Epoetin Alfa has not shown any adverse effect at doses as high as 500 Units/kg in pregnant rabbits (from day 6 to 18 of gestation).

Nursing Mothers: Postnatal observations of the live offspring (F1 generation) of female rats treated with Epoetin Alfa during gestation and lactation revealed no effect of Epoetin Alfa at doses of up to 500 Units/kg. There were, however, decreases in body weight gain, delays in appearance of abdominal hair, eyelid opening, and decreases in the number of caudal vertebrae in the F1 fetuses of the 500 Unit/kg group. There were no Epoetin Alfa related effects on the F2 generation fetuses.

It is not known whether Epoetin Alfa is excreted in human milk. Because many drugs are excreted in human milk, caution should be exercised when Epoetin Alfa is administered to a nursing woman.

Pediatric Use: The safety and effectiveness of Epoetin Alfa in children have not been established.

CHRONIC RENAL FAILURE PATIENTS
Patients with CRF Not Requiring Dialysis: Blood pressure and hematocrit should be monitored no less frequently than for patients maintained on dialysis. Renal function and fluid and electrolyte balance should be closely monitored, as an improved sense of well-being may obscure the need to initiate dialysis in some patients.

Hematology: In order to avoid reaching the target hematocrit too rapidly, or exceeding the target range (hematocrit of 30-33%), the guidelines for dose and frequency of dose adjustments (see *"Dosage and Administration"*) should be followed.

For patients who respond to Epoetin Alfa with a rapid increase in hematocrit (e.g., more than 4 points in any 2-week period), the dose of Epoetin Alfa should be reduced because of the possible association of excessive rate of rise of hematocrit with an exacerbation of hypertension.

The elevated bleeding time characteristic of CRF decreases toward normal after correction of anemia in Epoetin Alfa-treated patients. Reduction of bleeding time also occurs after correction of anemia by transfusion.

Sufficient time should be allowed to determine a patient's responsiveness to a dosage of Epoetin Alfa before adjusting the dose. Because of the time required for erythropoiesis and the red cell half-life, an interval of 2-6 weeks may occur between the time of a dose adjustment (initiation, increase, decrease, or discontinuation) and a significant change in hematocrit.

Laboratory Monitoring: The hematocrit should be determined twice a week until it has stabilized in the target range and the maintenance dose has been established. After any dose adjustment, the hematocrit should also be determined twice weekly for at least 2-6 weeks until it has been determined that the hematocrit has stabilized in response to the dose change. The hematocrit should then be monitored at regular intervals.

A complete blood count with differential and platelet count should be performed regularly. During clinical trials, modest increases were seen in platelets and white blood cell counts. While these changes were statistically significant, they were not clinically significant and the values remained within normal ranges. In patients with CRF, serum chemistry values [including blood urea nitrogen (BUN), uric acid, creatinine, phosphorus, and potassium] should be monitored regularly. During clinical trials in patients on dialysis, modest increases were seen in BUN, creatinine, phosphorus, and potassium. In some patients with CRF not on dialysis, treated with Epoetin Alfa, modest increases in serum uric acid and phosphorus were observed. While changes were statistically significant, the values remained within the ranges normally seen in patients with CRF.

Hypertension: Patients with uncontrolled hypertension should not be treated with Epoetin Alfa, blood pressure should be controlled adequately before initiation of therapy. Blood pressure may rise and episodes of hypertension may increase during Epoetin Alfa therapy in all CRF patients, whether or not they require dialysis, often during the early phase of treatment with the hematocrit is increasing. To prevent hypertension and sequelae, particular care needs to be taken in patients treated with Epoetin Alfa to monitor and aggressively control blood pressure. During the period when hematocrit is increasing, approximately 25% of patients on dialysis may require initiation of, or increases in, antihypertensive therapy. Patients should be advised as to the importance of compliance with antihypertensive therapy and dietary restrictions. For patients who respond to Epoetin Alfa with a rapid increase in hematocrit (e.g., more than 4 points in any 2-week period), the dose of Epoetin Alfa should be reduced because of the possible association of excessive rate of rise of hematocrit with an exacerbation of hypertension. If blood pressure is difficult to control, the dose of Epoetin Alfa should be reduced; if clinically indicated, Epoetin Alfa may be withheld until blood pressure control is re-establised.

Seizures: Seizures have occurred in patients with CRF participating in Epoetin Alfa clinical trials. In patients on dialysis, there was a higher incidence of seizures during the first 90 days of therapy (occurring in approximately 2.5% of patients), as compared with later timepoints.

Given the potential for an increased risk of seizures during the first 90 days of therapy, blood pressure and the presence of premonitory neurologic symptoms should be monitored closely. Patients should be cautioned to avoid potentially hazardous activities such as driving or operating heavy machinery during this period.

Thrombotic Events: During hemodialysis, patients treated with Epoetin Alfa may require increased anticoagulation with heparin to prevent clotting of the artificial kidney. Clotting of the vascular access has occurred at an annualized rate of about 0.25 events per patient-year on Epoetin Alfa therapy.

A relationship has not been established with statistical certainty between a rise in hematocrit and the rate of thrombotic events [including thrombosis of vascular access (A-V shunt)] in Epoetin Alfa-treated patients. Overall, for patients with CRF (whether on dialysis or not), other thrombotic events (e.g., myocardial infarction, cerebrovascular accident, transient ischemic attack) have occurred at an annualized rate of less than 0.04 events per patient-year of Epoetin Alfa therapy. Patients with pre-existing vascular disease should be monitored closely.

Diet: As the hematocrit increases and patients experience an improved sense of well-being and quality of life, the importance of compliance with dietary and dialysis prescriptions should be reinforced. In particular, hyperkalemia is not uncommon in patients with CRF. In U.S. studies in patients on dialysis, hyperkalemia has occurred at an annualized rate of approximately 0.11 episodes per patient-year of Epoetin Alfa therapy, often in association with poor compliance to medication, dietary and/or dialysis prescriptions.

Dialysis Management: Therapy with Epoetin Alfa results in an increase in hematocrit and a decrease in plasma volume which could affect dialysis efficiency. In studies to date, the resulting increase in hematocrit did not appear to adversely affect dialyzer function[9,10] or the efficiency of high-flux hemodialysis.[11] During hemodialysis, patients treated with Epoetin Alfa may require increased anticoagulation with heparin to prevent clotting of the artificial kidney.

Patients who are marginally dialyzed may require adjustments in their dialysis prescription. As with all patients on dialysis, the serum chemistry values [including blood urea nitrogen (BUN), creatinine, phosphorus, and potassium] in

► SHOWN IN PRODUCT IDENTIFICATION GUIDE

Epoetin Alfa-treated patients should be monitored regularly to assure the adequacy of the dialysis prescription.

Renal Function: In patients with CRF not on dialysis, renal function and fluid and electrolyte balance should be closely monitored, as an improved sense of well-being may obscure the need to initiate dialysis in some patients. In patients with CRF not on dialysis, placebo-controlled studies of progression of renal dysfunction over periods of greater than one year have not been completed. In shorter-term trials in patients with CRF not on dialysis, changes in creatinine and creatinine clearance were not significantly different in Epoetin Alfa-treated patients, compared with placebo-treated patients. Analysis of the slope of 1/serum creatinine vs. time plots in these patients indicates no significant change in the slope after the initiation of Epoetin Alfa therapy.

ZIDOVUDINE-TREATED HIV-INFECTED PATIENTS
Hypertension: Exacerbation of hypertension has not been observed in zidovudine-treated HIV-infected patients treated with Epoetin Alfa. However Epoetin Alfa should be withheld in these patients if pre-existing hypertension is uncontrolled, and should not be started until blood pressure is controlled. In double-blind studies, a single seizure has been experienced by an Epoetin Alfa-treated patient.[14]

CANCER PATIENTS ON CHEMOTHERAPY
Hypertension: Hypertension, associated with a significant increase in hematocrit, has been noted rarely in Epoetin Alfa-treated cancer patients. Nevertheless, blood pressure in Epoetin Alfa-treated patients should be monitored carefully, particularly in patients with an underlying history of hypertension or cardiovascular disease.

Seizures: In double-blind, placebo controlled trials, 3.2% (N = 2/63) of Epoetin Alfa-treated patients and 2.9% (N = 2/68) of placebo-treated patients had seizures. Seizures in 1.6% (N = 1/63) of Epoetin Alfa-treated patients occurred in the context of a significant increase in blood pressure and hematocrit from baseline values. However, both Epoetin Alfa-treated treated patients also had underlying CNS pathology which may have been related to seizure activity.

Thrombotic Events: In double-blind, placebo-controlled trials, 3.2% (N = 2/63) of Epoetin Alfa-treated patients and 11.8% (N = 8/68) of placebo-treated patients had thrombotic events (e.g., pulmonary embolism, cerebrovascular accident).

Growth Factor Potential: Epoetin Alfa is a growth factor that primarily stimulates red cell production. However, the possibility that Epoetin Alfa can act as a growth factor for any tumor type, particularly myeloid malignancies, cannot be excluded.

ADVERSE REACTIONS
CHRONIC RENAL FAILURE PATIENTS
Studies analyzed to date indicate that Epoetin Alfa is generally well-tolerated. The adverse events reported are frequent sequelae of CRF and are not necessarily attributable to Epoetin Alfa therapy. In double-blind, placebo-controlled studies involving over 300 patients with CRF, the events reported in greater than 5% of Epoetin Alfa-treated patients during the blinded phase were:

Event	Percent of Patients Reporting Event	
	Epoetin Alfa-Treated Patients (N = 200)	*Placebo-Treated Patients (N = 135)*
Hypertension	24%	19%
Headache	16%	12%
Arthralgias	11%	6%
Nausea	11%	9%
Edema	9%	10%
Fatigue	9%	14%
Diarrhea	9%	6%
Vomiting	8%	5%
Chest Pain	7%	9%
Skin Reaction (Administration Site)	7%	12%
Asthenia	7%	12%
Dizziness	7%	13%
Clotted Access	7%	2%

Significant adverse events of concern in patients with CRF treated in double-blind, placebo-controlled trials occurred in the following percent of patients during the blinded phase of the studies:

Seizure	1.1%	1.1%
CVA/TIA	0.4%	0.6%
MI	0.4%	1.1%
Death	0.0%	1.7%

In the U.S. Epoetin Alfa studies in patients on dialysis (over 567 patients) the incidence (number of events per patient-year) of the most frequently reported adverse events were: hypertension (0.75), headache (0.40), tachycardia (0.31), nausea/vomiting (0.26), clotted vascular access (0.25), shortness of breath (0.14), hyperkalemia (0.11), and diarrhea (0.11). Other reported events occurred at a rate of less than 0.10 events per patient per year.

Events reported to have occurred within several hours of administration of Epoetin Alfa were rare, mild and transient, and included flu-like symptoms such as arthralgias and myalgias.

In all studies analyzed to date, Epoetin Alfa administration was generally well tolerated, irrespective of the route of administration.

Allergic Reactions: There have been no reports of serious allergic reactions or anaphylaxis associated with Epoetin Alfa administration. Skin rashes and urticaria have been observed rarely and when reported have been mild and transient in nature. There has been no evidence for development of antibodies to erythropoietin in patients tested to date, including those receiving intravenous Epoetin Alfa for over two years. Nevertheless, if an anaphylactoid reaction occurs, Epoetin Alfa should be immediately discontinued and appropriate therapy initiated.

Seizures: The relationship, if any, of Epoetin Alfa therapy to seizures is uncertain. The baseline incidence of seizures in the untreated dialysis population is difficult to determine; it appears to be in the range of 5-10% per patient year.[15-17] There have been 47 seizures in 1,010 patients on dialysis, treated with Epoetin Alfa with an exposure of 986 patient-years for a rate of approximately 0.048 events per patient-year. However, there appeared to be a higher rate of seizures during the first 90 days of therapy (occurring in approximately 2.5% of patients), when compared to subsequent 90-day time periods. While the relationship between seizures and the rate of rise of hematocrit is uncertain, *it is recommended that the dose of Epoetin Alfa be decreased if the hematocrit increase exceeds 4 points in any 2-week period.*

Hypertension: Up to 80% of patients with CRF have a history of hypertension.[18] Blood pressure may rise during Epoetin Alfa therapy in CRF patients whether or not maintained on dialysis; during the early phase of treatment when hematocrit is increasing, approximately 25% of patients on dialysis may require initiation or increases in antihypertensive therapy. Hypertensive encephalopathy and seizures have been observed in patients with CRF treated with Epoetin Alfa. Increases in blood pressure may be associated with the rate of increase in hematocrit. *It is recommended that the dose of Epoetin Alfa be decreased if the hematocrit increase exceeds 4 points in any 2-week period.*

Increases in blood pressure have been reported in clinical trials, often during the first 90 days of therapy. When data from all patients in the U.S. Phase III multicenter trial were analyzed, there was an apparent trend of more reports of hypertensive adverse events in patients on dialysis with a faster rate of rise of hematocrit (greater than 4 hematocrit points in any two-week period). However, in a double-blind, placebo-controlled trial, hypertensive adverse events were not reported at an increased rate in the Epoetin Alfa-treated group (150 U/kg T.I.W.) relative to the placebo group. There do not appear to be any direct pressor effects of Epoetin Alfa. *Special care should be taken to closely monitor and control blood pressure in Epoetin Alfa treated patients with existing compromised cardiovasculature.*

Thrombotic Events: During hemodialysis, patients treated with Epoetin Alfa may require increased anticoagulation with heparin to prevent clotting of the artificial kidney. Clotting of the vascular access has occurred at an annualized rate of about 0.25 events per patient-year on Epoetin Alfa therapy.

A relationship has not been established with statistical certainty between a rise in hematocrit and the rate of thrombotic events [including thrombosis of vascular access (A-V shunt)] in Epoetin Alfa-treated patients. Overall for patients with CRF (whether on dialysis or not), other thrombotic events (e.g., myocardial infarction, cerebrovascular accident, transient ischemic attack) have occurred at an annualized rate of less than 0.04 events per patient-year of Epoetin Alfa therapy. Patients with pre-existing vascular disease should be monitored closely.

ZIDOVUDINE-TREATED HIV-INFECTED PATIENTS
Adverse events reported in clinical trials with Epoetin Alfa in zidovudine-treated HIV-infected patients were consistent with the progression of HIV infection. In double-blind, placebo-controlled studies of 3-months duration involving approximately 300 zidovudine-treated HIV-infected patients, adverse events with an incidence of ≥ 10% in either Epoetin Alfa-treated patients or placebo-treated patients were:

Event	Percent of Patients Reporting Events	
	Epoetin Alfa Treated Patients (N = 144)	*Placebo-Treated Patients (N = 153)*
Pyrexia	38%	29%
Fatigue	25%	31%
Headache	19%	14%
Cough	18%	14%
Diarrhea	16%	18%
Rash	16%	8%
Congestion, Respiratory	15%	10%
Nausea	15%	12%
Shortness of Breath	14%	13%
Asthenia	11%	14%
Skin Reaction, Medication Site	10%	7%
Dizziness	9%	10%

There were no statistically significant differences between treatment groups in the incidence of the above events.

In the 297 patients studied, Epoetin Alfa was not associated with significant increases in opportunistic infections or mortality.[14] In 71 patients from this group treated with Epoetin Alfa at 150 Units/kg T.I.W., serum p24 antigen levels did not

---

appear to increase.[14] Preliminary data showed no enhancement of HIV replication in infected cell lines in vitro.[14]

Peripheral white blood cell and platelet counts are unchanged following Epoetin Alfa therapy.

Allergic Reactions: Two zidovudine-treated HIV-infected patients had urticarial reactions within 48 hours of their first exposure to study medication. One patient was treated with Epoetin Alfa and one was treated with placebo (Epoetin Alfa vehicle alone). Both patients had positive immediate skin tests against their study medication with a negative saline control. The basis for this apparent pre-existing hypersensitivity to components of the Epoetin Alfa formulation is unknown, but may be related to HIV-induced immunosuppression or prior exposure to blood products.

Seizures: In double-blind and open-label trials of Epoetin Alfa in zidovudine-treated HIV-infected patients, 10 patients have experienced seizures.[14] In general, these seizures appear to be related to underlying pathology such as meningitis or cerebral neoplasms, not Epoetin Alfa therapy.

CANCER PATIENTS ON CHEMOTHERAPY
Adverse experiences reported in clinical trials with Epoetin Alfa in cancer patients were consistent with the underlying disease state. In double-blind, placebo-controlled studies of up to 3 months duration involving 131 cancer patients on chemotherapy, adverse events with an incidence > 10% in either Epoetin Alfa-treated or placebo-treated patients were as indicated below:

	Percent of Patients Reporting Event	
Event	*Epoetin Alfa-Treated Patients (N = 63)*	*Placebo-Treated Patients (N = 68)*
Pyrexia	29%	19%
Diarrhea	21%[a]	7%
Nausea	17%[b]	32%
Vomiting	17%	15%
Edema	17%[c]	1%
Asthenia	13%	16%
Fatigue	13%	15%
Shortness of Breath	13%	9%
Parasthesia	11%	6%
Upper Respiratory Infection	11%	4%
Dizziness	5%	12%
Trunk Pain	3%[d]	16%

[a] *p = 0.041*
[b] *p = 0.069*
[c] *p = 0.0016*
[d] *p = 0.017*

Although some statistically significant differences between Epoetin Alfa- and placebo-treated patients were noted, the overall safety profile of Epoetin Alfa appeared to be consistent with the disease process of advanced cancer. During double-blind and subsequent open label therapy in which patients (N=72 for total Epoetin Alfa exposure) were treated for up to 32 weeks with doses as high as 927 Units/kg, the adverse experience profile of Epoetin Alfa was consistent with the progression of advanced cancer.

Based on comparable survival data, and on the percentage of Epoetin Alfa- and placebo-treated patients who discontinued therapy due to death, disease progression, or adverse experiences (22% and 13%, respectively; p=0.25), the clinical outcome in the Epoetin Alfa- and placebo-treated patients appeared to be similar. Available data from animal tumor models and measurement of proliferation of solid tumor cells from clinical biopsy specimens in response to Epoetin Alfa suggest that Epoetin Alfa does not potentiate tumor growth. Nevertheless, as a growth factor, the possibility that Epoetin Alfa may potentiate growth of some tumors, particularly myeloid tumors, cannot be excluded. A randomized controlled Phase IV study is currently ongoing to further evaluate this issue.

The mean peripheral white blood cell count was unchanged following Epoetin Alfa therapy compared to the corresponding value in the placebo-treated group.

OVERDOSAGE
The maximum amount of Epoetin Alfa that can be safely administered in single or multiple doses has not been determined. Doses of up to 1500 Units/kg T.I.W. for 3-4 weeks have been administered without any direct toxic effects of Epoetin Alfa itself.[6]

Therapy with Epoetin Alfa can result in polycythemia if the hematocrit is not carefully monitored and the dose adjusted. If the target range is exceeded, Epoetin Alfa may be temporarily withheld until the hematocrit returns to the target range; Epoetin Alfa therapy may then be resumed using a lower dose (see *"Dosage and Administration"*). If polyeythemia is of concern, phlebotomy may be indicated to decrease the hematocrit.

DOSAGE AND ADMINISTRATION
CHRONIC RENAL FAILURE PATIENTS
Starting doses of Epoetin Alfa over the range of 50-100 Units/kg three times weekly (T.I.W.) have been shown to be safe and effective in increasing hematocrit and eliminating transfusion dependency in patients with CRF (see *"Clinical Experience"*). The dose of Epoetin Alfa should be reduced when the hematocrit reaches the target range of 30-33% or increases by more than 4 points in any 2-week period. The dosage of Epoetin Alfa must be individualized to maintain the

hematocrit within the target range. Dose changes should generally be in the range of 25 Units/kg, T.I.W. The table below provides general therapeutic guidelines.

Starting Dose:	50-100 Units/kg T.I.W.; IV: Dialysis Patients IV or SC: Non-dialysis CRF patients
Reduce Dose When:	1) Target range is reached, or 2) Hct. increases > 4 points in any 2-week period
Increase Dose If:	Hct. does not increase by 5-6 points after 8 weeks of therapy, and hct. is below target range
Maintenance Dose:	Individually titrate
Target Hct. Range:	30-33% (max. 36%)

In patients on dialysis, Epoetin Alfa usually has been administered as an IV bolus T.I.W. While the administration of Epoetin Alfa is independent of the dialysis procedure, Epoetin Alfa may be administered into the venous line at the end of the dialysis procedure to obviate the need for additional venous access. In patients with CRF not on dialysis, Epoetin Alfa may be given either as an intravenous or subcutaneous injection.

During therapy, hematological parameters should be monitored regularly (see *"Laboratory Monitoring"*).

Pre-Therapy Iron Evaluation: Prior to and during Epoetin Alfa therapy, the patient's iron stores, including transferrin saturation (serum iron divided by iron binding capacity) and serum ferritin, should be evaluated. Transferrin saturation should be at least 20%, and ferritin should be at least 100 ng/mL. Supplemental iron may be required to increase and maintain transferrin saturation to levels that will adequately support Epoetin Alfa-stimulated erythropoiesis.

Dose Adjustment:
■ When the hematocrit reaches 30-33%, the dosage should be decreased by approximately 25 Units/kg T.I.W., to avoid exceeding the target range. Once the hematocrit is within the target range, the maintenance dose must be individualized for each patient (see *"Maintenance Dose"*).
■ At any time, if the hematocrit increases by more than 4 points in a 2-week period, the dose should be immediately decreased. After the dose reduction, the hematocrit should be monitored twice weekly for 2-6 weeks, and further dose adjustments should be made as outlined in "Maintenance Dose."
■ As the hematocrit approaches, or if it exceeds 36%, Epoetin Alfa should be temporarily withheld until the hematocrit decreases to the target range of 30-33%; the dose should be reduced by approximately 25 Units/kg T.I.W. upon re-initiation of therapy.
■ If a hematocrit increase of 5-6 points is not achieved after an eight-week period and iron stores are adequate (see *"Delayed or Diminished Response"*), the dose of Epoetin Alfa may be increased in increments of 25 Units/kg T.I.W. Further increases of 25 Units/kg T.I.W. may be made at 4-6 week intervals until the desired response is attained.

Maintenance Dose: The maintenance dose must be individualized for each patient. As the hematocrit approaches, or if it exceeds, 36%, Epoetin Alfa should be temporarily withheld until the hematocrit is 33% or less. Upon re-initiation of therapy, the dose should be reduced by approximately 25 Units/kg T.I.W., or doses omitted, and an appropriate time interval (i.e., 2-6 weeks) allowed for stabilization of response.

If the hematocrit remains below, or falls below, the target range, iron stores should be re-evaluated. If the transferrin saturation is less than 20%, supplemental iron should be administered. If the transferrin saturation is greater than 20%, the dose of Epoetin Alfa may be increased by 25 Units/kg T.I.W. Such dose increases should not be made more frequently than once a month, unless clinically indicated, as the response time of the hematocrit to a dose increase can be 2-6 weeks. Hematocrit should be measured twice weekly for 2-6 weeks following dose increases.

In the U.S. Phase III multicenter trial in patients on hemodialysis, the median maintenance dose was 75 Units/kg T.I.W., with approximately 65% of the patients requiring doses of 100 Units/kg T.I.W., or less, to maintain their hematocrit within the range of 32-38% (maintenance doses ranged from 12.5 to 525 Units/kg T.I.W.). Almost 10% of the patients required a dose of 25 Units/kg T.I.W., or less, and approximately 10% of the patients required more than 200 Units/kg T.I.W. to maintain their hematocrit in this range.

In patients with CRF not on dialysis, the maintenance dose must also be individualized. Epoetin Alfa doses of 75-150 Units/kg per week have been shown to maintain hematocrits of 36-38% for up to six months.

Delayed or Diminished Response: Over 95% of patients with CRF responded with clinically significant increases in hematocrit, and virtually all patients were transfusion-independent within approximately 2 months of initiation of Epoetin Alfa therapy.

If a patient fails to respond or maintain a response, other etiologies should be considered and evaluated as clinically indicated. See *"Precautions"* section for discussion of delayed or diminished response.

ZIDOVUDINE-TREATED HIV-INFECTED PATIENTS
Prior to beginning Epoetin Alfa, it is recommended that the endogenous serum erythropoietin level be determined (prior to transfusion). Available evidence suggests that patients receiving zidovudine with endogenous serum erythropoietin levels > 500 mUnits/mL are unlikely to respond to therapy with Epoetin Alfa.

Starting Dose: For patients with serum erythropoietin levels ≤ 500 mUnits/mL who are receiving a dose of zidovudine ≤ 4200 mg/week, the recommended starting dose of Epoetin Alfa is 100 Units/kg as an intravenous or subcutaneous injection three times weekly (T.I.W.) for 8 weeks.

Increase Dose: During the dose adjustment phase of therapy, the hematocrit should be monitored weekly. If the response is not satisfactory in terms of reducing transfusion requirements or increasing hematocrit after 8 weeks of therapy, the dose of Epoetin Alfa can be increased by 50-100 Units/kg T.I.W. Response should be evaluated every 4-8 weeks thereafter and the dose adjusted accordingly by 50-100 Units/kg increments T.I.W. If patients have not responded satisfactorily to an Epoetin Alfa dose of 300 Units/kg T.I.W., it is unlikely that they will respond to higher doses of Epoetin Alfa.

Maintenance Dose: After attainment of the desired response (i.e., reduced transfusion requirements or increased hematocrit), the dose of Epoetin Alfa should be titrated to maintain the response based on factors such as variations in zidovudine dose and the presence of intercurrent infectious or inflammatory episodes. If the hematocrit exceeds 40%, the dose should be discontinued until the hematocrit drops to 36%. The dose should be reduced by 25% when treatment is resumed and then titrated to maintain the desired hematocrit.

CANCER PATIENTS ON CHEMOTHERAPY
Baseline endogenous serum erythropoietin levels varied among patients in these trials with approximately 75 percent (N = 88/110) having endogenous serum erythropoietin levels < 132 mUnits/mL, and approximately 4 percent (N = 4/110) of patients having endogenous serum erythropoietin levels > 500 mUnits/mL. In general patients with lower baseline serum erythropoietin levels responded more vigorously to Epoetin Alfa than patients with higher erythropoietin levels. Although no specific serum erythropoietin level can be stipulated above which patients would be unlikely to respond to Epoetin Alfa therapy, treatment of patients with grossly elevated serum erythropoietin levels (e.g., > 200 mUnits/mL) is not recommended. The hematocrit should be monitored on a weekly basis in patients receiving Epoetin Alfa therapy until hematocrit becomes stable.

Starting Dose: The recommended starting dose of Epoetin Alfa is 150 Units/kg subcutaneously T.I.W.

Dose Adjustment: If the response is not satisfactory in terms of reducing transfusions requirements or increasing hematocrit after 8 weeks of therapy, the dose of Epoetin Alfa can be increased up to 300 Units/kg T.I.W. If patients have not responded satisfactorily to an Epoetin Alfa dose of 300 Units/kg T.I.W., it is unlikely that they will respond to higher doses of Epoetin Alfa. If the hematocrit exceeds 40%, the dose of Epoetin Alfa should be withheld until the hematocrit falls to 36%. The dose of Epoetin Alfa should be reduced by 25% when treatment is resumed and titrated to maintain the desired hematocrit. If the initial dose of Epoetin Alfa includes a very rapid hematocrit response (e.g., an increase of more than 4 percentage points in any 2-week period), the dose of Epoetin Alfa should be reduced.

PREPARATION AND ADMINISTRATION OF EPOETIN ALFA
1. DO NOT SHAKE. Shaking may denature the glycoprotein, rendering it biologically inactive.
2. Parenteral drug products should be inspected visually for particulate matter and discoloration prior to administration. Do not use any vials exhibiting particulate matter or discoloration.
3. Using aseptic techniques, attach a sterile needle to a sterile syringe. Remove the flip top from the vial containing Epoetin Alfa, and wipe the septum with a disinfectant. Insert the needle into the vial, and withdraw into the syringe an appropriate volume of solution.
4. Use only one dose per vial; do not re-enter the vial. Discard unused portions. Contains no preservative.
5. Do not administer in conjunction with other drug solutions.

EPOETIN ALFA VIALS FOR INJECTION STORAGE
Store at 2° to 8°C (36° to 46°F). Do not freeze or shake.

REFERENCES
1. Egrie JC, Strickland TW, Lane J, *et al.*, (1986). "Characterization and Biological Effects of Recombinant Human Erythropoietin." *Immunobiol.* 72: 213-224. 2. Graber SE and Krantz SB, (1978). "Erythropoietin and the Control of Red Cell Production." *Ann. Rev. Med.* 29: 51-66. 3. Eschbach JW and Adamson JW, (1985). "Anemia of End-Stage Renal Disease (ESRD)." *Kidney Intl.* 28: 1-5. 4. Eschbach JW, Egrie JC, Downing MR, Browne JK, and Adamson JW, (1987). "Correction of the Anemia of End-Stage Renal Disease with Recombinant Human Erythropoietin." *NEJM* 316: 73-78. 5. Eschbach JW, Adamson JW, and Cooperative Multicenter r-HuEPO Trial Group, (1988). "Correction of the Anemia of Hemodialysis (HD) Patients with Recombinant Human Erythropoietin (r-HuEPO): Results of a Multicenter Study." *Kidney Intl.* 33: 189. 6. Eschbach JW, Egrie JC, Downing MR, Browne JK, Adamson JW, (1989). "The Use of Recombinant Human Erythropoietin (r-HuEPO): Effect in End-Stage Renal Disease (ESRD)." *Prevention of Chronic Uremia* (Friedman, Beyer, DeSanto, Giordano, eds.), Field and Wood Inc., Philadelphia, PA, pp 148-155. 7. Egrie JC, Eschbach JW, McGuire T, and Adamson JW, (1988). "Pharmacokinetics of Recombinant Human Erythropoietin (r-HuEPO) Administered to Hemodialysis (HD) Patients." *Kidney Intl.* 33: 262. 8. Lundin AP, Delano BG, Stein R, Quinn RM, and Friedman EA, (1988). "Recombinant Human Erythropoietin (r-HuEPO) Treatment Enhances Exercise Tolerance in Hemodialysis Patients." *Kidney Intl.* 33: 200. 9. Paganini E, Garcia J, Ellis P, Bodnar D, and Magnussen M, (1988). "Clinical Sequelae of Correction of Anemia with Recombinant Human Erythropoietin (r-HuEPO); Urea Kinetics, Dialyzer Function and Reuse." *Am. J. Kid. Dis.* 11: 16. 10. Delano BG, Lundin AP, Golansky R, Quinn RM, Rao TKS, and Friedman EA, (1988). "Dialyzer Urea and Creatinine Clearances Not Significantly Changed in r-HuEPO Treated Maintenance Hemodialysis (MD) Patients." *Kidney Intl.* 33: 219. 11. Stivelman J, Van Wyck D, and Ogden D, (1988). "Use of Recombinant Erythropoietin (r-HuEPO) with High Flux Dialysis (HFD) Does Not Worsen Azotemia or Shorten Access Survival." *Kidney Intl.* 33: 239. 12. Lim VS, DeGowin RL, Zavala D, Kirchner PT, Abels R, Perry P, and Fangman J, (1989). "Recombinant Human Erythropoietin Treatment in Pre-Dialysis Patients: A Double-Blind Placebo-Controlled Trial." *Ann. Int. Med.* 110: 108-114. 13. Stone WJ, Graber SE, Krantz SB, et al., (1988). "Treatment of the Anemia of Pre-Dialysis Patients with Recombinant Human Erythropoietin: A Randomized, Placebo-Controlled Trial." *Am. J. Med. Sci.* 296: 171-179. 14. Data on file, Ortho Biologics, Inc. 15. Raskin NH and Fishman RA, (1976). "Neurologic Disorders in Renal Failure (First of Two Parts)." *NEJM* 294: 143-148. 16. Raskin NH and Fishman RA, (1976). "Neurologic Disorders in Renal Failure (Second of Two Parts)." *NEJM* 294: 204-210. 17. Messing RO and Simon RP, (1986). "Seizures as a Manifestation of Systemic Disease." *Neurologic Clinics* 4: 563-584. 18. Kerr DN, (1979). "Chronic Renal Failure." *Cecil Textbook of Medicine,* (Beeson PB, McDermott W, Wyngaarden JB, eds.), W.B. Saunders, Philadelphia, PA, pp 1351-1367.

HOW SUPPLIED
INJECTION: 10,000 U/ML

BRAND/MANUFACTURER	NDC	SIZE	AWP
○ **BRAND**			
PROCRIT: Ortho Biotech	59676-0310-01	1 ml 6s	$684.00
EPOGEN: Amgen	55513-0144-10	1 ml 10s	$1200.00
PROCRIT: Ortho Biotech	59676-0310-02	1 ml 25s	$2850.00

INJECTION: 2000 U/ML

BRAND/MANUFACTURER	NDC	SIZE	AWP
○ **BRAND**			
PROCRIT: Ortho Biotech	59676-0302-01	1 ml 6s	$144.00
EPOGEN: Amgen	55513-0126-10	1 ml 10s	$240.00
PROCRIT: Ortho Biotech	59676-0302-02	1 ml 25s	$600.00

INJECTION: 3000 U/ML

BRAND/MANUFACTURER	NDC	SIZE	AWP
○ **BRAND**			
PROCRIT: Ortho Biotech	59676-0303-01	1 ml 6s	$216.00
EPOGEN: Amgen	55513-0267-10	1 ml 10s	$360.00
PROCRIT: Ortho Biotech	59676-0303-02	1 ml 25s	$900.00

INJECTION: 4000 U/ML

BRAND/MANUFACTURER	NDC	SIZE	AWP
○ **BRAND**			
PROCRIT: Ortho Biotech	59676-0304-01	1 ml 6s	$288.00
EPOGEN: Amgen	55513-0148-10	1 ml 10s	$480.00
PROCRIT: Ortho Biotech	59676-0304-02	1 ml 25s	$1200.00

Epogen *SEE* EPOETIN ALFA

Eppy/N *SEE* EPINEPHRINE, OPHTHALMIC

Equagesic *SEE* ASPIRIN WITH MEPROBAMATE

Equanil *SEE* MEPROBAMATE

Erex *SEE* YOHIMBINE HYDROCHLORIDE

Ergamisol *SEE* LEVAMISOLE HYDROCHLORIDE

Ergocalciferol

DESCRIPTION
Ergocalciferol Tablets USP contain 1.25 mg (50,000 USP units) of Ergocalciferol for oral administration.

Ergocalciferol is a Vitamin D analog (Vitamin D₂) used in the regulation of calcium. The empirical formula is $C_{28}H_{44}O$ and the molecular weight is 396.65. Chemically, it is 9,10-secoergosta-5,7,10(19), 22-tetraen-3-01,(3β,5Z,7E,22E).

◆ RATED THERAPEUTICALLY EQUIVALENT; ◇ THERAPEUTIC EQUIVALENCE UNCONFIRMED; ○ UNRATED

Following is its chemical structure:

CLINICAL PHARMACOLOGY

Vitamin D metabolites in their activated forms along with parathyroid hormone and calcitonin, regulate serum calcium concentrations. Vitamin D metabolites promote the active absorption of calcium and phosphorus by the small intestine, thus elevating serum calcium and phosphate levels sufficiently to permit bone mineralization. Also, they increase the rate of accretion and resorption of minerals in bone and promote the resorption of phosphate by the renal tubules. Vitamin D metabolites are also involved in magnesium metabolism.

Ergocalciferol is readily absorbed from the gastrointestinal tract, if fat absorption is normal. The presence of bile is necessary for absorption of Vitamin D and its analogs. Absorption is reduced in patients with liver disease and intestinal malabsorption syndrome. Once absorbed, Ergocalciferol is bound to α-globulins and albumin in the plasma. Ergocalciferol is stored primarily in the liver, but is also found in fat, muscle, skin, and bones. In the liver, Ergocalciferol is converted to 25-hydroxyergocalciferol. In the kidneys, 25-hydroxyergocalciferol is further hydroxylated to 1, 25-dihydroxyergocalciferol, the biologically active form of Ergocalciferol. The primary route of excretion is via the bile into the feces.

After oral administration, the onset of hypercalcemic action is 10-24 hours. Maximal hypercalcemic effects occur about four weeks after daily administration of a fixed dose and the duration of action can be two months or more.

INDICATIONS AND USAGE

Ergocalciferol is indicated for use in the treatment of refractory rickets (also known as Vitamin D resistant rickets), hypoparathyroidism, and familial hypophosphatemia.

UNLABELED USE

Ergocalciferol is used alone or as an adjunct in the treatment of deficiency of Vitamin D and osteodystrophy.

CONTRAINDICATIONS

Ergocalciferol Tablets are contraindicated in patients with hypercalcemia, malabsorption syndrome, abnormal sensitivity to the toxic effects of Vitamin D, hypervitaminosis D, and decreased renal function.

WARNINGS

Hypersensitivity to Vitamin D may be one etiologic factor in infants with idiopathic hypercalcemia. In these cases, Vitamin D must be severely restricted.

Overdosage of any form of Vitamin D is dangerous. Progressive hypercalcemia due to overdosage of Vitamin D and its metabolites may be so severe as to require emergency attention. Chronic hypercalcemia can lead to generalized vascular calcification, nephrocalcinosis, and other soft tissue calcification. Radiographic evaluation of suspect anatomical regions may be useful in the early detection of this condition.

PRECAUTIONS

GENERAL

Dosage levels must be individualized and great care exercised to prevent serious toxic effects. *The range between therapeutic and toxic doses is narrow.* When high therapeutic doses are used, progress should be followed with frequent serum and urinary calcium, phosphorus, and BUN determinations.

Vitamin D administration from fortified foods, dietary supplements, and other concomitantly administered drugs should be evaluated. Therapeutic dosage should be readjusted as soon as there is clinical improvement.

Adequate dietary calcium is necessary for clinical response to Vitamin D therapy.

In patients with hyperphosphatemia, normal serum phosphorus levels may be maintained by dietary phosphate restriction and/or administration of aluminum gels as intestinal phosphate binders, and is essential to prevent metastatic calcification. Hyperphosphatemia is frequently seen in patients with renal osteodystrophy.

In the treatment of hypoparathyroidism, calcium, parathyroid hormone, and/or dihydrotachysterol may be required.

Treatment of patients with coronary disease, impaired renal function, and arteriosclerosis, especially in the elderly, should be cautious.

LABORATORY TESTS

When starting treatment or during dosage adjustment, serum calcium should be determined twice weekly. Serum calcium levels should be maintained between 9 and 10 mg/dL. Similarly, phosphate, magnesium, and alkaline phosphatase and 24 hour urinary calcium and phosphate should be determined periodically. A fall in serum alkaline phosphatase levels usually precedes the appearance of hypercalcemia and may be an indication of impending hypercalcemia. Should hypercalcemia develop, the drug should be discontinued immediately.

DRUG INTERACTIONS

Mineral oil interferes with the absorption of fat-soluble vitamins, including Vitamin D preparations. Administer Ergocalciferol in the morning; mineral oil at night.

In hypoparathyroid patients being treated with Ergocalciferol the administration of thiazide diuretics may cause hypercalcemia.

CARCINOGENESIS, MUTAGENESIS, IMPAIRMENT OF FERTILITY

No long-term studies in animals have been performed to determine the carcinogenic, mutagenic or impairment of fertility potential of Ergocalciferol.

PREGNANCY - PREGNANCY CATEGORY C

Animal reproduction studies have shown fetal abnormalities in several species associated with hypervitaminosis D. These are similar to the supravalvular aortic stenosis syndrome described in infants by Black in England (1963). This syndrome was characterized by supravalvular aortic stenosis, elfin facies, and mental retardation. There are no adequate and well-controlled studies in pregnant women. The safety in excess of 400 units of Vitamin D daily during pregnancy has not been established. Therefore Ergocalciferol should be used during pregnancy only if the potential benefit justifies the potential risk to the fetus.

NURSING MOTHERS

Ergocalciferol is excreted in human milk. Caution should be exercised when Ergocalciferol is administered to a nursing woman. In a mother given large doses of Vitamin D, 25-hydroxycholecalciferol appeared in the milk and caused hypercalcemia in her child. Monitoring of the infant's serum calcium concentration is required in that case (Goldberg, 1972).

PEDIATRIC USE

Pediatric doses must be individualized and monitored under close medical supervision (see *"Dosage and Administration"*).

ADVERSE REACTIONS

Early: Weakness, headache, drowsiness, nausea, vomiting, dry mouth, constipation, muscle pain, bone pain, and metallic taste.

Late: Anorexia, irritability, weight loss, mild acidosis, polyuria, polydipsia, nocturia, reversible azotemia, generalized vascular calcification, nephrocalcinosis, hypertension, cardiac arrhythmias, and rarely, overt psychosis.

OVERDOSAGE

The effects of administered Vitamin D can persist for two or more months after cessation of treatment.

Hypervitaminosis D is characterized by:

Hypercalcemia with anorexia, nausea, weakness, weight loss, vague aches and stiffness, constipation, mental retardation, anemia, and mild acidosis.

Impairment of renal function with polyuria, nocturia, polydipsia, hypercalciuria, reversible azotemia, hypertension, nephrocalcinosis, generalized vascular calcification, or irreversible renal insufficiency which may result in death.

Widespread calcification of the soft tissues, including the heart, blood vessels, renal tubules, and lungs. Bone demineralization (osteoporosis) in adults occurs concomitantly.

Decline in the average rate of linear growth and increased mineralization of bones in infants and children (dwarfism).

The treatment of hypervitaminosis D with hypercalcemia consists of immediate withdrawal of the vitamin, a low calcium diet, generous intake of fluids, and acidification of the urine along with symptomatic and supportive treatment. Hypercalcemic crisis with dehydration, stupor, coma, and azotemia requires more vigorous treatment. The first step should be hydration of the patient. Intravenous saline may quickly and significantly increase urinary calcium excretion. A loop diuretic (furosemide or ethacrynic acid) may be given with the saline infusion to further increase renal calcium excretion. Other reported therapeutic measures include dialysis or the administration of citrates, sulfates, phosphates, corticosteroids, EDTA (ethylenediaminetraacetic acid), and mithramycin via appropriate regimens. With appropriate therapy, recovery is the usual outcome when no permanent damage has occurred.

The LD_{50} in animals is unknown.

DOSAGE AND ADMINISTRATION

Vitamin D - Resistant Rickets: 50,000 to 500,000 units daily.

Hypoparathyroidism: 50,000 to 200,000 units administered once daily plus 500 mg of elemental calcium administered 6 times daily.

Familial Hypophosphatemia: 10,000 to 80,000 units daily plus 1-2 gm of elemental phosphorus daily.

THE RANGE BETWEEN THERAPEUTIC AND TOXIC DOSES IS NARROW. DOSAGE MUST BE INDIVIDUALIZED UNDER CLOSE MEDICAL SUPERVISION. HIGH THERAPEUTIC DOSES MUST BE MONITORED CLOSELY. THERAPEUTIC DOSAGE SHOULD BE READJUSTED AS SOON AS THERE IS CLINICAL IMPROVEMENT.

Blood calcium, phosphorus, and BUN determinations must be made every 2 weeks or more frequently if necessary. The bones should be x-rayed every month until the condition is corrected and stabilized. Calcium intake should be adequate.

Store at controlled room temperature, 15°-30°C (59°-86°F). Protect from light.

➤ SHOWN IN PRODUCT IDENTIFICATION GUIDE

HOW SUPPLIED
CAPSULE: 50,000 U

BRAND/MANUFACTURER	NDC	SIZE	AWP
◆ GENERICS			
Rugby	00536-4783-01	100s	$3.30

CAPSULE: 50,000 IU

AVERAGE UNIT PRICE (AVAILABLE SIZES)		GENERIC A-RATED AVERAGE PRICE (GAAP)	
BRAND	$0.92	100s	$5.99
GENERIC	$0.06		
HCFA FUL (100s ea)	$0.03		

BRAND/MANUFACTURER	NDC	SIZE	AWP
◆ BRAND			
DRISDOL: Sanofi Winthrop	00024-0392-02	50s	$45.74
◆ GENERICS			
Richlyn	00115-0140-01	100s	$5.83
Major	00904-0291-60	100s	$6.15
Richlyn	00115-0140-03	1000s	$44.85

INJECTION: 500,000 IU/ML

BRAND/MANUFACTURER	NDC	SIZE	AWP
○ BRAND			
CALCIFEROL: Schwarz	00091-1150-05	1 ml 5s ud	$74.00

TABLETS: 50,000 IU

BRAND/MANUFACTURER	NDC	SIZE	AWP
○ BRAND			
CALCIFEROL: Schwarz	00091-3150-01	100s	$36.49

Ergoloid Mesylates

DESCRIPTION
Ergoloid Mesylates tablet 1 mg, Ergoloid Mesylates sublingual tablet 1 mg and Ergoloid Mesylates liquid capsule 1 mg, each contain: dihydroergocornine mesylate 0.333 mg, dihydroergocristine mesylate 0.333 mg, and dihydroergocryptine (dihydro-alpha-ergocryptine and dihydro-beta-ergocryptine in the proportion of 2:1) mesylate 0.333 mg, representing a total of 1 mg.

Ergoloid Mesylates: each sublingual tablet 0.5 mg contains dihydroergocornine mesylate 0.167 mg, dihydroergocristine mesylate 0.167 mg, and dihydroergocryptine (dihydro-alpha-ergocryptine and dihydro-beta-ergocryptine in the proportion of 2:1) mesylate 0.167 mg, representing a total of 0.5 mg.

Ergoloid Mesylates: liquid 1 mg/mL, contains dihydroergocornine mesylate 0.333 mg, dihydroergocristine mesylate 0.333 mg, and dihydroergocryptine (dihydro-alpha-ergocryptine and dihydro-beta-ergocryptine in the proportion of 2:1) mesylate 0.333 mg, representing a total of 1 mg; alcohol, 28.5% by volume.

PHARMACOKINETIC PROPERTIES
Pharmacokinetic studies have been performed in normal volunteers with the help of radiolabelled drug as well as employing a specific radioimmunoassay technique. From the urinary excretion quotient of orally and intravenously administered tritium-labelled Ergoloid Mesylates the absorption of Ergoloid was calculated to be 25%. Following oral administration, peak levels of 0.5 ng Eq/mL/mg were achieved within 1.5-3 hr. Bioavailability studies with the specific radioimmunoassay confirm that Ergoloid is rapidly absorbed from the gastrointestinal tract, with mean peak levels of 0.05-0.13 ng/mL/mg (with extremes of 0.03 and 0.18 ng/mL/mg) achieved within 0.6-1.3 hr. (with extremes of 0.4 and 2.8 hr.). The finding of lower peak levels of Ergoloid compared to the total drug-metabolite composite is consistent with a considerable first pass liver metabolism, with less than 50% of the therapeutic moiety reaching the systemic circulation. The elimination of radioactivity, representing Ergoloid plus metabolites bearing the radiolabel, was biphasic with half-lives of 4 and 13 hr. The mean half-life of unchanged Ergoloid in plasma is about 2.6-5.1 hr; after 3 half-lives Ergoloid plasma levels are less than 10% of radio activity levels, and by 24 hr no Ergoloid is detectable.

Bioequivalence studies were performed comparing Ergoloid Mesylates oral tablets (administered orally) with Ergoloid Mesylates sublingual tablets (administered sublingually), Ergoloid Mesylates oral tablets with Ergoloid Mesylates liquid and Ergoloid Mesylates oral tablets with Ergoloid Mesylates liquid capsules. The oral tablet, sublingual tablet and liquid capsule oral forms were shown to be bioequivalent. Within the bioequivalence limits, the liquid capsule showed a statistically significant (12%) greater bioavailability than the oral tablet. In the study comparing the oral tablet and liquid forms, both forms tested showed an equivalent rate of absorption and an equivalent peak plasma concentration (C_{max}).

Following is its chemical structure:

Dihydroergocornine	—CH(CH$_3$)$_2$
Dihydroergocristine	—CH$_2$C$_6$H$_5$
Dihydro-α-ergocryptine	—CH$_2$CH(CH$_3$)$_2$
Dihydro-β-ergocryptine	—CH(CH$_3$)CH$_2$CH$_3$

ACTIONS
There is no specific evidence which clearly establishes the mechanism by which Ergoloid Mesylates preparations produce mental effects, nor is there conclusive evidence that the drug particularly affects cerebral arteriosclerosis or cerebrovascular insufficiency.

INDICATIONS
A proportion of individuals over sixty who manifest signs and symptoms of an idiopathic decline in mental capacity (i.e., cognitive and interpersonal skills, mood, self-care, apparent motivation) can experience some symptomatic relief upon treatment with Ergoloid Mesylates preparations. The identity of the specific trait(s) or condition(s), if any, which would usefully predict a response to Ergoloid Mesylates therapy is not known. It appears, however, that those individuals who do respond come from groups of patients who would be considered clinically to suffer from some ill-defined process related to aging or to have some underlying dementing condition (i.e., primary progressive dementia, Alzheimer's dementia, senile onset, multi-infarct dementia).

Before prescribing Ergoloid Mesylates, the physician should exclude the possibility that the patient's signs and symptoms arise from a potentially reversible and treatable condition. Particular care should be taken to exclude delirium and dementiform illness secondary to systemic disease, primary neurological disease, or primary disturbance of mood. Ergoloid Mesylates preparations are not indicated in the treatment of acute or chronic psychosis, regardless of etiology (see *"Contraindications"*).

The decision to use Ergoloid Mesylates in the treatment of an individual with a symptomatic decline in mental capacity of unknown etiology should be continually reviewed since the presenting clinical picture may subsequently evolve sufficiently to allow a specific diagnosis and a specific alternative treatment. In addition, continued clinical evaluation is required to determine whether any initial benefit conferred by Ergoloid Mesylates therapy persists with time.

The efficacy of Ergoloid Mesylates was evaluated using a special rating scale known as the SCAG (Sandoz Clinical Assessment-Geriatric). The specific items on this scale on which modest but statistically significant changes were observed at the end of twelve weeks include: mental alertness, confusion, recent memory, orientation, emotional liability self-care, depression, anxiety/fears, cooperation, sociability, appetite, dizziness, fatigue, bothersome(ness), and an overall impression of clinical status.

CONTRAINDICATIONS
Ergoloid Mesylates preparations are contraindicated in individuals who have previously shown hypersensitivity to the drug. Ergoloid Mesylates preparations are also contraindicated in patients who have psychosis, acute or chronic, regardless of etiology.

PRECAUTIONS
Practitioners are advised that because the target symptoms are of unknown etiology, careful diagnosis should be attempted before prescribing Ergoloid Mesylates preparations.

ADVERSE REACTIONS
Ergoloid Mesylates preparations have not been found to produce serious side effects. Some sublingual irritation with the sublingual tablets, transient nausea, and gastric disturbances have been reported. Ergoloid Mesylates preparations do not possess the vasoconstrictor properties of the natural ergot alkaloids.

DOSAGE AND ADMINISTRATION
1 mg three times daily.

Alleviation of symptoms is usually gradual and results may not be observed for 3-4 weeks.

HOW SUPPLIED
CAPSULE: 1 MG

BRAND/MANUFACTURER	NDC	SIZE	AWP
○ BRAND			
HYDERGINE LC: Sandoz Pharm	00078-0101-05	100s	$68.28
	00078-0101-06	100s ud	$72.48
	00078-0101-08	500s	$333.36

LIQUID: 1 MG/ML

BRAND/MANUFACTURER		NDC	SIZE	AWP
○ BRAND				
HYDERGINE: Sandoz Pharm		00078-0100-36	100 ml	$53.46

TABLETS: 0.5 MG

AVERAGE UNIT PRICE (AVAILABLE SIZES)		GENERIC A-RATED AVERAGE PRICE (GAAP)	
GENERIC	$0.10	100s	$13.99
HCFA FUL (100s ea)	$0.13		

BRAND/MANUFACTURER	NDC	SIZE	AWP
◆ GENERICS			
Schein	00364-0415-01	100s	$12.22
Major	00904-0661-60	100s	$15.75
Major	00904-0661-40	500s	$16.25

TABLETS: 1 MG

AVERAGE UNIT PRICE (AVAILABLE SIZES)		GENERIC A-RATED AVERAGE PRICE (GAAP)	
BRAND	$0.65	100s	$19.64
GENERIC	$0.17	100s	$12.53
GENERIC	$0.11	500s	$73.94
HCFA FUL (100s ea)	$0.09	1000s	$149.56
		1000s	$86.21

BRAND/MANUFACTURER	NDC	SIZE	AWP
◆ BRAND			
HYDERGINE: Sandoz Pharm	00078-0070-05	100s	$64.98
	00078-0070-06	100s ud	$67.14
	00078-0070-08	500s	$310.26
◆ GENERICS			
Moore,H.L.	00839-6229-06	100s	$8.89
GERIMAL: Rugby	00536-3857-01	100s	$9.57
Zenith	00172-2959-60	100s	$11.10
Schein	00364-0446-01	100s	$12.73
Major	00904-0662-60	100s	$16.45
Goldline	00182-1059-01	100s	$16.45
Qualitest	00603-3527-21	100s	$17.40
Mason Dist	11845-0248-01	100s	$17.46
Parmed	00349-8071-01	100s	$18.12
Mutual	53489-0281-01	100s	$18.25
Schein	00364-0622-01	100s	$18.30
GERIMAL: Rugby	00536-3856-01	100s	$18.38
URL	00677-0782-01	100s	$18.40
Major	00904-0336-60	100s	$18.50
Goldline	00182-1518-01	100s	$18.50
Moore,H.L.	00839-6606-06	100s	$19.44
Aligen	00405-4384-01	100s	$20.80
U.S. Trading	56126-0252-11	100s ud	$13.50
UDL	51079-0110-20	100s ud	$21.75
Raway	00686-0110-20	100s ud	$23.50
Major	00904-0336-61	100s ud	$32.31
Major	00904-0662-70	250s	$20.25
Major	00904-0336-70	250s	$39.80
GERIMAL: Rugby	00536-3857-05	500s	$39.98
Schein	00364-0622-05	500s	$71.00
URL	00677-0782-05	500s	$71.50
Mutual	53489-0281-05	500s	$71.50
Major	00904-0336-40	500s	$74.95
Mason Dist	11845-0248-03	500s	$75.95
Aligen	00405-4384-02	500s	$76.20
Goldline	00182-1518-05	500s	$76.50
Major	00904-0662-80	1000s	$73.90
GERIMAL: Rugby	00536-3857-10	1000s	$78.45
Zenith	00172-2959-60	1000s	$96.25
Goldline	00182-1059-10	1000s	$96.25
Major	00904-0336-80	1000s	$135.50
Mutual	53489-0281-10	1000s	$140.00
Goldline	00182-1518-10	1000s	$147.00
Mason Dist	11845-0248-04	1000s	$154.77
Moore,H.L.	00839-6606-16	1000s	$157.34
GERIMAL: Rugby	00536-3856-10	1000s	$162.75

Ergostat SEE ERGOTAMINE TARTRATE

Ergotamine Tartrate

DESCRIPTION

Each sublingual tablet contains 2 mg Ergotamine Tartrate.

Pharmacological Category: Vasoconstrictor, uterine stimulant, alpha adrenoreceptor antagonist.

Therapeutic Class: Antimigraine.

Chemical Name: Ergotaman-3',6',18-trione,12'-hydroxy-2'-methyl-5'-(phenylmethyl)-,(5'α)-,[R-(R*, R*)]-2,3-dihydroxybutanedioate (2:1) salt.

Following is its chemical structure:

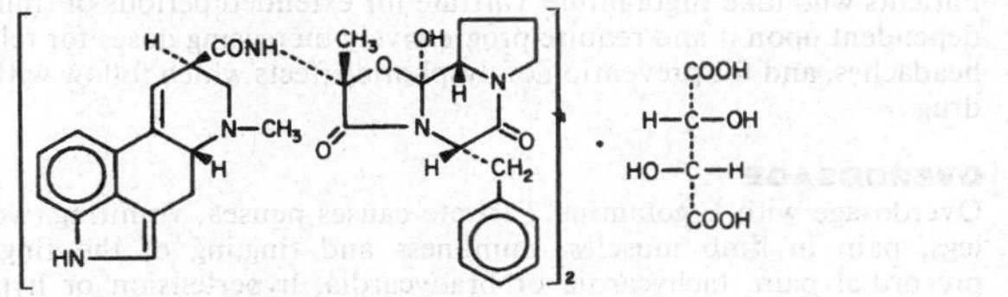

CLINICAL PHARMACOLOGY

The pharmacological properties of Ergotamine Tartrate are extremely complex; some of its actions are unrelated to each other, and even mutually antagonistic. The drug has partial agonist and/or antagonist activity against tryptaminergic, dopaminergic and alpha adrenergic receptors depending upon their site, and it is a highly active uterine stimulant. It causes constriction of peripheral and cranial blood vessels and produces depression of central vasomotor centers. The pain of a migraine attack is believed to be due to greatly increased amplitude of pulsations in the cranial arteries, especially the meningeal branches of the external carotid artery. Ergotamine Tartrate reduces extracranial blood flow, causes a decline in the amplitude of pulsation in the cranial arteries, and decreases hyperperfusion of the territory of the basilar artery. It does not reduce cerebral hemispheric blood flow. Long-term usage has established the fact that Ergotamine Tartrate is effective in controlling up to 70% of acute migraine attacks, so that it is now considered specific for the treatment of this headache syndrome. Ergotamine Tartrate produces constriction of both arteries and veins. In doses used in the treatment of vascular headaches, Ergotamine Tartrate usually produces only small increases in blood pressure, but it does increase peripheral resistance and decrease blood flow in various organs. Small doses of the drug increase the force and frequency of uterine contraction; larger doses increase the resting tone of the uterus also. The gravid uterus is particularly sensitive to these effects of Ergotamine. Although specific teratogenic effects attributable to Ergotamine Tartrate have not been found, the fetus suffers if Ergotamine Tartrate is given to the mother. Retarded fetal growth and an increase in intrauterine death and resorption have been seen in animals. These are thought to result from Ergotamine Tartrate induced increases in uterine motility and vasoconstriction in the placental vascular bed.

The bioavailability of sublingually administered Ergotamine Tartrate has not been determined.

Ergotamine Tartrate is metabolized in the liver by largely undefined pathways, and 90% of the metabolites are excreted in the bile. The unmetabolized drug is erratically secreted in the saliva, and only traces of unmetabolized drug appear in the urine and feces. Ergotamine Tartrate is secreted into breast milk. The elimination half-life of Ergotamine Tartrate from plasma is about 2 hours, but the drug may be stored in some tissues, which would account for its long-lasting therapeutic and toxic actions.

INDICATIONS AND USAGE

Ergotamine Tartrate is indicated as therapy to abort or prevent vascular headache, e.g., migraine, migraine variants, or so called "histaminic cephalalgia".

CONTRAINDICATIONS

Ergotamine Tartrate is contraindicated in peripheral vascular disease (thromboangiitis obliterans, luetic arteritis, severe arteriosclerosis, thrombophlebitis, Raynaud's disease), coronary heart disease, hypertension, impaired hepatic or renal function, severe pruritus, and sepsis. It is also contraindicated in patients who are hypersensitive to any of its components. Ergotamine Tartrate may cause fetal harm when administered to a pregnant woman by virtue of its powerful uterine stimulant actions. It is contraindicated in women who are, or may become, pregnant.

PRECAUTIONS

General: Although signs and symptoms of ergotism rarely develop even after long-term intermittent use of Ergotamine Tartrate, care should be exercised to remain within the limits of recommended dosage.

Drug Interactions: The effects of Ergotamine Tartrate may be potentiated by triacetyloleandomycin which inhibits the metabolism of Ergotamine. The pressor effects of Ergotamine Tartrate and other vasoconstrictor drugs can combine to cause dangerous hypertension.

Carcinogenesis: No studies have been performed to investigate Ergotamine Tartrate for carcinogenic effects.

Pregnancy: Pregnancy Category X— see "*Contraindications*".

Nursing Mothers: Ergotamine Tartrate is secreted into human milk. It can reach the breast-fed infant by this route and exert pharmacologic effects in it. Caution should be exercised when Ergotamine Tartrate is administered to a nursing woman. Excessive dosing or prolonged administration of Ergotamine Tartrate may inhibit lactation.

ADVERSE REACTIONS

Nausea and vomiting occur in up to 10% of patients after ingestion of therapeutic doses of Ergotamine. Weakness of the legs and pain in limb muscles are also frequent complaints. Numbness and tingling of the fingers and toes, precordial pain, transient changes in heart rate and localized edema and itching may also occur, particularly in patients who are sensitive to the drug.

➤ SHOWN IN PRODUCT IDENTIFICATION GUIDE

DRUG ABUSE AND DEPENDENCE

Patients who take Ergotamine Tartrate for extended periods of time may become dependent upon it and require progressively increasing doses for relief of vascular headaches, and for prevention of dysphoric effects which follow withdrawal of the drug.

OVERDOSAGE

Overdosage with Ergotamine Tartrate causes nausea, vomiting, weakness of the legs, pain in limb muscles, numbness and tingling of the fingers and toes, precordial pain, tachycardia or bradycardia, hypertension or hypotension and localized edema and itching together with signs and symptoms of ischemia due to vasoconstriction of peripheral arteries and arterioles.

The feet and hands become cold, pale and numb. Muscle pain occurs while walking and later at rest also. Gangrene may ensue. Confusion, depression, drowsiness, and convulsions are occasional signs of Ergotamine Tartrate toxicity. Overdosage is particularly likely to occur in patients with sepsis or impaired renal or hepatic function. Patients with peripheral vascular disease are especially at risk of developing peripheral ischemia following treatment with Ergotamine Tartrate. Some cases of Ergotamine Tartrate poisoning have been reported in patients who have taken less than 5 mg of the drug. Usually, however, toxicity is seen at doses of Ergotamine Tartrate in excess of about 15 mg in 24 hours or 40 mg in a few days.

Treatment of Ergotamine Tartrate overdosage consists of the withdrawal of the drug followed by symptomatic measures including attempts to maintain an adequate circulation in the affected parts. Anticoagulant drugs, low molecular weight dextran and potent vasodilator drugs may all be beneficial. Intravenous infusion of sodium nitroprusside has also been reported to be successful. Vasodilators must be used with special care in the presence of hypotension.

Nausea and vomiting may be relieved by atropine or antiemetic compounds of the phenothiazine group. Ergotamine Tartrate is dialyzable.

DOSAGE AND ADMINISTRATION

All efforts should be made to initiate therapy as soon as possible after the first symptoms of the attack are noted, because success is proportional to rapidity of treatment, and lower dosages will be effective. At the first sign of an attack or to relieve the symptoms of the full-blown attack, one sublingual tablet (2 mg) is placed under the tongue. Another sublingual tablet (2 mg) should be placed under the tongue at half-hourly intervals thereafter, if necessary, for a total of three tablets (6 mg). Dosage must not exceed three tablets (6 mg) in any 24-hour period. Limit dosage to not more than five tablets (10 mg) in any one week.

Store at controlled room temperature 15°-30°C (59°-86°F).

Protect from moisture and light.

HOW SUPPLIED
TABLETS: 2 MG

BRAND/MANUFACTURER	NDC	SIZE	AWP
◆ BRAND ERGOSTAT: Parke-Davis	00071-0111-13	24s	$17.72

Ergotamine Tartrate with Caffeine

DESCRIPTION

Each Ergotamine Tartrate/Caffeine Tablet contains:

Caffeine USP	100 mg
Ergotamine Tartrate USP	1 mg

Each Ergotamine Tartrate/Caffeine Suppository contains:

Caffeine USP	100 mg
Ergotamine Tartrate USP	2 mg

Ergotamine Tartrate/Caffeine suppositories contain the active ingredients in a synthetic cocoa butter base which melts rapidly at body temperature and are *sealed* in foil to afford protection from cocoa butter leakage. If an unavoidable period of exposure to heat softens the suppository, it should be chilled in ice-cold water to solidify it before removing the foil.

CLINICAL PHARMACOLOGY

Ergotamine is an alpha adrenergic blocking agent with a direct stimulating effect on the smooth muscle of peripheral and cranial blood vessels and produces depression of central vasomotor centers. The compound also has the properties of serotonin antagonism. In comparison to hydrogenated ergotamine, the adrenergic blocking actions are less pronounced and vasoconstrictive actions are greater.

Caffeine, also a cranial vasoconstrictor, is added to further enhance the vasoconstrictive effect without the necessity of increasing ergotamine dosage.

Many migraine patients experience excessive nausea and vomiting during attacks, making it impossible for them to retain any oral medication. In such cases, therefore, the only practical means of medication is through the rectal route where medication may reach the cranial vessels directly evading the splanchnic vasculature and the liver.

INDICATIONS AND USAGE

Indicated as therapy to abort or prevent vascular headache, e.g., migraine, migraine variants or so-called "histaminic cephalalgia".

CONTRAINDICATIONS

Ergotamine Tartrate/Caffeine may cause fetal harm when administered to pregnant women. It can produce prolonged uterine contractions which can result in abortion. Ergotamine Tartrate/Caffeine is contraindicated in women who are or may become pregnant. If this drug is used during pregnancy or if the patient becomes pregnant while taking this product, the patient should be apprised of the potential hazard to the fetus.

Peripheral vascular disease, coronary heart disease, hypertension, impaired hepatic or renal function and sepsis. Hypersensitivity to any of the components.

PRECAUTIONS
GENERAL

Although signs and symptoms of ergotism rarely develop even after long term intermittent use of the orally or rectally administered drugs, care should be exercised to remain within the limits of recommended dosage.

Ergotism is manifested by intense arterial vasoconstriction, producing signs and symptoms of peripheral vascular ischemia. Ergotamine induces vasoconstriction by a direct action on vascular smooth muscle. In chronic intoxication with ergot derivatives, headache, intermittent claudication, muscle pains, numbness, coldness and pallor of the digits may occur. If the condition is allowed to progress untreated, gangrene can result.

While most cases of ergotism associated with Ergotamine treatment result from frank overdosage, some cases have involved apparent hypersensitivity. There are few reports of ergotism among patients taking doses within the recommended limits or for brief periods of time. In rare instances, patients, particularly those who have used the medication indiscriminately over long periods of time, may display withdrawal symptoms consisting of rebound headache upon discontinuation of the drug.

Rare cases of a solitary rectal or anal ulcer have occurred from abuse of Ergotamine suppositories usually in higher than recommended doses or with continual use at the recommended dose for many years. Spontaneous healing occurs within usually 4-8 weeks after drug withdrawal.

INFORMATION FOR PATIENTS

Patients should be advised that two tablets or one suppository of Ergotamine Tartrate/Caffeine should be taken at the first sign of a migraine headache. No more than 6 tablets or 2 suppositories should be taken for any single migraine attack. No more than 10 tablets or 5 suppositories should be taken during any 7-day period. Ergotamine Tartrate/Caffeine should be used only for migraine headaches. It is not effective for other types of headaches and it lacks analgesic properties. Patients should be advised to report to the physician immediately any of the following: numbness or tingling in the fingers and toes, muscle pain in the arms and legs, weakness in the legs, pain in the chest or temporary speeding or slowing of the heart rate, swelling or itching.

DRUG INTERACTIONS

Ergotamine Tartrate/Caffeine should not be administered with other vasoconstrictors. Use with sympathomimetics (pressor agents) may cause extreme elevation of blood pressure. The beta blocker propranolol has been reported to potentiate the vasoconstrictive action of Ergotamine Tartrate/Caffeine by blocking the vasodilating property of epinephrine. Nicotine may provoke vasoconstriction in some patients, predisposing to a greater ischemic response to ergot therapy.

The blood levels of Ergotamine-containing drugs are reported to be elevated by the concomitant administration of macrolide antibiotics and vasospastic reactions have been reported with therapeutic doses of the Ergotamine-containing drugs when coadministered with these antibiotics.

PREGNANCY

Teratogenic Effects: Pregnancy Category X: There are no studies on the placental transfer or teratogenicity of the combined products of Ergotomine Tartrate/Caffeine. Caffeine is known to cross the placenta and has been shown to be teratogenic in animals. Ergotamine crosses the placenta in small amounts, although it does not appear to be embryotoxic in this quantity. However, prolonged vasoconstriction of the uterine vessels and/or increased myometrial tone leading to reduced myometrial and placental blood flow may have contributed to fetal growth retardation observed in animals. (See "*Contraindications*".)

Nonteracogenic Effects: Ergotamin Tartrate/Caffeine is contraindicated in pregnancy due to the oxytocic effects of Ergotamine. (See "*Contraindications*".)

LABOR AND DELIVERY

Ergotamine Tartrate/Caffeine is contraindicated in labor and delivery due to its oxytocic effect which is maximal in the third trimester. (See "*Contraindications*".)

NURSING MOTHERS

Ergot drugs are known to inhibit prolactin but there are no reports of decreased lactation with Ergotamine Tartrate/Caffeine. Ergotamine is excreted in breast milk and may cause symptoms of vomiting, diarrhea, weak pulse and unstable blood pressure in nursing infants. Because of the potential for serious adverse reactions in nursing infants from Ergotamine Tartrate/Caffeine, a decision should be made whether to discontinue nursing or discontinue the drug, taking into account the importance of the drug to the mother.

PEDIATRIC USE

Safety and effectiveness in children have not been established.

◆ RATED THERAPEUTICALLY EQUIVALENT; ◇ THERAPEUTIC EQUIVALENCE UNCONFIRMED; ○ UNRATED

ADVERSE REACTIONS

Cardiovascular: Vasoconstrictive complications of a serious nature may occur at times. These include ischemia, cyanosis, absence of pulse, cold extremities, gangrene, precordial distress and pain, EKG changes and muscle pains in the extremities. Although these effects occur most commonly with long-term therapy at relatively high doses, they have also been reported with short-term or normal doses. Other cardiovascular adverse effects include transient tachycardia or bradycardia and hypertension.

Gastrointestinal: Nausea and vomiting; rectal or anal ulcer (from overuse of suppositories), diarrhea.

Neurological: Paresthesias, numbness and tingling in fingers and toes, weakness in the legs, and vertigo.

Allergic: Localized edema and itching.

Miscellaneous: There have been a few reports of patients on Ergotamine Tartrate/Caffeine therapy developing retroperitoneal and/or pleuropulmonary fibroses.

DRUG ABUSE AND DEPENDENCE

There have been reports of drug abuse and psychological dependence in patients on Ergotamine Tartrate/Caffeine therapy. Due to the chronicity of vascular headaches, it is imperative that patients be advised not to exceed recommended dosages with long-term use to avoid ergotism. (See *"Precautions".*)

OVERDOSAGE

The toxic effects of an acute overdosage of Ergotamine Tartrate/Caffeine are due primarily to the Ergotamine component. The amount of Caffeine is such that its toxic effects will be overshadowed by those of Ergotamine. Symptoms include vomiting, numbness, tingling, pain and cyanosis of the extremities associated with diminished or absent peripheral pulses; hypertension or hypotension; drowsiness, stupor, coma, convulsions and shock. A case has been reported of reversible bilateral papillitis with ring scotomata in a patient who received five times the recommended daily adult dose over a period of 14 days.

Treatment consists of removal of the offending drug by induction of emesis, gastric lavage, and catharsis. Maintenance of adequate pulmonary ventilation, correction of hypotension, and control of convulsions and blood pressure are important considerations. Treatment of peripheral vasospasm should consist of warmth, but not heat, and protection of the ischemic limbs. Vasodilators may be beneficial but caution must be exercised to avoid aggravating an already existent hypotension. The LD50 limits of the various components as outlined in NIOSH 1978 Registry of Toxic Effects of Chemical Substances, published by U.S. Department of Health, Education and Welfare are as follows: Ergotamine Tartrate IV LD$_{50}$ in rats = 80mg/kg, Caffeine IV LD$_{50}$ in rats = 105mg/kg.

DOSAGE AND ADMINISTRATION
PROCEDURE

For the best results, dosage should start at the first sign of an attack. The average adult dose is 2 tablets at the start of a vascular headache (migraine) attack, followed by 1 additional tablet every ½ hour if needed, up to 6 tablets per attack. Total weekly dosage should not exceed 10 tablets.

MAXIMUM ADULT DOSAGE
ORALLY

Total dose for any one attack should not exceed 6 tablets.

RECTALLY

Two suppositories is the maximum dose for an individual attack.

Total weekly dosage should not exceed 10 tablets or 5 suppositories.
In carefully selected patients, with due consideration of maximum dosage recommendations, administration of the drug at bedtime may be an appropriate short-term preventive measure.

STORE AND DISPENSE TABLETS
Below 77-30°F (25°-80°C); tight, light-resistant container.

STORE AND DISPENSE SUPPOSITORIES
Below 77°F (25°C); tight container (sealed foil).

HOW SUPPLIED
SUPPOSITORY: 100 MG-2 MG

BRAND/MANUFACTURER	NDC	SIZE	AWP
◆ GENERICS			
MIGERGOT: Moore,H.L.	00839-7283-92	12s	$34.14

SUPPOSITORY: 100 MG-2 MG

BRAND/MANUFACTURER	NDC	SIZE	AWP
◇ BRAND			
CAFERGOT: Sandoz Pharm	00078-0033-02	12s	$44.64
◇ GENERICS			
CAFATINE: Major	00904-2595-12	12s	$32.95

SUPPOSITORY: 100 MG-2 MG

BRAND/MANUFACTURER	NDC	SIZE	AWP
○ BRAND			
MIGERGOT: G&W	00713-0166-12	12s	$29.30

BRAND/MANUFACTURER	NDC	SIZE	AWP
○ GENERICS			
CAFETRATE: Schein	00364-2177-12	12s	$33.25

TABLETS: 100 MG-1 MG

AVERAGE UNIT PRICE (AVAILABLE SIZES)

BRAND	$0.84

BRAND/MANUFACTURER	NDC	SIZE	AWP
◆ BRAND			
WIGRAINE: Organon	00052-0542-20	20s	$13.88
CAFERGOT: Sandoz Pharm	00078-0034-34	90s	$94.74
WIGRAINE: Organon	00052-0542-91	100s	$57.92
CAFERGOT: Sandoz Pharm	00078-0034-28	250s	$257.04
◆ GENERICS			
ERCAF: Geneva	00781-1995-01	100s	$56.10

Eryc SEE ERYTHROMYCIN, ORAL

Erycette SEE ERYTHROMYCIN, TOPICAL

Erygel SEE ERYTHROMYCIN, TOPICAL

EryPed SEE ERYTHROMYCIN, ORAL

Erythrityl Tetranitrate

DESCRIPTION

Erythrityl Tetranitrate is an antianginal drug that belongs to the organic nitrate class of pharmaceutical agents. Erythrityl Tetranitrate is soluble in alcohol, ether, and glycerol, but insoluble in water. It has the empirical formula $C_4H_6N_4O_{12}$, molecular weight of 302.12 and melting point of 61°C.

Erythrityl Tetranitrate is known chemically as ($R*S*$)-1,2,3,4-butanetetrol tetranitrate.

In the pure state, Erythrityl Tetranitrate will explode upon percussion, but properly diluted with lactose, as in the Erythrityl Tetranitrate tablets, it is nonexplosive. Since it is a low melting solid, Erythrityl Tetranitrate does not evaporate from the tablets.

The Erythrityl Tetranitrate Oral/Sublingual Tablets contain 10 mg Erythrityl Tetranitrate and the inactive ingredients lactose, magnesium stearate, and potato starch, with disintegration characteristics that permit sublingual or oral (swallowed) administration.

Following is its chemical structure:

$$\begin{array}{l} CH_2ONO_2 \\ H-C-ONO_2 \\ H-C-ONO_2 \\ CH_2ONO_2 \end{array}$$

CLINICAL PHARMACOLOGY

Erythrityl Tetranitrate exerts its effects by relaxation of vascular smooth muscle.[1] The action is maximal on the post-capillary vessels, including the large veins. Venodilatation results in peripheral blood pooling, which decreases venous return to the heart, central venous pressure, and pulmonary capillary wedge pressure (preload reduction).[2] Pulmonary arteriolar dilatation causes a reduction in pulmonary vascular resistance.[2] A decrease in systemic arterial pressure (afterload reduction) can also occur, but is usually less pronounced. Augmentation of cardiac output generally occurs in those patients with increased filling pressures and high resting systemic vascular resistance.[2]

Mechanism of Action: The inadequate myocardial oxygenation that precipitates angina can be corrected by: (1) increasing the supply of oxygen to ischemic myocardium through direct dilatation of the large coronary conductance vessels or (2) decreasing the myocardial oxygen demand secondary to a reduction of cardiac work (preload and afterload reduction).[3] The beneficial effect of Erythrityl Tetranitrate probably involves both mechanisms.

Pharmacokinetics and Metabolism: Erythrityl Tetranitrate is readily absorbed from the sublingual, buccal, and gastrointestinal mucosae. The peak effect from a swallowed dose is diminished but of longer duration when compared to the sublingual route.[4] The biotransformation of Erythrityl Tetranitrate is thought to occur by reductive hydrolysis catalyzed by the hepatic enzyme glutathione-organic nitrate reductase.[3] Differences in response among various nitrates may relate to both intrinsic potency at cardiovascular sites, as well as factors related to pharmacokinetics and biotransformation.[5]

Time to onset of effect is approximately 5 minutes for the sublingual route and 15 to 30 minutes for swallowed tablets, with peak effect in 15 minutes and 60 minutes, respectively. Duration of action will vary, but vasodilatory effects have been demonstrated for up to 3 hours after sublingual administration[4,6] and for 6 hours after the oral (swallowed) route.[4]

INDICATIONS AND USAGE

Erythrityl Tetranitrate is intended for the prophylaxis and long-term treatment of patients with frequent or recurrent anginal pain and reduced exercise tolerance associated with angina pectoris, rather than for the treatment of the acute attack of angina pectoris, since its onset is somewhat slower than that of nitroglycerin.

CONTRAINDICATIONS

Erythrityl Tetranitrate should not be administered to individuals with a known hypersensitivity or idiosyncratic reaction to organic nitrates.

WARNINGS

The use of nitrates in acute myocardial infarction or congestive heart failure should be undertaken only under close clinical observation and/or in conjunction with hemodynamic monitoring.

PRECAUTIONS

General: Erythrityl Tetranitrate should be used with caution in patients with severe liver or renal disease. Development of tolerance and cross-tolerance to the effects of Erythrityl Tetranitrate and other organic nitrates may occur. However, studies in patients with chronic heart failure[1] indicate that nitrates produce sustained beneficial hemodynamic effects.

Carcinogenesis, Mutagenesis, Impairment of Fertility: No long-term studies in animals have been performed.

Pregnancy: Teratogenic Effects: Pregnancy Category C. Animal reproduction studies have not been conducted with Erythrityl Tetranitrate. It is also not known whether Erythrityl Tetranitrate can cause fetal harm when administered to a pregnant woman or can affect reproduction capacity. Erythrityl Tetranitrate should be given to a pregnant woman only if clearly needed.

Nursing Mothers: It is not known whether this drug is excreted in human milk. Because many drugs are excreted in human milk, caution should be exercised when Erythrityl Tetranitrate is administered to a nursing woman.

Pediatric Use: Safety and effectiveness in children have not been established.

ADVERSE REACTIONS

The most frequent adverse reaction in patients treated with Erythrityl Tetranitrate is headache. Lowering the dose and the use of analgesics will help control headaches, which usually diminish or disappear as therapy is continued. Other adverse reactions occurring are the following: cutaneous vasodilatation with flushing, and transient episodes of dizziness and weakness, plus other signs of cerebral ischemia associated with postural hypotension. Occasional individuals exhibit marked sensitivity to the hypotensive effects of organic nitrates, and severe responses (e.g., nausea, vomiting, weakness, restlessness, pallor, perspiration, and collapse) can occur even with the usual therapeutic dose. Alcohol may enhance this effect. Drug rash and/or exfoliative dermatitis may occasionally occur.

OVERDOSAGE

Accidental overdosage of Erythrityl Tetranitrate may result in severe hypotension and reflex tachycardia, which can be treated by laying the patient down and elevating the legs. If further treatment is required, the administration of intravenous fluids or other means of treating hypotension should be considered.

DOSAGE AND ADMINISTRATION

The Erythrityl Tetranitrate Oral/Sublingual Tablet can be placed under the tongue or swallowed. Sublingual therapy may be initiated with a dose of 5 to 10 mg prior to each anticipated physical or emotional stress, and at bedtime for patients subject to nocturnal attacks of angina. The dose may be increased as needed.

If the patient is to swallow the tablet, therapy may be initiated with 10 mg before each meal, as well as mid-morning and mid-afternoon if needed, and at bedtime for patients subject to nocturnal attacks. The dose may be increased or decreased as needed.

Dosage titration up to 100 mg daily has been well tolerated, but temporary headache is more apt to occur with increasing doses. When headache occurs, the dose should be reduced for a few days. If headache is troublesome during adjustment of dosage, it may be effectively relieved with an analgesic.

Store at 15° to 25°C (59° to 77°F) in a dry place and dispense in glass.

REFERENCES

1. Chatterjee K. Parmley WW. Vasodilator therapy for chronic heart failure. *Ann Rev Pharmacol Toxicol.* 1980;20:475-512. 2. Goldberg S, Mann T, Grossman W. Nitrate therapy of heart failure in valvular heart disease. *Am J Med.* 1978;65:161-166. 3. Needleman P, Johnson EM. Vasodilators and the treatment of angina, in Gilman AG, Goodman LS, Gilman A (eds): *The Pharmacological Basis of Therapeutics,* ed 6. New York, Macmillan Publishing Co, Inc, 1980:819-833. 4. Hanneman RE, Erb RJ, Stoltman WP, et al. Digital plethysmography for assessing Erythrityl Tetranitrate bioavailability. *Clin Pharmacol Ther.* 1981;29:35-39. 5. Wastila WB, Namm DH, Maxwell RA. Comparison of the vascular effects of several organic nitrates in anesthetized rats and dogs after intravenous and intraportal administration, in *Second International Symposium on Vascular Neuroeffector Mechanisms, Odense,* 1975, Basel, Karger, 1976:216-225. 6. Haffty GB, Nakamura Y, Spodick DH, et al. Bioavailability of organic nitrates: A comparison of methods for evaluating plethysmographic responses. *J Clin Pharmacol.* 1982;22:117-124.

HOW SUPPLIED

Current prices are unavailable. Check wholesaler for further information.

Erythrocin Lactobionate *SEE* ERYTHROMYCIN, INJECTABLE

Erythrocin Stearate *SEE* ERYTHROMYCIN, ORAL

Erythromycin Ethylsuccinate with Sulfisoxazole Acetyl

DESCRIPTION

Erythromycin Ethylsuccinate/Sulfisoxazole Acetyl is a combination of Erythromycin Ethylsuccinate, USP, and Sulfisoxazole Acetyl, USP. When reconstituted with water as directed on the label, the granules form a suspension that provides the equivalent of 200 mg Erythromycin activity and the equivalent of 600 mg of Sulfisoxazole activity per teaspoonful (5 mL).

Erythromycin is produced by a strain of *Saccaropolyspora erythraea* and belongs to the macrolide group of antibiotics. It is basic and readily forms salts and esters. Erythromycin Ethylsuccinate is the 2'-ethylsuccinyl ester of Erythromycin. It is essentially a tasteless form of the antibiotic suitable for oral administration, particularly in suspension dosage forms. The chemical name is Erythromycin 2'-(ethylsuccinate).

Sulfisoxazole Acetyl or N^1-acetyl sulfisoxazole is an ester of Sulfisoxazole. Chemically, Sulfisoxazole is N^1-(3,4-dimethyl-5 -isoxazolyl) sulfanilamide.

CLINICAL PHARMACOLOGY

Orally administered Erythromycin Ethylsuccinate suspensions are readily and reliably absorbed. Erythromycin Ethylsuccinate products have demonstrated rapid and consistent absorption in both fasting and nonfasting conditions. However, higher serum concentrations are obtained when these products are given with food. Erythromycin is largely bound to plasma proteins. After absorption, Erythromycin diffuses readily into most body fluids. In the absence of meningeal inflammation, low concentrations are normally achieved in the spinal fluid, but the passage of the drug across the blood-brain barrier increases in meningitis. Erythromycin crosses the placental barrier and is excreted in human milk. Erythromycin is not removed by peritoneal dialysis or hemodialysis.

In the presence of normal hepatic function, Erythromycin is concentrated in the liver and is excreted in the bile; the effect of hepatic dysfunction on biliary excretion of Erythromycin is not known. After oral administration, less than 5% of the administered dose can be recovered in the active form in the urine.

Wide variation in blood levels may result following identical doses of a sulfonamide. Blood levels should be measured in patients receiving these drugs for serious infections. Free sulfonamide blood levels of 50 to 150 mcg/mL may be considered therapeutically effective for most infections, with blood levels of 120 to 150 mcg/mL being optimal for serious infections. The maximum sulfonamide level should be 200 mcg/mL, because adverse reactions occur more frequently above this concentration.

Following oral administration, Sulfisoxazole is rapidly and completely absorbed; the small intestine is the major site of absorption, but some of the drug is absorbed from the stomach. Sulfonamides are present in the blood as free, conjugated (acetylated and possibly other forms), and protein-bound forms. The amount present as "free" drug is considered to be the therapeutically active form. Approximately 85% of a dose of Sulfisoxazole is bound to plasma proteins, primarily to albumin; 65% to 72% of the unbound portion is in the nonacetylated form.

Maximum plasma concentrations of intact Sulfisoxazole following a single 2-g oral dose of Sulfisoxazole to healthy adult volunteers ranged from 127 to 211 mcg/mL (mean, 169 mcg/mL), and the time of peak plasma concentration ranged from 1 to 4 hours (mean, 2.5 hours). The elimination half-life of Sulfisoxazole ranged from 4.6 to 7.8 hours after oral administration. The elimination of Sulfisoxazole has been shown to be slower in elderly subjects (63 to 75 years) with diminished renal function (creatine clearance 37 to 68 mL/min).[1] After multiple-dose oral administration of 500 mg q.i.d. to healthy volunteers, the average steady-state plasma concentrations of intact Sulfisoxazole ranged from 49.9 to 88.8 mcg/mL (mean, 63.4 mcg/mL).[2]

Sulfisoxazole and its acetylated metabolites are excreted primarily by the kidneys through glomerular filtration. Concentrations of Sulfisoxazole are considerably higher in the urine than in the blood. The mean urinary recovery following oral administration of Sulfisoxazole is 97% within 48 hours; 52% of this is intact drug, and the remainder is the N^4-acetylated metabolite.

Sulfisoxazole is distributed only in extracellular body fluids. It is excreted in human milk. It readily crosses the placental barrier. In healthy subjects, cerebrospinal fluid concentrations of Sulfisoxazole vary; in patients with meningitis, however, concentrations of free drug in cerebrospinal fluid as high as 94 mcg/mL have been reported.

MICROBIOLOGY

Erythromycin Ethylsuccinate/Sulfisoxazole Acetyl has been formulated to contain Sulfisoxazole for concomitant use with Erythromycin.

Erythromycin acts by inhibition of protein synthesis by binding 50 S ribosomal subunits of susceptible organisms. It does not affect nucleic acid synthesis. Antagonism has been demonstrated in vitro between Erythromycin and clindamycin, lincomycin, and chloramphenicol.

The sulfonamides are bacteriostatic agents, and the spectrum of activity is similar for all. Sulfonamides inhibit bacterial synthesis of dihydrofolic acid by preventing the condensation of the pteridine with para-aminobenzoic acid through competitive inhibition of the enzyme dihydropteroate synthetase. Resistant strains have altered dihydropteroate synthetase with reduced affinity for sulfonamides or produce increased quantities of para-aminobenzoic acid.

SUSCEPTIBILITY TESTING

Quantitative methods that require measurement of zone diameter give the most precise estimates of the susceptibility of bacteria to antimicrobial agents. One such standardized single-disc procedure[3] has been recommended for use with discs to test susceptibility to Erythromycin and Sulfisoxazole. Interpretation involves correlation of the zone diameters obtained in the disc test with minimal inhibitory concentration (MIC) values for Erythromycin.

If the standardized procedure of disc susceptibility is used, a 15-mcg Erythromycin disc should give a zone diameter of at least 18 mm when tested against an Erythromycin-susceptible bacterial strain, and a 250-300 mcg Sulfisoxazole disc should give a zone diameter of at least 17 mm when tested against a Sulfisoxazole-susceptible bacterial strain.

In vitro sulfonamide susceptibility tests are not always reliable because media containing excessive amounts of thymidine are capable of reversing the inhibitory effect of sulfonamides, which may result in false resistant reports. The tests must be carefully coordinated with bacteriological and clinical responses. When the patient is already taking sulfonamides, follow-up cultures should have aminobenzoic acid added to the isolation media but not to subsequent susceptibility test media.

INDICATIONS AND USAGE

For treatment of Acute Otitis Media in children that is caused by susceptible strains of Haemophilus influenzae.

CONTRAINDICATIONS

Erythromycin Ethylsuccinate/Sulfisoxazole Acetyl is contraindicated in the following patient populations:

Patients with a known hypersensitivity to either of its components, children younger than 2 months, pregnant women at term, and mothers nursing infants less than 2 months of age.

Use in pregnant women at term, in children less than 2 months of age, and in mothers nursing infants less than 2 months of age is contraindicated because sulfonamides may promote kernicterus in the newborn by displacing bilirubin from plasma proteins.

Erythromycin is contraindicated in patients taking terfenadine. (See "Precautions—Drug Interactions".)

WARNINGS

FATALITIES ASSOCIATED WITH THE ADMINISTRATION OF SULFON-AMIDES, ALTHOUGH RARE, HAVE OCCURRED DUE TO SEVERE REACTIONS INCLUDING STEVENS-JOHNSON SYNDROME, TOXIC EPIDERMAL NECROLYSIS, FULMINANT HEPATIC NECROSIS, AGRANULOCYTOSIS, APLASTIC ANEMIA, AND OTHER BLOOD DYSCRASIAS. SULFONAMIDES, INCLUDING SULFONAMIDE-CONTAINING PRODUCTS SUCH AS ERYTHROMYCIN ETHYLSUCCINATE/SULFISOXAZOLE ACETYL, SHOULD BE DISCONTINUED AT THE FIRST APPEARANCE OF SKIN RASH OR ANY SIGN OF ADVERSE REACTION.

In rare instances, a skin rash may be followed by a more severe reaction, such as Stevens-Johnson syndrome, toxic epidermal necrolysis, hepatic necrosis, and serious blood disorders. (See "Precautions".)

Clinical signs such as sore throat, fever, pallor, rash, purpura, or jaundice may be early indications of serious reactions.

There have been reports of hepatic dysfunction with or without jaundice, occurring in patients receiving oral Erythromycin products.

Cough, shortness of breath, and pulmonary infiltrates are hypersensitivity reactions of the respiratory tract that have been reported in association with sulfonamide treatment.

The sulfonamides should not be used for the treatment of group A beta-hemolytic streptococcal infections. In an established infection, they will not eradicate the streptococcus and, therefore, will not prevent sequelae such as rheumatic fever.

Pseudomembranous colitis has been reported with nearly all antibacterial agents, including Erythromycin Ethylsuccinate/Sulfisoxazole Acetyl, and may range in severity from mild to life-threatening. Therefore, it is important to consider this diagnosis in patients who present with diarrhea subsequent to the administration of antibacterial agents.

Treatment with antibacterial agents alters the normal flora of the colon and may permit overgrowth of clostridia. Studies indicate that a toxin produced by Clostridium difficile is one primary cause of "antibiotic-associated colitis."

After diagnosis of pseudomembranous colitis has been established, therapeutic measures should be initiated. Mild cases of pseudomembranous colitis usually respond to drug discontinuation alone. In moderate to severe cases, consideration should be given to management with fluids and electrolytes, protein supplementation, and treatment with an antibacterial drug clinically effective against Clostridium difficile colitis.

There have been reports suggesting that Erythromycin does not reach the fetus in adequate concentration to prevent congenital syphilis. Infants born to women treated during pregnancy with Erythromycin for early syphilis should be treated with an appropriate penicillin regimen.

Rhabdomyolysis with or without renal impairment has been reported in seriously ill patients receiving Erythromycin concomitantly with lovastatin. Therefore, patients receiving concomitant lovastatin and Erythromycin should be carefully monitored for creatine kinase (CK) and serum transaminase levels. (See package insert for lovastatin.)

PRECAUTIONS

General: Erythromycin is principally excreted by the liver. Caution should be exercised when Erythromycin is administered to patients with impaired hepatic function. (See "Clinical Pharmacology" and "Warnings" sections.)

Prolonged or repeated use of Erythromycin may result in an overgrowth of nonsusceptible bacteria or fungi. If superinfection occurs, Erythromycin should be discontinued and appropriate therapy instituted.

There have been reports that Erythromycin may aggravate the weakness of patients with myasthenia gravis.

When indicated, incision and drainage or other surgical procedures should be performed in conjunction with antibiotic therapy.

Sulfonamides should be given with caution to patients with impaired renal or hepatic function and to those with severe allergy or bronchial asthma. In glucose-6-phosphate dehydrogenase-deficient individuals, hemolysis may occur; this reaction is frequently dose-related.

Information for Patients: Patients should maintain an adequate fluid intake to prevent crystalluria and stone formation.

Laboratory Test: Complete blood counts should be done frequently in patients receiving sulfonamides. If a significant reduction in the count of any formed blood element is noted, Erythromycin Ethylsuccinate/Sulfisoxazole Acetyl should be discontinued. Urinalysis with careful microscopic examination and renal function tests should be performed during therapy, particularly for those patients with impaired renal function. Blood levels should be measured in patients receiving a sulfonamide for serious infections. (See "Indications and Usage".)

Drug/Laboratory Test Interactions: Erythromycin interferes with the fluorometric determination of urinary catecholamines.

Drug Interactions: Erythromycin use in patients who are receiving high doses of theophylline may be associated with an increase in serum theophylline levels and potential theophylline toxicity. In case of theophylline toxicity and/or elevated serum theophylline levels, the dose of theophylline should be reduced while the patient is receiving concomitant Erythromycin therapy.

Concomitant administration of Erythromycin and Digoxin has been reported to result in elevated Digoxin serum levels. There have been reports of increased anticoagulant effects when Erythromycin and oral anticoagulants were used concomitantly. Increased anticoagulation effects due to this drug may be more pronounced in the elderly.

Concurrent use of Erythromycin and ergotamine or dihydroergotamine has been associated in some patients with acute ergot toxicity characterized by severe peripheral vasospasm and dysesthesia.

Erythromycin has been reported to decrease the clearance of triazolam and midazolam and thus may increase the pharmacologic effect of these benzodiazepines.

The use of Erythromycin in patients concurrently taking drugs metabolized by the cytochrome P450 system may be associated with elevations in serum levels of these other drugs. There have been reports of interactions of Erythromycin with arbamazepine, cyclosporine, hexobarbital, phenytoin, alfentanil, disopyramide, lovastatin, and bromocriptine. Serum concentrations of drugs metabolized by the cytochrome P450 system should be monitored closely in patients concurrently receiving Erythromycin.

Erythromycin significantly alters the metabolism of terfenadine when taken concomitantly. Rare cases of serious cardiovascular adverse events, including death, cardiac arrest, torsades de pointes, and other ventricular arrhythmias, have been observed (see "Contraindications").

It has been reported that Sulfisoxazole may prolong the prothrombin time in patients who are receiving the anticoagulant warfarin. This interaction should be kept in mind when Erythromycin Ethylsuccinate/Sulfisoxazole Acetyl is given to patients already on anticoagulant therapy, and the coagulation time should be reassessed.

It has been proposed that Sulfisoxazole competes with thiopental for plasma protein binding. In one study involving 48 patients, intravenous Sulfisoxazole resulted in a decrease in the amount of thiopenta required for anesthesia and in a shortening of the awakening time. It is not known whether chronic oral doses of Sulfisoxazole have a similar effect. Until more is known about this interaction, physicians should be aware that patients receiving Sulfisoxazole might require less thiopental for anesthesia.

Sulfonamides can displace methotrexate from plasma protein binding sites, thus increasing free methotrexate concentrations. Studies in man have shown Sulfisoxazole infusions to decrease plasma protein-bound methotrexate by one-fourth.

Sulfisoxazole can also potentiate the blood-sugar-lowering activity of sulfonylureas.

Carcinogenesis, Mutagenesis, Impairment of Fertility
Carcinogenesis: Erythromycin Ethylsuccinate/Sulfisoxazole Acetyl has not undergone adequate trials relating to carcinogenicity; each component, however, has been evaluated separately. Long-term (21 month) oral studies conducted in rats with Erythromycin Ethylsuccinate did not provide evidence of tumorigenicity. Sulfisoxazole was not carcinogenic in either sex when administered to mice by gavage for 103 weeks at dosages up to approximately 18 times the recommended human dose or to rats at 4 times the human dose. Rats appear to be especially susceptible to the goitrogenic effects of sulfonamides, and long-term administration of sulfonamides has resulted in thyroid malignancies in this species.

Mutagenesis: There are no studies available that adequately evaluate the mutagenic potential of Erythromycin Ethylsuccinate/Sulfisoxazole Acetyl or either of its components. However, Sulfisoxazole was not observed to be mutagenic in *E. coli* Sd-473 when tested in the absence of a metabolic activating system. There was no apparent effect on male or female fertility in rats fed Erythromycin (base) at levels up to 0.25% of diet.

Impairment of Fertility: Erythromycin Ethylsuccinate/Sulfisoxazole Acetyl has not undergone adequate trials relating to impairment of fertility. In a reproduction study in rats given 7 times the human dose per day of Sulfisoxazole no effects were observed regarding mating behavior, conception rate or fertility index (percent pregnant).

Pregnancy: Teratogenic Effects. Pregnancy Category C. At dosages 7 times the human daily dose, Sulfisoxazole was not teratogenic in either rats or rabbits. However, in two other teratogenicity studies, cleft palates developed in both rats and mice after administration of 5 to 9 times the human therapeutic dose of Sulfisoxazole.

There is no evidence of teratogenicity or any other adverse effect on reproduction in female rats fed Erythromycin base (up to 0.25% of diet) prior to and during mating, during gestation, and through weaning of two successive litters. There are, however, no adequate and well-controlled studies in pregnant women. Because animal reproduction studies are not always predictive of human response, this drug should be used during pregnancy only if clearly needed. Erythromycin has been reported to cross the placental barrier in humans, but fetal plasma levels are generally low.

There are no adequate or well-controlled studies of Erythromycin Ethylsuccinate/Sulfisoxazole Acetyl in either laboratory animals or in pregnant women. It is not known whether Erythromycin Ethylsuccinate/Sulfisoxazole Acetyl can cause fetal harm when administered to a pregnant woman prior to term or can affect reproduction capacity. Erythromycin Ethylsuccinate/Sulfisoxazole Acetyl should be used during pregnancy only if the potential benefit justifies the potential risk to the fetus.

Nonteratogenic Effects: Kernicterus may occur in the newborn as a result of treatment of a pregnant women *at term* with sulfonamides. (See *"Contraindications"*.)

Labor and Delivery: The effects of Erythromycin and Sulfisoxazole on labor and delivery are unknown.

Nursing Mothers: Both Erythromycin and Sulfisoxazole are excreted in human milk. **Because of the potential for the development of kernicterus in neonates due to the displacement of bilirubin from plasma proteins by Sulfisoxazole, a decision should be made whether to discontinue nursing or discontinue the drug, taking into account the importance of the drug to the mother.** (See *"Contraindications"*.)

Pediatric Use: See *"Indications and Usage"* and *"Dosage and Administration"* sections. Not for use in children under 2 months of age. (See *"Contraindications"*.)

ADVERSE REACTIONS

Erythromycin Ethylsuccinate: The most frequent side effects of oral Erythromycin preparations are gastrointestinal and are dose-related. They include nausea, vomiting, abdominal pain, diarrhea and anorexia. Symptoms of hepatic dysfunction and/or abnormal liver-function test results may occur (see *"Warnings"* section). Pseudomembranous colitis has been rarely reported in association with Erythromycin therapy.

Allergic reactions ranging from urticaria and mild skin eruptions to anaphylaxis have occurred.

There have been isolated reports of reversible hearing loss occurring chiefly in patients with renal insufficiency and in patients receiving high doses of Erythromycin.

Onset of pseudomembranous colitis symptoms may occur during or after antibiotic treatment. (See *"Warnings"*.)

Sulfisoxazole Acetyl: Included in the listing that follows are adverse reactions that have been reported with other sulfonamide products: pharmacologic similarities require that each of the reactions be considered with Erythromycin Ethylsuccinate/Sulfisoxazole Acetyl administration.

Allergic/Dermatologic: Anaphylaxis, erythema multiforme (Stevens-Johnson syndrome), toxic epidermal necrolysis (Lyell's syndrome), exfoliative dermatitis, angioedema, arteritis, vasculitis, allergic myocarditis, serum sickness, rash, urticaria, pruritus, photosensitivity, and conjunctival and scleral injection. In addition, periarteritis nodosa and systemic lupus erythematosus have been reported. (See *"Warnings"*.)

Cardiovascular: Tachycardia, palpitations, syncope, and cyanosis.

Rarely, Erythromycin has been associated with the production of ventricular arrhythmias, including ventricular tachycardia and torsade de pointes, in individuals with prolonged QT intervals.

Endocrine: The sulfonamides bear certain chemical similarities to some goitrogens, diuretics (acetazolamide and the thiazides) and oral hypoglycemic agents. Cross-sensitivity may exist with these agents. Developments of goiter, diuresis, and hypoglycemia have occurred rarely in patients receiving sulfonamides.

Gastrointestinal: Hepatitis, hepatocellular necrosis, jaundice, pseudomembranous colitis, nausea, emesis, anorexia, abdominal pain, diarrhea, gastrointestinal hemorrhage, melena, flatulence, glossitis, stomatitis, salivary gland enlargement, and pancreatitis. Onset of pseudomembranous colitis symptoms may occur during or after treatment with Sulfisoxazole, a component of Erythromycin Ethylsuccinate/Sulfisoxazole Acetyl. (See *"Warnings"*.)

The Sulfisoxazole Acetyl component of Erythromycin Ethylsuccinate/Sulfisoxazole Acetyl has been reported to cause increased elevation of liver-associated enzymes in patients with hepatitis.

Genitourinary: Crystalluria, hematuria, BUN and creatinine elevations, nephritis, and toxic nephrosis with oliguria and anuria. Acute renal failure and urinary retention have also been reported.

The frequency of renal complications, commonly associated with some sulfonamides, is lower in patients receiving the more soluble sulfonamides such as Sulfisoxazole.

Hematologic: Leukopenia, agranulocytosis, aplastic anemia, thrombocytopenia, purpura, hemolytic anemia, eosinophilia, clotting disorders including hypoprothrombinemia and hypofibrinogenemia, sulfhemoglobinemia, and methemoglobinemia.

Neurologic: Headache, dizziness, peripheral neuritis, paresthesia, convulsions, tinnitus, vertigo, ataxia, and intracranial hypertension.

Psychiatric: Psychosis, hallucinations, disorientation, depression, and anxiety.

Respiratory: Cough, shortness of breath, and pulmonary infiltrates. (See *"Warnings"*.)

Vascular: Angioedema, arteritis, and vasculitis.

Miscellaneous: Edema (including periorbital), pyrexia, drowsiness, weakness, fatigue, lassitude, rigors, flushing, hearing loss, insomnia, and pneumonitis.

OVERDOSAGE

No information is available on a specific result of overdose with Erythromycin Ethylsuccinate/Sulfisoxazole Acetyl. Overdosage of Erythromycin should be handled with the prompt elimination of unabsorbed drug and all other appropriate measures. Erythromycin is not removed by peritoneal dialysis or hemodialysis.

The amount of a single dose of Sulfisoxazole that is either associated with symptoms of overdosage or is likely to be life-threatening has not been reported. Signs and symptoms of overdosage reported with sulfonamides include anorexia, colic, nausea, vomiting, dizziness, headache, drowsiness and unconsciousness. Pyrexia, hematuria and crystalluria may be noted. Blood dyscrasias and jaundice are potential late manifestations of overdosage.

General principles of treatment include the immediate discontinuation of the drug, instituting gastric lavage or emesis, forcing oral fluids, and administering intravenous fluids if urine output is low and renal function is normal. The patient should be monitored with blood counts and appropriate blood chemistries, including electrolytes. If the patient becomes cyanotic, the possibility of methemoglobinemia should be considered and, if present, the condition should be treated appropriately with intravenous 1% methylene blue. If a significant blood dyscrasia or jaundice occurs, specific therapy should be instituted for these complications. Peritoneal dialysis is not effective, and hemodialysis is only moderately effective in removing sulfonamides.

The acute toxicity of Sulfisoxazole in animals is as follows:

Species	$LD_{50} \pm S.E.$ (mg/kg)
mouse	5700 ± 235
rats	> 10,000
rabbits	> 2000

DOSAGE AND ADMINISTRATION

ERYTHROMYCIN ETHYLSUCCINATE/SULFISOXAZOLE ACETYL SHOULD NOT BE ADMINISTERED TO INFANTS UNDER 2 MONTHS OF AGE BECAUSE OF CONTRAINDICATIONS OF SYSTEMIC SULFONAMIDES IN THIS AGE GROUP.

For Acute Otitis Media in Children: The dose of Erythromycin Ethylsuccinate/Sulfisoxazole Acetyl can be calculated based on the Erythromycin component (50 mg/kg/day) or the Sulfisoxazole component (150 mg/kg/day to a maximum of 6 g/day). The total daily dose of Erythromycin Ethylsuccinate/Sulfisoxazole Acetyl should be administered in equally divided doses three or four times a day for 10 days. Erythromycin Ethylsuccinate/Sulfisoxazole Acetyl may be administered without regard to meals.

The following approximate dosage schedules are recommended for using Erythromycin Ethylsuccinate/Sulfisoxazole Acetyl.

Children: Two months of age or older.

FOUR-TIMES-A-DAY SCHEDULE

Weight	Dose-every 6 hours
Less than 8 kg (< 18 lbs)	Adjust dosage by body weight
8 kg (18 lbs)	½ teaspoonful (2.5 mL)
16 kg (35 lbs)	1 teaspoonful (5 mL)
24 kg (53 lbs)	1 ½ teaspoonfuls (7.5 mL)
Over 32 kg (over 70 lbs)	2 teaspoonfuls (10 mL)

THREE-TIMES-A-DAY SCHEDULE

Weight	Dose-every 8 hours
Less than 6 kg (< 13 lbs)	Adjust dosage by body weight
6 kg (13 lbs)	½ teaspoonful (2.5 mL)
12 kg (26 lbs)	1 teaspoonful (5 mL)
18 kg (40 lbs)	1 ½ teaspoonfuls (7.5 mL)
24 kg (53 lbs)	2 teaspoonfuls (10 mL)
Over 30 kg (over 66 lbs)	2 ½ teaspoonfuls (12.5 mL)

Recommended storage: Before mixing, store below 86°F (30°C).

REFERENCES

1. Biovert A, Barbeau G. Belanger PM: Pharmacokinetics of Sulfisoxazole in young and elderly subjects. *Gerontology* 1984; 30:125-131. 2. Oie S. Gambertoglio JG. Fleckenstein L: Comparison of the disposition of total and unbound sulfisoxazole after single and multiple dosing. *J Pharmacokinet Biopharm* 1982; 10:157-172. 3. National Committee for Clinical Laboratory Standards: *Performance Standards for Antimicrobial Disk Susceptibility Tests*, ed. 4. Approved Standard NCCLS Document M2-A4, Vol 10, No. 7. Villanova, Pa: NCCLS, 1990.

HOW SUPPLIED
GRANULE FOR RECONSTITUTION: 200 MG-600 MG/5 ML

AVERAGE UNIT PRICE (AVAILABLE SIZES)

		GENERIC A-RATED AVERAGE PRICE (GAAP)	
BRAND	$0.16		
GENERIC	$0.12		
HCFA FUL (100 ml)	$0.09	100 ml	$11.45
HCFA FUL (150 ml)	$0.09	150 ml	$17.28
HCFA FUL (200 ml)	$0.09	200 ml	$23.11

BRAND/MANUFACTURER	NDC	SIZE	AWP
◆ BRAND			
PEDIAZOLE: Ross Nutr	00074-8030-13	100 ml	$16.02
	00074-8030-43	150 ml	$23.81
	00074-8030-53	200 ml	$31.26
	00074-8030-73	250 ml	$38.49
◆ GENERICS			
UDL	51079-0492-12	100 ml	$9.83
Schein	00364-2319-61	100 ml	$10.20
Goldline	00182-7063-70	100 ml	$10.50
Moore,H.L.	00839-7514-73	100 ml	$11.00
ERYZOLE: Alra	51641-0111-64	100 ml	$11.50
Qualitest	00603-6563-64	100 ml	$11.60
Geneva	00781-7043-46	100 ml	$11.80
URL	00677-1303-27	100 ml	$11.90
SULFIMYCIN: Rugby	00536-0050-82	100 ml	$11.93
Barr	00555-0445-22	100 ml	$11.93
Aligen	00405-2735-60	100 ml	$11.93
Warner Chilcott	00047-2545-17	100 ml	$11.93
Major	00904-2475-04	100 ml	$11.95
Lederle Std Prod	00005-3700-46	100 ml	$12.34
Schein	00364-2319-62	150 ml	$15.25
Goldline	00182-7063-72	150 ml	$15.75
ERYZOLE: Alra	51641-0111-66	150 ml	$17.25
SULFIMYCIN: Rugby	00536-0050-74	150 ml	$17.25
Major	00904-2475-07	150 ml	$17.30
Qualitest	00603-6563-66	150 ml	$17.40
Geneva	00781-7043-55	150 ml	$17.68
Barr	00555-0445-21	150 ml	$17.76
URL	00677-1303-28	150 ml	$17.79
Aligen	00405-2735-78	150 ml	$17.80
Moore,H.L.	00839-7514-75	150 ml	$17.81
Lederle Std Prod	00005-3700-49	150 ml	$18.29
Schein	00364-2319-63	200 ml	$19.85
Goldline	00182-7063-73	200 ml	$21.00
ERYZOLE: Alra	51641-0111-68	200 ml	$22.65
Warner Chilcott	00047-2545-20	200 ml	$22.84
SULFIMYCIN: Rugby	00536-0050-84	200 ml	$23.10
Qualitest	00603-6563-68	200 ml	$23.15
Geneva	00781-7043-48	200 ml	$23.24
Major	00904-2475-08	200 ml	$23.25
Barr	00555-0445-23	200 ml	$23.33
Aligen	00405-2735-70	200 ml	$23.34
Lederle Std Prod	00005-3700-60	200 ml	$24.04
URL	00677-1303-29	200 ml	$25.30
Moore,H.L.	00839-7514-78	200 ml	$25.37

POWDER FOR RECONSTITUTION: 200 MG-600 MG/5 ML

AVERAGE UNIT PRICE (AVAILABLE SIZES)

GENERIC	$0.13		

BRAND/MANUFACTURER	NDC	SIZE	AWP
◆ GENERICS			
Parmed	00349-8835-01	100 ml	$12.79
Parmed	00349-8835-05	150 ml	$18.91
Parmed	00349-8835-02	200 ml	$24.83

Erythromycin, Injectable

DESCRIPTION

Erythromycin is produced by a strain of *Streptomyces erythraeus* and belongs to the macrolide group of antibiotics. It is basic and readily forms salts with acids.

Erythromycin, Injectable, is available as the lactobionate and glucceptate salts suitable for intravenous administration. It is available as a sterile, lyophilized powder in vials containing the equivalent of 500 mg of Erythromycin activity or 1 g of Erythromycin activity.

ACTIONS/CLINICAL PHARMACOLOGY

Erythromycin diffuses readily into most body fluids. In the absence of meningeal inflammation, low concentrations are normally achieved in the spinal fluid but the passage of the drug across the blood-brain barrier increases in meningitis. Erythromycin crosses the placental barrier, but fetal plasma levels are low; it is excreted in breast milk. Erythromycin is not removed by peritoneal dialysis or hemodialysis.

In the presence of normal hepatic function, Erythromycin is concentrated in the liver and is excreted in the bile; the effect of hepatic dysfunction on biliary excretion of Erythromycin is not known. From 12 to 15 percent of intravenously administered Erythromycin is excreted in active form in the urine.

Intravenous infusion of 500 mg of Erythromycin Lactobionate at a constant rate over 1 hour in fasting adults produced a mean serum Erythromycin level of approximately 7 mcg/mL at 20 minutes, 10 mcg/mL at 1 hour, 2.6 mcg/mL at 2.5 hours, and 1 mcg/mL at 6 hours. Intravenous injection of 200 mg of Erythromycin produces peak serum levels of 3 to 4 μg/mL at 1 hour and 0.5 μg/mL at 6 hours.

MICROBIOLOGY

Erythromycin acts by inhibition of protein synthesis by binding 50 S ribosomal subunits of susceptible organisms. *It does not affect nucleic acid synthesis.* Antagonism has been demonstrated *in vitro* between Erythromycin and clindamycin, lincomycin and chloramphenicol.

Many strains of *Haemophilus influenzae* are resistant to Erythromycin alone, but are susceptible to Erythromycin and sulfonamides together.

Staphylococci resistant to Erythromycin may emerge during a course of therapy. Culture and susceptibility testing should be performed.

Erythromycin is usually active against the following organisms *in vitro* (prior to use, refer to "*Indications And Usage*" section):

Gram-positive Bacteria: Staphylococcus aureus (resistant organisms may emerge during treatment), Streptococcus pyogenes (Group A beta-hemolytic streptococcus), Alpha-hemolytic streptococcus (viridans group), Streptococcus (diplococcus) pneumoniae, Corynebacterium diphtheriae, Corynebacterium minutissimum.

Gram-negative Bacteria: Neisseria gonorrhoeae, Legionella pneumophila, Bordetella pertussis.

Mycoplasma: Mycoplasma pneumoniae, Ureaplasma urealyticum.

Other Microorganisms: Chlamydia trachomatis, Entamoeba histolytica, Treponema pallidum, Listeria monocytogenes.

SUSCEPTIBILITY TESTING

Quantitative methods that require measurement of zone diameters give the most precise estimates of antibiotic susceptibility. One such standardized single-disc procedure has been recommended for use with discs to test susceptibility to Erythromycin.[1] Interpretation involves correlation of the zone diameters obtained in the disc test with minimal inhibitory concentration (MIC) values for Erythromycin.

Reports from the laboratory giving results of the standardized single-disc susceptibility test using a 15 mcg Erythromycin disc should be interpreted according to the following criteria:

Susceptible organisms produce zones of 18 mm or greater, indicating that the tested organism is likely to respond to therapy.

Resistant organisms produce zones of 13 mm or less, indicating that other therapy should be selected.

Organisms of intermediate susceptibility produce zones of 14 to 17 mm. The "intermediate" category provides a "buffer zone" which should prevent small, uncontrolled technical factors from causing major discrepancies in interpretations; thus, when a zone diameter falls within the "intermediate" range, the results may be considered equivocal. If alternative drugs are not available, confirmation by dilution tests may be indicated.

Standardized procedures require the use of control organisms. The 15 mcg Erythromycin disc should give zone diameters between 22 and 30 mm for the *S. aureus* ATCC 25923 control strain.

A bacterial isolate may be considered susceptible if the MIC value[2] for Erythromycin is not more than 2 mcg/mL. Organisms are considered resistant if the MIC is 8 mcg/mL or higher. The MIC of Erythromycin for *S. aureus* ATCC 29213 control strain should be between 0.12 and 0.5 mcg/mL.

INDICATIONS AND USAGE

Erythromycin, Injectable, is indicated in the treatment of infections caused by susceptible strains of the designated organisms in the diseases listed below when oral administration is not possible or when the severity of the infection requires immediate high serum levels of Erythromycin. Intravenous therapy should be replaced by oral administration at the appropriate time.

Upper respiratory tract infections of mild to moderate degree caused by *Streptococcus pyogenes* (Group A beta-hemolytic streptococci); *Streptococcus pneumoniae (Diplococcus pneumoniae); Haemophilus influenzae* (when used concomitantly with adequate doses of sulfonamides, since many strains of *H. influenzae* are not susceptible to the Erythromycin concentrations ordinarily achieved). (See appropriate sulfonamide labeling for prescribing information.)

Lower respiratory tract infections of mild to moderate severity caused by *Streptococcus pyogenes* (Group A beta-hemolytic streptococci); *Streptococcus pneumoniae (Diplococcus pneumoniae).*

Respiratory tract infections due to *Mycoplasma pneumoniae.*

Skin and skin structure infections of mild to moderate severity caused by *Streptococcus pyogenes* and *Staphylococcus aureus* (resistant staphylococci may emerge during treatment).

Diphtheria: As an adjunct to antitoxin infections due to *Corynebacterium diphtheriae* to prevent establishment of carriers and to eradicate the organism in carriers.

Erythrasma: In the treatment of infections due to *Corynebacterium minutissimum.*

Acute pelvic inflammatory disease caused by *Neisseria gonorrhoeae*: Erythromycin, Injectable, followed by oral Erythromycin, as an alternative drug in treatment of acute pelvic inflammatory disease caused by *N. gonorrhoeae* in female patients with a history of sensitivity to penicillin.

Before treatment of gonorrhea, patients who are suspected of also having syphilis should have a microscopic examination for *T. pallidum* (by immunofluorescence or darkfield) before receiving Erythromycin and monthly serologic tests for a minimum of 4 months thereafter.

Infections due to *Listeria Monocytogenes* (glucceptate salt only).

Legionnaires' Disease caused by *Legionella pneumophila.* Although no controlled clinical efficacy studies have been conducted, *in vitro* and limited preliminary clinical data suggest that Erythromycin may be effective in treating Legionnaires' Disease.

Prevention of Initial Attacks of Rheumatic Fever: Penicillin is considered by the American Heart Association to be the drug of choice in the prevention of initial attacks of rheumatic fever (treatment of Group A beta-hemolytic streptococcal infections of the upper respiratory tract e.g., tonsillitis, or pharyngitis).[3] Erythromycin is indicated for the treatment of penicillin-allergic patients. The therapeutic dose should be administered for ten days.

Prevention of Recurrent Attacks of Rheumatic Fever: Penicillin or sulfonamides are considered by the American Heart Association to be the drugs of choice in the prevention of recurrent attacks of rheumatic fever. In patients who are allergic to penicillin and sulfonamides, oral Erythromycin is recommended by the American Heart Association in the long-term prophylaxis of streptococcal pharyngitis (for the prevention of recurrent attacks of rheumatic fever).[3]

Prevention of Bacterial Endocarditis: Although no controlled clinical efficacy trials have been conducted, oral Erythromycin has been recommended by the American Heart Association for prevention of bacterial endocarditis in penicillin-allergic patients with prosthetic cardiac valves, most congenital cardiac malformations, surgically constructed systemic pulmonary shunts, rheumatic or other acquired valvular dysfunction, idiopathic hypertrophic subaortic stenosis (IHSS), previous history of bacterial endocarditis and mitral valve prolapse with insufficiency when they undergo dental procedures and surgical procedures of the upper respiratory tract.[4]

UNLABELED USES

Erythromycin is used alone or as an adjunct in the treatment of Lyme disease and *Campylobacter jejuni* infections.

CONTRAINDICATIONS

Erythromycin is contraindicated in patients with known hypersensitivity to this antibiotic.

Erythromycin is contraindicated in patients taking terfenadine (see *"Precautions—Drug Interactions"*).

WARNINGS

Pseudomembranous colitis has been reported with virtually all broad-spectrum antibiotics (including macrolides, semisynthetic pencillins, and cephalosporins); therefore, it is important to consider its diagnosis in patients who develop diarrhea in association with the use of antibiotics. Such colitis may range in severity from mild to life threatening.

Treatment with broad-spectrum antibiotics alters the normal flora of the colon and may permit overgrowth of clostridia. Studies indicate that a toxin produced by *Clostridium difficile* is one primary cause of antibiotic-associated colitis. Mild cases of pseudomembraneous colitis usually respond to drug discontinuance alone. In moderate to severe cases, management should include sigmoidoscopy, appropriate bacteriologic studies, and fluid, electrolyte, and protein supplementation. When the colitis does not improve after the drug has been discontinued, or when it is severe, oral vancomycin is the drug of choice for antibiotic-associated

pseudomembranous colitis produced by *C. difficile.* Other causes should be ruled out.

There have been reports of hepatic dysfunction with or without jaundice occurring in patients receiving oral Erythromycin products.

Benzyl alcohol, contained in some brands of Erythromycin, Injectable, has been reported to be associated with a fatal "Gasping Syndrome" in premature infants.

PRECAUTIONS

General: Since Erythromycin is principally excreted by the liver, caution should be exercised when Erythromycin is administered to patients with impaired hepatic function. (See *"Clinical Pharmacology"* and *"Warnings"* sections).

Prolonged or repeated use of Erythromycin may result in an overgrowth of non-susceptible bacteria or fungi. If superinfection occurs, Erythromycin should be discontinued and appropriate therapy instituted.

When indicated, incision and drainage or other surgical procedures should be performed in conjunction with antibiotic therapy.

Laboratory Tests: Erythromycin interferes with the fluorometric determination of urinary catecholamines.

Drug Interactions: Erythromycin significantly alters the metabolism of terfenadine when taken concomitantly. Rare cases of serious cardiovascular adverse events, including death, cardiac arrest, torsades de pointes, and other ventricular arrhythmias, have been observed (see *"Contraindications"*).

Erythromycin use in patients who are receiving high doses of theophylline may be associated with an increase in serum theophyllin levels and potential theophylline toxicity. Serum theophylline levels should be monitored in patients receiving concomitant Erythromycin. The theophylline dose may need to be reduced in some patients.

There have been published reports suggesting that when oral Erythromycin is given concurrently with theophylline there is a significant decrease in Erythromycin serum concentrations. This decrease could result in subtherapeutic concentrations of Erythromycin.

Concurrent use of Erythromycin and ergotamine or dihydroergotamine has been associated in some patients with acute ergot toxicity characterized by severe peripheral vasospasm and dysesthesia.

Erythromycin has been reported to decrease the clearance of triazolam and midazolam and thus may increase the pharmacologic effect of these benzodiazepines.

The use of Erythromycin in patients concurrently taking drugs metabolized by the cytochrome P-450 system may be associated with elevations in serum concentrations of these other drugs. Elevated serum concentrations of the following drugs have been reported when administered concurrently with Erythromycin: carbamazepine, cyclosporine, hexobarbital, phenytoin, alfentanil, disopyramide, lovastatin, and bromocriptine. Serum concentrations of these and other drugs metabolized by the cytochrome P-450 system should be monitored closely in patients concurrently receiving Erythromycin.

Concomitant administration of Erythromycin and digoxin has been reported to result in elevated serum digoxin levels.

There have been reports of increased anticoagulant effects when Erythromycin and oral anticoagulants were used concomitantly. Increased anticoagulation effects due to this drug interaction may be more pronounced in the elderly.

Carcinogenesis, Mutagenesis, Impairment of Fertility: Long-term animal data with Erythromycin, Injectable, for use in determination of possible carcinogenic effects are not available. However, long-term oral studies in rats with Erythromycin Ethylsuccinate and Erythromycin base did not provide evidence of tumorigenicity. Mutagenicity studies have not been conducted. There was no apparent effect on male or female fertility in rats fed Erythromycin (base) at levels up to 0.25% of diet.

Pregnancy: Pregnancy Category B: There was no evidence of teratogenicity or any other adverse effect on reproduction in female rats fed Erythromycin base (up to 0.25% of diet) prior to and during mating, during gestation, and through weaning of two successive litters. There are, however, no adequate and well-controlled studies in pregnant women. Because animal reproduction studies are not always predictive of human response, this drug should be used during pregnancy only if clearly needed. Erythromycin has been reported to cross the placental barrier in humans, but fetal plasma levels are generally low.

Labor and Delivery: The effect of Erythromycin on labor and delivery is unknown.

Nursing Mothers: Erythromycin is excreted in breast milk. Caution should be exercised when Erythromycin is administered to a nursing woman.

Pediatric Use: See *"Indications and Usage"* and *"Dosage and Administration"* sections.

Some brands contain benzyl alcohol, which has been associated with a fatal gasping syndrome in infants.

ADVERSE REACTIONS

Side effects following the use of intravenous Erythromycin are rare. Occasional venous irritation has been encountered, but if the infusion is given slowly, in dilute solution, preferably by continuous intravenous infusion or intermittent infusion in no less than 20 to 60 minutes, pain and vessel trauma are minimized.

Occasional nausea, vomiting, abdominal cramping and abdominal pain have been reported.

Allergic reactions, ranging from urticaria and mild skin eruptions to anaphylaxis, have occurred with intravenously administered Erythromycin.

◆ RATED THERAPEUTICALLY EQUIVALENT; ◇ THERAPEUTIC EQUIVALENCE UNCONFIRMED; ○ UNRATED

Occasional case reports of cardiac arrhythmias such as ventricular tachycardia and torsade des pointes, in individuals with prolonged QT intervals, have been documented in patients receiving Erythromycin therapy.

Central nervous system side effects including seizures, hallucinations, confusion and vertigo have been reported in occasional patients; however, a cause and effect relationship has not been established.

There have been isolated reports of reversible hearing loss occurring chiefly in patients with renal insufficiency and in patients receiving high doses of Erythromycin.

Variations in liver function have been observed following daily doses at high levels or after prolonged therapy. Hepatic function tests should be performed when such therapy is given.

OVERDOSAGE

Signs and Symptoms: Experience with overdosage of Erythromycin, Injectable, is limited. Alterations in liver function tests and reversible hearing loss are possible, especially in patients with renal insufficiency.

Treatment: To obtain up-to-date information about the treatment of overdose, a good resource is your certified Regional Poison Control Center. Telephone numbers of certified poison control centers are listed in the *Physicians' Desk Reference (PDR)*. In managing overdosage, consider the possibility of multiple drug overdoses, interaction among drugs, and unusual drug kinetics in your patient.

Discontinue the Erythromycin infusion. Protect the patient's airway and support ventilation and perfusion. Meticulously monitor and maintain, within acceptable limits, the patient's vital signs, blood gases, serum electrolytes, etc.

Forced diuresis, peritoneal dialysis, hemodialysis, or charcoal hemoperfusion have not been established as beneficial for an overdose of Erythromycin.

DOSAGE AND ADMINISTRATION

For the treatment of severe infections in adults and children, the recommended intravenous dose of Erythromycin, Injectable, is 15 to 20 mg/kg/day. Higher doses, up to 4 g/day, may be given for very severe infections. Erythrocin lactobionate-I.V. must be administered by continuous or intermittent intravenous infusion only. Due to the irritative properties of Erythromycin, I.V. push is an unacceptable route of administration.

Continuous infusion of Erythromycin lactobionate is preferable due to the slower infusion rate and lower concentration of Erythromycin; however, intermittent infusion at six hour intervals is also effective. Intravenous Erythromycin should be replaced by oral Erythromycin as soon as possible.

For slow continuous infusion: The final diluted solution of Erythromycin lactobionate is prepared to give a concentration of 1 g per liter (1 mg/mL).

For intermittent infusion: Administer one-fourth the total daily dose of Erythromycin lactobionate by intravenous infusion in 20 to 60 minutes at intervals not greater than every six hours. The final diluted solution of Erythromycin lactobionate is prepared to give a concentration of 1 to 5 mg/mL. No less than 100 mL of I.V. diluent should be used. Infusion should be sufficiently slow to minimize pain along the vein.

For treatment of acute pelvic inflammatory disease caused by *N. gonorrhoeae*, in female patients hypersensitive to penicillins, administer 500 mg Erythromycin, Injectable, every six hours for three days, followed by oral administration of 250 mg Erythromycin every six hours for seven days.

For treatment of Legionnaires' Disease: Although optimal doses have not been established, doses utilized in reported clinical data were 1 to 4 grams daily in divided doses.

In the treatment of Group A beta-hemolytic streptococcal infections in the upper respiratory tract (e.g., tonsilitis or pharyngitis), the therapeutic dosage of Erythromycin should be administered for ten days. The American Heart Association suggests a dosage of 250 mg of Erythromycin orally, twice a day in long-term prophylaxis of streptococcal upper respiratory tract infections for the prevention of recurring attacks of rheumatic fever in patients allergic to penicillin and sulfonamides[3].

In prophylaxis against bacterial endocarditis (see *"Indications and Usage"* section), the oral regimen for penicillin allergic patients is Erythromycin 1 gram, 1 hour before the procedure followed by 500 mg six hours later[4].

PREPARATION OF SOLUTION

1. *Prepare the initial solution of erythromocin, injectable, by adding 10 ml of sterile water for injection, usp, to the 500 mg vial or 20 ml of sterile water for injection, usp, to the 1 g vial.* Shake the vial until all of the drug is dissolved. Use only Sterile Water for Injection, USP, as other diluents may cause precipitation during reconstitution. Do not use diluents containing preservatives or inorganic salts. Note: When the product is reconstituted as directed above, the resulting solution contains an effective antimicrobial preservative.

2. *Add the initial dilution to one of the following diluent before administration* to give a concentration of 1 g of Erythromycin activity per liter (1 mg/mL) for continuous infusion or 1 to 5 mg/mL for intermittent infusion:
0.9% Sodium chloride injection, usp lactated ringer's injection, usp normosol®-r

3. *The following solutions may also be used providing they are first buffered with 4% sodium bicarbonate by adding 1 mL per 100 mL of solution:*
5% Dextrose injection, USP
5% Dextrose and lactated Ringer's Injection (use with lactobionate salt only)
5% Dextrose and 0.9% Sodium Chloride Injection, USP.

IV fluid admixtures with a pH below 5.5 tend to lose potency rapidly. Therefore, such solutions should be administered completely within 4 hours after dilution.

If the period of administration is prolonged, the pH of the infusion fluid should be buffered to neutrality with a sterile agent such as Sodium Bicarbonate 4% Additive Solution or Phosphate-Carbonate Buffer. For administration of the antibiotic in 500 of 1,000 mL of 5% Dextrose in Water, add 1 ampoule full-strength Phosphate-Carbonate Buffer or 5 mL of Sodium Bicarbonate 4% Additive Solution; for administration of the antibiotic in the same volumes of 0.9% Sodium Chloride Injection, add 1 ampoule half-strength Phosphate-Carbonate Buffer or 5 mL of Sodium Bicarbonate 4% Additive Solution. These solutions should be completely administered within 24 hours after dilution.

If the medication is to be given in 100 to 250 mL of fluid by a volume control set, the IV fluid should be buffered in its primary container before being added to the volumetric administration set.

If the medication is to be given by intermittent injection, one-fourth of the total daily dose can be given in 20 to 60 minutes by slow intravenous injection of 250 to 500 mg in 100 to 250 mL of 0.9% Sodium Chloride Injection or 5% Dextrose in Water. Injection should be sufficiently slow to avoid pain along the vein.

No drug or chemical agent should be added to an Erythromycin, Injectable, fluid admixture unless its effect on the chemical and physical stability of the solution has first been determined.

STABILITY

The final diluted solution of Erythromycin, Injectable, should be completely administered within 8 hours, since it is not suitable for storage.

Parenteral drug products should be inspected visually for particulate matter and discoloration prior to administration, whenever solution and container permit.

STORAGE

Prior to reconstitution, store at controlled room temperature, 15° to 30° C (59° to 86° F). After reconstitution, store in a refrigerator and use within 7 or 14 days, depending on the brand. Some brands can be kept at room temperature for 24 hours.

REFERENCES

1. National Committee for Clinical Laboratory Standards, Approved Standard: *Performance Standards for Antimicrobial Disk Susceptibility Tests*, 3rd Edition, Vol. 4(16): M2-A3, Villanova, PA, December 1984. 2. Ericson, H.M. Sherris, J.C., Antibiotic Sensitivity Testing Report of an International Collaborative Study, *Acta Pathologica et Microbiologica Scandinavica* Section B. Suppl. 217:1-90, 1971. 3. Committee on Rheumatic Fever and Infective Endocarditis of the Council on Cardiovascular Disease of the Young: Prevention of Rheumatic Fever, *Circulation* 70(6):1118A-1122A, December 1984. 4. Committee on Rheumatic Fever and Infective Endocarditis of the Council on Cardiovascular Disease of the Young: Prevention of Bacterial Endocarditis, *Circulation* 70(6):1123A-1127A, December 1984.

J CODES

Up to 100 mg IM—J1350
Up to 500 mg IV—J1360

HOW SUPPLIED

ERYTHROMYCIN LACTOBIONATE
POWDER FOR INJECTION: 500 MG

AVERAGE UNIT PRICE (AVAILABLE SIZES)		GENERIC A-RATED AVERAGE PRICE (GAAP)	
BRAND	$12.92	1s	$6.48
GENERIC	$6.48		

BRAND/MANUFACTURER	NDC	SIZE	AWP
◆ BRAND			
ERYTHROCIN LACTOBIONATE: Abbott Hosp	00074-6368-13	5s	$53.62
	00074-6365-02	10s	$100.46
	00074-6476-44	10s	$105.09
	00074-3247-01	10s	$204.01
◆ GENERICS			
Elkins-Sinn	00641-2304-41	1s	$6.25
Elkins-Sinn	00641-2313-41	1s	$6.71

POWDER FOR INJECTION: 500 MG

BRAND/MANUFACTURER	NDC	SIZE	AWP
○ BRAND			
ERYTHROCIN LACTOBIONATE: Abbott Hosp	00074-6483-01	5s	$51.54
	00074-6482-01	10s	$96.78

POWDER FOR INJECTION: 1 GM

AVERAGE UNIT PRICE (AVAILABLE SIZES)	
BRAND	$21.58

BRAND/MANUFACTURER	NDC	SIZE	AWP
◆ BRAND			
ERYTHROCIN LACTOBIONATE: Abbott Hosp	00074-6342-05	10s	$182.16
	00074-6478-44	10s	$186.91
	00074-3246-01	10s	$278.35
◆ GENERICS			
Elkins-Sinn	00641-2309-41	1s	$11.59

► SHOWN IN PRODUCT IDENTIFICATION GUIDE

POWDER FOR INJECTION: 1 GM

BRAND/MANUFACTURER	NDC	SIZE	AWP
○ BRAND			
ERYTHROCIN LACTOBIONATE: Abbott Hosp	00074-6481-01	10s	$175.04

ERYTHROMYCIN GLUCEPTATE

POWDER FOR INJECTION: 1 GM

BRAND/MANUFACTURER	NDC	SIZE	AWP
○ BRAND			
ILOTYCIN GLUCEPTATE: Dista	00777-1441-01	1s	$22.45

Erythromycin, Ophthalmic

DESCRIPTION
Erythromycin USP belongs to the macrolide group of antibiotics. It is basic and readily forms a salt when combined with an acid. The base, as crystals or powder, is slightly soluble in water, moderately soluble in ether, and readily soluble in alcohol or chloroform. The empirical formula for Erythromycin is $C_{37}H_{67}NO_{13}$. Erythromycin-4-[(2,6-Dideoxy-3-C-methyl-3-O-methyl-α-L-$ribo$-hexopyranosyl])oxy]-14-ethyl-7, 12, 13-trihydroxy-3, 5, 7, 9,11,13-hexamethyl-6- [[3,4,6-trideoxy-3-(di- methylamino)-β-D-$xylo$-hexopyranosyl] oxy]oxacyclotetradecane-2,10-dione is an antibiotic produced from a strain of *Streptomyces erythraeus*.

Each gram contains 5 mg Erythromycin, USP, in a sterile ophthalmic base.

CLINICAL PHARMACOLOGY
Microbiology: Erythromycin inhibits protein synthesis without affecting nucleic acid synthesis. Erythromycin is usually active against the following organisms in vitro and in clinical infections:

Streptococcus pyogenes (group A β-hemolytic)
Alpha-hemolytic streptococci (viridans group)
Straphylococcus aureus, including penicillinase-producing strains (methicillin-resistant staphylococci are uniformly resistant to Erythromycin)
Streptococcus pneumoniae
Mycoplasma pneumoniae (Eaton Agent, PPLO)
Haemophilus influenzae (not all strains of this organism are susceptible at the Erythromycin concentrations ordinarily achieved)
Treponema pallidum
Corynebacterium diphtheriae
Neisseria gonorrhoeae
Chlamydia trachomatis

INDICATIONS AND USAGE
For the treatment of superficial ocular infections involving the conjunctiva and/or cornea caused by organisms susceptible to Erythromycin, USP.

For prophylaxis of ophthalmia neonatorum due to *N. gonorrhoeae* or *C. trachomatis*.

The effectiveness of Erythromycin in the prevention of ophthalmia caused by penicillinase-producing *N. gonorrhoeae* is not established.

For infants born to mothers with clinically apparent gonorrhea, intravenous or intramuscular injections of aqueous crystalline penicillin G should be given: a single dose of 50,000 units for term infants or 20,000 units for infants of low birth weight. Topical prophylaxis alone is inadequate for these infants.

CONTRAINDICATION
This drug is contraindicated in patients with a history of hypersensitivity to Erythromycin.

PRECAUTIONS
General: The use of antimicrobial agents may be associated with the overgrowth of nonsusceptible organisms including fungi; in such a case, antibiotic administration should be stopped and appropriate measures taken.

Information for Patients: Avoid contaminating the applicator tip with material from the eye, fingers, or other source.

Carcinogenesis Mutagenesis: Two year oral studies conducted in rats with Erythromycin did not provide evidence of tumorigenicity. Mutagenicity studies have not been conducted.

Pregnancy: Pregnancy Category B: Reproduction studies have been performed in rats, mice, and rabbits using Erythromycin and its various salts and esters, at doses that were several multiples of the usual human dose. No evidence of impaired fertility or harm to the fetus that appeared related to Erythromycin was reported in these studies. There are, however, no adequate and well-controlled studies in pregnant women. Because animal reproductive studies are not always predictive of human response, the Erythromycins should be used during pregnancy only if clearly needed.

Nursing Mothers: Caution should be exercised when Erythromycin is administered to a nursing woman.

Pediatric Use: (See "Indications and Usage" and "Dosage and Administrations.")

ADVERSE REACTIONS
The most frequently reported adverse reactions are minor ocular irritations, redness, and hypersensitivity reactions.

DOSAGE AND ADMINISTRATION
In the treatment of superficial ocular infections, Ophthalmic Ointment Erythromycin, USP approximately 1 cm in length should be applied directly to the infected structure up to 6 times daily, depending on the severity of the infection.

For prophylaxis of neonatal gonococcal or chlamydial conjunctivitis, a ribbon of ointment approximately 1 cm in length should be instilled into each lower conjunctival sac. The ointment should not be flushed from the eye following instillation. A new tube should be used for each infant.

Store at controlled room temperature, 59° to 86°F (15° to 30°C).

HOW SUPPLIED
OINTMENT: 5 MG/GM

AVERAGE UNIT PRICE (AVAILABLE SIZES)		GENERIC A-RATED AVERAGE PRICE (GAAP)	
BRAND	$1.43	3.5 gm	$2.98
GENERIC	$1.38	1 gm 50s	$140.25
HCFA FUL (3.5 gm)	$0.54		

BRAND/MANUFACTURER	NDC	SIZE	AWP
◆ BRAND			
ILOTYCIN: Dista	00777-1863-17	3.5 gm	$5.00
◆ GENERICS			
Logen	00820-0106-65	3.5 gm	$1.89
URL	00677-1017-18	3.5 gm	$2.35
Bausch&Lomb Pharm	24208-0910-55	3.5 gm	$2.93
Major	00904-2990-38	3.5 gm	$3.55
Moore,H.L.	00839-6767-43	3.5 gm	$4.17
Fougera	00168-0070-39	3.5 gm 24s	$100.08
Fougera	00168-0070-11	1 gm 50s	$208.50
Bausch&Lomb Pharm	24208-0910-19	1 gm 50s ud	$72.00

Erythromycin, Oral

WARNING

HEPATIC DYSFUNCTION WITH OR WITHOUT JAUNDICE HAS OCCURRED, CHIEFLY IN ADULTS, IN ASSOCIATION WITH ERYTHROMYCIN ESTOLATE ADMINISTRATION. IT MAY BE ACCOMPANIED BY MALAISE, NAUSEA, VOMITING, ABDOMINAL COLIC, AND FEVER. IN SOME INSTANCES, SEVERE ABDOMINAL PAIN MAY SIMULATE AN ABDOMINAL SURGICAL EMERGENCY.

IF THE ABOVE FINDINGS OCCUR, DISCONTINUE ERYTHROMYCIN ESTOLATE PROMPTLY.

ERYTHROMYCIN ESTOLATE IS CONTRAINDICATED FOR PATIENTS WITH A KNOWN HISTORY OF SENSITIVITY TO THIS DRUG AND FOR THOSE WITH PREEXISTING LIVER DISEASE.

DESCRIPTION
Erythromycin, Oral, is an antibacterial product available in several forms:

1. Erythromycin coated particles in tablets. The coating protects the antibiotic from the inactivating effects of gastric acidity and permits efficient absorption of the antibiotic in the small intestine.

It is available in two strengths: 333 mg or 500 mg Erythromycin base.

2. Erythromycin Stearate tablets, 250 mg or 500 mg.

3. Erythromycin Ethylsuccinate: granules for reconstitution, containing 200 mg Erythromycin/5 ml; ready-made suspension containing 200 mg or 400 mg Erythromycin/5 ml; film-coated tablets containing 400 mg Erythromycin.

4. Erythromycin Estolate: granules (Pulvules), 250 mg Erythromycin; tablets, 500 mg; suspension, 125 mg or 250 mg.

5. Erythromycin film-coated tablets, 250 mg and 500 mg.

6. Erythromycin delayed-release capsules, 250 mg.

7. Erythromycin Ethylsuccinate for oral suspension containing Erythromycin 200 mg/5 ml, 100 mg/2.5 ml, or 400 mg/5 ml; chewable tablets 200 mg.

Erythromycin is produced by a strain of *Streptomyces erythraeus* and belongs to the macrolide group of antibiotics. It is basic and readily forms salts with acids.

The base, the stearate salt, and the esters are poorly soluble in water, and are suitable for oral administration. Erythromycin Ethylsuccinate is an ester of Erythromycin suitable for oral administration. Erythromycin is a white to off-white powder, slightly soluble in water, and soluble in alcohol, chloroform, and ether. Erythromycin is known chemically as (3R*, 4S*, 5S*, 6R*, 7R*, 9R*, 11R*, 12R*, 13S*, 14R*)-4-[(2,6-Dideoxy-3-C-methyl-3-O-methyl-α-L- $ribo$- hexopyranosyl)oxy]-14-ethyl-7,12,13-trihydroxy-3,5,7,9,11,-13-hexamethyl-6-[[3,4,6-trideoxy-3-(dimethylamino)-β-D- $xylo$-hexopyranosyl]oxy]oxacyclotetradecane-2,10-dione.

The granules are intended for reconstitution with water. When reconstituted, they are palatable suspensions.

The liquids are supplied ready for oral administration.

Granules and ready-made suspensions are intended primarily for pediatric use but can also be used in adults.

The Erythromycin Ethylsuccinate film-coated tablets are intended primarily for adults or older children.

◆ RATED THERAPEUTICALLY EQUIVALENT; ◇ THERAPEUTIC EQUIVALENCE UNCONFIRMED; ○ UNRATED

CLINICAL PHARMACOLOGY

Orally administered Erythromycin base and its salts are readily absorbed in the microbiologically active form. Interindividual variations in the absorption of Erythromycin are, however, observed, and some patients do not achieve optimal serum levels. Erythromycin is largely bound to plasma proteins and the freely dissociating bound fraction after administration of Erythromycin base represents 90% of the total Erythromycin absorbed. After absorption, Erythromycin diffuses readily into most body fluids. In the absence of meningeal inflammation, low concentrations are normally achieved in the spinal fluid but the passage of the drug across the blood-brain barrier increases in meningitis. Erythromycin crosses the placental barrier and is excreted in breast milk. Erythromycin is not removed by peritoneal dialysis or hemodialysis.

In the presence of normal hepatic function, Erythromycin is concentrated in the liver and is excreted in the bile; the effect of hepatic dysfunction on biliary excretion of Erythromycin is not known. After oral administration, less than 5% of the administered dose can be recovered in the active form in the urine.

The Erythromycin particles in Enytromycin, Oral tablets are coated with a polymer whose dissolution is pH dependent. This coating allows for minimal release of Erythromycin in acidic environments, e.g., stomach. This delivery system is designed for optimal drug release and absorption in the small intestine.

In multiple-dose, steady-state studies, Erythromycin, Oral tablets have demonstrated rapid and generally adequate drug delivery in both fasting and nonfasting conditions. However, the presence of food results in lower blood levels, and optimal blood levels are obtained when Erythromycin, Oral tablets are given in the fasting state (at least ½ hour and preferably 2 hours before meals).

Orally administered Erythromycin is readily absorbed by most patients, especially on an empty stomach, but patient variation is observed. Enteric-coated Erythromycin tablets give reliable blood levels in the average subject; however, the levels may vary with the individual.

Orally administered Erythromycin Stearate is readily and reliably absorbed. Optimal serum levels of Erythromycin are reached when Erythromycin Stearate is taken in the fasting state or immediately before meals; comparable serum levels of Erythromycin are achieved with Erythromycin Ethylsuccinate or Erythromycin Estolate in the fasting and nonfasting states.

After a single 250-mg dose of Erythromycin Estolate, blood concentrations average 0.29, 1.2, and 1.2 μg/mL respectively at 2, 4, and 6 hours. Following a 500-mg dose, blood concentrations average 3, 1.9, and 0.7 μg/mL respectively at 2, 6, and 12 hours.

After oral administration of Erythromycin Estolate, serum antibiotic levels consist of Erythromycin base and propionyl Erythromycin ester. The propionyl ester continuously hydrolyzes to the base form of Erythromycin to maintain an equilibrium ratio of approximately 20% base and 80% ester in the serum.

The enteric coating of pellets in Erythromycin Delayed Release capsules protects the Erythromycin base from inactivation by gastric acidity. Because of their small size and enteric coating, the pellets readily pass intact from the stomach to the small intestine and dissolve efficiently to allow absorption of Erythromycin in a uniform manner. After administration of a single dose of a 250-mg Erythromycin Delayed Release capsule, peak serum levels in the range of 1:3 to 1.68 mcg/mL are attained in approximately 3 hours and decline to 0.30-0.42 mcg/mL in 6 hours. Optimal conditions for stability in the presence of gastric secretion and for complete absorption are attained when Erythromycin Delayed Release is taken on an empty stomach.

MICROBIOLOGY

Erythromycin acts by inhibition of protein synthesis by binding 50 S ribosomal subunits of susceptible organisms. It does not affect nucleic acid synthesis. Antagonism has been demonstrated *in vitro* between Erythromycin and clindamycin, lincomycin, and chloramphenicol.

Many strains of *Haemophilus influenzae* are resistant to Erythromycin alone, but are susceptible to erythromycin and sulfonamides together.

Staphylococci resistant to Erythromycin may emerge during a course of Erythromycin therapy. Culture and susceptibility testing should be performed.

Erythromycin is usually active against the following organisms *in vitro* **(prior to use, refer to** *"Indications and Usage"* **section):**

Gram-positive Bacteria: Staphylococcus aureus (resistant organisms may emerge during treatment), Streptococcus pyogenes (Group A beta-hemolytic streptococci), Alpha-hemolytic streptococci (viridans group), Streptococcus (diplococcus) pneumoniae, Corynebacterium diphtheriae, Corynebacterium minutissimum.

Gram-negative Bacteria: Moraxella (Branhamella) catarrhalis, Neisseria gonorrhoeae, Legionella pneumophila, Bordetella pertussis.

Myoplasma: Mycoplasma pneumoniae, Ureaplasma urealyticum.

Other Microorganisms: Chlamydia trachomatis, Entamoeba histolytica. Treponema pallidum, Listeria monocytogenes.

SUSCEPTIBILITY TESTING

Quantitative methods that require measurement of zone diameters give the most precise estimates of antibiotic susceptibility. One such standardized single-disc procedure has been recommended for use with discs to test susceptibility to Erythromycin.[1] Interpretation involves correlation of the zone diameters obtained in the disc test with minimal inhibitory concentration (MIC) values for Erythromycin.

Reports from the laboratory giving results of the standardized single-disc susceptibility test using a 15 mcg Erythromycin disc should be interpreted according to the following criteria:

Susceptible organisms produce zones of 18 mm or greater, indicating that the tested organism is likely to respond to therapy.

Resistant organisms produce zones of 13 mm or less, indicating that other therapy should be selected.

Organisms of intermediate susceptibility produce zones of 14 to 17 mm. The "intermediate" category provides a "buffer zone" which should prevent small, uncontrolled technical factors from causing major discrepancies in interpretations; thus, when a zone diameter falls within the "intermediate" range, the results may be considered equivocal. If alternative drugs are not available, confirmation by dilution tests may be indicated.

Standardized procedures require the use of control organisms. The 15 mcg Erythromycin disc should give zone diameters between 22 and 30 mm for the *S. aureus* ATCC 25923 control strain.

If the Bauer-Kirby method of disk susceptibility testing is used, a 15-μg Erythromycin disk should give a zone diameter of at least 18 mm when tested against an Erythromycin-susceptible organism.

A bacterial isolate may be considered susceptible if the MIC value[2] for Erythromycin is not more than 2 mcg/mL. Organisms are considered resistant if the MIC is 8 mcg/mL or higher. The MIC of Erythromycin for *S. aureus* ATCC 29213 control strain should be between 0.12 and 0.5 mcg/mL.

Disc Susceptibility Tests: Quantitative methods that require measurement of zone diameters give the most precise estimates of antibiotic susceptibility. One recommended procedure (21 CFR section 460.1) uses Erythromycin class discs for testing susceptibility; interpretations correlate zone diameters of this disc test with MIC values for Erythromycin. With this procedure, a report from the laboratory of "susceptible" indicates that the infecting organism is likely to respond to therapy. A report of "resistant" indicates that the infective organism is not likely to respond to therapy. A report of "intermediate susceptibility" suggests that the organism would be susceptible if higher doses were used.

INDICATIONS AND USAGE

Erythromycin, Oral tablets are indicated in the treatment of infections caused by susceptible strains of the designated microorganisms in the diseases listed below:

Upper respiratory tract infections of mild to moderate degree (e.g., otitis media, pharyngitis) caused by *Streptococcus pyogenes* (Group A beta-hemolytic streptococci); *Streptococcus pneumoniae (Diplococcus pneumoniae)*; *Haemophilus influenzae* (when used concomitantly with adequate doses of sulfonamides, since many strains of *H. influenzae* are not susceptible to the Erythromycin concentrations ordinarily achieved). (See appropriate sulfonamide labeling for prescribing information.)

Lower respiratory tract infections of mild to moderate severity (e.g., pneumonia) caused by *Streptococcus pyogenes* (Group A beta-hemolytic streptococci); *Streptococcus pneumoniae (Diplococcus pneumoniae)*.

Respiratory tract infections due to *Mycoplasma pneumoniae* (Eaton agent, PPLO).

Skin and skin structure infections of mild to moderate severity caused by *Streptococcus pyogenes* and *Staphylococcus aureus* (resistant staphylococci may emerge during treatment).

Pertussis (whooping cough) caused by *Bordetella pertussis*. Erythromycin is effective in eliminating the organism from the nasopharynx of infected individuals, rendering them noninfectious. Some clinical studies suggest that Erythromycin may be helpful in the prophylaxis of pertussis in exposed susceptible individuals.

Diphtheria—As an adjunct to antitoxin in infections due to *Corynebacterium diphtheriae*, to prevent establishment of carriers and to eradicate the organism in carriers.

Erythrasma—In the treatment of infections due to *Corynebacterium minutissimum*.

Intestinal amebiasis caused by *Entamoeba histolytica* (oral Erythromycins only). Extraenteric amebiasis requires treatment with other agents.

Acute pelvic inflammatory disease caused by *Neisseria gonorrhoeae*: Erythromycin Lactobionate for injection, USP followed by oral Erythromycin base, as an alternative drug in treatment of acute pelvic inflammatory disease caused by N. gonorrhoeae in female patients with a history of sensitivity to penicillin. Before treatment of gonorrhea, patients who are suspected of also having syphilis should have a microscopic examination for *T. pallidum* (by immunofluorescence or darkfield) before receiving Erythromycin and monthly serologic tests for a minimum of 4 months thereafter.

Erythromycins are indicated for treatment of the following infections caused by *Chlamydia trachomatis*: conjunctivitis of the newborn, pneumonia of infancy, and urogenital infections during pregnancy. When tetracyclines are contraindicated or not tolerated, Erythromycin is indicated for the treatment of uncomplicated urethral, endocervical, or rectal infections in adults due to *Chlamydia trachomatis*.[3]

When tetracyclines are contraindicated or not tolerated, Erythromycin is indicated for the treatment of nongonococcal urethritis caused by *Ureaplasma urealyticum*.[3]

Primary syphilis caused by *Treponema pallidum*. Erythromycin (oral forms only) is an alternative choice of treatment for primary syphilis in patients allergic to the penicillins. In treatment of primary syphilis, spinal fluid should be examined before treatment and as part of the follow-up after therapy.

Infections due to *Listeria monocytogenes*.

Legionnaires' Disease caused by *Legionella pneumophila*. Although no controlled clinical efficacy studies have been conducted, *in vitro* and limited preliminary clinical data suggest that Erythromycin may be effective in treating Legionnaires' Disease.

Therapy with Erythromycin should be monitored by bacteriological studies and by clinical response.

Prevention of Initial Attacks of Rheumatic Fever—Injectable benzathine penicillin G is considered by the American Heart Association to be the drug of choice in the treatment and prevention of initial attacks of rheumatic fever (treatment of Group A beta-hemolytic streptococcal infections of the upper respiratory tract e.g., tonsillitis, or pharyngitis).[4] Erythromycin is indicated for the treatment of penicillin-allergic patients. The therapeutic dose should be administered for ten days.

Prevention of Recurrent Attacks of Rheumatic Fever—Pencillin or sulfonamides are considered by the American Heart Association to be the drugs of choice in the prevention of recurrent attacks of rheumatic fever. In patients who are allergic to penicillin and sulfonamides, oral Erythromycin is recommended by the American Heart Association in the long-term prophylaxis of streptococcal pharyngitis (for the prevention of recurrent attacks of rheumatic fever).[4]

Prevention of Bacterial Endocarditis—Although no controlled clinical efficacy trials have been conducted, oral Erythromycin has been recommended by the American Heart Association and American Dental Association for prevention of bacterial endocarditis in penicillin-allergic patients with most congenital cardiac malformations, rheumatic or other acquired valvular dysfunction, idiopathic hypertrophic subaortic stenosis (IHSS), previous history of bacterial endocarditis and mitral valve prolapse with insufficiency when they undergo dental procedures and surgical procedures of the upper respiratory tract.[5]

Erythromycin is not suitable prior to genitourinary or gastrointestinal tract surgery. *Note*: When selecting antibiotics for the prevention of bacterial endocarditis the physician or dentist should read the full joint statement of the American Heart Association and the American Dental Association.[1]

CONTRAINDICATIONS

Erythromycin is contraindicated in patients with known hypersensitivity to this antibiotic.

Erythromycin is contraindicated in patients taking terfenadine (see *"Precautions—Drug Interactions"*).

WARNINGS

There have been reports of hepatic dysfunction with or without jaundice, occurring in patients receiving oral Erythromycin products.

(See boxed *"Warning".*) The administration of Erythromycin Estolate has been associated with the infrequent occurrence of cholestatic hepatitis. Laboratory findings have been characterized by abnormal hepatic function test values, peripheral eosinophilia, and leukocytosis. Symptoms may include malaise, nausea, vomiting, abdominal cramps, and fever. Jaundice may or may not be present. In some instances, severe abdominal pain may simulate the pain of biliary colic, pancreatitis, perforated ulcer, or an acute abdominal surgical problem. In other instances, clinical symptoms and results of liver function tests have resembled findings in extrahepatic obstructive jaundice.

Initial symptoms have developed in some cases after a few days of treatment but generally have followed 1 or 2 weeks of continuous therapy. Symptoms reappear promptly, usually within 48 hours after the drug is readministered to sensitive patients. The syndrome seems to result from a form of sensitization, occurs chiefly in adults, and has been reversible when medication is discontinued.

Pseudomembranous colitis has been reported with virtually all broad-spectrum antibiotics (including macrolides, semisynthetic penicillins, and cephalosporins); therefore, it is important to consider its diagnosis in patients who develop diarrhea in association with the use of antibiotics. Such colitis may range in severity from mild to life threatening.

Treatment with broad-spectrum antibiotics alters the normal flora of the colon and may permit overgrowth of clostridia. Studies indicate that a toxin produced by *Clostridium difficile* is a primary cause of antibiotic-associated colitis.

Mild cases of pseudomembraneous colitis usually respond to drug discontinuance alone. In moderate to severe cases, management should include sigmoidoscopy, appropriate bacteriologic studies, and fluid, electrolyte, and protein supplementation. When the colitis does not improve after the drug has been discontinued, or when it is severe, oral vancomycin is the drug of choice for antibiotic-associated pseudomembranous colitis produced by *C. difficile*. Other causes of colitis should be ruled out.

PRECAUTIONS

General: Erythromycin is principally excreted by the liver. Caution should be exercised when Erythromycin is administered to patients with impaired hepatic function. (See *"Clinical Pharmacology"* and *"Warnings"* sections).

Prolonged or repeated use of Erythromycin may result in an overgrowth of nonsusceptible bacteria or fungi. If superinfection occurs, Erythromycin should be discontinued and appropriate therapy instituted.

When indicated, incision and drainage or other surgical procedures should be performed in conjunction with antibiotic therapy.

The antibacterial activity of Erythromycin is markedly greater in alkaline than in neutral or acid media, and several investigators have recommended concomitant administration of urinary alkalinizing agents, such as sodium bicarbonate or acetazolamide, when Erythromycin is prescribed for treatment of urinary infections.

Laboratory Tests: Erythromycin interferes with the fluorometric determination of urinary catecholamines.

There are reports that Erythromycin interferes in some clinical laboratory tests and causes aberrant results. For example, evidence has been published indicating that high SGOT values recorded for some patients receiving Erythromycin Estolate may be artifacts and may not necessarily reflect changes in liver function.

Drug Interactions: Erythromycin use in patients who are receiving high doses of theophylline may be associated with an increase of serum theophylline levels and potential theophylline toxicity. In case of theophylline toxicity and/or elevated serum theophylline levels, the dose of theophylline should be reduced while the patient is receiving concomitant Erythromycin therapy.

Concomitant administration of Erythromycin and digoxin has been reported to result in elevated digoxin serum levels.

There have been reports of increased anticoagulant effects when erythromycin and oral anticoagulants were used concomitantly. Increased anticoagulation effects due to this drug interaction may be more pronounced in the elderly.

Concurrent use of Erythromycin and ergotamine or dihydroergotamine has been associated in some patients with acute ergot toxicity characterized by severe peripheral vasospasm and dysesthesia.

Erythromycin has been reported to decrease the clearance of triazolam and midazolam and thus may increase the pharmacologic effect of these benzodiazepines.

The use of Erythromycin in patients concurrently taking drugs metabolized by the cytochrome P450 system may be associated with elevations in serum Erythromycin with carbamazepine, cyclosporine, hexobarbital, phenytoin, alfentanil, disopyramide, lovastatin, bromocriptine, and valproate. Serum concentrations of drugs metabolized by the cytochrome P450 system should be monitored closely in patients concurrently receiving Erythromycin.

Troleandomycin significantly alters the metabolism of terfenadine when taken concomitantly; therefore, observe caution when Erythromycin and terfenadine are used concurrently.

Rare cases of serious cardiovascular adverse events, including death, cardiac arrest, torsades de pointes, and other ventricular arrhythmias, have been observed (see *"Contraindications"*).

Patients receiving concomitant lovastatin and Erythromycin should be carefully monitored; cases of rhabdomyolysis have been reported in seriously ill patients.

Since probenecid inhibits tubular reabsorption of Erythromycin in animals, it prolongs maintenance of plasma levels.

Erythromycin and lincomycin or clindamycin may under some conditions be antagonistic. Lincomycin or clindamycin therapy should be avoided in treatment of infections due to Erythromycin-resistant organisms.

Carcinogenesis, Mutagenesis, Impairment of Fertility: Long-term (2-year) oral studies conducted in rats with Erythromycin base did not provide evidence of tumorigenicity. Mutagenicity studies have not been conducted. There was no apparent effect on male or female fertility in rats fed Erythromycin (base) at levels up to 0.25 percent of diet.

Pregnancy: Pregnancy Category B: There is no evidence of teratogenicity or any other adverse effect on reproduction in female rats fed Erythromycin base (up to 0.25 percent of diet) prior to and during mating, during gestation, and through weaning of two successive litters. No evidence of impaired fertility or harm to the fetus was reported in studies performed in mice and rabbits. There are, however, no adequate and well-controlled studies in pregnant women. Because animal reproduction studies are not always predictive of human response, this drug should be used during pregnancy only if clearly needed. Erythromycin has been reported to cross the placental barrier in humans, but fetal plasma levels are generally low.

Labor and Delivery: The effect of Erythromycin on labor and delivery is unknown.

Nursing Mothers: Erythromycin is excreted in breast milk, therefore, caution should be exercised when Erythromycin is administered to a nursing woman.

Pediatric Use: See *"Indications and Usage"* and *"Dosage and Administration"* sections.

ADVERSE REACTIONS

The most frequent side effects of oral Erythromycin preparations are gastrointestinal and are dose-related. They include nausea, vomiting, abdominal pain, diarrhea and anorexia. Symptoms of hepatic dysfunction and/or abnormal liver function test results may occur (see *"Warnings"* section). Pseudomembranous colitis has been rarely reported in association with Erythromycin therapy.

There have been isolated reports of transient central nervous system side effects including confusion, hallucinations, seizures, and vertigo; however, a cause and effect relationship has not been established.

Occasional case reports of cardiac arrhythmias such as ventricular tachycardia and torsades de pointes have been documented in patients with prolonged QT intervals who are receiving Erythromycin therapy. There have been isolated reports of other cardiovascular symptoms such as chest pain, dizziness, and palpitations; however, a cause and effect relationship has not been established.

Allergic reactions ranging from urticaria and mild skin eruptions to anaphylaxis have occurred.

There have been isolated reports of hearing loss and/or tinnitus occurring chiefly in patients with renal or hepatic insufficiency and in patients receiving high doses of Erythromycin.

The ototoxic effect of the drug is usually reversible with drug discontinuance; however, in rare instances involving intravenous administration, the ototoxic effect has been irreversible.

◆ RATED THERAPEUTICALLY EQUIVALENT; ◇ THERAPEUTIC EQUIVALENCE UNCONFIRMED; ○ UNRATED

OVERDOSAGE

In case of overdosage, Erythromycin should be discontinued. Overdosage should be handled with the prompt elimination of unabsorbed drug and all other appropriate measures.

Erythromycin is not removed by peritoneal dialysis or hemodialysis.

Signs and Symptoms: Symptoms of oral overdose of Erythromycin Estolate may include nausea, vomiting, epigastric distress, and diarrhea. The severity of the epigastric distress and the diarrhea are dose related. Reversible mild acute pancreatitis has been reported. Hearing loss, with or without tinnitus and vertigo, may occur, especially in patients with renal or hepatic insufficiency.

Treatment: To obtain up-to-date information about the treatment of overdose, a good resource is your certified Regional Poison Control Center. Telephone numbers of certified poison control centers are listed in the *Physicians' Desk Reference (PDR)*. In managing overdosage, consider the possibility of multiple drug overdoses, interaction among drugs, and unusual drug kinetics in your patient.

Unless 5 times the normal single dose of Erythromycin Estolate has been ingested, gastrointestinal decontamination should not be necessary. An accidental ingestion of Erythromycin should not be predicted to have minimal toxicity unless there is a good approximation of how much was ingested and unless only a single medication was involved.

Protect the patient's airway and support ventilation and perfusion. Meticulously monitor and maintain, within acceptable limits, the patient's vital signs, blood gases, serum electrolytes, etc. Absorption of drugs from the gastrointestinal tract may be decreased by giving activated charcoal, which, in many cases, is more effective than emesis or lavage; consider charcoal instead of or in addition to gastric emptying. Repeated doses of charcoal over time may hasten elimination of some drugs that have been absorbed. Safeguard the patient's airway when employing gastric emptying or charcoal.

Forced diuresis, peritoneal dialysis, hemodialysis, or charcoal hemoperfusion have not been established as beneficial for an overdosage of Erythromycin Estolate.

DOSAGE AND ADMINISTRATION

In most patients Erythromycin, Oral tablets are well absorbed and may be dosed orally without regard to meals. However, optimal blood levels are obtained when Erythromycin, Oral is given in the fasting state (at least ½ hour and preferably 2 hours before meals). However, blood levels obtained upon administration of enteric-coated Erythromycin products in the presence of food are still above minimal inhibitory concentrations (MICs) of most organisms for which Erythromycin is indicated.

Adults: The usual dosage of Erythromycin, Oral is 333 mg every 8 hours, 500 mg every 12 hours or 500 mg every 12 hours, taken in the fasting state of immediately before meals. Up to 4 g per day may be administered depending upon the severity of the infection. Dosage may be increased up to 4 g per day according to the severity of the infection. However, twice-a-day dosing is not recommended when doses larger than 1 g daily are administered.

400 mg Erythromycin Ethylsuccinate every 6 hours is the usual dose. Dosage may be increased up to 4 g per day according to the severity of the infection. If twice-a-day dosage is desired, one-half of the total daily dose may be given every 12 hours. Doses may also be given three times daily by administering one-third of the total daily dose every 8 hours. For adult dosage calculation, use a ratio of 400 mg of Erythromycin activity as the Ethylsuccinate to 250 mg of Erythromycin activity as the stearate, base or estolate.

Children: Age, weight, and severity of the infection are important factors in determining the proper dosage. In mild to moderate infections, The usual dosage is 30 to 50 mg/kg/day, in equally divided doses.

When dosage is desired on a twice-a-day schedule, one-half of the total daily dose may be taken every 12 hours in the fasting state or immediately before meals. Twice a day dosing is not recommended when doses larger than 1 g daily are administered.

Doses may also be given three times daily by administering one-third of the total daily dose every 8 hours.

The following dosage schedule is suggested for mild to moderate infections:

Body Weight	Total Daily Dose
Under 10 lbs	30-50 mg/kg/day 15-25 mg/lb/day
10 to 15 lbs	200 mg
16 to 25 lbs	400 mg
26 to 50 lbs	800 mg
51 to 100 lbs	1200 mg
over 100 lbs	1600 mg

For more severe infections this dosage may be doubled but should not exceed 4 g per day.

In the treatment of Group A beta-hemolytic streptococcal infections of the upper respiratory tract (e.g., tonsillitis or pharyngitis), the therapeutic dosage of Erythromycin should be administered for at least ten days. The American Heart Association suggests a dosage of 250 mg of Erythromycin orally, twice a day, in long-term prophylaxis of streptococcal upper respiratory tract infections for the prevention of recurring attacks of rheumatic fever in patients allergic to penicillin and sulfonamides.[4]

For the treatment of streptococcal pharyngitis and tonsillitis, the usual dosage range of Erythromycin Estolate is 20 to 50 mg/kg/day in divided doses.

Body Weight	Total Daily Dose
10 kg or less (less than 25 lb)	250 mg
11-18 kg (25-40 lb)	375 mg
18-25 kg (40-55 lb)	500 mg
25-36 kg (55-80 lb)	750 mg
36 kg or more (more than 80 lb)	1,000 mg (adult dose).

In prophylaxis against bacterial endocarditis (see *"Indications and Usage"* section) the oral regimen for penicillin allergic patients is Erythromycin or Erythromycin Estolate 1 gram (20 mg/kg for children) 1 hour before the procedure followed by 500 mg (10 mg/kg for children) six hours later[5]

In patients with congenital heart disease, or rheumatic or other acquired valvular heart disease when undergoing dental procedures or surgical procedures of the upper respiratory tract, give 1 g (20 mg/kg for children) of some brands orally 1 ½ to 2 hours before the procedure, and then, 500 mg (10 mg/kg for children) orally every 6 hours for 8 doses, or give 1.6 g (20 mg/kg for children) of Erythromycin Ethylsuccinate orally 1½ to 2 hours before the procedure, and then, 800 mg (10 mg/kg for children) orally every 6 hours for 8 doses.

Conjunctivitis of the newborn caused by Chlamydia trachomatis: Oral Erythromycin suspension 50 mg/kg/day in 4 divided doses for at least 2 weeks.[3]

Pneumonia of infancy caused by Chlamydia trachomatis: Although the optimal duration of therapy has not been established, the recommended therapy is oral Erythromycin suspension 50 mg/kg/day in 4 divided doses for at least 3 weeks.[3]

Urogenital infections during pregnancy due to Chlamydia trachomatis: Although the optimal dose and duration of therapy have not been established, the suggested treatment is 500 mg of Erythromycin by mouth four times a day or two Erythromycin 333 mg tablets orally every 8 hours on an empty stomach for at least 7 days. For women who cannot tolerate this regimen, a decreased dose of one Erythromycin 500 mg tablet orally every 12 hours, one 333 mg tablet orally every 8 hours or 250 mg by mouth four times a day should be used for at least 14 days.[3,6]

For adults with uncomplicated urethral, endocervical, or rectal infections caused by Chlamydia trachomatis, when tetracycline is contraindicated or not tolerated: 500 mg of Erythromycin by mouth four times a day or two 333 mg Erythromycin tablets orally every 8 hours for at least 7 days.[3,6]

800 mg of Erythromycin Ethylsuccinate three times a day for 7 days.

For patients with nongonococcal urethritis caused by Ureaplasma urealyticum when tetracycline is contraindicated or not tolerated: 500 mg of Erythromycin by mouth four times a day or two 333 mg tablets orally every 8 hours for at least seven days.[3,6]

Primary syphilis: 30 to 40 g Erythromycin or Erythromycin Stearate given in divided doses over a period of 10 to 15 days, 48 to 64 g of Erythromycin Ethylsuccinate given in divided doses over a period of 10 to 15 days, 20 g of Erythromycin Estolate in divided doses over a period of 10 days.

Acute pelvic inflammatory disease caused by N gonorrhoeae: 500 mg Erythrocin Lactobionate for injection every 6 hours for 3 days, followed by 500 mg of Erythromycin base orally, every 12 hours or 333 mg of Erythromycin base orally every 8 hours or 250 mg of some brands of Erythromycin or Erythromycin Stearate, every 6 hours for 7 days.

Intestinal amebiasis: Adults: 500 mg every 12 hours, or 333 mg every 8 hours or 250 mg of Erythromycin, Erythromycin Stearate, or Erythromycin Estolate, or 400 mg Erythromycin Ethylsuccinate every 6 hours for 10 to 14 days. Children: 30 to 50 mg/kg/day in divided doses for 10 to 14 days.

Pertussis: Although optimal dosage and duration have not been established, doses of Erythromycin utilized in reported clinical studies were 40 to 50 mg/kg/day, given in divided doses for 5 to 14 days.

Legionnaires' Disease: Although optimal dosage has not been established, doses utilized in reported clinical data were 1 to 4 g daily in divided doses.

REFERENCES

1. National Committee for Clinical Laboratory Standards, Approved Standard: *Performance Standards for Antimicrobial Disk Susceptibility Tests,* 3rd Edition, Vol. 4(16)FD,2-A3, Villanova, PA. December 1984. 2. Ericson, H.M., Sherris, J.C., Antibiotic Sensitivity Testing; Report of an International Collaborative Study, *Acta Pathologica et Microbiologica Scandinavica* Section B Suppl. 217:1-90, 1971. 3. CDC Sexually Transmitted Diseases Treatment Guidelines 1985. 4. Committee on Rheumatic Fever and Infective Endocarditis of the Council on Cardiovascular Disease of the Young: Prevention of Rheumatic Fever, *Circulation* 70(6);118A-1122A, December 1984. 5. Committee on Rheumatic Fever and Infective Endocarditis of the Council on Cardiovascular Disease of the Young: Prevention of Bacterial Endocarditis. *Circulation* 70(6):1123A-1127A, December 1984. 6. Data on file, Abbott Laboratories. 7. American Heart Association. 1977. Prevention of bacterial endocarditis. Circulation 56: 139A-143A. 8. Sexually Transmitted Diseases Treatment Guidelines 1982. Centers for

➤ SHOWN IN PRODUCT IDENTIFICATION GUIDE

Disease Control, Morbidity and Mortality Weekly Report, US Department of Health and Human Services, Atlanta, 1982; 31 (suppl): 355.

HOW SUPPLIED

ERYTHROMYCIN
CAPSULE, EXTENDED RELEASE: 250 MG

AVERAGE UNIT PRICE (AVAILABLE SIZES)		GENERIC A-RATED AVERAGE PRICE (GAAP)	
BRAND	$0.41		
GENERIC	$0.29	100s	$26.45
HCFA FUL (100s ea)	$0.27	500s	$121.26

BRAND/MANUFACTURER	NDC	SIZE	AWP
◆ BRAND			
➤ ERYC: Parke-Davis	00071-0696-24	100s	$40.83
◆ GENERICS			
UDL	51079-0671-98	60s	$60.00
Major	00904-2465-60	100s	$24.00
Moore,H.L.	00839-7602-06	100s	$24.23
➤ Abbott Pharm	00074-6301-13	100s	$24.32
Major	00904-7743-60	100s	$25.25
Schein	00364-2425-01	100s	$26.00
Barr	00555-0584-02	100s	$26.65
Purepac	00228-2553-10	100s	$26.72
URL	00677-1381-01	100s	$27.85
Rugby	00536-0368-01	100s	$27.88
Aligen	00405-4399-01	100s	$28.05
Qualitest	00603-3548-21	100s	$28.80
Major	00904-2465-40	500s	$108.45
Major	00904-7743-40	500s	$114.20
Moore,H.L.	00839-7602-12	500s	$114.68
➤ Abbott Pharm	00074-6301-53	500s	$118.54
Barr	00555-0584-04	500s	$122.90
Purepac	00228-2553-50	500s	$122.92
Qualitest	00603-3548-28	500s	$124.60
Rugby	00536-0368-05	500s	$128.63
Aligen	00405-4399-02	500s	$129.37

CAPSULE, EXTENDED RELEASE: 333 MG

AVERAGE UNIT PRICE (AVAILABLE SIZES)		GENERIC A-RATED AVERAGE PRICE (GAAP)	
GENERIC	$0.27	100s	$29.32

BRAND/MANUFACTURER	NDC	SIZE	AWP
◆ GENERICS			
Major	00904-2474-60	100s	$24.90
Moore,H.L.	00839-7660-06	100s	$33.74
Major	00904-2474-40	500s	$116.90

ENTERIC COATED TABLETS: 250 MG

AVERAGE UNIT PRICE (AVAILABLE SIZES)		GENERIC A-RATED AVERAGE PRICE (GAAP)	
BRAND	$0.21	100s	$20.42
GENERIC	$0.20	500s	$82.90

BRAND/MANUFACTURER	NDC	SIZE	AWP
◆ BRAND			
➤ E-MYCIN: Boots Labs	00524-0207-99	40s	$9.45
	00524-0207-01	100s	$24.05
	00524-0207-21	100s ud	$12.90
	00524-0207-05	500s	$115.00
◆ GENERICS			
➤ ERY-TAB: Abbott Pharm	00074-6304-30	30s	$7.13
➤ ERY-TAB: Abbott Pharm	00074-6304-40	40s	$8.91
ROBIMYCIN: Robins Pharm	00031-8317-63	100s	$11.38
➤ ERY-TAB: Abbott Pharm	00074-6304-13	100s	$23.75
➤ ERY-TAB: Abbott Pharm	00074-6304-11	100s ud	$26.13
ROBIMYCIN: Robins Pharm	00031-8317-70	500s	$52.99
ERY-TAB: Abbott Pharm	00074-6304-53	500s	$112.81

ENTERIC COATED TABLETS: 333 MG

AVERAGE UNIT PRICE (AVAILABLE SIZES)		GENERIC A-RATED AVERAGE PRICE (GAAP)	
BRAND	$0.38	100s	$36.16
GENERIC	$0.36		

BRAND/MANUFACTURER	NDC	SIZE	AWP
◆ BRAND			
➤ E-MYCIN 333: Boots Labs	00524-0208-01	100s	$41.55
	00524-0208-21	100s ud	$34.40
	00524-0208-05	500s	$193.30
◆ GENERICS			
➤ ERY-TAB: Abbott Pharm	00074-6320-30	30s	$11.92
➤ ERY-TAB: Abbott Pharm	00074-6320-13	100s	$34.97
➤ ERY-TAB: Abbott Pharm	00074-6320-11	100s ud	$37.35
➤ ERY-TAB: Abbott Pharm	00074-6320-53	500s	$166.12

ENTERIC COATED TABLETS: 500 MG

AVERAGE UNIT PRICE (AVAILABLE SIZES)		GENERIC A-RATED AVERAGE PRICE (GAAP)	
GENERIC	$0.41	100s	$41.29

BRAND/MANUFACTURER	NDC	SIZE	AWP
◆ GENERICS			
➤ ERY-TAB: Abbott Pharm	00074-6321-13	100s	$40.10
➤ ERY-TAB: Abbott Pharm	00074-6321-11	100s ud	$42.48

GEL: 2%

AVERAGE UNIT PRICE (AVAILABLE SIZES)	
BRAND	$0.57
GENERIC	$0.43
GENERIC	$0.55

BRAND/MANUFACTURER	NDC	SIZE	AWP
◆ GENERICS			
Qualitest	00603-7735-78	30 gm	$13.27
Qualitest	00603-7735-88	60 gm	$24.89

TABLET, COATED PARTICLES: 333 MG

BRAND/MANUFACTURER	NDC	SIZE	AWP
○ BRAND			
➤ PCE DISPERTAB: Abbott Pharm	00074-6290-60	60s	$67.58

TABLET, COATED PARTICLES: 500 MG

BRAND/MANUFACTURER	NDC	SIZE	AWP
○ BRAND			
➤ PCE DISPERTAB: Abbott Pharm	00074-3389-13	100s	$148.50

TABLET, EXTENDED RELEASE: 250 MG

AVERAGE UNIT PRICE (AVAILABLE SIZES)	
GENERIC	$0.26

BRAND/MANUFACTURER	NDC	SIZE	AWP
◆ GENERICS			
Goldline	00182-1398-01	100s	$27.00
Goldline	00182-1398-05	500s	$120.00

TABLET, EXTENDED RELEASE: 333 MG

AVERAGE UNIT PRICE (AVAILABLE SIZES)		GENERIC A-RATED AVERAGE PRICE (GAAP)	
GENERIC	$0.30	100s	$32.45
HCFA FUL (100s ea)	$0.34	500s	$136.74

BRAND/MANUFACTURER	NDC	SIZE	AWP
◆ GENERICS			
Moore,H.L.	00839-7656-06	100s	$31.04
Major	00904-2472-60	100s	$31.10
Aligen	00405-4398-01	100s	$35.22
Moore,H.L.	00839-7656-12	500s	$99.89
Major	00904-2472-40	500s	$147.50
Aligen	00405-4398-02	500s	$162.82

ERYTHROMYCIN STEARATE
TABLETS: 250 MG

AVERAGE UNIT PRICE (AVAILABLE SIZES)		GENERIC A-RATED AVERAGE PRICE (GAAP)	
BRAND	$0.14	100s	$14.45
GENERIC	$0.14	500s	$64.97
HCFA FUL (100s ea)	$0.14	1000s	$121.29

BRAND/MANUFACTURER	NDC	SIZE	AWP
◆ BRAND			
➤ ERYTHROCIN STEARATE FILMTAB: Abbott Pharm			
	00074-6346-41	40s	$5.59
	00074-6346-20	100s	$13.75
	00074-6346-38	100s ud	$16.13
	00074-6346-53	500s	$65.31
	00074-6346-19	1000s	$126.71
◆ GENERICS			
Raway	00686-0106-01	100s	$9.22
Med-Derm	45565-0006-01	100s	$9.50
➤ Mylan	00378-0106-01	100s	$14.46
Aligen	00405-4411-01	100s	$14.92
Rugby	00536-0250-01	100s	$15.17
Parmed	00349-1011-01	100s	$15.18
URL	00677-0343-01	100s	$15.25
Zenith	00172-2458-60	100s	$15.45
Major	00904-2458-60	100s	$15.50
Goldline	00182-0538-01	100s	$15.75
MY-E: Seneca	47028-0013-01	100s	$16.86
Moore,H.L.	00839-5079-06	100s	$18.16
U.S. Trading	56126-0397-11	100s ud	$12.44
Rugby	00536-0250-05	500s	$56.19
Major	00904-2458-40	500s	$57.50

◆ RATED THERAPEUTICALLY EQUIVALENT; ◇ THERAPEUTIC EQUIVALENCE UNCONFIRMED; ○ UNRATED

BRAND/MANUFACTURER	NDC	SIZE	AWP
URL	00677-0343-05	500s	$57.95
Goldline	00182-0538-05	500s	$60.00
Qualitest	00603-3553-28	500s	$67.40
➤ Mylan	00378-0106-05	500s	$67.50
Parmed	00349-1011-05	500s	$71.68
Zenith	00172-2458-70	500s	$71.70
Aligen	00405-4411-02	500s	$74.84
Rugby	00536-0250-10	1000s	$109.00
Moore, H.L.	00839-5079-16	1000s	$133.58

TABLETS: 400 MG

AVERAGE UNIT PRICE (AVAILABLE SIZES)		GENERIC A-RATED AVERAGE PRICE (GAAP)	
BRAND	$0.22	100s	$22.64
GENERIC	$0.23	500s	$117.08
HCFA FUL (100s ea)	$0.22		

BRAND/MANUFACTURER	NDC	SIZE	AWP
◆ BRAND			
➤ E.E.S.-400 FILMTAB: Abbott Pharm	00074-5729-13	100s	$21.92
	00074-5729-11	100s ud	$24.30
	00074-5729-53	500s	$104.12
	00074-5729-19	1000s	$189.57
◆ GENERICS			
Major	00904-2464-39	40s	$11.30
Major	00904-2464-60	100s	$21.75
Abbott Pharm	00074-2589-13	100s	$21.92
Mylan	00378-6400-01	100s	$22.35
Qualitest	00603-3552-21	100s	$22.95
Aligen	00405-4406-01	100s	$23.80
Parmed	00349-8403-01	100s	$23.91
Moore, H.L.	00839-6588-06	100s	$25.77
U.S. Trading	56126-0387-11	100s ud	$18.66
Abbott Pharm	00074-2589-53	500s	$104.12
Mylan	00378-6400-05	500s	$106.15
Major	00904-2464-40	500s	$106.15
Qualitest	00603-3552-28	500s	$109.40
Parmed	00349-8403-05	500s	$133.55
Moore, H.L.	00839-6588-12	500s	$143.10

TABLETS: 500 MG

AVERAGE UNIT PRICE (AVAILABLE SIZES)		GENERIC A-RATED AVERAGE PRICE (GAAP)	
BRAND	$0.25	100s	$27.37
GENERIC	$0.27		
HCFA FUL (100s ea)	$0.22		

BRAND/MANUFACTURER	NDC	SIZE	AWP
◆ BRAND			
➤ ERYTHROCIN STEARATE FILMTAB: Abbott Pharm	00074-6316-13	100s	$24.85
◆ GENERICS			
Raway	00686-0107-01	100s	$17.00
Aligen	00405-4412-01	100s	$24.32
Rugby	00536-0265-01	100s	$25.38
Major	00904-2459-60	100s	$25.60
Goldline	00182-0539-01	100s	$27.00
Qualitest	00603-3554-21	100s	$27.40
➤ Mylan	00378-0107-01	100s	$28.62
Zenith	00172-2823-60	100s	$28.90
Parmed	00349-1010-01	100s	$29.95
URL	00677-0344-01	100s	$31.50
Moore, H.L.	00839-5185-06	100s	$40.84
U.S. Trading	56126-0391-11	100s ud	$21.96
Major	00904-2459-40	500s	$97.90

ERYTHROMYCIN ESTOLATE
CAPSULE: 250 MG

AVERAGE UNIT PRICE (AVAILABLE SIZES)		GENERIC A-RATED AVERAGE PRICE (GAAP)	
BRAND	$0.51	100s	$33.47
GENERIC	$0.34		
HCFA FUL (100s ea)	$0.19		

BRAND/MANUFACTURER	NDC	SIZE	AWP
◆ BRAND			
ILOSONE: Dista	00777-0809-02	100s	$50.97
◆ GENERICS			
Rugby	00536-0322-01	100s	$26.24
URL	00677-0653-01	100s	$27.70
Geneva	00781-2070-01	100s	$27.75
Schein	00364-0530-01	100s	$31.30
Barr	00555-0230-02	100s	$31.38
Qualitest	00603-3551-21	100s	$31.40
Aligen	00405-4401-01	100s	$43.32
Major	00904-2468-60	100s	$48.70

SUSPENSION: 125 MG/5 ML

AVERAGE UNIT PRICE (AVAILABLE SIZES)		GENERIC A-RATED AVERAGE PRICE (GAAP)	
BRAND	$0.09	480 ml	$28.37
GENERIC	$0.06		
HCFA FUL (480 ml)	$0.04		

BRAND/MANUFACTURER	NDC	SIZE	AWP
◆ BRAND			
ILOSONE LIQUID 125: Dista	00777-2315-05	480 ml	$42.09
◆ GENERICS			
Major	00904-2470-16	480 ml	$26.40
Goldline	00182-1560-40	480 ml	$26.40
Qualitest	00603-1202-58	480 ml	$28.08
Barre	00472-0977-16	480 ml	$28.60
URL	00677-0838-33	480 ml	$29.00
Schein	00364-2078-16	480 ml	$29.06
Rugby	00536-0335-85	480 ml	$31.05

SUSPENSION: 250 MG/5 ML

AVERAGE UNIT PRICE (AVAILABLE SIZES)		GENERIC A-RATED AVERAGE PRICE (GAAP)	
BRAND	$0.17	480 ml	$44.07
GENERIC	$0.09		
HCFA FUL (480 ml)	$0.07		

BRAND/MANUFACTURER	NDC	SIZE	AWP
◆ BRAND			
ILOSONE LIQUID 250: Dista	00777-2317-48	100 ml	$17.70
	00777-2317-05	480 ml	$75.76
◆ GENERICS			
Moore, H.L.	00839-6714-69	480 ml	$38.85
Rugby	00536-0337-85	480 ml	$41.18
Qualitest	00603-1203-58	480 ml	$41.85
Major	00904-2471-16	480 ml	$41.90
URL	00677-0839-33	480 ml	$45.85
Goldline	00182-1567-40	480 ml	$45.90
Barre	00472-0979-16	480 ml	$47.30
Schein	00364-2079-16	480 ml	$49.69

TABLETS: 500 MG

BRAND/MANUFACTURER	NDC	SIZE	AWP
○ BRAND			
ILOSONE: Dista	00777-2126-50	50s	$44.39

ERYTHROMYCIN ETHYLSUCCINATE
CHEW TABLET: 200 MG

BRAND/MANUFACTURER	NDC	SIZE	AWP
◆ BRAND			
➤ ERYPED: Abbott Pharm	00074-6314-40	40s	$19.64

CHEW TABLET: 400 MG

AVERAGE UNIT PRICE (AVAILABLE SIZES)	
GENERIC	$0.24

BRAND/MANUFACTURER	NDC	SIZE	AWP
◆ GENERICS			
Goldline	00182-1489-01	100s	$26.10
Goldline	00182-1489-05	500s	$110.00

DROP: 100 MG/2.5 ML

BRAND/MANUFACTURER	NDC	SIZE	AWP
○ BRAND			
ERYPED: Abbott Pharm	00074-6303-50	50 ml	$6.21

GRANULAR: 200 MG/5 ML

BRAND/MANUFACTURER	NDC	SIZE	AWP
◆ GENERICS			
Aligen	00405-2730-70	200 gm	$9.95

GRANULE FOR RECONSTITUTION: 200 MG/5 ML

AVERAGE UNIT PRICE (AVAILABLE SIZES)		GENERIC A-RATED AVERAGE PRICE (GAAP)	
BRAND	$0.08	100 gm	$7.35
GENERIC	$0.07	200 gm	$15.10
HCFA FUL (100 gm)	$0.07		
HCFA FUL (200 gm)	$0.07		

BRAND/MANUFACTURER	NDC	SIZE	AWP
◆ BRAND			
E.E.S. GRANULES: Abbott Pharm	00074-6369-02	100 gm	$7.91
	00074-6369-10	200 gm	$14.43

➤ SHOWN IN PRODUCT IDENTIFICATION GUIDE

BRAND/MANUFACTURER		NDC	SIZE	AWP
◆ **GENERICS**				
Aligen		00405-2730-60	100 gm	$5.14
Moore,H.L.		00839-6362-73	100 gm	$7.41
Rugby		00536-0318-82	100 gm	$8.18
Major		00904-2653-04	100 gm	$8.65
Moore,H.L.		00839-6362-78	200 gm	$13.89
Major		00904-2653-08	200 gm	$16.30

SUSPENSION: 200 MG/5 ML

AVERAGE UNIT PRICE (AVAILABLE SIZES)		GENERIC A-RATED AVERAGE PRICE (GAAP)	
BRAND	$0.08	100 ml	$6.62
GENERIC	$0.05	200 ml	$13.43
HCFA FUL (480 ml)	$0.02	480 ml	$20.05

BRAND/MANUFACTURER	NDC	SIZE	AWP
◆ **BRAND**			
E.E.S.-200: Abbott Pharm	00074-6306-13	100 ml	$4.50
ERYPED 200: Abbott Pharm	00074-6302-13	100 ml	$7.70
	00074-6302-53	200 ml	$14.02
E.E.S.-200: Abbott Pharm	00074-6306-16	480 ml	$19.59
ERYPED 200: Abbott Pharm	00074-6302-05	5 ml 100s ud	$74.00
◆ **GENERICS**			
Bausch&Lomb Pharm	24208-0965-39	100 ml	$5.05
Barr	00555-0215-22	100 ml	$7.01
Goldline	00182-1530-70	100 ml	$7.80
Barr	00555-0215-23	200 ml	$12.95
Goldline	00182-1530-73	200 ml	$13.90
Bausch&Lomb Pharm	24208-0965-94	480 ml	$16.80
Moore,H.L.	00839-6482-69	480 ml	$18.70
Goldline	00182-1371-40	480 ml	$19.00
Barre	00472-0971-16	480 ml	$19.04
Abbott Pharm	00074-3747-16	480 ml	$19.59
Qualitest	00603-1206-58	480 ml	$19.85
URL	00677-0673-33	480 ml	$20.65
Rugby	00536-0360-85	480 ml	$20.70
Major	00904-2462-16	480 ml	$20.95
Schein	00364-2067-16	480 ml	$22.00

SUSPENSION: 400 MG/5 ML

AVERAGE UNIT PRICE (AVAILABLE SIZES)		GENERIC A-RATED AVERAGE PRICE (GAAP)	
BRAND	$0.12	480 ml	$36.52
GENERIC	$0.08		
HCFA FUL (480 ml)	$0.04		

BRAND/MANUFACTURER	NDC	SIZE	AWP
◆ **BRAND**			
E.E.S.-400: Abbott Pharm	00074-6373-13	100 ml	$8.09
	00074-6373-16	480 ml	$36.49
ERYPED 400: Abbott Pharm	00074-6305-05	5 ml 100s ud	$108.00
◆ **GENERICS**			
Bausch&Lomb Pharm	24208-0970-39	100 ml	$9.10
Bausch&Lomb Pharm	24208-0970-94	480 ml	$30.45
Moore,H.L.	00839-6568-69	480 ml	$31.44
ERYTHRO: Mason Dist	11845-0422-13	480 ml	$32.60
Barre	00472-0974-16	480 ml	$33.39
Qualitest	00603-1207-58	480 ml	$34.90
Abbott Pharm	00074-3748-16	480 ml	$36.49
Goldline	00182-1773-40	480 ml	$37.45
URL	00677-1033-33	480 ml	$38.90
Schein	00364-2070-16	480 ml	$38.99
Major	00904-2463-16	480 ml	$39.75
Rugby	00536-0371-85	480 ml	$41.25

SUSPENSION: 400 MG/5 ML

BRAND/MANUFACTURER	NDC	SIZE	AWP
○ **BRAND**			
ERYPED 400: Abbott Pharm	00074-6305-60	60 ml	$7.78
	00074-6305-13	100 ml	$11.85
	00074-6305-53	200 ml	$21.62

Erythromycin, Topical

DESCRIPTION

Erythromycin, Topical, is a macrolide antibiotic produced from a strain of *Streptomyces erythraeus*. It is basic and readily forms salts with acids. Each mL of Erythromycin, Topical Solution or Gel contains 20 mg of Erythromycin base.

The empirical formula for Erythromycin is $C_{37}H_{67}NO_{13}$ and the molecular weight is 733.94.

Following is its chemical structure:

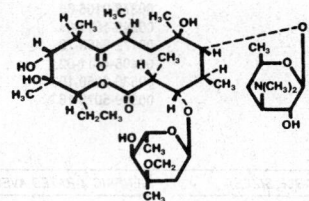

ACTIONS

Although the mechanism by which Erythromycin Topical Solution or Gel acts in reducing inflammatory lesions of acne vulgaris is unknown, it is presumably due to its antibiotic action.

Microbiology: Erythromycin appears to inhibit protein synthesis in susceptible organisms by reversibly binding to ribosomal subunits, thereby inhibiting translocation of aminoacyl transfer-RNA and inhibiting polypeptide synthesis. Antagonism has been demonstrated between Erythromycin, lincomycin, chloramphenicol, and clindamycin.

INDICATIONS

Erythromycin, Topical, is indicated for the topical treatment of acne vulgaris.

CONTRAINDICATIONS

Erythromycin, Topical, is contraindicated in persons who have shown hypersensitivity to any of its ingredients.

WARNING

The safe use of Erythromycin, Topical, during pregnancy or lactation has not been established.

PRECAUTIONS

General: The use of antibiotic agents may be associated with the overgrowth of antibiotic-resistant organisms. If this occurs, administration of the drug should be discontinued and appropriate measures taken.

Information for Patients: Erythromycin, Topical is for external use only and should be kept away from the eyes, nose, mouth, and other mucous membranes. Concomitant topical acne therapy should be used with caution because a cumulative irritant effect may occur, especially with the use of peeling, desquamating, or abrasive agents.

Carcinogenesis, Mutagenesis, Impairment of Fertility: Long-term animal studies to evaluate carcinogenic potential, mutagenicity, or the effect on fertility of Erythromycin have not been performed.

Pregnancy: Categories B and C.: There was no evidence of teratogenicity or any other adverse effect on reproduction in female rats fed Erythromycin base (up to 0.25% of diet) before and during mating, during gestation, and through weaning of two successive litters. There are, however, no adequate and well-controlled studies in pregnant women. Because animal reproduction studies are not always predictive of human response, this drug should be used in pregnancy only if clearly needed. Erythromycin has been reported to cross the placental barrier in humans, but fetal plasma levels are generally low.

Nursing Mothers: Erythromycin is excreted in breast milk. Caution should be exercised when Erythromycin is administered to a nursing woman.

Pediatric Use: Safety and effectiveness in children have not been established.

ADVERSE REACTIONS

Adverse conditions reported with the use of Erythromycin Topical solutions and gel include dryness, tenderness, pruritus, desquamation, erythema, oiliness, and burning sensation. Irritation of the eyes has also been reported. A case of generalized urticarial reaction, possibly related to the drug, which required the use of systemic steroid therapy has been reported.

Of a total of 90 patients exposed to Erythromycin, Topical during clinical effectiveness studies, 17 experienced some type of adverse effect. These included dry skin, scaly skin, pruritus, irritation of the eye, and burning sensation.

DOSAGE AND ADMINISTRATION

Erythromycin, Topical solution and gel should be applied as a thin layer to the affected area twice a day after the skin is thoroughly washed with warm water and soap and patted dry. Moisten the applicator or a pad with Erythromycin, Topical, then rub over the affected area. Acne lesions on the face, neck, shoulder, chest, and back may be treated in this manner.

The hands should be washed after application. If there has been no improvement after 6-8 weeks, or if the condition becomes worse, treatment should be discontinued, and the physician should be reconsulted. Spread the gel lightly rather than rubbing it in.

When using an applicator top, it should be moistened first by holding the bottle upside down and pressing once on the applicator surface with a clean finger. Then the solution can be applied with the applicator to the affected area(s) using a

---

◆ RATED THERAPEUTICALLY EQUIVALENT; ◇ THERAPEUTIC EQUIVALENCE UNCONFIRMED; ○ UNRATED

dabbing motion. To avoid excessive flow, the bottle should not be squeezed when applying medication. The bottle should be closed tightly after each use.

There are no data directly comparing the safety and efficacy of b.i.d. versus q.d. dosing.

Store at controlled room temperature (59-77°F).

Note: **FLAMMABLE: Keep away from heat and flame.**

HOW SUPPLIED
GEL: 2%

AVERAGE UNIT PRICE (AVAILABLE SIZES)	
BRAND	$0.57
GENERIC	$0.43
GENERIC	$0.55

BRAND/MANUFACTURER	NDC	SIZE	AWP
◆ BRAND			
A/T/S: Hoechst Derm	00039-0116-30	30 gm	$16.70
ERYGEL: Allergan Inc	00023-4312-30	30 gm	$17.83
	00023-4312-60	60 gm	$33.51
◆ GENERICS			
EMGEL: Glaxo Derm	00173-0440-01	27 gm	$18.08
Glades	59366-2462-03	30 gm	$15.16
EMGEL: Glaxo Derm	00173-0440-02	50 gm	$27.55
Glades	59366-2462-05	60 gm	$28.49

LIQUID: 2%

BRAND/MANUFACTURER	NDC	SIZE	AWP
◆ BRAND			
C-SOLVE-2: Syosset	47854-0668-19	30 ml	$2.95

OINTMENT: 2%

BRAND/MANUFACTURER	NDC	SIZE	AWP
◆ GENERICS			
AKNE-MYCIN: Hermal	48017-3501-01	25 gm	$18.00

SOLUTION: 1.5%

AVERAGE UNIT PRICE (AVAILABLE SIZES)		GENERIC A-RATED AVERAGE PRICE (GAAP)	
GENERIC	$0.21	60 ml	$12.87

BRAND/MANUFACTURER	NDC	SIZE	AWP
◆ GENERICS			
Major	00904-2844-03	60 ml	$5.25
STATICIN: Westwood-Squibb	00072-8000-60	60 ml	$20.48

SOLUTION: 2%

AVERAGE UNIT PRICE (AVAILABLE SIZES)		GENERIC A-RATED AVERAGE PRICE (GAAP)	
BRAND	$0.27	60 ml	$7.62
GENERIC	$0.13		
HCFA FUL (60 ml)	$0.07		

BRAND/MANUFACTURER	NDC	SIZE	AWP
◆ BRAND			
A/T/S: Hoechst Derm	00039-0016-60	60 ml	$16.40
◆ GENERICS			
ERYTHRA-DERM:	00574-0014-02	60 ml	$4.25
Clay-Park	45802-0038-46	60 ml	$4.32
Moore,H.L.	00839-7023-64	60 ml	$4.71
Schein	00364-2073-58	60 ml	$4.75
Pennex	00832-8671-60	60 ml	$4.80
Pennex	00426-8671-60	60 ml	$5.00
Rugby	00536-0292-96	60 ml	$5.18
Aligen	00405-2825-56	60 ml	$5.25
Major	00904-2845-03	60 ml	$5.25
Bausch&Lomb Pharm	24208-0551-67	60 ml	$5.25
URL	00677-1402-25	60 ml	$5.30
Qualitest	00603-7737-52	60 ml	$5.30
Raway	00686-1244-02	60 ml	$6.00
Barre	00472-1244-92	60 ml	$6.88
Geneva	00781-7013-61	60 ml	$7.49
Goldline	00182-1561-43	60 ml	$7.50
AKNE-MYCIN: Hermal	48017-9211-05	60 ml	$8.33
Syosset	47854-0668-20	60 ml	$12.00
ERYDERM: Abbott Pharm	00074-2698-02	60 ml	$15.84
T-STAT: Westwood-Squibb	00072-8300-60	60 ml	$15.84
ERYMAX: Allergan Inc	00023-0540-02	60 ml	$17.86
ERYMAX: Allergan Inc	00023-0540-04	120 ml	$31.56

SWAB: 2%

BRAND/MANUFACTURER	NDC	SIZE	AWP
◆ BRAND			
ERYCETTE: Ortho Pharm	00062-1185-01	60s	$18.78

Esidrix *SEE* HYDROCHLOROTHIAZIDE

Esimil *SEE* GUANETHIDINE MONOSULFATE WITH HYDROCHLOROTHIAZIDE

Eskalith *SEE* LITHIUM CARBONATE

Esmolol Hydrochloride

Not for direct intravenous injection. Must be diluted prior to its infusion. See *"Dosage and Administration"* section.

DESCRIPTION
Each ampule contains 250 mg of Esmolol Hydrochloride per mL (2.5 g per 10 mL ampule). Each single dose vial contains 10 mg of Esmolol Hydrochloride per mL (100 mg per 10 mL vial).

Following is its chemical structure:

$$CH_3OCCH_2CH_2 - \langle \text{ring} \rangle - OCH_2CHCH_2NHCH(CH_3)_2 \cdot HCl$$

INDICATIONS AND USAGE
SUPRAVENTRICULAR TACHYCARDIA
Esmolol HCl is indicated for the rapid control of ventricular rate in patients with atrial fibrillation or atrial flutter in perioperative, postoperative, or other emergent circumstances where short term control of ventricular rate with a short-acting agent is desirable. Esmolol HCl is also indicated in noncompensatory sinus tachycardia where, in the physician's judgment, the rapid heart rate requires specific intervention. Esmolol HCl is not intended for use in chronic settings where transfer to another agent is anticipated.

INTRAOPERATIVE AND POSTOPERATIVE TACHYCARDIA AND/OR HYPERTENSION
Esmolol HCl is indicated for the treatment of tachycardia and hypertension that occur during induction and tracheal intubation, during surgery, on emergence from anesthesia, and in the postoperative period, when in the physician's judgment such specific intervention is considered indicated.

Use of Esmolol HCl to prevent such events is not recommended.

UNLABELED USES
Esmolol HCl is used alone or as an adjunct in the treatment of thyrotoxicosis crisis, pheochromocytoma, unstable angina, and in myocardial infarction to improve postischemia recovery.

CONTRAINDICATIONS
Esmolol HCl is contraindicated in patients with sinus bradycardia, heart block greater than first degree, cardiogenic shock or overt heart failure (see *"Warnings"*).

WARNINGS
Hypotension: In clinical trials 20-50% of patients treated with Esmolol HCl have experienced hypotension, generally defined as systolic pressure less than 90 mmHg and/or diastolic pressure less than 50 mmHg. About 12% of the patients have been symptomatic (mainly diaphoresis or dizziness). Hypotension can occur at any dose but is dose-related so that doses beyond 200 mcg/kg/min (0.2 mg/kg/min) are not recommended. Patients should be closely monitored, especially if pretreatment blood pressure is low. Decrease of dose or termination of infusion reverses hypotension, usually within 30 minutes.

Cardiac Failure: Sympathetic stimulation is necessary in supporting circulatory function in congestive heart failure, and beta blockade carries the potential hazard of further depressing myocardial contractility and precipitating more severe failure. Continued depression of the myocardium with beta blocking agents over a period of time can, in some cases, lead to cardiac failure. At the first sign or symptom of impending cardiac failure, Esmolol HCl should be withdrawn. Although withdrawal may be sufficient because of the short elimination half-life of Esmolol HCl, specific treatment may also be considered. The use of Esmolol HCl for control of ventricular response in patients with supraventricular arrhythmias should be undertaken with caution when the patient is compromised hemodynamically or is taking other drugs that decrease any or all of the following: peripheral resistance, myocardial filling, myocardial contractility, or electrical impulse propagation in the myocardium. Despite the rapid onset and offset of Esmolol HCl's effects, several cases of death have been reported in complex clinical states where Esmolol HCl was presumably being used to control ventricular rate.

Intraoperative and Postoperative Tachycardia and/or Hypertension: Esmolol HCl should not be used as the treatment for hypertension in patients in whom the increased blood pressure is primarily due to the vasoconstriction associated with hypothemia.

Bronchospastic Diseases: PATIENTS WITH BRONCHOSPASTIC DISEASES SHOULD, IN GENERAL, NOT RECEIVE BETA BLOCKERS. Because of its relative beta$_1$ selectivity and titrability, Esmolol HCl may be used with caution in patients with bronchospastic diseases. However, since beta$_1$ selectivity is not absolute, Esmolol HCl should be carefully titrated to obtain the lowest possible effective dose. In the event of bronchospasm, the infusion should be terminated immediately; a beta$_2$ stimulating agent may be administered if conditions warrant but should be used with particular caution as patients already have rapid ventricular rates.

Diabetes Mellitus and Hypoglycemia: Esmolol HCl should be used with caution in diabetic patients requiring a beta blocking agent. Beta blockers may mask tachycardia occuring with hypoglycemia, but other manifestations such as dizziness and sweating may not be significantly affected.

PRECAUTIONS
GENERAL
Infusion concentrations of 20 mg/mL were associated with more serious venous irritation, including thrombophlebitis, than concentrations of 10 mg/mL. Extravasation of 20 mg/mL may lead to a serious local reaction and possible skin necrosis. Concentrations greater than 10 mg/mL or infusion into small veins or through a butterfly catheter should be avoided.

Because the acid metabolite of Esmolol HCl is primarily excreted unchanged by the kidney Esmolol HCl should be administered with caution to patients with impaired renal function. The elimination half-life of the acid metabolite was prolonged ten-fold and the plasma level was considerably elevated in patients with end-stage renal disease.

Care should be taken in the intravenous administration of Esmolol HCl as sloughing of the skin and necrosis have been reported in association with infiltration and extravasation of intravenous infusions.

DRUG INTERACTIONS
Catecholamine depleting drugs, e.g., reserpine, may have an additive effect when given with beta blocking agents. Patients treated concurrently with Esmolol HCl and a catecholamine depletor should therefore be closely observed for evidence of hypotension or marked bradycardia, which may result in vertigo, syncope, or postural hypotension.

A study of interaction between Esmolol HCl and warfarin showed that concomitant administration of Esmolol HCl and warfarin does not alter warfarin plasma levels. Esmolol HCl concentrations were equivocally higher when given with warfarin, but this is not likely to be clinically important.

When digoxin and Esmolol HCl were concomitantly administered intravenously to normal volunteers, there was a 10-20% increase in digoxin blood levels at some time points. Digoxin did not affect Esmolol HCl pharmacokinetics. When intravenous morphine and Esmolol HCl were concomitantly administered in normal subjects, no effect on Morphine blood levels was seen, but Esmolol HCl steady-state blood levels were increased by 46% in the presence of morphine. No other pharmacokinetic parameters were changed.

The effect of Esmolol HCl on the duration of succinylcholine-induced neuromuscular blockade was studied in patients undergoing surgery. The onset of neuromuscular blockade by succinylcholine was unaffected by Esmolol HCl, but the duration of neuromuscular blockade was prolonged from 5 minutes to 8 minutes.

Although the interactions observed in these studies do not appear to be of major clinical importance, Esmolol HCl should be titrated with caution in patients being treated concurrently with digoxin, morphine, succinylcholine or warfarin.

While taking beta-blockers, patients with a history of severe anaphylactic reaction to a variety of allergens may be more reactive to repeated challenge, either accidental, diagnostic, or therapeutic. Such patients may be unresponsive to the usual doses of Esmolol HCl used to treat allergic reaction.

Caution should be exercised when considering the use of Esmolol HCl and verapamil in patients with depressed myocardial function. Fatal cardiac arrests have occurred in patients receiving both drugs. Additionally, Esmolol HCl should not be used to control supraventricular tachycardia in the presence of agents which are vasoconstrictive and inotropic such as dopamine, epinephrine, and norepinephrine because of the danger of blocking cardiac contractility when systemic vascular resistance is high.

CARCINOGENESIS, MUTAGENESIS, IMPAIRMENT OF FERTILITY
Because of its short term usage no carcinogenicity, mutagenicity or reproductive performance studies have been conducted with Esmolol HCl.

PREGNANCY CATEGORY C
Teratogenicity studies in rats at intravenous dosages of Esmolol HCl up to 3000 mcg/kg/min (3 mg/kg/min) (ten times the maximum human maintenance dosage) for 30 minutes daily produced no evidence of maternal toxicity, embryotoxicity or teratogenicity, while a dosage of 10,000 mcg/kg/min (10 mg/kg/min) produced maternal toxicity and lethality. In rabbits, intravenous dosages up to 1000 mcg/kg/min (1 mg/kg/min) for 30 minutes daily produced no evidence of maternal toxicity, embryotoxicity or teratogenicity, while 2500 mcg/kg/min (2.5 mg/kg/min) produced minimal maternal toxicity and increased fetal resorptions.

Although there are no adequate and well-controlled studies in pregnant women, use of Esmolol in the last trimester of pregnancy or during labor delivery has been reported to cause fetal bradycardia, which continued after termination of drug infusion. Esmolol HCl should be used during pregnancy only if the potential benefit justifies the potential risk to the fetus.

NURSING MOTHERS
It is not known whether Esmolol HCl is excreted in human milk, however, caution should be exercised when Esmolol HCl is administered to a nursing woman.

PEDIATRIC USE
The safety and effectiveness of Esmolol HCl in children have not been established.

ADVERSE REACTIONS
The following adverse reaction rates are based on use of Esmolol HCl in clinical trials involving 369 patients with supraventricular tachycardia and over 600 intraoperative and postoperative patients enrolled in clinical trials. Most adverse effects observed in controlled clinical trial settings have been mild and transient. The most important adverse effect has been hypotension (see *"Warnings"*). Deaths have been reported in post-marketing experience occurring during complex clinical states where Esmolol HCl was presumably being used simply to control ventricular rate (see *"Warnings, Cardiac Failure"*).

Cardiovascular: Symptomatic hypotension (diaphoresis, dizziness) occurred in 12% of patients, and therapy was discontinued in about 11%, about half of whom were symptomatic. Asymptomatic hypotension occurred in about 25% of patients. Hypotension resolved during Esmolol HCl infusion in 63% of these patients and within 30 minutes after discontinuation of infusion in 80% of the remaining patients. Diaphoresis accompanied hypotension in 10% of patients. Peripheral ischemia occurred in approximately 1% of patients. Pallor, flushing, bradycardia (heart rate less than 50 beats per minute), chest pain, syncope, pulmonary edema and heart block have each been reported in less than 1% of patients. In two patients without supraventricular tachycardia but with serious coronary artery disease (post inferior myocardial infarction or unstable angina), severe bradycardia/sinus pause/asystole has developed, reversible in both cases with discontinuation of treatment.

Central Nervous System: Dizziness has occurred in 3% of patients; somnolence in 3%, confusion, headache, and agitation in about 2%, and fatigue in about 1% of patients. Paresthesia, asthenia, depression, abnormal thinking, anxiety, anorexia, and lightheadedness were reported in less than 1% of patients. Seizures were also reported in less than 1% of patients, with one death.

Respiratory: Bronchospasm, wheezing, dyspnea, nasal congestion, rhonchi, and rales have each been reported in less than 1% of patients.

Gastrointestinal: Nausea was reported in 7% of patients. Vomiting has occurred in about 1% of patients. Dyspepsia, constipation, dry mouth, and abdominal discomfort have each occurred in less than 1% of patients. Taste perversion has also been reported.

Skin (Infusion Site): Infusion site reactions including inflammation and induration were reported in about 8% of patients. Edema, erythema, skin discoloration, burning at the infusion site, thrombophlebitis, and local skin necrosis from extravasation have each occurred in less than 1% of patients.

Miscellaneous: Each of the following has been reported in less than 1% of patients: Urinary retention, speech disorder, abnormal vision, midscapular pain, rigors, and fever.

DOSAGE AND ADMINISTRATION
2.5 G AMPUL
THE 2.5 g AMPUL IS NOT FOR DIRECT INTRAVENOUS INJECTION. THIS DOSAGE FORM IS A CONCENTRATED, POTENT DRUG WHICH MUST BE DILUTED PRIOR TO ITS INFUSION. ESMOLOL HCl SHOULD NOT BE ADMIXED WITH SODIUM BICARBONATE. ESMOLOL HCl SHOULD NOT BE MIXED WITH OTHER DRUGS PRIOR TO DILUTION IN A SUITABLE INTRAVENOUS FLUID. (See *"Compatibility"* section below.)

Dilution: Aseptically prepare a 10 mg/mL infusion, by adding two 2.5 g ampuls to a 500 mL container, or one 2.5 g ampul to a 250 mL container, of a compatible intravenous solution listed below. (Remove overage prior to dilution as appropriate.) This yields a final concentration of 10 mg/mL. The diluted solution is stable for at least 24 hours at room temperature. Note: Concentrations of Esmolol HCl greater than 10 mg/mL are likely to produce irritation on continued infusion (see *"Precautions"*). Esmolol HCl has, however, been well tolerated when administered via a central vein.

100 MG VIAL
This dosage form is prediluted to provide a ready-to-use 10 mg/mL concentration recommended for Esmolol HCl intravenous administration. It may be used to administer the appropriate Esmolol HCl loading dosage infusions by handheld syringe while the maintenance infusion is being prepared.

When using the 100 mg vial, a loading dose of 0.5 mg/kg/min for a 70 kg patient would 3.5 mL.

SUPRAVENTRICULAR TACHYCARDIA
In the treatment of supraventricular tachycardia, responses to Esmolol HCl usually (over 95%) occur within the range of 50 to 200 mcg/kg/min (0.05 to 0.2 mg/kg/min). The average effective dosage is approximately 100 mcg/kg/min (0.1 mg/kg/min) although dosages as low as 25 mcg/kg/min (0.025 mg/kg/min) have been adequate in some patients. Dosages as high as 300 mcg/kg/min (0.3 mg/kg/min) have been used, but these provide little added effect and an increased rate of adverse effects, and are not recommended. Dosage of Esmolol HCl in supraventricular tachycardia must be individualized by titration in which each step consists of a loading dosage followed by a maintenance dosage.

To initiate treatment of a patient with supraventricular tachycardia, administer a loading infusion to 500 mcg/kg/min (0.5 mg/kg/min) over one minute followed by a four-minute maintenance infusion of 50 mcg/kg/min (0.05 mg/kg/min). If an adequate therapeutic effect is observed over the five minutes of drug administration, maintain the maintenance infusion dosage with periodic adjustments up or down as needed. If an adequate therapeutic effect is not observed, the same loading dosage is repeated over one minute followed by an increased maintenance rate infusion of 100 mcg/kg/min (0.1 mg/kg/min).

Continue titration procedure as above, repeating the original loading infusion of 500 mcg/kg/min (0.5 mg/kg/min) over 1 minute, but increasing the maintenance infusion rate over the subsequent four minutes by 50 mcg/kg/min (0.05 mg/kg/min) increments. As the desired heart rate or blood pressure is approached, omit subsequent loading doses and titrate the maintenance dosage up or down to endpoint. Also, if desired, increase the interval between steps from 5 to 10 minutes.

Time (minutes)	Loading Dose (over 1 minute)		Maintenance Dosage (over 4 minutes)	
	mcg/kg/min	mg/kg/min	mcg/kg/min	mg/kg/min
0-1	500	0.5		
1-5			50	0.05
5-6	500	0.5		
6-10			100	0.1
10-11	500	0.5		
11-15			150	0.15
15-16	*	*		
16-20			*200	*0.2
20-(24 hrs.)			Maintenance dose titrated to heart rate or other clinical endpoint.	

* *As the desired heart rate or endpoint is approached, the loading infusion may be omitted and the maintenance infusion titrated to 300 mcg/kg/min (0.3 mg/kg/min) or downward as appropriate. Maintenance dosages above 200 mcg/kg/min (0.2 mg/kg/min) have not been shown to have significantly increased benefits. The intervals between titration steps may be increased.*

This specific dosage regimen has not been studied intraoperatively and, because of the time required for titration, may not be optimal for intraoperative use.

The safety of dosages above 300 mcg/kg/min (0.3 mg/kg/min) has not been studied.

In the event of an adverse reaction, the dosage of Esmolol HCl may be reduced or discontinued. If a local infusion site reaction develops, an alternative infusion site should be used and caution should be taken to prevent extravasation. The use of butterfly needles should be avoided.

Abrupt cessation of Esmolol HCl in patients has not been reported to produce the withdrawal effects which may occur with abrupt withdrawal of beta blockers following chronic use in coronary artery disease (CAD) patients. However, caution should still be used in abruptly discontinuing infusions of Esmolol HCl in CAD patients.

After achieving an adequate control of the heart rate and a stable clinical status in patients with supraventricular tachycardia, transition to alternative antiarrhythmic agents such as propranolol, digoxin, or verapamil, may be accomplished. A recommended guideline for such a transition is given below but the physician should carefully consider the labeling instructions for the alternative agent selected:

Alternative Agent	Dosage
Propranolol hydrochloride	10-20 mg q 4-6 h
Digoxin	0.125-0.5 mg q 6 h (p.o. or i.v.)
Verapamil	80 mg q 6 h

The dosage of Esmolol HCl should be reduced as follows:

1. Thirty minutes following the first dose of the alternative agent, reduce the infusion rate of Esmolol HCl by one-half (50%).

2. Following the second dose of the alternative agent, monitor the patient's response and if satisfactory control is maintained for the first hour, discontinue Esmolol HCl.

The use of infusions of Emolol HCl up to 24 hours has been well documented: in addition, limited data from 24-48 hrs (N = 48) indicate that Esmolol HCl is well tolerated up to 48 hours.

INTRAOPERATIVE AND POSTOPERATIVE TACHYCARDIA AND/OR HYPERTENSION

In the intraoperative and postoperative settings it is not always advisable to slowly titrate the dose of Esmolol HCl to a therapeutic effect. Therefore, two dosing options are presented: immediate control dosing and a gradual control when the physician has time to titrate.

1. Immediate Control: For intraoperative treatment of tachycardia and/or hypertension give an 80 mg (approximately 1mg/kg) bolus dose over 30 seconds followed by a 150 mcg/kg/min infusion, if necessary. Adjust the infusion rate as required up to 300 mcg/kg/min to maintain desired heart rate and/or blood pressure.

2. Gradual Control: For postoperative tachycardia and hypertension, the dosing schedule is the same as that used in supraventricular tachycardia. To initiate

treatment, administer a loading dosage infusion of 500 mcg/kg/min Esmolol HCl for one minute followed by a four-minute maintenance infusion of 50 mcg/kg/min. If an adequate therapeutic effect is not observed within five minutes, repeat the same loading dosage and follow with a maintenance infusion increased to 100 mcg/kg/min (see above "*Supraventricular Tachycardia*").

Note: Higher dosages (250-300 mcg/kg/min) may be required for adequate control of blood pressure than those required for the treatment of atrial fibrillation, flutter and sinus tachycardia. One third of the postoperative hypertensive patients required these higher doses.

COMPATIBILITY WITH COMMONLY USED INTRAVENOUS FLUIDS

Esmolol HCl was tested for compatibility with ten commonly used intravenous fluids at a final concentration of 10 mg Esmolol HCl per mL. Esmolol HCl was found to be compatible with the following solutions and was stable for at least 24 hours at controlled room temperature or under refrigeration:

Dextrose (5%) Injection, USP
Dextrose (5%) in Lactated Ringer's Injection
Dextrose (5%) in Ringer's Injection
Dextrose (5%) and Sodium Chloride (0.45%) Injection, USP
Dextrose (5%) and Sodium Chloride (0.9%) Injection, USP
Lactated Ringer's Injection, USP
Potassium Chloride (40 mEq/liter) in Dextrose (5%) Injection, USP
Sodium Chloride (0.45%) Injection, USP
Sodium Chloride (0.9%) Injection, USP
Esmolol HCl was NOT compatible with Sodium Bicarbonate (5%) Injection, USP.

Note: Parenteral drug products should be inspected visually for particulate matter and discoloration prior to administration, whenever solution and container permit.

HOW SUPPLIED
INJECTION: 2.5 MG/10 ML

BRAND/MANUFACTURER	NDC	SIZE	AWP
○ **BRAND**			
BREVIBLOC: Du Pont Pharma	00590-0025-18	10 ml 10s	$557.50

INJECTION: 100 MG

BRAND/MANUFACTURER	NDC	SIZE	AWP
○ **BRAND**			
BREVIBLOC: Ohmeda	10019-0015-71	10 ml 20s	$11.20
BREVIBLOC: Du Pont Pharma	00590-0015-71	10 ml 20s	$234.72

INJECTION: 2.5 GM

BRAND/MANUFACTURER	NDC	SIZE	AWP
○ **BRAND**			
BREVIBLOC: Ohmeda	10019-0025-18	10 ml	$53.15

Esophotrast *SEE* BARIUM SULFATE

Espasmotex *SEE* HYOSCYAMINE SULFATE

Estazolam

DESCRPITION

Estazolam, a triazolobenzodiazepine derivative, is an oral hypnotic agent. Estazolam occurs as a fine, white, odorless powder that is soluble in alcohol and practically insoluble in water. The chemical name for Estazolam is 8-chloro-6-phenyl-4H-s-triazolo [4,3-α][1,4] benzodiazepine. The empirical formula is $C_{16}H_{11}ClN_4$.

Following is its chemical structure:

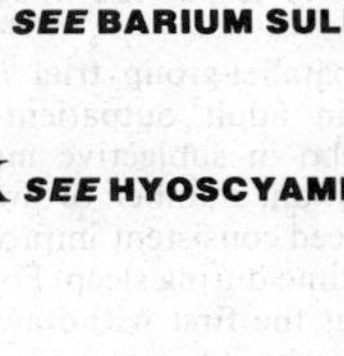

CLINICAL PHARMACOLOGY

Pharmacokinetics: Estazolam tablets have been found to be equivalent in absorption to an orally administered solution of Estazolam. Independent of concentration, Estazolam in plasma is 93% protein bound.

In healthy subjects who received up to three times the recommended dose of Estazolam, peak Estazolam plasma concentrations occurred within two hours after dosing (range 0.5 to 6.0 hours) and were proportional to the administered dose, suggesting linear pharmacokinetics over the dosage range tested.

The range of estimates for the mean elimination half-life of Estazolam varied from 10 to 24 hours. The clearance of benzodiazepines is accelerated in smokers compared to nonsmokers, and there is evidence that this occurs with Estazolam. This decrease in half-life, presumably due to enzyme induction by smoking, is consistent with other drugs with similar hepatic clearance characteristics. In all subjects and at all doses, the mean elimination half-life appeared to be independent of the dose.

In a small study (N = 8) using various doses in older subjects (59 to 68 years), peak Estazolam concentrations were found to be similar to those observed in younger subjects with a mean elimination half-life of 18.4 hours (range 13.5 to 34.6 hours). Estazolam is extensively metabolized, and the metabolites are excreted primarily in the urine. Less than 5% of a 2 mg dose of Estazolam is excreted unchanged in the urine, with only 4% of the dose appearing in the feces. 4'-hydroxy Estazolam is the major metabolite in plasma, with concentrations approaching 12% of those of the parent eight hours after administration. While it and the lesser metabolite, 1-oxo-estazolam, have some pharmacologic activity, their low potencies and low concentrations preclude any significant contribution to the hypnotic effect of Estazolam.

Postulated Relationship between Elimination Rate of Benzodiazepine Hypnotics and their Profile of Common untoward Effects: The type and duration of hypnotic effects and the profile of unwanted effects during administration of benzodiazepine drugs may be influenced by the biologic half-life of administered drug and any active metabolites formed. If half-lives are long, drug or metabolites may accumulate during periods of nightly administration and may be associated with impairments of cognitive and/or motor performance during waking hours; the possibility of interaction with other psychoactive drugs or alcohol will be increased. In contrast, if half-lives are short, drug and metabolites will be cleared before the next dose is ingested, and carry-over effects related to excessive sedation or CNS depression should be minimal or absent. However, during nightly use for an extended period, pharmacodynamic tolerance or adaptation to some effects of benzodiazepine hypnotics may develop. If the drug has a short elimination half-life, it is possible that a relative deficiency of the drug or its active metabolites (ie, in relationship to the receptor site) may occur at some point in the interval between each night's use. This sequence of events may account for two clinical findings reported to occur after several weeks of nightly use of rapidly eliminated benzodiazepine hypnotics, namely, increased wakefulness during the last third of the night and increased daytime anxiety in selected patients.

Controlled Trials Supporting Efficacy: In three 7-night, double-blind, parallel-group trials comparing Estazolam 1 mg and/or 2 mg with placebo in adult outpatients with chronic insomnia, Estazolam 2 mg was consistently superior to placebo in subjective measures of sleep induction (latency) and sleep maintenance (duration, number of awakenings, depth and quality of sleep); Estazolam 1 mg was similarly superior to placebo on all measures of sleep maintenance, however, it significantly improved sleep induction in only one of two studies. In a similarly designed trial comparing Estazolam 0.5 mg and 1 mg with placebo in geriatric outpatients with chronic insomnia, only the 1 mg Estazolam dose was consistently superior to placebo in sleep induction (latency) and in only one measure of sleep maintenance (ie, duration of sleep).

In a single-night, double-blind, parallel-group trial comparing Estazolam 2 mg and placebo in patients admitted for elective surgery and requiring sleep medications, Estazolam was superior to placebo in subjective measures of sleep induction and maintenance.

In a 12-week, double-blind, parallel-group trial including a comparison of Estazolam 2 mg and placebo in adult outpatients with chronic insomnia, Estazolam was superior to placebo in subjective measures of sleep induction (latency) and maintenance, (duration, number of awakenings, total wake time during sleep) at week 2, but produced consistent improvement over 12 weeks only for sleep duration and total wake time during sleep. Following withdrawal at week 12, rebound insomnia was seen at the first withdrawal week, but there was no difference between drug and placebo by the second withdrawal week in all parameters except latency, for which normalization did not occur until the fourth withdrawal week.

Adult outpatients with chronic insomnia were evaluated in a sleep laboratory trial comparing four doses of Estazolam (0.25, 0.50, 1.0 and 2.0 mg) and placebo, each administered for 2 nights in a crossover design. The higher Estazolam doses were superior to placebo in most EEG measures of sleep induction and maintenance, especially at the 2 mg dose, but only for sleep duration in subjective measures of sleep.

INDICATIONS AND USAGE

Estazolam is indicated for the short-term management of insomnia characterized by difficulty in falling asleep, frequent nocturnal awakenings, and/or early morning awakenings. Both outpatient studies and a sleep laboratory study have shown that Estazolam administered at bedtime improved sleep induction and sleep maintenance (see *"Clinical Pharmacology"*).

Because insomnia is often transient and intermittent, the prolonged administration of Estazolam is generally neither necessary nor recommended. Since insomnia may be a symptom of several other disorders, the possibility that the complaint may be related to a condition for which there is a more specific treatment should be considered.

There is evidence to support the ability of Estazolam to enhance the duration and quality of sleep for intervals up to 12 weeks (see *"Clinical Pharmacology"*).

CONTRAINDICATIONS

Benzodiazepines may cause fetal damage when administered during pregnancy. An increased risk of congenital malformations associated with the use of diazepam and chlordiazepoxide during the first trimester of pregnancy has been suggested in several studies. Transplacental distribution has resulted in neonatal CNS depression and also withdrawal phenomena following the ingestion of therapeutic doses of a benzodiazepine hypnotic during the last weeks of pregnancy. Estazolam is contraindicated in pregnant women. If there is a likelihood of the patient becoming pregnant while receiving Estazolam she should be warned of the potential risk to the fetus and instructed to discontinue the drug prior to becoming pregnant. The possibility that a woman of childbearing potential is pregnant at the time of institution of therapy should be considered.

WARNINGS

Estazolam like other benzodiazepines, has CNS depressant effects. For this reason, patients should be cautioned against engaging in hazardous occupations requiring complete mental alertness, such as operating machinery or driving a motor vehicle, after ingesting the drug, including potential impairment of the performance of such activities that may occur the day following ingestion of Estazolam. Patients should also be cautioned about possible combined effects with alcohol and other CNS depressant drugs.

As with all benzodiazepines, amnesia, paradoxical reactions (eg, excitement, agitation, etc.), and other adverse behavioral effects may occur unpredictably.

There have been reports of withdrawal signs and symptoms of the type associated with withdrawal from CNS depressant drugs following the rapid decrease or the abrupt discontinuation of benzodiazepines (see *"Drug Abuse and Dependence"*).

PRECAUTIONS

General: Impaired motor and/or cognitive performance attributable to the accumulation of benzodiazepines and their active metabolites following several days of repeated use at their recommended doses is a concern in certain vulnerable patients (eg, those especially sensitive to the effects of benzodiazepines or those with a reduced capacity to metabolize and eliminate them) (see *"Dosage and Administration"*).

Elderly or debilitated patients and those with impaired renal or hepatic function should be cautioned about these risks and advised to monitor themselves for signs of excessive sedation or impaired conditions.

Estazolam appears to cause dose related respiratory depression that is ordinarily not clinically relevant at recommended doses in patients with normal respiratory function. However, patients with normal respiratory function may be at risk and should be monitored appropriately. As a class, benzodiazepines have the capacity to depress respiratory drive; there are insufficient data available, however, to characterize their relative potency in depressing respiratory drive at clinically recommended doses.

As with other benzodiazepines, Estazolam should be administered with caution to patients exhibiting signs or symptoms of depression. Suicidal tendencies may be present in such patients and protective measures may be required. Intentional overdosage is more common in this group of patients; therefore, the least amount of drug that is feasible should be prescribed for the patient at any one time.

Information for Patients: To assure the safe and effective use of Estazolam the following information and instructions should be given to patients:

1. Inform your physician about any alcohol consumption and medicine you are taking now, including drugs you may buy without a prescription. Alcohol should not be used during treatment with hypnotics.

2. Inform your physician if you are planning to become pregnant, if you are pregnant, or if you become pregnant while you are taking this medicine.

3. You should not take this medicine if you are nursing, as the drug may be excreted in breast milk.

4. Until you experience the way this medicine affects you, do not drive a car, operate potentially dangerous machinery, or engage in hazardous occupations requiring complete mental alertness after taking this medicine.

5. Since benzodiazepines may produce psychological and physical dependence, you should not increase the dose before consulting your physician. In addition, since the abrupt discontinuation of Estazolam may be associated with temporary sleep disturbances, you should consult your physician before abruptly discontinuing doses of 2 mg per night or more.

Laboratory Tests: Laboratory tests are not ordinarily required in otherwise healthy patients. When treatment with Estazolam is protracted, periodic blood counts, urinalyses, and blood chemistry analyses are advisable.

Drug Interactions: If Estazolam is given concomitant with other drugs acting on the central nervous system, careful consideration should be given to the pharmacology of all agents. The action of the benzodiazepines may be potentiated by anticonvulsants, antihistamines, alcohol, barbiturates, monoamine oxidase inhibitors, narcotics, phenothiazines, psychotropic medications, or other drugs that produce CNS depression. Smokers have an increased clearance of benzodiazepines as compared to nonsmokers; this was seen in studies with Estazolam (see *"Clinical Pharmacology"*).

Carcinogenesis, Mutagenesis, Impairment of Fertility: Two-year carcinogenicity studies were conducted in mice and rats at dietary doses of 0.8, 3, and 10 mg/kg/day and 0.5, 2, and 10 mg/kg/day, respectively. Evidence of tumorigenicity was not observed in either study. Incidence of hyperplastic liver nodules increased in female mice given the mid- and high-dose levels. The significance of such modules in mice is not known at this time.

In vitro and *in vivo* mutagenicity tests including the Ames test, DNA repair in *B. subtilis*, *in vivo* cytogenetics in mice and rats, and the dominant lethal test in mice did not show a mutagenic potential for Estazolam.

◆ RATED THERAPEUTICALLY EQUIVALENT; ◇ THERAPEUTIC EQUIVALENCE UNCONFIRMED; ○ UNRATED

Fertility in male and female rats was not affected by doses up to 30 times the usual recommended human dose.

Pregnancy:
1. Teratogenic Effects: Pregnancy Category X (see *"Contraindications"*).
2. Nonteratogenic Effects: The child born of a mother taking benzodiazepines may be at some risk for withdrawal symptoms during the postnatal period. Neonatal flaccidity has been reported in an infant born of a mother who received benzodiazepines during pregnancy.

Labor and Delivery: Estazolam has no established use in labor or delivery.

Nursing Mothers: Human studies have not been conducted: however, studies in lactating rats indicate that Estazolam and/or its metabolites are secreted in the milk. The use of Estazolam in nursing mothers is not recommended.

Pediatric Use: Safety and effectiveness in children below the age of 18 have not been established.

Geriatric Use: Approximately 18% of individuals participating in the premarketing clinical trials of Estazolam were 60 years of age or older. Overall, the adverse event profile did not differ substantively from that observed in younger individuals. Care should be exercised when prescribing benzodiazepines to small or debilitated elderly patients (see *"Dosage and Administration"*).

ADVERSE REACTIONS
Commonly Observed: The most commonly observed adverse events associated with the use of Estazolam, not seen at an equivalent incidence among placebo-treated patients were somnolence, hypokinesia, dizziness, and abnormal coordination.

Associated with Discontinuation of Treatment: Approximately 3% of 1277 patients who received Estazolam in US premarketing clinical trials discontinued treatment because of an adverse clinical event. The only event commonly associated with discontinuation, accounting for 1.3% of the total, was somnolence.

Incidence in Controlled Clinical Trials: Table 1 enumerates adverse events that occurred at an incidence of 1% or greater among patients with insomnia who received Estazolam in 7-night, placebo-controlled trials. Events reported by investigators were classified into standard dictionary (COSTART) terms to establish event frequencies. Event frequencies reported were not corrected for the occurrence of these events at baseline. The frequencies were obtained from data pooled across six studies: Estazolam, N = 685; placebo, N = 433. The prescriber should be aware that these figures cannot be used to predict the incidence of side effects in the course of usual medical practice in which patient characteristics and other factors differ from those that prevailed in these six clinical trials. Similarly, the cited frequencies cannot be compared with figures obtained from other clinical investigators involving related drug products and uses, since each group of drug trials was conducted under a different set of conditions. However, the cited figures provide the physician with a basis of estimating the relative contribution of drug and nondrug factors to the incidence of side effects in the population studied.

Table 1
INCIDENCE OF ADVERSE EXPERIENCES IN PLACEBO-CONTROLLED CLINICAL TRIALS

	(Percentage of Patients Reporting)	
Body System/ *Adverse Event**	*Estazolam* *(N=685)*	*Placebo* *(N=433)*
Body as a Whole		
Headache	16	27
Asthenia	11	8
Malaise	5	5
Lower extremity pain	3	2
Back pain	2	2
Body pain	2	2
Abdominal pain	1	2
Chest pain	1	1
Digestive System		
Nausea	4	5
Dyspepsia	2	2
Musculoskeletal System		
Stiffness	1	—
Nervous System		
Somnolence	42	27
Hypokinesia	8	4
Nervousness	8	11
Dizziness	7	3
Coordination abnormal	4	1
Hangover	3	2
Confusion	2	—
Depression	2	3
Dream abnormal	2	1
Thinking abnormal	2	1
Respiratory System		
Cold symptoms	3	5
Pharyngitis	1	2

	(Percentage of Patients Reporting)	
Body System/ *Adverse Event**	*Estazolam* *(N=685)*	*Placebo* *(N=433)*
Skin and Appendages		
Pruritus	1	—

* *Events reported by at least 1% of Estazolam patients.*

Other Adverse Events: During clinical trials conducted by Abbott, some of which were not placebo-controlled, Estazolam was administered to approximately 1300 patients. Untoward events associated with this exposure were recorded by clinical investigators using terminology of their own choosing. To provide a meaningful estimate of the proportion of individuals experiencing adverse events, similar types of untoward events must be grouped into a smaller number of standardized event categories. In the tabulations that follow, a standard COSTART dictionary terminology has been used to classify reported adverse events. The frequencies presented, therefore, represent the proportion of the 1277 individuals exposed to Estazolam who experienced an event of the type cited on at least one occasion while receiving Estazolam. All reported events are included except those already listed in the previous table, those COSTART terms too general to be informative, and those events where a drug cause was remote. Events are further classified within body system categories and enumerated in order of decreasing frequency using the following definitions: frequent adverse events are defined as those occurring on one or more occasions in at least 1/100 patients; infrequent adverse events are those occurring in 1/100 to 1/1000 patients; rare events are those occurring in less than 1/1000 patients. It is important to emphasize that, although the events reported did occur during treatment with Estazolam, they were not necessarily caused by it.

Body as a Whole: Infrequent: allergic reaction, chills, fever, neck pain, upper extremity pain; Rare: edema, jaw pain, swollen breast.

Cardiovascular System: Infrequent: flushing, palpitation; Rare: arrhythmia, syncope.

Digestive System: Frequent: constipation, dry mouth; Infrequent: decreased appetite, flatulence, gastritis, increased appetite, vomiting; Rare: enterocolitis, melena, ulceration of the mouth.

Endocrine System: Rare: thyroid nodule.

Hematologic and Lymphatic System: Rare: leukopenia, purpura, swollen lymph nodes.

Metabolic/Nutritional Disorders: Infrequent: thirst; Rare: increased SGOT, weight gain, weight loss.

Musculoskeletal System: Infrequent: arthritis, muscle spasm, myalgia; Rare: arthralgia.

Nervous System: Frequent: anxiety; Infrequent: agitation, amnesia, apathy, emotional lability, euphoria, hostility, paresthesia, seizure, sleep disorder, stupor, twitch; Rare: ataxia, circumoral paresthesia, decreased libido, decreased reflexes, hallucinations, neuritis, nystagmus, tremor.

Minor changes in EEG patterns, usually low-voltage fast activity, have been observed in patients during Estazolam therapy or withdrawal and are of no known clinical significance.

Respiratory System: Infrequent: asthma, cough, dyspnea, rhinitis, sinusitis; Rare: epistaxis, hyperventilation, laryngitis.

Skin and Appendages: Infrequent: rash, sweating, urticaria; Rare: acne, dry skin.

Special Senses: Infrequent: abnormal vision, ear pain, eye irritation, eye pain, eye swelling, perverse taste, photophobia, tinnitus; Rare: decreased hearing, diplopia, scotomata.

Urogenital System: Infrequent: frequent urination, menstrual cramps, urinary hesitancy, urinary urgency, vaginal discharge/itching; Rare: hematuria, nocturia, oliguria, penile discharge, urinary incontinence.

Postintroduction Reports: Voluntary reports of non-US postmarketing experience with Estazolam have included rare occurrences of photosensitivity and agranulocytosis. Because of the uncontrolled nature of these spontaneous reports, a causal relationship to Estazolam treatment has not been determined.

DRUG ABUSE AND DEPENDENCE
Controlled Substance: Estazolam tablets are a controlled substance in Schedule IV.

Abuse and Dependence: Withdrawal symptoms similar to those noted with sedatives/hypnotics and alcohol have occurred following the abrupt discontinuation of drugs in the benzodiazepine class. The symptoms can range from mild dysphoria and insomnia to a major syndrome that may include abdominal and muscle cramps, vomiting, sweating, tremors, and convulsions.

Although withdrawal symptoms are more commonly noted after the discontinuation of higher than therapeutic doses of benzodiazepines, a proportion of patients taking benzodiazepines chronically at therapeutic doses may become physically dependent on them. Available data, however, cannot provide a reliable estimate of the incidence of dependency or the relationship of the dependency to dose and duration of treatment. There is some evidence to suggest that gradual reduction of dosage will attenuate or eliminate some withdrawal phenomena. In most instances, withdrawal phenomena are relatively mild and transient; however, life-threatening events (eg, seizures, delirium, etc.) have been reported. Gradual withdrawal is the preferred course for any patient taking benzodiazepines for a prolonged period. Patients with a history of seizures, regardless of their concomitant antiseizure drug therapy, should not be withdrawn abruptly from benzodiazepines.

Individuals with a history of addiction to or abuse of drugs or alcohol should be under careful surveillance when receiving benzodiazepines because of the risk of habituation and dependence to such patients.

OVERDOSAGE

As with other benzodiazepines, experience with Estazolam indicates that manifestations of overdosage include somnolence, respiratory depression, confusion, impaired coordination, slurred speech, and ultimately, coma. Patients have recovered from overdosage as high as 40 mg. As in the management of intentional overdose with any drug, the possibility should be considered that multiple agents may have been taken.

Gastric evacuation, either by the induction of emesis, lavage, or both, should be performed immediately. Maintenance of adequate ventilation is essential. General supportive care, including frequent monitoring of the vital signs and close observation of the patient, is indicated. Fluids should be administered intravenously to maintain blood pressure and encourage diuresis. The value of dialysis in treatment of benzodiazepine overdose has not been determined. The physician may wish to consider contacting a Poison Control Center for up-to-date information on the management of hypnotic drug product overdose.

DOSAGE AND ADMINISTRATION

The recommended initial dose for adults is 1 mg at bedtime; however, some patients may need a 2 mg dose. In healthy elderly patients, 1 mg is also the appropriate starting dose, but increases should be initiated with particular care. In small or debilitated older patients, a starting dose of 0.5 mg, while only marginally effective in the overall elderly population, should be considered.

Recommended Storage: Store below 86°F (30°C).

HOW SUPPLIED
TABLETS (C-IV): 1 MG

BRAND/MANUFACTURER	NDC	SIZE	AWP
○ BRAND			
▶ PROSOM: Abbott Pharm	00074-3735-13	100s	$85.21
	00074-3735-11	100s ud	$91.58

TABLETS (C-IV): 2 MG

BRAND/MANUFACTURER	NDC	SIZE	AWP
○ BRAND			
▶ PROSOM: Abbott Pharm	00074-3736-13	100s	$94.93
	00074-3736-11	100s ud	$101.80

Estinyl SEE ETHINYL ESTRADIOL

Estrace SEE ESTRADIOL

Estraderm SEE ESTRADIOL

Estradiol

> **ESTROGENS HAVE BEEN REPORTED TO INCREASE THE RISK OF ENDOMETRIAL CARCINOMA.**
> THREE INDEPENDENT CASE CONTROL STUDIES HAVE REPORTED AN INCREASED RISK OF ENDOMETRIAL CANCER IN POSTMENOPAUSAL WOMEN EXPOSED TO EXOGENOUS ESTROGENS FOR MORE THAN 1 YEAR. THIS RISK WAS INDEPENDENT OF THE OTHER KNOWN RISK FACTORS FOR ENDOMETRIAL CANCER. THESE STUDIES ARE FURTHER SUPPORTED BY THE FINDING THAT INCIDENCE RATES OF ENDOMETRIAL CANCER HAVE INCREASED SHARPLY SINCE 1969 IN EIGHT DIFFERENT AREAS OF THE UNITED STATES WITH POPULATION-BASED CANCER-REPORTING SYSTEMS, AN INCREASE WHICH MAY BE RELATED TO THE RAPIDLY EXPANDING USE OF ESTROGENS DURING THE LAST DECADE.
>
> THE THREE CASE CONTROL STUDIES REPORTED THAT THE RISK OF ENDOMETRIAL CANCER IN ESTROGEN USERS WAS ABOUT 4.5—13.9 TIMES GREATER THAN IN NONUSERS. THE RISK APPEARS TO DEPEND BOTH ON DURATION OF TREATMENT AND ON ESTROGEN DOSE. IN VIEW OF THESE FINDINGS, WHEN ESTROGENS ARE USED FOR THE TREATMENT OF MENOPAUSAL SYMPTOMS, THE LOWEST DOSE THAT WILL CONTROL SYMPTOMS SHOULD BE UTILIZED AND MEDICATION SHOULD BE DISCONTINUED AS SOON AS POSSIBLE.

> WHEN PROLONGED TREATMENT IS MEDICALLY INDICATED, THE PATIENT SHOULD BE REASSESSED ON AT LEAST A SEMIANNUAL BASIS TO DETERMINE THE NEED FOR CONTINUED THERAPY. ALTHOUGH THE EVIDENCE MUST BE CONSIDERED PRELIMINARY, ONE STUDY SUGGESTS THAT CYCLIC ADMINISTRATION OF LOW DOSES OF ESTROGEN MAY CARRY LESS RISK THAN CONTINUOUS ADMINISTRATION; IT THEREFORE APPEARS PRUDENT TO UTILIZE SUCH A REGIMEN.
>
> CLOSE CLINICAL SURVEILLANCE OF ALL WOMEN TAKING ESTROGENS IS IMPORTANT. IN ALL CASES OF UNDIAGNOSED PERSISTENT OR RECURRING ABNORMAL VAGINAL BLEEDING, ADEQUATE DIAGNOSTIC MEASURES, INCLUDING ENDOMETRIAL SAMPLING WHEN INDICATED, SHOULD BE UNDERTAKEN TO RULE OUT MALIGNANCY.
>
> THERE IS NO EVIDENCE AT PRESENT THAT "NATURAL" ESTROGENS ARE MORE OR LESS HAZARDOUS THAN "SYNTHETIC" ESTROGENS AT EQUIESTROGENIC DOSES.
>
> **ESTROGENS SHOULD NOT BE USED DURING PREGNANCY.**
> THE USE OF FEMALE SEX HORMONES, BOTH ESTROGENS AND PROGESTOGENS, DURING EARLY PREGNANCY MAY SERIOUSLY DAMAGE THE OFFSPRING. IT HAS BEEN SHOWN THAT WOMEN WHO HAD BEEN EXPOSED *IN UTERO* TO DIETHYLSTILBESTROL, A NONSTEROIDAL ESTROGEN, HAVE AN INCREASED RISK OF DEVELOPING IN LATER LIFE A FORM OF VAGINAL OR CERVICAL CANCER THAT IS ORDINARILY EXTREMELY RARE. THIS RISK HAS BEEN ESTIMATED AS NOT GREATER THAN 4 PER 1000 EXPOSURES.
>
> FURTHERMORE, A HIGH PERCENTAGE OF SUCH EXPOSED WOMEN (30—90%) HAVE BEEN BEEN FOUND TO HAVE VAGINAL ADENOSIS, EPITHELIAL CHANGES OF THE VAGINA AND CERVIX. ALTHOUGH THESE CHANGES ARE HISTOLOGICALLY BENIGN, IT IS NOT KNOWN WHETHER THEY ARE PRECURSORS OF MALIGNANCY. MALE OFFSPRING HAVE AN INCREASED RISK OF UROGENITAL ABNORMALITIES AND POSSIBLY TESTICULAR CANCER LATER IN LIFE. ALTHOUGH SIMILAR DATA ON THE USE OF OTHER ESTROGENS ARE NOT AVAILABLE, IT CANNOT BE PRESUMED THEY WOULD NOT INDUCE SIMILAR CHANGES.
>
> THE 1985 DES TASK FORCE CONCLUDED THAT USE OF DES DURING PREGNANCY IS ASSOCIATED WITH A SUBSEQUENT INCREASED RISK OF BREAST CANCER IN THE MOTHERS, ALTHOUGH A CAUSAL RELATIONSHIP REMAINS UNPROVEN AND THE OBSERVED LEVEL OF EXCESS RISK IS SIMILAR TO THAT FOR A NUMBER OF OTHER BREAST CANCER RISK FACTORS.
>
> SEVERAL REPORTS SUGGEST AN ASSOCIATION BETWEEN INTRAUTERINE EXPOSURE TO FEMALE SEX HORMONES AND CONGENITAL ANOMALIES, INCLUDING CONGENITAL HEART DEFECTS AND LIMB-REDUCTION DEFECTS. ONE CASE CONTROL STUDY ESTIMATED A 4.7-FOLD INCREASED RISK OF LIMB-REDUCTION DEFECTS IN INFANTS WHO HAD BEEN EXPOSED *IN UTERO* TO SEX HORMONES (ORAL CONTRACEPTIVES, HORMONE WITHDRAWAL TESTS FOR PREGNANCY, OR ATTEMPTED TREATMENT FOR THREATENED ABORTION). SOME OF THESE EXPOSURES WERE VERY SHORT AND INVOLVED ONLY A FEW DAYS OF TREATMENT. THE DATA SUGGEST THAT THE RISK OF LIMB-REDUCTION DEFECTS IN EXPOSED FETUSES IS SOMEWHAT LESS THAN 1 PER 1000.
>
> IN THE PAST, FEMALE SEX HORMONES HAVE BEEN USED DURING PREGNANCY IN AN ATTEMPT TO TREAT THREATENED OR HABITUAL ABORTION. THERE IS CONSIDERABLE EVIDENCE THAT ESTROGENS ARE INEFFECTIVE FOR THESE INDICATIONS, AND THERE IS NO EVIDENCE FROM WELL-CONTROLLED STUDIES THAT PROGESTOGENS ARE EFFECTIVE FOR THESE USES. ESTROGENS ARE NOT INDICATED FOR THE PREVENTION OF POSTPARTUM BREAST ENGORGEMENT.
>
> IF ESTRADIOL IS USED DURING PREGNANCY, OR IF THE PATIENT BECOMES PREGNANT WHILE TAKING THIS DRUG, SHE SHOULD BE APPRISED OF THE POTENTIAL RISKS TO THE FETUS AND OF THE ADVISABILITY OF CONTINUATION OF THE PREGNANCY.

DESCRIPTION

Estradiol transdermal system is designed to release 17β-estradiol through a rate-limiting membrane continuously upon application to intact skin.

Two systems are available to provide nominal *in vivo* delivery of 0.05 or 0.1 mg of Estradiol per day via skin of average permeability (interindividual variation in skin permeability is approximately 20%). Each corresponding system having a contact surface area of 10 or 20 cm^2 contains 4 or 8 mg of Estradiol USP and 0.3 or 0.6 ml of alcohol USP, respectively. Each gram of Estradiol Vaginal Cream contains 0.1 mg Estradiol. Estradiol tablets for oral administration contain 1 or 2 mg of micronized Estradiol per tablet.

Estradiol USP (17β-estradiol) is a white, crystalline powder, chemically described as estra-1,3,5(10)-triene-3, 17β-diol. It has an empirical formula of $C_{18}H_{24}O_2$ and molecular weight of 272.37.

Certain brands of Estradiol tablets may contain FD&C Yellow No. 5(tartrazine) which may cause allergic type reactions (including bronchial asthma) in certain susceptible individuals. Although the overall incidence of FD&C Yellow No. 5 (tartrazine) sensitivity in the general population is low, it is frequently seen in patients who also have aspirin hypersensitivity.

Following is its chemical structure:

CLINICAL PHARMACOLOGY

Estradiol is the major estrogenic hormone secreted by the human ovary. Estrogen drug products act by regulating the transcription of a limited number of genes. Estrogens diffuse through cell membranes, distribute themselves throughout the cell, and bind to and activate the nuclear estrogen receptor, a DNA-binding protein which is found in estrogen-responsive tissues. The activated estrogen receptor binds to specific DNA sequences, or hormone-response elements, which enhance the transcription of adjacent genes and in turn lead to the observed effects. Estrogen receptors have been identified in tissues of the reproductive tract, breast, pituitary, hypothalamus, liver, and bone of women.

Among numerous effects, Estradiol is largely responsible for the development and maintenance of the female reproductive system and of secondary sexual characteristics. It promotes growth and development of the vagina, uterus, and fallopian tubes. With other hormones, such as pituitary hormones and progesterone, they cause enlargement of the breasts through promotion of ductal growth, stromal development, and the accretion of fat. Indirectly, Estradiol contributes to the shaping of the skeleton, to the maintenance of tone and elasticity of urogenital structures, to changes in the epiphyses of the long bones that allow for the pubertal growth spurt and its termination, to the growth of axillary and pubic hair, and to the pigmentation of the nipples and genitals.

Estrogens are intricately involved with other hormones, especially progesterone, in the processes of the ovulatory menstrual cycle and pregnancy, and effect the release of pituitary gonadotropins.

Loss of ovarian Estradiol secretion after menopause can result in instability of thermoregulation, causing hot flushes associated with sleep disturbance and excessive sweating, and urogenital atrophy, causing dyspareunia and urinary incontinence. Estradiol replacement therapy alleviates many of these symptoms of Estradiol deficiency in the menopausal woman.

Estrogens occur naturally in several forms. The primary source of estrogen in normally cycling adult women is the ovarian follicle, which secretes 70 to 500 micrograms of Estradiol daily, depending on the phase of the menstrual cycle. This is converted primarily to estrone, which circulates in roughly equal proportion to Estradiol, and to small amounts of estriol. After menopause, most endogenous estrogen is produced by conversion of androstenedione, secreted by the adrenal cortex, to estrone by peripheral tissues. Thus, estrone—especially in its sulfate ester form—is the most abundant circulating estrogen in postmenopausal women. Although circulating estrogens exist in a dynamic equilibrium of metabolic interconversions, Estradiol is the principal intracellular human estrogen and is substantially more potent than estrone or estriol at the receptor.

Estrogens used in therapy are well absorbed through the skin, mucous membranes, and gastrointestinal tract. When applied for a local action, absorption is usually sufficient to cause systemic effects. When conjugated with aryl and alkyl groups for parenteral administration, the rate of absorption of oily preparations is slowed with a prolonged duration of action, such that a single intramuscular injection of Estradiol valerate or Estradiol cypionate is absorbed over several weeks.

Administered estrogens and their esters are handled within the body essentially the same as the endogenous hormones. Metabolic conversion of estrogens occurs primarily in the liver (first pass effect), but also at local target tissue sites. Complex metabolic processes result in a dynamic equilibrium of circulating conjugated and unconjugated estrogenic forms which are continually interconverted, especially between estrone and Estradiol and between esterified and unesterified forms. Although naturally-occurring estrogens circulate in the blood largely bound to sex hormone-binding globulin and albumin, only unbound estrogens enter target tissue cells. A significant proportion of the circulating estrogen exists as sulfate conjugates, especially estrone sulfate, which serves as a circulating reservoir for the formation of more active estrogenic species. A certain proportion of the estrogen is excreted into the bile and then reabsorbed from the intestine. During this enterohepatic recirculation, estrogens are desulfated and resulfated and undergo degradation through conversion to less active estrogens (estriol and other estrogens), oxidation to non-estrogenic substances (catecholestrogens), which interact with catecholamine metabolism, especially in the central nervous system), and conjugation with glucuronic acid (which is then rapidly excreted in the urine).

When given orally, naturally-occurring estrogens and their esters are extensively metabolized (first pass effect) and circulate primarily as estrone sulfate, with smaller amounts of other conjugated and unconjugated estrogenic species. This results in limited oral potency. By contrast, synthetic estrogens, such as ethinyl Estradiol and the nonsteroidal estrogens, are degraded very slowly in the liver and other tissues, which results in their high intrinsic potency. Estrogen drug products administered by nonoral routes are not subject to first-pass metabolism, but also undergo significant hepatic uptake, metabolism, and enterohepatic recycling.

The skin metabolizes Estradiol only to a small extent. Therefore, transdermal administration produces therapeutic serum levels of Estradiol with lower circulating levels of estrone and estrone conjugates, and requires smaller total doses than does oral therapy. Because Estradiol has a short half-life (~1 hour), transdermal administration of Estradiol allows a rapid decline in blood levels after an Estradiol transdermal system is removed, e.g., in a cycling regimen.

In a study using transdermally administered Estradiol, 0.1 mg daily, plasma levels increased by 66 pg/ml resulting in an average plasma level of 73 pg/ml. There were no significant increases in the concentration of renin substrate or other hepatic proteins (sex-hormone-binding globulin, thyroxine-binding globulin and corticosteroid-binding globulin).

PHARMACOKINETICS

Administration of Estradiol transdermal system produces mean serum concentrations of Estradiol comparable to those produced by a daily oral administration of Estradiol at about 20 times the daily transdermal dose. In single-application studies in 14 postmenopausal women using Estradiol transdermal systems that provided 0.05 and 0.1 mg of exogenous Estradiol per day, these systems produced increased blood levels within 4 hours and maintained respective mean serum Estradiol concentrations of 32 and 67 pg/ml above baseline over the application period. At the same time, increases in estrone serum concentration averaged only 9 and 27 pg/ml above baseline, respectively. Serum concentrations of Estradiol and estrone returned to preapplication levels within 24 hours after removal of the system. The estimated daily urinary output of Estradiol conjugates increased 5 to 10 times the baseline values and returned to near baseline within 2 days after removal of the system.

By comparison, Estradiol (2 mg per day) administered orally to postmenopausal women resulted in increases in mean serum concentration of 59 pg/ml of Estradiol and 302 pg/ml of estrone above baseline on the third consecutive day of dosing. Urinary output of Estradiol conjugates after oral administration increased to about 100 times the baseline values and did not approach baseline until 7–8 days after the last dose.

In a 3-week multiple-application study of 14 postmenopausal women in which Estradiol transdermal 0.05 was applied twice weekly, the mean increments in steady-state serum concentration were 30 pg/ml for Estradiol and 12 pg/ml for estrone. Urinary output of Estradiol conjugates returned to baseline within 3 days after removal of the last (6th) system, indicating little or no estrogen accumulation in the body.

INDICATIONS AND USAGE

Estradiol is indicated for the treatment of the following: moderate-to-severe vasomotor symptoms associated with menopause; (there is no adequate evidence that estrogens are effective for nervous symptoms or depression which might occur during menopause and they should not be used to treat these conditions); female hypogonadism; female castration; primary ovarian failure; and atrophic conditions caused by deficient endogenous estrogen production, such as atrophic vaginitis and kraurosis vulvae; and prevention of osteoporosis (loss of bone mass). Estradiol tablets are also used for treatment of breast cancer (for palliation only) in appropriately selected women and men with metastatic disease and treatment of advanced androgen-dependent carcinoma of the prostate (for palliation only).

Estradiol Vaginal Cream is indicated in the treatment of vulval and vaginal atrophy.

Estrogen replacement therapy is the most effective single modality for the prevention of postmenopausal osteoporosis in women. Since estrogen administration is associated with risk, selection of patients should ideally be based on prospective identification of risk factors for developing osteoporosis. Unfortunately, there is no certain way to identify those women who will develop osteoporotic fractures. Most prospective studies of efficacy for this indication have been carried out in white menopausal women, without stratification by other risk factors, and tend to show a universally salutary effect on bone. Thus, patient selection must be individualized based on the balance of risks and benefits. A more favorable risk/benefit ratio exists in a hysterectomized woman because she has no risk of endometrial cancer (see boxed "Warnings").

Estrogen replacement therapy reduces bone resorption and retards or halts post menopausal bone loss. Case-control studies have shown an approximately 60 percent reduction in hip and wrist fractures in women whose estrogen replacement was begun within a few years of menopause. Studies also suggest that estrogen reduces the rate of vertebral fractures. Even when started as late as 6 years after menopause, estrogen prevents further loss of bone mass for as long as the treatment is continued. When estrogen therapy is discontinued, bone mass declines at a rate comparable to the immediate postmenopausal period. There is no evidence that estrogen replacement therapy restores bone mass to premenopausal levels.

A recent, well-controlled, double-blind, prospective trial conducted at the Mayo Clinic has demonstrated that treatment with Estradiol transdermal system prevents bone loss in postmenopausal women at dosage of 0.05 mg per day.

Treatment with Estradiol transdermal system 0.05 mg showed full maintenance of bone density with a slight (0.8%), but not significant, increase. Placebo treatment resulted in a significant loss of more than 6% below baseline vertebral bone mass. Patients using either Estradiol transdermal system 0.1 mg, or 0.05 mg, had significantly greater bone densities than those using placebo. Other studies suggest that estrogen replacement therapy reduces the rate of vertebral fractures.

Peak bone mass is reached at age 30 to 35 and can best be maximized by adequate calcium intake and exercise during the adolescent and early adult years.

Early menopause is one of the best predictors for the development of osteoporosis. In addition, other factors affecting the skeleton which are associated with osteoporosis include genetic factors (small build, family history), and endocrine factors (nulliparity, thyrotoxicosis, hyperparathyroidism, Cushing's syndrome, hyperprolactinemia, Type I diabetes), lifestyle (cigarette smoking, alcohol abuse, sedentary exercise habits) and nutrition (below average body weight, dietary calcium intake).

At skeletal maturity there are sex and race differences in both the total amount of bone present and its density, in favor of men and blacks. Thus, women are at higher risk than men because they start with less bone mass and, for several years following natural or induced menopause, the rate of bone mass decline is accelerated. White and Asian women are at higher risk than black women.

Thin women are at higher risk than obese women. Cigarette smoking may be an additional risk factor. The mainstays of prevention and management of osteoporosis are estrogen, an adequate lifetime calcium intake, and exercise. Postmenopausal women absorb dietary calcium less efficiently than premenopausal women and require an average of 1500 mg/day of elemental calcium to remain in neutral calcium balance. By comparison, pre-menopausal women require about 1000 mg/day and the average calcium intake in the USA is 400-600 mg/day. Therefore, when not contraindicated, calcium supplementation may be helpful.

Weight-bearing exercise and nutrition may be important adjuncts to the prevention and management of osteoporosis.

Immobilization and prolonged bedrest produce rapid bone loss, while weight-bearing exercise has been shown to both reduce bone loss and to increase bone mass. The optimal type and amount of physical activity that might lower the risk for osteoporosis have not been established, however, in two studies an hour of walking and running exercise twice or three times weekly significantly increased lumbar spine bone mass.

UNLABELED USES
Estradiol is used alone or as an adjunct in the treatment of alopecia androgenetica, prophylaxis of cardiovascular disease, dyskinesia including chorea secondary to Huntington's disease and tardive dyskinesia, and levodopa-induced dyskinesia. It is also used to regress hirsutism due to polycystic ovaries, hyperlipidemia, hypersexuality, and induction of labor, premenstrual syndrome, including menstrual migraine. Estradiol is also prescribed in women with primary biliary cirrhosis, Turner's syndrome, abnormal uterine bleeding, and postcoital contraception.

CONTRAINDICATIONS
Patients with known hypersensitivity to any of the components of the therapeutic system should not use Estradiol transdermal system. Estrogens should not be used in women or men with any of the following conditions:
1. known or suspected cancer of the breast; except in appropriately selected patients being treated for metastatic disease.
2. known or suspected estrogen-dependent neoplasia;
3. known or suspected pregnancy (see boxed *"Warning"*); estrogens may cause fetal harm when administered to a pregnant woman;
4. undiagnosed abnormal genital bleeding;
5. active thrombophlebitis or thromboembolic disorders;
6. history of thrombophlebitis, thrombosis, or thromboembolic disorders associated with previous estrogen use.

WARNINGS
1. *Induction of Malignant Neoplasms.* Long-term continuous adminstration of natural and synthetic estrogens in certain animal species increases the frequency of carcinomas of the breast, cervix, vagina, and liver. There are now reports that estrogens increase the risk of carcinoma of the endometrium in humans. (See boxed *"Warning".*)

The reported endometrial cancer risk among unopposed estrogen users is about 2- to 12-fold greater than in non-users, and appears dependent on duration of treatment and on estrogen dose. Most studies show no significant increased risk associated with use of estrogens for less than one year. The greatest risk appears associated with prolonged use—with increased risks of 15- to 24-fold for five to ten years or more. In three studies, persistence of risk was demonstrated for 8 to over 15 years after cessation of estrogen treatment. In one study a significant decrease in the incidence of endometrial cancer occurred six months after estrogen withdrawal. Concurrent progestin therapy may offset this risk but the overall health impact in postmenopausal women is not known (see *"Precautions"*).

At the present time, there is no satisfactory evidence that estrogens given to postmenopausal women increase the risk of breast cancer, although a recent long-term followup study has raised this possibility. Some studies have reported a moderately increased risk (relative risks of 1.3—2.0) in those taking higher doses or those taking lower doses for prolonged periods of time, especially in excess of 10 years. Other studies have not shown this relationship. Because of the animal data, there is a need for caution in prescribing estrogens for women with a strong family history of breast cancer or who have breast nodules, fibrocystic disease, or abnormal mammograms.

Estrogen therapy during pregnancy is associated with an increased risk of fetal congenital reproductive tract disorders, and possibly other birth defects. Studies of women who received DES during pregnancy have shown that female offspring have an increased risk of vaginal adenosis, squamous cell dysplasia of the uterine cervix, and clear cell vaginal cancer later in life; male offspring have an increased risk of urogenital abnormalities and possibly testicular cancer later in life. Although some of these changes are benign, others are precursors of malignancy.

2. *Gallbladder Disease.* Two studies have reported a two- to fourfold increase in the risk of surgically confirmed gallbladder disease in postmenopausal women receiving oral estrogens, similar to the twofold increase previously noted in users of oral contraceptives.

3. *Effects Similar to Those Caused by Estrogen-Progestogen Oral Contraceptives.* There are several serious adverse effects of oral contraceptives and other high-dose oral estrogen treatments, most of which have not, up to now, been documented as consequences of postmenopausal estrogen replacement therapy. This may reflect the comparatively low doses of estrogen used in postmenopausal women.

a. *Thromboembolic Disease.* It is now well established that users of oral contraceptives have an increased risk of various thromboembolic and thrombotic vascular diseases, such as thrombophlebitis, pulmonary embolism, stroke, and myocardial infarction. Cases of retinal thrombosis, mesenteric thrombosis, and optic neuritis have been reported in oral contraceptive users. There is evidence that the risk of several of these adverse reactions is related to the dose of the drug. An increased risk of postsurgery thromboembolic complications has also been reported in users of oral contraceptives. If feasible, estrogen should be discontinued at least 4 weeks before surgery of the type associated with an increased risk of thromboembolism, or during periods of prolonged immobilization.

While an increased rate of thromboembolic and thrombotic disease in postmenopausal users of estrogens has not been found, this does not rule out the possibility that such an increase may be present or that subgroups of women who have underlying risk factors or who are receiving relatively large doses of estrogens may have increased risk. Therefore, estrogens should not be used in persons with active thrombophlebitis or thromboembolic disorders, and they should not be used in persons with a history of such disorders in association with estrogen use. They should be used with caution in patients with cerebral vascular or coronary artery disease and only for those in whom estrogens are clearly needed.

Large doses of estrogen (5 mg conjugated estrogens per day), comparable to those used to treat cancer of the prostate and breast, have been shown in a large prospective clinical trial in men to increase the risk of nonfatal myocardial infarction, pulmonary embolism, and thrombophlebitis. These risks cannot necessarily be extrapolated from men to women. However, to avoid the theoretical cardiovascular risk to women caused by high estrogen doses, the dose for estrogen replacement therapy should not exceed the lowest effective dose.

b. *Hepatic Adenoma.* Benign hepatic adenomas have been associated with the use of oral contraceptives. Although benign and rare, these tumors may rupture and cause death from intra-abdominal hemorrhage. Such lesions have not yet been reported in associated with other estrogen or progestogen preparations, but they should be considered if abdominal pain and tenderness, abdominal mass, or hypovolemic shock occurs in patients receiving estrogen. Hepatocellular carcinoma has also been reported in women taking estrogen-containing oral contraceptives. The causal relationship of this malignancy to these drugs is not known.

c. *Elevated Blood Pressure.* Women using oral contraceptives sometimes experience increased blood pressure which, in most cases, returns to normal upon discontinuing the drug. More often, blood pressure has remained the same or has dropped. One study showed that postmenopausal estrogen users have higher blood pressure than nonusers. Two other studies showed slightly lower blood pressure among estrogen users compared to nonusers. Postmenopausal estrogen use does not increase the risk of stroke. Nonetheless, blood pressure should be monitored at regular intervals with estrogen use. Ethinyl Estradiol and conjugated estrogens have been shown to increase renin substrate. In contrast to these oral estrogens, transdermally administered Estradiol does not affect renin substrate.

d. *Glucose Tolerance.* A worsening of glucose tolerance has been observed in a significant percentage of patients on estrogen-containing oral contraceptives. For this reason, diabetic patients should be carefully observed while receiving estrogen.

4. *Hypercalcemia.* Administration of high doses of estrogens may lead to severe hypercalcemia in patients with breast cancer and bone metastases. If hypercalcemia occurs, use of the drug should be stopped and appropriate measures should be taken to reduce the serum calcium level.

PRECAUTIONS
GENERAL
1. A complete medical and family history should be taken before initiation of any estrogen therapy. The pretreatment and periodic physical examinations should include special reference to blood pressure, breasts, abdomen, and pelvic organs, as well as a cervical Papanicolaou test. As a general rule, estrogen should not be prescribed for longer than 1 year without another physical examination being performed.

2. Because estrogens may cause some degree of fluid retention, careful observation is required when conditions that might be influenced by this factor are present (e.g., asthma, epilepsy, migraine, and cardiac or renal dysfunction).

3. Certain patients may develop undesirable manifestations of excessive estrogenic stimulation, such as uterine bleeding, mastodynia, etc.

4. Prolonged administration of unopposed estrogen therapy has been reported to increase the risk of endometrial hyperplasia in some patients. Estrogens should be used with caution in patients who have or have had endometriosis.

5. Studies of the addition of a progestin for 7 or more days of a cycle of estrogen administration have reported a lowered incidence of endometrial hyperplasia, which would otherwise be induced by estrogen treatment. Morphological and biochemical studies of endometrium suggest that 10 to 14 days of progestin are needed to provide maximal maturation of the endometrium and to eliminate any hyperplastic changes. Whether this will provide protection from

---

◆ RATED THERAPEUTICALLY EQUIVALENT; ◇ THERAPEUTIC EQUIVALENCE UNCONFIRMED; ○ UNRATED

endometrial carcinoma has not been clearly established. There are possible additional risks that may be associated with the inclusion of progestin in estrogen replacement regimens. The potential risks include (1) adverse effects on carbohydrate and lipid metabolism (lowering HDL and raising LDL) which may diminish the possible cardioprotective effect of estrogen therapy (see "Precautions" D.4., below); (2) impairment of glucose tolerance; and (3) possible enhancement of mitotic activity in breast epithelial tissue (although few epidemiological data are available to address this point). The choice of progestin and dosage may be important in minimizing these adverse effects.

6. Oral contraceptives appear to be associated with an increased incidence of mental depression. Although it is not clear whether this is due to the estrogenic or progestogenic component of the contraceptive, patients with a history of depression should be carefully observed.

7. Preexisting uterine leiomyomata may increase in size during prolonged estrogen use. If this occurs, estrogen therapy should be discontinued while the cause is investigated.

8. In patients with a history of jaundice during pregnancy, there is an increased risk that jaundice will recur with the use of estrogen-containing oral contraceptives. If jaundice develops in any patient receiving estrogen, the medication should be discontinued while the cause is investigated.

9. Estrogens may be poorly metabolized in patients with impaired liver function and should be administered with caution in such patients.

10. Because the prolonged use of estrogens influences the metabolism of calcium and phosphorus, estrogens should be used with caution in patients with metabolic bone diseases associated with hypercalcemia and in patients with renal insufficiency. Some studies have shown that women taking estrogen replacement therapy have hypercoagulability, primarily related to decreased antithrombin activity. This effect appears dose- and duration-dependent and is less pronounced than that associated with oral contraceptive use. Also, postmenopausal women tend to have increased coagulation parameters at baseline compared to premenopausal women. There is some suggestion that low dose postmenopausal mestranol may increase the risk of thromboembolism, although the majority of studies (of primarily conjugated estrogens users) report no such increase. There is insufficient information on hypercoagulability in women who have had previous thromboembolic disease.

Estrogen therapy may be associated with massive elevations of plasma triglycerides leading to pancreatitis and other complications in patients with familial defects of lipoprotein metabolism.

Some brands of Estradiol contain FD&C Yellow No. 5 (tartrazine) which may cause allergic-type reactions (including bronchial asthma) in certain susceptible individuals. Although the overall incidence of FD&C Yellow No. 5 (tartrazine) sensitivity in the general population is low, it is frequently seen in patients who also have aspirin hypersensitivity.

Laboratory Tests: Estrogen administration should generally be guided by clinical response at the smallest dose, rather than laboratory monitoring, for relief of symptoms for those indications in which symptoms are observable. For prevention and treatment of osteoporosis, however, see "Dosage and Administration" section.

DRUG/LABORATORY TEST INTERACTIONS
The results of certain endocrine and liver function tests may be affected by estrogen-containing oral contraceptives. The following changes have been observed with large doses of oral estrogen:

1. increased sulfobromophthalein retention;
2. accelerated prothrombin time, partial thromboplastin time, and platelet aggregation time; increased platelet count; increased factors II, VII antigen, VIII antigen, VIII coagulant activity, IX, X, XII, VII-X complex, II-VII-X complex, and beta-thromboglobulin; decreased levels of anti-factor Xa and antithrombin III, decreased antithrombin III activity; increased levels of fibrinogen and fibrinogen activity; increased plasminogen antigen and activity; increased norepinephrine-induced platelet aggregability;
3. increased thyroxine-binding globulin (TBG), leading to increased circulating total thyroid hormone as measured by protein-bound iodine (PBI), T_4 levels by column or radioimmunoassay or T_3 levels by radioimmunoassay; free T_3 resin uptake is decreased, reflecting the elevated TBG; free T_4 and T_3 concentrations are unaltered; TBG was not affected in clinical trials of Estradiol transdermal system;
4. reduced response to the metyrapone test;
5. reduced serum folate concentration;
6. increased serum triglyceride and phospholipid concentration, increased plasma HDL and HDL-2 subfraction concentrations, reduced LDL cholesterol concentration, and decreased pregnanediol excretion.
7. Other binding proteins may be elevated in serum, i.e., corticosteroid binding globulin (CBG), sex hormone-binding globulin (SHBG), leading to increased circulating corticosteroids and sex steroids, respectively. Free or biologically active hormone concentrations are unchanged. Other plasma proteins may be increased (angiotensinogen/renin substrate, alpha-1-antitrypsin, ceruloplasmin).
8. Impaired glucose tolerance.

The pathologist should be informed that the patient is receiving estrogen therapy when relevant specimens are submitted.

CARCINOGENESIS, MUTAGENESIS, IMPAIRMENT OF FERTILITY
See "Warnings" and boxed "Warning".

Long-term continuous administration of natural and synthetic estrogens in certain animal species increases the frequency of carcinomas of the breast, uterus, cervix, vagina, testis, and liver.

PREGNANCY CATEGORY X
See "Contraindications" and boxed "Warning". Estrogens should not be used during pregnancy.

NURSING MOTHERS
As a general principle, the administration of any drug to nursing mothers should be done only when clearly necessary since many drugs are excreted in human milk. In addition, estrogen administration to nursing mothers has been shown to decrease the quantity and quality of the milk.

ADVERSE REACTIONS
See "Warnings" and boxed "Warning" regarding potential adverse effects on the fetus, induction of malignant neoplasms, increased incidence of gallbladder disease, hypercalcemia, and adverse effects similar to those of oral contraceptives, including thromboembolism.

The most commonly reported adverse reaction to Estradiol transdermal system in clinical trials was redness and irritation at the application site. This occurred in about 17% of the women treated and caused approximately 2% to discontinue therapy. Reports of rash have been rare. There have also been rare reports of severe systemic allergic reactions.

The following additional adverse reactions have been reported with estrogenic therapy, including oral contraceptives:

Genitourinary System: Breakthrough bleeding, spotting, change in menstrual flow; increase in size of uterine fibromyomata; change in cervical erosion and amount of cervical secretion; vaginal candidiasis.

Endocrine: Breast tenderness, breast enlargement.

Gastrointestinal: Nausea, vomiting; abdominal cramps, bloating; cholestatic jaundice, increased incidence of gallbladder disease have been observed with oral estrogen therapy.

Eyes: Steepening of corneal curvature; intolerance to contact lenses.

Central Nervous System: Headache, migraine, dizziness, mental depression, chorea.

Skin: Chloasma or melasma which may persist when drug is discontinued; erythema multiforme; erythema nodosum; hemorrhagic eruption; loss of scalp hair; hirsutism.

Miscellaneous: Change in weight, edema, change in libido, reduced carbohydrate tolerance, aggravation of porphyria.

OVERDOSAGE
Numerous reports of ingestion of large doses of estrogen-containing oral contraceptives by young children indicate that acute serious ill effects do not occur. Overdosage with estrogen may cause nausea and vomiting, and withdrawal bleeding may occur in females.

DOSAGE AND ADMINISTRATION
ESTRADIOL TABLETS
The usual initial dosage range is 1 or 2 mg daily of Estradiol tablets adjusted as necessary to control presenting symptoms. The minimal effective dose for maintenance therapy should be determined by titration. Administration should be cyclic (e.g., 3 weeks on and 1 week off).

For Treatment of Female Hypoestrogenism Due to Hypogonadism, Castration, or Primary Ovarian Failure: Treatment is usually initiated with a dose of 1 or 2 mg daily of Estradiol tablets, adjusted as necessary to control presenting symptoms; the minimal effective dose for maintenance therapy should be determined by titration.

For Treatment of Breast Cancer, for Palliation Only, in Appropriately Selected Women and Men with Metastatic Disease: Suggested dosage is 10 mg three times daily for a period of at least three months.

For Treatment of Advanced Androgen-dependent Carcinoma of the Prostate, for Palliation Only: Suggested dosage is 1 to 2 mg three times daily. The effectiveness of therapy can be judged by phosphatase determinations as well as by symptomatic improvement of the patient.

For Prevention of Osteoporosis: Therapy with Estradiol tablets to prevent postmenopausal bone loss should be initiated with a daily dosage of 0.5 mg administered cyclically (e.g., 3 weeks on and 1 week off) as soon as possible after menopause. The dosage may be adjusted if necessary to control concurrent menopausal symptoms. Discontinuation of estrogen replacement therapy may reestablish the natural rate of bone loss.

ESTRADIOL VAGINAL CREAM
For treatment of vulval and vaginal atrophy associated with the menopause, the lowest dose and regimen that will control symptoms should be chosen and medication should be discontinued as promptly as possible.

Attempts to discontinue or taper medication should be made at 3-month to 6-month intervals.

Usual Dosage: The usual dosage range of Estradiol vaginal cream is 2 to 4 g (marked on the applicator) daily for one or two weeks, then gradually reduced to one half initial dosage for a similar period. A maintenance dosage of 1 g, one to three times a week, may be used after restoration of the vaginal mucosa has been achieved.

Patients with intact uteri should be monitored closely for signs of endometrial cancer and appropriate diagnostic measures should be taken to rule out malignancy in the event of persistent or recurring abnormal vaginal bleeding.

► SHOWN IN PRODUCT IDENTIFICATION GUIDE

ESTRADIOL TRANSDERMAL SYSTEM

The adhesive side of the Estradiol transdermal system should be placed on a clean, dry area of the skin on the trunk of the body (including the buttocks and abdomen.) The site selected should be one that is not exposed to sunlight. *Estradiol transdermal system should not be applied to the breasts.* The sites of application must be rotated, with an interval of at least 1 week allowed between applications to a particular site. The area selected should not be oily, damaged, or irritated. The waistline should be avoided, since tight clothing may rub the system off. The system should be applied immediately after opening the pouch and removing the protective liner. The system should be pressed firmly in place with the palm of the hand for about 10 seconds, making sure there is good contact, especially around the edges. In the unlikely event that a system should fall off, the same system may be reapplied. If necessary, a new system may be applied. In either case, the original treatment schedule should be continued.

INITIATION OF THERAPY

Treatment of menopausal symptoms is usually initiated with Estradiol transdermal system 0.05 mg applied to the skin twice weekly. The dosage should be adjusted as necessary to control symptoms. The lowest dosage necessary for the control of symptoms should be used, especially in women with an intact uterus. Attempts to taper or discontinue the medication should be made at 3-to-6-month intervals.

Prophylactic therapy with Estradiol transdermal system to prevent postmenopausal bone loss should be initiated with the 0.05 mg/day dosage as soon as possible after menopause. The dosage may be adjusted if necessary to control concurrent menopausal symptoms. Discontinuation of estrogen replacement therapy may reestablish the natural rate of bone loss.

In women not currently taking oral estrogens, treatment with Estradiol transdermal system can be initiated at once. In women who are currently taking oral estrogen, treatment with Estradiol transdermal system can be initiated 1 week after withdrawal of oral hormone replacement therapy, or sooner if menopausal symptoms reappear in less than 1 week.

THERAPEUTIC REGIMEN

Estradiol transdermal system therapy may be given continuously in patients who do not have an intact uterus. In those patients with an intact uterus, Estradiol transdermal system may be given on a cyclic schedule (e.g., 3 weeks on drug followed by 1 week off drug).

STORAGE

Store tablets at controlled room temperature 15°—30°C (59°—86°F). Store vaginal cream at room temperature; protect from temperatures in excess of 40°C (104°F). Do not store transdermal system above 30°C (86°F). Do not store unpouched. Apply immediately upon removal from the protective pouch.

HOW SUPPLIED
CREAM: 0.1 MG/GM

BRAND/MANUFACTURER	NDC	SIZE	AWP
○ **BRAND**			
ESTRACE: Mead Johnson Labs	00087-0754-42	42.5 gm	$25.68

FILM, EXTENDED RELEASE: 0.05 MG/24 HRS

BRAND/MANUFACTURER	NDC	SIZE	AWP
◇ **BRAND**			
ESTRADERM: Ciba Pharm	00083-2310-24	24s	$48.53
	00083-2310-62	48s	$100.04

FILM, EXTENDED RELEASE: 0.1 MG/24 HRS

BRAND/MANUFACTURER	NDC	SIZE	AWP
◇ **BRAND**			
ESTRADERM: Ciba Pharm	00083-2320-24	24s	$52.90
	00083-2320-62	48s	$109.05

TABLETS: 0.5 MG

BRAND/MANUFACTURER	NDC	SIZE	AWP
○ **BRAND**			
➤ ESTRACE: Mead Johnson Labs	00087-0021-41	100s	$24.64

TABLETS: 1 MG

BRAND/MANUFACTURER	NDC	SIZE	AWP
○ **BRAND**			
➤ ESTRACE: Mead Johnson Labs	00087-0755-01	100s	$32.84
	00087-0755-48	500s	$156.00

TABLETS: 2 MG

BRAND/MANUFACTURER	NDC	SIZE	AWP
○ **BRAND**			
➤ ESTRACE: Mead Johnson Labs	00087-0756-01	100s	$47.95
	00087-0756-48	500s	$227.73

Estradiol Cypionate and Testosterone Cypionate

WARNINGS

1. ESTROGENS HAVE BEEN REPORTED TO INCREASE THE RISK OF ENDOMETRIAL CARCINOMA IN POSTMENOPAUSAL WOMEN.

THREE INDEPENDENT CASE CONTROL STUDIES HAVE SHOWN AN INCREASED RISK OF ENDOMETRIAL CANCER IN POSTMENOPAUSAL WOMEN EXPOSED TO EXOGENOUS ESTROGENS FOR PROLONGED PERIODS. THIS RISK WAS INDEPENDENT OF THE OTHER KNOWN RISK FACTORS FOR ENDOMETRIAL CANCER. THESE STUDIES ARE FURTHER SUPPORTED BY THE FINDING THAT INCIDENCE RATES OF ENDOMETRIAL CANCER HAVE INCREASED SHARPLY SINCE 1969 IN EIGHT DIFFERENT AREAS OF THE UNITED STATES WITH POPULATION-BASED CANCER REPORTING SYSTEMS, AN INCREASE WHICH MAY BE RELATED TO THE RAPIDLY EXPANDING USE OF ESTROGENS DURING THE FIRST DECADE.

THE THREE CASE CONTROL STUDIES REPORTED THAT THE RISK OF ENDOMETRIAL CANCER IN ESTROGEN USERS WAS ABOUT 4.5 TO 13.9 TIMES GREATER THAN IN NONUSERS. THE RISK APPEARS TO DEPEND ON BOTH DURATION OF TREATMENT AND ON ESTROGEN DOSE. IN VIEW OF THESE FINDINGS, WHEN ESTROGENS ARE USED FOR THE TREATMENT OF MENOPAUSAL SYMPTOMS, THE LOWEST DOSE THAT WILL CONTROL SYMPTOMS SHOULD BE UTILIZED AND MEDICATION SHOULD BE DISCONTINUED AS SOON AS POSSIBLE. WHEN PROLONGED TREATMENT IS MEDICALLY INDICATED, THE PATIENT SHOULD BE REASSESSED ON AT LEAST A SEMI-ANNUAL BASIS TO DETERMINE THE NEED FOR CONTINUED THERAPY. ALTHOUGH THE EVIDENCE MUST BE CONSIDERED PRELIMINARY, ONE STUDY SUGGESTS THAT CYCLIC ADMINISTRATION OF LOW DOSES OF ESTROGEN MAY CARRY LESS RISK THAN CONTINUOUS ADMINISTRATION; IT THEREFORE APPEARS PRUDENT TO UTILIZE SUCH REGIMEN.

CLOSE CLINICAL SURVEILLANCE OF ALL WOMEN TAKING ESTROGENS IS IMPORTANT. ADEQUATE DIAGNOSTIC MEASURES, INCLUDING ENDOMETRIAL SAMPLING WHEN INDICATED, SHOULD BE UNDERTAKEN TO RULE OUT MALIGNANCY IN ALL CASES OF UNDIAGNOSED PERSISTENT OR RECURRING ABNORMAL VAGINAL BLEEDING. THERE IS NO EVIDENCE THAT "NATURAL" ESTROGENS ARE MORE OR LESS HAZARDOUS THAN "SYNTHETIC" ESTROGENS AT EQUI-ESTROGENIC DOSES.

2. ESTROGENS SHOULD NOT BE USED DURING PREGNANCY.

THERE IS NO INDICATION FOR ESTROGEN THERAPY DURING PREGNANCY OR DURING THE IMMEDIATE POSTPARTUM PERIOD. ESTROGENS ARE INEFFECTIVE FOR THE PREVENTION OR TREATMENT OF THREATENED OR HABITUAL ABORTION. ESTROGENS ARE NOT INDICATED FOR THE PREVENTION OF POSTPARTUM BREAST ENGORGEMENT.

SEVERAL REPORTS SUGGESTS AN ASSOCIATION BETWEEN INTRAUTERINE EXPOSURE TO FEMALE SEX HORMONES AND CONGENITAL ANOMALIES, INCLUDING CONGENITAL HEART DEFECTS AND LIMB REDUCTION DEFECTS. ONE CASE CONTROL STUDY ESTIMATED A 4.7 FOLD INCREASED RISK OF LIMB REDUCTION DEFECTS IN INFANTS EXPOSED IN UTERO TO SEX HORMONES (ORAL CONTRACEPTIVES, HORMONE WITHDRAWAL TESTS FOR PREGNANCY, OR ATTEMPTED TREATMENT FOR THREATENED ABORTION). SOME OF THESE EXPOSURES WERE VERY SHORT AND INVOLVED ONLY A FEW DAYS OF TREATMENT. THE DATA SUGGEST THAT THE RISK OF LIMB REDUCTION DEFECTS IN EXPOSED FETUSES IS SOMEWHAT LESS THAN 1 PER 1000.

ESTROGEN THERAPY DURING PREGNANCY IS ASSOCIATED WITH AN INCREASED RISK OF CONGENITAL DEFECTS IN THE REPRODUCTIVE ORGANS OF THE FETUS, AND POSSIBLY OTHER BIRTH DEFECTS. STUDIES OF WOMEN WHO RECEIVED DIETHYLSTILBESTROL (DES) DURING PREGNANCY HAVE SHOWN THAT FEMALE OFFSPRING HAVE AN INCREASED RISK OF VAGINAL ADENOSIS, SQUAMOUS CELL DYSPLASIA OF THE UTERINE CERVIX, AND CLEAR CELL VAGINAL CANCER LATER IN LIFE; MALE OFFSPRING HAVE AN INCREASED RISK OF UROGENITAL

◆ RATED THERAPEUTICALLY EQUIVALENT; ◇ THERAPEUTIC EQUIVALENCE UNCONFIRMED; ○ UNRATED

ABNORMALITIES AND POSSIBLY TESTICULAR CANCER LATER IN LIFE. THE 1985 DES TASK FORCE CONCLUDED THAT USE OF DES DURING PREGNANCY IS ASSOCIATED WITH A SUBSEQUENT INCREASED RISK OF BREAST CANCER IN THE MOTHERS, ALTHOUGH A CAUSAL RELATIONSHIP REMAINS UNPROVEN AND THE OBSERVED LEVEL OF EXCESS RISK IS SIMILAR TO THAT FOR A NUMBER OF OTHER BREAST CANCER RISK FACTORS.

IF TESTOSTERONE CYPIONATE AND ESTRADIOL CYPIONATE IS USED DURING PREGNANCY, OR IF THE PATIENT BECOMES PREGNANT WHILE TAKING THIS DRUG, SHE SHOULD BE APPRISED OF THE POTENTIAL RISKS TO THE FETUS, AND THE ADVISABILITY OF PREGNANCY CONTINUATION.

DESCRIPTION

Estradiol Cypionate/Testosterone Cypionate contains the androgenic hormone Testosterone Cypionate, and the estrogenic hormone, Estradiol Cypionate formulated for intramuscular administration only. Estradiol Cypionate/Testosterone Cypionate provides combined androgenic and estrogenic activity in the form of the long-acting esters of both components.

Each mL of Estradiol Cypionate/Testosterone Cypionate contains:
Testosterone . . . . .50 g
Estradiol Cypionate . . . . .2 mg

WARNING

Chlorobutanol is added as a presentative; chlorobutanol may be habit forming.

The chemical name for Testosterone Cypionate is androst-4-ene-3-one, 17-(3-cyclopentyl-1-oxopropoxy)-, (17β)-. Its molecular formula is $C_{27}H_{40}O_3$, and the molecular weight is 412.61.

Testosterone Cypionate occurs as a white or creamy white, crystalline powder. It is odorless or has a slight odor and is stable in air. It is insoluble in water, freely soluble in alcohol, chloroform, dioxane and ether, soluble in vegetable oils.

The chemical name for Estradiol Cypionate is Estra-1,3,5(10)-triene-3, 17-diol,(17-β)-, 17-cyclopentanepropriorate. Its molecular formula is $C_{26}H_{36}O_3$, and the molecular weight is 396.57.

Estradiol Cypionate occurs as a white to practically white, crystalline powder. It is odorless or has a slight odor. It is insoluble in water, soluble in alcohol, acetone, chloroform and dioxane; sparingly soluble in vegetable oils.

CLINICAL PHARMACOLOGY

The pharmacologic characteristics of Estradiol Cypionate/Testosterone Cypionate are indicated below:

Testosterone Cypionate: Androgen is responsible for the normal growth and development of the male sex organs and for the maintenance of secondary male characteristics. Androgens also cause retention of nitrogen, sodium, potassium, phosphorus, and decreased urinary excretion of calcium. Androgens have been reported to increase protein anabolism. Androgens have been reported to stimulate the production of red blood cells by enhancing the production or erythropoietic stimulating factor. Androgens also have a negative feedback relationship to pituitary luteinizing hormone (LH).

The half-life of Testosterone Cypionate when injected intramuscularly is approximately 8 days.

Estradiol Cypionate: Estrogen drug products act by regulating the transcription of a limited number of genes. Estrogens diffuse through cell membranes, distribute themselves throughout the cell, and bind to and activate the nuclear estrogen receptor, a DNA-binding protein which is found in estrogen-responsive tissues. The activated estrogen receptor binds to specific DNA sequences, or hormone-response elements, which enhance the transcription of adjacent genes and in turn lead to the observed effects. Estrogen receptors have been identified in tissues of the reproductive tract, breast, pituitary, hypothalamus, liver, and bone of women.

Estrogens are important in the development and maintenance of the female reproductive system and secondary sex characteristics. By a direct action, they cause growth and development of the uterus, Fallopian tubes, and vagina. With other hormones, such as pituitary hormones and progesterone, they cause enlargement of the breasts through promotion of ductal growth, stromal development, and the accretion of fat. Estrogens are intricately involved with other hormones, especially progesterone, in the processes of the ovulatory menstrual cycle and pregnancy, and affect the release of pituitary gonadotropins. They also contribute to the shaping of the skeleton, maintenance of tone and elasticity of urogenital structures, changes in the epiphyses of the long bones that allow for the pubertal growth spurt and its termination, and pigmentation of the nipples and genitals.

Estrogens occur naturally in several forms. The primary source of estrogen in normally cycling adult women is the ovarian follicle, which secretes 70 to 500 mcg of estradiol daily, depending on the phase of the menstrual cycle. This is converted primarily to estrone, which circulates in roughly equal proportion to estradiol, and to small amounts of estriol. After menopause, most endogenous estrogen is produced by conversion of androstenedione, secreted by the adrenal cortex, to estrone by peripheral tissues. Thus, estrone — especially in its sulfate ester form — is the most abundant circulating estrogen in postmenopausal women. Although circulating estrogens exist in a dynamic equilibrium of metabolic interconversions, estradiol is the principal intracellular human estrogen and is substantially more potent than estrone or estriol at the receptor.

Estrogens used in therapy are well absorbed through the skin, mucous membranes, and gastrointestinal tract. When applied for a local action, absorption is usually sufficient to cause systemic effects. When conjugated with aryl and alkyl groups for parenteral administration, the rate of absorption of oily preparations is slowed with a prolonged duration of action, such that a single intramuscular injection of estradiol is absorbed over several weeks.

Administered estrogens and their esters are handled within the body essentially the same as the endogenous hormones. Metabolic conversion of estrogens occurs primarily in the liver (first pass effect), but also at local target tissue sites. Complex metabolic processes result in a dynamic equilibrium of circulating conjugated and unconjugated estrogenic forms which are continually interconverted, especially between estrone and estradiol and between esterified and unesterified forms. Although naturally-occurring estrogens circulate in the blood largely bound to sex hormone-binding globulin and albumin, only unbound estrogens enter target tissue cells. A significant proportion of the circulating estrogen exists as sulfate conjugates, especially estrone sulfate, which serves as a circulating reservoir for the formation of more active estrogenic species. A certain proportion of the estrogen is excreted into the bile and then reabsorbed from the intestine. During this enterohepatic recirculation, estrogens are desulfated and resulfated and undergo degradation through conversion to less active estrogens (estriol and other estrogens), oxidation to nonestrogenic substances (catecholestrogens, which interact with catecholamine metabolism, especially in the central nervous system), and conjugation with glucuronic acids (which are then rapidly excreted in the urine).

When given orally, naturally-occurring estrogens and their esters are extensively metabolized (first pass effect) and circulate primarily as estrone sulfate, with smaller amounts of other conjugated and unconjugated estrogenic species. This results in limited oral potency. By contrast, synthetic estrogens, such as ethinyl estradiol and the nonsteroidal estrogens, are degraded very slowly in the liver and other tissues, which results in their high intrinsic potency. Estrogen drug products administered by non-oral routes are not subject to first-pass metabolism, but also undergo significant hepatic uptake, metabolism, and enterohepatic recycling.

The half-life of Estradiol Cypionate when injected intramuscularly is approximately 5 days.

INDICATIONS AND USAGE

Estradiol Cypionate/Testosterone Cypionate is indicated in the treatment of moderate to severe vasomotor symptoms associated with the menopause in those patients not improved by estrogen alone. There is no adequate evidence that estrogens are effective for nervous symptoms or depression which might occur during menopause and they should not be used to treat these conditions. The drugs should not be used to treat postpartum breast engorgement.

Estradiol Cypionate/Testosterone Cypionate has not been shown to be effective for any purpose during pregnancy and its use may cause severe harm to the fetus (See boxed *"Warnings"*).

CONTRAINDICATIONS

1. Known or suspected pregnancy (see boxed *"Warning"*). Estrogens may cause fetal harm when administered to a pregnant woman.

2. Undiagnosed abnormal genital bleeding.

3. Known or suspected cancer of the breast except in appropriately selected patients being treated for metastatic disease.

4. Known or suspected estrogen-dependent or androgen-dependent neoplasia.

5. Active thrombophlebitis or thromboembolic disorders.

6. Known hypersensitivity to the drugs.

7. A history of thrombophlebitis, thrombosis, or thromboembolic disorders associated with previous estrogen use (except when used in treatment of breast or prostatic malignancy).

8. Serious cardiac, hepatic or renal disease.

WARNINGS

1. Induction of malignant neoplasms.

Endometrial cancer: The reported endometrial cancer risk among unopposed estrogen users was about 2 to 12 fold greater than in non-users, and appears dependent on duration of treatment and on estrogen dose. Most studies show no significant increased risk associated with use of estrogens for less than one year. The greatest risk appears associated with prolonged use with increased risks of 15- to 24-fold for five to ten years or more. In three studies, persistence of risk was demonstrated for 8 to over 15 years after cessation of estrogen treatment. In one study a significant decrease in the incidence of endometrial cancer occurred six months after estrogen withdrawal. Concurrent progestin therapy may offset this risk but the overall health impact in postmenopausal women is not known (see *"Precautions"*).

Breast cancer: While the majority of studies have not shown an increased risk of breast cancer in women who have ever used estrogen replacement therapy, some have reported a moderately increased risk (relative risks of 1.3-2.0) in those taking higher doses or those taking lower doses for prolonged periods of time, especially in excess of 10 years. Other studies have not shown this relationship.

Congenital lesions with malignant potential: Estrogen therapy during pregnancy is associated with an increased risk of fetal congenital reproductive tract disorders, and possibly other birth defects. Studies of women who received DES during pregnancy have shown that female offspring have an increased risk of vaginal adenosis, squamous cell dysplasia of the uterine cervix, and clear cell vaginal cancer later in life; male offspring have an increased risk of urogenital abnormalities and possibly testicular cancer later in life. Although some of these changes are benign, others are precursors of malignancy.

2. *Gallbladder disease:* Two studies have reported a 2- to 4-fold increase in the risk of gallbladder disease requiring surgery in women receiving postmenopausal estrogens.

3. *Cardiovascular disease:* Large doses of estrogen (5 mg conjugated estrogens per day), comparable to those used to treat cancer of the prostate and breast, have been shown in a large prospective clinical trial in men to increase the risks of nonfatal myocardial infarction, pulmonary embolism, and thrombophlebitis. These risks cannot necessarily be extrapolated from men to women. However, to avoid the theoretical cardiovascular risk to women caused by high estrogen doses, the dose for estrogen replacement therapy should not exceed the lowest effective dose.

4. *Elevated blood pressure:* Occasional blood pressure increases during estrogen replacement therapy have been attributed to idiosyncratic reactions to estrogens. More often, blood pressure has remained the same or has dropped. One study showed that postmenopausal estrogen users have higher blood pressure than nonusers. Two other studies showed slightly lower blood pressure among estrogen users compared to nonusers. Postmenopausal estrogen use does not increase the risk of stroke. Nonetheless, blood pressure should be monitored at regular intervals with estrogen use.

5. *Hypercalcemia:* Administration of estrogens may lead to severe hypercalcemia in patients with breast cancer and bone metastases. If this occurs, the drug should be stopped and appropriate measures taken to reduce the serum calcium level.

6. *Virilization:* Female patients on androgen therapy should be watched closely for signs of virilization. Some effects such as voice changes may not be reversible even when the drug is stopped.

7. *Liver disease:* Androgens have been associated with the development of peliosis hepatitis, cholestatic hepatitis, jaundice and hepatocellular carcinoma. Peliosis hepatitis can be a life-threatening or fatal complication. If cholestatic hepatitis with jaundice appears, the androgen should be discontinued.

8. *Edema:* Edema with or without congestive heart failure, may occur in patients receiving androgens. This may be a serious complication in patients with preexisting cardiac, renal or hepatic disease. Diuretic therapy may be required if edema occurs.

9. *Glucose tolerance:* A worsening of glucose tolerance has been observed in a significant percentage of patients on estrogen-containing oral contraceptives. For this reason, diabetic patients should be carefully observed while receiving estrogen.

PRECAUTIONS
A. GENERAL
1. Addition of a progestin: Studies of the addition of a progestin for seven or more days of a cycle of estrogen administration have reported a lowered incidence of endometrial hyperplasia which would otherwise be induced by estrogen treatment. Morphological and biochemical studies of endometrium suggest that 10 to 14 days of progestin are needed to provide maximal maturation of the endometrium and to eliminate any hyperplastic changes. There are possible additional risks which may be associated with the inclusion of progestins in estrogen replacement regimens. These include: (1) adverse effects on lipoprotein metabolism (lowering HDL and raising LDL) which may diminish the possible cardioprotective effect of estrogen therapy, (see *"Precautions"* D.4., below); (2) impairment of glucose tolerance; and (3) possible enhancement of mitotic activity in breast epithelial tissue (although few epidemiological data are available to address this point). The choice of progestin, its dose, and its regimen may be important in minimizing these adverse effects, but these issues remain to be clarified.

2. Physical examination: A complete medical and family history should be taken prior to the initiation of any estrogen therapy. The pretreatment and periodic physical examinations should include special reference to blood pressure, breasts, abdomen, and pelvic organs, and should include a Papanicolaou smear. As a general rule, estrogen should not be prescribed for longer than one year without reexamining the patient.

3. Hypercoagulability: Some studies have shown that women taking estrogen replacement therapy have hypercoagulability, primarily related to decreased antithrombin activity. This effect appears dose- and duration-dependent and is less pronounced than that associated with oral contraceptive use. Also, postmenopausal women tend to have increased coagulation parameters at baseline compared to premenopausal women. There is some suggestion that low dose estrogens may increase the risk of thromboembolism. Patients with a past history of such disease may be at higher risk. The likelihood of thromboembolism has been reported to be increased when pharmacologic doses of estrogen are used to treat breast or prostatic cancer.

4. Familial hyperlipoproteinemia: Estrogen therapy may be associated with massive elevations of plasma triglycerides leading to pancreatitis and other complications in patients with familial defects of lipoprotein metabolism.

5. Fluid retention: Because estrogens may cause some degree of fluid retention, conditions which might be exacerbated by this factor, such as asthma, epilepsy, migraine, and cardiac or renal dysfunction, require careful observation.

6. Uterine bleeding and mastodynia: Certain patients may develop undesirable manifestations of estrogenic stimulation, such as abnormal uterine bleeding and mastodynia.

7. Impaired liver function: Estrogens may be poorly metabolized in patients with impaired liver function and should be administered with caution.

8. Because estrogens and/or androgens influence the metabolism of calcium and phosphorus, they should be used with caution in patients with metabolic bone diseases that are associated with hypercalcemia or in patients with renal insufficiency.

9. Androgen may increase sensitivity to oral anticoagulants. Dosage of the anticoagulant may require reduction in order to maintain a satisfactory therapeutic hypoprothrombinemia.

10. Serum cholesterol and/or bilirubin may increase during androgen therapy.

11. In diabetic patients the metabolic effect of androgens may result in a reduction of insulin requirements.

12. Oral contraceptives appear to be associated with an increased incidence of mental depression. Although it is not clear whether this is due to the estrogenic or progestogenic component of the contraceptive, patients with a history of depression should be carefully observed.

13. Preexisting uterine leiomyomata may increase in size during estrogen use.

14. The pathologist should be advised of estrogen therapy when relevant specimens are submitted.

15. Patients with a past history of jaundice during pregnancy have an increased risk of recurrence of jaundice while receiving estrogen-containing contraceptive therapy. If jaundice develops in any patient receiving estrogen, the medication should be discontinued while the cause is investigated.

B. INFORMATION FOR THE PATIENT
See text of patient package insert supplied with the product.

C. LABORATORY TESTS
Estrogen administration should generally be guided by clinical response at the smallest dose, rather than laboratory monitoring, for relief of symptoms for those indications in which symptoms are observable.

D. DRUG/LABORATORY TEST INTERACTIONS
1. Accelerated prothrombin time, partial thromboplastin time, and platelet aggregation time; increased platelet count; increased factors II, VII antigen; VIII antigen, VIII coagulant activity, IX, X, XII, VII-X complex, II-VII-X complex, and beta-thromboglobulin; decreased levels of anti-factor Xa and antithrombin III, decreased antithrombin III activity; increased levels of fibrinogen and fibrinogen activity; increased plasminogen antigen and activity.

2. Increased thyroid-binding globulin (TBG) leading to increased circulating total thyroid hormone, as measured by protein-bound iodine (PBI), T4 levels (by column or by radioimmunoassay) or T3 levels by radioimmunoassay. T3 resin uptake is decreased, reflecting the elevated TBG. Free T4 and free T3 concentrations are unaltered. The PBI may decrease during androgen therapy without clinical significance.

3. Other binding proteins may be elevated in serum, i.e., corticosteroid binding globulin (CBG), sex-hormone binding globulin (SHBG), leading to increased circulating corticosteroids and sex steroids respectively. Free or biologically active hormone concentrations are unchanged. Other plasma proteins may be increased (angiotensinogen/renin substrate, alpha-1-antitrypsin, ceruloplasmin).

4. Increased plasma HDL and HDL-2 subfraction concentrations increased serum cholesterol, reduced LDL cholesterol concentration, increased triglyceride and phospholipid levels.

5. Impaired glucose tolerance.

6. Reduced response to metyrapone test.

7. Reduced serum folate concentration.

8. The concomitant administration of an androgen, as in the case of Estrogen Cypionate/Testosterone Cypionate, may alter the estrogen effect on many of the above values.

9. Increased sulfobromophthalein retention.

10. Decreased pregnanediol excretion.

E. CARCINOGENESIS, MUTAGENESIS, AND IMPAIRMENT OF FERTILITY
Long term continuous administration of natural and synthetic estrogens in certain animal species increases the frequency of carcinomas of the breast, uterus, cervix, vagina, testis, and liver. See *"Contraindications"* and *"Warnings"*.

F. PREGNANCY CATEGORY X
Estrogens should not be used during pregnancy. See *"Contraindications"* and boxed *"Warnings"*.

G. LABOR AND DELIVERY
There is no reason why this drug should be administered during labor and delivery.

H. NURSING MOTHERS
As a general principle, the administration of any drug to nursing mothers should be done only when clearly necessary since many drugs are excreted in human milk. In addition, estrogen administration to nursing mothers has been shown to decrease the quantity and quality of the milk.

◆ RATED THERAPEUTICALLY EQUIVALENT; ◇ THERAPEUTIC EQUIVALENCE UNCONFIRMED; ○ UNRATED

I. HEMOGLOBIN AND HEMATOCRIT

An increase in red blood count, hemoglobin and hematocrit may occur in patients receiving large doses of androgen. Hemoglobin and hematocrit should be checked periodically for polycythemia in patients who are receiving high doses of androgens.

ADVERSE REACTIONS

The following additional adverse reactions have been reported with estrogen therapy (see *"Warnings"* regarding induction of neoplasia, adverse effects on the fetus, increased incidence of gallbladder disease, cardiovascular disease, elevated blood pressure, and hypercalcemia).

1. *Genitourinary System:* Changes in vaginal bleeding pattern and abnormal withdrawal bleeding or flow; breakthrough bleeding, spotting.
   Increase in size of uterine leiomyomata.
   Vaginal candidiasis.
   Change in amount of cervical secretion.
   Dysmenorrhea.
   Premenstrual-like syndrome.
   Amenorrhea during and after treatment.
   Cystitis-like syndrome.

2. *Breasts:* Tenderness, enlargement.

3. *Gastrointestinal:* Nausea, vomiting.
   Abdominal cramps, bloating.
   Cholestatic jaundice.
   Increased incidence of gallbladder disease.

4. *Skin:* Chloasma or melasma that may persist when drug is discontinued.
   Erythema multiforme.
   Erythema nodosum.
   Hemorrhagic eruption.
   Loss of scalp hair.
   Hirsutism.

5. *Eyes:* Steepening of corneal curvature.
   Intolerance to contact lenses.

6. *Central Nervous System:* Headache, migraine, dizziness.
   Mental depression.
   Chorea.

7. *Miscellaneous:* Increase or decrease in weight.
   Reduced carbohydrate tolerance.
   Aggravation of porphyria.
   Edema.
   Changes in libido.

Additional adverse reactions which have occurred with injectable androgen therapy alone include acne; hypersensitivity, including skin manifestations and anaphylactoid reactions; virilization; hypercalcemia (especially in immobilized patients); and local irritation.

DRUG ABUSE AND DEPENDENCE

Chlorobutanol anhydrous (chloral derivative) added as a preservative may be habit forming.

OVERDOSAGE

Serious ill effects have been reported following acute ingestion of large doses of estrogen-containing oral contraceptives by young children. Overdosage of estrogen may cause nausea and vomiting, and withdrawal bleeding may occur in females. The accidental injection of a large dose of Estrogen Cypionate/Testosterone Cypionate could produce androgenic or estrogenic effects, none of which would be expected to be life threatening.

DOSAGE AND ADMINISTRATION

Parenteral drug products should be inspected visually for particulate matter and discoloration prior to administration whenever solution and container permit.

Warming and shaking the vial should redissolve any crystals that may have formed during storage at temperatures lower than recommended.

Estrogen Cypionate/Testosterone Cypionate is for intramuscular use only.

Short-term cyclic use is for treatment of moderate to severe vasomotor symptoms associated with the menopause. The lowest dose and regimen that will control symptoms should be chosen and medication should be discontinued as promptly as possible.

Attempts to discontinue or taper medication should be made at 3 to 6 month intervals. The usual dosage is 1 mL injected at 4-week intervals.

Treated patients with an intact uterus should be monitored closely for signs of endometrial cancer and appropriate diagnostic measures should be taken to rule out malignancy in the event of persistent or recurring abnormal vaginal bleeding.

REFERENCES

1. Ziel HK, Finkle WD: Increased risk of endometrial carcinoma among users of conjugated estrogens. N Engl J Med 293:1167-1170, 1975. 2. Smith DC, Prentice R, Thompson DJ, et al: Association of exogenous estrogen and endometrial carcinoma. N Engl J Med 293:1164-1167, 1975. 3. Mack TM, Pike MC, Henderson BE, et al: Estrogens and endometrial cancer in a retirement community. N Engl J Med 294:1262-1267, 1976. 4. Weiss NS, Szekely DR, Austin DF: Increasing incidence of endometrial cancer in the United States. N Engl J Med 294:1259-1261, 1976. 5. Herbst AL, Ulfelder H, Poskanzer DC: Adenocarcinoma of the vagina. Association of maternal stilbestrol therapy with tumor appearance in young women. N Engl J Med 284:878-881, 1971. 6. Greenwald P, Barlow JJ, Nasca PC, Burnett WS: Vaginal cancer after maternal treatment with synthetic estrogens. N Engl J Med 285:390-392, 1971. 7. Lanier AP, Noller KL, Decker DG, Elveback LR, Kurland LT: Cancer and stilbestrol. A follow-up of 1,719 persons exposed to estrogens in utero and born 1943-1959. Mayo Clin Proc 48:793-799, 1973. 8. Herbst AL, Kurman RJ, Scully RE: Vaginal and cervical abnormalities after exposure to stilbestrol in utero. Obstet Gynecol 40:287-298, 1972. 9. Herbst AL, Robboy SJ, Macdonald GJ, Scully RE: The effects of local progesterone on stilbestrol-associated vaginal adenosis. Am J Obstet Gynecol 118:607-615, 1974. 10. Herbst AL, Poskanzer DC, Robboy SJ, Friedlander L, Scully RE: Prenatal exposure to stilbestrol. A prospective comparison of exposed female offspring with unexposed fetus. N Engl J Med 292:334-339, 1975. 11. Stafl A, Mattingly RF, Foley DV, Fetherston WC: Clinical diagnosis of vaginal adenosis. Obstet Gynecol 43:118-128, 1974. 12. Sherman AL, Goldrath M, Berlin A, et al: Cervical-vaginal adenosis after in utero exposure to synthetic estrogens. Obstet Gynecol 44:531-545, 1974. 13. Gall, Kirman B, Stern J: Hormonal pregnancy tests and congenital malformation. Nature 216:83, 1967. 14. Levy EP, Cohen A, Fraser FC: Hormone treatment during pregnancy and congenital heart defects. Lancet 1:611, 1973. 15. Nora JJ, Nora AH: Birth defects and oral contraceptives. Lancet 1:941-942, 1973. 16. Janerich DT, Piper JM, Glebatis DM: Oral contraceptives and congenital limb-reduction defects. N Engl J Med 291:697-700, 1974. 17. Boston Collaborative Drug Surveillance Program: Surgically confirmed gall bladder disease, venous thromboembolism, and breast tumors in relation to post-menopausal estrogen therapy. N Engl J Med 290:15-19, 1974. 18. Hoover R, Gray LA, Cole P. MacMahon B: Menopausal estrogens and breast cancer. N Engl J Med 295:401-405, 1976. 19. Boston Collaborative Drug Surveillance Program: Oral contraceptives and venous thromboembolism disease, surgically confirmed gall bladder disease and breast tumors. Lancet 1:1399-1404, 1973. 20. Daniel DG, Campbell H, Turnbull AC: Puerperal thromboembolism and suppression of lactation. Lancet 2:287-289, 1967. 21. The Veterans Administration Cooperative Urological Research Group: Carcinoma of the prostate: Treatment comparisons. J Urol 98:516-522, 1967. 22. Bailar JC: Thromboembolism and estrogen therapy. Lancet 2:560, 1967. 23. Blackard CE, Doe RP, Mellinger GT, Byar DP: Incidence of cardiovascular disease death in patients receiving diethylstilbestrol for carcinoma of the prostate. Cancer 26:249-256, 1970. 24. Royal College of General Practitioners: Oral contraception and thromboembolic disease. J R Coll Gen Pract 13:267-279, 1967. 25. Inman WHW, Vessey MP: Investigation of deaths from pulmonary, coronary, and cerebral thrombosis and embolism in women of child-bearing age. Br Med J 2:193-199, 1968. 26. Vessey MP, Doll R: Investigation of relation between use of oral contraceptives and thromboembolic disease. A further report. Br Med J 2:651-657, 1969. 27. Sartwell PE, Masi AT, Arthes FG, et al: Thromboembolism and oral contraceptives: An epidemiologic case-control study. Am J Epidemiol 90:365-380, 1969. 28. Collaborative Group for the Study of Stroke in Young Women: Oral contraception and increased risk of cerebral ischemia of thrombosis. N Engl J Med 288:871-878, 1973. 29. Collaborative Group for the Study of Stroke in Young Women: Oral contraceptives and stroke in young women: Associated risk factors. JAMA 231:718-722, 1975. 30. Mann JI, Inman WHW: Oral contraceptives and death from myocardial infarction. Br Med J 2:245-248, 1975. 31. Mann JI, Vessey MP, Thorogood M, Doll R: Myocardial infarction in young women with special reference to oral contraceptive practice. Br Med J 2:241-245, 1975. 32. Inman WHW, Vessey MP, Westerholm B, Engelund A: Thromboembolic disease and the steroidal content of oral contraceptives. Br Med J 2:203-209, 1970. 33. Stolley PD, Tonascia JA, Tockman MS, et al: Thrombosis with low-estrogen oral contraceptives. Am J Epidemiol 102:197-208, 1975. 34. Vessey MP, Doll R, Fairbairn AS, Glober G: Postoperative thromboembolism and the use of oral contraceptives. Br Med J 3:123-126, 1970. 35. Greene GR, Sartwell PE: Oral contraceptive use in patients with thromboembolism following surgery, trauma or infection. Am J Public Health 62:680-685, 1972. 36. Rosenberg L, Armstrong B, Phil D, Jick H: Myocardial infarction and estrogen therapy in post-menopausal women. N Engl J Med 294:1256-1259, 1976. 37. Coronary Drug Project Research Group: The Coronary Drug Project: Initial findings leading to modifications of its research protocol. JAMA 214:1303-1313, 1970. 38. Baum J, Holt F, Bookstein JJ, Klein EW: Possible association between benign hepatomas and oral contraceptives. Lancet 2:926-929, 1973. 39. Mays ET, Christopherson WM, Mahr MM, Williams HC: Hepatic changes in young women ingesting contraceptive steroids. Hepatic hemorrhage and primary hepatic tumors. JAMA 235:730-732, 1976. 40. Edmondson HA, Henderson B, Benton B: Liver-cell adenomas associated with use of oral contraceptives. N Engl J Med 294:470-472, 1976. 41. Pfeffer RI, VanDenNoort S: Estrogen use and stroke risk in post-menopausal women. Am J Epidemiol 103:445-456, 1976.

J CODES

Up to 1 ml IM—J1060

HOW SUPPLIED
INJECTION:

AVERAGE UNIT PRICE (AVAILABLE SIZES)		GENERIC A-RATED AVERAGE PRICE (GAAP)	
BRAND	$2.62	10 ml	$12.80
GENERIC	$1.28		

BRAND/MANUFACTURER	NDC	SIZE	AWP
◆ BRAND			
DEPO-TESTADIOL: Upjohn	00009-0253-02	10 ml	$26.15
◆ GENERICS			
DEPOTESTOGEN: Hyrex	00314-0875-70	10 ml	$10.90
Rugby	00536-9470-70	10 ml	$14.70

INJECTION: 50 MG/ML-2 MG/ML

BRAND/MANUFACTURER	NDC	SIZE	AWP
◆ GENERICS			
Steris	00402-0257-10	10 ml	$9.75

INJECTION: 50 MG-2 MG

BRAND/MANUFACTURER	NDC	SIZE	AWP
◆ GENERICS			
Goldline	00182-3069-63	10 ml	$13.50

➤ SHOWN IN PRODUCT IDENTIFICATION GUIDE

INJECTION (C-III):

AVERAGE UNIT PRICE (AVAILABLE SIZES)		GENERIC A-RATED AVERAGE PRICE (GAAP)	
BRAND	$2.62	10 ml	$12.80
GENERIC	$1.28		

BRAND/MANUFACTURER		NDC	SIZE	AWP
◆ **BRAND**				
DEPO-TESTADIOL: Upjohn		00009-0253-02	10 ml	$26.15
◆ **GENERICS**				
DEPOTESTOGEN: Hyrex		00314-0875-70	10 ml	$10.90
Rugby		00536-9470-70	10 ml	$14.70

Estradiol, Injectable

WARNING

1. ESTROGENS HAVE BEEN REPORTED TO INCREASE THE RISK OF ENDOMETRIAL CARCINOMA.

THREE INDEPENDENT CASE CONTROL STUDIES HAVE SHOWN AN INCREASED RISK OF ENDOMETRIAL CANCER IN POSTMENOPAUSAL WOMEN EXPOSED TO EXOGENOUS ESTROGENS FOR PROLONGED PERIODS.[1-3] THIS RISK WAS INDEPENDENT OF THE OTHER KNOWN RISK FACTORS FOR ENDOMETRIAL CANCER. THESE STUDIES ARE FURTHER SUPPORTED BY THE FINDING THAT INCIDENCE RATES OF ENDOMETRIAL CANCER HAVE INCREASED SHARPLY SINCE 1969 IN EIGHT DIFFERENT AREAS OF THE UNITED STATES WITH POPULATION-BASED CANCER REPORTING SYSTEMS, AN INCREASE WHICH MAY BE RELATED TO THE RAPIDLY EXPANDING USE OF ESTROGENS DURING THE LAST DECADE.[4]

THE THREE CASE CONTROL STUDIES REPORTED THAT THE RISK OF ENDOMETRIAL CANCER IN ESTROGEN USERS WAS ABOUT 4.5 TO 13.9 TIMES GREATER THAN IN NONUSERS. THE RISK APPEARS TO DEPEND ON BOTH DURATION OF TREATMENT[1] AND ON ESTROGEN DOSE.[3] IN VIEW OF THESE FINDINGS, WHEN ESTROGENS ARE USED FOR THE TREATMENT OF MENOPAUSAL SYMPTOMS, THE LOWEST DOSE THAT WILL CONTROL SYMPTOMS SHOULD BE UTILIZED AND MEDICATION SHOULD BE DISCONTINUED AS SOON AS POSSIBLE. WHEN PROLONGED TREATMENT IS MEDICALLY INDICATED, THE PATIENT SHOULD BE REASSESSED ON AT LEAST A SEMIANNUAL BASIS TO DETERMINE THE NEED FOR CONTINUED THERAPY. ALTHOUGH THE EVIDENCE MUST BE CONSIDERED PRELIMINARY, ONE STUDY SUGGESTS THAT CYCLIC ADMINISTRATION OF LOW DOSES OF ESTROGEN MAY CARRY LESS RISK THAN CONTINUOUS ADMINISTRATION;[3] IT THEREFORE APPEARS PRUDENT TO UTILIZE SUCH A REGIMEN.

CLOSE CLINICAL SURVEILLANCE OF ALL WOMEN TAKING ESTROGENS IS IMPORTANT. IN ALL CASES OF UNDIAGNOSED PERSISTENT OR RECURRING ABNORMAL VAGINAL BLEEDING, ADEQUATE DIAGNOSTIC MEASURES SHOULD BE UNDERTAKEN TO RULE OUT MALIGNANCY.

THERE IS NO EVIDENCE AT PRESENT THAT "NATURAL" ESTROGENS ARE MORE OR LESS HAZARDOUS THAN "SYNTHETIC" ESTROGENS AT EQUIESTROGENIC DOSES.

2. ESTROGENS SHOULD NOT BE USED DURING PREGNANCY.

THE USE OF FEMALE SEX HORMONES, BOTH ESTROGENS AND PROGESTOGENS, DURING EARLY PREGNANCY MAY SERIOUSLY DAMAGE THE OFFSPRING. AN ASSOCIATION HAS BEEN REPORTED BETWEEN *IN UTERO* EXPOSURE OF THE FEMALE FETUS TO DIETHYLSTILBESTROL, A NONSTEROIDAL ESTROGEN, AND AN INCREASED RISK OF THE POSTPUBERTAL DEVELOPMENT OF AN ORDINARILY EXTREMELY RARE FORM OF VAGINAL OR CERVICAL CANCER.[5,6] THIS RISK HAS RECENTLY BEEN ESTIMATED TO BE IN THE RANGE 0.14 TO 1.4 PER 1000 EXPOSED FEMALES, CONSISTENT WITH A PREVIOUS RISK ESTIMATE OF NOT GREATER THAN 4 PER 1000 EXPOSURES.[7] FURTHERMORE, A HIGH PERCENTAGE OF SUCH EXPOSED WOMEN (FROM 30 TO 90 PERCENT) HAVE BEEN FOUND TO HAVE VAGINAL ADENOSIS,[8-12] WITH EPITHELIAL CHANGES OF THE VAGINA AND CERVIX. ALTHOUGH THESE CHANGES ARE HISTOLOGICALLY BENIGN, IT IS NOT KNOWN WHETHER THEY ARE PRECURSORS OF MALIGNANCY. ALTHOUGH SIMILAR DATA ARE NOT AVAILABLE WITH THE USE OF OTHER ESTROGENS, IT CANNOT BE PRESUMED THEY WOULD NOT INDUCE SIMILAR CHANGES.

SEVERAL REPORTS SUGGEST AN ASSOCIATION BETWEEN INTRAUTERINE EXPOSURE TO FEMALE SEX HORMONES AND CONGENITAL ANOMALIES, INCLUDING CONGENITAL HEART DEFECTS AND LIMB REDUCTION DEFECTS.[13-16] ONE CASE CONTROL STUDY[16] ESTIMATED A 4.7-FOLD INCREASED RISK OF LIMB REDUCTION DEFECTS IN INFANTS EXPOSED *IN UTERO* TO SEX HORMONES (ORAL CONTRACEPTIVES, HORMONE WITHDRAWAL TESTS FOR PREGNANCY, OR ATTEMPTED TREATMENT FOR THREATENED ABORTION). SOME OF THESE EXPOSURES WERE VERY SHORT AND INVOLVED ONLY A FEW DAYS OF TREATMENT. THE DATA SUGGEST THAT THE RISK OF LIMB REDUCTION DEFECTS IN EXPOSED FETUSES IS SOMEWHAT LESS THAN 1 PER 1000.

IN THE PAST, FEMALE SEX HORMONES HAVE BEEN USED DURING PREGNANCY IN AN ATTEMPT TO TREAT THREATENED OR HABITUAL ABORTION. THERE IS NOW CONSIDERABLE LITERATURE TO THE EFFECT THAT ESTROGENS ARE INEFFECTIVE FOR THESE INDICATIONS, AND THE DATA ARE NOT NOW CONSIDERED ADEQUATE TO SUPPORT THE CONCLUSION THAT PROGESTOGENS ARE EFFECTIVE FOR THESE USES.

IF ESTRADIOL, INJECTABLE, IS USED DURING PREGNANCY OR IF THE PATIENT BECOMES PREGNANT WHILE TAKING THIS DRUG, SHE SHOULD BE APPRISED OF THE POTENTIAL RISKS TO THE FETUS AND THE ADVISABILITY OF PREGNANCY CONTINUATION.

DESCRIPTION

Estradiol, Injectable, is a sterile solution for intramuscular injection. Each ml contains Estradiol Valerate 10, 20, or 40 mg or Estradiol Cypionate 1 or 5 mg.

Estradiol valerate is a white, crystalline powder. It is usually odorless but may have a faint, fatty odor. It is practically insoluble in water; soluble in castor oil, methanol, benzyl benzoate and dioxane; sparingly soluble in sesame oil and in peanut oil. It is designated chemically as Estra-1,3,5(10)-triene-3,17-diol(17β)-, 17-pentanoate. Estradiol 17-valerate, and has the empirical formula $C_{23}H_{32}O_3$ and molecular weight 356.50.

Estradiol Cypionate is a white to practically white, crystalline powder. It is odorless or has a slight odor. It is insoluble in water, soluble in alcohol, in acetone, in chloroform, and in dioxane; sparingly soluble in vegetable oil. It is designated chemically as Estra-1,3,5(10)-triene-3,17-diol, (17β)-, 17-cyclopentane-propanoate. Estradiol 17-cyclopentanepropionate and has the empirical formula $C_{26}H_{36}O_3$ and molecular weight 396.57.

Following is its chemical structure:

$C_{23}H_{32}O_3$ MW 356.50 CAS-979-32-8

CLINICAL PHARMACOLOGY

Estradiol, Injectable, is a hormone with a potent and prolonged estrogenic effect. Estrogens are important in the development and maintenance of the female reproductive system and secondary sex characteristics. They promote growth and development of the vagina, uterus, and fallopian tubes, and enlargement of the breasts. Indirectly, they contribute to the shaping of the skeleton, maintenance of tone and elasticity of urogenital structures, changes in the epiphyses of the long bones that allow for the pubertal growth spurt and its termination, growth of axillary and pubic hair, and pigmentation of the nipples and genitals. Decline of estrogenic activity at the end of the menstrual cycle can bring on menstruation, although the cessation of progesterone secretion is the most important factor in the mature ovulatory cycle. However, in the preovulatory or nonovulatory cycle, estrogen is the primary determinant in the onset of menstruation. Estrogens also affect the release of pituitary gonadotropins.

The pharmacologic effects of conjugated estrogens are similar to those of endogenous estrogens. They are soluble in water and may be absorbed from mucosal surfaces after local administration. In estrogen-responsive tissues (female genital organs, breasts, hypothalamus, pituitary), estrogen binds to tissue-specific receptor proteins in the cytoplasm. The resulting estrogen-protein complex penetrates the nuclear membrane and ultimately binds to materials in the cell nucleus. Such binding activates the increased synthesis of DNA, RNA, and various proteins that in turn effect characteristic changes in responsive tissues. Estradiol promotes the growth of the endometrium; promotes thickening, stratification, and cornification of the vagina; causes growth of mammary gland ducts; and inhibits the anterior pituitary gland. These effects occur soon after administration and last for approximately two to three weeks after a single intramuscular injection.

About 80 percent of Estradiol is reported to be bound to sex hormone binding globulin; most of the remainder is loosely bound to albumin and about two percent is unbound. Some estrogens are excreted into the bile; however they are reabsorbed from the intestine and returned to the liver through the portal venous system. Water-soluble estrogen conjugates are strongly acidic and are ionized in body fluids, which favor excretion through the kidneys since tubular reabsorption is minimal. Estradiol is metabolized to a relatively inactive form in the liver and then excreted in the urine and the bile.

Estradiol Cypionate provides estradiol 17β, the most potent of the naturally occurring estrogens, in the form of a highly fat-soluble derivative with prolonged estrogenic effect.

Comparative clinical studies have demonstrated that Estradiol Cypionate produces estrogenic effects that are qualitatively the same as those produced by other estradiol esters. In menopausal women, the average duration of estrogenic effect (as measured by vaginal smear) following a single injection of 5 mg of Estradiol Cypionate was found to be approximately 3 to 4 weeks. Relief of vasomotor symptoms was observed to occur within 1 to 5 days and to be maintained for 1 to 8 weeks, with an average of approximately 5 weeks.

INDICATIONS AND USAGE

Estradiol, Injectable, is indicated in the treatment of moderate to severe *vasomotor* symptoms associated with the menopause. (There is no evidence that estrogens are effective for nervous symptoms or depression which might occur during menopause, and they should not be used to treat these conditions.) It is also indicated for the treatment of atrophic vaginitis, kraurosis vulvae, female hypogonadism, female castration, and primary ovarian failure. Estradiol, Injectable, may also be used for the palliative therapy of inoperable, progressing prostatic carcinoma.

ESTRADIOL INJECTABLE HAS NOT BEEN SHOWN TO BE EFFECTIVE FOR ANY PURPOSE DURING PREGNANCY, AND ITS USE MAY CAUSE SEVERE HARM TO THE FETUS (SEE BOXED "WARNING").

UNLABELED USES

Estradiol, Injectable is used alone or as an adjunct in the treatment of alopecia androgenetica, for prophylaxis of cardiovascular disease, and the treatment of dyskinesia including chorea secondary to Huntington's disease and tardive dyskinesia, and levodopa-induced dyskinesia. It is used to regress hirsutism due to polycystic ovaries. It is prescribed for hyperlipidemia, hypersexuality, and induction of labor. It is used in the treatment of premenstrual syndrome, including menstrual migraine and is prescribed for women with primary biliary cirrhosis, Turner's syndrome, or abnormal uterine bleeding. It is also used in postcoital contraception.

CONTRAINDICATIONS

Estrogens should not be used in women (or men) with any of the following conditions:

1. Known or suspected cancer of the breast except in appropriately selected patients being treated for metastatic disease.
2. Known or suspected estrogen-dependent neoplasia (e.g., genital malignancy).
3. Known or suspected pregnancy (see boxed "Warning").
4. Undiagnosed abnormal genital bleeding.
5. Active thrombophlebitis or thromboembolic disorders.
6. A past history of thrombophlebitis, thrombosis, or thromboembolic disorders associated with previous estrogen use (except when used in treatment of breast or prostatic malignancy).
7. A history of hypersensitivity to estradiol or any component of the preparation.

Contraindicated in those persons who have shown hypersensitivity to any component of this preparation.

WARNINGS

1. INDUCTION OF MALIGNANT NEOPLASMS

Long-term continuous administration of natural and synthetic estrogens in certain animal species increases the frequency of carcinomas of the breast, cervix, vagina, and liver. There is now evidence that estrogens increase the risk of carcinoma of the endometrium in humans (see boxed "Warning").

At the present time there is no satisfactory evidence that estrogens given to postmenopausal women increase the risk of cancer of the breast,[17] although a recent, long-term follow-up of a single physician's practice has raised this possibility.[18] Because of the animal data, there is a need for caution in prescribing estrogens for women with a strong family history of breast cancer or who have breast nodules, fibrocystic disease, or abnormal mammograms.

2. GALLBLADDER DISEASE

A recent study has reported a 2- to 3-fold increase in the risk of surgically confirmed gallbladder disease in women receiving postmenopausal estrogens[17] similar to the 2-fold increase previously noted in users of oral contraceptives.[19,24] In the case of oral contraceptives the increased risk appeared after two years of use.[24]

3. EFFECTS SIMILAR TO THOSE CAUSED BY ESTROGEN-PROGESTOGEN ORAL CONTRACEPTIVES

There are several serious adverse effects of oral contraceptives, most of which have not, up to now, been documented as consequences of postmenopausal estrogen therapy. This may reflect the comparatively low doses of estrogen used in postmenopausal women. It would be expected that the larger doses of estrogen used to treat prostatic or breast cancer or postpartum breast engorgement are more likely to result in these adverse effects, and, in fact, it has been shown that there is an increased risk of thrombosis in men receiving estrogens for prostatic cancer and women for postpartum breast engorgement.[20-23]

a. Thromboembolic disease: It is now well established that users of oral contraceptives have an increased risk of various thromboembolic and thrombotic vascular diseases, such as thrombophlebitis, pulmonary embolism, stroke, and myocardial infarction.[24-31] Cases of retinal thrombosis, mesenteric thrombosis, and optic neuritis have been reported in oral contraceptive users. There is evidence that the risk of several of these adverse reactions is related to the dose of the drug.[32,33] An increased risk of post-surgery thromboembolic complications has also been reported in users of oral contraceptives.[34,35] If feasible, estrogen

should be discontinued at least four weeks before, and not resumed until at least four weeks after, surgery of the type associated with an increased risk of thromboembolism or during periods of prolonged immobilization.

While an increased rate of thromboembolic and thrombotic disease in postmenopausal users of estrogens has not been found,[17,36] this does not rule out the possibility that such an increase may be present or that subgroups of women who have underlying risk factors or who are receiving relatively large doses of estrogens may have increased risk. Therefore, estrogens should not be used in persons with active thrombophlebitis or thromboembolic disorders, and they should not be used (except in treatment of malignancy) in persons with a history of such disorders in association with estrogen use. They should be used with caution in patients with cerebral vascular or coronary artery disease and only for those in whom estrogens are clearly needed.

Large doses of estrogen (5 mg conjugated estrogens per day), comparable to those used to treat cancer of the prostate and breast, have been shown in a large prospective clinical trial in men[37] to increase the risk of nonfatal myocardial infarction, pulmonary embolism, and thrombophlebitis. When estrogen doses of this size are used, any of the thromboembolic and thrombotic adverse effects associated with oral contraceptive use should be considered a clear risk.

b. Hepatic adenoma: Benign hepatic adenomas appear to be associated with the use of oral contraceptives.[38-40] Although benign, and rare, these may rupture and may cause death through intra-abdominal hemorrhage. Such lesions have not yet been reported in association with other estrogen or progestogen preparations but should be considered in estrogen users having abdominal pain and tenderness, abdominal mass, or hypovolemic shock. Hepatocellular carcinoma has also been reported in women taking estrogen-containing oral contraceptives.[39] The relationship of this malignancy to these drugs is not known at this time.

c. Elevated blood pressure: Increased blood pressure is not uncommon in women using oral contraceptives. There is now a report that this may occur with use of estrogens in the menopause,[41] and blood pressure should be monitored with estrogen use, especially if high doses are used.

d. Glucose tolerance: A worsening of glucose tolerance has been observed in a significant percentage of patients on estrogen-containing oral contraceptives. For this reason, diabetic patients should be carefully observed while receiving estrogen.

4. HYPERCALCEMIA

Administration of estrogens may lead to severe hypercalcemia in patients with breast cancer and bone metastases. If this occurs, the drug should be stopped and appropriate measures taken to reduce the serum calcium level.

PRECAUTIONS:

GENERAL

1. A complete medical and family history should be taken prior to the initiation of any estrogen therapy. The pretreatment and periodic physical examinations should include special reference to blood pressure, breasts, abdomen, and pelvic organs and should include a Papanicolaou smear. As a general rule, estrogen should not be prescribed for longer than 6 months to one year without another physical examination being performed.

2. Fluid retention—Because estrogens may cause some degree of fluid retention, conditions which might be influenced by this factor, such as epilepsy, migraine, and cardiac or renal dysfunction, require careful observation.

3. Certain patients may develop undesirable manifestations of excessive estrogenic stimulation, such as abnormal or excessive uterine bleeding, mastodynia, etc.

4. Oral contraceptives appear to be associated with an increased incidence of mental depression.[24] Although it is not clear whether this is due to the estrogenic or progestogenic component of the contraceptive, patients with a history of depression or other psychic abnormality should be carefully observed.

5. Preexisting uterine leiomyomata may increase in size during estrogen use.

6. The pathologist should be advised of estrogen therapy when relevant specimens are submitted.

7. Patients with a past history of jaundice during pregnancy have an increased risk of recurrence of jaundice while receiving estrogen-containing oral contraceptive therapy. If jaundice develops in any patient receiving estrogen, the medication should be discontinued while the cause is investigated.

8. Estrogens may be poorly metabolized in patients with impaired liver function, and they should be administered with caution in such patients.

9. Because estrogens influence the metabolism of calcium and phosphorus, they should be used with caution in patients with metabolic bone diseases that are associated with hypercalcemia or in patients with renal insufficiency.

10. The lowest effective dose appropriate for the specific indication should be utilized. Studies of the addition of a progestin for seven or more days of a cycle of estrogen administration have reported a lowered incidence of endometrial hyperplasia. Morphological and biochemical studies of endometrium suggest that 10 to 13 days of progestin are needed to provide maximal maturation of the endometrium and to eliminate any hyperplastic changes. Whether this will provide protection from endometrial carcinoma has not been clearly established. There are possible additional risks which may be associated with the inclusion of progestin in estrogen replacement regimens. The potential risks include adverse effects on carbohydrate and lipid metabolism. The choice of progestin and dosage may be important in minimizing these adverse effects.

INFORMATION FOR PATIENTS
See manufacturer's patient information.

LABORATORY TESTS

The following procedures may be helpful in monitoring the patient's response to therapy; physical examination at least every 6 to 12 months with special attention given to breast and pelvic organs, Papanicolaou test, and hepatic function determinations.

DRUG INTERACTIONS

Estrogens reduce the effect of oral anticoagulants; monitor prothrombin levels and increase anticoagulant dosage accordingly. Rifampin and anticonvulsant drugs may decrease the effect of estrogens by accelerating estrogen metabolism. Estrogens may increase the number of toxic reactions to tricyclic antidepressants.

DRUG/LABORATORY TEST INTERACTIONS

Certain endocrine and liver function tests may be affected by estrogen-containing oral contraceptives. The following similar changes may be expected with larger doses of estrogen:

1. Increased sulfobromophthalein retention.
2. Increased prothrombin and factors VII, VIII, IX, and X; decreased antithrombin 3; increased norepinephrine-induced platelet aggrega- bility.
3. Increased thyroid binding globulin (TBG) leading to increased circulating total thyroid hormone, as measured by PBI, T4 by column, or T4 by radioimmunoassay. Free T3 resin uptake is decreased, reflecting the elevated TBG; free T4 concentration is unaltered.
4. Impaired glucose tolerance.
5. Decreased pregnanediol excretion.
6. Reduced response to metyrapone test.
7. Reduced serum folate concentration.
8. Increased serum triglyceride and phospholipid concentration.

CARCINOGENESIS, MUTAGENESIS, IMPAIRMENT OF FERTILITY

In long-term studies in animals, continuous administration of estrogens increased the frequency of certain carcinomas (see "Warnings" section). There is evidence that estrogens increase the risk of endometrial carcinoma in postmenopausal women (see boxed "Warning"). Long-term studies in animals have not been performed to evaluate mutagenic potential or impairment of fertility in males or females.

PREGNANCY CATEGORY X

See "Contraindications" and boxed "Warning".

NURSING MOTHERS

As a general principle, the administration of any drug to nursing mothers should be done only when clearly necessary since many drugs including estrogens are excreted in human milk.

PEDIATRIC USE

Safety and effectiveness in children have not been established. Because of the effects of estrogens on epiphyseal closure, they should be used judiciously in young patients in whom bone growth is not complete.

ADVERSE REACTIONS

(See "Warnings" regarding induction of neoplasia, adverse effects on the fetus, increased incidence of gallbladder disease, and adverse effects similar to those of oral contraceptives, including thromboembolism.) The following additional adverse reactions have been reported with estrogenic therapy, including oral contraceptives:

1. *Genitourinary system:* breakthrough bleeding; spotting; change in menstrual flow; dysmenorrhea; premenstrual-like syndrome; amenorrhea during and after treatment; increase in size of uterine fibromyomata; vaginal candidiasis, change in cervical eversion and in degree of cervical secretion; cystitis-like syndrome.

2. *Breasts:* tenderness; enlargement; secretion.

3. *Gastrointestinal:* nausea; vomiting; abdominal cramps; bloating; cholestatic jaundice.

4. *Skin:* chloasma or melasma which may persist when drug is discontinued; erythema multiforme; erythema nodosum; hemorrhagic eruption; loss of scalp hair; hirsutism; localized dermatitis.

5. *Eyes:* steepening of corneal curvature; intolerance to contact lenses.

6. *CNS:* headache; migraine; dizziness; mental depression; chorea; convulsions.

7. *Miscellaneous:* increase or decrease in weight; reduced carbohydrate tolerance; aggravation of porphyria; edema; changes in libido; pain at the site of injection; sterile abscess; postinjection flare.

DRUG ABUSE AND DEPENDENCE

Chlorobutanol anhydrous (chloral derivative) added as a preservative to some brands may be habit-forming.

OVERDOSAGE

Numerous reports of ingestion of large doses of estrogen-containing oral contraceptives by young children indicate that serious ill effects do not occur.

Overdosage of estrogen may cause nausea; withdrawal bleeding may occur in females and mastodynia in females and males.

DOSAGE AND ADMINISTRATION

Care should be taken to inject deeply into the upper, outer quadrant of the gluteal muscle following the usual precautions for intramuscular administration.

Estradiol, Injectable, should be visually inspected for particulate matter and color prior to administration; the solution is clear, colorless to pale yellow.

Cyclic Regimens: For Short-Term Use Only: For the treatment of moderate to severe *vasomotor* symptoms, atrophic vaginitis, or kraurosis vulvae associated with the menopause: 10 to 20 mg Estradiol Valerate every 4 weeks; or 1 to 5 mg Estradiol Cypionate every 3 to 4 weeks or weekly for 3 to 4 weeks.

Given cyclically: For the treatment of female hypogonadism, female castration, or primary ovarian failure: 10 to 20 mg Estradiol Valerate every 4 weeks or 1.5 to 2 mg Estradiol Cypionate monthly.

If in the physician's judgment a patient requires cyclic estrogen-progesterone therapy, 10 to 20 mg Estradiol Valerate may be given as an initial injection followed two weeks later by 250 mg Hydroxyprogesterone Caproate Injection USP and 5 mg Estradiol Valerate. Four weeks after the initial injection, the cycle may be repeated starting with 10 to 20 mg of Estradiol Valerate.

The lowest dose that will control symptoms should be chosen, and medication should be discontinued as promptly as possible. Administration should be cyclic (e.g., 3 weeks on and 1 week off).

Attempts to discontinue or taper medication should be made at three- to six-month intervals.

Continuous therapy with estrogen alone may induce functional uterine bleeding.

Treated patients with an intact uterus should be monitored closely for signs of endometrial cancer, and appropriate diagnostic measures should be taken to rule out malignancy in the event of persistent or recurring abnormal vaginal bleeding.

Chronic Regimen: For the palliative treatment of inoperable, progressing prostatic carcinoma, the usual dosage is 30 mg of more of Estradiol Valerate administered every one or two weeks.

Parenteral drug products should be inspected visually for particulate matter and discoloration prior to administration, whenever the solution and container permit.

Warming and shaking the vial should redissolve any crystals that may have formed during storage at temperatures lower than recommended.

Storage: Store at controlled room temperature 15°—30°C (59°—86°F).

REFERENCES

1. Ziel HK, Finkle WD: Increased risk of endometrial carcinoma among users of conjugated estrogens. *N Engl J Med* 293:1167-1170, 1975. 2. Smith DC, Prentice R, Thompson DJ, et al: Association of exogenous estrogen and endometrial carcinoma. *N Engl J Med* 293:1164-1167, 1975. 3. Mack TM, Pike MC, Henderson BE, et al: Estrogens and endometrial cancer in a retirement community. *N Engl J Med* 294:1262-1267, 1976. 4. Weiss NS, Szekely DR, Austin DF: Increasing incidence of endometrial cancer in the United States. *N Engl J Med* 294:1259-1262, 1976. 5. Herbst AL, Ulfelder H, Poskanzer DC: Adenocarcinoma of the vagina. Association of maternal stilbestrol therapy with tumor appearance in young women. *N Engl J Med* 284:878-881, 1971. 6. Greenwald P, Barlow JJ, Nasca PC, Burnett WS: Vaginal cancer after maternal treatment with synthetic estrogens. *N Engl J Med* 285:390-392, 1971. 7. Lanier AP, Noller KL, Decker DG, Elveback LR, Kurland LT: Cancer and stilbestrol. A follow-up of 1,719 persons exposed to estrogens *in utero* and born 1943-1959. *Mayo Clin Proc* 48:793-799, 1973. 8. Herbst AL, Kurman RJ, Scully RE: Vaginal and cervical abnormalities after exposure to stilbestrol *in utero*. *Obstet Gynecol* 40:287-298, 1972. 9. Herbst AL, Robboy SJ, Macdonald GJ, Scully RE: The effects of local progesterone on stilbestrol-associated vaginal adenosis. *Am J Obstet Gynecol* 118:607-615, 1974. 10. Herbst AL, Poskanzer DC, Robboy SJ, Friedlander L, Scully RE: Prenatal exposure to stilbestrol. A prospective comparison of exposed female offspring with unexposed control. *N Engl J Med* 292:334-339, 1975. 11. Stafl A, Mattingly RF, Foley DV, Fetherston WC: Clinical diagnosis of vaginal adenosis. *Obstet Gynecol* 43:118-128, 1974. 12. Sherman AI, Goldrath M, Berlin A, et al: Cervical-vaginal adenosis after *in utero* exposure to synthetic estrogens. *Obstet Gynecol* 44:531-545, 1974. 13. Gall, Kirman B, Stern J: Hormonal pregnancy tests and congenital malformation. *Nature* 216:83, 1967. 14. Levy EP, Cohen A, Fraser FC: Hormone treatment during pregnancy and congenital heart defects. *Lancet* 1:611, 1973. 15. Nora JJ, Nora AH: Birth defects and oral contraceptives. *Lancet* 1:941-942, 1973. 16. Janerich DT, Piper JM, Glebatis DM: Oral contraceptives and congenital limb-reduction defects. *N Engl J Med* 291:697-700, 1974. 17. Boston Collaborative Drug Surveillance Program: Surgically confirmed gall bladder disease, venous thromboembolism, and breast tumors in relation to post-menopausal estrogen therapy. *N Engl J Med* 290:15-19, 1974. 18. Hoover R, Gray LA, Cole P, MacMahon B: Menopausal estrogens and breast cancer. *N Engl J Med* 295:401-405, 1976. 19. Boston Collaborative Drug Surveillance Program: Oral contraceptives and venous thromboembolic disease, surgically confirmed gall bladder disease, and breast tumors. *Lancet* 1:1399-1404, 1973. 20. Daniel DG, Campbell H, Turnbull AC: Puerperal thromboembolism and suppression of lactation. *Lancet* 2:287-289, 1967. 21. The Veterans Administration Cooperative Urological Research Group: Carcinoma of the prostate: Treatment comparisons. *J Urol* 98:516-522, 1967. 22. Bailar JC: Thromboembolism and estrogen therapy. *Lancet* 2:560, 1967. 23. Blackard CE, Doe RP, Mellinger GT, Byar DP: Incidence of cardiovascular disease and death in patients receiving diethylstilbestrol for carcinoma of the prostate. *Cancer* 26:249-256, 1970. 24. Royal College of General Practitioners: Oral contraception and thromboembolic disease. *J R Coll Gen Pract* 13:267-279, 1967. 25. Inman WHW, Vessey MP: Investigation of deaths from pulmonary, coronary, and cerebral thrombosis and embolism in women of child-bearing age. *Br Med J* 2:193-199, 1968. 26. Vessey MP, Doll R: Investigation of relation between use of oral contraceptives and thromboembolic disease. A further report. *Br Med J* 2:651-657, 1969. 27. Sartwell PE, Masi AT, Arthes FG, et al: Thromboembolism and oral contraceptives: An epidemiologic case-control study. *Am J Epidemiol* 90:365-380, 1969. 28. Collaborative Group for the Study of Stroke in Young Women: Oral contraception and increased risk of cerebral ischemia or thrombosis. *N Engl J Med* 288:871-878, 1973. 29. Collaborative Group for the Study of Stroke in Young Women: Oral contraceptives and stroke in young women: Associated risk factors. *JAMA* 231:718-722, 1975. 30. Mann JI, Inman WHW: Oral contraceptives and death from myocardial infarction. *Br Med J* 2:245-248, 1975. 31. Mann JI, Vessey MP, Thorogood M, Doll R: Myocardial infarction in young women with special reference to oral contraceptive practice. *Br Med J* 2:241-245, 1975. 32. Inman WHW, Vessey MP, Westerholm B, Engelund A: Thromboembolic disease and the steroidal

---

content of oral contraceptives. *Br Med J* 2:203-209, 1970. 33. Stolley PD, Tonascia JA, Tockman MS, et al: Thrombosis with low-estrogen oral contraceptives. *Am J Epidemiol* 102:197-208, 1975. 34. Vessey MP, Doll R, Fairbairn AS, Glober G: Postoperative thromboembolism and the use of oral contraceptives. *Br Med J* 3:123-126, 1970. 35. Greene GR, Sartwell PE: Oral contraceptive use in patients with thromboembolism following surgery, trauma or infection. *Am J Public Health* 62:680-685, 1972. 36. Rosenberg L, Armstrong B, Phil D, Jick H: Myocardial infarction and estrogen therapy in post-menopausal women. *N Engl J Med* 294:1256-1259, 1976. 37. Coronary Drug Project Research Group: The Coronary Drug Project: Initial findings leading to modifications of its research protocol. *JAMA* 214:1303-1313, 1970. 38. Baum J, Holtz F, Bookstein JJ, Klein EW: Possible association between benign hepatomas and oral contraceptives. *Lancet* 2:926-929, 1973. 39. Mays ET, Christopherson WM, Mahr MM, Williams HC: Hepatic changes in young women ingesting contraceptive steroids. Hepatic hemorrhage and primary hepatic tumors. *JAMA* 235:730-732, 1976. 40. Edmondson HA, Henderson B, Benton B: Liver-cell adenomas associated with use of oral contraceptives. *N Engl J Med* 294:470-472, 1976. 41. Pfeffer RI, VanDenNoort S: Estrogen use and stroke risk in post-menopausal women. *Am J Epidemiol* 103:445-456, 1976.

J CODES

Up to 20 mg IM—J1390
Up to 10 mg IM—J1380
Up to 5 mg IM—J1000
Up to 40 mg IM—J0970

HOW SUPPLIED

ESTRADIOL CYPIONATE
INJECTION: 5 MG/ML

AVERAGE UNIT PRICE (AVAILABLE SIZES)		GENERIC A-RATED AVERAGE PRICE (GAAP)	
BRAND	$2.96	10 ml	$7.94
GENERIC	$0.79		

BRAND/MANUFACTURER	NDC	SIZE	AWP
◆ BRAND			
DEPO-ESTRADIOL: Upjohn	00009-0271-01	5 ml	$14.79
◆ GENERICS			
Schein	00364-6608-54	10 ml	$5.67
Steris	00402-0254-10	10 ml	$5.67
Moore,H.L.	00839-5575-30	10 ml	$6.87
Major	00904-0840-10	10 ml	$7.50
DEPOGEN: Hyrex	00314-0855-70	10 ml	$8.70
Goldline	00182-0662-63	10 ml	$9.90
Rugby	00536-6851-70	10 ml	$11.25

ESTRADIOL VALERATE
INJECTION: 10 MG/ML

AVERAGE UNIT PRICE (AVAILABLE SIZES)		GENERIC A-RATED AVERAGE PRICE (GAAP)	
BRAND	$6.21	10 ml	$7.93
GENERIC	$0.79		

BRAND/MANUFACTURER	NDC	SIZE	AWP
◆ BRAND			
DELESTROGEN: Mead Johnson Labs	00003-0330-50	5 ml	$31.04
◆ GENERICS			
Major	00904-2909-10	10 ml	$7.45
VALERGEN: Hyrex	00314-0780-70	10 ml	$8.40

INJECTION: 20 MG/ML

AVERAGE UNIT PRICE (AVAILABLE SIZES)		GENERIC A-RATED AVERAGE PRICE (GAAP)	
BRAND	$12.008	10 ml	$11.81
GENERIC	$1.18		

BRAND/MANUFACTURER	NDC	SIZE	AWP
◆ BRAND			
DELESTROGEN: Mead Johnson Labs	00003-0343-50	5 ml	$43.73
	00003-0343-16	1 ml	$15.27
◆ GENERICS			
Schein	00364-6613-54	10 ml	$8.49
Steris	00402-0027-10	10 ml	$8.49
VALERGEN: Hyrex	00314-0782-70	10 ml	$14.50
Goldline	00182-1805-63	10 ml	$15.75

INJECTION: 40 MG/ML

AVERAGE UNIT PRICE (AVAILABLE SIZES)		GENERIC A-RATED AVERAGE PRICE (GAAP)	
BRAND	$14.51	10 ml	$15.15
GENERIC	$1.52		

BRAND/MANUFACTURER	NDC	SIZE	AWP
◆ BRAND			
DELESTROGEN: Mead Johnson Labs	00003-0251-50	5 ml	$72.55
◆ GENERICS			
Schein	00364-6614-54	10 ml	$10.50
Steris	00402-0244-10	10 ml	$10.50
Rugby	00536-1741-70	10 ml	$15.38

BRAND/MANUFACTURER	NDC	SIZE	AWP
VALERGEN: Hyrex	00314-0784-70	10 ml	$24.20

Estramustine Phosphate Sodium

DESCRIPTION
Estramustine Phosphate Sodium, an antineoplastic agent, is an off-white powder readily soluble in water. Estramustine Phosphate Sodium is available as white opaque capsules, each containing Estramustine Phosphate Sodium as the disodium salt monohydrate equivalent to 140 mg estramustine phosphate, for oral administration.

Chemically, Estramustine Phosphate Sodium is estra-1,3,5(10)-triene-3,17-diol(17β)-,3-[bis(2-chlorethyl) carbamate] 17-dihydrogen phosphate), disodium salt, monohydrate. It is also referred to as estradiol 3-[bis(2-chloroethyl) carbamate 17-(dihydrogen phosphate), disodium salt, monohydrate. Estramustine Phosphate Sodium has an empiric formula of $C_{23}H_{30}Cl_2NNa_2O_6P\cdot H_2O$ and a calculated molecular weight of 582.4.

Following is its chemical structure:

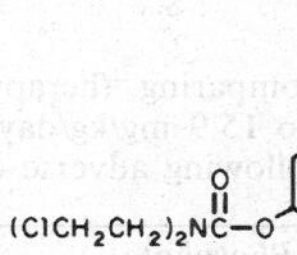

CLINICAL PHARMACOLOGY
Estramustine Phosphate is a molecule combining estradiol and nornitrogen mustard by a carbamate link. The molecule is phosphorylated to make it water soluble.

Estramustine Phosphate taken orally is readily dephosphorylated during absorption, and the major metabolites in plasma are estramustine, the estrone analog, estradiol and estrone.

Prolonged treatment with Estramustine Phosphate produces elevated total plasma concentrations of estradiol that fall within ranges similar to the elevated estradiol levels found in prostatic cancer patients given conventional estradiol therapy. Estrogenic effects, as demonstrated by changes in circulating levels of steroids and pituitary hormones, are similar in patients treated with either Estramustine Phosphate or conventional estradiol.

The metabolic urinary patterns of the estradiol moiety of Estramustine Phosphate and estradiol itself are very similar, although the metabolites derived from Estramustine Phosphate are excreted at a slower rate.

INDICATIONS AND USAGE
Estramustine Phosphate Sodium is indicated in the palliative treatment of patients with metastatic and/or progressive carcinoma of the prostate.

UNLABELED USES
Estramustine Phosphate Sodium is used alone or as an adjunct in the treatment of metastatic renal cell carcinoma.

CONTRAINDICATIONS
Estramustine Phosphate Sodium should not be used in patients with any of the following conditions:

1) Known hypersensitivity to either estradiol or to nitrogen mustard.
2) Active thrombophlebitis or thromboembolic disorders, except in those cases where the actual tumor mass is the cause of the thromboembolic phenomenon and the physician feels the benefits of therapy may outweigh the risks.

WARNINGS
It has been shown that there is an increased risk of thrombosis, including nonfatal myocardial infarction, in men receiving estrogens for prostatic cancer. Estramustine Phosphate Sodium should be used with caution in patients with a history of thrombophlebitis, thrombosis or thromboembolic disorders, especially if they were associated with estrogen therapy. Caution should also be used in patients with cerebral vascular or coronary artery disease.

Glucose Tolerance—Because glucose tolerance may be decreased, diabetic patients should be carefully observed while receiving Estramustine Phosphate Sodium.

Elevated Blood Pressure—Because hypertension may occur, blood pressure should be monitored periodically.

PRECAUTIONS
General: Fluid Retention—Exacerbation of preexisting or incipient peripheral edema or congestive heart disease has been seen in some patients receiving Estramustine Phosphate Sodium therapy. Other conditions which might be influenced by fluid retention, such as epilepsy, migraine or renal dysfunction, require careful observation.

Estramustine Phosphate Sodium may be poorly metabolized in patients with impaired liver function and should be administered with caution in such patients.

Because Estramustine Phosphate Sodium may influence the metabolism of calcium and phosphorus, it should be used with caution in patients with metabolic bone diseases that are associated with hypercalcemia or in patients with renal insufficiency.

➤ SHOWN IN PRODUCT IDENTIFICATION GUIDE

Information for the Patient: Because of the possibility of mutagenic effects, patients should be advised to use contraceptive measures.

Laboratory Tests: Certain endocrine and liver function tests may be affected by estrogen-containing drugs. Abnormalities of hepatic enzymes and of bilirubin have occurred in patients receiving Estramustine Phosphate Sodium but have seldom been severe enough to require cessation of therapy. Such tests should be done at appropriate intervals during therapy and repeated after the drug has been withdrawn for two months.

Food/Drug Interaction: Milk, milk products and calcium-rich foods or drugs may impair the absorption of Estramustine Phosphate Sodium.

Carcinogenesis, Mutagenesis, Impairment of Fertility: Long-term continuous administration of estrogen in certain animal species increases the frequency of carcinomas of the breast and liver. Compounds structurally similar to Estramustine Phosphate Sodium are carcinogenic in mice. Carcinogenic studies of Estramustine Phosphate Sodium have not been conducted in man. Although testing by the Ames method failed to demonstrate mutagenicity for Estramustine Phosphate Sodium, it is known that both estradiol and nitrogen mustard are mutagenic. For this reason and because some patients who had been impotent while on estrogen therapy have regained potency while taking Estramustine Phosphate Sodium, the patient should be advised to use contraceptive measures.

ADVERSE REACTIONS

In a randomized, double-blind trial comparing therapy with Estramustine Phosphate Sodium in 93 patients (11.5 to 15.9 mg/kg/day) or diethylstilbestrol (DES) in 93 patients (3.0 mg/day), the following adverse effects were reported:

	Estramustine Phosphate Sodium n = 93	DES n = 93
Cardiovascular-Respiratory		
Cardiac Arrest	0	2
Cerebrovascular Accident	2	0
Myocardial Infarction	3	1
Thrombophlebitis	3	7
Pulmonary Emboli	2	5
Congestive Heart Failure	3	2
Edema	19	17
Dyspnea	11	3
Leg Cramps	8	11
Upper Respiratory Discharge	1	1
Hoarseness	1	0
Gastrointestinal		
Nausea	15	8
Diarrhea	12	11
Minor Gastrointestinal Upset	11	6
Anorexia	4	3
Flatulence	2	0
Vomiting	1	1
Gastrointestinal Bleeding	1	0
Burning Throat	1	0
Thirst	1	0
Integumentary		
Rash	1	4
Pruritus	2	2
Dry Skin	2	0
Pigment Changes	0	1
Easy Bruising	3	0
Flushing	1	0
Night Sweats	0	1
Fingertip—Peeling Skin	1	0
Thinning Hair	1	1
Breast Changes		
Tenderness	66	64
Enlargement		
Mild	60	54
Moderate	10	16
Marked	0	5
Miscellaneous		
Lethargy Alone	4	3
Depression	0	2
Emotional Lability	0	1
Insomnia	3	0
Headache	1	1
Anxiety	1	0
Chest Pain	1	1
Hot Flashes	0	1
Pain in Eyes	0	1
Miscellaneous		
Tearing of Eyes	1	1
Tinnitus	0	1
Laboratory Abnormalities		
Hematologic		
Leukopenia	4	2
Thrombopenia	1	2
Hepatic		
Bilirubin Alone	1	5
Bilirubin and LDH	0	1
Bilirubin and SGOT	2	1
Bilirubin, LDH and SGOT	2	0
LDH and/or SGOT	31	28
Miscellaneous		
Hypercalemia— Transient	0	1

OVERDOSAGE

Although there has been no experience with overdosage to date, it is reasonable to expect that such episodes may produce pronounced manifestations of the known adverse reactions. In the event of overdosage, the gastric contents should be evacuated by gastric lavage and symptomatic therapy should be initiated. Hematologic and hepatic parameters should be monitored for at least six weeks after overdosage of Estramustine Phosphate Sodium.

DOSAGE AND ADMINISTRATION

The recommended daily dose is 14 mg per kg of body weight (*i.e.*, one 140 mg capsule for each 10 kg or 22 lb of body weight), given in 3 or 4 divided doses. Most patients in studies in the United States have been treated at a dosage range of 10 to 16 mg per kg per day.

Patients should be instructed to take Estramustine Phosphate Sodium at least one hour before or two hours after meals. Estramustine Phosphate Sodium should be swallowed with water. Milk, milk products and calcium-rich foods or drugs (such as calcium-containing antacids) must not be taken simultaneously with Estramustine Phosphate Sodium.

Patients should be treated for 30 to 90 days before the physician determines the possible benefits of continued therapy. Therapy should be continued as long as the favorable response lasts. Some patients have been maintained on therapy for more than three years at doses ranging from 10 to 16 mg per kg of body weight per day.

Procedures for proper handling and disposal of anticancer drugs should be considered. Several guidelines on this subject have been published.[1-6] There is no general agreement that all of the procedures recommended in the guidelines are necessary or appropriate.

Estramustine Phosphate Sodium should be stored in the refrigerator at 36° to 46°F (2° to 8°C).

REFERENCES

1. Recommendations for the safe handling of parenteral antineoplastic drugs. Washington, DC, U.S. Government Printing Office (NIH Publication No. 83-2621). 2. AMA Council Report. Guidelines for handling parenteral antineoplastics. *JAMA* 253:1590-1592, Mar. 15, 1985. 3. National Study Commission on Cytotoxic Exposure: Recommendations for handling cytotoxic agents. Available from Louis P. Jeffrey, ScD, Director of Pharmacy Services, Rhode Island Hospital, 593 Eddy Street, Providence, Rhode Island 02902. 4. Clinical Oncological Society of Australia: Guidelines and recommendations for safe handling of antineoplastic agents. *Med. J Aust 1*:426-428, Apr. 30, 1983. 5. Jones RB, Frank R, Mass T: Safe handling of chemotherapeutic agents: a report from the Mount Sinai Medical Center, *CA. 33*:258-263, Sept-Oct 1983. 6. ASHP technical assistance bulletin on handling cytotoxic drugs in hospitals. *Am J Hosp Pharm 42*:131-137, Jan 1985. 1991, Kabi Pharmacia text issued May, 1991

HOW SUPPLIED
CAPSULE: 140 MG

BRAND/MANUFACTURER	NDC	SIZE	AWP
○ **BRAND**			
EMCYT: Pharmacia	00016-0132-02	100s	$280.56

Estratab *SEE* ESTROGENS, ESTERIFIED

Estratest *SEE* ESTROGENS, ESTERIFIED AND METHYLTESTOSTERONE

Estrogens, Conjugated

1. ESTROGENS HAVE BEEN REPORTED TO INCREASE THE RISK OF ENDOMETRIAL CARCINOMA IN POSTMENOPAUSAL WOMEN.

◆ RATED THERAPEUTICALLY EQUIVALENT; ◇ THERAPEUTIC EQUIVALENCE UNCONFIRMED; ○ UNRATED

THREE INDEPENDENT, CASE-CONTROLLED STUDIES HAVE REPORTED AN INCREASED RISK OF ENDOMETRIAL CANCER IN POST-MENOPAUSAL WOMEN EXPOSED TO EXOGENOUS ESTROGENS FOR MORE THAN ONE YEAR.[1-3] THIS RISK WAS INDEPENDENT OF THE OTHER KNOWN RISK FACTORS FOR ENDOMETRIAL CANCER. THESE STUDIES ARE FURTHER SUPPORTED BY THE FINDING THAT INCIDENCE RATES OF ENDOMETRIAL CANCER HAVE INCREASED SHARPLY SINCE 1969 IN EIGHT DIFFERENT AREAS OF THE UNITED STATES WITH POPULATION-BASED CANCER-REPORTING SYSTEMS, AN INCREASE WHICH MAY BE RELATED TO THE RAPIDLY EXPANDING USE OF ESTROGENS DURING THE LAST DECADE.[4]

THE THREE CASE-CONTROLLED STUDIES REPORTED THAT THE RISK OF ENDOMETRIAL CANCER IN ESTROGEN USERS WAS ABOUT 4.5 TO 13.9 TIMES GREATER THAN IN NONUSERS. THE RISK APPEARS TO DEPEND ON BOTH DURATION OF TREATMENT[1] AND ON ESTROGEN DOSE.[3] IN VIEW OF THESE FINDINGS, WHEN ESTROGENS ARE USED FOR THE TREATMENT OF MENOPAUSAL SYMPTOMS, THE LOWEST DOSE THAT WILL CONTROL SYMPTOMS SHOULD BE UTILIZED AND MEDICATION SHOULD BE DISCONTINUED AS SOON AS POSSIBLE. WHEN PROLONGED TREATMENT IS MEDICALLY INDICATED, THE PATIENT SHOULD BE REASSESSED, ON AT LEAST A SEMI-ANNUAL BASIS, TO DETERMINE THE NEED FOR CONTINUED THERAPY. ALTHOUGH THE EVIDENCE MUST BE CONSIDERED PRELIMINARY, ONE STUDY SUGGESTS THAT CYCLIC ADMINISTRATION OF LOW DOSES OF ESTROGEN MAY CARRY LESS RISK THAN CONTINUOUS ADMINISTRATION.[3] IT THEREFORE APPEARS PRUDENT TO UTILIZE SUCH A REGIMEN.

CLOSE CLINICAL SURVEILLANCE OF ALL WOMEN TAKING ESTROGENS IS IMPORTANT. IN ALL CASES OF UNDIAGNOSED PERSISTENT OR RECURRING ABNORMAL VAGINAL BLEEDING, ADEQUATE DIAGNOSTIC MEASURES SHOULD BE UNDERTAKEN TO RULE OUT MALIGNANCY.

THERE IS NO EVIDENCE AT PRESENT THAT "NATURAL" ESTROGENS ARE MORE OR LESS HAZARDOUS THAN "SYNTHETIC" ESTROGENS AT EQUI-ESTROGENIC DOSES.

2. ESTROGENS SHOULD NOT BE USED DURING PREGNANCY.

ESTROGEN THERAPY DURING PREGNANCY IS ASSOCIATED WITH AN INCREASED RISK OF CONGENITAL DEFECTS IN THE REPRODUCTIVE ORGANS OF THE MALE AND FEMALE FETUS. IT HAS BEEN SHOWN THAT FEMALES EXPOSED *IN UTERO* TO DIETHYLSTILBESTROL, A NONSTEROIDAL ESTROGEN, HAVE AN INCREASED RISK OF DEVELOPING, IN LATER LIFE, A FORM OF VAGINAL OR CERVICAL CANCER THAT IS ORDINARILY EXTREMELY RARE.[5,6] THIS RISK HAS BEEN ESTIMATED AS NOT GREATER THAN 4 PER 1,000 EXPOSURES.[7] FURTHERMORE, A HIGH PERCENTAGE OF SUCH EXPOSED WOMEN (FROM 30% TO 90%) HAVE BEEN FOUND TO HAVE VAGINAL ADENOSIS,[8-12] EPITHELIAL CHANGES OF THE VAGINA AND CERVIX. ALTHOUGH THESE CHANGES ARE HISTOLOGICALLY BENIGN, IT IS NOT KNOWN WHETHER THEY ARE PRECURSORS OF MALIGNANCY. ALTHOUGH SIMILAR DATA ARE NOT AVAILABLE WITH THE USE OF OTHER ESTROGENS, IT CANNOT BE PRESUMED THEY WOULD NOT INDUCE SIMILAR CHANGES. THERE IS ALSO A RISK OF SQUAMOUS CELL DYSPLASIA OF THE UTERINE CERVIX. THE 1985 DES TASK FORCE CONCLUDED THAT WOMEN WHO USED DES DURING THEIR PREGNANCIES MAY SUBSEQUENTLY EXPERIENCE AN INCREASED RISK OF BREAST CANCER. HOWEVER, A CAUSAL RELATIONSHIP IS STILL UNPROVEN, AND THE OBSERVED LEVEL OF RISK IS SIMILAR TO THAT FOR A NUMBER OF OTHER BREAST-CANCER RISK FACTORS.

SEVERAL REPORTS SUGGEST AN ASSOCIATION BETWEEN INTRAUTERINE EXPOSURE TO FEMALE SEX HORMONES AND CONGENITAL ANOMALIES, INCLUDING CONGENITAL HEART DEFECTS AND LIMB-REDUCTION DEFECTS.[13-16] ONE CASE-CONTROLLED STUDY[16] ESTIMATED A 4.7-FOLD INCREASED RISK OF LIMB-REDUCTION DEFECTS IN INFANTS EXPOSED *IN UTERO* TO SEX HORMONES (ORAL CONTRACEPTIVES, HORMONE WITHDRAWAL TESTS FOR PREGNANCY, OR ATTEMPTED TREATMENT FOR THREATENED ABORTION). SOME OF THESE EXPOSURES WERE VERY SHORT AND INVOLVED ONLY A FEW DAYS OF TREATMENT. THE DATA SUGGEST THAT THE RISK OF LIMB-REDUCTION DEFECTS IN EXPOSED FETUSES IS SOMEWHAT LESS THAN 1 PER 1,000.

IN THE PAST, FEMALE SEX HORMONES HAVE BEEN USED DURING PREGNANCY IN AN ATTEMPT TO TREAT THREATENED OR HABITUAL ABORTION. THERE IS CONSIDERABLE EVIDENCE THAT ESTROGENS ARE INEFFECTIVE FOR THESE INDICATIONS, AND THERE IS NO EVIDENCE FROM WELL-CONTROLLED STUDIES THAT PROGESTOGENS ARE EFFECTIVE FOR THESE USES.

THERE IS NO INDICATION FOR ESTROGEN THERAPY DURING PREGNANCY.

IF ESTROGENS, CONJUGATED, TABLETS, VAGINAL CREAM, OR INJECTION IS USED DURING PREGNANCY, OR IF THE PATIENT BECOMES PREGNANT WHILE TAKING THIS DRUG, SHE SHOULD BE APPRISED OF THE POTENTIAL RISKS TO THE FETUS, AND THE ADVISABILITY OF PREGNANCY CONTINUATION.

DESCRIPTION

Estrogens, Conjugated, contain a mixture of estrogens obtained exclusively from natural sources, occurring as the sodium salts of water-soluble estrogen sulfates blended to represent the average composition of material derived from pregnant mares' urine. It contains estrone, equilin, and 17 α-dihydroequilin, together with smaller amounts of 17 α-estradiol, equilenin, and 17 α-dihydroequilenin as salts of their sulfate esters. Estrogens, Conjugated, are available as tablets, intravenous or intramuscular injection, and vaginal cream.

Tablets: For oral administration are available in 0.3 mg, 0.625 mg, 0.9 mg, 1.25 mg, and 2.5 mg strengths of Conjugated Estrogens.

Injection: Each vial contains 25 mg of Conjugated Estrogens in a sterile lyophilized cake.

Vaginal Cream: Each gram contains 0.625 mg Conjugated Estrogens.

CLINICAL PHARMACOLOGY

Estrogens are important in the development and maintenance of the female reproductive system and secondary sex characteristics. They promote growth and development of the vagina, uterus, and fallopian tubes, and enlargement of the breasts. Indirectly, they contribute to the shaping of the skeleton, maintenance of tone and elasticity of urogenital structures, changes in the epiphyses of the long bones that allow for the pubertal growth spurt and its termination, growth of axillary and pubic hair, and pigmentation of the nipples and genitals. Decline of estrogenic activity at the end of the menstrual cycle can bring on menstruation, although the cessation of progesterone secretion is the most important factor in the mature ovulatory cycle. However, in the preovulatory or nonovulatory cycle, Estrogen is the primary determinant in the onset of menstruation. Estrogens also affect the release of pituitary gonadotropins.

The pharmacologic effects of Conjugated Estrogens are similar to those of endogenous Estrogens. They are soluble in water and the tablets are well absorbed from the gastrointestinal tract; parenteral Estrogens may be administered by intravenous or intramuscular injection; the vaginal cream may be absorbed from mucosal surfaces after local administration. In responsive tissues (female genital organs, breasts, hypothalamus, pituitary) Estrogens enter the cell and are transported into the nucleus. As a result of Estrogen action, specific RNA and protein synthesis occurs.

Metabolism and inactivation occur primarily in the liver. Some Estrogens are excreted into the bile; however, they are reabsorbed from the intestine and returned to the liver through the portal venous system. Water-soluble Estrogen conjugates are strongly acidic and are ionized in body fluids, which favor excretion through the kidneys since tubular reabsorption is minimal.

INDICATIONS AND USAGE

Conjugated Estrogens tablets are indicated in the treatment of:

1. Moderate to severe vasomotor symptoms associated with the menopause. There is no adequate evidence that Estrogens are effective for nervous symptoms or depression which might occur during menopause and they should not be used to treat these conditions.
2. Atrophic vaginitis.
3. Osteoporosis (loss of bone mass). The mainstays of prevention and management of osteoporosis are Estrogen and calcium: exercise and nutrition may be important adjuncts. Estrogen replacement therapy is the most effective single modality for the prevention of osteoporosis in women. Estrogen reduces bone resorption and retards or halts postmenopausal bone loss. Case-controlled studies have shown an approximately 60-percent reduction in hip and wrist fractures in women whose Estrogen replacement was begun within a few years of menopause. Studies also suggest that Estrogen reduces the rate of vertebral fractures. Even when started as late as 6 years after menopause, Estrogen prevents further loss of bone mass but does not restore it to premenopausal levels. The lowest effective dose for prevention and treatment of osteoporosis should be utilized. (See *"Dosage and Administration."*)
Women are at higher risk than men because they have less bone mass, and for several years following natural or induced menopause, the rate of bone mass decline is accelerated. Early menopause is one of the strongest predictors for the development of osteoporosis. White women are at higher risk than black women, and white men are at higher risk than black men. Women who are underweight also have osteoporosis more often than overweight women. Cigarette smoking may be an additional factor in increasing risk. Calcium deficiency has been implicated in the pathogenesis of the disease. Therefore, when not contraindicated, it is recommended that postmenopausal women receive an elemental calcium intake of 1000 to 1500 mg/day.
Immobilization and prolonged bed rest produce rapid bone loss, while weight-bearing exercise has been shown both to reduce bone loss and to increase bone mass. The optimal type and amount of physical activity that would prevent osteoporosis have not been established.
4. Hypoestrogenism due to hypogonadism, castration, or primary ovarian failure.
5. Breast cancer (for palliation only) in appropriately selected women and men with metastatic disease.

6. Advanced androgen-dependent carcinoma of the prostate (for palliation only).

Conjugated Estrogens for injection is indicated in the treatment of abnormal uterine bleeding due to hormonal imbalance in the absence of organic pathology.

Conjugated Estrogens vaginal cream is indicated in the treatment of atrophic vaginitis and kraurosis vulvae. Conjugated Estrogens vaginal cream HAS NOT BEEN SHOWN TO BE EFFECTIVE FOR ANY PURPOSE DURING PREGNANCY AND ITS USE MAY CAUSE SEVERE HARM TO THE FETUS (SEE BOXED *"WARNING"*).

UNLABELED USES
Estrogens, Conjugated, are used alone or as an adjunct in the treatment of bleeding associated with renal failure (uremic bleeding), in prophylaxis of cardiovascular disease, and to prevent pregnancy as a postcoital contraceptive. They are used in the treatment of refractory depression and dyskinetic disorders, including chorea secondary to Huntington's disease and tardive dyskinesia, including levodopa-induced dyskinesia. They are used to normalize serum calcium levels in postmenopausal women with mild hyperparathyroidism and are prescribed in rheumatoid arthritis. They are also used to reduce the severity or frequency of epistaxis, gastrointestinal hemorrhage, and transfusion requirements in patients with bleeding telangiectasias, and are prescribed as an adjunctive therapy in premenstrual syndrome.

CONTRAINDICATIONS
Estrogens should not be used in women (or men) with any of the following conditions:
1. Known or suspected pregnancy (see boxed *"Warning"*). Estrogen may cause fetal harm when administered to a pregnant woman.
2. Known or suspected cancer of the breast except in appropriately selected patients being treated for metastatic disease.
3. Known or suspected estrogen-dependent neoplasia.
4. Undiagnosed abnormal genital bleeding.
5. Active thrombophlebitis or thromboembolic disorders.
6. A past history of thrombophlebitis, thrombosis, or thromboembolic disorders associated with previous estrogen use (except when used in treatment of breast malignancy). Women on Estrogen replacement therapy have not been reported to have an increased risk of thrombophlebitis and/or thromboembolic disease. However, there is insufficient information regarding women who have had previous thromboembolic disease.

Estrogens, Conjugated, tablets or vaginal cream should not be used in patients hypersensitive to their ingredients

WARNINGS
1. Induction of Malignant Neoplasms. Long-term, continuous administration of natural and synthetic estrogens in certain animal species increases the frequency of carcinomas of the breast, cervix, vagina, and liver. There are now reports that estrogens increase the risk of carcinoma of the endometrium in humans (see boxed *"Warning"*). The reported endometrial cancer risk among Estrogen users was about 4-fold or greater than in nonusers and appears dependent on duration of treatment and on estrogen dose. There is no significant increased risk associated with the use of Estrogens for less than one year. The greatest risk appears associated with prolonged use—five years or more. In one study, persistence of risk was demonstrated for 10 years after cessation of Estrogen treatment. In another study, a significant decrease in the incidence of endometrial cancer occurred six months after Estrogen withdrawal.

At the present time there is no satisfactory evidence that Estrogens given to postmenopausal women increase the risk of cancer of the breast,[17] although a recent long-term follow-up of a single physician's practice has raised this possibility.[18] Because of the animal data, there is a need for caution in prescribing Estrogens for women with a strong family history of breast cancer, or who have breast nodules, fibrocystic disease, or abnormal mammograms.

Estrogen therapy during pregnancy is associated with an increased risk of fetal congenital reproductive-tract disorders. In females there is an increased risk of vaginal adenosis, squamous-cell dysplasia of the cervix, and cancer later in life; in the male, urogenital abnormalities. Although some of these changes are benign, it is not known whether they are precursors of malignancy.

2. Gallbladder Disease. A recent study has reported a 2- to 3-fold increase in the risk of surgically confirmed gallbladder disease in women receiving postmenopausal Estrogens,[17] similar to the 2-fold increase previously noted in users of oral contraceptives.[19,24a]

3. Effects Similar to Those Caused by Estrogen-progestogen Oral Contraceptives. There are several serious adverse effects of oral contraceptives, most of which have not, up to now, been documented as consequences of postmenopausal Estrogen therapy. This may reflect the comparatively low doses of estrogen used in postmenopausal women. It would be expected that the larger doses of Estrogen used to treat prostatic or breast cancer are more likely to result in these adverse effects, and, in fact, it has been shown that there is an increased risk of thrombosis in men receiving Estrogens for prostatic cancer.[20-23]

a. Thromboembolic disease. It is now well established that users of oral contraceptives have an increased risk of various thromboembolic and thrombotic vascular diseases, such as thrombophlebitis, pulmonary embolism, stroke, and myocardial infarction.[24-31] Cases of retinal thrombosis, mesenteric thrombosis, and optic neuritis have been reported in oral-contraceptive users. There is evidence that the risk of several of these adverse reactions is related to the dose of the drug.[32,33] An increased risk of postsurgery thromboembolic complications has also been reported in users of oral contraceptives.[34,35] If feasible, Estrogen should be discontinued at least 4 weeks before surgery of the type associated with an increased risk of thromboembolism, or during periods of prolonged immobilization.

While an increased rate of thromboembolic and thrombotic disease in postmenopausal users of Estrogens has not been found,[17-24,25-36] this does not rule out the possibility that such an increase may be present, or that subgroups of women who have underlying risk factors, or who are receiving relatively large doses of Estrogens, may have increased risk. Therefore estrogens should not be used in persons with active thrombophlebitis or thromboembolic disorders, and they should not be used (except in treatment of malignancy) in persons with a history of such disorders in association with Estrogen use. They should be used with caution in patients with cerebral vascular or coronary artery disease and only for those in whom Estrogens are clearly needed.

Large doses of Estrogen (5 mg conjugated Estrogens per day), comparable to those used to treat cancer of the prostate and breast, have been shown in a large prospective clinical trial in men[37] to increase the risk of nonfatal myocardial infarction, pulmonary embolism, and thrombophlebitis. When Estrogen doses of this size are used, any of the thromboembolic and thrombotic adverse effects associated with oral-contraceptive use should be considered a clear risk.

b. Hepatic adenoma. Benign hepatic adenomas appear to be associated with the use of oral contraceptives.[38-40] Although benign, and rare, these may rupture and may cause death through intra-abdominal hemorrhage. Such lesions have not yet been reported in association with other Estrogen or progestogen preparations but should be considered in estrogen users having abdominal pain and tenderness, abdominal mass, or hypovolemic shock. Hepatocellular carcinoma has also been reported in women taking Estrogen-containing oral contraceptives.[39] The relationship of this malignancy to these drugs is not known at this time.

c. Elevated blood pressure. Women using oral contraceptives sometimes experience increased blood pressure which, in most cases, returns to normal on discontinuing the drug. There is now a report that this may occur with use of Estrogens in the menopause[41] and blood pressure should be monitored with estrogen use, especially if high doses are used.

d. Glucose tolerance. A worsening of glucose tolerance has been observed in a significant percentage of patients on Estrogen-containing oral contraceptives. For this reason, diabetic patients should be carefully observed while receiving Estrogen.

4. Hypercalcemia. Administration of Estrogens may lead to severe hypercalcemia in patients with breast cancer and bone metastases. If this occurs, the drug should be stopped and appropriate measures taken to reduce the serum calcium level.

PRECAUTIONS
A. GENERAL
1. Addition of a Progestin: The lowest effective dose appropriate for the specific indication should be utilized. Studies of the addition of a progestin for seven or more days of a cycle of Estrogen administration have reported a lowered incidence of endometrial hyperplasia. Morphological and biochemical studies of endometrium suggest that 10 to 13 days of progestin are needed to provide maximal maturation of the endometrium and to eliminate any hyperplastic changes. Whether this will provide protection from endometrial carcinoma has not been clearly established. There are possible additional risks which may be associated with the inclusion of progestin in Estrogen replacement regimens. The potential risks include adverse effects on carbohydrate and lipid metabolism. The choice of progestin and dosage may be important in minimizing these adverse effects.

2. Physical Examination: A complete medical and family history should be taken prior to the initiation of any Estrogen therapy. The pretreatment and periodic physical examinations should include special reference to blood pressure, breasts, abdomen, and pelvic organs, and should include a Papanicolaou smear. As a general rule, Estrogen should not be prescribed for longer than one year without another physical examination being performed.

3. Fluid Retention. Because Estrogens may cause some degree of fluid retention, conditions which might be influenced by this factor, such as asthma, epilepsy, migraine, and cardiac or renal dysfunction, require careful observation.

4. Uterine bleeding and mastodynia: Certain patients may develop undesirable manifestations of excessive estrogenic stimulation, such as abnormal or excessive uterine bleeding and mastodynia.

5. Uterine fibroids: Preexisting uterine leiomyomata may increase in size during prolonged high-dose Estrogen use.

6. Impaired liver function: Estrogens may be poorly metabolized in patients with impaired liver function and should be administered with caution.

7. Hypercalcemia and renal insufficiency: Prolonged use of Estrogens can alter the metabolism of calcium and phosphorus. Estrogens should be used with caution in patients with metabolic bone disease that is associated with hypercalcemia or in patients with renal insufficiency.

8. Oral contraceptives appear to be associated with an increased incidence of mental depression.[24a] Although it is not clear whether this is due to the estrogenic or progestogenic component of the contraceptive, patients with a history of depression should be carefully observed.

9. The pathologist should be advised of Estrogen therapy when relevant specimens are submitted.

---

10. Patients with a past history of jaundice during pregnancy have an increased risk of recurrence of jaundice while receiving Estrogen-containing oral contraceptive therapy. If jaundice develops in any patient receiving Estrogen, the medication should be discontinued while the cause is investigated.

11. Because of the effects of Estrogens on epiphyseal closure, they should be used judiciously in young patients in whom bone growth is not yet complete.

12. Prolonged administration of unopposed Estrogen therapy has been reported to increase the risk of endometrial hyperplasia in some patients.

C. LABORATORY TESTS
Clinical response at the smallest dose should generally be the guide to Estrogen administration for relief of symptoms for those indications in which symptoms are observable. However, for prevention and treatment of osteoporosis see *"Dosage and Administration"* section. Tests used to measure adequacy of Estrogen replacement therapy include serum estrone and estradiol levels and suppression of serum gonadotrophin levels.

D. DRUG/LABORATORY TEST INTERACTIONS
Certain endocrine and liver function tests may be affected by Estrogen-containing oral contraceptives. The following similar changes may be expected with larger doses of Estrogen.

Some of these drug/laboratory test interactions have been observed only with Estrogen-progestin combinations (oral contraceptives):

1. Increased prothrombin and factors VII, VIII, IX and X; decreased antithrombin 3; increased norepinephrine-induced platelet aggregability, decreased fibrinolysis.
2. Increased thyroid-binding globulin (TBG) leading to increased circulating total thyroid hormone, as measured by PB1 or T4 levels determined either by column or by radioimmunoassay. Free T3 resin uptake is decreased, reflecting the elevated TBG; free T4 concentration is unaltered.
3. Impaired glucose tolerance.
4. Reduced response to metyrapone test.
5. Reduced serum folate concentration.
6. Increased sulfobromophthalein retention.
7. Decreased pregnanediol excretion.
8. Increased serum triglyceride and phospholipid concentration.

E. MUTAGENESIS AND CARCINOGENESIS
Long-term, continuous administration of natural and synthetic Estrogens in certain animal species increases the frequency of carcinomas of the breast, cervix, vagina, and liver.

F. PREGNANCY CATEGORY X
Estrogens should not be used during pregnancy. See *"Contraindications"* and boxed *"Warning".*

G. NURSING MOTHERS
It is not known whether this drug is excreted in human milk. Because many drugs are excreted in human milk and because of the potential for serious adverse reactions in nursing infants from Estrogens, a decision should be made whether to discontinue nursing or to discontinue the drug, taking into account the importance of the drug to the mother.

H. PEDIATRIC USE.
Safety and effectiveness in children have not been established.

ADVERSE REACTIONS
(See *"Warnings"* regarding induction of neoplasia, adverse effects on the fetus, increased incidence of gallbladder disease, and adverse effects similar to those of oral contraceptives, including thromboembolism.) The following additional adverse reactions have been reported with estrogenic therapy, including oral contraceptives:

1. Genitourinary system: Changes in vaginal bleeding pattern and abnormal withdrawal bleeding or flow. Breakthrough bleeding, spotting. Dysmenorrhea. Premenstrual-like syndrome. Amenorrhea during and after treatment. Increase in size of uterine fibromyomata. Vaginal candidiasis. Change in cervical erosion and in degree of cervical secretion. Cystitis-like syndrome.

2. Breasts: Tenderness, enlargement, secretion.

3. Gastrointestinal: Nausea, vomiting; abdominal cramps, bloating; cholestatic jaundice.

4. Skin: Chioasma or melasma that may persist when drug is discontinued; erythema multiforme; erythema nodosum; hemorrhagic eruption; loss of scalp hair; hirsutism.

5. Eyes: Steepening of corneal curvature; intolerance of contact lenses.

6. CNS: Headache, migraine, dizziness, mental depression; chorea.

7. Miscellaneous: Increase or decrease in weight; reduced carbohydrate tolerance; aggravation of porphyria; edema; changes in libido.

ACUTE OVERDOSAGE
Numerous reports of ingestion of large doses of Estrogen-containing oral contraceptives by young children indicate that acute serious ill effects do not occur. Overdosage of Estrogen may cause nausea and vomiting, and withdrawal bleeding may occur in females.

DOSAGE AND ADMINISTRATION
TABLETS
1. For treatment of moderate to severe vasomotor symptoms, atrophic vaginitis, and atrophic urethritis associated with the menopause. The lowest dose that will control symptoms should be chosen, and medication should be discontinued as promptly as possible.

Attempts to discontinue or taper medication should be made at 3-month to 6-month intervals.

Usual dosage ranges: Vasomotor symptoms: 1.25 mg daily. If the patient has not menstruated within the last two months or more, cyclic administration is started arbitrarily. If the patient is menstruating, cyclic (e.g., three weeks on and one week off) administration is started on day 5 of bleeding.

Atrophic vaginitis and Atrophic urethritis—0.3 mg to 1.25 mg or more daily, depending upon the tissue response of the individual patient. Administer cyclically.

2. Hypoestrogenism due to:

a. Female hypogonadism: 2.5 mg to 7.5 mg daily, in divided doses for 20 days, followed by a rest period of 10 days' duration. If bleeding does not occur by the end of this period, the same dosage schedule is repeated. The number of courses of Estrogen therapy necessary to produce bleeding may vary depending on the responsiveness of the endometrium.

If bleeding occurs before the end of the 10-day period, begin a 20-day estrogen-progestin cyclic regimen with Estrogens, Conjugated, 2.5 mg to 7.5 mg daily in divided doses, for 20 days. During the last five days of Estrogen therapy, given an oral progestin. If bleeding occurs before this regimen is concluded, therapy is discontinued and may be resumed on the fifth day of bleeding.

b. Female castration or primary ovarian failure: 1.25 mg daily, cyclically. Adjust dosage, upward or downward, according to severity of symptoms and response of the patient. For maintenance, adjust dosage to lowest level that will provide effective control.

3. Osteoporosis (loss of bone mass): 0.625 mg daily. Administration should be cyclic (e.g., three weeks on and one week off).

4. Advanced androgen-dependent carcinoma of the prostate, for palliation only—1.25 mg to 2.5 mg three times daily. The effectiveness of therapy can be judged by phosphatase determinations as well as by symptomatic improvement of the patient.

5. Breast cancer (for palliation only) in appropriately selected women and men with metastatic disease. Suggested dosage is 10 mg three times daily for a period of at least three months.

Treated patients with an intact uterus should be monitored closely for signs of endometrial cancer, and appropriate diagnostic measures should be taken to rule out malignancy in the event of persistent or recurring abnormal vaginal bleeding.

STORAGE
Store at room temperature (approximately 25° C).

Dispense in a well-closed container as defined in the USP.

INJECTION
Abnormal Uterine Bleeding Due to Hormonal Imbalance: One 25 mg injection, intravenously or intramuscularly. Intravenous use is preferred since more rapid response can be expected from this mode of administration.

Repeat in 6 to 12 hours if necessary. The use of Estrogens, Conjugated, for injection does not preclude the advisability of other appropriate measures. The usual precautionary measures governing intravenous administration should be adhered to. Injection should be made SLOWLY to obviate the occurrence of flushes.

Infusion of Estrogens, Conjugated, for injection with other agents is not generally recommended. In emergencies, however, when an infusion has already been started it may be expedient to make the injection into the tubing just distal to the infusion needle. If so used, compatibility of solutions must be considered.

Compatibility of Solutions: Estrogens, Conjugated for injection is compatible with normal saline, dextrose, and invert sugar solutions. IT IS NOT COMPATIBLE WITH PROTEIN HYDROLYSATE, ASCORBIC ACID, OR ANY SOLUTION WITH AN ACID pH.

Treated patients with an intact uterus should be monitored closely for signs of endometrial cancer, and appropriate diagnostic measures should be taken to rule out malignancy in the event of persistent or recurring abnormal vaginal bleeding.

STORAGE AND RECONSTITUTION
Storage before reconstitution: Store package in refrigerator, 2°-8° C (36°-46° F).

To reconstitute: First withdraw air from vial so as to facilitate introduction of sterile diluent. Then, flow the sterile diluent slowly against side of vial and agitate gently. DO NOT SHAKE VIOLENTLY.

Storage after reconstitution: It is common practice to utilize the reconstituted solution within a few hours. If it is necessary to keep the reconstituted solution for more than a few hours, store the reconstituted solution under refrigeration (2°-8° C). Under these conditions, the solution is stable for 60 days, and is suitable for use unless darkening or precipitation occurs.

VAGINAL CREAM
Given Cyclically for Short-term Use Only: For treatment of atrophic vaginitis, or kraurosis vulvae. The lowest dose that will control symptoms should be chosen and medication should be discontinued as promptly as possible.

Administration should be cyclic (e.g., three weeks on and one week off).

➤ SHOWN IN PRODUCT IDENTIFICATION GUIDE

Attempts to discontinue or taper medication should be made at three- to six-month intervals.

Usual Dosage Range: 2 to 4 g (½ applicatorful to 1 applicatorful) daily, intravaginally, depending on the severity of the condition.

Treated patients with an intact uterus should be monitored closely for signs of endometrial cancer, and appropriate diagnostic measures should be taken to rule out malignancy in the event of persistent or recurring abnormal vaginal bleeding.

Instructions for Use of Applicator:

1. Remove cap from tube.
2. Screw nozzle end of applicator onto tube.
3. *Gently* squeeze tube from the *bottom* to force sufficient cream into the barrel to provide the prescribed dose.
4. Unscrew applicator from tube.
5. Lie on back with knees drawn up. To deliver medication, gently insert applicator deeply into vagina and press plunger downward to its original position.

To Cleanse: Pull plunger out from barrel. Wash with mild soap and warm water.
DO NOT BOIL OR USE HOT WATER.
Store at room temperature (approximately 25° C).

PHYSICIAN REFERENCES

1. Ziel, H. K., *et al.*: N Engl. J. Med. 293:1167-1170, 1975. 2. Smith, D. C., *et al.*: N. Engl. J. Med. 293:1164-1167, 1975. 3. Mack, T. M., *et al.*: N. Engl. J. Med. 294:1262-1267, 1976. 4. Weiss, N. S., *et al.*: N. Engl. J. Med. 294:1259-1262, 1976. 5. Herbst, A. L., *et al.*: N. Engl. J. Med. 284:878-881, 1971. 6. Greenwald, P., *et al.*: N. Engl. J. Med. 285:390-392, 1971. 7. Lanier, A., *et al.*: Mayo Clin. Proc. 48:793-799, 1973. 8. Herbst, A., *et al.*: Obstet. Gynecol. 40:287-298, 1972. 9. Herbst, A., *et al.*: Am. J. Obstet. Gynecol. 118:607-615, 1974. 10. Herbst, A., *et al.*: N. Engl. J. Med. 292:334-339, 1975. 11. Stafl, A., *et al.*: Obstet. Gynecol. 43:118-128, 1974. 12. Sherman, A. I., *et al.*: Obstet. Gynecol. 44:531-545, 1974. 13. Gal, I., *et al.*: Nature 216:83, 1967. 14. Levy, E. P., *et al.*: Lancet 1:611, 1973. 15. Nora, J., *et al.*: Lancet 1:941-942, 1973. 16. Janerich, D. T., *et al.*: N. Engl. J. Med. 291:697-700, 1974. 17. Boston Collaborative Drug Surveillance Program: N. Engl. J. Med. 290:15-19, 1974. 18. Hoover, R., *et al.*: N. Engl. J. Med. 295:401-405, 1976. 19. Boston Collaborative Drug Surveillance Program: Lancet 1:1399-1404, 1973. 20. Daniel, D. G., *et al.*: Lancet 2:287-289, 1967. 21. The Veterans Administration Cooperative Urological Research Group: J. Urol. 98:516-522, 1967. 22. Bailar, J. C.: Lancet 2:560, 1967. 23. Blackard, C., *et al.*: Cancer 26:249-256, 1970. 24. Royal College of General Practitioners: J. R. Coll. Gen. Pract. 13:267-279, 1967. 24a. Royal College of General Practitioners: Oral Contraceptives and Health, New York, Pitman Corp., 1974. 25. Inman, W. H. W., *et al.*: Br. Med. J. 2:193-199, 1968. 26. Vessey, M. P., *et al.*: Br. Med. J. 2:651-657, 1969. 27. Sartwell, P. E., *et al.*: Am. J. Epidemiol. 90:365-380, 1969. 28. Collaborative Group for the Study of Stroke in Young Women: N. Engl. J. Med. 288:871-878, 1973. 29. Collaborative Group for the Study of Stroke in Young Women: J.A.M.A. 231:718-722, 1975. 30. Mann, J. I., *et al.*: Br. Med. J. 2:245-248, 1975. 31. Mann, J. I., *et al.*: Br. Med. J. 2:241-245, 1975. 32. Inman, W. H. W., *et al.*: Br. Med. J. 2:203-209, 1970. 33. Stolley, P. D., *et al.*: Am. J. Epidemiol. 102:197-208, 1975. 34. Vessey, M. P., *et al.*: Br. Med. J. 3:123-126, 1970. 35. Greene, G. R., *et al.*: Am. J. Public Health 62:680-685, 1972. 36. Rosenberg, L., *et al.*: N. Engl. J. Med. 294:1256-1259, 1976. 37. Coronary Drug Project Research Group: J.A.M.A. 214:1303-1313, 1970. 38. Baum, J., *et al.*: Lancet 2:926-928, 1973. 39. Mays, E. T., *et al.*: J.A.M.A.. 235:730-732, 1976. 40. Edmondson, H. A., *et al.*: N. Engl. J. Med. 294:470-472, 1976. 41. Pfeffer, R. I., *et al.*: Am. J. Epidemiol. 103:445-456, 1976.

J CODES
Up to 2 mg or 20,000 units IV,IM—J1410

HOW SUPPLIED
CREAM: 0.625 MG/GM

BRAND/MANUFACTURER	NDC	SIZE	AWP
○ BRAND			
PREMARIN VAGINAL: Wyeth-Ayerst	00046-0872-01	42.5 gm	$27.40
	00046-0872-93	42.5 gm	$30.51

POWDER FOR INJECTION: 25 MG

BRAND/MANUFACTURER	NDC	SIZE	AWP
○ BRAND			
PREMARIN INTRAVENOUS: Wyeth-Ayerst	00046-0749-05	1s	$32.11

TABLETS: 0.3 MG

BRAND/MANUFACTURER	NDC	SIZE	AWP
○ BRAND			
▶ PREMARIN: Wyeth-Ayerst	00046-0868-81	100s	$26.61
	00046-0868-91	1000s	$256.63

TABLETS: 0.625 MG

BRAND/MANUFACTURER	NDC	SIZE	AWP
○ BRAND			
▶ PREMARIN: Wyeth-Ayerst	00046-0867-81	100s	$37.08
	00046-3867-81	100s	$37.08
	00046-0867-99	100s ud	$39.86
	00046-0867-91	1000s	$357.33
	00046-0867-95	5000s	$1742.98
○ GENERICS			
Southwood	58016-0925-00	100s	$24.47

TABLETS: 0.9 MG

BRAND/MANUFACTURER	NDC	SIZE	AWP
○ BRAND			
▶ PREMARIN: Wyeth-Ayerst	00046-0864-81	100s	$43.91

TABLETS: 1.25 MG

BRAND/MANUFACTURER	NDC	SIZE	AWP
○ BRAND			
▶ PREMARIN: Wyeth-Ayerst	00046-0866-81	100s	$50.74
	00046-0866-99	100s ud	$53.26
	00046-0866-91	1000s	$489.18
	00046-0866-95	5000s	$2386.18

TABLETS: 2.5 MG

BRAND/MANUFACTURER	NDC	SIZE	AWP
○ BRAND			
▶ PREMARIN: Wyeth-Ayerst	00046-0865-81	100s	$87.86
	00046-0865-91	1000s	$847.54

Estrogens, Conjugated and Meprobamate

1. ESTROGENS HAVE BEEN REPORTED TO INCREASE THE RISK OF ENDOMETRIAL CARCINOMA.

THREE INDEPENDENT, CASE-CONTROLLED STUDIES HAVE REPORTED AN INCREASED RISK OF ENDOMETRIAL CANCER IN POST-MENOPAUSAL WOMEN EXPOSED TO EXOGENOUS ESTROGENS FOR MORE THAN ONE YEAR.[1-3] THIS RISK WAS INDEPENDENT OF THE OTHER KNOWN RISK FACTORS FOR ENDOMETRIAL CANCER. THESE STUDIES ARE FURTHER SUPPORTED BY THE FINDING THAT INCIDENCE RATES OF ENDOMETRIAL CANCER HAVE INCREASED SHARPLY SINCE 1969 IN EIGHT DIFFERENT AREAS OF THE UNITED STATES WITH POPULATION-BASED CANCER REPORTING SYSTEMS, AN INCREASE WHICH MAY BE RELATED TO THE RAPIDLY EXPANDING USE OF ESTROGENS DURING THE LAST DECADE.[4]

THE THREE CASE-CONTROLLED STUDIES REPORTED THAT THE RISK OF ENDOMETRIAL CANCER IN ESTROGEN USERS WAS ABOUT 4.5 TO 13.9 TIMES GREATER THAN IN NONUSERS. THE RISK APPEARS TO DEPEND ON BOTH DURATION OF TREATMENT[1] AND ON ESTROGEN DOSE.[3] IN VIEW OF THESE FINDINGS, WHEN ESTROGENS ARE USED FOR THE TREATMENT OF MENOPAUSAL SYMPTOMS, THE LOWEST DOSE THAT WILL CONTROL SYMPTOMS SHOULD BE UTILIZED AND MEDICATION SHOULD BE DISCONTINUED AS SOON AS POSSIBLE. WHEN PROLONGED TREATMENT IS MEDICALLY INDICATED, THE PATIENT SHOULD BE REASSESSED, ON AT LEAST A SEMI-ANNUAL BASIS TO DETERMINE THE NEED FOR CONTINUED THERAPY. ALTHOUGH THE EVIDENCE MUST BE CONSIDERED PRELIMINARY, ONE STUDY SUGGESTS THAT CYCLIC ADMINISTRATION OF LOW DOSES OF ESTROGEN MAY CARRY LESS RISK THAN CONTINUOUS ADMINISTRATION.[3] IT THEREFORE APPEARS PRUDENT TO UTILIZE SUCH A REGIMEN.

CLOSE CLINICAL SURVEILLANCE OF ALL WOMEN TAKING ESTROGENS IS IMPORTANT. IN ALL CASES OF UNDIAGNOSED PERSISTENT OR RECURRING ABNORMAL VAGINAL BLEEDING, ADEQUATE DIAGNOSTIC MEASURES SHOULD BE UNDERTAKEN TO RULE OUT MALIGNANCY.

THERE IS NO EVIDENCE AT PRESENT THAT "NATURAL" ESTROGENS ARE MORE OR LESS HAZARDOUS THAN "SYNTHETIC" ESTROGENS AT EQUI-ESTROGENIC DOSES.

2. ESTROGENS SHOULD NOT BE USED DURING PREGNANCY.

THE USE OF FEMALE SEX HORMONES, BOTH ESTROGENS AND PROGESTOGENS, DURING EARLY PREGNANCY MAY SERIOUSLY DAMAGE THE OFFSPRING. IT HAS BEEN SHOWN THAT FEMALES EXPOSED IN UTERO TO DIETHYLSTILBESTROL, A NONSTEROIDAL ESTROGEN, HAVE AN INCREASED RISK OF DEVELOPING, IN LATER LIFE, A FORM OF VAGINAL OR CERVICAL CANCER THAT IS ORDINARILY EXTREMELY RARE.[5,6] THIS RISK HAS BEEN ESTIMATED AS NOT GREATER THAN 4 PER 1,000 EXPOSURES.[7] FURTHERMORE, A HIGH PERCENTAGE OF SUCH EXPOSED WOMEN (FROM 30% TO 90%) HAVE BEEN FOUND TO HAVE VAGINAL ADENOSIS,[8-12] EPITHELIAL CHANGES OF THE VAGINA AND CERVIX. ALTHOUGH THESE CHANGES ARE HISTOLOGICALLY BENIGN, IT IS NOT KNOWN WHETHER THEY ARE PRECURSORS OF MALIGNANCY. ALTHOUGH SIMILAR DATA ARE NOT AVAILABLE WITH THE USE OF OTHER ESTROGENS, IT CANNOT BE PRESUMED THEY WOULD NOT INDUCE SIMILAR CHANGES.

◆ RATED THERAPEUTICALLY EQUIVALENT; ◇ THERAPEUTIC EQUIVALENCE UNCONFIRMED; ○ UNRATED

SEVERAL REPORTS SUGGEST AN ASSOCIATION BETWEEN INTRAUTERINE EXPOSURE TO FEMALE SEX HORMONES AND CONGENITAL ANOMALIES, INCLUDING CONGENITAL HEART DEFECTS AND LIMB-REDUCTION DEFECTS.[13-16] ONE CASE-CONTROLLED STUDY[16] ESTIMATED A 4.7-FOLD INCREASED RISK OF LIMB-REDUCTION DEFECTS IN INFANTS EXPOSED IN UTERO TO SEX HORMONES (ORAL CONTRACEPTIVES, HORMONE WITHDRAWAL TESTS FOR PREGNANCY, OR ATTEMPTED TREATMENT FOR THREATENED ABORTION). SOME OF THESE EXPOSURES WERE VERY SHORT AND INVOLVED ONLY A FEW DAYS OF TREATMENT. THE DATA SUGGEST THAT THE RISK OF LIMB-REDUCTION DEFECTS IN EXPOSED FETUSES IS SOMEWHAT LESS THAN 1 PER 1,000.

IN THE PAST, FEMALE SEX HORMONES HAVE BEEN USED DURING PREGNANCY IN AN ATTEMPT TO THREAT THREATENED OR HABITUAL ABORTION. THERE IS CONSIDERABLE EVIDENCE THAT ESTROGENS ARE INEFFECTIVE FOR THESE INDICATIONS, AND THERE IS NO EVIDENCE FROM WELL-CONTROLLED STUDIES THAT PROGESTOGENS ARE EFFECTIVE FOR THESE USES.

IF PMB IS USED DURING PREGNANCY, OR IF THE PATIENT BECOMES PREGNANT WHILE TAKING THIS DRUG, SHE SHOULD BE APPRISED OF THE POTENTIAL RISKS TO THE FETUS, AND THE ADVISABILITY OF PREGNANCY CONTINUATION.

3. THIS FIXED-COMBINATION DRUG IS NOT INDICATED FOR INITIAL THERAPY.

IN CASES WHERE ESTROGEN GIVEN ALONE HAS NOT ALLEVIATED ANXIETY AND TENSION EXISTING AS PART OF THE MENOPAUSAL SYMPTOM COMPLEX, THERAPY MAY THEN CONSIST OF SEPARATE ADMINISTRATION OF ESTROGEN AND MEPROBAMATE IN ORDER TO DETERMINE THE APPROPRIATE DOSAGE OF EACH DRUG FOR THE PATIENT. IF THIS FIXED COMBINATION REPRESENTS THE DOSAGE SO DETERMINED, ITS USE MAY BE MORE CONVENIENT IN PATIENT MANAGEMENT. THE TREATMENT OF SUCH PATIENTS IS NOT STATIC, BUT MUST BE RE-EVALUATED AS CONDITIONS IN EACH PATIENT WARRANT.

DESCRIPTION

Estrogens, Conjugated USP is a mixture of Estrogens, obtained exclusively from natural sources, occuring as the sodium salts of water-soluble Estrogen sulfates blended to represent the average composition of material derived from pregnant mares' urine. It contains estrone, equilin, and 17α-dihydroequilin, together with smaller amounts of 17α-estradiol, equilenin, and 17α-dihydroequilenin as salts of their sulfate esters.

Meprobamate, USP, is the dicarbamic acid ester of 2-methyl-2-n-propyl-1,3-propanediol.

Estrogens, Conjugated/Meprobamate oral tablets contain: 0.45 mg of Conjugated Estrogens and 200 mg of Meprobamate, or 0.45 mg of Estrogens, Conjugated and 400 mg of Meprobamate.

CLINICAL PHARMACOLOGY

Estrogens are important in the development and maintenance of the female reproductive system and secondary sex characteristics. They promote growth and development of the vagina, uterus, and fallopian tubes, and enlargement of the breasts. Indirectly, they contribute to the shaping of the skeleton, maintenance of tone and elasticity of urogenital structures, changes in the epiphyses of the long bones that allow for the pubertal growth spurt and its termination, growth of axillary and pubic hair, and pigmentation of the nipples and genitals. Decline of estrogenic activity at the end of the menstrual cycle can bring on menstruation, although the cessation of progesterone secretion is the most important factor in the mature ovulatory cycle. However, in the pre-ovulatory or nonovulatory cycle, Estrogen is the primary determinant in the onset of menstruation. Estrogens also affect the release of pituitary gonadotropins.

The pharmacologic effects of Conjugated Estrogens are similar to those of endogenous Estrogens. They are soluble in water and are well absorbed from the gastrointestinal tract. In responsive tissues (female genital organs, breasts, hypothalamus, pituitary) Estrogens enter the cell and are transported into the nucleus. As a result of Estrogen action, specific RNA and protein synthesis occurs.

Metabolism and inactivation occur primarily in the liver. Some Estrogens are excreted into the bile; however, they are reabsorbed from the intestine and returned to the liver through the portal venous system. Water-soluble Estrogen Conjugates are strongly acidic and are ionized in body fluids, which favor excretion through the kidneys since tubular reabsorption is minimal.

Meprobamate is used clinically for the reduction of anxiety and tension. The precise mechanism(s) of its action is not known. It is well absorbed from the gastrointestinal tract and has a physiological half-life of about 10 hours. It is excreted in the urine primarily as hydroxymeprobamate and as a glucuronide.

The combination of Estrogens, Conjugated/Meprobamate relieves the underlying Estrogen deficiency and affords tranquilizing activity to ameliorate the anxiety and tension not due to Estrogen deficiency.

INDICATIONS AND USAGE

For the treatment of moderate-to-severe vasomotor symptoms of the menopause when anxiety and tension are part of the symptom complex and only in those cases in which the use of Estrogens alone has not resulted in alleviation of such symptoms.

ESTROGENS, CONJUGATED/MEPROBAMATE HAS NOT BEEN SHOWN TO BE EFFECTIVE FOR ANY PURPOSE DURING PREGNANCY AND ITS USE MAY CAUSE SEVERE HARM TO THE FETUS (see boxed *"Warning"*).

CONTRAINDICATIONS

Estrogens should not be used in women with any of the following conditions:

1. Known or suspected cancer of the breast except in appropriately selected patients being treated for metastatic disease.
2. Known or suspected Estrogen-dependent neoplasia.
3. Known or suspected pregnancy (see boxed *"Warning"*).
4. Undiagnosed abnormal genital bleeding.
5. Active thrombophlebitis or thromboembolic disorders.
6. A past history of thrombophlebitis, thrombosis, or thromboembolic disorders associated with previous estrogen use.

Meprobamate should not be used in patients with the following conditions:

1. A history of allergic or idiosyncratic reactions to meprobamate or related compounds such as carisoprodol, mebutamate, tybamate, or carbromal.
2. Acute intermittent porphyria.

WARNINGS

USAGE IN PREGNANCY AND LACTATION

An increased risk of congenital malformations associated with the use of minor tranquilizers (meprobamate, chlordiazepoxide, and diazepam) during the first trimester of pregnancy has been suggested in several studies. Because use of these drugs is rarely a matter of urgency, their use during this period should almost always be avoided. The possibility that a woman of childbearing potential may be pregnant at the time of institution of therapy should be considered. Patients should be advised that if they become pregnant during therapy or intend to become pregnant they should communicate with their physicians about the desirability of discontinuing the drug.

Meprobamate passes the placental barrier. It is present both in umbilical cord blood at or near maternal plasma levels and in breast milk of lactating mothers at concentrations two to four times that of maternal plasma. When use of meprobamate is contemplated in breast-feeding patients, the drug's higher concentrations in breast milk as compared to maternal plasma levels should be considered.

Usage in Children—Estrogens, Conjugated/Meprobamate is not intended for use in children.

ASSOCIATED WITH ESTROGEN ADMINISTRATION

1. Induction of Malignant Neoplasms: Estrogens have been reported to increase the risk of endometrial carcinoma. (See Boxed *"Warning"*). However, a recent, large, case-controlled study indicated no increase in risk of breast cancer in postmenopausal women.[18]

2. Gallbladder Disease: A recent study has reported a 2- to 3-fold increase in the risk of surgically confirmed gallbladder disease in women receiving postmenopausal Estrogen,[17] similar to the 2-fold increase previously noted in users of oral contraceptives.[19,24a]

3. Effects Similar to Those Caused by Estrogen-Progestogen Oral Contraceptives: There are several serious adverse effects of oral contraceptives, most of which have not, up to now, been documented as consequences of postmenopausal Estrogen therapy. This may reflect the comparatively low doses of Estrogen used in postmenopausal women. It would be expected that the larger doses of Estrogen used to treat prostatic or breast cancer are more likely to result in these adverse effects, and, in fact, it has been shown that there is an increased risk of thrombosis in men receiving Estrogens for prostatic cancer.[20-23]

a. Thromboembolic Disease: It is now well established that users of oral contraceptives have an increased risk of various thromboembolic and thrombotic vascular diseases, such as thrombophlebitis, pulmonary embolism, stroke, and myocardial infarction.[24-31] Cases of retinal thrombosis, mesenteric thrombosis, and optic neuritis have been reported in oral-contraceptive users. There is evidence that the risk of several of these adverse reactions is related to the dose of the drug.[32,33] An increased risk of postsurgery thromboembolic complications has also been reported in users of oral-contraceptives.[34,35] If feasible, Estrogen should be discontinued at least 4 weeks before surgery of the type associated with an increased risk of thromboembolism, or during periods of prolonged immobilization.

While an increased rate of thromboembolic and thrombotic disease in postmenopausal users of Estrogens has not been found,[17-24,25-36] this does not rule out the possibility that such an increase may be present or that subgroups of women who have underlying risk factors or who are receiving relatively large doses of Estrogens may have increased risk. Therefore Estrogens should not be used in persons with active thrombophlebitis or thromboembolic disorders, and they should not be used (except in treatment of malignancy) in persons with a history of such disorders in association with Estrogen use. They should be used with caution in patients with cerebral vascular or coronary artery disease and only for those in whom Estrogens are clearly needed.

Large doses of Estrogen (5 mg conjugated Estrogens per day), comparable to those used to treat cancer of the prostate and breast, have been shown in a large prospective clinical trial in men[37] to increase the risk of nonfatal myocardial infarction, pulmonary embolism, and thrombophlebitis. When Estrogen doses of this size are used, any of the thromboembolic and thrombotic adverse effects associated with oral contraceptive use should be considered a clear risk.

b. Hepatic Adenoma: Benign hepatic adenomas appear to be associated with the use of oral contraceptives.[38-40] Although benign, and rare, these may rupture and may cause death through intra-abdominal hemorrhage. Such lesions have not yet been reported in association with other Estrogen or progestogen preparations but should be considered in Estrogen users having abdominal pain and tenderness, abdominal mass, or hypovolemic shock. Hepatocellular carcinoma has also been reported in women taking Estrogen-containing oral contraceptives.[39] The relationship of this malignancy to these drugs is not known at this time.

c. Elevated Blood Pressure: Women using oral contraceptives sometimes experience increased blood pressure which, in most cases, returns to normal on discontinuing the drug. There is now a report that this may occur with use of Estrogens in the menopause[41] and blood pressure should be monitored with Estrogen use, especially if high doses are used.

d. Glucose Tolerance: A worsening of glucose tolerance has been observed in a significant percentage of patients on Estrogen-containing oral contraceptives. For this reason, diabetic patients should be carefully observed while receiving Estrogen.

4. Hypercalcemia: Administration of Estrogens may lead to severe hypercalcemia in patients with breast cancer and bone metastases. If this occurs, the drug should be stopped and appropriate measures taken to reduce the serum calcium level.

ASSOCIATED WITH MEPROBAMATE ADMINISTRATION

1. Drug Dependence: Physical dependence, psychological dependence, and abuse have occurred. When chronic intoxication from prolonged use occurs, it usually involves ingestion of greater than recommended doses and is manifested by ataxia, slurred speech, and vertigo. Therefore, careful supervision of dose and amounts prescribed is advised, as well as avoidance of prolonged administration, especially for alcoholics and other patients with a known propensity for taking excessive quantities of drugs.

Sudden withdrawal of the drug after prolonged and excessive use may precipitate recurrence of pre-existing symptoms, such as anxiety, anorexia, or insomnia, or withdrawal reactions, such as vomiting, ataxia, tremors, muscle twitching, confusional states, hallucinosis, and, rarely, convulsive seizures. Such seizures are more likely to occur in persons with central nervous system damage or pre-existent or latent convulsive disorders. Onset of withdrawal symptoms occurs usually within 12 to 48 hours after discontinuation of meprobamate; symptoms usually cease within the next 12 to 48 hours.

When excessive dosage has continued for weeks or months, dosage should be reduced gradually over a period of one or two weeks rather than abruptly stopped. Alternatively, a short-acting barbiturate may be substituted, then gradually withdrawn.

2. Potentially Hazardous Tasks: Patients should be warned that this drug may impair the mental and/or physical abilities required for the performance of potentially hazardous tasks such as driving a motor vehicle or operating machinery.

3. Additive Effects: Since the effects of Meprobamate and alcohol or Meprobamate and other CNS depressants or psychotropic drugs may be additive, appropriate caution should be exercised with patients who take more than one of these agents simultaneously.

PRECAUTIONS

A. GENERAL PRECAUTIONS

Associated with Estrogen: 1. A complete medical and family history should be taken prior to the initiation of any Estrogen therapy. The pretreatment and periodic physical examinations should include special reference to blood pressure, breasts, abdomen, and pelvic organs, and should include a Papanicolaou smear. As a general rule, Estrogen should not be prescribed for longer than one year without another physical examination being performed.

2. Fluid retention—Because Estrogens may cause some degree of fluid retention, conditions which might be influenced by this factor such as asthma, epilepsy, migraine, and cardiac or renal dysfunction, require careful observation.

3. Certain patients may develop undesirable manifestations of excessive estrogenic stimulation, such as abnormal or excessive uterine bleeding, mastodynia, etc.

4. Prolonged administration of unopposed Estrogen therapy has been reported to increase the risk of endometrial hyperplasia in some patients.

5. Oral contraceptives appear to be associated with an increased incidence of mental depression.[24a] Although it is not clear whether this is due to the estrogenic or progestogenic component of the contraceptive, patients with a history of depression should be carefully observed.

6. Pre-existing uterine leiomyomata may increase in size during Estrogen use.

7. The pathologist should be advised of Estrogen therapy when relevant specimens are submitted.

8. Patients with a past history of jaundice during pregnancy have an increased risk of recurrence of jaundice while receiving Estrogen-containing oral contraceptive therapy. If jaundice develops in any patient receiving Estrogen, the medication should be discontinued while the cause is investigated.

9. Estrogens may be poorly metabolized in patients with impaired liver function and should be administered with caution in such patients.

10. Because Estrogens influence the metabolism of calcium and phosphorus, they should be used with caution in patients with metabolic bone diseases that are associated with hypercalcemia or in patients with renal insufficiency.

11. Because of the effects of Estrogens on epiphyseal closure, they should be used judiciously in young patients in whom bone growth is not complete.

Concomitant Progestin Use: The lowest effective dose appropriate for the specific indication should be utilized. Studies of the addition of a progestin for 7 or more days of a cycle of Estrogen administration have reported a lowered incidence of endometrial hyperplasia. Morphological and biochemical studies of the endometrium suggest that 10 to 13 days of progestin are needed to provide maximal maturation of the endometrium and to eliminate any hyperplastic changes. Whether this will provide protection from endometrial carcinoma has not been clearly established. There are possible additional risks which may be associated with the inclusion of progestin in Estrogen replacement regimens. If concomitant progestin therapy is used, potential risks may include adverse effects on carbohydrate and lipid metabolism. The choice of progestin and dosage may be important in minimizing these adverse effects.

Associated with Meprobamate: 1. The lowest effective dose should be administered, particularly to debilitated patients, in order to preclude over-sedation.

2. The possibility of suicide attempts should be considered and the least amount of drug feasible should be dispensed at any one time.

3. Meprobamate is metabolized in the liver and excreted by the kidney; to avoid its excess accumulation, caution should be exercised in administration to patients with compromised liver or kidney function.

4. Meprobamate occasionally may precipitate seizures in epileptic patients.

B. INFORMATION FOR PATIENTS
See manufacturer's patient information.

C. DRUG/LABORATORY TEST INTERACTIONS
Certain endocrine and liver function tests may be affected by Estrogen-containing oral contraceptives. The following similar changes may be expected with larger doses of Estrogen.

a. Increased sulfobromophthalein retention.

b. Increased prothrombin and factors VII, VIII, IX, and X; decreased antithrombin 3; increased norepinephrine-induced platelet aggrega- bility.

c. Increased thyroid binding globulin (TBG) leading to increased circulating total thyroid hormone, as measured by PBI, T_4 by column or T_4 by radioimmunoassay. Free T_3 resin uptake is decreased, reflecting the elevated TBG; free T_4 concentration is unaltered.

d. Impaired glucose tolerance.

e. Decreased pregnanediol excretion.

f. Reduced response to metyrapone test.

g. Reduced serum folate concentration.

h. Increased serum triglyceride and phospholipid concentration.

D. MUTAGENESIS AND CARCINOGENESIS
Long-term, continuous administration of natural and synthetic Estrogens in certain animal species increases the frequency of carcinomas of the breast, cervix, vagina, and liver. However in a recent, large, case-controlled study of postmenopausal women, there was no increase in risk of breast cancer with use of conjugated Estrogens.[18]

E. PREGNANCY CATEGORY X
(See *"Contraindications"* and boxed *"Warning"*).

F. NURSING MOTHERS
Because of the potential for serious adverse reactions in nursing infants from PMB, a decision should be made whether to discontinue nursing or to discontinue the drugs, taking into account the importance of the drug to the mother. (See *"Warning"* section for information on use in pregnancy and lactation.)

G. PEDIATRIC USE
Safety and effectiveness in children have not been established.

ADVERSE REACTIONS

ASSOCIATED WITH ESTROGEN ADMINISTRATION
(See *"Warnings"* regarding induction of neoplasia, adverse effects on the fetus, increased incidence of gallbladder disease, and adverse effects similar to those of oral contraceptives, including thromboembolism.) The following additional adverse reactions have been reported with estrogenic therapy, including oral contraceptives:

1. Genitourinary System: Breakthrough bleeding, spotting, change in menstrual flow; dysmenorrhea; premenstrual-like syndrome; amenorrhea during and after treatment; increase in size of uterine fibromyomata; vaginal candidiasis; change in cervical erosion and in degree of cervical secretion; cystitis-like syndrome.

2. Breasts: Tenderness, enlargement, secretion.

3. Gastrointestinal: Nausea, vomiting, abdominal cramps, bloating; cholestatic jaundice.

4. Skin: Chloasma or melasma which may persist when drug is discontinued; erythema multiforme; erythema nodosum; hemorrhagic eruption; loss of scalp hair; hirsutism.

5. Eyes: Steepening of corneal curvature; intolerance to contact lenses.

6. CNS: Headache, migraine, dizziness; mental depression; chorea.

7. Miscellaneous: Increase or decrease in weight; reduced carbohydrate tolerance; aggravation of porphyria; edema; changes in libido.

◆ RATED THERAPEUTICALLY EQUIVALENT; ◇ THERAPEUTIC EQUIVALENCE UNCONFIRMED; ○ UNRATED

THE FOLLOWING HAVE BEEN REPORTED WITH MEPROBAMATE THERAPY

1. Central Nervous System: Drowsiness, ataxia, dizziness, slurred speech, headache, vertigo, weakness, paresthesias, impairment of visual accommodation, euphoria, overstimulation, paradoxical excitement, fast EEG activity.

2. Gastrointestinal: Nausea, vomiting, diarrhea.

3. Cardiovascular: Palpitations, tachycardia, various forms of arrhythmia, transient ECG changes, syncope; also, hypotensive crises (including one fatal case).

4. Allergic or Idiosyncratic: Allergic or idiosyncratic reactions are usually seen within the period of the first to fourth dose in patients having had no previous contact with the drug. Milder reactions are characterized by an itchy, urticarial, or erythematous maculopapular rash which may be generalized or confined to the groin. Other reactions have included leukopenia, acute nonthrombocytopenic purpura, petechiae, ecchymoses, eosinophilia, peripheral edema, adenopathy, fever, fixed drug eruption with cross reaction to carisoprodol, and cross sensitivity between meprobamate/mebutamate and meprobamate/carbromal.

More severe hypersensitivity reactions, rarely reported, include hyperpyrexia, chills, angioneurotic edema, bronchospasm, oliguria, and anuria. Also, anaphylaxis, erythema multiforme, exfoliative dermatitis, stomatitis, proctitis. Stevens-Johnson syndrome, and bullous dermatitis, including one fatal case of the latter, following administration of meprobamate in combination with prednisolone.

In case of allergic or idiosyncratic reactions to meprobamate, discontinue the drug and initiate appropriate symptomatic therapy, which may include epinephrine, antihistamines, and in severe cases corticosteroids. In evaluating possible allergic reactions, also consider allergy to excipients (information on excipients is available to physicians on request).

5. Hematologic (See also *"Allergic or Idiosyncratic"*): Agranulocytosis and aplastic anemia have been reported, although no causal relationship has been established. These cases rarely were fatal. Rare cases of thrombocytopenic purpura have been reported.

6. Other: Exacerbation of porphyric symptoms.

OVERDOSAGE

Acute Overdosage (Estrogen Alone): Numerous reports of ingestion of large doses of Estrogen-containing oral contraceptives by young children indicate that acute serious ill effects do not occur. Overdosage of estrogen may cause nausea, and withdrawal bleeding may occur in females.

Acute Simple Overdosage (Meprobamate Alone): Death has been reported with ingestion of as little as 12 grams meprobamate and survival with as much as 40 grams.

Blood Levels: 0.5-2.0 mg% represents the usual blood level range of meprobamate after therapeutic doses. The level may occasionally be as high as 3.0 mg%.

3-10 mg% usually corresponds to findings of mild-to-moderate symptoms of overdosage, such as stupor or light coma.

10-20 mg% usually corresponds to deeper coma, requiring more intensive treatment. Some fatalities occur.

At levels greater than 20 mg%, more fatalities than survivals can be expected.

Acute Combined (Alcohol or other CNS Depressants or Psychotropic Drugs) Overdosage: Since effects can be additive, a history of ingestion of a low dose of meprobamate plus any of these compounds (or of a relatively low blood or tissue level) cannot be used as a prognostic indicator.

In cases where excessive doses have been taken, sleep ensues rapidly and blood pressure, pulse, and respiratory rates are reduced to basal levels. Any drug remaining in the stomach should be removed and symptomatic therapy given. Should respiration or blood pressure become compromised, respiratory assistance, central nervous system stimulants, and pressor agents should be administered cautiously as indicated. Meprobamate is metabolized in the liver and excreted by the kidney. Diuresis, osmotic (mannitol) diuresis, peritoneal dialysis, and hemodialysis have been used successfully. Careful monitoring of urinary output is necessary and caution should be taken to avoid overhydration. Relapse and death, after initial recovery, have been attributed to incomplete gastric emptying and delayed absorption. Meprobamate can be measured in biological fluids by two methods: colorimetric[42] and gas chromatographic.[43]

DOSAGE AND ADMINISTRATION

Given Cyclically for Short-Term Use Only: For the treatment of moderate-to-severe vasomotor symptoms of the menopause when anxiety and tension are part of the symptom complex and only in those cases in which the use of Estrogens alone has not resulted in alleviation of such symptoms.

The lowest dose that will control symptoms should be chosen and medication should be discontinued as promptly as possible. The usual dosage of conjugated Estrogen is 1.25 milligrams daily. The usual dosage of meprobamate is 1,200 to 1,600 milligrams daily.

Administration should be cyclic (eg. three weeks on and one week off).

Attempts to discontinue or taper medication should be made at three- to six-month intervals.

The used dosage is one tablet of Estrogens, Conjugated 0.45 mg/Meprobamate 200 mg or Estrogens, Conjugated 0.45 mg/Meprobamate 400mg three times daily administered cyclically.

Use of Meprobamate during the rest period should be considered for those patients who may require continuing medication with tranquilizer. After the first few cycles of therapy, the patient's need for continuing the use of the Meprobamate component should be re-evaluated.

Daily dosage should be adjusted to individual requirements. The daily dosage should not exceed 6 tablets per day of Estrogens, Conjugated 0.45 mg/Meprobamate 200 mg or 4 tablets per day of Estrogens, Conjugated 0.45 mg/Meprobamate 400 mg.

Treated patients with an intact uterus should be monitored closely for signs of endometrial cancer and appropriate diagnostic measures should be taken to rule out malignancy in the event of persistent or recurring abnormal vaginal bleeding.

Storage: Store at room temperature (approximately 25°C).

Dispense in a well-closed container as defined in the USP.

PHYSICIAN REFERENCES
1. Ziel, H. K., *et al.:* N. Engl. J. Med. *293:*1167-1170, 1975. 2. Smith, D. C., *et al.:* N. Engl. J. Med. *293:*1164-1167, 1975. 3. Mack, T. M., *et al.:* N. Engl. J. Med. *294:*1262-1267, 1976. 4. Weiss, N. S., *et al.:* N. Engl. J. Med. *294:*1259-1262, 1976. 5. Herbst, A. L., *et al.:* N. Engl. J. Med. *284:*878-881, 1971. 6. Greenwald, P., *et al.:* N. Engl. J. Med. *285:*390-392, 1971. 7. Lanier, A., *et al.:* Mayo Clin. Proc. *48:*793-799, 1973. 8. Herbst, A., *et al.:* Obstet. Gynecol. *40:*287-298, 1972. 9. Herbst, A., *et al.:* Am. J. Obstet. Gynecol. *118:*607-615, 1974. 10. Herbst, A., *et al.:* N. Engl. J. Med. *292:*334-339, 1975. 11. Stafl, A., *et al.:* Obstet. Gynecol. *43:*118-128, 1974. 12. Sherman, A. I., *et al.:* Obstet. Gynecol. *44:*531-545, 1974. 13. Gal, I., *et al.:* Nature *216:*83, 1967. 14. Levy, E. P., *et al.:* Lancet *1:*611, 1973. 15. Nora, J., *et al.:* Lancet *1:*941-942, 1973. 16. Janerich, D. T., *et al.:* N. Engl. J. Med. *291:*697-700, 1974. 17. Boston Collaborative Drug Surveillance Program: N. Engl. J. Med. *290:*15-19, 1974. 18. Kaufman, D.W., *et al.:* J.A.M.A. 252:63-67, 1984. 19. Boston Collaborative Drug Surveillance Program: Lancet *1:*1399-1404, 1973. 20. Daniel, D. G., *et al.:* Lancet *2:*287-289, 1967. 21. The Veterans Administration Cooperative Urological Research Group: J. Urol. *98:*516-522, 1967. 22. Bailar, J. C.: Lancet *2:*560, 1967. 23. Blackard, C., *et al.:* Cancer *26:*249-256, 1970. 24. Royal College of General Practitioners: J. R. Coll. Gen. Pract. *13:*267-279, 1967. 24a. Royal College of General Practitioners: Oral Contraceptives and Health, New York, Pitman Corp., 1974. 25. Inman, W. H. W., *et al.:* Br. Med. J. *2:*193-199, 1968. 26. Vessey, M. P., *et al.:* Br. Med. J. *2:*651-657, 1969. 27. Sartwell, P. E., *et al.:* Am. J. Epidemiol. *90:*365-380, 1969. 28. Collaborative Group for the Study of Stroke in Young Women: N. Engl. J. Med. *288:*871-878, 1973. 29. Collaborative Group for the Study of Stroke in Young Women: J.A.M.A. *231:*718-722, 1975. 30. Mann, J. I., *et al.:* Br. Med. J. *2:*245-248, 1975. 31. Mann, J. I., *et al.:* Br. Med. J. *2:*241-245, 1975. 32. Inman, W. H. W., *et al.:* Br. Med. J. *2:*203-209, 1970. 33. Stolley, P. D., *et al.:* Am. J. Epidemiol. *102:*197-208, 1975. 34. Vessey, M. P., *et al.:* Br. Med. J. *3:*123-126, 1970. 35. Greene, G. R., *et al.:* Am. J. Public Health *62:*680-685, 1972. 36. Rosenberg, L., *et al.:* N. Engl. J. Med. *294:*1256-1259, 1976. 37. Coronary Drug Project Research Group: J.A.M.A. *214:*1303-1313, 1970. 38. Baum, J., *et al.:* Lancet *2:*926-928, 1973. 39. Mays, E. T., *et al.:* J.A.M.A. *235:*730-732, 1976. 40. Edmonson, H. A., *et al.:* N. Engl. J. Med. *294:*470-472, 1976. 41. Pfeffer, R. I., *et al.:* Am. J. Epidemiol. *103:*445-456, 1976. 42. Hoffman, A. J., *et al.:* J. Am. Pharm. Assoc. *48:*740, 1959. 43. Douglas, J. F., *et al.:* Anal. Chem. *39:*956,1967.

HOW SUPPLIED
TABLETS: 0.45 MG-200 MG

BRAND/MANUFACTURER	NDC	SIZE	AWP
◇ BRAND			
PMB-200: Wyeth-Ayerst	00046-0880-60	60s	$52.96

TABLETS: 0.45 MG-400 MG

BRAND/MANUFACTURER	NDC	SIZE	AWP
◇ BRAND			
PMB-400: Wyeth-Ayerst	00046-0881-60	60s	$62.78

Estrogens, Conjugated and Methyltestosterone

Each tablet contains:
1.25 mg of Estrogens, Conjugated
10 mg of Methyltestosterone
or
0.625 mg of Estrogens, Conjugated
5 mg of Methyltestosterone

---

1. ESTROGENS HAVE BEEN REPORTED TO INCREASE THE RISK OF ENDOMETRIAL CARCINOMA.

THREE INDEPENDENT, CASE-CONTROLLED STUDIES HAVE REPORTED AN INCREASED RISK OF ENDOMETRIAL CANCER IN POSTMENOPAUSAL WOMEN EXPOSED TO EXOGENOUS ESTROGENS FOR MORE THAN ONE YEAR.[1-3] THIS RISK WAS INDEPENDENT OF THE OTHER KNOWN RISK FACTORS FOR ENDOMETRIAL CANCER. THESE STUDIES ARE FURTHER SUPPORTED BY THE FINDING THAT INCIDENCE RATES OF ENDOMETRIAL CANCER HAVE INCREASED SHARPLY SINCE 1969 IN EIGHT DIFFERENT AREAS OF THE UNITED STATES WITH POPULATION-BASED CANCER REPORTING SYSTEMS, AN INCREASE WHICH MAY BE RELATED TO THE RAPIDLY EXPANDING USE OF ESTROGENS DURING THE LAST DECADE.[4]

THE THREE CASE-CONTROLLED STUDIES REPORTED THAT THE RISK OF ENDOMETRIAL CANCER IN ESTROGEN USERS WAS ABOUT 4.5 TO 13.9 TIMES GREATER THAN IN NONUSERS. THE RISK APPEARS TO DEPEND ON

BOTH DURATION OF TREATMENT[1] AND ON ESTROGEN DOSE.[3] IN VIEW OF THESE FINDINGS, WHEN ESTROGENS ARE USED FOR THE TREATMENT OF MENOPAUSAL SYMPTOMS, THE LOWEST DOSE THAT WILL CONTROL SYMPTOMS SHOULD BE UTILIZED AND MEDICATION SHOULD BE DISCONTINUED AS SOON AS POSSIBLE.

WHEN PROLONGED TREATMENT IS MEDICALLY INDICATED, THE PATIENT SHOULD BE REASSESSED, ON AT LEAST A SEMI-ANNUAL BASIS, TO DETERMINE THE NEED FOR CONTINUED THERAPY. ALTHOUGH THE EVIDENCE MUST BE CONSIDERED PRELIMINARY, ONE STUDY SUGGESTS THAT CYCLIC ADMINISTRATION OF LOW DOSES OF ESTROGEN MAY CARRY LESS RISK THAN CONTINUOUS ADMINISTRATION.[3] IT, THEREFORE, APPEARS PRUDENT TO UTILIZE SUCH A REGIMEN.

CLOSE CLINICAL SURVEILLANCE OF ALL WOMEN TAKING ESTROGENS IS IMPORTANT. IN ALL CASES OF UNDIAGNOSED PERSISTENT OR RECURRING ABNORMAL VAGINAL BLEEDING, ADEQUATE DIAGNOSTIC MEASURES SHOULD BE UNDERTAKEN TO RULE OUT MALIGNANCY.

THERE IS NO EVIDENCE AT PRESENT THAT "NATURAL" ESTROGENS ARE MORE OR LESS HAZARDOUS THAN "SYNTHETIC" ESTROGENS AT EQUI-ESTROGENIC DOSES.

2. ESTROGENS SHOULD NOT BE USED DURING PREGNANCY.

THE USE OF FEMALE SEX HORMONES, BOTH ESTROGENS AND PROGESTOGENS, DURING EARLY PREGNANCY MAY SERIOUSLY DAMAGE THE OFFSPRING. IT HAS BEEN SHOWN THAT FEMALES EXPOSED *IN UTERO* TO DIETHYLSTILBESTROL, A NONSTEROIDAL ESTROGEN, HAVE AN INCREASED RISK OF DEVELOPING, IN LATER LIFE, A FORM OF VAGINAL OR CERVICAL CANCER THAT IS ORDINARILY EXTREMELY RARE.[5,6] THIS RISK HAS BEEN ESTIMATED AS NOT GREATER THAN 4 PER 1,000 EXPOSURES.[7] FURTHERMORE, A HIGH PERCENTAGE OF SUCH EXPOSED WOMEN (FROM 30% TO 90%) HAVE BEEN FOUND TO HAVE VAGINAL ADENOSIS,[8-12] EPITHELIAL CHANGES OF THE VAGINA AND CERVIX. ALTHOUGH THESE CHANGES ARE HISTOLOGICALLY BENIGN, IT IS NOT KNOWN WHETHER THEY ARE PRECURSORS OF MALIGNANCY. ALTHOUGH SIMILAR DATA ARE NOT AVAILABLE WITH THE USE OF OTHER ESTROGENS, IT CANNOT BE PRESUMED THEY WOULD NOT INDUCE SIMILAR CHANGES.

SEVERAL REPORTS SUGGEST AN ASSOCIATION BETWEEN INTRA-UTERINE EXPOSURE TO FEMALE SEX HORMONES AND CONGENITAL ANOMALIES, INCLUDING CONGENITAL HEART DEFECTS AND LIMB-REDUCTION DEFECTS.[13-16] ONE CASE-CONTROLLED STUDY[16] ESTIMATED A 4.7-FOLD INCREASED RISK OF LIMB REDUCTION DEFECTS IN INFANTS EXPOSED *IN UTERO* TO SEX HORMONES (ORAL CONTRACEPTIVES, HORMONE WITHDRAWAL TESTS FOR PREGNANCY, OR ATTEMPTED TREATMENT FOR THREATENED ABORTION). SOME OF THESE EXPOSURES WERE VERY SHORT AND INVOLVED ONLY A FEW DAYS OF TREATMENT. THE DATA SUGGEST THAT THE RISK OF LIMB-REDUCTION DEFECTS IN EXPOSED FETUSES IS SOMEWHAT LESS THAN 1 PER 1,000.

IN THE PAST, FEMALE SEX HORMONES HAVE BEEN USED DURING PREGNANCY IN AN ATTEMPT TO TREAT THREATENED OR HABITUAL ABORTION. THERE IS CONSIDERABLE EVIDENCE THAT ESTROGENS ARE INEFFECTIVE FOR THESE INDICATIONS, AND THERE IS NO EVIDENCE FROM WELL-CONTROLLED STUDIES THAT PROGESTOGENS ARE EFFECTIVE FOR THESE USES.

IF CONJUGATED ESTROGENS/METHYLTESTOSTERONE IS USED DURING PREGNANCY, OR IF THE PATIENT BECOMES PREGNANT WHILE TAKING THIS DRUG, SHE SHOULD BE APPRISED OF THE POTENTIAL RISKS TO THE FETUS, AND THE ADVISABILITY OF PREGNANCY CONTINUATION.

DESCRIPTION

Conjugated Estrogens/Methyltestosterone is provided in tablets for oral administration.

Conjugated Estrogens, USP is a mixture of Estrogens, obtained exclusively from natural sources, occurring as the sodium salts of water-soluble Estrogen sulfates blended to represent the average composition of material derived from pregnant mares' urine. It contains estrone, equilin, and 17 α-dihydroequilin, together with smaller amounts of 17 α-estradiol, equilenin, and 17 α-dihydroequilenin as salts of their sulfate esters.

Methyltestosterone is an androgen.

Androgens are derivates of cyclopentano-perhydrophenanthrene. Endogenous androgens are C-19 steroids with a side chain at C-17, and with two angular methyl groups. Testosterone is the primary endogenous androgen. Fluoxymesterone and Methyltestosterone are synthetic derivatives of testosterone.

Methyltestosterone is a white to light-yellow crystalline substance that is virtually insoluble in water but soluble in organic solvents. It is stable in air but decomposes in light.

CLINICAL PHARMACOLOGY

ESTROGENS

Estrogens are important in the development and maintenance of the female reproductive system and secondary sex characteristics. They promote growth and development of the vagina, uterus, and fallopian tubes, and enlargement of the breasts. Indirectly, they contribute to the shaping of the skeleton, maintenance of tone and elasticity of urogenital structures, changes in the epiphyses of the long bones that allow for the pubertal growth spurt and its termination, growth of axillary and pubic hair, and pigmentation of the nipples and genitals. Decline of estrogenic activity at the end of the menstrual cycle can bring on menstruation, although the cessation of progesterone secretion is the most important factor in the mature ovulatory cycle. However, in the preovulatory or nonovulatory cycle, Estrogen is the primary determinant in the onset of menstruation. Estrogens also affect the release of pituitary gonadotropins.

The pharmacologic effects of conjugated Estrogens are similar to those of endogenous Estrogens. They are soluble in water and are well absorbed from the gastrointestinal tract. In responsive tissues (female genital organs, breasts, hypothalamus, pituitary) Estrogens enter the cell and are transported into the nucleus. As a result of Estrogen action, specific RNA and protein synthesis occurs.

Estrogen Pharmacokinetics: Metabolism and inactivation occur primarily in the liver. Some Estrogens are excreted into the bile; however, they are reabsorbed from the intestine and returned to the liver through the portal venous system. Water-soluble Estrogen conjugates are strongly acidic and are ionized in body fluids, which favor excretion through the kidneys since tubular reabsorption is minimal.

ANDROGENS

Endogenous androgens are responsible for the normal growth and development of the male sex organs and for maintenance of secondary sex characteristics. These effects include the growth and maturation of prostate, seminal vesicles, penis, and scrotum; the development of male hair distribution, such as beard, pubic, chest, and axillary hair, laryngeal enlargement, vocal chord thickening, alterations in body musculature, and fat distribution. Drugs in this class also cause retention of nitrogen, sodium, potassium, phosphorus, and decreased urinary excretion of calcium. Androgens have been reported to increase protein anabolism and decrease protein catabolism. Nitrogen balance is improved only when there is sufficient intake of calories and protein. Androgens are responsible for the growth spurt of adolescence and for the eventual termination of linear growth which is brought about by fusion of the epiphyseal growth centers. In children, exogenous androgens accelerate linear growth rates but may cause a disproportionate advancement in bone maturation. Use over long periods may result in fusion of the epiphyseal growth centers and termination of growth process. Androgens have been reported to stimulate the production of red blood cells by enhancing the production of erythropoietic stimulating factor.

Androgen Pharmacokinetics: Testosterone given orally is metabolized by the gut and 44% is cleared by the liver in the first pass. Oral doses as high as 400 mg per day are needed to achieve clinically effective blood levels for full replacement therapy. The synthetic androgens (Methyltestosterone and fluoxymesterone) are less extensively metabolized by the liver and have longer half-lives. They are more suitable than testosterone for oral administration. Testosterone in plasma is 98% bound to a specific testosterone-estradiol binding globulin, and about 2% is free. Generally, the amount of this sex-hormone-binding globulin in the plasma will determine the distribution of testosterone between free and bound forms, and the free testosterone concentration will determine its half-life.

About 90% of a dose of testosterone is excreted in the urine as glucuronic and sulfuric acid conjugates of testosterone and its metabolites; about 6% of a dose is excreted in the feces, mostly in the unconjugated form. Inactivation of testosterone occurs primarily in the liver. Testosterone is metabolized to various 17-keto steroids through two different pathways. There are considerable variations of the half-life of testosterone as reported in the literature, ranging from 10 to 100 minutes.

In many tissues the activity of testosterone appears to depend on reduction to dihydrotestosterone, which binds to cytosol receptor proteins. The steroid-receptor complex is transported to the nucleus where it initiates transcription events and cellular changes related to androgen action.

INDICATIONS

Conjugated Estrogens/Methyltestosterone is indicated in the treatment of:

Moderate to severe *vasomotor* symptoms associated with the menopause in those patients not improved by Estrogens alone. (There is no evidence that Estrogens are effective for nervous symptoms or depression without associated vasomotor symptoms, and they should not be used to treat such conditions.)

CONJUGATED ESTROGENS/METHYLTESTOSTERONE HAS NOT BEEN SHOWN TO BE EFFECTIVE FOR ANY PURPOSE DURING PREGNANCY, AND ITS USE MAY CAUSE SEVERE HARM TO THE FETUS (See Boxed *"Warning"*).

CONTRAINDICATIONS

Estrogens should not be used in women with any of the following conditions:
1. Known or suspected cancer of the breast, except in appropriately selected patients being treated for metastatic disease.
2. Known or suspected Estrogen-dependent neoplasia.
3. Known or suspected pregnancy (see Boxed *"Warning"*).
4. Undiagnosed abnormal genital bleeding.
5. Active thrombophlebitis or thromboembolic disorders.

◆ RATED THERAPEUTICALLY EQUIVALENT; ◇ THERAPEUTIC EQUIVALENCE UNCONFIRMED; ○ UNRATED

6. A past history of thrombophlebitis, thrombosis, or thromboembolic disorders associated with previous Estrogen use (except when used in treatment of breast malignancy).

Methyltestosterone should not be used in:

1. The presence of severe liver damage.

2. Pregnancy and in breast-feeding mothers because of the possibility of masculinization of the female fetus or breast-fed infant.

WARNINGS

ASSOCIATED WITH ESTROGENS

1. Induction of Malignant Neoplasms: Long-term continuous administration of natural and synthetic Eestrogens in certain animal species increases the frequency of carcinomas of the breast, cervix, vagina, and liver. There are now reports that Estrogens increase the risk of carcinoma of the endometrium in humans. (See Boxed *"Warning".*)

At the present time there is no satisfactory evidence that Estrogens given to postmenopausal women increase the risk of cancer of the breast,[17] although a recent, long-term follow-up of a single physician's practice has raised this possibility.[18] Because of the animal data, there is a need for caution in prescribing Estrogens for women with a strong family history of breast cancer or who have breast nodules, fibrocystic disease, or abnormal mammograms.

2. Gallbladder Disease: A recent study has reported a 2- to 3-fold increase in the risk of surgically confirmed gallbladder disease in women receiving postmenopausal estrogens,[17] similar to the 2-fold increase previously noted in users of oral contraceptives.[19,24a]

3. Effects Similar to Those Caused by Estrogen-progestogen Oral Contraceptives: There are several serious adverse effects of oral contraceptives, most of which have not, up to now, been documented as consequences of postmenopausal Estrogen therapy. This may reflect the comparatively low doses of Estrogen used in postmenopausal women. It would be expected that the larger doses of Estrogen used to treat prostatic or breast cancer are more likely to result in these adverse effects, and, in fact, it has been shown that there is an increased risk of thrombosis in men receiving Estrogens for prostatic cancer.[20-23]

a. Thromboembolic Disease: It is now well established that users of oral contraceptives have an increased risk of various thromboembolic and thrombotic vascular diseases, such as thrombophlebitis, pulmonary embolism, stroke, and myocardial infarction.[24-31] Cases of retinal thrombosis, mesenteric thrombosis, and optic neuritis have been reported in oral-contraceptive users. There is evidence that the risk of several of these adverse reactions is related to the dose of the drug.[32,33] An increased risk of postsurgery thromboembolic complications has also been reported in users of oral contraceptives.[34,35] If feasible, Estrogen should be discontinued at least 4 weeks before surgery of the type associated with an increased risk of thromboembolism, or during periods of prolonged immobilization.

While an increased rate of thromboembolic and thrombotic disease in postmenopausal users of Estrogens has not been found,[17-24,25-36] this does not rule out the possibility that such an increase may be present or that subgroups of women who have underlying risk factors or who are receiving relatively large doses of Estrogens may have increased risk. Therefore Estrogens should not be used in persons with active thrombophlebitis or thromboembolic disorders, and they should not be used (except in treatment of malignancy) in persons with a history of such disorders in association with Estrogen use. They should be used with caution in patients with cerebral-vascular or coronary-artery disease and only for those in whom Estrogens are clearly needed.

Large doses of Estrogen (5 mg conjugated Estrogens per day), comparable to those used to treat cancer of the prostate and breast, have been shown in a large prospective clinical trial in men[37] to increase the risk of nonfatal myocardial infarction, pulmonary embolism, and thrombophlebitis. When Estrogen doses of this size are used, any of the thromboembolic and thrombotic adverse effects associated with oral-contraceptive use should be considered a clear risk.

b. Hepatic Adenoma: Benign hepatic adenomas appear to be associated with the use of oral contraceptives.[38-40] Although benign, and rare, these may rupture and may cause death through intra-abdominal hemorrhage. Such lesions have not yet been reported in association with other Estrogen or progestogen preparations but should be considered in Estrogen users having abdominal pain and tenderness, abdominal mass, or hypovolemic shock. Hepatocellular carcinoma has also been reported in women taking Estrogen-containing oral contraceptives.[39] The relationship of this malignancy to these drugs is not known at this time.

c. Elevated Blood Pressure: Women using oral contraceptives sometimes experience increased blood pressure which, in most cases, returns to normal on discontinuing the drug. There is now a report that this may occur with use of Estrogens in the menopause,[41] and blood pressure should be monitored with Estrogen use, especially if high doses are used.

d. Glucose Tolerance: A worsening of glucose tolerance has been observed in a significant percentage of patients on Estrogen-containing oral contraceptives. For this reason, diabetic patients should be carefully observed while receiving Estrogens.

4. Hypercalcemia: Administration of Estrogens may lead to severe hypercalcemia in patients with breast cancer and bone metastases. If this occurs, the drug should be stopped and appropriate measures taken to reduce the serum calcium level.

ASSOCIATED WITH METHYLTESTOSTERONE

In patients with breast cancer, androgen therapy may cause hypercalcemia by stimulating osteolysis. In this case, the drug should be discontinued.

Prolonged use of high doses of androgens has been associated with the development of peliosis hepatis and hepatic neoplasms including hepatocellular carcinoma (see *"Precautions—Carcinogenesis"*). Peliosis hepatis can be a life-threatening or fatal complication.

Cholestatic hepatitis and jaundice occur with 17-alpha-alkylandrogens at a relatively low dose. If cholestatic hepatitis with jaundice appears or if liver function tests become abnormal, the androgen should be discontinued and the etiology should be determined. Drug-induced jaundice is reversible when the medication is discontinued.

Edema with or without heart failure may be a serious complication in patients with pre-existing cardiac, renal, or hepatic disease. In addition to discontinuation of the drug, diuretic therapy may be required.

PRECAUTIONS

ASSOCIATED WITH ESTROGENS

A. General:

1. Addition of a progestin—Studies of the addition of a progestin for 7 or more days of a cycle of Estrogen administration have reported a lowered incidence of endometrial hyperplasia. Morphological and biochemical studies of the endometrium suggest that 10 to 13 days of progestin are needed to provide maximal maturation of the endometrium and to eliminate any hyperplastic changes. Whether this will provide protection from endometrial carcinoma has not been clearly established. There are possible additional risks which may be associated with the inclusion of progestin in Estrogen-replacement regimens. The potential risks include adverse effects on carbohydrate and lipid metabolism. The choice of progestin and dosage may be important in minimizing these adverse effects.

2. Physical examination—A complete medical and family history should be taken prior to the initiation of any Estrogen therapy. The pretreatment and periodic physical examinations should include special reference to blood pressure, breasts, abdomen, and pelvic organs, and should include a Papanicolaou smear. As a general rule, Estrogen should not be prescribed for longer than one year without another physical examination being performed.

3. Fluid retention—Because Estrogens may cause some degree of fluid retention, conditions which might be influenced by this factor such as asthma, epilepsy, migraine, and cardiac or renal dysfunction, require careful observation.

4. Certain patients may develop undesirable manifestations of excessive Estrogenic stimulation, such as abnormal or excessive uterine bleeding, mastodynia, etc.

5. Prolonged administration of unopposed Estrogen therapy has been reported to increase the risk of endometrial hyperplasia in some patients.

6. Oral contraceptives appear to be associated with an increased incidence of mental depression.[24a] Although it is not clear whether this is due to the Estrogenic or progestogenic component of the contraceptive, patients with a history of depression should be carefully observed.

7. Preexisting uterine leiomyomata may increase in size during Estrogen use.

8. The pathologist should be advised of Estrogen therapy when relevant specimens are submitted.

9. Patients with a past history of jaundice during pregnancy have an increased risk of recurrence of jaundice while receiving Estrogen-containing oral contraceptive therapy. If jaundice develops in any patient receiving Estrogen, the medication should be discontinued while the cause is investigated.

10. Estrogens may be poorly metabolized in patients with impaired liver function and should be administered with caution in such patients.

11. Because Estrogens influence the metabolism of calcium and phosphorus, they should be used with caution in patients with metabolic bone diseases that are associated with hypercalcemia or in patients with renal insufficiency.

12. Because of the effects of Estrogens on epiphyseal closure, they should be used judiciously in young patients in whom bone growth is not yet complete.

13. Certain endocrine and liver function tests may be affected by Estrogen-containing oral contraceptives. The following similar changes may be expected with larger doses of Estrogen.

a. Increased sulfobromophthalein retention.

b. Increased prothrombin and factors VII, VIII, IX, and X; decreased antithrombin 3; increased norepinephrine-induced platelet aggrega- bility.

c. Increased thyroid binding globulin (TBG) leading to increased circulating total thyroid hormone, as measured by PBI, T_4 by column, or T_4 by radioimmunoassay. Free T_3 resin uptake is decreased, reflecting the elevated TBG; free T_4 concentration is unaltered.

d. Impaired glucose tolerance.

e. Decreased pregnanediol excretion.

f. Reduced response to metyrapone test.

g. Reduced serum folate concentration.

h. Increased serum triglyceride and phospholipid concentration.

B. Information for the Patient: See manufacturer's patient information.

C. Pregnancy Category X: (See *"Contraindications"* and Boxed *"Warning".*)

D. Nursing Mothers: As a general principle, the administration of any drug to nursing mothers should be done only when clearly necessary since many drugs are excreted in human milk.

ASSOCIATED WITH METHYLTESTOSTERONE

A. General Precautions:

1. Women should be observed for signs of virilization (deepening of the voice, hirsutism, acne, clitoromegaly, and menstrual irregularities). Discontinuation of drug therapy at the time of evidence of mild virilism is necessary to prevent

irreversible virilization. Such virilization is usual following androgen use at high doses.

2. Prolonged dosage of androgen may result in sodium and fluid retention. This may present a problem, especially in patients with compromised cardiac reserve or renal disease.

3. Hypersensitivity may occur rarely.

4. PBI may be decreased in patients taking androgens.

5. Hypercalcemia may occur. If this does occur, the drug should be discontinued.

B. Information for the Patient: The physician should instruct patients to report any of the following side effects of androgens:

Women: Hoarseness, acne, changes in menstrual periods, or more hair on the face.

All Patients: Any nausea, vomiting, changes in skin color or ankle swelling.

C. Laboratory Tests:

1. Women with disseminated breast carcinoma should have frequent determination of urine and serum calcium levels during the course of androgen therapy (see *"Warnings"*).

2. Because of the hepatotoxicity associated with the use of 17-alpha-alkylated androgens, liver-function tests should be obtained periodically.

3. Hemoglobin and hematocrit should be checked periodically for polycythemia in patients who are receiving high doses of androgens.

D. Drug Interactions

1. Anticoagulants: C-17 substituted derivatives of testosterone, such as methandrostenolone, have been reported to decrease the anticoagulant requirements of patients receiving oral anticoagulants. Patients receiving oral anticoagulant therapy require close monitoring, especially when androgens are started or stopped.

2. Oxyphenbutazone: Concurrent administration of oxyphenbutazone and androgens may result in elevated serum levels of oxyphenbutazone.

3. Insulin: In diabetic patients the metabolic effects of androgens may decrease blood glucose and insulin requirements.

E. Drug/Laboratory Test Interferences: Androgens may decrease levels of thyroxine-binding globulin, resulting in decreased T_4 serum levels and increased resin uptake of T_3 and T_4. Free thyroid hormone levels remain unchanged, however and there is no clinical evidence of thyroid dysfunction.

F. Carcinogenesis:

Animal Data: Testosterone has been tested by subcutaneous injection and implantation in mice and rats. The implant induced cervical-uterine tumors in mice, which metastasized in some cases. There is suggestive evidence that injection of testosterone into some strains of female mice increases their susceptibility to hepatoma. Testosterone is also known to increase the number of tumors and decrease the degree of differentiation of chemically induced carcinomas of the liver in rats.

Human Data: There are rare reports of hepatocellular carcinoma in patients receiving long-term therapy with androgens in high doses. Withdrawal of the drugs did not lead to regression of the tumors in all cases.

Geriatric patients treated with androgens may be at an increased risk for the development of prostatic hypertrophy and prostatic carcinoma.

G. Pregnancy:

Teratogenic Effects: Pregnancy Category X (see *"Contraindications"*).

H. Nursing Mothers: It is not known whether androgens are excreted in human milk. Because many drugs are excreted in human milk and because of the potential for serious adverse reactions in nursing infants from Estrogens, a decision should be made whether to discontinue nursing or to discontinue the drug, taking into account the importance of the drug to the mother.

ADVERSE REACTIONS
ASSOCIATED WITH ESTROGENS
(See *"Warnings"* regarding induction of neoplasia, adverse effects on the fetus, increased incidence of gallbladder disease, and adverse effects similar to those of oral contraceptives, including thromboembolism.) The following additional adverse reactions have been reported with Estrogenic therapy, including oral contraceptive:

1. Genitourinary System: Breakthrough bleeding, spotting, change in menstrual flow; dysmenorrhea; premenstrual-like syndrome; amenorrhea during and after treatment; increase in size of uterine fibromyomata; vaginal candidiasis; change in cervical erosion and in degree of cervical secretion: cystitis-like syndrome.

2. Breasts: Tenderness, enlargement, secretion.

3. Gastrointestinal: Nausea, vomiting; abdominal cramps, bloating; cholestatic jaundice.

4. Skin: Chloasma or melasma which may persist when drug is discontinued; erythema multiforme; erythema nodosum; hemorrhagic eruption; loss of scalp hair; hirsutism.

5. Eyes: Steepening of corneal curvature; intolerance to contact lenses.

6. CNS: Headache, migraine, dizziness; mental depression; chorea.

7. Miscellaneous: Increase or decrease in weight; reduced carbohydrate tolerance; aggravation of porphyria; edema; changes in libido.

ASSOCIATED WITH METHYLTESTOSTERONE
1. Endocrine and Urogenital, Female: The most common side effects of androgen therapy are amenorrhea and other menstrual irregularities, inhibition of gonadotropin secretion, and virilization, including deepening of the voice and clitoral enlargement. The latter ussually is not reversible after androgens are discontinued. When administered to a pregnant woman androgens cause virilization of external genitalia of the female fetus.

2. Skin and Appendages: Hirsutism, male pattern of baldness, and acne.

3. Fluid and Electrolyte Disturbances: Retention of sodium, chloride, water, potassium, calcium, and inorganic phosphates.

4. Gastrointestinal: Nausea, cholestatic jaundice, alterations in liver-function tests, rarely hepatocellular neoplasms, and peliosis hepatis (see *"Warnings"*).

5. Hematologic: Suppression of clotting factors II, V, VII, and X; bleeding in patients on concomitant anticoagulant therapy, and polycythemia.

6. Nervous System: Increased or decreased libido, headache, anxiety, depression, and generalized paresthesia.

7. Metabolic: Increased serum cholesterol.

8. Miscellaneous: Inflammation and pain at the site of intramuscular injection or subcutaneous implantation of testosterone-containing pellets, stomatitis with buccal preparations, and rarely anaphylactoid reactions.

ACUTE OVERDOSAGE
Numerous reports of ingestion of large doses of Estrogen-containing oral contraceptives by young children indicate that acute serious ill effects do not occur. Overdosage of Estrogens may cause nausea, and withdrawal bleeding may occur in females.

There have been no reports of acute overdosage with the androgens.

DOSAGE AND ADMINISTRATION
GIVEN CYCLICALLY FOR SHORT-TERM USE ONLY
For treatment of moderate-to-severe *vasomotor* symptoms associated with the menopause in patients not improved by Estrogen alone.

The lowest dose that will control symptoms should be chosen and medication should be discontinued as promptly as possible.

Administration should be cyclic (e.g., three weeks on and one week off).

Attempts to discontinue or taper medication should be made at 3- to 6-month intervals.

USUAL DOSAGE RANGE
1.25 mg conjugated Estrogens, USP, and 10.0 mg Methyltestosterone daily and cyclically.

Treated patients with an intact uterus should be monitored closely for signs of endometrial cancer and appropriate diagnostic measures should be taken to rule out malignancy in the event of persistent or recurring abnormal vaginal bleeding.

Store at room temperature (approximately 25°C).

Dispense in a well-closed container as defined in the USP.

PHYSICIAN REFERENCES
1. Ziel, H. K., *et al.:* N. Engl. J. Med. 293:1167-1170, 1975. 2. Smith, D. C., *et al.:* N. Engl. J. Med. 293:1164-1167, 1975. 3. Mack, T. M. *et al.:* N. Engl. J. Med. 294:1262-1267, 1976. 4. Weiss, N. S., *et al.:* N. Engl. J. Med. 294:1259-1262, 1976. 5. Herbst, A.L., *et al.:* N. Engl. J. Med. 284:878-881, 1971. 6. Greenwald, P., *et al.:* N. Engl. J. Med. 285:390-392, 1971. 7. Lanier, A. *et al.:* Mayo Clin. Proc. 48:793-799, 1973. 8. Herbst, A., *et al.:* Obstet. Gynecol. 40:287-298, 1972. 9. Herbst, A., *et al.:* Am. J. Obstet. Gynecol. 118:607-615, 1974. 10. Herbst, A., *et al.:* N. Engl. J. Med. 292:334-339, 1975. 11. Stafl, A., *et al.:* Obstet. Gynecol. 43:118-128, 1974. 12. Sherman, A. I., *et al.:* Obstet. Gynecol. 44:531-545, 1974. 13. Gal, I., *et al.:* Nature 216:83, 1967.> 14. Levy, E. P., *et al.:* Lancet 1:611, 1973. 15. Nora, J., *et al.:* Lancet 1:941-942, 1973. 16. Janerich, D. T., *et al.:* N. Engl. J. Med. 291:697-700, 1974. 17. Boston Collaborative Drug Surveillance Program: N. Engl. J. Med. 290:15-19, 1974. 18. Hoover, R., *et al.:* N. Engl. J. Med. 295: 401-405, 1976. 19. Boston Collaborative Drug Surveillance Program: Lancet 1:1399-1404, 1973. 20. Daniel, D. G., *et al.:* Lancet 2:287-289, 1967. 21. The Veterans Administration Cooperative Urological Research Group: J. Urol. 98:516-522, 1967. 22. Bailar, J. C.: Lancet 2:560, 1967. 23. Blackard, C., *et al.:* Cancer 26:249-256, 1970. 24. Royal College of General Practitioners: J. R. Coll. Gen. Pract. 13:267-279, 1967. 24a. Royal College of General Practitioners: Oral Contraceptives and Health, New York, Pitman Corp., 1974. 25. Inman, W. H. W., *et al.:* Br. Med. J. 2:193-199, 1968. 26. Vessey, M. P., *et al.:* Br. Med. J. 2:651-657, 1969. 27. Sartwell, P. E., *et al.:* Am. J. Epidemiol. 90:365-380, 1969. 28. Collaborative Group for the Study of Stroke in Young Women: N. Engl. J. Med. 288:871-878, 1973. 29. Collaborative Group for the Study of Stroke in Young Women: J.A.M.A. 231:718-722, 1975. 30. Mann, J. I., *et al.:* Br. Med. J. 2:245-248, 1975. 31. Mann, J. I., *et al.:* Br. Med. J. 2:241-245, 1975. 32. Inman, W. H. W., *et al.:* Br. Med. J. 2:203-209, 1970. 33. Stolley, P. D., *et al.:* Am. J. Epidemiol. 102:197-208, 1975. 34. Vessey, M. P., *et al.:* Br. Med. J. 3:123-126, 1970. 35. Greene, G. R., *et al.:* Am. J. Public Health 62:680-685, 1972. 36. Rosenberg, L., *et al.:* N. Engl. J. Med. 294:1256-1259, 1976. 37. Coronary Drug Project Research Group: J.A.M.A. 214:1303-1313, 1970. 38. Baum, J., *et al.:* Lancet 2:926-928, 1973. 39. Mays, E. T., *et al.:* J.A.M.A. 235:730-732, 1976. 40. Edmonson, H. A., *et al.:* N. Engl. J. Med. 294:470-472, 1976. 41. Pfeffer, R. I., *et al.:* Am. J. Epidemiol. 103:445-456, 1976.
Androgen references available upon request.

HOW SUPPLIED
TABLETS: 0.625 MG-5 MG

BRAND/MANUFACTURER	NDC	SIZE	AWP
○ BRAND			
PREMARIN W/METHYLTESTOSTERONE: Wyeth-Ayerst	00046-0878-81	100s	$74.66

TABLETS: 1.25 MG-10 MG

BRAND/MANUFACTURER	NDC	SIZE	AWP
○ **BRAND**			
PREMARIN W/METHYLTESTOSTERONE: Wyeth-Ayerst	00046-0879-81	100s	$125.60

Estrogens, Esterified

WARNINGS

1. ESTROGENS HAVE BEEN REPORTED TO INCREASE THE RISK OF ENDOMETRIAL CARCINOMA.

THREE INDEPENDENT CASE CONTROL STUDIES HAVE SHOWN AN INCREASED RISK OF ENDOMETRIAL CANCER IN POSTMENOPAUSAL WOMEN EXPOSED TO EXOGENOUS ESTROGENS FOR PROLONGED PERIODS.[1-3] THIS RISK WAS INDEPENDENT OF THE OTHER KNOWN RISK FACTORS FOR ENDOMETRIAL CANCER. THESE STUDIES ARE FURTHER SUPPORTED BY THE FINDING THAT INCIDENCE RATES OF ENDOMETRIAL CANCER HAVE INCREASED SHARPLY SINCE 1969 IN EIGHT DIFFERENT AREAS OF THE UNITED STATES WITH POPULATION-BASED CANCER REPORTING SYSTEMS, AN INCREASE WHICH MAY BE RELATED TO THE RAPIDLY EXPANDING USE OF ESTROGENS DURING THE LAST DECADE.[4]

THE THREE CASE CONTROL STUDIES REPORTED THAT THE RISK OF ENDOMETRIAL CANCER IN ESTROGEN USERS WAS ABOUT 4.5 TO 13.9 TIMES GREATER THAN IN NONUSERS. THE RISK APPEARS TO DEPEND ON BOTH DURATION OF TREATMENT[1] AND ON ESTROGEN DOSE.[3] IN VIEW OF THESE FINDINGS, WHEN ESTROGENS ARE USED FOR THE TREATMENT OF MENOPAUSAL SYMPTOMS, THE LOWEST DOSE THAT WILL CONTROL SYMPTOMS SHOULD BE UTILIZED AND MEDICATION SHOULD BE DISCONTINUED AS SOON AS POSSIBLE. WHEN PROLONGED TREATMENT IS MEDICALLY INDICATED, THE PATIENT SHOULD BE REASSESSED ON AT LEAST A SEMIANNUAL BASIS TO DETERMINE THE NEED FOR CONTINUED THERAPY. ALTHOUGH THE EVIDENCE MUST BE CONSIDERED PRELIMINARY, ONE STUDY SUGGESTS THAT CYCLIC ADMINISTRATION OF LOW DOSES OF ESTROGEN MAY CARRY LESS RISK THAN CONTINUOUS ADMINISTRATION;[3] IT THEREFORE APPEARS PRUDENT TO UTILIZE SUCH A REGIMEN.

CLOSE CLINICAL SURVEILLANCE OF ALL WOMEN TAKING ESTROGENS IS IMPORTANT. IN ALL CASES OF UNDIAGNOSED PERSISTENT OR RECURRING ABNORMAL VAGINAL BLEEDING, ADEQUATE DIAGNOSTIC MEASURES SHOULD BE UNDERTAKEN TO RULE OUT MALIGNANCY.

THERE IS NO EVIDENCE AT PRESENT THAT "NATURAL" ESTROGENS ARE MORE OR LESS HAZARDOUS THAN "SYNTHETIC" ESTROGENS AT EQUIESTROGENIC DOSES.

2. ESTROGENS SHOULD NOT BE USED DURING PREGNANCY.

THE USE OF FEMALE SEX HORMONES, BOTH ESTROGENS AND PROGESTAGENS, DURING EARLY PREGNANCY MAY SERIOUSLY DAMAGE THE OFFSPRING. IT HAS BEEN SHOWN THAT FEMALES EXPOSED IN UTERO TO DIETHYLSTILBESTROL, A NONSTEROIDAL ESTROGEN, HAVE AN INCREASED RISK OF DEVELOPING IN LATER LIFE A FORM OF VAGINAL OR CERVICAL CANCER THAT IS ORDINARILY EXTREMELY RARE.[5,6] THE RISK HAS BEEN ESTIMATED AS NOT GREATER THAN 4 PER 1000 EXPOSURES.[7] FURTHERMORE, A HIGH PERCENTAGE OF SUCH EXPOSED WOMEN (FROM 30 TO 90 PERCENT) HAVE BEEN FOUND TO HAVE VAGINAL ADENOSIS,[8-12] EPITHELIAL CHANGES OF THE VAGINA AND CERVIX. ALTHOUGH THESE CHANGES ARE HISTOLOGICALLY BENIGN, IT IS NOT KNOWN WHETHER THEY ARE PRECURSORS OF MALIGNANCY. ALTHOUGH SIMILAR DATA ARE NOT AVAILABLE WITH THE USE OF OTHER ESTROGENS, IT CANNOT BE PRESUMED THEY WOULD NOT INDUCE SIMILAR CHANGES. SEVERAL REPORTS SUGGEST AN ASSOCIATION BETWEEN INTRAUTERINE EXPOSURE TO FEMALE SEX HORMONES AND CONGENITAL ANOMALIES, INCLUDING CONGENITAL HEART DEFECTS AND LIMB REDUCTION DEFECTS.[13-16] ONE CASE CONTROL STUDY[16] ESTIMATED A 4.7-FOLD INCREASED RISK OF LIMB REDUCTION DEFECTS IN INFANTS EXPOSED IN UTERO TO SEX HORMONES (ORAL CONTRACEPTIVES, HORMONE WITHDRAWAL TESTS FOR PREGNANCY, OR ATTEMPTED TREATMENT FOR THREATENED ABORTION). SOME OF THESE EXPOSURES WERE VERY SHORT AND INVOLVED ONLY A FEW DAYS OF TREATMENT. THE DATA SUGGEST THAT THE RISK OF LIMB REDUCTION DEFECTS IN EXPOSED FETUSES IS SOMEWHAT LESS THAN 1 PER 1000. IN THE PAST, FEMALE SEX HORMONES HAVE BEEN USED DURING PREGNANCY IN AN ATTEMPT TO TREAT THREATENED OR HABITUAL ABORTION. THERE IS CONSIDERABLE EVIDENCE THAT ESTROGENS ARE INEFFECTIVE FOR THESE INDICATIONS, AND THERE IS NO EVIDENCE FROM WELL-CONTROLLED STUDIES THAT PROGESTAGENS ARE EFFECTIVE FOR THESE USES. IF ESTROGENS, ESTERIFIED TABLETS IS USED DURING PREGNANCY, OR IF THE PATIENT BECOMES PREGNANT WHILE TAKING THIS DRUG, SHE SHOULD BE APPRISED OF THE POTENTIAL RISKS TO THE FETUS, AND THE ADVISABILITY OF PREGNANCY CONTINUATION.

DESCRIPTION

Estrogens, Esterified is a mixture of the sodium salts of the sulfate esters of the estrogenic substances, principally estrone, that are of the type excreted by pregnant mares. The content of total Estrogens, Esterified is not less than 90 percent and not more than 110 percent of the labeled amount. Estrogens, Esterified contain not less than 75 percent and not more than 85 percent of sodium estrone sulfate, and not less than 6 percent and not more than 15 percent of sodium equilin sulfate, in such proportion that the total of these two components is not less than 90 percent, all percentages being calculated on the basis of the total Estrogens, Esterified content.

Following is its chemical structure:

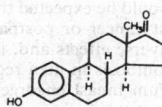

CLINICAL PHARMACOLOGY

Estrogens are important in the development and maintenance of the female reproductive system and secondary sex characteristics. They promote growth and development of the vagina, uterus, and fallopian tubes, and enlargement of the breasts. Indirectly, they contribute to the shaping of the skeleton, maintenance of tone and elasticity of urogenital structures, changes in the epiphyses of the long bones that allow for the pubertal growth spurt and its termination, growth of axillary and pubic hair, and pigmentation of the nipples and genitals. Decline of estrogenic activity at the end of the menstrual cycle can bring on menstruation, although the cessation of progesterone secretion is the most important factor in the mature ovulatory cycle. However, in the preovulatory or nonovulatory cycle, estrogen is the primary determinant in the onset of menstruation. Estrogens also affect the release of pituitary gonadotropins. The pharmacologic effects of Estrogens, Esterified are similar to those of endogenous estrogens. They are soluble in water and are well absorbed from the gastrointestinal tract.

In responsive tissues (female genital organs, breasts, hypothalamus, pituitary) Estrogens enter the cell and are transported into the nucleus. As a result of Estrogen action, specific RNA and protein synthesis occurs. Metabolism and inactivation occur primarily in the liver. Some Estrogens are excreted into the bile; however, they are reabsorbed from the intestine and returned to the liver through the portal venous system. Water soluble Estrogen conjugates are strongly acidic and are ionized in body fluids, which favor excretion through the kidneys since tubular reabsorption is minimal.

INDICATIONS AND USAGE

Estrogens, Esterified tablets is indicated in the treatment of:

1. Moderate to severe *vasomotor* symptoms associated with the menopause. (There is no evidence that Estrogens are effective for nervous symptoms or depression which might occur during menopause, and they should not be used to treat these conditions.)
2. Atrophic vaginitis.
3. Kraurosis vulvae.
4. Female hypogonadism.
5. Female castration.
6. Primary ovarian failure.
7. Breast cancer (for palliation only) in appropriately selected women and men with metastatic disease.
8. Prostatic carcinoma—palliative therapy of advanced disease.

Estrogens, Esterified HAVE NOT BEEN SHOWN TO BE EFFECTIVE FOR ANY PURPOSE DURING PREGNANCY AND ITS USE MAY CAUSE SEVERE HARM TO THE FETUS (see Boxed *"Warning"*).

UNLABELED USES

Estrogens, Esterified are used alone or as an adjunct in the treatment of postmenopausal osteoporosis and to reduce the risk of coronary artery disease in postmenopausal women.

CONTRAINDICATIONS

Estrogens should not be used in women (or men) with any of the following conditions:

1. Known or suspected cancer of the breast except in appropriately selected patients being treated for metastatic disease.
2. Known or suspected Estrogen-dependent neoplasia.
3. Known or suspected pregnancy (See Boxed *"Warning"*).
4. Undiagnosed abnormal genital bleeding.
5. Active thrombophlebitis or thromboembolic disorders.
6. A past history of thrombophlebitis, thrombosis or thromboembolic disorders associated with previous estrogen use (except when used in treatment of breast or prostatic malignancy).

► SHOWN IN PRODUCT IDENTIFICATION GUIDE

WARNINGS

1. Induction of Malignant Neoplasms: Long-term continuous administration of natural and synthetic estrogens in certain animal species increases the frequency of carcinomas of the breast, cervix, vagina, and liver. There is now evidence that estrogens increase the risk of carcinoma of the endometrium in humans. (See Boxed *"Warning"*). At the present time there is no satisfactory evidence that estrogens given to postmenopausal women increase the risk of cancer of the breast[18] although a recent long-term followup of a single physician's practice has raised this possibility.[18a] Because of the animal data, there is a need for caution in prescribing Estrogens for women with a strong family history of breast cancer or who have breast nodules, fibrocystic disease, or abnormal mammograms.

2. Gallbladder Disease: A recent study has reported a 2- to 3-fold increase in the risk of surgically confirmed gallbladder disease in women receiving postmenopausal estrogens,[18] similar to the 2-fold increase previously noted in users of oral contraceptives.[19-24] In the case of oral contraceptives the increased risk appeared after 2 years of use.[24]

3. Effects Similar to Those Caused by Estrogen-progestagen Oral Contraceptives: There are several serious adverse effects of oral contraceptives, most of which have not, up to now, been documented as consequences of postmenopausal Estrogen therapy. This may reflect the comparatively low doses of Estrogen used in post-menopausal women. It would be expected that the larger doses of Estrogen used to treat prostatic or breast cancer or postpartum breast engorgement are more likely to result in these adverse effects and, in fact, it has been shown that there is an increased risk of thrombosis in men receiving Estrogens for prostatic cancer and women for postpartum breast engorgement.[20-23]

a. Thromboembolic Disease: It is now well established that uses of oral contraceptives have an increased risk of various thromboembolic and thrombotic vascular diseases, such as thrombophlebitis, pulmonary embolism, stroke, and myocardial infarction.[24-31] Cases of retinal thrombosis, mesenteric thrombosis, and optic neuritis have been reported in oral contraceptive users. There is evidence that the risk of several of these adverse reactions is related to the dose of the drug.[32,33] An increased risk of post-surgery thromboembolic complications has also been reported in users of oral contraceptives.[34,35] If feasible, estrogen should be discontinued at least 4 weeks before surgery of the type associated with an increased risk of thromboembolism, or during periods of prolonged immobilization.

While an increased rate of thromboembolic and thrombotic disease in postmenopausal users of Estrogens has not been found,[18-36] this does not rule out the possibility that such an increase may be present or that subgroups of women who have underlying risk factors or who are receiving relatively large doses of Estrogens may have increased risk.

Therefore Estrogens should not be used in persons with active thrombophlebitis or thromboembolic disorders, and they should not be used (except in treatment of malignancy) in persons with a history of such disorders in association with Estrogen use. They should be used with caution in patients with cerebral vascular or coronary artery disease and only for those in whom Estrogens are clearly needed.

Large doses of estrogen (5 mg Estrogens, Esterified per day), comparable to those used to treat cancer of the prostate and breast, have been shown in a large prospective clinical trial in men[37] to increase the risk of nonfatal myocardial infarction, pulmonary embolism and thrombophlebitis. When Estrogen doses of this size are used, any of the thromboembolic and thrombotic adverse effects associated with oral contraceptive use should be considered a clear risk.

b. Hepatic Adenoma: Benign hepatic adenomas appear to be associated with the use of oral contraceptives.[38-40] Although benign, and rare, these may rupture and may cause death through intra-abdominal hemorrhage. Such lesions have not yet been reported in association with other Estrogen or progestagen preparations but should be considered in estrogen users having abdominal pain and tenderness, abdominal mass, or hypovolemic shock. Hepatocellular carcinoma has also been reported in women taking estrogen-containing oral contraceptives.[39] The relationship of this malignancy to these drugs is not known at this time.

c. Elevated Blood Pressure: Increased blood pressure is not uncommon in women using oral contraceptives. There is now a report that this may occur with use of Estrogens in the menopause[41] and blood pressure should be monitored with Estrogen use, especially if high doses are used.

d. Glucose Tolerance: A worsening of glucose tolerance has been observed in a significant percentage of patients on estrogen-containing oral contraceptives. For this reason, diabetic patients should be carefully observed while receiving Estrogen.

4. Hypercalcemia: Administration of Estrogens may lead to severe hypercalcemia in patients with breast cancer and bone metastases. If this occurs, the drug should be stopped and appropriate measures taken to reduce the serum calcium level.
    See footnotes at end of article.

PRECAUTIONS

A. General Precautions:

1. A complete medical and family history should be taken prior to the initiation of any Estrogen therapy. The pretreatment and periodic physical examinations should include special reference to blood pressure, breast, abdomen, and pelvic organs, and should include a Papanicolau smear. As a general rule, estrogen should not be prescribed for longer than 1 year without another physical examination being performed.

2. Fluid retention—Because Estrogens may cause some degree of fluid retention, conditions which might be influenced by this factor, such as epilepsy, migraine, and cardiac or renal dysfunction, require careful observation.

3. Certain patients may develop undesirable manifestations of excessive estrogenic stimulation, such as abnormal or excessive uterine bleeding, mastodynia, etc.

4. Oral contraceptives appear to be associated with an increased incidence of mental depression.[24] Although it is not clear whether this is due to the estrogenic or progestagenic component of the contraceptive, patients with a history of depression should be carefully observed.

5. Pre-existing uterine leiomyomata may increase in size during estrogen use.

6. The pathologist should be advised of estrogen therapy when relevant specimens are submitted.

7. Patients with a past history of jaundice during pregnancy have an increased risk of recurrence of jaundice while receiving Estrogen-containing oral contraceptive therapy. If jaundice develops in any patient receiving Estrogen, the medication should be discontinued while the cause is investigated.

8. Estrogens may be poorly metabolized in patients with impaired liver function and they should be administered with caution in such patients.

9. Because Estrogens influence the metabolism of calcium and phosphorus, they should be used with caution in patients with metabolic bone diseases that are associated with hypercalcemia or in patients with renal insufficiency.

10. Because of the effects of Estrogens on epiphyseal closure, they should be used judiciously in young patients in whom bone growth is not complete.

11. The lowest effective dose appropriate for the specific indication should be utilized. Studies of the addition of a progestin for 7 or more days of a cycle of Estrogen administration have reported a lowered incidence of endometrial hyperplasia. Morphological and biochemical studies of endometrium suggest that 10 to 13 days of progestin are needed to provide maximal maturation of the endometrium and to eliminate any hyperplastic changes. Whether this will provide protection from endometrial carcinoma has not been clearly established. There are possible additional risks which may be associated with the inclusion of progestin in Estrogen replacement regimens. The potential risks include adverse effects on carbohydrate and lipid metabolism. The choice of progestin and dosage may be important in minimizing these adverse effects.

12. Certain endocrine and liver function tests may be affected by estrogen-containing oral contraceptives. The following similar changes may be expected with larger doses of estrogen:

a. Increased sulfobromophthalein retention.

b. Increased prothrombin and factors VII, VIII, IX, and X; decreased antithrombin 3; increased norepinephrine-induced platelet aggreg- ability.

c. Increased thyroid binding globulin (TBG) leading to increased circulating total thyroid hormone, as measured by PBI, T4 by column or T4 by radioimmunoassay. Free T3 resin uptake is decreased, reflecting the elevated TBG; free T4 concentration is unaltered.

d. Impaired glucose tolerance.

e. Decreased pregnanediol excretion.

f. Reduced response to metyrapone test.

g. Reduced serum folate concentration.

h. Increased serum triglyceride and phospholipid concentration.

B. Information for Patients: See manufacturer's patient information.

C. Pregnancy Category X: See *"Contraindications"* and Boxed *"Warning"*.

D. Nursing Mothers: As a general principle, the administration of any drug to nursing mothers should be done only when clearly necessary since many drugs are excreted in human milk.

ADVERSE REACTIONS

(See *"Warnings"* regarding induction of neoplasia, adverse effects on the fetus, increased incidence of gall bladder disease, and adverse effects similar to those of oral contraceptives, including thromboembolism.) The following additional adverse reactions have been reported with estrogenic therapy, including oral contraceptives.

1. Genitourinary System: Breakthrough bleeding, spotting, change in
    menstrual flow.
    Dysmenorrhea.
    Premenstrual-like syndrome.
    Amenorrhea during and after treatment.
    Increase in size of uterine fibromyomata.
    Vaginal candidiasis.
    Change in cervical eversion and in degree of cervical secretion.
    Cystitis-like syndrome.

2. Breasts: Tenderness, enlargement, secretion.

3. Gastrointestinal: Nausea, vomiting.
    Abdominal cramps, bloating.
    Cholestatic jaundice.

4. Skin: Chloasma or melasma which may persist when drug is
    discontinued.
    Erythema multiforme.
    Erythema nodosum.
    Hemorrhagic eruption.
    Loss of scalp hair.
    Hirsutism.

◆ RATED THERAPEUTICALLY EQUIVALENT; ◇ THERAPEUTIC EQUIVALENCE UNCONFIRMED; ○ UNRATED

5. *Eyes:* Steepening of corneal curvature.
Intolerance to contact lenses.
6. *CNS:* Headache, migraine, dizziness.
Mental depression.
Chorea.
7. *Miscellaneous:* Increase or decrease in weight.
Reduced carbohydrate tolerance.
Aggravation of porphyria.
Edema.
Changes in libido.

ACUTE OVERDOSAGE

Numerous reports of ingestion of large doses of Estrogen-containing oral contraceptives by young children indicate that serious ill effects do not occur. Overdosage of Estrogen may cause nausea, and withdrawal bleeding may occur in females.

DOSAGE AND ADMINISTRATION

1. Given Cyclically for Short-term Use Only: For treatment of moderate to severe *vasomotor symptoms, atrophic vaginitis* or *kraurosis vulvae* associated with the menopause.

The lowest dose that will control symptoms should be chosen and medication should be discontinued as promptly as possible.

Administration should be cyclic (e.g., 3 weeks on and 1 week off).

Attempts to discontinue or taper medication should be made at 3 to 6 month intervals.

USUAL DOSAGE RANGES:
Vasomotor Symptoms: 1.25 mg daily. If the patient has not menstruated within the last 2 months or more, cyclic administration is started arbitrarily. If the patient is menstruating, cyclic administration is started on day 5 of bleeding.

Atrophic Vaginitis and Kraurosis Vulvae: 0.3 mg to 1.25 mg or more daily, depending upon the tissue response of the individual patient. Administer cyclically.

2. Given Cyclically: Female hypogonadism; female castration; primary ovarian failure.

USUAL DOSAGE RANGES:
Female Hypogonadism: 2.5 to 7.5 mg daily, in divided doses for 20 days, followed by a rest period of 10 days' duration. If bleeding does not occur by the end of this period, the same dosage schedule is repeated. The number of courses of estrogen therapy necessary to produce bleeding may vary depending on responsiveness of the endometrium.

If bleeding occurs before the end of the 10 day period, begin a 20 day estrogen-progestin cyclic regimen with Estrogens, Esterified tablets, 2.5 to 7.5 mg daily in divided doses, for 20 days. During the last 5 days of Estrogen therapy, give an oral progestin. If bleeding occurs before this regimen is concluded, therapy is discontinued and may be resumed on the fifth day of bleeding.

Female Castration and Primary Ovarian Failure: 1.25 mg daily, cyclically. Adjust dosage upward or downward according to severity of symptoms and response of the patient. For maintenance, adjust dosage to lowest level that will provide effective control.

3. Given Chronically: Inoperable progressing prostatic cancer—1.25 to 2.5 mg three times daily. The effectiveness of therapy can be judged by phosphatase determinations as well as by symptomatic improvement of the patient.

Inoperable progressing breast cancer in appropriately selected men and postmenopausal women. (See *"Indications and Usage")*—Suggested dosage is 10 mg three times daily for a period of at least 3 months.

Treated patients with an intact uterus should be monitored closely for signs of endometrial cancer and appropriate diagnostic measures should be taken to rule out malignancy in the event of persistent or recurring abnormal vaginal bleeding.

PHYSICIAN REFERENCES

1. Ziel HK, Finkel WD: Increased Risk of Endometrial Carcinoma Among Users of Conjugated Estrogens, *New England Journal of Medicine* 293:1167-1170, 1975. 2. Smith DC, Prentic R, Thompson DJ, Hermann WL: Association of Exogenous Estrogen and Endometrial Carcinoma, *New England Journal of Medicine* 293:1164-1167, 1975. 3. Mack TM, Pike MC, Henderson BE, et al: Estrogens and Endometrial Cancer in a Retirement Community, *New England Journal of Medicine* 294:1262-1267, 1976. 4. Weiss NS, Szekely DR, Austin DF: Increasing Incidence of Endometrial Cancer in the United States, *New England Journal of Medicine* 294:1259-1262, 1976. 5. Herbst AL, Ulfelder H, Poskanzer DC: Adenocarcinoma of Vagina, *New England Journal of Medicine* 284:878-881, 1971. 6. Greenwald P, Barlow J, Nasca P, Burnett W: Vaginal Cancer After Maternal Treatment with Synthetic Estrogens, *New England Journal of Medicine* 285:390-392, 1971. 7. Lanier A, Noller K, Decker D, et al: Cancer and Stilbestrol. A Follow-up of 1719 Persons Exposed to Estrogens in Utero and Born 1943-1959, *Mayo Clinic Proceedings* 48:793-799, 1973. 8. Herbst A, Kurman R, Scully R: Vaginal and Cervical Abnormalities After Exposure to Stilbestrol In Utero, *Obstetrics and Gynecology* 40:287-298, 1972. 9. Herbst A, Robboy S, Macdonald G, Scully R: The Effects of Local Progesterone on Stilbestrol-Associated Vaginal Adenosis, *American Journal of Obstetrics and Gynecology* 118:607-615, 1974. 10. Herbst A, Poskanzer D,

Robboy S, et al: Prenatal Exposure to Stilbestrol, A Prospective Comparison of Exposed Female Offspring with Unexposed Controls, *New England Journal of Medicine* 292:334-339, 1975. 11. Stafl A, Mattingly R, Foley D, Fetherston W: Clinical Diagnosis of Vaginal Adenosis, *Obstetrics and Gynecology* 43:118-128, 1974. 12. Sherman AI, Goldrath M, Berlin A, et al: Cervical-Vaginal Adenosis After *In Utero* Exposure to Synthetic Estrogens, *Obstetrics and Gynecology* 44:531-545, 1974. 13. Gal I, Kirman B, Stern J: Hormone Pregnancy Tests and Congenital Malformation, *Nature* 216:83, 1967. 14. Levy EP, Cohen A, Fraser FC: Hormone Treatment During Pregnancy and Congenital Heart Defects, *Lancet* 1:611, 1973. 15. Nora J, Nora A: Birth Defects and Oral Contraceptives, *Lancet* 1:941-942, 1973. 16. Janerich DT, Piper JM, Glebatis, DM: Oral Contraceptives and Congenital Limb-Reduction Defects, *New England Journal of Medicine* 291:697-700, 1974. 17. Estrogens for Oral or Parental Use, *Federal Register* 40:8212, 1975. 18. Boston Collaborative Drug Surveillance Program: Surgically Confirmed Gall Bladder Disease, Venous Thromboembolism and Breast Tumors in Relations to Post-Menopausal Estrogen Therapy, *New England Journal of Medicine* 290:15-19, 1974. 18a. Hoover R, Gray LA Sr, Cole P, MacMahon B: Menopausal Estrogens and Breast Cancer, *New England Journal of Medicine* 295:401-405, 1976. 19. Boston Collaborative Drug Surveillance Program: Oral Contraceptives and Venous Thromboembolic Disease, Surgically Confirmed Gall Bladder Disease, and Breast Tumors, *Lancet* 1:1399-1404, 1973. 20. Daniel DG, Campbell H, Turnbull AC: Puerperal Thromboembolism and Suppression of Lactation, *Lancet* 2:287-289, 1967. 21. The Veterans Administration Cooperative Urological Research Group: Carcinoma of the Prostate: Treatment Comparisons, *Journal of Urology* 98:516-522, 1967. 22. Bailar JC: Thromboembolism and Oestrogen Therapy, *Lancet* 2:560, 1967. 23. Blackard C, Doe R, Mellinger G, Byar D: Incidence of Cardiovascular Disease and Death in Patients Receiving Diethylstilbestrol for Carcinoma of the Prostate, *Cancer* 26:249-256, 1970. 24. Royal College of General Practitioners: Oral Contraception and Thromboembolic Disease, *Journal of the Royal College of General Practitioners* 13:267-279, 1967. 25. Inman WHW, Vessey MP: Investigation of Deaths from Pulmonary, Coronary and Cerebral Thrombosis and Embolism in Women of Child-Bearing Age, *British Medical Journal* 2:193-199, 1968. 26. Vessey MP, Doll R: Investigation of Relation Between Use of Oral Contraceptives and Thromboembolic Disease. A Further Report, *British Medical Journal* 2:651-657, 1969. 27. Sartwell PE, Masi AT, Arthes FG, et al: Thromboembolism and Oral Contraceptives: An Epidemiological Case Control Study, *American Journal of Epidemiology* 90:365-380, 1969. 28. Collaborative Group for the Study of Stroke in Young Women: Oral Contraception and Increased Risk of Cerebral Ischemia or Thrombosis, *New England Journal of Medicine* 288:871-878, 1973. 29. Collaborative Group for the Study of Stroke in Young Women: Oral Contraceptives and Stroke in Young Women: Associated Risk Factors, *Journal of the American Medical Association* 231:718-722, 1975. 30. Mann JI, Inman WHW: Oral Contraceptives and Death from Myocardial Infarction, *British Medical Journal* 2:245-248, 1975. 31. Mann JI, Vessey MP, Thorogood M, Doll R: Myocardial Infarction in Young Women with Special Reference to Oral Contraceptive Practice, *British Medical Journal* 2:241-245, 1975. 32. Inman WHW, Vessey VP, Westerholm B, Engelund A: Thromboembolic Disease and the Steroidal Content of Oral Contraceptives, *British Medical Journal* 2:203-209, 1970. 33. Stolley PD, Tonascia JA, Tockman MS, et al: Thrombosis with Low-Estrogen Oral Contraceptives, *American Journal of Epidemiology* 102:197-208, 1975. 34. Vessey MP, Doll R, Fairbairn AS, Glober G: Post-Operative Thromboembolism and the Use of the Oral Contraceptives, *British Medical Journal* 3:123-126, 1970. 35. Greene GR. Sartwell PE: Oral Contraceptive Use in Patients with Thromboembolism Following Surgery, Trauma or Infection, *American Journal of Public Health* 62:680-685, 1972. 36. Rosenberg L, Armstrong MB, Jick H: Myocardial Infarction and Estrogen Therapy in Postmenopausal Women. *New England Journal of Medicine* 294:1256-1259, 1976. 37. Coronary Drug Project Research Group: The Coronary Drug Project: Initial Findings Leading to Modification of Its Research Protocol, *Journal of the American Medical Association* 214:1303-1313, 1970. 38. Baum J, Holtz F, Bookstein JJ, Klein EW: Possible Association Between Benign Hepatomas and Oral Contraceptives, *Lancet* 2:926-928, 1973. 39. Mays ET, Christopherson WM, Mahr MM, Williams HC: Hepatic Changes in Young Women Ingesting Contraceptive Steroids, Hepatic Hemorrhage and Primary Hepatic Tumors, *Journal of the American Medical Association* 235:730-782, 1976. 40. Edmondson HA, Henderson B, Benton B: Liver Cell Adenomas with the Use of Oral Contraceptives, *New England Journal of Medicine* 294:470-472, 1976. 41. Pfeffer RI, Van Den Noort S: Estrogen Use and Stroke Risk in Postmenopausal Women, *American Journal of Epidemiology* 103:445-456, 1976.

HOW SUPPLIED
TABLETS: 0.3 MG

BRAND/MANUFACTURER	NDC	SIZE	AWP
◇ BRAND			
MENEST: SK Beecham Pharm	00029-2800-30	100s	$11.65
ESTRATAB: Solvay	00032-1014-01	100s	$20.80

TABLETS: 0.625 MG

BRAND/MANUFACTURER	NDC	SIZE	AWP
◇ BRAND			
MENEST: SK Beecham Pharm	00029-2810-30	100s	$16.45
ESTRATAB: Solvay	00032-1022-01	100s	$28.97
	00032-1022-10	1000s	$275.26

TABLETS: 1.25 MG

BRAND/MANUFACTURER	NDC	SIZE	AWP
◇ BRAND			
MENEST: SK Beecham Pharm	00029-2820-30	100s	$27.70
ESTRATAB: Solvay	00032-1024-01	100s	$39.64
	00032-1024-10	1000s	$377.83
◇ GENERICS			
Cheshire	55175-2092-00	30s	$19.01

➤ SHOWN IN PRODUCT IDENTIFICATION GUIDE

TABLETS: 2.5 MG

BRAND/MANUFACTURER	NDC	SIZE	AWP
◇ **BRAND**			
MENEST: SK Beecham Pharm	00029-2830-29	50s	$25.80
ESTRATAB: Solvay	00032-1025-01	100s	$68.65

Estrogens, Esterified and Methyltestosterone

WARNING

1. ESTROGENS HAVE BEEN REPORTED TO INCREASE THE RISK OF ENDOMETRIAL CARCINOMA.

THREE INDEPENDENT CASE CONTROL STUDIES HAVE REPORTED AN INCREASED RISK OF ENDOMETRIAL CANCER IN POSTMENOPAUSAL WOMEN EXPOSED TO EXOGENOUS ESTROGENS FOR PROLONGED PERIODS.[1-3] THIS RISK WAS INDEPENDENT OF THE OTHER KNOWN RISK FACTORS FOR ENDOMETRIAL CANCER. THESE STUDIES ARE FURTHER SUPPORTED BY THE FINDING THAT INCIDENCE RATES OF ENDOMETRIAL CANCER HAVE INCREASED SHARPLY SINCE 1969 IN EIGHT DIFFERENT AREAS OF THE UNITED STATES WITH POPULATION-BASED CANCER REPORTING SYSTEMS, AN INCREASE WHICH MAY BE RELATED TO THE RAPIDLY EXPANDING USE OF ESTROGENS DURING THE LAST DECADE.[4]

THE THREE CASE CONTROL STUDIES REPORTED THAT THE RISK OF ENDOMETRIAL CANCER IN ESTROGEN USERS WAS ABOUT 4.5 TO 13.9 TIMES GREATER THAN IN NONUSERS. THE RISK APPEARS TO DEPEND ON BOTH DURATION OF TREATMENT[1] AND ON ESTROGEN DOSE.[3] IN VIEW OF THESE FINDINGS, WHEN ESTROGENS ARE USED FOR THE TREATMENT OF MENOPAUSAL SYMPTOMS, THE LOWEST DOSE THAT WILL CONTROL SYMPTOMS SHOULD BE UTILIZED AND MEDICATION SHOULD BE DISCONTINUED AS SOON AS POSSIBLE. WHEN PROLONGED TREATMENT IS MEDICALLY INDICATED, THE PATIENT SHOULD BE REASSESSED ON AT LEAST A SEMIANNUAL BASIS TO DETERMINE THE NEED FOR CONTINUED THERAPY. ALTHOUGH THE EVIDENCE MUST BE CONSIDERED PRELIMINARY, ONE STUDY SUGGESTS THAT CYCLIC ADMINISTRATION OF LOW DOSES OF ESTROGEN MAY CARRY LESS RISK THAN CONTINUOUS ADMINISTRATION;[3] IT THEREFORE APPEARS PRUDENT TO UTILIZE SUCH A REGIMEN.

CLOSE CLINICAL SURVEILLANCE OF ALL WOMEN TAKING ESTROGENS IS IMPORTANT. IN ALL CASES OF UNDIAGNOSED PERSISTENT OR RECURRING ABNORMAL VAGINAL BLEEDING, ADEQUATE DIAGNOSTIC MEASURES SHOULD BE UNDERTAKEN TO RULE OUT MALIGNANCY.

THERE IS NO EVIDENCE AT PRESENT THAT "NATURAL" ESTROGENS ARE MORE OR LESS HAZARDOUS THAN "SYNTHETIC" ESTROGENS AT EQUIESTROGENIC DOSES.

2. ESTROGENS SHOULD NOT BE USED DURING PREGNANCY.

THE USE OF FEMALE SEX HORMONES, BOTH ESTROGENS AND PROGESTOGENS, DURING EARLY PREGNANCY MAY SERIOUSLY DAMAGE THE OFFSPRING. IT HAS BEEN SHOWN THAT FEMALES EXPOSED IN UTERO TO DIETHYLSTILBESTROL, A NON-STEROIDAL ESTROGEN, HAVE AN INCREASED RISK OF DEVELOPING IN LATER LIFE A FORM OF VAGINAL OR CERVICAL CANCER THAT IS ORDINARILY EXTREMELY RARE.[5,6] THIS RISK HAS BEEN ESTIMATED AS NOT GREATER THAN 4 PER 1000 EXPOSURES.[7] FURTHERMORE, A HIGH PERCENTAGE OF SUCH EXPOSED WOMEN (FROM 30 TO 90 PERCENT) HAVE BEEN FOUND TO HAVE VAGINAL ADENOSIS,[8-12] EPITHELIAL CHANGES OF THE VAGINA AND CERVIX. ALTHOUGH THESE CHANGES ARE HISTOLOGICALLY BENIGN, IT IS NOT KNOWN WHETHER THEY ARE PRECURSORS OF MALIGNANCY. ALTHOUGH SIMILAR DATA ARE NOT AVAILABLE WITH THE USE OF OTHER ESTROGENS, IT CANNOT BE PRESUMED THEY WOULD NOT INDUCE SIMILAR CHANGES.

SEVERAL REPORTS SUGGEST AN ASSOCIATION BETWEEN INTRAUTERINE EXPOSURE TO FEMALE SEX HORMONES AND CONGENITAL ANOMALIES, INCLUDING CONGENITAL HEART DEFECTS AND LIMB REDUCTION DEFECTS.[13-16] ONE CASE CONTROL STUDY[16] ESTIMATED A 4.7 FOLD INCREASED RISK OF LIMB REDUCTION DEFECTS IN INFANTS EXPOSED IN UTERO TO SEX HORMONES (ORAL CONTRACEPTIVES, HORMONE WITHDRAWAL TESTS FOR PREGNANCY, OR ATTEMPTED TREATMENT FOR THREATENED ABORTION). SOME OF THESE EXPOSURES WERE VERY SHORT AND INVOLVED ONLY A FEW DAYS OF TREATMENT. THE DATA SUGGEST THAT THE RISK OF LIMB REDUCTION DEFECTS IN EXPOSED FETUSES IS SOMEWHAT LESS THAN 1 PER 1000.

IN THE PAST, FEMALE SEX HORMONES HAVE BEEN USED DURING PREGNANCY IN AN ATTEMPT TO TREAT THREATENED OR HABITUAL ABORTION. THERE IS CONSIDERABLE EVIDENCE THAT ESTROGENS ARE INEFFECTIVE FOR THESE INDICATIONS, AND THERE IS NO EVIDENCE FROM WELL CONTROLLED STUDIES THAT PROGESTOGENS ARE EFFECTIVE FOR THESE USES.

IF ESTROGENS, ESTERIFIED/METHYLTESTOSTERONE IS USED DURING PREGNANCY, OR IF THE PATIENT BECOMES PREGNANT WHILE TAKING THIS DRUG, SHE SHOULD BE APPRISED OF THE POTENTIAL RISKS TO THE FETUS, AND THE ADVISABILITY OF PREGNANCY CONTINUATION.

DESCRIPTION

Estrogens, Esterified/Methyltestosterone oral tablets contain: 1.25 mg of Estrogens, Esterified USP and 2.5 mg of Methyltestosterone, or 0.625 mg of Estrogens, Esterified USP and 1.25 mg of Methyltestosterone.

ESTERIFIED ESTROGENS

Estrogens, Esterified USP is a mixture of the sodium salts of the sulfate esters of the estrogenic substances, principally estrone, that are of the type excreted by pregnant mares. Estrogens Esterified contain not less than 75.0 percent and not more than 85.0 percent of sodium estrone sulfate, and not less than 6.0 percent and not more than 15.0 percent of sodium equilin sulfate, in such proportion that the total of these two components is not less than 90.0 percent.

Category: Estrogens

METHYLTESTOSTERONE

Methyltestosterone is an androgen.

Androgens are derivatives of cyclopentano-perhydro-phenanthrene. Endogenous androgens are C-19 steroids with a side chain at C-17, and with two angular methyl groups. Testosterone is the primary endogenous androgen. Fluoxymesterone and methyltestosterone are synthetic derivatives of testosterone.

Methyltestosterone is a white to light yellow crystalline substance that is virtually insoluble in water but soluble in organic solvents. It is stable in air but decomposes in light.

Its molecular formula is: $C_{20}H_{30}O_2$. Its molecular weight is 302.46.

Androst-4-en-3-one, 17-hydroxy-17-methyl-, (17B)-

Category: Androgen.

CLINICAL PHARMACOLOGY

ESTROGENS

Estrogens are important in the development and maintenance of the female reproductive system and secondary sex characteristics. They promote growth and development of the vagina, uterus, and fallopian tubes, and enlargement of the breasts. Indirectly, they contribute to tne shaping of the skeleton, maintenance of tone and elasticity of urogenital structures, changes in the epiphyses of the long bones that allow for the pubertal growth spurt and its termination, growth of axillary and pubic hair, and pigmentation of the nipples and genitals. Decline of Estrogenic activity at the end of the menstrual cycle can bring on menstruation, although the cessation of progesterone secretion is the most important factor in the mature ovulatory cycle. However, in the preovulatory or nonovulatory cycle, Estrogen is the primary determinant in the onset of menstruation. Estrogens also affect the release of pituitary gonadotropins.

The pharmacologic effects of Esterifed Estrogens are similar to those of endogenous Estrogens. They are soluble in water and are well absorbed from the gastrointestinal tract.

In responsive tissues (female genital organs, breasts, hypothalamus, pituitary) Estrogens enter the cell and are transported into the nucleus. As a result of Estrogen action, specific RNA and protein synthesis occurs.

ESTROGEN PHARMACOKINETICS

Metabolism and inactivation occur primarily in the liver. Some Estrogens are excreted into the bile; however they are reabsorbed from the intestine and returned to the liver through the portal venous system. Water soluble Esterifed Estrogens are strongly acidic and are ionized in body fluids, which favor excretion through the kidneys since tubular reabsorption is minimal.

Androgens: Endogenous androgens are responsible for the normal growth and development of the male sex organs and for maintenance of secondary sex characteristics. These effects include the growth and maturation of prostate, seminal vesicles, penis, and scrotum; the development of male hair distribution, such as beard, pubic, chest, and axillary hair, laryngeal enlargement, vocal cord thickening, alterations in body musculature, and fat distribution. Drugs in this class also cause retention of nitrogen, sodium, potassium, phosphorus, and decreased urinary excretion of calcium. Androgens have been reported to increase protein anabolism and decrease protein catabolism. Nitrogen balance is improved only when there is sufficient intake of calories and protein. Androgens are responsible for the growth spurt of adolescence and for the eventual termination of linear growth which is brought about by fusion of the epiphyseal growth centers. In children, exogenous androgens accelerate linear growth rates, but may cause a disproportionate advancement in bone maturation. Use over long periods may result in fusion of the epiphyseal growth centers and termination of growth process. Androgens have been reported to stimulate the production of red blood cells by enhancing the production of erythropoietic stimulating factor.

ANDROGEN PHARMACOKINETICS

Testosterone given orally is metabolized by the gut and 44 percent is cleared by the liver in the first pass. Oral doses as high as 400 mg per day are needed to achieve clinically effective blood levels for full replacement therapy. The synthetic androgens (methyltestosterone and fluoxymesterone) are less extensively metabolized by the liver and have longer half-lives. They are more suitable than testosterone for oral administration.

Testosterone in plasma is 98 percent bound to a specific testosterone-estradiol binding globulin, and about 2 percent is free. Generally, the amount of this sex-hormone binding globulin in the plasma will determine the distribution of testosterone between free and bound forms, and the free testosterone concentration will determine its half-life.

About 90 percent of a dose of testosterone is excreted in the urine as glucuronic and sulfuric acid conjugates of testosterone and its metabolites; about 6 percent of a dose is excreted in the feces, mostly in the unconjugated form. Inactivation of testosterone occurs primarily in the liver. Testosterone is metabolized to various 17-keto steroids through two different pathways. There are considerable variations of the half-life of testosterone as reported in the literature, ranging from 10 to 100 minutes.

In many tissues the activity of testosterone appears to depend on reduction to dihydrotestosterone, which binds to cytosol receptor proteins. The steroid-receptor complex is transported to the nucleus where it initiates transcription events and cellular changes related to androgen action.

INDICATIONS

Estrogens, Esterified/Methyltestosterone is indicated in the treatment of:

Moderate to severe *vasomotor* symptoms associated with the menopause in those patients not improved by Estrogens alone. (There is no evidence that Estrogens are effective for nervous symptoms or depression without associated vasomotor symptoms, and they should not be used to treat such conditions.)

ESTROGENS, ESTERIFIED/METHYLTESTOSTERONE HAS NOT BEEN SHOWN TO BE EFFECTIVE FOR ANY PURPOSE DURING PREGNANCY AND ITS USE MAY CAUSE SEVERE HARM TO THE FETUS (See Boxed *"Warning"*).

CONTRAINDICATIONS

Estrogens should not be used in women with any of the following conditions:
1. Known or suspected cancer of the breast except in appropriately selected patients being treated for metastatic disease.
2. Known or suspected Estrogen-dependent neoplasia.
3. Known or suspected pregnancy (See Boxed *"Warning"*).
4. Undiagnosed abnormal genital bleeding.
5. Active thrombophlebitis or thromboembolic disorders.
6. A past history of thrombophlebitis, thrombosis, or thromboembolic disorders associated with previous Estrogen use (except when used in treatment of breast malignancy).

Methyltestosterone should not be used in:
1. The presence of severe liver damage.
2. Pregnancy and in breast-feeding mothers because of the possibility of masculinization of the female fetus or breast-fed infant.

WARNINGS

ASSOCIATED WITH ESTROGENS

1. *Induction of Malignant Neoplasms:* Long term continuous administration of natural and synthetic Estrogens in certain animal species increases the frequency of carcinomas of the breast, cervix, vagina, and liver. There is now evidence that Estrogens increase the risk of carcinoma of the endometrium in humans (See Boxed *"Warning"*).

At the present time there is no satisfactory evidence that Estrogens given to postmenopausal women increase the risk of cancer of the breast,[18] although a recent long-term follow-up of a single physician's practice has raised the possibility.[18a] Because of the animal data, there is a need for caution in prescribing Estrogens for women with a strong family history of breast cancer or who have breast nodules, fibrocystic disease, or abnormal mammograms.

2. *Gallbladder Disease:* A recent study has reported a 2 to 3-fold increase in the risk of surgically confirmed gallbladder disease in women receiving postmenopausal Estrogen,[18] similar to the 2-fold increase previously noted in users of oral contraceptives.[19-24a] In the case of oral contraceptives the increased risk appeared after two years of use.[24]

3. *Effects Similar to Those Caused by Estrogen-Progestogen Oral Contraceptives:* There are several serious adverse effects of oral contra- ceptives, most of which have not, up to now, been documented as consequences of postmenopausal Estrogen therapy. This may reflect the comparatively low doses of Estrogen used in postmenopausal women. It would be expected that the larger doses of Estrogen used to treat prostatic or breast cancer or postpartum breast engorgement are more likely to result in these adverse effects, and, in fact, it has been shown that there is an increased risk of thrombosis in men receiving Estrogens for prostatic cancer and women for postpartum breast engorgement.[20-23]

a. *Thromboembolic Disease:* It is now well established that users of oral contraceptives have an increased risk of various thromboembolic and thrombotic vascular diseases, such as thrombophlebitis, pulmonary embolism, stroke, and myocardial infarction.[24-31] Cases of retinal thrombosis, mesenteric thrombosis, and optic neuritis have been reported in oral contraceptive users. There is evidence that the risk of several of these adverse reactions is related to the dose of the drug.[32,33] An increased risk of postsurgery thromboembolic complications has

also been reported in users of oral contraceptives.[34,35] If feasible, Estrogen should be discontinued at least 4 weeks before surgery of the type associated with an increased risk of thromboembolism, or during periods of prolonged immobolization.

While an increased rate of thromboembolic and thrombotic disease in postmenopausal users of Estrogen has not been found,[18-36] this does not rule out the possibility that such an increase may be present or that subgroups of women who have underlying risk factors or who are receiving relatively large doses of Estrogens may have increased risk. Therefore Estrogens should not be used in persons with active thrombophlebitis or thromboembolic disorders, and they should not be used (except in treatment of malignancy) in persons with a history of such disorders in association with Estrogen use. They should be used with caution in patients with cerebral vascular or coronary artery disease and only for those in whom Estrogens are clearly needed.

Large doses of Estrogen (5 mg Esterifed Estrogens per day), comparable to those used to treat cancer of the prostate and breast, have been shown in a large prospective clinical trial in men[37] to increase the risk of nonfatal myocardial infarction, pulmonary embolism and thrombophlebitis. When Estrogen doses of this size are used, any of the thromboembolic and thrombotic adverse effects associated with oral contraceptive use should be considered a clear risk.

b. *Hepatic Adenoma:* Benign hepatic adenomas appear to be associated with the use of oral contraceptives.[38-40] Although benign and rare, these may rupture and may cause death through intra-abdominal hemorrhage. Such lesions have not yet been reported in association with other Estrogen or progestogen preparations but should be considered in Estrogen users having abdominal pain and tenderness, abdominal mass, or hypovolemic shock. Hepatocellular carcinoma has also been reported in women taking Estrogen-containing oral contraceptives.[39] The relationship of this malignancy to these drugs is not known at this time.

c. *Elevated Blood Pressure:* Increased blood pressure is not uncommon in women using oral contraceptives. There is now a report that this may occur with use of Estrogens in the menopause[41] and blood pressure should be monitored with Estrogen use, especially if high doses are used.

d. *Glucose Tolerance:* A worsening of glucose tolerance has been observed in a significant percentage of patients on Estrogen-containing oral contraceptives. For this reason, diabetic patients should be carefully observed while receiving Estrogens.

4. *Hypercalcemia:* Administration of Estrogens may lead to severe hypercalcemia in patients with breast cancer and bone metastases. If this occurs, the drug should be stopped and appropriate measures taken to reduce the serum calcium level.

ASSOCIATED WITH METHYLTESTOSTERONE

In patients with breast cancer, androgen therapy may cause hypercalcemia by stimulating osteolysis. In this case, the drug should be discontinued.

Prolonged use of high doses of androgens has been associated with the development of peliosis, hepatis and hepatic neoplasms including hepatocellular carcinoma. (See *"Precautions—Carcinogenesis"*). Peliosis hepatis can be a life-threatening or fatal complication.

Cholestatic hepatitis and jaundice occur with 17-alpha-alkylandrogens at a relatively low dose. If cholestatic hepatitis with jaundice appears or if liver function tests become abnormal, the androgen should be discontinued and the etiology should be determined. Drug-induced jaundice is reversible when the medication is discontinued.

Edema with or without heart failure may be a serious complication in patients with preexisting cardiac, renal, or hepatic disease. In addition to discontinuation of the drug, diuretic therapy may be required.

PRECAUTIONS

ASSOCIATED WITH ESTROGENS

A. *General Precautions:* 1. A complete medical and family history should be taken prior to the initiation of any Estrogen therapy. The pretreatment and periodic physical examinations should include special reference to blood pressure, breasts, abdomen, and pelvic organs, and should include a Papanicolaou smear. As a general rule, Estrogen should not be prescribed for longer than one year without another physical examination being performed.

2. Fluid retention—Because Estrogens may cause some degree of fluid retention, conditions which might be influenced by this factor such as asthma, epilepsy, migraine, and cardiac or renal dysfunction, require careful observation.

3. Certain patients may develop undesirable manifestations of excessive Estrogenic stimulation, such as abnormal or excessive uterine bleeding, mastodynia, etc.

4. Oral contraceptives appear to be associated with an increased incidence of mental depression.[24] Although it is not clear whether this is due to the Estrogenic or progestogenic component of the contraceptive, patients with a history of depression should be carefully observed.

5. Preexisting uterine leiomyomata may increase in size during Estrogen use.

6. The pathologist should be advised of Estrogen therapy when relevant specimens are submitted.

7. Patients with a past history of jaundice during pregnancy have an increased risk of recurrence of jaundice while receiving Estrogen-containing oral contraceptive therapy. If jaundice develops in any patient receiving Estrogen, the medication should be discontinued while the cause is investigated.

8. Estrogens may be poorly metabolized in patients with impaired liver function and they should be administered with caution in such patients.

9. Because Estrogens influence the metabolism of calcium and phosphorus, they should be used with caution in patients with metabolic bone diseases that are associated with hypercalcemia or in patients with renal insufficiency.

10. Because of the effects of Estrogens on epiphyseal closure, they should be used judiciously in young patients in whom bone growth is not complete.

11. Certain endocrine and liver function tests may be affected by Estrogen-containing oral contraceptives. The following similar changes may be expected with larger doses of Estrogen:

a. Increased sulfobromophthalein retention.

b. Increased prothrombin and factors VII, VIII, IX and X; decreased antithrombin 3; increased norepinephrine-induced platelet aggregability.

c. Increased thyroid binding globulin (TBG) leading to increased circulating total thyroid hormone, as measured by PBI, T_4 by column, or T_4 by radioimmunoassay. Free T_3 resin uptake is decreased, reflecting the elevated TBG; free T_4 concentration is unaltered.

d. Impaired glucose tolerance.

e. Decreased pregnanediol excretion.

f. Reduced response to metyrapone test.

g. Reduced serum folate concentration.

h. Increased serum triglyceride and phospholipid concentration.

B. Information for the Patient: See manufacturer's patient information.

C. Pregnancy Category X: See "Contraindications" and Boxed "Warning".

D. Nursing Mothers: As a general principle, the administration of any drug to nursing mothers should be done only when clearly necessary since many drugs are excreted in human milk.

ASSOCIATED WITH METHYLTESTOSTERONE

A. General Precautions:

1. Women should be observed for signs of virilization (deepening of the voice, hirsutism, acne, clitoromegaly, and menstrual irregularities). Discontinuation of drug therapy at the time of evidence of mild virilism is necessary to prevent irreversible virilization. Such virilization is usual following androgen use at high doses.

2. Prolonged dosage of androgen may result in sodium and fluid retention. This may present a problem, especially in patients with compromised cardiac reserve or renal disease.

3. Hypersensitivity may occur rarely.

4. PBI may be decreased in patients taking androgens.

5. Hypercalcemia may occur. If this does occur, the drug should be discontinued.

B. Information for the Patient: The physician should instruct patients to report any of the following side effects of androgens:

Women: Hoarseness, acne, changes in menstrual periods, or more hair on the face.

All Patients: Any nausea, vomiting, changes in skin color or ankle swelling.

C. Laboratory tests: 1. Women with disseminated breast carcinoma should have frequent determination of urine and serum calcium levels during the course of androgen therapy (see "Warnings").

2. Because of the hepatotoxicity associated with the use of 17-alpha-alkylated androgens, liver function tests should be obtained periodically.

3. Hemoglobin and hematocrit should be checked periodically for polycythemia in patients who are receiving high doses of androgens.

D. Drug Interactions: 1. *Anticoagulants* C-17 substituted derivatives of testosterone, such as methandrostenolone, have been reported to decrease the anticoagulant requirements of patients receiving oral anticoagulants. Patients receiving oral anticoagulant therapy require close monitoring, especially when androgens are started or stopped.

2. *Oxyphenbutazone.* Concurrent administration of oxyphenbutazone and androgens may result in elevated serum levels of oxyphenbutazone.

3. *Insulin.* In diabetic patients the metabolic effects of androgens may decrease blood glucose and insulin requirements.

E. Drug/Laboratory Test Interferences: Androgens may decrease levels of thyroxine-binding globulin, resulting in decreased T_4 serum levels and increased resin uptake of T_3 and T_4. Free thyroid hormone levels remain unchanged, however, and there is no clinical evidence of thyroid dysfunction.

F. Carcinogenesis: Animal Data. Testosterone has been tested by subcutaneous injection and implantation in mice and rats. The implant induced cervical-uterine tumors in mice, which metastasized in some cases. There is suggestive evidence that injection of testosterone into some strains of female mice increases their susceptibility to hepatoma. Testosterone is also known to increase the number of tumors and decrease the degree of differentiation of chemically induced carcinomas of the liver in rats.

Human Data. There are rare reports of hepatocellular carcinoma in patients receiving long-term therapy with androgens in high doses. Withdrawal of the drugs did not lead to regression of the tumors in all cases.

Geriatric patients treated with androgens may be at an increased risk for the development of prostatic hypertrophy and prostatic carcinoma.

G. Pregnancy: Teratogenic Effects. Pregnancy Category X (see "Contraindications").

H. Nursing Mothers: It is not known whether androgens are excreted in human milk. Because many drugs are excreted in human milk and because of the potential for serious adverse reactions in nursing infants from androgens, a decision should be made whether to discontinue nursing or to discontinue the drug, taking into account the importance of the drug to the mother.

ADVERSE REACTIONS
ASSOCIATED WITH ESTROGENS

(See "Warnings" regarding induction of neoplasia, adverse effects on the fetus, increased incidence of gallbladder disease, and adverse effects similar to those of oral contraceptives, including thromboembolism).

The following additional adverse reactions have been reported with Estrogenic therapy, including oral contraceptives:

1. *Genitourinary system:*
   Breakthrough bleeding, spotting, change in menstrual flow.
   Dysmenorrhea.
   Premenstrual-like syndrome.
   Amenorrhea during and after treatment.
   Increase in size of uterine fibromyomata.
   Vaginal candidiasis.
   Change in cervical erosion and in degree of cervical secretion.
   Cystitis-like syndrome.

2. *Breasts:*
   Tenderness, enlargement, secretion.

3. *Gastrointestinal:*
   Nausea, vomiting.
   Abdominal cramps, bloating.
   Cholestatic jaundice.

4. *Skin:*
   Chloasma or melasma which may persist when drug is discontinued.
   Erythema multiforme.
   Erythema nodosum.
   Hemorrhagic eruption.
   Loss of scalp hair.
   Hirsutism.

5. *Eyes:*
   Steepening of corneal curvatures.
   Intolerance to contact lenses.

6. *CNS:*
   Headache, migraine, dizziness.
   Mental depression.
   Chorea.

7. *Miscellaneous:*
   Increase or decrease in weight.
   Reduced carbohydrate tolerance.
   Aggravation of porphyria.
   Edema.
   Changes in libido.

ASSOCIATED WITH METHYLTESTOSTERONE

1. Endocrine and Urogenital, Female: The most common side effects of androgen therapy are amenorrhea and other menstrual irregularities, inhibition of gonadotropin secretion, and virilization, including deepening of the voice and clitoral enlargement. The latter usually is not reversible after androgens are discontinued. When administered to a pregnant woman androgens cause virilization of external genitalia of the female fetus.

2. Skin and Appendages: Hirsutism, male pattern of baldness, and acne.

3. Fluid and Electrolyte Disturbances: Retention of sodium, chloride, water, potassium, calcium, and inorganic phosphates.

4. Gastrointestinal: Nausea, cholestatic jaundice, alterations in liver function test, rarely hepatocellular neoplasms, and peliosis hepatis (see "Warnings").

5. Hematologic: Suppression of clotting factors II, V, VII, and X, bleeding in patients on concomitant anticoagulant therapy, and polycythemia.

6. Nervous System: Increased or decreased libido, headache, anxiety, depression, and generalized paresthesia.

7. Metabolic: Increased serum cholesterol.

8. Miscellaneous: Inflammation and pain at the site of intramuscular injection or subcutaneous implantation of testosterone containing pellets, stomatitis with buccal preparations, and rarely anaphylactoid reactions.

OVERDOSAGE

Numerous reports of ingestion of large doses of Estrogen-containing oral contraceptives by young children indicate that serious ill effects do not occur. Overdosage of Estrogen may cause nausea, and withdrawal bleeding may occur in females.

There have been no reports of acute overdosage with the androgens.

DOSAGE AND ADMINISTRATION

Given cyclically for short-term use only:

For treatment of moderate to severe *vasomotor* symptoms associated with the menopause in patients not improved by Estrogen alone.

The lowest dose that will control symptoms should be chosen and medication should be discontinued as promptly as possible.

Administration should be cyclic (e.g., three weeks on and one week off).

Attempts to discontinue or taper medication should be made at three to six month intervals.

◆ **RATED THERAPEUTICALLY EQUIVALENT**; ◇ **THERAPEUTIC EQUIVALENCE UNCONFIRMED**; ○ **UNRATED**

Usual Dosage Range: 1 or 2 tablets daily as recommended by the physician. Treated patients with an intact uterus should be monitored closely for signs of endometrial cancer and appropriate diagnostic measures should be taken to rule out malignancy in the event of persistent or recurring abnormal vaginal bleeding.

Store at controlled room temperature, 15°-30°C (59°-86°F).

REFERENCES

1. Ziel, H.K. *et al.*: N. Engl. J. Med. *293*:1167-1170, 1975. 2. Smith, D.C., *et al.*: N. Engl. J. Med. *293*:1164-1167, 1975. 3. Mack, T.M., *et al.*: N. Engl. J. Med. *294*:1262-1267, 1976. 4. Weiss, N.S., *et al.*: N. Engl. J. Med. *294*:1259-1262, 1976. 5. Herbst, A.L., *et al.*: N. Engl. J. Med. *284*:878-881, 1971. 6. Greenwald, P., *et al.*: N. Engl. J. Med. *285*:390-392, 1971. 7. Lanier, A., *et al.*: Mayo Clin. Proc. *48*:793-799, 1973. 8. Herbst, A., *et al.*: Obstet. Gynecol. *40*:287-298, 1972. 9. Herbst, A., *et al.*: Am. J. Obstet. Gynecol. *118*:607-615, 1974. 10. Herbst, A., *et al.*: N. Engl. J. Med. *292*:334-339, 1975. 11. Stafl, A., *et al.*: Obstet. Gynecol. *43*-128, 1974. 12. Sherman, A.I., *et al.*: Obstet. Gynecol. *44*:531-545, 1974. 13. Gal, I., *et al.*: Nature *216*:83, 1967. 14. Levy, E.P., *et al.*: Lancet *1*:611, 1973. 15. Nora, J., *et al.*: Lancet *1*:941-942, 1973. 16. Janerich, D.T., *et al.*: N. Engl. J. Med. *291*:697-700, 1974. 17. Estrogens for Oral or Parenteral Use: Federal Register *40*:8212, 1975. 18. Boston Collaborative Drug Surveillance Program: N. Engl. J. Med. *290*:15-19, 1974. 18a. Hoover, R., *et al.*: N. Engl. J. Med. *295*:401-405, 1976. 19. Boston Collaborative Drug Surveillance Program: Lancet *1*:1399-1404, 1973. 20. Daniel, D.G., *et al.*: Lancet *2*:287-289, 1967. 21. The Veterans Administration Cooperative Urological Research Group: J. Urol. *98*:516-522, 1967. 22. Bailar, J. C.: Lancet *2*:560, 1967. 23. Blackard, C., *et al.*: Cancer *26*:249-256, 1970. 24. Royal College of General Practitioners: J.R. Coll, Gen. Pract. *13*:267-279, 1967. 25. Inman, W.H.W., *et al.*: Br. Med. J. *2*:193-199, 1968. 26. Vessey, M.P., *et al.*: Br. Med. J. *2*:651-657, 1969. 27. Sartwell, P.E., *et al.*: Am. J. Epidemiol, *90*:365-380, 1969. 28. Collaborative Group for the Study of Stroke in Young Women: N. Engl. J. Med. *288*:871-878, 1973. 29. Collaborative Group for the Study of Stroke in Young Women: J.A.M.A. *231*:718-722, 1975. 30. Mann, J.I., *et al.*: Br. Med. J. *2*:245-248, 1975. 31. Mann, J.I., *et al.*: Br. Med. J. *2*:241-245, 1975. 32. Inman, W.H.W., *et al.*: Br. Med. J. *2*:203-209, 1970. 33. Stolley, P.D., *et al.*: Am. J. Epidemiol, *102*:197-208, 1975. 34. Vessey, M.P., *et al.*: Br. Med. J. *3*:123-126, 1970. 35. Greene, G.R., *et al.*: Am. J. Public Health *62*:680-685, 1972. 36. Rosenberg, L., *et al.*: N. Engl. J. Med. *294*:1256-1259, 1976. 37. Coronary Drug Project Research Group: J.A.M.A. *214*:1303-1313, 1970. 38. Baum, J., *et al.*: Lancet *2*:926-928, 1973. 39. Mays, E.T., *et al.*: J.A.M.A. *235*:730-732, 1976. 40. Edmondson, H.A., *et al.*: N. Engl. J. Med. *294*:470-472, 1976. 41. Pfeffer, R.I., *et al.*: Am. J. Epidemiol, *103*:445-456, 1976.

HOW SUPPLIED
TABLETS: 0.625 MG-5 MG

BRAND/MANUFACTURER	NDC	SIZE	AWP
○ **BRAND**			
ESTRATEST H.S.: Solvay	00032-1023-01	100s	$59.43

TABLETS: 1.25 MG-2.5 MG

BRAND/MANUFACTURER	NDC	SIZE	AWP
○ **BRAND**			
ESTRATEST: Solvay	00032-1026-01	100s	$73.98
	00032-1026-10	1000s	$696.08

Estrone

WARNING

1. ESTROGENS HAVE BEEN REPORTED TO INCREASE THE RISK OF ENDOMETRIAL CARCINOMA.

THREE INDEPENDENT CASE CONTROL STUDIES HAVE SHOWN AN INCREASED RISK OF ENDOMETRIAL CANCER IN POSTMENOPAUSAL WOMEN EXPOSED TO EXOGENOUS ESTROGENS FOR PROLONGED PERIODS. THIS RISK WAS INDEPENDENT OF THE OTHER KNOWN RISK FACTORS FOR ENDOMETRIAL CANCER. THESE STUDIES ARE FURTHER SUPPORTED BY THE FINDING THAT INCIDENCE RATES OF ENDOMETRIAL CANCER HAVE INCREASED SHARPLY SINCE 1969 IN EIGHT DIFFERENT AREAS OF THE UNITED STATES WITH POPULATION-BASED CANCER REPORTING SYSTEMS, AN INCREASE WHICH MAY BE RELATED TO THE RAPIDLY EXPANDING USE OF ESTROGENS DURING THE LAST DECADE.

THE THREE CASE CONTROL STUDIES REPORTED THAT THE RISK OF ENDOMETRIAL CANCER IN ESTROGEN USERS WAS ABOUT 4.5 TO 13.9 TIMES GREATER THAN IN NONUSERS. THE RISK APPEARS TO DEPEND ON BOTH DURATION OF TREATMENT AND ON ESTROGEN DOSE. IN VIEW OF THESE FINDINGS, WHEN ESTROGENS ARE USED FOR THE TREATMENT OF MENOPAUSAL SYMPTOMS, THE LOWEST DOSE THAT WILL CONTROL SYMPTOMS SHOULD BE UTILIZED AND MEDICATION SHOULD BE DISCONTINUED AS SOON AS POSSIBLE. WHEN PROLONGED TREATMENT IS MEDICALLY INDICATED, THE PATIENT SHOULD BE REASSESSED ON AT LEAST A SEMI-ANNUAL BASIS TO DETERMINE THE NEED FOR CONTINUED THERAPY. ALTHOUGH THE EVIDENCE MUST BE CONSIDERED PRELIMINARY, ONE STUDY SUGGESTS THAT CYCLIC ADMINISTRATION OF LOW DOSES OF ESTROGEN MAY CARRY LESS RISK THAN CONTINUOUS ADMINISTRATION; IT THEREFORE APPEARS PRUDENT TO UTILIZE SUCH A REGIMEN.

CLOSE CLINICAL SURVEILLANCE OF ALL WOMEN TAKING ESTROGENS IS IMPORTANT. IN ALL CASES OF UNDIAGNOSED PERSISTENT OR RECURRING ABNORMAL VAGINAL BLEEDING, ADEQUATE DIAGNOSTIC MEASURES SHOULD BE UNDERTAKEN TO RULE OUT MALIGNANCY.

THERE IS NO EVIDENCE AT PRESENT THAT "NATURAL" ESTROGENS ARE MORE OR LESS HAZARDOUS THAN "SYNTHETIC" ESTROGENS AT EQUIESTROGENIC DOSES.

2. ESTROGENS SHOULD NOT BE USED DURING PREGNANCY.

THE USE OF FEMALE SEX HORMONES, BOTH ESTROGENS AND PROGESTOGENS, DURING EARLY PREGNANCY MAY SERIOUSLY DAMAGE THE OFFSPRING. IT HAS BEEN SHOWN THAT FEMALES EXPOSED *IN UTERO* TO DIETHYLSTILBESTROL, A NON-STEROIDAL ESTROGEN, HAVE AN INCREASED RISK OF DEVELOPING IN LATER LIFE A FORM OF VAGINAL OR CERVICAL CANCER THAT IS ORDINARILY EXTREMELY RARE. THIS RISK HAS BEEN ESTIMATED AS NOT GREATER THAN 4 PER 1000 EXPOSURES. FURTHERMORE, A HIGH PERCENTAGE OF SUCH EXPOSED WOMEN (FROM 30 TO 90 PERCENT) HAVE BEEN FOUND TO HAVE VAGINAL ADENOSIS WITH EPITHELIAL CHANGES OF VAGINA AND CERVIX. ALTHOUGH THESE CHANGES ARE HISTOLOGICALLY BENIGN, IT IS NOT KNOWN WHETHER THEY ARE PRECURSORS OF MALIGNANCY. ALTHOUGH SIMILAR DATA ARE NOT AVAILABLE WITH THE USE OF OTHER ESTROGENS, IT IS REASONABLE TO PRESUME THEY WOULD INDUCE SIMILAR CHANGES.

SEVERAL REPORTS SUGGEST AN ASSOCIATION BETWEEN INTRAUTERINE EXPOSURE TO FEMALE SEX HORMONES AND CONGENITAL ANOMALIES, INCLUDING CONGENITAL HEART DEFECTS AND LIMB REDUCTION DEFECTS. ONE CASE CONTROL STUDY ESTIMATED A 4.7 FOLD INCREASED RISK OF LIMB REDUCTION DEFECTS IN INFANTS EXPOSED *IN UTERO* TO SEX HORMONES (ORAL CONTRACEPTIVES, HORMONE WITHDRAWAL TESTS FOR PREGNANCY, OR ATTEMPTED TREATMENT FOR THREATENED ABORTION). SOME OF THESE EXPOSURES WERE VERY SHORT AND INVOLVED ONLY A FEW DAYS OF TREATMENT. THESE DATA SUGGEST THAT THE RISK OF LIMB REDUCTION DEFECTS IN EXPOSED FETUSES IS SOMEWHAT LESS THAN 1 PER 1000.

IN THE PAST, FEMALE SEX HORMONES HAVE BEEN USED DURING PREGNANCY IN AN ATTEMPT TO TREAT THREATENED OR HABITUAL ABORTION. THERE IS CONSIDERABLE EVIDENCE THAT ESTROGENS ARE INEFFECTIVE FOR THESE INDICATIONS, AND THERE IS NO EVIDENCE FROM WELL CONTROLLED STUDIES THAT PROGESTOGENS ARE EFFECTIVE FOR THESE USES.

IF THIS DRUG IS USED DURING PREGNANCY, OR IF THE PATIENT BECOMES PREGNANT WHILE TAKING THIS DRUG, SHE SHOULD BE APPRISED OF THE POTENTIAL RISKS TO THE FETUS, AND THE ADVISABILITY OF PREGNANCY CONTINUATION.

DESCRIPTION

Sterile Estrone occurs as small, white crystals or as a white to creamy white, crystalline powder. It is odorless, and is stable in air. It melts at about 260° C. Estrone is practically insoluble in water. It is soluble in alcohol, in acetone, in dioxane, and in vegetable oils. It is slightly soluble in solutions of fixed alkali hydroxides.

Estrone has the chemical formula:

$C_{18}H_{22}O_2$ Estra-1,3,5(10)-trien-17-one,3-hydroxy-3-Hydroxyestra-1, 3,5(10)-trien-17-one

Molecular weight: 270.37

Category: Estrogen

Available as: Sterile aqueous suspension of Estrone for intramuscular injection containing Estrone 2 mg or 5 mg per mL.

Following is its chemical structure:

CLINICAL PHARMACOLOGY

Estrogens are important in the development and maintenance of the female reproductive system and secondary sex characteristics. They promote growth and development of the vagina, uterus, and fallopian tubes, and enlargement of the breasts. Indirectly, they contribute to the shaping of the skeleton, maintenance of tone and elasticity of urogenital structures, changes in the epiphyses of the long bones that allow for the pubertal growth spurt and its termination, growth of axillary and pubic hair, and pigmentation of the nipples and genitals. Decline of estrogenic activity at the end of the menstrual cycle can bring on menstruation, although the cessation of progesterone secretion is the most important factor in the mature ovulatory cycle. However, in the preovulatory or nonovulatory cycle, estrogen is the primary determination in the onset of menstruation. Estrogens also affect the release of pituitary gonadotropins.

In responsive tissues (female genital organs, breasts, hypothalamus, pituitary) estrogens enter the cell and are transported into the nucleus. As a result of estrogen action, specific RNA and DNA syntheses occur. Metabolism and inactivation occur primarily in the liver. Some estrogens are excreted into the bile, however they are reabsorbed from the intestine and returned to the liver through the portal venous system.

INDICATIONS AND USAGE

Sterile Estrone Suspension is indicated in the treatment of:

1. Moderate to severe vasomotor symptoms associated with the menopause. (There is no evidence that estrogens are effective for nervous symptoms or depression which might occur during menopause, and they should not be used to treat these conditions.)
2. Atrophic vaginitis.
3. Kraurosis vulvae.
4. Female hypogonadism.
5. Female castration.
6. Primary ovarian failure.
7. Breast cancer (for palliation only) in appropriately selected women and men with metastatic disease.
8. Prostatic carcinoma — palliative therapy of advanced disease.

UNLABELED USES

Estrone is used alone or as an adjunct in the treatment of dyskinesia including chorea secondary to Huntington's disease and tardive dyskinesia, and levodopa-induced dyskinesia, osteoporosis, male hypersexuality including deviant sexual behavior, and prophylaxis of cardiovascular disease.

STERILE ESTRONE SUSPENSION HAS NOT BEEN SHOWN TO BE EFFECTIVE FOR ANY PURPOSE DURING PREGNANCY AND ITS USE MAY CAUSE SEVERE HARM TO THE FETUS (see boxed *"Warning"*).

CONTRAINDICATIONS

Estrogens should not be used in women (or men) with any of the following conditions:

1. Known or suspected cancer of the breast except in appropriately selected patients being treated for metastatic disease.
2. Known or suspected estrogen-dependent neoplasia.
3. Known or suspected pregnancy (see boxed *"Warning"*).
4. Undiagnosed abnormal genital bleeding.
5. Active thrombophlebitis or thromboembolic disorders.
6. A past history of thrombophlebitis, thrombosis or thromboembolic disorders associated with previous estrogen use (except when used in treatment of breast or prostatic malignancy).

Hypersensitivity to any of the components of the product.

WARNINGS

1. Induction of Malignant Neoplasms: Long term continuous administration of natural and synthetic estrogens in certain animal species increases the frequency of carcinomas of the breast, cervix, vagina, and liver. There is now evidence that estrogens increase the risk of carcinoma of the endometrium in humans (see boxed *"Warning"*). At the present time there is no satisfactory evidence that estrogens given to postmenopausal women increase the risk of cancer of the breast, although a recent long-term follow-up of a single physician's practice has raised this possibility. Because of the animal data, there is a need for caution in prescribing estrogens for women with a strong family history of breast cancer or who have breast nodules, fibrocystic disease, or abnormal mammograms.

2. Gallbladder Diseases: A recent study has reported a 2- to 3-fold increase in the risk of surgically confirmed gallbladder disease in women receiving postmenopausal estrogens, similar to the 2-fold increase previously noted in users of oral contraceptives. In the case of oral contraceptives the increased risk appeared after two years of use.

3. Effects Similar to Those Caused by Estrogen-Progestogen Oral Contraceptives: There are several serious adverse effects of oral contraceptives, most of which have not, up to now, been documented as consequences of postmenopausal estrogen therapy. This may reflect the comparatively low doses of estrogen used in postmenopausal women. It would be expected that the larger doses of estrogen used to treat prostatic or breast cancer are more likely to result in these adverse effects, and, in fact, it has been shown that there is an increased risk of thrombosis in men receiving estrogens for prostatic cancer and women for postpartum breast engorgement.

a. Thromboembolic disease. It is now well established that users of oral contraceptives have an increased risk of various thromboembolic and thrombotic disease, such as thrombophlebitis, pulmonary embolism, stroke, and myocardial infarction. Cases of retinal thrombosis, mesenteric thrombosis and optic neuritis have been reported in oral contraceptive users. There is evidence that the risk of several of these adverse reactions is related to the dose of the drug. An increased risk of post-surgery thromboembolic complications has also been reported in users of oral contraceptives. If feasible, estrogen should be discontinued at least 4 weeks before surgery of the type associated with an increased risk of thromboembolism, or during periods of prolonged immobilization.

While an increased rate of thromboembolic and thrombotic disease in postmenopausal users of estrogens has not been found, this does not rule out the possibility that such an increase may be present or that subgroups of women who have under-lying risk factors or who are receiving relatively large doses of estrogens may have increased risk. Therefore estrogens should not be used in persons with active thrombophlebitis or thromboembolic disorders, and they should not be used (except in treatment of malignancy) in persons with a history of such disorders in association with estrogen use. They should be used with caution in patients with cerebral vascular or coronary artery disease and only for those in whom estrogens are clearly needed.

Large doses of estrogen (5 mg conjugated estrogens per day), comparable to those used to treat cancer of the prostate and breast, have been shown in a large prospective clinical trial in men to increase the risk of nonfatal myocardial infarction, pulmonary embolism and thrombophlebitis. When estrogen doses of this size are used, any of the thromboembolic and thrombotic adverse effects associated with oral contraceptive use should be considered a clear risk.

b. Hepatic adenoma. Benign hepatic adenomas appear to be associated with the use of oral contraceptives. Although benign, and rare, these may rupture and cause death through intra-abdominal hemorrhage. Such lesions have not yet been reported in association with other estrogen or progestogen preparations but should be considered in estrogen users having abdominal pain and tenderness, abdominal mass, or hypovolemic shock. Hepatocellular carcinoma has also been reported in women taking estrogen-containing oral contraceptives. The relationship of this malignancy to these drugs is not known at this time.

c. Elevated blood pressure. Increased blood pressure is not uncommon in women using oral contraceptives. There is now a report that this may occur with use of estrogens in the menopause and blood pressure should be monitored with estrogen use, especially if high doses are used.

d. Glucose tolerance. A worsening of glucose tolerance has been observed in a significant percentage of patients on estrogen-containing oral contraceptives. For this reason, diabetic patients should be carefully observed while receiving estrogen.

4. Hypercalcemia: The administration of estrogens may lead to severe hypercalcemia in patients with breast cancer and bone metastases. If this occurs, the drug should be stopped and appropriate measures taken to reduce the serum calcium level.

PRECAUTIONS

A. General Precautions: 1. A complete medical and family history should be taken prior to the initiation of any estrogen therapy. The pre-treatment and periodic physical examinations should include special reference to blood pressure, breasts, abdomen, and pelvic organs, and should include a Papanicolaou smear. As a general rule, estrogen should not be prescribed for longer than one year without another physical examination being performed.

2. Fluid retention — Because estrogens may cause some degree of fluid retention, conditions that might be influenced by this factor such as epilepsy, migraine, and cardiac or renal dysfunction, require careful observation.

3. Certain patients may develop undesirable manifestations of excessive estrogenic stimulation, such as abnormal or excessive uterine bleeding, mastodynia, etc.

4. Oral contraceptives appear to be associated with an increased incidence of mental depression. Although it is not clear whether this is due to the estrogenic or progestogenic component of the contraceptive, patients with a history of depression should be carefully observed.

5. Preexisting uterine leiomyomata may increase in size during estrogen use.

6. The pathologist should be advised of estrogen therapy when relevant specimens are submitted.

7. Patients with a past history of jaundice during pregnancy have an increased risk of recurrence of jaundice while receiving estrogen-containing oral contraceptive therapy. If jaundice develops in any patient receiving estrogen, the medication should be discontinued while the cause is investigated.

8. Estrogens may be poorly metabolized in patients with impaired liver function and they should be administered with caution in such patients.

9. Because estrogens influence the metabolism of calcium and phosphorus, they should be used with caution in patients with metabolic bone diseases that are associated with hypercalcemia or in patients with renal insufficiency.

10. Because of the effects of estrogens on epiphyseal closure, they should be used judiciously in young patients in whom bone growth is not complete.

11. Certain endocrine and liver function tests may be affected by estrogen-containing oral contraceptives. The following similar changes may be expected with larger doses of estrogen.

a. Increased sulfobromophthalein retention.

b. Increased prothrombin and factors VII, VIII, IX, and X; decreased antithrombin 3; increased norepinephrine-induced platelet aggregability.

c. Increased thyroid binding globulin (TBG) leading to increased circulating total thyroid hormone, as measured by PBI, T4 by column, or T4 by radioimmunoassay. Free T3 resin uptake is decreased, reflecting the elevated TBG; free T4 concentration is unaltered.

d. Impaired glucose tolerance.

e. Decreased pregnanediol excretion.

f. Reduced response to metyrapone test.

g. Reduced serum folate concentration.

h. Increased serum triglyceride and phospholipid concentration.

12. The lowest effective dose appropriate for the specific indication should be utilized. Studies of the addition of a progestin for seven or more days of cycle of estrogen administration have reported a lowered incidence of endometrial hyperplasia. Morphological and biochemical studies of endometrium suggest that 10 to 13 days of progestin are needed to provide maximal maturation of the endometrium and to eliminate any hyperplastic changes. Whether this will provide protection from endometrial carcinoma has not been clearly established.

There are possible additional risks which may be associated with the inclusion of progestin in estrogen replacement regimens. The potential risks include adverse effects on carbohydrate and lipid metabolism. The choice of progestin and dosage may be important in minimizing these adverse effects.

B. Information for Patients: See manufacturer's patient information.

C. Pregnancy Category X: See "Contraindications" and boxed "Warning."

D. Nursing Mothers: As a general principle, the administration of any drug to nursing mothers should be done only when clearly necessary since many drugs are excreted in human milk.

ADVERSE REACTIONS

(See "Warnings" regarding induction of neoplasia, adverse effects on the fetus, increased incidence of gallbladder disease, and adverse effects similar to those of oral contraceptives including thromboembolism). The following additional adverse reactions have been reported with estrogenic therapy, including oral contraceptives.

1. Genitourinary System: Breakthrough bleeding, spotting, change in menstrual flow; dysmenorrhea; premenstrual-like syndrome; amenorrhea during and after treatment; increase in size of uterine fibromyomata; vaginal candidiasis; change in cervical eversion and in degree of cervical secretion; cystitis-like syndrome.

2. Breasts: Tenderness, enlargement, secretion.

3. Gastrointestinal: Nausea, vomiting; abdominal cramps, bloating; cholestatic jaundice.

4. Skin: Chloasma or melasma which may persist when drug is discontinued; erythema multiforme; erythema nodosum; hemorrhagic eruption; loss of scalp hair; hirsutism.

5. Eyes: Steepening of corneal curvature; intolerance to contact lenses.

6. CNS: Headache, migraine, dizziness; mental depression; chorea.

7. Miscellaneous: Increase or decrease in weight; reduced carbohydrate tolerance; aggravation of porphyria; edema; changes in libido.

ACUTE OVERDOSAGE

Numerous reports of ingestion of large doses of estrogen-containing oral contraceptives by young children indicate that serious ill effects do not occur. Overdosage of estrogen may cause nausea, and withdrawal bleeding may occur in females.

DOSAGE AND ADMINISTRATION

Shake vial and syringe well prior to withdrawal and injection (using a 21-23 gauge needle) to properly suspend medication.

1. Replacement Therapy of Estrogen-Deficiency Associated Conditions: The lowest dose that will control symptoms should be chosen and medication should be discontinued as promptly as possible.

Administration should be cyclic (e.g., 3 weeks on and 1 week off).

Attempts to discontinue or taper medication should be made at 3 to 6 month intervals.

Initial relief of symptoms may be achieved through the administration of 0.1 mg to 1 mg of estrone weekly in single or divided doses. Some patients may require 0.5 mg to 2 mg weekly.

Note: Continual therapy with Estrogen alone may induce functional uterine bleeding.

2. Senile Vaginitis and Kraurosis Vulvae: Will generally respond to injection of 0.1 mg to 0.5 mg of estrone two or three times weekly. Administration should be cyclic (e.g. 3 weeks on and 1 week off).

3. Abnormal Uterine Bleeding Due to Hormone Imbalance: May respond to brief courses of intensive estrogen therapy. Dosage in the range of 2 mg to 5 mg daily for several days.

4. Given Chronically: Inoperable progressing prostatic cancer.

For palliation in prostatic cancer, estrone may be employed at a dosage level of 2 mg to 4 mg two or three times weekly. If a response to estrogen therapy is going to occur, it should be apparent within 3 months of the beginning of therapy. If a response does occur, the hormone should be continued until the disease is again progressive.

Inoperable progressing breast cancer in appropriately selected men and post-menopausal women. (See "Indications").

The usual dosage is 5 mg 3 or more times weekly according to severity of pain.

Treated patients with an intact uterus should be monitored closely for signs of endometrial cancer and appropriate diagnostic measures should be taken to rule out malignancy in the event of persistent or recurring abnormal vaginal bleeding.

Parenteral drug products should be inspected visually for particulate matter and discoloration prior to administration, whenever the solution and container permit.

Storage: Store at controlled room temperature 15°-30° C (59°-86° F). DO NOT PERMIT TO FREEZE.

J CODES
IM—J1435

HOW SUPPLIED
INJECTION: 2 MG/ML

BRAND/MANUFACTURER	NDC	SIZE	AWP
◇ GENERICS			
Major	00904-0911-10	10 ml	$5.95
KESTRIN: Hyrex	00314-0638-70	10 ml	$9.50
Rugby	00536-5501-75	30 ml	$2.06

INJECTION: 5 MG/ML

BRAND/MANUFACTURER	NDC	SIZE	AWP
◇ GENERICS			
Schein	00364-6601-54	10 ml	$8.02
Steris	00402-0041-10	10 ml	$8.02
KESTRONE 5: Hyrex	00314-0644-70	10 ml	$9.60
Moore,H.L.	00839-5585-30	10 ml	$10.38
URL	00677-0274-21	10 ml	$12.10
Rugby	00536-5602-70	10 ml	$15.45

INJECTION: 5 MG

BRAND/MANUFACTURER	NDC	SIZE	AWP
◇ GENERICS			
Goldline	00182-3027-63	10 ml	$12.15

Estropipate

WARNINGS

1. ESTROGENS HAVE BEEN REPORTED TO INCREASE THE RISK OF ENDOMETRIAL CARCINOMA IN POST-MENOPAUSAL WOMEN.

THREE INDEPENDENT CASE CONTROL STUDIES HAVE SHOWN AN INCREASED RISK OF ENDOMETRIAL CANCER IN POST-MENOPAUSAL WOMEN EXPOSED TO EXOGENOUS ESTROGENS FOR PROLONGED PERIODS. THIS RISK WAS INDEPENDENT OF THE OTHER KNOWN RISK FACTORS FOR ENDOMETRIAL CANCER. THESE STUDIES ARE FURTHER SUPPORTED BY THE FINDING THAT INCIDENCE RATES OF ENDOMETRIAL CANCER HAVE INCREASED SHARPLY SINCE 1969 IN EIGHT DIFFERENT AREAS OF THE UNITED STATES WITH POPULATION-BASED CANCER REPORTING SYSTEMS, AN INCREASE WHICH MAY BE RELATED TO THE RAPIDLY EXPANDING USE OF ESTROGENS DURING THE LAST DECADE.

THE THREE CASE CONTROL STUDIES REPORTED THAT THE RISK OF ENDOMETRIAL CANCER IN ESTROGEN USERS WAS ABOUT 4.5 TO 13.9 TIMES GREATER THAN IN NONUSERS. THE RISK APPEARS TO DEPEND ON BOTH DURATION OF TREATMENT AND ON ESTROGEN DOSE. IN VIEW OF THESE FINDINGS, WHEN ESTROGENS ARE USED FOR THE TREATMENT OF MENOPAUSAL SYMPTOMS, THE LOWEST DOSE THAT WILL CONTROL SYMPTOMS SHOULD BE UTILIZED AND MEDICATION SHOULD BE DISCONTINUED AS SOON AS POSSIBLE. WHEN PROLONGED TREATMENT IS MEDICALLY INDICATED, THE PATIENT SHOULD BE REASSESSED ON AT LEAST A SEMIANNUAL BASIS TO DETERMINE THE NEED FOR CONTINUED THERAPY. ALTHOUGH THE EVIDENCE MUST BE CONSIDERED PRELIMINARY, ONE STUDY SUGGESTS THAT CYCLIC ADMINISTRATION OF LOW DOSES OF ESTROGEN MAY CARRY LESS RISK THAN CONTINUOUS ADMINISTRATION; IT THEREFORE APPEARS PRUDENT TO UTILIZE SUCH A REGIMEN.

CLOSE CLINICAL SURVEILLANCE OF ALL WOMEN TAKING ESTROGENS IS IMPORTANT. ADEQUATE DIAGNOSTIC MEASURES, INCLUDING ENDOMETRIAL SAMPLING WHEN INDICATED, SHOULD BE UNDERTAKEN TO RULE OUT MALIGNANCY IN ALL CASES OF UNDIAGNOSED PERSISTENT OR RECURRING ABNORMAL VAGINAL BLEEDING. THERE IS NO EVIDENCE THAT "NATURAL" ESTROGENS ARE MORE OR LESS HAZARDOUS THAN "SYNTHETIC" ESTROGENS AT EQUI-ESTROGENIC DOSES.

2. ESTROGENS SHOULD NOT BE USED DURING PREGNANCY.

ACCORDING TO SOME INVESTIGATORS, THE USE OF FEMALE SEX HORMONES, BOTH ESTROGENS AND PROGESTOGENS, DURING EARLY PREGNANCY MAY SERIOUSLY DAMAGE THE OFFSPRING. STUDIES HAVE REPORTED THAT FEMALES EXPOSED IN UTERO TO DIETHYLSTILBESTROL, A NON-STEROIDAL ESTROGEN, HAVE AN INCREASED RISK OF DEVELOPING IN LATER LIFE A FORM OF VAGINAL OR CERVICAL CANCER THAT IS ORDINARILY EXTREMELY RARE. IN ONE OF THESE STUDIES, THIS RISK WAS ESTIMATED AS NOT GREATER THAN 4 PER 1000 EXPOSURES. FURTHERMORE, THERE ARE REPORTS THAT A HIGH PERCENTAGE OF SUCH EXPOSED WOMEN (FROM 30 TO 90 PERCENT) HAVE BEEN FOUND TO HAVE VAGINAL ADENOSIS, SQUAMOUS CELL DYSPLASIA OF THE UTERINE CERVIX, AND CLEAR CELL VAGINAL

CANCER LATER IN LIFE. ALTHOUGH THESE REPORTED CHANGES ARE HISTOLOGICALLY BENIGN, THE INVESTIGATORS HAVE NOT DETERMINED WHETHER THEY ARE PRECURSORS OF ADENOCARCINOMA.

MALE OFFSPRING HAVE AN INCREASED RISK OF UROGENITAL ABNORMALITIES AND POSSIBLY TESTICULAR CANCER LATER IN LIFE. THE 1985 DES TASK FORCE CONCLUDED THAT USE OF DES DURING PREGNANCY IS ASSOCIATED WITH A SUBSEQUENT INCREASED RISK OF BREAST CANCER IN THE MOTHERS, ALTHOUGH A CAUSAL RELATIONSHIP REMAINS UNPROVEN AND THE OBSERVED LEVEL OF EXCESS RISK IS SIMILAR TO THAT FOR A NUMBER OF OTHER BREAST CANCER RISK FACTORS.

ALTHOUGH SIMILAR DATA ARE NOT AVAILABLE WITH THE USE OF OTHER ESTROGENS, IT CANNOT BE PRESUMED THEY WOULD NOT INDUCE SIMILAR CHANGES.

SEVERAL REPORTS SUGGEST AN ASSOCIATION BETWEEN INTRAUTERINE EXPOSURE TO FEMALE SEX HORMONES AND CONGENITAL ANOMALIES IN THE OFFSPRING, INCLUDING CONGENITAL HEART DEFECTS AND LIMB REDUCTION DEFECTS. ONE CASE CONTROL STUDY ESTIMATED A 4.7-FOLD INCREASED RISK OF LIMB REDUCTION DEFECTS IN INFANTS EXPOSED IN UTERO TO SEX HORMONES (ORAL CONTRACEPTIVES, HORMONE WITHDRAWAL TESTS FOR PREGNANCY, OR ATTEMPTED TREATMENT FOR THREATENED ABORTION). SOME OF THESE EXPOSURES WERE VERY SHORT AND INVOLVED ONLY A FEW DAYS OF TREATMENT. THE DATA SUGGEST THAT THE RISK OF LIMB REDUCTION DEFECTS IN EXPOSED FETUSES IS SOMEWHAT LESS THAN 1 PER 1000.

IN THE PAST, FEMALE SEX HORMONES HAVE BEEN USED DURING PREGNANCY IN AN ATTEMPT TO TREAT THREATENED OR HABITUAL ABORTION. ESTROPIPATE HAS NOT BEEN STUDIED FOR THESE USES, AND THEREFORE, SHOULD NOT BE USED DURING PREGNANCY. THERE IS NO EVIDENCE FROM WELL-CONTROLLED STUDIES THAT PROGESTOGENS ARE EFFECTIVE FOR THESE USES. IF ESTROPIPATE IS USED DURING PREGNANCY, OR IF THE PATIENT BECOMES PREGNANT WHILE TAKING THIS DRUG, SHE SHOULD BE APPRISED OF THE POTENTIAL RISKS TO THE FETUS, AND THE QUESTION OF CONTINUATION OF THE PREGNANCY SHOULD BE ADDRESSED.

DESCRIPTION

Estropipate (formerly piperazine estrone sulfate), is a natural estrogenic substance prepared from purified crystalline estrone, solubilized as the sulfate and stabilized with piperazine. It is appreciably soluble in water and has almost no odor or taste. The amount of piperazine in Estropipate is not sufficient to exert a pharmacological action. Its addition ensures solubility, stability, and uniform potency of the estrone sulfate. Chemically Estropipate, molecular weight: 436.56, is represented by estra-1,3,5(10)-trien-17-one,3-(sulfooxy)-, compound with piperazine (1:1).

Estropipate is available as tablets for oral administration containing either 0.75 mg, 1.5 mg, or 3 mg Estropipate (calculated as sodium estrone sulfate 0.625 mg, 1.25 mg, and 2.5 mg respectively). Each gram of Estropipate cream contains 1.5 mg Estropipate USP.

Following is its chemical structure:

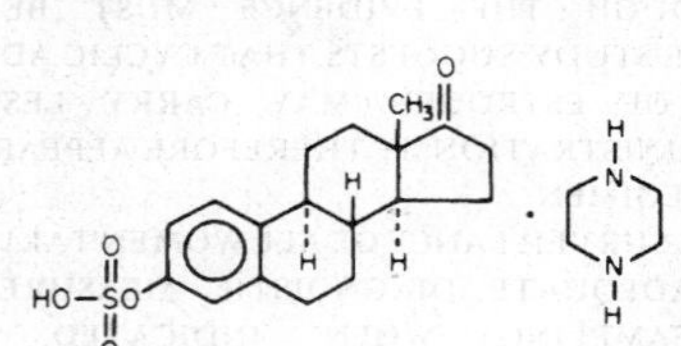

CLINICAL PHARMACOLOGY

Estrogen drug products act by regulating the transcription of a limited number of genes. Estrogens diffuse through cell membranes, distribute themselves throughout the cell, and bind to and activate the nuclear estrogen receptor, a DNA-binding protein which is found in estrogen-responsive tissues. The activated estrogen receptor binds to specific CNA sequences, or hormone-response elements, which enhance the transcription of adjacent genes and in turn lead to the observed effects. Estrogen receptors have been identified in tissues of the reproductive tract, breast, pituitary, hypothalamus, liver, and bone of women.

Estrogens are important in the development and maintenance of the female reproductive system and secondary sex characteristics. By a direct action, they cause growth and development of the uterus, fallopian tubes, and vagina. With other hormones, such as pituitary hormones and progesterone, they cause enlargement of the breasts through promotion of ductal growth, stromal development, and the accretion of fat. Estrogens are intricately involved with other hormones, especially progesterone, in the processes of the ovulatory menstrual cycle and pregnancy, and affect the release of pituitary gonadotropins. They also contribute to the shaping of the skeleton, maintenance of tone and elasticity of urogenital structures, changes in the epiphyses of the long bones that

allow for the pubertal growth spurt and its termination, growth of axillary and pubic hair, and pigmentation of the nipples and genitals.

Estrogens occur naturally in several forms. The primary source of estrogen in normally cycling adult women is the ovarian follicle, which secretes 70 to 500 micrograms of estradiol daily, depending on the phase of the menstrual cycle. Estradiol is rapidly hydrolyzed in the body to estrone, which in turn may be hydrated to the less active estriol. These transformations occur readily, mainly in the liver, where there is also free interconversion between estrone and estradiol.

A depletion of endogenous estrogens occurs postmenopausally as a result of a decline in ovarian function, and may cause symptomatic vulvovaginal epithelial atrophy. The signs and symptoms of these atrophic changes in the vaginal and vulval epithelia may be alleviated by the topical application of an estrogenic hormone such as Estropipate Cream.

After menopause, most endogenous estrogen is produced by conversion of androstenedione, secreted by the adrenal cortex, to estrone by peripheral tissues. Thus, estrone—especially in its sulfate ester form—is the most abundant circulating estrogen in postmenopausal women. Although circulating estrogens exist in a dynamic equilibrium of metabolic interconversions, estradiol is the principal intracellular human estrogen and is substantially more potent than estrone or estriol as the receptor.

Estrogens used in therapy are well absorbed through the skin, mucous membranes, and gastrointestinal tract. When applied for a local action, absorption is usually sufficient to cause systemic effects. When conjugated with aryl and alkyl groups for parenteral administration, the rate of absorption of oily preparations is slowed with a prolonged duration of action, such that a single intramuscular injection of estradiol valerate or estradiol cypionate is absorbed over several weeks.

Administered estrogens and their esters are handled within the body essentially the same as the endogenous hormones. Metabolic conversion of estrogens occurs primarily in the liver (first pass effect), but also at local target tissue sites. Complex metabolic processes result in a dynamic equilibrium of circulating conjugated and unconjugated estrogenic forms which are continually interconverted, especially between estrone and estradiol and between esterified and unesterified forms. Although naturally-occurring estrogens circulate in the blood largely bound to sex hormone-binding globulin and albumin, only unbound estrogens enter target tissue cells. A significant proportion of the circulating estrogen exists as sulfate conjugates, especially estrone sulfate, which serves as a circulating reservoir for the formation of more active estrogenic species. A certain proportion of the estrogen is excreted into the bile and then reabsorbed from the intestine. During this enterohepatic recirculation, estrogens are desulfated and resulfated and undergo degradation through conversion to less active estrogens (estriol and other estrogens), oxidation to nonestrogenic substances (catecholestrogens, which interact with catecholamine metabolism, especially in the central nervous system), and conjugation with glucoronic acids (which are then rapidly excreted in the urine).

When given orally, naturally-occurring estrogens and their esters are extensively metabolized (first pass effect) and circulate primarily as estrone sulfate, with smaller amounts of other conjugated and unconjugated estrogenic species. This results is limited oral potency. By contrast, synthetic estrogens, such as ethinyl estradiol and the nonsteroidal estrogens, are degraded very slowly in the liver and other tissues, which results in their high intrinsic potency. Gastrointestinal absorption of orally administered estrogens is usually prompt and complete. Estrogen drug products administered by non-oral routes are not subject to first-pass metabolism.

Estropipate Vaginal Cream may be absorbed transmucosally and may produce systemic estrogenic effects. Inactivation of estrogens in the body occurs mainly in the liver. During cyclic passage through the liver, estrogens are degraded to less active estrogenic compounds and conjugated with sulfuric and glucuronic acids. Estrone is 50-80% bound to proteins as it circulates in the blood, principally as a conjugate with sulfate.

INDICATIONS AND USAGE

Estrogen drug products are indicated in the:
1. Treatment of moderate to severe vasomotor symptoms associated with the menopause. There is no adequate evidence that estrogens are effective for nervous symptoms or depression which might occur during menopause and they should not be used to treat these conditions.
2. Treatment of vulval and vaginal atrophy.
3. Treatment of hypoestrogenism due to hypogonadism, castration or primary ovarian failure.
4. Prevention of osteoporosis.
5. Kraurosis vulvae.
6. Female hypogonadism.
7. Female castration.

Since estrogen administration is associated with risk, selection of patients should ideally be based on prospective identification of risk factors for developing osteoporosis. Unfortunately, there is no certain way to identify those women who will develop osteoporotic fractures. Most prospective studies of efficacy for this indication have been carried out in white menopausal women, without stratification by other risk factors, and tend to show a universally salutary effect on bone. Thus, patient selection must be individualized based on the balance of risks and benefits. A more favorable risk/benefit ratio exists in a hysterectomized woman because she has no risk of endometrial cancer (see Boxed "Warning").

Estrogen replacement therapy reduces bone resorption and retards or halts postmenopausal bone loss. Case-control studies have shown an approximately 60 percent reduction in hip and wrist fractures in women whose estrogen replacement was begun within a few years of menopause. Studies also suggest that estrogen reduces the rate of vertebral fractures. Even when started as late as 6 years after menopause, estrogen prevents further loss of bone mass for as long as the treatment is continued. The results of a double-blind, placebo-controlled two year study have shown that treatment with one tablet of Estropipate 0.75 mg daily for 25 days (of a 31-day cycle per month) prevents vertebral bone mass loss in postmenopausal women. When estrogen therapy is discontinued, bone mass declines at a rate comparable to the immediate postmenopausal period. There is no evidence that estrogen replacement therapy restores bone mass to premenopausal levels.

At skeletal maturity there are sex and race differences in both the total amount of bone present and its density, in favor of men and blacks. Thus, women are at higher risk than men because they start with less bone mass and, for several years following natural or induced menopause, the rate of bone mass decline is accelerated. White and Asian women are at higher risk than black women.

Early menopause is one of the strongest predictors for the development of osteoporosis. In addition, other factors affecting the skeleton which are associated with osteoporosis include genetic factors (small build, family history), endocrine factors (nulliparity, thyrotoxicosis, hyperparathyroidism, Cushing's syndrome, hyperprolactinemia, Type I diabetes), lifestyle (cigarette smoking, alcohol abuse, sedentary exercise habits) and nutrition (below average body weight, dietary calcium intake).

The mainstays of prevention and management of osteoporosis are estrogen, an adequate lifetime calcium intake, and exercise. Postmenopausal women absorb dietary calcium less efficiently than premenopausal women and require an average of 1500 mg/day of elemental calcium to remain in neutral calcium balance. By comparison, premenopausal women require about 100 mg/day and the average calcium intake in the USA is 400-600 mg/day. Therefore, when not contraindicated, calcium supplementation may be helpful. Weight-bearing exercise and nutrition may be important adjuncts to the prevention and management of osteoporosis. Immobilization and prolonged bed rest produce rapid bone loss, while weight-bearing exercise has been shown both to reduce bone loss and to increase bone mass. The optimal type and amount of physical activity that would prevent osteoporosis have not been established, however in two studies an hour of walking and running exercises twice or three times weekly significantly increased lumbar spine bone mass.

ESTROPIPATE VAGINAL CREAM HAS NOT BEEN TESTED FOR EFFICACY FOR ANY PURPOSE DURING PREGNANCY. SINCE ITS EFFECT UPON THE FETUS IS UNKNOWN, IT CANNOT BE RECOMMENDED FOR ANY CONDITION DURING PREGNANCY (See Boxed "Warning").

UNLABELED USES
Estropipate is used in the treatment of dysfunctional uterine bleeding associated with estrogen and progesterone imbalance.

CONTRAINDICATIONS
Estrogens should not be used in individuals with any of the following conditions:
1. Known or suspected pregnancy (see Boxed *"Warning"*). Estrogens may cause fetal harm when administered to a pregnant woman.
2. Undiagnosed abnormal genital bleeding.
3. Known or suspected cancer of the breast except in appropriately selected patients being treated for metastatic disease.
4. Known or suspected estrogen-dependent neoplasis.
5. Active thrombophlebitis or thromboembolic disorders.
6. Known or suspected cancer of the breast.
7. A past history of thrombophtebitis, thrombosis, or thromboembolic disorders associated with previous estrogen use.

WARNINGS
1. Induction of Malignant Neoplasms: Long-term continuous administration of natural and synthetic estrogens in certain animal species has been reported by some investigators to increase the frequency of carcinomas of the breast, cervix, vagina, and liver. There is now evidence that estrogens increase the risk of carcinoma of the endometrium in humans. (See Boxed *"Warning"*).

Endometrial Cancer: The reported endometrial cancer risk among unopposed estrogen users is about 2 to 12 fold greater than in non-users, and appears dependent on duration of treatment and on estrogen dose. Most studies show no significant increased risk associated with use of estrogens for less than one year. The greatest risk appears associated with prolonged use-with increased risks of 15 to 24-fold for five to ten years or more. In three studies, persistence of risk was demonstrated for 8 to over 15 years after cessation of estrogen treatment. In one study a significant decrease in the incidence of endometrial cancer occurred six months after estrogen withdrawal. Concurrent progestin therapy may offset this risk but the overall health impact in postmenopausal women is not known (see *"Precautions"*).

Breast Cancer: While the majority of studies have not shown an increased risk of breast cancer in women who have ever used estrogen replacement therapy, some have reported a moderately increased risk (relative risks of 1.3-2.0) in those taking higher doses or those taking lower doses for prolonged periods of time, especially in excess of 10 years. Other studies have not shown this relationship. Therefore, caution should be exercised when administering estrogens to women with a strong family history of breast cancer or who have breast nodules, fibrocystic disease, or abnormal mammograms. Careful breast examinations should be performed periodically.

Congenital Lesions with Malignant Potential: Estrogen therapy during pregnancy is associated with an increased risk of fetal congenital reproductive tract

disorders, and possibly other birth defects. Studies of women who received DES during pregnancy have shown that female offspring have an increased risk of vaginal adenosis, squamous cell dysplasia of the uterine cervix, and clear cell vaginal cancer later in life; male offspring have an increased risk of urogenital abnormalities and possibly testicular cancer later in life. Although some of these changes are benign, others are precursors of malignancy.

2. Gallbladder Disease: Two studies have reported a 2- to 4-fold increase in the risk of gallbladder disease requiring surgery in women receiving postmenopausal estrogen similar to the 2-fold increase previously noted in users of oral contraceptives. In the case of oral contraceptives, the increased risk appeared after two years of use.

3. Effects Similar to Those Caused by Estrogen-Progestogen Oral Contraceptives: There are several serious adverse effects of oral contraceptives, most of which have not, up to now, been documented as consequences of postmenopausal estrogen therapy. This may reflect the comparatively low doses of estrogen used in postmenopausal women. It would be expected that the larger doses of estrogen used to treat postpartum breast engorgement would be more likely to result in these adverse effects, and, in, fact, it has been shown that there is an increased risk of thrombosis in women receiving estrogens for postpartum breast engorgement.

a. Throembolic disease: It is now well established that users of oral contraceptives have an increased risk of various thromboembolic and thrombotic vascular diseases such as thrombophlebitis, pulmonary embolism, stroke, and myocardial infarction. Cases of retinal thrombosis, mesenteric thrombosis and optic neuritis have been reported in oral contraceptive users. There is evidence that the risk of several of these adverse reactions is related to the dose of the drug. An increased risk of post-surgery thromboembolic complications has also been reported in users of oral contraceptives. If feasible, estrogen should be discontinued at least 4 weeks before surgery of the type associated with an increased risk of thromboembolism; it should also be discontinued during periods of prolonged immobilization.

While an increased rate of thromboembolic and thrombotic disease in postmenopausal users of estrogens has not been found, this does not rule out the possibility that such an increase may be present or that subgroups of women who have underlying risk factors or who are receiving relatively large doses of estrogens may have increased risk. Therefore, estrogens should not be used in persons with active thrombophlebitis or thromboembolic disorders, and they should not be used in persons with a history of such disorders in association with estrogen use. They should be used with caution in patients with cerebral vascular or coronary artery disease and only for those in whom estrogens are clearly needed. Large doses of estrogen (5 mg conjugated estrogens per day), comparable to those used to treat cancer of the prostate and breast, have been shown in a large prospective clinical trial in men to increase the risk of nonfatal myocardial infarction, pulmonary embolism and thrombophlebitis. When estrogen doses of this size are used, any of the thromboembolic and thrombotic adverse effects associated with oral contraceptive use should be considered a clear risk. These risks cannot necessarily be extrapolated from men to women. However, to avoid the theoretical cardiovascular risk to women caused by high estrogen doses, the dose for estrogen replacement therapy should not exceed the lowest effective dose.

b. Hepatic adenoma: Benign hepatic adenomas appear to be associated with the use of oral contraceptives. Although benign, and rare, these may rupture and cause death through intra-abdominal hemorrhage. Such lesions have not yet been reported in association with other estrogen or progestogen preparations but should be considered in estrogen users having abdominal pain and tenderness, abdominal mass, or hypovolemic shock. Hepatocellular carcinoma has also been reported in women taking estrogen-containing oral contraceptives. The relationship of this malignancy to these drugs is not known at this time.

c. Elevated blood pressure: Occasional blood pressure increases during estrogen replacement therapy have been attributed to idiosyncratic reactions to estrogens. More often, blood pressure has remained the same or has dropped. One study showed that postmenopausal estrogen users have higher blood pressure than nonusers. Two other studies showed slightly lower blood pressure among estrogen users compared to nonusers. Postmenopausal estrogen use does not increase the risk of stroke. Nonetheless, blood pressure should be monitored at regular intervals with estrogen use.

d. Glucose tolerance: A worsening of glucose tolerance has been observed in a significant percentage of patients on estrogen-containing oral contraceptives. For this reason, diabetic patients should be carefully observed while receiving estrogen.

4. Hypercalcemia: Administration of estrogens may lead to severe hypercalcemia in patients with breast cancer and bone metastases. If this occurs, the drug should be stopped and appropriate measures taken to reduce the serum calcium level.

PRECAUTIONS
A. GENERAL
1. Addition of a Progestin: The lowest effective dose appropriate for the specific indication should be utilized. Studies of the addition of a progestin for seven or more days of a cycle of estrogen administration have reported a lowered incidence of endometrial hyperplasia which would otherwise be induced by estrogen treatment. Morphological and biochemical studies of endometrium suggest that 10 to 14 days of progestin are needed to provide maximal maturation of the endometrium and to eliminate any hyperplastic changes. Whether this will provide protection from endometrial carcinoma has not been clearly established.

There are possible additional risks which may be associated with the inclusion of progestins in estrogen replacement regimens. These include: (1) adverse effects on lipoprotein metabolism (lowering HDL and raising LDL) which may diminish the possible cardioprotective effect of estrogen therapy (see "Precautions": D.4., below); (2) impairment of glucose tolerance; and (3) possible enhancement of mitotic activity in breast epithelial tissue (although few epidemiological data are available to address this point). The choice of progestin, its dose, and its regimen may be important in minimizing these adverse effects, but these issues remain to be clarified.

2. Physical Examination: A complete medical and family history should be taken prior to the initiation of any estrogen therapy. The pretreatment and periodic physical examinations should include special reference to blood pressure, breasts, abdomen, and pelvic organs, and should include a Papanicolaou smear. As a general rule, estrogen should not be prescribed for longer than one year without reexamining the patient.

3. Diagnostic Measures should be taken to rule out gonorrhea or neoplasia before prescribing Estropipate Virginal Cream. Trichomonal, monilial, or bacterial infection should be treated by appropriate anti-microbial therapy.

4. Hypercoagulability: Some studies have shown that women taking estrogen replacement therapy have hypercoagulability, primarily related to decreased antithrombin activity. This effect appears dose- and duration-dependent and is less pronounced than that associated with oral contraceptive use. Also, postmenopausal women tend to have increased coagulation parameters at baseline compared to premenopausal women. There is some suggestion that low dose postmenopausal mestranol may increase the risk of thromboembolism, although the majority of studies (of primarily conjugated estrogens users) report no such increase. There is insufficient information on hypercoagulability in women who have had previous thromboembolic disease.

5. Familial Hyperlipoproteinemia: Estrogen therapy may be associated with massive elevations of plasma triglycerides leading to pancreatitis and other complications in patients with familial defects of lipoprotein metabolism.

6. Fluid Retention: Because estrogens may cause some degree of fluid retention, conditions which might be exacerbated by this factor, such as asthma, epilepsy, migraine, and cardiac or renal dysfunction, require careful observation.

7. Uterine Bleeding and Mastodynia: Certain patients may develop undesirable manifestations of excessive estrogenic stimulation, such as abnormal or excessive uterine bleeding and mastodynia.

8. Impaired liver function: Estrogen may be poorly metabolized in patients with impaired liver function and should be administered with caution.

9. Oral contraceptives appear to be associated with an increased incidence of mental depression. Although it is not clear whether this is due to the estrogenic or progestogenic component of the contraceptive, patients with a history of depression should be carefully observed.

10. Preexisting uterine leiomyomata may increase in size during estrogen use.

11. The pathologist should be advised of the patient's use of estrogen therapy when relevant specimens are submitted.

12. Patients with a past history of jaundice during pregnancy have an increased risk of recurrence of jaundice while receiving estrogen-containing oral contraceptive therapy. If jaundice develops in any patient receiving estrogen, the medication should be discontinued while the cause is investigated.

13. Because estrogens influence the metabolism of calcium and phosphorus, they should be used with caution in patients with metabolic bone diseases that are associated with hypercalcemia or in patients with renal insufficiency.

INFORMATION FOR THE PATIENT
See manufacturer's patient information.

DRUG INTERACTIONS
The concomitant use of any drugs which can induce hepatic microsomal enzymes with estrogens may produce estrogen levels which are lower than would be expected from the dose of estrogen administered. The use of **broad spectrum antibiotics** which profoundly affect intestinal flora may influence the absorption of steriodal compounds including the estrogens.

Diabetics receiving **insulin** may have increased insulin requirements when receiving estrogens.

LABORATORY TESTS
Estrogen administration should generally be guided by clinical response at the smallest dose, rather than laboratory monitoring, for relief of symptoms for those indications in which symptoms are observable. For prevention and treatment of osteoporosis, however, see "Dosage and Administration" section.

DRUG/LABORATORY TEST INTERACTIONS
1. Accelerated prothrombin time, partial thromboplastin time, and platelet aggregation time; increased platelet count; increased factors II, VII antigen, VIII antigen, VIII coagulant activity, IX, X, XII, VII—X complex. II—VII—X complex, and betathromboglobulin; decreased levels of anti-factor Xa and antithrombin III, decreased antithrombin III activity; increased levels of fibrinogen and fibrinogen activity; increased plasminogen antigen and activity.

2. Increased thyroid-binding globulin (TBG) leading to increased circulating total thyroid hormone, as measured by protein-bound iodine (PBI). T4 levels (by column or by radioimmunoassay) or T3 levels by radioimmunoassay). T3 resin uptake is decreased, reflecting the elevated TBG. Free T4 and free T3 concentrations are unaltered.

3. Other binding proteins may be elevated in serum, i.e., corticosteroid binding globulin (CBG), sex hormone-binding globulin (SHBG), leading to increased circulating corticosteroids and sex steroids respectively. Free or biologically active hormone concentrations are unchanged. Other plasma proteins may be increased (angiotensinogen/renin substrate, alpha-1-antitrypsin, ceruloplasmin).

4. Increased plasma HDL and HDL-2 subfraction concentrations, reduced LDL cholesterol concentration, increased triglycerides levels.

5. Impaired glucose tolerance.

6. Reduced response to metyrapone test.

7. Reduced serum folate concentration.

8. Decreased pregnanediol excretion.

9. Increased sulfobromophthalein retention.

CARCINOGENESIS, MUTAGENESIS, AND IMPAIRMENT OF FERTILITY
Long term continuous administration of natural and synthetic estrogens in certain animal species increases the frequency of carcinomas of the breast, uterus, cervix, vagina, testis, and liver. Studies have shown an increased risk of endometrial cancer in postmenopausal women exposed to exogenous estrogens for prolonged periods (see boxed "Warning"). At the present time there is no conclusive evidence that estrogens given to postmenopausal women increase the risk of cancer of the breast. There are, however, a few retrospective studies which suggest a small but statistically significant increase in the risk factor for breast cancer among these women. See "Contraindications" and "Warnings" sections.

PREGNANCY CATEGORY X
Estrogens should not be used during pregnancy. See "Contraindications" and boxed "Warning".

NURSING MOTHERS
Estrogens have been reported to be excreted in human breast milk. As a general principle, the administration of any drug to nursing mothers should be done only when clearly necessary since many drugs are excreted in human milk. In addition, estrogen administration to nursing mothers has been shown to decrease the quantity and quality of the milk.

PEDIATRIC USE
Because of the effects of estrogens on epiphyseal closure, they should be used judiciously in young patients in whom bone growth is not complete.

ADVERSE REACTIONS
The following additional adverse reactions have been reported with estrogen therapy in decreasing order of severity within each category (see "Warnings" regarding induction of neoplasia, adverse effects on the fetus, increased incidence of gallbladder disease, cardiovascular disease, elevated blood pressure, and hypercalcemia).

1. GENITOURINARY SYSTEM
Increase in size of uterine fibromyomata
Vaginal candidiasis
Cystitis-like syndrome
Dysmenorrhea
Amenorrhea during and after treatment
Change in cervical erosion and in degree of cervical secretion
Breakthrough bleeding, spotting, change in menstrual flow an abnormal withdrawal bleeding
Premenstrual-like syndrome

2. BREAST
Tenderness, enlargement, secretion

3. GASTROINTESTINAL
Cholestatic jaundice
Vomiting, nausea
Abdominal cramps, bloating
Increased incidence of gallbladder disease

4. SKIN
Hemorrhagic eruption
Erythema nodosum
Erythema multiforme
Hirsutism
Chloasma or melasma which may persist when drug is discontinued
Loss of scalp hair

5. EYES
Steepening of corneal curvature
Intolerance to contact lenses

6. CENTRAL NERVOUS SYSTEM
Chorea
Mental depression
Migraine, dizziness, headache

7. MISCELLANEOUS
Aggravation of porphyria
Edema
Reduced carbohydrate tolerance
Increase or decrease in weight

◆ RATED THERAPEUTICALLY EQUIVALENT; ◇ THERAPEUTIC EQUIVALENCE UNCONFIRMED; ○ UNRATED

Changes in libido

Hypersensitivity reactions, systemic effects such as breast tenderness, and rarely, withdrawal bleeding, have occurred with the use of topical estrogens. Local irritation (especially when prior inflammation is present) has occurred at initiation of therapy.

OVERDOSAGE

Serious ill effects have not been reported following acute ingestion of large doses of estrogen-containing oral contraceptives by young children. Overdosage of estrogen may cause nausea and vomiting, and withdrawal bleeding may occur in females.

DOSAGE AND ADMINISTRATION

ESTROPIPATE TABLETS

1. For treatment of moderate to severe vasomotor symptoms, vulval and vaginal atrophy associated with the menopause, the lowest dose and regimen that will control symptoms should be chosen and medication should be discontinued as promptly as possible.

Administration should be cyclic (e.g., 3 weeks on and 1 week off).

Attempts to discontinue or taper medication should be made at 3-month to 6-month intervals.

Usual dosage ranges:

Vasomotor Symptoms: 0.75 mg to 6 mg Estropipate per day. The lowest dose that will control symptoms should be chosen. If the patient has not menstruated within the last two months or more, cyclic administration is started arbitrarily. If the patient is menstruating, cyclic administration is started on day 5 of bleeding.

Vulval and Vaginal Atropy: 0.75 mg to 3 mg Estropipate per day, depending upon the tissue response of the individual patient. The lowest dose that will control symptoms should be chosen. Administer cyclically.

Atropic Vaginitis and Kraurosis Vulvae: 0.75 mg to 6 mg Estropipate daily, depending upon the tissue response of the individual patient. The lowest dose that will control symptoms should be chosen. Administer cyclically.

2. For treatment of female hypoestrogenism due to hypogonadism, castration, or primary ovarian failure. Usual dosage ranges:

Female Hypogonadism: 1.5 mg-9 mg Estropipate per day may be given for the first three weeks of a theoretical cycle, followed by a rest period of eight to ten days. The lowest dose that will control symptoms should be chosen. If bleeding does not occur by the end of this period, the same dosage schedule is repeated. The number of courses of estrogen therapy necessary to produce bleeding may vary depending on the responsiveness of the endometrium. If satisfactory withdrawal bleeding does not occur, an oral progestogen may be given in addition to estrogen during the third week of the cycle.

Female Castration or Primary Ovarian Failure: 1.5 mg-9 mg Estropipate per day may be given for the first three weeks of a theoretical cycle, followed by a rest period of eight to ten days. Adjust dosage upward or downward according to severity of symptoms and response of the patient. For maintenance, adjust dosage to lowest level that will provide effective control.

Treated patients with an intact uterus should be monitored closely for signs of endometrial cancer and appropriate diagnostic measures should be taken to rule out malignancy in the event of persistent or recurring abnormal vaginal bleeding.

3. For prevention of esteoporosis. A daily dose of 0.75 mg Estropipate for 25 days of a 31 day cycle per month.

ESTROPIPATE VAGINAL CREAM

For treatment of atrophic vaginitis or kraurosis vulvae.

The lowest dose that will control symptoms should be chosen and medication should be discontinued as promptly as possible.

Administration should be cyclic (e.g., three weeks on and one week off).

Attempts to discontinue or taper medication should be made at three to six-month intervals.

Treated patients with an intact uterus should be monitored closely for signs of endometrial cancer and appropriate diagnostic measures should be taken to rule out malignancy in the event of persistent or recurring abnormal vaginal bleeding.

Usual dosage: Intravaginally, 2 to 4 grams of Estropipate vaginal cream daily, depending upon the severity of the condition. The following instructions for use are intended for the patient and are printed on the carton label for Estropipate vaginal cream.

1. Remove cap from tube.
2. Make sure plunger of applicator is all the way into the barrel.
3. Screw nozzle end of applicator onto the tube.
4. Squeeze tube to force sufficient cream into applicator so that number on plunger indicating prescribed dose is level with top of barrel.
5. Unscrew applicator from tube and replace cap on tube.
6. To deliver medication, insert end of applicator into vagina and push plunger all the way down.

Between uses, pull plunger out of barrel and wash applicator in warm, soapy water. DO NOT PUT APPLICATOR IN HOT OR BOILING WATER.

TABLETS AND CREAM

Recommended storage: Store below 77°F (25°C).

REFERENCES

1. Ziel, H.K., Finkle, W.D., "Increased Risk of Endometrial Carcinoma Among Users of Conjugated Estrogens," New England Journal of Medicine. 293:1167—1170, 1975. 2. Smith, D.C., Prentic, R., Thompson, D.J., et al., "Association of Exogenous Estrogen and Endometrial Carcinoma," New England Journal of Medicine, 293:1164-1167, 1975. 3. Mack, T.M., Pike, M.C., Henderson, B.E., et al., "Estrogens and Endometrial Cancer in a Retirement Community," New Engalnd Journal of Medicine, 294:1262—1267, 1976. 4. Weiss, N.S., Szekely, D.R., Austin, D.F., "Increasing Incidence of Endometrial Cancer in the United States," New England Journal of Medicine, 294:1259—1262, 1976. 5. Herbst, A.L., Ulfielder, H., Poskanzer, D.C., "Adenocarcinoma of the Vagina," New England Journal of Medicine, 284:878—881, 1971. 6. Greenwald, P., Barlow, J., Nasca, P., et al., 'Vaginal Cancer after Maternal Treatment with Synthetic Estrogens," New England Journal of Medicine, 285:390—392, 1971. 7. Lanier, A., Noller, K., Decker, D., et al., "Cancer and Stilbestrol, A Follow-up of 1719 Persons Exposed to Estrogens in Utero and Born 1943-1959," Mayo Clinic Proceedings, 48:793—799, 1973. 8. Herbst, A., Kurman, R., Scully, R., "Vaginal and Cervical Abnormalities After Exposure to Stilbestrol In Utero," Obstetrics and Gynecology, 40:287—298, 1972. 9. Herbst, A., Robboy, S., Macdonald, G., et al., 'The Effects of Local Progestrone on Stilbestrol-Associated Vaginal Adenosis," American Journal of Obstetrics and Gynecology, 118:607—615, 1974. 10. Herbst, A., Poskanzer, D., Robboy, S., et al., "Prenatal Exposure to Stilbestrol, A Prospective Comparison to Exposed Female Offspring with Unexposed Controls," New England Journal of Medicine, 292:334—339, 1975. 11. Stafl, A., Mattingly, R., Foley, D., et al., "Clinical Diagnosis of Vaginal Adenosis," Obstetrics and Gynecology, 44:531—545, 1974. 13. Gal, I., Kirman, B., Stern, J., "Hormone Pregnancy Tests and Congenital Malformation," Nature, 216:83, 1967. 14. Levy, E.P., Cohen, A., Fraser, F.C., "Hormone Treatment During Pregnancy and Congenital Heart Defects," Lancet, 1:611, 1973. 15. Nora, J., Nora, A., "Birth Defects and Oral Contraceptives," Lancet, 1:941—942, 1973. 16. Janerich, D.T., Piper, J.M., Glebatis, D.M., "Oral Contraceptives and Congenital Limb-Reduction Defects," New England Journal of Medicine, 291:697—700, 1974. 17. Boston Collaborative Drug Surveillance Program, "Surgically Confirmed Gallbladder Disease, Venous Thromboembolism and Breast Tumors in Relation to Post-Menopausal Estrogen Therapy," New England Journal of Medicine, 290:15—19, 1974. 18. Brinton, L.A., Hoover, R.N., Szklo, M., et al., "Menopausal Estrogen Use and Risk of Breast Cancer," Cancer, 47(10):2517—2522, 1981. 19. Boston Collaborative Drug Surveillance Program, "Oral Contraceptives and Venous Thromboembolic Disease, Surgically Confirmed Gallbladder Disease and Breast Tumors," Lancet, 1:1399—1404, 1973. 20. Daniel, D.G., Campbell, H., Turnbull, A.C., "Puerperal Thromboembolism and Suppression of Lactation," Lancet, 2:287—289, 1967. 21. Bailar, J.C., "Thromboembolism and Oestrogen Therapy," Lancet, 2:560, 1967. 22. Royal College of General Practitioner, "Oral Contraception and Thromboembolic Disease," Journal of the Royal College of General Practitioners, 13:267—279, 1967. 23. Inman, W.H.W., Vessey, M.P., "Investigations of Deaths from Pulmonary, Coronary and Cerebral Thrombosis and Embolism in Women of Childbearing Age," British Medical Journal, 2:193—199, 1968. 24. Vessey, M.P., Doll, R., "Investigation of Relation Between Use of Oral Contraceptives and Thromboembolic Disease. A Further Report," British Medical Journal, 2:651—657, 1969. 25. Sartwell, P.E., Masi, A.T., Arthes, F.G., et al., "Thromboembolism and Oral Contraceptives: An Epidimiological Case Control Study," American Journal of Epidimiology, 90:365—380, 1969. 26. Collaborative Group for the Study of stroke in Young Women, "Oral Contraception and Increased Risk of Cerebral Ischemia or Thrombosis," New England Journal of Medicine, 288:871—878, 1973. 27. Collaborative Group for the Study of stroke in Young Women, "Oral Contraceptives and Stroke in Young Women: Associated Risk Factors," Journal of the American Medical Association, 231:718—722, 1975. 28. Mann, J.I., Inman, W.H.W., "Oral Contraceptives and Death from Myocardial Infarction," British Medical Journal, 2:245—248, 1975. 29. Mann, J.I., Vessey, M.P., Thorogood, M., et al., "Myocardial Infarction in Young Women with Special Reference to Oral contraceptive Practice," British Medical Journal, 2:241—245, 1975. 30. Inman, W.H.W., Vessey, M.P., Westerholm, B., et al., "Thromboembolic Disease and the Steroidal Content of Oral Contraceptive," British Medical Journal, 2:203—209, 1970. 31. Stolley, P.D., Tonascia, J.A., Tockman, M.S., et al., Thrombosis with Low-Estrogen Oral Contraceptives," American Journal of Epidimiology, 102:197—208, 1975. 32. Vessey, M.P., Doll, R., Fairbairn, A.S., et al., "Post Operative Thromboembolism and the Use of the Oral Contraceptives," British Medical Journal, 3:123—126, 1970. 33. Greene, G.R., Sartwell, P.E., "Oral Contraceptive Use in Patients with Thromoboembolism Following Surgery, Trauma or Infection," American Journal of Public Health, 62:680—685, 1972. 34. Rosenberg, L., Armstrong, M.B., Jick, H., "Myocardial Infarction and Estrogen Therapy in Postmenopausal Women," New England Journal of Medicine, 294:1256—1259, 1976. 35. Coronary Drug Project Research Group, "The Coronary Drug Project: Initial Findings Leading to Modifications of Its Research Protocol," Journal of the American Medical Association, 214:1303—1313, 1970. 36. Baum, J., Holtz, F., Bookstein, J.J., et al., "Possible Association Between Benign Hepatomas and Oral Contraceptives," Lancet, 2:926—928, 1973. 37. Mays, E.T., Christopherson, W.M., Mahr, M.M., et al., "Hepatic Changes in Young Women Ingesting Contraceptive Steroids, Hepatic Hemorrhage and Primary Hepatic Tumors," Journal of the American Medical Association, 235:730—782, 1976. 38. Edmondson, H.A., Henderson, B., Benton, B., "Liver Cell Adenomas Associated with the Use of Oral Contraceptives," New England Journal of Medicine, 294:470—472, 1976. 39. Pfeffer, R.I., Van Den Noort, S., "Estrogen Use and Stroke Risk in Postmenopausal Women," American Journal of Epidimiology, 103:445—456, 1976. 40. Gambrell, R.D., Massey, F.M., Castaneda, T.A., et al., "Estrogen Therapy and Breast Cancer in Postmenopausal Women," Journal of the American Geriatrics Society, 28(6):251—257, 1980. 41. Kelsey, J.L., Fischer, D.B., Holford, T.R., et al., "Exogenous Estrogen and Other Factors in the Epidimiology of Breast Cancer," Journal of the National Cancer Institute, 57(2):327—333, 1981. 42. Ross, R.K., Paganini-Hill, A., Gerkins, V., et al., "A Case-Control Study of Menopausal Estrogen Therapy and Breast Cancer," Journal of the American Medical Association, 243(16):1635—1639, 1980. 43. Hoover, R., Glass, A., Finkle, W.D., et al., "Conjugated Estrogens and Breast Cancer Risk in Women," Journal of the National Cancer Institute, 67(4):815—820, 1981. 44. Lawson, D.H., Jick, H., Hunter, J.R., et al., "Exogenous Estrogens and Breast Cancer," American Journal of Epidimiology, 114(5):710, 1981.

HOW SUPPLIED

CREAM: 1.5 MG/GM

BRAND/MANUFACTURER	*NDC*	*SIZE*	*AWP*
○ **BRAND**			
OGEN: Upjohn	00009-3776-01	42.5 gm	$37.61

➤ SHOWN IN PRODUCT IDENTIFICATION GUIDE

TABLETS: 0.625 MG

AVERAGE UNIT PRICE (AVAILABLE SIZES)

BRAND	$0.42

BRAND/MANUFACTURER	NDC	SIZE	AWP
◆ BRAND			
➤ ORTHO-EST: Ortho Pharm	00062-1801-01	100s	$33.16
OGEN .625: Upjohn	00009-3772-01	100s	$51.13
◆ GENERICS			
Rugby	00536-3560-01	100s	$46.05

TABLETS: 0.75 MG

AVERAGE UNIT PRICE (AVAILABLE SIZES)

GENERIC	$0.43	GENERIC A-RATED AVERAGE PRICE (GAAP)	
		100s	$43.15

BRAND/MANUFACTURER	NDC	SIZE	AWP
◆ GENERICS			
Duramed	51285-0875-02	100s	$40.90
Schein	00364-2600-01	100s	$41.28
Watson	52544-0414-01	100s	$41.28
URL	00677-1508-01	100s	$43.00
Qualitest	00603-3559-01	100s	$43.12
Goldline	00182-1976-01	100s	$43.71
Warner Chilcott	00047-0124-24	100s	$45.95
Geneva	00781-1543-01	100s	$45.97

TABLETS: 1.25 MG

AVERAGE UNIT PRICE (AVAILABLE SIZES)

BRAND	$0.58

BRAND/MANUFACTURER	NDC	SIZE	AWP
◆ BRAND			
➤ ORTHO-EST: Ortho Pharm	00062-1800-01	100s	$45.37
OGEN 1.25: Upjohn	00009-3773-01	100s	$71.43
◆ GENERICS			
Rugby	00536-3561-01	100s	$64.46

TABLETS: 1.5 MG

AVERAGE UNIT PRICE (AVAILABLE SIZES)

GENERIC	$0.60	GENERIC A-RATED AVERAGE PRICE (GAAP)	
		100s	$60.27

BRAND/MANUFACTURER	NDC	SIZE	AWP
◆ GENERICS			
Duramed	51285-0876-02	100s	$57.14
Schein	00364-2601-01	100s	$57.67
Watson	52544-0415-01	100s	$57.67
URL	00677-1509-01	100s	$60.00
Qualitest	00603-3560-21	100s	$60.35
Goldline	00182-1977-01	100s	$61.07
Warner Chilcott	00047-0126-24	100s	$64.00
Geneva	00781-1553-01	100s	$64.22

TABLETS: 2.5 MG

BRAND/MANUFACTURER	NDC	SIZE	AWP
◆ BRAND			
OGEN 2.5: Upjohn	00009-3774-01	100s	$124.33

TABLETS: 3 MG

AVERAGE UNIT PRICE (AVAILABLE SIZES)

GENERIC	$1.05	GENERIC A-RATED AVERAGE PRICE (GAAP)	
		100s	$104.91

BRAND/MANUFACTURER	NDC	SIZE	AWP
◆ GENERICS			
Qualitest	00603-3561-21	100s	$100.35
Watson	52544-0416-01	100s	$100.39
Warner Chilcott	00047-0128-24	100s	$105.75
Goldline	00182-1978-01	100s	$106.30
Geneva	00781-1563-01	100s	$111.77

TABLETS: 6 MG

BRAND/MANUFACTURER	NDC	SIZE	AWP
◆ GENERICS			
Goldline	00182-1979-17	100s	$157.84

Estrovis SEE QUINESTROL

Ethacrynic Acid

Ethacrynic Acid is a potent diuretic which, if given in excessive amounts, may lead to profound diuresis with water and electrolyte depletion. Therefore, careful medical supervision is required, and dose and dose schedule must be adjusted to the individual patient's needs (see *"Dosage and Administration"*).

DESCRIPTION

Ethacrynic Acid is an unsaturated ketone derivative of an aryloxyacetic acid. It is designated chemically as [2,3-dichloro-4-(2-methylene-1-oxobutyl)phenoxy] acetic acid, and has a molecular weight of 303.14. Ethacrynic Acid is a white, or practically white, crystalline powder, very slightly soluble in water, but soluble in most organic solvents such as alcohols, chloroform, and benzene. Its empirical formula is $C_{13}H_{12}Cl_2O_4$:

Ethacrynate sodium, the sodium salt of Ethacrynic Acid, is soluble in water at 25°C to the extent of about 7 percent. Solutions of the sodium salt are relatively stable at about pH 7 at room temperature for short periods, but as the pH or temperature increases the solutions are less stable. The molecular weight of Ethacrynate sodium is 325.12. Its empirical formula is $C_{13}H_{11}Cl_2NaO_4$.

Ethacrynic Acid is supplied as 25 mg and 50 mg tablets for oral use. Intravenous Ethacrynate sodium is a sterile freeze-dried powder and is supplied in a vial containing Ethacrynate sodium equivalent to Ethacrynic acid, 50.0 mg

Following is its chemical structure:

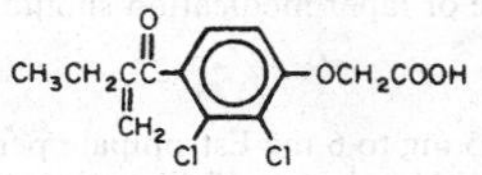

$$CH_3CH_2C \cdots \cdots OCH_2COOH$$
$$CH_2 \quad Cl \quad Cl$$

CLINICAL PHARMACOLOGY

Pharmacokinetics and Metabolism: Ethacrynic Acid acts on the ascending limb of the loop of Henle and on the proximal and distal tubules. Urinary output is usually dose dependent and related to the magnitude of fluid accumulation. Water and electrolyte excretion may be increased several times over that observed with thiazide diuretics, since Ethacrynic Acid inhibits reabsorption of a much greater proportion of filtered sodium than most other diuretic agents. Therefore, Ethacrynic Acid is effective in many patients who have significant degrees of renal insufficiency (see *"Warnings"* concerning deafness). Ethacrynic Acid has little or no effect on glomerular filtration or on renal blood flow, except following pronounced reductions in plasma volume when associated with rapid diuresis.

The electrolyte excretion pattern of ethacrynic acid varies from that of the thiazides and mercurial diuretics. Initial sodium and chloride excretion is usually substantial and chloride loss exceeds that of sodium. With prolonged administration, chloride excretion declines, and potassium and hydrogen ion excretion may increase. Ethacrynic Acid is effective whether or not there is clinical acidosis or alkalosis.

Although Ethacrynic Acid in carefully controlled studies in animals and experimental subjects produces a more favorable sodium/potassium excretion ratio than the thiazides, in patients with increased diuresis excessive amounts of potassium may be excreted.

Onset of action is rapid, usually within 30 minutes after an oral dose of Ethacrynic Acid or within 5 minutes after an intravenous injection of Ethacrynate sodium. After oral use, diuresis peaks in about 2 hours and lasts about 6 to 8 hours.

The sulfhydryl binding propensity of ethacrynic acid differs somewhat from that of the organomercurials. Its mode of action is not by carbonic anhydrase inhibition.

Ethacrynic Acid does not cross the blood-brain barrier.

INDICATIONS AND USAGE

Ethacrynic Acid is indicated for treatment of edema when an agent with greater diuretic potential than those commonly employed is required.

1. Treatment of the edema associated with congestive heart failure, cirrhosis of the liver, and renal disease, including the nephrotic syndrome.

2. Short-term management of ascites due to malignancy, idiopathic edema, and lymphedema.

3. Short-term management of hospitalized pediatric patients, other than infants, with congenital heart disease or the nephrotic syndrome.

4. Intravenous Ethacrynate sodium is indicated when a rapid onset of diuresis is desired, e.g., in acute pulmonary edema, or when gastrointestinal absorption is impaired or oral medication is not practicable.

UNLABELED USES
Ethacrynic Acid is used alone or as an adjunct in the treatment of bromide intoxication, diabetes insipidus, hypercalcemia, and hypertension.

CONTRAINDICATIONS

All diuretics, including ethacrynic acid, are contraindicated in anuria. If increasing electrolyte imbalance, azotemia, and/or oliguria occur during treatment of severe, progressive renal disease, the diuretic should be discontinued.

In a few patients this diuretic has produced severe, watery diarrhea. If this occurs, it should be discontinued and not used again.

Until further experience in infants is accumulated, therapy with oral and parenteral Ethacrynic Acid is contraindicated.

Hypersensitivity to any component of this product.

WARNINGS

The effects of Ethacrynic Acid on electrolytes are related to its renal pharmacologic activity and are dose dependent. The possibility of profound electrolyte and

---

◆ RATED THERAPEUTICALLY EQUIVALENT; ◇ THERAPEUTIC EQUIVALENCE UNCONFIRMED; ○ UNRATED

water loss may be avoided by weighing the patient throughout the treatment period, by careful adjustment of dosage, by initiating treatment with small doses, and by using the drug on an intermittent schedule when possible. When excessive diuresis occurs, the drug should be withdrawn until homeostasis is restored. When excessive electrolyte loss occurs, the dosage should be reduced or the drug temporarily withdrawn.

Initiation of diuretic therapy with Ethacrynic Acid in the cirrhotic patient with ascites is best carried out in the hospital. When maintenance therapy has been established, the individual can be satisfactorily followed as an outpatient.

Ethacrynic Acid should be given with caution to patients with advanced cirrhosis of the liver, particularly those with a history of previous episodes of electrolyte imbalance or hepatic encephalopathy. Like other diuretics it may precipitate hepatic coma and death.

Too vigorous a diuresis, as evidenced by rapid and excessive weight loss, may induce an acute hypotensive episode. In elderly cardiac patients, rapid contraction of plasma volume and the resultant hemoconcentration should be avoided to prevent the development of thromboembolic episodes, such as cerebral vascular thromboses and pulmonary emboli which may be fatal. Excessive loss of potassium in patients receiving digitalis glycosides may precipitate digitalis toxicity. Care should also be exercised in patients receiving potassium-depleting steroids.

A number of possibly drug-related deaths have occurred in critically ill patients refractory to other diuretics. These generally have fallen into two categories: (1) patients with severe myocardial disease who have been receiving digitalis and presumably developed acute hypokalemia with fatal arrhythmia; (2) patients with severely decompensated hepatic cirrhosis with ascites, with or without accompanying encephalopathy, who were in electrolyte imbalance and died because of intensification of the electrolyte defect.

Deafness, tinnitus, and vertigo with a sense of fullness in the ears have occurred, most frequently in patients with severe impairment of renal function. These symptoms have been associated most often with intravenous administration and with doses in excess of those recommended. The deafness has usually been reversible and of short duration (one to 24 hours). However, in some patients the hearing loss has been permanent. A number of these patients were also receiving drugs known to be ototoxic. Ethacrynic Acid may increase the ototoxic potential of other drugs (see *"Precautions"*, subsection *"Drug Interactions"*).

Lithium generally should not be given with diuretics (see *"Precautions"*, subsection *"Drug Interactions"*).

PRECAUTIONS

General: Weakness, muscle cramps, paresthesias, thirst, anorexia, and signs of hyponatremia, hypokalemia, and/or hypochloremic alkalosis may occur following vigorous or excessive diuresis and these may be accentuated by rigid salt restriction. Rarely tetany has been reported following vigorous diuresis. *During therapy with ethacrynic acid, liberalization of salt intake and supplementary potassium chloride are often necessary.*

When a metabolic alkalosis may be anticipated, e.g., in cirrhosis with ascites, the use of potassium chloride or a potassium-sparing agent before and during therapy with Ethacrynic Acid may mitigate or prevent the hypokalemia.

Loop diuretics have been shown to increase the urinary excretion of magnesium; this may result in hypomagnesemia. The safety and efficacy of Ethacrynic Acid in hypertension have not been established. However, the dosage of coadministered antihypertensive agents may require adjustment.

Orthostatic hypotension may occur in patients receiving other antihypertensive agents when given ethacrynic acid. Ethacrynic Acid has little or no effect on glomerular filtration or on renal blood flow, except following pronounced reductions in plasma volume when associated with rapid diuresis. A transient increase in serum urea nitrogen may occur. Usually, this is readily reversible when the drug is discontinued. As with other diuretics used in the treatment of renal edema, hypoproteinemia may reduce responsiveness to Ethacrynic Acid and the use of salt-poor albumin should be considered. A number of drugs, including Ethacrynic Acid, have been shown to displace warfarin from plasma protein; a reduction in the usual anticoagulant dosage may be required in patients receiving both drugs.

Ethacrynic Acid may increase the risk of gastric hemorrhage associated with corticosteroid treatment.

Laboratory Tests: Frequent serum electrolyte, CO_2 and BUN determinations should be performed early in therapy and periodically thereafter during active diuresis. Any electrolyte abnormalities should be corrected or the drug temporarily withdrawn. Increases in blood glucose and alterations in glucose tolerance tests have been observed in patients receiving Ethacrynic Acid.

Drug Interactions: Lithium generally should not be given with diuretics because they reduce its renal clearance and add a high risk of lithium toxicity. Read circulars for lithium preparations before use of such concomitant therapy.

Ethacrynic Acid may increase the ototoxic potential of other drugs such as aminoglycoside and some cephalosporin antibiotics. Their concurrent use should be avoided.

A number of drugs, including ethacrynic acid, have been shown to displace warfarin from plasma protein; a reduction in the usual anticoagulant dosage may be required in patients receiving both drugs.

In some patients, the administration of a nonsteroidal anti-inflammatory agent can reduce the diuretic, natriuretic, and antihypertensive effects of loop, potassium-sparing and thiazide diuretics. Therefore, when Ethacrynic Acid and non-steroidal anti-inflammatory agents are used concomitantly, the patient should be observed closely to determine if the desired effect of the diuretic is obtained.

Carcinogenesis, Mutagenesis, Impairment of Fertility: There was no evidence of a tumorigenic effect in a 79-week oral chronic toxicity study in rats at doses up to 45 times the human dose.

Ethacrynic acid had no effect on fertility in a two-litter study in rats or a two-generation study in mice at 10 times the human dose.

Pregnancy Category B: Reproduction studies in the mouse and rabbit at doses up to 50 times the human dose showed no evidence of external abnormalities of the fetus due to Ethacrynic Acid.

In a two-litter study in the dog and rat, oral doses of 5 or 20 mg/kg/day (2 ½ or 10 times the human dose), respectively, did not interfere with pregnancy or with growth and development of the pups. Although there was reduction in the mean body weights of the fetuses in a teratogenic study in the rat at a dose level of 100 mg/kg (50 times the human dose), there was no effect on mortality or postnatal development. Functional and morphologic abnormalities were not observed.

There are, however, no adequate and well-controlled studies in pregnant women. Since animal reproduction studies are not always predictive of human response Ethacrynic Acid should be used during pregnancy only if clearly needed.

Nursing Mothers: It is not known whether this drug is excreted in human milk. Because many drugs are excreted in human milk and because of the potential for serious adverse reactions in nursing infants from Ethacrynic Acid, a decision should be made whether to discontinue nursing or to discontinue the drug, taking into account the importance of the drug to the mother.

Pediatric Use: For information on oral use in pediatrics, other than infants, see *"Indications and Usage"* and *"Dosage and Administration"*.

Safety and effectiveness in infants have not been established (see *"Contraindications"*).

Safety and effectiveness of intravenous use in children have not been established (see *"Dosage and Administration, Intravenous Use"*).

ADVERSE REACTIONS

Gastrointestinal: Anorexia, malaise, abdominal discomfort or pain, dysphagia, nausea, vomiting, and diarrhea have occurred. These are more frequent with large doses or after one to three months of continuous therapy. A few patients have had sudden onset of profuse, watery diarrhea. Discontinue Ethacrynic Acid if diarrhea is severe and do not give it again. Gastrointestinal bleeding has occurred in some patients. Rarely, acute pancreatitis has been reported.

Metabolic: Reversible hyperuricemia and acute gout have been reported. Acute symptomatic hypoglycemia with convulsions occurred in two uremic patients who received doses above those recommended. Hyperglycemia has been reported. Rarely, jaundice and abnormal liver function tests have been reported in seriously ill patients receiving multiple drug therapy, including Ethacrynic Acid.

Hematologic: Agranulocytosis or severe neutropenia has been reported in a few critically ill patients also receiving agents known to produce this effect. Thrombocytopenia has been reported rarely. Henoch-Schonlein purpura has been reported rarely in patients with rheumatic heart disease receiving multiple drug therapy, including Ethacrynic Acid.

Special Senses (see "Warnings"): Deafness, tinnitus and vertigo with a sense of fullness in the ears, and blurred vision have occurred.

Central Nervous System: Headache, fatigue, apprehension, confusion.

Miscellaneous: Skin rash, fever, chills, hematuria. Ethacrynate sodium occasionally has caused local irritation and pain after intravenous use.

OVERDOSAGE

Overdosage may lead to excessive diuresis with electrolyte depletion and dehydration.

In the event of overdosage, symptomatic and supportive measures should be employed. Emesis should be induced or gastric lavage performed. Correct dehydration, electrolyte imbalance, hepatic coma, and hypotension by established procedures. If required, give oxygen or artificial respiration for respiratory impairment.

In the mouse, the oral LD_{50} of Ethacrynic Acid is 627 mg/kg and the intravenous LD_{50} of ethacrynate sodium is 175 mg/kg.

DOSAGE AND ADMINISTRATION

Dosage must be regulated carefully to prevent a more rapid or substantial loss of fluid or electrolyte than is indicated or necessary . The magnitude of diuresis and natriuresis is largely dependent on the degree of fluid accumulation present in the patient. Similarly, the extent of potassium excretion is determined in large measure by the presence and magnitude of aldosteronism.

Oral Use: Ethacrynic Acid is available for oral use as 25 mg and 50 mg tablets.

Dosage: To Initiate Diuresis:

In Adults: The smallest dose required to produce gradual weight loss (about 1 to 2 pounds per day) is recommended. Onset of diuresis usually occurs at 50 to 100 mg for adults. After diuresis has been achieved, the minimally effective dose (usually from 50 to 200 mg daily) may be given on a continuous or intermittent dosage schedule. Dosage adjustments are usually in 25 to 50 mg increments to avoid derangement of water and electrolyte excretion.

The patient should be weighted under standard conditions before and during the institution of diuretic therapy with this compound. Small alterations in dose should effectively prevent a massive diuretic response. The following schedule may be helpful in determining the smallest effective dose.

Day 1—50 mg (single dose) after a meal
Day 2—50 mg twice daily after meals, if necessary
Day 3—100 mg in the morning and 50 to 100 mg following the afternoon or evening meal, depending upon response to the morning dose.

A few patients may require initial and maintenance doses as high as 200 mg twice daily. These higher doses, which should be achieved gradually, are most often required in patients with severe, refractory edema.

In children: (excluding infants, see "Contraindications"): The initial dose should be 25 mg. Careful stepwise increments in dosage of 25 mg should be made to achieve effective maintenance.

Maintenance Therapy: It is usually possible to reduce the dosage and frequency of administration once dry weight has been achieved.

Ethacrynic Acid may be given intermittently after an effective diuresis is obtained with the regimen outlined above. Dosage may be on an alternate daily schedule or more prolonged periods of diuretic therapy may be interspersed with rest periods. Such an intermittent dosage schedule allows time for correction of any electrolyte imbalance and may provide a more efficient diuretic response.

The chloruretic effect of this agent may give rise to retention of bicarbonate and a metabolic alkalosis. This may be corrected by giving chloride (ammonium chloride or arginine chloride). Ammonium chloride should not be given to cirrhotic patients.

Ethacrynic Acid has additive effects when used with other diuretics. For example, a patient who is on maintenance dosage of an oral diuretic may require additional intermittent diuretic therapy, such as an organomercurial, for the maintenance of basal weight. The intermittent use of Ethacrynic Acid orally may eliminate the need for injections of organomercurials. Small doses of Ethacrynic Acid may be added to existing diuretic regimens to maintain basal weight. This drug may potentiate the action of carbonic anhydrase inhibitors, with augmentation of natriuresis and kaluresis. Therefore, when adding Ethacrynic Acid the initial dose and changes of dose should be in 25 mg increments, to avoid electrolyte depletion. Rarely, patients who failed to respond to ethacrynic acid have responded to older established agents.

While many patients do not require supplemental potassium, the use of potassium chloride or potassium-sparing agents, or both, during treatment with Ethacrynic Acid is advisable, especially in cirrhotic or nephrotic patients and in patients receiving digitalis.

Salt liberalization usually prevents the development of hyponatremia and hypochloremia. During treatment with Ethacrynic Acid salt may be liberalized to a greater extent than with other diuretics. Cirrhotic patients, however, usually require at least moderate salt restriction concomitant with diuretic therapy.

Intravenous Use: Intravenous Ethacrynate sodium is for intravenous use when oral intake is impractical or in urgent conditions, such as acute pulmonary edema.

The usual intravenous dose for the average sized adult is 50 mg, or 0.5 to 1.0 mg per kg of body weight. Usually only one dose has been necessary; occasionally a second dose at a new injection site, to avoid possible thrombophlebitis, may be required. A single intravenous dose not exceeding 100 mg has been used in critical situations.

Insufficient pediatric experience precludes recommendation for this age group.

To reconstitute the dry material, add 50 mL of 5 percent Dextrose Injection, or Sodium Chloride Injection to the vial. Occasionally, some 5 percent Dextrose Injection solutions may have a low pH (below 5). The resulting solution with such a diluent may be hazy or opalescent. Intravenous use of such a solution is not recommended. Inspect the vial containing Intravenous Ethacrynate sodium for particulate matter and discoloration before use.

The solution may be given slowly through the tubing of a running infusion or by direct intravenous injection over a period of several minutes. Do not mix this solution with whole blood or its derivatives. Discard unused reconstituted solution after 24 hours.

Ethacrynate sodium should not be given subcutaneously or intramuscularly because of local pain and irritation.

HOW SUPPLIED
POWDER FOR INJECTION: 50 MG

BRAND/MANUFACTURER	NDC	SIZE	AWP
○ **BRAND**			
EDECRIN SODIUM: Merck	00006-3330-50	1s	$18.25

TABLETS: 25 MG

BRAND/MANUFACTURER	NDC	SIZE	AWP
○ **BRAND**			
EDECRIN: Merck	00006-0065-68	100s	$28.61

TABLETS: 50 MG

BRAND/MANUFACTURER	NDC	SIZE	AWP
○ **BRAND**			
EDECRIN: Merck	00006-0090-68	100s	$40.78

Ethambutol Hydrochloride

DESCRIPTION
Ethambutol Hydrochloride is an oral chemotherapeutic agent which is specifically effective against actively growing microorganisms of the genus *Mycobacterium*, including *M tuberculosis*.

Ethambutol Hydrochloride is available in 100 mg and 400 mg oral tablets.

Following is its chemical structure:

$$CH_3CH_2-\underset{\underset{H}{|}}{\overset{\overset{CH_2OH}{|}}{C}}-NHCH_2CH_2NH-\underset{\underset{CH_2OH}{|}}{\overset{\overset{H}{|}}{C}}-CH_2CH_3 \cdot 2HCl$$

ACTION
Ethambutol Hydrochloride, following a single oral dose of 25 mg/kg of body weight, attains a peak of 2 to 5 micrograms/mL in serum 2 to 4 hours after administration. When the drug is administered daily for longer periods of time at this dose, serum levels are similar. The serum level of Ethambutol Hydrochloride falls to undetectable levels by 24 hours after the last dose except in some patients with abnormal renal function. The intracellular concentrations of erythrocytes reach peak values approximately twice those of plasma and maintain this ratio throughout the 24 hours.

During the 24-hour period following oral administration of Ethambutol Hydrochloride approximately 50% of the initial dose is excreted unchanged in the urine, while an additional 8% to 15% appears in the form of metabolites. The main path of metabolism appears to be an initial oxidation of the alcohol to an aldehydic intermediate, followed by conversion to a dicarboxylic acid. From 20% to 22% of the initial dose is excreted in the feces as unchanged drug. No drug accumulation has been observed with consecutive single daily doses of 25 mg/kg in patients with normal kidney function, although marked accumulation has been demonstrated in patients with renal insufficiency.

Ethambutol Hydrochloride diffuses into actively growing *mycobacterium* cells such as tubercle bacilli. Ethambutol Hydrochloride appears to inhibit the synthesis of one or more metabolites, thus causing impairment of cell metabolism, arrest of multiplication, and cell death. No cross resistance with other available antimycobacterial agents has been demonstrated.

Ethambutol Hydrochloride has been shown to be effective against strains of *Mycobacterium tuberculosis* but does not seem to be active against fungi, viruses, or other bacteria. *Mycobacterium tuberculosis* strains previously unexposed to Ethambutol Hydrochloride have been uniformly sensitive to concentrations of 8 or less micrograms/mL, depending on the nature of the culture media. When Ethambutol Hydrochloride has been used alone for treatment of tuberculosis, tubercle bacilli from these patients have developed resistance to Ethambutol Hydrochloride by *in vitro* susceptibility tests; the development of resistance has been unpredictable and appears to occur in a step-like manner. No cross resistance between Ethambutol Hydrochloride and other antituberculous drugs has been reported.

Ethambutol Hydrochloride has reduced the incidence of the emergence of mycobacterial resistance to isoniazid when both drugs have been used concurrently.

An agar diffusion microbiologic assay, based upon inhibition of *Mycobacterium smegmatis* (ATCC 607) may be used to determine concentrations of Ethambutol Hydrochloride in serum and urine. This technique has not been published, but further information can be obtained upon inquiry to Lederle Laboratories.

ANIMAL PHARMACOLOGY
Toxicological studies in dogs on high prolonged doses produced evidence of myocardial damage and failure, and depigmentation of the tapetum lucidum of the eyes, the significance of which is not known. Degenerative changes in the central nervous system, apparently not dose-related, have also been noted in dogs receiving Ethambutol Hydrochloride over a prolonged period.

In the rhesus monkey, neurological signs appeared after treatment with high doses given daily over a period of several months. These were correlated with specific serum levels of Ethambutol Hydrochloride and with definite neuroanatomical changes in the central nervous system. Focal interstitial carditis was also noted in monkeys which received Ethambutol Hydrochloride in high doses for a prolonged period.

When pregnant mice or rabbits were treated with high doses of Ethambutol Hydrochloride, fetal mortality was slightly but not significantly ($P > 0.05$) increased. Female rats treated with Ethambutol Hydrochloride displayed slight but insignificant ($P > 0.05$) decreases in fertility and litter size.

In fetuses born of mice treated with high doses of Ethambutol Hydrochloride during pregnancy, a low incidence of cleft palate, exencephaly and abnormality of the vertebral column were observed. Minor abnormalities of the cervical vertebra were seen in the newborn of rats treated with high doses of Ethambutol Hydrochloride during pregnancy. Rabbits receiving high doses of Ethambutol Hydrochloride during pregnancy gave birth to two fetuses with monophthalmia, one with a shortened right forearm accompanied by bilateral wrist-joint contracture and one with hare lip and cleft palate.

◆ RATED THERAPEUTICALLY EQUIVALENT; ◇ THERAPEUTIC EQUIVALENCE UNCONFIRMED; ○ UNRATED

INDICATIONS

Ethambutol Hydrochloride is indicated for the treatment of pulmonary tuberculosis. It should not be used as the sole antituberculous drug, but should be used in conjunction with at least one other antituberculous drug. Selection of the companion drug should be based on clinical experience, considerations of comparative safety and appropriate *in vitro* susceptibility studies. In patients who have not received previous antituberculous therapy, ie, initial treatment, the most frequently used regimens have been the following.

　　Ethambutol Hydrochloride plus isoniazid
　　Ethambutol Hydrochloride plus isoniazid plus streptomycin.

In patients who have received previous antituberculous therapy, mycobacterial resistance to other drugs used in initial therapy is frequent. Consequently, in such retreatment patients, Ethambutol Hydrochloride should be combined with at least one of the second line drugs not previously administered to the patient and to which bacterial susceptibility has been indicated by appropriate *in vitro* studies. Antituberculous drugs used with Ethambutol Hydrochloride have included cycloserine, ethionamide, pyrazinamide, viomycin, and other drugs. Isoniazid, aminosalicylic acid, and streptomycin have also been used in multiple drug regimens. Alternating drug regimens have also been utilized.

UNLABELED USES

Ethambutol Hydrochloride is used as an adjunct in the treatment of atypical mycobacterial infections including Mycobacterium Kansasii and Micobacterium Avium Complex (MAC).

CONTRAINDICATIONS

Ethambutol Hydrochloride is contraindicated in patients who are known to be hypersensitive to this drug. It is also contraindicated in patients with known optic neuritis unless clinical judgment determines that it may be used.

PRECAUTIONS

The effects of combinations of Ethambutol Hydrochloride with other antituberculous drugs on the fetus is not known. While administration of this drug to pregnant human patients has produced no detectable effect upon the fetus, the possible teratogenic potential in women capable of bearing children should be weighed carefully against the benefits of therapy. There are published reports of five women who received the drug during pregnancy without apparent adverse effect upon the fetus.

Ethambutol Hydrochloride is not recommended for use in children under 13 years of age since safe conditions for use have not been established.

Patients with decreased renal function need the dosage reduced as determined by serum levels of Ethambutol Hydrochloride since the main path of excretion of this drug is by the kidneys.

Because this drug may have adverse effects on vision, physical examination should include ophthalmoscopy, finger perimetry, and testing of color discrimination. In patients with visual defects such as cataracts, recurrent inflammatory conditions of the eye, optic neuritis, and diabetic retinopathy, the evaluation of changes in visual acuity is more difficult, and care should be taken to be sure the variations in vision are not due to the underlying disease conditions. In such patients, consideration should be given to relationship between benefits expected and possible visual deterioration since evaluation of visual changes is difficult. (For recommended procedures, see next paragraphs under *"Adverse Reactions".*)

As with any potent drug, periodic assessment of organ system functions, including renal, hepatic, and hematopoietic, should be made during long-term therapy.

ADVERSE REACTIONS

Ethambutol Hydrochloride may produce decreases in visual acuity which appear to be due to optic neuritis and to be related to dose and duration of treatment. The effects are generally reversible when administration of the drug is discontinued promptly. In rare cases recovery may be delayed for up to 1 year or more and the effect may possibly be irreversible in these cases.

Patients should be advised to report promptly to their physician any change of visual acuity.

The change in visual acuity may be unilateral or bilateral and hence *each eye must be tested separately and both eyes tested together.* Testing of visual acuity should be performed before beginning Ethambutol Hydrochloride therapy and periodically during drug administration, except that it should be done monthly when a patient is on a dosage of more than 15 mg per kilogram per day. Snellen eye charts are recommended for testing of visual acuity. Studies have shown that there are definite fluctuations of one or two lines of the Snellen chart in the visual acuity of many tuberculous patients *not* receiving Ethambutol Hydrochloride.

The following table may be useful in interpreting possible changes in visual acuity attributable to Ethambutol Hydrochloride.

Initial Snellen Reading	Reading Indicating Significant Decrease	Significant Number of Lines	Decrease Number of Points
20/13	20/25	3	12
20/15	20/25	2	10
20/20	20/30	2	10
20/25	20/40	2	15
20/30	20/50	2	20
20/40	20/70	2	30
20/50	20/70	1	20

In general, changes in visual acuity less than those indicated under "Significant Number of Lines" and "Decrease-Number of Points," may be due to chance variation, limitations of the testing method or physiologic variability. Conversely, changes in visual acuity equaling or exceeding those under "Significant Number of Lines" and "Decrease-Number of Points" indicate need for retesting and careful evaluation of the patient's visual status. If careful evaluation confirms the magnitude of visual change and fails to reveal another cause, Ethambutol Hydrochloride should be discontinued and the patient reevaluated at frequent intervals. Progressive decreases in visual acuity during therapy must be considered to be due to Ethambutol Hydrochloride.

If corrective glasses are used prior to treatment, these must be worn during visual acuity testing. During 1 to 2 years of therapy, a refractive error may develop which must be corrected in order to obtain accurate test results. Testing the visual acuity through a pinhole eliminates refractive error. Patients developing visual abnormality during Ethambutol Hydrochloride treatment may show subjective visual symptoms before, or simultaneously with, the demonstration of decreases in visual acuity, and all patients receiving Ethambutol Hydrochloride should be questioned periodically about blurred vision and other subjective eye symptoms.

Recovery of visual acuity generally occurs over a period of weeks to months after the drug has been discontinued. Patients have then received Ethambutol Hydrochloride again without recurrence of loss of visual acuity.

Other adverse reactions reported include: anaphylactoid reactions, dermatitis pruritus and joint pain; anorexia, nausea, vomiting, gastrointestinal upset, abdominal pain; fever, malaise, headache, and dizziness; mental confusion, disorientation and possible hallucinations. Numbness and tingling of the extremities due to peripheral neuritis have been reported infrequently.

Elevated serum uric acid levels occur and precipitation of acute gout has been reported. Transient impairment of liver function as indicated by abnormal liver function tests is not an unusual finding. Since Ethambutol Hydrochloride is recommended for therapy in conjunction with one or more other antituberculous drugs, these changes may be related to the concurrent therapy.

DOSAGE AND ADMINISTRATION

Ethambutol Hydrochloride should not be used alone, in initial treatment or in retreatment. Ethambutol Hydrochloride should be administered on a once every 24-hour basis only. Absorption is not significantly altered by administration with food. Therapy, in general, should be continued until bacteriological conversion has become permanent and maximal clinical improvement has occurred.

Ethambutol Hydrochloride is not recommended for use in children under 13 years of age since safe conditions for use have not been established.

Initial Treatment: In patients who have not received previous antituberculous therapy, administer Ethambutol Hydrochloride 15 mg per kilogram (7 mg per pound) of body weight, as a single oral dose once every 24 hours. In the more recent studies, isoniazid has been administered concurrently in a single, daily, oral dose.

Retreatment: In patients who have received previous antituberculous therapy, administer Ethambutol Hydrochloride 25 mg per kilogram (11 mg per pound) of body weight, as a single oral dose once every 24 hours. Concurrently administer at least one other antituberculous drug to which the organisms have been demonstrated to be susceptible by appropriate *in vitro* tests. Suitable drugs usually consist of those not previously used in the treatment of the patient. After 60 days of Ethambutol Hydrochloride administration, decrease the dose to 15 mg per kilogram (7 mg per pound) of body weight, and administer as a single oral dose once every 24 hours.

During the period when a patient is on a daily dose of 25 mg/kg, monthly eye examinations are advised. See Table for easy selection of proper weight-dose tablet(s).

WEIGHT-DOSE TABLE

15 mg/kg (7 mg/lb) Schedule		
Weight Range		Daily Dose
Pounds	Kilograms	In mg
Under 85 lbs	Under 37 kg	500
85-94.5	37-43	600
95-109.5	43-50	700
110-124.5	50-57	800
125-139.5	57-64	900
140-154.5	64-71	1000
155-169.5	71-79	1100
170-184.5	79-84	1200
185-199.5	84-90	1300
200-214.5	90-97	1400
215 and Over	Over 97	1500

➤ SHOWN IN PRODUCT IDENTIFICATION GUIDE

25 mg/kg (11 mg/lb) Schedule

Under 85 lbs	Under 38 kg	900
85-92.5	38-42	1000
93-101.5	42-45.5	1100
102-109.5	45.5-50	1200
110-118.5	50-54	1300
119-128.5	54-58	1400
129-136.5	58-62	1500
137-146.5	62-67	1600
147-155.5	67-71	1700
156-164.5	71-75	1800
165-173.5	75-79	1900
174-182.5	79-83	2000
183-191.5	83-87	2100
192-199.5	87-91	2200
200-209.5	91-95	2300
210-218.5	95-99	2400
219 and Over	Over 99	2500

Storage: Store at controlled room temperature, 15°-30°C (59°-86°F).

HOW SUPPLIED
TABLETS: 100 MG

BRAND/MANUFACTURER	NDC	SIZE	AWP
○ BRAND			
MYAMBUTOL: Lederle Labs	00005-5015-23	100s	$41.88

TABLETS: 400 MG

BRAND/MANUFACTURER	NDC	SIZE	AWP
○ BRAND			
MYAMBUTOL: Lederle Labs	00005-5084-62	100s	$140.11
	00005-5084-60	100s ud	$145.13
	00005-5084-34	1000s	$1276.75

Ethamolin SEE ETHANOLAMINE OLEATE

Ethanolamine Oleate

DESCRIPTION
Ethanolamine Oleate Injection is a mild sclerosing agent. Chemically it is $C_{17}H_{33}COOH.NH_2CH_2CH_2OH$.

The empirical formula is $C_{20}H_{41}NO_3$, representing a molecular weight of 343.55.

Ethanolamine Oleate Injection consists of Ethanolamine, a basic substance, which when combined with oleic acid forms a clear, straw to pale yellow colored, deliquescent oleate. The pH ranges from 8.0 to 9.0.

Ethanolamine Oleate Injection is a sterile, apyrogenic, aqueous solution containing in each ml approximately 50 mg of Ethanolamine Oleate.

Following is its chemical structure:

CLINICAL PHARMACOLOGY
When injected intravenously, Ethanolamine Oleate acts primarily by irritation of the intimal endothelium of the vein and produces a sterile dose-related inflammatory response. This results in fibrosis and possible occlusion of the vein. Ethanolamine Oleate also rapidly diffuses through the venous wall and produces a dose-related extravascular inflammatory reaction.

The oleic acid component of the Ethanolamine Oleate is responsible for the inflammatory response, and may also activate coagulation *in vivo* by release of tissue factor and activation of Hageman factor. The Ethanolamine component, however, may inhibit fibrin clot formation by chelating calcium, so that a procoagulant action of Ethanolamine Oleate has not been demonstrated.

After injection, Ethanolamine Oleate disappears from the injection site within five minutes via the portal vein. When volumes larger than 20 ml are injected, some Ethanolamine Oleate also flows into the azygos vein through the periesophageal vein. In human autopsy studies it was found that within four days after injection there is neutrophil infiltration of the esophageal wall and hemorrhage within six days. Granulation tissue is first seen at ten days, red thrombi obliterating the varices by twenty days, and sclerosis of the varices by two and a half months. The time course of these findings suggests that sclerosis of esophageal varices will be a delayed rather than an immediate effect of the drug.

The minimum lethal dose of Ethanolamine Oleate administered intravenously to rabbits is 130 mg/kg.

In dogs, Ethanolamine Oleate injected into the right atrium at a dose of 1 ml/kg over one minute has been shown to increase extravascular lung water. The maximum recommended human dose is 20 ml, or 0.4 ml/kg for a 50-kg person. The concentration of Ethanolamine Oleate reaching the lung in human treatment will be less than in the dog studies, but pleural effusions, pulmonary edema, pulmonary infiltration, and pneumonitis have been reported in clinical trials, and minimizing the total per session dose, especially in patients with concomitant cardiopulmonary disease, is recommended (see "Precautions").

INDICATIONS AND USAGE
Ethanolamine Oleate is indicated for the treatment of patients with esophageal varices that have recently bled, to prevent rebleeding.

Ethanolamine Oleate is not indicated for the treatment of patients with esophageal varices that have not bled. There is no evidence that treatment of this population decreases the likelihood of bleeding.

Sclerotherapy with Ethanolamine Oleate has no beneficial effect upon portal hypertension, the cause of esophageal varices, so that recanalization and collateralization may occur, necessitating reinjection.

UNLABELED USES
Ethanolamine Oleate is used alone or as an adjunct in the treatment of testicular hydroceles and epididymal cysts.

CONTRAINDICATIONS
Ethanolamine Oleate should not be administered to subjects with a known hypersensitivity to ethanolamine, oleic acid, or ethanolamine oleate.

WARNINGS
Ethanolamine Oleate should be used in pregnant women only when clearly needed (see "Precautions").

The practice of injecting varicosities of the leg with Ethanolamine Oleate is not supported by adequately controlled clinical trials. Therefore, such use is not recommended.

PRECAUTIONS
Fatal anaphylactic shock was reported following injection of a larger than normal volume of Ethanolamine Oleate into a male who had a known allergic disposition. Although there are only three known reports of anaphylaxis, the possibility of an anaphylactic reaction should be kept in mind, and the physician should be prepared to treat it appropriately. In extreme emergencies, 0.25 ml of a 1:1,000 intravenous solution of epinephrine (0.25 mg) should be used and allergic reactions should be controlled with antihistamines.

Acute renal failure with spontaneous recovery followed injection of 15 to 20 ml of Ethanolamine Oleate into two women.

The physician should bear in mind that severe injection necrosis may result from direct injection of sclerosing agents, especially if excessive volumes are used. At least one fatal case of extensive esophageal necrosis and death has been reported. The drug should be administered by physicians who are familiar with an acceptable injection technique.

Patients in Child Class C are more likely to develop esophageal ulceration than those in Classes A and B. Complications of ulceration, necrosis, and delayed esophageal perforation appear to occur more frequently when Ethanolamine Oleate is injected submucosally. This route is not recommended.

In patients with concomitant cardiorespiratory disease, careful monitoring and minimization of the total dose per session is recommended.

Fatal aspiration pneumonia has occurred in elderly patients undergoing esophageal variceal sclerotherapy with Ethanolamine Oleate. This adverse event appears to be procedure-related rather than drug-related, but as aspiration of blood and/or stomach contents is not uncommon in patients with bleeding esophageal varices, special precautions should be taken to prevent its occurrence, especially in the elderly and critically ill subjects.

Pregnancy: Teratogenic Effects: Pregnancy Category C: Animal reproduction reproduction studies have not been conducted with Ethanolamine Oleate. It is also not known whether Ethanolamine Oleate can cause fetal harm when administered to a pregnant woman or can affect reproduction capacity. Ethanolamine Oleate should be given to a pregnant woman only if clearly needed.

Nursing Mothers: It is not known whether this drug is excreted in human milk. Because many drugs are excreted in human milk, caution should be exercised when Ethanolamine Oleate is administered to a nursing woman.

Pediatric Use: Safety and effectiveness in children have not been established.

ADVERSE REACTIONS
The reported frequency of complications/adverse events per injection session was 13%. The most common complications were pleural effusion/infiltration (2.1%), esophageal ulcer (2.1%), pyrexia (1.8%), retrosternal pain (1.6%), esophageal stricture (1.3%), and pneumonia (1.2%).

Other adverse local esophageal reactions have also been reported at rates of 0.1 to 0.4%, including esophagitis, tearing of the esophagus, sloughing of the mucosa overlying the injected varix, ulceration, stricture, necrosis, periesophageal abscess and perforation (see "Precautions"). These complications appear to be dependent upon the dose and the patient's clinical state.

Bacteremia has been observed in patients following injection of esophageal varices with Ethanolamine Oleate. Pyrexia and retrosternal pain are not infrequently observed during the post-injection period. Fatal aspiration pneumonia has occurred in patients with esophageal varices who underwent Ethanolamine Oleate sclerotherapy (see "Precautions"). Anaphylactic shock and acute renal failure with spontaneous recovery have occurred (see "Precautions").

Spinal cord paralysis due to occlusion of the anterior spinal artery has been reported in one child eight hours after Ethanolamine Oleate sclerotherapy.

◆ RATED THERAPEUTICALLY EQUIVALENT; ◇ THERAPEUTIC EQUIVALENCE UNCONFIRMED; ○ UNRATED

OVERDOSAGE

Overdosage of Ethanolamine Oleate can result in severe intramural necrosis of the esophagus. Complications resulting from such overdosage have resulted in death.

DOSAGE AND ADMINISTRATION

Local Ethanolamine Oleate sclerotherapy of esophageal varices should be performed by physicians who are familiar with an acceptable technique. The usual intravenous dose is 1.5 to 5 ml per varix. The maximum total dose per treatment session should not exceed 20 ml. Patients with significant liver dysfunction (Child Class C) or concomitant cardiopulmonary disease should usually receive less than the recommended maximum dose. Submucosal injections are not recommended as they are reportedly more likely to result in ulceration at the site of injection.

To obliterate the varix, injections may be made at the time of the acute bleeding episode and then after one week, six weeks, three months, and six months as indicated.

Note: Parenteral drug products should be inspected visually for particulate matter and discoloration before administration whenever solution and container permit.

Store at controlled room temperature, 15°-30°C (59°-86°F). Protect from light.

HOW SUPPLIED
INJECTION: 5%

BRAND/MANUFACTURER	NDC	SIZE	AWP
○ **BRAND**			
ETHAMOLIN: Reed & Carnrick	00021-4790-06	2 ml 10s	$240.00

Ethaquin SEE ETHAVERINE HYDROCHLORIDE

Ethatab SEE ETHAVERINE HYDROCHLORIDE

Ethaverine Hydrochloride

DESCRIPTION

Each tablet contains Ethaverine Hydrochloride 100 mg.

ACTION

Ethaverine Hydrochloride acts directly on the smooth muscle cells without involving the autonomic nervous system or its receptors. It produces smooth muscle relaxation, particularly where spasm exists, affecting the larger blood vessels, especially systemic, peripheral, and pulmonary vessels, and smooth muscle of the intestines, biliary tree, and ureters.

INDICATIONS AND USAGE

In peripheral and cerebral vascular insufficiency associated with arterial spasm; also useful as a smooth muscle spasmolytic in spastic conditions of the gastrointestinal and genitourinary tracts.

CONTRAINDICATIONS

The use of Ethaverine Hydrochloride is contraindicated in the presence of complete atrioventricular dissociation.

PRECAUTIONS

As with all vasodilators, Ethaverine Hydrochloride should be administered with caution to patients with glaucoma. The safety of Ethaverine Hydrochloride during pregnancy or lactation has not been established; therefore, it should not be used in pregnant women or in women of childbearing age unless, in the judgment of the physician, its use is deemed essential to the welfare of the patient.

ADVERSE REACTIONS

Even though the incidence of adverse reactions as reported in the literature is very low, it is possible for a patient to evidence nausea; anorexia; abdominal distress, including diarrhea; dryness of the throat; hypotension; malaise; lassitude; drowsiness; flushing; sweating; vertigo; respiratory depression; cardiac depression; cardiac arrhythmia; and headache. If these adverse reactions occur, reduce dosage or discontinue medication.

DOSAGE AND ADMINISTRATION

In mild or moderate disease, the usual dosage for adults is one tablet three times a day. In more difficult cases, dosage may be increased to two tablets three times a day. It is most effective given early in the course of the vascular disorder. Because of the chronic nature of the disease, long-term therapy is required.

HOW SUPPLIED
CAPSULE: 100 MG

BRAND/MANUFACTURER	NDC	SIZE	AWP
○ **GENERICS**			
ISOVEX: U.S. Pharm	52747-0204-60	100s	$24.84
ISOVEX: U.S. Pharm	52747-0204-80	1000s	$148.34

TABLETS: 100 MG

BRAND/MANUFACTURER	NDC	SIZE	AWP
○ **BRAND**			
ETHAQUIN: Ascher	00225-0250-15	100s	$38.52
ETHATAB: Whitby	50474-0281-43	100s	$43.79
ETHAQUIN: Ascher	00225-0250-20	500s	$187.80
	00225-0250-25	1000s	$365.94
	00225-0250-60	2500s	$629.10
	00225-0250-65	5000s	$1188.30
○ **GENERICS**			
Major	00904-2213-60	100s	$9.75
Sidmak	50111-0336-01	100s	$10.73
ETHAVEX-100: EconoMed	38130-0011-01	100s	$14.94
ETHAVEX-100: EconoMed	38130-0011-10	1000s	$114.90

Ethchlorvynol

DESCRIPTION

Ethchlorvynol is a tertiary carbinol. It is chemically designated as 1-chloro-3-ethyl-1-penten-4-yl-3-ol. Ethchlorvynol occurs as a liquid which is immiscible with water and miscible with most organic solvents.

Ethchlorvynol is an oral hypnotic available in capsule form containing either 200 mg, 500 mg or 750 mg.

WARNING

MANUFACTURED WITH CARBON TETRACHLORIDE, A SUBSTANCE WHICH HARMS PUBLIC HEALTH AND ENVIRONMENT BY DESTROYING OZONE IN THE UPPER ATMOSPHERE.

Following is its chemical structure:

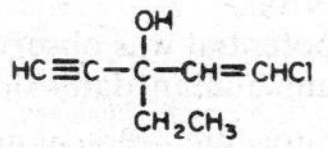

$$HC\equiv C-\underset{\underset{CH_2CH_3}{|}}{\overset{\overset{OH}{|}}{C}}-CH=CHCl$$

CLINICAL PHARMACOLOGY

The usual hypnotic dose of Ethchlorvynol induces sleep within 15 minutes to one hour. The duration of the hypnotic effect is about five hours. The mechanism of action is unknown.

Ethchlorvynol is rapidly absorbed from the gastrointestinal tract with peak plasma concentrations usually occurring within two hours after a single oral fasting dose. Plasma concentrations required for hypnotic effects are unknown. The plasma half-life ($t\frac{1}{2}$, β) of the parent compound is approximately ten to twenty hours. Studies with ^{14}C-Ethchlorvynol have demonstrated that within 24 hours, 33% of a single 500 mg dose is excreted in the urine mostly as metabolites. The major plasma and urinary metabolite is the secondary alcohol of Ethchlorvynol. The free and conjugated forms of this metabolite in the urine account for about 40% of the dose. Other minor metabolites have been identified as the primary alcohol and a secondary alcohol with an altered acetylene group. Studies with ^{14}C-Ethchlorvynol in animals indicate that the parent compound and its metabolites undergo extensive enterophepatic recirculation.

Distribution studies indicate that there is extensive tissue localization of Ethchlorvynol, particularly in adipose tissue. Ethchlorvynol and/or its metabolites have also been detected in liver, kidneys, spleen, brain, bile and cerebrospinal fluid.

INDICATIONS AND USAGE

Ethchlorvynol is indicated as short-term hypnotic therapy for periods up to one week in duration for the management of insomnia. If retreatment becomes necessary, after drug-free intervals of one or more weeks, it should only be undertaken upon further evaluation of the patient.

CONTRAINDICATIONS

Ethchlorvynol is contraindicated in patients with known hypersensitivity to the drug and in patients with porphyria.

WARNINGS

ETHCHLORVYNOL SHOULD BE ADMINISTERED WITH CAUTION TO MENTALLY DEPRESSED PATIENTS WITH OR WITHOUT SUICIDAL TENDENCIES. IT SHOULD ALSO BE ADMINISTERED WITH CAUTION TO THOSE WHO HAVE A PSYCHOLOGICAL POTENTIAL FOR DRUG DEPENDENCE. THE LEAST AMOUNT OF DRUG THAT IS FEASIBLE SHOULD BE PRESCRIBED FOR THESE PATIENTS.

Psychological and Physical Dependence: PROLONGED USE OF ETHCHLORVYNOL MAY RESULT IN TOLERANCE AND PSYCHOLOGICAL AND PHYSICAL DEPENDENCE. PROLONGED ADMINISTRATION OF THE DRUG IS NOT RECOMMENDED. (See *"Drug Abuse and Dependence"* section.)

PRECAUTIONS

General: Elderly or debilitated patients should receive the smallest effective amount of Ethchlorvynol.

Caution should be exercised when treating patients with impaired hepatic or renal function.

➤ SHOWN IN PRODUCT IDENTIFICATION GUIDE

Patients who exhibit unpredictable behavior, or paradoxical restlessness or excitement in response to barbiturates or alcohol may react in this manner to Ethchlorvynol.

Ethchlorvynol should not be used for the management of insomnia in the presence of pain unless insomnia persists after pain is controlled with analgesics.

Certain brands of Ethchlorvynol contain FD&C Yellow No. 5 (tartrazine) which may cause allergic-type reactions (including bronchial asthma) in certain susceptible individuals. Although the overall incidence of FD&C Yellow No. 5 (tartrazine) sensitivity in the general population is low, it is frequently seen in patients who also have aspirin hypersensitivity.

Information for Patients: The use of Ethchlorvynol carries with it an associated risk of psychological and/or physical dependence. The patient should be warned against increasing the dose of the drug without consulting a physician.

Patients should be advised that, for the duration of the effect of Ethchlorvynol, mental and/or physical abilities required for the performance of potentially hazardous tasks such as the operation of dangerous machinery including motor vehicles, may be impaired.

Patients should be cautioned to avoid the concomitant use of Ethchlorvynol with alcohol, barbiturates, other CNS depressants, or MAO inhibitors.

Drug Interactions: The concomitant use of Ethchlorvynol with alcohol, barbiturates, other CNS depressants, or MAO inhibitors may produce exaggerated depressant effects.

Ethchlorvynol may cause a decreased prothrombin time response to coumarin anticoagulants; therefore, the dosage of these drugs may require adjustment when therapy with Ethchlorvynol is initiated and after it is discontinued.

Transient delirium has been reported with the concomitant use of Ethchlorvynol and amitriptyline; therefore, Ethchlorvynol should be administered with caution to patients receiving tricyclic antidepressants.

Carcinogenesis: A study in mice receiving oral doses of Ethchlorvynol up to 7 times the maximum human daily dose for 22 to 24 months produced equivocal results. When compared to controls, a statistically significant increase in total lung tumors was found in female mice given the high dose of Ethchlorvynol. However, the 48% incidence is not substantially higher than the high value (39%) reported for the historical laboratory controls.

No evidence of carcinogenic potential was observed in rats given Ethchlorvynol at 5 to 15 times the maximum human daily dose for up to 2 years.

Usage During Pregnancy: 1. Teratogenic—Pregnancy Category C. Ethchlorvynol has been associated with a higher percentage of stillbirths and a lower survival rate of progeny among rats given 40 mg/kg/day. There are no adequate and well-controlled studies in pregnant women. Therefore, Ethchlorvynol is not recommended for use during the first and second trimesters of pregnancy. Ethchlorvynol should be used during pregnancy only if the potential benefit justifies the potential risk to the fetus.

2. Non-teratogenic—Clinical experience has indicated that Ethchlorvynol taken during the third trimester of pregnancy may produce CNS depression and transient withdrawal symptoms in the newborn. These symptoms resemble congenital narcotic withdrawal symptoms (See *"Drug Abuse and Dependence"* section).

Nursing Mothers: It is not known whether this drug is excreted in breast milk. Because many drugs are excreted in human milk and because of the potential for serious adverse reactions in nursing infants from Ethchlorvynol a decision should be made whether to discontinue nursing or to discontinue the drug, taking into account the importance of the drug to the mother.

Pediatric Use: Ethchlorvynol is not recommended for use in children since its safety and effectiveness in the pediatric age group has not been determined.

ADVERSE REACTIONS

Adverse effects in decreasing order of severity within each of the following categories are:

Hypersensitivity: cholestatic jaundice, urticaria and rash.

Hematologic: thrombocytopenia—one case of fatal immune thrombocytopenia due to Ethchlorvynol has been reported.

Gastrointestinal: vomiting, gastric upset, nausea and aftertaste.

Neurologic: dizziness and facial numbness.

Miscellaneous: blurred vision, hypotension and mild "hangover".

The following idiosyncratic responses have been reported occasionally: syncope without marked hypotension, profound muscular weakness, hysteria, marked excitement, prolonged hypnosis and mild stimulation.

Transient ataxia and giddiness have occurred in patients in whom absorption of the drug is especially rapid. These effects can sometimes be controlled by giving Ethchlorvynol with food.

(See *"Drug Abuse and Dependence"* section for the signs and symptoms of chronic intoxication).

DRUG ABUSE AND DEPENDENCE

Ethchlorvynol is subject to control by the Federal Controlled Substances Act under DEA schedule IV.

Abuse: Pulmonary edema of rapid onset has resulted from the I.V. abuse of Ethchlorvynol.

Dependence: Signs and symptoms of intoxication have been reported with the prolonged use of doses as low as 1 g/day. Signs and symptoms of chronic intoxication may include incoordination, tremors, ataxia, confusion, slurred speech, hyperreflexia, diplopia, and generalized muscle weakness. Toxic amblyopia, scotoma, nystagmus, and peripheral neuropathy have also been reported with prolonged use of Ethchlorvynol; these symptoms are usually reversible.

Severe withdrawal symptoms similar to those seen during barbiturate and alcohol withdrawal have been reported following abrupt discontinuance of prolonged use of Ethchlorvynol. These symptoms may appear as late as nine days after sudden withdrawal of the drug. Signs and symptoms of Ethchlorvynol withdrawal may include convulsions, delirium, hallucinations, schizoid reaction, perceptual distortions, memory loss, ataxia, insomnia, slurring of speech, unusual anxiety, irritability, agitation, and tremors. Other signs and symptoms may include anorexia, nausea, vomiting, weakness, dizziness, sweating, muscle twitching, and weight loss.

Management of a patient who manifests withdrawal symptoms from Ethchlorvynol involves readministration of the drug to approximately the same level of chronic intoxication which existed before the abrupt discontinuance. (Phenobarbital may be substituted for Ethchlorvynol.) A gradual, stepwise reduction of dosage may then be made over a period of days or weeks. A phenothiazine compound may be used in addition to this regimen for those patients who exhibit psychotic symptoms during the withdrawal period. The patient undergoing withdrawal from Ethchlorvynol must be hospitalized or closely observed, and given general supportive care as indicated.

In one report an infant born to a mother who received 500 mg Ethchlorvynol at bedtime daily throughout the third trimester, exhibited withdrawal symptoms on the second day of life. The symptoms included episodic jitteriness, hyperactivity, restlessness, irritability, disturbed sleep and hunger. The neonate responded to a single oral dose of phenobarbital (3 mg/kg). The withdrawal symptoms gradually decreased and completely disappeared by the tenth day of life.

OVERDOSAGE

Acute intoxication is characterized by prolonged deep coma, severe respiratory depression, hypothermia, hypotension, and relative bradycardia. Nystagmus and pancytopenia resulting from acute Ethchlorvynol overdose have been reported. Although death has occurred following the ingestion of 6 g of Ethchlorvynol, there have been reports of patients who have survived overdoses of 50 g and more with intensive care. Fatal blood concentrations usually range from 20 to 50 µg/mL.[1] Because large amounts of Ethchlorvynol are taken up by adipose tissue, the blood concentration is an unreliable indicator of the magnitude of overdose.

Management of acute Ethchlorvynol intoxication is similar to that of acute barbiturate intoxication.[2] Gastric evacuation should be performed immediately. (In the unconscious patient, gastric lavage should be preceded by tracheal intubation with a cuffed tube.) Supportive care (assisted ventilation, frequent and careful monitoring of vital signs, control of blood pressure) is essential. Emphasis should be placed on pulmonary care and monitoring of blood gases. Hemoperfusion utilizing the Amberlite column technique has been reported in the literature to be the most effective method in the management of acute Ethchlorvynol overdose.[3] In addition, hemodialysis and peritoneal dialysis have each been reported to be of some value. (Aqueous and oil dialysates have been used. Forced diuresis with maintenance of a high urinary output has also been reported of some value.) (See *"Drug Abuse and Dependence"* section for the signs and symptoms of chronic intoxication).

DOSAGE AND ADMINISTRATION

The usual adult hypnotic dose of Ethchlorvynol is 500 mg taken orally at bedtime. A dose of 750 mg may be required for patients whose sleep response to a 500 mg capsule is inadequate, or for patients being changed from barbiturates or other nonbarbiturate hypnotics. Up to 1000 mg may be given as a single bedtime dose when insomnia is unusually severe. A single supplemental dose of 200 mg may be given to reinstitute sleep in patients who may awaken after the original bedtime dose of 500 or 750 mg.

For patients whose insomnia is characterized only by untimely awakening during the early morning hours, a single dose of 200 mg taken upon awakening may be adequate for relief.

The smallest effective dose of Ethchlorvynol should be given to elderly or debilitated patients.

Ethchlorvynol should not be prescribed for periods exceeding one week. (See *"Drug Abuse and Dependence"* section).

Recommended storage: 59°-77° F (15°-25° C).

REFERENCES

1. AMA Dept. of Drugs, *AMA Drug Evaluations,* Massachusetts: Publishing Sciences Group, Inc., 1980. 2. Khantzian, E. J., McKenna, E. J., Jr., Acute Toxic and Withdrawal Reactions Associated with Drug Abuse, *Annals of Internal Medicine,* 90:361-372, 1979. 3. Lynn, R.I. et al., Resin Hemoperfusion for Treatment of Ethchlorvynol Overdose, *Annals of Internal Medicine,* 91:549-553, 1979.

HOW SUPPLIED
CAPSULE (C-IV): 200 MG

BRAND/MANUFACTURER	NDC	SIZE	AWP
◆ BRAND			
PLACIDYL: Abbott Pharm	00074-6661-08	100s	$101.13

◆ RATED THERAPEUTICALLY EQUIVALENT; ◇ THERAPEUTIC EQUIVALENCE UNCONFIRMED; ○ UNRATED

CAPSULE (C-IV): 500 MG

AVERAGE UNIT PRICE (AVAILABLE SIZES)

BRAND		$1.29	

BRAND/MANUFACTURER	NDC	SIZE	AWP
◆ **BRAND**			
PLACIDYL: Abbott Pharm	00074-6685-15	100s	$124.58
	00074-6685-10	100s ud	$133.01

CAPSULE (C-IV): 750 MG

BRAND/MANUFACTURER	NDC	SIZE	AWP
◆ **BRAND**			
PLACIDYL: Abbott Pharm	00074-6630-01	100s	$165.34
◆ **GENERICS**			
Major	00904-3391-60	100s	$66.50

Ethinyl Estradiol

WARNINGS

1 ESTROGENS HAVE BEEN REPORTED TO INCREASE THE RISK RATIO OF ENDOMETRIAL CARCINOMA.

THREE INDEPENDENT CASE CONTROL STUDIES HAVE REPORTED AN INCREASED RISK RATIO OF ENDOMETRIAL CANCER IN POSTMENOPAUSAL WOMEN EXPOSED TO EXOGENOUS ESTROGENS FOR PROLONGED PERIODS.[1-3] THIS RISK RATIO WAS INDEPENDENT OF THE OTHER RISK FACTORS FOR ENDOMETRIAL CANCER. THESE STUDIES ARE FURTHER SUPPORTED BY THE REPORT THAT INCIDENCE RATES OF ENDOMETRIAL CANCER HAVE INCREASED SHARPLY SINCE 1969 IN EIGHT DIFFERENT AREAS OF THE UNITED STATES WITH POPULATION-BASED CANCER REPORTING SYSTEMS, AN INCREASE WHICH MAY BE RELATED TO THE RAPIDLY EXPANDING USE OF ESTROGENS DURING THE LAST DECADE.[4]

THE THREE CASE CONTROL STUDIES REPORTED THAT THE RISK RATIO OF ENDOMETRIAL CANCER IN ESTROGEN USERS WAS ABOUT 4.5 TO 13.9 TIMES GREATER THAN IN NONUSERS. THE RISK RATIO APPEARS TO DEPEND ON BOTH DURATION OF TREATMENT[1] AND ON ESTROGEN DOSE.[3] IN VIEW OF THESE REPORTS, WHEN ESTROGENS ARE USED FOR THE TREATMENT OF MENOPAUSAL SYMPTOMS, THE LOWEST DOSE THAT WILL CONTROL SYMPTOMS SHOULD BE UTILIZED AND MEDICATION SHOULD BE DISCONTINUED AS SOON AS POSSIBLE. WHEN PROLONGED TREATMENT IS MEDICALLY INDICATED, THE PATIENT SHOULD BE REASSESSED ON AT LEAST A SEMI-ANNUAL BASIS TO DETERMINE THE NEED FOR CONTINUED THERAPY. ALTHOUGH THE EVIDENCE MUST BE CONSIDERED PRELIMINARY, ONE STUDY SUGGESTS THAT CYCLIC ADMINISTRATION OF LOW DOSES OF ESTROGEN MAY CARRY LESS RISK THAN CONTINUOUS ADMINISTRATION[3]: IT THEREFORE APPEARS PRUDENT TO UTILIZE SUCH A REGIMEN.

CLOSE CLINICAL SURVEILLANCE OF ALL WOMEN TAKING ESTROGENS IT IS IMPORTANT. IN ALL CASES OF UNDIAGNOSED PERSISTENT OR RECURRING ABNORMAL VAGINAL BLEEDING, ADEQUATE DIAGNOSTIC MEASURES SHOULD BE UNDERTAKEN TO RULE OUT MALIGNANCY.

THERE IS NO EVIDENCE AT PRESENT THAT 'NATURAL' ESTROGENS ARE MORE OR LESS HAZARDOUS THAN 'SYNTHETIC' ESTROGENS AT EQUI-ESTROGENIC DOSES

2 ESTROGENS SHOULD NOT BE USED DURING PREGNANCY

THE USE OF ESTROGENS DURING EARLY PREGNANCY MAY SERIOUSLY DAMAGE THE OFFSPRING. IT HAS BEEN REPORTED THAT FEMALES EXPOSED IN UTERO TO DIETHYLSTILBESTROL, A NONSTEROIDAL ESTROGEN, MAY HAVE AN INCREASED RISK OF DEVELOPING IN LATER LIFE A FORM OF VAGINAL OR CERVICAL CANCER THAT IS ORDINARILY EXTREMELY RARE.[5,6] THIS RISK HAS BEEN ESTIMATED STATISTICALLY AS NOT GREATER THAN 4 PER 1000 EXPOSURES.[7] IN CERTAIN STUDIES, A HIGH PERCENTAGE OF SUCH EXPOSED WOMEN (FROM 30% TO 90%) HAVE BEEN FOUND TO HAVE VAGINAL ADENOSIS,[8-11] EPITHELIAL CHANGES OF THE VAGINA AND CERVIX. ALTHOUGH THESE CHANGES ARE HISTOLOGICALLY BENIGN, IT IS NOT KNOWN WHETHER THEY ARE PRECURSORS OF MALIGNANCY. ALTHOUGH SIMILAR DATA ARE NOT AVAILABLE WITH THE USE OF OTHER ESTROGENS, IT CANNOT BE PRESUMED THEY WOULD NOT INDUCE SIMILAR CHANGES. EXPOSURE TO DIETHYLSTILBESTROL HAS ALSO BEEN ASSOCIATED WITH ADVERSE EFFECTS ON REPRODUCTIVE PERFORMANCE, INCLUDING INCREASED RATES OF SPONTANEOUS ABORTION, ECTOPIC PREGNANCY, PREMATURE DELIVERIES, AND PERINATAL DEATHS.

SEVERAL REPORTS SUGGEST AN ASSOCIATION BETWEEN INTRAUTERINE FETAL EXPOSURE TO FEMALE SEX HORMONES AND CONGENITAL ANOMALIES, INCLUDING CONGENITAL HEART DEFECTS AND LIMB REDUCTION DEFECTS.[12-15] ONE CASE CONTROL STUDY[15] ESTIMATED A 4.7-FOLD INCREASED RISK OF LIMB REDUCTION DEFECTS IN INFANTS EXPOSED IN UTERO TO SEX HORMONES (ORAL CONTRACEPTIVES, HORMONE WITHDRAWAL TESTS FOR PREGNANCY, OR ATTEMPTED TREATMENT FOR THREATENED ABORTION). SOME OF THESE EXPOSURES WERE VERY SHORT AND INVOLVED ONLY A FEW DAYS OF TREATMENT. THE DATA SUGGESTS THAT THE RISK OF LIMB REDUCTION DEFECTS IN EXPOSED FETUSES IS SOMEWHAT LESS THAN 1 PER 1000.

IN THE PAST, ESTROGENS HAVE BEEN USED DURING PREGNANCY IN AN ATTEMPT TO TREAT THREATENED OR HABITUAL ABORTION. THERE IS CONSIDERABLE EVIDENCE THAT ESTROGENS ARE INEFFECTIVE FOR THESE INDICATIONS.

IF ETHINYL ESTRADIOL TABLETS ARE USED DURING PREGNANCY, OR IF THE PATIENT BECOMES PREGNANT WHILE TAKING THIS DRUG, SHE SHOULD BE APPRISED OF THE POTENTIAL RISKS TO THE FETUS, AND THE ADVISABILITY OF PREGNANCY CONTINUATION.

DESCRIPTION

Ethinyl Estradiol tablets contain Ethinyl Estradiol, USP, a potent synthetic estrogen, having the chemical name 19-Nor-17α-pregna-1.3.5(10)-trien-20-yne-3.17-diol: the chemical formula $C_{20}H_{24}O_2$, molecular weight of 296.41.

Ethinyl Estradiol is a white to creamy white, odorless, crystalline powder. It is insoluble in water, soluble in alcohol, chloroform, ether, and vegetable oils.

Biologically, estrogens may be defined as compounds capable of stimulating female secondary sex characteristics. Chemically, there are different groups of estrogens, depending on whether they are natural or synthetic, steroidal or non-steroidal. Natural human estrogens are ultimately formed from either androstenedione or testosterone as immediate precursors. Ethinyl Estradiol is a synthetic, steroidal estrogen.

Ethinyl Estradiol for oral administration, is available in tablets containing 0.02, 0.05, or 0.5 mg Ethinyl Estradiol, USP.

Following is its chemical structure:

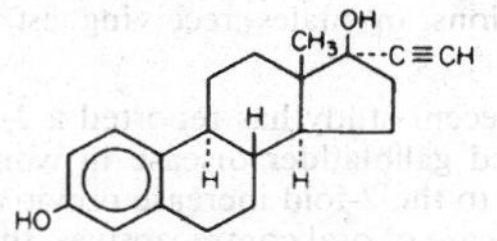

CLINICAL PHARMACOLOGY

Ethinyl Estradiol is a synthetic derivative of the natural estrogen, Estradiol.

Ethinyl Estradiol, like Estradiol, promotes growth of the endometrium and thickening, stratification, and cornification of the vagina. It causes growth of the ducts of the mammary glands, but inhibits lactation. It also inhibits the anterior pituitary and causes capillary dilatation, fluid retention, and protein anabolism.

Estradiol is the major estrogen in premenopausal women, with up to 100 to 600 mcg being secreted daily by the ovary. Natural estrogens are poorly effective when given by mouth. Apparently this is due to rapid clearance of the endogenous hormone from blood, along with a first-pass-effect after oral administration. The addition of a 17-alpha-ethinyl group to Estradiol increases potency and enhances oral activity by impeding hepatic degradation. The oral efficacy of Ethinyl Estradiol is related to slower elimination than Estradiol from the circulation. A part of ingested Ethinyl Estradiol is excreted in glucuronide form via urine in animals and in man, but also extensive metabolism of the steroid nucleus occurs. The major metabolism takes place mainly in the liver. Large amounts of Ethinyl Estradiol metabolites are excreted via human bile, much similar to what has been reported for Estradiol. However, unlike Estradiol, Ethinyl Estradiol metabolites do not exclusively leave via urine. Urinary recovery is much less than that of Estradiol and substantial amounts of Ethinyl Estradiol metabolites appear in human feces. Quantitatively, the major metabolic pathway for Ethinyl Estradiol, both in rats and in humans, is aromatic hydroxylation as it is for the natural estrogens.

Rapid and complete absorption follows oral intake of Ethinyl Estradiol. Elimination of Ethinyl Estradiol from plasma proceeds slower than that of Estradiol. After oral administration, an initial peak occurs in plasma at 2 to 3 hours, with a secondary peak at about 12 hours after dosing; the second peak is interpreted as evidence for extensive enterohepatic circulation of Ethinyl Estradiol.

INDICATIONS AND USAGE

Ethinyl Estradiol Tablets are indicated in the treatment of: 1) Moderate to severe *vasomotor* symptoms associated with the menopause. (There is no evidence that estrogens are effective for nervous symptoms or depression which might occur during menopause, and they should not be used to treat these conditions.) 2) Female hypogonadism. 3) Prostatic carcinoma-palliative therapy of advanced disease. 4) Breast cancer (for palliation only) in appropriately selected women, such as those who are more than 5 years postmenopausal with progressing inoperable or radiation-resistant disease.

➤ SHOWN IN PRODUCT IDENTIFICATION GUIDE

ETHINYL ESTRADIOL HAS NOT BEEN SHOWN TO BE EFFECTIVE FOR ANY PURPOSE DURING PREGNANCY AND ITS USE MAY CAUSE SEVERE HARM TO THE FETUS (See boxed *"Warnings"*).

The lowest effective dose appropriate for the specific indication should be used. Studies of the addition of a progestin for seven or more days of a cycle of Estrogen administration have reported a lowered incidence of endometrial hyperplasia. Morphological and biochemical studies of endometrium suggest that 10 to 13 days of progestin are needed to provide maximal maturation of the endometrium and to eliminate any hyperplastic changes. Whether this will provide protection from endometrial carcinoma has not been clearly established. There are possible additional risks which may be associated with the inclusion of progestin in estrogen replacement regimens. The potential risks include adverse effects on carbohydrate and lipid metabolism. The choice of progestin and dosage may be important in minimizing these adverse effects.

CONTRAINDICATIONS
Estrogens should not be used in women (or men) with any of the following conditions:

1. Known or suspected cancer of the breast except in appropriately selected patients being treated for metastatic disease.
2. Known or suspected estrogen-dependent neoplasia.
3. Known or suspected pregnancy (see boxed *"Warnings"*).
4. Undiagnosed abnormal genital bleeding.
5. Active thrombophlebitis or thromboembolic disorders.
6. A past history of thrombophlebitis, thrombosis, or thromboembolic disorders associated with previous estrogen use (except when used in treatment of breast or prostatic malignancy).

WARNINGS
1. Induction of malignant neoplasms: Long-term continuous administration of natural and synthetic estrogens in certain animal species increases the frequency of carcinomas of the breast, cervix, vagina, and liver. There is now evidence that estrogens increase the risk of carcinoma of the endometrium in humans. (See boxed *"Warnings"*).

At the present time there is no satisfactory evidence that estrogens given to postmenopausal women increase the risk of cancer of the breast,[16] although a recent long-term follow-up of a single physician's practice has raised this possibility.[17] Because of the animal data, there is a need for caution in prescribing estrogens for women with a strong family history of breast cancer or who have breast nodules, fibrocystic disease, or abnormal mammograms.

Estrogens have been reported to be associated with carcinoma of the male breast and suspicious lesions in males receiving estrogen therapy should be investigated accordingly.

2. Gallbladder disease: A recent study has reported a 2- to 3-fold increase in the risk of surgically confirmed gallbladder disease in women receiving postmenopausal estrogens,[16] similar to the 2-fold increase previously noted in users of oral contraceptives.[18,22] In the case of oral contraceptives, the increased risk appeared after two years of use.[22]

3. Effects similar to those caused by estrogen-progestagen oral contraceptives: There are several serious adverse effects of oral contraceptives, most of which have not, up to now, been documented as consequences of postmenopausal estrogen therapy. This may reflect the comparatively low doses of estrogen used in postmenopausal women. It would be expected that the larger doses of estrogen used to treat prostatic or breast cancer are more likely to result in these adverse effects, and, in fact, it has been shown that there is an increased risk of thrombosis in men receiving estrogens for prostatic cancer.[19-22]

a. Thromboembolic disease: It is now well established that users of oral contraceptives have an increased risk of various thromboembolic and thrombotic vascular diseases, such as thrombophlebitis, pulmonary embolism, stroke, and myocardial infarction.[22-29] Cases of retinal thrombosis, mesenteric thrombosis, and optic neuritis have been reported in oral contraceptive users. There is evidence that the risk of several of these adverse reactions is related to the dose of the drug.[30,31] An increased risk of postsurgery thromboembolic complications has also been reported in users of oral contraceptives.[32,33] If feasible, estrogen should be discontinued at least 4 weeks before surgery of the type associated with an increased risk of thromboembolism, or during periods of immobilization.

While an increased rate of thromboembolic and thrombotic disease in postmenopausal users of estrogen has not been found,[16,34] this does not rule out the possibiity that such an increase may be present or that subgroups of women who have underlying risk factors or who are receiving relatively large doses of estrogens may have increased risk. Therefore, estrogens should not be used in persons with active thrombophlebitis or thromboembolic disorders, and they should not be used (except in treatment of malignancy) in persons with a history of such disorders in association with estrogen use. They should be used with caution in patients with cerebral vascular or coronary artery disease and only for those in whom estrogens are clearly needed.

Large doses of estrogen (5 mg conjugated estrogens per day), comparable to those used to treat cancer of the prostate and breast, have been shown in a large prospective clinical trial in men[35] to increase the risk of nonfatal myocardial infarction, pulmonary embolism and thrombophlebitis. When estrogen doses of this size are used, any of the thromboembolic and thrombotic adverse effects associated with oral contraceptive use should be considered a clear risk.

b. Hepatic adenoma: Benign hepatic adenomas appear to be associated with the use of oral contraceptives.[36,38] Although benign, and rare, these may rupture and may cause death through intra-abdominal hemorrhage. Such lesions have not yet been reported in association with other estrogen or progestagen preparations, but should be considered in estrogen users having abdominal pain and tenderness, abdominal mass, or hypovolemic shock. Hepatocellular carcinoma has also been reported in women taking estrogen-containing oral contraceptives.[37] The relationship of this malignancy to these drugs is not known at this time.

c. Elevated blood pressure: Increased blood pressure is not uncommon in women using oral contraceptives. There is now a report that this may occur with use of estrogens in the menopause[39] and blood pressure should be monitored with estrogen use, especially if high doses are used.

d. Glucose tolerance: A worsening of glucose tolerance has been observed in a significant percentage of patients on estrogen-containing oral contraceptives. For this reason, diabetic patients should be carefully observed while receiving estrogen.

4. Hypercalcemia: Administration of estrogens may lead to severe hypercalcemia in patients with breast cancer and bone metastases. If this occurs, the drug should be stopped and appropriate measures taken to reduce the serum calcium level.

PRECAUTIONS
General: A complete medical and family history should be taken prior to the initiation of any estrogen therapy. The pretreatment and periodic physical examinations should include special reference to blood pressure, breasts, abdomen, and pelvic organs, and should include a Papanicolaou smear. As a general rule, estrogen should not be prescribed for longer than one year without another physical examination being performed.

2. Fluid retention: Because estrogens may cause some degree of fluid retention, conditions which might be influenced by this factor, such as epilepsy, migraine, and cardiac or renal dysfunction, require careful observation.

3. Certain patients may develop undesirable manifestations of excessive estrogenic stimulation, such as abnormal or excessive uterine bleeding, mastodynia, etc.

4. Oral contraceptives appear to be associated with an increased incidence of mental depression.[22] Although it is not clear whether this is due to the estrogenic or progestagenic component of the contraceptive, patients with a history of depression should be carefully observed.

5. Preexisting uterine leiomyomata may increase in size during estrogen use.

6. The pathologist should be advised of estrogen therapy when relevant specimens are submitted.

7. Patients with a past history of jaundice during pregnancy have an increased risk of recurrence of jaundice while receiving estrogen-containing oral contraceptive therapy. If jaundice develops in any patient receiving estrogen, the medication should be discontinued while the cause is investigated.

8. Estrogens may be poorly metabolized in patients with impaired liver function and they should be administered with caution in such patients.

9. Because estrogens influence the metabolism of calcium and phosphorus, they should be used with caution in patients with metabolic bone diseases that are associated with hypercalcemia or in patients with renal insufficiency.

10. Because of the effects of estrogens on epiphyseal closure, they should be used judiciously in young patients in whom bone growth is not complete.

11. Ethinyl Estradiol Tablets, 0.02 mg, contain FD&C Yellow No. 5 (tartrazine) which may cause allergic-type reactions (including bronchial asthma) in certain susceptible individuals. Although the overall incidence of FD&C Yellow No. 5 (tartrazine) sensitivity in the general population is low, it is frequently seen in patients who also have aspirin hypersensitivity.

Information for the Patient: See manufacturer's patient information..

Drug/Laboratory Test Interactions: Certain endocrine and liver function tests may be affected by estrogen-containing oral contraceptives. The following similar changes may be expected with larger doses of estrogen:

Increased sulfobromophthalein retention; increased prothrombin and factors VII. VIII. IX. and X; decreased antithrombin 3; increased norepinephrine-induced platelet aggregation; increased thyroid binding globulin (TBG) leading to increased circulating total thyroid hormone, as measured by PBI, T_4 by column, or T_4 by radioimmunoassay. Free T_3 resin uptake is decreased, reflecting the elevated TBG; free T_4 concentration is unaltered; impaired glucose tolerance; decreased pregnanediol excretion; reduced response to metyrapone test; reduced serum folate concentration; increased serum triglyceride and phospholipid concentration.

Carcinogenesis, Mutagenesis, Impairment of Fertility: See boxed *"Warnings"*.

Pregnancy Category X: See *"Contraindications"* and boxed *"Warnings"*.

Nursing Mothers: Because of the potential for tumorigenicity should be made whether to discontinue nursing or to discontinue the drug, taking into account the importance of the drug to the mother.

Pediatric Use: Safety and effectiveness in children have not been established.

ADVERSE REACTIONS
(See *"Warnings"* regarding induction of reobiasia, adverse effects on the fetus, increased incidence of gallbladder disease, and adverse effects similar to those of oral contraceptives, including thromboembolism.) The following additional adverse reactions have been reported with estrogenic therapy, including oral contraceptives:

Genitourinary system: Breakthrough bleeding, spotting, change in menstrual flow: dysmenorrhea; premenstrual-like syndrome; amenorrhea during and after treatment; increase in size of uterine fibromyomata; vaginal candidiasis; change in cervical eversion and in degree of cervical secretion; cystitis-like syndrome.

◆ RATED THERAPEUTICALLY EQUIVALENT; ◇ THERAPEUTIC EQUIVALENCE UNCONFIRMED; ○ UNRATED

Breasts: Tenderness, enlargement, secretion.

Gastrointestinal: Nausea, vomiting; abdominal cramps, bloating; cholestatic jaundice.

Skin: Chloasma or melasma which may persist when drug is discontinued; erythema multiforme; erythema nodosum; hemorrhagic eruption; loss of scalp hair; hirsutism.

Eyes: Steepening of corneal curvature; intolerance to contact lenses.

CNS: Headache, migraine, dizziness; mental depression; chorea.

Miscellaneous: Increase or decrease in weight; reduced carbohydrate tolerance; aggravation of porphyria; edema; changes in libido.

ACUTE OVERDOSAGE
Numerous reports of ingestion of large doses of estrogen-containing oral contraceptives by young children indicate that serious ill effects do not occur. Overdosage of estrogen may cause nausea, and withdrawal bleeding may occur in females.

DOSAGE AND ADMINISTRATION
1. GIVEN CYCLICALLY FOR SHORT-TERM USE ONLY
For treatment of moderate to severe vasomotor symptoms associated with the menopause. The lowest dose that will control symptoms should be chosen and medication should be discontinued as promptly as possible. Administration should be cyclic (e.g., 3 weeks on and 1 week off). Attempts to discontinue or taper medication should be made at 3-to 6-month intervals. The usual dosage range is one 0.02 mg or 0.05 mg tablet daily. In some instances the effective dose may be as low as one 0.02 mg tablet every other day. A useful dosage schedule for early menopause, while spontaneous menstruation continues, is 0.05 mg once a day for twenty-one days and then a rest period for seven days. For the initial treatment of the late menopause, the same regimen is indicated with the 0.02 mg Ethinyl Estradiol Tablet for the first few cycles, after which the 0.05 mg dosage may be substituted. In more severe cases, such as those due to surgical and roentgenologic castration, one 0.05 mg tablet may be administered three times daily at the start of treatment. With adequate clinical improvement, usually obtainable in a few weeks, the dosage may be reduced to one 0.05 mg tablet daily and the patient continued thereafter on a maintenance dosage as in the average case.

2. GIVEN CYCLICALLY
Female hypogonadism: One 0.05 mg tablet is given one to three times daily during the first 2 weeks of a theoretical menstrual cycle. This is followed by progesterone during the last half of the arbitrary cycle. This regimen is continued for 3 to 6 months. The patient is then allowed to go untreated for 2 months to determine whether or not she can maintain the cycle without hormonal therapy. If not, additional courses of therapy may be prescribed.

3. GIVEN CHRONICALLY
Inoperable progressing prostatic cancer: From three 0.05 mg to four 0.5 mg tablets may be administered daily for palliation.

Inoperable progressing breast cancer in appropriately selected postmenopausal women (see *"Indications and Usage"*): Two 0.5 mg tablets three times daily for palliation.

Treated patients with an intact uterus should be monitored closely for signs of endometrial cancer and appropriate diagnostic measures should be taken to rule out malignancy in the event of persistent or recurring abnormal vaginal bleeding.

STORAGE
Store between 2° and 30°C (36° and 86°F).

PHYSICIAN REFERENCES
1. Ziel, H. K. and W. D. Finkle, "Increased Risk of Endometrial Carcinoma Among User of Conjugated Estrogens," *N Engl J Med.* 293:1167-1170. 1975. 2. Smith, D. C., R. Prentic, D. J. Thompson, and W. L. Hermann, "Association of Exogenous Estrogen and Endometrial Carcinoma," *N Engl J Med.* 293:1164-1167, 1975. 3. Mack. T. M., M. C. Pike, B. E. Henderson, et al. "Estrogens and Endometrial Cancer in a Retirement Community," *N Engl J Med.* 294:1262-1267, 1976. 4. Weiss, N.S., D.R. Szekely and D.F. Austin, "Increasing Incidence of Endomotrial Cancer in the United States," N Engl J med. 294: 1259—1262. 1976. 5. Herbst. A. L. H., Ulfelder and D. C. Poskanzer. "Adeno-carcinoma of Vagina," *N Engl J Med.* 284:878-881, 1971. 6. Greenwald, P., J. Barlow, P. Nasca, and W. Burnett, "Vaginal Cancer after Maternal Treatment with Synthetic Estrogens," *N Engl J Med.* 285:390-392, 1971. 7 Lanier A. K. Noller, D. Decker, L Elveback, and L. Kurland. "Cancer and Stilbestrol. A Follow-up of 1.719 Persons Exposed to Estrogens in Utero and Born 1943-1959," *Mayo Clin Proc.* 48:793-799, 1973. 8 Herbst. A. R. Kurman, and R. Scully. "Vaginal and Cervical Abnormalities After Exposure to Stilbestrol in Utero," *Obstet Gynecol.* 40:287-298, 1972. 9. Herbst A. D. Poskanzer, S. Robboy. L. Friedlander, and R. Scully, "Prenatal Exposure to Stilbestrol. A Prospective Comparison of Exposed Female Offspring with Unexposed Controls," *N Engl J Med.* 292:334-339, 1975. 10. Staft. A. R. Mattingly. D. Foley, and W. Fetherston, "Clinical Diagnosis of Vaginal Adenosis," *Obstet Gynecol,* 43:118-128, 1974. 11. Sherman A. I. M Goldrath. A Berlin, et al. "Cervical-Vaginal Aderosis After *in Utero* Exposure to Synthetic Estrogens." *Obstet Gynecol* 44:531-545, 1974. 12. Gal. I. B. Kirman, and J. Stern, "Hormone Pregnancy Tests and Congenital Malformation," *Nature,* 216:83, 1967. 13. Levy, E. P. A. Cohen, and F. C. Fraser, "Hormone Treatment During Pregnancy and Congenital Heart Defects," *Lancet,* 1:611, 1973. 14. Nora, J. and A. Nora, "Birth Defects and Oral Contraceptives," *Lancet,* 1:941-942, 1973. 15. Janerich, D.T.J.M. Piper, and D. M. Glebatis, "Oral Contraceptives and Congenital Limb-Reduction Defects," *N Engl J Med.* 291:697-700, 1974. 16. Boston Collaborative Drug Surveillance Program, "Surgically Confirmed Gall Bladder Disease. Venous Thromboembolism and Breast Tumors in Relation to Post-Menopausal Estrogen Therapy," *N Engl J Med.* 290:15-19, 1974. 17. Hoover, R., L.A. Gray, Sr., P. Cole, and B. MacMahon, "Menopausal Estrogens and Breast Cancer," N Engl J Med. 295:401-405, 1976. 18. Boston Collaborative Drug Surveillance Program. "Oral Contraceptives and Venous Thromboembolic Disease. Surgically Confirmed Gallbladder Disease, and Breast Tumors," *Lancet.* 1:1399-1404, 1973. 19. The Veterans Administration Cooperative Urological Research Group. "Carcinoma of the Prostate: Treatment Comparisons," *J Urol.* 98:516-522, 1967. 20. Bailar, J.C., "Thromboembolism and Oestrogen Therapy," *Lancet.* 2:560. 1967. 21. Blackard, C., R. Doe. G. Mellinger, and D. Byar, "Incidence of Cardiovascular Disease and Death in Patients Receiving Diethylstilbestrol for Carcinoma of the Prostate." *Cancer.* 26:249-256. 1970. 22. Royal College of General Practitioners. "Oral Contraception and Thromboembolic Disease," *J R Coll Gen Pract.* 13:267-279. 1967. 23. Inman, W.H.W. and M.P. Vessey, "Investigation of Deaths from Pulmonary, Coronary, and Cerebral Thrombosis and Embolism in Women of Child-Bearing Age," *Br Med J.* 2:193-199, 1968. 24. Vessey, M.P. and R. Doll. "Investigation of Relation Between Use of Oral Contraceptives and Thromboembolic Disease. A Further Report." *Br Med J.* 2:651-657, 1969. 25. Sartwell, P.E., A.T. Masi, F.G. Arthes, G.R. Greene, and H.E. Smith, "Thromboembolism and Oral Contraceptives: An Epidemiological Case Control Study." *Am J Epidemiol,* 90:365-380, 1969. 26. Collaborative Group for the Study of Stroke in Young Women. "Oral Contraception and Increased Risk of Cerebral Ischemia or Thrombosis," *N Engl J Med.* 288:871-878, 1973. 27. Collaborative Group for the Study of Stroke in Young Women. "Oral Contraceptives and Stroke in Young Women Associated Risk Factors." *JAMA* 231:718-722, 1975. 28. Mann J.I. and W.H.W. Inman. "Oral Contraceptives and Death from Myocardial Infarction," *Br Med J.* 2:245-248, 1975. 29. Mann, J.I. M.P. Vessey, M. Thorogood, and R Doll, "Myocardial Infarction in Young Women with Special Reference to Oral Contraceptive Practice," *Br Med J.* 2:241-245, 1975. 30. Inman, W.H.W. M.P. Vessey, B. Westerholm, and A Engelund. "Thromboembolic Disease and the Steroidal Content of Oral Contraceptives," *Br Med J.* 2:203-209, 1970. 31. Stolley, P.D. J.A. Tonascia, M.S. Tockman, P.E. Sartwell, A.H. Rutledge, and M.P. Jacobs, "Thrombosis with Low-Estrogen Oral Contraceptives," *Am J Epidemiol,* 102:197-208, 1975. 32. Vessey, M.P.R. Doll, A.S. Fairbairn, and G. Glober, "Post-Operative Thromboembolism and the Use of the Oral Contraceptives," *Br Med J.* 3:123-126, 1970. 33. Greene, G.R. and P.E. Sartwell, "Oral Contraceptive Use in Patients with Thromboembolism Following Surgery. Trauma or Infection," *Am J Public Health* 62:680-685, 1972. 34. Rosenberg, L., M.B. Armstrong and H. Jick, "Myocardial Infarction and Estrogen Therapy in Postmenopausal Women," *N Engl J Med.* 294:1256-1259, 1976. 35. Coronary Drug Project Research Group. "The Coronary Drug Project: Initial Findings Leading to Modifications of its Research Protocol," *JAMA.* 214:1303-1313, 1970. 36. Baum, J., F. Holtz, J.J. Bookstein, and E.W. Klein, "Possible Association between Benign Hepatomas and Oral Contraceptives," *Lancet,* 2:926-928, 1973. 37. Mays, E.T., W.M. Christopherson, M.M. Mahr, and H.C. Williams, "Hepatic Changes in Young Women Ingesting Contraceptive Steroids: Hepatic Hemorrhage and Primary Hepatic Tumors," *JAMA,* 235:730-782, 1976. 38. Edmondson, H.A.B. Henderson, and B. Benton, "Liver Cell Adenomas Associated with the Use of Oral Contraceptives," *N Engl J Med.* 294:470-472, 1976. 39. Pfeffer, R.I. and S. Van Den Noort, "Estrogen Use and Stroke Risk in Postmenopausal Women," *Am J Epidemiol,* 103:445-456, 1976.

HOW SUPPLIED
TABLETS: 0.02 MG

BRAND/MANUFACTURER	NDC	SIZE	AWP
○ **BRAND**			
ESTINYL: Schering	00085-0298-03	100s	$26.99
	00085-0298-06	250s	$63.46

TABLETS: 0.05 MG

BRAND/MANUFACTURER	NDC	SIZE	AWP
◇ **BRAND**			
ESTINYL: Schering	00085-0070-03	100s	$45.48
	00085-0070-06	250s	$106.13

TABLETS: 0.5 MG

BRAND/MANUFACTURER	NDC	SIZE	AWP
○ **BRAND**			
ESTINYL: Schering	00085-0150-03	100s	$91.92

Ethinyl Estradiol and Norgestrel

Patients should be counseled that this product does not protect against HIV infection (AIDS) and other sexually transmitted diseases.

DESCRIPTION
Each Ethinyl Estradiol/Norgestrel tablet contains 0.3 or 0.5 mg of norgestrel (*dl*-13-beta-ethyl-17-alpha-ethinyl-17-beta-hydrogen-4-en-3-one), a totally synthetic progestogen, and 0.03 or 0.05 mg of ethinyl estradiol (19-nbr-17α-pregna-1,3,5 (10)-trien-20-yne-3,17-diol). The package also contains 7 inert tablets.

CLINICAL PHARMACOLOGY
Combination oral contraceptives act by suppression of gonadotropins. Although the primary mechanism of this action is inhibition of ovulation, other alterations include changes in the cervical mucus (which increase the difficulty of sperm entry into the uterus) and the endometrium (which reduce the likelihood of implantation).

INDICATIONS AND USAGE
Oral contraceptives are indicated for the prevention of pregnancy in women who elect to use this product as a method of contraception.

Oral contraceptives are highly effective. Table I lists the typical accidental pregnancy rates for users of combination oral contraceptives and other methods of contraception. The efficacy of these contraceptive methods, except sterilization and the IUD, depends upon the reliability with which they are used. Correct and consistent use of methods can result in lower failure rates.

Table 1
LOWEST EXPECTED AND TYPICAL FAILURE RATES DURING THE FIRST YEAR OF CONTINUOUS USE OF A METHOD
% of Women Experiencing an Accidental Pregnancy in the First Year of Continuous Use

Method	Lowest Expected*	Typical**
(No Contraception)	(89)	(89)
Oral contraceptives		3
combined	0.1	N/A***
progestin only	0.5	N/A***
Diaphragm with spermicidal cream or jelly	3	18
Spermicides alone (foam, creams, jellies and vaginal suppositories)	3	21
Vaginal Sponge nulliparous	5	18
multiparous	>8	>28
IUD (medicated)	1	6#
Condom without spermicides	2	12
Periodic abstinence (all methods)	2-10	20
Female sterilization	0.2	0.4
Male sterilization	0.1	0.15

Adapted from J. Trussell and K. Kost, Table 11, Studies in Family Planning, 18(5), Sept.-Oct. 1987.

* *The authors' best guess of the percentage of women expected to experience an accidental pregnancy among couples who initiate a method (not necessarily for the first time) and who use it consistently and correctly during the first year if they do not stop for any other reason.*

** *This term represents "typical" couples who initiate use of a method (not necessarily for the first time), who experience an accidental pregnancy during the first year if they do not stop use for any other reason.*

*** *N/A—Data not available.*

\# *Combined typical rate for both medicated and non-medicated IUD. The rate for medicated IUD alone is not available.*

CONTRAINDICATIONS
Oral contraceptives should not be used in women with any of the following conditions:

Thrombophlebitis or thromboembolic disorders
A past history of deep-vein thrombophlebitis or thromboembolic disorders
Cerebral-vascular or coronary-artery disease
Known or suspected carcinoma of the breast
Carcinoma of the endometrium or other known or suspected estrogen-dependent neoplasia
Undiagnosed abnormal genital bleeding
Cholestatic jaundice of pregnancy or jaundice with prior pill use
Hepatic adenomas or carcinomas
Known or suspected pregnancy

WARNINGS

> CIGARETTE SMOKING INCREASES THE RISK OF SERIOUS CARDIOVASCULAR SIDE EFFECTS FROM ORAL-CONTRACEPTIVE USE. THIS RISK INCREASES WITH AGE AND WITH HEAVY SMOKING (15 OR MORE CIGARETTES PER DAY) AND IS QUITE MARKED IN WOMEN OVER 35 YEARS OF AGE. WOMEN WHO USE ORAL CONTRACEPTIVES SHOULD BE STRONGLY ADVISED NOT TO SMOKE.

The use of oral contraceptives is associated with increased risks of several serious conditions including myocardial infarction, thromboembolism, stroke, hepatic neoplasia, gallbladder disease, and hypertension, although the risk of serious morbidity or mortality is very small in healthy women without underlying factors. The risk of morbidity and mortality increases significantly in the presence of other underlying risk factors such as hypertension, hyperlipidemias, obesity, and diabetes.

Practitioners prescribing oral contraceptives should be familiar with the following information relating to these risks. The information contained in this package insert is based principally on studies carried out in patients who used oral contraceptives with higher formulations of estrogens and progestogens than those in common use today. The effect of long-term use of the oral contraceptives with lower formulations of both estrogens and progestogens remains to be determined.

Throughout this labeling, epidemiological studies reported are of two types: retrospective or case control studies and prospective or cohort studies. Case control studies provide a measure of the relative risk of disease, namely, a ratio of the incidence of a disease among oral-contraceptive users to that among nonusers. The relative risk does not provide information on the actual clinical occurrence of a disease. Cohort studies provide a measure of attributable risk, which is the difference in the incidence of disease between oral-contraceptive users and nonusers. The attributable risk does provide information about the actual occurrence of a disease in the population. For further information, the reader is referred to a text on epidemiological methods.

1. THROMBOEMBOLIC DISORDERS AND OTHER VASCULAR PROBLEMS
a. Myocardial Infarction: An increased risk of myocardial infarction has been attributed to oral-contraceptive use. This risk is primarily in smokers or women with other underlying risk factors for coronary-artery disease such as hypertension, hypercholesterolemia, morbid obesity, and diabetes. The relative risk of heart attack for current oral-contraceptive users has been estimated to be two to six. The risk is very low under the age of 30.

Smoking in combination with oral-contraceptive use has been shown to contribute substantially to the incidence of myocardial infarctions in women in their mid-thirties or older with smoking accounting for the majority of excess cases. Mortality rates associated with circulatory disease have been shown to increase substantially in smokers over the age of 35 and nonsmokers over the age of 40 (Table 2) among women who use oral contraceptives.

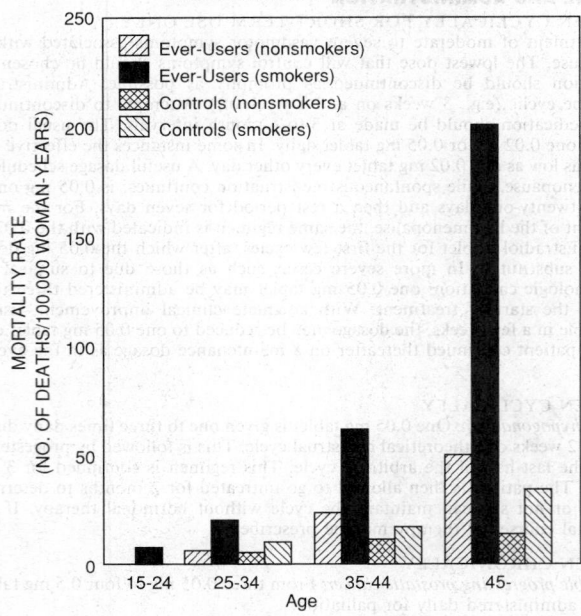

CIRCULATORY DISEASE MORTALITY RATES PER 100,000 WOMAN-YEARS BY AGE, SMOKING STATUS AND ORAL CONTRACEPTIVE USE

Table 2: (Adapted from P.M. Layde and V. Beral, Lancet. 1:541-546, 1981.)

Oral contraceptives may compound the effects of well-known risk factors, such as hypertension, diabetes, hyperlipidemias, age, and obesity. In particular, some progestogens are known to decrease HDL cholesterol and cause glucose intolerance, while estrogens may create a state of hyperinsulinism. Oral contraceptives have been shown to increase blood pressure among users (see section 9 in *"Warnings"*). Similar effects on risk factors have been associated with an increased risk of heart disease. Oral contraceptives must be used with caution in women with cardiovascular disease risk factors.

b. Thromboembolism: An increased risk of thromboembolic and thrombotic disease associated with the use of oral contraceptives is well established. Case control studies have found the relative risk of users compared to nonusers to be 3 for the first episode of superficial venous thrombosis, 4 to 11 for deep vein thrombosis or pulmonary embolism, and 1.5 to 6 for women with predisposing conditions for venous thromboembolic disease. Cohort studies have shown the relative risk to be somewhat lower, about 3 for new cases and about 4.5 for new cases requiring hospitalization. The risk of thromboembolic disease due to oral contraceptives is not related to length of use and disappears after pill use is stopped.

A two- to four-fold increase in relative risk of postoperative thromboembolic complications has been reported with the use of oral contraceptives. The relative risk of venous thrombosis in women who have predisposing conditions is twice that of women without such medical conditions. If feasible, oral contraceptives should be discontinued at least four weeks prior to and for two weeks after elective surgery of a type associated with an increase in risk of thromboembolism and during and following prolonged immobilization. Since the immediate postpartum period is also associated with an increased risk of thromboembolism, oral contraceptives should be started no earlier than four to six weeks after delivery in women who elect not to breast-feed, or a midtrimester pregnancy termination.

c. Cerebrovascular Diseases: Oral contraceptives have been shown to increase both the relative and attributable risks of cerebrovascular events (thrombotic and hemorrhagic strokes), although, in general, the risk is greatest among older (> 35 years), hypertensive women who also smoke. Hypertension was found to be a risk factor for both users and nonusers, for both types of strokes, while smoking interacted to increase the risk for hemorrhagic strokes.

In a large study, the relative risk of thrombotic strokes has been shown to range from 3 for normotensive users to 14 for users with severe hypertension. The relative risk of hemorrhagic stroke is reported to be 1.2 for nonsmokers who used oral contraceptives, 2.6 for smokers who did not use oral contraceptives, 7.6 for smokers who used oral contraceptives, 1.8 for normotensive users, and 25.7 for users with severe hypertension. The attributable risk is also greater in older women.

d. Dose Related Risk of Vascular Disease from Oral Contraceptives: A positive association has been observed between the amount of estrogen and progestogen in oral contraceptives and the risk of vascular disease. A decline in serum high-density lipoproteins (HDL) has been reported with many progestational agents. A decline in serum high-density lipoproteins has been associated with an increased incidence of ischemic heart disease. Because estrogens increase HDL cholesterol, the net effect of an oral contraceptive depends on a balance achieved between doses of estrogen and progestogen and the nature and absolute amount of progestogen used in the contraceptive. The amount of both hormones should be considered in the choice of an oral contraceptive.

Minimizing exposure to estrogen and progestogen is in keeping with good principles of therapeutics. For any particular estrogen/progestogen combination, the dosage regimen prescribed should be one which contains the least amount of estrogen and progestogen that is compatible with a low failure rate and the needs of the individual patient. New acceptors of oral-contraceptive agents should be started on preparations containing less than 50 mcg of estrogen.

e. Persistence of Risk of Vascular Disease: There are two studies which have shown persistence of risk of vascular disease for ever-users of oral contraceptives. In a study in the United States, the risk of developing myocardial infarction after discontinuing oral contraceptives persists for at least 9 years for women 40 to 49 years who had used oral contraceptives for five or more years, but this increased risk was not demonstrated in other age groups. In another study in Great Britain, the risk of developing cerebrovascular disease persisted for at least 6 years after discontinuation of oral contraceptives, although excess risk was very small. However, both studies were performed with oral-contraceptive formulations containing 50 mcg or higher of estrogens.

2. ESTIMATES OF MORTALITY FROM CONTRACEPTIVE USE

One study gathered data from a variety of sources which have estimated the mortality rate associated with different methods of contraception at different ages (Table 3). These estimates include the combined risk of death associated with contraceptive methods plus the risk attributable to pregnancy in the event of method failure. Each method of contraception has its specific benefits and risks. The study concluded that with the exception of oral-contraceptive users 35 and older who smoke and 40 and older who do not smoke, mortality associated with all methods of birth control is less than that associated with childbirth. The observation of a possible increase in risk of mortality with age for oral-contraceptive users is based on data gathered in the 1970's—but not reported until 1983. However, current clinical practice involves the use of lower estrogen dose formulations combined with careful restriction of oral contraceptive use to women who do not have the various risk factors listed in this labeling.

Because of these changes in practice and, also, because of some limited new data which suggest that the risk of cardiovascular disease with the use of oral contraceptives may now be less than previously observed, the Fertility and Maternal Health Drugs Advisory Committee was asked to review the topic in 1989. The Committee concluded that although cardiovascular disease risks may be increased with oral-contraceptive use after age 40 in healthy nonsmoking women (even with the newer low-dose formulations), there are greater potential health risks associated with pregnancy in older women and with the alternative surgical and medical procedures which may be necessary if such women do not have access to effective and acceptable means of contraception. Therefore, the Committee recommended that the benefits of oral-contraceptive use by healthy nonsmoking women over 40 may outweigh the possible risks. Of course, older women, as all women who take oral contraceptives, should take the lowest possible dose formulation that is effective. (See related table).

3. CARCINOMA OF THE REPRODUCTIVE ORGANS

Numerous epidemiological studies have been performed on the incidence of breast, endometrial, ovarian, and cervical cancer in women using oral contraceptives. The overwhelming evidence in the literature suggests that use of oral

contraceptives is not associated with an increase in the risk of developing breast cancer, regardless of the age and parity of first use or with most of the marketed brands and doses. The Cancer and Steroid Hormone (CASH) study also showed no latent effect on the risk of breast cancer for at least a decade following long-term use. A few studies have shown a slightly increased relative risk of developing breast cancer, although the methodology of these studies, which included differences in examination of users and nonusers and differences in age at start of use, has been questioned.

Some studies suggest that oral-contraceptive use has been associated with an increase in the risk of cervical intraepithelial neoplasia in some populations of women. However, there continues to be controversy about the extent to which such findings may be due to differences in sexual behavior and other factors.

In spite of many studies of the relationship between oral-contraceptive use and breast and cervical cancers, a cause-and-effect relationship has not been established.

4. HEPATIC NEOPLASIA

Benign hepatic adenomas are associated with oral-contraceptive use, although the incidence of benign tumors is rare in the United States. Indirect calculations have estimated the attributable risk to be in the range of 3.3 cases/100,000 for users, a risk that increases after four or more years of use. Rupture of rare, benign, hepatic adenomas may cause death through intra-abdominal hemorrhage.

Studies from Britain have shown an increased risk of developing hepatocellular carcinoma in long-term (> 8 years) oral-contraceptive users. However, these cancers are extremely rare in the U.S., and the attributable risk (the excess incidence) of liver cancers in oral contraceptive users approaches less than one per million users.

5. OCULAR LESIONS

There have been clinical case reports of retinal thrombosis associated with the use of oral contraceptives. Oral contraceptives should be discontinued if there is unexplained partial or complete loss of vision; onset of proptosis or diplopia; papilledema; or retinal vascular lesions. Appropriate diagnostic and therapeutic measures should be undertaken immediately.

6. ORAL-CONTRACEPTIVE USE BEFORE OR DURING EARLY PREGNANCY

Extensive epidemiological studies have revealed no increased risk of birth defects in women who have used oral contraceptives prior to pregnancy. Studies also do not suggest a teratogenic effect, particularly insofar as cardiac anomalies and limb reduction defects are concerned, when taken inadvertently during early pregnancy.

The administration of oral contraceptives to induce withdrawal bleeding should not be used as a test for pregnancy: Oral contraceptives should not be used during pregnancy to treat threatened or habitual abortion.

It is recommended that for any patient who has missed two consecutive periods, pregnancy should be ruled out before continuing oral contraceptive use. If the patient has not adhered to the prescribed schedule, the possibility of pregnancy should be considered at the time of the first missed period. Oral contraceptive use should be discontinued if pregnancy is confirmed.

7. GALLBLADDER DISEASE

Earlier studies have reported an increased lifetime relative risk of gallbladder surgery in users of oral contraceptives and estrogens. More recent studies, however, have shown that the relative risk of developing gallbladder disease among oral-contraceptive users may be minimal. The recent findings of minimal risk may be related to the use of oral-contraceptive formulations containing lower hormonal doses of estrogens and progestogens.

8. CARBOHYDRATE AND LIPID METABOLIC EFFECTS

Oral contraceptives have been shown to cause glucose intolerance in a significant percentage of users. Oral contraceptives containing greater than 75 mcg of estrogens cause hyperinsulinism, while lower doses of estrogen cause less glucose intolerance. Progestogens increase insulin secretion and create insulin resistance, this effect varying with different progestational agents. However, in the nondiabetic woman, oral contraceptives appear to have no effect on fasting blood glucose. Because of these demonstrated effects, prediabetic and diabetic women should be carefully observed while taking oral contraceptives.

Table 3

ANNUAL NUMBER OF BIRTH-RELATED OR METHOD-RELATED DEATHS ASSOCIATED WITH CONTROL OF FERTILITY PER 100,000 NONSTERILE WOMEN, BY FERTILITY-CONTROL METHOD ACCORDING TO AGE

Method of control and outcome	*15-19*	*20-24*	*25-29*	*30-34*	*35-39*	*40-44*
No fertility-control methods*	7.0	7.4	9.1	14.8	25.7	28.2
Oral contraceptives nonsmoker**	0.3	0.5	0.9	1.9	13.8	31.6
Oral contraceptives smoker**	2.2	3.4	6.6	13.5	51.1	117.2
IUD**	0.8	0.8	1.0	1.0	1.4	1.4
Condom*	1.1	1.6	0.7	0.2	0.3	0.4
Diaphragm/spermicide*	1.9	1.2	1.2	1.3	2.2	2.8
Periodic abstinence*	2.5	1.6	1.6	1.7	2.9	3.6

* *Deaths are birth related*
** *Deaths are method related*
Adapted from H.W. Ory, Family Planning Perspectives, 15:57-63, 1983.

A small proportion of women will have persistent hypertriglyceridemia while on the pill. As discussed earlier (see *"Warnings,"* 1a and 1d), changes in serum triglycerides and lipoprotein levels have been reported in oral-contraceptive users.

9. ELEVATED BLOOD PRESSURE

An increase in blood pressure has been reported in women taking oral contraceptives, and this increase is more likely in older oral-contraceptive users and with continued use. Data from the Royal College of General Practitioners and subsequent randomized trials have shown that the incidence of hypertension increases with increasing quantities of progestogens.

Women with a history of hypertension or hypertension-related diseases, or renal disease, should be encouraged to use another method of contraception. If women with hypertension elect to use oral contraceptives, they should be monitored closely, and if significant elevation of blood pressure occurs, oral contraceptives should be discontinued. For most women, elevated blood pressure will return to normal after stopping oral contraceptives, and there is no difference in the occurrence of hypertension among ever-and never-users.

10. HEADACHE

The onset or exacerbation of migraine or development of headache with a new pattern that is recurrent, persistent, or severe requires discontinuation of oral contraceptives and evaluation of the cause.

11. BLEEDING IRREGULARITIES

Breakthrough bleeding and spotting are sometimes encountered in patients on oral contraceptives, especially during the first three months of use. The type and dose of progestogen may be important. Non-hormonal causes should be considered and adequate diagnostic measures taken to rule out malignancy or pregnancy in the event of breakthrough bleeding, as in the case of any abnormal vaginal bleeding. If pathology has been excluded, time or a change to another formulation may solve the problem. In the event of amenorrhea, pregnancy should be ruled out.

Some women may encounter post-pill amenorrhea or oligomenorrhea, especially when such a condition was preexistent.

PRECAUTIONS

Patients should be counseled that this product does not protect against HIV infection (AIDS) and other sexually transmitted diseases.

1. PHYSICAL EXAMINATION AND FOLLOW-UP

A complete medical history and physical examination should be taken prior to the initiation or reinstitution of oral contraceptives and at least annually during use of oral contraceptives. These physical examinations should include special reference to blood pressure, breasts, abdomen and pelvic organs, including cervical cytology, and relevant laboratory tests. In case of undiagnosed, persistent or recurrent abnormal vaginal bleeding, appropriate diagnostic measures should be conducted to rule out malignancy. Women with a strong family history of breast cancer or who have breast nodules should be monitored with particular care.

2. LIPID DISORDERS

Women who are being treated for hyperlipidemias should be followed closely if they elect to use oral contraceptives. Some progestogens may elevate LDL levels and may render the control of hyperlipidemias more difficult. (See *"Warnings,"* 1d.).

3. LIVER FUNCTION

If jaundice develops in any woman receiving such drugs, the medication should be discontinued. Steroid hormones may be poorly metabolized in patients with impaired liver function.

4. FLUID RETENTION

Oral contraceptives may cause some degree of fluid retention. They should be prescribed with caution, and only with careful monitoring, in patients with conditions which might be aggravated by fluid retention.

5. EMOTIONAL DISORDERS

Patients becoming significantly depressed while taking oral contraceptives should stop the medication and use an alternate method of contraception in an attempt to determine whether the symptom is drug related. Women with a history of depression should be carefully observed and the drug discontinued if depression recurs to a serious degree.

6. CONTACT LENSES

Contact lens wearers who develop visual changes or changes in lens tolerance should be assessed by an ophthalmologist.

7. DRUG INTERACTIONS

Reduced efficacy and increased incidence of breakthrough bleeding and menstrual irregularities have been associated with concomitant use of rifampin. A similar association, though less marked, has been suggested with barbiturates, phenylbutazone, phenytoin sodium, and possibly with griseofulvin, ampicillin, and tetracyclines.

8. INTERACTIONS WITH LABORATORY TESTS

Certain endocrine- and liver-function tests and blood components may be affected by oral contraceptives:

a. Increased prothrombin and factors VII, VIII, IX, and X; decreased antithrombin 3; increased norepinephrine-induced platelet aggregability.

b. Increased thyroid-binding globulin (TBG) leading to increased circulating total thyroid hormone, as measured by protein-bound iodine (PBI), T4 by column or by radioimmunoassay. Free T3 resin uptake is decreased, reflecting the elevated TBG; free T4 concentration is unaltered.

c. Other binding proteins may be elevated in serum.

d. Sex-binding globulins are increased and result in elevated levels of total circulating sex steroids and corticoids; however, free or biologically active levels remain unchanged.

e. Triglycerides may be increased.

f. Glucose tolerance may be decreased.

g. Serum folate levels may be depressed by oral-contraceptive therapy. This may be of clinical significance if a woman becomes pregnant shortly after discontinuing oral contraceptives.

9. CARCINOGENESIS

See *"Warnings"* section.

10. PREGNANCY

Pregnancy Category X. See *"Contraindications"* and *"Warnings"* sections.

11. NURSING MOTHERS

Small amounts of oral-contraceptive steroids have been identified in the milk of nursing mothers, and a few adverse effects on the child have been reported, including jaundice and breast enlargement. In addition, oral contraceptives given in the postpartum period may interfere with lactation by decreasing the quantity and quality of breast milk. If possible, the nursing mother should be advised not to use oral contraceptives but to use other forms of contraception until she has completely weaned her child.

INFORMATION FOR THE PATIENT

See manufacturer's patient information.

ADVERSE REACTIONS

An increased risk of the following serious adverse reactions has been associated with the use of oral contraceptives (see *"Warnings"* section):

Thrombophlebitis.
Arterial thromboembolism.
Pulmonary embolism.
Myocardial infarction.
Cerebral hemorrhage.
Cerebral thrombosis.
Hypertension.
Gallbladder disease.
Hepatic adenomas or benign liver tumors.

There is evidence of an association between the following conditions and the use of oral contraceptives, although additional confirmatory studies are needed:

Mesenteric thrombosis.
Retinal thrombosis.

The following adverse reactions have been reported in patients receiving oral contraceptives and are believed to be drug related:

Nausea.
Vomiting.
Gastrointestinal symptoms (such as abdominal cramps and bloating).
Breakthrough bleeding.
Spotting.
Change in menstrual flow.
Amenorrhea.
Temporary infertility after discontinuation of treatment.
Edema.
Melasma which may persist.
Breast changes: tenderness, enlargement, secretion.
Change in weight (increase or decrease).
Change in cervical erosion and secretion.
Diminution in lactation when given immediately postpartum.
Cholestatic jaundice.
Migraine.
Rash (allergic).
Mental depression.
Reduced tolerance to carbohydrates.
Vaginal candidiasis.
Change in corneal curvature (steepening).
Intolerance to contact lenses.

The following adverse reactions have been reported in users of oral contraceptives and the asociation has been neither confirmed nor refuted:

Congenital anomalies.
Premenstrual syndrome.
Cataracts.
Optic neuritis.
Changes in appetite.
Cystitis-like syndrome.
Headache.
Nervousness.
Dizziness.
Hirsutism.
Loss of scalp hair.

◆ RATED THERAPEUTICALLY EQUIVALENT; ◇ THERAPEUTIC EQUIVALENCE UNCONFIRMED; ○ UNRATED

Erythema multiforme.
Erythema nodosum.
Hemorrhagic eruption.
Vaginitis.
Porphyria.
Impaired renal function.
Hemolytic uremic syndrome.
Budd-Chiari syndrome.
Acne.
Changes in libido.
Colitis.
Sickle cell disease.
Cerebral-vascular disease with mitral valve prolapse.
Lupus-like syndromes.

OVERDOSAGE

Serious ill effects have not been reported following acute ingestion of large doses of oral contraceptives by young children. Overdosage may cause nausea, and withdrawal bleeding may occur in females.

NONCONTRACEPTIVE HEALTH BENEFITS

The following noncontraceptive health benefits related to the use of oral contraceptives are supported by epidemiological studies which largely utilized oral contraceptive formulations containing doses exceeding 0.035 mg of ethinyl estradiol or 0.05 mg of mestranol.
Effects on menses:

Increased menstrual cycle regularity.
Decreased blood loss and decreased incidence of iron-deficiency anemia.
Decreased incidence of dysmenorrhea.

Effects related to inhibition of ovulation:

Decreased incidence of functional ovarian cysts.
Decreased incidence of ectopic pregnancies.

Effects from long-term use:

Decreased incidence of fibroadenomas and fibrocystic disease of the breast.
Decreased incidence of acute pelvic inflammatory disease.
Decreased incidence of endometrial cancer.
Decreased incidence of ovarian cancer.

DOSAGE AND ADMINISTRATION

To achieve maximum contraceptive effectiveness, Ethinyl Estradiol/Norgestrel must be taken exactly as directed and at intervals not exceeding 24 hours.

The dosage of Ethinyl Estradiol/Norgestrel is one tablet daily for 21 consecutive days per menstrual cycle according to prescribed schedule. Tablets are then discontinued for 7 days (three weeks on, one week off).

It is recommended that Ethinyl Estradiol/Norgestrel tablets be taken at the same time each day, preferably after the evening meal or at bedtime.

During the first cycle of medication, the patient is instructed to take one Ethinyl Estradiol/Norgestrel tablet daily for twenty-one consecutive days, beginning on day five of her menstrual cycle. (The first day of menstruation is day one.) The tablets are then discontinued for one week (7 days). Withdrawal bleeding should usually occur within 3 days following discontinuation of Ethinyl Estradiol/Norgestrel. (If Ethinyl Estradiol/Norgestrel is first taken later than the fifth day of the first menstrual cycle of medication or post-partum, contraceptive reliance should not be placed on Ethinyl Estradiol/Norgestrel until after the first seven consecutive days of administration. The possibility of ovulation and conception prior to initiation of medication should be considered.) The patient begins her next and all subsequent 21-day courses of Ethinyl Estradiol/Norgestrel tablets on the same day of the week that she began her first course, following the same schedule: 21 days on—7 days off. She begins taking her tablets on the 8th day after discontinuance, regardless of whether or not a menstrual period has occurred or is still in progress. Any time a new cycle of Ethinyl Estradiol/Norgestrel is started later than the 8th day, the patient should be protected by another means of contraception until she has taken a tablet daily for seven consecutive days.

If spotting or breakthrough bleeding occurs, the patient is instructed to continue on the same regimen. This type of bleeding is usually transient and without significance; however, if the bleeding is persistent or prolonged, the patient is advised to consult her physician. Although the occurrence of pregnancy is highly unlikely if Ethinyl Estradiol/Norgestrel is taken according to directions, if withdrawal bleeding does not occur, the possibility of pregnancy must be considered. If the patient has not adhered to the prescribed schedule (missed one or more tablets or started taking them on a day later than she should have), the probability of pregnancy should be considered at the time of the first missed period and appropriate diagnostic measures taken before the medication is resumed. If the patient has adhered to the prescribed regimen and misses two consecutive periods, pregnancy should be ruled out before continuing the contraceptive regimen.

The patient should be instructed to take a missed tablet as soon as it is remembered. If two consecutive tablets are missed, they should both be taken as soon as remembered. The next tablet should be taken at the usual time.

Any time the patient misses one or two tablets, she should also use another method of contraception until she has taken a tablet daily for seven consecutive days. If breakthrough bleeding occurs following missed tablets, it will usually be transient and of no consequence. While there is little likelihood of ovulation occurring if only one or two tablets are missed, the possibility of ovulation increases with each successive day that scheduled tablets are missed. If three consecutive tablets are missed, all medication should be discontinued and the remainder of the package discarded. A new tablet cycle should be started on the 8th day after the last tablet was taken, and an alternate means of contraception should be prescribed during the seven days without tablets and until the patient has taken a tablet daily for seven consecutive days.

In the nonlactating mother, Ethinyl Estradiol/Norgestrel may be initiated postpartum, for contraception. When the tablets are administered in the postpartum period, the increased risk of thromboembolic disease associated with the postpartum period must be considered (see *"Contraindications," "Warnings,"* and *"Precautions,"* concerning thromboembolic disease). It is to be noted that early resumption of ovulation may occur if bromocriptine mesylate has been used for the prevention of lactation.

REFERENCES

Available Upon Request.

HOW SUPPLIED

TABLETS: 0.3 MG-30 MCG

BRAND/MANUFACTURER	NDC	SIZE	AWP
○ **BRAND**			
LO/OVRAL-28: Wyeth-Ayerst	00008-2514-01	28s	$22.30
► LO/OVRAL: Wyeth-Ayerst	00008-0078-01	126s	$149.03
LO/OVRAL-28: Wyeth-Ayerst	00008-2514-02	168s	$150.83

TABLETS: 0.5 MG-50 MCG

BRAND/MANUFACTURER	NDC	SIZE	AWP
○ **BRAND**			
► OVRAL: Wyeth-Ayerst	00008-0056-02	21s	$32.90
OVRAL-28: Wyeth-Ayerst	00008-2511-01	28s	$33.27
► OVRAL: Wyeth-Ayerst	00008-0056-01	126s	$226.44
OVRAL-28: Wyeth-Ayerst	00008-2511-02	168s	$228.95

Ethinyl Estradiol and Norethindrone

Patients should be counseled that this product does not protect against HIV infection (AIDS) and other sexually transmitted diseases.

DESCRIPTION

Each brown tablet contains:
Fe 1/20 Ferrous Fumarate ....75 mg
Fe 1.5/30 Ferrous Fumarate ....75 mg

Each green tablet contains:
1.5/30 Ethinyl Estradiol ....30 mcg
Norethindrone ....1.5 mg

Each white tablet contains:
1/20 Ethinyl Estradiol ....20 mcg
Norethindrone ....1 mg

Ethinyl Estradiol/Norethindrone/Fe is a progestogen-estrogen combination.

Ethinyl Estradiol/Norethindrone/Fe 1/20 and 1.5/30 provides a continuous dosage regimen consisting of 21 oral contraceptive tablets and seven Ferrous Fumarate tablets. The Ferrous Fumarate tablets are present to facilitate ease of drug administration via a 28-day regimen and do not serve any therapeutic purpose.

21-DAY
Ethinyl Estradiol/Norethindrone 35 and Ethinyl Estradiol/Norethindrone 50 tablets provide a regimen for oral contraception derived from 21 tablets.

28-DAY
Ethinyl Estradiol/Norethindrone 35 and Ethinyl Estradiol/Norethindrone 50 tablets provide a continuous regimen for oral contraception derived from 21 tablets composed of Ethinyl Estradiol/Norethindrone to be followed by 7 green tablets of inert ingredients.

The active Ethinyl Estradiol/Norethindrone 35 tablets contain 0.4 mg Norethindrone and 0.035 mg Ethinyl Estradiol. The active Ethinyl Estradiol/Norethindrone 50 tablets contain 1 mg Norethindrone and 0.05 mg Ethinyl Estradiol. The green tablets contain inert ingredients.

CLINICAL PHARMACOLOGY

Combination oral contraceptives act by suppression of gonadotropins. Although the primary mechanism of this action is inhibition of ovulation, other alterations include changes in the cervical mucus (which increase the difficulty of sperm entry into the uterus) and the endometrium (which reduce the likelihood of implantation).

INDICATIONS AND USAGE

Ethinyl Estradiol/Norethindrone Acetate 21 and Ethinyl Estradiol/Norethindrone Acetate/Fe are indicated for the prevention of pregnancy in women who elect to use oral contraceptives as a method of contraception.

Oral contraceptives are highly effective. Table 1 lists the typical accidental pregnancy rates for users of combination oral contraceptives and other methods of contraception. The efficacy of these contraceptive methods, except sterilization, depends upon the reliability with which they are used. Correct and consistent use of methods can result in lower failure rates. (See related table).

CONTRAINDICATIONS

Oral contraceptives should not be used in women who currently have the following conditions:

- Thrombophlebitis or thromboembolic disorders
- A past history of deep vein thrombophlebitis or thromboembolic disorders
- Cerebral vascular or coronary artery disease
- Known or suspected carcinoma of the breast
- Carcinoma of the endometrium or other known or suspected estrogen-dependent neoplasia
- Undiagnosed abnormal genital bleeding
- Cholestatic jaundice of pregnancy or jaundice with prior pill use
- Hepatic adenomas or carcinomas
- Known or suspected pregnancy

WARNINGS

> CIGARETTE SMOKING INCREASES THE RISK OF SERIOUS CARDIOVASCULAR SIDE EFFECTS FROM ORAL CONTRACEPTIVE USE. THIS RISK INCREASES WITH AGE AND WITH HEAVY SMOKING (15 OR MORE CIGARETTES PER DAY) AND IS QUITE MARKED IN WOMEN OVER 35 YEARS OF AGE. WOMEN WHO USE ORAL CONTRACEPTIVES SHOULD BE STRONGLY ADVISED NOT TO SMOKE.

The use of oral contraceptives is associated with increased risks of several serious conditions including myocardial infarction, thromboembolism, stroke, hepatic neoplasia, and gallbladder disease, although the risk of serious morbidity or mortality is very small in healthy women without underlying risk factors. The risk of morbidity and mortality increases significantly in the presence of other underlying risk factors such as hypertension, hyperlipidemias, obesity and diabetes.

Practitioners prescribing oral contraceptives should be familiar with the following information relating to these risks. The information contained in this package insert is principally based on studies carried out in patients who used oral contraceptives with higher formulations of estrogens and progestogens than those in common use today. The effect of long-term use of the oral contraceptives with lower formulations of both estrogens and progestogens remains to be determined.

Throughout this labeling, epidemiological studies reported are of two types: retrospective or case control studies and prospective or cohort studies. Case control studies provide a measure of the relative risk of a disease, namely, a *ratio* of the incidence of a disease among oral contraceptive users to that among nonusers. The relative risk does not provide information on the actual clinical occurrence of a disease. Cohort studies provide a measure of attributable risk, which is the *difference* in the incidence of disease between oral contraceptive users and nonusers. The attributable risk does provide information about the actual occurrence of a disease in the population (adapted from refs. 2 and 3 with the author's permission). For further information, the reader is referred to a text on epidemiological methods.

1. THROMBOEMBOLIC DISORDERS AND OTHER VASCULAR PROBLEMS

The physician should be alert to the earliest manifestations of thromboembolic thrombotic disorders as discussed below. Should any of these occur or be suspected the drug should be discontinued immediately.

a. Myocardial Infarction: An increased risk of myocardial infarction has been attributed to oral contraceptive use. This risk is primarily in smokers or women with other underlying risk factors for coronary artery disease such as hypertension, hypercholesterolemia, morbid obesity, and diabetes. The relative risk of heart attack for current oral contraceptive users has been estimated to be two to six (4-10). The risk is very low under the age of 30.

Smoking in combination with oral contraceptive use has been shown to contribute substantially to the incidence of myocardial infarctions in women in their mid-thirties or older with smoking accounting for the majority of excess cases (11). Mortality rates associated with circulatory disease have been shown to increase substantially in smokers over the age of 35 and nonsmokers over the age of 40 (Table 2) among women who use oral contraceptives.

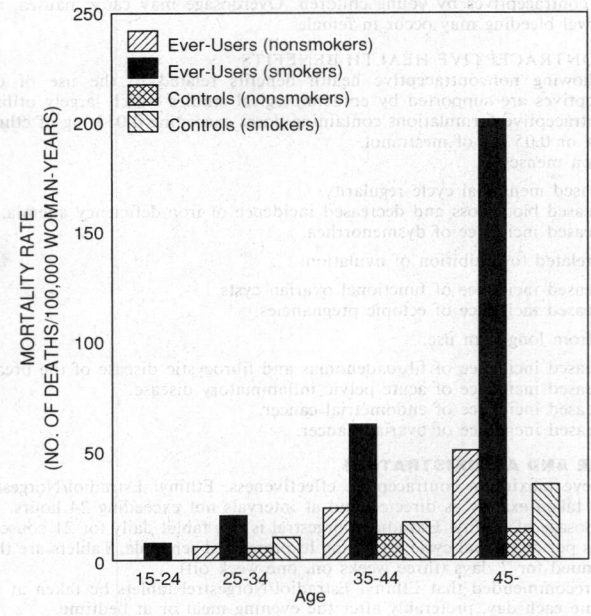

CIRCULATORY DISEASE MORTALITY RATES PER 100,000 WOMAN-YEARS BY AGE, SMOKING STATUS AND ORAL CONTRACEPTIVE USE

Oral contraceptives may compound the effects of well-known risk factors, such as hypertension, diabetes, hyperlipidemias, age and obesity (13). In particular, some progestogens are known to decrease HDL cholesterol and cause glucose intolerance, while estrogens may create a state of hyperinsulinism (14-18). Oral contraceptives have been shown to increase blood pressure among users (see section 9 in *"Warnings"*). Similar effects on risk factors have been associated with an increased risk of heart disease and the risk increases with the number of risk

Table 1
LOWEST EXPECTED AND TYPICAL FAILURE RATES DURING THE FIRST YEAR OF CONTINUOUS USE OF A METHOD
% OF WOMEN EXPERIENCING AN ACCIDENTAL PREGNANCY IN THE FIRST YEAR OF CONTINUOUS USE

Method	Lowest Expected*	Typical**
(No contraception)	(89)	(89)
Oral contraceptives		3
combined	0.1	N/A***
progestin only	0.5	N/A***
Diaphragm with spermicidal cream or jelly	3	18
Spermicides alone		
(foam, creams, jellies and vaginal suppositories)	3	21
Vaginal sponge		
nulliparous	5	18
multiparous	> 8	> 28
IUD (medicated)	1	6†
Condom without spermicides	2	12
Periodic abstinence (all methods)	2-10	20
Female sterilization	0.2	0.4
Male sterilization	0.1	0.15

Adapted from J. Trussell and K. Kost, Table 11, ref. #1.
* *The authors' best guess of the percentage of women expected to experience an accidental pregnancy among couples who initiate a method (not necessarily for the first time) and who use it consistently and correctly during the first year if they do not stop for any other reason.*
** *This term represents "typical" couples who initiate use of a method (not necessarily for the first time), who experience an accidental pregnancy during the first year if they do not stop use for any other reason.*
*** *N/A—Data not available*
† *Combined typical rate for both medicated and non-medicated IUD. The rate for medicated IUD alone is not available.*

factors present. Oral contraceptives must be used with caution in women with cardiovascular disease risk factors.

b. Thromboembolism: An increased risk of thromboembolic and thrombotic disease associated with the use of oral contraceptives is well established. Case control studies have found the relative risk of users compared to non-users to be 3 for the first episode of superficial venous thrombosis, 4 to 11 for deep vein thrombosis or pulmonary embolism, and 1.5 to 6 for women with predisposing conditions for venous thromboembolic disease (2,3,19-24). Cohort studies have shown the relative risk to be somewhat lower, about 3 for new cases and about 4.5 for new cases requiring hospitalization (25). The risk of thromboembolic disease due to oral contraceptives is not related to length of use and disappears after pill use is stopped. (2).

A two- to four-fold increase in relative risk of postoperative thromboembolic complications has been reported with the use of oral contraceptives (9,26). The relative risk of venous thrombosis in women who have predisposing conditions is twice that of women without such medical conditions. (9,26). If feasible, oral contraceptives should be discontinued at least four weeks prior to and for two weeks after elective surgery of a type associated with an increase in risk of thromboembolism and during and following prolonged immobilization. Since the immediate post partum period is also associated with an increased risk of thromboembolism, oral contraceptives should be started no earlier than four to six weeks after delivery in women who elect not to breastfeed.

c. Cerebrovascular Diseases: Oral contraceptives have been shown to increase both the relative and attributable risks of cerebrovascular events (thrombotic and hemorrhagic strokes), although, in general, the risk is greatest among older (> 35 years), hypertensive women who also smoke. Hypertension was found to be a risk factor for both users and non-users, for both types of strokes, while smoking interacted to increase the risk for hemorrhagic strokes (27-29).

In a large study, the relative risk of thrombotic strokes has been shown to range from 3 for normotensive users to 14 for users with severe hypertension (30). The relative risk of hemorrhagic stroke is reported to be 1.2 for nonsmokers who used oral contraceptives, 2.6 for smokers who did not use oral contraceptives, 7.6 for smokers who used oral contraceptives, 1.8 for normotensive users and 25.7 for users with severe hypertension(30). The attributable risk is also greater in older women (3).

d. Dose-related Risk of Vascular Disease from Oral Contraceptives: A positive association has been observed between the amount of estrogen and progestogen in oral contraceptives and the risk of vascular disease. (31-33). A decline in serum high density lipoproteins (HDL) has been reported with many progestational agents (14-16). A decline in serum high density lipoproteins has been associated with an increased incidence of ischemic heart disease. Because estrogens increase HDL cholesterol, the net effect of an oral contraceptive depends on a balance achieved between doses of estrogen and progestogen and the nature and absolute amount of progestogens used in the contraceptive. The amount of both hormones should be considered in the choice of an oral contraceptive.

Minimizing exposure to estrogen and progestogen is in keeping with good principles of therapeutics. For any particular estrogen/progestogen combination, the dosage regimen prescribed should be one which contains the least amount of estrogen and progestogen that is compatible with a low failure rate and the needs of the individual patient. New acceptors of oral contraceptive agents should be started on preparations containing the lowest dose of estrogen which produces satisfactory results for the patient (0.05 mg or less).

e. Persistence of Risk of Vascular Disease: There are two studies which have shown persistence of risk of vascular disease for ever-users of oral contraceptives. In a study in the United States, the risk of developing myocardial infarction after discontinuing oral contraceptives persists for at least 9 years for women 40-49 years who had used oral contraceptives for 5 or more years, but this increased risk was not demonstrated in other age groups (8). In another study in Great Britain, the risk of developing cerebrovascular disease persisted for at least 6 years after discontinuation of oral contraceptives, although excess risk was very small (34). However, both studies were performed with oral contraceptive formulations containing 50 micrograms or higher of estrogens.

2. ESTIMATES OF MORTALITY FROM CONTRACEPTIVE USE

One study gathered data from a variety of sources which have estimated the mortality rate associated with different methods of contraception at different ages (Table III). These estimates include the combined risk of death associated with contraceptive methods plus the risk attributable to pregnancy in the event of method failure. Each method of contraception has its specific benefits and risks. The study concluded that with the exception of oral contraceptive users 35 and older who smoke and 40 and older who do not smoke, mortality associated with all methods of birth control is low and below that associated with childbirth. The observation of a possible increase in risk of mortality with age for oral contraceptive users is based on data gathered in the 1970's—but not reported until 1983 (35). However, current clinical practice involves the use of lower estrogen dose formulations combined with careful restriction of oral contraceptive use to women who do not have the various risk factors listed in this labeling.

Because of these changes in practice and, also, because of some limited new data which suggest that the risk of cardiovascular disease with the use of oral contraceptives may now be less than previously observed, the Fertility and Maternal Health Drugs Advisory Committee was asked to review the topic in 1989. The Committee concluded that although cardiovascular disease risk may be increased with oral contraceptive use after age 40 in healthy nonsmoking women (even with the newer low-dose formulations), there are greater potential health risks associated with pregnancy in older women and with the alternative surgical

and medical procedures which may be necessary if such women do not have access to effective and acceptable means of contraception.

Therefore, the Committee recommended that the benefits of oral contraceptive use by healthy non-smoking women over 40 may outweigh the possible risks. Of course, older women, as all women who take oral contraceptives, should take the lowest possible dose formulation that is effective. (See related table).

3. CARCINOMA OF THE REPRODUCTIVE ORGANS

Numerous epidemiological studies have been performed on the incidence of breast, endometrial, ovarian and cervical cancer in women using oral contraceptives. Most of the studies on breast cancer and oral contraceptive use report that the use of oral contraceptives is not associated with an increase in the risk of developing breast cancer, regardless of the age and parity of first use or with most of the marketed brands and doses. The Cancer and Steroid Hormone (CASH) study also showed no latent effect on the risk of breast cancer for at least a decade following long-term use (36, 38, 83). Some studies have reported an increased risk of developing breast cancer in certain sub-groups of oral contraceptive users but the findings reported in these studies are not consistent, and the methodology of these studies, which included differences in examination of users and nonusers and differences in age at start of use, has been questioned. (37, 39, 43, 79-82).

Some studies suggest that oral contraceptive use has been associated with an increase in the risk of cervical intraepithelial neoplasia in some populations of women (45-48). However, there continues to be controversy about the extent to which such findings may be due to differences in sexual behavior and other factors.

In spite of many studies of the relationship between oral contraceptive use and breast and cervical cancers, a cause and effect relationship has not been established.

4. HEPATIC NEOPLASIA

Benign hepatic adenomas are associated with oral contraceptive use, although the incidence of benign tumors is rare in the United States. Indirect calculations have estimated the attributable risk to be in the range of 3.3 cases/100,000 for users, a risk that increases after four or more years of use (49). Rupture of rare, benign, hepatic adenomas may cause death through intra-abdominal hemorrhage (50,51).

Studies from Britain have shown an increased risk of developing hepatocellular carcinoma (52-54) in long-term (> 8 years) oral contraceptive users. However, these cancers are extremely rare in the U.S., and the attributable risk (the excess incidence) of liver cancers in oral contraceptive users approaches less than one per million users.

5. OCULAR LESIONS

There have been clinical case reports of retinal thrombosis associated with the use of oral contraceptives. Oral contraceptives should be discontinued if there is unexplained partial or complete loss of vision; onset of proptosis or diplopia; papilledema; or retinal vascular lesions. Appropriate diagnostic and therapeutic measures should be undertaken immediately.

6. ORAL CONTRACEPTIVE USE BEFORE OR DURING EARLY PREGNANCY

Extensive epidemiological studies have revealed no increased risk of birth defects in women who have used oral contraceptives prior to pregnancy (55-57). Studies also do not suggest a teratogenic effect, particularly insofar as cardiac anomalies and limb reduction defects are concerned (55,56,58,59), when taken inadvertently during early pregnancy.

The administration of oral contraceptives to induce withdrawal bleeding should not be used as a test for pregnancy. Oral contraceptives should not be used during pregnancy to treat threatened or habitual abortion.

It is recommended that for any patient who has missed two consecutive periods, pregnancy should be ruled out before continuing oral contraceptive use. If the patient has not adhered to the prescribed schedule, the possibility of pregnancy should be considered at the time of the first missed period. Oral contraceptive use should be discontinued if pregnancy is confirmed.

7. GALLBLADDER DISEASE

Earlier studies have reported an increased lifetime relative risk of gallbladder surgery in users of oral contraceptives and estrogens (60,61). More recent studies, however, have shown that the relative risk of developing gallbladder disease among oral contraceptive users may be minimal (62-64). The recent findings of minimal risk may be related to the use of oral contraceptive formulations containing lower hormonal doses of estrogens and progestogens.

8. CARBOHYDRATE AND LIPID METABOLIC EFFECTS

Oral contraceptives have been shown to cause glucose intolerance in a significant percentage of users (17). Oral contraceptives containing greater than 75 micrograms of estrogens cause hyperinsulinism, while lower doses of estrogen cause less glucose intolerance (65). Progestogens increase insulin secretion and create insulin resistance, this effect varying with different progestational agents (17,66). However, in the non-diabetic woman, oral contraceptives appear to have no effect on fasting blood glucose (67). Because of these demonstrated effects, prediabetic and diabetic women should be carefully observed while taking oral contraceptives.

A small proportion of women will have persistent hypertriglyceridemia while on the pill. As discussed earlier (see "Warnings", 1a. and 1d.), changes in serum triglycerides and lipoprotein levels have been reported in oral contraceptive users.

9. ELEVATED BLOOD PRESSURE

An increase in blood pressure has been reported in women taking oral contraceptives (68) and this increase is more likely in older oral contraceptive users (69) and with continued use (68). Data from the Royal College of General Practitioners (12) and subsequent randomized trials have shown that the incidence of hypertension increases with increasing concentrations of progestogens.

Women with a history of hypertension or hypertension-related diseases, or renal disease (70) should be encouraged to use another method of contraception. If women elect to use oral contraceptives, they should be monitored closely and if significant elevation of blood pressure occurs, oral contraceptives should be discontinued. For most women, elevated blood pressure will return to normal after stopping oral contraceptives (69), and there is no difference in the occurrence of hypertension among ever and never users (68,70,71).

10. HEADACHE

The onset or exacerbation of migraine or development of headache of a new pattern which is recurrent, persistent or severe requires discontinuation of oral contraceptives and evaluation of the cause.

11. BLEEDING IRREGULARITIES

Breakthrough bleeding and spotting are sometimes encountered in patients on oral contraceptives, especially during the first three months of use. Non-hormonal causes should be considered and adequate diagnostic measures taken to rule out malignancy or pregnancy in the event of break-through bleeding, as in the case of any abnormal vaginal bleeding. If pathology has been excluded, time or a change to another formulation may solve the problem. In the event of amenorrhea, pregnancy should be ruled out.

Women with a history of oligomenorrhea or secondary amenorrhea or young women without regular cycles prior to taking oral contraceptives may again have irregular bleeding or amenorrhea after discontinuation of oral contraceptives.

PRECAUTIONS

1. SEXUALLY-TRANSMITTED DISEASES

Patients should be counseled that this product does not protect against HIV infection (AIDS) and other sexually transmitted diseases.

2. PHYSICAL EXAMINATION AND FOLLOW-UP

A complete medical history and physical examination should be taken prior to the initiation or reinstitution of oral contraceptives and at least annually during use of oral contraceptives. These physical examinations should include special reference to blood pressure, breasts, abdomen and pelvic organs, including cervical cytology, and relevant laboratory tests. In case of undiagnosed, persistent or recurrent abnormal vaginal bleeding, appropriate diagnostic measures should be conducted to rule out malignancy. Women with a strong family history of breast cancer or who have breast nodules should be monitored with particular care.

3. LIPID DISORDERS

Women who are being treated for hyperlipidemias should be followed closely if they elect to use oral contraceptives. Some progestogens may elevate LDL levels and may render the control of hyperlipidemias more difficult.

4. LIVER FUNCTION

If jaundice develops in any woman receiving such drugs, the medication should be discontinued. Steroid hormones may be poorly metabolized in patients with impaired liver function.

5. FLUID RETENTION

Oral contraceptives may cause some degree of fluid retention. They should be prescribed with caution, and only with careful monitoring, in patients with conditions which might be aggravated by fluid retention.

6. EMOTIONAL DISORDERS

Women with a history of depression should be carefully observed and the drug discontinued if depression recurs to a serious degree.

Patients becoming significantly depressed while taking oral contraceptives should stop the medication and use an alternate method of contraception in an attempt to determine whether the symptom is drug-related.

7. CONTACT LENSES

Contact lens wearers who develop visual changes or changes in lens tolerance should be assessed by an ophthalmologist.

8. DRUG INTERACTIONS

Reduced efficacy and increased incidence of breakthrough bleeding and menstrual irregularities have been associated with concomitant use of rifampin. A similar association, though less marked, has been suggested with barbiturates, phenylbutazone, phenytoin sodium, and possibly with griseofulvin, ampicillin and tetracyclines (72).

9. INTERACTIONS WITH LABORATORY TESTS

Certain endocrine and liver function tests and blood components may be affected by oral contraceptives:

a. Increased prothrombin and factors VII, VIII, IX, and X; decreased antithrombin 3; increased norepinephrine-induced platelet aggregability.
b. Increased thyroid binding globulin (TBG) leading to increased circulating total thyroid hormone, as measured by protein-bound iodine (PBI), T4 by column, or by radioimmunoassay. Free T3 resin uptake is decreased, reflecting the elevated TBG; free T4 concentration is unaltered.
c. Other binding proteins may be elevated in serum.
d. Sex-binding globulins are increased and result in elevated levels of total circulating sex steroids and corticoids; however, free or biologically active levels remain unchanged.
e. Triglycerides may be increased.
f. Glucose tolerance may be decreased.
g. Serum folate levels may be depressed by oral contraceptive therapy. This may be of clinical significance if a woman becomes pregnant shortly after discontinuing oral contraceptives.

10. CARCINOGENESIS

See *"Warnings"* section.

11. PREGNANCY

Pregnancy Category X. See *"Contraindications"* and *"Warnings"* sections.

12. NURSING MOTHERS

Small amounts of oral contraceptive steroids have been identified in the milk of nursing mothers and a few adverse effects on the child have been reported, including jaundice and breast enlargement. In addition, oral contraceptives given in the postpartum period may interfere with lactation by decreasing the quantity and quality of breast milk. If possible, the nursing mother should be advised not to use oral contraceptives but to use other forms of contraception until she has completely weaned her child.

13. VOMITING AND/OR DIARRHEA

Although a cause-and-effect relationship has not been clearly established, several cases of oral contraceptive failure have been reported in association with vomiting and/or diarrhea. If significant gastrointestinal disturbance occurs in any woman receiving contraceptive steroids, the use of a back-up method of contraception for the remainder of that cycle is recommended.

ADVERSE REACTIONS

An increased risk of the following serious adverse reactions has been associated with the use of oral contraceptives (see "Warnings" section).

- Thrombophlebitis
- Arterial thromboembolism
- Pulmonary embolism
- Myocardial infarction
- Cerebral hemorrhage
- Cerebral thrombosis
- Hypertension
- Gallbladder disease
- Hepatic adenomas or benign liver tumors

There is evidence of an association between the following conditions and the use of oral contraceptives, although additional confirmatory studies are needed:

- Mesenteric thrombosis
- Retinal thrombosis

Table 3

ANNUAL NUMBER OF BIRTH-RELATED OR METHOD-RELATED DEATHS ASSOCIATED WITH CONTROL OF FERTILITY PER 100,000 NONSTERILE WOMEN, BY FERTILITY CONTROL METHOD ACCORDING TO AGE

Method of control and outcome	15-19	20-24	25-29	30-34	35-39	40-44
No fertility control methods*	7.0	7.4	9.1	14.8	25.7	28.2
Oral contraceptives non-smoker**	0.3	0.5	0.9	1.9	13.8	31.6
Oral contraceptives smoker**	2.2	3.4	6.6	13.5	51.1	117.2
IUD**	0.8	0.8	1.0	1.0	1.4	1.4
Condom*	1.1	1.6	0.7	0.2	0.3	0.4
Diaphragm/spermicide*	1.9	1.2	1.2	1.3	2.2	2.8
Periodic abstinence*	2.5	1.6	1.6	1.7	2.9	3.6

* *Deaths are birth related*
** *Deaths are method related*
Adapted from HW Ory, ref. #35.

The following adverse reactions have been reported in patients receiving oral contraceptives and are believed to be drug related:

- Nausea
- Vomiting
- Gastrointestinal symptoms (such as abdominal cramps and bloating)
- Breakthrough bleeding
- Spotting
- Change in menstrual flow
- Amenorrhea
- Temporary infertility after discontinuation of treatment
- Edema
- Melasma which may persist
- Breast changes: tenderness, enlargement, secretion
- Change in weight (increase or decrease)
- Change in cervical erosion and secretion
- Diminution in lactation when given immediately postpartum
- Cholestatic jaundice
- Migraine
- Rash (allergic)
- Mental depression
- Reduced tolerance to carbohydrates
- Vaginal candidiasis
- Change in corneal curvature (steepening)
- Intolerance to contact lenses

The following adverse reactions have been reported in users of oral contraceptives and the association has been neither confirmed nor refuted:

- Pre-menstrual syndrome
- Cataracts
- Changes in appetite
- Cystitis-like syndrome
- Headache
- Nervousness
- Dizziness
- Hirsutism
- Loss of scalp hair
- Erythema multiforme
- Erythema nodosum
- Hemorrhagic eruption
- Vaginitis
- Porphyria
- Impaired renal function
- Hemolytic uremic syndrome
- Budd-Chiari syndrome
- Acne
- Changes in libido
- Colitis

OVERDOSAGE

Serious ill effects have not been reported following acute ingestion of large doses of oral contraceptives by young children. Overdosage may cause nausea, and withdrawal bleeding may occur in females.

NONCONTRACEPTIVE HEALTH BENEFITS

The following non-contraceptive health benefits related to the use of oral contraceptives are supported by epidemiological studies which largely utilized oral contraceptive formulations containing estrogen doses exceeding 0.035 mg of Ethinyl Estradiol or 0.05 mg of mestranol exceeding 0.035 mg of Ethinyl Estradiol or 0.05 mg of mestranol (73-78).

Effects on menses:

- Increased menstrual cycle regularity
- Decreased blood loss and decreased incidence of iron deficiency anemia
- Decreased incidence of dysmenorrhea

Effects related to inhibition of ovulation:

- Decreased incidence of functional ovarian cysts
- Decreased incidence of ectopic pregnancies

Effects from long-term use:

- Decreased incidence of fibroadenomas and fibrocystic disease of the breast
- Decreased incidence of acute pelvic inflammatory disease
- Decreased incidence of endometrial cancer
- Decreased incidence of ovarian cancer

DOSAGE AND ADMINISTRATION

The tablet dispenser has been designed to make oral contraceptive dosing as easy and as convenient as possible. The tablets are arranged in either three or four rows of seven tablets each, with the days of the week appearing on the tablet dispenser above the first row of tablets.

Important Notes: The patient should be instructed to use an additional method of protection until after the first week of administration in the initial cycle if utilizing the Sunday-Start Regimen.

The possibility of ovulation and conception prior to initiation of use should be considered.

The patient is told (a) that she should take one pill every day at the same time, (b) many women have spotting or light bleeding or gastric distress during the first one to three cycles, (c) missing pills can also cause spotting or light bleeding, (d) she should use a back-up method for contraception if she has vomiting or diarrhea or takes some concomitant medications, and/or if she has trouble remembering the pill, (e) if she has any other questions she should consult her physician.

DOSAGE AND ADMINISTRATION FOR 21-DAY DOSAGE REGIMEN
To achieve maximum contraceptive effectiveness Ethinyl Estradiol/Norethindrone 21 must be taken exactly as directed and at intervals not exceeding 24 hours. Ethinyl Estradiol/Norethindrone 21 provides the patient with a convenient tablet schedule of "3 weeks on—1 week off." Two dosage regimens are described, one of which may be more convenient or suitable than the other for an individual patient. For the initial cycle of therapy, the patient begins her therapy according to the Day-5 or Sunday-Start Regimen. With either regimen, the patient takes one tablet daily for 21 consecutive days followed by one week of no tablets.

A. Sunday-Start Regimen: The patient begins taking tablets on the first Sunday after menstrual flow begins. When menstrual flow begins on Sunday, the first tablet is taken on the same day. The last tablet in the dispenser will then be taken on a Saturday, followed by no tablets for a week (7 days). For all subsequent cycles the patient then begins a new 21-tablet regimen on the eighth day, Sunday, after taking her last tablet. Following this regimen, of 21 days on—7 days off, the patient will start all subsequent cycles on a Sunday.

B. Day-5 Regimen: The first day of menstrual flow is Day 1. On Day 5 of her menstrual flow, the patient starts taking 1 tablet daily, beginning with the tablet that corresponds to Day 5 of her flow. After the last tablet (Saturday) has been taken, if any tablets remain, the patient completes her 21-tablet regimen starting with the Sunday tablet, followed by no tablets for a week (7 days). For all subsequent cycles, the patient begins a new 21 tablet regimen on the eighth day after taking her last tablet, again beginning on the same day of the week on which she began her first course. Following this regimen of 21 days on—7 days off, the patient will start all subsequent cycles on the same day of the week as the first course. Likewise, the interval of no tablets will always start on the same day of the week.

Whether utilizing the Sunday-Start or Day-5 Regimen, all tablets should be taken regularly with a meal or at bedtime. It should be stressed that efficacy of medication depends on strict adherence to the dosage schedule.

SPECIAL NOTES ON ADMINISTRATION
Menstruation usually begins two or three days, but may begin as late as the fourth or fifth day, after discontinuing medication. If spotting occurs while on the usual regimen of one tablet daily, the patient should continue medication without interruption.

If a patient forgets to take one or more tablets, the following is suggested: If one tablet is missed, take it as soon as remembered, or take two tablets the next day. If two consecutive tablets are missed, take two tablets daily for the next two days, then resume the regular schedule. While there is little likelihood of pregnancy occurring if the patient misses only one or two tablets, the possibility of pregnancy increases with each successive day that tablets are missed. *However if the patient is taking Ethinyl Estradiol/Norethindrone 21 1/20 in addition to taking two white tablets a day for two days, the patient should use an additional means of contraception for seven consecutive days.* If three consecutive tablets are missed, the patient starts a new course of tablets in the following manner: If the patient is on the Sunday-Start Regimen, a new course of tablets is started on the first Sunday following the last missed tablet, whether or not she is still menstruating. If the patient is on the Day 5-Regimen, a new course of tablets is started on the eighth day after the last tablet was taken. For example, if the patient took her last tablet on Monday, she should start her new course of tablets the following Monday. The patient should also use an additional method of birth control during the seven days without tablets, and until she has taken a tablet daily for seven consecutive days.

The possibility of ovulation occurring increases with each successive day that scheduled tablets are missed. While there is little likelihood of ovulation occurring if only one tablet is missed, the possibility of spotting or bleeding is increased. This is particularly likely to occur if two or more consecutive tablets are missed.

In the rare case of bleeding which resembles menstruation, the patients should be advised to discontinue medication and then begin taking tablets from a dispenser on the next Sunday or the fifth day (Day 5) depending on their regimen. Persistent bleeding which is not controlled by this method indicates the need for reexamination of the patient, at which time nonfunctional causes should be borne in mind.

DOSAGE AND ADMINISTRATION FOR 28-DAY DOSAGE REGIMEN
To achieve maximum contraceptive effectiveness, Ethinyl Estradiol/Norethindrone/Fe must be taken exactly as directed and at intervals not exceeding 24 hours.

Ethinyl Estradiol/Norethindrone/Fe provides a continuous administration regimen consisting of 21 *light-colored* (white or green) tablets of Ethinyl Estradiol/Norethindrone and 7 *brown* tablets of ferrous fumarate. The ferrous fumarate tablets are present to facilitate ease of drug administration via a 28-day regimen and do not serve any therapeutic purpose. There is no need for the patient to count days between cycles because there are no "off-tablet days."

The patient begins taking *light-colored* tablets from the top row on the first Sunday after menstrual flow begins. When menstrual flow begins on Sunday, the first *light-colored* tablet is taken on the same day. The patient takes one *light-colored* tablet daily for 21 days. The last *light-colored* tablet taken is the Saturday tablet. Upon completion of all 21 tablets, and without interruption, the patient takes one *brown* tablet daily for 7 days. Upon completion of this first course of tablets, the patient begins a second course of 28 tablets without interruption, the next day, Sunday, starting with the Sunday *light-colored* tablet in the top row. Adhering to this regimen, of one *light-colored* tablet daily for 21 days, followed without interruption by one *brown* tablet daily for seven days, the patient will start all subsequent cycles on a Sunday.

Tablets should be taken regularly with a meal or at bedtime. It should be stressed that efficacy of medication depends on strict adherence to the dosage schedule.

SPECIAL NOTES ON ADMINISTRATION

Menstruation usually begins two or three days, but may begin as late as the fourth or fifth day, after the *brown* tablets have been started. In any event, the next course of tablets should be started without interruption. There should never be a day when the patient is not taking a tablet.

If spotting occurs while the patient is taking *light-colored* tablets, continue medication without interruption.

If a patient forgets to take one or more *light-colored* tablets, the following is suggested. If one *light-colored* tablet is missed, take it as soon as remembered, or take two *light-colored* tablets the next day. If two consecutive *light-colored* tablets are missed, take two *light-colored* tablets daily for the next two days, then resume the regular schedule. While there is little likelihood of pregnancy occurring if the patient misses only one or two *light-colored* tablets, the possibility of pregnancy increases with each successive day that *light-colored* tablets are missed. *However, if the patient is taking Ethinyl Estradiol/Norethindnone/Fe 1/20 in addition to taking two white tablets a day for two days, the patient should use an additional means of contraception for seven consecutive days.* If three consecutive tablets are missed, the patient starts a new course of tablets the first Sunday following the last missed tablet, whether or not she is still menstruating. The patient should also use an additional method of birth control during the days without tablets, and until she has taken a tablet daily for seven consecutive days.

The possibility of ovulation occurring increases with each successive day that scheduled *light-colored* tablets are missed. While there is little likelihood of ovulation occurring if only one *light-colored* tablet is missed, the possibility of spotting or bleeding is increased. This is particularly likely to occur if two or more consecutive *light-colored* tablets are missed.

If one or more *brown* tablets are missed, the *light-colored* tablets should be started no later than the eighth day after the last *light-colored* tablet was taken. The possibility of conception occurring is not increased if *brown* tablets are missed.

In the rare case of bleeding which resembles menstruation, the patient should be advised to discontinue medication and then begin taking tablets from a dispenser on the next Sunday. Persistent bleeding which is not controlled by this method indicates the need for reexamination of the patient, at which time nonfunctional causes should be borne in mind.

USE OF ORAL CONTRACEPTIVES IN THE EVENT OF A MISSED MENSTRUAL PERIOD

1. If the patient has not adhered to the prescribed dosage regimen, the possibility of pregnancy should be considered after the first missed period and oral contraceptives should be withheld until pregnancy has been ruled out.

2. If the patient has adhered to the prescribed regimen and misses two consecutive periods, pregnancy should be ruled out before continuing the contraceptive regimen.

After several months on treatment, bleeding may be reduced to a point of virtual absence. This reduced flow may occur as a result of medication, in which event it is not indicative of pregnancy.

Store below 30°C (86°F).

REFERENCES

1. Reproduced with permission of the Population Council from J. Trussell and K. Kost: Contraceptive failure in the United States: A critical review of the literature. *Studies in Family Planning*, 18 (5), September-October 1987. 2. Stadel, BV: Oral contraceptives and cardiovascular disease, (Pt. 1). *New England Journal of Medicine*, 305:612-618, 1981. 3. Stadel, B.V.: Oral contraceptives and cardiovascular disease. (Pt. 2). *New England Journal of Medicine*, 305:672-677, 1981. 4. Adam, S.A., and M. Thorogood: Oral contraception and myocardial infarction revisited: The effects of new preparations and prescribing patterns. *Brit. J. Obstet. and Gynec.*, 88:838-845, 1981. 5. Mann, J.I., and W.H. Inman: Oral contraceptives and death from myocardial infarction. *Brit. Med. J.*, 2(5965): 245-248, 1975. 6. Mann, J.I., M.P. Vessey, M. Thorogood, and R. Doll: Myocardial infarction in young women with special reference to oral contraceptive practice. *Brit. Med. J.*, 2(5956):241-245, 1975. 7. Royal College of General Practitioners' Oral Contraception Study: Further analyses of mortality in oral contraceptive users. *Lancet* 1:541-546, 1981. 8. Slone, D., S. Shapiro, D.W. Kaufman, L. Rosenberg, O.S. Miettinen, and P.D. Stolley: Risk of myocardial infarction in relation to current and discontinued use of oral contraceptives. *N.E.J.M.*, 305:420-424, 1981. 9. Vessey, M.P.: Female hormones and vascular disease: An epidemiological overview, *Brit. J. Fam. Plann.*, 6:1-12, 1980. 10. Russell-Brief, R.G., T.M. Ezzati, R. Fulwood, J.A. Perlman, and R.S. Murphy; Cardiovascular risk status and oral contraceptive use, United States, 1976-80. *Preventive Medicine*, 15:352-362, 1986. 11. Goldbaum, G.M., J.S. Kendrick, G.C. Hogelin, and E.M. Gentry: The relative impact of smoking and oral contraceptive use on women in the United States. *J.A.M.A.*, 258:1339-1342, 1987. 12. Layde, P.M., and V. Beral: Further analyses of mortality in oral contraceptive users: Royal College General Practitioners' Oral Contraception Study. (Table 5) *Lancet*, 1:541-546, 1981. 13. Knopp, R.H.: Arteriosclerosis risk: The roles of oral contraceptives and postmenopausal estrogens. *J. of Reprod. Med.*, 31(9)(Supplement): 913-921, 1986. 14. Krauss, R.M., S. Roy, D.R. Mishell, J. Casagrande, and M.C. Pike: Effects of two low-dose oral contraceptives on serum lipids and lipoproteins: Differential changes in high-density lipoprotein subclasses. *Am. J. Obstet. Gyn*, 145:446-452, 1983. 15. Wahl, P., C. Walden, R. Knopp, J. Hoover, R. Wallace, G. Heiss, and B. Rifkind: Effect of estrogen/progestin potency on lipid/lipoprotein cholesterol, *N.E.J.M.*, 308:862-867, 1983. 16. Wynn, V., and R. Niththyananthan: The effect of progestin in combined oral contraceptives on serum lipids with special reference to high-density lipoproteins. *Am. J. Obstet. and Gyn.*, 142:766-771, 1982. 17. Wynn, V., and I. Godsland: Effects of oral contraceptives on carbohydrate metabolism. *J. Reprod. Medicine*, 31(9)(Supplement): 892-897, 1986. 18. LaRosa, J.C.: Atherosclerotic risk factors in cardiovascular disease. *J. Reprod. Med*, 31(9)(Supplement): 906-912, 1986. 19. Inman, W.H., and M.P. Vessey: Investigations of death from pulmonary, coronary, and cerebral thrombosis and embolism in women of child-bearing age. *Brit. Med. J.*, 2(5599): 193-199, 1968. 20. Maguire, M.G., J. Tonascia, P.E. Sartwell, P.D. Stolley, and M.S. Tockman: Increased risk of thrombosis due to oral contraceptives: A further report. *Am. J. Epidemiology*, 110(2):188-195, 1979. 21. Pettiti, D.B., J. Wingerd, F. Pellegrin, and S. Ramacharan: Risk of vascular disease in women: Smoking, oral contraceptives, noncontraceptive estrogens, and other factors, *J.A.M.A.*, 242:1150-1154, 1979. 22. Vessey, M.P., and R. Doll: Investigation of relation between use of oral contraceptives and thromboembolic disease. *Brit. Med. J.*, 2(5599): 199-205, 1968. 23. Vessey, M.P., and R. Doll: Investigation of relation between use of oral contraceptives and thromboembolic disease: A further report. *Brit. Med. J.*, 2(5658): 651-657, 1969. 24. Porter, J.B., J.R. Hunter, D.A. Danielson, H. Jick, and A. Stergachis: Oral contraceptives and non-fatal vascular disease: Recent experience. *Obstet. and Gyn.*, 59(3):299-302, 1982. 25. Vessey, M., R. Doll, R. Peto, B. Johnson, and P. Wiggins: A long-term follow-up study of women using different methods of contraception: An interim report. *J. Biosocial. Sci.*, 8:375-427, 1976. 26. Royal College of General Practitioners: Oral contraceptives, venous thrombosis, and varicose veins. *J. of Royal College of General Practitioners*, 28:393-399, 1978. 27. Collaborative Group for the study of stroke in young women: Oral contraception and increased risk of cerebral ischemia or thrombosis. *N.E.J.M.*, 288:871-878, 1973. 28. Petitti, D.B., and J. Wingerd: Use of oral contraceptives, cigarette smoking, and risk of subarachnoid hemorrhage. *Lancet*, 2:234-236, 1978. 29. Inman, W.H.: Oral contraceptives and fatal subarachnoid hemorrhage. *Brit. Med. J.*, 2(6203): 1468-70, 1979. 30. Collaborative Group for the study of stroke in young women: Oral contraceptives and stroke in young women: Associated risk factors. *J.A.M.A.*, 231:718-722, 1975. 31. Inman, W.H., M.P. Vessey, B. Westerholm, and A. Engelund: Thromboembolic disease and the steroidal content of oral contraceptives. A report to the Committee on Safety of Drugs. *Brit. Med. J.*, 2:203-209, 1970. 32. Meade, T.W., G. Greenberg, and S.G. Thompson: Progestogens and cardiovascular reactions associated with oral contraceptives and a comparison of the safety of 50- and 35-mcg oestrogen preparations. *Brit. Med. J.*, 280(6224): 1157-1161, 1980. 33. Kay, C.R.: Progestogens and arterial disease: Evidence from the Royal College of General Practitioners' study. *Amer. J. Obstet. Gyn.*, 142:762-765, 1982. 34. Royal College of General Practitioners: Incidence of arterial disease among oral contraceptive users. *J. Coll. Gen. Pract.*, 33:75-82, 1983. 35. Ory, H.W.: Mortality associated with fertility and fertility control: 1983. *Family Planning Perspectives*, 15:50-56, 1983. 36. The Cancer and Steroid Hormone Study of the Centers for Disease Control and the National Institute of Child Health and Human Development: Oral-contraceptive use and the risk of breast cancer. *N.E.J.M.*, 315:405-411, 1986. 37. Pike, M.C., B.E. Henderson, M.D. Krailo, A. Duke, and S. Roy: Breast cancer in young women and use of oral contraceptives: Possible modifying effect of formulation and age at use. *Lancet*, 2:926-929. 1983. 38. Paul, C., D.G. Skegg, G.F.S. Spears, and J.M. Kaldor: Oral contraceptives and breast cancer: A national study. *Brit. Med. J.*, 293:723-725, 1986. 39. Miller, D.R., L. Rosenberg, D.W. Kaufman, D. Schottenfeld, P.D. Stolley, and S. Shapiro: Breast cancer risk in relation to early oral contraceptive use. *Obstet. Gynec.*, 68:863-868, 1986. 40. Olson, H., K.L. Olson, T.R. Moller, J. Ranstam, P. Holm: Oral contraceptive use and breast cancer in young women in Sweden (letter). *Lancet*, 2:748-749, 1985. 41. McPherson, K., M. Vessey, A. Neil, R. Doll, L. Jones, and M. Roberts: Early contraceptive use and breast cancer: Results of another case-control study. *Brit. J. Cancer*, 56: 653-660, 1987. 42. Huggins, C.R., and P.F. Zucker: Oral contraceptives and neoplasia: 1987 update. *Fertil. Steril.*, 47:733-761, 1987. 43. McPherson, K., and J.O. Drife: The pill and breast cancer: Why the uncertainty? *Brit. Med. J.*, 293:709-710, 1986. 44. Shapiro, S.: Oral contraceptives: Time to take stock. *N.E.J.M.*, 315:450-451, 1987. 45. Ory, I.I., Z. Naib, S.B. Conger, R.A. Hatcher, and C.W. Tyler: Contraceptive choice and prevalence of cervical dysplasia and carcinoma in situ. *Am. J. Obstet. Gynec.*, 124:573-577, 1976. 46. Vessey, M.P., M. Lawless, K. McPherson, D. Yeates: Neoplasia of the cervix uteri and contraception: A possible adverse effect of the pill. *Lancet*, 2:930, 1983. 47. Brinton, L.A., G.R. Huggins, H.F. Lehman, K. Malli, D.A. Savitz, E. Trapido, J. Rosenthal, and R. Hoover: Long-term use of oral contraceptives and risk of invasive cervical cancer. *Int. J. Cancer*, 38:339-344, 1986. 48. WHO Collaborative Study of Neoplasia and Steroid Contraceptives: Invasive cervical cancer and combined oral contraceptives. *Brit. Med. J.*, 290:961-965, 1985. 49. Rooks, J.B., H.W. Ory, K.G. Ishak, L.T. Strauss, J.R. Greenspan, A.P. Hill, and C.W. Tyler: Epidemiology of hepatocellular adenoma: The role of oral contraceptive use, *J.A.M.A.*, 242:644-648, 1979. 50. Bein, N.N., and H.S. Goldsmith: Recurrent massive hemorrhage from benign hepatic tumors secondary to oral contraceptives. *Brit. J. Surg.*, 64:433-435, 1977. 51. Klatskin, G.: Hepatic tumors: Possible relationship to use of oral contraceptives. *Gastroenterology*, 73:386-394, 1977. 52. Henderson, B.E., S. Preston-Martin, H.A. Edmondson, R.L. Peters, and M.C. Pike: Hepatocellular carcinoma and oral contraceptives. *Brit. J. Cancer*, 48:437-440, 1983. 53. Neuberger, J., D. Forman, R. Doll, and R. Williams: Oral contraceptives and hepatocellular carcinoma, *Brit. Med. J.*, 292:1355-1357, 1986. 54. Forman, D., T.J. Vincent, and R. Doll: Cancer of the liver and oral contraceptives. *Brit. Med. J.*, 292:1357-1361, 1986. 55. Harlap, S., and J. Eldor: Births following oral contraceptive failures. *Obstet. Gynec.*, 55:447-452, 1980. 56. Savolainen, E., E. Saksela, and L. Saxen: Teratogenic hazards of oral contraceptives analyzed in a national malformation register. *Amer. J. Obstet. Gynec.*, 140:521-524, 1981. 57. Janerich, D.T., J.M. Piper, and D.M. Glebatis: Oral contraceptives and birth defects. *Am. J. Epidemiology*, 112:73-79, 1980. 58. Ferencz, C., G.M. Matanoski, P.D. Wilson, J.D. Rubin, C.A. Neill, and R. Gutherlet: Maternal hormone therapy and congenital heart disease. *Teratology*, 21:225-239, 1980. 59. Rothman, K.J., D.C. Fyler, A. Goldbatt, and M.B. Kreidberg: Exogenous hormones and other drug exposures of children with congenital heart disease. *Am. J. Epidemiology*, 109:433-439, 1979. 60. Boston Collaborative Drug Surveillance Program: Oral contraceptives and venous thromboembolic disease, surgically confirmed gallbladder disease, and breast tumors. *Lancet*, 1:1399-1404, 1973. 61. Royal College of General Practitioners: *Oral Contraceptives and Health*. New York, Pittman, 1974, 100p. 62. Layde, P.M., M.P. Vessey, and D. Yeates: Risk of gallbladder disease: A cohort study of young women attending family planning clinics. *J. of Epidemiol. and Comm. Health*, 36: 274-278, 1982. 63. Rome Group for the Epidemiology and Prevention of Cholelithiasis (GREPCO): Prevalence of gallstone disease in an Italian adult female population, *Am. J. Epidemiol.*, 119:796-805, 1984. 64. Strom, B.L., R.T. Tamragouri, M.L. Morse, E.L. Lazar, S.L. West, P.D. Stolley, and J.K. Jones: Oral contraceptives and other risk factors for gallbladder disease. *Clin. Pharmacol. Ther.*, 39:335-341, 1986. 65. Wynn, V., P.W. Adams, I.F. Godsland, J. Melrose, R. Niththyananthan, N.W. Oakley, and A. Seedj:

Comparison of effects of different combined oral-contraceptive formulations on carbohydrate and lipid metabolism. *Lancet*, 1:1045-1049, 1979. 66. Wynn, V.: Effect of progesterone and progestins on carbohydrate metabolism. In Progesterone and Progestin. Edited by C.W. Bardin, E. Milgrom, P. Mauvis-Jarvis. New York, *Raven Press*, pp. 395-410, 1983. 67. Perlman, J.A., R.G Roussell-Briefel, T.M. Ezzati, and G. Lieberknecht: Oral glucose tolerance and the potency of oral contraceptive progestogens. *J. Chronic Dis.*, 38:857-864, 1985. 68. Royal College of General Practitioners' Oral Contraception Study: Effect on hypertension and benign breast disease of progestogen component in combined oral contraceptives. *Lancet*, 1:624, 1977. 69. Fisch, I.R., and J. Frank. Oral contraceptives and blood pressure. *J.A.M.A.* 237:2499-2503, 1977. 70. Laragh, A.J.: Oral contraceptive induced hypertension: Nine years later. *Amer. J. Obstet. Gynecol.*, 126:141-147, 1976. 71. Ramcharan, S., E. Peritz., F.A. Pellegrin, and W.T. Williams: Incidence of hypertension in the Walnut Creek Contraceptive Drug Study cohort. In Pharmacology of Steroid Contraceptive Drugs. Edited by S. Garattini and H.W. Berendes, New York. *Raven Press*, pp. 277-288, 1977. (Monographs of the Mario Negri Institute for Pharmacological Research, Milan). 72. Stockley, I.: Interactions with oral contraceptives. *Pharm. J.* 216:140-143, 1976. 73. The Cancer and Steroid Hormone Study of the Centers for Disease Control and the National Institute of Child Health and Human Development: Oral contraceptive use and the risk of ovarian cancer. *J.A.M.A.*, 249:1596-1599, 1983. 74. The Cancer and Steroid Hormone Study of the Centers for Disease Control and the National Institute of Child Health and Human Development: Combination oral contraceptive use and the risk of endometrial cancer. *J.A.M.A.*, 257:796-800, 1987. 75. Ory, H.W.: Functional ovarian cysts and oral contraceptives: Negative association confirmed surgically. *J.A.M.A.*, 228:68-69, 1974. 76. Ory, H.W., P. Cole, B. Macmahon, and R. Hoover: Oral contraceptives and reduced risk of benign breast disease. *N.E.J.M.*, 294:41-422, 1976. 77. Ory, H.W.: The noncontraceptive health benefits from oral contraceptive use. *Fam. Plann. Perspectives*, 14:182-184, 1982. 78. Ory, H.W., J.D. Forrest, and R. Lincoln: Making Choices: Evaluating the health risks and benefits of birth control methods. New York, The Alan Guttmacher Institute, p.1, 1983. 79. Miller, D.R., L. Rosenberg, D. W. Kaufman, P. Stolley, M.E. Warshauer and S. Shapiro: Breast Cancer Before Age 45 and Oral Contraceptive Use: New Findings. *Am. J. Epidemiol.*, 129:269-280, 1989. 80. Kay, C. R. and P.C. Hannaford: Breast Cancer and the Pill; A Further Report from The Royal College of General Practitioners Oral Contraception Study *Br. J. Cancer*, 48:675-680, 1988. 81. Stadel, B.V., S. Lai, J.J. Schlesselman and P. Murray: Oral Contraceptives and Premenopausal Breast Cancer in Nulliparous Women. *Contraception.* 38:287-299, 1988. 82. UK National Case - Control Study Group: Oral Contraceptive Use and Breast Cancer Risk in Young Women. *Lancet*, 973-982, 1989. 83. Romieu, I., W.C. Willett, G.A. Colditz, M.J. Stampfer, B. Rosner, C.H. Hennekens, F.E. Speizer Prospective Study of Oral Contraceptive Use and Risk of Breast Cancer in Women. *J. Natl. Cancer Inst.* 81:1313-1321, 1989.

HOW SUPPLIED

ETHINYL ESTRADIOL/NORETHINDRONE
TABLETS: 0.4 MG-35 MCG

BRAND/MANUFACTURER	NDC	SIZE	AWP
○ BRAND			
➤ OVCON 35: Mead Johnson Labs	00087-0583-42	126s	$147.77
	00087-0578-41	168s	$147.77

TABLETS: 0.5 MG-1 MG-35 MCG

AVERAGE UNIT PRICE (AVAILABLE SIZES)			
BRAND	$1.01		

BRAND/MANUFACTURER	NDC	SIZE	AWP
◆ BRAND			
➤ ORTHO-NOVUM 10/11: Ortho Pharm	00062-1770-15	126s	$145.02
	00062-1771-15	168s	$145.98
◆ GENERICS			
NELOVA 10/11: Warner Chilcott	00047-0944-35	168s	$83.81

TABLETS: 0.5 MG-1 MG-35 MCG

BRAND/MANUFACTURER	NDC	SIZE	AWP
○ BRAND			
➤ TRI-NORINYL: Syntex/F.P.	42987-0114-27	126s	$126.89
	42987-0114-23	126s	$128.28
	42987-0115-28	168s	$126.89
	42987-0115-24	168s	$128.28
	42987-0115-61	672s	$543.97

TABLETS: 0.5 MG-35 MCG

AVERAGE UNIT PRICE (AVAILABLE SIZES)			
BRAND	$0.95		
GENERIC	$0.41		
HCFA FUL (21s ea)	$0.51		

BRAND/MANUFACTURER	NDC	SIZE	AWP
◆ BRAND			
BREVICON: Syntex/F.P.	42987-0108-13	63s	$68.82
	42987-0110-14	84s	$68.82
MODICON: Ortho Pharm	00062-1712-15	126s	$145.02
	00062-1714-15	168s	$145.98
BREVICON: Syntex/F.P.	42987-0110-61	672s	$533.93
◆ GENERICS			
GENORA 0.5/35: Rugby	00536-4057-48	84s	$27.17
NELOVA 0.5/35: Warner Chilcott	00047-0926-35	168s	$83.81

TABLETS: 0.5, 0.75, 1 MG-35 MCG

BRAND/MANUFACTURER	NDC	SIZE	AWP
○ BRAND			
➤ ORTHO-NOVUM 7/7/7: Ortho Pharm	00062-1780-15	126s	$133.20
	00062-1781-15	168s	$133.86
	00062-1780-22	252s	$264.12
	00062-1781-22	336s	$265.74

TABLETS: 0.5 MG-35 MCG

BRAND/MANUFACTURER	NDC	SIZE	AWP
○ BRAND			
MODICON: Ortho Pharm	00062-1714-20	28s	$23.28

TABLETS: 1 MG-20 MCG

BRAND/MANUFACTURER	NDC	SIZE	AWP
○ BRAND			
➤ LOESTRIN 21 1/20: Parke-Davis	00071-0915-47	105s	$126.20

TABLETS: 1.5 MG-30 MCG

BRAND/MANUFACTURER	NDC	SIZE	AWP
○ BRAND			
➤ LOESTRIN 21 1.5/30: Parke-Davis	00071-0916-47	105s	$126.20

TABLETS: 20 MCG-1 MG

BRAND/MANUFACTURER	NDC	SIZE	AWP
○ BRAND			
LOESTRIN FE 1/20: Parke-Davis	00071-0913-47	140s	$126.20

TABLETS: 30 MCG-1.5 MG

BRAND/MANUFACTURER	NDC	SIZE	AWP
○ BRAND			
LOESTRIN FE 1.5/30: Parke-Davis	00071-0917-47	140s	$126.20

TABLETS: 35 MCG-1 MG

AVERAGE UNIT PRICE (AVAILABLE SIZES)		GENERIC A-RATED AVERAGE PRICE (GAAP)	
BRAND	$0.88	126s	$67.90
GENERIC	$0.48	168s	$69.61
HCFA FUL (21s ea)	$0.49		

BRAND/MANUFACTURER	NDC	SIZE	AWP
◆ BRAND			
➤ ORTHO-NOVUM 1/35: Ortho Pharm	00062-1760-15	126s	$132.36
➤ NORINYL 1/35: Syntex/F.P.	42987-0109-23	126s	$133.45
	42987-0111-28	168s	$132.01
ORTHO-NOVUM 1/35: Ortho Pharm	00062-1761-15	168s	$133.08
➤ NORINYL 1/35: Syntex/F.P.	42987-0111-24	168s	$133.45
	42987-0111-61	672s	$533.93
◆ GENERICS			
GENORA 1/35: Rugby	00536-4058-44	63s	$36.30
N.E.E. 1/35: Lexis	00454-3521-21	126s	$61.50
NELOVA 1/35: Warner Chilcott	00047-0930-11	126s	$74.30
N.E.E. 1/35: Lexis	00454-3528-28	168s	$61.50
➤ GENORA 1/35: Rugby	00536-4055-48	168s	$72.60
NELOVA 1/35: Warner Chilcott	00047-0927-35	168s	$74.74

TABLETS: 35 MCG-1 MG

BRAND/MANUFACTURER	NDC	SIZE	AWP
○ BRAND			
➤ JENEST-28: Organon	00052-0269-06	168s	$105.14

TABLETS: 50 MCG-1 MG

AVERAGE UNIT PRICE (AVAILABLE SIZES)			
GENERIC	$0.43		

BRAND/MANUFACTURER	NDC	SIZE	AWP
◆ GENERICS			
N.E.E. 1/50: Lexis	00454-5021-21	126s	$61.50
N.E.E. 1/50: Lexis	00454-5028-28	168s	$61.50

TABLETS: 50 MCG-1 MG

BRAND/MANUFACTURER	NDC	SIZE	AWP
○ BRAND			
➤ OVCON 50: Mead Johnson Labs	00087-0579-41	168s	$163.05

Ethinyl Estradiol and Norgestimate

DESCRIPTION
Ethinyl Estradiol/Norgestimate Tablets are a combination oral contraceptive. Each white tablet contains 0.180 mg of the progestational compound, Norgestimate (18,19-Dinor-17-pregn-4-en-20-yn-3-one, 17-(acetyl-oxy)-13-ethyl-,oxime,

(17α)-(+)-) and 0.035 mg of the estrogenic compound, Ethinyl Estradiol (19-nor-17α-pregna, 1,3,5(10)-trien-20-yne-3,17-diol).

Each light blue tablet contains 0.125 mg of Norgestimate with 0.035 mg of Ethinyl Estradiol. Each blue tablet contains 0.250 mg of Norgestimate together with 0.035 mg of Ethinyl Estradiol.

Ethinyl Estradiol/Norgestimate is administered on a 21 day on medication, and 7 day off medication cyclic regimen.

Each green tablet in the Ethinyl Estradiol/Norgestimate 28 package contains only inert ingredients.

CLINICAL PHARMACOLOGY

Combination oral contraceptives act by suppression of gonadotropins. Although the primary mechanism of this action is inhibition of ovulation, other alterations include changes in the cervical mucus (which increase the difficulty of sperm entry into the uterus) and the endometrium (which reduce the likelihood of implantation).

Norgestimate and Ethinyl Estradiol are well absorbed following oral administration of Ethinyl Estradiol/Norgestimate. On the average, peak serum concentrations of Norgestimate and Ethinyl Estradiol are observed within two hours (0.5-2.0 hr for Norgestimate and 0.75-3.0 hr for Ethinyl Estradiol) after administration followed by a rapid decline due to distribution and elimination. Although Norgestimate serum concentrations following single or multiple dosing were generally below assay detection within 5 hours, a major Norgestimate serum metabolite, 17-deacetyl Norgestimate (which exhibits a serum half-life ranging from 12 to 30 hours), appears rapidly in serum with concentrations greatly exceeding that of Norgestimate. The 17-deacetylated metabolite is pharmacologically active and the pharmacologic profile is similar to that of Norgestimate. The elimination half-life of Ethinyl Estradiol ranges from approximately 6 to 14 hours.

Both Norgestimate and Ethinyl Estradiol are extensively metabolized and eliminated by renal and fecal pathways. Following administration of ^{14}C-Norgestimate, 47% (45-49%) and 37% (16-49%) of the administered radioactivity was eliminated in the urine and feces, respectively. Unchanged Norgestimate was not detected in the urine. In addition to 17-deacetyl Norgestimate, a number of metabolites of Norgestimate have been identified in human urine following administration of radiolabeled Norgestimate. These include 18,19-Dinor-17-pregn-4-en-20-yn-3-one,17-hydroxy-13-ethyl,(17α)-(-);18,19-Dinor-5β-17-pregnan-20-yn,3α,17β-dihydroxy-13-ethyl,(17α), various hydroxylated meta- bolites and conjugates of these metabolites. Ethinyl Estradiol is metabolized to various hydroxylated products and their glucuronide and sulfate conjugates.

INDICATIONS AND USAGE

Ethinyl Estradiol/Norgestimate Tablets are indicated for the prevention of pregnancy in women who elect to use oral contraceptives as a method of contraception.

Oral contraceptives are highly effective. Table 1 lists the typical accidental pregnancy rates for users of combination oral contraceptives and other methods of contraception. The efficacy of these contraceptive methods, except sterilization, depends upon the reliability with which they are used. Correct and consistent use of methods can result in lower failure rates.

Table 1:
LOWEST EXPECTED AND TYPICAL FAILURE RATES DURING THE FIRST YEAR OF CONTINUOUS USE OF A METHOD

% of Women Experiencing an Accidental Pregnancy in the First Year of Continuous Use

Method	Lowest Expected*	Typical**
(No contraception)	(89)	(89)
Oral contraceptives		3
combined	0.1	N/A***
progestin only	0.5	N/A***
Diaphragm with spermicidal cream or jelly	3	18
Spermicides alone (foam, creams, jellies and vaginal suppositories)	3	21
Vaginal sponge		
nulliparous	5	18
multiparous	> 8	> 28
IUD (medicated)	1	6#
Condom without spermicides	2	12
Periodic abstinence (all methods)	2-10	20
Female sterilization	0.2	0.4
Male sterilization	0.1	0.15

Adapted from J. Trussel and K. Kost, Table 2, ref. # 1.

* *The authors' best guess of the percentage of women expected to experience an accidental pregnancy among couples who initiate a method (not necessarily for the first time) and who use it consistently and correctly during the first year if they do not stop for any other reason.*

** *This term represents "typical" couples who initiate use of a method (not necessarily for the first time), who experience an accidental pregnancy during the first year if they do not stop use for any other reason.*

*** *N/A—Data not available*

\# *Combined typical rate for both medicated and non-medicated IUD. The rate for medicated IUD alone is not available.*

In four clinical trials with Ethinyl Estradiol/Norgestimate, the use-efficacy pregnancy rate ranged from 0.68 to 1.47 per 100 women-years. In total, 4,756 subjects completed 45,244 cycles and a total of 42 pregnancies were reported. This represents an overall use-efficacy rate of 1.21 per 100 women-years. One of these 4 studies was a randomized comparative clinical trial in which 4,633 subjects completed 22,312 cycles. Of the 2,312 patients on Ethinyl Estradiol/Norgestimate, 8 pregnancies were reported. This represents an overall use-efficacy pregnancy rate of 0.94 per 100 women-years.

In clinical trials with Ethinyl Estradiol/Norgestimate 0.250 mg, 1,651 subjects completed 24,272 cycles and a total of 18 pregnancies were reported. This represents an overall use-efficacy (typical user efficacy) pregnancy rate of 0.96 per 100 woman-years. This rate includes patients who did not take the drug correctly.

CONTRAINDICATIONS

Oral contraceptives should not be used in women who currently have the following conditions.

- Thrombophlebitis or thromboembolic disorders
- A past history of deep vein thrombophlebitis or thromboembolic disorders
- Cerebral vascular or coronary artery disease
- Known or suspected carcinoma of the breast
- Carcinoma of the endometrium or other known or suspected estrogen-dependent neoplasia
- Undiagnosed abnormal genital bleeding
- Cholestatic jaundice of pregnancy or jaundice with prior pill use
- Hepatic adenomas or carcinomas
- Known or suspected pregnancy

WARNINGS

CIGARETTE SMOKING INCREASES THE RISK OF SERIOUS CARDIOVASCULAR SIDE EFFECTS FROM ORAL CONTRACEPTIVE USE. THIS RISK INCREASES WITH AGE AND WITH HEAVY SMOKING (15 OR MORE CIGARETTES PER DAY) AND IS QUITE MARKED IN WOMEN OVER 35 YEARS OF AGE. WOMEN WHO USE ORAL CONTRACEPTIVES ARE STRONGLY ADVISED NOT TO SMOKE.

The use of oral contraceptives is associated with increased risks of several serious conditions including myocardial infarction, thromboembolism, stroke, hepatic neoplasia, and gallbladder disease, although the risk of serious morbidity or mortality is very small in healthy women without underlying risk factors. The risk of morbidity and mortality increases significantly in the presence of other underlying risk factors such as hypertension, hyperlipidemia, obesity and diabetes.

Practitioners prescribing oral contraceptives should be familiar with the following information relating to these risks. The information contained in this package insert is principally based on studies carried out in patients who use oral contraceptives with higher formulations of estrogens and progestogens than those in common use today. The effect of long term use of the oral contraceptives with lower formulations of both estrogens and progestogens remains to be determined.

Throughout this labeling, epidemiological studies reported are of two types: retrospective or case control studies, and prospective or cohort studies. Case control studies provide a measure of the relative risk of a disease, namely, a *ratio* of the incidence of a disease among oral contraceptive users to that among non-users. The relative risk does not provide information on the actual clinical occurrence of a disease. Cohort studies provide a measure of attributable risk, which is the *difference* in the incidence of disease between oral contraceptive users and non-users. The attributable risk does provide information about the actual occurrence of a disease in the population (adapted from refs. 2 and 3 with the author's permission). For further information, the reader is referred to a text on epidemiological methods.

1. THROMBOEMBOLIC DISORDERS AND OTHER VASCULAR PROBLEMS

a. Myocardial Infarction

An increased risk of myocardial infarction has been associated with oral contraceptive use. This risk is primarily in smokers or women with other underlying risk factors for coronary artery disease such as hypertension, hypercholesterolemia, morbid obesity, and diabetes. The relative risk of heart attack for current oral contraceptive users has been estimated to be two to six.[4-10] The risk is very low under the age of 30.

Smoking in combination with oral contraceptive use has been shown to contribute substantially to the incidence of myocardial infarctions in women in their mid-thirties or older, with smoking accounting for the majority of excess cases.[11] Mortality rates associated with circulatory disease have been shown to increase substantially in smokers, especially in those 35 years of age and older among women who use oral contraceptives.

CIRCULATORY DISEASE MORTALITY RATES PER 100,000 WOMAN-YEARS BY AGE, SMOKING STATUS AND ORAL CONTRACEPTIVE USE

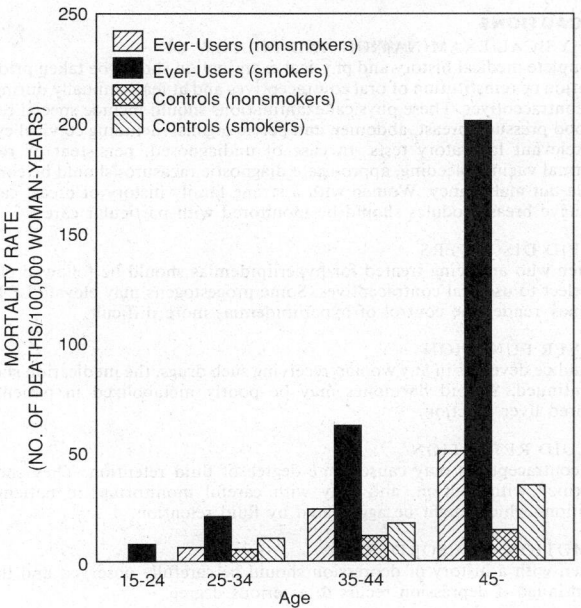

TABLE 2. (Adapted from P.M. Layde and V. Beral, ref. # 12.)

Oral contraceptives may compound the effects of well-known risk factors, such as hypertension, diabetes, hyperlipidemias, age and obesity.[13] In particular, some progestogens are known to decrease HDL cholesterol and cause glucose intolerance, while estrogens may create a state of hyperinsulinism.[14-18] Oral contraceptives have been shown to increase blood pressure among users (see Section 9 in "Warnings"). Similar effects on risk factors have been associated with an increased risk of heart disease. Oral contraceptives must be used with caution in women with cardiovascular disease risk factors.

b. Thromboembolism

An increased risk of thromboembolic and thrombotic disease associated with the use of oral contraceptives is well established. Case control studies have found the relative risk of users compared to non-users to be 3 for the first episode of superficial venous thrombosis, 4 to 11 for deep vein thrombosis or pulmonary embolism, and 1.5 to 6 for women with predisposing conditions for venous thromboembolic disease.[2,3,19-24] Cohort studies have shown the relative risk to be somewhat lower, about 3 for new cases and about 4.5 for new cases requiring hospitalization.[25] The risk of thromboembolic disease associated with oral contraceptives is not related to length of use and disappears after pill use is stopped.[2]

A two- to four-fold increase in relative risk of postoperative thromboembolic complications has been reported with the use of oral contraceptives.[9] The relative risk of venous thrombosis in women who have predisposing conditions is twice that of women without such medical conditions.[26] If feasible, oral contraceptives should be discontinued at least four weeks prior to and for two weeks after elective surgery of a type associated with an increase in risk of thromboembolism, and during and following prolonged immobilization. Since the immediate postpartum period is also associated with an increased risk of thromboembolism, oral contraceptives should be started no earlier than four weeks after delivery in women who elect not to breast feed.

c. Cerebrovascular diseases

Oral contraceptives have been shown to increase both the relative and attributable risks of cerebrovascular events (thrombotic and hemorrhagic strokes), although, in general, the risk is greatest among older (> 35 years), hypertensive women who also smoke. Hypertension was found to be a risk factor for both users and non-users, for both types of strokes, and smoking interacted to increase the risk of stroke.[27-29]

In a large study, the relative risk of thrombotic strokes has been shown to range from 3 for normotensive users to 14 for users with severe hypertension.[30] The relative risk of hemorrhagic stroke is reported to be 1.2 for non-smokers who used oral contraceptives, 2.6 for smokers who did not use oral contraceptives, 7.6 for smokers who used oral contraceptives, 1.8 for normotensive users and 25.7 for users with severe hypertension.[30] The attributable risk is also greater in older women.[3]

d. Dose-related risk of vascular disease from oral contraceptives

A positive association has been observed between the amount of estrogen and progestogen in oral contraceptives and the risk of vascular disease.[31-33] A decline in serum high density lipoproteins (HDL) has been reported with many progestational agents.[14-16] A decline in serum high density lipoproteins has been associated with an increased incidence of ischemic heart disease. Because

estrogens increase HDL cholesterol, the net effect of an oral contraceptive depends on a balance achieved between doses of estrogen and progestogen and the activity of the progestogen used in the contraceptive. The activity and amount of both hormones should be considered in the choice of an oral contraceptive.

Minimizing exposure to estrogen and progestogen is in keeping with good principles of therapeutics. For any particular estrogen/progestogen combination, the dosage regimen prescribed should be one which contains the least amount of estrogen and progestogen that is compatible with a low failure rate and the needs of the individual patient. New acceptors of oral contraceptive agents should be started on preparations containing 0.035 mg or less of estrogen.

e. Persistence of risk of vascular disease

There are two studies which have shown persistence of risk of vascular disease for ever-users of oral contraceptives. In a study in the United States, the risk of developing myocardial infarction after discontinuing oral contraceptives persists for at least 9 years for women 40-49 years who had used oral contraceptives for five or more years, but this increased risk was not demonstrated in other age groups.[8] In another study in Great Britain, the risk of developing cardiovascular disease persisted for at least 6 years after discontinuation of oral contraceptives, although excess risk was very small.[34] However, both studies were performed with oral contraceptive formulations containing 50 micrograms or higher of estrogens.

2. ESTIMATES OF MORTALITY FROM CONTRACEPTIVE USE

One study gathered data from a variety of sources which have estimated the mortality rate associated with different methods of contraception at different ages (Table 3). These estimates include the combined risk of death associated with contraceptive methods plus the risk attributable to pregnancy in the event of method failure. Each method of contraception has its specific benefits and risks. The study concluded that with the exception of oral contraceptive users 35 and older who smoke, and 40 and older who do not smoke, mortality associated with all methods of birth control is low and below that associated with childbirth. The observation of an increase in risk of mortality with age for oral contraceptive users is based on data gathered in the 1970's.[35] Current clinical recommendation involves the use of lower estrogen dose formulations and a careful consideration of risk factors. In 1989, the Fertility and Maternal Health Drugs Advisory Committee was asked to review the use of oral contraceptives in women 40 years of age and over. The Committee concluded that although oral contraceptive disease risks may be increased with oral contraceptive use after age 40 in healthy non-smoking women (even with the newer low-dose formulations), there are also greater potential health risks associated with pregnancy in older women and with the alternative surgical and medical procedures which may be necessary if such women do not have access to effective and acceptable means of contraception. The Committee recommended that the benefits of low-dose oral contraceptive use by healthy non-smoking women over 40 may outweigh the possible risks.

Of course, older women, as all women, who take oral contraceptives, should take an oral contraceptive which contains the least amount of estrogen and progestogen that is compatible with a low failure rate and individual patient needs. (See related table).

Adapted from H.W. Ory, ref. #35.

3. CARCINOMA OF THE REPRODUCTIVE ORGANS

Numerous epidemiological studies have been performed on the incidence of breast, endometrial, ovarian, and cervical cancer in women using oral contraceptives. While there are conflicting reports, most studies suggest that use of oral contraceptives is not associated with an overall increase in the risk of developing breast cancer. Some studies have reported an increased relative risk of developing breast cancer, particularly at a younger age. This increased relative risk appears to be related to duration of use.[36-44,79-89]

Some studies suggest that oral contraceptive use has been associated with an increase in the risk of cervical intraepithelial neoplasia in some populations of women.[45-48] However, there continues to be controversy about the extent to which such findings may be due to differences in sexual behavior and other factors.

4. HEPATIC NEOPLASIA

Benign hepatic adenomas are associated with oral contraceptive use, although the incidence of benign tumors is rare in the United States. Indirect calculations have estimated the attributable risk to be in the range of 3.3 cases/100,000 for users, a risk that increases after four or more years of use especially with oral contraceptives of higher dose.[49] Rupture of benign, hepatic adenomas may cause death through intra-abdominal hemorrhage.[50,51]

Studies from Britain have shown an increased risk of developing hepatocellular carcinoma[52-54] in long-term (> 8 years) oral contraceptive users. However, these cancers are rare in the U.S. and the attributable risk (the excess incidence) of liver cancers in oral contraceptive users approaches less than one per million users.

5. OCULAR LESIONS

There have been clinical case reports of retinal thrombosis associated with the use of oral contraceptives. Oral contraceptives should be discontinued if there is unexplained partial or complete loss of vision; onset of proptosis or diplopia; papilledema; or retinal vascular lesions. Appropriate diagnostic and therapeutic measures should be undertaken immediately.

6. ORAL CONTRACEPTIVE USE BEFORE OR DURING EARLY PREGNANCY

Extensive epidemiological studies have revealed no increased risk of birth defects in women who have used oral contraceptives prior to pregnancy.[56,57] The majority of recent studies also do not indicate a teratogenic effect, particularly in so far as cardiac anomalies and limb reduction defects are concerned,[55,56,58,59] when taken inadvertently during early pregnancy.

The administration of oral contraceptives to induce withdrawal bleeding should not be used as a test for pregnancy. Oral contraceptives should not be used during pregnancy to treat threatened or habitual abortion.

It is recommended that for any patient who has missed two consecutive periods, pregnancy should be ruled out before continuing oral contraceptive use. If the patient has not adhered to the prescribed schedule, the possibility of pregnancy should be considered at the time of the first-missed period. Oral contraceptive use should be discontinued until pregnancy is ruled out.

7. GALLBLADDER DISEASE

Earlier studies have reported an increased lifetime relative risk of gallbladder surgery in users of oral contraceptives and estrogens.[60,61] More recent studies, however, have shown that the relative risk of developing gallbladder disease among oral contraceptive users may be minimal.[62-64] The recent findings of minimal risk may be related to the use of oral contraceptive formulations containing lower hormonal doses of estrogens and progestogens.

8. CARBOHYDRATE AND LIPID METABOLIC EFFECTS

Oral contraceptives have been shown to cause a decrease in glucose tolerance in a significant percentage of users.[17] This effect has been shown to be directly related to estrogen dose.[65] Progestogens increase insulin secretion and create insulin resistance, this effect varying with different progestational agents.[17,66] However, in the non-diabetic woman, oral contraceptives appear to have no effect on fasting blood glucose.[67] Because of these demonstrated effects, prediabetic and diabetic women in particular should be carefully monitored while taking oral contraceptives.

A small proportion of women will have persistent hypertriglyceridemia while on the pill. As discussed earlier (see "Warnings" 1a and 1d), changes in serum triglycerides and lipoprotein levels have been reported in oral contraceptive users.

In clinical studies with Ethinyl Estradiol/Norgestimate there were no clinically significant changes in fasting blood glucose levels. Minimal statistically significant changes were noted in glucose levels over 24 cycles of use; no statistically significant changes in mean fasting blood glucose levels were observed over 24 cycles of use with Ethinyl Estradiol/Norgestimate 0.250 mg. Glucose tolerance tests showed no or minimal clinically significant changes from baseline to cycles 3, 12, and 24.

9. ELEVATED BLOOD PRESSURE

An increase in blood pressure has been reported in women taking oral contraceptives[68] and this increase is more likely in older oral contraceptive users[69] and with extended duration of use.[61]

Data from the Royal College of General Practitioners[12] and subsequent randomized trials have shown that the incidence of hypertension increases with increasing progestational activity.

Women with a history of hypertension or hypertension-related diseases, or renal disease[70] should be encouraged to use another method of contraception. If women elect to use oral contraceptives, they should be monitored closely and if significant elevation of blood pressure occurs, oral contraceptives should be discontinued. For most women, elevated blood pressure will return to normal after stopping oral contraceptives, and there is no difference in the occurrence of hypertension between former and never users.[68-71] It should be noted that in two separate large clinical trials (N = 633 and N = 911), no statistically significant changes in mean blood pressure were observed with Ethinyl Estradiol/Norgestimate 0.250 mg.

10. HEADACHE

The onset or exacerbation of migraine or development of headache with a new pattern which is recurrent, persistent or severe requires discontinuation of oral contraceptives and evaluation of the cause.

11. BLEEDING IRREGULARITIES

Breakthrough bleeding and spotting are sometimes encountered in patients on oral contraceptives, especially during the first three months of use. Nonhormonal causes should be considered and adequate diagnostic measures taken to rule out malignancy or pregnancy in the event of breakthrough bleeding, as in the case of any abnormal vaginal bleeding. If pathology has been excluded, time or a change to another formulation may solve the problem. In the event of amenorrhea, pregnancy should be ruled out.

Some women may encounter post-pill amenorrhea or oligomenorrhea, especially when such a condition was preexistent.

12. ECTOPIC PREGNANCY

Ectopic as well as intrauterine pregnancy may occur in contraceptive failures.

PRECAUTIONS

1. PHYSICAL EXAMINATION AND FOLLOW UP

A complete medical history and physical examination should be taken prior to the initiation or reinstitution of oral contraceptives and at least annually during use of oral contraceptives. These physical examinations should include special reference to blood pressure, breast, abdomen and pelvic organs, including cervical cytology, and relevant laboratory tests. In case of undiagnosed, persistent or recurrent abnormal vaginal bleeding, appropriate diagnostic measures should be conducted to rule out malignancy. Women with a strong family history of breast cancer or who have breast nodules should be monitored with particular care.

2. LIPID DISORDERS

Women who are being treated for hyperlipidemias should be followed closely if they elect to use oral contraceptives. Some progestogens may elevate LDL levels and may render the control of hyperlipidemias more difficult.

3. LIVER FUNCTION

If jaundice develops in any woman receiving such drugs, the medication should be discontinued. Steroid hormones may be poorly metabolized in patients with impaired liver function.

4. FLUID RETENTION

Oral contraceptives may cause some degree of fluid retention. They should be prescribed with caution, and only with careful monitoring, in patients with conditions which might be aggravated by fluid retention.

5. EMOTIONAL DISORDERS

Women with a history of depression should be carefully observed and the drug discontinued if depression recurs to a serious degree.

6. CONTACT LENSES

Contact lens wearers who develop visual changes or changes in lens tolerance should be assessed by an ophthalmologist.

7. DRUG INTERACTIONS

Reduced efficacy and increased incidence of breakthrough bleeding and menstrual irregularities have been associated with concomitant use of rifampin. A similar association, though less marked, has been suggested with barbiturates, phenylbutazone, phenytoin sodium, and possibly with griseofulvin, ampicillin and tetracyclines.[72]

8. INTERACTIONS WITH LABORATORY TESTS

Certain endocrine and liver function tests and blood components may be affected by oral contraceptives:

a. Increased prothrombin and factors VII, VIII, IX, and X; decreased antithrombin 3; increased norepinephrine-induced platelet aggregability.

b. Increased thyroid binding globulin (TBG) leading to increased circulating total thyroid hormone, as measured by protein-bound iodine (PBI), T4 by column or by radio-immunoassay. Free T3 resin uptake is decreased, reflecting the elevated TBG, free T4 concentration is unaltered.

c. Other binding proteins may be elevated in serum.

d. Sex-binding globulins are increased and result in elevated levels of total circulating sex steroids and corticoids; however, free or biologically active levels remain unchanged.

e. Triglycerides may be increased.

f. Glucose tolerance may be decreased.

g. Serum folate levels may be depressed by oral contraceptive therapy. This may be of clinical significance if a woman becomes pregnant shortly after discontinuing oral contraceptives.

9. CARCINOGENESIS

See "Warnings" Section.

10. PREGNANCY

Pregnancy Category X. (See "Contraindications" and "Warnings" sections.)

Table 3
ANNUAL NUMBER OF BIRTH-RELATED OR METHOD-RELATED DEATHS ASSOCIATED WITH CONTROL OF FERTILITY PER 100,000 NONSTERILE WOMEN, BY FERTILITY CONTROL METHOD ACCORDING TO AGE

Method of control and outcome	15-19	20-24	25-29	30-34	35-39	40-44
No fertility control methods*	7.0	7.4	9.1	14.8	25.7	28.2
Oral contraceptives nonsmoker**	0.3	0.5	0.9	1.9	13.8	31.6
Oral contraceptives smoker**	2.2	3.4	6.6	13.5	51.1	117.2
IUD**	0.8	0.8	1.0	1.0	1.4	1.4
Condom*	1.1	1.6	0.7	0.2	0.3	0.4
Diaphragm/spermicide*	1.9	1.2	1.2	1.3	2.2	2.8
Periodic abstinence*	2.5	1.6	1.6	1.7	2.9	3.6

* *Deaths are birth-related*
** *Deaths are method-related*

11. NURSING MOTHERS
Small amounts of oral contraceptive steroids have been identified in the milk of nursing mothers and a few adverse effects on the child have been reported, including jaundice and breast enlargement. In addition, oral contraceptives given in the postpartum period may interfere with lactation by decreasing the quantity and quality of breast milk. If possible, the nursing mother should be advised not to use oral contraceptives but to use other forms of contraception until she has completely weaned her child.

INFORMATION FOR THE PATIENT
See manufacturer's patient information.

ADVERSE REACTIONS
An increased risk of the following serious adverse reactions has been associated with the use of oral contraceptives (see *"Warnings"* section).

- Thrombophlebitis and venous thrombosis with or without embolism
- Arterial thromboembolism
- Pulmonary embolism
- Myocardial infarction
- Cerebral hemorrhage
- Cerebral thrombosis
- Hypertension
- Gallbladder disease
- Hepatic adenomas or benign liver tumors

The following adverse reactions have been reported in patients receiving oral contraceptives and are believed to be drug-related:

- Nausea
- Vomiting
- Gastrointestinal symptoms (such as abdominal cramps and bloating)
- Breakthrough bleeding
- Spotting
- Change in menstrual flow
- Amenorrhea
- Temporary infertility after discontinuation of treatment
- Edema
- Melasma which may persist
- Breast changes: tenderness, enlargement, secretion
- Change in weight (increase or decrease)
- Change in cervical erosion and secretion
- Diminution in lactation when given immediately postpartum
- Cholestatic jaundice
- Migraine
- Rash (allergic)
- Mental depression
- Reduced tolerance to carbohydrates
- Vaginal candidiasis
- Change in corneal curvature (steepening)
- Intolerance to contact lenses

The following adverse reactions have been reported in users of oral contraceptives and the association has been neither confirmed nor refuted:

- Pre-menstrual syndrome
- Cataracts
- Changes in appetite
- Cystitis-like syndrome
- Headache
- Nervousness
- Dizziness
- Hirsutism
- Loss of scalp hair
- Erythema multiforme
- Erythema nodosum
- Hemorrhagic eruption
- Vaginitis
- Porphyria
- Impaired renal function
- Hemolytic uremic syndrome
- Acne
- Changes in libido
- Colitis

OVERDOSAGE
Serious ill effects have not been reported following acute ingestion of large doses of oral contraceptives by young children. Overdosage may cause nausea and withdrawal bleeding may occur in females.

NONCONTRACEPTIVE HEALTH BENEFITS
The following non-contraceptive health benefits related to the use of combination oral contraceptives are supported by epidemiological studies which largely utilized oral contraceptive formulations containing estrogen doses exceeding 0.035 mg of estrogen.[73-78]

Effects on menses:

- increased menstrual cycle regularity
- decreased blood loss and decreased incidence of iron deficiency anemia
- decreased incidence of dysmenorrhea

Effects related to inhibition of ovulation:

- decreased incidence of functional ovarian cysts
- decreased incidence of ectopic pregnancies

Other effects:

- decreased incidence of fibroadenomas and fibrocystic disease of the breast
- decreased incidence of acute pelvic inflammatory disease
- decreased incidence of endometrial cancer
- decreased incidence of ovarian cancer

DOSAGE AND ADMINISTRATION
To achieve maximum contraceptive effectiveness, Ethinyl Estradiol/Norgestimate Tablets must be taken exactly as directed and at intervals not exceeding 24 hours.

21-DAY REGIMEN (DAY 1 START)
The dosage of Ethinyl Estradiol/Norgestimate 21 for the initial cycle of therapy is one tablet administered daily from the 1st day through the 21st day of the menstrual cycle, counting the first day of menstrual flow as "Day 1." Tablets are taken without interruption for 21 days as follows: One Norgestimate 0.180 mg tablet daily for 7 days, then one Norgestimate 0.215 mg tablet daily for 7 days, then one Norgestimate 0.250 mg tablet daily for 7 days or one 0.250 mg tablet a day for 21 days. For subsequent cycles, no tablets are taken for 7 days, then a new course is started of one tablet a day for 21 days. The dosage regimen then continues with 7 days of no medication, followed by 21 days of medication, instituting a three-weeks-on, one-week-off dosage regimen.

The use of Ethinyl Estradiol/Norgestimate 21 for contraception may be initiated postpartum. When the tablets are administered during the postpartum period, the increased risk of thromboembolic disease associated with the postpartum period must be considered. (See *"Contraindications"* and *"Warnings"* concerning thromboembolic disease.) The possibility of ovulation and conception prior to initiation of medication should be considered. If the patient misses two (2) active tablets in Week 1 or Week 2, the patient should take two (2) tablets the day she remembers and two (2) tablets the next day; and then continue taking one (1) tablet a day until she finishes the pack. The patient should be instructed to use a back-up method of birth control if she has sex in the seven (7) days after missing pills. If the patient misses two (2) active tablets in the 3rd week or misses three (3) or more active tablets in a row, the patient should throw out the rest of the pack and start a new pack that same day. The patient should also be instructed to use a back-up method of birth control if she has sex in the seven (7) days after missing pills.

21-DAY REGIMEN (SUNDAY START)
When taking Ethinyl Estradiol/Norgestimate 21, the first Norgestimate 0.180 mg or the first Norgestimate 0.250 mg tablet should be taken on the first Sunday after menstruation begins. If period begins on Sunday, the first Norgestimate 0.180 mg or the first Norgestimate 0.250 mg tablet is taken on that day. If switching directly from another oral contraceptive, the first Norgestimate 0.180 mg or the first Norgestimate 0.250 mg tablet should be taken on the first Sunday after the last ACTIVE tablet of the previous product. Tablets are taken without interruption for 21 days as follows: One Norgestimate 0.180 mg tablet daily for 7 days, then one Norgestimate 0.215 mg tablet daily for 7 days, then one Norgestimate 0.250 mg Tablet for 7 days, one Norgestimate 0.250 mg tablet daily for 21 days. For subsequent cycles, no tablets are taken for 7 days, then a new course is started of one tablet a day for 21 days, instituting a 3-weeks-on, one-week-off dosage regimen.

The use of Ethinyl Estradiol/Norgestimate 21 Tablets for contraception may be initiated postpartum. When tablets are administered during the postpartum period, the increased risk of thromboembolic disease associated with the postpartum period must be considered. (See *"Contraindications"* and *"Warnings"* concerning thromboembolic disease.) The possibility of ovulation and conception prior to initiation of medication should be considered. If the patient misses two (2) active tablets in Week 1 or Week 2, the patient should take two (2) tablets the day she remembers and two (2) tablets the next day; and then continue taking one (1) tablet a day until she finishes the pack. The patient should be instructed to use a back-up method of birth control if she has sex in the seven (7) days after missing pills. If the patient misses two (2) active tablets in the 3rd week or misses three (3) or more tablets in a row, the patient should continue taking one tablet every day until Sunday. On Sunday the patient should throw out the rest of the pack and start a new pack that same day. The patient should be instructed to use a back-up method of birth control if she has sex in the seven (7) days after missing pills.

28-DAY REGIMEN (DAY 1 START)
The dosage of Ethinyl Estradiol/Norgestimate 28 for the initial cycle of therapy is one tablet administered daily from the 1st day through the 21st day of the menstrual cycle, counting the first day of menstrual flow as "Day 1." Tablets are taken without interruption as follows: One Norgestimate 0.180 mg tablet daily for 7 days, then one Norgestimate 0.215 mg tablet daily for 7 days, then one Norgestimate 0.250 mg tablet daily for 7 days, or one Norgestimate 0.250 mg daily for 21 days, then one inert tablet daily for 7 days. After 28 tablets have been taken, a new course is started and a Norgestimate 0.180 mg or Norgestimate 0.250 mg tablet is taken the next day.

The use of Ethinyl Estradiol/Norgestimate 28 for contraception may be initiated postpartum. When the tablets are administered during the postpartum period, the increased risk of thromboembolic disease associated with the postpartum period must be considered. (See *"Contraindications"* and *"Warnings"* concerning thromboembolic disease.) The possibility of ovulation and conception prior to initiation of medication should be considered. If the patient misses two (2) active tablets in Week 1 or Week 2, the patient should take two (2) tablets the day she remembers and two (2) tablets the next day; and then continue taking one (1) tablet a day until she finishes the pack. The patient should be instructed to use a back-up method of birth control if she has sex in the seven (7) days after missing pills. If the patient misses two (2) active tablets in the 3rd week or misses three (3) or more active tablets in a row, the patient should throw out the rest of the pack and start a new pack that same day. The patient should be instructed to use a back-up method of birth control if she has sex in the seven (7) days after missing pills.

28-DAY REGIMEN (SUNDAY START)

When taking Ethinyl Estradiol/Norgestimate 28, the first Norgestimate 0.180 mg or the first Norgestimate 0.250 mg tablet should be taken on the first Sunday after menstruation begins. If period begins on Sunday the first Norgestimate 0.180 mg or the first Norgestimate 0.250 mg tablet is taken on that day. If switching directly from another oral contraceptive, the first Norgestimate 0.180 mg or the first Norgestimate 0.250 mg tablet should be taken on the first Sunday after the last ACTIVE tablet of the previous product. The tablets are taken without interruption as follows: one Norgestimate 0.180 mg tablet daily for 7 days, then one Norgestimate 0.215 mg tablet daily for 7 days, then one Norgestimate 0.250 mg tablet daily for 7 days or one Norgestimate 0.250 mg tablet daily for 21 days, then one inert tablet daily for 7 days. After 28 tablets have been taken, a new course is started and a Norgestimate 0.180 mg or a Norgestimate 0.250 mg tablet is taken the next day (Sunday).

The use of Ethinyl Estradiol/Norgestimate 28 for contraception may be initiated postpartum. When the tablets are administered during the postpartum period, the increased risk of thromboembolic disease associated with the postpartum period must be considered. (See *"Contraindications"* and *"Warnings"* concerning thromboembolic disease). The possibility of ovulation and conception prior to initiation of medication should be considered. If the patient misses two (2) active tablets in Week 1 or Week 2, the patient should take two (2) tablets the day she remembers and two (2) tablets the next day; and then continue taking one (1) tablet a day until she finishes the pack. The patient should be instructed to use a back-up method of birth control if she has sex in the seven (7) days after missing pills. If the patient misses two (2) active tablets in the 3rd week or misses three (3) or more tablets in a row, the patient should continue taking one tablet every day until Sunday. On Sunday the patient should throw out the rest of the pack and start a new pack that same day. The patient should be instructed to use a back-up method of birth control if she has sex in the seven (7) days after missing pills.

ADDITIONAL INSTRUCTIONS FOR ALL DOSING REGIMENS

Breakthrough bleeding, spotting, and amenorrhea are frequent reasons for patients discontinuing oral contraceptives. In breakthrough bleeding, as in all cases of irregular bleeding from the vagina, nonfunctional causes should be borne in mind. In undiagnosed persistent or recurrent abnormal bleeding from the vagina, adequate diagnostic measures are indicated to rule out pregnancy or malignancy. If pathology has been excluded, time or a change to another formulation may solve the problem. Changing to an oral contraceptive with a higher estrogen content, while potentially useful in minimizing menstrual irregularity, should be done only if necessary since this may increase the risk of thromboembolic disease.

Use of oral contraceptives in the event of a missed menstrual period:

1. If the patient has not adhered to the prescribed schedule, the possibility of pregnancy should be considered at the time of the first missed period and oral contraceptive use should be discontinued until pregnancy is ruled out.

2. If the patient has adhered to the prescribed regimen and misses two consecutive periods, pregnancy should be ruled out before continuing oral contraceptive use.

REFERENCES

1. Reproduced with permission of the Population Council from J. Trussell and K. Kost: Contraceptive failure in the United States: A critical review of the literature. Studies in Family Planning, 18(5), September-October 1987. 2. Stadel BV, Oral contraceptives and cardiovascular disease. (Pt.1). N Engl J Med 1981; 305:612-618. 3. Stadel BV, Oral contraceptives and cardiovascular disease. (Pt 2). N Engl J Med 1981; 305:672-677. 4. Adam SA, Thorogood M. Oral contraception and myocardial infarction revisited: The effects of new preparations and prescribing patterns. Br J Obstet Gynecol 1981:88:838-845. 5. Mann JI, Inman WH. Oral contraceptives and death from myocardial infarction. Br Med J 1975; 2(5965):245-248. 6. Mann JI, Vessey MP, Thorogood M, Doll R. Myocardial infarction in young women with special reference to oral contraceptive practice. Br Med J 1975; 2(5956):241-245. 7. Royal College of General Practioners' Oral Contraception Study: Further analyses of mortality in oral contraceptive users. Lancet 1981; 1:541-546. 8. Slone D, Shapiro S, Kaufman DW, Rosenberg L, Miettinen OS, Stolley PD. Risk of myocardial infarction in relation to current and discontinued use of oral contraceptives. N Engl J Med 1981; 305:420-424. 9. Vessey MP. Female hormones and vascular disease—an epidemiological overview. Br J Fam Plann 1980; 6 (Supplement): 1-12. 10. Russell-Briefel RG, Ezzati TM, Fulwood R, Perlman JA, Murphy RS. Cardiovascular risk status and oral contraceptive use, United States, 1976-80. Prevent Med 1986; 15:352-362. 11. Goldbaum GM, Kendrick JS, Hogelin GC, Gentry EM. The relative impact of smoking and oral contraceptive use on women in the United States. JAMA 1987; 258:1339-1342. 12. Layde PM, Beral V. Further analyses of mortality in oral contraceptive users; Royal College of General Practitioners' Oral Contraception Study. (Table 5) Lancet 1981; 1:541-546. 13. Knopp RH. Arteriosclerosis risk: the roles of oral contraceptives and postmenopausal estrogens. J Reprod Med 1986; 31(9)(Supplement):913-921. 14. Krauss RM, Roy S, Mishell DR, Casagrande J, Pike MC. Effects of two low-dose oral contraceptives on serum lipids and lipoproteins: Differential changes in high-density lipoproteins subclasses. Am J Obstet 1983; 145:446-452. 15. Wahl P, Walden C, Knopp R, Hoover J, Wallace R, Heiss G, Rifkind B. Effect of estrogen/progestin potency on lipid/lipoprotein cholesterol. N Engl J Med 1983; 308:862-867. 16. Wynn V, Niththyananthan R. The effect of progestin in combined oral contraceptives on serum lipids with special reference to high density lipoproteins. Am J Obstet Gynecol 1982; 142:766-771. 17. Wynn V, Godsland I. Effects of oral contraceptives on carbohydrate metabolism. J Reprod Med 1986; 31(9)(Supplement):892-897. 18. LaRosa JC. Atherosclerotic risk factors in cardiovascular disease. J Reprod Med 1986; 31(9)(Supplement):906-912. 19. Inman WH, Vessey MP. Investigation of death from pulmonary, coronary, and cerebral thrombosis and embolism in women of child-bearing age. Br Med J 1968; 2(5599):193-199. 20. Maguire MG, Tonascia J, Sartwell PE, Stolley PD, Tockman MS. Increased risk of thrombosis due to oral contraceptives: a further report. Am J Epidemiol 1979; 110(2): 188-195. 21. Petitti DB, Wingerd J, Pellegrin F, Ramacharan S. Risk of vascular disease in women: smoking, oral contraceptives, noncontraceptive estrogens, and other factors. JAMA 1979; 242:1150-1154. 22. Vessey MP, Doll R. Investigation of relation between use of oral contraceptives and thromboembolic disease. Br Med J 1968; 2(5599):199-205. 23. Vessey MP, Doll R. Investigation of relation between use of oral contraceptives and thromboembolic disease. A further report. Br Med J 1969; 2(5658):651-657. 24. Porter JB, Hunter JR, Danielson DA, Jick H, Stergachis A. Oral contraceptives and nonfatal vascular disease—recent experience. Obstet Gynecol 1982;59(3):299-302. 25. Vessey M, Doll R, Johnson B, Wiggins P. A long-term follow-up study of women using different methods of contraception: an interim report. J Biosocial Sci 1976: 8:375-427. 26. Royal College of General Practitioners: Oral Contraceptives, venous thrombosis, and varicose veins. J Royal Coll Gen Pract 1978; 28:393-399. 27. Collaborative Group for the Study of Stroke in Young Women: Oral contraception and increased risk of cerebral ischemia or thrombosis. N Engl J Med 1973; 288:871-878. 28. Petitti DB, Wingerd J. Use of oral contraceptives, cigarette smoking, and risk of subarachnoid hemorrhage. Lancet 1978; 2:234-236. 29. Inman WH. Oral contraceptives and fatal subarachnoid hemorrhage. Br Med J 1979; 2(6203):1468-1470. 30. Collaborative Group for the Study of Stroke in Young Women: Oral Contraceptives and stroke in young women: associated risk factors. JAMA 1975; 231:718-722. 31. Inman WH, Vessey MP, Westerholm B, Engelund A. Thromboembolic disease and the steroidal content of oral contraceptives. A report to the Committee on Safety of Drugs. Br Med J 1970; 2:203-209. 32. Meade TW, Greenberg G, Thompson SG. Progestogens and cardiovascular reactions associated with oral contraceptives and a comparison of the safety of 50- and 35-mcg oestrogen preparations. Br Med J 1980; 280(6224):1157-1161. 33. Kay CR. Progestogens and arterial disease—evidence from the Royal College of General Practitioners' Study. Am J Obstet Gynecol 1982; 142:762-765. 34. Royal College of General Practitioners: Incidence of arterial disease among oral contraceptive users. J Royal Coll Gen Pract 1983; 33: 75-82. 35. Ory HW. Mortality associated with fertility and fertility control: 1983. Family Planning Perspectives 1983; 15:50-56. 36. The Cancer and Steroid Hormone Study of the Centers for Disease Control and the National Institute of Child Health and Human Development: Oral contraceptive use and the risk of breast cancer. N Engl J Med 1986; 315:405-411. 37. Pike MC, Henderson BE, Krailo MD, Duke A, Roy S. Breast cancer in young women and use of oral contraceptives: possible modifying effect of formulation and age at use. Lancet 1983; 2:926-929. 38. Paul C. Skegg DG, Spears GFS, Kaldor JM. Oral contraceptives and breast cancer: A national study. Br Med J 1986; 293:723-725. 39. Miller DR, Rosenberg L, Kaufman DW, Schottenfeld D, Stolley PD, Shapiro S. Breast cancer risk in relation to early oral contraceptive use. Obstet Gynecol 1986; 68:863-868. 40. Olson H, Olson KL, Moller TR, Ranstam J, Holm P. Oral contraceptive use and breast cancer in young women in Sweden (letter). Lancet 1985; 2:748-749. 41. McPherson K, Vessey M, Neil A, Doll R, Jones L, Roberts M. Early contraceptive use and breast cancer: Results of another case-control study. Br J Cancer 1987; 56:653-660. 42. Huggins GR, Zucker PF. Oral contraceptives and neoplasia: 1987 update. Fertil Steril 1987; 47:733-761. 43. McPherson K, Drife JO. The pill and breast cancer: why the uncertainty? Br Med J 1986; 293:709-710. 44. Shapiro S. Oral contraceptives—time to take stock. N Engl J Med 1987; 315:450-451. 45. Ory H, Haib Z, Conger SB, Hatcher RA, Tyler CW. Contraceptive choice and prevalence of cervical dysplasia and carcinoma in situ. Am J Obstet Gynecol 1976; 124:573-577. 46. Vessey MP, Lawless M, McPherson K, Yeates D. Neoplasia of the cervix uteri and contraception: a possible adverse effect of the pill. Lancet 1983; 2:930. 47. Brinton LA, Huggins GR, Lehman HF, Malli K, Savitz DA, Trapido E, Rosenthal J, Hoover R. Long term use of oral contraceptives and risk of invasive cervical cancer. Int J Cancer 1986; 38:339-344. 48. WHO Collaborative Study of Neoplasia and Steroid Contraceptives: Invasive cervical cancer and combined oral contraceptives. Br Med J 1985; 290:961-965. 49. Rooks JB, Ory HW, Ishak KG, Strauss LT, Greenspan JR, Hill AP, Tyler CW. Epidemiology of hepatocellular adenoma: the role of oral contraceptive use. JAMA 1979; 242:644-648. 50. Bein NN, Goldsmith HS. Recurrent massive hemorrhage from benign hepatic tumors secondary to oral contraceptives. Br J Surg 1977; 64:433-435. 51. Klatskin G. Hepatic tumors: possible relationship to use of oral contraceptives. Gastroenterology 1977; 73:386-394. 52. Henderson BE, Preston-Martin S, Edmondson HA, Peters RL, Pike MC. Hepatocellular carcinoma and oral contraceptives. Br J Cancer 1983; 48:437-440. 53. Neuberger J, Forman D, Doll R, Williams R. Oral contraceptives and hepatocellular carcinoma. Br Med J 1986; 292:1355-1357. 54. Forman D, Vincent TJ, Doll R. Cancer of the liver and oral contraceptives. Br Med J 1986; 292:1357-1361. 55. Harlap S. Eldor J. Births following oral contraceptive failures. Obstet Gynecol 1980; 55:447-452. 56. Savolainen E, Saksela E, Saxen L. Teratogenic hazards of oral contraceptives analyzed in a national malformation register. Am J Obstet Gynecol 1981; 140:521-524. 57. Janerich DT, Piper JM, Glebatis DM. Oral contraceptives and birth defects. Am J Epidemiol 1980; 112:73-79. 58. Ferencz C, Matanoski GM, Wilson PD, Rubin JD, Neill CA, Gutberlet R. Maternal hormone therapy and congenital heart disease. Teratology 1980; 21:225-239. 59. Rothman KJ, Fyler DC, Goldblatt A, Kreidberg MB. Exogenous hormones and other drug exposures of children with congenital heart disease. Am J Epidemiol 1979; 109:433-439. 60. Boston Collaborative Drug Surveillance Program: Oral contraceptives and venous thromboembolic disease, surgically confirmed gallbladder disease, and breast tumors. Lancet 1973; 1:1399-1404. 61. Royal College of General Practitioners: Oral contraceptives and health. New York, Pittman 1974. 62. Layde PM, Vessey MP, Yeates D. Risk of gallbladder disease: a cohort study of young women attending family planning clinics. J Epidemiol Community Health 1982; 36:274-278. 63. Rome Group for Epidemiology and Prevention of Cholelithiasis (GREPCO): Prevalence of gallstone disease in an Italian adult female population. Am J Epidemiol 1984; 119:796-805. 64. Storm BL, Tamragouri RT, Morse ML, Lazar EL, West SL, Stolley PD, Jones JK. Oral contraceptives and other risk factors for gallbladder disease. Clin Pharmacol Ther 1986; 39:335-341. 65. Wynn V, Adams PW, Godsland IF, Melrose J, Niththyananthan R, Oakley NW, Seedj A. Comparison of effects of different combined oral-contraceptive formulations on carbohydrate and lipid metabolism. Lancet 1979; 1:1045-1049. 66. Wynn V. Effect of progesterone and progestins on carbohydrate metabolism. In: Progesterone and Progestin. Bardin CW, Milgrom E, Mauvis-Jarvis P. eds. New York, Raven Press 1983; pp. 395-410. 67. Perlman JA, Roussell-Briefel RG, Ezzati TM, Lieberknecht G. Oral glucose tolerance and the potency of oral contraceptive progestogens. J Chronic Dis 1985; 38:857-864. 68. Royal

College of General Practitioners' Oral Contraception Study: Effect on hypertension and benign breast disease of progestogen component in combined oral contraceptives. Lancet 1977; 1:624. 69. Fisch IR, Frank J. Oral contraceptives and blood pressure. JAMA 1977; 237:2499-2503. 70. Laragh AJ. Oral contraceptive induced hypertension—nine years later. Am J Obstet Gynecol 1976; 126:141-147. 71. Ramcharan S, Peritz, E, Pellegrin FA, Williams WT. Incidence of hypertension in the Walnut Creek Contraceptive Drug Study cohort; In: Pharmacology of steroid contraceptive drugs. Garattini S, Berendes HW, eds. New York, Raven Press, 1977; pp. 277-288, (Monographs of the Mario Negri Institute for Pharmacological Research Milan.) 72. Stockley I. Interactions with oral contraceptives. J Pharm 1976: 216:140-143. 73. The Cancer and Steroid Hormone Study of the Centers for Disease Control and the National Institute of Child Health and Human Development: Oral contraceptive use and the risk of ovarian cancer. JAMA 1983; 249:1596-1599. 74. The Cancer and Steroid Hormone Study of the Centers for Disease Control and the National Institute of Child Health and Human Development: Combination oral contraceptive use and the risk of endometrial cancer. JAMA 1987; 257:796-800. 75. Ory HW. Functional ovarian cysts and oral contraceptives: negative association confirmed surgically. JAMA 1974; 228:68-69. 76. Ory HW, Cole P, MacMahon B, Hoover R. Oral contraceptives and reduced risk of benign breast disease. N Engl J Med 1976; 294:419-422. 77. Ory HW. The noncontraceptive health benefits from oral contraceptive use. Fam Plann Perspect 1982; 14:182-184. 78. Ory HW, Forrest JD, Lincoln R. Making choices: evaluating the health risks and benefits of birth control methods. New York, The Alan Guttmacher Institute, 1983; p. 1. 79. Schlesselman J, Stadel BV, Murray P, Lai S. Breast cancer in relation to early use of oral contraceptives. JAMA 1988; 259:1828-1833. 80. Hennekens CH, Speizer FE, Lipnick RJ, Rosner B, Bain C, Belanger C, Stampfer MJ, Willett W, Peto R. A case-control study of oral contraceptive use and breast cancer. JNCI 1984; 72:39-42. 81. LaVecchia C, Decarli A, Fasoli M, Franceschi S, Gentile A, Negri E, Parazzini F, Tognoni G. Oral contraceptives and cancers of the breast and of the female genital tract. Interim results from a case-control study. Br J Cancer 1986: 54:311-317. 82. Meirik O, Lund E, Adami H, Bergstrom R, Christoffersen T, Bergsjo P. Oral contraceptive use and breast cancer in young women. A Joint National Case-control study in Sweden and Norway. Lancet 1986; 11:650-654. 83. Kay CR, Hannaford PC. Breast cancer and the pill—A further report from the Royal College of General Practitioners' oral contraception study. Br J Cancer 1988; 58:675-680. 84. Stadel BV, Lai S, Schlesselman JJ. Murray P. Oral contraceptives and premenopausal breast cancer in nulliparous women. Contraception 1988; 38:287-299. 85. Miller DR, Rosenberg L. Kaufman DW, Stolley P, Warshauer ME, Shapiro S. Breast cancer before age 45 and oral contraceptive use: New findings. Am J Epidemiol 1989; 129:269-280. 86. The UK National Case-Control Study Group, Oral contraceptive use and breast cancer risk in young women. Lancet 1989; 1:973-982. 87. Schlesselman JJ. Cancer of the breast and reproductive tract in relation to use of oral contraceptives. Contraception 1989; 40:1-38. 88. Vessey MP. McPherson K, Villard-Mackintosh L, Yeates D. Oral contraceptives and breast cancer: latest findings in a large cohort study. Br. J Cancer 1989; 59:613-617. 89. Jick SS, Walker AM, Stergachis A, Jick H. Oral contraceptives and breast cancer, Br J Cancer 1989; 59:618-621.

HOW SUPPLIED
TABLETS:

BRAND/MANUFACTURER	NDC	SIZE	AWP
○ **BRAND**			
➤ ORTHO TRI-CYCLEN: Ortho Pharm	00062-1902-15	126s	$133.20
	00062-1903-15	168s	$133.86

TABLETS: 0.25 MG-35 MCG

BRAND/MANUFACTURER	NDC	SIZE	AWP
○ **BRAND**			
➤ ORTHO CYCLEN: Ortho Pharm	00062-1900-15	126s	$133.20
	00062-1901-15	168s	$133.86

Ethinyl Estradiol with Ethynodiol Diacetate

DESCRIPTION

Each tablet contains:

1/35 Ethynodiol Diacetate	1 mg
Ethinyl Estradiol	35 mcg
1/50 Ethynodiol Diacetate	1 mg
Ethinyl Estradiol	50 mcg

The chemical name for Ethynodiol Diacetate is 19-nor-17α-pregn-4-en-zo-yne-3β, 17-diol diacetate, and for Ethinyl Estradiol it is 19-nor-17α-pregna-1,3,5(10)-trien-zo-yne-3,17-diol.

Therapeutic class: Oral contraceptive.

CLINICAL PHARMACOLOGY

Combination oral contraceptives act primarily by suppression of gonadotropins. Although the primary mechanism of this action is inhibition of ovulation, other alterations in the genital tract, including changes in the cervical mucus (which increase the difficulty of sperm entry into the uterus) and the endometrium (which may reduce the likelihood of implantation) may also contribute to contraceptive effectiveness.

INDICATIONS AND USAGE

Ethynodiol Diacetate with Ethinyl Estradiol is indicated for the prevention of pregnancy in women who elect to use oral contraceptives as a method of contraception.

Oral contraceptives are highly effective. Table 1 lists the typical accidental pregnancy rates for users of combination oral contraceptives and other methods of contraception. The efficacy of these contraceptive methods, except sterilization, depends upon the reliability with which they are used. Correct and consistent use of methods can result in lower failure rates.

Table 1

LOWEST EXPECTED AND TYPICAL FAILURE RATES DURING THE FIRST YEAR OF CONTINUOUS USE OF A METHOD. PERCENT OF WOMEN EXPERIENCING AN ACCIDENTAL PREGNANCY IN THE FIRST YEAR OF CONTINUOUS USE.[1]

Method	Lowest Expected*	Typical**
No contraception	85	85
Oral contraceptives		
Combined	0.1	N/A***
Progestogen only	0.5	N/A***
Diaphragm with spermicidal cream or jelly	6	18
Spermicides alone (foam, creams, jellies and vaginal suppositories)	3	21
Vaginal sponge		
Nulliparous	6	18
Parous	9	28
IUD (medicated)		
Progesterone	2	N/A***
Copper T 380A	0.8	N/A***
Condom without spermicides	2	12
Periodic abstinence (all methods)	1-9	20
Female sterilization	0.2	0.4
Male sterilization	0.1	0.15

Adapted from Trussell et al.[1]
* The authors' best guess of the percentage of women expected to experience an accidental pregnancy among couples who initiate a method (not necessarily for the first time) and who use it consistently and correctly during the first year if they do not stop for any other reason.
** This term represents "typical" couples who initiate use of a method (not necessarily for the first time), who experience an accidental pregnancy during the first year if they do not stop for any other reason.
*** N/A—Data not available.

CONTRAINDICATIONS

Oral contraceptives should not be used in women who have the following conditions:

■ Thrombophlebitis or thromboembolic disorders
■ A past history of deep vein thrombophlebitis or thromboembolic disorders
■ Cerebral vascular disease, myocardial infarction, or coronary artery disease, or a past history of these conditions
■ Known or suspected carcinoma of the breast, or a history of this condition
■ Known or suspected carcinoma of the female reproductive organs or suspected estrogen-dependent neoplasia, or a history of these conditions
■ Undiagnosed abnormal genital bleeding
■ History of cholestatic jaundice of pregnancy or jaundice with prior oral contraceptive use
■ Past or present, benign or malignant liver tumors
■ Known or suspected pregnancy.

WARNINGS

> CIGARETTE SMOKING INCREASES THE RISK OF SERIOUS CARDIOVASCULAR SIDE EFFECTS FROM ORAL CONTRACEPTIVE USE. THIS RISK INCREASES WITH AGE AND WITH HEAVY SMOKING (15 OR MORE CIGARETTES PER DAY) AND IS QUITE MARKED IN WOMEN OVER 35 YEARS OF AGE. WOMEN WHO USE ORAL CONTRACEPTIVES SHOULD BE STRONGLY ADVISED NOT TO SMOKE.

The use of oral contraceptives is associated with increased risk of several serious conditions including venous and arterial thromboembolism, thrombotic and hemorrhagic stroke, myocardial infarction, liver tumors or other liver lesions, and gallbladder disease. The risk of morbidity and mortality increases significantly in the presence of other risk factors such as hypertension, hyperlipidemia, obesity, and diabetes mellitus.

Practitioners prescribing oral contraceptives should be familiar with the following information relating to these and other risks.

The information contained herein is principally based on studies carried out in patients who used oral contraceptives with formulations containing higher amounts of estrogens and progestogens than those in common use today. The effect of long-term use of the oral contraceptives with lesser amounts of both estrogens and progestogens remains to be determined.

Throughout this labeling, epidemiological studies reported are of two types: retrospective case-control studies and prospective cohort studies. Case-control studies provide an estimate of the relative risk of a disease, which is defined as the *ratio* of the incidence of a disease among oral contraceptive users to that among nonusers. The relative risk (or odds ratio) does not provide information about the actual clinical occurrence of a disease. Cohort studies provide a measure of both the relative risk and the attributable risk. The latter is the *difference* in the incidence of disease between oral contraceptive users and nonusers. The attributable risk does provide information about the actual occurrence or incidence of a disease in the subject population. For further information, the reader is referred to a text on epidemiological methods.

1. THROMBOEMBOLIC DISORDERS AND OTHER VASCULAR PROBLEMS

a. Myocardial Infarction: An increased risk of myocardial infarction has been associated with oral contraceptive use.[2-21] This increased risk is primarily in smokers or in women with other underlying risk factors for coronary artery disease such as hypertension, obesity, diabetes, and hypercholesterolemia. The relative risk for myocardial infarction in current oral contraceptive users has been estimated to be 2 to 6. The risk is very low under the age of 30. However, there is the possibility of a risk of cardiovascular disease even in very young women who take oral contraceptives.

Smoking in combination with oral contraceptive use has been reported to contribute substantially to the risk of myocardial infarction in women in their mid-thirties or older, with smoking accounting for the majority of excess cases.[22] Mortality rates associated with circulatory disease have been shown to increase substantially in smokers, especially in those 35 years of age and older among women who use oral contraceptives (see Figure 1, Table 2).

Figure 1. Circulatory disease mortality rates per 100,000 woman-years by age, smoking status, and oral contraceptive use.[14]

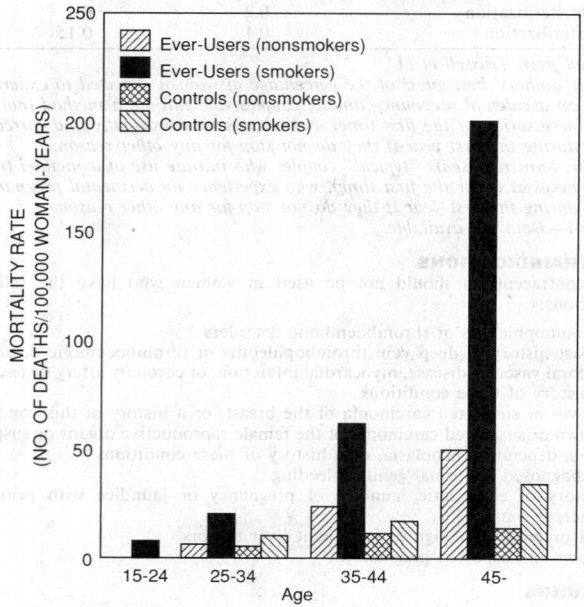

CIRCULATORY DISEASE MORTALITY RATES PER 100,000
WOMAN-YEARS BY AGE, SMOKING STATUS
AND ORAL CONTRACEPTIVE USE

Legend:
- Ever-Users (nonsmokers)
- Ever-Users (smokers)
- Controls (nonsmokers)
- Controls (smokers)

Y-axis: MORTALITY RATE (NO. OF DEATHS/100,000 WOMAN-YEARS)
X-axis: Age — 15-24, 25-34, 35-44, 45-

Adapted from Layde and Beral.[14]

Oral contraceptives may compound the effects of well-known cardiovascular risk factors such as hypertension, diabetes, hyperlipidemias, hypercholesterolemia, age, cigarette smoking, and obesity. In particular, some progestogens decrease HDL cholesterol[23-31] and cause glucose intolerance, while estrogens may create a state of hyperinsulinism.[32] Oral contraceptives have been shown to increase blood pressure among some users (see *"Warning"* No. 9). Similar effects on risk factors have been associated with an increased risk of heart disease.

b. Thromboembolism: An increased risk of thromboembolic and thrombotic disease associated with the use of oral contraceptives is well established.[17,33-51] Case-control studies have estimated the relative risk to be 3 for the first episode of superficial venous thrombosis, 4 to 11 for deep vein thrombosis or pulmonary embolism, and 1.5 to 6 for women with predisposing conditions for venous thromboembolic disease.[34-37,45,46] Cohort studies have shown the relative risk to be somewhat lower, about 3 for new cases (subjects with no past history of venous thrombosis or varicose veins) and about 4.5 for new cases requiring hospitalization.[42,47,48] The risk of venous thromboembolic disease associated with oral contraceptives is not related to duration of use.

A two- to seven-fold increase in relative risk of postoperative thromboembolic complications has been reported with the use of oral contraceptives.[38,39] The relative risk of venous thrombosis in women who have predisposing conditions is about twice that of women without such medical conditions.[43] If feasible, oral contraceptives should be discontinued at least 4 weeks prior to and for 2 weeks after elective surgery of a type associated with an increased risk of thromboembolism, and also during and following prolonged immobilization. Since the

immediate postpartum period is also associated with an increased risk of thromboembolism, oral contraceptives should be started no earlier than 4 to 6 weeks after delivery in women who elect not to breast feed.

c. Cerebrovascular Diseases: Both the relative and attributable risks of cerebrovascular events (thrombotic and hemorrhagic strokes) have been reported to be increased with oral contraceptive use,[14,17,18,34,42,46,52-59] although, in general, the risk was greatest among older (over 35 years), hypertensive women who also smoked. Hypertension was reported to be a risk factor for both users and nonusers, for both types of strokes, while smoking increased the risk for hemorrhagic strokes.

In one large study,[52] the relative risk for thrombotic stroke was reported as 9.5 times greater in users than in nonusers. It ranged from 3 for normotensive users to 14 for users with severe hypertension.[54] The relative risk for hemorrhagic stroke was reported to be 1.2 for nonsmokers who used oral contraceptives, 1.9 to 2.6 for smokers who did not use oral contraceptives, 6.1 to 7.6 for smokers who used oral contraceptives, 1.8 for normotensive users, and 25.7 for users with severe hypertension. The risk is also greater in older women and among smokers.

d. Dose-related Risk of Vascular Disease with Oral Contraceptives: A positive association has been reported between the amount of estrogen and progestogen in oral contraceptives and the risk of vascular disease.[41,43,53,59-64] A decline in serum high density lipoproteins (HDL) has been reported with many progestogens.[23-31] A decline in serum high density lipoproteins has been associated with an increased incidence of ischemic heart disease.[65] Because estrogens increase HDL-cholesterol, the net effect of an oral contraceptive depends on the balance achieved between doses of estrogen and progestogen and the nature and absolute amount of progestogens used in the contraceptives. The amount of both steroids should be considered in the choice of an oral contraceptive.

Minimizing exposure to estrogen and progestogen is in keeping with good principles of therapeutics. For any particular estrogen-progestogen combination, the dosage regimen prescribed should be one that contains the least amount of estrogen and progestogen that is compatible with a low failure rate and the needs of the individual patient. New acceptors of oral contraceptives should be started on preparations containing the lowest estrogen content that produces satisfactory results in the individual.

e. Persistence of Risk of Vascular Disease: There are three studies that have shown persistence of risk of vascular disease for users of oral contraceptives. In a study in the United States, the risk of developing myocardial infarction after discontinuing oral contraceptives persisted for at least 9 years for women 40-49 years old who had used oral contraceptives for 5 or more years, but this increased risk was not demonstrated in other age groups.[16] Another American study reported former use of oral contraceptives was significantly associated with increased risk of subarachnoid hemorrhage.[57] In another study, in Great Britain, the risk of developing nonrheumatic heart disease plus hypertension, subarachnoid hemorrhage, cerebral thrombosis, and transient ischemic attacks persisted for at least 6 years after discontinuation of oral contraceptives, although the excess risk was small.[14,18,66] It should be noted that these studies were performed with oral contraceptive formulations containing 50 mcg or more of estrogens.

2. ESTIMATES OF MORTALITY FROM CONTRACEPTIVE USE

One study[67] gathered data from a variety of sources that have estimated the mortality rates associated with different methods of contraception at different ages (Table 2). These estimates include the combined risk of death associated with contraceptive methods plus the risk attributable to pregnancy in the event of method failure. Each method of contraception has its specific benefits and risks. The study concluded that, with the exception of oral contraceptive users 35 and older who smoke and 40 or older who do not smoke, mortality associated with all methods of birth control is low and below that associated with childbirth. The observation of a possible increase in risk of mortality with age for oral contraceptive users is based on data gathered in the 1970's, but not reported until 1983.[67] However, current clinical practice involves the use of lower estrogen dose formulations combined with careful restriction of oral contraceptive use to women who do not have the various risk factors listed in this labeling.

Because of these changes in practice and, also, because of some limited new data that suggest that the risk of cardiovascular disease with the use of oral contraceptives may now be less than previously observed,[48,152] the Fertility and Maternal Health Drugs Advisory Committee was asked to review the topic in 1989. The Committee concluded that, although cardiovascular disease risks may be increased with oral contraceptive use after age 40 in healthy nonsmoking women (even with the newer low-dose formulations), there are greater potential health risks associated with pregnancy in older women and with the alternative surgical and medical procedures that may be necessary if such women do not have access to effective and acceptable means of contraception.

Therefore, the Committee recommended that the benefits of oral contraceptive use by healthy nonsmoking women over 40 may outweigh the possible risks. Of course, older women, as all women who take oral contraceptives, should take the lowest dose formulation that is effective. (See related table).

3. CARCINOMA OF THE BREAST AND REPRODUCTIVE ORGANS

Numerous epidemiological studies have been performed on the incidence of breast, endometrial, ovarian, and cervical cancer in women using oral contraceptives. While there are conflicting reports, most studies suggest that the use of oral contraceptives is not associated with an overall increase in the risk of developing breast cancer.[17,40,68-78] Some studies have reported an increased relative risk of developing breast cancer, particularly at a young age.[79-102,151] This increased relative risk appears to be related to duration of use.

Some studies suggested that oral contraceptive use was associated with an increase in the risk of cervical intraepithelial neoplasia, dysplasia, erosion, carcinoma, or microglandular dysplasia in some populations of women.[17,50,103-115] However, there continues to be controversy about the extent to which such findings may be due to differences in sexual behavior and other factors.

In spite of many studies of the relationship between oral contraceptive use and breast and cervical cancers, a cause and effect relationship has not been established.

4. HEPATIC NEOPLASIA
Benign hepatic adenomas and other hepatic lesions have been associated with oral contraceptive use,[116-121] although the incidence of such benign tumors is rare in the United States. Indirect calculations have estimated the attributable risk to be in the range of 3.3 cases per 100,000 users, a risk that increases after 4 or more years of use.[120] Rupture of benign, hepatic adenomas or other lesions may cause death through intra-abdominal hemorrhage. Therefore, such lesions should be considered in women presenting with abdominal pain and tenderness, abdominal mass, or shock. About one quarter of the cases presented because of abdominal masses; up to one half had signs and symptoms of acute intraperitoneal hemorrhage.[121] Diagnosis may prove difficult.

Studies from the U.S.,[122,150] Great Britain,[123,124] and Italy[125] have shown an increased risk of hepatocellular carcinoma in long-term (> 8 years; relative risk of 7-20) oral contraceptive users. However, these cancers are rare in the United States, and the attributable risk (the excess incidence) of liver cancers in oral contraceptive users approaches less than 1 per 1,000,000 users.

5. OCULAR LESIONS
There have been reports of retinal thrombosis and other ocular lesions associated with the use of oral contraceptives. Oral contraceptives should be discontinued if there is unexplained, gradual or sudden, partial or complete loss of vision; onset of proptosis or diplopia; papilledema; or any evidence of retinal vascular lesions. Appropriate diagnostic and therapeutic measures should be undertaken immediately.

6. ORAL CONTRACEPTIVE USE BEFORE OR DURING PREGNANCY
Extensive epidemiological studies have revealed no increased risk of birth defects in women who have used oral contraceptives prior to pregnancy.[126,129] The majority of recent studies also do not suggest a teratogenic effect, particularly insofar as cardiac anomalies and limb reduction defects are concerned,[126-129] when the pill is taken inadvertently during early pregnancy.

The administration of oral contraceptives to induce withdrawal bleeding should not be used as a test for pregnancy. Oral contraceptives should not be used during pregnancy to treat threatened or habitual abortion. It is recommended that for any patient who has missed two consecutive periods, pregnancy should be ruled out before continuing oral contraceptive use. If the patient has not adhered to the prescribed schedule, the possibility of pregnancy should be considered at the time of the first missed period and further use of oral contraceptives should be withheld until pregnancy has been ruled out. Oral contraceptive use should be discontinued if pregnancy is confirmed.

7. GALLBLADDER DISEASE
Earlier studies reported an increased lifetime relative risk of gallbladder surgery in users of oral contraceptives and estrogens.[40,42,53,70] More recent studies, however, have shown that the relative risk of developing gallbladder disease among oral contraceptive users may be minimal.[130-132] The recent findings of minimal risk may be related to the use of oral contraceptive formulations containing lower doses of estrogens and progestogens.

8. CARBOHYDRATE AND LIPID METABOLIC EFFECTS
Oral contraceptives have been shown to cause a decrease in glucose tolerance in a significant percentage of users.[32] This effect has been shown to be directly related to estrogen dose.[133] Progestogens increase insulin secretion and create insulin resistance, the effect varying with different progestational agents.[32,134] However, in the nondiabetic woman, oral contraceptives appear to have no effect on fasting blood glucose. Because of these demonstrated effects, prediabetic and diabetic women should be carefully observed while taking oral contraceptives.

Some women may have persistent hypertriglyceridemia while on the pill. As discussed earlier (see "Warnings" 1a and 1d), changes in serum triglycerides and lipoprotein levels have been reported in oral contraceptive users.[23-31,135,136]

9. ELEVATED BLOOD PRESSURE
An increase in blood pressure has been reported in women taking oral contraceptives[50,53,137-139] and this increase is more likely in older oral contraceptive users[137] and with extended duration of use.[53] Data from the Royal College of General Practitioners[138] and subsequent randomized trials have shown that the incidence of hypertension increases with increasing concentrations of progestogens.

Women with a history of hypertension or hypertension-related diseases, or renal disease[139] should be encouraged to use another method of contraception. If such women elect to use oral contraceptives, they should be monitored closely and if significant elevation of blood pressure occurs, oral contraceptives should be discontinued. For most women, elevated blood pressure will return to normal after stopping oral contraceptives,[137] and there is no difference in the occurrence of hypertension among ever- and never-users.[140]

10. HEADACHE
The onset or exacerbation of migraine or the development of headache of a new pattern that is recurrent, persistent, or severe requires discontinuation of oral contraceptives and evaluation of the cause.

11. BLEEDING IRREGULARITIES
Breakthrough bleeding and spotting are sometimes encountered in patients on oral contraceptives, especially during the first three months of use. Nonhormonal causes should be considered and adequate diagnostic measures taken to rule out malignancy or pregnancy in the event of breakthrough bleeding, as in the case of any abnormal vaginal bleeding. If a pathologic basis has been excluded, time alone or a change to another formulation may solve the problem. In the event of amenorrhea, pregnancy should be ruled out.

PRECAUTIONS
1. Physical Examination and Follow-up: A complete medical history and physical examination should be completed prior to the initiation or reinstitution of oral contraceptives and at least annually during the use of oral contraceptives. These physical examinations should include special reference to blood pressure, breasts, abdomen, and pelvic organs, including cervical cytology, and relevant laboratory tests. In case of undiagnosed, persistent, or recurrent abnormal vaginal bleeding, appropriate diagnostic measures should be conducted to rule out malignancy. Women with a strong family history of breast cancer or who have breast nodules should be monitored with particular care.

2. Lipid Disorders: Women who are being treated for hyperlipidemias should be followed closely if they elect to use oral contraceptives. Some progestogens may elevate LDL levels and may render the control of hyperlipidemias more difficult.

3. Liver Function: If jaundice develops in any woman receiving oral contraceptives, they should be discontinued. Steroids may be poorly metabolized in patients with impaired liver function and should be administered with caution in such patients. Cholestatic jaundice has been reported after combined treatment with oral contraceptives and troleandomycin. Hepatotoxicity following a combination of oral contraceptives and cyclosporine has also been reported.

4. Fluid Retention: Oral contraceptives may cause some degree of fluid retention. They should be prescribed with caution, and only with careful monitoring, in patients with conditions that might be aggravated by fluid retention, such as convulsive disorders, migraine syndrome, asthma, or cardiac, hepatic, or renal dysfunction.

5. Emotional Disorders: Women with a history of depression should be carefully observed and the drug discontinued if depression recurs to a serious degree.

6. Contact Lenses: Contact lens wearers who develop visual changes or changes in lens tolerance should be assessed by an opthalmologist.

7. Drug Interactions: Reduced efficacy and increased incidence of breakthrough bleeding and menstrual irregularities have been associated with concomitant use of rifampin. A similar association, though less marked, has been suggested for

Table 2.
ANNUAL NUMBER OF BIRTH-RELATED OR METHOD-RELATED DEATHS ASSOCIATED WITH CONTROL OF FERTILITY PER 100,000 NONSTERILE WOMEN, BY FERTILITY CONTROL METHOD ACCORDING TO AGE.[67]

Method of control	Age					
	15-19	20-24	25-29	30-34	35-39	40-44
No fertility control methods*	7.0	7.4	9.1	14.8	25.7	28.2
Oral contraceptives						
nonsmoker**	0.3	0.5	0.9	1.9	13.8	31.6
smoker**	2.2	3.4	6.6	13.5	51.1	117.2
IUD**	0.8	0.8	1.0	1.0	1.4	1.4
Condom*	1.1	1.6	0.7	0.2	0.3	0.4
Diaphragm/spermicide*	1.9	1.2	1.2	1.3	2.2	2.8
Periodiodic abstinence*	2.5	1.6	1.6	1.7	2.9	3.6

* *Deaths are birth-related*
** *Deaths are method-related*
Adapted from Ory.[67]

barbiturates, phenylbutazone, phenytoin sodium, and possibly with griseofulvin, ampicillin, and tetracyclines.

8. Laboratory Test Interactions: Certain endocrine and liver function tests and blood components may be affected by oral contraceptives:

a. Increased prothrombin and factors VII, VIII, IX, and X; decreased antithrombin III; increased platelet aggregability.

b. Increased thyroid binding globulin (TBG), leading to increased circulating total thyroid hormone as measured by protein-bound iodine (PBI), T_4 by column or by radioimmunoassay. Free T_3 resin uptake is decreased, reflecting the elevated TBG; free T_4 concentration is unaltered.

c. Other binding proteins may be elevated in the serum.

d. Sex-steroid binding globulins are increased and result in elevated levels of total circulating sex steroids and corticoids; however, free or biologically active levels remain unchanged.

e. Triglycerides and phospholipids may be increased.

f. Glucose tolerance may be decreased.

g. Serum folate levels may be depressed. This may be of clinical significance if a woman becomes pregnant shortly after discontinuing oral contraceptives.

h. Increased sulfobromophthalein and other abnormalities in liver function tests may occur.

i. Plasma levels of trace minerals may be altered.

j. Response to the metyrapone test may be reduced.

9. Carcinogenesis: See *"Warnings".*

10. Pregnancy: Pregnancy Category X. See *"Contraindications"* and *"Warnings".*

11. Nursing Mothers: Small amounts of oral contraceptive steroids have been identified in the milk of nursing mothers[141-143] and a few adverse effects on the child have been reported, including jaundice and breast enlargement. In addition, oral contraceptives given in the postpartum period may interfere with lactation by decreasing the quantity and quality of breast milk. If possible, the nursing mother should be advised not to use oral contraceptives, but to use other forms of contraception until she has completely weaned her child.

12. Venereal Diseases: Oral contraceptives are of no value in the prevention or treatment of venereal disease. The prevalence of cervical *Chlamydia trachomatis* and *Neisseria gonorrhoeae* in oral contraceptive users is increased several-fold.[144,145] It should not be assumed that oral contraceptives afford protection against pelvic inflammatory disease from chlamydia.[144]

13. General:

a. The pathologist should be advised of oral contraceptive therapy when relevant specimens are submitted.

b. Treatment with oral contraceptives may mask the onset of the climacteric. (See *"Warnings"* regarding risks in this age group).

INFORMATION FOR THE PATIENT

See manufacturer's patient information.

ADVERSE REACTIONS

An increased risk of the following serious adverse reactions has been associated with the use of oral contraceptives (see *"Warnings"*):

- Thrombophlebitis and thrombosis
- Arterial thromboembolism
- Pulmonary embolism
- Myocardial infarction and coronary thrombosis
- Cerebral hemorrhage
- Cerebral thrombosis
- Hypertension
- Gallbladder disease
- Benign and malignant liver tumors, and other hepatic lesions.

There is evidence of an association between the following conditions and the use of oral contraceptives, although additional confirmatory studies are needed:

- Mesenteric thrombosis
- Neuro-ocular lesions (eg, retinal thrombosis and optic neuritis)

The following adverse reactions have been reported in patients receiving oral contraceptives and are believed to be drug-related:

- Nausea
- Vomiting
- Gastrointestinal symptoms (such as abdominal cramps and bloating)
- Breakthrough bleeding
- Spotting
- Change in menstrual flow
- Amenorrhea during or after use
- Temporary infertility after discontinuation of use
- Edema
- Chloasma or melasma, which may persist
- Breast changes: tenderness, enlargement, secretion
- Change in weight (increase or decrease)
- Change in cervical erosion or secretion
- Diminution in lactation when given immediately post-partum
- Cholestatic jaundice
- Migraine
- Rash (allergic)
- Mental depression
- Reduced tolerance to carbohydrates

- Vaginal candidiasis
- Change in corneal curvature (steepening)
- Intolerance to contact lenses

The following adverse reactions or conditions have been reported in users of oral contraceptives and the association has been neither confirmed nor refuted:

- Premenstrual syndrome
- Cataracts
- Changes in appetite
- Cystitis-like syndrome
- Headache
- Nervousness
- Dizziness
- Hirsutism
- Loss of scalp hair
- Erythema multiforme
- Erythema nodosum
- Hemorrhagic eruption
- Vaginitis
- Porphyria
- Impaired renal function
- Hemolytic uremic syndrome
- Acne
- Changes in libido
- Colitis
- Budd-Chiari syndrome
- Endocervical hyperplasia or ectropion

OVERDOSAGE

Serious ill effects have not been reported following acute ingestion of large doses of oral contraceptives by young children.[180,181] Overdosage may cause nausea, and withdrawal bleeding may occur in females.

NONCONTRACEPTIVE HEALTH BENEFITS

The following non-contraceptive health benefits related to the use of oral contraceptives are supported by epidemiological studies that largely utilized oral contraceptive formulations containing estrogen doses exceeding 35 mcg of ethinyl estradiol or 50 mcg of mestranol.[148,149]

EFFECTS ON MENSES

- Increased menstrual cycle regularity
- Decreased blood loss and decreased risk of iron-deficiency anemia
- Decreased frequency of dysmenorrhea.

EFFECTS RELATED TO INHIBITION OF OVULATION

- Decreased risk of functional ovarian cysts
- Decreased risk of ectopic pregnancies

EFFECTS FROM LONG-TERM USE

- Decreased risk of fibroadenomas and fibrocystic disease of the breast
- Decreased risk of acute pelvic inflammatory disease
- Decreased risk of endometrial cancer
- Decreased risk of ovarian cancer
- Decreased risk of uterine fibroids

DOSAGE AND ADMINISTRATION

To achieve maximum contraceptive effectiveness, oral contraceptives must be taken exactly as directed and at intervals of 24 hours.

Important: The patient should be instructed to use an additional method of protection until after the first week of administration *in the initial cycle.* The possibility of ovulation and conception prior to initiation of use should be considered.

Two dosage schedules are described, one of which may be more convenient or suitable than the other for an individual patient.

Schedule #1: Sunday start: The patient begins taking Ethynodiol Diacetate and Ethinyl Estradiol from the first row of her package, one tablet daily, starting on the first Sunday after the onset of menstruation. If the patient's period begins on a Sunday she takes her first tablet that very same day. The 21st tablet or the 28th tablet, depending on whether the patient is taking the 21- or 28-tablet course, will then be taken on a Saturday.

Subsequent cycles:

21-tablet course—The patient begins a new 21-tablet course on the eighth day, Sunday, after taking her last tablet. All subsequent cycles will also begin on Sunday, one tablet being taken each day for 3 weeks followed by a week of no pill-taking.

28-tablet course—The patient begins a new 28-tablet course on the next day, Sunday, and all subsequent cycles will also begin on Sunday, one tablet being taken each and every day.

With a Sunday-start schedule, a woman whose period begins on the day of or 1 to 4 days before taking the first tablet should expect a diminution of flow and fewer menstrual days. The initial cycle will likely be shortened by from 1 to 5 days. Thereafter, cycles are about 28 days in length.

Schedule #2: Day 5 start: The patient begins taking Ethynodiol Diacetate and Ethinyl Estradiol from the first row of her package, one tablet daily, starting with the pill day which corresponds to day 5 of her menstrual cycle: the first day of menstruation is counted as day 1. After the last (Saturday) tablet in row #3 has been taken, if any remain in the first row, the patient completes her 21-tablet schedule starting with Sunday in row #1.

Subsequent cycles: The patient begins a new 21-tablet course on the eighth day after taking her last tablet, again starting the same day of the week on which she began her first course. All subsequent cycles will also begin on that same day, one tablet being taken each day for 3 weeks followed by a week of no pill-taking.

SPECIAL NOTES

Spotting or breakthrough bleeding: If spotting (bleeding insufficient to require a pad) or breakthrough bleeding (heavier bleeding similar to a menstrual flow) occurs when these products are used for contraception, the patient should continue taking her tablets as directed. The incidence of spotting or breakthrough bleeding is minimal, most frequently occurring in the first cycle. Ordinarily spotting or breakthrough bleeding will stop within a week. Usually the patient will begin to cycle regularly within two or three courses of tablet-taking. In the event of spotting or breakthrough bleeding organic causes should be borne in mind. (See *"Warning"* No. 11.)

Missed menstrual periods: Withdrawal flow will normally occur 2 or 3 days after the last active tablet is taken. Failure of withdrawal bleeding ordinarily does not mean that the patient is pregnant, providing the dosage schedule has been correctly followed. (See *"Warning"* No. 6.)

If the patient has *not* adhered to the prescribed dosage regimen, the possibility of pregnancy should be considered after the first missed period, and oral contraceptives should be withheld until pregnancy has been ruled out.

If the patient has adhered to the prescribed regimen and misses two consecutive periods, pregnancy should be ruled out before continuing the contraceptive regimen.

The first intermenstrual interval after discontinuing the tablets is usually prolonged; consequently, a patient for whom a 28-day cycle is usual might not begin to menstruate for 35 days or longer. Ovulation in such prolonged cycles will occur correspondingly later in the cycle. Posttreatment cycles after the first one, however, are usually typical for the individual woman prior to taking tablets. (See *"Warning"* No. 11.)

Missed tablets: If a woman misses taking one active tablet the missed tablet should be taken as soon as it is remembered. In addition, the next tablet should be taken at the usual time. If two consecutive active tablets are missed the dosage should be doubled for the next 2 days. The regular schedule should then be resumed, but an additional method of protection is recommended for the remainder of the cycle.

While there is little likelihood of ovulation if only one active tablet is missed, the possibility of spotting or breakthrough bleeding is increased and should be expected if two or more successive active tablets are missed. However, the possibility of ovulation increases with each successive day that scheduled active tablets are missed.

If one or more placebo tablets of Ethynodiol Diacetate and Ethinyl Estradiol 28 day are missed, Ethynodiol Diacetate and Ethinyl Estradiol 28 day schedule should be resumed on the following Sunday (the eighth day after the last white tablet was taken). Omission of placebo tablets in the 28-tablet courses does not increase the possibility of conception provided that this schedule is followed.

REFERENCES

1. Trussel J, et al. *Stud Fam Plann.* 1987;18(Sept-Oct):237; and 1990:21(Jan-Feb):51. 2. Mann JI, et al. *Br Med J.* 1975;2(May 3):241. 3. Mann JI, et al. *Br Med J.* 1975;3(Sept 13):631. 4. Mann JI, et al. *Br Med J.* 1975;2(May 3):245. 5. Mann JI, et al. *Br Med J.* 1976;2(Aug 21):445. 6. Arthes FG, et al. *Chest.* 1976:70(Nov):574. 7. Jain AK. *Am J Obstet Gynecol.* 1976:301(Oct 1):126; and *Stud Fam Plann.* 1977;8(March) 50. 8. Ory HW. *JAMA.* 1977;237(June 13):2619. 9. Jick H, et al. *JAMA.* 1978;239(April 3):1403, 1407. 10. Jick H, et al. *JAMA.* 1978;240(Dec 1):2548. 11. Shapiro S, et al. *Lancet.* 1979; 1(April 7):743. 12. Rosenberg L, et al. *Am J Epidemiol.* 1980;111(Jan):59. 13. Krueger DE, et al. *Am J Epidemiol.* 1980;111(June):655. 14. Layde P, et al. *Lancet.* 1981;1(March 7):541. 15. Adam SA, et al. *Br J Obstet Gynaecol.* 1981; 88(Aug):838. 16. Slone D, et al. *N Engl J Med.* 1981; 305(Aug 20):420. 17. Ramcharan S, et al. *The Walnut Creek Contraceptive Drug Study.* Vol 3. US Govt Ptg Off; 1981; and *J Reprod Med.* 1980;25(Dec):346. 18. Layde PM, et al. *J R Coll Gen Pract.* 1983;33(Feb):75. 19. Rosenberg L, et al. *JAMA.* 1985;253(May 24/31):2965. 20. Mant D, et al. *J Epidemiol Community Health.* 1987;41(Sept):215. 21. Croft P, et al. *Br Med J.* 1989;298(Jan 21):165. 22. Goldbaum GM, et al. *JAMA.* 1987;258(Sept 11):1339. 23. Bradley DD, et al. *N Engl J Med.* 1978;299(July 6):17. 24. Tikkanen MJ, *J Reprod Med.* 1986;31(Sept suppl):898. 25. Lipson A, et al. *Contraception.* 1986;34(Aug):121. 26. Burkman RT, et al. *Obstet Gynecol.* 1988;71(Jan):33. 27. Knopp RH, *J Reprod Med.* 1986;31(Sept suppl):913. 28. Krauss RM, et al. *Am J Obstet Gynecol.* 1983; 145(Feb 15):446. 29. Wahl P, et al. *N Engl J Med.* 1983;308(April 14):862. 30. Wynn V, et al. *Am J Obstet Gynecol.* 1982;142(March 15):766. 31. LaRosa JC. *J Reprod Med.* 1986;31(Sept suppl):906. 32. Wynn V, et al. *J Reprod Med.* 1986;31(Sept suppl):892. 33. Royal College of General Practitioners. *J R Coll Gen Pract.* 1967;13(May):267. 34. Inman WHW, et al. *Br Med J.* 1968;2(April 27):193. 35. Vessey MP, et al. *Br Med J.* 1968;2(April 27):199. 36. Vessey MP, et al. *Br Med J.* 1969;2(June 14):651. 37. Sartwell PE, et al. *Am J Epidemiol.* 1969;90(Nov):365. 38. Vessey MP, et al. *Br Med J.* 1970;3(July 18):123. 39. Greene GR, et al. *Am J Public Health.* 1972;62(May):680. 40. Boston Collaborative Drug Surveillance Programme, *Lancet.* 1973;1(June 23):1399. 41. Stolley PD, et al. *Am J Epidemiol.* 1975;102(Sept):197. 42. Vessey MP, et al. *J Biosoc Sci.* 1976;8(Oct):373. 43. Kay CR, *J R Coll Gen Pract.* 1978;28(July):393. 44. Petitti DB, et al. *Am J Epidemiol.* 1978;108(Dec):480. 45. Maquire MG, et al. *Am J Epidemiol.* 1979;110(Aug):188. 46. Petitti DB, et al. *JAMA.* 1979:242(Sept 14):1150. 47. Porter JB, et al. *Obstet Gynecol.* 1982:59(March):299. 48. Porter JB, et al. *Obstet Gynecol.* 1985;66(July):1. 49. Vessey MP, et al. *Br Med J.* 1986:292(Feb 22):526. 50. Hoover R, et al. *Am J Public Health.* 1978:68(April):335. 51. Vessey MP. *Br J Fam Plann.* 1980;6(Oct suppl):1. 52. Collaborative Group for the Study of Stroke in Young Women. *N Engl J Med.* 1973;288(April 26):871. 53. Royal College of General Practitioners. *Oral Contraceptives and Health.* New York, NY: Pitman Publ Corp; May 1974. 54. Collaborative Group for the Study of Stroke in Young Women. *JAMA.* 1975;231(Feb 17):718. 55. Beral V. *Lancet.* 1976;2(Nov 13):1047. 56. Vessey MP, et al. *Lancet.* 1977;2(Oct 8):731; and 1981;1(March 7):549. 57. Petitti DB, et al. *Lancet.* 1978;2(July 29):234. 58. Inman WHW. *Br Med J.* 1979;2(Dec 8):1468. 59. Vessey MP, et al. *Br Med J.* 1984:289(Sept 1):530. 60. Inman WHW, et al. *Br Med J.* 1970;2(April 25):203. 61. Meade TW, et al. *Br Med J.* 1980;280(May 10):1157. 62. Böttiger LE, et al. *Lancet.* 1980;1(May 24):1097. 63. Kay CR, *Am J Obstet Gynecol.* 1982;142(March 15):762. 64. Vessey MP, et al. *Br Med J.* 1986;292(Feb 22):526. 65. Gordon T, et al. *Am J Med.* 1977;62(May): 707. 66. Beral V, et al. *Lancet.* 1977;2(Oct 8): 727. 67. Ory H. *Fam Plann Perspect.* 1983;15(March April):57. 68. Arthes FG, et al. *Cancer, 1971,28(Dec):1391. 69. Vessey MP, et al. Br Med J.* 1972;3(Sept 23):719. 70. Boston Collaborative Drug Surveillance Program. *N Engl J Med.* 1974;290(Jan 3):15. 71. Vessey MP, et al. *Lancet.* 1975; 1(April 26):941. 72. Casagrande J. et al. *J Natl Cancer Inst.* 1976;56(April):839. 73. Kelsey JL, et al. *Am J Epidemiol.* 1978;107(March):236. 74. Kay CR. *Br Med J.* 1981;282(June 27);2089. 75. Vessey MP, et al. *Br Med J.* 1981;282(June 27):2093. 76. The Cancer and Steroid Hormone Study of the Centers for Disease Control and the National Institute of Child Health and Human Development. Oral contraceptive use and the risk of breast cancer. *N Engl J Med.* 1986;315(Aug 14):405. 77. Paul C, et al. *Br Med J.* 1986:293(Sept 20):723. 78. Miller DR, et al. *Obstet Gynecol.* 1986;68(Dec):863. 79. Pike MC, et al. *Lancet.* 1983;2(Oct 22);926. 80. McPherson K, et al. *Br J Cancer.* 1978:56(Nov):653. 81. Hoover R. et al. *N Engl J Med.* 1976,295(Aug 19):401. 82. Lees AW, et al. *Int J Cancer.* 1978;22(Dec):700. 83. Brinton LA, et al. *J Natl Cancer Inst.* 1979;62(Jan):37. 84. Black MM. *Pathol Res Pract.* 1980;166:491; and *Cancer.* 1980;46(Dec):2747; and *Cancer.* 1983;51(June):2147. 85. Clavel F, et al. *Bull Cancer (Paris).* 1981;68(Dec):449. 86. Brinton LA, et al. *Int J Epidemiol.* 1982;11(Dec):316. 87. Harris NV, et al. *Am J Epidemiol.* 1982;116(Oct):643. 88. Jick H. et al. *Am J Epidemiol.* 1980;112(Nov):577. 89. McPherson K, et al. *Lancet.* 1983;2(Dec 17):1414. 90. Hoover R. et al. *J Natl Cancer Inst.* 1981;67(Oct):815. 91. Jick H, et al. *Am J Epidemiol.* 1980;112(Nov):586. 92. Meirik O, et al. *Lancet.* 1986;2(Sept 20):650. 93. Fasal E, et al. *J Natl Cancer Inst.* 1975;55(Oct):767. 94. Paffenbarger RS, et al. *Cancer.* 1977; 39(April suppl):1887. 95. Stadel BV, et al. *Contraception.* 1988;38(Sept):287. 96. Miller DR, et al. *Am J Epidemiol.* 1989;129(Feb):269. 97. Kay CR, et al. *Br J Cancer.* 1988:58(Nov): 675. 98. Miller DR, et al. *Obstet Gynecol.*1986;68(Dec):863. 99. Olsson H, et al. *Lancet.* 1985;1(March 30):748. 100. Chilvers C, et al. *Lancet.* 1989;1(May 6):973. 101. Huggins GR, et al. *Fertil Steril.* 1987;47(May):733. 102. Pike MC, et al. *Br J Cancer.* 1981;43(Jan):72. 103. Ory H, et al. *Am J Obstet Gynecol.* 1976:124(March 15):573. 104. Stern E, et al. *Science.* 1977;196(June 24):1460. 105. Peritz E, et al. *Am J Epidemiol.* 1977;106(Dec):462. 106. Ory HW, et al. In: Garattini S, Berendes H, eds. *Pharmacology of Steroid Contraceptive Drugs.* New York, NY: Raven Press; 1977:211-224. 107. Meisels A, et al. *Cancer.* 1977;40(Dec):3076. 108. Goldacre MJ, et al. *Br Med J.* 1978;1(March 25):748. 109. Swan SH, et al. *Am J Obstet Gynecol.* 1981;139(Jan 1):52. 110. Vessey MP, et al. *Lancet.* 1983;2(Oct 22):930. 111. Dallenbach-Hellweg G. *Pathol Res Pract.* 1984;179:38. 112. Thomas DB, et al. *Br Med J.* 1985:290(March 30):961. 113. Brinton LA, et al. *Int J Cancer.* 1986;38(Sept):339. 114. Ebeling K, et al. *Int J Cancer.* 1987;39(April):427. 115. Beral V. et al. *Lancet.* 1988;2(Dec 10):1331. 116. Baum JK, et al. *Lancet.* 1973;2(Oct 27):926. 117. Edmondson HA, et al. *N Engl J Med.* 1976;294(Feb 26):470. 118. Bein NN, et al. *Br J Surg.* 1977;64(June):433. 119. Klatskin G. *Gastroenterology,* 1977;73(Aug):386. 120. Rooks JB, et al. *JAMA.* 1979;242(Aug 17):644. 121. Sturtevant FM. In: Moghissi K. ed. *Controversies in Contraception.* Baltimore, MD; Williams & Wilkins; 1979:93-150. 122. Henderson BE, et al. *Br J Cancer.* 1983;48(July):437. 123. Neuberger J, et al. *Br Med J.* 1986;292(May 24):1355. 124. Forman D, et al. *Br Med J.* 1986;292(May 24):1357. 125. La Vecchia C, et al. *Br J Cancer.* 1989;59(March):460. 126. Savolainen E, et al. *Am J Obstet Gynecol.* 1981;140(July 1):521. 127. Ferencz C, et al. *Teratology.* 1980;21(April):225. 128. Rothman KJ, et al. *Am J Epidemiol.* 1979;109(April):433. 129. Harlap S, et al. *Obstet Gynecol.* 1980;55(April):447. 130. Layde PM, et al. *J Epidemiol Community Health.* 1982;36(Dec):274. 131. Rome Group for the Epidemiology and Prevention of Cholelithiasis (GREPCO). *Am J Epidemiol.* 1984;119(May):796. 132. Strom BL, et al. *Clin Pharmacol Ther.* 1986;39(March):335. 133. Wynn V. In: Bardin CE, et al. eds. *Progesterone and Progestins.* New York. NY: Raven Press: 1983:395-410. 134. Perlman JA, et al. *J Chron Dis.* 1985;38(Oct):857. 135. Powell MG, et al. *Obstet Gynecol.* 1984;63(June):764. 136. Wynn V, et al. *Lancet.* 1966:2(Oct 1):720. 137. Fisch IR, et al. *JAMA.* 1977:237(June 6):2499. 138. Kay CR, *Lancet.* 1977;1(March 19):624. 139. Laragh JH. *Am J Obstet Gynecol.* 1976:126(Sept 1):141. 140. Ramcharan S. In: Garattini S. Berendes HW, eds. *Pharmacology of Steroid Contraceptive Drugs.* New York, NY: Raven Pres; 1977:277-288. 141. Laumas KR, et al. *Am J Obstet Gynecol.* 1967;98(June 1):411. 142. Saxena BN, et al. *Contraception.* 1977;16(Dec):605. 143. Nilsson S, et al. *Contraception.* 1978;17(Feb):131. 144. Washington AE, et al. *JAMA.* 1985;253(April 19):2246. 145. Louv WC, et al. *Am J Obstet Gynecol.* 1989;160(Feb):396. 146. Francis WG, et al. *Can Med Assoc J.* 1965;92(Jan 23):191. 147. Verhulst HL, et al. *J Clin Pharmacol.* 1967:7(Jan-Feb):9. 148. Ory HW. *Fam Plann Perspect.* 1982;14(July-Aug):182. 149. Ory HW, et al. *Making Choices: Evaluating the Health Risks and Benefits of Birth Control Methods.* New York, NY: The Alan Guttmacher Institute; 1983. 150. Palmer JR, et al. *Am J Epidemiol.* 1989;130(Nov):878. 151. Romieu I, et al. *J Natl Cancer Inst.* 1989;81(Sept):1313. 152. Porter JB, et al.*Obstet Gynecol.* 1987;70(July):29.

HOW SUPPLIED

TABLETS: 35 MCG-1 MG

BRAND/MANUFACTURER	NDC	SIZE	AWP
○ **BRAND**			
DEMULEN 1/35-21: Searle	00025-0151-07	126s	$139.91
➤ DEMULEN 1/35-28: Searle	00025-0161-09	168s	$141.34
DEMULEN 1/35-21: Searle	00025-0151-24	504s	$531.85
➤ DEMULEN 1/35-28: Searle	00025-0161-24	672s	$537.31

TABLETS: 50 MCG-1 MG

BRAND/MANUFACTURER	NDC	SIZE	AWP
○ **BRAND**			
➤ DEMULEN 1/50-21: Searle	00025-0071-07	126s	$156.02
➤ DEMULEN 1/50-28: Searle	00025-0081-09	168s	$157.46
➤ DEMULEN 1/50-21: Searle	00025-0071-24	504s	$541.63

➤ SHOWN IN PRODUCT IDENTIFICATION GUIDE

BRAND/MANUFACTURER	NDC	SIZE	AWP
▶ DEMULEN 1/50-28: Searle	00025-0081-24	672s	$546.86

Ethinyl Estradiol with Levonorgestrel

Patients should be counseled that this product does not protect against HIV infection (AIDS) and other sexually transmitted diseases.

DESCRIPTION

ETHINYL ESTRADIOL/LEVONORGESTREL—
TRIPHASIC REGIMEN 21 TABLETS
Each cycle of Ethinyl Estradiol/Levonorgestrel—Triphasic Regimen 21 tablets consists of three different drug phases as follows: Phase 1 comprised of 6 brown tablets, each containing 0.050 mg of Levonorgestrel ($\underline{d}$(-)-13 beta-ethyl-17-alpha-Ethinyl-17-beta-hydroxygon-4-en-3-one), a totally synthetic progestogen, and 0.030 mg of Ethinyl Estradiol (19-nor-17 α-pregna-1,3,5(10)-trien-20-yne-3,17-diol); phase 2 comprised of 5 white tablets, each containing 0.075 mg Levonorgestrel and 0.40 mg Ethinyl Estradiol; and, phase 3 comprised of 10 light yellow tablets, each containing 0.125 mg Levonorgestrel and 0.030 mg Ethinyl Estradiol.

ETHINYL ESTRADIOL/LEVONORGESTREL—
TRIPHASIC REGIMEN 28 TABLETS
Each cycle of Ethinyl Estradiol/Levonorgestrel—Triphasic Regimen tablets consists of three different drug phases as follows: Phase 1 comprised of 6 brown tablets, each containing 0.050 mg of Levonorgestrel ($\underline{d}$(-)-13 beta-ethyl-17-alpha-Ethinyl-17-beta-hydroxygon-4-en-3-one), a totally synthetic progestogen, and 0.030 mg of Ethinyl Estradiol (19-nor-17 α-pregna-1,3,5(10)-trien-20-yne-3, 17-diol); phase 2 comprised of 5 white tablets, each containing 0.075 mg Levonorgestrel and 0.040 mg Ethinyl Estradiol; and phase 3 comprised of 10 light yellow tablets, each containing 0.125 mg Levonorgestrel and 0.030 mg Ethinyl Estradiol; then followed by 7 light-green inert tablets.

ETHINYL ESTRADIOL/LEVONORGESTREL 21 TABLETS
Each Ethinyl Estradiol/Levonorgestrel 21 tablet contains 0.15 mg of Levonorgestrel ($\underline{d}$(-)-13 beta-ethyl-17-alpha-Ethinyl-17-beta-hydroxygon-4-en-3-one), a totally synthetic progestogen, and 0.03 mg of Ethinyl Estradiol (19-nor-17 α-pregna-1,3,5(10)-trien-20-yne-3, 17-diol).

ETHINYL ESTRADIOL/LEVONORGESTREL 28 TABLETS
21 Ethinyl Estradiol/Levonorgestrel tablets light orange, each containing 0.15 mg of Levonorgestrel ($\underline{d}$(-)-13 beta-ethyl-17-alpha-Ethinyl-17-beta-hydroxygon-4-en-3-one), a totally synthetic progestogen, and 0.03 mg of Ethinyl Estradiol (19-nor-17 α-pregna-1,3,5(10)-trien-20-yne-3, 17-diol), and 7 inert tablets.

CLINICAL PHARMACOLOGY

Combination oral contraceptives act by suppression of gonadotropins. Although the primary mechanism of this action is inhibition of ovulation, other alterations include changes in the cervical mucus (which increase the difficulty of sperm entry into the uterus) and the endometrium (which reduce the likelihood of implantation).

INDICATIONS AND USAGE

Oral contraceptives are indicated for the prevention of pregnancy in women who elect to use this product as a method of contraception.

Oral contraceptives are highly effective. Table I lists the typical accidental pregnancy rates for users of combination oral contraceptives and other methods of contraception. The efficacy of these contraceptive methods, except sterilization and the IUD, depends upon the reliability with which they are used. Correct and consistent use of methods can result in lower failure rates.

Table 1
LOWEST EXPECTED AND TYPICAL FAILURE RATES DURING THE FIRST YEAR OF CONTINUOUS USE OF A METHOD

% of Women Experiencing an Accidental Pregnancy in the First Year of Continuous Use

Method	Lowest Expected*	Typical**
(No Contraception)	(89)	(89)
Oral contraceptives		
combined	0.1	3
progestin only	0.5	N/A***
Diaphragm with spermicidal cream or jelly	3	18
Spermicides alone (foam, creams, jellies and vaginal suppositories)	3	21
Vaginal Sponge		
nulliparous	5	18
multiparous	> 8	> 28
IUD (medicated)	1	6#

% of Women Experiencing an Accidental Pregnancy in the First Year of Continuous Use

Method	Lowest Expected*	Typical**
Condom without spermicides	2	12
Periodic abstinence (all methods)	2-10	20
Female sterilization	0.2	0.4
Male sterilization	0.1	0.15

Adapted from J. Trussell and K. Kost. Table II, Studies in Family Planning, 18(5), Sept.-Oct. 1987.
* The authors' best guess of the percentage of women expected to experience an accidental pregnancy among couples who initiate a method (not necessarily for the first time) and who use it consistently and correctly during the first year if they do not stop for any other reason.
** This term represents "typical" couples who initiate use of a method (not necessarily for the first time), who experience an accidental pregnancy during the first year if they do not stop use for any other reason.
*** N/A — Data not available.
# Combined typical rate for both medicated and nonmedicated IUD. The rate for medicated IUD alone is not available.

CONTRAINDICATIONS

Oral contraceptives should not be used in women with any of the following conditions:
Thrombophlebitis or thromboembolic disorders.
A past history of deep-vein thrombophlebitis or thromboembolic disorders.
Cerebral-vascular or coronary-artery disease.
Known or suspected carcinoma of the breast.
Carcinoma of the endometrium or other known or suspected estrogen-dependent neoplasia.
Undiagnosed abnormal genital bleeding.
Cholestatic jaundice of pregnancy or jaundice with prior pill use.
Hepatic adenomas or carcinomas.
Known or suspected pregnancy.

WARNINGS

CIGARETTE SMOKING INCREASES THE RISK OF SERIOUS CARDIOVASCULAR SIDE EFFECTS FROM ORAL-CONTRACEPTIVE USE. THIS RISK INCREASES WITH AGE AND WITH HEAVY SMOKING (15 OR MORE CIGARETTES PER DAY) AND IS QUITE MARKED IN WOMEN OVER 35 YEARS OF AGE. WOMEN WHO USE ORAL CONTRACEPTIVES SHOULD BE STRONGLY ADVISED NOT TO SMOKE.

The use of oral contraceptives is associated with increased risks of several serious conditions including myocardial infarction, thromboembolism, stroke, hepatic neopiasia, gall-bladder disease, and hypertension, although the risk of serious morbidity or mortality is very small in healthy women without underlying risk factors. The risk of morbidity and mortality increases significantly in the presence of other underlying risk factors such as hypertension, hyperlipidemias, obesity and diabetes.

Practitioners prescribing oral contraceptives should be familiar with the following information relating to these risks. The information contained here is based principally on studies carried out in patients who used oral contraceptives with higher formulations of estrogens and progestogens than those in common use today. The effect of long-term use of the oral contraceptives with lower formulations of both estrogens and progestogens remains to be determined.

Throughout this prescribing information, epidemiological studies reported are of two types: retrospective or case control studies and prospective or cohort studies. Case control studies provide a measure of the relative risk of disease, namely, a ratio of the incidence of a disease among oral-contraceptive users to that among nonusers. The relative risk does not provide information on the actual clinical occurrence of a disease. Cohort studies provide a measure of attributable risk, which is the difference in the incidence of disease between oral-contraceptive users and nonusers. The attributable risk does provide information about the actual occurrence of a disease in the population. For further information, the reader is referred to a text on epidemiological methods.

1. THROMBOEMBOLIC DISORDERS AND OTHER VASCULAR PROBLEMS

a. Myocardial Infarction: An increased risk of myocardial infarction has been attributed to oral-contraceptive use. This risk is primarily in smokers or women with other underlying risk factors for coronary-artery disease such as hypertension, hypercholesterolemia, morbid obesity, and diabetes. The relative risk of heart attack for current oral-contraceptive users has been estimated to be two to six. The risk is very low under the age of 30.

Smoking in combination with oral-contraceptive use has been shown to contribute substantially to the incidence of myocardial infarctions in women in their mid-thirties or older with smoking accounting for the majority of excess cases. Mortality rates associated with circulatory disease have been shown to increase substantially in smokers over the age of 35 and nonsmokers over the age of 40 (Table 2) among women who use oral contraceptives.

◆ RATED THERAPEUTICALLY EQUIVALENT; ◇ THERAPEUTIC EQUIVALENCE UNCONFIRMED; ○ UNRATED

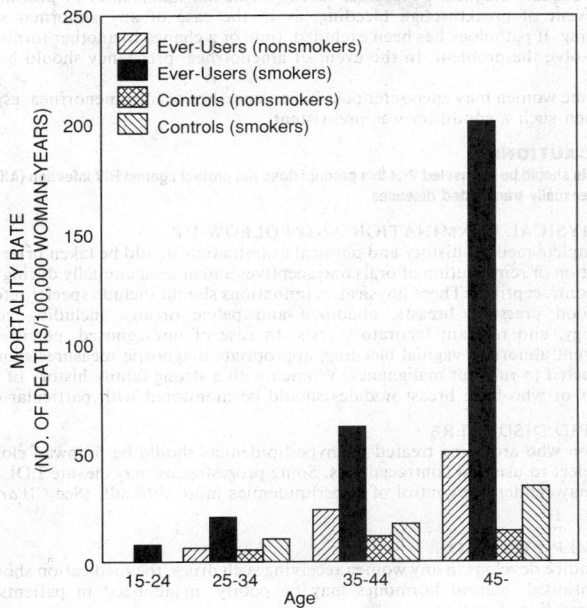

CIRCULATORY DISEASE MORTALITY RATES PER 100,000
WOMAN-YEARS BY AGE, SMOKING STATUS
AND ORAL CONTRACEPTIVE USE

Legend:
- Ever-Users (nonsmokers)
- Ever-Users (smokers)
- Controls (nonsmokers)
- Controls (smokers)

Y-axis: MORTALITY RATE (NO. OF DEATHS/100,000 WOMAN-YEARS)
X-axis: Age — 15-24, 25-34, 35-44, 45-

Oral contraceptives may compound the effects of well-known risk factors, such as hypertension, diabetes, hyperlipidemias, age and obesity. In particular, some progestogens are known to decrease HDL cholesterol and cause glucose intolerance, while estrogens may create a state of hyperinsulinism. Oral contraceptives have been shown to increase blood pressure among users (see section 9 in "Warnings"). Similar effects on risk factors have been associated with an increased risk of heart disease. Oral contraceptives must be used with caution in women with cardiovascular disease risk factors.

b. Thromboembolism: An increased risk of thromboembolic and thrombotic disease associated with the use of oral contraceptives is well established. Case control studies have found the relative risk of users compared to nonusers to be 3 for the first episode of superficial venous thrombosis, 4 to 11 for deep vein thrombosis or pulmonary embolism, and 1.5 to 6 for women with predisposing conditions for venous thromboembolic disease. Cohort studies have shown the relative risk to be somewhat lower, about 3 for new cases and about 4.5 for new cases requiring hospitalization. The risk of thromboembolic disease due to oral contraceptives is not related to length of use and disappears after pill use is stopped.

A two- to four-fold increase in relative risk of postoperative thromboembolic complications has been reported with the use of oral contraceptives. The relative risk of venous thrombosis in women who have predisposing conditions is twice that of women without such medical conditions. If feasible, oral contraceptives should be discontinued at least four weeks prior to and for two weeks after elective surgery of a type associated with an increase in risk of thromboembolism and during and following prolonged immobilization. Since the immediate post partum period is also associated with an increased risk of thromboembolism, oral contraceptives should be started no earlier than four to six weeks after delivery in women who elect not to breast-feed, or a midtrimester pregnancy termination.

c. Cerebrovascular Diseases: Oral contraceptives have been shown to increase both the relative and attributable risks of cerebrovascular events (thrombotic and hemorrhagic strokes), although, in general, the risk is greatest among older (> 35 years), hypertensive women who also smoke. Hypertension was found to be a risk factor for both users and nonusers, for both types of strokes, while smoking interacted to increase the risk for hemorrhagic strokes.

In a large study, the relative risk of thrombotic strokes has been shown to range from 3 for normotensive users to 14 for users with severe hypertension. The relative risk of hemorrhagic stroke is reported to be 1.2 for nonsmokers who used oral contraceptives, 2.6 for smokers who did not use oral contraceptives, 7.6 for smokers who used oral contraceptives, 1.8 for normotensive users and 25.7 for users with severe hypertension. The attributable risk is also greater in older women.

d. Dose-related Risk of Vascular Disease from Oral Contraceptives: A positive association has been observed between the amount of estrogen and progestogen in oral contraceptives and the risk of vascular disease. A decline in serum high-density lipoproteins (HDL) has been reported with many progestational agents. A decline in serum high-density lipoproteins has been associated with an increased incidence of ischemic heart disease. Because estrogens increase HDL cholesterol, the net effect of an oral contraceptive depends on a balance achieved between

doses of estrogen and progestogen and the nature and absolute amount of progestogen used in the contraceptive. The amount of both hormones should be considered in the choice of an oral contraceptive.

Minimizing exposure to estrogen and progestogen is in keeping with good principles of therapeutics. For any particular estrogen/progestogen combination, the dosage regimen prescribed should be one which contains the least amount of estrogen and progestogen that is compatible with a low failure rate and the needs of the individual patient. New acceptors of oral-contraceptive agents should be started on preparations containing less than 50 mcg of estrogen.

e. Persistence of Risk of Vascular Disease: There are two studies which have shown persistence of risk of vascular disease for ever-users of oral contraceptives. In a study in the United States, the risk of developing myocardial infarction after discontinuing oral contraceptives persists for at least 9 years for women 40-49 years who had used oral contraceptives for five or more years, but this increased risk was not demonstrated in other age groups. In another study in Great Britain, the risk of developing cerebrovascular disease persisted for at least 6 years after discontinuation of oral contraceptives, although excess risk was very small. However, both studies were performed with oral contraceptive formulations containing 50 micrograms or higher of estrogens.

2. ESTIMATES OF MORTALITY FROM CONTRACEPTIVE USE
One study gathered data from a variety of sources which have estimated the mortality rate associated with different methods of contraception at different ages (Table 3). These estimates include the combined risk of death associated with contraceptive methods plus the risk attributable to pregnancy in the event of method failure. Each method of contraception has its specific benefits and risks. The study concluded that with the exception of oral-contraceptive users 35 and older who smoke and 40 and older who do not smoke, mortality associated with all methods of birth control is less than that associated with childbirth. The observation of a possible increase in risk of mortality with age for oral-contraceptive users is based on data gathered in the 1970s—but not reported until 1983. However, current clinical practice involves the use of lower estrogen dose formulations combined with careful restriction of oral-contraceptive use to women who do not have the various risk factors listed in this prescribing information.

Because of these changes in practice and, also, because of some limited new data which suggest that the risk of cardiovascular disease with the use of oral contraceptives may now be less than previously observed, the Fertility and Maternal Health Drugs Advisory Committee was asked to review the topic in 1989. The Committee concluded that although cardiovascular disease risks may be increased with oral-contraceptive use after age 40 in healthy nonsmoking women (even with the newer low-dose formulations), there are greater potential health risks associated with pregnancy in older women and with the alternative surgical and medical procedures which may be necessary if such women do not have access to effective and acceptable means of contraception.

Therefore, the Committee recommended that the benefits of oral-contraceptive use by healthy nonsmoking women over 40 may outweigh the possible risks. Of course, older women, as all women who take oral contraceptives, should take the lowest possible dose formulation that is effective.

Table 3
ANNUAL NUMBER OF BIRTH-RELATED OR METHOD-RELATED DEATHS ASSOCIATED WITH CONTROL OF FERTILITY PER 100,000 NONSTERILE WOMEN, BY FERTILITY-CONTROL METHOD ACCORDING TO AGE

Method of control and outcome	15-19	20-24	25-29	30-34	35-39	40-44
No fertility control methods*	7.0	7.4	9.1	14.8	25.7	28.2
Oral contraceptives nonsmoker**	0.3	0.5	0.9	1.9	13.8	31.6
Oral contraceptives smoker**	2.2	3.4	6.6	13.5	51.1	117.2
IUD**	0.8	0.8	1.0	1.0	1.4	1.4
Condom*	1.1	1.6	0.7	0.2	0.3	0.4
Diaphragm/ spermicide*	1.9	1.2	1.2	1.3	2.2	2.8
Periodic abstinence*	2.5	1.6	1.6	1.7	2.9	3.6

* Deaths are birth related
** Deaths are method related
Adapted from H.W. Ory, Family Planning Perspectives 15:57-63, 1983.

3. CARCINOMA OF THE REPRODUCTIVE ORGANS
Numerous epidemiological studies have been performed on the incidence of breast, endometrial, ovarian and cervical cancer in women using oral contraceptives. The overwhelming evidence in the literature suggests that use of oral contraceptives is not associated with an increase in the risk of developing breast cancer, regardless of the age and parity of first use or with most of the marketed brands and doses. The Cancer and Steroid Hormone (CASH) study also showed no latent effect on the risk of breast cancer for at least a decade following long-term use. A few studies have shown a slightly increased relative risk of developing

breast cancer, although the methodology of these studies, which included differences in examination of users and nonusers and differences in age at start of use, has been questioned.

Some studies suggest that oral-contraceptive use has been associated with an increase in the risk of cervical intraepithelial neoplasia in some populations of women. However, there continues to be controversy about the extent to which such findings may be due to differences in sexual behavior and other factors.

In spite of many studies of the relationship between oral-contraceptive use and breast and cervical cancers, a cause-and-effect relationship has not been established.

4. HEPATIC NEOPLASIA
Benign hepatic adenomas are associated with oral-contraceptive use, although the incidence of benign tumors is rare in the United States. Indirect calculations have estimated the attributable risk to be in the range of 3.3 cases/100,000 for users, a risk that increases after four or more years of use. Rupture of rare, benign, hepatic adenomas may cause death through intra-abdominal hemorrhage.

Studies from Britain have shown an increased risk of developing hepatocellular carcinoma in long-term (> 8 years) oral-contraceptive users. However, these cancers are extremely rare in the U.S. and the attributable risk (the excess incidence) of liver cancers in oral-contraceptive users approaches less than one per million users.

5. OCULAR LESIONS
There have been clinical case reports of retinal thrombosis associated with the use of oral contraceptives. Oral contraceptives should be discontinued if there is unexplained partial or complete loss of vision; onset of proptosis or diplopia; papilledema; or retinal vascular lesions. Appropriate diagnostic and therapeutic measures should be undertaken immediately.

6. ORAL-CONTRACEPTIVE USE BEFORE OR DURING EARLY PREGNANCY
Extensive epidemiological studies have revealed no increased risk of birth defects in women who have used oral contraceptives prior to pregnancy. Studies also do not suggest a teratogenic effect, particularly insofar as cardiac anomalies and limb-reduction defects are concerned, when taken inadvertently during early pregnancy.

The administration of oral contraceptives to induce withdrawal bleeding should not be used as a test for pregnancy. Oral contraceptives should not be used during pregnancy to treat threatened or habitual abortion.

It is recommended that for any patient who has missed two consecutive periods, pregnancy should be ruled out before continuing oral-contraceptive use. If the patient has not adhered to the prescribed schedule, the possibility of pregnancy should be considered at the time of the first missed period. Oral-contraceptive use should be discontinued if pregnancy is confirmed.

7. GALLBLADDER DISEASE
Earlier studies have reported an increased lifetime relative risk of gallbladder surgery in users of oral contraceptives and estrogens. More recent studies, however, have shown that the relative risk of developing gallbladder disease among oral-contraceptive users may be minimal. The recent findings of minimal risk may be related to the use of oral-contraceptive formulations containing lower hormonal doses of estrogens and progestogens.

8. CARBOHYDRATE AND LIPID METABOLIC EFFECTS
Oral contraceptives have been shown to cause glucose intolerance in a significant percentage of users. Oral contraceptives containing greater than 75 micrograms of estrogens cause hyperinsulinism, while lower doses of estrogen cause less glucose intolerance. Progestogens increase insulin secretion and create insulin resistance, this effect varying with different progestational agents. However, in the nondiabetic woman, oral contraceptives appear to have no effect on fasting blood glucose. Because of these demonstrated effects, prediabetic and diabetic women should be carefully observed while taking oral contraceptives.

A small proportion of women will have persistent hypertriglyceridemia while on the pill. As discussed earlier (see "Warnings, 1a. and 1d."), changes in serum triglycerides and lipoprotein levels have been reported in oral-contraceptive users.

9. ELEVATED BLOOD PRESSURE
An increase in blood pressure has been reported in women taking oral contraceptives and this increase is more likely in older oral-contraceptives users and with continued use. Data from the Royal College of General Practitioners and subsequent randomized trials have shown that the incidence of hypertension increases with increasing quantities of progestogens.

Women with a history of hypertension or hypertension-related diseases, or renal disease should be encouraged to use another method of contraception. If women with hypertension elect to use oral contraceptives, they should be monitored closely, and if significant elevation of blood pressure occurs, oral contraceptives should be discontinued. For most women, elevated blood pressure will return to normal after stopping oral contraceptives, and there is no difference in the occurrence of hypertension among ever- and never-users.

10. HEADACHE
The onset of exacerbation of migraine or development of headache with a new pattern that is recurrent, persistent, or severe requires discontinuation of oral contraceptives and evaluation of the cause.

11. BLEEDING IRREGULARITIES
Breakthrough bleeding and spotting are sometimes encountered in patients on oral contraceptives, especially during the first three months of use. The type and dose of progestogen may be important. Nonhormonal causes should be considered and adequate diagnostic measures taken to rule out malignancy or pregnancy in the event of breakthrough bleeding, as in the case of any abnormal vaginal bleeding. If pathology has been excluded, time or a change to another formulation may solve the problem. In the event of amenorrhea, pregnancy should be ruled out.

Some women may encounter post-pill amenorrhea or oligomenorrhea, especially when such a condition was preexistent.

PRECAUTIONS
Patients should be counseled that this product does not protect against HIV infection (AIDS) and other sexually transmitted diseases.

1. PHYSICAL EXAMINATION AND FOLLOW-UP
A complete medical history and physical examination should be taken prior to the initiation or reinstitution of oral contraceptives and at least annually during use of oral contraceptives. These physical examinations should include special reference to blood pressure, breasts, abdomen and pelvic organs, including cervical cytology, and relevant laboratory tests. In case of undiagnosed, persistent, or recurrent abnormal vaginal bleeding, appropriate diagnostic measures should be conducted to rule out malignancy. Women with a strong family history of breast cancer or who have breast nodules should be monitored with particular care.

2. LIPID DISORDERS
Women who are being treated for hyperlipidemias should be followed closely if they elect to use oral contraceptives. Some progestogens may elevate LDL levels and may render the control of hyperlipidemias more difficult. (See "Warnings, 1d.")

3. LIVER FUNCTION
If jaundice develops in any women receiving such drugs, the medication should be discontinued. Steroid hormones may be poorly metabolized in patients with impaired liver function.

4. FLUID RETENTION
Oral contraceptives may cause some degree of fluid retention. They should be prescribed with caution, and only with careful monitoring, in patients with conditions which might be aggravated by fluid retention.

5. EMOTIONAL DISORDERS
Patients becoming significantly depressed while taking oral contraceptives should stop the medication and use an alternate method of contraception in an attempt to determine whether the symptom is drug related. Women with a history of depression should be carefully observed and the drug discontinued if depression recurs to a serious degree.

6. CONTACT LENSES
Contact-lens wearers who develop visual changes or changes in lens tolerance should be assessed by an ophthalmologist.

7. DRUG INTERACTIONS
Reduced efficacy and increased incidence of breakthrough bleeding and menstrual irregularities have been associated with concomitant use of rifampin. A similar association, though less marked, has been suggested with barbiturates, phenylbutazone, phenytoin sodium, and possibly with griseofulvin, ampicillin, and tetracyclines.

8. INTERACTIONS WITH LABORATORY TESTS
Certain endocrine and liver-function tests and blood components may be affected by oral contraceptives:

a. Increased prothrombin and factors VII, VIII, IX, and X; decreased antithrombin 3; increased norepinephrine-induced platelet aggregability.

b. Increased thyroid-binding globulin (TBG) leading to increased circulating total thyroid hormone, as measured by protein-bound iodine (PBI), T4 by column or by radioimmunoassay. Free T3 resin uptake is decreased, reflecting the elevated TBG; free T4 concentration is unaltered.

c. Other binding proteins may be elevated in serum.

d. Sex-binding globulins are increased and result in elevated levels of total circulating sex steroids and corticoids; however, free or biologically active levels remain unchanged.

e. Triglycerides may be increased.

f. Glucose tolerance may be decreased.

g. Serum folate levels may be depressed by oral-contraceptive therapy. This may be of clinical significance if a woman becomes pregnant shortly after discontinuing oral contraceptives.

9. CARCINOGENESIS
See "Warnings" section.

10. PREGNANCY
Pregnancy Category X. See "Contraindications" and "Warnings" sections.

11. NURSING MOTHERS
Small amounts of oral-contraceptive steroids have been identified in the milk of nursing mothers and a few adverse effects on the child have been reported, including jaundice and breast enlargement. In addition, oral contraceptives given

in the postpartum period may interfere with lactation by decreasing the quantity and quality of breast milk. If possible, the nursing mother should be advised not to use oral contraceptives but to use other forms of contraception until she has completely weaned her child.

INFORMATION FOR THE PATIENT
See manufacturer's patient information.

ADVERSE REACTIONS
An increased risk of the following serious adverse reactions has been associated with the use of oral contraceptives (see *"Warnings"* section).

Thrombophlebitis
Arterial thromboembolism
Pulmonary embolism
Myocardial infarction
Cerebral hemorrhage
Cerebral thrombosis
Hypertension
Gallbladder disease
Hepatic adenomas or benign liver tumors

There is evidence of an association between the following conditions and the use of oral contraceptives, although additional confirmatory studies are needed:
Mesenteric thrombosis
Retinal thrombosis

The following adverse reactions have been reported in patients receiving oral contraceptives and are believed to be drug related:
Nausea
Vomiting
Gastrointestinal symptoms (such as abdominal cramps and bloating)
Breakthrough bleeding
Spotting
Change in menstrual flow
Amenorrhea
Temporary infertility after discontinuation of treatment
Edema
Melasma which may persist
Breast changes: tenderness, enlargement, and secretion
Change in weight (increase or decrease)
Change in cervical erosion and cervical secretion
Diminution in lactation when given immediately postpartum
Cholestatic jaundice
Migraine
Rash (allergic)
Mental depression
Reduced tolerance to carbohydrates
Vaginal candidiasis
Change in corneal curvature (steepening)
Intolerance to contact lenses

The following adverse reactions have been reported in users of oral contraceptives and the association has been neither confirmed nor refuted:
Congenital anomalies
Premenstrual syndrome
Cataracts
Optic neuritis
Changes in appetite
Cystitis-like syndrome
Headache
Nervousness
Dizziness
Hirsutism
Loss of scalp hair
Erythema multiforme
Cerebral-vascular disease with mitral valve prolapse
Lupus-like Syndromes
Erythema nodosum
Hemorrhagic eruption
Vaginitis
Porphyria
Impaired renal function
Hemolytic uremic syndrome
Budd-Chiari syndrome
Acne
Changes in libido
Colitis
Sickle-Cell Disease

OVERDOSAGE
Serious ill effects have not been reported following acute ingestion of large doses of oral contraceptives by young children. Overdosage may cause nausea, and withdrawal bleeding may occur in females.

NONCONTRACEPTIVE HEALTH BENEFITS
The following noncontraceptive health benefits related to the use of combination oral contraceptives are supported by epidemiological studies which largely

utilized oral-contraceptive formulations containing doses exceeding 0.035 mg of Ethinyl Estradiol or 0.05 mg of mestranol.

Effects on menses:
increased menstrual cycle regularity
decreased blood loss and decreased incidence of iron deficiency anemia
decreased incidence of dysmenorrhea

Effects related to inhibition of ovulation:
decreased incidence of functional ovarian cysts
decreased incidence of ectopic pregnancies

Effects from long-term use:
decreased incidence of fibroadenomas and fibrocystic disease of the breast
decreased incidence of acute pelvic inflammatory disease
decreased incidence of endometrial cancer
decreased incidence of ovarian cancer

DOSAGE AND ADMINISTRATION
ETHINYL ESTRADIOL/LEVONORGESTREL—
TRIPHASIC REGIMEN 21 TABLETS
To achieve maximum contraceptive effectiveness, Ethinyl Estradiol/Levonorgestrel—Triphasic Regimen 21 Tablets must be taken exactly as directed and at intervals not exceeding 24 hours.

Ethinyl Estradiol/Levonorgestrel—Triphasic Regimen 21 Tablets are a three-phase preparation. The dosage of Ethinyl Estradiol/Levonorgestrel—Triphasic Regimen 21 Tablets is *one tablet* daily for 21 consecutive days per menstrual cycle in the following order: 6 brown tablets (phase 1), followed by 5 white tablets (phase 2), and then followed by the last 10 light-yellow tablets (phase 3), according to the prescribed schedule. Tablets are then discontinued for 7 days (three weeks on, one week off).

It is recommended that Ethinyl Estradiol/Levonorgestrel—Triphasic Regimen 21 Tablets be taken at the same time each day, preferably after the evening meal or at bedtime. During the first cycle of medication, the patient should be instructed to take one Ethinyl Estradiol/Levonorgestrel—Triphasic Regimen 21 Tablet daily in the order of 6 brown, 5 white and, finally, 10 light-yellow tablets for twenty-one (21) consecutive days, beginning on day one (1) of her menstrual cycle. (The first day of menstruation is day one.) The tablets are then discontinued for one week (7 days). Withdrawal bleeding usually occurs within 3 days following discontinuation of Ethinyl Estradiol/Levonorgestrel—Triphasic Regimen 21 Tablets. (If an alternate starting regimen is used [Sunday Start or postpartum], contraceptive reliance should not be placed on Ethinyl Estradiol/Levonorgestrel—Triphasic Regimen 21 Tablets until after the first 7 consecutive days of administration. The possibility of ovulation and conception prior to initiation of medication should be considered.)

The patient begins her next and all subsequent 21-day courses of Ethinyl Estradiol/Levonorgestrel—Triphasic Regimen 21 Tablets on the same day of the week that she began her first course, following the same schedule: 21 days on—7 days off. She begins taking her brown tablets on the 8th day after discontinuance, regardless of whether or not a menstrual period has occurred or is still in progress. Any time the next cycle of Ethinyl Estradiol/Levonorgestrel—Triphasic Regimen 21 Tablets is started later than the 8th day, the patient should be protected by another means of contraception until she has taken a tablet daily for seven consecutive days.

If spotting or breakthrough bleeding occurs, the patient is instructed to continue on the same regimen. This type of bleeding is usually transient and without significance; however, if the bleeding is persistent or prolonged, the patient is advised to consult her physician. Although the occurrence of pregnancy is highly unlikely if Ethinyl Estradiol/Levonorgestrel—Triphasic Regimen 21 Tablets are taken according to directions, if withdrawal bleeding does not occur, the possibility of pregnancy must be considered. If the patient has not adhered to the prescribed schedule (missed one or more tablets or started taking them on a day later than she should have), the probability of pregnancy should be considered at the time of the first missed period and appropriate diagnostic measures taken before the medication is resumed. If the patient has adhered to the prescribed regimen and misses two consecutive periods, pregnancy should be ruled out before continuing the contraceptive regimen.

The risk of pregnancy increases with each tablet missed. If the patient misses one tablet, she should be instructed to take it as soon as she remembers and also to take her next two tablets on that day. If she misses two active tablets consecutively, she should take the second missed tablet as soon as she remembers, discard the first missed tablet and take her regular tablet for that day at the proper time. Furthermore, she should use an additional method of birth control until menses has appeared or pregnancy has been excluded. If breakthrough bleeding occurs following missed tablets, it will usually be transient and of no consequence. If three consecutive tablets are missed, all medication should be discontinued and the remainder of the package discarded. A new package should be started on the first day of the patient's next bleed after the last tablet was taken. An alternative means of birth control should be prescribed during the days without tablets and continued until the patient has taken a tablet daily for seven consecutive days (six brown, and one white).

In the nonlactating mother, Ethinyl Estradiol/Levonorgestrel—Triphasic Regimen 21 Tablets may be initiated postpartum, for contraception. When the tablets are administered in the postpartum period, the increased risk of thromboembolic disease associated with the postpartum period must be considered. (See *"Contraindications"*, *"Warnings"*, and *"Precautions"* concerning thromboembolic disease.) It is to be noted that early resumption of ovulation may occur if bromocriptine mesylate has been used for the prevention of lactation.

► SHOWN IN PRODUCT IDENTIFICATION GUIDE

ETHINYL ESTRADIOL/LEVONORGESTREL—TRIPHASIC REGIMEN 28 TABLETS

To achieve maximum contraceptive effectiveness. Ethinyl Estradiol/Levonorgestrel—Triphasic Regimen 28 Tablets must be taken exactly as directed and at intervals not exceeding 24 hours.

Ethinyl Estradiol/Levonorgestrel—Triphasic Regimen 28 Tablets are a three-phase preparation plus 7 inert tablets. The dosage of Ethinyl Estradiol/Levonorgestrel—Triphasic Regimen 28 Tablets is one tablet daily for 28 consecutive days per menstrual cycle in the following order: 6 brown tablets (phase 1), followed by 5 white tablets (phase 2), followed by 10 light-yellow tablets (phase 3), plus 7 light-green inert tablets according to the prescribed schedule.

It is recommended that Ethinyl Estradiol/Levonorgestrel—Triphasic Regimen 28 Tablets be taken at the same time each day, preferably after the evening meal or at bedtime. During the first cycle of medication, the patient should be instructed to take one Ethinyl Estradiol/Levonorgestrel—Triphasic Regimen 28 Tablet daily in the order of 6 brown, 5 white, 10 light-yellow tablets and then 7 light-green inert tablets for twenty-eight (28) consecutive days, beginning on day one (1) of her menstrual cycle. (The first day of menstruation is day one.) Withdrawal bleeding usually occurs within 3 days following the last light-yellow tablet. (If an alternate starting regimen is used [Sunday Start or postpartum], contraceptive reliance should not be placed on Ethinyl Estradiol/Levonorgestrel—Triphasic Regimen 28 Tablets until after the first 7 consecutive days of administration. The possibility of ovulation and conception prior to initiation of medication should be considered.)

The patient begins her next and all subsequent 28-day courses of Ethinyl Estradiol/Levonorgestrel—Triphasic Regimen 28 Tablets on the same day of the week that she began her first course, following the same schedule. She begins taking her brown tablets on the next day after ingestion of the last light-green tablet, regardless of whether or not a menstrual period has occurred or is still in progress. Any time a subsequent cycle of Ethinyl Estradiol/Levonorgestrel—Triphasic Regimen 28 Tablets is started later than the next day, the patient should be protected by another means of contraceptive until she has taken a tablet daily for seven consecutive days.

If spotting or breakthrough bleeding occurs, the patient is instructed to continue on the same regimen. This type of bleeding is usually transient and without significance; however, if the bleeding is persistent or prolonged, the patient is advised to consult her physician. Although the occurrence of pregnancy is highly unlikely if Ethinyl Estradiol/Levonorgestrel—Triphasic Regimen 28 Tablets are taken according to directions, if withdrawal bleeding does not occur, the possibility of pregnancy must be considered. If the patient has not adhered to the prescribed schedule (missed one or more active tablets or started taking them on a day later than she should have), the probability of pregnancy should be considered at the time of the first missed period and appropriate diagnostic measures taken before the medication is resumed. If the patient has adhered to the prescribed regimen and misses two consecutive periods, pregnancy should be ruled out before continuing the contraceptive regimen.

The risk of pregnancy increases with each active (brown, white, or light-yellow) tablet missed. If the patient misses one active tablet, she should be instructed to take it as soon as she remembers, and also to take her next tablet at the regular time, which means that she will be taking two tablets on that day. If she misses two active tablets consecutively, she should take the second missed tablet as soon as she remembers, discard the first missed tablet and take her regular tablet for that day at the proper time. Furthermore, she should use an additional method of birth control in addition to taking Ethinyl Estradiol/Levonorgestrel—Triphasic Regimen 28 Tablets until menses has appeared or pregnancy has been excluded. If breakthrough bleeding occurs following missed active tablets, it will usually be transient and of no consequence. If three consecutive active tablets are missed, all medication should be discontinued and the remainder of the package discarded. A new package of Ethinyl Estradiol/Levonorgestrel—Triphasic Regimen 28 Tablets should be started on the first day of the patient's next bleed after the last tablet was taken. An alternate means of birth control should be prescribed during the days without tablets and continued until the patient has taken a tablet daily for seven consecutive days (six brown, and one white).

In the nonlactating mother, Ethinyl Estradiol/Levonorgestrel—Triphasic Regimen 28 Tablets may be initiated postpartum, for contraception. When the tablets are administered in the postpartum period, the increased risk of thromboembolic disease associated with the postpartum period must be considered. (see *"Contraindications"*, *"Warnings"*, and *"Precautions"* concerning thromboembolic disease.) It is to be noted that early resumption of ovulation may occur if bromocriptine mesylate has been used for the prevention of lactation.

ETHINYL ESTRADIOL/LEVONORGESTREL 21 TABLETS

To achieve maximum contraceptive effectiveness, Ethinyl Estradiol/Levonorgestrel 21 Tablets must be taken exactly as directed and at intervals not exceeding 24-hours.

The dosage of Ethinyl Estradiol/Levonorgestrel 21 Tablets is *one tablet* daily for 21 consecutive days per menstrual cycle according to the prescribed schedule. Tablets are then discontinued for 7 days (three weeks on, one week off).

It is recommended that Ethinyl Estradiol/Levonorgestrel 21 Tablets be taken at the same time each day, preferably after the evening meal or at bedtime. During the first cycle of medication, the patient should be instructed to take one Ethinyl Estradiol/Levonorgestrel 21 Tablet daily for twenty-one (21) consecutive days, beginning on day one (1), or day five for some brands, of her menstrual cycle. (The first day of menstruation is day one.) The tablets are then discontinued for one week (7 days). Withdrawal bleeding usually occurs within 3 days following discontinuation of Ethinyl Estradiol/Levonorgestrel 21 Tablets. (If an alternate starting regimen is used [Sunday Start or postpartum], contraceptive reliance should not be placed on Ethinyl Estradiol/Levonorgestrel 21 Tablets until after the first 7 consecutive days of administration. The possibility of ovulation and conception prior to initiation of medication should be considered.)

The patient begins her next and all subsequent 21-day courses of Ethinyl Estradiol/Levonorgestrel 21 Tablets on the same day of the week that she began her first course, following the same schedule: 21 days on—7 days off. She begins taking her tablets on the 8th day after discontinuance, regardless of whether or not a menstrual period has occurred or is still in progress. Any time the next cycle of Ethinyl Estradiol/Levonorgestrel 21 Tablets is started later than the 8th day, the patient should be protected by another means of contraception until she has taken a tablet daily for seven consecutive days.

If spotting or breakthrough bleeding occurs, the patient is instructed to continue on the same regimen. This type of bleeding is usually transient and without significance; however, if the bleeding is persistent or prolonged, the patient is advised to consult her physician. Although the occurrence of pregnancy is highly unlikely if Ethinyl Estradiol/Levonorgestrel 21 Tablets are taken according to directions, if withdrawal bleeding does not occur, the possibility of pregnancy must be considered. If the patient has not adhered to the prescribed schedule (missed one or more tablets or started taking them on a day later than she should have), the probability of pregnancy should be considered at the time of the first missed period and appropriate diagnostic measures taken before the medication is resumed. If the patient has adhered to the prescribed regimen and misses two consecutive periods, pregnancy should be ruled out before continuing the contraceptive regimen.

The patient should be instructed to take a missed tablet as soon as it is remembered. If two consecutive tablets are missed, they should both be taken as soon as remembered. The next tablet should be taken at the usual time.

Any time the patient misses one or two tablets she should also use another method of contraception until she has taken a tablet daily for seven consecutive days. If breakthrough bleeding occurs following missed tablets it will usually be transient and of no consequence. While there is little likelihood of ovulation occurring if only one or two tablets are missed, the possibility of ovulation increases with each successive day that scheduled tablets are missed. If three consecutive tablets are missed, all medication should be discontinued and the remainder of the package discarded. A new tablet cycle should be started on the 8th day after the last tablet was taken, and an alternate means of contraception should be prescribed during the seven days without tablets and until the patient has taken a tablet daily for seven consecutive days.

In the nonlactating mother, Ethinyl Estradiol/Levonorgestrel 21 Tablets may be initiated postpartum, for contraception. When the tablets are administered in the postpartum period, the increased risk of thromboembolic disease associated with the postpartum period must be considered. (See *"Contraindications"*, *"Warnings"*, and *"Precautions"* concerning thromboembolic disease.) It is to be noted that early resumption of ovulation may occur if bromocriptine mesylate has been used for the prevention of lactation.

ETHINYL ESTRADIOL/LEVONORGESTREL 28 TABLETS

To achieve maximum contraceptive effectiveness, Ethinyl Estradiol/Levonorgestrel 28 Tablets must be taken exactly as directed as directed at intervals not exceeding 24 hours.

The dosage of Ethinyl Estradiol/Levonorgestrel 28 Tablets is one light-orange tablet daily for 21 consecutive days per menstrual cycle, followed by 7 inert tablets according to the prescribed schedule. It is recommended that Ethinyl Estradiol/Levonorgestrel 28 Tablets be taken at the same time each day, preferably after the evening meal or at bedtime. During the first cycle of medication with some brands, the patient should be instructed to take one Ethinyl Estradiol/Levonorgestrel 28 Tablet daily in light-orange and then 7 inert tablets for twenty-eight (28) consecutive days, beginning on day one (1) of her menstrual cycle. (The first day of menstruation is day one.) During the first cycle of medication with other brands, the patient is instructed to begin taking Ethinyl Estradiol/Levonogestrel 28 Tablet on the first Sunday after the onset of menstruation. If menstruation begins on a Sunday, the first tablet (light-orange) is taken that day. One light-orange tablet should be taken daily for 21 consecutive days, followed by one inert tablet daily for 7 consecutive days. Withdrawal bleeding usually occurs within 3 days following the last light-orange tablet. (If an alternate starting regimen is used [Sunday Start or postpartum], contraceptive reliance should not be placed on Ethinyl Estradiol/Levonorgestrel 28 Tablets until after the first 7 consecutive days of administration. The possibility of ovulation and conception prior to initiation of medication should be considered.)

The patient begins her next and all subsequent 28-day courses of Ethinyl Estradiol/Levonorgestrel 28 Tablets on the same day of the week that she began her first course, following the same schedule. She begins taking her light-orange tablets on the next day after ingestion of the last inert tablet, regardless of whether or not a menstrual period has occurred or is still in progress. Any time a subsequent cycle of Ethinyl Estradiol/Levonorgestrel 28 Tablets is started later than the next day, the patient should be protected by another means of contraception until she has taken a light-orange tablet daily for seven consecutive days.

If spotting or breakthrough bleeding occurs, the patient is instructed to continue on the same regimen. This type of bleeding is usually transient and without significance; however, if the bleeding is persistent or prolonged, the patient is advised to consult her physician. Although the occurrence of pregnancy is highly unlikely if Ethinyl Estradiol/Levonorgestrel 28 Tablets are taken according to directions, if withdrawal bleeding does not occur, the possibility of pregnancy must be considered. If the patient has not adhered to the prescribed schedule (missed one or more active tablets or started taking them on a day later than she should have), the probability of pregnancy should be considered at the time of the first period and appropriate diagnostic measures taken before the medication is resumed. If the patient has adhered to the prescribed regimen and misses two consecutive periods, pregnancy should be ruled out before continuing the contraceptive regimen.

The patient should be instructed to take a missed light-orange tablet as soon as it is remembered. If two consecutive light-orange tablets are missed, they should both be taken as soon as remembered. The next tablet should be taken at the usual time.

Any time the patient misses two or more light-orange tablets, she should also use another method of contraception until she has taken a tablet daily for seven consecutive days. If breakthrough bleeding occurs following missed active tablets, it usually will be transient and of no consequence. If the patient misses one or more inert tablets, she is still protected against pregnancy provided she begins taking the light-orange tablets again on the proper day.

While there is little likelihood of ovulation occurring if only one or two light-orange tablets are missed, the possibility of ovulation increases with each successive day that scheduled light-orange tablets are missed. If three consecutive light-orange Ethinyl Estradiol/Levonorgestrel Tablets are missed, all medication should be discontinued and the remainder of the 28-day package discarded. A new tablet cycle should be started on the first Sunday following the last missed tablet, and an alternate means of contraception should be prescribed during the days without tablets and until the patient has taken a light-orange tablet daily for 7 consecutive days.

In the nonlactating mother, Ethinyl Estradiol/Levonorgestrel 28 Tablets may be initiated postpartum, for contraception. When the tablets are administered in the postpartum period, the increased risk of thromboembolic disease associated with the postpartum period must be considered. (See *"Contraindications"*, *"Warnings"*, and *"Precautions"* concerning thromboembolic disease.) It is to be noted that early resumption of ovulation may occur if bromocriptine mesylate has been used for the prevention of lactation.

HOW SUPPLIED
TABLETS:

BRAND/MANUFACTURER	NDC	SIZE	AWP
○ **BRAND**			
➤ TRI-LEVLEN: Berlex Labs	50419-0432-03	63s	$57.60
➤ TRIPHASIL-21: Wyeth-Ayerst	00008-2535-01	63s	$70.56
➤ TRI-LEVLEN: Berlex Labs	50419-0433-03	84s	$57.60
➤ TRIPHASIL-28: Wyeth-Ayerst	00008-2536-01	84s	$71.40
➤ TRI-LEVLEN: Berlex Labs	50419-0432-06	126s	$109.85
➤ TRIPHASIL-21: Wyeth-Ayerst	00008-2535-02	126s	$128.18
➤ TRI-LEVLEN: Berlex Labs	50419-0433-06	168s	$109.85

TABLETS: 0.15 MG-30 MCG

AVERAGE UNIT PRICE (AVAILABLE SIZES)

GENERIC	$0.85

BRAND/MANUFACTURER	NDC	SIZE	AWP
◆ **GENERICS**			
LEVORA: Hamilton	60322-0145-21	21s	$20.39
LEVORA: Hamilton	60322-0147-28	28s	$20.39

TABLETS: 30 MCG-0.15 MG

BRAND/MANUFACTURER	NDC	SIZE	AWP
○ **BRAND**			
➤ NORDETTE-21: Wyeth-Ayerst	00008-0075-02	21s	$21.03
NORDETTE-28: Wyeth-Ayerst	00008-2533-01	28s	$21.29
➤ LEVLEN: Berlex Labs	50419-0410-21	63s	$61.75
	50419-0411-28	84s	$61.75
➤ NORDETTE-21: Wyeth-Ayerst	00008-0075-01	126s	$148.45
NORDETTE-28: Wyeth-Ayerst	00008-2533-02	168s	$150.31

Ethiodized Oil

DESCRIPTION
Ethiodized Oil is a sterile injectable radio-opaque diagnostic agent for use in hysterosalpingography and lymphography. It contains 37% iodine (475 mg/mL) organically combined with ethyl esters of the fatty acids (primarily as ethyl monoiodostearate and ethyl diiodosterate) of poppyseed oil. Stabilized with poppyseed oil, 1%. The precise structure of Ethiodized Oil is unknown at this time. Ethiodized Oil is a straw to amber colored, oily fluid, which because of simplified molecular structure, possesses a greatly reduced viscosity (1.280 specific gravity at 15°C yields viscosity of 0.5 - 1.0 poise). This high fluidity provides a new flexibility for radiographic exploration.

CLINICAL PHARMACOLOGY
There has been little detailed investigation of the metabolic fate of Ethiodized Oil in either man or animals. However, the fate of Ethiodized Oil following lymphangiography in dogs has been reported.[1] Koehler et al. employed I[131]-tagged Ethiodized Oil for lymphangiography in dogs and analyses of individual organs at various time intervals were done. The investigators reported an average of only 25% of the injected medium was retained in the lymphatics at the end of

three days. An average of 50% was recovered from the lungs. They found the remainder of injected activity was fairly uniformly distributed throughout the body. Urinary excretion in the form of inorganic iodine was revealed as the chief mode of iodine loss from the system.

INDICATIONS
Ethiodized Oil is indicated for use as a radio-opaque medium for hysterosalpingography and lymphography.

UNLABELED USES
Ethiodized Oil is used alone or as an adjunct for hepatic computed tomography and spleen imaging. Ethiodized Oil is also used to promote conception in females with unexplained infertility.

IN HYSTEROSALPINGOGRAPHY

CONTRAINDICATIONS
Ethiodized Oil is contraindicated in patients hypersensitive to it. Ethiodized Oil should not be injected intrathecally or intravascularly, or used in bronchography. A history of sensitivity to iodine contraindicates the use of Ethiodized Oil; iodine is split off from fatty compounds and becomes free iodine in the body. Hysterosalpingography is contraindicated in intrauterine pregnancy, acute pelvic inflammatory disease, marked cervical erosion, endocervicitis in the presence of intrauterine bleeding in the immediate pre- or postmenstrual phase, or within 30 days of curettage or conization.

WARNINGS
Ethiodized Oil is not intended for use in bronchography and, therefore, is not to be introduced into the bronchial tree. A history of sensitivity to iodine or to other contrast materials is not an absolute contraindication to Ethiodized Oil, but calls for extreme caution. All procedures utilizing contrast media carry a definite risk of adverse reactions. While most reactions are minor, life threatening and fatal reactions may occur without warning. The risk/benefit factor should always be carefully evaluated. At all times a fully equipped emergency cart and resuscitation equipment should be readily available, and personnel competent in recognizing and treating reactions of all severity should be on hand.

PRECAUTIONS
General: Since iodine-containing contrast materials may alter the results of certain thyroid function tests, such tests, if indicated, should be performed prior to the administration of this drug. Pulmonary embolization of the contrast material may occur if hysterosalpingography is performed under conditions which may lead to intravasation of the contrast materials. These conditions include uterine bleeding, recent curettage or conization and injection of the contrast material under excessive pressure.

Carcinogenesis, Mutagenesis, and Impairment of Fertility: Long-term studies in animals have not been performed to evaluate carcinogenic potential, mutagenesis, or whether Ethiodized Oil can affect fertility in males or females.

Pregnancy Category C: Animal reproduction studies have not been conducted with Ethiodized Oil. It is also not known whether Ethiodized Oil can cause fetal harm when administered to a pregnant woman or can affect reproduction capacity. Ethiodized Oil should be administered to a pregnant woman only if clearly needed.

Nursing Mothers: It is not known whether this drug is excreted in human milk. Because many drugs are excreted in human milk and because of the potential for serious adverse reactions in nursing infants from Ethiodized Oil, a decision should be made whether to discontinue nursing or to discontinue the drug, taking into account the importance of the drug to the mother.

ADVERSE REACTIONS
Hypersensitivity reactions, foreign body reactions and exacerbation of pelvic inflammatory disease, although infrequent, have been reported. In an occasional patient, abdominal pains may occur. Such pains may be the result of tubal torsion, or possibly due to too rapid a rate of instillation or excessive pressure, or both. The condition is usually only transitory, lasting one or two hours at most, and may be relieved by the administration of any of the commonly used analgesics.

DOSAGE AND ADMINISTRATION
The hysterosalpingogram is preferably taken during the patient's preovulatory phase (as determined from her basal body temperature record) and not less than two days after cessation of her menstrual flow. It has been frequently observed that some bleeding will occur during or after the onset of pregnancy which cannot be distinguished by the patient from a normal menstrual period. In such cases a basal body temperature record will reveal a sustained high temperature phase, and thus enable an operator to avoid hysterosalpingography when a pregnancy may exist. Salpingography should not be performed if the blood is exuding from the cervical os (which occasionally occurs without the patient being aware of it) or if any gross evidence of endocervicitis exists.

Careful aseptic technique should be employed as for any operative procedure in which the uterus is entered. A self-retaining cannula should be used thereby permitting removal of the vaginal speculum so that the outline of the cervical canal may be seen in the film. The use of a radio-opaque aluminum speculum may be employed in patients where a lacerated or patulous cervix does not permit the use of a retaining cannula.

The radio-opaque agent is introduced under pressure and preferably with fluoroscopic control. A preliminary film is exposed and a skiagram is made after the injection of 5 mL of the agent The pressure is raised to 80-90 mm Hg. In cases of normal bilateral tubal patency, the pressure falls immediately to below 60 mm Hg. The wet film may be viewed immediately and if both tubes are seen to "fill", the apparatus is removed and the procedure is finished, except for the 24 hour follow-up to establish whether or not "spill" into the peritoneal cavity has occurred.

Increments of 2 mL of the agent are injected and successive films exposed until tubal patency is established or until the patient's limit of tolerance to discomfort is reached. Few patients will complain of discomfort at pressures under 200 mm Hg.

IN LYMPHOGRAPHY

CONTRAINDICATIONS
Ethiodized Oil is contraindicated in patients hypersensitive to it. Ethiodized Oil should not be injected intrathecally or intravascularly or introduced into the bronchial tree. Patients with known sensitivity to iodine should not have lymphography performed. Iodine is spit off from fatty compounds and becomes free iodine in the body. Lymphography is contraindicated in patients with a right to left cardiac shunt, in patients with advanced pulmonary disease, especially those with alveolar-capillary block, and in patients who have had radiotherapy to the lungs.

WARNINGS
The use of intralymphatic Ethiodized Oil presents a significant hazard in patients with pre-existing pulmonary disease characterized by a decrease in pulmonary diffusing capacity and/or pulmonary blood flow. A few fatalities have been noted in such patients. With reference to this potential complication, recent studies indicate a significant decrease in both pulmonary diffusing capacity and pulmonary capillary blood flow following Ethiodized Oil lymphography without appreciable concomitant clinical manifestations. Also care should be exercised in patients with other types of pulmonary disease in view of the more frequent incidence of overt pulmonary complications such as pulmonary infarction, in these groups. However, it is to be noted that pulmonary infarction, although rare, has occurred in patients without evidence of pre-existing pulmonary disease.

The safety of intralymphatic Ethiodized Oil has not been established in pregnant women, and accordingly, its use should be restricted to such situations where it is deemed necessary.

PRECAUTIONS
General: Although subclinical pulmonary embolization occurs in a majority of patients following Ethiodized Oil lymphography, clinical evidence of such embolization is infrequent and is usually of a transient nature. Such clinical manifestations are usually immediate, but may be delayed from a few hours to days. It would appear that it is advantageous to use the smallest volume of Ethiodized Oil necessary for radiographic visualization. For this reason, and to prevent inadvertent venous administration, radiographic monitoring of patients is recommended during the injection of Ethiodized Oil.

The timing and choice of anesthesia following Ethiodized Oil injection may be influenced by consideration of the above noted decrease in pulmonary and capillary blood flow and diffusing capacity. It should be noted that although an average of 2 to 3 days was required for complete reversibility for such tests, an occasional patient required up to 12 days to return to baseline values.

PBI determination of thyroid uptake studies should be carried out prior to the lymphographic procedure because interference with these tests may be anticipated for as long as one year. In the presence of known iodine sensitivity, Ethiodized Oil lymphography should be carried out with greatest precaution.

Carcinogenesis, Mutagenesis, and Impairment of Fertility: Long-term studies in animals have not been performed to evaluate carcinogenic potential, mutagenesis, or whether Ethiodized Oil can affect fertility in males or females.

Pregnancy Category C: Animal reproduction studies have not been conducted with Ethiodized Oil. It is also not known whether Ethiodized Oil can cause fetal harm when administered to a pregnant women or can affect reproduction capacity. Ethiodized Oil should be administered to a pregnant woman only if clearly needed.

Nursing Mothers: It is not known whether this drug is excreted in human milk. Because many drugs are excreted in human milk and because of the potential for serious adverse reactions in nursing infants from Ethiodized Oil, a decision should be made whether to discontinue nursing or to discontinue the drug, taking into account the importance of the drug to the mother.

ADVERSE REACTIONS
The occasional observation of pulmonary Ethiodized Oil embolization (infarction) several hours after injection has been reported. This was noticed more frequently when excessive amounts of Ethiodized Oil have been injected, in the presence of marked lymphatic obstruction or through accidental intravenous injection. Radiologic manifestations are fine, granular stippling throughout both lung fields. The clinical symptoms usually noted have been mild, consisting of moderate temperature elevation, dyspnea, and cough. However, severe acute symptoms developed in two patients both of whom were severely ill and required extensive care.[2] Fuchs[3] experienced 1 severe and 3 minor complications in a series of 20 bilateral procedures. Two are described by the author as cardiovascular collapse occurring at two hours respectively following the completion of the procedure. It was postulated that minute emboli may have been causative. Recovery was rapid and complete in both instances.

The occurrence of pulmonary invasion may be minimized if radiographic confirmation of intralymphatic (rather than venous) injection is secured, and the

procedure discontinued when the medium becomes visible in the thoracic duct or the presence of lymphatic obstruction is noticed.

While rare, other side effects reported include transient fever, lymphangitis, iodism (headache, soreness of mouth and pharynx, coryza and skin rash), allergic dermatitis, and lipogranuloma formation. Delayed wound healing at the site of incision and secondary infection are occasionally seen, and can be prevented or minimized by adhering to a strict sterile technique.

Transient edema or temporary exacerbation of preexisting lymphedema, as well as thrombophlebitis have also been reported. In the extremely rare presence of concomitant lymphatic and inferior vena cava obstruction the contrast medium may be shunted partially to the liver, resulting in hepatic embolization. Also, when accidental intravenous administration of Ethiodized Oil results in a considerable amount of this medium entering the circulation, embolization other than pulmonary may occur as reported in 2 cases[4]. Both cases developed a transient, psychotic-like manifestation, which in all probability stemmed from the entrance of fine oil droplets into the cerebral circulation. Recovery was uneventful and complete without evidence of neurological sequelae.

DOSAGE AND ADMINISTRATION
This method applies for both the upper and lower extremities. A lymphatic vessel is selected for cannulization.

The patient should be comfortably arranged in a supine position on a portable stretcher or an x-ray table. When available, a radiolucent pad will add to the patient's comfort during the one to two hours required for completion of the examination. It is important that the patient be in a cooperative state. Premedication might be advisable in the unusually apprehensive patient.

In the unusually restless patient, the extremities should be immobilized during the entire procedure to prevent displacement of the needle. Thomas splints have been satisfactorily employed for the legs and simple arm boards for the upper extremities. The cut-down and injection instruments and materials include the following:

Sterile pediatric cut-down set;
Sterile towels for draping, sponges, etc.;
Local anesthetic, such as procaine hydrochloride, and a syringe;
Bactericidal painting solution;
20 mL syringe containing 15 mL of Ethiodized Oil with an 18 inch catheter to which is affixed a 27 or 30 gauge needle. (If bilateral lymphography is scheduled, two syringes should be prepared.)
A manually driven or motorized unit (a pressure regulated pump) to provide for slow injection.

Under local infiltration anesthesia, a transverse, curvilinear or longitudinal small skin incision should be made near the ankle or wrist (just lateral and distal to the first metatarsal head on the dorsum of the foot, or just over the "snuff-box" in the dorsum of the hand).

Upon superficial dissection (but not penetrating the subcutaneous layer of tissue) lymph vessels will be noted in the immediate subcutaneous tissue, while larger lymph vessel trunks are found in the extrafascial plane. The deeper lymph trunks will be easier to cannulate.

One lymph vessel is then exposed, avoiding circumferential dissection. The less manipulation performed, the better the results that will be obtained. The lymphatic, thus isolated, is then cannulated with a 27 or 30 gauge ⅝ inch needle, depending upon the size of the lymphatic selected for injection. It is rarely possible to cannulate with a needle greater than 27 gauge. Insertion of the needle through the skin flap before cannulating the lymphatic serves to reduce the movement of the needle with the vessel. Additional security of the needle in the lymphatic is obtained by strapping, with sterile tape, the polyethylene tubing to the patient's foot.

The injection should be started at a slow rate, i.e., 0.1 mL to 0.2 mL per minute. Radiographic monitoring either by fluoroscopy or serial radiographs after 1 mL to 2 mL has been injected, will confirm the proper intralymphatic placement of the needle, and rule out accidental intravenous injection or extravasation of the medium by perforation or rupture of the lymphatic. Monitoring will also permit prompt termination of the procedure in the event that lymphatic blockade is present. In such situations, continuation of the injection will result in unnecessary introduction of contrast material in the venous system via the lymphovenous communication channels. If the injection is satisfactory, approximately 6 to 8 mL, are then injected. However, as soon as it becomes radiographically evident that Ethiodized Oil has entered the thoracic duct, the procedure should be terminated to minimize entry of the contrast material into the subclavian vein. Two to four mL of Ethiodized Oil injected into the upper extremity will suffice to demonstrate the axillary and supraclavicular nodes. In penile lymphography approximately 2 to 3 mL of Ethiodized Oil is required. In infants and children, a minimum of 1 mL to a maximum of 6 mL should be employed.

The rate of speed at which the contrast material may be introduced varies and is dependent upon receptivity of the lymphatics in the individual patient. If the injection is proceeding at too rapid a rate, extravasation will be noted and the patient may refer to pain in the foot, leg or arm.

At the completion of the injection, anteroposterior roentgenograms are obtained of the legs of arms, thighs, pelvis, abdomen and chest (dorsal spine technique). Lateral or oblique views as well as laminograms are obtained when indicated. Follow-up films at 24 or 48 hours provide better demonstration of lymph nodes and permit more concise evaluation of nodal architecture.

As a general rule, the smallest possible amount of Ethiodized Oil should be employed according to the anatomical area to be visualized. Therefore, and to

---

prevent inadvertent venous administration, fluoroscopic monitoring or serial radiographic guidance of patients is recommended during the injection of Ethiodized Oil.

Average dose in the adult patient for unilateral lymphography of the upper extremities is 2 to 4 mL; of lower extremities, 6 to 8 mL; of penile lymphography, 2 to 3 mL; of cervical lymphography, 1 to 2 mL.

In the pediatric patient, a minimum of 1 mL to a maximum of 6 mL may be employed according to the anatomical area to be visualized.

SUMMARY OF STEPS TO AVOID COMPLICATIONS IN LYMPHOGRAPHY[5]

1. Contraindicate patients:

   A. With a known hypersensitivity to Ethiodized Oil
   B. With a right to left cardiac shunt
   C. With advanced pulmonary disease, especially those with alveolar-capillary block. Pulmonary gas difusion studies should be done if in doubt.
   D. Who have had radiation therapy to the lungs

2. Proceed with caution:

   A. Patients having markedly advanced neoplastic disease with expected lymphatic obstruction.
   B. Patients having undergone previous surgery interrupting the lymphatic system.
   C. Patients having had deep radiation therapy to the examined area.

If in those cases in which extreme caution should be exercised, lymphography is still necessary, a smaller dose of oily contrast medium with protracted injection time with less pressure and careful monitoring is required.

3. Skin testing should be done on all patients before submitting them to lymphography. Be aware of possible hypersensitivity to local anesthetics and skin disinfectants. Careful history taking is important.

4. Technique of cannulation: extravasation is to be avoided and/or detected early. The injection site should be included on the "scout film" or observed under image amplification fluoroscopy. The needle tip must remain visible in the incision wound.

5. Oily contrast materials: once opened, ampules should be discarded. Ampules of Ethiodized Oil should not be used if the color has darkened or if particulate matter is present. The average dose for each foot in an adult is 5 to 6 mL; one-half as much for the upper extremity. The amount for children should be determine by careful monitoring. It should stay below 0.25 mL/kg.

6. Injection pressure should be regulated to deliver the average dose in no less than 1¼ hours. Continuous monitoring helps to determine the speed most appropriate for each individual. Sensation of pain is a warming of too high pressure.

7. Scout roentgenograms: If scout roentgenograms are used for monitoring, they should be developed and viewed immediately in order to apply corrective measures when needed; e.g., discontinuation of the study when one sees intravenous injection or lymphatico-venous anastomosis. Reduction of injection speed is needed if evidence of collateral circulation occurs or if the higher abdomino-aortic nodes do not opacify in spite of the usual injection pressure. This is highly suggestive of lymphatic obstruction. Scout roentgenograms should be taken more frequently in such cases.

8. Surgical technique: strict aseptic surgical technique is followed including the weaning of a face mask. Before suturing the incision wound, the remnants of the lymphatic vessels and loose tissue are removed and the wound well washed with saline to remove any possible oil. In case of reflux type lymphedema, the cannulated large lymphatic vessel may have to be closed by catgut to avoid development of a lymphocyst.

The patient is instructed to elevate the legs as often as possible to promote healing. The sutures are removed from the feet on the 10th day, and on the 5th or 6th from the hands.

Store at controlled room temperature 15°-30°C (59°-86°F). Protect from light. Remove from carton only upon use.

Parenteral drug products should be inspected visually for particulate matter and discoloration prior to administration, whenever solution and container permit. Ethiodized Oil for injection is straw to amber color under normal conditions. (See "Description".)

BIBLIOGRAPHY
1. P. Ruben Koehler, M.D. et al.: "Body Distribution of Ethiodol Following Lymphangiography", Radiology, 1964, 82, 5 866-871. 2. Bronk, et al.: "Oil Embolism in Lymphography", Radiation, 80: 194, February 1963. 3. Fuchs, S.A., "Complications in Lymphography With Oily Contrast Media", Acta Radiol., 57:247, November 1962. 4. Viamonte, M. Jr., University of Miami, Jackson Memorial Hospital, Miami, Florida, Private Communication. 5. Kuisk, H., "Techniques of Lymphography and Principles of Interpretation", 1971, Warren H. Green, Inc., St. Louis, Missouri, 63105.

HOW SUPPLIED
INJECTION:

BRAND/MANUFACTURER	NDC	SIZE	AWP
○ **BRAND**			
ETHIODOL: Savage	00281-7062-37	10 ml 2s	$66.91

Ethiodol *SEE* ETHIODIZED OIL

Ethionamide

DESCRIPTION

Ethionamide is used in the treatment of tuberculosis. The chemical name for Ethionamide is 2-ethyl-thioisonicotinamide.

Ethionamide is a yellow, crystalline, nonhygroscopic compound with a faint-to-moderate sulfide odor. It is practically insoluble in water and ether but soluble in methanol and ethanol. It melts at about 162° C and is stable at ordinary temperatures and humidities.

Tablets contain 250 mg of Ethionamide.

Following is its chemical structure:

ACTION

Bacteriostatic against *Mycobacterium tuberculosis*.

INDICATIONS

Failure after adequate treatment with primary drugs (i.e., isoniazid, streptomycin, aminosalicylic acid) in any form of active tuberculosis. Ethionamide should only be given with other effective antituberculous agents.

CONTRAINDICATIONS

Severe hypersensitivity.
Severe hepatic damage.

WARNING

USE IN PREGNANCY
Teratogenic effects have been demonstrated in animals (rabbits, rats) receiving doses in excess of those recommended in humans. Use of the drug should be avoided during pregnancy or in women of childbearing potential unless the benefits outweigh its possible hazard.

USE IN CHILDREN
Optimum dosage for children has not been established. This, however, does not preclude use of the drug when its use is crucial to therapy.

PRECAUTIONS

Pretreatment examinations should include *in vitro* susceptibility tests of recent cultures of *M. tuberculosis* from the patient as measured against Ethionamide and the usual primary antituberculous drugs.

Determinations of serum transaminase (SGOT, SGPT) should be made prior to and every 2 to 4 weeks during therapy.

In patients with diabetes mellitus, management may be more difficult and hepatitis occurs more frequently.

Ethionamide may intensify the adverse effects of the other antituberculous drugs administered concomitantly. Convulsions have been reported, and special care should be taken, particularly when Ethionamide is administered with cycloserine.

ADVERSE REACTIONS

The most common side effect is gastrointestinal intolerance. Other adverse effects similar to those seen with isoniazid have been reported: peripheral neuritis, optic neuritis, psychic disturbances (including mental depression), postural hypotension, skin rashes, thrombocytopenia, pellagralike syndrome, jaundice and/or hepatitis, increased difficulty in management of diabetes mellitus, stomatitis, gynecomastia, and impotence.

DOSAGE AND ADMINISTRATION

Ethionamide should be administered with at least one other effective antituberculous drug.

Average Adult Dose: 0.5 gram to 1.0 gram/day in divided doses.
Concomitant administration of pyridoxine is recommended.

Storage: Store at room temperature, approximately 25°C (77°F). Keep tightly closed. Dispense in tight container.

HOW SUPPLIED
TABLETS: 250 MG

BRAND/MANUFACTURER	NDC	SIZE	AWP
○ **BRAND**			
TRECATOR-SC: Wyeth-Ayerst	00008-4130-01	100s	$159.91

Ethosuximide

DESCRIPTION

Ethosuximide is an anticonvulsant succinimide, chemically designated as alpha-ethyl-alpha-methyl-succinimide.

Each Ethosuximide capsule contains 250 mg Ethosuximide, USP. Each teaspoonful (5 mL), for oral administration, contains 250 mg Ethosuximide, USP.

➤ SHOWN IN PRODUCT IDENTIFICATION GUIDE

Following is its chemical structure:

$$\text{(chemical structure of ethosuximide, with H, CH}_3\text{, C}_2\text{H}_5\text{ groups)}$$

CLINICAL PHARMACOLOGY

Ethosuximide suppresses the paroxysmal three cycle per second spike and wave activity associated with lapses of consciousness which is common in absence (petit mal) seizures. The frequency of epileptiform attacks is reduced, apparently by depression of the motor cortex and elevation of the threshold of the central nervous system to convulsive stimuli.

INDICATIONS AND USAGE

Ethosuximide is indicated for the control of absence (petit mal) epilepsy.

UNLABELED USES

Ethosuximide is used alone or as an adjunct in improving learning problems in children 6 to 18 years of age.

CONTRAINDICATION

Ethosuximide should not be used in patients with a history of hypersensitivity to succinimides.

WARNINGS

Blood dyscrasias including some with fatal outcome, have been reported to be associated with the use of Ethosuximide; therefore, periodic blood counts should be performed. Should signs and/or symptoms of infection (eg, sore throat, fever) develop, blood counts should be considered at that point.

Ethosuximide is capable of producing morphological and functional changes in the animal liver. In humans, abnormal liver and renal function studies have been reported.

Ethosuximide should be administered with extreme caution to patients with known liver or renal disease. Periodic urinalysis and liver function studies are advised for all patients receiving the drug.

Cases of systemic lupus erythematosus have been reported with the use of Ethosuxide. The physician should be alert to this possibility.

Usage in Pregnancy: Reports suggest an association between the use of anticonvulsant drugs by women with epilepsy and an elevated incidence of birth defects in children born to these women. Data are more extensive with respect to phenytoin and phenobarbital, but these are also the most commonly prescribed anticonvulsants; less systematic or anecdotal reports suggest a possible similar association with the use of all known anticonvulsant drugs.

The reports suggesting an elevated incidence of birth defects in children of drug-treated epileptic women cannot be regarded as adequate to prove a definite cause and effect relationship. There are intrinsic methodological problems in obtaining adequate data on drug teratogenicity in humans; the possibility also exists that other factors, eg, genetic factors or the epileptic condition itself, may be more important than drug therapy in leading to birth defects. The great majority of mothers on anticonvulsant medication deliver normal infants. It is important to note that anticonvulsant drugs should not be discontinued in patients in whom the drug is administered to prevent major seizures because of the strong possibility of precipitating status epilepticus with attendant hypoxia and threat to life. In individual cases where the severity and frequency of the seizure disorder are such that the removal of medication does not pose a serious threat to the patient, discontinuation of the drug may be considered prior to and during pregnancy, although it cannot be said with any confidence that even minor seizures do not pose some hazard to the developing embryo or fetus.

The prescribing physician will wish to weight these considerations in treating or counseling epileptic women of childbearing potential.

PRECAUTIONS

GENERAL

Ethosuximide, when used alone in mixed types of epilepsy, may increase the frequency of grand mal seizures in some patients.

As with other anticonvulsants, it is important to proceed slowly when increasing or decreasing dosage, as well as when adding or eliminating other medication. Abrupt withdrawal of anticonvulsant medication may precipitate absence (petit mal) status.

INFORMATION FOR PATIENTS

Ethosuximide may impair the mental and/or physical abilities required for the performance of potentially hazardous tasks, such as driving a motor vehicle or other such activity requiring alertness; therefore, the patient should be cautioned accordingly.

Patients taking Ethosuximide should be advised of the importance of adhering strictly to the prescribed dosage regimen. Patients should be instructed to promptly contact their physician if they develop signs and/or symptoms (eg, sore throat, fever) suggesting an infection.

DRUG INTERACTIONS

Since Ethosuximide may interact with concurrently administered antiepileptic drugs, periodic serum level determinations of these drugs may be necessary (eg, Ethosuximide may elevate phenytoin serum levels and valproic acid has been reported to both increase and decrease Ethosuximide levels).

PREGNANCY
See "Warnings".

ADVERSE REACTIONS

Gastrointestinal System: Gastrointestinal symptoms occur frequently and include anorexia, vague gastric upset, nausea and vomiting, cramps, epigastric and abdominal pain, weight loss, and diarrhea. There have been reports of gum hypertrophy and swelling of the tongue.

Hemopoietic System: Hemopoietic complications associated with the administration of Ethosuximide have included leukopenia, agranulocytosis, pancytopenia, with or without bone marrow suppression, and eosinophilia.

Nervous System: Neurologic and sensory reactions reported during therapy with Ethosuximide have included drowsiness, headache, dizziness, euphoria, hiccups, irritability, hyperactivity, lethargy, fatigue, and ataxia. Psychiatric or psychological aberrations associated with Ethosuximide administration have included disturbances of sleep, night terrors, inability to concentrate, and aggressiveness. These effects may be noted particularly in patients who have previously exhibited psychological abnormalities. There have been rare reports of paranoid psychosis, increased libido, and increased state of depression with overt suicidal intentions.

Integumentary System: Dermatologic manifestations which have occurred with the administration of Ethosuximide have included urticaria, Stevens-Johnson syndrome, systemic lupus erythematosus, pruritic erythematous rashes, and hirsutism.

Special Senses: Myopia.

Genitourinary System: Vaginal bleeding, microscopic hematuria.

OVERDOSAGE

Acute overdoses may produce nausea, vomiting, and CNS depression including coma with respiratory depression. A relationship between Ethosuximide toxicity and its plasma levels has not been established. The therapeutic range of serum levels is 40 mcg/mL to 100 mcg/mL, although levels as high as 150 mcg/mL have been reported without signs of toxicity.

TREATMENT

Treatment should include emesis (unless the patient is or could rapidly become obtunded, comatose, or convulsing) or gastric lavage, activated charcoal, cathartics and general supportive measures. Hemodialysis may be useful to treat Ethosuximide overdose. Forced diuresis and exchange transfusions are ineffective.

DOSAGE AND ADMINISTRATION

Ethosuximide is administered by the oral route. The *initial* dose of capsules for patients 3 to 6 years of age is one capsule (250 mg) per day; for patients 6 years of age and older, 2 capsules (500 mg) per day. The *initial* dose of syrup for patients 3 to 6 years of age is one teaspoonful (250 mg) per day; for patients 6 years of age and older, 2 teaspoonfuls (500 mg) per day. The dose thereafter must be individualized according to the patient's response. Dosage should be increased by small increments. One useful method is to increase the daily dose by 250 mg every four to seven days until control is achieved with minimal side effects. Dosages exceeding 1.5 g daily, in divided doses, should be administered only under the strictest supervision of the physician. The *optimal* dose for most children is 20 mg/kg/day. This dose has given average plasma levels within the accepted therapeutic range of 40 to 100 mcg/mL. Subsequent dose schedules can be based on effectiveness and plasma level determinations.

Ethosuximide may be administered in combination with other anticonvulsants when other forms of epilepsy coexist with absence (petit mal). The *optimal* dose for most children is 20 mg/kg/day.

Store capsules at controlled room temperature, 15°-30°C (59°-86°F).

Store syrup below 30°C (86°F). Protect from freezing and light.

HOW SUPPLIED
CAPSULE: 250 MG

BRAND/MANUFACTURER	NDC	SIZE	AWP
○ BRAND			
▶ ZARONTIN: Parke-Davis	00071-0237-24	100s	$71.72

SYRUP: 250 MG/5 ML

BRAND/MANUFACTURER	NDC	SIZE	AWP
○ BRAND			
ZARONTIN: Parke-Davis	00071-2418-23	480 ml	$75.44
○ GENERICS			
Copley	38245-0660-07	480 ml	$63.20

Ethotoin

DESCRIPTION

Ethotoin is an oral antiepileptic of the hydantoin series and is chemically identified as 3-ethyl-5-phenyl-2, 4-imidazolidinedione. Ethotoin tablets are available in two dosage strengths of 250 mg and 500 mg respectively.

Following is its chemical structure:

CLINICAL PHARMACOLOGY

Ethotoin exerts an antiepileptic effect without causing general central nervous system depression. The mechanism of action is probably very similar to that of phenytoin. The latter drug appears to stabilize rather than to raise the normal seizure threshold, and to prevent the spread of seizure activity rather than to abolish the primary focus of seizure discharges.

In laboratory animals, the drug was found effective against electroshock convulsions, and to a lesser extent, against complex partial (psychomotor) and pentylenetetrazol-induced seizures.

In mice, the duration of antiepileptic activity was prolonged by hepatic injury but not by bilateral nephrectomy; the drug is apparently biotransformed by the liver.

Ethotoin is fairly rapidly absorbed; the extent of oral absorption is not known. The drug exhibits saturable metabolism with respect to the formation of N-deethyl and p-hydroxyl-Ethotoin, the major metabolites. Where plasma concentrations are below about 8 mcg/mL, the elimination half-life of Ethotoin is in the range of 3 to 9 hours. A study comparing single doses of 500 mg, 1000 mg, and 1500 mg of Ethotoin demonstrated that Ethotoin, and to a lesser extent 5-phenylhydantoin, a major metabolite, exhibits substantial nonlinear kinetics. The degree of nonlinearity with multiple dosing may be increased over that seen after a single dose, given the likelihood of plasma accumulation based on a reported elimination half-life of 6 to 9 hours and a dosing interval of 4 to 6 hours. Experience suggests that therapeutic plasma concentrations fall in the range of 15 to 50 mcg/mL; however, this range is not as extensively documented as those quoted for other antiepileptics.

INDICATIONS AND USAGE

Ethotoin is indicated for the control of tonic-clonic (grand mal) and complex partial (psychomotor) seizures.

CONTRAINDICATIONS

Ethotoin is contraindicated in patients with hepatic abnormalities or hematologic disorders.

WARNINGS

USAGE DURING PREGNANCY—THERE ARE MULTIPLE REPORTS IN THE CLINICAL LITERATURE WHICH INDICATE THAT THE USE OF ANTIEPILEPTIC DRUGS DURING PREGNANCY RESULTS IN AN INCREASED INCIDENCE OF BIRTH DEFECTS IN THE OFFSPRING. ALTHOUGH DATA ARE MORE EXTENSIVE WITH RESPECT TO TRIMETHADIONE, PARAMETHADIONE, PHENYTOIN, AND PHENOBARBITAL, REPORTS INDICATE A POSSIBLE SIMILAR ASSOCIATION WITH THE USE OF OTHER ANTIEPILEPTIC DRUGS. THEREFORE, ANTIEPILEPTIC DRUGS SHOULD BE ADMINISTERED TO WOMEN OF CHILDBEARING POTENTIAL ONLY IF THEY ARE CLEARLY SHOWN TO BE ESSENTIAL IN THE MANAGEMENT OF THEIR SEIZURES.

ANTIEPILEPTIC DRUGS SHOULD NOT BE DISCONTINUED IN PATIENTS IN WHOM THE DRUG IS ADMINISTERED TO PREVENT MAJOR SEIZURES BECAUSE OF THE STRONG POSSIBILITY OF PRECIPITATING STATUS EPILEPTICUS WITH ATTENDANT HYPOXIA AND RISK TO BOTH MOTHER AND THE UNBORN CHILD. CONSIDERATION SHOULD, HOWEVER, BE GIVEN TO DISCONTINUATION OF ANTIEPILEPTICS PRIOR TO AND DURING PREGNANCY WHEN THE NATURE, FREQUENCY AND SEVERITY OF THE SEIZURES DO NOT POSE A SERIOUS THREAT TO THE PATIENT. IT IS NOT, HOWEVER, KNOWN WHETHER EVEN MINOR SEIZURES CONSTITUTE SOME RISK TO THE DEVELOPING EMBRYO OR FETUS.

REPORTS HAVE SUGGESTED THAT THE MATERNAL INGESTION OF ANTIEPILEPTIC DRUGS, PARTICULARLY BARBITURATES, IS ASSOCIATED WITH A NEONATAL COAGULATION DEFECT THAT MAY CAUSE BLEEDING DURING THE EARLY (USUALLY WITHIN 24 HOURS OF BIRTH) NEONATAL PERIOD. THE POSSIBILITY OF THE OCCURRENCE OF THIS DEFECT WITH THE USE OF ETHOTOIN SHOULD BE KEPT IN MIND. THE DEFECT IS CHARACTERIZED BY DECREASED LEVELS OF VITAMIN K-DEPENDENT CLOTTING FACTORS, AND PROLONGATION OF EITHER THE PROTHROMBIN TIME OR THE PARTIAL THROMBOPLASTIN TIME, OR BOTH. IT HAS BEEN SUGGESTED THAT VITAMIN K BE GIVEN PROPHYLACTICALLY TO THE MOTHER ONE MONTH PRIOR TO, AND DURING DELIVERY, AND TO THE INFANT, INTRAVENOUSLY, IMMEDIATELY AFTER BIRTH.

THE PHYSICIAN SHOULD WEIGH THESE CONSIDERATIONS IN TREATMENT AND COUNSELING OF EPILEPTIC WOMEN OF CHILDBEARING POTENTIAL.

PRECAUTIONS

General: Blood dyscrasias have been reported in patients receiving Ethotoin. Although the etiologic role of Ethotoin has not been definitely established, physicians should be alert for general malaise, sore throat and other symptoms indicative of possible blood dyscrasia.

There is some evidence suggesting that hydantoin-like compounds may interfere with folic acid metabolism, precipitating a megaloblastic anemia. If this should occur during gestation, folic acid therapy should be considered.

Information for Patients: Patients should be advised to report immediately such signs and symptoms as sore throat, fever, malaise, easy bruising, petechiae, epistaxis, or others that may be indicative of an infection or bleeding tendency.

Laboratory Tests: Liver function tests should be performed if clinical evidence suggests the possibility of hepatic dysfunction. Signs of liver damage are indication for withdrawal of the drug.

It is recommended that blood counts and urinalyses be performed when therapy is begun and at monthly intervals for several months thereafter. As in patients receiving other hydantoin compounds and other antiepileptic drugs, blood dyscrasias have been reported in patients receiving Ethotoin. Marked depression of the blood count is indication for withdrawal of the drug.

Drug Interactions: Ethotoin used in combination with other drugs known to adversely affect the hematopoietic system should be avoided if possible.

Considerable caution should be exercised if Ethotoin is administered concurrently with *phenacemide* since paranoid symptoms have been reported during therapy with this combination.

A two-way interaction between the hydantoin antiepileptic, *phenytoin*, and the *coumarin anticoagulants* has been suggested. Presumably, phenytoin acts as a stimulator of coumarin metabolism and has been reported to cause decreased serum levels of the coumarin anticoagulants and increased prothrombin-proconvertin concentrations. Conversely, the coumarin anticoagulants have been reported to increase the serum levels and prolong the serum half-life of phenytoin by inhibiting its metabolism. Although there is no documentation of such, a similar interaction between Ethotoin and the coumarin anticoagulants may occur. Caution is therefore advised when administering Ethotoin to patients receiving coumarin anticoagulants.

Carcinogenesis: No data are available on long-term potential for carcinogenicity in animals or humans.

Pregnancy: Pregnancy Category C. See *"Warnings"* section.

Nursing Mothers: Ethotoin is excreted in breast milk. Because of the potential for serious adverse reactions in nursing infants from Ethotoin, a decision should be made whether to discontinue nursing or to discontinue the drug, taking into account the importance of the drug to the mother.

ADVERSE REACTIONS

Adverse reactions associated with Ethotoin in decreasing order of severity, are:

Isolated cases of lymphadenopathy and systemic lupus erythematosus have been reported in patients taking hydantoin compounds, and lymphadenopathy has occurred with Ethotoin. Withdrawal of therapy has resulted in remission of the clinical and pathological findings. Therefore, if a lymphoma-like syndrome develops, the drug should be withdrawn and the patient should be closely observed for regression of signs and symptoms before treatment is resumed.

Ataxia and gum hypertrophy have occurred only rarely—usually only in patients receiving an additional hydantoin derivative. It is of interest to note that ataxia and gum hypertrophy have subsided in patients receiving other hydantoins when Ethotoin was given as a substitute antiepileptic.

Occasionally, vomiting or nausea after ingestion of Ethotoin has been reported, but if the drug is administered after meals, the incidence of gastric distress is reduced. Other side effects have included chest pain, nystagmus, diplopia, fever, dizziness, diarrhea, headache, insomnia, fatigue, numbness and skin rash.

OVERDOSAGE

Symptoms of acute overdosage include drowsiness, visual disturbance, nausea and ataxia. Coma is possible at very high dosage.

Treatment should be begun by inducing emesis; gastric lavage may be considered as an alternative. General supportive measures will be necessary. A careful evaluation of blood-forming organs should be made following recovery.

DOSAGE AND ADMINISTRATION

Ethotoin is administered orally in 4 to 6 divided doses daily. The drug should be taken after food, and doses should be spaced as evenly as practicable. Initial dosage should be conservative. For adults, the initial daily dose should be 1 g or less, with subsequent gradual dosage increases over a period of several days. The optimum dosage must be determined on the basis of individual response. The usual adult maintenance dose is 2 to 3 g daily. Less than 2 g daily has been found ineffective in most adults.

Pediatric dosage depends upon the age and weight of the patient. The initial dose should not exceed 750 mg daily. The usual maintenance dose in children ranges from 500 mg to 1 g daily, although occasionally 2 or (rarely) 3 g daily may be necessary.

If a patient is receiving another antiepileptic drug, it should not be discontinued when Ethotoin therapy is begun. The dosage of the other drug should be reduced gradually as that of Ethotoin is increased. Ethotoin may eventually replace the other drug or the optimal dosage of both antiepileptics may be established.

Ethotoin is compatible with all commonly employed antiepileptic medications with the possible exception of phenacemide. In tonic-clonic (grand mal) seizures, use of the drug with phenobarbital may be beneficial. Ethotoin may be used in combination with drugs such as trimethadione or paramethadione as an adjunct in those patients with absence (petit mal) associated with tonic-clonic (grand mal).

Tablets (Recommended Storage): Store below 77°F (25°C)

▶ SHOWN IN PRODUCT IDENTIFICATION GUIDE

HOW SUPPLIED
TABLETS: 250 MG

BRAND/MANUFACTURER	NDC	SIZE	AWP
○ **BRAND**			
PEGANONE: Abbott Pharm	00074-6902-01	100s	$39.74

TABLETS: 500 MG

BRAND/MANUFACTURER	NDC	SIZE	AWP
○ **BRAND**			
PEGANONE: Abbott Pharm	00074-6905-04	100s	$74.56

Ethrane SEE ENFLURANE

Ethyl Chloride

INDICATIONS AND USAGE
Ethyl Chloride is a vapocoolant intended for topical application to control pain associated with minor surgical procedures (such as lancing boils, or incision and drainage of small abscesses), athletic injuries, injections, and for treatment of myofascial pain, restricted motion, and muscle spasm.

PRECAUTIONS
Inhalation of Ethyl Chloride should be avoided as it may produce narcotic and general anesthetic effects, and may produce deep anesthesia or fatal coma with respiratory or cardiac arrest. Ethyl Chloride is flammable and should never be used in the presence of an open flame, or electrical cautery equipment. When used to produce local freezing of tissues, adjacent skin areas should be protected by application of petrolatum. The thawing process may be painful, and freezing may lower local resistance to infection and delay healing.

ADVERSE REACTIONS
Cutaneous sensitization may occur, but appears to be extremely rare. Freezing can occasionally alter pigmentation.

CONTRAINDICATIONS
Ethyl Chloride is contraindicated in individuals with a history of hypersensitivity to it. This product should not be used on patients having vascular impairment of the extremities.

WARNINGS
For external use only.

Skin absorption of Ethyl Chloride can occur; no cases of chronic poisoning have been reported. Ethyl Chloride is known as a liver and kidney toxin; long term exposure may cause liver or kidney damage.

DOSAGE AND ADMINISTRATION
To apply Ethyl Chloride from metal tube, invert nozzle 12 inches (30 cm.) above the treatment area. Open adjustable dispensing valve until the spray flows freely.

To apply Ethyl Chloride from amber bottle with dispensal valve, invert over the treatment area approximately 12 inches (30 cm.) away from site of application. Open dispenseal spring valve completely allowing Ethyl Chloride to flow in a stream from the bottle.

1. TOPICAL ANESTHESIA IN MINOR SURGERY
The operative site should be cleansed with a suitable antiseptic. Apply petrolatum to protect the adjacent area. Spray Ethyl Chloride for a few seconds to the point of frost formation, when the tissue becomes white. Avoid prolonged spraying of skin beyond this state. The anesthetic action of Ethyl Chloride rarely lasts more than a few seconds to a minute. Quickly swab operative site with antiseptic and promptly make incision. Reapply as needed.

2. SPORTS INJURIES
The pain of bruises, contusions, abrasions, swelling, and minor sprains may be controlled with Ethyl Chloride.

Spray affected area for a few seconds until the tissue begins to frost and turn white. Avoid spraying of skin beyond this state. Use as you would ice. The amount of cooling depends on the dosage. The smallest dose needed to produce the desired effect should be used. Dosage varies with the nozzle size and duration of application.

Determine the extent of injury (fracture, sprain, etc.). The anesthetic effect of Ethyl Chloride rarely lasts more than a few seconds to a minute. This time interval is usually sufficient to help reduce or relieve the initial trauma of the injury.

3. FOR PRE-INJECTION ANESTHESIA
Prepare syringe and have it ready. Spray skin with Ethyl Chloride from a distance of about 12 inches (30 cm.) continuously for 3 to 5 seconds; do not frost skin. Swab skin with alcohol and quickly introduce needle with skin taut.

4. SPRAY AND STRETCH TECHNIQUE FOR MYOFASCIAL PAIN
Ethyl Chloride may be used as a counterirritant in the management of myofascial pain, restricted motion, and muscle spasm. Clinical conditions that may respond to Ethyl Chloride include low back pain (due to muscle spasm), acute stiff neck, torticollis, acute bursitis of the shoulder, muscle spasm associated with osteoarthritis, tight hamstring, sprained ankle, masseter muscle spasm, certain types of headache, and referred pain due to irritated trigger point. Relief of pain facilitates early mobilization in restoration of muscle function. The Spray and Stretch technique is a therapeutic system which involves three stages: EVALUATION, SPRAYING, and STRETCHING.

The therapeutic value of Spray and Stretch becomes most effective when the practitioner has mastered all stages and applies them in the proper sequence.

I. EVALUATION
During the evaluation phase the cause of pain is determined as local spasm or an irritated trigger point. The method of applying the spray to a muscle spasm differs slightly from application to a trigger point. A trigger point is a deep hypersensitive localized spot in a muscle which causes a referred pain pattern. With trigger points the source of pain is seldom the site of the pain. A trigger point may be detected by a snapping palpation over the muscle, causing the muscle in which the irritated trigger point is situated to "jump".

II. SPRAYING
A. Patient should assume a comfortable position.

B. Take precautions to cover the patient's eyes, nose, mouth, if spraying near face.

C. Hold bottle in an upside down position 12 to 18 inches (30 to 45 cm.) away from the treatment surface allowing the jet stream of vapocoolant to meet the skin at an acute angle to lessen the shock of impact.

D. The spray is directed in parallel sweeps 1.5 to 2 cm. apart. The rate of spraying is approximately 10 cm/sec. and is continued until the entire muscle has been covered. The number of sweeps is determined by the size of the muscle. In the case of trigger point, the spray should be applied over the trigger point, through and over the reference zone. In the case of muscle spasm, the spray should be applied from origin to insertion.

III. STRETCHING
During application of the spray, the muscle is passively stretched. Force is gradually increased with successive sweeps, and the slack is smoothly taken up as the muscle relaxes, establishing a new stretch length.

Reaching the full normal length of the muscle is necessary to completely inactivate trigger points and relieve pain.

After rewarming, the procedure may be repeated as necessary. Moist heat should be applied for 10 to 15 minutes following treatment. For lasting benefit, any factors that perpetuate the trigger mechanism must be eliminated.

Contents under pressure. Store in a cool place. Do not store above 120° F. Do not store on or near high frequency ultrasound equipment.

HOW SUPPLIED
POWDER:

BRAND/MANUFACTURER	NDC	SIZE	AWP
○ **GENERICS**			
Lannett	00527-0747-85	100 gm	$8.25
	17137-0754-04	125 gm	$12.60

SPRAY:

BRAND/MANUFACTURER	NDC	SIZE	AWP
○ **GENERICS**			
Gebauer	00386-0001-01	105 ml	$9.09
Gebauer	00386-0001-05	105 ml	$18.11
Allscrips	54569-2302-00	120 ml	$5.85
Gebauer	00386-0001-02	120 ml	$8.77
Gebauer	00386-0001-03	120 ml	$8.77
Gebauer	00386-0001-04	120 ml	$8.77

Etidocaine Hydrochloride

DESCRIPTION
Etidocaine Hydrochloride Injections are sterile aqueous solutions that contain a local anestheic agent and are administered parenterally by injection See "Indications and Usage" for specific uses. The specific quantitative composition of each available solution is shown in Table 1. Etidocaine HCl is chemically designated as butanamide, N-(2,6-dimethylphenyl)-2-(ethylpropylamine)-, monohydrochloride.

Epinephrine is (-)-3, 4-Dihydroxy-α-[(methylamino)methyl] benzyl alcohol.

The pK_a of Etidocaine (7.74) is similar to that of lidocaine (7.86). However, Etidocaine possesses a greater degree of lipid solubility and protein binding capacity than does lidocaine. Etidocaine Hydrochloride Injections are sterile and, except for the 1.5% concentration, are available with or without epinephrine 1:200,000. Single dose containers of Etidocaine Hydrochloride Injection without epinephrine may be reautoclaved if necessary.

See Table 1 for composition of available injections. (See related table).

CLINICAL PHARMACOLOGY
Mechanism of Action: Etidocaine stabilizes the neuronal membrane by inhibiting the ionic fluxes required for the initiation and conduction of impulses, thereby effecting local anesthetic action.

Onset and Duration of Action: In vivo animal studies have shown that Etidocaine has a rapid onset (3-5 minutes) and a prolonged duration of action (5-10 hours).

Based on comparative clinical studies of lidocaine and Etidocaine, the anesthetic properties of Etidocaine in man may be characterized as follows: Initial onset of sensory analgesia and motor blockade is rapid (usually 3-5 minutes) and similar to that produced by lidocaine. Duration of sensory analgesia is 1.5 to 2 times longer than that of lidocaine by the peridural route. The difference in analgesic duration between Etidocaine and lidocaine may be even greater following peripheral nerve blockade than following central neural block. Duration of analgesia in excess of 9 hours is not infrequent when Etidocaine is used for peripheral nerve blocks such as brachial plexus blockade. Etidocaine produces a profound degree of motor blockade and abdominal muscle relaxation when used for peridural analgesia.

Hemodynamics: Excessive blood levels may cause changes in cardiac output, total peripheral resistance, and mean arterial pressure. With central neural blockade these changes may be attributable to block of autonomic fibers, a direct depressant effect of the local anesthetic agent on various components of the cardiovascular system, and/or the beta-adrenergic receptor stimulating action of epinephrine when present. The net effect is normally a modest hypotension when the recommended dosages are not exceeded.

Pharmacokinetics and Metabolism: Information derived from diverse formulations, concentrations and usages reveals that Etidocaine is completely absorbed following parenteral administration, its rate of absorption depending, for example, upon such factors as the site of administration and the presence or absence of a vasoconstrictor agent. Except for intravenous administration, the highest blood levels are obtained following intercostal nerve block and the lowest after subcutaneous administration.

The plasma binding of Etidocaine is dependent on drug concentration, and the fraction bound decreases with increasing concentration. At 0.5-1.0 µg/mL, 95% is bound to plasma protein.

Etidocaine crosses the blood-brain and placental barriers, presumably by passive diffusion.

Etidocaine is metabolized rapidly by the liver, and metabolites and unchanged drug are excreted by the kidney. Biotransformation includes oxidative N-dealkylation, ring hydroxylation, cleavage of the amide linkage, and conjugation. To date, approximately 20 metabolites of Etidocaine have been found in the urine. The percent of dose excreted as unchanged drug is less than 10%.

The mean elimination half-life of Etidocaine following a bolus intravenous injection is about 2.5 hours. Because of the rapid rate at which Etidocaine is metabolized, any condition that affects liver function may alter Etidocaine kinetics. Renal dysfunction may not affect Etidocaine kinetics but may increase the accumulation of metabolites.

Factors such as acidosis and the concomitant use of CNS stimulants and depressants affect the CNS levels of Etidocaine required to produce overt systemic effects. In the rhesus monkey, arterial blood levels of 4.5 µg/mL have been shown to be threshold for convulsive activity.

INDICATIONS AND USAGE
Etidocaine Hydrochloride Injections are indicated for infiltration anesthesia, peripheral nerve blocks (e.g., brachial plexus, intercostal, retrobulbar, ulnar, inferior alveolar), and central neural block (i.e., lumbar or caudal epidural blocks).

UNLABELED USES
Etidocaine is also used alone or as an adjunct in reducing postoperative analgesic requirements following fallopian tube banding and laproscopic tubal occlusion.

CONTRAINDICATIONS
Etidocaine is contraindicated in patients with a known history of hypersensitivity to local anesthetics of the amide type.

WARNINGS
ETIDOCAINE HYDROCHLORIDE INJECTIONS FOR INFILTRATION AND NERVE BLOCK SHOULD BE EMPLOYED ONLY BY CLINICIANS WHO ARE WELL VERSED IN DIAGNOSIS AND MANAGEMENT OF DOSE-RELATED TOXICITY AND OTHER ACUTE EMERGENCIES THAT MIGHT ARISE FROM THE BLOCK TO BE EMPLOYED AND THEN ONLY AFTER ENSURING THE *IMMEDIATE* AVAILABILITY OF OXYGEN, OTHER RESUSCITATIVE DRUGS, CARDIOPULMONARY EQUIPMENT, AND THE PERSONNEL NEEDED FOR PROPER MANAGEMENT OF TOXIC REACTIONS AND RELATED EMERGENCIES (see also *"Adverse Reactions"* and *"Precautions"*). DELAY IN PROPER MANAGEMENT OF DOSE-RELATED TOXICITY, UNDERVENTILATION FROM ANY CAUSE AND/OR ALTERED SENSITIVITY MAY LEAD TO THE DEVELOPMENT OF ACIDOSIS, CARDIAC ARREST, AND, POSSIBLY DEATH.

To avoid intravascular injection, aspiration should be performed before the local anesthetic solution is injected. The needle must be repositioned until no return of blood can be elicited by aspiration. Note, however, that the absence of blood in the syringe does not guarantee that intravascular injection has been avoided.

Local anesthetic solutions containing antimicrobial preservatives (e.g., methylparaben) should not be used for epidural anesthesia because the safety of these agents has not been established with regard to intrathecal injection, either intentional or accidental.

Vasopressor agents administered for the treatment of hypotension related to caudal or other epidural blocks should not be used in the presence of ergot-type oxytocic drugs, since severe persistent hypertension and even rupture of cerebral blood vessels may occur.

Etidocaine Hydrochloride with epinephrine solutions contain sodium metabisulfite, a sulfite that may cause allergic-type reactions including anaphylactic symptoms and life-threatening or less severe asthmatic episodes in certain susceptible people. The overall prevalence of sulfite sensitivity in the general population is unknown and probably low. Sulfite sensitivity is seen more frequently in asthmatic than in nonasthmatic people.

PRECAUTIONS
General: The safety and effectiveness of Etidocaine depend on proper dosage, correct technique, adequate precautions, and readiness for emergencies. Standard textbooks should be consulted for specific techniques and precautions for various regional anesthetic procedures. Resuscitative equipment, oxygen, and other resuscitative drugs should be available for immediate use. (See *"Warnings and Adverse Reactions"*.) The lowest dosage that results in effective anesthesia should be used to avoid high plasma levels and serious adverse effects. Syringe aspirations should also be performed before and during each supplemental injection when using indwelling catheter techniques. During the administration of epidural anesthesia, it is recommended that a test dose be administered initially and that the patient be monitored for central nervous system toxicity and cardiovascular toxicity, as well as for signs of unintended intrathecal administration, before proceeding. When clinical conditions permit, consideration should be given to employing local anesthetic solutions that contain epinephrine for the test dose because circulatory changes compatible with epinephrine may also serve as a warning sign of unintended intravascular injection. An intravascular injection is still possible even if aspirations for blood are negative. Repeated doses of Etidocaine may cause significant increases in blood levels with each repeated dose because of slow accumulation of the drug or its metabolites. Tolerance to elevated blood levels varies with the status of the patient. Debilitated, elderly patients, acutely ill patients, and children should be given reduced doses commensurate with their age and physical condition. Etidocaine should also be used with caution in patients with severe shock or heart block.

Lumbar and caudal epidural anesthesia should be used with extreme caution in persons with the following conditions: existing neurological disease, spinal deformities, septicemia, and severe hypertension.

Local anesthetic solutions containing a vasoconstrictor should be used cautiously and in carefully circumscribed quantities in areas of the body supplied by end arteries or having otherwise compromised blood supply. Patients with peripheral vascular disease and those with hypertensive vascular disease may exhibit exaggerated vasoconstrictor response. Ischemic injury or necrosis may result. Preparations containing a vasoconstrictor should be used with caution in patients during or following the administration of potent general anesthetic agents, since cardiac arrhythmias may occur under such conditions.

Careful and constant monitoring of cardiovascular and respiratory (adequacy of ventilation) vital signs and the patient's state of consciousness should be accomplished after each local anesthetic injection. It should be kept in mind at such times that restlessness, anxiety, tinnitus, dizziness, blurred vision, tremors, depression or drowsiness may be early warning signs of central nervous system toxicity.

Since amide-type local anesthetics are metabolized by the liver, Etidocaine Hydrochloride Injections should be used with caution in patients with hepatic disease.

Patients with severe hepatic disease, because of their inability to metabolize local anesthetics normally, are a greater risk of developing toxic plasma concentrations. Etidocaine Hydrochloride Injection should also be used with caution in patients with impaired cardiovascular function since they may be less able to compensate for functional changes associated with the prolongation of A-V conduction produced by these drugs. Many drugs used during the conduct of anesthesia are considered potential triggering agents for familial malignant

Table 1.
COMPOSITION OF AVAILABLE INJECTIONS

Etidocaine Hydrochloride Concentration %	Production Identification			Formula		
	Epinephrine Dilution (as the bitartrate)	pH	Sodium chloride (mg/mL)	Single Dose Vials/ Dental Cartridge Sodium metabisulfite (mg/mL)	Citric acid (mg/mL)	
1.0	None	4.0-5.0	7.1	None	—	
1.0	1:200,000	3.0-4.5	7.1	0.5	0.2	
1.5	1:200,000	3.0-4.5	6.2	0.5	0.2	

Note: pH of all solutions adjusted with sodium hydroxide and/or hydrochloric acid. Duranest dental cartridges are only available as 1.5% solution with epinephrine 1:200,000. Filled under nitrogen.

hyperthermia. Since it is not known whether amide-type local anesthetics may trigger this reaction and since the need for supplemental general anesthesia cannot be predicted in advance, it is suggested that a standard protocol for the management of malignant hyperthermia should be available. Early unexplained signs of tachycardia, tachypnea, labile blood pressure and metabolic acidosis may precede temperature elevation. Successful outcome is dependent on early diagnosis, prompt discontinuance of the suspect triggering agent(s) and institution of treatment, including oxygen therapy, indicated supportive measures and dantrolene (consult dantrolene sodium intravenous package insert before using).

Etidocaine should be used with caution in persons with known drug sensitivities. Patients allergic to para-aminobenzoic acid derivatives (procaine, tetracaine, benzocaine, etc.) have not shown cross sensitivity to Etidocaine.

Use in the Head and Neck Area: Small doses of local anesthetics injected into the head and neck area, including retrobulbar, dental and stellate ganglion blocks, may produce adverse reactions similar to systemic toxicity seen with unintentional intravascular injections of larger doses. The injection procedures require the utmost care. Confusion, convulsions, respiratory depression and/or respiratory arrest, and cardiovascular stimulation or depression have been reported. These reactions may be due to intra-arterial injection of the local anesthetic with retrograde flow to the cerebral circulation. They may also be due to puncture of the dural sheath of the optic nerve during retrobulbar block with diffusion of any local anesthetic along the subdural space to the midbrain. Patients receiving these blocks should have their circulation and respiration monitored and be constantly observed. Resuscitative equipment and personnel for treating adverse reactions should be immediately available. Dosage recommendations should not be exceeded. (See *"Dosage and Administration".*)

Use in Ophthalmic Surgery: When local anesthetic injections are employed for retrobulbar block, lack of corneal sensation should not be relied upon to determine whether or not the patient is ready for surgery. This is because complete lack of corneal sensation usually precedes clinically acceptable external ocular muscle akinesia.

Use in Dentistry: Because of the long duration of anesthesia, when Etidocaine Hydrochloride 1.5% with epinephrine is used for dental injections, patients should be cautioned about the possibility of inadvertent trauma to tongue, lips and buccal mucosa and advised not to chew solid foods or test the anesthetized area by biting or probing.

Information for Patient: When appropriate, patients should be informed in advance that they may experience temporary loss of sensation and motor activity, usually in the lower half of the body, following proper administration of epidural anesthesia.

Clinically Significant Drug Interactions: The administration of local anesthetic solutions containing epinephrine or norepinephrine to patients receiving monoamine oxidase inhibitors, tricyclic antidepressants or phenothiazines may produce severe, prolonged hypotension or hypertension. Concurrent use of these agents should generally be avoided. In situations when concurrent therapy is necessary, careful patient monitoring is essential.

Concurrent administration of vasopressor drugs (for the treatment of hypotension related to epidural blocks) and ergot-type oxytocic drugs may cause severe, persistent hypertension or cerebrovascular accidents.

Drug/Laboratory Test Interactions: The intramuscular injection of Etidocaine may result in an increase in creatine phosphokinase levels. Thus, the use of this enzyme determination, without isoenzyme separation, as a diagnostic test for the presence of acute myocardial infarction may be compromised by the intramuscular injection of Etidocaine.

Carcinogenesis, Mutagenesis, Impairment of Fertility: Studies of Etidocaine in animals to evaluate the carcinogenic and mutagenic potential have not been conducted. Studies in rats at 1.7 times the maximum recommended human dose have revealed no impairment of fertility.

Use in Pregnancy: Teratogenic Effects. Pregnancy Category B. Reproduction studies have been performed in rats and rabbits at doses up to 1.7 times the human dose and have revealed no evidence of harm to the fetus caused by Etidocaine. There are, however, no adequate and well-controlled studies in pregnant women. Animal reproduction studies are not always predictive of human response. General consideration should be given to this fact before administering Etidocaine to women of childbearing potential, especially during early pregnancy when maximum organogenesis takes place.

Labor and Delivery: Local anesthetics rapidly cross the placenta and when used for epidural, paracervical, pudendal or caudal block anesthesia, can cause varying degrees of maternal, fetal and neonatal toxicity. (See *"Clinical Pharmacology— Pharmacokinetics".*) The incidence and degree of toxicity depend upon the procedure performed, the type and amount of drug used, and the technique of drug administration. Adverse reactions in the parturient, fetus and neonate involve alterations of the central nervous system, peripheral vascular tone and cardiac function.

Maternal hypotension has resulted from regional anesthesia. Local anesthetics produce vasodilation by blocking sympathetic nerves. Elevating the patient's legs and positioning her on her left side will help prevent decreases in blood pressure. The fetal heart rate also should be monitored continuously and electronic fetal monitoring is highly advisable.

Epidural anesthesia may alter the forces of parturition through changes in uterine contractility or maternal expulsive efforts. Because Etidocaine Hydrochloride Injection may produce profound motor block, it is not recommended for

epidural anesthesia in normal delivery. Etidocaine Hydrochloride Injection is, however, recommended for epidural anesthesia when caesarean section is to be performed.

The use of some local anesthetic drug products during labor and delivery may be followed by diminished muscle strength and tone for the first day or two of life. The long-term significance of these observations is unknown.

Fetal bradycardia may occur in 20 to 30 percent of patients receiving paracervical nerve block anesthesia with the amide-type local anesthetics and may be associated with fetal acidosis. Fetal heart rate should always be monitored during paracervical anesthesia. The physician should weigh the possible advantages against risks when considering paracervical block in prematurity, toxemia of pregnancy, and fetal distress. Careful adherence to recommended dosage is of the utmost importance in obstetrical paracervical block. Failure to achieve adequate analgesia with recommended doses should arouse suspicion of intravascular or fetal intracranial injection. Cases compatible with unintended fetal intracranial injection of local anesthetic solution have been reported following intended paracervical or pudendal block or both. Babies so affected present with unexplained neonatal depression at birth, which correlates with high local anesthetic serum levels, and often manifest seizures within six hours. Prompt use of supportive measures combined with forced urinary excretion of the local anesthetic has been used successfully to manage this complication. Case reports of maternal convulsions and cardiovascular collapse following use of some local anesthetics for paracervical block in early pregnancy (as anesthesia for elective abortion) suggest that systemic absorption under these circumstances may be rapid. There are inadequate data in support of safe and effective use of Etidocaine for obstetrical or non-obstetrical paracervical block, therefore, such use is not recommended.

Nursing Mothers: It is not known whether this drug is excreted in human milk. Because many drugs are excreted in human milk, caution should be exercised when Etidocaine is administered to a nursing woman.

Pediatric Use: No information is currently available on appropriate pediatric doses.

ADVERSE REACTIONS

Systemic: Adverse experiences following the administration of Etidocaine are similar in nature to those observed with other amide local anesthetic agents. These adverse experiences are, in general, dose-related and may result from high plasma levels caused by excessive dosage, rapid absorption or unintended intravascular injection, or may result from a hypersensitivity, idiosyncrasy or diminished tolerance on the part of the patient. Serious adverse experiences are generally systemic in nature. The following types are those most commonly reported:

Central Nervous System: CNS manifestations are excitatory and/or depressant and may be characterized by lightheadedness, nervousness, apprehension, euphoria, confusion, dizziness, drowsiness, tinnitus, blurred or double vision, vomiting, sensations of heat, cold or numbness, twitching, tremors, convulsions, unconsciousness, respiratory depression and arrest. The excitatory manifestations may be very brief or may not occur at all, in which case the first manifestation of toxicity may be drowsiness merging into unconsciousness and respiratory arrest.

Drowsiness following the administration of Etidocaine is usually an early sign of a high blood level of the drug and may occur as a consequence of rapid absorption.

Cardiovascular System: Cardiovascular manifestations are usually depressant and are characterized by bradycardia, hypotension, and cardiovascular collapse, which may lead to cardiac arrest.

Allergic: Allergic reactions are characterized by cutaneous lesions, urticaria, edema or anaphylactoid reactions. Allergic reactions may occur as a result of sensitivity either to local anesthetic agents or to the methylparaben used as a preservative in multiple dose vials. The detection of sensitivity by skin testing is of doubtful value.

Neurologic: The incidences of adverse reactions associated with the use of local anesthetics may be related to the total dose of local anesthetic administered and are also dependent upon the particular drug used, the route of administration and the physical status of the patient.

In the practice of caudal or lumbar epidural block, occasional unintentional penetration of the subarachnoid space by the catheter may occur. Subsequent adverse effects may depend partially on the amount of drug administered subdurally. These may include spinal block of varying magnitude (including total spinal block), hypotension secondary to spinal block, loss of bladder and bowel control, and loss of perineal sensation and sexual function. Persistent motor, sensory and/or autonomic (sphincter control) deficit of some lower spinal segments with slow recovery (several months) or incomplete recovery have been reported in rare instances when caudal or lumbar epidural block has been attempted. Backache and headache have also been noted following use of these anesthetic procedures.

Other: There have been rare reports of TRISMUS in patients who have received Etidocaine Hydrochloride for dental anesthesia. Onset of symptoms occurs within hours or days upon resolution of blockade. No correlation has been demonstrated with dosage, administration technique or dental procedure. In most patients, symptoms resolved within days to weeks, although some reports have suggested that symptoms were present for many months. Symptomatic treatment with analgesics, moist heat and physiotherapy was helpful in some cases.

◆ RATED THERAPEUTICALLY EQUIVALENT; ◇ THERAPEUTIC EQUIVALENCE UNCONFIRMED; ○ UNRATED

OVERDOSAGE

Acute emergencies from local anesthetics are generally related to high plasma levels encountered during therapeutic use of local anesthetics or to unintended subarachnoid injection of local anesthetic solution (see "Adverse Reactions, Warnings," and "Precautions").

Management of Local Anesthetic Emergencies: The first consideration is prevention, best accomplished by careful and constant monitoring of cardiovascular and respiratory vital signs and the patient's state of consciousness after each local anesthetic injection. At the first sign of change, oxygen should be administered.

The first step in the management of convulsions, as well as underventilation or apnea due to unintentional subarachnoid injection of drug solution, consists of immediate attention to the maintenance of a patent airway and assisted or controlled ventilation with oxygen and a delivery system capable of permitting immediate positive airway pressure by mask. Immediately after the institution of these ventilatory measures, the adequacy of the circulation should be evaluated, keeping in mind that drugs used to treat convulsions sometimes depress the circulation when administered intravenously. Should convulsions persist despite adequate respiratory support, and if the status of the circulation permits, small increments of an ultra-short acting barbiturate (such as thiopental or thiamylal) or a benzodiazepine (such as diazepam) may be administered intravenously. The clinician should be familiar, prior to use of local anesthetics, with these anticonvulsant drugs. Supportive treatment of circulatory depression may require administration of intravenous fluids and, when appropriate, a vasopressor as directed by the clinical situation (e.g., ephedrine).

If not treated immediately, both convulsions and cardiovascular depression can result in hypoxia, acidosis, bradycardia, arrhythmias and cardiac arrest. Underventilation or apnea due to unintentional subarachnoid injection of local anesthetic solution may produce these same signs and also lead to cardiac arrest if ventilatory support is not instituted. If cardiac arrest should occur, standard cardiopulmonary resuscitative measures should be instituted.

Endotracheal intubation, employing drugs and techniques familiar to the clinician, may be indicated, after initial administration of oxygen by mask, if difficulty is encountered in the maintenance of a patent airway or if prolonged ventilatory support (assisted or controlled) is indicated.

Dialysis is of negligible value in the treatment of acute overdosage with Etidocaine.

The intravenous LD$_{50}$ of Etidocaine Hydrochloride in female mice is 7.6 (6.6-8.5) mg/kg and the subcutaneous LD$_{50}$ is 112 (96-166) mg/kg.

DOSAGE AND ADMINISTRATION

As with all local anesthetic agents, the dose of Etidocaine Hydrochloride Injection to be employed will depend upon the area to be anesthetized, the vascularity of the tissues, the number of neuronal segments to be blocked, the type of regional anesthetic technique, and the physical condition and tolerance of the individual patient.

The maximum dose to be employed as a single injection should be determined on the basis of the status of the patient and the type of regional anesthetic technique to be performed. Although single injections of 450 mg have been employed for regional anesthesia without adverse effects, at present it is strongly recommended that the maximal dose as a single injection should not exceed 400 mg (approximately 8.0 mg/kg or 3.6 mg/lb based on a 50 kg person) with epinephrine 1:200,000 and 300 mg (approximately 6 mg/kg or 2.7 mg/lb based on a 50 kg person) without epinephrine. Because Etidocaine has been shown to disappear quite rapidly from blood, toxicity is influenced by rapidity of administration, and therefore, slow injection in vascular areas is highly recommended. Incremental doses of Etidocaine Hydrochloride Injection may be repeated at 2-3 hour intervals.

Caudal and Lumbar Epidural Block: As a precaution against the adverse experiences sometimes observed following unintentional penetration of the subarachnoid space, a test dose of 2-5 mL should be administered at least 5 minutes prior to injecting the total volume required for a lumbar or caudal epidural block. The test dose should be repeated if the patient is moved in a manner that may have displaced the catheter. Epinephrine, if contained in the test dose (10-15μg have been suggested), may serve as a warning of unintentional intravascular injection. If injected into a blood vessel, this amount of epinephrine is likely to produce a transient "epinephrine response" within 45 seconds, consisting of an increase in heart rate and systolic blood pressure, circumoral pallor, palpitations and nervousness in the unsedated patient. The sedated patient may exhibit only a pulse rate increase of 20 or more beats per minute for 15 or more seconds. Patients on beta-blockers may not manifest changes in heart rate, but blood pressure monitoring can detect an evanescent rise in systolic blood pressure. Adequate time should be allowed for onset of anesthesia after administration of each test dose. The rapid injection of a large volume of Etidocaine Hydrochloride Injection through the catheter should be avoided, and when feasible, fractional doses should be administered.

In the event of the known injection of a large volume of local anesthetic solution into the subarachnoid space, after suitable resuscitation; and if the catheter is in place, consider attempting the recovery of drug by draining a moderate amount of cerebrospinal fluid (such as 10 mL) through the epidural catheter.

Use in Dentistry: When used for local anesthesia in dental procedures the dosage of Etidocaine Hydrochloride Injection depends on the physical status of the patient, the area of the oral cavity to be anesthetized, the vascularity of the oral tissues, and the technique of anesthesia. The least volume of solution that results in effective local anesthesia should be administered. For specific techniques and procedures of local anesthesia in the oral cavity, refer to standard textbooks.

Dosage requirements should be determined on an individual basis. In maxillary infiltration and/or inferior alveolar nerve block, initial dosages of 1.0-5.0 mL (1/2-2 1/2 cartridges) of Etidocaine Hydrochloride Injection 1.5% with epinephrine 1:200,000 are usually effective.

Aspiration is recommended since it reduces the possibility of intravascular injection, thereby keeping the incidence of side effects and anesthetic failures to a minimum.

The following dosage recommendations are intended as guides for the use of Etidocaine Hydrochloride Injection in the average adult patient. As indicated previously, the dosage should be reduced for elderly or debilitated patients or patients with severe renal disease.

NOTE

Parenteral drug products should be inspected visually for particulate matter and discoloration prior to administration whenever the solution and container permit. The Injection is not to be used if its color is pinkish or darker than slightly yellow or if it contains a precipitate.

Store at controlled room temperature 15°-30°C (59°-86°F).

Table 2.
DOSAGE RECOMMENDATIONS

Procedure	Etidocaine Hydrochloride with epinephrine 1:200,000		
	Conc. (%)	Vol. (mL)	Total Dose (mg)
Peripheral Nerve Block	1.0	5-40	50-400
Central Neural Block Lumbar Peridural Intraabdominal or Pelvic Surgery	1.0	10-30	100-300
Lower Limb Surgery or Caesarean Section	1.5	10-20	150-300
Caudal	1.0	10-30	100-300
Retrobulbar	1.0 or 1.5	2-4	20-60
Maxillary Infiltration and/or Inferior Alveolar Nerve Block	1.5	1-5	15-75

HOW SUPPLIED

ETIDOCAINE HYDROCHLORIDE

INJECTION: 1%

BRAND/MANUFACTURER	NDC	SIZE	AWP
○ BRAND DURANEST: Astra	00186-0820-01	30 ml	$17.26

EPINEPHRINE BITARTRATE/ETIDOCAINE HYDROCHLORIDE

INJECTION:

BRAND/MANUFACTURER	NDC	SIZE	AWP
○ BRAND DURANEST W/EPINEPHRINE: Astra	00186-0836-03	20 ml	$20.10
	00186-0825-01	30 ml	$18.78
	00186-0840-14	1.8 ml 100s	$62.50

Etidronate Disodium, Injectable

DESCRIPTION

Etidronate Disodium I.V. Infusion is a clear, colorless, sterile solution, the disodium salt of (1-hydroxyethylidene) diphosphonic acid. Each 6-ml ampule contains a 5% solution of 300 mg Etidronate Disodium in water for injection for slow intravenous infusion.

Etidronate Disodium is a white powder, highly soluble in water, with a molecular weight of 250.

Following is its chemical structure:

$$\begin{array}{c} O \\ \parallel \\ P-OH \\ \mid \\ ONa \\ CH_3-C-\\ \mid \\ ONa \\ \mid \\ P \\ \parallel \quad OH \\ O \end{array}$$

CLINICAL PHARMACOLOGY

Etidronate Disodium acts primarily on bone. Its major pharmacologic action is the reduction of normal and abnormal bone resorption. Secondarily, it reduces bone formation since formation is coupled to resorption. This reduces bone turnover, but the reduction of bone turnover, *per se*, is not the important action in the reduction of hypercalcemia.

Etidronate Disodium's reduction of abnormal bone resorption is responsible for its therapeutic benefit in hypercalcemia. The antiresorptive action of Etidronate Disodium has been demonstrated under a variety of conditions, although the exact mechanism(s) is not fully understood. It may be related to the drug's inhibition of hydroxyapatite crystal dissolution and/or its action on bone resorbing cells. The number of osteoclasts in active bone turnover sites is substantially reduced after Etidronate Disodium therapy is administered. Etidronate Disodium also can inhibit the formation and growth of hydroxyapatite crystals and their amorphous precursors at concentrations in excess of those required to inhibit crystal dissolution.

Etidronate Disodium is not metabolized. A large fraction of the infused dose is excreted rapidly and unchanged in the urine. The mean residence time in the exchangeable pool is approximately 8.7 ± 1.0 hours. The mean volume of distribution at steady-state in normal humans is 1370 ± 203 ml/kg while the plasma half-life ($t\frac{1}{2}$) is 6.0 ± 0.7 hours. In these same subjects, nonrenal clearance from the exchangeable pool amounts to 30-50% of the infused dose. This nonrenal clearance is considered to be due to uptake of the drug by bone; subsequently the drug is slowly eliminated through bone turnover. The half-life of the dose on bone is in excess of 90 days.

Hyperphosphatemia, which is often observed in association with oral Etidronate Disodium medication at doses of 10-20 mg/kg/day, occurs less frequently, in association with intravenous medication of patients with hypercalcemia of malignancy.

Hyperphosphatemia is apparently due to increased tubular reabsorption of phosphate by the kidney. No adverse effects have been associated with Etidronate Disodium-related hyperphosphatemia and its occurrence is not a contraindication to therapy. Serum phosphate elevations usually return to normal 2-4 weeks after medication is discontinued.

The responsiveness of animal tumors susceptible to four commonly employed classes or subclasses of chemotherapeutic agents, antitumor antibiotics (doxorubicin), a classic alkylating agent (cyclosphosphamide), a nitrosourea (carmustine), and a pyrimidine antagonist (5-fluorouracil), were not adversely altered by the concurrent administration of intravenous Etidronate Disodium.

Hypercalcemia of Malignancy: Hypercalcemia of malignancy is usually related to increased bone resorption associated with the presence of neoplastic tissue. It occurs in 8 to 20% of patients with malignant disease. Whereas hypercalcemia is more often seen in patients with demonstrable osteolytic, osteoblastic, or mixed metastatic tumors in bone, discrete skeletal lesions cannot be demonstrated in at least 30% of patients.

Patients with certain types of neoplasms, such as carcinoma of the breast, bronchogenic carcinoma, renal cell carcinoma, cancers of the head and neck, lymphomas, and multiple myeloma, are especially prone to developing hypercalcemia.

As hypercalcemia of malignancy evolves, the renal tubules develop a diminished capacity to concentrate urine. The resultant polyuria and nocturia decrease the extracellular fluid volume. This decrease may be aggravated by vomiting and reduced fluid intake. Thus, the ability of the kidney to eliminate excess calcium is compromised. Renal impairment can eventually cause nitrogen retention, acidosis, renal failure, and further decrease in excretion of calcium. Etidronate Disodium I.V. Infusion, by inhibiting excessive bone resorption, interrupts this process. Salt loading and use of "high ceiling" or "loop" diuretics may be used to promote calcium excretion, because the rate of renal calcium excretion is directly related to the rate of sodium excretion.

The physiologic derangements induced by excessive serum calcium are due to increased levels of ionized calcium. The pathophysiologic effects of excessive serum calcium are heightened by reductions in serum albumin which normally binds a fraction (about 40%) of the total serum calcium. In patients with hypercalcemia of malignancy, serum albumin is often reduced and this tends to mask the magnitude of the increase in the level of ionized calcium. By reducing the flow of calcium from resorbing bone, Etidronate Disodium I.V. Infusion effectively reduces total and ionized serum calcium.

In the principal clinical study of Etidronate Disodium for hypercalcemia of malignancy, patients with elevated calcium levels (10.1-17.4 mg/dl) were treated simultaneously with daily administrations of intravenous Etidronate Disodium over a 3-day period and up to 3000 ml of saline and 80 mg of loop diuretic. The response to treatment for these patients was compared with that from patients treated with saline and loop diuretics alone. In terms of total serum calcium changes, 88% of patients treated with Etidronate Disodium I.V. Infusion as described, had reductions of serum calcium of 1 mg/dl or more. Total serum calcium returned to normal in 63% of patients within 7 days compared to 33% of patients treated with hydration alone.

Reductions in urinary calcium excretion, which accompany reductions in excessive bone resorption, became apparent after 24 hours. This was accompanied or followed by maximum decreases in serum calcium which were observed, most frequently, 72 hours after the first infusion. The physiologically important component of serum calcium is the ionized portion. In most institutions, this cannot be measured directly. It is important to recognize that factors influencing the ratio of free and bound calcium such as serum proteins, particularly albumin, may complicate the interpretation of total serum calcium measurements. If indicated, a corrected serum calcium value should be calculated using an established algorithm.

When the total serum calcium values are adjusted for serum albumin levels, there was a return to normocalcemia in 24% of Etidronate Disodium-treated patients and in 7% of patients treated with saline infusion. Eighty-seven percent of patients receiving Etidronate Disodium and 67% of patients on saline had albumin-adjusted serum calcium levels returned to normal or reduced by at least 1 mg/dl.

In the above mentioned study, a second course of Etidronate Disodium I.V. Infusion was tried in a small number of patients who had a recurrence of hypercalcemia following an initial response to a 3-day infusion of the drug. All patients who received a second 3-day course of Etidronate Disodium I.V. Infusion showed a decrease of total serum calcium of at least 1 mg/dl. Normalization of total serum calcium occurred in 11 out of 14 patients.

Etidronate Disodium I.V. Infusion does not appear to alter renal tubular reabsorption of calcium, and does not affect hypercalcemia in patients with hyperparathyroidism where increased calcium reabsorption may be a factor in the hypercalcemia.

Limited clinical study results suggest that continuation of Etidronate Disodium therapy with oral tablets may maintain clinically acceptable serum calcium levels and prolong normocalcemia.

INDICATIONS AND USAGE

Etidronate Disodium I.V. Infusion, together with achievement and maintenance of adequate hydratio, is indicated for the treatment of hypercalcemia of malignancy inadequately managed by dietary modification and/or oral hydration.

In the treatment of hypercalcemia of malignancy, it is important to initiate rehydration with saline together with "high ceiling" or "loop" diuretics if indicated to restore urine output. This also is intended to increase the renal excretion of calcium and initiate a reduction in serum calcium. Since increased bone resorption is usually the underlying cause of an increased flux of calcium into the vascular compartment, concurrent therapy with Etidronate Disodium I.V. Infusion is recommended as soon as there is a restoration of urine output. Since Etidronate Disodium is excreted by the kidney, it is important to know that renal function is adequate to handle not only the increased fluid load but also the excretion of the drug itself. (See *"Warnings".*)

Etidronate Disodium I.V. Infusion is also indicated for the treatment of hypercalcemia of malignancy which persists after adequate hydration has been restored. Patients with and without metastases and with a variety of tumors have been responsive to treatment with Etidronate Disodium I.V. Infusion. Adequate hydration of patients should be maintained, but in aged patients and in those with cardiac failure, care must be taken to avoid overhydration.

CONTRAINDICATIONS

In patients with Class Dc and higher renal functional impairment (serum creatinine greater than 5.0 mg/dl) Etidronate Disodium I.V. Infusion should be withheld.

WARNINGS

Occasional mild to moderate abnormalities in renal function (elevated BUN and/or serum creatinine) have been observed when Etidronate Disodium I.V. Infusion was given as directed to patients with hypercalcemia of malignancy. These changes were reversible or remained stable, without worsening, after completion of the course of Etidronate Disodium I.V. Infusion. In some patients with pre-existing renal impairment or in those who had received potentially nephrotoxic drugs, further depression of renal function was sometimes seen. This suggests that Etidronate Disodium I.V. Infusion may produce or aggravate the depression of renal function in approximately 8 of 203 treatment courses when used to treat hypercalcemia of malignancy. Therefore, it is recommended that appropriate monitoring of renal function with serum creatinine and/or BUN be carried out with Etidronate Disodium I.V. Infusion treatment.

The effects of Etidronate Disodium I.V. Infusion administration on renal function in patients with serum creatinine greater than 2.5 mg/dl (Class Cc and higher, Classification of Renal Functional Impairment, Council on the Kidney in Cardiovascular Disease, American Heart Association, Ann. Int. Med. 75:251-52, 1971) has not been systematically examined in controlled trials.

Since Etidronate Disodium is excreted by the kidney, it is important to know that renal function is adequate to handle not only the increased fluid load but also the excretion of the drug itself. Since these capacities are impaired in patients with underlying renal disease and since experience with Etidronate Disodium I.V. Infusion in patients with serum creatinine > 2.5 mg/dl is limited, the use of Etidronate Disodium I.V. Infusion in such patients should occur only after a careful assessment of renal status or potential risks and potential benefits.

Reduction of the dose of Etidronate Disodium I.V. Infusion, if used at all, may be advisable in Class Cc renal functional impairment (serum creatinine 2.5 to 4.9 mg/dl); and, Etidronate Disodium I.V. Infusion be used only if the potential benefit of hypercalcemia correction will substantially exceed the potential for worsening of renal function. In patients with Class Dc and higher renal functional impairment (serum creatinine greater than 5.0 mg/dl) Etidronate Disodium I.V. Infusion should be withheld.

PRECAUTIONS
General: Hypercalcemia may cause or exacerbate impaired renal function. In clinical trials, while elevations of serum creatinine or blood urea nitrogen were seen in patients with hypercalcemia of malignancy prior to treatment with Etidronate Disodium I.V. Infusion, these measurements improved in some patients or remained unchanged in most patients. Nevertheless, elevations in serum creatinine during treatment with Etidronate Disodium I.V. Infusion have been observed in approximately 10% of patients.

Rare cases of acute renal failure have been reported in association with the use of Etidronate Disodium I.V. Infusion (see also *"Warnings"*). Concomitant use of non-steroidal anti-inflammatory drugs and diuretics in these patients may have contributed to the renal failure.

In animal preclinical studies, administration of Etidronate Disodium I.V. Infusion in amounts or at rates in excess of those recommended produced transient hypocalcemia or induced proximal renal tubular damage.

In the principal clinical trial of Etidronate Disodium I.V. Infusion, 33 of 185 patients (18%) treated one or more times with Etidronate Disodium I.V. Infusion had serum calcium values below the lower limits of normal. When adjusted for levels of reduced serum albumin, less than 1% of the 185 patients are estimated to have hypocalcemic ionized serum calcium levels. No adverse effects have been traced to hypocalcemia.

The hypercalcemia of hyperparathyroidism is refractory to Etidronate Disodium I.V. Infusion. It is possible for this disease to coexist in patients with malignancy.

Carcinogenesis, Mutagenesis, Impairment of Fertility: Longterm studies in rats indicate that Etidronate Disodium is not carcinogenic.

Pregnancy: Teratogenic Effects: Pregnancy Category C. Animal reproduction studies have not been conducted with Etidronate Disodium I.V. Infusion. It is also not known whether Etidronate Disodium I.V. Infusion can cause fetal harm when administered to a pregnant woman or can affect reproduction capacity. Etidronate Disodium I.V. Infusion should be given to a pregnant woman only if clearly needed.

Nursing Mothers: It is not known whether this drug is excreted in human milk. Because many drugs are excreted in human milk, caution should be exercised when Etidronate Disodium I.V. Infusion is administered to a nursing woman.

Pediatric Use: Safety and effectiveness in children have not been established.

ADVERSE REACTIONS
Hypercalcemia of malignancy is frequently associated with abnormal elevations of serum creatinine and BUN. One-third of the patients participating in multiclinic trials had such elevations before receiving Etidronate Disodium I.V. Infusion. In these trials, the elevations of BUN or serum creatinine improved in some patients, or remained unchanged in most patients; however, in approximately 10% of patients, occational mild to moderate abnormalities in renal function (increases of > 0.5 mg/dl serum creatinine) were observed during or immediately after treatment. The possibility that Etidronate Disodium I.V. Infusion contributed to these changes cannot be excluded (see *"Warnings"*).

Of patients who participated in the controlled hypercalcemia trials, 10 of 221 (5%) treatment courses reported a metallic or altered taste, or loss of taste, which usually disappeared within hours, during and/or shortly after Etidronate Disodium I.V. Infusion. A few patients with Paget's Disease of bone have reported allergic skin rashes in association with oral Etidronate Disodium medication.

OVERDOSAGE
Rapid intravenous administration of Etidronate Disodium at doses above 27 mg/kg has produced ECG changes and bleeding problems in animals. These abnormalities are probably related to marked and/or rapid decreases in ionized calcium levels in blood and tissue fluids. They are thought to be due to chelation of calcium by massive amounts of diphosphonate. These abnormalities have been shown to be reversible in animal studies by the administration of ionizable calcium salts.

Similar problems are not expected to occur in humans treated with Etidronate Disodium I.V. Infusion used as recommended (see *"Dosage and Administration"*). Moreover, signs and symptoms of hypocalcemia such as paresthesias and carpopedal spasms have not been reported. The chelation effects of the diphosphonate, should they occur in man, should be reversible with the intravenous administration of calcium gluconate.

Administration of intravenous etidronate disodium at doses and possibly at rates in excess of those recommended has been reported to be associated with renal insufficiency.

DOSAGE AND ADMINISTRATION
Etidronate Disodium I.V. Infusion: The recommended dose of Etidronate Disodium I.V. Infusion is 7.5 mg/kg body weight/day for three successive days. **This daily dose must be diluted in at least 250 ml of sterile normal saline.** Stability studies show that diluted solution stored at controlled room temperature (59°F to 86°F or 15°C to 30°C) shows no loss of drug for a 48-hour period. THE DILUTED DOSE OF ETIDRONATE DISODIUM I.V. INFUSION SHOULD BE ADMINISTERED INTRAVENOUSLY OVER A PERIOD OF AT LEAST 2 HOURS. Etidronate Disodium I.V. Infusion may be added to volumes of fluid greater than 250 ml when this is convenient.

REGARDLESS OF THE VOLUME OF SOLUTION IN WHICH ETIDRONATE DISODIUM I.V. INFUSION IS DILUTED, SLOW INFUSION IS

IMPORTANT TO SAFETY. The minimum infusion time of two hours at the recommended dose, or smaller doses, should be observed. The usual course of treatment is one infusion of 7.5 mg/kg body weight/day on each of 3 consecutive days but some patients have been treated for up to 7 days. When patients are treated for more than 3 days, there may be an increased possibility of producing hypocalcemia.

Retreatment with Etidronate Disodium I.V. Infusion may be appropriate if hypercalcemia recurs. There should be at least a seven-day interval between courses of treatment with Etidronate Disodium I.V. Infusion. The dose and manner of retreatment is the same as that for initial treatment. Retreatment for more than three days has not been adequately studied. The safety and efficacy of more than two courses of therapy with Etidronate Disodium I.V. Infusion have not been studied. In the presence of renal impairment, reduction of the dose may be advisable.

Parenteral drug products should be inspected visually for particulate matter and discoloration prior to administration whenever solution and container permit.

Etidronate Disodium Oral Tablets: Etidronate Disodium tablets may be started on the day following the last dose of Etidronate Disodium I.V. Infusion. The recommended oral dose of Etidronate Disodium for patients who have hypercalcemia is 20 mg/kg body weight/day for 30 days. If serum calcium levels remain normal or at clinically acceptable levels, treatment may be extended. Treatment for more than 90 days has not been adequately studied and is not recommended. Please consult the package insert pertaining to oral Etidronate Disodium tablets for additional prescribing information.

Avoid excessive heat (over 104°F or 40°C) for undiluted product.

HOW SUPPLIED
INJECTION: 300 MG/6 ML

BRAND/MANUFACTURER	NDC	SIZE	AWP
○ **BRAND**			
DIDRONEL I.V.: MGI	58063-0457-01	6 ml 6s	$381.60

Etidronate Disodium, Oral

DESCRIPTION
Etidronate Disodium tablets contain either 200 mg or 400 mg of the disodium salt of (1-hydroxyethylidene) diphosphonic acid, for oral administration. This compound, also known as EHDP, regulates bone metabolism. It is a white powder, highly soluble in water, with a molecular weight of 250.

Following is its chemical structure:

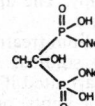

CLINICAL PHARMACOLOGY
Etidronate Disodium acts primarily on bone. It can inhibit the formation, growth and dissolution of hydroxyapatite crystals and their amorphous precursors by chemisorption to calcium phosphate surfaces. Inhibition of crystal resorption occurs at lower doses than are required to inhibit crystal growth. Both effects increase as the dose increases.

Etidronate Disodium is not metabolized. Absorption averages about 1% of an oral dose of 5 mg/kg body weight/day. This increases to about 2.5% at 10 mg/kg/day and 6% at 20 mg/kg/day. Most of the absorbed drug is cleared from the blood within 6 hours. Within 24 hours about half of the absorbed dose is excreted in the urine. The remainder is chemically adsorbed to bone, especially to areas of elevated osteogenesis, and is slowly eliminated. Unabsorbed drug is excreted intact in the feces.

Etidronate Disodium therapy does not adversely affect serum levels of parathyroid hormone or calcium. Hyperphosphatemia has been observed in Etidronate Disodium patients, usually in association with doses of 10-20 mg/kg/day. No adverse effects have been traced to this, and it is not a contraindication for therapy. It is apparently due to drug-related increased tubular reabsorption of phosphate by the kidney. Serum phosphate levels generally return to normal 2-4 weeks posttherapy.

Paget's Disease: Paget's disease of bone (osteitis deformans) is an idiopathic, progressive disease characterized by abnormal and accelerated bone metabolism in one or more bones. Signs and symptoms may include bone pain and/or deformity, neurologic disorders, elevated cardiac output and other vascular disorders, and increased serum alkaline phosphatase and/or urinary hydroxyproline levels. Bone fractures are common in patients with Paget's disease.

Etidronate Disodium slows accelerated bone turnover (resorption and accretion) in pagetic lesions and, to a lesser extent, in normal bone. This has been demonstrated histologically, scintigraphically, biochemically, and through calcium kinetic and balance studies. Reduced bone turnover is often accompanied by symptomatic improvement, including reduced bone pain. Also, the incidence of pagetic fractures may be reduced, and elevated cardiac output and other vascular disorders may be improved by Etidronate Disodium therapy.

Heterotopic Ossification: Heterotopic ossification, also referred to as myositis ossificans (circumscripta, progressiva or traumatica), ectopic calcification, periarticular ossification, or paraosteoarthropathy, is characterized by metaplastic osteogenesis. It usually presents with signs of localized inflammation or pain, elevated skin temperature, and redness. When tissues near joints are involved, functional loss may also be present.

Heterotopic ossification may occur for no known reason as in myositis ossificans progressiva or may follow a wide variety of surgical, occupational, and sports trauma (*e.g.* hip arthroplasty, spinal cord injury, head injury, burns, and severe thigh bruises). Heterotopic ossification has also been observed in nontraumatic conditions (*e.g.* infections of the central nervous system, peripheral neuropathy, tetanus, biliary cirrhosis, Peyronie's disease, as well as in association with a variety of benign and malignant neoplasms).

Clinical trials have demonstrated the efficacy of Etidronate Disodium in heterotopic ossification following total hip replacement, or due to spinal cord injury.

— *Heterotopic ossification complicating total hip replacement* typically develops radiographically 3-8 weeks postoperatively in the pericapsular area of the affected hip joint. The overall incidence is about 50%; about one-third of these cases are clinically significant.

— *Heterotopic ossification due to spinal cord injury* typically develops radiographically 1-4 months after injury. It occurs below the level of injury, usually at major joints. The overall incidence is about 40%; about one-half of these cases are clinically significant.

Etidronate Disodium chemisorbs to calcium hydroxyapatite crystals and their amorphous precursors, blocking the aggregation, growth and mineralization of these crystals. This is thought to be the mechanism by which Etidronate Disodium prevents or retards heterotopic ossification. There is no evidence Etidronate Disodium affects mature heterotopic bone.

INDICATIONS AND USAGE

Paget's Disease: Etidronate Disodium is indicated for the treatment of symptomatic Paget's disease of bone. Etidronate Disodium therapy usually arrests or significantly impedes the disease process as evidenced by:

— Symptomatic relief, including decreased pain and/or increased mobility (experienced by 3 out of 5 patients).

— Reductions in serum alkaline phosphatase and urinary hydroxyproline levels (30% or more in 4 out of 5 patients).

— Histomorphometry showing reduced numbers of osteoclasts and osteoblasts, and more lamellar bone formation.

— Bone scans showing reduced radionuclide uptake at paget lesions.

In addition, reductions in pagetically elevated cardiac output and skin temperature have been observed in some patients. Also, the incidence of pagetic fractures may be reduced when Etidronate Disodium is administered intermittently over a period of years.

In many patients, the disease process will be suppressed for a period of at least one year following cessation of therapy. The upper limit of this period has not been determined.

The effects of the Etidronate Disodium treatment in patients with asymptomatic Paget's disease have not been studied. However, Etidronate Disodium treatment of such patients may be warranted if extensive involvement threatens irreversible neurologic damage, major joints, or major weight-bearing bones.

Heterotopic Ossification: Etidronate Disodium is indicated in the prevention and treatment of heterotopic ossification following total hip replacement or due to spinal cord injury. Etidronate Disodium reduces the incidence of clinically important heterotopic bone by about two-thirds. Among those patients who form heterotopic bone, Etidronate Disodium retards the progression of immature lesions and reduces the severity by at least half. Follow-up data (at least nine months posttherapy) suggest these benefits persist.

In Total Hip Replacement Patients: Etidronate Disodium does not promote loosening of the prosthesis or impede trochanteric reattachment.

In Spinal Cord Injury Patients: Etidronate Disodium does not inhibit fracture healing or stabilization of the spine.

UNLABELED USES
Etidronate Disodium is used alone or as an adjunct in the treatment of postmenopausal osteoporosis.

CONTRAINDICATIONS
None known.

WARNINGS
In Paget's Patients: the response to therapy may be of slow onset and continue for months after Etidronate Disodium therapy is discontinued. Dosage should not be increased prematurely. A 90-day drug-free interval should be provided between courses of therapy.

Heterotopic Ossification: No specific warnings.

PRECAUTIONS
General: Patients should maintain an adequate nutritional status, particularly an adequate intake of calcium and vitamin D.

Therapy has been withheld from some patients with enterocolitis since diarrhea may be experienced, particularly at higher doses.

Etidronate Disodium is not metabolized and is excreted intact via the kidney. There is no experience to specifically guide treatment in patients with impaired renal function. Etidronate Disodium dosage should be reduced when reductions

in glomerular filtration rates are present. Patients with renal impairment should be closely monitored. In approximately 10% of patients in clinical trials of Etidronate Disodium I.V. Infusion for hypercalcemia of malignancy, occasional, mild-to-moderate abnormalities in renal function (increases of > 0.5 mg/dl serum creatinine) were observed during or immediately after treatment.

Etidronate Disodium suppresses bone turnover, and may retard mineralization of osteoid laid down during the bone accretion process. These effects are dose and time dependent. Osteoid, which may accumulate noticeably at doses of 10-20 mg/kg/day, mineralizes normally posttherapy. In patients with fractures, especially of long bones, it may be advisable to delay or interrupt treatment until callus is evident.

In Paget's Patients: treatment regimens exceeding the recommended (see *"Dosage and Administration"*) daily maximum dose of 20 mg/kg or continuous administration of medication for periods greater than 6 months may be associated with an increased risk of fracture.

Long bones predominantly affected by lytic lesions, particularly in those patients unresponsive to Etidronate Disodium therapy, may be especially prone to fracture. Patients with predominantly lytic lesions should be monitored radiographically and biochemically to permit termination of Etidronate Disodium in those patients unresponsive to treatment.

Carcinogenesis: Long-term studies in rats have indicated that Etidronate Disodium is not carcinogenic.

Pregnancy: Teratogenic Effects: Pregnancy Category C. In teratology and developmental toxicity studies conducted in rats and rabbits treated with dosages of up to 100 mg/kg (5-20 times the clinical dose), no adverse or teratogenic effects have been observed in the offspring. Etidronate Disodium has been shown to cause skeletal abnormalities in rats when given at oral dose levels of 300 mg/kg (15-60 times the human dose). Other effects on the offspring (including decreased live births) are at dosages that cause significant toxicity in the parent generation and are 25 to 200 times the human dose. The skeletal effects are thought to be the result of the pharmacological effects of the drug on bone.

There are no adequate and well-controlled studies in pregnant women. Etidronate Disodium should be used during pregnancy only if the potential benefit justifies the potential risk to the fetus.

Nursing Mothers: It is not known whether this drug is excreted in human milk. Because many drugs are excreted in human milk, caution should be exercised when Etidronate Disodium is administered to a nursing woman.

Pediatric Use: Safety and effectiveness in children have not been established. Children have been treated with Etidronate Disodium, at doses recommended for adults, to prevent heterotopic ossifications or soft tissue calcifications. A rachitic syndrome has been reported infrequently at doses of 10 mg/kg/day and more for prolonged periods approaching or exceeding a year. The epiphyseal radiologic changes associated with retarded mineralization of new osteoid and cartilage, and occasional symptoms reported, have been reversible when medication is discontinued.

ADVERSE REACTIONS
The incidence of gastrointestinal complaints (diarrhea, nausea) is the same for Etidronate Disodium at 5 mg/kg/day as for placebo, about 1 patient in 15. At 10-20 mg/kg/day the incidence may increase to 2 or 3 in 10. These complaints are often alleviated by dividing the total daily dose.

In Paget's Patients: Increased or recurrent bone pain at pagetic sites, and/or the onset of pain at previously asymptomatic sites has been reported. At 5 mg/kg/day about 1 patient in 10 (versus 1 in 15 in the placebo group) report these phenomena. At higher doses the incidence rises to about 2 in 10. When therapy continues, pain resolves in some patients but persists in others.

Heterotopic Ossification: No specific adverse reactions.

Worldwide Postmarketing Experience: The worldwide postmarketing experience for Etidronate Disodium reflects its use in the following indications: Paget's disease, heterotopic ossification, hypercalcemia of malignancy, and osteoporosis. Other adverse events that have been reported and were thought to be possibly related to Etidronate Disodium include the following: alopecia; arthropathies, including arthralgia and arthritis; bone fracture; esophagitis; glossitis; hypersensitivity reactions, including angioedema, follicular eruption, macular rash, maculopapular rash, pruritus, a single case of Stevens Johnson syndrome, and urticaria; osteomalacia; neuropsychiatric events, including amnesia, confusion, depression, and hallucination; and paresthesias.

In patients receiving Etidronate Disodium, there have been rare reports of agranulocytosis, pancytopenia, and a report of leukopenia with recurrence on rechallenge. In addition, exacerbation of existing peptic ulcer disease has been reported in a few patients. In one patient, perforation also occurred.

OVERDOSAGE
Clinical experience with acute Etidronate Disodium overdosage is extremely limited. Decreases in serum calcium following substantial overdosage may be expected in some patients. Signs and symptoms of hypocalcemia also may occur in some of these patients. Some patients may develop vomiting. In one event, an 18-year-old female who ingested an estimated single dose of 4,000-6,000 mg (67-100 mg/kg) of Etidronate Disodium was reported to be mildly hypocalcemic (7.52 mg/dl) and experienced paresthesia of the fingers. Hypocalcemia resolved 6 hours after lavage and treatment with intravenous calcium gluconate. A 92-year-old female who accidentally received 1,600 mg of Etidronate Disodium per day for 3.5 days experienced marked diarrhea and required treatment for electrolyte

imbalance. Orally administered Etidronate Disodium may cause hematologic abnormalities in some patients (see "Adverse Reactions").

Etidronate Disodium suppresses bone turnover and may retard mineralization of osteoid laid down during the bone accretion process. These effects are dose and time dependent. Osteoid which may accumulate noticeably at doses of 10-20 mg/kg/day of chronic, continuous dosing mineralizes normally posttherapy.

Prolonged continuous treatment (chronic overdosage) has been reported to cause nephrotic syndrome and fracture. Gastric lavage may remove unabsorbed drug. Standard procedures for treating hypocalcemia, including the administration of Ca^{++} intravenously, would be expected to restore physiologic amounts of ionized calcium and relieve signs and symptoms of hypocalcemia. Such treatment has been effective.

DOSAGE AND ADMINISTRATION

Etidronate Disodium should be taken as a single, oral dose. However, should gastrointestinal discomfort occur, the dose may be divided. To maximize absorption, patients should avoid taking the following items within two hours of dosing:

—Food, especially food high in calcium, such as milk or milk products.

—Vitamins with mineral supplements or antacids which are high in metals such as calcium, iron, magnesium or aluminum.

PAGET'S DISEASE

Initial Treatment Regimens: 5-10 mg/kg/day, not to exceed 6 months, or 11-20 mg/kg/day, not to exceed 3 months.

The recommended initial dose is 5 mg/kg/day for a period not to exceed six months. Doses above 10 mg/kg/day should be reserved for when 1) lower doses are ineffective or 2) there is an overriding need to suppress rapid bone turnover (especially when irreversible neurologic damage is possible) or reduce elevated cardiac output. Doses in excess of 20 mg/kg/day are not recommended.

Retreatment Guidelines: Retreatment should be initiated only after 1) a Etidronate Disodium-free period of at least 90 days and 2) there is biochemical, symptomatic or other evidence of active disease process. It is advisable to monitor patients every 3-6 months although some patients may go drug free for extended periods. Retreatment regimens are the same as for initial treatment. For most patients the original dose will be adequate for retreatment. If not, consideration should be given to increasing the dose within the recommended guidelines.

HETEROTOPIC OSSIFICATION

The following treatment regimens have been shown to be effective:

—Total Hip Replacement Patients: 20 mg/kg/day for 1 month before and 3 months after surgery (4 months total).

—Spinal Cord Injured Patients: 20 mg/kg/day for 2 weeks followed by 10 mg/kg/day for 10 weeks (12 weeks total).

Etidronate Disodium therapy should begin as soon as medically feasible following the injury, preferably prior to evidence of heterotopic ossification.

Retreatment has not been studied.

STORAGE

Avoid excessive heat (over 104°F or 40°C).

HOW SUPPLIED
TABLETS: 200 MG

BRAND/MANUFACTURER	NDC	SIZE	AWP
○ **BRAND** DIDRONEL: P&G Pharm	00149-0405-60	60s	$104.70

TABLETS: 400 MG

BRAND/MANUFACTURER	NDC	SIZE	AWP
○ **BRAND** DIDRONEL: P&G Pharm	00149-0406-60	60s	$209.40

Etodolac

DESCRIPTION

Etodolac is a pyranocarboxylic acid chemically designated as (±) 1,8-diethyl-1,3,4,9-tetrahydropyrano-[3,4-b]indole-1-acetic acid.

The empirical formula for Etodolac is $C_{17}H_{21}NO_3$. The molecular weight of the base is 287.37. It has a pKa of 4.65 and an n-octanol:water partition coefficient of 11.4 at pH 7.4. Etodolac is a white crystalline compound insoluble in water but soluble in alcohols, chloroform, dimethyl sulfoxide, and aqueous polyethylene glycol.

Etodolac is available in 200 and 300 mg capsules and 400 mg tablets for oral administration.

Following is its chemical structure:

CLINICAL PHARMACOLOGY
PHARMACOLOGY

Etodolac is a nonsteroidal anti-inflammatory drug (NSAID) that exhibits anti-inflammatory, analgesic and antipyretic activities in animal models. The mechanism of action of Etodolac, like that of other NSAIDs, is not known but is believed to be associated with the inhibition of prostaglandin biosynthesis.

Etodolac is a racemic mixture of R- and S-Etodolac. As with other NSAIDs, it has been demonstrated in animals that the S-form is biologically active and the R-form is not. Both enantiomers are stable and there is no R-to-S conversion *in vivo*.

PHARMACODYNAMICS

Analgesia was demonstrable by 1/2 hour following single doses of 200 to 400 mg Etodolac with the peak effect occurring in 1 to 2 hours. The analgesic effect generally lasts for 4 to 6 hours (with some patients maintaining analgesia up to 8 to 12 hours: see "Analgesia" and "Osteoarthritis" sections under "Clinical Trials" below.)

PHARMACOKINETICS

The pharmacokinetics of Etodolac have been evaluated in 267 normal subjects, 44 elderly patients (> 65 years old), 19 patients with renal failure (creatinine clearance 37 to 88 mL/min), 9 patients on hemodialysis, and 10 patients with compensated hepatic cirrhosis. Etodolac is well absorbed and had a relative bioavailability of 100% when 200 mg capsules were compared with a solution of Etodolac. Based on mass balance studies, the systemic availability of Etodolac is at least 80%, and Etodolac does not undergo significant first-pass metabolism following oral administration. The dose-proportionality based on AUC (the area under the plasma concentration-time curve) is linear following doses up to 600 mg every 12 hours. Peak concentrations are dose-proportional for both total and free Etodolac following doses up to 400 mg every 12 hours, but following a 600 mg dose, the peak is about 20% higher than predicted on the basis of lower doses. As shown on the graphs below, Etodolac plasma concentrations, after multiple-dose administration, are slightly higher than after single doses, as predicted, indicating no change in pharmacokinetics with multiple dose use. Etodolac is more than 99% bound to plasma proteins. The free fraction is less than 1% and is independent of Etodolac total concentration over the dose range studied.

Etodolac, when administered orally, exhibits characteristics which are well described by a two-compartment model with first-order absorption. Mean (± 1 SD) peak plasma concentrations range from approximately 14±4 to 37±9 µg/mL after 200 to 600 mg single doses and are reached in 80±30 minutes. The mean plasma clearance of Etodolac is 47 (± 16) mL/h/kg, and terminal disposition half-life is 7.3 (± 4.0) hours (see table for summary of pharmacokinetic parameters).

As with many drugs which are hepatically metabolized and not dosed on a mg/kg basis, the intersubject variability of Etodolac plasma levels, achieved after recommended doses, is substantial. The graph of simulated curves below demonstrates the range of plasma concentrations that would be expected for 95% of the patients following 200 or 400 mg single doses on the top and on t.i.d. regimens on the bottom (at steady-state). The cross-hatched area represents the over-lap in plasma levels following 200 or 400 mg of Etodolac orally as single or multiple doses. The area above the upper 95% C.L. lines represents blood levels which would be achieved by larger doses or in individuals with decreased clearance in whom one should anticipate increased adverse reactions. The area below the 95% C.L. lines represents blood levels following lower doses or in individuals with high clearance of Etodolac, and one would expect less effectiveness in such patients. The data used to produce these simulations were derived from the mean ± 2 SD of the plasma concentrations at each time point from a total of 267 normal subjects following multiple dosing. As with other drugs, including NSAIDs, greater variability is to be expected in patients, particularly those with GI problems and those taking other drugs affecting the GI tract, protein binding, or hepatic or renal function. (See graphs and table on following page).

Etodolac is extensively metabolized in the liver, with renal elimination of Etodolac and its metabolites being the primary route of excretion. Approximately 72% of the administered dose is recovered in the urine as the following, indicated as % of the administered dose:

—Etodolac, unchanged — 1%
—Etodolac glucuronide — 13%
—hydroxylated metabolites (6,7-and 8-OH) — 5%
—hydroxylated metabolite glucuronides — 20%
—unidentified metabolites — 33%

Fecal excretion accounted for 16% of the dose. Therefore, enterohepatic circulation, if present, is not extensive.

The extent of absorption of Etodolac is not affected when Etodolac is administered after a meal or with an antacid. Food intake, however, reduces the peak concentration reached by approximately one half, and increases the time-to-peak concentration by 1.4 to 3.8 hours. Coadministration with an antacid decreases the peak concentration reached by about 15 to 20%, with no measurable effect on time-to-peak.

In studies in the elderly, age was found to have no effect on Etodolac $t_{1/2}$ or protein binding, and there was no drug accumulation. Etodolac clearance was reduced by about 15%. Because the reduction in clearance is small, no dosage adjustment is generally necessary in the elderly on the basis of pharmacokinetics. The elderly may need dosage adjustment, however, on the basis of body size (See "Geriatric Population"), and they may be more sensitive to antiprostaglandin effects than younger patients (See "Precautions").

ETODOLAC PLASMA CONCENTRATIONS
UPPER AND LOWER 95% CONFIDENCE LIMITS
FOLLOWING SINGLE 200 AND 400 MG ORAL DOSES

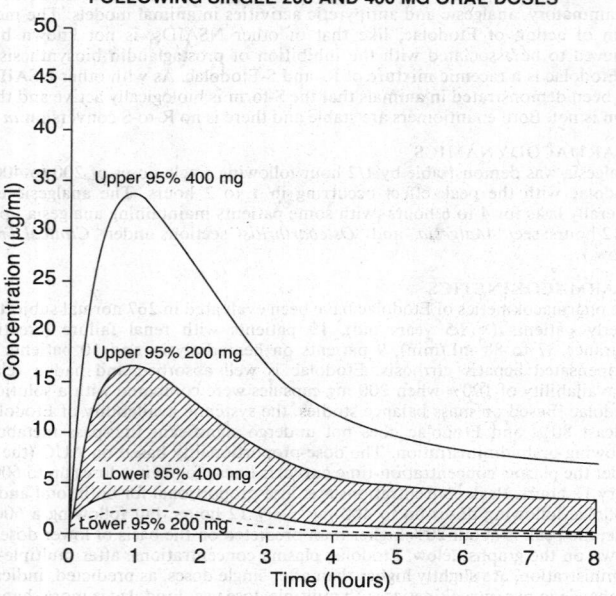

ETODOLAC PLASMA CONCENTRATIONS
UPPER AND LOWER 95% CONFIDENCE LIMITS
FOLLOWING 200 AND 400 MG T.I.D. ORAL DOSES

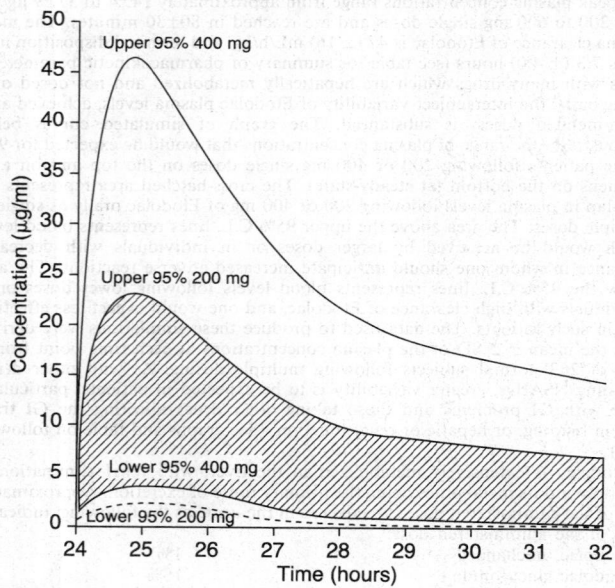

ETODOLAC
STEADY-STATE PHARMACOKINETIC PARAMETERS (N = 267)

Kinetic Parameters	Scientific Notation (units)	Mean ± SD
Extent of oral absorption (bioavailability)	F (%)	≥ 80
Peak concentration time	t_{max} (h)	1.7 ± 1.3
Oral-dose clearance	CL/F (mL/h/kg)	47 ± 16
Central compartment volume	V_c/F (mL/kg)	132 ± 47
Steady-state volume	V_{ss}/F (mL/kg)	362 ± 129
Distribution half-life	$t_{1/2,\alpha}$ (h)	0.71 ± 0.50
Terminal half-life	$t_{1/2,\beta}$ (h)	7.3 ± 4.0

In studies of the effects of mild-to-moderate renal impairment, no significant differences in the disposition of total and free Etodolac were observed. In patients undergoing hemodialysis, there was a 50% greater apparent clearance of total Etodolac, due to a 50% greater unbound fraction. Free Etodolac clearance was not altered, indicating the importance of protein binding in Ethodolac's disposition. Nevertheless Etodolac is not dialyzable. No dosage adjustment of Etodolac is generally required in patients with mild-to-moderate renal impairment; however Etodolac should be used with caution in such patients because, as with other NSAIDs, it may further decrease renal function in some patients with impaired renal function (See "Precautions").

In patients with compensated hepatic cirrhosis, the disposition of total and free Etodolac is not altered. Although no dosage adjustment is generally required in this patient population, Etodolac clearance is dependent on hepatic function and could be reduced in patients with severe hepatic failure.

SPECIAL STUDIES
Etodolac was compared with other NSAIDs in inducing gastrointestinal (GI) microbleeding. Etodolac 1200 mg/day caused less GI blood loss than ibuprofen 2400 mg/day, indomethacin 200 mg/day, or naproxen 750 mg/day. Etodolac was also compared with piroxicam 20 mg/day in two studies: piroxicam caused more blood loss than Etodolac in one of these studies but not the other.

Etodolac was also compared to other NSAIDs in GI endoscopic studies. Endoscopic scores in studies of 12 healthy subjects following 1 week of Etodolac 1200 mg/day showed significantly fewer GI mucosal erosions with Etodolac than with aspirin 3900 mg/day. In another study performed in healthy males 18 to 41 years of age, 12 subjects treated with Etodolac 1000 mg/day for one week had lower endoscopic scores than 12 subjects treated with indomethacin 200 mg/day, naproxen 1000 mg/day, or ibuprofen 2400 mg/day. Another endoscopic study comparing effects of Etodolac 1000 mg/day with piroxicam 20 mg/day, each administered to 12 normal volunteers for one month, yielded equivocal results, with both treatments showing higher scores than the 12-subject placebo-treated group.

The clinical significance of these findings is unknown.

CLINICAL TRIALS
ANALGESIA
Controlled clinical trials in analgesia were single dose, randomized, double-blind, parallel studies in 3 pain models (dental extractions, post-general surgery, and post-episiotomy pain). In these studies there were patients treated with placebo, 2 or more doses of Etodolac, and varying combinations of aspirin, acetaminophen with codeine (oral surgery only), or zomepirac. The analgesic effective dose for Etodolac established in these acute pain models was 200 to 400 mg. The onset of analgesia occurred approximately 30 minutes after oral administration and was comparable for Etodolac (200 to 400 mg), aspirin (650 mg), acetaminophen with codeine (600 mg - 60 mg), and zomepirac (100 mg). The peak analgesic effect was between 1 to 2 hours. Duration of relief averaged 4 to 5 hours for 200 mg of Etodolac and 5 to 6 hours for 400 mg of Etodolac as measured by when approximately half of the patients required remediation. However, in some studies there were still statistically significant differences between the degree of pain relief experienced by patients treated with 200 and 400 mg of Etodolac and placebo-treated patients at 8 hours.

OSTEOARTHRITIS
The use of Etodolac in managing the signs and symptoms of osteoarthritis of the hip or knee, was assessed in double-blind, randomized, controlled clinical trials in 341 patients. In patients with osteoarthritis of the knee, Etodolac in doses of 600 to 1000 mg/day was better than placebo in 2 studies. The clinical trials in osteoarthritis used b.i.d. dosage regimens. The initial dosing recommendation for Etodolac in patients with osteoarthritis is t.i.d. administration, due to Etodolac's pharmacokinetic profile (see "Pharmacokinetics" and "Individualization of Dosage").

RHEUMATOID ARTHRITIS
Etodolac is not recommended for the treatment of patients with rheumatoid arthritis because in controlled clinical trials, although Etodolac treatment was sometimes better than placebo treatment, it was generally not as effective as treatment with other marketed NSAIDs.

INDIVIDUALIZATION OF DOSAGE
Etodolac, like other NSAIDs, shows considerable interindividual variation in response. Consequently, the recommended strategy for initiating therapy is to use a starting dose likely to be effective for the majority of patients and to adjust dosage thereafter based on observations of Etodolac beneficial and adverse effects.

The effectiveness of Etodolac in otherwise healthy, young to middle-aged adults in acute pain studies showed symptom relief to last approximately 5 to 6 hours following single 400 mg doses and 4 to 5 hours following 200 mg doses as judged by the time by which approximately half of the patients needed remediation. In dental extraction studies, hourly comparisons were made of the number of placebo-treated patients versus the number of Etodolac-treated patients who needed to be remediated. In these studies, the 200 mg Etodolac group had significantly fewer patients who needed remediation up to 6 hours than the placebo group, while the 400 mg Etodolac group had significantly fewer patients who required remediation for up to 12 hours.

These results suggest an initial Etodolac dose of 400 mg for acute pain followed by doses of 200 to 400 mg every 6 to 8 hours, as needed, not to exceed a maximum total daily dose of 1200 mg. If a patient taking 400 mg doses has adequate pain relief that does not last 8 hours, then 300 mg every 6 hours (q.i.d.) is a reasonable schedule to try. As with all NSAIDs, if symptoms are still not adequately controlled by recommended doses, another analgesic should be tried.

In osteoarthritis, the recommended starting dose of Etodolac is 800 to 1200 mg/day in divided doses: 400 mg t.i.d. or b.i.d. or 300 mg q.i.d. or t.i.d. which is derived from pharmacokinetic and single-dose analgesic trial data. In controlled

◆ RATED THERAPEUTICALLY EQUIVALENT; ◇ THERAPEUTIC EQUIVALENCE UNCONFIRMED; ○ UNRATED

clinical trials in patients with osteoarthritis, total daily doses of 600 to 1000 mg of Etodolac were successfully given on a b.i.d. schedule. In one study some patients were apparently adequately treated with as little as 200 mg Etodolac b.i.d. The pharmacokinetic profile of Etodolac and the results of single-dose analgesia studies suggest, however, that the drug may provide greater benefit when given on a t.i.d. schedule. As with other NSAIDs, the lowest dose and longest dosing interval should be sought for each patient. Therefore, after observing the response to initial therapy with Etodolac, the dose and frequency should be adjusted to suit individual patient's needs. The recommended total daily dose of Etodolac is 600 to 1200 mg/day given in divided doses: 400 mg t.i.d. or b.i.d.: 300 mg q.i.d., t.i.d. or b.i.d.; 200 mg q.i.d. or t.i.d.

Total daily doses of Etodolac above 20 mg/kg/day have not been studied. Therefore, in patients weighing less than 60 kg (132 lbs), or where the severity of the disease, concomitant medications, or other diseases warrant, the maximum recommended total daily dose of 1200 mg should be reduced. (See "Precautions".)

INDICATIONS AND USAGE
Etodolac is indicated for acute and long-term use in the management of signs and symptoms of osteoarthritis. Etodolac is also indicated for the management of pain.

UNLABELED USES
Etodolac is used alone or as an adjunct in the treatment of rheumatoid arthritis.

CONTRAINDICATIONS
Etodolac is contraindicated in patients who have previously shown hypersensitivity to it. Etodolac should not be given to patients in whom Etodolac, aspirin, other NSAIDs induce asthma, rhinitis, urticaria, or other allergic reactions. Fatal asthmatic reactions have been reported in such patients receiving NSAIDs.

WARNINGS
RISK OF GASTROINTESTINAL (GI) ULCERATION, BLEEDING, AND PERFORATION WITH NONSTEROIDAL ANTI-INFLAMMATORY DRUG THERAPY
Serious GI toxicity, such as bleeding, ulceration, and perforation, can occur at any time, with or without warning symptoms, in patients treated chronically with NSAIDs. Although minor upper GI problems, such as dyspepsia, are common, usually developing early in therapy, physicians should remain alert for ulceration and bleeding in patients treated chronically with NSAIDs even in the absence of previous GI-tract symptoms. In patients observed in clinical trials of such agents for several months to 2 years' duration, symptomatic upper GI ulcers, gross bleeding, or perforation appear to occur in approximately 1% of patients treated for 3 to 6 months and in about 2% to 4% of patients treated for 1 year. Physicians should inform patients about the signs and/or symptoms of serious GI toxicity and what steps to take if they occur.

Studies to date have not identified any subset of patients not at risk of developing peptic ulceration and bleeding. Except for a prior history of serious GI events and other risk factors known to be associated with peptic ulcer disease, such as alcoholism, smoking, etc., no risk factors (e.g., age, sex) have been associated with increased risk. Elderly or debilitated patients seem to tolerate ulceration or bleeding less well than other individuals, and most spontaneous reports of fatal GI events are in this population. Studies to date are inconclusive concerning the relative risk of various NSAIDs in causing such reactions. High doses of any NSAID probably carry a greater risk of these reactions, although controlled clinical trials showing this do not exist in most cases. In considering the use of relatively large doses (within the recommended dosage range), sufficient benefit should be anticipated to offset the potential increased risk of GI toxicity.

PRECAUTIONS
GENERAL PRECAUTIONS
Renal Effects: As with other NSAIDs, long-term administration of Etodolac to rats has resulted in renal papillary necrosis and other renal medullary changes. Renal pelvic transitional epithelial hyperplasia, a spontaneous change occurring with variable frequency, was observed with increased frequency in treated male rats in a 2-year chronic study. The cause-effect relationship to Etodolac has not been established.

A second form of renal toxicity encountered with Etodolac as with other NSAIDs, is seen in patients with conditions in which renal prostaglandins have a supportive role in the maintenance of renal perfusion. In these patients, administration of a nonsteroidal anti-inflammatory drug may cause a dose-dependent reduction in prostaglandin formation and, secondarily, in renal blood flow, which may precipitate overt renal decompensation. Patients at greatest risk of this reaction are those with impaired renal function, heart failure, liver dysfunction, those taking diuretics, and the elderly. Discontinuation of nonsteroidal anti-inflammatory drug therapy is usually followed by recovery to the pretreatment state.

Etodolac metabolites are eliminated primarily by the kidneys. The extent to which the inactive glucuronide metabolites may accumulate in patients with renal failure has not been studied. As with other drugs whose metabolites are excreted by the kidney, the possibility that adverse reactions (not listed in "Adverse Reactions") may be attributable to these metabolites should be considered.

Hepatic Effects: As with all NSAIDs, borderline elevations of one or more liver tests may occur in up to 15% of patients. These abnormalities may disappear, remain essentially unchanged, or progress with continued therapy. Meaningful elevations of ALT or AST (approximately three or more times the upper limit of normal) have been reported in approximately 1% of patients in clinical trials with Etodolac. A patient with symptoms and/or signs suggesting liver dysfunction, or

in whom an abnormal liver test has occurred, should be evaluated for evidence of the development of a more severe hepatic reaction while on therapy with Etodolac. Although such reactions are rare, if abnormal liver tests persist or worsen, if clinical signs and symptoms consistent with liver disease develop, or if systemic manifestations occur (e.g., eosinophilia, rash, etc.), Etodolac should be discontinued.

Hematological Effect: Anemia is sometimes seen in patients receiving Etodolac or other NSAIDs. This may be due to fluid retention, gastrointestinal blood loss, or an incompletely described effect upon erythropoiesis. Patients on long-term treatment with NSAIDs, including Etodolac, should have their hemoglobin or hematocrit checked if they develop signs or symptoms of anemia.

All drugs which inhibit the biosynthesis of prostaglandins may interfere to some extent with platelet function and vascular responses to bleeding. Patients receiving Etodolac who may be adversely affected by such actions should be carefully observed.

Fluid Retention and Edema: Fluid retention and edema have been observed in some patients taking Etodolac. Therefore, as with other NSAIDs, Etodolac should be used with caution in patients with fluid retention, hypertension, or heart failure.

INFORMATION FOR PATIENTS
Etodolac, like other NSAIDs (Nonsteroidal Anti-inflammatory Drugs), is not free of side effects. The side effects of these drugs can cause discomfort and, rarely, there may be serious side effects, such as GI bleeding, that may result in hospitalization and even fatal outcomes.

NSAIDs are often essential agents in the management of arthritis and have a major role in the treatment of pain, but they also may be commonly employed for conditions that are less serious.

Physicians may wish to discuss with their patients the potential risks (see "Warnings," "Precautions", and "Adverse Reactions" sections) and likely benefits of Etodolac treatment, particularly when it may be used for less serious conditions in which treatment without Etodolac may represent an acceptable alternative to both the patient and physician.

LABORATORY TESTS
Because serious GI-tract ulceration and bleeding can occur without warning symptoms, physicians should observe chronically treated patients for the signs and symptoms of ulceration and bleeding and should inform them of the importance of this follow-up (see "Risk of GI Ulcerations, Bleeding, and Perforation with NSAID Therapy").

DRUG INTERACTIONS
Antacids: The concomitant administration of antacids has no apparent effect on the extent of absorption of Etodolac. However, antacids can decrease the peak concentration reached by 15 to 20% but have no detectable effect on the time-to-peak.

Aspirin: When Etodolac is administered with aspirin, its protein binding is reduced, although the clearance of free Etodolac is not altered. The clinical significance of this interaction is not known: however, as with other NSAIDs, concomitant administration of Etodolac and aspirin is not generally recommended because of the potential of increased adverse effects.

Warfarin: Short-term pharmacokinetic studies have demonstrated that concomitant administration of warfarin and Etodolac results in reduced protein binding of warfarin, but there was no change in the clearance of free warfarin. There was no significant difference in the pharmacodynamic effect of warfarin administered alone and warfarin administered with Etodolac as measured by prothrombin time. Thus, concomitant therapy with warfarin and Etodolac should not require dosage adjustment of either drug. However, following US market introduction of Etodolac, there have been a few spontaneous reports of prolonged prothrombin times in Etodolac-treated patients receiving concomitant warfarin therapy. Caution should be exercised because interactions have been seen with other NSAIDs.

Phenytoin: Etodolac has no apparent pharmacokinetic interaction when administered with phenytoin.

Glyburide: Etodolac has no apparent pharmacokinetic or pharmacodynamic interaction when administered with glyburide.

Diuretics: Etodolac has no apparent pharmacokinetic interaction when administered with furosemide or hydrochlorothiazide; nor does Etodolac attenuate the diuretic response of either of these drugs in normal volunteers. Etodolac and other NSAIDs, nevertheless, should be used with caution in patients receiving diuretics, who have cardiac, renal, or hepatic failure (see "Renal Effects").

Cyclosporine, Digoxin, Lithium, Methotrexate: Etodolac, like other NSAIDs, through effects on renal prostaglandins, may cause changes in the elimination of these drugs leading to elevated serum levels of digoxin, lithium, and methotrexate and increased toxicity. Nephrotoxicity associated with cyclosporine may also be enhanced. Patients receiving these drugs who are given Etodolac, or any other NSAID, and particularly those patients with altered renal function, should be observed for the development of the specific toxicities of these drugs.

Protein Binding: Data from *in vitro* studies, using peak serum concentrations at reported therapeutic doses in humans, show that the Etodolac free fraction is not significantly altered by acetaminophen, ibuprofen, indomethacin, naproxen, piroxicam, chlorpropamide, glipizide, glyburide, phenytoin, and probenecid. In contrast, phenylbutazone causes an increase (by about 80%) in the free fraction of

Etodolac. Although *in vivo* studies have not been done to see if Etodolac clearance is changed by coadministration of phenylbutazone, it is not recommended that they be coadministered.

DRUG/LABORATORY TEST INTERACTIONS
The urine of patients who take Etodolac can give a false-positive reaction for urinary bilirubin (urobilin) due to the presence of phenolic metabolites of Etodolac.

Diagnostic dip-stick methodology, used to detect ketone bodies in urine, has resulted in false-positive findings in some patients treated with Etodolac. Generally, this phenomenon has not been associated with other clinically significant events. No dose-relationship has been observed.

Etodolac treatment is associated with a small decrease in serum uric acid levels. In clinical trials, mean decreases of 1 to 2 mg/dL were observed in arthritic patients receiving Etodolac (600 mg to 1000 mg/day) after 4 weeks of therapy. These levels then remained stable for up to one year of therapy.

CARCINOGENESIS, MUTAGENESIS, AND IMPAIRMENT OF FERTILITY
No carcinogenic effect of Etodolac was observed in mice or rats receiving oral doses of 15 mg/kg/day (45 to 89 mg/m^2, respectively) or less for periods of 2 years or 18 months, respectively. Etodolac was not mutagenic in *in vitro* tests performed with S. typhimurium and mouse lymphoma cells as well as in an *in vivo* mouse micronucleus test. However, data from the *in vitro* human peripheral lymphocyte test showed an increase (p = 0.06) in the number of gaps (3.0 to 5.3% unstained regions in the chromatid without dislocation) among the Etodolac-treated cultures (50 to 200 µg/mL) compared to negative controls (2.0%); no other difference was noted between the controls and drug-treated groups. Etodolac showed no impairment of fertility in male and female rats up to oral doses of 16 mg/kg (94 mg/m^2). However, reduced implantation of fertilized eggs occurred in the 8 mg/kg group.

TERATOGENIC EFFECTS: PREGNANCY CATEGORY C
In teratology studies, isolated occurrences of alterations in limb development were found and included polydactyly, oligodactyly, syndactyly, and unossified phalanges in rats and oligodactyly and synostosis of metatarsals in rabbits. These were observed at dose levels (2 to 14 mg/kg/day) close to human clinical doses. However, the frequency and the dosage group distribution of these findings in initial or repeated studies did not establish a clear drug or dose-response relationship.

There are no adequate or well-controlled studies in pregnant women. Etodolac should be used during pregnancy only if the potential benefits justifies the potential risk of the fetus. Because of the known effects of NSAIDs on parturition and on the human fetal cardiovascular system with respect to closure of the ductus arteriosus, use during late pregnancy should be avoided.

LABOR AND DELIVERY
In rat studies with Etodolac, as with other drugs known to inhibit prostaglandin synthesis, an increased incidence of dystocia, delayed parturition, and decreased pup survival occurred. The effects of Etodolac on labor and delivery in pregnant women are unknown.

NURSING MOTHERS
Caution should be exercised if Etodolac is administered to a nursing woman, because many drugs are excreted in human milk. It is not known whether Etodolac is excreted in human milk.

PEDIATRIC USE
Safety and effectiveness in children have not been established.

GERIATRIC POPULATION
In patients 65 years and older, no substantial differences in the pharmacokinetics or the side-effect profile of Etodolac were seen compared with the general population. Therefore, no dosage adjustment is generally necessary in the elderly. As with any NSAID, however, caution should be exercised in treating the elderly, and when individualizing their dosage, extra care should be taken when increasing the dose because the elderly seem to tolerate NSAID side effects less well than younger patients (see *"Pharmacokinetics"*).

ADVERSE REACTIONS
Adverse-reaction information for Etodolac was derived from 2,629 arthritic patients treated with Etodolac in double-blind and open-label clinical trials of 4 to 320 weeks in duration and worldwide postmarketing surveillance studies in approximately 60,000 patients.

In clinical trials, most adverse reactions were mild and transient. The discontinuation rate in controlled clinical trials, because of adverse events, was 9% for patients treated with Etodolac.

New patient complaints (with an incidence greater than or equal to 1%) are listed below by body system. The incidences were determined from clinical trials involving 465 patients with osteoarthritis treated with 300 to 500 mg of Etodolac b.i.d. (i.e., 600 to 1000 mg per day).

INCIDENCE GREATER THAN OR EQUAL TO 1%—
PROBABLY CAUSALLY RELATED
Body as a whole—Chills and fever.

Digestive system—Dyspepsia (10%), abdominal pain*, diarrhea*, flatulence*, nausea*, constipation, gastritis, melena, vomiting.
Nervous system—Asthenia/malaise*, dizziness*, depression, nervousness.
Skin and appendages—Pruritus, rash.
Special senses—Blurred vision, tinnitus.
Urogenital system—Dysuria, urinary frequency.

INCIDENCE LESS THAN 1%—
PROBABLY CAUSALLY RELATED
(Adverse reactions reported only in worldwide postmarketing experience, not seen in clinical trials, are considered rarer and are italicized.)
Cardiovascular system—Hypertension, congestive heart failure, flushing, palpitations, syncope.
Digestive system—Thirst, dry mouth, ulcerative stomatitis, anorexia, eructation, elevated liver enzymes, *cholestatic hepatitis*, hepatitis, *cholestatic jaundice, jaundice*, PUB (i.e., peptic ulcer with or without bleeding and/or perforation) *pancreatitis.*
Hemic and lymphatic system—Ecchymosis, anemia, thrombocytopenia, bleeding time increased, *agranulocytosis, hemolytic anemia, neutropenia, pancytopenia.*
Metabolic and nutritional—Edema, serum creatinine increase, *hyperglycemia in previously controlled diabetic patients.*
Nervous system—Insomnia, somnolence.
Respiratory system—Asthma.
Skin and appendages—Angioedema, sweating, urticaria, vesiculobullous rash, *cutaneous vasculitis with purpura, Stevens-Johnson Syndrome*, hyperpigmentation, *erythema multiforme.*
Special senses—Photophobia, transient visual disturbances.
Urogenital system—*Elevated BUN, renal failure, renal insufficiency, renal papillary necrosis.*

INCIDENCE LESS THAN 1%—
CAUSAL RELATIONSHIP UNKNOWN
(Medical events occurring under circumstances where causal relationship to Etodolac is uncertain. These reactions are listed as alerting information for physicians):
Body as a whole—Infection.
Cardiovascular system—Arrhythmias, myocardial infarction.
Digestive system—Esophagitis with or without stricture or cardiospasm, colitis.
Hemic and lympathic system—Leukopenia.
Metabolic and nutritional—Change in weight.
Nervous system—Paresthesia, confusion.
Respiratory system—Bronchitis, dyspnea, pharyngitis, rhinitis, sinusitis.
Skin and appendages—Maculopapular rash, alopecia, skin peeling, photosensitivity.
Special senses—Conjunctivitis, deafness, taste perversion.
Urogenital system—Cystitis, hematuria, leukorrhea, renal calculus, interstitial nephritis, uterine bleeding irregularities.

DRUG ABUSE AND DEPENDENCE
Etodolac is a nonnarcotic drug. Several predictive animal studies indicated that Etodolac has no addiction potential in humans.

OVERDOSAGE
Symptoms following acute NSAID overdose are usually limited to lethargy, drowsiness, nausea, vomiting, and epigastric pain which are generally reversible with supportive care. Gastrointestinal bleeding can occur and coma has occurred following massive ibuprofen or mefenamic-acid overdose. Hypertension, acute renal failure, and respiratory depression may occur but are rare. Anaphylactoid reactions have been reported with therapeutic ingestion of NSAIDs, and may occur following overdose.

Patients should be managed by symptomatic and supportive care following an NSAID overdose. There are no specific antidotes. Gut decontamination may be indicated in patients seen within 4 hours of ingestion with symptoms or following a large overdose (5 to 10 times the usual dose). This should be accomplished via emesis and/or activated charcoal (60 to 100 g in adults, 1 to 2 g/kg in children) with an osmotic cathartic. Forced diuresis, alkalinization of the urine, hemodialysis or hemoperfusion would probably not be useful due to Etodolac's high protein binding.

One case of intentional Etodolac overdosage has been reported (Human Toxicol. 1988; 7:203-4). This 53-year-old female ingested from 15 to 46 two-hundred mg Etodolac capsules (3 to 8.6 grams). Plasma Etodolac concentrations were measured frequently over the next 4 days. At 5 hours after ingestion (3 hours after gastric lavage) the plasma Etodolac level was 22 µg/mL. These plasma levels and her subsequent recovery with no signs or symptoms of Etodolac toxicity were consistent with systemic absorption of 600 to 800 mg. Her laboratory tests on admission showed a prolonged prothrombin time and a false-positive urine bilirubin (attributed to the phenolic Etodolac metabolites).

DOSAGE AND ADMINISTRATION
ANALGESIA
The recommended dose of Etodolac for acute pain is 200 to 400 mg every 6 to 8 hours, as needed, not to exceed a total daily dose of 1200 mg. For patients

---

* Drug-related patient complaints occurring in 3% to 9% of patients treated with Etodolac. Drug-related patient complaints occurring in fewer than 3%, but more than 1%, are unmarked.

---

weighing 60 kg or less, the total daily dose of Etodolac should not exceed 20 mg/kg. For more details see *"Individualization of Dosage."*

OSTEOARTHRITIS

The recommended dose of Etodolac for the management of the signs and symptoms of osteoarthritis is initially 800 to 1200 mg/day in divided doses, followed by dosage adjustment within the range of 600 to 1200 mg/day given in divided doses: 400 mg t.i.d. or b.i.d.: 300 mg q.i.d., t.i.d., or b.i.d.: 200 mg q.i.d. or t.i.d.. The total daily dose of Etodolac should not exceed 1200 mg. For patients weighing 60 kg or less, the total daily dose of Etodolac should not exceed 20 mg/kg. For more details see *"Individualization Of Dosage."*

CAPSULES IN BOTTLES
Store at 15°-30°C (59°-86°F), protected from moisture.

CAPSULES IN UNIT-DOSE PACKAGES
Store at 15°-25°C (59°-77°F), protected from moisture.

TABLETS IN BOTTLES
Store at 15°-30°C (59°-86°F).

TABLETS IN UNIT-DOSE PACKAGES
Store at 15°-30°C (59°-36°F).

HOW SUPPLIED
CAPSULE: 200 MG

BRAND/MANUFACTURER	NDC	SIZE	AWP
○ **BRAND**			
➤ LODINE: Wyeth-Ayerst	00046-0738-81	100s	$97.21
	00046-0738-99	100s ud	$101.79

CAPSULE: 300 MG

BRAND/MANUFACTURER	NDC	SIZE	AWP
○ **BRAND**			
➤ LODINE: Wyeth-Ayerst	00046-0739-81	100s	$110.10
	00046-0739-99	100s ud	$114.59

TABLETS: 400 MG

BRAND/MANUFACTURER	NDC	SIZE	AWP
○ **BRAND**			
➤ LODINE: Wyeth-Ayerst	00046-0761-81	100s	$116.38
	00046-0761-99	100s ud	$116.38

Etomidate

DESCRIPTION
Etomidate is a sterile, nonpyrogenic solution.

It is intended for the induction of general anesthesia by intravenous injection.

The drug Etomidate is chemically identified as (R)-(+)-ethyl-1-(1-phenylethyl)-1H-imidazole-5-carboxylate.

Following is its chemical structure:

CLINICAL PHARMACOLOGY
Etomidate is a hypnotic drug without analgesic activity. Intravenous injection of Etomidate produces hypnosis characterized by a rapid onset of action, usually within one minute. Duration of hypnosis is dose dependent but relatively brief, usually three to five minutes when an average dose of 0.3 mg/kg is employed. Immediate recovery from anesthesia (as assessed by awakening time, time needed to follow simple commands and time to perform simple tests after anesthesia as well as they were performed before anesthesia), based upon data derived from short operative procedures where intravenous Etomidate was used for both induction and maintenance of anesthesia, is about as rapid as, or slightly faster than, immediate recovery after similar use of thiopental. These same data revealed that the immediate recovery period will usually be shortened in adult patients by the intravenous administration of approximately 0.1 mg of intravenous fentanyl, one or two minutes before induction of anesthesia, probably because less Etomidate is generally required under these circumstances (consult the package insert for fentanyl before using).

The most characteristic effect of intravenous Etomidate on the respiratory system is a slight elevation in arterial carbon dioxide tension ($PaCO_2$). See also *"Adverse Reactions".*

Reduced cortisol plasma levels have been reported with induction doses of 0.3 mg/kg Etomidate. These persist for approximately 6 to 8 hours and appear to be unresponsive to ACTH administration.

The intravenous administration of up to 0.6 mg/kg of Etomidate to patients with severe cardiovascular disease has little or no effect on myocardial metabolism, cardiac output, peripheral circulation or pulmonary circulation. The hemodynamic effects of Etomidate have in most cases been qualitatively similar to those of thiopental sodium, except that the heart rate tended to increase by a moderate amount following administration of thiopental under conditions where there was little or no change in heart rate following administration of Etomidate. There are insufficient data concerning use of Etomidate in patients with recent severe trauma or hypovolemia to predict cardiovascular response under such circumstances.

Clinical experience and special studies to date suggest that standard doses of intravenous Etomidate ordinarily neither elevate plasma histamine nor cause signs of histamine release.

Limited clinical experience, as well as animal studies, suggests that inadvertent intra-arterial injection of Etomidate, unlike thiobarbiturates, will not usually be followed by necrosis of tissue distal to the injection site. Intra-arterial injection of Etomidate is, however, not recommended.

Etomidate induction is associated with a transient 20-30% decrease in cerebral blood flow. This reduction in blood flow appears to be uniform in the absence of intracranial space occupying lesions. As with other intravenous induction agents, reduction in cerebral oxygen utilization is roughly proportional to the reduction in cerebral blood flow. In patients with and without intracranial space occupying lesions, Etomidate induction is usually followed by a moderate lowering of intracranial pressure, lasting several minutes. All of these studies provided for avoidance of hypercapnia. Information concerning regional cerebral perfusion in patients with intracranial space occupying lesions is too limited to permit definitive conclusions.

Preliminary data suggests that Etomidate will usually lower intraocular pressure moderately.

Etomidate is rapidly metabolized in the liver. Minimal hypnotic plasma levels of unchanged drug are equal to or higher than 0.23 µg/mL; they decrease rapidly up to 30 minutes following injection and thereafter more slowly with a half-life value of about 75 minutes. Approximately 75% of the administered dose is excreted in the urine during the first day after injection. The chief metabolite is R-(+)-1-(1-phenylethyl)-1H-imidazole-5-carboxylic acid, resulting from hydrolysis of Etomidate, and accounts for about 80% of the urinary excretion. Limited pharmacokinetic data in patients with cirrhosis and esophageal varices suggest that the volume of distribution and elimination half-life of Etomidate are approximately double that seen in healthy subjects. (Reference: H. Van Beem, et. al., Anaesthesia 38 (Supp 38:61-62, July 1983).

Reduced plasma cortisol and aldosterone levels have been reported following induction doses of Etomidate. These results persist for approximately 6-8 hours and appear to be unresponsive to ACTH stimulation. This probably represents blockage of 11 beta-hydroxylation within the adrenal cortex. (References: 1. R.J. Fragen, et. al., Anesthesiology 61:652-656, 1984. 2. R.L. Wagner & P.F. White, Anesthesiology 61:647-651, 1984. 3. F.H. DeJong, et. al., Clin. Endocrinology and Metabolism 59:(6):1143-1147, 1984, and three additional drafts of Metabolic Studies, all submitted to NDA 18-228 on April 1, 1985).

INDICATIONS AND USAGE
Etomidate is indicated by intravenous injection for the induction of general anesthesia. When considering use of Etomidate, the usefulness of its hemodynamic properties (see *"Clinical Pharmacology"*) should be weighed against the high frequency of transient skeletal muscle movements (see *"Adverse Reactions"*).

Intravenous Etomidate is also indicated for the supplementation of subpotent anesthetic agents, such as nitrous oxide in oxygen, during maintenance of anesthesia for short operative procedures such as dilation and curettage or cervical conization.

UNLABELED USE

Etomidate is used alone or as an adjunct in the treatment of status epilepticus resistant to standard therapy.

CONTRAINDICATIONS
Etomidate is contraindicated in patients who have shown hypersensitivity to it.

WARNINGS
INTRAVENOUS ETOMIDATE SHOULD BE ADMINISTERED ONLY BY PERSONS TRAINED IN THE ADMINISTRATION OF GENERAL ANESTHETICS AND IN THE MANAGEMENT OF COMPLICATIONS ENCOUNTERED DURING THE CONDUCT OF GENERAL ANESTHESIA.

BECAUSE OF THE HAZARDS OF PROLONGED SUPPRESSION OF ENDOGENOUS CORTISOL AND ALDOSTERONE PRODUCTION, THIS FORMULATION IS NOT INTENDED FOR ADMINISTRATION BY PROLONGED INFUSION.

PRECAUTIONS
Do not administer unless solution is clear and container is undamaged. Discard unused portion (see *"Dosage and Administration"*).

1. Carcinogenesis, Mutagenesis, Impairment of Fertility: No carcinogenesis or mutagenesis studies have been carried out on Etomidate. The results of reproduction studies showed no impairment of fertility in male and female rats when Etomidate was given prior to pregnancy at 0.31, 1.25 and 5 mg/kg (approximately 1X, 4X and 16X human dosage).

2. Pediatric Use: There are inadequate data to make dosage recommendations for induction of anesthesia in patients below the age of ten (10) years; therefore, such use is not recommended (see also *"Dosage and Administration"*).

3. Pregnancy Category C. Etomidate has been shown to have an embryocidal effect in rats when given in doses 1 and 4 times the human dose. There are no adequate and well-controlled studies in pregnant women. Etomidate should be used during pregnancy only if the potential benefit justifies the potential risks to

➤ SHOWN IN PRODUCT IDENTIFICATION GUIDE

1348 / PRODUCT INFORMATION

the fetus. Etomidate has not been shown to be teratogenic in animals. Reproduction studies with Etomidate have been shown to:

a. Decrease pup survival at 0.3 and 5 mg/kg in rats (approximately 1X and 16X human dosage) and at 1.5 and 4.5 mg/kg in rabbits (approximately 5X and 15X human dosage). No clear dose-related pattern was observed.

b. Increase slightly the number of stillborn fetuses in rats at 0.3 and 1.25 mg/kg (approximately 1X and 4X human dosage).

c. Cause maternal toxicity with deaths of 6/20 rats at 5 mg/kg (approximately 16X human dosage) and 6/20 rabbits at 4.5 mg/kg (approximately 15X human dosage).

4. Labor and Delivery: There are insufficient data to support use of intravenous Etomidate in obstetrics, including Caesarean section deliveries. Therefore, such use is not recommended.

5. Nursing Mothers: It is not known whether this drug is excreted in human milk. Because many drugs are excreted in human milk, caution should be exercised when Etomidate is administered to a nursing mother.

6. Plasma Cortisol Levels: Induction doses of Etomidate have been associated with reduction in plasma cortisol and aldosterone concentrations (see *"Clinical Pharmacology"*). These have not been associated with changes in vital signs or evidence of increased mortality; however, where concern exists for patients undergoing severe stress, exogenous replacement should be considered.

ADVERSE REACTIONS

The most frequent adverse reactions associated with use of intravenous Etomidate are transient venous pain on injection and transient skeletal muscle movements, including myoclonus:

1. Transient venous pain was observed immediately following intravenous injection of Etomidate in about 20% of the patients, with considerable difference in the reported incidence (1.2% to 42%). This pain is usually described as mild to moderate in severity but it is occasionally judged disturbing. The observation of venous pain is not associated with a more than usual incidence of thrombosis or thrombophlebitis at the injection site. Pain also appears to be less frequently noted when larger, more proximal arm veins are employed and it appears to be more frequently noted when smaller, more distal, hand or wrist veins are employed.

2. Transient skeletal muscle movements were noted following use of intravenous Etomidate in about 32% of the patients, with considerable difference in the reported incidence (22.7% to 63%). Most of these observations were judged mild to moderate in severity but some were judged disturbing. The incidence of disturbing movements was less when 0.1 mg of fentanyl was given immediately before induction. These movements have been classified as myoclonic in the majority of cases (74%), but averting movements (7%), tonic movements (10%), and eye movements (9%) have also been reported. No exact classification is available, but these movements may also be placed into three groups by location:

a. Most movements are bilateral. The arms, legs, shoulders, neck, chest wall, trunk and all four extremities have been described in some cases, with one or more of these muscle groups predominating in each individual case. Results of electroencephalographic studies suggest that these muscle movements are a manifestation of disinhibition of cortical activity; cortical electroencephalograms, taken during periods when these muscle movements were observed, have failed to reveal seizure activity.

b. Other movements are described as either unilateral or having a predominance of activity of one side over the other. These movements sometimes resemble a localized response to some stimuli, such as venous pain on injection, in the lightly anesthetized patient (averting movements). Any muscle group or groups may be involved, but a predominance of movement of the arm in which the intravenous infusion is started is frequently noted.

c. Still other movements probably represent a mixture of the first two types.

Skeletal muscle movements appear to be more frequent in patients who also manifest venous pain on injection.

OTHER ADVERSE OBSERVATIONS

Respiratory System: Hyperventilation, hypoventilation, apnea of short duration (5 to 90 seconds with spontaneous recovery), laryngospasm, hiccup and snoring suggestive of partial upper airway obstruction have been observed in some patients. These conditions were managed by conventional countermeasures.

Circulatory System: Hypertension, hypotension, tachycardia, bradycardia and other arrhythmias have occasionally been observed during induction and maintenance of anesthesia. One case of severe hypotension and tachycardia, judged to be anaphylactoid in character, has been reported. (Reference: M. Sold and A. Rothhammer, Anaesthesist 34:208-210, 1985. Submitted to NDA 18-228 on 16 May 1985).

Gastrointestinal System: Postoperative nausea and/or vomiting following induction of anesthesia with Etomidate is probably no more frequent than the general incidence. When Etomidate was used for both induction and maintenance of anesthesia in short procedures such as dilation and curettage, or when insufficient analgesia was provided, the incidence of postoperative nausea and/or vomiting was higher than that noted in control patients who received thiopental.

OVERDOSAGE

Overdosage may occur from too rapid or repeated injections. Too rapid injection may be followed by a fall in blood pressure. No adverse cardiovascular or respiratory effects attributable to Etomidate overdose have been reported.

In the event of suspected or apparent overdosage, the drug should be discontinued, a patent airway established (intubate, if necessary) or maintained and oxygen administered with assisted ventilation, if necessary.

The LD_{50} of Etomidate administered intravenously to rats is 20.4 mg/kg.

DOSAGE AND ADMINISTRATION

Etomidate injection is intended for administration only by the intravenous route (see *"Clinical Pharmacology"*). The dose for induction of anesthesia in adult patients and in children above the age of ten (10) years will vary between 0.2 and 0.6 mg/kg of body weight, and it must be individualized in each case. The usual dose for induction in these patients is 0.3 mg/kg, injected over a period of 30 to 60 seconds. There are inadequate data to make dosage recommendations for induction of anesthesia in patients below the age of ten (10) years; therefore, such use is not recommended.

Smaller increments of intravenous Etomidate may be administered to adult patients during short operative procedures to supplement subpotent anesthetic agents, such as nitrous oxide. The dosage employed under these circumstances, although usually smaller than the original induction dose, must be individualized. There are insufficient data to support this use of Etomidate for longer adult procedures or for any procedures in children; therefore, such use is not recommended. The use of intravenous fentanyl and other neuroactive drugs employed during the conduct of anesthesia may alter the Etomidate dosage requirements. Consult the prescribing information for all other such drugs before using.

Premedication: Etomidate injection is compatible with commonly administered pre-anesthetic medications, which may be employed as indicated. See also *"Clinical Pharmacology"*, *"Adverse Reactions"*, and dosage recommendations for maintenance of anesthesia.

Etomidate hypnosis does not significantly alter the usual dosage requirements of neuromuscular blocking agents employed for endotracheal intubation or other purposes shortly after induction of anesthesia.

Parenteral drug products should be inspected visually for particulate matter and discoloration prior to administration, whenever solution and container permit.

To prevent needle-stick injuries, needles should not be recapped, purposely bent, or broken by hand.

Storage: Store at controlled room temperature 15° to 30°C (59° to 86° F).

HOW SUPPLIED
INJECTION: 2 MG/ML

BRAND/MANUFACTURER	NDC	SIZE	AWP
○ BRAND			
AMIDATE: Abbott Hosp	00074-8062-01	10 ml 5s	$112.58
	00074-8061-01	20 ml 5s	$128.90
	00074-8060-01	20 ml 10s	$260.78
	00074-8060-03	20 ml 10s	$274.08

Etoposide

> ## WARNINGS
> ETOPOSIDE SHOULD BE ADMINISTERED UNDER THE SUPERVISION OF A QUALIFIED PHYSICIAN EXPERIENCED IN THE USE OF CANCER CHEMOTHERAPEUTIC AGENTS. SEVERE MYELOSUPPRESSION WITH RESULTING INFECTION OR BLEEDING MAY OCCUR.

DESCRIPTION

Etoposide (also commonly known as VP-16) is a semisynthetic derivative of podophyllotoxin used in the treatment of certain neoplastic diseases. It is 4'-demethylepipodophyllotoxin 9-[4,6-0-(R)-ethylidene-β-D-glucopryanoside]. It is very soluble in methanol and chloroform, slightly soluble in ethanol, and sparingly soluble in water and ether. It is made more miscible with water by means of organic solvents. It has a molecular weight of 588.58 and a molecular formula of $C_{29}H_{32}O_{13}$.

Etoposide may be administered either intravenously or orally. Etoposide for injection is available in 100 mg (5 mL) or 150 mg (7.5 mL), sterile, multiple dose vials. The pH of the clear yellow solution is 3 to 4. Each mL contains 20 mg Etoposide, 2 mg citric acid, 30 mg benzyl alcohol, 80 mg modified polysorbate 80/tween 80, 650 mg polyethylene glycol 300, and 30.5 percent (v/v) alcohol. Vial headspace contains nitrogen.

Etoposide is also available as 50 mg pink capsules. Each liquid filled, soft gelatin capsule contains 50 mg of Etoposide in a vehicle consisting of citric acid, glycerin, purified water, and polyethylene glycol 400.

◆ RATED THERAPEUTICALLY EQUIVALENT; ◇ THERAPEUTIC EQUIVALENCE UNCONFIRMED; ○ UNRATED

Following is its chemical structure:

CLINICAL PHARMACOLOGY

Etoposide has been shown to cause metaphase arrest in chick fibroblasts. Its main effect, however, appears to be at the G_2 portion of the cell cycle in mammalian cells. Two different dose-dependent responses are seen. At high concentrations (10 µ/mL or more), lysis of cells entering mitosis is observed. At low concentrations (0.3 to 10 µg/mL), cells are inhibited from entering prophase. It does not interfere with microtubular assembly. The predominant macromolecular effect of Etoposide appears to be DNA synthesis inhibition.

Pharmacokinetics: On intravenous administration, the disposition of Etoposide is best described as a biphasic process with a distribution half-life of about 1.5 hours and terminal elimination half-life ranging from 4 to 11 hours. Total body clearance values range from 33 to 48 mL/min or 16 to 36 mL/min/m^2 and, like the terminal elimination half-life, are independent of dose over a range 100-600 mg/m^2. Over the same dose range, the areas under the plasma concentration vs. time curves (AUC) and the maximum plasma concentration (Cmax) values increase linearly with dose. Etoposide does not accumulate in the plasma following daily administration of 100 mg/m^2 for 4 to 5 days.

The mean volumes of distribution at steady state fall in the range of 18 to 29 liters or 7 to 17 L/m^2. Etoposide enters the CSF poorly. Although it is detectable in CSF and intracerebral tumors, the concentrations are lower than in extracerebral tumors and in plasma. Etoposide concentrations are higher in normal lung than in lung metastases and are similar in primary tumors and normal tissues of the myometrium. In vitro, Etoposide is highly protein bound (97%) to human plasma proteins. An inverse relationship between plasma albumin levels and Etoposide renal clearance is found in children. In a study determining the effect of other therapeutic agents on the *in vitro* binding of carbon-14 labeled Etoposide to human serum proteins, only phenylbutazone, sodium salicylate and aspirin displaced protein-bound Etoposide at concentrations achieved *in vivo*.[1]

Etoposide binding ratio correlates directly with serum albumin in patients with cancer and in normal volunteers. The unbound fraction of Etoposide significantly correlated with bilirubin in a population of cancer patients.[2,3]

After intravenous administration of ^{3}H-Etoposide (70-290 mg/m^2), mean recoveries of radioactivity in the urine range from 42 to 67%, and fecal recoveries range from 0 to 16% of the dose. Less than 50% of an intravenous dose is excreted in the urine as Etoposide with mean recoveries of 8 to 35% within 24 hours.

In children, approximately 55% of the dose is excreted in the urine as Etoposide in 24 hours. The mean renal clearance of Etoposide is 7 to 10 mL/min/m^2 or about 35% of the total body clearance over a dose range of 80 to 600 mg/m^2. Etoposide, therefore, is cleared by both renal and nonrenal processes, ie, metabolism and biliary excretion. The effect of renal disease on plasma Etoposide clearance is not known. Biliary excretion appears to be a minor route of Etoposide elimination. Only 6% or less of an intravenous dose is recovered in the bile as Etoposide. Metabolism accounts for most of the nonrenal clearance of Etoposide. The major urinary metabolite of Etoposide in adults and children is the hydroxy acid [4'-demethylepipodophyllic acid-9-(4, 6-0-(R)-ethylidene-β-D-glucopyranoside)], formed by opening of the lactone ring. It is also present in human plasma, presumably as the *trans* isomer. Glucuronide and/or sulfate conjugates of Etoposide are excreted in human urine and represent 5 to 22% of the dose.

After either intravenous infusion or oral capsule administration, the Cmax and AUC values exhibit marked intra- and inter-subject variability. This results in variability in the estimates of the absolute oral bioavailability of Etoposide oral capsules.

Cmax and AUC values for orally administered Etoposide capsules consistently fall in the same range as the Cmax and AUC values for an intravenous dose of one-half the size of the oral dose. The overall mean value of oral capsule bioavailability is approximately 50% (range 25-75%). The bioavailability of Etoposide capsules appears to be linear up to a dose of at least 250 mg/m^2.

There is no evidence of a first-pass effect for Etoposide. For example, no correlation exists between the absolute oral bioavailability of Etoposide capsules and nonrenal clearance. No evidence exists for any other differences in Etoposide metabolism and excretion after administration of oral capsules as compared to intravenous infusion.

In adults, the total body clearance of Etoposide is correlated with creatinine clearance, serum albumin concentration, and nonrenal clearance. In children, elevated serum SGPT levels are associated with reduced drug total body clearance. Prior use of cisplatin may also result in a decrease of Etoposide total body clearance in children.

INDICATION AND USAGE

Etoposide is indicated in the management of the following neoplasms:

Refractory Testicular Tumors: Etoposide for injection in combination therapy with other approved chemotherapeutic agents in patients with refractory testicular tumors who have already received appropriate surgical, chemotherapeutic, and radiotherapeutic therapy.

Adequate data on the use of Etoposide capsules in the treatment of testicular cancer are not available.

Small Cell Lung Cancer: Etoposide for injection and/or capsules in combination with other approved chemotherapeutic agents as first line treatment in patients with small cell lung cancer.

UNLABELED USES

Etoposide is used alone or as an adjunct in the treatment of choriocarcinoma, chorioadenoma destruens, Ewing's sarcoma, Kaposi sarcoma in patients with acquired immunodeficiency syndrome (AIDS), neuroblastoma, rhabdomyosarcoma, ovarian cancer, glioma, refractory advanced breast carcinoma, and hydatiform moles.

CONTRAINDICATIONS

Etoposide is contraindicated in patients who have demonstrated a previous hypersensitivity to Etoposide or any component of the formulation.

WARNINGS

Patients being treated with Etoposide must be frequently observed for myelosuppression both during and after therapy. Dose-limiting bone marrow suppression is the most significant toxicity associated with Etoposide therapy. Therefore, the following studies should be obtained at the start of therapy and prior to each subsequent dose of Etoposide platelet count, hemoglobin, white blood cell count and differential. The occurrence of a platelet count below 50,000/mm^3 or an absolute neutrophil count below 500/mm^3 is an indication to withhold further therapy until the blood counts have sufficiently recovered.

Physicians should be aware of the possible occurrence of an anaphylactic reaction manifested by chills, fever, tachycardia, bronchospasm, dyspnea, and hypotension. (See *"Adverse Reactions"* section.) Treatment is symptomatic. The infusion should be terminated immediately followed by the administration of pressor agents, corticosteroids, antihistamines, or volume expanders at the discretion of the physician.

For parenteral administration, Etoposide should be given only by slow intravenous infusion (usually over a 30 to 60 minute period) since hypotension has been reported as a possible side effect of rapid intravenous injection.

Pregnancy: Pregnancy "Category D." Etoposide can cause fetal harm when administered to a pregnant woman. Etoposide has been shown to be teratogenic in mice and rats. There are no adequate and well-controlled studies in pregnant women. If this drug is used during pregnancy, or if the patient becomes pregnant while receiving this drug, the patient should be apprised of the potential hazard to the fetus. Women of childbearing potential should be advised to avoid becoming pregnant.

Etoposide is teratogenic and embryocidal in rats and mice at doses of 1 to 3% of the recommended clinical dose based on body surface area.

In a teratology study in SPF rats, Etoposide was administered intravenously at doses of 0.13, 0.4, 1.2, and 3.6 mg/kg/day on days 6 to 15 of gestation. Etoposide caused dose-related maternal toxicity; embryotoxicity, and teratogenicity at dose levels of 0.4 mg/kg/day and higher. Embryonic resorptions were 90 and 100% at the 2 highest dosages. At 0.4 and 1.2 mg/kg, fetal weights were decreased and fetal abnormalities including decreased weight, major skeletal abnormalities, exencephaly, encephalocele, and anophthalmia occurred. Even at the lowest dose tested, 0.13 mg/kg, a significant increase in retarded ossification was observed.

Etoposide administered as a single intraperitoneal, injection in Swiss-Albino mice at dosages of 1, 1.5 and 2 mg/kg on days 6, 7, or 8 of gestation caused dose-related embryotoxicity, cranial abnormalities, and major skeletal malformations.

PRECAUTIONS

General: In all instances where the use of Etoposide is considered for chemotherapy, the physician must evaluate the need and usefulness of the drug against the risk of adverse reactions. Most such adverse reactions are reversible if detected early. If severe reactions occur, the drug should be reduced in dosage or discontinued and appropriate corrective measures should be taken according to the clinical judgment of the physician. Reinstitution of Etoposide therapy should be carried out with caution, and with adequate consideration of the further need for the drug and alertness as to possible recurrence of toxicity.

Laboratory Tests: Periodic complete blood counts should be done during the course of Etoposide treatment. They should be performed prior to therapy and appropriate intervals during and after therapy. At least one determination should be done prior to each dose of Etoposide.

Carcinogenesis, Mutagenesis, Impairment of Fertility: Carcinogenicity tests with Etoposide have not been conducted in laboratory animals. Etoposide should be considered a potential carcinogen in humans. The occurrence of acute leukemia with or without a preleukemic phase has been reported rarely in patients treated with Etoposide in association with other antineoplastic agents.

The mutagenic and genotoxic potential of Etoposide has been established in mammalian cells. Etoposide caused aberrations in chromosome number and structure in embryonic murine cells and human hematopoietic cells; gene mutations in Chinese hamster ovary cells; and DNA damage by strand breakage and DNA-protein cross-links in mouse leukemia cells. Etoposide also caused a dose-related increase in sister chromatid exchanges in Chinese hamster ovary cells.

Treatment of Swiss-Albino mice with 1.5 mg/kg IP of Etoposide on day 7 of gestation increased the incidence of intrauterine death and fetal malformations as well as significantly decreased the average fetal body weight. Maternal weight gain was not affected.

Treatment of pregnant SPF rats with 1.2 mg/kg/day IV of Etoposide for 10 days led to a prenatal mortality of 92%, and 50% of the implanting fetuses were abnormal.

Pregnancy: Pregnancy "Category D." (See "*Warnings*") section.

Nursing Mothers: It is not known whether this drug is excreted in human milk. Because many drugs are excreted in human milk and because of the potential for serious adverse reactions in nursing infants from Etoposide, a decision should be made whether to discontinue nursing or to discontinue the drug, taking into account the importance of the drug to the mother.

Pediatric Use: Safety and effectiveness in children have not been established.

Etoposide for injection contains polysorbate 80. In premature infants, a life-threatening syndrome consisting of liver and renal failure, pulmonary deterioration, thrombocytopenia, and ascites has been associated with an injectable vitamin E product containing polysorbate 80.

ADVERSE REACTIONS

The following data on adverse reactions are based on both oral and intravenous administration of Etoposide as a single agent, using several different dose schedules for treatment of a wide variety of malignancies.

Hematologic Toxicity: Myelosuppression is dose related and dose limiting, with granulocyte nadirs occurring 7 to 14 days after drug administration and platelet nadirs occurring 9 to 16 days administration. Bone marrow recovery is usually complete by day 20, and no cumulative toxicity has been reported.

The occurrence of acute leukemia with or without a preleukemic phase has been reported rarely in patients treated with Etoposide in association with other antineoplastic agents.

Gastrointestinal Toxicity: Nausea and vomiting are the major gastrointestinal toxicities. The severity of such nausea and vomiting is generally mild to moderate with treatment discontinuation required in 1% of patients. Nausea and vomiting can usually be controlled with standard antiemetic therapy. Gastrointestinal toxicities are slightly more frequent after oral administration than after intravenous infusion.

Hypotension: Transient hypotension following rapid intravenous administration has been reported in 1% to 2% of patients. It has not been associated with cardiac toxicity or electrocardiographic changes. No delayed hypotension has been noted. To prevent this rare occurrence, it is recommended that Etoposide administered by slow intravenous infusion over a 30- to 60-minute period. If hypotension occurs, it usually responds to cessation of the infusion and administration of fluids or other supportive therapy as appropriate. When restarting the infusion, a slower administration rate should be used.

Allergic Reactions: Anaphylactic-like reactions characterized by chills, fever, tachycardia, bronchospasm, dyspnea and/or hypotension have been reported to occur in 0.7% to 2% of patients receiving intravenous Etoposide and in less than 1% of the patients treated with the oral capsules. These reactions have usually responded promptly to the cessation of the infusion and administration of pressor agents, corticosteroids, antihistamines, or volume expanders as appropriate; however, the reactions can be fatal. Hypertension and/or flushing have also been reported. Blood pressure usually normalizes within a few hours after cessation of the infusion. Anaphylatic-like reactions have occurred during the initial infusion of Etoposide.

Facial/tongue swelling, coughing, diaphoresis, cyanosis, tightness in throat, laryngospasm, back pain and/or loss of consciousness have sometimes occurred in association with the above reactions. In addition, an apparent hypersensitivity-associated apnea has been reported rarely.

Rash, urticaria, and/or pruritus have infrequently been reported at recommended doses. At investigational doses, a generalized pruritic erythematous maculopapular rash, consistent with perivasculitis, has been reported.

Alopecia: Reversible alopecia, sometimes progressing to total baldness, was observed in up to 66% of patients.

Other Toxicities: The following adverse reactions have been infrequently reported: aftertaste, fever, pigmentation, abdominal pain, constipation, dysphagia, transient cortical blindness, and optic neuritis, and a single report of radiation recall dermatitis.

Hepatic toxicity, generally in patients receiving higher doses of the drug than those recommended, has been reported with Etoposide. Metabolic acidosis has also been reported in patients receiving higher doses.

The incidences of adverse reactions in the table that follows are derived from multiple data bases from studies in 2,081 patients when Etoposide was used either orally or by injection as a single agent.

Adverse Drug Effect	Percent Range of Reported Incidence
Hematologic toxicity	
Leukopenia (less than 1,000 WBC/mm^3)	3-17
Leukopenia (less than 4,000 WBC/mm^3)	60-91
Thrombocytopenia (less than 50,000 platelets/mm^3)	1-20
Thrombocytopenia (less than 100,000 platelets/mm^3)	22-41
Anemia	0-33
Gastrointestinal toxicity	
Nausea and vomiting	31-43
Abdominal pain	0-2
Anorexia	10-13
Diarrhea	1-13
Stomatitis	1-6
Hepatic	0-3
Alopecia	8-66
Peripheral neurotoxicity	1-2
Hypotension	1-2
Allergic reaction	1-2

OVERDOSAGE

No proven antidotes have been established for Etoposide dosage.

DOSAGE AND ADMINISTRATION

Note: Plastic devices made of acrylic or ABS (a polymer composed of acrylonitrile, butadiene, and styrene) have been reported to crack and leak when used with *undiluted* Etoposide for Injection.

Etoposide for Injection: The usual dose of Etoposide for injection in testicular cancer in combination with other approved chemotherapeutic agents ranges from 50 to 100 mg/m^2/day on days 1 through 5 to 100 mg/m^2/day on days 1, 3, and 5. In small cell lung cancer, the Etoposide for injection dose in combination with other approved chemotherapeutic drugs ranges from 35 mg/m^2/day for 4 days to 50 mg/m^2/day for 5 days.

Chemotherapy courses are repeated at 3-to 4-week intervals after adequate recovery from any toxicity.

Etoposide Capsules: In small cell lung cancer, the recommended dose of Etoposide Capsules is two times the IV dose rounded to the nearest 50 mg.

The dosage, by either route, should be modified to take into account the myelosuppressive effects of other drugs in the combination or the effects of prior x-ray therapy or chemotherapy which may have compromised bone marrow reserve.

Administration Precautions: As with other potentially toxic compounds, caution should be exercised in handling and preparing the solution of Etoposide. Skin reactions associated with accidental exposure to Etoposide may occur. The use of gloves is recommended. If Etoposide solution contacts the skin or mucosa, immediately wash the skin or mucosa thoroughly with soap and water.

Preparation for Intravenous Administration: Etoposide for injection must be diluted prior to use with either 5% Dextrose Injection, USP, or 0.9% Sodium Chloride Injection, USP, to give a final concentration of 0.2 or 0.4 mg/mL. If solutions are prepared at concentrations above 0.4 mg/mL, precipitation may occur. Hypotension following rapid intravenous administration has been reported hence, it is recommended that the Etoposide solution be administered over a 30- to 60-minute period. A longer duration of administration may be used if the volume of fluid to be infused is a concern.

Etoposide should not be given by rapid intravenous injection: Parenteral drug products should be inspected visually for particulate matter and discoloration (see "*Description*" section) prior to administration whenever solution and container permit.

Stability: Unopened vials of Etoposide for injection are stable for 24 months at room temperature (25°C). Vials diluted as recommended to a concentration of 0.2 or 0.4 mg/mL are stable for 96 and 24 hours, respectively, at room temperature (25°C) under normal room fluorescent light in both glass and plastic containers.

Etoposide capsules must be stored under refrigeration 2°-8°C (36°-46°F). The capsules are stable for 24 months under such refrigeration conditions.

Procedures for proper handling and disposal of anticancer drugs should be considered. Several guidelines on this subject have been published[4-10]. There is no general agreement that all of the procedures recommended in the guidelines are necessary or appropriate.

Capsules are to be stored under refrigeration 2°-8°C (36°-46°F).
Do Not Freeze.
Dispense in child-resistant containers.

REFERENCES

1. Gaver RC; Deeb G; "The effect of other drugs on the *in vitro* binding of 14C-Etoposide to human serum proteins." *Pro Am Assoc Cancer Res.* 30132, 1989. 2. Stewart CF; Pieper JA; Arbuck SG; Evans WE; "Altered protein binding of Etoposide in patients with cancer." *Clin Pharmacol Ther.* 45:49-55 1989. 3. Stewart CF; Arbuck SG; Fleming RA; Evans WE; "Prospective evaluation of a model for predicting Etoposide plasma protein binding in cancer patients." *Proc Am Assoc Cancer Res.* 30-A958 1989. 4. Recommendations for the Safe Handling of Parenteral Antineoplastic Drugs, NIH Publication No. 83-2621. For sale by the Superintendent of Documents, US Government Printing Office, Washington, D.C. 20402. 5. AMA Council Report. Guidelines for Handling Parenteral Antineoplastics. *JAMA.* 1985; 253 (11): 1590-1592. 6. National Study Commission on Cytotoxic Exposure—Recommendations for Handling Cytotoxic Agents. Available from Louis P. Jeffrey, Sc.D., Chairman, National Study Commission on Cytotoxic Exposure, Massachusetts College of Pharmacy and Allied Health Sciences, 179 Longwood Avenue, Boston, Massachusetts 02115. 7. Clinical

Oncological Society of Australia. Guidelines and Recommendations for Safe Handling of Antineoplastic Agents. *Med J Australia.* 1983; 1:426-428. 8. Jones RB, et al; Safe handling of chemotherapeutic agents: A report from the Mount Sinai Medical Center. *CA-A Cancer Journal for Clinicians.* 1983; (Sept/Oct) 258-263. 9. American Society of Hospital Pharmacists Technical Assistance Bulletin on Handling Cytotoxic and Hazardous Drugs. *Am J Hosp Pharm.* 1990; 47:1033-1049. 10. OSHA Work-Practice Guidelines for Personnel Dealing with Cytotoxic (Antineoplastic) Drugs. *Am J Hosp Pharm.* 1986; 43:1193-1204.

J CODES
100 mg IV—J9182
10 mg IV—J9181

HOW SUPPLIED
CAPSULE: 50 MG

BRAND/MANUFACTURER	NDC	SIZE	AWP
○ **BRAND**			
VEPESID: Bristol-Myer Onc/Hiv	00015-3091-45	20s ud	$674.68

INJECTION: 20 MG/ML

BRAND/MANUFACTURER	NDC	SIZE	AWP
○ **BRAND**			
VEPESID: Bristol-Myer Onc/Hiv	00015-3095-20	5 ml	$136.49
	00015-3084-20	7.5 ml	$204.74
○ **GENERICS**			
Gensia	00703-5643-01	5 ml	$131.30
Gensia	00703-5646-01	25 ml	$638.76

INJECTION: 500 MG

BRAND/MANUFACTURER	NDC	SIZE	AWP
○ **BRAND**			
VEPESID: Bristol-Myer Onc/Hiv	00015-3061-20	25 ml	$665.38

INJECTION: 1 GM

BRAND/MANUFACTURER	NDC	SIZE	AWP
○ **BRAND**			
VEPESID: Bristol-Myer Onc/Hiv	00015-3062-20	50 ml	$1296.64

Etrafon *SEE* AMITRIPTYLINE HYDROCHLORIDE WITH PERPHENAZINE

Etretinate

CONTRAINDICATION

ETRETINATE MUST NOT BE USED BY FEMALES WHO ARE PREGNANT, WHO INTEND TO BECOME PREGNANT, OR WHO ARE UNRELIABLE OR MAY NOT USE RELIABLE CONTRACEPTION WHILE UNDERGOING TREATMENT. THE PERIOD OF TIME DURING WHICH PREGNANCY MUST BE AVOIDED AFTER TREATMENT IS CONCLUDED HAS NOT BEEN DETERMINED. ETRETINATE BLOOD LEVELS OF 0.5 TO 12 NG/ML HAVE BEEN REPORTED IN 5 OF 47 PATIENTS IN THE RANGE OF 2.1 TO 2.9 YEARS AFTER TREATMENT WAS CONCLUDED. THE LENGTH OF TIME NECESSARY TO WAIT AFTER DISCONTINUATION OF TREATMENT TO ASSURE THAT NO DRUG WILL BE DETECTABLE IN THE BLOOD HAS NOT BEEN DETERMINED. THE SIGNIFICANCE OF UNDETECTABLE BLOOD LEVELS RELATIVE TO THE RISK OF TERATOGENICITY IS UNKNOWN.

MAJOR HUMAN FETAL ABNORMALITIES RELATED TO ETRETINATE ADMINISTRATION HAVE BEEN REPORTED, INCLUDING MENINGOMYELOCOELE, MENINGOENCEPHALOCOELE, MULTIPLE SYNOSTOSES, FACIAL DYSMORPHIA, SYNDACTYLIES, ABSENCE OF TERMINAL PHALANGES, MALFORMATIONS OF HIP, ANKLE AND FOREARM, LOW SET EARS, HIGH PALATE, DECREASED CRANIAL VOLUME, AND ALTERATIONS OF THE SKULL AND CERVICAL VERTEBRAE ON X-RAY.

WOMEN OF CHILDBEARING POTENTIAL MUST NOT BE GIVEN ETRETINATE UNTIL PREGNANCY IS EXCLUDED. IT IS STRONGLY RECOMMENDED THAT A PREGNANCY TEST BE PERFORMED WITHIN TWO WEEKS PRIOR TO INITIATING ETRETINATE THERAPY. ETRETINATE THERAPY SHOULD START ON THE SECOND OR THIRD DAY OF THE NEXT NORMAL MENSTRUAL PERIOD. AN EFFECTIVE FORM OF CONTRACEPTION MUST BE USED FOR AT LEAST ONE MONTH BEFORE ETRETINATE THERAPY, DURING THERAPY AND FOLLOWING DISCONTINUATION OF ETRETINATE THERAPY FOR AN INDEFINITE PERIOD OF TIME.

FEMALES SHOULD BE FULLY COUNSELED ON THE SERIOUS RISKS TO THE FETUS SHOULD THEY BECOME PREGNANT WHILE UNDERGOING TREATMENT OR AFTER DISCONTINUATION OF THERAPY. IF PREGNANCY DOES OCCUR, THE PHYSICIAN AND PATIENT SHOULD DISCUSS THE DESIRABILITY OF CONTINUING THE PREGNANCY.

DESCRIPTION

Etretinate, a retinoid, is available in 10-mg and 25-mg gelatin capsules for oral administration. Chemically, etretinate is ethyl (*all-E*)-9-(4-methoxy-2,3,6-trimethylphenyl)-3,7-dimethyl-2,4,6,8-nonate traenoate and is related to both retinoic acid and retinol (vitamin A). It is a greenish-yellow to yellow powder with a calculated molecular weight of 354.5.

Following is its chemical structure:

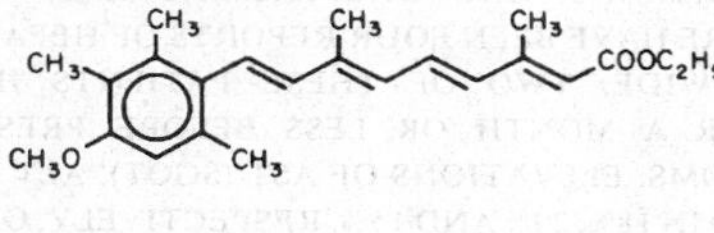

CLINICAL PHARMACOLOGY

The mechanism of action of Etretinate is unknown.

Clinical: Improvement in psoriatic patients occurs in association with a decrease in scale, erythema and thickness of lesions, as well as histological evidence of normalization of epidermal differentiation, decreased stratum corneum thickness and decreased inflammation in the epidermis and dermis.

Pharmacokinetics: The pharmacokinetic profile of Etretinate is predictable and is linear following single and multiple doses. Etretinate is extensively metabolized following oral dosing, with significant first-pass metabolism to the acid form, which also has the all-*trans* structure and is pharmacologically active. Subsequent metabolism results in the 13-*cis* acid form, chain-shortened breakdown products and conjugates that are ultimately excreted in the bile and urine.

After a six-month course of therapy with doses ranging from 25 mg once daily to 25 mg four times daily, Cmax values ranged from 102 to 389 ng/mL and occurred at Tmax values of two to six hours. In one study the apparent terminal half-life after six months of therapy was approximately 120 days. In another study of 47 patients treated chronically with Etretinate, 5 had detectable serum drug levels (in the range of 0.5 to 12 ng/mL) 2.1 to 2.9 years after therapy was discontinued. The long half-life appears to be due to storage of Etretinate in adipose tissue.

Etretinate is more than 99% bound to plasma proteins, predominantly lipoproteins, whereas its active metabolite, the all-*trans* acid form, is predominantly bound to albumin. Concentrations of Etretinate in blister fluid after six weeks of dosing were approximately one-tenth of those observed in plasma. Concentrations of Etretinate and its all-*trans* acid metabolite in epidermal specimens obtained after 1 to 36 months of therapy were a function of location; subcutis > > serum > epidermis > dermis. Similarly, liver concentrations of Etretinate in patients receiving therapy for six months were generally higher than concomitant plasma concentrations and tended to be higher in livers with a higher degree of fatty infiltration.

Studies in normal volunteers indicated that, when compared with the fasting state, the absorption of Etretinate was increased by whole milk or a high-lipid diet.

INDICATIONS AND USAGE

Etretinate indicated for the treatment of severe recalcitrant psoriasis, including the erythrodermic and generalized pustular types. Because of significant adverse effects associated with its use, Etretinate should be prescribed only by physicians knowledgeable in the systemic use of retinoids and reserved for patients with severe recalcitrant psoriasis who are unresponsive to or intolerant of standard therapies: topical tar plus UVB light; psoralens plus UVA light; systemic corticosteroids; and methotrexate.

The use of Etretinate resulted in clinical improvement in the majority of patients treated. Complete clearing of the disease was observed after four to nine months of therapy in 13% of all patients treated for severe psoriasis. This included complete clearing in 16% of patients with erythrodermic psoriasis and 37% of patients with generalized pustular psoriasis.

After discontinuation of Etretinate the majority of patients experience some degree of relapse by the end of two months. After relapse, subsequent four- to nine-month courses of Etretinate therapy resulted in approximately the same clinical response as experienced during the initial course of therapy.

UNLABELED USES

Etretinate is used alone or as an adjunct in the treatment of actinic keratosis, Darier's disease, lamellar ichthyosis, and X-linked ichthyosis. It is also used in the treatment of erythrokeratoderma variabilis, lichen planus and porokeratosis mibelli.

CONTRAINDICATIONS

Pregnancy: Category X. See boxed "*Contraindication*." (See related table).

WARNINGS

> *PSEUDOTUMOR CEREBRI:* ETRETINATE AND OTHER RETINOIDS HAVE BEEN ASSOCIATED WITH CASES OF PSEUDOTUMOR CEREBRI (BENIGN INTRACRANIAL HYPERTENSION). EARLY SIGNS AND SYMPTOMS OF PSEUDOTUMOR CEREBRI INCLUDE PAPILLEDEMA, HEADACHE, NAUSEA AND VOMITING, AND VISUAL DISTURBANCES. PATIENTS WITH THESE SYMPTOMS SHOULD BE EXAMINED FOR PAPILLEDEMA AND, IF PRESENT, THEY SHOULD DISCONTINUE ETRETINATE IMMEDIATELY AND BE REFERRED FOR NEUROLOGIC DIAGNOSIS AND CARE.
>
> *HEPATOXICITY:* OF THE 652 PATIENTS TREATED IN U.S. CLINICAL TRIALS, TEN HAD CLINICAL OR HISTOLOGIC HEPATITIS CONSIDERED POSSIBLY OR PROBABLY RELATED TO ETRETINATE TREATMENT. LIVER FUNCTION TESTS RETURNED TO NORMAL IN EIGHT OF THESE PATIENTS AFTER ETRETINATE WAS DISCONTINUED; ONE PATIENT HAD HISTOLOGIC CHANGES RESEMBLING CHRONIC ACTIVE HEPATITIS SIX MONTHS OFF THERAPY, AND ONE PATIENT HAD NO FOLLOW-UP AVAILABLE. THERE HAVE BEEN FOUR REPORTS OF HEPATITIS-RELATED DEATHS WORLDWIDE; TWO OF THESE PATIENTS HAD RECEIVED ETRETINATE FOR A MONTH OR LESS BEFORE PRESENTING WITH HEPATIC SYMPTOMS. ELEVATIONS OF AST (SGOT), ALT (SGPT) OR LDH HAVE OCCURRED IN 18%, 23% AND 15%, RESPECTIVELY, OF INDIVIDUALS TREATED WITH ETRETINATE. CASES WITH PATHOLOGY FINDINGS OF HEPATIC FIBROSIS, NECROSIS AND/OR CIRRHOSIS WHICH MAY BE RELATED TO ETRETINATE THERAPY HAVE BEEN REPORTED. IF HEPATOXICITY IS SUSPECTED DURING TREATMENT WITH ETRETINATE, THE DRUG SHOULD BE DISCONTINUED AND THE ETIOLOGY FURTHER INVESTIGATED.

Ophthalmic Effects: Corneal erosion, abrasion, irregularity and punctuate staining have occurred in patients treated with Etretinate although these effects were absent or improved after therapy was stopped in those patients who had follow-up examinations. Corneal opacities have occurred in patients receiving isotretinoin; they had either completely resolved or were resolving at follow-up six to seven weeks after discontinuation of the drug. Other ophthalmic effects that have occurred in Etretinate patients include decreased visual acuity and blurring of vision, minimal posterior subcapsular cataract, iritis, blot retinal hemorrhage, scotoma and photophobia. A number of cases of decreased night vision have occurred during Etretinate therapy. Because the onset in some patients was sudden, patients should be advised of this potential problem and warned to be cautious when driving or operating any vehicle at night. Any Etretinate patient experiencing visual difficulties should discontinue the drug and have an ophthalmological examination.

Hyperostosis: There is a very high likelihood of the development of hyperostosis with Etretinate therapy. In one clinical trial, 45 patients with a mean age of 40 years were retrospectively evaluated for evidence of hyperostosis. They had received Etretinate at a mean dose of 0.8 mg/kg for a mean duration of 33 months at the time of x-ray. Eleven patients had psoriasis, while 34 patients had a disorder of keratinization. Of these, 38 patients who continued to receive Etretinate at an average dose of 0.8 mg/kg/day for an average duration of 60 months, 32 (84%) had radiographic evidence of extraspinal tendon and ligament calcification. The most common sites of involvement were the ankles (76%), pelvis (53%) and knees (42%); spinal changes were uncommon. Involvement tended to be bilateral and multifocal. There were no bone or joint symptoms at the sites of radiographic abnormalities in 47% of the affected patients.

Lipids: Blood lipid determinations should be performed before Etretinate is administered and then at intervals of one or two weeks until the lipid response to Etretinate is established; this usually occurs within four to eight weeks.

Approximately 45% of patients receiving Etretinate during clinical trials experienced an elevation of plasma triglycerides. Approximately 37% developed a decrease in high density lipoproteins and about 16% showed an increase in cholesterol levels. These effects on triglycerides, HDL and cholesterol were reversible after cessation of Etretinate therapy. Patients with an increased tendency to develop hypertriglyceridemia include those with diabetes mellitus, obesity, increased alcohol intake or a familial history of these conditions.

Hypertriglyceridemia, hypercholesterolemia and lowered HDL may increase a patient's cardiovascular risk status. In addition, elevation of serum triglycerides in excess of 800 mg/dL has been associated with acute pancreatitis. Therefore, every attempt should be made to control significant elevations of triglycerides or cholesterol or significant decreases in HDL. Some patients have been able to reverse triglyceride and cholesterol elevations or HDL decrease by reduction in weight or restriction of dietary fat and alcohol while continuing Etretinate therapy.

Cardiovascular Effects: During clinical trials of 652 patients, 21 significant cardiovascular adverse incidents were reported, all in patients who had a strong history of cardiovascular risk. These incidents were not considered related to Etretinate therapy except for two cases of myocardial infarction: one which was considered possibly related to Etretinate therapy and one for which a relationship was not specified.

Animal Studies: In general, the signs of Etretinate toxicity in rats, mice and dogs are dose-related with respect to incidence, onset and severity. In rodents, the most striking manifestations of this toxicity are bone fractures; no evidence of fractures was observed in a one-year dog study. Other dose-related changes in some animals treated with Etretinate in subchronic or chronic toxicity studies include alopecia, erythema, reductions in body weight and food consumption, stiffness, altered gait, hematologic changes, elevations in serum alkaline phosphatase and testicular atrophy with microscopic evidence of reduced spermatogenesis.

PRECAUTIONS

Information for Patients: Women of childbearing potential should be advised that they must not be pregnant when Etretinate therapy is initiated, and that they should use an effective form of contraception for one month prior to Etretinate therapy, while taking Etretinate and after Etretinate has been discontinued. Etretinate has been found in the blood of some patients two to three years after the drug was discontinued. See boxed *"Contraindication."*

Because of the relationship of Etretinate to vitamin A, patients should be advised against taking vitamin A supplements to avoid possible additive toxic effects.

Patients should be advised that transient exacerbation of psoriasis is commonly seen during the initial period of therapy.

Patients should be informed that they may experience decreased tolerance to contact lenses during and after therapy.

Laboratory Tests: See *"Warnings"* section. In clinical studies, the incidence of hypertriglyceridemia was one patient in two, that of hypercholesterolemia one

Table 1

ADVERSE EVENTS FREQUENTLY REPORTED DURING CLINICAL TRIALS PERCENT OF PATIENTS REPORTING

Body System	> 75%	50-75%	25-50%	10-25%
Mucocutaneous	Dry nose Chapped lips	Excessive thirst Sore mouth	Nosebleed	Cheilitis Sore tongue
Dermatologic	Loss of hair Palm/sole/ fingertip peeling	Dry skin	Bruising	Nail disorder
		Itching Rash Red scaly face Skin fragility	Sunburn	Skin peeling
Musculoskeletal	Hyperostosis*	Bone/joint pain	Muscle cramps	
Central Nervous		Fatigue	Headache	Fever
Special Senses		Irritation of eyes	Eyeball pain Eyelid abnormalities	Abnormalities of: —conjunctiva —cornea —lens —retina Conjunctivitis Decrease in visual acuity Double vision
Gastrointestinal			Abdominal pain Changes in appetite	Nausea

* *In a retrospective study of 45 patients, 38 of whom received long-term Etretinate therapy, 32 (84%) had radiographic evidence of hyperotosis. See "Warnings."*

◆ RATED THERAPEUTICALLY EQUIVALENT; ◇ THERAPEUTIC EQUIVALENCE UNCONFIRMED; ○ UNRATED

patient in six, and that of decreased HDL one patient in three during Etretinate therapy. Pretreatment and follow-up blood lipids should be obtained under fasting conditions. If alcohol has been consumed, at least 36 hours should elapse before these determinations are made. It is recommended that these tests be performed at weekly or biweekly intervals until the lipid response to Etretinate is established.

Elevations of AST (SGOT), ALT (SGPT) or LDH have occurred in 18%, 23% and 15%, respectively, of individuals treated with Etretinate. It is recommended that these tests be performed prior to initiation of Etretinate therapy, at one to two week intervals for the first one to two months of therapy and thereafter at intervals of one to three months, depending on the response to Etretinate administration.

Drug Interactions: Little information is available on drug interactions with Etretinate; however, concomitant consumption of milk increases the absorption of etretinate. See *"Pharmacokinetics"* and *"Dosage and Administration"* sections.

Carcinogenesis, Mutagenesis, Impairment of Fertility:

Carcinogenesis: In a two-year study, male or female Sprague-Dawley rats given Etretinate by dietary admixture at doses up to 3 mg/kg/day (two times the maximum recommended human therapeutic dose) had no increase in tumor incidence. In an 80-week study, Crl:CD-1 (1CR) BR mice were given Etretinate by dietary admixture at doses of 1 to 5 mg/kg/day. An increased incidence of blood vessel tumors (hemangiomas and hemangiosarcomas in several different tissue sites) was noted in the high-dose male group (4 to 5 mg/kg/day) but not in the female group.

Mutagenesis: Etretinate was evaluated by the Ames test in a host-mediated assay, in the micronucleus test, and in a "treat and plate" test using the diploid yeast strain *S. cerevisiae* D7. Except for a weakly positive response in the Ames test using the tester strain TA 100, there was no evidence of genotoxicity. No differences in the rate of sister chromatid exchange (SCE) were noted in lymphocytes of patients before and after four weeks of treatment with therapeutic doses of Etretinate.

Impairment of Fertility: In a study of fertility and general reproductive performance in rats, no Etretinate-related effects were observed at doses up to 2.5 mg/kg/day. At a dose of 5 mg/kg/day (approximately three times the maximum recommended human therapeutic dose) the readiness of the treated animals to copulate was reduced but the pregnancy rate was unaffected. The number of viable young at birth and their postnatal weight gain and survival were adversely affected at the high dose. The pregnancy rate of the untreated first generation animals and postnatal weight gain of the untreated second generation animals were also reduced. No adverse effects on sperm production were noted in 12 psoriatic patients given 75 mg/day of Etretinate for one month and 50 mg/day for an additional two months. However, testicular atrophy was noted in subchronic and chronic rat studies and in a chronic dog study, in some cases at doses approaching those recommended for use in humans. Decreased sperm counts were reported in a 13-week dog study at doses as low as 3 mg/kg/day (approximately twice the maximum recommended human dose). Spermatogenic arrest also was reported with chronic administration of the all-*trans* metabolite to dogs.

Pregnancy: Category X. See boxed *"Contraindication."*
The following limited preliminary data must not be read or understood to diminish the serious risk of teratogenicity set forth in the boxed pregnancy *"Contraindication"*.

Thirty women worldwide have been reported as having taken one or more doses of Etretinate during pregnancy. In 29 cases in which information was available, there were a total of ten congenital abnormalities. The occurrence of congenital abnormalities was four of 20 among delivered infants, two of two among spontaneously aborted fetuses, and four of seven among induced abortions.

A further 38 women are reported to have become pregnant within 24 months after discontinuing Etretinate therapy. Because congenital abnormalities have been reported in these pregnancies, it cannot be stated that there is a "safe" time to become pregnant after Etretinate therapy. In 37 cases in which information was available, there were a total of three congenital abnormalities. The occurrence of congenital abnormalities was two of 29 among delivered infants, zero of one among spontaneously aborted fetuses, and one of five among induced abortions. Two stillbirths with no apparent congenital abnormalities were attributed to other causes.

Nonteratogenic Effects: No adverse effects on various parameters of late gestation and lactation were observed in rats at doses of Etretinate up to 4 mg/kg/day (approximately three times the maximum human recommended dose). At doses of 8 mg/kg/day (approximately five times the maximum human recommended dose) of Etretinate, the rate of stillbirths was increased and neonatal weight gain and survival rate were markedly reduced.

Nursing Mothers: Studies have shown that Etretinate is excreted in the milk of lactating rats; however, it is not known whether this drug is excreted in human milk. Because of the potential for adverse effects, nursing mothers should not receive Etretinate.

Pediatric Use: No clinical studies have been conducted in the U.S. using Etretinate in children. Ossification of interosseous ligaments and tendons of the extremities has been reported. Two children showed x-ray changes suggestive of premature epiphyseal closure during treatment with Etretinate. Skeletal hyperostosis has also been reported after treatment with isotretinoin. It is not known if any of these effects occur more commonly in children, but concern should be greater because of the growth process. Pretreatment x-rays for bone age including x-rays of the knees, followed by yearly monitoring, are advised. In addition, pain or limitation of motion should be evaluated with appropriate radiological examination. Because of the lack of data on the use of Etretinate in children and the possibility of their being more sensitive to effects of the drug, this product should be used only when all alternative therapies have been exhausted.

ADVERSE EVENTS
Clinical: Hepatitis was observed in about 1.5% of patients treated with Etretinate in clinical trials. Pathology findings of hepatic fibrosis, necrosis and/or cirrhosis have been reported. See *"Warnings"* section.

Etretinate has been associated with pseudotumor cerebri. See *"Warnings"* section.

Hypervitaminosis A produces a wide spectrum of signs and symptoms of primarily the mucocutaneous, musculoskeletal, hepatic and central nervous systems. Nearly all of the clinical adverse events reported to date with Etretinate administration resemble those of the hypervitaminosis A syndrome. Table 1 lists the adverse events frequently reported during clinical trials in which 652 patients were treated either for psoriasis (591 patients) or a disorder of keratinization (61 patients). Table 2 lists less frequently reported adverse events in these same patients. However the number of patients evaluated for each adverse event was not 652 in every case. (See table on next page).

Laboratory: Etretinate therapy induces change in serum lipids in a significant number of treated patients. Approximately 45% of patients experienced elevation in serum triglycerides, 37% a decrease in high density lipoproteins and 16% an increase in cholesterol levels.

Approximately 46% of patients had elevations of triglycerides above 250 mg/dL, 54% had decreases of HDL below 36 mg%, and 19% had elevations of cholstrerol above 300 mg%. One case of eruptive xanthomas associated with triglyceride levels greater than 1000 mg% has been reported. Elevations of AST (SGOT), ALT (SGPT) or LDH were experienced by 18%, 23% and 15%, respectively, of individuals treated with Etretinate. In most of the patients, the elevations were slight to moderate and became normal either during therapy or after cessation of treatment. See *"Warnings"* section.

Table 3 lists the laboratory abnormalities reported during clinical trials. Data for patients who received intermittent courses of therapy for periods up to five years are included. Any instance of two consecutive values outside the range of normal, or an abnormal value with no follow-up during therapy, was considered to be possibly related to Etretinate. (See related table).

OVERDOSAGE
There has been no experience with acute overdosage in humans.

The acute oral and intraperitoneal toxicities (LD$_{50}$) of Etretinate capsules in mice and rats were greater than 4000 mg/kg. The acute oral toxicity (LD$_{50}$) of Etretinate substance in 4% solution was 2300 mg/kg in mice and 1300 mg/kg in rats.

DOSAGE AND ADMINISTRATION
There is intersubject variation in the absorption and the rate of metabolism of Etretinate. Individualization of dosage is required to achieve the maximal therapeutic response with a tolerable degree of side effects. Therapy with Etretinate should generally be initiated at a dosage of 0.75 to 1 mg/kg of body weight/day taken in divided doses. A maximum dose of 1.5 mg/kg/day should not be exceeded. Erythrodermic psoriasis may respond to lower intial doses of 0.25 mg/kg/day increased by 0.25 mg/kg/day each week until optimal initial response is attained.

Maintenance doses of 0.5 to 0.75 mg/kg/day may be initiated after initial response, generally after 8 to 16 weeks of therapy. In general, therapy should be terminated in patients whose lesions have sufficiently resolved. Relapses may be treated as outlined for initial therapy.

Etretinate should be administered with food.

Store at 59° to 86°F; (15° to 30°C). Protect from light.

HOW SUPPLIED

CAPSULE: 10 MG

BRAND/MANUFACTURER	NDC	SIZE	AWP
○ **BRAND**			
TEGISON: Roche Labs	00004-0177-57	30s	$56.67

CAPSULE: 25 MG

BRAND/MANUFACTURER	NDC	SIZE	AWP
○ **BRAND**			
TEGISON: Roche Labs	00004-0179-57	30s	$88.65

➤ SHOWN IN PRODUCT IDENTIFICATION GUIDE

Table 2
LESS FREQUENT ADVERSE EVENTS REPORTED DURING CLINICAL TRIALS (SOME OF WHICH MAY BEAR NO RELATIONSHIP TO THERAPY)

	Percent of Patients Reporting	
Body System	*1-10%*	*< 1%*
Mucocutaneous	Dry eyes Mucous membrane abnormalities Dry mouth Gingival bleeding/inflammation	Decreased mucous secretion Rhinorrhea
Dermatologic	Hair abnormalities Bullous eruption Cold/clammy skin Onycholysis Paronychia Pyogenic granuloma Changes in perspiration	Abnormal skin odor Granulation tissue Healing impairment Herpes simplex Hirsutism Increased pore size Sensory skin changes Skin atrophy Skin fissures Skin infection Skin nodule Skin ulceration Urticaria
Musculoskeletal	Myalgia	Gout Hyperkinesia Hypertonia
Central Nervous System	Dizziness Lethargy Changes in sensation Pain Rigors	Abnormal thinking Amnesia Anxiety Depression Pseudotumor cerebri Emotional lability Faint feeling Flu-like symptoms
Special Senses	Abnormal lacrimation Abnormal vision Abnormalities of: —Extraocular musculature —Ocular tension —Pupil —Vitreous Earache Otitis externa	Change in equilibrium Ear drainage Ear infection Hearing change Night vision decrease Photophobia Visual change Scotoma
Gastrointestinal	Hepatitis	Constipation Diarrhea Melena Flatulence Weight loss Oral ulcers Taste perversion Tooth caries
Cardiovascular	Cardiovascular thrombotic or obstructive events Edema	Atrial fibrillation Chest pain Coagulation disorder Phlebitis Postural hypotension Syncope
Respiratory	Dyspnea	Coughing Increased sputum Dysphonia Pharyngitis
Renal		Kidney stones
Urogenital		Abnormal menses Atrophic vaginitis Dysuria Polyuria Urinary retention
Other	Malignant neoplasms	

Table 3
LABORATORY ABNORMALITIES REPORTED DURING CLINICAL TRIALS

	Percent of Patients Reporting		
Body System	*25-50%*	*10-25%*	*1-10%*
Hematologic	Increased: —MCHC (60%) —MCH —Reticulocytes —PTT	Decreased: —Hemoglobin/HCT —RBC —MCV Increased platelets	Decreased: —Platelets —MCH —MCHC —PTT

◆ RATED THERAPEUTICALLY EQUIVALENT; ◇ THERAPEUTIC EQUIVALENCE UNCONFIRMED; ○ UNRATED

Body System	Percent of Patients Reporting		
	25-50%	10-25%	1-10%
	—ESR	Increased or decreased: —WBC and components —Prothrombin time	Increased: —Hemoglobin/HCT —RBC
Urinary		WBC in urine	Proteinuria Glycosuria Microscopic hematuria Casts in urine Acetonuria Hemoglobinuria
Hepatic	Increased triglycerides	Increased: —AST (SGOT) —ALT (SGPT) —Alkaline phosphatase —GGTP —Globulin —Cholesterol	Increased bilirubin Increased or decreased: —Total protein —Albumin
Renal			Increased: —BUN —Creatinine
Electrolytes	Increased or decreased potassium	Increased or decreased: —Venous CO_2 —Sodium —Chloride	
Miscellaneous	Increased or decreased: FBS —Calcium —Phosphorus	Increased or decreased	Increased CPK

Eulexin SEE FLUTAMIDE

Eurax SEE CROTAMITON

Exelderm SEE SULCONAZOLE NITRATE

Exna SEE BENZTHIAZIDE

Exosurf Neonatal SEE COLFOSCERIL PALMITATE

Exsel SEE SELENIUM SULFIDE

Extendryl SEE CHLORPHENIRAMINE MALEATE/METHSCOPOLAMINE/PHENYLEPHRINE HYDROCHLORIDE

EZ III SEE ACETAMINOPHEN WITH CODEINE PHOSPHATE

Ezol SEE ACETAMINOPHEN/BUTALBITAL/CAFFEINE

Factor IX (Human)

DESCRIPTION

Coagulation Factor IX (Human) is a sterile, stable, lyophilized concentrate of Factor IX prepared from pooled human plasma and is intended for use in therapy of Factor IX deficiency, known as Hemophilia B or Christmas disease. Coagulation Factor IX (Human) is purified of extraneous plasma-derived proteins, including Factors II, VII and X, by use of immunoaffinity chromatography. A murine monoclonal antibody to Factor IX is used as an affinity ligand to isolate Factor IX from the source material. Factor IX is then dissociated from the monoclonal antibody, recovered, purified further, formulated and provided as a sterile, lyophilized powder. The immunoaffinity protocol utilized results in a highly pure Factor IX preparation. It shows predominantly a single component by SDS polyacrylamide electrophoretic evaluation and has a specific activity of not less than 150 Factor IX units per mg total protein. This concentrate has been processed by monoclonal antibody immunoaffinity chromatography during its manufacturer which has been shown to be capable of reducing the risk of viral transmission. Additionally, a chemical treatment protocol and an ultrafiltration step used in its manufacture have also been shown to be capable of significant viral reductions. However, no procedure has been shown to be totally effective in removing viral infectivity from coagulation factor concentrates (See "Clinical Pharmacology" and "Warnings").

Coagulation Factor IX (Human) is a highly purified preparation of Factor IX. When stored as directed, it will maintain its labeled potency for the period indicated on the container and package labels. Each vial contains the labeled amount of Factor IX activity expressed in International Units (I.U.) One I.U. represents the activity of Factor IX present in 1 mL of normal, pooled plasma. When reconstituted as recommended, the resulting solution is a clear, colorless, isotonic preparation of neutral pH, containing approximately 100 times the Factor IX potency found in an equal volume of plasma. Each mL of the reconstituted concentrate contains approximately 100 I.U. of Factor IX and non-detectable levels of Factors II, VII and X (< 0.0025 units per Factor IX unit using standard coagulation assays). It also contains histidine (approx. 10mM), sodium chloride (approx. 0.066M) and mannitol (approximatel 3%). Hydrochloric acid and/or sodium hydroxide may have been used to adjust pH. Coagulation Factor IX (Human) also contains trace amounts (≤ ng mouse protein/100 Factor IX activity units) of the murine monoclonal antibody used in its purification (see "Clinical Pharmacology").

Coagulation Factor IX (Human) is to be administered only intravenously.

CLINICAL PHARMACOLOGY

Hemophilia B, or Christmas disease, is an X-linked recessively inherited disorder of blood coagulation characterized by insufficient or abnormal synthesis of the clotting protein Factor IX. Factor IX is a vitamin K-dependent coagulation factor which is synthesized in the liver. Factor IX is activated by Factor XIa in the intrinsic coagulation pathway. Activated Factor IX (IXa), in combination with Factor VIII:C, activates Factor X to Xa, resulting ultimately in the convesion of prothrombin to thrombin and the formation of a fibrin clot. The infusion of exogenous Factor IX to replace the deficiency present in Hemophilia B temporarily restores hemostasis. Depending upon the patient's level of biologically active Factor IX, clinical symptoms range from moderate skin bruising or excessive hemorrhage after trauma or surgery to spontaneous hemorrhage into joints, muscles or internal organs including the brain. Severe or recurring hemorrhages can produce death, organ dysfunction or orthopedic defomity.

Infusion of Factor IX Complex concentrates which contain varying but significant amounts of the other liver-dependent blood coagulation proteins, Factor II, VII and X, into patients with Hemophilia B results in Factor IX recoveries ranging from approximately 0.57-1.1 1U/dL rise per IU/Kg body weight infused with plasma half-lives for Factor IX ranging from approximately 23 hours to 31 hours.[1,2] Infusion of Coagulation Factor IX (Human) into ten patients with severe or moderate Hemophilia B has shown a mean recovery of 0.67 IU/dL rise per IU/Kg body weight infused and a mean half-life 22.6 hours.[7] After six months of experience with repeated infusions performed on the nine patients who remained in the study, it was shown that the half-life and recovery was maintained at a level comparable to that found with the initial infusion. The six-month data showed a mean recovery of 0.68 IU/dL rise per IU/Kg body weight infused and a mean half-life of 25.3 hours.[7] The data show no statistically significant differences between the initial and six-month values.

The manufacturing procedure for Coagulation Factor IX (Human) includes multiple processing steps which have been designed to reduce the risk of viral transmission. Validation studies of the monoconal antibody (MAb) immunoaffinity chromatography/chemical treatment steps and an ultrafiltration step used in the production of Coagulation Factor IX (Human), document the viral reduction capacity of the processes employed. These studies were conducted using the Human immunodeficiency Virus (HIV) and four model viruses representing a broad range of viral characteristics, i.e., Sindbis, Vaccinia, Vesicular Stomatitis (VSV) and Murine Encephalomyocarditis (EMC), a non-lipid encapsulated model virus. The results of these validation studies (see table below) document an HIV viral reduction capacity of ≥ 11.56 log_{10} and a viral reduction capacity of 10.24 log_{10} for Sindbis, 11.64 log_{10} for EMC, ≥ 14.23 log_{10} for VSV, and ≥ 10.90 log_{10} for Vaccinia. (See related table).

The viral safety of Coagulation Factor IX (Human) is being studied in clinical trials of two cohorts of hemophilia B patients previously unexposed to blood or blood products. One cohort of patients includes those with moderate to severe Factor IX deficiency requiring chronic replacement therapy and the second cohort of patients includes those with a mild deficiency requiring Factor IX replacement for surgical procedures. These patients are being followed for serum ALT levels as well as for a range of viral serologies. Available serum ALT data, representing 22 patients, 13 of whom were followed for 6-15 months and 9 of whom were followed for less than 6 months, and available serology results, representing 19 patients, have continued to show no evidence of transmission of hepatitis or HIV. Although these studies are ongoing, these preliminary results show no evidence of viral transmission resulting from the infusion of Coagulation Factor IX (Human) (see *"Warnings"*).

Coagulation Factor IX (Human) contains trace amounts of the murine monoclonal antibody used in its purification (≤ 50 ng mouse protein per 100 Factor IX activity units). Using another murine monoclonal antibody purified concentrate, Antihemophilic Factor (Human) Factor VIII:C, Heat Treated, also containing trace amounts of murine protein (≤ 50 ng per 100 AHF activity units), a number of patients seronegative for Anti-HIV-1 were monitored to determine whether they would develop antibody to mouse protein or experience adverse reactions as a result of repeated exposure. Pre-study serum measurements of 27 patients for human anti-mouse IgG showed that, prior to treatment, 6 of them had either detectable antibody to mouse proteins or cross-reactive proteins. These patients continued to demonstrate similar or lower antibody levels during the study. Of the remaining 21 patients, 6 were shown to have low antibody level on one or more occasions. In no case was observance of low antibody level associated with an anamnestic response or with any clinical adverse reaction. Patients were observed for time periods ranging from 2 to 30 months.

In similar clinical studies with Coagulation Factor IX (Human) a cohort of nine Anti-HIV seropositive hemophilia B patients were administered Coagulation Factor IX (Human) for periods of 15-24 months. No appreciable increases in levels of IgG, IgM or IgE Human Anti-Mouse Antibodies (HAMA) were observed when compared with pre-study levels.

In clinical studies of Coagulation Factor IX (Human) patients were monitored for evidence of disseminated intravascular coagulation. In six patients evaluated after infusion, fibrinogen levels and platelet counts were unchanged, and fibrin degradation products did not appear.[7]

In further clinical evaluations of Factor IX (Human) Coagulation in a crossover study with a Factor IX Complex concentrate was not associated with the formation of prothrombin activation fragment (F_{1+2}) whereas the Factor IX Complex was.[7,8] Prothrombin activation fragment (F_{1+2}) is indicative of activation of prothrombin.

INDICATIONS AND USAGE

Coagulation Factor IX (Human) is indicated for the prevention and control of bleeding in Factor IX deficiency, also known as Hemophilia B or Christmas disease.

Coagulation Factor IX (Human) is not indicated in the treatment or prophylaxis of Hemophilia A patients with inhibitors to Factor VIII.

Coagulation Factor IX (Human) contains non-detectable levels of Factors II, VII and X (< 0.0025 units per Factor IX unit using standard coagulation assays) and is, therefore, not indicated for replacement therapy of these clotting factors.

Coagulation Factor IX (Human) is also not indicated in the treatment or reversal of coumarin-induced anticoagulation or in a hemorrhagic state caused by hepatitis-induced lack of production of liver dependent coagulation factors.

UNLABELED USES

Coagulation Factor IX (Human) is used alone or as an adjunct in the treatment of hemophiliac arthropathy and severe hepatic dysfunction.

CONTRAINDICATIONS

Known hypersensitivity to mouse protein is a contraindication to Coagulation Factor IX (Human).

WARNINGS

This product is prepared from pooled human plasma which may contain the causative agents of hepatitis and other viral diseases. Prescribed manufacturing procedures utilized at the plasma collection centers, plasma testing laboratories, and the fractionation facilities are designed to reduce the risk of transmitting viral infection. However, the risk of viral infectivity from this product cannot be totally eliminated. Accordingly, the benefits and risks of treatment with this concentrate should be carefully assessed prior to use. Individuals who receive infusions of blood or plasma products may develop signs and/or symptoms of some viral infections, particularly nonA, nonB hepatitis.

Since the use of Factor IX Complex concentrates has historically been associated with the development of thromboembolic complications, the use of Factor IX-containing products may be potentially hazardous in patients with signs of fibrinolysis and in patients with disseminated intravascular coagulation (DIC).

PRECAUTIONS

The administration of Factor IX Complex concentrates, containing Factors II, VII, IX and X, has been associated with the development of thromboembolic complications. Although Coagulation Factor IX (Human) contains highly purified Factor IX, the potential risk of thrombosis or disseminated intravascular coagulation observed with the use of other products containing Factor IX should be recognized. Patients given Coagulation Factor IX (Human) should be observed closely for signs or symptoms of intravascular coagulation or thrombosis. Because of the potential risk of thromboembolic complications, caution should be exercised when administering this concentrate to patients with liver disease, to patients post-operatively, to neonates, or to patients at risk of thromboembolic phenomena or disseminated intravascular coagulation.[3,4] In each of these situations, the potential benefit of treatment with Coagulation Factor IX (Human) should be weighed against the risk of these complications.

Coagulation Factor IX (Human) should be administered intravenously at a rate that will permit observation of the patient for any immediate reactions. Rates of infusion of up to 225 units per minute have been regularly tolerated with no adverse reactions. If any reaction takes place that is thought to be related to the administration of Coagulation Factor IX (Human) the rate of infusion should be decreased or the infusion stopped, as dictated by the response of the patient. During the course of treatment, determination of daily Factor IX levels is advised to guide the dose to be administered and the frequency of repeated infusions. Individual patients may vary in their response to Coagulation Factor IX (Human) achieving different levels of *in vivo* recovery and demonstrating different half-lives.

The use of high doses of Factor IX Complex concentrates has been reported to be associated with instances of myocardial infarction, disseminated intravascular coagulation, venous thrombosis and pulmonary embolism. Generally a Factor IX level of 25% to 50% is considered adequate for hemostasis, including major hemorrhages and surgery. Attempting to maintain Factor IX levels of $> 75\%$ to 100% during treatment is not recommended. To achieve Factor IX levels that will remain above 25% between once a day administrations, each daily dose should attempt to raise the level to 50-60%. (See *"Dosage and Administration"*).

No data are available regarding the use of E-amino caproic acid following an initial infusion of Coagulation Factor IX (Human) for the prevention or treatment of oral bleeding following trauma or dental procedures such as extractions.

Formation of Antibodies to Mouse Protein: Although no hypersensitivity reactions have been observed, because Coagulation Factor IX (Human) contains trace amounts of mouse protein (≤ 50 ng per 100 Factor IX activity units), the possibility exists that patients treated with Coagulation Factor IX (Human) may develop hypersensitivity to the mouse protein.

INFORMATION FOR PATIENTS

Patients should be informed of the early signs of hypersensitivity reactions including hives, generalized urticaria, tightness of the chest, wheezing, hypotension, and anaphylaxis, and should be advised to discontinue use of the concentrate and contact their physician if these symptoms occur.

SUMMARY OF VIRUS REDUCTION STUDIES (LOG$_{10}$ REDUCTION)

Processing Step	HIV	Sindbis	EMC	VSV	Vaccinia
MAb Chromatography	*	2.76	3.89	≥ 7.18**	≥ 3.60
Sodium Thiocyanate Chemical Treatment	≥ 4.16	0	0	**	0
Ultrafiltration	≥ 7.4	7.48	7.75	7.05	≥ 7.30
Total Log$_{10}$ Reduction	≥ 11.56	10.24	11.64	≥ 14.23	≥ 10.90

* *MAb Chromatography not studied*
** *Results are for combined MAb chromatography/sodium thiocyanate step.*

◆ RATED THERAPEUTICALLY EQUIVALENT; ◇ THERAPEUTIC EQUIVALENCE UNCONFIRMED; ○ UNRATED

PREGNANCY CATEGORY C

Animal reproduction studies have not been conducted with Coagulation Factor IX (Human). It is also not known whether Coagulation Factor IX (Human) can cause fetal harm when administered to a pregnant woman or can affect reproduction capacity. Coagulation Factor IX (Human) should be given to a pregnant woman only if clearly needed.

ADVERSE REACTIONS

As with the administration of any product intravenously, the following reactions may be observed following administration: headache, fever, chills, flushing, nausea, vomiting, tingling, lethargy, hives, stinging or burning at the infusion site or other manifestations of allergic reactions.

There is a potential risk of thromboembolic episodes following the administration of Coagulation Factor IX (Human) (see *"Warnings and Precautions."*.)

The patient should be monitored closely during the infusion of Coagulation Factor IX (Human) to observe for the development of any reaction. If any reaction takes place that is thought to be related to the administration of Coagulation Factor IX (Human) the rate of infusion should be decreased or the infusion stopped, as dictated by the response of the patient.

DOSAGE AND ADMINISTRATION

Coagulation Factor IX (Human) is intended for intravenous administration only. It should be reconstituted with the volume of Sterile Water for Injection, USP supplied with the lot, and administered within three hours of reconstitution. Do not refrigerate after reconstitution. After administration, any unused solution and the administration equipment should be discarded.

As a general rule, 1 unit of Factor IX activity per Kg can be expected to increase the circulating level of Factor IX by 1% of normal. The following formula provides a guide to dosage calculations: (See related table).

The amount of Coagulation Factor IX (Human), to be infused, as well as the frequency of infusions, will vary with each patient and with the clinical situation.(5,6)

As a general rule, the level of Factor IX required for treatment of different conditions is as follows: (See related table).

Recovery of the loading dose varies from patient to patient. Doses administered should be titrated to the patient's response.

In the presence of an inhibitor to Factor IX, higher doses of Coagulation Factor IX (Human) might be necessary to overcome the inhibitor (see *"Precautions"*). No data on the treatment of patients with inhibitors to Factor IX with Coagulation Factor IX (Human) are available. For information on rate of administration, see *"Rate of Administration,"* below.

RECONSTITUTION

1. Warm both the diluent and Coagulation Factor IX (Human) in unopened vials to room temperature [not above 37℃ (98°F)].
2. Remove the caps from both vials to expose the central portions of the rubber stoppers.
3. Treat the surface of the rubber stoppers with antiseptic solution and allow them to dry.
4. Using aseptic technique, insert one end of the double-end needle into the rubber stopper of the diluent vial. Invert the diluent vial and insert the other end of the double-end needle into the rubber stopper of the Coagulation Factor IX (Human) vial. Direct the diluent, which will be drawn in by vacuum, over the entire surface of the Coagulation Factor IX (Human) cake. (In order to assure transfer of all the diluent, adjust the position of the tip of the needle in the diluent vial to the inside edge of the diluent stopper.) Rotate the vial to ensure complete wetting of the cake during the transfer process.
5. Remove the diluent vial to release the vacuum, *then remove the double-end needle* from the Coagulation Factor IX (Human) vial.
6. Gently swirl the vial until the powder is dissolved and the solution is ready for administration. The concentrate routinely and easily reconstitutes within one minute. To assure sterility, Coagulation Factor IX (Human) should be administered within three hours after reconstitution.
7. Product should be filtered prior to use as described under Administration. Parenteral drug preparations should be inspected visually for particulate matter and discoloration prior to administration, whenever solution and container permit.

ADMINISTRATION
INTRAVENOUS INJECTION

Plastic disposable syringes are recommended with Coagulation Factor IX (Human) solution. The ground glass surface of all-glass syringes tend to stick with solutions of this type. Please note, this concentrate is supplied with a SELF-VENTING filter spike.

1. Using aseptic technique, attach the vented filter spike to a sterile disposable syringe.

Caution: The use of other, nonvented filter needles or spikes without the proper procedure may result in an air lock and prevent the complete transfer of the concentrate.

Caution: DO NOT INJECT AIR INTO THE COAGULATION FACTOR IX (HUMAN) VIAL. The self-venting feature of the vented filter spike precludes the need to inject air in order to facilitate withdrawal of the reconstituted solution. The injection of air could cause partial product loss through the vent filter.
2. Insert the vented filter spike into the stopper of the Coagulation Factor IX (Human) vial, invert the vial, and position the filter spike so that the orifice is at the inside edge of the stopper.
3. Withdraw the reconstituted solution into the syringe.
4. Discard the filter spike. Perform venipuncture using the enclosed winged needle with microbore tubing. Attach the syringe to the luer end of the tubing.

Caution: Use of other winged needles without microbore tubing, although compatible with the concentrate, will result in a larger retention of solution within the winged infusion set.

RATE OF ADMINISTRATION

The rate of administration should be determined by the response and comfort of the patient; intravenous dosage administration rates of up to 225 units/minute have been regularly tolerated without incident. When reconstituted as directed, i.e., to approximately 100 units/mL, Coagulation Factor IX (Human) should be administered at a rate of approximately 2.0 mL per minute.

STORAGE

When stored at refrigerator temperature 2°-8℃ (36°-46°F), Coagulation Factor IX (Human), is stable for the period indicated by the expiration date on its label. Within this period, Coagulation Factor IX (Human) may be stored at room temperature not to exceed 30℃ (86°F), for up to one month. Avoid freezing which may damage container for the diluent.

REFERENCES

1. Zauber NP, Levin J: Factor IX levels in patients with hemophilia B (Christmas disease) following transfusion with concentrates of Factor IX or fresh frozen plasma (FFP). *Medicine* (Baltimore) 56(3): 213-24, 1977. 2. Smith KJ, Thompson AR: Labeled Factor IX Kinetics in Patients with Hemophilia-B. *Blood* 58(3): 625-629, 1981. 3. Aledort LM: Factor IX and Thrombosis. *Scand. J. Haematology* Suppl. 30:40, 1977. 4. Cederbaum AI, Blatt PM, Roberts HR: Intravascular coagulation with use of human prothrombin complex concentrates. *Ann. Intern. Med.* 84:683-687, 1976. 5. Kasper CK, Dietrich SL: Comprehensive Management of Hemophilia. *Clin Haematol* 14(2): 489-512, 1985. 6. Johnson AJ, Aronson DL, Williams WJ: Preparation and clinical use of plasma and plasma fractions. Chap. 167 in *Hematology* 3rd Edition, Williams WJ, Beutler E, Erslev AJ, Lichtman MA (Eds.), McGraw Hill Book Co., New York: pp 1563-1583, 1983. 7. Kim HC, McMillan CW, White GC, Bergman GE, Horton MW, Saidi P: Purified Factor IX Using Monoclonal Immunoaffinity Technique: Clinical Trials in Hemophilia B and Comparison to Prothrombin Complex Concentrates. *Blood* 79, No. 3: pp 568-575, 1992. 8. Kim HC, Matts L, Eisele J, Czachur M, Saidi P: Monoclonal Antibody Purified Factor IX—Comparative Thrombogenicity to Prothrombin Complex Concentrate. Seminars in Hematology, Vol. 28, No. 3, Suppl. 6, July, 1991, pp. 15-20.

J CODES

Per IU IV—J7196

HOW SUPPLIED
POWDER FOR INJECTION: 1 I.U.

BRAND/MANUFACTURER	NDC	SIZE	AWP
○ **BRAND**			
ALPHANINE SD: Alpha Therapeutic	49669-3800-01	1s	$1.00

POWDER FOR INJECTION: 250 IU

BRAND/MANUFACTURER	NDC	SIZE	AWP
○ **BRAND**			
MONONINE: Armour	00053-7668-01	1s	$1.10

Number of Factor IX I.U. required	= Body Weight (in Kg)	× desired Factor IX increase (% normal)	× 1.0 unit/Kg

	Minor Spontaneous Hemorrhage, Prophylaxis	Major Trauma or Surgery
Desired levels of Factor IX for Hemostasis	15-25%	25-50%
Initial loading dose to achieve desired level	up to 20-30 units/kg	up to 75 units/kg
Frequency of dosing	once; repeated in 24 hours if necessary	every 18-30 hours, depending on T$_{1/2}$ and measured Factor IX levels
Duration of treatment	once; repeated if necessary	up to ten days, depending upon nature of insult

➤ SHOWN IN PRODUCT IDENTIFICATION GUIDE

POWDER FOR INJECTION: 500 IU

BRAND/MANUFACTURER		NDC	SIZE	AWP
○ BRAND MONONINE: Armour		00053-7668-02	1s	$1.10

POWDER FOR INJECTION: 1000 I.U.

BRAND/MANUFACTURER		NDC	SIZE	AWP
○ BRAND MONONINE: Armour		00053-7668-04	1s	$1.10

Factor IX Complex, Human

DESCRIPTION

Factor IX Complex heat-treated at 80°C for 72 hours is a sterile, dried, plasma fraction comprising coagulation factors II, IX, X and low levels of factor VII.

NOMENCLATURE

Factor	Synonyms:
II	prothrombin
VII	proconvertin
IX	plasma thromboplastin component, PTC, Christmas factor
X	Stuart-Prower factor

Factor IX Complex, Human, is standardized in terms of Factor IX content and each vial of Factor IX Complex, Human is labeled for Factor IX. One international unit (IU) of Factor IX as defined by the World Health Organization standard for blood coagulation Factor IX is approximately equal to the level of Factor IX found in 1.0 mL of fresh, normal plasma.

The Factor IX content is approximately 50 times purified over whole plasma, and when reconstituted as directed, Factor IX Complex, Human contains 25 times as much Factor IX as an equal volume of fresh plasma. Factor IX Complex, Human containing approximately 1000 IU of Factor IX administered in 40 mL, contains the Factor IX content of 1 liter of fresh plasma. Factor IX Complex, Human must be administered intravenously.

CLINICAL PHARMACOLOGY

Factor IX Complex raises the plasma level of Factor IX and restores hemostasis in patients with Factor IX deficiency. In general, a level of Factor IX less than 5% of normal will give rise to spontaneous hemorrhage, while levels greater than 20% of normal will lead to satisfactory hemostasis even in the face of trauma or surgery. Approximately 30% to 50% of the Factor IX activity can be detected in a hemophilia B (Factor IX deficiency) recipient's plasma immediately after infusion.[1,2] The biological activity of the infused Factor IX disappears from the plasma with a half-life of approximately 24 hours.[2] It must be noted that administration of Factor IX Complex causes an increase in blood levels of Factors II, VII, IX and X.

Factors II, VII, IX and X are the vitamin K dependent coagulation factors and are synthesized in the liver. Congenital deficiencies of each of the four factors do occur and may result in a bleeding tendency. Naturally low levels of the vitamin K dependent factors may also be found in vitamin K deficiency and in severe liver disease.

This product has been heated at 80°C for 72 hours and there is no evidence of adverse effects upon the product. In a study[3] designed to assess the effectiveness of heat treatment at 68°C for 72 hours, hepatitis naive chimpanzees were inoculated with heated antihemophilic factor (human) and Factor IX Complex preparations to which had been previously added non-A, non-B hepatitis Hutchinson Strain[4] to a total level of 2500 chimpanzee infectious doses (CID). The chimpanzees receiving heated preparations failed to exhibit any symptoms of non-A, non-B hepatitis. In contrast, one chimpanzee receiving antihemophilic factor (human) concentrate which was not heated after the non-A, non-B inoculum was added, developed abnormally elevated alanine aminotransferase (ALT) levels beginning 10 weeks postinoculation and liver histopathology at 6 weeks. From these results, it was concluded that the heat treatment employed inactivated a known quantity of non-A, non-B hepatitis at least 2500 CID. Additional *in vitro* studies[5] on the effect of heating Factor IX Complex, Human, in a dried state at 80°C for 72 hours, on virus inactivation were carried out with a number of viruses, including human immunodeficiency virus (HIV), added to Factor IX Complex, Human, prior to heating. The following table shows the amount of each model virus inactivated by the process:

Virus	Starting Amount Logs*	Logs Inactivated
Vesicular Stomatitis Virus	8.0	≥7.5
Vaccinia Virus	5.75	1.0
Sindbis Virus	7.25	≥ 6.75
Bovine Parvovirus	4.5	3.5
Human Immunodeficiency Virus (HIV) HIV-1	4.8	≥ 4.3

* $\log_{10} TCID_{50}/mL$ (for HiV-1, $\log_{10} TCID_{50}$)

INDICATIONS AND USAGE

Factor IX Complex, Human, is indicated for the prevention and control of bleeding caused by Factor IX deficiency due to hemophilia B.

Factor IX Complex, Human, is not indicated for use in the treatment of factor VII deficiency.

Factor IX Complex, Human, is appropriate for use in:

1. Hemophilia B (Christmas disease); demonstrated Factor IX deficiency in children or adults with real or impending bleeding episodes. Spontaneous bleeding can occur even in the absence of any trauma.

2. Reversal of coumarin anticoagulant induced hemorrhage; in situations where prompt reversal is required (e.g., preceding emergency surgery, trauma, etc.), administration of fresh-frozen plasma should be initially considered as treatment; however, Factor IX Complex, Human may be considered as a secondary approach if the risk of transmitting hepatitis is considered justifiable in the face of a life-threatening situation.[6-8]

3. Treatment of bleeding episodes in patients with hemophilia A (Factor VIII deficiency) who have inhibitors to Factor VIII.[9]

In addition to coumarin anticoagulant induced deficiencies, low levels of Factors II, VII, IX and X may be found in vitamin K deficiency, in patients with liver disease, and in those with nephrotic syndrome. However, Factor IX Complex, Human, is not indicated in these situations and treatment should be aimed at correcting the primary condition.

Note: For publications on the clinical use of Factor IX Complex, Human, please refer to references 1, 2, 6-17.

UNLABELED USES

Factor IX Complex, Human, is used alone or as an adjunct in the treatment and prophylaxis of hemophilic arthropathy (hemarthrosis) in patients with hemophilia. It is also used in the treatment of clotting factor deficiency secondary to severe liver disease.

CONTRAINDICATIONS

None known.

WARNINGS

1. HEPATITIS AND VIRAL DISEASES

THIS PRODUCT IS PREPARED FROM POOLED HUMAN PLASMA WHICH MAY CONTAIN THE CAUSATIVE AGENTS OF HEPATITIS AND OTHER VIRAL DISEASES. PRESCRIBED MANUFACTURING PROCEDURES UTILIZED AT THE PLASMA COLLECTION CENTERS, PLASMA TESTING LABORATORIES, AND THE FRACTIONATION FACILITIES ARE DESIGNED TO REDUCE THE RISK OF TRANSMITTING VIRAL INFECTION. HOWEVER, THE RISK OF VIRAL INFECTIVITY FROM THIS PRODUCT CANNOT BE TOTALLY ELIMINATED.

INDIVIDUALS WHO RECEIVE INFUSIONS OF BLOOD OR PLASMA PRODUCTS MAY DEVELOP SIGNS AND/OR SYMPTOMS OF SOME VIRAL INFECTIONS, PARTICULARLY NON-A, NON-B HEPATITIS.[18] IT IS EMPHASIZED THAT HEPATITIS B VACCINATION IS ESSENTIAL FOR PATIENTS WITH HEMOPHILIA AND IT IS RECOMMENDED THAT THIS BE DONE AT BIRTH OR DIAGNOSIS.[19]

FACTOR IX COMPLEX, HUMAN, IS A PLASMA FRACTION OBTAINED FROM MANY PAID DONORS. THE PRESENCE OF HEPATITIS VIRUSES SHOULD BE ASSUMED AND THE HAZARD OF ADMINISTERING FACTOR IX COMPLEX, HUMAN SHOULD BE WEIGHED AGAINST THE MEDICAL CONSEQUENCES OF WITHHOLDING IT, PARTICULARLY IN PERSONS WITH FEW PREVIOUS TRANSFUSIONS OF BLOOD OR BLOOD PRODUCTS.

2. THROMBOSIS

CASES OF PATIENTS DEVELOPING POSTOPERATIVE THROMBOSIS AFTER TREATMENT WITH FACTOR IX COMPLEX, HUMAN, HAVE BEEN DESCRIBED. ALTHOUGH THROMBOSIS IS A WELL-KNOWN RISK OF THE POSTOPERATIVE PERIOD, IT IS FOUND TO BE GREATER IN THESE PATIENTS.[13-15] NO OTHER DATA ARE PRESENTLY AVAILABLE. UNTIL FURTHER SURVEYS AND MORE CONCLUSIVE STUDIES ARE AVAILABLE, FACTOR IX COMPLEX, HUMAN IS ONLY ADVISED FOR PATIENTS UNDERGOING ELECTIVE SURGERY WHERE THE EXPECTED BENEFICIAL EFFECTS OF ITS USE OUTWEIGH THE INCREASED RISK OF THE POSSIBILITY OF THROMBOSIS. THIS APPLIES ESPECIALLY TO THOSE WHO MAY BE PREDISPOSED TO THROMBOSIS. DO NOT USE IN CASES OF KNOWN LIVER DISEASE WHERE THERE IS ANY SUSPICION OF INTRAVASCULAR COAGULATION OR FIBRINOLYSIS.

PRECAUTIONS

GENERAL

1. Reconstitute only with Sterile Water for Injection, USP.

2. Administer within 3 hours after reconstitution. Do not refrigerate after reconstitution.

3. Administer only by the intravenous route.

4. The administration equipment and any reconstituted Factor IX Complex, Human, not immediately used should be discarded.

5. E-aminocaproic acid should not be administered with Factor IX Complex, Human, as this may increase the risk of thrombosis.

6. Patients who receive Factor IX Complex, Human, either postoperatively or with known liver disease should be kept under close observation for signs and symptoms of intravascular coagulation or thrombosis. Any suspicious findings of this nature indicate the dosage should be markedly decreased if the patient's conditions are such that the treatment cannot be discontinued entirely. In the event of thrombohemorrhagic disorders occurring, reduction in dosage should be considered, and treatment with heparin may be warranted. Although this preparation does not contain heparin, it has been suggested that reconstitution with heparin in a concentration of 2-5 IU per mL may reduce the risk of development of thrombosis.[17] However, thrombosis can occur even in the presence of heparin.

7. Patients receiving Factor IX Complex, Human, for prolonged periods should be continually monitored at least for levels of Factors II, IX and X. The same comments as in No. 6 above are indicated. Half-lives of Factors II and X are considerably longer than the half-life of Factor IX. Hence frequent repeated high-dose administration may result in build-up of Factors II and X, with increasing risk of thrombotic side effects.

PREGNANCY CATEGORY C
Animal reproduction studies have not been conducted with Factor IX Complex, Human. It is also known whether Factor IX Complex, Human can cause fetal harm when administered to a pregnant woman or can affect reproduction capacity. Factor IX Complex, Human, should be given to a pregnant woman only if clearly needed.

ADVERSE REACTIONS
In some patients the rapid administration of Factor IX Complex, Human can cause transient fever, chills, headache, flushing or tingling.

DOSAGE AND ADMINISTRATION
Each bottle of Factor IX Complex, Human, has the Factor IX activity, in IU, stated on the bottle label. One IU is defined as the activity present in 1 mL of fresh, normal plasma. The potency is standardized in terms of Factor IX content.

The amount of Factor IX Complex, Human, required for normalizing hemostasis will depend upon the patient and upon the circumstances. Sufficient Factor IX Complex, Human, should be administered to achieve and maintain a plasma level of at least 20% until hemostasis is achieved.

Levels of Factor IX of 30 to 40 percent are considered effective in stopping hemorrhages.[1] Bleeds in life- or limb-threatening areas require Factor IX levels of 50 to 80 percent which should be maintained at 30 to 40 percent for a few days.[1] The desired hemostatic plasma level in surgical patients for minor procedures or invasive dental surgery is between 30 and 40 percent of normal.[1] This can be achieved by a dosage not exceeding 30 to 40 units per kg body weight. In major hemorrhage, as during surgery or severe accidental trauma, plasma levels of 60 to 80 percent just prior to surgery, maintained above 30 percent for a further 5 to 7 days and then above 15 to 20 percent for 7 to 10 additional days, until healing occurs, are required.[1]

While the range of values in normal clinical practice is likely to vary depending upon differences between patients, their clinical condition and the type of assay employed, it is again stressed that high dosages, especially if frequently repeated (e.g., more than once per day) are hazardous. Such regimens can induce major thrombotic complications and hence must be avoided.

The following formulas may be used as guidelines to calculate an appropriate dose or to estimate the expected percentage increase obtained from a given dose:

$$\text{Expected Factor IX increase (in \% of normal)} = \frac{\text{IU administered} \times 1.0}{\text{body weight (in kg)}}$$

IU required = body weight (kg) × desired Factor IX increase (% normal) × 1.0

Thus, in order to bring a 70 kg patient from 0% to 50% of normal, the patient would require 70 × 50 × 1.0 = 3500 IU or 50 IU/kg body weight.

PROPHYLAXIS
The ideal treatment for proven congenital deficiency of pro-coagulants is prophylactic administration. For prophylaxis against hemorrhage during times of extensive physical activity, the plasma Factor IX levels should be raised to 15 to 30 percent. Maintenance dosage should be adapted to the individual patient's needs. Additional Factor IX Complex, Human, should be administered when a patient on prophylaxis is exposed to trauma or surgery.

MAINTENANCE DOSE
Maintenance dosage should be administered according to the clinical response and the Factor IX level achieved. Such dosage is usually about 10-20 IU per kg body weight per day.

INHIBITOR PATIENTS
For treatment of bleeding episodes in patients with hemophilia A (Factor VIII deficiency) who have inhibitors to Factor VIII, the recommended dose should be 75 IU/kg. A second dose may be administered after 12 hours if necessary.[9]

RECONSTITUTION
Vacuum Transfer

1. Warm the unopened diluent and concentrate to room temperature (NMT 37°C, 99°F).

2. After removing the plastic flip-top caps, aseptically cleanse the rubber stoppers of both bottles.

3. Remove the protective cover from the plastic transfer-needle cartridge with tamper-proof seal and penetrate the stopper of the diluent bottle.

4. Remove the remaining portion of the cartridge. Invert the diluent bottle and penetrate the rubber seal on the concentrate bottle with the needle at an angle. Alternate method of transferring sterile water: With a sterile needle and syringe, withdraw the appropriate volume of diluent and transfer to the bottle of lyophilized concentrate.

5. Hold the diluent bottle at an angle to the concentrate bottle in order to direct the jet of diluent against the wall of the concentrate bottle. The vacuum will draw the diluent into the concentrate bottle. Avoid excessive foaming. Do not shake the concentrate bottle.

6. After removing the diluent bottle and transfer-needle, optimal reconstitution time is achieved by swirling continuously until completely dissolved. Reconstitution can also be achieved by very gently agitating until dissolved.

Parenteral drug products should be inspected visually for particulate matter and discoloration prior to administration, whenever solution and container permit.

7. After the concentrate powder is completely dissolved, withdraw the Factor IX Complex, Human, solution into the syringe through the filter needle which is supplied in the package. Replace the filter needle with an appropriate sterile injection needle, e.g., 21 gauge × 1 inch, and inject intravenously.

8. If the same patient is to receive more than one bottle of Factor IX Complex, Human, the contents of two bottles may be drawn into the same syringe through filter needles before attaching the vein needle.

RATE OF ADMINISTRATION
The rate of administration should be adapted to the response of the individual patient, but is generally well-tolerated at a rate of approximately 100 IU per minute.

STORAGE
Factor IX Complex, Human, should be stored under refrigeration (2°-8°C; 35°-46°F). Freezing should be avoided as breakage of the diluent bottle might occur.

Factor IX Complex, Human, concentrate may be stored for a period of up to 1 month at temperatures not to exceed 25°C (77°F) during travel.

REFERENCES
1. Johnson AJ, Aronson DL, Williams WJ; Preparation and clinical use of plasma and plasma fractions. In: Williams WJ (ed): *Hematology*, 4th ed, New York, McGraw-Hill, 1990, ch 170, pp 1659-1673. 2. Zauber NP, Levin J: Factor IX levels in patients with hemophilia B (Christmas disease) following transfusion with concentrates of factor IX or fresh frozen plasma (FFP). *Medicine* (Baltimore) 56(3): 213-24, 1977. 3. Mozen MM, Louie RE, Mitra G: Heat inactivation of viruses in antihemophilic factor concentrates. Abstracts, XVIth International Congress of the World Federation of Hemophilia, Rio de Janeiro, Aug. 24-28, 1984. Number 240. 4. Feinstone SM, Alter HJ, Dienes HP, et al: Non-A, non-B hepatitis in chimpanzees and marmosets. *J Infect Dis* 144(6):588-98, 1981. 5. Unpublished data in files of Miles Inc., Cutter Biological. 6. Taberner DA, Thompson JM, Poller L: Comparison of prothrombin complex concentrate and vitamin K₁ in oral anticoagulant reversal. *Br Med J* 2(6027):83-5, 1976. 7. Menache D. Roberts HR: Summary report and recommendations of the task force members and consultants. *Thromb Diath Haemorrh* 33:645-7, 1975. 8. Aronson DL: Factor IX Complex. *Semin Thromb Hemostas* 6(1):28-43, 1979. 9. Lusher JM, Shapiro SS, Palascak JE, et al: Efficacy of prothrombin-complex concentrates in hemophiliacs with antibodies to factor VIII: a multicenter therapeutic trial. *N Engl J Med* 303(8):421-5, 1980. 10. Hoag MS, Johnson FF, Robinson AJ, et al: Treatment of hemophilia B with a new clotting-factor concentrate. *N Engl J Med* 280(11):581-6, 1969. 11. Hoag MS, Johnson FF, Robinson AJ, et al: Use of plasma concentrate in congenital factor VII and IX deficiencies. *Clin Res* 17:152, 1969. 12. Breen FA Jr, Tullis JL: Prothrombin concentrates in treatment of Christmas disease and allied disorders. *JAMA* 208(10):1848-52, 1969. 13. Kasper CK: Postoperative thrombosis in hemophilia. *N Engl J Med* 289(3):160, 1973. 14. Kasper CK: Surgical operation in hemophilia B. Use of factor IX concentrate. *Calif Med* 113(1):4-8, 1970. 15. George JN, Breckenridge RT: The use of factor VIII and factor IX concentrates during surgery. *JAMA* 214(9):1673-6, 1970. 16. Gunay U, Choi HS, Maurer HS, et al: Commercial preparations of prothrombin complex. A clinical comparison. *Am J Dis Child* 126(6):775-7, 1973. 17. White GC 2d, Lundblad RL, Kingdon HS: Prothrombin complex concentrates: preparation, properties, and clinical uses. *Curr Top Hematol* 2:203-44, 1979. 18. Colombo M. Mannucci PM, Carnelli V, et al: Transmission of non-A, non-B hepatitis by heat-treated factor VIII concentrate. *Lancet* 2(8445):1-4, 1985. 19. National Hemophilia Foundation Medical and Scientific Advisory Council. Hemophilia Information Exchange—AIDS Update: Recommendations concerning AIDS and the treatment of hemophilia. HIV infection, Section I.G. (Rev. Jan., 1988).

J CODES
Per IU IV—J7194

HOW SUPPLIED
POWDER FOR INJECTION:

BRAND/MANUFACTURER	NDC	SIZE	AWP
○ GENERICS			
PROFILNINE: Alpha Therapeutic	49669-3700-01	1s	$0.35
PROFILNINE: Alpha Therapeutic	49669-3700-02	1s	$0.35
BEBULIN VH: Immuno-U.S.	54129-0244-02	1s	$0.55

► SHOWN IN PRODUCT IDENTIFICATION GUIDE

POWDER FOR INJECTION: 1 U

BRAND/MANUFACTURER	NDC	SIZE	AWP
○ GENERICS			
KONYNE-80: Miles Biol	00192-0626-20	1s	$0.35
KONYNE-80: Miles Biol	00192-0626-50	1s	$0.35

POWDER FOR INJECTION: 700 U-3,900 U

BRAND/MANUFACTURER	NDC	SIZE	AWP
○ GENERICS			
PROPLEX T: Baxter Biotech	00944-0581-01	1s	$0.25

Factrel *SEE* GONADORELIN HYDROCHLORIDE

Famciclovir

DESCRIPTION

Famciclovir is an orally administered prodrug of the antiviral agent penciclovir. Chemically, Famciclovir is known as 3-[2-(2-amino-9 *H*-purin-9-yl)ethyl]-1,3-propanediol diacetate. Its molecular formula is $C_{14}H_{19}N_5O_4$: its molecular weight is 321.3. It is a synthetic acyclic guanine derivative.

Famciclovir is a white to pale yellow solid. It is freely soluble in acetone and methanol, and sparingly soluble in ethanol and isopropanol. At 25°C Famciclovir is freely soluble (> 25% w/v) in water initially, but rapidly precipitates as the sparingly soluble (2-3% w/v) monohydrate. Famciclovir is not hygroscopic below 85% relative humidity. Partition coefficients are: octanol/water (pH 4.8) $P = 1.09$ and octanol/phosphate buffer (pH 7.4) $P = 2.08$.

Tablets for Oral Administration: Each white, oval, film-coated tablet contains 500 mg of Famciclovir.

Following is its chemical structure:

CLINICAL PHARMACOLOGY

MICROBIOLOGY

Mechanism of Antiviral Activity: Famciclovir undergoes rapid biotransformation to the active antiviral compound penciclovir, which has inhibitory activity against herpes simplex virus types 1 (HSV-1) and 2 (HSV-2) and varicella zoster virus (VZV). In HSV-1-, HSV-2- and VZV-infected cells, viral thymidine kinase phosphorylates penciclovir to a monophosphate form which, in turn, is converted to penciclovir triphosphate by cellular kinases. *In vitro* studies demonstrate that penciclovir triphosphate inhibits HSV-2 polymerase competitively with deoxyguanosine triphosphate. Consequently, herpes viral DNA synthesis and, therefore, replication are selectively inhibited.

In uninfected cells, penciclovir does not affect DNA synthesis at concentrations ≥ 20 times those achieved in clinical usage, because it is phosphorylated only in virus-infected cells. Penciclovir triphosphate has an intracellular half-life of 10 hours in HSV-1-, 20 hours in HSV-2- and 7 hours in VZV-infected cells. The long intracellular half-life of penciclovir triphosphate may ensure prolonged antiviral activity in virus-infected cells.

Antiviral Activity In Vitro and In Vivo: In cell culture studies, penciclovir has antiviral activity against the following herpesviruses (listed in decreasing order of potency): HSV-1, HSV-2 and VZV. However, the degree of inhibition is dependent upon a number of variables, including the assay method, the host cell, virus type and multiplicity of infection (MOI). See Table 1.

Table 1

Method of Assay	Virus Type	Cell Type	IC_{50}	IC_{99} (mcg/mL)
Plaque Reduction	VZV (c.i.)	MRC-5	5.0 ± 3.0	
	VZV (c.i.)	Hs68	0.9 ± 0.4	
	HSV-1 (c.i.)	MRC-5	0.2 — 0.6	
	HSV-1 (c.i.)	WISH	0.04 — 0.5	
	HSV-2 (c.i.)	MRC-5	0.9 — 2.1	
	HSV-2 (c.i.)	WISH	0.1 — 0.8	
Virus Yield Reduction	HSV-1 (c.i.)	MRC-5		0.4-0.5
	HSV-2 (c.i.)	MRC-5		0.6-0.7
DNA Synthesis Inhibition	VZV (Ellen)	MRC-5	0.1	
	HSV-1 (SC16)	MRC-5	0.04	
	HSV-2 (MS)	MRC-5	0.05	

(c.i.) = clinical isolates.

Short-term treatment of HSV-1 or HSV-2-infected MRC-5 cells with 1 mcg/mL penciclovir reduced rival DNA by 76% and 52%, respectively. Studies of VZV-infected MRC-5 cells exposed to pulse-treatment with penciclovir for 8 hours on days 0, 1, 2, and 3 produced an IC_{50} of 5 mcg/mL.

As there is no appropriate animal model that mimics VZV infection in humans, the antiviral activity of penciclovir has not been evaluated in animals infected with VZV. However, penciclovir has been shown to have inhibitory activity against HSV-1 and HSV-2 infections in mice and guinea pigs. The level of antiviral activity depends on a number of factors, including the route of infection, route of administration of penciclovir, and time between virus infection and treatment with penciclovir.

The clinical significance of inhibitory activity of penciclovir against HSV-1 and HSV-2 in *in vitro* animal studies is unknown at this time.

PHARMACOKINETICS

Absorption and Bioavailability: Famciclovir is the diacetyl 6-deoxy analog of the active antiviral compound penciclovir. Following oral administration, little or no Famciclovir is detected in plasma or urine.

The absolute bioavailability of Famciclovir is 77 ± 8% as determined following the administration of a 500 mg Famciclovir oral dose and a 400 mg penciclovir intravenous dose to 12 healthy male subjects.

Following single oral-dose administration of 500 mg Famciclovir to 124 healthy male volunteers across 10 studies, the mean ± SD area under the plasma concentration-time profile (AUC) was 8.6 ± 1.9 mcg•hr/mL. The maximum concentration (C_{max}) was 3.3 ± 0.8 mcg/mL and the time to C_{max} (T_{max}) was 0.9 ± 0.5 hours.

Following single oral-dose administration of 500 mg Famciclovir to seven patients with herpes zoster, the mean ± SD AUC, C_{max}, and T_{max} were 12.1 ± 1.7 mcg•hr/mL, 4.0 ± 0.7 mcg/mL, and 0.7 ± 0.2 hours, respectively. The AUC of penciclovir was approximately 35% greater in patients with herpes zoster as compared to healthy volunteers. Some of this difference may be due to differences in renal function between the two groups.

There is no accumulation of penciclovir after the administration of 500 mg Famciclovir t.i.d. for 7 days.

Penciclovir concentrations increased in proportion to dose over a Famciclovir dose range of 125 mg to 750 mg administered as a single dose.

Penciclovir C_{max} decreased approximately 50% and T_{max} was delayed by 1.5 hours when a capsule formulation of Famciclovir was administered with food (nutritional content was approximately 910 Kcal and 26% fat). There was no effect on the extent of availability (AUC) of penciclovir. There was an 18% decrease in C_{max} and a delay in T_{max} of about 1 hour when Famciclovir was given 2 hours after a meal as compared to its administration 2 hours before a meal. Because there was no effect on the extent of systemic availability of penciclovir, it appears that Famciclovir can be taken without regard to meals.

Distribution: After a 1-hour intravenous infusion of penciclovir at doses of 5 mg/kg to 20 mg/kg, the volume of distribution (Vdβ) of penciclovir in 18 and 12 healthy male volunteers who received a dose of 5 mg/kg and 400 mg, respectively, was 83.1 ± 7.7 L (1.13 ± 0.11 L/kg) and 125 ± 21.3 L (1.55 ± 0.28 L/kg). Vd$_{ss}$ was 72.6 ± 11.5 L (0.98 ± 0.13 L/kg) and 85.3 ± 10.8 L (1.08 ± 0.17 L/kg).

Penciclovir is < 20% bound to plasma proteins over the concentration range of 0.1 to 20 mcg/mL. The blood/plasma ratio of penciclovir is approximately 1.

Metabolism: Following oral administration, Famciclovir is deacetylated and oxidized to form penciclovir. Metabolites that are inactive include 6-deoxy penciclovir, monoacetylated penciclovir, and 6-deoxy monoacetylated penciclovir (each < 0.5% of the dose). Little or no Famciclovir is detected in plasma or urine.

An *in vitro* study using human liver microsomes demonstrated that cytochrome P450 does not play an important role in Famciclovir metabolism. The conversion of 6-deoxy penciclovir to penciclovir is catalyzed by aldehyde oxidase.

Elimination: Approximately 94% of administered radioactivity was recovered in urine over 24 hours (83% of the dose was excreted in the first 6 hours) after the administration of 5 mg/kg radiolabeled penciclovir as a 1-hour infusion to three healthy male volunteers. Penciclovir accounted for 91% of the radioactivity excreted in the urine.

Following the oral administration of a single 500-mg dose of radiolabeled Famciclovir to three healthy male volunteers. 73% and 27% of administered radioactivity were recovered in urine and feces over 72 hours, respectively. Penciclovir accounted for 82% and 6-deoxy penciclovir accounted for 7% of the radioactivity excreted in the urine. Approximately 60% of the administered radiolabeled dose was collected in urine in the first 6 hours.

After intravenous administration of penciclovir in 48 healthy male volunteers, mean ± SD total plasma clearance of penciclovir was 36.6 ± 6.3 L/hr (0.48 ± 0.09 L/hr/kg). Penciclovir renal clearance accounted for 74.5 ± 8.8% of total plasma clearance.

Renal clearance of penciclovir following the oral administration of a single 500 mg dose of Famciclovir to 109 healthy male volunteers was 27.7 ± 7.6 L/hr.

The plasma elimination half-life of penciclovir was 2.0 ± 0.3 hours after intravenous administration of penciclovir to 48 healthy male volunteers and 2.3 ± 0.4 hours after oral administration of 500 mg Famciclovir to 124 male volunteers. The half-life in seven patients with herpes zoster was 3.0 ± 1.1 hours.

Renal Insufficiency: Apparent plasma clearance, renal clearance, and the plasma-elimination rate constant of penciclovir decreased linearly with reductions in renal function. After the administration of a single 500 mg Famciclovir oral dose (n = 27) to healthy volunteers and to volunteers with varying degrees of renal insufficiency (CL_{CR} ranged from 6.4 to 138.8 mL/min.), the following results were obtained (Table 2): (See related table).

A dosage adjustment is recommended for patients with renal insuffi- ciency (see "Dosage and Administration").

Hepatic Insufficiency: Well-compensated chronic liver disease (chronic hepatitis [n = 6], chronic ethanol abuse [n = 8], or primary biliary cirrhosis [n = 1] had no effect on the extent of availability (AUC) of penciclovir following a single dose of 500 mg Famciclovir. However, there was a 44% decrease in penciclovir mean maximum plasma concentration and the time to maximum plasma concentration was increased by 0.75 hours in patients with hepatic insufficiency compared to normal volunteers. No dosage adjustment is recommended for patients with well-compensated hepatic impairment. The pharmacokinetics of penciclovir have not been evaluated in patients with severe uncompensated hepatic impairment.

Elderly Subjects: Based on cross-study comparisons, mean penciclovir AUC was 40% larger and penciclovir renal clearance was 22% lower after the oral administration of Famciclovir in elderly volunteers (n = 18, age 65 to 79 years) compared to younger volunteers. Some of this difference may be due to differences in renal function between the two groups.

Gender: The pharmacokinetics of penciclovir was evaluated in 18 healthy male and 18 healthy female volunteers after single-dose oral administration of 500 mg Famciclovir. AUC of penciclovir was 9.3 ± 1.9 mcg•hr/mL and 11.1 ± 2.1 mcg•hr/mL in males and females, respectively. Penciclovir renal clearance was 28.5 ± 8.9 L/hr and 21.8 ± 4.3 L/hr, respectively. These differences were attributed to differences in renal function between the two groups. No Famciclovir dosage adjustment based on gender is recommended.

Pediatric Patients: The pharmacokinetics of Famciclovir or penciclovir have not been evaluated in patients < 18 years of age.

Race: The pharmacokinetics of Famciclovir or penciclovir with respect to race have not been evaluated.

DRUG INTERACTIONS
Cimetidine: Penciclovir AUC and urinary recovery increased $18 \pm 12\%$ (mean $\pm$ SD) and $12 \pm 16\%$, respectively, in 12 healthy volunteers following the administration of a single 500 mg Famciclovir dose after pre-treatment with cimetidine 400 mg b.i.d. for 7 days. The magnitude of this effect is considered to be of no clinical importance.

Allopurinol: The pharmacokinetics of penciclovir were not altered following a single oral dose of 500 mg Famciclovir in 12 healthy volunteers after pretreatment with allopurinol 300 mg once daily for 7 days.

Theophylline: Penciclovir AUC and C_{max} increased $22 \pm 9\%$ and $26 \pm 27\%$, respectively, following a single oral dose of 500 mg Famciclovir in 12 healthy volunteers who were pre-treated with theophylline 300 mg b.i.d. for 7 days. Renal clearance of penciclovir decreased by $12 \pm 14\%$ (n = 10). The magnitude of this effect is considered to be of no clinical importance.

Digoxin: After single-dose administration of digoxin and Famciclovir in 12 healthy male volunteers, the C_{max} of digoxin increased $19 \pm 18\%$ as compared to digoxin administered alone. There was no change in digoxin AUC O-t where t ranged from 10 to 72 hours.

CLINICAL TRIALS
PLACEBO-CONTROLLED TRIAL
Famciclovir was studied in a placebo-controlled, double-blind trial of 419 otherwise healthy patients with uncomplicated herpes zoster who were treated with Famciclovir 500 mg t.i.d. (n = 138), Famciclovir 750 mg t.i.d. (n = 135) or placebo (n = 146). Treatment was begun within 72 hours of initial lesion appearance and therapy was continued for 7 days.

Dermatology and Virology: The times to full crusting, loss of vesicles, loss of ulcers, and loss of crusts were shorter for Famciclovir 500 mg-treated patients than for placebo-treated patients in the overall study population. The median time to full crusting in Famciclovir 500 mg-treated patients was 5 days compared to 7 days in placebo-treated patients. No additional efficacy was demonstrated with the higher dose of Famciclovir (750 mg t.i.d.), when compared to Famciclovir 500 mg t.i.d. In the total population, 65.2% of patients had a positive viral culture at some time during their acute infection. Patients treated with Famciclovir 500 mg had a shorter median duration of viral shedding (time to last positive viral culture) than did placebo-treated patients (1 day and 2 days, respectively).

Acute Pain and Postherpetic Neuralgia: There were no overall differences in the duration of acute pain (i.e., pain before rash healing) between Famciclovir and placebo-treated groups. In addition, there was no difference in the incidence of postherpetic neuralgia (i.e., pain after rash healing) between the treatment groups.

In the 186 patients (44.4% of total study population) who did develop postherpetic neuralgia, the median duration of postherpetic neuralgia was shorter in patients treated with Famciclovir 500 mg than in those treated with placebo (63 days and 119 days, respectively).

ACTIVE-CONTROL TRIAL
A second double-blind controlled trial in 545 otherwise healthy patients with uncomplicated herpes zoster treated within 72 hours of initial lesion appearance compared Famciclovir 250 mg t.i.d. (n = 134), Famciclovir 500 mg t.i.d. (n = 134), Famciclovir 750 mg t.i.d. (n = 138), and acyclovir 800 mg 5 times per day (n = 139) for 7 days. In this study, patients treated with Famciclovir at each dose and acyclovir had comparable times to full lesion crusting and times to loss of acute pain. There were no statistically significant differences in the time to loss of postherpetic neuralgia between Famciclovir and acyclovir-treated groups.

INDICATIONS AND USAGE
Famciclovir is indicated for the management of acute herpes zoster (shingles).

UNLABELED USES
Famciclovir is used alone or as an adjunct in the treatment of herpes simplex virus infections.

CONTRAINDICATIONS
Famciclovir is contraindicated in patients with known hypersensitivity to the product.

PRECAUTIONS
GENERAL
The efficacy of Famciclovir has not been studied in ophthalmic zoster, disseminated zoster, or in immunocompromised patients.

Dosage adjustment is recommended when administering Famciclovir to patients with creatinine clearance values < 60 mL/min. (see "Dosage and Administration"). There is no information from clinical trials about the safety of administering Famciclovir to patients with renal dysfunction.

DRUG INTERACTIONS
No clinically significant alterations in penciclovir pharmacokinetics were observed following single-dose administration of 500 mg Famciclovir after pre-treatment with multiple doses of cimetidine, allopurinol, or theophylline (see "Clinical Pharmacology").

Concurrent use with probenecid or other drugs significantly eliminated by active renal tubular secretion may result in increased plasma concentrations of penciclovir.

The conversion of 6-deoxy penciclovir is catalyzed by aldehyde oxidase. Interactions with other drugs metabolized by this enzyme could potentially occur.

CARCINOGENESIS, MUTAGENESIS, IMPAIRMENT OF FERTILITY
Famciclovir was administered orally unless otherwise stated.

Carcinogenesis: Two-year dietary carcinogenicity studies of Famciclovir were conducted in rats and mice. The high dose tested in rats and mice was lowered after 7 to 8 months of drug administration to ensure long-term survival (female rats and male/female mice from 750 to 600-mg/kg/day; male rats from 300 to 240 mg/kg/day). A significant increase in the incidence of mammary adenocarcinoma was seen in female rats receiving 600 mg/kg/day (1.5 times the human systemic exposure at the recommended oral dose of 500 mg t.i.d. based on area under the plasma concentration curve comparisons [24 hr AUC] for penciclovir). Marginal increases in the incidence of subcutaneous tissue fibrosarcomas or squamous cell carcinomas of the skin were seen in female rats (dosed at 600 mg/kg/day) and male mice (dosed at 600 mg/kg/day: 0.4x the human systemic exposure, based on 24 hr AUC for penciclovir), respectively. No increases in tumor incidence were reported for male rats treated at doses up to 240 mg/kg/day (0.9x the human AUC), or in female mice at doses up to 600 mg/kg/day (0.4x the human AUC).

Mutagenesis: Famciclovir and penciclovir (the active metabolite of Famciclovir) were tested for genotoxic potential in a battery of *in vitro* and *in vivo* assays. Famciclovir and penciclovir were negative in *in vitro* tests for gene mutations in bacteria (S. *typhimurium* and *E. coli*) and unscheduled DNA synthesis in mammalian HeLa 83 cells (at doses up to 10,000 and 5000 mcg/plate, respectively). Famciclovir was also negative in the L5178Y mouse lymphoma assay (5000 mcg/mL), the *in vivo* mouse micronucleus test (4800 mg/kg), and rat dominant lethal study (5000 mg/kg). Famciclovir induced increases in polyploidy in human lymphocytes *in vitro* in the absence of chromosomal damage (1200 mcg/mL). Penciclovir was positive in the L5178Y mouse lymphoma assay for gene mutation/chromosomal aberrations, with and without metabolic activation (1000 mcg/mL). In human lymphocytes, penciclovir caused chromosomal aberrations in

Table 2

Parameter (mean ± S.D.)	Cl_{CR}* ≥ 60 (mL/min.)	CL_{CR} 40-59 (mL/min.)	CL_{CR} 20-39 (mL/min.)	CL_{CR} < 20 (mL/min.)
CL_{CR}(mL/min)	88.1 ± 20.6	49.3 ± 5.9**	26.5 ± 5.3	12.7 ± 5.9
CL_R(L/hr)	30.1 ± 10.6	13.0 ± 1.3**	4.2 ± 0.9	1.6 ± 1.0
CL/F***(L/hr)	66.9 ± 27.5	27.3 ± 2.8	12.8 ± 1.3	5.8 ± 2.8
Half-life (hr)	2.3 ± 0.5	3.4 ± 0.7	6.2 ± 1.6	13.4 ± 10.2
n	15	5	4	3

*CL_{CR} is measured creatinine clearance.
**n = 4.
*** CL/F consists of bioavailability factor and Famciclovir to penciclovir conversion factor.

the absence of metabolic activation (250 mcg/mL). Penciclovir caused an increased incidence of micronuclei in mouse bone marrow *in vivo* when administered intravenously at doses highly toxic to bone marrow (500 mg/kg), but not when administered orally.

Impairment of Fertility: Testicular toxicity was observed in rats, mice, and dogs following repeated administration of Famciclovir or penciclovir. Testicular changes included atrophy of the seminiferous tubules, reduction in sperm count, and/or increased incidence of sperm with abnormal morphology or reduced motility. The degree of toxicity to male reproduction was related to dose and duration of exposure. In male rats, decreased fertility was observed after 10 weeks of dosing at 500 mg/kg/day (1.9x the human AUC). The no observable effect level for sperm and testicular toxicity in rats following chronic administration (26 weeks) was 50 mg/kg/day (0.2x the human systemic exposure based on AUC comparisons). Testicular toxicity was observed following chronic administration to mice (104 weeks) and dogs (26 weeks) at doses of 600 mg/kg/day (0.4x the human AUC) and 150 mg/kg/day (1:7x the human AUC), respectively.

Famciclovir had no effect on general reproductive performance or fertility in female rats at doses up to 1000 mg/kg/day (3.6x the human AUC).

PREGNANCY

Teratogenic Effects: Pregnancy Category B: Famciclovir was tested for effects on embryo-fetal development in rats and rabbits at oral doses up to 1000 mg/kg/day (approximately 3.6x and 1.8x the human systemic exposure to penciclovir based on AUC comparisons for the rat and rabbit, respectively) and intravenous doses of 360 mg/kg/day in rats (2x the human dose based on body surface area [BSA] comparisons or 120 mg/kg/day in rabbits (1:5 × the human dose [BSA]). No adverse effects were observed on embryo-fetal development. Similarly, no adverse effects were observed following intravenous administration of penciclovir to rats (80 mg/kg/day. 0.4 × the human dose [BSA] or rabbits (60 mg/kg/day, 0.7 × the human dose [BSA]). There are, however, no adequate and well-controlled studies in pregnant women. Because animal reproduction studies are not always predictive of human response, Famciclovir should be used during pregnancy only if the benefit to the patient clearly exceeds the potential risk to the fetus.

NURSING MOTHERS

Following oral administration of Famciclovir to lactating rats, penciclovir was excreted in breast milk at concentrations higher than those seen in the plasma. It is not known whether it is excreted in human milk. Because of the potential for tumorigenicity shown for Famciclovir in rats, a decision should be made whether to discontinue nursing or to discontinue the drug, taking into account the importance of the drug to the mother.

USAGE IN CHILDREN

Safety and efficacy in children under the age of 18 years have not been established.

GERIATRIC USE

Of 816 patients with herpes zoster in clinical studies who were treated with Famciclovir 248 (30.4%) were > 65 years of age and 103 (13%) were ≥ 75 years of age. No overall differences were observed in the incidence or types of adverse events between younger and older patients.

ADVERSE REACTIONS

In four clinical studies involving 816 Famciclovir treated patients with herpes zoster (Famciclovir 250 mg t.i.d. to 750 mg t.i.d.), the most frequent adverse events associated with Famciclovir were headache, nausea and fatigue, which occurred in similar frequencies in placebo-treated patients. Table 3 lists adverse events occurring on-therapy with an incidence of ≥ 2% per treatment group in the placebo-controlled Famciclovir trial 008. The frequency and types of reported adverse events in trial 008 were representative of the safety experience in the active-controlled herpes zoster Famciclovir trials (007 and 094).

Table 3

ADVERSE EVENTS REPORTED BY ≥ 2% OF TREATMENT GROUP IN PATIENTS IN FAMCICLOVIR 008 HERPES ZOSTER TRIAL

	Incidence	
Event	Famciclovir (n = 273) %	Placebo (n = 146) %
Body as a Whole		
Fatigue	4.4	3.4
Fever	3.3	4.1
Injury	2.6	0.0
Pain	2.6	2.7
Rigors	1.5	2.7
Gastrointestinal		
Nausea	12.5	11.6
Diarrhea	7.7	4.8
Vomiting	4.8	3.4
Constipation	4.4	4.8
Anorexia	2.6	4.1
Abdominal Pain	1.1	3.4
Musculoskeletal		
Back Pain	1.5	2.7
Arthralgia	1.5	2.1
Nervous System		
Headache	22.7	17.8
Dizziness	3.3	4.1
Paresthesia	2.6	0.0
Somnolence	2.6	2.7
Respiratory		
Pharyngitis	2.6	4.8
Sinusitis	2.6	1.4
Skin and Appendages		
Pruritus	3.7	2.7
Zoster-related Signs		
Symptoms/Complications	2.9	3.4

* *There were no statistically significant differences in adverse event reporting rates between Famciclovir and placebo-treated patients.*

OVERDOSAGE

No acute overdosage has been reported. Appropriate symptomatic and supportive therapy should be given.

It is not known if hemodialysis removes penciclovir from the blood. However, hemodialysis does enhance the elimination of acyclovir, a related nucleoside analog.

DOSAGE AND ADMINISTRATION

The recommended dosage is 500 mg every 8 hours for 7 days. Therapy should be initiated promptly as soon as herpes zoster is diagnosed. In clinical trials, the effect of Famciclovir on rash resolution was more pronounced in patients age 50 years and older. Treatment was begun within 72 hours of rash onset in these studies and was more useful if started within the first 48 hours. The efficacy of Famciclovir initiated more than 72 hours after rash onset has not been studied. When Famciclovir was administered with food, penciclovir C_{max} decreased approximately 50%. Because the systemic availability of penciclovir (AUC) was not altered, it appears that Famciclovir may be taken without regard to meals.

In patients with reduced renal function, dosage reduction is recommended:

Table 4

Creatinine Clearance (mL/min.)	Dose Regimen
≥ 60	500 mg every 8 hours
40-59	500 mg every 12 hours
20-39	500 mg every 24 hours

There are insufficient data to recommend a dosage for patients with creatinine clearance < 20 mL/min.

Store at controlled room temperature, (15° to 30°C; 59° to 86°F).

HOW SUPPLIED
TABLETS: 500 MG

BRAND/MANUFACTURER	NDC	SIZE	AWP
○ **BRAND**			
▶ FAMVIR: SK Beecham Pharm	00007-4117-13	30s	$184.50
	00007-4117-19	50s	$340.07

Famotidine

DESCRIPTION

The active ingredient in Famotidine is a histamine H_2-receptor antagonist. Famotidine is *N'*-(aminosulfonyl)-3-[[[2-[(diaminomethylene)amino]-4-thiazolyl]methyl]thio]propanimidamide. The empirical formula of Famotidine is $C_8H_{15}N_7O_2S_3$ and its molecular weight is 337.43.

Famotidine is a white to pale yellow crystalline compound that is freely soluble in glacial acetic acid, slightly soluble in methanol, very slightly soluble in water, and practically insoluble in ethanol.

Famotidine is supplied in three dosage forms: Famotidine tablets, Famotidine oral suspension, and Famotidine injection. The solution for intravenous injection also comes premixed in single dose containers.

Each tablet for oral administration contains either 20 mg or 40 mg of Famotidine.

Each 5 mL of the oral suspension when prepared as directed contains 40 mg of Famotidine.

Each mL of the solution for intravenous injection contains 10 mg of Famotidine.

Each 50 mL of the premixed intravenous injection contains 20 mg Famotidine.

Following is its chemical structure:

$$H_2N\text{-}C\text{-}N \quad CH_2SCH_2CH_2C\text{-}NSO_2NH_2$$

CLINICAL PHARMACOLOGY
GI EFFECTS

Famotidine is a competitive inhibitor of histamine H_2-receptors. The primary clinically important pharmacologic activity of Famotidine is inhibition of gastric secretion. Both the acid concentration and volume of gastric secretion are

---

◆ RATED THERAPEUTICALLY EQUIVALENT; ◇ THERAPEUTIC EQUIVALENCE UNCONFIRMED; ○ UNRATED

suppressed by Famotidine, while changes in pepsin secretion are proportional to volume output.

In normal volunteers and hypersecretors, Famotidine inhibited basal and nocturnal gastric secretion, as well as secretion stimulated by food and pentagastrin. After oral administration, the onset of the antisecretory effect occurred within one hour; the maximum effect was dose-dependent, occurring within one to three hours. Duration of inhibition of secretion by doses of 20 and 40 mg was 10 to 12 hours.

After intravenous administration, the maximum effect was achieved within 30 minutes. Single intravenous doses of 10 and 20 mg inhibited nocturnal secretion for a period of 10 to 12 hours. The 20 mg dose was associated with the longest duration of action in most subjects.

Single evening oral doses of 20 and 40 mg inhibited basal and nocturnal acid secretion in all subjects; mean nocturnal gastric acid secretion was inhibited by 86% and 94%, respectively, for a period of at least 10 hours. The same doses given in the morning suppressed food-stimulated acid secretion in all subjects. The mean suppression was 76% and 84% respectively 3 to 5 hours after administration, and 25% and 30% respectively 8 to 10 hours after administration. In some subjects who received the 20 mg dose, however, the antisecretory effect was dissipated within 6-8 hours. There was no cumulative effect with repeated doses. The nocturnal intragastric pH was raised by evening doses of 20 and 40 mg of Famotidine to mean values of 5.0 and 6.4, respectively. When Famotidine was given after breakfast, the basal daytime interdigestive pH at 3 and 8 hours after 20 or 40 mg of Famotidine was raised to about 5.

Famotidine had little or no effect on fasting or postprandial serum gastrin levels. Gastric emptying and exocrine pancreatic function were not affected by Famotidine.

OTHER EFFECTS
Systemic effects of Famotidine in the CNS, cardiovascular, respiratory or endocrine systems were not noted in clinical pharmacology studies. Also, no antiandrogenic effects were noted. (See "Adverse Reactions".) Serum hormone levels, including prolactin, cortisol, thyroxine (T_4), and testosterone, were not altered after treatment with Famotidine.

PHARMACOKINETICS
Orally administered Famotidine is incompletely absorbed. The bioavailability of oral doses is 40-45%. Famotidine Tablets and Famotidine Oral Suspension are bioequivalent. Bioavailability may be slightly increased by food, or slightly decreased by antacids; however, these effects are of no clinical consequence. Famotidine undergoes minimal first-pass metabolism. After oral doses, peak plasma levels occur in 1-3 hours. Plasma levels after multiple doses are similar to those after single doses. Fifteen to 20% of Famotidine in plasma is protein bound. Famotidine has an elimination half-life of 2.5-3.5 hours. Famotidine is eliminated by renal (65-70%) and metabolic (30-35%) routes. Renal clearance is 250-450 mL/min, indicating some tubular excretion. Twenty-five to 30% of an oral dose and 65-70% of an intravenous dose are recovered in the urine as unchanged compound. The only metabolite identified in man is the S-oxide.

There is a close relationship between creatinine clearance values and the elimination half-life of Famotidine. In patients with severe renal insufficiency, i.e., creatinine clearance less than 10 mL/min, Famotidine elimination half-life may exceed 20 hours and adjustment of dose or dosing intervals may be necessary (see "Precautions", "Dosage and Administration").

In elderly patients, there are no clinically significant age-related changes in the pharmacokinetics of Famotidine.

CLINICAL STUDIES: DUODENAL ULCER
The majority of clinical study experience involved oral administration of Famotidine Tablets.

In a U.S. multicenter, double-blind study in outpatients with endoscopically confirmed duodenal ulcer, orally administered Famotidine was compared to placebo. As shown in Table 1, 70% of patients treated with Famotidine 40 mg h.s. were healed by week 4.

Table 1
OUTPATIENTS WITH ENDOSCOPICALLY CONFIRMED HEALED DUODENAL ULCERS

	Famotidine 40 mg h.s. (N = 89)	Famotidine 20 mg b.i.d. (N = 84)	Placebo h.s. (N = 97)
Week 2	*32%	*38%	17%
Week 4	*70%	*67%	31%

* Statistically significantly different than placebo (p < 0.001)

Patients not healed by week 4 were continued in the study. By week 8, 83% of patients treated with Famotidine had healed versus 45% of patients treated with placebo. The incidence of ulcer healing with Famotidine was significantly higher than with placebo at each time point based on proportion of endoscopically confirmed healed ulcers.

In this study, time to relief of daytime and nocturnal pain was significantly shorter for patients receiving Famotidine than for patients receiving placebo; patients receiving Famotidine also took less antacid than the patients receiving placebo.

LONG TERM MAINTENANCE TREATMENT OF DUODENAL ULCERS
Famotidine, 20 mg p.o. h.s. was compared to placebo h.s. as maintenance therapy in two double-blind, multicenter studies of patients with endoscopically confirmed healed duodenal ulcers. In the U.S. study the observed ulcer incidence within 12 months in patients treated with placebo was 2.4 times greater than in the patients treated with Famotidine. The 89 patients treated with Famotidine had a cumulative observed ulcer incidence of 23.4% compared to an observed ulcer incidence of 56.6% in the 89 patients receiving placebo (p < 0.01). These results were confirmed in an international study where the cumulative observed ulcer incidence within 12 months in the 307 patients treated with Famotidine was 35.7%, compared to an incidence of 75.5% in the 325 patients treated with placebo (p < 0.01).

GASTRIC ULCER
In both a U.S. and an international multicenter, double-blind study in patients with endoscopically confirmed active benign gastric ulcer, orally administered Famotidine, 40 mg h.s., was compared to placebo h.s. Antacids were permitted during the studies, but consumption was not significantly different between the Famotidine and placebo groups. As shown in Table 2, the incidence of ulcer healing (dropouts counted as unhealed) with Famotidine was statistically significantly better than placebo at weeks 6 and 8 in the U.S. study, and at weeks 4, 6 and 8 in the international study, based on the number of ulcers that healed, confirmed by endoscopy.

Table 2
PATIENTS WITH ENDOSCOPICALLY CONFIRMED HEALED GASTRIC ULCERS

	U.S. Study		International Study	
	Famotidine 40 mg h.s. (N = 74)	Placebo h.s. (N = 75)	Famotidine 40 mg h.s. (N = 149)	Placebo h.s. (N = 145)
Week 4	45%	39%	**47%	31%
Week 6	**66%	44%	**65%	46%
Week 8	*78%	64%	**80%	54%

*,** Statistically significantly better than placebo (p ≤ 0.05, p ≤ 0.01 respectively)

Time to complete relief of daytime and nighttime pain was statistically significantly shorter for patients receiving Famotidine than for patients receiving placebo; however, in neither study was there a statistically significant difference in the proportion of patients whose pain was relieved by the end of the study (week 8).

GASTROESOPHAGEAL REFLUX DISEASE (GERD)
Famotidine was compared to placebo in a U.S. study that enrolled patients with symptoms of GERD and without endoscopic evidence of erosion or ulceration of the esophagus. Famotidine 20 mg b.i.d. was statistically significantly superior to 40 mg h.s. and to placebo in providing a successful symptomatic outcome, defined as moderate or excellent improvement of symptoms (Table 3).

Table 3
% SUCCESSFUL SYMPTOMATIC OUTCOME

	Famotidine 20 mg b.i.d. (N = 154)	Famotidine 40 mg h.s. (N = 149)	Placebo (N = 73)
Week 6	82**	69	62

** p ≤ 0.01 vs Placebo

By two weeks of treatment, symptomatic success was observed in a greater percentage of patients taking Famotidine 20 mg b.i.d. compared to placebo (p ≤ 0.01).

Symptomatic improvement and healing of endoscopically verified erosion and ulceration were studied in two additional trials. Healing was defined as complete resolution of all erosions or ulcerations visible with endoscopy. The U.S. study comparing Famotidine 40 mg b.i.d. to placebo and Famotidine 20 mg b.i.d., showed a significantly greater percentage of healing for Famotidine 40 mg b.i.d. at weeks 6 and 12 (Table 4).

Table 4
% ENDOSCOPIC HEALING—U.S. STUDY

	Famotidine 40 mg b.i.d. (N = 127)	Famotidine 20 mg b.i.d. (N = 125)	Placebo (N = 66)
Week 6	48**, ++	32	18
Week 12	69**,+	54**	29

** p ≤ 0.01 vs Placebo
+ p ≤ 0.05 vs Famotidine 20 mg b.i.d.
++ p ≤ 0.01 vs Famotidine 20 mg b.i.d.

As compared to placebo, patients who received Famotidine had faster relief of daytime and nighttime heartburn and a greater percentage of patients experienced complete relief of nighttime heartburn. These differences were statistically significant.

➤ SHOWN IN PRODUCT IDENTIFICATION GUIDE

In the international study, when Famotidine 40 mg b.i.d., was compared to ranitidine 150 mg b.i.d., a statistically significantly greater percentage of healing was observed with Famotidine 40 mg b.i.d. at week 12 (Table 5). There was, however, no significant difference among treatments in symptom relief.

Table 5

% ENDOSCOPIC HEALING—INTERNATIONAL STUDY

	Famotidine 40 mg b.i.d. (N = 175)	Famotidine 20 mg b.i.d. (N = 93)	Ranitidine 150 mg b.i.d. (N = 172)
Week 6	48	52	42
Week 12	71*	68	60

* $p \leq 0.05$ vs ranitidine 150 mg b.i.d.

Pathological Hypersecretory Conditions (e.g., Zollinger-Ellison Syndrome, Multiple Endocrine Adenomas): In studies of patients with pathological hypersecretory conditions such as Zollinger-Ellison Syndrome with or without multiple endocrine adenomas, Famotidine significantly inhibited gastric acid secretion and controlled associated symptoms. Doses from 20 to 160 mg q 6 h maintained basal acid secretion below 10 mEq/hr; initial doses were titrated to the individual patient need and subsequent adjustments were necessary with time in some patients. Famotidine was well tolerated at these high dose levels for prolonged periods (greater than 12 months) in eight patients, and there were no cases reported of gynecomastia, increased prolactin levels, or impotence which were considered to be due to the drug.

INDICATIONS AND USAGE
Famotidine Injection Premixed, supplied as a premixed solution in plastic containers, and Famotidine Injection, supplied as a concentrated solution for intravenous injection, are intended for intravenous use only. Famotidine Injection Premixed and Famotidine Injection are indicated in some hospitalized patients with pathological hypersecretory conditions or intractable ulcers, or as an alternative to the oral dosage forms for short term use in patients who are unable to take oral medication.

Famotidine is indicated in:

1. Short term treatment of active duodenal ulcer. Most patients heal within 4 weeks; there is rarely reason to use Famotidine at full dosage for longer than 6 to 8 weeks. Studies have not assessed the safety of Famotidine in uncomplicated active duodenal ulcer for periods of more than eight weeks.

2. Maintenance therapy for duodenal ulcer patients at reduced dosage after healing of an active ulcer. Controlled studies have not extended beyond one year.

3. Short term treatment of active benign gastric ulcer. Most patients heal within 6 weeks. Studies have not assessed the safety or efficacy of Famotidine in uncomplicated active benign gastric ulcer for periods of more than 8 weeks.

4. Short term treatment of gastroesophageal reflux disease (GERD). Famotidine is indicated for short term treatment of patients with symptoms of GERD (see "Clinical Pharmacology, Clinical Studies").

Famotidine is also indicated for the short term treatment of esophagitis due to GERD including erosive or ulcerative disease diagnosed by endoscopy (see "Clinical Pharmacology, Clinical Studies").

5. Treatment of pathological hypersecretory conditions (e.g., Zollinger-Ellison Syndrome, multiple endocrine adenomas). Famotidine Injection is indicated in some hospitalized patients with pathological hypersecretory conditions or intractable ulcers, or as an alternative to the oral dosage forms for short-term use in patients who are unable to take oral medication.

UNLABELED USES
Famotidine is used alone or as an adjunct in the treatment of gastritis.

CONTRAINDICATIONS
Hypersensitivity to any component of these products.

PRECAUTIONS
GENERAL
Symptomatic response to therapy with Famotidine does not preclude the presence of gastric malignancy.

PATIENTS WITH SEVERE RENAL INSUFFICIENCY
Longer intervals between doses or lower doses may need to be used in patients with severe renal insufficiency (creatinine clearance < 10 mL/min) to adjust for the longer elimination half-life of Famotidine. (See "Clinical Pharmacology" and "Dosage and Administration".) However, currently, no drug-related toxicity has been found with high plasma concentrations of Famotidine.

INFORMATION FOR PATIENTS
The patient should be instructed to shake the oral suspension vigorously for 5-10 seconds prior to each use. Unused constituted oral suspension should be discarded after 30 days.

DRUG INTERACTIONS
No drug interactions have been identified. Studies with Famotidine in man, in animal models, and *in vitro* have shown no significant interference with the disposition of compounds metabolized by the hepatic microsomal enzymes, e.g., cytochrome P450 system. Compounds tested in man include warfarin, theophylline, phenytoin, diazepam, aminopyrine and antipyrine. Indocyanine green as an index of hepatic drug extraction has been tested and no significant effects have been found.

CARCINOGENESIS, MUTAGENESIS, IMPAIRMENT OF FERTILITY
In a 106 week study in rats and a 92 week study in mice given oral doses of up to 2000 mg/kg/day (approximately 2500 times the recommended human dose for active duodenal ulcer), there was no evidence of carcinogenic potential for Famotidine.

Famotidine was negative in the microbial mutagen test (Ames test) using *Salmonella typhimurium* and *Escherichia coli* with or without rat liver enzyme activation at concentrations up to 10,000 mcg/plate. In *in vivo* studies in mice, with a micronucleus test and a chromosomal aberration test, no evidence of a mutagenic effect was observed.

In studies with rats given oral doses of up to 2000 mg/kg/day or intravenous doses of up to 200 mg/kg/day fertility and reproductive performance were not affected.

PREGNANCY
PREGNANCY CATEGORY B
Reproductive studies have been performed in rats and rabbits at oral doses of up to 2000 and 500 mg/kg/day respectively and in both species at I.V. doses of up to 200 mg/kg/day, and have revealed no significant evidence of impaired fertility or harm to the fetus due to Famotidine. While no direct fetotoxic effects have been observed, sporadic abortions occurring only in mothers displaying marked decreased food intake were seen in some rabbits at oral doses of 200 mg/kg/day (250 times the usual human dose) or higher. There are, however, no adequate or well-controlled studies in pregnant women. Because animal reproductive studies are not always predictive of human response, this drug should be used during pregnancy only if clearly needed.

NURSING MOTHERS
Studies performed in lactating rats have shown that Famotidine is secreted into breast milk. Transient growth depression was observed in young rats suckling from mothers treated with maternotoxic doses of at least 600 times the usual human dose. It is not known whether this drug is secreted into human milk. Because many drugs are secreted into human milk and because of the potential for serious adverse reactions in nursing infants from Famotidine, a decision should be made whether to discontinue nursing or discontinue the drug, taking into account the importance of the drug to the mother.

PEDIATRIC USE
Safety and effectiveness in children have not been established.

USE IN ELDERLY PATIENTS
No dosage adjustment is required based on age (see "Clinical Pharmacology, Pharmacokinetics"). Dosage adjustment in the case of severe renal impairment may be necessary.

ADVERSE REACTIONS
The adverse reactions listed below have been reported during domestic and international clinical trials in approximately 2500 patients. In those controlled clinical trials in which Famotidine Tablets were compared to placebo, the incidence of adverse experiences in the group which received Famotidine Tablets, 40 mg at bedtime, was similar to that in the placebo group.

The following adverse reactions have been reported to occur in more than 1% of patients on therapy with Famotidine in controlled clinical trials, and may be causally related to the drug: headache (4.7%), dizziness (1.3%), constipation (1.2%) and diarrhea (1.7%).

The following other adverse reactions have been reported infrequently in clinical trials or since the drug was marketed. The relationship to therapy with Famotidine has been unclear in many cases. Within each category the adverse reactions are listed in order of decreasing severity:

Body as a Whole: fever, asthenia, fatigue

Cardiovascular: arrhythmia, AV block, palpitation

Gastrointestinal: cholestatic jaundice, liver enzyme abnormalities, vomiting, nausea, abdominal discomfort, anorexia, dry mouth

Hematologic: rare cases of agranulocytosis, pancytopenia, leukopenia, thrombocytopenia

Hypersensitivity: anaphylaxis, angioedema, orbital or facial edema, urticaria, rash, conjunctival injection

Musculoskeletal: musculoskeletal pain, arthralgia

Nervous System/Psychiatric: grand mal seizure; psychic disturbances, which were reversible in cases for which follow-up was obtained, including hallucinations, confusion, agitation, depression, anxiety, decreased libido; paresthesia; insomnia; somnolence

Respiratory: bronchospasm

Skin: alopecia, acne, pruritus, dry skin, flushing

Special Senses: tinnitus, taste disorder

Other: rare cases of impotence have been reported; however, in controlled clinical trials, the incidence was not greater than that seen with placebo.

The adverse reactions reported for Famotidine Tablets may also occur with Famotidine Oral Suspension or Famotidine Injection or Injection Premixed. In addition, transient irritation at the injection site has been observed with Famotidine Injection.

OVERDOSAGE

There is no experience to date with deliberate overdosage. Doses of up to 640 mg/day have been given to patients with pathological hypersecretory conditions with no serious adverse effects. In the event of overdosage, treatment should be symptomatic and supportive. Unabsorbed material should be removed from the gastrointestinal tract, the patient should be monitored, and supportive therapy should be employed.

The oral LD$_{50}$ of Famotidine in male and female rats and mice was greater than 3000 mg/kg and the minimum lethal acute oral dose in dogs exceeded 2000 mg/kg. Famotidine did not produce overt effects at high oral doses in mice, rats, cats and dogs, but induced significant anorexia and growth depression in rabbits starting with 200 mg/kg/day orally. The intravenous LD$_{50}$ of Famotidine for mice and rats ranged from 254-563 mg/kg and the minimum lethal single I.V. dose in dogs was approximately 300 mg/kg. Signs of acute intoxication in I.V. treated dogs were emesis, restlessness, pallor of mucous membranes or redness of mouth and ears, hypotension, tachycardia and collapse.

DOSAGE AND ADMINISTRATION

DUODENAL ULCER

Acute Therapy: The recommended adult oral dosage for active duodenal ulcer is 40 mg once a day at bedtime. Most patients heal within 4 weeks; there is rarely reason to use Famotidine at full dosage for longer than 6 to 8 weeks. A regimen of 20 mg b.i.d. is also effective.

Maintenance Therapy: The recommended oral dose is 20 mg once a day at bedtime.

BENIGN GASTRIC ULCER

Acute Therapy: The recommended adult oral dosage for active benign gastric ulcer is 40 mg once a day at bedtime.

GASTROESOPHAGEAL REFLUX DISEASE (GERD)

The recommended oral dosage for treatment of patients with symptoms of GERD is 20 mg b.i.d. for up to 6 weeks. The recommended oral dosage for the treatment of patients with esophagitis including erosions and ulcerations and accompanying symptoms due to GERD is 20 or 40 mg b.i.d. for up to 12 weeks (see *"Clinical Pharmacology, Clinical Studies"*).

PATHOLOGICAL HYPERSECRETORY CONDITIONS (E.G., ZOLLINGER-ELLISON SYNDROME, MULTIPLE ENDOCRINE ADENOMAS)

The dosage of Famotidine in patients with pathological hypersecretory conditions varies with the individual patient. The recommended adult oral starting dose for pathological hypersecretory conditions is 20 mg q 6 h. The recommended adult intravenous dose is 20 mg q 12h. In some patients, a higher starting dose may be required. Doses should be adjusted to individual patient needs and should continue as long as clinically indicated. Oral doses up to 160 mg q 6 h have been administered to some patients with severe Zollinger-Ellison Syndrome.

ORAL SUSPENSION

Famotidine Oral Suspension may be substituted for Famotidine Tablets in any of the above indications. Each five mL contains 40 mg of Famotidine after constitution of the powder with 46 mL of Purified Water as directed.

DIRECTIONS FOR PREPARING FAMOTIDINE ORAL SUSPENSION

Prepare suspension at time of dispensing. Slowly add 46 mL of Purified Water. Shake vigorously for 5-10 seconds immediately after adding the water and immediately before use.

STABILITY OF FAMOTIDINE ORAL SUSPENSION

Unused constituted oral suspension should be discarded after 30 days.

INTRAVENOUS ADMINISTRATION

In some hospitalized patients with pathological hypersecretory conditions or intractable ulcers, or in patients who are unable to take oral medication, Famotidine Injection or Injection Premixed may be administered until oral therapy can be instituted.

FAMOTIDINE INJECTION

The recommended dosage is 20 mg q 12 h.

FAMOTIDINE INJECTION PREMIXED

The recommended dosage is 20 mg q 12 h, administered as an infusion over a 15—30 minute period.

The doses and regimen for parenteral administration in patients with GERD have not been established.

PREPARATION OF FAMOTIDINE INTRAVENOUS SOLUTIONS

Dilute 2 mL of Famotidine Injection (solution containing 10 mg/mL) with 0.9% Sodium Chloride Injection or other compatible intravenous solution to a total volume of either 5 mL or 10 mL and inject over a period of not less than 2 minutes.

PREPARATION OF FAMOTIDINE INTRAVENOUS INFUSION SOLUTIONS

Famotidine Injection may also be administered as an infusion, 2 mL diluted with 100 mL of 5% dextrose or other compatible solution, and infused over a 15-30 minute period.

PREPARATION OF FAMOTIDINE INJECTION PREMIXED

Famotidine Injection Premixed is a 50 mL iso-osmotic solution premixed with 0.9% sodium chloride for administration as an infusion over a 15—30 minute period. *This premixed solution is for intravenous use only using sterile equipment.*

Check the container for minute leaks prior to use by squeezing the bag firmly. If leaks are found, discard solution as sterility may be impaired. Do not add supplementary medication. Do not use unless solution is clear and seal is intact. CAUTION: Do not use plastic containers in series connections. Such use could result in air embolism due to residual air being drawn from the primary container before administration of the fluid from the secondary container is complete. Preparation for administration:
1. Suspend container from eyelet support.
2. Remove plastic protector from outlet port at bottom of container.
3. Attach administration set. Refer to complete directions accompanying set.

STABILITY OF FAMOTIDINE INJECTION

Famotidine Injection is stable for 48 hours at room temperature when added to or diluted with most commonly used intravenous solutions, e.g., Water for Injection, 0.9% Sodium Chloride Injection, 5% and 10% Dextrose Injection, Lactated Ringer's Injection, or Sodium Bicarbonate Injection, 5%.

Parenteral drug products should be inspected visually for particulate matter and discoloration prior to administration whenever solution and container permit.

STABILITY OF FAMOTIDINE INJECTION PREMIXED

Famotidine Injection Premixed, as supplied premixed in 0.9% sodium choloride, is stable through the labeled expiration date when stored under the recommended conditions.

CONCOMITANT USE OF ANTACIDS

Antacids may be given concomitantly if needed.

DOSAGE ADJUSTMENT FOR PATIENTS WITH SEVERE RENAL INSUFFICIENCY

In patients with severe renal insufficiency, i.e., with a creatinine clearance less than 10 mL/min, the elimination half-life of Famotidine may exceed 20 hours, reaching approximately 24 hours in anuric patients. Although no relationship of adverse effects to high plasma levels has been established, to avoid excess accumulation of the drug, the dose of Famotidine may be reduced to 20 mg h.s. or the dosing interval may be prolonged to 36-48 hours as indicated by the patient's clinical response.

STORAGE

Avoid storage of Famotidine Tablets at temperatures above 40°C (104°F).

Avoid storage of the powder for oral suspension at temperatures above 40°C (104°F). After constitution store the suspension below 30°C (86°F). Do not freeze. Discard unused suspension after 30 days.

Store Famotidine Injection at 2-8°C (36-46°F). If solution freezes, bring to room temperature; allow sufficient time to solubilize all the components.

When diluted as recommended (see *"Dosage and Administration"*) Famotidine Injection is stable for 48 hours at room temperature.

Store Famotidine Injection Premixed at room temperature (25°C, 77°F). Exposure of the premixed product to excessive heat should be avoided. Brief exposure to temperatures up to 35°C (95°F) does not adversely affect the product.

HOW SUPPLIED
INJECTION: 10 MG/ML

BRAND/MANUFACTURER	NDC	SIZE	AWP
BRAND			
PEPCID: Merck	00006-3541-14	4 ml	$6.93
	00006-3539-04	2 ml 10s	$34.68

INJECTION: 20 MG

BRAND/MANUFACTURER	NDC	SIZE	AWP
BRAND			
PEPCID: Merck	00006-3537-50	50 ml 24s	$147.00

POWDER FOR RECONSTITUTION: 400 MG

BRAND/MANUFACTURER	NDC	SIZE	AWP
BRAND			
PEPCID: Merck	00006-3538-92	50 ml	$78.84

TABLETS: 20 MG

BRAND/MANUFACTURER	NDC	SIZE	AWP
BRAND			
PEPCID: Merck	00006-0963-31	30s	$44.54
	00006-0963-58	100s	$148.49
	00006-0963-28	100s ud	$151.11

➤ SHOWN IN PRODUCT IDENTIFICATION GUIDE

BRAND/MANUFACTURER	NDC	SIZE	AWP
	00006-0963-82	1000s	$1484.95
	00006-0963-94	1080s	$1603.84
	00006-0963-98	2160s	$3207.69
	00006-0963-70	4500s	$6682.29
	00006-0963-87	10000s	$14849.50

TABLETS: 40 MG

BRAND/MANUFACTURER	NDC	SIZE	AWP
○ **BRAND**			
▶ PEPCID: Merck	00006-0964-31	30s	$86.06
	00006-0964-58	100s	$286.88
	00006-0964-28	100s ud	$292.05
	00006-0964-82	1000s	$2868.83
	00006-0964-94	1080s	$3098.44
	00006-0964-70	4500s	$12909.75
	00006-0964-87	10000s	$28688.33

Famvir SEE FAMCICLOVIR

Fansidar SEE PYRIMETHAMINE AND SULFADOXINE

Fastin SEE PHENTERMINE

Fat Emulsion

DESCRIPTION

Fat Emulsion is a sterile, nonpyrogenic preparation for intravenous administration. It is supplied in both a 10% and 20% concentration.

Fat Emulsion 10% contains 10g of Fat per 100 mL. The major components are 5% safflower oil, 5% soybean oil. Fat Emulsion 10% has an osmolarity of 276 mOsmol/liter (actual). The total caloric value of Fat Emulsion 10% including Fat, phospholipid and glycerol is 1.1 kcal/mL. Of this total, approximately 0.6 kcal/mL is supplied by linoleic acid.

Fat Emulsion 20% contains 20g of Fat per 100 mL. The major components are 10% safflower oil, 10% soybean oil. Fat Emulsion 20% has an osmolarity of 258 mOsmol/liter (actual). The total caloric value of Fat Emulsion 20% including Fat, phospholipid and glycerol is 2.0 kcal/mL. Of this total, approximately 1.2 kcal/mL are supplied by linoleic acid.

Both Fat Emulsion 10% and Fat Emulsion 20% contain emulsified Fat particles of approximately 0.4 micron in diameter, similar to naturally occurring chylomicrons.

$R_1C—$, $R_2C—$ and $R_3C—$ are saturated and unsaturated fatty acid residues. The major component fatty acids of the 50/50 safflower/soybean oil mixture are approximately 65.8% linoleic, 17.7% oleic, 8.8% palmitic, 3.4% stearic, and 4.2% linolenic acid.

Egg phosphatides, purified, are primarily a mixture of naturally occurring phospholipids which are isolated from the egg yolk.

$R_1C—$ and $R_2C—$ are the same saturated and unsaturated fatty acid residues that abound in neutral fats. R_3 is primarily either the choline [$HOCH_2CH_2N(CH_3)_3OH$] ester or ethanolamine ($HOCH_2CH_2NH_2$) ester of phosphoric acid (H_3PO_4).

Glycerol, USP is chemically designated $C_3H_8O_3$ and is a clear colorless, hygroscopic syrupy liquid.

CLINICAL PHARMACOLOGY

Fat Emulsion provides the patient requiring parenteral nutrition with a source of calories and the essential fatty acids normally obtained from a nutritionally complete oral diet. The supplemental polyunsaturated Fat prevents biochemical changes of essential fatty acid deficiency (EFAD) and prevents and reverses EFAD clinical manifestations (e.g., scaliness of skin, growth retardation, poor wound healing and sparse hair growth).

The infused Fat particles are cleared from the bloodstream in a manner thought to be similar to the clearing of chylomicrons. Following infusion, there is a transient increase in plasma triglycerides. The triglycerides are hydrolyzed to free fatty acids and glycerol by the enzyme, lipoprotein lipase. The free fatty acids either enter the tissues (where they may be oxidized or resynthesized into triglycerides and stored) or circulate in the plasma, bound to albumin. In the liver, circulating free fatty acids are oxidized or converted to very low density lipoproteins that re-enter the bloodstream.

Phosphatides are the hydrophobic components of membranes and provide electrically insulated layers. They are involved in the formation of membrane structures. Choline prevents the deposition of Fat in the liver.

Glycerol is metabolized to carbon dioxide and glycogen or is used in the synthesis of body fats.

INDICATIONS AND USAGE

Fat Emulsion is indicated as a source of calories for patients requiring parenteral nutrition. Where such nutrition is required for extended periods of time (more than 5 days), Fat Emulsion is also indicated as a source of essential fatty acids to prevent or reverse biochemical changes in fatty acid composition of plasma lipids (elevated triene/tetraene ratio) and the clinical manifestations of EFAD.

UNLABELED USES

Fat Emulsion is used alone or as an adjunct in the treatment of adult respiratory distress syndrome and as energy replenishment in burn patients.

CONTRAINDICATIONS

The administration of Fat Emulsion is contraindicated in patients demonstrating disturbances in normal Fat metabolism such as pathologic hyperlipemia, lipoid nephrosis or acute pancreatitis if accompanied by hyperlipemia.

With the exception of heparin at 1 to 2 units/mL of Fat Emulsion, additives to the Fat Emulsion II bottle are contraindicated.

Partly used containers must not be stored for later use. Filters must not be used with Fat Emulsion. Do not use any bottle in which there appears to be an oiling out of the Emulsion.

WARNINGS

DEATHS IN PRETERM INFANTS AFTER INFUSION OF INTRAVENOUS FAT EMULSIONS HAVE BEEN REPORTED IN THE MEDICAL LITERATURE.[1,2] AUTOPSY FINDINGS INCLUDED INTRAVASCULAR FAT ACCUMULATION IN THE LUNGS. TREATMENT OF PREMATURE AND LOW BIRTH WEIGHT INFANTS WITH INTRAVENOUS FAT EMULSION MUST BE BASED UPON CAREFUL BENEFIT-RISK ASSESSMENT. STRICT ADHERENCE TO THE RECOMMENDED TOTAL DAILY DOSE IS MANDATORY; HOURLY INFUSION RATE SHOULD BE AS SLOW AS POSSIBLE IN EACH CASE AND SHOULD NOT IN ANY CASE EXCEED 1 G/KG IN FOUR HOURS. PREMATURE AND SMALL FOR GESTATIONAL AGE INFANTS HAVE POOR CLEARANCE OF INTRAVENOUS FAT EMULSION AND INCREASED FREE FATTY ACID PLASMA LEVELS FOLLOWING FAT EMULSION INFUSION; THEREFORE, SERIOUS CONSIDERATION MUST BE GIVEN TO ADMINISTRATION OF LESS THAN THE MAXIMUM RECOMMENDED DOSES IN THESE PATIENTS IN ORDER TO DECREASE THE LIKELIHOOD OF INTRAVENOUS FAT OVERLOAD. THE INFANT'S ABILITY TO ELIMINATE INFUSED FAT FROM THE CIRCULATION MUST BE CAREFULLY MONITORED (SUCH AS TRIGLYCERIDE AND/OR PLASMA FREE FATTY ACID LEVELS). THE LIPEMIA MUST CLEAR BETWEEN DAILY INFUSIONS.

Caution should be exercised in administering Fat Emulsion to patients with severe liver damage, pulmonary disease, anemia or blood coagulation disorders or when there is danger of fat embolism. The too rapid administration of Fat Emulsion can cause fluid and/or fat overloading resulting in dilution of serum electrolyte concentrations, overhydration, congested states, pulmonary edema, impaired pulmonary diffusion capacity or metabolic acidosis.

Caution should be exercised when admixing Fat Emulsion. Studies have documented the stability of Fat Emulsion 10% and 20% with necessary electrolytes, trace metals, and 10% through 70% Dextrose Injection, USP in a TPN admixture container (See *"Note"*) with the following amino acid solutions:

Concentrations	Aminosyn (pH 6)	Aminosyn II	Aminosyn II w/ Electrolytes
7%	X	X	X
8.5%	X	X	X
10%	X	X	X

(Also see *"Mixing Instructions for Combined Administration"* under *"Dosage and Administration"*). Compounded admixtures may be stored under refrigeration for up to 24 hours. Administration of admixtures should be completed within 24 hours after removal from refrigeration. Reference should be made to the individual package inserts for detailed information on each component.

The prime destabilizers of emulsions are excessive acidity (low pH) and inappropriate electrolyte content. Careful consideration should be given to the dosage levels of the divalent cations (Ca^{++} and Mg^{++}) administered, as these have been shown to cause emulsion instability. Amino acid solutions exert a buffering effect, protecting the emulsion.

Note: The TPN admixture containers used in the stability studies were formulated to minimize lipid/container interactions. The principal bag materials were a nonphthalate polyvinylchloride (PVC) or ethylene vinyl acetate (EVA). The only significant leachable from EVA is acetate. Acetate is found in total parenteral nutrition (TPN) admixtures as acetic acid, used for adjusting the pH of amino acid solutions, and as lysine acetate. The level of leachable acetate from EVA is not sufficient to alter the final acetate concentration significantly.

PRECAUTIONS

Because free fatty acids displace bilirubin bound to albumin, the use of lipid infusions in jaundiced or premature infants should be undertaken with caution.

During Fat Emulsion administration, the patient's hemogram, blood coagulation, liver function, platelet count and plasma lipid profile must be closely monitored. The lipemia must clear between daily infusions. Fat Emulsion should be discontinued should a significant abnormality in any one of these parameters be attributed to the infusion.

◆ RATED THERAPEUTICALLY EQUIVALENT; ◇ THERAPEUTIC EQUIVALENCE UNCONFIRMED; ○ UNRATED

Pregnancy Category C: Animal reproduction studies have not been conducted with Fat Emulsion. It is also not known whether Fat Emulsion can cause fetal harm when administered to a pregnant woman or can affect reproduction capacity. Fat Emulsion should be given to a pregnant woman only if clearly needed.

Fat Emulsion is supplied in single-dose containers. Partially used containers must be discarded and should not be stored or resterilized for later use. Do not administer the contents of any container in which the emulsion appears to be oiling out.

ADVERSE REACTIONS

Sepsis due to contamination of administration equipment and thrombophlebitis due to vein irritation from concurrently administered hypertonic solutions have been encountered. These are attributable to I.V. therapy in general or to the type of infusion administered.

Adverse reactions directly related to Fat Emulsions are of two types: (1) immediate (acute) and (2) long term (chronic). In studies of lipid products in general, the following immediate reactions have been noted: Allergic reactions, hyperlipemia, dyspnea, cyanosis, flushing, dizziness, headache, sleepiness, nausea, vomiting, hyperthermia, sweating, chest and back pain, thrombocytopenia (rarely in neonates), hypercoagulability and transient increases in liver enzymes.

The following reactions have been noted with long-term therapy with lipid infusions in general: Hepatomegaly, jaundice due to central lobular cholestasis, splenomegaly, thrombocytopenia, leucopenia, transient increases in liver function tests, overloading syndrome and deposition of brown pigment ("fat pigment") in the reticuloendothelial tissue of the liver. The significance of this last occurrence and its cause are unknown.

OVERDOSAGE

In the event of Fat overload during therapy, stop the infusion of Fat Emulsion until visual inspection of the plasma, determination of triglyceride concentrations, or measurement of plasma light-scattering activity by nephelometry indicates the lipid has cleared. Re-evaluate the patient and institute appropriate corrective measures. See *"Warnings"* and *"Precautions"*.

DOSAGE AND ADMINISTRATION

Fat Emulsion should be administered as part of an intravenous total nutrition program via peripheral vein or central venous catheter.

ADULT PATIENTS

Fat Emulsion can provide up to 60% of daily calories at a dose not to exceed 3 g/kg of body weight per day. The other 40% should be provided by carbohydrate and amino acids.

For the prevention of essential fatty acid deficiency, the recommended daily requirement is approximately 4% of the caloric intake as linoleate. In most adult patients, this can be supplied as 500 mL of Fat Emulsion 10% or 250 mL of Fat Emulsion 20% administered twice weekly.

The initial infusion rate for the first 15 minutes should be 1.0 mL/minute for Fat Emulsion 10% and 0.5 mL/minute for Fat Emulsion 20%. If no adverse effects are observed during this initial infusion, the rate can be increased to allow no more than 500 mL of Fat Emulsion 10% or 250 mL of Fat Emulsion 20% to be given over a period of four to six hours.

PEDIATRIC PATIENTS

Fat Emulsion can provide up to 60% of daily calories at a dose not to exceed 4 g/kg of body weight per day. The other 40% should be provided by carbohydrate and amino acids.

For the prevention of essential fatty acid deficiency, the recommended daily requirement is approximately 4% of the caloric intake as linoleate. The daily dosage of Fat Emulsion ranges from 5 mL to 10 mL per kilogram for the 10% Emulsion and 2.5 mL to 5 mL per kilogram for the 20% Emulsion, depending upon the size and maturity of the patient.

The infusion should be started at a rate of 0.1 mL/minute for the first 15 minutes. If no adverse effects are observed during this initial infusion, the rate can be increased to allow no more than 100 mL of Fat Emulsion 10% or 50 mL of Fat Emulsion 20% per hour.

For infants who require small volumes of Fat Emulsion at slow, controlled administration rates, consider using a Syringe Pump Unit.

ADMINISTRATION

See *"Contraindications"* regarding mixing this Emulsion with other I.V. fluids or additives.

Fat Emulsion can be infused into the same central or peripheral vein as the carbohydrate/amino acid solutions by means of a short Y-connector near the infusion site. This allows for mixing of the solutions immediately before entering the vein or for alternation of each solution. Flow rates of each solution should be controlled separately by infusion pumps, if these are used. Fat Emulsion may also be infused through a separate peripheral site. If desired, heparin may be added to Fat Emulsion at a concentration of 1 to 2 units per mL prior to administration. Alternatively, studies have documented the stability of Fat Emulsion 10% and 20%, necessary electrolytes, trace metals, and 10% through 70% Dextrose Injection, USP in a TPN admixture container with the following amino acid solutions:

Concentrations	Aminosyn (pH 6)	Aminosyn II	Aminosyn II w/ Electrolytes
7%	X	X	X

Concentrations	Aminosyn (pH 6)	Aminosyn II	Aminosyn II w/ Electrolytes
8.5%	X	X	X
10%	X	X	X

Admixtures were compounded in either a nonphthalate polyvinylchloride (PVC) or an ethylene vinyl acetate (EVA) container. (See *"Note"* under *"Warnings"*.) See *"Mixing Instructions for Combined Administration"*. Compounded admixtures may be stored under refrigeration for up to 24 hours. Administration of admixtures should be completed within 24 hours after removal from refrigeration. Conventional administration sets contain polyvinyl chloride (PVC) components that have DEHP (diethylhexyl phthalate) as a plasticizer. Fat-containing fluids such as Fat Emulsion extract DEHP from this PVC component, and it may be advisable to consider infusion of Fat Emulsion or the 3-in-1 admixture through a non-DEHP administration set.

Filters should not be used for administration of the Emulsion. Parenteral drug products should be inspected visually for particulate matter and discoloration prior to administration, whenever solution and container permit.

MIXING INSTRUCTIONS FOR COMBINED ADMINISTRATION

Caution should be exercised when admixing Fat Emulsion.

It is absolutely essential that the admixture be prepared using strict aseptic techniques as this nutrient mixture is a good growth media for microorganisms.

Studies have documented the stability of Fat Emulsion 10% and 20% with necessary electrolytes, trace metals, and 10% through 70% Dextrose Injection, USP in a TPN admixture container with the following amino acid solutions:

Concentrations	Aminosyn (pH 6)	Aminosyn II	Aminosyn II w/ Electrolytes
7%	X	X	X
8.5%	X	X	X
10%	X	X	X

(See *"Note"* under *"Warnings"*.) Compounded admixtures may be stored under refrigeration for up to 24 hours. Administration of admixtures should be completed within 24 hours after removal from refrigeration. Reference should be made to the individual package inserts for detailed information on each component.

The prime destabilizers of Emulsions are excessive acidity (low pH) and inappropriate electrolyte content. Careful consideration should be given to the dosage levels of the divalent cations (Ca^{++} and Mg^{++}) administered, as these have been shown to cause Emulsion instability. Amino acid solutions exert a buffering effect, protecting the Emulsion.

The following proper mixing sequence must be followed to minimize pH-related problems by ensuring that typically acidic dextrose injections are not mixed with lipid Emulsion alone:

1. Transfer Fat Emulsion to the TPN admixture container.
2. Transfer an amino acid injection.
3. Transfer Dextrose Injection, USP.
4. Perform addition of necessary electrolyte and trace metal additives.

Admixing should be accompanied by gentle agitation to avoid localized concentration effects. *Note*: Simultaneous or sequential mixing of Fat Emulsion with other nutritional substrates using an automated, gravimetric pumping system is considered an acceptable method for admixture compounding, especially for institutions with a high volume of 3-in-1 admixtures.

STORAGE

Exposure of pharmaceutical products to heat should be minimized. Protect from freezing. It is recommended that the product be stored at room temperature (25°C). Do not store above 30°C (86°F). However, brief exposure up to 40°C does not adversely affect the product.

REFERENCES

1. Levene M, Wigglesworth J, Desai R. Pulmonary fat accumulation after Intralipid infusion in the preterm infant. *Lancet II*: 815-818, (Oct. 18), 1980. 2. Dahms B, Halpin T. Pulmonary arterial lipid deposit in newborn infants receiving intravenous lipid infusion. *J. Pediatrics*: 97:800-805, (Nov.), 1980.

HOW SUPPLIED
INJECTION: 10%

AVERAGE UNIT PRICE (AVAILABLE SIZES)		GENERIC A-RATED AVERAGE PRICE (GAAP)	
		100 ml 12s	$433.63
BRAND	$0.22	200 ml 12s	$473.17
GENERIC	$0.27	500 ml 12s	$765.58

BRAND/MANUFACTURER	NDC	SIZE	AWP
◆ BRAND			
INTRALIPID: Clintec	00338-0490-41	50 ml 10s	$131.88
	00338-0490-48	100 ml 10s	$298.49
	00338-0490-96	100 ml 10s	$373.62
	00338-0490-02	250 ml 10s	$375.48
	00338-0490-03	500 ml 10s	$607.68
	00338-0490-98	500 ml 10s	$672.28

➤ SHOWN IN PRODUCT IDENTIFICATION GUIDE

BRAND/MANUFACTURER		NDC	SIZE	AWP
◆ **GENERICS**				
LIPOSYN II: Abbott Hosp		00074-9794-01	500 ml 8s	$590.62
LIPOSYN II: Abbott Hosp		00074-9784-02	50 ml 12s	$364.94
LIPOSYN II: Abbott Hosp		00074-9786-21	100 ml 12s	$380.19
LIPOSYN III: Abbott Hosp		00074-9790-21	100 ml 12s	$487.07
LIPOSYN III: Abbott Hosp		00074-9790-01	200 ml 12s	$459.28
LIPOSYN II: Abbott Hosp		00074-9786-01	200 ml 12s	$487.07
LIPOSYN III: Abbott Hosp		00074-9790-03	500 ml 12s	$743.28
LIPOSYN II: Abbott Hosp		00074-9786-03	500 ml 12s	$787.88

INJECTION: 20%

AVERAGE UNIT PRICE (AVAILABLE SIZES)		GENERIC A-RATED AVERAGE PRICE (GAAP)	
BRAND	$0.34	500 ml 12s	$1104.45
GENERIC	$0.34		

BRAND/MANUFACTURER	NDC	SIZE	AWP
◆ **BRAND**			
INTRALIPID: Clintec	00338-0491-41	50 ml 10s	$313.64
	00338-0491-48	100 ml 10s	$367.71
	00338-0491-96	100 ml 10s	$442.91
	00338-0491-02	250 ml 10s	$536.97
	00338-0491-03	500 ml 10s	$885.24
	00338-0491-98	500 ml 10s	$997.60
◆ **GENERICS**			
LIPOSYN II: Abbott Hosp	00074-9792-03	200 ml 8s	$550.24
LIPOSYN II: Abbott Hosp	00074-9793-01	500 ml 8s	$854.24
LIPOSYN II: Abbott Hosp	00074-9787-02	50 ml 12s	$478.94
LIPOSYN II: Abbott Hosp	00074-9789-01	200 ml 12s	$696.11
LIPOSYN II: Abbott Hosp	00074-9791-03	500 ml 12s	$1082.72
LIPOSYN II: Abbott Hosp	00074-9789-03	500 ml 12s	$1126.18

INJECTION: 30%

BRAND/MANUFACTURER	NDC	SIZE	AWP
◆ **BRAND**			
INTRALIPID: Clintec	00338-0495-03	500 ml	$132.79

VIAL: 20%

BRAND/MANUFACTURER	NDC	SIZE	AWP
◆ **GENERICS**			
LIPOSYN III: Abbott Hosp	00074-9791-01	200 ml 12s	$656.78

Fedahist SEE CHLORPHENIRAMINE MALEATE AND PSEUDOEPHEDRINE HYDROCHLORIDE

Felbamate

WARNING

THE USE OF FELBAMATE IS ASSOCIATED WITH A MARKED INCREASE IN THE INCIDENCE OF APLASTIC ANEMIA. ACCORDINGLY, FELBAMATE SHOULD ONLY BE USED IN PATIENTS WHOSE EPILEPSY IS SO SEVERE THAT THAT RISK OF APLASTIC ANEMIA IS DEEMED ACCEPTABLE IN LIGHT OF THE BENEFITS CONFERRED BY ITS USE (SEE ''INDICATIONS''). ORDINARILY, A PATIENT SHOULD NOT BE PLACED ON AND/OR CONTINUED ON FELBAMATE WITHOUT CONSIDERATION OF APPROPRIATE EXPERT HEMATOLOGIC CONSULTATION.

AMONG FELBAMATE TREATED PATIENTS, APLASTIC ANEMIA (PANCYTOPENIA IN THE PRESENCE OF A BONE MARROW LARGELY DEPLETED OF HEMATOPOIETIC PRECURSORS) OCCURS AT AN INCIDENCE THAT MAY BE MORE THAN A 100 FOLD GREATER THAN THAT SEEN IN THE UNTREATED POPULATION (I.E., 2 TO 5 PER MILLION PERSONS PER YEAR). THE RISK OF DEATH IN PATIENTS WITH APLASTIC ANEMIA GENERALLY VARIES AS A FUNCTION OF ITS SEVERITY AND ETIOLOGY; CURRENT ESTIMATES OF THE OVERALL CASE FATALITY RATE ARE IN THE RANGE OF 20 TO 30%, BUT RATES AS HIGH AS 70% HAVE BEEN REPORTED IN THE PAST.

THERE ARE TOO FEW FELBAMATE ASSOCIATED CASES, AND TOO LITTLE KNOWN ABOUT THEM TO PROVIDE A RELIABLE ESTIMATE OF THE SYNDROME'S INCIDENCE OR ITS CASE FATALITY RATE OR TO IDENTIFY THE FACTORS, IF ANY, THAT MIGHT CONCEIVABLY BE USED TO PREDICT WHO IS AT GREATER OR LESSER RISK.

IN MANAGING PATIENTS ON FELBAMATE, IT SHOULD BE BORNE IN MIND THAT THE CLINICAL MANIFESTATION OF APLASTIC ANEMIA MAY NOT BE SEEN UNTIL AFTER A PATIENT HAS BEEN ON FELBAMATE FOR SEVERAL MONTHS (E.G., ONSET OF APLASTIC ANEMIA AMONG FELBAMATE EXPOSED PATIENTS FOR WHOM DATA ARE AVAILABLE HAS RANGED FROM 5 TO 30 WEEKS). HOWEVER, THE INJURY TO BONE MARROW STEM CELLS THAT IS HELD TO BE ULTIMATELY RESPONSIBLE FOR THE ANEMIA MAY OCCUR WEEKS TO MONTHS EARLIER. ACCORDINGLY, PATIENTS WHO ARE DISCONTINUED FROM FELBAMATE REMAIN AT RISK FOR DEVELOPING ANEMIA FOR A VARIABLE, AND UNKNOWN, PERIOD AFTERWARDS.

IT IS NOT KNOWN WHETHER OR NOT THE RISK OF DEVELOPING APLASTIC ANEMIA CHANGES WITH DURATION OF EXPOSURE. CONSEQUENTLY, IT IS NOT SAFE TO ASSUME THAT A PATIENT WHO HAS BEEN ON FELBAMATE WITHOUT SIGNS OF HEMATOLOGIC ABNORMALITY FOR LONG PERIODS OF TIME IS WITHOUT RISK. IT IS NOT KNOWN WHETHER OR NOT THE DOSE OF FELBAMATE AFFECTS THE INCIDENCE OF APLASTIC ANEMIA.

IT IS NOT KNOWN WHETHER OR NOT CONCOMITANT USE OF ANTIEPILEPTIC DRUGS AND/OR OTHER DRUGS AFFECTS THE INCIDENCE OF APLASTIC ANEMIA.

APLASTIC ANEMIA TYPICALLY DEVELOPS WITHOUT PREMONITORY CLINICAL OR LABORATORY SIGNS, THE FULL BLOWN SYNDROME PRESENTING WITH SIGNS OF INFECTION, BLEEDING, OR ANEMIA. ACCORDINGLY, ROUTINE BLOOD TESTING CANNOT BE RELIABLY USED TO REDUCE THE INCIDENCE OF APLASTIC ANEMIA. BUT, IT WILL, IN SOME CASES, ALLOW THE DETECTION OF THE HEMATOLOGIC CHANGES BEFORE THE SYNDROME DECLARES ITSELF CLINICALLY. FELBAMATE SHOULD BE DISCONTINUED IF ANY EVIDENCE OF BONE MARROW DEPRESSION OCCURS.

DESCRIPTION

Felbamate is an antiepileptic available as 400 mg and 600 mg tablets and as a 600 mg/5 mL suspension for oral administration. Its chemical name is 2-phenyl-1,3-propanediol dicarbamate.

Felbamate is a white to off-white crystalline powder with a characteristic odor. It is very slightly soluble in water, slightly soluble in ethanol, sparingly soluble in methanol, and freely soluble in dimethyl sulfoxide. The molecular weight is 238.24; Felbamate's molecular formula is $C_{11}H_{14}N_2O_4$.

Following is its chemical structure:

$$CH_2OCONH_2$$
$$CH$$
$$CH_2OCONH_2$$

CLINICAL PHARMACOLOGY

MECHANISM OF ACTION

The mechanism by which Felbamate exerts its anticonvulsant activity is unknown, but in animal test systems designed to detect anticonvulsant activity, Felbamate has properties in common with other marketed anticonvulsants. Felbamate is effective in mice and rats in the maximal electroshock test, the subcutaneous pentylenetetrazol seizure test, and the subcutaneous picrotoxin seizure test. Felbamate also exhibits anticonvulsant activity against seizures induced by intracerebroventricular administration of glutamate in rats and N-methyl-D,L-aspartic acid in mice. Protection against maximal electroshock-induced seizures suggests that Felbamate may reduce seizure spread, an effect possibly predictive of efficacy in generalized tonic-clonic or partial seizures. Protection against pentylenetetrazol-induced seizures suggests that Felbamate may increase seizure threshold, an effect considered to be predictive of potential efficacy in absence seizures.

Receptor-binding studies in vitro indicate that Felbamate has weak inhibitory effects on GABA-receptor binding, benzodiazepine receptor binding, and is devoid of activity at the MK-801 receptor binding site of the NMDA receptor-ionophore complex. However, Felbamate does interact as an antagonist at the strychnine-insensitive glycine recognition site of the NMDA receptor-inophore complex. Felbamate is not effective in protecting chick embryo retina tissue against the neurotoxic effects of the excitatory amino acid agonists NMDA, kainate, or quisqualate in vitro.

The monocarbamate, p-hydroxy, and 2-hydroxy metabolites were inactive in the maximal electroshock-induced seizure test in mice. The monocarbamate and p-hydroxy metabolites had only weak (0.2 to 0.6) activity compared with Felbamate in the subcutaneous pentylenetetrazol seizure test. These metabolites did not contribute significantly to the anticonvulsant action of Felbamate.

PHARMACOKINETICS

The numbers in the pharmacokinetic section are mean ± standard deviation.

Felbamate is well-absorbed after oral administration. Over 90% of the radioactivity after a dose of 1000 mg [14]C Felbamate was found in the urine. Absolute bioavailability (oral vs. parenteral) has not been measured. The tablet and suspension were each shown to be bioequivalent to the capsule used in clinical trials, and pharmacokinetic parameters of the tablet and suspension are similar. There was no effect of food on absorption of the tablet; the effect of food on absorption of the suspension has not been evaluated.

Following oral administration, Felbamate is the predominant plasma species (about 90% of plasma radioactivity). About 40-50% of absorbed dose appears unchanged in urine, and an additional 40% is present as unidentified metabolites and conjugates. About 15% is present as parahydroxyfelbamate, 2-hydroxyfelbamate, and Felbamate monocarbamate, none of which have significant anticonvulsant activity.

Binding of Felbamate to human plasma protein was independent of Felbamate concentrations between 10 and 310 micrograms/mL. Binding ranged from 22% to 25%, mostly to albumin, and was dependent on the albumin concentration. Felbamate is excreted with a terminal half-life of 20-23 hours, which is unaltered after multiple doses. Clearance after a single 1200 mg dose is 26±3 mL/hr/kg, and after multiple daily doses of 3600 mg is 30±8 mL/hr/kg. The apparent volume of distribution was 756±82 mL/kg after a 1200 mg dose. Felbamate Cmax, and AUC are proportionate to dose after single and multiple doses over a range of 100-800 mg single doses and 1200-3600 mg daily doses. Cmin (trough) blood levels are also dose proportional. Multiple daily doses of 1200, 2400, and 3600 mg gave Cmin values of 30±5, 55±8, and 83±21 micrograms/mL (N=10 patients). Felbamate gave dose proportional steady-state peak plasma concentrations in children age 4-12 over a range of 15, 30, and 45 mg/kg/day with peak concentrations of 17, 32, and 49 micrograms/mL.

The effects of race and gender on Felbamate pharmacokinetics have not been systematically evaluated, but plasma concentrations in males (N=5) and females (N=4) given Felbamate have been similar. The effects of Felbamate kinetics on renal and hepatic functional impairment have not been evaluated.

PHARMACODYNAMICS
TYPICAL PHYSIOLOGIC RESPONSES
1. Cardiovascular: In adults, there is no effect of Felbamate on blood pressure. Small but statistically significant mean increases in heart rate were seen during adjunctive therapy and monotherapy; however, these mean increases of up to 5 bpm were not clinically significant. In children, no clinically relevant changes in blood pressure or heart rate were seen during adjunctive therapy or monotherapy with Felbamate.

2. Other Physiologic Effects: The only other change in vital signs was a mean decrease of approximately 1 respiration per minute in respiratory rate during adjunctive therapy in children. In adults, statistically significant mean reductions in body weight were observed during Felbamate monotherapy and adjunctive therapy. In children, there were mean decreases in body weight during adjunctive therapy and monotherapy; however, these mean changes were not statistically significant. These mean reductions in adults and children were approximately 5% of the mean weights at baseline.

CLINICAL STUDIES
The results of controlled clinical trials established the efficacy of Felbamate as monotherapy and adjunctive therapy in adults with partial-onset seizures with or without secondary generalization and in partial and generalized seizures associated with Lennox-Gastaut syndrome in children.

FELBAMATE MONOTHERAPY TRIALS IN ADULTS
Felbamate (3600 mg/day given QID) and low-dose valproate (15 mg/kg/day) were compared as monotherapy during a 112-day treatment period in a multicenter and a single-center double-blind efficacy trial. Both trials were conducted according to an identical study design. During a 56-day baseline period, all patients had at least four partial-onset seizures per 28 days and were receiving one antiepileptic drug at a therapeutic level, the most common being carbamazepine. In the multicenter trial, baseline seizure frequencies were 12.4 per 28 days in the Felbamate group and 21.3 per 28 days in the low-dose valproate group. In the single-center trial, baseline seizure frequencies were 18.1 per 28 days in the Felbamate group and 15.9 per 28 days in the low-dose valproate group. Patients were converted to monotherapy with Felbamate or low-dose valproic acid during the first 28 days of the 112-day treatment period. Study endpoints were completion of 112 study days or fulfilling an escape criterion. Criteria for escape relative to baseline were: (1) twofold increase in monthly seizure frequency, (2) twofold increase in highest 2-day seizure frequency, (3) single generalized tonic-clonic seizure (GTC) if none occurred during baseline, or (4) significant prolongation of GTCs. The primary efficacy variable was the number of patients in each treatment group who met escape criteria.

In the multicenter trial, the percentage of patients who met escape criteria was 40% (18/45) in the Felbamate group and 78% (39/50) in the low-dose valproate group. In the single-center trial, the percentage of patients who met escape criteria was 14% (3/21) in the Felbamate group and 90% (19/21) in the low-dose valproate group. In both trials, the difference in the percentage of patients meeting escape criteria was statistically significant (P < .001) in favor of Felbamate. These two studies by design were intended to demonstrate the effectiveness of Felbatol monotherapy. The studies were not designed or intended to demonstrate comparative efficacy of the two drugs. For example, valproate was not used at the maximally effective dose.

FELBAMATE ADJUNCTIVE THERAPY TRIALS IN ADULTS
A double-blind, placebo-controlled crossover trial consisted of two 10-week outpatient treatment periods. Patients with refractory partial-onset seizures who were receiving phenytoin and carbamazepine at therapeutic levels were administered Felbamate as add-on therapy at a starting dosage of 1400 mg/day in three divided doses, which was increased to 2600 mg/day in three divided doses. Among the 56 patients who completed the study, the baseline seizure frequency was 20 per month. Patients treated with Felbamate had fewer seizures than patients treated with placebo for each treatment sequence. There was a 23% (P=.018) difference in percentage seizure frequency reduction in favor of Felbamate.

Felbamate 3600 mg/day given QID and placebo were compared in a 28-day double-blind add-on trial in patients who had their standard antiepileptic drugs reduced while undergoing evaluations for surgery of intractable epilepsy. All patients had confirmed partial-onset seizures with or without generalization, seizure frequency during surgical evaluation not exceeding an average of four partial seizures per day or more than one generalized seizure per day, and a minimum average of one partial or generalized tonic-clonic seizure per day for the last 3 days of the surgical evaluation. The primary efficacy variable was time to fourth seizure after randomization to treatment with Felbamate or placebo. Thirteen (46%) of 28 patients in the Felbamate group versus 29 (88%) of 33 patients in the placebo group experienced a fourth seizure. The median times to fourth seizure were greater than 28 days in the Felbamate group and 5 days in the placebo group. The difference between Felbamate and placebo in time to fourth seizure was statistically significant (P=.002) in favor of Felbamate.

FELBAMATE ADJUNCTIVE THERAPY TRIAL IN CHILDREN WITH LENNOX-GASTAUT SYNDROME
In a 70-day double-blind, placebo-controlled add-on trial in the Lennox-Gastaut syndrome, Felbamate 45 mg/kg/day given QID was superior to placebo in controlling the multiple seizure types associated with this condition. Patients had at least 90 atonic and/or atypical absence seizures per month while receiving therapeutic dosages of one or two other antiepileptic drugs. Patients had a past history of using an average of eight antiepileptic drugs. The most commonly used antiepileptic drug during the baseline period was valproic acid. The frequency of all types of seizures during the baseline period was 1617 per month in the Felbamate group and 716 per month in the placebo group. Statistically significant differences in the effect on seizure frequency favored Felbamate over placebo for total seizures (26% reduction vs 5% increase, P<.001), atonic seizures (44% reduction vs 7% reduction, P=.002), and generalized tonic-clonic seizures (40% reduction vs 12% increase, P=.017). Parent/guardian global evaluations based on impressions of quality of life with respect to alertness, verbal responsiveness, general well-being, and seizure control significantly (P<.001) favored Felbamate over placebo.

When efficacy was analyzed by gender in four well-controlled trials of Felbamate as adjunctive and monotherapy for partial-onset seizures and Lennox-Gastaut syndrome, a similar response was seen in 122 males and 142 females.

INDICATIONS AND USAGE
Felbamate is not indicated as a first line antiepileptic treatment (see *"Warnings"*). Felbamate is recommended for use only in those patients who respond inadequately to alternative treatments and whose epilepsy is so severe that a substantial risk of aplastic anemia is deemed acceptable in light of the benefits conferred by its use.

If these criteria are met, Felbamate can be considered for either monotherapy and adjunctive therapy in the treatment of partial seizures with and without generalization in adults with epilepsy and as adjunctive therapy in the treatment of partial and generalized seizures associated with Lennox-Gastaut syndrome in children.

CONTRAINDICATIONS
Felbamate is contraindicated in patients with known hypersensitivity to Felbamate or its ingredients and it should not be used in patients with a history of previous bone marrow depression, hypersensitivity to the drug, or known sensitivity to other carbamates.

WARNINGS
See Boxed *"Warning"* regarding aplastic anemia.

Antiepileptic drugs should not be suddenly discontinued because of the possibility of increasing seizure frequency.

PRECAUTIONS
Information for Patients: Patients should be informed that the use of Felbamate is associated with aplastic anemia, a potentially fatal condition acutely or over a long term.

Aplastic anemia in the general population is relatively rare. The absolute risk for the individual patient is not known with any degree of reliability, but patients on Felbamate may be at more than a 100 fold greater risk for developing the syndrome than the general population.

The long term outlook for patients with aplastic anemia is variable. Although many patients are apparently cured, others require repeated transfusions and other treatments for relapses, and some, although surviving for years, ultimately develop serious complications that sometimes prove fatal (e.g., leukemia).

At present there is no way to predict who is likely to get aplastic anemia, nor is there a documented effective means to monitor the patient so as to avoid and/or reduce the risk. Patients should be advised to be alert for signs of infection, bleeding, easy bruising, or signs of anemia (fatigue, weakness, lassitude, etc.), and should be advised to report to the physician immediately if any such signs or symptoms appear.

Laboratory Tests: Full hematologic evaluations should be performed before Felbamate therapy, frequently during therapy, and for a significant period of time after discontinuation of Felbamate therapy. While it might appear prudent to perform frequent CBCs in patients continuing on Felbamate, there is no evidence that such monitoring will allow early detection of marrow suppression before aplastic anemia occurs. (See *"Boxed Warnings"*) Complete pretreatment blood counts, including platelets and reticulocytes should be obtained as a baseline. If any hematologic abnormalities are detected during the course of treatment, immediate consultation with a hematologist is advised. Felbamate should be discontinued if any evidence of bone marrow depression occurs.

DRUG INTERACTIONS

The drug interaction data described in this section were obtained from controlled clinical trials and studies involving otherwise healthy adults with epilepsy.

Use in Conjunction with Other Antiepileptic Drugs: (see "*Dosage and Administration*"):

The addition of Felbamate to antiepileptic drugs (AEDs) affects the steady-state plasma concentrations of AEDs. The net effect of these interactions is summarized in the following table:

AED Coadministered	AED Concentration	Felbamate Concentration
Phenytoin	↑	
Valproate	↑	**
Carbamazepine (CBZ)	↑	
* CBZ epoxide		

* *Not administered, but an active metabolite of carbamazepine.*

** *No significant effect.*

SPECIFIC EFFECTS OF FELBAMATE ON OTHER ANTIEPILEPTIC DRUGS

Phenytoin: Felbamate causes an increase in steady-state phenytoin plasma concentrations. In 10 otherwise healthy subjects with epilepsy ingesting phenytoin, the steady-state trough (Cmin) phenytoin plasma concentration was 17±5 micrograms/mL. The steady-state Cmin increased to 21±5 micrograms/mL when 1200 mg/day of Felbamate was coadministered. Increasing the Felbamate dose to 1800 mg/day in six of these subjects increased the steady-state phenytoin Cmin to 25±7 micrograms/mL. In order to maintain phenytoin levels, limit adverse experiences, and achieve the Felbamate dose of 3600 mg/day, a phenytoin dose reduction of approximately 40% was necessary for eight of these 10 subjects.

In a controlled clinical trial, a 20% reduction of the phenytoin dose at the initiation of Felbamate therapy resulted in phenytoin levels comparable to those prior to Felbamate administration.

Carbamazepine: Felbamate causes a decrease in the steady-state carbamazepine plasma concentrations and an increase in the steady-state carbamazepine epoxide plasma concentration. In nine otherwise healthy subjects with epilepsy ingesting carbamazepine, the steady-state trough (Cmin) carbamazepine concentration was 8±2 micrograms/mL. The carbamazepine steady-state Cmin decreased 31% to 5±1 micrograms/mL when Felbamate (3000 mg/day, divided into three doses) was coadministered. Carbamazepine epoxide steady-state Cmin concentrations increased 57% from 1.0±0.3 to 1.6±0.4 micrograms/mL with the addition of Felbamate.

In clinical trials, similar changes in carbamazepine and carbamazepine epoxide were seen.

Valproate: Felbamate causes an increase in steady-state valproate concentrations. In four subjects with epilepsy ingesting valproate, the steady-state trough (Cmin) valproate plasma concentration was 63±16 micrograms/mL. The steady-state Cmin increased to 78±14 micrograms/mL when 1200 mg/day of Felbamate was coadministered. Increasing the Felbamate dose to 2400 mg/day increased the steady-state valproate Cmin to 96±25 micrograms/mL. Corresponding values for free valproate Cmin concentrations were 7±3, 9±4, and 11±6 micrograms/mL for 0, 1200, and 2400 mg/day Felbamate, respectively. The ratios of the AUCs of unbound valproate to the AUCs of the total valproate were 11.1%, 13.0%, and 11.5%, with coadministration of 0, 1200, and 2400 mg/day of Felbamate, respectively. This indicates that the protein binding of valproate did not change appreciably with increasing doses of Felbamate.

EFFECTS OF OTHER ANTIEPILEPTIC DRUGS ON FELBAMATE

Phenytoin: Phenytoin causes an approximate doubling of the clearance of Felbamate at steady state and, therefore, the addition of phenytoin causes an approximate 45% decrease in the steady-state trough concentrations of Felbamate as compared to the same dose of Felbamate given as monotherapy.

Carbamazepine: Carbamazepine causes an approximate 50% increase in the clearance of Felbamate at steady state and, therefore, the addition of carbamazepine results in an approximate 40% decrease in the steady-state trough concentrations of Felbamate as compared to the same dose of Felbamate given as monotherapy.

Valproate: Available data suggest that there is no significant effect of valproate on the clearance of Felbamate at steady state. Therefore, the addition of valproate is not expected to cause a clinically important effect on Felbamate plasma concentrations.

EFFECTS OF ANTACIDS ON FELBAMATE

The rate and extent of absorption of a 2400 mg dose of Felbamate as monotherapy given as tablets was not affected when coadministered with antacids.

Drug/Laboratory Test Interactions: There are no known interactions of Felbamate with commonly used laboratory tests.

Carcinogenesis, Mutagenesis, Impairment of Fertility: Carcinogenicity studies were conducted in mice and rats. Mice received Felbamate as a feed admixture for 92 weeks at doses of 300, 600, and 1200 mg/kg and rats were also dosed by feed admixture for 104 weeks at doses of 30, 100, and 300 (males) or 10, 30, and 100 (females) mg/kg. The maximum doses in these studies produced steady-state plasma concentrations that were equal to or less than the steady-state plasma concentrations in epileptic patients receiving 3600 mg/day. There was a statistically significant increase in hepatic cell adenomas in high-dose male and female mice and in high-dose female rats. Hepatic hypertrophy was significantly increased in a dose-related manner in mice, primarily males, but also in females. Hepatic hypertrophy was not found in female rats. The relationship between the occurrence of benign hepatocellular adenomas and the finding of liver hypertrophy resulting from liver enzyme induction has not been examined. There was a statistically significant increase in benign interstitial cell tumors of the testes in high-dose male rats receiving Felbamate. The relevance of these findings to humans is unknown.

As a result of the synthesis process, Felbamate could contain small amounts of two known animal carcinogens, the genotoxic compound ethyl carbamate (urethane) and the non-genotoxic compound methyl carbamate. It is theoretically possible that a 50 kg patient receiving 3600 mg of Felbamate could be exposed to up to 0.72 micrograms of urethane and 1800 micrograms of methyl carbamate. These daily doses are approximately 1/35,000 (urethane) and 1/5,500 (methyl carbamate) on a mg/kg basis, and 1/10,000 (urethane) and 1/1,600 (methyl carbamate) on a mg/m^2 basis, of the dose levels shown to be carcinogenic in rodents. Any presence of these two compounds in Felbamate used in the lifetime carcinogenicity studies was inadequate to cause tumors.

Microbial and mammalian cell assays revealed no evidence of mutagenesis in the Ames *Salmonella*/microsome plate test, CHO/HGPRT mammalian cell forward gene mutation assay, sister chromatid exchange assay in CHO cells, and bone marrow cytogenetics assay.

Reproduction and fertility studies in rats showed no effects on male or female fertility at oral doses of up to 13.9 times the human total daily dose of 3600 mg on a mg/kg basis, or up to 3 times the human total daily dose on a mg/m^2 basis.

Pregnancy: Pregnancy Category C. The incidence of malformations was not increased compared to control in offspring of rats or rabbits given doses up to 13.9 times (rat) and 4.2 times (rabbit) the human daily dose on a mg/kg basis, or 3 times (rat) and less than 2 times (rabbit) the human daily dose on a mg/m^2 basis. However, in rats, there was a decrease in pup weight and an increase in pup deaths during lactation. The cause for these deaths is not known. The no effect dose for rat pup mortality was 6.9 times the human dose on a mg/kg basis or 1.5 times the human dose on a mg/m^2 basis.

Placental transfer of Felbamate occurs in rat pups. There are, however, no studies in pregnant women. Because animal reproduction studies are not always predictive of human response, this drug should be used during pregnancy only if clearly needed.

Labor and Delivery: The effect of Felbamate on labor and delivery in humans is unknown.

Nursing Mothers: Felbamate has been detected in human milk. The effect on the nursing infant is unknown (see "*Pregnancy*" section).

Pediatric Use: The safety and effectiveness of Felbamate in children other than those with Lennox-Gastaut syndrome has not been established.

Geriatric Use: No systematic studies in geriatric patients have been conducted. Clinical studies of Felbamate did not include sufficient numbers of patients aged 65 and over to determine whether they respond differently from younger patients. Other reported clinical experience has not identified differences in responses between the elderly and younger patients. In general, dosage selection for an elderly patient should be cautious, usually starting at the low end of the dosing range, reflecting the greater frequency of decreased hepatic, renal, or cardiac function, and of concomitant disease or other drug therapy.

ADVERSE REACTIONS

The most common adverse reactions seen in association with Felbamate in adults during monotherapy are anorexia, vomiting, insomnia, nausea, and headache. The most common adverse reactions seen in association with Felbamate in adults during adjunctive therapy are anorexia, vomiting, insomnia, nausea, dizziness, somnolence and headache.

The most common adverse reactions seen in association with Felbamate in children during adjunctive therapy are anorexia, vomiting, insomnia, headache, and somnolence.

The dropout rate because of adverse experiences or intercurrent illness among adult Felbamate patients was 12 percent (120/977). The dropout rate because of adverse experiences or intercurrent illnesses among pediatric Felbamate patients was six percent (22/357). In adults, the body systems associated with causing these withdrawals in order of frequency were: digestive (4.3%), psychological (2.2%), whole body (1.7%), neurological (1.5%), and dermatological (1.5%). In children, the body systems associated with causing these withdrawals in order of frequency were: digestive (1.7%), neurological (1.4%), dermatological (1.4%), psychological (1.1%), and whole body (1.0%). In adults, specific events with an incidence of 1% or greater associated with causing these withdrawals, in order of frequency were: anorexia (1.6%), nausea (1.4%), rash (1.2%), and weight decrease (1.1%). In children, the specific event with an incidence of 1% or greater associated with causing these withdrawals was rash (1.1%).

INCIDENCE IN CLINICAL TRIALS

The prescriber should be aware that the figures cited in the following table cannot be used to predict the incidence of side effects in the course of usual medical practice where patient characteristics and other factors differ from those which prevailed in the clinical trials. Similarly, the cited frequencies cannot be compared with figures obtained from other clinical investigations involving different investigators, treatments, and uses including the use of Felbamate as adjunctive therapy where the incidence of adverse events may be higher due to drug interactions. The cited figures, however, do provide the prescribing physician with some basis for estimating the relative contribution of drug and nondrug factors to the side effect incidence rate in the population studied.

ADULTS
INCIDENCE IN CONTROLLED CLINICAL TRIALS—MONOTHERAPY STUDIES IN ADULTS

The table that follows enumerates adverse events that occurred at an incidence of 2% or more among 58 adult patients who received Felbamate monotherapy at dosages of 3600 mg/day in double-blind controlled trials. Reported adverse events were classified using standard WHO-based dictionary terminology.

ADULTS
TREATMENT-EMERGENT ADVERSE EVENT
INCIDENCE IN CONTROLLED MONOTHERAPY TRIALS

Body System/Event	Felbamate* (N=58) %	Low Dose Valproate** (N=50) %
Body as a Whole		
Fatigue	6.9	4.0
Weight Decrease	3.4	0
Face Edema	3.4	0
Central Nervous System		
Insomnia	8.6	4.0
Headache	6.9	18.0
Anxiety	5.2	2.0
Dermatological		
Acne	3.4	0
Rash	3.4	0
Digestive		
Dyspepsia	8.6	2.0
Vomiting	8.6	2.0
Constipation	6.9	2.0
Diarrhea	5.2	2.0
SGPT Increased	5.2	2.0
Metabolic/Nutritional		
Hypophosphatemia	3.4	0
Respiratory		
Upper Respiratory Tract Infection	8.6	4.0
Rhinitis	6.9	4.0
Special Senses		
Diplopia	3.4	4.0
Otitis Media	3.4	0
Urogenital		
Intramenstrual Bleeding	3.4	0
Urinary Tract Infection	3.4	2.0

* 3600 mg/day; ** 15 mg/kg/day

INCIDENCE IN CONTROLLED ADD-ON CLINICAL STUDIES IN ADULTS

The table that follows enumerates adverse events that occurred at an incidence of 2% or more among 114 adult patients who received Felbamate adjunctive therapy in add-on controlled trials at dosages up to 3600 mg/day. Reported adverse events were classified using standard WHO-based dictionary terminology.

Many adverse experiences that occurred during adjunctive therapy may be a result of drug interactions. Adverse experiences during adjunctive therapy typically resolved with conversion to monotherapy, or with adjustment of the dosage of other antiepileptic drugs.

ADULTS
TREATMENT-EMERGENT ADVERSE EVENT
INCIDENCE IN CONTROLLED ADD-ON TRIALS

Body System/Event	Felbamate (N=114) %	Placebo (N=43) %
Body as a Whole		
Fatigue	16.8	7.0
Fever	2.6	4.7
Chest Pain	2.6	0
Central Nervous System		
Headache	36.8	9.3
Somnolence	19.3	7.0
Dizziness	18.4	14.0
Insomnia	17.5	7.0
Nervousness	7.0	2.3
Tremor	6.1	2.3
Anxiety	5.3	4.7
Gait Abnormal	5.3	0
Depression	5.3	0
Paresthesia	3.5	2.3
Ataxia	3.5	0
Mouth Dry	2.6	0
Stupor	2.6	0
Dermatological		
Rash	3.5	4.7
Digestive		
Nausea	34.2	2.3
Anorexia	19.3	2.3
Vomiting	16.7	4.7
Dyspepsia	12.3	7.0
Constipation	11.4	2.3
Diarrhea	5.3	2.3
Abdominal Pain	5.3	0
SGPT Increased	3.5	0
Musculoskeletal		
Myalgia	2.6	0
Respiratory		
Upper Respiratory Tract Infection	5.3	7.0
Sinusitis	3.5	0
Pharyngitis	2.6	0
Special Senses		
Diplopia	6.1	0
Taste Perversion	6.1	0
Vision Abnormal	5.3	2.3

CHILDREN
INCIDENCE IN A CONTROLLED ADD-ON TRIAL IN CHILDREN WITH LENNOX-GASTAUT SYNDROME

The table that follows enumerates adverse events that occurred more than once among 31 pediatric patients who received Felbamate up to 45 mg/kg/day or a maximum of 3600 mg/day. Reported adverse events were classified using standard WHO-based dictionary terminology.

CHILDREN
TREATMENT-EMERGENT ADVERSE EVENT
INCIDENCE IN A CONTROLLED ADD-ON LENNOX-GASTAUT TRIAL

Body System/Event	Felbamate (N=31) %	Placebo (N=27) %
Body as a Whole		
Fever	22.6	11.1
Fatigue	9.7	3.7
Weight Decrease	6.5	0
Pain	6.5	0
Central Nervous System		
Somnolence	48.4	11.1
Insomnia	16.1	14.8
Nervousness	16.1	18.5
Gait Abnormal	9.7	0
Headache	6.5	18.5
Thinking Abnormal	6.5	3.7
Ataxia	6.5	3.7
Urinary Incontinence	6.5	7.4
Emotional Lability	6.5	0
Miosis	6.5	0
Dermatological		
Rash	9.7	7.4
Digestive		
Anorexia	54.8	14.8
Vomiting	38.7	14.8
Constipation	12.9	0
Hiccup	9.7	3.7
Nausea	6.5	0
Dyspepsia	6.5	3.7
Hematologic		
Purpura	12.9	7.4
Leukopenia	6.5	0
Respiratory		
Upper Respiratory Tract Infection	45.2	25.9
Pharyngitis	9.7	3.7
Coughing	6.5	0
Special Senses		
Otitis Media	9.7	0

OTHER EVENTS OBSERVED IN ASSOCIATION WITH THE ADMINISTRATION OF FELBAMATE

In the paragraphs that follow, the adverse clinical events, other than those in the preceding tables, that occurred in a total of 977 adults and 357 children exposed to Felbamate and that are reasonably associated with its use are presented. They are listed in order of decreasing frequency. Because he reports cite events observed in open-label and uncontrolled studies, the role of Felbamate in their causation cannot be reliably determined.

DOSAGE TABLE (ADULTS)

	Week 1	Week 2	Week 3
Dosage reduction of concomitant AEDs	REDUCE original dose by 20-33%*	REDUCE original dose by up to an additional 1/3*	REDUCE as clinically indicated
Felbamate Dosage	1200 mg/day Initial dose	2400 mg/day Therapeutic dosage range	3600 mg/day Therapeutic dosage range

* See "Adjunctive" and "Conversion to Monotherapy" sections.

Events are classified within body system categories and enumerated in order of decreasing frequency using the following definitions: frequent adverse events are defined as those occurring on one or more occasions in at least 1/100 patients; infrequent adverse events are those occurring in 1/100-1/1000 patients; and rare events are those occurring in fewer than 1/1000 patients.

Event frequencies are calculated as the number of patients reporting an event divided by the total number of patients (N=1334) exposed to Felbamate.

Body as a Whole: Frequent: Weight increase, asthenia, malaise, influenza-like symptoms; *Rare*: anaphylactoid reaction, chest pain substernal.

Cardiovascular: Frequent: Palpitation, tachycardia; *Rare*: supraventricular tachycardia.

Central Nervous System: Frequent: Agitation, psychological disturbance, aggressive reaction; *Infrequent*: hallucination, euphoria, suicide attempt, migraine.

Digestive: Frequent: SGOT increased; *Infrequent*: esophagitis, appetite increased; *Rare*: GGT elevated.

Hematologic: Infrequent: Lymphadenopathy, leukopenia, leukocytosis, thrombocytopenia, granulocytopenia; *Rare*: antinuclear factor test positive, qualitative platelet disorder, agranulocytosis.

Metabolic/Nutritional: Infrequent: Hypokalemia, hyponatremia, LDH increased, alkaline phosphatase increased, hypophosphatemia; *Rare*: creatinine phosphokinase increased.

Musculoskeletal: Infrequent: Dystonia.

Dermatological: Frequent: Pruritus; *Infrequent*: urticaria, bullous eruption; *Rare*: buccal mucous membrane swelling, Stevens-Johnson Syndrome.

Special Senses: Rare: Photosensitivity allergic reaction.

POST-MARKETING ADVERSE EVENT REPORTS:
Voluntary reports of adverse events in patients taking Felbamate (usually in conjunction with other drugs) have been received since market introduction and may have no causal relationship with the drug(s). These include the following by body system:

Body as a Whole: edema, hypothermia, rigors.

Central & Peripheral Nervous System: paranoid reaction, nystagmus, choreoathetosis, extrapyramidal disorder, confusion, psychosis, status epilepticus, dyskinesia, dysarthria.

Digestive: stomatitis, glossitis, dysphagia, jaundice.

Cardiovascular: hypotesion, hypertension, flushing.

Hematologic: (Refer to "Warnings") increased and decreased prothrombin time, anemia, hypochromic anemia, aplastic anemia, pancytopenia.

Metabolic/Nutritional: hypomagnesemia.

Dermatological: abnormal body order, sweating, liche planus, livedo reticularis, alopecia, toxic epidermal necrolysis.

Urogenital: menstrual disorder.

DRUG ABUSE AND DEPENDENCE
Abuse: Abuse potential was not evaluated in human studies.

Dependence: Rats administered Felbamate orally at doses 8.3 times the recommended human dose 6 days each week for 5 consecutive weeks demonstrated no signs of physical dependence as measured by weight loss following drug withdrawal on day 7 of each week.

OVERDOSAGE
Four subjects inadvertently received Felbamate as adjunctive therapy in dosages ranging from 5400 to 7200 mg/day for durations between 6 and 51 days. One subject who received 5400 mg/day as monotherapy for 1 week reported no adverse experiences. Another subject attempted suicide by ingesting 12,000 mg of Felbamate in a 12-hour period. The only adverse experiences reported were mild gastric distress and a resting heart rate of 100 bpm. No serious adverse reactions have been reported.

General supportive measures should be employed if overdosage occurs. It is not known if Felbamate is dialyzable.

DOSAGE AND ADMINISTRATION
Felbamate has been studied as monotherapy and adjunctive therapy in adults and as adjunctive therapy in children with seizures associated with Lennox-Gastaut syndrome. As Felbamate is added to or substituted for existing AEDs, it is necessary to reduce the dosage of those AEDs in the range of 20-33% to minimize side effects (see "*Drug Interactions*" subsection).

ADULTS (14 YEARS OF AGE AND OVER)
The majority of patients received 3600 mg/day in clinical trials evaluating its use as both monotherapy and adjunctive therapy.

Monotherapy: (Initial therapy) Felbamate has not been systematically evaluated as initial monotherapy. Initiate Felbamate at 1200 mg/day in divided doses three or four times daily. The prescriber is advised to titrate previously untreated patients under close clinical supervision, increasing the dosage in 600-mg increments every 2 weeks to 2400 mg/day based on clinical response and thereafter to 3600 mg/day if clinically indicated.

Conversion to Monotherapy: Initiate Felbamate at 1200 mg/day in divided doses three or four times daily. Reduce the dosage of concomitant AEDs by one-third at initiation of Felbamate therapy. At week 2, increase the Felbamate dosage to 2400 mg/day while reducing the dosage of other AEDs up to an additional one-third of their original dosage. At week 3, increase the Felbamate dosage up to 3600 mg/day and continue to reduce the dosage of other AEDs as clinically indicated.

Adjunctive Therapy: Felbamate should be added at 1200 mg/day in divided doses three or four times daily while reducing present AEDs by 20% in order to control plasma concentrations of concurrent phenytoin, valproic acid, and carbamazepine and its metabolites. Further reductions of the concomitant AEDs dosage may be necessary to minimize side effects due to drug interactions. Increase the dosage of Felbamate by 1200 mg/day increments at weekly intervals to 3600 mg/day. Most side effects seen during Felbamate adjunctive therapy resolve as the dosage of concomitant AEDs is decreased. (See related table).

While the above Felbamate conversion guidelines may result in a Felbamate 3600 mg/day dose within 3 weeks, in some patients titration to a 3600 mg/day Felbamate dose has been achieved in as little as 3 days with appropriate adjustment of other AEDs.

CHILDREN WITH LENNOX-GASTAUT SYNDROME (AGES 2-14 YEARS)
Adjunctive Therapy: Felbamate should be added at 15 mg/kg/day in divided doses three or four times daily while reducing present AEDs by 20% in order to control plasma levels of concurrent phenytoin, valproic acid, and carbamazepine and its metabolites. Further reductions of the concomitant AED dosage may be necessary to minimize side effects due to drug interactions. Increase the dosage of Felbamate by 15 mg/kg/day increments at weekly intervals to 45 mg/kg/day. Most side effects seen during Felbamate adjunctive therapy resolve as the dosage of concomitant AEDs is decreased.

STORAGE
Shake suspension well before using.
Store at controlled room temperature 15°-30°C (59°-86°F).
Dispense in tight container.

HOW SUPPLIED
SUSPENSION: 600 MG/5 ML

BRAND/MANUFACTURER	NDC	SIZE	AWP
○ BRAND			
FELBATOL: Wallace	00037-0442-67	240 ml	$70.80
	00037-0442-17	960 ml	$273.00

TABLETS: 400 MG

BRAND/MANUFACTURER	NDC	SIZE	AWP
○ BRAND			
▶ FELBATOL: Wallace	00037-0430-01	100s	$57.60
	00037-0430-11	100s ud	$57.60

TABLETS: 600 MG

BRAND/MANUFACTURER	NDC	SIZE	AWP
○ BRAND			
▶ FELBATOL: Wallace	00037-0431-01	100s	$66.00
	00037-0431-11	100s ud	$66.00

Felbatol SEE FELBAMATE

Feldene SEE PIROXICAM

Felodipine

DESCRIPTION
Felodipine is a calcium antagonist (calcium channel blocker). Felodipine is a dihydropyridine derivative that is chemically described as ± ethyl methyl 4-(2, 3-

dichlorophenyl)-1, 4-dihydro-2,6-dimethyl-3,5-pyridine-dicarboxylate. Its empirical formula is $C_{18}H_{19}Cl_2NO_4$.

Felodipine is a slightly yellowish, crystalline powder with a molecular weight of 384.26. It is insoluble in water and is freely soluble in dichloromethane and ethanol. Felodipine is a racemic mixture.

Tablets provide extended release of Felodipine. They are available as tablets containing 5 mg or 10 mg of Felodipine for oral administration.

Following is its chemical structure:

CLINICAL PHARMACOLOGY

MECHANISM OF ACTION
Felodipine is a member of the dihydropyridine class of calcium channel antagonists (calcium channel blockers). It reversibly competes with nitrendipine and/or other calcium channel blockers for dihydropyridine binding sites, blocks voltage-dependent Ca++ currents in vascular smooth muscle and cultured rabbit atrial cells and blocks potassium-induced contracture of the rat portal vein.

In vitro studies show that the effects of Felodipine on contractile processes are selective, with greater effects on vascular smooth muscle than cardiac muscle. Negative inotropic effects can be detected *in vitro*, but such effects have not been seen in intact animals.

The effect of Felodipine on blood pressure is principally a consequence of a dose-related decrease of peripheral vascular resistance in man, with a modest reflex increase in heart rate (see *"Cardiovascular Effects"*). With the exception of a mild diuretic effect seen in several animal species and man, the effects of Felodipine are accounted for by its effects on peripheral vascular resistance.

PHARMACOKINETICS AND METABOLISM
Following oral administration, Felodipine is almost completely absorbed and undergoes extensive first-pass metabolism. The systemic bioavailability of Felodipine is approximately 20 percent. Mean peak concentrations following the administration of Felodipine are reached in 2.5 to 5 hours. Both peak plasma concentration and the area under the plasma concentration time curve (AUC) increase linearly with doses up to 20 mg. Felodipine is greater than 99 percent bound to plasma proteins.

Following intravenous administration, the plasma concentration of Felodipine declined triexponentially with mean disposition half-lives of 4.8 minutes, 1.5 hours and 9.1 hours. The mean contributions of the three individual phases to the overall AUC were 15, 40 and 45 percent, respectively, in the order of increasing $t_{1/2}$.

Following oral administration of the immediate-release formulation, the plasma level of felodipine also declined polyexponentially with a mean terminal $t_{1/2}$ of 11 to 16 hours. The mean peak and trough steady-state plasma concentrations achieved after 10 mg of the immediate-release formulation given once a day to normal volunteers, were 20 and 0.5 nmol/L, respectively. The trough plasma concentration of Felodipine in most individuals was substantially below the concentration needed to effect a half-maximal decline in blood pressure (EC_{50}) [4-6 nmol/L for Felodipine], thus precluding once a day dosing with the immediate-release formulation.

Following administration of a 10-mg dose of Felodipine, the extended-release formulation, to young, healthy volunteers, mean peak and trough steady-state plasma concentrations of Felodipine were 7 and 2 nmol/L, respectively. Corresponding values in hypertensive patients (mean age 64) after a 20-mg dose of Felodipine were 23 and 7 nmol/L. Since the EC_{50} for Felodipine is 4 to 6 nmol/L, a 5 to 10-mg dose of Felodipine in some patients, and a 20-mg dose in others, would be expected to provide an antihypertensive effect that persists for 24 hours (see *"Cardiovascular Effects"* below and *"Dosage And Administration"*).

The systemic plasma clearance of Felodipine in young healthy subjects is about 0.8 L/min and the apparent volume of distribution is about 10 L/kg.

Following an oral or intravenous dose of ^{14}C-labeled Felodipine in man, about 70 percent of the dose of radioactivity was recovered in urine and 10 percent in the feces. A negligible amount of intact Felodipine is recovered in the urine and feces (< 0.5%). Six metabolites, which account for 23 percent of the oral dose, have been identified; none has significant vasodilating activity.

Following administration of Felodipine to hypertensive patients, mean peak plasma concentrations at steady state are about 20 percent higher than after a single dose. Blood pressure response is correlated with plasma concentrations of Felodipine.

The bioavailability of Felodipine is not influenced by the presence of food in the gastrointestinal tract. In a study of six patients, the bioavailability of Felodipine was increased more than two-fold when taken with doubly concentrated grape-fruit juice, compared to when taken with water or orange juice. A similar finding has been seen with some other dihydropyridine calcium antagonists, but to a lesser extent than that seen with Felodipine.

Age Effects: Plasma concentrations of Felodipine, after a single dose and at steady state, increase with age. Mean clearance of Felodipine in elderly hypertensives (mean age 74) was only 45 percent of that of young volunteers (mean age 26). At

steady state mean AUC for young patients was 39 percent of that for the elderly. Data for intermediate age ranges suggest that the AUC's fall between the extremes of the young and the elderly.

Hepatic Dysfunction: In patients with hepatic disease, the clearance of Felodipine was reduced to about 60 percent of that seen in normal young volunteers.

Renal impairment does not alter the plasma concentration profile of Felodipine; although higher concentrations of the metabolites are present in the plasma due to decrease urinary excretion, these are inactive.

Animal studies have demonstrated that Felodipine crosses the blood-brain barrier and the placenta.

CARDIOVASCULAR EFFECTS
Following administration of Felodipine, a reduction in blood pressure generally occurs within two to five hours. During chronic administration, substantial blood pressure control lasts for 24 hours, with trough reductions in diastolic blood pressure approximately 40-50 percent of peak reductions.

The antihypertensive effect is dose-dependent and correlates with the plasma concentration of Felodipine.

A reflex increase in heart rate frequently occurs during the first week of therapy; this increase attenuates over time. Heart rate increases of 5-10 beats per minute may be seen during chronic dosing. The increase is inhibited by beta-blocking agents.

The P-R interval of the ECG is not affected by Felodipine when administered alone or in combination with a beta-blocking agent. Felodipine alone or in combination with a beta-blocking agent has been shown, in clinical and electrophysiologic studies, to have no significant effect on cardiac conduction (P-R, P-Q and H-V intervals).

In clinical trials in hypertensive patients without clinical evidence of left ventricular dysfunction, no symptoms suggestive of a negative inotropic effect were noted; however none would be expected in this population (see *"Precautions"*).

RENAL/ENDOCRINE EFFECTS
Renal vascular resistance is decreased by Felodipine while glomerular filtration rate remains unchanged. Mild diuresis, natriuresis and kalliuresis have been observed during the first week of therapy. No significant effects on serum electrolytes were observed during short- and long-term therapy. In clinical trials increases in plasma noradrenaline levels have been observed.

CLINICAL STUDIES
Felodipine produces dose-related decreases in systolic and diastolic blood pressure as demonstrated in six placebo-controlled, dose response studies using either immediate-release or extended-release dosage forms. These studies enrolled over 800 patients on active treatment, at total daily doses ranging from 2.5 to 20 mg. In those studies Felodipine was administered either as monotherapy or was added to beta blockers. The results of the two studies with Felodipine once daily as monotherapy are shown in the table below:

MEAN REDUCTIONS IN BLOOD PRESSURE (MMHG)* SYSTOLIC/DIASTOLIC

Dose	N	Mean Peak Response	Mean Trough Response	Trough/Peak Ratios (%s)
		Study 1 (8 weeks)		
2.5 mg	68	9.4/4.7	2.7/2.5	29/53
5 mg	68	9.5/6.3	2.4/3.7	25/59
10 mg	67	18.0/10.8	10.0/6.0	56/56
		Study 2 (4 weeks)		
10 mg	50	5.3/7.2	1.5/3.2	33/40**
20 mg	50	11.3/10.2	4.5/3.2	43/34**

* *Placebo response subtracted*
** *Different number of patients available for peak and trough measurements*

INDICATIONS AND USAGE
Felodipine is indicated for the treatment of hypertension. Felodipine may be used alone or concomitantly with other antihypertensive agents.

UNLABELED USES
Felodipine is used alone or as an adjunct in the treatment of angina pectoris.

CONTRAINDICATIONS
Felodipine is contraindicated in patients who are hypersensitive to this product.

PRECAUTIONS

GENERAL
Hypotension: Felodipine, like other calcium antagonists, may occasionally precipitate significant hypotension and rarely syncope. It may lead to reflex tachycardia which in susceptible individuals may precipitate angina pectoris. (See *"Adverse Reactions"*.)

Heart Failure: Although acute hemodynamic studies in a small number of patients with NYHA Class II or III heart failure treated with Felodipine have not demonstrated negative inotropic effects, safety in patients with heart failure has not been established. Caution therefore should be exercised when using Felodipine in patients with heart failure or compromised ventricular function, particularly in combination with a beta blocker.

► SHOWN IN PRODUCT IDENTIFICATION GUIDE

Elderly Patients or Patients with Impaired Liver Function: Patients over 65 years of age or patients with impaired liver function may have elevated plasma concentrations of felodipine and may therefore respond to lower doses of Felodipine. These patients should have their blood pressure monitored closely during dosage adjustment of Felodipine and should rarely require dose above 10 mg. (See "*Clinical Pharmacology*" and "*Dosage and Administration*".)

Peripheral Edema: Peripheral edema, generally mild and not associated with generalized fluid retention, was the most common adverse event in the clinical trials. The incidence of peripheral edema was both dose- and age-dependent. Frequency of peripheral edema ranged from about 10 percent in patients under 50 years of age taking 5 mg daily to about 30 percent in those over 60 years of age taking 20 mg daily. This adverse effect generally occurs within 2-3 weeks of the initiation of treatment.

INFORMATION FOR PATIENTS
Patients should be instructed to take Felodipine whole and not to crush or chew the tablets. They should be told that mild gingival hyperplasia (gum swelling) has been reported. Good dental hygiene decreases its incidence and severity.

Note: As with many other drugs, certain advice to patients being treated with Felodipine is warranted. This information is intended to aid in the safe and effective use of this medication. It is not a disclosure of all possible adverse or intended effects.

DRUG INTERACTIONS
Beta-Blocking Agents: A pharmacokinetic study of Felodipine in conjunction with metoprolol demonstrated no significant effects on the pharmacokinetics of elodipine. The AUC and C_{max} of metoprolol, however, were increased approximately 31 and 38 percent, respectively. In controlled clinical trials, however, beta blockers including metoprolol were concurrently administered with Felodipine and were well tolerated.

Cimetidine: In healthy subjects pharmacokinetic studies showed an approximately 50 percent increase in the area under the plasma concentration time curve (AUC) as well as the C_{max} of Felodipine when given concomitantly with cimetidine. It is anticipated that a clinically significant interaction may occur in some hypertensive patients. Therefore, it is recommended that low doses of Felodipine be used when given concomitantly with cimetidine.

Digoxin: When given concomitantly with Felodipine the peak plasma concentration of digoxin was significantly increased. There was, however, no significant change in the AUC of digoxin.

Anticonvulsants: In a pharmacokinetic study, maximum plasma concentrations of Felodipine were considerably lower in epileptic patients on long-term anticonvulsant therapy (e.g., phenytoin, carbamazepine, or phenobarbital) than in healthy volunteers. In such patients, the mean area under the Felodipine plasma concentration-time curve was also reduced to approximately six percent of that observed in healthy volunteers. Since a clinically significant interaction may be anticipated, alternative antihypertensive therapy should be considered in these patients.

Other Concomitant Therapy: In healthy subjects there were no clinically significant interactions when Felodipine was given concomitantly with indomethacin or spironolactone.

Interaction with Food: See "*Clinical Pharmacology, Pharmacokinetics and Metabolism*".

CARCINOGENESIS, MUTAGENESIS, IMPAIRMENT OF FERTILITY
In a two-year carcinogenicity study in the rats fed Felodipine at doses of 7.7, 23.1 or 69.3 mg/kg/day (up to 28 times* the maximum recommended human dose on a mg/m² basis), a dose-related increase in the incidence of benign interstitial cell tumors of the testes (Leydig cell tumors) was observed in treated male rats. These tumors were not observed in a similar study in mice at doses up to 138.6 mg/kg/day (28 times* the maximum recommended human dose on a mg/m² basis). Felodipine, at the doses employed in the two-year rat study, has been shown to lower testicular testosterone and to produce a corresponding increase in serum luteinizing hormone in rats. The Leydig cell tumor development is possibly secondary to these hormonal effects which have not been observed in man.

In this same rate study a dose-related increase in the incidence of focal squamous cell hyperplasia compared to control was observed in the esophageal groove of male and female rats in all dose groups. No other drug-related esophageal or gastric pathology was observed in the rats or with chronic administration in mice and dogs. The latter species, like man, has no anatomical structure comparable to the esophageal groove.

Felodipine was not carcinogenic when fed to mice at doses of up to 138.6 mg/kg/day (28 times* the maximum recommended human dose on a mg/m² basis) for periods of up to 80 weeks in males and 99 weeks in females.

Felodipine did not display any mutagenic activity *in vitro* in the Ames microbial mutagenicity test or in the mouse lymphoma forward mutation assay. No elastogenic potential was seen *in vivo* in the mouse micronucleus test at oral doses up to 2500 mg/kg (506 times* the maximum recommended human dose on a mg/m² basis) or *in vitro* in a human lymphocyte chromosome aberration assay.

A fertility study in which male and female rats were administered doses of 3.8, 9.6 or 26.9 mg/kg/day showed no significant effect of Felodipine on reproductive performance.

PREGNANCY
PREGNANCY CATEGORY C
Teratogenic Effects: Studies in pregnant rabbits administered doses of 0.46, 1.2, 2.3 and 4.6 mg/kg/day (from 0.4 to 4 times* the maximum recommended human dose on a mg/m² basis) showed digital anomalies consisting of reduction in size and degree of ossification of the terminal phalanges in the fetuses. The frequency and severity of the changes appeared dose-related and were noted even at the lowest dose. These changes have been shown to occur with other members of the dihydropyridine class and are possibly a result of compromised uterine blood flow. Similar fetal anomalies were not observed in rats given Felodipine.

In a teratology study in cynomolgus monkeys no reduction in the size of the terminal phalanges was observed but an abnormal position of the distal phalanges was noted in about 40 percent of the fetuses.

Nonteratogenic Effects: A prolongation of parturition with difficult labor and an increased frequency of fetal and early postnatal deaths were observed in rats administered doses of 9.6 mg/kg/day (4 times* the maximum human dose on a mg/m² basis) and above.

Significant enlargement of the mammary glands in excess of the normal enlargement for pregnant rabbits was found with doses greater than or equal to 1.2 mg/kg/day (equal to the maximum human dose on a mg/m² basis). This effect occurred only in pregnant rabbits and regressed during lactation. Similar changes in the mammary glands were not observed in rats or monkeys.

There are no adequate and well-controlled studies in pregnant woman. If Felodipine is used during pregnancy, or if the patient becomes pregnant while taking this drug, she should be apprised of the potential hazard to the fetus, possible digital anomalies of the infant, and the potential effects of Felodipine on labor and delivery, and on the mammary glands of pregnant females.

NURSING MOTHERS
It is not known whether this drug is secreted in human milk and because of the potential for serious adverse reactions from Felodipine in the infant, a decision should be made whether to discontinue nursing or to discontinue the drug, taking into account the importance of the drug to the mother.

PEDIATRIC USE
Safety and effectiveness in children have not been established.

ADVERSE REACTIONS
In controlled studies in the United States and overseas approximately 3000 patients were treated with Felodipine as either the extended-release or the immediate-release formulation.

The most common clinical adverse experiences reported with Felodipine administered as monotherapy in all settings and with all dosage forms of Felodipine were peripheral edema and headache. Peripheral edema was generally mild, but it was age- and dose-related and resulted in discontinuation of therapy in about 4 percent of the enrolled patients. Discontinuation of therapy due to any clinical adverse experience occurred in about 9 percent of the patients receiving Felodipine, principally for peripheral edema, headache, or flushing.

Adverse experiences that occurred with an incidence of 1.5 percent or greater during monotherapy with Felodipine without regard to causality are compared to placebo in the table below.

PERCENT OF PATIENTS WITH ADVERSE EFFECTS IN CONTROLLED TRIALS OF FELODIPINE AS MONOTHERAPY (INCIDENCE OF DISCONTINUATIONS SHOWN IN PARENTHESES)

Adverse Effect	Felodipine % N = 730	Placebo % N = 283
Peripheral Edema	22.3 (4.2)	3.5
Headache	18.6 (2.1)	10.6
Flushing	6.4 (1.0)	1.1
Dizziness	5.8 (0.8)	3.2
Upper Respiratory Infection	5.5 (0.1)	1.1
Asthenia	4.7 (0.1)	2.8
Cough	2.9 (0.0)	0.4
Paresthesia	2.5 (0.1)	1.8
Dyspepsia	2.3 (0.0)	1.4
Chest Pain	2.1 (0.1)	1.4
Nausea	1.9 (0.8)	1.1
Muscle Cramps	1.9 (0.0)	1.1
Palpitation	1.8 (0.5)	2.5
Abdominal Pain	1.8 (0.3)	1.1
Constipation	1.6 (0.1)	1.1
Diarrhea	1.6 (0.1)	1.1
Pharyngitis	1.6 (0.0)	0.4
Rhinorrhea	1.6 (0.0)	0.0
Back Pain	1.6 (0.0)	1.1
Rash	1.5 (0.1)	1.1

In the two dose response studies using Felodipine as monotherapy, the following table describes the incidence (percent) of adverse experiences that were dose-related. The incidence of discontinuations due to these adverse experiences are shown in parentheses.

* Based on patient weight of 50 kg

◆ RATED THERAPEUTICALLY EQUIVALENT; ◇ THERAPEUTIC EQUIVALENCE UNCONFIRMED; ○ UNRATED

Adverse Effect	Placebo N = 121	2.5 mg N = 71	5.0 mg N = 72	10.0 mg N = 123	20 mg N = 50
Peripheral Edema	2.5 (1.6)	1.4 (0.0)	13.9 (2.8)	19.5 (2.4)	36.0 (10.0)
Palpitation	0.8 (0.8)	1.4 (0.0)	0.0 (0.0)	2.4 (0.8)	12.0 (8.0)
Headache	12.4 (0.0)	11.3 (1.4)	11.1 (0.0)	18.7 (4.1)	28.0 (18.0)
Flushing	0.0 (0.0)	4.2 (0.0)	2.8 (0.0)	8.1 (0.8)	20.0 (0.0)

In addition, adverse experiences that occurred in 0.5 up to 1.5 percent of patients who received Felodipine in all controlled clinical studies (listed in order of decreasing severity within each category) and serious adverse events that occurred at a lower rate or were found during marketing experience (those lower rate events are in italics) were:

Body as a Whole: Facial edema, warm sensation;

Cardiovascular: Tachycardia, *myocardial infarction, hypotension, syncope, angina pectoris,* arrhythmia;

Digestive: Vomiting, dry mouth, flatulence;

Hematologic; Anemia; Musculoskeletal: Athralgia, arm pain, knee pain, leg pain, foot pain, hip pain, myalgia;

Nervous/Psychiatric: Depression, anxiety disorders, insomnia, irritability, nervousness, somnolence;

Respiratory: Bronchitis, influenza, sinusitis, dyspnea, epistaxis, respiratory infection, sneezing;

Skin: Contusion, erythema, urticaria;

Urogenital: Decreased libido, impotence, urinary frequency, urinary urgency, dysuria.

Felodipine, as an immediate release formulation, has also been studied as monotherapy in 680 patients with hypertension in U.S. and overseas controlled clinical studies. Other adverse experiences not listed above and with an incidence of 0.5 percent or greater include:

Body as a Whole: Fatigue;

Digestive: Gastrointestinal pain;

Musculoskeletal: Arthritis, local weakness, neck pain, shoulder pain, ankle pain;

Nervous/Psychiatric: Tremor;

Respiratory: Rhinitis;

Skin: Hyperhidrosis, pruritus;

Special Senses: Blurred vision, tinnitus;

Urogenital: Nocturia.

Gingival Hyperplasia: Gingival hyperplasia, usually mild, occurred in < 0.5 percent of patients in controlled studies. This condition may be avoided or may regress with improved dental hygiene. (See *"Precautions", "Information for Patients".*)

CLINICAL LABORATORY TEST FINDINGS
Serum Electrolytes: No significant effects on serum electrolytes were observed during short- and long-term therapy (see *"Clinical Pharmacology, Renal/Endocrine Effects"*).

Serum Glucose: No significant effects on fasting serum glucose were observed in patients treated with Felodipine in the U.S. controlled study.

Liver Enzymes: One of two episodes of elevated serum transaminases decreased once drug was discontinued in clinical studies; no follow-up was available for the other patient.

OVERDOSAGE
Oral doses of 240 mg/kg and 264 mg/kg in male and female mice, respectively and 2390 mg/kg and 2250 mg/kg in male and female rats, respectively, caused significant lethality.

In a suicide attempt, one patient took 150 mg Felodipine together with 15 tablets each of atenolol and spironolactone and 20 tablets of nitrazepam. The patient's blood pressure and heart rate were normal on admission to hospital; he subsequently recovered without significant sequelae.

Overdosage might be expected to cause excessive peripheral vasodilation with marked hypotension and possibly bradycardia.

If severe hypotension occurs, symptomatic treatment should be instituted. The patient should be placed supine with the legs elevated. The administration of intravenous fluids may be useful to treat hypotension due to overdosage with calcium antagonists. In case of accompanying bradycardia, atropine (0.5-1 mg) should be administered intravenously. Sympathomimetic drugs may also be given if the physician feels they are warranted.

It has not been established whether Felodipine can be removed from the circulation by hemodialysis.

DOSAGE AND ADMINISTRATION
The recommended initial dose is 5 mg once a day. Therapy should be adjusted individually according to patient response, generally at intervals of not less than two weeks. The usual dosage range is 5-10 mg once daily. The maximum recommended daily dose is 20 mg once a day. That dose in clinical trials showed an increased blood pressure response but a large increase in the rate of peripheral

edema and other vasodilatory adverse events (See *"Adverse Reactions"*). Modification of the recommended dosage is usually not required in patients with renal impairment.

Felodipine should be swallowed whole and not crushed or chewed.

Use in the Elderly or Patients with Impaired Liver Function: Patients over 65 years of age or patients with impaired liver function, because they may develop higher plasma concentrations of Felodipine, should have their blood pressure monitored closely during dosage adjustment (see *"Precautions"*). In general, doses above 10 mg should not be considered in these patients.

Store below 30°C (86°F). Keep container tightly closed. Protect from light.

HOW SUPPLIED
TABLET, EXTENDED RELEASE: 2.5 MG

BRAND/MANUFACTURER	NDC	SIZE	AWP
○ **BRAND**			
PLENDIL: Merck	00006-0450-31	30s	$26.69
	00006-0450-58	100s	$88.94
	00006-0450-28	100s ud	$93.39

TABLET, EXTENDED RELEASE: 5 MG

BRAND/MANUFACTURER	NDC	SIZE	AWP
○ **BRAND**			
▶ PLENDIL: Merck	00006-0451-31	30s	$26.69
	00006-0451-58	100s	$88.94
	00006-0451-28	100s ud	$93.39

TABLET, EXTENDED RELEASE: 10 MG

BRAND/MANUFACTURER	NDC	SIZE	AWP
○ **BRAND**			
▶ PLENDIL: Merck	00006-0452-31	30s	$47.93
	00006-0452-58	100s	$159.81
	00006-0452-28	100s ud	$167.80

Femstat *SEE* BUTOCONAZOLE NITRATE

Fenex-PSE *SEE* GUAIFENESIN AND PSEUDOEPHEDRINE HYDROCHLORIDE

Fenfluramine Hydrochloride

DESCRIPTION
Fenfluramine Hydrochloride is an anoretic drug for oral administration. It is available in immediate release tablets containing 20 mg Fenfluramine Hydrochloride.

Following is its chemical structure:

$$F_3C-\bigcirc-CH_2CHNHC_2H_5 \cdot HCl$$
$$CH_3$$

CLINICAL PHARMACOLOGY
Fenfluramine is a sympathomimetic amine, the pharmacologic activity of which differs somewhat from that of the prototype drugs of this class used in obesity, the amphetamines, in appearing to produce more central nervous system depression than stimulation.

The mechanism of action of Fenfluramine Hydrochloride is unclear but may be related to brain levels (or turnover rates) of serotonin or to increased glucose utilization. The antiappetite effects of Fenfluramine Hydrochloride are suppressed by serotonin-blocking drugs and by drugs that lower brain levels of the amine. Furthermore, decreased serotonin levels produced by selective brain lesions suppress the action of Fenfluramine Hydrochloride.

In a study of 20 normal males, Fenfluramine increased glucose utilization, resulting in decreased blood glucose levels. Experimental work in animals suggested that increased glucose utilization activated the satiety center and decreased the activity of the feeding center. Perhaps by this mechanism Fenfluramine Hydrochloride inhibits appetite. The relationship between glucose utilization and serotonin has not been clarified. Fenfluramine is well-absorbed from the gastrointestinal tract, and a maximal anorectic effect is generally seen after 2 to 4 hours. In man, Fenfluramine is de-ethylated to norfenfluramine which is subsequently oxidized to m-trifluoromethyl benzoic acid and excreted as the glycine conjugate, m-trifluoromethylhippuric acid. Other compounds found in the urine include unchanged Fenfluramine and norfenfluramine.

The rate of excretion of Fenfluramine is pH dependent, with much smaller amounts appearing in an alkaline than in an acid urine.

The half-life of Fenfluramine is said to be about 20 hours, compared with 5 hours for amphetamines; however, if urinary excretion is rapid and the pH maintained in the acidic range (below pH 5), half-life can be reduced to 11 hours.

▶ SHOWN IN PRODUCT IDENTIFICATION GUIDE

Fenfluramine and norfenfluramine reach steady state concentrations in plasma within 3 to 4 days following chronic dosage.

The greatest weight loss is seen in those patients who maintain the highest levels of Fenfluramine Hydrochloride. A 2-to-3-kg weight loss over 6 weeks is associated with a plasma level of 0.1 mcg/mL (or 10 mcg/100 mL).

Fenfluramine is widely distributed in almost all body tissues. It is soluble in lipids and crosses the blood-brain barrier. Fenfluramine crosses the placenta readily in monkeys.

INDICATIONS AND USAGE

Fenfluramine Hydrochloride is indicated in the management of exogenous obesity as a short-term (a few weeks) adjunct in a regimen of weight reduction based on caloric restriction.

Drugs of this class used in obesity are commonly known as "anorectics" or "anorexigenics." It has not been established, however, that the action of such drugs in treating obesity is primarily one of appetite suppression. Other central nervous system actions or metabolic effects may be involved.

Adult obese subjects instructed in dietary management and treated with "anorectic" drugs, lose more weight on the average than those treated with placebo and diet, as determined in relatively short-term trials.

The average magnitude of increased weight loss of drug-treated patients over placebo-treated is only a fraction of a pound a week. The rate of weight loss is greatest in the first weeks of therapy for both drug and placebo subjects and tends to decrease in succeeding weeks. The possible origins of the increased weight loss due to the various drug effects are not established. The average amount of weight loss associated with the use of an "anorectic" drug varies from trial to trial, and the increased weight loss appears to be related in part to variables other than the drug prescribed such as the physician-investigator, the population treated and the diet prescribed. Studies do not permit conclusions as to the relative importance of the drug and non-drug factors on weight loss.

The natural history of obesity is measured in years, whereas the studies cited are restricted to a few weeks duration; thus, the total impact of drug-induced weight loss over that of diet alone must be considered clinically limited.

CONTRAINDICATIONS

Fenfluramine is contraindicated in patients with glaucoma or with hypersensitivity to Fenfluramine or other sympathomimetic amines. Do not administer Fenfluramine during or within 14 days following the administration of monoamine oxidase inhibitors, since hypertensive crises may result. Patients with a history of drug abuse should not receive the drug.

Do not administer Fenfluramine to patients with alcoholism since psychiatric symptoms (paranoia, depression, psychosis) have been reported in a few such patients who had been administered this drug.

Fenfluramine should also generally be avoided in patients with psychotic illness. There have been reports of schizophrenic patients who have become agitated, delusional, and assaultive.

A fatal cardiac arrest has been reported shortly after the induction of anesthesia in a patient who had been taking Fenfluramine prior to surgery. Fenfluramine may have a catecholamine-depleting effect when administered for prolonged periods of time; therefore, potent anesthetic agents should be administered with caution to patients taking Fenfluramine. If general anesthesia cannot be avoided, full cardiac monitoring and facilities for instant resuscitative measures are a minimum necessity.

WARNINGS

When tolerance to the "anorectic" effect develops, the maximum recommended dose should not be exceeded in an attempt to increase the effect; rather, the drug should be discontinued.

PRECAUTIONS

General: Fenfluramine differs in its pharmacological profile from other "anorectic" drugs with which the prescribing practitioner may be familiar. Correspondingly, there are possible adverse effects not associated with other "anorectics"; such effects include those of diarrhea, sedation, and depression. The possibility of these effects should be weighed against the possible advantage of decreased central nervous system stimulation and/or abuse potential.

There have been four cases of pulmonary hypertension reported in association with Fenfluramine use. Two cases were apparently reversible after discontinuation of Fenfluramine, but evidence of pulmonary hypertension recurred in one of these patients upon rechallenge with Fenfluramine. A third patient was initially improved with nifedipine treatment, but was noted to have increased pulmonary arterial pressure again at a four month follow-up visit. Finally, an irreversible and fatal case of pulmonary hypertension has been reported in a patient who had seven 1-month courses of Fenfluramine in the twelve years prior to death. Patients taking Fenfluramine should be advised to report immediately any deterioration in exercise tolerance.

Use only with caution in hypertension, with monitoring of blood pressure, since evidence is insufficient to rule out a possible adverse effect on blood pressure in some hypertensive patients. The drug is not recommended in severely hypertensive patients. The drug is not recommended for patients with symptomatic cardiovascular disease including arrhythmias.

Caution should be exercised in prescribing Fenfluramine for patients with a history of mental depression. Further depression of mood may become evident while the patient is on Fenfluramine or following withdrawal of Fenfluramine. Symptoms of depression occurring immediately following abrupt withdrawal can be readily controlled by reinstituting Fenfluramine Hydrochloride, followed by a gradual tapering off of the daily dose.

Information for Patients: Fenfluramine may impair the ability of the patient to engage in potentially hazardous activities such as operating machinery or driving a motor vehicle (see "*Adverse Reactions*") the patient should be cautioned accordingly. Patient should also be advised to avoid alcoholic beverages while taking Fenfluramine Hydrochloride.

Drug Interactions. Fenfluramine may increase slightly the effect of antihypertensive drugs, e.g., guanethidine, methyldopa, reserpine.

Other CNS depressant drugs should be used with caution in patients taking Fenfluramine, since the effects may be additive.

Carcinogenesis, Mutagenesis: No carcinogenic studies or mutagenic studies have been undertaken with this drug.

Pregnancy Category C: Fenfluramine Hydrochloride was shown to produce a questionable embryotoxic effect in rats and a reduced conception rate when given in a dose of 20 times the human dose. However, additional reproduction studies in rats, rabbits, mice, and monkeys at doses up to, respectively, 5 times, 20 times, 1 time, and 5 times the human dose yielded negative results.

There are no adequate and well-controlled studies in pregnant women. Fenfluramine Hydrochloride should be used during pregnancy only if the potential benefit justifies the potential risk to the fetus.

Labor and Delivery: The effect of Fenfluramine during labor or delivery on the mother and the fetus is unknown. The effect on later growth, development, and functional maturation of the child is unknown.

Nursing Mothers: It is not known whether this drug is excreted in human milk. Because many drugs are excreted in human milk, caution should be exercised when Fenfluramine is administered to a nursing mother.

Pediatric Use: Safety and effectiveness in children below the age of 12 years have not been established.

ADVERSE REACTIONS

The most common adverse reactions of Fenfluramine are drowsiness, diarrhea, and dry mouth. Less frequent adverse reactions reported in association with Fenfluramine are:

Central Nervous System: Dizziness; confusion; incoordination; headache; elevated mood; depression; anxiety, nervousness, or tension; insomnia; weakness or fatigue; increased or decreased libido; agitation, dysarthria.

Gastrointestinal: Constipation; abdominal pain; nausea.

Autonomic: Sweating; chills; blurred vision.

Genitourinary: Dysuria; urinary frequency.

Cardiovascular: Palpitation; hypotension; hypertension; fainting; pulmonary hypertension.

Skin: Rash; urticaria; burning sensation.

Miscellaneous: Eye irritation; myalgia; fever; chest pain; bad taste.

DRUG ABUSE AND DEPENDENCE

Fenfluramine Hydrochloride is a controlled substance in Schedule IV. Fenfluramine is related chemically to the amphetamines, although it differs somewhat pharmacologically. The amphetamines and related stimulant drugs have been extensively abused and can produce tolerance and severe psychological dependence, as well as other adverse organic and mental changes. In this regard, there has been a report of abuse of Fenfluramine by subjects with a history of abuse of other drugs. Abuse of 80 to 400 milligrams of the drug has been reported to be associated with euphoria, derealization, and perceptual changes. Fenfluramine did not produce signs of dependence in animals and appears to produce sedation more often than CNS stimulation at therapeutic doses. Its abuse potential appears qualitatively different from that of amphetamines. The possibility that Fenfluramine may induce dependence should be kept in mind when evaluating the desirability of including the drug in the weight reduction programs of individual patients.

OVERDOSAGE

Signs and Symptoms: Only limited data have been reported concerning clinical effects and management of over-dosage of Fenfluramine.

Agitation and drowsiness, confusion, flushing, tremor (or shivering), fever, sweating, abdominal pain, hyperventilation, and dilated non-reactive pupils seem frequent in Fenfluramine overdosage. Reflexes may be either exaggerated or depressed and some patients may have rotary nystagmus. Tachycardia may be present, but blood pressure may be normal or only slightly elevated. Convulsions, coma, and ventricular extrasystoles, culminating in ventricular fibrillation, and cardiac arrest, may occur at higher dosages.

Human Toxicity: Less than 5 mg/kg are toxic to humans. Five-ten mg/kg may produce coma and convulsions. Reported single overdoses have ranged from 300 to 2000 mg; the lowest reported fatal dose was a few hundred mg in a small child, and the highest reported nonfatal dose was 1800 mg in an adult. Most deaths were apparently due to respiratory failure and cardiac arrest.

Toxic effects will appear within 30 to 60 minutes and may progress rapidly to potentially fatal complications in 90 to 240 minutes. Symptoms may persist for extended periods depending upon the dose ingested.

Management: After overdosage, only a small percentage of the drug is excreted in the urine. Forced acid diuresis has been recommended only in extreme cases in which the patient survives the early hours of intoxication but fails to show decisive improvement from other measures. Hemodialysis and peritoneal dialysis are of theoretical advantage but have not been used clinically.

Reportedly the treatment of Fenfluramine intoxication should include:

- *Gastric lavage* (but not drug-induced emesis because the patient may become unconscious at a very early stage.)
- In the event that gastric lavage is not feasible due to trismus, consult an anesthesiologist for endotracheal intubation after administration of muscle relaxants; only then gastric evacuation should be tried.
- Administration of activated charcoal after emesis or lavage may reduce absorption of drug.
- *Monitoring of vital functions.* If necessary, mechanical respiration, defibrillation, or "cardioversion" should be instituted.
- *Drug therapy.* Diazepam or phenobarbital for convulsions or muscular hyperactivity. In the presence of extreme tachycardia; propranolol; in the presence of ventricular extrasystoles; lidocaine; in the presence of hyperpyrexia; chlorpromazine.

Since Fenfluramine has been shown to have a slight lowering effect on blood sugar in some patients, the theoretical possibility of hypoglycemia should be borne in mind although this effect has not been reported in cases of clinical overdosage.

DOSAGE AND ADMINISTRATION
The usual dose is one 20 mg tablet three times daily before meals. Depending on the degree of effectiveness and side effects, the dosage may be increased at weekly intervals by one tablet (20 mg) daily until a maximum dosage of two tablets three times daily is attained. Total dosage of Fenfluramine should not exceed 120 mg per day.

Store at controlled room temperature, between 15°C and 30°C (59°F and 86°F). Dispense in well-closed container.

HOW SUPPLIED
TABLETS (C-IV): 20 MG

BRAND/MANUFACTURER	NDC	SIZE	AWP
BRAND			
PONDIMIN: Robins Pharm	00031-6447-63	100s	$29.16
	00031-6447-70	500s	$139.09

Fenoprofen Calcium

DESCRIPTION
Fenoprofen Calcium is a nonsteroidal, anti-inflammatory, antiarthritic drug. Fenoprofen Calcium Capsules contain Fenoprofen Calcium as the dihydrate in an amount equivalent to 200 mg (0.826 mmol) or 300 mg (1.24 mmol) of Fenoprofen.

Fenoprofen Calcium Tablets contain Fenoprofen Calcium as the dihydrate in an amount equivalent to 600 mg (2.48 mmol) of Fenoprofen.

Chemically, Fenoprofen Calcium is an arylacetic acid derivative Benzeneacetic acid, α-methyl-3-phenoxy-, calcium salt dihydrate (±)- Fenoprofen Calcium is a white crystalline powder with a molecular weight of 558.64. At 25°C, it dissolves to a 15 mg/mL solution in alcohol (95%). It is slightly soluble in water and insoluble in benzene.

The *p*Ka of Fenoprofen Calcium is 4.5 at 25°C.

Following is its chemical structure:

CLINICAL PHARMACOLOGY
Fenoprofen Calcium is a nonsteroidal, anti-inflammatory, antiarthritic drug that also possesses analgesic and antipyretic activities. Its exact mode of action is unknown, but it is thought that prostaglandin synthetase inhibition is involved. Fenoprofen Calcium has been shown to inhibit prostaglandin synthetase isolated from bovine seminal vesicles. Reproduction studies in rats have shown Fenoprofen Calcium to be associated with prolonged labor and difficult parturition when given during late pregnancy. Evidence suggests that this may be due to decreased uterine contractility resulting from the inhibition of prostaglandin synthesis. Its action is not mediated through the adrenal gland.

Fenoprofen shows anti-inflammatory effects in rodents by inhibiting the development of redness and edema in acute inflammatory conditions and by reducing soft-tissue swelling and bone damage associated with chronic inflammation. It exhibits analgesic activity in rodents by inhibiting the writhing response caused by the introduction of an irritant into the peritoneal cavities of mice and by elevating pain thresholds that are related to pressure in edematous hind-paws of rats. In rats made febrile by the subcutaneous administration of brewer's yeast, Fenoprofen produces antipyretic action. These effects are characteristic of nonsteroidal, anti-inflammatory, antipyretic, analgesic drugs.

The results in humans confirmed the anti-inflammatory and analgesic actions found in animals. The emergence and degree of erythemic response were measured in adult male volunteers exposed to ultraviolet irradiation. The effects

of Fenoprofen Calcium, aspirin, and indomethacin were each compared with those of a placebo. All 3 drugs demonstrated anti-erythemic activity.

In patients with rheumatoid arthritis, the anti-inflammatory action of Fenoprofen Calcium has been evidenced by relief of pain, increase in grip strength, and reductions in joint swelling, duration of morning stiffness, and disease activity (as assessed by both the investigator and the patient). The anti-inflammatory action of Fenoprofen Calcium has also been evidenced by increased mobility (ie, a decrease in the number of joints having limited motion).

The use of Fenoprofen Calcium in combination with gold salts or corticosteroids has been studied in patients with rheumatoid arthritis. The studies, however, were inadequate in demonstrating whether further improvement is obtained by adding Fenoprofen Calcium to maintenance therapy with gold salts or steroids. Whether or not Fenoprofen Calcium used in conjunction with partially effective doses of a corticosteroid has a "steroid-sparing" effect is unknown.

In patients with osteoarthritis, the anti-inflammatory and analgesic effects of Fenoprofen Calcium have been demonstrated by reduction in tenderness as a response to pressure and reductions in night pain, stiffness, swelling, and overall disease activity (as assessed by both the patient and the investigator). These effects have also been demonstrated by relief of pain with motion and at rest and increased range of motion in involved joints.

In patients with rheumatoid arthritis and osteoarthritis clinical studies have shown Fenoprofen Calcium to be comparable to aspirin in controlling the aforementioned measures of disease activity, but mild gastrointestinal reactions (nausea, dyspepsia) and tinnitus occurred less frequently in patients treated with Fenoprofen Calcium than in aspirin-treated patients. It is not known whether Fenoprofen Calcium causes less peptic ulceration than does aspirin.

In patients with pain, the analgesic action of Fenoprofen Calcium has produced a reduction in pain intensity, an increase in pain relief, improvement in total analgesia scores, and a sustained analgesic effect.

Under fasting conditions, Fenoprofen Calcium is rapidly absorbed, and peak plasma levels of 50 μg/mL are achieved within 2 hours after oral administration of 600-mg doses. Good dose proportionality was observed between 200-mg and 600-mg doses in fasting male volunteers. The plasma half-life is approximately 3 hours. About 90% of a single oral dose is eliminated within 24 hours as Fenoprofen Glucuronide and 4'-hydroxy-Fenoprofen glucuronide, the major urinary metabolites of Fenoprofen. Fenoprofen is highly bound (99%) to albumin. The concomitant administration of antacid (containing both alumium and magnesium hydroxide) does not interfere with absorption of Fenoprofen Calcium.

There is less suppression of collagen-induced platelet aggregation with single doses of Fenoprofen Calcium than there is with aspirin.

INDICATIONS AND USAGE
Fenoprofen Calcium is indicated for relief of the signs and symptoms of rheumatoid arthritis and osteoarthritis. It is recommended for the treatment of acute flareups and exacerbations and for the long-term management of these diseases.

Fenoprofen Calcium is also indicated for the relief of mild to moderate pain.

UNLABELED USES
Fenoprofen Calcium is used alone or as an adjunct in the treatment of acute gout, episiotomy pain, and migraine headache.

CONTRAINDICATIONS
Fenoprofen Calcium is contraindicated in patients who have shown hypersensitivity to it.

The drug should not be administered to patients with a history of significantly impaired renal function.

Fenoprofen Calcium should not be given to patients in whom aspirin and other nonsteroidal anti-inflammatory drugs induce the symptoms of asthma, rhinitis, or urticaria, because cross-sensitivity to these drugs occurs in a high proportion of such patients.

WARNINGS
Risk of GI Ulceration, Bleeding, and Perforation with NSAID Therapy: Serious gastrointestinal toxicity, such as bleeding, ulceration, and perforation, can occur at any time, with or without warning symptoms, in patients treated chronically with NSAID therapy. Although minor upper gastrointestinal problems, such as dyspepsia, are common, usually developing early in therapy, physicians should remain alert for ulceration and bleeding in patients treated chronically with NSAIDs, even in the absence of previous GI tract symptoms. In patients observed in clinical trials of several months to 2 years duration, symptomatic upper GI ulcers, gross bleeding, or perforation appear to occur in approximately 1% of patients treated for 3 to 6 months, and in about 2% to 4% of patients treated for 1 year. Physicians should inform patients about the signs and/or symptoms of serious GI toxicity and what steps to take if they occur.

Studies to date have not identified any subset of patients not at risk of developing peptic ulceration and bleeding. Except for a prior history of serious GI events and other risk factors known to be associated with peptic ulcer disease, such as alcoholism, smoking, etc, no risk factors (eg, age, sex) have been associated with increased risk. Elderly or debilitated patients seem to tolerate ulceration or bleeding less well than other individuals and most spontaneous reports of fatal GI events are in this population. Studies to date are inconclusive concerning the relative risk of various NSAIDs in causing such reactions. High doses of any NSAID probably carry a greater risk of these reactions, although controlled clinical trials showing this do not exist in most cases. In considering the use of relatively large doses (within the recommended dosage range), sufficient benefit should be anticipated to offset the potential increased risk of GI toxicity.

Since Fenoprofen Calcium has been marketed, there have been reports of genitourinary tract problems in patients taking it. The most frequently reported problems have been episodes of dysuria, cystitis, hematuria, interstitial nephritis, and nephrotic syndrome. This syndrome may be preceded by the appearance of fever, rash, arthralgia, oliguria, and azotemia and may progress to anuria. There may also be substantial proteinuria, and, on renal biopsy, electron microscopy has shown foot process fusion and T-lymphocyte infiltration in the renal interstitium. Early recognition of the syndrome and withdrawal of the drug have been followed by rapid recovery. Administration of steroids and the use of dialysis have also been included in the treatment. Because a syndrome with some of these characteristics has also been reported with other nonsteroidal anti-inflammatory drugs, it is recommended that patients who have had these reactions with other such drugs not be treated with Fenoprofen Calcium. In patients with possibly compromised renal function, periodic renal function examinations should be done.

PRECAUTIONS
General—Renal Effects: There have been reports of acute interstitial nephritis and nephrotic syndrome (see "Contraindications" and "Warnings").

A second form of renal toxicity has been seen in patients with prerenal conditions leading to a reduction in renal blood flow or blood volume, in which renal prostaglandins play a supportive role in the maintenance of renal perfusion. In these patients, administration of an NSAID may cause a dose-dependent reduction in prostaglandin formation and may precipitate overt renal decompensation at any time. Patients at greatest risk for this reaction are those with impaired renal function, heart failure, liver dysfunction, those taking diuretics, and the elderly. Discontinuation of NSAID therapy is typically followed by recovery to the pretreatment state.

Since Fenoprofen Calcium is primarily eliminated by the kidneys, patients with possibly compromised renal function (such as the elderly) should be monitored periodically, especially during long-term therapy. For such patients, it may be anticipated that a lower daily dosage will avoid excessive drug accumulation.

Miscellaneous: Peripheral edema has been observed in some patients taking Fenoprofen Calcium therefore, Fenoprofen Calcium, should be used with caution in patients with compromised cardiac function or hypertension. The possibility of renal involvement should be considered.

Studies to date have not shown changes in the eyes attributable to the administration of Fenoprofen Calcium. However, adverse ocular effects have been observed with other anti-inflammatory drugs. Eye examinations, therefore, should be performed if visual disturbances occur in patients taking Fenoprofen Calcium.

Caution should be exercised by patients whose activities require alertness if they experience CNS side effects while taking Fenoprofen Calcium.

Since the safety of Fenoprofen Calcium has not been established in patients with impaired hearing, these patients should have periodic tests of auditory function during prolonged therapy with Fenoprofen Calcium.

Information for Patients: Fenoprofen Calcium like other drugs of its class, is not free of side effects. The side effects of these drugs can cause discomfort and, rarely, there are more serious side effects, such as gastrointestinal bleeding, which may result in hospitalization and even fatal outcomes.

NSAIDs (Nonsteroidal Anti-Inflammatory Drugs) are often essential agents in the management of arthritis and have a major role in the treatment of pain, but they also may be commonly employed for conditions which are less serious. Physicians may wish to discuss with their patients the potential risks (see "Warnings", "Precautions", and "Adverse Reactions" sections) and likely benefits of NSAID treatment, particularly when the drugs are used for less serious conditions where treatment without NSAIDs may represent an acceptable alternative to both the patient and physician.

Laboratory Tests: In chronic studies in rats, high doses of Fenoprofen Calcium caused elevation of serum transaminase and hepatocellular hypertrophy. In clinical trials, some patients developed elevation of serum transaminase, LDH, and alkaline phosphatase that persisted for some months and usually, but not always, declined despite continuation of the drug. The significance of this is unknown. It is recommended, therefore, that Fenoprofen Calcium be discontinued if any significant liver abnormality occurs.

As with other nonsteroidal anti-inflammatory drugs, border-line elevations in 1 or more liver tests may occur in up to 15% of patients. These abnormalities may progress, may remain essentially unchanged, or may be transient with continued therapy. The SGPT (ALT) test is probably the most sensitive indicator of liver dysfunction. Meaningful (ie, 3 times the upper limit of normal) elevations of SGPT or SGOT (AST) occurred in controlled clinical trials in less than 1% of patients. A patient with symptoms and/or signs suggesting liver dysfunction, or in whom an abnormal liver test has occurred, should be evaluated for evidence of the development of more severe hepatic reactions while using Fenoprofen Calcium. Severe hepatic reactions, including jaundice and cases of fatal hepatitis, have been reported with Fenoprofen Calcium, as with other nonsteroidal anti-inflammatory drugs. As a result, during long-term therapy, liver function tests should be monitored periodically. Although such reactions are rare, if liver tests continue to be abnormal or worsen, if clinical signs and symptoms consistent with liver disease develop, or if systemic manifestations occur (eg, eosinophilia and rash), Fenoprofen Calcium should be discontinued. If this drug is to be used in the presence of impaired liver function, it must be done under strict observation.

Patients with initial low hemoglobin values who are receiving long-term therapy with Fenoprofen Calcium should have a hemoglobin determination made at reasonable intervals.

Fenoprofen Calcium decreases platelet aggregation and may prolong bleeding time. Patients who may be adversely affected by prolongation of the bleeding time should be carefully observed when Fenoprofen Calcium is administered.

Because serious GI tract ulceration and bleeding can occur without warning symptoms, physicians should follow chronically treated patients for the signs and symptoms of ulceration and bleeding and should inform them of the importance of this follow-up (see "Risk of GI Ulceration, Bleeding, and Perforation with NSAID Therapy" under "Warnings").

Laboratory Test Interactions: Amerlex-M kit assay values of total and free triiodothyronine in patients receiving Fenoprofen Calcium have been reported as falsely elevated on the basis of a chemical cross-reaction that directly interferes with the assay. Thyroid-stimulating hormone, total thyroxine, and thyrotropin-releasing hormone response are not affected.

Drug Interactions: The coadministration of aspirin decreases the biologic half-life of Fenoprofen because of an increase in metabolic clearance that results in a greater amount of hydroxylated Fenoprofen in the urine. Although the mechanism of interaction between Fenoprofen and aspirin is not totally known, enzyme induction and displacement of Fenoprofen from plasma albumin binding sites are possibilities. Because Fenoprofen has not been shown to produce any additional effect beyond that obtained with aspirin alone and because aspirin increases the rate of excretion of Fenoprofen Calcium, the concomitant use of Fenoprofen Calcium and salicylates is not recommended.

Chronic administration of phenobarbital, a known enzyme inducer, may be associated with a decrease in the plasma half-life of Fenoprofen. When phenobarbital is added to or withdrawn from treatment, dosage adjustment of Fenoprofen Calcium may be required.

In vitro studies have shown that Fenoprofen, because of its affinity for albumin, may displace from their binding sites other drugs that are also albumin bound, and this may lead to drug interaction. Theoretically, Fenoprofen could likewise be displaced. Patients receiving hydantoin, sulfonamides, or sulfonylureas should be observed for increased activity of these drugs and, therefore, signs of toxicity from these drugs. In patients receiving coumarin-type anticoagulants, the addition of Fenoprofen Calcium to therapy could prolong the prothrombin time. Patients receiving both drugs should be under careful observation. Patients treated with Fenoprofen Calcium may be resistant to the effects of loop diuretics.

In patients receiving Fenoprofen Calcium and a steroid concomitantly, any reduction in steroid dosage should be gradual in order to avoid the possible complications of sudden steroid withdrawal.

Usage in Pregnancy: Safe use of Fenoprofen Calcium during pregnancy and lactation has not been established: therefore, administration to pregnant patients and nursing mothers is not recommended. Reproduction studies have been performed in rats and rabbits. When Fenoprofen was given to rats during pregnancy and continued until the time of labor, parturition was prolonged. Similar results have been found with other nonsteroidal anti-inflammatory drugs that inhibit prostaglandin synthetase.

Usage in Children: Fenoprofen Calcium is not recommended for use in children because documented clinical experience has been insufficient to establish safety and a suitable dosage regimen in the pediatric age group.

ADVERSE REACTIONS
During clinical studies for rheumatoid arthritis, osteoarthritis, or mild to moderate pain and studies of pharmacokinetics, complaints were compiled from a checklist of potential adverse reactions, and the following data emerged. These encompass observations in 6,786 patients, including 188 observed for at least 52 weeks. For comparison, data are also presented from complaints received from 266 patients who received placebo in these same trials. During short-term studies for analgesia, the incidence of adverse reactions was markedly lower than that seen in longer-term studies.

INCIDENCE GREATER THAN 1% PROBABLE CAUSAL RELATIONSHIP
Digestive System: During clinical trials with Fenoprofen Calcium the most common adverse reactions were gastrointestinal in nature and occurred in 20.8% of patients receiving Fenoprofen Calcium as compared to 16.9% of patients receiving placebo. In descending order of frequency, these reactions included dyspepsia (10.3%, Nalfon, vs 2.3%, placebo), nausea (7.7% vs 7.1%), constipation (7% vs 1.5%), vomiting (2.6% vs 1.9%), abdominal pain (2% vs 1.1%), and diarrhea (1.8% vs 4.1%).

The drug was discontinued because of adverse gastrointestinal reactions in less than 2% of patients during premarketing studies.

Nervous System: The most frequent adverse neurologic reactions were headache (8.7% treated vs 7.5% placebo) and somnolence (8.5% vs 6.4%). Dizziness (6.5% vs 5.6%), tremor (2.2% vs 0.4%), and confusion (1.4% vs none) were noted less frequently.

Fenoprofen Calcium was discontinued in less than 0.5% of patients because of these side effects during premarketing studies.

Skin and Appendages: Increased sweating (4.6% vs 0.4%), pruritus (4.2% vs 0.8%), and rash (3.7% vs 0.4%) were reported.

Fenoprofen Calcium was discontinued in about 1% of patients because of an adverse effect related to the skin during premarketing studies.

Special Senses: Tinnitus (4.5% vs 0.4%), blurred vision (2.2% vs none), and decreased hearing (1.6% vs none) were reported.

◆ **RATED THERAPEUTICALLY EQUIVALENT;** ◇ **THERAPEUTIC EQUIVALENCE UNCONFIRMED;** ○ **UNRATED**

Fenoprofen Calcium was discontinued in less than 0.5% of patients because of these side effects during premarketing studies.

Cardiovascular: Palpitations (2.5% vs 0.4%).

Fenoprofen Calcium was discontinued in about 0.5% of patients because of adverse cardiovascular reactions during premarketing studies.

Miscellaneous: Nervousness (5.7% vs 1.5%), asthenia (5.4% vs 0.4%), peripheral edema (5.0% vs 0.4%), dyspnea (2.8% vs none), fatigue (1.7% vs 1.5%), upper respiratory infection (1.5% vs 5.6%), and nasopharyngitis (1.2% vs none).

INCIDENCE LESS THAN 1%
PROBABLE CAUSAL RELATIONSHIP
The following adverse reactions, occurring in less than 1% of patients, were reported in controlled clinical trials and voluntary reports made since Fenoprofen Calcium was initially marketed. The probability of a causal relationship exists between Fenoprofen Calcium and these adverse reactions:

Digestive System: Gastritis, peptic ulcer with/without perforation, gastrointestinal hemorrhage, anorexia, flatulence, dry mouth, and blood in the stool. Increases in alkaline phosphatase, LDH, and SGOT, jaundice and cholestatic hepatitis were observed (see *"Precautions"*).

Genitourinary Tract: Dysuria, cystitis, hematuria, oliguria, azotemia, anuria, interstitial nephritis, nephrosis, and papillary necrosis (see *"Warnings"*).

Hypersensitivity: Angioedema (angioneurotic edema).

Hematologic: Purpura, bruising, hemorrhage, thrombocytopenia, hemolytic anemia, aplastic anemia, agranulocytosis, and pancytopenia.

Miscellaneous: Anaphylaxis, urticaria, malaise, insomnia, and tachycardia.

INCIDENCE LESS THAN 1%
CAUSAL RELATIONSHIP UNKNOWN
Other reactions reported either in clinical trials or spontaneously, occurred in circumstances in which a causal relationship could not be established. However, with these rarely reported reactions, the possibility of such a relationship cannot be excluded. Therefore, these observations are listed to alert the physician.

Skin and Appendages: Exfoliative dermatitis, toxic epidermal necrolysis, Stevens-Johnson syndrome, and alopecia.

Digestive System: Aphthous ulcerations of the buccal mucosa, metallic taste, and pancreatitis.

Cardiovascular: Atrial fibrillation, pulmonary edema, electrocardiographic changes, and supraventricular tachycardia.

Nervous System: Depression, disorientation, seizures, and trigeminal neuralgia.

Special Senses: Burning tongue, diplopia, and optic neuritis.

Miscellaneous: Personality change, lymphadenopathy, mastodynia, and fever.

OVERDOSAGE
Signs and Symptoms: Symptoms of overdose appear within several hours and generally involve the gastrointestinal and central nervous systems. They include dyspepsia, nausea, vomiting, abdominal pain, dizziness, headache, ataxia, tinnitus, tremor, drowsiness, and confusion. Hyperpyrexia, tachycardia, hypotension, and acute renal failure may occur rarely following overdose. Respiratory depression and metabolic acidosis have also been reported following overdose with certain NSAIDs.

Treatment: To obtain up-to-date information about the treatment of overdose, a good resource is your certified Regional Poison Control Center. Telephone numbers of certified poison control centers are listed in the *Physicians' Desk Reference (PDR)*. In managing overdosage, consider the possibility of multiple drug overdoses, interaction among drugs, and unusual drug kinetics in your patient.

Protect the patient's airway and support ventilation and perfusion. Meticulously monitor and maintain, within acceptable limits, the patient's vital signs, blood gases, serum electrolytes, etc. Absorption of drugs from the gastrointestinal tract may be decreased by giving activated charcoal, which, in many cases, is more effective than emesis or lavage; consider charcoal instead of or in addition to gastric emptying. Repeated doses of charcoal over time may hasten elimination of some drugs that have been absorbed. Safeguard the patient's airway when employing gastric emptying or charcoal.

Alkalinization of the urine, forced diuresis, peritoneal dialysis, hemodialysis, and charcoal hemoperfusion do not enhance systemic drug elimination.

DOSAGE AND ADMINISTRATION
Analgesia: For the treatment of mild to moderate pain, the recommended dosage is 200 mg every 4 to 6 hours, as needed.

Rheumatoid Arthritis and Osteoarthritis: The suggested dosage is 300 to 600 mg, 3 or 4 times a day. The dose should be tailored to the needs of the patient and may be increased or decreased depending on the severity of the symptoms. Dosage adjustments may be made after initiation of drug therapy or during exacerbations of the disease. Total daily dosage should not exceed 3,200 mg.

If gastrointestinal complaints occur, Fenoprofen Calcium may be administered with meals or with milk. Although the total amount absorbed is not affected, peak blood levels are delayed and diminished.

Patients with rheumatoid arthritis generally seem to require larger doses of Fenoprofen Calcium than do those with osteoarthritis. The smallest dose that yields acceptable control should be employed.

Although improvement may be seen in a few days in many patients, an additional 2 to 3 weeks may be required to gauge the full benefits of therapy.

Store at controlled room temperature, 59° to 86°F (15° to 30°C).

HOW SUPPLIED
CAPSULE: 200 MG

AVERAGE UNIT PRICE (AVAILABLE SIZES)		GENERIC A-RATED AVERAGE PRICE (GAAP)	
BRAND	$0.48	100s	$28.15
GENERIC	$0.28		
HCFA FUL (100s ea)	$0.33		

BRAND/MANUFACTURER	NDC	SIZE	AWP
◆ BRAND			
NALFON 200: Dista	00777-0876-02	100s	$48.42
◆ GENERICS			
Watson	52544-0367-01	100s	$23.60
Major	00904-3778-60	100s	$29.15
Moore,H.L.	00839-7511-06	100s	$30.63
Major	00904-3778-61	100s ud	$29.21

CAPSULE: 300 MG

AVERAGE UNIT PRICE (AVAILABLE SIZES)		GENERIC A-RATED AVERAGE PRICE (GAAP)	
BRAND	$0.39	100s	$33.08
GENERIC	$0.32		
HCFA FUL (100s ea)	$0.31		

BRAND/MANUFACTURER	NDC	SIZE	AWP
◆ BRAND			
NALFON: Dista	00777-0877-02	100s	$38.76
◆ GENERICS			
Watson	52544-0368-01	100s	$27.37
Warner Chilcott	00047-0081-24	100s	$31.04
Schein	00364-2315-01	100s	$33.75
Major	00904-3785-60	100s	$33.85
Geneva	00781-2862-01	100s	$35.38
Moore,H.L.	00839-7512-06	100s	$35.49
Major	00904-3785-61	100s ud	$34.69
Watson	52544-0368-05	500s	$132.65

CAPSULE: 600 MG

AVERAGE UNIT PRICE (AVAILABLE SIZES)	
GENERIC	$0.46

BRAND/MANUFACTURER	NDC	SIZE	AWP
◆ GENERICS			
Major	00904-3786-60	100s	$46.70
Major	00904-3786-40	500s	$226.80

TABLETS: 600 MG

AVERAGE UNIT PRICE (AVAILABLE SIZES)		GENERIC A-RATED AVERAGE PRICE (GAAP)	
GENERIC	$0.45	100s	$45.71
HCFA FUL (100s ea)	$0.21	500s	$213.42

BRAND/MANUFACTURER	NDC	SIZE	AWP
◆ GENERICS			
Watson	52544-0366-01	100s	$37.80
Warner Chilcott	00047-0077-24	100s	$40.86
Zenith	00172-4141-60	100s	$43.40
Schein	00364-2316-01	100s	$44.00
Geneva	00781-1863-01	100s	$44.46
Martec	52555-0473-01	100s	$44.70
Qualitest	00603-3578-21	100s	$44.80
Rugby	00536-3813-01	100s	$44.85
Mutual	53489-0287-01	100s	$45.00
Goldline	00182-1902-01	100s	$45.00
Mylan	00378-0471-01	100s	$45.36
Purepac	00228-2317-10	100s	$45.65
URL	00677-1308-01	100s	$45.75
Moore,H.L.	00839-7513-06	100s	$46.29
Lederle Std Prod	00005-3559-43	100s	$47.19
Aligen	00405-4424-01	100s	$47.80
Raway	00686-0477-20	100s ud	$39.25
Goldline	00182-1902-89	100s ud	$40.00

► SHOWN IN PRODUCT IDENTIFICATION GUIDE

BRAND/MANUFACTURER	NDC	SIZE	AWP
Vangard	00615-3507-13	100s ud	$49.93
Auro	55829-0252-10	100s ud	$56.15
UDL	51079-0477-20	100s ud	$61.70
Watson	52544-0366-05	500s	$183.60
Schein	00364-2316-05	500s	$198.00
Qualitest	00603-3578-28	500s	$198.53
Goldline	00182-1902-05	500s	$210.00
Zenith	00172-4141-70	500s	$210.55
Geneva	00781-1863-05	500s	$216.98
Purepac	00228-2317-50	500s	$219.25
Mutual	53489-0287-05	500s	$220.00
Mylan	00378-0471-05	500s	$220.33
Rugby	00536-3813-05	500s	$221.70
Aligen	00405-4424-02	500s	$221.97
Moore,H.L.	00839-7513-12	500s	$224.36
Lederle Std Prod	00005-3559-31	500s	$229.21
Purepac	00228-2317-96	1000s	$438.50

Fentanyl

BECAUSE SERIOUS OR LIFE-THREATENING HYPOVENTILATION COULD OCCUR, FENTANYL TRANSDERMAL SYSTEM IS CONTRAINDICATED:

- *IN THE MANAGEMENT OF ACUTE OR POST-OPERATIVE PAIN, INCLUDING USE IN OUTPATIENT SURGERIES*
- *IN THE MANAGEMENT OF MILD OR INTERMITTENT PAIN RESPONSIVE TO PRN OR NON-OPIOID THERAPY*
- *IN DOSES EXCEEDING 25 MCG/HOUR AT THE INITIATION OF OPIOID THERAPY*

(SEE "CONTRAINDICATIONS" FOR FURTHER INFORMATION.) FENTANYL TRANSDERMAL SYSTEM SHOULD NOT BE ADMINISTERED TO CHILDREN UNDER 12 YEARS OF AGE OR PATIENTS UNDER 18 YEARS OF AGE WHO WEIGH LESS THAN 50 KG (110 LBS) EXCEPT IN AN AUTHORIZED INVESTIGATIONAL RESEARCH SETTING. (SEE "PRECAUTIONS, PEDIATRIC USE.")

FENTANYL TRANSDERMAL SYSTEM IS INDICATED FOR TREATMENT OF CHRONIC PAIN (SUCH AS THAT OF MALIGNANCY) THAT:

- *CANNOT BE MANAGED BY LESSER MEANS SUCH AS ACETAMINOPHEN-OPIOID COMBINATIONS, NON-STEROIDAL ANALGESICS, OR PRN DOSING WITH SHORT-ACTING OPIOIDS AND*
- *REQUIRES CONTINUOUS OPIOID ADMINISTRATION.*

THE 50, 75, AND 100 MCG/HOUR DOSAGES SHOULD ONLY BE USED IN PATIENTS WHO ARE ALREADY ON AND ARE TOLERANT TO OPIOID THERAPY.

WARNING:

FENTANYL ORAL TRANSMUCOSAL CONTAINS THE POTENT NARCOTIC FENTANYL CITRATE IN A FORMULATION WHICH:

- CARRIES A RISK OF HYPOVENTILATION WITH ITS USE WHICH MAY RESULT IN DEATH IF NOT MONITORED BY TRAINED PERSONNEL SUPPORTED BY APPROPRIATE, IMMEDIATELY AVAILABLE EQUIPMENT.
- SHOULD ONLY BE USED AS AN ANETHETIC PREMEDICATION OR FOR INDUCING CONSCIOUS SEDATION PRIOR TO A DIAGNOSTIC OR THERAPEUTIC PROCEDURE IN A MONITORED ANESTHESIA CARE SETTING.
- SHOULD ONLY BE ADMINISTERED IN HOSPITAL SETTINGS SUCH AS THE OPERATING ROOM, EMERGENCY DEPARTMENT, ICU OR OTHER MONITORED ANESTHESIA CARE SETTINGS IN HOSPITALS WHERE THERE IS IMMEDIATE ACCESS TO LIFE SUPPORT EQUIPMENT, OXYGEN, FACILITIES FOR ENDOTRACHEAL INTUBATION, INTRAVENOUS FLUIDS, AND OPIOID ANTAGONISTS.
- CAN ONLY BE USED SAFELY IN PATIENTS BEING MONITORED BY BOTH (1) DIRECT VISUAL OBSERVATION BY A HEALTH PROFESSIONAL WHOSE SOLE RESPONSIBILITY IS OBSERVATION OF THE PATIENT AND BY (2) SOME MEANS OF MEASURING RESPIRATORY FUNCTION SUCH AS PULSE OXIMETRY UNTIL THEY ARE COMPLETELY RECOVERED.
- SHOULD ONLY BE ADMINISTERED BY PERSONS SPECIFICALLY TRAINED IN THE USE OF ANESTHETIC DRUGS AND THE MANAGEMENT OF THE RESPIRATORY EFFECTS OF POTENT OPIOIDS, INCLUDING RESPIRATORY AND CARDIAC RESUSCITATION OF PATIENTS IN THE AGE GROUP BEING TREATED, SUCH TRAINING MUST INCLUDE THE ESTABLISHMENT AND MAINTENANCE OF A PATENT AIRWAY AND ASSISTED VENTILATION.
- SHOULD ONLY BE USED BY HEALTH CARE PRACTITIONERS CREDENTIALED TO USE THE PRODUCT BY THE DIRECTOR OF ANESTHESIA OF THE INSTITUTION IN WHICH THE PRODUCT WILL BE USED.
- IS CONTRAINDICATED FOR USE AT ANY OTHER SETTING OUTSIDE A HOSPITAL

FENTANYL ORAL TRANSMUCOSAL

- IS CONTRAINDICATED IN CHILDREN WHO WEIGH LESS THAN 15 KILOGRAMS (33 POUNDS).
- IS CONTRAINDICATED FOR THE TREATMENT OF ACUTE OR CHRONIC PAIN BECAUSE THE SAFETY OF THIS PRODUCT FOR USE IN THESE INDICATIONS HAS NOT BEEN ESTABLISHED.
- IS CONTRAINDICATED IN DOSES ABOVE 15 µG/KG IN CHILDREN, AND IN DOSES ABOVE 5 µG/KG IN ADULTS. BECAUSE OF THE EXCESSIVE FREQUENCY OF SIGNIFICANT HYPOVENTILATION AT HIGHER DOSES, THE MAXIMUM DOSE ANY CHILD OR ADULT SHOULD RECEIVE IS 400 µG REGARDLESS OF WEIGHT.

Warning: May be habit forming.

DESCRIPTION

Fentanyl Transdermal System provides continuous systemic delivery of Fentanyl, a potent opioid analgesic, for 72 hours. The chemical name is N-Phenyl-N-(1-2-phenyl-ethyl-4-piperidyl) propanamide.

The molecular weight of Fentanyl base is 336.5, and the empirical formula is $C_{22}H_{28}N_2O$. The n-octanol:water partition coefficient is 860:1. The pKa is 8.4.

SYSTEM COMPONENTS AND STRUCTURE
The amount of Fentanyl released from each system per hour is proportional to the surface area (25 µg/h per 10 cm^2). The composition per unit area of all system sizes is identical. Each system also contains 0.1 mL of alcohol USP per 10 cm^2.

Dose* (µg/h)	Size (cm^2)	Fentanyl Content (mg)
25	10	2.5
50**	20	5
75**	30	7.5
100**	40	10

* *Nominal delivery rate per hour*
** *FOR USE ONLY IN OPIOID TOLERANT PATIENTS*

The active component of the system is Fentanyl. The remaining components are pharmacologically inactive. Less than 0.2 ml of alcohol is also released from the system during use. Do not cut or damage Fentanyl Transdermal System. If the Fentanyl Transdermal System is cut or damaged, controlled drug delivery will not be possible.

Fentanyl Citrate is available as an injection and an oral transmucosal lozenge, which is sucked in the mouth. Fentanyl Citrate is a potent narcotic analgesic. Each milliliter of solution for injection contains Fentanyl Citrate equivalent to 50 µg of fentanyl base, adjusted to pH 4.0-7.5 with sodium hydroxide. Each lozenge contains the equivalent of 200, 300, or 400 µg of Fentanyl base. Fentanyl Citrate is chemically identified as N-(1-phenethyl-4-piperidyl) propionanilide citrate (1:1) with a molecular weight of 528.60. The empirical formula is $C_{22}H_{28}N_2O.C_6H_8O_7$.

Fentanyl Citrate is a sterile, non-pyrogenic, preservative free aqueous solution for intravenous or intramuscular injection.

CLINICAL PHARMACOLOGY

PHARMACOLOGY
Fentanyl is an opioid analgesic. Fentanyl interacts predominately with the opioid µ-receptor. These µ-binding sites are discretely distributed in the human brain, spinal cord, and other tissues.

Fentanyl citrate is a narcotic analgesic. A dose of 100 µg (0.1 mg) (2.0 ml) is approximately equivalent in analgesic activity to 10 mg of morphine or 75 mg of meperidine. The principal actions of therapeutic value are analgesia (reduced pain) and sedation (reduced activity and reduced apprehension). Alterations in respiratory rate and alveolar ventilation, associated with narcotic analgesics, may last longer than the analgesic effect. As the dose of narcotic is increased, the decrease in pulmonary exchange becomes greater. Large doses may produce apnea. Fentanyl citrate appears to have less emetic activity than either morphine or meperidine.

In clinical settings, Fentanyl exerts its principal pharmacologic effects on the central nervous system. Its primary actions of therapeutic value are analgesia and sedation. Fentanyl may increase the patient's tolerance for pain and decrease the perception of suffering, although the presence of the pain itself may still be recognized.

In addition to analgesia, alterations in mood, euphoria and dysphoria, and drowsiness commonly occur, as do hypoventilation, pruritus, dizziness, diaphoresis, flushing, confusion, and difficulty in concentrating. Fentanyl depresses the respiratory centers, depresses the cough reflex, and constricts the pupils. Fentanyl given rapidly in large doses may also interfere with respiration by causing muscle rigidity which may affect the muscles of respiration. Analgesic blood levels of Fentanyl may cause nausea and vomiting directly by stimulating the chemorecep-

◆ RATED THERAPEUTICALLY EQUIVALENT; ◇ THERAPEUTIC EQUIVALENCE UNCONFIRMED; ○ UNRATED

tor trigger zone, but nausea and vomiting are significantly more common in ambulatory than in recumbent patients, as is postural syncope.

Opioids increase the tone and decrease the propulsive contractions of the smooth muscle of the gastrointestinal tract. The resultant prolongation in gastrointestinal transit time may be responsible for the constipating effect of Fentanyl. Because opioids may increase biliary tract pressure, some patients with biliary colic may experience worsening rather than relief of pain.

While opioids generally increase the tone of urinary tract smooth muscle, the net effect tends to be variable, in some cases producing urinary urgency, in others, difficulty in urination.

At therapeutic dosages, Fentanyl usually does not exert major effects on the cardiovascular system. However, some patients may exhibit orthostatic or postural hypotension, bradycardia, and fainting.

Histamine assays and skin wheal testing in man indicate that clinically significant histamine release rarely occurs with Fentanyl administration. Assays in man show no clinically significant histamine release in dosages up to 50 µg/kg (0.05 mg/kg) (1 ml/kg). Fentanyl citrate preserves cardiac stability and blunts stress-related hormonal changes at higher doses.

PHARMACOKINETICS (SEE TABLE AND GRAPH)
Fentanyl Transdermal System releases Fentanyl from the reservoir at a nearly constant amount per unit time. The concentration gradient existing between the saturated solution of drug in the reservoir and the lower concentration in the skin drives drug release. Fentanyl moves in the direction of the lower concentration at a rate determined by the copolymer release membrane and the diffusion of Fentanyl through the skin layers. While the actual rate of Fentanyl delivery to the skin varies over the 72 hour application period, each system is labeled with a nominal flux which represents the average amount of drug delivered to the systemic circulation per hour across average skin.

While there is variation in dose delivered among patients, the nominal flux of the systems (25, 50, 75, and 100 µg of Fentanyl per hour) are sufficiently accurate as to allow individual titration of dosage for a given patient. The small amount of alcohol which has been incorporated into the system enhances the rate of drug flux through the rate-limiting copolymer membrane and increases the permeability of the skin to Fentanyl.

Following Fentanyl Transdermal System application, the skin under the system absorbs Fentanyl, and a depot of Fentanyl concentrates in the upper skin layers. Fentanyl then becomes available to the systemic circulation. Serum Fentanyl concentrations increase gradually following initial Fentanyl Transdermal System application, generally leveling off between 12 and 24 hours and remaining relatively constant, with some fluctuation, for the remainder of the 72 hour application period. Peak serum levels of Fentanyl generally occur between 24 and 72 hours after initial application. Serum Fentanyl concentrations achieved are proportional to the Fentanyl Transdermal System delivery rate. With continuous use, serum Fentanyl concentrations continue to rise for the first few system applications. After several sequential 72-hour applications, patients reach and maintain a steady state serum concentration that is determined by individual variation in skin permeability and body clearance of Fentanyl (see graph and Table A).

After system removal, serum Fentanyl concentrations decline gradually, falling about 50% in approximately 17 (range 13-22) hours. Continued absorption of Fentanyl from the skin accounts for a slower disappearance of the drug from the serum than is seen after an IV infusion, where the apparent half-life ranges from 3-12 hours. (See related table).

The plasma protein binding of Fentanyl is 80 to 85%. The main binding protein is alpha-1-acid glycoprotein, but both albumin and lipoproteins contribute to some extent. The free fraction of Fentanyl increases with acidosis. Following an IV dose, Fentanyl is rapidly redistributed from the blood to lung tissue and skeletal muscle and then more slowly to deeper fat compartments. It is then slowly released into the blood from the tissues during its metabolic elimination. Large single doses or many repeated doses can result in the accumulation of a large body burden of Fentanyl that may take many hours to clear.

The average volume of distribution for Fentanyl is 6 L/kg (range 3-8, N = 8). The average clearance in patients undergoing various surgical procedures is 46 L/h (range 27-75, N = 8). The kinetics of Fentanyl in geriatric patients has not been well studied, but in geriatric patients the clearance of IV Fentanyl may be reduced and the terminal half-life greatly prolonged (see "Precautions"). The absorption, distribution, and metabolism of Fentanyl have been shown to be relatively constant over the age range intended for Fentanyl citrate oral transmucosal, although elderly patients have been shown to be approximately twice as sensitive to the same blood level of the drug as younger patients. Although Fentanyl kinetics are known to be altered in both hepatic and renal disease due to alterations in metabolic clearance and plasma proteins, individualized doses of Fentanyl have been used successfully in anesthesia in both kinds of disorders. This is because the duration of effect for the initial dose of Fentanyl is determined by redistribution of the drug, such that diminished metabolic clearance will only become significant with repeated dosing or with excessively large single doses. For these reasons, reduced doses titrated to clinical effect are recommended in the elderly, and in patients with severe hepatic and/or renal disease.

Fentanyl is metabolized primarily in the liver. In humans the drug appears to be metabolized primarily by N-dealkylation to norfentanyl and other inactive metabolites that do not contribute materially to the observed activity of the drug. Fentanyl Citrate demonstrates a high first pass clearance. Within 72 hours of IV Fentanyl administration, approximately 75% of the dose is excreted in urine, mostly as metabolites with less than 10% representing unchanged drug. Approximately 9% of the dose is recovered in the feces, primarily as metabolites. Less than 7% of the oral dose is excreted unchanged in the urine, and only about 1% is excreted unchanged in the feces. The metabolites are mainly excreted in the urine, while fecal excretion is less important. Mean values for unbound fractions of Fentanyl in plasma are estimated to be between 13 and 21%.

Skin does not appear to metabolize Fentanyl delivered transdermally. This was determined in a human keratinocyte cell assay and in clinical studies in which 92% of the dose delivered from the system was accounted for as unchanged Fentanyl that appeared in the systemic circulation.

The pharmacokinetics of Fentanyl Citrate can be described as a three-compartment model, with a distribution time of 1.7 minutes, redistribution of 13 minutes and a terminal elimination half life of 219 minutes. The volume of distribution for Fentanyl Citrate is 4 L/kg.

The onset of action of Fentanyl citrate is almost immediate when the drug is given intravenously; however, the maximal analgesic and respiratory depressant effect may not be noted for several minutes. The usual duration of action of the analgesic effect is 30 to 60 minutes after a single intravenous dose of up to 100 µg (0.1 mg) (2.0 ml). Following intramuscular administration, the onset of action is from seven to eight minutes, and the duration of action is one to two hours. The onset of effects begins 5 to 15 minutes from the start of administration when the drug is delivered as Fentanyl Citrate oral transmucosal. Maximum effects are typically noted 20 to 30 minutes from the start of administration. Complete consumption of the Fentanyl citrate oral transmucosal usually occurs in 10 to 20 minutes.

The absorption pharmacokinetics of Fentanyl from the oral transmucosal dosage form are a combination of the initial rapid absorption from the buccal mucosa and a more prolonged absorption of swallowed Fentanyl from the GI tract. Both the blood Fentanyl profile and the bioavailability of Fentanyl will vary depending on the fraction of the dose that is absorbed through the oral mucosa and the fraction swallowed.

Table A
RANGE OF PHARMACOKINETIC PARAMETERS OF FENTANYL IN PATIENTS

	Clearance (L/h) Range (70 kg)	Volume of Distribution V_{ss} (L/kg) Range	Half Life $t_{1/2}$ (h) Range	Maximal Concentration C_{max} (ng/mL) Range	Time to Maximal Concentration (h) Range	Bio-availability %
IV Fentanyl Surgical Patients	27-75	3-8	3-12			
Hepatically Impaired Patients	3-80†	0.8-8†	4-12†			
Renally Impairred Patients	30-78					
Fentanyl Transdermal System						
25 µg/h			*	0.3-1.2	26-78	
50 µg/h			*	0.6-1.8†	24-72†	
75 µg/h			*	1.1-2.6	24-48	
100 µg/h			*	1.9-3.8	25-72	
Oral Fentanyl 15µg/kg			5-15	1.4-4.6	19-30 (min.)	36-71

† Estimated
* After system removal there is continued systemic absorption from residual Fentanyl in the skin so that serum concentrations fall 50%, on average, in 17 hours.

➤ SHOWN IN PRODUCT IDENTIFICATION GUIDE

Normally, approximately 25% of the total dose is rapidly absorbed from the buccal mucosa and becomes systemically available. The remaining 75% is swallowed with the saliva and then is slowly absorbed from the GI tract. About ⅓ of this amount (25% of the total dose) escapes hepatic first-pass elimination and becomes systemically available. Therefore, the generally observed 50% bioavailability of Fentanyl citrate oral transmucosal is divided equally between rapid transmucosal and slower GI absorption. Chewed or swallowed Fentanyl contributes little to the peak concentration, but is responsible for the prolonged "tail" on the blood level profile as it is slowly absorbed.

Dose proportionality among the three available strengths of Fentanyl citrate oral transmucosal (200, 300, and 400 μg) has not been demonstrated. As portrayed in Table A, there is a wide variability in the range of the pharmacokinetic parameters of this dosing form of Fentanyl, especially in C_{max}, T_{max}, and $t_{1/2}$. Because of the absorption characteristics of this product in this dosage form, there is a sustained plasma level of the drug. *Those who administer this product must be cognizant of the clinical implications of this pharmacokinetic characteristic and continue to monitor and observe the patient until he/she is fully recovered.*

In healthy male volunteers given 15 μg/kg, the mean C_{max} after Fentanyl citrate oral transmucosal is 2.7 ng/mL (see Table A). The median time of maximum plasma concentration (T_{max}) with Fentanyl citrate oral transmucosal is 23 minutes. Absolute bioavailability, as determined by area under the concentration-time curve, of 15 μg/kg of Fentanyl citrate oral transmucosal in 12 healthy male volunteers was 50% compared to intravenous Fentanyl. The mean volume of distribution at steady state (V_{ss}) was 4 L/kg and the total plasma clearance of Fentanyl was 0.5 L/hr/kg (range 0.3 to 0.7 L/hr/kg).

In clinical studies in children, a single dose of 10 to 20 (mean 16.5) μg/kg Fentanyl citrate oral transmucosal resulted in a mean peak plasma Fentanyl level (C_{max}) of 2 ng/mL that occurred about 20 minutes from the start of administration. In these studies, the C_{max} increased with increasing dose while the T_{max} increased (slower absorption) with longer consumption times (time to consume the dosage form). In general, the pharmacokinetic profile of Fentanyl citrate oral transmucosal was similar in adults and children. As with longer acting narcotic analgesics, the duration of the respiratory depressant effect of Fentanyl Citrate may be longer than the analgesic effect. The following observations have been reported concerning altered respiratory response to CO_2 stimulation following administration of Fentanyl citrate to man.

1. *Diminished sensitivity to CO_2 stimulation may persist longer than depression of respiratory rate.* (Altered sensitivity to CO_2 stimulation has been demonstrated for up to four hours following a single intravenous dose of 600 μg (0.6 mg) (12 ml) Fentanyl citrate to healthy volunteers and up to eight hours after 5 mg of transmucosal Fentanyl citrate.) Fentanyl Citrate frequently slows the respiratory rate, duration and degree of respiratory depression being dose related.

2. *Prolonged effects on respiration are possible.* The peak respiratory depressant effect of a single intravenous dose of Fentanyl citrate is noted 5 to 15 minutes following injection. See also *"Warnings"* and *"Precautions"* concerning respiratory depression. The peak respiratory depressant effects of a Fentanyl citrate oral transmucosal dose (10 to 20 μg/kg) occur 15 to 30 minutes following initiation of administration, but respiratory effects may persist for several hours, especially when Fentanyl citrate oral transmucosal is given in conjunction with other anesthetic agents.

3. *Serious respiratory depression can occur, even with proper doses, in vulnerable individuals.* As with other potent anesthetic agents, Fentanyl has been associated with cases of serious respiratory depression in individuals with respiratory disorders, cases of excessive or improper dosage, in individuals with unsuspected abnormalities of absorption or metabolism of the drug, and in rare cases where no specific etiology can be identified. Fentanyl citrate oral transmucosal should be administered only in specifically monitored settings and by persons specifically trained in the use of anesthetics and the management of the respiratory effects of potent opioids, including establishment and maintenance of a patent airway and assisted ventilation (see also box *"Warnings"* and *"Precautions"*.)

PHARMACODYNAMICS

Analgesia: Fentanyl is a strong opioid analgesic. In controlled clinical trials in non-opioid tolerant patients, 60 mg/day IM morphine was considered to provide analgesia approximately equivalent to Fentanyl 100 μg/h in an acute pain model. The analgesic and anesthetic effects of Fentanyl are related to the blood level of the drug, if proper allowance is made for the delay into and out of the CNS (a process with a 3 to 5 minute half-life). Minimum effective analgesic serum concentrations of Fentanyl in opioid naive patients range from 0.2 to 1.2 ng/mL; side effects increase in frequency at serum levels above 2 ng/mL. Respiratory depression and surgical anesthesia occur at levels of 10 to 20 ng/mL. Both the minimum effective concentration and the concentration at which toxicity occurs rise with increasing tolerance. The rate of development of tolerance varies widely among individuals.

Fentanyl redistributes into muscle and fat like most other highly lipophilic drugs, and the duration of the effects of Fentanyl depends on the route of administration, the duration of administration and the total cumulative dose. Initially, the effects of small single doses are short-lived because the drug is rapidly redistributed into peripheral tissues. With large or repeated doses these tissues begin to accumulate Fentanyl. Eventually, the duration of Fentanyl effects becomes dependent on clearance of the drug from these tissue reservoirs by metabolic elimination, a slower process than redistribution (see *"Pharmacokinetics"*).

In clinical studies of Fentanyl citrate oral transmucosal, both the beneficial effect of the medication and the adverse effect of opioid-induced hypoventilation were related to the dose of Fentanyl administered.

Ventilatory Effects: In both children and adults, respiratory rate and oxygen saturation typically decrease as Fentanyl concentration increases. At equivalent analgesic serum concentrations, Fentanyl and morphine produce a similar degree of hypoventilation. A small number of patients have experienced clinically significant hypoventilation with Fentanyl. Hypoventilation was manifest by respiratory rates of less than 8 breaths/minute or a pCO_2 greater than 55 mm Hg. In clinical trials of 357 postoperative (acute pain) patients treated with Fentanyl, 13 patients experienced hypoventilation. As a consequence, 10 of these 13 patients received naloxone, two patients had their dose reduced and one patient required no treatment beyond verbal stimulation. Of the 13 events, seven were associated with Fentanyl 100 μg/h and six were associated with Fentanyl 75 μg/h. In these studies the incidence of hypoventilation was higher in nontolerant women (10) than in men (3) and in patients weighing less than 63 kg (9 of 13). Although patients with impaired respiration were not common in the trials, they had higher rates of hypoventilation.

While most patients using Fentanyl Transdermal System chronically develop tolerance to Fentanyl induced hypoventilation, episodes of slowed respirations may occur at any time during therapy; medical intervention generally was not required in these instances.

Typically, peak respiratory depressant effects (decrease in respiratory rate) are seen 15 to 30 minutes from the start of Fentanyl citrate oral transmucosal administration, but such effects may persist for several hours.

Hypoventilation can occur throughout the therapeutic range of Fentanyl serum concentrations. However, the risk of hypoventilation increases at serum Fentanyl concentrations greater than 2 ng/mL in non opioid-tolerant patients, especially for patients who have an underlying pulmonary condition or who receive usual doses of opioids or other CNS drugs associated with hypoventilation in addition to Fentanyl. The use of Fentanyl transdermal system should be monitored by clinical evaluation. As with other drug level measurements, serum Fentanyl concentrations may be useful clinically, although they do not reflect patient sensitivity to Fentanyl and should not be used by physicians as a sole indicator of effectiveness or toxicity.

See *"Warnings," "Precautions"* and *"Overdosage"* for additional information on hypoventilation.

Cardiovascular Effects: Intravenous Fentanyl may infrequently produce bradycardia. The incidence of bradycardia in clinical trials with Fentanyl Transdermal System was less than 1%.

CNS Effects: In opioid naive patients, central nervous system effects increase when serum Fentanyl concentrations are greater than 3 ng/mL.

CLINICAL TRIALS

Fentanyl Transdermal System was studied in patients with acute and chronic pain (postoperative and cancer pain models).

The analgesic efficacy of Fentanyl was demonstrated in an acute pain model with surgical procedures expected to produce various intensities of pain (eg hysterectomy, major orthopedic surgery). Clinical use and safety was evaluated in patients experiencing chronic pain due to malignancy. Based on the results of these trials, Fentanyl was determined to be effective in both populations, but safe only for use in patients with chronic pain. Because of the risk of hypoventilation (4% incidence) in postoperative patients with acute pain, Fentanyl Transdermal System should not be used for postoperative analgesia. (See box *"Warning"* and *"Contraindications"*.)

Fentanyl Transdermal System as therapy for pain due to cancer has been studied in 153 patients. In this patient population, Fentanyl has been administered in doses of 25 μg/h to 600 μg/h. Individual patients have used Fentanyl continuously for up to 866 days. At one month after initiation of Fentanyl therapy, patients generally reported lower pain intensity scores as compared to a prestudy analgesic regimen of oral morphine.

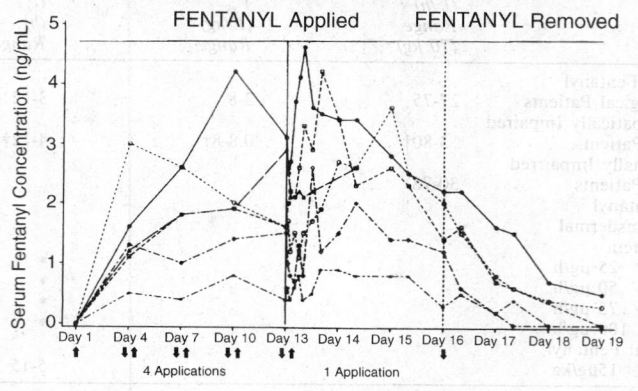

Serum Fentanyl Concentrations Following Multiple Applications of Fentanyl 100 μg/h

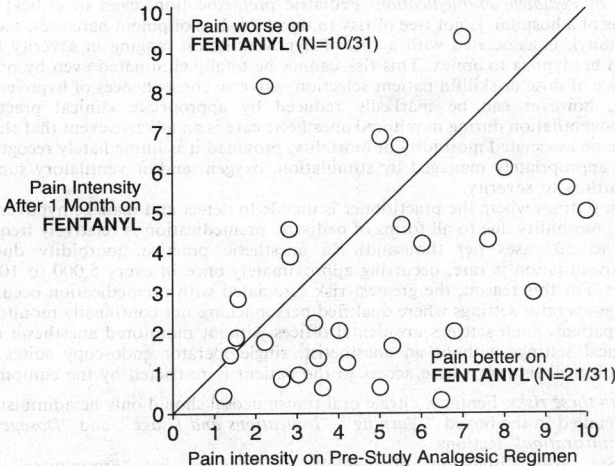

Visual Analogue Score of Pain Intesity Rating at Entry in the Study and After One Month of Fentanyl Use.

Anesthetic Premedication: The efficacy of Fentanyl citrate oral transmucosal was investigated in five randomized, placebo-controlled, clinical trials as premedication for various pediatric surgical procedures (cardiovascular, orthopedic, urological, and general surgery). Single Fentanyl citrate oral transmucosal doses of 5 to 20 µg/kg (18 to 30 patients per treatment group) were compared to placebo in patients 2 to 18 years old. Patients receiving Fentanyl citrate oral transmucosal were significantly more sedated than patients receiving placebo. Median time to peak sedative effect was 30 minutes. Generally, intraoperative and postoperative analgesics were less frequently required in the Fentanyl citrate oral transmucosal group.

The efficacy of Fentanyl citrate oral transmucosal was also compared to an oral solution of meperidine 1.5 mg/kg, diazepam 0.2 mg/kg, and atropine 0.02 mg/kg (MDA solution) as premedication in pediatric patients undergoing cardiovascular surgery. In a study with 20 patients per treatment group, Fentanyl citrate oral transmucosal 20 to 25 µg/kg was compared to MDA solution. In that study, a high incidence of nausea and vomiting suggested that **20 to 25 µg/kg was an excessive Fentanyl citrate oral transmucosal dose.** A second study in patients with Fentanyl citrate oral transmucosal dose of 15 to 20 µg/kg found that Fentanyl citrate oral transmucosal was similar in efficacy to MDA solution without the excessive vomiting seen in the first study.

The efficacy of Fentanyl citrate oral transmucosal with and without droperidol was also compared to placebo in pediatric general surgery patients. Fentanyl citrate oral transmucosal was administered in doses of 15 to 20 µg/kg with and without droperidol 50 µg/kg versus placebo (also with and without droperidol). Use of Fentanyl citrate oral transmucosal was associated with improved induction and a reduced use of post operative opioids. Droperidol reduced the incidence of nausea and vomiting associated with Fentanyl citrate oral transmucosal, but the combination of droperidol and Fentanyl citrate oral transmucosal resulted in a significantly delayed awakening (the combination of droperidol and Fentanyl citrate oral transmucosal doubled the awakening time after surgery from that of Fentanyl citrate oral transmucosal alone) (see *"Precautions, Drug Interactions"*).

Despite the provision of gentle, non-pharmacologic reassurance to all patients, in placebo-controlled studies of a total of 496 children, 42% of patients administered placebo remained apprehensive 30 minutes following administration of the placebo. Doses of 5 to 10 µg/kg of Fentanyl citrate oral transmucosal reduced the number of apprehensive patients at 30 minutes post drug administration from 42% in the placebo group to about 7% in the Fentanyl citrate oral transmucosal group. Larger doses provided no apparent gain in efficacy, but substantially increased the frequency of adverse events.

About 10 to 20% of the patients who were studied pre-operatively had symptoms of apprehension that were so severe as to unequivocally need premedication. In those cases, Fentanyl citrate oral transmucosal, in doses of 5 to 15 µg/kg produced a dose-related reduction in apprehension that was suffficient to allow a calm, manageable induction of anesthesia within 20 to 30 minutes. Doses above 5 µg/kg (10 and 15 µg/kg) were more effective in managing the already apprehensive patient but were associated with a dose-dependent increase in pruritus, vomiting and hypoventilation.

Conscious Sedation In a Monitored Anesthesia Care Setting: Conscious sedation in a monitored anesthesia care setting in the hospital is commonly required in a patient needing to undergo a painful diagnostic or therapeutic procedure. Fentanyl citrate oral transmucosal has been evaluated for such monitored anesthesia care outside the operating room environment in two open trials. Eight (8) adult and 34 pediatric patients have been administered Fentanyl citrate oral transmucosal 10 to 20 µg/kg as a premedicant in the emergency room. Patients who were administered 10 to 15 µg/kg had increased levels of sedation similar to patients administered 15 to 20 µg/kg. However, the lower dose range of 10 to 15 µg/kg was associated with a lower risk of adverse effects. Onset of analgesia occurred at approximately 6 to 8 minutes following Fentanyl citrate oral transmucosal.

In a double-blind, placebo-controlled trial, Fentanyl citrate oral transmucosal 15 to 20 µg/kg was administered to 31 pediatric oncology patients prior to undergoing a painful diagnostic or therapeutic procedure. Some of these children had previous opioid experience. Of the patients who received Fentanyl citrate oral transmucosal, 68% became more sedate over 30 minutes compared to 26% of the patients who received placebo. Median time to peak effect in these patients was 20 minutes.

Because of the risk of hypoventilation, the lowest effective dose of Fentanyl citrate oral transmucosal should be used, and it should be administered only in monitored settings and by persons specifically trained in the use of anesthetics and the mangement of the respiratory effects of potent opioids, including the establishment and maintenance of a patent airway and assisted ventilation.

INDICATIONS AND USAGE
Fentanyl Transdermal System is indicated in the management of chronic pain in patients who require continuous opioid analgesia for pain that cannot be managed by lesser means such as acetaminophen-opioid combinations, non-steroidal analgesics, or PRN dosing with short-acting opioids.

Fentanyl should not be used in the management of acute or postoperative pain because serious or life-threatening hypoventilation could result. (See box *"Warning"* and *"Contraindications"*.)

In patients with chronic pain, it is possible to individually titrate the dose of the transdermal system to minimize the risk of adverse effects while providing analgesia. In properly selected patients, Fentanyl is a safe and effective alternative to other opioid regimens. (See *"Dosage and Administration"*.)

Fentanyl Citrate injection is indicated:

—for analgesic action of short duration during the anesthetic periods, premedication, induction and maintenance, and in the immediate postoperative period (recovery room) as the need arises.

—for use as a narcotic analgesic supplement in general or regional anesthesia.

—for administration with a neuroleptic such as droperidol injection as an anesthetic premedication, for the induction of anesthesia and as an adjunct in the maintenance of general and regional anesthesia.

—for use as an anesthetic agent with oxygen in selected high risk patients, such as those undergoing open heart surgery or certain complicated neurological or orthopedic procedures.

Fentanyl citrate oral transmucosal is only indicated for use in a hospital setting (1) as an anesthetic premedication in the operating room setting or (2) to induce conscious sedation prior to a diagnostic or therapeutic procedure in other monitored anesthesia care settings in the hospital. Appropriate monitored anesthesia care settings are described immediately below and in the boxed *"Warning"*. Doses must be chosen that minimize the risk of hypoventilation (see *"Dosage and Administration"* and *"Warnings"*.)

Caution: BEFORE ADMINISTERING THIS PRODUCT, PLEASE NOTE THE FOLLOWING INSTRUCTIONS ON THE PROPER USE OF THIS PRODUCT:

Fentanyl citrate oral transmucosal should only be administered in hospital settings such as the operating room, emergency department, ICU, or other monitored anesthesia care settings in hospitals where there is immediate access to life support equipment, including oxygen, facilities for endotracheal intubation, intravenous fluids, and opioid antagonists.

Fentanyl citrate oral transmucosal must be given only to patients being monitored by both (1) direct visual observation by a health professional whose sole responsibility is observation of the patient and also by (2) some means of measuring respiratory functon such as pulse oximetry until they are completely recovered.

Fentanyl citrate oral transmucosal should only be administered by persons specifically trained in the use of anesthetic drugs and the management of the respiratory effects of potent opioids, including respiratory and cardiac resuscitation of patients in the age group being treated. Such training must include the establishment and maintenance of a patent airway and assisted ventilation. This product should only be used by health care practitioners credentialed to use the product by the director of anesthesia of the institution in which the product will be used.

(See also box *"Warnings"*, *"Clinical Pharmacology"*, and *"Precautions"*.)

CONTRAINDICATIONS
BECAUSE SERIOUS OR LIFE-THREATENING HYPOVENTILATION COULD OCCUR, FENTANYL TRANSDERMAL SYSTEM IS CONTRAINDICATED:

■ in the management of acute or postoperative pain, including use in outpatient surgeries because there is no opportunity for proper dose titration. (See *"Clinical Pharmacology"* and *"Dosage and Administration."*)

■ in the management of mild or intermittent pain that can otherwise be managed by lesser means such as acetaminophen-opioid combinations, nonsteroidal analgesics, or PRN dosing with short-acting opioids, and

■ in doses exceeding 25 µg/hour at the initiation of opioid therapy because of the need to individualize dosing by titrating to the desired analgesic effect.

Fentanyl Transdermal System is also contraindicated in patients with known hypersensitivity to Fentanyl or adhesives.

Fentanyl Citrate Injection is contraindicated in patients with known intolerance to the drug.

Fentanyl citrate oral transmucosal is contraindicated:

■ in children who weigh less than 15 kg (33 lb.).

■ for use at home or in any other setting outside a hospital.

■ for the treatment of acute or chronic pain because the safety of this product for use in these indications has not been established.

■ in doses above 15 µg/kg in children, and in doses above 5 µg/kg in adults. Because of the excessive frequency of significant hypoventilation at higher doses, the maximum dose any child or adult should receive is 400 µg, regardless of weight.

■ in patients with known intolerance or hypersensitivity to any of its components or the drug Fentanyl.

WARNINGS

FENTANYL TRANSDERMAL SYSTEM SHOULD NOT BE ADMINISTERED TO CHILDREN UNDER 12 YEARS OF AGE OR PATIENTS UNDER 18 YEARS OF AGE WHO WEIGH LESS THAN 50 KG (110 LBS) EXCEPT IN AN AUTHORIZED INVESTIGATIONAL RESEARCH SETTING. (SEE "PRECAUTIONS, PEDIATRIC USE.")
PATIENTS WHO HAVE EXPERIENCED ADVERSE EVENTS SHOULD BE MONITORED FOR AT LEAST 12 HOURS AFTER FENTANYL TRANSDERMAL SYSTEM REMOVAL SINCE SERUM FENTANYL CONCENTRATIONS DECLINE GRADUALLY AND REACH AN APPROXIMATE 50% REDUCTION IN SERUM CONCENTRATIONS 17 HOURS AFTER SYSTEM REMOVAL.

FENTANYL TRANSDERMAL SYSTEM SHOULD BE PRESCRIBED ONLY BY PERSONS KNOWLEDGEABLE IN THE CONTINUOUS ADMINISTRATION OF POTENT OPIOIDS, IN THE MANAGEMENT OF PATIENTS RECEIVING POTENT OPIOIDS FOR TREATMENT OF PAIN, AND IN THE DETECTION AND MANAGEMENT OF HYPOVENTILATION INCLUDING THE USE OF OPIOID ANTAGONISTS.

THE CONCOMITANT USE OF OTHER CENTRAL NERVOUS SYSTEM DEPRESSANTS, INCLUDING OTHER OPIOIDS, SEDATIVES OR HYPNOTICS, GENERAL ANESTHETICS, PHENOTHIAZINES, TRANQUILIZERS, SKELETAL MUSCLE RELAXANTS, SEDATING ANTIHISTAMINES, AND ALCOHOLIC BEVERAGES WITH FENTANYL TRANSDERMAL SYSTEM OR FENTANYL CITRATE INJECTION MAY PRODUCE ADDITIVE DEPRESSANT EFFECTS. HYPOVENTILATION, HYPOTENSION AND PROFOUND SEDATION OR COMA MAY OCCUR. WHEN SUCH COMBINED THERAPY IS CONTEMPLATED, THE DOSE OF ONE OR BOTH AGENTS SHOULD BE REDUCED BY AT LEAST 50%.

ALL PATIENTS SHOULD BE ADVISED TO AVOID EXPOSING THE FENTANYL TRANSDERMAL SYSTEM APPLICATION SITE TO DIRECT EXTERNAL HEAT SOURCES, SUCH AS HEATING PADS OR ELECTRIC BLANKETS, HEAT LAMPS, SAUNAS AND HOT TUBS, ETC, WHILE WEARING THE SYSTEM. THERE IS A POTENTIAL FOR TEMPERATURE-DEPENDENT INCREASES IN FENTANYL RELEASE FROM THE SYSTEM. (See "Precautions, Patients with Fever/External Heat.").

FENTANYL CITRATE SHOULD BE ADMINISTERED ONLY BY PERSONS SPECIFICALLY TRAINED IN THE USE OF INTRAVENOUS ANESTHETICS AND MANAGEMENT OF THE RESPIRATORY EFFECTS OF POTENT OPIOIDS.

AN OPIOID ANTAGONIST, RESUSCITATIVE AND INTUBATION EQUIPMENT AND OXYGEN SHOULD BE READILY AVAILABLE.

See also discussion of narcotic antagonists in "Precautions" and "Overdosage".

If Fentanyl Citrate is administered with a tranquilizer such as droperidol or a sedative, the user should become familiar with the special properties of each drug or the combinations of opioids and other CNS depressants, particularly the widely differing or extended duration of action. In addition, when such a combination is used, fluids and other countermeasures to manage hypotension should be available.

As with other potent narcotics, the respiratory depressant effect of Fentanyl Citrate may persist longer than the measured analgesic effect. The total dose of all narcotic analgesics administered should be considered by the practitioner before ordering narcotic analgesics during recovery from anesthesia. It is recommended that narcotics, when required, should be used in reduced doses initially, as low as ¼ to ⅓ those usually recommended.

Fentanyl Citrate may cause muscle rigidity, particularly involving the muscles of respiration. This rigidity has been reported to occur or recur infrequently in the extended postoperative period usually following high dose intravenous administration. In addition, skeletal muscle movements of various groups in the extremities, neck and external eye have been reported during induction of anesthesia with Fentanyl; these reported movements have, on rare occasions, been strong enough to pose patient management problems. This effect is related to the dose and speed of injection and its incidence can be reduced by: 1) administration of up to ¼ of the full paralyzing dose of a nondepolarizing neuromuscular blocking agent just prior to intravenous administration of Fentanyl citrate; 2) administration of a full paralyzing dose of a neuromuscular blocking agent following loss of eyelash reflex when Fentanyl citrate is used in anesthetic doses titrated by slow intravenous infusion; or, 3) simultaneous intravenous administration of Fentanyl citrate and a full paralyzing dose of a neuromuscular blocking agent when Fentanyl citrate is used in rapidly administered anesthetic dosages. The neuromuscular blocking agent used should be compatible with the patient's cardiovascular status.

Although muscle rigidity interfering with respiration has not been seen following the use of Fentanyl citrate oral transmucosal, the possibility of it happening should be kept in mind. If it occurs, it should be managed by the use of assisted or controlled respiration, by an opioid antagonist, and as a final alternative, by a neuromuscular blocking agent.

Adequate facilities should be available for postoperative monitoring and ventilation of patients administered anesthetic doses of Fentanyl citrate. Where moderate or high doses are used (above 10 µg/kg), there must be adequate facilities for postoperative observation, and ventilation if necessary, of patients who have received Fentanyl Citrate. It is essential that these facilities be fully equipped to handle all degrees of respiratory depression.

Use in Pediatric Premedication: Pediatric premedication, even in critical care areas of a hospital, is not free of risk to the child. Use of potent narcotics, such as Fentanyl, is associated with a risk of hypoventilation ranging in severity from mild bradypnea to apnea. This risk cannot be totally eliminated even by proper choice of dose or skillful patient selection. Adverse consequences of hypoventilation, however can be markedly reduced by appropriate clinical practices. Hypoventilation during monitored anesthetic care is an adverse event that should have no associated morbidity or mortality, provided it is immediately recognized and appropriately managed by stimulation, oxygen, and/or ventilatory support according to severity.

In settings where the practitioner is unable to detect and manage hypoventilation, morbidity due to all forms of pediatric premedication is relatively frequent (10 to 50 cases per thousand). In anesthetic practice, morbidity due to hypoventilation is rare, occurring approximately once in every 5,000 to 10,000 cases. For this reason, the greatest risk associated with premedication occurs in single-operator settings where qualified personnel are not continually monitoring the patient. Such settings are dental offices without monitored anesthesia care, surgical settings without an anesthetist, single-operator endoscopy suites and radiological settings where access to the patient is restricted by the equipment.

Given these risks: Fentanyl citrate oral transmucosal should only be administered as detailed in the boxed "Warning", "Indications and Usage", and "Dosage and Administration" sections.

(See also discussion of narcotic antagonists in "Precautions" and "Overdosage".)

Fentanyl citrate may also produce other signs and symptoms characteristic of narcotic analgesics including euphoria, miosis, bradycardia and bronchoconstriction.

Severe and unpredictable potentiation by MAO inhibitors has been reported for other narcotic analgesics. Although this has not been reported for Fentanyl, there are insufficient data to establish that this does not occur with Fentanyl. Therefore, when Fentanyl is administered to patients who have received MAO inhibitors within 14 days, appropriate monitoring and ready availability of vasodilators and beta-blockers for the treatment of hypertension is indicated.

Cases of self-administration of Fentanyl by health care professionals, including fatalities, have been reported with all Fentanyl products. The handling of Fentanyl Citrate oral transmucosal should be managed to minimize the risk of diversion, including restriction of access to the appropriate clinical setting and accounting procedures as required by law.

Head Injuries and Increased Intracranial Pressure: Fentanyl citrate should be used with caution in patients who may be particularly susceptible to respiratory depression, such as comatose patients who may have a head injury or brain tumor. In addition, Fentanyl citrate may obscure the clinical course of patients with head injury.

PRECAUTIONS
GENERAL
Fentanyl doses greater than 25 µg/h are too high for initiation of therapy in non opioid-tolerant patients and should not be used to begin Fentanyl transdermal system therapy in these patients. (See box "Warning.")

The initial dose of Fentanyl citrate oral transmucosal should be appropriately individualized by assessing the clinical status of the patient in regard to the desired clinical effect(s). The effect(s) of the initial dose should be considered in subsequent administration of any additional CNS depressive agents.

Fentanyl may impair mental and/or physical ability required for the performance of potentially hazardous tasks (e.g. driving, operating machinery). Patients who have been given Fentanyl should not drive or operate dangerous machinery unless they are tolerant to the side effects of the drug.

Patients should be instructed to keep both used and unused transdermal systems out of the reach of children. Used systems should be folded so that the adhesive side of the system adheres to itself and flushed down the toilet immediately upon removal. Patients should be advised to dispose of any systems remaining from a prescription as soon as they are no longer needed. Unused systems should be removed from their pouch and flushed down the toilet.

The initial dose of Fentanyl citrate should be appropriately reduced in elderly and debilitated patients. The effect of the initial dose should be considered in determining incremental doses.

Nitrous oxide has been reported to produce cardiovascular depression when given with higher doses of Fentanyl citrate. Certain forms of conduction anesthesia, such as spinal anesthesia and some peridural anesthetics, can alter respiration by blocking intercostal nerves. Through other mechanisms (see "Clinical Pharmacology") Fentanyl citrate can also alter respiration. Therefore, when Fentanyl citrate is used to supplement these forms of anesthesia, the anesthetist should be familiar with the physiological alterations involved, and be prepared to manage them in the patients selected for these forms of anesthesia.

When a tranquilizer such as droperidol is used with Fentanyl citrate, pulmonary arterial pressure may be decreased. This fact should be considered by those who conduct diagnostic and surgical procedures where interpretation of pulmonary arterial pressure measurements might determine final management of the patient. When high dose or anesthetic dosages of Fentanyl citrate are employed, even relatively small dosages of diazepam may cause cardiovascular depression.

When Fentanyl citrate is used with a tranquilizer such as droperidol, hypotension can occur. If it occurs, the possibility of hypovolemia should also be considered and managed with appropriate parenteral fluid therapy. Repositioning the patient to improve venous return to the heart should be considered when operative conditions permit. Care should be exercised in moving and positioning of patients because of the possibility of orthostatic hypotension. If volume expansion with fluids plus other countermeasures do not correct hypotension, the administration of pressor agents other than epinephrine should be considered. Because of the alpha-adrenergic blocking action of droperidol, epinephrine may paradoxically decrease the blood pressure in patients treated with droperidol.

Elevated blood pressure, with and without pre-existing hypertension, has been reported following administration of Fentanyl citrate combined with droperidol. This might be due to unexplained alterations in sympathetic activity following large doses; however, it is also frequently attributed to anesthetic and surgical stimulation during light anesthesia.

When droperidol is used with Fentanyl Citrate and the EEG is used for postoperative monitoring, it may be found that the EEG pattern returns to normal slowly.

Vital signs should be monitored routinely.

Respiratory depression caused by opioid analgesics can be reversed by opioid antagonists such as naloxone. Because the duration of respiratory depression produced by Fentanyl citrate may last longer than the duration of the opioid antagonist action, appropriate surveillance should be maintained. As with all potent opioids, profound analgesia is accompanied by respiratory depression and diminished sensitivity to CO_2 stimulation which may persist into or recur in the postoperative period. Respiratory depression secondary to chest wall rigidity has been reported in the postoperative period. Intraoperative hyperventilation may further alter postoperative response to CO_2. Appropriate postoperative monitoring should be employed to ensure that adequate spontaneous breathing is established and maintained in the absence of stimulation prior to discharging the patient from the recovery area.

Rare cases of unexplained clinically significant methemoglobinemia have been reported in premature neonates undergoing emergency anesthesia and surgery which included combined use of Fentanyl, pancuronium and atropine. A direct cause and effect relationship between the combined use of these drugs and the reported cases of methemoglobinemia has not been established.

HYPOVENTILATION (RESPIRATORY DEPRESSION)
Hypoventilation may occur at any time during the use of Fentanyl transdermal system.

Because significant amounts of Fentanyl are absorbed from the skin for 17 hours or more after the system is removed, hypoventilation may persist beyond the removal of Fentanyl transdermal system. Consequently, patients with hypoventilation should be carefully observed for degree of sedation and their respiratory rate monitored until respiration has stabilized.

The use of concomitant CNS active drugs requires special patient care and observation. See "Warnings".

CHRONIC PULMONARY DISEASE
Because potent opioids can cause hypoventilation, Fentanyl Transdermal System should be administered with caution to patients with preexisting medical conditions predisposing them to hypoventilation. Similarly, Fentanyl citrate oral transmucosal should be used with caution in patients with chronic obstructive pulmonary disease, patients with decreased respiratory reserve, and others with potentially compromised respiration. In all such patients, normal analgesic doses of opioids may further increase airway resistance and decrease respiratory drive to the point of respiratory failure. During anesthesia, this can be managed by assisted or controlled respiration. As with many opioid drugs, Fentanyl can cause histamine release in some patients, which may be of clinical significance in patients with asthma or other reactive airway disorders.

HEAD INJURIES AND INCREASED INTRACRANIAL PRESSURE
Fentanyl should not be used in patients who may be particularly susceptible to the intracranial effects of CO_2 retention such as those with evidence of increased intracranial pressure, impaired consciousness, or coma. Opioids may obscure the clinical course of patients with head injury. Fentanyl should be used with caution in patients with brain tumors.

CARDIAC DISEASE
Intravenous Fentanyl may produce bradycardia, which may be treated with atropine. Fentanyl and Fentanyl citrate should be administered with caution to patients with bradyarrhythmias. As with other opioids, orthostatic hypotension is possible.

HEPATIC OR RENAL DISEASE
At the present time insufficient information exists to make recommendations regarding the use of Fentanyl in patients with impaired renal or hepatic function. If the drug is used in these patients, it should be used with caution because of the hepatic metabolism and renal excretion of Fentanyl.

PATIENTS WITH FEVER/EXTERNAL HEAT
Based on a pharmacokinetic model, serum Fentanyl concentrations could theoretically increase by approximately one third for patients with a body temperature of 40°C (102°F) due to temperature-dependent increases in Fentanyl release from the system and increased skin permeability. Therefore, patients wearing Fentanyl systems who develop fever should be monitored for opioid side effects and the Fentanyl dose should be adjusted if necessary.

ALL PATIENTS SHOULD BE ADVISED TO AVOID EXPOSING THE DURAGESIC APPLICATION SITE TO DIRECT EXTERNAL HEAT SOURCES, SUCH AS HEATING PADS OR ELECTRIC BLANKETS, HEAT LAMPS, SAUNAS AND HOT TUBS, ETC. WHILE WEARING THE SYSTEM. THERE IS A POTENTIAL FOR TEMPERATURE-DEPENDENT INCREASES IN FENTANYL RELEASE FROM THE SYSTEM.

USE OF ANESTHESIA
Certain forms of conduction anesthesia, such as spinal anesthesia and some peridural anesthetics can alter respiration by blocking intercostal nerves. Through other mechanisms (see "Clinical Pharmacology") Fentanyl can also alter respiration. Therefore, when Fentanyl citrate oral transmucosal is used before these forms of anesthesia, the anesthesia provider must be familiar with the physiological alterations involved, and be prepared to manage them in the patients selected for these forms of anesthesia.

Nitrous oxide has been reported to produce cardiovascular depression when given with higher doses of IV Fentanyl.

Elevated blood pressure in patients with and without preexisting hypertension has been reported following administration of Fentanyl Citrate combined with droperidol. This might be due to unexplained alterations in sympathetic activity following large doses; however, it is also frequently attributed to anesthesia and surgical stimulation during light anesthesia.

USE IN AMBULATORY SURGERY
Orthostatic hypotension has been observed following the use of Fentanyl in the ambulatory setting. Therefore, if Fentanyl citrate oral transmucosal is used, care should be exercised in moving and positioning patients preoperatively, intraoperatively, and postoperatively, and fluid status should be evaluated prior to discharge.

USE OF NARCOTIC ANTAGONISTS
Respiratory depression caused by opioid analgesics can be reversed by opioid antagonists. Because the duration of respiratory depression may be longer than the duration of the narcotic antagonist action, appropriate surveillance should be maintained. (Consult relevant prescribing information before employing narcotic antagonists.) Opioid analgesia is often accompanied by respiratory depression and diminished sensitivity to CO_2 stimulation that may persist into or recur in the postoperative period. Intraoperative hyperventilation may further alter postoperative response to CO_2. Appropriate postoperative monitoring should be employed to ensure that adequate spontaneous breathing is established and maintained in the absence of stimulation prior to discharging the patient from the recovery area.

CENTRAL NERVOUS SYSTEM DEPRESSANTS
When patients are receiving Fentanyl, the dose of additional opioids or other CNS depressant drugs (including benzodiazepines) should be reduced by at least 50%. With the concomitant use of CNS depressants, hypotension may occur.

DRUG OR ALCOHOL DEPENDENCE
Use of Fentanyl in combination with alcoholic beverages and/or other CNS depressants can result in increased risk to the patient. Fentanyl should be used with caution in individuals who have a history of drug or alcohol abuse, especially if they are outside a medically controlled environment.

AMBULATORY PATIENTS
Strong opioid analgesics impair the mental or physical abilities required for the performance of potentially dangerous tasks such as driving a car or operating machinery. Patients who have been given Fentanyl should not drive or operate dangerous machinery unless they are tolerant to the effects of the drug.

LABORATORY TEST
Fentanyl citrate oral transmucosal is without known effect on common laboratory tests, but may produce hypoxia, respiratory acidosis, and hypercarbia if given in doses that depress respiration.

DRUG INTERACTIONS
For use with other potent narcotics, please see "Warnings."

Fentanyl is not recommended for use in patients who have received MAO inhibitors within 14 days, because severe and unpredictable potentiation by MAO inhibitors has been reported with narcotic analgesics.

Other CNS depressant drugs (e.g., barbiturates, tranquilizers, narcotics and general anesthetics) have additive or potentiating effect with Fentanyl. When patients have received such drugs, the dose of Fentanyl required may be less than usual. Likewise, following the administration of Fentanyl, the dose of other CNS depressant drugs should be reduced.

The particular enzyme(s) responsible for Fentanyl biotransformation has (have) not been identified even though the major metabolites are well known. Because swallowed Fentanyl is known to undergo extensive hepatic first-pass metabolism, Fentanyl Citrate oral transmucosal has the potential to have an increased bioavailability in the presence of an inhibitor of drug metabolism, e.g., a food component or another drug. Caution should therefore be exercised in such cases.

The combination of droperidol and Fentanyl Citrate oral transmucosal results in a significantly delayed awakening (the combination of droperidol and Fentanyl Citrate oral transmucosal doubled the awakening time after surgery from that of Fentanyl Citrate oral transmucosal alone.)

Nitrous oxide has been reported to produce cardiovascular depression when given with higher doses of IV Fentanyl.

CARCINOGENESIS, MUTAGENESIS, AND IMPAIRMENT OF FERTILITY

Because long-term animal studies have not been conducted, the potential carcinogenic effects of Fentanyl are unknown. There was no evidence of mutagenicity in the Ames Salmonella mutagenicity assay, the primary rat hepatocyte unscheduled DNA synthesis assay, the BALB/c-3T3 transformation test, and the human lymphocyte and CHO chromosomal aberration *in-vitro* assays.

In the mouse lymphoma assay, Fentanyl concentrations 2000 times greater than those seen with chronic Fentanyl use were only mutagenic in the presence of metabolic activation.

Reproduction studies in rats revealed a significant decrease in the pregnancy rate of all experimental groups. This decrease was most pronounced in the high dose group (1.25 mg/kg—12.5 × human dose) in which one of twenty animals became pregnant. This high dose is approximately 180 × the maximum recommended human dose of 400 mcg for a 60-kg patient.

PREGNANCY—PREGNANCY CATEGORY C

Fentanyl has been shown to impair fertility and to have an embryocidal effect in rats when given for a period of 12 to 21 days in doses of 30 μg/kg IV or 160 μg/kg SC, equivalent to 4 and 23 times, respectively, the maximum recommended human dose. No evidence of teratogenic effects has been observed after administration of Fentanyl to rats. There are no adequate and well-controlled studies in pregnant women. Fentanyl should be used during pregnancy only if the potential benefit justifies the potential risk to the fetus.

LABOR AND DELIVERY

Fentanyl is not recommended for analgesia during labor and delivery.

NURSING MOTHERS

Fentanyl is excreted in human milk; therefore Fentanyl is not recommended for use in nursing women because of the possibility of effects in their infants.

PEDIATRIC USE

The safety and efficacy of Fentanyl Transdermal System in children, or of Fentanyl citrate injection or oral transmucosal in children under 2 years of age, have not been established. (See box *"Warning"* and *"Contraindications."*)

Fentanyl transdermal system should not be administered to children under 12 years of age or patients under 18 years of age who weight less than 50 kg (110 lbs) except in an authorized investigational research setting.

Use of Fentanyl citrate oral transmucosal in children than 15 kg weight is contraindicated as an appropriate dose cannot be administered with the present presentations of this product.

Safety and effectiveness of Fentanyl citrate oral transmucosal in children who weigh less than 15 kilograms have not been established (see *"Dosage and Administration."*)

GERIATRIC USE

Information from a pilot study of the pharmacokinetics of IV Fentanyl in geriatric patients indicates that the clearance of Fentanyl may be greatly decreased in the population above the age of 60. The relevance of these findings to transdermal Fentanyl is unknown at this time.

Since elderly, cachectic, or debilitated patients may have altered pharmacokinetics due to poor fat stores, muscle wasting or altered clearance, they should not be started on Fentanyl doses higher than 25 μg/h unless they are already taking more than 135 mg of oral morphine a day or an equivalent dose of another opioid (see *"Dosage and Administration"*).

If Fentanyl citrate oral transmucosal is to be used in patients over age 65, the dose should be reduced to 2.5 to 5 μg/kg. Although studies of Fentanyl citrate oral transmucosal in the elderly have not been conducted, elderly patients have been shown to be twice as sensitive as the younger population to the effects of the forms of Fentanyl. Caution is indicated because, like all potent opioids, Fentanyl citrate oral transmucosal has the ability to depress respiration and reduce ventilatory drive to a clinically significant extent.

INFORMATION FOR PATIENTS

Instructions for the application, removal, and disposal of Fentanyl transdermal system are provided in each carton.

DISPOSAL OF FENTANYL TRANSDERMAL SYSTEM

Fentanyl transdermal system should be kept out of the reach of children. Fentanyl Transdermal Systems should be folded so that the adhesive side of the system adheres to itself, then the system should be flushed down the toilet immediately upon removal. Patients should dispose of any systems remaining from a prescription as soon as they are no longer needed. Unused systems should be removed from their pouch and flushed down the toilet.

If the gel from the drug reservoir accidentally contacts the skin, the area should be washed with clear water.

ADVERSE REACTIONS

FENTANYL TRANSDERMAL SYSTEM

In post-marketing experience, deaths from hypoventilation due to inappropriate use of Fentanyl Transdermal System have been reported.

(See box *"Warning"* and *"Contraindications."*)

PREMARKETING CLINICAL TRIAL EXPERIENCE

The safety of Fentanyl Transdermal System has been evaluated in 357 postoperative patients and 153 cancer patients for a total of 510 patients. Patients with acute pain used Fentanyl Transdermal System for 1 to 3 days. The duration of Fentanyl Transdermal System use varied in cancer patients. 56% of patients used Fentanyl Transdermal System for over 30 days, 28% continued treatment for more than 4 months, and 10% used Fentanyl Transdermal System for more than 1 year.

Hypoventilation was the most serious adverse reaction observed in 13 (4%) postoperative patients and in 3 (2%) of the cancer patients. Hypotension and hypertension were observed in 11 (3%) and 4 (1%) of the opioid-naive patients.

Various adverse events were reported; a causal relationship to Fentanyl Transdermal System was not always determined. The frequencies presented here reflect the actual frequency of each adverse effect in patients who received Fentanyl. There has been no attempt to correct for a placebo effect, concomitant use of other opioids, or to subtract the frequencies reported by placebo-treated patients in controlled trials.

The following adverse reactions were reported in 153 cancer patients at a frequency of 1% or greater; similar reactions were seen in the 357 postoperative patients studied.

Body as a Whole: abdominal pain*, headache*

Cardiovascular: arrhythmia, chest pain

Digestive: nausea**, vomiting**, constipation**, dry mouth**, anorexia*, diarrhea*, dyspepsia*, flatulence

Nervous: somnolence**, confusion,** asthenia**, dizziness*, nervousness*, hallucinations*, anxiety*, depression*, euphoria*, tremor, abnormal coordination, speech disorder, abnormal thinking, abnormal gait, abnormal dreams, agitation, paresthesia, amnesia, syncope, paranoid reaction

Respiratory: dyspnea*, hypoventilation*, apnea*, hemoptysis, pharyngitis, hiccups

Skin and Appendages: sweating**, pruritus*, rash, application site reaction - erythema, papules, itching, edema

Urogenital: urinary retention*

The following adverse effects have been reported in less than 1% of the 510 postoperative and cancer patients studied; the association between these events and Fentanyl Transdermal System administration is unknown. This information is listed to serve as alerting information for the physician.

Digestive: abdominal distention

Nervous: aphasia, hypertonia, vertigo, stupor, hypotonia, depersonalization, hostility

Respiratory: stertorous breathing, asthma, respiratory disorder

Skin and Appendages, General: exfoliative dermatitis, pustules

Special Senses: amblyopia

Urogenital: bladder pain, oliguria, urinary frequency

FENTANYL CITRATE INJECTION

As with other narcotic analgesics, the most common serious adverse reactions reported to occur with Fentanyl citrate are respiratory depression, apnea, rigidity, and bradycardia; if these remain untreated, respiratory arrest, circulatory depression or cardiac arrest could occur. Other adverse reactions that have been reported are hypertension, hypotension, dizziness, blurred vision, nausea, emesis, laryngospasm, and diaphoresis.

It has been reported that secondary rebound respiratory depression may occasionally occur postoperatively. Patients should be monitored for this possibility and appropriate countermeasures taken as necessary.

When a tranquilizer such as droperidol is used with Fentanyl citrate the following adverse reactions can occur: chills and/or shivering, restlessness, and postoperative hallucinatory episodes (sometimes associated with transient periods of mental depression); extrapyramidal symptoms (dystonia, akathisia, and oculogyric crisis) have been observed up to 24 hours postoperatively. When they occur, extrapyramidal symptoms can usually be controlled with anti-parkinson agents. Postoperative drowsiness is also frequently reported following the use of droperidol.

FENTANYL CITRATE ORAL TRANSMUCOSAL

The safety of Fentanyl citrate oral transmucosal has been formally evaluated across a broad range of doses in a total of 825 patients in clinical trials. *The primary adverse event of concern is opioid-induced hypoventilation, the severity of which is related to the patient's age, physical condition, the dose employed, and the clinical setting.*

Ventilatory response to Fentanyl citrate oral transmucosal was examined over doses ranging from 5 to 25 μg/kg in both clinical and pharmacokinetic studies. Hypoventilation, usually defined as either desaturation (85 to 90%) or by clinical observation, was the most common potentially serious adverse event and occurred during the first 30 minutes following administration in 6% of patients

---

* Reactions occurring in 3%-10% of Fentanyl Transdermal System patients
** Reactions occurring in 10% or more of Fentanyl Transdermal System patients

---

(14% of adults and 5% of children) participating in clinical trials investigating premedication.

Desaturation and/or hypoventilation was generally dose-related, occurring in 0 to 7% of children across the dose range from 5 to 20 µg/kg and 25 to 42% of adults across the dose range of 5 to 15 µg/kg.

The hypoventilation observed in clinical studies was usually mild, owing in part to prompt response by the monitoring physician, usually responding to gentle stimulation or administration of oxygen. Cases of serious hypoventilation (delayed onset of respirations, and apnea) were observed but were uncommon under the conditions of the clinical trials (8 of 825 cases). All cases of apnea involved doses greater than 15 µg/kg and readily responded to a single dose of naloxone.

Doses above 15 µg/kg are contraindicated regardless of age, and doses above 5 µg/kg (400 µg maximum regardless of weight) are contraindicated in adults, because of this excessive frequency of significant hypoventilation at higher doses.

Besides hypoventilation, other dose-related adverse events occurring in the first 30 minutes following administration in premedication studies included flushing in adults and pruritus in children. Pruritus occurred in over half of the cases studied, and was manifested by the children touching their face and/or complaining of mild itching. Urticaria or generalized pruritus was uncommon.

Common Adverse Events (> 1%, probably causally related): The following adverse events were reported at a frequency of 1% or more in 189 patients who received Fentanyl citrate oral transmucosal as premedication in anesthesia or in monitored anesthetic care settings at the recommended doses. No adjustment has been made for the rate at which events were observed in placebo treated patients, for causality, or for severity. It should be noted that the reported adverse events include the intraoperative and postoperative period for patients undergoing surgery.

Body as a Whole: headache

Cardiovascular: bradycardia, flushing*, hypotension, palor, ventricular extrasystole

Digestive: nausea (17%), vomiting (34%)

Nervous: apathy, dizziness (15%), euphoria*, paresthesia

Respiratory: hypoventilation (11%)

Skin: pruritus (56%), rash

Special Senses: vision abnormality

(%) = adverse reaction above 10%; (*) = adverse reactions 3-9%; all others 1-3%

Uncommon Adverse Events Related to Fentanyl citrate oral transmucosal (< 1%, probably causally related):

The following adverse events occurred in less than 1% of patients who received Fentanyl citrate oral transmucosal in the recommended doses, or were only observed in patients who were studied outside the recommended dosage range and indication (N=636).

Body as a Whole: asthenia, hypertonia, spasm

Digestive: anorexia, dyspepsia, dysphagia, gastrointestinal disorder

Musculoskeletal: myasthenia

Nervous: agitation, anxiety, confusion, dry mouth, emotional lability, miosis, somnolence, speech disorder, stupor, urinary retention, vertigo

Respiration: airway obstruction, apnea, exacerbation of asthma

Skin: urticaria

Special Senses: accommodation abnormality

Uncommon Adverse Events (< 1%, Relationship Unknown):

The following adverse events were uncommon, usually occurred during or after surgery, and their relationship to Fentanyl citrate oral transmucosal administration is unknown.

They are provided as alerting information for the physician.

Body as a Whole: abdominal pain, anaphylactoid reaction, back pain, chest pain, chills, fever

Cardiovascular: bigeminy, tachycardia, ventricular fibrillation

Metabolism and Nutrition: dehydration, hypoglycemia

Musculoskeletal: myalgia

Nervous: abnormal dreams, dystonia, hostility, hypertension, hysteria, nystagmus, twitch

Respiratory: dyspnea, hiccup, increase cough, laryngismus, pharyngitis, rhinitis, voice alteration

Special Senses: ear disorder, lacrimation disorder, photophobia, perverse taste

DRUG ABUSE AND DEPENDENCE

Fentanyl is a Schedule II controlled substance and can produce drug dependence similar to that produced by morphine. Fentanyl and Fentanyl Citrate therefore have the potential for abuse. Tolerance, physical and psychological dependence may develop upon repeated administration of opioids. Iatrogenic addiction following opioid administration is relatively rare. Physicians should not let concerns of physical dependence deter them from using adequate amounts of opioids in the management of severe pain when such use is indicated.

The handling of Fentanyl should be managed to minimize the risk of diversion, including restriction of access and accounting procedures as appropriate to the clinical setting and as required by law.

OVERDOSAGE

Clinical Presentation: The manifestations of Fentanyl overdosage are an extension of its pharmacologic actions with the most serious significant effect being hypoventilation.

The intravenous LD_{50} of Fentanyl Citrate is 3 mg/kg in rats, 1 mg/kg in cats, 14 mg/kg in dogs and 0.03 mg/kg in monkeys.

Treatment: For the management of hypoventilation immediate counter-measures include removing the Fentanyl transdermal system and physically or verbally stimulating the patient. These actions can be followed by administration of a specific narcotic antagonist such as naloxone. The duration of hypoventilation following an overdose may be longer than the effects of the narcotic antagonist's action (the half-life of naloxone ranges from 30 to 81 minutes). The interval between IV antagonist doses should be carefully chosen because of the possibility of re-narcotization after system removal; repeated administration of naloxone may be necessary. Reversal of the narcotic effect may result in acute onset of pain and the release of catecholamines.

If the clinical situation warrants, or in the presence of hypoventilation or apnea, ensure a patent airway is established and maintained, administer oxygen and assist or control respiration as indicated and use an orophyaryngeal airway or endotracheal tube if necessary. Conduct GI decontamination with lavage and/or activated charcoal once the patient's airway is secure. Adequate body temperature and fluid intake should be maintained.

If severe or persistent hypotension occurs, the possibility of hypovolemia should be considered and managed with appropriate parenteral fluid therapy.

If depressed respiration is associated with muscular rigidity, an intravenous neuromuscular blocking agent might be required to facilitate assisted or controlled respiration. The patient should be carefully observed for 24 hours. Although muscle rigidity interfering with respiration has not been seen following the use of Fentanyl citrate oral transmucosal, this is always possible with Fentanyl and other opioids. A specific narcotic antagonist such as nalorphine, levallorphan or naloxone should be available for use as indicated to manage respiratory depression. This does not preclude the use of more immediate countermeasures. The duration of respiratory depression following overdosage of Fentanyl citrate may be longer than the duration of narcotic antagonist action. Consult the package insert of the individual narcotic antagonists for details about use.

Dialysis is not likely to be effective because of the large volume of distribution and high lipid solubility of Fentanyl.

DOSAGE AND ADMINISTRATION

FENTANYL TRANSDERMAL SYSTEM

With all opioids, the safety of patients using the products is dependent on health care practitioners prescribing them in strict conformity with their approved labeling with respect to patient selection, dosing, and proper conditions for use.

As with all opioids, dosage should be individualized. The most important factor to be considered in determining the appropriate dose is the extent of preexisting opioid tolerance. (See box *"Warning"* and *"Contraindications."*) Initial doses should be reduced in elderly or debilitated patients (see *"Precautions"*).

Fentanyl transdermal system should be applied to non-irritated and nonirradiated skin on a flat surface such as chest, back, flank or upper arm. Hair at the application site should be clipped (not shaved) prior to system application. If the site of Fentanyl transdermal system application must be cleansed prior to application of the system, do so with clear water. Do not use soaps, oils, lotions, alcohol, or any other agents that might irritate the skin or alter its characteristics. Allow the skin to dry completely prior to system application.

Fentanyl transdermal system should be applied immediately upon removal from the sealed package. Do not alter the system, e.g., cut, in any way prior to application.

The transdermal system should be pressed firmly in place with the palm of the hand for 30 seconds, making sure the contact is complete, especially around the edges.

Each Fentanyl Transdermal System may be worn continuously for 72 hours. If analgesia for more than 72 hours is required, a new system should be applied to a different skin site after removal of the previous transdermal system.

Fentanyl Transdermal System should be kept out of the reach of children. Used systems should be folded so that the adhesive side of the system adheres to itself, then the system should be flushed down the toilet immediately upon removal. Patients should dispose of any systems remaining from a prescription as soon as they are no longer needed. Unused systems should be removed from their pouch and flushed down the toilet.

DOSE SELECTION

DOSES MUST BE INDIVIDUALIZED BASED UPON THE STATUS OF EACH PATIENT AND SHOULD BE ASSESSED AT REGULAR INTERVALS AFTER FENTANYL TRANSDERMAL SYSTEM APPLICATION. REDUCED DOSES OF FENTANYL TRANSDERMAL SYSTEM ARE SUGGESTED FOR THE ELDERLY AND OTHER GROUPS DISCUSSED IN *"PRECAUTIONS."*

FENTANYL TRANSDERMAL SYSTEM DOSES GREATER THAN 25 µG/H SHOULD NOT BE USED FOR INITIATION OF FENTANYL THERAPY IN NONOPIOID TOLERANT PATIENTS.

In selecting an initial Fentanyl dose, attention should be given to 1) the daily dose, potency, and characteristics of the opioid the patient has been taking previously (eg whether it is a pure agonist or mixed agonist-antagonist), 2) the reliability of the relative potency estimates used to calculate the Fentanyl dose needed (potency estimates may vary with the route of administration), 3) the degree of opioid tolerance, if any, and 4) the general condition and medical status of the patient. Each patient should be maintained at the lowest dose providing acceptable pain control.

INITIAL FENTANYL DOSE SELECTION

There has been no systematic evaluation of Fentanyl as an initial opioid analgesic in the management of chronic pain, since most patients in the clinical trials were converted to Fentanyl from other narcotics. Therefore, unless the patient has pre-existing opioid tolerance, the lowest Fentanyl dose, 25 µg/h, should be used as the initial dose.

To convert patients from oral or parenteral opioids to Fentanyl Transdermal System use the following methodology:

1. Calculate the previous 24-hour analgesic requirement.
2. Convert this amount to the equianalgesic oral morphine dose using Table B.
3. Table C displays the range of 24-hour oral morphine doses that are recommended for conversion to each Fentanyl dose. Use this table to find the calculated 24-hour morphine dose and the corresponding Fentanyl dose. Initiate Fentanyl treatment using the recommended dose and titrate patients upwards (no more frequently than every 3 days after the initial dose or than every 6 days thereafter) until analgesic efficacy is attained. For delivery rates in excess of 100 µg/h, multiple systems may be used.

Table B
EQUIANALGESIC POTENCY CONVERSION

Name	IM^a	Equianalgesic Dose (mg) PO
morphine	10	60 (30)^b
hydromorphone	1.5	7.5
methadone	10	20
oxycodone	15	30
levorphanol	2	4
oxymorphone	1	10 (PR)
heroin	5	60
meperidine	75	—
codeine	130	200

Note: All IM and PO doses in this chart are considered equivalent to 10 mg of IM morphine in analgesic effect. IM denotes intramuscular, PO oral, and PR rectal.
^{a} *Based on single-dose studies in which an intramuscular dose of each drug listed was compared with morphine to establish the relative potency. Oral doses are those recommended when changing from parenteral to an oral route.*
^{b} *The oral/IM potency ratio of 1:3 for morphine is based on clinical experience in patients with chronic pain.*

Reference:
^{a} Foley, K.M. (1985) *The treatment of cancer pain.* NEJM 313(2):84-95.
^{b} Ashburn and Lipman (1993) *Management of pain in the cancer patient.* Anesth Analg 76: 402-416.

Table C
RECOMMENDED FENTANYL DOSE BASED UPON DAILY ORAL MORPHINE DOSE

Oral 24-hour Morphine (mg/day)	Fentanyl Dose (µg/hr)
45- 134	25
135- 224	50
225- 314	75
315- 404	100
405- 494	125
495- 584	150
585- 674	175
675- 764	200
765- 854	225
855- 944	250
945-1034	275
1035-1124	300

Note: In clinical trials these ranges of daily oral morphine doses were used as a basis for conversion to Fentanyl. Although controlled studies are not available, in clinical practice it is customary to consider the doses of opioid given IM, IV or subcutaneously to be equivalent. There may be some differences in pharmacokinetic parameters such as C_{max} and T_{max}.

The majority of patients are adequately maintained with Fentanyl administered every 72 hours. A small number of patients may not achieve adequate analgesia using this dosing interval and may require systems to be applied every 48 hours rather than every 72 hours. An increase in the Fentanyl dose should be evaluated before changing dosing intervals in order to maintain patients on a 72-hour regimen.

Because of the increase in serum Fentanyl concentration over the first 24 hours following initial system application, the initial evaluation of the maximum

analgesic effect of Fentanyl cannot be made before 24 hours of wearing. The initial Fentanyl dosage may be increased after 3 days (see *"Dose Titration"*).

During the initial application of Fentanyl, patients should use short-acting analgesics for the first 24 hours as needed until analgesic efficacy with Fentanyl is attained. Thereafter, some patients still may require periodic supplemental doses of other short-acting analgesics for "breakthrough" pain.

DOSE TITRATION

The conversion ratio from oral morphine to Fentanyl transdermal system is conservative, and 50% of patients are likely to require a dose increase after initial application of Fentanyl transdermal system. The initial Fentanyl dosage may be increased after 3 days, based on the daily dose of supplemental analgesics required by the patient in the second or third day of the initial application.

Physicians are advised that it may take up to 6 days after increasing the dose of Fentanyl for the patient to reach equilibrium on the new dose (see graph in *"Clinical Pharmacology"*). Therefore, patients should wear a higher dose through two applications before any further increase in dosage is made on the basis of the average daily use of a supplemental analgesic.

Appropriate dosage increments should be based on the daily dose of supplementary opioids, using the ratio of 90 mg/24 hours of oral morphine to a 25 µg/h increase in Fentanyl dose.

DISCONTINUATION OF FENTANYL TRANSDERMAL SYSTEM

To convert patients to another opioid, remove Fentanyl Transdermal System and titrate the dose of the new analgesic based upon the patient's report of pain until adequate analgesia has been attained. Upon system removal, 17 hours or more are required for a 50% decrease in serum Fentanyl concentrations. For patients requiring discontinuation of opioids, a gradual downward titration is recommended since it is not known at what dose level the opioid may be discontinued without producing the signs and symptoms of abrupt withdrawal.

SAFETY AND HANDLING

Fentanyl is supplied in sealed transdermal systems which pose little risk of exposure to health care workers. If the gel from the drug reservoir accidentally contacts the skin, the area should be washed with copious amounts of water. Do not use soap, alcohol, or other solvents to remove the gel because they may enhance the drug's ability to penetrate the skin. Do not cut or damage Fentanyl transdermal system. If the Fentanyl system is cut or damaged, controlled drug delivery will not be possible.

Do not store Fentanyl transdermal system above 86°F (30°C). Apply immediately after removal from individually sealed package. Do not use if the seal is broken. *For transdermal use only.*

DEA order form required. A schedule CII narcotic.

FENTANYL CITRATE INJECTION

50 µg = 0.05 mg = 1 mL

Dosage should be individualized. Some of the factors to be considered in determining the dose are age, body weight, physical status, underlying pathological condition, use of other drugs, type of anesthesia to be used and the surgical procedure involved. Dosage should be reduced in elderly or debilitated patients (see *"Precautions"*).

Vital signs should be monitored routinely.

I. Premedication—Premedication (to be appropriately modified in the elderly, debilitated and those who have received other depressant drugs)—50 to 100 µg (0.05 to 0.1 mg) (1 to 2 ml) may be administered intramuscularly 30 to 60 minutes prior to surgery.
II. Adjunct to General Anesthesia—See Dosage Range Chart
III. Adjunct to Regional Anesthesia—50 to 100 µg (0.05 to 0.1 mg) (1 to 2 ml) may be administered intramuscularly or slowly intravenously, over one to two minutes, when additional analgesia is required.
IV. Postoperatively (recovery room)—50 to 100 µg (0.05 to 0.1 mg) (1 to 2 ml) may be administered intramuscularly for the control of pain, tachypnea and emergence delirium. The dose may be repeated in one to two hours as needed.

Usage in Children: For induction and maintenance in children 2 to 12 years of age, a reduced dose as low as 2 to 3 µg/kg is recommended. (See related table).

AS A GENERAL ANESTHETIC

When attenuation of the responses to surgical stress is especially important, doses of 50 to 100 µg/kg (0.05 to 0.1 mg/kg) (1 to 2 ml/kg) of Fentanyl citrate may be administered with oxygen and a muscle relaxant. This technique has been reported to provide anesthesia without the use of additional anesthetic agents. In certain cases, doses up to 150 µg/kg (0.15 mg/kg) (3 ml/kg) may be necessary to produce this anesthetic effect. It has been used for open heart surgery and certain other major surgical procedures in patients for whom protection of the myocardium from excess oxygen demand is particularly indicated, and for certain complicated neurological and orthopedic procedures.

As noted above, it is essential that qualified personnel and adequate facilities be available for the management of respiratory depression.

See *"Warnings"* and *"Precautions"* for use of Fentanyl citrate with other CNS depressants, and in patients with altered response.

Parenteral drug products should be inspected visually for particulate matter and discoloration prior to administration, whenever solution and container permit.

STORAGE

Protect from light. Store at room temperature 15°-30°C (59°-86°F).

◆ RATED THERAPEUTICALLY EQUIVALENT; ◇ THERAPEUTIC EQUIVALENCE UNCONFIRMED; ○ UNRATED

FENTANYL CITRATE ORAL TRANSMUCOSAL:
WARNING: BEFORE PRESCRIBING THIS PRODUCT, PLEASE NOTE THE FOLLOWING INSTRUCTIONS ON THE PROPER USE OF THIS PRODUCT:

Fentanyl citrate oral transmucosal should only be administered in hospital settings such as the operating room, emergency department, ICU, or other monitored anesthesia care settings in hospitals where there is immediate access to life support equipment, including oxygen, facilities for endotracheal intubation, intravenous fluids, and opioid antagonists.

Fentanyl citrate oral transmucosal must be given only to patients being monitored by both (1) direct visual observation by a health professional whose sole responsibility is observation of the patient and also by (2) some means of measuring respiratory function such as pulse oximetry until they are completely recovered.

Fentanyl citrate oral transmucosal should only be administered by persons specifically trained in the use of anesthetic drugs and the management of the respiratory effects of potent opioids, including respiratory and cardiac resuscitation of patients in the age group being treated. Such training must include the establishment and maintenance of a patent airway and assisted ventilation.

Fentanyl citrate oral transmucosal should only be used by health care practitioners credentialed to use the product by the director of anesthesia of the institution in which the product will be used. (See also box "Warnings", "Clinical Pharmacology", "Indications and Usage," and "Precautions".)

DOSES SHOULD BE INDIVIDUALIZED BASED UPON THE STATUS OF EACH PATIENT, THE CLINICAL ENVIRONMENT, AND THE DESIRED THERAPEUTIC EFFECT. DOSAGE SHOULD BE REDUCED IN ELDERLY, DEBILITATED, OR OTHER VULNERABLE PATIENTS (see "Precautions").

Some of the factors to be considered in determining an individualized dose are age, body weight, physical status, general condition and medical status, underlying pathological condition, use of other drugs, type of anesthesia to be used, and the type and length of the procedure. Fentanyl citrate oral transmucosal doses of 5 µg/kg provide effects similar to the usual doses of Fentanyl given IM (0.75-1.25 µg/kg). Larger doses have not been shown to increase efficacy. As with all opioids, the dosage should be reduced in vulnerable patients (see *"Precautions"*). The magnitude of the expected effect will vary from mild with doses of 5 µg/kg to marked with doses of 15 µg/kg. Adults should not receive doses larger than 5 µg/kg (400 µg), and most children not apprehensive at onset may be managed with the same 5 µg/kg dose. Children apprehensive at onset, and some younger children may need doses of 5 to 15 µg/kg, with an attendant increased risk of hypoventilation.

1. Normal Children:

Because of the excessive frequency of significant hypoventilation at higher doses, doses above 15 µg/kg (maximum dose 400 µg) are contraindicated in children.
Selection of dosage strength based on patient weight with a dose range of 5 to 15 µg/kg is recommended. Premedication of children below 40 kg may require doses of 10 to 15 µg/kg.

Patient Weight kg	5 to 10 µg/kg	10 to 15 µg/kg
< 15 kg	contraindicated	contraindicated
15 kg	not available	200 µg
20 kg	200 µg	200 or 300 µg
25 kg	200 µg	300 µg
30 kg	300 µg	300 or 400 µg
35 kg	300 µg	400 µg
40 kg and over	400 µg	Use 400 µg (see Section II Normal Adults)

II. Normal Adults:

Because of the excessive frequency of significant hypoventilation at higher doses, doses above 5 µg/kg (maximum dose 400 µg) are contraindicated in adults.

III. Vulnerable Patients:
Selection of lower dose should be considered for vulnerable patients, for example: patients with head injury, cardiovascular or pulmonary disease, hepatic disease, or liver dysfunction. If signs of excessive opioid effects appear before the unit is consumed, the dosage unit should be removed from the patient's mouth immediately.

IV. Elderly Patients:
If Fentanyl citrate oral transmucosal is to be used in patients over age 65, the dose should be reduced to 2.5 to 5 µg/kg. Although studies of Fentanyl citrate oral transmucosal in the elderly have not been conducted, elderly patients have been shown to be twice as sensitive to the effects of other forms of Fentanyl as the younger population. Like all potent opioid analgesics, Fentanyl citrate oral transmucosal has the ability to depress respiration and reduce ventilatory drive to a clinically significant extent.

ADMINISTRATION OF FENTANYL CITRATE ORAL TRANSMUCOSAL
The patient should be instructed to place the Fentanyl citrate oral transmucosal unit in his/her mouth and to suck (not chew) it. Chewed or swallowed Fentanyl contributes little to the peak concentration, but is responsible for a prolonged "tail" on the blood level profile as it is slowly absorbed.
The Fentanyl citrate oral transmucosal unit should be removed after it is consumed or if the patient has achieved an adequate effect and/or shows signs of respiratory depression. Place any remaining portion of the Fentanyl citrate oral transmucosal unit in the cap and dispose of the unit appropriately as for Schedule II drugs.
Administration of the Fentanyl citrate oral transmucosal unit should begin 20 to 40 minutes prior to the anticipated need of desired effect. Patients typically take 10 to 20 minutes for complete consumption. Peak effect occurs approximately 20 to 30 minutes after the start of Fentanyl citrate oral transmucosal administration. In the event that hypoventilation or some other adverse effect

FENTANYL CITRATE DOSAGE RANGE CHART

Total Dosage

Low Dose	Moderate Dose	High Dose
2 µg/kg (0.002 mg/kg) (0.04 ml/kg) Fentanyl citrate.	2-20 µg/kg (0.002-0.02 mg/kg) (0.04-0.4 ml/kg) Fentanyl citrate.	20-50 µg/kg (0.02-0.05 mg/kg) (0.4-1 ml/kg) Fentanyl Citrate.
Fentanyl citrate in small doses is most useful for minor, but painful, surgical procedures. In addition to the analgesia during surgery, Fentanyl Citrate may also provide some pain relief in the immediate postoperative period.	Where surgery becomes more major, a larger dose is required. With this dose, in addition to adequate analgesia, one would expect to see some abolition of the stress response. However, respiratory depression will be such that artificial ventilation during anesthesia is necessary and careful observation of ventilation postoperatively is essential.	During open heart surgery and certain more complicated neurosurgical and orthopedic procedures where surgery is more prolonged, and in the opinion of the anesthesiologist, the stress response to surgery would be detrimental to the well-being of the patient, dosages of 20-50 µg/kg (0.02-0.05 mg) (0.4-1 ml) of Fentanyl citrate with nitrous oxide/oxygen have been shown to attenuate the stress response as defined by increased levels of circulating growth hormone, catecholamine, ADH and prolactin. When dosages in this range have been used during surgery, postoperative ventilation and observation are essential due to extended postoperative respiratory depression. The main objective of this technique would be to produce "stress free" anesthesia.

Maintenance Dose

Low Dose	Moderate Dose	High Dose
2 µg/kg (0.002 mg/kg) (0.04 ml/kg) Fentanyl Citrate.	2-20 µg/kg (0.002-0.02 mg/kg) (0.04-0.4 ml/kg) Fentanyl Citrate.	20-50 µg/kg (0.02-0.05 mg/kg) (0.4-1.0 ml/kg) Fentanyl Citrate.
Additional dosages of Fentanyl Citrate are frequently needed in these minor procedures.	25 to 100 µg (0.025-0.1 mg) (0.5-2.0 ml) may be administered intravenously or intramuscularly when movement and/or changes in vital signs indicate surgical stress or lightening of analgesia.	Maintenance dosage (ranging from 25 µg (0.025 mg) (0.5 ml) to one-half the initial loading dose) will be dictated by the changes in vital signs which indicate stress and lightening of analgesia. However, the additional dosage selected must be individualized especially if the anticipated remaining operative time is short.

► SHOWN IN PRODUCT IDENTIFICATION GUIDE

occurs before the dosage unit is consumed, the unit should be removed from the patient's mouth immediately.

The patient should be attended at all times by a health care professional skilled in airway management and resuscitative measures. Fentanyl citrate oral transmucosal should be administered only in monitored settings and by persons specifically trained in the use of anesthetics and the management of the respiratory effects of potent opioids, including maintenance of a patent airway and assisted ventilation. Some means for measuring respiratory function is recommended, such as pulse oximetry (see boxed *"Warnings"*).

SAFETY AND HANDLING
Accidental dermal exposure to Fentanyl citrate oral transmucosal should be treated by rinsing the affected area with cool water.

Fentanyl citrate oral transmucosal should be protected from freezing and moisture. Do not store above 30°C (86°F). Cases of self-administration of Fentanyl by health care professionals, including fatalities, have been reported with all Fentanyl products. The handling of Fentanyl citrate oral transmucosal should be managed to minimize the risk of diversion, including restriction of access to the appropriate clinical use setting and accounting procedures as required by law.

DISPOSAL OF FENTANYL CITRATE ORAL TRANSMUCOSAL
The disposal of Schedule II controlled substances must be consistent with State and Federal Regulations.

Flush the drug matrix down the toilet. During the disposal process, avoid contact of the drug matrix with the skin, eyes, or mucous membranes. Wash hands thoroughly when complete.

J CODES
Up to 2 ml IM,IV—J3010

HOW SUPPLIED
FENTANYL
FILM, EXTENDED RELEASE (C-II): 25 MCG/HR

BRAND/MANUFACTURER	NDC	SIZE	AWP
○ BRAND			
DURAGESIC: Janssen	50458-0033-05	5s	$49.97

FILM, EXTENDED RELEASE (C-II): 50 MCG/HR

BRAND/MANUFACTURER	NDC	SIZE	AWP
○ BRAND			
DURAGESIC: Janssen	50458-0034-05	5s	$74.92

FILM, EXTENDED RELEASE (C-II): 75 MCG/HR

BRAND/MANUFACTURER	NDC	SIZE	AWP
○ BRAND			
DURAGESIC: Janssen	50458-0035-05	5s	$114.42

FILM, EXTENDED RELEASE (C-II): 100 MCG/HR

BRAND/MANUFACTURER	NDC	SIZE	AWP
○ BRAND			
DURAGESIC: Janssen	50458-0036-05	5s	$142.56

FENTANYL CITRATE
INJECTION (C-II): 0.05 MG/ML

AVERAGE UNIT PRICE (AVAILABLE SIZES)		GENERIC A-RATED AVERAGE PRICE (GAAP)	
BRAND	$1.00	2 ml 10s	$14.99
GENERIC	$1.97	5 ml 10s	$26.94
		2 ml 50s	$569.60
		5 ml 50s	$505.28

BRAND/MANUFACTURER	NDC	SIZE	AWP
◆ BRAND			
SUBLIMAZE: Janssen	50458-0030-10	10 ml 5s	$44.58
	50458-0030-20	20 ml 5s	$86.66
	50458-0030-02	2 ml 10s	$25.81
	50458-0030-05	5 ml 10s	$46.92
◆ GENERICS			
Elkins-Sinn	00641-1118-34	10 ml 5s	$35.50
Elkins-Sinn	00641-1119-34	20 ml 5s	$69.88
Sanofi Winthrop	00024-0682-02	2 ml 10s	$9.35
Elkins-Sinn	00641-1116-33	2 ml 10s	$20.63
Sanofi Winthrop	00024-0682-05	5 ml 10s	$16.07
Elkins-Sinn	00641-1117-33	5 ml 10s	$37.81
Abbott Hosp	00074-9096-10	10 ml 10s	$194.28
Abbott Hosp	00074-9096-20	20 ml 10s	$388.08
Abbott Hosp	00074-9093-26	10 ml 25s	$323.00
Abbott Hosp	00074-9093-28	20 ml 25s	$633.83
Abbott Hosp	00074-9093-22	2 ml 50s	$183.47
Abbott Hosp	00074-9094-12	2 ml 50s	$368.13
Abbott Hosp	00074-9095-02	2 ml 50s	$1157.22
Abbott Hosp	00074-9093-25	5 ml 50s	$337.25
Abbott Hosp	00074-9094-15	5 ml 50s	$673.31

BRAND/MANUFACTURER	NDC	SIZE	AWP
Abbott Hosp	00074-9094-18	10 ml 50s	$646.00
Abbott Hosp	00074-9094-21	20 ml 50s	$1267.66
Abbott Hosp	00074-9094-51	50 ml 50s	$3168.84

LOZENGE (C-II): 200 MCG

BRAND/MANUFACTURER	NDC	SIZE	AWP
○ GENERICS			
FENTANYL ORALET: Abbott Hosp.	00074-2444-05	5s	4.54

LOZENGE (C-II): 300 MCG

BRAND/MANUFACTURER	NDC	SIZE	AWP
○ GENERICS			
FENTANYL ORALET: Abbott Hosp.	00074-2445-05	5s	4.54

LOZENGE (C-II): 400 MCG

BRAND/MANUFACTURER	NDC	SIZE	AWP
○ GENERICS			
FENTANYL ORALET: Abbott Hosp.	00074-2446-05	5s	4.54

Fentex *SEE* GUAIFENESIN/PHENYLEPHRINE HYDROCHLORIDE/PHENYLPROPANOLAMINE HYDROCHLORIDE

Fero-Folic 500 *SEE* FERROUS SULFATE/FOLIC ACID/ VITAMINS, MULTI

Ferric Pyrophosphate/Folic Acid/ Vitamin B Complex

Each 5 mL (one teaspoonful) contains:

Ferric Pyrophosphate, soluble (10.4 mg Element of Iron)	100.00 mg
Folic Acid	0.25 mg
Niacinamide	13.3 mg
Vitamin B_6, (Pyridoxine Hydrochloride)	2.0 mg
Vitamin B_{12}, crystalline	8.34 mcg

INDICATIONS
For the prevention of Vitamin B_{12}, Vitamin B_6 and iron deficiencies.

CONTRAINDICATIONS
This product should not be used in patients with pernicious anemia. In the recommended dosage this product supplies 0.75 mg of Folic Acid daily. The use of Folic Acid in patients who have or may develop pernicious anemia involves a serious hazard of permitting progressive degeneration of the spinal cord while treating the anemia characteristic of the disease.

Furthermore the absorption of the vitamin B_{12} in this product is not enhanced in patients with pernicious anemia. Parenterally administered cyanocobalamine (Vitamin B_{12}) is the therapy of choice in pernicious anemia and should be employed in patients receiving Folic Acid unless pernicious anemia has been ruled out.

DOSAGE AND ADMINISTRATION
In both adults and older children, one teaspoonful (5 mL) three times daily or one tablespoonful (15 mL) once a day if preferred. Children up to 2 years of age may be given one teaspoonful (5 mL) twice daily.

IMPORTANT
Dispense only in amber bottle. This product is light sensitive.
Shake well before using.

Note: In some infants large doses of this product may produce the diarrhea often associated with concentrated sugars.

IMPORTANT
If particularly rapid B_{12} response is desired, an injection of 100 mcg B_{12} intramuscularly can be given initially. Oral use of this product on a daily basis will then maintain the levels quickly achieved with B_{12} injections.

WARNING
Like other iron preparations, this preparation should be stored out of reach of children to guard against accidental iron poisoning.

HOW SUPPLIED
SYRUP:

BRAND/MANUFACTURER	NDC	SIZE	AWP
○ GENERICS			
VITAFOL: Everett	00642-0074-16	480 ml	$25.50

◆ RATED THERAPEUTICALLY EQUIVALENT; ◇ THERAPEUTIC EQUIVALENCE UNCONFIRMED; ○ UNRATED

Ferrous Fumarate with Folic Acid

Oral iron supplement containing 324 mg Ferrous Fumarate and 1 mg Folic Acid. For any patient needing iron supplementation for documented iron deficiency. Suitable for certain patients undergoing therapy with erythropoietin.

DESCRIPTION

Each tablet contains:

Ferrous Fumarate element iron ....106.5 mg
Folic Acid ....1 mg

Ferrous Fumarate may be better tolerated than ferrous sulfate in some patients.

INDICATIONS

Renal failure patients and patients not on dialysis who have documented iron deficiency. Patients undergoing erythropoietin therapy who risk iron deficiency as reflected by low transferrin saturation and low serum ferritin.

DOSAGE

One to three tablets daily between meals in increments throughout the day, as required to correct iron deficiency condition. The total amount of elemental iron prescribed should be titrated to the amount of iron assessed to provide adequate iron for red blood cell synthesis and replacement of iron body stores, particularly preceding or during erythropoietin therapy.

SIDE EFFECTS

Transient bloating, flatulence, constipation, and diarrhea. Ingestion of greater than 400 mg per day of elemental iron can result in nausea and vomiting.

PRECAUTION

Folic Acid can mask the symptoms of anemia. A careful assessment of the patient should precede prescribing this medication.

HOW SUPPLIED
TABLETS:

BRAND/MANUFACTURER	NDC	SIZE	AWP
◆ GENERICS			
NEPHRO-FER RX: R&D	54391-1313-06	120s	$21.20

Ferrous Fumarate/Folic Acid/ Minerals/Vitamins, Multi

DESCRIPTION

Ferrous Fumarate/Folic Acid/Minerals/Vitamins, Multi is a therapeutic iron-containing multivitamin with minerals tablet for oral administration.

Graphic formulas and physical/chemical information for the vitamins may be found in the US Pharmacopeia XX.

Ferrous Fumarate/Folic Acid/Minerals/Vitamin, Multi tablets supply:

Active Ingredients	Each Tablet	3 Tablets (usual daily dose)
Vitamin A (as Acetate)	(1400 IU) 0.42 mg	4200 IU
Vitamin D (Ergocalciferol)	(140 IU) 3.5 mcg	420 IU
Thiamine Mononitrate	3.3 mg	10 mg
Riboflavin	3.3 mg	10 mg
Pyridoxine Hydrochloride	3.3 mg	10 mg
Niacinamide	33.3 mg	100 mg
Calcium Pentothenate	11.7 mg	35 mg
Vitamin E (di-α-Tocopheryl Acetate)	(5 IU) 5 mg	15 IU
Copper (as Sulfate)	0.67 mg	2 mg
Magnesium (as Carbonate)	41.7 mg	125 mg
Iron, elemental (as Ferrous Fumarate)	66.7 mg	200 mg
Vitamin B_{12} (as Cyanocobalamin)	50 mcg	150 mcg
Folic Acid	0.33 mg	1 mg
Vitamin C (as Sodium Ascorbate)	100 mg	300 mg

CLINICAL PHARMACOLOGY

Vitamins and dietary minerals are fundamentally involved in vital metabolic processes, where they usually serve as oxidizing and reducing agents and as factors in various enzyme systems. These essential micronutrients are so closely interrelated that the lack of any one may affect the body requirements of others.

METABOLIC FUNCTIONS OF INORGANIC IONS

Iron: plays an important role in oxygen and electron transport. Iron may be functional (in hemoglobin, myoglobin, heme enzymes, and cofactor and transport iron) or stored as ferritin and hemosiderin in the liver, spleen, bone marrow, and reticuloendothelial system. The hemoglobin (0.34 percent iron) content of blood is about 14 to 17 g per 100 mL in adult males; in adult females it ranges between 12 and 14 g. Following ingestion, ferrous iron forms low molecular chelates with amino acids, ascorbic acid, and sugars which may be solubilized and absorbed before they reach the distal small intestine. Iron is probably absorbed passively into the mucosal layer of the small intestine, then transferred actively to transferrin where it is incorporated into red blood cells in bone marrow or into all body cells. Transferrin iron may also be stored in bone marrow, liver and spleen. Iron is removed from the body in the urine, bile, sweat, feces, and via desquamation of cells.

Copper: an essential enzyme cofactor in the utilization of iron in hemoglobin synthesis.

Magnesium: an enzyme activator — certain peptidases and phosphatases require magnesium for maximal activity as do virtually all reactions involving adenosine triphosphate.

METABOLIC FUNCTIONS OF THE VITAMINS
FAT SOLUBLE VITAMINS

These tend to be stored in the body; their precise mode of action is largely unknown.

Vitamin A: essential to the production and regeneration of the visual purple of the retina; maintenance of the integrity of epithelial tissue; lysosome stability.

Vitamin D: functions in bone metabolism by regulating the intestinal absorption of calcium and phosphorus.

Vitamin E: intracellular antioxidant, important to the stability of biologic membranes.

WATER SOLUBLE VITAMINS

Except for vitamin B_{12}, these micronutrients are not stored in the body.

B Complex Vitamins (thiamine, riboflavin, pyridoxine, niacinamide, pantothenic acid, vitamin B_{12}, Folic Acid): these function, either alone or as structural components of more complex molecules, in catalytic systems where they usually function as coenzymes in carbohydrate, protein, or amino acid metabolism, synthesis of DNA and other molecules, maturation of RBCs, nerve cell function, or oxidation-reduction reactions.

Vitamin C: a coenzyme, essential to osteoid tissue; collagen formation; vascular function; tissue respiration and wound healing; facilitates absorption of iron.

INDICATIONS AND USAGE

Ferrous Fumarate/Folic Acid/Minerals/Vitamins, Multi tablets are indicated in the treatment of many of the common iron-deficiency anemias, particularly those associated with nutritional deficiency states or when nutritional requirements are high, and tropical and nontropical sprue. These iron-deficiency states include anemias associated with dietary inadequacy, convalescence, those frequently encountered in late childhood, early adolescence and old age, menorrhagia, and the anemias of women from menarche to menopause including macrocytic or microcytic anemia of pregnancy.

Iron deficiency may result in fatigue, palpitation, smooth and sore tongue, angular stomatitis, dysphagia, gastritis enteropathy, and koilonychia, as well as anemia. In young children, depressed growth and impaired mental performance occur.

CONTRAINDICATIONS

Hemochromatosis and hemosiderosis are contraindications to iron therapy.

WARNINGS

Folic Acid alone is improper therapy in the treatment of pernicious anemia and other megaloblastic anemias where vitamin B_{12} is deficient.

Ferrous Fumarate/Folic Acid/Minerals/Vitamins, Multi tablets contains sodium bisulfite, a sulfite that may cause allergic-type reactions including anaphylactic symptoms and life-threatening or less severe asthmatic episodes in certain susceptible people. The overall prevalence of sulfite sensitivity in the general population is unknown and probably low. Sulfite sensitivity is seen more frequently in asthmatic than in nonasthmatic people.

PRECAUTIONS
GENERAL

The use of niacin-containing preparations in patients with gastritis, peptic ulcer, or asthma should be undertaken carefully.

Since iron-deficiency anemia may be a manifestation of a basic systemic disturbance such as recurrent blood loss, the underlying cause of the anemia should be determined and corrected if possible.

The ingredients in Ferrous Fumarate/Folic Acid/Minerals/Vitamin, multi are not sufficient nor are they intended for the treatment of pernicious anemia. Folic acid in doses above 0.1 mg daily may obscure pernicious anemia in that hematologic remission can occur while neurological manifestations remain progressive; therefore, the possibility of pernicious anemia should be excluded before treatment with this preparation. Parenteral use of vitamin B_{12} is recommended to assure essential medical supervision of the patient (see *"Warnings"*).

INFORMATION FOR THE PATIENT

Keep Ferrous Fumarate/Folic Acid/Minerals/Vitamins, Multi and all other medication out of the reach of children.

Patients should be informed of symptoms of intolerance to components of this preparation: if any of these symptoms appear the patient should be advised to discontinue dosing, and to notify the physician.

Recommended dosage should not be exceeded unless directed by the physician.

LABORATORY TESTS

Periodic hematologic studies should be performed.

DRUG INTERACTIONS

Since oral iron products interfere with absorption of oral tetracyclines, these products should not be taken within two hours of each other.

Mineral oil and bile-acid sequestrants such as cholestyramine and colestipol hydrochloride in long term therapy have been shown to decrease the absorption of fat-soluble vitamins.

Pyridoxine hydrochloride may act as an antagonist to levodopa.

Hydralazine hydrochloride, penicillamine, isoniazid, and cycloserine may antagonize pyridoxine hydrochloride.

Phenytoin, methotrexate, and pyrimethamine may interfere with folic acid absorption.

Colestipol hydrochloride may decrease the bioavailability of niacin.

Vitamin C may decrease the hypoprothrombinemic effect of oral anticoagulants; prothrombin levels should be monitored.

Neomycin and colchicine may impair cyanocobalamin absorption.

CARCINOGENESIS, MUTAGENESIS, IMPAIRMENT OF FERTILITY

Long-term studies in animals have not been performed.

PREGNANCY CATEGORY C

Animal reproduction studies have not been conducted with therapeutic formula vitamin tablets with hematinics. Controlled clinical studies have not been performed to determine if therapeutic formula vitamin tablets with hematinics can cause fetal harm when administered to a pregnant woman or can affect reproduction capacity. The tablets should be given to a pregnant woman only if clearly needed.

NURSING MOTHERS

It is not known whether components of this product are excreted in human milk. Because many substances are excreted in human milk, caution should be exercised when these tablets are administered to a nursing woman.

PEDIATRIC USE

Safety and effectiveness in children have not been established.

ADVERSE REACTIONS

Allergic reactions, skin rashes, and gastrointestinal disturbances, such as nausea, vomiting, diarrhea, or constipation may occur.

A generalized flushing and a feeling of warmth has been reported following niacinamide therapy.

Allergic sensitization has been reported following both oral and parenteral administration of folic acid.

DOSAGE AND ADMINISTRATION

The usual adult dose is one tablet three times daily. When prescribed in late childhood and early adolescence, dosage reduction according to the size and weight of the child should be considered by the physician. Dosage may be adjusted according to the response of the patient. Since Ferrous Fumarate is not likely to cause gastric upsets, dosage need not be given at meal-time.

Store at room temperature; avoid excessive heat.

HOW SUPPLIED
CAPSULE:

BRAND/MANUFACTURER	NDC	SIZE	AWP
○ BRAND			
TRINSICON: Whitby	50474-0364-22	60s	$26.69
	50474-0364-27	100s ud	$46.77
	50474-0364-24	500s ud	$211.18
○ GENERICS			
PROMAR: Marlop	12939-0315-30	30s	$14.50
PRONEMIA: Lederle Labs	00005-5150-13	30s	$24.66
MARTINIC: Marlop	12939-0305-41	60s	$13.00
MORTRINSIC: Moore,H.L.	00839-6738-06	100s	$4.45
FOLTRIN: Eon	00185-5380-01	100s	$7.75
LIVITRINSIC-F: Goldline	00182-0651-01	100s	$8.85
TRIFAC: Major	00904-0171-60	100s	$8.95
INTRINSIC FACTOR: Dixon-Shane	17236-0181-01	100s	$9.00
CONTRIN: Geneva	00781-2025-01	100s	$9.69
INTRINSITINIC: Schein	00364-1057-01	100s	$10.35
FEROCON: Econolab	55053-0121-01	100s	$11.45
FEROTRINSIC: Rugby	00536-3804-01	100s	$11.69
FUMATINIC: Laser	00277-0172-01	100s	$22.59
ANEMATRINSIC: Richwood	58521-0121-01	100s	$36.10
FEROTRINSIC: Rugby	00536-3804-10	1000s	$70.88
FOLTRIN: Eon	00185-5380-10	1000s	$72.05
INTRINSIC FACTOR: Dixon-Shane	17236-0181-10	1000s	$77.90
TRIFAC: Major	00904-0171-80	1000s	$80.95

CAPSULE: 240 MG

BRAND/MANUFACTURER	NDC	SIZE	AWP
○ GENERICS			
FERCON: Aligen	00405-4432-01	100s	$11.45

CAPSULE, EXTENDED RELEASE:

BRAND/MANUFACTURER	NDC	SIZE	AWP
○ GENERICS			
CEVI-FER: Geriatric	59441-0134-30	30s	$12.78
CEVI-FER: Geriatric	59441-0134-01	100s	$34.99

ELIXIR:

BRAND/MANUFACTURER	NDC	SIZE	AWP
○ GENERICS			
HEMOCYTE PLUS: U.S. Pharm	52747-0309-90	240 ml	$14.84

TABLETS:

BRAND/MANUFACTURER	NDC	SIZE	AWP
○ BRAND			
TRIHEMIC 600: Lederle Labs	00005-4590-13	30s	$23.84
THERAGRAN HEMATINIC: Apothecon	00003-0535-40	90s	$30.66
TRIHEMIC 600: Lederle Labs	00005-4590-31	500s	$357.88
○ GENERICS			
THERA HEMATINIC: Dixon-Shane	17236-0449-01	100s	$4.20
MORGRAN HEMATINIC: Moore,H.L.	00839-5174-06	100s	$4.45
VITAFOL: Everett	00642-0072-10	100s	$16.80
HEMOCYTE PLUS: U.S. Pharm	52747-0308-60	100s	$32.99
THERA HEMATINIC: Dixon-Shane	17236-0449-10	1000s	$33.90
VITAFOL: Everett	00642-0072-11	1000s	$161.28

Ferrous Fumarate/Stomach Substance, Desiccated/Vitamin B_{12}/ Vitamin C

DESCRIPTION

Contents: Each capsule contains: Ferrous Fumarate USP 200 mg, ascorbic acid USP 250 mg, cyanocobalamin USP 10 mcg, Desiccated Stomach Substance 100 mg.

Discussion: The amount of elemental iron and the absorption of the iron components of commercial iron preparations vary widely. It is further established that certain "accessory components" may be included to enhance absorption and utilization of iron.

ACTIONS

High Elemental Iron Content: Ferrous Fumarate is an organic iron complex which has a higher elemental iron content than any other hematinic salt—33%. This compares with 20% for Ferrous sulfate and 12% for Ferrous gluconate.[1,2]

More Complete Absorption: It has been repeatedly shown that ascorbic acid, when given in sufficient amounts, can increase the absorption of Ferrous iron from the gastrointestinal tract.[3,4,5,6,7,8,9] The absorption-promoting effect is mainly due to the reducing action of ascorbic acid within the gastrointestinal lumen, which helps to prevent or delay the formation of insoluble or less dissociated ferric compounds.[3] Iron absorption has been shown to increase sharply with increasing amounts of ascorbic acid, showing a gain in absorption of approximately 40% at 250 mg. Above 250 mg, the gain becomes insignificant, with an additional gain of only approximately 8% at 500 mg.[3] Each capsule contains 250 mg of ascorbic acid, believed to be the optimal amount.

Promotes Movement of Plasma Iron: Ascorbic acid also plays an important role in the movement of plasma iron to storage depots in the tissues.[10] The action, which leads to the transport of plasma iron to ferritin, presumably involves its reducing effect, converting transferrin iron from the ferric to the Ferrous state.[5] There is also evidence that ascorbic acid improves iron utilization, presumably as a further result of its reducing action,[6,9] and some evidence that it may have a direct effect upon erythropoiesis. Ascorbic acid is further alleged to enhance the conversion of folic acid to a more physiologically active form, folinic acid, which would make it even more important in the treatment of anemia since it would aid in the utilization of dietary folic acid.[11]

Excellent Oral Toleration: Ferrous Fumarate is used in capsule because it is less likely to cause the gastric disturbances so often associated with oral iron therapy. Ferrous Fumarate has a low ionization constant and high solubility in the entire pH range of the gastrointestinal tract. It does not precipitate proteins or have the astringency of more ionizable forms of iron, and does not interfere with proteolytic or diastatic activities of the digestive system. Because of excellent oral toleration, capsule can usually be administered between meals when iron absorption is maximal.

Facilitates Absorption of Vitamin B_{12}: It is now known that "Intrinsic Factor" is essential for the adequate alimentary absorption of Vitamin B_{12}.[12,13,14,15] The

---

◆ RATED THERAPEUTICALLY EQUIVALENT; ◇ THERAPEUTIC EQUIVALENCE UNCONFIRMED; ○ UNRATED

chemical structure of intrinsic factor is still undertermined and it has not yet been isolated in pure form;[16] however, the inclusion of Stomach Substance, Desiccated with oral Vitamin B_{12} will furnish sufficient intrinsic factor to assure absorption of the vitamin.

Toxicity: Ferrous Fumarate was found to be the least toxic of three popular oral iron salts, with an oral LD_{50} of 630 mg/kg. In the same report, the LD_{50} of Ferrous gluconate was reported to be 320 mg/kg and Ferrous sulfate 230 mg/kg.[1,17]

INDICATIONS
For the treatment of all anemias responsive to oral iron therapy, such as hypochromic anemia associated with pregnancy, chronic or acute blood loss, dietary restriction, metabolic disease and post-surgical convalescence.

CONTRAINDICATIONS
Hemochromatosis and hemosiderosis are contraindications to iron therapy.

SIDE EFFECTS
Average doses in sensitive individuals or excessive dosage may cause nausea, skin rash, vomiting, diarrhea, precordial pain, or flushing of the face and extremities.

DOSAGE AND ADMINISTRATION
Usual adult dose is 1 capsule daily or as recommended by physician.

Capsules
Store at controlled room temperature 15°-30°C (59°-86°F).

BIBLIOGRAPHY
1. Berk. M.S. and Novich, M.A.: "Treatment of Iron Deficiency Anemia With Ferrous Fumarate," Am. J. Obst. & Gynec., 203-206, 1962. 2. Shapleigh, J.B., and Montgomery, A.; Am. Pract & Dig. Treat 10-461, 1959. 3. Brise, H. and Hallberg. L.: "Effect of Ascorbic Acid on Iron Absorption," Acta. Med. Scand. 171:376, 51-58, 1962. 4. New Drugs, p.309, AMA, Chicago, 1966. 5.Mazur, A., Green, S. and Carleton, A.: "Mechanism of Plasma Iron Incorporation into Hepatic Ferritin," J. of Bio. Chem. 3:595-603, 1960. 6. Greenberg, S.M., Tucker, A.E., Mathues, H. and J.D.: "Iron Absorption and Metabolism, I. Interrelationship of Ascorbic Acid and Vitamin E", J. Nutrition 63:19-31, 1957. 7. Moore, C.V., and Dubach, R.: "Observations on the Absorption of Iron From Foods Tagged with Radioiron," Trans. Assoc. Amer. Physic. 64:245, 1951. 8. Steinkamp, R., Dubach, R. and Moore, C.V.: "Studies in Iron Transportation and Metabolism," Arch. Int. Med. 95:181, 1955. 9. Gorten, M.K. and Bradley, J.E.: "The Treatment of Nutritional Anemia in Infancy and Childhood with Oral Iron and Ascorbic Acid," J. Pediatrics, 45:1, 1954. 10. Mazur, A.: "Role of Ascorbic Acid in the Incorportion of Plasma Iron into Ferritin," An. N.Y. Acad. Sci. 92:223-229, 1961. 11. Cox, E.V. et al.: "The Anemia of Scurvy," Amer. J. Med. 42:220-227, 1967. 12. Berk, L. et al.: "Observations on the Etiologic Relationship of Achylia Gastrica to Pernicious Anemia, X," N. Eng. J. Med. 239:911-913, 1948. 13. Hall, B.E.: "Studies on the Nature of the Intrinsic Factor of Castle," Brit. Med. J. 2:585-589, 1950. 14. Wallerstein, R.O. et al.: "Observations on the Etiologic Relationship of Achylia Gastrica to Pernicious Anemia, XV," J. Lab & Clin. Med. 41:363-375, 1953. 15. Castle, W.B.: "Observations on the Etiologic Relationship of Achylia Gastrica to Pernicious Anemia, 1," Am. J. Med. Sc. 178:748-764, 1929. 16. Goodman, L.S. and Gilman, A.: The Pharmacological Basis of Therapeutics, 2 ed., P. 1482, N.Y., 1958. 17. Berenbaum, M.C. et al.: Blood, 15:540, 1960.

HOW SUPPLIED
CAPSULE:

BRAND/MANUFACTURER	NDC	SIZE	AWP
○ **GENERICS**			
HEM FE: Wakefield	59310-0105-10	100s	$10.58
CHROMAGEN: Savage	00281-4285-53	100s	$25.70
CHROMAGEN: Savage	00281-4285-56	500s	$114.79

Ferrous Fumarate/Vitamin B Complex/Vitamin C

DESCRIPTION
The process of hemodialysis and CAPD causes vitamin losses necessitating the regular replacement of the water soluble vitamins. It is important not to over supplement some vitamins. Vitamin A should not be supplemented and Vitamin C supplementation should be limited to 60 mg per day to avoid the risk of increased oxalate formation*.

Each tablet provides:

Vitamin C	.60 mg
Vitamin B_1	1.5 mg
Vitamin B_2	1.7 mg
Niacinamide	20 mg
Vitamin B_6	10 mg
Vitamin B_{12}	6 mg
Folic Acid	0.8 or 1 mg
Pantothenic Acid	10 mg
Biotin	300 mg
Ferrous Fumarate	304 mg (100 mg elemental iron)

*Formulated to provide optimum one-a-day vitamin replacement amounts daily as suggested by latest literature on the subject. Please ask for R & D's review of the literature on this subject.

INDICATIONS
For any patient needing vitamin and iron supplementation for documented iron deficiency. Suitable for patients with end stage renal disease.
Dialysis patients. Azotemic patients not on dialysis who eat poorly.

PRECAUTION
Folic acid may partially correct the hematological damage due to vitamin B_{12} deficiency of pernicious anemia while the associated neurological damage progresses.

ADVERSE REACTIONS
Allergic sensitization has been reported following administration of folic acid. Iron sensitivity to low doses of iron has been reported and high doses result in iron toxicity. Transient bloating, flatulence, constipation and diarrhea. Ingestion of greater than 400 mg/day of iron can result in nausea and vomiting.

DOSAGE
One tablet daily.

HOW SUPPLIED
TABLETS:

BRAND/MANUFACTURER	NDC	SIZE	AWP
◆ **GENERICS**			
NEPHRO-VITE RX & FE: R&D	54391-2213-06	120s	$68.25

Ferrous Fumarate/Vitamin B₁₂/ Vitamin C

DESCRIPTION
Each dark-brown, film-coated tablet contains Ferrous Fumarate 600 mg (providing 200 mg elemental iron), Ascorbic Acid 100 mg, and vitamin B (Cyanocobalamin) 25 mcg (anhydrous). Ferrous Fumarate/Vitamin B_{12}/Vitamin C is a hematinic iron and vitamin B supplement. The chemical names are 2-butenedioic acid. (E)-, iron (2+) salt (Ferrous Fumarate). L-Ascorbic Acid, and a-(5, 6-Dimethylbenzimidazolyl) cobamide cyanide Cyanocobalamin).

CLINICAL PHARMACOLOGY
Iron and vitamin B are essential factors for normal hemoglobin synthesis and proper red blood cell maturation. Absorption of iron from the gastrointestinal tract is controlled by an active transport system that limits absorption to 5-10% of the ingested amount in normal individuals, increasing to 10-30% in iron-deficient individuals. For therapy of iron-deficiency anemia, a daily intake of approximately 200 mg of elemental iron should be maintained for approximately 6 months to insure proper replenishment of body iron stores. Vitamin B is a cofactor in many human metabolic systems and is essential for a normal growth, hematopoiesis, production of all epithelial cells and maintenance of myelin throughout the nervous system. In addition to megaloblastic anemia, vitamin B deficiency can result in neurologic damage due to deficient synthesis of the lipoprotein myelin sheaths of nerves. The recommended daily dietary intake for vitamin B is 6 mcg for adults, 3 mcg for infants and 8 mcg during pregnancy and lactation. The absorption of vitamin B from the gastrointestinal tract is complex and requires the presence of "intrinsic factor" which is secreted by the gastric mucosa. Vitamin B forms a complex with intrinsic factor and is absorbed in the ileum via a carrier process which additionally requires the presence of calcium at a pH of approximately 6. Pernicious anemia is usually due to inadequate absorption of vitamin B from the gastrointestinal tract secondary to a lack of intrinsic factor. Ferrous Fumarate/Vitamin B_{12}/Vitamin C contains sufficient vitamin B to correct dietary deficiencies in patients with normal intrinsic factor and absorptive function.

INDICATIONS AND USAGE
For the prevention and treatment of iron-deficiency anemia and nutritional Vitamin B deficiency.

CONTRAINDICATIONS
Ferrous Fumarate/Vitamin B_{12}/Vitamin C is contraindicated in children under the age of 12 years or weighing less than 50 kg. Hypersensitivity to Ferrous Fumarate, iron, Ascorbic Acid, cobalt or Cyanocobalamin. Hemochromatosis or other iron storage diseases are contraindications for iron therapy.

WARNING
Patients with pernicious anemia are usually unable to absorb orally administered Vitamin B_{12}. Parenterally administered Vitamin B_{12} is the therapy of choice in pernicious anemia.

PRECAUTIONS
General: Oral iron can be irritating to the GI mucosa and this product should be used with caution in patients with peptic ulcer disease, regional enteritis, ulcerative colitis and other forms of active gastrointestinal disease. Black, tarry stools may be the result of oral iron therapy or occult gastrointestinal bleeding. Any evidence of blood loss from the gastrointestinal tract should be thoroughly investigated.

Information For Patients: Oral iron therapy may cause black, tarry stools. Gastrointestinal intolerance may be decreased by taking the tablet with meals. Do not take within one hour of taking tetracycline, antacids or cholestyramine.

Laboratory Tests: Numerous laboratory tests may be employed to ascertain the cause and presence of iron-deficiency anemia. Once the diagnosis of iron-deficiency anemia has been established and appropriate therapy is initiated, response to oral iron therapy can be adequately monitored by periodic hemoglobin determinations. With adequate response to oral iron therapy, the hemoglobin concentration should increase by at least 2 grams over baseline in 3-4 weeks. Failure to achieve such a response indicates the need for further investigation to determine the cause of failure to respond to iron therapy.

Drug Interactions: The concomitant administration of oral iron with antacids, cholestyramine or tetracycline may result in decreased bioavailability of the iron due to the formation of insoluble chelates. The oral bioavailability of tetracycline is also decreased. This interaction can be avoided by giving the iron one hour before or two hours after the administration of antacids, tetracycline or cholestyramine. Concomitant administration of iron and penicillamine results in the formation of an insoluble chelate, which inhibits the absorption of penicillamine. Iron should be administered one hour before or two hours after the dose of penicillamine, in order to avoid the interaction. Concomitant administration of chloramphenicol in high doses (serum levels of 25 mcg/ml) inhibits the bone marrow response to iron by blocking the activity of the ferrochelatase enzyme. This effect is usually reversible and the response to iron returns to normal upon discontinuation of the chloramphenicol. The absorption of Vitamin B_{12} from the gastrointestinal tract is inhibited by concomitant administration of neomycin and colchicine. Parenteral administration of Vitamin B_{12} may be necessary to correct deficiencies in patients taking neomycin or colchicine chronically. Very high doses of Ascorbic Acid have been reported to impair the clinical response to warfarin. This interaction has not been reported to occur with the amount contained in Ferrous Fumarate/Vitamin B_{12}/Vitamin C.

Drug/Laboratory Test Interactions: The presence of Ascorbic Acid in the urine may result in false negative reactions to urine glucose determinations by the glucose oxidase method (Diastix®, Clinistix® and Tes-Tape®). The validity of glucose oxidase tests for urine glucose should be validated by an alternate method (e.g., copper reduction method) in patients taking Ascorbic Acid.

Carcinogenesis, Mutagenesis, Impairment of Fertility: Long-term studies in animals have not been performed to evaluate the carcinogenic potential of Ferrous Fumarate/Vitamin B_{12}/Vitamin C.

Pregnancy: Teratogenic Effects—Pregnancy Category C. Animal reproduction studies have not been conducted with Ferrous Fumarate/Vitamin B_{12}/Vitamin C. It is also not known whether Ferrous Fumarate/Vitamin B_{12}/Vitamin C can cause fetal harm when administered to a pregnant woman or can affect reproductive capacity. Ferrous Fumarate/Vitamin B_{12}/Vitamin C should be given to a pregnant woman only if clearly needed.

Nursing Mothers: Caution should be exercised when Ferrous Fumarate/Vitamin B_{12}/Vitamin C is administered to a nursing woman.

Pediatric Use: The safety and effectiveness in children below the age of 12 have not been established. See *"Contraindications"*. Ferrous Fumarate/Vitamin B_{12}/Vitamin C contains 200 mg of elemental iron per tablet. This amount of iron may cause iron overload or intoxication in children under the age of 12 or weighing less than 50 kg.

ADVERSE REACTIONS
The primary adverse reaction to oral iron therapy in therapeutic doses is gastrointestinal intolerance. The frequency of gastrointestinal intolerance appears to be causally related to the concentration of elemental iron in the preparation. The most common symptoms of gastrointestinal intolerance include pain, diarrhea, nausea, vomiting or constipation.

OVERDOSAGE
The principal concern with an overdose of Ferrous Fumarate/Vitamin B_{12}/Vitamin C is iron poisoning. The toxicity or iron overdose is directly related to the amount of elemental iron ingested and the size of the patient. Each Ferrous Fumarate/Vitamin B_{12}/Vitamin C tablet contains 200 mg of elemental iron. The range of toxic doses of iron is 20-60 mg/kg of elemental iron. Ingestion of 60 mg/kg (elemental iron) is potentially lethal and 150 mg/kg (elemental iron) will almost certainly produce serious toxicity. As few as two Ferrous Fumarate/Vitamin B_{12}/Vitamin C tablets may produce serious toxicity in a small child. Serum iron concentrations are a useful indicator of potential toxicity when combined with clinical findings. Serum iron concentrations of 150-350 mcg/100 ml indicate toxicity and levels greater than 350 mcg/100 ml indicate definite poisoning. Iron is not effectively removed by dialysis in the setting of an acute overdose. The toxicity of iron overdose is related to direct hemorrhagic necrosis of the GI tract (primarily stomach and upper small intestine) and cellular toxicity in various organs including the liver, spleen, brain, kidney, heart and cardiovascular system. The clinical course of iron poisoning is divided into four stages.

Stage 1: (less than 6 hours): Onset of symptoms in 30 minutes to 2 hours post-ingestion. GI: nausea, vomiting, diarrhea, abdominal pain and hemorrhage. Cardiovascular, hypotension, shock. CNS: lethargy, coma.

Stage 2: (6-12 hours): General clinical improvement, persisting lethargy.

Stage 3: (12-24 hours): Onset of stage 3 may be precipitous. GI: hemorrhage. Cardiovascular: collapse, shock. CNS: lethargy, coma, convulsions. Other: hepatic and renal failure, fever, metabolic acidosis, leukocytosis, coagulopathy.

Stage 4: (greater than 4 weeks): Sequalae of GI damage: gastric scarring, pyloric or duodenal obstruction.

In the initial management, removal of unabsorbed tablets from the GI tract should be performed, preferably with syrup-of-ipecac-induced emesis. Emesis is preferred over lavage due to the difficulty of removing iron tablets by lavage. Lavage should be done with a 1-5% solution of sodium bicarbonate or a 1:4 dilution of disodium phosphate (phosphate enema) in water. This aids in the formation of insoluble iron precipitates in the GI tract, to prevent further absorption of the iron. Following emesis or lavage, administer 50-100 ml of the phosphate solution for catharsis and further iron precipitation. Large quantities of the phosphate solution should be avoided to prevent possible hyperphosphatemia and hypocalcemia. There is no adequate physiologic mechanism for iron removal, so chelation therapy with intravenous or intramuscular deferoxamine should be started immediately if the serum iron concentration is greater than 500 mcg/100 ml. The use of deferoxamine may be indicated at lower serum iron concentrations if the clinical situation dictates. The iron-deferoxamine chelate is dialyzable. A radiograph of the abdomen should be obtained following emesis or lavage to identify iron tablets remaining in the GI tract. Vigorous fluid and electrolyte therapy and other symptomatic support is indicated based on the patient's clinical condition. Correction of blood, fluid and electrolyte losses from the GI tract and close monitoring of the patient's cardiovascular and renal status are of paramount importance. Exchange transfusion has been life-saving in some cases of severe intoxication.

DOSAGE AND ADMINISTRATION
The recommended adult dose is one tablet daily for 3 to 6 months depending on the patient's hematologic response. The dose may be increased to 2 tablets daily in the treatment of iron-deficiency anemia. For children, age 12 years and older, weighing more than 50 kg, the dose is one tablet daily.

HOW SUPPLIED
CAPSULE, EXTENDED RELEASE:

BRAND/MANUFACTURER	NDC	SIZE	AWP
○ BRAND FETRIN: Lunsco	10892-0114-10	100s	$34.38

TABLETS:

BRAND/MANUFACTURER	NDC	SIZE	AWP
○ GENERICS TOLFRINIC: Ascher	00225-0105-15	100s	$31.56

Ferrous Gluconate/Liver Extract/ Vitamin B Complex

DESCRIPTION
A sterile aqueous solution of liver, iron and vitamins with preservatives.

Each mL contains: Cyanocobalamin 15 mcg, Liver Injection equivalent to Vitamin B_{12} activity 1 mcg, Ferrous Gluconate 25 mg, Riboflavin 0.75 mg, Calcium Pantothenate 1.25 mg, Niacinamide 50 mg.

CLINICAL PHARMACOLOGY
This product provides a combination of the hematinic effect of parenteral iron with the hematopoetic effects of liver injection. Ferric iron administered parenterally is transported by transferrin and incorporated into hemoglobin.

INDICATIONS AND USAGE
For the treatment of iron deficiency and nutritional macrocytic anemias.

Intramuscular injections of iron are advisable solely for use in those patients in whom iron deficiency anemia is present, its cause has been determined and, if possible, corrected and in whom oral administration of iron is unsatisfactory or impossible; for example:

Intolerance to oral preparations; resistance to oral iron therapy; rapid replenishment of iron stores in selected patients in whom oral therapy is ineffective, such as hypochromic anemia of the last trimesters of pregnancy; selected hemorrhagic cases (appropriate steps should be taken to correct and prevent any excessive blood loss that may have been revealed as an etiologic factor); to replace postoperative transfusion to some degree; in those patients who cannot be relied upon to take oral medication.

CONTRAINDICATIONS
Hypersensitivity to any of the components of the product. This product is not recommended for use in infants or young children. Benzyl Alcohol has been reported to be associated with a fatal "Gasping Syndrome" in premature infants.

WARNINGS
This preparation should be used with extreme care in the presence of serious impairment of liver function. The patient must be treated with continuous and ample quantities of parenteral vitamin B_{12} whenever pernicious anemia is suspected.

PRECAUTIONS
The usual precautions for parenteral therapy should be observed. Do not inject intravenously.

Improper therapy with these agents will cause storage of iron with the consequent possibility of exogenous hemosiderosis. Such iron overload is

---

◆ RATED THERAPEUTICALLY EQUIVALENT; ◇ THERAPEUTIC EQUIVALENCE UNCONFIRMED; ○ UNRATED

particularly apt to occur with patients with hemoglobinopathies and other refractory anemias which might be erroneously diagnosed as iron deficiency anemia.

ADVERSE REACTIONS
Untoward reactions, although rare, have been reported. They include nausea, urticaria, tachycardia and possibly syncope. Variable degree of soreness and inflammation; brownish discoloration in the area of injection; anaphylactoid and anaphylactic reactions, including fatal anaphylactic reactions; severe febrile reactions. These reactions are more likely to occur in children than in adults and are generally dosage related. Reactions to the local anesthetic may include drowsiness, nervousness, dizziness, blurred vision, nausea, tremors, convulsions, respiratory arrest, cardiovascular collapse and cardiac arrest. Although local anesthetics have been shown to be relatively free from allergic and/or sensitizing properties these possibilities should not be overlooked, and appropriate precautions should be observed.

DOSAGE AND ADMINISTRATION
Intramuscularly only, 1 mL -2 mL two to three times weekly, depending upon the response of the individual patient, until the blood count and color index obtained reach normal levels. Maintenance therapy may be instituted by administration of 1 mL weekly as determined by the physician. It should be kept in mind that periodic hematologic determinations are to be used as a guide to therapy since iron storage may lag behind the appearance of normal blood morphology.

Parenteral drug products should be inspected visually for particulate matter and discoloration prior to administration whenever the solution and container permit.

Refrigerate at 2° - 8° C (36° - 46° F).

HOW SUPPLIED
INJECTION:

BRAND/MANUFACTURER	NDC	SIZE	AWP
◆ GENERICS			
Rugby	00536-1201-75	30 ml	$9.75

Ferrous Gluconate/Liver Extract/ Vitamins, Multi

DESCRIPTION
A sterile aqueous solution of liver, iron and vitamins with preservatives.

Each mL contains:

Cyanocobalamin	15 mcg
Liver Injection equivalent to Vitamin B-12 activity	1 mcg
Ferrous Gluconate	25 mg
Riboflavin	0.75 mg
Calcium Panthothenate	1.25 mg
Niacinamide	50 mg
Citric Acid	8.2 mg
Sodium Citrate	11.8 mg
Procaine HCl	2%
Benzyl Alcohol	2%

as preservative in Water for Injection.
Sodium Hydroxide to adjust pH.

CLINICAL PHARMACOLOGY
This product provides a combination of the hematinic effect of parenteral iron with the hematopoetic effects of liver injection. Ferric iron administered parenterally is transported by transferrin and incorporated into hemoglobin.

INDICATIONS AND USAGE
For the treatment of iron deficiency and nutritional macrocytic anemias.

Intramuscular injections of iron are advisable solely for use in those patients in whom iron deficiency anemia is present, its cause has been determined and, if possible, corrected and in whom oral administration of iron is unsatisfactory or impossible; for example:

Intolerance to oral preparations; resistance to oral iron therapy; rapid replenishment of iron stores in selected patients in whom oral therapy is ineffective, such as hypochromic anemia of the last trimester of pregnancy; selected hemorrhagic cases (appropriate steps should be taken to correct and prevent any excessive blood loss that may have been revealed as an etiologic factor); to replace postoperative transfusion to some degree; in those patients who cannot be relied upon to take oral medication.

CONTRAINDICATIONS
Hypersensitivity to any of the components of the product. This product is not recommended for use in infants or young children. Benzyl Alcohol has been reported to be associated with a fatal "Gasping Syndrome" in premature infants.

WARNINGS
This preparation should be used with extreme care in the presence of serious impairment of liver function. The patient must be treated with continuous and

ample quantities of parenteral vitamin B-12 whenever pernicious anemia is suspected.

PRECAUTIONS
The usual precautions for parenteral therapy should be observed. Do not inject intravenously.

Improper therapy with these agents will cause storage of iron with the consequent possibility of exogenous hemosiderosis. Such iron overload is particularly apt to occur with patients with hemoglobinopathies and other refractory anemias which might be erroneously diagnosed as iron deficiency anemia.

ADVERSE REACTIONS
Untoward reactions, although rare, have been reported. They include nausea, urticaria, tachycardia and possibly syncope. Variable degree of soreness and inflammation; brownish discoloration in the area of injection; anaphylactoid and anaphylactic reactions, including fatal anaphylactic reactions; severe febrile reactions. These reactions are more likely to occur in children than in adults and are generally dosage related. Reactions to the local anesthetic may include drowsiness, nervousness, dizziness, blurred vision, nausea, tremors, convulsions, respiratory arrest, cardiovascular collapse and cardiac arrest. Although local anesthetics have been shown to be relatively free from allergic and/or sensitizing properties these possibilities should not be overlooked, and appropriate precautions should be observed.

DOSAGE AND ADMINISTRATION
Intramuscularly only, 1 mL - 2 mL two to three times weekly depending upon the response of the individual patient until the blood count and color index obtained reach normal levels. Maintenance therapy may be instituted by administration of 1 mL weekly as determined by the physician. It should be kept in mind that periodic hematologic determinations are to be used as a guide to therapy since iron storage may lag behind the appearance of normal blood morphology.

Parenteral drug products should be inspected visually for particulate matter and discoloration prior to administration whenever the solution and container permit.

Refrigerate at 2° - 8°C (36° - 46°F).

HOW SUPPLIED
INJECTION:

BRAND/MANUFACTURER	NDC	SIZE	AWP
○ GENERICS			
Schein	00364-2258-56	30 ml	$5.44
Steris	00402-0024-30	30 ml	$5.44
Major	00904-0879-30	30 ml	$6.55
Allscrips	54569-3384-00	30 ml	$6.59
FERBEE: Truxton	00463-1031-30	30 ml	$7.50
CMC-Cons	00223-7950-00	30 ml	$7.50
Moore,H.L.	00839-7658-36	30 ml	$8.22
L.I.B.: Merit	30727-0333-80	30 ml	$11.85
Goldline	00182-0570-66	30 ml	$13.05

Ferrous Sulfate/Folic Acid/ Vitamins, Multi

DESCRIPTION
Ferrous Sulfate/Folic Acid/Vitamins, Multi is a hematinic for oral administration containing 525 mg of Ferrous Sulfate (equivalent to 105 mg of elemental iron) in a unique controlled-release vehicle. In addition, this product contains 800 mcg of Folic Acid and 500 mg of ascorbic acid present as sodium ascorbate.

A preparation containing iron in a controlled-release vehicle; Vitamin C for enhancement of iron absorption; and the B-Complex Vitamins including Folic Acid is also available.

Each tablet provides:

*Ferrous Sulfate	525 mg
(equivalent to 105 mg of elemental iron)	
Ascorbic Acid (present as sodium ascorbate) (C)	500 mg
Niacinamide	30 mg
Calcium Pantothenate	10 mg
Thiamine Mononitrate (B_1)	6 mg
Riboflavin (B_2)	6 mg
Pyridoxine Hydrochloride (B_6)	5 mg
Folic Acid	800 mcg
Cyanocobalamin (B_{12})	25 mcg

* *In controlled-release form.*

CLINICAL PHARMACOLOGY
Oral iron is absorbed most efficiently when it is administered between meals. Conventional iron preparations, however, frequently cause gastric irritation when taken on an empty stomach. Studies with iron in controlled release vehicle have indicated that relatively little of the iron is released in the stomach, gastric intolerance is seldom encountered, and hematologic response ranks with that obtained from plain Ferrous Sulfate. Iron is found in the body principally as

---

➤ **SHOWN IN PRODUCT IDENTIFICATION GUIDE**

hemoglobin. Storage in the form of ferritin occurs in the liver, spleen, and bone marrow. Concentrations of plasma iron and the total iron-binding capacity of plasma vary greatly in different physiological conditions and disease states.

Large amounts of ascorbic acid administered orally with Ferrous Sulfate have been shown to enhance iron absorption. Apparently this is due to the ability of ascorbic acid to prevent the oxidation of Ferrous iron to the less effectively absorbed ferric form.

Folic Acid and iron are absorbed in the proximal small intestine, particularly the duodenum. Folic Acid is absorbed maximally and rapidly at this site, and iron is absorbed in a descending gradient from the duodenum distally.

After absorption Folic Acid is rapidly converted into its metabolically active forms. Approximately two-thirds is bound to plasma protein. Half of the Folic Acid stored in the body is found in the liver. Folic Acid is also concentrated in spinal fluid.

Except for the folates ingested in liver, yeast, and egg yolk, the percentage of absorption of food folates averages about 10%.

The B-complex Vitamins are absorbed by the active transport process. B-complex Vitamins are rapidly eliminated and therefore are not stored in the body.

Calcium pantothenate is absorbed readily from the gastrointestinal tract and distributed to all body tissues.

INDICATIONS AND USAGE

Controlled Release Iron with Folic Acid and Vitamin C (Film-coated) is indicated for the treatment of iron deficiency and prevention of concomitant Folic Acid deficiency in non-pregnant adults. Controlled Release Iron with Folic Acid and Vitamin C (Film-coated) is also indicated in pregnancy for the prevention and treatment of iron deficiency and to supply a maintenance dosage of Folic Acid.

Controlled Release Iron with Vitamin C and B-Complex, including Folic Acid (Film-coated) is indicated in non pregnant adults for the treatment of iron deficiency and prevention of concomitant Folic Acid deficiency where there is an associated deficient intake of increased need for the B-complex Vitamins. Controlled Release Iron with Vitamin C and B-Complex including Folic Acid (Film-coated) is also indicated in pregnancy for the prevention and treatment of iron deficiency where there is a concomitant deficient intake or increased need for the B-complex Vitamins (including Folic Acid).

CONTRAINDICATIONS

These products are contraindicated in patients with pernicious anemia.

These products are also contraindicated in the rare instance of hypersensitivity to Folic Acid.

WARNINGS

Folic Acid alone is improper therapy in the treatment of pernicious anemia and other megaloblastic anemias where Vitamin B_{12} is deficient.

PRECAUTIONS

Where anemia exists, its nature should be established and underlying causes determined.

These products contain 800 mcg of Folic Acid per tablet. Folic Acid especially in doses above 0.1 mg daily may obscure pernicious anemia, in that hematologic remission may occur while neurological manifestations remain progressive. Concomitant parenteral therapy with Vitamin B_{12} may be necessary in patients with deficiency of Vitamin B_{12}. Pernicious anemia is rare in women of childbearing age, and the likelihood of its occurrence along with pregnancy is reduced by the impairment of fertility associated with Vitamin B_{12} deficiency.

Like other oral iron preparations, these products should be stored out of the reach of children to guard against accidental iron poisoning (see *"Overdosage"*).

Laboratory Tests: In older patients and those with conditions tending to lead to Vitamin B_{12} depletion, serum B_{12} levels should be regularly assessed during treatment with these products.

Drug Interactions: Absorption of iron is inhibited by *magnesium trisilicate* and *antacids containing carbonates.*

Ferrous Sulfate may interfere with the absorption of *tetracyclines.*

The antiparkinsonism effects of *levodopa* may be reversed by pyridoxine.

Iron absorption is inhibited by the ingestion of eggs or milk.

Carcinogenesis: Adequate data are not available on long-term potential for carcinogenesis in animals or humans.

Pregnancy: Pregnancy Category A. Studies in pregnant women have not shown that these products increase the risk of fetal abnormalities if administered during pregnancy. If either of these drugs is used during pregnancy, the possibility of fetal harm appears remote. Because studies cannot rule out the possibility of harm, however, these products should be used during pregnancy only if clearly needed.

Nursing Mothers: Folic Acid, ascorbic acid, and B-complex Vitamins are excreted in breast milk.

ADVERSE REACTIONS

The likelihood of gastric intolerance to iron in the controlled-release vehicle is remote. If such should occur, the tablet may be taken after a meal. Allergic sensitization has been reported following both oral and parenteral administration of Folic Acid.

OVERDOSAGE

Signs of serious toxicity may be delayed because the iron is in a controlled-release dose form. Increased capillary permeability, reduced plasma volume, increased cardiac output, and sudden cardiovascular collapse may occur in acute iron intoxication. In overdosage, efforts should be made to hasten the elimination of the tablets ingested. An emetic should be administered as soon as possible, followed by gastric lavage if indicated. Immediately following emesis, a large dose of a saline cathartic should be used to speed passage through the intestinal tract. X-ray examination may then be considered to determine the position and number of tablets remaining in the gastrointestinal tract.

DOSAGE AND ADMINISTRATION

Controlled Release Iron with Folic Acid and Vitamin C (Film-coated) is administered orally and may be taken on an empty stomach.

Adults: For treatment of iron deficiency and prevention of Folic Acid deficiency, the recommended dose is one tablet daily.

Pregnant Adults: For prevention and treatment of iron deficiency and to supply a maintenance dosage of Folic Acid, the recommended dose is one tablet daily.

Controlled Release Iron with Vitamin C and B-complex including Folic Acid (Film-coated) is administered orally and may be taken on an empty stomach.

Adults: For the treatment of iron deficiency and prevention of concomitant Folic Acid deficiency where there is an associated deficient intake or increased need for the B-complex Vitamins, the recommended dose is one tablet daily.

Pregnant Adults: For the prevention and treatment of iron deficiency where there is a concomitant deficient intake or increased need for the B-complex Vitamins including Folic Acid, the recommended dose is one tablet daily.

Recommended storage: Store tablets below 77°F (25°C).

HOW SUPPLIED
TABLET, EXTENDED RELEASE:

BRAND/MANUFACTURER	NDC	SIZE	AWP
○ **BRAND**			
IBERET-FOLIC-500: Abbott Pharm	00074-7125-60	60s	$38.14
FERO-FOLIC 500: Abbott Pharm	00074-7079-13	100s	$34.75
	00074-7079-53	500s	$168.51

TABLETS:

BRAND/MANUFACTURER	NDC	SIZE	AWP
○ **GENERICS**			
VITA-RET-FOLIC 500: Rugby	00536-4758-08	60s	$6.43
MULTI-FERROUS FOLIC 500: URL	00677-0657-06	60s	$7.37
IBC 500: Moore,H.L.	00839-6433-05	60s	$7.41
MULTI-FERROUS FOLIC 500: URL	00677-0990-06	60s	$7.60
MULTIRET FOLIC-500: Amide	52152-0048-01	60s	$7.90
GENERET-500: Goldline	00182-4333-26	60s	$9.00
FERRO BC-500: Major	00904-0391-60	100s	$12.40
FERRO BC-500: Major	00904-0391-40	500s	$53.05
MULTIRET FOLIC-500: Amide	52152-0048-04	500s	$57.90

Ferrous Sulfate/Sodium Fluoride/ Vitamins, Multi

DESCRIPTION

Each 1.0 ml supplies:		Percentage of U.S. Recommended Daily Allowance	
		Infants	Children Under 4
Vitamin A, IU	1500	100	60
Vitamin D, IU	400	100	100
Vitamin E, IU	5	100	50
Vitamin C, mg	35	100	88
Thiamine, mg	0.5	100	71
Riboflavin, mg	0.6	100	75
Niacin, mg	8	100	89
Vitamin B_6, mg	0.4	100	57
Iron, mg	10	67	100
Fluoride, mg	0.5 or 0.25	*	*

*U.S. Recommended Daily Allowance has not been established.

See *"Indications and Usage"* section below for use by infants and children under two years of age.

This product does not contain the essential vitamins folic acid and B_{12}.

Active ingredient for caries prophylaxis: Each 1 ml contains 0.5 mg or 0.25 mg fluoride as Sodium Fluoride.

◆ RATED THERAPEUTICALLY EQUIVALENT; ◇ THERAPEUTIC EQUIVALENCE UNCONFIRMED; ○ UNRATED

CLINICAL PHARMACOLOGY

It is well established that fluoridation of the water supply (1 ppm fluoride) during the period of tooth development leads to a significant decrease in the incidence of dental caries.

Hydroxyapatite is the principal crystal for all calcified tissue in the human body. The fluoride ion reacts with the *hydroxyapatite* in the tooth as it is formed to produce the more caries-resistant crystal, *fluorapatite*. The reaction may be expressed by the equation:

$$Ca_{10}(PO_4)_6(OH)_2 + 2F - CA_{10}(PO_4)_6F_2 + 2OH-$$

(Hydroxyapatite)   (Fluorapatite)

Three stages of fluoride deposition in tooth enamel can be distinguished.

1. Small amounts (reflecting the low levels of fluoride in tissue fluids) are incorporated into the enamel crystals while they are being formed.

2. After enamel has been laid down, fluoride deposition continues in the surface enamel. Diffusion of fluoride from the surface inward is apparently restricted.

3. After eruption, the surface enamel acquires fluoride from water, food, supplementary fluoride and smaller amounts from saliva.

INDICATIONS AND USAGE

Supplementation of the diet with eight essential vitamins and iron.

Supplementation of the diet with fluoride for caries prophylaxis.

The American Academy of Pediatrics recommends that children up to age 16, in areas where drinking water contains less than optimal levels of fluoride, receive daily fluoride supplementation.

Ferrous Sulfate/Sodium Fluoride/Vitamins, Multi 0.25 mg drops provide fluoride in drop form for children ages 2-3 years in areas where the drinking water contains less than 0.3 ppm fluoride; and for children over 3 years in areas where the drinking water contains 0.3 thru 0.7 ppm of fluoride. Each 1.0 ml provides Sodium Fluoride (0.25 mg fluoride) plus eight essential vitamins and iron.

Ferrous Sulfate/Sodium Fluoride/Vitamins, Multi 0.5 mg drops provide fluoride in drop form for children ages 2-3 years in areas where the drinking water contains less than 0.3 ppm fluoride; and for children over 3 years in areas where the drinking water contains 0.3 through 0.7 ppm of fluoride. Each 1.0 ml provides Sodium Fluoride (0.50 mg fluoride) plus eight essential vitamins and iron.

The American Academy of Pediatrics and the American Dental Association currently recommend that infants and children under 2 years of age, in areas where drinking water contains less than 0.3 ppm of fluoride, and children 2-3, in areas where the drinking water contains 0.3 through 0.7 ppm of fluoride, receive 0.25 mg of supplemental fluoride daily which is provided in a full dose (1 ml) of Ferrous Sulfate/Sodium Fluoride/Vitamins, Multi 0.25 mg drops. A half dose (0.5 mg) of Ferrous Sulfate/Sodium Fluoride/Vitamins, Multi 0.5 mg drops could also provide a daily fluoride intake of 0.25 mg; however, this dosage reduces vitamin supplementation by half.

Ferrous Sulfate/Sodium Fluoride/Vitamins, Multi 0.5 mg or 0.25 mg supply significant amounts of vitamins A, D, E, C, thiamine, riboflavin, niacin, pyridoxine, and Ferrous Sulfate to supplement the diet, and to help assure that nutritional deficiencies of these vitamins will not develop. Thus, in a single easy-to-use preparation, children obtain eight essential vitamins and iron, plus fluoride.

WARNINGS

As in the case of all medications, keep out of the reach of children.

PRECAUTIONS

The suggested dose should not be exceeded since dental fluorosis may result from continued ingestion of large amounts of fluoride.

When prescribing multivitamin and fluoride products, the physician should:

1. Determine the fluoride content of the drinking water.

2. Make sure the child is not receiving significant amounts of fluoride from other medications.

3. Periodically check to make sure that the child does not develop significant dental fluorosis.

Ferrous Sulfate/Sodium Fluoride/Vitamins, Multi 0.25 mg and 0.5 mg should be dispensed in the original plastic container, since contact with glass leads to instability and precipitation. (The amount of sodium fluoride in the 50 ml size is well below the maximum to be dispensed at one time according to recommendations of the American Dental Association.)

ADVERSE REACTIONS

Allergic rash and other idiosyncrasies have been reported rarely.

DOSAGE AND ADMINISTRATION

Ferrous Sulfate/Sodium Fluoride/Vitamins, Multi 0.25 mg: 1.0 ml daily for infants and children under 2 years of age, or as prescribed by physician.

Ferrous Sulfate/Sodium Fluoride/Vitamins, Multi 0.5 mg: 1.0 ml daily for children 2 years of age and older, or as prescribed by physician.

Both products may be dropped directly into mouth with dropper or mixed with fruit juice, cereal or other food.

Store at room temperature, protect from light.

HOW SUPPLIED

CHEW TABLET: 0.25 MG

BRAND/MANUFACTURER	NDC	SIZE	AWP
○ **BRAND**			
POLY-VI-FLOR W/IRON: Mead Johnson Nutr	00087-0488-41	100s	$15.65

CHEW TABLET: 0.5 MG

BRAND/MANUFACTURER	NDC	SIZE	AWP
○ **BRAND**			
POLY-VI-FLOR W/IRON: Mead Johnson Nutr	00087-0482-41	100s	$15.65
○ **GENERICS**			
MULTI-VITE & FLUORIDE W/IRON: Moore,H.L.	00839-7719-06	100s	$3.85
Copley	38245-0197-10	100s	$4.00
Balan,J.J.	00304-1248-01	100s	$5.18
Rugby	00536-4475-01	100s	$5.55
Schein	00364-2506-01	100s	$9.50
FLORVITE PLUS IRON: Everett	00642-0088-10	100s	$11.50

CHEW TABLET: 1 MG

BRAND/MANUFACTURER	NDC	SIZE	AWP
○ **BRAND**			
POLY-VI-FLOR W/IRON: Mead Johnson Nutr	00087-0476-03	100s	$15.65
VI-DAYLIN/F PLUS IRON: Ross Pharm	00074-7621-13	100s	$15.93
○ **GENERICS**			
Copley	38245-0159-10	100s	$4.00
Moore,H.L.	00839-7052-06	100s	$4.25
Amide	52152-0038-02	100s	$4.50
Rugby	00536-4308-01	100s	$5.25
POLY-VITA W/FLUORIDE & IRON: Allscrips	54569-4021-00	100s	$5.25
Southwood	58016-0904-00	100s	$9.22
Schein	00364-0770-01	100s	$10.04
FLORVITE PLUS IRON: Everett	00642-0086-10	100s	$11.50
Copley	38245-0159-20	1000s	$39.00
Amide	52152-0038-05	1000s	$39.95

Fetrin *SEE* **FERROUS FUMARATE/VITAMIN B₁₂/VITAMIN C**

Filgrastim

DESCRIPTION

Filgrastim is a human granulocyte colony stimulating factor (G-CSF), produced by recombinant DNA technology. G-CSF regulates the production of neutrophils within the bone marrow; endogenous G-CSF is a glycoprotein produced by monocytes, fibroblasts, and endothelial cells.[1-5] G-CSF is a colony stimulating factor which has been shown to have minimal direct *in vivo* or *in vitro* effects on the production of other hematopoietic cell types.[5,6] Filgrastim has been selected as the name for recombinant methionyl human granulocyte colony stimulating factor (r-metHuG-CSF).

Filgrastim[7] is a 175 amino acid protein manufactured by recombinant DNA technology.[7] Filgrastim is produced by *Escherichia coli* (*E. coli*) bacteria into which has been inserted the human granulocyte colony stimulating factor gene. Filgrastim has a molecular weight of 18,800 daltons. The protein has an amino acid sequence that is identical to the natural sequence predicted from human DNA sequence analysis, except for the addition of an N-terminal methionine necessary for expression in *E. coli*. Because Filgrastim is produced in *E. coli*, the product is nonglycosylated and thus differs from G-CSF isolated from a human cell.

Filgrastim is a sterile, clear, colorless, preservative-free liquid for parenteral administration. Each single-use vial of Filgrastim contains 300 mcg/mL at a specific activity of $1.0 \pm 0.6 \times 10^8$ U/mg, (as measured by a cell mitogenesis assay).

Manufacture is initiated from a master seed lot of *E. coli* containing the gene for r-metHuG-CSF. The *E. coli* are grown and the product is purified by conventional means. Prior to final purification, r-metHuG-CSF is allowed to oxidize to its native state and its final purity is achieved by sequential passage over a series of chromatography columns.

➤ **SHOWN IN PRODUCT IDENTIFICATION GUIDE**

Following is its chemical structure:

```
                                        H — Met — Thr — Pro — Leu — Gly — Pro — Ala — Ser — Ser — Leu —
                                          |     1     2     3     4     5     6     7     8     9
  Pro — Gln — Ser — Phe — Leu — Leu — Lys — Cys — Leu — Glu — Gln — Val — Arg — Lys — Ile — Gln — Gly — Asp —
   10    11    12    13    14    15    16    17    18    19    20    21    22    23    24    25    26    27
                                                                                   s
                                                                              s
  Gly — Ala — Ala — Leu — Gln — Glu — Lys — Leu — Cys — Ala — Thr — Tyr — Lys — Leu — Cys — His — Pro — Glu —
   28    29    30    31    32    33    34    35    36    37    38    39    40    41    42    43    44    45
  Glu — Leu — Val — Leu — Leu — Gly — His — Ser — Leu — Gly — Ile — Pro — Trp — Ala — Pro — Leu — Ser — Ser —
   46    47    48    49    50    51    52    53    54    55    56    57    58    59    60    61    62    63
     s                                           s
   s                                           s
  Cys — Pro — Ser — Gln — Ala — Leu — Gln — Leu — Ala — Gly — Cys — Leu — Ser — Gln — Leu — His — Ser — Gly —
   64    65    66    67    68    69    70    71    72    73    74    75    76    77    78    79    80    81
  Leu — Phe — Leu — Tyr — Gln — Gly — Leu — Leu — Gln — Ala — Leu — Glu — Gly — Ile — Ser — Pro — Glu — Leu —
   82    83    84    85    86    87    88    89    90    91    92    93    94    95    96    97    98    99
  Gly — Pro — Thr — Leu — Asp — Thr — Leu — Gln — Leu — Asp — Val — Ala — Asp — Phe — Ala — Thr — Thr — Ile —
  100   101   102   103   104   105   106   107   108   109   110   111   112   113   114   115   116   117
  Trp — Gln — Gln — Met — Glu — Glu — Leu — Gly — Met — Ala — Pro — Ala — Leu — Gln — Pro — Thr — Gln — Gly —
  118   119   120   121   122   123   124   125   126   127   128   129   130   131   132   133   134   135
  Ala — Met — Pro — Ala — Phe — Ala — Ser — Ala — Phe — Gln — Arg — Arg — Ala — Gly — Gly — Val — Leu — Val —
  136   137   138   139   140   141   142   143   144   145   146   147   148   149   150   151   152   153
  Ala — Ser — His — Leu — Gln — Ser — Phe — Leu — Glu — Val — Ser — Tyr — Arg — Val — Leu — Arg — His — Leu —
  154   155   156   157   158   159   160   161   162   163   164   165   166   167   168   169   170   171
  Ala — Gln — Pro — OH
  172   173   174
```

CLINICAL PHARMACOLOGY

COLONY STIMULATING FACTORS

Colony stimulating factors are glycoproteins which act on hematopoietic cells by binding to specific cell surface receptors and stimulating proliferation, differentiation commitment, and some end-cell functional activation.

Endogenous G-CSF is a lineage-specific colony stimulating factor with selectivity for the neutrophil lineage. G-CSF is not species specific and has been shown to primarily affect neutrophil progenitor proliferation,[8,9] differentiation,[8,10] and selected end-cell functional activation (including enhanced phagocytic ability,[11] priming of the cellular metabolism associated with respiratory burst,[12] antibody dependent killing,[13] and the increased expression of some functions associated with cell surface antigens[14]).

PRE-CLINICAL EXPERIENCE

Filgrastim was administered to monkeys, dogs, hamsters, rats, and mice as part of a comprehensive pre-clinical toxicology program which included single-dose acute, repeated-dose subacute, and chronic studies. Single-dose administration of Filgrastim by the oral, intravenous, subcutaneous, or intraperitoneal routes resulted in no significant toxicity in mice, rats, hamsters, or monkeys. Although no deaths were observed in mice, rats, or monkeys at dose levels up to 3450 mcg/kg and in hamsters using single doses up to approximately 860 mcg/kg, deaths were observed in a subchronic (13 week) study in monkeys. In this study, evidence of neurological symptoms was seen in monkeys treated with doses of Filgrastim greater than 1150 mcg/kg/day for up to 18 days. Deaths were seen in 5 of the 8 treated animals and were associated with 15- to 28-fold increases in peripheral leukocyte counts, and neutrophil-infiltrated hemorrhagic foci were seen in both the cerebrum and cerebellum. In contrast, no monkeys died following 13 weeks of daily intravenous administration of Filgrastim at a dose level of 115 mcg/kg.

In subacute, repeated-dose studies, changes observed were attributable to the expected pharmacological actions of Filgrastim (i.e., dose-dependent increases in white cell counts, increased circulating segmented neutrophils, and increased myeloid:erythroid ratio in bone marrow). In all species, histo-pathologic examination of the liver and spleen revealed evidence of ongoing extramedullary granulopoiesis; increased spleen weights were seen in all species and appeared to be dose-related. A dose-dependent increase in serum alkaline phosphatase was observed in rats, and may reflect increased activity of osteoblasts and osteoclasts. Changes in serum chemistry values were reversible following discontinuation of treatment.

In rats treated at doses of 1150 mcg/kg/day for four weeks (5 of 32 animals) and for 13 weeks at doses of 100 mcg/kg/day (4 of 32 animals) and 500 mcg/kg/day (6 of 32 animals) articular swelling of the hind legs was observed. Some degree of hind leg dysfunction was also observed; however, symptoms reversed following cessation of dosing. In rats, osteoclasis and osteoanagenesis were found in the femur, humerus, coccyx and hind legs (where they were accompanied by synovitis) after intravenous treatment for four weeks (115 to 1150 mcg/kg/day), and in the sternum after intravenous treatment for 13 weeks (115 to 575 mcg/kg/day). These effects reversed to normal within 4 to 5 weeks following cessation of treatment.

PHARMACOLOGIC EFFECTS OF FILGRASTIM

In Phase I studies involving 96 patients with various non-myeloid malignancies, Filgrastim administration resulted in a dose-dependent increase in circulating neutrophil counts over the dose range of 1-70 mcg/kg/day.[15-17] This increase in neutrophil counts was observed whether Filgrastim was administered intravenously (1-70 mcg/kg twice daily),[15] subcutaneously (1-3 mcg/kg once daily),[17] or by continuous subcutaneous infusion (3-11 mcg/kg/day).[16] With discontinuation of Filgrastim therapy, neutrophil counts returned to baseline, in most cases within four days. Isolated neutrophils displayed normal phagocytic (measured by zymosan-stimulated chemoluminescence) and chemotactic [measured by migration under agarose using N-formyl-methionyl-leucyl-phenylalanine (fMLP) as the chemotaxin] activity *in vitro*.

The absolute monocyte count was reported to increase in a dose-dependent manner in most patients receiving Filgrastim, however, the percentage of monocytes in the differential count remained within the normal range. In all studies to date, absolute counts of both eosinophils and basophils did not change and were within the normal range following administration of Filgrastim. Increases in lymphocyte counts following Filgrastim administration have been reported in some normal subjects and cancer patients. White blood cell differentials obtained during clinical trials have demonstrated a shift towards earlier granulocyte progenitor cells (left shift), including the appearance of promyelocytes and myeloblasts, usually during neutrophil recovery following the chemotherapy-induced nadir. In addition, Dohle bodies, increased granulocyte granulation, as well as hypersegmented neutrophils have been observed. Such changes were transient, and were not associated with clinical sequelae nor were they necessarily associated with infection.

PHARMACOKINETICS

Absorption and clearance of Filgrastim follows first-order pharmacokinetic modeling without apparent concentration dependence. A positive linear correlation occurred between the parenteral dose and both the serum concentration and area under the concentration-time curve. Continuous intravenous infusion of 20 mcg/kg of Filgrastim over 24 hours resulted in mean and median serum concentrations of approximately 48 and 56 ng/mL, respectively. Subcutaneous administration of 3.45 mcg/kg and 11.5 mcg/kg resulted in maximum serum concentrations of 4 and 49 ng/mL, respectively, within 2 to 8 hours. The volume of distribution averaged 150 mL/kg in both normal subjects and cancer patients. The elimination half-life, in both normal subjects and cancer patients was approximately 3.5 hours. Clearance rate of Filgrastim were approximately 0.5-0.7 mL/min/kg. Single parenteral doses or daily intravenous doses, over a 14 day period, resulted in comparable half-lives. The half-lives were similar for intravenous administration (231 minutes, following doses of 34.5 mcg/kg) and for subcutaneous administration (210 minutes, following Filgrastim doses of 3.45 mcg/kg). Continous 24-hour intravenous infusions at 20 mcg/kg over an 11 to 20 day period produced steady state serum concentrations of Filgrastim with no evidence of drug accumulation over the time period investigated.

INDICATIONS AND USAGE

Filgrastim is indicated to decrease the incidence of infection, as manifested by febrile neutropenia, in patients with non-myeloid malignancies receiving myelosuppressive anti-cancer drugs associated with a significant incidence of severe neutropenia with fever (see *"Clinical Experience"*). A complete blood count and platelet count should be obtained prior to chemotherapy, and twice per week (see *"Laboratory Monitoring"*) during Filgrastim therapy to avoid leukocytosis and to monitor the neutrophil count. In Phase III clinical studies, Filgrastim therapy was discontinued when the absolute neutrophil count (ANC) was $\geq 10,000/mm^3$ after the expected chemotherapy-induced nadir.

CLINICAL EXPERIENCE: RESPONSE TO FILGRASTIM

Filgrastim has been shown to be safe and effective in accelerating the recovery of neutrophil counts following a variety of chemotherapy regimens. In a Phase III clinical trial in small cell lung cancer, patients received subcutaneous administration of Filgrastim (4 to 8 mcg/kg/day, days 4-17) or placebo. In this study, the benefits of Filgrastim therapy where shown to be prevention of infection as manifested by febrile neutropenia, decreased hospitalization, and decreased intravenous antibiotic usage. No difference in survival or disease progression was demonstrated. In the Phase III, randomized, double-blind, placebo-controlled trial conducted in patients with small cell lung cancer, patients were randomized to receive Filgrastim (n = 99) or placebo (n = 111) starting on day 4, after receiving standard dose chemotherapy with cyclophosphomide, doxorubicin, and etoposide. A total of 210 patients were evaluated for efficacy and 207 evaluated for safety. Treatment with Filgrastim resulted in a clinically and statistically significant reduction in the incidence of infection, as manifested by febrile neutropenia: the incidence of at least one infection over all cycles of chemotherapy was 76% (84/111) for placebo-treated patients, versus 40% (40/99) for Filgrastim treated patients (p < 0.001). The following secondary analyses were also performed. The requirements for in-patient hospitalization and antibiotic use were also significantly decreased during the first cycle of chemotherapy; incidence of hospitalization was 69% (77/111) for placebo-treated patients in cycle one, versus 52% (51/99) for Filgrastim treated patients (p = 0.032). The incidence of intravenous antibiotic usage was 60% (67/111) for placebo-treated patients in cycle one, versus 38% (38/99) for Filgrastim treated patients (p = 0.003). The incidence, severity, and duration of severe neutropenia (ANC < 500/mm^3) following chemotherapy were all significantly reduced. The incidence of severe neutropenia in cycle one was 84% (83/99) for patients receiving Filgrastim versus 96% (106/110) for patients receiving placebo (p = 0.004). Over all cycles, patients randomized to Filgrastim had a 57% (286/500 cycles) rate of severe neutropenia versus 77% (416/543 cycles) for patients randomized to placebo. The median duration of severe neutropenia in cycle one was reduced from 6 days (range 0-10 days) for patients receiving placebo to 2 days (range 0-9 days) for patients receiving Filgrastim (p < 0.001). The mean duration of neutropenia in cycle one was 5.64 ± 2.27 for patients receiving placebo versus 2.44 ± 1.90 days for patients receiving Filgrastim. Over all cycles, the median duration of neutropenia was 3 days for patients randomized to placebo to 1 day for patients randomized to Filgrastim. The median severity of neutropenia (as measured by ANC nadir) was 72/mm^3 (range 0/mm^3-7912/mm^3) in cycle one for patients receiving Filgrastim versus 38/mm^3 (range 0/mm^3-9520/mm^3) for patients receiving placebo (p = 0.012). The mean severity of neutropenia in cycle one was 496/mm^3±1382/mm^3 for patients receiving Filgrastim versus 204/mm^{3}953/mm^3 for patients receiving placebo. Over all cycles, the ANC nadir for patients randomized to Filgrastim was 403/mm^3 versus 161/mm^3 for patients randomized to placebo. Administration of Filgrastim resulted in an earlier ANC nadir following chemotherapy than was experienced by patients receiving placebo (day 10 versus day 12 Filgrastim was well tolerated when given subcutaneously daily at doses of 4 to 8 mcg/kg for up to 14 consecutive days following each cycle of chemotherapy (see "Adverse Reactions").

Several other Phase I/II studies, which did not directly measure the incidence of infection, but which did measure increases in neutrophils, support the efficacy of Filgrastim. The regimens are presented to provide some background on the clinical experience with Filgrastim. No claim regarding the safety or efficacy of the chemotherapy regimens is made. The effects of Filgrastim on tumor growth or on the antitumor activity of the chemotherapy were not assessed. The doses of Filgrastim used in these studies are considerably greater than those found to be effective in the Phase III study described above. Such Phase I/II studies are summarized in the following table. (See related table).

UNLABELED USES
Filgrastim is also used alone or as an adjunct in the treatment of agranulocytosis and AIDS-related complex.

CONTRAINDICATIONS
Filgrastim is contraindicated in patients with known hypersensitivity to *E. coli*-derived proteins, Filgrastim, or any component of the product.

WARNINGS
Since commercial introduction, there have been rare reports (< 1 in 4,000 patients) of allergic-type reactions in patients treated with Filgrastim. These have generally been characterized by systemic symptoms involving at least two body systems, most often skin (rash, urticaria, facial edema), respiratory (wheezing, dyspnea), and cardiovascular (hypotension, tachycardia). Some reactions occurred on initial exposure. Reactions tended to occur within the first 30 minutes after administration and appeared to occur more frequently in patients receiving Filgrastim intravenously. Rapid resolution of symptoms occurred in most cases after administration of antihistamines, steroids, bronchodilators, and/or epinephrine. Symptoms recurred in more than half the patients who were rechallenged.

PRECAUTIONS
GENERAL
SIMULTANEOUS USE WITH CHEMORADIATION
The safety and efficacy of Filgrastim given simultaneously with cytotoxic chemotherapy have not been established. Because of the potential sensitivity of rapidly dividing myeloid cells to cytotoxic chemotherapy, do not use Filgrastim in the period 24 hours before through 24 hours after the administration of cytotoxic chemotherapy (see "Dosage and Administration"). Simultaneous use of Filgrastim with chemoradiation should be avoided. The efficacy of Filgrastim has not been evaluated in patients receiving chemotherapy associated with delayed myelosuppression (e.g., nitrosources) or with mitomycin C or with myelosuppressive doses of antimetabolites such as 5-fluorouracil or cytosine arabinoside.

GROWTH FACTOR POTENTIAL
Filgrastim is a growth factor that primarily stimulates neutrophils. However, the possibility that Filgrastim can act as a growth factor for any tumor type, particularly myeloid malignancies, cannot be excluded. Therefore, because of the possibility of tumor growth, precaution should be exercised in using this drug in any malignancy with myeloid characteristics.

LEUKOCYTOSIS
White blood cell counts of 100,000/mm^3 or greater were observed in approximately 2% of patients receiving Filgrastim at doses above 5 mcg/kg/day. There

Type of Malignancy	Regimen	Chemotherapy Dose	Number of Pts.	Trial Phase	Filgrastim Daily Dose[a]
Small Cell Lung Cancer	Cyclophosphamide Doxorubicin Etoposide	1 g/m^2/day 50 mg/m^2/day 120 mg/m^2/day x3 q 21 days	210	III	4-8 mcg/kg SC days 4-17
Small Cell Lung Cancer[17]	Ifosfamide Doxorubicin Etoposide Mesna	5 g/m^2/day 50 mg/m^2/day 120 mg/m^2/day x3 8 g/m^2 /day q 21 days	12	I/II	5.75-46 mcg/kg IV days 4-17
Urothelial Cancer[18]	Methotrexate Vinblastine Doxorubicin Cisplatin	30 mg/m^{2}day x2 3mg/m^2/day x2 30 mg/m^2/day 70 mg/m^2/day q 28 days	40	I/II	3.45-69 mcg/kg IV days 4-11
Various Non-Myeloid Malignancies[19]	Cyclophosphamide Etoposide Cisplatin	2.5 g/m^2/day x2 500 mg/m^2/day x3 50 mg/m^2/day x3 q 28 days	18	I/II	23-69 mcg/kg[b] IV days 8-28
Breast/ Ovarian Cancer[20]	Doxorubicin[c]	75 mg/m^2 100 mg/m^2 125 mg/m^2 150 mg/m^2 q 14 days	21	II	11.5 mcg/kg days 2-9 IV 5.75 mcg/kg days 10-12 IV
Neuroblastoma	Cyclophosphamide Doxorubicin Cisplatin	150 mg/m^2 x7 35 mg/m^2 90 mg/m^2 q 28 days (cycles 1,3,5)[d]	12	II	5.45-17.25 mcg/kg SC days 6-19

[a] Filgrastim doses were those that accelerated neutrophil production. Doses which provided no additional acceleratrion beyond that achieved at the next lower dose are not reported.
[b] Lowest dose(s) tested in the study.
[c] Patients received doxorubicin at either 75, 100, 125 or 150 mg/m^2.
[d] Cycles 2,6 = cyclophospamide 150 mg/m^2 × 7 and etoposide 280 mg/m^2 × 3 Cycle 4 = cisplatin 90 mg/m^2 × 1 and etoposide 280 mg/m^2 × 3

➤ SHOWN IN PRODUCT IDENTIFICATION GUIDE

were no reports of adverse events associated with this degree of leukocytosis. In order to avoid the potential complications of excessive leukocytosis, a complete blood count (CBC) is recommended twice per week during Filgrastim therapy (see *"Laboratory Monitoring"*).

PREMATURE DISCONTINUATION OF FILGRASTIM THERAPY
A transient increase in neutrophil counts is typically seen 1 to 2 days after initiation of Filgrastim therapy. However, for a sustained therapeutic response, Filgrastim therapy should be continued until the post nadir ANC reaches 10,000/mm^3. Therefore, the premature discontinuation of Filgrastim therapy, prior to the time of recovery from the expected neutrophil nadir, is generally not recommended (see *"Dosage and Administration"*).

CHRONIC ADMINISTRATION
The safety and efficacy of chronic administration of Filgrastim have not been established. Preliminary investigational studies with Filgrastim have been conducted in 224 patients with severe chronic neutropenia, 13 of whom have been treated for up to three years. In these patients, subclinical splenomegaly (detected by CT or MRI scanning) was the most frequently observed adverse effect, occurring in approximately one third of patients receiving chronic administration of Filgrastim; 3% of patients were noted to have clinical splenomegaly. Other infrequently observed adverse events included exacerbation of some pre-existing skin disorders (e.g., psoriasis), alopecia, hematuria/ proteinuria with or without elevated creatinine, thrombocytopenia (platelets less than 50,000/mm^3) and osteoporosis.

OTHER
In studies of Filgrastim administration following chemotherapy, most reported side effects were consistent with those usually seen as a result of cytotoxic chemotherapy (see *"Adverse Reactions"*). Because of the potential of receiving higher doses of chemotherapy (i.e., full doses on the prescribed schedule), the patient may be at greater risk of thrombocytopenia, anemia, and non-hematologic consequences of increased chemotherapy doses (please refer to the prescribing information of the specific chemotherapy agents used). Regular monitoring of the hematocrit and platelet count is recommended. Furthermore, care should be exercised in the administration of Filgrastim in conjunction with other drugs known to lower the platelet count. In septic patients receiving Filgrastim the physican should be alert to the theoretical possibility of adult respiratory distress syndrome, due to the possible influx of neutrophils at the site of inflammation. Cardiac events (myocardial infarctions, arrhythmias) have been reported in 11 of 375 cancer patients receiving Filgrastim in clinical studies; the relationship to Filgrastim therapy is unknown. However, patients with pre-existing cardiac conditions receiving Filgrastim should be monitored closely.

There have been rare reports (< 1 in 7,000 patients) of cutaneous vasculitis in patients treated with Filgrastim. In most cases, the severity of cutaneous vasculitis was moderate or severe. Most of the reports involved patients with severe chronic neutropenia receiving long term Filgrastim therapy. Symptoms of vasculitis generally developed simultaneously with an increase in the ANC and abated when the ANC decreased. Many patients were able to continue Filgrastim at a reduced dose.

INFORMATION FOR PATIENTS
In those situations in which the physician determines that the patient can safely and effectively self-administer Filgrastim, the patient should be instructed as to the proper dosage and administration. Patients should be referred to the full "Information for Patients" section attached; it is not a disclosure of all, or possible, intended effects. The most common adverse experience occurring with Filgrastim therapy is bone pain. If home use is prescribed, patients should be thoroughly instructed in the importance of proper disposal and cautioned against the reuse of needles, syringes, or drug product. A puncture-resistant container for the disposal of used syringes and needles should be available to the patient. The full container should be disposed of according to the directions provided by the physician.

LABORATORY MONITORING
A CBC and platelet count should be obtained prior to chemo-therapy, and at regular intervals (twice per week) during Filgrastim therapy. Following cytotoxic chemotherapy, the neutrophil nadir occurred earlier during cycles when Filgrastim was administered, and white cell differentials demonstrated a left shift, including the appearance of promyelocytes and myeloblasts. In addition, the duration of severe neutropenia was reduced, and was followed by an accelerated recovery in the neutrophil counts. Therefore, regular monitoring of white blood cell counts, particularly at the time of the recovery from the post chemotherapy nadir, is recommended in order to avoid excessive leukocytosis.

DRUG INTERACTION
Drug interactions between Filgrastim and other drugs have not been fully evaluated. Drugs which may potentiate the release of neutrophils, such as lithium, should be used with caution.

CARCINOGENESIS, MUTAGENESIS, IMPAIRMENT OF FERTILITY
The carcinogenic potential of Filgrastim has not been studied Filgrastim failed to induce bacterial gene mutations in either the presence or absence of a drug metabolizing enzyme system. Filgrastim had no observed effect on the fertility of male or female rats, or on gestation at doses up to 500 mcg/kg.

PREGNANCY CATEGORY C
Filgrastim has been shown to have adverse effects in pregnant rabbits when given in doses 2 to 10 times the human dose. There are no adequate and well controlled studies in pregnant women. Filgrastim should be used during pregnancy only if the potential benefit justifies the potential risk to the fetus.

In rabbits, increased abortion and embryolethality were observed in animals treated with Filgrastim at 80 mcg/kg/day. Filgrastim administered to pregnant rabbits at doses of 80 mcg/kg/day during the period of organogenesis was associated with increased fetal resorption, genitourinary bleeding, developmental abnormalities, and decreased body weight, live births, and food consumption. External abnormalities were not observed in the fetuses of dams treated at 80 mcg/kg/day. Reproductive studies in pregnant rats have shown that Filgrastim was not associated with lethal, teratogenic, or behavioral effects on fetuses when administered by daily intravenous injection during the period of organogensis at dose levels up to 575 mcg/kg/day.

In Segment III studies in rats, offspring of dams treated at > 20 mcg/kg/day exhibited a delay in external differentiation (detachment of auricles and descent of testes) and slight growth retardation, possibly due to lower body weight of females during rearing and nursing. Offspring of dams treated at 100 mcg/kg/day exhibited decreased body weights at birth, and a slightly reduced four day survival rate.

NURSING MOTHERS
It is not known whether Filgrastim is excreted in human milk. Because many drugs are excreted in human milk, caution should be exercised if Filgrastim is administered to a nursing woman.

PEDIATRIC USE
Although efficacy of Filgrastim has not been demonstrated in a pediatric population, safety data indicate that Filgrastim does not exhibit any greater toxicity in children than in adults. Filgrastim has been used to treat 128 pediatric severe chronic neutropenia patients; such patients ranged in age from 3 months to 18 years and were treated with Filgrastim at 0.6-120 mcg/kg/day for up to three years. Such doses were well tolerated, and the overall pattern of adverse events in children and adults appeared to be similar. While subclinical increases in spleen size, detected by imaging studies (CT or MRI) were reported more often in children than in adults, the clinical significance of these radiographic findings relative to normal growth and development is not known. No hematologic abnormalities were noted which were unique to children treated with Filgrastim. In addition, 12 pediatric patients with neuroblastoma have received up to six cycles of cyclophosphamide, cisplatin, doxorubicin, and etoposide chemotherapy concurrently with Filgrastim; in this population, Filgrastim was well tolerated. There was one report of palpable splenomegaly associated with Filgrastim therapy, however, the only consistently reported adverse event was musculoskeletal pain, which is no different from the experience in the adult population.

ADVERSE REACTIONS
In clinical trials involving over 350 patients receiving Filgrastim following cytotoxic chemotherapy, most adverse experiences were the sequelae of the underlying malignancy or cytotoxic chemotherapy. In all Phase II and III trials, medullary bone pain, reported in 24% of patients, was the only consistently observed adverse reaction attributed to Filgrastim therapy. This bone pain was generally reported to be of mild-to-moderate severity, and could be controlled in most patients with non-narcotic analgesics; infrequently, bone pain was severe enough to require narcotic analgesics. Bone pain was reported more frequently in patients treated with higher doses (20-100 mcg/kg/day) administered intravenously, and less frequently in patients treated with lower subcutaneous doses of Filgrastim (3-10 mcg/kg/day).

In the randomized, double-blind, placebo-controlled trial of Filgrastim therapy following combination chemotherapy in patients (n = 207) with small cell lung cancer, the following adverse events were reported during blinded cycles of study medication (placebo or Filgrastim at 4 to 8 mcg/kg/day). Events are reported as exposure adjusted since patients remained on double-blind Filgrastim a median of three cycles versus one cycle for placebo.

Event	% of Blinded Cycles with Events	
	Filgrastim N = 384 patient cycles	Placebo N = 257 patient cycles
Nausea/Vomiting	57	64
Skeletal Pain	22	11
Alopecia	18	27
Diarrhea	14	23
Neutropenic Fever	13	35
Mucositis	12	20
Fever	12	11
Fatigue	11	16
Anorexia	9	11
Dyspnea	9	11
Headache	7	9
Cough	6	8
Skin Rash	6	9
Chest Pain	5	6
Generalized Weakness	4	7
Sore Throat	4	9
Stomatitis	5	10

Event	% of Blinded Cycles with Events	
	Filgrastim N = 384 patient cycles	Placebo N = 257 patient cycles
Constipation	5	10
Pain (Unspecfied)	2	7

In this study, there were no serious, life-threatening, or fatal adverse reactions attributed to Filgrastim therapy. Specifically, there were no reports of flu-like symptoms, pleuritis, pericarditis, or other major systemic reactions to Filgrastim.

Spontaneously reversible elevations in uric acid, lactate dehydrogenase, and alkaline phosphatase occurred in 27% to 58% of 98 patients receiving blinded Filgrastim therapy following cytotoxic chemotherapy; increases were generally mild to moderate. Transient decreases in blood pressure ($< 90/60$ mmHg), which did not require clinical treatment, were reported in 7 to 176 patients in Phase III clinical studies following administration of Filgrastim. No evidence of interaction of Filgrastim with other drugs was observed in the course of clinical trials (see *"Precautions—Simultaneous Use with Chemoradiation"*).

There has been no evidence for the development of antibodies or of a blunted or diminished response to Filgrastim in treated patients, including those receiving Filgrastim daily for almost two years.

OVERDOSAGE

The maximum tolerated dose of Filgrastim has not been determined. Twenty-seven patients have been treated at Filgrastim doses of ≥ 69 mcg/kg/day. Of those, six patients have been treated at 115 mcg/kg/day with no toxic effects attributable to Filgrastim. Efficacy has been demonstrated using much lower doses. (Doses of 4 to 8 mcg/kg/day showed efficacy in the Phase III study.) Doses of Filgrastim which increase the ANC beyond 10,000/mm^3 may not result in any additional clinical benefit.

In Filgrastim clinical trials, white blood cell counts $> 100,000$/mm^3 have been reported in less than 5% of patients, but were not associated with any reported adverse clinical effects.

It is recommended, to avoid the potential risks of excessive leukocytosis, that Filgrastim therapy should be discontinued if the ANC surpasses 10,000/mm^3 after the ANC nadir has occurred.

Discontinuation of Filgrastim therapy usually results in a 50% decrease in circulating neutrophils within 1 to 2 days, with a return to pretreatment levels in 1 to 7 days.

DOSAGE AND ADMINISTRATION

The recommended starting dose of Filgrastim is 5 mcg/kg/day, administered as a single daily injection by subcutaneous bolus injection, by short intravenous infusion (15-30 minutes), or by continuous subcutaneous or continuous intravenous infusion. A CBC and platelet count should be obtained before instituting Filgrastim therapy, and monitored twice weekly during therapy. Doses may be increased in increments of 5 mcg/kg for each chemotherapy cycle, according to the duration and severity of the ANC nadir.

Filgrastim should be administered no earlier than 24 hours after the administration of cytotoxic chemotherapy. Filgrastim should not be administered in the period 24 hours before the administration of chemotherapy (see *"Precautions"*). Filgrastim should be administered daily for up to two weeks, until the ANC has reached 10,000/mm^3 following the expected chemotherapy-induced neutrophil nadir. The duration of Filgrastim therapy needed to attenuate chemotherapy-induced-neutropenia may be dependent on the myelosuppressive potential of the chemotherapy regimen employed. Filgrastim therapy should be discontinued if the ANC surpasses 10,000/mm^3 after the expected chemotherapy-induced neutrophil nadir (see *"Precautions"*). In Phase III trials, efficacy was observed at doses of 4 to 8 mcg/kg/day.

DILUTION

If required Filgrastim may be diluted in 5% dextrose. Filgrastim diluted to concentrations between 5 and 15 mcg/mL should be protected from adsorption to plastic materials by addition of Albumin (Human) to a final concentration of 2 mg/mL. When diluted in 5% dextrose or 5% dextrose plus Albumin (Human), Filgrastim is compatible with glass bottles, PVC and polyolefin IV bags, and polypropylene syringes.

Dilution of Filgrastim to a final concentration of less than 5 mcg/mL is not recommended at any time. *Do not dilute with saline at any time; product may precipitate.*

Injectable solution: Each 1 mL of Filgrastim contains 300 mcg of Filgrastim in a preservative-free solution containing 0.59 mg acetate, 50 mg mannitol, 0.004% Tween® 80, 0.035 mg sodium, and 1 mL water for injection, USP, pH 4.0. Each 1.6 mL of Filgrastim contains 480 mcg of Filgrastim in a preservative-free solution containing 0.94 mg acetate, 80 mg mannitol, 0.004% Tween 80, 0.056 mg sodium, and 1.6 mL water for injection, USP, pH 4.0.

Filgrastim should be stored in the refrigerator at 2-8 degrees Centigrade (39-46 degrees Fahrenheit). Do not freeze. Avoid shaking. Prior to injection, Filgrastim may be allowed to reach room temperature for a maximum of 24 hours. Any vial left at room temperature for greater than 24 hours should be discarded.

Parenteral drug products should be inspected visually for particulate matter and discoloration prior to administration, whenever solution and container permit; if particulates or discoloration are observed, the container should not be used.

REFERENCES

1. Zsebo KM, Yuschenkoff VN, Schiffer S, *et al.* Vascular endothelial cells and granulopoiesis: Interleukin-1 stimulates release of G-CSF and GM-CSF. *Blood* 71:99-103 (1988) 2. Souza LM, Boone TC, Gabrilove J, *et al.* Recombinant human granulocyte colony-stimulating factor: effects on normal and leukemic myeloid cells. *Science* 232:61-65 (1986). 3. Koeffler HP, Gasson J, Raynard J, Souza LM, Shephard M, and Munker R. Recombinant human TNF stimulates production of granulocyte colony-stimulating factor. *Blood* 70:55-59 (1987). 4. Seelentag WK, Mermod JJ, Montesano R, and Vassalli P. Additive effects of interleukin 1 and tumor necrosis factor-alpha on the accumulation of three granulocyte and macrophage colony-stimulating factor mRNAs in human endothelial cells. *EMBO J.* 6:2261-2265 (1987). 5. Metcalf D. The Haemopoietic colony stimulating factors. *Elsevier Sci. Pub.* Chp. 13:55-92 (1984). 6. Burgess AW and Metcalf D. Characterization of a serum factor stimulating the differentiation of myelomonocytic leukemic cells. *Int. J. Cancer* 26:647-654 (1980). 7. Zsebo KM, Cohen AM, Murdock DC, Boone TC, Inque H, Chazin VR, Hines D, and Souza LM. Recombinant human granulocyte colony-stimulating factor: Molecular and biological characterization. *Immunobiol.* 172:175-184 (1986). 8. Welte K, Bonilla MA, Gillio AP, *et al.* Recombinant human G-CSF: Effects on hematopoiesis in normal and cyclophosphamide treated primates. *J. Exp. Med.* 165:941-948 (1987). 9. Duhrsen U, Villefal JL, Boyd J, *et al.* Effects of recombinant human granulocyte colony-stimulating factor on hematopoietic progenitor cells in cancer patients. *Blood* 72:2074-2081 (1988). 10. Souza LM, Boone TC, Gabrilove J, *et al.* Recombinant human granulocyte colony-stimulating factor: Effects on normal and leukemic myeloid cells. *Science* 232:61-65 (1986). 11. Weisbart RH, Kacena A, Schuh A, Golde DW. GM-CSF induces human neutrophil IgA-mediated phagocytosis by an IgA Fc receptor activation mechanism. *Nature* 332:647-648 (1988). 12. Kitagawa S, Yuo A, Souza LM, Saito M, Miura Y, Takaku F. Recombinant human granulocyte colony-stimulating factor enhances superoxide release in human granulocytes stimulated by chemotactic peptide. *Biochem. Biophys. Res. Commun.* 144: 1143 (1987). 13. Glaspy JA, Baldwin GC, Robertson PA, *et al.* Therapy for neutropenia in hairy cell leukemia with recombinant human granulocyte colony-stimulating factor. *Ann. Int. Med.* 109:789-795 (1988). 14. You A, Kitagawa S, Ohsaka A, *et al.* Recombinant human granulocyte colony-stimulating factor as an activator of human granulocytes: potentiation of responses triggered by receptor-mediated agonists and stimulation of C3bi receptor expression and adherence. *Blood* 74:2144-2149 (1989). 15. Gabrilove JL, Jakubowski A, Fain K, *et al.* Phase I study of granulocyte colony-stimulating factor in patients with transitional cell carcinoma of the urothelium. *J. Clin. Invest.* 82:1454-1461 (1988). 16. Morstyn G, Souza L, Keech J, *et al.* Effect of granulocyte colony-stimulating factor on neutropenia induced by cytotoxic chemotherapy. *Lancet* March 26:667-672 (1988). 17. Bronchud MH, Scarffe JH, Thatcher N, *et al.* Phase I/II study of recombinant human granulocyte colony-stimulating factor in patients receiving intensive chemotherapy for small cell lung cancer. *Br. J. Cancer* 56:809-813 (1987). 18. Gabrilove JL, Jakubowski A, Scher H, *et al.* Effect of granulocyte colony-stimulating factor on neutropenia and associated morbidity due to chemotherapy for transitional cell carcinoma of the urothelium. *N. Engl. J. Med.* 318:1414-1422 (1988). 19. Neidhart J, Mangalik A, Kohler W, *et al.* Granulocyte colony-stimulating factor stimulates recovery of granulocytes in patients receiving dose-intensive chemotherapy without bone-marrow transplantation. *J. Clin. Oncol.* 7:1685-1691 (1981). 20. Bronchud MH, Howell A, Crowther D, *et al.* The use of granulocyte colony-stimulating factor to increase the intensity of treatment with doxorubicin in patients with advanced breast and ovarian cancer. *Br. J. Cancer* 60:121-128 (1989).

J CODES
300 mcg SC,IV—J1440

HOW SUPPLIED
INJECTION: 300 MCG/ML

BRAND/MANUFACTURER	NDC	SIZE	AWP
○ **BRAND**			
NEUPOGEN: Amgen	55513-0347-01	1 ml	$148.30
	55513-0348-01	1.6 ml	$236.20
	55513-0347-10	1 ml 10s	$1483.00
	55513-0348-10	1.6 ml 10s	$2362.00

Finasteride

DESCRIPTION

Finasteride, a synthetic 4-azasteroid compound, is a specific inhibitor of steroid 5α-reductase, an intracellular enzyme that converts testosterone into the potent androgen 5α-dihydrotestosterone (DHT).

Finasteride is 4-azaandrost-1-ene-17-carboxamide, *N*-(1,1-dimethylethyl)-3-oxo-,(5α, 17β)-. The empirical formula of finasteride is $C_{23}H_{36}N_2O_2$ and its molecular weight is 372.55.

Finasteride is a white crystalline powder with a melting point near 250°C. It is freely soluble in chloroform and in lower alcohol solvents, but is practically insoluble in water.

Following is its chemical structure:

CLINICAL PHARMACOLOGY

Progressive enlargement of the prostate gland is often associated with urinary symptoms and a decrease in urine flow, although a precise correlation between increased gland size and symptoms has not been demonstrated. Benign prostatic hyperplasia (BPH) produces symptoms in the majority of men over the age of 50 and its prevalence increases with age. The development of the prostate gland is dependent on the potent androgen, 5α-dihydrotestosterone (DHT). The enzyme 5α-reductase metabolizes testosterone to DHT in the prostate gland, liver and skin. DHT induces androgenic effects by binding to androgen receptors in the cell nuclei of these organs.

Finasteride is a competitive and specific inhibitor of 5α-reductase. This has been demonstrated both *in vivo* and *in vitro*. Finasteride has no affinity for the androgen receptor. In man, the 5α-reduced steroid metabolites in blood and urine are decreased after administration of Finasteride.

In man, a single 5-mg oral dose of Finasteride produces a rapid reduction in serum DHT concentration, with the maximum effect observed 8 hours after the first dose. The suppression of DHT is maintained throughout the 24-hour dosing interval and with continued treatment. Daily dosing of Finasteride at 5 mg/day for up to 24 months has been shown to reduce the serum DHT concentration by approximately 70%. The median circulating level of testosterone increased by 10% but remained within the physiologic range.

Adult males with genetically inherited 5α-reductase deficiency also have decreased levels of DHT. Except for the associated urogenital defects present at birth, no other clinical abnormalities related to 5α-reductase deficiency have been observed in these individuals. These individuals have a small prostate gland throughout life and do not develop BPH.

In patients with BPH treated with Finasteride (1-100 mg/day) for 7-10 days prior to prostatectomy, an approximate 80% lower DHT content was measured in prostatic tissue removed at surgery, compared to placebo; testosterone tissue concentration was increased up to 10 times over pretreatment levels, relative to placebo. Intraprostatic content of prostate-specific antigen (PSA) was also decreased.

In healthy male volunteers treated with Finasteride for 14 days, discontinuation of therapy resulted in a return of DHT levels to pretreatment levels in approximately 2 weeks.

In patients with BPH, Finasteride had no effect on circulating levels of cortisol, estradiol, prolactin, thyroid-stimulating hormone, or thyroxine. Nor did it affect the plasma lipid profile (i.e. total cholesterol, low density lipoproteins, high density lipoproteins and triglycerides) of 56 patients receiving Finasteride for 12 weeks. The effects of long-term administration of Finasteride on the plasma lipid profile are unknown. Increases of about 10% were observed in luteinizing hormone (LH), follicle-stimulating hormone (FSH) and testosterone levels in patients receiving Finasteride but levels remained within the normal range. In healthy volunteers, treatment with Finasteride did not alter the response of LH and FSH to gonadotropin-releasing hormone, indicating that the hypothalamic-pituitary-testicular axis was not affected.

PHARMACOKINETICS

Following an oral dose of ^{14}C-Finasteride in man, a mean of 39% (range, 32-46%) of the dose was excreted in the urine in the form of metabolites: 57% (range, 51-64%) was excreted in the feces. The major compound isolated from urine was the monocarboxylic acid metabolite: virtually no unchanged drug was recovered. The t-butyl side chain monohydroxylated metabolite has been isolated from plasma. These metabolites possess no more than 20% of the 5α-reductase inhibitory activity of Finasteride.

In a study in 15 healthy male subjects, the mean bioavailability of a 5-mg Finasteride tablet was 63% (range, 34-108%), based on the ratio of AUC relative to a 5-mg intravenous dose infused over 60 minutes. Maximum Finasteride plasma concentration averaged 37 ng/mL (range, 27-49 ng/mL) and was reached 1 to 2 hours postdose. The mean plasma half-life of elimination was 6 hours (range, 3-16 hours). Following the intravenous infusion, mean plasma clearance was 165 mL/min (range, 70-279 mL/min) and mean steady-state volume of distribution was 76 liters (range, 44-96 liters). In a separate study, the bioavailability of finasteride was not affected by food.

Approximately 90% of circulating Finasteride is bound to plasma proteins. Finasteride has been found to cross the blood-brain barrier.

There is a slow accumulation phase for finasteride after multiple dosing. After dosing with 5 mg/day of Finasteride for 17 days, plasma concentrations of Finasteride were 47% and 54% higher than after the first dose in men 45-60 years old (n = 12) and ≥ 70 years old (n = 12), respectively. Mean trough concentrations after 17 days of dosing were 6.2 ng/mL (range, 24-9.8 ng/mL) and 8.1 ng/mL (range, 1.8-19.7 ng/mL), respectively in the two age groups. Although steady state was not reached in this study, mean trough plasma concentration in another study in patients with BPH (mean age, 65 years) receiving 5 mg/day was 9.4 ng/mL (range, 7.1-13.3 ng/mL; n = 22) after over a year of dosing.

The elimination rate of Finasteride is decreased in the elderly, but no dosage adjustment is necessary. The mean terminal half-life of Finasteride in subjects ≥ 70 years of age was approximately 8 hours (range, 6-15 hours) compared to 6 hours (range, 4-12 hours) in subjects 45-60 years of age. As a result, mean AUC (0-24 hr) after 17 days of dosing was 15% higher in subjects ≥ 70 years of age (p = 0.02).

No dosage adjustment is necessary in patients with renal insufficiency. In patients with chronic renal impairment, with creatinine clearances ranging from 9.0 to 55 mL/min, area under the curve, maximum plasma concentration, half-life, and protein binding after a single dose of ^{14}C-Finasteride were similar to values obtained in healthy volunteers. Urinary excretion of metabolites was decreased in patients with renal impairment. This decrease was associated with an increase in fecal excretion of metabolites. Plasma concentrations of metabolites were significantly higher in patients with renal impairment (based on a 60% increase in total radioactivity AUC). However, Finasteride has been well tolerated in BPH patients with normal renal function receiving up to 80 mg/day for 12 weeks where exposure of these patients to metabolites would presumably be much greater. In 16 subjects receiving Finasteride 5 mg/day, Finasteride concentrations in semen ranged from undetectable (< 1 ng/mL) to 21 ng/mL. Based on a 5 mL ejaculate volume, the amount of Finasteride in ejaculate was estimated to be less than 1/50 of the dose of Finasteride (5 mcg) that had no effect on circulating DHT levels in adults.

CLINICAL STUDIES

TWELVE-MONTH CONTROLLED CLINICAL TRIALS

In a North American and in an international multicenter, double-blind, placebo-controlled 12-month study in patients with BPH treated with Finasteride 5 mg/day, statistically significant regression of the enlarged prostate gland was noted at the first evaluation at 3 months and was maintained during the studies (Table 1). In both studies, the maximum urinary flow rates showed statistically significant increases from baseline in patients treated with Finasteride from week 2 throughout the 12-month studies. Compared to placebo, statistically significant increases in maximum urinary flow rates were maintained in the North American study from month 4 through 12 in patients treated with Finasteride. The maximum urinary flow rates in the international study were statistically significantly greater than placebo at months 7, 8, 11 and 12 (Figures 1-3 and Table 2).

Table 1
MEDIAN % CHANGE IN PROSTATE VOLUME† FROM BASELINE

	North American Study		International Study	
	Finasteride 5 mg (n = 297)[a]	Placebo (n = 300)[a]	Finasteride 5 mg (n = 246)[a]	Placebo (n = 255)[a]
Baseline volume (cc)	52.1	50.0	45.5	41.5
	%	%	%	%
Month 3	12.1***	-2.4	-19.1***	-6.0
Month 6	-17.4***	-2.8	-21.9***	-5.5
Month 12	-19.2***	-3.0	-24.0***	-6.1

† Prostate volume was measured by magnetic resonance imaging (N. Am.) and ultrasound (Int'l). (Prostate volume was not measured at month 9.)
[a] Enrolled at baseline
*** p < 0.001 vs placebo

Figure 1
MAXIMUM URINARY FLOW RATE†

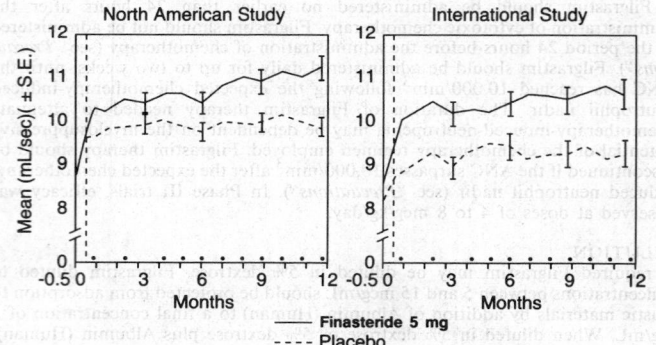

* p < 0.05 vs Placebo
† Maximum urinary flow rates (voided volumes ≥ 150 mL) were measured with a non-invasive urinary flow meter.
NOTE: Area of the graph to the left of time 0 is a two-week placebo run-in period.

Table 2
MEAN INCREASE IN MAXIMUM URINARY FLOW RATE (ML/SEC)†0 FROM BASELINE

	North American Study		International Study	
	Finasteride 5 mg (n = 297)	Placebo (n = 300)	Finasteride 5 mg (n = 246)	Placebo (n = 255)
Baseline flow rate (mL/ sec)	9.6	9.6	9.2	8.6
Week 2	0.5*	-0.2	0.6	0.2

		North American Study		International Study	
		Finasteride 5 mg (n = 297)	Placebo (n = 300)	Finasteride 5 mg (n = 246)	Placebo (n = 255)
Month	1	0.5	0.2	0.7	0.3
Month	2	0.9*	0.3	1.1	0.6
Month	3	0.8	0.3	0.8	0.2
Month	4	1.0*	0.4	1.0	0.6
Month	5	1.0**	0.2	0.9	0.8
Month	6	0.8*	0.1	1.1	0.7
Month	7	1.2**	0.4	1.3*	0.4
Month	8	1.4***	0.4	1.3*	0.5
Month	9	1.3**	0.3	1.2	0.4
Month	10	1.5***	0.5	1.3	0.7
Month	11	1.4***	0.3	1.5**	0.4
Month	12	1.6***	0.2	1.3*	0.4

† *Maximum urinary flow rates (voided volumes < 150 mL) were measured with a non-invasive urinary flow meter.*

*, **, *** $p < 0.05$, $p < 0.01$, $p < 0.001$ vs placebo, respectively

Figure 2
**MEAN INCREASE IN MAXIMUM URINARY FLOW RATE (mL/sec)†
(POOLED DATA)**

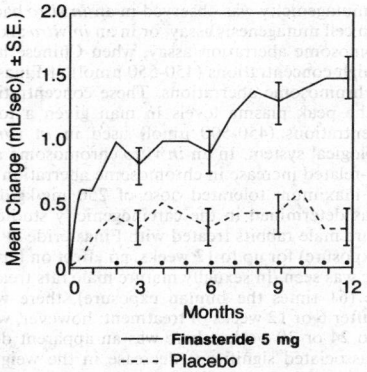

* $p < 0.05$ vs Placebo

† Maximum urinary flow rates (voided volumes ≥ 150 mL) were measured with a non invasive urinary flow meter.

Figure 3
**PERCENT OF PATIENTS WITH A MAXIMUM URINARY FLOW
RATE INCREASE ≥ 3 ML/SEC**

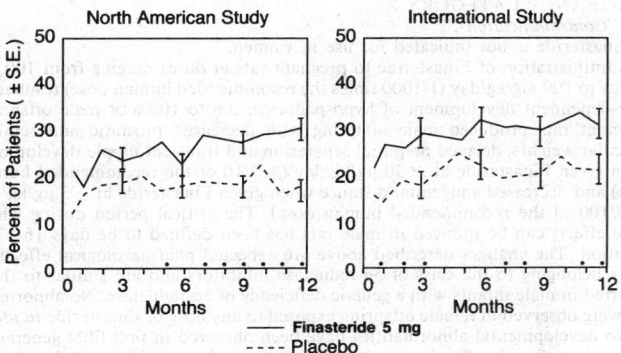

* $p < 0.05$ vs Placebo

Symptomatic improvement was also evaluated in these multicenter studies. Obstructive and total symptom scores were calculated based on patient responses to a validated questionnaire. The obstructive symptoms evaluated were hesitancy, feeling of incomplete bladder emptying, interruption of urinary stream, impairment of size and force of urinary stream and terminal urinary dribbling. The total symptom score also included straining to start urinary flow, dysuria, frequency of clothes wetting and urgency to urinate. On a scale of 0 (absence of all symptoms) to 36 (worst response for all symptoms), the mean baseline total symptom scores for the North American and international studies were 10.1 and 10.6, respectively.

The mean total symptom scores of patients in the North American and international studies decreased from baseline starting at week 2 of treatment with either Finasteride or placebo; from week 2 the scores of the patients treated with Finasteride were numerically lower than those of placebo and remained so

throughout the 12-month study. These scores became statistically significantly lower than placebo ($p < 0.05$) starting at month 7 in the international study and at month 10 in the North American study (Figure 4). Similar results were observed with the obstructive symptom scores.

Figure 4
**MEAN CHANGE IN TOTAL SYMPTOM SCORES
FROM BASELINE**

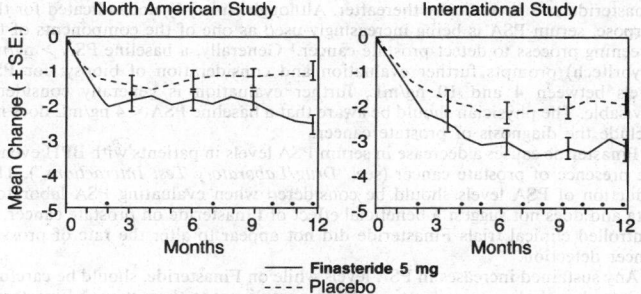

* $p < 0.05$ vs Placebo

Blinded global assessments of overall urinary function and symptoms were performed. Greater improvement in patients treated with Finasteride as compared to placebo was demonstrated by both the investigator's assessment (N.Am. and Int'l, $p \leq 0.01$) and the patient's own assessment (N. Am., $p \leq 0.01$; Int'l, $p \leq 0.01$).

In both of these 12-month studies, patients treated with Finasteride 5 mg had progressively decreasing prostate volumes, increasing maximum urinary flow rates and improvement of symptoms associated with BPH, suggesting an arrest in the disease process. Controlled clinical data beyond 12 months are not available.

LONG-TERM OPEN EXTENSIONS
In long-term uncontrolled extensions of these studies in approximately 300 patients receiving Finasteride 5 mg/day for 24 months, prostate volume was reduced by a median of 25.5% (baseline, 52.2 cc), maximum flow rate increased by a mean of 2.2 mL/sec (baseline, 11.3 mL/sec) and the total symptom score improved by a mean of 3.4 points (baseline, 9.6 points).

In addition, regression of the enlarged prostate gland and a decrease in PSA levels were maintained in approximately 50 patients who were treated with Finasteride for 36 months.

INDICATIONS AND USAGE
Finasteride is indicated for the treatment of symptomatic benign prostatic hyperplasia (BPH). Although there is a rapid regression of the enlarged prostate gland in most treated patients, less than 50% of patients experience an increase in urinary flow and improvement in symptoms of BPH when treated with Finasteride for 12 months. (See "Clinical Pharmacology".)

The long-term effects of Finasteride on the incidence of surgery, acute urinary obstruction or other complications of BPH are yet to be determined.

A minimum of 6 months treatment may be necessary to determine whether an individual will respond to Finasteride. It is not possible to identify prospectively those patients who will respond.

Prior to initiating therapy with Finasteride appropriate evaluation should be performed to identify other conditions, such as infection, prostate cancer, stricture disease, hypotonic bladder or other neurogenic disorders, that might mimic BPH.

CONTRAINDICATIONS
Finasteride is contraindicated in the following:
Hypersensitivity to any component of this medication.

Pregnancy: Finasteride is contraindicated in women who are or may become pregnant. Because of the ability of 5α-reductase inhibitors to inhibitors to the conversion of testosterone to DHT, Finasteride may cause abnormalities of the external genitalia of a male fetus of a pregnant woman who receives Finasteride. If this drug is used during pregnancy, or if pregnancy occurs while taking this drug, the pregnant woman should be apprised of the potential hazard to the male fetus. (See also "Warnings, Exposure of Women—Risk to Male Fetus" and "Precautions, Information for Patients and Pregnancy.") In female rats, low doses of Finasteride administered during pregnancy have produced abnormalities of the external genitalia in male offspring.

WARNINGS
Finasteride is not indicated for use in children (see "Precautions, Pediatric Use") or women (see also "Clinical Pharmacology, Pharmacokinetics", "Warnings, Exposure of Women—Risk to Male Fetus," "Precautions, Information for Patients, Pregnancy", and "How Supplied".).

Exposure of Women—Risk to Male Fetus: It is not known whether the amont of Finasteride that could potentially be absorbed by a pregnant woman through either direct contact with crushed Finasteride tablets or from the semen of a patient taking Finasteride can adversely affect a developing male fetus (see "Clinical Pharmacology, Pharmacokinetics," "Contraindications"; "Precautions, Information for Patients, Pregnancy," and "How Supplied". Therefore, because of the potential risk to a male fetus, a woman who is pregnant or who may become pregnant should not handle crushed Finasteride tablets; in addition, when the patient's sexual partner is or may become pregnant, the patient should either avoid exposure of his partner to semen or he should discontinue Finasteride.

PRECAUTIONS

GENERAL
Digital rectal examinations, as well as other evaluations for prostate cancer, should be performed on patients with BPH prior to initiating therapy with Finasteride and periodically thereafter. Although currently not indicated for this purpose, serum PSA is being increasingly used as one of the components of the screening process to detect prostate cancer.[1] Generally, a baseline PSA > ng/mL (Hybritech) prompts further evaluation and consideration of biopsy; for PSA levels between 4 and 10 ng/mL, further evaluation is generally considered advisable. The physician should be aware that a baseline PSA < 4 ng/mL does not exclude the diagnosis of prostate cancer.

Finasteride causes a decrease in serum PSA levels in patients with BPH even in the presence of prostate cancer (see "Drug/Laboratory Test Interactions"). This reduction of PSA levels should be considered when evaluating PSA laboratory data and does not suggest a beneficial effect of Finasteride on prostate cancer. In controlled clinical trials Finasteride did not appear to alter the rate of prostate cancer detection.

Any sustained increases in PSA levels while on Finasteride, should be carefully evaluated. including consideration of non-compliance to therapy with Finasteride (see "Drug/Laboratory Test Interactions").

Since not all patients demonstrate a response to Finasteride, patients with a large residual urinary volume and/or severely diminished urinary flow should be carefully monitored for obstructive uropathy. These patients may not be candidates for this therapy.

Caution should be used in the administration of Finasteride in those patients with liver function abnormalities, as Finasteride is metabolized extensively in the liver.

INFORMATION FOR PATIENTS
Crushed Finasteride tablets should not be handled by a woman who is pregnant or who may become pregnant because of the potential for absorption of Finasteride and the subsequent potential risk to the male fetus. Similarly, when the patient's sexual partner is or may become pregnant, the patient should either avoid exposure of his partner to semen or he should discontinue Finasteride (see "Clinical Pharmacology, Pharmacokinetics", "Contraindications", "Warnings, Exposure of Women—Risk to Male Fetus", "Precautions, Pregnancy", and "How Supplied").

Physicians should inform patients that the volume of ejaculate may be decreased in some patients during treatment with Finasteride. This decrease does not appear to interfere with normal sexual function. However, impotence and decreased libido may occur in patients treated with Finasteride (see "Adverse Reactions, Twelve-Month Controlled Clinical Trials").

Physicians should instruct their patients to read the patient package insert before starting therapy with Finasteride and to reread it each time the prescription is renewed so that they are aware of current information for patients regarding Finasteride.

DRUG/LABORATORY TEST INTERACTIONS
When PSA laboratory determinations are evaluated, consideration should be given to the fact that PSA levels are decreased in patients treated with Finasteride. In controlled clinical trials in patients with BPH treated with Finasteride PSA levels decreased from baseline by a median of 41% (95% confidence interval of the median: 38-45%) at month 6 and by a median of 48% (95% confidence interval of the median: 45-52%) at month 12.

DRUG INTERACTIONS
Antipyrine: Antipyrine is used as a model for drugs that are metabolized by the same isoenzymatic cytochrome P450 system. In 12 subjects receiving Finasteride 10 mg/day for 28 days, Finasteride had no effect on the pharmacokinetic parameters of antipyrine or its metabolites.

Propranolol: In 19 normal volunteers receiving Finasteride 5 mg/day for 10 days, Finasteride did not affect the beta-adrenergic blocking activity or plasma concentrations of propranolol enantiomers after a single dose of propranolol.

Digoxin: In 17 normal volunteers receiving Finasteride 5 mg/day for 10 days, concomitant administration of multiple doses of Finasteride and a single dose of digoxin resulted in no effect on plasma concentrations of digoxin and its immunoreactive metabolites.

Theophylline: In 12 normal volunteers receiving Finasteride 5 mg/day for 8 days, Finasteride significantly increased theophylline clearance by 7% and decreased its half-life by 10% after intravenous administration of aminophylline. These changes were not clinically significant.

Warfarin: In 12 patients chronically treated with warfarin, the prothrombin times and plasma concentrations of warfarin enantiomers were not altered after treatment with Finasteride 5 mg/day for 14 days.

Other Concomitant Therapy: Although specific interaction studies were not performed, Finasteride was concomitantly used in clinical studies with α-blockers,

---

[1] Catalona, W.J.; Smith, D.S.; Ratliff, T.L.; Dodds, K.M.; Coplen, M.D.; Yuan, J.J.J.; Petros, J.A.; Andriole, G.L.; Measurement of prostate-specific antigen in serum as a screening test for prostate cancer, N.Eng.J.Med. *324* (17); 1156-1161, April 25, 1991.

angiotensin-converting enzyme (ACE) inhibitors, analgesics, anticonvulsants, beta-adrenergic blocking agents, diuretics, calcium channel blockers, cardiac nitrates, HMG-CoA reductase inhibitors, nonsteroidal anti-inflammatory drugs (NSAIDs), benzodiazepines, H_2 antagonists and quinolone anti-infectives without evidence of clinically significant adverse interactions.

CARCINOGENESIS, MUTAGENESIS, IMPAIRMENT OF FERTILITY
No evidence of a tumorigenic effect was observed in a 24-month study in Sprague-Dawley rats receiving doses of finasteride up to 160 mg/kg/day in males and 320 mg/kg/day in females. These doses produced respective systemic exposure in rats of 111 and 274 times those observed in man receiving the recommended human dose of 5 mg/day. All exposure calculations were based on calculated AUC(0-24hr) for animals and mean AUC(0-24hr) for man (0.4 µg · hr/mL).

In a 19-month carcinogenicity study in CD-1 mice, a statistically significant (p ≤ 0.05) increase in the incidence of testicular Leydig cell adenomas was observed at a dose of 250 mg/kg/day (228 times the human exposure). In mice at a dose of 25 mg/kg/day (23 times the human exposure, estimated) and in rats at a dose of ≥ 40 mg/kg/day (39 times the human exposure) an increase in the incidence of Leydig cell hyperplasia was observed. A positive correlation between the proliferative changes in the Leydig cells and an increase in serum LH levels (2-3 fold above control) has been demonstrated in both rodent species treated with high doses of Finasteride. No drug-related Leydig cell changes were seen in either rats or dogs treated with Finasteride for 1 year at doses of 20 mg/kg/day and 45 mg/kg/day (30 and 350 times, respectively, the human exposure) or in mice treated for 19 months at a dose of 2.5 mg/kg/day (2.3 times the human exposure, estimated).

No evidence of mutagenicity was observed in an *in vitro* bacterial mutagenesis assay, a mammalian cell mutagenesis assay, or in an *in vitro* alkaline elution assay. In an *in vitro* chromosome aberration assay, when Chinese hamster ovary cells were treated with high concentrations (450-550 µmol) of Finasteride, there was a slight increase in chromosome aberrations. These concentrations correspond to 4000-5000 times the peak plasma levels in man given a total dose of 5 mg. Further, the concentrations (450-500 µmol) used in *in vitro* studies are not achievable in a biological system. In an *in vitro* chromosome aberration assay in mice, no treatment-related increase in chromosome aberration was observed with Finasteride at the maximum tolerated dose of 250 mg/kg/day (228 times the human exposure) as determined in the carcinogenicity studies.

In sexually mature male rabbits treated with Finasteride at 80 mg/kg/day (543 times the human exposure) for up to 12 weeks, no effect on fertility, sperm count, or ejaculate volume was seen. In sexually mature male rats treated with 80 mg/kg/day of Finasteride (61 times the human exposure), there were no significant effects on fertility after 6 or 12 weeks of treatment; however, when treatment was continued for up to 24 or 30 weeks, there was an apparent decrease in fertility, fecundity and an associated significant decrease in the weights of the seminal vesicles and prostate. All these effects were reversible within 6 weeks of discontinuation of treatment. No drug-related effect on testes or on mating performance has been seen in rats or rabbits. This decrease in fertility in Finasteride-treated rats is secondary to its effect on accessory sex organs (prostate and seminal vesicles) resulting in failure to form a seminal plug. The seminal plug is essential for normal fertility in rats and is not relevant in man.

PREGNANCY
PREGNANCY CATEGORY X
See "Contraindications."

Finasteride is not indicated for use in women.

Administration of Finasteride to pregnant rats at doses ranging from 100 µg/kg/day to 100 mg/kg/day (1-1000 times the recommended human dose) resulted in dose-dependent development of hypospadias in 3.6 to 100% of male offspring. Pregnant rats produced male offspring with decreased prostatic and seminal vesicular weights, delayed preputial separation and transient nipple development when given Finasteride at ≥ 30 µg/kg/day (≥ 3/10 of the recommended human dose) and decreased anogenital distance when given Finasteride at ≥ 3 µg/kg/day (≥ 3/100 of the recommended human dose). The critical period during which these effects can be induced in male rats has been defined to be days 16-17 of gestation. The changes described above are expected pharmacological effects of drugs belonging to the class of 5α-reductase inhibitors and are similar to those reported in male infants with a genetic deficiency of 5α-reductase. No abnormalities were observed in female offspring exposed to any dose of Finasteride *in utero*.

No developmental abnormalities have been observed in first filial generation (F_1) male or female offspring resulting from mating Finasteride-treated male rats (80 mg/kg/day; 61 times the human exposure) with untreated females. Administration of Finasteride at 3 mg/kg/day (30 times the recommended human dose) during the late gestation and lactation period resulted in slightly decreased fertility in F_1 male offspring. No effects were seen in female offspring. No evidence malformations has been observed in rabbit fetuses exposed to Finasteride *in utero* from days 6-18 of gestation at doses up to 100 mg/kg/day (1000 times the recommended human dose). However, effects on male genitalia would not be expected since the rabbits were not exposed during the critical period of genital system development.

NURSING MOTHERS
Finasteride is not indicated for use in women.

It is not known whether Finasteride is excreted in human milk.

PEDIATRIC USE
Finasteride is not indicated for use in children.

Safety and effectiveness in children have not been established.

◆ RATED THERAPEUTICALLY EQUIVALENT; ◇ THERAPEUTIC EQUIVALENCE UNCONFIRMED; ○ UNRATED

ADVERSE REACTIONS

Finasteride is generally well tolerated; adverse reactions usually have been mild and transient.

TWELVE-MONTH CONTROLLED CLINICAL TRIALS

In North American and international clinical trials, 543 patients were treated with 5 mg of Finasteride for 12 months. Seven of these patients (1.3%) were discontinued due to adverse experiences that were considered to be possibility, probably or definitely drug-related; only 1 of these patients (0.2%) discontinued therapy with Finasteride because of a sexual adverse experience.

The following clinical adverse reactions were reported as possibly, probably or definitely drug-related in ≥ 1% of patients treated for 12 months with 5 mg/day of Finasteride or placebo, respectively: impotence (3.7%, 1.1%), decreased libido (3.3%, 1.6%), decreased volume of ejaculate (2.8%, 0.9%).

The adverse experience profile for an additional 547 patients treated with 1 mg/day of Finasteride for 12 months was similar to that observed in patients treated for 12 months with 5 mg/day of Finasteride.

LONG-TERM OPEN EXTENSIONS

The adverse experience profile for approximately 300 patients who were maintained on Finasteride 5 mg/day for 24 months was similar to that observed in the controlled studies. In addition, a similar safety profile was observed in 50 patients treated with Finasteride 5 mg/day for 36 months.

The following additional adverse effects have been reported in post-marketing experience:
—breast tenderness and enlargement
—hypersensitivity reactions, including lip swelling and skin rash

OVERDOSAGE

Patients have received single doses of Finasteride up to 400 mg and multiple doses of Finasteride up to 80 mg/day for three months without adverse effects. Until further experience is obtained, no specific treatment for an overdose with Finasteride can be recommended.

Significant lethality was observed in male and female mice at single oral doses of 1500 mg/m^2 (500 mg/kg) and in female and male rats at single oral doses of 2360 mg/m^2 (400 mg/kg) and 5900 mg/m^2 (1000 mg/kg), respectively.

DOSAGE AND ADMINISTRATION

The recommended dose is 5 mg once a day.

Although early improvement may be seen, at least 6-12 months of therapy with Finasteride may be necessary in some patients to assess whether a beneficial response has been achieved. Periodic follow-up evaluations should be performed to determine whether a clinical response has occurred.

Finasteride may be administered with or without meals. No dosage adjustment is necessary for patients with renal impairment or for the elderly (see *"Clinical Pharmacology, Pharmacokinetics"*).

Store at room temperatures below 30°C (86°F). Protect from light and keep container tightly closed.

If the film coating of Finasteride tablets has been broken (e.g., crushed), the tablets should not be handled by a woman who is pregnant or who may become pregnant because of the potential for absorption of finasteride and the subsequent potential risk to a male fetus (see *"Clinical Pharmacology, Pharmacokinetics"*, *"Warnings, Exposure of Women—Risk to Male Fetus"*, *"Precautions, Information for Patients*, and *Pregnancy"*).

HOW SUPPLIED
TABLETS: 5 MG

BRAND/MANUFACTURER	NDC	SIZE	AWP
○ **BRAND**			
➤ PROSCAR: Merck	00006-0072-31	30s	$56.55
	00006-0072-58	100s	$188.50
	00006-0072-28	100s ud	$188.50

Fioricet *SEE* ACETAMINOPHEN/BUTALBITAL/CAFFEINE

Fioricet with Codeine *SEE* ACETAMINOPHEN/BUTALBITAL/CAFFEINE/CODEINE PHOSPHATE

Fiorinal *SEE* ASPIRIN/BUTALBITAL/CAFFEINE

Fiorinal with Codeine *SEE* ASPIRIN/BUTALBITAL/CAFFEINE/CODEINE PHOSPHATE

Flagyl *SEE* METRONIDAZOLE, SYSTEMIC

Flarex *SEE* FLUOROMETHOLONE

Flavoxate Hydrochloride

DESCRIPTION

Flavoxate tablets contain Flavoxate Hydrochloride, a synthetic urinary tract spasmolytic.

Chemically, Flavoxate Hydrochloride is 2-piperidinoethyl 3-methyl-4-oxo-2-phenyl-4 H-1-benzopyran-8-carboxylate Hydrochloride. The empirical formula of Flavoxate Hydrochloride is $C_{24}H_{25}NO_4 \cdot HCl$. The molecular weight is 427.94. Flavoxate is available as a 100 mg tablet for oral administration.

Following is its chemical structure:

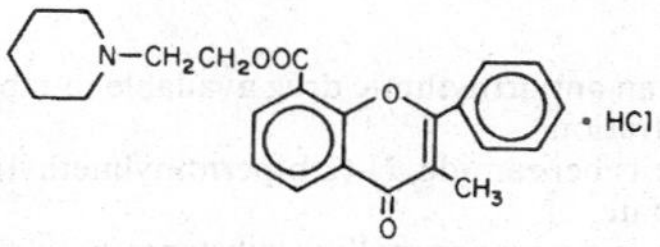

CLINICAL PHARMACOLOGY

Flavoxate Hydrochloride (Flavoxate HCl) counteracts smooth muscle spasm of the urinary tract and exerts its effect directly on the muscle.

In a single study of 11 normal male subjects, the time to onset of action was 55 minutes. The peak effect was observed at 112 minutes, 57% of the Flavoxate HCl was excreted in the urine within 24 hours.

INDICATIONS AND USAGE

Flavoxate is indicated for symthomatic relief of dysuria, urgency, nocturia, suprapubic pain, frequency and incontinence as may occur in cystitis, prostatitis, urethritis, urethrocystitis/urethrotrigonitis. Flavoxate is not indicated for definitive treatment, but is compatible with drugs used for the treatment of urinary tract infections.

CONTRAINDICATIONS

Flavoxate is contraindicated in patients who have any of the following obstructive conditions: pyloric or duodenal obstruction, obstructive intestinal lesions or ileus, achalasia, gastrointestinal hemorrhage and obstructive uropathies of the lower urinary tract.

WARNINGS

Flavoxate should be given cautiously in patients with suspected glaucoma.

PRECAUTIONS

Information for Patients: Patients should be informed that if drowsiness and blurred vision occur, they should not operate a motor vehicle or machinery or participate in activities where alertness is required.

Carcinogenesis, Mutagenesis, Impairment of Fertility: Mutagenicity studies and long-term studies in animals to determine the carcinogenic potential of Flavoxate have not been performed.

Pregnancy: Teratogenic Effects—Pregnancy Category B. Reproduction studies have been performed in rats and rabbits at doses up to 34 times the human dose and revealed no evidence of impaired fertility or harm to the fetus due to Flavoxate HCl. There are, however, no well-controlled studies in pregnant women. Because animal reproduction studies are not always predictive of human response, this drug should be used during pregnancy only if clearly needed.

Nursing Mothers: It is not known whether this drug is excreted in human milk. Because many drugs are excreted in human milk, caution should be exercised when Flavoxate in administered to a nursing woman.

Pediatric Use: Safety and effectiveness in children below the age of 12 years have not been established.

ADVERSE REACTIONS

The following adverse reactions have been observed, but there are not enough data to support an estimate of their frequency.

Gastrointestinal: Nausea, vomiting, dry mouth.

CNS: Vertigo, headache, mental confusion, especially in the elderly, drowsiness, nervousness.

Hematologic: Leukopenia (1 case which was reversible upon discontinuation of the drug).

Cardiovascular: Tachycardia and palpitation.

Allergic: Urticaria and other dermatoses, eosinophilia and hyperpyrexia.

Ophthalmic: Increased ocular tension, blurred vision, disturbance in eye accommodation.

Renal: Dysuria.

OVERDOSAGE

The oral LD_{50} for Flavoxate HCl in rats is 4273 mg/kg. The oral LD_{50} for Flavoxate HCl in mice is 1837 mg/kg.

It is not known whether Flavoxate HCl is dialyzable.

➤ SHOWN IN PRODUCT IDENTIFICATION GUIDE

DOSAGE AND ADMINISTRATION

Adults and children over 12 years of age: One or two 100 mg tablets 3 or 4 times a day. With improvement of symptoms, the dose may be reduced. This drug cannot be recommended for infants and children under 12 years of age because safety and efficacy have not been demonstrated in this age group.

HOW SUPPLIED
TABLETS: 100 MG

BRAND/MANUFACTURER	NDC	SIZE	AWP
○ **BRAND**			
URISPAS: SK Beecham Pharm	00007-5290-20	100s	$71.70
	00007-5290-21	100s ud	$73.95

Flecainide Acetate

DESCRIPTION

Flecainide Acetate is an antiarrhythmic drug available in tablets of 50, 100 or 150 mg for oral administration.

Flecainide Acetate is benzamide, N-(2-piperidinylmethyl)-2,5-bis(2,2,2-trifluoroethoxy)-, monoacetate.

Flecainide Acetate is a white crystalline substance with a pK_a of 9.3. It has an aqueous solubility of 48.4 mg/mL at 37°C.

Following is its chemical structure:

$$CF_3CH_2O \qquad CONHCH_2 \qquad N-H \cdot CH_3COOH \qquad OCH_2CF_3$$

CLINICAL PHARMACOLOGY

Flecainide Acetate has local anesthetic activity and belongs to the membrane stabilizing (Class 1) group of antiarrhythmic agents; it has electrophysiologic effects characteristic of the IC class of antiarrhythmics.

Electrophysiology: In man, Flecainide Acetate produces a dose-related decrease in intracardiac conduction in all parts of the heart with the greatest effect on the His-Purkinje system (H-V conduction). Effects upon atrioventricular (AV) nodel conduction time and intra-atrial conduction times, although present, are less pronounced than those on ventricular conduction velocity. Significant effects on refractory periods were observed only in the ventricle. Sinus node recovery times (corrected) following pacing and spontaneous cycle lengths are somewhat increased. This latter effect may become significant in patients with sinus node dysfunction. (See *"Warnings"*.)

Flecainide Acetate causes a dose-related and plasma-level related decrease in single and multiple PVCs and can suppress recurrence of ventricular tachycardia. In limited studies of patients with a history of ventricular tachycardia, Flecainide Acetate has been successful 30-40% of the time in fully suppressing the inducibility of arrhythmias by programmed electrical stimulation. Based on PVC suppression, it appears that plasma levels of 0.2 to 1.0 µg/mL may be needed to obtain the maximal therapeutic effect. It is more difficult to assess the dose needed to suppress serious arrhythmias, but trough plasma levels in patients successfully treated for recurrent ventricular tachycardia were between 0.2 and 1.0 µg/mL. Plasma levels above 0.7-1.0 µg/mL are associated with a higher rate of cardiac adverse experiences such as conduction defects or bradycardia. The relation of plasma levels to proarrhythmic events is not established, but dose reduction in clinical trials of patients with ventricular tachycardia appears to have led to a reduced frequency and severity of such events.

Hemodynamics: Flecainide Acetate does not usually alter heart rate, although bradycardia and tachycardia have been reported occasionally.

In animals and isolated myocardium, a negative inotropic effect of Flecainide has been demonstrated. Decreases in ejection fraction, consistent with a negative inotropic effect, have been observed after single administration of 200 to 250 mg of the drug in man; both increases and decreases in ejection fraction have been encountered during multidose therapy in patients at usual therapeutic dose. (See *"Warnings"*.)

Metabolism in Humans: Following oral administration, the absorption of Flecainide Acetate is nearly complete. Peak plasma levels are attained at about three hours in most individuals (range, 1 to 6 hours). Flecainide does not undergo any consequential presystemic biotransformation (first-pass effect). Food or antacid do not affect absorption.

The apparent plasma half-life averages about 20 hours and is quite variable (range, 12 to 27 hours) after multiple oral doses in patients with premature ventricular contractions (PVCs). With multiple dosing, plasma levels increase because of its long half-life with steady-state levels approached in 3 to 5 days; once at steady-state, no additional (or unexpected) accumulation of drug in plasma occurs during chronic therapy. Over the usual therapeutic range, data suggest that plasma levels in an individual are approximately proportional to dose, deviating upwards from linearity only slightly (about 10 to 15% per 100 mg on average).

In healthy subjects, about 30% of a single oral dose (range, 10 to 50%) is excreted in urine as unchanged drug. The two major urinary metabolites are meta-O-dealkylated Flecainide (active, but about one-fifth as potent) and the meta-O-dealkylated lactam of Flecainide (non-active metabolite). These two metabolites (primarily conjugated) account for most of the remaining portion of the dose. Several minor metabolites (3% of the dose or less) are also found in urine; only 5% of an oral dose is excreted in feces. In patients, free (unconjugated) plasma levels of the two major metabolites are very low (less than 0.05 µg/mL).

When urinary pH is very alkaline (8 or higher), as may occur in rare conditions (e.g., renal tubular acidosis, strict vegetarian diet), Flecainide elimination from plasma is much slower. The elimination of Flecainide from the body depends on renal function (i.e., 10 to 50% appears in urine as unchanged drug). With increasing renal impairment, the extent of unchanged drug excretion in urine is reduced and the plasma half-life of Flecainide is prolonged. Since Flecainide is also extensively metabolized, there is no simple relationship between creatinine clearance and the rate of Flecanide elimination from plasma. (See *"Dosage and Administration"*.)

In patients with NYHA class III congestive heart failure (CFH), the rate of Flecainide elimination from plasma (mean half-life, 19 hours) is moderately slower than for healthy subjects (mean half-life, 14 hours), but similar to the rate for patients with PVCs without CHF. The extent of excretion of unchanged drug in urine is also similar. (See *"Dosage and Administration"*.)

From age 20 to 80, plasma levels are only slightly higher with advancing age; Flecainide elimination from plasma is somewhat slower in elderly subjects than in younger subjects. Patients up to age 80 + have been safely treated with usual dosages.

The extent of Flecainide binding to human plasma proteins is about 40% and is independent of plasma drug level over the range of 0.015 to about 3.4 µg/mL. Thus, clinically significant drug interactions based on protein binding effects would not be expected.

Hemodialysis removes only about 1% of an oral dose as unchanged Flecainide. Small increases in plasma digoxin levels are seen during coadministration of Flecainide Acetate with digoxin. Small increases in both Flecainide and propranolol plasma levels are seen during coadministration of these two drugs. (See *"Precautions, Drugs Interactions"*.)

Clinical Trials: In two randomized, crossover, placebo-controlled clinical trials of 16 weeks double-blind durations, 79% of patients with paroxysmal supraventricular tachycardia (PSVT) receiving Flecainide were attack free, whereas 15% of patients receiving placebo remained attack free. The median time-before-recurrence of PSVT in patients receiving placebo was 11 to 12 days, whereas over 85% of patients receiving Flecainide had no recurrence at 60 days.

In two randomized, crossover, placebo-controlled clinical trials of 16 weeks double-blind duration, 31% of patients with paroxysmal atrial fibrillation/flutter (PAF) receiving Flecainide were attack free, whereas 8% receiving placebo remained attack free. The median time-before-recurrence of PAF in patients receiving placebo was about 2 to 3 days, whereas for those receiving Flecainide the median time-before recurrence was 15 days.

INDICATIONS AND USAGE

In patients without structural heart disease, Flecainide Acetate is indicated for the prevention of

—paroxysmal supraventricular tachycardias (PSVT), including atrioventricular nodal reentrant tachycardia, atrioventricular reentrant tachycardia and other supraventricular tachycardias of unspecified mechanism associated with disabling symptoms

—paroxysmal atrial fibrillation/flutter (PAF) associated with disabling symptoms

Flecainide Acetate is also indicated for the prevention of

— documented ventricular arrhythmias, such as *sustained* ventricular tachycardia (*sustained* VT), that in the judgement of the physician, are life-threatening.

Use of Flecainide Acetate for the treatment of *sustained* VT, like other antiarrhythmics, should be initiated in the hospital. The use of Flecainide Acetate is not recommended in patients with less severe ventricular arrhythmias even if the patients are symptomatic.

Because of the proarrhythmic effects of Flecainide Acetate, its use should be reserved for patients in whom, in the opinion of the physician, the benefits of treatment outweight the risks. Flecainide Acetate should not be used in patients with recent myocardial infarction. (See *"Boxed Warnings"*.)

Use of Flecainide Acetate in chronic atrial fibrillation has not been adequately studied and is not recommended. (See *"Boxed Warnings"*.)

As is the case for other antiarrhythmic agents, there is no evidence from controlled trials that the use of Flecainide Acetate favorably affects survival or the incidence of sudden death.

CONTRAINDICATIONS

Flecainide Acetate is contraindicated in patients with pre-existing second- or third-degree AV block, or with right bundle branch block when associated with a left hemiblock (bifascicular block), unless a pacemaker is present to sustain the cardiac rhythm should complete heart block occur. Flecainide Acetate is also contraindicated in the presence of cardiogenic shock or known hypersensitivity to the drug.

WARNINGS

MORTALITY. FLECAINIDE ACETATE WAS INCLUDED IN THE NATIONAL HEART LUNG AND BLOOD INSTITUTE'S CARDIAC ARRHYTHMIA SUPPRESSION TRIAL (CAST), A LONG-TERM, MULTICENTER, RANDOMIZED, DOUBLE-BLIND STUDY IN PATIENTS WITH ASYMPTOMATIC NON-LIFE-THREATENING VENTRICULAR ARRHYTHMIAS WHO HAD A MYOCARDIAL INFARCTION MORE THAN SIX DAYS, BUT LESS THAN TWO YEARS PREVIOUSLY. AN EXCESSIVE MORTALITY OR NON-FATAL CARDIAC ARREST

RATE WAS SEEN IN PATIENTS TREATED WITH FLECAINIDE ACETATE COMPARED WITH THAT SEEN IN A CAREFULLY MATCHED PLACEBO-TREATED GROUP. THIS RATE WAS 16/315 (5.1%) FOR FLECAINIDE ACETATE AND 7/309 (2.3%) FOR ITS MATCHED PLACEBO. THE AVERAGE DURATION OF TREATMENT WITH FLECAINIDE ACETATE IN THIS STUDY WAS 10 MONTHS.

VENTRICULAR PROARRHYTHMIC EFFECTS IN PATIENTS WITH ATRIAL FIBRILLA-TION/FLUTTER. A REVIEW OF THE WORLD LITERATURE REVEALED REPORTS OF 568 PATIENTS TREATED WITH ORAL FLECAINIDE ACETATE FOR PAROXYSMAL ATRIAL FIBRILLATION/FLUTTER (PAF). VENTRICULAR TACHYCARDIA WAS EXPERI-ENCED IN 0.4% (2/568) OF THESE PATIENTS. OF 19 PATIENTS IN THE LITERATURE WITH CHRONIC ATRIAL FIBRILLATION (CAF), 10.5% (2) EXPERIENCED VT OR VF. FLECAINIDE IS NOT RECOMMENDED FOR USE IN PATIENTS WITH CHRONIC ATRIAL FIBRILLATION. CASE REPORTS OF VENTRICULAR PROARRHYTHMIC EFFECTS IN PATIENTS TREATED WITH FLECAINIDE ACETATE FOR ATRIAL FIBRILLATION/FLUT-TER HAVE INCLUDED INCREASED PVCS, VT, VENTRICULAR FIBRILLATION (VF), AND DEATH.

AS WITH OTHER CLASS I AGENTS, PATIENTS TREATED WITH FLECAINIDE ACETATE FOR ATRIAL FLUTTER HAVE BEEN REPORTED WITH 1:1 ATRIOVENTRICU-LAR CONDUCTION DUE TO SLOWING THE ATRIAL RATE. A PARADOXICAL IN-CREASE IN THE VENTRICULAR RATE ALSO MAY OCCUR IN PATIENTS WITH ATRIAL FIBRILLATION WHO RECEIVE FLECAINIDE ACETATE CONCOMITANT NEGATIVE CHRONOTROPIC THERAPY SUCH AS DIGOXIN OR BETA-BLOCKERS MAY LOWER THE RISK OF THIS COMPLICATION.

The applicability of the CAST results to other populations (e.g., those without recent infarction) is uncertain, but at present it is prudent to consider the risks of Class IC agents, coupled with the lack of any evidence of improved survival, generally unacceptable in patients whose ventricular arrhythmias are not life-threatening, even if the patients are experiencing unpleasant, but not life-threatening, symptoms or signs.

PROARRHYTHMIC EFFECTS

Flecainide Acetate, like other antiarrhythmic agents, can cause new or worsened supraventricu-lar or ventricular arrhythmias. Ventricular proarrhythmic effects range from an increase in frequency of PVCs to the development of more severe ventricular tachycardia, e.g., tachycardia that is more sustained or more resistant to conversion to sinus rhythm, with potentially fatal consequences. In studies of ventricular arrhythmia patients treated with Flecainide Acetate three-fourths of proarrhythmic events were new or worsened ventricular tachyarrhythmias, the remainder being increased frequency of PVCs or new supraventricular arrhythmias. In patients treated with Flecainide for *sustained* ventricular tachycardia, 80% (51/54) of proarrhythmic events occurred within 14 days of the onset of therapy. In studies of 225 patients with supraventricular arrhythmias (108 with paroxysmal supraventricular tachycardia and 117 with paroxysmal atrial fibrillation), there were 9 (4 %) proarrhythmic events, 8 of them in patients with paroxysmal atrial fibrillation. Of the 9, 7 (including the one in a PSVT patient) were exacerbations of supraventricular arrhythmias (longer duration, more rapid rate, harder to reverse) while 2 were ventricular arrhythmias, including one fatal case of VT/VF and one wide complex VT (the patient showed inducible VT, however, after withdrawal of Flecainide), both in patients with paroxysmal atrial fibrillation and known coronary artery disease.

It is uncertain Flecainide Acetate's risk of proarrhythmia is exaggerated in patients with chronic atrial fibrillation (CAF), high ventricular rate, and/or exercise. Wide complex tachycardia and ventricular fibrillation have been reported in two of 12 CAF patients undergoing maximal exercise tolerance testing.

In patients with complex ventricular arrhythmias, it is often difficult to distinguish a spontaneous variation in the patient's underlying rhythm disorder from drug-induced worsening, so that the following occurrence rates must be considered approximations. Their frequency appears to be related to dose and to the underlying cardiac disease.

Among patients treated for *sustained* VT (who frequently also had CHF, a low ejection fraction, a history of myocardial infarction and/or an episode of cardiac arrest), the incidence of proarrhythmic events was 13% when dosage was initiated at 200 mg/day with slow upward titration, and did not exceed 300 mg/day in most patients. In early studies in patients with *sustained* VT utilizing a higher initial dose (400 mg/day) the incidence of proarrhythmic events was 26%; moreover, in about 10% of the patients treated proarrhythmic events resulting in death, despite prompt medical attention. With lower initial doses, the incidence of proarrhythmic events resulting in death decreased to 0.5% of these patients. Accordingly, it is extremely important to follow the recommended dosage schedule. (See *"Dosage and Administration".)*

The relatively high frequency of proarrhythmic events in patients with *sustained* VT and serious underlying heart disease, and the need for careful titration and monitoring, requires that therapy of patients with *sustained* VT be started in the hospital. (See *"Dosage and Administra-tion".)*

HEART FAILURE

Flecainide Acetate has a negative inotropic effect and may cause or worsen CHF, particularly in patients with cardiomyopathy, preexisting severe heart failure (NYHA functional class III or IV) or low ejection fractions (less than 30%). In patients with supraventricular arrhythmias new or worsened CHF developed in 0.4% (1/225) of patients. In patients with *sustained* ventricular tachycardia during a mean duration of 7.9 months Flecainide Acetate therapy, 6.3% (20/317) developed new CHF. In patients with *sustained* ventricular tachycardia and a history of CHF, during a mean duration of 5.4 months of Flecainide Acetate therapy, 25.7% (78/304) developed worsened CHF. Exacerbation of preexisting CHF occurred more commonly in studies which included patients with class III or IV failure than in studies which excluded such patients. Flecainide Acetate should be used cautiously in patients who are known to have a history of CHF or myocardial dysfunction. The initial dosage in such patients should be no more than 100 mg bid (see *"Dosage and Administration")* and patients should be monitored carefully. Close attention must be given to maintenance of cardiac function, including optimization of digitalis,

diuretic, or other therapy. In cases where CHF has developed or worsened during treatment with Flecainide Acetate, the time of onset has ranged from a few hours to several months after starting therapy. Some patients who develop evidence of reduced myocardial function while on Flecainide Acetate can continue on Flecainide Acetate with adjustment of digitalis or diuretics, others may require dosage reduction or discontinuation of Flecainide Acetate. When feasible, it is recommended that plasma Flecainide levels be monitored. Attempts should be made to keep trough plasma levels below 0.7 to 1.0 µg/mL.

Effects on Cardiac Conduction: Flecainide Acetate slows cardiac conduction in most patients to produce dose-related increases in PR, QRS, and QT intervals.

PR interval increases on average about 25% (0.04 seconds) and as much as 118% in some patients. Approximately one-third of patients may develop new first-degree AV heart block (PR interval $\geq$ 0.20 seconds). The QRS complex increases on average about 25% (0.02 seconds) and as much as 150% in some patients. Many patients develop QRS complexes with a duration of 0.12 seconds or more. In one study, 4% of patients developed new bundle branch block while on Flecainide Acetate. The degree of lengthening of PR and QRS intervals does not predict either efficacy or the development of cardiac adverse effects. In clinical trials, it was unusual for PR intervals to increase to 0.30 seconds or more, or for QRS intervals to increase to 0.18 seconds or more. Thus, caution should be used when such intervals occur, and dose reductions may be considered. The QT interval widens about 8%, but most of this widening (about 60% to 90%) is due to widening of the QRS duration. The JT interval (QT minus QRS) only widens about 4% on the average. Significant JT prolongation occurs in less than 2% of patients. There have been rare cases of Torsade de Pointes-type arrhythmia associated with Flecainide Acetate therapy.

Clinically significant conduction changes have been observed at these rates: sinus node dysfunction such as sinus pause, sinus arrest and symptomatic bradycardia (1.2%), second-degree AV block (0.5%) and third-degree AV block (0.4%). An attempt should be made to manage the patient on the lowest effective dose in an effort to minimize these effects. (See *"Dosage and Administration".)* If second- or third-degree AV block, or right bundle branch block associated with a left hemiblock occur, Flecainide Acetate therapy should be discontinued unless a temporary or implanted ventricular pacemaker is in place to ensure an adequate ventricular rate.

Sick Sinus Syndrome (Bradycardia-Tachycardia Syndrome): Flecainide Acetate should be used only with extreme caution in patients with sick sinus syndrome because it may cause sinus bradycardia, sinus pause, or sinus arrest.

Effects on Pacemaker Thresholds: Flecainide Acetate is known to increase endocardial pacing thresholds and may suppress ventricular escape rhythms. These effects are reversible if Flecainide is discontinued. It should be used with caution in patients with permanent pacemakers or temporary pacing electrodes and should not be administered to patients with existing poor thresholds or nonprogrammable pacemakers unless suitable pacing rescue is available.

The pacing threshold in patients with pacemakers should be determined prior to instituting therapy with Flecainide Acetate again after one week of administra-tion and at regular intervals thereafter. Generally threshold changes are within the range of multiprogrammable pacemakers and, when these occur, a doubling of either voltage or pulse width is usually sufficient to regain capture.

Electrolyte Disturbances: Hypokalemia or hyperkalemia may alter the effects of Class I antiarrhythmic drugs. Preexisting hypokalemia or hyperkalemia should be corrected before administration of Flecainide Acetate.

PRECAUTIONS

Drug Interactions: Flecainide Acetate has been administered to patients receiving **digitalis** preparations or **beta-adrenergic blocking agents** without adverse effects. During administration of multiple oral doses of Flecainide Acetate to healthy subjects stabilized on a maintenance dose of **digoxin**, a 13%-19% increase in plasma **digoxin** levels occurred at six hours postdose.

In a study involving healthy subjects receiving Flecainide Acetate and **propranol-ol** concurrently, plasma Flecainide levels were increased about 20% and propranolol levels were increased about 30% compared to control values. In this formal interaction study, Flecainide Acetate and **propranolol** were each found to have negative inotropic effects; when the drugs were administered together, the effects were additive. The effects of concomitant administration of Flecainide Acetate and **propranolol** on the PR interval were less than additive. In Flecainide Acetate clinical trials, patients who were receiving **beta blockers** concurrently did not experience an increased incidence of side effects. Nevertheless, the possibility of additive negative inotropic effects of **beta blockers** and Flecainide should be recognized.

Flecainide is not extensively bound to plasma proteins. In vitro studies with several drugs which may be administered concomitantly showed that the extent of Flecainide binding to human plasma proteins is either unchanged or only slightly less. Consequently, interactions with other drugs which are highly protein bound (e.g., **anticoagulants**) would not be expected. Flecainide Acetate has been used in a large number of patients receiving **diuretics** without apparent interaction. Limited data in patients receiving known enzyme inducers (**phenytcin, phenobarbital, carbam-azepine**) indicate only a 30% increase in the rate of Flecainide elimination. In healthy subjects receiving **cimetidine** (1 gm daily) for one week, plasma Flecainide levels increased by about 30% and half-life increased by about 10%.

When **amiodarone** is added to Flecainide therapy, plasma Flecainide levels may increase two-fold or more in some patients, if Flecainide dosage is not reduced. (See *"Dosage and Administration".)*

There has been little experience with the coadministration of Flecainide Acetate and either **disopyramide** or **verapamil**. Because both of these drugs have negative inotropic properties and the effects of coadministration with Flecainide

Acetate are unknown, neither **disopyramide** nor **verapamil** should be administered concurrently with Flecainide Acetate unless, in the judgment of the physician, the benefits of this combination outweigh the risks. There has been too little experience with the coadministration of Flecainide Acetate with **nifedipine** or **diltiazem** to recommend concomitant use.

Carcinogenesis, Mutagenesis, Impairment of Fertility: Long-term studies with Flecainide in rats and mice at doses up 60 mg/kg/day have not revealed any compound-related carcinogenic effects. Mutagenicity studies (Ames test, mouse lymphoma and in vivo cytogenetics) did not reveal any mutagenic effects. A rat reproduction study at doses up to 50 mg/kg/day (seven times the usual human dose) did not reveal any adverse effect on male or female fertility.

Pregnancy: Pregnancy Category C. Flecainide has been shown to have teratogenic effects (club paws, sternebrae and vertebrae abnormalities, pale hearts with contracted ventricular septum) and an embryotoxic effect (increased resorptions) in one breed of rabbit (New Zealand White) when given doses of 30 and 35 mg/kg/day, but not in another breed of rabbit (Dutch Belted) when given up to 30 mg/kg/day. No teratogenic effects were observed in rats and mice given doses up to 50 and 80 mg/kg/day, respectively; however, delayed sternebral and vertebral ossification was observed at the high dose in rats. Because there are no adequate and well-controlled studies in pregnant women, Flecainide Acetate should be used during pregnancy only if the potential benefit justifies the potential risk to the fetus.

Labor and Delivery: It is not known whether the use of Flecainide Acetate during labor or delivery has immediate or delayed adverse effects on the mother or fetus, affects the duration of labor or delivery, or increases the possibility of forceps delivery or other obstetrical intervention.

Nursing Mothers: Results from a multiple dose study conducted in mothers soon after delivery indicates that Flecainide is excreted in human breast milk in concentrations as high as 4 times (with average levels about 2.5 times) corresponding plasma levels; assuming a maternal plasma level at the top of the therapeutic range (1 μg/mL), the calculated daily dose to a nursing infant (assuming about 700 mL breast milk over 24 hours) would be less than 3 mg. Because of the drug's potential for serious adverse effects in nursing infants, a decision should be made whether to discontinue nursing or discontinue the drug, taking into account the importance of the drug to the mother.

Pediatric Use: The safety and effectiveness of Flecainide Acetate in children less than 18 years of age have not been established.

Hepatic Impairment: Since Flecainide elimination from plasma can be markedly slower in patients with significant hepatic impairment, Flecainide Acetate should not be used in such patients unless the potential benefits clearly outweigh the risks. If used, frequent and early plasma level monitoring is required to guide dosage (see *"Plasma Level Monitoring"*): dosage increases should be made very cautiously when plasma levels have plateaued (after more than four days).

ADVERSE REACTIONS
In post-myocardial infarction patients with asymptomatic PVCs and non-sustained ventricular tachycardia, Flecainide Acetate therapy was found to be associated with a 5.1% rate of death and non-fatal cardiac arrest, compared with a 2.3% rate in a matched placebo group. (see "Warnings".)

Adverse effects reported for Flecainide Acetate described in detail in the Warnings section, were new or worsened arrhythmias which occurred in 1% of 108 patients with PSVT and in 7% of 117 patients with PAF; and new or exacerbated ventricular arrhythmias which occurred in 7% of 1330 patients with PVCs, non-sustained or *sustained* VT. In patients treated with Flecainide for *sustained* VT, 80% (51/64) of proarrhythmic events occurred within 14 days of the onset of therapy. 198 patients with *sustained* VT experienced a 13% incidence of new or exacerbated ventricular arrhythmias when dosage was initiated at 200 mg/day with slow upward titration, and did not exceed 300 mg/day in most patients. In some patients, Flecainide Acetate treatment has been associated with episodes of unresuscitatable VT or ventricular fibrillation (cardiac arrest). (See *"Warnings"*.) New or worsened CHF occurred in 6.3% of 1046 patients with PVCs, non-sustained or *sustained* VT. Of 297 patients with *sustained* VT, 9.1% experienced new or worsened CHF. New or worsened CHF was reported in 0.4% of 225 patients with supraventricular arrhythmias. There have also been instances of second-(0.5%) or third-degree (0.4%) AV block. Patients have developed sinus bradycardia, sinus pause, or sinus arrest, about 1.2% altogether (see *"Warnings"*). The frequency of most of these serious adverse events probably increases with higher trough plasma levels, especially when these trough levels exceed 1.0 μg/mL.

There have been rare reports of isolated elevations of serum alkaline phosphatase and isolated elevations of serum transaminase levels. These elevations have been asymptomatic and no cause and effect relationship with Flecainide Acetate has been established. In foreign postmarketing surveillance studies, there have been rare reports of hepatic dysfunction including reports of cholestasis and hepatic failure, and extremely rare reports of blood dyscrasias. Although no cause and effect relationship has been established, it is advisable to discontinue Flecainide Acetate in patients who develop unexplained jaundice or signs of hepatic dysfunction or blood dyscrasias in order to eliminate Flecainide Acetate as the possible causative agent.

Incidence figures for other adverse effects in patients with ventricular arrhythmias are based on a multicenter efficacy study, utilizing starting doses of 200 mg/day with gradual upward titration to 400 mg/day. Patients were treated for an average of 4.7 months, with some receiving up to 22 months of therapy. In this trial, 5.4% of patients discontinued due to non-cardiac adverse effects.

Table 1
MOST COMMON NONCARDIAC ADVERSE EFFECTS IN VENTRICULAR ARRHYTHMIA PATIENTS TREATED WITH FLECAINIDE ACETATE IN THE MULTICENTER STUDY

Adverse Effect	Incidence in All 429 Patients at Any Dose	*Incidence By Dose During Upward Titration*		
		200 mg/Day (N = 426)	300 mg/Day (N = 293)	400 mg/Day (N = 100)
Dizziness*	18.9%	11.0%	10.6%	13.0%
Visual Disturbance†	15.9%	5.4%	12.3%	18.0%
Dyspnea	10.3%	5.2%	7.5%	4.0%
Headache	9.6%	4.5%	6.1%	9.0%
Nausea	8.9%	4.9%	4.8%	6.0%
Fatigue	7.7%	4.5%	4.4%	3.0%
Palpitation	6.1%	3.5%	2.4%	7.0%
Chest Pain	5.4%	3.1%	3.8%	1.0%
Asthenia	4.9%	2.6%	2.0%	4.0%
Tremor	4.7%	2.4%	3.4%	2.0%
Constipation	4.4%	2.8%	2.1%	1.0%
Edema	3.5%	1.9%	1.4%	2.0%
Abdominal pain	3.3%	1.9%	2.4%	1.0%

* *Dizziness includes reports of dizziness, light-headedness, faintness, unsteadiness, near syncope, etc.*
† *Visual disturbance includes reports of blurred vision, difficulty in focusing, spots before eyes, etc.*

The following additional adverse experiences, possibly related to Flecainide Acetate therapy and occurring in 1% to less than 3% of patients, have been reported in acute and chronic studies:

Body as a Whole—malaise, fever;

Cardiovascular—tachycardia, sinus pause or arrest;

Gastrointestinal—vomiting, diarrhea, dyspepsia, anorexia;

Skin—rash;

Visual—diplopia;

Nervous System—hypoesthesia, paresthesia, paresis, ataxia, flushing, increased sweating, vertigo, syncope, somnolence, tinnitus;

Psychiatric—anxiety, insomnia, depression.

The following additional adverse experiences, possibly related to Flecainide Acetate, have been reported in less than 1% of patients:

Body as a Whole—swollen lips, tongue and mouth; arthralgia, bronchospasm, myalgia;

Cardiovascular—angina pectoris, second-degree and third-degree AV block, bradycardia, hypertension, hypotension;

Gastrointestinal—flatulence;

Urinary System—polyuria, urinary retention;

Hematologic: leukopenia, thrombocytopenia;

Skin—urticaria, exfoliative dermatitis, pruritus, alopecia;

Visual—eye pain or irritation, photophobia, nystagmus;

Nervous System—twitching, weakness, change in taste, dry mouth, convulsions, impotence, speech disorder, stupor, neuropathy;

Psychiatric: amnesia, confusion, decreased libido, depersonalization, euphoria, morbid dreams, apathy.

For patients with supraventricular arrhythmias, the most commonly reported noncardiac adverse experiences remain consistent with those known for patients treated with Flecainide Acetate for ventricular arrhythmias. Dizziness is possibly more frequent in PAF patients.

OVERDOSAGE
No specific antidote has been identified for the treatment of Flecainide Acetate overdosage. Animal studies suggest that the following events might occur with overdosage: lengthening of the PR interval; increase in the QRS duration, QT interval and amplitude of the T-wave; a reduction in myocardial rate and contractility; conduction disturbances; hypotension; and death from respiratory failure or asystole. Treatment of overdosage should be supportive and may include the following: removal of unabsorbed drug from the gastrointestinal tract, administration of inotropic agents or cardiac stimulants such as dopamine, dobutamine or isoproterenol; mechanically assisted respiration; circulatory assists such as intra-aortic balloon pumping; and transvenous pacing in the event of conduction block. Because of the long plasma half-life of Flecainide (12 to 27 hours in patients receiving usual doses), and the possibility of markedly non-linear elimination kinetics at very high doses, these supportive treatments may need to be continued for extended periods of time.

Hemodialysis is not an effective means of removing Flecainide from the body. Since Flecainide elimination is much slower when urine is very alkaline (pH 8 or higher), theoretically, acidification of urine to promote drug excretion may be beneficial in overdose cases with very alkaline urine. There is no evidence that acidification from normal urinary pH increases excretion.

DOSAGE AND ADMINISTRATION

FOR PATIENTS WITH *SUSTAINED* VT, NO MATTER WHAT THEIR CARDIAC STATUS, FLECAINIDE ACETATE, LIKE OTHER ANTIARRHYTHMICS, SHOULD BE INITIATED IN-HOSPITAL WITH RHYTHM MONITORING.

Flecainide has a long half-life (12 to 27 hours in patients). Steady-state plasma levels, in patients with normal renal and hepatic function, may not be achieved until the patient has received 3 to 5 days of therapy at a given dose. Therefore, INCREASES IN DOSAGE SHOULD BE MADE NO MORE FREQUENTLY THAN ONCE EVERY FOUR DAYS since during the first 2 to 3 days of therapy the optimal effect of a given dose may not be achieved. For patients with PSVT and patients with PAF the recommended starting dose is 50 mg every 12 hours. Flecainide Acetate doses may be increased in increments of 50 mg bid every four days until efficacy is achieved. For PAF patients, a substantial increase in efficacy without a substantial increase in discontinuations for adverse experiences may be achieved by increasing the Flecainide Acetate dose from 50 mg to 100 mg bid. The maximum recommended dose for patients with paroxysmal supraventricular arrhythmias is 300 mg/day.

For *sustained* VT the recommended starting dose is 100 mg every 12 hours. This dose may be increased in increments of 50 mg bid every four days until efficacy is achieved. Most patients with *sustained* VT do not require more than 150 mg every 12 hours (300 mg/day), and the maximum dose recommended is 400 mg/day.

In patients with *sustained* VT, the use of higher initial doses and more rapid dosage adjustments have resulted in an increased incidence of proarrhythmic events and CHF, particularly during the first few days of dosing (see *"Warnings"*). Therefore, a loading dose is not recommended.

Intravenous lidocaine has been used occasionally with Flecainide Acetate while awaiting the therapeutic effect of Flecainide Acetate. No adverse drug interactions were apparent. However, no formal studies have been performed to demonstrate the usefulness of this regimen.

An occasional patient not adequately controlled by (or intolerant to) a dose given at 12-hour intervals may be dosed at eight-hour intervals.

Once adequate control of the arrhythmia has been achieved, it may be possible in some patients to reduce the dose as necessary to minimize side effects or effects on conduction. In such patients, efficacy at the lower dose should be evaluated. Flecainide Acetate should be used cautiously in patients with a history of CHF or myocardial dysfunction (see *"Warnings"*). In patients with severe renal impairment (creatinine clearance of 35 mL/min/1.73 square meters or less), the initial dosage should be 100 mg once daily (or 50 mg bid); when used in such patients, frequent plasma level monitoring is required to guide dosage adjustments (see *"Plasma Level Monitoring"*). In patients with less severe renal disease, the initial dosage should be 100 mg every 12 hours; plasma level monitoring may also be useful in these patients during dosage adjustment. In both groups of patients, dosage increases should be made very cautiously when plasma level have plateaued (after more than four days), observing the patient closely for signs of adverse cardiac effects or other toxicity. It should be borne in mind that in these patients it may take longer than four days before a new steady-state plasma level is reached following a dosage change.

Based on theoretical considerations, rather than experimental data, the following suggestion is made: when transferring patients from another antiarrhythmic drug to Flecainide Acetate allow at least two to four plasma half-lives to elapse for the drug being discontinued before starting Flecainide Acetate at the usual dosage. In patients where withdrawal of a previous antiarrhythmic agent is likely to produce life-threatening arrhythmias, the physician should consider hospitalizing the patient.

When Flecainide is given in the presence of amiodarone, reduce the usual Flecainide dose by 50% and monitor the patient closely for adverse effects. Plasma level monitoring is strongly recommended to guide dosage with such combination therapy (see below).

Plasma Level Monitoring. The large majority of patients successfully treated with Flecainide Acetate were found to have trough plasma levels between 0.2 and 1.0 µg/mL. The probability of adverse experiences, especially cardiac, may increase with higher trough plasma levels, especially when these exceed 1.0 µg/mL. Periodic monitoring of trough plasma levels may be useful in patient management. Plasma level monitoring is required in patients with severe renal failure or severe hepatic disease, since elimination of Flecainide from plasma may be markedly slower. Monitoring of plasma levels is strongly recommended in patients on concurrent amiodarone therapy and may also be helpful in patients with CHF and in patients with moderate renal disease.

Store at controlled room temperature 15°-30°C (59°-86°F) in a tight, light-resistant container.

HOW SUPPLIED
TABLETS: 50 MG

BRAND/MANUFACTURER	NDC	SIZE	AWP
○ BRAND			
TAMBOCOR: 3M Pharm	00089-0305-10	100s	$63.42
	00089-0305-16	100s ud	$66.66

TABLETS: 100 MG

BRAND/MANUFACTURER	NDC	SIZE	AWP
○ BRAND			
TAMBOCOR: 3M Pharm	00089-0307-10	100s	$115.14
	00089-0307-16	100s ud	$126.72

TABLETS: 150 MG

BRAND/MANUFACTURER	NDC	SIZE	AWP
○ BRAND			
TAMBOCOR: 3M Pharm	00089-0314-10	100s	$158.46

Flexeril SEE CYCLOBENZAPRINE HYDROCHLORIDE

Florinef Acetate SEE FLUDROCORTISONE ACETATE

Florone SEE DIFLORASONE DIACETATE

Floropryl SEE ISOFLUROPHATE

Floxin SEE OFLOXACIN, SYSTEMIC

Floxuridine

WARNING

IT IS RECOMMENDED THAT FLOXURIDINE BE GIVEN ONLY BY OR UNDER THE SUPERVISION OF A QUALIFIED PHYSICIAN WHO IS EXPERIENCED IN CANCER CHEMOTHERAPY AND INTRA-ARTERIAL DRUG THERAPY AND IS WELL VERSED IN THE USE OF POTENT ANTIMETABOLITES.

BECAUSE OF THE POSSIBILITY OF SEVERE TOXIC REACTIONS, ALL PATIENTS SHOULD BE HOSPITALIZED FOR INITIATION OF THE FIRST COURSE OF THERAPY.

DESCRIPTION

Sterile Floxuridine, an antineoplastic antimetabolite, is available as a sterile, nonpyrogenic, lyophilized powder for reconstitution. Each vial contains 500 mg of Floxuridine which is to be reconstituted with 5 mL of sterile water for injection. An appropriate amount of reconstituted solution is then diluted with a parenteral solution for intra-arterial infusion (see *"Dosage And Administration"* section).

Floxuridine is a fluorinated pyrimidine. Chemically, Floxuridine is 2'-deoxy-5-fluorouridine with an empirical formula of $C_9H_{11}FN_2O_5$. It is a white to off-white odorless solid which is freely soluble in water.

The 2% aqueous solution has a pH of between 4.0 to 5.5. The molecular weight of Floxuridine is 246.19.

Following is its chemical structure:

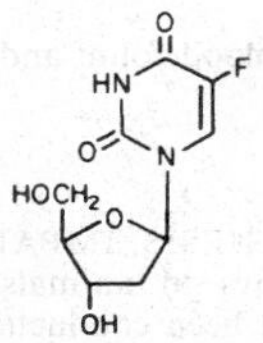

CLINICAL PHARMACOLOGY

When Floxuridine is given by rapid intra-arterial injection it is apparently rapidly catabolized to 5-fluorouracil. Thus, rapid injection of Floxuridine produces the same toxic and antimetabolic effects as does 5-fluorouracil. The primary effect is to interfere with the synthesis of deoxyribonucleic acid (DNA) and to a lesser extent inhibit the formation of ribonucleic acid (RNA). However, when Floxuridine is given by continuous intra-arterial infusion its direct anabolism to Floxuridine is enhanced, thus increasing the inhibition of DNA.

Floxuridine is metabolized in the liver. The drug is excreted intact and as urea, fluorouracil, α-fluoro-β-ureidopropionic acid, dihydrofluorouracil, α-fluoro-β-guanidopropionic acid and α-fluoro-β-alanine in the urine; it is also expired as respiratory carbon dioxide. Pharmacokinetic data on intra-arterial infusion of Floxuridine are not available.

INDICATIONS AND USAGE

Floxuridine is effective in the palliative management of gastrointestinal adenocarcinoma metastatic to the liver, when given by continuous regional intra-arterial infusion in carefully selected patients who are considered incurable by surgery or other means. Patients with known disease extending beyond an area capable of infusion via a single artery should, except in unusual circumstances, be considered for systemic therapy with other chemotherapeutic agents.

UNLABELED USES

Floxuridine is used alone or as an adjunct in the treatment of carcinoma of the gallbladder and liver.

CONTRAINDICATIONS

Floxuridine therapy is contraindicated for patients in a poor nutritional state, those with depressed bone marrow function or those with potentially serious infections.

WARNINGS

BECAUSE OF THE POSSIBILITY OF SEVERE TOXIC REACTIONS, ALL PATIENTS SHOULD BE HOSPITALIZED FOR THE FIRST COURSE OF THERAPY.

Floxuridine should be used with extreme caution in poor risk patients with impaired hepatic or renal function or a history of high-dose pelvic irradiation or previous use of alkylating agents. The drug is not intended as an adjuvant to surgery. Floxuridine may cause fetal harm when administered to a pregnant woman. It has been shown to be teratogenic in the chick embryo, mouse (at doses of 2.5 to 100 mg/kg) and rat (at doses of 75 to 150 mg/kg). Malformations included cleft palates; skeletal defects; and deformed appendages, paws and tails. The dosages which were teratogenic in animals are 4.2 to 125 times the recommended human therapeutic dose.

There are no adequate and well-controlled studies with Floxuridine in pregnant women. If this drug is used during pregnancy or if the patient becomes pregnant while taking (receiving) this drug, the patient should be apprised of the potential hazard to the fetus. Women of childbearing potential should be advised to avoid becoming pregnant.

Combination Therapy: Any form of therapy which adds to the stress of the patient, interferes with nutrition or depresses bone marrow function will increase the toxicity of Floxuridine.

PRECAUTIONS

GENERAL

Sterile Floxuridine is a highly toxic drug with a narrow margin of safety. Therefore, patients should be carefully supervised since therapeutic response is unlikely to occur without some evidence of toxicity. Severe hematological toxicity, gastrointestinal hemorrhage and even death may result from the use of Floxuridine despite meticulous selection of patients and careful adjustment of dosage. Although severe toxicity is more likely in poor risk patients, fatalities may be encountered occasionally even in patients in relatively good condition.

Therapy is to be discontinued promptly whenever one of the following signs of toxicity appears:

Myocardial ischemia
Stomatitis or esophagopharyngitis, at the first visible sign
Leukopenia (WBC under 3500) or a rapidly falling white blood count
Vomiting, intractable
Diarrhea, frequent bowel movements or watery stools
Gastrointestinal ulceration and bleeding
Thrombocytopenia (platelets under 100,000).
Hemorrhage from any site

INFORMATION FOR PATIENTS

Patients should be informed of expected toxic effects, particularly oral manifestations. Patients should be alerted to the possibility of alopecia as a result of therapy and should be informed that it is usually a transient effect.

LABORATORY TESTS:

Careful monitoring of the white blood count and platelet count is recommended.

DRUG INTERACTIONS

See *"Warnings"* section.

CARCINOGENESIS, MUTAGENESIS, IMPAIRMENT OF FERTILITY:

Carcinogenesis: Long-term studies in animals to evaluate the carcinogenic potential of Floxuridine have not been conducted. On the basis of the available data no evaluation can be made of the carcinogenic risk of Floxuridine to humans.

Mutagenesis: Oncogenic transformation of fibroblasts from mouse embryo has been induced *in vitro* by Floxuridine, but the relationship between oncogenicity and mutagenicity is not clear. Floxuridine has also been shown to be mutagenic in human leukocytes *in vitro* and in the *Drosophila* test system. In addition, 5-fluorouracil, to which Floxuridine is catabolized when given by intra-arterial injection, has been shown to be mutagenic in *in vitro* tests.

Impairment of Fertility: The effects of Floxuridine on fertility and general reproductive performance have not been studied in animals. However, because Floxuridine is catabolized to 5-fluorouracil, it should be noted that 5-fluorouracil has been shown to induce chromosomal aberrations and changes in chromosome organization of spermatogonia in rats at doses of 125 or 250 mg/kg, administered intraperitoneally.

Spermatogonial differentiation was also inhibited by fluorouracil, resulting in transient infertility. In female rats, fluorouracil, administered intraperitoneally at doses of 25 or 50 mg/kg during the preovulatory phase of oogenesis, significantly reduced the incidence of fertile matings, delayed the development of pre- and postimplantation embryos, increased the incidence of preimplantation lethality and induced chromosomal anomalies in these embryos. Compounds such as Floxuridine which interfere with DNA, RNA and protein synthesis, might be expected to have adverse effects on gametogenesis.

PREGNANCY

Teratogenic effects: Pregnancy category D. See *"Warnings"* section. Floxuridine has been shown to be teratogenic in the chick embryo, mouse (at doses of 2.5 to 100 mg/kg) and rat (at doses of 75 to 150 mg/kg). Malformations included cleft palates, skeletal defects and deformed appendages, paws and tails. The dosages which were teratogenic in animals are 4.2 to 125 times the recommended human therapeutic dose.

There are no adequate and well-controlled studies with Floxuridine in pregnant women. While there is no evidence of teratogenicity in humans due to Floxuridine, it should be kept in mind that other drugs which inhibit DNA synthesis (*e.g.,* methotrexate and aminopterin) have been reported to be teratogenic in humans. Floxuridine should be used during pregnancy only if the potential benefit justifies the potential risk to the fetus.

Nonteratogenic Effects: Floxuridine has not been studied in animals for its effects on peri- and postnatal development. However, compounds which inhibit DNA, RNA and protein synthesis might be expected to have adverse effects on peri- and postnatal development.

Nursing Mothers: It is not known whether Floxuridine is excreted in human milk. Because Floxuridine inhibits DNA and RNA synthesis, mothers should not nurse while receiving this drug.

Pediatric Use: Safety and effectiveness in children have not been established.

ADVERSE REACTIONS

Adverse reactions to the arterial infusion of Floxuridine are generally related to the procedural complications of regional arterial infusion.

The more common adverse reactions to the drug are nausea, vomiting, diarrhea, enteritis, stomatitis and localized erythema. The more common laboratory abnormalities are anemia, leukopenia, thrombocytopenia and elevations of alkaline phosphatase, serum transaminase, serum bilirubin and lactic dehydrogenase.

Other adverse reactions are:

Gastrointestinal: duodenal ulcer, duodenitis, gastritis, bleeding, gastroenteritis, glossitis, pharyngitis, anorexia, cramps, abdominal pain; possible intra- and extrahepatic biliary sclerosis, as well as acalculous cholecystitis.

Dermatologic: alopecia, dermatitis, nonspecific skin toxicity, rash.

Cardiovascular: myocardial ischemia.

Miscellaneous clinical reactions: fever, lethargy, malaise, weakness.

Laboratory abnormalities: BSP, prothrombin, total proteins, sedimentation rate and thrombopenia.

Procedural complications of regional arterial infusion: arterial aneurysm; arterial ischemia; arterial thrombosis; embolism; fibromyositis; thrombophlebitis; hepatic necrosis; abscesses; infection at catheter site; bleeding at catheter site; catheter blocked, displaced or leaking.

The following adverse reactions have not been reported with Floxuridine but have been noted following the administration of 5-fluorouracil. While the possibility of these occurring following Floxuridine therapy is remote because of its regional administration, one should be alert for these reactions following the administration of Floxuridine because of the pharmacological similarity of these two drugs: pancytopenia, agranulocytosis, myocardial ischemia, angina, anaphylaxis, generalized allergic reactions, acute cerebellar syndrome, nystagmus, headache, dry skin, fissuring, photosensitivity, pruritic masculopapular rash, increased pigmentation of the skin, vein pigmentation, lacrimal duct stenosis, visual changes, lacrimation, photophobia, disorientation, confusion, euphoria, epistaxis and nail changes, including loss of nails.

OVERDOSAGE

The possibility of overdosage with Floxuridine is unlikely in view of the mode of administration. Nevertheless, the anticipated manifestations would be nausea, vomiting, diarrhea, gastrointestinal ulceration and bleeding, bone marrow depression (including thrombocytopenia, leukopenia and agranulocytosis).

No specific antidotal therapy exists. Patients who have been exposed to an overdosage of Floxuridine should be monitored hematologically for at least four weeks. Should abnormalities appear, appropriate therapy should be utilized.

The acute intravenous toxicity of Floxuridine is as follows:

Species	LD_{50} (mg/kg ± S.E.)
Mouse	880 ± 51
Rat	670 ± 73
Rabbit	94 ± 19.6
Dog	157 ± 46

◆ RATED THERAPEUTICALLY EQUIVALENT; ◇ THERAPEUTIC EQUIVALENCE UNCONFIRMED; ○ UNRATED

DOSAGE AND ADMINISTRATION

Each vial must be reconstituted with 5 mL of sterile water for injection to yield a solution containing approximately 100 mg of Floxuridine/mL. The calculated daily dose(s) of the drug is then diluted with 5% dextrose or 0.9% sodium chloride injection to a volume appropriate for the infusion apparatus to be used. The administration of Floxuridine is best achieved with the use of an appropriate pump to overcome pressure in large arteries and to ensure a uniform rate of infusion.

Parenteral drug products should be inspected visually for particulate matter and discoloration prior to administration whenever solution and container permit.

The recommended therapeutic dosage schedule of Floxuridine by continuous arterial infusion is 0.1 to 0.6 mg/kg/day. The higher dosage ranges (0.4 to 0.6 mg) are usually employed for hepatic artery infusion because the liver metabolizes the drug, thus reducing the potential for systemic toxicity. Therapy can be given until adverse reactions appear. (See "Precautions" section.) When these side effects have subsided, therapy may be resumed. The patient should be maintained on therapy as long as response to Floxuridine continues.

Procedures for proper handling and disposal of anticancer drugs should be considered. Several guidelines on this subject have been published.[1-6] There is no general agreement that all of the procedures recommended in the guidelines are necessary or appropriate.

The sterile powder should be stored at 59° to 86°F (15° to 30°C). Reconstituted vials should be stored under refrigeration (36° to 46°F, 2° to 8°C) for not more than two weeks.

REFERENCES

1. Recommendations for the safe handling of parenteral antineoplastic drugs. Washington, DC, U.S. Government Printing Office (NIH Publication No. 83-2621). 2. AMA Council Report. Guidelines for handling parenteral antineoplastics. *JAMA* 253: 1590-1592, Mar 15, 1985. 3. National Study Commission on Cytotoxic Exposure: Recommendations for handling cytotoxic agents. Available from Louis P. Jeffrey, ScD, Director of Pharmacy Services, Rhode Island Hospital, 593 Eddy Street, Providence, Rhode Island 02902. 4. Clinical Oncological Society of Australia: Guidelines and recommendations for safe handling of antineoplastic agents. *Med J Aust 1*: 426-428, Apr 30, 1983. 5. Jones RB, Frank R, Mass T: Safe handling of chemotherapeutic agents: a report from the Mount Sinai Medical Center. *CA 33*: 258-263, Sept-Oct 1983. 6. ASHP technical assistance bulletin on handling cytotoxic drugs in hospitals. *Am J Hosp Pharm 42*: 131-137, Jan 1985.

J CODES

500 mg IV—J9200

HOW SUPPLIED

POWDER FOR INJECTION: 0.5 GM

BRAND/MANUFACTURER	NDC	SIZE	AWP
◆ BRAND			
FUDR: Roche Labs	00004-1935-08	1s	$121.72

Fluconazole

DESCRIPTION

Fluconazole is the first of a new class of synthetic broad-spectrum bis-triazole antifungal agents, available as an oral tablet, as a powder for oral suspension and as a sterile solution for intravenous use.

Fluconazole is designated chemically as 2,4-difluoro-α,α^1-bis(1H-1,2,4-triazol-1-ylmethyl)benzyl alcohol with an empirical formula of $C_{13}H_{12}F_2N_6O$ and molecular weight 306.3.

Fluconazole is a white crystalline solid which is slightly soluble in water and saline.

Fluconazole is available for oral administration as 50- mg, 100- mg, and 200-mg tablets.

Fluconazole is available as an oral suspension containing 350 mg or 1400 mg of Fluconazole.

Fluconazole is available as an injection. Each ml contains 2 mg of Fluconazole. Injection volumes of 100 ml and 200 ml are packaged in glass and in Viaflex®. Plus plastic containers.

Following is its chemical structure:

CLINICAL PHARMACOLOGY

MODE OF ACTION

Fluconazole is a highly selective inhibitor of fungal cytochrome P-450 sterol C-14 alpha-demethylation. Mammalian cell demethylation is much less sensitive to Fluconazole inhibition. The subsequent loss of normal sterols correlates with the accumulation of 14 alpha-methyl sterols in fungi and may be responsible for the fungistatic activity of Fluconazole.

PHARMACOKINETICS AND METABOLISM

The pharmacokinetic properties of Fluconazole are similar following administration by the intravenous or oral routes. In normal volunteers, the bioavailability of orally administered Fluconazole is over 90% compared with intravenous administration. Bioequivalence was established between the 100 mg tablet and both suspension strengths when administered as a single 200 mg dose.

Peak plasma concentrations (Cmax) in fasted normal volunteers occur between 1 and 2 hours with a terminal plasma elimination half-life of approximately 30 hours (range 20-50 hours) after oral administration.

In fasted normal volunteers, administration of a single oral 400 mg dose of Fluconazole leads to a mean Cmax of 6.72 µg/mL (range: 4.12 to 8.08 µg/mL) and after single oral doses of 50-400 mg, Fluconazole plasma concentrations and AUC (area under the plasma concentration-time curve) are dose proportional.

Steady-state concentrations are reached within 5-10 days following oral doses of 50-400 mg given once daily. Administration of a loading dose (on Day 1) of twice the usual daily dose results in plasma concentrations close to steady state by the second day. The apparent volume of distribution of Fluconazole approximates that of total body water. Plasma protein binding is low (11-12%). Following either single- or multiple-oral doses for up to 14 days, Fluconazole penetrates into all body fluids studied (see table below). In normal volunteers, saliva concentrations of Fluconazole were equal to or slightly greater than plasma concentrations regardless of dose, route, or duration of dosing. In patients with bronchiectasis, sputum concentrations of Fluconazole following a single 150 mg oral dose were equal to plasma concentrations at both 4 and 24 hours post dose. In patients with fungal meningitis, Fluconazole concentrations in the CSF are approximately 80% of the corresponding plasma concentrations.

Tissue or Fluid	Ratio of Fluconazole Tissue (Fluid)/Plasma Concentration*
Cerebrospinal fluid†	.5-.9
Saliva	1
Sputum	1
Blister fluid	1
Urine	10
Normal skin	10
Nails	1
Blister skin	2

* *Relative to concurrent concentrations in plasma in subjects with normal renal function.*
† *Independent of degree of meningeal inflammation.*

In normal volunteers, Fluconazole is cleared primarily by renal excretion, with approximately 80% of the administered dose appearing in the urine as unchanged drug. About 11% of the dose is excreted in the urine as metabolites.

The pharmacokinetics of Fluconazole are markedly affected by reduction in renal function. There is an inverse relationship between the elimination half-life and creatinine clearance. The dose of Fluconazole may need to be reduced in patients with impaired renal function (see "Dosage and Administration"). A 3-hour hemodialysis session decreases plasma concentrations by approximately 50%.

In normal volunteers, Fluconazole administration (doses ranging from 200 mg to 400 mg once daily for up to 14 days) was associated with small and inconsistent effects on testosterone concentrations, endogenous corticosteroid concentrations, and the ACTH-stimulated cortisol response.

DRUG INTERACTION STUDIES

Oral Contraceptives: Oral contraceptives were administered as a single dose both before and after the oral administration of Fluconazole 50 mg once daily for 10 days in 10 healthy women. There was no significant difference in ethinyl estradiol or levonorgestrel AUC after the administration of Fluconazole. This mean increase in ethinyl estradiol AUC was 6% (range: −47 to 108%) and levonorgestrel AUC increased 17% (range: −33 to 141%).

Cimetidine: Fluconazole 100 mg was administered as a single dose alone and two hours after a single dose of cimetidine 400 mg to six healthy male volunteers. After the administration of cimetidine, there was a significant decrease in fluconazole AUC and Cmax. There was a mean ± SD decrease in Fluconazole AUC of 14% ± 11% (range: −3.4 to −31%) and Cmax decreased 19% ± 14% (range: −5 to −40%). However, the administration of cimetidine 600 mg to 900 mg intravenously over a four hour period (from one hour before to 3 hours after a single oral dose of Fluconazole 200 mg) did not affect the bioavailability or pharmacokinetics of Fluconazole in 24 healthy male volunteers.

Antacid: Administration of Maalox (20 ml) to 14 normal male volunteers immediately prior to a single dose of Fluconazole 100 mg had no effect on the absorption or elimination of Fluconazole.

Hydrochlorothiazide: Concomitant oral administration of 100 mg Fluconazole and 50 mg hydrochlorothiazide for 10 days in 13 normal volunteers resulted in a significant increase in Fluconazole AUC and Cmax compared to Fluconazole given alone. There was a mean ± SD increase in Fluconazole AUC and Cmax of 45% ± 31% (range: 19 to 114%) and 43% ± 31% (range: 19 to 122%), respectively. These changes are attributable to a mean ± SD reduction in renal clearance of 30% ± 12% (range: −10 to −50%).

Rifampin: Administration of a single oral 200 mg dose of Fluconazole after 15 days of rifampin administered as 600 mg daily in eight healthy male volunteers resulted in a significant decrease in Fluconazole AUC and a significant increase in apparent oral clearance of Fluconazole. There was a mean ± SD reduction in Fluconazole AUC of 23% ± 9% (range: −13 to −42%). Apparent oral clearance of Fluconazole increased 32% ± 17% (range: 16 to 72%). Fluconazole half-life decreased from 33.4 ± 4.4 hours to 26.8 ± 3.9 hours. (See "Precautions".)

Warfarin: There was a significant increase in prothrombin time response (area under the prothrombin time—time curve) following a single dose of warfarin (15 mg) administered to 13 normal male volunteers following oral Fluconazole 200 mg administered daily for 14 days as compared to the administration of warfarin alone. There was a mean ± SD increase in the prothrombin time response (area under the prothrombin time—time curve) of 7% ± 4% (range: −2 to 13%). (See "Precautions".) Mean is based on data from 12 subjects as one of 13 subjects experienced a 2-fold increase in his prothrombin time response.

Phenytoin: Phenytoin AUC was determined after 4 days of phenytoin dosing (200 mg daily, orally for 3 days followed by 250 mg intravenously for one dose) both with and without the administration of fluconazole (oral Fluconazole 200 mg daily for 16 days) in 10 normal male volunteers. There was a significant increase in phenytoin AUC. The mean ± SD increase in phenytoin AUC was 88% ± 68% (range: 16 to 247%). The absolute magnitude of this interaction is unknown because of the intrinsically nonlinear disposition of phenytoin. (See "Precautions".)

Cyclosporine: Cyclosporine AUC and Cmax were determined before and after the administration of Fluconazole 200 mg daily for 14 days in eight renal transplant patients who had been on cyclosporine therapy for at least 6 months and on a stable cyclosporine dose for at least 6 weeks. There was a significant increase in cyclosporine AUC, Cmax, Cmin (24 hour concentration), and a significant reduction in apparent oral clearance following the administration of Fluconazole. The mean ± SD increase in AUC was 92% ± 43% (range: 18 to 147%). The Cmax increased 60% ± 48% (range: −5 to 133%). The Cmin increased 157% ± 96% (range: 33 to 360%). The apparent oral clearance decreased 45% ± 15% (range: −15 to −60%). (See "Precautions".)

Zidovudine: Plasma zidovudine concentrations were determined on two occasions (before and following Fluconazole 200 mg daily for 15 days) in 13 volunteers with AIDS or ARC who were on a stable zidovudine dose for at least two weeks. There was a significant increase in zidovudine AUC following the administration of Fluconazole. The mean ± SD increase in AUC was 20% ± 32% (range: −27 to 104%). The metabolite, GZDV, to parent drug ratio significantly decreased after the administration of Fluconazole, from 7.6 ± 3.6 to 5.7 ± 2.2.

Theophylline: The pharmacokinetics of theophylline were determined from a single intravenous dose of aminophylline (6 mg/kg) before and after the oral administration of Fluconazole 200 mg daily for 14 days in 16 normal male volunteers. There were significant increases in theophylline AUC, Cmax, and half-life with a corresponding decrease in clearance. The mean ± SD theophylline AUC increased 21% ± 16% (range: −5 to 48%). The Cmax increased 13% ± 17% (range: −13 to 40%). Theophylline clearance decreased 16% ± 11% (range: −32 to 5%). The half-life of theophylline increased from 6.6 ± 1.7 hours to 7.9 ± 1.5 hours.

Terfenadine: Six healthy volunteers received terfenadine 60 mg BID for 15 days. Fluconazole 200 mg was administered daily from days 9 through 15. Fluconazole did not affect terfenadine plasma concentrations. Terfenadine acid metabolite AUC increased 36% ± 36% (range: 7 to 102%) from day 8 to day 15 with the concomitant administration of Fluconazole. There was no change in cardiac repolarization as measured by Holter QTc intervals.

Oral Hypoglycemics: The effects of Fluconazole on the pharmacokinetics of the sulfonylurea oral hypoglycemic agents tolbutamide, glipizide, and glyburide were evaluated in three placebo-controlled studies in normal volunteers. All subjects received the sulfonylurea alone as a single dose and again as a single dose following the administration of Fluconazole 100 mg daily for 7 days. In these three studies 22/46 (47.8%) of Fluconazole treated patients and 9/22 (40.1%) of placebo treated patients experienced symptoms consistent with hypoglycemia. (See "Precautions".)

Tolbutamide: In 13 normal male volunteers, there was a significant increase in tolbutamide (500 mg single dose) AUC and Cmax following the administration of Fluconazole. There was a mean ± SD increase in tolbutamide AUC of 26% ± 9% (range: 12 to 39%). Tolbutamide Cmax increased 11% ± 9% (range: −6 to 27%). (See "Precautions".)

Glipizide: The AUC and Cmax of glipizide (2.5 mg single dose) were significantly increased following the administration of Fluconazole in 13 normal male volunteers. There was a mean ± SD increase in AUC of 49% ± 13% (range: 27 to 73%) and an increase in Cmax of 19% ± 23% (range: −11 to 79%). (See "Precautions".)

Glyburide: The AUC and Cmax of glyburide (5 mg single dose) were significantly increased following the administration of Fluconazole in 20 normal male volunteers. There was a mean ± SD increase in AUC of 44% ± 29% (range: −13 to 115%) and Cmax increased 19% ± 19% (range: −23 to 62%). Five subjects required oral glucose following the ingestion of glyburide after 7 days of Fluconazole administration. (See "Precautions".)

MICROBIOLOGY

Fluconazole exhibits *in vitro* activity against *Cryptococcus neoformans* and *Candida spp.* Fungistatic activity has also been demonstrated in normal and immunocompromised animal models for systemic and intracranial fungal infec-

tions due to *Cryptococcus neoformans* and for systemic infections due to *Candida albicans.* Development of resistance to Fluconazole has not been studied.

In common with other azole antifungal agents, most fungi show a higher apparent sensitivity to Fluconazole *in vivo* than *in vitro.* Fluconazole administered orally and/or intravenously was active in a variety of animal models of fungal infection using standard laboratory strains of fungi. Activity has been demonstrated against fungal infections caused by *Aspergillus flavus* and *Aspergillus fumigatus* in normal mice. Fluconazole has also been shown to be active in animal models of endemic mycoses, including one model of *Blastomyces dermatitidis* pulmonary infections in normal mice; one model of *Coccidioides immitis* intracranial infections in normal mice; and several models of *Histoplasma capsulatum* pulmonary infection in normal and immunosuppressed mice. The clinical significance of results obtained in these studies is unknown.

Concurrent administration of Fluconazole and amphotericin B in infected normal and immunosuppressed mice showed the following results: a small additive antifungal effect in systemic infection with *C. albicans,* no interaction in intracranial infection with *Cr. neoformans,* and antagonism of the two drugs in systemic infection with *Asp. fumigatus.* The clinical significance of results obtained in these studies is unknown.

Development of resistance to Fluconazole has not been studied; however, there have been reports of cases of superinfection with candida species other than *C. albicans,* which are often inherently not susceptible to Fluconazole (e.g., *Candida krusei*). Such cases may require alternative antifungal therapy.

INDICATIONS AND USAGE

Fluconazole is indicated for the treatment of:

1. Oropharyngeal and esophageal candidiasis. In open comparative studies of relatively small numbers of patients, Fluconazole was also effective for the treatment of candidal urinary tract infections, peritonitis, and systemic candidal infections including candidemia, disseminated candidiasis, and pneumonia.
2. Cryptococcal meningitis. Before prescribing Fluconazole for AIDS patients with cryptococcal meningitis, please see "Clinical Studies" section. Studies comparing Fluconazole to amphotericin B in non-HIV infected patients have not been conducted.

Prophylaxis Fluconazole is also indicated to decrease the incidence of candidiasis in patients undergoing bone marrow transplantation who receive cytotoxic chemotherapy and/or radiation therapy.

Specimens for fungal culture and other relevant laboratory studies (serology, histopathology) should be obtained prior to therapy to isolate and identify causative organisms. Therapy may be instituted before the results of the cultures and other laboratory studies are known; however, once these results become available, anti-infective therapy should be adjusted accordingly.

UNLABELED USES

Fluconazole is used alone or as an adjunct in the treatment of fungal infections in patients with acquired immunodeficiency syndrome, chronic mucocutaneous candidiasis, systemic candidiasis, vaginal candidiasis, and fungal meningitis.

CLINICAL STUDIES

Cryptococcal meningitis: In a large multicenter study comparing Fluconazole (200 mg/day) to amphotericin B (0.3 mg/kg/day) for treatment of cryptococcal meningitis in patients with AIDS, a multivariate analysis revealed three pretreatment factors that predicted death during the course of therapy: abnormal mental status, cerebrospinal fluid cryptococcal antigen titer greater than 1:1024, and cerebrospinal fluid white blood cell count of less than 20 cells/mm^3. Mortality among high risk patients was 33% and 40% for amphotericin B and Fluconazole patients, respectively (p=0.58), with overall deaths 14% (9 of 63 subjects) and 18% (24 of 131 subjects) for the 2 arms of the study (p=0.48). Optimal doses and regimens for patients with acute cryptococcal meningitis and at high risk for treatment failure remain to be determined. (Saag, *et al.* N Engl J Med 1992; 326:83-9)

Development of resistance to fluconazole has not been studied; however, there have been reports of cases of superinfection with candida species other than *C. albicans,* which are often inherently not susceptible to Fluconazole (e.g., *Candida krusei*). Such cases may require alternative antifungal therapy.

CONTRAINDICATIONS

Fluconazole is contraindicated in patients who have shown hypersensitivity to Fluconazole or to any of its excipients. There is no information regarding cross hypersensitivity between Fluconazole and other azole antifungal agents. Caution should be used in prescribing Fluconazole to patients with hypersensitivity to other azoles.

WARNINGS

(1) Hepatic injury: Fluconazole has been associated with rare cases of serious hepatic toxicity, including fatalities primarily in patients with serious underlying medical conditions. In cases of Fluconazole associated hepatotoxicity, no obvious relationship to total daily dose duration of therapy, sex or age of the patient has been observed. Fluconazole hepatotoxicity has usually, but not always, been reversible on discontinuation of therapy. Patients who develop abnormal liver function tests during Fluconazole therapy should be monitored for the development of more severe hepatic injury. Fluconazole should be discontinued if clinical signs and symptoms consistent with liver disease develop that may be attributable to Fluconazole.

(2) Anaphylaxis: In rare cases, anaphylaxis has been reported.

(3) *Dermatologic:* Patients have rarely developed exfoliative skin disorders during treatment with Fluconazole. In patients with serious underlying diseases (predominantly AIDS and malignancy) these have rarely resulted in a fatal outcome.

Patients who develop rashes during treatment with Fluconazole should be monitored closely and the drug discontinued if lesions progress. (See *"Adverse Reactions."*)

PRECAUTIONS
DRUG INTERACTIONS
(See *"Clinical Pharmacology."*)

Prothrombin time may be increased in patients receiving concomitant Fluconazole and coumarin-type anticoagulants. Careful monitoring of prothrombin time in patients receiving Fluconazole and coumarin-type anticoagulants is recommended.

Fluconazole increased the plasma concentrations of phenytoin. Careful monitoring of phenytoin concentrations in patients receiving Fluconazole and phenytoin is recommended.

Fluconazole may significantly increase cyclosporine levels in renal transplant patients with or without impaired renal function. Careful monitoring of cyclosporine concentrations in patients receiving Fluconazole and cyclosporine is recommended.

Clinically significant hypoglycemia may be precipitated by the use of Fluconazole with oral hypoglycemic agents; one fatality has been reported from hypoglycemia in association with combined Fluconazole and glyburide use. Fluconazole increased the plasma concentrations and reduced the metabolism of tolbutamide, glyburide and glipizide. When Fluconazole is used concomitantly with these or other sulfonylurea oral hypoglycemic agents, blood glucose concentrations should be carefully monitored, and the dose of the sulfonylurea should be adjusted as necessary.

Rifampin enhances the metabolism of concurrently administered Fluconazole. Depending on clinical circumstances, consideration should be given to increasing the dose of Fluconazole when it is administered with rifampin.

Fluconazole increases the serum concentrations of theophylline. Careful monitoring of serum theophylline concentrations in patients receiving Fluconazole and theophylline is recommended.

Because of the occurrence of serious cardiac dysrhythmias in patients receiving other azole antifungals in conjunction with terfenadine, an interaction study has been performed (see *"Drug Interaction Studies"*) and failed to demonstrate a clinically significant drug interaction. Although these events have not been observed in patients receiving Fluconazole, the co-administration of Fluconazole and terfenadine should be carefully monitored.

Physicians should be aware that drug-drug interaction studies with other medications have not been conducted, but such interactions may occur.

CARCINOGENESIS, MUTAGENESIS AND IMPAIRMENT OF FERTILITY
Fluconazole showed no evidence of carcinogenic potential in mice and rats treated orally for 24 months at doses of 2.5, 5 or 10 mg/kg/day (approximately 2-7 × the recommended human dose). Male rats treated with 5 and 10 mg/kg/day had an increased incidence of hepatocellular adenomas.

Fluconazole, with or without metabolic activation, was negative in tests for mutagenicity in 4 strains of *S. typhimurium*, and in the mouse lymphoma L5178Y system. Cytogenetic studies *in vivo* (murine bone marrow cells, following oral administration of Fluconazole) and *in vitro* (human lymphocytes exposed to Fluconazole at 1000 μg/mL) showed no evidence of chromosomal mutations.

Fluconazole did not affect the fertility of male or female rats treated orally with daily doses of 5, 10 or 20 mg/kg or with parenteral doses of 5, 25 or 75 mg/kg, although the onset of parturition was slightly delayed at 20 mg/kg p.o. In an intravenous perinatal study in rats at 5, 20 and 40 mg/kg, dystocia and prolongation of parturition were observed in a few dams at 20 mg/kg (approximately 5-15 × the recommended human dose) and 40 mg/kg, but not at 5 mg/kg. The disturbances in parturition were reflected by a slight increase in the number of still-born pups and decrease of neonatal survival at these dose levels. The effects on parturition in rats are consistent with the species specific estrogen-lowering property produced by high doses of Fluconazole. Such a hormone change has not been observed in women treated with Fluconazole. (See *"Clinical Pharmacology."*)

PREGNANCY
Teratogenic Effects. Pregnancy Category C: Fluconazole was administered orally to pregnant rabbits during organogenesis in two studies, at 5, 10 and 20 mg/kg and at 5, 25, and 75 mg/kg respectively. Maternal weight gain was impaired at all dose levels, and abortions occurred at 75 mg/kg (approximately 20-60 × the recommended human dose); no adverse fetal effects were detected. In several studies in which pregnant rats were treated orally with Fluconazole during organogenesis, maternal weight gain was impaired and placental weights were increased at 25 mg/kg. There were no fetal effects at 5 or 10 mg/kg; increases in fetal anatomical variants (supernumerary ribs, renal pelvis dilation) and delays in ossification were observed at 25 and 50 mg/kg and higher doses. At doses ranging from 80 mg/kg (approximately 20-60 × the recommended human dose) to 320 mg/kg, embryolethality in rats was increased and fetal abnormalities included wavy ribs, cleft palate and abnormal cranio-facial ossification. These effects are consistent with the inhibition of estrogen synthesis in rats and may be a result of known effects of lowered estrogen on pregnancy, organogenesis and parturition.

There are no adequate and well controlled studies in pregnant women. Fluconazole should be used in pregnancy only if the potential benefit justifies the possible risk to the fetus.

NURSING MOTHERS
Fluconazole is secreted in human milk at concentrations similar to plasma. Therefore, the use of Fluconazole in nursing mothers is not recommended.

PEDIATRIC USE
Efficacy of Fluconazole has not been established in children. A small number of patients from age 3 to 13 years have been treated safely with Fluconazole using doses of 3-6 mg/kg daily.

ADVERSE REACTIONS
Sixteen percent of over 4000 patients treated with Fluconazole in clinical trials of 7 days or more experienced adverse events. Treatment was discontinued in 1.5% of patients due to adverse clinical events and in 1.3% of patients due to laboratory test abnormalities.

In combined clinical trials and marketing experience, there have been rare cases of serious hepatic reactions during treatment with Fluconazole (see *"Warnings"*). The spectrum of these hepatic reactions has ranged from mild transient elevations in transaminases to clinical hepatitis, cholestasis and fulminant hepatic failure, including fatalities. Instances of fatal hepatic reactions were noted to occur primarily in patients with serious underlying medical conditions (predominantly AIDS or malignancy) and often while taking multiple concomitant medications. Transient hepatic reactions, including hepatitis and jaundice have occurred among patients with no other identifiable risk factors. In each of these cases, liver function returned to baseline on discontinuation of Fluconazole.

Clinical adverse events were reported more frequently in HIV infected patients (21%) than in non-HIV infected patients (13%); however, the patterns in HIV infected and non-HIV infected patients were similar. The proportions of patients discontinuing therapy due to clinical adverse events were similar in the two groups (1.5%).

The following treatment-related clinical adverse events occurred at an incidence of 1% or greater in 4048 patients receiving Fluconazole for 7 or more days in clinical trials: nausea 3.7%, headache 1.9%, skin rash 1.8%, vomiting 1.7%, abdominal pain 1.7%, and diarrhea 1.5%.

In two comparative trials evaluating the efficacy of Fluconazole for the suppression of relapse of cryptococcal meningitis, a statistically significant increase was observed in median AST (SGOT) levels from a baseline value of 30 IU/L to 41 IU/L in one trial and 34 IU/L to 66 IU/L in the other. The overall rate of serum transaminase elevations of more than 8 times the upper limit of normal was approximately 1% in Fluconazole-treated patients in clinical trials. These elevations occurred in patients with severe underlying disease, predominantly AIDS or malignancies, most of whom were receiving multiple concomitant medications, including many known to be hepatotoxic. The incidence of abnormally elevated serum transaminases was greater in patients taking Fluconazole concomitantly with one or more of the following medications: rifampin, phenytoin, isoniazid, valproic acid, or oral sulfonylurea hypoglycemic agents.

In rare cases, anaphylaxis has been reported.

The following adverse experiences occurred under conditions (e.g. open trials, marketing experience) where a causal association is uncertain.

Central Nervous System: seizures

Dermatologic: exfoliative skin disorders including Stevens-Johnson Syndrome and toxic epidermal necrolysis (see *"Warnings"*), alopecia.

Hematopoietic and Lymphatic: leukopenia, thrombocytopenia.

Metabolic: hypercholesterolemia, hypertriglyceridemia, hypokalemia.

OVERDOSAGE
There has been one reported case of overdosage with Fluconazole. A 42-year-old patient infected with human immunodeficiency virus developed hallucinations and exhibited paranoid behavior after reportedly ingesting 8,200 mg of Fluconazole. The patient was admitted to the hospital, and his condition resolved within 48 hours.

In the event of overdose, symptomatic treatment (with supportive measures and gastric lavage if clinically indicated) should be instituted.

Fluconazole is largely excreted in urine. A three hour hemodialysis session decreases plasma levels by approximately 50%.

In mice and rats receiving very high doses of Fluconazole, clinical effects, in both species, included decreased motility and respiration, ptosis, lacrimation, salivation, urinary incontinence, loss of righting reflex and cyanosis; death was sometimes preceded by clonic convulsions.

DOSAGE AND ADMINISTRATION
SINCE ORAL ABSORPTION IS RAPID AND ALMOST COMPLETE, THE DAILY DOSE OF FLUCONAZOLE IS THE SAME FOR ORAL (TABLETS AND SUSPENSION) AND INTRAVENOUS ADMINISTRATION.

In general, a loading dose of twice the daily dose is recommended on the first day of therapy to result in plasma concentrations close to steady state by the second day of therapy.

TABLETS AND SUSPENSION
The daily dose of Fluconazole should be based on the infecting organism and the patient's response to therapy. Treatment should be continued until clinical parameters or laboratory tests indicate that active fungal infection has subsided. An inadequate period of treatment may lead to recurrence of active infection. Patients with AIDS and cryptococcal meningitis or recurrent oropharyngeal candidiasis usually require maintenance therapy to prevent relapse.

The recommended dosage of Fluconazole for oropharyngeal candidiasis is 200 mg on the first day, followed by 100 mg once daily. Clinical evidence of oropharyngeal candidiasis generally resolves within several days, but treatment should be continued for at least 2 weeks to decrease the likelihood of relapse.

The recommended dosage of Fluconazole for esophageal candidiasis is 200 mg on the first day, followed by 100 mg once daily. Doses up to 400 mg/day may be used, based on medical judgment of the patient's response to therapy. Patients with esophageal candidiasis should be treated for a minimum of three weeks and for at least two weeks following resolution of symptoms.

For the treatment of candidal urinary tract infections and peritonitis, daily doses of 50-200 mg have been used in open, noncomparative studies of small numbers of patients. For systemic candidal infections including candidemia, disseminated candidiasis, and pneumonia, optimal therapeutic dosage and duration of therapy have not been established. In open, noncomparative studies of small numbers of patients, doses of up to 400 mg daily have been used.

For cryptococcal meningitis, the recommended dosage of Fluconazole is 400 mg on the first day, followed by 200 mg once daily. A dosage of 400 mg once daily may be used, based on medical judgment of the patient's response to therapy. The recommended duration of treatment for initial therapy of cryptococcal meningitis is 10-12 weeks after the cerebrospinal fluid becomes culture negative. The recommended dosage of Fluconazole for suppression of relapse of cryptococcal meningitis in patients with AIDS is 200 mg once daily.

The recommended Fluconazole daily dosage for the prevention of candidiasis of patients undergoing bone marrow transplantation is 400 mg, once daily. Patients who are anticipated to have severe granulocytopenia (less than 500 neutrophils per cu mm) should start Fluconazole prophylaxis several days before the anticipated onset of neutropenia and continue for 7 days after the neutrophil count rises above 1000 cells per cu mm.

DOSAGE IN PATIENTS WITH IMPAIRED RENAL FUNCTION

Fluconazole is cleared primarily by renal excretion as unchanged drug. In patients with impaired renal function, an initial loading dose of 50 to 400 mg should be given. After the loading dose, the daily dose (according to indication) should be based on the following table:

FLUCONAZOLE

Creatinine Clearance (mL/min)	Percent of Recommended Dose
> 50	100%
11-50	50%
Patients receiving regular hemodialysis	one recommended dose after each dialysis

These are suggested dose adjustments based on pharmacokinetics following administration of multiple doses. Further adjustment may be needed depending upon clinical condition.

When serum creatinine is the only measure of renal function available, the following formula (based on sex, weight, and age of the patient) should be used to estimate the creatinine clearance.

Males:
$$\frac{\text{Weight (kg)} \times (140 - \text{age})}{72 \times \text{serum creatinine (mg/100 mL)}}$$

Females: $0.85 \times$ above value

Fluconazole may be administered either orally or by intravenous infusion. Fluconazole injection has been used safely for up to fourteen days of intravenous therapy. The intravenous infusion of Fluconazole should be administered at a maximum rate of approximately 200 mg/hour, given as a continuous infusion.

Fluconazole injections in glass and Viaflex® Plus plastic containers are intended only for intravenous administration using sterile equipment.

Parenteral drug products should be inspected visually for particulate matter and discoloration prior to administration whenever solution and container permit.

Do not use if the solution is cloudy or precipitated or if the seal is not intact.

DIRECTIONS FOR MIXING THE ORAL SUSPENSION

Prepare a suspension at time of dispensing as follows: tap bottle until all the powder flows freely. To reconstitute, add 24 mL of distilled water or Purified Water (USP) to Fluconazole bottle and shake vigorously to suspend powder. Each bottle will deliver 35 mL of suspension. The concentrations of the reconstituted suspensions are as follows:

Fluconazole Content per bottle	Concentration of Reconstituted Suspension
350 mg	10 mg/mL
1400 mg	40 mg/mL

Note: Shake oral suspension well before using. Store reconstituted suspension between 86°F (30°C) and 41°F (5°C) and discard unused portion after 2 weeks. Protect from freezing.

DIRECTIONS FOR IV USE OF FLUCONAZOLE IN VIAFLEX® PLUS PLASTIC CONTAINERS

Do not remove unit from overwrap until ready for use. The overlap is a moisture barrier. The inner bag maintains the sterility of the product.

Caution: Do not use plastic containers in series connections. Such use could result in air embolism due to residual air being drawn from the primary container before administration of the fluid from the secondary container is completed.

TO OPEN

Tear overwrap down side at slit and remove solution container. Some opacity of the plastic due to moisture absorption during the sterilization process may be observed. This is normal and does not affect the solution quality or safety. The opacity will diminish gradually. After removing overwrap, check for minute leaks by squeezing inner bag firmly. If leaks are found, discard solution as sterility may be impaired.

DO NOT ADD SUPPLEMENTARY MEDICATION.

PREPARATION FOR ADMINISTRATION

1. Suspend container from eyelet support.
2. Remove plastic protector from outlet port at bottom of container.
3. Attach administration set. Refer to complete directions accompanying set.

Storage
Tablets: Store below 86°F (30°C)
Injections: Store between 77°F (25°C) and 41°F (5°C). Brief exposure up to 104°F (40°C) does not adversely affect the product. Protect from freezing.

HOW SUPPLIED
INJECTION: 200 MG

BRAND/MANUFACTURER	NDC	SIZE	AWP
○ **BRAND**			
DIFLUCAN IV: Roerig,J.B.	00049-3371-26	100 ml 6s	$487.50
	00049-3435-26	100 ml 6s	$487.50
	00049-3437-26	100 ml 6s	$487.50

INJECTION: 400 MG

BRAND/MANUFACTURER	NDC	SIZE	AWP
○ **BRAND**			
DIFLUCAN IV: Roerig,J.B.	00049-3372-26	200 ml 6s	$712.50
	00049-3436-26	200 ml 6s	$712.50
	00049-3438-26	200 ml 6s	$712.50

TABLETS: 50 MG

BRAND/MANUFACTURER	NDC	SIZE	AWP
○ **BRAND**			
▶ DIFLUCAN: Roerig,J.B.	00049-3410-30	30s	$131.25

TABLETS: 100 MG

BRAND/MANUFACTURER	NDC	SIZE	AWP
○ **BRAND**			
▶ DIFLUCAN: Roerig,J.B.	00049-3420-30	30s	$206.25
	00049-3420-41	100s ud	$687.50

TABLETS: 150 MG

BRAND/MANUFACTURER	NDC	SIZE	AWP
○ **BRAND**			
DIFLUCAN: Roerig,J.B.	00049-3500-79	12s	$127.50

TABLETS: 200 MG

BRAND/MANUFACTURER	NDC	SIZE	AWP
○ **BRAND**			
▶ DIFLUCAN: Roerig,J.B.	00049-3430-30	30s	$337.50
	00049-3430-41	100s ud	$1125.00

Flucytosine

WARNING
USE WITH EXTREME CAUTION IN PATIENTS WITH IMPAIRED RENAL FUNCTION. CLOSE MONITORING OF HEMATOLOGIC, RENAL AND HEPATIC STATUS OF ALL PATIENTS IS ESSENTIAL. THESE INSTRUCTIONS SHOULD BE THOROUGHLY REVIEWED BEFORE ADMINISTRATION OF FLUCYTOSINE.

DESCRIPTION
Flucytosine is an antifungal agent available as 250 mg and 500 mg capsules for oral administration. Chemically, Flucytosine is 5-fluorocytosine, a fluorinated pyrimidine which is related to fluorouracil and floxuridine. It is a white to off-white crystalline powder with a molecular weight of 129.09.

◆ RATED THERAPEUTICALLY EQUIVALENT;   ◇ THERAPEUTIC EQUIVALENCE UNCONFIRMED;   ○ UNRATED

Following is its chemical structure:

CLINICAL PHARMACOLOGY

Flucytosine is rapidly and virtually completely absorbed following oral administration. Bioavailability estimated by comparing the area under the curve of serum concentrations after oral and intravenous administration showed 78% to 89% absorption of the oral dose. Peak blood concentrations of 30 to 40 mcg/mL were reached within two hours of administration of a 2-Gm oral dose to normal subjects. The mean blood concentrations were approximately 70 to 80 mcg/mL one to two hours after a dose in patients with normal renal function who received a six-week regimen of Flucytosine (150 mg/kg/day given in divided doses every 6 hours) in combination with amphotericin B. The half-life in the majority of normal subjects ranged between 2.4 and 4.8 hours. Flucytosine is excreted via the kidneys by means of glomerular filtration without significant tubular reabsorption. More than 90% of the total radioactivity after oral administration was recovered in the urine as intact drug. Approximately 1% of the dose is present in the urine as the α-fluoro-β-ureido-propionic acid metabolite. A small portion of the dose is excreted in the feces.

The half-life of Flucytosine is prolonged in patients with renal insufficiency; the average half-life in nephrectomized or anuric patients was 85 hours (range: 29.9 to 250 hours). A linear correlation was found between the elimination rate constant of Flucytosine and creatinine clearance.

In vitro studies have shown that 2.9% to 4% of Flucytosine is protein-bound over the range of therapeutic concentrations found in the blood. Flucytosine readily penetrates the blood-brain barrier, achieving clinically significant concentrations in cerebrospinal fluid. Studies in pregnant rats have shown that Flucytosine injected intraperitoneally crosses the placental barrier (see "*Precautions*").

MICROBIOLOGY

Flucytosine has *in vitro* and *in vivo* activity against Candida and Cryptococcus. Although the exact mode of action is unknown, it has been proposed that Flucytosine acts directly on fungal organisms by competitive inhibition of purine and pyrimidine uptake and indirectly by intracellular metabolism to 5-fluorouracil. Flucytosine enters the fungal cell via cytosine permease; thus, Flucytosine is metabolized to 5-fluorouracil within in fungal organisms. The 5-fluorouracil is extensively incorporated into fungal RNA and inhibits synthesis of both DNA and RNA. The result is unbalanced growth and death of the fungal organism. Antifungal synergism between Flucytosine and polyene antibiotics, particularly amphotericin B; has been reported.

ACTIONS

Flucytosine has *in vitro* and *in vivo* activity against Candida and Cryptococcus. The exact mode of action against these fungi is not known Flucytosine is not metabolized significantly when given orally to man.

SUSCEPTIBILITY

Cryptococcus: Most strains initially isolated from clinical material have shown Flucytosine minimal inhibitory concentrations (MIC's) ranging from .46 to 7.8 mcg/mL. Any isolate with an MIC greater than 12.5 mcg/mL is considered resistant. *In vitro* resistance has developed in originally susceptible strains during therapy. It is recommended that clinical cultures for susceptibility testing be taken initially and at weekly intervals during therapy. The initial culture should be reserved as a reference in susceptibility testing of subsequent isolates.

Candida: As high as 40 to 50 percent of the pretreatment clinical isolates of Candida have been reported to be resistant to Flucytosine. It is recommended that susceptibility studies be performed as early as possible and be repeated during therapy. An MIC value greater than 100 mcg/mL is considered resistant.

Interference with *in vitro* activity of Flucytosine occurs in complex or semisynthetic media. In order to rely upon the recommended *in vitro* interpretations of susceptibility, it is essential that the broth medium and the testing procedure used be that described by Shadomy.[1]

INDICATIONS AND USAGE

Flucytosine is indicated only in the treatment of serious infections caused by susceptible strains of Candida and/or Cryptococcus. *Candida:* Septicemia, endocarditis and urinary system infections have been effectively treated with Flucytosine. Limited trials in pulmonary infections justify the use of Flucytosine. *Cryptococcus:* Meningitis and pulmonary infections have been treated effectively. Studies in septicemias and urinary tract infections are limited, but good responses have been reported.

UNLABELED USES

Flucytosine is used alone or as an adjunct in the treatment of aspergillosis.

CONTRAINDICATIONS

Flucytosine should not be used in patients with a known hypersensitivity to the drug.

WARNINGS

Flucytosine must be given with extreme caution to patients with impaired renal function. Since Flucytosine is excreted primarily by the kidneys, renal impairment may lead to accumulation of the drug. Flucytosine blood concentrations should be monitored to determine the adequacy of renal excretion in such patients.[1] Dosage adjustments should be made in patients with renal insufficiency to prevent progressive accumulation of active drug.

Flucytosine must be given with extreme caution to patients with bone marrow depression. Patients may be more prone to depression of bone marrow function if they: 1) have a hematologic disease, 2) are being treated with radiation or drugs which depress bone marrow, or 3) have a history of treatment with such drugs or radiation. Frequent monitoring of hepatic function and of the hematopoietic system is indicated during therapy.

PRECAUTIONS

General: Before therapy with Flucytosine is instituted, electrolytes (because of hypokalemia) and the hematologic and renal status of the patient should be determined (see "*Warnings*"). Close monitoring of the patient during therapy is essential.

Laboratory Tests: Since renal impairment can cause progressive accumulation of the drug, blood concentrations and kidney function should be monitored during therapy. Hematologic status (leucocyte and thrombocyte count) and liver function (alkaline phosphatase, SGOT and SGPT) should be determined at frequent intervals during treatment as indicated.

Drug Interactions: Cytosine arabinoside, a cytostatic agent, has been reported to inactivate the antifungal activity of Flucytosine by competitive inhibition. Drugs which impair glomerular filtration may prolong the biological half-life of Flucytosine. Antifungal synergism between Flucytosine and polyene antibiotics particularly amphotericin B, has been reported.

Drug/Laboratory Test Interactions: Measurement of serum creatinine levels should be determined by the Jaffe method, since Flucytosine does not interfere with the determination of creatinine values by this method, as it does when the dry-slide enzymatic method with the Kodak Ektachem analyzer is used.

Carcinogenesis, Mutagenesis, Impairment of Fertility: Flucytosine has not undergone adequate animal testing to evaluate carcinogenic potential. The mutagenic potential of Flucytosine was evaluated in Ames-type studies with five different mutants of *S. typhimurium* and no mutagenicity was detected in the presence or absence of activating enzymes. Flucytosine was nonmutagenic in three different repair assay systems.

There have been no adequate trials in animals on the effects of Flucytosine on fertility or reproductive performance. The fertility and reproductive performance of the offspring (F_1 generation) of mice treated with 100, 200 or 400 mg/kg/day of Flucytosine on days 7 to 13 of gestation was studied; the *in utero* treatment had no adverse effect on the fertility or reproductive performance of the offspring.

Pregnancy: Teratogenic effects. Pregnancy Category C. Flucytosine has been shown to be teratogenic in the rat and mouse at doses of 40 mg/kg/day (*i.e.*, 0.27 times the maximum recommended human dose). There are no adequate and well-controlled studies in pregnant women. Flucytosine should be used during pregnancy only if the potential benefit justifies the potential risk to the fetus.

The teratogenicity of Flucytosine is apparently species-related. Although there is confirmation of rat teratogenicity in the published literature, three studies in the mouse and studies in the rabbit and monkey have failed to reveal a teratogenic liability.

Nursing Mothers: It is not known whether this drug is excreted in human milk. Because many drugs are excreted in human milk and because of the potential for serious adverse reactions in nursing infants from Flucytosine a decision should be made whether to discontinue nursing or to discontinue the drug, taking into account the importance of the drug to the mother.

Pediatric Use: Safety and effectiveness in children have not been established.

ADVERSE REACTIONS

The adverse reactions which have occurred during treatment with Flucytosine are grouped according to organ system affected.

Cardiovascular: Cardiac arrest.

Respiratory: Respiratory arrest, chest pain, dyspnea.

Dermatologic: Rash, pruritus, urticaria, photosensitivity.

Gastrointestinal: Nausea, emesis, abdominal pain, diarrhea, anorexia, dry mouth, duodenal ulcer, gastrointestinal hemorrhage, hepatic dysfunction, jaundice, ulcerative colitis, bilirubin elevation.

Genitourinary: Azotemia, creatinine and BUN elevation, crystalluria, renal failure.

Hematologic: Anemia, agranulocytosis, aplastic anemia, eosinophilia, leukopenia, pancytopenia, thrombocytopenia.

Neurologic: Ataxia, hearing loss, headache, paresthesia, parkinsonism, peripheral neuropathy, pyrexia, vertigo, sedation.

Psychiatric: Confusion, hallucinations, psychosis.

Miscellaneous: Fatigue, hypoglycemia, hypokalemia, weakness.

OVERDOSAGE

There is no experience with intentional overdosage. It is reasonable to expect that overdosage may produce pronounced manifestations of the known clinical adverse reactions. Prolonged serum concentrations in excess of 100 mcg/mL may be associated with an increased incidence of toxicity, especially gastrointestinal (diarrhea, nausea, vomiting), hematologic (leukopenia, thrombocytopenia) and hepatic (hepatitis).

In the management of overdosage, prompt gastric lavage or the use of an emetic is recommended. Adequate fluid intake should be maintained, by the intravenous route if necessary, since Flucytosine is excreted unchanged via the renal tract. The hematologic parameters should be monitored frequently; liver and kidney function should be carefully monitored. Should any abnormalities appear in any of these parameters, appropriate therapeutic measures should be instituted. Since hemodialysis has been shown to rapidly reduce serum concentrations in anuric patients, this method may be considered in the management of overdosage.

DOSAGE AND ADMINISTRATION

The usual dosage of Flucytosine is 50 to 150 mg/kg/day administered in divided doses at 6-hour intervals. Nausea or vomiting may be reduced or avoided if the capsules are given a few at a time over a 15-minute period. If the BUN or the serum creatinine is elevated, or if there are other signs of renal impairment, the initial dose should be at the lower level (see "Warnings").

REFERENCE

1. Shadomy S: *Appl Microbiol* 17:871-877, June 1969.

HOW SUPPLIED
CAPSULE: 250 MG

BRAND/MANUFACTURER	NDC	SIZE	AWP
○ BRAND			
ANCOBON: Roche Labs	00004-0077-01	100s	$102.32

CAPSULE: 500 MG

BRAND/MANUFACTURER	NDC	SIZE	AWP
○ BRAND			
ANCOBON: Roche Labs	00004-0079-01	100s	$196.95

Fludara *SEE* FLUDARABINE PHOSPHATE

Fludarabine Phosphate

> **WARNING:**
> FLUDARABINE PHOSPHATE SHOULD BE ADMINISTERED UNDER THE SUPERVISION OF A QUALIFIED PHYSICIAN EXPERIENCED IN THE USE OF ANTINEOPLASTIC THERAPY. FLUDARABINE PHOSPHATE CAN SEVERELY SUPPRESS BONE MARROW FUNCTION. WHEN USED AT HIGH DOSES IN DOSE-RANGING STUDIES IN PATIENTS WITH ACUTE LEUKEMIA, FLUDARABINE PHOSPHATE WAS ASSOCIATED WITH SEVERE NEUROLOGIC EFFECTS, INCLUDING BLINDNESS, COMA, AND DEATH. THIS SEVERE CENTRAL NERVOUS SYSTEM TOXICITY OCCURRED IN 36% OF PATIENTS TREATED WITH DOSES APPROXIMATELY FOUR TIMES GREATER (96 MG/M^2/DAY FOR 5-7 DAYS) THAN THE RECOMMENDED DOSE. SIMILAR SEVERE CENTRAL NERVOUS SYSTEM TOXICITY HAS BEEN RARELY ($\leq 0.2\%$) REPORTED IN PATIENTS TREATED AT DOSES IN THE RANGE OF THE DOSE RECOMMENDED FOR CHRONIC LYMPHOCYTIC LEUKEMIA. IN A CLINICAL INVESTIGATION USING FLUDARABINE PHOSPHATE IN COMBINATION WITH PENTOSTATIN (DEOXYCOFORMYCIN) FOR THE TREATMENT OF REFRACTORY CHRONIC LYMPHOCYTIC LEUKEMIA (CLL), THERE WAS AN UNACCEPTABLY HIGH INCIDENCE OF FATAL PULMONARY TOXICITY. THEREFORE, THE USE OF FLUDARABINE PHOSPHATE IN COMBINATION WITH PENTOSTATIN IS NOT RECOMMENDED.

DESCRIPTION

Fludarabine Phosphate is a fluorinated nucleotide analog of the antiviral agent vidarabine, 9-β-D-arabinofuranosyladenine (ara-A) that is relatively resistant to deamination by adenosine deaminase. Each vial of sterile lyophilized solid cake contains 50 mg of the active ingredient Fludarabine Phosphate. The pH range for the final product is 7.2-8.2. Reconstitution with 2 mL of Sterile Water for Injection USP results in a solution containing 25 mg/mL of Fludarabine Phosphate intended for intravenous administration.

The chemical name for Fludarabine Phosphate is 9H-Purin-6-amine, 2-fluoro-9-(5-O-phosphono-β-D-arabinofuranosyl). The molecular formula of Fludarabine Phosphate is $C_{10}H_{13}FN_5O_7P$ (MW 365.2).

Following is its chemical structure:

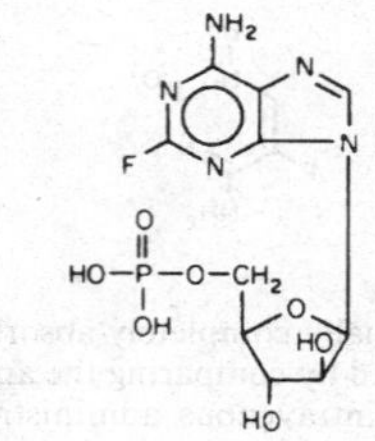

CLINICAL PHARMACOLOGY

Fludarabine Phosphate is rapidly dephosphorylated to 2-fluoro-ara-A and then phosphorylated intracellularly by deoxycytidine kinase to the active triPhosphate, 2-fluoro-ara-ATP. This metabolite appears to act by inhibiting DNA polymerase alpha, ribonucleotide reductase and DNA primase, thus inhibiting DNA synthesis. The mechanism of action of this antimetabolite is not completely characterized and may be multifaceted.

Phase I studies in humans have demonstrated that Fludarabine Phosphate is rapidly converted to the active metabolite, 2-fluoro-ara-A, within minutes after intravenous infusion. Consequently, clinical pharmacology studies have focused on 2-fluoro-ara-A pharmacokinetics. In a study with 4 patients treated with 25 mg/m^2/day for 5 days, the half-life of 2-fluoro-ara-A was approximately 10 hours. The mean total plasma clearance was 8.9 L/hr/m^2 and the mean volume of distribution was 98 L/m^2. Approximately 23% of the dose was excreted in the urine as unchanged 2-fluoro-ara-A. The mean C_{max} after the Day 1 dose was 0.57 mcg/mL and after the Day 5 dose was 0.54 mcg/mL. No information is available on pharmacokinetic parameters, other than C_{max}, following the Day 5 dose of 25 mg/m^2. Total body clearance of 2-fluoro-ara-A has been shown to be inversely correlated with serum creatinine, suggesting renal elimination of the compound. A correlation was noted between the degree of absolute granulocyte count nadir and increased area under the concentration $\times$ time curve (AUC).

Two single-arm open-label studies of Fludarabine Phosphate have been conducted in patients with CLL refractory to at least one prior standard alkylating-agent containing regimen. In a study conducted by M.D. Anderson Cancer Center (MDAH), 48 patients were treated with a dose of 22-40 mg/m^2 daily for 5 days every 28 days. Another study conducted by the Southwest Oncology Group (SWOG) involved 31 patients treated with a dose of 15-25 mg/m^2 daily for 5 days every 28 days. The overall objective response rates were 48% and 32% in the MDAH and SWOG studies, respectively. The complete response rate in both studies was 13%: the partial response rate was 35% in the MDAH study and 19% in the SWOG study. These response rates were obtained using standardized response criteria developed by the National Cancer Institute CLL Working Group[1] and were achieved in heavily pre-treated patients. The ability of Fludarabine Phosphate to induce a significant rate of response in refractory patients suggests minimal cross-resistance with commonly used anti-CLL agents.

The median time to response in the MDAH and SWOG studies was 7 weeks (range of 1 to 68 weeks) and 21 weeks (range of 1 to 53 weeks) respectively. The median duration of disease control was 91 weeks (MDAH) and 65 weeks (SWOG). The median survival of all refractory CLL patients treated with Fludarabine Phosphate was 43 weeks and 52 weeks in the MDAH and SWOG studies, respectively.

Rai stage improved to Stage II or better in 7 of 12 MDAH responders (58%) and in 5 of 7 SWOG responders (71%) who were Stage III or IV at baseline. In the combined studies, mean hemoglobin concentration improved from 9.0 g/dL at baseline to 11.8 g/dL at the time of response, in a subgroup of anemic patients. Similarly, average platelet count improved from 63,500/mm^3 to 103,300/mm^3 at the time of response in a subgroup of patients who were thrombocytopenic at baseline.

INDICATIONS AND USAGE

Fludarabine Phosphate is indicated for the treatment of patients with B-cell chronic lymphocytic leukemia (CLL) who have not responded to or whose disease has progressed during treatment with at least one standard alkylating-agent containing regimen. The safety and effectiveness of Fludarabine Phosphate is previously untreated or non-refractory patients with CLL have not been established.

UNLABELED USES

Fludarabine Phosphate is used in the treatment of mycosis fungoidas and nonHodgkin's lymphoma.

CONTRAINDICATIONS

Fludarabine Phosphate is contraindicated in those patients who are hypersensitive to this drug or its components.

WARNINGS

(SEE BOXED WARNING.)
There are clear dose dependent toxic effects seen with Fludarabine Phosphate. Dose levels approximately 4 times greater (96 mg/m^2/day for 5 to 7 days) than that recommended for CLL (25 mg/m^2/day for 5 days) were associated with a syndrome characterized by delayed blindness, coma and death. Symptoms appeared from 21 to 60 days following the last dose. Thirteen of 36 patients (36%) who received Fludarabine Phosphate at high doses (96 mg/m^2/day for 5 to 7 days)

◆ RATED THERAPEUTICALLY EQUIVALENT; ◇ THERAPEUTIC EQUIVALENCE UNCONFIRMED; ○ UNRATED

developed this severe neurotoxicity. This syndrome has been reported rarely in patients treated with doses in the range of the recommended CLL dose of 25 mg/m²/day for 5 days every 28 days. The effect of chronic administration of Fludarabine Phosphate on the central nervous system is unknown, however, patients have received the recommended dose for up to 15 courses of therapy.

Severe bone marrow suppression, notably anemia, thrombocytopenia and neutropenia has been reported in patients treated with Fludarabine Phosphate. In a Phase I study in solid tumor patients, the median time to nadir counts was 13 days (range, 3-25 days) for granulocytes and 16 days (range 2-32) for platelets. Most patients had hematologic impairment at baseline either as a result of disease or as a result of prior myelosuppressive therapy. Cumulative myelosuppression may be seen. While chemotherapy-induced myelosuppression is often reversible, administration of Fludarabine Phosphate requires careful hematologic monitoring.

Rare instances of clinically significant hemolytic anemia have been reported to occur after one (or more cycles of treatment with Fludarabine Phosphate in patients with or without a previous history of autoimmune hemolytic anemia or a positive Coombs' test. Severe anemia led to hospitalization and transfusion in some patients and a fatal outcome in one patient.

In a clinical investigation using Fludarabine Phosphate in combination with pentostatin (deoxycoformycin) for the treatment of refractory chronic lymphocytic leukemia (CLL), there was an unacceptably high incidence of fatal pulmonary toxicity. Therefore, the use of Fludarabine Phosphate in combination with pentostatin is not recommended.

Of the 133 CLL patients in the two trials, there were 29 fatalities during study. Approximately 50% of the fatalities were due to infection and 25% due to progressive disease.

Pregnancy Category D: Fludarabine Phosphate may cause fetal harm when administered to a pregnant woman. Fludarabine Phosphate was teratogenic in rats and in rabbits. Fludarabine Phosphate was administered intravenously at doses of 0, 1, 10 or 30 mg/kg/day to pregnant rats on days 6 to 15 of gestation. At 10 and 30 mg/kg/day in rats, there was an increased incidence of various skeletal malformations. Fludarabine Phosphate was administered intravenously at doses of 0, 1, 5 or 8 mg/kg/day to pregnant rabbits on days 6 to 15 of gestation. Dose-related teratogenic effects manifested by external deformities and skeletal malformations were observed in the rabbits at 5 and 8 mg/kg/day. Drug-related deaths or toxic effects on maternal and fetal weights were not observed. There are no adequate and well-controlled studies in pregnant women.

If Fludarabine Phosphate is used during pregnancy, or if the patient becomes pregnant while taking this drug, the patient should be apprised of the potential hazard to the fetus. Women of childbearing potential should be advised to avoid becoming pregnant.

PRECAUTIONS
General: Fludarabine Phosphate is a potent antineoplastic agent with potentially significant toxic side effects. Patients undergoing therapy should be closely observed for signs of hematologic and nonhematologic toxicity. Periodic assessment of peripheral blood counts is recommended to detect the development of anemia, neutropenia and thrombocytopenia.

Tumor lysis syndrome associated with Fludarabine Phosphate treatment has been reported in CLL patients with large tumor burdens. Since Fludarabine Phosphate can induce a response as early as the first week of treatment, precautions should be taken in those patients at risk of developing this complication.

There are inadequate data on dosing of patients with renal insufficiency Fludarabine Phosphate must be administered cautiously in patients with renal insufficiency. The total body clearance of 2-fluoro-ara-A has been shown to be inversely correlated with serum creatinine, suggesting renal elimination of the compound.

Laboratory Tests: During treatment, the patient's hematologic profile (particularly neutrophils and platelets) should be monitored regularly to determine the degree of hematopoietic suppression.

Drug Interaction: The use of Fludarabine Phosphate in combination with pentostatin is not recommended due to the risk of severe pulmonary toxicity (see "Warnings" section).

Carcinogenesis: No animal carcinogenicity studies with Fludarabine Phosphate have been conducted.

Mutagenesis: Fludarabine Phosphate has been shown to be non-mutagenic to several strains of Salmonella typhimurium, including TA-98, TA-100, TA-1535 and TA-1537. In addition Fludarabine Phosphate was non-mutagenic to Chinese hamster ovary (CHO) cells at the hypoxanthine-guanine-phosphoribosyltransferase (HGPRT) locus under both activated and non-activated metabolic conditions. Chromosomal aberrations were observed in an in vitro assay using CHO cells under metabolically activated conditions. In addition, Fludarabine Phosphate was determined to cause increased sister chromatid exchanges using an in vitro sister chromatid exchange (SCE) assay under both metabolically activated and non-activated conditions.

Impairment of Fertility: Studies in mice, rats and dogs have demonstrated dose-related adverse effects on the male reproductive system. Observations consisted of a decrease in mean testicular weights in mice and rats with a trend toward decreased testicular weights in dogs and degeneration and necrosis of spermatogenic epithelium of the testes in mice, rats and dogs. The possible adverse effects on fertility in humans have not been adequately evaluated.

Pregnancy: Pregnancy Category D: (see "Warnings" section).

Nursing Mothers: It is not known whether this drug is excreted in human milk. Because many drugs are excreted in human milk and because of the potential for serious adverse reactions in nursing infants from Fludarabine Phosphate a decision should be made to discontinue nursing or discontinue the drug, taking into account the importance of the drug for the mother.

Pediatric Use: The safety and effectiveness of Fludarabine Phosphate in children have not been established.

ADVERSE REACTIONS:
The most common adverse events include myelosuppression (neutropenia, thrombocytopenia and anemia), fever and chills, infection, and nausea and vomiting. Other commonly reported events include malaise, fatigue, anorexia, and weakness. Serious opportunistic infections have occurred in CLL patients treated with Fludarabine Phosphate. The most frequently reported adverse events and those reactions which are more clearly related to the drug are arranged below according to body system.

Hematopoietic Systems: Hematologic events (neutropenia, thrombocytopenia, and/or anemia) were reported in the majority of CLL patients treated with Fludarabine Phosphate. During Fludarabine Phosphate treatment of 133 patients with CLL, the absolute neutrophil count decreased to less than 500/mm³ in 59% of patients, hemoglobin decreased from pretreatment values by at least 2 grams percent in 60%, and platelet count decreased from pretreatment values by at least 50% in 55%. Myelosuppression may be severe and cumulative. Bone marrow fibrosis occurred in one CLL patient treated with Fludarabine Phosphate. Clinically significant hemolytic anemia has been rarely reported in patients receiving Fludarabine Phosphate (see "Warnings" section).

Metabolic: Tumor lysis syndrome has been reported in CLL patients treated with Fludarabine Phosphate. This complication may include hyperuricemia, hyperphosphatemia, hypocalcemia, metabolic acidosis, hyperkalemia, hematuria, urate crystalluria, and renal failure. The onset of this syndrome may be heralded by flank pain and hematuria.

Nervous System: (see "Warnings" section). Objective weakness, agitation, confusion, visual disturbances, and coma have occurred in CLL patients treated with Fludarabine Phosphate at the recommended dose. Peripheral neuropathy has been observed in patients treated with Fludarabine Phosphate and one case of wrist-drop was reported.

Pulmonary System: Pneumonia, a frequent manifestation of infection in CLL patients, occurred in 16% and 22% of those treated with Fludarabine Phosphate in the MDAH and SWOG studies, respectively. Pulmonary hypersensitivity reactions to Fludarabine Phosphate characterized by dyspnea, cough and interstitial pulmonary infiltrate have been observed.

Gastrointestinal System: Gastrointestinal disturbances such as nausea and vomiting, anorexia, diarrhea, stomatitis and gastrointestinal bleeding have been reported in patients treated with Fludarabine Phosphate.

Cardiovascular: Edema has been frequently reported. One patient developed a pericardial effusion possibly related to treatment with Fludarabine Phosphate. No other severe cardiovascular events were considered to be drug related.

Genitourinary System: Rare cases of hemorrhagic cystitis have been reported in patients treated with Fludarabine Phosphate.

Skin: Skin toxicity, consisting primarily of skin rashes, has been reported in patients treated with Fludarabine Phosphate.

Data in the following table are derived from the 133 patients with CLL who received Fludarabine Phosphate in the MDAH and SWOG studies.

PERCENT OF CLL PATIENTS REPORTING NONHEMATOLOGIC ADVERSE EVENTS

Adverse Events	MDAH (N = 101)	SWOG (N = 32)
Any Adverse Event	88%	91%
Body as a Whole	72	84
Fever	60	69
Chills	11	19
Fatigue	10	38
Infection	33	44
Pain	20	22
Malaise	8	6
Diaphoresis	1	13
Alopecia	0	3
Anaphylaxis	1	0
Hemorrhage	1	0
Hyperglycemia	1	6
Dehydration	1	0
Neurological	21	69
Weakness	9	65
Paresthesia	4	12
Headache	3	0
Visual Disturbance	3	15
Hearing Loss	2	6
Sleep Disorder	1	3
Depression	1	0
Cerebellar Syndrome	1	0
Impaired Mentation	1	0

Adverse Events	MDAH (N = 101)	SWOG (N = 32)
Pulmonary	35	69
Cough	10	44
Pneumonia	16	22
Dyspnea	9	22
Sinusitis	5	0
Pharyngitis	0	9
Upper Respiratory Infection	2	16
Allergic Pneumonitis	0	6
Epistaxis	1	0
Hemoptysis	1	6
Bronchitis	1	0
Hypoxia	1	0
Gastrointestinal	46	63
Nausea/Vomiting	36	31
Diarrhea	15	13
Anorexia	7	34
Stomatitis	9	0
GI Bleeding	3	13
Esophagitis	3	0
Mucositis	2	0
Liver Failure	1	0
Abnormal Liver Function Test	1	3
Cholelithiasis	0	3
Constipation	1	3
Dysphacia 1		
Cutaneous	17	18
Rash	15	15
Pruritus	1	3
Seborrhea	1	0
Genitourinary	12	22
Dysuria	4	3
Urinary Infection	2	15
Hematuria	2	3
Renal Failure	1	0
Abnormal Renal Function Test	1	0
Proteinuria	1	0
Hesitancy	0	3
Cardiovascular	12	38
Edema	8	19
Angina	0	6
Congestive Heart Failure	0	3
Arrhythmia	0	3
Supraventricular Tachycardia	0	3
Myocardial Infarction	0	3
Deep Venous Thrombosis	1	0
Phlebitis	1	3
Transient Ischemic Attach	1	0
Aneurysm	1	0
Cerebrovascular Accident	0	3
Musculoskeletal	7	16
Myalgia	4	16
Osteoporosis	2	0
Arthralgia	1	0
Tumor Lysis Syndrome	1	0

More than 3000 patients received Fludarabine Phosphate in studies of other leukemias, lymphomas, and other solid tumors. The spectrum of adverse effects reported in these studies was consistent with the data presented above.

OVERDOSAGE

High doses of Fludarabine Phosphate (see *"Warnings"*) have been associated with an irreversible central nervous system toxicity characterized by delayed blindness, coma and death. High doses are also associated with severe thrombocytopenia and neutropenia due to bone marrow suppression. There is no known specific antidote for Fludarabine Phosphate overdosage. Treatment consists of drug discontinuation and supportive therapy.

DOSAGE AND ADMINISTRATION

USUAL DOSE

The recommended dose of Fludarabine Phosphate is 25 mg/m² administered intravenously over a period of approximately 30 minutes daily for five consecutive days. Each 5 day course of treatment should commence every 28 days. Dosage may be decreased or delayed based on evidence of hematologic or nonhematologic toxicity. Physicians should consider delaying or discontinuing the drug if neurotoxicity occurs.

A number of clinical settings may predispose to increased toxicity from Fludarabine Phosphate. These include advanced age, renal insufficiency, and bone marrow impairment. Such patients should be monitored closely for excessive toxicity and the dose modified accordingly.

The optimal duration of treatment has not been clearly established. It is recommended that three additional cycles of Fludarabine Phosphate be administered following the achievement of a maximal response and then the drug should be discontinued.

PREPARATION OF SOLUTIONS

Fludarabine Phosphate should be prepared for parenteral use by aseptically adding Sterile Water for Injection USP. When reconstituted with 2 mL of Sterile Water for Injection, USP, the solid cake should fully dissolve in 15 seconds or less; each mL of the resulting solution will contain 25 mg of Fludarabine Phosphate, 25 mg of mannitol, and sodium hydroxide to adjust the pH to 7.7. The pH range for the final product is 7.2-8.2. In clinical studies, the product has been diluted in 100 cc or 125 cc of 5% Dextrose Injection USP or 0.9% Sodium Chloride USP.

Reconstituted Fludarabine Phosphate contains no antimicrobial preservative and thus should be used within 8 hours of reconstitution. Care must be taken to assure the sterility of prepared solutions. Parenteral drug products should be inspected visually for particulate matter and discoloration prior to administration.

HANDLING AND DISPOSAL

Procedures for proper handling and disposal should be considered. Consideration should be given to handling and disposal according to guidelines issued for cytotoxic drugs. Several guidelines on this subject have been published. [2-8] There is no general agreement that all of the procedures recommended in the guidelines are necessary or appropriate.

Caution should be exercised in the handling and preparation of Fludarabine Phosphate solution. The use of latex gloves and safety glasses is recommended to avoid exposure in case of breakage of the vial or other accidental spillage. If the solution contacts the skin or mucous membranes, wash thoroughly with soap and water; rinse eyes thoroughly with plain water. Avoid exposure by inhalation or by direct contact of the skin or mucous membranes.

STORAGE

Store under refrigeration between 2°-8°C (36°-46°F).

REFERENCES

1. Cheson B.D., Bennett J.M., Rai K.R. et al. Guidelines for clinical protocols for chronic lymphocytic leukemia: Recommendations of the National Cancer Institute-Sponsored Working Group. Amer J Hematol 29:152-163, 1988. 2. Recommendations for the Safe Handling of Parenteral Antineoplastic Drugs. NIH Publication No. 83-2621. For sale by the Superintendent of Documents, U.S. Government Printing Office, Washington, D.C. 20402. 3. AMA Council Report. Guidelines for Handling Parenteral Antineoplastics, JAMA, 1985; March 15. 4. National Study Commission on Cytotoxic Exposure—Recommendations for Handling Cytotoxic Agents. Available from Louis P. Jeffrey, Sc.D., Chairman, National Study Commission on Cytotoxic Exposure, Massachusetts College of Pharmacy and Allied Health Sciences, 179 Longwood Avenue, Boston, Massachusetts 02115. 5. Clinical Oncological Society of Australia: Guidelines and Recommendations for Safe Handling of Antineoplastic Agents, Med. J. Australia 1983;1:426-428. 6. Jones, R.B. et al. Safe Handling of Chemotherapeutic Agents: A Report from the Mount Sinai Medical Center, Ca—A Cancer Journal for Clinicians 1983; Sept/Oct. 258-263. 7. American Society of Hospital Pharmacists Technical Assistance Bulletin on Handling Cytotoxic Drugs in Hospitals, Am. J. Hosp. Pharm. 1985;42:131-137. 8. OSHA Work-Practice Guidelines for Personnel Dealing with Cytotoxic (antineoplastic) Drugs. Am. J. Hosp. Pharm. 1986;43-1193-1204.

J CODES

50 mg IV—J9185

HOW SUPPLIED

POWDER FOR INJECTION: 50 MG

BRAND/MANUFACTURER	NDC	SIZE	AWP
○ **BRAND**			
FLUDARA: Berlex Labs	50419-0511-06	1s	$169.35

Fludrocortisone Acetate

DESCRIPTION

Fludrocortisone Acetate USP is a synthetic adrenocortical steroid possessing very potent mineralocorticoid properties and high glucocorticoid activity; it is used only for its mineralocorticoid effects. The chemical name for Fludrocortisone Acetate is 9-fluoro-11β, 17, 21-trihydroxypregn-4-ene-3,20-dione 21-Acetate. Its molecular formula is $C_{23}H_{31}FO_6$ and its molecular weight is 422.49 (CAS 514363).

Fludrocortisone Acetate is available for oral administration as scored tablets providing 0.1 mg Fludrocortisone Acetate per tablet.

Following is its chemical structure:

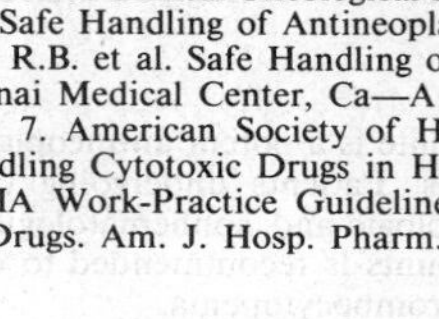

CLINICAL PHARMACOLOGY

Corticosteroids are thought to act, at least in part, by controlling the rate of synthesis of proteins. Although there are a number of instances in which the synthesis of specific proteins is known to be induced by corticosteroids, the links between the initial actions of the hormones and the final metabolic effects have not been completely elucidated.

◆ RATED THERAPEUTICALLY EQUIVALENT; ◇ THERAPEUTIC EQUIVALENCE UNCONFIRMED; ○ UNRATED

The physiologic action of Fludrocortisone Acetate is similar to that of hydrocortisone. However, the effects of Fludrocotisone Acetate, particularly on electrolyte balance, but also on carbohydrate metabolism, are considerably heightened and prolonged. Mineralocorticoids act on the distal tubules of the kidney to enhance the reabsorption of sodium ions from the tubular fluid into the plasma; they increase the urinary excretion of both potassium and hydrogen ions. The consequence of these three primary effects together with similar actions on cation transport in other tissues appear to account for the entire spectrum of physiological activities that are characteristic of mineralocorticoids. In small oral doses, Fludrocortisone Acetate produces marked sodium retention and increased urinary potassium excretion. It also causes a rise in blood pressure, apparently because of these effects on electrolyte levels.

In larger doses Fludrocortisone Acetate inhibits endogenous adrenal cortical secretion, thymic activity, and pituitary corticotropin excretion; promotes the deposition of liver glycogen; and, unless protein intake is adequate, induces negative nitrogen balance.

The approximate plasma half-life of Fludrocortisone (fluorohydrocortisone) is 3.5 hours or more and the biological half-life is 18 to 36 hours.

INDICATIONS AND USAGE
Fludrocortisone Acetate is indicated as partial replacement therapy for primary and secondary adrenocortical insufficiency in Addison's disease and for the treatment of salt-losing adrenogenital syndrome.

UNLABELED USES
Fludrocortisone Acetate is used alone or as an adjunct in the treatment of orthostatic hypotension and hypovolemia.

CONTRAINDICATIONS
Corticosteroids are contraindicated in patients with systemic fungal infections and in those with a history of possible or known hypersensitivity to these agents.

WARNINGS
BECAUSE OF ITS MARKED EFFECT ON SODIUM RETENTION, THE USE OF FLUDROCORTISONE ACETATE IN THE TREATMENT OF CONDITIONS OTHER THAN THOSE INDICATED HEREIN IS NOT ADVISED.

Corticosteroids may mask some signs of infection, and new infections may appear during their use. There may be decreased resistance and inability to localize infection when corticosteroids are used. If an infection occurs during Fludrocortisone Acetate therapy, it should be promptly controlled by suitable antimicrobial therapy.

Prolonged use of corticosteroids may produce posterior subcapsular cataracts, glaucoma with possible damage to the optic nerves, and may enhance the establishment of secondary ocular infections due to fungi or viruses.

Average and large doses of hydrocortisone or cortisone can cause elevation of blood pressure, salt and water retention, and increased excretion of potassium. These effects are less likely to occur with the synthetic derivatives except when used in large doses. However, since Fludrocortisone Acetate is a potent mineralocorticoid, both the dosage and salt intake should be carefully monitored in order to avoid the development of hypertension, edema, or weight gain. **Periodic checking of serum electrolyte levels is advisable during prolonged therapy; dietary salt restriction and potassium supplementation may be necessary.** All corticosteroids increase calcium excretion.

Patients should not be vaccinated against smallpox while on corticosteroid therapy. Other immunization procedures should not be undertaken in patients who are on corticosteroids, especially on high dose, because of possible hazards of neurological complications and a lack of antibody response. The use of Fludrocortisone Acetate Tablets USP in patients with active tuberculosis should be restricted to those cases of fulminating or disseminated tuberculosis in which the corticosteroid is used for the management of the disease in conjunction with an appropriate anti-tuberculous regimen. If corticosteroids are indicated in patients with latent tuberculosis or tuberculin reactivity, close observation is necessary since reactivation of the disease may occur. During prolonged corticosteroid therapy these patients should receive chemoprophylaxis.

Children who are on immunosuppressant drugs are more susceptible to infections than healthy children. Chicken pox and measles, for example, can have a more serious or even fatal course in children on immunosuppressant corticosteroids. In such children, or in adults who have not had these diseases, particular care should be taken to avoid exposure. If exposed, therapy with varicella zoster immune globulin (VZIG) or pooled intravenous immunoglobulin (IVIG), as appropriate, may be indicated. If chicken pox develops, treatment with antiviral agents may be considered.

PRECAUTIONS
GENERAL
Adverse reactions to corticosteroids may be produced by too rapid withdrawal or by continued use of large doses. To avoid drug-induced adrenal insufficiency, supportive dosage may be required in times of stress (such as trauma, surgery, or severe illness) both during treatment with Fludrocortisone Acetate and for a year afterwards.

There is an enhanced corticosteroid effect in patients with hypothyroidism and in those with cirrhosis.

Corticosteroids should be used cautiously in patients with ocular herpes simplex because of possible corneal perforation.

The lowest possible dose of corticosteroid should be used to control the condition being treated. A gradual reduction in dosages should be made when possible.

Psychic derangements may appear when corticosteroids are used. These may range from euphoria, insomnia, mood swings, personality changes, and severe depression to frank psychotic manifestations. Existing emotional instability or psychotic tendencies may also be aggravated by corticosteroids.

Aspirin should be used cautiously in conjunction with corticosteroids in patients with hypoprothrombinemia.

Corticosteroids should be used with caution in patients with nonspecific ulcerative colitis if there is a probability of impending perforation, abscess, or other pyogenic infection. Corticosteroids should also be used cautiously in patients with diverticulitis, fresh intestinal anastomoses, active or latent peptic ulcer, renal insufficiency, hypertension, osteoporosis, and myasthenia gravis.

INFORMATION FOR PATIENTS
The physician should advise the patient to report any medical history of heart disease, high blood pressure, or kidney or liver disease and to report current use of any medicines to determine if these medicines might interact adversely with Fludrocortisome Acetate (see "Drug Interactions").

Patients who are on immunosuppressant doses of corticosteroids should be warned to avoid exposure to chicken pox or measles and, if exposed, to obtain medical advice.

The patient's understanding of his steroid-dependent status and increased dosage requirement under widely variable conditions of stress is vital. Advise the patient to carry medical identification indicating his dependence on steroid medication and, if necessary, instruct him to carry an adequate supply of medication for use in emergencies.

Stress to the patient the importance of regular follow-up visits to check his progress and the need to promptly notify the physician of dizziness, severe or continuing headaches, swelling of feet or lower legs, or unusual weight gain.

Advise the patient to use the medicine only as directed, to take a missed dose as soon as possible, unless it is almost time for the next dose, and not to double the next dose.

Inform the patient to keep this medication and all drugs out of the reach of children.

LABORATORY TESTS
Patients should be monitored regularly for blood pressure determination and serum electrolyte determinations (see "Warnings").

DRUG INTERACTIONS
When administered concurrently, the following drugs may interact with adrenal corticosteroids.

Amphotericin B or Potassium-depleting Diuretics: (benzothiadiazines and related drugs, ethacrynic acid and furosemide) —enhanced hypokalemia. Check serum potassium levels at frequent intervals; use potassium supplements if necessary (see "Warnings").

Digitalis Glycosides: enhanced possibility of arrhythmias or digitalis toxicity associated with hypokalemia. Monitor serum potassium levels; use potassium supplements if necessary.

Oral Anticoagulants: decreased prothrombin time response. Monitor prothrombin levels and adjust anticoagulant dosage accordingly.

Antidiabetic Drugs: (oral agents and insulin): diminished antidiabetic effect. Monitor for symptoms of hyperglycemia; adjust dosage of antidiabetic drug upward if necessary.

Aspirin: increased ulcerogenic effect; decreased pharmacologic effect of aspirin. Rarely salicylate toxicity may occur in patients who discontinue steroids after concurrent high-dose aspirin therapy. Monitor salicylate levels or the therapeutic effect for which aspirin is given; adjust salicylate dosage accordingly if effect is altered (see "Precautions, General").

Barbiturates, Phenytoin, or Rifampin: increased metabolic clearance of Fludrocortisone Acetate because of the induction of hepatic enzymes. Observe the patient for possible diminished effect of steroid and increase the steroid dosage accordingly.

Anabolic Steroids: particularly C-17 alkylated androgens such as oxymetholone, methandrostenolone, norethandrolone, and similar compounds): enhanced tendency toward edema. Use caution when giving these drugs together, especially in patients with hepatic or cardiac disease.

Vaccines: neurological complications and lack of antibody response (see "Warnings").

Estrogen: increased levels of corticosteroid-binding globulin, thereby increasing the bound (inactive) fraction; this effect is at least balanced by decreased metabolism of corticosteroids. When estrogen therapy is initiated, a reduction in corticosteroid dosage may be required, and increased amounts may be required when estrogen is terminated.

DRUG/LABORATORY TEST INTERACTIONS
Corticosteroids may affect the nitrobluetetrazolium test for bacterial infection and produce false-negative results.

CARCINOGENESIS, MUTAGENESIS, IMPAIRMENT OF FERTILITY
Adequate studies have not been performed in animals to determine whether Fludrocortisone Acetate has carcinogenic or mutagenic activity or whether it affects fertility in males or females.

PREGNANCY

Category C: Adequate animal reproduction studies have not been conducted with Fludrocortisone Acetate. However, many corticosteroids have been shown to be teratogenic in laboratory animals at low doses. Teratogenicity of these agents in man has not been demonstrated. It is not known whether Fludrocortisone Acetate can cause fetal harm when administered to a pregnant woman or can affect reproduction capacity. Fludrocortisone Acetate should be given to a pregnant woman only if clearly needed.

PREGNANCY

Nonteratogenic Effects: Infants born of mothers who have received substantial doses of Fludrocortisone Acetate during pregnancy should be carefully observed for signs of hypoadrenalism.

Maternal treatment with corticosteroids should be carefully documented in the infant's medical records to assist in follow up.

NURSING MOTHERS

Corticosteroids are found in the breast milk of lactating women receiving systemic therapy with these agents. Caution should be exercised when Fludrocortisone Acetate is administered to a nursing woman.

PEDIATRIC USE

Safety and effectiveness in children have not been established.

Growth and development of infants and children on prolonged corticosteroid therapy should be carefully observed.

ADVERSE REACTIONS

Most adverse reactions are caused by the drug's mineralocorticoid activity (retention of sodium and water) and include hypertension, edema, cardiac enlargement, congestive heart failure, potassium loss, and hypokalemic alkalosis.

When Fludrocortisone Acetate is used in the small dosages recommended, the glucocorticoid side effects often seen with cortisone and its derivatives are not usually a problem; however the following untoward effects should be kept in mind, particularly when Fludrocortisone Acetate is used over a prolonged period of time or in conjunction with cortisone or a similar glucocorticoid.

Musculoskeletal: muscle weakness, steroid myopathy, loss of muscle mass, osteoporosis, vertebral compression fractures, aseptic necrosis of femoral and humeral heads, pathologic fracture of long bones, and spontaneous fractures.

Gastrointestinal: peptic ulcer with possible perforation and hemorrhage, pancreatitis, abdominal distention, and ulcerative esophagitis.

Dermatologic: impaired wound healing, thin fragile skin, bruising, petechiae and ecchymoses, facial erythema, increased sweating, subcutaneous fat atrophy, purpura, striae, hyperpigmentation of the skin and nails, hirsutism, acneiform eruptions, and hives and/or allergic skin rash; reactions to skin tests may be suppressed.

Neurological: convulsions, increased intracranial pressure with papilledema (pseudotumor cerebri) usually after treatment, vertigo, headache, and severe mental disturbances.

Endocrine: menstrual irregularities, development of the cushingoid state: suppression of growth in children; secondary adrenocortical and pituitary unresponsiveness, particularly in times of stress (e.g., trauma, surgery, or illness); decreased carbohydrate tolerance; manifestations of latent diabetes mellitus; and increased requirements for insulin or oral hypoglycemic agents in diabetics.

Ophthalmic: posterior subcapsular cataracts, increased intraocular pressure, glaucoma, and exophthalmos.

Metabolic: hyperglycemia, glycosuria, and negative nitrogen balance due to protein catabolism.

Other adverse reactions that may occur following the administration of a corticosteroid are necrotizing angiitis, thrombophlebitis, aggravation or masking of infections, insomnia, syncopal episodes, and anaphylactoid reactions.

OVERDOSAGE

Development of hypertension, edema, hypokalemia, excessive increase in weight, and increase in heart size are signs of overdosage of Fludrocortisone Acetate. When these are noted, administration of the drug should be discontinued, after which the symptoms will usually subside within several days; subsequent treatment with Fludrocortisone Acetate should be with a reduced dose. Muscular weakness may develop due to excessive potassium loss and can be treated by administering a potassium supplement. Regular monitoring of blood pressure and serum electrolytes can help to prevent overdosage (see *"Warnings"*).

DOSAGE AND ADMINISTRATION

Dosage depends on the severity of the disease and the response of the patient. Patients should be continually monitored for signs that indicate dosage adjustment is necessary, such as remissions or exacerbations of the disease and stress (surgery, infection, trauma) (see *"Warnings"* and *"Precautions, General"*).

ADDISON'S DISEASE

In Addison's disease, the combination of Fludrocortisone Acetate Tablets USP with a glucocorticoid such as hydrocortisone or cortisone provides substitution therapy approximating normal adrenal activity with minimal risks of unwanted effects.

The usual dose is 0.1 mg of Fludrocortisone Acetate daily, although dosage ranging from 0.1 mg three times a week to 0.2 mg daily has been employed. In the event transient hypertension develops as a consequence of therapy, the dose

should be reduced to 0.05 mg daily. Fludrocortisone Acetate is preferably administered in conjunction with cortisone (10 mg to 37.5 mg daily in divided doses) or hydrocortisone (10 mg to 30 mg daily in divided doses).

SALT-LOSING ADRENOGENITAL SYNDROME

The recommended dosage for treating the salt-losing adrenogenital syndrome is 0.1 mg to 0.2 mg of Fludrocortisone Acetate daily.

Tablets:

Store at room temperature; avoid excessive heat.

HOW SUPPLIED

TABLETS: 0.1 MG

BRAND/MANUFACTURER	NDC	SIZE	AWP
○ BRAND			
FLORINEF ACETATE: Apothecon	00003-0429-50	100s	$40.82

Flumadine *SEE* RIMANTADINE HYDROCHLORIDE
Flumazenil

DESCRIPTION

Flumazenil is a benzodiazepine receptor antagonist. Chemically, Flumazenil is ethyl 8-fluoro-5,6-dihydro-5-methyl-6-oxo-4H-imidazo [1,5-a](1,4) benzodiazepine-3-carboxylate. Flumazenil has an imidazobenzodiazepine structure, a calculated molecular weight of 303.3.

Flumazenil is a white to off-white crystalline compound with an octanol:buffer partition coefficient of 14 to 1 at pH 7.4. It is insoluble in water but slightly soluble in acidic aqueous solutions. Flumazenil is available as a sterile parenteral dosage form for intravenous administration.

Following is its chemical structure:

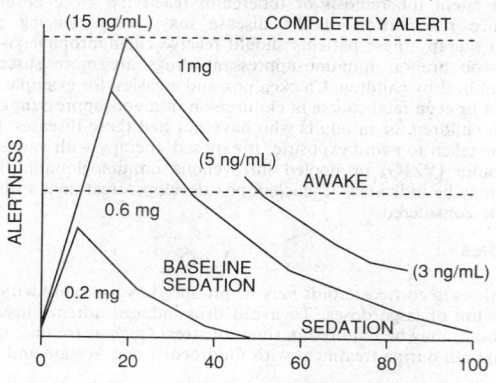

CLINICAL PHARMACOLOGY

Flumazenil, an imidazobenzodiazepine derivative, antagonizes the actions of benzodiazepines on the central nervous system. Flumazenil competitively inhibits the activity at the benzodiazepine recognition site on the GABA/benzodiazepine receptor complex. Flumazenil is a weak partial agonist in some animal models of activity, but has little or no agonist activity in man. Flumazenil does not antagonize the central nervous system effects of drugs affecting GABA-ergic neurons by means other than the benzodiazepine receptor (including ethanol, barbiturates, or general anesthetics) and does not reverse the effects of opioids.

Pharmacodynamics: Intravenous Flumazenil has been shown to antagonize sedation, impairment of recall and psychomotor impairment produced by benzodiazepines in healthy human volunteers.

The duration and degree of reversal of benzodiazepine effects are related to the dose and plasma concentrations of Flumazenil as shown in the following data from a study in normal volunteers.

Magnitude and Duration of Reversal of Sedation as a Function of Flumazenil Dose* Flumazenil Doses of 0.2, 0.6 & 1 mg (blood level in ng/mL)

Generally, doses of approximately 0.1 to 0.2 mg (corresponding to peak plasma levels of 3 to 6 ng/mL) produce partial antagonism, whereas higher doses of 0.4 to 1 mg (peak plasma levels of 12 to 28 ng/mL) usually produce complete antagonism in patients who have received the usual sedating doses of benzodiazepines. The onset of reversal is usually evident within 1 to 2 minutes after the injection is completed. Eighty percent response will be reached within 3 minutes, with the peak effect occurring at 6 to 10 minutes. The duration and degree of reversal are related to the plasma concentration of the sedating benzodiazepine as well as the dose of Flumazenil given.

In healthy volunteers, Flumazenil did not alter intraocular pressure when given alone and reversed the decrease in intraocular pressure seen after administration of midazolam.

Pharmacokinetics: After IV administration, plasma concentrations of flumazenil follow a two compartment open pharmacokinetic model with an initial distribution half-life of 7 to 15 minutes and a terminal half-life of 41 to 79 minutes. Peak concentrations of Flumazenil are proportional to dose, with an apparent initial volume of distribution of 0.5 L/kg. After redistribution the apparent volume of distribution (V_{ss}) ranges from 0.77 to 1.60L/kg. Protein binding is approximately 50% and the drug shows no preferential partitioning into red blood cells.

Flumazenil is a highly extracted drug. Clearance of Flumazenil occurs primarily by hepatic metabolism and is dependent on hepatic blood flow. In pharmacokinetic studies of normal volunteers, total clearance ranges from 0.7 to 1.3 L/hr/kg, with less than 1% of the administered dose eliminated unchanged in the urine. The major metabolites of Flumazenil identified in urine are the de-ethylated free acid and its glucuronide conjugate. In preclinical studies there was no evidence of pharmacologic activity exhibited by the de-ethylated free acid. Elimination of radiolabelled drug is essentially complete within 72 hours, with 90% to 95% of the radioactivity appearing in urine and 5% to 10% in the feces. Pharmacokinetic Parameters Following a 5-minute infusion of a total of 1 mg of Flumazenil Mean (Coefficient of variation, Range).

C_{max}(ng/mL)	24 (38%, 11-43)
AUC (ng* hr/mL)	15 (22%, 10-22)
V_{ss}(L/kg)	1 (24%, 0.8-1.6)
Cl (L/hr/kg)	1 (20%, 0.7-1.4)
Half-life (min)	54 (21%, 41-79)

The pharmacokinetics of Flumazenil are not significantly affected by gender, age, renal failure (creatinine clearance < 10mL/min), or hemodialysis beginning 1 hour after drug administration. Mean total clearance is decreased to 40% to 60% of normal in patients with moderate liver dysfunction and to 25% of normal in patients with severe liver dysfunction compared with age-matched healthy subjects. This results in a prolongation of the half-life from 0.8 hours in healthy subjects to 1.3 hours in patients with moderate hepatic impairment and 2.4 hours in severely impaired patients. Ingestion of food during an intravenous infusion of the drug results in a 50% increase in clearance, most likely due to the increased hepatic blood flow that accompanies a meal. The pharmacokinetic profile of Flumazenil is unaltered in the presence of benzodiazepine agonists and the kinetic profiles of these benzodiazepines are unaltered by Flumazenil.

CLINICAL TRIALS

Flumazenil has been administered to reverse the effects of benzodiazepines in conscious sedation, general anesthesia, and the management of suspected benzodiazepine overdose.

Conscious Sedation: Flumazenil was studied in four trials in 970 patients who received an average of 30 mg diazepam or 10 mg midazolam for sedation (with or without a narcotic) in conjunction with both inpatient and outpatient diagnostic or surgical procedures. Flumazenil was effective in reversing the sedating and psychomotor effects of the benzodiazepines, however, amnesia was less completely and less consistently reversed. In these studies, Flumazenil was administered as an initial dose of 0.4 mg I.V. (two doses of 0.2 mg) with additional 0.2 mg doses as needed to achieve complete awakening, up to a maximum total dose of 1 mg. Seventy-eight percent of patients receiving Flumazenil responded by becoming completely alert. Of those patients, approximately half responded to doses of 0.4 to 0.6 mg, while the other half responded to doses of 0.8 to 1 mg. Adverse effects were infrequent in patients who received 1 mg of Flumazenil or less, although injection site pain, agitation and anxiety did occur. Reversal of sedation was not associated with any increase in the frequency of inadequate analgesia or increase in narcotic demand in these studies. While most patients remained alert throughout the 3 hour post-procedure observation period, resedation was observed to occur in 3% to 9% of the patients, and was most common in patients who had received high doses of benzodiazepine. (See *"Precautions"*.)

General Anesthesia: Flumazenil was studied in four trials in 644 patients who received midazolam as an induction and/or maintenance agent in both balanced and inhalational anesthesia. Midazolam was generally administered in doses ranging from 5 to 80 mg, alone and/or in conjunction with muscle relaxants, nitrous oxide, regional or local anesthetics, narcotics and/or inhalational anesthetics. Flumazenil was given as an initial dose of 0.2 mg IV, with additional 0.2 mg doses as needed to reach a complete response, up to a maximum total dose of 1 mg. These doses were effective in reversing sedation and restoring psychomotor function, but did not completely restore memory as tested by picture recall. Flumazenil was not as effective in the reversal of sedation in patients who had received multiple anesthetic agents in addition to benzodiazepines.

Eighty-one percent of patients sedated with midazolam responded to Flumazenil by becoming completely alert or just slightly drowsy. Of those patients, 36% responded to doses of 0.4 to 0.6 mg, while 64% responded to doses of 0.8 to 1 mg. Resedation in patients who responded to Flumazenil occurred in 10% to 15% of patients studied and was more common with larger doses of midazolam (> 20 mg), long procedures (> 60 minutes) and use of neuromuscular blocking agents. (See *"Precautions"*.)

Management of Suspected Benzodiazepine Overdose: Flumazenil was studied in two trials in 497 patients who were presumed to have taken an overdose of a benzodiazepine, either alone or in combination with a variety of other agents. In these trials, 299 patients were proven to have taken a benzodiazepine as part of the overdose, and 80% of the 148 who received Flumazenil responded by an improvement in level of consciousness. Of the patients who responded to Flumazenil, 75% responded to a total dose of 1 to 3 mg.

Reversal of sedation was associated with an increased frequency of symptoms of CNS excitation. Of the patients treated with Flumazenil, 1% to 3% were treated for agitation or anxiety. Serious side effects were uncommon, but six seizures were observed in 446 patients treated with Flumazenil in these studies. Four of these 6 patients had ingested a large dose of cyclic antidepressants, which increased the risk of seizures. (See *"Warnings."*)

INDIVIDUALIZATION OF DOSAGE

General Principles: The serious adverse effects of Flumazenil are related to the reversal of benzodiazepine effects. Using more than the minimally effective dose of Flumazenil is tolerated by most patients but may complicate the management of patients who are physically dependent on benzodiazepines or patients who are depending on benzodiazepines for therapeutic effect (such as suppression of seizures in cyclic antidepressant overdose).

In high-risk patients, it is important to administer the smallest amount of Flumazenil that is effective. The 1-minute wait between individual doses in the dose-titration recommended for general clinical populations may be too short for high-risk patients. This is because it takes 6 to 10 minutes for any single dose of Flumazenil to reach full effects. Practitioners should slow the rate of administration of Flumazenil administered to high-risk patients as recommended below.

Anesthesia and Conscious Sedation: Flumazenil is well tolerated at the recommended doses in individuals who have no tolerance to (or dependence on) benzodiazepines. The recommended dosages and titration rates in anesthesia and conscious sedation (0.2 to 1 mg given at 0.2 mg/min) are well tolerated in patients receiving the drug for reversal of a single benzodiazepine exposure in most clinical settings (see *"Adverse Events"*). The major risk will be resedation because the duration of effect of a long-acting (or large dose of a short-acting) benzodiazepine may exceed that of Flumazenil. Resedation may be treated by giving a repeat dose at no less than 20-minute intervals. For repeat treatment, no more than 1 mg (at 0.2 mg/min doses) should be given at any one time and no more than 3 mg should be given in any one hour.

Overdose Patients: The risk of confusion, agitation, emotional lability and perceptual distortion with the doses recommended in patients with benzodiazepine overdose (3 to 5 mg administered as 0.5 mg/min) may be greater than that expected with lower doses and slower administration. The recommended doses represent a compromise between a desirable slow awakening and the need for prompt response and a persistent effect in the overdose situation. If circumstances permit, the physician may elect to use the 0.2 mg/minute titration rate to slowly awaken the patient over 5 to 10 minutes, which may help to reduce signs and symptoms on emergence.

Flumazenil has no effect in cases where benzodiazepines are not responsible for sedation. Once doses of 3 to 5 mg have been reached without clinical response, additional Flumazenil is likely to have no effect.

Patients Tolerant to Benzodiazepines: Flumazenil may cause benzodiazepine withdrawal symptoms in individuals who have been taking benzodiazepines long enough to have some degree of tolerance. Patients who had been taking benzodiazepines prior to entry into the Flumazenil trials who were given Flumazenil in doses over 1 mg experienced withdrawal-like events 2 to 5 times more frequently than patients who received less than 1 mg.

In patients who may have tolerance to benzodiazepines, as indicated by clinical history or by the need for larger than usual doses of benzodiazepine, slower titration rates of 0.1 mg/min and lower total doses may help reduce the frequency of emergent confusion and agitation. In such cases special care must be taken to monitor the patients for resedation because of the lower doses of Flumazenil used.

Patients Physically Dependent on Benzodiazepines: Flumazenil is known to precipitate withdrawal seizures in patients who are physically dependent on benzodiazepines, even if such dependence was established in a relatively few days of high dose sedation in Intensive Care Unit environments. The risk of either seizures or resedation in such cases is high and patients have experienced seizures before regaining consciousness. Flumazenil should be used in such settings with extreme caution, since the use of Flumazenil in this situation has not been studied and no information as to dose and rate of titration is available. Flumazenil should be used in such patients only if the potential benefits of using the drug outweigh the risks of precipitated seizures. Physicians are directed to the scientific literature for the most current information in this area.

INDICATIONS AND USAGE

Flumazenil is indicated for the complete or partial reversal of the sedative effects of benzodiazepines in cases where general anesthesia has been induced and/or maintained with benzodiazepines, where sedation has been produced with benzodiazepines for diagnostic and therapeutic procedures, and for the management of benzodiazepine overdose.

UNLABELED USES

Flumazenil is used in the treatment of acute alcohol withdrawal and the management of alcohol intoxication.

CONTRAINDICATIONS

Flumazenil is contraindicated:

■ in patients with a known hypersensitivity to Flumazenil or to benzodiazepines.

■ in patients who have been given a benzodiazepine for control of a potentially life-threatening condition (*e.g.* control of intracranial pressure or status epilepticus).

■ in patients who are showing signs of serious cyclic antidepressant overdose. (See *"Warnings"*.)

WARNINGS

THE USE OF FLUMAZENIL HAS BEEN ASSOCIATED WITH THE OCCURRENCE OF SEIZURES.

THESE ARE MOST FREQUENT IN PATIENTS WHO HAVE BEEN ON BENZODIAZEPINES FOR LONG-TERM SEDATION OR IN OVERDOSE CASES WHERE PATIENTS ARE SHOWING SIGNS OF SERIOUS CYCLIC ANTIDEPRESSANT OVERDOSE.

PRACTITIONERS SHOULD INDIVIDUALIZE THE DOSAGE OF FLUMAZENIL AND BE PREPARED TO MANAGE SEIZURES.

Risk of Seizures: The reversal of benzodiazepine effects may be associated with the onset of seizures in certain high risk populations. Possible risk factors for seizures include: concurrent major sedative-hypnotic drug withdrawal, recent therapy with repeated doses of parenteral benzodiazepines, myoclonic jerking or seizure activity prior to Flumazenil administration in overdose cases, or concurrent cyclic anti-depressant poisoning.

Flumazenil is not recommended in cases of serious cyclic antidepressant poisoning, as manifested by motor abnormalities (twitching, rigidity, focal seizure), dysrhythmia (wide QRS, ventricular dysrhythmia, heart block), anticholinergic signs (mydriasis, dry mucosa, hypoperistalsis), and cardiovascular collapse at presentation. In such cases Flumazenil should be withheld and the patient should be allowed to remain sedated (with ventilatory and circulatory support as needed) until the signs of antidepressant toxicity have subsided. Treatment with Flumazenil has no known benefit to the seriously ill mixed-overdose patient other than reversing sedation and should not be used in cases where seizures (from any cause) are likely.

Most convulsions associated with Flumazenil administration require treatment and have been successfully managed with benzodiazepines phenytoin or barbiturates. Because of the presence of Flumazenil, higher than usual doses of benzodiazepines may be required.

Hypoventilation: Patients who have received Flumazenil for the reversal of benzodiazepine effects (after conscious sedation or general anesthesia) should be monitored for resedation, respiratory depression, or other residual benzodiazepine effects for an appropriate period (up to 120 minutes) based on the dose and duration of effect of the benzodiazepine employed.

This is because Flumazenil has not been established as an effective treatment for hypoventilation due to benzodiazepine administration. The availability of Flumazenil does not diminish the need for prompt detection of hypoventilation and the ability to effectively intervene by establishing an airway and assisting ventilation.

Flumazenil may not fully reverse postoperative airway problems or ventilatory insufficiency induced by benzodiazepines. In addition, even if Flumazenil is initially effective, such problems may recur because the effects of Flumazenil wear off before the effects of many benzodiazepines.

Overdose cases should always be monitored for resedation until the patients are stable and resedation in unlikely.

PRECAUTIONS

Return of Sedation: Flumazenil may be expected to improve the alertness of patients recovering from a procedure involving sedation or anesthesia with benzodiazepines, but should not be substituted for an adequate period of postprocedure monitoring. The availability of Flumazenil does not reduce the risks associated with the use of large doses of benzodiazepines for sedation.

Patients should be monitored for resedation, respiratory depression (see *"Warnings"*), or other persistent or recurrent agonist effects for an adequate period of time after administration of Flumazenil.

Resedation is least likely in cases where Flumazenil is administered to reverse a low dose of a short acting benzodiazepine (< 10 mg midazolam). It is most likely in cases where a large single or cumulative dose of a benzodiazepine has been given in the course of a long procedure along with neuromuscular blocking agents and multiple anesthetic agents.

Profound resedation was observed in 1% to 3% of patients in the clinical studies. In clinical situations where resedation must be prevented, physicians may wish to repeat the initial dose (up to 1 mg of Flumazenil given at 0.2 mg/min) at 30 minutes and possibly again at 60 minutes. This dosage schedule, although not studied in clinical trials, was effective in preventing resedation in a pharmacologic study in normal volunteers.

Use In The ICU: Flumazenil should be used with caution in the Intensive Care Unit because of the increased risk of unrecognized benzodiazepine dependence in such settings. Flumazenil may produce convulsions in patients physically dependent on benzodiazepines. (See *"Individualization of Dosage"* and *"Warnings"*.)

Administration of Flumazenil to diagnose benzodiazepine-induced sedation in the Intensive Care Unit is not recommended due to the risk of adverse events as described above. In addition, the prognostic significance of a patient's failure to respond to Flumazenil in cases confounded by metabolic disorder, traumatic injury, drugs other than benzodiazepines, or any other reasons not associated with benzodiazepine receptor occupancy is not known.

Use In Overdose: Flumazenil is intended as an adjunct to, not as a substitute for, proper management of airway, assisted breathing, circulatory access and support,

internal decontamination by lavage and charcoal, and adequate clinical evaluation.

Necessary measures should be instituted to secure airway, ventilation and intravenous access prior to administering Flumazenil. Upon arousal patients may attempt to withdraw endotracheal tubes and/or intravenous lines as the result of confusion and agitation following awakening.

Head Injury: Flumazenil should be used with caution in patients with head injury as it may be capable of precipitating convulsions or altering cerebral blood flow in patients receiving benzodiazepines. It should be used only by practitioners prepared to manage such complications should they occur.

Use With Neuromuscular Blocking Agents: Flumazenil should not be used until the effects of neuromuscular blockade have been fully reversed.

Use in Psychiatric Patients: Flumazenil has been reported to provoke panic attacks in patients with a history of panic disorder.

Pain On Injection: To minimize the likelihood of pain or inflammation at the injection site, Flumazenil should be administered through a freely flowing intravenous infusion into a large vein. Local irritation may occur following extravasation into perivascular tissues.

Use In Respiratory Disease: The primary treatment of patients with serious lung disease who experience serious respiratory depression due to benzodiazepines should be appropriate ventilatory support (see *"Precautions"*) rather than the administration of Flumazenil. Flumazenil is capable of partially reversing benzodiazepine-induced alterations in ventilatory drive in healthy volunteers, but has not been shown to be clinically effective.

Use In Cardiovascular Disease: Flumazenil did not increase the work of the heart when used to reverse benzodiazepines in cardiac patients when given at a rate of 0.1 mg/min in total doses of less than 0.5 mg in studies reported in the clinical literature. Flumazenil alone had no significant effects on cardiovascular parameters when administered to patients with stable ischemic heart disease.

Use In Liver Disease: The clearance of Flumazenil is reduced to 40% to 60% of normal in patients with mild to moderate hepatic disease and to 25% of normal in patients with severe hepatic dysfunction. (See *"Pharmacokinetics"*.) While the dose of Flumazenil used for initial reversal of benzodiazepine effects is not affected, repeat doses of the drug in liver disease should be reduced in size or frequency.

Use In Drug and Alcohol Dependent Patients: Flumazenil should be used with caution in patients with alcoholism and other drug dependencies due to the increased frequency of benzodiazepine tolerance and dependence observed in these patient populations.

Flumazenil is not recommended either as a treatment for benzodiazepine dependence or for the management of protracted benzodiazepine abstinence syndromes, as such use has not been studied. The administration of Flumazenil can precipitate benzodiazepine withdrawal in animals and man. This has been seen in healthy volunteers treated with therapeutic doses of oral lorazepam for up to 2 weeks who exhibited effects such as hot flushes, agitation and tremor when treated with cumulative doses of up to 3 mg doses of Flumazenil.

Similar adverse experiences suggestive of Flumazenil precipitation of benzodiazepine withdrawal have occurred in some patients in clinical trials. Such patients had a short-lived syndrome characterized by dizziness, mild confusion, emotional lability, agitation (with signs and symptoms of anxiety), and mild sensory distortions. This response was dose-related, most common at doses above 1 mg, rarely required treatment other than reassurance and was usually short lived. When required (5 to 10 cases), these patients were successfully treated with usual doses of a barbiturate, a benzodiazepine, or other sedative drug.

Practitioners should assume that Flumazenil administration may trigger dose-dependent withdrawal syndromes in patients with established physical dependence on benzodiazepines and may complicate the management of withdrawal syndromes for alcohol, barbiturates and cross-tolerant sedatives.

Drug Interactions: Interaction with central nervous system depressants other than benzodiazepines has not been specifically studied; however, no deleterious interactions were seen when Flumazenil was administered after narcotics, inhalational anesthetics, muscle relaxants and muscle relaxant antagonists administered in conjunction with sedation or anesthesia.

Particular caution is necessary when using Flumazenil in cases of mixed drug overdosage since the toxic effects (such as convulsions and cardiac dysrhythmias) of other drugs taken in overdose (especially cyclic antidepressants) may emerge with the reversal of the benzodiazepine effect by Flumazenil. (See *"Warnings"*.)

The pharmacokinetics of benzodiazepines are unaltered in the presence of Flumazenil.

Use in Ambulatory Patients: The effects of Flumazenil may wear off before a long-acting benzodiazepine is completely cleared from the body. In general, if a patient shows no signs of sedation within 2 hours after a 1 mg dose of Flumazenil, serious resedation at a later time is unlikely. An adequate period of observation must be provided for any patient in whom either long-acting benzodiazepines (such as diazepam) or large doses of short-acting benzodiazepines (such as > 10 mg of midazolam) have been used. (See *"Individualization of Dosage"*.)

Because of the increased risk of adverse reactions in patients who have been taking benzodiazepines on a regular basis, it is particularly important that physicians query carefully about benzodiazepine, alcohol and sedative use as part of the history prior to any procedure in which the use of Flumazenil is planned. (See *"Drug and Alcohol Dependent Patients"*.)

Information For Patients: Flumazenil does not consistently reverse amnesia. Patients cannot be expected to remember information told to them in the postprocedure period and instructions given to patients should be reinforced in writing or given to a responsible family member. Physicians are advised to discuss with their patients, both before surgery and at discharge, that although the patient may feel alert at the time of discharge, the effects of the benzodiazepine may recur. As a result, the patient should be instructed, preferably in writing, that their memory and judgment may be impaired and specifically advised:

1. Not to engage in any activities requiring complete alertness, and not to operate hazardous machinery or a motor vehicle until at least 18 to 24 hours after discharge, and it is certain no residual sedative effects of the benzodiazepine remain.

2. Not to take any alcohol or non-prescription drugs for 18 to 24 hours after Flumazenil administration or if the effects of the benzodiazepine persist.

Laboratory Tests: No specific laboratory tests are recommended to follow the patient's response or to identify possible adverse reactions.

Drug/Laboratory Test Interactions: The possible interaction of Flumazenil with commonly used laboratory tests has not been evaluated.

Carcinogenesis, Mutagenesis, Impairment of Fertility:

Carcinogenesis: No studies in animals to evaluate the carcinogenic potential of Flumazenil have been conducted.

Mutagenesis: No evidence for mutagenicity was noted in the Ames test using five different tester strains. Assays for mutagenic potential in *S. cerevisiae* D7 and in Chinese hamster cells were considered to be negative as were blastogenesis assays *in vitro* in peripheral human lymphocytes and *in vivo* in a mouse micronucleus assay. Flumazenil caused a slight increase in unscheduled DNA synthesis in rat hepatocyte culture at concentrations which were also cytotoxic; no increase in DNA repair was observed in male mouse germ cells in an *in vivo* DNA repair assay.

Impairment of fertility: A reproduction study in male and female rats did not show any impairment of fertility at oral dosages of 125 mg/kg/day. From the available data on the area under the curve (AUC) in animals and man the dose represented 120 × the human exposure from a maximum recommended intravenous dose of 5 mg.

Pregnancy: Category C. There are no adequate and well-controlled studies of the use of Flumazenil in pregnant women. Flumazenil should be used during pregnancy only if the potential benefit justifies the potential risk to the fetus.

Teratogenic Effects: Flumazenil has been studied for teratogenicity in rats and rabbits following oral treatments of up to 150 mg/kg/day. The treatments during the major organogenesis were on days 6 to 15 of gestation in the rat and days 6 to 18 of gestation in the rabbit. No teratogenic effects were observed in rats or rabbits at 150 mg/kg; the dose, based on the available data on the area under the plasma concentration-time curve (AUC) represented 120 × to 600 × the human exposure from a maximum recommended intravenous dose of 5 mg in humans. In rabbits, embryocidal effects (as evidenced by increased pre-implantation and post-implantation losses) were observed at 50 mg/kg or 200 × the human exposure from a maximum recommended intravenous dose of 5 mg. The no-effect dose of 15 mg/kg in rabbits represents 60 × the human exposure.

Nonteratogenic Effects: An animal reproduction study was conducted in rats at oral dosages of 5, 25 and 125 mg/kg/day of Flumazenil. Pup survival was decreased during the lactating period, pup liver weight at weaning was increased for the high-dose group (125 mg/kg/day) and incisor eruption and ear opening in the offspring were delayed; the delay in ear opening was associated with a delay in the appearance of the auditory startle response. No treatment-related adverse effects were noted for the other dose groups. Based on the available data from AUC, the effect level (125 mg/kg), represents 120 × the human exposure from 5 mg, the maximum recommended intravenous dose in humans. The no-effect level represents 24 × the human exposure from an intravenous dose of 5 mg.

Labor and Delivery: The use of Flumazenil to reverse the effects of benzodiazepines used during labor and delivery is not recommended because the effects of the drug in the newborn are unknown.

Nursing Mothers: Caution should be exercised when deciding to administer Flumazenil to a nursing woman because it is not known whether Flumazenil is excreted in human milk.

Pediatric Use: Flumazenil is not recommended for use in children (either for the reversal of sedation, the management of overdose or the resuscitation of the newborn), as no clinical studies have been performed to determine the risks, benefits and dosages to be used.

Geriatric Use: The pharmacokinetics of Flumazenil have been studied in the elderly and are not significantly different from younger patients. Several studies of Flumazenil in patients over the age of 65 and one study in patients over the age of 80 suggest that while the doses of benzodiazepine used to induce sedation should be reduced, ordinary doses of Flumazenil may be used for reversal.

ADVERSE REACTIONS

Serious Adverse Reactions. Deaths have occurred in patients who received Flumazenil in a variety of clinical settings. The majority of deaths occurred in patients with serious underlying disease or in patients who had ingested large amounts of non-benzodiazepine drugs, (usually cyclic antidepressants) as part of an overdose.

Serious adverse events have occurred in all clinical settings, and convulsions are the most common serious adverse event reported. Flumazenil administration has been associated with the onset of convulsions in patients who are relying on

benzodiazepine effects to control seizures, are physically dependent on benzodiazepines, or who have ingested large doses of other drugs. (See "Warnings".)

Two of the 446 patients who received Flumazenil in controlled clinical trials for the management of a benzodiazepine overdosage had cardiac dysrhythmias (1 ventricular tachycardia, 1 junctional tachycardia).

Adverse Events in Clinical Studies: The following adverse reactions were considered to be related to Flumazenil administration (both alone and for the reversal of benzodiazepine effects) and were reported in studies involving 1875 individuals who received Flumazenil in controlled trials. Adverse events most frequently associated with Flumazenil alone were limited to dizziness, injection site pain, increased sweating, headache and abnormal or blurred vision (3% to 9%).

Body as a Whole: Fatigue (asthenia, malaise), Headache, Injection Site Pain*, Injection Site Reaction (thrombophlebitis, skin abnormality, rash).

Cardiovascular System: Cutaneous vasodilation (sweating, flushing, hot flushes).

Digestive System: Nausea and Vomiting (11%)

Nervous System: Agitation (anxiety, nervousness, dry mouth, tremor, palpitations, insomnia, dyspnea, hyperventilation)*, Dizziness (vertigo, ataxia) (10%), Emotional lability (crying abnormal, depersonalization, euphoria, increased tears, depression, dysphoria, paranoia).

Special Senses: Abnormal Vision (visual field defect, diplopia), Paresthesia (sensation abnormal, hypoesthesia)

All adverse reactions occurred in 1% to 3% of cases unless otherwise marked. Observed percentage reported if greater than 9%.

The following adverse events were observed infrequently (less than 1%) in the clinical studies, but were judged as probably related to Flumazenil administration and/or reversal of benzodiazepine effects:

Nervous System: Confusion (difficulty concentrating, delirium), Convulsions (See "Warnings"), Somnolence (stupor).

Special Senses: Abnormal Hearing (transient hearing impairment, hyperacusis, tinnitus).

The following adverse events occurred with frequencies less than 1% in the clinical trials. Their relationship to Flumazenil administration is unknown, but they are included as alerting information for the physician.

Body as a Whole: Rigors, shivering.

Cardiovascular: Arrythmia (atrial, nodal, ventricular extrasystoles), bradycardia, tachycardia, hypertension, chest pain.

Digestive System: Hiccup.

Nervous System: Speech disorder (dysphonia, thick tongue).

Not included in this list is operative site pain that occurred with the same frequency in patients receiving placebo as in patients receiving Flumazenil for reversal of sedation following a surgical procedure.

DRUG ABUSE AND DEPENDENCE

Flumazenil acts as a benzodiazepine antagonist, blocks the effects of benzodiazepines in animals and man, antagonizes benzodiazepine reinforcement in animal models, produces dysphoria in normal subjects, and has had no reported abuse in foreign marketing. Although Flumazenil has a benzodiazepine-like structure it does not act as a benzodiazepine agonist in man and is not a controlled substance.

OVERDOSAGE

Large intravenous doses of Flumazenil, when administered to healthy normal volunteers in the absence of a benzodiazepine agonist, produced no serious adverse reactions, severe signs or symptoms, or clinically significant laboratory test abnormalities. In clinical studies, most adverse reactions to Flumazenil were an extension of the pharmacologic effects of the drug in reversing benzodiazepine effects.

Reversal with an excessively high dose of Flumazenil may produce anxiety, agitation, increased muscle tone, hyperesthesia and possibly convulsions. Convulsions have been treated with barbiturates, benzodiazepines and phenytoin, generally with prompt resolution of the seizures. (See "Warnings".)

DOSAGE AND ADMINISTRATION

Flumazenil is recommended for intravenous use only. It is compatible with 5% dextrose in water, lactated Ringer's and normal saline solutions. If Flumazenil is drawn into a syringe or mixed with any of these solutions, it should be discarded after 24 hours. For optimum sterility, Flumazenil should remain in the vial until just before use. As with all parenteral drug products, Flumazenil should be inspected visually for particulate matter and discoloration prior to administration, whenever solution and container permit.

To minimize the likelihood of pain at the injection site, Flumazenil should be administered through a freely running intravenous infusion into a large vein.

Reversal of Conscious Sedation or in General Anesthesia: For the reversal of the sedative effects of benzodiazepines administered for conscious sedation or general anesthesia, the recommended initial dose of Flumazenil is 0.2 mg (2 mL) administered intravenously over 15 seconds. If the desired level of consciousness is not obtained after waiting an additional 45 seconds, a further dose of 0.2 mg (2

---

* indicates reaction in 3% to 9% of cases

mL) can be injected and repeated at 60-second intervals where necessary (up to a maximum of 4 additional times) to a maximum total dose of 1 mg (10 mL). The dose should be individualized based on the patient's response, with most patients responding to doses of 0.6 to 1 mg. (See *"Individualization of Dosage"*.)

In the event of resedation, repeated doses may be administered at 20 minute intervals as needed. For repeat treatment, no more than 1 mg (given as 0.2 mg/min) should be administered at any one time, and no more than 3 mg should be given in any one hour.

It is recommended that Flumazenil be administered as the series of small injections described (not as a single bolus injection) to allow the practitioner to control the reversal of sedation to the approximate endpoint desired and to minimize the possibility of adverse effects. (See *"Individualization of Dosage"*.)

Management of Suspected Benzodiazepine Overdose: For initial management of a known or suspected benzodiazepine overdose, the recommended initial dose of Flumazenil is 0.2 mg (2 mL) administered intravenously over 30 seconds. If the desired level of consciousness is not obtained after waiting 30 seconds, a further dose of 0.3 mg (3 mL) can be administered over another 30 seconds. Further doses of 0.5 mg (5 mL) can be administered over 30 seconds at 1-minute intervals up to a cumulative dose of 3 mg. Do not rush the administration of Flumazenil. Patients should have a secure airway and intravenous access before administration of the drug and be awakened gradually. (See *"Precautions"*.)

Most patients with benzodiazepine overdose will respond to a cumulative dose of 1-3 mg of Flumazenil, and doses beyond 3 mg do not reliably produce additional effects. On rare occasions, patients with a partial response at 3 mg may require additional titration up to a total dose of 5 mg (administered slowly in the same manner).

If a patient has not responded 5 minutes after receiving a cumulative dose of 5 mg Flumazenil the major cause of sedation is likely not to be due to benzodiazepines, and additional Flumazenil is likely to have no effect.

In the event of resedation, repeated doses may be given at 20-minutes intervals if needed. For repeat treatment, no more than 1 mg (given as 0.5 mg/min) should be given at any one time and no more than 3 mg should be given in any one hour.

Safety and Handling: Flumazenil poses no known risk to the health care provider. Routine care should be taken to avoid aerosol generation when preparing syringes for injection, and spilled medication should be rinsed from the skin with cool water.

Store at 59° to 86°F (15° to 30°C).

HOW SUPPLIED
INJECTION: 0.1 MG/ML

BRAND/MANUFACTURER	NDC	SIZE	AWP
○ **BRAND**			
ROMAZICON: Roche Labs	00004-6911-06	5 ml 10s	$269.28
	00004-6912-06	10 ml 10s	$428.40

Flunisolide

DESCRIPTION

Flunisolide is an anti-inflammatory steroid having the chemical name 6α-fluoro-11β, 16α, 17, 21-tetrahydroxypregna-1, 4-diene-3, 20-dione cyclic-16, 17-acetal with acetone.

Flunisolide is a white to creamy white crystalline powder with a molecular weight of 434.49. It is soluble in acetone, sparingly soluble in chloroform, slightly soluble in methanol, and practically insoluble in water. It has a melting point of about 245°C.

Flunisolide inhaler is delivered in a metered-dose aerosol system containing a microcrystalline suspension of Flunisolide as the hemihydrate in propellants (trichloromonofluoromethane, dichlorodifluoromethane and dichlorotetrafluoroethane) with sorbitan trioleate as a dispersing agent. Each activation delivers approximately 250 mcg of Flunisolide to the patient. One Flunisolide inhaler is designed to deliver at least 100 metered inhalations.

Flunisolide nasal solution is intended for administration as a spray to the nasal mucosa.

Each 25 mL spray bottle contains Flunisolide 6.25 mg (0.25 mg/mL). It contains no fluorocarbons.

After priming the delivery system for Flunisolide nasal solution, each actuation of the unit delivers a metered droplet spray containing approximately 25 mcg of Flunisolide. The size of the droplets produced by the unit is in excess of 8 microns to facilitate deposition on the nasal mucosa. The contents of one nasal spray bottle deliver at least 200 sprays.

Following is its chemical structure:

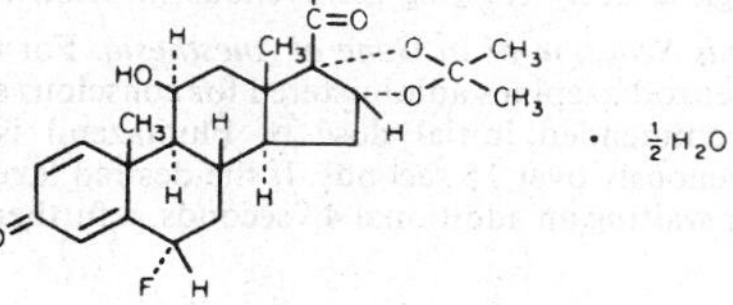

CLINICAL PHARMACOLOGY

Flunisolide has demonstrated marked anti-inflammatory and anti-allergic activity in classical test systems. It is a corticosteroid that is several hundred times more potent in animal anti-inflammatory assays than the cortisol standard. The molar dose of each activation of Flunisolide in this preparation is approximately 2 ½ to 7 times that of comparable inhaled corticosteroid products marketed for the same indication. The dose of Flunisolide delivered per activation in this preparation is 10 times that per activation of Flunisolide nasal solution. Clinical studies have shown therapeutic activity on bronchial mucosa with minimal evidence of systemic activity at recommended doses.

After oral inhalation of 1 mg Flunisolide, total systemic availability was 40%. The Flunisolide that is swallowed is rapidly and extensively converted to the 6β-OH metabolite and to water-soluble conjugates during the first pass through the liver. This offers a metabolic explanation for the low systemic activity of oral Flunisolide itself since the metabolite has low corticosteroid potency (on the order of the cortisol standard). The inhaled Flunisolide absorbed through the bronchial tree is converted to the same metabolites. Repeated inhalation of 2.0 mg of Flunisolide per day (the maximum recommended dose) for 14 days did not show accumulation of the drug in plasma. The plasma half-life of Flunisolide is approximately 1.8 hours.

The following observations relevant to systemic absorption were made in clinical studies. In one uncontrolled study a statistically significant decrease in responsiveness to metyrapone was noted in 15 adult steroid-independent patients treated with 2.0 mg of Flunisolide per day (the maximum recommended dose) for 3 months. A small but statistically significant drop in eosinophils from 11.5% to 7.4% of total circulating leucocytes was noted in another study in children who were not taking oral corticosteroids simultaneously. A 5% incidence of menstrual disturbances was reported during open studies, in which there were no control groups for comparison.

Aerosol administration of Flunisolide 2.0 mg twice daily for one week to 6 healthy male subjects revealed neither suppression of adrenal function as measured by early morning cortisol levels nor impairment of HPA axis function as determined by insulin hypoglycemia tests.

Controlled clinical studies have included over 500 patients with asthma, among them 150 children age 6 and over. More than 120 patients have been treated in open trials for two years or more. No significant adrenal suppression attributed to Flunisolide was seen in these studies.

Significant decreases of systemic steroid dosages have been possible in Flunisolide-treated patients. Asthma patients have had further symptomatic improvement with Flunisolide treatment even while reducing concomitant medication.

A study in approximately 100 patients which compared the recommended dose of Flunisolide nasal solution with an oral dose providing equivalent systemic amounts of Flunisolide has shown that the clinical effectiveness of Flunisolide nasal solution when used topically as recommended, is due to its direct local effect and not to an indirect effect through systemic absorption.

Following administration of Flunisolide to man, approximately half of the administered dose is recovered in the urine and half in the stool; 65-70% of the dose recovered in urine is the primary metabolite, which has undergone loss of the 6α fluorine and addition of a 6β hydroxy group. Flunisolide is well absorbed but is rapidly converted by the liver to the much less active primary metabolite and to glucuronate and/or sulfate conjugates. Because of first-pass liver metabolism, only 20% of the Flunisolide reaches the systemic circulation when it is given orally whereas 50% of the Flunisolide administered intranasally reaches the systemic circulation unmetabolized. The plasma half-life of Flunisolide is 1-2 hours.

The effects of Flunisolide on hypothalamic-pituitary-adrenal (HPA) axis function have been studied in adult volunteers. Flunisolide nasal solution was administered intranasally as a spray in total doses over 7 times the recommended dose (2200 mcg, equivalent to 88 sprays/day) in 2 subjects for 4 days, about 3 times the recommended dose (800 mcg, equivalent to 32 sprays/day) in 4 subjects for 4 days, and over twice the recommended dose (700 mcg, equivalent to 28 sprays/day) in 6 subjects for 10 days. Early morning plasma cortisol concentrations and 24-hour urinary 17-ketogenic steroids were measured daily. There was evidence of decreased endogenous cortisol production at all three doses.

In controlled studies, Flunisolide nasal solution was found to be effective in reducing symptoms of stuffy nose, runny nose and sneezing in most patients. These controlled clinical studies have been conducted in 488 adult patients at doses ranging from 8 to 16 sprays (200-400 mcg) per day and 127 children at doses ranging from 6 to 8 sprays (150-200 mcg) per day for periods as long as 3 months. In 170 patients who had cortisol levels evaluated at baseline and after 3 months or more of Flunisolide treatment, there was no unequivocal Flunisolide-related depression of plasma cortisol levels.

The mechanisms responsible for the anti-inflammatory action of corticosteroids and for the activity of the aerosolized drug on the nasal mucosa are unknown.

INDICATIONS AND USAGE

Flunisolide inhaler is indicated only for patients who require chronic treatment with corticosteroids for control of the symptoms of bronchial asthma. Such patients would include those already receiving systemic corticosteroids, and selected patients who are inadequately controlled on a non-steroid regimen and in whom steroid therapy has been withheld because of concern over potential adverse effects.

As with any topically applied medication. Flunisolide is absorbed through the mucous membrane and is systemically available. For these reasons, Flunisolide inhaler should be used with caution for initial therapy and the recommended

---

◆ RATED THERAPEUTICALLY EQUIVALENT; ◇ THERAPEUTIC EQUIVALENCE UNCONFIRMED; ○ UNRATED

dosage should not be exceeded. When the drug is used chronically at 2 mg/day, patients should be monitored periodically for effects on the hypothalamic-pituitary-adrenal axis.

Flunisolide inhalers are NOT indicated:

1. For relief of asthma that can be controlled by bronchodilators and other non-steroid medications.

2. In patients who require systemic corticosteroid treatment infrequently.

3. In the treatment of nonasthmatic bronchitis.

Insufficient information is available to warrant use in children under the age of 6.

Flunisolide nasal solution is indicated for the topical treatment of the symptoms of seasonal or perennial rhinitis when effectiveness of or tolerance to conventional treatment is unsatisfactory.

Clinical studies have shown that improvement is based on a local effect rather than systemic absorption, and is usually apparent within a few days after starting Flunisolide nasal solution. However, symptomatic relief may not occur in some patients for as long as two weeks. Although systemic effects are minimal at recommended doses, Flunisolide nasal solution should not be continued beyond 3 weeks in the absence of significant symptomatic improvement.

Flunisolide nasal solution should not be used in the presence of untreated localized infection involving nasal mucosa.

CONTRAINDICATIONS

Flunisolide inhaler is contraindicated in the primary treatment of status asthmaticus or other acute episodes of asthma where intensive measures are required.

Hypersensitivity to any of the ingredients of these preparations contraindicates the use of either Flunisolide inhaler or Flunisolide nasal solution.

WARNINGS

PARTICULAR CARE IS NEEDED IN PATIENTS WHO ARE TRANSFERRED FROM SYSTEMICALLY ACTIVE CORTICOSTEROIDS TO A FLUNISOLIDE INHALER OR FLUNISOLIDE NASAL SOLUTION BECAUSE DEATHS DUE TO ADRENAL INSUFFICIENCY HAVE OCCURRED IN ASTHMATIC PATIENTS DURING AND AFTER TRANSFER FROM SYSTEMIC CORTICOSTEROIDS TO AEROSOL CORTICOSTEROIDS. AFTER WITHDRAWAL FROM SYSTEMIC CORTICOSTEROIDS, A NUMBER OF MONTHS ARE REQUIRED FOR RECOVERY OF HYPOTHALAMIC-PITUITARY-ADRENAL (HPA) FUNCTION. DURING THIS PERIOD OF HPA SUPPRESSION, PATIENTS MAY EXHIBIT SIGNS AND SYMPTOMS OF ADRENAL INSUFFICIENCY WHEN EXPOSED TO TRAUMA, SURGERY OR INFECTIONS, PARTICULARLY GASTROENTERITIS. ALTHOUGH A FLUNISOLIDE INHALER MAY PROVIDE CONTROL OF ASTHMATIC SYMPTOMS DURING THESE EPISODES, IT DOES **NOT** PROVIDE THE SYSTEMIC STEROID THAT IS NECESSARY FOR COPING WITH THESE EMERGENCIES.

DURING PERIODS OF STRESS OR A SEVERE ASTHMATIC ATTACK, PATIENTS WHO HAVE BEEN WITHDRAWN FROM SYSTEMIC CORTICOSTEROIDS SHOULD BE INSTRUCTED TO RESUME SYSTEMIC STEROIDS (IN LARGE DOSES) IMMEDIATELY AND TO CONTACT THEIR PHYSICIAN FOR FURTHER INSTRUCTION. THESE PATIENTS SHOULD ALSO BE INSTRUCTED TO CARRY A WARNING CARD INDICATING THAT THEY MAY NEED SUPPLEMENTARY SYSTEMIC STEROIDS DURING PERIODS OF STRESS OR A SEVERE ASTHMA ATTACK. TO ASSESS THE RISK OF ADRENAL INSUFFICIENCY IN EMERGENCY SITUATIONS, ROUTINE TESTS OF ADRENAL CORTICAL FUNCTION, INCLUDING MEASUREMENT OF EARLY MORNING RESTING CORTISOL LEVELS, SHOULD BE PERFORMED PERIODICALLY IN ALL PATIENTS. AN EARLY MORNING RESTING CORTISOL LEVEL MAY BE ACCEPTED AS NORMAL IF IT FALLS AT OR NEAR THE NORMAL MEAN LEVEL.

The use of Flunisolide nasal solution with alternate-day prednisone systemic treatment could increase the likelihood of HPA suppression compared to a therapeutic dose of either one alone. Therefore Flunisolide nasal solution treatment should be used with caution in patients already on alternate-day prednisone regimens for any disease.

Localized infections with *Candida albicans* or *Aspergillus niger* have occurred in the mouth and pharynx and occasionally in the larynx. Positive cultures for oral *Candida* may be present in up to 34% of patients. Although the frequency of clinically apparent infection is considerably lower, these infections may require treatment with appropriate antifungal therapy or discontinuance of treatment with Flunisolide inhaler.

Flunisolide inhaler is not to be regarded as a bronchodilator and is not indicated for rapid relief of bronchospasm.

Patients should be instructed to contact their physician immediately when episodes of asthma that are not responsive to bronchodilators occur during the course of treatment. During such episodes, patients may require therapy with systemic corticosteroids.

There is no evidence that control of asthma can be achieved by administration of the drug in amounts greater than the recommended doses, which appear to be the therapeutic equivalent of approximately 10 mg/day of oral prednisone. Theoretically, the use of inhaled corticosteroids with alternate day prednisone

systemic treatment should be accompanied by more HPA suppression than a therapeutically equivalent regimen of either alone.

Transfer of patients from systemic steroid therapy to a Flunisolide inhaler may unmask allergic conditions previously suppressed by the systemic steroid therapy, e.g., rhinitis, conjunctivitis, and eczema.

Children who are on immunosuppressant drugs are more susceptible to infections than healthy children. Chickenpox and measles, for example, can have a more serious or even fatal course in children on immunosuppressant corticosteroids. In such children, or in adults who have not had these diseases, particular care should be taken to avoid exposure. If exposed, therapy with varicella zoster immune globulin (VZIG) or pooled intravenous immunoglobulin (IVIG), as appropriate, may be indicated. If chickenpox develops, treatment with antiviral agents may be considered.

PRECAUTIONS

General: Because of the relatively high molar dose of Flunisolide per activation in this preparation, and because of the evidence suggesting higher levels of systemic absorption with Flunisolide than with other comparable inhaled corticosteroids (see *"Clinical Pharmacology"* section), patients treated with Flunisolide inhaler should be observed carefully for any evidence of systemic corticosteroid effect, including suppression of bone growth in children. Particular care should be taken in observing patients postoperatively or during periods of stress for evidence of a decrease in adrenal function. During withdrawal from oral steroids, some patients may experience symptoms of systemically active steroid withdrawal, e.g., joint and/or muscular pain, lassitude and depression, despite maintenance or even improvement of respiratory function (see *"Dosage and Administration"* for details).

In responsive patients, Flunisolide may permit control of asthmatic symptoms without suppression of HPA function. Since Flunisolide is absorbed into the circulation and can be systemically active, the beneficial effects of Flunisolide inhaler in minimizing or preventing HPA dysfunction may be expected only when recommended dosages are not exceeded. The long-term effects of the drug in human subjects are still unknown. In particular, the local effects of the agent on developmental or immunologic processes in the mouth, pharynx, trachea, and lung are unknown. There is also no information about the possible long-term systemic effects of the agent.

The potential effects of the drug on acute, recurrent, or chronic pulmonary infections, including active or quiescent tuberculosis, are not known. Similarly, the potential effects of long-term administration of the drug on lung or other tissues are unknown.

Pulmonary infiltrates with eosinophilia may occur in patients on Flunisolide inhaler therapy. Although it is possible that in some patients this state may become manifest because of systemic steroid withdrawal when inhalational steroids are administered, a causative role for the drug and/or its vehicle cannot be ruled out.

In clinical studies with Flunisolide administered intranasally, the development of localized infections of the nose and pharynx with *Candida albicans* has occurred only rarely. When such an infection develops it may require treatment with appropriate local therapy or discontinuance of treatment with Flunisolide nasal solution.

Flunisolide is absorbed into the circulation. Use of excessive doses of Flunisolide nasal solution may suppress hypothalamic-pituitary-adrenal function.

Flunisolide should be used with caution, if at all, in patients with active or quiescent tuberculosis infections of the respiratory tract or in untreated fungal, bacterial or systemic viral infections or ocular herpes simplex.

Because of the inhibitory effect of corticosteroids on wound healing, in patients who have experienced recent nasal septal ulcers, recurrent epistaxis, nasal surgery or trauma, a nasal corticosteroid should be used with caution until healing has occurred.

Although systemic effects have been minimal with recommended doses, this potential increases with excessive dosages. Therefore, larger than recommended doses should be avoided.

INFORMATION FOR PATIENTS

There is no evidence that better control of asthma can be achieved by the administration of Flunisolide inhaler in amounts greater than the recommended doses; higher doses may induce adrenal suppression.

Since the relief from Flunisolide inhaler depends on its regular use and on proper inhalation technique, patients must be instructed to take inhalations at regular intervals. They should also be instructed in the correct method of use (See *"Patient Instruction Leaflet"*).

Patients receiving bronchodilators by inhalation should be advised to use the bronchodilator before Flunisolide inhaler in order to enhance penetration of Flunisolide into the bronchial tree. After use of an aerosol bronchodilator, several minutes should elapse before using the Flunisolide inhaler.

Patients whose systemic corticosteroids have been reduced or withdrawn should be instructed to carry a warning card indicating that they may need supplemental systemic steroids during periods of stress or a severe asthmatic attack that is not responsive to bronchodilators.

Patients who are on immunosuppressant doses of corticosteroids should be warned to avoid exposure to chickenpox or measles and, if exposed, to obtain medical advice.

An illustrated leaflet of patient instructions for proper use accompanies each Flunisolide inhaler.

➤ SHOWN IN PRODUCT IDENTIFICATION GUIDE

CONTENTS UNDER PRESSURE.
Do not puncture. Do not use or store near heat or open flame. Exposure to temperatures above 120°F (49°C) may cause container to explode. Never throw container into fire or incinerator. Keep out of reach of children.

Patients should use Flunisolide nasal solution at regular intervals since its effectiveness depends on its regular use. The patient should take the medication as directed. It is not acutely effective and the prescribed dosage should not be increased. Instead, nasal vasoconstrictors or oral antihistamines may be needed until the effects of Flunisolide nasal solution are fully manifested. One to two weeks may pass before full relief is obtained. The patient should contact the physician if symptoms do not improve, or if the condition worsens, or if sneezing or nasal irritation occurs.

For the proper use of this unit and to attain maximum improvement, the patient should read and follow the accompanying Patient Instructions carefully.

Carcinogenesis: Long-term studies were conducted in mice and rats using oral administration to evaluate the carcinogenic potential of the drug. There was an increase in the incidence of pulmonary adenomas in mice, but not in rats.

Female rats receiving the highest oral dose had an increased incidence of mammary adenocarcinoma compared to control rats. An increased incidence of this tumor type has been reported for other corticosteroids.

Impairment of Fertility: Female rats receiving high doses of Flunisolide (200 mcg/kg/day) showed some evidence of impaired fertility. Reproductive performance in the low (8 mcg/kg/day) and mid-dose (40 mcg/kg/day) groups was comparable to controls.

Pregnancy: Pregnancy Category C. As with other corticosteroids Flunisolide has been shown to be teratogenic in rabbits and rats at doses of 40 and 200 mcg/kg/day respectively. It was also fetotoxic in these animal reproductive studies. There are no adequate and well-controlled studies in pregnant women. Flunisolide should be used during pregnancy only if the potential benefit justifies the potential risk to the fetus.

Nursing Mothers: It is not known whether this drug is excreted in human milk. Because other corticosteroids are excreted in human milk, caution should be exercised when Flunisolide is administered to nursing women.

ADVERSE REACTIONS
Adverse events reported in controlled clinical trials and long-term open studies in 514 patients treated with Flunisolide inhaler are described below. Of those patients, 463 were treated for 3 months or longer, 407 for 6 months or longer, 287 for 1 year or longer, and 122 for 2 years or longer.

Musculoskeletal reactions were reported in 35% of steroid-dependent patients in whom the dose of oral steroid was being tapered. This is a well-known effect of steroid withdrawal.

INCIDENCE 10% OR GREATER
Gastrointestinal: diarrhea (10%), nausea and/or vomiting (25%), upset stomach (10%)

General: flu (10%)

Mouth and Throat: sore throat (20%)

Nervous system: headache (25%)

Respiratory: cold symptoms (15%), nasal congestion (15%) upper respiratory infection (25%)

Special Senses: unpleasant taste (10%)

INCIDENCE 3-9%
Cardiovascular: palpitations

Gastrointestinal: abdominal pain, heartburn

General: chest pain, decreased appetite, edema, fever

Mouth and Throat: Candida infection

Nervous System: dizziness, irritability, nervousness, shakiness

Reproductive: menstrual disturbances

Respiratory: chest congestion, cough,* hoarseness, rhinitis, runny nose, sinus congestion, sinus drainage, sinus infection, sinusitis, sneezing, sputum, wheezing*

Skin: eczema, itching (pruritus), rash

Special Senses: ear infection, loss of smell or taste

INCIDENCE 1-3%
General: chills, increased appetite and weight gain, malaise, peripheral edema, sweating, weakness

Cardiovascular: hypertension, tachycardia

Gastrointestinal: constipation, dyspepsia, gas

Hemic/Lynch: dry throat, glossitis, mouth irritation, pharyngitis, phlegm, throat irritation.

---

* The incidences as shown of cough, wheezing, and chest tightness were judged by investigators to be possibly or probably drug-related. In placebo-controlled trials, the *overall* incidences of these adverse events (regardless of investigators' judgment of drug relationship) were similar for drug and placebo-treated groups. They may be related to the vehicle or delivery system.

Nervous System: anxiety, depression, faintness, fatigue, hyperactivity, hypoactivity, insomnia, moodiness, numbness, vertigo.

Respiratory: bronchitis, chest tightness*, dyspnea, epistaxis, head stuffiness, laryngitis, nasal irritation, pleurisy, pneumonia, sinus discomfort

Skin: acne, hives, or urticaria

Special Senses: blurred vision, earache, eye discomfort, eye infection

INCIDENCE LESS THAN 1%
Judged by investigators as possibly or probably drug related: abdnormal fullness, shortness of breath.

Adverse reactions reported in controlled clinical trials and long-term open studies in 595 patients treated with Flunisolide nasal solution are described below. Of these patients, 409 were treated for 3 months or longer, 323 for 6 months or longer, 259 for 1 year or longer, and 91 for 2 years or longer.

In general, side effects elicited in the clinical studies have been primarily associated with the nasal mucous membranes. The most frequent complaints were those of mild transient nasal burning and stinging, which were reported in approximately 45% of the patients treated with Flunisolide nasal solution in placebo-controlled and long-term studies. These complaints do not usually interfere with treatment; in only 3% of patients was it necessary to decrease dosage or stop treatment because of these symptoms. Approximately the same incidence of mild transient nasal burning and stinging was reported in patients on placebo as was reported in patients treated with Flunisolide nasal solution in controlled studies, implying that these complaints may be related to the vehicle or the delivery system. The incidence of complaints of nasal burning and stinging decreased with increasing duration of treatment.

Other side effects reported at a frequency of 5% or less were nasal congestion, sneezing, epistaxis and/or bloody mucus, nasal irritation, watery eyes, sore throat, nausea and/or vomiting, headaches and loss of sense of smell and taste. As is the case with other nasally inhaled corticosteriods, nasal septal perforations have been observed in rare instances.

Systemic corticesteroid side effects were not reported during the controlled clinical trials. If recommended doses are exceeded, or if individuals are particularly sensitive, symptoms of hypercorticism, i.e., Cushing's syndrome, could occur.

OVERDOSAGE
I.V. Flunisolide in animals at doses up to 4 mg/kg showed no effect. One spray bottle contains 6.25 mg of Flunisolide nasal solution; therefore acute overdosage is unlikely.

DOSAGE AND ADMINISTRATION
Flunisolide inhaler:

Adults: The recommended starting dose is 2 inhalations twice daily morning and evening for a total daily dose of 1 mg. The maximum daily dose should not exceed 4 inhalations twice a day for a total daily dose of 2 mg. When the drug is used chronically at 2 mg/day, patients should be monitored periodically for effects on the hypothalamic-pituitary-adrenal axis.

Children: For children 6-15 years of age, two inhalations may be administered twice daily for a total daily dose of 1 mg. Higher doses have not been studied. Insufficient information is available to warrant use in children under age 6. With chronic use, children should be monitored for growth as well as for effects on the HPA axis.

Rinsing the mouth after inhalation is advised. Patients receiving bronchodilators by inhalation should be advised to use the bronchodilator before Flunisolide inhaler in order to enhance penetration of Flunisolide into the bronchial tree. After use of an aerosol bronchodilator, several minutes should elapse before use of the Flunisolide inhaler to reduce the potential toxicity from the inhaled fluorocarbon propellants in the two aerosols.

Different considerations must be given to the following groups of patients in order to obtain the full therapeutic benefit of Flunisolide inhaler.

Patients not receiving systemic steroids: The use of Flunisolide inhaler is straightforward in patients who are inadequately controlled with non-steroid medications but in whom systemic steroid therapy has been withheld because of concern over potential adverse reactions. In patients who respond to the drug, an improvement in pulmonary function is usually apparent within one to four weeks after the start of treatment.

Patients receiving systemic steroids: In those patients dependent on systemic steroids, transfer to Flunisolide inhaler and subsequent management may be more difficult because recovery from impaired adrenal function is usually slow. Such supression has been known to last for up to 12 months. Clinical studies, however, have demonstrated that Flunisolide inhaler may be effective in the management of these asthmatic patients and may permit replacement or significant reduction in the dosage of systemic corticosteroids.

Inhaled corticosteroids generally are not recommended for chronic use with alternate day prednisone regimens (see "Warnings").

The patient's asthma should be reasonably stable before treatment with Flunisolide inhaler is started. Initially, the aerosol should be used concurrently with the patient's usual maintenance dose of systemic steroid. After approximately one week, gradual withdrawal of the systemic steroid is started by reducing the daily or alternate daily dose. The next reduction is made after an interval of one or two weeks, depending on the response of the patient. Generally, these decrements should not exceed 2.5 mg of prednisone or its equivalent. A slow rate of withdrawal cannot be overemphasized. During withdrawal, some patients may

---

experience symptoms of systemically active steroid withdrawal, e.g., joint and/or muscular pain, lassitude and depression, despite maintenance or even improvement of respiratory function. Such patients should be encouraged to continue with the inhaler but should be watched carefully for objective signs of adrenal insufficiency, such as hypotension and weight loss. If evidence of adrenal insufficiency occurs, the systemic steroid dose should be boosted temporarily and thereafter further withdrawal should continue more slowly. *During periods of stress or a severe asthma attack, transfer patients will require supplementary treatment with systemic steroids.* Exacerbations of asthma that occur during the course of treatment with Flunisolide inhaler should be treated with a short course of systemic steroid that is gradually tapered as these symptoms subside. There is no evidence that control of asthma can be achieved by administration of the drug in amounts greater than the recommended doses.

The therapeutic effects of corticosteroids, unlike those of decongestants, are not immediate. This should be explained to the patient in advance in order to ensure cooperation and continuation of treatment with the prescribed dosage regimen. Full therapeutic benefit requires regular use, and is usually evident within a few days. However, a longer period of therapy may be required for some patients to achieve maximum benefit (up to 3 weeks). If no improvement is evident by that time, Flunisolide nasal solution should not be continued.

Patients with blocked nasal passages should be encouraged to use a decongestant just before Flunisolide nasal solution administration to ensure adequate penetration of the spray. Patients should also be advised to clear their nasal passages of secretions prior to use.

Adults: The recommended starting dose of Flunisolide nasal solution is 2 sprays (50 mcg) in each nostril 2 times a day (total dose 200 mcg/day). If needed, this dose may be increased to 2 sprays in each nostril 3 times a day (total dose 300 mcg/day).

Children 6 to 14 years: The recommended starting dose of Flunisolide nasal solution is one spray (25 mcg) in each nostril 3 times a day or two sprays (50 mcg) in each nostril 2 times a day (total dose 150-200 mcg/day. Flunisolide nasal solution is not recommended for use in children less than 6 years of age as safety and efficacy studies, including possible adverse effects on growth, have not been conducted.

Maximum total daily doses should not exceed 8 sprays in each nostril for adults (total dose 400 mcg/day) and 4 sprays in each nostril for children under 14 years of age (total dose 200 mcg/day). Since there is no evidence that exceeding the maximum recommended dosage is more effective and increased systemic absorption would occur, higher doses should be avoided.

After the desired clinical effect is obtained, the maintenance dose should be reduced to the smallest amount necessary to control the symptoms. Approximately 15% of patients with perennial rhinitis may be maintained on as little as 1 spray in each nostril per day.

Store at controlled room temperature, 15°-30°C (59°-86°F).

HOW SUPPLIED
AEROSOL LIQUID W/ADAPTER: 0.25 MG/INH

BRAND/MANUFACTURER	NDC	SIZE	AWP
○ **BRAND**			
AEROBID-M: Forest Pharm	00456-0670-99	7 ml	$47.59
AEROBID: Forest Pharm	00456-0672-99	7 ml	$47.59

SPRAY: 0.025%

BRAND/MANUFACTURER	NDC	SIZE	AWP
○ **BRAND**			
NASALIDE: Syntex	00033-2906-40	25 ml	$26.52

Fluocinolone Acetonide

DESCRIPTION
Fluocinolone Acetonide creams are intended for topical administration. The active component is the corticosteroid Fluocinolone Acetonide, which has the chemical name pregna-1,4-diene-3,20-dione,6,9-difluoro-11,21-dihydroxy-16, 17-[(1-methylethylidene)bis(oxy)]-,(6α,11β,16α)-.

The creams contain Fluocinolone Acetonide 0.25 mg/g or 0.1 mg/g in a water-washable aqueous base; the high potency cream contains Fluocinolone Acetonide 2 mg/g.

Following is its chemical structure:

CLINICAL PHARMACOLOGY
Topical corticosteroids share anti-inflammatory, antipruritic and vasoconstrictive actions.

The mechanism of anti-inflammatory activity of the topical corticosteroids is unclear. Various laboratory methods, including vasoconstrictor assays, are used to compare and predict potencies and/or clinical efficacies of the topical corticosteroids. There is some evidence to suggest that a recognizable correlation exists between vasoconstrictor potency and therapeutic efficacy in man.

PHARMACOKINETICS
The extent of percutaneous absorption of topical corticosteroids is determined by many factors including the vehicle, the integrity of the epidermal barrier, and the use of occlusive dressings.

Topical corticosteroids can be absorbed from normal intact skin. Inflammation and/or other disease processes in the skin increase percutaneous absorption. Occlusive dressings substantially increase the percutaneous absorption of topical corticosteroids. Thus, occlusive dressings may be a valuable therapeutic adjunct for treatment of resistant dermatoses. (See *"Dosage and Administration."*)

Once absorbed through the skin, topical corticosteroids are handled through pharmacokinetic pathways similar to systemically administered corticosteroids. Corticosteroids are bound to plasma proteins in varying degrees. Corticosteroids are metabolized primarily in the liver and are then excreted by the kidneys. Some of the topical corticosteroids and their metabolites are also excreted into the bile.

INDICATIONS AND USAGE
Fluocinolone Acetonide creams are indicated for the relief of the inflammatory and pruritic manifestations of corticosteroid-responsive dermatoses.

UNLABELED USES
Fluocinolone topical is used alone or as an adjunct in the treatment of alopecia areata.

CONTRAINDICATIONS
Topical corticosteroids are contraindicated in those patients with a history of hypersensitivity to any of the components of the preparation.

PRECAUTIONS
GENERAL
Systemic absorption of topical corticosteroids has produced reversible hypothalamic-pituitary-adrenal (HPA) axis suppression, manifestations of Cushing's syndrome, hyperglycemia, and glucosuria in some patients.

Conditions which augment systemic absorption include the application of the more potent steroids, use over large surface areas, prolonged use, and the addition of occlusive dressings.

Therefore, patients receiving a large dose of a potent topical steroid applied to a large surface area or under an occlusive dressing should be evaluated periodically for evidence of HPA axis suppression by using the urinary free cortisol and ACTH stimulation tests. If HPA axis suppression is noted, an attempt should be made to withdraw the drug, to reduce the frequency of application, or to substitute a less potent steroid.

Recovery of HPA axis function is generally prompt and complete upon discontinuation of the drug. Infrequently, signs and symptoms of steroid withdrawal may occur, requiring supplemental systemic corticosteroids.

Children may absorb proportionally larger amounts of topical corticosteroids and thus be more susceptible to systemic toxicity. (See *"Precautions—Pediatric Use."*)

If irritation develops, topical corticosteroids should be discontinued and appropriate therapy instituted.

As with any topical corticosteroid product, prolonged use may produce atrophy of the skin and subcutaneous tissues. When used on intertriginous or flexor areas, or on the face, this may occur even with short-term use.

In the presence of dermatological infections, the use of an appropriate antifungal or antibacterial agent should be instituted. If a favorable response does not occur promptly, the corticosteroid should be discontinued until the infection has been adequately controlled.

Fluocinolone Acetonide high potency cream should not be used for prolonged periods and the quantity per day should not exceed 2 g of formulated material.

INFORMATION FOR THE PATIENT
Patients using topical corticosteroids should receive the following information and instructions:

1. This medication is to be used as directed by the physician. It is for external use only. Avoid contact with the eyes.
2. Patients should be advised not to use this medication for any disorder other than for which it was prescribed.
3. The treated skin area should not be bandaged or otherwise covered or wrapped as to be occlusive unless directed by the physician.
4. Patients should report any signs of local adverse reactions especially under occlusive dressing.
5. Parents of pediatric patients should be advised not to use tight-fitting diapers or plastic pants on a child being treated in the diaper area, as these garments may constitute occlusive dressings.

LABORATORY TESTS
The following tests may be helpful in evaluating the HPA axis suppression:

Urinary free cortisol test
ACTH stimulation test

CARCINOGENESIS, MUTAGENESIS, AND IMPAIRMENT OF FERTILITY

Long-term animal studies have not been performed to evaluate the carcinogenic potential or the effect on fertility of topical corticosteroids.

Studies to determine mutagenicity with prednisolone and hydrocortisone have revealed negative results.

PREGNANCY CATEGORY C

Corticosteroids are generally teratogenic in laboratory animals when administered systemically at relatively low dosage levels. The more potent corticosteroids have been shown to be teratogenic after dermal application in laboratory animals. There are no adequate and well-controlled studies in pregnant women on teratogenic effects from topically applied corticosteroids. Therefore, topical corticosteroids should be used during pregnancy only if the potential benefit justifies the potential risk to the fetus. Drugs of this class should not be used extensively on pregnant patients, in large amounts, or for prolonged periods of time.

NURSING MOTHERS

It is not known whether topical administration of corticosteroids could result in sufficient systemic absorption to produce detectable quantities in breast milk. Systematically administered corticosteroids are secreted into breast milk in quantities *not* likely to have a deleterious effect on the infant. Nevertheless, caution should be exercised when topical corticosteroids are administered to a nursing woman.

PEDIATRIC USE

Fluocinolone Acetonide high potency cream should not be used on infants up to two years of age.

Pediatric patients may demonstrate greater susceptibility to topical corticosteroid-induced HPA axis suppression and Cushing's syndrome than mature patients because of a larger skin surface area to body weight ratio.

Hypothalamic-pituitary-adrenal (HPA) axis suppression, Cushing's syndrome, and intracranial hypertension have been reported in children receiving topical corticosteroids. Manifestations of adrenal suppression in children include linear growth retardation, delayed weight gain, low plasma cortisol levels, and absence of response to ACTH stimulation. Manifestations of intracranial hypertension include bulging fontanelles, headaches, and bilateral papilledema.

Administration of topical corticosteroids to children should be limited to the least amount compatible with an effective therapeutic regimen. Chronic corticosteroid therapy may interfere with the growth and development of children.

ADVERSE REACTIONS

The following local adverse reactions are reported infrequently with topical corticosteroids, but may occur more frequently with the use of occlusive dressings. These reactions are listed in an approximate decreasing order of occurrence:

Burning
Itching
Irritation
Dryness
Folliculitis
Hypertrichosis
Acneiform eruptions
Hypopigmentation
Perioral dermatitis
Allergic contact dermatitis
Maceration of the skin
Secondary infection
Skin atrophy
Striae
Miliaria

OVERDOSAGE

Topically applied corticosteroids can be absorbed in sufficient amounts to produce systemic effects. (See *"Precautions."*)

DOSAGE AND ADMINISTRATION

Fluocinolone Acetonide creams are generally applied to the affected area as a thin film from two to four times daily depending on the severity of the condition. In hairy sites, the hair should be parted to allow direct contact with the lesion.

Occlusive dressing may be used for the management of psoriasis or recalcitrant conditions. Some plastic films may be flammable and due care should be exercised in their use. Similarly, caution should be employed when such films are used on children or left in their proximity, to avoid the possibility of accidental suffocation.

If an infection develops, the use of occlusive dressings should be discontinued and appropriate antimicrobial therapy instituted.

Store tubes at room temperature; avoid freezing and excessive heat, above 40°C (104°F).

Store jars at controlled room temperature, 15°-30°C (59°-86°F).

HOW SUPPLIED

CREAM: 0.01%

AVERAGE UNIT PRICE (AVAILABLE SIZES)		GENERIC A-RATED AVERAGE PRICE (GAAP)	
BRAND	$0.47	15 gm	$1.75
GENERIC	$0.08	60 gm	$3.80
HCFA FUL (15 gm)	$0.08	425 gm	$11.83
HCFA FUL (60 gm)	$0.04		

BRAND/MANUFACTURER	NDC	SIZE	AWP
◆ BRAND			
SYNALAR: Syntex	00033-2502-13	15 gm	$9.41
	00033-2502-17	60 gm	$18.95
◆ GENERICS			
Clay-Park	45802-0067-35	15 gm	$1.34
Schein	00364-7262-72	15 gm	$1.45
Thames	49158-0142-20	15 gm	$1.50
Moore,H.L.	00839-6346-47	15 gm	$1.60
Qualitest	00603-7747-74	15 gm	$1.66
FLUROSYN: Rugby	00536-4431-20	15 gm	$1.69
Major	00904-2660-36	15 gm	$1.80
URL	00677-0713-40	15 gm	$2.00
G&W	00713-0223-15	15 gm	$2.00
Fougera	00168-0058-15	15 gm	$2.04
UDL	51079-0266-61	15 gm	$2.19
Clay-Park	45802-0067-37	60 gm	$2.86
Thames	49158-0142-24	60 gm	$3.20
Moore,H.L.	00839-6346-50	60 gm	$3.36
Qualitest	00603-7747-88	60 gm	$3.74
FLUROSYN: Rugby	00536-4431-25	60 gm	$4.06
URL	00677-0713-43	60 gm	$4.06
Major	00904-2660-02	60 gm	$4.10
G&W	00713-0223-60	60 gm	$4.20
Fougera	00168-0058-60	60 gm	$4.20
Goldline	00182-1149-52	60 gm	$4.20
Major	00904-2660-27	425 gm	$10.45
FLUROSYN: Rugby	00536-4431-98	425 gm	$11.00
Clay-Park	45802-0067-38	425 gm	$11.88
Thames	49158-0142-23	425 gm	$14.00

CREAM: 0.025%

AVERAGE UNIT PRICE (AVAILABLE SIZES)		GENERIC A-RATED AVERAGE PRICE (GAAP)	
BRAND	$0.75	15 gm	$2.47
GENERIC	$0.12	60 gm	$5.16
HCFA FUL (15 gm)	$0.11	425 gm	$26.73
HCFA FUL (60 gm)	$0.06		

BRAND/MANUFACTURER	NDC	SIZE	AWP
◆ BRAND			
SYNALAR: Syntex	00033-2501-13	15 gm	$13.72
SYNEMOL: Syntex	00033-2509-13	15 gm	$14.44
SYNALAR: Syntex	00033-2501-17	60 gm	$32.24
SYNEMOL: Syntex	00033-2509-17	60 gm	$33.86
◆ GENERICS			
Moore,H.L.	00839-6347-47	15 gm	$1.61
Thames	49158-0143-20	15 gm	$1.80
Clay-Park	45802-0068-35	15 gm	$1.80
Major	00904-2659-36	15 gm	$2.35
FLUROSYN: Rugby	00536-4401-20	15 gm	$2.44
G&W	00713-0222-15	15 gm	$2.60
URL	00677-0712-40	15 gm	$2.65
Goldline	00182-1150-51	15 gm	$2.70
Qualitest	00603-7748-74	15 gm	$2.90
Fougera	00168-0060-15	15 gm	$3.05
UDL	51079-0268-61	15 gm	$3.23
Moore,H.L.	00839-6347-50	60 gm	$3.50
Thames	49158-0143-24	60 gm	$4.20
Clay-Park	45802-0068-37	60 gm	$4.32
Qualitest	00603-7748-88	60 gm	$4.41
URL	00677-0712-43	60 gm	$5.10
Goldline	00182-1150-52	60 gm	$5.10
G&W	00713-0222-60	60 gm	$5.35
FLUROSYN: Rugby	00536-4401-25	60 gm	$5.81
Major	00904-2659-02	60 gm	$6.58
Fougera	00168-0060-60	60 gm	$7.20
Clay-Park	45802-0068-38	425 gm	$25.38
Major	00904-2659-27	425 gm	$26.55
Thames	49158-0143-23	425 gm	$27.50
Moore,H.L.	00839-6347-99	425 gm	$27.50

CREAM: 0.05%

BRAND/MANUFACTURER	NDC	SIZE	AWP
◆ GENERICS			
Major	00904-0770-36	15 gm	$7.30

LOTION: 0.01%

BRAND/MANUFACTURER	NDC	SIZE	AWP
◆ GENERICS			
Raway	00686-0067-37	60 ml	$2.98

◆ RATED THERAPEUTICALLY EQUIVALENT; ◇ THERAPEUTIC EQUIVALENCE UNCONFIRMED; ○ UNRATED

OIL:

BRAND/MANUFACTURER	NDC	SIZE	AWP
◇ BRAND			
DERMA-SMOOTHE/FS: Hill Derm	28105-0149-04	120 ml	$17.00

OINTMENT: 0.025%

AVERAGE UNIT PRICE (AVAILABLE SIZES)		GENERIC A-RATED AVERAGE PRICE (GAAP)	
BRAND	$0.73	15 gm	$3.57
GENERIC	$0.19	60 gm	$8.58
HCFA FUL (15 gm)	$0.26		
HCFA FUL (60 gm)	$0.13		

BRAND/MANUFACTURER	NDC	SIZE	AWP
◆ BRAND			
SYNALAR: Syntex	00033-2504-13	15 gm	$13.72
	00033-2504-17	60 gm	$32.25
◆ GENERICS			
G&W	00713-0224-15	15 gm	$2.60
Fougera	00168-0064-15	15 gm	$3.53
Major	00904-2580-36	15 gm	$4.00
FLUROSYN: Rugby	00536-4462-20	15 gm	$4.15
G&W	00713-0224-60	60 gm	$5.35
Fougera	00168-0064-60	60 gm	$9.08
FLUROSYN: Rugby	00536-4462-25	60 gm	$9.95
Major	00904-2580-02	60 gm	$9.95

SHAMPOO:

BRAND/MANUFACTURER	NDC	SIZE	AWP
◇ BRAND			
FS SHAMPOO: Hill Derm	28105-0249-04	120 ml	$12.35

SOLUTION: 0.01%

AVERAGE UNIT PRICE (AVAILABLE SIZES)		GENERIC A-RATED AVERAGE PRICE (GAAP)	
BRAND	$0.66	20 ml	$4.25
GENERIC	$0.18	60 ml	$9.51
HCFA FUL (20 ml)	$0.18		
HCFA FUL (60 ml)	$0.12		

BRAND/MANUFACTURER	NDC	SIZE	AWP
◆ BRAND			
SYNALAR: Syntex	00033-2506-44	20 ml	$17.18
FLUONID: Allergan Inc	00023-0878-60	60 ml	$33.03
SYNALAR: Syntex	00033-2506-46	60 ml	$34.03
◆ GENERICS			
Thames	49158-0209-40	20 ml	$3.50
Major	00904-2661-55	20 ml	$3.95
Moore,H.L.	00839-6660-97	20 ml	$4.17
Schein	00364-7343-55	20 ml	$4.25
Bausch&Lomb Pharm	24208-0465-63	20 ml	$4.40
Goldline	00182-1564-65	20 ml	$4.45
Qualitest	00603-1231-43	20 ml	$4.45
Rugby	00536-0720-73	20 ml	$4.79
Thames	49158-0209-32	60 ml	$7.30
Schein	00364-7343-58	60 ml	$8.38
Qualitest	00603-1231-49	60 ml	$8.64
Bausch&Lomb Pharm	24208-0465-67	60 ml	
Moore,H.L.	00839-6660-64	60 ml	$9.30
Fougera	00168-0059-60	60 ml	$9.99
URL	00677-0790-25	60 ml	$10.50
Rugby	00536-0720-61	60 ml	$10.57
Major	00904-2661-03	60 ml	$10.60
Goldline	00182-1564-68	60 ml	$10.80

SOLUTION: 0.025%

BRAND/MANUFACTURER	NDC	SIZE	AWP
◆ GENERICS			
Goldline	00182-5015-52	60 gm	$12.30

Fluocinonide

DESCRIPTION
Fluocinonide cream and ointment are intended for topical administration. The active component is the corticosteroid Fluocinonide, which is the 21-acetate ester of Fluocinonide acetonide and has the chemical name pregna-1,4-diene-3,20-dione,21-(acetyloxy)-6, 9-difluoro-11-hydroxy-16,17-[(methylethylidene)bis(oxy)]-,(6α, 11β, 16α)-.

Following is its chemical structure:

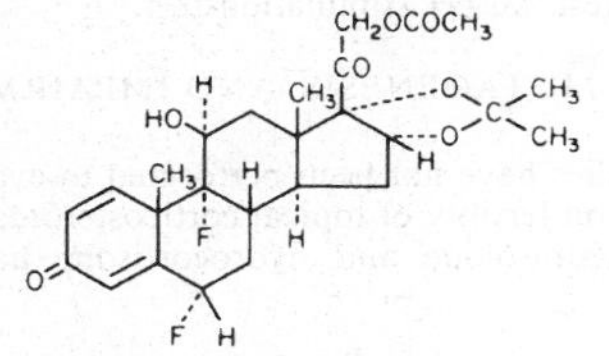

CLINICAL PHARMACOLOGY
Topical corticosteroids share anti-inflammatory, anti-pruitic and vasconstrictive actions.

The mechanism of anti-inflammatory activity of the topical corticosteroids is unclear. Various laboratory methods, including vasoconstrictor assays, are used to compare and predict potencies and/or clinical efficacies of the topical corticosteroids. There is some evidence to suggest that a recognizable correlation exists between vasconstrictor potency and therapeutic efficacy in man.

PHARMACOKINETICS
The extent of percutaneous absorption of topical corticosteroids is determined by many factors including the vehicle, the integrity of the epidermal barrier, and the use of occlusive dressings.

Topical corticosteroids can be absorbed from normal intact skin. Inflammation and/or other disease processes in the skin increase percutaneous absorption. Occlusive dressings substantially increase the percutaneous absorption of topical corticosteroids. Thus, occlusive dressings may be a valuable therapeutic adjunct for treatment of resistant dermatoses. (See *"Dosage and Administration"*).

Once absorbed through the skin, topical corticosteroids are handled through pharmacokinetic pathways similar to systemically administered corticosteroids. Corticosteroids are bound to plasma proteins in varying degrees. Corticosteroids are metabolized primarily in the liver and are then excreted by the kidneys. Some of the topical corticosteroids and their metabolites are also excreted into the bile.

INDICATIONS AND USAGE
Fluocinonide cream and ointment are indicated for the relief of the inflammatory and pruritic manifestations of corticosteroid-responsive dermatoses.

CONTRAINDICATIONS
Topical corticosteroids are contraindicated in those patients with a history of hypersensitivity to any of the components of the preparation.

PRECAUTIONS
GENERAL
Systemic absorption of topical corticosteroids has produced reversible hypothalamic-pituitary-adrenal (HPA) axis suppression, manifestations of Cushing's syndrome, hyperglycemia, and glucosuria in some patients.

Conditions which augment systemic absorption include the application of the more potent steroids, use over large surface areas, prolonged use, and the addition of occlusive dressings.

Therefore, patients receiving a large dose of potent topical steroid applied to a large surface area or under an occlusive dressing should be evaluated periodically for evidence of HPA axis suppression by using the urinary free cortisol and ACTH stimulation tests. If HPA axis suppression is noted, an attempt should be made to withdraw the drug, to reduce the frequency of application, or to substitute a less potent steroid. Recovery of HPA axis function is generally prompt and complete upon discontinuation of the drug. Infrequently, signs and symptoms of steroid withdrawal may occur, requiring supplemental systemic corticosteroids.

Children may absorb proportionally larger amounts of topical corticosteroids and thus be more susceptible to systemic toxicity. (See *"Precautions - Pediatric Use"*). If irritation develops, topical corticosteroids should be discontinued and appropriate therapy instituted.

As with any topical corticosteroid product, prolonged use may produce atrophy of the skin and subcutaneous tissues. When used on intertriginous or flexor areas, or on the face, this may occur even with short-term use.

In the presence of dermatological infections, the use of an appropriate antifungal or antibacterial agent should be instituted. If a favorable response does not occur promptly, the corticosteroid should be discontinued until the infection has been adequately controlled.

INFORMATION FOR THE PATIENT
Patients using topical corticosteroids should receive the following information and instructions:

1. This medication is to be used as directed by the physician. It is for external use only. Avoid contact with the eyes.
2. Patients should be advised not to use this medication for any disorder other than for which it was prescribed.
3. The treated skin area should not be bandaged or otherwise covered or wrapped as to be occlusive unless directed by the physician.
4. Patients should report any signs of local adverse reactions especially under occlusive dressing.
5. Parents of pediatric patients should be advised not to use tight-fitting diapers or plastic pants on a child being treated in the diaper area, as these garments may constitute occlusive dressings.

➤ SHOWN IN PRODUCT IDENTIFICATION GUIDE

LABORATORY TESTS

The following tests may be helpful in evaluating the HPA axis suppression: Urinary free cortisol test ACTH stimulation test.

CARCINOGENESIS, MUTAGENESIS, AND IMPAIRMENT OF FERTILITY

Long-term animal studies have not been performed to evaluate the carcinogenic potential or the effect on fertility of topical corticosteroids. Studies to determine mutagenicity with prednisolone and hydrocortisone have revealed negative results.

PREGNANCY CATEGORY C

Corticosteroids are generally teratogenic in laboratory animals when administered systemically at relatively low dosage levels. The more potent corticosteroids have been shown to be teratogenic after dermal application in laboratory animals. There are no adequate and well-controlled studies in pregnant women on teratogenic effects from topically applied corticosteroids. Therefore, topical corticosteroids should be used during pregnancy only if the potential benefit justifies the potential risk to the fetus. Drugs of this class should not be used extensively on pregnant patients, in large amounts, or for prolonged periods of time.

NURSING MOTHERS

It is not known whether topical administration of corticosteroids could result in sufficient systemic absorption to produce detectable quantities in breast milk. Systemically administered corticosteroids are secreted into breast milk in quantities not likely to have a deleterious effect on the infant. Nevertheless, caution should be exercised when topical corticosteroids are administered to a nursing woman.

PEDIATRIC USE

Pediatric patients may demonstrate greater susceptibility to topical corticosteroid-induced HPA axis suppression and Cushing's syndrome than mature patients because of a larger skin surface to body weight ratio.

Hypothalamic-pituitary-adrenal (HPA) axis suppression, Cushing's syndrome, and intracranial hypertension have been reported in children receiving topical corticosteroids. Manifestations of adrenal suppression in children include linear growth retardation, delayed weight gain, low plasma cortisol levels, and absence of response to ACTH stimulation. Manifestations of intracranial hypertension include bulging fontanelles, headaches, and bilateral papilledema.

Administration of topical corticosteroids to children should be limited to the least amount compatible with an effective therapeutic regimen. Chronic corticosteroid therapy may interfere with the growth and development of children.

ADVERSE REACTIONS

The following local adverse reactions are reported infrequently with topical corticosteroids, but may occur more frequently with the use of occlusive dressings. These reactions are listed in an approximate decreasing order of occurrence:

Burning	Perioral dermatitis
Itching	Allergic contact dermatitis
Irritation	Maceration of the skin
Dryness	Secondary infection
Folliculitis	Skin atrophy
Hypertrichosis	Striae
Acneiform eruptions	Miliaria
Hypopigmentation	

OVERDOSAGE

Topically applied corticosteroids can be absorbed in sufficient amounts to produce systemic effects. (See *"Precautions"*.)

DOSAGE AND ADMINISTRATION

Fluocinonide cream and ointment are generally applied to the affected area as a thin film from two to four times daily depending on the severity of the condition.

Occlusive dressings may be used for the management of psoriasis or recalcitrant conditions.

If an infection develops, the use of occlusive dressings should be discontinued and appropriate antimicrobial therapy instituted.

Store at room temperature. Avoid temperatures above 30°C (86°F) for the ointment, 40°C (104°F) for the cream.

HOW SUPPLIED
CREAM: 0.05%

AVERAGE UNIT PRICE (AVAILABLE SIZES)		GENERIC A-RATED AVERAGE PRICE (GAAP)	
BRAND	$0.82	30 gm	$10.73
GENERIC	$0.41		
HCFA FUL (15 gm)	$0.30		
HCFA FUL (30 gm)	$0.22		
HCFA FUL (60 gm)	$0.17		
HCFA FUL (120 gm)	$0.20		

BRAND/MANUFACTURER	NDC	SIZE	AWP
◆ **BRAND**			
LIDEX: Syntex	00033-2511-13	15 gm	$17.80
LIDEX-E: Syntex	00033-2513-13	15 gm	$17.80
LIDEX: Syntex	00033-2511-14	30 gm	$24.67

BRAND/MANUFACTURER	NDC	SIZE	AWP
LIDEX-E: Syntex	00033-2513-14	30 gm	$24.67
LIDEX: Syntex	00033-2511-17	60 gm	$41.36
LIDEX-E: Syntex	00033-2513-17	60 gm	$41.36
LIDEX: Syntex	00033-2511-22	120 gm	$69.54
LIDEX-E: Syntex	00033-2513-22	120 gm	$69.54
◆ **GENERICS**			
Thames	49158-0212-20	15 gm	$4.80
NMC	23317-0390-15	15 gm	$6.24
Schein	00364-0857-72	15 gm	$6.50
Moore,H.L.	00839-7698-47	15 gm	$6.60
Genetco	00302-3010-15	15 gm	$6.89
Mason Dist	11845-0383-01	15 gm	$6.90
Rugby	00536-4350-20	15 gm	$7.00
Major	00904-0770-36	15 gm	$7.30
Qualitest	00603-7759-74	15 gm	$7.32
Moore,H.L.	00839-7013-47	15 gm	$7.90
Taro	51672-1253-01	15 gm	$8.25
Lemmon	00093-0262-15	15 gm	$8.25
Hamilton	60322-0511-13	15 gm	$8.25
URL	00677-0735-40	15 gm	$8.50
Geneva	00781-7008-27	15 gm	$8.55
Goldline	00182-1731-51	15 gm	$8.85
Taro	51672-1254-01	15 gm	$9.50
Major	00904-0773-36	15 gm	$10.45
Moore,H.L.	00839-7758-47	15 gm	$11.95
Hamilton	60322-0513-13	15 gm	$12.35
Lemmon	00093-0263-15	15 gm	$12.50
Thames	49158-0212-68	30 gm	$7.30
NMC	23317-0390-30	30 gm	$8.58
Schein	00364-0857-56	30 gm	$8.68
Mason Dist	11845-0383-02	30 gm	$9.46
Qualitest	00603-7759-78	30 gm	$9.68
Rugby	00536-4350-28	30 gm	$9.75
LICON: Major	00904-0770-31	30 gm	$10.15
Moore,H.L.	00839-7013-49	30 gm	$10.25
Moore,H.L.	00839-7698-49	30 gm	$10.25
Taro	51672-1253-02	30 gm	$11.25
Lemmon	00093-0262-30	30 gm	$11.25
Genetco	00302-3010-31	30 gm	$11.25
FLUEX: Ocusoft	54799-0801-30	30 gm	$11.30
URL	00677-1404-45	30 gm	$12.40
Goldline	00182-1731-56	30 gm	$12.40
Geneva	00781-7008-30	30 gm	$12.45
Taro	51672-1254-02	30 gm	$14.16
Major	00904-0773-31	30 gm	$15.75
Goldline	00182-5051-56	30 gm	$16.50
Moore,H.L.	00839-7758-49	30 gm	$17.48
Lemmon	00093-0263-30	30 gm	$17.50
Thames	49158-0212-24	60 gm	$12.40
Schein	00364-0857-58	60 gm	$12.75
Moore,H.L.	00839-7698-50	60 gm	$13.37
Geneva	00781-7008-35	60 gm	$14.44
Mason Dist	11845-0383-04	60 gm	$15.86
Moore,H.L.	00839-7013-50	60 gm	$16.05
Taro	51672-1253-03	60 gm	$16.25
Genetco	00302-3010-02	60 gm	$16.25
Qualitest	00603-7759-88	60 gm	$16.26
Rugby	00536-4350-25	60 gm	$16.38
Major	00904-0770-02	60 gm	$16.50
Lemmon	00093-0262-92	60 gm	$19.00
Hamilton	60322-0511-17	60 gm	$19.00
Goldline	00182-1731-52	60 gm	$20.85
Taro	51672-1254-03	60 gm	$22.60
URL	00677-0735-43	60 gm	$25.63
Geneva	00781-7103-35	60 gm	$25.68
Moore,H.L.	00839-7589-50	60 gm	$25.91
URL	00677-1404-43	60 gm	$26.90
Goldline	00182-5051-52	60 gm	$27.75
Rugby	00536-0781-25	60 gm	$28.00
Major	00904-0773-02	60 gm	$28.35
Hamilton	60322-0513-17	60 gm	$28.65
Lemmon	00093-0263-92	60 gm	$28.70
Moore,H.L.	00839-7698-53	120 gm	$21.99
Thames	49158-0212-25	120 gm	$24.60
Major	00904-0770-22	120 gm	$26.95
Rugby	00536-4350-31	120 gm	$27.25
Taro	51672-1254-04	120 gm	$30.33
Goldline	00182-1731-57	120 gm	$35.05
Major	00904-0773-22	120 gm	$44.65

CREAM: 0.05%

BRAND/MANUFACTURER	NDC	SIZE	AWP
◇ **BRAND**			
DERMACIN: Pedinol	00884-5793-01	30 gm	$12.00
◇ **GENERICS**			
Interstate	00814-3200-93	15 gm	$5.93
Cheshire	55175-2193-05	15 gm	$7.44
Allscrips	54569-7062-00	15 gm	$7.55
Allscrips	54569-2177-00	15 gm	$8.57
Cheshire	55175-2454-05	15 gm	$9.59
Southwood	58016-3042-01	15 gm	$11.60
Southwood	58016-3121-04	30 gm	$15.64
Cheshire	55175-2193-06	60 gm	$13.78
Interstate	00814-3200-91	60 gm	$14.93
Allscrips	54569-2275-00	60 gm	$19.84

◆ RATED THERAPEUTICALLY EQUIVALENT; ◇ THERAPEUTIC EQUIVALENCE UNCONFIRMED; ○ UNRATED

GEL: 0.05%

AVERAGE UNIT PRICE (AVAILABLE SIZES)		GENERIC A-RATED AVERAGE PRICE (GAAP)	
BRAND	$0.82	60 gm	$34.51
GENERIC	$0.58		
HCFA FUL (60 gm)	$0.71		

BRAND/MANUFACTURER	NDC	SIZE	AWP
◆ **BRAND**			
LIDEX: Syntex	00033-2507-13	15 gm	$17.80
	00033-2507-14	30 gm	$24.67
	00033-2507-17	60 gm	$41.36
	00033-2507-22	120 gm	$69.54
◆ **GENERICS**			
Lemmon	00093-0265-92	60 gm	$30.68
Moore,H.L.	00839-7590-50	60 gm	$38.33

For additional alternatives, turn to the section beginning on page 2859.

Fluogen SEE INFLUENZA VIRUS VACCINE

Fluonid SEE FLUOCINOLONE ACETONIDE

Fluor-I-Strip SEE FLUORESCEIN SODIUM

Fluor-Op SEE FLUOROMETHOLONE

Fluorescein Sodium

DESCRIPTION

Fluorescein Sodium is a dye used as a diagnostic acid. It is available as a sterile, aqueous solution for intravenous use and as ophthalmic strips.

Its chemical name is Spiro [isobenzofuran•1 (3H), 9′•[9H]xanthene]-3-one, 3′6′-dihydroxy, disodium salt.

Each ml of injection contains:
Fluorescein Sodium ....100 mg or 250 mg

Each strip contains:
Fluorescein Sodium ....1mg or 9mg

Following is its chemical structure:

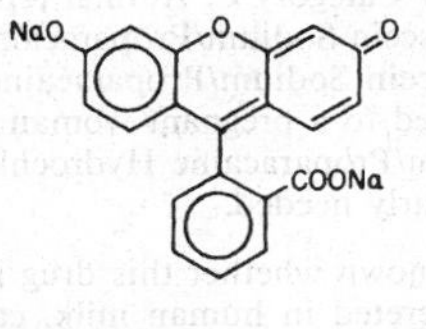

CLINICAL PHARMACOLOGY

The yellowish-green fluorescence of the injection demarcates the vascular area under observation, distinguishing it from adjacent areas.

INDICATIONS

I. Some brands of injection are indicated for angiography of retinal vessels. To detect occlusion or obliteration of retinal vessels, vascular malformations, neovascularization, changes in vascular permeability, ocular tumors and defects in the retinal pigment epithelium.

II. Other brands of injection are indicated in diagnostic fluorescein angiography or angioscopy of the fundus and of the iris vasculature.

The strips are indicated for staining the anterior segment of the eye when:
a) delineating a corneal injury, herpetic lesion or foreign body,
b) determining the site of an intraocular injury,
c) fitting contact lenses,
d) making the Fluorescein test to ascertain postoperative closure of the sclerocorneal (also referred to as corneoscleral) wound in delayed anterior chamber reformation,
e) making the lacrimal drainage test.

CONTRAINDICATIONS

Known hypersensitivity to any of the components.

WARNING

The injection is for ophthalmic use only—not for intrathecal injection. Care must be taken to avoid extravasation during injection as the high pH of Fluorescein solution can result in severe local tissue damage. The following complications resulting from extravasation of Fluorescein have been noted to occur; sloughing of the skin, superficial phlebitis, subcutaneous granuloma, and toxic neuritis along the median curve in the antecubital area. Complications from extravasation can cause severe pain in the arm for up to several hours. When significant extravasation occurs, the injection should be discontinued and conservative measures to treat damaged tissue and to relieve pain should be implemented.

Never use Fluorescein while the patient is wearing *soft contact lenses* because the lenses may become stained. Whenever Fluorescein is used, flush the eyes with sterile, normal saline solution, and wait at least one hour before replacing the lenses.

PRECAUTIONS

General: Caution is to be exercised in patients with a history of allergy or bronchial asthma. An emergency tray including such items as 0.1% epinephrine for intravenous or intramuscular use; an antihistamine, soluble steroid, and aminophyllenl for IV use; and oxygen should always be available in the event of possible reaction to Fluorescein injection[1].

Information for Patients: Skin will attain a temporary yellowish discoloration. Urine attains a bright yellow color. Discoloration of the skin fades in 6 to 12 hours; urine fluorescence in 24 to 36 hours.

Carcinogenesis, Mutagenesis, Impairment of Fertility: There have been no long-term studies done using Fluorescein in animals to evaluate carcinogenic potential.

Use in Pregnancy: Avoid angiography on patients who are pregnant, especially those in the first trimester. There have been no reports of fetal complications from using Fluorescein Sodium injection during pregnancy.

Nursing Mothers: Fluorescein has been demonstrated to be excreted in human milk. Caution should be exercised when Fluorescein is administered to a nursing woman.

Pediatric Use: Safety and effectiveness in children have not been established.

ADVERSE REACTIONS

Nausea, vomiting, headache, gastrointestinal distress, syncope, hypotension, and other symptoms and signs of hypersensitivity have occurred. Cardiac arrest, basilar artery ischemia, severe shock, convulsions, thrombophlebitis at the injected site and rare cases of death have been reported. Following systemic absorption, this dye causes transient fluorescence of the skin and appears in the urine. Discoloration of the skin fades in 6 to 12 hours, urine fluorescence in approximately 24 to 36 hours.

Extravasation of the solution at the injection site causes intense pain at the site and a dull aching pain in the injected arm. (See *"Warning"*.) Generalized hives and itching, bronchospasm and anaphylaxis have been reported. A strong taste may develop after injection. The most common reaction is nausea.

DOSAGE AND ADMINISTRATION

INDICATION I
10% Fluorescein Sodium Injection—Sterile

Adults: 5 mL (500 mg) injected rapidly into the antecubital vein.

Children: 0.035 mL (3.5 mg) for each pound of body weight, injected rapidly into the antecubital vein.
25% Fluorescein Sodium Injection—Sterile

Adults: 2 mL (500 mg) (3 mL = 750 mg) injected rapidly into the antecubital vein.

Children: 0.02 mL (5 mg) for each pound of body weight, injected rapidly into the antecubital vein.

Fluorescence of the retinal vessels should occur within 12 seconds.
IN CASE OF EMERGENCY, INTRAVENOUS EPINEPHRINE 1:10 SHOULD BE AVAILABLE AT THE TIME OF DRUG ADMINISTRATION. AN ANTIHISTAMINE SHOULD ALSO BE AVAILABLE.
Inject rapidly into the antecubital vein. The dye should appear in the central retinal artery in 9 to 15 seconds. This may be observed with standard viewing equipment. At the time of administration, an emergency tray including such items as 0.1% epinephrine for intravenous or intramuscular use, an antihistamine, soluble steroid aminophylline for intravenous use, and oxygen should be available in the event of possible reaction to Fluorescein Sodium injection.[1]

In patients with inaccessible veins where early phases of an angiogram are not necessary, such as cystoid macular edema, one gram of Fluorescein Sodium has been administered orally. Ten to fifteen minutes is usually required before evidence of dye appears in the fundus.

INDICATION II
Inject the contents of the ampule, vial, or pre-filled syringe rapidly into the antecubital vein, *after taking precautions to avoid extravasation.* A syringe, filled with Fluorescein, is attached to transparent tubing and a 25 gauge scalp vein needle for injection. Insert the needle and draw the patient's blood to the hub of

the syringe so that a *small* air bubble separates the patient's blood in the tubing from the Fluorescein. With the room lights on, slowly inject the blood back into the vein while watching the skin over the needle tip. If the needle has extravasated, the patient's blood will be seen to bulge the skin and the injection should be stopped before any Fluorescein is injected. When assured that extravasation has not occurred, the room light may be turned off and the Fluorescein injection completed. Luminescence appears in the retina and choroidal vessels in 9 to 14 seconds and can be observed by standard viewing equipment. If potential allergy is suspected, an intradermal skin test may be performed prior to intravenous administration, i.e., 0.05 mL injected intradermally to be evaluated 30 to 60 minutes following injection. For children, the dose is calculated on the basis of 35 mg for each ten pounds of body weight.

Parenteral drug products should be inspected visually for particulate matter and discoloration, whenever solution and container permit.

To open envelope, grasp pull-tabs firmly and separate slowly. Separate the two strips by tearing off white tab end. Moisten end of strip with a drop of sterile water. Place moistened strip at the fornix in the lower cul-de-sac close to the punctum. For best results, patient should close lid tightly over strip until desired amount of staining is obtained. Another method is to anesthetize the eyes and retract upper lid and touch tip of strip to the bulbar conjunctiva on the temporal side until an adequate amount of stain is available for a clearly defined end point reading.

STORAGE

Injection: Protect from light. Store at 80° F (27° C) or below. Do not freeze.

Strips: Store at room temperature (approximately 25° C).

REFERENCES

1. Schatz, Burton, Yannuzzi and Rabb. Interpretation of Fundus Fluorescein Angiography, Page 38, C.V. Mosby Co., St. Louis, MO, 1978

HOW SUPPLIED
ACCESSORIES:

BRAND/MANUFACTURER	NDC	SIZE	AWP
○ BRAND			
FUL-GLO: Akorn	00077-0631-93	300s	$36.44

DROP: 2%

BRAND/MANUFACTURER	NDC	SIZE	AWP
○ GENERICS			
Alcon Labs	00065-0003-15	15 ml	$12.44
Iolab	00058-0776-12	1 ml 12s	$24.96
Allscrips	54569-2073-00	1 ml 12s	$24.96
Alcon Surg	00065-0781-12	2 ml 12s	$37.80

DROP: 10%

BRAND/MANUFACTURER	NDC	SIZE	AWP
○ BRAND			
OCU-FLUR 10: Ocumed	51944-4700-35	5 ml 10s	$2.50

INJECTION: 10%

BRAND/MANUFACTURER	NDC	SIZE	AWP
○ BRAND			
FUNDUSCEIN: Iolab	00058-0300-40	5 ml 12s	$88.08
FLUORESCITE: Alcon Labs	00065-0092-05	5 ml 12s	$136.56
	00065-0093-05	10 ml 12s	$264.00
○ GENERICS			
AK-FLUOR: Akorn	17478-0253-10	5 ml 12s	$6.00
AK-FLUOR: Akorn	17478-0254-10	5 ml 25s	$6.00

INJECTION: 25%

BRAND/MANUFACTURER	NDC	SIZE	AWP
○ BRAND			
FLUORESCITE: Alcon Labs	00065-0094-02	2 ml 12s	$165.00
FUNDUSCEIN: Iolab	00058-0305-40	3 ml 12s	$108.54
○ GENERICS			
AK-FLUOR: Akorn	17478-0250-20	2 ml 12s	$6.00
AK-FLUOR: Akorn	17478-0251-20	2 ml 12s	$6.00

SOLUTION: 2%

BRAND/MANUFACTURER	NDC	SIZE	AWP
○ GENERICS			
Southwood	58016-6286-01	15 ml	$23.99

SWAB:

BRAND/MANUFACTURER	NDC	SIZE	AWP
○ BRAND			
FLUOR-I-STRIP: Wyeth-Ayerst	00046-1028-83	300s	$58.45
FLUOR I-STRIP-A.T.: Wyeth-Ayerst	00046-1048-83	300s	$58.45

TEST: 1 MG

BRAND/MANUFACTURER	NDC	SIZE	AWP
○ GENERICS			
FLUORETS: Akorn	17478-0400-01	100s	$11.88

Fluorescein Sodium and Proparacaine Hydrochloride

DESCRIPTION

Fluorescein Sodium/Proparacaine Hydrochloride is a sterile ophthalmic solution combining the disclosing action of Fluorescein with the anesthetic action of Proparacaine Hydrochloride.

Established name: Fluorescein Sodium.

Chemical name: Spiro[isobenzofuran-1(3H), 9'-[9H]xanthene]-3-one, 3'6'-dihydroxy, disodium salt.

Established name: Proparacaine Hydrochloride.

Chemical name: Benzoic acid, 3-amino-4-propoxy-, 2-(diethyl-amino)ethylester, monohydrochloride.

Each mL contains: Actives: Proparacaine Hydrochloride 0.5%, Fluorescein Sodium 0.25%.

CLINICAL PHARMACOLOGY

Fluorescein Sodium/Proparacaine Hydrochloride is the combination of a disclosing agent with a rapidly acting anesthetic agent of short duration.

INDICATIONS AND USAGE

For procedures requiring a disclosing agent in combination with an anesthetic agent such as tonometry, gonioscopy, removal of corneal foreign bodies and other short corneal or conjunctival procedures.

CONTRAINDICATIONS

Known hypersensitivity to any component of this product.

WARNINGS

Prolonged use of a topical ocular anesthetic is not recommended. It may produce permanent corneal opacification with accompanying visual loss.

PRECAUTIONS

Fluorescein Sodium/Proparacaine Hydrochloride should be used cautiously and sparingly in patients with known allergies, cardiac disease, or hyperthyroidism. The long-term toxicity is unknown; prolonged use may possibly delay wound healing. Although exceedingly rare in ophthalmic application of local anesthetics, systemic toxicity (manifested by central nervous system stimulation followed by depression) may occur. Protection of the eye from irritating chemicals, foreign bodies and rubbing during the period of anesthesia is very important. Tonometers soaked in sterilizing or detergent solutions should be thoroughly rinsed with sterile distilled water prior to use. Patients should be advised to avoid touching the eye until the anesthesia has worn off.

Use in Pregnancy: Pregnancy Category C. Animal reproduction studies have not been conducted with Fluorescein Sodium/Proparacaine Hydrochloride. It is also not known whether Fluorescein Sodium/Proparacaine Hydrochloride can cause fetal harm when administered to a pregnant woman or can affect reproduction capacity. Fluorescein Sodium/Proparacaine Hydrochloride should be given to a pregnant woman only if clearly needed.

Nursing Mothers: It is not known whether this drug is excreted in human milk. Because many drugs are excreted in human milk, caution should be exercised when Fluorescein Sodium/Proparacaine Hydrochloride is administered to a nursing woman.

Pediatric Use: Safety and effectiveness in children have not been established.

ADVERSE REACTION

Occasional temporary stinging, burning, and conjunctival redness have been reported after use of ocular anesthetics, as well as rare, severe, immediate-type, apparently hyperallergic corneal reaction, with acute, intense and diffuse epithelial keratitis, a gray, ground glass appearance, sloughing of large areas of necrotic epithelium corneal filaments and sometimes, iritis with descemetitis.

Allergic contact dermatitis with drying and fissuring of the fingertips has been reported.

DOSAGE AND ADMINISTRATION

Removal of foreign bodies and sutures, and for tonometry: 1 to 2 drops (in single instillations) in each eye before operating.

Deep ophthalmic anesthesia: 1 drop in each eye every 5 to 10 minutes for 5-7 doses.

Note: The use of an eye patch is recommended.

Refrigerate at 2°-8°C (35°-46°F) before and after opening. Protect from light.

◆ RATED THERAPEUTICALLY EQUIVALENT; ◇ THERAPEUTIC EQUIVALENCE UNCONFIRMED; ○ UNRATED

HOW SUPPLIED
DROP:

BRAND/MANUFACTURER	NDC	SIZE	AWP
◆ **GENERICS**			
Bausch&Lomb Pharm	24208-0733-60	5 ml	$8.24

Fluorescite *SEE* FLUORESCEIN SODIUM

Fluorinse *SEE* SODIUM FLUORIDE

Fluorometholone

DESCRIPTION
Fluorometholone sterile ophthalmic suspension and ointment are topical anti-inflammatory agents for ophthalmic use.

Fluorometholone Acetate is a corticosteroid prepared as a sterile topical ophthalmic suspension. The active ingredient, Fluorometholone Acetate, is a white to creamy white powder with an empirical formula of $C_{24}H_{31}FO_5$ and a molecular weight of 418.5.

Chemical Name: Fluorometholone: 9-Fluoro-11β,17-dihydroxy-6α-methylpregna-1,4-diene-3,20-dion e.

Fluorometholone Acetate: 9-fluoro-11β, 17-dihydroxy-α-methylpregna-1, 4-diene-3, 20-dione 17-acetate.

Sulfacetamide sodium: N-Sulfanilylacetamide monosodium salt monohydrate.

Each mL of opthalmic suspension contains:

Fluorometholone	0.1%
or	
Fluorometholone Acetate	0.1% or 0.25%

Ophthalmic ointment contains:

Fluorometholone	0.1%

An anti-inflammatory/anti-infective combination product is also available.

Each mL of the combination opthalmic suspension contains:

Fluorometholone	0.1%
Sulfacetamide Sodium	10%

Following is its chemical structure:

CLINICAL PHARMACOLOGY
Corticosteroids inhibit the inflammatory response to a variety of inciting agents and probably delay or slow healing. They inhibit the edema, fibrin deposition, capillary dilation, leukocyte migration, capillary proliferation, fibroblast proliferation, deposition of collagen, and scar formation associated with inflammation. Clinical studies demonstrate that Fluorometholone Acetate is significantly more efficacious than Fluorometholone for the treatment of external ocular inflammation.

There is no generally accepted explanation for the mechanism of action of ocular corticosteroids. However, corticosteroids are thought to act by the induction of phospholipase A_2 inhibitory proteins, collectively called lipocortins. It is postulated that these proteins control the biosynthesis of potent mediators of inflammation such as prostaglandins and leukotrienes by inhibiting the release of their common precursor arachidonic acid. Arachidonic acid is released from membrane phospholipids by phospholipase A_2.

Corticosteroids are capable of producing a rise in intraocular pressure. Since corticosteroids may inhibit the body's defense mechanism against infection, a concomitant antimicrobial drug may be used when this inhibition is considered to be clinically significant in a particular case. In clinical studies on patients' eyes treated with both dexamethasone and Fluorometholone 0.1% suspensions, Fluorometholone demonstrated a lower propensity to increase intraocular pressure than did dexamethasone; however, in a small percentage of individuals a significant rise in intraocular pressure occurred within one week. The ultimate magnitude of the rise was equivalent for both drugs.

However, in a small percentage of individuals, a significant rise in intraocular pressure occurred within one week. The ultimate magnitude of the rise was equivalent for both drugs.

In a small study, Fluorometholone Acetate ophthalmic suspension demonstrated a significantly longer average time to produce a rise in intraocular pressure than did dexamethasone phosphate; however, the ultimate magnitude of the rise was equivalent for both drugs and in a small percentage of individuals a significant rise in intraocular pressure occurred within three days.

Sulfacetamide Sodium, the anti-infective component in the combination product, is included to provide action against specific organisms susceptible to it. Sulfacetamide Sodium is active *in vitro* against susceptible strains of the following microorganisms: *Escherichia coli, Staphylococcus aureus, Streptococcus pneumoniae, Streptococcus* (viridans group), *Haemophilus influenzae, Klebsiella* species, and *Enterobacter* species. Some strains of these bacteria may be resistant to sulfacetamide or resistant strains may emerge *in vivo*. When a decision to administer both a corticosteroid and an antimicrobial is made, the administration of such drugs in combination has the advantage of greater patient compliance and convenience, with the added assurance that the appropriate dosage of both drugs is administered. When both types of drugs are in the same formulation, compatibility of ingredients is assured and the correct volume of drug is delivered and retained.

The relative potency of corticosteroid formulations depends on the molecular structure, concentration, and release from the vehicle.

INDICATIONS AND USAGE
Fluorometholone suspension and ointment are indicated for the treatment of corticosteroid-responsive inflammation of the palpebral and bulbar conjunctiva, cornea and anterior segment of the globe.

Fluorometholone with Sulfacetamide Sodium is indicated for steroid-responsive inflammatory ocular conditions for which a corticosteroid is indicated and where superficial bacterial ocular infection or a risk of bacterial ocular infection exists.

Ocular steroids are indicated in inflammatory conditions of the palpebral and bulbar conjunctiva, cornea, and anterior segment of the globe where the inherent risk of steroid use in certain infective conjuctivitides is accepted to obtain a diminution in edema and inflammation. They are also indicated in chronic anterior uveitis and corneal injury from chemical, radiation or thermal burns or penetration of foreign bodies.

The use of a combination drug with an anti-infective component is indicated where the risk of superficial ocular infection is high or where there is an expectation that potentially dangerous numbers of bacterial will be present in the eye.

The anti-infective drug in this product, sulfacetamide, is active against the following common bacterial eye pathogens: *Escherichia coli, Staphylococcus aureus, Streptococcus pneumoniae, Streptococcus* (viridans group), *Haemophilus influenzae, Klebsiella* species, and *Enterobacter* species.

The product does not provide adequate coverage against: *Neisseria* species and *Serratia marcescens.* A significant percentage of Staphylococcal isolates are completely resistant to sulfa drugs.

CONTRAINDICATIONS
Fluorometholone suspension and ointment are contraindicated in most viral diseases of the cornea and conjunctiva, including epithelial herpes simplex keratitis (dendritic keratitis), vaccinia, and varicella and also in mycobacterial infection of the eye; tuberculosis; acute purulent untreated infections which, like other diseases caused by microorgansms, may be masked or enhanced by the presence of the steroid; and fungal disease of ocular structures. Fluorometholone suspension and ointment are also contraindicated in individuals with known or suspected hypersensitivity to any of the ingredients of this preparation and to other corticosteroids.

WARNINGS
NOT FOR INJECTION INTO THE EYE.

Prolonged use of corticosteroids may result in glaucoma with damage to the optic nerve, defects in visual acuity and fields of vision, and/or in posterior subcapsular cataract formation. If used for longer than 10 days, intraocular pressure should be routinely monitored even though it may be difficult in children and uncooperative patients. Prolonged use may also suppress the host immune response in ocular tissues and thus increase the hazard of secondary ocular infections.

Various ocular disease and long-term use of topical corticosteroids have been known to cause corneal and scleral thinning. Use of topical corticosteroids in the presence of thin corneal or scleral tissue may lead to perforation. It is advisable that the intraocular pressure be checked frequently. Acute purulent untreated infections of the eye may be masked or activity enhanced by presence of corticosteroid medication.

Use of ocular steroids may prolong the course and may exacerbate the severity of many viral infections of the eye.

Employment of a corticosteroid medication in the treatment of patients with a history of herpes simplex requires great caution.

Fatalities have occurred, although rarely, due to severe reactions to sulfonamides including Stevens-Johnson syndrome, toxic epidermal necrolysis, fulminant hepatic necrosis, agranulocytosis, aplastic anemia, and other blood dyscrasias. Sensitizations may recur when a sulfonamide is readministered, irrespective of the route of administration. If signs of hypersensitivity or other serious reactions occur, discontinue use of this preparation (see *"Adverse Reactions").* Cross-sensitivity among corticosteroids has been demonstrated.

A significant percentage of staphylococcal isolates are completely resistant to sulfa drugs.

If this product is used for 10 days or longer, intraocular pressure should be routinely monitored even though it may be difficult in children and uncooperative patients. Steroids should be used with caution in the presence of glaucoma. Intraocular pressure should be checked frequently.

The use of steroids after cataract surgery may delay healing and increase the incidence of bleb formation.

Use of ocular steroids may prolong the course and may exacerbate the severity of many viral infections of the eye (including herpes simplex). Employment of a corticosteroid medication in the treatment of patients with a history of herpes simplex requires great caution; frequent slit lamp microscopy is recommended.

Corticosteroids are not effective in mustard gas keratitis and Sjogren's keratocon junctivitis.

PRECAUTIONS

General: The initial prescription and renewal of the medication order beyond 20 milliliters of Fluorometholone suspension or 8 gm of Fluorometholone Ointment should be made by a physician only after evaluation of the patient's intraocular pressure, examination of the patient with the aid of magnification, such as slit lamp biomicroscopy and, where appropriate, fluorescein staining. If signs and symptoms fail to improve after two days, the patient should be re-evaluated.

As fungal infections of the cornea are particularly prone to develop coincidentally with long-term local corticosteroid applications, fungal invasion must be suspected in any persistent corneal ulceration where a corticosteroid has been used or is in use. Fungal cultures should be taken when appropriate.

If this product is used for 10 days or longer, intraocular pressure should be monitored (see *"Warnings"*).

Ophthalmic ointments may retard corneal healing.

Information for Patients: If inflammation or pain persists longer than 48 hours or becomes aggravated, the patient should be advised to discontinue use of the medication and consult a physician.

This product is sterile when packaged. To prevent contamination, care should be taken to avoid touching the bottle, tube, or dropper tip to eyelids or to any other surface. The use of this bottle, tube, or dropper by more than one person may spread infection. Keep bottle or tube tightly closed when not in use. Keep out of the reach of children.

Drug Interactions: Sulfacetamide preparations are incompatible with silver preparations.

Carcinogenesis, Mutagenesis, Impairment of Fertility: No studies have been conducted in animals or in humans to evaluate the possibility of these effects with Fluorometholone or Sulfacetamide.

Pregnancy: Teratogenic Effects. Pregnancy Category C: Animal studies have not been conducted with Fluorometholone with Sulfacetamide Sodium ophthalmic suspension. Fluorometholone has been shown to be embryocidal and teratogenic in rabbits when administered at low multiples of the human ocular dose. Fluorometholone was applied ocularly to rabbits daily on days 6-18 of gestation, and dose-related fetal loss and fetal abnormalities including cleft palate, deformed rib cage, anomalous limbs and neural abnormalities such as encephalocele, craniorachischisis, and spina bifida were observed. Kernicterus may be precipitated in infants by sulfonamides being given systemically during the third trimester of pregnancy.

There are no adequate and well-controlled studies of Fluorometholone in pregnant women, and it is not known whether Fluorometholone can cause fetal harm when administered to a pregnant woman. Fluorometholone should be used during pregnancy only if the potential benefit justifies the potential risk to the fetus.

Nursing Mothers: It is not known whether topical ophthalmic administration of corticosteroids could result in sufficient systemic absorption to produce detectable quantities in breast milk. Systemically administered corticosteroids appear in human milk and could suppress growth, interfere with endogenous corticosteroid production or cause other untoward effects. Systemically administered sulfonamides are capable of producing kernicterus in infants of lactating women. Because of the potential for serious adverse reactions in nursing infants from Fluorometholone, a decision should be made whether to discontinue nursing or to discontinue the drug, taking into account the importance of the drug to the mother.

Pediatric Use: Safety and effectiveness of the 0.1% suspension in children have not been established; safety and effectiveness of the ointment and the 0.25% suspension in children below the age of two years have not been established.

ADVERSE REACTIONS

Adverse reactions include, in decreasing order of frequency, elevation of intraocular pressure (IOP) with possible development of glaucoma and infrequent optic nerve damage, posterior subcapsular cataract formation, and delayed wound healing.

Although systemic effects are extremely uncommon, there have been rare occurrences of systemic hypercorticoidism after use of topical steroids.

Corticosteroid-containing preparations have also been reported to cause acute anterior uveitis and perforation of the globe. Keratitis, conjunctivitis, corneal ulcers, mydriasis, conjunctival hyperemia, loss of accommodation and ptosis have occasionally been reported following local use of corticosteroids.

Fluorometholone with Sulfacetamide Sodium: Adverse reactions have occurred with corticosteroid/anti-infective combination drugs which can be attributed to the corticosteroid component, the anti-infective component, or the combination. Exact incidence figures are not available since no denominator of

treated patients is available. Reactions occurring most often from the presence of the anti-infective ingredient are allergic sensitizations. Fatalities have occurred, although rarely, due to severe reactions to sulfonamides including Stevens-Johnson syndrome, toxic epidermal necrolysis, fulminant hepatic necrosis, agranulocytosis, aplastic anemia, and other blood dyscrasias (see *"Warnings"*). Sulfacetamide Sodium may cause local irritation.

The development of secondary ocular infection (bacterial, fungal and viral) following suppression of the host response has occurred. Fungal and viral infections of the cornea are particularly prone to develop coincidentally with long-term applications of steriods. The possibility of fungal invasion should be considered in any persistent corneal ulceration where steroid treatment has been used (see *"Warnings"*).

DOSAGE AND ADMINISTRATION

Instill one drop of ophthalmic suspension into the conjunctival sac two to four times daily. A small amount (approximately 1/2 inch ribbon) of ointment should be applied in the conjunctival sac one to three times daily. During the initial 24 to 48 hours, the dosage may be increased to one application every four hours. One drop of Fluorometholone with Sulfacetamide Sodium suspension should be instilled into the conjunctival sac four times daily. One to two drops of Fluorometholone Acetate suspension should be instilled into the conjunctival sac(s) four times daily. During the initial 24 to 48 hours the dosage may be safely increased to two drops every two hours. Care should be taken not to discontinue therapy prematurely.

If signs and symptoms fail to improve after two days, with Fluorometholone suspension or ointment or after two weeks with Fluorometholone Acetate Suspension, the patient should be re-evaluated (see *"Precautions"*).

The dosing of Fluorometholone suspension or ointment may be reduced, but care should be taken not to discontinue therapy prematurely. In chronic conditions, withdrawal of treatment should be carried out by gradually decreasing the frequency of applications.

Not more than 20 milliliters of Fluorometholone with Sulfacetamide Sodium should be prescribed initially and the prescription should not be refilled without further evaluation as outlined in *"Precautions"* above.

Note: Store at or below 25°C (77°F); protect from freezing. Avoid exposure of the ointment to temperatures above 40°C (104°F).

Store Fluorometholone with Sulfacetamide Sodium at controlled room temperature, 15°-30° C (59°-86°F). Protect from freezing and light.

Store Fluorometholone Acetate suspension upright between 36° and 80°F. **Shake the suspenion well before using.** Do not use suspension if it is dark brown.

HOW SUPPLIED
DROP: 0.1%

AVERAGE UNIT PRICE (AVAILABLE SIZES)

BRAND	$2.38

BRAND/MANUFACTURER	NDC	SIZE	AWP
◆ **BRAND**			
FML LIQUIFILM: Allergan Optical	11980-0211-01	1 ml	$4.69
FLUOR-OP: Iolab	00058-2358-05	5 ml	$9.36
FLAREX: Alcon Ophthalmic	00065-0096-05	5 ml	$14.13
FML LIQUIFILM: Allergan Optical	11980-0211-05	5 ml	$14.50
FLUOR-OP: Iolab	00058-2358-10	10 ml	$15.06
FLAREX: Alcon Ophthalmic	00065-0096-10	10 ml	$21.69
FML LIQUIFILM: Allergan Optical	11980-0211-10	10 ml	$21.98
FLUOR-OP: Iolab	00058-2358-15	15 ml	$18.72
FML LIQUIFILM: Allergan Optical	11980-0211-15	15 ml	$30.73

DROP: 0.1%

BRAND/MANUFACTURER	NDC	SIZE	AWP
○ **BRAND**			
FML-S LIQUIFILM: Allergan Optical	11980-0422-05	5 ml	$13.75
	11980-0422-10	10 ml	$18.53

DROP: 0.25%

BRAND/MANUFACTURER	NDC	SIZE	AWP
○ **BRAND**			
FML FORTE LIQUIFILM: Allergan Optical	11980-0228-02	2 ml	$5.40
	11980-0228-05	5 ml	$12.89
	11980-0228-10	10 ml	$21.10
	11980-0228-15	15 ml	$29.61

OINTMENT: 0.1%

BRAND/MANUFACTURER	NDC	SIZE	AWP
○ **BRAND**			
FML S.O.P.: Allergan Optical	00023-0316-04	3.5 gm	$17.25

Fluoroplex *SEE FLUOROURACIL, SYSTEMIC AND FLUOROURACIL, TOPICAL*

◆ RATED THERAPEUTICALLY EQUIVALENT; ◇ THERAPEUTIC EQUIVALENCE UNCONFIRMED; ○ UNRATED

Fluorouracil, Systemic

DESCRIPTION

Fluorouracil Injection, an antineoplastic antimetabolite, is a colorless to faint yellow aqueous, sterile, nonpyrogenic injectable solution for intravenous administration. Each 10 mL contains 500 mg Fluorouracil; pH is adjusted to 8.6-9.4 with sodium hydroxide and hydrochloric acid if necessary.

Chemically, Fluorouracil, a fluorinated pyrimidine, is 5-fluoro-2,4(1 H, 3 H)-pyrimidinedione. It is a white to practically white crystalline powder which is sparingly soluble in water.

Following is its chemical structure:

CLINICAL PHARMACOLOGY

There is evidence that the metabolism of Fluorouracil in the anabolic pathway blocks the methylation reaction of deoxyuridylic acid to thymidylic acid. In this manner, Fluorouracil interferes with the synthesis of deoxyribonucleic acid (DNA) and to a lesser extent inhibits the formation of ribonucleic acid (RNA). Since DNA and RNA are essential for cell division and growth, the effect of Fluorouracil may be to create a thymine deficiency which provokes unbalanced growth and death of the cell. The effects of DNA and RNA deprivation are most marked in those cells which grow more rapidly and which take up Fluorouracil at a more rapid rate.

Following intravenous injection, Fluorouracil distributes into tumors, intestinal mucosa, bone marrow, liver and other tissues throughout the body. In spite of its limited lipid solubility, Fluorouracil diffuses readily across the blood-brain barrier and distributes into cerebrospinal fluid and brain tissue.

Seven to twenty percent of the parent drug is excreted unchanged in the urine in six hours; of this over 90% is excreted in the first hour. The remaining percentage of the administered dose is metabolized, primarily in the liver. The catabolic metabolism of Fluorouracil results in degradation products (e.g., CO_2, urea and α-fluoro-β-alanine) which are inactive. The inactive metabolites are excreted in the urine over the next 3 to 4 hours. When Fluorouracil is labeled in the six carbon position. thus preventing the ^{14}C metabolism to CO_2, approximately 90% of the total radioactivity is excreted in the urine. When Fluorouracil is labeled in the two carbon position approximately 90% of the total radioactivity is excreted in expired CO_2. Ninety percent of the dose is accounted for during the first 24 hours following intravenous administration.

Following intravenous administration of Fluorouracil, the mean half-life of elimination from plasma is approximately 16 minutes, with a range of 8 to 20 minutes, and is dose dependent. No intact drug can be detected in the plasma three hours after an intravenous injection.

INDICATIONS AND USAGE

Fluorouracil Injection is effective in the palliative management of carcinoma of the colon, rectum, breast, stomach and pancreas.

UNLABELED USES

Fluorouracil is used as an adjunct in the treatment of lung cancer.

CONTRAINDICATIONS

Fluorouracil Injection therapy is contraindicated for patients in a poor nutritional state, those with depressed bone marrow function, those with potentially serious infections or those with a known hypersensitivity to Fluorouracil Injection.

WARNINGS

The daily dose of Fluorouracil Injection is not to exceed 800 mg. It is recommended that patients be hospitalized during their first course of treatment.

Fluorouracil Injection should be used with extreme caution in poor risk patients with a history of high-dose pelvic irradiation or previous use of alkylating agents, those who have a widespread invovement of bone marrow by metastatic tumors or those with impaired hepatic or renal function.

Pregnancy: Teratogenic effects: Pregnancy Category D. Fluorouracil may cause fetal harm when administered to a pregnant woman. Fluorouracil has been shown to be teratogenic in laboratory animals. Fluorouracil exhibited maximum teratogenicity when given to mice as single intraperitoneal injections of 10 to 40 mg/kg on day 10 or 12 of gestation. Similarly, intraperitoneal doses of 12 to 37 mg/kg given to rats between days 9 and 12 of gestation and intramuscular doses of 3 to 9 mg given to hamsters between days 8 and 11 of gestation were teratogenic. Malformations included cleft palates, skeletal defects and deformed appendages, paws and tails. The dosages which were teratogenic in animals are 1 to 3 times the maximum recommended human therapeutic dose. In monkeys, divided doses of 40 mg/kg given between days 20 and 24 of gestation were not teratogenic.

There are no adequate and well-controlled studies with Fluorouracil Injection in pregnant women. While there is no evidence of teratogenicity in humans due to Fluorouracil Injection, it should be kept in mind that other drugs which inhibit DNA synthesis (e.g., methotrexate and aminoptern) have been reported to be teratogenic in humans. Women of childbearing potential should be advised to avoid becoming pregnant. If the drug is used during pregnancy, or if the patient becomes pregnant while taking the drug, the patient should be told of the potential hazard to the fetus. Fluorouracil Injection should be used during pregnancy only if the potential benefit justifies the potential risk to the fetus.

Combination Therapy: Any form of therapy which adds to the stress of the patient, interferes with nutrition or depresses bone marrow function will increase the toxicity of Fluorouracil Injection.

PRECAUTIONS

General: Fluorouracil Injection is a highly toxic drug with a narrow margin of safety. Therefore, patients should be carefully supervised, since therapeutic response is unlikely to occur without some evidence of toxicity. Severe hematological toxicity, gastrointestinal hemorrhage and even death may result from the use of Flourouracil despite meticulous selection of patients and careful adjustment of dosage. Although severe toxicity is more likely in poor risk patients, fatalities may be encountered occasionally even in patients of relatively good condition.

Therapy is to be discontinued promptly whenever one of the following signs of toxicity appears:

Stomatitis or esophagopharyngitis, at the first visible sign.
Leukopenia (WBC under 3500) or a rapidly falling white blood count.
Vomiting, intractable.
Diarrhea, frequent bowel movements or watery stools.
Gastrointestinal ulceration and bleeding.
Thrombocytopenia (platelets under 100,000).
Hemorrhage from any site.

Information for Patients: Patients should be informed of expected toxic effects, particularly oral manifestations. Patients should be alerted to the possibility of alopecia as a result of therapy and should be informed that it is usually a transient effect.

Laboratory Tests: White blood counts with differential are recommended before each dose.

Drug Interactions: Leucovorin calcium may enhance the toxicity of Fluorouracil Injection.

Also see "*Warnings*" section.

Carcinogenesis, Mutagenesis, Impairment of Fertility:

Carcinogenesis: Long-term studies in animals to evaluate the carcinogenic potential of Fluorouracil have not been conducted. However, there was no evidence of carcinogenicity in small groups of rats given Fluorouracil orally at doses of 0.01, 0.3, 1 or 3 mg per rat 5 days per week for 52 weeks, followed by a six-month observation period. Also, in other studies, 33 mg/kg of Fluorouracil was administered intravenously to male rats once a week for 52 weeks followed by observation for the remainder of their lifetimes with no evidence of carcinogenicity. Female mice were given 1 mg of Fluorouracil intravenously once a week for 16 weeks with no effect on the incidence of lung adenomas. On the basis of the available data, no evaluation can be made of the carcinogenic risk of Fluorouracil to humans.

Mutagenesis: Oncogenic transformation of fibroblasts from mouse embryo has been induced *in vitro* by Fluorouracil, but the relationship between oncogenicity and mutagenicity is not clear. Fluorouracil has been shown to be mutagenic to several strains of *Salmonella typhimurium*, including TA 1535, TA 1537 and TA 1538, and to Saccharomyces cerevisiae, although no evidence of of mutagenicity was found with *Salmonella typhimurium* strains TA 92, TA 98 and TA 100. In addition, a positive effect was observed in the micronucleus test on bone marrow cells of the mouse, and Fluorouracil at very high concentrations produced chromosomal breaks in hamster fibroblasts *in vitro*.

Impairment of fertility: Fluorouracil Injection has not been adequately studied in animals to permit an evaluation of its effects on fertility and general reproductive performance. However, doses of 125 or 250 mg/kg administered intraperitoneally, have been shown to induce chromosomal aberrations and changes in chromosomal organization of spermatogonia in rats. Spermatogonial differentiation was also inhibited by Fluorouracil, resulting in transient infertility. However, in studies with a strain of mouse which is sensitive to the induction of sperm head abnormalities after exposure to a range of chemical mutagens and carcinogens, Fluorouracil did not produce any abnormalities at oral doses of up to 80 mg/kg/day. In female rats, Fluorouracil, administered intraperitoneally at weekly doses of 25 or 50 mg/kg for three weeks during the pre-ovulatory phase of oogenesis, significantly reduced the incidence of fertile matings, delayed the development of pre- and postimplantation embryos, increased the incidence of preimplantation lethality and induced chromosomal anomalies in these embryos. In a limited study in rabbits, a single 25 mg/kg dose of Fluorouracil or 5 daily doses of 5 mg/kg had no effect on ovulation, appeared not to affect implantation and had only limited effect in producing zygote destruction. Compounds such as

Fluorouracil, which interfere with DNA, RNA and protein synthesis, might be expected to have adverse effects on gametogenesis.

Pregnancy: Pregnancy Category D. See *"Warnings"* section.

Nonteratogenic effects: Fluorouracil Injection has not been studied in animals for its effects on peri- and postnatal development. However, Fluorouracil has been shown to cross the placenta and enter into fetal circulation in the rat. Administration of Fluorouracil has resulted in increased resorptions and embryolethality in rats. In monkeys, maternal doses higher than 40 mg/kg resulted in abortion of all embryos exposed to Fluorouracil. Compounds which inhibit DNA, RNA and protein synthesis might be expected to have adverse effects on peri- and postnatal development.

Nursing Mothers: It is not known whether Fluorouracil is excreted in human milk. Because Fluorouracil inhibits DNA, RNA and protein synthesis, mothers should not nurse while receiving this drug.

Pediatric Use: Safety and effectiveness in children have not been established.

ADVERSE REACTIONS

Stomatitis and esophagopharyngitis (which may lead to sloughing and ulceration), diarrhea, anorexia, nausea and emesis are commonly seen during therapy.

Leukopenia usually follows every course of adequate therapy with Fluorouracil. The lowest white blood cell counts are commonly observed between the 9th and 14th days after the first course of treatment, although uncommonly the maximal depression may be delayed for as long as 20 days. By the 30th day the count has usually returned to the normal range.

Alopecia and dermatitis may be seen in a substantial number of cases. The dermatitis most often seen is a pruritic maculopapular rash usually appearing on the extremities and less frequently on the trunk. It is generally reversible and usually responsive to symptomatic treatment.

Other adverse reactions are:

Hematologic: pancytopenia, thrombocytopenia, agranulocytosis, anemia.

Cardiovascular: myocardial ischemia, angina.

Gastrointestinal: gastrointestinal ulceration and bleeding.

Allergic reactions: anaphylaxis and generalized allergic reactions.

Neurologic: acute cerebellar syndrome (which may persist following discontinuance of treatment), nystagmus, headache.

Dermatologic: dry skin, fissuring, photosensitivity, as manifested by erythema or increased pigmentation of the skin; vein pigmentation.

Ophthalmic: lacrimal duct stenosis, visual changes, lacrimation, photophobia.

Psychiatric: disorientation, confusion, euphoria.

Miscellaneous: thrombophlebitis, epistaxis, nail changes (including loss of nails).

OVERDOSAGE

The possibility of overdosage with Fluorouracil is unlikely in view of the mode of administration. Nevertheless, the anticipated manifestations would be nausea, vomiting, diarrhea, gastrointestinal ulceration and bleeding, bone marrow depression (including thrombocytopenia, leukopenia and granulocytosis). No specific antidotal therapy exists. Patients who have been exposed to an overdose of Fluorouracil should be monitored hematologically for at least four weeks. Should abnormalities appear, appropriate therapy should be utilized.

The acute intravenous toxicity of Fluorouracil is as follows:

Species	LD_{50} (mg/kg $\pm$ S.E.)
Mouse	340 ± 17
Rat	165 ± 26
Rabbit	27 ± 5.1
Dog	31.5 ± 3.8

DOSAGE AND ADMINISTRATION

General Instructions: Fluorouracil Injection should be administered only intravenously, using care to avoid extravasation. No dilution is required.

All dosages are based on the patient's actual weight. However, the estimated lean body mass (dry weight) is used if the patient is obese or if there has been a spurious weight gain due to edema, ascites or other forms of abnormal fluid retention.

It is recommended that prior to treatment each patient be carefully evaluated in order to estimate as accurately as possible the optimum initial dosage of Fluorouracil Injection.

Dosage: Twelve mg/kg are given intravenously once daily for four successive days. The daily dose should not exceed 800 mg. *If no toxicity is observed,* 6 mg/kg are given on the 6th, 8th, 10th and 12th days *unless toxicity occurs.* No therapy is given on the 5th, 7th, 9th or 11th days. *Therapy is to be discontinued at the end of the 12th day, even if no toxicity has become apparent.* (See *"Warnings"* and *"Precautions"* sections.)

Poor risk patients or those who are not in an adequate nutritional state (see *"Contraindications"* and *"Warnings"* sections) should receive 6 mg/kg/day for three days. *If no toxicity is observed,* 3 mg/kg may be given on the 5th, 7th and 9th days *unless toxicity occurs.* No therapy is given on the 4th, 6th or 8th days. The daily dose should not exceed 400 mg.

A sequence of injections on either schedule constitutes a "course of therapy."

Maintenance Therapy: In instances where toxicity has not been a problem, it is recommended that therapy be continued using either of the following schedules:

1. Repeat dosage of first course every 30 days after the last day of the previous course of treatment.

2. When toxic signs resulting from the initial course of therapy have subsided, administer a maintenance dosage of 10 to 15 mg/kg/week as a single dose. Do not exceed 1 g per week.

The patient's reaction to the previous course of therapy should be taken into account in determining the amount of the drug to be used, and the dosage should be adjusted accordingly. Some patients have received from 9 to 45 courses of treatment during periods which ranged from 12 to 60 months.

HANDLING AND DISPOSAL

Procedures for proper handling and disposal of anticancer drugs should be considered. Several guidelines on this subject have been published.[1-7] There is no general agreement that all of the procedures recommended in the guidelines are necessary or appropriate.

Note: Parenteral drug products should be inspected visually for particulate matter and discoloration prior to administration, whenever solution and container permit. If a precipitate occurs due to exposure to low temperatures, resolubilize by heating to 140°F and shaking vigorously; allow to cool to body temperature before using.

STORAGE

Note: Although Fluorouracil solution may discolor slightly during storage, the potency and safety are not adversely affected.

Store at controlled room temperature 15°-30°C (59°-86°F). Protect from light. Retain in carton until time of use. Discard unused portion.

REFERENCES
1. Recommendations for the Safe Handling of Parenteral Antineoplastics Drugs. NIH Publication No. 83-2621. For sale by the Superintendent of Documents, U.S. Government Printing Office, Washington, D.C. 20402. 2. AMA Council Report. Guidelines for Handling Parenteral Antineoplastics. JAMA, March 15, 1985. 3. National Study Commission on Cytotoxic Exposure — Recommendations for Handling Cytotoxic Agents. Available from Louis P. Jeffrey, Sc.D., Director of Pharmacy Services, Rhode Island Hospital, 593 Eddy Street, Providence, Rhode Island 02902. 4. Clinical Oncological Society of Australia: Guidelines and recommendations for safe handling of antineoplastic agents. Med J Australia 1:426-428 1983. 5. Jones R.B., et al. Safe handling of chemotherapeutic agents: A report from the Mount Sinai Medical Center, Ca — A Cancer Journal for Clinicians Sept/Oct, 258-263 1983. 6. American Society of Hospital Pharmacists technical assistance bulletin on handling cytotoxic drugs in hospitals. Am J Hosp Pharm 42:131-137, 1985. 7. OSHA Work-Practice Guidelines for Personnel Dealing with Cytotoxic (Antineoplastic) Drugs. Am J Hosp Pharm 1986; 43:1193-1204.

J CODES
500 mg IV—J9190

HOW SUPPLIED
CREAM: 1%

BRAND/MANUFACTURER	NDC	SIZE	AWP
○ BRAND			
FLUOROPLEX: Allergan Herbert	00023-0812-30	30 gm	$31.50

CREAM: 5%

BRAND/MANUFACTURER	NDC	SIZE	AWP
○ BRAND			
EFUDEX: Roche Labs	00004-1506-03	25 gm	$33.70

INJECTION: 500 MG/10 ML

AVERAGE UNIT PRICE (AVAILABLE SIZES)		GENERIC A-RATED AVERAGE PRICE (GAAP)	
GENERIC	$0.21	10 ml 10s	$22.41
		100 ml 10s	$201.88

BRAND/MANUFACTURER	NDC	SIZE	AWP
◆ GENERICS			
ADRUCIL: Pharmacia	00013-1046-94	50 ml 5s	$38.45
Roche Labs	00004-1977-01	10 ml 10s	$14.34
ADRUCIL: Pharmacia	00013-1036-91	10 ml 10s	$15.38
Solo Pak	39769-0012-10	10 ml 10s	$37.50
ADRUCIL: Pharmacia	00013-1056-94	100 ml 10s	$153.75
Solo Pak	39769-0012-90	100 ml 10s	$250.00

SOLUTION: 1%

BRAND/MANUFACTURER	NDC	SIZE	AWP
○ BRAND			
FLUOROPLEX: Allergan Herbert	00023-0810-30	30 ml	$31.50

SOLUTION: 2%

BRAND/MANUFACTURER	NDC	SIZE	AWP
○ BRAND			
EFUDEX: Roche Labs	00004-1704-06	10 ml	$20.97

◆ RATED THERAPEUTICALLY EQUIVALENT; ◇ THERAPEUTIC EQUIVALENCE UNCONFIRMED; ○ UNRATED

SOLUTION: 5%

BRAND/MANUFACTURER	NDC	SIZE	AWP
○ BRAND EFUDEX: Roche Labs	00004-1705-06	10 ml	$29.73

Fluorouracil, Topical

DESCRIPTION
Fluorouracil solutions and cream are topical preparations containing the fluorinated pyrimidine 5-fluorouracil, an antineoplastic antimetabolite.

Following is its chemical structure:

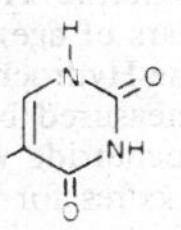

ACTIONS
There is evidence that the metabolism of Fluorouracil in the anabolic pathway blocks the methylation reaction of deoxyuridylic acid to thymidylic acid. In this fashion Fluorouracil interferes with the synthesis of deoxyribonucleic acid (DNA) and to a lesser extent inhibits the formation of ribonucleic acid (RNA). Since DNA and RNA are essential for cell division and growth, the effect of Fluorouracil may be to create a thymine deficiency which provokes unbalanced growth and death of the cell. The effects of DNA and RNA deprivation are most marked on those cells which grow more rapidly and which take up Fluorouracil at a more rapid pace. The catabolic metabolism of Fluorouracil results in degradative products (e.g., CO_2, urea, α-fluoro-β-alamine) which are inactive. Studies in man with topical application of ^{14}C-labeled Efudex demonstrated insignificant absorption as measured by ^{14}C content of plasma, urine and respiratory CO_2.

INDICATIONS
Topical Fluorouracil is recommended for the topical treatment of multiple actinic or solar keratoses. In the 5% strength it is also useful in the treatment of superficial basal cell carcinomas, when conventional methods are impractical, such as with multiple lesions or difficult treatment sites. The diagnosis should be established prior to treatment, since this new method has not been proven effective in other types of basal cell carcinomas. With isolated, easily accessible lesions, conventional techniques are preferred since success with such lesions is almost 100% with these methods. The success rate with Fluorouracil cream and solution is approximately 93%. This 93% success rate is based on 113 lesions in 54 patients. Twenty-five lesions treated with the solution produced one failure and 88 lesions treated with the cream produced 7 failures.

UNLABELED USES
Topical Fluorouracil is used alone in the treatment of condyloma acuminata.

CONTRAINDICATIONS
Topical Fluorouracil is contraindicated in patients with known hypersensitivity to any of its components.

WARNINGS
If an occlusive dressing is used, there may be an increase in the incidence of inflammatory reactions in the adjacent normal skin. A porous gauze dressing may be applied for cosmetic reasons without increase in reaction.

Prolonged exposure to ultraviolet rays should be avoided while under treatment with Fluorouracil because the intensity of the reaction may be increased.

Usage in Pregnancy: Safety for use in pregnancy has not been established.

PRECAUTIONS
If topical Fluorouracil is applied with the fingers, the hands should be washed immediately afterward. Topical Fluorouracil should be applied with care near the eyes, nose and mouth. Solar keratoses which do not respond should be biopsied to confirm the diagnosis. Patients should be forewarned that the reaction in the treated areas may be unsightly during therapy, and, in some cases, for several weeks following cessation of therapy.

Follow-up biopsies should be performed as indicated in the management of superficial basal cell carcinoma.

ADVERSE REACTIONS
The most frequently encountered local reactions are pain, pruritus, hyperpigmentation and burning at the site of application. Other local reactions include allergic contact dermatitis, scarring, soreness, tenderness, suppuration, scaling and swelling.

Also reported are alopecia, insomnia, stomatitis, irritability, medicinal taste, photosensitivity, lacrimation, telangiectasia and urticaria, although a causal relationship is remote.

Laboratory abnormalities reported are leukocytosis, thrombocytopenia, toxic granulation and eosinophilia.

DOSAGE AND ADMINISTRATION
When Fluorouracil is applied to a lesion, a response occurs with the following sequence: erythema, usually followed by vesiculation, erosion, ulceration, necrosis and epithelization.

Actinic or Solar Keratosis: Apply cream or solution twice daily in an amount sufficient to cover the lesions. Medication should be continued until the inflammatory response reaches the erosion, necrosis and ulceration stage, at which time use of the drug should be terminated. The usual duration of therapy is from two to four weeks. Complete healing of the lesions may not be evident for one to two months following cessation of topical Fluorouracil therapy.

Superficial Basal Cell Carcinomas: Only the 5% strength is recommended. Apply cream or solution twice daily in an amount sufficient to cover the lesions. Treatment should be continued for at least three to six weeks. Therapy may be required for as long as 10 to 12 weeks before the lesions are obliterated. As in any neoplastic condition, the patient should be followed for a reasonable period of time to determine if a cure has been obtained.

HOW SUPPLIED
CREAM: 1%

BRAND/MANUFACTURER	NDC	SIZE	AWP
○ BRAND FLUOROPLEX: Allergan Herbert	00023-0812-30	30 gm	$31.50

CREAM: 5%

BRAND/MANUFACTURER	NDC	SIZE	AWP
○ BRAND EFUDEX: Roche Labs	00004-1506-03	25 gm	$33.70

SOLUTION: 1%

BRAND/MANUFACTURER	NDC	SIZE	AWP
○ BRAND FLUOROPLEX: Allergan Herbert	00023-0810-30	30 ml	$31.50

SOLUTION: 2%

BRAND/MANUFACTURER	NDC	SIZE	AWP
○ BRAND EFUDEX: Roche Labs	00004-1704-06	10 ml	$20.97

SOLUTION: 5%

BRAND/MANUFACTURER	NDC	SIZE	AWP
○ BRAND EFUDEX: Roche Labs	00004-1705-06	10 ml	$29.73

Fluothane SEE HALOTHANE

Fluoxetine Hydrochloride

DESCRIPTION
Fluoxetine Hydrochloride is an antidepressant for oral administration; it is chemically unrelated to tricyclic, tetracyclic, or other available antidepressant agents. It is designated (±)-N-methyl-3-phenyl-3-[(α,α,α-trifluoro-p-tolyl)oxy] propylamine hydrochloride and has the empirical formula of $C_{17}H_{18}F_3NO \cdot HCl$. Its molecular weight is 345.79.

Fluoxetine Hydrochloride is a white to off-white crystalline solid with a solubility of 14 mg/mL in water.

Each capsule contains Fluoxetine Hydrochloride equivalent to 10 mg (32.3 μmol) or 20 mg (64.7 μmol) of Fluoxetine.

The oral solution contains Fluoxetine Hydrochloride equivalent to 20 mg/5 mL (64.7 μmol) of Fluoxetine.

Following is its chemical structure:

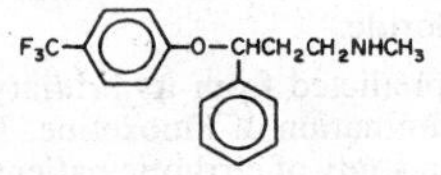

CLINICAL PHARMACOLOGY
Pharmacodynamics: The antidepressant and antiobessive-compulsive action of Fluoxetine is presumed to be linked to its inhibition of CNS neuronal uptake of serotonin. Studies at clinically relevant doses in man have demonstrated that Fluoxetine blocks the uptake of serotonin into human platelets. Studies in animals also suggest that Fluoxetine is a much more potent uptake inhibitor of serotonin than of norepinephrine.

Antagonism of muscarinic, histaminergic, and α_1-adrenergic receptors has been hypothesized to be associated with various anticholinergic, sedative, and cardiovascular effects of classical tricyclic antidepressant drugs. Fluoxetine binds to these and other membrane receptors from brain tissue much less potently *in vitro* than do the tricyclic drugs.

➤ SHOWN IN PRODUCT IDENTIFICATION GUIDE

Absorption, Distribution, Metabolism, and Excretion: Systemic Bioavailability: In man, following a single oral 40 mg dose, peak plasma concentrations of Fluoxetine from 15 to 55 ng/mL are observed after 6 to 8 hours.

The capsule and oral solution dosage forms of Fluoxetine are bioequivalent. Food does not appear to affect the systemic bioavailability of Fluoxetine, although it may delay its absorption inconsequentially. Thus, Fluoxetine may be administered with or without food.

Protein Binding: Over the concentration range from 200 to 1,000 ng/mL, approximately 94.5% of Fluoxetine is bound *in vitro* to human serum proteins, including albumin and α_1-glycoprotein. The interaction between Fluoxetine and other highly protein-bound drugs has not been fully evaluated, but may be important (see *"Precautions"*).

Enantiomers: Fluoxetine is a racemic mixture (50/50) of *R*-Fluoxetine and *S*-Fluoxetine enantiomers. In animal models, both enantiomers are specific and potent serotonin uptake inhibitors with essentially equivalent pharmacologic activity. The *S*-Fluoxetine enantiomer is eliminated more slowly and is the predominant enantiomer present in plasma at steady state.

Metabolism: Fluoxetine is extensively metabolized in the liver to norfluoxetine and a number of other, unidentified metabolites. The only identified active metabolite, norfluoxetine, is formed by demethylation of Fluoxetine. In animal models, *S*-norfluoxetine is a potent and selective inhibitor of serotonin uptake and has activity essentially equivalent to *R*- or *S*-Fluoxetine. *R*-norfluoxetine is significantly less potent than the parent drug in the inhibition of serotonin uptake. The primary route of elimination appears to be hepatic metabolism to inactive metabolites excreted by the kidney.

Clinical Issues Related to Metabolism/Elimination: The complexity of the metabolism of Fluoxetine has several consequences that may potentially affect Fluoxetine's clinical use.

Variability in Metabolism: A subset (about 7%) of the population has reduced activity of the drug metabolizing enzyme cytochrome PA45011D6. Such individuals are referred to as 'poor metabolizers' of drugs such as debrisoquin, dextromethorphan, and the tricyclic antidepressants. In a study involving labeled and unlabeled enantiomers administered as a racemate, these individuals metabolized *S*-Fluoxetine at a slower rate and thus achieved higher concentrations of *S*-Fluoxetine. Consequently, concentrations of *S*-norfluoxetine at steady state were lower. The metabolism of *R*-Fluoxetine in these poor metabolizers appears normal. When compared with normal metabolizers, the total sum at steady state of the plasma concentrations of the 4 active enantiomers was not significantly greater among poor metabolizers. Thus, the net pharmacodynamic activities were essentially the same. Alternative, nonsaturable pathways (non-IID6) also contribute to the metabolism of Fluoxetine. This explains how Fluoxetine achieves a steady-state concentration rather than increasing without limit.

Because Fluoxetine's metabolism, like that of a number of other compounds including tricyclic and other selective serotonin antidepressants, involves the P450IID6 system, concomitant therapy with drugs also metabolized by this enzyme system (such as the tricyclic antidepressants) may lead to drug interactions (see *"Drug Interactions"* under *"Precautions"*).

Accumulation and Slow Elimination: The relatively slow elimination of Fluoxetine (elimination half-life of 1 to 3 days after acute administration and 4 to 6 days after chronic administration) and its active metabolite, norfluoxetine (elimination half-life of 4 to 16 days after acute and chronic administration), leads to significant accumulation of these active species in chronic use. After 30 days of dosing at 40 mg/day, plasma concentrations of Fluoxetine in the range of 91 to 302 ng/mL and norfluoxetine in the range of 72 to 258 ng/mL have been observed. Plasma concentrations of Fluoxetine were higher than those predicted by single-dose studies, because Fluoxetine's metabolism is not proportional to dose. Norfluoxetine, however, appears to have linear pharmacokinetics. Its mean terminal half-life after after a single dose was 8.6 days and after multiple dosing was 9.3 days. Steady state levels after prolonged dosing are similar to levels seen at 4-5 weeks.

The long elimination half-lives of Fluoxetine and norfluoxetine assure that, even when dosing is stopped, active drug substance will persist in the body for weeks (primarily depending on individual patient characteristics, previous dosing regimen, and length of previous therapy at discontinuation). This is of potential consequence when drug discontinuation is required or when drugs are prescribed that might interact with Fluoxetine and norfluoxetine following the discontinuation of Fluoxetine Hydrochloride.

Liver Disease: As might be predicted from its primary site of metabolism, liver impairment can affect the elimination of Fluoxetine. The elimination half-life of Fluoxetine was prolonged in a study of cirrhotic patients, with a mean of 7.6 days compare to the range of 2 to 3 days seen in subjects without liver disease; norfluoxetine elimination was also delayed, with a mean duration of 12 days for cirrhotic patients compared to the range of 7 to 9 days in normal subjects. This suggests that the use of Fluoxetine in patients with liver disease must be approached with caution. If Fluoxetine is administered to patients with liver disease, a lower or less frequent dose should be used (see *"Precautions"* and *"Dosage and Administration"*).

Renal Disease: In single dose studies, the pharmacokinetics of Fluoxetine and norfluoxetine were similar among subjects with all levels of impaired renal function including anephric patients on chronic hemodialysis. However, with chronic administration, additional accumulation of Fluoxetine or its metabolites (possibly including some not yet identified) may occur in patients with severely impaired renal function and use of a lower or less frequent dose is advised (see *"Precautions"*).

Age: The disposition of single doses of Fluoxetine in healthy elderly subjects (greater than 65 years of age) did not differ significantly from that in younger normal subjects. However, given the long half-life and nonlinear disposition of the drug, a single-dose study is not adequate to rule out the possibility of altered pharmacokinetics in the elderly, particularly if they have systemic illness or are receiving multiple drugs for concomitant diseases. The effects of age upon the metabolism of Fluoxetine have been investigated in 260 elderly but otherwise healthy depressed patients ($\geq$ 60 years of age) who received 20 mg Fluoxetine for 6 weeks. Combined Fluoxetine plus norfluoxetine plasma concentrations were 209.3 $\pm$ 85.7 ng/mL at the end of 6 weeks. No unusual age-associated pattern of adverse events was observed in those elderly patients.

CLINICAL TRIALS

Depression: The efficacy of Fluoxetine Hydrochloride for the treatment of patients with depression ($\geq$ 18 years of age) has been studied in 5- and 6-week placebo-controlled trials. Fluoxetine Hydrochloride was shown to be significantly more effective than placebo as measured by the Hamilton Depression Rating Scale (HAM-D). Fluoxetine Hydrochloride was also significantly more effective than placebo on the HAM-D subscores for depressed mood, sleep disturbance, and the anxiety subfactor.

Two 6-week controlled studies comparing Fluoxetine Hydrochloride, 20 mg, and placebo have shown Fluoxetine Hydrochloride, 20 mg daily, to be effective in the treatment of elderly patients ($\geq$ 60 years of age) with depression. In these studies, Fluoxetine Hydrochloride produced a significantly higher rate of response and remission as defined respectively by a 50% decrease in the HAM-D score and a total endpoint HAM-D score of $\leq$ 7. Fluoxetine Hydrochloride was well tolerated and the rate of treatment discontinuations due to adverse events did not differ between Fluoxetine Hydrochloride (12%) and placebo (9%).

Obsessive Compulsive Disorder: The effectiveness of Fluoxetine Hydrochloride for the treatment for obsessive compulsive disorder (OCD) was demonstrated in two 13-week, multicenter, parallel group studies (Studies 1 and 2) of adult outpatients who received fixed Fluoxetine Hydrochloride doses of 20, 40, or 60 mg/day (on a once a day schedule, in the morning) or placebo. Patients in both studies had moderate to severe OCD (DSM-III-R), with mean baseline ratings on the Yale-Brown Obsessive Compulsive Scale (YBOCS,total score) ranging from 22 to 26. In Study 1, patients receiving Fluoxetine Hydrochloride experienced mean reductions of approximately 4 to 6 units on the YBOCS total score, compared to a 1-unit reduction for placebo patients. In Study 2, patients receiving Fluoxetine Hydrochloride experienced mean reductions of approximately 4 to 6 units on the YBOCS total score, compared to a 1-unit reduction for placebo patients. While there was no indication of a dose response relationship for effectiveness in Study 1, a dose response relationship was observed in Study 2, with numerically better responses in the 2 higher dose groups. The following table provides the outcome classification by treatment group on the CGI improvement scale for studies 1 and 2 combined.

OUTCOME CLASSIFICATION (%) ON CGI IMPROVEMENT SCALE FOR COMPLETERS IN POOL OF TWO OCD STUDIES

Classification	Placebo	Fluoxetine Hydrochloride		
		20 mg	40 mg	60 mg
Worse	8%	0%	0%	0%
No Change	64%	41%	33%	29%
Minimally Improved	17%	23%	28%	24%
Much Improved	8%	28%	27%	28%
Very Much Improved	3%	8%	12%	19%

Exploratory analyses for age and gender effects on outcome did not suggest any differential responsiveness on the basis of age or sex.

INDICATIONS AND USAGE

Depression: Fluoxetine Hydrochloride is indicated for the treatment of depression. The efficacy of Fluoxetine Hydrochloride was established in 5- and 6-week trials with depressed outpatients ($\geq$ 18 years of age) whose diagnoses corresponded most closely to the DSM-III category of major depressive disorder. (see *"Clinical Trials"* under *"Clinical Pharmacology"*).

A major depressive episode implies a prominent and relatively persistent depressed or dysphoric mood that usually interferes with daily functioning (nearly every day for at least 2 weeks); it should include at least 4 of the following 8 symptoms: change in appetite, change in sleep, psychomotor agitation or retardation, loss of interest in usual activities or decrease in sexual drive, increased fatigue, feelings of guilt or worthlessness, slowed thinking or impaired concentration, and a suicide attempt or suicidal ideation.

The antidepressant action of Fluoxetine Hydrochloride in hospitalized depressed patients has not been adequately studied.

The effectiveness of Fluoxetine Hydrochloride in long-term use that is for more than 5 to 6 weeks, has not been systematically evaluated in controlled trials. Therefore, the physician who elects to use Fluoxetine Hydrochloride for extended periods should periodically reevaluate the long-term usefulness of the drug for the individual patient.

Obsessive-Compulsive Disorder: Fluoxetine Hydrochloride is indicated for the treatment of obsessions and compulsions in patients with obsessive-compulsive disorder (OCD), as defined in the DSM-III-R.-; i.e., the obsessions or compulsions cause marked distress, are time-consuming, or significantly interfere with social or occupational functioning.

The efficacy of Fluoxetine Hydrochloride was established in 13-week trials with obsessive-compulsive outpatients whose diagnoses corresponded most closely to the DSM-III-R category of obsessive-compulsive disorder (see *"Clinical Trials"* under *"Clinical Pharmacology"*).

Obsessive-compulsive disorder is characterized by recurrent and persistent ideas, thoughts, impulses, or images (obsessions) that are ego-dystonic and/or repetitive, purposeful, and intentional behaviors (compulsions) that are recognized by the person as excessive or unreasonable.

The effectiveness of Fluoxetine Hydrochloride in long-term use, i.e., for more than 13 weeks, has not been systematically evaluated in placebo-controlled trials. Therefore, the physician who elects to use Fluoxetine Hydrochloride for extended periods should periodically reevaluate the long-term usefulness of the drug for the individual patient (see *"Dosage and Administration"*).

UNLABELED USES

Fluoxetine is used alone or as an adjunct in the treatment of panic attacks, diabetic neuropathy, and kleptomania. It is also used in the treatment of eating disorders, including obesity and bulimia nervosa.

CONTRAINDICATIONS

Fluoxetine Hydrochloride is contraindicated in patients known to be hypersensitive to it.

Monoamine Oxidase Inhibitors: There have been reports of serious, sometimes fatal, reactions (including hyperthermia, rigidity, myoclonus, autonomic instability with possible rapid fluctuations of vital signs, and mental status changes that include extreme agitation progressing to delirium and coma) in patients receiving Fluoxetine in combination with a monoamine oxidase inhibitor (MAOI), and in patients who have recently discontinued Fluoxetine and are then started on an MAOI. Some cases presented with features resembling neuroleptic malignant syndrome. Therefore Fluoxetine Hydrochloride should not be used in combination with an MAOI, or within 14 days of discontinuing therapy with an MAOI. Since Fluoxetine and its major metabolite have very long elimination half-lives, at least 5 weeks (perhaps longer, especially if Fluoxetine has been prescribed chronically and/or at higher doses [see *"Accumulation and Slow Elimination"* under *"Clinical Pharmacology"*]) should be allowed after stopping Fluoxetine Hydrochloride before starting an MAOI.

WARNINGS

Rash and Possibly Allergic Events: During premarketing testing of more than 5,600 US patients given Fluoxetine, approximately 4% developed a rash and/or urticaria. Among these cases, almost a third were withdrawn from treatment because of the rash and/or systemic signs or symptoms associated with the rash. Clinical findings reported in association with rash include fever, leukocytosis, arthralgias, edema, carpal tunnel syndrome, respiratory distress, lymphadenopathy, proteinuria, and mild transaminase elevation. Most patients improved promptly with discontinuation of Fluoxetine and/or adjunctive treatment with antihistamines or steroids, and all patients experiencing these events were reported to recover completely.

In premarketing clinical trials, 2 patients are known to have developed a serious cutaneous systemic illness. In neither patient was there an unequivocal diagnosis, but 1 was considered to have a leukocytoclastic vasculitis, and the other, a severe desquamating syndrome that was considered variously to be a vasculitis or erythema multiforme. Other patients have had systemic syndrome suggestive of serum sickness.

Since the introduction of Fluoxetine Hydrochloride, systemic events, possibly related to vasculitis, have developed in patients with rash. Although these events are rare, they may be serious, involving the lung, kidney, or liver. Death has been reported to occur in association with these systemic events.

Anaphylactoid events, including bronchospasm, angioedema, and urticaria alone and in combination, have been reported.

Pulmonary events, including inflammatory processes of varying histopathology and/or fibrosis, have been reported rarely. These events have occurred with dyspnea as the only preceding symptom.

Whether these systemic events and rash have a common underlying cause or are due to different etiologies or pathogenic processes is not known. Furthermore, a specific underlying immunologic basis for these events has not been identified. Upon the appearance of rash or of other possibly allergic phenomena for which an alternative etiology cannot be identified, Fluoxetine Hydrochloride should be discontinued.

PRECAUTIONS

General: Anxiety and Insomnia: Anxiety, nervousness, and insomnia were reported by 10% to 15% of patients treated with Fluoxetine Hydrochloride. These symptoms led to drug discontinuation in 5% of patients treated with Fluoxetine Hydrochloride.

In controlled clinical trials for obsessive-compulsive disorder, insomnia was reported in 30% of patients treated with Fluoxetine Hydrochloride and in 22% of patients treated with placebo. Anxiety was reported in 14% of patients treated with Fluoxetine Hydrochloride and in 7% of patients treated with placebo. These 2 symptoms led to drug discontinuation in 2% of patients treated with Fluoxetine Hydrochloride and no patients treated with placebo.

Altered Appetite and Weight: Significant weight loss, especially in underweight depressed patients, may be an undesirable result of treatment with Fluoxetine Hydrochloride.

In controlled clinical trials, approximately 9% of patients treated with Fluoxetine Hydrochloride experienced anorexia. This incidence is approximately sixfold that seen in placebo controls. A weight loss of greater than 5% of body weight occurred in 13% of patients treated with Fluoxetine Hydrochloride compared to 4% of placebo and 3% of patients treated with tricyclics. However, only rarely have patients discontinued treatment with Fluoxetine Hydrochloride because of weight loss.

In controlled clinical trials for OCD, 17% of patients treated with Fluoxetine Hydrochloride and 10% of patients treated with placebo reported anorexia. One patient discontinued treatment with Fluoxetine Hydrochloride because of anorexia.

Activation of Mania/Hypomania: During premarketing testing, hypomania or mania occurred in approximately 1% of Fluoxetine treated patients. Activation of mania/hypomania has also been reported in a small proportion of patients with Major Affective Disorder treated with other marketed antidepressants.

Mania/hypomania was reported in 1% of patients treated with Fluoxetine in controlled clinical OCD trials.

Seizures: Twelve patients among more than 6,000 evaluated worldwide in the course of premarketing development of Fluoxetine experienced convulsions (or events described as possibly having been seizures), a rate of 0.2% that appears to be similar to that associated with other marketed antidepressants. Fluoxetine Hydrochloride should be introduced with care in patients with a history of seizures.

In controlled clinical trials for OCD, 1 patient treated with Fluoxetine experienced a seizure.

Suicide: The possibility of a suicide attempt is inherent in depression and may persist until significant remission occurs. Close supervision of high risk patients should accompany initial drug therapy. Prescriptions for Fluoxetine Hydrochloride should be written for the smallest quantity of capsules consistent with good patient management, in order to reduce the risk of overdose.

The Long Elimination Half-Lives of Fluoxetine and Its Metabolites: Because of the long elimination half-lives of the parent drug and its major active metabolite, changes in dose will not be fully reflected in plasma for several weeks, affecting both strategies for titration to final dose and withdrawal from treatment (see *"Clinical Pharmacology"* and *"Dosage and Administration"*).

Use in Patients With Concomitant Illness: Clinical experience with Fluoxetine Hydrochloride in patients with concomitant systemic illness is limited. Caution is advisable in using Fluoxetine Hydrochloride in patients with diseases or conditions that could affect metabolism or hemodynamic responses.

Fluoxetine has *not* been evaluated or used to any appreciable extent in patients with a recent history of myocardial infarction or unstable heart disease. Patients with these diagnoses were systematically excluded from clinical studies during the product's premarket testing. However, the electrocardiograms of 312 patients who received Fluoxetine Hydrochloride in double-blind trials were retrospectively evaluated; no conduction abnormalities that resulted in heart block were observed. The mean heart rate was reduced by approximately 3 beats/min. In subjects with cirrhosis of the liver, the clearances of Fluoxetine and its active metabolite, norfluoxetine, were decreased, thus increasing the elimination half-lives of these substances. A lower or less frequent dose should be used in patients with cirrhosis.

Since Fluoxetine is extensively metabolized, excretion of unchanged drug in urine is a minor route of elimination. However, until adequate numbers of patients with severe renal impairment have been evaluated during chronic treatment with Fluoxetine, it should be used with caution in such patients.

In patients with diabetes, Fluoxetine Hydrochloride may alter glycemic control. Hypoglycemia has occurred during therapy with Fluoxetine Hydrochloride and hyperglycemia has developed following discontinuation of the drug. As is true with many other types of medication when taken concurrently by patients with diabetes, insulin and/or oral hypoglycemic dosage may need to be adjusted when therapy with Fluoxetine Hydrochloride is instituted or discontinued.

Interference with Cognitive and Motor Performance: Any psychoactive drug may impair judgment, thinking, or motor skills, and patients should be cautioned about operating hazardous machinery, including automobiles, until they are reasonably certain that the drug treatment does not affect them adversely.

Information for Patients: Physicians are advised to discuss the following issues with patients for whom they prescribe Fluoxetine Hydrochloride:

Because Fluoxetine Hydrochloride may impair judgment, thinking, or motor skills, patients should be advised to avoid driving a car or operating hazardous machinery until they are reasonably certain that their performance is not affected.

Patients should be advised to inform their physician if they are taking or plan to take any prescription or over-the-counter drugs, or alcohol.

Patients should be advised to notify their physician if they become pregnant or intend to become pregnant during therapy.

Patients should be advised to notify their physician if they are breast feeding an infant.

Patients should be advised to notify their physician if they develop a rash or hives.

Laboratory Tests: There are no specific laboratory tests recommended.

Drug Interactions: As with all drugs, the potential for interaction by a variety of mechanisms (eg, pharmacodynamic, pharmacokinetic drug inhibition or enhancement, etc.) is a possibility (see *"Accumulation and Slow Elimination"* under *"Clinical Pharmacology"*).

Drugs Metabolized by P450IID6: Approximately 7% of the normal population has a genetic defect that leads to reduced levels of activity of the cytochrome P450 isoenzyme P450IID6. Such individuals have been referred to as "poor metabolizers" of drugs such as debrisoquin, dextromethorphan, and tricyclic antidepressants. Many drugs, such as most antidepressants including Fluoxetine and other selective uptake inhibitors of serotonin, are metabolized by this isoenzyme; thus, both the pharmacokinetic properties and relative proportion of metabolites are altered in poor metabolizers. However, for Fluoxetine and its metabolite the sum of the plasma concentrations of the 4 active enantiomers is comparable between poor and extensive metabolizers (see *"Variability in Metabolism"* under *"Clinical Pharmacology"*).

Fluoxetine, like other agents that are metabolized by P450IID6, inhibits the activity of this isoenzyme, and thus may make normal metabolizers resemble "poor metabolizers." Therapy with medications that are predominantly metabolized by the P450IID6 system and that have a relatively narrow therapeutic index (see list below), should be initiated at the low end of the dose range if a patient is receiving Fluoxetine concurrently or has taken it in the previous 5 weeks. Thus, his/her dosing requirements resemble those of "poor metabolizers." If Fluoxetine is added to the treatment regimen of a patient already receiving a drug metabolized by P450IID6, the need for decreased dose of the original medication, should be considered. Drugs with a narrow therapeutic index represent the greatest concern (eg, flecainide, vinblastine, carbamazepine, and tricyclic antidepressants).

Tryptophan: Five patients receiving Fluoxetine Hydrochloride in combination with tryptophan experienced adverse reactions, including agitation, restlessness, and gastrointestinal distress.

Monoamine Oxidase Inhibitors: See *"Contraindications"*.

Other Antidepressants: There have been greater than 2-fold increases of previously stable plasma levels of other antidepressants when Fluoxetine Hydrochloride has been administered in combination with these agents (see *"Accumulation and Slow Elimination"* under *"Clinical Pharmacology"*).

Lithium: There have been reports of both increased and decreased lithium levels when lithium was used concomitantly with Fluoxetine. Cases of lithium toxicity have been reported. Lithium levels should be monitored when these drugs are administered concomitantly.

Diazepam Clearance: The half-life of concurrently administered diazepam may be prolonged in some patients (see *"Accumulation and Slow Elimination"* under *"Clinical Pharmacology"*).

Phenytoin: Patients on stable doses of phenytoin have developed elevated plasma phenytoin concentrations and clinical phenytoin toxicity following initiation of concomitant Fluoxetine treatment.

Potential Effects of Coadministration of Drugs Tightly Bound to Plasma Proteins: Because Fluoxetine is tightly bound to plasma protein, the administration of Fluoxetine to a patient taking another drug that is tightly bound to protein (e.g., Coumadin, digitoxin) may cause a shift in plasma concentrations potentially resulting in an adverse effect. Conversely, adverse effects may result from displacement of protein bound Fluoxetine by other tightly bound drugs (see *"Accumulation and Slow Elimination"* under *"Clinical Pharmacology"*).

CNS Active Drugs: The risk of using Fluoxetine Hydrochloride in combination with other CNS active drugs has not been systematically evaluated. Consequently, caution is advised if the concomitant administration of Fluoxetine Hydrochloride and such drugs is required (see *"Accumulation and Slow Elimination"* under *"Clinical Pharmacology"*).

Electroconvulsive Therapy: There are no clinical studies establishing the benefit of the combined use of ECT and Fluoxetine. There have been rare reports of prolonged seizures in patients on Fluoxetine receiving ECT treatment.

Carcinogenesis, Mutagenesis, Impairment of Fertility: There is no evidence of carcinogenicity, mutagenicity, or impairment of fertility with Fluoxetine Hydrochloride.

The dietary administration of Fluoxetine to rats and mice for 2 years at levels equivalent to approximately 7.5 and 9.0 times the maximum human dose (80 mg) respectively produced no evidence of carcinogenicity.

Fluoxetine and norfluoxetine have been shown to have no genotoxic effects based on the following assays: bacterial mutation assay, DNA repair assay in cultured rat hepatocytes, mouse lymphoma assay, and in vivo sister chromatid exchange assay in Chinese hamster bone marrow cells.

Two fertility studies conducted in rats at doses of approximately 5 and 9 times the maximum human dose (80 mg) indicated that Fluoxetine had no adverse effects on fertility. A slight decrease in neonatal survival was noted, but this was probably associated with depressed maternal food consumption and suppressed weight gain.

Pregnancy: Teratogenic Effects: Pregnancy Category B: Reproduction studies have been performed in rats and rabbits at doses 9 and 11 times the maximum daily human dose (80 mg) respectively and have revealed no evidence of harm to the fetus due to Fluoxetine Hydrochloride. There are, however, no adequate and well-controlled studies in pregnant women. Because animal reproduction studies are not always predictive of human response, this drug should be used during pregnancy only if clearly needed.

Labor and Delivery: The effect of Fluoxetine Hydrochloride on labor and delivery in humans is unknown.

Nursing Mothers: Because Fluoxetine Hydrochloride is excreted in human milk, nursing while on Fluoxetine Hydrochloride is not recommended. In 1 breast milk sample, the concentration of Fluoxetine plus norfluoxetine was 70.4 ng/mL. The concentration in the mother's plasma was 295.0 ng/mL. No adverse effects on the infant were reported.

In another case, an infant nursed by a mother on Fluoxetine Hydrochloride developed crying, sleep disturbance, vomiting, and watery stools. The infant's plasma drug levels were 240 ng/mL of Fluoxetine and 208 ng/mL of norfluoxetine on the second day of feeding.

Usage in Children: Safety and effectiveness in children have not been established.

Usage in the Elderly: Evaluation of patients over the age of 60 who received Fluoxetine Hydrochloride 20 mg daily revealed no unusual pattern of adverse events relative to the clinical experience in younger patients.

However, these data are insufficient to rule out possible age-related differences during chronic use, particularly in elderly patients who have concomitant systemic illnesses or who are receiving concomitant drugs (see *"Age"* under *"Clinical Pharmacology"*).

Hyponatremia: Several cases of hyponatremia (some with serum sodium lower than 110 mmol/L) have been reported. The hyponatremia appeared to be reversible when Fluoxetine Hydrochloride was discontinued. Although these cases were complex with varying possible etiologies, some were possibly due to the syndrome of inappropriate antidiuretic hormone secretion (SIADH). The majority of these occurrences have been in older patients and in patients taking diuretics or who were otherwise volume depleted.

In a placebo-controlled, double-blind trial, 10 of 313 Fluoxetine patients and 6 of 320 placebo recipients had a lowering of serum sodium below the reference range; this difference was not statistically significant. The lowest observed concentration was 129 mmol/L. The observed decreases were not clinically significant.

Platelet Function: There have been rare reports of alterd platelet function and/or abnormal results from laboratory studies in patients taking Fluoxetine. While there have been reports of abnormal bleeding in several patients taking Fluoxetine, it is unclear whether Fluoxetine had a causative role.

ADVERSE REACTIONS

Commonly Observed: The most commonly observed adverse events associated with the use of Fluoxetine Hydrochloride and not seen at an equivalent incidence among placebo-treated patients were: nervous system complaints, including anxiety, nervousness, and insomnia; drowsiness and fatigue or asthenia; tremor; sweating; gastrointestinal complaints, including anorexia, nausea, and diarrhea; and dizziness or lightheadedness.

In controlled clinical trials for OCD using fixed doses of 20, 40, or 60 mg daily, adverse events observed at an incidence of at least 5% for Fluoxetine Hydrochloride and for which the incidence was approximately twice or more the incidence among placebo-treated patients included: somnolence, anxiety, tremor, nausea, dyspepsia, gastrointestinal disorder, vasodilatation, dry mouth, sweating, rash, abnormal vision, yawn, decreased libido, and abnormal ejaculation.

Associated With Discontinuation of Treatment: Fifteen percent of approximately 4,000 patients who received Fluoxetine Hydrochloride in US premarketing clinical trials discontinued treatment due to an adverse event. The more common events causing discontinuation included: psychiatric (5.3%), primarily nervousness, anxiety, and insomnia; digestive (3.0%), primarily nausea; nervous system (1.6%), primarily dizziness; body as a whole (1.5%), primarily asthenia and headache; and skin (1.4%), primarily rash and pruritus.

In controlled clinical trials for OCD, 12% of patients treated with Fluoxetine Hydrochloride discontinued treatment due to adverse events. The most common events were anxiety (2%) and rash/urticaria (2%).

Incidence in Controlled Clinical Trials: Depression: Table 1 enumerates adverse events that occurred at a frequency of 1% or more among patients treated with Fluoxetine Hydrochloride who participated in controlled trials comparing Fluoxetine Hydrochloride with placebo.

Obsessive-Compulsive Disorder: Table 2 enumerates adverse events that occurred at a frequency of 2% or more among patients on Fluoxetine Hydrochloride who participated in controlled trials comparing Fluoxetine Hydrochloride with placebo in the treatment of OCD.

The prescriber should be aware that the figures in Tables 1 and 2 cannot be used to predict the incidence of side effects in the course of usual medical practice where patient characteristics and other factors differ from those that prevailed in the clinical trials. Similarly, the cited frequencies cannot be compared with figures obtained from other clinical investigations involving different treatments, uses, and investigators. The cited figures, however, do provide the prescribing physician with some basis for estimating the relative contribution of drug and nondrug factors to the side effect incidence rate in the population studied. (See related tables.)

Other Events Observed During Premarketing Evaluation of Fluoxetine Hydrochloride: During clinical testing in the US, multiple doses of Fluoxetine Hydrochloride were administered to approximately 5,600 subjects. Untoward events associated with this exposure were recorded by clinical investigators using descriptive terminology of their own choosing. Consequently, it is not possible to provide a meaningful estimate of the proportion of individuals experiencing adverse events without first grouping similar types of untoward events into a limited (i.e., reduced) number of standardized event categories.

◆ RATED THERAPEUTICALLY EQUIVALENT; ◇ THERAPEUTIC EQUIVALENCE UNCONFIRMED; ○ UNRATED

In the tabulations that follow, a standard COSTART Dictionary terminology has been used to classify reported adverse events. The frequencies presented, therefore, represent the proportion of the 5,600 individuals exposed to Fluoxetine Hydrochloride who experienced an event of the type cited on at least 1 occasion while receiving Fluoxetine Hydrochloride. All reported events are included except those already listed in Table 1, those COSTART terms so general as to be uninformative, and those events where a drug cause was remote. It is important to emphasize that, although the events reported did occur during treatment with Fluoxetine Hydrochloride they were not necessarily caused by it.

Events are further classified within body system categories and enumerated in order of decreasing frequency using the following definitions: frequent adverse events are defined as those occurring on 1 or more occasions in at least 1/100 patients; infrequent adverse events are those occurring in 1/100 to 1/1,000 patients; rare events are those occurring in less than 1/1,000 patients.

Body as a Whole: Frequent: chills; *Infrequent*: chills and fever, cyst, face edema, hangover effect, jaw pain, malaise, neck pain, neck rigidity, and pelvic pain; *Rare*: abdomen enlarged, cellulitis, hydrocephalus, hypothermia, LE syndrome, moniliasis, and serum sickness.

Cardiovascular System: Infrequent: angina pectoris, arrhythmia, hemorrhage, hypertension, hypotension, migraine, postural hypotension, syncope, and tachycardia; *Rare*: AV block first degree, bradycardia, bundle branch block, cerebral ischemia, myocardial infarct, thrombophlebitis, vascular headache, and ventricular arrhythmia.

Digestive System: Frequent: increased appetite; *Infrequent*: aphthous stomatitis, dysphagia, eructation, esophagitis, gastritis, gingivitis, glossitis, liver function tests abnormal, melena, stomatitis, thirst; *Rare*: bloody diarrhea, cholecystitis, cholelithiasis, colitis, duodenal ulcer, enteritis, fecal incontinence, hematemesis, hepatitis, hepatomegaly, hyperchlorhydria, increased salivation, jaundice, liver tenderness, mouth ulceration, salivary gland enlargement, stomach ulcer, tongue discoloration, and tongue edema.

Endocrine System: Infrequent: hypothyroidism; *Rare*: goiter and hyperthyroidism.

Hemic and Lymphatic System: Infrequent: anemia and lymphadenopathy; *Rare*: bleeding time increased, blood dyscrasia, leukopenia, lymphocytosis, petechia, purpura, sedimentation rate increased, and thrombocythemia.

Metabolic and Nutritional: Frequent: weight loss; *Infrequent*: generalized edema, hypoglycemia, peripheral edema, and weight gain; *Rare*: dehydration, gout, hypercholesteremia, hyperglycemia, hyperlipemia, hypoglycemic reaction, hypokalemia, hyponatremia, and iron deficiency anemia.

Musculoskeletal System: Infrequent: arthritis, bone pain, bursitis, tenosynovitis, and twitching; *Rare*: bone necrosis, chondrodystrophy, muscle hemorrhage, myositis, osteoporosis, pathological fracture, and rheumatoid arthritis.

Nervous System: Frequent: abnormal dreams and agitation; *Infrequent*: abnormal gait, acute brain syndrome, akathisia, amnesia, apathy, ataxia, buccoglossal syndrome, CNS stimulation, convulsion, delusions, depersonalization, emotional lability, euphoria, hallucinations, hostility, hyperkinesia, hypesthesia, incoordination, libido increased, manic reaction, neuralgia, neuropathy, paranoid reaction, psychosis, and vertigo; *Rare*: abnormal electroencephalogram, antisocial reaction, chronic brain syndrome, circumoral paresthesia, CNS depression, coma, dysarthria, dystonia, extrapyramidal syndrome, hypertonia, hysteria, myoclonus, nystagmus, paralysis, reflexes decreased, stupor, and torticollis.

Respiratory System: Frequent: bronchitis, rhinitis, and yawn; *Infrequent*: asthma, epistaxis, hiccup, hyperventilation, and pneumonia; *Rare*: apnea, hemoptysis, hypoxia, larynx edema, lung edema, lung fibrosis/alveolitis, and pleural effusion.

Skin and Appendages: Infrequent: acne, alopecia, contact dermatitis, dry skin, herpes simplex, maculopapular rash, and urticaria; *Rare*: eczema, erythema multiforme, fungal dermatitis, herpes zoster, hirsutism, psoriasis, purpuric rash, pustular rash, seborrhea, skin discoloration, skin hypertrophy, subcutaneous nodule, and vesiculobullous rash.

Table 1

TREATMENT-EMERGENT ADVERSE EXPERIENCE INCIDENCE IN PLACEBO-CONTROLLED CLINICAL TRIALS

Body System/Preferred Term*	*Percentage of Patients Reporting Event*		Body System/Preferred Term*	*Percentage of Patients Reporting Event*	
	Fluoxetine Hydrochloride (N = 1,730)	Placebo (N = 799)		Fluoxetine Hydrochloride (N = 1,730)	Placebo (N = 799)
Nervous			**Body as a Whole**		
Headache	20.3	15.5	Asthenia	4.4	1.9
Nervousness	14.9	8.5	Infection, viral	3.4	3.1
Insomnia	13.8	7.1	Pain, limb	1.6	1.1
Drowsiness	11.6	6.3	Fever	1.4	—
Anxiety	9.4	5.5	Pain, chest	1.3	1.1
Tremor	7.9	2.4	Allergy	1.2	1.1
Dizziness	5.7	3.3	Influenza	1.2	1.5
Fatigue	4.2	1.1	**Respiratory**		
Sedated	1.9	1.3	Upper respiratory infection	7.6	6.0
Sensation disturbance	1.7	2.0	Flu-like syndrome	2.8	1.9
Libido, decreased	1.6	—	Pharyngitis	2.7	1.3
Light headedness	1.6	—	Nasal congestion	2.6	2.3
Concentration, decreased	1.5	—	Headache, sinus	2.3	1.8
Digestive			Sinusitis	2.1	2.0
Nausea	21.1	10.1	Cough	1.6	1.6
Diarrhea	12.3	7.0	Dyspnea	1.4	—
Mouth dryness	9.5	6.0	**Cardiovascular**		
Anorexia	8.7	1.5	Hot flushes	1.8	1.0
Dyspepsia	6.4	4.3	Palpitations	1.3	1.4
Constipation	4.5	3.3	**Musculoskeletal**		
Pain, abdominal	3.4	2.9	Pain, back	2.0	2.4
Vomiting	2.4	1.3	Pain, joint	1.2	1.1
Taste change	1.8	—	Pain, muscle	1.2	1.0
Flatulence	1.6	1.1	**Urogenital**		
Gastroenteritis	1.0	1.4	Menstruation, painful†	2.6	2.1
Skin and Appendages			Sexual dysfunction	1.9	—
Sweating, excessive	8.4	3.8	Impotence, sexual‡	1.7	0.4
			Frequent micturition	1.6	—
Rash	2.7	1.8	Urinary tract infection	1.2	—
Pruritus	2.4	1.4	**Special Senses**		
			Vision disturbance	2.8	1.8

* Events reported by at least 1% of patients treated with Fluoxetine Hydrochloride are included.
† Denominator used was females only (N = 1,210 Fluoxetine Hydrochloride; N = 523 placebo).
‡ Denominator used was male only (N = 520 Fluoxetine Hydrochloride; N = 276 placebo).

— Incidence less than 1%.

Special Senses: Infrequent: amblyopia, conjunctivitis, ear pain, eye pain, mydriasis, photophobia, and tinnitus; *Rare*: blepharitis, cataract, corneal lesion, deafness, diplopia, eye hemorrhage, glaucoma, iritis, ptosis, strabismus, and taste loss.

Urogenital System: Infrequent: abnormal ejaculation, amenorrhea, breast pain, cystitis, dysuria, fibrocystic breast, impotence, leukorrhea, menopause, menorrhagia, ovarian disorder, urinary incontinence, urinary retention, urinary urgency, urination impaired, and vaginitis; *Rare*: abortion, albuminuria, breast enlargement, dyspareunia, epididymitis, female lactation, hematuria, hypomenorrhea, kidney calculus, metrorrhagia, orchitis, polyuria, pyelonephritis, pyuria, salpingitis, urethral pain, urethritis, urinary tract disorder, urolithiasis, uterine hemorrhage, uterine spasm, and vaginal hemorrhage.

Postintroduction Reports: Voluntary reports of adverse events temporally associated with Fluoxetine Hydrochloride that have been received since market introduction that are not listed above, and that may have no causal relationship with the drug include the following: aplastic anemia, cerebral vascular accident, confusion, dyskinesia (including, for example, a case of buccal-lingual-masticatory syndrome with involuntary tongue protrusion reported to develop in a 77-year-old female after 5 weeks of Fluoxetine therapy and which completely resolved over the next few months following drug discontinuation), eosinophilic pneumonia, hyperprolactinemia, immune-related hemoly- tic anemia, movement disorders developing in patients with risk factors including drugs associated with such events and worsening of preexisting movement disorders, neuroleptic malignant syndrome-like events, pancreatitis, pancytopenia, suicidal ideation, thrombocytopenia, thrombocytopenic purpura, vaginal bleeding after drug withdrawal, and violent behaviors.

DRUG ABUSE AND DEPENDENCE
Controlled Substance Class: Fluoxetine Hydrochloride is not a controlled substance.

Physical and Psychological Dependence: Fluoxetine Hydrochloride has not been systematically studied, in animals or humans, for its potential for abuse, tolerance, or physical dependence. While the premarketing clinical experience with Fluoxetine Hydrochloride did not reveal any tendency for a withdrawal syndrome or any drug seeking behavior, these observations were not systematic and it is not possible to predict on the basis of this limited experience the extent to which a CNS active drug will be misused, diverted, and/or abused once marketed. Consequently, physicians should carefully evaluate patients for history of drug abuse and follow such patients closely, observing them for signs of misuse or abuse of Fluoxetine Hydrochloride (eg, development of tolerance, incrementation of dose, drug-seeking behavior).

OVERDOSAGE
Human Experience: As of December 1987, there were 2 deaths among approximately 38 reports of acute overdose with Fluoxetine, either alone or in combination with other drugs and/or alcohol. One death involved a combined overdose with approximately 1,800 mg of Fluoxetine and an undetermined amount of maprotiline. Plasma concentrations of Fluoxetine and maprotiline were 4.57 mg/L and 4.18 mg/L, respectively. A second death involved 3 drugs yielding plasma concentrations as follows: Fluoxetine, 1.93 mg/L; norfluoxetine, 1.10 mg/L; codeine, 1.80 mg/L; and temazepam, 3.80 mg/L.

One other patient who reportedly took 3,000 mg of Fluoxetine experienced 2 grand mal seizures that remitted spontaneously without specific anticonvulsant treatment (see *"Management of Overdose"*). The actual amount of drug absorbed may have been less due to vomiting.

Nausea and vomiting were prominent in overdoses involving higher Fluoxetine doses. Other prominent symptoms of overdose included agitation, restlessness, hypomania, and other signs of CNS excitation. Except for the 2 deaths noted above, all other overdose cases recovered without residua.

Since introduction, reports of death attributed to overdosage of Fluoxetine alone have been extremely rare.

Animal Experience: Studies in animals do not provide precise or necessarily valid information about the treatment of human overdose. However, animal experiments can provide useful insights into possible treatment strategies.

The oral median lethal dose in rats and mice was found to be 452 and 248 mg/kg respectively. Acute high oral doses produced hyperirritability and convulsions in several animal species.

Among 6 dogs purposely overdosed with oral Fluoxetine, 5 experienced grand mal seizures. Seizures stopped immeidiately upon the bolus intravenous administration of a standard veterinary dose of diazepam. In this short term study, the lowest plasma concentration at which a seizure occurred was only twice the maximum plasma concentration seen in humans taking 80 mg/day, chronically.

Table 2
TREATMENT EMERGENT ADVERSE EXPERIENCE INCIDENCE OF PLACEBO-CONTROLLED CLINICAL TRIALS FOR OBSESSIVE-COMPULSIVE DISORDER

Body System/Preferred Term	Percent of Patients Reporting Events		Body System/Preferred Term	Percent of Patients Reporting Events	
	Fluoxetine Hydrochloride (N = 264)	Placebo (N = 89)		Fluoxetine Hydrochloride (N = 264)	Placebo (N = 89)
Nervous			**Body as a Whole**		
Insomnia	30	22	Headache	33	24
Somnolence	17	7	Asthenia	15	10
Anxiety	14	7	Flu syndrome	10	7
Dizziness	13	11	Pain	6	4
Libido, decreased	11	2	Injury, accidental	4	2
Tremor	9	1	Surgical procedure	—	
Abnormal dreams	5	2	Chest pain	3	1
Thinking, abnormal	4	2	Allergic reaction	3	—
Sleep disorder	3	1	Fever	2	1
Confusion	2	1	**Respiratory**		
Myoclonus	2	—	Pharyngitis	11	9
Agitation	2	1	Yawn	7	—
Amnesia	2	1	Sinusitis	5	2
Digestive			Cough, increased	3	2
Nausea	27	13	**Cardiovascular**		
Diarrhea	18	13	Vasodilatation	5	—
Anorexia	17	10	Palpitations	2	1
Dry mouth	12	3	**Musculoskeletal**		
Dyspepsia	10	4	Myalgia	5	4
Gastrointestinal disorder	6	1	Arthralgia	3	2
Melena	2	—	**Urogenital**		
Skin and Appendages			Urinary frequency	4	1
Sweating	7	—	Abnormal ejaculation†	7	—
Rash	6	3	**Hemic and Lymphatic**		
Pruritus	3	1	Lymphadenopathy	2	—
Acne	2	1	**Metabolic and Nutritional**		
			Weight loss	5	3
			Special Senses		
			Amblyopia	3	1
			Abnormal vision	2	—
			Taste perversion	2	1
			Tinnitus	2	—

* Events reported by at least 2% of patients treated with Fluoxetine Hydrochloride are included, except the following events which had an incidence on placebo ≥ Fluoxetine Hydrochloride abdominal pain, back pain, constipation, depression, dysmenorrhea, flatulence, infection, menstrual disorder, nervousness, rhinitis, tooth disorder, and twitching.
† Denominator used was males only (N = 116 Fluoxetine Hydrochloride; N = 43 placebo).
— Adverse event not reported by placebo-treated patients.

◆ RATED THERAPEUTICALLY EQUIVALENT; ◇ THERAPEUTIC EQUIVALENCE UNCONFIRMED; ○ UNRATED

In a separate single-dose study, the ECG in dogs given high doses did not reveal prolongation of the PR, QRS, or QT intervals. Tachycardia and an increase in blood pressure were observed. Consequently, the value of the ECG in predicting cardiac toxicity is unknown. Nonetheless, the ECG should ordinarily be monitored in cases of human overdose (see *"Management of Overdose"*).

Management of Overdose: Establish and maintain an airway; ensure adequate oxygenation and ventilation. Activated charcoal, which may be used with sorbitol, may be as or more effective than emesis or lavage, and should be considered in treating overdose.

Cardiac and vital signs monitoring is recommended, along with general symptomatic and supportive measures. Based on experience in animals, which may not be relevant to humans Fluoxetine-induced seizures that fail to remit spontaneous may respond to diazepam.

There are no specific antidotes for Fluoxetine Hydrochloride.

Due to the large volume of distribution of Fluoxetine Hydrochloride uresis, dialysis, hemoperfusion, and exchange transfusion are unlikely to be of benefit.

In managing overdosage, consider the possibility of multiple drug involvement. A specific caution involves patients taking or recently having taken Fluoxetine who might ingest by accident or intent, excessive quantitities of a tricyclic antidepressant. In such a case, accumulation of the parent tricyclic and an active metabolite may increase the possibility of clinically significant sequelae and extend the time needed for close medical observation (see *"Other Antidepressants"* under *"Precautions"*).

The physician should consider contacting a poison control center on the treatment of any overdose. Telephone numbers of certified poison control centers are listed in the *Physicians' Desk Reference (PDR)*.

DOSAGE AND ADMINISTRATION

DEPRESSION

Initial Treatment: In controlled trials used to support the efficacy of Fluoxetine, patients were administered morning doses ranging from 20 mg to 80 mg/day. Studies comparing Fluoxetine 20, 40, and 60 mg/day to placebo indicate that 20 mg/day is sufficient to obtain a satisfactory antidepressant response. Consequently, a dose of 20 mg/day, administered in the morning, is recommended as the initial dose.

A dose increase may be considered after several weeks if no clinical improvement is observed. Doses above 20 mg/day may be administered on a once a day (morning) or b.i.d. schedule (ie, morning and noon) and should not exceed a maximum dose of 80 mg/day. As with other antidepressants, the full antidepressant effect may be delayed until 4 weeks of treatment or longer.

As with many other medications, a lower or less frequent dosage should be used in patients with renal and/or hepatic impairment. A lower or less frequent dosage should also be considered for patients, such as the elderly with concurrent disease or on multiple medications. (see *"Usage in the Elderly"* under *"Precautions"*).

Maintenance/Continuation/Extended Treatment: There is no body of evidence available to answer the question of how long the patient treated with Fluoxetine should remain on it. It is generally agreed among expert psychopharmacologists (circa 1987) that acute episodes of depression require several months or longer of sustained pharmacologic therapy. Whether the dose of antidepressant needed to induce remission is identical to the dose needed to maintain and/or sustain euthymia is unknown.

OBSESSIVE-COMPULSIVE DISORDER

Initial Treatment: In the controlled clinical trials of Fluoxetine supporting its effectiveness in the treatment of obsessive-compulsive disorder, patients were administered fixed daily doses of 20, 40, or 60 mg of Fluoxetine or placebo (see *"Clinical Trials"* under *"Clinical Pharmacology"*). In one of these studies, no dose response relationship for effectiveness was demonstrated. Consequently, a dose of 20 mg/day, administered in the morning, is recommended as the initial dose. Since there was a suggestion of a possible dose response relationship for effectiveness in the second study, a dose increase may be considered after several weeks if insufficient clinical improvement is observed. The full therapeutic effect may be delayed until 5 weeks of treatment or longer.

Doses above 20 mg/day may be administered on a once a day (i.e., morning) or b.i.d. schedule (i.e., morning and noon). A dose range of 20 to 60 mg/day is recommended, however, doses of up to 80 mg/day have been well tolerated in open studies of OCD. The maximum Fluoxetine dose should not exceed 80 mg/day.

As with the use of Fluoxetine Hydrochloride in depression, a lower or less frequent dosage should be used in patients with renal and/or hepatic impairment. A lower or less frequent dosage should also be considered for patients, such as the elderly (see *"Usage in the Elderly"* under *"Precautions"*), with concurrent disease or on multiple medications.

Maintenance/Continuation Treatment: While there are no systematic studies that answer the question of how long to continue Fluoxetine Hydrochloride, OCD is a chronic condition and it is reasonable to consider continuation for a responding patient. Although the efficacy of Fluoxetine Hydrochloride after 13 weeks has not been documented in controlled trials, patients have been continued in therapy under double-blind conditions for up to an additional 6 months without loss of benefit. However, dosage adjustments should be made to maintain the patient on the lowest effective dosage, and patients should be periodically reassessed to determine the need for treatment.

ANIMAL TOXICOLOGY

Phospholipids are increased in some tissues of mice, rats, and dogs given Fluoxetine chronically. This effect is reversible after cessation of Fluoxetine treatment. Phospholipid accumulation in animals has been observed with many cationic amphiphilic drugs, including fenfluramine, imipramine, and ranitidine. The significance of this effect in humans is unknown.

STORAGE

Dispense in a tight, light-resistant container.

Store at controlled room temperature, 59° to 86°F (15° to 30°C).

HOW SUPPLIED

CAPSULE: 10 MG

BRAND/MANUFACTURER	NDC	SIZE	AWP
○ **BRAND**			
▶ PROZAC PULVULES: Dista	00777-3104-02	100s	$210.41

CAPSULE: 20 MG

BRAND/MANUFACTURER	NDC	SIZE	AWP
○ **BRAND**			
▶ PROZAC PULVULES: Dista	00777-3105-02	100s	$215.82
	00777-3105-33	100s ud	$220.20

LIQUID: 20 MG/5 ML

BRAND/MANUFACTURER	NDC	SIZE	AWP
○ **BRAND**			
PROZAC: Dista	00777-5120-58	120 ml	$95.83

Fluoxymesterone

DESCRIPTION

Fluoxymesterone, an androgenic hormone, is a white or practically white odorless, crystalline powder, melting at about 240° C, with some decomposition. It is practically insoluble in water, sparingly soluble in alcohol and slightly soluble in chloroform.

The chemical name for Fluoxymesterone is androst-4-en-3-one, 9-fluoro-11, 17- dihydroxy-17- methyl-,(11β,17β). The molecular formula is $C_{20}H_{29}FO_3$ and the molecular weight 336.45.

Each Fluoxymesterone tablet, for oral administration, contains 2 mg, 5 mg or 10 mg Fluoxymesterone.

Following is its chemical structure:

CLINICAL PHARMACOLOGY

Endogenous androgens are responsible for normal growth and development of the male sex organs and for maintenance of secondary sex characteristics. These effects include growth and maturation of the prostate, seminal vesicles, penis, and scrotum; development of male hair distribution, such as beard, pubic, chest, and axillary hair; laryngeal enlargement, vocal cord thickening, and alterations in body musculature and fat distribution. Drugs in this class also cause retention of nitrogen, sodium, potassium, and phosphorus, and decreased urinary excretion of calcium. Androgens have been reported to increase protein anabolism and decrease protein catabolism. Nitrogen balance is improved only when there is sufficient intake of calories and protein. Androgens are responsible for the growth spurt of adolescence and for eventual termination of linear growth, brought about by fusion of the epiphyseal growth centers. In children, exogenous androgens accelerate linear growth rates, but may cause disproportionate advancement in bone maturation. Use over long periods may result in fusion of the epiphyseal growth centers and termination of the growth process. Androgens have been reported to stimulate production of red blood cells by enhancing production of erythropoietic stimulation factor.

During exogenous administration of androgens, endogenous testosterone release is inhibited through feedback inhibition of pituitary luteinizing hormone (LH). At large doses of exogenous androgen, spermatogenesis may also be suppressed through feedback inhibition of pituitary follicle stimulating hormone (FSH).

Inactivation of testosterone occurs primarily in the liver. The half-life of Fluoxymesterone after oral administration is approximately 9.2 hours.

INDICATIONS AND USAGE

In the male: Fluoxymesterone tablets are indicated for:

1. Replacement therapy in conditions associated with symptoms of deficiency or absence of endogenous testosterone:

   a. Primary hypogonadism (congenital or acquired)—testicular failure due to cryptorchidism, bilateral torsion, orchitis, vanishing testis syndrome; or orchidectomy.

b. Hypogonadotropic hypogonadism (congenital or acquired)—idiopathic gonadotropin or LHRH deficiency, or pituitary-hypothalamic injury from tumors, trauma, or radiation.

2. Delayed puberty, provided it has been definitely established as such, and is not just a familial trait.

In the female: Fluoxymesterone tablets are indicated for palliation of androgen-responsive recurrent mammary cancer in women who are more than one year but less than five years postmenopausal, or who have been proven to have a hormone-dependent tumor as shown by previous beneficial response to castration.

UNLABELED USES
Fluoxymesterone is used alone or as an adjunct to increase erythropoiesis in patients with anemia associated with chronic renal failure.

CONTRAINDICATIONS

1. Known hypersensitivity to the drug
2. Males with carcinoma of the breast
3. Males with known or suspected carcinoma of the prostate gland
4. Women known or suspected to be pregnant
5. Patients with serious cardiac, hepatic or renal disease

WARNINGS

Hypercalcemia may occur in immobilized patients and in patients with breast cancer. If this occurs, the drug should be discontinued.

Prolonged use of high doses of androgens (principally the 17α alkyl-androgens) has been associated with development of hepatic adenomas, hepatocellular carcinoma, and peliosis hepatis—all potentially life-threatening complications.

Cholestatic hepatitis and jaundice may occur with 17α-alkyl-androgens. Should this occur, the drug should be discontinued. This is reversible with discontinuation of the drug. Geriatric patients treated with androgens may be at an increased risk of developing prostatic hypertrophy and prostatic carcinoma although conclusive evidence to support this concept is lacking.

Edema, with or without congestive heart failure, may be a serious complication in patients with pre-existing cardiac, renal or hepatic disease.

Gynecomastia may develop and occasionally persists in patients being treated for hypogonadism.

Androgen therapy should be used cautiously in males with delayed puberty. Androgens can accelerate bone maturation without producing compensatory gain in linear growth. The effect on bone maturation should be monitored by assessing bone age of the wrist and hand every six months.

This drug has not been shown to be safe and effective for the enhancement of athletic performance. Because of the potential risk of serious adverse health effects, this drug should not be used for such purpose.

PRECAUTIONS

GENERAL

Women should be observed for signs of virilization which is usual following androgen use at high doses. Discontinuation of drug therapy at the time of evidence of mild virilism is necessary to prevent irreversible virilization. A decision may be made by the patient and the physician that some virilization will be tolerated during treatment for breast carcinoma. Patients with benign prostatic hypertrophy may develop acute urethral obstruction. Priapism or excessive sexual stimulation may develop. Oligospermia may occur after prolonged administration or excessive dosage. If any of these effects appear, the androgen should be stopped and if restarted, a lower dosage should be utilized.

Certain brands of Fluoxymesterone contain FD&C Yellow No. 5 (tartrazine) which may cause allergic-type reactions (including bronchial asthma) in certain susceptible individuals. Although the overall incidence of FD&C Yellow No. 5 (tartrazine) sensitivity in the general population is low, it is frequently seen in patients who also have aspirin hypersensitivity.

INFORMATION FOR PATIENTS

Patients should be instructed to report any of the following: nausea, vomiting, changes in skin color, and ankle swelling. Males should be instructed to report too frequent or persistent erections of the penis and females any hoarseness, acne, changes in menstrual periods or increase in facial hair.

LABORATORY TESTS

Women with disseminated breast carcinoma should have frequent determination of urine and serum calcium levels during the course of androgen therapy (see *"Warnings"*). Because of the hepatotoxicity associated with the use of 17-alpha-alkylated androgens, liver function tests should be obtained periodically.

Periodic (every six months) x-ray examinations of bone age should be made during treatment of prepubertal males to determine the rate of bone maturation and the effects of androgen therapy on the epiphyseal centers.

Hemoglobin and hematocrit levels (to detect polycythemia) should be checked periodically in patients receiving long-term androgen administration.

Serum cholesterol may increase during androgen therapy.

DRUG INTERACTIONS

Androgens may increase sensitivity to oral anticoagulants. Dosage of the anticoagulant may require reduction in order to maintain satisfactory therapeutic hypoprothrombinemia. Concurrent administration of oxyphenbutazone and androgens may result in elevated serum levels of oxyphenbutazone.

In diabetic patients, the metabolic effects of androgens may decrease blood glucose and, therefore, insulin requirements.

DRUG/LABORATORY TEST INTERFERENCES

Androgens may decrease levels of thyroxine-binding globulin, resulting in decreased total T_4 serum levels and increased resin uptake of T_3 and T_4. Free thyroid hormone levels remain unchanged, however, and there is no clinical evidence of thyroid dysfunction.

CARCINOGENESIS, MUTAGENESIS, IMPAIRMENT OF FERTILITY

Animal Data: Testosterone has been tested by subcutaneous injection and implantation in mice and rats. The implant induced cervical-uterine tumors in mice, which metastasized in some cases. There is suggestive evidence that injection of testosterone into some strains of female mice increases their susceptibility to hepatoma. Testosterone is also known to increase the number of tumors and decrease the degree of differentiation of chemically-induced carcinomas of the liver in rats.

Human Data: There are rare reports of hepatocellular carcinoma in patients receiving long-term therapy with androgens in high doses. Withdrawal of the drugs did not lead to regression of the tumors in all cases.

Geriatric patients treated with androgens may be at an increased risk of developing prostatic hypertrophy and prostatic carcinoma although conclusive evidence to support this concept is lacking.

This compound has not be tested for mutagenic potential. However, as noted above, carcinogenic effects have been attributed to treatment with androgenic hormones. The potential carcinogenic effects likely occur through a hormonal mechanism rather than by a direct chemical interaction mechanism.

Impairment of fertility was not tested directly in animal species. However, as noted below under *"Adverse Reactions,"* oligospermia in males and amenorrhea in females are potential adverse effects of treatment with Fluoxymesterone tablets. Therefore, impairment of fertility is a possible outcome of treatment with Fluoxymesterone.

PREGNANCY

Teratogenic Effects: Pregnancy Category X (see *"Contraindications"*).

NURSING MOTHERS

Fluoxymesterone tablets are not recommended for use in nursing mothers.

PEDIATRIC USE

Androgen therapy should be used very cautiously in children and only by specialists aware of the adverse effects on bone maturation. Skeletal maturation must be monitored every six months by an x-ray of the hand and wrist (see *"Warnings"*).

ADVERSE REACTIONS

Endocrine and Urogenital:

Female: The most common side effects of androgen therapy are amenorrhea and other menstrual irregularities; inhibition of gonadotropin secretion; and virilization, including deepening of the voice and clitoral enlargement. The latter usually is not reversible after androgens are discontinued. When administered to a pregnant woman, androgens can cause virilization of external genitalia of the female fetus.

Male: Gynecomastia, and excessive frequency and duration of penile erections. Oligospermia may occur at high dosage.

Skin and Appendages: Hirsutism, male pattern of baldness, seborrhea, and acne.

Fluid and Electrolyte Disturbances: Retention of sodium, chloride, water, potassium, calcium, and inorganic phosphates.

Gastrointestinal: Nausea, cholestatic jaundice, alterations in liver function tests, rarely hepatocellular neoplasms and peliosis hepatis (see *"Warnings"*).

Hematologic: Suppression of clotting factors II, V, VII, and X, bleeding in patients on concomitant anticoagulant therapy, and polycythemia.

Nervous System: Increased or decreased libido, headache, anxiety, depression, and generalized paresthesia.

Allergic: Hypersensitivity, including skin manifestations and anaphylactoid reactions.

DRUG ABUSE AND DEPENDENCE

Controlled Substance Class: Fluoxymesterone is a controlled substance under the Anabolic Steroids Control Act, and Fluoxymesterone tablets has been assigned to Schedule III.

OVERDOSAGE

There have been no reports of acute overdosage with the androgens.

DOSAGE AND ADMINISTRATION

The dosage will vary depending upon the individual, the condition being treated, and its severity. The total daily oral dose may be administered singly or in divided (three or four) doses.

Male Hypogonadism: For complete replacement in the hypogonadal male, a daily dose of 5 to 20 mg will suffice in the majority of patients. It is usually preferable to begin treatment with full therapeutic doses which are later adjusted to individual requirements. Priapism is indicative of excessive dosage and is indication for temporary withdrawal of the drug.

Delayed Puberty: Dosage should be carefully titrated utilizing a low dose, appropriate skeletal monitoring, and by limiting the duration of therapy to four to six months.

◆ RATED THERAPEUTICALLY EQUIVALENT; ◇ THERAPEUTIC EQUIVALENCE UNCONFIRMED; ○ UNRATED

Inoperable Carcinoma of the Breast in the Female: The recommended total daily dose for palliative therapy in advanced inoperable carcinoma of the breast is 10 to 40 mg. Because of its short action, Fluoxymesterone should be administered to patients in divided, rather than single, daily doses to ensure more stable blood levels. In general, it appears necessary to continue therapy for at least one month for a satisfactory subjective response, and for two to three months for an objective response.

HOW SUPPLIED
TABLETS (C-III): 2 MG

BRAND/MANUFACTURER	NDC	SIZE	AWP
◇ **BRAND**			
HALOTESTIN: Upjohn	00009-0014-01	100s	$41.28

TABLETS (C-III): 5 MG

BRAND/MANUFACTURER	NDC	SIZE	AWP
◇ **BRAND**			
HALOTESTIN: Upjohn	00009-0019-06	100s	$101.26

TABLETS (C-III): 10 MG

BRAND/MANUFACTURER	NDC	SIZE	AWP
◇ **BRAND**			
HALOTESTIN: Upjohn	00009-0036-03	30s	$46.31
	00009-0036-04	100s	$150.59
◇ **GENERICS**			
Rosemont	00832-0086-00	100s	$65.00
Qualitest	00603-3645-21	100s	$65.00
URL	00677-0934-01	100s	$82.38
Major	00904-1218-60	100s	$95.95
Rugby	00536-3826-01	100s	$138.71

Fluphenazine

DESCRIPTION
Fluphenazine is a trifluoromethyl phenothiazine derivative intended for the management of schizophenia. Fluphenazine hydrochloride injection is available in multiple dose vials providing 2.5 mg of Fluphenazine hydrochloride per mL. Fluphenazine hydrochloride oval solution contains 5 mg Fluphenazine hydrochloride per mL.

Fluphenazine hydrochloride tablets contain 1, 2.5, 5, and 10 mg Fluphenazine hydrochloride per tablet.

Fluphenazine hydrochloride elixir contains 0.5 mg Fluphenazine hydrochloride per mL.

Fluphenazine decanoate is the decanoate ester of a trifluoromethyl phenothiazine derivative. It is a highly potent behavior modifier with a markedly extended duration of effect. Fluphenazine decanoate is available for intramuscular or subcutaneous administration, providing 25 mg fluphenazine decanoate per mL.

Fluphenazine enanthate injection is an esterified trifluoromethyl phenothiazine derivative, chemically designated as 2-[4-[3-[2-(Trifluoromethyl)-phenothiazin-10-yl]propyl] -1-piperazinyl]ethyl heptanoate. It is a highly potent behavior modifier with a markedly extended duration of effect. Fluphenazine enanthate is available for intramuscular or subcutaneous administration, providing 25 mg Fluphenazine enan- thate per mL.

Following is its chemical structure:

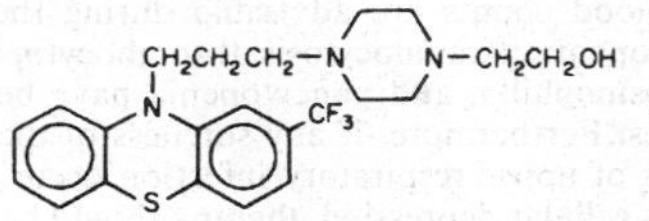

CLINICAL PHARMACOLOGY
Fluphenazine has activity at all levels of the central nervous system as well as on multiple organ systems. The mechanism whereby its therapeutic action is exerted is unknown.

The basic effects of Fluphenazine decanoate appear to be no different from those of Fluphenazine hydrochloride, with the exception of duration of action. The esterification of Fluphenazine markedly prolongs the drug's duration of effect without unduly attenuating its beneficial action.

The basic effects of Fluphenazine enanthate appear to be no different from those of Fluphenazine hydrochloride, with the exception of duration of action. The esterification of Fluphenazine markedly prolongs the drug's duration of effect without unduly attenuating its beneficial action. The onset of action generally appears between 24 to 72 hours after injection, and the effects of the drug on psychotic symptoms become significant within 48 to 96 hours. Amelioration of symptoms then continues for one to three weeks or longer, with an average duration of effect of about two weeks.

Fluphenazine differs from other phenothiazine derivatives in several respects: it is more potent on a milligram basis, it has less potentiating effect on central nervous system depressants and anesthetics than do some of the phenothiazines and appears to be less sedating, and it is less likely than some of the older phenothiazines to produce hypotension (nevertheless, appropriate cautions should be observed— see sections on *"Precautions"* and *"Adverse Reactions"*).

INDICATIONS AND USAGE
Fluphenazine is indicated in the management of manifestations of psychotic disorders.

Fluphenazine decanoate and Fluphenazine enanthate injections are long-acting parenteral antipsychotic drugs intended for use in the management of patients requiring prolonged parenteral neuroleptic therapy (e.g., chronic schizophrenics).

Fluphenazine has not been shown effective in the management of behavorial complications in patients with mental retardation.

UNLABELED USES
Fluphenazine is used alone or as an adjunct in the treatment of cancer chemotherapy-induced vomiting, Huntington's chorea, and irritable bladder syndrome. Fluphenazine is also used in the treatment of diabetic neuropathy, multifocal tic disorders, Gilles de la Tourette syndrome, and in the treatment of hypersexuality including sexual deviant behavior.

CONTRAINDICATIONS
Phenothiazines are contraindicated in patients with suspected or established subcortical brain damage, in patients receiving large doses of hypnotics, and in comatose or severely depressed states. The presence of blood dyscrasia or liver damage precludes the use of Fluphenazine decanoate, enanthate, or hydrochloride. Fluphenazine is contraindicated in patients who have shown hypersensitivity to Fluphenazine; cross-sensitivity to phenothiazine derivatives may occur.

Fluphenazine decanoate and Fluphenazine enanthate are not intended for use in children under 12 years of age.

Fluphenazine enanthate is contraindicated in comatose or severely depressed states.

WARNINGS
TARDIVE DYSKINESIA
Tardive dyskinesia, a syndrome consisting of potentially irreversible, involuntary, dyskinetic movements may develop in patients treated with neuroleptic (antipsychotic) drugs. Although the prevalence of the syndrome appears to be highest among the elderly, especially elderly women, it is impossible to rely upon prevalence estimates to predict, at the inception of neuroleptic treatment, which patients are likely to develop the syndrome. Whether neuroleptic drug products differ in their potential to cause tardive dyskinesia is unknown.

Both the risk of developing the syndrome and the likelihood that it will become irreversible are believed to increase as the duration of treatment and the total cumulative dose of neuroleptic drugs administered to the patient increase. However, the syndrome can develop, although much less commonly, after relatively brief treatment periods at low doses.

There is no known treatment for established cases of tardive dyskinesia, although the syndrome may remit, partially or completely, if neuroleptic treatment is withdrawn. Neuroleptic treatment, itself, however, may suppress (or partially suppress) the signs and symptoms of the syndrome and thereby may possibly mask the underlying disease process. The effect that symptomatic suppression has upon the long-term course of the syndrome is unknown.

Given these considerations, neuroleptics should be prescribed in a manner that is most likely to minimize the occurrence of tardive dyskinesia. Chronic neuroleptic treatment should generally be reserved for patients who suffer from a chronic illness that, 1) is known to respond to neuroleptic drugs, and, 2) for whom alternative, equally effective, but potentially less harmful treatments are *not* available or appropriate. In patients who do require chronic treatment, the smallest dose and the shortest duration of treatment producing a satisfactory clinical response should be sought. The need for continued treatment should be reassessed periodically.

If signs and symptoms of tardive dyskinesia appear in a patient on neuroleptics, drug discontinuation should be considered. However, some patients may require treatment despite the presence of the syndrome.

(For further information about the description of tardive dyskinesia and its clinical detection, please refer to the sections on *"Precautions, Information for Patients"* and *"Adverse Reactions, Tardive Dyskinesia."*)

NEUROLEPTIC MALIGNANT SYNDROME (NMS)
A potentially fatal symptom complex sometimes referred to as Neuroleptic Malignant Syndrome (NMS) has been reported in association with antipsychotic drugs. Clinical manifestations of NMS are hyperpyrexia, muscle rigidity, altered mental status and evidence of autonomic instability (irregular pulse or blood pressure, tachycardia, diaphoresis, and cardiac dysrhythmias).

The diagnostic evaluation of patients with this syndrome is complicated. In arriving at a diagnosis, it is important to identify cases where the clinical presentation includes both serious medical illness (e.g., pneumonia, systemic infection, etc.) and untreated or inadequately treated extrapyramidal signs and symptoms (EPS). Other important considerations in the differential diagnosis include central anticholinergic toxicity, heat stroke, drug fever and primary central nervous system (CNS) pathology.

The management of NMS should include: 1) immediate discontinuation of antipsychotic drugs and other drugs not essential to concurrent therapy; 2) intensive symptomatic treatment and medical monitoring; and 3) treatment of any concomitant serious medical problems for which specific treatments are available. There is no general agreement about specific pharmacological treatment regimens for uncomplicated NMS.

If a patient requires antipsychotic drug treatment after recovery from NMS, the potential reintroduction of drug therapy should be carefully considered. The patient should be carefully monitored, since recurrences of NMS have been reported.

The use of this drug may impair the mental and physical abilities required for driving a car or operating heavy machinery.

Physicians should be alert to the possibility that severe adverse reactions may occur which require immediate medical attention.

Potentiation of the effects of alcohol may occur with the use of this drug.

Since there is no adequate experience in children who have received this drug, safety and efficacy in children have not been established.

USAGE IN PREGNANCY
The safety for the use of this drug during pregnancy has not been established; therefore, the possible hazards should be weighed against the potential benefits when administering this drug to pregnant patients.

PRECAUTIONS
GENERAL
Because of the possibility of cross-sensitivity, Fluphenazine should be used cautiously in patients who have developed cholestatic jaundice, dermatoses or other allergic reactions to phenothiazine derivatives.

Certain brands of Fluphenazine tablets may contain FD&C Yellow No. 5 (tartrazine) which may cause allergic-type reactions (including bronchial asthma) in certain susceptible individuals. Although the overall incidence of FD&C Yellow No. 5 (tartrazine) sensitivity in the general population is low, it is frequently seen in patients who also have aspirin hypersensitivity.

Psychotic patients on large doses of a phenothiazine drug who are undergoing surgery should be watched carefully for possible hypotensive phenomena. Moreover, it should be remembered that reduced amounts of anesthetics or central nervous system depressants may be necessary.

The effects of atropine may be potentiated in some patients receiving Fluphenazine because of added anticholinergic effects.

Fluphenazine should be used cautiously in patients exposed to extreme heat or phosphorus insecticides; in patients with a history of convulsive disorders, since grand mal convulsions have been known to occur; and in patients with special medical disorders, such as mitral insufficiency or other cardiovascular diseases and pheochromocytoma.

The possibility of liver damage, pigmentary retinopathy, lenticular and corneal deposits, and development of irreversible dyskinesia should be remembered when patients are on prolonged therapy.

Neuroleptic drugs elevate prolactin levels; the elevation persists during chronic administration. Tissue culture experiments indicate that approximately one-third of human breast cancers are prolactin dependent *in vitro*, a factor of potential importance if the prescription of these drugs is contemplated in a patient with a previously detected breast cancer. Although disturbances such as galactorrhea, amenorrhea, gynecomastia, and impotence have been reported, the clinical significance of elevated serum prolactin levels is unknown for most patients. An increase in mammary neoplasms has been found in rodents after chronic administration of neuroleptic drugs. Neither clinical studies nor epidemiologic studies conducted to date, however, have shown an association between chronic administration of these drugs and mammary tumorigenesis; the available evidence is considered too limited to be conclusive at this time.

INFORMATION FOR PATIENTS
Given the likelihood that some patients exposed chronically to neuroleptics will develop tardive dyskinesia, it is advised that all patients in whom chronic use is contemplated be given, if possible, full information about this risk. The decision to inform patients and/or their guardians must obviously take into account the clinical circumstances and the competency of the patient to understand the information provided.

ABRUPT WITHDRAWAL
In general, phenothiazines do not produce psychic dependence; however, gastritis, nausea and vomiting, dizziness, and tremulousness have been reported following abrupt cessation of high dose therapy. Reports suggest that these symptoms can be reduced if concomitant antiparkinsonian agents are continued for several weeks after the phenothiazine is withdrawn.

Outside state hospitals or other psychiatric institutions, Fluphenazine decanoate or enanthate should be administered under the direction of a physician experienced in the clinical use of psychotropic drugs, particularly phenothiazine derivatives.

Facilities should be available for periodic checking of hepatic function, renal function and the blood picture. Renal function of patients on long-term therapy should be monitored; if BUN (blood urea nitrogen) becomes abnormal, treatment should be discontinued.

As with any phenothiazine, the physician should be alert to the possible development of "silent pneumonias" in patients under treatment with Fluphenazine.

ADVERSE REACTIONS
Central Nervous System: The side effects most frequently reported with phenothiazine compounds are extrapyramidal symptoms including pseudoparkinsonism, dystonia, dyskinesia, akathisia, oculogyric crises, opisthotonos, and hyperreflexia. Muscle rigidity sometimes accompanied by hyperthermia has been reported following use of Fluphenazine decanoate. Most often these extrapyramidal symptoms are reversible; however, they may be persistent (see below). The frequency of such reactions is related in part to chemical structure: one can expect a higher incidence with Fluphenazine decanoate or enanthate than with less potent piperazine derivatives or with straight-chain phenothiazines such as chlorpromazine. With any given phenothiazine derivative, the incidence and severity of such reactions depend more on individual patient sensitivity than on other factors, but dosage level and patient age are also determinants.

Extrapyramidal reactions may be alarming, and the patient should be forewarned and reassured. These reactions can usually be controlled by administration of antiparkinsonian drugs such as Benztropine Mesylate or intravenous Caffeine and Sodium Benzoate Injection, and by subsequent reductions in dosage.

Tardive Dyskinesia: See *"Warnings"*. The syndrome is characterized by involuntary choreoathetoid movements which variously involve the tongue, face, mouth, lips, or jaw (e.g. protrusion of the tongue, puffing of cheeks, puckering of the mouth, chewing movements), trunk and extremities. The severity of the syndrome and the degree of impairment produced vary widely.

The syndrome may become clinically recognizable either during treatment, upon dosage reduction, or upon withdrawal of treatment. Early detection of tardive dyskinesia is important. To increase the likelihood of detecting the syndrome at the earliest possible time, the dosage of neuroleptic drug should be reduced periodically (if clinically possible) and the patient observed for signs of the disorder. This maneuver is critical, since neuroleptic drugs may mask the signs of the syndrome.

Other CNS Effects: Occurrences of neuroleptic malignant syndrome (NMS) have been reported in patients on neuroleptic therapy (see *"Warnings, Neuroleptic Malignant Syndrome"*). Leukocytosis, elevated CPK, liver function abnormalities, and acute renal failure may also occur with NMS. Drowsiness or lethargy, if they occur, may necessitate a reduction in dosage; the induction of a catatonic-like state has been known to occur with dosages of Fluphenazine far in excess of the recommended amounts. As with other phenothiazine compounds, reactivation or aggravation of psychotic processes may be encountered.

Phenothiazine derivatives have been known to cause, in some patients, restlessness, excitement, or bizarre dreams.

Autonomic Nervous System: Hypertension and Fluctuations in blood pressure have been reported with Fluphenazine.

Hypotension has rarely presented a problem with Fluphenazine. However, patients with pheochromocytoma, cerebral vascular or renal insufficiency, or a severe cardiac reserve deficiency (such as mitral insufficiency) appear to be particularly prone to hypotensive reactions with phenothiazine compounds, and should therefore be observed closely when the drug is administered. If severe hypotension should occur, supportive measures including the use of intravenous vasopressor drugs should be instituted immediately. Levarterenol Bitartrate Injection is the most suitable drug for this purpose; *epinephrine should not be used* since phenothiazine derivatives have been found to reverse its action, resulting in a further lowering of blood pressure.

Autonomic reactions including nausea and loss of appetite, salivation, polyuria, perspiration, dry mouth, headache, and constipation may occur. Autonomic effects can usually be controlled by reducing or temporarily discontinuing dosage. In some patients, phenothiazine derivatives have caused blurred vision, glaucoma, bladder paralysis, fecal impaction, paralytic ileus, tachycardia, or nasal congestion.

Metabolic and Endocrine: Weight change, peripheral edema, abnormal lactation, gynecomastia, menstrual irregularities, false results on pregnancy tests, impotency in men and increased libido in women have all been known to occur in some patients on phenothiazine therapy.

Allergic Reactions: Skin disorders such as itching, erythema, urticaria, seborrhea, photosensitivity, eczema and even exfoliative dermatitis have been reported with phenothiazine derivatives. The possibility of anaphylactoid reactions occurring in some patients should be borne in mind.

Hematologic: Routine blood counts are advisable during therapy since blood dyscrasias including leukopenia, agranulocytosis, thrombocytopenic or nonthrombocytopenic purpura, eosinophilia, and pancytopenia have been observed with phenothiazine derivatives. Furthermore, if any soreness of the mouth, gums, or throat, or any symptoms of upper respiratory infection occur and confirmatory leukocyte count indicates cellular depression, therapy should be discontinued and other appropriate measures instituted immediately.

Hepatic: Liver damage as manifested by cholestatic jaundice may be encountered, particularly during the first months of therapy; treatment should be discontinued if this occurs. An increase in cephalin flocculation, sometimes accompanied by alterations in other liver function tests, has been reported in patients receiving Fluphenazine who have had no clinical evidence of liver damage.

Others: Sudden, unexpected and unexplained deaths have been reported in hospitalized psychotic patients receiving phenothiazines. Previous brain damage or seizures may be predisposing factors; high doses should be avoided in known seizure patients. Several patients have shown sudden flare-ups of psychotic behavior patterns shortly before death. Autopsy findings have usually revealed acute fulminating pneumonia or pneumonitis, aspiration of gastric contents, or intramyocardial lesions.

Although this is not a general features of Fluphenazine, potentiation of central nervous system depressants (opiates, analgesics, antihistamines, barbiturates, alcohol) may occur.

The following adverse reactions have also occurred with phenothiazine derivatives: systemic lupus erythematosus-like syndrome, hypotension severe enough to cause fatal cardiac arrest, altered electrocardiographic and electroencephalographic tracings, altered cerebrospinal fluid proteins, cerebral edema, asthma, laryngeal edema and angioneurotic edema; with long-term use—skin pigmentation, and lenticular and corneal opacities.

Injections of Fluphenazine decanoate or enanthate are extremely well tolerated, local tissue reactions occurring only rarely.

DOSAGE AND ADMINISTRATION

FLUPHENAZINE INJECTION

The average well-tolerated starting dose for adult psychotic patients is 1.25 mg (0.5 mL) intramuscularly. Depending on the severity and duration of symptoms, initial total daily dosage may range from 2.5 to 10.0 mg and should be divided and given at six- to eight-hour intervals.

The smallest amount that will produce the desired results must be carefully determined for each individual, since optimal dosage levels of this potent drug vary from patient to patient. In general, the parenteral dose for Fluphenazine has been found to be approximately ⅓ to ½ the oral dose. Treatment may be instituted with a *low initial dosage,* which may be increased, if necessary, until the desired clinical effects are achieved. Dosages exceeding 10.0 mg daily should be used with caution.

When symptoms are controlled, oral maintenance therapy can generally be instituted, often with single daily doses. Continued treatment, by the oral route if possible, is needed to achieve maximum therapeutic benefits; further adjustments in dosage may be necessary during the course of therapy to meet the patient's requirements.

FLUPHENAZINE ORAL CONCENTRATE

Depending on the severity and duration of symptoms, total daily dosage for *adult* psychotic patients may range initially from 2.5 to 10.0 mg and should be divided and given at six- to eight-hour intervals.

The smallest amount that will produce the desired results must be carefully determined for each individual, since optimal dosage levels of this potent drug vary from patient to patient. In general, the oral dose has been found to be approximately two to three times the parenteral dose of Fluphenazine. Treatment is best instituted with a *low initial dosage,* which may be increased, if necessary, until the desired clinical effects are achieved. Therapeutic effect is often achieved with doses under 20 mg daily. Patients remaining severely disturbed or inadequately controlled may require upward titration of dosage. Daily doses up to 40 mg may be necessary; controlled clinical studies have not been performed to demonstrate safety of prolonged administration of such doses.

When symptoms are controlled, dosage can generally be reduced gradually to daily maintenance doses of 1.0 or 5.0 mg, often given as a single daily dose. Continued treatment is needed to achieve maximum therapeutic benefits; further adjustments in dosage may be necessary during the course of therapy to meet the patient's requirements.

For psychotic patients who have been stabilized on a fixed daily dosage of orally administered Fluphenazine hydrochloride dosage forms, conversion to the long-acting injectable Fluphenazine decanoate may be indicated [see package insert for Fluphenazine decanoate injection for conversion information]. For *geriatric* patients, the suggested starting dose is 1.0 to 2.5 mg daily, adjusted according to the response of the patient. When the oral concentrate dosage form is to be used, the desired dose (measured by calibrated device only) should be added to at least 60 mL (2 fl oz) of a suitable diluent *just prior to administration* to insure palatability and stability. Suggested diluents include tomato or fruit juice, milk, and uncaffeinated soft drinks. The oral concentrate should not be mixed with beverages containing caffeine (coffee, cola), tannics (tea), or pectinates (apple juice) because of potential incompatibility.

Fluphenazine hydrochloride injection is useful when psychotic patients are unable or unwilling to take oral therapy.

FLUPHENAZINE TABLETS AND ELIXIR

Fluphenazine tablets and elixir should be inspected prior to use. Upon standing a slight wispy precipitate or globular material may develop due to the flavoring oils separating from the solution (potency is not affected). Gentle shaking redisperses the oils and the solution becomes clear. Solutions that do not clarify should not be used.

Depending on the severity and duration of symptoms, total daily dosage for *adult* psychotic patients may range initially from 2.5 to 10.0 mg and should be divided and given at six-to eight-hour intervals.

The smallest amount that will produce the desired results must be carefully determined for each individual, since optimal dosage levels of this potent drug vary from patient to patient. In general, the oral dose has been found to be approximately two to three times the parenteral dose of Fluphenazine. Treatment is best instituted with a *low initial dosage,* which may be increased, if necessary, until the desired clinical effects are achieved. Therapeutic effect is often achieved with doses under 20 mg daily. Patients remaining severely disturbed or inadequately controlled may require upward titration of dosage. Daily doses up to 40 mg may be necessary; controlled clinical studies have not been performed to demonstrate safety of prolonged administration of such doses.

When symptoms are controlled, dosage can generally be reduced gradually to daily maintenance doses of 1.0 or 5.0 mg, often given as a single daily dose. Continued treatment is needed to achieve maximum therapeutic benefits; further adjustments in dosage may be necessary during the course of therapy to meet the patient's requirements.

For psychotic patients who have been stabilized on a fixed daily dosage of orally administered Fluphenazine hydrochloride dosage forms, conversion to the long-acting injectable Fluphenazine decanoate may be indicated [see package insert for Fluphenazine decanoate injection for conversion information]. For *geriatric* patients, the suggested starting dose is 1.0 to 2.5 mg daily, adjusted according to the response of the patient. Fluphenazine hydrochloride injection is useful when psychotic patients are unable or unwilling to take oral therapy.

FLUPHENAZINE DECANOATE

Parenteral drug products should be inspected visually for particulate matter and discoloration prior to administration, whenever solution and container permit.

Fluphenazine decanoate injection may be given intramuscularly or subcutaneously. A dry syringe and needle of at least 21 gauge should be used. Use of a wet needle or syringe may cause the solution to become cloudy.

To begin therapy with Fluphenazine decanoate the following regimens are suggested:

For *most patients,* a dose of 12.5 to 25 mg (0.5 to 1 mL) may be given to initiate therapy. The onset of action generally appears between 24 and 72 hours after injection and the effects of the drug on psychotic symptoms become significant within 48 to 96 hours. Subsequent injections and the dosage interval are determined in accordance with the patient's response. When administered as maintenance therapy, a single injection may be effective in controlling schizophrenic symptoms up to four weeks or longer. The response to a single dose has been found to last as long as six weeks in a few patients on maintenance therapy.

It may be advisable that patients who have no history of taking phenothiazines should be treated initially with a shorter-acting form of Fluphenazine before administering the decanoate to determine the patient's response to Fluphenazine and to establish appropriate dosage. For psychotic patients who have been stabilized on a fixed daily dosage of Fluphenazine hydrochloride tablets, Fluphenazine hydrochloride elixir, or Fluphenazine hydrochloride oral solution, conversion of therapy from these short-acting oral forms to the long-acting injectable Fluphenazine decanoate may be indicated.

Appropriate dosage of Fluphenazine decanoate should be individualized for each patient and responses carefully monitored. No precise formula can be given to convert to use of Fluphenazine decanoate; however, a controlled multicentered study,[*] in patients receiving oral doses from 5 to 60 mg Fluphenazine hydrochloride daily, showed that 20 mg Fluphenazine hydrochloride daily was equivalent to 25 mg (1 mL) Fluphenazine decanoate every three weeks. This represents an approximate conversion ratio of 0.5 mL (12.5 mg) of decanoate every three weeks for every 10 mg of Fluphenazine hydrochloride daily.

Once conversion to Fluphenazine decanoate is made, careful clinical monitoring of the patient and appropriate dosage adjustment should be made at the time of each injection. *Severely agitated patients* may be treated initially with a rapid-acting phenothiazine compound such as Fluphenazine hydrochloride injection. When acute symptoms have subsided, 25 mg (1 mL) of Fluphenazine decanoate may be administered; subsequent dosage is adjusted as necessary.

"Poor risk" patients (those with known hypersensitivity to phenothiazines, or with disorders that predispose to undue reactions): Therapy may be initiated cautiously with oral or parenteral Fluphenazine hydrochloride (see package inserts accompanying these products for complete information). When the pharmacologic effects and an appropriate dosage are apparent, an equivalent dose of Fluphenazine decanoate may be administered. Subsequent dosage adjustments are made in accordance with the response of the patient. The optimal amount of the drug and the frequency of administration must be determined for each patient, since dosage requirements have been found to vary with clinical circumstances as well as with individual response to the drug.

Dosage should not exceed 100 mg. If doses greater than 50 mg are deemed necessary, the next dose and succeeding doses should be increased cautiously in increments of 12.5 mg.

FLUPHENAZINE ENANTHATE

Fluphenazine enanthate injection may be given intramuscularly or subcutaneously.

A dry syringe and needle of at least 21 gauge should be used. Use of a wet needle or syringe may cause the solution to become cloudy.

To begin therapy with Fluphenazine enanthate the following regimens are suggested:

For *most patients* a dose of 25 mg (1 mL) every two weeks should prove to be adequate, and therapy may be started on that basis. Subsequent adjustments in the amount and the dosage interval may be made, if necessary, in accordance with the patient's response.

It may be advisable that patients who have no history of taking phenothiazines should be treated initially with a shorter-acting form of Fluphenazine before administering the enanthate to determine the patient's response to Fluphenazine and to establish appropriate dosage. Since the dosage comparability of the shorter-acting forms of Fluphenazine to the longer-acting enanthate is not known, special caution should be exercised when switching from the shorter-acting forms to the enanthate.

Severely agitated patients may be treated initially with a rapid-acting phenothiazine compound such as Fluphenazine hydrochloride injection. When acute symptoms have subsided, 25 mg (1 mL) of Fluphenazine enanthate may be administered; subsequent dosage is adjusted as necessary.

"Poor risk" patients (those with known hypersensitivity to phenothiazines, or with disorders that predispose to undue reactions): Therapy may be initiated cautiously with oral or parenteral Fluphenazine hydrochloride. (See package inserts accompanying these products for complete information.) When the pharmacologic effects and an appropriate dosage are apparent, an equivalent dose of Fluphenazine enanthate may be administered. Subsequent dosage adjustments are made in accordance with the response of the patient.

---

* The Initiation of Long-Term Pharmacotherapy in Schizophrenia: Dosage and Side Effect Comparisons Between Oral and Depot Fluphenazine; N.R. Schooler; Pharmakopsych. 91:159-169, 1976.

The optimal amount of the drug and the frequency of administration must be determined for each patient, since dosage requirements have been found to vary with clinical circumstances as well as with individual response to the drug. Although in a large series of patients the optimal dose was usually 25 mg every two weeks, the amount required ranged from 12.5 to 100 mg (0.5 to 4 mL). The interval between doses ranged from one to three weeks in most instances. The response to a single dose was found to last as long as six weeks in a few patients on maintenance therapy.

Dosage should not exceed 100 mg. If doses greater than 50 mg are deemed necessary, the next dose and succeeding doses should be increased cautiously in increments of 12.5 mg.

STORAGE

Solutions should be protected from exposure to light. Parenteral solutions may vary in color from essentially colorless to light amber. If a solution has become any darker than light amber or is discolored in any other way, it should not be used. Keep tightly closed. Store tablets and solutions at room temperature; avoid freezing and avoid excessive heat. Protect from light.

J CODES

Up to 25 mg IM,SC—J2680

HOW SUPPLIED

FLUPHENAZINE DECANOATE
INJECTION: 25 MG/ML

AVERAGE UNIT PRICE (AVAILABLE SIZES)

BRAND	$20.03

BRAND/MANUFACTURER	NDC	SIZE	AWP
◆ **BRAND**			
PROLIXIN DECANOATE: Apothecon	00003-0569-02	1 ml ud	$21.18
	00003-0569-15	5 ml	$94.40
◆ **GENERICS**			
Fujisawa	00469-2720-20	5 ml	$74.18

FLUPHENAZINE ENANTHATE
INJECTION: 25 MG/ML

BRAND/MANUFACTURER	NDC	SIZE	AWP
○ **BRAND**			
PROLIXIN ENANTHATE: Apothecon	00003-0824-05	5 ml	$100.57

FLUPHENAZINE HYDROCHLORIDE
CONCENTRATE: 5 MG/ML

AVERAGE UNIT PRICE (AVAILABLE SIZES)

BRAND	$0.73

BRAND/MANUFACTURER	NDC	SIZE	AWP
◆ **BRAND**			
PERMITIL: Schering	00085-0296-05	118 ml	$65.82
PROLIXIN: Apothecon	00003-0801-10	120 ml	$109.16

ELIXIR: 0.5 MG/ML

BRAND/MANUFACTURER	NDC	SIZE	AWP
○ **BRAND**			
PROLIXIN: Apothecon	00003-0820-30	60 ml	$17.35
	00003-0820-50	473 ml	$138.35

INJECTION: 2.5 MG/ML

BRAND/MANUFACTURER	NDC	SIZE	AWP
◆ **BRAND**			
PROLIXIN: Apothecon	00003-0586-30	10 ml	$53.87

INJECTION: 2.5 MG

BRAND/MANUFACTURER	NDC	SIZE	AWP
◆ **GENERICS**			
Fujisawa	00469-2810-30	10 ml	$42.57

SOLUTION: 5 MG/ML

BRAND/MANUFACTURER	NDC	SIZE	AWP
◆ **GENERICS**			
Copley	38245-0630-14	120 ml	$91.15

TABLETS: 1 MG

AVERAGE UNIT PRICE (AVAILABLE SIZES)		GENERIC A-RATED AVERAGE PRICE (GAAP)	
BRAND	$0.81	100s	$49.82
GENERIC	$0.48	500s	$186.45
HCFA FUL (100s ea)	$0.25		

BRAND/MANUFACTURER	NDC	SIZE	AWP
◆ **BRAND**			
PROLIXIN: Apothecon	00003-0863-50	100s	$79.70
	00003-0863-55	100s ud	$87.84
	00003-0863-70	500s	$377.11
◆ **GENERICS**			
Geneva	00781-1436-50	50s	$24.21
Rugby	00536-3805-01	100s	$36.45
Qualitest	00603-3666-21	100s	$42.80
Schein	00364-2265-01	100s	$43.05
Goldline	00182-1365-01	100s	$45.00
URL	00677-1217-01	100s	$45.65
Par	49884-0061-01	100s	$45.90
Mason Dist	11845-0337-01	100s	$45.90
Major	00904-3673-60	100s	$47.05
Mylan	00378-6004-01	100s	$47.42
Geneva	00781-1436-01	100s	$47.45
Parmed	00349-8802-01	100s	$47.95
Parmed	00349-8983-01	100s	$47.95
Moore,H.L.	00839-6440-06	100s	$48.18
Aligen	00405-4439-01	100s	$48.31
Goldline	00182-1365-89	100s ud	$58.40
UDL	51079-0485-20	100s ud	$62.40
Geneva	00781-1436-13	100s ud	$62.40
Major	00904-3673-61	100s ud	$74.43
Major	00904-3673-40	500s	$139.80
Mylan	00378-6004-05	500s	$188.24
Geneva	00781-1436-05	500s	$188.25
Par	49884-0061-01	500s	$229.50
Par	49884-0061-10	1000s	$550.00

TABLETS: 2.5 MG

AVERAGE UNIT PRICE (AVAILABLE SIZES)		GENERIC A-RATED AVERAGE PRICE (GAAP)	
BRAND	$1.15	100s	$71.10
GENERIC	$0.68	500s	$266.02
HCFA FUL (100s ea)	$0.37		

BRAND/MANUFACTURER	NDC	SIZE	AWP
◆ **BRAND**			
PROLIXIN: Apothecon	00003-0864-50	100s	$113.03
	00003-0864-52	100s ud	$124.25
	00003-0864-70	500s	$533.26
◆ **GENERICS**			
Geneva	00781-1437-50	50s	$34.36
Rugby	00536-3806-01	100s	$51.90
Qualitest	00603-3667-21	100s	$60.80
Schein	00364-2266-01	100s	$61.05
Goldline	00182-1366-01	100s	$64.00
URL	00677-1218-01	100s	$64.70
Par	49884-0062-01	100s	$64.98
Mason Dist	11845-0338-01	100s	$64.98
Major	00904-3674-60	100s	$67.25
Mylan	00378-6009-01	100s	$67.34
Geneva	00781-1437-01	100s	$67.35
Moore,H.L.	00839-6441-06	100s	$68.24
Parmed	00349-8803-01	100s	$68.95
Parmed	00349-8981-01	100s	$68.95
Aligen	00405-4440-01	100s	$75.42
Goldline	00182-1366-89	100s ud	$83.00
UDL	51079-0486-20	100s ud	$89.60
Geneva	00781-1437-13	100s ud	$89.60
Major	00904-3674-61	100s ud	$101.67
Major	00904-3674-40	500s	$198.45
Mylan	00378-6009-05	500s	$270.35
Geneva	00781-1437-05	500s	$270.37
Par	49884-0062-05	500s	$324.90
Par	49884-0062-10	1000s	$640.00

TABLETS: 2.5 MG

BRAND/MANUFACTURER	NDC	SIZE	AWP
◇ **BRAND**			
PERMITIL: Schering	00085-0442-04	100s	$92.08

TABLETS: 5 MG

AVERAGE UNIT PRICE (AVAILABLE SIZES)		GENERIC A-RATED AVERAGE PRICE (GAAP)	
BRAND	$1.53	100s	$90.57
GENERIC	$0.86	500s	$361.97
HCFA FUL (100s ea)	$0.45		

BRAND/MANUFACTURER	NDC	SIZE	AWP
◆ **BRAND**			
PROLIXIN: Apothecon	00003-0877-50	100s	$145.80
	00003-0877-52	100s ud	$160.68

◆ RATED THERAPEUTICALLY EQUIVALENT; ◇ THERAPEUTIC EQUIVALENCE UNCONFIRMED; ○ UNRATED

BRAND/MANUFACTURER	NDC	SIZE	AWP
◆ GENERICS			
Geneva	00781-1438-50	50s	$44.26
Rugby	00536-3807-01	100s	$66.90
Qualitest	00603-3668-21	100s	$78.74
Schein	00364-2267-01	100s	$78.90
Goldline	00182-1367-01	100s	$83.00
URL	00677-1219-01	100s	$83.25
Mason Dist	11845-0339-01	100s	$83.65
Par	49884-0076-01	100s	$83.75
Aligen	00405-4441-01	100s	$83.88
Major	00904-3675-60	100s	$84.25
Mylan	00378-6074-01	100s	$86.74
Geneva	00781-1438-01	100s	$86.75
Parmed	00349-8804-01	100s	$87.95
Parmed	00349-8982-01	100s	$87.95
Moore,H.L.	00839-6442-06	100s	$87.95
Goldline	00182-1367-89	100s ud	$97.60
Geneva	00781-1438-13	100s ud	$99.70
UDL	51079-0487-20	100s ud	$132.74
Major	00904-3675-61	100s ud	$136.49
Major	00904-3675-40	500s	$300.55
Mylan	00378-6074-05	500s	$329.85
Geneva	00781-1438-05	500s	$329.95
Qualitest	00603-3668-28	500s	$373.95
Par	49884-0076-05	500s	$418.75
Mason Dist	11845-0339-03	500s	$418.75
Par	49884-0076-10	1000s	$910.00

TABLETS: 5 MG

BRAND/MANUFACTURER	NDC	SIZE	AWP
◇ BRAND			
PERMITIL: Schering	00085-0550-04	100s	$122.92

TABLETS: 10 MG

AVERAGE UNIT PRICE (AVAILABLE SIZES)		GENERIC A-RATED AVERAGE PRICE (GAAP)	
BRAND	$2.00	100s	$121.73
GENERIC	$1.14	500s	$463.19
HCFA FUL (100s ea)	$0.67		

BRAND/MANUFACTURER	NDC	SIZE	AWP
◆ BRAND			
PROLIXIN: Apothecon	00003-0956-50	100s	$189.77
	00003-0956-52	100s ud	$209.22
◆ GENERICS			
Geneva	00781-1439-50	50s	$57.58
Rugby	00536-3808-01	100s	$86.85
Qualitest	00603-3669-21	100s	$102.36
Schein	00364-2268-01	100s	$102.60
Goldline	00182-1368-01	100s	$108.00
URL	00677-1220-01	100s	$108.45
Par	49884-0064-01	100s	$109.05
Aligen	00405-4442-01	100s	$109.05
Mason Dist	11845-0340-01	100s	$109.05
Parmed	00349-8805-01	100s	$109.95
Parmed	00349-8979-01	100s	$110.15
Major	00904-3676-60	100s	$111.40
Mylan	00378-6097-01	100s	$112.84
Geneva	00781-1439-01	100s	$112.85
Moore,H.L.	00839-7452-06	100s	$114.48
Goldline	00182-1368-89	100s ud	$167.50
UDL	51079-0488-20	100s ud	$168.50
Geneva	00781-1439-13	100s ud	$168.55
Major	00904-3676-61	100s ud	$179.57
Major	00904-3676-40	500s	$339.45
Mylan	00378-6097-05	500s	$431.60
Geneva	00781-1439-05	500s	$431.70
Qualitest	00603-3669-28	500s	$485.90
Par	49884-0064-05	500s	$545.25
Mason Dist	11845-0340-03	500s	$545.25
Par	49884-0064-10	1000s	$1080.00

TABLETS: 10 MG

BRAND/MANUFACTURER	NDC	SIZE	AWP
◇ BRAND			
PERMITIL: Schering	00085-0316-05	1000s	$1458.51

Flurandrenolide

DESCRIPTION
Flurandrenolide, USP is a potent corticosteroid intended for topical use. It occurs as white to off-white, fluffy, crystalline powder and is ordorless. Flurandrenolide is practically insoluble in water and in ether. One g dissolves in 72 mL of alcohol and in 10 mL of chloroform. The molecular weight of Flurandrenolide is 436.52.

The chemical name of Flurandrenolide is pregn-4-ene-3,20-dione, 6-fluoro-11,21-dihydroxy-16,17-[(1-methylethylidene)-bis (oxy)]-, (6α, 11β, 16α)-; its empirical formula is $C_{24}H_{33}FO_6$.

Each g of Flurandrenolide Cream USP contains 0.5 mg (1.145 μmol; 0.05%) or 0.25 mg (0.57 μmol; 0.025%) Flurandrenolide.

Each g of Flurandrenolide Ointment, USP contains 0.5 mg (1.145 μmol; 0.05%) or 0.25 mg (0.57 μmol: 0.025% Flurandrenolide.

Each mL of Flurandrenolide Lotion contains 0.5 mg (1.145 μmol) (0.05%) Flurandrenolide.

Each square centimeter of Flurandrenolide Tape contains 4 μg (0.00916 μmol) Flurandernolide uniformly distributed in the adhesive layer. The tape is made of a thin, matte-finish polyethylene film that is slightly elastic and highly flexible. The adhesive is a synthetic copolymer of acrylate ester and acrylic acid is free from substances of plant origin. The pressure-sensitive adhesive surface is covered with a protective paper liner to permit handling and trimming before application.

Following is its chemical structure:

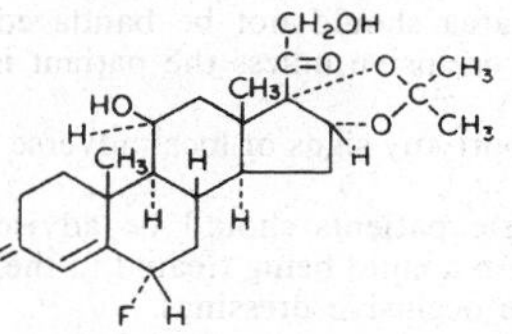

CLINICAL PHARMACOLOGY
Flurandrenolide is primarily effective because of its anti-inflammatory, antipruritic, and vasconstrictive actions.

The mechanism of the anti-inflammatory effect of topical corticosteroids is not completely understood. Various laboratory methods, including vasconstrictor assays, are used to compare and predict potencies and/or clinical efficacies of the topical corticosteroids. There is some evidence to suggest that a recognizable correlation exists between vasconstrictor potency and therapeutic efficacy in man. Corticosteroids with anti-inflammatory activity may stabilize cellular and lysosomal membranes. There is also the suggestion that the effect on the membranes of lysosomes prevents the release of proteolytic enzymes and, thus, plays a part in reducing inflammation.

Evaporation of water from the Flurandrenolide Lotion vehicle produces a cooling effect, which is often desirable in the treatment of acutely inflamed or weeping lesions.

Flurandrenolide Tape serves as both a vehicle and an occlusive dressing. Retention of insensible perspiration by the tape results in hydration of the stratum corneum and improved diffusion of the medication. The skin is protected from scratching, rubbing, desiccation, and chemical irritation. The tape acts as a mechanical splint to fissured skin. Since it prevents removal of the medication by washing or the rubbing action of clothing, the tape formulation provides a sustained action.

Pharmacokinetics: The extent of percutaneous absorption of topical corticosteroids is determined by many factors, including the vehicle, the integrity of the epidermal barrier, and the use of occlusive dressings.

Topical corticosteroids can be absorbed from normal intact skin. Inflammation and/or other disease processes in the skin increase percutaneous absorption. Occlusive dressings substantially increase the percutaneous absorption of topical corticosteroids. Thus, occlusive dressings may be a valuable therapeutic adjunct for treatment of resistant dermatoses (see *"Dosage and Administration"*).

Once absorbed through the skin, topical corticosteroids are handled through pharmacokinetic pathways similar to systematically administered corticosteroids. Corticosteroids are bound to plamsa proteins in varying degrees. They are metabolized primarily in the liver and then excreted in the kidneys. Some of the topical corticosteroids and their metabolites are also excreted into the bile.

INDICATIONS AND USAGE
Flurandrenolide is indicated for the relief of the inflammatory and pruritic manifestations of corticosteroid-responsive dermatoses. Flurandrenolide Tape is indicated particularly for dry, scaling localized lesions.

CONTRAINDICATIONS
Topical corticosteroids are contraindicated in patients with a history of hypersensitivity to any of the components of these preparations.

Use of Flurandrenolide Tape is not recommended for lesions exuding serum or in intertriginous areas.

PRECAUTIONS
General: Systemic absorption of topical corticosteroids has produced reversible hypothalamic-pituitary-adrenal (HPA) axis suppression, manifestations of Cushing's syndrome, hyperglycemia, and glucosuria in some patients.

Conditions that augment systemic absorption include application of the more potent steroids, use over large surface areas, prolonged use, and the addition of occlusive dressings. Therefore, patients receiving a large dose of a potent topical steroid, applied to a large surface area or under an occlusive dressing should be evaluated periodically for evidence of HPA axis suppression using urinary-free cortisol and ACTH stimulation tests. If HPA axis suppression is noted, an attempt should be made to withdraw the drug, to reduce the frequency of application, or to substitute a less potent steroid.

Recovery of HPA axis function is generally prompt and complete on discontinuation of the drug. Infrequently, signs and symptoms of steroid withdrawal may occur, so that supplemental systemic corticosteroids are required.

Children may absorb proportionately large amounts of topical corticosteroids and thus be more susceptible to systemic toxicity (see *"Usage in Children"* under *"Precautions"*).

If irritation develops, topical corticosteroids should be discontinued and appropriate therapy instituted.

In the presence of dermatologic infections, the use of an appropriate antifungal or antibacterial agent should be instituted. If a favorable responses does not occur promptly, Flurandrenolide should be discontinued until the infection has been adequately controlled.

Information for the Patients: Patients using topical corticosteroids should receive the following information and instructions:

1. This medication is to be used as directed by the physician. It is for external use only. Avoid contact with the eyes.

2. Patients should be advised not to use this medication for any disorder other than that for which it was prescribed.

3. The treated skin area should not be bandaged or otherwise covered or wrapped in order to be occlusive unless the patient is directed to do so by the physician.

4. Patients should report any signs of local adverse reactions, especially under occlusive dressing.

5. Parents of pediatric patients should be advised not to use tight-fitting diapers or plastic pants on a child being treated in the diaper area, because these garments may constitute occlusive dressings.

Laboratory Tests: The following tests may be helpful in evaluating the HPA axis suppression:
    Urinary-free cortisol test
    ACTH stimulation test

Carcinogenesis, Mutagenesis, and Impairment of Fertility: Long-term animal studies have not been performed to evaluate the carcinogenic potential or the effect on fertility of topical corticosteroids.

Studies to determine mutagenicity with prednisolone and hydrocortisone have revealed negative results.

Usage in Pregnancy—Pregnancy Category C: Corticosteroids are generally teratogenic in laboratory animals when administered systemically at relatively low dosage levels. The more potent corticosteroids have been shown to be teratogenic after dermal application in laboratory animals. There are no adequate and well-controlled studies in pregnant women on teratogenic effects from topically applied corticosteroids. Therefore, topical corticosteroids should be used during pregnancy only if the potential benefit justifies the potential risk to the fetus. Drugs of this class should not be used extensively for pregnant patients or in large amounts or for prolonged periods of time.

Nursing Mothers: It is not known whether topical administration of corticosteroids could result in sufficient systemic absorption to produce detectable quantities in breast milk. Systemically administered corticosteroids are secreted into breast milk in quantities *not* likely to have a deleterious effect on the infant. Nevertheless, caution should be exercised when topical corticosteroids are administered to a nursing woman.

Usage in Children: Pediatric patients may demonstrate greater susceptibility to topical corticosteroid-induced HPA axis suppression and Cushing's syndrome than do mature patients because of a larger skin surface area to body weight ratio.

Hypothalamic-pituitary-adrenal (HPA) axis suppression, Cushing's syndrome, and intracranial hypertension have been reported in children receiving topical corticosteroids. Manifestations of adrenal suppression in children include linear growth retardation, delayed weight gain, low plasma cortisol levels, and absence of response to ACTH stimulation. Manifestations of intracranial hypertension include bulging fontanelles, headaches, and bilateral papilledema.

Administration of topical corticosteroids to children should be limited to the least amount compatible with an effective therapeutic regimen. Chronic corticosteroid therapy may interfere with the growth and development of children.

ADVERSE REACTIONS

The following local adverse reactions are reported infrequently with topical corticosteroids but may occur more frequently with the use of occlusive dressings. These reactions are listed in an approximate decreasing order of occurrence:
    Burning
    Itching
    Irritation
    Dryness
    Folliculitis
    Hypertrichosis
    Acneform eruptions
    Hypopigmentation
    Perioral dermatitis
    Allergic contact dermatitis
    The following may occur more frequently with occlusive dressings:
    Maceration of the skin
    Secondary infection
    Skin atrophy
    Striae
    Miliaria

OVERDOSAGE

Topically applied corticosteroids can be absorbed in sufficient amounts to produce systemic effects (see *"Precautions"*).

DOSAGE AND ADMINISTRATION

Topical corticosteroids are generally applied to the affected area as a thin film 1 to 4 times daily, depending on the severity of the condition.

For moist lesions, a small quantity of Flurandrenolide Cream should be rubbed gently into the affected areas 2 or 3 times a day. For dry, scaly lesions, Flurandrenolide Ointment is applied as a thin film to affected areas 2 or 3 times daily.

A small quantity of Flurandrenolide Lotion should be rubbed gently into the affected area 2 or 3 times daily.

Occlusive dressings may be used for the management of psoriasis or recalcitrant conditions.

If an infection develops, the use of Flurandrenolide Tape and other occlusive dressings should be discontinued and appropriate antimicrobial therapy instituted.

USE WITH OCCLUSIVE DRESSINGS; FLURANDRENOLIDE CREAM, OINTMENT, AND LOTION

The technique of occlusive dressings (for management of psoriasis and other persistant dermatoses) is as follows:

1. Remove as much as possible of the superficial scaling before applying Flurandrenolide Cream, Ointment, or Lotion. Soaking in a bath will help soften the scales and permit easier removal by brushing, picking, or rubbing.

2. Rub the Flurandrenolide product thoroughly into the affected areas.

3. Cover with an occlusive plastic film, such as polyethylene or a commercial plastic food wrap. (When Flurandrenolide Cream or Lotion is used, added moisture may be provided by placing a slightly dampened cloth or gauze over the lesion before the plastic film is applied.)

4. Seal the edges to adjacent normal skin with tape or hold in place by a gauze wrapping.

5. For convenience, the patient may remove the dressing during the day. The dressing should then be reapplied each night.

6. For daytime therapy, the condition may be treated by rubbing Flurandrenolide Cream, Ointment, or Lotion sparingly into the affected areas.

7. In more resistant cases, leaving the dressing in place for 3 to 4 days at a time may result in a better response.

8. Thin polyethylene gloves are suitable for treatment of the hands and fingers; plastic garment bags may be utilized for treating lesions on the trunk or buttocks. A tight shower cap is useful in treating lesions on the scalp.

Occlusive Dressings Have the Following Advantages:

1. Percutaneous penetration of the corticosteroid is enhanced.

2. Medication is concentrated on the areas of skin where it is most needed.

3. This method of administration frequently is more effective in very resistant dermatoses than is the conventional application of Flurandrenolide.

Precautions to Be Observed in Therapy With Occlusive Dressings: Treatment should be continued for at least a few days after clearing of the lesions. If it is stopped too soon, a relapse may occur. Reinstitution of treatment frequently will cause remission.

Because of the increased hazard of secondary infection from resistant strains of staphylococci among hospitalized patients, it is suggested that the use of occlusive plastic films for corticosteroid therapy in such cases be restricted.

Generally, occlusive dressings should not be used on weeping, or exudative, lesions.

When large areas of the body are covered, thermal homeostasis may be impaired. If elevation of body temperature occurs, use of the occlusive dressing should be discontinued.

Rarely, a patient may develop miliaria, folliculitis, or a sensitivity to either the particular dressing material or a combination of Flurandrenolide and the occlusive dressing. If miliaria or folliculitis occurs, use of the occlusive dressing should be discontinued. Treatment by inunction with a corticosteroid such as Flurandrenolide may be continued. If the sensitivity is caused by the particular material of the dressing, substitution of a different material may be tried.

Warnings: Some plastic films are readily flammable. Patients should be cautioned against the use of any such material.

When plastic films are used on infants and children, the persons caring for the patients must be reminded of the danger of suffocation if the plastic material accidentally covers the face.

Replacement of Flurandrenolide Tape every 12 hours produces the lowest incidence of adverse reactions, but it may be left in place for 24 hours if it is well tolerated and adheres satisfactorily. When necessary, the tape may be used at night only and removed during the day.

If ends of the tape loosen prematurely, they may be trimmed off and replaced with fresh tape.

The directions given below are included on a separate package insert for the patient to follow unless otherwise instructed by the physician.

APPLICATION OF FLURANDRENOLIDE TAPE

IMPORTANT: SKIN SHOULD BE CLEAN AND *DRY* BEFORE TAPE IS APPLIED. TAPE SHOULD ALWAYS BE CUT, NEVER TORN.

Directions For Use

1. Prepare skin as directed by your physician or as follows: Gently clean the area to be covered to remove scales, crusts, dried exudates, and any previously

used ointments or creams. A germicidal soap or cleanser should be used to prevent the development of odor under the tape. Shave or clip the hair in the treatment area to allow good contact with the skin and comfortable removal. If shower or tub bath is to be taken, it should be completed before the tape is applied. The skin should be dry before application of the tape.

2. Remove tape from package and cut a piece slightly larger than area to be covered. Round off corners.

3. Pull white paper from transparent tape. Be careful that tape does not stick to itself.

4. Apply tape, keeping skin smooth; press tape into place.

REPLACEMENT OF TAPE
Unless instructed otherwise by your physician, replace tape after 12 hours. Cleanse skin and allow it to dry for 1 hour before applying new tape.

IF IRRITATION OR INFECTION DEVELOPS, REMOVE TAPE AND CONSULT PHYSICIAN.

HOW SUPPLIED
CREAM: 0.025%

BRAND/MANUFACTURER		NDC	SIZE	AWP
○ **BRAND**				
CORDRAN SP: Oclassen		55515-0034-30	30 gm	$13.03
		55515-0034-60	60 gm	$18.41

CREAM: 0.05%

BRAND/MANUFACTURER		NDC	SIZE	AWP
○ **BRAND**				
CORDRAN SP: Oclassen		55515-0035-15	15 gm	$11.76
		55515-0035-30	30 gm	$16.63
		55515-0035-60	60 gm	$30.90

LOTION: 0.05%

AVERAGE UNIT PRICE (AVAILABLE SIZES)				
BRAND	$0.65			

BRAND/MANUFACTURER		NDC	SIZE	AWP
◆ **BRAND**				
CORDRAN: Oclassen		55515-0052-15	15 ml	$11.76
		55515-0052-60	60 ml	$30.90

OINTMENT: 0.025%

BRAND/MANUFACTURER		NDC	SIZE	AWP
○ **BRAND**				
CORDRAN: Oclassen		55515-0024-30	30 gm	$13.03
		55515-0024-60	60 gm	$18.41

OINTMENT: 0.05%

BRAND/MANUFACTURER		NDC	SIZE	AWP
○ **BRAND**				
CORDRAN: Oclassen		55515-0026-15	15 gm	$11.76
		55515-0026-30	30 gm	$16.63
		55515-0026-60	60 gm	$30.90

TAPE: 4 MCG/CM2

BRAND/MANUFACTURER		NDC	SIZE	AWP
○ **BRAND**				
CORDRAN TAPE: Oclassen		55515-0014-24	1s	$12.91
		55515-0014-80	1s	$27.74
		55515-0014-12	12s	$12.91

Flurazepam Hydrochloride

DESCRIPTION
Flurazepam Hydrochloride is available as capsules containing 15 mg or 30 mg Flurazepam Hydrochloride. Flurazepam Hydrochloride is chemically 7-chloro-1-[2-(diethylamino)ethyl]-5-(o-fluorophenyl)-1, 3-dihydro-2H-1, 4-benzodiazepin-2-one dihydrochloride. It is a pale yellow, crystalline compound, freely soluble in U.S.P. alcohol and very soluble in water. It has a molecular weight of 460.826.

Following is its chemical structure:

CLINICAL PHARMACOLOGY
Flurazepam Hydrochloride is rapidly absorbed from the G.I. tract. Flurazepam is rapidly metabolized and is excreted primarily in the urine. Following a single oral dose, peak Flurazepam plasma concentrations ranging from 0.5 to 4.0 ng/mL occur at 30 to 60 minutes post-dosing. The harmonic mean apparent half-life of Flurazepam is 2.3 hours. The blood level profile of Flurazepam HCl and its major metabolites was determined in man following the oral administration of 30 mg daily for 2 weeks. The N_1-hydroxyethyl-flurazepam was measurable only during the early hours after a 30-mg dose and was not detectable after 24 hours. The major metabolite in blood was N_1-desalkyl-flurazepam, which reached steady-state (plateau) levels after 7 to 10 days of dosing, at levels approximately 5- to 6-fold greater than the 24-hour levels observed on Day 1. The half-life of elimination of N_1-desalkyl-flurazepam ranged from 47 to 100 hours. The major urinary metabolite is conjugated N_1-hydroxyethyl-flurazepam which accounts for 22% to 55% of the dose. Less than 1% of the dose is excreted in the urine as N_1-desalkylflurazepam.

This pharmacokinetic profile may be responsible for the clinical observation that Flurazepam HCl is increasingly effective on the second or third night of consecutive use and that for 1 or 2 nights after the drug is discontinued both sleep latency and total wake time may still be decreased.

INDICATIONS
Flurazepam HCl is a hypnotic agent useful for the treatment of insomnia characterized by difficulty in falling asleep, frequent nocturnal awakenings, and/or early morning awakening. Flurazepam HCl can be used effectively in patients with recurring insomnia or poor sleeping habits, and in acute or chronic medical situations requiring restful sleep. Sleep laboratory studies have objectively determined that Flurazepam HCl is effective for at least 28 consecutive nights of drug administration. Since insomnia is often transient and intermittent, short-term use is usually sufficient. Prolonged use of hypnotics is usually not indicated and should only be undertaken concomitantly with appropriate evaluation of the patient.

CONTRAINDICATIONS
Flurazepam HCl is contraindicated in patients with known hypersensitivity to the drug.

Usage in Pregnancy: Benzodiazepines may cause fetal damage when administered during pregnancy. An increased risk of congenital malformations associated with the use of diazepam and chlordiazepoxide during the first trimester of pregnancy has been suggested in several studies.

Flurazepam HCl is contraindicated in pregnant women. Symptoms of neonatal depression have been reported; a neonate whose mother received 30 mg of Flurazepam HCl nightly for insomnia during the 10 days prior to delivery appeared hypotonic and inactive during the first 4 days of life. Serum levels of N_1-desalkyl-flurazepam in the infant indicated transplacental circulation and implicate this long-acting metabolite in this case. If there is a likelihood of the patient becoming pregnant while receiving Flurazepam HCl, she should be warned of the potential risks to the fetus. Patients should be instructed to discontinue the drug prior to becoming pregnant. The possibility that a woman of childbearing potential may be pregnant at the time of institution of therapy should be considered.

WARNINGS
Patients receiving Flurazepam HCl should be cautioned about possible combined effects with alcohol and other CNS depressants. Also, caution patients that an additive effect may occur if alcoholic beverages are consumed during the day following the use of Flurazepam HCl for nighttime sedation. The potential for this interaction continues for several days following discontinuance of Flurazepam HCl, until serum levels of psychoactive metabolites have declined.

Patients should also be cautioned about engaging in hazardous occupations requiring complete mental alertness such as operating machinery or driving a motor vehicle after ingesting the drug, including potential impairment of the performance of such activities which may occur the day following ingestion of Flurazepam HCl.

Usage in Children: Clinical investigations of Flurazepam HCl have not been carried out in children. Therefore, the drug is not currently recommended for use in persons under 15 years of age.

Withdrawal symptoms of the barbiturate type have occurred after the discontinuation of benzodiazepines. (See *"Drug Abuse and Dependence"* section.)

PRECAUTIONS
Since the risk of the development of oversedation, dizziness, confusion and/or ataxia increases substantially with larger doses in elderly and debilitated patients, it is recommended that in such patients the dosage be limited to 15 mg. If Flurazepam HCl is to be combined with other drugs having known hypnotic properties or CNS-depressant effects, due consideration should be given to potential additive effects.

The usual precautions are indicated for severely depressed patients or those in whom there is any evidence of latent depression; particularly the recognition that suicidal tendencies may be present and protective measures may be necessary.

The usual precautions should be observed in patients with impaired renal or hepatic function and chronic pulmonary insufficiency.

Information for Patients: To assure the safe and effective use of benzodiazepines, patients should be informed that since benzodiazepines may produce psychological and physical dependence, it is advisable that they consult with their physician before either increasing the dose or abruptly discontinuing this drug.

ADVERSE REACTIONS

Dizziness, drowsiness, light-headedness, staggering, ataxia and falling have occurred, particularly in elderly or debilitated persons. Severe sedation, lethargy, disorientation and coma, probably indicative of drug intolerance or overdosage, have been reported.

Also reported were headache, heartburn, upset stomach, nausea, vomiting, diarrhea, constipation, gastrointestinal pain, nervousness, talkativeness, apprehension, irritability, weakness, palpitations, chest pains, body and joint pains and genitourinary complaints. There have also been rare occurrences of leukopenia, granulocytopenia, sweating, flushes, difficulty in focusing, blurred vision, burning eyes, faintness, hypotension, shortness of breath, pruritus, skin rash, dry mouth, bitter taste, excessive salivation, anorexia, euphoria, depression, slurred speech, confusion, restlessness, hallucinations, and elevated SGOT, SGPT, total and direct bilirubins, and alkaline phosphatase. Paradoxical reactions, eg, excitement, stimulation and hyperactivity, have also been reported in rare instances.

DRUG ABUSE AND DEPENDENCE

Withdrawal symptoms, similar in character to those noted with barbiturates and alcohol (convulsions, tremor, abdominal and muscle cramps, vomiting and sweating), have occurred following abrupt discontinuance of benzodiazepines. The more severe withdrawal symptoms have usually been limited to those patients who had received excessive doses over an extended period of time. Generally milder withdrawal symptoms (eg, dysphoria and insomnia) have been reported following abrupt discontinuance of benzodiazepines taken continuously at therapeutic levels for several months. Consequently, after extended therapy, abrupt discontinuation should generally be avoided and a gradual dosage tapering schedule followed. Addiction-prone individuals (such as drug addicts or alcoholics) should be under careful surveillance when receiving Flurazepam HCl or other psychotropic agents because of the predispostion of such patients to habituation and dependence.

DOSAGE AND ADMINISTRATION

Dosage should be individualized for maximal beneficial effects. The usual adult dosage is 30 mg before retiring. In some patients, 15 mg may suffice. In elderly and/or debilitated patients, 15 mg is usually sufficient for a therapeutic response and it is therefore recommended that therapy be initiated with this dosage.

OVERDOSAGE

Manifestations of Flurazepam HCl overdosage include somnolence, confusion and coma. Respiration, pulse and blood pressure should be monitored as in all cases of drug overdosage. General supportive measures should be employed, along with immediate gastric lavage. Intravenous fluids should be administered and an adequate airway maintained. Hypotension and CNS depression may be combated by judicious use of appropriate therapeutic agents. The value of dialysis has not been determined. If excitation occurs in patients following Flurazepam HCl overdosage, barbiturates should not be used. As with the management of intentional overdosage with any drug, it should be borne in mind that multiple agents may have been ingested.

Flumazenil, a specific benzodiazepine-receptor antagonist, is indicated for the complete or partial reversal of the sedative effects of benzodiazepines and may be used in situations when an overdose with a benzodiazepine is known or suspected. Prior to the administration of flumazenil, necessary measures should be instituted to secure airway, ventilation, and intravenous access. Flumazenil is intended as an adjunct to, not as a substitute for, proper management of benzodiazepine overdose. Patients treated with flumazenil should be monitored for resedation, respiratory depression and other residual benzodiazepine effects for an appropriate period after treatment. **The prescriber should be aware of a risk of seizure in association with flumazenil treatment, particularly in long-term benzodiazepine users and in cyclic anti-depressant overdose.** The complete flumazenil package insert, including "Contraindications", "Warnings" and "Precautions", should be consulted prior to use.

HOW SUPPLIED
CAPSULE (C-IV): 15 MG

AVERAGE UNIT PRICE (AVAILABLE SIZES)		GENERIC A-RATED AVERAGE PRICE (GAAP)	
BRAND	$0.53	100s	$24.14
GENERIC	$0.22	500s	$97.62
HCFA FUL (100s ea)	$0.05		

BRAND/MANUFACTURER	NDC	SIZE	AWP
◆ BRAND			
▶ DALMANE: Roche Prod	00140-0065-01	100s	$53.18
	00140-0065-14	500s	$264.76
◆ GENERICS			
West-Ward	00143-3367-01	100s	$15.00
Qualitest	00603-3691-21	100s	$19.91
Rugby	00536-3795-01	100s	$19.94
Goldline	00182-1817-01	100s	$20.00
Major	00904-2800-60	100s	$21.50
Schein	00364-0801-01	100s	$21.50
Warner Chilcott	00047-0988-24	100s	$21.60
Geneva	00781-2806-01	100s	$21.65
Halsey Pharm	00879-0534-01	100s	$22.00
Par	49884-0193-01	100s	$22.10
Aligen	00405-0085-01	100s	$22.10
Purepac	00228-2021-10	100s	$22.10

BRAND/MANUFACTURER	NDC	SIZE	AWP
URL	00677-1065-01	100s	$22.75
Moore,H.L.	00839-7154-06	100s	$22.80
▶ Mylan	00378-4415-01	100s	$23.38
West-Ward	00143-3367-52	100s	$32.95
Vangard	00615-0460-13	100s ud	$26.17
Vangard	00615-0460-47	100s ud	$26.17
UDL	51079-0302-20	100s ud	$26.94
Auro	55829-0836-10	100s ud	$28.85
UDL	51079-0302-21	100s ud	$29.33
West-Ward	00143-3367-25	100s ud	$32.00
Major	00904-2800-61	100s ud	$34.46
Schein	00364-0801-05	500s	$67.10
West-Ward	00143-3367-05	500s	$75.00
Moore,H.L.	00839-7154-12	500s	$96.51
Rugby	00536-3795-05	500s	$96.88
Major	00904-2800-40	500s	$96.95
Goldline	00182-1817-05	500s	$96.95
Geneva	00781-2806-05	500s	$97.75
Purepac	00228-2021-50	500s	$98.63
Aligen	00405-0085-02	500s	$103.82
Par	49884-0193-05	500s	$104.35
Mason Dist	11845-0201-03	500s	$104.35
Halsey Pharm	00879-0534-05	500s	$105.22
▶ Mylan	00378-4415-05	500s	$111.26
Parmed	00349-8465-05	500s	$111.90

CAPSULE (C-IV): 30 MG

AVERAGE UNIT PRICE (AVAILABLE SIZES)		GENERIC A-RATED AVERAGE PRICE (GAAP)	
BRAND	$0.58	100s	$26.32
GENERIC	$0.25	500s	$108.55
HCFA FUL (100s ea)	$0.07		

BRAND/MANUFACTURER	NDC	SIZE	AWP
◆ BRAND			
▶ DALMANE: Roche Prod	00140-0066-01	100s	$57.84
	00140-0066-14	500s	$288.15
◆ GENERICS			
West-Ward	00143-3370-01	100s	$15.00
Qualitest	00603-3692-21	100s	$21.86
Rugby	00536-3796-01	100s	$21.88
Goldline	00182-1818-01	100s	$21.95
Schein	00364-0802-01	100s	$23.50
Major	00904-2801-60	100s	$23.85
Geneva	00781-2807-01	100s	$24.00
Warner Chilcott	00047-0989-24	100s	$24.00
Aligen	00405-0086-01	100s	$24.55
Purepac	00228-2022-10	100s	$24.55
Par	49884-0194-01	100s	$24.65
Halsey Pharm	00879-0533-01	100s	$24.70
URL	00677-1066-01	100s	$25.05
Moore,H.L.	00839-7155-06	100s	$25.10
▶ Mylan	00378-4430-01	100s	$26.50
West-Ward	00143-3370-52	100s	$35.95
Vangard	00615-0461-13	100s ud	$29.92
Vangard	00615-0461-47	100s ud	$29.92
UDL	51079-0303-20	100s ud	$31.58
UDL	51079-0303-21	100s ud	$31.58
West-Ward	00143-3370-25	100s ud	$34.00
Major	00904-2801-61	100s ud	$34.87
Schein	00364-0802-05	500s	$74.60
West-Ward	00143-3370-05	500s	$85.00
Moore,H.L.	00839-7155-12	500s	$103.94
Rugby	00536-3796-05	500s	$106.13
Goldline	00182-1818-05	500s	$106.20
Qualitest	00603-3692-28	500s	$106.80
Major	00904-2801-40	500s	$110.50
Purepac	00228-2022-50	500s	$113.59
Par	49884-0194-05	500s	$116.35
Geneva	00781-2807-05	500s	$116.35
Mason Dist	11845-0202-03	500s	$116.35
Halsey Pharm	00879-0533-05	500s	$117.75
Aligen	00405-0086-02	500s	$119.57
▶ Mylan	00378-4430-05	500s	$126.50

Flurbiprofen Sodium, Ophthalmic

DESCRIPTION
Flurbiprofen Sodium ophthalmic solution is a topical nonsteroidal anti-inflammatory product for ophthalmic use.

Chemical Name: Sodium (±)2-fluoro-α-methyl-4-biphenyl-acetate dihydrate.

Contains: Flurbiprofen Sodium 0.03%

Following is its chemical structure:

◆ RATED THERAPEUTICALLY EQUIVALENT; ◇ THERAPEUTIC EQUIVALENCE UNCONFIRMED; ○ UNRATED

CLINICAL PHARMACOLOGY

Flurbiprofen Sodium is one of a series of phenylalkanoic acids that have shown analgesic, antipyretic, and anti-inflammatory activity in animal inflammatory diseases. Its mechanism of action is believed to be through inhibition of the cyclooxygenase enzyme that is essential in the biosynthesis of prostaglandins.

Prostaglandins have been shown in many animal models to be mediators of certain kinds of intraocular inflammation. In studies performed on animal eyes, prostaglandins have been shown to produce disruption of the blood-aqueous humor barrier, vasodilatation, increased vascular permeability, leukocytosis, and increased intraocular pressure.

Prostaglandins also appear to play a role in the miotic response produced during ocular surgery by constricting the iris sphincter independently of cholinergic mechanisms. In clinical studies, Flurbiprofen Sodium, Ophthalmic, has been shown to inhibit the miosis induced during the course of cataract surgery.

Results from clinical studies indicate that Flurbiprofen Sodium has no significant effect upon intraocular pressure.

INDICATIONS AND USAGE

Flurbiprofen Sodium, Ophthalmic, is indicated for the inhibition of intraoperative miosis.

CONTRAINDICATIONS

Flurbiprofen Sodium, Ophthalmic, is contraindicated in individuals who are hypersensitive to any components of the medication.

WARNING

With nonsteroidal anti-inflammatory drugs, there exists the potential for increased bleeding due to interference with thrombocyte aggregation. There have been reports that Flurbiprofen Sodium, Ophthalmic, may cause increased bleeding of ocular tissues (including hyphemas) in conjunction with ocular surgery. There exists the potential for cross-sensitivity to acetylsalicylic acid and other nonsteroidal anti-inflammtory drugs. Therefore, caution should be used when treating individuals who have previously exhibited sensitivities to these drugs.

PRECAUTIONS

General: Wound healing may be delayed with the use of Flurbiprofen Sodium, Ophthalmic. It is recommended that Flurbiprofen Sodium, Ophthalmic, solution be used with caution in surgical patients with known bleeding tendencies or who are receiving other medications which may prolong bleeding time.

Drug Interactions: Interaction of Flurbiprofen Sodium, Ophthalmic, with other topical ophthalmic medications has not been fully investigated.

Although clinical studies with acetylcholine chloride and animal studies with acetylcholine chloride or carbachol revealed no interference, and there is no known pharmacological basis for an interaction, there have been reports that acetylcholine chloride, and carbachol have been ineffective when used in patients treated with Flurbiprofen Sodium, Ophthalmic.

Carcinogenesis, Mutagenesis, Impairment of Fertility: Long-term studies in mice and/or rats have shown no evidence of carcinogenicity or impairment of fertility with Flurbiprofen.

Long-term mutagenicity studies in animals have not been performed.

Pregnancy: Pregnancy Category C.: Flurbiprofen has been shown to be embryocidal, delay parturition, prolong gestation, reduce weight, and/or slightly retard growth of fetuses when given to rats in daily oral doses of 0.4 mg/kg (approximately 185 times the human daily topical dose) and above. There are no adequate and well-controlled studies in pregnant women. Flurbiprofen Sodium, Ophthalmic, should be used during pregnancy only if the potential benefit justifies the potential risk to the fetus.

Nursing Mothers: It is not known whether this drug is excreted in human milk. Because many drugs are excreted in human milk and because of the potential for serious adverse reactions in nursing infants from Flurbiprofen Sodium, a decision should be made whether to discontinue nursing or to discontinue the drug, taking into account the importance of the drug to the mother.

Pediatric Use: Safety and effectiveness in children have not been established.

ADVERSE REACTIONS

The most frequent adverse reactions reported with the use of Flurbiprofen Sodium, Ophthalmic, are transient burning and stinging upon instillation and other minor symptoms of ocular irritation.

Increased bleeding tendency of ocular tissues in conjunction with ocular surgery has also been reported.

OVERDOSAGE

Overdosage will not ordinarily cause acute problems. If accidentally ingested, drink fluids to dilute.

DOSAGE AND ADMINISTRATION

A total of four (4) drops of Flurbiprofen Sodium, Opthalmic, should be administered by instilling 1 drop approximately every ½ hour beginning 2 hours before surgery.

Store at room temperature.

HOW SUPPLIED

DROP: 0.03%

BRAND/MANUFACTURER	NDC	SIZE	AWP
○ **BRAND**			
OCUFEN: Allergan Pharm	11980-0801-03	2.5 ml	$13.88

Flurbiprofen, Oral

DESCRIPTION

Flurbiprofen, a nonsteroidal anti-inflammatory agent. Flurbiprofen is a phenylalkanoic acid derivative designated chemically as [1,1'-biphenyl]-4-acetic acid, 2-fluoro-alphamethyl-, (±)-. The empirical formula is $C_{15}H_{13}FO_2$, with a molecular weight of 244.26. Flurbiprofen is a white or slightly yellow crystalline powder. It is slightly soluble in water at pH 7.0 and readily soluble in most polar solvents.

Flurbiprofen is available as 50 mg and 100 mg tablets for oral administration.

Following is its chemical structure:

CLINICAL PHARMACOLOGY

Flurbiprofen is a nonsteroidal anti-inflammatory agent which has shown anti-inflammatory, analgesic, and antipyretic properties in pharmacologic studies. As with other such drugs, its mode of action is not known. However, it is a potent prostaglandin synthesis inhibitor, and this property may be involved in its anti-inflammatory effect.

Flurbiprofen is well absorbed after oral administration, reaching peak blood levels in approximately 1.5 hours (range 0.5 to 4 hours). Administration with food alters the rate of absorption but does not affect the extent of drug availability. The elimination half-life is 5.7 hours with 90% of the half-life values from 3 to 9 hours. Individual half-life values ranged from 2.8 to 12 hours. There is no evidence of drug accumulation and Flurbiprofen does not induce enzymes that alter its metabolism. Excretion of Flurbiprofen is 88% to 98% complete 24 hours after the last dose.

Flurbiprofen is extensively metabolized and excreted primarily in the urine, about 20% as free and conjugated drug and about 50% as hydroxylated metabolites. About 90% of the Flurbiprofen in urine is present as conjugates. The major metabolite, 4'-hydroxyl Flurbiprofen, has been detected in human plasma, but in animal models of inflammation this metabolite showed little anti-inflammatory activity. Flurbiprofen is more than 99% bound to human serum proteins. The average maximum serum concentration of Flurbiprofen, following a 100 mg oral dose of Flurbiprofen Tablets in normal volunteers (n = 184), was 15.2 µg/ml, with 90% of the values between 10 and 22 µg/ml. In geriatric subjects (n = 7) between the ages of 58 and 77 years, 100 mg Flurbiprofen Tablets resulted in an average peak drug level of 18.0 µg/ml and an average elimination half-life of 6.5 hours (range 3-10 hours). In geriatric rheumatoid arthritis patients (n = 13) between the ages of 65 and 83 years receiving 100 mg Flurbiprofen Tablets, the average maximum blood level was 12.7 µg/ml and the average elimination half-life was 5.6 hours (range 4-10 hours).

In a study assessing Flurbiprofen pharmacokinetics in end stage renal disease (ESRD), mean urinary recovery of a 100 mg dose was 73% in 48 hours for 9 normal subjects and 17% in 96 hours for 8 ESRD patients undergoing continuous ambulatory peritoneal dialysis. Plasma concentrations of Flurbiprofen were about 40% lower in the ESRD patients; the elimination half-life of Flurbiprofen was unchanged. Elimination of the 4'-hydroxy Flurbiprofen metabolite was markedly reduced in the ESRD patients. The pharmacokinetics of Flurbiprofen in patients with decreased renal function but not ESRD have not been determined.

The pharmacokinetics of Flurbiprofen in patients with hepatic disease have not been determined.

The efficacy of Flurbiprofen has been demonstrated in patients with rheumatoid arthritis and osteoarthritis. Using standard assessments of therapeutic response, Flurbiprofen (200-300 mg/day) demonstrated effectiveness comparable to aspirin (2000-4000 mg/day), ibuprofen (2400-3200 mg/day), and indomethacin (75-150 mg/day).

In patients with rheumatoid arthritis, Flurbiprofen may be used in combination with gold salts or corticosteroids.

INDICATIONS AND USAGE

Flurbiprofen Tablets are indicated for the acute or long-term treatment of the signs and symptoms of rheumatoid arthritis and osteorthritis.

UNLABELED USES

Florbiproten is used alone or as an adjunct in the treatment of dental pain, primary dysmenorrhea, and acute gout.

CONTRAINDICATIONS

Flurbiprofen Tablets are contraindicated in patients who have previously demonstrated hypersensitivity to it. Flurbiprofen should not be given to patients in whom Flurbiprofen, aspirin, or other nonsteroidal anti-inflammatory drugs induce asthma, urticaria, or other allergic-type reactions. Fatal asthmatic reactions have been reported in such patients receiving this type of drug.

► SHOWN IN PRODUCT IDENTIFICATION GUIDE

WARNINGS

RISK OF GASTROINTESTINAL (GI) ULCERATIONS, BLEEDING AND PERFORATION WITH NONSTEROIDAL ANTI-INFLAMMATORY THERAPY

Serious gastrointestinal toxicity, such as bleeding, ulceration, and perforation, can occur at any time, with or without warning symptoms, in patients treated chronically with nonsteroidal anti-inflammatory drugs. Although minor upper GI problems, such as dyspepsia, are common, usually developing early in therapy, physicians should remain alert for ulceration and bleeding in patients treated chronically with nonsteroidal anti-inflammatory drugs, even in the absence of previous GI tract symptoms. In patients observed in clinical trials of such agents for several months to two years, symptomatic upper GI ulcers, gross bleeding, or perforation appear to occur in approximately 1% of patients treated for 3-6 months, and in about 2-4% of patients treated for one year. Physicians should inform patients about the signs and/or symptoms of serious GI toxicity and what steps to take if they occur.

Studies to date have not identified any subset of patients not at risk of developing peptic ulceration and bleeding. Except for a prior history of serious GI events and other risk factors known to be associated with peptic ulcer disease, such as alcoholism, smoking, etc., no risk factors (e.g., age, sex) have been associated with increased risk. Elderly or debilitated patients seem to tolerate ulceration or bleeding less well than other individuals and most spontaneous reports of fatal GI events are in this population. Studies to date are inconclusive concerning the relative risk of various nonsteroidal anti-inflammatory agents in causing such reactions. High doses of any such agent probably carry a greater risk of these reactions, although controlled clinical trials showing this do not exist in most cases. In considering the use of relatively large doses (within the recommended dosage range), sufficient benefit should be anticipated to off-set the potential increased risk of GI toxicity.

Because serious GI tract ulceration and bleeding can occur without warning symptoms, physicians should follow chronically treated patients for the signs and symptoms of ulceration and bleeding and should inform the patients of the importance of this follow-up.

PRECAUTIONS

GENERAL PRECAUTIONS

Impaired Renal or Hepatic Function: As with other nonsteroidal anti-inflammatory drugs, Flurbiprofen Tablets should be used with caution in patients with impaired renal or hepatic function, or a history of kidney or liver disease. Studies to assess the pharmacokinetics of Flurbiprofen in patients with decreased liver function have not been done.

Renal Effects: Toxicology studies in rats have shown renal papillary necrosis at dosage levels equivalent on a mg/kg basis to those used clinically in humans. Similar findings were seen in monkeys given high doses (50-100 mg/kg, or approximately 20-40 times the human therapeutic dose) for 90 days.

In Upjohn clinical studies, kidney function tests were done at least monthly in patients taking Flurbiprofen. In these studies, renal effects of Flurbiprofen were similar to those seen with other nonsteroidal anti-inflammatory drugs.

A second form of renal toxicity has been seen in patients with prerenal conditions leading to a reduction in renal blood flow or blood volume, where the renal prostaglandins have a supportive role in the maintenance of renal perfusion. In these patients administration of a nonsteroidal anti-inflammatory drug may cause a dose-dependent reduction in prostaglandin formation, which may precipitate overt renal decompensation. Patients at greatest risk of this reaction are those with impaired renal function, heart failure, liver dysfunction, those taking diuretics, and the elderly. Discontinuation of nonsteroidal anti-inflammatory drug therapy is typically followed by recovery of the pretreatment state. Those patients at high risk who chronically take Flurbiprofen should have renal function monitored if they have signs or symptoms that may be consistent with mild azotemia, such as malaise, fatigue, loss of appetite, etc. Occasional patients may develop some elevation of serum creatinine and BUN levels without signs or symptoms.

The elimination half-life of Flurbiprofen was unchanged in patients with end stage renal disease (ESRD). Flurbiprofen metabolites are primarily eliminated by the kidneys and elimination of 4-hydroxy-Flurbiprofen was markedly reduced in ESRD patients. Therefore, patients with significantly impaired renal function may require a reduction of dosage to avoid accumulation of Flurbiprofen metabolites and should be monitored. (See also the *"Clinical Pharmacology"* section.)

Liver Tests: As with other nonsteroidal anti-inflammatory drugs, borderline elevations of one or more liver tests may occur in up to 15% of patients. These abnormalities may progress, may remain essentially unchanged, or may disappear with continued therapy. The ALT (SGPT) test is probably the most sensitive indicator of liver injury. Meaningful (3 times the upper limit of normal) elevations of ALT or AST (SGOT) have been reported in controlled clinical trials in less than 1% of patients. A patient with symptoms and/or signs suggesting liver dysfunction, or in whom an abnormal liver test has occurred, should be evaluated for evidence of the development of a more severe hepatic reaction while on therapy with Flurbiprofen.

Anemia: Anemia is commonly observed in rheumatoid arthritis and is sometimes aggravated by nonsteroidal anti-inflammatory drugs, which may produce fluid retention or minor gastrointestinal blood loss in some patients. Therefore, patients who have initial hemoglobin values of 10 g/dL or less, and who are to receive long-term therapy, should have hemoglobin values determined periodically.

Fluid Retention and Edema: Fluid retention and edema have been reported; therefore, Flurbiprofen should be used with caution in patients with cardiac decompensation, hypertension, or similar conditions.

Vision Changes: Blurred and/or diminished vision has been reported with the use of Flurbiprofen and other nonsteroidal anti-inflammatory drugs. Patients experiencing eye complaints should have ophthalmologic examinations.

Effect on Platelets and Coagulation: Flurbiprofen inhibits collagen-induced platelet aggregation. Prolongation of bleeding time by Flurbiprofen has been demonstrated in humans after single and multiple oral doses. Patients who may be adversely affected by prolonged bleeding time should be carefully observed when Flurbiprofen is administered.

Information for Patients: Flurbiprofen like other drugs of its class, is not free of side effects. The side effects of these drugs can cause discomfort and, rarely, there are more serious side effects, such as gastrointestinal bleeding, which may result in hospitalization and even fatal outcomes. Nonsteroidal anti-inflammatory drugs are often essential agents in the management of arthritis, but they also may be commonly employed for conditions which are less serious. Physicians may wish to discuss with their patients the potential risks (see *"Warnings," "Precautions,"* and *"Adverse Reactions"* sections) and likely benefits of nonsteroidal anti-inflammatory drug treatment, particularly when the drugs are used for less serious conditions where treatment without such agents may represent an acceptable alternative to both the patient and the physician.

DRUG INTERACTIONS

Antacids: Administration of Flurbiprofen to volunteers under fasting conditions, or with antacid suspension, yielded similar serum Flurbiprofen-time profiles in young subjects (n = 12). In geriatric subjects (n = 7) there was a reduction in the rate but not the extent of Flurbiprofen absorption.

Anticoagulants: Flurbiprofen, like other nonsteroidal anti-inflammatory drugs, has been shown to affect bleeding parameters in patients receiving anticoagulants, and serious clinical bleeding has been reported. The physician should be cautious when administering Flurbiprofen to patients taking anticoagulants.

Aspirin: Concurrent administration of aspirin and Flurbiprofen resulted in 50% lower serum Flurbiprofen concentrations. This effect of aspirin (which also lowers serum concentrations of other nonsteroidal anti-inflammatory drugs given with it) has been demonstrated in patients with rheumatoid arthritis (n = 15) as well as normal volunteers (n = 16). Concurrent use of Flurbiprofen and aspirin is therefore not recommended.

Beta-adrenergic Blocking Agents: The effect of Flurbiprofen on blood pressure response to propranolol and atenolol was evaluated in men with mild uncomplicated hypertension (n = 10). Flurbiprofen pretreatment attenuated the hypotensive effect of a single dose of propranolol but not atenolol. Flurbiprofen did not appear to affect the beta-blocker-mediated reduction in heart rate. Flurbiprofen did not affect the pharmacokinetic profile of either drug, and the mechanism underlying the interference with propranolol's hypotensive effect is unknown. Patients taking both Flurbiprofen and a beta-blocker should be monitored to ensure that a satisfactory hypotensive effect is achieved.

Cimetidine, Ranitidine: In normal volunteers (n = 9), pretreatment with cimetidine or ranitidine did not affect Flurbiprofen pharmacokinetics, except that a small (13%) but statistically significant increase in the area under the serum concentration curve of Flurbiprofen resulted with cimetidine.

Digoxin: Studies of concomitant administration of Flurbiprofen and digoxin to healthy men (n = 14) did not show a change in the steady state serum levels of either drug.

Diuretics: Studies in normal volunteers have shown that Flurbiprofen, like other nonsteroidal anti-inflammatory drugs, can interfere with the effects of furosemide. Although results have varied from study to study, effects have been shown on furosemide-stimulated diuresis, natriuresis, and kaliuresis. Other nonsteroidal anti-inflammatory drugs that inhibit prostaglandin synthesis have been shown to interfere with thiazide diuretics in some studies, and with potassium-sparing diuretics. Patients receiving Flurbiprofen and furosemide or other diuretics should be observed closely to determine if the desired effect is obtained.

Oral Hypoglycemia Agents: In one study Flurbiprofen was given to adult diabetics who were already receiving glyburide (n = 4), metformin (n = 2), chlorpropamide with phenformin (n = 3), or glyburide with phenformin (n = 6). Although there was a slight reduction in blood sugar concentrations during concomitant administration of Flurbiprofen and hypoglycemic agents, there were no signs or symptoms of hypoglycemia.

Carcinogenesis, Mutagenesis, Impairment of Fertility: An 80-week study in mice at doses of 2, 5, and 12/mg/kg/day and a 2-year study in rats at doses of 0.5, 2, and 4 mg/kg/day did not show evidence of carcinogenicity at maximum tolerated doses of Flurbiprofen.

Flurbiprofen did not impair the fertility of male or female rats treated orally at 2.25 mg/kg/day for 65 days and 16 days, respectively, before mating.

Teratogenic Effects: Pregnancy Category B: In teratology studies Flurbiprofen, given to mice in doses up to 12 mg/kg/day, to rats in doses up to 25 mg/kg/day, and to rabbits in doses up to 7.5 mg/kg/day, showed no teratogenic effects.

Because there are no adequate and well-controlled studies in pregnant women, and animal teratology studies do not always predict human response, Flurbiprofen is not recommended for use in pregnancy.

Labor and Delivery: The effects of Flurbiprofen on labor and delivery in women are not known. As with other drugs known to inhibit prostaglandin synthesis, an increased incidence of dystocia and delayed parturition occurred in rats treated throughout pregnancy. Because of the known effects of prostaglandin-inhibiting drugs on the fetal cardiovascular system (closure of the ductus arteriosus), use of Flurbiprofen during late pregnancy is not recommended.

Nursing Mothers: Concentrations of Flurbiprofen in breast milk and plasma of nursing mothers suggested that a nursing infant could receive approximately 0.10 mg Flurbiprofen per day in the established milk of a woman taking 200 mg/day. Because of possible adverse effects of prostaglandin-inhibiting drugs on neonates Flurbiprofen is not recommended for use in nursing mothers.

Pediatric Use: Safety and effectiveness in children have not been established.

ADVERSE REACTIONS

Adverse reaction information was derived from patients who received Flurbiprofen in blinded-controlled and open-label clinical trials, and from worldwide marketing experience and from publications. In the description below, rates of the more common events (greater than 1%) and many of the less common events (less than 1%) represent clinical study results. For rarer events that were derived principally from worldwide marketing experience and the literature (printed in *italics*), accurate rate estimates are generally impossible. Of the 4123 patients in premarketing studies, 2954 were treated for at least 1 month, 1448 for at least 3 months, 948 for at least 6 months, 356 for at least 1 year, and 100 for at least 2 years. Of the 4123 patients, 9.4% dropped out of the studies because of an adverse drug reaction, principally involving the gastrointestinal tract (5.8%) central nervous system and special senses (1.4%), skin (0.6%) and genitourinary tract (0.5%).

INCIDENCE GREATER THAN 1%
An asterisk after a reaction identifies reactions which occurred in 3-9% of patients treated with Flurbiprofen. Reactions occurring in 1-3% of the patients are unmarked.

Gastrointestinal: Dyspepsia*, diarrhea*, abdominal pain*, nausea*, constipation, GI bleeding, flatulence, elevated liver enzymes, and vomiting.

Central Nervous System: Headache, nervousness, and other manifestations of CNS "stimulation" (e.g., anxiety, insomnia, reflexes increased, and tremor), and symptoms associated with CNS "inhibition" (e.g., amnesia, asthenia, somnolence malaise, and depression).

Respiratory: Rhinitis.

Dermatological: Rash.

Special Senses: Dizziness, tinnitus, and changes in vision.

Genitourinary: Signs and symptoms suggesting urinary tract infection*.

Body as a Whole: Edema*.

Metabolic/Nutritional: Body weight changes.

INCIDENCE LESS THAN 1% (CAUSAL RELATIONSHIP PROBABLE)
The reactions listed in this category occurred in < 1% of patients in the clinical trials or were reported during postmarketing experience from other countries. Adverse reactions reported only in worldwide postmarketing experience or the literture (which presumably indicates that they are rarer) are italicized.

Gastrointestinal: Peptic ulcer disease (see also *"Warnings, Risk of Gastrointestinal, (GI) Ulcerations, Bleeding and Perforation with Nonsteroidal Anti-inflammatory Therapy"*), gastritis, bloody diarrhea, stomatitis, esophageal disease, hematemesis, and hepatitis; *cholestatic and non-cholestatic jaundice.*

Central Nervous System: Ataxia, cerebrovascular ischemia, confusion, parethesia, and twitching.

Hematologic: Decrease in hemoglobin and hematocrit, iron deficiency anemia, *hemolytic anemia* and *a plastic anemia:* leukopenia; eosinophilia; ecchymosis and *thrombocytopenia.* (See also *"Precautions, Effect On Platelets and Coagulation.")*

Respiratory: Asthma and epistaxis.

Dermatological: Angioedema, urticaria, eczema, and pruritus; *photosensitivity, toxic epidermal necrolysis,* and *exfoliative dermatitis.*

Special Senses: Conjunctivitis and parosmia.

Genitourinary: Hematuria and renal failure; *interstititial nephritis.*

Body as a Whole: Chills and fever; *anaphylactic reaction.*

Metabolic/Nutritional: Hyperuricemia.

Cardiovascular: Heart failure, hypertension, vascular diseases and vasodilation.

INCIDENCE LESS THAN 1% (CAUSAL RELATIONSHIP UNKNOWN)
The following reactions have been reported in patients taking Flurbiprofen under circumstances that do not permit a clear attribution of the reaction to Flurbiprofen. These reactions are being included as alerting information for physicians. Adverse reactions reported only in worldwide postmarketing experience or the literature (which presumably indicates that they are rarer) are italicized.

Gastrointestinal: Periodontal abscess, appetite changes, cholecystitis, and dry mouth.

Central Nervous System: Convulsion, meningitis, hypertonia, cerebrovascular accident, emotional lability, and subarachnoid hemorrhage.

Hematologic: Lymphadenopathy.

Respiratory: Bronchitis, laryngitis, dyspenea, pulmonary embolism, pulmonary infarct, and hyperventilation.

Dermatological: Alopecia, nail disorder, herpes simplex, zoster, dry skin, and sweating.

Special Senses: Ear disease, corneal opacity, glaucoma, retrobulbar neuritis, changes in taste, and transient hearing loss; *retinal hemorrhage.*

Genitourinary: Menstrual disturbances, vaginal and uterine hemorrhage, vulvovaginitis, and prostate disease.

Metabolic/Nutritional: Hyperkalemia.

Cardiovascular: Arrhythmias, angina pectoris, and myocardial infarction.

Musculoskeletal: Myasthenia.

DRUG ABUSE AND DEPENDENCE
No drug abuse or drug dependence has been observed with Flurbiprofen.

OVERDOSAGE
Information on overdosage is available for 13 children and 12 adults. Nine of the 13 children were less than 6 years old. Drowsiness occurred after doses of 150 to 800 mg in 3 of these young children (with dilated pupils in 1), and in a 2-year-old who also had semi-consciousness, pinpoint pupils, diminished tone, and elevated liver enzymes. Other children who ingested doses of 200 mg to 2.5 g showed no symptoms.

Among the adults, a 70-year-old man with a history of chronic obstructive airway disease died. Toxicological analysis showed acute Flurbiprofen overdose and a blood ethanol concentration of 100 mg/dL. In the other cases, symptoms were as follows: coma and respiratory depression after 3-6 g; drowsiness, nausea and epigastric pain after 2.5-5 g; epigastric pain and dizziness after 3 g; headache and nausea after $\leq$ 2 g; agitation after 1.5 g; and drowsiness after 1.0 g. One patient, who took 200-400 mg Flurbiprofen and 2.4 g fenoprofen, had disorientation and diplopia. Three adults had no symptoms after 3-5 g Flurbiprofen.

Treatment of an overdose: the stomach should be emptied by vomiting or lavage, though little drug will likely be recovered if more than an hour has elapsed since ingestion. Supportive treatment should be instituted as necessary. Some patients have been given supplemental oral or intravenous fluids and required no other treatment.

In mice, the Flurbiprofen LD_{50} was 750 mg/kg when administered orally and 200 mg/kg when administered intraperitoneally. The primary signs of toxicity were prostration, ataxia, loss of righting reflex, labored respiration, twitches, convulsions, CNS depression, and splayed hind limbs. In rats, the Flurbiprofen LD_{50} was 160 mg/kg when administered orally and 400 mg/kg when administered intraperitoneally. The primary signs of toxicity were tremors, convulsions, labored respiration, and prostration. These were observed mostly in the intraperitoneal studies.

DOSAGE AND ADMINISTRATION
Flurbiprofen Tablets are administered orally.

Rheumatoid arthritis and osteoarthritis: Recommended starting dose is 200 to 300 mg total daily dose administered BID, TID, or QID. (Most experience in rheumatoid arthritis has been with TID or QID dosage.) The largest recommended single dose in a multiple-dose daily regimen is 100 mg. The dose should be tailored to each patient according to the severity of the symptoms and the response to therapy.

Although a few patients have received higher doses, doses above 300 mg per day are not recommended until more clinical experience with Flurbiprofen is obtained.

Store at controlled room temperature 15° to 30°C (59° to 86°F).

HOW SUPPLIED
TABLET: 50 MG

AVERAGE UNIT PRICE (AVAILABLE SIZES)		GENERIC A-RATED AVERAGE PRICE (GAAP)	
BRAND	$0.78	100s	$68.35
GENERIC	$0.68		

BRAND/MANUFACTURER	NDC	SIZE	AWP
◆ BRAND			
➤ ANSAID: Upjohn	00009-0170-07	100s	$76.58
	00009-0170-08	100s ud	$82.19
	00009-0170-09	500s	$371.41
◆ GENERICS			
Allscrips	54569-3857-00	30s	$20.56
Greenstone	59762-3723-01	100s	$68.15
Mylan	00378-0076-01	100s	$68.54

TABLET: 50 MG

BRAND/MANUFACTURER	NDC	SIZE	AWP
○ GENERICS			
Geneva	00781-1031-01	100s	$68.59

For additional alternatives, turn to the section beginning on page 2859.

➤ SHOWN IN PRODUCT IDENTIFICATION GUIDE

Fluress SEE BENOXINATE HYDROCHLORIDE AND FLUORESCEIN SODIUM

Fluro-Ethyl SEE DICHLOROTETRAFLUOROETHANE AND ETHYL CHLORIDE

Flu-Shield SEE INFLUENZA VIRUS VACCINE

Flutamide

DESCRIPTION
Flutamide is an acetanilid, nonsteroidal, orally active antiandrogen having the chemical name, 2-methyl-*N*-[4-nitro-3-(trifluoromethyl)phenyl] propanamide.

Each capsule contains 125 mg Flutamide. The compound is a buff to yellow powder with a molecular weight of 276.2.

Following is its chemical structure:

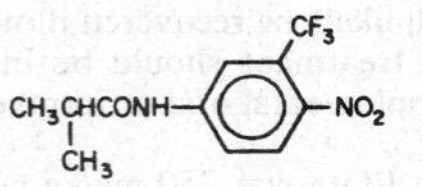

CLINICAL PHARMACOLOGY
General: In animal studies Flutamide demonstrates potent antiandrogenic effects. It exerts its antiandrogenic action by inhibiting androgen uptake and/or by inhibiting nuclear binding of androgen in target tissues or both. Prostatic carcinoma is known to be androgen-sensitive and responds to treatment that counteracts the effect of androgen and/or removes the source of androgen, e.g., castration.

Pharmacokinetics: Analysis of plasma, urine, and feces following a single oral 200 mg dose of tritium-labeled Flutamide to human volunteers showed that the drug is rapidly and completely absorbed. It is excreted mainly in the urine with only 4.2% of the dose excreted in the feces over 72 hours. The composition of plasma radioactivity showed that Flutamide is rapidly and extensively metabolized, with Flutamide comprising only 2.5% of plasma radioactivity one hour after administration. At least six metabolites have been identified in plasma. The major plasma metabolite is a biologically active alpha-hydroxylated derivative which accounts for 23% of the plasma tritium one hour after drug administration.

The major urinary metabolite is 2-amino-5-nitro-4-(trifluoromethyl)phenol.

Following a single 250 mg oral dose to normal adult volunteers, low plasma levels of varying amounts of Flutamide were detected. The biologically active alpha-hydroxylated metabolite reaches maximum plasma levels in about two hours, indicating that it is rapidly formed from Flutamide. The plasma half-life for this metabolite is about 6 hours.

Following multiple oral dosing of 250 mg t.i.d. in normal geriatric volunteers, Flutamide and its active metabolite approached steady-state plasma levels (based on pharmacokinetic simulations) after the fourth Flutamide dose. The half-life of the active metabolite in geriatric volunteers after a single Flutamide dose is about 8 hours and at steady-state is 9.6 hours.

Flutamide, *in vivo*, at steady-state plasma concentrations of 24 to 78 ng/mL is 94% to 96% bound to plasma proteins. The active metabolite of Flutamide, *in vivo*, at steady-state plasma concentrations of 1556 to 2284 ng/mL, is 92% to 94% bound to plasma proteins.

In male rats neither Flutamide nor any of its metabolites is preferentially accumulated in any tissue except the prostate after an oral 5 mg/kg dose of ^{14}C-flutamide. Total drug levels were highest 6 hours after drug administration in all tissues. Levels declined at roughly similar rates to low levels at 18 hours. The major metabolite was present at higher concentrations than Flutamide in all tissues studied.

Elevations of plasma testosterone and estradiol levels have been noted following Flutamide administration.

Clinical Studies: Flutamide has been demonstrated to interfere with testosterone at the cellular level. This can complement medical castration achieved with leuprolide, which suppresses testicular androgen production by inhibiting luteinizing horome secretion.

To study the effects of combination therapy, 617 patients (311 leuprolide + Flutamide, 306 leuprolide + placebo) with previously untreated advanced prostatic carcinoma were enrolled in a large multi-centered, controlled clinical trial. Three and one-half years after the study was initiated, median survival had been reached. The median actuarial survival time was 34.9 months for patients treated with leuprolide and Flutamide versus 27.9 months for patients treated with leuprolide alone. This seven month increment represents a 25% improvement in overall survival with the Flutamide therapy. Analysis of progression free survival showed a 2.6 month improvement in patients who received leuprolide plus Flutamide, a 19% increment over leuprolide and placebo.

INDICATIONS AND USAGE
Flutamide is indicated for use in combination with LHRH agonistic analogues (such as leuprolide acetate) for the treatment of metastatic prostatic carcinoma (stage D_2). To achieve the benefit of the adjunctive therapy with Flutamide, treatment must be started simultaneously using both drugs.

UNLABELED USES
Flutamide is used alone or as an adjunct in the symptomatic treatment of benign prostatic hyperplasia.

CONTRAINDICATIONS
Flutamide is contraindicated in patients who are hypersensitive to Flutamide or any component of this preparation.

WARNINGS
Gynecomastia occurred in 9% of patients receiving Flutamide together with medical castration.

Flutamide may cause fetal harm when administered to a pregnant woman. There was decreased 24-hour survival in the offspring of rats treated with Flutamide at doses of 30, 100, or 200 mg/kg/day (approximately 3, 9, and 19 times the human dose) during pregnancy. A slight increase in minor variations in the development of the sternebrae and vertebrae was seen in fetuses of rats at the two higher doses. Feminization of the males also occurred at the two higher dose levels. There was a decreased survival rate in the offspring of rabbits receiving the highest dose (15 mg/kg/day; equal to 1.4 times the human dose).

Hepatic Injury: Since transaminase abnormalities, cholestatic jaundice, hepatic necrosis, and hepatic encephalopathy have been reported with the use of Flutamide, periodic liver function tests should be considered. (See *"Adverse Reactions"* section.) Appropriate laboratory testing should be done at the first symptom/sign of liver dysfunction (e.g., pruritus, dark urine, persistent anorexia, jaundice, right upper quadrant tenderness or unexplained "flu-like" symptoms). If the patient has jaundice or laboratory evidence of liver injury in the absence of biopsy-confirmed liver metastases, Flutamide therapy should be discontinued or the dosage reduced. The hepatic injury is usually reversible after discontinuation of therapy and in some patients, after dosage reduction. However, there have been reports of death following severe hepatic injury associated with use of Flutamide.

PRECAUTIONS
Information for Patients: Patients should be informed that Flutamide and the drug used for medical castration should be administered concomitantly, and that they should not interrupt their dosing or stop taking these medications without consulting their physician.

Laboratory Tests: See *"Warnings, Hepatic Injury"* above.

Drug Interactions: Interactions between Flutamide and leuprolide have not occurred. Increases in prothrombin time have been noted in patients receiving longterm warfarin therapy after Flutamide was initiated. Therefore close monitoring of prothrombin time is recommended and adjustment of the anticoagulant dose may be necessary when Flutamide administered concomitantly with warfarin.

Carcinogenesis, Mutagenesis, Impairment of Fertility: No carcinogenicity studies were performed with Flutamide. However, daily administration of Flutamide to rats for 52 weeks at doses of 30, 90, or 180 mg/kg/day (approximately 3, 8, or 17 times the human dose) produced testicular interstitial cell adenomas at all doses.

Flutamide did not demonstrate DNA modifying activity in the Ames *Salmonella*/microsome Mutagenesis Assay. Dominant lethal tests in rats were negative.

Reduced sperm counts were observed during a six-week study of Flutamide monotherapy in normal human volunteers.

Flutamide did not affect estrous cycles or interfere with the mating behavior of male and female rats when the drug was administered at 25 and 75 mg/kg/day prior to mating. Males treated with 150 mg/kg/day (30 times the minimum effective antiandrogenic dose) failed to mate; mating behavior returned to normal after dosing was stopped. Conception rates were decreased in all dosing groups. Suppression of spermatogenesis was observed in rats dosed for 52 weeks at approximately 3, 8, or 17 times the human dose and in dogs dosed for 78 weeks at 1.4, 2.3, and 3.7 times the human dose.

Pregnancy: Pregnancy Category D. See *"Warnings"* section.

ADVERSE REACTIONS
The following adverse experiences were reported during a multicenter clinical trial comparing Flutamide + LHRH agonist versus placebo + LHRH agonist.

The most frequently reported (greater than 5%) adverse experiences during treatment with Flutamide in combination with a LHRH agonist are listed in the table below. For comparison, adverse experiences seen with a LHRH agonist and placebo are also listed in the following table.

◆ RATED THERAPEUTICALLY EQUIVALENT; ◇ THERAPEUTIC EQUIVALENCE UNCONFIRMED; ○ UNRATED

	(n = 294) Flutamide + LHRH agonist % All	(n = 285) Placebo + LHRH agonist % All
Hot Flashes	61	57
Loss of Libido	36	31
Impotence	33	29
Diarrhea	12	4
Nausea/Vomiting	11	10
Gynecomastia	9	11
Other	7	9
Other GI	6	4

As shown in the table, for both treatment groups, the most frequently occurring adverse experiences (hot flashes, impotence, loss of libido) were those known to be associated with low serum androgen levels and known to occur with LHRH agonists alone.

The only notable difference was the higher incidence of diarrhea in the Flutamide + LHRH agonist group (12%), which was severe in five percent as opposed to the placebo + LHRH agonist (4%), which was severe in less than one percent.

In addition, the following adverse reactions were reported during treatment with Flutamide + LHRH agonist. No causal relatedness of these reactions to drug treatment has been made, and some of the adverse experiences reported are those that commonly occur in elderly patients.

Cardiovascular System: hypertension in 1% of patients.

Central Nervous System: CNS (drowsiness/confusion/depression/anxiety/nervousness) reactions occurred in 1% of patients.

Gastrointestinal System: anorexia 4%, and other GI disorders occurred in 6% of patients.

Hematopoietic System: anemia occurred in 6%, leukopenia in 3%, and thrombocytopenia in 1% of patients.

Liver and Biliary System: hepatitis and jaundice in less than 1% of patients.

Skin: irritation at the injection site and rash occurred in 3% of patients.

Other: edema occurred in 4%, genitourinary and neuromuscular symptoms in 2%, and pulmonary symptoms in less than 1% of patients.

In addition, the following spontaneous adverse experiences have been reported during the marketing of Flutamide: hemolytic anemia, macrocytic anemia, methemoglobinemia, photosensitivity reactions (including erythema, ulceration, bullous eruptions, and epidermal necrolysis) and urine discoloration. The urine was noted to change to an amber or yellow-green appearance which can be attributed to the Flutamide and/or its metabolites. Also reported were cholestatic jaundice, hepatic encephalopathy, and hepatic necrosis. The hepatic conditions were usually reversible after discontinuing therapy; however, there have been reports of death following severe hepatic injury associated with use of Flutamide.

Abnormal Laboratory Test Values: Laboratory abnormalities including elevated SGOT, SGPT, bilirubin values. SGGT, BUN and serum creatinine have been reported.

OVERDOSAGE

In animal studies with Flutamide alone, signs of overdose included hypoactivity, piloerection, slow respiration, ataxia, and/or lacrimation, anorexia, tranquilization, emesis, and methemoglobinemia.

Clinical trials have been conducted with Flutamide in doses up to 1500 mg per day for periods up to 36 weeks with no serious adverse effects reported. Those adverse reactions reported included gynecomastia, breast tenderness and some increases in SGOT. The single dose of Flutamide ordinarily associated with symptoms of overdose or considered to be life-threatening has not been established.

Since Flutamide is highly protein bound, dialysis may not be of any use as treatment for overdose. As in the management of overdosage with any drug, it should be borne in mind that multiple agents may have been taken. If vomiting does not occur spontaneously, it should be induced if the patient is alert. General supportive care, including frequent monitoring of the vital signs and close observation of the patient, is indicated.

DOSAGE AND ADMINISTRATION

The recommended dosage is two capsules three times a day at eight hour intervals for a total daily dosage of 750 mg.

Store between 2° and 30°C (36° and 86°F).

Protect the unit dose packages from excessive moisture.

HOW SUPPLIED
CAPSULE: 125 MG

BRAND/MANUFACTURER	NDC	SIZE	AWP
○ BRAND			
EULEXIN: Schering	00085-0525-03	100s ud	$158.22
	00085-0525-06	180s	$268.64
	00085-0525-05	500s	$746.35

Fluticasone Propionate

DESCRIPTION

Fluticasone Propionate Cream and Ointment contain Fluticasone Propionate [(6α,11β,16α,17α)-6,9-difluoro-11-hydroxy-16-methyl-3-oxo-17 -(1-oxopropoxy) androsta-1,4-diene-17-carbothioic acid, S-fluoromethyl ester], a synthetic fluorinated corticosteroid, for topical dermatologic use. The topical corticosteroids constitute a class of primarily synthetic steroids used as anti-inflammatory and anti-pruritic agents.

Chemically, Fluticasone Propionate is $C_{25}H_{31}F_3O_5S$.

Fluticasone Propionate has a molecular weight of 500.6. It is a white to off-white powder and is insoluble in water.

Each gram of Fluticasone Propionate Cream, 0.05% contains Fluticasone Propionate 0.5 mg.

Each gram of Fluticasone Propionate ointment 0.005% contains Fluticasone Propionate 0.05 mg.

Following is its chemical structure:

CLINICAL PHARMACOLOGY

Like other topical corticosteroids, Fluticasone Propionate has anti-inflammatory, antipruritic, and vasoconstrictive properties. The mechanism of the anti-inflammatory activity of the topical steroids, in general, is unclear. However, corticosteroids are thought to act by the induction of phospholipase A_2 inhibitory proteins, collectively called lipocortins. It is postulated that these proteins control the biosynthesis of potent mediators of inflammation such as prostaglandins and leukotrienes by inhibiting the release of their common precursor, arachidonic acid, which is released from membrane phospholipids by phospholipase A_2.

Pharmacokinetics: The extent of percutaneous absorption of topical corticosteroids is determined by many factors, including the vehicle and the integrity of the epidermal barrier. Occlusive dressing with hydrocortisone for up to 24 hours has not been demonstrated to increase penetration; however, occlusion of hydrocortisone for 96 hours markedly enhances penetration. Topical corticosteroids can be absorbed from normal intact skin, while inflammation and/or other disease processes in the skin increase percutaneous absorption.

Studies performed with Fluticasone Propionate indicate that it is in the medium range of potency as compared with other topical corticosteroids.

INDICATIONS AND USAGE

Fluticasone Propionate is a medium potency corticosteroid indicated for the relief of the inflammatory and pruritic manifestations of corticosteroid-responsive dermatoses.

CONTRAINDICATIONS

Fluticasone Propionate is contraindicated in those patients with a history of hypersensitivity to any of the components of the preparation.

PRECAUTIONS

General: Systemic absorption of topical corticosteroids can produce reversible hypothalamic-pituitary-adrenal (HPA) axis suppression with the potential for glucocorticosteroid insufficiency after withdrawal from treatment. Manifestations of Cushing's syndrome, hyperglycemia, and glucosuria can also be produced in some patients by systemic absorption of topical corticosteroids while on therapy.

Patients receiving a large dose of a potent topical steroid applied to a large surface area or under an occlusive dressing should be evaluated periodically for evidence of HPA axis suppression. This may be done by using the ACTH stimulation, a.m. plasma cortisol, and urinary free cortisol tests.

Fluticasone Propionate Cream 0.05% produced HPA axis suppression within 7 days when used at a dose of 30 g per day in diseased patients. In a study of the effects of Fluticasone Propionate Cream 0.05% on the HPA axis, a total of 30 g per day was used in two applications daily for 7 days to six patients with psoriasis or atopic dermatitis involving at least 30% of the body surface. One patient developed evidence of adrenal suppression after 6 days of treatment with a below normal plasma cortisol level that returned to low normal levels the following day. Another patient developed a 60% decrease (although never below normal) in the plasma cortisol level from pretreatment values after 2 days of treatment. This suppression persisted at this level for 48 hours before recovering by day 6 of treatment. The results of this study indicate that Fluticasone Propionate Cream

0.05% may be able to suppress the HPA axis within a few days with a dose of 30 g per day.

Fluticasone Propionate Ointment, 0.05% (a concentration 10 times that of Fluticasone Propionate Ointment, 0.005%) did not suppress plasma cortisol in any of six patients but did moderately suppress 24-hour urinary free cortisol levels in two of six patients when used at dose of 30 g per day for a week in patients with psoriasis or eczema. In a second study, Fluticasone Propionate ointment, 0.05% caused a minimal depression of a.m. plasma cortisol levels in 3 of 12 normal volunteers when applied at doses of 50 g per day for 21 days. Morning plasma levels returned to normal levels within the first week upon discontinuation of Fluticasone Propionate. In this study there was no corresponding decrease in 24-hour urinary free cortisol levels.

If HPA axis suppression is noted, an attempt should be made to withdraw the drug, to reduce the frequency of application, or to substitute a less potent steroid. Recovery of HPA axis function is generally prompt and complete upon discontinuation of topical corticosteroids. Infrequently, signs and symptoms of glucocorticosteroid insufficiency may occur that require supplemental systemic corticosteroids. For information on systemic supplementation, see prescribing information for those products.

Children may be more susceptible to systemic toxicity from equivalent doses due to their larger skin surface to body mass ratios (see *"Precautions: Pediatric Use"*).

If irritation develops, Fluticasone Propionate should be discontinued and appropriate therapy instituted. Allergic contact dermatitis with corticosteroids is usually diagnosed by observing *failure to heal* rather than noting a clinical exacerbation as with most topical products not containing corticosteroids. Such an observation should be corroborated with appropriate diagnostic patch testing.

If concomitant skin infections are present or develop, an appropriate antifungal or antibacterial agent should be used. If a favorable response does not occur promptly, use of Fluticasone Propionate should be discontinued until the infection has been adequately controlled.

Fluticasone Propionate should not be used in the treatment of rosacea and perioral dermatitis.

Information for Patients: Patients using topical corticosteroids should receive the following information and instructions:

1. This medication is to be used as directed by the physician. It is for external use only. Avoid contact with the eyes.

2. This medication should not be used for any disorder other than that for which it was prescribed.

3. The treated skin area should not be bandaged or otherwise covered or wrapped so as to be occlusive unless directed by the physician.

4. Patients should report to their physician any signs of local adverse reactions.

Laboratory Tests: The following tests may be helpful in evaluating patients for HPA axis suppression:

ACTH stimulation test
A.M. plasma cortisol test
Urinary free cortisol test

Carcinogenesis, Mutagenesis, Impairment of Fertility: Long-term animal studies have not been performed to evaluate the carcinogenic potential of Fluticasone Propionate.

Fluticasone Propionate was not mutagenic in the standard Ames test, *E. coli* fluctuation test, *S. cerevisiae* gene conversion test or Chinese Hamster ovarian cell assay. It was not clastogenic in mouse micronucleus or cultured human lymphocyte tests.

In a fertility and general reproductive performance study in rats, Fluticasone Propionate administered subcutaneously to females at up to 50 µg/kg per day and to males at up to 100 µg/kg per day (later reduced to 50 µg/kg per day) had no effect upon mating performance or fertility. These doses are approximately 15 and 30 times, respectively, the human systemic exposure following use of the recommended human topical dose of Fluticasone Propionate Cream 0.05%, and 150 and 300 times, respectively, the human systemic exposure following use of the recommended human topical dose of Fluticasone Propionate Ointment 0.005%, assuming human percutaneous absorption of approximately 3% and the use in a 70-kg person of 15 g per day.

Pregnancy Teratogenic Effects; Pregnancy Category C: Corticosteroids have been shown to be teratogenic in laboratory animals when administered systemically at relatively low dosage levels. The more potent corticosteroids have been shown to be teratogenic after dermal application in laboratory animals. Teratology studies in the mouse demonstrated Fluticasone Propionate to be teratogenic (cleft palate) when administered subcutaneously in doses of 45 µg/kg per day and 150 µg/kg per day. This dose is approximately 14 and 45 times, respectively, the human topical dose of Fluticasone Propionate Cream 0.05%, approximately 140 and 450 times, respectively, the human topical dose of Fluticasone Propionate Ointment, 0.005%. There are no adequate and well-controlled studies in pregnant women. Fluticasone Propionate should be used during pregnancy only if the potential benefit justifies the potential risk to the fetus.

Nursing Mothers: Systemically administered corticosteroids appear in human milk and could suppress growth, interfere with endogenous corticosteroid production, or cause other untoward effects. It is not known whether topical administration of corticosteroids could result in sufficient systemic absorption to produce detectable quantities in human milk. Because many drugs are excreted in human milk, caution should be exercised when Fluticasone Propionate is administered to a nursing woman.

Pediatric Use: Safety and effectiveness in children and infants have not been established. Because of a higher ratio of skin surface area to body mass, children are at a greater risk than adults of HPA axis suppression when they are treated with topical corticosteroids. They are therefore also at greater risk of glucocorticosteroid insufficiency after withdrawal of treatment and of Cushing's syndrome while on treatment. Adverse effects including striae have been reported with inappropriate use of topical corticosteroids in infants and children (see *"Precautions"*).

HPA axis suppression, Cushing's syndrome, and intracranial hypertension have been reported in children receiving topical corticosteroids. Manifestations of adrenal suppression in children include linear growth retardation, delayed weight gain, low plasma cortisol levels, and absence of response to ACTH stimulation. Manifestations of intracranial hypertension include bulging fontanelles, headaches, and bilateral papilledema.

ADVERSE REACTIONS

In controlled clinical trials, the total incidence of adverse reactions associated with the use of Fluticasone Propionate Cream, 0.05% was approximately 4%. These adverse reactions were mild, usually self-limiting, and consisted primarily of pruritus, dryness, numbness of fingers, and burning. These events occurred in 2.9%, 1.2%, 1.0%, and 0.6% of patients, respectively.

In controlled clinical trials, the total incidence of adverse reactions associated with the use of Fluticasone Propionate Ointment, 0.005% was approximately 4%. These adverse reactions were mild, usually self-limiting, and consisted primarily of pruritus, burning, hypertrichosis, increased erythema, hives, irritation, and light-headedness. Each of these events occurred individually in less than 1% of patients.

The following additional local adverse reactions have been reported infrequently with other topical corticosteroids, and they may occur more frequently with the use of occlusive dressings, especially with higher potency corticosteroids. These reactions are listed in an approximately decreasing order of occurrence: irritation, folliculitis, acneiform eruptions, hypopigmentation, perioral dermatitis, allergic contact dermatitis, secondary infection, skin atrophy, striae, and miliaria. Also, there are reports of the development of pustular psoriasis from chronic plaque psoriasis following reduction or discontinuation of potent topical corticosteroid products.

OVERDOSAGE

Topically applied Fluticasone Propionate can be absorbed in sufficient amounts to produce systemic effects (see *"Precautions"*).

DOSAGE AND ADMINISTRATION

Apply a thin film of Fluticasone Propionate to the affected skin areas twice daily. Rub in gently.

Store between 2° and 30°C (36° and 86°F).

HOW SUPPLIED
CREAM: 0.05%

BRAND/MANUFACTURER	NDC	SIZE	AWP
○ BRAND			
CUTIVATE: Glaxo Derm	00173-0430-00	15 gm	$11.84
	00173-0430-01	30 gm	$18.25
	00173-0430-02	60 gm	$27.76

OINTMENT: 0.005%

BRAND/MANUFACTURER	NDC	SIZE	AWP
○ BRAND			
CUTIVATE: Glaxo Derm	00173-0431-00	15 gm	$11.84
	00173-0431-01	30 gm	$18.25
	00173-0431-02	60 gm	$27.76

Fluvastatin Sodium

DESCRIPTION

Fluvastatin Sodium, is a water soluble cholesterol lowering agent which acts through the inhibition of 3-hydroxy-3-methylglutaryl-coenzyme A (HMG-CoA) reductase. Fluvastatin Sodium is $[R^*, S^*,-(E)]-(\pm)-7-[3-(4-fluorophenyl)-1-(1-methylethyl)-1 H-indol-2-yl]-3,5-dihydroxy-6-heptenoic acid, monosodium salt. Its molecular formula is $C_{24}H_{25}FNO_4$. Na and its molecular weight is 433.46.

This molecular entity is the first entirely synthetic HMG-CoA reductase inhibitor, and is in part structurally distinct from the fungal derivatives of this therapeutic class.

Following is its chemical structure:

CLINICAL PHARMACOLOGY

A variety of clinical studies have demonstrated that elevated levels of total cholesterol (Total-C), low density lipoprotein cholesterol (LDL-C), and apolipoprotein B (a membrane transport complex for LDL-C) promote human atherosclerosis. Similarly, decreased levels of HDL-cholesterol (HDL-C) and its transport complex, apolipoprotein A, are associated with the development of atherosclerosis. Epidemiologic investigations have established that cardiovascular morbidity and mortality vary directly with the level of Total-C and LDL-C and inversely with the level of HDL-C. The Lipid Research Clinics Coronary Primary Prevention Trial (LRC-CPPT) was a multicenter, randomized, doubleblind study involving 3,806 asymptomatic middle-aged men in the United States with Type II hyperlipoproteinemia treated with diet and cholestyramine. Results of this trial demonstrated that a statistically significant reduction of 19% in the incidence of definite myocardial infarction and/or coronary heart disease death was associated with an 8% decrease in blood cholesterol and 11% decrease in LDL-C levels. In other multicenter clinical trials, those pharmacologic and/or nonpharmacologic interventions that simultaneously lowered LDL-C and increased HDL-C also have reduced the rate of cardiovascular events (both fatal and nonfatal myocardial infarctions).

In patients with hypercholesterolemia, treatment with Fluvastatin Sodium reduced Total-C, LDL-C, and apolipoprotein B. Fluvastatin Sodium also moderately reduced triglycerides (TG) while producing an increase in HDL-C of variable magnitude. The agent had no consistent effect on either Lp(a) or fibrinogen. The effect of Fluvastatin Sodium-induced changes in lipoprotein levels on the evolution of atherosclerosis has not been established.

MECHANISM OF ACTION

Fluvastatin Sodium is a competitive inhibitor of HMG-CoA reductase, which is responsible for the conversion of 3-hydroxy-3-methyl-glutaryl-coenzyme A (HMG-CoA) to mevalonate, a precursor of sterols, including cholesterol. The inhibition of cholesterol biosynthesis reduces the cholesterol in hepatic cells, which stimulates the synthesis of LDL receptors and thereby increases the uptake of LDL particles. The end result of these biochemical processes is a reduction of the plasma cholesterol concentration.

PHARMACOKINETICS/METABOLISM

Fluvastatin Sodium is administered orally in the active form. Fluvastatin is absorbed rapidly and completely (98%) following oral administration to fasted volunteers. In a fed state, even up to 4 hours post prandial, the drug is also completely absorbed, but at a reduced rate (C_{max} is reduced by 40%-70%). The action of HMGR inhibitors occurs within the liver. The absolute systemic bioavailability for this drug class is low. The absolute systemic bioavailability of Fluvastatin following a 10 mg oral dose was 24% (range 9%-50%). At doses above 20 mg, Fluvastatin exhibits nonlinear kinetics, at least in the fasting state, resulting in dose normalized AUC values 20%-40% higher than expected for the 40 mg dose. The volume of distribution (VD_{ss}) for the drug is calculated to be 34.4 liters. More than 98% of the circulating drug is bound to plasma proteins, and this binding is unaffected by drug concentration.

Biotransformation pathways for Fluvastatin include: a) hydroxylation of the indole ring at the 5- and 6-positions; b) N-dealkylation; and c) beta-oxidation. The major circulating blood components are Fluvastatin and the pharmacologically inactive N-desisopropyl-propionic acid metabolite. The hydroxylated metabolites have pharmacological activity but do not circulate systemically. Both enantiomers of Fluvastatin are metabolized in a similar manner resulting in only minor differences in systemic exposure.

Following administration of ^{3}H-Fluvastatin Sodium to healthy volunteers, excretion of radioactivity was about 5% in the urine and 90% in the feces, with the parent Fluvastatin, accounting for less than 2% of the total radioactivity excreted. The plasma clearance for Fluvastatin in man is calculated to be 39.2 ± 4.4 liters per hour. Steady-state plasma concentrations show no evidence of Fluvastatin accumulation following administration of 40 mg daily; however, after 6 days of dosing with 40 mg ^{3}H-Fluvastatin Sodium solution, total radioactivity—which includes parent compound and pharmacologically inactive metabolites—accumulated by a factor of 2 based on C_{min} values. Following oral administration of 20 mg of Fluvastatin Sodium the beta elimination half-life for Fluvastatin is 1.2 hours (range of 0.53-3.1 hours). The bioavailability of Fluvastatin Sodium 20 mg capsules is equivalent to a solution of Fluvastatin Sodium except that the time to peak under fasted conditions is about 0.7 hours following administration of the capsule compared to about 0.4 hours for the solution. Following ingestion of a single 20 mg Fluvastatin Sodium capsule under fasted conditions, measurable plasma concentrations of Fluvastatin appear systemically within 10 minutes after dosing and reach a peak of 147 ± 86 ng/mL at 0.66 ± 0.3 hours. Fluvastatin Sodium, like the other HMGR inhibitors, has variable systemic bioavailability. The coefficient of variation (based on the inter-subject variability) was 47%-57% for AUC, and 58%-69% for C_{max}.

Results from an overnight pharmacokinetic evaluation following steady-state administration of Fluvastatin Sodium with the evening meal or 4 hours after the evening meal for 15 weeks showed that administration of Fluvastatin Sodium with the evening meal results in a two-fold decrease in C_{max} and more than a two-fold increase in t_{max} as compared to patients receiving the drug 4 hours after the evening meal. No significant difference in AUC was observed between the 2 treatment groups, and there were no differences in the lipid-lowering effects of Fluvastatin Sodium administered with the evening meal or 4 hours after the evening meal.

The effects of gender and age on the pharmacokinetics of Fluvastatin Sodium were evaluated in 4 patient subgroups; young and elderly males and females. All patients were administered 20 mg Fluvastatin daily, at least 2 hours after the evening meal, for 21 days. Results from an overnight pharmacokinetic evaluation indicate that for the general patient population plasma concentrations of Fluvastatin do not vary either as a function of age or gender. Due to their generally smaller body weight, young female patients show higher Fluvastatin plasma concentrations after administration of 10-40 mg of Fluvastatin compared to young males.

Since Fluvastatin is eliminated primarily via the biliary route and is subject to significant presystemic metabolism, the potential exists for drug accumulation in patients with hepatic insufficiency. In a single-dose study the kinetics of Fluvastatin Sodium in subjects with cirrhosis (n = 11) and in healthy age- and sex-matched subjects (n = 11) were compared. The mean AUC and C_{max} parameters were about 2.5 times higher in the subjects with hepatic insufficiency. There was a 28% decrease in plasma clearance and a 31% smaller volume of distribution. No apparent difference was observed in the plasma elimination half-lives for the 2 groups. Caution should be exercised when fluvastatin sodium is administered to patients with a history of liver disease or heavy alcohol ingestion (see "Warnings").

CLINICAL STUDIES

Fluvastatin Sodium has been studied in 4 controlled Phase 3 trials. These studies involved 1605 North American patients with Type IIa or IIb hyperlipoproteinemia. Fluvastatin Sodium was administered to 946 patients in these trials of 24-54 weeks duration. In the largest single randomized study, with Fluvastatin Sodium (n = 292), treatment at a dose of 20 mg QPM resulted in a highly significant decrease in LDL-C of 22.2% after 9 weeks of study. In the largest single study (n = 210) of patients randomized to 40 mg daily and limited to FH patients, a mean LDL-C reduction of 24.0% was observed. Reductions in Apo B were also seen as a result of treatment with Fluvastatin Sodium. Small but statistically significant increases in HDL-C and corresponding decreases in TG were also noted. No consistent effect on Lp(a) was found.

INDICATIONS AND USAGE

Fluvastatin Sodium is indicated as an adjunct to diet in the treatment of elevated total cholesterol (total-C) and LDL-C levels in patients with primary hypercholesterolemia (Type IIa and IIb) whose response to dietary restriction of saturated fat and cholesterol and other nonpharmacological measures has not been adequate.

Therapy with lipid-altering agents should be considered only after secondary causes for hyperlipidemia such as poorly controlled diabetes mellitus, hypothyroidism, nephrotic syndrome, dysproteinemias, obstructive liver disease, other medication, or alcoholism, have been excluded. Prior to initiation of Fluvastatin Sodium, a lipid profile should be performed to measure Total-C, HDL-C and TG. For patients with TG < 400mg/dL (< 4.5 mmol/L), LDL-C can be estimated using the following equation:

$$LDL\text{-}C = Total\text{-}C - HDL\text{-}C - 1/5 \ TG$$

For TG levels > 400 mg/dL (> 4.5 mmol/L), this equation is less accurate and LDL-C concentrations should be determined by ultracentrifugation. In many hypertriglyceridemic patients LDL-C may be low or normal despite elevated Total-C. In such cases, Fluvastatin Sodium is not indicated.

Lipid determinations should be performed at intervals of no less than 4 weeks and dosage adjusted according to the patient's response to therapy.

The National Cholesterol Education Program (NCEP) Treatment Guidelines are summarized below:

		LDL-Cholesterol mg/dL (mmol/L)	
Definite Atherosclerotic Disease*	Two or More Other Risk Factors**	Initiation Level	Goal
No	No	≥ 190 (≥ 4.9)	< 160 (< 4.1)
No	Yes	≥ 160 (≥ 4.1)	< 130 (< 3.4)
Yes	Yes or No	≥ 130 (≥ 3.4)	≤ 100 (≤ 2.6)

* *Coronary heart disease or peripheral vascular disease (including symptomatic carotid artery disease).*

** *Other risk factors for coronary heart disease (CHD) include: age (males ≥ 45 years; females: ≥ 55 years or premature menopause without estrogen replacement therapy); family history of premature CHD; current cigarette smoking; hypertension; confirmed HDL-C < 35 mg/dL (< 0.91 mmol/L); and diabetes mellitus. Subtract one risk factor if HDL-C is ≥ 60 mg/dL (≥ 1.6 mmol/L).*

Since the goal of treatment is to lower LDL-C, the NCEP recommends that the LDL-C levels be used to initiate and assess treatment response. Only if LDL-C levels are not available, should the Total-C be used to monitor therapy.

CLASSIFICATION OF HYPERLIPOPROTEINEMIAS

		Lipid Elevations	
Type	Lipoproteins Elevated	Major	Minor
I (rare)	Chylomicrons	TG	↑ → C
IIa	LDL	C	—
IIb	LDL, VLDL	C	TG

Type	Lipoproteins Elevated	Lipid Elevations	
		Major	Minor
III (rare)	IDL	C/TG	—
IV	VLDL	TG	$\uparrow \rightarrow C$
V (rare)	Chylomicrons, VLDL	TG	$\uparrow \rightarrow C$

C = cholesterol
TG = triglycerides
LDL = low density lipoprotein
VLDL = very low density lipoprotein
IDL = intermediate density lipoprotein

Fluvastatin Sodium has not been studied in conditions where the major abnormality is elevation of chylomicrons, VLDL, or IDL (i.e. hypolipoproteinemia Types I, III, IV, or V).

The effect of Fluvastatin Sodium-induced changes in lipoprotein levels on cardiovascular morbidity or mortality has not been established.

CONTRAINDICATIONS

Hypersensitivity to any component of this medication. Fluvastatin Sodium is contraindicated in patients with active liver disease or unexplained, persistent elevations in serum transaminases (see "Warnings").

PREGNANCY AND LACTATION

Atherosclerosis is a chronic process and discontinuation of lipid-lowering drugs during pregnancy should have little impact on the outcome of long-term therapy of primary hypercholesterolemia. Cholesterol and other products of cholesterol biosynthesis are essential components for fetal development (including synthesis of steroids and cell membranes). Since HMG-CoA reductase inhibitors decrease cholesterol synthesis and possibly the synthesis of other biologically active substances derived from cholesterol, they may cause fetal harm when administered to pregnant women. Therefore, HMG-CoA reductase inhibitors are contraindicated during pregnancy and in nursing mothers. **Fluvastatin Sodium should be administered to women of childbearing age only when such patients are highly unlikely to conceive and have been informed of the potential hazards.** If the patient becomes pregnant while taking this class of drug, therapy should be discontinued and the patient apprised of the potential hazard to the fetus.

WARNINGS

LIVER ENZYMES

Biochemical abnormalities of liver function have been associated with HMG-CoA reductase inhibitors and other lipid-lowering agents. A small number of patients treated with Fluvastatin Sodium in United States controlled trials (N = 17, 1.1%) developed persistent elevations of transaminase levels to more than 3 times the upper limit of normal. Ten of these patients (0.7%) were discontinued from therapy. Most of these (10/17) abnormalities occurred within the first 6 weeks of treatment and resolved rapidly to pretreatment values. In a long-term open-label extension study, 5 of 824 (0.6%) patients exposed to Fluvastatin Sodium at a dose of 40 mg developed persistent transaminase elevations. Only 2 of these patients were discontinued from the study. The majority of these abnormal biochemical findings were asymptomatic.

It is recommended that liver function tests be performed before the initiation of treatment, at 6 and 12 weeks after initiation of therapy or elevation in dose, and periodically thereafter (e.g., semiannually). Liver enzyme changes generally occur in the first 3 months of treatment with Fluvastatin Sodium. Patients who develop increased transaminase levels should be monitored with a second liver function evaluation to confirm the finding and be followed thereafter with frequent liver function tests until the abnormality(ies) return to normal. Should an increase in AST or ALT of three times the upper limit of normal or greater persist, withdrawal of Fluvastatin Sodium therapy is recommended. Active liver disease or unexplained transaminase elevations are contraindications to the use of Fluvastatin Sodium (see "Contraindications"). Caution should be exercised when Fluvastatin Sodium is administered to patients with a history of liver disease or heavy alcohol ingestion (see "Clinical Pharmacology: Pharmacokinetics/Metabolism"). Such patients should be closely monitored.

SKELETAL MUSCLE

Rhabdomyolysis with renal dysfunction secondary to myoglobinuria has been reported with other drugs in this class. To date, this has not occurred with Fluvastatin Sodium. Myopathy, defined as muscle aching or muscle weakness in conjunction with increases in creatine phosphokinase (CPK) values to greater than 10 times the upper limit of normal, has been reported in 1 Fluvastatin Sodium patient to date and was related to physical exertion. An additional case was reported in a patient receiving placebo.

Myopathy should be considered in any patients with diffuse myalgias, muscle tenderness or weakness, and/or marked elevation of CPK. Patients should be advised to report promptly unexplained muscle pain, tenderness or weakness, particularly if accompanied by malaise or fever. Fluvastatin Sodium therapy should be discontinued if markedly elevated CPK levels occur or myopathy is diagnosed or suspected. Fluvastatin sodium therapy should also be temporarily withheld in any patient experiencing an acute or serious condition predisposing to the development of renal failure secondary to rhabdomyolysis, e.g., sepsis; hypotension; major surgery; trauma; severe metabolic, endocrine, or electrolyte disorders; or uncontrolled epilepsy.

The risk of myopathy during treatment with another HMG-CoA reductase inhibitor was found to be increased if therapy with either cyclosporine, gemfibrozil, erythromycin, or niacin is administered concurrently. Myopathy was not observed in a clinical trial in 74 patients involving patients who were treated with Fluvastatin Sodium together with niacin.

Uncomplicated myalgia has been observed infrequently in patients treated with Fluvastatin Sodium at rates indistinguishable from placebo.

The use of fibrates alone may occasionally be associated with myopathy. The combined use of HMG-CoA inhibitors and fibrates should generally be avoided.

PRECAUTIONS

GENERAL

Before instituting therapy with Fluvastatin Sodium, an attempt should be made to control hypercholesterolemia with appropriate diet, exercise, and weight reduction in obese patients, and to treat other underlying medical problems (see "Indications and Usage").

The HMG-CoA reductase inhibitors may cause elevation of creatine phosphokinase and transaminase levels (see "Warnings" and "Adverse Reactions"). This should be considered in the differential diagnosis of chest pain in a patient on therapy with Fluvastatin Sodium.

HOMOZYGOUS FAMILIAL HYPERCHOLESTEROLEMIA

HMG-CoA reductase inhibitors are reported to be less effective in patients with rare homozygous familial hypercholesterolemia, possibly because these patients have few functional LDL receptors.

INFORMATION FOR PATIENTS

Patients should be advised to report promptly unexplained muscle pain, tenderness or weakness, particularly if accompanied by malaise or fever.

DRUG INTERACTIONS

Immunosuppressive Drugs, Gemfibrozil, Niacin (Nicotinic Acid, Erythromycin: See "Warnings: Skeletal Muscle.")

Antipyrine: Administration of Fluvastatin Sodium does not influence the metabolism and excretion of antipyrine, either by induction or inhibition. Antipyrine is a model for drugs metabolized by the microsomal hepatic enzyme system; therefore, interactions with other drugs metabolized by this mechanism are not expected.

Niacin/Propranolol: Concomitant administration of Fluvastatin Sodium with niacin or propranolol has no effect on the bioavailability of Fluvastatin Sodium.

Cholestyramine: Administration of Fluvastatin Sodium concomitantly with, or up to 4 hours after cholestyramine results in Fluvastatin decreases of more than 50% for AUC and 50%-80% for C_{max}. However, administration of Fluvastatin Sodium 4 hours after cholestyramine resulted in a clinically significant additive effect compared with that achieved with either component drug.

Digoxin: In a crossover study involving 18 patients chronically receiving digoxin, a single 40 mg dose of Fluvastatin had no effect on digoxin AUC, but had an 11% increase in digoxin C_{max} and small increase in digoxin urinary clearance. Patients taking digoxin should be monitored appropriately when Fluvastatin therapy is initiated.

Clinetidine/Ranitidine/Omeprazole: Concomitant administration of Fluvastatin Sodium with cimetidine, ranitidine and omeprazole results in a significant increase in the Fluvastatin C_{max} (43%, 70% and 50%, respectively) and AUC (24%-33%), with an 18%-23% decrease in plasma clearance.

Rifampicin: Administration of Fluvastatin Sodium to subjects pretreated with rifampicin results in significant reduction in C_{max} (59%) and AUC (51%), with a large increase (95%) in plasma clearance.

Warfarin: In vitro protein binding studies demonstrated no interaction at therapeutic concentrations.

Other Concomitant Therapy: Although specific interaction studies were not performed, in clinical studies, Fluvastatin Sodium was used concomitantly with angiotensin-converting enzyme (ACE) inhibitors, beta blockers, calcium-channel blockers, diuretics and nonsteroidal anti-inflammatory drugs (NSAIDs) without evidence of clinically significant adverse interactions.

ENDOCRINE FUNCTION

HMG-CoA reductase inhibitors interfere with cholesterol synthesis and lower circulating cholesterol levels and, as such, might theoretically blunt adrenal or gonadal steroid hormone production.

Fluvastatin exhibited no effect upon non-stimulated cortisol levels and demonstrated no effect upon thyroid metabolism as assessed by TSH. Small declines in total testosterone have been noted in treated groups, but no commensurate elevation in LH occurred, suggesting that the observation was not due to a direct effect upon testosterone production. No effect upon FSH in males was noted. Due to the limited number of premenopausal females studied to date, no conclusions regarding the effect of Fluvastatin upon female sex hormones may be made.

Two investigational clinical studies in patients receiving Fluvastatin at doses up to 80 mg daily (twice the recommended dose) for periods of 24-28 weeks demonstrated no effect of treatment upon the adrenal response to ACTH stimulation. A clinical study evaluated the effect of Fluvastatin at doses up to 80 mg daily for 28 weeks upon the gonadal response to HCG stimulation. Although the mean total testosterone response was significantly reduced (p < 0.05) relative to baseline in the 80 mg group, it was not significant in comparison to the changes noted in groups receiving either 40 mg of Fluvastatin or placebo.

Patients treated with Fluvastatin Sodium develop clinical evidence of endocrine dysfunction should be evaluated appropriately. Caution should be exercised if an HMG-CoA reductase inhibitor or other agent used to lower cholesterol levels is administered to patients receiving other drugs (e.g. ketoconazole, spironolactone, or cimetidine) that may decrease the levels of endogenous steroid hormones.

CNS TOXICITY
CNS effects, as evidenced by decreased activity, ataxia, loss or righting reflex, and ptosis were seen in the following animal studies; the 18-month mouse carcinogenicity study at 50 mg/kg/day, the 6-month dog study at 36 mg/kg/day, the 6-month hamster study at 40 mg/kg/day, and in acute, high-dose studies in rats and hamsters (50 mg/kg), rabbits (300 mg/kg) and mice (1500 mg/kg). CNS toxicity in the acute high-dose studies was characterized (in mice) by conspicuous vacuolation in the ventral white columns of the spinal cord at a dose of 5000 mg/kg and (in rat) by edema with separation of myelinated fibers of the ventral spinal tracts and sciatic nerve at a dose of 1500 mg/kg. CNS toxicity, characterized by periaxonal vacuolization, was observed in the medulla of dogs that died after treatment for 5 weeks with 48 mg/kg/day; this finding was not observed in the remaining dogs when the dose level was lowered to 36 mg/kg/day. CNS vascular lesions, characterized by perivascular hemorrhages, edema, and mononuclear cell infiltration of perivascular spaces, have been observed in dogs treated with other members of this class. No CNS lesions have been observed after chronic treatment for up to 2 years with Fluvastatin in the mouse (at doses up to 350 mg/kg/day), rat (up to 24 mg/kg/day), or dog (up to 16 mg/kg/day).

CARCINOGENESIS, MUTAGENESIS, IMPAIRMENT OF FERTILITY
A 2-year study was performed in rats at dose levels of 6, 9, and 18-24 (escalated after 1 year) mg/kg/day. These treatment levels represented plasma drug levels of approximately 9, 13, and 26-35 times the mean human plasma drug concentration after a 40 mg oral dose. A low incidence of fore-stomach squamous papillomas and 1 carcinoma of the fore-stomach at the 24 mg/kg/day dose level was considered to reflect the prolonged hyperplasia induced by direct contact exposure to Fluvastatin Sodium rather than to a systemic effect of the drug. In addition, an increased incidence of thyroid follicular cell adenomas and carcinomas was recorded for males treated with 18-24 mg/kg/day. The increased incidence of thyroid follicular cell neoplasm in male rats with Fluvastatin Sodium appears to be consistent with species specific findings from other HMG-CoA reductase inhibitors. In contrast to other HMG-CoA reductase inhibitors, no hepatic adenomas or carcinomas were observed.

The carcinogenicity study conducted in mice at dose levels of 0.3, 15 and 30 mg/kg/day revealed, as in rats, a statistically significant increase in forestomach squamous cell papillomas in males and females at 30 mg/kg/day and in females at 15 mg/kg/day. These treatment levels represented plasma drug levels of approximately, 0.05, 2, and 7 times the mean human plasma drug concentration after a 40 mg oral dose.

No evidence of mutagenicity was observed in vitro, with or without ratliver metabolic activation, in the following studies: microbial mutagen test using mutant strains of Salmonella typhimurium or Escherichia coli; malignant transformation assay in BALB/3T3 cells; unscheduled DNA synthesis in rat primary hepatocytes; chromosomal aberrations in V79 Chinese Hamster cells; HGPRT V79 Chinese Hamster cells. In addition, there was no evidence of mutagenicity in vivo in either a rat or mouse micronucleus test.

In a study in rats at dose levels for females of 0.6, 2 and 6 mg/kg/day and for males at 2, 10 and 20 mg/kg/day Fluvastatin Sodium had no adverse effects on the fertility or reproductive performance at any of the dose levels studied. A study in which female rats were dosed during the third trimester at 12 and 24 mg/kg/day resulted in maternal mortality at or near term and postpartum. In addition, fetal and neonatal lethality were apparent. No effects on the dam or fetus occurred at the low dose level of 2 mg/kg/day. A second study at levels of 2, 6, 12 and 24 mg/kg/day confirmed the findings in the first study. A modified Segment III study was performed at dose levels of 12 or 24 mg/kg/day with or without the presence of concurrent supplementation with mevalonic acid, a product of HMG-CoA reductase which is essential for cholesterol biosynthesis. The concurrent administration of mevalonic acid completely prevented the maternal and neonatal mortality. Therefore, the maternal and neonatal lethality observed with Fluvastatin Sodium reflect its exaggerated pharmacologic effect during pregnancy.

PREGNANCY
Pregnancy Category X: See "Contraindications."

Fluvastatin Sodium was not teratogenic rats at doses up to 36 mg/kg daily or in rabbits at doses of up to 10 mg/kg/day. There are no data in pregnant women.

NURSING MOTHERS
Based on preclinical data, drug is present in breast milk in a 2:1 ratio (milk; plasma). Because of the potential for serious adverse reactions in nursing infants nursing women should not take Fluvastatin Sodium (see "Contraindications").

PEDIATRIC USE
Safety and effectiveness in individuals less than 18 years old have not been established. Treatment in patients less than 18 years of age is not recommended at this time.

GERIATRIC USE
The effect of age on the pharmacokinetics of Fluvastatin Sodium was evaluated. Results indicate that for the general patient population plasma concentrations of Fluvastatin Sodium do not vary either as a function of age or gender. (See also "Clinical Pharmacology: Pharmacokinetics/Metabolism.") Elderly patients (≥ 65 years of age) demonstrated a greater treatment response in respect to LDL-C, Total-C and LDL/HDL ratio than patients < 65 years of age.

ADVERSE REACTIONS
In the controlled clinical studies and their open extensions, Fluvastatin Sodium was discontinued in 1.0% of 1881 patients due to adverse experiences (mean exposure approximately 14 months ranging in duration from 1- > 24 months). This results in an exposure adjusted rate of 0.9% per patient-year in Fluvastatin patients compared to an incidence of 1.3% in placebo patients. Fluvastatin Sodium has been studied in more than 2200 patients. Adverse reactions have usually been mild and similar in incidence to placebo.

Adverse experiences occurring with a frequency > 2% regardless of causality include the following:

Adverse Event	Fluvastatin Sodium (%) (N = 620)	Placebo (%) (N = 411)
Integumentary		
Rash	2.7	3.6
Musculoskeletal		
Back Pain	6.1	8.5
Arthropathy	4.0	3.2
Exercise-Related Muscle Pain	3.4	2.4
Respiratory		
Upper Respiratory Tract Infection	11.6	15.3
Pharyngitis	4.5	4.9
Rhinitis	4.5	6.1
Sinusitis	2.7	1.5
Coughing	2.6	3.2
Bronchitis	2.3	1.2
Gastrointestinal		
Dyspepsia	8.1	4.9
Diarrhea	6.0	5.6
Abdominal Pain	5.5	4.1
Nausea	3.2	2.4
Constipation	2.6	4.9
Flatulence	2.6	4.1
Misc. Tooth Disorder	2.1	1.9
Central Nervous System		
Dizziness	2.6	2.9
Psychiatric Disorders		
Insomnia	2.6	1.7
Miscellaneous		
Headache	8.7	8.8
Influenza-Like Symptoms	5.3	5.4
Accidental Trauma	5.3	5.1
Fatigue	3.5	3.4
Allergy	2.6	3.6

The following effects have been reported with drugs in this class. Not all the effects listed below have necessarily been associated with Fluvastatin Sodium therapy.

Skeletal: myopathy, rhabdomyolysis, arthralgias.

Neurological: dysfunction of certain cranial nerves (including alteration of taste, impairment of extra-ocular movement, facial paresis), tremor, vertigo, memory loss, paresthesia, peripheral neuropathy, peripheral nerve palsy, anxiety, insomnia, depression.

Hypersensitivity Reactions: An apparent hypersensitivity syndrome has been reported rarely which has included one or more of the following features: anaphylaxis, angioedema, lupus erythematosus-like syndrome, polymyalgia rheumatica, vasculitis, purpura, thrombocytopenia, leukopenia, hemolytic anemia, positive ANA, ESR increase, eosinophilia, arthritis, arthralgia, urticaria, asthenia, photosensitivity, fever, chills, flushing, malaise, dyspnea, toxic epidermal necrolysis, erythema multiforme, including Stevens-Johnson syndrome.

Gastrointestinal: pancreatitis, hepatitis, including chronic active hepatitis, cholestatic jaundice, fatty change in liver, and, rarely, cirrhosis, fulminant hepatic necrosis, and hepatoma; anorexia, vomiting.

Skin: alopecia, pruritus. A variety of skin changes (e.g., nodules, discoloration, dryness of skin/mucous membranes, changes to hair/nails) have been reported.

Reproductive: gynecomastia, loss of libido, erectile dysfunction.

Eye: progression of cataracts (lens opacities), ophthalmoplegia.

Laboratory Abnormalities: elevated transaminases, alkaline phosphatase, and bilirubin; thyroid function abnormalities.

CONCOMITANT THERAPY
Fluvastatin Sodium has been administered concurrently with cholestyramine and nicotinic acid. No adverse reactions unique to the combination or in addition to those previously reported for this class of drugs alone have been reported. Myopathy and rhabdomyolysis (with or without acute renal failure) have been reported when another HMG-CoA reductase inhibitor was used in combination with immunosuppressive drugs, gemfibrozil, erythromycin, or lipid-lowering

doses of nicotinic acid. Concomitant therapy with HMG-CoA reductase inhibitors and these agents is generally not recommended. (See *"Warnings: Skeletal Muscle."*)

OVERDOSAGE

The approximate oral LD$_{50}$ is greater than 2 g/kg in mice and greater than 0.7 g/kg in rats.

The maximum single oral dose received by healthy volunteers was 60 mg. No clinically significant adverse experiences were seen at this dose. There has been a single report of 2 children, one 2 years old and the other 3 years of age, either of whom may have possibly ingested Fluvastatin Sodium. The maximum amount of Fluvastatin Sodium that could have been ingested was 80 mg (4 × 20 mg capsules). Vomiting was induced by ipecac in both children and no capsules were noted in their emesis. Neither child experienced any adverse symptoms and both recovered from the incident without problems.

No specific information on the treatment of overdosage can be recommended. Should an accidental overdose occur, treat symptomatically and institute supportive measures as required. The dialyzability of Fluvastatin Sodium and of its metabolites in humans is not known at present.

DOSAGE AND ADMINISTRATION

The patient should be placed on a standard cholesterol-lowering diet before receiving Fluvastin Sodium and should continue on this diet during treatment with Fluvastin Sodium. (See *"NCEP Treatment Guidelines"* for details on dietary therapy.)

The recommended starting dose for the majority of patients is 20 mg once daily at bedtime. The recommended dosing range is 20-40 mg/day as a single dose in the evening. Splitting the 40 mg QPM dose into a BID regimen provides a modest improvement in LDL-C response Fluvastatin Sodium may be taken without regard to meals, since there are no apparent differences in the lipid-lowering effects of Fluvastatin Sodium administered with the evening meal or 4 hours after the evening meal. Since the maximal reductions in LDL-C of a given dose are seen within 4 weeks, periodic lipid determinations should be performed during this time with dosage adjusted according to the patient's response to therapy and established treatment guidelines. The therapeutic effect of Fluvastatin Sodium is maintained with prolonged administration.

CONCOMITANT THERAPY

Lipid-lowering effects on total cholesterol and LDL cholesterol are additive when Fluvastatin Sodium is combined with a bile-acid binding resin or niacin. When administering a bile-acid resin (e.g., cholestyramine) and Fluvastatin Sodium, Fluvastatin Sodium should be administered at bedtime, at least 2 hours following the resin to avoid a significant interaction due to drug binding to resin. (See also *"Adverse Reactions: Concomitant Therapy."*)

DOSAGE IN PATIENTS WITH RENAL INSUFFICIENCY

Since Fluvastatin Sodium is cleared hepatically with less than 5% of the administered dose excreted into the urine, dose adjustments for mild to moderate renal impairment are not necessary. Caution should be exercised with severe impairment.

STORE AND DISPENSE

Below 86°F (30°C) in a tight container. Protect from light.

HOW SUPPLIED
CAPSULE: 20 MG

BRAND/MANUFACTURER	NDC	SIZE	AWP
○ BRAND			
▶ LESCOL: Sandoz Pharm	00078-0176-15	30s	$30.60
	00078-0176-05	100s	$102.00

CAPSULE: 40 MG

BRAND/MANUFACTURER	NDC	SIZE	AWP
○ BRAND			
▶ LESCOL: Sandoz Pharm	00078-0234-15	30s	$34.20
	00078-0234-05	100s	$114.00

Fluvirin SEE INFLUENZA VIRUS VACCINE

Fluzone SEE INFLUENZA VIRUS VACCINE

FML SEE FLUOROMETHOLONE

Folex Pfs SEE METHOTREXATE

Folic Acid

DESCRIPTION

Folic Acid, N-[4[[(2-Amino-1,4-dihydro-4-oxo-6-ptendinyl) methyl]-amino]benzoyl]-L-glutamic acid, is a complex organic compound present in liver, yeast, and natural sources; it also may be prepared synthetically. Each tablet, for oral administration, contains 1 mg of Folic Acid. Each mL of Folic Acid injection contains sodium folate equivalent to 5 mg of Folic Acid.

Following is its chemical structure:

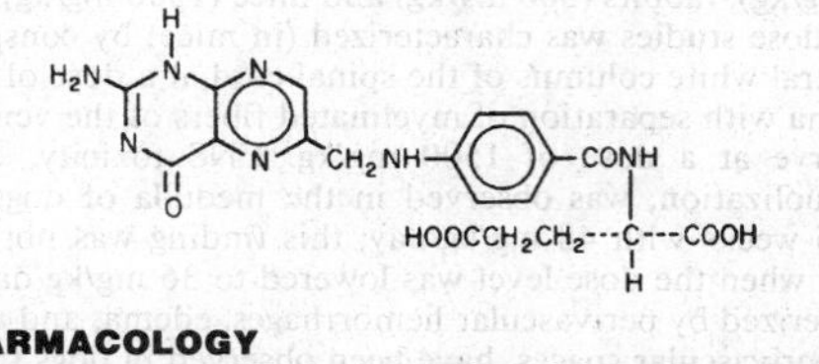

CLINICAL PHARMACOLOGY

In man, an exogenous source of folate is required for nucleo-protein synthesis and maintenance of normal erthropoiesis. Folic Acid, whether given by mouth or parenterally, stimulates specifically the production of red blood cells, white blood cells, and platelets in persons suffering from certain megaloblastic anemias.

INDICATIONS AND USAGE

Folic Acid is effective in the treatment of megaloblastic anemias due to a deficiency of Folic Acid (as may be seen in tropical or non-tropical sprue) in anemias of nutritional origin, pregnancy, infancy, or childhood.

WARNINGS

Administration of Folic Acid alone is improper therapy in the treatment of pernicious anemia and other megaloblastic anemias where Vitamin B$_{12}$ is deficient.

PRECAUTIONS

Folic Acid in doses above 0.1 mg daily may obscure pernicious anemia in that hematologic remission can occur while neurological manifestations remain progressive.

ADVERSE REACTIONS

Allergic sensitization has been reported following both oral and parenteral administration of Folic Acid.

DOSAGE AND ADMINISTRATION

Oral Administration: Folic Acid is well absorbed and may be administered orally with satisfactory results except in severe instances of intestinal malabsorption.

Parenteral Administration: Intramuscular, intravenous, and subcutaneous routes may be used if the disease is exceptionally severe, or if gastrointestinal absorption may be, or is known to be, impaired.

Usual Therapeutic Dosage: In adults and children (regardless of age) up to 1 mg daily. Resistant cases may require larger doses.

Maintenance Level: When clinical symptoms have subsided and the blood picture has become normal, a daily maintenance level should be used, i.e., 0.1 mg for infants and up to 0.3 mg for children under four years of age, 0.4 mg for adults and children four or more years of age, and 0.8 mg for pregnant and lactating women, per day, but never less than 0.1 mg per day Patients should be kept under close supervision and adjustment of the maintenance level made if relapse appears imminent in the presence of alcoholism, hemolytic anemia, anticonvulsant therapy, or chronic infection, the maintenance level may need to be increased.

Storage: Store at controlled room temperature, 15°-30°C (59°-86°F). Protect from light and moisture. Dispense in a tight, light-resistant container as defined in the USP using a child-resistant closure.

HOW SUPPLIED
INJECTION: 5 MG/ML

AVERAGE UNIT PRICE (AVAILABLE SIZES)		GENERIC A-RATED AVERAGE PRICE (GAAP)	
GENERIC	$1.34	10 ml	$13.37

BRAND/MANUFACTURER	NDC	SIZE	AWP
◆ GENERICS			
Raway	00686-1840-30	10 ml	$12.50
Fujisawa	00469-1840-30	10 ml	$13.27
Lederle Std Prod	00205-4154-34	10 ml	$14.33

TABLETS: 1 MG

AVERAGE UNIT PRICE (AVAILABLE SIZES)		GENERIC A-RATED AVERAGE PRICE (GAAP)	
GENERIC	$0.04	30s	$3.24
HCFA FUL (1000s ea)	$0.01	100s	$6.07
		1000s	$11.52

BRAND/MANUFACTURER	NDC	SIZE	AWP
◆ GENERICS			
Major	00904-0625-46	30s	$1.85
Medirex	57480-0327-06	30s	$4.62
Richlyn	00115-3585-01	100s	$1.31

◆ RATED THERAPEUTICALLY EQUIVALENT; ◇ THERAPEUTIC EQUIVALENCE UNCONFIRMED; ○ UNRATED

BRAND/MANUFACTURER	NDC	SIZE	AWP
	00574-0060-01	100s	$2.10
Pioneer	60104-6004-02	100s	$2.31
➤ Schein	00364-0137-01	100s	$2.72
Major	00904-0625-60	100s	$2.80
West-Ward	00143-1248-01	100s	$3.00
Moore,H.L.	00839-5066-06	100s	$3.09
	00574-0060-11	100s ud	$4.30
Major	00904-0625-61	100s ud	$5.89
Raway	00686-0041-20	100s ud	$6.50
➤ Schein	00364-0137-90	100s ud	$7.25
Vangard	00615-0664-13	100s ud	$7.85
West-Ward	00143-1248-25	100s ud	$8.50
Goldline	00182-0507-89	100s ud	$8.60
Medirex	57480-0327-01	100s ud	$15.40
UDL	51079-0041-20	100s ud	$15.44
➤ Schein	00364-0137-02	1000s	$8.28
West-Ward	00143-1248-10	1000s	$8.90
Pioneer	60104-6004-08	1000s	$9.02
Richlyn	00115-3585-03	1000s	$10.05
Qualitest	00603-3714-32	1000s	$10.80
Parmed	00349-2069-10	1000s	$12.31
Major	00904-0625-80	1000s	$12.90
Rugby	00536-3845-10	1000s	$13.04
URL	00677-0449-10	1000s	$13.17
Aligen	00405-4447-03	1000s	$13.17
Moore,H.L.	00839-5066-16	1000s	$13.22
Goldline	00182-0507-10	1000s	$13.35

Folic Acid/Liver Extract/Vitamin B12

DESCRIPTION

A sterile solution of Liver injection, Vitamin B_{12} and Folic Acid for intramuscular injection.

Liver injection is that soluble thermostable fraction of mammalian livers standardized to its Vitamin B_{12} activity equivalent.

Vitamin B_{12} occurs as dark red crystals or amorphous or crystalline red powder, very hygroscopic and sparingly soluble in water (1:80). The activity is destroyed by heavy metals (Iron) and strong oxidizing or reducing agents (vitamin C), but not by autoclaving for short periods at 121 degrees C. The Vitamin B_{12} coenzymes are very unstable in light.

Vitamin B_{12} is also known as the "extrinsic factor" and the "antipernicious anemia principle of Castle". Hydroxocobalamin is equally effective and shares the cobalamin molecular structure with Vitamin B_{12}.

Folic Acid is a yellowish-orange crystal, slightly soluble in water but soluble in solutions of alkali hydroxides and bicarbonates.

Each mL contains: Liver Injection equivalent to Vitamin B_{12} 10 mcg, Folic Acid 0.4 mg, 100 mcg, Phenol 0.5% as preservative in Water for Injection q.s. Sodium Hydroxide and/or Hydrochloric Acid may have been used to adjust pH.

CLINICAL PHARMACOLOGY

Vitamin B_{12} is found almost exclusively in foods of animal origin, bound to protein. Prior to absorption this bond must be split by heat or gastric pepsin in an acid medium. In man synthesis of the vitamin occurs by bacteria in the colon, from which site it is not absorbed. Absorption is 30 to 70% in normal persons. Vitamin B_{12} is poorly absorbed by mass-action diffusion. Normally, Vitamin B_{12} is bound to gastric intrinsic factor (absent in pernicious anemia) for safe transit and attachment to the ileum mucosa with the aid of calcium and a pH above 6. Colchicine and para-amino salicylic drugs are known to interfere with Vitamin B_{12} absorption. Heavy alcohol intake longer than 2 weeks may produce malabsorption of vitamin B_{12}. Vitamin B_{12} is released into the mucosal cells and passes into the portal circulation where it is 90 to 99% bound to the plasma beta-globulins. The maximum total body stores are 5 to 11 mg. The liver contains 50 to 90% of this amount. The time to deplete the body stores is 2 to 3 years. The plasma concentration normal range is 140 to 190 picograms (micro-micrograms) per mL using the *Euglena Gracilis* assay method. Persons taking antibiotics invalidate Folic Acid and Vitamin B_{12} diagnostic blood assays. Persons with P.A. may develop "precipitating antibodies" to the intrinsic factor, which are found in the circulating blood, gastric juice, and saliva.

Vitamin B_{12} is essential to nucleoprotein synthesis, growth, hematopoiesis and myelin synthesis. Hematopoiesis is suppressed by infection, uremia, chloramphenicol and other factors. The only step in protein metabolism proven to require cobalamin, the conversion of homocystine to methionine, also requires folate.

The minimum daily requirement is less than one microgram. The National Academy of Sciences "Recommended Dietary Allowances" are up to 5 micrograms daily for adults, 6 micrograms for the elderly and lactating women, and 8 micrograms for pregnancy. Fifteen micrograms daily are recommended to saturate the body stores. At birth the blood level of Vitamin B_{12} in the newborn is 3 to 5 times that in the mother.

Methylmalonic aciduria, an inborn error of metabolism, appears to be Vitamin B_{12} dependent.

The approximate daily Vitamin B_{12} excretion is 3 to 7 micrograms in the bile and 0 to 0.25 micrograms in the urine.

Though no active fraction other than the cobalamins has been isolated from liver injection and, in fact, liver injection is now standardized in terms of Vitamin B_{12} by microbiological assay, many clinicians are of the opinion that the administration of liver injection is preferable to Vitamin B_{12} in the treatment of macrocytic anemias of various etiologies.

INDICATIONS AND USAGE

Folic Acid is effective in the treatment of megaloblastic anemias due to deficiency of Folic Acid as may be seen in tropical or non-tropical sprue, in anemias of nutritional origin or pregnancy, and in vitamin B_{12} deficiency due to:

1. Inadequate dietary intake as may be seen in poverty, famine, ignorance, vegans, alcoholics, and edentulous persons.

2. Malabsorption occurring in pernicious anemia (P.A.); gastric pathology, dysfunction or surgery; fish tapeworm infestation, blind loop of small intestine; ileal functional damage, (gluten enteropathy, sprue, regional enteritis) and resection of ileum; diarrhea; laxative habit and accompanying Folic Acid deficiency.

3. Increased requirements occur in pregnancy, thyrotoxicosis, hemolytic anemia, hemorrhage, malignancy, hepatic and renal disease.

This combination of anti-anemic vitamins is indicated in a wide variety of macrocytic anemias including Addisonian pernicious anemia, the macrocytic anemias of sprue, pellagra and pregnancy, as well as macrocytic anemias caused by gastrointestinal disturbances. It is not indicated in the treatment of microcytic anemia due to iron deficiency.

CONTRAINDICATIONS

Sensitivity to cobalt and/or Vitamin B_{12}, Folic Acid, Liver injection, phenol.

WARNINGS

Protect product from light. This preparation should not be administered to patients having an established or suspected allergy to liver extracts.

Indiscriminate administration may mask the true diagnosis. Patients with Vitamin B_{12} deficiency have shown neurologic disease and psychotic behavior without anemia.

Vitamin B_{12} deficiency allowed to progress over 3 months may produce permanent degenerative lesions of the spinal cord, as observed when folic acid therapy is used.

Folic Acid alone is improper therapy in the treatment of pernicious anemia and other megaloblastic anemias where Vitamin B_{12} is deficient.

PRECAUTIONS

An intradermal test dose is recommended prior to administration to patients suspected to be sensitive to the cobalamines. Patients with early Leber's disease, hereditary optic nerve atrophy, treated with Vitamin B_{12}, have been found to suffer severe and swift optic atrophy. In megaloblastic anemia, treatment with Vitamin B_{12} returns normal hematopoiesis, producing a sudden increase in the potassium requirements. Hypokalemia has been reported and serum potassium levels should be monitored early in the treatment.

Single Vitamin B_{12} deficiency is rare. Multiple vitamin deficiency is expected in any dietary deficiency.

Folic Acid in doses above 0.1 mg daily may obscure pernicious anemia in that hematologic remission can occur while neurological manifestations remain progressive.

ADVERSE REACTIONS

Mild transient diarrhea, polycythemia vera, peripheral vascular thrombosis, itching transitory exanthema, feeling of swelling of entire body, anaphylactic shock and death.

Allergic sensitization has been reported following both oral and parenteral administration of Folic Acid.

OVERDOSAGE

(See *"Warnings"*.) When injected amount of vitamin B_{12} exceeds the binding capacity of plasma, liver, and other tissues, it is free in the blood and available for urine excretion.

Within 48 hours after injection of 100 to 1000 micrograms of Vitamin B_{12} from 50 to 98% of the injected dose may appear in the urine. The major portion is excreted within the first 8 hours.

DOSAGE AND ADMINISTRATION

For intramuscular use only. NOT FOR INTRAVENOUS USE.

Pernicious Anemia: The recommended regimen is the injection of 1 mL daily for three days followed by 1 mL once a week until the erythrocyte count becomes normal. The dosage may then be reduced to 1 mL once or twice a month. This dosage schedule must be adjusted by the physician to the needs and response of the patient. Do not use more than 1 mL daily.

Other Macrocytic Anemias: The dosage in the macrocytic anemias of sprue, pellagra and pregnancy must be adjusted according to the needs and response of the patient. It is recommended that the initial dosage be intensive, as for pernicious anemia, reduced as allowed by the condition and response of the patient. Do not use more than 1 mL daily.

In patients with Addisonian pernicious anemia, vitamin B_{12} is required for life. Oral therapy is undependable.

In malabsorption, a clinical evaluation of the patient is essential to the future course of treatment.

Follow up with an oral therapeutic multivitamin preparation, containing 15 mcg Vitamin B_{12} daily for one month is recommended in patients having normal

➤ SHOWN IN PRODUCT IDENTIFICATION GUIDE

intestinal absorption. Poor dietary habits should be corrected and an abundant and well balanced dietary intake should be prescribed.

Parenteral drug products should be inspected visually for particulate matter and discoloration prior to administration, whenever the solution and container permit.

Refrigerate at 2°-8°C (36°-46°F). Protect from light. Keep in opaque container until used.

HOW SUPPLIED
INJECTION:

BRAND/MANUFACTURER	NDC	SIZE	AWP
○ GENERICS			
Schein	00364-2257-54	10 ml	$3.70
Veratex	17022-2365-03	10 ml	$3.95
LIVIFOL: Dunhall	00217-8808-08	10 ml	$4.00
HEPFOMIN-R: Keene	00588-5443-70	10 ml	$4.50
LIVER FOLIC: Major	00904-0878-10	10 ml	$6.40
LIVERFOL-B12: Truxton	00463-1039-10	10 ml	$7.20
CMC-Cons	00223-7956-10	10 ml	$7.50
LIVERFOL-B12: Allscrips	54569-2561-00	10 ml	$7.95
LIFOLEX-PLUS: Bolan	44437-0777-10	10 ml	$8.00
HYLIVER-PLUS: Hyrex	00314-0666-70	10 ml	$9.90
TRI-HEMATINIC-R: Merit	30727-0655-70	10 ml	$14.85

Folic Acid/Polysaccharide-Iron Complex/Vitamin B₁₂

DESCRIPTION

Each capsule contains:
Iron (elemental) (as Polysaccharide-Iron Complex) .... 150 mg
Folic Acid .... 1 mg
Vitamin B_{12} .... 25 mcg

Each teaspoon (5 ml) Folic Acid/Polysaccharide-Iron Complex/Vitamin B_{12} Forte Elixir contains:
Iron (Elemental) (as Polysaccharide-Iron Complex) .... 100 mg
Folic Acid .... 1 mg
Vitamin B_{12} .... 25 mcg

CHEMISTRY
Folic Acid/Polysaccharide-Iron Complex/Vitamin $_{12}$ is the product of iron complexed to a low molecular weight polysaccharide. This polysaccharide is produced by the drastic hydrolysis of starch. Folic Acid/Polysaccharide-Iron Complex/Vitamin B_{12} is a dark brown powder which dissolves in water to form a very dark brown solution. It is virtually tasteless and odorless. Because it is an organic complex, it contains no free ions, either ferric or ferrous. Folic Acid/Polysaccharide-Iron Complex Vitamin B_{12} is clinically non-toxic. Studies in rats demonstrate an LD 50 of greater than 2800 mg of iron per kilogram. Chronic toxicity studies in rats and dogs demonstrate that a daily dosage of 250 mg of iron per kilogram for three months had no adverse effects. In spite of this extreme safety, radioisotope tracer studies in man demonstrate that Folic Acid/Polysaccharide Iron-Complex Vitamin B_{12} is absorbed as well as ferrous sulfate. Clinical studies demonstrate that Folic Acid/Polysaccharide Iron-Complex Vitamin B_{12} gives good hematopoietic response with almost complete absence of the side effects usually associated with oral iron therapy.

INDICATIONS
Iron deficiency anemia and/or nutritional megaloblastic anemias due to inadequate diet.

WARNINGS
Folic acid alone is improper therapy in the treatment of pernicious anemia and other megaloblastic anemias where vitamin B_{12} is deficient.

PRECAUTION
Folic acid in doses above 0.1 mg-0.4 mg daily may obscure pernicious anemia in that hematologic remission can occur while neurological manifestations remain progressive.

ADVERSE REACTIONS
Allergic sensitization has been reported following both oral and parenteral administration of folic acid.

DOSAGE AND ADMINISTRATION
One capsule daily or as directed by a physician.
One or two teaspoonfuls of elixir daily or as prescribed by a physician.
Store at controlled room temperature, 15°-30°C (59°-86°F).
Dispense in a tight, light-resistant container as defined in the USP/NF with a child-resistant closure.

HOW SUPPLIED
CAPSULE:

BRAND/MANUFACTURER	NDC	SIZE	AWP
○ BRAND			
NIFEREX-150 FORTE: Central	00131-4330-37	100s	$23.20
	00131-4330-43	1000s	$215.30

ELIXIR:

BRAND/MANUFACTURER	NDC	SIZE	AWP
○ BRAND			
NIFEREX FORTE: Central	00131-5065-64	120 ml	$9.80
○ GENERICS			
NU-IRON PLUS: Mayrand	00259-0342-08	240 ml	$14.00

Forane *SEE* ISOFLURANE

Forma-Ray *SEE* FORMALDEHYDE

Formaldehyde

COMPOSITION
Active: 10% Formaldehyde.

INDICATIONS
Drying Agent for pre and post surgical removal of warts or for non-surgical laser treatment of warts where dryness is required. Safeguards against offensive odor and dries excessive moisture of feet.

CONTRAINDICATIONS
Do not use in patients known to be sensitive to Formaldehyde. Check skin for sensitivity to Formaldehyde prior to application.

PRECAUTIONS
FOR EXTERNAL USE ONLY: HARMFUL IF SWALLOWED. CONTACT A LOCAL POISON CONTROL CENTER IMMEDIATELY. KEEP OUT OF THE REACH OF CHILDREN. Avoid contact with eyes or mucous membranes. Check skin for sensitivity to Formaldehyde prior to application since it may be irritating and sensitizing to the skin of some patients. If redness or irritation persists, consult your PODIATRIST, DERMATOLOGIST or PHYSICIAN.

ADMINISTRATION
Apply with *roll-on* applicator once a day to affected areas or as directed by your podiatrist or physician. Do not shake the bottle with cap removed. Keep cap closed tightly.

HOW SUPPLIED
LIQUID: 10%

BRAND/MANUFACTURER	NDC	SIZE	AWP
○ GENERICS			
FORMADON: Gordon	10481-1050-05	60 ml dozdoz	$55.00
FORMADON: Gordon	10481-1050-02	120 ml dozdoz	$68.75
FORMADON: Gordon	10481-1050-03	1920 ml	$33.75
FORMADON: Gordon	10481-1050-04	3840 ml	$51.25

SOLUTION: 10%

BRAND/MANUFACTURER	NDC	SIZE	AWP
○ BRAND			
LAZERFORMALYDE: Pedinol	00884-3986-03	90 ml	$5.50

SOLUTION: 20%

BRAND/MANUFACTURER	NDC	SIZE	AWP
○ BRAND			
FORMA-RAY: Gordon	10481-3015-05	60 ml doz	$70.00
	10481-3015-02	120 ml doz	$82.50

SPRAY: 10%

BRAND/MANUFACTURER	NDC	SIZE	AWP
○ GENERICS			
FORMALYDE-10 SPRAY: Pedinol	00884-4789-02	60 ml	$4.25

Fortaz *SEE* CEFTAZIDIME

◆ RATED THERAPEUTICALLY EQUIVALENT; ◇ THERAPEUTIC EQUIVALENCE UNCONFIRMED; ○ UNRATED

Foscarnet Sodium

RENAL IMPAIRMENT IS THE MAJOR TOXICITY OF FOSCARNET SODIUM, AND OCCURS TO SOME DEGREE IN MOST PATIENTS, CONSEQUENTLY, CONTINUAL ASSESSMENT OF A PATIENT'S RISK AND FREQUENT MONITORING OF SERUM CREATININE WITH DOSE ADJUSTMENT FOR CHANGES IN RENAL FUNCTION ARE IMPERATIVE.

FOSCARNET SODIUM HAS BEEN SHOWN TO CAUSE ALTERATIONS IN PLASMA MINERALS AND ELECTROLYTES THAT HAVE LED TO SEIZURES. THEREFORE, PATIENTS MUST BE MONITORED FREQUENTLY FOR SUCH CHANGES AND THEIR POTENTIAL SEQUELAE.

DESCRIPTION

The chemical name of Foscarnet Sodium is phosphonoformic acid, trisodium salt. Foscarnet Sodium is a white, crystalline powder containing 6 equivalents of water of hydration with an empirical formula of $Na_3CO_5P.6\ H_2O$, and a molecular weight of 300.1.

Foscarnet Sodium has the potential to chelate divalent metal ions, such as calcium and magnesium, to form stable coordination compounds. Foscarnet Sodium injection is a sterile, isotonic aqueous solution for intravenous administration only. The solution is clear and colorless. Each milliliter of Foscarnet Sodium injection contains 24 mg of Foscarnet Sodium hexahydrate in Water for Injection, USP. Hydrochloric acid and/or sodium hydroxide may have been added to adjust the pH of the solution to 7.4. Foscarnet Sodium Injection contains no preservatives.

Following is its chemical structure:

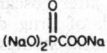

$(NaO)_2PCOONa$

CLINICAL PHARMACOLOGY

MICROBIOLOGY:

Foscarnet Sodium is an organic analogue of inorganic pyrophosphate that inhibits replication of all known herpesviruses *in vitro* including cytomegalovirus (CMV), herpes simplex virus types 1 and 2 (HSV-1, HSV-2), human herpesvirus 6 (HHV-6), Epstein-Barr virus (EBV), and varicella-zoster virus (VZV).

Foscarnet Sodium exerts its antiviral activity by a selective inhibition at the pyrophosphate binding site on virus-specific DNA polymerases and reverse transcriptases at concentrations that do not affect cellular DNA polymerases. Foscarnet Sodium does not require activation (phosphorylation) by thymidine kinase or other kinases, and therefore is active *in vitro* against HSV mutants deficient in thymidine kinase (TK). CMV strains resistant to ganciclovir may be sensitive to Foscarnet Sodium. No controlled trials have been completed involving Foscarnet Sodium treatment of patients with CMV resistant to ganciclovir.

The quantitative relationship between the *in vitro* susceptibility of human cytomegalovirus (CMV) to Foscarnet Sodium and clinical response to therapy has not been clearly established in man and virus sensitivity testing has not been standardized. Sensitivity test results, expressed as the concentration of drug required to inhibit by 50% the growth of virus in cell culture (IC_{50}) vary greatly depending on the assay method used, cell type employed and the laboratory performing the test. A number of sensitive viruses and their IC_{50} values are listed below.

Table 1
FOSCARNET SODIUM INHIBITION OF VIRUS MULTIPLICATION IN CELL CULTURE

Virus	$IC_{50}(\mu M)$
CMV	50-800*
HSV-1, HSV-2	10-130
VZV	48-90
EBV	< 500**
HHV-6	< 67***
Ganciclovir-resistant CMV	190
HSV-TK minus mutant	67
HSV-DNA polymerase mutants	5-443

* *Mean = 269 μM*
** *97% of viral antigen synthesis inhibited at 500 μM*
*** *IC_{100} = 67 μM*

Clinical isolates of CMV taken from patients show different sensitivities to Foscarnet Sodium *in vitro*. Statistically significant decreases in positive CMV cultures from blood and urine have been demonstrated in two studies (FOS-03 and ACTG-015/915) of patients treated with Foscarnet Sodium. Although median time to progression of CMV retinitis was reduced in patients treated with the drug, reductions in positive blood or urine cultures have not been shown to correlate with clinical efficacy in individual patients.

Table 2
BLOOD AND URINE CULTURE RESULTS FROM CMV RETINITIS PATIENTS*

Blood	+ CMV	− CMV
Baseline	27	34
End of Induction**	1	60
Urine	+ CMV	− CMV
Baseline	52	6
End of Induction**	21	37

* *A combined total of 77 patients were treated with Foscarnet Sodium in two clinical trials (FOS-03 and ACTG-015/915). Not all patients had blood or urine cultures done and some patients had results from both cultures.*
** *(60 mg/kg Foscarnet Sodium TID for 2-3 weeks).*

If no clinical response to Foscarnet Sodium is observed, viral isolate should be tested for sensitivity to Foscarnet Sodium as naturally resistant mutants may emerge under selective pressure both *in vitro* and *in vivo*. The latent state of any of the human herpesviruses is not known to be sensitive to Foscarnet Sodium and viral reactivation of CMV occurs after Foscarnet Sodium therapy is terminated.

PHARMACOKINETICS

Protein Binding: *In vitro* studies have shown that 14-17% of Foscarnet is bound to plasma protein at plasma drug concentrations of 1-1000 μM. *Plasma Concentrations:* The pharmacokinetics of Foscarnet Sodium infusions have been determined when administered as an intermittent infusion during induction therapy in AIDS patients with CMV retinitis. Observed plasma Foscarnet concentrations in two studies (FOS-01 and ACTG-015 respectively) are summarized in the following table:

Table 3

Mean ±SD Dose mg/kg* (Infusion Time)	Day of Sampling	Mean Plasma Concentration (μM)	
		CMAX**[range]	CMIN***[range]
FOS-01 57±6 q 8 hr (1 hour)	1	573 [213-1305]	78 [± 33-139]
47±12 q 8 hr (1 hour)	14 or 15	579 [246-922]	110 [<33-148]
ACTG-015 55±6 q 8 hr (2 hours)	3	445 [306-720]	88 [<33-162]
57±7 q 8 hr (2 hours)	14 or 15	517 [348-789]	105 [43-205]

* *Planned dose = 60 mg/kg q8hr in both studies.*
** *Observed Maximum Concentration:*
  FOS-01:
  Day 1 (N=14): Observed 0.9-2.0 hr after start of infusion.
  Day 14/15 (N=10): Observed 0.8-1.3 hr after start of infusion.
  ACTG-015:
  Day 3 (N=12): Observed 1.8-2.4 hr after start of infusion.
  Day 14/15 (N=12): Observed 1.7-2.6 hr after start of infusion.
*** *Observed Minimum Concentration:*
  FOS-01:
  Day 1 (N=13): Observed 4-8 hr after start of infusion.
  (Mean represents 5/13 observations, 8/13 <33 μM)
  Day 14/15 (N=10): Observed 6,3-8 hr after start of infusion.
  (Mean represents 9/10 observations, 1/10 <33 μM)
  ACTG-015:
  Day 3 (N=12): Observed 7.8-8.1 hr after start of infusion.
  (Mean represents 9/12 observations, 3/12 <33 μM)
  Day 14/15 (N=12): Observed 6.4-8.7 hr after start of infusion.
  (Means represents 12/12 observations)

Clearance: Mean (±SD) plasma clearances were 130 ± 44 and 178 ± 48 mL/min in two studies in which Foscarnet Sodium was given by intermittent infusion (ACTG-015 and FOS-01 respectively), and 152 ± 59 and 214 ± 25 mL/min/1.73 m^2 in two studies using continuous infusion. Approximately 80-90% of IV Foscarnet Sodium is excreted unchanged in the urine of patients with normal renal function. Urinary excretion data suggest that both tubular secretion and glomerular filtration account for urinary elimination of Foscarnet Sodium. In one study, plasma clearance was less than creatinine clearance, suggesting that Foscarnet Sodium may also undergo tubular reabsorption. In three studies, decreases in plasma clearance of Foscarnet Sodium were proportional to decreases in creatinine clearance.

Half-life: Two studies (FOS-01 and ACTG-015) in patients with initially normal renal function who were treated with intermittant infusions of Foscarnet Sodium showed average drug plasma half-lives of about three hours determined on days 1 or 3 of therapy. This may be an underestimate of the effective half-life of Foscarnet Sodium due to the limited duration of the observation period. The plasma half-life of Foscarnet Sodium increases with the severity of renal impairment. Half-lives of 2-8 hours have been reported in patients having estimated or measured 24-hour creatinine clearances of 44-90 mL/min. Careful

➤ SHOWN IN PRODUCT IDENTIFICATION GUIDE

monitoring of renal function and dose adjustment in patients on Foscarnet Sodium is imperative (see *"Warnings"* and *"Dosage and Administration"*).

Following the continuous infusion of Foscarnet Sodium for 72 hours in six HIV + patients, plasma half-lives of 0.45 ± 0.32 and 3.3 ± 1.3 hours were determined. A terminal half-life of 18 ± 2.8 hours was estimated from the urinary excretion of Foscarnet over 48 hours after stopping the infusion. When Foscarnet Sodium was administered as a continuous infusion to 13 patients with HIV infection for 8 to 21 days, plasma half-lives of 1.4 ± 0.6 and 6.8 ± 5.0 hours were determined. A terminal half-life of 87.5 ± 41.8 hours was estimated from the urinary excretion of Foscarnet Sodium over six days after the last infusion; however, the renal function of these patients at the time of discontinuing the Foscarnet Sodium infusion was not known.

Measurements of urinary excretion are required to detect the longer terminal half-life assumed to represent release of Foscarnet Sodium from bone. In animal studies (mice), 40% of an intravenous dose of Foscarnet Sodium is deposited in bone in young animals and 7% in adults. Postmortem data on several patients in European clinical trials provide evidence that Foscarnet Sodium does accumulate in bone in humans: however, the extent to which this occurs has not been determined.

Volume of Distribution: Mean volumes of distribution at steady state range from 0.3-0.6 L/kg.

Cerebrospinal Fluid: Variable penetration of Foscarnet Sodium into cerebrospinal fluid has been observed. Intermittent infusion of 50 mg/kg of Foscarnet Sodium every 8 hours for 28 days in 9 patients produced Foscarnet Sodium CSF levels 3 hours after the end of the infusion of 150-260 µM or 39-103% of plasma levels. In another 4 patients, the CSF concentrations of Foscarnet Sodium were 35-69% of the plasma drug level after a dose of 230 mg/kg/day by continuous infusion for 2-13 days; however, the CSF: plasma ratio was only 13% in one patient while receiving a continuous infusion of Foscarnet Sodium at a rate of 274 mg/kg/day. Disease-related defects in the blood-brain barrier may be responsible for the variations seen.

PHARMACODYNAMICS

A pharmacodynamic analysis of patient data from one U.S. clinical trial (FOS-01) revealed a relationship between cumulative exposure to Foscarnet Sodium (product of plasma Foscarnet concentration x time) and changes in renal function (serum creatinine) during induction. All patients had their doses adjusted according to the recommended Foscarnet Sodium dosing nomogram. Seventeen of 24 patients (72%) showed evidence of renal impairment (> 20% suppression from baseline estimated creatinine clearance) during induction. This occurred in 3 patients on days 5-6, in 11 patients on days 7-14 and in 3 patients after day 14. Eleven patients had at least 40% suppression from baseline estimated creatinine clearance and six patients had more than 50% suppression, demonstrating that patients vary in their degree of sensitivity to Foscarnet Sodium-induced renal impairment. No specific factors were identified that predicted patients at higher risk. No relationship was found between a patient's initial creatinine clearance or initial drug clearance and renal impairment. Thus initial renal function may not be predictive of a patient's potential for renal impairment induced by Foscarnet Sodium.

CLINICAL TRIALS

Controlled clinical trials of Foscarnet Sodium have been conducted in the treatment of CMV retinitis. In most studies, treatment was begun with an induction dosage regimen of 60 mg/kg every 8 hours for the first 2-3 weeks, followed by a once-daily maintenance regimen at doses ranging from 60-120 mg/kg. No studies of Foscarnet Sodium as a treatment for other manifestations of CMV disease (i.e., viremia, pneumonitis, or gastroenteritis) have been conducted.

A prospective, randomized, masked, controlled clinical trial (FOS-03) was conducted in 24 patients with AIDS and CMV retinitis. All diagnoses and determinations of retinitis progression were made from retinal photographs by ophthalmologists who were masked to the patient's treatment assignment. Patients received induction treatment of Foscarnet Sodium, 60 mg/kg every 8 hours for 3 weeks, followed by maintenance treatment with 90 mg/kg/day until retinitis progression (appearance of a new lesion or advancement of the border of a posterior lesion greater than 750 microns in diameter). The 13 patients randomized to treatment with Foscarnet Sodium had a significant delay in progression of CMV retinitis compared to untreated controls. Median times to retinitis progression from study entry were 93 days (range 21- > 364) and 22 days (range 7-42), respectively, p < 0.001. In another prospective clinical trial of CMV retinitis in patients with AIDS (ACTG-915), 33 patients were treated with two to three weeks of Foscarnet Sodium induction (60 mg/kg TID) and then randomized to two maintenance dose groups, 90 entry to retinitis progression were 96 (range 14- > 176) days and 140 (range 16- > 233) days, respectively (FDA analysis). This difference was not statistically significant. The same criteria for retinitis progression were used as described above for FOS-03.

INDICATIONS

Foscarnet Sodium is indicated for the treatment of CMV retinitis in patients with acquired immunodeficiency syndrome (AIDS). SAFETY AND EFFICACY OF FOSCARNET SODIUM HAVE NOT BEEN ESTABLISHED FOR TREATMENT OF OTHER CMV INFECTIONS (e.g., PNEUMONITIS, GASTRONTERITIS); CONGENITAL OR NEONATAL CMV DISEASE: OR NON-IMMUNO- COMPROMISED INDIVIDUALS.

The diagnosis of CMV retinitis should be made by indirect ophthalmoscopy. Other conditions in the differential diagnosis of CMV retinitis include candidiasis, toxoplasmosis and other diseases producing a similar retinal pattern, any of

which may produce a retinal appearance similar to CMV. For this reason it is essential that the diagnosis of CMV retinitis be established by an ophthalmologist familiar with the retinal presentation of these conditions. The diagnosis of CMV retinitis may be supported by culture of CMV from urine, blood, throat, or other sites, but a negative CMV culture does not rule out CMV retinitis.

CONTRAINDICATIONS

Foscarnet Sodium is contraindicated in patients with clinically significant hypersensitivity to Foscarnet Sodium.

WARNINGS

RENAL IMPAIRMENT

THE MAJOR TOXICITY OF FOSCARNET SODIUM IS RENAL IMPAIRMENT, WHICH OCCURS TO SOME DEGREE IN MOST PATIENTS. Approximately 33% of 189 patients with AIDS and CMV retinitis who received intravenous Foscarnet Sodium in clinical studies developed significant impairment of renal function, manifested by a rise in serum creatinine concentration to 2.0 mg/dL or greater. Foscarnet Sodium must therefore be used with caution in all patients, especially those with a history of impairment of renal function. Patients vary in their sensitivity to nephrotoxicity induced by Foscarnet Sodium and initial renal function may not be predictive of the potential for drug induced renal impairment (see Pharmacodynamics). Foscarnet Sodium has not been studied in patients with baseline serum creatinine levels greater than 2.8 mg/dL or measured 24-hour creatinine clearances < 50 mL/min.

Analysis of data in one clinical trial (FOS-01) demonstrated renal impairment is most likely to become clinically evident, as assessed by increasing serum creatinine, during the second week of induction therapy at 60 mg/kg TID (see Pharmacodynamics). Renal impairment, however, may occur at any time in any patient during Foscarnet Sodium treatment and renal function should therefore be monitored especially carefully (see *"Patient Monitoring"*).

Elevations in serum creatinine are usually, but not uniformly, reversible following discontinuation or dose adjustment of Foscarnet Sodium. In the U.S. studies, recovery of renal function after Foscarnet Sodium induced impairment usually occurred within one week of drug discontinuation. However, of 35 patients in the U.S. controlled clinical studies who experienced grade II renal impairment (serum creatinine 2-3 times the upper limit of normal), two died with renal failure within four weeks of stopping Foscarnet Sodium, and three others died with renal insufficiency still present less than four weeks after the drug cessation.

BECAUSE OF FORSCARNET SODIUM'S POTENTIAL TO CAUSE RENAL IMPAIRMENT, DOSE ADJUSTMENT FOR DECREASED BASELINE RENAL FUNCTION AND ANY CHANGE IN RENAL FUNCTION DURING TREATMENT IS NECESSARY. In addition, it may be beneficial for adequate hydration to be established (e.g., by inducing diuresis) prior to and during Foscarnet Sodium administration.

MINERAL AND ELECTROLYTE IMBALANCES:

Foscarnet Sodium has been associated with changes in serum electrolytes including hypocalcemia (15%), hypophosphatemia (8%) and hyperphosphatemia (6%), hypomagnesemia (15%), and hypokalemia (16%). Administration of Foscarnet Sodium has been shown to be associated with a transient, dose-related decrease in ionized serum calcium, which may not be reflected in total serum calcium. This effect most likely is related to Foscarnet's chelation of divalent metal ions such as calcium. Therefore, patients should be advised to report symptoms of low ionized calcium such as perioral tingling, numbness in the extremities and paresthesias. Physicians should be prepared to treat these as well as severe manifestations of electrolyte abnormalities such as tetany and seizures. The rate of Foscarnet Sodium infusion may affect the transient decrease in ionized clacium. Slowing the rate may decrease or prevent symptoms.

Transient changes in calcium or other electrolytes (including magnesium, potassium or phosphate) may also contribute to a patient's risk for cardiac disturbances and seizures (see below). Therefore, particular caution is advised in patients with altered calcium or other electrolyte levels before treatment, especially those with neurologic or cardiac abnormalities and those receiving other drugs known to influence minerals and electrolytes (see *"Patient Monitoring"* and *"Drug Interactions"*).

NEUROTOXICITY AND SEIZURES:

Foscarnet Sodium treatment has been associated with seizures in 18/189 (10%) of AIDS patients in five controlled studies. Three patients were not taking Foscarnet Sodium at the time of seizure. In most cases (15/18), the patients had an active CNS condition (e.g., toxoplasmosis, HIV encephalopathy) or a history of CNS diseases. The rate of seizures did not increase with duration of treatment. These cases were associated with overdose of Foscarnet Sodium (see *"Overdosage"*).

A logistic regression analysis was performed comparing the 18 patients in these five studies who had seizures with the 161 who did not. Statistically significant (p < 0.05) risk factors associated with seizures were low baseline absolute neutrophil count (ANC), impaired baseline renal function, and low total serum calcium. Several cases of seizures were associated with death. However, occurrence of seizures did not always necessitate discontinuation of Foscarnet Sodium ten of fifteen patients with seizures that occurred while receiving the drug continued or resumed Foscarnet Sodium following treatment of their underlying disease, electrolyte disturbances, and/or dose decreases. If factors predisposing a patient to seizures are present, electrolytes, including calcium and magnesium, must be monitored especially carefully (see *"Patient Monitoring"*).

◆ RATED THERAPEUTICALLY EQUIVALENT; ◇ THERAPEUTIC EQUIVALENCE UNCONFIRMED; ○ UNRATED

PRECAUTIONS

GENERAL:
In controlled clinical studies with Foscarnet Sodium the maximum single dose administered was 120 mg/kg by intravenous infusion over 2 hours. It is likely that larger doses, or more rapid infusions, would result in increased toxicity. Care must be taken to infuse solutions containing Foscarnet Sodium only into veins with adequate blood flow to permit rapid dilution and distribution, and avoid local irritation (see *"Dosage and Administration"*). Local irritation and ulceration of penile epithelium have been reported in male patients receiving Foscarnet Sodium, possibly related to the presence of drug in urine. One case of vulvovaginal ulcerations in a female receiving Foscarnet Sodium has been reported. Adequate hydration with close attention to personal hygiene may minimize the occurrence of such events.

HEMOPOIETIC SYSTEM:
Anemia has been reported in 33% of patients receiving Foscarnet Sodium in controlled studies. This anemia was usually manageable with transfusions and required discontinuation of Foscarnet Sodium in less than 1% (1/189) of patients in the studies. Granulocytopenia has been reported in 17% of patients receiving Foscarnet Sodium in controlled studies; however, only 1% (2/189) were terminated from these studies because of neutropenia.

INFORMATION FOR PATIENTS
Patients should be advised that Foscarnet Sodium is not a cure for CMV retinitis, and that they may continue to experience progression of retinitis during or following treatment. They should be advised to have regular ophthalmologic examinations. They should be informed that the major toxicities of Foscarnet Sodium are renal impairment, electrolyte disturbances, and seizures, and that dose modifications and possibly discontinuation may be required. The importance of close monitoring while on therapy must be emphasized. Patients should be advised of the importance of perioral tingling, numbness in the extremities or paresthesias during or after infusion or possible symptoms of electrolyte abnormalities. Should such symptoms occur, the infusion of Foscarnet Sodium should be stopped, appropriate laboratory samples for assessment of electrolyte concentrations obtained, and a physician consulted before resuming treatment. The rate of infusion must be no more than 1 mg/kg/minute. The potential for renal impairment may be minimized by accompanying Foscarnet Sodium administration with hydration adequate to establish and maintain a diuresis during dosing.

DRUG INTERACTIONS
Coadministration of Foscarnet Sodium with other drugs could theoretically alter its antiviral activity, toxicity, or pharmacokinetics.

A possible drug interaction of Foscarnet Sodium and intravenous pentamidine has been described. Concomitant treatment of four patients in the United Kingdom with Foscarnet Sodium and intravenous pentamidine may have caused hypocalcemia; one patient died with severe hypocalcemia. Toxicity associated with concomitant use of aerosolized pentamidine has not been reported.

The elimination of Foscarnet Sodium may be impaired by drugs that inhibit renal tubular secretion; however, no studies have been conducted to determine whether this occurs. Nonetheless because of Foscarnet Sodium's tendency to cause renal impairment, the use of Foscarnet Sodium should be avoided in combination with potentially nephrotoxic drugs such as aminoglycosides, amphotericin B and intravenous pentamidine (see above) unless the potential benefits outweigh the risks to the patient.

Since Foscarnet Sodium decreases serum levels of ionized calcium, concurrent treatment with other drugs known to influence serum calcium levels should be used with particular caution. Foscarnet Sodium was used concomitantly with zidovudine in approximately one-third of patients in the U.S. studies. Although the combination was generally well tolerated, additive effects on anemia may have occurred. In one study of 24 patients (FOS-03), anemia was reported as an adverse event in 60% (3/5) patients receiving Foscarnet Sodium only, 88% (7/8) of patients receiving both zidovudine and Foscarnet Sodium 29% (2/7) of patients receiving only zidovudine and 25% (1/4) of patients receiving neither drug. However, no evidence of increased myelosuppression was seen with Foscarnet Sodium in combination with zidovudine.

CARCINOGENESIS, MUTAGENESIS, IMPAIRMENT OF FERTILITY
Carcinogenicity studies were conducted in rats and mice at oral doses of 500 mg/kg/day and 250 mg/kg/day. Oral bioavailability in unfasted rodents is < 20%. No evidence of oncogenicity was reported at plasma drug levels equal to 1/3 and 1/5, respectively, of those in humans (at the maximum recommended human daily dose) as measured by the area-under-the-time/ concentration curve (AUC).

Foscarnet Sodium showed genotoxic effects in the BALB/3T3 *in vitro* transformation assay at concentrations greater than 0.5 mcg/mL and an increased frequency of chromosome aberrations in the sister chromatid exchange assay at 1000 mcg/mL. A high dose of Foscarnet Sodium (350 mg/kg) caused an increase in micronucleated polychromatic erythrocytes *in vivo* in mice at doses that produced exposures (Area Under Curve) comparable to that anticipated clinically.

PREGNANCY: TERATOGENIC EFFECT
Pregnancy Category C: Foscarnet Sodium did not adversely affect fertility and general reproductive performance in rats. The results of peri- and post-natal studies in rats were also negative. However, these studies used exposures that are inadequate to define the potential for impairment of fertility at human drug exposure levels.

Daily subcutaneous doses up to 75 mg/kg administered to female rats prior to and during mating, during gestation, and 21 days postpartum caused a slight increase (< 5%) in the number of skeletal anomalies compared with the control group. Daily subcutaneous doses up to 75 mg/kg administered to rabbits and 150 mg/kg administered to rats during gestation caused an increase in the frequency of skeletal anomalies/variations.

On the basis of estimated drug exposure (as measured by AUC), the 150 mg/kg dose in rats and 75 mg/kg dose in rabbits were approximately one-eighth (rat) and one-third (rabbit) the estimated maximal daily human exposure. These studies are inadequate to define the potential teratogenicity at levels to which women will be exposed. There are no adequate and well controlled studies in pregnant women. Because animal reproductive studies are not always predictive of human response, Foscarnet Sodium should be used during pregnancy only if clearly needed.

NURSING MOTHERS
It is not known whether Foscarnet Sodium is excreted in human milk; however, in lactating rats administered 75 mg/kg, Foscarnet Sodium was excreted in maternal milk at concentrations three times higher than peak maternal blood concentrations. Because many drugs are excreted in human milk, caution should be exercised if Foscarnet Sodium is administered to a nursing woman.

PEDIATRIC USE
The safety and effectiveness of Foscarnet Sodium in children have not been studied. Foscarnet Sodium is deposited in teeth and bone and deposition is greater in young and growing animals. Foscarnet Sodium has been demonstrated to adversely affect development of tooth enamel in mice and rats. The effects of this deposition on skeletal development have not been studied. Since deposition in human bone also occurs, it is likely that it does so to a greater degree in developing bone in children. Administration to children should be undertaken only after careful evaluation and only if the potential benefits for treatment outweigh the risks.

USE IN THE ELDERLY
No studies of the efficacy or safety of Foscarnet Sodium in persons over age 65 have been conducted. Since these individuals frequently have reduced glomerular filtration, particular attention should be paid to assessing renal function before and during Foscarnet Sodium administration (see *"Dosage and Administration"*).

ADVERSE REACTIONS
In five controlled U.S. clinical trials in which 189 patients with AIDS and CMV retinitis were treated with Foscarnet Sodium, the most frequently reported events were the following: fever 65% (123/189), nausea 47% (88/189), anemia 33% (63/189), diarrhea 30% (57/189), abnormal renal function including acute renal failure, decreased creatinine clearance and increased serum creatinine 27% (51/189), vomiting 26% (50, 189), headache 26% (49/189), and seizure 10% (18/189) (see *"Warnings"* and *"Precautions"*). These incidence figures were calculated without reference to drug relationship or severity.

From the same controlled studies, adverse events categorized by investigator as "severe" were death (14%), abnormal renal function (14%), marrow suppression (10%), anemia (9%), and seizures (7%). Although death was specifically attributed to Foscarnet Sodium in only one case, other complications of Foscarnet Sodium (i.e., renal impairment, electrolyte abnormalities, and seizures) may have contributed to patient deaths (see *"Warnings"* and *"Precautions"*).

The types and incidences of adverse events reported worldwide with Foscarnet Sodium have not been different from, or greater in frequency, than those observed in the U.S. trials. From the five U.S. controlled clinical trials of Foscarnet Sodium, the following list of adverse events has been compiled regardless of casual relationship to Foscarnet Sodium. Evaluation of these reports was difficult because of the diverse manifestations of the underlying disease and because most patients received numerous concomitant medications.

INCIDENCE 5% OR GREATER
Body as a Whole: fever, fatigue, rigors, asthenia, malaise, pain, infection, sepsis, death

Central and Peripheral Nervous System: headache, paresthesia, dizziness, involuntary muscle contractions, hypoesthesia, neuropathy, seizures including grand mal seizures (see *"Warnings"*)

Gastrointestinal System: anorexia, nausea, diarrhea, vomiting, abdominal pain

Hematologic: anemia, granulocytopenia, leukopenia (see *"Precautions"*)

Metabolic and Nutritional: mineral and electrolyte imbalances (see *"Warnings"*) including hypokalemia, hypocalcemia, hypomagnesemia, hypophosphatemia, hyperphosphatemia

Psychiatric: depression, confusion, anxiety

Respiratory System: coughing, dyspnea

Skin and Appendages: rash, increased sweating

Urinary: alterations in renal function including increased serum creatinine, decreased creatinine clearance, and abnormal renal function (see *"Warnings"*)

Special Senses: vision abnormalities

INCIDENCE BETWEEN 1% AND 5%
Application Site: injection site pain, injection site inflammation

Body as a Whole: back pain, chest pain, edema, influenza-like symptoms, bacterial infections, moniliasis, fungal infections, abscess

Cardiovascular: hypertension, palpitations, ECG abnormalities including sinus tachycardia, first degree AV block and non-specific ST-T segment changes, hypotension, flushing, cerebrovascular disorder (see *"Warnings"*)

Central and Peripheral Nervous System: tremor, ataxia, dementia, stupor, generalized spasms, sensory disturbances, meningitis, aphasia, abnormal coordination, leg cramps, EEG abnormalities (see *"Warnings"*)

Gastrointestinal: constipation, dysphagia, dyspepsia, rectal hemorrhage, dry mouth, melena, flatulence, ulcerative stomatitis, pancreatitis

Hematologic: thrombocytopenia, platelet abnormalities, thrombosis, white blood cell abnormalities, lymphadenopathy

Liver and Biliary: abnormal A-G ratio, abnormal hepatic function, increased SGPT, increased SGOT

Metabolic and Nutritional: hyponatremia, decreased weight, increased alkaline phosphatase, increased LDH, increased BUN, acidosis, cachexia, thirst, hypercalcemia (see *"Warnings"*)

Musculo-Skeletal: arthralgia, myalgia

Neoplasms: lymphoma-like disorder, sarcoma

Psychiatric: insomnia, somnolence, nervousness, amnesia, agitation, aggressive reaction, hallucination

Respiratory System: pneumonia, sinusitis, pharyngitis, rhinitis, respiratory disorders, respiratory insufficiency, pulmonary infiltration, stridor, pneumothorax, hemoptysis, bronchospasm

Skin and Appendages: pruritus, skin ulceration, seborrhea, erythematous rash, maculo-papular rash, skin discoloration

Special Senses: taste perversions, eye abnormalities, eye pain, conjunctivitis

Urinary System: albuminuria, dysuria, polyuria, urethral disorder, urinary retention, urinary tract infections, acute renal failure, nocturia, facial edema

INCIDENCE LESS THAN 1%
Body as a Whole: hypothermia, leg edema, peripheral edema, syncope, ascites, substernal chest pain, abnormal crying, malignant hyperpyrexia, herpes simplex, viral infection, toxoplasmosis

Cardiovascular: cardiomyopathy, cardiac failure, cardiac arrest, bradycardia, extrasystole, arrhythmias, atrial arrhythmias, atrial fibrillation, phlebitis, superficial thrombophlebitis of the arm, mesenteric vein thrombophlebitis

Central and Peripheral Nervous System: vertigo, coma, encephalopathy, abnormal gait, hyperesthesia, hypertonia, visual field defects, dyskinesia, extrapyramidal disorders, hemiparesis, hyperkinesia, vocal cord paralysis, paralysis, paraplegia, speech disorders, tetany, hyporeflexia, neuralgia, neuritis, peripheral neuropathy, hyperreflexia, cerebral edema, nystagmus

Endocrine: antidiuretic hormone disorders, decreased gonadotropins, gynecomastia

Gastrointestinal System: enteritis, enterocolitis, glossitis, proctitis, stomatitis, tenesmus, increased amylase, pseudomembranous colitis, gastroenteritis, oral leukoplakia, oral hemorrhage, rectal disorders, colitis, duodenal ulcer, hematemesis, paralytic ileus, esophageal ulceration, ulcerative proctitis, tongue ulceration

Hematologic: pulmonary embolism, coagulation disorders, decreased coagulation factors, epistaxis, decreased prothrombin, hypochromic anemia, pancytopenia, hemolysis, leukocytosis, cervical lymphadenopathy, lymphopenia

Special Senses: deafness, earache, tinnitus, otitis

Liver and Biliary System: cholecystitis, cholelithiasis, hepatitis, cholestatic hepatitis, hepatosplenomegaly, jaundice

Metabolic and Nutritional: dehydration, glycosuria, increased creatine phosphokinase, diabetes mellitus, abnormal glucose tolerance, hypervolemia, hypochloremia, periorbital edema, hypoproteinemia

Musculo-Skeletal System: arthrosis, synovitis, torticollis

Neoplasms: malignant lymphoma, skin hypertrophy

Psychiatric: impaired concentration, emotional lability, psychosis, suicide attempt, delirium, personality disorders, sleep disorders

Reproductive: perineal pain in women, penile inflammation

Respiratory System: bronchitis, laryngitis, respiratory depression, abnormal chest x-ray, pleural effusion, lobar pneumonia, pulmonary hemorrhage, pneumonitis

Skin and Appendages: acne, alopecia, dermatitis, anal pruritis, genital pruritis, aggravated psoriasis, psoriaform rash, skin disorders, dry skin, urticaria, verruca

Urinary System: hematuria, glomerulonephritis, micturition disorders, micturition frequency, toxic nephropathy, nephrosis, urinary incontinence, renal tubular disorders, pyelonephritis, urethral irritation, uremia

Special Senses: diplopia, blindness, retinal detachment, mydriasis, photophobia

OVERDOSAGE
In controlled clinical trials performed in the United States, overdosage with Foscarnet Sodium was reported in 10 patients. All 10 patients experienced adverse events and all except one made a complete recovery. One patient died after receiving a total daily dose of 12.5 g for three days instead of the intended 10.9 g. The patient suffered a grand mal seizure and become comatose. Three days later the patient expired with the cause of death listed as respiratory/cardiac

arrest. The other nine patients received doses ranging from 1.14 times to 8 times their recommended doses with an average of 4 times their recommended doses. Overall, three patients had seizures, three patients had renal function impairment, four patients had paresthesis either in limbs or periorally, and five patients had documented electrolyte disturbances primarily involving calcium and phosphate.

There is no specific antidote for Foscarnet Sodium overdose. Hemodialysis and hydration may be of benefit in reducing drug plasma levels in patients who receive an overdosage of Foscarnet Sodium, but these have not been evaluated in a clinical trial setting. The patient should be observed for signs and symptoms of renal impairment and electrolyte imbalance. Medical treatment should be instituted if clinically warranted.

DOSAGE AND ADMINISTRATION
CAUTION—DO NOT ADMINISTER FOSCARNET SODIUM BY RAPID OR BOLUS INTRAVENOUS INJECTION. THE TOXICITY OF FOSCARNET SODIUM MAY BE INCREASED AS A RESULT OF EXCESSIVE PLASMA LEVELS. CARE SHOULD BE TAKEN TO AVOID UNINTENTIONAL OVERDOSE BY CAREFULLY CONTROLLING THE RATE OF INFUSION. THEREFORE, AN INFUSION PUMP MUST BE USED. IN SPITE OF THE USE OF AN INFUSION PUMP, OVERDOSES HAVE OCCURRED.

ADMINISTRATION
Foscarnet Sodium is administered by controlled intravenous infusion, either by using a central venous line or by using a peripheral vein. The standard 24 mg/mL solution may be used without dilution when using a central venous catheter for infusion. When a peripheral vein catheter is used, the 24 mg/mL solution **must** be diluted to 12 mg/mL with 5% dextrose in water or with a normal saline solution prior to administration to avoid local irritation of peripheral veins. Since the dose of Foscarnet Sodium is calculated on the basis of body weight, it may be desirable to remove and discard any unneeded quantity from the bottle before starting with the infusion to avoid overdosage. Dilutions and/or removals of excess quantities should be accomplished under aseptic conditions. Solutions thus prepared should be used within 24 hours of first entry into a sealed bottle.

Other drugs and supplements can be administered to a patient receiving Foscarnet Sodium. However, care must be taken to ensure that Foscarnet Sodium is only administered with normal saline or 5% dextrose solution and that no other drug or supplement is administered concurrently via the same catheter. Foscarnet Sodium has been reported to be chemically incompatible with 30% dextrose, amphotericin B, and solutions containing calcium such as Ringer's lactate and TPN. Physical incompatibility with other IV drugs has also been reported including acyclovir sodium, ganciclovir, trimetrexate glucuronate, pentamidine isethionate, vancomycin, trimethoprim/sulfamethoxazole, diazepam, midazolam, digoxin, phenytoin, leucovorin, and prochlorperazine. Because of Foscarnet Sodium's chelating properties, a precipitate can potentially occur when divalent cations are administered concurrently in the same catheter.

Parenteral drug products must be inspected visually for particulate matter and discoloration prior to administration whenever the solution and container permit. Solutions that are discolored or contain particulate matter should not be used.

DOSAGE
THE RECOMMENDED DOSAGE, FREQUENCY, OR INFUSION RATES SHOULD NOT BE EXCEEDED. ALL DOSES MUST BE INDIVIDUALIZED FOR PATIENTS' RENAL FUNCTION.
INDUCTION TREATMENT:
The recommended initial dose of Foscarnet Sodium for patients with normal renal function is 60 mg/kg, adjusted for individual patients' renal function, given intravenously at a constant rate over a minimum of one hour every 8 hours for 2-3 weeks depending on clinical response. An infusion pump must be used to control the rate of infusion. Adequate hydration is recommended to establish a diuresis, both prior to and during treatment to minimize renal toxicity (see *"Warnings"*), provided there are no clinical contraindications.

MAINTENANCE TREATMENT:
Following induction treatment the recommended maintenance dose of Foscarnet Sodium is 90 mg/kg/day to 120 mg/kg/day (individualized for renal function) given as an intravenous infusion over 2 hours. Because the superiority of the 120 mg/kg/day has not been established in controlled trials, and given the likely relationship of higher plasma Foscarnet Sodium levels to toxicity, it is recommended that most patients be started on maintenance treatment with a dose of 90 mg/kg/day. Escalation to 120 mg/kg/day may be considered should early reinduction be required because of retinitis progression. Some patients who show excellent tolerance to Foscarnet Sodium may benefit from initiation of maintenance treatment at 120 mg/kg/day earlier in their treatment. An infusion pump must be used to control the rate of infusion with all doses. Again, hydration to establish diuresis both prior to and during treatment is recommended to minimize renal toxicity, provided there are no clinical contraindications (see *"Warnings"*).

Patients who experience progression of retinitis while receiving Foscarnet Sodium maintenance therapy may be retreated with the induction and maintenance regimens given above.

USE IN PATIENTS WITH ABNORMAL RENAL FUNCTION:
Foscarnet Sodium should be used with caution in patients with abnormal renal function because reduced plasma clearance of Foscarnet Sodium will result in elevated plasma levels (see *"Clinical Pharmacology"*). In addition, Foscarnet Sodium has the potential to further impair renal function (see *"Warnings"*). Foscarnet Sodium has not been specifically studied in patients with creatinine clearances < 50 mL/min or serum creatinines > 2.8 mg/dL. Renal function must

be monitored carefully at baseline and during induction and maintenance therapy with appropriate dose adjustments for Foscarnet Sodium as outlined below (see "Dose Adjustment" and "Patient Monitoring"). During Foscarnet Sodium therapy if creatinine clearance falls below the limits of the dosing nomograms (0.4 mL/min/kg), Foscarnet Sodium should be discontinued and the patient monitored daily until resolution of renal impairment is ensured.

DOSE ADJUSTMENT

Foscarnet Sodium dosing must be individualized according to the patient's renal function status. Refer to *Table 4* below for recommended doses and adjust the dose as indicated.

To use this dosing guide, actual 24-hour creatinine clearance (mL/min) must be divided by body weight (kg), or the estimated creatinine clearance in mL/min/kg can be calculated from serum creatinine (mg/dL) using the following formula (modified Cockcroft and Gault equation):

For males:

$$\frac{140 - \text{age}}{\text{serum creatinine} \times 72} \quad (\text{x } 0.85 \text{ for females})$$

Table 4

FOSCARNET SODIUM DOSING GUIDE INDUCTION

CrCl (mL/min/kg)	Equivalent to 60 mg/kg Dose Q8H
≥ 1.6	60
1.5	57
1.4	53
1.3	49
1.2	46
1.1	42
1.0	39
0.9	35
0.8	32
0.7	28
0.6	25
0.5	21
0.4	18

MAINTENANCE

CrCl (mL/min/kg)	Equivalent to 90 mg/kg Dose Q24H	Equivalent to 120 mg/kg Dose Q24H
≥ 1.4	90	120
1.2–1.4	78	104
1.0–1.2	75	100
0.8–1.0	71	94
0.6–0.8	63	84
0.4–0.6	57	76

PATIENT MONITORING

The majority of patients will experience some decrease in renal function due to Foscarnet Sodium administration. Therefore, it is recommended that creatinine clearance, either measured or estimated using the modified Cockcroft and Gault equation based on serum creatinine, be determined at baseline, 2-3 times per week during induction therapy and at least once every one to two weeks during maintenance therapy, with Foscarnet Sodium dose adjusted accordingly (see "Dose Adjustment"). More frequent monitoring may be required for some patients. It is also recommended that a 24-hour creatinine clearance be determined at baseline and periodically thereafter to ensure correct dosing (assuming verification of an adequate collection using creatinine index) Foscarnet Sodium should be discontinued if creatinine clearance drops below 0.4 mL/min/kg.

Due to Foscarnet Sodium propensity to chelate divalent metal ions and alter levels of serum electrolytes, patients must be monitored closely for such changes. It is recommended that a schedule similar to that recommended for serum creatinine (see above) be used to monitor serum calcium, magnesium, potassium and phosphorus. Particular caution is advised in patients with decreased total serum calcium or other electrolyte levels before treatment, as well as patients with neurologic or cardiac abnormalities, and in patients receiving other drugs known to influence serum calcium levels. Any clinically significant metabolic changes should be corrected. Also patients who experience mild (e.g., perioral numbness or paresthesias) or severe (e.g., seizures) symptoms of electrolyte abnormalities should have serum electrolyte and mineral levels assessed as close in time to the event as possible. Careful monitoring and appropriate management of electrolytes, calcium, magnesium and creatinine are of particular importance in patients with conditions that may predispose them to seizures (see "Warnings").

Foscarnet Sodium Injection should be stored at controlled room temperature 15°-30°C (59°-86°F), and should be protected from excessive heat (above 40°C) and from freezing. Foscarnet Sodium Injection should be used only if the bottle and seal are intact, a vacuum is present, and the solution is clear and colorless.

J CODES

Per 1,000 mg IV—J1455

HOW SUPPLIED
INJECTION: 24 MG/ML

BRAND/MANUFACTURER	NDC	SIZE	AWP
○ BRAND			
FOSCAVIR: Astra	00186-1905-01	250 ml	$73.28
	00186-1906-01	500 ml	$145.93

Foscavir *SEE* FOSCARNET SODIUM

Fosinopril Sodium

USE IN PREGNANCY

WHEN USED IN PREGNANCY DURING THE SECOND AND THIRD TRIMESTERS, ACE INHIBITORS CAN CAUSE INJURY AND EVEN DEATH TO THE DEVELOPING FETUS.

WHEN PREGNANCY IS DETECTED, FOSINOPRIL SODIUM SHOULD BE DISCONTINUED AS SOON AS POSSIBLE. SEE *"WARNINGS"*: FETAL/NEONATAL MORBIDITY AND MORTALITY.

DESCRIPTION

Fosinopril Sodium is the sodium salt of Fosinopril, the ester prodrug of an angiotensin converting enzyme (ACE) inhibitor, fosinoprilat. Fosinopril Sodium is designated chemically as: L-proline, 4-cyclohexyl-1-[[[2-methyl-1-(1-oxopropoxy)propoxy](4-phenylbutyl) phosphinyl]acetyl]-, sodium salt, *trans*-.

Fosinopril Sodium is a white to off-white crystalline powder. It is soluble in water (100 mg/mL), methanol, and ethanol and slightly soluble in hexane.

Its empiric formula is $C_{30}H_{45}NNaO_7P$, and its molecular weight is 585.65.

Fosinopril Sodium is available for oral administration as 10 mg and 20 mg tablets.

Following is its chemical structure:

CLINICAL PHARMACOLOGY

MECHANISM OF ACTION

In animals and humans, Fosinopril Sodium is hydrolyzed by esterases to the pharmacologically active form, fosinoprilat, a specific competitive inhibitor of angiotensin converting enzyme (ACE).

ACE is a peptidyl dipeptidase that catalyzes the conversion of angiotensin I to the vasoconstrictor substance, angiotensin II. Angiotensin II also stimulates aldosterone secretion by the adrenal cortex. Inhibition of ACE results in decreased plasma angiotensin II, which leads to decreased vasopressor activity and to decreased aldosterone secretion. The latter decrease may result in a small increase of serum potassium. In 647 hypertensive patients treated with Fosinopril alone for an average of 29 weeks, mean increases in serum potassium of 0.1 mEq/L were observed. Similar increases were observed among all patients treated with Fosinopril Sodium, including those receiving concomitant diuretic therapy. Removal of angiotensin II negative feedback on renin secretion leads to increased plasma renin activity.

ACE is identical to kininase, an enzyme that degrades bradykinin. Whether increased levels of bradykinin, a potent vasodepressor peptide, play a role in the therapeutic effects of Fosinopril Sodium remains to be elucidated.

While the mechanism through which Fosinopril Sodium lowers blood pressure is believed to be primarily suppression of the renin-angiotensin-aldosterone system, Fosinopril Sodium has an antihypertensive effect even in patients with low-renin hypertension. Although Fosinopril Sodium was antihypertensive in all races studied, black hypertensive patients (usually a low-renin hypertensive population) had a smaller average response to ACE inhibitor monotherapy than non-black patients.

PHARMACOKINETIC AND METABOLISM

Following oral administration, Fosinopril Sodium (the prodrug) is absorbed slowly. The absolute absorption of Fosinopril Sodium averaged 36% of an oral dose. The primary site of absorption is the proximal small intestine (duodenum/jejunum). While the rate of absorption may be slowed by the presence of food in the gastrointestinal tract, the extent of absorption of Fosinopril Sodium is essentially unaffected.

Fosinoprilat is highly protein-bound (≥ 95%), has a relatively small volume of distribution, and has negligible binding to cellular components in blood. After single and multiple oral doses, plasma levels, areas under plasma concentration-time curves (AUCs) and peak concentrations (Cmaxs) are directly proportional to the dose of Fosinopril Sodium. Times to peak concentrations are independent of dose and are achieved in approximately 3 hours.

After an oral dose of radiolabeled Fosinopril Sodium, 75% of radioactivity in plasma was present as active fosinoprilat, 20-30% as a glucuronide conjugate of fosinoprilat, and 1-5% as a *p*-hydroxy metabolite of fosinoprilat. Since fosinoprilat is not biotransformed after intravenous administration, Fosinopril Sodium, not fosinoprilat, appears to be the precursor for the glucuronide and *p*-hydroxy metabolites. In rats, the *p*-hydroxy metabolite of fosinoprilat is as potent an inhibitor of ACE as fosinoprilat; the glucuronide conjugate is devoid of ACE inhibitory activity.

After intravenous administration, fosinoprilat was eliminated approximately equally by the liver and kidney. After oral administration of radiolabeled Fosinopril Sodium, approximately half of the absorbed dose is excreted in the urine and the remainder is excreted in the feces. In two studies involving healthy subjects, the mean body clearance of intravenous fosinoprilat was between 26 and 39 mL/min.

In healthy subjects, the terminal elimination half-life (t1/2) of an intravenous dose of radiolabeled fosinoprilat is approximately 12 hours. In hypertensive patients with normal renal and hepatic function, who received repeated doses of Fosinopril Sodium, the effective t1/2 for accumulation of fosinoprilat averaged 11.5 hours.

In Patients with Renal Insufficiency: (creatinine clearance < 80 mL/min/1.73m^2), the total body clearance of fosinoprilat is approximately one-half of that in patients with normal renal function, while absorption, bioavailability, and protein-binding are not appreciably altered. The clearance of fosinoprilat does not differ appreciably with degree of renal insufficiency, because the diminished renal elimination is offset by increased hepatobiliary elimination. A modest increase in plasma AUC levels (less than two times that in normals) was observed in patients with various degrees of renal insufficiency, including end-stage renal failure (creatinine clearance < 10 mL/min/1.73m^2). (See *"Dosage And Administration"*.)

Fosinopril Sodium is not well dialyzed. Clearance of fosinoprilat by hemodialysis and peritoneal dialysis averages 2% and 7%, respectively, of urea clearances.

In patients with hepatic insufficiency (alcoholic or biliary cirrhosis), the extent of hydrolysis of Fosinopril Sodium is not appreciably reduced, although the rate of hydrolysis may be slowed: the apparent total body clearance of fosinoprilat is approximately one-half of that in patients with normal hepatic function.

In Elderly (Male) Subjects: (65-74 years old) with clinically normal renal and hepatic function, there appear to be no significant differences in pharmacokinetic parameters for fosinoprilat compared to those of younger subjects (20-35 years old).

Fosinoprilat was found to cross the placenta of pregnant animals.

Studies in animals indicate that Fosinopril Sodium and fosinoprilat do not cross the blood-brain barrier.

PHARMACODYNAMICS AND CLINICAL EFFECTS

Serum ACE activity was inhibited by $\geq 90\%$ at 2 to 12 hours after single doses of 10 to 40 mg of Fosinopril Sodium. At 24 hours, serum ACE activity remained suppressed by 85%. 93%, and 93% in the 10, 20, and 40 mg dose groups, respectively.

Administration of Fosinopril Sodium to patients with mild to moderate hypertension results in a reduction of both supine and standing blood pressure to about the same extent with no compensatory tachycardia. Symptomatic postural hypotension is infrequent, although it can occur in patients who are salt- and/or volume-depleted (see *"Warnings"*). Use of Fosinopril Sodium in combination with thiazide diuretics gives a blood pressure-lowering effect greater than that seen with either agent alone.

Following oral administration of single doses of 10-40 mg, Fosinopril Sodium lowered blood pressure within one hour, with peak reductions achieved 2-6 hours after dosing. The antihypertensive effect of a single dose persisted for 24 hours. Following four weeks of monotherapy in placebo-controlled trials in patients with mild to moderate hypertension, once daily doses of 20-80 mg lowered supine or seated systolic and diastolic blood pressures 24 hours after dosing by an average of 8-9/6-7 mmHg more than placebo. The trough effect was about 50-60% of the peak diastolic response and about 80% of the peak systolic response.

In most trials, the antihypertensive effect of Fosinopril Sodium increased during the first several weeks of repeated measurements. The antihypertensive effect of Fosinopril Sodium has been shown to continue during long-term therapy for at least 2 years. Abrupt withdrawal of Fosinopril Sodium has not resulted in a rapid increase in blood pressure. Limited experience in controlled and uncontrolled trials combining Fosinopril Sodium with a calcium channel blocker or a loop diuretic has indicated no unusual drug-drug interactions. Other ACE inhibitors have had less than additive effects with beta-adrenergic blockers, presumably because both drugs lower blood pressure by inhibiting parts of the renin-angiotensin system.

ACE inhibitors are generally less effective in blacks than in non-blacks. The effectiveness of Fosinopril Sodium was not influenced by age, sex, or weight.

In hemodynamic studies in hypertensive patients, after three months of therapy, responses (changes in BP, heart rate, cardiac index, and PVR) to various stimuli (e.g., isometric exercise, 45° head-up tilt, and mental challenge) were unchanged compared to baseline, suggesting that Fosinopril Sodium does not affect the activity of the sympathetic nervous system. Reduction in systemic blood pressure appears to have been mediated by a decrease in peripheral vascular resistance without reflex cardiac effects. Similarly, renal, splanchnic, cerebral, and skeletal muscle blood flow were unchanged compared to baseline, as was glomerular filtration rate.

INDICATIONS AND USAGE

Fosinopril Sodium is indicated for the treatment of hypertension. It may be used alone or in combination with thiazide diuretics.

In using Fosinopril Sodium, consideration should be given to the fact that another angiotensin converting enzyme inhibitor, captopril, has caused agranulocytosis, particularly in patients with renal impairment or collagen-vascular disease. Available data are insufficient to show that Fosinopril Sodium does not have a similar risk (see *"Warnings"*).

UNLABELED USES

Fosinopril Sodium is also used alone or as an adjunct in the treatment of congestive heart failure.

CONTRAINDICATIONS

Fosinopril Sodium is contraindicated in patients who are hypersensitive to this product or to any other angiotensin converting enzyme inhibitor (e.g., a patient who has experienced angioedema with any other ACE inhibitor therapy).

WARNINGS

ANGIOEDEMA

Angioedema involving the extremities, face, lips, mucous membranes, tongue, glottis or larynx have been reported in patients treated with ACE inhibitors. If angioedema involves the tongue, glottis or larynx, airway obstruction may occur and be fatal. If laryngeal stridor or angioedema of the face, lips, mucous membranes, tongue, glottis or extremities occurs, treatment with Fosinopril Sodium should be discontinued and appropriate therapy instituted immediately. **Where there is involvement of the tongue, glottis, or larynx, likely to cause airway obstruction, appropriate therapy, e.g., subcutaneous epinephrine solution 1: 1000 (0.3 mL to 0.5 mL) should be promptly administered** (see *"Precautions: Information for Patients"* and *"Adverse Reactions"*).

HYPOTENSION

Fosinopril Sodium can cause symptomatic hypotension. Like other ACE inhibitors, Fosinopril Sodium has been only rarely associated with hypotension in uncomplicated hypertensive patients. Symptomatic hypotension is most likely to occur in patients who have been volume- and/or salt-depleted as a result of prolonged diuretic therapy, dietary salt restriction, dialysis, diarrhea, or vomiting. Volume and/or salt depletion should be corrected before initiating therapy with Fosinopril Sodium.

In patients with congestive heart failure, with or without associated renal insufficiency, ACE inhibitor therapy may cause excessive hypotension, which may be associated with oliguria or azotemia and, rarely, with acute renal failure and death. In such patients, Fosinopril Sodium therapy should be started under close medical supervision; they should be followed closely for the first 2 weeks of treatment and whenever the dose of Fosinopril Sodium or diuretic is increased.

If hypotension occurs, the patient should be placed in a supine position and, if necessary, treated with intravenous infusion of physiological saline. Fosinopril Sodium treatment usually can be continued following restoration of blood pressure and volume.

NEUTROPENIA/AGRANULOCYTOSIS

Another angiotensin converting enzyme inhibitor, captopril, has been shown to cause agranulocytosis and bone marrow depression, rarely in uncomplicated patients, but more frequently in patients with renal impairment, especially if they also have a collagen-vascular disease such as systemic lupus erythematosus or scleroderma. Available data from clinical trials of fosinopril are insufficient to show that Fosinopril Sodium does not cause agranulocytosis at similar rates. Monitoring of white blood cell counts should be considered in patients with collagen-vascular disease, especially if the disease is associated with impaired renal function.

FETAL/NEONATAL MORBIDITY AND MORTALITY

ACE inhibitors can cause fetal and neonatal morbidity and death when administered to pregnant women. Several dozen cases have been reported in the world literature. When pregnancy is detected, ACE inhibitors should be discontinued as soon as possible.

The use of ACE inhibitors during the second and third trimesters of pregnancy has been associated with fetal and neonatal injury, including hypotension, neonatal skull hypoplasia, anuria, reversible or irreversible renal failure, and death. Oligohydramnios has also been reported, presumably resulting from decreased fetal renal function; oligohydramnios in this setting has been associated with fetal limb contractures, craniofacial deformation, and hypoplastic lung development. Prematurity, intrauterine growth retardation, and patent ductus arteriosus have also been reported, although it is not clear whether these occurrences were due to the ACE-inhibitor exposure.

These adverse effects do not appear to have resulted from intrauterine ACE-inhibitor exposure that has been limited to the first trimester. Mothers whose embryos and fetuses are exposed to ACE inhibitors only during the first trimester should be so informed. Nonetheless, when patients become pregnant, physicians should make every effort to discontinue the use of Fosinopril Sodium as soon as possible.

Rarely (probably less often than once in every thousand pregnancies), no alternative to ACE inhibitors will be found. In these rare cases, the mothers should be apprised of the potential hazards to their fetuses, and serial ultrasound examinations should be performed to assess the intraamniotic environment.

If oligohydramnios is observed, Fosinopril Sodium should be discontinued unless it is considered life-saving for the mother. Contraction stress testing (CST), a nonstress test (NST), or biophysical profiling (BPP) may be appropriate, depending upon the week of pregnancy. Patients and physicians should be aware, however, that oligohydramnios may not appear until after the fetus has sustained irreversible injury.

Infants with histories of *in utero* exposure to ACE inhibitors should be closely observed for hypotension, oliguria, and hyperkalemia. If oliguria occurs, attention should be directed toward support of blood pressure and renal perfusion. Exchange transfusion or dialysis may be required as a means of reversing hypotension and/or substituting for disordered renal function. Fosinopril Sodium is poorly dialyzed from the circulation of adults by hemodialysis and peritoneal dialysis. There is no experience with any procedure for removing Fosinopril Sodium from the neonatal circulation.

When Fosinopril Sodium was given to pregnant rats at doses about 80 to 250 times (on a mg/kg basis) the maximum recommended human dose, three similar orofacial malformations and one fetus with *situs inversus* were observed among the offspring. No teratogenic effects of Fosinopril Sodium were seen in studies in pregnant rabbits at doses up to 25 times (on a mg/kg basis) the maximum recommended human dose.

PRECAUTIONS
GENERAL
Impaired Renal Function: As a consequence of inhibiting the renin-angiotensin-aldosterone system, changes in renal function may be anticipated in susceptible individuals. In patients with severe congestive heart failure whose renal function may depend on the activity of the renin-angioten-sin-aldosterone system, treatment with angiotensin converting enzyme inhibitors, including Fosinopril Sodium, may be associated with oliguria and/or progressive azotemia and (rarely) with acute renal failure and/or death. In hypertensive patients with renal artery stenosis in a solitary kidney or bilateral renal artery stenosis, increases in blood urea nitrogen and serum creatinine may occur. Experience with another angiotensin converting enzyme inhibitor suggests that these increases are usually reversible upon discontinuation of ACE inhibitor and/or diuretic therapy. In such patients, renal function should be monitored during the first few weeks of therapy. Some hypertensive patients with no apparent pre-existing renal vascular disease have developed increases in blood urea nitrogen and serum creatinine, usually minor and transient, especially when Fosinopril Sodium has been given concomitantly with a diuretic. This is more likely to occur in patients with pre-existing renal impairment. Dosage reduction of Fosinopril Sodium and/or discontinuation of the diuretic may be required.

EVALUATION OF THE HYPERTENSIVE PATIENT SHOULD ALWAYS INCLUDE ASSESSMENT OF RENAL FUNCTION (SEE *"DOSAGE AND ADMINISTRATION".)*
Impaired renal function decreases total clearance of fosinoprilat and approximately doubles AUC. In general, however, no adjustment of dosing is needed (see *"Clinical Pharmacology"*).

Hyperkalemia: In clinical trials, hyperkalemia (serum potassium greater than 10% above the upper limit of normal) has occurred in approximately 2.6% of hypertensive patients receiving Fosinopril Sodium. In most cases, these were isolated values which resolved despite continued therapy. In clinical trials, 0.1% of patients (two patients) were discontinued from therapy due to an elevated serum potassium. Risk factors for the development of hyperkalemia include renal insufficiency, diabetes mellitus, and the concomitant use of potassium-sparing diuretics, potassium supplements, and/or potassium-containing salt substitutes, which should be used cautiously, if at all, with Fosinopril Sodium (see *"Precautions: Drug Interactions"*).

Cough: Cough has been reported with the use of ACE inhibitors. Characteristically, the cough is nonproductive, persistent, and resolves after discontinuation of therapy. ACE inhibitor-induced cough should be considered as part of the differential diagnosis of cough.

Impaired Liver Function: Since Fosinopril Sodium is primarily metabolized by hepatic and gut wall esterases to its active moiety, fosinoprilat, patients with impaired liver function could develop elevated plasma levels of unchanged Fosinopril Sodium. In a study in patients with alcoholic or biliary cirrhosis, the extent of hydrolysis was unaffected, although the rate was slowed. In these patients, the apparent total body clearance of fosinoprilat was decreased and the plasma AUC approximately doubled.

Surgery/Anesthesia: In patients undergoing surgery or during anesthesia with agents that produce hypotension, Fosinopril Sodium will block the angiotensin II formation that could otherwise occur secondary to compensatory renin release. Hypotension that occurs as a result of this mechanism can be corrected by volume expansion.

HEMODIALYSIS
Recent clinical observations have shown an association of hypersensitivity-like (anaphylactoid) reactions during hemodialysis with high-flux dialysis membranes (e.g., AN69) in patients receiving ACE inhibitors. In these patients, consideration should be given to using a different type of dialysis membrane or a different class of medication.

INFORMATION FOR PATIENTS
Angioedema: Angioedema, including laryngeal edema, can occur with treatment with ACE inhibitors, especially following the first dose. Patients should be advised to immediately report to their physician any signs or symptoms suggesting angioedema (e.g., swelling of face, eyes, lips, tongue, larynx, mucous

membranes, and extremities; difficulty in swallowing or breathing; hoarseness) and to discontinue therapy. (See *"Warnings"* and *"Adverse Reactions"*.)

Symptomatic Hypotension: Patients should be cautioned that light-headedness can occur, especially during the first days of therapy, and it should be reported to a physician. Patients should be told that if syncope occurs Fosinopril Sodium should be discontinued until the physician has been consulted.

All patients should be cautioned that inadequate fluid intake or excessive perspiration, diarrhea, or vomiting can lead to an excessive fall in blood pressure, with the same consequences of light-headedness and possible syncope.

Hyperkalemia: Patients should be told not to use potassium supplements or salt substitutes containing potassium without consulting the physician.

Neutropenia: Patients should be told to promptly report any indication of infection (e.g., sore throat, fever), which could be a sign of neutropenia.

Pregnancy: Female patients of childbearing age should be told about the consequences of second- and third-trimester exposure to ACE inhibitors, and they should also be told that these consequences do not appear to have resulted for intrauterine ACE-inhibitor exposure that has been limited to the first trimester. These patients should be asked to report pregnancies to their physicians as soon as possible.

DRUG INTERACTIONS
With Diuretics: Patients on diuretics, especially those with intravascular volume depletion, may occasionally experience an excessive reduction of blood pressure after initiation of therapy with Fosinopril Sodium. The possibility of hypotensive effects with Fosinopril Sodium can be minimized by either discontinuing the diuretic or increasing salt intake prior to initiation of treatment with Fosinopril Sodium. If this is not possible, the starting dose should be reduced and the patient should be observed closely for several hours following an initial dose and until blood pressure has stabilized (see *"Dosage and Administration"*).

With Potassium Supplements and Potassium-Sparing Diuretics: Fosinopril Sodium can attenuate potassium loss caused by thiazide diuretics. Potassium-sparing diuretics (spironolactone, amiloride, triamterene, and others) or potassium supplements can increase the risk of hyperkalemia. Therefore, if concomitant use of such agents is indicated, they should be given with caution, and the patient's serum potassium should be monitored frequently.

With Lithium: Increased serum lithium levels and symptoms of lithium toxicity have been reported in patients receiving ACE inhibitors during therapy with lithium. These drugs should be coadministered with caution, and frequent monitoring of serum lithium levels is recommended. If a diuretic is also used, the risk of lithium toxicity may be increased.

With Antacids: In a clinical pharmacology study, coadministration of an antacid (aluminum hydroxide, magnesium hydroxide, and simethicone) with Fosinopril Sodium reduced serum levels and urinary excretion of fosinoprilat as compared with Fosinopril Sodium administrated alone, suggesting that antacids may impair absorption of Fosinopril Sodium. Therefore, if concomitant administration of these agents is indicated, dosing should be separated by 2 hours.

Other: Neither Fosinopril Sodium nor its metabolites have been found to interact with food. In separate single or multiple dose pharmacokinetic interaction studies with chlorthalidone, nifedipine, propranolol, hydrochlorothiazide, cimetidine, metoclopramide, propantheline, digoxin, and warfarin, the bioavailability of fosinoprilat was not altered by coadministration of Fosinopril Sodium with any one of these drugs. In a study with concomitant administration of aspirin and Fosinopril Sodium, the bioavailability of unbound fosinoprilat was not altered.

In a pharmacokinetic interaction study with warfarin, bioavailability parameters, the degree of protein binding, and the anticoagulant effect (measured by prothrombin time) of warfarin were not significantly changed.

DRUG/LABORATORY TEST INTERACTION
Fosinopril Sodium may cause a false low measurement of serum digoxin levels with the Digi-Tab® RIA Kit for Digoxin. Other kits, such as the Coat-A-Count® RIA Kit, may be used.

CARCINOGENESIS, MUTAGENESIS, AND IMPAIRMENT OF FERTILITY
No evidence of a carcinogenic effect was found when Fosinopril Sodium was given in the diet to mice and rats for up to 24 months at doses up to 400 mg/kg/day. On a body weight basis, the highest dose in mice and rats is about 250 times the maximum human dose of 80 mg, assuming a 50 kg subject. On a body surface area basis, in mice, this dose is 20 times the maximum human dose; in rats, this dose is 40 times the maximum human dose. Male rats given the highest dose level had a slightly higher incidence of mesentery/omentum lipomas.

Neither Fosinopril Sodium nor the active fosinoprilat was mutagenic in the Ames microbial mutagen test, the mouse lymphoma forward mutation assay, or a mitotic gene conversion assay. Fosinopril Sodium was also not genotoxic in a mouse micronucleus test *in vivo* and a mouse bone marrow cytogenetic assay *in vivo*.

In the Chinese hamster ovary cell cytogenetic assay Fosinopril Sodium increased the frequency of chromosomal aberrations when tested without metabolic activation at a concentration that was toxic to the cells. However, there was no increase in chromosomal aberrations at lower drug concentrations without metabolic activation or at any concentration with metabolic activation.

There were no adverse reproductive effects in male and female rats treated with 15 or 60 mg/kg daily. On a body weight basis, the high dose of 60 mg/kg is about 38 times the maximum recommended human dose. On a body surface area basis, this dose is 6 times the maximum recommended human dose. There was no effect on pairing time prior to mating in rats until a daily dose of 240 mg/kg, a toxic dose, was given; at this dose, a slight increase in pairing time was observed. On a body weight basis, this dose is 150 times the maximum recommended human dose. On a body surface area basis, this dose is 24 times the maximum recommended human dose.

PREGNANCY CATEGORIES C (FIRST TRIMESTER) AND D (SECOND AND THIRD TRIMESTERS)
See *"Warnings: Fetal/Neonatal Mobility and Mortality."*

NURSING MOTHERS
Ingestion of 20 mg daily for three days resulted in detectable levels of fosinoprilat in breast milk. Fosinopril Sodium should not be administered to nursing mothers.

GERIATRIC USE
Of the total number of patients who receiving Fosinopril Sodium in US clinical studies of Fosinopril Sodium 13% were 65 and older while 1.3% were 75 and older. No overall differences in effectiveness or safety were observed between these patients and younger patients, and other reported clinical experience has not identified differences in response between the elderly and younger patients, but greater sensitivity of some older individuals cannot be ruled out.

In a pharmacokinetic study comparing elderly (65-74 years old) and non-elderly (20-35 years old) healthy volunteers, there were no differences between the groups in peak fosinoprilat levels or area under the plasma concentration time curve (AUC).

PEDIATRIC USE
Safety and effectiveness in children have not been established

ADVERSE REACTIONS
Fosinopril Sodium has been evaluated for safety in more than 1500 individuals in hypertension trials, including approximately 450 patients treated for a year or more. Generally adverse events were mild and transient, and their frequency was not prominently related to dose within the recommended daily dosage range.

In placebo-controlled clinical trials (688 Fosinopril Sodium-treated patients), the usual duration of therapy was two to three months. Discontinuations due to any clinical or laboratory adverse event were 4.1 and 1.1 percent in Fosinopril Sodium-treated and placebo-treated patients, respectively. The most frequent reasons (0.4 to 0.9%) were headache, elevated transaminases, fatigue, cough (See *"Precautions: General: Cough"*), diarrhea, and nausea and vomiting.

During clinical trials with any Fosinopril Sodium regimen, the incidence of adverse events in the elderly ($\geq$ 65 years old) was similar to that seen in younger patients.

Clinical adverse events probably or possibly related or of uncertain relationship to therapy, occurring in at least 1% of patients treated with Fosinopril Sodium alone in placebo-controlled clinical trials are shown in the table below.

CLINICAL ADVERSE EVENTS IN PLACEBO-CONTROLLED TRIALS

	Fosinopril Sodium (N = 688) Incidence (Discontinuation)	Placebo (N = 184) Incidence (Discontinuation)
Headache	3.2 (0.9)	3.3
Cough	2.2 (0.4)	0.0
Dizziness	1.6	0.0
Diarrhea	1.5 (0.4)	1.6
Fatigue	1.5 (0.6)	1.6
Nausea/Vomiting	1.2 (0.4)	0.5
Sexual Dysfunction	1.0 (0.1)	1.1 (0.5)

Other clinical events probably or possibly related, or of uncertain relationship to therapy occurring in 0.2 to 1.0% of patients (except as noted) treated with Fosinopril Sodium in controlled or uncontrolled clinical trials (N = 1479) and less frequent, clinically significant events include (listed by body system):

General: Chest pain, edema, weakness, excessive sweating.

Cardiovascular: Angina/myocardial infarction, cerebrovascular accident, hypertensive crisis, rhythm disturbances, palpitations, hypotension, syncope, flushing, claudication. Orthostatic hypotension occurred in 1.4% of patients treated with fosinopril monotherapy. Hypotension or orthostatic hypotension was a cause for discontinuation of therapy in 0.1% of patients.

Dermatologic: Urticaria, rash, photosensitivity, pruritus.

Endocrine/Metabolic: Gout, decreased libido.

Gastrointestinal: Pancreatitis, hepatitis, dysphagia, abdominal distention, abdominal pain, flatulence, constipation, heartburn, appetite/weight change, dry mouth.

Hematologic: Lymphadenopathy.

Immunologic: Angioedema.

Musculoskeletal: Arthralgia, musculoskeletal pain, myalgia/muscle cramp.

Nervous/Psychiatric: Memory disturbance, tremor, confusion, mood change, paresthesia, sleep disturbance, drowsiness, vertigo.

Respiratory: Bronchospasm, pharyngitis, sinusitis/rhinitis, laryngitis/hoarseness, epistaxis. A symptom-complex of cough, bronchospasm, and eosinophilia has been observed in two patients treated with Fosinopril Sodium.

Special Senses: Tinnitus, vision disturbance, taste disturbance, eye irritation.

Urogenital: Renal insufficiency, urinary frequency.

FETAL/NEONATAL MORBIDITY AND MORTALITY
See *"Warnings: Fetal/Neonatal Morbidity and Mortality."*

POTENTIAL ADVERSE EFFECTS REPORTED WITH ACE INHIBITORS
Body as a Whole: Anaphylactoid reactions (see *"Precautions: Hemodialysis"*).

Other medically important adverse effects reported with ACE inhibitors include: Cardiac arrest: eosinophilic pneumonitis; neutropenia/agranulocytosis; pancytopenia, anemia (including hemolytic and aplastic); thrombocytopenia; acute renal failure; hepatic failure, jaundice (hepatocellular or cholestatic); symptomatic hyponatremia; bullous pemphigus, exfoliative dermatitis; a syndrome which may include: arthralgia/arthritis, vasculitis, serositis, myalgia, fever, rash or other dermatologic manifestations, a positive ANA, leukocytosis, eosinophilia, or an elevated ESR.

LABORATORY TEST ABNORMALITIES
Serum Electrolytes: Hyperkalemia, (see *"Precautions"*); hyponatremia, (see *"Precautions: Drug Interactions, With Diuretics"*).

BUN/Serum Creatinine: Elevations, usually transient and minor, of BUN or serum creatinine have been observed. In placebo-controlled clinical trials, there were no significant differences in the number of patients experiencing increases in serum creatinine (outside the normal range of 1.33 times the pre-treatment value) between the Fosinopril Sodium and placebo treatment groups. Rapid reduction of longstanding or markedly elevated blood pressure by any antihypertensive therapy can result in decreases in the glomerular filtration rate and, in turn, lead to increases in BUN or serum creatinine. (See *"Precautions: General."*)

Hematology: In controlled trials, a mean *hemoglobin* decrease of 0.01 g/dL was observed in Fosinopril-treated patients. In individual patients decreases in hemoglobin or hematocrit were usually transient, small, and not associated with symptoms. No patient was discontinued from therapy due to the development of anemia. *Other:* Neutropenia (see *"Warnings"*), leukopenia and eosinophilia.

Liver Function Tests: Elevations of transaminases, LDH, alkaline phosphatase and serum bilirubin have been reported. Fosinopril Sodium therapy was discontinued because of serum transaminase elevations in 0.7% of patients. In the majority of cases, the abnormalities were either present at baseline or were associated with other etiologic factors. In those cases which were possibly related to Fosinopril Sodium therapy, the elevations were generally mild and transient and resolved after discontinuation of therapy.

OVERDOSAGE
Oral doses of Fosinopril Sodium at 2600 mg/kg in rats were associated with significant lethality. Human overdoses of Fosinopril Sodium have not been reported, but the most common manifestation of human Fosinopril Sodium overdosage is likely to be hypotension. Laboratory determinations of serum levels of fosinoprilat and its metabolites are not widely available, and such determinations have, in any event, no established role in the management of Fosinopril Sodium overdose. No data are available to suggest physiological maneuvers (e.g., maneuvers to change the pH of the urine) that might accelerate elimination of fosinopril and its metabolites. Fosinoprilat is poorly removed from the body by both hemodialysis and peritoneal dialysis.

Angiotensin II could presumably serve as a specific antagonist-antidote in the setting of fosinopril overdose, but angiotensin II is essentially unavailable outside of scattered research facilities. Because the hypotensive effect of Fosinopril Sodium is achieved through vasodilation and effective hypovolemia, it is reasonable to treat Fosinopril Sodium overdose by infusion of normal saline solution.

DOSAGE AND ADMINISTRATION
The recommended initial dose of Fosinopril Sodium is 10 mg once a day, both as monotherapy and when the drug is added to a diuretic. Dosage should then be adjusted according to blood pressure response at peak (2-6 hours) and trough (about 24 hours after dosing) blood levels. The usual dosage range needed to maintain a response at trough is 20-40 mg but some patients appear to have a further response to 80 mg. In some patients treated with once daily dosing, the antihypertensive effect may diminish toward the end of the dosing interval. If trough response is inadequate, dividing the daily dose should be considered. If blood pressure is not adequately controlled with Fosinopril Sodium alone, a diuretic may be added.

Concomitant administration of Fosinopril Sodium with potassium supplements, potassium salt substitutes, or potassium-sparing diuretics can lead to increases of serum potassium (see *"Precautions"*).

In patients who are currently being treated with a diuretic, symptomatic hypotension occasionally can occur following the initial dose of Fosinopril Sodium. To reduce the likelihood of hypotension, the diuretic should, if possible, be discontinued two to three days prior to beginning therapy with Fosinopril Sodium (see *"Warnings"*). Then, if blood pressure is not controlled with Fosinopril Sodium alone, diuretic therapy should be resumed. If diuretic therapy cannot be discontinued, an initial dose of 10 mg of Fosinopril Sodium should be used with careful medical supervision for several hours and until blood pressure has stabilized. (See *"Warnings"*; *"Precautions: Information for Patients"* and *"Drug Interactions"*).

Since concomitant administration of Fosinopril Sodium with potassium supplements, or potassium-containing salt substitutes or potassium-sparing diuretics may lead to increases in serum potassium, they should be used with caution.

For Hypertensive Patients With Renal Impairment: In patients with impaired renal function, the total body clearance of fosinoprilat is approximately 50% slower than in patients with normal renal function. Since hepatobiliary elimination partially compensates for diminished renal elimination, the total body clearance of fosinoprilat does not differ appreciably with any degree of renal insufficiency (creatinine clearances < 80 mL/min/1.73m^2), including end-stage renal failure (creatinine clearance < 10 mL/min/1.73m^2). This relative constancy of body clearance of active fosinoprilat, resulting from the dual route of elimination, permits use of the usual dose in patients with any degree of renal impairment. (See also "*Precautions: Hemodialysis*").

Storage

Store between 15°C (59°F) and 30°C (86°F). Avoid prolonged exposure to temperatures above 30°C (86°F). Keep bottles tightly closed (protect from moisture).

HOW SUPPLIED
TABLETS: 10 MG

BRAND/MANUFACTURER	NDC	SIZE	AWP
○ **BRAND**			
▶ MONOPRIL: Mead Johnson Pharm	00087-0158-50	100s	$70.87
	00087-0158-45	100s ud	$70.87
	00087-0158-85	1000s	$708.66

TABLETS: 20 MG

BRAND/MANUFACTURER	NDC	SIZE	AWP
○ **BRAND**			
▶ MONOPRIL: Mead Johnson Pharm	00087-0609-50	100s	$75.84
	00087-0609-45	100s ud	$75.84
	00087-0609-85	1000s	$758.43

FreAmine *SEE* AMINO ACIDS WITH ELECTROLYTES, INJECTABLE, AMINO ACIDS, INJECTABLE *AND* AMINO ACIDS/CALCIUM CHLORIDE/DEXTROSE/ELECTROLYTES

FS Shampoo *SEE* FLUOCINOLONE ACETONIDE

FUDR *SEE* FLOXURIDINE

Ful-Glo *SEE* FLUORESCEIN SODIUM

Fulvicin *SEE* GRISEOFULVIN

Funduscein *SEE* FLUORESCEIN SODIUM

Fungizone *SEE* AMPHOTERICIN B, INJECTABLE *AND* AMPHOTERICIN B, TOPICAL

Fungoid *SEE* MICONAZOLE NITRATE

Furacin *SEE* NITROFURAZONE, TOPICAL

Furadantin *SEE* NITROFURANTOIN

Furazolidone

DESCRIPTION
Furazolidone is one of the synthetic antimicrobial nitrofurans. It is a stable, yellow, crystalline compound.

Following is its chemical structure:

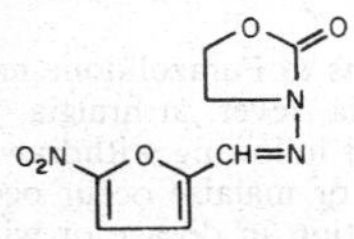

ACTION
Furazolidone has a broad antibacterial spectrum covering the majority of gastrointestinal tract pathogens including *E. coli*, staphylococci, *Salmonella, Shigella, Proteus, Aerobacter aerogenes, Vibrio cholerae*[9,10,11] and *Giardia lamblia*.[5,6] Its bactericidal activity is based upon its interference with several bacterial enzyme systems; this antimicrobial action minimizes the development of resistant organisms. It neither significantly alters the normal bowel flora nor results in fungal overgrowth. The brown color found in the urine with adequate dosage is of no clinical significance.

INDICATIONS
Indicated in the specific and symptomatic treatment of bacterial or protozoal diarrhea and enteritis caused by susceptible organisms. Furazolidone products are well tolerated, have a very low incidence of adverse reactions.

UNLABELED USES
Furazolidine is used alone or as an adjunct in the treatment of traveler's diarrhea and peptic ulcers.

CONTRAINDICATIONS
Furazolidone is contraindicated in patients with known hypersensitivity to Furazolidone and in patients with glucose and phosphate dehydrogenase deficiency. It is contraindicated in infants under one month.

WARNINGS
Use in Pregnancy: The safety of Furazolidone during the childbearing age has not been established; as with any potent antibacterial, Furazolidone must be administered with caution during the childbearing age. However, animal breeding studies have revealed no evidence of teratogenicity following the administration of Furazolidone for long periods of time and at doses far in excess of those recommended for the human. There have been no clinical reports regarding this possible adverse effect on the fetus or the newborn infant.

Furazolidone concentration in breast milk of lactating mothers has not been established, therefore safety of this drug in this circumstance has not been established. Caution should be exercised while prescribing Furazolidone to nursing mothers.

PRECAUTIONS AND DRUG INTERACTIONS
A disulfiram-like reaction may occur in patients ingesting alcohol while taking Furazolidone. Alcohol should be avoided during or within four days after Furazolidone therapy.

Monoamine Oxidase Inhibition:[7] Effective inhibition of monoamine oxidase by Furazolidone has been demonstrated experimentally in man by the enhancement of tyramine and amphetamine sensitivity and by the directly measured monoamine oxidase inhibition.

A period of five days of Furazolidone administration in the recommended doses in these patients was required to give an enhancement of the tyramine and amphetamine sensitivities by two to threefold. Administration of Furazolidone in the recommended dose of 400 mg/day for a period of five days should not subject the adult patient to an undue hazard of hypertensive crisis due to monoamine oxidase inhibition. Hypertensive crises have never been reported even after the peroral administration of larger doses and/or for doses given over longer periods of time. Controlled studies reveal no signs or symptoms of hypertensive crisis even after the peroral administration of Furazolidone in doses of 400 mg/day in excess of 48 consecutive months.[8]

If administered in doses larger than recommended or in excess of five days, the indications must be weighed against the possible hazards of hypertensive crisis related to the accumulation of monoamine oxidase inhibition. If indications are sufficient, the patients should be informed of drugs and foods which predispose to hypertensive crises:

(A) Other known MAOI drugs; however, when indicated they should be prescribed with caution and at a reduced dosage.
(B) Tyramine-containing foods such as broad beans, yeast extracts, strong unpasteurized cheeses, beer, wine, pickled herring, chicken livers, and fermented products are contraindicated.
(C) Indirectly-acting sympathomimetic amines such as those found in nasal decongestants (phenylephrine, ephedrine) and anorectics (amphetamines) are contraindicated.
(D) Likewise, sedatives, antihistamines, tranquilizers, and narcotics should be used in reduced dosages and with caution.

Orthostatic hypotension and hypoglycemia may occur.

Carcinogenesis, Mutagenesis, Impairment of Fertility: Furazolidone has shown evidence of tumorigenic activity in several studies involving chronic, high-dose oral administration to rodents. Promotion of the development of mammary neoplasia has been demonstrated in rats of two strains. Prominent among the findings in mice was that Furazolidone caused significant increases in malignant lung tumors. The relevance of these animal findings, particularly in relationship to short-term therapy in humans, is not established.

ADVERSE REACTIONS

A few hypersensitivity reactions to Furazolidone have been reported including a fall in blood pressure, urticaria, fever, arthralgia, and a vesicular morbilliform rash. These reactions subsided following withdrawal of the drug.

Nausea, emesis, headache, or malaise occur occasionally and may be minimized or eliminated by reduction in dosage or withdrawal of the drug.

Rarely, individuals receiving Furazolidone have exhibited an Antabuse® (disulfiram)-like reaction to alcohol characterized by flushing, slight temperature elevation, dyspnea, and in some instances, a sense of constriction within the chest. All symptomatology disappeared within 24 hours with no lasting ill effects. During nine years of clinical use and approximately 3.5 million courses of therapy (in the U.S.A. alone) in the published literature and documented case reports 43 cases have been reported—of which 14 were produced under experimental conditions with planned doses of the compound in excess of those recommended. Three of these experienced a fall in blood pressure necessitating active therapy. Indications are that levarterenol (Levophed®) may be used to combat such hypotensive episodes since human studies show that this drug is not potentiated in patients treated with Furazolidone (Indirectly acting pressor agents should be avoided.) The ingestion of alcohol in any form should be avoided during Furazolidone therapy and for four days thereafter to prevent this reaction.

Furazolidone may cause mild reversible intravascular hemolysis in certain ethnic groups of Mediterranean and Near-Eastern origin, and Negroes.[1,3] This is due to an intrinsic defect of red blood cell metabolism in a small percentage of these ethnic groups, making them unusually susceptible to hemolysis by numerous compounds.[2] It is necessary to observe such patients closely while receiving Furazolidone and to discontinue its use if there is any indication of hemolysis.

Should not be administered to infants under 1 month of age because of the possibility of producing a hemolytic anemia due to immature enzyme systems (glutathione instability) in the early neonatal period.[4]

Colitis, proctitis, anal pruritus, staphylococcic enteritis and renal or hepatic toxicity have not been a significant problem with Furazolidone.

OVERDOSAGE

In case of accidental overdosage, supportive and or symptomatic therapy should be provided. Induction of vomiting or gastric lavage may be required. Vomiting should not be induced in unconscious patients or in children under one year of age.

DOSAGE AND ADMINISTRATION

Average Adult Dosage: One 100 mg tablet four times daily.

Average Dosage for Children: Those 5 years of age or older should receive 25 to 50 mg (¼ to ½ tablet) four times daily. The tablet dosage may be crushed and given in a spoonful of corn syrup.

Furazolidone Liquid composition: each 15 ml tablespoonful contains Furazolidone 50 mg per 15 ml (3.33 mg per ml) in a light-yellow aqueous vehicle. It is stable in storage. Prior to administering Furazolidone liquid shake the bottle vigorously. It should be dispensed in amber bottles.

Average Adult Dosage: Two tablespoonfuls four times daily.

Average Dosage for Children:

5 years or older—½ to 1 tablespoonful four times daily (7.5-15.0 ml)
1 to 4 years old—1 to 1½ teaspoonfuls four times daily (5.0-7.5 ml)
1 month to 1 year—½ to 1 teaspoonful four times daily 2.5-5.0 ml)

In Giardiasis the usual adult dose is 100mg four times daily for 7 to 10 days. Children may be given 1.25mg/Kg body weight four times daily.

This dosage is based on an average dose of 5 mg of Furazolidone per Kg (2.3 mg per lb) of body weight given in four equally divided doses during 24 hours. The maximal dose of 8.8 mg of Furazolidone per Kg (4 mg per lb) of body weight per 24 hours should probably not be exceeded because of the possibility of producing nausea or emesis. If these are severe, the dosage should be reduced.

The average case of diarrhea treated with Furazolidone will respond within 2 to 5 days of therapy. Occasional patients may require a longer term of therapy. If satisfactory clinical response is not obtained within 7 days it indicates that the pathogen is refractory to Furazolidone and the drug should be discontinued. Adjunctive therapy with other antibacterial agents or bismuth salts is not contraindicated. (See "Warnings.')

In order to administer Furazolidone in doses larger than recommended or in excess of five days the indications must be weighed against the possible hazards of hypertensive crisis related to the accumulation of monoamine oxidase inhibition. If indications are sufficient, the patient should be informed of drugs and foods which predispose to hypertensive crises. (See "Precautions.')

REFERENCES

1. Kellermeyer, R.S., Tarlov, A.R., Schrier, S.L., and Alving, A.S.J. Lab. Clin. Med. 52:827-828 (Nov) 1958. 2. Tarlov et al. Arch. Int. Med. 109:209-204, 1962. 3. Kellermeyer et al. J.A.M.A. 180: No. 5, 388-394, 1962. 4. Zinkham, Pediatrics 23:18-32, 1959; Gross & Hurwitz, Pediatrics 22:453, 1958. 5. Fallas Vargas, M. un Nuevo Tratamiento para la Giardiasis (A New Treatment for Giardiasis). Rev. Med. Costa Rica 19:269-284 (July) 1962. 6. Webster, B. H. Furazolidone in the Treatment of Giardiasis. Amer. J. Dig. Diseases 5:618-622 (July) 1960. 7. Oates, J.A., Pettinger, W.A. Inhibition of Monoamine Oxidase by Furazolidone in Man. Data on file: Office of the Medical Director, Roberts Pharmaceutical, Corp. Available upon request. 8. Kirsner, Joseph B., M.D., Ph.D. Data on file: Office of the Medical Director, Roberts Pharmaceutical, Corp. Available upon request. 9. Neogy, K.N., et al. Furazolidone in

Chloera, Journ. Indian Med. Assoc. 48:137, 1967. 10. Chaudhuri, R.N. et al. Furazolidone in Cholera, Lancet 2:909 (Oct 30) 1965. 11. Curlin, G. Comparison of Antibiotic Regimens in Cholera. Abstracts of papers, Epidemiological Intelligence Service Conference, Atlanta, Ga., April 11-14, 1967, p. 11.

HOW SUPPLIED
LIQUID: 50 MG/15 ML

BRAND/MANUFACTURER	NDC	SIZE	AWP
○ BRAND			
FUROXONE: Roberts Pharm	54092-0430-60	60 ml	$11.19
	54092-0430-16	473 ml	$69.63

TABLETS: 100 MG

BRAND/MANUFACTURER	NDC	SIZE	AWP
○ BRAND			
FUROXONE: Roberts Pharm	54092-0130-20	20s	$39.56
	54092-0130-01	100s	$190.98

Furosemide

WARNING

Furosemide is a potent diuretic which, if given in excessive amounts, can lead to a profound diuresis with water and electrolyte depletion. Therefore, careful medical supervision is required, and dose and dose schedule must be adjusted to the individual patient's needs. (See "Dosage And Administration".)

DESCRIPTION

Furosemide is a diuretic which is an anthranilic acid derivative. Chemically, it is 4-chloro-N-furfuryl-5-sulfamoy-lanthranilic acid. Furosemide is available in 20 mg, 40 mg and 80 mg tablets and a 10 mg per 1 ml and 40 mg per 5 ml oral solution. The injection is available as 10 mg per 1 mL in a 10 mL and 2,4, and 10 mL single dose vial.

Furosemide is a white to off-white odorless crystalline powder. It is practically insoluble in water, sparingly soluble in alcohol, freely soluble in dilute alkali solutions and insoluble in dilute acids.

The CAS Registry Number is 54-31-9.

Following is its chemical structure:

CLINICAL PHARMACOLOGY

Investigations into the mode of action of Furosemide have utilized micropuncture studies in rats, stop flow experiments in dogs, and various clearance studies in both humans and experimental animals. It has been demonstrated that Furosemide inhibits primarily the absorption of sodium and chloride not only in the proximal and distal tubules but also in the loop of Henle. The high degree of efficacy is largely due to this unique site of action. The action on the distal tubule is independent of any inhibitory effect on carbonic anhydrase and aldosterone.

Recent evidence suggests that furosemide glucuronide is the only or at least the major bio-transformation product of furosemide in man. Furosemide is extensively bound to plasma proteins, mainly to albumin. Plasma concentrations ranging from 1 to 400 µg/mL are 91 to 99% bound in healthy individuals. The unbound fraction averages 2.3 to 4.1% at therapeutic concentrations.

The onset of diuresis following oral administration is within 1 hour. The peak effect occurs within the first or second hour. The duration of diuretic effect is 6 to 8 hours.

In fasted normal men, the mean bioavailability of Furosemide from Furosemide Tablets and Furosemide Oral Solution is 64% and 60%, respectively, of that from an intravenous injection of the drug. Although Furosemide is more rapidly absorbed from the oral solution (50 minutes) than from the tablet (87 minutes), peak plasma levels and area under the plasma concentration-time curves do not differ significantly. Peak plasma concentrations increase with increasing dose but times-to-peak do not differ among doses. The terminal half-life of Furosemide is approximately 2 hours.

Significantly more Furosemide is excreted in urine following the IV injection than after the tablet or oral solution. There are no significant differences between the two oral formulations in the amount of unchanged drug excreted in urine.

INDICATIONS AND USAGE
EDEMA

Furosemide is indicated in adults, infants, and children for the treatment of edema associated with congestive heart failure, cirrhosis of the liver, and renal disease, including the nephrotic syndrome. Furosemide is particularly useful when an agent with greater diuretic potential is desired.

HYPERTENSION

Oral Furosemide may be used in adults for the treatment of hypertension alone or in combination with other antihypertensive agents. Hypertensive patients who cannot be adequately controlled with thiazides will probably also not be adequately controlled with Furosemide alone.

UNLABELED USES
Furosemide is used alone or as an adjunct in the treatment of chronic bronchopulmonary dysplasia, refractory congestive heart failure, inapporiate secretion of antidiuretic hormone, patent ductus, and respiratory distress syndrome.

CONTRAINDICATIONS
Furosemide is contraindicated in patients with anuria and in patients with a history of hypersensitivity to Furosemide.

WARNINGS
In patients with hepatic cirrhosis and ascites, Furosemide therapy is best initiated in the hospital. In hepatic coma and in states of electrolyte depletion, therapy should not be instituted until the basic condition is improved. Sudden alterations of fluid and electrolyte balance in patients with cirrhosis may precipitate hepatic coma; therefore, strict observation is necessary during the period of diuresis. Supplemental potassium chloride and, if required, an aldosterone antagonist are helpful in preventing hypokalemia and metabolic alkalosis.

If increasing azotemia and oliguria occur during treatment of severe progressive renal disease, Furosemide should be discontinued.

Cases of tinnitus and reversible or irreversible hearing impairment have been reported. Usually, reports indicate that Furosemide ototoxicity is associated with rapid injection, severe renal impairment, doses exceeding several times the usual recommended dose, or concomitant therapy with aminoglycoside antibiotics, ethacrynic acid, or other ototoxic drugs. If the physician elects to use high dose parenteral therapy, controlled intravenous infusion is advisable (for adults, an infusion rate not exceeding 4 mg Furosemide per minute has been used).

PRECAUTIONS
GENERAL
Excessive diuresis may cause dehydration and blood volume reduction with circulatory collapse and possibly vascular thrombosis and embolism, particularly in elderly patients. As with any effective diuretic, electrolyte depletion may occur during Furosemide therapy, especially in patients receiving higher doses and a restricted salt intake. Hypokalemia may develop with Furosemide, especially with brisk diuresis, inadequate oral electrolyte intake, when cirrhosis is present, or during concomitant use of corticosteroids or ACTH. Digitalis therapy may exaggerate metabolic effects of hypokalemia, especially myocardial effects.

All patients receiving Furosemide therapy should be observed for these signs or symptoms of fluid or electrolyte imbalance (hyponatremia, hypochloremic alkalosis, hypokalemia, hypomagnesemia or hypocalcemia): dryness of mouth, thirst, weakness, lethargy, drowsiness, restlessness, muscle pains or cramps, muscular fatigue, hypotension, oliguria, tachycardia, arrhythmia, or gastrointestinal disturbances such as nausea and vomiting.

Increases in blood glucose and alterations in glucose tolerance tests (with abnormalities of the fasting and 2-hour postprandial sugar) have been observed, and rarely, precipitation of diabetes mellitus has been reported.

Asymptomatic hyperuricemia can occur and gout may rarely be precipitated. Patients allergic to sulfonamides may also be allergic to Furosemide. The possibility exists of exacerbation or activation of systemic lupus erythematosus.

As with many other drugs, patients should be observed regularly for the possible occurrence of blood dyscrasias, liver or kidney damage, or other idiosyncratic reactions.

INFORMATION FOR PATIENTS
Patients receiving Furosemide should be advised that they may experience symptoms from excessive fluid and/or electrolyte losses. The postural hypotension that sometimes occurs can usually be managed by getting up slowly. Potassium supplements and/or dietary measures may be needed to control or avoid hypokalemia.

Patients with diabetes mellitus should be told that Furosemide may increase blood glucose levels and thereby affect urine glucose tests. The skin of some patients may be more sensitive to the effects of sunlight while taking Furosemide. Hypertensive patients should avoid medications that may increase blood pressure, including over-the-counter products for appetite suppression and cold symptoms.

LABORATORY TESTS
Serum electrolytes (particularly potassium), CO_2, creatinine and BUN should be determined frequently during the first few months of Furosemide therapy and periodically thereafter. Serum and urine electrolyte determinations are particularly important when the patient is vomiting profusely or receiving parenteral fluids. Abnormalities should be corrected or the drug temporarily withdrawn. Other medications may also influence serum electrolytes.

Reversible elevations of BUN may occur and are associated with dehydration, which should be avoided, particularly in patients with renal insufficiency.

Urine and blood glucose should be checked periodically in diabetics receiving Furosemide even in those suspected of latent diabetes.

Furosemide may lower serum levels of calcium (rarely cases of tetany have been reported) and magnesium. Accordingly, serum levels should be determined periodically.

DRUG INTERACTIONS
Furosemide may increase the ototoxic potential of aminoglycoside antibiotics, especially in the presence of impaired renal function. Except in life-threatening situations, avoid this combination.

Furosemide should not be used concomitantly with ethacrynic acid because of the possibility of ototoxicity. Patients receiving high doses of salicylates concomitantly with Furosemide, as in rheumatic disease, may experience salicylate toxicity at lower doses because of competitive renal excretory sites.

Furosemide has a tendency to antagonize the skeletal muscle relaxing effect of tubocurarine and may potentiate the action of succinylcholine.

Lithium generally should not be given with diuretics because they reduce lithium's renal clearance and add a high risk of lithium toxicity.

Furosemide may add to or potentiate the therapeutic effect of other antihypertensive drugs. Potentiation occurs with ganglionic or peripheral adrenergic blocking drugs.

Furosemide may decrease arterial responsiveness to norepinephrine. However, norepinephrine may still be used effectively. Simultaneous administration of sucralfate and Furosemide tablets may reduce the nutriuretic and antihypertensive effects of Furosemide. Patients receiving both drugs should be observed closely to determine if the desired diuretic and/or antihypertensive affect of Furosemide is achieved. The intake of Furosemide and sucralfate should be separated by at least two hours.

One study in six subjects demonstrated that the combination of Furosemide and acetylsalicylic acid temporarily reduced creatinine clearance in patients with chronic renal insufficiency. There are case reports of patients who developed increased BUN, serum creatinine and serum potassium levels, and weight gain when Furosemide was used in conjunction with NSAIDs.

Literature reports indicate that coadministration of indomethacin may reduce the natriuretic and antihypertensive effects of Furosemide. In some patients by inhibiting prostaglandin synthesis. Indomethacin may also affect plasma renin levels, aldosterone excretion, and renin profile evaluation. Patients receiving both indomethacin and Furosemide should be observed closely to determine if the desired diuretic and/or antihypertensive effect of Furosemide is achieved.

CARCINOGENESIS, MUTAGENESIS, IMPAIRMENT OF FERTILITY
No carcinogenic or mutagenic studies have been conducted with Furosemide.

Furosemide produced no impairment of fertility in male or female rats, at 100 mg/kg/day (the maximum effective diuretic dose in the rat and 8 times the maximal human dose of 600 mg/day).

PREGNANCY
Pregnancy Category C: Furosemide has been shown to cause unexplained maternal deaths and abortions in rabbits at 2, 4, and 8 times the maximal recommended human dose. There are no adequate and well-controlled studies in pregnant women. Furosemide should be used during pregnancy only if the potential benefit justifies the potential risk to the fetus.

The effects of Furosemide on embryonic and fetal development and on pregnant dams were studied in mice, rats and rabbits.

Furosemide caused unexplained maternal deaths and abortions in the rabbit at the lowest dose of 25 mg/kg (2 times the maximal recommended human dose of 600 mg/day). In another study, a dose of 50 mg/kg (4 times the maximal recommended human dose of 600 mg/day) also caused maternal deaths and abortions when administered to rabbits between Days 12 and 17 of gestation. In a third study, none of the pregnant rabbits survived a dose of 100 mg/kg. Data from the above studies indicate fetal lethality that can precede maternal deaths.

The results of the mouse study and one of the three rabbit studies also showed an increased incidence and severity of hydronephrosis (distention of the renal pelvis and, in some cases, of the ureters) in fetuses derived from treated dams as compared to the incidence in fetuses from the control group.

NURSING MOTHERS
Because it appears in breast milk, caution should be exercised when Furosemide is administered to a nursing mother.

ADVERSE REACTIONS
Adverse reactions are categorized below by organ system and listed by decreasing severity.

GASTROINTESTINAL SYSTEM REACTIONS
1. pancreatitis
2. jaundice (intrahepatic cholestatic jaundice)
3. anorexia
4. oral and gastric irritation
5. cramping
6. diarrhea
7. constipation
8. nausea
9. vomiting

SYSTEMATIC HYPERSENSITIVITY REACTIONS
1. systemic vasculitis
2. interstitial nephritis
3. necrotizing angiitis

CENTRAL NERVOUS SYSTEM REACTIONS
1. tinnitus and hearing loss
2. paresthesias
3. vertigo
4. dizziness
5. headache
6. blurred vision
7. xanthopsia

► SHOWN IN PRODUCT IDENTIFICATION GUIDE

HEMATOLOGIC REACTIONS

1. asplastic anemia (rare)
2. thrombocytopenia
3. agranulocytosis (rare)
4. hemolytic anemia
5. leukopenia
6. anemia

DERMATOLOGIC REACTIONS

1. exfoliative dermatitis
2. erythema multiforme
3. purpura
4. photosensitivity
5. urticaria
6. rash
7. pruritus

CARDIOVASCULAR REACTION

Orthostatic hypotension may occur and be aggravated by alcohol, barbiturates or narcotics.

OTHER REACTIONS

1. hyperglycemia
2. glycosuria
3. hyperuricemia
4. muscle spasm
5. weakness
6. restlessness
7. urinary bladder spasm
8. thrombophlebitis
9. fever

Whenever adverse reactions are moderate or severe, Furosemide dosage should be reduced or therapy withdrawn.

OVERDOSAGE

The principal signs and symptoms of overdose with Furosemide are dehydration, blood volume reduction, hypotension, electrolyte imbalance, hypokalemia and hypochloremic alkalosis, and are extension of its diuretic action.

The acute toxicity of Furosemide has been determined in mice, rats and dogs. In all three, the oral LD_{50} exceeded 1000 mg/kg body weight, while the intravenous LD_{50} ranged from 300 to 680 mg/kg. The acute intragastric toxicity in neonatal rats is 7 to 10 times that of adult rats.

The concentration of Furosemide in biological fluids associated with toxicity or death is not known.

Treatment of overdose is supportive and consists of replacement of excessive fluid and electrolyte losses. Serum electrolytes, carbon dioxide level and blood pressure should be determined frequently. Adequate drainage must be assured in patients with urinary bladder outlet obstruction (such as prostatic hypertrophy).

Hemodialysis does not accelerate Flurosemide elimination.

DOSAGE AND ADMINISTRATION

EDEMA

Therapy should be individualized according to patient response to gain maximal therapeutic response and to determine the minimal dose needed to maintain that response.

Adults: The usual initial dose of Furosemide is 20 to 80 mg given as a single dose. Ordinarily a prompt diuresis ensues. If needed, the same dose can be administered 6 to 8 hours later or the dose may be increased. The dose may be raised by 20 or 40 mg and given not sooner than 6 to 8 hours after the previous dose until the desired diuretic effect has been obtained. This individually determined single dose should then be given once or twice daily (eg, at 8 am and 2 pm). The dose of Furosemide may be carefully titrated up to 600 mg/day in patients with clinically severe edematous states.

Edema may be most efficiently and safely mobilized by giving Furosemide on 2 to 4 consecutive days each week.

When doses exceeding 80 mg/day are given for prolonged periods, careful clinical observation and laboratory monitoring are particularly advisable. (See *"Precautions: Laboratory Tests".*):

Infants and Children: The usual initial dose of oral Furosemide in infants and children is 2 mg/kg body weight, given as a single dose. If the diuretic response is not satisfactory after the initial dose, dosage may be increased by 1 or 2 mg/kg no sooner than 6 to 8 hours after the previous dose. Doses greater than 6 mg/kg body weight are not recommended. For maintenance therapy in infants and children, the dose should be adjusted to the minimum effective level.

HYPERTENSION

Therapy should be individualized according to the patient's response to gain maximal therapeutic response and to determine the minimal dose needed to maintain that therapeutic response.

Adults: The usual initial daily dose of Furosemide for hypertension is 80 mg, usually divided into 40 mg twice a day. Dosage should be adjusted according to response. If response is not satisfactory, add other antihypertensive agents.

Changes in blood pressure must be carefully monitored when Furosemide is used with other antihypertensive drugs, especially during initial therapy. To prevent excessive drop in blood pressure, the dosage of other agents should be reduced by at least 50 percent when Furosemide is added to the regimen. As the

blood pressure falls under the potentiating effect of Furosemide, a further reduction in dosage or even discontinuation of other antihypertensive drugs may be necessary.

Furosemide Tablets should be dispensed in a well-closed, light-resistant container.

Exposure to light might cause a slight discoloration. Discolored tablets should not be dispensed.

Furosemide Oral Solution should be dispensed in a light-resistant container.

Note: Store at controlled room temperature (59°-86°F).
Discard opened bottle after 60 days.

Furosemide Injection: Store at controlled room temperature (59°-86°F). Do not use if solution is discolored.
Protect syringes from light.

J CODES

Up to 20 mg IM,IV—J1940

HOW SUPPLIED

INJECTION: 10 MG/ML

AVERAGE UNIT PRICE (AVAILABLE SIZES)		GENERIC A-RATED AVERAGE PRICE (GAAP)	
BRAND	$0.55	10 ml	$3.71
GENERIC	$0.63	4 ml 10s	$36.46
		10 ml 10s	$93.64
		2 ml 25s	$40.40
		4 ml 25s	$51.23
		10 ml 25s	$110.24

BRAND/MANUFACTURER	NDC	SIZE	AWP
◆ **BRAND**			
LASIX: Hoechst	00039-0061-15	2 ml 5s	$5.50
	00039-0062-08	2 ml 5s	$8.30
	00039-0061-45	4 ml 5s	$9.25
	00039-0064-08	4 ml 5s	$11.00
	00039-0061-08	10 ml 5s	$26.15
	00039-0069-08	10 ml 5s	$27.50
	00039-0162-25	2 ml 25s	$33.70
	00039-0061-65	4 ml 25s	$45.00
	00039-0163-25	4 ml 25s	$51.50
	00039-0061-25	10 ml 25s	$126.50
	00039-0164-25	10 ml 25s	$132.00
	00039-0061-05	2 ml 50s	$51.50
◆ **GENERICS**			
Moore,H.L.	00839-6677-30	10 ml	$2.36
Major	00904-1485-10	10 ml	$5.05
Astra	00186-0635-01	4 ml 10s	$26.25
Abbott Hosp	00074-6055-04	4 ml 10s	$46.67
Abbott Hosp	00074-6056-20	8 ml 10s	$67.57
Astra	00186-0636-01	10 ml 10s	$68.88
Abbott Hosp	00074-6056-10	10 ml 10s	$118.39
Elkins-Sinn	00641-1425-35	2 ml 25s	$13.18
Elkins-Sinn	00641-0382-25	2 ml 25s	$19.76
Amer Regent	00517-5702-25	2 ml 25s	$22.19
Astra	00186-1114-13	2 ml 25s	$34.38
Abbott Hosp	00074-6101-02	2 ml 25s	$48.69
Abbott Hosp	00074-6102-02	2 ml 25s	$59.08
Abbott Hosp	00074-6054-02	2 ml 25s	$85.50
Elkins-Sinn	00641-1426-35	4 ml 25s	$19.76
Sanofi Winthrop	00024-0609-25	4 ml 25s	$20.46
Elkins-Sinn	00641-2311-25	4 ml 25s	$29.65
Amer Regent	00517-5704-25	4 ml 25s	$35.94
Astra	00186-1115-13	4 ml 25s	$57.75
Abbott Hosp	00074-6101-04	4 ml 25s	$94.11
Abbott Hosp	00074-6102-04	4 ml 25s	$100.94
Astra	00186-1116-12	8 ml 25s	$108.29
Schein	00364-6763-34	10 ml 25s	$44.00
Amer Regent	00517-5710-25	10 ml 25s	$57.19
Elkins-Sinn	00641-1427-35	10 ml 25s	$59.31
Elkins-Sinn	00641-2312-25	10 ml 25s	$72.49
Astra	00186-1117-12	10 ml 25s	$105.00
Intl Med Sys	00548-1431-00	10 ml 25s	$194.70
Abbott Hosp	00074-6101-10	10 ml 25s	$238.98

INJECTION: 20 MG

AVERAGE UNIT PRICE (AVAILABLE SIZES)	
GENERIC	$0.36

BRAND/MANUFACTURER	NDC	SIZE	AWP
◆ **GENERICS**			
Sanofi Winthrop	00024-0611-03	2 ml 10s	$7.12
Sanofi Winthrop	00024-0611-50	2 ml 50s	$35.59

INJECTION: 40 MG

BRAND/MANUFACTURER	NDC	SIZE	AWP
◆ **GENERICS**			
Sanofi Winthrop	00024-0609-40	4 ml 10s	$8.19

◆ RATED THERAPEUTICALLY EQUIVALENT; ◇ THERAPEUTIC EQUIVALENCE UNCONFIRMED; ○ UNRATED

INJECTION: 100 MG

BRAND/MANUFACTURER		NDC	SIZE	AWP
◆ GENERICS				
Abbott Hosp		00074-6102-11	10 ml 25s	$271.94

SOLUTION:

AVERAGE UNIT PRICE (AVAILABLE SIZES)		GENERIC A-RATED AVERAGE PRICE (GAAP)	
GENERIC	$0.12	60 ml	$8.20
		120 ml	$11.75

BRAND/MANUFACTURER	NDC	SIZE	AWP
◆ GENERICS			
Pennex	00832-8613-60	60 ml	$7.80
Pennex	00426-8613-60	60 ml	$8.60
Pennex	00832-8613-04	120 ml	$11.50
Pennex	00426-8613-04	120 ml	$12.00

SOLUTION: 10 MG/ML

AVERAGE UNIT PRICE (AVAILABLE SIZES)		GENERIC A-RATED AVERAGE PRICE (GAAP)	
BRAND	$0.17	60 ml	$9.17
GENERIC	$0.14	120 ml	$15.29

BRAND/MANUFACTURER	NDC	SIZE	AWP
◆ BRAND			
LASIX: Hoechst	00039-0063-06	60 ml	$11.10
	00039-0063-40	120 ml	$18.40
◆ GENERICS			
Moore,H.L.	00839-7431-64	60 ml	$7.14
Qualitest	00603-1250-52	60 ml	$8.88
Roxane	00054-3294-46	60 ml	$9.10
Major	00904-1477-03	60 ml	$9.75
Rugby	00536-0709-96	60 ml	$9.87
Goldline	00182-6053-68	60 ml	$10.00
Major	00904-1477-20	120 ml	$12.60
Goldline	00182-6053-37	120 ml	$12.90
Roxane	00054-3294-50	120 ml	$17.67

SOLUTION: 10 MG

AVERAGE UNIT PRICE (AVAILABLE SIZES)		GENERIC A-RATED AVERAGE PRICE (GAAP)	
GENERIC	$0.15	60 ml	$8.77

BRAND/MANUFACTURER	NDC	SIZE	AWP
◆ GENERICS			
Geneva	00781-6302-02	60 ml	$7.71
URL	00677-1423-25	60 ml	$9.82

SYRUP: 10 MG/ML

BRAND/MANUFACTURER	NDC	SIZE	AWP
◆ GENERICS			
Aligen	00405-2832-56	60 ml	$9.05

TABLETS: 20 MG

AVERAGE UNIT PRICE (AVAILABLE SIZES)		GENERIC A-RATED AVERAGE PRICE (GAAP)	
BRAND	$0.15	30s	$2.76
GENERIC	$0.05	90s	$3.38
HCFA FUL (100s ea)	$0.02	100s	$6.28
		500s	$17.06
		1000s	$28.00

BRAND/MANUFACTURER	NDC	SIZE	AWP
◆ BRAND			
➤ LASIX: Hoechst	00039-0067-10	100s	$15.75
	00039-0067-11	100s ud	$16.65
	00039-0067-50	500s	$74.40
	00039-0067-70	1000s	$141.35
◆ GENERICS			
Major	00904-1580-46	30s	$1.85
Vangard	00615-1569-30	30s	$2.89
Medirex	57480-0328-06	30s	$3.53
Major	00904-1580-89	90s	$2.80
Allscrips	54569-8557-00	90s	$3.95
Zenith	00172-2908-60	100s	$3.05
➤ Rugby	00536-3840-01	100s	$3.90
Major	00904-1480-60	100s	$3.90
Major	00904-1580-60	100s	$3.90
Watson	52544-0300-01	100s	$3.95
Watson	52544-0311-01	100s	$3.95
Goldline	00182-1170-01	100s	$4.00
URL	00677-0662-01	100s	$4.15
➤ Mylan	00378-0208-01	100s	$4.15
Qualitest	00603-3736-21	100s	$4.15
Schein	00364-0568-01	100s	$4.20
➤ Geneva	00781-1818-01	100s	$4.20
Moore,H.L.	00839-6345-06	100s	$4.25
Moore,H.L.	00839-7782-06	100s	$4.25
Aligen	00405-4452-01	100s	$4.98
Roxane	00054-4297-25	100s	$5.25
Parmed	00349-8486-01	100s	$8.79
Lederle Std Prod	00005-3708-23	100s	$11.36
Raway	00686-0072-20	100s ud	$5.00
Major	00904-1480-61	100s ud	$6.39
Major	00904-1580-61	100s ud	$6.39
Roxane	00054-8297-25	100s ud	$7.57
Goldline	00182-1170-89	100s ud	$7.65
Schein	00364-0568-90	100s ud	$8.75
Vangard	00615-1569-13	100s ud	$9.11
➤ Geneva	00781-1818-13	100s ud	$9.95
Auro	55829-0265-10	100s ud	$11.30
UDL	51079-0072-20	100s ud	$11.75
Medirex	57480-0328-01	100s ud	$11.75
➤ Rugby	00536-3840-05	500s	$10.45
Zenith	00172-2908-70	500s	$10.70
Watson	52544-0300-05	500s	$18.75
Watson	52544-0311-05	500s	$18.75
Lederle Std Prod	00005-3708-31	500s	$26.64
➤ Rugby	00536-3840-10	1000s	$17.32
Zenith	00172-2908-80	1000s	$18.50
Schein	00364-0568-02	1000s	$19.75
Qualitest	00603-3736-32	1000s	$19.75
Major	00904-1480-80	1000s	$19.90
Major	00904-1580-80	1000s	$19.90
Goldline	00182-1170-10	1000s	$24.00
➤ Geneva	00781-1818-10	1000s	$25.49
URL	00677-0662-10	1000s	$25.50
➤ Mylan	00378-0208-10	1000s	$25.55
Moore,H.L.	00839-6345-16	1000s	$25.65
Moore,H.L.	00839-7782-16	1000s	$25.65
Martec	52555-0274-10	1000s	$26.10
Watson	52544-0300-10	1000s	$34.95
Watson	52544-0311-10	1000s	$34.95
Aligen	00405-4452-03	1000s	$36.02
Roxane	00054-4297-31	1000s	$36.05
Parmed	00349-8486-10	1000s	$69.05

TABLETS: 40 MG

AVERAGE UNIT PRICE (AVAILABLE SIZES)		GENERIC A-RATED AVERAGE PRICE (GAAP)	
BRAND	$0.22	30s	$3.35
GENERIC	$0.06	90s	$4.10
HCFA FUL (100s ea)	$0.03	100s	$8.00
		500s	$14.94
		1000s	$39.99

BRAND/MANUFACTURER	NDC	SIZE	AWP
◆ BRAND			
➤ LASIX: Hoechst	00039-0060-13	100s	$22.10
	00039-0060-11	100s ud	$23.00
➤ LASIX: Hoechst	00039-0060-50	500s	$104.75
	00039-0060-70	1000s	$199.00
◆ GENERICS			
Major	00904-1481-46	30s	$1.90
Medirex	57480-0329-06	30s	$4.80
Major	00904-1481-89	90s	$2.95
Allscrips	54569-8523-00	90s	$5.25
Zenith	00172-2907-60	100s	$3.50
➤ Mylan	00378-0216-01	100s	$4.73
➤ Rugby	00536-3841-01	100s	$4.73
Major	00904-1481-60	100s	$4.85
Watson	52544-0301-01	100s	$5.00
➤ Goldline	00182-1161-01	100s	$5.05
URL	00677-0659-01	100s	$5.05
➤ Schein	00364-0514-01	100s	$5.10
Aligen	00405-4453-01	100s	$5.32
➤ Geneva	00781-1966-01	100s	$5.54
Moore,H.L.	00839-6323-06	100s	$5.66
Moore,H.L.	00839-7783-06	100s	$5.66
➤ Roxane	00054-4299-25	100s	$5.98
➤ Lederle Std Prod	00005-3709-23	100s	$13.56
Major	00904-1481-61	100s ud	$6.61
Raway	00686-0073-20	100s ud	$7.00
Roxane	00054-8299-25	100s ud	$8.49
➤ Goldline	00182-1161-89	100s ud	$8.75
Vangard	00615-0446-13	100s ud	$11.33
➤ Geneva	00781-1966-13	100s ud	$11.90
➤ Schein	00364-0514-90	100s ud	$12.10
Auro	55829-0266-10	100s ud	$14.10
Medirex	57480-0329-01	100s ud	$16.00
UDL	51079-0073-20	100s ud	$16.10
Allscrips	54569-8523-01	180s	$10.49
➤ Rugby	00536-3841-05	500s	$10.67
Zenith	00172-2907-70	500s	$12.25
Major	00904-1481-40	500s	$13.10
Watson	52544-0301-05	500s	$23.75
➤ Rugby	00536-3841-10	1000s	$20.63
Zenith	00172-2907-80	1000s	$21.55
➤ Schein	00364-0514-02	1000s	$21.75

BRAND/MANUFACTURER	NDC	SIZE	AWP
Qualitest	00603-3737-32	1000s	$21.85
Major	00904-1481-80	1000s	$23.75
➤ Goldline	00182-1161-10	1000s	$30.00
Martec	52555-0275-10	1000s	$38.05
➤ Geneva	00781-1966-10	1000s	$42.49
➤ Mylan	00378-0216-10	1000s	$42.57
URL	00677-0659-10	1000s	$43.14
Moore,H.L.	00839-6323-16	1000s	$43.19
Moore,H.L.	00839-7783-16	1000s	$43.19
Watson	52544-0301-10	1000s	$44.95
Aligen	00405-4453-03	1000s	$44.98
➤ Roxane	00054-4299-31	1000s	$45.25
➤ Lederle Std Prod	00005-3709-34	1000s	$59.46
Parmed	00349-2337-10	1000s	$93.09

TABLETS: 80 MG

AVERAGE UNIT PRICE (AVAILABLE SIZES)		GENERIC A-RATED AVERAGE PRICE (GAAP)	
BRAND	$0.35	100s	$16.24
GENERIC	$0.15	500s	$64.74
HCFA FUL (100s ea)	$0.05		

BRAND/MANUFACTURER	NDC	SIZE	AWP
◆ BRAND			
➤ LASIX: Hoechst	00039-0066-05	50s	$17.95
➤ LASIX: Hoechst	00039-0066-11	100s ud	$36.55
	00039-0066-50	500s	$169.30
◆ GENERICS			
Medirex	57480-0330-06	30s	$6.67
Raway	00686-0527-20	100s	$9.75
➤ Rugby	00536-3835-01	100s	$11.52
Major	00904-1482-60	100s	$11.75
Schein	00364-0700-01	100s	$11.75
Mylan	00378-0232-01	100s	$11.82
Goldline	00182-1736-01	100s	$12.00
Qualitest	00603-3738-21	100s	$12.20
Martec	52555-0276-01	100s	$12.24
➤ Geneva	00781-1446-01	100s	$12.50
URL	00677-0976-01	100s	$13.02
Moore,H.L.	00839-6777-06	100s	$13.07
Roxane	00054-4301-25	100s	$13.49
Watson	52544-0302-01	100s	$19.95
Aligen	00405-4454-01	100s	$19.98
Lederle Std Prod	00005-3100-23	100s	$20.69
Parmed	00349-8353-01	100s	$24.56
Major	00904-1482-61	100s ud	$17.31
Roxane	00054-8301-25	100s ud	$17.54
Goldline	00182-1736-89	100s ud	$18.70
➤ Geneva	00781-1446-13	100s ud	$18.75
Vangard	00615-1571-13	100s ud	$18.78
Schein	00364-0700-90	100s ud	$19.15
Auro	55829-0267-10	100s ud	$21.50
UDL	51079-0527-20	100s ud	$21.93
Medirex	57480-0330-01	100s ud	$22.00
➤ Geneva	00781-1446-05	500s	$52.50
Mylan	00378-0232-05	500s	$54.06
Schein	00364-0700-05	500s	$54.50
Qualitest	00603-3738-28	500s	$54.70
➤ Rugby	00536-3835-05	500s	$54.81
Goldline	00182-1736-05	500s	$54.85
Major	00904-1482-40	500s	$54.95
Moore,H.L.	00839-6777-12	500s	$56.16
Moore,H.L.	00839-7697-12	500s	$56.16
Lederle Std Prod	00005-3100-31	500s	$65.13
Roxane	00054-4301-29	500s	$67.47
Parmed	00349-8353-05	500s	$91.49
Watson	52544-0302-05	500s	$94.75
Aligen	00405-4454-02	500s	$94.80

Furoxone *SEE* FURAZOLIDONE

G Bid *SEE* GUAIFENESIN

Gabapentin

DESCRIPTION
Gabapentin is supplied as imprinted hard shell capsules containing 100 mg, 300 mg, and 400 mg.

Gabapentin is described as 1-(aminomethyl)cyclohexaneacetic acid with an empirical formula of $C_9H_{17}NO_2$ and a molecular weight of 171.24.

Gabapentin is a white to off-white crystalline solid. It is freely soluble in water and both basic and acidic aqueous solutions.

Following is its chemical structure:

H_2N ——— $COOH$

CLINICAL PHARMACOLOGY
MECHANISM OF ACTION
The mechanism by which Gabapentin exerts its anticonvulsant action is unknown, but in animal test systems designed to detect anticonvulsant activity, Gabapentin prevents seizures as do other marketed anticonvulsants. Gabapentin exhibits antiseizure activity in mice and rats in both the maximal electroshock and pentylenetetrazole seizure models and other preclinical models (e.g., strains with genetic epilepsy, etc.). The relevance of these models to human epilepsy is not known.

Gabapentin is structurally related to the neurotransmitter GABA (gamma-aminobutyric acid) but it does not interact with GABA receptors, it is not converted metabolically into GABA or a GABA agonist, and it is not an inhibitor of GABA uptake or degradation. Gabapentin was tested in radioligand binding assays at concentrations up to 100 μM and did not exhibit affinity for a number of other common receptor sites, including benzodiazepine, glutamate, N-methyl-D-aspartate (NMDA), quisqualate, kainate, strychnine-insensitive or strychnine-sensitive glycine, alpha 1, alpha 2, or beta adrenergic, adenosine A1 or A2, cholinergic muscarinic or nicotinic, dopamine D1 or D2, histamine H1, serotonin S1 or S2, opiate mu, delta or kappa, voltage-sensitive calcium channel sites labeled with nitrendipine or diltiazem, or at voltage-sensitive sodium channel sites with batrachotoxinin A 20-alpha-benzoate.

Several test systems ordinarily used to assess activity at the NMDA receptor have been examined. Results are contradictory. Accordingly, no general statement about the effects, if any, of Gabapentin at the NMDA receptor can be made.

In vitro studies with radiolabeled Gabapentin have revealed a Gabapentin binding site in areas of rat brain including neocortex and hippocampus. The identity and function of this binding site remain to be elucidated.

PHARMACOKINETICS AND DRUG METABOLISM
All pharmacological actions following Gabapentin administration are due to the activity of the parent compound; Gabapentin is not appreciably metabolized in humans.

Oral Bioavailability: Gabapentin bioavailability is not dose proportional; i.e., as dose is increased, bioavailability decreases. A 400-mg dose, for example, is about 25% less bioavailable than a 100-mg dose. Over the recommended dose range of 300 to 600 mg T.I.D., however, the differences in bioavailability are not large, and bioavailability is about 60 percent. Food has no effect on the rate and extent of absorption of Gabapentin.

Distribution: Gabapentin circulates largely unbound (< 3%) to plasma protein. The apparent volume of distribution of Gabapentin after 150 mg intravenous administration is 58 ± 6 L (Mean ± SD). In patients with epilepsy, steady-state predose (Cmin) concentrations of Gabapentin in cerebrospinal fluid were approximately 20% of the corresponding plasma concentrations.

Elimination: Gabapentin is eliminated from the systemic circulation by renal excretion as unchanged drug. Gabapentin is not appreciably metabolized in humans.

Gabapentin elimination half-life is 5 to 7 hours and is unaltered by dose or following multiple dosing. Gabapentin elimination rate constant, plasma clearance, and renal clearance are directly proportional to creatinine clearance (see "Special Populations: Patients With Renal Insufficiency" below). In elderly patients, and in patients with impaired renal function, Gabapentin plasma clearance is reduced. Gabapentin can be removed from plasma by hemodialysis.

Dosage adjustment in patients with compromised renal function or undergoing hemodialysis is recommended (see "Dosage and Administration", Table 2).

Special Populations: Patients With Renal Insufficiency: Subjects (N = 60) with renal insufficiency (mean creatinine clearance ranging from 13-114 mL/min) were administered single 400-mg oral doses of Gabapentin. The mean Gabapentin half-life ranged from about 6.5 hours (patients with creatinine clearance > 60 mL/min) to 52 hours (creatinine clearance < 30 mL/min) and Gabapentin renal clearance from about 90 mL/min (> 60 mL/min group) to about 10 mL/min (< 30 mL/min). Mean plasma clearance (CL/F) decreased from approximately 190 mL/min to 20 mL/min.

Dosage adjustment in patients with compromised renal function is necessary (see "Dosage and Administration").

Hemodialysis: In a study in anuric subjects (N = 11), the apparent elimination half-life of Gabapentin on nondialysis days was about 132 hours; dialysis three times a week (4 hours duration) lowered the apparent half-life of Gabapentin by about 60%, from 132 hours to 51 hours. Hemodialysis thus has a significant effect on Gabapentin elimination in anuric subjects.

Dosage adjustment in patients undergoing hemodialysis is necessary (see "Dosage and Administration").

Hepatic Disease: Because Gabapentin is not metabolized, no study was performed in patients with hepatic impairment.

Age: The effect of age was studied in subjects 20-80 years of age. Apparent oral clearance (CL/F) of Gabapentin decreased as age increased, from about 225 mL/min in those under 30 years of age to about 125 mL/min in those over 70 years of age. Renal clearance (CLr) and CLr adjusted for body surface area also declined with age; however, the decline in the renal clearance of Gabapentin with age can largely be explained by the decline in renal function. Reduction of Gabapentin dose may be required in patients who have age related compromised renal function. (See *"Precautions, Geriatric Use"* and *"Dosage and Administration"*.)

Pediatric: No pharmacokinetic data are available in children below the age of 18 years.

Gender: Although no formal study has been conducted to compare the pharmacokinetics of Gabapentin in men and women, it appears that the pharmacokinetic parameters for males and females are similar and there are no significant gender differences.

Race: Pharmacokinetic differences due to race have not been studied. Because Gabapentin is primarily renally excreted and there are no important racial differences in creatinine clearance, pharmacokinetic differences due to race are not expected.

CLINICAL STUDIES

The effectiveness of Gabapentin as adjunctive therapy (added to other antiepileptic drugs) was established in three multicenter placebo-controlled, double-blind, parallel-group clinical trials in 705 adults with refractory partial seizures. The patients enrolled had a history of at least 4 partial seizures per month in spite of receiving one or more antiepileptic drugs at therapeutic levels and were observed on their established antiepileptic drug regimen during a 12-week baseline period. In patients continuing to have at least 2 (or 4 in some studies) seizures per month, Gabapentin or placebo was then added on to the existing therapy during a 12-week treatment period. Effectiveness was assessed primarily on the basis of the percent of patients with a 50% or greater reduction in seizure frequency from baseline to treatment (the "responder rate") and a derived measure called response ratio, a measure of change defined as $(T - B)/(T + B)$, where B is the patient's baseline seizure frequency and T is the patient's seizure frequency during treatment. Response ratio is distributed within the range -1 to +1. A zero value indicates no change while complete elimination of seizures would give a value of -1; increased seizure rates would give positive values. A response ratio of -0.33 corresponds to a 50% reduction in seizure frequency. The results given below are for all partial seizures in the intent-to-treat (all patients who received any doses of treatment) population in each study, unless otherwise indicated.

One study compared Gabapentin 1200 mg/day t.i.d. with placebo. Responder rate was 23% (14/61) in the Gabapentin group and 9% (6/66) in the placebo group; the difference between groups was statistically significant. Response ratio was also better in the Gabapentin group (-0.199) than in the placebo group (-0.044), a difference that also achieved statistical significance.

A second study compared primarily 1200 mg/day t.i.d. Gabapentin (N = 101) with placebo (N = 98). Additional smaller Gabapentin dosage groups (600 mg/day, N = 53; 1800 mg/day, N = 54) were also studied for information regarding dose response. Responder rate was higher in the Gabapentin 1200 mg/day group (16%) than in the placebo group (8%), but the difference was not statistically significant. The responder rate at 600 mg (17%) was also not significantly higher than in the placebo, but the responder rate in the 1800 mg group (26%) was statistically significantly superior to the placebo rate. Response ratio was better in the Gabapentin 1200 mg/day group (-0.103) than in the placebo group (-0.022); but this difference was also not statistically significant (p = 0.0224). A better response was seen in the Gabapentin 600 mg/day group (-0.105) and 1800 mg/day group (-0.222) than in the 1200 mg/day group, with the 1800 mg/day group achieving statistical significance compared to the placebo group.

A third study compared Gabapentin 900 mg/day t.i.d. (N = 111) and placebo (N = 109). An additional Gabapentin 1200 mg/day dosage group (N = 52) provided dose-response data. A statistically significant difference in responder rate was seen in the Gabapentin 900 mg/day group (22%) compared to that in the placebo group (10%). Response ratio was also statistically significantly superior in the Gabapentin 900 mg/day group (-0.119) compared to that in the placebo group (-0.027), as was response ratio in 1200 mg/day Gabapentin (-0.184) compared to placebo.

Analyses were also performed in each study to examine the effect of Gabapentin on preventing secondarily generalized tonic-clonic seizures. Patients who experienced a secondarily generalized tonic-clonic seizure in either the baseline or in the treatment period in all three placebo-controlled studies were included in these analyses. There were several response ratio comparisons that showed a statistically significant advantage for Gabapentin compared to placebo and favorable trends for almost all comparisons.

Analysis of responder rate using combined data from all three studies and all doses (N = 162, Gabapentin; N = 89, placebo) also showed a significant advantage for Gabapentin over placebo in reducing the frequency of secondarily generalized tonic-clonic seizures.

In two of the three controlled studies, more than one dose of Gabapentin was used. Within each study the results did not show a consistently increased response to dose. However, looking across studies, a trend toward increasing efficacy with increasing dose is evident (see Figure 1).

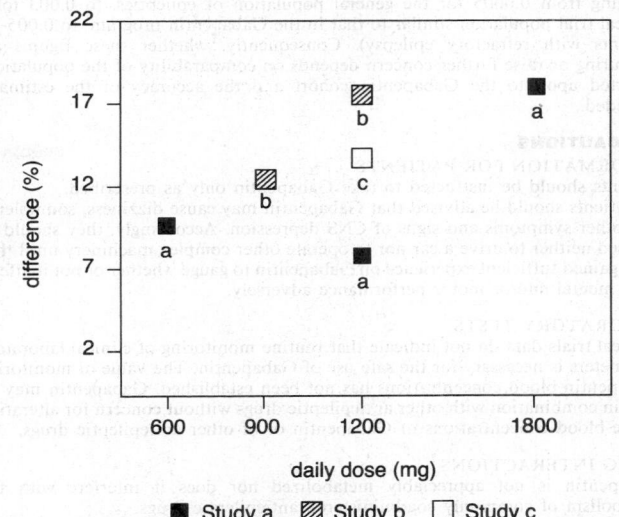

FIGURE 1. Responder rate in patients receiving Gabapentin expressed as a difference from placebo by dose and study

In the figure, treatment effect magnitude, measured on the Y axis in terms of the difference in the proportion of Gabapentin and placebo assigned patients attaining a 50% or greater reduction in seizure frequency from baseline, is plotted against the daily dose of Gabapentin administered (X axis).

Although no formal analysis by gender has been performed, estimates of response (Response Ratio) derived from clinical trials (398 men, 307 women) indicate no important gender differences exist. There was no consistent pattern indicating that age had any effect on the response to Gabapentin. There were insufficient numbers of patients of races other than Caucasian to permit a comparison of efficacy among racial groups.

INDICATIONS AND USAGE

Gabapentin is indicated as adjunctive therapy in the treatment of partial seizures with and without secondary generalization in adults with epilepsy.

CONTRAINDICATIONS

Gabapentin is contraindicated in patients who have demonstrated hypersensitivity to the drug or its ingredients.

WARNINGS

WITHDRAWAL PRECIPITATED SEIZURE, STATUS EPILEPTICUS

Antiepileptic drugs should not be abruptly discontinued because of the possibility of increasing seizure frequency.

In the placebo-controlled studies, the incidence of status epilepticus in patients receiving Gabapentin was 0.6% (5 of 543) versus 0.5% in patients receiving placebo (2 of 378). Among the 2074 patients treated with Gabapentin across all studies (controlled and uncontrolled) 31 (1.5%) had status epilepticus. Of these, 14 patients had no prior history of status epilepticus either before treatment or while on other medications. Because adequate historical data are not available, it is impossible to say whether or not treatment with Gabapentin is associated with a higher or lower rate of status epilepticus than would be expected to occur in a similar population not treated with Gabapentin.

TUMORIGENIC POTENTIAL

In standard preclinical *in vivo* lifetime carcinogenicity studies, an unexpectedly high incidence of pancreatic acinar adenocarcinomas was identified in male, but not female, rats. (See *"Precautions": Carcinogenesis, Mutagenesis, Impairment of Fertility.*) The clinical significance of this finding is unknown. Clinical experience during Gabapentin's premarketing development provides no direct means to assess its potential for inducing tumors in humans.

In clinical studies comprising 2085 patient-years of exposure, new tumors were reported in 10 patients (2 breast, 3 brain, 2 lung, 1 adrenal, 1 non-Hodgkin's lymphoma, 1 endometrial carcinoma *in situ*), and preexisting tumors worsened in 11 patients (9 brain, 1 breast, 1 prostate) during or up to 2 years following discontinuation of Gabapentin. Without knowledge of the background incidence and recurrence in a similar population not treated with Gabapentin it is impossible to know whether the incidence seen in this cohort is or is not affected by treatment.

SUDDEN AND UNEXPLAINED DEATHS

During the course of premarketing development of Gabapentin, 8 sudden and unexplained deaths were recorded among a cohort of 2203 patients treated (2103 patient-years of exposure).

Some of these could represent seizure-related deaths in which the seizure was not observed, e.g., at night. This represents an incidence of 0.0038 deaths per patient-year. Although this rate exceeds that expected in a healthy population matched for age and sex, it is within the range of estimates for the incidence of sudden unexplained deaths in patients with epilepsy not receiving Gabapentin (ranging from 0.0005 for the general population of epileptics, to 0.003 for a clinical trial population similar to that in the Gabapentin program, to 0.005 for patients with refractory epilepsy). Consequently, whether these figures are reassuring or raise further concern depends on comparability of the populations reported upon to the Gabapentin cohort and the accuracy of the estimates provided.

PRECAUTIONS

INFORMATION FOR PATIENTS
Patients should be instructed to take Gabapentin only as prescribed.

Patients should be advised that Gabapentin may cause dizziness, somnolence and other symptoms and signs of CNS depression. Accordingly, they should be advised neither to drive a car nor to operate other complex machinery until they have gained sufficient experience on Gabapentin to gauge whether or not it affects their mental and/or motor performance adversely.

LABORATORY TESTS
Clinical trials data do not indicate that routine monitoring of clinical laboratory parameters is necessary for the safe use of Gabapentin. The value of monitoring Gabapentin blood concentrations has not been established. Gabapentin may be used in combination with other antiepileptic drugs without concern for alteration of the blood concentrations of Gabapentin or of other antiepileptic drugs.

DRUG INTERACTIONS
Gabapentin is not appreciably metabolized nor does it interfere with the metabolism of commonly coadministered antiepileptic drugs.

The drug interaction data described in this section were obtained from studies involving healthy adults and patients with epilepsy.

Phenytoin: In a single and multiple dose study of Gabapentin (400 mg tid) in epileptic patients (N = 8) maintained on phenytoin monotherapy for at least 2 months, Gabapentin had no effect on the steady-state trough plasma concentrations of phenytoin and phenytoin had no effect on Gabapentin pharmacokinetics.

Carbamazepine: Steady-state trough plasma carbamazepine and carbamazepine 10, 11 epoxide concentrations were not affected by concomitant Gabapentin (400 mg tid; N = 12) administration. Likewise Gabapentin pharmacokinetics were unaltered by carbamazepine administration.

Valproic Acid: The mean steady-state trough serum valproic acid concentrations prior to and during concomitant Gabapentin administration (400 mg tid; N = 17) were not different and neither were Gabapentin pharmacokinetic parameters affected by valproic acid.

Phenobarbital: Estimates of steady-state pharmacokinetic parameters for phenobarbital or Gabapentin (300 mg tid; N = 12) are identical whether the drugs are administered alone or together.

Cimetidine: In the presence of cimetidine at 300 mg qid (N = 12) the mean apparent oral clearance of Gabapentin fell by 14% and creatinine clearance fell by 10%. Thus cimetidine appeared to alter the renal excretion of both Gabapentin and creatinine, an endogenous marker of renal function. This small decrease in excretion of Gabapentin by cimetidine is not expected to be of clinical importance. The effect of Gabapentin on cimetidine was not evaluated.

Oral Contraceptive: Based on AUC and half-life, multiple-dose pharmacokinetic profiles of norethindrone and ethinyl estradiol following administration of tablets containing 2.5 mg of norethindrone acetate and 50 mcg of ethinyl estradiol were similar with and without coadministration of Gabapentin (400 mg tid; N = 13). The Cmax of norethindrone was 13% higher when it was coadministered with Gabapentin; this interaction is not expected to be of clinical importance.

Antacid (Maalox®): Maalox reduced the bioavailability of Gabapentin (N = 16) by about 20%. This decrease in bioavailability was about 5% when Gabapentin was administered 2 hours after Maalox. It is recommended that Gabapentin be taken at least 2 hours following Maalox administration.

Effect of Probenecid: Probenecid is a blocker of renal tubular secretion. Gabapentin pharmacokinetic parameters without and with probenecid were comparable. This indicates that Gabapentin does not undergo renal tubular secretion by the pathway that is blocked by probenecid.

DRUG/LABORATORY TESTS INTERACTIONS
Because false positive readings were reported with the Ames N-Multistix SG® dipstick test for urinary protein when Gabapentin was added to other antiepileptic drugs, the more specific sulfiosalicylic acid precipitation procedure is recommended to determine the presence of urine protein.

CARCINOGENESIS, MUTAGENESIS, IMPAIRMENT OF FERTILITY
Gabapentin was given in the diet to mice at 200, 600, and 2000 mg/kg/day and to rats at 250, 1000, and 2000 mg/kg/day for 2 years. A statistically significant increase in the incidence of pancreatic acinar cell adenomas and carcinomas was found in male rats receiving the high dose; the no-effect dose for the occurrence of carcinomas was 1000 mg/kg/day. Peak plasma concentrations of Gabapentin in rats receiving the high dose of 2000 mg/kg were 10 times higher than plasma concentrations in humans receiving 3600 mg per day, and in rats receiving 1000 mg/kg/day peak plasma concentrations were 6.5 times higher than in humans receiving 3600 mg/day. The pancreatic acinar cell carcinomas did not affect survival, did not metastasize and were not locally invasive. Studies to attempt to define a mechanism by which this relatively rare tumor type is occurring are in progress. The relevance of this finding to carcinogenic risk in humans is unclear.

Gabapentin did not demonstrate mutagenic or genotoxic potential in three *in vitro* and two *in vivo* assays. It was negative in the Ames test and the *in vitro* HGPRT forward mutation assay in Chinese hamster lung cells; it did not produce significant increases in chromosomal aberrations in the *in vitro* Chinese hamster lung cell assay; it was negative in the *in vivo* chromosomal aberration assay and in the *in vivo* micronucleus test in Chinese hamster bone marrow.

No adverse effects on fertility or reproduction were observed in rats at doses up to 2000 mg/kg (approximately 5 times the maximum recommended human dose on an mg/m² basis).

PREGNANCY
Pregnancy Category C: Gabapentin has been shown to be fetotoxic in rodents, causing delayed ossification of several bones in the skull, vertebrae, forelimbs, and hindlimbs. These effects occurred when pregnant mice received oral doses of 1000 or 3000 mg/kg/day during the period of organogenesis, or approximately 1 to 4 times the maximum dose of 3600 mg/day given to epileptic patients on a mg/m² basis. The no-effect level was 500 mg/kg/day or approximately 1/2 of the human dose on a mg/m² basis.

When rats were dosed prior to and during mating, and throughout gestation, pups from all dose groups (500, 1000 and 2000 mg/kg/day) were affected. These doses are equivalent to less than approximately 1 to 5 times the maximum human dose on a mg/m² basis. There was an increased incidence of hydroureter and/or hydronephrosis in rats in a study of fertility and general reproductive performance at 2000 mg/kg/day with no effect at 1000 mg/kg/day, in a teratology study at 1500 mg/kg/day with no effect at 300 mg/kg/day, and in a perinatal and postnatal study at all doses studied (500, 1000 and 2000 mg/kg/day). The doses at which the effects occurred are approximately 1 to 5 times the maximum human dose of 3600 mg/day on a mg/m² basis; the no-effect doses were approximately 3 times (Fertility and General Reproductive Performance study) and approximately equal to (Teratogenicity study) the maximum human dose on a mg/m² basis. Other than hydroureter and hydronephrosis, the etiologies of which are unclear, the incidence of malformations was not increased compared to controls in offspring of mice, rats, or rabbits given doses up to 50 times (mice), 30 times (rats), and 25 times (rabbits) the human daily dose on a mg/kg basis, or 4 times (mice) 5 times (rats), or 8 times (rabbits) the human daily dose on a mg/m² basis.

In a teratology study in rabbits, an increased incidence of postimplantation fetal loss occurred in dams exposed to 60, 300 and 1500 mg/kg/day, or less than approximately 1/4 to 8 times the maximum human dose on a mg/m² basis. There are no adequate and well-controlled studies in pregnant women. Because animal reproduction studies are not always predictive of human response, this drug should be used during pregnancy only if the potential benefit justifies the potential risk to the fetus.

USE IN NURSING MOTHERS
It is not known if Gabapentin is excreted in human milk and the effect on the nursing infant is unknown. However, because many drugs are excreted in human milk, Gabapentin should be used in women who are nursing only if the benefits clearly outweigh the risks.

PEDIATRIC USE
Safety and effectiveness in children below the age of 12 years have not been established.

GERIATRIC USE
No systematic studies in geriatric patients have been conducted. Adverse clinical events reported among 59 Gabapentin exposed patients over age 65 did not differ in kind from those reported for younger individuals. The small number of older individuals evaluated, however, limits the strength of any conclusions reached about the influence, if any, of age on the kind and incidence of adverse events or laboratory abnormality associated with the use of Gabapentin.

Because Gabapentin is eliminated primarily by renal excretion, the dose of Gabapentin should be adjusted as noted in *"Dosage and Administration"* (Table 2) for elderly patients with compromised renal function. Creatinine clearance is difficult to measure in outpatients and serum creatinine may be reduced in the elderly because of decreased muscle mass. Creatinine clearance (C_{cr}) can be reasonably well estimated using the equation of Cockcroft and Gault:

for females C_{cr} = (0.85) (140-age) (wt)/[(72) (S_{Cr})]
for males C_{cr} = (140-age) (wt)/[(72) (S_{Cr})]

where age is in years, wt is in kilograms and S_{Cr} is serum creatinine in mg/dL.

ADVERSE REACTIONS
The most commonly observed adverse events associated with the use of Gabapentin in combination with other antiepileptic drugs, not seen at an equivalent frequency among placebo-treated patients, were somnolence, dizziness, ataxia, fatigue, and nystagmus.

Approximately 7% of the 2074 individuals who received Gabapentin in premarketing clinical trials discontinued treatment because of an adverse event. The adverse events most commonly associated with withdrawal were somnolence (1.2%), ataxia (0.8%), fatigue (0.6%), nausea and/or vomiting (0.6%), and dizziness (0.6%).

INCIDENCE IN CONTROLLED CLINICAL TRIALS
Table 1 lists treatment-emergent signs and symptoms that occurred in at least 1% of Gabapentin treated patients with epilepsy participating in placebo-controlled trials and were numerically more common in the Gabapentin group. In these studies, either Gabapentin or placebo was added to the patients current

antiepileptic drug therapy. Adverse events were usually mild to moderate in intensity.

The prescriber should be aware that these figures, obtained when Gabapentin was added to concurrent antiepileptic drug therapy, cannot be used to predict the frequency of adverse events in the course of usual medical practice where patient characteristics and other factors may differ from those prevailing during clinical studies. Similarly, the cited frequencies cannot be directly compared with figures obtained from other clinical investigations involving different treatments, uses, or investigators. An inspection of these frequencies, however, does provide the prescribing physician with one basis to estimate the relative contribution of drug and nondrug factors to the adverse event incidences in the population studied.

Table 1.

TREATMENT-EMERGENT ADVERSE EVENT INCIDENCE IN CONTROLLED ADD-ON TRIALS (EVENTS IN AT LEAST 1% OF GABAPENTIN PATIENTS AND NUMERICALLY MORE FREQUENT THAN IN THE PLACEBO GROUP)

Body System/ Adverse Event	Gabapentin N = 543 %	Placebo[a] N = 378 %
Body As A Whole		
Fatigue	11.0	5.0
Weight Increase	2.9	1.6
Back Pain	1.8	0.5
Peripheral Edema	1.7	0.5
Cardiovascular		
Vasodilatation	1.1	0.3
Digestive System		
Dyspepsia	2.2	0.5
Mouth or Throat		
Dry	1.7	0.5
Constipation	1.5	0.8
Dental		
Abnormalities	1.5	0.3
Increased		
Appetite	1.1	0.8
Hematologic and Lymphatic Systems		
Leukopenia	1.1	0.5
Musculoskeletal System		
Myalgia	2.0	1.9
Fracture	1.1	0.8
Nervous System		
Somnolence	19.3	8.7
Dizziness	17.1	6.9
Ataxia	12.5	5.6
Nystagmus	8.3	4.0
Tremor	6.8	3.2
Nervousness	2.4	1.9
Dysarthria	2.4	0.5
Amnesia	2.2	0.0
Depression	1.8	1.1
Thinking		
Abnormal	1.7	1.3
Twitching	1.3	0.5
Coordination		
Abnormal	1.1	0.3
Respiratory System		
Rhinitis	4.1	3.7
Pharyngitis	2.8	1.6
Coughing	1.8	1.3
Skin and Appendages		
Abrasion	1.3	0.0
Pruritus	1.3	0.5
Urogenital System		
Impotence	1.5	1.1
Special Senses		
Diplopia	5.9	1.9
Amblyopia[b]	4.2	1.1
Laboratory Deviations		
WBC Decreased	1.1	0.5

[a] *Plus background antiepileptic drug therapy*
[b] *Amblyopia was often described as blurred vision.*

Other events in more than 1% of patients but equally or more frequent in the placebo group included: headache, viral infection, fever, nausea and/or vomiting, abdominal pain, diarrhea, convulsions, confusion, insomnia, emotional lability, rash, acne.

Among the treatment-emergent adverse events occuring at an incidence of at least 10% of Gabapentin treated patients, somnolence and ataxia appeared to exhibit a positive dose-response relationship.

The overall incidence of adverse events and the types of adverse events seen were similar among men and women treated with Gabapentin. The incidence of adverse events increased slightly with increasing age in patients treated with either Gabapentin or placebo. Because only 3% of patients (28/921) in placebo-

controlled studies were identified as nonwhite (black or other), there are insufficient data to support a statement regarding the distribution of adverse events by race.

OTHER ADVERSE EVENTS OBSERVED DURING ALL CLINICAL TRIALS

Gabapentin has been administered to 2074 individuals during all clinical trials, only some of which were placebo-controlled. During these trials, all adverse events were recorded by the clinical investigators using terminology of their own choosing. To provide a meaningful estimate of the proportion of individuals having adverse events, similar types of events were grouped into a smaller number of standardized categories using modified COSTART dictionary terminology. These categories are used in the listing below. The frequencies presented represent the proportion of the 2074 individuals exposed to Gabapentin who experienced an event of the type cited on at least one occasion while receiving Gabapentin. All reported events are included except those already listed in the previous table, those too general to be informative, and those not reasonably associated with the use of the drug.

Events are further classified within body system categories and enumerated in order of decreasing frequency using the following definitions: frequent adverse events are defined as those occurring in at least 1/100 patients; infrequent adverse events are those occurring in 1/100 to 1/1000 patients; rare events are those occurring in fewer than 1/1000 patients.

Body as a Whole: Frequent: asthenia, malaise, face edema; *Infrequent*: allergy, generalized edema, weight decrease, chill; *Rare*: strange feelings, lastitude alcohol intolerance, hangover effect.

Cardiovascular System: Frequent: hypertension; *Infrequent*: hypotension, angina pectoris, peripheral vascular disorder, palpitation, tachycardia, migraine, murmur; *Rare*: atrial fibrillation, heart failure, thrombophlebitis, deep thrombophlebitis, myocardial infarction, cerebrovascular accident, pulmonary thrombosis, ventricular extrasystoles, bradycardia, premature atrial contraction, pericardial rub, heart block, pulmonary embolus, hyperlipidemia, hypercholesterolemia, pericardial effusion, pericarditis.

Digestive System: Frequent: anorexia, flatulence, gingivitis; *Infrequent*: glossitis, gum hemorrhage, thirst, stomatitis, increased salivation, gastroenteritis, hemorrhoids, bloody stools, fecal incontinence, hepatomegaly; *Rare*: dysphagia, eructation, pancreatitis, peptic ulcer, colitis, blisters in mouth, tooth discolor, perleche, salivary gland enlarged, lip hemorrhage, esophagitis, hiatal hernia, hematemesis, proctitis, irritable bowel syndrome, rectal hemorrhage, esophageal spasm.

Endocrine System: Rare: hyperthyroid, hypothyroid, goiter, hypoestrogen, ovarian failure, epididymitis, swollen testicle, cushingoid appearance.

Hematologic and Lymphatic System: Frequent: purpura most often described as bruises resulting from physical trauma; *Infrequent*: anemia, thrombocytopenia, lymphadenopathy; *Rare*: WBC count increased, lymphocytosis, non-Hodgkin's lymphoma, bleeding time increased.

Musculoskeletal System: Frequent: arthralgia; *Infrequent*: tendinitis, arthritis, joint stiffness, joint swelling, positive Romberg test; *Rare*: costochondritis, osteoporosis, bursitis, contracture.

Nervous System: Frequent: Vertigo, hyperkinesia, paresthesia, decreased or absent reflexes, increased reflexes, anxiety, hostility; *Infrequent*: CNS tumors, syncope, dreaming abnormal, aphasia, hypesthesia, intracranial hemorrhage, hypotonia, dysesthesia, paresis, dystonia, hemiplegia, facial paralysis, stupor, cerebellar dysfunction, positive Babinski sign, decreased position sense, subdural hematoma, apathy, hallucination, decrease or loss of libido, agitation, paranoia, depersonalization, euphoria, feeling high, doped-up sensation, suicidal, psychosis; *Rare*: choreoathetosis orofacial dyskinesia, encephalopathy, nerve palsy, personality disorder, increased libido, subdued temperament, apraxia, fine motor control disorder, meningismus, local myoclonus, hyperesthesia, hypokinesia, mania, neurosis, hysteria, antisocial reaction, suicide gesture.

Respiratory System: Frequent: pneumonia; *Infrequent*: epistaxis, dyspnea, apnea; *Rare*: mucositis, aspiration pneumonia, hyperventilation, hiccup, laryngitis, nasal obstruction, snoring, bronchospasm, hypoventilation, lung edema.

Dermatological: Infrequent alopecia, eczema, dry skin, increased sweating, urticaria, hirsutism, seborrhea, cyst, herpes simplex; *Rare*: herpes zoster, skin discolor; skin papules, photosensitive reaction, leg ulcer, scalp seborrhea, psoriasis, desquamation, maceration, skin nodules, subcutaneous nodule, melanosis, skin necrosis, local swelling.

Urogenital System: Infrequent: hematuria, dysuria, urination frequency, cystitis, urinary retention, urinary incontinence, vaginal hemorrhage, amenorrhea, dysmenorrhea, menorrhagia, breast cancer, unable to climax, ejaculation abnormal; *Rare*: kidney pain, leukorrhea, pruritius genital, renal stone, acute renal failure, anuria, glycosuria, nephrosis, nocturia, pyuria, urination urgency, vaginal pain, breast pain, testicle pain.

Special Senses: Frequent: abnormal vision; *Infrequent*: cataract, conjunctivitis, eyes dry, eye pain, visual field defect, photophobia, bilateral or unilateral ptosis, eye hemorrhage, hordeolum, hearing loss, earache, tinnitus, inner ear infection, otitis, taste loss, unusual taste, eye twitching, ear fullness; *Rare*: eye itching, abnormal accommodation, perforated ear drum, sensitivity to noise, eye focusing problem, watery eyes, retinopathy, glaucoma, iritis, corneal disorders, lacrimal dysfunction, degenerative eye changes, blindness, retinal degeneration, miosis, chorioretinitis, strabismus, eustachian tube dysfunction, labyrinithitis, otitis externa, odd smell.

DRUG ABUSE AND DEPENDENCE

The abuse and dependence potential of Gabapentin has not been evaluated in human studies.

OVERDOSAGE

A lethal dose of Gabapentin was not identified in mice and rats receiving single oral doses as high as 8000 mg/kg. Signs of acute toxicity in animals included ataxia, labored breathing, ptosis, sedation, hypoactivity, or excitation.

Acute oral overdoses of Gabapentin up to 49 grams have been reported. In these cases, double vision, slurred speech, drowsiness, lethargy and diarrhea were observed. All patients recovered with supportive care.

Gabapentin can be removed by hemodialysis. Although hemodialysis has not been performed in the few overdose cases reported, it may be indicated by the patient's clinical state or in patients with significant renal impairment.

DOSAGE AND ADMINISTRATION

Gabapentin is recommended for add-on therapy in patients over 12 years of age. Evidence bearing on its safety and effectiveness in children is not available.

Gabapentin is given orally with or without food.

The effective dose of Gabapentin is 900 to 1800 mg/day and given in divided doses (three times a day) using 300- or 400-mg capsules. Titration to an effective dose can take place rapidly, over a few days, giving 300 mg on Day 1, 300 mg twice a day on Day 2, and 300 mg three times a day on Day 3. To minimize potential side effects, especially somnolence, dizziness, fatigue, and ataxia, the first dose on Day 1 may be administered at bedtime. If necessary, the dose may be increased using 300- or 400-mg capsules three times a day up to 1800 mg/day. Dosages up to 2400 mg/day have been well tolerated in long-term clinical studies. Doses of 3600 mg/day have also been administered to a small number of patients for a relatively short duration, and have been well tolerated. The maximum time between doses in the tid schedule should not exceed 12 hours.

It is not necessary to monitor Gabapentin plasma concentrations to optimize Gabapentin therapy. Further, because there are no significant pharmacokinetic interactions among Gabapentin and other commonly used antiepileptic drugs, the addition of Gabapentin does not after the plasma levels of these drugs appreciably.

If Gabapentin is discontinued and/or an alternate anticonvulsant medication is added to the therapy, this should be done gradually over a minimum of 1 week.

Dosage adjustment in patients with compromised renal function or undergoing hemodialysis is recommended as follows:

Table 2

GABAPENTIN DOSAGE BASED ON RENAL FUNCTION

Renal Function Creatinine Clearance (mL/min)	Total Daily Dose (mg/day)	Dose Regimen (mg)
> 60	1200	400 tid
30-60	600	300 bid
15-30	300	300 qd
> 15	150	300 qod[a]
Hemodialysis	-	200-300[b]

[a] *Every other day*
[b] *Loading dose of 300 to 400 mg in patients who have never received Gabapentin then 200 to 300 mg Gabapentin following each 4 hours of hemodialysis.*

Store at controlled room temperature, 15°-30°C (59°-86°F).

HOW SUPPLIED
CAPSULE: 100 MG

BRAND/MANUFACTURER	NDC	SIZE	AWP
○ BRAND			
► NEURONTIN: Parke-Davis	00071-0803-40	50s ud	$24.00
	00071-0803-24	100s	$36.00

CAPSULE: 300 MG

BRAND/MANUFACTURER	NDC	SIZE	AWP
○ BRAND			
► NEURONTIN: Parke-Davis	00071-0805-40	50s ud	$54.00
	00071-0805-24	100s	$90.00

CAPSULE: 400 MG

BRAND/MANUFACTURER	NDC	SIZE	AWP
○ BRAND			
► NEURONTIN: Parke-Davis	00071-0806-40	50s ud	$60.00
	00071-0806-24	100s	$108.00

Gadodiamide

DESCRIPTION

Gadodiamide Injection is the formulation of the gadolinium complex of diethylenetriamine pentaacetic acid bismethylamide, and is an injectable, nonionic extracellular enhancing agent for magnetic resonance imaging. Gadodiamide is to be administered by intravenuous injection. Each mL contains 287 mg of Gadodiamide. Gadodiamide is a 0.5 mol/L solution of aqua [5,8-bis (carboxymethyl)-11-[2-(methylamino)-2-oxoethyl] -3-oxo-2, 5,8,11-tetraazatridecan-13-oato (3-)-N^5, N^{-8},N^{-11},O^3,O^5,O^8,O^{11},O^{13}] gadolinium hydrate, with a molecular weight of 573.66 (anhydrous), an empirical formula of $C_{16}H_{28}GdN_5O_9.xH_2O$.

Pertinent physiochemical data for Gadodiamide are noted below:

PARAMETER

Osmolality (mOsm/kg water)	@ 37°C	789
Viscosity (cp)	@ 20°C	2.0
	@ 37°C	1.4
Density (g/cm³)	@ 20°C	1.13

Gadodiamide has an osmolality 2.8 times that of plasma (285 mOsm/kg water) at 37°C and is hypertonic under conditions of use.

Following is its chemical structure:

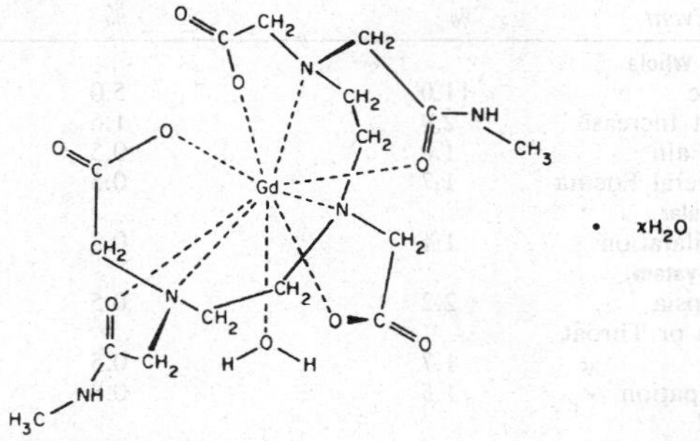

CLINICAL PHARMACOLOGY

The pharmacokinetics of intravenously administered Gadodiamide in normal subjects conforms to an open, two-compartment model with mean distribution and elimination half-lives (reported as mean±SD) of 3.7±2.7 minutes and 77.8±16 minutes, respectively.

Gadodiamide is eliminated primarily in the urine with 95.4±5.5% (mean±SD) of the administered dose eliminated by 24 hours. There is no detectable biotransformation or decomposition of Gadodiamide. The renal and plasma clearance rates of Gadodiamide are nearly identical (1.7 and 1.8 mL/min/kg, respectively), and are similar to that of substances excreted primarily by glomerular filtration. The volume of distribution of Gadodiamide (200±61 mL/kg) is equivalent to that of extracellular water. The potential for protein binding is unknown.

In magnetic resonance imaging, visualization of normal and pathological brain and spinal tissue depends in part on variations in the radiofrequency signal intensity. These variations occur due to: changes in proton density; alteration of the spin-lattice or longitudinal relaxation time (T_1); and variation of the spin-spin or transverse relaxation time (T_2). Gadodiamide is a paramagnetic agent with unpaired electron spins which generate a local magnetic field. As water protons move through this local magnetic field, the changes in magnetic field experienced by the protons reorient them with the main magnetic field more quickly than in the absence of a paramagnetic agent.

Therefore, by increasing the relaxation rate, Gadodiamide decreases both the T_1 and T_2 relaxation times in tissues where it is distributed. At clinical doses, the effect is primarily on the T_1 relaxation time, and produces an increase in signal intensity. Gadodiamide does not cross the intact blood-brain barrier and, therefore, does not accumulate in normal brain or in lesions that do not have an abnormal blood-brain barrier e.g., cysts, mature post-operative scars, etc. However, disruption of the blood-brain barrier or abnormal vascularity allows accumulation of Gadodiamide in lesions such as neoplasms, abscesses, subacute infarcts.

The extended time for Gadodiamide to be accumulated in the lesions is unknown.

INDICATIONS AND USAGE

Gadodiamide is indicated for intravenous administration with magnetic resonance imaging in adult patients to provide contrast enhancement in those central nervous system lesions with abnormal vascularity or those thought to cause abnormalities in the blood-brain barrier. Gadodiamide Injection has been shown to facilitate visualization of central nervous system lesion including but not limited to tumors.

CONTRAINDICATIONS

None known.

WARNINGS

Deoxygenated sickle erythrocytes have been shown to *in vitro* studies to align perpendicular to a magnetic field which may result in vaso-occlusive complications *in vivo*. The enhancement of magnetic moment by Gadodiamide may possibly potentiate sickle erythrocyte alignment. Gadodiamide Injection in patients with sickle cell anemia and other hemoglobinopathies has not been studied.

◆ RATED THERAPEUTICALLY EQUIVALENT; ◇ THERAPEUTIC EQUIVALENCE UNCONFIRMED; ○ UNRATED

Patients with other hemolytic anemias have not been adequately evaluated following administration of Gadodiamide Injection to exclude the possibility of increased hemolysis. Patients with history of allergy or drug reaction should be observed for several hours after drug administration.

PRECAUTIONS
GENERAL
Diagnostic procedures involving the use of contrast agents should be conducted under supervision of a physician with the prerequisite training and a thorough knowledge of the procedure to be performed.

Since Gadodiamide is cleared from the body by glomerular filtration, caution should be exercised in patients with impaired renal function. An alternate route of excretion frequently observed in patients with severe renal impairment receiving iodinated contrast media, is the hepatobiliary enteric pathway, although this has not been demonstrated with Gadodiamide. However, caution should be exercised in patients with renal insufficiency with or without hepatic impairment.

The possibility of a reaction, including serious, life-threatening, fatal, anaphylactoid or cardiovascular reactions or other idiosyncratic reactions should always be considered (see "Adverse Reactions") especially in those patients with a known clinical hypersensitivity.

Gadodiamide should be drawn into the syringe and used immediately. If nondisposable equipment is used, scrupulous care should be taken to prevent residual contamination with traces of cleansing agents.

Repeat Procedures: Data for repeated injections are not available. If the physician determines sequential or repeat examinations are required, a suitable interval of time between administrations should be observed to allow for normal clearance of the drug from the body.

INFORMATION FOR PATIENTS
Patients receiving Gadodiamide should be instructed to:
1. Inform their physician if they are pregnant or breast feeding.
2. Inform their physician if they have anemia or diseases that affect red blood cells.
3. Inform their physician if they have a history of renal or hepatic disease, seizure, asthma or allergic respiratory disorders.

LABORATORY TEST FINDINGS
Asymptomatic transitory changes in serum iron have been observed. The clinical significance is unknown.

CARCINOGENESIS, MUTAGENESIS, IMPAIRMENT OF FERTILITY
No long-term animal studies have been performed to evaluate the carcinogenic potential of Gadodiamide. The results of three *in vitro* and one *in vivo* short-term genotoxicity assays were negative.

PREGNANCY CATEGORY C
Gadodiamide has been shown to increase the incidence of skeletal and visceral abnormalities in the offspring of rabbits administered 0.5 mmol/kg/day (5 times the recommended human dose of 0.1 mmol/kg). This may have been related to maternal toxicity. There are no adequate and well-controlled studies in pregnant women. Gadodiamide should be used during pregnancy only if the potential benefit justifies the potential risk to the fetus.

NURSING MOTHERS
It is not known whether this drug is excreted in human milk. Because many drugs are excreted in human milk, caution should be exercised when Gadodiamide is administered to a nursing woman.

PEDIATRIC USE
Safety and effectiveness of Gadodiamide in children have not been established.

ADVERSE REACTIONS
The most frequent adverse reactions observed in patients during Gadodiamide clinical trials were nausea, headache and dizziness with an incidence of 3% or less. The majority of these adverse reactions were of mild to moderate intensity. The following adverse reactions occurred in less than 1% of the patients:

Body as a Whole: Chest pain, fatigue, fever, rigors, asthenia, hot flushes, malaise, pain.

Cardiovascular: Warmth.

Digestive: Vomiting, abdominal pain, diarrhea, eructation, melena.

Musculoskeletal: Arthralgia.

Nervous System: Paresthesia, convulsion including generalized seizure, abnormal coordination, anorexia, anxiety, syncope, tremor, ataxia, dry mouth, personality disorder, somnolence.

Respiratory System: Rhinitis.

Skin and Appendages: Flushing, pruritus, urticaria, rash erythematous, bruise, erythema, myalgia, skin discoloration, sweating (increased), swelling.

Special Senses: Taste perversion, tinnitus, vision abnormality, taste loss.

Urinary: Renal failure (reversible).

OVERDOSAGE
The minimum lethal dose of intravenously administered Gadodiamide in rats and mice is greater than 20 mmol/kg (200 times the recommended human dose of 10.1 mmol/kg).

DOSAGE AND ADMINISTRATION
The recommended dosage of Gadodiamide is 0.2 mL/kg (0.1 mmol/kg), administered as a bolus intravenous injection. The maximum total dose should not exceed 20 mL. Any unused portion must be discarded.

DOSAGE CHART

Body Weight		Dose
(kg)	(lbs)	(mL)
40	88	8.0
50	110	10.0
60	132	12.0
70	154	14.0
80	176	16.0
90	198	18.0
100	220	20.0

To ensure complete injection of the contrast medium, the injection should be followed by a 5 mL normal saline flush. The imaging procedure should be completed within 1 hour of administration of Gadodiamide.

Parenteral products should be inspected visually for particulate matter and discoloration prior to administration, whenever solution and container permit. Do not use the solution if it is discolored or particulate matter is present.

Gadodiamide should be stored at controlled room temperature 59°F-86°F (15°C-30°C).

Protect from light: Do not freeze. Freezing could cause small cracks in the vials which would compromise the sterility of the product. Do not use if the product is inadvertently frozen.

HOW SUPPLIED
INJECTION:

BRAND/MANUFACTURER	NDC	SIZE	AWP
○ **BRAND**			
OMNISCAN: Sanofi Winthrop	00024-1900-01	10 ml 10s	$711.76
	00024-1920-01	15 ml 10s	$1029.41
	00024-1940-01	20 ml 10s	$1264.71

INJECTION: 287 MG/ML

BRAND/MANUFACTURER	NDC	SIZE	AWP
○ **BRAND**			
OMNISCAN: Sanofi Winthrop	00024-0690-10	10 ml 10s	$682.35
	00024-0690-15	15 ml 10s	$1000.00
	00024-0690-20	20 ml 10s	$1235.29

Gadopentetate Dimeglumine

DESCRIPTION
Gadopentetate Dimeglumine Injection is the N-methylglucamine salt of the gadolinium complex of diethylenetriamine pentaacetic acid, and is an injectable contrast medium for magnetic resonance imaging (MRI). Gadopentetate Dimeglumine is is to be administered by intravenous injection.

Each mL of Gadopentetate Injection contains 469.01 mg of Gadopentetate Dimeglumine.

Gadopentetate Dimeglumine Injection is a 0.5 mol/L solution of 1-deoxy-1-(methylamino)-D-glucitol dihydrogen [N,N-bis[2-[bis(carboxymethyl) amino] ethyl] glycinato-(5-)] gadolinate(2-)(2:1) with a molecular weight of 938.

Gadopentetate Dimeglumine Injection has a pH of 6.5 to 8.0. Pertinent physicochemical data are noted below:

PARAMETER	
Osmolality (mOsmol/kg water) @ 37° C	1,960
Viscosity	
(cP) @ 20° C	4.9
@ 37° C	2.9
Density (g/mL)	1.195

Gadopentetate Dimeglumine Injection has an osmolality 6.9 times that of plasma (285 mOsmol/kg water) and is hypertonic under conditions of use.

Following is its chemical structure:

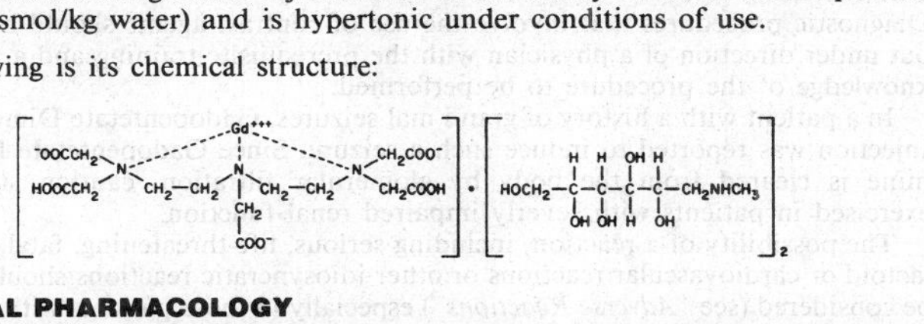

CLINICAL PHARMACOLOGY
The pharmacokinetics of intravenously administered Gadopentetate Dimeglumine in normal subjects conforms to a two compartment open-model with mean distribution and elimination half-lives (reported as mean ± SD) of about 0.2 ± 0.13 hours and 1.6 ± 0.13 hours, respectively. Upon injection, the meglumine salt is completely dissociated from the Gadopentetate Dimeglumine complex. Gadopentetate is exclusively eliminated in the urine with 83 ± 14% (mean ± SD) of the dose excreted within 6 hours, and 91 ± 13% (mean ± SD) by 24 hours, post-

injection. There was no detectable biotransformation or decomposition of Gadopentetate Dimeglumine.

The urinary and plasma clearance rates (1.76 ± 0.39 mL/min/kg 1.94 ± 0.28 mL/min/kg, respectively) of Gadopentetate are essentially identical, indicating no alteration in elimination kinetics on passage through the kidneys and that the drug is essentially cleared through the kidney. The volume of distribution (266 ± 43 mL/kg) is equal to that of extracellular water, and clearance is similar to that of substances which are subject to glomerular filtration.

The extent of protein binding and blood cell partitioning of Gadopentetate Dimeglumine is not known.

Gadopentetate Dimeglumine is a paramagnetic agent and, as such, it develops a magnetic moment when placed in a magnetic field. The relatively large magnetic moment produced by the paramagnetic agent results in a relatively large local magnetic field, which can enhance the relaxation rates of water protons in the vicinity of the paramagnetic agent.

In magnetic resonance imaging (MRI), visualization of normal and pathological brain tissue depends in part on variations in the radiofrequency signal intensity that occur with 1) changes in proton density; 2) alteration of the spin-lattice or longitudinal relaxation time (T1); and 3) variation of the spin-spin or transverse relaxation time (T2). When placed in a magnetic field, Gadopentetate Dimeglumine decreases the T1 and T2 relaxation time in tissues where it accumulates. At usual doses the effect is primarily on the T1 relaxation time.

Gadopentetate Dimeglumine does not cross the intact blood-brain barrier and, therefore, does not accumulate in normal brain or in lesions that do not have an abnormal blood-brain barrier, e.g., cysts, mature postoperative scars, etc. However, disruption of the blood-brain barrier or abnormal vascularity allows accumulation of Gadopentetate Dimeglumine in lesions such as neoplasms, abscesses, subacute infarcts.

INDICATIONS AND USAGE

Gadopentetate Dimeglumine Injection is indicated for use with magnetic resonance imaging (MRI) in adults and children (2 years of age and older) to provide contrast enhancement in those intracranial lesions with abnormal vascularity or those thought to cause an abnormality in the blood-brain barrier. Gadopentetate Dimeglumine Injection has been shown to facilitate visualization of intracranial lesions including but not limited to tumors.

Gadopentetate Dimeglumine Injection is also indicated for use with MRI in adults and children (2 years of age and older) to provide contrast enhancement and facilitate visualization of lesions in the spine and associated tissues. There is, however, only limited clinical experience in children for this indication.

CONTRAINDICATIONS
None known.

WARNINGS

The accepted safety considerations and procedures that are required for magnetic resonance imaging are applicable when Gadopentetate Dimeglumine Injection is used for contrast enhancement. In addition, deoxygenated sickle erythrocytes have been shown in *in vitro* studies to align perpendicular to a magnetic field which may result in vaso-occlusive complications *in vivo*. The enhancement of magnetic moment by Gadopentetate Dimeglumine may possibly potentiate sickle erythrocyte alignment Gadopentetate Dimeglumine Injection in patients with sickle cell anemia and other hemoglobinopathies has not been studied.

Patients with other hemolytic anemias have not been adequately evaluated following administration of Gadopentetate Dimeglumine Injection to exclude the possibility of increased hemolysis.

Hypotension may occur in some patients after injection of Gadopentetate Dimeglumine Injection. In clinical trials two cases were reported and in addition, there was one case of a vasovagal reaction and two cases of pallor with dizziness, sweating and nausea in one and substernal pain and flushing in the other. These were reported within 25 to 85 minutes after injection except for the vasovagal reaction which was described as mild by the patient and occurred after 6-1/2 hours. In a study in normal volunteers one subject experienced syncope after arising from a sitting position two hours after administration of the drug. Although the relationship of Gadopentetate Dimeglumine to these events is uncertain, patients should be observed for several hours after drug administration.

PRECAUTIONS
GENERAL
Diagnostic procedures that involve the use of contrast agents should be carried out under direction of a physician with the prerequisite training and a thorough knowledge of the procedure to be performed.

In a patient with a history of grand mal seizures, Gadopentetate Dimeglumine Injection was reported to induce such a seizure. Since Gadopentetate Dimeglumine is cleared from the body by glomerular filtration, caution should be exercised in patients with severly impaired renal function.

The possibility of a reaction, including serious, life-threatening, fatal, anaphylactoid or cardiovascular reactions or other idiosyncratic reactions should always be considered (see *"Adverse Reactions"*) especially in those patients with a known clinical hypersensitivity or a history of asthma or other allergic respiratory disorders.

Animal studies suggest that Gadopentetate Dimeglumine may alter red cell membrane morphology resulting in a slight degree of extravascular (splenic) hemolysis. In clinical trials 15-30% of the patients experienced an asymptomatic transient rise in serum iron. Serum bilirubin levels were slightly elevated in approximately 3.4% of patients. Levels generally returned to baseline within 24 to

48 hours. Hematocrit and red blood cell count were unaffected and liver enzymes were not elevated in these patients. While the effects of Gadopentetate Dimeglumine on serum iron and bilirubin have not been associated with clinical manifestations, the effect of the drug in patients with hepatic disease is not known and caution is therefore advised.

When Gadopentetate Dimeglumine Injection is to be injected using plastic disposable syringe, the contrast medium should be drawn into the syringe and used immediately.

If nondisposable equipment is used, scrupulous care should be taken to prevent residual contamination with traces of cleansing agents.

Repeat Procedures: If in the clinical judgement of the physician sequential or repeat examinations are required, a suitable interval of time between administrations should be observed to allow for normal clearance of the drug from the body.

Information for Patients: Patients receiving Gadopentetate Dimeglumine Injection should be instructed to:
1. Inform your physician if you are pregnant or breast feeding.
2. Inform your physician if you have anemia or any diseases that affect red blood cells.
3. Inform your physician if you have asthma or other allergic respiratory disorders.

LABORATORY TEST FINDINGS
Transitory changes in serum iron and bilirubin levels have been reported in patients with normal and abnormal liver function (see *"Precautions—General"*).

CARCINOGENESIS, MUTAGENESIS, AND IMPAIRMENT OF FERTILITY
No animal studies have been performed to evaluate the carcinogenic potential of Gadopentetate Dimeglumine.

Gadopentetate Dimeglumine did not evoke any evidence of mutagenic potential in the Ames test (histidine-dependent *Salmonella typhimurium*) nor in a reverse mutation assay using tryptophan-dependent *Escherichia coli*. Gadopentetate Dimeglumine did not induce a positive response in the (C3H 10T1/2) mouse embryo fibroblast cellular transformation assay, nor did not it induce unscheduled DNA repair synthesis in primary cultures of rat hepatocytes at concentrations up to 5000 μg/mL. However, the drug did show some evidence of mutagenic potential *in vivo* in the mouse dominant lethal assay at doses of 6 mmol/kg, but did not show any such potential in the mouse and dog micronucleus tests at intravenous doses of 9 mmol/kg and 2.5 mmol/kg, respectively.

The results of a reproductive study in rats showed that Gadopentetate Dimeglumine when administered in daily doses of 0.1-2.5 mmol/kg, did not cause a significant change in the pregnancy rate in comparison to a control group. However, suppression of body weight gain and food consumption and a decrease in the mean weights of testis and epididymis occurred in male rats at the 2.5 mmol/kg dose. In female rats a decrease in the number of corpora lutea at the 0.1 mmol/kg dose and the suppression of body weight gain and food consumption at the 2.5 mmol/kg dose were observed.

In a separate experiment, 16 daily intravenous injections were administered to male rats. At a dose of 5 mmol/kg of Gadopentetate Dimeglumine, spermatogenic cell atrophy was observed. This atrophy was not reversed within a 16-day observation period following the discontinuation of the drug. This effect was not observed at a dose of 2.5 mmol/kg.

PREGNANCY CATEGORY C.
Gadopentetate Dimeglumine has been shown to retard development slightly in rats when given in doses 2.5 times the human dose, and in rabbits when given in doses of 7.5 and 12.5 times the human dose. The drug did not exhibit this effect in rabbits when given in doses 2.5 times the human dose. No congenital anomalies were noted in either species. There are no adequate and well-controlled studies in pregnant women. Gadopentetate Dimeglumine Injection should be used during pregnancy only if the potential benefit justifies the potential risk to the fetus.

NURSING MOTHERS
C[14] labelled Gadopentetate Dimeglumine was administered intravenously to lactating rats at a dose of 0.5 mmol/kg. Less than 0.2% of the total dose was transferred to the neonate via the milk during the 24-hour evaluation period. It is not known to what extent Gadopentetate Dimeglumine Injection is excreted in human milk. Because many drugs are excreted in human milk, caution should be exercised when the drug is administered to a nursing mother and consideration should be given to temporarily discontinuing nursing.

PEDIATRIC USE
Safety and efficacy in children under the age of 2 years have not been established. (See *"Indications and Usage"* and *"Dosage and Administration"* sections).

ADVERSE REACTIONS
The most commonly noted adverse experience is headache with an incidence of 8.7%. The majority of headaches are transient and of mild to moderate severity. In 42.3% of the cases it was felt that the headaches were not related to Gadopentetate Dimeglumine Injection. Injection site coldness/localized coldness is the second most common adverse experience at 4.8%. Nausea occurs in 3.2% of the patients.

Localized pain, vomiting, paresthesia, dizziness and localized warmth occur in less than 2% of the patients.

The following additional adverse events occur in less than 1% of the patients:

Body as a Whole: Injection site symptoms, namely, pain, warmth, burning; localized burning sensation, substernal chest pain, fever, weakness, generalized coldness, localized edema, tiredness, chest tightness, regional lymphangitis, and anaphylactoid reactions (characterized by cardiovascular, respiratory and cutaneous symptoms) rarely resulting in death.

Cardiovascular: Hypotension, vasodilation, pallor, non-specific ECG changes, angina pectoris, phlebitis.

Digestive: Gastrointestinal distress, stomach pain, teeth pain, increased salivation.

Nervous System: Agitation, thirst, convulsions (including grand mal).

Respiratory System: Throat irritation, rhinorrhea, sneezing, dyspnea, wheezing, laryngismus, cough.

Skin: Rash, sweating, pruritus, urticaria (hives).

Special Senses: Tinnitus, conjunctivitis, visual field defect, taste abnormality, dry mouth, lacrimation disorder (tearing), eye irritation.

Laboratory: Transient elevation of serum transaminases. The following other adverse events were reported. A casual relationship has neither been established nor refuted.

Body as a Whole: Back pain, pain, generalized warmth.

Cardiovascular: Hypertension, tachycardia, migraine, syncope, death related to myocardial infarction or other undetermined causes.

Digestive: Constipation, diarrhea.

Nervous System: Anxiety, anorexia, nystagmus, drowsiness, diplopia, stupor.

Skin: facial edema, erythema multiforme, epidermal necrolysis.

Special Senses: Eye pain, ear pain. Data from foreign studies did not reveal any additional adverse experiences.

OVERDOSAGE

The LD_{50} of intravenously administered Gadopentetate Dimeglumine injection in mice is 5-12.5 mmol/kg and in rats it is 10-15 mmol/kg. The LD_{50} of intravenously administered Gadopentetate Dimeglumine Injection in dogs is greater than 6 mmol/kg.

Clinical consequences of overdose with Gadopentetate Dimeglumine Injection have not been reported.

DOSAGE AND ADMINISTRATION

The recommended dosage of Gadopentetate Dimeglumine Injection is 0.2 mL/kg (0.1 mmol/kg), administered intravenously, at a rate not to exceed 10 mL per minute. More rapid injection rates may be associated with nausea. The maximum total dose is 20 mL. Any unused portion must be discarded.

DOSAGE CHART

Body Weight (kg)	Dose in mL	Approx. Duration of Injection in Seconds
10	2.0	20
20	4.0	30
30	6.0	40
40	8.0	50
50	10.0	60
60	12.0	70
70	14.0	80
80	16.0	95
90	18.0	110
100	20.0	120

To ensure complete injection of the contrast medium, the injection should be followed by a 5-mL normal saline flush. The imaging procedure should be completed within 1 hour of injection of Gadopentetate Dimeglumine Injection.

Parenteral products should be inspected visually for particulate matter and discoloration prior to administration, whenever solution and container permit.

Gadopentetate Dimeglumine Injection should be stored at controlled room temperature, between 15°-30°C (59°-86°F) and protected from light. DO NOT FREEZE. Should solidification occur in the vial because of exposure to the cold. Gadopentetate Dimeglumine Injection should be brought to room temperature before use. If allowed to stand at room temperature for a minimum of 90 minutes, Gadopentetate Dimeglumine Injection will return to a clear, colorless to slightly yellow solution. Before use, examine the product to assure that all solids are redissolved and that the container and closure have not been damaged.

HOW SUPPLIED

Current prices are unavailable. Check wholesaler for further information.

Gadoteridol

DESCRIPTION

Gadoteridol Injection is a nonionic contrast medium for magnetic resonance imaging (MRI), available as a 0.5M sterile clear colorless to slightly yellow aqueous solution in vials for intravenous injection.

Gadoteridol is the gadolinium complex of 10-(2-hydroxypropyl)-1,4,7,10-tetraazacyclododecane-1,4,7-triacetic acid with a molecular weight of 558.7 and an empirical formula of $C_{17}H_{29}N_4O_7Gd$.

Each mL contains 279.3 mg Gadoteridol.

Gadoteridol has a pH of 6.5 to 8.0. Pertinent physicochemical data are noted below:

PARAMETER	
Osmolality (mOsmol/kg water)	
@37°C	630
Viscosity	
(cP) @20°C	2.0
@37°C	1.3
Specific Gravity	
@25°C	1.140

Gadoteridol has an osmolality 2.2 times that of plasma (285 mOsmol/kg water) and is hypertonic under conditions of use.

Following is its chemical structure:

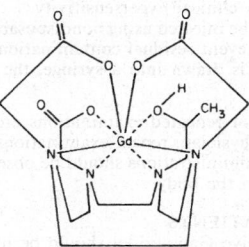

CLINICAL PHARMACOLOGY

The pharmacokinetics of intravenously administered Gadoteridol in normal subjects conforms to a two-compartment open model with mean distribution and elimination half-lives (reported as mean ± SD) of about 0.20 ± 0.04 hours and 1.57 ± 0.08 hours, respectively.

Gadoteridol is eliminated in the urine with 94.4 ± 4.8% (mean ± SD) of the dose excreted within 24 hours post-injection. It is unknown if biotransformation or decomposition of Gadoteridol occurs *in vivo*.

The renal and plasma clearance rates (1.41 ± 0.33 mL/min/kg and 1.50 ± 0.35 mL/min/kg, respectively) of Gadoteridol are essentially identical, indicating no alteration in elimination kinetics on passage through the kidneys and that the drug is essentially cleared through the kidney. The volume of distribution (204 ± 58 mL/kg) is equal to that of extracellular water, and clearance is similar to that of substances which are subject to glomerular filtration.

It is unknown if protein binding of Gadoteridol occurs *in vivo*.

Gadoteridol is a paramagnetic agent and, as such, develops a magnetic moment when placed in a magnetic field. The relatively large magnetic moment produced by the paramagnetic agent results in a relatively large local magnetic field, which can enhance the relaxation rates of water protons in the vicinity of the paramagnetic agent.

In magnetic resonance imaging (MRI), visualization of normal and pathologic brain tissue depends in part on variations in the radiofrequency signal intensity that occur with 1) differences in proton density; 2) differences of the spin-lattice or longitudinal relaxation times (T1); and 3) differences in the spin-spin or transverse relaxation time (T2). When placed in a magnetic field, Gadoteridol decreases T1 relaxation times in the target tissues. At recommended doses, the effect is observed with greatest sensitivity in the T1-weighted sequences.

Gadoteridol does not cross the intact blood-brain barrier and, therefore, does not accumulate in normal brain or in lesions that have a normal blood-brain barrier, e.g., cysts, mature post-operative scars, etc. However, disruption of the blood-brain barrier or abnormal vascularity allows accumulation of Gadoteridol in lesions such as neoplasms, abscesses, and subacute infarcts. The pharmacokinetics of Gadoteridol in various lesions is not known.

INDICATIONS AND USAGE

Using magnetic resonance imaging (MRI), Gadoteridol Injection provides contrast enhancement of the brain, spine and surrounding tissues, resulting in improved visualization (compared with unenhanced MRI) of lesions with abnormal vascularity or those thought to cause a disruption of the normal blood-brain barrier. Gadoteridol Injection has been shown to facilitate visualization of central nervous system lesions, including, but not limited to, tumors.

CONTRAINDICATIONS

None known.

WARNINGS

Deoxygenated sickle erythrocytes have been shown in *in vitro* studies to align perpendicular to a magnetic field which may result in vaso-occlusive complications *in vivo* . The enhancement of magnetic moment by Gadoteridol may possibly potentiate sickle erythrocyte alignment. Gadoteridol in patients with sickle cell anemia and other hemoglobinopathies has not been studied.

Patients with other hemolytic anemias have not been adequately evaluated following administration of Gadoteridol to exclude the possibility of increased hemolysis.

Patients with a history of allergy or drug reaction should be observed for several hours after drug administration.

PRECAUTIONS
GENERAL
Diagnostic procedures that involve the use of contrast agents should be carried out under the direction of a physician with the prerequisite training and a thorough knowledge of the procedure to be performed. In a patient with a history of grand mal seizure, the possibility of inducing such a seizure by Gadoteridol is unknown.

Since Gadoteridol is cleared from the body by glomerular filtration, caution should be exercised in patients with severely impaired renal function. An alternate route of excretion frequently observed in patients with severe renal impairment receiving iodinated contrast media, is the hepato-biliary enteric pathway, although this has not been demonstrated with Gadoteridol. However, caution should be exercised in patients with either renal or hepatic impairment.

The possibility of a reaction, including serious life threatening or fatal anaphylaxis or cardiovascular reactions or other idiosyncratic reactions (see "Adverse Reactions"), should always be considered, especially in those patients with a history of a known clinical hypersensitivity.

When Gadoteridol is to be injected using nondisposable equipment, scrupulous care should be taken to prevent residual contamination with traces of cleansing agents. After Gadoteridol is drawn into a syringe, the solution should be used immediately.

Repeat Procedures: Data for repeated examinations are not available. If in the clinical judgment of the physician, repeat examinations are required, a suitable interval of time between administrations should be observed to allow for normal clearance of the drug from the body.

INFORMATION FOR PATIENTS
Patients scheduled to receive Gadoteridol should be instructed to:
1. Inform their physician if they are pregnant or breast feeding.
2. Inform their physician if they have anemia or diseases that affect the red blood cells.
3. Inform their physician if they have a history of renal or hepatic disease, seizure, asthma or allergic respiratory diseases.

CARCINOGENESIS, MUTAGENESIS, AND IMPAIRMENT OF FERTILITY
No animal studies have been performed to evaluate the carcinogenic potential of Gadoteridol or potential effects on fertility.

Gadoteridol did not demonstrate genotoxic activity in bacterial reverse mutation assays using *Salmonella typhimurium* and *Escherichia coli*, in a mouse lymphoma forward mutation assay, in an *in vitro* cytogenetic assay measuring chromosomal aberration frequencies in Chinese hamster ovary cells, or in an *in vivo* mouse micronucleus assay at intravenous doses as high as 5.0 mmol/kg.

PREGNANCY CATEGORY C
Gadoteridol administered to rats at 10 mmol/kg/day (33 times the maximum recommended human dose of 0.3 mmol/kg) for 12 days during gestation doubled the incidence of postimplantation loss. This may have been related to maternal toxicity.

When rats were administered 6.0 or 10.0 mmol/kg/day for 12 days, an increase in spontaneous locomotor activity was observed in the offspring.

Gadoteridol increased the incidence of spontaneous abortion and early delivery in rabbits administered 6 mmol/kg/day (20 times the maximum recommended human dose) for 13 days during gestation. This may have been related to maternal toxicity.

There are no adequate and well-controlled studies in pregnant women. Gadoteridol Injection should be used during pregnancy only if the potential benefit justifies the potential risk to the fetus.

NURSING MOTHERS
It is not known whether this drug is excreted in human milk. Because many drugs are excreted in human milk, caution should be exercised when Gadoteridol is administered to a nursing woman.

PEDIATRIC USE
Safety and effectiveness of Gadoteridol in children have not been established.

ADVERSE REACTIONS
The most commonly noted adverse experiences were nausea and taste perversion with an incidence of 1.4%. These events were mild to moderate in severity.

The following additional adverse events occurred in fewer than 1% of the patients:

Body as a Whole: Facial edema; neck rigidness; pain; pain at injection site; injection site reaction; chest pain; headache; fever; itching, watery eyes; abdominal cramps; tingling sensation in throat; laryngismus; flushed feeling; vasovagal reaction; anaphylactoid reactions (characterized by cardiovascular, respiratory and cutaneous symptoms)

Cardiovascular: Prolonged P-R interval; hypotension; elevated heart rate; A-V nodal rhythm

Digestive: Edema-tongue; gingivitis; dry mouth; loose bowel; vomiting; itching tongue

Nervous System: Anxiety; dizziness; paresthesia; mental status decline; loss of coordination in arm; staring episode; seizure; syncope

Respiratory System: Dyspnea; rhinitis; cough

Skin and Appendages: Pruritus; rash; rash macular, papular; urticaria; hives; tingling sensation of extremity and digits

Special Senses: Tinnitus

OVERDOSAGE
The minimal lethal single dose of Gadoteridol in mice was found to be between 7 and 10 mmol/kg (23 to 33 times the maximum recommended human dose of 0.3 mmol/kg). Overt clinical signs noted prior to death included ataxia, convulsions, collapse, bloody exudate from nares and decreased activity. Gadoteridol Injection was not lethal to rats at single doses up to 10 mmol/kg.

DOSAGE AND ADMINISTRATION
The recommended dose of Gadoteridol is 0.1 mmol/kg (0.2 mL/kg) administered as a rapid intravenous infusion or bolus. However, in patients suspected of having cerebral metastases or other poorly enhancing lesions, in the presence of negative or equivocal scans, after 0.1 mmol/kg injection, at the clinician's discretion, a second dose of 0.2 mmol/kg (0.4 mL/kg) can be administered up to 30 minutes after the first dose for further evaluation. Any unused portion must be discarded.

To ensure complete injection of the contrast medium, the injection should be followed by a 5 mL normal saline flush. The imaging procedure should be completed within 1 hour of the first injection of Gadoteridol.

Parenteral products should be inspected visually for particulate matter and discoloration prior to administration. Do not use the solution if it is discolored or particulate matter is present.

Gadoteridol should be stored at controlled room temperature, between 15° and 30° C (59°–86° F) and protected from light. Do not freeze. Should freezing occur in the vial, Gadoteridol should be brought to room temperature before use. If allowed to stand at room temperature for a minimum of 60 minutes, Gadoteridol should return to a clear, colorless to slightly yellow solution. Before use, examine the product to assure that all solids are redissolved and that the container and closure have not been damaged. Should solids persist, discard vial.

HOW SUPPLIED
INJECTION: 279.3 MG/ML

BRAND/MANUFACTURER	NDC	SIZE	AWP
○ BRAND			
PROHANCE: Bracco Diag	00003-1111-04	5 ml 5s	$189.06
	00003-1111-01	10 ml 5s	$370.94
	00003-1111-02	15 ml 5s	$542.81
	00003-1111-03	20 ml 5s	$670.31

Gallium Nitrate

> ### WARNING
> CONCURRENT USE OF GALLIUM NITRATE WITH OTHER POTENTIALLY NEPHROTOXIC DRUGS (E.G., AMINOGLYCOSIDES, AMPHOTERICIN B) MAY INCREASE THE RISK FOR DEVELOPING SEVERE RENAL INSUFFICIENCY IN PATIENTS WITH CANCER-RELATED HYPERCALCEMIA. IF USE OF A POTENTIALLY NEPHROTOXIC DRUG IS INDICATED DURING GALLIUM NITRATE THERAPY, GALLIUM NITRATE ADMINISTRATION SHOULD BE DISCONTINUED AND IT IS RECOMMENDED THAT HYDRATION BE CONTINUED FOR SEVERAL DAYS AFTER ADMINISTRATION OF THE POTENTIALLY NEPHROTOXIC DRUG. SERUM CREATININE AND URINE OUTPUT SHOULD BE CLOSELY MONITORED DURING AND SUBSEQUENT TO THIS PERIOD. GALLIUM NITRATE THERAPY SHOULD BE DISCONTINUED IF THE SERUM CREATININE LEVEL EXCEEDS 2.5 MG/DL.

DESCRIPTION
Gallium Nitrate injection is a clear, colorless, odorless, sterile, solution of Gallium Nitrate, a hydrated Nitrate salt of the group IIIa element, Gallium. Gallium Nitrate is formed by the reaction of elemental Gallium with nitric acid, followed by crystallization of the drug from the solution. The stable, nonanhydrate, $[Ga(NO_3)_3 \cdot 9(H_2O)]$ is a white, slightly hygroscopic, crystalline powder of molecular weight 417.87, that is readily soluble in water.

Each mL of Gallium Nitrate injection contains 25mg of Gallium Nitrate.

Following is its chemical structure:

$$Ga(NO_3)_3 \cdot 9H_2O$$

CLINICAL PHARMACOLOGY
MECHANISM OF ACTION
Gallium Nitrate exerts a hypocalcemic effect by inhibiting calcium resorption from bone, possibly by reducing increased bone turnover. Although *in vitro* and

animal studies have been performed to investigate the mechanism of action of Gallium Nitrate, the precise mechanism for inhibiting calcium resorption has not been determined. No cytotoxic effects were observed on bone cells in drug-treated animals.

PHARMACOKINETICS

Gallium Nitrate was infused at a daily dose of 200 mg/m^2 for 5 (n=2) or 7 (n=10) consecutive days to 12 cancer patients. In most patients, apparent steady-state is achieved by 24 to 48 hours. The range of average steady-state plasma levels of Gallium observed among 7 fully evaluable patients was between 1134 and 2399 ng/mL. The average plasma clearance of Gallium (n=7) following daily infusion of Gallium Nitrate at a dose of 200 mg/m^2 for 5 or 7 days was 0.15 L/hr/kg (range: 0.12 to 0.20 L/hr/kg). In one patient who received daily infusion doses of 100, 150 and 200 mg/m^2, the apparent steady-state levels of Gallium did not increase proportionally with an increase in dose. Gallium Nitrate is not metabolized either by the liver or the kidney and appears to be significantly excreted via the kidney. Urinary excretion data for a dose of 200 mg/m^2 has not been determined.

CANCER-RELATED HYPERCALCEMIA

Hypercalcemia is a common problem in hospitalized patients with malignancy. It may affect 10-20% of patients with cancer. Different types of malignancy seem to vary in their propensity to cause hypercalcemia. A higher incidence of hypercalcemia has been observed in patients with non-small-cell lung cancer, breast cancer, multiple myeloma, kidney cancer, and cancer of head and neck. Hypercalcemia of malignancy seems to result from an imbalance between the net resorption of bone and urinary excretion of calcium. Patients with extensive osteolytic bone metastases frequently develop hypercalcemia; this type of hypercalcemia is common with primary breast cancer. Some of these patients have been reported to have increased renal tubular calcium resorption. Breast cancer cells have been reported to produce several potential bone-resorbing factors which stimulate the local osteoclast activity. Humoral hypercalcemia is common with the solid tumors of the lung, head and neck, kidney, and ovaries. Systemic factors (e.g., PTH-rP) produced either by the tumor or host cells have been implicated in the altered calcium fluxes between the extracellular fluid, the kidney, and the skeleton. About 30% of patients with myeloma develop hypercalcemia associated with extensive osteolytic lesions and impaired glomerular filtration. Myeloma cells have been reported to produce local factors that stimulate adjacent osteoclasts.

Hypercalcemia may produce a spectrum of signs and symptoms including: anorexia, lethargy, fatigue, nausea, vomiting, constipation, dehydration, renal insufficiency, impaired mental status, coma and cardiac arrest. A rapid rise in serum calcium may cause more severe symptoms for a given level of hypercalcemia. Since calcium is bound to serum proteins, which may fluctuate in concentration as a response to changes in blood volume, changes in total serum calcium (especially during rehydration) may not accurately reflect changes in the concentration of free-ionized calcium. In the absence of a direct measurement of free-ionized calcium, measurement of the serum albumin concentration and correction of the total serum calcium concentration may help in assessing the severity of hypercalcemia. The patient's acid-base status should also be taken into consideration while assessing the degree of hypercalcemia. Mild or asymptomatic hypercalcemia may be treated with conservative measures (i.e., saline hydration, with or without diuretics). The patient's cardiovascular status should be taken into consideration in the use of saline. In patients who have an underlying cancer type that may be sensitive to corticosteroids (e.g., hematologic cancers), the use or addition of corticosteroid therapy may be indicated.

HYPOCALCEMIC ACTIVITY

A randomized double-blind clinical study comparing Gallium Nitrate with calcitonin was conducted in patients with a serum calcium concentration (corrected for albumin) $\geq$ 12.0 mg/dL following 2 days of hydration. Gallium Nitrate was given as a continuous intravenous infusion at a dose of 200 mg/m^2 for 5 days and calcitonin was given intramuscularly at a dose of 8 I.U./kg every 6 hours for 5 days. Elevated serum calcium (corrected for albumin) was normalized in 75% (18 of 24) of the patients receiving Gallium Nitrate and in 27% (7 of 26) of the patients receiving calcitonin (p=0.0016). The time-course effect on serum calcium (corrected for albumin) is summarized in the following table.

CHANGE IN CORRECTED SERUM CALCIUM BY TIME FROM INITIATION OF TREATMENT

Time Period[1] (hours)	Mean Change in Serum Calcium (mg/dL)[2]	
	Gallium Nitrate	Calcitonin
24	−0.4	−1.6*
48	−0.9	−1.4
72	−1.5	−1.1
96	−2.9*	−1.1
120	−3.3*	−1.3

[1] Time after initiation of therapy in hours.
[2] Change from baseline in serum calcium (corrected for albumin).
* Comparison between treatment groups (p < 0.01).

The median duration of normocalcemia/hypocalcemia was 7.5 days for patients treated with Gallium Nitrate and 1 day for patients treated with calcitonin. A total of 92% of patients treated with Gallium Nitrate had a decrease in serum calcium (corrected for albumin) $\geq$ 2.0 mg/dL as compared to 54% of the patients treated with calcitonin (p=0.004).

An open-label, non-randomized study was conducted to examine a range of doses and dosing schedules of Gallium Nitrate for control of cancer-related hypercalcemia. The principal dosing regimens were 100 and 200 mg/m^2/day, administered as continuous intravenous infusions for 5 days. Gallium Nitrate at a dose of 200 mg/m^2/day for 5 days was found to normalize elevated serum calcium levels (corrected for albumin) in 83% of patients as compared to 50% of patients receiving a dose of 100 mg/m^2/day for 5 days. A decrease in serum calcium (corrected for albumin) $\geq$ 2.0 mg/dL was observed in 83% and 94% of patients treated with Gallium Nitrate at dosages of 100 and 200 mg/m^2/day for 5 days, respectively. There were no significant differences in the proportion of patients responding to Gallium Nitrate when considering either the presence or absence of bone metastasis, or whether the tumor histology was epidermoid or nonepidermoid.

INDICATIONS AND USAGE

Gallium Nitrate is indicated for the treatment of clearly symptomatic cancer-related hypercalcemia that has not responded to adequate hydration. In general, patients with a serum calcium (corrected for albumin) < 12 mg/dL would not be expected to be symptomatic. Mild or asymptomatic hypercalcemia may be treated with conservative measures (i.e., saline hydration, with or without diuretics). In the treatment of cancer-related hypercalcemia, it is important first to establish adequate hydration, preferably with intravenous saline, in order to increase the renal excretion of calcium and correct dehydration caused by hypercalcemia.

CONTRAINDICATIONS

Gallium Nitrate should not be administered to patients with severe renal impairment (serum creatinine > 2.5 mg/dL).

WARNINGS

(see boxed "Warning").

The hypercalcemic state in cancer patients is commonly associated with impaired renal function. Abnormalities in renal function (elevated BUN and/or serum creatinine) have been observed in clinical trials with Gallium Nitrate. *It is strongly recommended that serum creatinine be monitored during Gallium Nitrate therapy.* Since patients with cancer-related hypercalcemia are frequently dehydrated, it is important that such patients be adequately hydrated with oral and/or intravenous fluids (preferably saline) and that a satisfactory urine output (2 L/day is recommended) be established before therapy with Gallium Nitrate is started. Adequate hydration should be maintained throughout the treatment period, with careful attention to avoid overhydration in patients with compromised cardiovascular status. Diuretic therapy should not be employed prior to correction of hypovolemia. Gallium Nitrate therapy should be discontinued if the serum creatinine level exceeds 2.5 mg/dL.

The use of Gallium Nitrate in patients with marked renal insufficiency (serum creatinine > 2.5 mg/dL) has not been systematically examined. If therapy is undertaken in patients with moderately impaired renal function (serum creatinine 2.0 to 2.5 mg/dL), frequent monitoring of the patient's renal status is recommended. Treatment should be discontinued if the serum creatinine level exceeds 2.5 mg/dL.

Combined use of Gallium Nitrate with other potentially nephrotoxic drugs (e.g., aminoglycosides, amphotericin B) may increase the risk for developing renal insufficiency in patients with cancer-related hypercalcemia (see boxed "Warnings").

PRECAUTIONS

GENERAL

Asymptomatic or mild to moderate hypocalcemia (6.5-8.0 mg/dL, corrected for serum albumin) occurred in approximately 38% of patients treated with Gallium Nitrate in a controlled clinical trial. One patient exhibited a positive Chvostek's sign. If hypocalcemia occurs, Gallium Nitrate therapy should be stopped and short-term calcium therapy may be necessary.

LABORATORY TESTS

Renal function (serum creatinine and BUN) and serum calcium must be closely monitored during Gallium Nitrate therapy. In addition to baseline assessment, the suggested frequency of calcium and phosphorus determinations is daily and twice weekly, respectively. Gallium Nitrate should be discontinued if the serum creatinine exceeds 2.5 mg/dL.

DRUG INTERACTIONS

The concomitant use of highly nephrotoxic drugs in combination with Gallium Nitrate may increase the risk for development of renal insufficiency (see "Warnings"). Available information does not indicate any adverse interaction with diuretics such as furosemide.

CARCINOGENESIS, MUTAGENESIS, IMPAIRMENT OF FERTILITY

Long-term studies in animals have not been performed to evaluate the carcinogenic potential of Gallium Nitrate. Gallium Nitrate is not mutagenic in standard tests (i.e., Ames test and chromosomal aberration studies on human lymphocytes).

USE IN PREGNANCY

PREGNANCY CATEGORY C

Animal reproduction studies have not been conducted with Gallium Nitrate. It is also not known whether Gallium Nitrate can cause fetal harm when administered to a pregnant woman or can affect reproductive capacity. Gallium Nitrate should be administered to a pregnant woman only if clearly needed.

NURSING MOTHERS

It is not known whether Gallium Nitrate is excreted in human milk. Because of the potential for serious adverse reactions in nursing infants from Gallium Nitrate, a decision should be made whether to discontinue nursing or discontinue the drug, taking into account the importance of the drug to the mother.

PEDIATRIC USE

The safety and effectiveness of Gallium Nitrate in children have not been established.

ADVERSE REACTIONS
KIDNEY

Adverse renal effects, as demonstrated by rising BUN and creatinine, have been reported in about 12.5% of patients treated with Gallium Nitrate. In a controlled clinical trial of patients with cancer-related hypercalcemia, two patients receiving Gallium Nitrate and one patient receiving calcitonin developed acute renal failure. Due to the serious nature of the patients' underlying conditions, the relationship of these events to the drug was unclear. Gallium Nitrate should not be administered to patients with serum creatinine > 2.5 mg/dL (see "Contraindications" and "Warnings").

METABOLIC

Hypocalcemia may occur after Gallium Nitrate treatment (see "Precautions").

PRECAUTIONS

Transient hypophosphatemia of mild-to-moderate degree may occur in up to 79% of hypercalcemic patients following treatment with Gallium Nitrate. In a controlled clinical trial, 33% of patients had at least 1 serum phosphorus measurement between 1.5-2.4 mg/dL, while 46% of patients had at least 1 serum phosphorus value < 1.5 mg/dL. Severe hypophosphatemia was also reported in 7% of patients in controlled clincial trials (see "Warnings"). Patients who develop hypophosphatemia may require oral phosphorus therapy.

Decreased serum bicarbonate, possibly secondary to mild respiratory alkalosis, was reported in 40-50% of cancer patients treated with Gallium Nitrate. The cause for this effect is not clear. This effect has been asymptomatic and has not required specific treatment.

HEMATOLOGIC

The use of very high doses of Gallium Nitrate (up to 1400 mg/m^2) in treating patients for advanced cancer has been associated with anemia, and several patients have received red blood cell transfusions. Due to the serious nature of the underlying illness, it is uncertain whether the anemia was caused by Gallium Nitrate.

BLOOD PRESSURE

A decrease in mean systolic and diastolic blood pressure was observed several days after treatment with Gallium Nitrate in a controlled clinical trial. The decrease in blood pressure was asymptomatic and did not require specific treatment.

VISUAL AND AUDITORY

In cancer chemotherapy trials, a small proportion (< 1%) of patients treated with multiple high doses of Gallium Nitrate combined with other investigational anticancer drugs, have developed acute optic neuritis. While these patients were critically ill and had received multiple drugs, a reaction to high-dose Gallium Nitrate is possible. Most patients had full visual recovery; however, at least one case of persistent visual impairment has been reported. One patient with cancer-related hypercalcemia was reported to develop decreased hearing following Gallium Nitrate administration. Due to the patient's underlying condition and concurrent therapies, the relationship of this event to Gallium Nitrate administration is unclear. Tinnitus and partial loss of auditory acuity have been reported rarely (<1%) in patients who received high-dose Gallium Nitrate as anticancer treatment.

MISCELLANEOUS

Other clinical events reported in association with Gallium Nitrate treatment for cancer as well as cancer-related hypercalcemia include: nausea and/or vomiting, tachycardia, lethargy, confusion, diarrhea, constipation, lower extremity edema, hypothermia, fever, dyspnea, rales and rhonchi, anemia, leukopenia, paresthesia, skin rash, pleural effusion, pulmonary infiltrates, and seizures. Due to the serious nature of the underlying condition of these patients, the relationship of these events to therapy with Gallium Nitrate is unknown.

OVERDOSAGE

Rapid intravenous infusion of Gallium Nitrate or use of doses higher than recommended (200 mg/m^2) may cause nausea and vomiting and a substantially increased risk of renal insufficiency. In the event of overdosage, further drug administration should be discontinued, serum calcium should be monitored, and the patient should receive vigorous intravenous hydration, with or without diuretics, for 2-3 days. During this time period, renal function and urinary output should be carefully monitored so that fluid intake and output are balanced.

DOSAGE AND ADMINISTRATION

The usual recommended dose of Gallium Nitrate is 200 mg per square meter of body surface area (200 mg/m^2) daily for 5 consecutive days. In patients with mild hypercalcemia and few symptoms, a lower dosage of 100 mg/m^2/day for 5 days may be considered. If serum calcium levels are lowered into the normal range in less than 5 days, treatment may be discontinued early. The daily dose must be administered as an intravenous infusion over 24 hours. The daily dose should be diluted, preferably in 1,000 mL of 0.9% Sodium Chloride injection, USP, or 5% Dextrose Injection, USP, for administration as an intravenous infusion over 24 hours. Adequate hydration must be maintained throughout the treatment period, with careful attention to avoid overhydration in patient with compromised cardiovascular status. Controlled studies have not been undertaken to evaluate the safety and effectiveness of retreatment with Gallium Nitrate.

When Gallium Nitrate is added to either 0.9% sodium chloride injection, USP, or 5% dextrose injection, USP, it is stable for at least 48 hours at room temperature (15°-30°C) and for seven (7) days if stored under refrigeration (2°-8°C). Parenteral drug products should be inspected visually for particulate matter and discoloration prior to administration whenever solution and container permit.

Store at controlled room temperature 15°-30°C (59°-86°F).
Contains no preservative. Discard unused portion.

HOW SUPPLIED
INJECTION: 500 MG/ML

BRAND/MANUFACTURER	NDC	SIZE	AWP
○ BRAND			
GANITE: Fujisawa	57317-0243-20	20 ml	$102.66

Gamastan *SEE* GLOBULIN, IMMUNE

Gamimune *SEE* GLOBULIN, IMMUNE

Gammagard S/D *SEE* GLOBULIN, IMMUNE

Gammar *SEE* GLOBULIN, IMMUNE

Gamulin Rh *SEE* GLOBULIN, IMMUNE RHO$_O$(D) *AND* RH$_O$(D) IMMUNE GLOBULIN

Ganciclovir Sodium

> THE CLINICAL TOXICITY OF GANCICLOVIR SODIUM INCLUDES GRANULOCYTOPENIA AND THROMBOCYTOPENIA. IN ANIMAL STUDIES GANCICLOVIR SODIUM WAS CARCINOGENIC, TERATOGENIC, AND CAUSED ASPERMATOGENESIS. GANCICLOVIR SODIUM IS INDICATED FOR USE *ONLY* IN THE TREATMENT OF CYTOMEGALOVIRUS (CMV) RETINITIS IN IMMUNOCOMPROMISED PATIENTS AND FOR THE PREVENTION OF CMV DISEASE IN TRANSPLANT PATIENTS AT RISK FOR CMV DISEASE. (SEE "INDICATIONS AND USAGE" SECTION.)

DESCRIPTION

Ganciclovir Sodium is an antiviral drug active against cytomegalovirus. Reconstituted Ganciclovir Sodium Sterile Powder is for intravenous administration only. Each vial of Ganciclovir Sodium Sterile Powder contains the equivalent of 500 mg Ganciclovir as the sodium salt (46 mg sodium). Reconstitution with 10 mL of Sterile Water for Injection, USP, yields a solution with pH 11 and a Ganciclovir Sodium concentration of approximately 50 mg/mL. Further dilution in an appropriate intravenous solution must be performed before infusion (see "Dosage and Administration" section). All doses in this insert are specified in terms of Ganciclovir Sodium. The chemical name of Ganciclovir Sodium is 9-(1,3-dihydroxy-2-propoxymethyl) guanine, monosodium salt, with a molecular formula of $C_9H_{12}N_5NaO_4$ and a molecular weight of 277.21.

Ganciclovir Sodium, as a white lyophilized powder, has an aqueous solubility of greater than 50 mg/mL at 25°C. At physiological pH, Ganciclovir Sodium exists as the unionized form with an aqueous solubility of 3.65 mg/mL at 25°C.

Following is its chemical structure:

◆ RATED THERAPEUTICALLY EQUIVALENT; ◇ THERAPEUTIC EQUIVALENCE UNCONFIRMED; ○ UNRATED

CLINICAL PHARMACOLOGY
VIROLOGY
Mechanism of Action: Ganciclovir Sodium is a synthetic nucleoside analogue of 2'-deoxyguanosine that inhibits replication of herpes viruses both *in vitro* and *in vivo*. Sensitive human viruses include cytomegalovirus (CMV), herpes simplex virus -1 and -2 (HSV-1, HSV-2), Epstein-Barr virus (EBV) and varicella zoster virus (VZV). Clinical studies have been limited to assessment of efficacy in patients with CMV infection. Available evidence indicates that upon entry into host cells, cytomegaloviruses induce one or more cellular kinases that phosphorylate Ganciclovir to its triphosphate. It has been shown that there is approximately a 10-fold greater concentration of Ganciclovir-triphosphate in CMV-infected cells than in uninfected cells, indicating a preferential phosphorylation of Ganciclovir in virus-infected cells. *In vitro*, Ganciclovir-triphosphate is catabolized slowly, with 60 to 70% of the original level remaining in the infected cells 18 hours after removal of Ganciclovir from the extracellular medium.[1] The antiviral activity of Ganciclovir-triphosphate is believed to be the result of inhibition of viral DNA synthesis by two known modes: (1) competitive inhibition of viral DNA polymerases (2) direct incorporation into viral DNA, resulting in eventual termination of viral DNA, resulting in eventual termination of viral DNA elongation. The cellular DNA polymerase alpha is also inhibited, but at a higher concentration than required for viral DNA polymerase.

Antiviral Activity: Median effective inhibitory doses (ED_{50}) of Ganciclovir Sodium for human CMV isolates tested *in vitro* in several cell lines ranged from 0.2 to 3.0 µg/mL. The relationship between *in vitro* sensitivity of CMV to Ganciclovir Sodium and clinical response has not been established. Ganciclovir Sodium inhibits mammalian cell proliferation *in vitro* at higher concentrations (10 to 60 µg/mL) with bone marrow colony forming cells being the most sensitive ($ID_{50} \geq 10$ µg/mL) of those cell types tested.

Ganciclovir Sodium has shown antiviral activity *in vivo* in several animal CMV infection models. Both normal and immuno-suppressed mice had reduced titers of murine CMV when treated with Ganciclovir Sodium at 5 to 50 mg/kg/day.[2] Normal mice had increased survival as well, when treated with doses of 3 mg/kg/day. Immunosuppressed mice did not show increased survival until they received doses of at least 10 mg/kg/day.[3] In guinea pigs infected with cavian CMV and treated with Ganciclovir Sodium at 50 mg/kg/day for 7 days, viral titers in the salivary glands were reduced approximately 50% at day 28 post-infection as compared to sham-treated controls.[4]

Of 314 immunocompromised patients enrolled in an open label study of the treatment of life- or sight-threatening CMV disease, 121 patients were identified who had a positive culture for CMV within 7 days prior to treatment and had sequential viral cultures after treatment with Ganciclovir Sodium.[5] Post-treatment virologic response was defined as conversion to culture negativity, or a greater than 100-fold decrease in CMV infectious units, as shown in the following table:

VIROLOGIC RESPONSE

Culture Source	No. Patients Cultured	No. (%) Patients Responding	Median Days to Response
Urine	107	93 (87)	8
Blood	41	34 (83)	8
Throat	21	19 (90)	7
Semen	6	6 (100)	15

The antiviral activity of Ganciclovir Sodium has been confirmed in two separate placebo-controlled studies for the prevention of CMV disease in transplant recipients. One hundred forty-nine CMV seropositive heart allograft[6] recipients were randomized to treatment with Ganciclovir Sodium (5 mg/kg BID for 14 days followed by 6 mg/kg QD for 5 days/week for an additional 14 days) or placebo. Seventy-two CMV culture positive allogeneic bone marrow[7] transplant recipients were randomized to treatment with Ganciclovir Sodium (5 mg/kg BID for 7 days followed by 5 mg/kg QD) or placebo until day 100 post-transplant. Ganciclovir Sodium prevented recrudescence of CMV shedding in heart allograft recipients and suppressed CMV shedding in bone marrow allograft recipients. The antiviral effect of Ganciclovir Sodium in these patients is summarized in the following table: (See related table).

Viral Resistance: Viral resistance has been observed with appreciable frequency ($\geq$ 8%) in patients receiving prolonged treatment with Ganciclovir Sodium.[9,10] There is also a possibility that some patients may be infected with strains of CMV that are resistant to Ganciclovir prior to treatment with Ganciclovir Sodium.[8] In one report, 72 AIDS patients treated with Ganciclovir Sodium were prospectively monitored for viral shedding and drug resistance (defined as $ID_{50} \geq 3.0$ µg/mL).[8] All patients were shedding Ganciclovir Sodium sensitive CMV pre-treatment. During 7 months of therapy with Ganciclovir Sodium, approximately 80% of patients were culture negative and 20% continued to shed CMV. No resistant CMV strains were isolated during the first 3 months of treatment. After 3 months,

38% of patients shedding CMV (7.6% of all treated patients) had resistant strains isolated, all of which were associated with clinical progression of CMV retinitis. Therefore, the possibility of viral resistance should be considered in patients who show poor clinical response or experience persistent viral excretion during therapy.

PHARMACOKINETICS
The pharmacokinetics of Ganciclovir Sodium have been evaluated in immuno-compromised adults with serious CMV disease. The Pharmacokinetics of Ganciclovir Sodium in children are under investigation. Twenty-two adults with normal renal function, enrolled in open-label treatment at different study centers, received 5 mg/kg doses of Ganciclovir Sodium each dose infused intravenously over one hour. The plasma level of Ganciclovir Sodium at the end of the first one hour infusion (Cmax) was 8.3 ± 4.0 µg/mL (mean ± SD) and the plasma level 11 hours after the start of infusion (Cmin) was 0.56 ± 0.66 µg/mL. The plasma half-life was 2.9 ± 1.3 hours and the systemic clearance was 3.64 ± 1.86 mL/kg/min (approximately 250 mL/min/$1.73M^2$). Dose-independent kinetics were demonstrated over the range of 1.6 to 5.0 mg/kg. Multiple-dose kinetics were measured in eight patients with normal renal function who received Ganciclovir Sodium 5 mg/kg twice daily for 12-14 days. After the first dose and after multiple dosing, plasma levels of Ganciclovir at the end of infusion were 7.1 µg/mL (3.1 to 14.0 µg/mL) and 9.5 µg/mL (2.7 to 24.2 µg/mL), respectively. At 7 hours after infusion, plasma levels after the first dose were 0.85 µg/mL (0.2 to 1.8 µg/mL) and were 1.2 µg/mL (0.6 to 1.8 µg/mL) after multiple dosing.

Renal excretion of unchanged drug by glomerular filtration is the major route of elimination of Ganciclovir Sodium. In patients with normal renal function, more than 90% of the administered Ganciclovir Sodium was recovered unmetabolized in the urine. The pharmacokinetic analysis in 10 patients with renal impairment showed that in 4 patients with mild impairment (creatinine clearance 50 to 79 mL/min/$1.73M^2$) the systemic clearance of Ganciclovir Sodium was 128 ± 63 mL/min/$1.73M^2$, and the plasma half-life was 4.6 ± 1.4 hours. In 3 patients with moderate impairment (creatinine clearance 25 to 49 mL/min/$1.73M^2$) the systemic clearance of Ganciclovir Sodium was 57 ± 8 mL/min/$1.73M^2$, and the plasma half-life was 4.4 ± 0.4 hours. In 3 patients with severe impairment (creatinine clearance less than 25 mL/min/$1.73M^2$) the systemic clearance was 30 ± 13 mL/min/$1.73M^2$, and the plasma half-life was 10.7 ± 5.7 hours. There was positive correlation between systemic clearance of Ganciclovir Sodium and creatinine clearance (r = 0.90).

Data from 4 patients with severe renal impairment showed that hemodialysis reduced plasma drug levels by approximately 50%.

BECAUSE THE MAJOR EXCRETION PATHWAY FOR GANCICLOVIR SODIUM IS RENAL, DOSAGE MUST BE REDUCED ACCORDING TO CREATININE CLEARANCE. FOR DOSING INSTRUCTIONS IN RENAL IMPAIRMENT, REFER TO THE SECTION ON *"Dosage and Administration."*

There is limited evidence to suggest that Ganciclovir crosses the blood-brain barrier. Cerebrospinal fluid (CSF) concentrations have been measured in three patients who received 2.5 mg/kg Ganciclovir intravenously q8 or q12 hours. The results are shown in the following table:

CSF CONCENTRATIONS[11,12]

Patient	CSF Conc. (µg/mL)	Plasma Conc. (µg/mL)	Hr after dose	CSF/Plasma Ratio
1	0.62	0.92*	5.67	.67
	0.68	2.20	3.5	.31
	0.51	1.96	2.75	.26
2	0.50	2.05*	0.25	.24
3	0.31	0.44	5.5	.70

* *Estimation (model-predicted values)*

Binding of Ganciclovir Sodium to plasma proteins is 1-2%. Drug interactions involving binding site displacement are not expected.

INDICATIONS AND USAGE
Ganciclovir Sodium is indicated for the treatment of CMV retinitis in immuno-compromised individuals, including patients with acquired immunodeficiency syndrome (AIDS) Ganciclovir Sodium is also indicated for the prevention of CMV disease in transplant patients at risk for CMV disease (See *"Clinical Trials"* section below). SAFETY AND EFFICACY OF GANCICLOVIR SODIUM HAVE NOT BEEN ESTABLISHED FOR CONGENITAL OR NEONATAL CMV DISEASE; NOR FOR TREATMENT OF ESTABLISHED CMV DISEASE OTHER THAN RETINITIS (SUCH AS PNEUMONITIS OR COLITIS); NOR FOR USE IN NONIMMUNOCOMPROMISED INDIVI- DUALS.

The diagnosis of CMV retinitis is ophthalmologic and should be made by indirect ophthalmoscopy. Other conditions in the differential diagnosis of CMV retinitis include candidiasis, toxoplasmosis, histoplasmosis, retinal scars, and cotton wool spots, any of which may produce a retinal appearance similar to

PATIENTS WITH POSITIVE CMV CULTURES

Time	Heart Allograft		Bone Marrow Allograft	
	Ganciclovir Sodium	Placebo	Ganciclovir Sodium	Placebo
Pre-Treatment	2% (1/67)	8% (5/64)	100% (37/37)	100% (35/35)
Week 2	3% (2/75)	16% (11/67)	6% (2/31)	68% (19/28)
Week 4	5% (3/66)	43% (28/66)	0% (0/24)	80% (16/20)

CMV. For this reason it is essential that the diagnosis of CMV be established by an ophthalmologist familiar with the retinal presentation of these conditions. The diagnosis of CMV retinitis may be supported by culture of CMV from urine, blood, throat, or other sites, but a negative CMV culture does not rule out CMV retinitis.

UNLABELED USES

Ganciclovir Sodium is used alone or as an adjunct to reduce the incidence of cytomegalovirus disease in bone marrow and liver transplant patients. It is also used in the treatment of gastrointestinal cytomegalovirus infections in AIDS patients and in combination with immune globulin to treat cytomegalovirus pneumonia.

CLINICAL TRIALS

1. CMV RETINITIS
In a retrospective, nonrandomized, single-center analysis[13,14] of 41 patients with AIDS and CMV retinitis, treatment with Ganciclovir Sodium resulted in a significant delay in median to first retinitis progression compared to untreated controls (71 days from diagnosis versus 29 days from diagnosis). Patients in this series received induction treatment of Ganciclovir Sodium 5 mg/kg BID for 14-21 days followed by maintenance treatment with either 5 mg/kg once per day, seven days per week or 6 mg/kg once per day, five days each week. (See "Dosage and Administration" section.)

2. PREVENTION OF CMV DISEASE IN TRANSPLANT RECIPIENTS
Ganciclovir Sodium was evaluated in three randomized, controlled trials of prevention of CMV disease in organ transplant recipients.

ICM 1496: In a randomized, double-blind, placebo-controlled study of 149 heart transplant recipients[6] at risk for CMV infection (CMV seropositive, or a seronegative recipient of an organ from a CMV seropositive donor), there was a statistically significant reduction in the overall incidence of CMV disease in patients treated with Ganciclovir Sodium. Immediately post-transplant, patients received Ganciclovir Sodium 5 mg/kg BID for 14 days followed by 6 mg/kg QD for 5 days/week for an additional 14 days. Twelve of the 76 (16%) patients treated with Ganciclovir Sodium versus 31 of the 73 (43%) placebo treated patients developed CMV disease during the 120 day post-transplant observation period. No significant differences in hematologic toxicities were seen between the two treatment groups, (refer to table in *Adverse Reactions* section).

ICM 1689: In a randomized double-blind, placebo-controlled study of 72 bone marrow transplant recipients[7] with asymptomatic CMV infection (CMV positive culture of urine, throat or blood) there was a statistically significant reduction in the incidence of CMV disease in patients treated with Ganciclovir Sodium following successful hematopoietic engraftment. Patients with virologic evidence of CMV infection received Ganciclovir Sodium 5 mg/kg BID for 7 days followed by 5 mg/kg QD daily through day 100 post-transplant. One of the 37 (3%) of the patients treated with Ganciclovir Sodium versus 15 of the 35 (43%) placebo patients developed CMV disease during the study. At six months post-transplant, there continued to be a statistically significant reduction in the incidence of CMV disease in patients treated with Ganciclovir Sodium. Six of 37 (16%) of the patients treated with Ganciclovir Sodium versus 15 of the 35 (43%) placebo patients developed disease through six months post-transplant. The overall rate of survival was statistically significantly higher in the group treated with Ganciclovir Sodium, both at day 100 and day 180 post-transplant. Although the differences in hematologic toxicities were not statistically significant, the incidence of neutropenia was higher in the group treated with Ganciclovir Sodium (refer to table in "Adverse Reactions" section).

A second, randomized unblinded, bone marrow transplant study[15] was performed, evaluating 40 allogeneic transplant recipients at risk for CMV disease. Patients underwent bronchoscopy and bronchoalveolar lavage (BAL) on day 35 post-transplant. Patients with histologic, immunologic, or virologic evidence of CMV infection in the lung were then randomized to observation or treatment with Ganciclovir Sodium (5 mg/kg BID for 14 days followed by 5 mg/kg QD 5 days/week until day 120). Four of 20 (20%) patients treated with Ganciclovir Sodium and 14 of 20 (70%) control patients developed interstitial pneumonia. The incidence of CMV disease was significantly lower in the group treated with Ganciclovir Sodium, consistent with the results observed in ICM 1689.

CONTRAINDICATIONS

Ganciclovir Sodium is contraindicated in patients with hypersensitivity to Ganciclovir or acyclovir.

WARNINGS

Hematologic: **Ganciclovir Sodium should not be administered if the absolute neutrophil count is less than 500 cells/mm³ or the platelet count is less than 25,000 cells/mm³.** Granulocytopenia (neutropenia) and the thrombocytopenia have been observed in patients treated with Ganciclovir Sodium. The frequency and severity of these events vary widely in different patient populations (see "Adverse Reactions" section). Ganciclovir Sodium should, therefore, be used with caution in patients with pre-existing cytopenia, or with a history of cytopenic reactions to other drugs, chemicals or irradiation. Granulocytopenia usually occurs during the first or second week of treatment, but may occur at any time during treatment. Cell counts usually begin to recover within 3 to 7 days of discontinuing drug.

Impairment of Fertility: Animal data indicate that administration of Ganciclovir Sodium causes inhibition of spermatogenesis and subsequent infertility. These effects were reversible at lower doses and irreversible at higher doses (see "Carcinogenesis, Mutagenesis, and Impairment of Fertility" sections in "Precau-

tions"). *Although data in humans have not been obtained regarding this effect, it is considered probable that intravenous Ganciclovir Sodium at the recommended doses causes temporary or permanent inhibition of spermatogenesis. Animal data also indicate that suppression of fertility in females may occur.*

Teratogenic: Because of the mutagenic potential of Ganciclovir Sodium, women of childbearing potential should be advised to use effective contraception during treatment. Similarly, male patients should be advised to practice barrier contraception during and for at least 90 days following treatment with Ganciclovir Sodium (see "Pregnancy: Category C").

PRECAUTIONS

GENERAL
In clinical studies with Ganciclovir Sodium the maximum single dose administered was 6 mg/kg by intravenous infusion over one hour. It is likely that larger doses, or more rapid infusions, result in increased toxicity (see "Overdosage" section).

Administration of Ganciclovir Sodium by intravenous infusion should be accompanied by adequate hydration, since Ganciclovir Sodium is excreted by the kidneys and normal clearance depends on adequate renal function. **IF RENAL FUNCTION IS IMPAIRED, DOSAGE ADJUSTMENTS ARE REQUIRED.** Such adjustments should be based on measured or estimated creatinine clearance (see "Dosage and Administration" section).

INFORMATION FOR PATIENTS
All patients should be informed that the major toxicities of Ganciclovir are granulocytopenia (neutropenia) and thrombocytopenia discontinuation. The importance of close monitoring of blood counts while on therapy should be emphasized. Patients should be advised that Ganciclovir Sodium has caused decreased sperm production in animals and may cause infertility in humans. Women of childbearing potential should be advised that Ganciclovir Sodium causes birth defects in animals and should not be used during pregnancy. Women of child bearing potential should be advised to use effective contraception during treatment with Ganciclovir Sodium. Similarly, men should be advised to practice barrier contraception during and for at least 90 days following treatment with Ganciclovir Sodium.

Patients should be advised that Ganciclovir Sodium causes tumors in animals. Although there is no information from human studies, Ganciclovir Sodium should be considered a potential carcinogen.

Patients with AIDS and CMV Retinitis: Ganciclovir Sodium is not a cure for CMV retinitis, and immunocompromised patients may continue to experience progression of retinitis during or following treatment. Patients should be advised to have ophthalmologic follow-up examinations at a minimum of every six weeks while being treated with Ganciclovir Sodium. (Many patients will require more frequent follow-up.)

Patients with AIDS may be receiving zidovudine (Retrovir). Patients should be counseled that treatment with both Ganciclovir Sodium and zidovudine simultaneously will not be tolerated by many patients, and may result in severe granulocytopenia (neutropenia).

Transplant Recipients: Transplant recipients should be counseled regarding the high frequency of impaired renal function in transplant recipients who received Ganciclovir Sodium in controlled clinical trials, particularly in patients receiving concomitant administration of nephrotoxic agents such as cyclosporine and amphotericin B. Although the specific mechanism of this toxicity, which in most cases was reversible, has not been determined, the higher rate of renal impairment in patients receiving Ganciclovir Sodium compared to those who received placebo in the same trials may indicate that Ganciclovir Sodium played a significant role.

LABORATORY TESTING
Due to the frequency of granulocytopenia and thrombocytopenia, in patients receiving Ganciclovir Sodium (see "Adverse Reactions" section), it is recommended that neutrophil counts and platelet counts be performed every two days during BID dosing of Ganciclovir Sodium and at least weekly thereafter. Neutrophil counts should be monitored daily in patients in whom Ganciclovir Sodium or other nucleoside analogues have previously resulted in leukopenia, or in whom neutrophil counts are less than 1,000 cells/mm³ at the beginning of treatment. Because dosing must be modified in patients with renal impairment, and because of the incidence of increased serum creatinine levels that have been observed in transplant recipients treated with Ganciclovir Sodium patients should have serum creatinine or creatinine clearance monitored at least once every two weeks. The incidence of increased serum creatinine levels observed in heart and bone marrow transplant recipients treated with Ganciclovir Sodium is shown in the table in the "Adverse Reactions, Renal Toxicity" section.

DRUG INTERACTIONS
It is possible that probenecid, as well as other drugs that inhibit renal tubular secretion or resorption, may reduce renal clearance of Ganciclovir Sodium. It is also possible that drugs that inhibit replication of rapidly dividing cell populations such as bone marrow, spermatogonia, and germinal layers of skin and gastrointestinal mucosa may have additive toxicity when administered concomitantly with Ganciclovir Sodium. Therefore, drugs such as dapsone, pentamidine, flucytosine, vincristine, vinblastine, adriamycin, amphotericin B, trimethoprim/sulfa combinations or other nucleoside analogues, should be considered for concomitant use with Ganciclovir Sodium only if the potential benefits are judged to outweigh the risks.

◆ RATED THERAPEUTICALLY EQUIVALENT; ◇ THERAPEUTIC EQUIVALENCE UNCONFIRMED; ○ UNRATED

Patients with AIDS may be receiving, or have received, treatment with zidovudine (Retrovir). *Since both zidovudine and Ganciclovir Sodium have the potential to cause granulocytopenia (neutropenia), many patients will not tolerate combination therapy with those two drugs at full dosage strength.* Data from 41 patients indicate that treatment with Ganciclovir plus zidovudine at the recommended doses is not tolerated.[16] Generalized seizures have been reported in seven patients who received Ganciclovir Sodium and imipenem-cilastatin. These drugs should not be used concomitantly with Ganciclovir Sodium unless the potential benefits outweigh the risks.

No formal drug interaction studies of Ganciclovir Sodium and drugs commonly used in transplant recipients have been conducted. Allograft recipients treated with Ganciclovir Sodium in three controlled clinical studies also received a variety of concomitant medications, including amphotericin B, azathioprine, cyclosporine, muromonab-CD3 (OKT3), and/or prednisone. Increases in serum creatinine were observed in patients treated with Ganciclovir Sodium plus either cyclosporine or amphotericin B, drugs with known potential for nephrotoxicity (see *"Adverse Reactions"* section).

CARCINOGENESIS, MUTAGENESIS*
Ganciclovir Sodium was carcinogenic in the mouse at oral doses of 20 and 1000 mg/kg/day (approximately 0.1× and 1.4×, respectively, the mean drug exposure in humans following the recommended intravenous dose of 5 mg/kg, based on area under the plasma concentration curve (AUC) comparisons). At the dose of 1000 mg/kg/day there was a significant increase in the incidence of tumors of the preputial gland in males, forestomach (nonglandular mucosa) in males and females, and reproductive tissues, (ovaries, uterus, mammary gland, clitoral gland and vagina) and liver in females. At the dose of 20 mg/kg/day, a slightly increased incidence of tumors was noted in the preputial and harderian glands in males, forestomach in males and females, and liver in females. No carcinogenic effect was observed in mice administered Ganciclovir at 1 mg/kg/day (estimated as 0.01x the human dose based on AUC comparison). Except for histiocytic sarcoma of the liver, Ganciclovir induced tumors were generally of epithelia or vascular origin. Although the preputial and clitoral glands, forestomach, and harderian glands of mice do not have human counterparts, Ganciclovir Sodium should be considered a potential carcinogen in humans.

Ganciclovir increased mutations in mouse lymphoma cells and DNA damage in human lymphocytes in vitro at concentrations between 50-500 and 250-2000 µg/mL, respectively. In the mouse micronucleus assay, Ganciclovir was clastogenic at doses of 150 and 500 mg/kg (IV) (2.8-10× human exposure based on AUC) but not 50 mg/kg (exposure approximately comparable to the human based on AUC). Ganciclovir was not mutagenic in the Ames Salmonella assay at concentrations of 500-5000 µg/mL.

IMPAIRMENT OF FERTILITY*
Ganciclovir caused decreased mating behavior, decreased fertility, and an increased incidence of embryolethality in female mice following intravenous doses of 90 mg/kg/day (approximately 1.7× the mean drug exposure in humans following the dose of 5 mg/kg, based on AUC comparisons). Ganciclovir caused decreased fertility in male mice and hypospermatogenesis in mice and dogs following daily oral or intravenous administration of doses ranging from 0.2-10 mg/kg. Systemic drug exposure (AUC) at the lowest dose showing toxicity in each species ranged from 0.03-0.1× the AUC of the recommended human intravenous dose.

PREGNANCY: CATEGORY C*
Ganciclovir Sodium has been shown to be embryotoxic in rabbits and mice following intravenous administration. Fetal resorptions were present in at least 85% of rabbits and mice administered 60 mg/kg/day and 108 mg/kg/day (2× the human exposure based on AUC comparisons), respectively. Effects observed in rabbits included: fetal growth retardation, embryolethality, teratogenicity, and/or maternal toxicity. Teratogenic changes included cleft palate, anophthalmia/microphthalmia, aplastic organs (kidney and pancreas), hydrocephaly, and brachygnathia. In mice, effects observed were maternal/fetal toxicity and embryolethality.

Daily intravenous dose of 90 mg/kg administered to female mice prior to mating, during gestation, and during lactation caused hypoplasia of the testes and seminal vesicles in the month-old male offspring, as well as pathologic changes in the nonglandular region of the stomach (see *"Carcinogensis, Mutagenesis"* section). The drug exposure in mice as estimated by the AUC is approximately 1.7× the human AUC. Ganciclovir Sodium may be teratogenic or embryotoxic at dose levels recommended for human use. There are no adequate and well-controlled studies in pregnant women. Ganciclovir Sodium should be used during pregnancy only if the potential benefits justifies the potential risk to the fetus.

NURSING MOTHERS
It is not known if Ganciclovir Sodium is excreted in human milk. However, many drugs are excreted in human milk and, because carcinogenic and teratogenic effects occurred in animals treated with Ganciclovir, the possibility of serious adverse reactions from Ganciclovir in nursing infants is considered likely (see *"Pregnancy: Category C"* section). Mothers should be instructed to discontinue nursing if they are receiving Ganciclovir Sodium. The minimum interval before

nursing can safely be resumed after the last dose of Ganciclovir Sodium is unknown.

PEDIATRIC USE
SAFETY AND EFFICACY OF GANCICLOVIR SODIUM® IN CHILDREN HAVE NOT BEEN ESTABLISHED. THE USE OF GANCICLOVIR SODIUM IN CHILDREN WARRANTS EXTREME CAUTION DUE TO THE PROBABILITY OF LONG-TERM CARCINOGENICITY AND REPRODUCTIVE TOXICITY. ADMINISTRATION TO CHILDREN SHOULD BE UNDERTAKEN ONLY AFTER CAREFUL EVALUATION AND ONLY IF THE POTENTIAL BENEFITS OF TREATMENT OUTWEIGH THE RISKS.

Adverse events reported in 120 immunocompromised children with serious CMV infections receiving Ganciclovir were similar to those reported in adults. Granulocytopenia (17%) and thrombocytopenia (10%) were the most common adverse events reported.

There has been very limited clinical experience in treating cytomegalovirus retinitis in patients under the age of 12 years. Two children (ages 9 and 5 years) showed improvement or stabilization of retinitis for 23 and 9 months, respectively. These children received induction treatment with 2.5 mg/kg TID followed by maintenance therapy with 6-6.5 mg/kg once per day, five to seven days per week. When retinitis progressed during once daily maintenance therapy, both children were treated with 5 mg/kg BID regimen. Two other children (ages 2.5 and 4 years) who received similar induction regimens showed only partial or no response to treatment. Another child, a six year old with T-cell dysfunction, showed stabilization of retinitis for 3 months while receiving continuous infusions of Ganciclovir Sodium at doses of 2-5 mg/kg/24 hours. Continuous infusion treatment was discontinued due to granulocytopenia. The pharmacokinetics of Ganciclovir Sodium in children are under investigation.

Eleven of the 72 patients in the placebo-controlled trial in bone marrow transplant recipients were children, ranging in age from 3 to 10 years of age (5 treated with Ganciclovir Sodium and 6 placebo-treated). Five of the pediatric patients treated with Ganciclovir Sodium received 5 mg/kg BID for up to 7 days; 4 patients went on to receive 5 mg/kg QD up to day 100 post-transplant. Results were similar to those observed in adult transplant patients treated with Ganciclovir Sodium. Two of the 6 placebo-treated pediatric patients developed CMV pneumonia, versus none of the 5 patients treated with Ganciclovir Sodium. Toxicity in the pediatric group was similar to that observed in the adult patients.

USE IN PATIENTS WITH RENAL IMPAIRMENT
Ganciclovir Sodium should be used with caution in patients with impaired renal function because the plasma half-life and peak plasma levels of Ganciclovir Sodium will be increased due to reduced renal clearance (see *"Dosage and Administration"* and *"Adverse Reactions: Renal Toxicity"* sections).

Data from 4 patients indicate that plasma levels of Ganciclovir Sodium are reduced approximately 50% following hemodialysis.

USE IN THE ELDERLY
No studies of the efficacy or safety of Ganciclovir Sodium in elderly patients have been conducted. Since elderly individuals frequently have reduced glomerular filtration, particular attention should be paid to assessing renal function before and during Ganciclovir Sodium administration (see *"Dosage and Administration"* section).

ADVERSE REACTIONS
During clinical trials Ganciclovir Sodium was withdrawn or interrupted in approximately 32% of patients because of adverse events. In some instances treatment was restarted and the reappearance of adverse events again necessitated withdrawal or interruption.

Hematologic Toxicity: The most frequent adverse events seen in patients treated with Ganciclovir Sodium are granulocytopenia/neutropenia and thrombocytopenia.

In most cases, withdrawal of Ganciclovir Sodium resulted in increased neutrophil or platelet counts. While granulocytopenia was generally reversible with discontinuation of treatment, some patients experienced irreversible neutropenia or died with severe bacterial or fungal infections during neutropenia episodes.

The following table shows the frequency of granulocytopenia and thrombocytopenia observed in clinical trials with Ganciclovir Sodium. (See related table). *(See discussion of clinical trials under "Indications and Usage" section.)*

Adverse events other than granulocytopenia and thrombocytopenia were reported as "probably related", "probably not related", and "unknown" in relationship to therapy with Ganciclovir Sodium. Evaluation of these reports was difficult because of the protean manifestations of the underlying disease, and because most patients received numerous concomitant medications.

Renal Toxicity: The following table shows the frequency of elevated serum creatinine in clinical trials of Ganciclovir Sodium for the prevention of CMV disease in transplant recipients: (See related table).

In a placebo-controlled clinical trial conducted in heart allograft recipients (ICM 1496), more patients receiving Ganciclovir Sodium had elevation of serum creatinine to values exceeding 2.5 mg/dL than patients receiving placebo (18% vs. 4%, respectively). These increases in serum creatinine, up to 5.5 mg/dL in one patient, were transient and occurred primarily during the first week of treatment with Ganciclovir Sodium. In a randomized, but unblinded study of Ganciclovir Sodium in bone marrow allograft recipients (ICM 1570), more patients treated with Ganciclovir Sodium experienced serum creatinine values exceeding 1.5 mg/dL than patients who were not treated (70% vs. 35%, respectively). These

---

* All dose comparisons presented in the *Carcinogenesis, Mutagenesis, Impairment of Fertility,* and *Pregnancy* sections are based on the human AUC following administration of a single 5 mg/kg intravenous infusion as used during the maintenance phase of treatment. Because human exposure is approximately doubled during the induction phase of treatment (5 mg/kg, BID) the cross-species dose comparisons should be divided by 2.

➤ SHOWN IN PRODUCT IDENTIFICATION GUIDE

elevations in serum creatinine, up to 3.2 mg/dL in one patient, were transient and occurred intermittently throughout the 3 month study. Most patients in these studies also received cyclosporine. In a second study in bone marrow transplant patients that was placebo-controlled (ICM 1689), no differences in elevations of serum creatinine were seen between the patients receiving Ganciclovir Sodium and those receiving placebo. The mechanism of impairment of renal function (whether it is the result of an interaction between Ganciclovir Sodium and cyclosporine or other nephrotoxic agents) is not known. However, careful monitoring of renal function during therapy with Ganciclovir Sodium is essential, especially for those patients receiving concomitant agents that may cause nephrotoxicity.

CNS Toxicity: In two placebo-controlled trials in transplant recipients, headache (17% vs. 11%, respectively), and confusion (6% vs. 1%, respectively) were noted to occur more frequently in patients treated with Ganciclovir Sodium than in placebo-treated patients.

Other Toxicities: In the same two studies, sepsis was observed more frequently in the patients treated with Ganciclovir Sodium than in the placebo-treated patients (6% vs 2%, respectively).

RETINAL DETACHMENT
Retinal detachment has been observed in patients with CMV retinitis both before and after initiation of therapy with Ganciclovir Sodium. The relationship of retinal detachment to therapy with Ganciclovir Sodium is unknown. Patients with CMV retinitis should have frequent ophthalmologic evaluations to monitor the status of their retinitis and detect any other retinal lesions.

General: Other than leukopenia and thrombocytopenia, the most frequent adverse events observed in over 5,000 patients who received Ganciclovir Sodium were anemia, fever, rash, and abnormal liver function values, each of which was reported in approximately 2% of treated patients. Adverse events that were thought to be possibly related to drug and occurred in 1% or fewer patients who received Ganciclovir Sodium were:

Body as a Whole: chills, edema, infections, malaise.

Cardiovascular System: arrhythmia, hypertension, hypotension.

Central Nervous System: abnormal thoughts or dreams, ataxia, coma, confusion, dizziness, headache, nervousness, paresthesia, psychosis, somnolence, tremor (Overall, neurologic system events occurred in 5% of patients).

Digestive System: nausea, vomiting, anorexia, diarrhea, hemorrhage, abdominal pain.

Hematologic System: eosinophilia

Laboratory Abnormalities: decrease in blood glucose

Respiratory System: dyspnea

Skin and Appendages: alopecia, pruritus, urticaria

Urogenital System: hematuria, increased blood urea nitrogen (BUN)

Injection Site: Inflammation, pain, phlebitis

OVERDOSAGE
Overdosage with Ganciclovir Sodium has been reported in eleven patients. In three of these patients, no adverse events were observed after the overdosage. (The doses received were: 7 doses of 11 mg/kg over a 3-day period, 9 mg/kg BID for 3 days, and 2 doses of 500 mg given to a 21-month old child.) An 18-month old child received a single dose of approximately 60 mg/kg and was given an exchange transfusion. No adverse events were noted. A 4-month old child received a 500 mg dose (72.5 mg/kg) and no adverse events were noted. The child underwent 48 hours of peritoneal dialysis and was doing well at the completion.

Irreversible pancytopenia was reported following overdose in one 28 years old AIDS patient with CMV colitis and abdominal pain who inadvertently received 3,000 mg of Ganciclovir Sodium on each of two consecutive days. After the second dosage the patient became anorexic and had more severe abdominal pain, substernal pain, vomiting, and lethargy. The patient was dialyzed twice for acute renal failure. Two weeks following the overdose he was noted to be pancytopenic. The patient continued to have persistent bone marrow suppression and pancytopenia, until his death from a malignancy several months later.

Reversible neutropenia was reported following overdoses in three patients: one patient had a history of bone marrow depression prior to treatment and received Ganciclovir Sodium 5 mg/kg for 14 days followed by 8 mg/kg given as single daily doses for 4 days; one patient received a single dose of 1,675 mg (approximately 24 mg/kg); and a 60 year old man with preexisting neutropenia received a single dose of 20 mg/kg Ganciclovir Sodium. In all cases the neutropenia was reversible (after 17 days, 1 day, and 9 days, respectively) following discontinuation of Ganciclovir Sodium.

A 19-year old patient with a history of renal insufficiency and hematuria received a single dose of 500 mg Ganciclovir Sodium and developed a worsening of the hematuria, which resolved in 2 days. During evaluation for renal insufficiency (creatinine 5.2 mg/dL), a 33 year old patient reported that 4 days prior to the evaluation, he had intentionally self administered a single dose of 5 to 7 g of Ganciclovir Sodium; no hematologic abnormalities were noted and the relationship of the overdosage to his renal insufficiency is unknown.

Hemodialysis and hydration may be of benefit in reducing drug plasma levels in patients who receive an overdosage of Ganciclovir Sodium.

DOSAGE AND ADMINISTRATION
CAUTION—DO NOT ADMINISTER GANCICLOVIR SODIUM BY RAPID OR BOLUS INTRAVENOUS INJECTION. THE TOXICITY OF GANCICLOVIR SODIUM MAY BE INCREASED AS A RESULT OF EXCESSIVE PLASMA LEVELS.

CAUTION—INTRAMUSCULAR OR SUBCUTANEOUS INJECTION OF RECONSTITUTED GANCICLOVIR SODIUM MAY RESULT IN SEVERE TISSUE IRRITATION DUE TO HIGH pH (11).

| | Uncontrolled Trials | | Controlled Trials—Transplant Recipients | | | |
| | Persons w/AIDS | Transplant Recipients | Heart Allograft* | | Bone Marrow Allograft** | |
	Ganciclovir Sodium (n = 532)	Ganciclovir Sodium (n = 207)	Ganciclovir Sodium (n = 76)	Placebo (n = 73)	Ganciclovir Sodium (n = 57)	Control (n = 55)
Granulocytopenia/Neutropenia						
ANC < 500/µL	18%	11%	4%	3%	12%	6%
ANC 500-1000/µL	24%	10%	3%	8%	29%	17%
Total ANC ≤ 1,000 µL	42%	21%	7%	11%	41%	23%
Thrombocytopenia						
Platelet counts < 25,000/µL	4%	22%	3%	1%	32%	28%
Platelet counts 25,000-50,000/µL	9%	23%	5%	3%	25%	37%
Total Platelets ≤ 50,000 µL	13%	45%	8%	4%	57%	65%

* Mean duration of treatment = 28 days
** Mean duration of treatment = 45 days

	Controlled Trials—Transplant Recipients					
	Heart Allograft		Bone Marrow Allograft			
	ICM 1496		ICM 1570		ICM 1689	
Maximum Serum Creatinine Levels	Ganciclovir Sodium (n = 76)	Placebo (n = 73)	Ganciclovir Sodium (n = 20)	Control (n = 20)	Ganciclovir Sodium (n = 37)	Placebo (n = 35)
Serum Creatinine ≥ 2.5 mg/dL	18%	4%	20%	0%	0%	0%
Serum Creatinine ≥ 1.5	58%	69%	50%	35%	43%	44%

◆ RATED THERAPEUTICALLY EQUIVALENT; ◇ THERAPEUTIC EQUIVALENCE UNCONFIRMED; ○ UNRATED

DOSAGE

The Recommended Dosage, Frequency, Or Infusion Rates Should Not Be Exceeded.

FOR TREATMENT OF CMV RENTINITIS:

1. Induction Treatment: The recommended initial dose for patients with normal renal function is 5 mg/kg (given intravenously at a constant rate over 1 hour) every 12 hours for 14-21 days.

2. Maintenance Treatment: Following induction treatment the recommended dose of Ganciclovir Sodium is 5 mg/kg given as an intravenous infusion over one hour once per day on seven days each week, or 6 mg/kg once per day on five days each week. Patients who experience progression of retinitis while receiving maintenance therapy may be retreated with the BID regimen.

FOR THE PREVENTION OF CMV DISEASE IN TRANSPLANT RECIPIENTS

The recommended initial dose for patient with normal renal function is 5 mg/kg (given intravenously at the constant rate over 1 hour) every 12 hours for 7 to 14 days, followed by 5 mg/kg once per day on seven days each week, or 6 mg/kg once per day on five days each week.

The duration of treatment with Ganciclovir Sodium in transplant recipients is dependent upon the duration and degree of immunosuppression. In controlled clinical trials in bone marrow allograft recipients, treatment was continued until day 100 to 120 post-transplantation. CMV disease occurred in several patients who discontinued treatment with Ganciclovir Sodium prematurely. In heart allograft recipients, the onset of newly diagnosed CMV disease occurred after treatment with Ganciclovir Sodium was stopped at day 28 post-transplant, suggesting that continued dosing may be necessary to prevent late occurrence of CMV disease in this patient population. (See *"Indications and Usage"* section for a more detailed discussion.)

RENAL IMPAIRMENT

For patients with impairment of renal function, refer to the table below for recommended doses during the induction phase of treatment, and adjust the dosing interval as indicated.

Creatinine Clearance* (mL/min)	Ganciclovir Sodium Dose (mg/kg)	Dosing Interval (hours)
≥ 80	5.0	12
50-79	2.5	12
25-49	2.5	24
< 25	1.25	24

* Creatinine clearance can be related to serum creatinine by the following formulae:

Creatinine clearance for males $= \dfrac{(140 - \text{age [yrs]}) (\text{body wt [kg]})}{(72) (\text{serum creatinine [mg/dL]})}$

Creatinine clearance for females $= 0.85 \times$ male value

The optimal maintenance dose for patients with renal impairment is not known. Physicians may elect to reduce the dose to 50% of the induction dose and monitor the patient for disease progression.

Only limited data are available on elimination of Ganciclovir Sodium in patients undergoing hemodialysis. Dosing for these patients should not exceed 1.25 mg/kg/24 hours. On days when hemodialysis is performed, the dose should be given shortly after the completion of the hemodialysis session, since hemodialysis has been shown to reduce plasma levels by approximately 50%. Neutrophil and platelet counts should be monitored daily.

PATIENT MONITORING

Due to the frequency of granulocytopenia and thrombocytopenia in patients receiving Gancyclovin Sodium (see *"Adverse Reactions"* section), it is recommended that neutrophil counts and platelet counts be performed every two days during BID dosing of Ganciclovir Sodium and at least weekly thereafter. In patients in whom Ganciclovir Sodium or other nucleoside analogues have previously resulted in leukopenia, or in whom neutrophil counts are less than 1,000 cells/mm^3 at the beginning of treatment, neutrophil counts should be monitored daily. Because dosing must be modified in patients with renal impairment, and because of the incidence of increased serum creatinine levels that have been observed in transplant recipients treated with Ganciclovir Sodium, patients should have serum creatinine or creatinine clearance monitored at least once every two weeks. The incidence of increased serum creatinine levels observed in heart and bone marrow transplant recipients treated with Ganciclovir Sodium is shown in the table in the *"Adverse Reactions—Renal Toxicity"* section.

REDUCTION OF DOSE

The most frequently observed adverse event following treatment with Ganciclovir Sodium is leukopenia/neutropenia (see *"Adverse Reaction"* section).

Therefore, frequent white blood cell counts should be performed. Severe neutropenia (ANC less than 500/mm^3) or severe thrombocytopenia (platelets less than 25,000/mm^3) requires a dose interruption until evidence of marrow recovery is observed (ANC ≥ 750/mm^3).

METHOD OF PREPARATION

Each 10 mL clear glass vial contains Ganciclovir Sodium equivalent to 500 mg of the free base form of Ganciclovir Sodium and 46 mg of Sodium. The contents of the vial should be prepared for administration in the following manner:

1. RECONSTITUTED SOLUTION:

a. Lyophilized Ganciclovir Sodium should be reconstituted by injecting 10 mL of Sterile Water for Injection, USP, into the vial.
DO NOT USE BACTERIOSTATIC WATER FOR INJECTION CONTAINING PARABENS. IT IS INCOMPATIBLE WITH GANCICLOVIR SODIUM STERILE POWDER AND MAY CAUSE PRECIPITATION.
b. The vial should be shaken to dissolve the drug.
c. Reconstituted solution should be inspected visually for particulate matter and discoloration prior to proceeding with infusion solution. If particulate matter or discoloration is observed, the vial should be discarded.
d. Reconstituted solution in the vial is stable at room temperature for 12 hours. It should not be refrigerated.

2. INFUSION SOLUTION

Based on patient weight, the appropriate volume of the reconstituted solution (Ganciclovir Sodium concentration 50 mg/mL) should be removed from the vial and added to an acceptable (see below) infusion fluid (typically 100 mL) for delivery over the course of one hour. Infusion concentrations greater than 10 mg/mL are not recommended. The following infusion fluids have been determined to be chemically and physically compatible with Ganciclovir Sodium 0.9% Sodium Chloride, 5% Dextrose, Ringer's Injection, and Lactated Ringer's Injection, USP.

Note: Because non-bacteriostatic infusion fluid must be used with Ganciclovir Sodium, the infusion solution must be used within 24 hours of dilution to reduce the risk of bacterial contamination. The infusion solution should be refrigerated. Freezing is not recommended.

HANDLING AND DISPOSAL

Caution should be exercised in the handling and preparation of solutions of Ganciclovir Sodium Solutions of Ganciclovir Sodium are alkaline (pH 11). Avoid direct contact with the skin or mucous membranes. If such contact occurs, wash thoroughly with soap and water, rinse eyes thoroughly with plain water. Because Ganciclovir Sodium shares some of the properties of anti-tumor agents (i.e., carcinogenicity and mutagenicity), consideration should be given to handling and disposal according to guidelines issued for antineoplastic drugs. Several guidelines on this subject have been published.[17-22]

There is no general agreement that all of the procedures recommended in the guidelines are necessary or appropriate.

Store below 40°C (104°F).

REFERENCES

1. Smee D.F., Boehme R. Chernow M., et al: Intracellular metabolism and enzymatic phosphorylation of 9-(1,3-dihydroxy-2-propoxymethyl) guanine and acyclovir in herpes simplex virus-infected and uninfected cells. *Biochemical Pharmacol* 1985; 34:1049-1056. 2. Shanley J.D., Morningstar J., Jordan M.C.: Inhibition of murine cytomegalovirus lung infection and interstitial pneumonitis by acyclovir and 9-(1,3-dihydroxy-2-propoxymethyl) guanine. *Antimicrob Agents Chemother* 1985; 28: 172-175. 3. Wilson E.J., Medearis D.N. Jr., Hansen L.A., et al: 9-(1,3-dihydroxy-2-propoxymethyl) guanine prevents death but not immunity in murine cytomegalovirus-infected normal and immunosuppressed BALB/c mice, *Antimicrob Agents Chemother* 1987; 31:1017-1020. 4. Fong C.K.Y., Cohen S.D., McCormick S., Hsiung G.D.: Antiviral Effect of 9-(1,3-dihydroxy-2-propoxymethyl) guanine against cytomegalovirus infection in a guinea pig model. *Antiviral Res* 1987; 7: 11-23. 5. Buhles W.C., Mastre B.J., Tinker A.J., et al: Ganciclovir Treatment of Life- or Sight-Threatening Cytomegalovirus Infection: Experience in 314 immunocompromised Patients. *Rev Inf Dis* 1987; 10:495-506. 6. Merigan, T.C., Renlund, D.G., et al: A Controlled Trial of Ganciclovir to Prevent Cytomegalovirus Disease After Heart Transplantation. *NEJM* 1992; 326: 1182-1186. 7. Goodrich, J.M., Mori, M., et al: Early Treatment With Ganciclovir To Prevent Cytomegalovirus Disease After Allogenic Bone Marow Transplantation. *NEJM* 1991; 325: 1601-1607. 8. Erice A., Chou S., Byron K.K., et al: Progressive disease due to Ganciclovir-resistant cytomegalovirus in immunocompromised patients. *NEJM* 1989; 320:289-293. 9. Drew, W.L., Miner, R.C., et al: Prevalence of Resistance In Patients Receiving Ganciclovir For Serious Cytomegalovirus Infection. *J. Infect. Dis.* 1991; 716-719. 10. Jacobson, M.A., Drew, W.L., Feinberg, J., et al.: Foscarnet Therapy for Ganciclovir-Resistant Cytomegalovirus Retinitis in AIDS. *J. Infect. Dis.* 1991; 163: 1348-1351. 11. Fletcher C., Balfour H.: Evaluation of Ganciclovir for cytomegalovirus disease. *DICP, Ann Pharmacother* 1989; 23:5-12. 12. Fletcher C., Sawchuk R., Chinnock B., et al: Human pharmacokinetics of the antiviral drug DHPG. *Clin Pharmacol Ther* 1986; 40:281-286. 13. Jabs D., Enger E., Bartlett J.: Cytomegalovirus retinitis and acquired immunodeficiency syndrome. *Arch Ophthalmol* 1989; 107:75-80. 14. Updated unpublished data on file with Syntex Corp. 15. Schmidt, G., Horak, D., et al: A Randomized, Controlled Trial of Prophylactic Ganciclovir For Cytomegalovirus Pulmonary Infection In Recipients of Allogenic Bone Marrow Transplants *NEJM* 1991; 15: 1005-1011. 16. Hochster, H., et al: Toxicity of Combined Ganciclovir and Zidovudine for Cytomegalovirus Disease Associated with AIDS. *Annuals of Internal Medicine*, 1990; 113: 111-117. 17. Recommendations for the Safe Handling of Parenteral Antineoplastic Drugs. NIH Publication No. 83-2621. For sale by the Superintendent of Documents, U.S. Government Printing Office, Washington, D.C. 20402. 18. AMA Council Report. Guidelines for Handling Parenteral Antineoplastics. *JAMA*, March 15, 1985. 19. National Study Commission on Cytotoxic Exposure-Recommendations for Handling Cytotoxic Agents. Available from Louis P. Jeffrey, Sc. D., Director of Pharmacy Services, Rhode Island Hospital, 593 Eddy Street, Providence, Rhode Island 02902. 20. Clinical Oncological Society of Australia: Guidelines and recommendations for safe handling of antineoplastic agents. *Med J Australia* 1983; 1:426-428. 21. Jones R.B., et al: Safe handling of chemotherapeutic agents: A report from the Mount Sinai Medical Center, GA—A *Cancer Journal for Clinicians* 1983; 33: 258-263. 22. American Society of Hospital Pharmacists technical assistance bulletin on handling cytotoxic drugs in hospitals. *Am J Hosp Pharm* 1985; 42:131-137.

► SHOWN IN PRODUCT IDENTIFICATION GUIDE

J CODES
500 mg IV—J1570

HOW SUPPLIED
POWDER FOR INJECTION: 500 MG

BRAND/MANUFACTURER	NDC	SIZE	AWP
○ BRAND			
CYTOVENE: Syntex/F.P.	00033-2903-48	25s	$870.00

Ganite SEE GALLIUM NITRATE

Gantanol SEE SULFAMETHOXAZOLE

Gantrisin SEE SULFISOXAZOLE, ORAL

Gantrisin Ophthalmic SEE SULFISOXAZOLE
DIOLAMINE, OPHTHALMIC

Garamycin SEE GENTAMICIN SULFATE, INJECTABLE,
GENTAMICIN SULFATE, OPHTHALMIC AND GENTAMICIN SULFATE,
TOPICAL

Gastrocrom SEE CROMOLYN SODIUM, ORAL

Gel-Kam SEE STANNOUS FLUORIDE

Gelatin, Absorbable

DESCRIPTION
Gelatin, Absorbable, is a medical device intended for application to bleeding surfaces as a hemostatic. Gelatin, Absorbable, is available as a sterile powder and as compressed sponges. Gelatin, Absorbable, is a water-insoluble, off-white, nonelastic, porous, pliable product able to absorb and hold within its interstices, many times its weight of blood and other fluids. Gelatin Sterile Powder is a fine, dry, heat-sterilized light powder prepared by milling absorbable gelatin sponge.
   Gelatin Sterile Compressed Sponges are sterile, pliable, surgical sponges.

ACTION
Gelatin, Absorbable, has hemostatic properties. While its mode of action is not fully understood, its effect appears to be more physical than the result of altering the blood clotting mechanism.
   When not used in excessive amounts Gelatin, Absorbable, is absorbed completely, with little tissue reaction. This absorption is dependent on several factors, including the amount used, degree of saturation with blood or other fluids, and the site of use. When placed in soft tissues, Gelatin, Absorbable, is usually absorbed completely in from four to six weeks, without inducing excessive scar tissue. When applied to bleeding nasal, rectal or vaginal mucosa, it liquefies within two to five days.

INDICATIONS
Hemostasis: Gelatin, Absorbable, Sterile Powder and Compressed Sponges, are indicated in surgical procedures as a hemostatic device, when control of capillary, venous, and arteriolar bleeding by pressure, ligature, and other conventional procedures is either ineffective or impractical. The sponges are designed especially for application in the dry state.

DIRECTIONS FOR USE
Gelatin, Absorbable, Sterile Powder can be saturated with sterile, isotonic sodium chloride solution (sterile saline), before use as an adjunct to hemostasis. The jar of Gelatin, Absorbable, Sterile Powder should be opened and the contents (1 gram) poured carefully into a sterile beaker, avoiding contamination. Using sterile technique, a putty-like paste is prepared by adding a total of approximately 3-4 mL of sterile saline to the Gelatin, Absorbable. Dispersion of the powder can be avoided by initially compressing it with the gloved fingers into the bottom of the beaker and then kneading it into the desired consistency. The resulting doughy paste may be smeared or pressed against the bleeding surface to control bleeding. When bleeding stops, the excess should be removed. Pieces of Gelatin, Absorbable, Sterile Compressed Sponge, cut to desired size, are applied dry to the bleeding surface and held in place with moderate pressure for 10 to 15 seconds. Suction may be applied if desired to draw blood into the Gelatin, Absorbable, sponge.

While suction hastens clotting, it is not essential, since Gelatin, Absorbable, sponge will draw up blood by capillary attraction and cause clotting satisfactorily. Usually the first application of Gelatin, Absorbable, sponge will control bleeding, but if not, additional applications should be made using fresh pieces of sponge.
   Use only the minimum amount of Gelatin, Absorbable, necessary to produce hemostasis. The Gelatin, Absorbable, may be left in place at the bleeding site, when necessary; otherwise, bleeding may start again. Since Gelatin, Absorbable, causes little more cellular reaction than does the blood clot, the wound may be closed over it. Gelatin, Absorbable, may be left in place when applied to mucosal surfaces until it liquefies.

CONTRAINDICATIONS
Gelatin, Absorbable, should not be used in closure of skin incisions because it may interfere with healing of the skin edges. This is due to mechanical interposition of Gelatin and is not secondary to intrinsic interference with wound healing.
   Gelatin, Absorbable, should not be placed in intravascular compartments, because of the risk of embolization.

WARNINGS
Gelatin, Absorbable, is not intended as a substitute for meticulous surgical technique and the proper application of ligatures, or other conventional procedures for hemostasis.
   Gelatin, Absorbable, Sterile Powder is supplied as a sterile product and cannot be resterilized. Gelatin, Absorbable, Sterile Compressed Sponge should not be resterilized by heat, because heating may change absorption time. Ethylene oxide is not recommended for resterilization because it may be trapped in the interstices of the foam. Although not reported for Gelatin, Absorbable, Sterile Compressed Sponge, the gas is toxic to tissue, and in trace amounts may cause burns or irritation. Unused, opened jars of Gelatin, Absorbable, Sterile Powder should be discarded.
   Only the minimum amount of Gelatin, Absorbable, necessary to achieve hemostasis should be used. Once hemostasis is attained, excess Gelatin, Absorbable, should be carefully removed.
   The use of Gelatin, Absorbable, is not recommended in the presence of infection. Gelatin, Absorbable, should be used with caution in contaminated areas of the body. If signs of infection of abscess develop where Gelatin, Absorbable, has been positioned, reoperation may be necessary in order to remove the infected material and allow drainage.
   The safety and efficacy of the combined use of Gelatin, Absorbable, with other agents such as topical thrombin has not been evaluated in controlled clinical trials and therefore cannot be recommended. If in the physician's judgment concurrent use of topical thrombin or other agents are medically advisable, the product literature for that agent should be consulted for complete prescribing information.
   While packing a cavity for hemostasis is sometimes surgically indicated, Gelatin, Absorbable Sterile Powder should not be used in this manner unless excess product not needed to maintain hemostasis is removed.
   Whenever possible, it should be removed after use in laminectomy procedures and from foramina in bone, once hemostasis is achieved. This is because Gelatin, Absorbable, may swell on absorbing fluids, and produce nerve damage by pressure within confined bony spaces.
   The packing of Gelatin, Absorbable, Sterile Powder, particularly within bony cavities, should be avoided, since swelling may interfere with normal function and/or possibly result in compression necrosis of surrounding tissues. By absorbing fluid, Gelatin, Absorbable, sponges may expand and impinge on neighboring structures. Therefore, when placed into cavities or closed tissue spaces, care should be exercised to avoid overpacking.

PRECAUTIONS
The minimum amount of Gelatin, Absorbable, needed for hemostasis should be applied together with pressure until the bleeding stops. The excess should then be removed.
   Gelatin, Absorbable, should not be used for controlling postpartum hemorrhage or menorrhagia.
   It has been demonstrated that fragments of another hemostatic agent, microfibrillar collagen, pass through the 40μ transfusion filters of blood scavenging systems. Gelatin, Absorbable, should not be used in conjunction with autologous blood salvage circuits since the safety of this use has not been evaluated in controlled clinical trials.
   Microfibrillar collagen has been reported to reduce the strength of methylmethacrylate adhesives used to attach prosthetic devices to bone surfaces. As a precaution, Gelatin, Absorbable, should not be used in conjunction with such adhesives.
   Gelatin, Absorbable, is not recommended for the primary treatment of coagulation disorders. It is not recommended that Gelatin, Absorbable, be saturated with an antibiotic solution or dusted with antibiotic powder.

ADVERSE REACTIONS
There have been reports of fever associated with the use of Gelatin, Absorbable, without demonstrable infection. Gelatin, Absorbable, may serve as a nidus for infection and abscess formation[1], and has been reported to potentiate bacterial growth. Giant-cell granuloma has been reported at the implantation site of absorbable gelatin product in the brain[2], as has compression of the brain and spinal cord resulting from the accumulation of sterile fluid.[3]
   Foreign body reactions, "encapsulation" of fluid and hematoma have also been reported.

◆ RATED THERAPEUTICALLY EQUIVALENT; ◇ THERAPEUTIC EQUIVALENCE UNCONFIRMED; ○ UNRATED

When Gelatin, Absorbable, Sterile Powder was used in laminectomy operations, multiple neurologic events were reported, including but not limited to cauda equina syndrome, spinal stenosis, meningitis, arachnoiditis, headaches, paresthesias, pain, bladder and bowel dysfunction, and impotence.

Excessive fibrosis and prolonged fixation of a tendon have been reported when absorbable gelatin products were used in severed tendon repair.

Toxic shock syndrome has been reported in association with the use of Gelatin, Absorbable, Sterile Powder in nasal surgery.

Fever, failure of absorption, and hearing loss have been reported in association with the use of Gelatin, Absorbable, Sterile Powder during tympanoplasty.

ADVERSE REACTIONS REPORTED FROM UNAPPROVED USES
Gelatin, Absorbable, is not recommended for use other than as an adjunct for hemostatis.

While some adverse medical events following the unapproved use of Gelatin, Absorbable, have been reported (see "Adverse Reactions"), other hazards associated with such use may not have been reported.

When Gelatin, Absorbable, has been used during intravascular catheterization for the purpose of producing vessel occlusion, the following adverse events have been reported; fever, duodenal and pancreatic infarct, embolization of lower extremity vessels, pulmonary embolization, splenic abscess, necrosis of specific anatomic areas, asterixis, and death.

These adverse medical events have been associated with the use of Gelatin, Absorbable, for repair of dural defects encountered during laminectomy and craniotomy operations: fever, infection, leg paresthesias, neck and back pain, bladder and bowel incontinence, cauda equina syndrome, neurogenic bladder, impotence, and paresis.

DOSAGE AND ADMINISTRATION
Sterile technique should always be used. The minimum amount of Gelatin, Absorbable, should be applied to the bleeding site (see *"Directions For Use"*) with pressure until hemostasis is observed. Opened jars and packages of unused Gelatin, Absorbable, should always be discarded.

Gelatin, Absorbable, Sterile Powder and Compressed Sponges should be stored at controlled room temperature 15°-30°C (59°-86°F). Once the jar and/or packages are opened, contents are subject to contamination. It is recommended that Gelatin, Absorbable, be used as soon as the jar and/or package is opened and unused contents discarded.

CLINICAL STUDIES
Gelatin, Absorbable, Sterile Sponge is a water-insoluble, hemostatic device capable of absorbing up to 45 times its weight of whole blood.[4] The absorptive capacity of Gelatin, Absorbable, is a function of its physical size, increasing as the size of the gelatin sponge increases.[5]

The mechanism of action of surface-mediated hemostatic devices is supportive and mechanical.[5] Surface-acting devices, when applied directly to bleeding surfaces, arrest bleeding by the formation of an artificial clot and by producing a mechanical matrix that facilitates clotting.[6] Jenkins et al[7] have theorized that the clotting effect of Gelatin, Absorbable, may be due to release of thromboplastin from platelets, occurring when platelets entering the sponge become damaged by contact with the walls of its myriad of interstices. Thromboplastin interacts with prothrombin and calcium to produce thrombin, and this sequence of events initiates the clotting reaction. The authors suggest that the physiologic formation of thrombin in the sponge is sufficient to produce formation of a clot, by its action on the fibrinogen in blood.[7] The spongy physical properties of the gelatin sponge hasten clot formation and provide structural support for the forming clot.[6,8]

ANIMAL PHARMACOLOGY
Surface-acting hemostatic devices, when applied directly to bleeding surfaces, arrest bleeding by providing a mechanical matrix that facilitates clotting.[6,8,15,16] Due to their bulk, surface-acting hemostatic agents slow the flow of blood, protect the forming clot, and offer a framework for deposition of the cellular elements of blood.[6,7,8,15]

MacDonald and Mathews[14] studied Gelatin, Absorbable, implants in canine kidneys and reported that it assisted in healing, with no marked inflammatory or foreign-body reactions.

Jenkins and Janda[15] studied the use of Gelatin, Absorbable, in canine liver resections and noted that the gelatin sponge appeared to offer a protective cover and provide structural support for the reparative process.

Correll et al[16] studied the histology of Gelatin, Absorbable, Sterile Sponge when implanted in rat muscle and reported no significant tissue reaction.

REFERENCES
1. Lindstrom PA: Complications from the use of absorbable hemostatic sponges. *AMA Arch Surg* 1956;73:133-141. 2. Knowlson GTG: Gelfoam granuloma in the brain. *J Neuro Neurosurg Psychiatry* 1974;37:971-973. 3. Herndon JH, Grillo HC, Riseborough EJ, et al: Compression of the brain and spinal cord following use of GELFOAM. *Arch Surg* 1972;104:107. 4. Council on Pharmacy and Chemistry: Absorbable Gelatin sponge- new and nonofficial remedies, *JAMA* 1947; 135:921. 5. Goodman LS, Gilman A: Surface-acting drugs, in *The Pharmacologic Basis of Therapeutics*, ed 6. New York, MacMillan Publishing Co. 1980, p 955. 6. Guralnick W, Berg L: GELFOAM in oral surgery. *Oral Surg* 1948; *1*:629-632. 7. Jenkins HP, Senz EH, Owen H, et al: Present status of gelatin sponge for control of hemorrhage. *JAMA* 1946;132:614-619. 8. Jenkins HP, Janda R, Clarke J: Clinical and experimental observations on the use of gelatin sponge or foam. *Surg* 1946;20:124-132. 9. Treves N: Prophylaxis of post mammectomy lymphedema by the use of GELFOAM laminated rolls. *Cancer* 1952;5:73-83. 10. Barnes AC: The use of gelatin foam sponges in obstetrics and gynecology. *Am J Obstet Gynecol* 1963;86:105-107. 11. Rarig HR: Successful use of gelatin foam sponge in surgical restoration of fertility. *Am J Obstet Gynecol* 1963;86:136. 12. Jacobs BJ, Rafel

SS: Pharmacology and Therapeutics: Absorbable hemostatic agents. *Oral Surg* 1950;2:356-377. 13. Nishimura S: The fate of a gelatin sponge introduced into the fourth ventricle: Experiments in dogs. *Arch Jap Chir* 1954; *23*:310-319. 14. MacDonald SA, Mathews WH: Fibrin foam and GELFOAM in experimental kidney wounds. *Annual American Urological Association*, July 1946. 15. Jenkins HP, Janda R: Studies on the use of gelatin sponge or foam as a hemostatic agent in experimental liver resections and injuries to large veins. *Ann Surg* 1946;*124*:952-961. 16. Correll JT, Prentice HR, Wise EC: Biologic investigations of a new absorbable sponge, *Surg Gynecol Obstet* 1945:181:585-589.

HOW SUPPLIED

GELATIN
ACCESSORIES:

BRAND/MANUFACTURER	NDC	SIZE	AWP
BRAND			
GELFILM: Upjohn	00009-0283-01	1s	$158.43
GELFILM, OPHTHALMIC: Upjohn	00009-0297-01	6s	$95.08

POWDER:

BRAND/MANUFACTURER	NDC	SIZE	AWP
BRAND			
GELFOAM: Upjohn	00009-0433-01	1 gm	$32.81

GELATIN SPONGE
SPONGE:

BRAND/MANUFACTURER	NDC	SIZE	AWP
BRAND			
GELFOAM: Upjohn	00009-0364-01	1s	$26.31
	00009-0301-01	4s	$19.46
	00009-0315-02	4s	$20.83
	00009-0323-01	4s	$69.10
	00009-0353-01	6s	$154.66
	00009-0342-01	6s	$154.96
	00009-0449-01	6s	$202.79
	00009-0349-01	6s	$237.41
	00009-0371-01	6s	$371.90
	00009-0457-01	6s	$391.29
	00009-0315-03	12s	$57.74
	00009-0396-01	15s	$20.40

Gemfibrozil

DESCRIPTION
Gemfibrozil is a lipid regulating agent. It is available as tablets for oral administration. Each tablet contains 600 mg Gemfibrozil. The chemical name is 5-(2,5-dimethylphenoxy)-2,2-dimethylpentanoic acid.

The empirical formula is $C_{15}H_{22}O_3$ and the molecular weight is 250.35; the solubility in water and acid is 0.0019% and in dilute base it is greater than 1%. The melting point is 58°-61°C. Gemfibrozil is a white solid which is stable under ordinary conditions.

Following is its chemical structure:

$$CH_3$$
$$O(CH_2)_3C(CH_3)_2COOH$$
$$CH_3$$

CLINICAL PHARMACOLOGY
Gemfibrozil is a lipid regulating agent which decreases serum triglycerides and very low density lipoprotein (VLDL) cholesterol, and increases high density lipoprotein (HDL) cholesterol. While modest decreases in total and low density lipoprotein (LDL) cholesterol may be observed with Gemfibrozil therapy, treatment of patients with elevated triglycerides due to Type IV hyperlipoproteinemia often results in a rise in LDL-cholesterol. LDL-cholesterol levels in Type IIb patients with elevations of both serum LDL-cholesterol and triglycerides are, in general, minimally affected by Gemfibrozil treatment; however Gemfibrozil usually raises HDL-cholesterol significantly in this group. Gemfibrozil increases levels of high density lipoprotein (HDL) subfractions HDL_2 and HDL_3, as well as apolipoproteins AI and AII. Epidemiological studies have shown that both low HDL-cholesterol and high LDL-cholesterol are independent risk factors for coronary heart disease.

In the primary prevention component of the Helsinki Heart Study (refs. 1, 2), in which 4081 male patients between the ages of 40 and 55 were studied in a randomized, double-blind, placebo-controlled fashion, Gemfibrozil therapy was associated with significant reductions in total plasma triglycerides and a significant increase in high density lipoprotein cholesterol. Moderate reductions in total plasma cholesterol and low density lipoprotein cholesterol were observed for the Gemfibrozil treatment group as a whole, but the lipid response was heterogeneous, especially among different Fredrickson types. The study involved subjects with serum non-HDL-cholesterol of over 200 mg/dL and no previous history of coronary heart disease. Over the 5-year study period, the Gemfibrozil group experienced a 1.4% absolute (34% relative) reduction in the rate of serious coronary events (sudden cardiac deaths plus fatal and nonfatal myocardial infarctions) compared to placebo, p = 0.04 (see Table 1). There was a 37% relative reduction in the rate of nonfatal myocardial infarction compared to placebo, equivalent to a treatment-related difference of 13.1 events per thousand persons. Deaths from any cause during the double-blind portion of the study totaled 44 (2.2%) in the Gemfibrozil randomization group and 43 (2.1%) in the placebo group. (See related table).

Among Fredrickson types, during the 5-year double-blind portion of the primary prevention component of the Helsinki Heart Study, the greatest reduction in the incidence of serious coronary events occured in Type IIb patients who had elevations of both LDL-cholesterol and total plasma triglycerides. This subgroup of Type IIb Gemfibrozil group patients had a lower mean HDL-cholesterol level at baseline than the Type IIa subgroup that had elevations of LDL-cholesterol and normal plasma triglycerides. The mean increase in HDL-cholesterol among the Type IIb patients in this study was 12.6% compared to placebo. The mean change in LDL-cholesterol among Type IIb patients was −4.1% with Gemfibrozil compared to a rise of 3.9% in the placebo subgroup. The Type IIb subjects in the Helsinki Heart Study had 26 fewer coronary events per thousand persons over 5 years in the Gemfibrozil group compared to placebo. The difference in coronary events was substantially greater between Gemfibrozil and placebo for that subgroup of patients with the triad of LDL-cholesterol > 175 mg/dL (> 4.5 mmol), triglycerides > 200 mg/dL (> 2.2 mmol), and HDL-cholesterol < 35 mg/dL (< 0.90 mmol) (see Table I).

Further information is available from a 3.5 year (8.5 year cumulative) follow-up of all subjects who had participated in the Helsinki Heart Study. At the completion of the Helsinki Heart study, subjects could choose to start, stop, or continue to receive Gemfibrozil; without knowledge of their own lipid values or double-blind treatment, 60% of patients originally randomized to placebo began therapy with Gemfibrozil and 60% of patients originally randomized to Gemfibrozil continued medication. After approximately 6.5 years following randomization, all patients were informed of their original treatment group and lipid values during the 5 years of the double-blind treatment. After further elective changes in Gemfibrozil treatment status, 61% of patients in the group originally randomized to Gemfibrozil were taking the drug; in the group originally randomized to placebo, 65% were taking Gemfibrozil. The event rate per 1000 occurring during the open-label follow-up period is detailed in Table 2. (See related table).

Cumulative mortality through 8.5 years showed a 20% relative excess of deaths in the group originally randomized to Gemfibrozil versus the originally randomized placebo group and a 20% relative decrease in cardiac events in the group originally randomized to Gemfibrozil versus the originally randomized placebo group (see Table 3). This analysis of the originally randomized "intent-to-treat" population neglects the possible complicating effects of treatment switching during the open-label phase. Adjustment of hazard ratios taking into account open-label treatment status from year 6.5 to 8.5 could change the reported hazard ratios for mortality toward unity.

Table 3

CARDIAC EVENTS, CARDIAC DEATHS, NON-CARDIAC DEATHS AND ALL-CAUSE MORTALITY IN THE HELSINKI HEART STUDY. YEARS 5.0-8.5[1]

Event	Gemfibrozil at Study Start	Placebo at Study Start	Placebo Hazard Ratio[2]	Cl Hazard Ratio
Cardiac Events[4]	110	131	0.80	0.62-1.03
Cardiac Deaths	36	38	0.98	0.63-1.54
Non-Cardiac Deaths	65	45	1.40	0.95-2.05
All-Cause Mortality	101	83	1.20	0.90-1.61

[1] *Intention-to-Treat Analysis of originally randomized patients neglecting the open-label treatment switches and exposure to study conditions.*
[2] *Hazard ratio for risk of event in the group originally randomized to Gemfibrozil compared to the group originally randomized to placebo neglecting open-label treatment switch and exposure to study condition.*
[3] *95% confidence intervals of Gemfibrozil placebo group hazard ratio.*
[4] *Fatal and nonfatal myocardial infarctions plus sudden cardiac deaths over the 8.5 year period.*

It is not clear to what extent the findings of the primary prevention component of the Helsinki Heart Study can be extrapolated to other segments of the dyslipidemic population not studied (such as women, younger or older males, or those with lipid abnormalities limited solely to HDL-cholesterol) or to other lipid-altering drugs.

The secondary prevention component of the Helsinki Heart Study was conducted over 5 years in parallel and at the same centers in Finland in 628 middle-aged males excluded from the primary prevention component of The Helsinki Heart Study because of a history of angina, myocardial infarction or unexplained ECG changes (ref. 3). The primary efficacy endpoint of the study was cardiac events (the sum of fatal and non-fatal myocardial infarctions and sudden cardiac deaths). The hazard ratio (Gemfibrozil: placebo) for cardiac events was 1.47 (95% confidence limits 0.88-2.48, p = 0.14). Of the 35 patients in the Gemfibrozil group who experienced cardiac events, 12 patients suffered events after discontinuation from the study. Of the 24 patients in the placebo group with cardiac events, 4 patients suffered events after discontinuation from the study. There were 17 cardiac deaths in the Gemfibrozil group and 8 in the placebo group (hazard ratio 2.18; 95% confidence limits 0.94-5.05, p = 0.06). Ten of these deaths in the Gemfibrozil group and 3 in the placebo group occurred after discontinuation from therapy. In this study of patients with known or suspected coronary heart disease, no benefit from Gemfibrozil treatment was observed in reducing cardiac events or cardiac deaths. Thus, Gemfibrozil has shown benefit only in selected dyslipidemic patients *without* suspected or established coronary heart disease. Even in patients with coronary heart disease and the trial of elevated LDL-cholesterol, elevated triglycerides, plus low HDL-cholesterol, the possible effect of Gemfibrozil on coronary events has not been adequately studied.

No efficacy in the patients with established coronary heart disease was observed during the Coronary Drug Project with the chemically and pharmacologically related drug, clofibrate. The Coronary Drug Project was a 6-year randomized, double-blind study involving 1000 clofibrate, 1000 nicotinic acid, and 3000 placebo patients with known coronary heart disease. A clinically and statistically

Table 1

REDUCTION IN CHD RATES (EVENTS PER 1000 PATIENTS) BY BASELINE LIPIDS[1] IN THE HELSINKI HEART STUDY, YEARS 0-5[2]

	All Patients			LDL-C > 175; HDL-C > 46.4			LDL-C > 175; TG > 177			LDL-C > 175; TG > 200; HDL-C < 35		
	P	G	Dif[3]	P	G	Dif	P	G	Dif	P	G	Dif
Incidence of Evidents[4]	41	27	14	32	29	3	71	44	27	149	64	85

[1] *lipid values in mg/dL at baseline*
[2] *P = placebo group; G = Gemfibrozil group*
[3] *difference in rates between placebo and Gemfibrozil groups*
[4] *fatal and nonfatal myocardial infarctions plus sudden cardiac deaths (events per 1000 patients over 5 years)*

Table 2

CARDIAC EVENTS AND ALL-CAUSE MORTALITY (EVENTS PER 1000 PATIENTS) OCCURRING DURING THE 3.5 YEAR OPEN LABEL FOLLOW-UP TO THE HELSINKI HEART STUDY[1]

Group:	PDrop N = 215	PN N = 494	PG N = 1283	GDrop N = 221	GN N = 574	GL N = 1207
Cardiac Events	38.8	22.9	22.5	37.2	28.3	25.4
All-Cause Mortality	41.9	22.3	15.6	72.3	19.2	24.9

[1] *The six open-label groups are designated first by the original randomization (P = placebo, G = Gemfibrozil) and then by the drug taken in the follow-up period (N = Attended clinic but took no drug G = Gemfibrozil, Drop = No attendance at clinic during open-label).*

♦ RATED THERAPEUTICALLY EQUIVALENT; ◇ THERAPEUTIC EQUIVALENCE UNCONFIRMED; ○ UNRATED

significant reduction in myocardial infarctions was seen in the concurrent nicotinic acid group compared to placebo; no reduction was seen with clofibrate.

The mechanism of action of Gemfibrozil has not been definitely established. In man, Gemfibrozil has been shown to inhibit peripheral lipolysis and to decrease the hepatic extraction of free fatty acids, thus reducing hepatic triglyceride production. Gemfibrozil inhibits synthesis and increases clearance of VLDL carrier apolipoprotein B, leading to a decrease in VLDL production.

Animal studies suggest that Gemfibrozil may, in addition to elevating HDL-cholesterol, reduce incorporation of long-chain fatty acids into newly formed triglycerides, accelerate turnover and removal of cholesterol from the liver, and increase excretion of cholesterol in the feces. Gemfibrozil is well absorbed from the gastrointestinal tract after oral administration. Peak plasma levels occur in 1 to 2 hours with a plasma half-life of 1.5 hours following multiple doses. Plasma levels appear proportional to dose and do not demonstrate accumulation across time following multiple doses.

Gemfibrozil mainly undergoes oxidation of a ring methyl group to successively form a hydroxymethyl and a carboxyl metabolite. Approximately seventy percent of the administered human dose is excreted in the urine, mostly as the glucuronide conjugate, with less than 2% excreted as unchanged Gemfibrozil. Six percent of the dose is accounted for in the feces.

INDICATIONS AND USAGE

Gemfibrozil tablets are indicated as adjunctive therapy to diet for:

1. Treatment of adult patients with very high elevations of serum triglyceride levels (Types IV and V hyperlipidemia) who present a risk of pancreatitis and who do not respond adequately to a determined dietary effort to control them. Patients who present such risk typically have serum triglycerides over 2000 mg/dL and have elevations of VLDL-cholesterol as well as fasting chylomicrons (Type V hyperlipidemia). Subjects who consistently have total serum or plasma triglycerides below 1000 mg/dL are unlikely to present a risk of pancreatitis. Gemfibrozil therapy may be considered for those subjects with triglyceride elevations between 1000 and 2000 mg/dL who have a history of pancreatitis or of recurrent abdominal pain typical of pancreatitis. It is recognized that some Type IV patients with triglycerides under 1000 mg/dL may, through dietary or alcoholic indiscretion, convert to a Type V pattern with massive triglyceride elevations accompanying fasting chylomicronemia, but the influence of Gemfibrozil therapy on the risk of pancreatitis in such situations has not been adequately studied. Drug therapy is not indicated for patients with Type I hyperlipoproteinemia, who have elevations of chylomicrons and plasma triglycerides, but who have normal levels of very low density lipoprotein (VLDL). Inspection of plasma refrigerated for 14 hours is helpful in distinguishing Types I, IV, and V hyperlipoproteinemia (ref. 4).

2. Reducing the risk of developing coronary heart disease *only* in Type IIb patients without history of or symptoms of existing coronary heart disease who have had an inadequate response to weight loss, dietary therapy, exercise, and other pharmacologic agents (such as bile acid sequestrants and nicotinic acid, known to reduce LDL-and raise HDL-cholesterol *and* who have the following triad of lipid abnormalities: low HDL-cholesterol levels in addition to elevated LDL-cholesterol and elevated triglycerides (see *"Warnings," "Precautions"*, and *"Clinical Pharmacology"*). The National Cholesterol Education Program has defined a serum HDL-cholesterol value that is consistently below 35 mg/dL as constituting an independent risk factor for coronary heart disease (ref. 5). Patients with significantly elevated triglycerides should be closely observed when treated with Gemfibrozil. In some patients with high triglyceride levels, treatment with Gemfibrozil is associated with a significant increase in LDL-cholesterol. BECAUSE OF POTENTIAL TOXICITY SUCH AS MALIGNANCY, GALLBLADDER DISEASE, ABDOMINAL PAIN LEADING TO APPENDECTOMY AND OTHER ABDOMINAL SURGERIES, AN INCREASED INCIDENCE IN NONCORONARY MORTALITY, AND THE 44% RELATIVE INCREASE DURING THE TRIAL PERIOD IN AGE-ADJUSTED ALL-CAUSE MORTALITY SEEN WITH THE CHEMICALLY AND PHARMACOLOGICALLY RELATED DRUG, CLOFIBRATE, THE POTENTIAL BENEFIT OF GEMFIBROZIL IN TREATING TYPE IIA PATIENTS WITH ELEVATIONS OF LDL-CHOLESTEROL ONLY IS NOT LIKELY TO OUTWEIGH THE RISKS. GEMFIBROZIL IS ALSO NOT INDICATED FOR THE TREATMENT OF PATIENTS WITH LOW HDL-CHOLESTEROL AS THEIR ONLY LIPID ABNORMALITY.

In a subgroup analysis of patients in the Helsinki Heart Study with above-median HDL-cholesterol values at baseline (greater than 46.4 mg/dL), the incidence of serious coronary events was similar for Gemfibrozil and placebo subgroups (see Table 1).

The initial treatment for dyslipidemia is dietary therapy specific for the type of lipoprotein abnormality. Excess body weight and excess alcohol intake may be important factors in hypertriglyceridemia and should be managed prior to any drug therapy. Physical exercise can be an important ancillary measure, and has been associated with rises in HDL-cholesterol. Diseases contributory to hyperlipidemia such as hypothyroidism or diabetes mellitus should be looked for and adequately treated. Estrogen therapy is sometimes associated with massive rises in plasma triglycerides, especially in subjects with familial hypertriglyceridemia. In such cases, discontinuation of estrogen therapy may obviate the need for specific drug therapy of hypertriglyceridemia. The use of drugs should be considered only when reasonable attempts have been made to obtain satisfactory results with nondrug methods. If the decision is made to use drugs, the patient should be instructed that this does not reduce the importance of adhering to diet.

CONTRAINDICATIONS

1. Hepatic or severe renal dysfunction, including primary biliary cirrhosis.
2. Preexisting gallbladder disease (see *"Warnings"*).
3. Hypersensitivity to Gemfibrozil.

WARNINGS

1. Because of chemical, pharmacological, and clinical similarities between Gemfibrozil and clofibrate, the adverse findings with clofibrate in two large clinical studies may also apply to Gemfibrozil. In the first of those studies, the Coronary Drug Project, 1000 subjects with previous myocardial infarction were treated for 5 years with clofibrate. There was no difference in mortality between the clofibrate-treated subjects and 3000 placebo-treated subjects, but twice as many clofibrate-treated subjects developed cholelithiasis and cholecystitis requiring surgery. In the other study, conducted by the World Health Organization (WHO), 5000 subjects without known coronary heart disease were treated with clofibrate for 5 years and followed one year beyond. There was a statistically significant, 44%, higher age-adjusted total mortality in the clofibrate-treated than in a comparable placebo-treated control group during the trial period. The excess mortality was due to a 33% increase in noncardiovascular causes, including malignancy, post-cholecystectomy complications, and pancreatitis. The higher risk of clofibrate-treated subjects for gallbladder disease was confirmed.

Because of the more limited size of the Helsinki Heart Study, the observed difference in mortality from any cause between the Gemfibrozil and placebo group is not statistically significantly different from the 29% excess mortality reported in the clofibrate group in the separate WHO study at the 9 year follow-up (see *"Clinical Pharmacology"*). Noncoronary heart disease related mortality showed an excess in the group originally randomized to Gemfibrozil primarily due to cancer deaths observed during the open-label extension.

During the 5 year primary prevention component of the Helsinki Heart Study mortality from any cause was 44 (2.2%) in the Gemfibrozil group and 43 (2.1%) in the placebo group; including the 3.5 year follow-up period since the trial was completed, cumulative mortality from any cause was 101 (4.9%) in the Gemfibrozil group and 83 (4.1%) in the group originally randomized to placebo (hazard ratio 1.20 in favor of placebo). Because of the more limited size of the Helsinki Heart Study, the observed difference in mortality from any cause between the Gemfibrozil and placebo groups at year-5 or at year-8.5 is not statistically significantly different from the 29% excess mortality reported in the clofibrate group in the separate WHO study at the 9 year follow-up. Noncoronary heart disease related mortality showed an excess in the group originally randomized to Gemfibrozil at the 8.5 year follow-up (65 Gemfibrozil versus 45 placebo noncoronary deaths).

The incidence of cancer (excluding basal cell carcinoma) discovered during the trial and in the 3.5 years after the trial was completed was 51 (2.5%) in both originally randomized groups. In addition, there were 16 basal cell carcinomas in the group originally randomized to Gemfibrozil and 9 in the group randomized to placebo ($p = 0.22$). There were 30 (1.5%) deaths attributed to cancer in the group originally randomized to Gemfibrozil and 18 (0.9%) in the group originally randomized to placebo ($p = 0.11$). Adverse outcomes, including coronary events, were higher in Gemfibrozil patients in a corresponding study in men with a history of known or suspected coronary heart disease in the secondary prevention component of the Helsinki Heart Study. (See *"Clinical Pharmacology"*).

2. A gallstone prevalence substudy of 450 Helsinki Heart Study participants showed a trend toward a greater prevalence of gallstones during the study within the Gemfibrozil treatment group (7.5% vs 4.9% for the placebo group, a 55% excess for the Gemfibrozil group). A trend toward a greater incidence of gallbladder surgery was observed for the Gemfibrozil group (17 vs 11 subjects, a 54% excess). This result did not differ statistically from the increased incidence of cholecystectomy observed in the WHO study in the group treated with clofibrate. Both clofibrate and Gemfibrozil may increase cholesterol excretion into the bile leading to cholelithiasis. If cholelithiasis is suspected, gallbladder studies are indicated Gemfibrozil therapy should be discontinued if gallstones are found.

3. Since a reduction of mortality from coronary artery disease has not been demonstrated and because liver and interstitial cell testicular tumors were increased in rats, Gemfibrozil should be administered only to those patients described in the *"Indications and Usage"* section. If a significant serum lipid response is not obtained, Gemfibrozil should be discontinued.

4. Concomitant Anticoagulants—Caution should be exercised when anticoagulants are given in conjunction with Gemfibrozil. The dosage of the anticoagulant should be reduced to maintain the prothrombin time at the desired level to prevent bleeding complications. Frequent prothrombin determinations are advisable until it has been definitely determined that the prothrombin level has stabilized.

5. Concomitant therapy with Gemfibrozil and lovastatin has been associated with rhabdomyolysis, markedly elevated creatine kinase (CK) levels and myoglobinuria, leading in a high proportion of cases to acute renal failure. IN VIRTUALLY ALL PATIENTS WHO HAVE HAD AN UNSATISFACTORY LIPID RESPONSE TO EITHER DRUG ALONE, ANY POTENTIAL LIPID BENEFIT OF COMBINED THERAPY WITH LOVASTATIN AND GEMFIBROZIL DOES NOT OUTWEIGH THE RISKS OF SEVERE MYOPATHY, RHABDOMYOLYSIS, AND ACUTE RENAL FAILURE (see *"Drug Interactions"*). The use of fibrates alone, including Gemfibrozil may occasionally be associated with myositis. Patients receiving Gemfibrozil and complaining of muscle pain, tenderness, or weakness should have prompt medical evaluation for myositis, including serum creatine kinase level determination. If myositis is suspected or diagnosed, Gemfibrozil therapy should be withdrawn.

6. Cataracts—Subcapsular bilateral cataracts occurred in 10% and unilateral in 6.3% of male rats treated with Gemfibrozil at 10 times the human dose.

PRECAUTIONS

1. Initial Therapy: Laboratory studies should be done to ascertain that the lipid levels are consistently abnormal. Before instituting Gemfibrozil therapy, every attempt should be made to control serum lipids with appropriate diet, exercise, weight loss in obese patients, and control of any medical problems such as diabetes mellitus and hypothrryoidism that are contributing to the lipid abnormalities.

2. Continued Therapy: Periodic determination of serum lipids should be obtained, and the drug withdrawn if lipid response is inadequate after 3 months of therapy.

3. Drug Interactions: (A) HMG-CoA reductase inhibitors: Rhabdomyolysis has occurred with combined Gemfibrozil and lovastatin therapy. It may be seen as early as 3 weeks after initiation of combined therapy or after several months. In most subjects who have had an unsatisfactory lipid response to either drug alone, the possible benefit of combined therapy with lovastatin (or other HMG-CoA reductase inhibitors) and Gemfibrozil does not outweigh the risks of severe myopathy, rhabdomyolysis, and acute renal failure. There is no assurance that periodic monitoring of creatine kinase will prevent the occurrence of severe myopathy and kidney damage.

(B) Anticoagulants: CAUTION SHOULD BE EXERCISED WHEN ANTICO-AGULANTS ARE GIVEN IN CONJUNCTION WITH GEMFIBROZIL. THE DOSAGE OF THE ANTICOAGULANT SHOULD BE REDUCED TO MAINTAIN THE PROTHROMBIN TIME AT THE DESIRED LEVEL TO PREVENT BLEEDING COMPLICATIONS. FREQUENT PROTHROMBIN DETERMINATIONS ARE ADVISABLE UNTIL IT HAS BEEN DEFINITELY DETERMINED THAT THE PROTHROMBIN LEVEL HAS STABILIZED.

4. Carcinogenesis, Mutagenesis, Impairment of Fertility: Long-term studies have been conducted in rats at 0.2 and 2 times the human dose (based on surface area, mg/meter^2). Based on two-week toxicokinetic studies, exposure (AUC) of the dose groups was estimated to be 0.2 and 1.3 times the human exposure. The incidence of benign liver nodules and liver carcinomas was significantly increased in high dose male rats. The incidence of liver carcinomas increased also in low dose males, but this increase was not statistically significant ($p = 0.1$). Male rats had a dose-related and statistically significant increase of benign Leydig cell tumors. The higher dose female rats had a significant increase in the combined incidence of benign and malignant liver neoplasms.

Long-term studies have been conducted in mice at 0.1 and 1 times the human dose (based on surface area). Based on two-week toxicokinetic studies, exposure (AUC) of the two dose groups was estimated to be 0.1 and 0.7 times the human exposure. There were no statistically significant differences from controls in the incidence of liver tumors, but the doses tested were lower than those shown to be carcinogenic with other fibrates. Electron microscopy studies have demonstrated a florid hepatic peroxisome proliferation following Gemfibrozil administration to the male rat. An adequate study to test for peroxisome proliferation has been shown to occur in humans with either of two other drugs of the fibrate class when liver biopsies were compared before and after treatment in the same individual.

Administration of approximately 0.6 and 2 times the human dose (based on surface area) to male rats for 10 weeks resulted in a dose-related decrease of fertility. Subsequent studies demonstrated that this effect was reversed after a drug-free period of about eight weeks, and it was not transmitted to the offspring.

5. Pregnancy Category C: Gemfibrozil has been shown to produce adverse effects in rats and rabbits at doses between 0.5 and 3 times the human dose (based on surface area) but no developmental toxicity or teratogenicity among offspring of either species. There are no adequate and well-controlled studies in pregnant women. Gemfibrozil should be used during pregnancy only if the potential benefit justifies the potential risk to the fetus.

Administration of Gemfibrozil to female rats at 0.6 and 2 times the human dose (based on surface area) before and throughout gestation caused a dose-related decrease in conception rate and, at the high dose, an increase in still-borns and a slight reduction in pup weight during lactation. There were also dose-related increased skeletal variations. Anophthalmia occurred, but rarely.

Administration of 0.6 and 2 times the human dose (based on surface area) of Gemfibrozil to female rats from gestation day 15 through weaning caused dose-related decreases in birth weight and suppressions of pup growth during lactation.

Administration of 1 and 3 times the human dose (based on surface area) of Gemfibrozil to female rabbits during organogenesis caused a dose-related decrease in litter size and, at the high dose, an increased incidence of parietal bone variations.

6. Nursing Mothers: It is not known whether this drug is excreted in human milk. Because many drugs are excreted in human milk and because of the potential for tumorigenicity shown for Gemfibrozil in animal studies, a decision should be made whether to discontinue nursing or to discontinue the drug, taking into account the importance of the drug to the mother.

7. Hematologic Changes: Mild hemoglobin, hematocrit and white blood cell decreases have been observed in occasional patients following initiation of Gemfibrozil therapy. However, these levels stabilize during long-term administration. Rarely, severe anemia, leukopenia, thrombocytopenia, and bone marrow hypoplasia have been reported. Therefore, periodic blood counts are recommended during the first 12 months of Gemfibrozil administration.

8. Liver Function: Abnormal liver function tests have been observed occasionally during Lopid administration, including elevations of AST (SGOT), ALT (SGPT), LDH, bilirubin, and alkaline phosphatase. These are usually reversible when Gemfibrozil is discontinued. Therefore periodic liver function studies are

recommended and Gemfibrozil therapy should be terminated if abnormalities persist.

9. Kidney Function: There have been reports of worsening renal insufficiency upon the addition of Gemfibrozil therapy in individuals with baseline plasma creatinine > 2.0 mg/dL. In such patients, the use of alternative therapy should be considered against the risks and benefits of a lower dose of Gemfibrozil.

10. Use in Children: Safety and efficacy in children have not been established.

ADVERSE REACTIONS

In the double-blind controlled phase of the primary prevention component of the Helsinki Heart Study, 2046 patients received Gemfibrozil for up to 5 years. In that study, the following adverse reactions were statistically more frequent in subjects in the Gemfibrozil group:

	Gemfibrozil (N = 2046)	Placebo (N = 2035)
	Frequency in percent of subjects	
Gastrointestinal reactions	34.2	23.8
Dyspepsia	19.6	11.9
Abdominal pain	9.8	5.6
Acute appendicitis (histologically confirmed in most cases where data were available)	1.2	0.6
Atrial fibrillation	0.7	0.1

Adverse events reported by more than 1% of subjects, but without a significant difference between groups:

Diarrhea	7.2	6.5
Fatigue	3.8	3.5
Nausea/Vomiting	2.5	2.1
Eczema	1.9	1.2
Rash	1.7	1.3
Vertigo	1.5	1.1
Constipation	1.4	1.3
Headache	1.2	1.1

Gallbladder surgery was performed in 0.9% of Gemfibrozil and 0.5% of placebo subjects in the primary prevention component, a 64% excess, which is not statistically different from the excess of gallbladder surgery observed in the clofibrate compared to the placebo group of the WHO study. Gallbladder surgery was also performed more frequently in the Gemfibrozil group compared to placebo (1.9% vs 0.3%, p = 0.07) in the secondary prevention component. A statistically significant increase in appendectomy in the Gemfibrozil group was seen also in the secondary prevention component (6 on Gemfibrozil vs 0 on placebo, p = 0.014).

Nervous system and special senses adverse reactions were more common in the Gemfibrozil group. These included hypesthesia, paresthesias, and taste perversion. Other adverse reactions that were more common among Gemfibrozil treatment group subjects but where a causal relationship was not established include cataracts, peripheral vascular disease, and intracerebral hemorrhage.

From other studies it seems probable that Gemfibrozil is causally related to the occurrence of *Musculoskeletal Symptoms* (See *"Warnings"*), and to *Abnormal Liver Function Tests* and *Hematologic Changes* (See *"Precautions"*).

Reports of viral and bacterial infections (common cold, cough, urinary tract infections) were more common in Gemfibrozil treated patients in other controlled clinical trials of 805 patients. Additional adverse reactions that have been reported for Gemfibrozil are listed below by system. These are categorized according to whether a causal relationship to treatment with Gemfibrozil is probable or not established:

	Causal Relationship Probable	Causal Relationship Not Established
General:		weight loss
Cardiac:		extrasystoles
Gastrointestinal:	cholestatic jaundice	pancreatitis
		hepatoma
		colitis
Central Nervous System:	dizziness	confusion
	somnolence	convulsions
	paresthesia	syncope
	peripheral neuritis	
	decreased libido	
	depression	
	headache	
Eye:	blurred vision	retinal edema
Genitourinary:	impotence	decreased male fertility
		renal dysfunction
Musculoskeletal:	myopathy	
	myasthenia	

	Causal Relationship Probable	Causal Relationship Not Established
	myalgia	
	painful extremities	
	arthralgia	
	synovitis	
	rhabdomyolysis (See "Warnings" and Drug Interactions under "Precautions")	
Clinical Laboratory:	increased creatine phosphokinase	positive antinuclear antibody
	increased bilirubin	
	increased liver transaminases (AST [SGOT], ALT [SGPT])	
	increased alkaline phosphatase	
Hematopoietic:	anemia	thrombocytopenia
	leukopenia	
	bone marrow hypoplasia	
	eosinophilia	
Immunologic:	angioedema	anaphylaxis
	laryngeal edema	Lupus-like syndrome
	urticaria	vasculitis
Integumentary:	exfoliative dermatitis	alopecia
	rash	
	dermatitis	
	pruritus	

OVERDOSAGE

There have been reported cases of overdosage with Gemfibrozil. In one case a 7-year-old child recovered after ingesting up to 9 grams of Gemfibrozil. Symptomatic supportive measures should be taken should an overdose occur.

DOSAGE AND ADMINISTRATION

The recommended dose for adults is 1200 mg administered in two divided doses 30 minutes before the morning and evening meal.

Store below 30°C (86°F).

REFERENCES

1. Frick MH, Elo O, Haapa K, et al: Helsinki Heart Study: Primary prevention trial with gemfibrozil in middle-aged men with dyslipidemia. N Engl J Med 1987; 317:1237-1245. 2. Manninen V, Elo O, Frick MH, et al: Lipid alterations and decline in the incidence of coronary heart disease in the Helsinki Heart Study. JAMA 1988; 260:641-651. 3. Frick MH, Heinonen OP, et al: Efficacy of Gemfibrozil in Dyslipidemic Subjects with Suspected Heart Disease. An Ancillary Study in the Helsinki Heart Study Frame Population. Annals of Medicine 1993; 25:41-45. 4. Nikkila EA: Familial lipoprotein lipase deficiency and related disorders of chylomicron metabolism. In Stanbury J.B. et al. (eds.): The Metabolic Basis of Inherited Disease, 5th ed., McGraw-Hill, 1983, Chap. 30, pp. 622-642. 5. Report of the National Cholesterol Education Program Expert Panel on Detection, Evaluation, and Treatment of High Blood Cholesterol. Arch Int Med 1988;148:36-69.

HOW SUPPLIED
TABLET: 600 MG

AVERAGE UNIT PRICE (AVAILABLE SIZES)		GENERIC A-RATED AVERAGE PRICE (GAAP)	
BRAND	$1.15	60s	$55.76
GENERIC	$0.95	100s	$97.69
HCFA FUL (60s ea)	$0.68	180s	$166.95
		500s	$461.90
		750s	$739.72

BRAND/MANUFACTURER	NDC	SIZE	AWP
◆ BRAND			
➤ LOPID: Parke-Davis	00071-0737-20	60s	$65.74
	00071-0737-40	100s ud	$125.98
	00071-0737-30	500s	$547.83
◆ GENERICS			
Allscrips	54569-3695-01	6s	$5.57
Medirex	57480-0809-06	30s	$32.85
Major	00904-7732-52	50s	$57.20
Sidmak	50111-0857-04	60s	$51.00
Lemmon	00093-0670-06	60s	$54.00
Purepac	00228-2552-06	60s	$54.05
Qualitest	00603-3750-20	60s	$54.92
URL	00677-1473-06	60s	$55.50
Schein	00364-2566-06	60s	$55.65
GEMCOR: Upsher-Smith	00245-0670-60	60s	$55.65
Allscrips	54569-3695-00	60s	$55.65
West Point	59591-0017-68	60s	$55.65
Geneva	00781-1056-60	60s	$56.31
➤ Lederle Std Prod	00005-3160-32	60s	$56.60
Rugby	00536-5554-08	60s	$59.95
Rugby	00536-5668-08	60s	$59.95
Allscrips	54569-8511-01	90s	$83.48
Vangard	00615-3559-13	100s ud	$79.74

BRAND/MANUFACTURER	NDC	SIZE	AWP
UDL	51079-0787-20	100s ud	$103.82
Medirex	57480-0809-01	100s ud	$109.50
Allscrips	54569-8016-00	180s	$166.95
Allscrips	54569-8511-00	180s	$166.95
Sidmak	50111-0857-02	500s	$418.00
Purepac	00228-2552-50	500s	$447.35
Lemmon	00093-0670-05	500s	$450.00
Qualitest	00603-3750-28	500s	$456.90
Schein	00364-2566-05	500s	$461.95
GEMCOR: Upsher-Smith	00245-0670-15	500s	$461.95
Geneva	00781-1056-05	500s	$466.56
Major	00904-7732-40	500s	$469.10
➤ Lederle Std Prod	00005-3160-31	500s	$471.14
Rugby	00536-5554-05	500s	$489.00
Rugby	00536-5668-05	500s	$489.00
Glasgow	60809-0122-55	750s ud	$739.72
Glasgow	60809-0122-72	750s ud	$739.72

Genoptic SEE GENTAMICIN SULFATE, OPHTHALMIC

Gentacidin SEE GENTAMICIN SULFATE, OPHTHALMIC

Gentamicin Sulfate and Prednisolone Acetate

DESCRIPTION

Gentamicin Sulfate/Prednisolone Acetate is a topical anti-infective/anti-inflammatory combination product for ophthalmic use available as an ointment and a suspension.

The ointment contains:

Gentamicin Sulfate equivalent to ....0.3% Gentamicin base
Prednisolone Acetate 0.6%

The suspension contains:

Gentamicin Sulfate equivalent to ....0.3% Gentamicin Base
Prednisolone Acetate 1.0%

Chemical Names: Prednisolone Acetate: 11β, 17,21-Trihydroxypregna-1,4-diene-3,20-dione 21-acetate.

Gentamicin Sulfate is the sulfate salt of Gentamicin C_1, Gentamicin C_2, and Gentamicin C_{1A} which are produced by the growth of *Micromonospora purpurea.*

CLINICAL PHARMACOLOGY

Corticosteroids suppress the inflammatory response to a variety of agents and they probably delay or slow healing. Since corticosteroids may inhibit the body's defense mechanism against infection, a concomitant antimicrobial drug may be used when this inhibition is considered to be clinically significant in a particular case.

The anti-infective component in Gentamicin Sulfate/Prednisolone Acetate is included to provide action against specific organisms susceptible to it Gentamicin Sulfate is active *in vitro* against susceptible strains of the following microorganisms: coagulase-positive and coagulase-negative staphylococci, including *S. aureus,* and certain strains that are resistant to penicillin; Group A beta-hemolytic and non-hemolytic streptococci, and *Streptococcus pneumoniae; Escherichia coll; Haemophilus influenzae; Klebsiella/Enterobacter* species; *Neisseria* species, including *Neisseria gonorrhoeae; Pseudomonas aeruginosa;* indole-positive and indole-negative *Proteus* species; and *Serratia marcescens.*

When a decision to administer both a corticosteroid and an antimicrobial is made, the administration of such drugs in combination has the advantage of greater patient compliance and convenience, with the added assurance that the appropriate dosage of both drugs is administered. When both types of drugs are in the same formulation, compatibility of ingredients is assured and the correct volume of drug is delivered and retained.

The relative potency of corticosteroids depends on the molecular structure, concentration, and release from the vehicle.

INDICATIONS AND USAGE

Gentamicin Sulfate/Prednisolone Acetate is indicated for steroid-responsive inflammatory ocular conditions for which a corticosteroid is indicated and where superficial bacterial ocular infection or a risk of bacterial ocular infection exists.

Ocular steroids are indicated in inflammatory conditions of the palpebral and bulbar conjunctiva, cornea, and anterior segment of the globe where the inherent risk of steroid use in certain infective conjunctivitides is accepted to obtain a diminution in edema and inflammation. They are also indicated in chronic anterior uveitis and corneal injury from chemical, radiation, or thermal burns or penetration of foreign bodies.

The use of a combination drug with an anti-infective component is indicated where the risk of superficial ocular infection is high or where there is an expectation that potentially dangerous numbers of bacteria will be present in the eye.

The particular anti-infective drug in this product is active against the following common eye pathogens: coagulase-positive and coagulase-negative staphylococci, including *Staphylococcus aureus,* and certain strains that are resistant to

➤ SHOWN IN PRODUCT IDENTIFICATION GUIDE

penicillin; Group A beta-hemolytic and nonhemolytic streptococci, and *Streptococcus pneumoniae; Escherichia coli; Haemophilus influenzae; Klebsiella/Enterobacter* species; *Neisseria* species, including *Neisseria gonorrhoeae; Pseudomonas aeruginosa;* indole-positive and indole-negative *Proteus* species; and *Serratia marcescens.*

CONTRAINDICATIONS
Epithelial herpes simplex keratitis (dendritic keratitis), vaccinia, varicella, and many other viral diseases of the cornea and conjunctiva. Mycobacterial infection of the eye. Fungal diseases of the ocular structures. Hypersensitivity to a component of the medication. (Hypersensitivity to the antibiotic component occurs at a higher rate than for other components.)

Gentamicin Sulfate/Prednisolone Acetate is always contraindicated after uncomplicated removal of a corneal foreign body.

WARNINGS
Prolonged use may result in glaucoma, with damage to the optic nerve, defects in visual acuity and fields of vision, and in posterior subcapsular cataract formation. Prolonged use may suppress the host immune response and thus increase the hazard of secondary ocular infections. In those diseases causing thinning of the cornea or sclera, perforations have been known to occur with the use of topical steroids. In acute purulent conditions of the eye, steroids may mask infection or enhance existing infection. If these products are used for 10 days or longer, intraocular pressure should be routinely monitored even though it may be difficult in children and uncooperative patients.

Employment of a steroid medication in the treatment of patients with a history of herpes simplex requires great caution.

Gentamicin Sulfate/Prednisolone Acetate is contraindicated in patients with active herpes simplex keratitis.

Gentamicin Sulfate/Prednisolone Acetate suspension is not for injection. It should never be injected subconjunctivally, nor should it be directly introduced into the anterior chamber of the eye.

PRECAUTIONS
General: Ocular irritation and punctate keratitis have been associated with the use of Gentamicin Sulfate/Prednisolone Acetate. The initial prescription and renewal of the medication order beyond 8 gm of ointment or 20 ml of suspension should be made by a physician only after examination of the patient's intraocular pressure, examination of the patient with the aid of magnification, such as slit lamp biomicroscopy and, where appropriate, fluorescein staining.

The possibility of fungal infections of the cornea should be considered after prolonged steroid dosing.

Carcinogenesis, Mutagenesis, Impairment of Fertility: There are no published carcinogenicity or impairment of fertility studies on Gentamicin. Aminoglycoside antibiotics have been found to be nonmutagenic.

There are no published mutagenicity or impairment of fertility studies on Prednisolone. Prednisolone has been reported to be non-carcinogenic.

Pregnancy: Pregnancy Category C: Gentamicin has been shown to depress newborn body weights, kidney weights, nephron counts and shows evidence of glomeruli and proximal tubule nephrotoxicity in rats when administered systemically in daily doses of approximately 500 times the maximum recommended ophthalmic dose in humans.

Prednisolone has been shown to be teratogenic in mice when given in doses 1-10 times the human dose. Dexamethasone, hydrocortisone and Prednisolone were ocularly applied to both eyes of pregnant mice five times per day on days 10 through 13 of gestation. A significant increase in the incidence of cleft palate was observed in the fetuses of the treated mice. There are no adequate well-controlled studies in pregnant women. Gentamicin Sulfate/Prednisolone Acetate should be used during pregnancy only if the potential benefit justifies the potential risk to the fetus.

Nursing Mothers: It is not known whether topical administration of corticosteroids could result in sufficient systemic absorption to produce detectable quantities in breast milk. Systemically administered corticosteroids appear in breast milk and could suppress growth, interfere with endogenous corticosteroid production, or cause other untoward effects. Because of the potential for serious adverse reactions in nursing infants from Gentamicin Sulfate/Prednisolone Acetate, a decision should be made whether to discontinue nursing or to discontinue the medication.

Pediatric Use: Safety and effectiveness in children have not been established.

ADVERSE REACTIONS
Adverse reactions have occurred with steroid/anti-infective combination drugs which can be attributed to the steroid component, the anti-infective component, or the combination. Exact incidence figures are not available since no denominator of treated patients is available.

The most frequent reactions observed include ocular discomfort, burning, stinging, and other symptoms of irritation upon instillation of the medication and, typically after several days of use, punctate keratitis. These reactions have resolved upon discontinuation of the medication.

Reactions occurring most often from the presence of the anti-infective ingredient are allergic sensitizations. The reactions due to the steroid component in decreasing order of frequency are: elevation of intraocular pressure (IOP) with possible development of glaucoma, and infrequent optic nerve damage; posterior subcapsular cataract formation; and delayed wound healing.

Secondary Infection: The development of secondary infection has occurred after use of combinations containing steroids and antimicrobials. Fungal infections of the cornea are particularly prone to develop coincidentally with long-term applications of steroid. The possibility of fungal invasion must be considered in any persistent corneal ulceration where steroid treatment has been used.

Secondary bacterial ocular infection following suppression of host responses also occurs.

DOSAGE AND ADMINISTRATION
A small amount (½ inch ribbon) of ointment should be applied in the conjunctival sac one to three times daily. Care should be taken not to discontinue therapy prematurely.

Not more than 8 gm should be prescribed initially and the prescription should not be refilled without further evaluation as outlined in *"Precautions"* above.

Instill one drop into the conjunctival sac two to four times daily. During the initial 24 to 48 hours, the dosing frequency may be increased if necessary. Care should be taken not to discontinue therapy prematurely.

Not more than 20 ml should be prescribed initially and the prescription should not be refilled without further evaluation as outlined in *"Precautions"* above.

Note: Store the ointment at controlled room temperature between 15°-30° C (59°-86° F).

Note: Store the suspension at room temperature. Avoid excessive heat, 40° C (104° F) and above. Protect from freezing. Shake well before using.

HOW SUPPLIED
DROP: 1%-0.3%

BRAND/MANUFACTURER	NDC	SIZE	AWP
○ **BRAND**			
PRED-G: Allergan Optical	00023-0106-02	2 ml	$6.69
	00023-0106-05	5 ml	$18.29
	00023-0106-10	10 ml	$33.11

OINTMENT:

BRAND/MANUFACTURER	NDC	SIZE	AWP
○ **BRAND**			
PRED-G S.O.P.: Allergan Optical	00023-0066-04	3.5 gm	$17.78

Gentamicin Sulfate, Injectable

WARNINGS
PATIENTS TREATED WITH AMINOGLYCOSIDES SHOULD BE UNDER CLOSE CLINICAL OBSERVATION BECAUSE OF THE POTENTIAL TOXICITY ASSOCIATED WITH THEIR USE.

AS WITH OTHER AMINOGLYCOSIDES, GENTAMICIN SULFATE, INJECTABLE IS POTENTIALLY NEPHROTOXIC. THE RISK OF NEPHROTOXICITY IS GREATER IN PATIENTS WITH IMPAIRED RENAL FUNCTION AND IN THOSE WHO RECEIVE HIGH DOSAGE OR PROLONGED THERAPY.

NEUROTOXICITY MANIFESTED BY OTOTOXICITY, BOTH VESTIBULAR AND AUDITORY, CAN OCCUR IN PATIENTS TREATED WITH GENTAMICIN SULFATE, INJECTABLE PRIMARILY IN THOSE WITH PREEXISTING RENAL DAMAGE AND IN PATIENTS WITH NORMAL RENAL FUNCTION TREATED WITH HIGHER DOSES AND/OR FOR LONGER PERIODS THAN RECOMMENDED. AMINOGLYCOSIDE-INDUCED OTOTOXICITY IS USUALLY IRREVERSIBLE. OTHER MANIFESTATIONS OF NEUROTOXICITY MAY INCLUDE NUMBNESS, SKIN TINGLING, MUSCLE TWITCHING AND CONVULSIONS.

RENAL AND EIGHTH CRANIAL NERVE FUNCTION SHOULD BE CLOSELY MONITORED, ESPECIALLY IN PATIENTS WITH KNOWN OR SUSPECTED REDUCED RENAL FUNCTION AT ONSET OF THERAPY, AND ALSO IN THOSE WHOSE RENAL FUNCTION IS INITIALLY NORMAL BUT WHO DEVELOP SIGNS OF RENAL DYSFUNCTION DURING THERAPY. URINE SHOULD BE EXAMINED FOR DECREASED SPECIFIC GRAVITY, INCREASED EXCRETION OF PROTEIN, AND THE PRESENCE OF CELLS OR CASTS. BLOOD UREA NITROGEN, SERUM CREATININE, OR CREATININE CLEARANCE SHOULD BE DETERMINED PERIODICALLY. WHEN FEASIBLE, IT IS RECOMMENDED THAT SERIAL AUDIOGRAMS BE OBTAINED IN PATIENTS OLD ENOUGH TO BE TESTED, PARTICULARLY HIGH-RISK PATIENTS. EVIDENCE OF OTOTOXICITY (DIZZINESS, VERTIGO, ATAXIA TINNITUS, ROARING IN THE EARS OR HEARING LOSS) OR NEPHROTOXICITY REQUIRES DOSAGE ADJUSTMENT OR DISCONTINUANCE OF THE DRUG. AS WITH THE OTHER AMINOGLYCOSIDES, ON RARE OCCASIONS CHANGES IN RENAL AND EIGHTH CRANIAL NERVE FUNCTION MAY NOT BECOME MANIFEST UNTIL SOON AFTER COMPLETION OF THERAPY.

SERUM CONCENTRATIONS OF AMINOGLYCOSIDES SHOULD BE MONITORED WHEN FEASIBLE TO ASSURE ADEQUATE LEVELS AND TO

AVOID POTENTIALLY TOXIC LEVELS. WHEN MONITORING GENTAMICIN PEAK CONCENTRATIONS, DOSAGE SHOULD BE ADJUSTED SO THAT PROLONGED LEVELS ABOVE 12 MCG/ML ARE AVOIDED. WHEN MONITORING GENTAMICIN TROUGH CONCENTRATIONS, DOSAGE SHOULD BE ADJUSTED SO THAT LEVELS ABOVE 2 MCG/ML ARE AVOIDED. EXCESSIVE PEAK AND/OR TROUGH SERUM CONCENTRATIONS OF AMINOGLYCOSIDES MAY INCREASE THE RISK OF RENAL AND EIGHTH CRANIAL NERVE TOXICITY. IN THE EVENT OF OVERDOSE OR TOXIC REACTIONS, HEMODIALYSIS MAY AID IN THE REMOVAL OF GENTAMICIN FROM THE BLOOD, ESPECIALLY IF RENAL FUNCTION IS, OR BECOMES, COMPROMISED. THE RATE OF REMOVAL OF GENTAMICIN IS CONSIDERABLY LESS BY PERITONEAL DIALYSIS THAN BY HEMODIALYSIS. IN THE NEWBORN INFANT, EXCHANGE TRANSFUSIONS MAY ALSO BE CONSIDERED.

CONCURRENT AND/OR SEQUENTIAL SYSTEMIC OR TOPICAL USE OF OTHER POTENTIALLY NEUROTOXIC AND/OR NEPHROTOXIC DRUGS, SUCH AS CISPLATIN, CEPHALORIDINE, KANAMYCIN, AMIKACIN, NEOMYCIN, POLYMYXIN B, COLISTIN, PAROMOMYCIN, STREPTOMYCIN, TOBRAMYCIN, VANCOMYCIN, AND VIOMYCIN, SHOULD BE AVOIDED. OTHER FACTORS WHICH MAY INCREASE PATIENT RISK OF TOXICITY ARE ADVANCED AGE AND DEHYDRATION.

THE CONCURRENT USE OF GENTAMICIN WITH POTENT DIURETICS, SUCH AS ETHACRYNIC ACID OR FUROSEMIDE, SHOULD BE AVOIDED, SINCE CERTAIN DIURETICS BY THEMSELVES MAY CAUSE OTOTOXICITY. IN ADDITION, WHEN ADMINISTERED INTRAVENOUSLY, DIURETICS MAY ENHANCE AMINOGLYCOSIDE TOXICITY BY ALTERING THE ANTIBIOTIC CONCENTRATION IN SERUM AND TISSUE.

GENTAMICIN SULFATE INTRATHECAL INJECTION IS INTENDED AS ADJUNCTIVE THERAPY IN PATIENTS WITH CENTRAL NERVOUS SYSTEM INFECTIONS.

SINCE PATIENTS CONSIDERED FOR TREATMENT WITH GENTAMICIN SULFATE INTRATHECAL INJECTION WILL USUALLY BE RECEIVING CONCOMITANT TREATMENT WITH INTRAMUSCULAR OR INTRAVENOUS GENTAMICIN SULFATE, ALL WARNINGS AND PRECAUTIONS FOR THIS OR OTHER CONCOMITANTLY ADMINISTERED AGENTS MUST BE OBSERVED. MOREOVER, WHEN THE DRUG IS ADMINISTERED BY MORE THAN ONE ROUTE, ADDITIVE EFFECTS MUST BE CONSIDERED.

LABORATORY STUDIES IN ANIMALS HAVE SHOWN THAT GENTAMICIN SULFATE, WHEN ADMINISTERED DIRECTLY INTO THE CENTRAL NERVOUS SYSTEM, HAS CAUSED NEUROLOGIC DISTURBANCES, INCLUDING ADVERSE EFFECTS ON THE EIGHTH CRANIAL NERVE. THE RISK OF DIRECT ADMINISTRATION OF A POTENTIALLY NEUROTOXIC DRUG INTO THE CEREBROSPINAL FLUID SPACES OF THE CENTRAL NERVOUS SYSTEM MUST BE WEIGHED AGAINST THE POTENTIAL BENEFIT TO BE DERIVED FROM THIS ROUTE OF ADMINISTRATION.

DESCRIPTION

Gentamicin Sulfate, USP, a water-soluble antibiotic of the aminoglycoside group, is derived from *Micromonospora purpurea*, an actinomycete. Gentamicin Sulfate, Injectable is a sterile, aqueous solution for parenteral administration. The chemical name of Gentamicin Sulfate is 0-2-Amino-2,3,4,6-tetradeoxy.

Gentamicin Sulfate intrathecal injection is a sterile, aqueous solution for direct administration into the cerebrospinal fluid spaces of the central nervous system.

Each ml contains Gentamicin Sulfate equivalent to:

Gentamicin base ....40 mg
Gentamicin base (pediatric) ....10 mg
Gentamicin base (intrathecal) ....2 mg

Following is its chemical structure:

Gentamicin	R
C_1	$H_3C-HN-\overset{CH_3}{\underset{H}{C}}-H$
C_2	$H_2N-\overset{CH_3}{\underset{H}{C}}-H$
C_{1A}	CH_2NH_2

CLINICAL PHARMACOLOGY

After intramuscular administration of Gentamicin Sulfate, Injectable peak serum concentrations usually occur between 30 and 60 minutes and serum levels are measurable for six to eight (12 for the pediatric formulation) hours. In infants, a single dose of 2.5 mg/kg usually provides a peak serum level in the range of 3 to 5 mcg/ml. When Gentamicin is administered by intravenous infusion over a two-

hour period, the serum concentrations are similar to those obtained by intramuscular administration.

In patients with normal renal function, peak serum concentrations of Gentamicin (mcg/ml) are usually up to four times the single intramuscular dose (mg/kg); for example, a 1.0 mg/kg injection in adults may be expected to result in a peak serum concentration up to 4 mcg/ml; a 1.5 mg/kg dose may produce levels up to 6 mcg/ml. While some variation is to be expected due to a number of variables such as age, body temperature, surface area and physiologic differences, the individual patient given the same dose tends to have similar levels in repeated determinations. Gentamicin administered at 1.0 mg/kg every eight hours for the usual 7- to 10-day treatment period to patients with normal renal function does not accumulate in serum. Age markedly affects the peak concentrations; in one report, a 1 mg/kg dose produced mean peak concentrations of 1.58, 2.03, and 2.81 mcg/mL in patients 6 months to 5 years old, 5 to 10 years old, and over 10 years old, respectively.

In infants 1 week to 6 months of age, the half-life is 3 to 3½ hours. In full-term and large premature infants less than 1 week old, the approximate serum half-life of Gentamicin is 5½ hours. In small premature infants, the half-life is inversely related to birth weight. In premature infants weighing less than 1500 grams, the half-life is 11½ hours; in those weighing 1500 to 2000 grams, the half-life is 8 hours; in those weighing over 2000 grams, the half-life is approximately 5 hours. While some variation is to be expected due to a number of variables such as age, body temperature, surface area, and physiologic differences, the individual patient given the same dose tends to have similar levels in repeated determinations.

Gentamicin, like all aminoglycosides, may accumulate in the serum and tissues of patients treated with higher doses and/or for prolonged periods, particularly in the presence of impaired or immature renal function. In adult patients, treatment with Gentamicin dosages of 4 mg/kg/day or higher for seven to ten days may result in a slight, progressive rise in both peak and trough concentrations. In patients with immature or impaired renal function, Gentamicin is cleared from the body more slowly than in patients with normal renal function. The more severe the impairment, the slower the clearance. (Dosage must be adjusted.)

Since Gentamicin is distributed in extracellular fluid, peak serum concentrations may be lower than usual in adult patients who have a large volume of this fluid. Serum concentrations of Gentamicin in febrile patients may be lower than those in afebrile patients given the same dose. When body temperature returns to normal, serum concentrations of the drug may rise. Febrile and anemic states may be associated with a shorter than usual serum half-life. (Dosage adjustment is usually not necessary.) In severely burned patients, the half-life may be significantly decreased and resulting serum concentrations may be lower than anticipated from the mg/kg dose.

Protein-binding studies have indicated that the degree of Gentamicin binding is low; depending upon the methods used for testing, this may be between 0 and 30%.

After initial administration to patients with normal renal function, generally 70% or more of the Gentamicin dose is recoverable in the urine in 24 hours; concentrations in urine above 100 mcg/ml may be achieved. Little, if any, metabolic transformation occurs; the drug is excreted principally by glomerular filtration. After several days of treatment, the amount of Gentamicin excreted in the urine approaches the daily dose administered.

In neonates less than 3 days old, approximately 10% of the administered dose is excreted in 12 hours; in infants 5 to 40 days old, approximately 40% is excreted over the same period. Excretion of Gentamicin correlates with postnatal age and creatinine clearance. Thus, with increasing postnatal age and concomitant increase in renal maturity, Gentamicin is excreted more rapidly. Little, if any, metabolic transformation occurs; the drug is excreted principally by glomerular filtration. After several days of treatment, the amount of Gentamicin excreted in the urine approaches, but does not equal, the daily dose administered.

As with other aminoglycosides, a small amount of the Gentamicin dose may be retained in the tissues, especially in the kidneys. Minute quantities of aminoglycosides have been detected in the urine of some patients weeks after drug administration was discontinued. Renal clearance of Gentamicin is similar to that of endogenous creatinine.

In patients with marked impairment of renal function, there is a decrease in the concentration of aminoglycosides in urine and in their penetration into defective renal parenchyma. This decreased drug excretion, together with the potential nephrotoxicity of aminoglycosides, should be considered when treating such patients who have urinary tract infections.

Probenecid does not affect renal tubular transport of Gentamicin.

The endogenous creatinine clearance rate and the serum creatinine level have a high correlation with the half-life of Gentamicin in serum. Results of these tests may serve as guides for adjusting dosage in patients with renal impairment (see *"Dosage and Administration"*).

Following parenteral administration, Gentamicin can be detected in serum, lymph, tissues, sputum, and in pleural, synovial, and peritoneal fluids. Concentrations in renal cortex sometimes may be eight times higher than the usual serum levels. Concentrations in bile, in general, have been low and have suggested minimal biliary excretion. Gentamicin crosses the peritoneal as well as the placental membranes. Since aminoglycosides diffuse poorly into the subarachnoid space after parenteral administration, concentrations of Gentamicin in cerebrospinal fluid are often low and dependent upon dose, rate of penetration, and degree of meningeal inflammation. There is minimal penetration of Gentamicin into ocular tissues following intramuscular or intravenous administration.

Since Gentamicin Sulfate and other aminoglycosides diffuse poorly into the subarachnoid space after systemic administration, concentrations of these antibiotics in the lumbar or ventricular cerebrospinal fluid (CSF) are often low. Following intramuscular or intravenous administration of the usual dose, Gentamicin concentrations in CSF in the absence of infection are usually less than 1 mcg/ml. In acute meningitis, slightly higher concentrations are obtained but these vary and are usually well below the peak serum concentration. CSF concentrations which are attained following intravenous or intramuscular administration of Gentamicin Sulfate tend to become lower as meningeal inflammation subsides Gentamicin Sulfate intrathecal injections are intended to increase the concentration of Gentamicin in the CSF when used as part of the management of patients with central nervous system infections.

When Gentamicin Sulfate intrathecal injection is given concomitantly with systemically administered Gentamicin Sulfate the CSF levels are substantially increased depending upon the location of the injection. Peak CSF concentrations which follow intralumbar administration generally occur at 1 to 6 hours after injection.

Factors which affect the concentration of Gentamicin in the CSF following injection into cerebrospinal fluid spaces are the dose administered, the site of the injection (intralumbar, intraventricular), the volume in which the dose is diluted, and the presence or absence of obstruction to the CSF flow. There appears to be considerable inter-patient variation.

The half-life of Gentamicin in the CSF of adults who received intralumbar injections is approximately 5.5 hours; this is somewhat longer than that in serum.

In one pharmacokinetic study in adults, a 3 to 4 mg intralumbar injection resulted in a mean CSF concentration of 6.2 mcg/ml 24 hours after injection. The mean CSF concentration was noted to decrease with time: during days 1 through 6 of treatment with Gentamicin Sulfate intrathecal injection by the intralumbar route, the mean 24-hour concentration was 9.9 mcg/ml, while during days 7 through 13, the mean concentration was 3.7 mcg/ml.

In another study in adults, CSF levels were measured at varying intervals after intralumbar administration of Gentamicin sulfate. During days 1 through 6 of treatment, a 4 mg dose produced a mean CSF level of 2.4 mcg/ml 24 hours after injection, while during days 7 through 13, the same dose produced a mean 24-hour level of 0.5 mcg/ml.

Following intralumbar administration there may be limited upward diffusion of the drug, presumably because of the direction of the CSF flow. Intraventricular administration produces high concentrations in the ventricles and throughout the central nervous system. Adequate levels will usually result from dosing every 24 hours, but it is desirable to manage each patient's infection with serial monitoring of Gentamicin serum and CSF concentrations.

Microbiology: In vitro tests have demonstrated that Gentamicin is a bactericidal antibiotic which acts by inhibiting normal protein synthesis in susceptible microorganisms. It is active against a wide variety of pathogenic bacteria including *Escherichia coli, Proteus* species, (indole-positive and indole-negative), *Pseudomonas aeruginosa,* species of the *Klebsiella-Enterobacter-Serratia* group. *Citrobacter* species and *Staphylococcus* species (including penicillin- and methicillin-resistant strains). Gentamicin is also active *in vitro* against species of *Salmonella* and *Shigella.* The following bacteria are usually resistant to aminoglycosides: *Streptococcus pneumoniae,* most species of streptococci, particularly group D and anaerobic organisms, such as *Bacteroides* species or *Clostridium* species.

In vitro studies have shown that an aminoglycoside combined with an antibiotic that interferes with cell wall synthesis may act synergistically against some group D streptococcal strains. The combination of Gentamicin and penicillin G has a synergistic bactericidal effect against virtually all strains of *Streptococcus faecalis* and its varieties (*S. faecalis* var. *liquifaciens, S. faecalis* var. *zymogenes), S. faecium* and *S. durans.* An enhanced killing effect against many of these strains has also been shown *in vitro* with combinations of Gentamicin and ampicillin, carbenicillin, nafcillin, or oxacillin.

The combined effect of Gentamicin and carbenicillin is synergistic for many strains of *Pseudomonas aeruginosa. In vitro* synergism against other gram-negative organisms has been shown with combinations of Gentamicin and cephalosporins. Gentamicin may be active against clinical isolates of bacteria resistant to other aminoglycosides. Bacteria resistant to one aminoglycoside may be resistant to one or more other aminoglycosides. Bacterial resistance to Gentamicin is generally developed slowly.

Susceptibility Testing: If the disc method of susceptibility testing used is that described by Bauer *et al. (Am. J Clin Path* 45:493, 1966; *Federal Register* 37:20525-20529, 1972), a disc containing 10 mcg of Gentamicin should give a zone of inhibition of 15 mm or more to indicate susceptibility of the infecting organism. A zone of 12 mm or less indicates that the infecting organism is likely to be resistant. Zones greater than 12 mm and less than 15 mm indicate intermediate susceptibility. In certain conditions it may be desirable to do additional susceptibility testing by the tube or agar dilution method; Gentamicin substance is available for this purpose.

INDICATIONS AND USAGE

Gentamicin Sulfate, Injectable, is indicated in the treatment of serious infections caused by susceptible strains of the following microorganisms: *Pseudomonas aeruginosa, Proteus* species (indole-positive and indole-negative), *Escherichia coli, Klebsiella-Enterobacter-Serratia* species, *Citrobacter* species and *Staphylococcus* species (coagulase-positive and coagulase-negative).

Intrathecal Gentamicin Sulfate is indicated as adjunctive therapy to systemically administered Gentamicin Sulfate in the treatment of serious central nervous system infections (meningitis, ventriculitis) caused by susceptible *Pseudomonas* species.

Bacteriologic tests should be performed to determine that the causative organisms are *Pseudomonas* species susceptible to Gentamicin.

Clinical studies have shown Gentamicin Sulfate, Injectable, to be effective in bacterial neonatal sepsis; bacterial septicemia; and serious bacterial infections of the central nervous system (meningitis), urinary tract, respiratory tract, gastrointestinal tract (including peritonitis), skin, bone and soft tissue (including burns). Aminoglycosides, including Gentamicin, are not indicated in uncomplicated initial episodes of urinary tract infections unless the causative organisms are susceptible to these antibiotics and are not susceptible to antibiotics having less potential for toxicity.

Specimens for bacterial culture should be obtained to isolate and identify causative organisms and to determine their susceptibility to Gentamicin.

Gentamicin may be considered as initial therapy in suspected or confirmed gram-negative infections, and therapy may be instituted before obtaining results of susceptibility testing. The decision to continue therapy with this drug should be based on the results of susceptibility tests, the severity of the infection, and the important additional concepts contained in the *"Warnings"* box above. If the causative organisms are resistant to Gentamicin other appropriate therapy should be instituted.

In serious infections when the causative organisms are unknown Gentamicin Sulfate, Injectable, may be administered as initial therapy in conjunction with a penicillin-type or cephalosporin-type drug before obtaining results of susceptibility testing. If anaerobic organisms are suspected as etiologic agents, consideration should be given to using other suitable antimicrobial therapy in conjunction with Gentamicin. Following identification of the organism and its susceptibility, appropriate antibiotic therapy should then be continued.

Gentamicin Sulfate, Injectable, has been used effectively in combination with carbenicillin for the treatment of life-threatening infections caused by *Pseudomonas aeruginosa.* It has also been found effective when used in conjunction with a penicillin-type drug for the treatment of endocarditis caused by group D streptococci.

Gentamicin Sulfate, Injectable, has also been shown to be effective in the treatment of serious staphylococcal infections. While not the antibiotic of first choice, Gentamicin Sulfate, Injectable, may be considered when penicillins or other less potentially toxic drugs are contraindicated and bacterial susceptibility tests and clinical judgment indicate its use. It may also be considered in mixed infections caused by susceptible strains of staphylococci and gram-negative organisms.

In the neonate with suspected bacterial sepsis or staphylococcal pneumonia, a penicillin-type drug is also usually indicated as concomitant therapy with Gentamicin.

UNLABELED USES

Gentamicin Sulfate is used alone or as an adjunct in the treatment of gangrenous or perforated appendicitis, to eliminate or suppress sputum bacteria in cystic fibrosis patients, endophthalmitis, and penicillin sensitive or penicillin resistant enterococcal endocarditis. It is also used in gonorrhea, infantile diarrhea, pelvic inflammatory disease, campylobacter jejuni infections, and febrile neutropenia in immunocompromised patients. Gentamicin is also prescribed, via local intratympanic administration, in the treatment of Ménière's disease.

CONTRAINDICATIONS

Hypersensitivity to Gentamicin is a contraindication to its use. A history of hypersensitivity or serious toxic reactions to other aminoglycosides may contraindicate use of Gentamicin because of the known cross-sensitivity of patients to drugs in this class.

WARNINGS

(See boxed *"Warnings".*) Aminoglycosides can cause fetal harm when administered to a pregnant woman. Aminoglycoside antibiotics cross the placenta, and there have been several reports of total irreversible bilateral congenital deafness in children whose mothers received streptomycin during pregnancy. Serious side effects to mother, fetus, or newborn have not been reported in the treatment of pregnant women with other aminoglycosides. Animal reproduction studies conducted on rats and rabbits did not reveal evidence of impaired fertility or harm to the fetus due to Gentamicin Sulfate.

It is not known whether Gentamicin Sulfate can cause fetal harm when administered to a pregnant woman or can affect reproduction capacity. If Gentamicin is used during pregnancy or if the patient becomes pregnant while taking Gentamicin, she should be apprised of the potential hazard to the fetus.

Some brands of Gentamicin Sulfate, Injectable, contain sodium bisulfite, a sulfite that may cause allergic-type reactions including anaphylactic symptoms and life-threatening or less severe asthmatic episodes in certain susceptible people. The overall prevalence of sulfite sensitivity in the general population is unknown and probably low. Sulfite sensitivity is seen more frequently in asthmatic than in nonasthmatic people.

PRECAUTIONS

Neurotoxic and nephrotoxic antibiotics may be absorbed in significant quantities from body surfaces after local irrigation or application. The potential toxic effect of antibiotics administered in this fashion should be considered.

Increased nephrotoxicity has been reported following concomitant administration of aminoglycoside antibiotics and cephalosporins.

Neuromuscular blockade and respiratory paralysis have been re- ported in the cat receiving high doses (40 mg/kg) of Gentamicin. The possibility of these phenomena occurring in man should be considered if aminoglycosides are administered by any route to patients receiving anesthetics, or to patients receiving neuromuscular blocking agents, such as succinylcholine, tubocurarine, or decamethonium, or in patients receiving massive transfusions of citrate-anticoagulated blood. If neuromuscular blockade occurs, calcium salts may reverse it.

Aminoglycosides should be used with caution in patients with neuromuscular disorders, such as myasthenia gravis, since these drugs may aggravate muscle weakness because of their potential curare-like effects on the neuromuscular junction. During or following Gentamicin therapy, paresthesias, tetany, positive Chvostek and Trousseau signs, and mental confusion have been described in patients with hypomagnesemia, hypocalcemia, and hypokalemia. When this has occurred in infants, tetany and muscle weakness have been described. Both adults and infants required appropriate corrective electrolyte therapy.

Elderly patients may have reduced renal function which may not be evident in the results of routine screening tests, such as BUN or serum creatinine. A creatinine clearance determination may be more useful. Monitoring of renal function during treatment with Gentamicin, as with other aminoglycosides, is particularly important in such patients. A Fanconi-like syndrome, with aminoaciduria and metabolic acidosis, has been reported in some adults and infants being given Gentamicin injections.

Cross-allergenicity among aminoglycosides has been demonstrated.

Patients should be well hydrated during treatment.

Although the *in vitro* mixing of Gentamicin and carbenicillin results in a rapid and significant inactivation of Gentamicin, this interaction has not been demonstrated in patients with normal renal function who received both drugs by different routes of administration. A reduction in Gentamicin serum half-life has been reported in patients with severe renal impairment receiving carbenicillin concomitantly with Gentamicin.

Treatment with Gentamicin may result in overgrowth of nonsusceptible organisms. If this occurs, appropriate therapy is indicated.

See *"Warnings"* box regarding concurrent use of potent diuretics and regarding concurrent and/or sequential use of other neurotoxic and/or nephrotoxic antibiotics and for other essential information.

Usage in Pregnancy: Safety for use in pregnancy has not been established.

In a patient with a seven-year history of multiple sclerosis who was treated with Gentamicin Sulfate by intralumbar injection, disseminated microscopic lesions of the brain stem were reported at autopsy. Lesions observed were: tissue rarefaction with loss and marked swelling of axis cylinders with occasional calcification, loss of oligodendroglia and astroglia, and a poor inflammatory response.

Safety and efficacy of intrathecal Gentamicin Sulfate in children below the age of three months have not been established.

ADVERSE REACTIONS

Nephrotoxicity: Adverse renal effects, as demonstrated by the presence of casts, cells, or protein in the urine or by rising BUN, NPN, serum creatinine or oliguria, have been reported. They occur more frequently in patients with a history of renal impairment and in patients treated for longer periods or with larger dosages than recommended.

Neurotoxicity: Serious adverse effects on both vestibular and auditory branches of the eighth cranial nerves have been reported, primarily in patients with renal impairment (especially if dialysis is required), and in patients on high doses and/ or prolonged therapy. Symptoms include dizziness, vertigo, ataxia, tinnitus, roaring in the ears and hearing loss, which, as with the other aminoglycosides, may be irreversible. Hearing loss is usually manifested initially by diminution of high-tone acuity. Other factors which may increase the risk of toxicity include excessive dosage, dehydration and previous exposure to other ototoxic drugs.

Peripheral neuropathy or encephalopathy, including numbness, skin tingling, muscle twitching, convulsions, and a myasthenia gravis-like syndrome, have been reported.

Note: The risk of toxic reactions is low in patients with normal renal function who do not receive Gentamicin Sulfate, Injectable, at higher doses or for longer periods of time than recommended.

Other reported adverse reactions possibly related to Gentamicin include: respiratory depression, lethargy, confusion, depression, visual disturbances, decreased appetite, weight loss, and hypotension and hypertension; rash, itching, urticaria, generalized burning, laryngeal edema, anaphylactoid reactions, fever, and headache; nausea, vomiting, increased salivation, and stomatitis; purpura, pseudotumor cerebri, acute organic brain syndrome, pulmonary fibrosis, alopecia, joint pain, transient hepatomegaly, and splenomegaly.

Laboratory abnormalities possibly related to Gentamicin include: increased levels of serum transaminase (SGOT, SGPT), serum LDH and bilirubin; decreased serum calcium, magnesium, sodium and potassium; anemia, leukopenia, granulocytopenia, transient agranulocytosis, eosinophilia, increased and decreased reticulocyte counts, and thrombocytopenia. While clinical laboratory test abnormalities may be isolated findings, they may also be associated with clinically related signs and symptoms. For example, tetany and muscle weakness may be associated with hypomagnesemia, hypocalcemia, and hypokalemia.

While local tolerance of Gentamicin Sulfate, Injectable, is generally excellent, there has been an occasional report of pain at the injection site. Subcutaneous atrophy or fat necrosis suggesting local irritation has been reported rarely.

Local tolerance to Gentamicin Sulfate intrathecal injection has been good. Local reactions of arachnoiditis or burning at the injection site have been reported rarely.

Because the recommended dosage of Gentamicin Sulfate intrathecal injection is low, the potential for systemic adverse effects is minimal. However, Gentamicin Sulfate intrathecal injection is recommended as adjunctive therapy with other antibiotics, such as parenteral Gentamicin Sulfate, which should be administered in full therapeutic dosages. Evidence of eighth nerve dysfunction, changes in renal function, leg cramps, rash, fever, convulsions, and an increase in cerebrospinal fluid protein have been reported in patients who were treated concomitantly with Gentamicin Sulfate intrathecal injection and the parenteral preparation of Gentamicin.

Administration of excessive (40 to 160 mg) doses of the parenteral formulation of Gentamicin (which contains a preservative system) by the various intrathecal routes has been reported to produce neuromuscular disturbances, e.g., ataxia, paresis, and incontinence.

OVERDOSAGE

In the event of overdose or toxic reactions, hemodialysis may aid in the removal of Gentamicin from the blood, and is especially important if renal function is, or becomes, compromised. The rate of removal of Gentamicin is considerably less by peritoneal dialysis than it is by hemodialysis. In the newborn infant, exchange transfusions may also be considered.

DOSAGE AND ADMINISTRATION

Gentamicin Sulfate, Injectable, may be given intramuscularly or intravenously. The patient's pretreatment body weight should be obtained for calculation of correct dosage. The dosage of aminoglycosides in obese patients should be based on an estimate of the lean body mass. It is desirable to limit the duration of treatment with aminoglycosides to short term.

DOSAGE FOR PATIENTS WITH NORMAL RENAL FUNCTION

Adults: The recommended dosage of Gentamicin Sulfate, Injectable, for patients with serious infections and normal renal function is 3 mg/kg/day, administered in three equal doses every eight hours (Table 1).

For patients with life-threatening infections, dosages up to 5 mg/kg/day may be administered in three or four equal doses. This dosage should be reduced to 3 mg/kg/day as soon as clinically indicated (Table 1).

It is desirable to measure periodically both peak and trough serum concentrations of Gentamicin when feasible during therapy to assure adequate but not excessive drug levels. For example, the peak concentration (at 30 to 60 minutes after intramuscular injection) is expected to be in the range of 4 to 6 mcg/ml (3 to 5 mcg/mL in children). When monitoring peak concentrations after intramuscular or intravenous administration, dosage should be adjusted so that prolonged levels above 12 mcg/ml are avoided. When monitoring trough concentrations (just prior to the next dose); dosage should be adjusted so that levels above 2 mcg/ml are avoided. Determination of the adequacy of a serum level for a particular patient must take into consideration the susceptibility of the causative organism, the severity of the infection, and the status of the patient's host-defense mechanisms.

In patients with extensive burns, altered pharmacokinetics may result in reduced serum concentrations of aminoglycosides. In such patients treated with Gentamicin, measurement of serum concentrations is recommended as a basis for dosage adjustment.

Table 1

DOSAGE SCHEDULE GUIDE FOR ADULTS WITH NORMAL RENAL FUNCTION

(Dosage at Eight-Hour Intervals) 40 mg per ml

Patient's Weight*		Usual Dose For Serious Infections 1 mg/kg q8h (3 mg/kg/day)		Dose for Life-Threatening Infections (Reduce as Soon as Clinically Indicated) 1.7 mg/kg q8h** (5 mg/kg/day)	
kg	(lb)	mg/dose	ml/dose	mg/dose	ml/dose
		q8h		q8h	
40	(88)	40	1.0	66	1.6
45	(99)	45	1.1	75	1.9
50	(110)	50	1.25	83	2.1
55	(121)	55	1.4	91	2.25
60	(132)	60	1.5	100	2.5
65	(143)	65	1.6	108	2.7
70	(154)	70	1.75	116	2.9
75	(165)	75	1.9	125	3.1
80	(176)	80	2.0	133	3.3
85	(187)	85	2.1	141	3.5
90	(198)	90	2.25	150	3.75
95	(209)	95	2.4	158	4.0
100	(220)	100	2.5	166	4.2

* *The dosage of aminoglycosides in obese patients should be based on an estimate of the lean body mass.*
** *For q6h schedules, dosage should be recalculated.*

Children: 6 to 7.5 mg/kg/day. (2.0 to 2.5 mg/kg administered every 8 hours.)

Infants and Neonates: 7.5 mg/kg/day. (2.5 mg/kg administered every 8 hours.)

Premature or Full-Term Neonates One Week of Age or Less: 5 mg/kg/day. (2.5 mg/kg administered every 12 hours).

The usual duration of treatment for all patients is seven to ten days. In difficult and complicated infections, a longer course of therapy may be necessary. In such cases, monitoring of renal, auditory, and vestibular functions is recommended, since toxicity is more apt to occur with treatment extended for more than ten days. Dosage should be reduced if clinically indicated.

FOR INTRAVENOUS ADMINISTRATION
The intravenous administration of Gentamicin may be particularly useful for treating patients with bacterial septicemia or those in shock. It may also be the preferred route of administration for some patients with congestive heart failure, hematologic disorders, severe burns, or those with reduced muscle mass. For intermittent intravenous administration in adults a single dose of Gentamicin Sulfate, Injectable, may be diluted in 50 to 200 ml of sterile isotonic saline solution or in a sterile solution of dextrose 5% in water; in infants and children, the volume of diluent should be less. The solution may be infused over a period of one-half to two hours.

The recommended dosage for intravenous and intramuscular administration is identical.

Gentamicin Sulfate, Injectable, should not be physically premixed with other drugs, but should be administered separately in accordance with the recommended route of administration and dosage schedule.

DOSAGE FOR PATIENTS WITH IMPAIRED RENAL FUNCTION
Dosage must be adjusted in patients with impaired renal function to assure therapeutically adequate, but not excessive, blood levels. Whenever possible, serum concentrations of Gentamicin should be monitored. One method of dosage adjustment is to increase the interval between administration of the usual doses. Since the serum creatinine concentration has a high correlation with the serum half-life of Gentamicin, this laboratory test may provide guidance for adjustment of the interval between doses. In adults, the interval between doses (in hours) may be approximated by multiplying the serum creatinine level (mg/100 ml) by 8. For example, a patient weighing 60 kg with a serum creatinine level of 2.0 mg/100 ml could be given 60 mg (1 mg/kg) every 16 hours (2 × 8). These guidelines may be considered when treating infants and children with serious renal impairment.

In patients with serious systemic infections and renal impairment, it may be desirable to administer the antibiotic more frequently but in reduced dosage. In such patients, serum concentrations of Gentamicin should be measured so that adequate but not excessive levels result. A peak and trough concentration measured intermittently during therapy will provide optimal guidance for adjusting dosage. After the usual initial dose, a rough guide for determining reduced dosage at eight-hour intervals is to divide the normally recommended dose by the serum creatinine level (Table 2). For example, after an initial dose of 60 mg (1 mg/kg), a patient weighing 60 kg with a serum creatinine level of 2.0 mg/100 ml could be given 30 mg every eight hours (60 ÷ 2); after an initial dose of 20 mg (2.0 mg/kg), a child weighing 10 kg with a serum creatinine level of 2.0 mg/100 mL could be given 10 mg every 8 hours (20 ÷ 2). It should be noted that the status of renal function may be changing over the course of the infectious process.

It is important to recognize that deteriorating renal function may require a greater reduction in dosage than that specified in the above guidelines for patients with stable renal impairment.

Table 2
DOSAGE ADJUSTMENT GUIDE FOR PATIENTS WITH RENAL IMPAIRMENT
(Dosage at Eight-Hour Intervals After The Usual Initial Dose)

Serum Creatinine (mg %)	Approximate Creatinine Clearance Rate (ml/min/1.73M²)	Percent of Usual Doses Shown in Table 1
≤1.0	>100	100
1.1-1.3	70-100	80
1.4-1.6	55-70	65
1.7-1.9	45-55	55
2.0-2.2	40-45	50
2.3-2.5	35-40	40
2.6-3.0	30-35	35
3.1-3.5	25-30	30
3.6-4.0	20-25	25
4.1-5.1	15-20	20
5.2-6.6	10-15	15
6.7-8.0	<10	10

In patients with renal failure undergoing hemodialysis, the amount of Gentamicin removed from the blood may vary depending upon several factors including the dialysis method used. An eight-hour hemodialysis may reduce serum concentrations of Gentamicin by approximately 50%. The recommended dosage at the end of each dialysis period is 1 to 1.7 mg/kg depending upon the severity of infection. In children the recommended dose at the end of each dialysis period is 2.0 to 2.5 mg/kg depending upon the severity of infection.

The above dosage schedules are not intended as rigid recommendations but are provided as guides to dosage when the measurement of Gentamicin serum levels is not feasible.

A variety of methods are available to measure Gentamicin concentrations in body fluids; these include microbiologic, enzymatic and radioimmunoassay techniques.

Gentamicin Sulfate intrathecal injection is intended for administration directly into the cerebrospinal fluid spaces of the central nervous system.

The dosage will vary depending upon factors, such as age and weight of the patient, site of injection, degree of obstruction to cerebrospinal fluid flow and the amount of cerebrospinal fluid estimated to be present. In general, the recommended dose for infants 3 months of age and older (see *"Precautions"*) and children is 1 to 2 mg once a day. For adults, 4 to 8 mg may be administered once a day.

Administration of Gentamicin Sulfate intrathecal injection should be continued as long as sensitive organisms are demonstrated in the cerebrospinal fluid. Since the intralumbar or intraventricular dose is administered immediately after specimens are taken for laboratory study, treatment should usually be continued for at least one day after negative results have been obtained from CSF cultures and/or stained smears.

The suggested method for administering Gentamicin Sulfate intrathecal injection into the lumbar area is as follows: the desired quantity of Gentamicin Sulfate intrathecal injection is drawn up carefully from the ampule into a 5- or 10-ml sterile syringe. After the lumbar puncture is performed and a specimen of the spinal fluid is removed for laboratory tests, the syringe containing Gentamicin Sulfate intrathecal injection is inserted into the hub of the spinal needle. A quantity of cerebrospinal fluid (approximately 10% of the estimated total CSF volume) is allowed to flow into the syringe and mix with the Gentamicin Sulfate intrathecal injection. The resultant solution is then injected over a period of 3 to 5 minutes with the bevel of the needle directed upward.

If the cerebrospinal fluid is grossly purulent, or if it is unobtainable, Gentamicin Sulfate intrathecal injection may be diluted with sterile normal saline before injection.

Gentamicin Sulfate intrathecal injection may also be administered directly into the subdural space or directly into the ventricles, including administration by use of an implanted reservoir.

STORAGE
Store between 2° and 30°C (36° and 86°F).
Store intrathecal Gentamicin Sulfate below 30°C (86°F).

Note: Some intrathecal preparations do not contain any preservative. Once opened, contents should be used immediately and unused portions should be discarded.

ANIMAL PHARMACOLOGY AND TOXICOLOGY — INTRATHECAL GENTAMICIN SULFATE
In dogs, an 8-hour perfusion of the ventriculosubarchnoid system with a solution containing 40 mcg/ml (~5 mg or ~0.3 mg/kg) Gentamicin produced no seizure activity or change in vital signs during administration. No morphological changes were observed when the dogs were sacrificed at 10 and 90 days following infusion.

The effects of repeated intrathecal injections of Gentamicin at 0.1 and 0.3 mg/kg were evaluated in tranquilized beagle puppies. Transient flaccid paralysis was observed on the first day when the drug was administered rapidly (i.e., in less than 5 seconds), but no adverse effects were observed thereafter when the drug was administered less rapidly (i.e., over a period of approximately 30 seconds). No drug-related changes were found on histological examination of the cerebellum, brain stem or cephalic cord. In cats, Gentamicin administered intracisternally at one-hour intervals in doses of up to 50 mg/kg did not produce any abnormalities in the electroencephalogram. In another study in cats, Gentamicin Sulfate given daily by the intracisternal route for up to 7 days caused neurological disturbances, including adverse effects on the eighth cranial nerve.

In rabbits intracisternal injection of Gentamicin at doses 50 and 100 times the therapeutic dose produced peak CSF concentrations of 160 and 180 mcg/ml, respectively. These doses were associated with changes in the myelin sheath predominantly of the lateral columns of the upper cervical cord, and some changes in glial cells and lesions in the medulla oblongata. In addition to a high incidence of mortality, the animals demonstrated weakness, ataxia and paralysis. At doses of one and ten times the therapeutic dose (providing peak levels of 16.5 and 40 mcg/ml CSF), no morphologic changes occurred and there were no drug-related symptoms identified.

J CODES
Up to 80 mg IM,IV—J1580

◆ RATED THERAPEUTICALLY EQUIVALENT; ◇ THERAPEUTIC EQUIVALENCE UNCONFIRMED; ○ UNRATED

HOW SUPPLIED
INJECTION: 2 MG/ML

BRAND/MANUFACTURER	NDC	SIZE	AWP
◆ **BRAND**			
GARAMYCIN: Schering	00085-0337-03	2 ml 25s	$63.47

INJECTION: 10 MG/ML

AVERAGE UNIT PRICE (AVAILABLE SIZES)		GENERIC A-RATED AVERAGE PRICE (GAAP)	
BRAND	$1.06	2 ml	$1.46
GENERIC	$0.66	2 ml 25s	$26.01

BRAND/MANUFACTURER	NDC	SIZE	AWP
◆ **BRAND**			
GARAMYCIN: Schering	00085-0013-06	2 ml 10s	$21.16
◆ **GENERICS**			
Fujisawa	00469-1730-10	2 ml	$1.46
Fujisawa	00469-5130-25	2 ml	$1.46
Elkins-Sinn	00641-0394-25	2 ml 25s	$17.71
Gensia	00703-9642-04	2 ml 25s	$27.50
Solo Pak	39769-0001-02	2 ml 25s	$32.81
Abbott Hosp	00074-3400-01	6 ml 25s	$134.48
Abbott Hosp	00074-3401-01	8 ml 25s	$143.69
Abbott Hosp	00074-3402-01	10 ml 25s	$154.38

INJECTION: 10 MG/ML

BRAND/MANUFACTURER	NDC	SIZE	AWP
○ **GENERICS**			
CMC-Cons	00223-7715-02	2 ml	$1.75
CMC-Cons	00223-7714-02	2 ml 25s	$35.00

INJECTION: 40 MG/ML

AVERAGE UNIT PRICE (AVAILABLE SIZES)		GENERIC A-RATED AVERAGE PRICE (GAAP)	
BRAND	$2.12	2 ml	$2.88
GENERIC	$0.86	20 ml	$9.80
		2 ml 25s	$42.89
		20 ml 25s	$260.32

BRAND/MANUFACTURER	NDC	SIZE	AWP
◆ **BRAND**			
GARAMYCIN: Schering	00085-0069-05	1.5 ml	$3.61
	00085-0069-06	2 ml	$4.02
	00085-0069-04	2 ml 25s	$96.88

BRAND/MANUFACTURER	NDC	SIZE	AWP
◆ **GENERICS**			
Moore,H.L.	00839-6503-23	2 ml	$2.15
Fujisawa	00469-1000-10	2 ml	$2.26
Steris	00402-0559-02	2 ml	$2.32
Insource	58441-1125-02	2 ml	$2.62
Goldline	00182-1424-61	2 ml	$3.00
Rugby	00536-4690-67	2 ml	$4.95
Schein	00364-6739-55	20 ml	$8.33
Steris	00402-0559-20	20 ml	$8.33
Insource	58441-1125-06	20 ml	$8.77
Goldline	00182-1424-65	20 ml	$9.45
Rugby	00536-4690-73	20 ml	$11.25
Fujisawa	00469-1000-40	20 ml	$12.64
Fujisawa	00469-1000-60	50 ml	$32.59
Elkins-Sinn	00641-2331-43	20 ml 10s	$104.13
Elkins-Sinn	00641-0395-25	2 ml 25s	$26.04
Gensia	00703-9652-04	2 ml 25s	$27.81
Abbott Hosp	00074-1207-03	2 ml 25s	$51.06
Solo Pak	39769-0014-02	2 ml 25s	$51.56
Schein	00364-6739-48	2 ml 25s	$58.00
Gensia	00703-9665-04	20 ml 25s	$133.13
Solo Pak	39769-0014-20	20 ml 25s	$387.50

INJECTION: 40 MG/ML

BRAND/MANUFACTURER	NDC	SIZE	AWP
○ **GENERICS**			
CMC-Cons	00223-7719-02	2 ml	$1.75
G-MYCIN: Bolan	44437-0559-02	2 ml	$3.00
CMC-Cons	00223-7717-20	20 ml	$7.50
A-MYCIN: Clint	55553-0559-20	20 ml	$9.00
JENAMICIN: Roberts/Hauck	59441-0604-20	20 ml	$9.95
Allscrips	54569-3149-00	2 ml 25s	$26.04
CMC-Cons	00223-7719-25	2 ml 25s	$52.50

Gentamicin Sulfate, Ophthalmic

DESCRIPTION
Gentamicin Sulfate, Ophthalmic, is a sterile, topical anti-infective agent for ophthalmic use. The active ingredient, Gentamicin Sulfate, is a water-soluble antibiotic of the aminoglycoside group.

Gentamicin is obtained from cultures of *Micromonospora purpurea*. It is a mixture of the sulfate salts of Gentamicin C_1, C_2, and C_{1A}. All three components appear to have similar antimicrobial activities. Gentamicin Sulfate occurs as a white to buff powder and is soluble in water but insoluble in alcohol.

Each mL of solution contains Gentamicin Sulfate equivalent to 3 mg (0.3%) Gentamicin base. Each gram of ointment contains Gentamicin Sulfate, USP (equivalent to 3.0 mg Gentamicin).

Following is its chemical structure:

CLINICAL PHARMACOLOGY
Microbiology: Gentamicin Sulfate is active *in vitro* against many strains of the following microorganisms:

Staphylococcus aureus, Staphylococcus epidermidis, Streptococcus pyogenes, Streptococcus pneumoniae, Enterobacter aerogenes, Escherichia coli, Haemophilus influenzae, Klebsiella pneumoniae, Neisseria gonorrhoeae, Pseudomonas aeruginosa, and Serratia marcescens.

INDICATIONS AND USAGE
Gentamicin Sulfate, Ophthalmic, is indicated in the topical treatment of ocular bacterial infections including conjunctivitis, keratitis keratoconjunctivitis, corneal ulcers, blepharitis, blepharocon junctivitis, acute meibomianitis, and dacryocystitis, caused by susceptible strains of the following microorganisms: Staphylococcus aureus, Staphylococcus epidermidis, Streptococcus pyogenes, Stereptococcus pneumoniae, Enterobacter aerogenes, Escherichia coli, Haemophilus influenzae, Klebsiella pneumoniae, Neisseria gonorrhoeae, Pseudomonas Aeruginosa, and Serratia marcescens.

CONTRAINDICATIONS
Gentamicin Sulfate, Ophthalmic, is contraindicated in patients with known hypersensitivity to any of the components.

WARNINGS
Not For Injection Into The Eye: Gentamicin Sulfate, Ophthalmic, is not for injection. It should never be injected subconjunctivally, nor should it be introduced directly into the anterior chamber of the eye.

PRECAUTIONS
General: Prolonged use of topical antibiotics may give rise to overgrowth of nonsusceptible microorganisms, including fungi. Bacterial resistance to Gentamicin may also develop. If purulent discharge occurs, inflammation or pain becomes aggravated, the patient should discontinue use of the medication and consult a physician.

If irritation or hypersensitivity to any component of the drug develops, the patient should discontinue use of this preparation and appropriate therapy should be instituted. Ophthalmic ointments may retard corneal healing.

Information for Patients: To avoid contamination, do not touch tip of container to the eye, eyelid or any surface.

Carcinogenesis, Mutagenesis, Impairment of Fertility: There are no published carcinogenicity or impairment of fertility studies on Gentamicin. Aminoglycoside antibiotics have been found to be non-mutagenic.

Pregnancy Category C: Gentamicin has been shown to depress body weights, kidney weights and median glomerular counts in newborn rats when administered systemically to pregnant rats in daily doses approximately 500 times the maximum recommended ophthalmic human dose. There are no adequate and well-controlled studies in pregnant women. Gentamicin should be used during pregnancy only if the potential benefit justifies the potential risk to the fetus.

ADVERSE REACTIONS

Bacterial and fungal corneal ulcers have developed during treatment with Gentamicin ophthalmic preparations.

The most frequently reported adverse reactions are ocular burning and irritation upon drug instillation, non-specific conjunctivitis, conjunctival epithelial defects and conjunctival hyperemia.

Other adverse reactions which have occurred rarely are allergic reactions, thrombocytopenic purpura and hallucinations.

DOSAGE AND ADMINISTRATION

Solution: Instill one or two drops into the affected eye(s) every four hours. In severe infections, dosage may be increased to as much as two drops every hour.

Ointment: Apply a small amount (about 1/2 inch) to the affected eye two to three times a day.

Note: Store solution at or below 25°C (77°F). Avoid exposure to excessive heat (104°F/40°C or above).

Note: Store ointment between 2° and 30°C (36° and 86°F).

HOW SUPPLIED
DROP: 3 MG/ML

AVERAGE UNIT PRICE (AVAILABLE SIZES)		GENERIC A-RATED AVERAGE PRICE (GAAP)	
BRAND	$2.47	5 ml	$5.48
GENERIC	$0.87	15 ml	$6.73

BRAND/MANUFACTURER	NDC	SIZE	AWP
◆ **BRAND**			
GENOPTIC: Allergan Inc	11980-0117-01	1 ml	$2.96
GENTACIDIN: Iolab	00058-2365-05	5 ml	$7.26
GENOPTIC: Allergan Inc	11980-0117-05	5 ml	$13.43
GARAMYCIN: Schering	00085-0899-05	5 ml	$13.98
◆ **GENERICS**			
Schein	00364-7388-53	5 ml	$4.90
Steris	00402-0749-05	5 ml	$4.90
Bausch&Lomb Pharm	24208-0580-60	5 ml	$4.95
Raway	00686-0580-60	5 ml	$5.10
Geneva	00781-7110-75	5 ml	$5.10
GENTAK: Akorn	17478-0283-10	5 ml	$5.31
GENTAFAIR: Qualitest	00603-7158-37	5 ml	$5.40
Moore,H.L.	00839-6745-25	5 ml	$5.52
URL	00677-0901-20	5 ml	$5.55
Goldline	00182-1695-62	5 ml	$5.55
Major	00904-1907-05	5 ml	$5.60
Parmed	00349-8579-75	5 ml	$5.89
Rugby	00536-0925-65	5 ml	$5.99
Aligen	00405-6060-05	5 ml	$6.14
GENTASOL: Ocusoft	54799-0510-05	5 ml	$6.35
Bausch&Lomb Pharm	24208-0580-64	15 ml	$5.53
Schein	00364-7388-72	15 ml	$5.63
Steris	00402-0749-15	15 ml	$5.63
Raway	00686-0580-64	15 ml	$6.00
GENTAK: Akorn	17478-0283-12	15 ml	$7.19
Rugby	00536-0925-72	15 ml	$7.35
Aligen	00405-6060-15	15 ml	$7.52
Geneva	00781-7110-85	15 ml	$8.95

DROP: 3%

AVERAGE UNIT PRICE (AVAILABLE SIZES)	
GENERIC	$0.41

BRAND/MANUFACTURER	NDC	SIZE	AWP
◆ **GENERICS**			
Paco	52967-0505-35	5 ml	$2.95
Paco	52967-0505-45	15 ml	$3.45

OINTMENT:

BRAND/MANUFACTURER	NDC	SIZE	AWP
◆ **GENERICS**			
Bausch&Lomb Pharm	24208-0575-55	3.5 gm	$5.49

OINTMENT: 3 MG/GM

BRAND/MANUFACTURER	NDC	SIZE	AWP
◆ **BRAND**			
GENOPTIC S.O.P.: Allergan Inc	00023-0320-04	3.5 gm	$13.51

OINTMENT: 3 MG

BRAND/MANUFACTURER	NDC	SIZE	AWP
◆ **BRAND**			
GARAMYCIN: Schering	00085-0151-05	3.5 gm	$13.98

Gentamicin Sulfate, Topical

DESCRIPTION
For Dermatologic Use Only—Not For Ophthalmic Use.

Each gram of Gentamicin Sulfate cream 0.1% contains 1.7 mg gentamicin sulfate, USP, equivalent to 1.0 mg Gentamicin base.

Each gram of Gentamicin Sulfate ointment 0.1% contains 1.7 mg Gentamicin Sulfate, USP, equivalent to 1.0 mg Gentamicin base.

Following is its chemical structure:

ACTIONS
Gentamicin Sulfate, a wide-spectrum antibiotic, provides highly effective topical treatment in primary and secondary bacterial infections of the skin. Gentamicin Sulfate may clear infections that have not responded to other topical antibiotic agents. In impetigo contagiosa and other primary skin infections, treatment three or four times daily with Gentamicin Sulfate usually clears the lesions promptly.

In secondary skin infections, Gentamicin Sulfate facilitates the treatment of the underlying dermatosis by controlling the infection. Bacteria susceptible to the action of Gentamicin Sulfate include sensitive strains of streptococci (group A beta-hemolytic, alpha-hemolytic), *Staphylococcus aureus* (coagulase-positive, coagulase-negative, and some penicillinase-producing strains), and the gram-negative bacteria, *Pseudomonas aeruginosa, Aerobacter aerogenes, Escherichia coli, Proteus vulgaris,* and *Klebsiella pneumoniae.*

INDICATIONS
Primary skin infections: Impetigo contagiosa, superficial folliculitis, ecthyma, furunculosis, sycosis barbae, and pyoderma gangrenosum. *Secondary skin infections:* Infectious eczematoid dermatitis, pustular acne, pustular psoriasis, infected seborrheic dermatitis, infected contact dermatitis (including poison ivy), infected excoriations, and bacterial superinfections of fungal or viral infections. *Note:* Gentamicin Sulfate is a bactericidal agent that is not effective against viruses or fungi in skin infections. Gentamicin Sulfate is useful in the treatment of infected skin cysts and certain other skin abscesses when preceded by incision and drainage to permit adequate contact between the antibiotic and the infecting bacteria. Good results have been obtained in the treatment of infected stasis and other skin ulcers, infected superficial burns, paronychia, infected insect bites and stings, infected lacerations and abrasions, and wounds from minor surgery. Patients sensitive to neomycin can be treated with Gentamicin, although regular observation of patients sensitive to topical antibiotics is advisable when such patients are treated with any topical antibiotic. Gentamicin Sulfate ointment helps retain moisture and has been useful in infection on dry eczematous or psoriatic skin. Gentamicin Sulfate cream is recommended for wet, oozing primary infections and greasy, secondary infections, such as pustular acne or infected seborrheic dermatitis. If a water-washable preparation is desired, Gentamicin Sulfate cream is preferable. Gentamicin Sulfate ointment and cream have been used successfully in infants over one year of age, as well as in adults and children.

◆ **RATED THERAPEUTICALLY EQUIVALENT;** ◇ **THERAPEUTIC EQUIVALENCE UNCONFIRMED;** ○ **UNRATED**

CONTRAINDICATIONS

This drug is contraindicated in individuals with a history of sensitivity reactions to any of its components.

PRECAUTIONS

Use of topical antibiotics occassionally allows overgrowth of nonsusceptible organisms, including fungi. If this occurs, or if irritation, sensitization, or superinfection develops, treatment with Gentamicin should be discontinued and appropriate therapy instituted.

ADVERSE REACTIONS

In patients with dermatoses treated with Gentamicin, irritation (erythema and pruritus) that did not usually require discontinuance of treatment has been reported in a small percentage of cases. There was no evidence of irritation or sensitization, however, in any of these patients patch-tested subsequently with Gentamicin on normal skin. Possible photosensitization has been reported in several patients but could not be elicited in these patients by reapplication of Gentamicin followed by exposure to ultraviolet radiation.

DOSAGE AND ADMINISTRATION

A small amount of Gentamicin Sulfate cream or ointment should be applied gently to the lesions three or four times daily. The area treated may be covered with a gauze dressing if desired. In impetigo contagiosa, the crusts should be removed before application of Gentamicin Sulfate to permit maximum contact between the antibiotic and the infection. Care should be exercised to avoid further contamination of the infected skin. Infected stasis ulcers have responded well to Gentamicin Sulfate under gelatin packing.

  Store between 2° and 30° C (36° and 86° F).

HOW SUPPLIED
CREAM: 0.1%

AVERAGE UNIT PRICE (AVAILABLE SIZES)		GENERIC A-RATED AVERAGE PRICE (GAAP)	
BRAND	$1.03	15 gm	$3.35
GENERIC	$0.18	30 gm	$4.88

BRAND/MANUFACTURER	NDC	SIZE	AWP
◆ BRAND			
GARAMYCIN: Schering	00085-0008-05	15 gm	$15.44
◆ GENERICS			
Geneva	00781-7310-27	15 gm	$3.10
Fougera	00168-0071-15	15 gm	$3.60
Clay-Park	45802-0056-11	30 gm	$4.00
Schein	00364-7305-56	30 gm	$4.75
Rugby	00536-4470-28	30 gm	$5.88
Thames	49158-0162-16	454 gm	$70.00
Clay-Park	45802-0056-05	454 gm	$86.40

CREAM: 1%

BRAND/MANUFACTURER	NDC	SIZE	AWP
◆ GENERICS			
Goldline	00182-1403-51	15 gm	$3.75

CREAM: 1 MG

AVERAGE UNIT PRICE (AVAILABLE SIZES)		GENERIC A-RATED AVERAGE PRICE (GAAP)	
GENERIC	$0.21	15 gm	$3.07
HCFA FUL (15 gm)	$0.14		

BRAND/MANUFACTURER	NDC	SIZE	AWP
◆ GENERICS			
Raway	00686-0056-35	15 gm	$2.10
Thames	49158-0162-20	15 gm	$2.40
Clay-Park	45802-0056-35	15 gm	$2.59
Schein	00364-7305-72	15 gm	$2.88
Qualitest	00603-7769-74	15 gm	$2.90
Rugby	00536-4470-20	15 gm	$2.94
Major	00904-2663-36	15 gm	$3.10
URL	00677-0709-40	15 gm	$3.20
Moore,H.L.	00839-6492-47	15 gm	$3.23
Parmed	00349-8760-35	15 gm	$3.40
G-MYTICIN: Pedinol	00884-3684-15	15 gm	$3.75
UDL	51079-0157-61	15 gm	$4.35

OINTMENT: 0.1%

AVERAGE UNIT PRICE (AVAILABLE SIZES)		GENERIC A-RATED AVERAGE PRICE (GAAP)	
BRAND	$1.03	15 gm	$3.23
GENERIC	$0.20	30 gm	$4.86

BRAND/MANUFACTURER	NDC	SIZE	AWP
◆ BRAND			
GARAMYCIN: Schering	00085-0343-05	15 gm	$15.44
◆ GENERICS			
Thames	49158-0191-20	15 gm	$2.40
Clay-Park	45802-0046-35	15 gm	$2.60
Schein	00364-7338-72	15 gm	$2.88
Qualitest	00603-7770-74	15 gm	$2.90
Major	00904-2664-36	15 gm	$3.10
Geneva	00781-7320-27	15 gm	$3.10
Rugby	00536-4480-20	15 gm	$3.12
URL	00677-0710-40	15 gm	$3.20
Moore,H.L.	00839-6599-47	15 gm	$3.23
Fougera	00168-0078-15	15 gm	$3.60
G-MYTICIN: Pedinol	00884-3784-15	15 gm	$3.75
Goldline	00182-1474-51	15 gm	$3.75
UDL	51079-0158-61	15 gm	$4.35
Clay-Park	45802-0046-11	30 gm	$4.00
Goldline	00182-1474-56	30 gm	$4.50
Schein	00364-7338-56	30 gm	$4.75
Rugby	00536-4480-28	30 gm	$6.19
Thames	49158-0191-16	454 gm	$70.00
Clay-Park	45802-0046-05	454 gm	$86.40

OINTMENT: 0.3%

BRAND/MANUFACTURER	NDC	SIZE	AWP
◆ GENERICS			
GENTASOL: Ocusoft	54799-0510-35	3.5 gm	$6.35

Gentran SEE DEXTRAN 40

Geocillin SEE CARBENICILLIN INDANYL SODIUM

Geref SEE SERMORELIN ACETATE

Glaucon SEE EPINEPHRINE, OPHTHALMIC

Glipizide

DESCRIPTION

Glipizide is an oral blood-glucose-lowering drug of the sulfonylurea class.

  The Chemical Abstracts name of Glipizide is 1-cyclohexyl-3-[[p-[2-(5-methyl-pyrazinecarboxamido)ethyl]phenyl] sulfonyl]urea. The molecular formula is $C_{21}H_{27}N_5O_4S$; the molecular weight is 445.55.

  Glipizide is a whitish, odorless powder with a pKa of 5.9. It is insoluble in water and alcohols, but soluble in 0.1 N NaOH; it is freely soluble in dimethylformamide. Glipizide immediate release and extended release tablets for oral use are available in 5 and 10 mg strengths.

  The Glipizide extended release tablet is designed to provide a controlled rate of delivery of Glipizide into the gastrointestinal lumen which is independent of pH or gastrointestinal motility. The function of the Glipizide extended release tablet depends upon the existence of an osmotic gradient between the contents of the bi-layer core and fluid in the GI tract. Drug delivery is essentially constant as long as the osmotic gradient remains constant, and then gradually falls to zero. The biologically inert components of the tablet remain intact during GI transit and are eliminated in the feces as an insoluble shell.

  Following is its chemical structure:

CLINICAL PHARMACOLOGY

Mechanism of Action: The primary mode of action of Glipizide in experimental animals appears to be the stimulation of insulin secretion from the beta cells of pancreatic islet tissue and is thus dependent on functioning beta cells in the pancreatic islets. In humans Glipizide appears to lower the blood glucose acutely by stimulating the release of insulin from the pancreas, an effect dependent upon functioning beta cells in the pancreatic islets. The mechanism by which Glipizide lowers blood glucose during long-term administration has not been clearly established. In man, stimulation of insulin secretion by Glipizide in response to a meal is undoubtedly of major importance. Fasting insulin levels are not elevated even on long-term Glipizide administration, but the postprandial insulin and C peptide responses continue to be enhanced after at least 6 months of treatment. In 2 randomized, double-blind, dose-response studies comprising a total of 347 patients, there was no significant increase in fasting insulin in all Glipizide extended release-treated patients combined compared to placebo, although minor elevations were observed at some doses. The insulinotropic response to a meal occurs within 30 minutes after an oral dose of Glipizide in diabetic patients, but elevated insulin levels do not persist beyond the time of the meal challenge. The insulinotropic response to a meal is enhanced with Glipizide extended release administration in diabetic patients. Extrapancreatic effects may play a part in the mechanism of action of oral sulfonylurea hypoglycemic drugs. Two extrapancreatic effects shown to be important in the action of glipizide are an increase in insulin sensitivity and a decrease in hepatic glucose production.

Blood sugar control persists in some patients for up to 24 hours after a single dose of Glipizide, even though plasma levels have declined to a small fraction of peak levels by that time (see *"Pharmacokinetics"* below).

Some patients fail to respond initially, or gradually lose their responsiveness to sulfonylurea drugs, including Glipizide. Alternatively, Glipizide may be effective in some patients who have not responded or have ceased to respond to other sulfonylureas.

Effects on Blood Glucose: The effectiveness of Glipizide extended release tablets in NIDDM at doses from 5-60 mg once daily has been evaluated in 4 therapeutic clinical trials each with long-term open extensions involving a total of 598 patients. Once daily administration of 5, 10 and 20 mg produced statistically significant reductions from placebo in hemoglobin A_{1C}, fasting plasma glucose and postprandial glucose in mild to severe NIDDM patients. In a pooled analysis of the patients treated with 5 mg and 20 mg, the relationship between dose and Glipizide extended release effect of reducing hemoglobin A_{1C} was not established. However, in the case of fasting plasma glucose patients treated with 20 mg had a statistically significant reduction of fasting plasma glucose compared to the 5 mg-treated group.

The reductions in hemoglobin A_{1C} and fasting plasma glucose were similar in younger and older patients. Efficacy of Glipizide extended release was not affected by gender, race or weight (as assessed by body mass index). In long term extension trials, efficacy, of Glipizide extended release was maintained in 81% of patients for up to 12 months.

In an open, two-way crossover study 132 patients were randomly assigned to either Glipizide extended release or Glipizide immediate release for 8 weeks and then crossed over to the other drug for an additional 8 weeks. Glipizide extended release administration resulted in significantly lower fasting plasma glucose levels and equivalent hemoglobin A_{1C} levels, as compared to Glipizide immediate release.

Other Effects: It has been shown that Glipizide therapy is effective in controlling blood sugar without deleterious changes in the plasma lipoprotein profiles of patients treated for NIDDM.

In a placebo-controlled, crossover study in normal volunteers, Glipizide had no anti-diuretic activity, and, in fact, led to a slight increase in free water clearance.

Pharmacokinetics: Gastrointestinal absorption of Glipizide immediate release in man is uniform, rapid, and essentially complete. The absolute bioavailability of glipizide was 100% after single oral doses in patients with NIDDM. Peak plasma concentrations occur 1-3 hours after a single oral dose. The half-life of elimination ranges from 2-4 hours in normal subjects, whether given intravenously or orally and from 2-5 hours after single or multiple doses in patients with NIDDM. The metabolic and excretory patterns are similar with the two routes of administration, indicating that first-pass metabolism is not significant. Glipizide does not accumulate in plasma on repeated oral administration. Total absorption and disposition of an oral dose was unaffected by food in normal volunteers, but absorption was delayed by about 40 minutes. Thus Glipizide was more effective when administered about 30 minutes before, rather than with, a test meal in diabetic patients. Protein binding was studied in serum from volunteers who received either oral or intravenous Glipizide and found to be 98-99% one hour after either route of administration. The apparent volume of distribution of Glipizide after intravenous administration was 10-11 liters, indicative of localization within the extracellular fluid compartment. In mice no Glipizide or metabolites were detectable autoradiographically in the brain or spinal cord of males or females, nor in the fetuses of pregnant females. In another study, however, very small amounts of radioactivity were detected in the fetuses of rats given labelled drug.

Beginning 2 to 3 hours after administration of Glipizide extended release tablets, plasma drug concentrations gradually rise reaching maximum concentrations within 6 to 12 hours after dosing. With subsequent once daily dosing of Glipizide extended release tablets, effective plasma Glipizide concentrations are maintained throughout the 24 hour dosing interval with less peak to trough fluctuation than that observed with twice daily dosing of immediate release Glipizide. The mean relative bioavailability of Glipizide in 21 males with NIDDM after administration of 20 mg Glipizide extended release tablets, compared to immediate release Glipizide (10 mg given twice daily), was 90% at steady state. Steady state plasma concentrations were achieved by at least the fifth day of dosing with Glipizide extended release tablets in 21 males with NIDDM and patients younger than 65 years. Approximately 1 to 2 days longer were required to reach steady state in 24 elderly (≥65 years) males and females with NIDDM. No accumulation of drug was observed in patients with NIDDM during chronic dosing with Glipizide extended release tablets. Administration of Glipizide extended release with food has no effect on the 2 to 3 hour lag time in drug absorption. In a single dose, food effect study in 21 healthy male subjects, the administration of Glipizide extended release immediately before a high fat breakfast resulted in a 40% increase in the Glipizide mean Cmax value, which was significant, but the effect on the AUC was not significant. There was no change in glucose response between the fed and fasting state. Markedly reduced GI retention times of the Glipizide extended release tablets over prolonged periods (e.g., short bowel syndrome) may influence the pharmacokinetic profile of the drug and potentially result in lower plasma concentrations. In a multiple dose study in 26 males with NIDDM, the pharmacokinetics of Glipizide were linear over the dose range of 5 to 60 mg of Glipizide extended release in that the plasma drug concentrations increased proportionately with dose. In a single dose study in 24 healthy subjects, four 5 mg, two 10 mg, and one 20 mg Glipizide extended release tablets were bioequivalent.

Glipizide is eliminated primarily by hepatic biotransformation; less than 10% of a dose is excreted as unchanged drug in urine and feces; approximately 90% of a dose is excreted as biotransformation products in urine (80%) and feces (10%). The major metabolites of Glipizide are products of aromatic hydroxylation and have no hypoglycemic activity. A minor metabolite which accounts for less than 2% of a dose, an acetylamino-ethyl benzine derivative, is reported to have 1/10 to 1/3 as much hypoglycemic activity as the parent compound. The mean total body clearance of Glipizide was approximately 3 liters per hour after single intravenous doses in patients with NIDDM. There were no significant differences in the pharmacokinetics of Glipizide after single dose administration to older diabetic subjects compared to younger healthy subjects. There is only limited information regarding the effects of renal impairment on the disposition of Glipizide, and no information regarding the effects of hepatic disease. However, since Glipizide is highly protein bound and hepatic biotransformation is the predominant route of elimination, the pharmacokinetics and/or pharmacodynamics of Glipizide may be altered in patients with renal or hepatic impairment.

INDICATIONS AND USAGE

Glipizide is indicated as an adjunct to diet for the control of hyperglycemia and its associated symptomatology in patients with non-insulin-dependent diabetes mellitus (NIDDM; type II), formerly known as maturity-onset diabetes, after an adequate trial of dietary therapy has proved unsatisfactory. Glipizide extended release is indicated when diet alone has been unsuccessful in correcting hyperglycemia, but even after the introduction of the drug in the patient's regimen, dietary measures should continue to be considered as important. In 12 week, well-controlled studies there was a maximal average net reduction in hemoglobin A_{1C} of 1.7% in absolute units between placebo-treated and Glipizide extended release-treated patients.

In initiating treatment for non-insulin-dependent diabetes, diet should be emphasized as the primary form of treatment. Caloric restriction and weight loss are essential in the obese diabetic patient. Proper dietary management alone may be effective in controlling the blood glucose and symptoms of hyperglycemia. The importance of regular physical activity should also be stressed, and cardiovascular risk factors should be identified, and corrective measures taken where possible.

If this treatment program fails to reduce symptoms and/or blood glucose, the use of an oral sulfonylurea should be considered. If additional reduction of symptoms and/or blood glucose is required, the addition of insulin to the treatment regimen should be considered. Use of Glipizide must be viewed by both the physician and patient as a treatment in addition to diet, and not as a substitute for diet or as a convenient mechanism for avoiding dietary restraint. Furthermore, loss of blood glucose control on diet alone also may be transient, thus requiring only short-term administration of Glipizide.

During maintenance programs, Glipizide should be discontinued if satisfactory lowering of blood glucose is no longer achieved. Judgments should be based on regular clinical and laboratory evaluations. Hemoglobin A_{1C} levels may be useful.

In considering the use of Glipizide in asymptomatic patients, it should be recognized that controlling blood glucose in non-insulin-dependent diabetes has not been definitely established to be effective in preventing the long-term cardiovascular or neural complications of diabetes. However, in insulin-dependent diabetes mellitus controlling blood glucose has been effective in slowing the progression of diabetic retinopathy, nephropathy, and neuropathy.

UNLABELED USES

Glipizide is used alone or as an adjunct in the treatment of diabetic microangiopathy.

CONTRAINDICATIONS

Glipizide is contraindicated in patients with:

1. Known hypersensitivity to the drug.
2. Diabetic ketoacidosis, with or without coma. This condition should be treated with insulin.

WARNINGS

SPECIAL WARNING ON INCREASED RISK OF CARDIOVASCULAR MORTALITY: The administration of oral hypoglycemic drugs has been reported to be associated with increased cardiovascu-

lar mortality as compared to treatment with diet alone or diet plus insulin. This warning is based on the study conducted by the University Group Diabetes Program (UGDP), a long-term prospective clinical trial designed to evaluate the effectiveness of glucose-lowering drugs in preventing or delaying vascular complications in patients with non-insulin-dependent diabetes. The study involved 823 patients who were randomly assigned to one of four treatment groups (*Diabetes*, 19, supp. 2: 747-830, 1970). UGDP reported that patients treated for 5 to 8 years with diet plus a fixed dose of tolbutamide (1.5 grams per day) had a rate of cardiovascular mortality approximately 2½ times that of patients treated with diet alone. A significant increase in total mortality was not observed, but the use of tolbutamide was discontinued based on the increase in cardiovascular mortality, thus limiting the opportunity for the study to show an increase in overall mortality. Despite controversy regarding the interpretation of these results, the findings of the UGDP study provide an adequate basis for this warning. The patient should be informed of the potential risks and advantages of Glipizide and of alternative modes of therapy.

Although only one drug in the sulfonylurea class (tolbutamide) was included in this study, it is prudent from a safety standpoint to consider that this warning may also apply to other oral hypoglycemic drugs in this class, in view of their close similarities in mode of action and chemical structure.

As with any other non-deformable material, caution should be used when administering Glipizide extended release tablets in patients with preexisting severe gastrointestinal narrowing (pathologic or iatrogenic). There have been rare reports of obstructive symptoms in patients with known strictures in association with the ingestion of another drug in this non-deformable sustained release formulation.

PRECAUTIONS
GENERAL
Renal and Hepatic Disease: The pharmacokinetics and/or pharmacodynamics of Glipizide may be affected in patients with impaired renal and/or hepatic function. If hypoglycemia should occur in such patients, it may be prolonged and appropriate management should be instituted.

GI Disease: Markedly reduced GI retention times of the Glipizide extended release tablets may influence the pharmacokinetic profile and hence the clinical efficacy of the drug.

Hypoglycemia: All sulfonylurea drugs are capable of producing severe hypoglycemia. Proper patient selection, dosage, and instructions are important to avoid hypoglycemic episodes. Renal or hepatic insuffi- ciency may cause elevated blood levels of Glipizide and the latter may also diminish gluconeogenic capacity, both of which increase the risk of serious hypoglycemic reactions. Elderly, debilitated or malnourished patients, and those with adrenal or pituitary insufficiency are particularly susceptible to the hypoglycemic action of glucose-lowering drugs. Hypoglycemia may be difficult to recognize in the elderly, and in people who are taking beta-adrenergic blocking drugs. Hypoglycemia is more likely to occur when caloric intake is deficient, after severe or prolonged exercise, when alcohol is ingested, or when more than one glucose-lowering drug is used.

Loss of Control of Blood Glucose: When a patient stabilized on any diabetic regimen is exposed to stress such as fever, trauma, infection, or surgery, a loss of control may occur. At such times, it may be necessary to discontinue Glipizide and administer insulin.

The effectiveness of any oral hypoglycemic drug, including Glipizide, in lowering blood glucose to a desired level decreases in many patients over a period of time, which may be due to progression of the severity of the diabetes or to diminished responsiveness to the drug. This phenomenon is known as secondary failure, to distinguish it from primary failure in which the drug is ineffective in an individual patient when first given. Adequate adjustment of dose and adherence to diet should be assessed before classifying a patient as a secondary failure.

Laboratory Tests: Blood and urine glucose should be monitored periodically. Measurement of hemoglobin A_{1C} may be useful.

Information for Patients: Patients should be informed of the potential risks and advantages of Glipizide and of alternative modes of therapy. They should also be informed about the importance of adhering to dietary instructions, of a regular exercise program, and of regular testing of urine and/or blood glucose.

The risks of hypoglycemia, its symptoms and treatment, and conditions that predispose to its development should be explained to patients and responsible family members. Primary and secondary failure should also be explained.

Patients should be informed that Glipizide extended release tablets should be swallowed whole. Patients should not chew, divide or crush tablets. Patients should not be concerned if they occasionally notice in their stool something that looks like a tablet. In the Glipizide extended release tablet, the medication is contained with a nonabsorbable shell that has been designed to slowly release the drug so the body can absorb it. When this process is completed, the empty tablet is eliminated from the body.

Drug Interactions: The hypoglycemic action of sulfonylureas may be potentiated by certain drugs including nonsteroidal anti-inflammatory agents, some azoles, and other drugs that are highly protein bound, salicylates, sulfonamides, chloramphenicol, probenecid, coumarins, monoamine oxidase inhibitors, and beta-adrenergic blocking agents. When such drugs are administered to a patient receiving Glipizide, the patient should be observed closely for hypoglycemia. When such drugs are withdrawn from a patient receiving Glipizide, the patient should be observed closely for loss of control. *In vitro* binding studies with human serum proteins indicate that Glipizide binds differently than tolbutamide and does not interact with salicylate or dicumarol. However, caution must be exercised in extrapolating these findings to the clinical situation and in the use of Glipizide with these drugs.

Certain drugs tend to produce hyperglycemia and may lead to loss of control. These drugs include the thiazides and other diuretics, corticosteroids, phenothiazines, thyroid products, estrogens, oral contraceptives, phenytoin, nicotinic acid, sympathomimetics, calcium channel blocking drugs, and isoniazid. When such drugs are administered to a patient receiving Glipizide, the patient should be closely observed for loss of control. When such drugs are withdrawn from a patient receiving Glipizide, the patient should be observed closely for hypoglycemia.

A potential interaction between oral miconazole and oral hypoglycemic agents leading to severe hypoglycemia has been reported. Whether this interaction also occurs with the intravenous, topical, or vaginal preparations of miconazole is not known. The effect of concomitant administration of fluconazole and Glipizide has been demonstrated in a placebo-controlled crossover study in normal volunteers. All subjects received Glipizide alone and following treatment with 100 mg of fluconazole as a single daily oral dose for 7 days. The mean percentage increase in the Glipizide AUC after fluconazole administration was 56.9% (range: 35 to 81%).

Carcinogenesis, Mutagenesis, Impairment of Fertility: A twenty month study in rats and an eighteen month study in mice at doses up to 75 times the maximum human dose revealed no evidence of drug-related carcinogenicity. Bacterial and *in vivo* mutagenicity tests were uniformly negative. Studies in rats of both sexes at doses up to 75 times the human dose showed no effects on fertility.

Pregnancy: Pregnancy Category C: Glipizide was found to be mildly fetotoxic in rat reproductive studies at all dose levels (5-50 mg/kg). This fetotoxicity has been similarly noted with other sulfonylureas, such as tolbutamide and tolazamide. The effect is perinatal and believed to be directly related to the pharmacologic (hypoglycemic) action of Glipizide. In studies in rats and rabbits no teratogenic effects were found. There are no adequate and well controlled studies in pregnant women. Glipizide should be used during pregnancy only if the potential benefit justifies the potential risk to the fetus.

Because recent information suggests that abnormal blood glucose levels during pregnancy are associated with a higher incidence of congenital abnormalities, many experts recommend that insulin be used during pregnancy to maintain blood glucose levels as close to normal as possible.

Nonteratogenic Effects: Prolonged severe hypoglycemia (4 to 10 days) has been reported in neonates born to mothers who were receiving a sulfonylurea drug at the time of delivery. This has been reported more frequently with the use of agents with prolonged half-lives. If Glipizide is used during pregnancy, it should be discontinued at least one month before the expected delivery date.

Nursing Mothers: Although it is not known whether Glipizide is excreted in human milk, some sulfonylurea drugs are known to be excreted in human milk. Because the potential for hypoglycemia in nursing infants may exist, a decision should be made whether to discontinue nursing or to discontinue the drug, taking into account the importance of the drug to the mother. If the drug is discontinued and if diet alone is inadequate for controlling blood glucose, insulin therapy should be considered.

Pediatric Use: Safety and effectiveness in children have not been established.

Geriatric Use: Of the total number of patients in clinical studies of Glipizide extended release 33 percent were 65 and over. No overall differences in effectiveness or safety were observed between these patients and younger patients, but greater sensitivity of some individuals cannot be ruled out. Approximately 1-2 days longer were required to reach steady state in the elderly. (See *"Clinical Pharmacology"* and *"Dosage and Administration"*).

ADVERSE REACTIONS
GLIPIZIDE IMMEDIATE RELEASE
In U.S. and foreign controlled studies, the frequency of serious adverse reactions reported was very low. Of 702 patients, 11.8% reported adverse reactions and in only 1.5% was Glipizide discontinued.

Hypoglycemia: See *"Precautions"* and *"Overdosage"* sections.

Gastrointestinal: Gastrointestinal disturbances are the most common reactions. Gastrointestinal complaints were reported with the following approximate incidence: nausea and diarrhea, one in seventy; constipation and gastralgia, one in one hundred. They appear to be dose-related and may disappear on division or reduction of dosage. Cholestatic jaundice may occur rarely with sulfonylureas; Glipizide should be discontinued if this occurs.

Dermatologic: Allergic skin reactions including erythema, morbilliform or maculopapular eruptions, urticaria, pruritus, and eczema have been reported in about one in seventy patients. These may be transient and may disappear despite continued use of Glipizide; if skin reactions persist, the drug should be discontinued. Porphyria cutanea tarda and photosensitivity reactions have been reported with sulfonylureas.

Hematologic: Leukopenia, agranulocytosis, thrombocytopenia, hemolytic anemia, aplastic anemia, and pancytopenia have been reported with sulfonylureas.

Metabolic: Hepatic porphyria and disulfiram-like reactions have been reported with sulfonylureas. In the mouse, Glipizide pretreatment did not cause an accumulation of acetaldehyde after ethanol administration. Clinical experience to date has shown that Glipizide has an extremely low incidence of disulfiram-like alcohol reactions.

➤ SHOWN IN PRODUCT IDENTIFICATION GUIDE

Endocrine Reactions: Cases of hyponatremia and the syndrome of inappropriate antidiuretic hormone (SIADH) secretion have been reported with this and other sulfonylureas.

Miscellaneous: Dizziness, drowsiness, and headache have each been reported in about one in fifty patients treated with Glipizide. They are usually transient and seldom require discontinuance of therapy.

Laboratory Tests: The pattern of laboratory test abnormalities observed with Glipizide was similar to that for other sulfonylureas. Occasional mild to moderate elevations of SGOT, LDH, alkaline phosphatase, BUN and creatinine were noted. One case of jaundice was reported. The relationship of these abnormalities to Glipizide is uncertain, and they have rarely been associated with clinical symptoms.

GLIPIZIDE EXTENDED RELEASE:

In U.S. controlled studies the frequency of serious adverse experiences reported was very low and causal relationship has not been established.

The 580 patients from 31 to 87 years of age who received Glipizide extended release tablets in doses from 5 mg to 60 mg in both controlled and open trials were included in the evaluation of adverse experiences. All adverse experiences reported were tabulated independently of their possible causal relation to medication.

Hypoglycemia: See *"Precautions"* and *"Overdosage"* sections.

Only 3.4% of patients receiving Glipizide extended release tablets had hypoglycemia documented by a blood glucose measurement < mg/dL and/or symptoms believed to be associated with hypoglycemia. In a comparative efficacy study of Glipizide extended release and Glipizide immediate release hypoglycemia occurred rarely with an incidence of less than 1% with both drugs.

In double-blind, placebo-controlled studies the adverse experiences reported with an incidence of 3% or more in Glipizide extended release-treated patients include:

Adverse Effect	Glipizide extended release (%) (N=278)	Placebo (%) (N=69)
Asthenia	10.1	13.0
Headache	8.6	8.7
Dizziness	6.8	5.8
Nervousness	3.6	2.9
Tremor	3.6	0.0
Diarrhea	5.4	0.0
Flatulence	3.2	1.4

The following adverse experiences occurred with an incidence of less than 3% in Glipizide extended release-treated patients:

Body as a whole: pain

Nervous system: insomnia, paresthesia, anxiety, depression and hypesthesia

Gastrointestinal: nausea, dyspepsia, constipation and vomiting

Metabolic: hypoglycemia

Musculoskeletal: arthralgia, leg cramps and myalgia

Cardiovascular: syncope

Skin: sweating and pruritus

Respiratory: rhinitis

Special senses: blurred vision

Urogenital: polyuria

Other adverse experiences occurred with an incidence of less than 1% in Glipizide extended release-treated patients:

Body as a whole: chills

Nervous system: hypertonia, confusion, vertigo, somnolence, gait abnormality and decreased libido

Gastrointestinal: anorexia and trace blood in stool

Metabolic: thirst and edema

Cardiovascular: arrhythmia, migraine, flushing and hypertension

Skin: rash and urticaria

Respiratory: pharyngitis and dyspnea

Special senses: pain in the eye, conjunctivitis and retinal hemorrhage

Urogenital: dysuria

Although these adverse experiences occurred in patients treated with Glipizide extended release, a causal relationship to the medication has not been established in all cases.

There have been rare reports of gastrointestinal irritation and gastrointestinal bleeding with use of another drug in this non-deformable sustained release formulation, although causal relationship to the drug is uncertain.

OVERDOSAGE

There is no well documented experience with Glipizide overdosage. There have been no known suicide attempts associated with purposeful overdosing with Glipizide extended release. The acute oral toxicity was extremely low in all species tested (LD$_{50}$ greater than 4 g/kg).

Overdosage of sulfonylureas including Glipizide can produce hypoglycemia. Mild hypoglycemic symptoms without loss of consciousness or neurologic findings should be treated aggressively with oral glucose and adjustments in drug dosage and/or meal patterns. Close monitoring should continue until the physician is assured that the patient is out of danger. Severe hypoglycemic reactions with coma, seizure, or other neurological impairment occur infrequently, but constitute medical emergencies requiring immediate hospitalization. If hypoglycemic coma is diagnosed or suspected, the patient should be given a rapid intravenous injection of concentrated (50%) glucose solution. This should be followed by a continuous infusion of a more dilute (10%) glucose solution at a rate that will maintain the blood glucose at a level above 100 mg/dL. Patients should be closely monitored for a minimum of 24 to 48 hours since hypoglycemia may recur after apparent clinical recovery. Clearance of Glipizide from plasma may be prolonged in persons with liver disease. Because of the extensive protein binding of Glipizide, dialysis is unlikely to be of benefit.

DOSAGE AND ADMINISTRATION

There is no fixed dosage regimen for the management of diabetes mellitus with Glipizide or any other hypoglycemic agent. In addition to the usual monitoring of urinary glucose, glycemic control should be monitored with hemoglobin A$_{1c}$ and/or blood glucose levels to determine the minimum effective dose for the patient; to detect primary failure, i.e., inadequate lowering of blood glucose at the maximum recommended dose of medication; and to detect secondary failure, i.e., loss of an adequate blood-glucose-lowering response after an initial period of effectiveness. Home blood glucose monitoring may also provide useful information to the patient and physician.

Short-term administration of Glipizide may be sufficient during periods of transient loss of control in patients usually controlled well on diet.

In general, Glipizide should be given approximately 30 minutes before a meal to achieve the greatest reduction in postprandial hyperglycemia; Glipizide extended release should be given with breakfast.

Initial Dose: The recommended starting dose of Glipizide immediate release is 5 mg, given before breakfast. Geriatric patients or those with liver disease may be started on 2.5 mg. The recommended starting dose of Glipizide extended release is 5 mg per day, given with breakfast. The recommended dose for geriatric patients is also 5 mg per day.

Titration: Dosage adjustments of Glipizide immediate release should ordinarily be in increments of 2.5-5 mg, as determined by blood glucose response. At least several days should elapse between titration steps. If response to a single dose is not satisfactory, dividing that dose may prove effective. The maximum recommended once daily dose is 15 mg. Doses above 15 mg should ordinarily be divided and given before meals of adequate caloric content. The maximum recommended total daily dose is 40 mg.

Dosage adjustment of Glipizide extended release should be based on laboratory measures of glycemic control. While fasting blood glucose levels generally reach steady state following initiation or change in Glipizide extended release dosage, a single fasting glucose determination may not accurately reflect the response to therapy. In most cases, hemoglobin A$_{1C}$ level measured at three month intervals is the preferred means of monitoring response to therapy.

Hemoglobin A$_{1C}$ should be measured as Glipizide extended release therapy is initiated at the 5 mg dose and repeated approximately three months later. If the result of this test suggests that glycemic control over the preceding three months was inadequate, the Glipizide extended release dose may be increased to 10 mg. Subsequent dosage adjustments should be made on the basis of hemoglobin A$_{1C}$ levels measured at three month intervals. If no improvement is seen after three months of therapy with a higher dose, the previous dose should be resumed. Decisions which utilize fasting blood glucose to adjust Glipizide extended release therapy should be based on at least two or more similar, consecutive values obtained seven days or more after the previous dose adjustment.

Maintenance: Some patients may be effectively controlled on a once-a-day regimen of Glipizide immediate release, while others show better response with divided dosing. Total daily doses above 15 mg should ordinarily be divided. Total daily doses above 30 mg have been safely given on a b.i.d. basis to long-term patients.

Most patients will be controlled with 5 mg or 10 mg of Glipizide extended release taken once daily. However, some patients may require up to the maximum recommended daily dose of 20 mg. While the glycemic control of selected patients may improve with doses which exceed 10 mg, clinical studies conducted to date have not demonstrated an additional group average reduction of hemoglobin A$_{1C}$ beyond what was achieved with the 10 mg dose.

Based on the results of a randomized crossover study patients receiving immediate release glipizide may be switched safely to Glipizide extended release tablets once-a-day at the nearest equivalent total daily dose. Patients receiving immediate release Glipizide also may be titrated to the appropriate dose of Glipizide extended release starting with 5 mg once daily. The decision to switch to the nearest equivalent dose or to titrate should be based on clinical judgment.

In elderly patients, debilitated or malnourished patients, and patients with impaired renal or hepatic function, the initial and maintenance dosing should be conservative to avoid hypoglycemic reactions (see *"Precautions"* section).

Patients Receiving Insulin: As with other sulfonylurea-class hypoglycemics, many stable non-insulin-dependent diabetic patients receiving insulin may be safely placed on Glipizide. When transferring patients from insulin to Glipizide the following general guidelines should be considered:

◆ RATED THERAPEUTICALLY EQUIVALENT; ◇ THERAPEUTIC EQUIVALENCE UNCONFIRMED; ○ UNRATED

For patients whose daily insulin requirement is 20 units or less, insulin may be discontinued and Glipizide therapy may begin at usual dosages. Several days should elapse between Glipizide titration steps.

For patients whose daily insulin requirement is greater than 20 units, the insulin dose should be reduced by 50% and Glipizide therapy may begin at usual dosages. Subsequent reductions in insulin dosage should depend on individual patient response. Several days should elapse between Glipizide titration steps.

During the insulin withdrawal period, the patient should test urine samples for sugar and ketone bodies at least three times daily. Patients should be instructed to contact the prescriber immediately if these tests are abnormal. In some cases, especially when the patient has been receiving greater than 40 units of insulin daily, it may be advisable to consider hospitalization during the transition period.

Patients Receiving Other Oral Hypoglycemic Agents: As with other sulfonylurea-class hypoglycemics, no transition period is necessary when transferring patients to Glipizide. Patients should be observed carefully (1-2 weeks) for hypoglycemia when being transferred from longer half-life sulfonylureas (e.g., chlorpropamide) to Glipizide due to potential overlapping of drug effect.

Recommended Storage: Store Glipizide immediate release tablets below 86°F (30°C). Store Glipizide extended release tablets at controlled room temperature, 59° to 86°F (15° to 30°C); protect from moisture and humidity.

HOW SUPPLIED
TABLET: 5 MG

AVERAGE UNIT PRICE (AVAILABLE SIZES)		GENERIC A-RATED AVERAGE PRICE (GAAP)	
GENERIC	$0.31	100s	$31.25
		500s	$146.16

BRAND/MANUFACTURER	NDC	SIZE	AWP
◆ GENERICS			
Schein	00364-2604-01	100s	$30.25
Endo	60951-0711-70	100s	$30.62
Mylan	00378-1105-01	100s	$30.67
Rugby	00536-5697-01	100s	$30.67
Rugby	00536-5702-01	100s	$30.67
Aligen	00405-5380-01	100s	$30.67
Moore,H.L.	00839-7939-06	100s	$31.85
UDL	51079-0810-20	100s ud	$34.60
Schein	00364-2604-05	500s	$144.00
Qualitest	00603-3755-28	500s	$144.05
Mylan	00378-1105-05	500s	$145.71
Aligen	00405-5380-02	500s	$145.73
Moore,H.L.	00839-7939-12	500s	$151.29

TABLET: 5 MG

BRAND/MANUFACTURER	NDC	SIZE	AWP
○ BRAND			
GLUCOTROL:	00662-4110-41	100s ud	$37.23
	59012-0411-41	100s ud	$37.23
	00662-4110-73	500s	$168.39
○ GENERICS			
Allscrips	54569-3841-00	30s	$9.10
Qualitest	00603-3755-21	100s	$30.35
Major	00904-7924-60	100s	$30.65
Goldline	00182-1994-01	100s	$30.67
Major	00904-7924-40	500s	$145.70
Goldline	00182-1994-05	500s	$145.73

TABLET: 10 MG

AVERAGE UNIT PRICE (AVAILABLE SIZES)		GENERIC A-RATED AVERAGE PRICE (GAAP)	
GENERIC	$0.56	100s	$57.06
		500s	$267.75

BRAND/MANUFACTURER	NDC	SIZE	AWP
◆ GENERICS			
Schein	00364-2605-01	100s	$55.50
Qualitest	00603-3756-21	100s	$55.70
Endo	60951-0714-70	100s	$56.22
Mylan	00378-1110-01	100s	$56.31
Rugby	00536-5698-01	100s	$56.31
Rugby	00536-5703-01	100s	$56.31
Aligen	00405-5381-01	100s	$56.31
Moore,H.L.	00839-7940-06	100s	$58.47
UDL	51079-0811-20	100s ud	$62.40
Schein	00364-2605-05	500s	$264.50
Qualitest	00603-3756-28	500s	$264.50
Aligen	00405-5381-02	500s	$264.52
Mylan	00378-1110-05	500s	$267.49
Moore,H.L.	00839-7940-12	500s	$277.75

For additional alternatives, turn to the section beginning on page 2859.

Globulin, Immune

DESCRIPTION
Globulin, Immune is a sterile solution of human protein, primarily immunoglobulin G (IgG), for intravenous (IV) or intramuscular (IM) use. The distribution of IgG subclasses is similar to that found in normal serum. The product is made by cold ethanol fractionation of large pools of human plasma.

CLINICAL PHARMACOLOGY
PRIMARY HUMORAL IMMUNODEFICIENCY
Globulin, Immune supplies a broad spectrum of opsonic and neutralizing IgG antibodies for the prevention or attenuation of a wide variety of infectious diseases. If Globulin, Immune is administered intravenously, essentially 100% of the infused IgG antibodies are immediately available in the recipient's circulation. After approximately 6 days, an equilibrium is reached between the intra- and extravascular compartments, with IgG being distributed approximately 50% intravascular and 50% extravascular. Therefore, a rapid initial drop in serum IgG levels is to be expected.[1] In comparison, after the intramuscular injection of immune globulin, the IgG requires 2-5 days to reach its maximum concentration in the intravascular compartment. This concentration corresponds to about 40% of the injected dose.[2] Peak blood levels of IgG are obtained approximately 2 days after intramuscular injection of Globulin, Immune.[3] Studies using a modified intravenous immunoglobulin have shown that approximately 30% of the infused IgG disappeared from the circulation in the first 24 hours, due primarily to equilibration of the IgG between the plasma and the extravascular space.[4-6] A further decline to about 40% of the peak level found immediately post-infusion is to be expected during the first week.[4-6] The *in vivo* half-life of Globulin, Immune, 5% Globulin, Immune, 5% equals or exceeds the 3-week half-life reported for IgG in the literature. Recent studies show that the half-life of IgG is approximately 37.7 ± 15 days.[7] The half-life of IgG can vary considerably from person to person, however. In particular, high concentrations of IgG and hypermetabolism associated with fever and infection have been seen to coincide with a shortened half-life of IgG.[1,8,9,10] This variable as well as the amount of immune globulin administered per dose is important in determining the frequency of administration of the drug for each individual patient.

Passive immunization with Globulin, Immune modifies hepatitis A, prevents or modifies measles, and provides replacement therapy in persons with hypo- or agammaglobulinemia. Globulin, Immune is not standardized with respect to antibody titers against hepatitis B surface antigen (HBsAg) and should not be used for prophylaxis of viral hepatitis type B. Prophylactic treatment to prevent hepatitis B can best be accomplished with the use of hepatitis B immune globulin, often in combination with hepatitis B vaccine.[11]

Globulin, Immune may be of benefit in women who have been exposed to rubella in the first trimester of pregnancy and who would not consider a therapeutic abortion.[12] Globulin, Immune may also be considered for use in immunocompromised patients for passive immunization against varicella if varicella zoster immune globulin (human) is not available.[13]

Globulin, Immune is not indicated for routine prophylaxis or treatment of rubella, poliomyelitis, mumps or varicella. It is not indicated for allergy or asthma in patients who have normal levels of immunoglobulin.[14]

IDIOPATHIC THROMBOCYTOPENIC PURPURA
While Globulin, Immune has been shown to be effective in some cases of idiopathic thrombocytopenic Purpura (ITP) (see *"Indications and Usage"*), the mechanism of action has not been fully elucidated.

BONE MARROW TRANSPLANTATION
Clinical studies with Globulin, Immune have shown that it is effective in bone marrow transplant patients ≥ 20 years of age in the first 100 days posttransplant for the following: prevention of systemic and local infections, interstitial pneumonia of infectious and idiopathic etiologies and acute graft-versus-host disease (AGVHD)[15] (see *"Indications and Usage"*). Administration of Globulin, Immune to bone marrow transplant patients significantly increased IgG and IgG subclass levels while those seen in the control group fell below predicted levels. The mechanism of action of Globulin, Immune in reducing the incidence of AGVHD is presently unknown.

PEDIATRIC HIV INFECTION
Children infected with human immunodeficiency virus (HIV) may display defects in both cellular and humoral immunity.[16-19] As a result, some children with HIV-1 infection experience serious, potentially life-threatening recurrent bacterial infections.[20-22] In one retrospective report, among 71 HIV-infected children observed over 3.5 years, 27 (37%) experienced serious documented bacterial infections.[21] The types of bacterial and viral infections observed in HIV-infected children are similar to those seen in children with primary hypogammaglobulinemia.[23] The replacement of opsonic and neutralizing IgG antibodies has been shown to reduce serious and minor bacterial infection in HIV-infected children.[24,25]

In a randomized, double-blind, placebo-controlled, multicenter study performed between March 7, 1988 and January 15, 1991, the efficacy of Globulin, Immune in pediatric HIV disease to decrease the frequency of serious and minor bacterial infections and the frequency of hospitalization, and to increase the time free of serious bacterial infection was documented in children with clinical or immunologic evidence of HIV disease (see *"Indications and Usage"*). The primary endpoint of this study was prospectively defined as a significant reduction in the proportion of subjects who develop at least one serious bacterial infection when compared to the control group of HIV-infected children who received placebo. Serious bacterial infections were defined as laboratory-proven and clinically diagnosed (i.e., radiologically proven acute pneumonia and sinusitis) infections. The Data Safety and Monitoring Board (DSMB) recommended early termination of the study based on data presented to them from an interim analysis in December 1990 which showed that treatment with Globulin, Immune 5% increased the time free from serious infections in children with CD4 + counts $\geq 200/m^3$.

▶ SHOWN IN PRODUCT IDENTIFICATION GUIDE

GENERAL

Glycine (aminoacetic acid) is a nonessential amino acid normally present in the body.[26] Glycine is a major ingredient in some amino acid solutions employed in intravenous alimentation.[27] Toxic effects of glycine administration have been reported.[28] The buffer capacity of Globulin, Immune is 16.5 or 35.0 mEq/L (approximately 0.3 or 0.35 mEq/g protein). A dose of 1,000 mg/kg body weight therefore represents an acid load of 0.33 or 0.35 mEq/kg body weight. The total buffering capacity of whole blood in a normal individual is 45-50 mEq/L of blood, or 3.6 mEq/kg body weight.[29] Thus, the acid load delivered with a dose of 1,000 mg/kg of Globulin, Immune, would be neutralized by the buffering capacity of whole blood alone, even if the dose were infused instantaneously. (An infusion usually lasts several hours.)

In patients with limited or compromised acid-base compensatory mechanisms, consideration should be given to the effect of the additional acid load Globulin, Immune might present.

Some preparations contain added sucrose. Because sucrose, when given intravenously, is excreted unchanged in the urine, such Globulin, Immune products may be given to diabetics without compensatory changes in insulin dosage regimen.

INDICATIONS AND USAGE

PRIMARY HUMORAL IMMUNODEFICIENCY

Globulin, Immune is efficacious in the treatment of primary immunodeficiency states in which severe impairment of antibody forming capacity has been shown, such as: congenital agammaglobulinemias, common variable immunodeficiency, Wiskott-Aldrich syndrome, x-linked immunodeficiency with hyper IgM, and severe combined immunodeficiencies.[6,30-32]

In patients with immunoglobulin deficiencies, Globulin, Immune, may prevent serious infection. However, Globulin, Immune, may not prevent chronic infections of the external secretory tissues such as the respiratory and gastrointestinal tract.

Globulin, Immune is preferable to intramuscular in treating patients who require an immediate and large increase in the intravascular immunoglobulin level,[2] in patients with limited muscle mass, and in patients with bleeding tendencies for whom intramuscular injections are contraindicated. The infusions must be repeated at regular intervals.

B-CELL CHRONIC LYMPHOCYTIC LEUKEMIA (CLL)

Globulin, Immune is indicated for prevention of bacterial infections in patients with hypogammaglobulinemia and/or recurrent bacterial infections associated with B-cell chronic lymphocytic leukemia (CLL). In a study of 81 patients, 41 of whom were treated with Globulin, Immune bacterial infections were significantly reduced in the treatment group.[3,5] In this study, the placebo group had approximately twice as many bacterial infections as the Globulin, Immune group. The median time to first bacterial infection for the Globulin, Immune group was greater than 365 days. By contrast, the time to first bacterial infection in the placebo group was 192 days. The number of viral and fungal infections, which were for the most part minor, was not statistically different between the two groups.

IDIOPATHIC THROMBOCYTOPENIC PURPURA (ITP)

In clinical situations in which a rapid rise in platelet count is needed to control bleeding or to allow a patient with ITP to undergo surgery, administration of Globulin, Immune, should be considered. Studies with Globulin, Immune, demonstrate that in patients in whom a response was achieved, the rise of platelets was generally rapid (within 1-5 days), transient (most often lasting from several days to several weeks) and were not considered curative. It is presently not possible to predict which patients with ITP will respond to therapy, although the increase in platelet counts in children seems to be better than that in adults. Childhood ITP may, however, respond spontaneously without treatment.

In children with chronic ITP, Globulin, Immune therapy resulted in a mean rise in platelet count of 312,000/μl with a duration of increase ranging from 2-6 months,[33,34] Globulin, Immune, therapy may be considered as a means to defer or avoid splenectomy.[34] In adults, Globulin, Immune therapy has been shown to be effective in maintaining the platelet count in an acceptable range with or without periodic booster therapy. The mean rise in platelet count was 93,000/μl and the average duration of the increase was 20-24 days.[33,37] However, it should be noted that not all patients will respond. Even in those patients who do respond, this treatment should not be considered to be curative.

Globulin, Immune, has been studied in 31 adult and pediatric subjects with ITP using a dosage of 1,000 mg/kg body weight on either 1 day or 2 consecutive days. Fourteen of 16 children (87.5%) and 9 of 10 adults with platelet follow-up (90%) responded to treatment with clinically significant platelet increments of ≥ 30,000/mm³. In the 12 children with acute ITP, there was an average increase in platelet count above baseline of 274,000/mm³ (range 33,000-529,000/mm³).

A controlled study was performed in children in which Globulin, Immune, was compared with steroids for the treatment of acute (defined as less than 6 months duration) ITP. In this study sequential platelet levels of 30,000, 100,000, and 150,000/μl were all achieved faster with Globulin, Immune, than with steroids and without any of the side effects associated with steroids.[38,39] However, it should be noted that many cases of acute ITP in childhood resolve spontaneously within weeks to months. Globulin, Immune, has been used with good results in the treatment of acute ITP in adult patients.[40,41,42] In a study involving 10 adults with ITP of less than 16 weeks duration, Globulin, Immune, therapy raised the platelet count to the normal range after a 5 day course. This effect lasted a mean of over 173 days, ranging from 30-372 days.[37]

Two different dosing regimens of Globulin, Immune have been studied in clinical investigations: a regimen consisting of 400 mg/kg body weight daily for 5 consecutive days, and a high dose treatment regimen consisting of 1,000 mg/kg body weight administered on either 1 day or 2 consecutive days (these studies are summarized below).

In clinical studies of Globulin, Immune, five of six (83.3%) children and 12 of 16 (75%) adults with acute or chronic ITP treated with 400 mg/kg body weight for 5 consecutive days demonstrated clinically significant platelet increments of ≥ 30,000/mm³ over baseline. The mean platelet count in children with ITP rose from 27,800/mm³ at baseline to 297,000/mm³ (range 50,000-455,000/mm³) and the mean platelet count in adults with ITP rose from 27,900/mm³ at baseline to 124,900/mm³ (range 11,000-341,000/mm³). Two of three children with acute ITP rapidly went into complete remission.

Thirteen of 14 children (92.9%) and 26 of 29 adults (89.7%) with acute or chronic ITP treated with Globulin, Immune, 1,000 mg/kg body weight administered on either 1 day or 2 consecutive days responded to treatment with clinically significant platelet increments of ≥ 30,000/mm³ over baseline. This included three of three patients with ITP that were human immunodeficiency virus (HIV) antibody positive and two of two patients with ITP that were pregnant. The mean platelet count in children with ITP treated with Globulin, Immune, 1,000 mg/kg body weight on 1 day or 2 consecutive days rose from 44,400/mm³ at baseline to 285,600/mm³ (range 89,000-473,000/mm³), and the mean platelet count in adults with ITP treated with the regimen rose from 23,400/mm³ at baseline to 173,100/mm³ (range 28,000-709,000/mm³). Two patients, one each with acute adult and chronic childhood ITP, entered complete remission with treatment. Six of the 29 adult patients with ITP received Globulin, Immune, 1,000 mg/kg on 1 day or 2 consecutive days to increase the platelet count prior to splenectomy. Mean platelet counts rose from 14.500/mm³ at baseline to 129,300/mm³ (range 51,000-242,000/mm³) prior to surgery.

The duration of the platelet rise following treatment of ITP with either treatment regimen of Globulin, Immune, was variable, ranging from several days to 12 months or more. Some ITP patients have demonstrated continuing responsiveness over many months to intermittent infusions of Globulin, Immune, 400-1,000 mg/kg body weight, administered as a single maintenance dose, at intervals as indicated by the platelet count.

Of 16 patients in a clinical study, 13 had chronic ITP (11 adults, 2 children), and 3 patients had acute ITP (one adult, 2 children). All 16 patients (100%) demonstrated a clinically significant rise in platelet count to a level greater than 40,000/mm³ following the administration of Globulin, Immune. Ten of the 16 patients (62.5%) exhibited a significant rise to greater than 80,000 platelets/mm³. Of these 10 patients, 7 had chronic ITP (5 adults, 2 children), and 3 patients had acute ITP (one adult, 2 children).

The rise in platelet count to greater than 40,000/mm³ occurred after a single I g/kg infusion of Globulin, Immune, in 8 patients with chronic ITP (6 adults, 2 children), and in 2 patients with acute ITP (one adult, one child). A similar response was observed after two I g/kg infusions in 3 adults patients with chronic ITP, and one child with acute ITP. The remaining 2 adult patients with chronic ITP received more than two I g/kg infusions before achieving a platelet count greater than 40,000/mm³. The rise in platelet count was generally rapid, occurring within 5 days. However, this rise was transient and not considered curative. Platelet count rises lasted 2 to 3 weeks, with a range of 12 days to 6 months.

BONE MARROW TRANSPLANTATION (BMT)

In clinical studies in bone marrow transplant patients ≥ 20 years of age, Globulin, Immune, decreased the risk of septicemia and other infections, interstitial pneumonia of infectious or idiopathic etiologies and acute graft-versus-host disease (AGVHD) in the first 100 days posttransplant. Globulin, Immune, is not indicated in bone marrow transplant patients below 20 years of age. In a controlled study of 369 evaluable BMT patients (184 treated and 185 controls) who either did or did not receive Globulin, Immune, in doses of 500 mg/kg body weight on days −7 and −2 pretransplant, then weekly through day 90 posttransplant, posttransplant complications were evaluated in the entire study group and in patients under age 20 and age 20 or older. For patients ≥ 20 years of age (128 patients in the control group and 119 patients in the treated group), there was a statistically significant reduction in interstitial pneumonia from 21% in the control group to 9% in the treated group (p = 0.0032) during the first 100 days posttransplant. Also significantly reduced in this age group were: overall septicemia from 53 infections in the 128 patient control group to 26 infections in the 119 patient treated group (relative risk control treated [RR] 2.36, p = 0.0025); gram-negative septicemia from 24 infections in the 128 patient control group to 9 infections in the 119 patient treated group (RR 2.53, p = 0.0015); gram-positive septicemia from 16 infections in the 128 patient control group to 8 infections in the 119 patient treated group (RR 2.73, p = 0.046); and Grade II to IV AGVHD from an incidence of 58 of 110 in the control group to 38 of 108 in the treated group (p = 0.0051).

The given p-values do not take into account multiple end-points and subset analyses. Therefore, some of the p-values could occur by chance alone. There was no significant improvement in overall mortality in this study.

In patients below age 20, there appeared to be no benefit from treatment with Globulin, Immune, either in reducing the incidence of infections or the incidence of AGVHD.

PEDIATRIC HIV INFECTION

Globulin, Immune, 400 mg/kg every 28 days significantly decreased the frequency of serious and minor bacterial infections (laboratory-proven and clinically diagnosed) and the frequency of hospitalization, and increased the time free of serious bacterial infection. The effect of Globulin, Immune, in preventing serious bacterial infections was especially apparent in preventing primary bacteremia (including *Streptococcus pneumoniae* bacteremia) and acute pneumonia.

In a randomized, double-blind, placebo-controlled, multicenter study, 394 HIV-infected, non-hemophilic, children less than 13 years of age were randomized. Of the children randomized, 369 were included in the efficacy analysis and 376 in the safety analysis. The study population had 1) a mean age of 40 months (range 2.4-136.8 months), 2) acquired HIV primarily through vertical transmission (91%), 3) a majority (87%) of CDC Class P-2 (symptomatic), and 4) had a median CD4+ count of 937 cells/mm^3 (range 0-6660 cells/mm^3). At the time of study entry, 14% (52 of 369) were receiving *Pneumocystis carinii* pneumonia (PCP) prophylaxis. During the course of the study, 51% (189 of 369) received PCP prophylaxis and 44% (164 of 369) received zidovudine (ZDV). Children with HIV-1 infection were initially stratified into two groups based upon CD4- count (< 200 cells/mm^3 versus ≥ 200 cells/mm^3) and CDC classification of pediatric HIV disease (history of opportunistic infections [P-2-D-1] and recurrent serious bacterial infections [P-2-D-2] versus others). Subjects received Globulin, Immune, (400 mg/kg = 8 mL/kg) (n = 185) or an equivalent volume of placebo (0.1% albumin [human]) (n = 184) every 28 days. The mean followup for subjects receiving Globulin, Immune, was 17.9 months and 17.8 months for patients on placebo.

The number of subjects who had at least one serious bacterial infection was 86 of 184 (47%) in the placebo group and 55 of 185 (30%) in the Globulin, Immune group (p = 0.0009). All p-values reported are two-sided. Treatment with Globulin, Immune, compared to placebo was also associated with a significant reduction in both the number of subjects with at least one laboratory-proven infection (36 of 184 vs. 18 of 185, p = 0.0081), and the number of subjects with at least one clinically diagnosed infection (71 of 184 vs. 45 of 185, p = 0.0036).

Efficacy in patients with CD4- counts < 200/mm^3 was not established, possibly because of the small number of subjects in this category.

The 2-year treatment period defined in the protocol was truncated for some patients by the DSMB based on data from the interim analysis. Rates of serious bacterial infections per 100 patient-years were computed and analyzed to take into account both the unequal duration of treatment and followup, as well as recurrent infections in individual subjects. Children treated with Globulin, Immune, experienced a 50.5% lower frequency of laboratory-proven serious bacterial infection compared to the group treated with placebo (9.1 vs. 18.2 infections per 100 patient-years, p = 0.031), a 36.0% lower frequency of clinically diagnosed serious infections (24.0 vs. 37.5 infections per 100 patient-years, p = 0.013), a 40.6% reduction in total serious infections (laboratory-proven and clinically diagnosed) (33.1 vs. 55.7 infections per 100 patient-years, p = 0.003), a 60% lower frequency of primary bacteremias (5.8 vs. 14.5 infections per 100 patient-years, p = 0.009), a 75.6% lower frequency of *Streptococcus pneumoniae* bacteremia (1.1 vs. 4.5 bacteremias per 100 patient-years, p = 0.026), a 54.3% lower frequency of clinically diagnosed pneumonia (12.7 vs. 27.8 infections per 100 patient-years, p = 0.001), and a 22.5% lower frequency of minor bacterial infections (including otitis media, skin and soft tissue infections, and upper respiratory tract infections) (123.6 vs. 159.5 infections per 100 patient-years, p = 0.033).

In addition to a reduced frequency of infection, children treated with Globulin, Immune, had a 36.8% lower number of hospitalizations per 100 patient-years (72 vs. 114 per 100 patient-years, p = 0.002) and a reduced number of hospital days (6.9 vs. 10.5 per patient-year, p = 0.030) than patients treated with placebo. Patients treated with Globulin, Immune, had a higher probability of remaining free of laboratory-proven infections (p = 0.0093) and combined laboratory-proven and clinically diagnosed infections (p = 0.0015) for 24 months than the group of children treated with placebo. At 24 months, the estimated probabilities of remaining infection-free for the Globulin, Immune, and placebo arms were 87.8% vs. 76.1%, respectively, for laboratory-proven infections and 63.5% vs. 44.5%, respectively, for combined laboratory-proven and clinically diagnosed infections.

There was no effect of Globulin, Immune, therapy on mortality, which was low in both treatment groups (17%), or on the frequency of opportunistic or viral infections during the period of study.

Since antibacterial prophylaxis could also account for the observed reduction in the rate of serious bacterial infections, further analysis was performed to evaluate the role of *Pneumocystis carinii* pneumonia (PCP) prophylaxis on the efficacy of Globulin, Immune. PCP prophylaxis consisted primarily (96%) of trimethoprim/sulfamethoxazole given 3 successive days each week. This antibiotic combination could be active against the bacteria commonly encountered in this patient population. In the subgroup of patients receiving PCP prophylaxis at study entry, treatment with Globulin, Immune, was associated with 44.0 infections per 100 patient-years, whereas placebo recipients had 64.7 infections per 100 patient-years (p = 0.047). In the subgroup of patients not receiving PCP prophylaxis at study entry, treatment with Globulin, Immune, was associated with 22.1 infections per 100 patient-years, whereas placebo recipients had 44.9 infections per 100 patient-years (p = 0.024). Thus, Globulin, Immune, benefitted patients by reducing the rate of serious bacterial infections whether or not they were receiving PCP prophylactic treatment at study entry. However, it should be noted that the use of PCP prophylactic treatment in this study was not randomized and specific guidelines for its administration were not identified.

Hepatitis A: The prophylactic value of Globulin, Immune, is greatest when given before or soon after exposure to hepatitis A. Globulin, Immune, is not indicated in persons with clinical manifestations of hepatitis A or in those exposed more than 2 weeks previously.

Measles (Rubeola): Globulin, Immune, should be given to prevent or modify measles in a susceptible person exposed less than 6 days previously.[43] (A susceptible person is one who has not been vaccinated and has not had measles previously). Globulin, Immune, may be especially indicated for susceptible household contacts of measles patients, particularly contacts under one year of age, for whom the risk of complications is highest.[43] Globulin, Immune, IM, *and measles vaccine should not be given at the same time.*[43] If a child is older than 12 months and has received Globulin, Immune, IM, he should be given measles vaccine about 3 months later, when the measles antibody titer will have disappeared.

If a susceptible child exposed to measles is immunocompromised, Globulin, Immune, IM, should be given immediately.[44] Children who are immunocompromised should not receive measles vaccine or any other live viral vaccine.

Varicella: Passive immunization against varicella in immunosuppressed patients is best accomplished by use of varicella-zoster immune globulin (human) (VZIG). If VZIG is unavailable, Globulin, Immune, IM, promptly given, may also modify varicella.[13]

Rubella: The routine use of Globulin, Immune, IM, for prophylaxis of rubella in early pregnancy is of dubious value and cannot be justified.[13] Some studies suggest that the use of Globulin, Immune, IM, in exposed susceptible women can lessen the likelihood of infection and fetal damage. Globulin, Immune, IM, may benefit those women who will not consider a therapeutic abortion.[12]

UNLABELED USES

Globulin, Immune, is used alone or as an adjunct in the treatment of juvenile rheumatoid arthritis, polymyositis, dermatomyositis, and acute myocarditis. It is also used in the treatment of autoimmune hemolytic anemia, severe aplastic anemia with bleeding problems, asthma, and Crohn's disease. In addition, Globulin, Immune, is used in the early treatment of pulmonary exacerbations of cystic fibrosis, and in cytomegalovirus interstitial pneumonitis following allogeneic bone marrow transplantation. It is also prescribed for Guillain-Barre syndrome, hemophilia A, chronic inflammatory demyelinating polyneuropathy, Kawasaki disease, and to slow or delay the progression of disease in patients with relapsing-remitting multiple sclerosis. It is used in generalized myasthenia gravis, and necrotizing enterocolitis, to prevent infections in high-risk preterm very-low birth weight infants, and to treat autoimmune neutropenia of infancy. It is also used in the treatment of respiratory syncytial virus, and is prescribed, systemic vasculitis, and severe neonatal autoimmune thrombocytopenia. It is also used in children with intractable epilepsy.

CONTRAINDICATIONS

Globulin, Immune, is contraindicated in individuals who are known to have had an anaphylactic or severe systemic response to it. Individuals with selective IgA deficiencies should not receive Globulin, Immune.

Such persons have the potential for developing antibodies to IgA and could have anaphylactic reactions to subsequent administration of blood products that contain IgA.[45]

Globulin, Immune, IM, should not be administered to patients who have severe thrombocytopenia or any coagulation disorder that would contraindicate intramuscular injections.

WARNINGS

Globulin, Immune, should be given with caution to patients with a history of prior systemic allergic reactions following the administration of human immunoglobulin preparations.[45]

Globulin, Immune, has, on rare occasions, caused a precipitous fall in blood pressure and a clinical picture of anaphylaxis, even when the patient is not known to be sensitive to immune globulin preparations. These reactions may be related to the rate of infusion. Accordingly, the infusion rate given under *"Dosage and Administration"* for Globulin, Immune, should be closely followed, at least until the physician has had sufficient experience with a given patient. The patient's vital signs should be monitored continuously and careful observation made for any symptoms throughout the entire infusion. If anaphylactic or severe anaphylactoid reactions occur, discontinue infusion immediately. Epinephrine should be available for the treatment of any acute anaphylactoid reactions.

Patients with agammaglobulinemia or extreme hypogammaglobulinemia who have never received immunoglobulin therapy or who have not received immunoglobulin therapy within the preceding 8 weeks may be at risk of developing inflammatory reactions upon the infusion of human immunoglobulins. These reactions are manifested by a rise in temperature, chills, nausea and vomiting, and appear to be related to the rate of infusion.

Infusion rates and the patient's clinical state should be monitored closely during infusion, since these reactions on rare occasions may lead to shock. (See *"Administration"* section under *"Dosage and Administration"*.)

Particular care should be exercised when Globulin, Immune, is administered to patients with paraproteins.[46]

PRECAUTIONS

GENERAL

Any vial that has been entered should be used promptly. Partially used vials should be discarded. Do not use if turbid. Solution which has been frozen should not be used.

Globulin, Immune, IM, should not be administered intravenously because of the potential for serious reactions. Injections should be made intramuscularly, and care should be taken to draw back on the plunger of the syringe before injection in order to be certain that the needle is not in a blood vessel.

DRUG INTERACTIONS

Antibodies in Globulin, Immune, may interfere with the response to live viral vaccines such as measles, mumps and rubella. Therefore, use of such vaccines should be deferred until approximately 3 (IM) to 6 months after administration.

Please see *"Dosage and Administration"* for other drug interactions.

PREGNANCY CATEGORY C

Animal reproduction studies have not been conducted with Globulin, Immune. It is not known whether Globulin, Immune can cause fetal harm when administered to a pregnant woman or can affect reproduction capacity. Globulin, Immune should be given to a pregnant woman only if clearly needed.

Intact immune globulins cross the placenta from maternal circulation increasingly after 30 weeks gestation.[47,48] In cases of maternal ITP where Globulin, Immune, was administered to the mother prior to delivery, the platelet response and clinical effect were similar in the mother and neonate.[42,48-57]

ADVERSE REACTIONS

PRIMARY HUMORAL IMMUNODEFICIENCY

Symptoms related to the infusion of Globulin, Immune were observed in 9 (3.5%) of 255 infusions. These symptoms were all mild to moderate in severity and included chills, fever, headache and emesis.

In a study of 37 patients with immunodeficiency syndromes receiving Globulin, Immune, in a monthly dose of 400 mg/kg body weight, reactions were seen in 5.2% of the infusion. Symptoms reported included malaise, a feeling of faintness, fever, chills, headache, nausea, vomiting, fatigue, leg cramps, urticaria, flushing, slight elevation of blood pressure, chest tightness, dyspnea and chest, back or hip pain. Mild erythema following infiltration of Globulin, Immune, at the infusion site was reported in some cases.

Twenty-one adverse reactions occurred in 341 infusions (6%), when using Globulin, Immune, in a clinical trial of 17 patients with primary immunodeficiency. Of the 17 patients, 12 (71%) were adults, and 5 (29%) were children (16 years or younger).

In another study, local pain or irritation was experienced during 35 (16%) of 219 infusions. Application of a warm compress to the infusion site alleviated local symptoms. These local reactions tended to be associated with hand vein infusions and their incidence may be reduced by infusions via the antecubital vein.

B-CELL CHRONIC LYMPHOCYTIC LEUKEMIA (CLL)

In the study of patients with B-cell chronic lymphocytic leukemia the incidence of adverse reactions associated with Globulin, Immune, infusions was approximately 1.3% while that associated with placebo (normal saline) infusions was 0.6%.[58]

IDIOPATHIC THROMBOCYTOPENIC PURPURA

An investigation of Globulin, Immune, in 31 adult and pediatric subjects with ITP encountered side effects in 17 of 119 (14.3%) infusions. The dosage in these studies was 1,000 mg/kg body weight for 1 day or 2 consecutive days. However, in the adult study, an induction dosage of 500 mg/kg body weight for 1 day or 2 consecutive days was associated with 17 of these infusions. Of those 17 infusions, three had adverse events. Overall, side effects included mild chest pain, mild and moderate emesis, moderate fever, mild or moderate headache (severe on one occasion) and a single incidence of hives, pruritus and rash. At least 17 of the 50 infusions in the pediatric study were given at rates of ≤ 0.1 mL/kg body weight per minute as part of a rate escalation investigation. Maximum infusion rates obtained were not limited by or interrupted due to adverse effects.

In studies of Globulin, Immune, administered at a dose of 400 mg/kg body weight in the treatment of adult and pediatric patients with ITP, systemic reactions were noted in only 4 of 154 (2.6%) infusions, and all but one occurred at rates of infusion greater than 0.04 mL/kg body weight per minute. The symptoms reported included chest tightness, a sense of tachycardia (pulse was 84 beats per minute), and a burning sensation in the head: these symptoms were all mild and transient.

In studies of Globulin, Immune administered at a dose of 1,000 mg/kg body weight either as a single dose or as two doses on consecutive days in the treatment of adult and pediatric patients with ITP, adverse reactions were noted in 25 of 251 (10%) infusions. Symptoms reported included headache, nausea, fever, chills, back pain, chest tightness, and shortness of breath. In children, the high dose regimen has been well-tolerated at the highest rates of infusion. In adults, however, the frequency of adverse reactions tended to increase with infusion rates in excess of 0.06 mL/kg body weight per minute. In general, reactions reported with infusion of Globulin, Immune, in these studies were reported as mild or moderate, and responded to slowing of the infusion rate.

BONE MARROW TRANSPLANTATION

In studies of Globulin, Immune, administered to 185 bone marrow transplant recipients at doses of 500 mg/kg body weight on day −7 and day −2 pretransplant, then weekly through day 90 posttransplant, adverse reactions were noted in 12 (6.5%) of the 185 patients that received Globulin, Immune, and in 14 (0.6%) of 2176 infusions. All reactions reported were rate-related and classified as mild. Chills were the most common symptom reported, occurring in nine patients. The other symptoms reported included headache, flushing, fever, pruritus and slight back discomfort. All reactions resolved satisfactorily, usually without treatment or decreasing the infusion rate.

PEDIATRIC HIV INFECTION

Three hundred seventy-six (376) patients, 187 treated with Globulin, Immune, and 189 treated with placebo (0.1% albumin [human]), were included in the safety analysis. Adverse reactions occurred during or within 24 hours of an infusion in 50 of 3,451 (1.4%) infusions of Globulin, Immune, and 62 of 3,447 (1.8%) infusions of placebo. Fever was the most common adverse reaction and occurred in 30 of 105 (28.6%) patients receiving placebo and 19 of 78 (24.4%) patients treated with Globulin, Immune. Irratability was the second most common symptom reported, with 10 of 105 (9.5%) reports for the placebo group and 9 of 78 (11.5%) for the group treated with Globulin, Immune. A large number of diverse adverse reactions accounted for the remaining adverse reactions reported in both study groups. In general, the number of adverse events reported was comparable in both the placebo and Globulin, Immune, treated groups. Three serious adverse reactions were reported. One patient experienced a hypersensitivity reaction and did not receive further Globulin, Immune, treatment. A second patient developed tachycardia and was admitted to an intensive care unit, but later continued treatment with Globulin, Immune. A third patient had skin infiltration during infusion and developed a full thickness skin slough over the dorsum of the hand that required skin grafting.

GENERAL

In the studies undertaken to date, other types of reactions have not been reported with Globulin, Immune. It may be, however, that adverse effects will be similar to those previously reported with intravenous and intramuscular immunoglobulin administration. Potential reactions, therefore, may also include local pain and tenderness at the injection site, urticaria, angioedema, anxiety, flushing, wheezing, abdominal cramps, myalgias, arthralgia, headache, backache, pyrexia, hypotension, chills, nausea, and dizziness; rash has been reported only rarely. Reactions to intravenous immunoglobulin tend to be related to the rate of infusion. Infusion rates and clinical state should be monitored closely during infusion. If an adverse reaction occurs, the infusion rate should be reduced or the infusion stopped until the symptoms have subsided. (See *"Dosage and Administration".)*

True anaphylactic reactions to Globulin, Immune, may occur in recipients with documented prior histories of severe allergic reactions to intramuscular immunoglobulin, but some patients may tolerate cautiously administered intravenous immunoglobulin without adverse effects.[59] Very rarely an anaphylactoid reaction may occur in patients with no prior history of severe allergic reactions to either intramuscular or intravenous immunoglobulin.

Patients previously sensitized to certain antigens, most commonly IgA, may be at risk of immediate anaphylactoid and hypersensitivity reactions. Epinephrine should be available for the treatment of any acute anaphylactoid reaction. (See *"Warning and Contraindications".)*

DOSAGE AND ADMINISTRATION

GENERAL

The usual dose of Globulin, Immune, is directed toward restoration of the immune deficient patient's circulating IgG level to near-normal levels. Use of 100-200 mg/kg body weight every three to four weeks is recommended for some brands. An initial loading dose of at least 200 mg/kg at more frequent intervals, proceeding to 100-200 mg/kg at three week intervals once a therapeutic plasma level has been established can be used. However, treatment must be individualized for each patient due to variation among patients in catabolic rate of IgG. Investigations indicate that Globulin, Immune, is well-tolerated and less likely to produce side effects when infused at the indicated rate. A rate of administration which is too rapid may cause flushing and changes in pulse rate and blood pressure. Slowing or stopping the infusion usually allows the symptoms to disappear promptly. If side effects occur, the rate may be reduced, or the infusion interrupted until symptoms subside. The infusion may then be resumed at the rate which is comfortable for the patient. Parenteral drug products should be inspected visually for particulate matter and discoloration prior to administration, whenever solution and container permit.

It is recommended that infusion of Globulin, Immune, be given by a separate line, by itself, without mixing with other intravenous fluids or medications the patient might be receiving. Some brands are not compatible with saline. If dilution is required, Globulin, Immune, may be diluted with 5% dextrose in water (D5/W). No other drug interactions or compatibilities have been evaluated.

Based upon other compatibility studies, Globulin, Immune, may be infused sequentially into a primary IV line containing either 0.9% sodium chloride injection or 5% dextrose injection or flushed with 0.9% sodium chloride injection or 5% dextrose injection. *Do not mix products of differing formulations.* If several doses of Globulin, Immune, are to be administered, several reconstituted vials of identical formulation and diluent may be pooled, using proper aseptic technique. Do not shake or cause excessive foaming. Swirl gently to mix. Filtration is acceptable but not required: pore sizes of greater than or equal to 15 microns will be less likely to slow infusion.

PRIMARY HUMORAL IMMUNODEFICIENCY

The usual dosage of Globulin, Immune, for prophylaxis in primary immunodeficiency syndromes is 100-200 mg/kg of body weight administered approximately once a month by intravenous infusion. The dosage may be given more frequently or increased as high as 400 mg/kg body weight, if the clinical response is inadequate, or the level of IgG achieved in the circulation is felt to be insufficient. The minimum level of IgG required for protection has not been determined.

Globulin, Immune, IM, may prevent serious infection in patients with immunoglobulin deficiencies if circulating IgG levels of approximately 200 mg/ 100 mL plasma are maintained. The recommended dosage is 0.66 mL/kg (at least 100 mg/kg) given every 3 to 4 weeks.[14] A double dose is given at onset of therapy; some patients may require more frequent injections.

B-CELL CHRONIC LYMPHOCYTIC LEUKEMIA (CLL)

For patients with hypogammaglobulinemia and/or recurrent bacterial infections due to B-cell chronic lymphocytic leukemia, a dose of 400 mg/kg every 3 to 4 weeks is recommended.

Globulin, Immune, in previously untreated agammaglobulinemic and hypogammaglobulinemic patients may lead to systemic side effects. Some of the effects may occur as a result of the reaction between the antibodies administered and free antigens in the blood and tissues of the immunodeficient recipient.[60,61]. When free antigen is no longer present, further administration of Globulin, Immune, to immunodeficient patients as well as to normal individuals usually does not cause further untoward side effects.

IDIOPATHIC THROMBOCYTOPENIC PURPURA (ITP)

Induction: An increase in platelet count has been observed in children and some adults with acute or chronic ITP receiving Globulin, Immune, 400 mg/kg body weight daily for 5 days. In acute ITP of childhood, if an initial platelet count response to the first two doses is adequate (30-50,000/μl), therapy may be discontinued after the second day of the 5 day course.[39] Alternatively, studies in adults and children with Globulin, Immune, using a dose of 1,000 mg/kg body weight daily for 1 day or 2 consecutive days have also shown increases in platelet count. In the latter treatment regimen, if an adequate increase in the platelet count is observed at 24 hours, the second dose of 1,000 mg/kg body weight may be withheld. The high dose regimen (1,000 mg/kg x 1-2 days) is not recommended for individuals with expanded fluid volumes or where fluid volume may be a concern. With both treatment regimens, a response usually occurs within several days and is maintained for a variable period of time. In general, a response is seen less often in adults than in children.

Maintenance: In adults and children with ITP, if after induction therapy the platelet count falls to less than 30,000/mm^3 and/or the patient manifests clinically significant bleeding, Globulin, Immune, 400 mg/kg body weight may be given as a single infusion. If an adequate response does not result, the dose can be increased to 800-1,000 mg/kg of body weight given as a single infusion. Maintenance infusions may be administered intermittently as clinically indicated to maintain a platelet count greater than 30,000/mm^3.

BONE MARROW TRANSPLANTATION

A reduction in posttransplant complications has been observed served in bone marrow transplant patients ≥ 20 years of age receiving Globulin, Immune, 500 mg/kg body weight beginning on days −7 and −2 pretransplant (or at the time conditioning therapy for transplantation is begun), then weekly through day 90 posttransplant. Globulin, Immune should be administered by itself through a Hickman line while it is in place and thereafter through a peripheral vein. Please see *"Dosage and Administration"* for other drug interactions.

PEDIATRIC HIV INFECTION

A reduction in bacterial infections has been observed in children infected with HIV-1 receiving Globulin, Immune, in doses of 400 mg/kg body weight every 28 days.

Hepatitis A: Globulin, Immune, IM, in a dose of 0.01 mL/lb (0.02 mL/kg) is recommended for household and institutional hepatitis A contacts.

The following doses of Globulin, Immune, IM, are recommended for persons who plan to travel in ares where hepatitis A is common[62].

Length of Stay	Dose Volume
Less than 3 months	0.02 mL/kg
3 months or longer	0.06 mL/kg (repeat every 4-6 months)

Measles (Rubeola): Globulin, Immune, IM, should be given in a dose of 0.11 mL/lb (0.25 mL/kg) to prevent or modify measles in a susceptible person exposed less than 6 days previously[43].

If a susceptible child who is also immunocompromised is exposed, Globulin, Immune, IM, in a dose of 0.5 mL/kg (maximum 15 mL) should be given immediately[44].

Varicella: If varicella-zoster immune globulin (human) is unavailable, Globulin, Immune, IM, at a dose of 0.6 to 1.2 mL/kg given promptly, is the recommended dose[13].

Rubella: The recommended dose of 0.55 mL/kg Globulin, Immune, IM, may benefit women who will not consider a therapeutic abortion[12].

ADMINISTRATION

Globulin, Immune, IM, is administered intramuscularly (see *"Precautions"*), preferably in the gluteal region. Doses over 10 mL should be divided and injected into several muscle sites to reduce local pain and discomfort.

Parenteral drug products should be inspected visually for particulate matter and discoloration prior to administration whenever solution and container permit.

STORAGE

Store at 2-8°C (35-46°). Some brands may be stored at temperatures up to 30°C (86°F). Do not freeze. Do not use after expiration date.

REFERENCES

1. Waldmann TA. Storber W: Metabolism of immunoglobulins. Prog Allergy 13:1-110, 1969. 2. Morell A, Schurch B, Ryser D, et al: In vivo behavior of gamma globulin preparations. *Vax Sang* 38:272, 1980. 3. Smith GN, Mollison, D. Griffiths, B. and Mollison, PL; Uptake of IgG after intramuscular and subcutaneous injection. Lancet i:1208-1212, 1972. 4. Pirofsky B. Campbell SM, Montanaro A: Individual patient variations in the kinetics of intravenous immunoglobulin administration. *J Clin Immunol* 2(2). 7S-14S, 1982. 5. Pirofsky B: Intravenous immune globulin therapy in hypogammaglobulinemia. *Amer J Med* 76(3r. 53-60, 1984. 6. Pirofsky B, Anderson CJ, Bardana EJ Jr.: Therapeutic section. and detrimental effects of intravenous immunoglobulin therapy. In: Alving BM (ed.): *Immunoglobulins: characteristics and uses of intravenous preparations.* Washington. D.C., U.S. Government Printing Office (1980). pp. 15-22. 7. Unpublished data in the files of Baxter Healthcare Corporation. 8. Morell A. Riesen W: Structure, function and catabolism of immunoglobulins in Immunohemotherapy. Nydegger UE (ed), London, Academic Press, 1981, pp 17-26 9. Stiehm ER: Standard and special human immune serum globulins as therapeutic agents. Pediatrics 83:301-319, 1979 10. Buckley RH: Immunoglobulin replacement therapy: Indications and contraindications for use and variable Ig G levels achieved in Immunoglobulins: Characteristics and Use of Intravenous Preparations. Alving BM, Finlayson JS (eds), Washington, DC, U.S. Department of Health and Human Services, 1979, pp 3-8. 11. Morbidity and Mortality Weekly Report, June 1, 1984 (Vol. 33, No. 21). Revised: October, 1990 12. Report of the Committee on Infectious Diseases, American Academy of Pediatrics, 1982, Red Book p. 231. 13. Gershon, AA, Pelmelli, S, Karpatkin., M, Smithwick, E, and Steinberg, S: Antibody to varicella-zoster virus after passive immunization against chickenpox. J. Clin. Microbiol. 8:733-735, 1978. 14. Report of the Committee on Infectious Diseases, American Academy of Pediatrics, 1982, Red Book pp. 34-36. 15. Sullivan K.M. Kopecky KJ. Jocom J. et al: Immunomodulatory and antimicrobial efficacy of intravenous immunoglobulin in bone marrow transplantation. *N Engl J Med* 323(11):705-12. 1990. 16. Bernstein LJ, Ochs HD. Wedgwood RJ, et al. Defective humoral immunity in pediatric acquired immune deficiency syndrome. *J Pediatr* 107(3):352-7, 1985. 17. Borkowsky W. Steele CJ. Grubman S, et al: Antibody responses to bacterial toxoids in children infected with human immunodeficiency virus. *J Pediatr* 110(4):563-6. 1987. 18. Blanche S, Le Deist F, Fischer A, et al: Longitudinal study of 18 children with perinatal LAV/HTLV III infection: attempt at prognostic evaluation. *J Pediatr* 109(6):965-70, 1986. 19. Pahwa S, Fikrig S, Menez R, et al: Pediatric acquired immunodeficiency syndrome demonstration of B-lymphocyte defects in vitro. *Diagn Immunol* 4(1)24-30, 1986. 20. Bernstein LJ, Krieger BZ, Novick B, et al: Bacterial infections in the acquired immunodeficiency syndrome of children. *Pediatr Infect Dis* 4(5):472-5, 1985. 21. Krasinski K, Borkowsky W, Bonk S, et al: Bacterial infections in human immunodeficiency virus-infected children. *Pediatr Infect Dis J* 4(5):323-8, 1988. 22. Scott GB, Buck BE. Leterman JG, et al: Acquired immunodeficiency syndrome in infants, *N Engl J Med* 310(2):76-81, 1984. 23. Mofenson LM. Willoughby A. Passive immunization. In: Pizzo PA, Wilfert CM, (eds.) *Pediatric AIDS: the challenge of HIV infection in infants, children and adolescents.* Baltimore: Williams & Wilkins (1991) pp 633-50. 24. National Institute of Child Health and Human Development Intravenous Immunoglobulin Study Group. Intravenous immune globulin for the prevention of bacterial infections in children with symptomatic human immunodeficiency virus infection. *N Engl J Med* 325(2):73-80, 1991. 25. Mofenson LM, Moye J Jr, Bethel J. et al: Prophylactic intravenous immunoglobulin in HIV-infected children with CD4+ counts of 0.20×10^9/L or more. Effect on viral, opportunistic, and bacterial infections. *JAMA* 268(4):483-88, 1992. 26. Glycine. In: Budavari S, O'Neil MJ, Smith A. et al, eds.: *Merck Index.* 11th ed. Rahway, NJ, Merck & Co., 1989, p. 706. 27. Wretlind. A: Complete intravenous nutrition: theoretical and experimental background. *Nutr Metab* 14(Suppl):1-57, 1972. 28. Hahn RG. Stalberg HP, Gustafsson SA: Intravenous infusion of irrigating fluids containing glycine or mannitol with and without ethanol. *J Urol* 142(4):1102-1105, 1989. 29. Guyton *AC: Textbook of Medical Physiology.* 5th ed. Philadelphia, W.B. Saunders, 1976, pp. 499-500. 30. Nolte MT. Pirofsky B, Gerritz GA, et al: intravenous immunoglobulin therapy for antibody deficiency. *Clin Exp Immunol* 36: 237-43, 1979. 31. Buckley RH: Immunoglobulin replacement therapy: indications and contraindications for use and variable IgG levels achieved. In: Alving BM (ed): *Immunoglobulins: characteristics and uses of intravenous preparations.* Washington. D.C., U.S. Government Printing Office. (1980), pp. 3-8. 32. Ochs HD: Intravenous immunoglobulin therapy of patients with primary immunodeficiency syndromes: efficacy and safety of a new modified immune globulin preparation. In: Alving BM (ed): *Immunoglobulins: characteristic and uses of intravenous preparations.* Washington, D.C., U.S. Government Printing Office, (1980), pp. 9-14. 33. Bussel JB, Kimberly RP, Inman RD, et al: Intravenous gammaglobulin for chronic idiopathic thrombocytopenic purpura. *Blood* 62:480-486, 1983. 34. Imholz B, et al: Intravenous immunoglobulin (i.v. IgG) for previously treated acute or for chronic idiopathic thrombocytopenic purpura (ITP) in childhood: A prospective multicenter study. *Blut* 56:63-68. 1988. 35. Bussel JB, Schulman I, Hilgartner MW, et al: Intravenous use of gamma globulin in the treatment of chronic immune thrombocytopenic purpura as a means to defer splenectomy. *J Pediatr* 103:651-654, 1983. 36. Lusher JM, and Warrier I: Use of intravenous gammaglobulin in children with idiopathic thrombocytopenic purpura and other immune thrombocytopenias. *Am J Med* 83(suppl 4A): 10-16, 1987. 37. Newland AC, Treleaven JG, Minchinton B, et al: High-dose intravenous IgG in adults with autommune thrombocytopenia. *Lancet* 1:84-87, 1983. 38. Imbach P, Barandum S, d' Apuzzo V, et al: High-dose intravenous gamma globulin for idiopathic thrombocytopenic purpura in childhood. *Lancet* 1: 1228, 1981. 39. Imbach P, Wagner HP, Berchtold W, et al: Intravenous immunoglobulin versus oral corticosteroids in acute immune thrombocytopenic purpura in childhood. *Lancet* 2:464, 1985. 40. Fehr J, Hofmann V, Kappeler U: Transient reversal of thrombocytopenia in idiopathic thrombocytopenic purpura by high-dose intravenous gamma globulin. *N Engl J Med* 306:1254, 1982. 41. Mueller-Eckhardt C, Kuenzlen E, Thilo-Korner D, et al: High-dose intravenous immunoglobulin for posttransfusion purpura. *N Engl J Med* 308:287, 1983. 42. Wenske G, Gaedicke G, Kuenzlen E, et al: Treatment of idiopathic thrombocytopenic purpura in pregnancy by high-dose intravenous immunoglobulin. *Blut* 46:347-353, 1983. 43. Morbidity and Mortality Weekly Report, May 7, 1982 (Vol. 31, No. 17). 44. Report of the Committee on Infectious Diseases, American Academy of Pediatrics, 1982, Red Book pp. 134-135. 45. Fudenberg, HH: Sensitization to immunoglobulins and hazards of gamma globulin therapy, in Immunoglobulins. Biologic Aspects and Clinical Uses. Edited by Ezio Merler, National Academy of Sciences, Washington, D.C., 1970, pp. 211-220. 46. Cunningham-Rundles C, Smithwick EM, Siegal FP, et al: Treatment of primary humoral immunodeficiency disease with intravenous (pH 4.0 treated) gamma globulin, in Nydegger UE (ed): *Immunohemotherapy: A Guide to Immunoglobulin Prophylaxis and Therapy.* London, Academic Press, 1981, p 283. 47. Hammarstrom L, and Smith CI: Placental transfer of intravenous immunoglobulin. *Lancet* 1:681, 1986. 48. Sidiropoulos D, et al: Transplacental passage of intravenous immunoglobulin in the last trimester of pregnancy. *J Pediatr* 109:505-508, 1986. 49. Wenske G, et al: Idiopathic thrombocytopenic purpura in pregnancy and neonatal period. *Blut* 48:377-382, 1984. 50. Fabris P, et al: Successful treatment of a steroid-resistant form of idiopathic

thrombocytopenic purpura in pregnancy with high doses of intravenous immunoglobulins. *Acta Haemat* **77**:107-110, 1987. 51. Coller BS, et al: Management of severe ITP during pregnancy with intravenous immunoglobulin (IVIgG). *Clin Res* 33:545A, 1985. 52. Tchernia G, et al: Management of immune thrombocytopenia in pregnancy: Response to infusions of immunoglobulins. *Am J Obstet Gynecol* 148:225-226, 1984. 53. Newland AC, et al: Intravenous IgG for autoimmune thrombocytopenia in pregnancy. *N Engl J Med* **310**:261-262, 1984. 54. Morgenstern GR, et al: Autoimmune thrombocytopenia in pregnancy: New approach to management. *Br Med J* 287:584, 1983. 55. Ciccimarra F, et al: Treatment of neonatal passive immune thrombocytopenia. *J Pediat* 105:677-678, 1984. 56. Rose VL, and Gordon LI: Idiopathic thrombocytopenic purpura in pregnancy. Successful management with immunoglobulin infusion. *JAMA* 254:2626-2628, 1985. 57. Gounder MP, et al: Intravenous gammaglobulin therapy in the management of a patient with idiopathic thrombocytopenic purpura and a warm autoimmune erythrocyte panagglutinin during pregnancy. *Obstet Gynecol* 67:741-746, 1986. 58. Cooperative Group for the Study of Immunoglobulin in Chronic Lymphocytic Leukemia: Intravenous immunoglobulin for the prevention of infection in Chronic Lymphocytic Leukemia: A randomized, controlled clinical trial. N Eng J Med 319:902-907, 1988 59. Peerless AG, Stiehm ER: Intravenous gammaglobulin for reaction to intramuscular preparation. [letter] *Lancet* 2(8347): 461, 1983. 60. Cunningham-Rundles C, Day NK, Wahn V, et al: Reactions to intravenous gamma globulin infusions and immune complex formation, in Nydegger UE (ed): *Immunohemotherapy: A Guide to Immunoglobulin Prophylaxis and Therapy*. London, Academic Press, 1981, p 447. 61. Barandum S, Morell A: Adverse reactions to immunoglobulin preparations, in Nydegger UE (ed): *Immunohemotherapy: A Guide to Immunoglobulin Prophylaxis and Therapy*. London, Academic Press, 1981, p 223. 62. Morbidity and Mortality Weekly Report, September 4, 1981 (Vol. 30, No. 34).

J CODES
Per 500 mg IV—J1561

HOW SUPPLIED
INJECTION:

BRAND/MANUFACTURER	NDC	SIZE	AWP
○ **BRAND**			
GAMMAR I.M.: Armour	00053-7595-01	2 ml	$10.62
	00053-7595-02	10 ml	$16.86
GAMASTAN: Miles Biol	00192-0615-12	10 ml	$18.00

INJECTION: 2.5 GM (5%)

BRAND/MANUFACTURER	NDC	SIZE	AWP
○ **GENERICS**			
VENOGLOBULIN-S: Alpha Therapeutic	49669-1612-01	50 ml	$190.38

INJECTION: 5 GM (5%)

BRAND/MANUFACTURER	NDC	SIZE	AWP
○ **GENERICS**			
VENOGLOBULIN-S: Alpha Therapeutic	49669-1613-01	100 ml	$380.75

INJECTION: 10 GM (5%)

BRAND/MANUFACTURER	NDC	SIZE	AWP
○ **GENERICS**			
VENOGLOBULIN-S: Alpha Therapeutic	49669-1614-01	200 ml	$761.50

INJECTION: 125 U

BRAND/MANUFACTURER	NDC	SIZE	AWP
○ **BRAND**			
VARICELLA ZOSTER IMMUNE GLOBULIN: Amer Red Cr-Blood	14362-0118-02	2.5 ml	$83.00

POWDER FOR INJECTION: 2.5 MG

BRAND/MANUFACTURER	NDC	SIZE	AWP
○ **BRAND**			
GAMIMUNE N- 5 %: Miles Biol	00192-0640-20	1s	$142.80
GAMMAR I.V.: Armour	00053-7490-02	1s	$155.00
○ **GENERICS**			
IVEEGAM: Immuno-U.S.	54129-0233-25	1s	$162.50

POWDER FOR INJECTION: 0.5 GM

BRAND/MANUFACTURER	NDC	SIZE	AWP
○ **BRAND**			
GAMIMUNE N- 5 %: Miles Biol	00192-0640-12	1s	$45.60
GAMMAGARD S/D: Baxter Biotech	00944-2620-01	1s	$54.92

POWDER FOR INJECTION: 1 GM

BRAND/MANUFACTURER	NDC	SIZE	AWP
○ **BRAND**			
GAMMAR I.V.: Armour	00053-7490-01	1s	$62.00
SANDOGLOBULIN: Sandoz Pharm	00078-0120-58	1s	$70.02
GAMIMUNE N- 10 %: Miles Biol	00192-0649-12	1s	$75.00
○ **GENERICS**			
IVEEGAM: Immuno-U.S.	54129-0233-10	1s	$65.00

POWDER FOR INJECTION: 2.5 GM

BRAND/MANUFACTURER	NDC	SIZE	AWP
○ **BRAND**			
GAMMAGARD S/D: Baxter Biotech	00944-2620-02	1s	$156.62
○ **GENERICS**			
VENOGLOBULIN-I: Alpha Therapeutic	49669-1602-01	1s	$152.05

POWDER FOR INJECTION: 3 GM

BRAND/MANUFACTURER	NDC	SIZE	AWP
○ **BRAND**			
SANDOGLOBULIN: Sandoz Pharm	00078-0122-59	1s	$133.20
	00078-0122-19	10s	$1305.00

POWDER FOR INJECTION: 5 GM

BRAND/MANUFACTURER	NDC	SIZE	AWP
○ **BRAND**			
GAMIMUNE N- 5 %: Miles Biol	00192-0640-71	1s	$285.60
GAMMAR I.V.: Armour	00053-7490-05	1s	$310.00
GAMMAGARD S/D: Baxter Biotech	00944-2620-03	1s	$317.98
GAMIMUNE N- 10 %: Miles Biol	00192-0649-20	1s	$375.00
GAMMAR I.V.: Armour	00053-7490-06	6s	$1767.00
○ **GENERICS**			
VENOGLOBULIN-I: Alpha Therapeutic	49669-1603-01	1s	$304.10
IVEEGAM: Immuno-U.S.	54129-0233-50	1s	$325.00

POWDER FOR INJECTION: 6 GM

BRAND/MANUFACTURER	NDC	SIZE	AWP
○ **BRAND**			
SANDOGLOBULIN: Sandoz Pharm	00078-0124-60	1s	$252.00
	00078-0124-19	10s	$2484.00

POWDER FOR INJECTION: 10 GM

BRAND/MANUFACTURER	NDC	SIZE	AWP
○ **BRAND**			
GAMMAR I.V.: Armour	00053-7490-10	1s	$620.00
GAMMAGARD S/D: Baxter Biotech	00944-2620-04	1s	$640.71
GAMIMUNE N- 10 %: Miles Biol	00192-0649-71	1s	$750.00
○ **GENERICS**			
VENOGLOBULIN-I: Alpha Therapeutic	49669-1604-01	1s	$608.20

POWDER FOR INJECTION: 12 GM

BRAND/MANUFACTURER	NDC	SIZE	AWP
○ **BRAND**			
SANDOGLOBULIN: Sandoz Pharm	00078-0244-93	1s	$504.00
	00078-0244-19	10s	$4956.00

POWDER FOR INJECTION: 12.5 GM

BRAND/MANUFACTURER	NDC	SIZE	AWP
○ **BRAND**			
GAMIMUNE N- 5 %: Miles Biol	00192-0640-25	1s	$714.00

POWDER FOR INJECTION: 20 GM

BRAND/MANUFACTURER	NDC	SIZE	AWP
○ **BRAND**			
GAMIMUNE N- 10 %: Miles Biol	00192-0649-24	1s	$1500.00

Globulin, Immune Rho$_o$(D)

DESCRIPTION
Globulin, Immune Rho$_o$ (D), is a sterile solution containing IgG anti-Rho$_o$(D) for use in preventing Rh immunization in Rh negative individuals exposed to Rh positive red blood cells. A single dose of Globulin, Immune Rho$_o$(D), microdose contains sufficient anti-Rho$_o$(D) (approximately 50 μg)[†] to suppress the immune response to 2.5 mL (or less) of Rh positive red blood cells; a single full dose of Globulin, Immune Rho$_o$(D) contains sufficient anti-Rho$_o$(D) (approximately 300 μg)[†] to suppress the immune response to 15 mL (or less) of Rh positive red blood cells.

All donors are carefully screened to eliminate those in high risk groups for disease transmission. Fractionation of the plasma is done by a modification of the cold alcohol procedure.

This product is for intramuscular injection only.

† A full dose of Globulin, Immune Rho$_o$(D), has traditionally been referred to as a "300 μg" dose and this usage is employed here for convenience in terminology. *It should not be construed as the actual anti-D content.* Each full dose of Globulin, Immune Rho$_o$(D), must contain at least as much anti-D as 1 ml of the U.S. Reference Rho$_o$(D) Immune Globulin (Human). Studies performed at the Food and Drug Administration have shown that the U.S. Reference contains 820 international units (IU) of anti-D per ml. When the conversion factor determined for the International (WHO) Reference Preparation is used, 820 IU per ml is equivalent to 164 μg per ml of anti-D. Globulin, Immune Rho$_o$(D), microdose contains approximately one-sixth the amount of anti-D contained in the full dose.

◆ RATED THERAPEUTICALLY EQUIVALENT; ◇ THERAPEUTIC EQUIVALENCE UNCONFIRMED; ○ UNRATED

CLINICAL PHARMACOLOGY

Human immune globulins prepared by cold alcohol fractionation have not been reported to transmit hepatitis or other infectious diseases.

Globulin, Immune $Rh_o(D)$ acts by suppressing the immune response of Rh negative individuals to Rh positive red blood cells. The obstetrical patient may be exposed to red blood cells from her Rh positive fetus during the normal course of pregnancy. The risk of immunization is related to the number of Rh positive red cells received. The risk was found to be 3% when 0.1 mL of fetal red blood cells is present in the mother and 65% when 5 mL is present. In the first 12 weeks of gestation the total volume of red blood cells in the fetus is estimated at less than 2.5 mL.

Clinical studies demonstrated that administration of Globulin, Immune $Rh_o(D)$, microdose, within three (3) hours following abortion was 100% effective in preventing Rh immunization. Studies in male volunteers showed Globulin, Immune $Rh_o(D)$, microdose, to be effective when given as long as 72 hours after the infusion of Rh positive red cells. A lesser degree of protection is afforded if the antibody is administered beyond this time period.

Clinical studies proved that the incidence of Rh immunization as a result of pregnancy was reduced to 1% to 2% from 12% to 13% when Globulin, Immune $Rh_o(D)$, full dose, was given within 72 hours following delivery. Further studies in which patients received Rh immune globulin, antepartum at 28 to 32 weeks and postpartum, reduced the risk of immunization to less than 0.1%.

An Rh negative individual transfused with one unit of Rh positive red blood cells has about an 80% likelihood of producing anti-$Rh_o(D)$. Protection from Rh immunization is accomplished by administering the appropriate dose of Globulin, Immune $Rh_o(D)$, full dose.

INDICATIONS AND USAGE

Globulin, Immune $Rh_o(D)$, microdose, is indicated for an Rh negative woman following spontaneous or induced abortion or termination of ectopic pregnancy up to and including 12 weeks' gestation, unless the father is conclusively shown to be Rh negative.

Globulin, Immune $Rh_o(D)$, full dose, is indicated whenever it is known or suspected that fetal red cells have entered the circulation of an Rh negative mother unless the fetus or the father can be shown conclusively to be Rh negative.

TRANSFUSION

Globulin, Immune $Rh_o(D)$, full dose is indicated for any Rh negative female of childbearing age who receives any Rh positive red blood cells or component such as platelets or granulocytes prepared from Rh positive blood.

CONTRAINDICATIONS

Globulin, Immune $Rh_o(D)$, microdose, must not be used for genetic amniocentesis at 15 to 18 weeks' gestation or antepartum prophylaxis at 28 weeks' gestation. Globulin, Immune $Rh_o(D)$, full dose, is recommended for any indication beyond 12 weeks' gestation.

Individuals known to have had an anaphylactic or severe systemic reaction to human globulin should not receive Globulin, Immune $Rh_o(D)$.

WARNINGS

Do not inject infants.
Do not inject intravenously.

PRECAUTIONS

The presence of passively acquired anti-$Rh_o(D)$ in the maternal serum may cause a positive antibody screening test. This does not preclude further antepartum or postpartum prophylaxis.

Some babies born of women given Globulin, Immune $Rh_o(D)$ antepartum have weakly positive direct antiglobulin tests at birth.

Late in pregnancy or following delivery there may be sufficient fetal red blood cells in the maternal circulation to cause a positive result if one tests for the $Rh_o(D)$ variant known as D^u. When there is any doubt as to the patient's Rh type, Globulin, Immune $Rh_o(D)$ should be administered.

Pregnancy Category C: Animal reproduction studies have not been conducted with Globulin, Immune $Rh_o(D)$. It is also not known whether Globulin, Immune $Rh_o(D)$, can cause fetal harm when administered to a pregnant woman or can affect reproduction capacity. Globulin, Immune $Rh_o(D)$ should be given to a pregnant woman only if clearly needed. However, use of Rh antibody during the third trimester in full doses of antibody has been reported to produce no evidence of hemolysis in the infant.

ADVERSE REACTIONS

Systemic reactions associated with administration of Globulin, Immune $Rh_o(D)$, are extremely rare. Discomfort at the site of injection has been reported and a small number of women have noted a slight elevation in temperature.

About one-quarter of a group of 22 individuals who were given multiple doses of Globulin, Immune $Rh_o(D)$, full dose, to treat mismatched transfusions noted fever, myalgia and lethargy. Bilirubin levels of 0.4 to 6.8 mg/dL were observed in some of the treated individuals and one had splenomegaly.

DOSAGE AND ADMINISTRATION

Parenteral drug products should be inspected visually for particulate matter and discoloration prior to administration, whenever solution and container permit.

A single dose (approximately 50 µg)† of Globulin, Immune $Rh_o(D)$, microdose, will completely suppress the immune response to 2.5 ml of Rh positive red blood cells (packed cells, not whole blood).

Administer a single dose of Globulin, Immune $Rh_o(D)$, microdose, intramuscularly as soon as possible after termination of a pregnancy up to and including 12 weeks' gestation.

A single dose (approximately 300 µg)† of Globulin, Immune $Rh_o(D)$, full dose, is the usual dose for the indications associated with pregnancy unless there is clinical or laboratory evidence of a fetal-maternal hemorrhage in excess of 15 ml of Rh positive red blood cells. The indications and recommended dosage for Globulin, Immune $Rh_o(D)$, full dose, are summarized in the following table.

INDICATIONS AND RECOMMENDED DOSAGE

Indication	Dose (approximately)
Threatened abortion at any stage of gestation with continuation of pregnancy	300 µg†
Abortion or termination of pregnancy at or beyond 13 weeks' gestation	300 µg
Genetic amniocentesis, chorionic villus sampling (CVS) and percutaneous umbilical blood sampling (PUBS)	300 µg
Abdominal trauma	300 µg
Antepartum prophylaxis at 26 to 28 weeks' gestation‡	300 µg
Postpartum (if newborn Rh positive)	300 µg

† *See footnote under Description*
‡ *If antepartum prophylaxis is indicated, it is essential that the mother receive a postpartum dose if the infant is Rh positive.*

If an adverse event requires the administration of Globulin, Immune $Rh_o(D)$, full dose, early in the pregnancy, there is an obligation to maintain a level of passively acquired anti-$Rh_o(D)$ by administration of Globulin, Immune $Rh_o(D)$, full dose, at 12-week intervals. Globulin, Immune $Rh_o(D)$, full dose, should be given within 72 hours after delivery if the baby is Rh positive. If delivery occurs within three weeks after the last antepartum dose, the postpartum dose may be withheld, but a test for fetal-maternal hemorrhage (FMH) should still be performed to determine a bleed greater than 15 mL of packed red blood cells.

Whenever there is a fetal-maternal hemorrhage in excess of 15 ml of Rh positive red blood cells, multiple doses of Globulin, Immune $Rh_o(D)$, full dose, are required. A fetal-maternal hemorrhage of this magnitude is unlikely prior to the last trimester of pregnancy. Patients who may need multiple doses of Globulin, Immune $Rh_o(D)$, full dose, can be identified by a fetal-maternal hemorrhage screening test. If the test is positive, the volume of the fetal-maternal hemorrhage should be determined by a quantitative method. A single dose of Globulin, Immune $Rh_o(D)$, full dose, should be administered for every 15 ml of fetal red blood cells. If the dose calculation results in a fraction administer the next number of whole syringes of Globulin, Immune $Rh_o(D)$, full dose.

Multiple doses of Globulin, Immune $Rh_o(D)$, full dose, are usual for indications associated with transfusion. For every 15 ml of Rh positive red blood cells transfused, the patient should receive a single dose of Globulin, Immune $Rh_o(D)$, full dose. If multiple doses are required, consult your pharmacy for pooling directions.

Administer Globulin, Immune $Rh_o(D)$, full dose, intramuscularly. Do not inject intravenously. Multiple doses may be administered at the same time or at spaced intervals, as long as the total dose is administered within three days of exposure.

Store at 2 to 8°C. DO NOT FREEZE.

J CODES
1 dose package IM—J2790

HOW SUPPLIED
INJECTION:

BRAND/MANUFACTURER	NDC	SIZE	AWP
○ **BRAND**			
MINI-GAMULIN RH: Armour	00053-7591-04	1 ml 6s	$86.80
GAMULIN RH: Armour	00053-7590-02	3 ml 6s	$351.68
MINI-GAMULIN RH: Armour	00053-7591-06	1 ml 10s	$168.00
GAMULIN RH: Armour	00053-7590-06	3 ml 10s	$546.14
MINI-GAMULIN RH: Armour	00053-7591-03	1 ml 25s	$370.00
GAMULIN RH: Armour	00053-7590-03	3 ml 25s	$1167.00

INJECTION: 50 U/GM

BRAND/MANUFACTURER	NDC	SIZE	AWP
○ **BRAND**			
HYPRHO-D MINI-DOSE: Miles Biol	00192-0621-05	0.17 ml 10s	$262.50

INJECTION: 50 MCG

BRAND/MANUFACTURER	NDC	SIZE	AWP
○ **BRAND**			
MICRHOGAM: Ortho Diagnostic	00562-8080-80	1 ea 5s	$140.00
	00562-8080-82	1 ea 25s	$650.00

INJECTION: 300 U/GM

BRAND/MANUFACTURER	NDC	SIZE	AWP
○ **BRAND**			
HYPRHO-D MINI-DOSE: Miles Biol	00192-0621-01	1 ml	$43.88
	00192-0621-10	1 ml 10s	$438.75
	00192-0621-22	1 ml 10s	$438.75

► SHOWN IN PRODUCT IDENTIFICATION GUIDE

INJECTION: 300 MCG

BRAND/MANUFACTURER	NDC	SIZE	AWP
○ **BRAND**			
RHOGAM: Ortho Diagnostic	00562-8070-20	1 ea 25s	$1125.00
	00562-8070-90	1 ea 100s	$4265.00

Glucagon

DESCRIPTION

Glucagon is extracted from beef and pork pancreas.

Chemically unrelated to insulin, Glucagon is a single-chain polypeptide containing 29 amino acid residues and having a molecular weight of 3,483.

The empirical formula is $C_{153}H_{225}N_{43}O_{49}S$.

Crystalline Glucagon is a white powder containing less than 0.05% zinc. It is relatively insoluble in water but is soluble at a pH of less than 3 or more than 9.5. Glucagon is stable in lyophilized form at room temperatures.

Glucagon for Injection, USP, contains Glucagon as the hydrochloride. The 1-mg vials contain 1 mg (1 unit) of Glucagon. The 10-mg vial contains 10 mg (10 units) of Glucagon. One USP unit of Glucagon is equivalent to 1 International Unit of Glucagon and also to about 1 mg of Glucagon.[1]

Following is its chemical structure:

His - Ser - Gln - Gly - Thr - Phe - Thr - Ser - Asp - Tyr - Ser - Lys - Tyr - Leu - Asp - Ser -
1   2   3   4   5   6   7   8   9   10   11   12   13   14   15   16

Arg - Arg - Ala - Gln - Asp - Phe - Val - Gln - Trp - Leu - Met - Asn - Thr
17   18   19   20   21   22   23   24   25   26   27   28   29

CLINICAL PHARMACOLOGY

Glucagon causes an increase in blood glucose concentration and is used in the treatment of hypoglycemia. It is effective in small doses, and no evidence of toxicity has been reported with its use. Glucagon acts only on liver glycogen, converting it to glucose.

Parenteral administration of Glucagon produces relaxation of the smooth muscle of the stomach, duodenum, small bowel, and colon.

The half-life of Glucagon in plasma is approximately 3 to 6 minutes, which is similar to that of insulin.

INDICATIONS AND USAGE

For the Treatment of Hypoglycemia: Glucagon is useful in counteracting severe hypoglycemic reactions.

The patient with type I diabetes does not have as great a response in blood glucose levels as does the type II stable patient. Therefore, supplementary carbohydrate should be given as soon as possible, especially to the child or adolescent patient.

For Use as a Diagnostic Aid: Glucagon is indicated as a diagnostic aid in the radiologic examination of the stomach, duodenum, small bowel, and colon when a hypotonic state would be advantageous.

Glucagon is as effective for this examination as are the anticholinergic drugs, but it has fewer side effects. When Glucagon is administered concomitantly with an anticholinergic agent, the response is not significantly greater than when either drug is used alone. However, the addition of the anticholinergic agent results in increased side effects.

UNLABELED USES

Glucagon is used alone or as adjunct in the treatment of biliary tract pain, endoscopy, and esophageal obstruction.

CONTRADICTIONS

Glucagon is contraindicated in patients with known hypersensitivity to it or in patients with pheochromocytoma.

WARNINGS

Glucagon should be administered cautiously to patients with a history suggestive of insulinoma and/or pheochromocytoma. In patients with insulinoma, intravenous administration of Glucagon will produce an initial increase in blood glucose; however, because of Glucagon's insulin-releasing effect, it may cause the insulinoma to release its insulin and subsequently cause hypoglycemia. A patient developing symptoms of hypoglycemia after a dose of Glucagon should be given glucose orally, intravenously, or by gavage, whichever is more appropriate.

Exogenous Glucagon also stimulates the release of catecholamines. In the presence of pheochromocytoma, Glucagon can cause the tumor to release catecholamines, which results in a sudden and marked increase in blood pressure. If a patient suddenly develops a marked increase in blood pressure, 5 to 10 mg of phentolamine mesylate may be administered intravenously in an attempt to control the blood pressure.

Generalized allergic reactions, including urticaria, respiratory distress, and hypotension, have been reported in patients who received Glucagon by injection.

PRECAUTIONS

General: Glucagon is helpful in hypoglycemia only if liver glycogen is available. Because Glucagon is of little or no help in states of starvation, adrenal insufficiency, or chronic hypoglycemia, glucose should be considered for the treatment of hypoglycemia.

Laboratory Test: Blood glucose determinations may be obtained to follow the patient in hypoglycemia shock until he or she is asymptomatic.

Carcinogenesis, Mutagenesis, Impairment of Fertility: Because Glucagon is usually given in a single dose and has a very short half-life (3 to 6 minutes), no studies have been done regarding carcinogenesis.

Reproduction studies have been performed in rats at doses up to 2 mg/kg b.i.d. (up 120 times the human dose) and have revealed no evidence of impaired fertility.

Usage in Pregnancy: Pregnancy Category B: Reproduction studies have been performed in rats at doses up to 2 mg/kg b.i.d. (up to 120 times the human dose), and have revealed no evidence of harm to the fetus due to Glucagon. There are, however, no adequate and well-controlled studies in pregnant women. Because animal reproduction studies are not always predictive of human response, this drug should be used during pregnancy only if clearly needed.

Nursing Mothers: It is not known whether this drug is excreted in human milk. Because many drugs are excreted in human milk, caution should be exercised when Glucagon is administered to a nursing woman. If the drug is excreted in human milk during its short half-life, it will be handled like any other polypeptide, i.e., it will be hydrolyzed and absorbed. Glucagon is not active when taken orally because it is destroyed in the gastrointestinal tract before it can be absorbed.

ADVERSE REACTIONS

Glucagon is relatively free of adverse reactions except for occasional nausea and vomiting, which may also occur with hypoglycemia. Generalized allergic reactions have been reported (see *"Warnings"*).

OVERDOSAGE

Signs and Symptoms: No cases of human overdosage of Glucagon have been reported. Glucagon is generally well tolerated. If overdosage occurred, it would not be expected to cause consequential toxicity but would be expected to be associated with nausea, vomiting, gastric hypotonicity, and diarrhea.

Intravenous administration of Glucagon has been shown to have a positive inotropic and chronotropic effect. A transient increment in both blood pressure and pulse rate may occur following the administration of Glucagon. Patients taking B-blockers might be expected to have a greater increment in both pulse and blood pressure. This increase will be transient because of Glucagon's short half-life. The increase in blood pressure and pulse rate may require therapy in patients with pheochromocytoma or coronary artery disease.

When Glucagon was given in large doses to cardiac patients, investigators reported a positive inotropic effect. These investigators administered Glucagon in doses of 0.5 to 16 mg/hour by continuous infusion for periods of 5 to 166 hours. Total doses ranged from 25 to 996 mg, and a 21-month child received approximately 8.25 mg in 165 hours. Side effects included nausea, vomiting, and decreasing serum potassium concentration. Serum potassium concentration could be maintained within normal limits with supplemental potassium.

The intravenous median lethal dose for Glucagon in mice is approximately 300 mg/kg.

Because Glucagon is a polypeptide, it would be rapidly destroyed in the gastrointestinal tract if it were to be accidentally ingested.

Treatment: To obtain up-to-date information about the treatment of overdose, a good resource is your certified Regional Poison Control Center. Telephone numbers of certified poison control centers are listed in the *Physicians' Desk Reference (PDR).* In managing overdosage, consider the possibility of multiple drug overdoses, interaction among drugs, and unusual drug kinetics in your patient.

In view of the extremely short half-life of Glucagon and its prompt destruction and excretion, the treatment of overdosage is symptomatic, primarily for nausea, vomiting, and possible hypokalemia.

If the patient develops a dramatic increase in blood pressure, 5 mg to 10 mg of phentolamine has been shown to be effective in lowering blood pressure for the short time that control would be needed.

Forced diuresis, peritoneal dialysis, hemodialysis, or charcoal hemoperfusion have not been established as beneficial for an overdose of Glucagon; it is extremely unlikely that one of these procedures would ever be indicated.

DOSAGE AND ADMINISTRATION

For the Treatment of Hypoglycemia: The diluent is provided for use only in the preparation of Glucagon for *intermittent* parenteral injection and for no other use.

If Glucagon is to be given at doses higher than 2 mg, it should be reconstituted with Sterile Water for Injection instead of the supplied diluting solution and used immediately.

Directions for Use of Glucagon: 1. Dissolve the lyophilized Glucagon in the accompanying diluent.

2. Glucagon should not be used at concentrations greater than 1 mg (1 unit/mL).

3. Glucagon solutions should not be used unless they are clear and of a water-like consistency.

4. For adults and for children weighing more than 20 kg, give 1 mg (1 unit) by subcutaneous, intramuscular, or intravenous injection.

5. For children weighing less than 20 kg, give 0.5 mg (0.5 unit) or a dose equivalent to 20-30 μg/kg.[2,3,4,5,6]

6. The patient will usually awaken within 15 minutes. If the response is delayed, there is no contraindication to the administration of 1 or 2 additional doses of Glucagon; however, in view of the deleterious effects of cerebral hypoglycemia and depending on the duration and depth of coma, the use of parenteral glucose *must* be considered by the physician.

◆ RATED THERAPEUTICALLY EQUIVALENT; ◇ THERAPEUTIC EQUIVALENCE UNCONFIRMED; ○ UNRATED

7. Intravenous glucose *must* be given if the patient fails to respond to Glucagon.

8. When the patient responds, give supplemental carbohydrate to restore the liver glycogen and prevent secondary hypoglycemia.

Instructions to the Family: Instructions describing the method of using this preparation are included in the literature that accompanies the patient's package. It is advisable for the patient and family members to become familiar with the technique of preparing Glucagon for Injection before an emergency arises. Patients are instructed to use 1 mg (1 unit) for adults and, if recommended by a doctor, 1/2 the adult dose (0.5 mg) [0.5 unit]) for children weighing less than 44 lb (20 kg).

General Management of Hypoglycemia: The following are helpful measures in the prevention of hypoglycemic reactions due to insulin:

1. Reasonable uniformity from day to day with regard to diet, insulin, and exercise.

2. Careful adjustment of the insulin program so that the type (or types) of insulin, dose, and time (or times) of administration are suited to the individual patient.

3. Frequent testing of the blood or urine so that a change in insulin requirements can be foreseen.

4. Routine carrying of sugar, candy, or other readily absorbable carbohydrate by the patient so that it may be taken at the first warning of an oncoming reaction.

If the patient is unaware of the symptoms of hypoglycemia, he/she may lapse into insulin shock; therefore, the physician should instruct the patient in this regard when feasible.

It is important that the patient be aroused as quickly as possible, because prolonged hypoglycemic reactions may result in cortical damage. Glucagon or intravenous glucose will awaken the patient sufficiently so that oral carbohydrates may be taken.

Caution—Although the patient may use Glucagon for the treatment of hypoglycemia during an emergency, the physician must still be notified when hypoglycemic reactions occur so that the dose of insulin may be adjusted if necessary.

For Use as a Diagnostic Aid: Dissolve the lyophilized Glucagon in the accompanying diluting solution.

Glucagon should not be used at concentration greater than 1 mg (1 unit/mL).

The following doses may be administered for relaxation of the stomach, duodenum, and small bowel, depending on the time of onset of action and the duration of effect required for the examination. Since the stomach is less sensitive to the effect of Glucagon, 0.5 mg (0.5 units) IV or 2 mg (2 units) IM are recommended.

Dose	Route of Administration	Time of Onset of Action	Approximate Duration of Effect
0.25-0.5 mg	IV	1 minute	9-17 minutes
1 mg	IM	8-10 minutes	12-27 minutes
2 mg*	IV	1 minute	22-25 minutes
2mg*	IM	4-7 minutes	21-32 minutes

* *Administration of 2-mg (2 units) doses produces a higher incidence of nausea and vomiting than do lower doses.*

For examination of the colon, it is recommended that a 2-mg (2 units) dose be administered intramuscularly approximately 10 minutes prior to initiation of the procedure. Relaxation of the colon and reduction of discomfort to the patient will allow the radiologist to perform a more satisfactory examination.

STABILITY AND STORAGE

Before Reconstitution: Vials of Glucagon as well as the Diluting Solution for Glucagon for Injection, USP, may be stored at controlled room temperature, 59° to 86°F (15° to 30°C).

After Reconstitution: Glucagon in 1-mL vials or Hyporets should be used immediately. Glucagon reconstituted with the Diluting Solution for Glucagon for Injection in multiple-dose vials may be stored at 41°F (5°C) for up to 48 hours if necessary. Glucagon reconstituted with Sterile Water for Injection should be used immediately.

1. *Drug Information for the Health Care Professional.* 11th ed. Rockville, Maryland: The United States Pharmacopeial Convention, Inc; 1991; IA: 1380. 2. Gibbs et al: Use of Glucagon to terminate insulin reactions in diabetic children. *Nebr Med J* 1958;43:56-57. 3. Cornblath M, et al: Studies of carbohydrate metabolism in the newborn: Effect of Glucagon on concentration of sugar in capillary blood of newborn infant. *Pediatrics* 1958;21:885-892. 4. Carson MJ, Koch R, Clinical studies with Glucagon in children. *J Pediatr* 1955;47:167-170 5. Shipp JC, et al: Treatment of insulin hypoglycemia in diabetic campers. *Diabetes* 1964;13:645-648. 6. Amos J, Wranne L: Hypoglycemia in childhood diabetes II: Effect of subcutaneous or intramuscular injection of different doses of Glucagon. *Acta Pediatr Scand* 1988;77:548-553.

HOW SUPPLIED
POWDER FOR INJECTION: 1 MG

BRAND/MANUFACTURER	NDC	SIZE	AWP
○ GENERICS			
Lilly	00002-1450-01	1s	$27.07
Allscrips	54569-2239-00	1s	$27.07
Lilly	00002-8030-01	1s	$34.55

POWDER FOR INJECTION: 10 MG

BRAND/MANUFACTURER	NDC	SIZE	AWP
○ GENERICS			
Lilly	00002-1451-01	1s	$257.20

Glucotrol *SEE* GLIPIZIDE

Glukor *SEE* GONADOTROPIN, CHORIONIC

Glyburide

DESCRIPTION
Glyburide is an oral blood-glucose-lowering drug of the sulfonylurea class. Glyburide is a white, crystalline compound available as tablets and as micronized (smaller particle size) tablets.

Regular Glyburide tablets contain: Glyburide 1.25, 2.5, or 5 mg.

Glyburide micronized tablets contain: Glyburide 1.5, 3, or 6 mg.

The chemical name for Glyburide is 1-[[p-[2-(5-chloro-o-anisamido)ethyl] phenyl]-sulfonyl]-3-cyclohexylurea and the molecular weight is 493.99.

Following is its chemical structure:

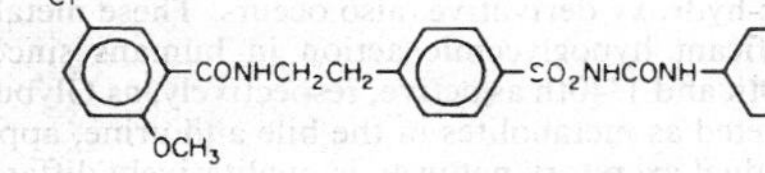

CLINICAL PHARMACOLOGY
ACTIONS
Glyburide appears to lower the blood glucose acutely by stimulating the release of insulin from the pancreas, an effect dependent upon functioning beta cells in the pancreatic islets. The mechanism by which Glyburide lowers blood glucose during long-term administration has not been clearly established. With chronic administration in Type II diabetic patients, the blood glucose lowering effect persists despite a gradual decline in the insulin secretory response to the drug. Extrapancreatic effects may be involved in the mechanism of action of oral sulfonylurea hypoglycemic drugs.

Some patients who are initially responsive to oral hypoglycemic drugs, including Glyburide, may become unresponsive or poorly responsive over time. Alternatively, Glyburide may be effective in some patients who have become unresponsive to one or more other sulfonylurea drugs.

In addition to its blood glucose lowering actions, Glyburide produces a mild diuresis by enhancement of renal free water clearance. Disulfiram-like reactions have very rarely been reported in patients treated with Glyburide.

PHARMACOKINETICS
Single dose studies with Glyburide tablets in normal subjects demonstrate significant absorption of Glyburide within one hour, peak drug levels at about four hours for regular Glyburide and two to three hours for Glyburide, micronized, and low but detectable levels at twenty-four hours.

Bioavailability studies have demonstrated that Glyburide micronized tablets 3 mg provide serum Glyburide concentrations that are not bioequivalent to those from Glyburide tablets 5 mg. Therefore, the patient should be retitrated.

In a single-dose bioavailability study in which subjects received Glyburide micronized tablets 3 mg and regular Glyburide tablets 5 mg with breakfast, the peak of the mean serum Glyburide concentration-time curve was 97.2 ng/mL for Glyburide micronized tablets 3 mg and 87.5 ng/mL for regular Glyburide tablets 5 mg. The mean of the individual maximum serum concentration values of Glyburide (Cmax) from Glyburide micronized tablets 3 mg was 106 ng/mL and that from regular Glyburide Tablets 5 mg was 104 ng/mL. The mean Glyburide area under the serum concentration-time curve (AUC) for this study was 568 ng x hr/mL for Glyburide micronized tablets 3 mg and 746 ng x hr/mL for regular Glyburide tablets 5 mg.

➤ SHOWN IN PRODUCT IDENTIFICATION GUIDE

Figure A

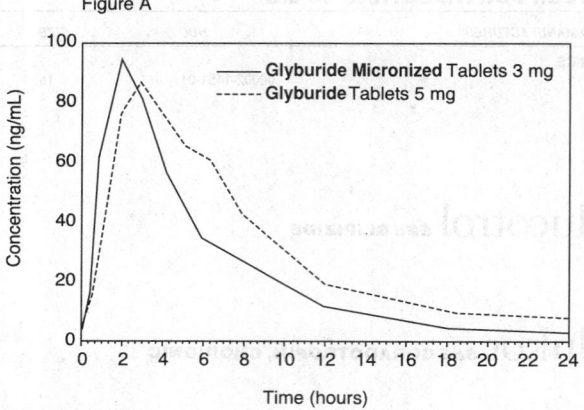

In a single-dose study, *in fasting healthy subjects,* two Glyburide micronized tablets 1.5 mg were shown to be bioequivalent to one Glyburide micronized tablet 3 mg. Mean serum levels of Glyburide, as reflected by areas under the serum concentration-time curve, increase in proportion to corresponding increases in dose. Multiple dose studies with Glyburide in diabetic patients demonstrate drug level concentration-time curves similar to single dose studies, indicating no buildup of drug in tissue depots. The decrease of Glyburide in the serum of normal healthy individuals is biphasic; the terminal half-life is about 10 hours. The serum concentration of Glyburide in normal subjects decreased with a half-life of about four hours. In single dose studies in fasting normal subjects, the degree and duration of blood glucose lowering is proportional to the dose administered and to the area under the drug level concentration-time curve. The blood glucose lowering effect persists for 24 hours following single morning doses in nonfasting diabetic patients. Under conditions of repeated administration in diabetic patients, however, there is no reliable correlation between blood drug levels and fasting blood glucose levels. A one year study of diabetic patients treated with Glyburide showed no reliable correlation between administered dose and serum drug level.

The major metabolite of Glyburide is the 4-trans-hydroxy derivative. A second metabolite, the 3-cis-hydroxy derivative, also occurs. These metabolites probably contribute no significant hypoglycemic action in humans since they are only weakly active (1/400th and 1/40th as active, respectively, as Glyburide) in rabbits.

Glyburide is excreted as metabolites in the bile and urine, approximately 50% by each route. This dual excretory pathway is qualitatively different from that of other sulfonylureas, which are excreted primarily in the urine.

Sulfonylurea drugs are extensively bound to serum proteins. Displacement from protein binding sites by other drugs may lead to enhanced hypoglycemic action. *In vitro,* the protein binding exhibited by Glyburide is predominantly nonionic, whereas that of other sulfonylureas (chlorpropamide, tolbutamide, tolazamide) is predominantly ionic. Acidic drugs such as phenylbutazone, warfarin, and salicylates displace the ionic-binding sulfonylureas from serum proteins to a far greater extent than the non-ionic binding Glyburide. It has not been shown that this difference in protein binding will result in fewer drug-drug interactions with Glyburide in clinical use.

INDICATIONS AND USAGE
Glyburide tablets are indicated as an adjunct to diet to lower the blood glucose in patients with noninsulin-dependent diabetes mellitus (type II) whose hyperglycemia cannot be satisfactorily controlled by diet alone. In initiating treatment for non insulin-dependent diabetes, diet should be emphasized as the primary form of treatment. Caloric restriction and weight loss are essential in the obese diabetic patient. Proper dietary management alone may be effective in controlling the blood glucose and symptoms of hyperglycemia. The importance of regular physical activity should also be stressed, and cardiovascular risk factors should be identified and corrective measures taken where possible. If this treatment program fails to reduce symptoms and/or blood glucose, the use of an oral sulfonylurea or insulin should be considered. Use of Glyburide must be viewed by both the physician and patient as a treatment in addition to diet and not as a substitution or as a convenient mechanism for avoiding dietary restraint. Furthermore, loss of blood glucose control on diet alone may be transient, thus requiring only short-term administration of Glyburide. During maintenance programs, Glyburide should be discontinued if satisfactory lowering of blood glucose is no longer achieved. Judgment should be based on regular clinical and laboratory evaluations. In considering the use of Glyburide in asymptomatic patients, it should be recognized that controlling blood glucose in non-insulin-dependent diabetes has not been definitely established to be effective in preventing the long-term cardiovascular or neural complications of diabetes.

CONTRAINDICATIONS
Glyburide tablets are contraindicated in patients with:

1. Known hypersensitivity or allergy to the drug.
2. Diabetic ketoacidosis, with or without coma. This condition should be treated with insulin.
3. Type I diabetes mellitus, as sole therapy.

Special Warning on Increased Risk of Cardiovascular Mortality: The administration of oral hypoglycemic drugs has been reported to be associated with increased cardiovascular mortality as compared to treatment with diet alone or diet plus insulin. This warning is based on the study conducted by the University Group Diabetes Program (UGDP), a long-term prospective clinical trial designed to evaluate the effectiveness of glucose-lowering drugs in preventing or delaying vascular complications in patients with non-insulin-dependent diabetes. The study involved 823 patients who were randomly assigned to one of four treatment groups (*Diabetes,* 19 (Suppl. 2):747-830, 1970.)

UGDP reported that patients treated for 5 to 8 years with diet plus a fixed dose of tolbutamide (1.5 grams per day) had a rate of cardiovascular mortality approximately 2 1/2 times that of patients treated with diet alone. A significant increase in total mortality was not observed, but the use of tolbutamide was discontinued based on the increase in cardiovascular mortality, thus limiting the opportunity for the study to show an increase in overall mortality. Despite controversy regarding the interpretation of these results, the findings of the UGDP study provide an adequate basis for this warning. The patient should be informed of the potential risks and advantages of Glyburide and of alternative modes of therapy.

Although only one drug in the sulfonylurea class (tolbutamide) was included in this study, it is prudent from a safety standpoint to consider that this warning may also apply to other oral hypoglycemic drugs in this class, in view of their close similarities in mode of action and chemical structure.

PRECAUTIONS
GENERAL
Bioavailability studies have demonstrated that Glyburide micronized tablets 3 mg provide serum Glyburide concentrations that are not bioequivalent to those from regular Glyburide tablets 5 mg. Therefore, patients should be retitrated when transferred from regular Glyburide or other oral hypoglycemic agents to Glyburide micronized.

Hypoglycemia: All sulfonylureas are capable of producing severe hypoglycemia. Proper patient selection and dosage and instructions are important to avoid hypoglycemic episodes. Renal or hepatic insufficiency may cause elevated drug levels of Glyburide and the latter may also diminish gluconeogenic capacity, both of which increase the risk of serious hypoglycemic reactions. Elderly, debilitated or malnourshed patients, and those with adrenal or pituitary insufficiency, are particularly susceptible to the hypoglycemic action of glucose-lowering drugs. Hypoglycemia may be difficult to recognize in the elderly and in people who are talking beta-adrenergic blocking drugs. Hypoglycemia is more likely to occur when caloric intake is deficient, after severe or prolonged exercise, when alcohol is ingested, or when more than one glucose lowering drug is used.

Loss of Control of Blood Glucose: When a patient stabilized on any diabetic regimen is exposed to stress such as fever, trauma, infection or surgery, a loss of control may occur. At such times it may be necessary to discontinue Glyburide and administer insulin.

The effectiveness of any hypoglycemic drug, including Glyburide, in lowering blood glucose to a desired level decreases in many patients over a period of time which may be due to progression of the severity of diabetes or to diminished responsiveness to the drug. This phenomenon is known as secondary failure, to distinguish it from primary failure in which the drug is ineffective in an individual patient when Glyburide is first given. Adequate adjustment of dose and adherence to diet should be assessed before classifying a patient as a secondary failure.

Information for Patients: Patients should be informed of the potential risks and advantages of Glyburide and of alternative modes of therapy. They also should be informed about the importance of adherence to dietary instructions, of a regular exercise program, and of regular testing of urine and/or blood glucose.

The risks of hypoglycemia, its symptoms and treatment, and conditions that predispose to its development should be explained to patients and responsible family members. Primary and secondary failure also should be explained.

LABORATORY TESTS
Therapeutic response to Glyburide tablets should be monitored by frequent urine glucose tests and periodic blood glucose tests. Measurement of glycosylated hemoglobin levels may be helpful in some patients.

DRUG INTERACTIONS
The hypoglycemic action of sulfonylureas may be potentiated by certain drugs including nonsteroidal anti-inflammatory agents and other drugs that are highly protein bound, salicylates, sulfonamides, chloramphenicol, probenecid, coumarins, monoamine oxidase inhibitors, and beta adrenergic blocking agents. When such drugs are administered to a patient receiving Glyburide, the patient should be observed closely for hypoglycemia. When such drugs are withdrawn from a patient receiving Glyburide the patient should be observed closely for loss of control.

Certain drugs tend to produce hyperglycemia and may lead to loss of control. These drugs include the thiazides and other diuretics, corticosteroids, phenothiazines, thyroid products, estrogens, oral contraceptives, phenytoin, nicotinic acid, sympathomimetics, calcium channel blocking drugs, and isoniazid. When such drugs are administered to a patient receiving Glyburide, the patient should be closely observed for loss of control. When such drugs are withdrawn from a patient receiving Glyburide, the patient should be observed closely for hypoglycemia.

A possible interaction between Glyburide and ciprofloxacin, a fluoroquinolone antibiotic, has been reported, resulting in a potentiation of the hypoglycemic action of Glyburide. The mechanism for this interaction is not known.

◆ RATED THERAPEUTICALLY EQUIVALENT; ◇ THERAPEUTIC EQUIVALENCE UNCONFIRMED; ○ UNRATED

A potential interaction between oral miconazole and oral hypoglycemic agents leading to severe hypoglycemia has been reported. Whether this interaction also occurs with the intravenous, topical or vaginal preparations of miconazole is not known.

CARCINOGENESIS, MUTAGENESIS, AND IMPAIRMENT OF FERTILITY
Studies in rats at doses up to 300 mg/kg/day for 18 months showed no carcinogenic effects. Glyburide is nonmutagenic when studied in the Salmonella microsome test (Ames test) and in the DNA damage/alkaline elution assay.

No drug-related effects were noted in any of the criteria evaluated in the two-year oncogenicity study of Glyburide in mice.

PREGNANCY
Teratogenic Effects: Pregnancy Category B Reproduction studies have been performed in rats and rabbits at doses up to 500 times the human dose and have revealed no evidence of impaired fertility or harm to the fetus due to Glyburide. There are, however, no adequate and well controlled studies in pregnant women. Because animal reproduction studies are not always predictive of human response, this drug should be used during pregnancy only if clearly needed.

Because recent information suggests that abnormal blood glucose levels during pregnancy are associated with a higher incidence of congenital abnormalities, many experts recommend that insulin be used during pregnancy to maintain blood glucose as close to normal as possible.

Nonteratogenic Effects: Prolonged severe hypoglycemia (4 to 10 days) has been reported in neonates born to mothers who were receiving a sulfonylurea drug at the time of delivery. This has been reported more frequently with the use of agents with prolonged half-lives. If Glyburide is used during pregnancy, it should be discontinued at least two weeks before the expected delivery date.

NURSING MOTHERS
Although it is not known whether Glyburide is excreted in human milk, some sulfonylurea drugs are known to be excreted in human milk. Because the potential for hypoglycemia in nursing infants may exist, a decision should be made whether to discontinue nursing or to discontinue the drug, taking into account the importance of the drug to the mother. If the drug is discontinued, and if diet alone is inadequate for controlling blood glucose, insulin therapy should be considered.

PEDIATRIC USE
Safety and effectiveness in children have not been established.

ADVERSE REACTIONS
Hypoglycemia: See "Precautions" and "Overdose" sections.

Gastrointestinal Reactions: Cholestatic jaundice and hepatitis may occur rarely: Glyburide Tablets should be discontinued if this occurs.

Liver function abnormalities, including isolated transaminase elevations, have been reported.

Gastrointestinal disturbances, e.g., nausea, epigastric fullness, and heartburn are the most common reactions, having occurred in 1.8% of treated patients during clinical trials. They tend to be dose related and may disappear when dosage is reduced.

Dermatologic Reactions: Allergic skin reactions, e.g., pruritus, erythema, urticaria, and morbilliform or maculopapular eruptions occurred in 1.5% of treated patients during clinical trials. These may be transient and may disappear despite continued use of Glyburide; if skin reactions persist, the drug should be discontinued.

Porphyria cutanea tarda and photosensitivity reactions have been reported with sulfonylureas.

Hematologic Reactions: Leukopenia, agranulocytosis, thrombocytopenia, hemolytic anemia, aplastic anemia, and pancytopenia have been reported with sulfonylureas.

Metabolic Reactions: Hepatic porphyria and disulfiram-like reactions have been reported with sulfonylureas; however, hepatic porphyria has not been reported with Glyburide and disulfiram-like reactions have been reported very rarely.

Cases of hyponatremia have been reported with Glyburide and all other sulfonylureas, most often in patients who are on other medications or have medical conditions known to cause hyponatremia or increase release of antidiuretic hormone. The syndrome of inappropriate antidiuretic hormone (SIADH) secretion has been reported with certain other sulfonylureas, and it has been suggested that these sulfonylureas may augment the peripheral (antidiuretic) action of ADH and/or increase release of ADH.

Other Reactions: Changes in accommodation and/or blurred vision have been reported with Glyburide and other sulfonylureas. These are thought to be related to fluctuation in glucose levels.

In addition to dermatologic reactions, allergic reactions such as angioedema, arthralgia, myalgia and vasculitis have been reported.

OVERDOSAGE
Overdosage of sulfonylureas, including Glyburide, can produce hypoglycemia. Mild hypoglycemic symptoms, without loss of consciousness or neurological findings, should be treated aggressively with oral glucose and adjustments in drug dosage and/or meal patterns. Close monitoring should continue until the physician is assured that the patient is out of danger. Severe hypoglycemic reactions with coma, seizure, or other neurological impairment occur infrequently, but constitute medical emergencies requiring immediate hospitalization. If hypoglycemic coma is diagnosed or suspected, the patient should be given a rapid intravenous injection of concentrated (50%) glucose solution. This should be followed by a continuous infusion of a more dilute (10%) glucose solution at a rate which will maintain the blood glucose at a level above 100 mg/dL. Patients should be closely monitored for a minimum of 24 to 48 hours, since hypoglycemia may recur after apparent clinical recovery.

DOSAGE AND ADMINISTRATION
Patients should be retitrated when transferred from regular Glyburide or other oral hypoglycemic agents to Glyburide micronized.

There is no fixed dosage regimen for the management of diabetes mellitus with Glyburide Tablets or any other hypoglycemic agent. In addition to the usual monitoring of urinary glucose, the patient's blood glucose must also be monitored periodically to determine the minimum effective dose for the patient; to detect primary failure, i.e., inadequate lowering of blood glucose at the maximum recommended dose of medication; and to detect secondary failure, i.e., loss of adequate blood glucose lowering response after an initial period of effectiveness. Glycosylated hemoglobin levels may also be of value in monitoring the patient's response to therapy.

Short-term administration of Glyburide may be sufficient during periods of transient loss of control in patients usually controlled well on diet.

USUAL STARTING DOSE
The usual starting dose of regular Glyburide tablets is 2.5 to 5 mg daily and of Glyburide micronized tablets 1.5 to 3 mg daily, administered with breakfast or the first main meal. Those patients who may be more sensitive to hypoglycemic drugs should be started at 1.25 mg regular Glyburide or 0.75 mg Glyburide micronized daily. (See "Precautions" section for patients at increased risk.) Failure to follow an appropriate dosage regimen may precipitate hypoglycemia. Patients who do not adhere to their prescribe dietary and drug regimen are more prone to exhibit unsatisfactory response to therapy.

TRANSFER FROM OTHER HYPOGLYCEMIC THERAPY PATIENTS RECEIVING OTHER ORAL ANTIDIABETIC THERAPY
Transfer of patients from other oral antidiabetic regimens to Glyburide should be done conservatively and the initial daily dose should be 2.5 to 5 mg of regular Glyburide and 1.5 to 3 mg of Glyburide micronized. When transferring patients from oral hypoglycemic agents other than chlorpropamide to Glyburide, no transition period and no initial or priming dose are necessary. When transferring patients from chlorpropamide, particular care should be exercised during the first two weeks because the prolonged retention of chlorpropamide in the body and subsequent overlapping drug effects may provoke hypoglycemia.

Patients Receiving Insulin: Some type II diabetic patients being treated with insulin may respond satisfactorily to Glyburide. If the insulin dose is less than 20 units daily, substitution of regular Glyburide tablets 2.5 to 5 mg or Glyburide micronized tablets 1.5 to 3 mg as a single daily dose may be tried. If the insulin dose is between 20 and 40 units daily, the patient may be placed directly on regular Glyburide tablets 5 mg or Glyburide micronized 3 mg daily as a single dose. If the insulin dose is more than 40 units daily, a transition period is required for conversion to Glyburide. In these patients, insulin dosage is decreased by 50% and regular Glyburide tablets 5 mg or Glyburide micronized tablets 3 mg daily is started.

TITRATION TO MAINTENANCE DOSE
The usual maintenance dose is in the range of 1.25 to 20 mg regular Glyburide or 0.75 to 12 mg Glyburide micronized daily, which may be given as a single dose or in divided doses (see "Dosage Interval" section). Dosage increases should be made in increments of no more than 2.5 mg regular Glyburide or 1.5 mg Glyburide micronized at weekly intervals based upon the patient's blood glucose response.

No exact dosage relationship exists between Glyburide and the other oral hypoglycemic agents. Although patients may be transferred from the maximum dose of other sulfonylureas, the maximum starting dose of 5 mg regular Glyburide or 3 mg Glyburide micronized should be observed. A maintenance dose of 5 mg of regular Glyburide tablets or 3 mg of Glyburide micronized tablets provides approximately the same degree of blood glucose control as 250 to 375 mg chlorpropamide, 250 to 375 mg tolazamide, 500 to 750 mg acetohexamide, or 1000 to 1500 mg tolbutamide.

When transferring patients receiving more than 40 units of insulin daily, they may be started on a daily dose of regular Glyburide tablets 5 mg or Glyburide micronized 3 mg concomitantly with a 50% reduction in insulin dose. Progressive withdrawal of insulin and increase of regular Glyburide in increments of insulin and increase of regular Glyburide in increments of 1.25 to 2.5 mg or of Glyburide micronized in increments of 0.75 to 1.5 mg every 2 to 10 days is then carried out. During this conversion period when both insulin and Glyburide are being used, hypoglycemia may rarely occur. During insulin withdrawal, patients should test their urine for glucose and acetone at least three times daily and report results to their physician. The appearance of persistent acetonuria with glycosuria indicates that the patient is a type I diabetic who requires insulin therapy.

EQUIVALENT DOSES

Glyburide	Glyburide, Micronized
1.25 mg	0.75 mg
2.5 mg	1.5 mg
5 mg	3 mg
10 mg	6 mg

* *Both dosage forms may be given in single or divided doses. Once a day therapy is usually satisfactory*

MAXIMUM DOSE

Daily doses of more than 20 mg of regular Glyburide or 12mg Glyburide micronized are not recommended.

DOSAGE INTERVAL

Once-a-day therapy is usually satisfactory. Some patients, particularly those receiving more than 10 mg of regular Glyburide or 6mg of Glyburide micronized daily, may have a more satisfactory response with twice-a-day dosage.

SPECIFIC PATIENT POPULATIONS

Glyburide is not recommended for use in pregnancy or for use in children.

In elderly patients, debilitated or malnourished patients, and patients with impaired renal or hepatic function, the initial and maintenance dosing should be conservative to avoid hypoglycemic reactions. (See "Precautions" section.)

Store at controlled room temperature, 15° to 30° C (59° to 86° F). Dispensed in well closed containers with safety closures. Keep container tightly closed.

HOW SUPPLIED

TABLETS: 1.25 MG

BRAND/MANUFACTURER	NDC	SIZE	AWP
◇ BRAND			
DIABETA: Hoechst	00039-0053-05	50s	$8.30
▶ MICRONASE: Upjohn	00009-0131-01	100s	$20.58
◇ GENERICS			
Allscrips	54569-3832-00	30s	$4.30
Rugby	00536-5641-06	50s	$7.20
Goldline	00182-1219-19	50s	$7.20

TABLETS: 1.5 MG

BRAND/MANUFACTURER	NDC	SIZE	AWP
○ BRAND			
▶ GLYNASE PRES-TAB: Upjohn	00009-0341-01	100s	$30.96
	00009-0341-02	100s ud	$30.96

TABLETS: 2.5 MG

BRAND/MANUFACTURER	NDC	SIZE	AWP
◇ BRAND			
▶ DIABETA: Hoechst	00039-0051-03	30s	$8.60
▶ MICRONASE: Upjohn	00009-0141-06	30s	$10.33
▶ DIABETA: Hoechst	00039-0051-06	60s	$16.75
▶ MICRONASE: Upjohn	00009-0141-07	60s	$20.58
▶ DIABETA: Hoechst	00039-0051-10	100s	$32.10
▶ MICRONASE: Upjohn	00009-0141-01	100s	$34.30
▶ DIABETA: Hoechst	00039-0051-11	100s ud	$32.10
▶ MICRONASE: Upjohn	00009-0141-02	100s ud	$34.30
▶ DIABETA: Hoechst	00039-0051-50	500s	$137.10
◇ GENERICS			
Allscrips	54569-3830-00	30s	$8.38
Rugby	00536-5642-01	100s	$27.77
Goldline	00182-1220-01	100s	$27.77
Aligen	00405-5361-01	100s	$28.40
Goldline	00182-1220-05	500s	$118.67
Aligen	00405-5361-02	500s	$130.32
Goldline	00182-1220-10	1000s	$235.00

TABLETS: 3 MG

BRAND/MANUFACTURER	NDC	SIZE	AWP
○ BRAND			
▶ GLYNASE PRES-TAB: Upjohn	00009-0352-01	100s	$52.33
	00009-0352-02	100s ud	$52.33
	00009-0352-03	500s	$229.44
	00009-0352-04	1000s	$443.61

TABLETS: 5 MG

BRAND/MANUFACTURER	NDC	SIZE	AWP
◇ BRAND			
▶ DIABETA: Hoechst	00039-0052-03	30s	$14.85
▶ MICRONASE: Upjohn	00009-0171-11	30s	$17.36
▶ DIABETA: Hoechst	00039-0052-06	60s	$29.35
▶ MICRONASE: Upjohn	00009-0171-12	60s	$34.78
	00009-0171-13	90s	$52.15
	00009-0171-05	100s	$57.96
▶ DIABETA: Hoechst	00039-0052-10	100s	$58.90
▶ MICRONASE: Upjohn	00009-0171-03	100s ud	$57.96
▶ DIABETA: Hoechst	00039-0052-11	100s ud	$58.90
	00039-0052-50	500s	$246.70
▶ MICRONASE: Upjohn	00009-0171-06	500s	$254.61
▶ DIABETA: Hoechst	00039-0052-70	1000s	$441.30
▶ MICRONASE: Upjohn	00009-0171-07	1000s	$492.78
◇ GENERICS			
Allscrips	54569-3831-00	30s	$15.28
Allscrips	54569-3831-02	60s	$30.56
Allscrips	54569-3831-01	100s	$50.93
Goldline	00182-1221-01	100s	$50.99
Rugby	00536-5643-01	100s	$51.17
Rugby	00536-5643-05	500s	$213.48

BRAND/MANUFACTURER	NDC	SIZE	AWP
Goldline	00182-1221-05	500s	$213.48
Goldline	00182-1221-10	1000s	$381.87
Aligen	00405-5362-03	1000s	$423.00

TABLETS: 6 MG

BRAND/MANUFACTURER	NDC	SIZE	AWP
○ BRAND			
GLYNASE PRES-TAB: Upjohn	00009-3449-01	100s	$78.49
	00009-3449-03	500s	$344.16

Glycerin

Glycerin Oral Osmotic Agent is a 50% v/v (0.628 g/mL) solution of Glycerin. It is administered orally, thereby avoiding the hazards of hypertonic agents that must be given intravenously.

DESCRIPTION

Active: Glycerin 50% v/v (0.628 g/mL).

Linear structure of Glycerin is: $CH_2OH \cdot CHOH \cdot CH_2OH$.

Chemical name: 1,2,3-Propanetriol.

Following is its chemical structure:

$$CH_2OH.CHOH.CH_2OH$$

CLINICAL PHARMACOLOGY

An oral osmotic agent for reducing intraocular pressure. It adds to the tonicity of the blood until metabolized and eliminated by the kidneys.

INDICATIONS AND USAGE

For the short term reduction of intraocular pressure. May be used prior to and after intraocular surgery. May be used to interrupt an acute attack of glaucoma. Glycerin suppositories are used in the treatment of constipation.

UNLABELED USES

Glycerin is used alone or as an adjunct in the treatment of cerebral edema when administered IV or PO. It is also used in nasal hemorrhage and Reye's syndrome, and in diagnosis of perilymphatic fistula. Glycerin injection is also used in the treatment of trigeminal neuralgia.

CONTRAINDICATIONS

Contraindicated in patients with well-established anuria; severe dehydration; frank or impending acute pulmonary edema; severe cardiac decompensation; and in those with hypersensitivity to any component of this preparation.

WARNINGS

For oral use only. Not for injection. Caution should be exercised in hypervolemia, confused mental states, and congestive heart disease; and in the dehydrated patient, e.g., certain diabetics.

PRECAUTIONS

When administered prior to surgery, ensure that the patient's bladder is emptied. Prolonged use may cause excess weight gain. Glycerin should be administered with caution to patients with cardiac, renal or hepatic diseases. Altered hydration may lead to pulmonary edema and/or congestive heart failure.

Pregnancy Category C: Animal reproduction studies have not been conducted with Glycerin. It is also not known whether Glycerin can cause fetal harm when administered to a pregnant woman or can affect reproduction capacity. This drug should be given to a pregnant woman only if clearly needed.

ADVERSE REACTIONS

Nausea, vomiting, headache, confusion, and disorientation may occur. Severe dehydration, cardiac arrhythmia, or hyperosmolar nonketotic coma which can result in death have been reported.

DOSAGE AND ADMINISTRATION

Usual dosage is 2 to 3 mL of Glycerin per kg of body weight (approximately 4 to 6 oz. per individual), given 1 to 1 1/2 hours prior to surgery.

Serving over cracked ice with a soda straw improves palatability.

Store at room temperature.

HOW SUPPLIED

SOLUTION: 50%

BRAND/MANUFACTURER	NDC	SIZE	AWP
○ BRAND			
OSMOGLYN: Alcon Surg	00065-0035-08	220 ml 12s	$203.40

Glycine

DESCRIPTION

Nonelectrolyte irrigating fluid for transurethral surgical procedures. For urologic irrigation only; not for injection by usual parenteral routes.

◆ RATED THERAPEUTICALLY EQUIVALENT; ◇ THERAPEUTIC EQUIVALENCE UNCONFIRMED; ○ UNRATED

1.5% Glycine is a sterile, nonpyrogenic, hypotonic, aqueous solution of Glycine intended only for urologic irrigation during transurethral surgical procedures.

Each 100 mL contains 1.5 g of Glycine in water for injection. The solution is nonelectrolytic, hypotonic, and has an osmolarity of 200 mOsmol/liter (calc.); pH 6.0 (4.5 to 6.5).

The solution contains no bacteriostat, antimicrobial agent or added buffer and is intended only for use as a single-dose irrigation. When smaller volumes are required, the unused portion should be discarded.

1.5% Glycine is a urologic nonelectrolyte irrigant.

Glycine is chemically designated aminoacetic acid ($C_2H_5NO_2$), a white crystalline powder freely soluble in water.

Water for Injection is chemically designated H_2O.

CLINICAL PHARMACOLOGY

Glycine is an amino acid and a nonelectrolyte. A solution of Glycine in water is therefore nonconductive and suitable for urologic irrigation during electrosurgical procedures. A 1.5% concentration of Glycine in water (200 mOsmol/liter calc.) is sufficient to minimize the risk of intravascular hemolysis which can occur from absorption of plain water through open prostatic veins during transurethral resection (TUR). It is hypotonic in relation to the extracellular fluid (280 mOsmol/liter). Any solution absorbed intravascularly during transurethral prostatic or bladder surgery, although variable in amount depending primarily on the extent of surgery, will be excreted by the kidney. Studies have shown that the absorption of Glycine does not cause significant hemolysis (increase of free hemoglobin) or release significant amounts of free ammonia in the blood. Glycine is rapidly degraded in the liver by Glycine oxidase.

Water is an essential constituent of all body tissues and accounts for approximately 70% of total body weight. Average normal adult daily requirement ranges from two to three liters (1.0 to 1.5 liters each for insensible water loss by perspiration and urine production).

Water balance is maintained by various regulatory mechanisms. Water distribution depends primarily on the concentration of electrolytes in the body compartments and sodium (Na+) plays a major role in maintaining physiologic equilibrium.

INDICATIONS AND USAGE

1.5% Glycine is indicated for use as irrigating fluid during transurethral prostatic resection and other transurethral surgical procedures.

CONTRAINDICATIONS

Not for injection by usual parenteral routes. Do not use in patients with anuria.

WARNINGS

For urologic irrigation only.

Solutions for urologic irrigation must be used with caution in patients with severe cardiopulmonary or renal dysfunction. Irrigating fluids used during transurethral prostatectomy have been demonstrated to enter the systemic circulation in relatively large volumes. Thus, Glycine irrigating solution must be regarded as a systemic drug. Absorption of large amounts of fluids containing Glycine may significantly alter cardiopulmonary and renal dynamics.

Do not heat container over 66°C (150°F).

PRECAUTIONS

Cardiovascular status, especially of the patient with cardiac disease, should be carefully observed before and during transurethral resection of the prostate when using Glycine irrigating solution, because the quantity of fluid absorbed into the systemic circulation by opened prostatic veins may produce significant expansion of the extracellular fluid and lead to fulminating congestive heart failure. Shift of sodium free intracellular fluid into the extracellular compartment following systemic absorption of solution may lower serum sodium concentration and aggravate pre-existing hyponatremia.

Care should be exercised if impaired liver function is known or suspected. Under such conditions, ammonia resulting from metabolism of Glycine may accumulate in the blood.

Aseptic technique is essential with the use of sterile solutions for irrigation. The administration set should be attached promptly. Unused portions should be discarded and a fresh container of appropriate size used for the start-up of each cycle or repeat procedure.

Do not administer unless solution is clear, seal is intact and container is undamaged. Discard unused portion.

ADVERSE REACTIONS

Adverse reactions may result from intravascular absorption of Glycine. Large intravenous doses of Glycine are known to cause salivation, nausea and light-headedness. Other consequences of absorption of urologic irrigating solutions include fluid and electrolyte disturbances such as acidosis, electrolyte loss, marked diuresis, urinary retention, edema, dryness of mouth, thirst, dehydration, coma from hyponatremia, secondary hyponatremia due to fluid overload, and hyperammonemia with resultant coma and/or encephalopathy; cardiovascular disorders such as hypotension, tachycardia, angina-like pains; pulmonary disorders such as pulmonary congestion; and other general reactions such as blurred vision, convulsions, nausea, vomiting, rhinitis, chills, vertigo, backache, transient blindness and urticaria. Allergic reactions from Glycine are unknown or exceedingly rare.

Should any adverse reaction occur, discontinue the irrigant, evaluate the patient, institute appropriate therapeutic countermeasures and save the remainder of the fluid for examination if deemed necessary.

OVERDOSAGE

In the event of overhydration or solute overload, re-evaluate the patient and institute appropriate corrective measures. (See *"Warnings," "Precautions"* and *"Adverse Reactions".*)

DOSAGE AND ADMINISTRATION

1.5% Glycine should be administered only by transurethral instillation with appropriate urologic instrumentation. A disposable irrigation set should be used. The total volume of solution used for irrigation is solely at the discretion of the surgeon.

Height of container(s) above the operating table in excess of 60 cm (approx. 2 ft.) has been reported to increase intravascular absorption of the irrigating fluid.

DRUG INTERACTIONS

Additives may be incompatible. Consult with pharmacist, if available. When introducing additives, use aseptic technique, mix thoroughly and do not store.

Parenteral drug products should be inspected visually for particulate matter and discoloration prior to administration, whenever solution container permits. (See *"Precautions".*)

Exposure of pharmaceutical products to heat should be minimized. Avoid excessive heat. Protect from freezing. It is recommended that the product be stored at room temperature (25°C); however, brief exposure up to 40°C does not adversely affect the product.

HOW SUPPLIED
SOLUTION: 1.5%

AVERAGE UNIT PRICE (AVAILABLE SIZES)			
GENERIC		$0.008	
BRAND/MANUFACTURER	*NDC*	*SIZE*	*AWP*
◆ **GENERICS**			
Baxter	00338-0289-08	3000 ml 4s	$39.16
McGaw	00264-2302-70	4000 ml 4s	$97.92
Baxter	00338-0291-04	1000 ml 6s	$101.16
McGaw	00264-2302-50	2000 ml 8s	$160.42
Baxter	00338-0288-05	1000 ml 12s	$57.00

Glycopyrrolate

DESCRIPTION

Glycopyrrolate is a quaternary ammonium compound with the following chemical name: 3-[(cyclopentylhydroxyphenylacetyl)oxy]-1,1-dimethylpyrrolidinium bromide.

Glycopyrrolate is available as a 1mg and 2mg tablet for oral administration and a 0.2 mg/1mL injection for intramuscular or intravenous administration.

Following is its chemical structure:

ACTIONS

Glycopyrrolate, like other anticholinergic (antimuscarinic) agents, inhibits the action of acetylcholine on structures innervated by postganglionic cholinergic nerves and on smooth muscles that respond to acetylcholine but lack cholinergic innervation. These peripheral cholinergic receptors are present in the autonomic effector cells of smooth muscle, cardiac muscle, the sino-atrial node, the atrioventricular node, exocrine glands, and, to a limited degree, in the autonomic ganglia. Thus, it diminishes the volume and free acidity of gastric secretions and controls excessive pharyngeal, tracheal, and bronchial secretions.

Glycopyrrolate antagonizes muscarinic symptoms (e.g., bronchorrhea, bronchospasm, bradycardia, and intestinal hypermotility) induced by cholinergic drugs such as the anticholinesterases.

The highly polar quaternary ammonium group of Glycopyrrolate limits its passage across lipid membranes, such as the blood-brain barrier, in contrast to atropine sulfate and scopolamine hydrobromide, which are non-polar tertiary amines which penetrate lipid barriers easily.

Peak effects occur approximately 30 to 45 minutes after intramuscular administration. The vagal blocking effects persist for 2 to 3 hours and the antisialagogue effects persist up to 7 hours, periods longer than for atropine. With intravenous injection, the onset of action is generally evident within one minute.

INDICATIONS

In Anesthesia: Glycopyrrolate Injectable is indicated for use as a preoperative antimuscarinic to reduce salivary, tracheobronchial, and pharyngeal secretions; to reduce the volume and free acidity of gastric secretions; and, to block cardiac vagal inhibitory reflexes during induction of anesthesia and intubation. When indicated Glycopyrrolate Injectable may be used intraoperatively to counteract drug-induced or vagal traction reflexes with the associated arrhythmias. Glycopyrrolate protects against the peripheral muscarinic effects (e.g., bradycardia and excessive secretions) of cholinergic agents such as neostigmine and pyridostigmine given to reverse the neuromuscular blockade due to non-depolarizing muscle relaxants.

In Peptic Ulcer: For use in adults as adjunctive therapy for the treatment of peptic ulcer when rapid anticholinergic effect is desired or when oral medication is not tolerated.

UNLABELED USES

Glycopyrrolate is used alone or as an adjunct in the treatment of bronchial asthma and Frey syndrome. It is also used for idiopathic hyperhidrosis and myasthenia gravis.

CONTRAINDICATIONS

Known hypersensitivity to Glycopyrrolate.

Due to its benzyl alcohol content, Glycopyrrolate Injectable should not be used in newborns (children less than 1 month of age).

Glaucoma: obstructive uropathy (for example, bladder neck obstruction due to prostatic hypertrophy); obstructive disease of the gastrointestinal tract (as in achalasia, pyloroduodenal stenosis, etc.); paralytic ileus; intestinal atony of the elderly or debilitated patient; unstable cardiovascular status in acute hemorrhage: severe ulcerative colitis: toxic megacolon complicating ulcerative colitis; myasthenia gravis. Glycopyrrolate is contraindicated in those patients with a hypersensitivity to Glycopyrrolate.

WARNINGS

This drug should be used with great caution, if at all, in patients with glaucoma or asthma.

In the presence of a high environmental temperature, heat prostration (fever and heat stroke due to decreased sweating) can occur with use of Glycopyrrolate.

Diarrhea may be an early symptom of incomplete intestinal obstruction, especially in patients with ileostomy or colostomy. In this instance treatment with this drug would be inappropriate and possibly harmful.

Glycopyrrolate may produce drowsiness or blurred vision. In this event, the patient should be warned not to engaged in activities requiring mental alertness such as operating a motor vehicle or other machinery, or performing hazardous work while taking this drug.

Theoretically, with overdosage, a curare-like action may occur, i.e., neuromuscular blockade leading to muscular weakness and possible paralysis.

Pregnancy: The safety of this drug during pregnancy has not been established. The use of any drug during pregnancy requires that the potential benefits of the drug be weighed against possible hazards to mother and child. Reproduction studies in rats revealed no teratogenic effects from Glycopyrrolate: however, the potent anticholinergic action of this agent resulted in diminished rates of conception and of survival at weaning, in a dose-related manner. Other studies in dogs suggest that this may be due to diminished seminal secretion which is evident at high doses of Glycopyrrolate. Information on possible adverse effects in the pregnant female is limited to uncontrolled data derived from marketing experience. Such experience has revealed no reports of teratogenic or other fetus-damaging potential. No controlled studies to establish the safety of the drug in pregnancy have been performed.

Nursing mothers: It is not known whether this drug is secreted in human milk. As a general rule, nursing should not be undertaken while a patient is on a drug since many drugs are excreted in human milk.

Pediatric Use: Since there is no adequate experience in children who have received this drug, safety and efficacy in children have not been established.

PRECAUTIONS

Use Glycopyrrolate with caution in the elderly and in all patients with:

- Autonomic neuropathy.
- Hepatic or renal disease.
- Ulcerative colitis—large doses may suppress intestinal motility to the point of producing a paralytic ileus and for this reason may precipitate or aggravate "toxic megacolon," a serious complication of the disease.
- Hyperthyroidism, coronary heart disease, congestive heart failure, cardiac tachyarrhythmias, tachycardia, hypertension and prostatic hypertrophy.
- Hiatal hernia associated with reflux esophagitis, since anticholinergic drugs may aggravate this condition.

Drug Interactions: The intravenous administration of any anticholinergic in the presence of cyclopropane anesthesia can result in ventricular arrhythmias; therefore, caution should be observed if Glycopyrrolate Injectable is used during cyclopropane anesthesia. If the drug is given in small incremental doses of 0.1 mg or less, the likelihood of producing ventricular arrhythmias is reduced.

Carcinogenesis, Mutagenesis, Impairment of Fertility: Long-term studies in animals have not been performed to evaluate carcinogenic potential. In the teratology studies, diminished rates of conception and of survival at weaning were observed in rats, in a dose-related manner. Studies in dogs suggest that this may be due to diminished seminal secretion which is evident at high doses of Glycopyrrolate.

Pregnancy Category B: Reproduction studies have been performed in rats and rabbits up to 1000 times the human dose and have revealed no teratogenic effects from Glycopyrrolate. There are, however, no adequate and well-controlled studies in pregnant women. Because animal reproduction studies are not always predictive of human response, this drug should be used during pregnancy only if clearly needed.

Nursing Mothers: It is not known whether this drug is excreted in human milk. Because many drugs are excreted in human milk, caution should be exercised when Glycopyrrolate is administered to a nursing woman.

Pediatric Use: Safety and effectiveness in children below the age of 12 years have not been established for the management of peptic ulcer.

ADVERSE REACTIONS

Anticholinergics produce certain effects, most of which are extensions of their fundamental pharmacological actions. Adverse reactions to anticholinergics in general may include xerostomia; decreased sweating; urinary hesitancy and retention; blurred vision; tachycardia; palpitations; dilatation of the pupil; cycloplegia; increased ocular tension; loss of taste; headaches; nervousness; mental confusion; drowsiness; weakness; dizziness; insomnia; nausea; vomiting; constipation; bloated feeling; impotence; suppression of lactation; severe allergic reaction or drug idiosyncrasies including anaphylaxis, urticaria and other dermal manifestations.

Glycopyrrolate is chemically a quaternary ammonium compound; hence, its passage across lipid membranes, such as the blood-brain barrier, is limited in contrast to atropine sulfate and scopolamine hydrobromide. For this reason the occurrence of CNS related side effects is lower, in comparison to their incidence following administration of anticholinergics which are chemically tertiary amines that can cross this barrier readily.

OVERDOSAGE

The symptoms of overdosage of Glycopyrrolate are peripheral in nature rather than central.

To guard against further oral absorption of the drug—use gastric lavage, cathartics and/or enemas.

To combat peripheral anticholinergic effects, a quaternary ammonium anticholinesterase such as neostigmine methylsulfate (which does not cross the blood-brain barrier) may be given intravenously in increments of 0.25 mg in adults. This dosage may be repeated every five to ten minutes until anticholinergic overactivity is reversed or up to a maximum of 2.5 mg. Proportionately smaller doses should be used in children. Indication for repetitive doses of neostigmine should be based on close monitoring of the decrease in heart rate and the return of bowel sounds.

In the unlikely event that CNS symptoms (excitement, restlessness, convulsions, psychotic behavior) occur, physostigmine (which does cross the blood-brain barrier) should be used. Physostigmine 0.5 to 2 mg should be slowly administered intravenously and repeated as necessary up to a total of 5 mg in adults. Proportionately smaller doses should be used in children.

Fever should be treated symptomatically. In the event of a curare-like effect on respiratory muscles, artificial respiration should be instituted and maintained until effective respiratory action returns.

DOSAGE AND AMINISTRATION

TABLETS

The dosage of Glycopyrrolate oral should be adjusted to the needs of the individual patient to assure symptomatic control with a minimum of adverse reactions. The presently recommended maximum daily dosage of Glycopyrrolate is 8 mg.

Glycopyrrolate, 1 mg tablets. The recommended initial dosage of Glycopyrrolate for adults is one tablet three times daily (in the morning, early afternoon, and at bedtime). Some patients may require two tablets at bedtime to assure overnight control of symptoms. For maintenance, a dosage of one tablet twice a day is frequently adequate.

Glycopyrrolate, 2 mg tablets. The recommended dosage of Glycopyrrolate for adults is one tablet two or three times daily at equally spaced intervals.

Glycopyrrolate tablets are not recommended for use in children under the age of 12 years.

INJECTABLE

Glycopyrrolate Injectable may be administered intramuscularly, or intravenously, without dilution, in the following indications:

Adults:

Preanesthetic Medication: The recommended dose of Glycopyrrolate Injectable is 0.002 mg (0.01 mL) per pound of body weight by intramuscular injection, given 30 to 60 minutes prior to the anticipated time of induction of anesthesia or at the time the preanesthetic narcotic and/or sedative are administered.

Intraoperative Medication: Glycopyrrolate Injectable may be used during surgery to counteract drug induced or vagal traction reflexes with the associated arrhythmias (e.g., bradycardia). It should be administered intravenously as single doses of 0.1 mg (0.5 mL) and repeated, as needed, at intervals of 2-3 minutes. The usual attempts should be made to determine the etiology of the arrhythmia, and the surgical or anesthetic manipulations necessary to correct parasympathetic imbalance should be performed.

Reversal of Neuromuscular Blockade: The recommended dose of Glycopyrrolate Injectable is 0.2 mg (1.0 mL) for each 1.0 mg of neostigmine or 5.0 mg of pyridostigmine. In order to minimize the appearance of cardiac side effects, the drugs may be administered simultaneously by intravenous injection and may be mixed in the same syringe.

Children: (Read "Contraindications".)

Preanesthetic Medication: The recommended dose of Glycopyrrolate Injectable in children 1 month to 12 years of age is 0.002 mg (0.01 mL) per pound of body weight intramuscularly, given 30 to 60 minutes prior to the anticipated time of induction of anesthesia or at the time the preanesthetic narcotic and/or sedative are administered.

Children 1 month to 2 years of age may require up to 0.004 mg (0.02 mL) per pound of body weight.

Intraoperative Medication: Because of the long duration of action of Glycopyrrolate if used as preanesthetic medication, additional Glycopyrrolate Injectable for anticholinergic effect intraoperatively is rarely needed; in the event it is required the recommended pediatric dose is 0.002 mg (0.01 mL) per pound of body weight intravenously, not to exceed 0.1 mg (0.5 mL) in a single dose which may be repeated, as needed, at intervals of 2-3 minutes. The usual attempts should be made to determine the etiology of the arrhythmia, and the surgical or anesthetic manipulations necessary to correct parasympathetic imbalance should be performed.

Reversal of Neuromuscular Blockade: The recommended pediatric dose of Glycopyrrolate Injectable is 0.2 mg (1.0 mL) for each 1.0 mg of neostigmine or 5.0 mg of pyridostigmine. In order to minimize the appearance of cardiac side effects, the drugs may be administered simultaneously by intravenous injection and may be mixed in the same syringe.

Adults:

Peptic Ulcer: The usual recommended dose of Glycopyrrolate Injectable is 0.1 mg (0.5 mL) administered at 4-hour intervals, 3 or 4 times daily intravenously or intramuscularly. Where more profound effect is required, 0.2 mg (1.0 mL) may be given. Some patients may need only a single dose, and frequency of administration should be dictated by patient response up to a maximum of four times daily.

Glycopyrrolate Injectable is not recommended for peptic ulcers in children under 12 years of age. (See *"Precautions"*.)

NOTE: Parenteral drug products should be inspected visually for particulate matter and discoloration prior to administration whenever solution and container permit.

Admixture Compatibilities: Glycopyrrolate Injectable is compatible for mixing and injection with the following injectable dosage forms: 5% and 10% glucose in water or saline; atropine sulfate, USP; physostigmine salicylate; diphenhydramine HCl; codeine phosphate, USP; benzquinamide HCl; hydromorphone HCl, USP; droperidol; droperidol and fentanyl citrate; propiomazine HCl; levorphanol tartrate lidocaine, USP; meperidine and promethazine HCls; meperidine HCl, USP; pyridostigmine bromide; morphine sulfate, USP; alphaprodine HCl; nalbuphine HCl; oxymorphone HCl; opium alkaloids HCls; procaine HCl, USP; promethazine HCl, USP; neostigmine methylsulfate, USP; scopolamine HBr, USP; promazine HCl; butorphanol tartrate; fentanyl citrate); pentazocine lactate; trimethobenzamide HCl; triflupromazine HCl; and hydroxyzine HCl. Glycopyrrolate Injectable may be administered via the tubing of a running infusion of physiological saline or lactated Ringer's solution.

Since the stability of Glycopyrrolate is questionable above a pH of 6.0, do *not* combine Glycopyrrolate Injectable in the same syringe with methohexital Na; chloramphenicol Na succinate; dimenhydrinate; pentobarbital Na; thiopental Na; secobarbital Na; sodium bicarbonate; diazepam. A gas will evolve or a precipitate may form. Mixing with dexamethasone Na phosphate or buffered solution of lactated Ringer's solution will result in a pH higher than 6.0. Mixing chlorpromazine HCl, USP, or prochlorperazine with other agents in a syringe is not recommended by the manufacturer, although the mixture with Glycopyrrolate Injectable is physically compatible.

DRUG INTERACTIONS
There are no known drug interactions.

HOW SUPPLIED
INJECTION: 0.2 MG/ML

AVERAGE UNIT PRICE (AVAILABLE SIZES)		GENERIC A-RATED AVERAGE PRICE (GAAP)	
BRAND	$0.49	1 ml 25s	$19.90
GENERIC	$0.58	5 ml 25s	$64.22

BRAND/MANUFACTURER	NDC	SIZE	AWP
◆ BRAND			
ROBINUL: Robins Pharm	00031-7890-93	5 ml	$2.86
	00031-7890-83	20 ml	$4.59
	00031-7890-11	1 ml 25s	$14.69
	00031-7890-95	2 ml 25s	$26.66
	00031-7890-06	5 ml 25s	$65.00
◆ GENERICS			
Gensia	00703-2635-01	20 ml	$3.00
Gensia	00703-2601-04	1 ml 25s	$15.63
Gensia	00703-2612-04	1 ml 25s	$21.88
Amer Regent	00517-4601-25	1 ml 25s	$22.19
Amer Regent	00517-4602-25	2 ml 25s	$35.94
Gensia	00703-2623-04	5 ml 25s	$50.00
Amer Regent	00517-4605-25	5 ml 25s	$78.44
Amer Regent	00517-4620-25	20 ml 25s	$155.94

TABLETS: 1 MG

BRAND/MANUFACTURER	NDC	SIZE	AWP
◆ BRAND			
ROBINUL: Robins Pharm	00031-7824-63	100s	$16.50

TABLETS: 2 MG

BRAND/MANUFACTURER	NDC	SIZE	AWP
◆ BRAND			
ROBINUL FORTE: Robins Pharm	00031-7840-63	100s	$26.28

Glynase Pres-Tab *SEE* GLYBURIDE

Gold Sodium Thiomalate

PHYSICIANS PLANNING TO USE GOLD SODIUM THIOMALATE SHOULD THOROUGHLY FAMILIARIZE THEMSELVES WITH ITS TOXICITY AND ITS BENEFITS. THE POSSIBILITY OF TOXIC REACTIONS SHOULD ALWAYS BE EXPLAINED TO THE PATIENT BEFORE STARTING THERAPY. PATIENTS SHOULD BE WARNED TO REPORT PROMPTLY ANY SYMPTOMS SUGGESTING TOXICITY. BEFORE EACH INJECTION OF GOLD SODIUM THIOMALATE, THE PHYSICIAN SHOULD REVIEW THE RESULTS OF LABORATORY WORK, AND SEE THE PATIENT TO DETERMINE THE PRESENCE OR ABSENCE OF ADVERSE REACTIONS SINCE SOME OF THESE CAN BE SEVERE OR EVEN FATAL.

DESCRIPTION
Gold Sodium Thiomalate is a sterile aqueous solution. The pH of the product is 5.8-6.5.

Gold Sodium Thiomalate is a mixture of the mono- and disodium salts of gold thiomalic acid.

Chemically, Gold Sodium Thiomalate is mercaptobutanedioic acid, monogold (1-) sodium salt.

The molecular weight for $C_4H_3AuNa_2O_4S$ (the disodium salt) is 390.07 and for $C_4H_4AuNaO_4S$ (the monosodium salt) is 368.09.

Gold Sodium Thiomalate is supplied as a solution for intramuscular injection containing 25 mg or 50 mg of Gold Sodium Thiomalate per mL.

Following is its chemical structure:

$$\begin{array}{c} CH_2COO^- \\ | \\ Au-S-CHCOO^- \end{array} \cdot \ xNa^+ \cdot (2-x)H^+$$

CLINICAL PHARMACOLOGY
The mode of action of Gold Sodium Thiomalate is unknown. The predominant action appears to be a suppressive effect on the synovitis of active rheumatoid disease.

INDICATIONS AND USAGE
Gold Sodium Thiomalate is indicated in the treatment of selected cases of active rheumatoid arthritis—both adult and juvenile type. The greatest benefit occurs in the early active stage. In late stages of the illness when cartilage and bone damage have occurred, gold can only check the progression of rheumatoid arthritis and prevent further structural damage to joints. It cannot repair damage caused by previously active disease.

Gold Sodium Thiomalate should be used only as *one part* of a complete program of therapy; alone it is not a complete treatment.

UNLABELED USES
If Gold Sodium Thiomalate is used alone or as an adjunct in the treatment of psoriatic Arthritis, Bronchial Asthma, Felty's Syndrome, and Pemphigus.

CONTRAINDICATIONS
Hypersensitivity to any component of this product.
Severe toxicity resulting from previous exposure to gold or other heavy metals.
Severe debilitation.
Systemic lupus erythematosus.

WARNINGS
Before treatment is started, the patient's hemoglobin, erythrocyte, white blood cell, differential and platelet counts should be determined, and urinalysis should be done to serve as basic reference. Urine should be analyzed for protein and sediment changes prior to each injection. Complete blood counts including platelet estimation should be made before every second injection throughout treatment. The occurrence of purpura or ecchymoses at any time always requires a platelet count.

Danger signals of possible gold toxicity include: rapid reduction of hemoglobin, leukopenia below 4000 WBC/mm^3, eosinophilia above 5 percent, platelet decrease below 100,000/mm^3, albuminuria, hematuria, pruritus, skin eruption, stomatitis, or persistent diarrhea. No additional injections of Gold Sodium Thiomalate should be given unless further studies show these abnormalities to be caused by conditions other than gold toxicity.

PRECAUTIONS
GENERAL
Gold salts should not be used concomitantly with penicillamine.
The safety of coadministration with cytotoxic drugs has not been established.

➤ SHOWN IN PRODUCT IDENTIFICATION GUIDE

Caution is indicated in the use of Gold Sodium Thiomalate in patients with the following:

1. a history of blood dyscrasias such as granulocytopenia or anemia caused by drug sensitivity,
2. allergy or hypersensitivity to medications,
3. skin rash,
4. previous kidney or liver disease,
5. marked hypertension,
6. compromised cerebral or cardiovascular circulation.

Diabetes mellitus or congestive heart failure should be under control before gold therapy is instituted.

CARCINOGENICITY

Renal adenomas have been reported in long-term toxicity studies of rats receiving Gold Sodium Thiomalate at high dose levels (2 mg/kg weekly for 45 weeks, followed by 6 mg/kg daily for 47 weeks), approximately 2 to 42 times the usual human dose. These adenomas are histologically similar to those produced in rats by chronic administration of experimental gold compounds and other heavy metals, such as lead. No reports have been received of renal adenomas in man in association with the use of Gold Sodium Thiomalate.

PREGNANCY

PREGNANCY CATEGORY C

Gold Sodium Thiomalate has been shown to be teratogenic during the organogenetic period in rats and rabbits when given in doses, respectively, of 140 and 175 times the usual human dose. Hydrocephaly and microphthalmia were the malformations observed in rats when Gold Sodium Thiomalate was administered subcutaneously at a dose of 25 mg/kg/day from day 6 through day 15 of gestation. In rabbits, limb malformations and gastroschisis were the malformations observed when Gold Sodium Thiomalate was administered subcutaneously at doses of 20-45 mg/kg/day from day 6 through day 18 of gestation. There are no adequate and well-controlled studies in pregnant women. Gold Sodium Thiomalate should be used during pregnancy only if the potential benefit to the mother justifies the potential risk of the fetus.

NURSING MOTHERS

The presence of gold has been demonstrated in the milk of lactating mothers. In addition, gold has been found in the serum and red blood cells of a nursing infant. In view of the above findings and because of the potential for serious adverse reactions in nursing infants from Gold Sodium Thiomalate a decision should be made whether to discontinue nursing or to discontinue the drug, taking into account the importance of the drug to the mother. The slow excretion and persistence of gold in the mother, even after therapy is discontinued, must also be kept in mind.

ADVERSE REACTIONS

A variety of adverse reactions may develop during the initial phase (weekly injections) of therapy or during maintenance treatment. Adverse reactions are observed most frequently when the cumulative dose of Gold Sodium Thiomalate administered is between 400 and 800 mg. Very uncommonly, complications occur days to months after cessation of treatment.

Cutaneous Reactions: Dermatitis is the most common reaction. *Any eruption, especially if pruritic, that develops during treatment with* Gold Sodium Thiomalate *should be considered a reaction to gold until proven otherwise.* Pruritus often exists before dermatitis becomes apparent, and therefore should be considered a warning signal of impending cutaneous reaction. The most serious form of cutaneous reaction is generalized exfoliative dermatitis which may lead to alopecia and shedding of nails. Gold dermatitis may be aggravated by exposure to sunlight or an actinic rash may develop.

Mucous Membrane Reactions: Stomatitis is the second most common adverse reaction. Shallow ulcers on the buccal membranes, on the borders of the tongue, and on the palate or in the pharynx may occur as the only adverse reaction, or along with dermatitis. Sometimes diffuse glossitis or gingivitis develops. A metallic taste may precede these oral mucous membrane reactions and should be considered a warning signal.

Conjunctivitis is a rare reaction.

Renal Reactions: Gold may be toxic to the kidney and produce a nephrotic syndrome or glomerulitis with hematuria. These renal reactions are usually relatively mild and subside completely if recognized early and treatment is discontinued. They may become severe and chronic if treatment is continued after onset of the reaction. Therefore, it is important to perform a *urinalysis before every injection,* and to discontinue treatment promptly if proteinuria or hematuria develops.

Hematologic Reactions: Blood dyscrasia due to gold toxicity is rare, but because of the potential serious consequences it must be constantly watched for and recognized early by frequent blood examinations done throughout treatment. Granulocytopenia; thrombocytopenia, with or without purpura; hypoplastic and aplastic anemia; and eosinophilia have all been reported. These hematologic disorders may occur separately or in combinations.

Nitritoid and Allergic Reactions: Reactions of the "nitritoid type" which may resemble anaphylactoid effects have been reported. Flushing, fainting, dizziness and sweating are most frequently reported. Other symptoms that may occur include: nausea, vomiting, malaise, headache, and weakness. More severe, but less common effects include: anaphylactic shock, syncope, bradycardia, thickening of the tongue, difficulty in swallowing and breathing, and angioneurotic edema. These effects may occur almost immediately after injection or as late as 10 minutes following injection. They may occur at any time during the course of therapy and if observed, treatment with Gold Sodium Thiomalate should be discontinued.

Miscellaneous Reactions: Gastrointestinal reactions have been reported, including nausea, vomiting, anorexia, abdominal cramps and diarrhea. Ulcerative enterocolitis, which can be severe or even fatal, has been reported rarely.

There have been rare reports of reactions involving the eye such as iritis, corneal ulcers, and gold deposits in ocular tissues. Peripheral and central nervous system complications have been reported rarely. Peripheral neuropathy, with or without fasciculations, sensorimotor effects (including Guillain-Barré syndrome) and elevated spinal fluid protein have been reported. Central nervous system complications have included confusion, hallucinations and seizures. Usually these signs and symptoms cleared upon discontinuation of gold therapy.

Hepatitis, jaundice, with or without cholestasis, gold bronchitis, pulmonary injury manifested by interstitial pneumonitis and fibrosis, partial or complete hair loss and fever have also been reported.

Sometimes arthralgia occurs for a day or two after an injection Gold Sodium Thiomalate; this reaction usually subsides after the first few injections.

MANAGEMENT OF ADVERSE REACTIONS

Treatment with Gold Sodium Thiomalate should be discontinued immediately when toxic reactions occur. Minor complications such as localized dermatitis, mild stomatitis, or slight proteinuria generally require no other therapy and resolve spontaneously with suspension of Gold Sodium Thiomalate. Moderately severe skin and mucous membrane reactions often benefit from topical corticosteroids, oral antihistaminics, and soothing or anesthetic lotions.

If stomatitis or dermatitis becomes severe or more generalized, systemic corticosteroids (generally, prednisone 10 to 40 mg daily in divided doses) may provide symptomatic relief. For serious renal, hematologic, pulmonary, and enterocolitic complications, high doses of systemic corticosteroids (prednisone 40 to 100 mg daily in divided doses) are recommended. The optimum duration of corticosteroid treatment varies with the response of the individual patient. Therapy may be required for many months when adverse effects are unusually severe or progressive.

In patients whose complications do not improve with high-dose corticosteroid treatment, or who develop significant steroid-related adverse reactions, a chelating agent may be given to enhance gold excretion. Dimercaprol (BAL) has been used successfully, but patients must be monitored carefully as numerous untoward reactions may attend its use. Corticosteroids and a chelating agent may be used concomitantly.

Gold Sodium Thiomalate *should not be reinstituted after severe or idiosyncratic reactions.*

Gold Sodium Thiomalate may be readministered following resolution of mild reactions, using a reduced dosage schedule. If an initial test dose of 5 mg Gold Sodium Thiomalate is well-tolerated, progressively larger doses (5 to 10 mg increments) may be given at weekly to monthly intervals until a dose of 25 to 50 mg is reached.

DOSAGE AND ADMINISTRATION

Gold Sodium Thiomalate should be administered only by intramuscular injection, preferably intragluteally. It should be given with the patient lying down. He should remain recumbent for approximately 10 minutes after the injection.

Therapeutic effects from Gold Sodium Thiomalate occur slowly. Early improvement, often limited to a reduction in morning stiffness, may begin after six to eight weeks of treatment, but beneficial effects may not be observed until after months of therapy.

Parenteral drug products should be inspected visually for particulate matter and discoloration prior to administration. Do not use if material has darkened. Color should not exceed pale yellow.

For the adult of average size the following dosage schedule is suggested:

WEEKLY INJECTIONS

1st injection	10 mg
2nd injection	25 mg
3rd and subsequent injections	25 to 50 mg until there is toxicity or major clinical improvement, or, in the absence of either of these, the cumulative dose of Gold Sodium Thiomalate reaches one gram.

Gold Sodium Thiomalate is continued until the cumulative dose reaches one gram unless toxicity or major clinical improvement occurs. If significant clinical improvement occurs before a cumulative dose of one gram has been administered, the dose may be decreased or the interval between injections increased as with maintenance therapy. Maintenance doses of 25 to 50 mg every other week for two to 20 weeks are recommended. If the clinical course remains stable, injections of 25 to 50 mg may be given every third and subsequently every fourth week indefinitely. Some patients may require maintenance treatment at intervals of one to three weeks. Should the arthritis exacerbate during maintenance therapy, weekly injections may be resumed temporarily until disease activity is suppressed.

Should a patient fail to improve during initial therapy (cumulative dose of one gram), several options are available:

◆ RATED THERAPEUTICALLY EQUIVALENT; ◇ THERAPEUTIC EQUIVALENCE UNCONFIRMED; ○ UNRATED

1. the patient may be considered to be unresponsive and Gold Sodium Thiomalate is discontinued

2. the same dose (25 to 50 mg) of Gold Sodium Thiomalate may be continued for approximately ten additional weeks

3. the dose of Gold Sodium Thiomalate may be increased by increments of 10 mg every one to four weeks, not to exceed 100 mg in a single injection.

If significant clinical improvement occurs using option 2 or 3, the maintenance schedule described above should be initiated. If there is no significant improvement or if toxicity occurs, therapy with Gold Sodium Thiomalate should be stopped. The higher the individual dose of Gold Sodium Thiomalate the greater the risk of gold toxicity. Selection of one of these options for chrysotherapy should be based upon a number of factors, including the physician's experience with gold salt therapy, the course of the patient's condition, the choice of alternative treatments, and the availability of the patient for the close supervision required.

JUVENILE RHEUMATOID ARTHRITIS

The pediatric dose of Gold Sodium Thiomalate is proportional to the adult dose on a weight basis. After the initial test dose of 10 mg, the recommended dose for children is one mg per kilogram body weight, not to exceed 50 mg for a single injection. Otherwise, the guidelines given above for administration to adults also apply to children.

Concomitant Drug Therapy: Gold salts should not be used concomitantly with penicillamine.

The safety of coadministration with cytotoxic drugs has not been established. Other measures, such as salicylates, other non-steroidal anti-inflammatory drugs, or systemic corticosteroids, may be continued when Gold Sodium Thiomalate is initiated. After improvement commences, analgesic and anti-inflammatory drugs may be discontinued slowly as symptoms permit.

STORAGE

Protect from light.

Store container in carton until contents have been used.

J CODES

Up to 50 mg IM—J1600

HOW SUPPLIED
INJECTION:

BRAND/MANUFACTURER	NDC	SIZE	AWP
○ **BRAND**			
AUROLATE: Pasadena	00418-4450-10	10 ml	$67.74
	00418-4450-01	1 ml 6s	$45.81

INJECTION: 50 MG/ML

BRAND/MANUFACTURER	NDC	SIZE	AWP
○ **BRAND**			
MYOCHRYSINE: Merck	00006-7762-10	10 ml	$100.39
	00006-7762-64	1 ml 6s	$64.30
○ **GENERICS**			
King Pharm	60793-0109-10	10 ml	$82.97

GoLYTELY *SEE* ELECTROLYTES AND POLYETHYLENE
GLYCOL 3350

Gonadorelin Acetate

DESCRIPTION

Gonadorelin Acetate for Injection is used for the induction of ovulation in women with primary hypothalamic amenorrhea. Gonadorelin Acetate is a synthetic deca-peptide that is identical in amino acid sequence to endogenous gonadotropin-releasing hormone (GnRH) synthesized in the human hypothalamus and in various neurons terminating in the hypothalamus. The molecular formula of Gonadorelin Acetate is:

$C_{55}H_{75}N_{17}O_{13} \cdot xC_2H_4O_2 \cdot yH_2O$

Its molecular weight is $1182.3 + x60 + y18$, where x and y represent a non-stoichiometric ratio of acetate and water associated with the peptide, and x ranges from 1-2 and y ranges from 2-3. The amino acid sequence of GnRH is:

5-oxPro-His-Trp-Ser-Tyr-Glv-Leu-Arg-Pro-Gly-NH₂

Gonadorelin Acetate for Injection is a sterile, lyophilized powder intended for intravenous pulsatile injection after reconstitution. It is white and very soluble in water. Vials are available containing 0.8 mg or 3.2 mg Gonadorelin Acetate (expressed as the diacetate) and 10.0 mg mannitol as a carrier. After reconstituting with 8 mL of diluent (sterile 0.9% Sodium Chloride Solution and hydrochloric acid to adjust the pH) for Gonadorelin Acetate for Injection, the concentration of Gonadorelin Acetate is 5 μg per 50 μl in each vial containing 0.8 mg lyophilized hormone, and 20 μg per 50 μl in each vial containing 3.2 mg lyophilized hormone. Gonadorelin Acetate for Injection is intended for use with the Gonadorelin Acetate for Injection KITS. The volumes and concentrations are specific for use with the Gonadorelin Acetate PUMP for appropriate dosing.

Following is its chemical structure:

5-oxoPro-His-Trp-Ser-Tyr-Gly-Leu-Arg-Pro-Gly-NH₂ · xC₂H₄O₂ · yH₂O
1 2 3 4 5 6 7 8 9 10

CLINICAL PHARMACOLOGY

Under physiologic conditions, gonadotropin-releasing hormone (GnRH) is released by the hypothalamus in a pulsatile fashion. The primary effect of GnRH is the synthesis and release of luteinizing hormone (LH) in the anterior pituitary gland. GnRH also stimulates the synthesis and release of follicle stimulating hormone (FSH), but this effect is less pronounced. LH and FSH subsequently stimulate the gonads to produce steroids which are instrumental in regulating reproductive hormonal status. Unlike human menopausal gonadotropin (hMG) which supplies pituitary hormones, pulsatile administration of Gonadorelin Acetate for Injection replaces defective hypothalamic secretion of GnRH. The pulsatile administration of Gonadorelin Acetate for Injection approximates the natural hormonal secretory pattern, causing pulsatile release of pituitary gonadotropins. Accordingly, Gonadorelin Acetate for Injection is useful in treating conditions of infertility caused by defective GnRH stimulation from the hypothalamus (see *"Indications and Usage"*). The following information summarizes clinical efficacy of Gonadorelin Acetate administered by pulsatile intravenous injection to patients with primary hypothalamic amenorrhea.

44 patients with primary hypothalamic amenorrhea (HA)
93% (41/44) patients ovulatory with Gonadorelin Acetate therapy
62% (24/39)* patients pregnant
100% (7/7) of those failing past attempts at ovulation induction by other methods were ovulatory on Gonadorelin Acetate.

Following intravenous injection of GnRH into normal subjects and/or hypogonadotropic patients, plasma GnRH concentrations rapidly decline with initial and terminal half-lives of 2-10 min. and 10-40 min., respectively. In these studies, high clearance values (500-1500 L/day) and low volumes of distribution (10-15 L) were calculated. The pharmacokinetics of GnRH in normal subjects and in hypogonadotropic patients were similar. GnRH was rapidly metabolized to various biologically inactive peptide fragments which are readily excreted in urine. Renal failure, but not hepatic disease, prolonged the half-life land reduced the clearance of GnRH.

INDICATIONS AND USAGE

Gonadorelin Acetate for Injection is indicated in the treatment of primary hypothalamic amenorrhea.

Differential Diagnosis: Proper diagnosis is critical for successful treatment with Gonadorelin Acetate for Injection. It must be established that hypothalamic amenorrhea or hypogonadism is, in fact, due to a deficiency in quantity or pulsing of endogenous GnRH. The diagnosis of hypothalamic amenorrhea or hypogonadism is based on the exclusion of other causes of the dysfunction, since there is currently no practical technique to directly assess hypothalamic function. Prior to initiation of therapy with Gonadorelin Acetate for Injection, the physician should rule out disorders of general health, reproductive organs, anterior pituitary, and central nervous system, other than abnormalities of GnRH secretion.

UNLABELED USES

Gonadorelin Acetate is used to induce ovulation in cases of female infertility and to increase sperm count in men with idiopathic oligospermia. It is used to treat hypogonadotropic hypogonadism and is also prescribed for treatment of cryptorchidism in prepubertal boys.

CONTRAINDICATIONS

Gonadorelin Acetate for Injection is contraindicated in women with any condition that could be exacerbated by pregnancy. For example, pituitary prolactinoma should be considered one such condition. Additionally, any history of sensitivity to Gonadorelin Acetate, Gonadorelin hydrochloride or any component of Gonadorelin Acetate for Injection is a contraindication. Patients who have ovarian cysts or causes of anovulation other than those of hypothalamic origin should not receive Gonadorelin Acetate for Injection.

Gonadorelin Acetate for Injection is intended to initiate events including the production of reproductive hormones (e.g. estrogens and progestins). Therefore, any condition that may be worsened by reproductive hormones, such as hormonally-dependent tumor, is a contraindication to the use of Gonadorelin Acetate for Injection.

WARNINGS

Therapy with Gonadorelin Acetate for Injection should be conducted by physicians familiar with pulsatile GnRH delivery and the clinical ramifications of ovulation induction. While there have been few cases of hyper-stimulation (< 1%) this possibility must be considered. If hyperstimulation should occur, therapy should be discontinued and spontaneous resolution can be expected. The preservation of the endogenous feedback mechanisms makes severe hyperstimulation (with ascites and pleural effusion) rare. However, the physician shoud be aware of the possibility and be alert for any evidence of ascites, pleural effusion, hemoconcentration, rupture of a cyst, fluid or electrolyte imbalance, or sepsis.

Multiple pregnancy is a possibility that can be minimized by careful attention to the recommended doses and ultrasonographic monitoring of the ovarian

---

* Five patients did not desire pregnancy.

response to therapy. Following a baseline pelvic ultrasound, follow-up studies should be conducted at a minimum on day 7 and day 14 of therapy.

Serious hypersensitivity reactions (anaphylaxis) have been reported following gonadotropin-releasing hormone administration, including Gonadorelin Acetate. Clinical manifestations may include: cardiovascular collapse, hypotension, tachycardia, loss of consciousness, angioedema, bronchospasm, dyspnea, urticaria, flushing and pruritus. If any allergic reaction occurs, therapy with Gonadorelin should be discontinued. Serious acute hypersensitivity reactions may require emergency medical treatment.

As with any intravenous medication, scrupulous attention to asepsis is important. The infusion area must be monitored as with all indwelling parenteral approaches. The cannula and IV site should be changed at 48-hour intervals.

PRECAUTIONS

General: Ovarian hyperstimulation has been reported. This may be related to pulse dosage or concomitant use of other ovulation stimulators. Hyperstimulation may be a greater risk in patients where spontaneous variations in endogenous GnRH secretion occur. Multiple follicle development, multiple pregnancy, and spontaneous termination of pregnancy have been reported. Multiple pregnancy can be minimized by appropriate monitoring of follicle formation; nonetheless, the patient and her partner should be advised of the frequency (12%) and potential risks of multiple pregnancy before starting treatment.

Ovarian hyperstimulation, a syndrome of sudden ovarian enlargement, ascites with or without pain, and/or pleural effusion, is rare with pulsatile GnRH therapy. Among 268 patients participating in clinical trials, one case of moderate hyperstimulation has been reported, but this cycle included the concomitant use of clomiphene citrate.

Antibody formation (IgE and IgG) has been reported following administration of Gonadorelin. The safety and efficacy implication of antibody development are uncertain (see *"Warnings"*).

Gonadorelin Acetate for Injection should be administered only with the Gonadorelin Acetate Pump. The patient should be provided with detailed oral and written instructions regarding infusion pump usage and potential sepsis in order to minimize the frequency of infusion pump malfunction and inflammation, infection, mild phlebitis, or hematoma at the catheter site.

Information for Patients: The patients should be advised to discontinue the drug and seek medical attention at the first sign of skin rash, urticaria, rapid heart beat, difficulty in swallowing and breathing, or any swelling which may suggest angioedema (see *"Warnings"* and *"Adverse Reactions"*).

Laboratory Tests: Following a diagnosis of primary hypothalamic amenorrhea, initiation of Gonadorelin Acetate for Injection therapy may be monitored by the following:

1) Ovarian ultrasound—baseline, therapy day 7, therapy day 14.
2) Mid-luteal phase serum progesterone.
3) Clinical observation of infusion site at each visit as needed.
4) Physical examination including pelvic at regularly scheduled visits.

Drug Interactions: None are known. Gonadorelin Acetate for Injection should not be used concomitantly with other ovulation stimulators.

Drug/Laboratory Test Interactions: None are known.

Carcinogenesis, Mutagenesis, Impairment of Fertility: Since GnRH is a natural substance normally present in humans, long-term studies in animals have not been performed to evaluate carcinogenic potential. Mutagenicity testing was not done.

Pregnancy: Pregnancy Category B

Reproduction studies (teratology and embryo-toxicity) performed in rats and rabbits have not revealed any evidence of harm to the fetus due to Gonadorelin Acetate. There was no evidence of teratogenicity when Gonadorelin Acetate was administered intravenously up to 120 µg/kg/day (> 70 times the recommended human dose of 5 µg per pulse) in rats and rabbits.

Studies in pregnant women have shown that Gonadorelin Acetate does not increase the risk of abnormalities when administered during the first trimester of pregnancy. It appears that the possibility of fetal harm is remote, if the drug is used during pregnancy. In clinical studies, 47 pregnant patients have used Gonadorelin Acetate during the first trimester of pregnancy (51 pregnancies) and the drug had no apparent adverse effect on the course of pregnancy. Available follow-up reports on infants born to these women reveal no adverse effects or complications that were attributable to Gonadorelin Acetate. Nevertheless, because the studies in humans cannot rule out the possibility of harm, Gonadorelin Acetate should be used during pregnancy only for maintenance of the corpus luteum in ovulation induction cycles.

Nursing Mothers: It is not known whether this drug is excreted in human milk. There is no indication for use of Gonadorelin Acetate for Injection in a nursing woman.

Pediatric Use: Safety and effectiveness in children under the age of 18 have not been established.

ADVERSE REACTIONS

Adverse reactions have been reported in approximately 10% of treatment regimens. Ten of 268 patients interrupted therapy because of an adverse reaction but subsequently resumed treatment. One other subject did not resume treatment.

In clinical studies involving 268 women, one case of moderate ovarian hyperstimulation has been reported. This cycle included concomitant use of clomiphene citrate. This low incidence of hyperstimulation appears to be due to the preservation of normal feedback mechanisms of the pituitary-ovarian axis.

Despite the preservation of feedback mechanisms, some incidents of multiple follicle development, multiple pregnancy, and spontaneous termination of pregnancy have been reported. Multiple pregnancy can be minimized by appropriate monitoring of follicle formation; nonetheless, the patient and her partner should be advised of the frequency and potential hazards of multiple pregnancy before starting treatment. In clinical studies involving 142 pregnancies, delivery information was available on 89 pregnancies. Eleven of these Gonadorelin Hydrochloride for Injection-induced pregnancies (12%) were multiple (10 sets of twins, 1 set of triplets).

The following adverse reactions have occurred at the injection site: urticaria, pruritus, inflammation, infection, mild phlebitis, or hematoma at the catheter site. Additionally, infusion set malfunction and interruption of infusion may occur; this has no known adverse effect other than interruption of therapy. Acute generalized (anaphylaxis, angioedema, urticaria, etc.) hypersensitivity reactions have been reported (see *"Warnings"* and *"Precautions"*).

Anaphylaxis (bronchospasm, tachycardia, flushing, urticaria, induration at injection site) has also been reported with the related polypeptide hormone Gonadorelin Hydrochloride.

OVERDOSAGE

Continuous, non-pulsatile exposure to gonadorelin acetate could temporarily reduce pituitary responsiveness. If the pump should malfunction and deliver the entire contents of the 3.2 mg system, no harmful effects would be expected. Bolus doses as high as 3000 µg of Gonadorelin Hydrochloride have not been harmful. Pituitary hyperstimulation and multiple follicle development can be minimized by adhering to recommended doses, and appropriate monitoring of follicle formation (see *"Precautions"*).

Administration of 640 µg/kg in monkeys as a single intravenous bolus resulted in no compound-related effects in clinical observations or gross morphologic evaluations.

DOSAGE AND ADMINISTRATION

Dosage: Dosages between 1 and 20 µg have been successfully used in clinical studies. The recommended dose in primary hypothalamic amenorrhea is 5 µg every 90 minutes. This is delivered by Gonadorelin Acetate Pump using the 0.8 mg solution at 50 µl per pulse (see physician pump manual). Sixty-eight percent of the 5 µg every 90 minute regimens induced ovulation in patients with primary hypothalamic amenorrhea.

The Gonadorelin Acetate Pump is capable of delivering 2.5, 5, 10, or 20 µg of Gonadorelin Acetate every 90 minutes. Some women may require a reduction in the recommended dose of 5 µg should laboratory testing and patient monitoring indicate an inappropriate response. While most primary hypothalamic amenorrhea patients will ovulate during the first cycle of 5 µg therapy, some may be refractory to this dose. The recommended treatment interval is 21 days. It may be necessary to raise the dose cautiously, and in stepwise fashion if there is no response after three treatment intervals. All dose changes should be carefully monitored for inappropriate response.

The following table can be used to calculate the dose per pulse when individualizing treatment:

Vial	Diluent	Volume/pulse	Dose/pulse
0.8 mg	8 mL	25 µL	2.5 µg
0.8 mg	8 mL	50 µL	5 µg
3.2 mg	8 mL	25 µL	10 µg
3.2 mg	8 mL	50 µL	20 µg

The response to Gonadorelin Acetate for Injection usually occurs within two to three weeks after therapy initiation. When ovulation occurs with the Gonadorelin Acetate Pump in place, therapy should be continued for another two weeks to maintain the corpus luteum. A comparison of Gonadorelin Acetate for Injection to hCG or hCG + Gonadorelin Acetate for Injection for corpus luteum maintenance revealed the following information:

hCG
Delivered = 43/63 = 68%
Aborted = 20/63 = 32%

Gonadorelin Acetate for Injection
Delivered = 19/26 = 73%
Aborted = 7/26 = 27%

hCG + Gonadorelin Acetate for Injection
Delivered = 19/25 = 76%
Aborted = 6/26 = 24%

Gonadorelin Acetate for Injection alone was able to maintain the corpus luteum during pregnancy.

Administration: Gonadorelin Acetate for Injection is to be reconstituted aseptically with 8 mL of diluent for Gonadorelin Acetate for Injection. *The drug product should be reconstituted immediately prior to use and transferred to the plastic reservoir.* First withdraw 8 mL of the saline diluent and then inject it onto the lyophile (drug product) cake. The product is shaken for a few seconds to produce a solution which should be clear, colorless, and free of particulate matter. Parenteral drug products should be inspected visually for particulate matter and discoloration prior to administration, whenever solution and container permit. If particulate matter or discoloration are present, the solution should not be used. A presterilized reservoir (bag) with the infusion catheter set supplied with the Gonadorelin Acetate for Injection is filled with the reconstituted solution, and administered intravenously using the Gonadorelin Acetate Pump. The pump should be set to deliver 25 or 50 μL of solution, based upon the dose selected, over a pulse period of one minute and at a pulse frequency of 90 minutes. The 8 mL of solution will supply 90 minute pulsatile doses for approximately 7 consecutive days.

HOW SUPPLIED
KIT: 0.8 MG

BRAND/MANUFACTURER	NDC	SIZE	AWP
○ **BRAND** LUTREPULSE: Ferring	55566-7208-05	1s	$271.14

KIT: 3.2 MG

BRAND/MANUFACTURER	NDC	SIZE	AWP
○ **BRAND** LUTREPULSE: Ferring	55566-7232-05	1s	$551.94

POWDER FOR INJECTION: 0.8 MG

BRAND/MANUFACTURER	NDC	SIZE	AWP
○ **BRAND** LUTREPULSE: Ferring	55566-7208-00	1s	$139.14

POWDER FOR INJECTION: 3.2 MG

BRAND/MANUFACTURER	NDC	SIZE	AWP
○ **BRAND** LUTREPULSE: Ferring	55566-7232-00	1s	$419.94

Gonadorelin Hydrochloride

DESCRIPTION
An agent for use in evaluating hypothalamic-pituitary gonadotropic function. Gonadorelin Hydrochloride injectable is available as a sterile lyophilized powder for reconstitution and administration by subcutaneous or intravenous routes.

Chemical Name: 5-oxo-L-prolyl-L-histidyl-L-tryptophyl-L-seryl -L-tyrosyl-glycyl-L-lecyl-L-arginyl-L-prolyl glycinamide hydrochloride.

Gonadorelin Hydrochloride is $C_{55}H_{75}N_{17}O_{13}HCL$, as the mono- or dihydrochloride, or their mixture. The Gonadorelin base has a molecular weight of 1182.33. It is a white powder, soluble in alcohol and water, bygroscopic and moisture-sensitive, and stable at room temperature. The synthetic decapeptide, Gonadorelin Hydrochloride has a chemical composition and structure identical to the natural hormone, identified from porcine or ovine hypothalami.

Each vial of Gonadorelin Hydrochloride contains 100 or 500 mcg Gonadorelin as the Hydrochloride.

CLINICAL PHARMACOLOGY
Gonadorelin Hydrochloride has been shown to have gonadotropin-releasing effects upon the anterior pituitary. The range for normal baseline LH levels, as determined from the literature, is 5-25 mIU/mL in postpubertal males, and postpubertal and premenopausal females. The standard used in is the Second International Reference Preparation—HMC. This range may not correspond in each laboratory performing the assay since the concentration of LH in normal individuals varies with different assay methods. The normal responses to Gonadorelin Hydrochloride analyzed from the results of clinical studies included:

(1) LH peak (mIU/mL) (highest LH value post-FACTREL administration)
(2) Maximum LH increase (mIU/mL) (peak LH value—LH baseline value)
(3) LH percent response
(peak LH—baseline LH)/baseline LH x 100%
(4) Time to peak (minutes) (time required to reach LH peak value)
Normal adult subjects were shown to have these LH responses following Gonadorelin Hydrochloride administration by subcutaneous or intravenous routes.

I. MALE ADULTS:
A) Subcutaneous Administration:
The results are based on 18 tests in males between the ages of 18-42 years, inclusive:

(1) LH peak: mean 60.3 ± 26.2 mIU/mL 100% $\geq$ 24.0 mIU/mL 90% $\geq$ 32.8 mIU/mL
(2) Maximum LH increase: mean 46.7 ± 20.8 mIU/mL 100% $\geq$ 12.3 mIU/mL 90% $\geq$ 20.9 mIU/mL
(3) LH percent response: mean 437 + 243% range: 66-1853% 90% $\geq$ 188%
(4) Time to peak: mean 34 ± 13 min

B) Intravenous Administration:
The results are based on 26 tests in males between the ages of 19-58 years, inclusive:

(1)LH peak: mean 63.8 ± 40.3 mIU/mL 100% $\geq$ 12.6 mIU/mL 90% $\geq$ 26.0 mIU/mL

(2) Maximum LH increase: mean 51.3 ± 35.2 mIU/mL 100% $\geq$ 7.4 mIU/mL 90% $\geq$ 14.8 mIU/mL
(3) LH percent response: mean $481 \pm 184\%$ range: 67-2139% 90% $\geq$ 142%
(4) Time to peak: mean 27 ± 14 min
In males older than 50 years, the LH baseline and peak levels tend to be higher; however, the maximum LH increases do not differ in regard to age.

II. FEMALE ADULTS
A) Sucutaneous Administration:
The results are based on 38 tests in females between the ages of 19-36 years, inclusive:

(1) LH peak: mean 67.9 ± 27.5 mIU/mL 100% $\geq$ 12.5 mIU/mL 90% $\geq$ 39.0 mIU/mL
(2) Maximum LH increase: mean 52.8 ± 26.4 mIU/mL 100% $\geq$ 7.5 mIU/mL 90% $\geq$ 23.8 mIU/mL
(3) LH percent response: mean $374 \pm 221\%$ range: 108-981% 90% $\geq$ 185%
(4) Time to peak: mean 71.5 ± 49.6 min

(B) Intravenous Administration:
The results are based on 31 tests in females between the ages of 20-35 years inclusive:

(1) LH peak: mean 57.6 ± 36.7 mIU/ml 100% $\geq$ 20.0 mIU/mL 90% $\geq$ 24.6 mIU/mL
(2) Maximum LH increase: mean 44.5 ± 31.8 mIU/mL 100% $\geq$ 7.5 mIU/mL 90% $\geq$ 16.2 mIU/mL
(3) LH percent response: mean $356 \pm 282\%$ range: 60-1300% 90% $\geq$ 142%
(4) Time to peak: mean 36 ± 24 min

The Gonadorelin Hydrochloride tests on which the normal female responses are based were performed in the early follicular phase of the menstrual cycle (Days 1-7).

In menopausal and postmenopausal females, the baseline LH levels are elevated and the maximum LH increases are exaggerated when compared with the premenopausal levels.

Patients with clinically diagnosed or suspected pituitary and/or hypothalamic dysfunction were often shown to have subnormal or no LH responses following Gonadorelin Hydrochloride administration. For example, in clinical tests of 6 patients with known postpubertal panhypopituitarism, and 11 patients with Prader-Willi syndrome, 100% showed subnormal responses or no rise in LH. Subnormal responses to the Gonadorelin Hydrochloride test also were observed in 21 (95% of 22 patients with prepubertal panhypopituitarism. In 19 patients with Sheehan's syndrome, 16 (84%) had a subnormal response. In the Gonadorelin Hydrochloride test in 44 patients with Kallmann's syndrome, 33 (77%) had subnormal LH responses.

INDICATIONS AND USAGE
Gonadorelin Hydrochloride as a single injection is indicated for evaluating the functional capacity and response of the gonadotropes of the anterior pituitary. This single-injection test does not measure pituitary gonadotropic reserve, for which more prolonged or repeated administration may be required. The LH response is useful in testing patients with suspected gonadotropin deficiency, whether due to the hypothalamus alone or in combination with anterior pituitary failure. Gonadorelin Hydrochloride is also indicated for evaluating residual gonadotropic function of the pituitary following removal of a pituitary tumor by surgery and/or irradiation. In clinical studies to date, however, the single-injection test has not been useful in differentiating pituitary disorders from hypothalamic disorders. The Gonadorelin Hydrochloride test can be performed concomitantly with other post-treatment evaluations. The results of the Gonadorelin Hydrochloride test complement the clinical examination and other laboratory tests used to confirm or substantiate hypogonadotropic hypogonadism.

In cases where there is a normal response, it indicates the presence of functional pituitary gonadotropes. The single-injection test does not measure pituitary gonadotropic reserve.

CONTRAINDICATIONS
Hypersensitivity to Gonadorelin Hydrochloride or any of the components.

PRECAUTIONS
Although allergic and hypersensitivity reactions have been observed with other polypeptide hormones, and rarely with multiple doses of Gonadorelin Hydrochloride to date no such reactions have been reported following the administration of a single 100 mcg dose of Gonadorelin Hydrochloride.

Antibody formation has been reported rarely after chronic administration of large doses of Gonadorelin Hydrochloride.

The Gonadorelin Hydrochloride test should be conducted in the absence of other drugs which directly affect the pituitary secretion of the gonadotropins. These would include a variety of preparations which contain androgens, estrogens, progestins, or glucocorticoids. The gonadotropin levels may be transiently elevated by spironolactone, minimally elevated by levodopa, and suppressed by oral contraceptives and digoxin. The response to Gonadorelin Hydrochloride may be blunted by phenothiazines and dopamine antagonists which cause a rise in prolactin.

Pregnancy Category B: Reproduction studies have been performed in mice, rats, and rabbits at doses up to 50 times the human dose and have revealed no evidence of harm to the fetus due to Gonadorelin Hydrochloride. There are, however, no adequate and well-controlled studies in pregnant women. Because

▶ SHOWN IN PRODUCT IDENTIFICATION GUIDE

animal reproduction studies are not always predictive of human response, this drug should be used during pregnancy only if clearly needed.

Appropriate precautions should be taken because the effects of LH-RH on the fetus and developing offspring have not been adequately evaluated. Repetitive, high doses of Gonadorelin Hydrochloride may cause luteolysis and inhibition of spermatogenesis.

ADVERSE REACTIONS

Systemic complaints such as headaches, nausea, light-headedness, abdominal discomfort, and flushing have been reported rarely following administration of 100 meg of Gonadorelin Hydrochloride. Local swelling, occasionally with pain and pruritus, at the injection site may occur if Gonadorelin Hydrochloride is administered subcutaneously. Local and generalized skin rash have been noted after chronic subcutaneous administration.

Rare instances of hypersensitivity reaction (bronchospasm, tachycardia, flushing, urticaria, induration at injection site) and anaphylactic reactions have been reported following multiple-dose administration.

OVERDOSAGE

Gonadorelin Hydrochloride has been administered parenterally in doses up to 3 mg bid for 28 days without any signs or symptoms of over-dosage. In case of overdosage or idiosyncrasy, symptomatic treatment should be administered as required.

DOSAGE AND ADMINISTRATION

Parenteral drug products should be inspected visually for particulate matter and discoloration prior to administration, whenever solution and container permit.

Adults: 100 mcg dose, subcutaneously or intravenously. In females for whom the phase of the menstrual cycle can be established, the test should be performed in the early follicular phase (Days 1-7).

TEST METHODOLOGY
To determine the status of the gonadotropin secretory capacity of the anterior pituitary, a test procedure requiring seven venous blood samples for LH is recommended.

Procedure:

1. Venous blood samples should be drawn at -15 minutes and immediately prior to Gonadorelin Hydrochloride administration. The LH baseline is obtained by averaging the LH values of the two samples.
2. Administer a bolus of 100 meg of Gonadorelin Hydrochloride subcutaneously or intravenously.
3. Draw venous blood samples at 15, 30, 45, 60, and 120 minutes after administration.
4. Blood samples should be handled as recommended by the laboratory that will determine the LH content. It must be emphasized that the reliability of the test is directly related to the inter-assay and intra-assay reliability of the laboratory performing the assay.

INTERPRETATION OF TEST RESULTS
Interpretation of the LH response to Gonadorelin Hydrochloride requires an understanding of the hypothalamic-pituitary physiology, knowledge of the clinical status of the individual patient, and familiarity with the normal ranges and the standards used in the laboratory performing the LH assays.

Figures 1 through 4 represent the LH response curves after Gonadorelin Hydrochloride administration in normal subjects. The normal LH response curves were established between the 10th percentile (B line) and 90th percentile (A line) of all LH responses in normal subjects analyzed from the results of clinical studies. LH values are reported in units of mIU/mL and time is displayed in minutes. Individual patient responses should be plotted on the appropriate curve. A subnormal response in patients is defined as three or more LH values which fall below the B line of the normal LH response curve. In cases where there is a blunted or borderline response, the Gonadorelin Hydrochloride test should be repeated.

The Gonadorelin Hydrochloride test complements the clinical assessment of patients with a variety of endocrine disorders involving the hypothalamic-pituitary axis. In cases where there is a normal response, it indicates the presence of functional pituitary gonadotropes. The single-injection test does not determine the pathophysiological cause for the subnormal response and does not measure pituitary gonadotropic reserve.

DIRECTIONS

Store at room temperature (approximately 25°C).
Reconstitute 100 mcg vial with 1.0 mL of the accompanying sterile diluent.
Reconstitute 500 mcg vial with 2.0 mL of the accompanying sterile diluent.
Prepare solution immediately before use.
After reconstitution, store at room temperature and use within 1 day.
Discard unused reconstituted solution and diluent.

HOW SUPPLIED
POWDER FOR INJECTION: 100 MCG

BRAND/MANUFACTURER	NDC	SIZE	AWP
○ **BRAND**			
FACTREL: Wyeth-Ayerst	00046-0507-05	1s	$65.26

POWDER FOR INJECTION: 500 MCG

BRAND/MANUFACTURER	NDC	SIZE	AWP
○ **BRAND**			
FACTREL: Wyeth-Ayerst	00046-0509-05	1s	$108.75

Gonadotropin, Chorionic

DESCRIPTION
Human Chorionic Gonadotropin (HCG), a polypeptide hormone produced by the human placenta, is composed of an alpha and a beta sub-unit. The alpha sub-unit is essentially identical to the alpha sub-units of the human pituitary gonadotropins, luteinizing hormone (LH) and follicle-stimulating hormone (FSH), as well as to the alpha sub-unit of human thyroid-stimulating hormone (TSH). The beta sub-units of these hormones differ in amino acid sequence.

Chorionic Gonadotropin is a water soluble glycoprotein derived from human pregnancy urine. The sterile lyophilized powder is stable. When reconstituted the solution should be refrigerated and should be used within 30 days.

Each vial when reconstituted with provided diluent (bacteriostatic water for injection, USP), will contain:

Chorionic Gonadotropin: 5,000 USP Units, 10,000 USP Units, or 20,000 USP Units.

For intramuscular injection only.

CLINICAL PHARMACOLOGY
The action of HCG is virtually identical to that of pituitary LH, although HCG appears to have a small degree of FSH activity as well. It stimulates production of gonadal steroid hormones by stimulating the interstitial cells (Leydig cells) of the testis to produce androgens and the corpus luteum of the ovary to produce progesterone. Androgen stimulation in the male leads to the development of secondary sex characteristics and may stimulate testicular descent when no anatomical impediment to descent is present. This descent is usually reversible when HCG is discontinued. During the normal menstrual cycle, LH participates with FSH in the development and maturation of the normal ovarian follicle, and the mid-cycle LH surge triggers ovulation. HCG can substitute for LH in this function.

During a normal pregnancy, HCG secreted by the placenta maintains the corpus luteum after LH secretion decreases, supporting continued secretion of estrogen and progesterone and preventing menstruation. HCG HAS NO KNOWN EFFECT ON FAT MOBILIZATION, APPETITE OR SENSE OF HUNGER, OR BODY FAT DISTRIBUTION.

Following intramuscular injection, a detectable rise in serum HCG levels is seen in 2 hours; peak levels are reached in 6 hours and remain at this level for 36 hours. HCG levels begin to decline at 48 hours and approach baseline (undetectable) levels at 72 hours.

INDICATIONS AND USAGE
HCG HAS NOT BEEN DEMONSTRATED TO BE EFFECTIVE ADJUNCTIVE THERAPY IN THE TREATMENT OF OBESITY. THERE IS NO SUBSTANTIAL EVIDENCE THAT IT INCREASES WEIGHT LOSS BEYOND THAT RESULTING FROM CALORIC RESTRICTION, THAT IT CAUSES A MORE ATTRACTIVE OR "NORMAL" DISTRIBUTION OF FAT, OR THAT IT DECREASES THE HUNGER AND DISCOMFORT ASSOCIATED WITH CALORIE-RESTRICTED DIETS.

1. Prepubertal cryptorchidism not due to anatomical obstruction. In general, HCG is thought to induce testicular descent in situations when descent would have occurred at puberty. HCG thus may help predict whether or not orchiopexy will be needed in the future. Although, in some cases, descent following HCG administration is permanent, in most cases, the response is temporary. Therapy, is usually instituted between the ages of 4 and 9.

2. Selected cases of hypogonadotropic hypogonadism (hypogonadism secondary to a pituitary deficiency) in males.

3. Induction of ovulation and pregnancy in the anovulatory, infertile woman in whom the cause of anovulation is secondary and not due to primary ovarian failure, and who has been appropriately pre-treated with human menotropins.

CONTRAINDICATIONS
Precocious puberty, prostatic carinoma or other androgen-dependent neoplasm, prior allergic reaction to HCG.

Pregnancy: HCG may cause fetal harm when administered to a pregnant woman. Combined HCG/PMS (pregnant mare's serum) therapy has been noted to induce high incidences of external congenital anomalies in the offspring of mice, in a dose-dependent manner. The potential extrapolation to humans has not been determined.

WARNINGS
HCG should be used in conjunction with human menopausal gonadotropins only by physicians experienced with infertility problems who are familiar with the criteria for patient selection, contraindications, warnings, precautions, and adverse reactions described in the package insert for menotropins. The principal serious adverse reactions during this use are: (1) Ovarian hyperstimulation, a syndrome of sudden ovarian enlargement, ascites with or without pain, and/or pleural effusion, (2) Enlargement or rupture of ovarian cysts with resultant hemoperitoneum, (3) Multiple births, and (4) Arterial thromboembolism secondary to hyperestrogenism.

◆ RATED THERAPEUTICALLY EQUIVALENT; ◇ THERAPEUTIC EQUIVALENCE UNCONFIRMED; ○ UNRATED

The diluent (bacteriostatic water for injection, USP) used for reconstitution contains benzyl alcohol. Benzyl alcohol has been reported to be associated with a fatal "Gasping Syndrome" in premature infants.

PRECAUTIONS
GENERAL
1. Induction of androgen secretion by HCG may induce precocious puberty (phallic enlargement, testicular enlargement and redness, development of pubic hair, aggressive behavior) in patients treated for cryptorchidism. Therapy should be discontinued if signs of precocious puberty occur. These changes are reversible within four weeks of the last injection.

2. Since adrogens may cause fluid retention, HCG should be used with caution in patients with cardiac or renal disease, epilepsy, migraine, or asthma.

Laboratory Tests: In adult males and females, the following hormone levels may be monitored depending on the nature of the diagnostic and therapeutic purpose: testosterone, dihydrotesterone, 17β-estradiol, 17β-hydroxyprogesterone, progesterone, androstenedione. In prepubertal males, testosterone and dihydrotestosterone should be followed.

Drug/Laboratory Test Interactions: HCG can cross-react in the radio-immunoassay of gonadotropins, especially luteinizing hormone. Each individual laboratory should establish the degree of cross-reactivity with their gonadotropin assay. Physicians should make the laboratory aware of patients on HCG if gonadotropin levels are requested.

Carcinogenesis, Mutagenesis, Impairment of Fertility: There have been sporadic reports of testicular tumors in otherwise healthy young men receiving HCG for secondary infertility. A causative relationship between HCG and tumor development in these men has not been established.

Defects of forelimbs and of the central nervous system, as well as alterations in sex ratio, have been reported in mice on combined gonadotropin and HCG regimens. The dose of gonadotropins used was intended to induce superovulation. No mutagenic effect has been clearly established in humans. Fertility— see *"Indications and Usage".*

PREGNANCY
Pregnancy Category C: Animal reproduction studies have not been conducted with Human Chorionic Gondotropin. It is also not known whether Human Chorionic Gonadotropin can cause fetal harm when administered to a pregnant woman or can affect reproduction capacity. Human Chorionic Gonadotropin should be given to a pregnant woman only if clearly needed.

Tetratogenic effects—Category X: see *"Contraindications"* section. Combined HCG/PMS (pregnant mare's serum) therapy has been noted to induce high incidences of external congenital anomalies in the offspring of mice, in a dose-dependent manner. The potential extrapolation to humans has not been determined.

Nursing Mothers: It is not known whether this drug is excreted in human milk. Because many drugs are excreted in human milk, caution should be exercised when HCG is administered to a nursing woman.

Pediatric Use: Safety and effectiveness in children below the age of 4 have not been established.

ADVERSE REACTIONS
Headache, irritability, restlessness, depression, fatigue, edema, precocious puberty, gynecomastia, pain at the site of injection, aggressive behavior, ovarian hyperstimulation syndrome, enlargement of preexisting ovarian cysts and possible rupture, phallic or testicular enlargement, growth of pubic hair, signs or symptoms of androgen excess, arterial thromboembolism.

Hypersensitivity reactions both localized and systemic in nature, including erythema, urticaria, rash, angioedema, dyspnea and shortness of breath, have been reported. The relationship of these allergic-like events to the polypeptide hormone or the diluent containing benzyl alcohol is not clear.

OVERDOSAGE
There is no experience to date with deliberate overdosage of HCG.
Treatment must be symptomatic and supportive.

DOSAGE AND ADMINISTRATION
For intramuscular use only. The dosage regimen employed in any particular case will depend upon the indication for use, the age and weight of the patient, and the physician's preference. The following regimens have been advocated by various authorities.
Prepubertal cryptorchidism not due to anatomical obstruction:
1. 4,000 USP Units three times weekly for three weeks.
2. 5,000 USP Units every second day for four injections.
3. 15 injections of 500 to 1,000 USP Units over a period of six weeks.
4. 500 USP Units three times weekly for four to six weeks. If this course of treatment is not successful, another is begun one month later, giving 1,000 USP Units per injection.
Selected cases of hypogonadotropic hypogonadism in males:
1. 500 to 1,000 USP Units three times a week for three weeks, followed by the same dose twice a week for three weeks.
2. 1,000 to 2,000 USP Units three times weekly (for some brands).
3. 4,000 USP Units three times weekly for six to nine months, following which the dosage may be reduced to 2,000 USP Units three times weekly for an additional three months.

Induction of ovulation and pregnancy in the anovulatory, infertile woman in whom the cause of anovulation is secondary and not due to primary ovarian failure and who has been appropriately pre-treated with human menotropins (see prescribing information for menotropins for dosage and administration for that drug product):
5,000 to 10,000 USP Units one day following the last dose of menotropins (a dosage of 10,000 USP Units is recommended in the labeling for menotropins).

Parenteral drug products should be inspected visually for particulate matter and discoloration prior to administration, whenever solution and container permit.

DIRECTIONS FOR RECONSTITUTION
Two Vial Package: Withdraw sterile air from lyophilized vial and inject into diluent vial. Remove up to 10 mL of diluent and add to lyophilized vial, agitate gently until solution is complete.

Store dry product at controlled room temperature 15°-30°C (59°-86°F) or in the refrigerator, depending on the brand. AFTER RECONSTITUTION, REFRIGERATE THE PRODUCT AT 2°-8°C (36°-46°F) AND USE WITHIN 30 to 60 DAYS depending on the brand.

J CODES
IM—J0725

HOW SUPPLIED
POWDER FOR INJECTION: 10,000 U

AVERAGE UNIT PRICE (AVAILABLE SIZES)		GENERIC A-RATED AVERAGE PRICE (GAAP)	
BRAND	$72.46	1s	$25.15
GENERIC	$25.15		

BRAND/MANUFACTURER	NDC	SIZE	AWP
◆ BRAND			
PREGNYL: Organon	00052-0315-10	1s	$30.97
PROFASI: Serono	44087-8010-03	1s	$41.20
A.P.L.: Wyeth-Ayerst	00046-0971-10	1s	$145.20
◆ GENERICS			
Schein	00364-6584-54	1s	$21.30
Schein	00364-6706-54	1s	$21.30
Steris	00402-0126-10	1s	$21.30
Steris	00402-0126-11	1s	$21.30
Rugby	00536-0500-70	1s	$23.13
Rugby	00536-5130-70	1s	$23.13
Goldline	00182-0805-63	1s	$31.50
Goldline	00182-1165-63	1s	$31.50
CHOREX: Hyrex	00314-0618-70	1s	$31.90

POWDER FOR INJECTION: 20,000 U

BRAND/MANUFACTURER	NDC	SIZE	AWP
◆ BRAND			
A.P.L.: Wyeth-Ayerst	00046-0972-10	1s	$295.58

POWDER FOR INJECTION: 200 U

BRAND/MANUFACTURER	NDC	SIZE	AWP
○ BRAND			
GLUKOR: Hyrex	00314-1015-25	1s	$29.90

POWDER FOR INJECTION: 5000 U

AVERAGE UNIT PRICE (AVAILABLE SIZES)		GENERIC A-RATED AVERAGE PRICE (GAAP)	
BRAND	$49.47	1s	$16.22
GENERIC	$16.22		

BRAND/MANUFACTURER	NDC	SIZE	AWP
◆ BRAND			
PROFASI: Serono	44087-8005-03	1s	$21.27
A.P.L.: Wyeth-Ayerst	00046-0970-10	1s	$77.66
◆ GENERICS			
Steris	00402-0125-10	1s	$13.95
Rugby	00536-0400-70	1s	$16.81
CHOREX: Hyrex	00314-0617-70	1s	$17.90

Gordochom SEE CHLOROXYLENOL AND UNDECYLENIC ACID

Goserelin Acetate

DESCRIPTION
Goserelin Acetate implant contains a potent synthetic decapeptide analogue of luteinizing hormone-releasing hormone (LHRH), also known as a gonadotropin releasing hormone (GnRH) agonist analogue. Goserelin Acetate is chemically described as an acetate salt of [D-Ser(Bu^t)^6,Azgly^{10}]LHRH. Its chemical structure is pyro-Glu-His-Trp-Ser-Tyr-D-Ser(Bu^t)-Leu-Arg-Pro-Azgly-NH$_2$ acetate [C$_{59}$H$_{84}$N$_{18}$O$_{14}$·(C$_2$H$_4$O$_2$)$_x$ where x = 1 to 2.4].

➤ SHOWN IN PRODUCT IDENTIFICATION GUIDE

Goserelin Acetate is an off-white powder with a molecular weight of 1269 Daltons (free base). It is freely soluble in glacial acetic acid. It is soluble in water, 0.1M hydrochloric acid, 0.1M sodium hydroxide, dimethylformamide and dimethyl sulfoxide. Goserelin Acetate is practically insoluble in acetone chloroform and ether.

Goserelin Acetate is supplied as a sterile, biodegradable product containing Goserelin Acetate equivalent to 3.6 mg of Goserelin. Goserelin Acetate is designed for subcutaneous injection with continuous release over a 28-day period.

Following is its chemical structure:

$$H-5\text{-oxoPro-His-Trp-Ser-Tyr-D-Ser}(t\text{-Bu})\text{-Leu-Arg-Pro-NH-NH-C-NH}_2$$
$$\quad\quad 1\quad 2\quad 3\quad 4\quad 5\quad 6\quad\quad 7\quad 8\quad 9$$

CLINICAL PHARMACOLOGY

Mechanism of Action: Goserelin Acetate is a synthetic decapeptide analogue of LHRH Goserelin Acetate acts as a potent inhibitor of pituitary gonadotropin secretion when administered in the biodegradable formulation. Following initial administration in males, Goserelin Acetate causes an initial increase in serum luteinizing hormone (LH) and follicle stimulating hormone (FSH) levels with subsequent increases in serum levels of testosterone. Chronic administration of Goserelin Acetate leads to sustained suppression of pituitary gonadotropins, and serum levels of testosterone consequently fall into the range normally seen in surgically castrated men approximately 2-4 weeks after initiation of therapy. This leads to accessory sex organ regression. In animal and in vitro studies, administration of Goserelin resulted in the regression or inhibition of growth of the hormonally sensitive dimethylbenzanthracene (DMBA)-induced rat mammary tumor and Dunning R3327 prostate tumor. In clinical trials with follow-up of more than 2 years, suppression of serum testosterone to castrate levels has been maintained for the duration of therapy.

In females, a similar down-regulation of the pituitary gland by chronic exposure to Goserelin Acetate leads to suppression of gonadotropin secretion, a decrease in serum estradiol to levels consistent with the postmenopausal state, and would be expected to lead to a reduction of ovarian size and function, reduction in the size of the uterus and mammary gland, as well as a regression of sex hormone-responsive tumors, if present. Serum estradiol is suppressed to levels similar to those observed in postmenopausal women within 3 weeks following initial administration; this suppression is sustained upon continued administration of the drug for at least 6 months. Serum LH and FSH are suppressed to follicular phase levels within 4 weeks after initial administration and are maintained in that range during at least 6 months of continuous Goserelin Acetate administration. Rarely, in certain individuals, suppression of these hormones to such levels may not be achieved with Goserelin Acetate. Estradiol, LH and FSH levels return to pretreatment values within 12 weeks following the last implant administration in all but rare cases.

Pharmacokinetics and Metabolism: In clinical trials using the 3.6 mg formulation of Goserelin Acetate in males, peak concentrations in serum were achieved 12 to 15 days after subcutaneous administration. The mean peak serum concentration was approximately 2.6 and 1.6 mg/mL in males and females respectively, and the corresponding area under the serum concentration-time curves for males and females were appproximately 26.7 and 18.3 ng/day/mL due to the higher total body clearance found in females. Pharmacokinetic data were obtained using a nonspecific RIA method.

Goserelin is released from the depot at a much slower rate initially for the first 8 days, and then there is more rapid and continuous release for the remainder of the 28-day dosing period. Despite the change in the releasing rate of Goserelin, administration of Goserelin Acetate every 28 days resulted in testosterone levels that were suppressed to and maintained in the range normally seen in surgically castrated men.

Administration of the 3.6 mg formulation of Goserelin Acetate results in measurable concentrations of the drug in serum throughout the 28-day dosing period. Goserelin does not accumulate in serum following a second administration 1 month after the first injection, nor does it accumulate following six sequential monthly administrations.

When Goserelin Acetate 3.6 mg depot was used for treating male and female patients with normal renal and hepatic function, there was no significant evidence of drug accumulation. However, in clinical trials the C_{min} levels of a few patients were increased. These levels can be attributed to interpatient variation.

In clinical trials with the solution formulation of Goserelin, male subjects with impaired renal function (creatinine clearance less than 20 mL/min) had a serum elimination half-life of 12.1 hours compared to 4.2 hours for subjects with normal renal function (creatinine clearance greater than 70 mL/min). However, in clinical trials with the monthly formulation of Goserelin Acetate for treating prostate cancer in males, the incidence of adverse events was not increased in patients with impaired renal function.

Pharmacokinetic studies in patients with renal or hepatic impairment using the aqueous formulation of Goserelin do not indicate a need for dose adjustment with the use of the depot formulation.

Clearance of Goserelin following subcutaneous administration of the solution formulation of Goserelin is very rapid and occurs via a combination of hepatic metabolism and urinary excretion. The metabolism of Goserelin Acetate in humans yields a similar but narrow profile of metabolites to that found in other species. All metabolites found in humans have also been found in toxicology studies.

In controlled clinical studies using the 3.6 mg formulation every 28 days for 6 months, Goserelin Acetate was shown to be as effective as danazol therapy in relieving clinical symptoms (dysmenorrhea, dyspareunia and pelvic pain) and signs (pelvic tenderness, pelvic induration) of endometriosis and decreasing the size of endometrial lesions as determined by laparoscopy. In one study comparing Goserelin Acetate with danazol (800 mg/day), 63% of Goserelin Acetate treated patients and 42% of danazol-treated patients had a greater than or equal to 50% reduction in the extent of endometrial lesions. In the second study comparing Goserelin Acetate with danazol (600 mg/day), 62% of Goserelin Acetate-treated and 51% of danazol-treated patients had a greater than or equal to 50% reduction in the extent of endometrial lesions. The clinical significance of a decrease in endometriotic lesions is not known at this time; and in addition, laparoscopic staging of endometriosis does not necessarily correlate with severity of symptoms.

In these two studies, Goserelin Acetate led to amenorrhea in 92% and 80%, respectively, of all treated women within 8 weeks after initial administration. Menses usually resumed within 8 weeks following completion of therapy.

Within 4 weeks following initial administration, clinical symptoms were significantly reduced, and at the end of treatment were, on average, reduced by approximately 84%.

During the first two months of Goserelin Acetate use, some women experience vaginal bleeding of variable duration and intensity. In all likelihood, this bleeding represents estrogen withdrawal bleeding, and is expected to stop spontaneously.

This is insufficient evidence to determine whether pregnancy rates are enhanced or adversely affected by the use of Goserelin Acetate.

INDICATIONS AND USAGE

Prostatic Carcinoma: Goserelin Acetate is indicated to the palliative treatment of advanced carcinoma of the prostate. Goserelin Acetate offers an alternative treatment of prostatic cancer when orchiectomy or estrogen administration are either not indicated or unacceptable to the patient.

In controlled studies of patients with advanced prostatic cancer comparing Goserelin Acetate to orchiectomy, the long-term endocrine responses and objective responses were similar between the two treatment arms. Additionally, duration of survival was similar between the two treatment arms in a major comparative trial.

Endometriosis: Goserelin Acetate is indicated for the management of endometriosis, including pain relief and reduction of endometriotic lesions for the duration of therapy. Experience with Goserelin Acetate for the management of endometriosis has been limited to women 18 years of age and older treated for 6 months.

UNLABELED USES
Goserelin Acetate is used alone or as an adjunct in the treatment of breast cancer.

CONTRAINDICATIONS

Goserelin Acetate is contraindicated in those patients who have a known hypersensitivity to LHRH, LHRH agonist analogues or any of the components in Goserelin Acetate.

Goserelin Acetate is contraindicated in women who are or may become pregnant while receiving the drug. In studies in rats and rabbits, Goserelin Acetate increased preimplantation loss, resorptions, and abortions (see *"Pregnancy"* section). In rats and dogs, Goserelin Acetate suppressed ovarian function, decreased ovarian weight and size, and led to atrophic changes in secondary sex organs. Further evidence suggests that fertility was reduced in female rats that became pregnant after Goserelin Acetate was stopped. These effects are an expected consequence of the hormonal alterations produced by Goserelin Acetate in humans. If a patient becomes pregnant during treatment, the drug must be discontinued and the patient must be apprised of the potential risk for loss of the pregnancy due to possible hormonal imbalance as a result of the expected pharmacologic action of Goserelin Acetate treatment. In animals studies, there was no evidence that Goserelin Acetate possessed the potential to cause teratogenicity in rabbits; however, in rats the incidence of umbilical hernia was significantly increased with treatment. (See *"Pregnancy, Teratogenic Effects"*.)

Goserelin Acetate is contraindicated in women who are breast feeding and/or lactating (see *"Nursing Mothers"* section).

WARNINGS

Males: Initially, Goserelin Acetate like other LHRH agonists, causes transient increases in serum levels of testosterone. Transient worsening of symptoms, or the occurrence of additional signs and symptoms of prostatic cancer, may occasionally develop during the first few weeks of Goserelin Acetate treatment. A small number of patients may experience a temporary increase in bone pain, which can be managed symptomatically. As with other LHRH agonists, isolated cases of ureteral obstruction and spinal cord compression have been observed. If spinal cord compression or renal impairment develops, standard treatment of these complications should be instituted, and in extreme cases an immediate orchiectomy considered.

Females: Before starting treatment with Goserelin Acetate, pregnancy must be excluded. (See *"Contraindications"*.) Safe use of Goserelin Acetate in pregnancy has not been established clinically.

When used every 28 days Goserelin Acetate usually inhibits ovulation and stops menstruation. Contraception is not ensured, however, by taking Goserelin Acetate. During treatment, pregnancy must be avoided by the use of nonhormonal methods of contraception. If however, a patient becomes pregnant during treatment, the drug must be discontinued and the patient must be apprised of the potential risk for loss of the pregnancy due to possible hormonal imbalance as a result of the expected pharmacologic action of Goserelin Acetate treatment. Following the last Goserelin Acetate injection, nonhormonal methods of contraception must be continued until the return of menses or for at least 12 weeks. (See "Contraindications".)

PRECAUTIONS

General: Hypersensitivity, antibody formation and anaphylactic reactions have been reported with LHRH agonist analogues. Currently, no anaphylactic reactions have been reported with the use of Goserelin Acetate.

Of 115 women worldwide treated with Goserelin Acetate and tested for development of binding to Goserelin following treatment with Goserelin Acetate, one patient showed low-titer binding to Goserelin. On further testing of this patient's plasma obtained following treatment, her Goserelin binding component was found not be precipitated with rabbit antihuman immunoglobulin polyvalent sera. These findings suggest the possibility of antibody formation.

INFORMATION FOR PATIENTS

Males: The use of Goserelin Acetate in patients at particular risk of developing ureteral obstruction or spinal cord compression should be considered carefully and the patients monitored closely during the first month of therapy. Patients with ureteral obstruction or spinal cord compression should have appropriate treatment prior to initiation of Goserelin Acetate therapy.

Females: Patients must be made aware of the following information:

1. Since menstruation should stop with effective doses of Goserelin Acetate the patient should notify her physician if regular menstruation persists. Patients missing one or more successive doses of Goserelin Acetate may experience breakthrough menstrual bleeding.

2. Goserelin Acetate should not be prescribed if the patient is pregnant, breast feeding, lactating, has nondiagnosed abnormal vaginal bleeding, or is allergic to any of the components of Goserelin Acetate.

3. Use of Goserelin Acetate in pregnancy is contraindicated. Therefore, a nonhormonal method of contraception should be used during treatment. Patients should be advised that if they miss one or more successive doses of Goserelin Acetate, breakthrough menstrual bleeding or ovulation may occur with the potential for conception. If a patient becomes pregnant during treatment, Goserelin Acetate treatment should be discontinued and the patient should be advised of the possible risks to the pregnancy and fetus. (See "Contraindications".)

4. Those adverse events occuring most frequently in clinical studies with Goserelin Acetate are associated with hypoestrogenism; of these the most frequently reported are hot flashes (flushes), headaches, vaginal dryness, emotional lability, change in libido, depression, sweating and change in breast size.

5. As with other LHRH agonist analogues, treatment with Goserelin Acetate induces a hypoestrogenic state which results in a loss of bone mineral density (BMD) over the course of treatment, some of which may not be reversible. In patients with a history of prior treatment that may have resulted in bone mineral density loss and/or in patients with major risk factors for decreased bone mineral density such as chronic alcohol abuse and/or tobacco abuse, significant family history of osteoporosis, or chronic use of drugs that can reduce bone density such as anticonvulsants or corticosteroids. Goserelin Acetate therapy may pose an additional risk. In these patients the risks and benefits must be weighed carefully before therapy with Goserelin Acetate is instituted.

6. Currently, there are no clinical data on the effects of retreatment or treatment of benign gynecological conditions with Goserelin Acetate for periods in excess of 6 months.

7. As with other hormonal interventions that disrupt the pituitary-gonadal axis, some patients may have delayed return to menses. The rare patient, however, may experience persistent amenorrhea.

Drug Interactions: No drug interaction studies with other drugs have been conducted with Goserelin Acetate. No confirmed interactions have been reported between Goserelin Acetate and other drugs.

Drug/Laboratory Test Interactions: Administration of Goserelin Acetate in therapeutic doses results in suppression of the pituitary-gonadal system. Because of this suppression, diagnostic tests of pituitary-gonadotropic and gonadal functions conducted during treatment and until the resumption of menses may show results which are misleading. Normal function is usually restored within 12 weeks after treatment is discontinued.

Carcinogenesis, Mutagenesis, Impairment of Fertility: After subcutaneous implant injections once every 4 weeks for 1 year at two dose levels to male and female rats equivalent to 31.5 (22.5) and 62.4 (44.6) times, and 21.5 (15.4) and 42.4 (30.3) times the recommended monthly dose for a 70 kg (50 kg) human, respectively, an increased incidence of benign pituitary macroadenomas was found. No increase in pituitary adenomas was seen in mice receiving injections of Goserelin every 3 weeks for 2 years at doses up to 2,400 μ/kg/day (1,200 times the recommended 70 kg human dose and 850 times the 50 kg human dose). An increased incidence of histiocytic sarcomas of the bone marrow in vertebral column and femur were observed at both doses in mice. No evidence of pituitary adenomas was seen in a 1 year study in dogs at doses up to 100 times the 70 kg human dose (70 times the dose for a 50 kg human) or in a 6 month study in monkeys at doses up to 200 times the 70 kg human dose (140 times the dose for a 50 kg human.) The relevance of rat pituitary tumors to humans has not been established.

Mutagenicity tests using bacterial and mammalian systems for point mutations and cytogenetic effects have provided no evidence for mutagenic potential.

Administration of Goserelin led to changes that were consistent with gonadal suppression in both male and female rats as a result of its endocrine action. In male rats treated at 30—60 times the recommended monthly dose for a 70 kg human, a decrease in weight and atrophic histological changes were observed in the testes, epididymis, seminal vesicle, and prostate gland with complete suppression of spermatogenesis. In female rats treated with 20—40 times (15—30) times the recommended monthly dose for a 70 kg (50 kg) human, suppression of ovarian function led to decreased size and weight of ovaries and secondary sex organs; follicular development was arrested at the antral stage and the corpora lutea were reduced in size and number. Except for the testes, almost complete histologic reversal of these effects in males and females were observed several weeks after dosing was stopped; however, fertility and general reproductive performance were reduced in those that became pregnant after Goserelin was discontinued. Fertile matings occurred within 2 weeks after cessation of dosing, even though total recovery of reproductive function may not have occurred before mating took place; and, the ovulation rate, the corresponding implantation rate, and number of live fetuses were reduced. Based on histological examination, drug effects on reproductive organs seemed to be completely reversible in male and female dogs when drug treatment was stopped after continuous administration for 1 year at 100 times the recommended monthly dose.

Pregnancy, Teratogenic Effects: Pregnancy Category X: see "Contraindications" section. Studies in both rats and rabbits at doses of 2, 10, 20, and 50 μg/kg/day and 20, 250, and 1,000 μg/kg/day, respectively (up to 25 times and 500 times the maximum recommended dose to a 70 kg human and 17.8 and 357 times for a 50 kg human), given during the period of organogenesis, have confirmed that Goserelin Acetate will increase pregnancy loss in a dose-related manner. While there was no evidence that Goserelin Acetate possessed the potential to cause teratogenicity in rabbits, in rats the incidence of umbilical hernia was significantly increased with treatment.

Nursing Mothers: It is not known if this drug is excreted in human milk. Many drugs are excreted in human milk and there is a potential for serious adverse reactions in nursing infants of mothers receiving Goserelin Acetate. Thus Goserelin Acetate is contraindicated in nursing/lactating women and should not be administered.

Pediatric Use: The safety and efficacy of Goserelin Acetate in children have not been established.

ADVERSE REACTIONS

As with other endocrine therapies, hypercalcemia (increased calcium) has rarely been reported in cancer patients with bone metastases following initiation of treatment with Goserelin Acetate or other LHRH agonists.

Males: Goserelin Acetate has been found to be generally well tolerated in clinical trials. Adverse reactions reported in these trials were rarely severe enough to result in the patients' withdrawal from Goserelin Acetate treatment. As seen with other hormonal therapies, the most commonly observed adverse events during Goserelin Acetate therapy were due to the expected physiological effects from decreased testosterone levels. These included hot flashes, sexual dysfunction and decreased erections.

Initially, Goserelin Acetate like other LHRH agonists, causes transient increases in serum levels of testosterone. A small percentage of patients experienced a temporary worsening of signs and symptoms (see "Warnings" section), usually manifested by an increase in cancer-related pain which was managed symptomatically. Isolated cases of exacerbation of disease symptoms, either ureteral obstruction or spinal cord compression, occurred at similar rates in controlled clinical trials with both Goserelin Acetate and orchiectomy. The relationship of these events to therapy is uncertain.

In the controlled clinical trials of Goserelin Acetate versus orchiectomy, the following events were reported as adverse reactions in greater than 5% of the patients.

TREATMENT RECEIVED

Adverse Reaction	Goserelin Acetate (n = 242) %	Orchiectomy (n = 254) %
Hot Flashes	62	53
Sexual Dysfunction	21	15
Decreased Erections	18	16
Lower Urinary Tract Symptoms	13	8
Lethargy	8	4
Pain (worsened in the first 30 days)	8	3
Edema	7	8
Upper Respiratory Infection	7	2
Rash	6	1
Sweating	6	4
Anorexia	5	2
Chronic Obstructive Pulmonary Disease	5	3
Congestive Heart Failure	5	1
Dizziness	5	4
Insomnia	5	1
Nausea	5	2
Complications of Surgery	0	18*

* *Complications related to surgery were reported in 18% of the orchiectomy patients, while only 3% of Goserelin Acetate patients reported adverse reactions at the injection site. The surgical complications included scrotal infection (5.9%), groin pain (4.7%), wound seepage (3.1%), scrotal hematoma (2.8%), incisional discomfort (1.6%) and skin necrosis (1.2%).*

The following additional adverse reactions were reported in greater than 1% but less than 5% of the patients treated with Goserelin Acetate.

Cardiovascular: arrhythmia, cerebrovascular accident, hypertension, myocardial infarction, peripheral vascular disorder, chest pain.

Central Nervous System: anxiety, depression, headache.

Gastrointestinal: constipation, diarrhea, ulcer, vomiting.

Hematologic: anemia.

Metabolic/Nutritional: gout, hyperglycemia, weight increase.

Miscellaneous: chills, fever.

Urogenital: renal insufficiency, urinary obstruction, urinary tract infection, breast swelling and tenderness.

Females: As would be expected with a drug that results in hypoestrogenism, the most frequently reported adverse reactions were those related to this effect.

In controlled clinical trials compring Goserelin Acetate every 28 days and danazol daily for the treatment of endometriosis, the following events were reported at a frequency of 5% or greater:

TREATMENT RECEIVED

Adverse Reaction	Goserelin Acetate (n = 411) %	Danazol (n = 207) %
Hot Flushes	96	67
Vaginitis	75	43
Headache	75	63
Emotional Liability	60	56
Libido Decreased	61	44
Sweating	45	30
Depression	54	48
Acne	42	55
Breast Atrophy	33	42
Sbeorrhea	26	52
Peripheral Edema	21	34
Breast Enlargement	18	15
Pelvic Symptoms	18	23
Pain	17	16
Dyspareunia	14	5
Libido Increased	12	19
Infection	13	11
Asthenia	11	13
Nausea	8	14
Hirsutism	7	15
Insomnia	11	7
Breast Pain	7	4
Abdominal Pain	7	7
Back Pain	7	13
Flu Syndrome	5	5
Dizziness	6	4
Application Site Reaction	6	—
Voice Alterations	3	8
Pharyngitis	5	2
Hair Disorders	4	11
Myalgia	3	11
Nervousness	3	5
Weight Gain	3	23
Leg Cramps	2	6
Increased Appetite	2	5
Pruritis	2	6
Hypertonia	1	10

The following adverse events not already listed above were reported at a frequency of 1% or greater, regardless of causality, in Goserelin Acetate-treated women from all clinical trials.

Whole Body: allergic reaction, chest pain, fever, malaise.

Cardiovascular: hemorrhage, hypertension, migraine, palpitations, tachycardia:

Digestive: anorexia, constipation, diarrhea, dry mouth, dyspepsia, flatulence:

Hematologic: ecchymosis:

Metabolic And Nutritional: edema:

Musculoskeletal: arthralgia, joint disorder; CNS—anxiety, paresthesia, somnolence, thinking abnormal:

Respiratory: bronchitis, cough increased, epistaxis, rhinitis; sinusitis:

Skin: alopecia, dry skin, rash, skin discoloration:

Special Senses: amblyopia, dry eyes:

Urogenital: dysmenorrhea, urinary frequency, urinary tract infection, vaginal hemorrhage.

Changes in Bone Mineral Density: After 6 months of Goserelin Acetate treatment, 109 female patients treated with Goserelin Acetate showed an average 4.3% decrease in vertebral trabecular bone mineral density (BMD) as compared to pretreatment values. BMD was measured by dual-photon absorptiometry or dual energy x-ray absorptometry. Sixty-six of these patients were assessed for BMD loss 6 months after the completion (posttherapy) of the 6-month therapy period. Data from these patients showed an average 2.4% BMD loss compared to pretreatment values. Twenty-eight of the 109 patients were assessed for BMD at 12 months posttherapy. Data from these patients showed an average decrease of 2.5% in BMD compared to pretreatment values. These data suggest a possibility of partial reversibility.

CHANGES IN LABORATORY VALUES DURING TREATMENT

Plasma Enzymes: Elevation of liver enzymes (AST, ALT) have been reported in female patients exposed to Goserelin Acetate (representing less than 1% of all patients). There was no other evidence of abnormal liver function. Causality between these changes and Goserelin Acetate have not been established.

Lipids: In a controlled trial, Goserelin Acetate therapy resulted in a minor, but statistically significant effect on serum lipids. In patients treated for endometriosis at 6 months following initiation of therapy, danazol treatment resulted in a mean increase in LDL cholesterol of 33.3 mg/dL and a decrease in HDL cholesterol of 21.3 mg/dL compared to increases of 21.3 and 2.7 mg/dL in LDL cholesterol and HDL cholesterol, respectively, for Goserelin Acetate-treated patients. Triglycerides increased by 8.0 mg/dL in Goserelin Acetate-treated patients compared to a decrease of 8.9 mg/dL in danazol-treated patients. In patients treated for endometriosis, Goserelin Acetate increased total cholesterol and LDL cholesterol during 6 months of treatment. However, Goserelin Acetate therapy resulted in HDL cholesterol levels which were significantly higher relative to danazol therapy. At the end of 6 months of treatment, HDL cholesterol fractions (HDL_2 and HDL_3) were decreased by 13.5 and 7.7 mg/dL, respectively, for danazol-treated patients compared to treatment increases of 1.9 and 0.8 mg/dL, respectively, for Goserelin Acetate treated patients.

OVERDOSAGE

The pharmacologic properties of Goserelin Acetate and its mode of administration make accidental or intentional overdosage unlikely. There is no experience of overdosage from clinical trials. Animal studies indicate that no increased pharmacologic effect occurred at higher doses or more frequent administration. Subcutaneous doses of the drug as high as 1 mg/kg/day in rats and dogs did not produce any nonendocrine related sequelae; this dose is greater than 400 times that proposed for human use. If overdosage occurs, it should be managed symptomatically.

DOSAGE AND ADMINISTRATION

Goserelin Acetate, at a dose of 3.6 mg, should be administered subcutaneously every 28 days into the upper abdominal wall using sterile technique under the supervision of a physician. While a delay of a few days is permissible, every effort should be made to adhere to the 28-day schedule.

For the management of advanced prostate cancer, Goserelin Acetate is intended for long-term administration unless clinically inappropriate.

For the management of endometriosis, the recommended duration of administration is 6 months.

Currently, there are no clinical data on the effect of treatment of benign gynecological conditions with Goserelin Acetate for periods in excess of 6 months.

Retreatment cannot be recommended for the management of endometriosis since safety data for retreatment are not available. If the symptoms of endometriosis recur after a course of therapy, and further treatment with Goserelin Acetate is contemplated, consideration should be given to monitoring bone mineral density.

No dosage adjustment is necessary for patients with renal or hepatic impairment.

Administration Technique: The proper method of administration of Goserelin Acetate is described in the instructions that follow.

1. The package should be inspected for damage prior to opening. If the package is damaged, the syringe should not be used. Do not remove the sterile syringe from the package until immediately before use. Examine the syringe for damage, and check that Goserelin Acetate is visible in the translucent chamber.

2. Clean an area of skin of the upper abdominal wall with an alcohol swab. (A local anesthetic may be used in the normal fashion at the option of the administrator or patient.)

3. Grasp red plastic safety clip tab, pull out and away from needle, and discard immediately. Then remove needle cover.

4. Using an aseptic technique, stretch or pinch the patient's skin with one hand, and grip the needle with your fingers around the barrel. Insert the hypodermic needle into the subcutaneous tissue.

Note: The Goserelin Acetate syringe cannot be used for aspiration. If the hypodermic needle penetrates a large vessel, blood will be seen instantly in the syringe chamber. If a vessel is penetrated, withdraw the needle and inject with a new syringe elsewhere.

5. Change the direction of the needle so it parallels the abdominal wall. Push the needle in until the barrel hub touches the patient's skin. Withdraw the needle one centimeter to create a space to discharge Goserelin Acetate. Fully depress the plunger to discharge Goserelin Acetate.

6. Withdraw the needle. Then bandage the site. Confirm discharge of Goserelin Acetate by ensuring tip of the plunger is visible within the tip of the needle. Dispose of the used needle and syringe in a safe manner.

Note: In the unlikely event of the need to surgically remove Goserelin Acetate, it may be localized by ultrasound.

Storage: Store at room temperature (do not exceed 25°C).

◆ RATED THERAPEUTICALLY EQUIVALENT; ◇ THERAPEUTIC EQUIVALENCE UNCONFIRMED; ○ UNRATED

J CODES
Per 3.6 mg SC—J9202

HOW SUPPLIED
IMPLANT: 3.6 MG

BRAND/MANUFACTURER	NDC	SIZE	AWP
○ BRAND			
ZOLADEX: Zeneca	00310-0960-36	1s	$344.76

Gramicidin/Neomycin Sulfate/ Polymyxin B Sulfate, Ophthalmic

DESCRIPTION
Gramicidin/Neomycin Sulfate/Polymyxin B Sulfate Ophthalmic Solution is a sterile antimicrobial solution for ophthalmic use. Each mL contains: Polymyxin B Sulfate 10,000 units, Neomycin Sulfate equivalent to 1.75 mg Neomycin base and Gramicidin 0.025 mg. The vehicle contains alcohol 0.5% and thimerosal 0.001% (added as a preservative).

Polymyxin B Sulfate is the Sulfate salt of Polymyxin B_1 and B_2 which are produced by the growth of *Bacillus polymyxa* (Prazmowski) Migula (Fam. Bacillaceae). It has a potency of not less than 6,000 Polymyxin B units per mg, calculated on an anhydrous basis.

Neomycin Sulfate is the Sulfate salt of Neomycin B and C, which are produced by the growth of *Streptomyces fradiae* Waksman (Fam. Streptomycetaceae). It has a potency equivalent of not less than 600 μg of Neomycin standard per mg, calculated on an anhydrous basis.

Gramicidin (also called Gramicidin D) is a mixture of three pairs of antibacterial substances (Gramicidin A, B and C) produced by the growth of *Bacillus brevis* Dubos (Fam. Bacillaceae). It has a potency of not less than 900 μg of standard Gramicidin per mg.

CLINICAL PHARMACOLOGY
A wide range of antibacterial action is provided by the overlapping spectra of Polymyxin B Sulfate, Neomycin and Gramicidin. The spectrum of action encompasses most bacterial pathogens capable of causing external infections of the eye and its adnexa.

Polymyxin B is bactericidal for a variety of gram-negative organisms. It increases the permeability of the bacterial cell membrane by interacting with the phospholipid components of the membrane.

Neomycin is bactericidal for many gram-positive and gram-negative organisms. It is an aminoglycoside antibiotic which inhibits protein synthesis by binding with ribosomal RNA and causing misreading of the bacterial genetic code.

Gramicidin is bactericidal for a variety of gram-positive organisms. It increases the permeability of the bacterial cell membrane to inorganic cations by forming a network of channels through the normal lipid bilayer of the membrane. When used topically, Polymyxin B, Neomycin and Gramicidin are rarely irritating, and absorption from the intact skin or mucous membrane is insignificant. The incidence of skin sensitization to this combination has been shown to be low on normal skin.[1,2] Since these antibiotics are seldom used systemically, the patient is spared sensitization to those antibiotics which might later be required systemically.

Microbiology: Polymyxin B Sulfate, Neomycin Sulfate and Gramicidin together are considered active against the following microorganisms: *Staphylococcus aureus*, streptococci, including *Streptococcus pneumoniae, Escherichia coli, Haemophilus influenzae, Klebsiella-Enterobacter* species, *Neisseria* species and *Pseudomonas aeruginosa*. The product does not provide adequate coverage against *Serratia marcescens.*

INDICATIONS AND USAGE
Gramicidin/Neomycin Sulfate/Polymyxin B Sulfate Ophthalmic Solution is indicated in the short-term treatment of superficial external ocular infections caused by organisms susceptible to one or more of the antibiotics contained therein.

CONTRAINDICATIONS
This product is contraindicated in those individuals who have shown hypersensitivity to any of its components.

WARNINGS
The manifestations of sensitization to Neomycin are usually itching, reddening and edema of the conjunctiva and eyelid. It may be manifest simply as a failure to heal. During long-term use of Neomycin-containing products, periodic examination for such signs is advisable, and the patient should be told to discontinue the product if they are observed. These symptoms subside quickly on withdrawing the medication. Neomycin-containing applications should be avoided for the patient thereafter.

PRECAUTIONS
General: As with other antibiotic preparations, prolonged use may result in overgrowth of nonsusceptible organisms including fungi. Appropriate measures should be taken if this occurs.

Allergic cross-reactions may occur which could prevent the use of any or all of the following antibiotics for the treatment of future infections: kanamycin, paromomycin, streptomycin, and possibly gentamicin.

Information for Patients: If redness, irritation, swelling or pain persists or increases, discontinue use and contact your physician.

Avoid contaminating the applicator tip with material from the eye, fingers, or other source. This caution is necessary if the sterility of the drops is to be preserved.

ADVERSE REACTIONS
Neomycin Sulfate may cause cutaneous and conjunctival sensitization. A precise incidence of hypersensitivity reactions (primarily skin rash) due to topical Neomycin is not known.

DOSAGE AND ADMINISTRATION
The suggested dosage is one or two drops in the affected eye two to four times daily, or more frequently as required, for 7 to 10 days. In acute infections, initiate therapy with one or two drops every 15 to 30 minutes, reducing the frequency of instillation gradually as the infection is controlled.

Store at 15°-25°C (59°-77°F) and protect from light.

REFERENCES
1. Leyden JJ, and Kligman AM. Contact Dermatitis to Neomycin Sulfate. JAMA 242(12): 1276-1278, 1979. 2. Prystowsky SD, Allen AM, Smith RW, Nonomura JH, Odom RB and Akers WA. Allergic Contact Hypersensitivity to Nickel, Neomycin, Ethylenediamine, and Benzocaine. Arch Dermatol 115:959-962, 1979.

HOW SUPPLIED
DROP:

BRAND/MANUFACTURER	NDC	SIZE	AWP
◆ GENERICS			
AK-SPORE: Akorn	17478-0790-11	10 ml	$8.69

DROP: 25 MCG-1.75 MG-10,000 U

AVERAGE UNIT PRICE (AVAILABLE SIZES)		GENERIC A-RATED AVERAGE PRICE (GAAP)	
BRAND	$1.55	10 ml	$6.50
GENERIC	$0.75		

BRAND/MANUFACTURER	NDC	SIZE	AWP
◆ BRAND			
NEOSPORIN: Burr Wellcome	00081-0728-69	10 ml	$15.50
◆ GENERICS			
OCUTRICIN: Bausch&Lomb Pharm	24208-0790-62	10 ml	$4.34
URL	00677-0906-21	10 ml	$4.45
NEOCIDIN: Major	00904-3016-10	10 ml	$4.50
OCUTRICIN HC: Moore,H.L.	00839-6662-90	10 ml	$4.52
Parmed	00349-8328-70	10 ml	$4.60
Geneva	00781-7250-70	10 ml	$7.31
Steris	00402-0747-10	10 ml	$7.90
Schein	00364-7375-54	10 ml	$7.90
Goldline	00182-1549-63	10 ml	$8.10
Aligen	00405-6110-10	10 ml	$8.32
Rugby	00536-1890-70	10 ml	$9.56
OCUTRICIN: Bausch&Lomb Pharm	24208-0790-59	2 ml 12s	$44.88

Granisetron Hydrochloride

DESCRIPTION
Granisetron Hydrochloride Injection is an antinauseant and antiemetic agent. Chemically it is endo-N-(9 methyl-9-azabicyclo [3.3.1] non-3-yl)-1-methyl-1H-indazole-3-carboxamide hydrochloride with a molecular weight of 348.9 (312.4 free base).

Granisetron Hydrochloride is a white to off-white solid that is readily soluble in water and normal saline at 20°C. Granisetron Hydrochloride Injection is a clear, colorless, sterile, nonpyrogenic, aqueous solution for intravenous administration.

Each 1 mL of preservative free aqueous solution contains 1.12 mg Granisetron Hydrochloride equivalent to granisetron, 1.0 mg and sodium chloride, 9.0 mg. The solution's pH ranges from 4.7 to 7.3.

Following is its chemical structure:

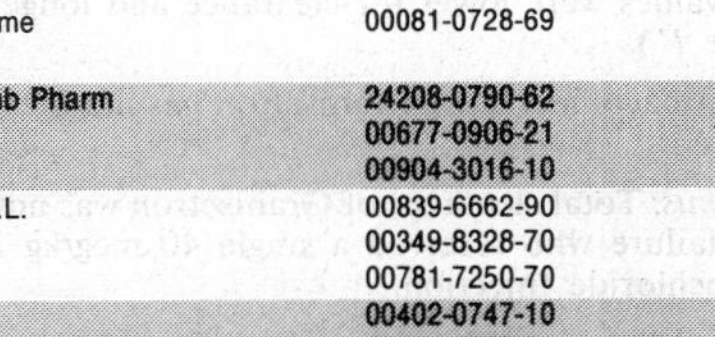

CLINICAL PHARMACOLOGY
Granisetron is a selective 5-hydroxytryptamine₃ (5-HT₃) receptor antagonist with little or no affinity for other serotonin receptors, including 5-HT₁; 5-HT₁A; 5-HT₁B/C; 5-HT₂; for alpha₁; alpha₂- or beta-adrenoreceptors; for dopamine-D₂; or for histamine-H₁; benzodiazepine; picrotoxin, or opioid receptors.

Serotonin receptors of the 5-HT$_3$ type are located peripherally on vagal nerve terminals and centrally in the chemoreceptor trigger zone of the area postrema. During chemotherapy-induced vomiting, mucosal enterochromaffin cells release serotonin, which stimulates 5-HT$_3$ receptors. This evokes vagal afferent discharge, inducing vomiting. Animal studies demonstrate that, in binding to 5-HT$_3$ receptors, Granisetron blocks serotonin stimulation and subsequent vomiting after emetogenic stimuli such as cisplatin. In the ferret animal model, a single granisetron injection prevented vomiting due to high-dose cisplatin or arrested vomiting within 5 to 30 seconds.

In most human studies, Granisetron has had little effect on blood pressure, heart rate or ECG. No evidence of an effect on plasma prolactin or aldosterone concentrations has been found in other studies.

Granisetron Hydrochloride Injection exhibited no effect on oro-cecal transit time in normal volunteers given a single intravenous infusion of 50 mcg/kg or 200 mcg/kg. Single and multiple oral doses slowed colonic transit in normal volunteers.

PHARMACOKINETICS
In adult cancer patients undergoing chemotherapy and in volunteers, infusion of a single 40 mcg/kg dose of Granisetron Hydrochloride Injection produced the following mean pharmacokinetic data: (See related table).

There was high inter and intrasubject variability noted in these studies. No difference in mean AUC was found between males and females, although males had a higher C$_{max}$ generally.

Granisetron metabolism involves N-demethylation and aromatic ring oxidation followed by conjugation. Animal studies suggest that some of the metabolites may also have 5-HT$_3$ receptor antagonist activity.

Clearance is predominantly by hepatic metabolism. In normal volunteers, approximately 12% of the administered dose is eliminated unchanged in the urine in 48 hours. The remainder of the dose is excreted as metabolites, 49% in the urine and 34% in the feces.

In vitro liver microsomal studies show that Granisetron's major route of metabolism is inhibited by ketoconazole, suggestive of metabolism mediated by the cytochrome P-450 3A subfamily.

Plasma protein binding is approximately 65% and Granisetron distributes freely between plasma and red blood cells.

Elderly: The ranges of the pharmacokinetic parameters in elderly volunteers (mean age 71 years), given a single 40 mcg/kg intravenous dose of Granisetron Hydrochloride Injection, were generally similar to those in younger healthy volunteers; mean values were lower for clearance and longer for half-life in the elderly (see "Table 1").

Pediatrics: The pharmacokinetics of Granisetron has not been adequately studied in children.

Renal Failure Patients: Total clearance of Granisetron was not affected in patients with severe renal failure who received a single 40 mcg/kg intravenous dose of Granisetron Hydrochloride Injection.

Hepatically Impaired Patients: A pharmacokinetic study in patients with hepatic impairment due to neoplastic liver involvement showed that total clearance was approximately halved compared to patients without hepatic impairment. Given the wide variability in pharmacokinetic parameters noted in patients and the good tolerance of doses well above the recommended 10 mcg/kg dose, dosage adjustment in patients with possible hepatic, functional impairment is not necessary.

CLINICAL TRIALS
Granisetron Hydrochloride Injection has been shown to prevent nausea and vomiting associated with single-day and repeat cycle cancer chemotherapy.

SINGLE-DAY CHEMOTHERAPY
Cisplatin-Based Chemotherapy: In a double-blind, placebo controlled study in 28 cancer patients, Granisetron Hydrochloride Injection, administered as a single intravenous infusion of 40 mcg/kg, was significantly more effective than placebo in preventing nausea and vomiting induced by cisplatin chemotherapy. See Table 2.

Table 2

PREVENTION OF CHEMOTHERAPY-INDUCED NAUSEA AND VOMITING—SINGLE-DAY CISPLATIN THERAPY[1]

	Granisetron Hydrochloride Injection	Placebo	P-Value
Number of Patients	14	14	
Response Over 24 Hours			
Complete Response[2]	93%	7%	<0.001
No Vomiting	93%	14%	<0.001
No More Than Mild Nausea	93%	7%	<0.001

1. Cisplatin administration began within 10 minutes of Granisetron Hydrochloride Injection infusion and continued for 1.5 to 3.0 hours. Mean cisplatin dose was 86 mg/m^2 in the Granisetron Hydrochloride Injection group and 80 mg/m^3 in the placebo group.
2. No vomiting and no moderate or severe nausea.

Granisetron Hydrochloride Injection was also evaluated in a randomized dose response study of cancer patients receiving cisplatin $\geq$ 75 mg/m^2. Additional chemotherapeutic agents included: anthracyclines, carboplatin, cytostatic antibiotics, folic acid derivatives, methylhydrazine, nitrogen mustard analogs, podophyllotoxin derivatives, pyrimidine analogs and vinca alkaloids. Granisetron Hydrochloride Injection doses of 10 and 40 mcg/kg were superior to 2 mcg/kg in preventing cisplatin-induced nausea and vomiting, but 40 mcg/kg was not significantly superior to 10 mcg/kg. See Table 3. (See related table).

Granisetron Hydrochloride Injection was also evaluated in a double-blind, randomized dose response study of 353 patients stratified for high ($\geq$ 80 to 120 mg/m^2) or low (50 to 79 mg/m^2) cisplatin dose. Response rates of patients for both cisplatin strata are given in Table 4. (See related table).

For both the low and high cisplatin strata, the 10, 20 and 40 mcg/kg doses were more effective than the 5 mcg/kg dose in preventing nausea and vomiting within 24 hours of chemotherapy administration. The 10 mcg/kg dose was at least as effective as the higher doses.

Moderately Emetogenic Chemotherapy: Granisetron Hydrochloride Injection, 40 mcg/kg, was compared with the combination of chlorpromazine (50 to 200 mg/24 hours) and dexamethasone (12 mg) in patients treated with moderately emetogenic chemotherapy, including primarily carboplatin > 300 mg/m^2, cisplatin 20 to 50 mg/m^2 and cyclophosphamide > 600 mg/m^2. Granisetron Hydrochloride Injection was superior to the chlorpromazine regimen in preventing nausea and vomiting. See Table 5.

Table 5

PREVENTION OF CHEMOTHERAPY-INDUCED NAUSEA AND VOMITING—SINGLE-DAY MODERATELY EMETOGENIC CHEMOTHERAPY

	Granisetron Hydrochloride Injection	Chlorpromazine[1]	P-Value
Number of Patients	133	133	
Response Over 24 hours			
Complete Response[2]	68%	47%	<0.001
No Vomiting	73%	53%	<0.001
No More Than Mild Nausea	77%	59%	<0.001

1. Patients also received dexamethasone, 12 mg.
2. No vomiting and no moderate or severe nausea.

Table 1

PHARMACOKINETIC PARAMETERS IN ADULT CANCER PATIENTS UNDERGOING CHEMOTHERAPY AND IN VOLUNTEERS FOLLOWING A SINGLE INTRAVENOUS 40 MCG/KG DOSE OF GRANISETRON HYDROCHLORIDE INJECTION

	Peak Plasma Concentration (ng/mL)	Terminal Phase Plasma Half-life (h)	Total Clearance (L/h/kg)	Volume of Distribution (L/kg)
Cancer Patients				
Mean	63.8*	8.95*	0.38*	3.07*
Range	18.0 to 176	0.90 to 31.1	0.14 to 1.54	0.85 to 10.4
Volunteers				
21 to 42 years				
Mean	64.3†	4.91†	0.79†	3.04†
Range	11.2 to 182	0.88 to 15.2	0.20 to 2.56	1.68 to 6.13
65 to 81 years				
Mean	57.0†	7.69†	0.44†	3.97†
Range	14.6 to 153	2.65 to 17.7	0.17 to 1.06	1.75 to 7.01

* 5 - minute infusion.
† 3 - minute infusion.

In other studies of moderately emetogenic chemotherapy, no significant difference in efficacy was found between Granisetron Hydrochloride doses of 40 mcg/kg and 160 mcg/kg doses.

REPEAT-CYCLE CHEMOTHERAPY
In an uncontrolled trial, 512 cancer patients received Granisetron Hydrochloride Injection, 40 mcg/kg, prophylactically, for two cycles of chemotherapy, 224 patients received it for at least four cycles and 108 patients received it for at least six cycles. Granisetron Hydrochloride Injection efficacy remained relatively constant over the first six repeat cycles, with complete response rates (no vomiting and no moderate or severe nausea in 24 hours) of 60% to 69%. No patients were studied for more than 15 cycles.

PEDIATRIC STUDIES
A randomized double-blind study evaluated the 24-hour response of 80 pediatric cancer patients (age 2 to 16 years) to Granisetron Hydrochloride Injection 10, 20 or 40 mcg/kg. Patients were treated with cisplatin $\geq$ 60 mg/m^2, cytarabine $\geq$ 3 g/m^2, cyclophosphamide $\geq$ 1 g/m^2 or nitrogen mustard $\geq$ 6 mg/m^2. See Table 6.

Table 6
PREVENTION OF CHEMOTHERAPY-INDUCED NAUSEA AND VOMITING IN PEDIATRIC PATIENTS

	Granisetron Hydrochloride Injection Dose (mcg/kg)		
	10	20	40
Number of Patients	29	26	25
Median Number of Vomiting Episodes	2	3	1
Complete Response Over 24 Hours[1]	21%	31%	32%

1. No vomiting and no moderate or severe nausea.

Table 3
PREVENTION OF CHEMOTHERAPY-INDUCED NAUSEA AND VOMITING—SINGLE-DAY HIGH-DOSE CISPLATIN THERAPY[1]

	Granisetron Hydrochloride Injection (mcg/kg)			P-Value (vs. 2 mcg/kg)	
	2	10	40	10	40
Number of Patients	52	52	53		
Response Over 24 Hours					
Complete Response[2]	31%	62%	68	<0.002	<0.001
No Vomiting	38%	65%	74%	<0.001	<0.001
No More Than Mild Nausea	58%	75%	79%	NS	0.007

1. Cisplatin administration began within 10 minutes of Granisetron Hydrochloride Injection infusion and continued for 2.6 hours (mean). Mean cisplatin doses were 96 to 99 mg/m^2.
2. No vomiting and no moderate or severe nausea.

Table 4.
PREVENTION OF CHEMOTHERAPY-INDUCED NAUSEA AND VOMITING—SINGLE-DAY HIGH-DOSE AND LOW-DOSE CISPLATIN THERAPY[1]

	Granisetron Hydrochloride Injection (mcg/kg)				P-Value (vs. 5 mcg/kg)		
	5	10	20	40	10	20	40
High-Dose Cisplatin							
Number of Patients	40	49	48	47			
Response Over 24 Hours							
Complete Response[2]	18%	41%	40%	47%	0.018	0.025	0.004
No Vomiting	28%	47%	44%	53%	NS	NS	0.016
No Nausea	15%	35%	38%	43%	0.036	0.019	0.005
Low-Dose Cisplatin							
Number of Patients	42	41	40	46			
Response Over 24 Hours							
Complete Response[2]	29%	56%	58%	41%	0.012	0.009	NS
No Vomiting	36%	63%	65%	43%	0.012	0.008	NS
No Nausea	29%	56%	38%	33%	0.012	NS	NS

1. Cisplatin administration began within 10 minutes of Granisetron Hydrochloride Injection infusion and continued for 2 hours (mean). Mean cisplatin doses were 64 and 98 mg/m^2 for low and high strata.
2. No vomiting and no use of rescue antiemetic.

A second pediatric study compared Granisetron Hydrochloride Injection 20 mcg/kg to chlorpromazine plus dexamethasone in 88 patients treated with ifosfamide > 3 g/m^2/day for two or three days. Granisetron Hydrochloride Injection was administered on each day of ifosfamide treatment. At 24 hours, 22% of Granisetron Hydrochloride Injection patients achieved complete response (no vomiting and no moderate or severe nausea in 24 hours) compared with 10% on the chlorpromazine regimen. The median number of vomiting episodes with Granisetron Hydrochloride Injection was 1.5; with chlorpromazine it was 7.0.

INDICATIONS AND USAGE
Granisetron Hydrochloride Injection is indicated for the prevention of nausea and vomiting associated with initial and repeat courses of emetogenic cancer therapy, including high-dose cisplatin.

UNLABELED USES
Granisetron Hydrochloride is used alone or as an adjunct in the treatment of postoperative nausea.

CONTRAINDICATIONS
Granisetron Hydrochloride Injection is contraindicated in patients with known hypersensitivity to the drug.

PRECAUTIONS
DRUG INTERACTIONS
Granisetron does not induce or inhibit the cytochrome P-450 drug-metabolizing enzyme system. There have been no definitive drug-drug interaction studies to examine pharmacokinetic or pharmacodynamic interaction with other drugs, but in humans, Granisetron Hydrochloride Injection has been safely administered with drugs representing benzodiazepines, neuroleptics and anti-ulcer medications commonly prescribed with antiemetic treatments. Granisetron Hydrochloride Injection also does not appear to interact with emetogenic cancer chemotherapies. Because Granisetron is metabolized by hepatic cytochrome P-450 drug-metabolizing enzymes, inducers or inhibitors of these enzymes may change the clearance and, hence, the half-life of Granisetron.

CARCINOGENESIS, MUTAGENESIS, IMPAIRMENT OF FERTILITY
In a 24-month carcinogenicity study, rats were treated orally with Granisetron 1, 5 or 50 mg/kg/day (6, 30 or 300 mg/m^2/day). The 50 mg/kg/day dose was reduced

to 25 mg/kg/day (150 mg/m^2/day) during week 59 due to toxicity. For a 50 kg person of average height (1.46m^2 body surface area), these doses represent 16, 81 and 405 times the recommended clinical dose (0.37 mg/m^2, i.v.) on a body surface area basis. There was a statistically significant increase in the incidence of hepatocellular carcinomas and adenomas in males treated with 5 mg/kg/day (30 mg/m^2/day, 81 times the recommended human dose based on body surface area) and above, and in females treated with 25 mg/kg/day (150 mg/m^2/day, 405 times the recommended human dose based on body surface area). No increase in liver tumors was observed at a dose of 1 mg/kg/day (6 mg/m^2/day, 16 times the recommended human dose based on body surface area) in males and 5 mg/kg/day (30 mg/m^2/day, 81 times the recommended human dose based on body surface area) in females. In a 12-month oral toxicity study, treatment with Granisetron 100 mg/kg/day (600 mg/m^2/day, 1622 times the recommended human dose based on body surface area) produced hepatocellular adenomas in male and female rats while no such tumors were found in the control rats. A 24-month mouse carcinogenicity study of Granisetron did not show a statistically significant increase in tumor incidence, but the study was not conclusive.

Because of the tumor findings in rat studies, Granisetron Hydrochloride Injection should be prescribed only at the dose and for the indication recommended (see "Indications And Usage" and "Dosage and Administration").

Granisetron was not mutagenic in in vitro Ames test and mouse lymphoma cell forward mutation assay, and in vivo mouse micronucleus test and in vitro and ex vivo rat hepatocyte UDS assays. It, however, produced a significant increase in UDS in HeLa cells in vitro and a significant increased incidence of cells with polyploidy in an in vitro human lymphocyte chromosomal aberration test.

Granisetron at subcutaneous doses up to 6 mg/kg/day (36 mg/m^2/day, 97 times the recommended human dose based on body surface area) was found to have no effect on fertility and reproductive performance of male and female rats.

PREGNANCY
Teratogenic Effects: Pregnancy Category B: Reproduction studies have been performed in pregnant rats at intravenous doses up to 9 mg/kg/day (54 mg/m^2/day, 146 times the recommended human dose based on body surface area) and pregnant rabbits at intravenous doses up to 3 mg/kg/day (35.4 mg/m^2/day, 96 times the recommended human dose based on body surface area) and have revealed no evidence of impaired fertility or harm to the fetus due to Granisetron. There are, however, no adequate and well-controlled studies in pregnant women. Because animal reproduction studies are not always predictive of human response, this drug should be used during pregnancy only if clearly needed.

NURSING MOTHERS
It is not known whether Granisetron is excreted in human milk. Because many drugs are excreted in human milk, caution should be exercised when Granisetron Hydrochloride Injection is administered to a nursing woman.

PEDIATRIC USE
See "Dosage And Administration" for use in children 2 to 16 years of age. Safety and effectiveness in children under 2 years of age have not been established.

GERIATRIC USE
During clinical trials, 713 patients 65 years of age or older received Granisetron Hydrochloride Injection. Effectiveness and safety were similar in patients of various ages.

ADVERSE REACTIONS
Table 7 gives the comparative frequencies of the five most commonly reported adverse events (>3%) in patients, receiving Granisetron Hydrochloride Injection, in single-day chemotherapy trials. These patients received chemotherapy, primarily cisplatin, and intravenous fluids during the 24-hour period following Granisetron Hydrochloride Injection administration. Events were generally recorded over seven days post-Granisetron Hydrochloride Injection administration. In the absence of a placebo group, there is uncertainty as to how many of these events should be attributed to Granisetron Hydrochloride except for headache, which was clearly more frequent than in comparison groups.

Table 7
PRINCIPAL ADVERSE EVENTS IN CLINICAL TRIALS—
SINGLE-DAY CHEMOTHERAPY

	Number of Patients with Event	
	Granisetron Hydrochloride Injection 40 mcg/kg (n = 1,268)	Comparator[1] (n = 422)
Headache	14%	6%
Asthenia	5%	6%
Somnolence	4%	15%
Diarrhea	4%	6%
Constipation	3%	3%

1. Metoclopramide/dexamethasone and phenothiazines/dexamethasone.
In over 3,000 patients receiving Granisetron Hydrochloride Injection (2 to 160 mcg/kg) in single-day and multiple-day clinical trials with emetogenic cancer therapies, adverse events, other than those in Table 7, were observed; attribution of many of these events to Granisetron Hydrochloride is uncertain:

Hepatic: In comparative trials, mainly with cisplatin regimens, elevations of AST and ALT (> 2 times the upper limit of normal) following administration of Granisetron Hydrochloride Injection occurred in 2.8% and 3.3% of patients, respectively. These frequencies were not significantly different from those seen with comparators (AST: 2.1%; ALT: 2.4%).

Cardiovascular: Hypertension (2%); hypotension, arrhythmias such as sinus bradycardia, atrial fibrillation, varying degrees of A-V block, ventricular ectopy including non-sustained tachycardia, and ECG abnormalities have been observed rarely.

Central Nervous System: Agitation, anxiety, CNS stimulation and insomnia were seen in less than 2% of patients. Extrapyramidal syndrome occurred rarely and only in the presence of other drugs associated with this syndrome.

Hypersensitivity: Rare cases of anaphylactoid reactions, other allergic reactions and skin rashes have been reported.

Other: Taste disorder (2%), fever (3%). In multiple-day comparative studies, fever occurred more frequently with Granisetron Hydrochloride Injection (8.6%) than with comparative drugs (3.4%, P < 0.014), which usually included dexamethasone.

OVERDOSAGE
There is no specific antidote for Granisetron Hydrochloride Injection overdosage. In case of overdosage, symptomatic treatment should be given. Overdosage of up to 38.5 mg of Granisetron Hydrochloride Injection has been reported without symptoms or only the occurrence of a slight headache.

DOSAGE AND ADMINISTRATION
The recommended dosage for Granisetron Hydrochloride Injection is 10 mcg/kg infused intravenously over 5 minutes, beginning within 30 minutes before initiation of chemotherapy, and only on the day(s) chemotherapy is given.

Pediatric Use: The recommended dose in children 2 to 16 years of age is 10 mcg/kg (see "Clinical Trials"). Children under 2 years of age have not been studied.

Use in the Elderly, Renal Failure Patients or Hepatically Impaired Patients: No dosage adjustment is recommended. (See "Clinical Pharmacology Pharmacokinetics".)

INFUSION PREPARATION
Granisetron Hydrochloride Injection should be diluted in 0.9% Sodium Chloride or 5% Dextrose to a total volume of 20 to 50 mL.

STABILITY
Intravenous infusion of Granisetron Hydrochloride Injection should be prepared at the time of administration. However, Granisetron Hydrochloride Injection has been shown to be stable for at least 24 hours when diluted in 0.9% Sodium Chloride or 5% Dextrose and stored at room temperature under normal lighting conditions.

As a general precaution Granisetron Hydrochloride Injection should not be mixed in solution with other drugs. Parenteral drug products should be inspected visually for particulate matter and discoloration before administration whenever solution and container permit.

Store vials at 30°C (86°F) or below. Do not freeze. Protect from light.

HOW SUPPLIED
INJECTION:

BRAND/MANUFACTURER	NDC	SIZE	AWP
○ BRAND KYTRIL: SK Beecham Pharm	00029-4149-01	1 ml	$166.00

Granulex SEE CASTOR OIL/PERU BALSAM/TRYPSIN

GranuMed SEE CASTOR OIL/PERU BALSAM/TRYPSIN

Grass Treatment Set SEE ALLERGENIC EXTRACTS

Grifulvin V SEE GRISEOFULVIN

Grisactin SEE GRISEOFULVIN

Griseofulvin

DESCRIPTION
Griseofulvin is an oral fungistatic antibiotic for the treatment of superficial mycoses. It is derived from a species of Penicillium.

◆ RATED THERAPEUTICALLY EQUIVALENT; ◇ THERAPEUTIC EQUIVALENCE UNCONFIRMED; ○ UNRATED

Each capsule contains Griseofulvin:
250 mg crystalized/particulate

Each 5 mL of suspension contains Griseofulvin:
125 mg microsize

Each tablet contains Griseofulvin:
125 mg ultramicrosize
250 mg microsize
250 mg ultramicrosize
330 mg ultramicrosize
500 mg crystalized/particulate
500 mg microsize

Following is its chemical structure:

CLINICAL PHARMACOLOGY

Griseofulvin microsize acts systemically to inhibit the growth of *Trichophyton*, *Microsporum* and *Epidermophyton* genera of fungi. It has no effect on bacteria or on other genera of fungi. Following oral administration, fungistatic amounts are deposited in the keratin precursor cells. Griseofulvin has a greater affinity for diseased tissue. The drug is tightly bound to the new keratin which becomes highly resistant to fungal invasions.

Griseofulvin absorption from the gastrointestinal tract varies considerably among individuals, mainly because of insolubility of the drug in aqueous media of the upper G.I. tract. The peak serum level found in fasting adults given 0.5 g occurs at about four hours and ranges between 0.5 and 2.0 mcg/mL.

It should be noted that some individuals are consistently "poor absorbers" and tend to attain lower blood levels at all times. This may explain unsatisfactory therapeutic results in some patients. Better blood levels can probably be attained in most patients if the tablets are administered after a meal with a high fat content.

The efficiency of gastrointestinal absorption of ultramicrocrystalline Griseofulvin is approximately one and one-half times that of the conventional microsize Griseofulvin. This factor permits the oral intake of two-thirds as much ultramicrocrystalline Griseofulvin as the microsize form. However, there is currently no evidence that this lower dose confers any significant clinical difference with regard to safety and/or efficacy.

INDICATIONS AND USAGE

Major indications for Griseofulvin are:
Tinea capitis (ringworm of the scalp)
Tinea corporis (ringworm of the body)
Tinea pedis (athlete's foot)
Tinea unguium (onychomycosis ringworm of the nails):
Tinea cruris (ringworm of the thigh)
Tinea barbae (barber's itch)
Griseofulvin inhibits the growth of those genera of fungi that commonly cause ringworm infections of the hair, skin, and nails, such as:
Trichophyton rubrum
Trichophyton tonsurans
Trichophyton mentagrophytes
Trichophyton interdigitalis
Trichophyton verrucosum
Trichophyton sulphureum
Trichophyton schoenleini
Microsporum audouini
Microsporum canis
Microsporum gypseum
Epidermophyton floccosum
Trichophyton megnini
Trichophyton gallinae
Trichophyton crateriform

Note: Prior to therapy, the type of fungi responsible for the infection should be identified. The use of the drug is not justified in minor or trivial infections which will respond to topical antifungal agents alone.
It is *not* effective in:
Bacterial infections
Candidiasis (Moniliasis)
Histoplasmosis
Actinomycosis
Sporotrichosis
Chromoblastomycosis
Coccidioidomycosis
North American Blastomycosis
Cryptococcosis (Torulosis)
Tinea versicolor
Nocardiosis

UNLABELED USES
Griseofulvin is used alone or as an adjunct in the treatment of shingles (herpes zoster infection), cutaneous lichen planus, and to retard the progression of progressive systemic sclerosis.

CONTRAINDICATIONS

This drug is contraindicated in patients with porphyria, hepatocellular failure, and in individuals with a history of hypersensitivity to Griseofulvin.

Two cases of conjoined twins have been reported in patients taking Griseofulvin during the first trimester of pregnancy. Griseofulvin should not be prescribed to pregnant patients or to women contemplating pregnancy.

WARNINGS

Prophylactic Usage: Safety and efficacy of Griseofulvin for prophylaxis of fungal infections have not been established.

Animal Toxicology: Chronic feeding of Griseofulvin, at levels ranging from 0.5-2.5% of the diet, resulted in the development of liver tumors in several strains of mice, particularly in males. Smaller particle sizes result in an enhanced effect. Lower oral dosage levels have not been tested. Subcutaneous administration of relatively small doses of Griseofulvin once a week during the first three weeks of life has also been reported to induce hepatomata in mice. Thyroid tumors, mostly adenomas but some carcinomas, have been reported in male rats receiving Griseofulvin at levels of 2.0%, 1.0%, and 0.2% of the diet, and in female rats receiving the two higher dose levels. Although studies in other animal species have not yielded evidence of tumorigenicity, these studies were not of adequate design to form a basis for conclusions in this regard.

In subacute toxicity studies, orally administered Griseofulvin produced hepatocellar necrosis in mice, but this has not been seen in other species. Disturbances in porphyrin metabolism have been reported in Griseofulvin-treated laboratory animals. Griseofulvin has been reported to have a colchicine-like effect on mitosis and cocarcinogenicity with methylcholanthrene in cutaneous tumor induction in laboratory animals.

Usage in Pregnancy: The safety of this drug during pregnancy has not been established.

Animal Reproduction Studies: Reports of animal studies in the Soviet literature state that a Griseofulvin preparation was found to be embryotoxic and teratogenic on oral administration to pregnant Wistar rats. Rat reproduction studies done thus far in the United States and Great Britain have been inconclusive in this regard, and additional animal reproduction studies are under way. Pups with abnormalities have been reported in the litters of a few bitches treated with Griseofulvin.

Suppression of spermatogenesis has been reported to occur in rats but investigation in man failed to confirm this.

PRECAUTIONS

Patients on prolonged therapy with any potent medication should be under close observation. Periodic monitoring of organ system function, including renal, hepatic and hemopoietic, should be done.

Since Griseofulvin is derived from species of Penicillium, the possibility of cross sensitivity with penicillin exists; however, known penicillin-sensitive patients have been treated without difficulty.

Since a photosensitivity reaction is occasionally associated with Griseofulvin therapy, patients should be warned to avoid exposure to intense natural or artificial sunlight. Should a photosensitivity reaction occur, lupus erythematosus may be aggravated. Lupus erythematosus, lupus-like syndromes, or exacerbation of existing lupus erythematosus have been reported in patients receiving Griseofulvin.

Drug Interactions: Griseofulvin decreases the activity of warfarin-type anticoagulants so that patients on warfarin-type anticoagulant therapy may require dosage adjustment of the anticoagulant during and after Griseofulvin therapy. Concomitant use of barbiturates usually depresses Griseofulvin activity and may necessitate raising the dosage.

Griseofulvin may potentiate an increase in hepatic enzymes that metabolize estrogens at an increased rate, including the estrogen component of oral contraceptives, thereby reducing the efficacy of oral contraceptives and increasing the incidence of breakthrough bleeding.

The effect of alcohol may be potentiated by Griseofulvin, producing such effects as tachycardia and flush.

ADVERSE REACTIONS

When adverse reactions occur, they are most commonly of the hypersensitivity type such as skin rashes, urticaria and rarely, angioneurotic edema, and may necessitate withdrawal of therapy and appropriate countermeasures. Paresthesias of the hands and feet have been reported rarely after extended therapy. Other side effects reported occasionally are oral thrush, nausea, vomiting, epigastric distress, diarrhea, headache, fatigue, dizziness, insomnia, mental confusion and impairment of performance of routine activities.

Proteinuria, nephrosis, leukopenia, hepatic toxicity, GI bleeding and menstrual irregularities have been reported rarely. Administration of the drug should be discontinued if granulocytopenia occurs.

When rare, serious reactions occur with griseofulvin, they are usually associated with high dosages, and/or long periods of therapy.

➤ SHOWN IN PRODUCT IDENTIFICATION GUIDE

DOSAGE AND ADMINISTRATION

Accurate diagnosis of the infecting organism is essential. Identification should be made either by direct microscopic examination of a mounting of infected tissue in a solution of potassium hydroxide or by culture on an appropriate medium.

Medication must be continued until the infecting organism is completely eradicated as indicated by appropriate clinical or laboratory examination. Representative treatment periods are tinea capitis, 4 to 6 weeks; tinea corporis, 2 to 4 weeks; tinea pedis, 4 to 8 weeks; tinea unguium—depending on rate of growth—fingernails, at least 4 months; toenails, at least 6 months.

General measures in regard to hygiene should be observed to control sources of infection or reinfection. Concomitant use of appropriate topical agents is usually required, particularly in treatment of tinea pedis since in some forms of athlete's foot, yeast and bacteria may be involved as well as fungi. Griseofulvin will not eradicate the bacterial or monilial infection.

DOSE

Microsize and crystalized particulate forms

Adults:	500 mg/day (125 mg q.i.d., 250 mg b.i.d., 500 mg once a day)	tinea corporis, tinea cruris, and tinea capitis
	(750 mg-1g/day)	for more difficult infections such as tinea pedis and tinea unguium
Children:	5 mg/lb/day (10 mg/kg/day)	
	30-50 lb — 125 mg - 250 mg	
	50+ lb — 250 mg - 500 mg (divided)	

Ultramicrosize form

Adults:	330-375 mg/day (single or divided)	tinea corporis, tinea cruris and tinea capitis
	660-750 mg/day	for more difficult infections such as tinea pedis and tinea unguium
Children:	3.3 mg/lb/day (6.6 mg/kg/day)	
	35-50 lb — 125 mg - 165 mg	
	50-75 lb — 165 mg - 250 mg	
	75 + lb — 250 mg - 330 mg	
with some brands,	35-60 lb — 125 mg - 187.5 mg	
	60 + lb — 187.5 mg - 375mg	

Children 2 years of age and younger: dosage has not been established.

Clinical experience with Griseofulvin in children with tinea capitis indicates that a single daily dose is effective. Clinical relapse will occur if the medication is not continued until the infecting organism is eradicated.

STORE AT ROOM TEMPERATURE
Dispense in a well-closed container as defined in the USP.

HOW SUPPLIED

GRISEOFULVIN, MICROCRYSTALLINE
CAPSULE: 250 MG

AVERAGE UNIT PRICE (AVAILABLE SIZES)

BRAND	$0.63

BRAND/MANUFACTURER	NDC	SIZE	AWP
◆ **BRAND**			
GRISACTIN 250: Wyeth-Ayerst	00046-0443-81	100s	$65.51
	00046-0443-85	500s	$306.50

SUSPENSION: 125 MG/5 ML

BRAND/MANUFACTURER	NDC	SIZE	AWP
○ **BRAND**			
GRIFULVIN V: Ortho Pharm	00062-0206-04	120 ml	$21.36

TABLETS: 250 MG

AVERAGE UNIT PRICE (AVAILABLE SIZES)

BRAND	$0.65

BRAND/MANUFACTURER	NDC	SIZE	AWP
◆ **BRAND**			
FULVICIN-U/F: Schering	00085-0948-03	60s	$39.95
GRIFULVIN V: Ortho Pharm	00062-0211-60	100s	$65.58
FULVICIN-U/F: Schering	00085-0948-06	250s	$157.67

TABLETS: 500 MG

AVERAGE UNIT PRICE (AVAILABLE SIZES)

BRAND	$1.03

BRAND/MANUFACTURER	NDC	SIZE	AWP
◆ **BRAND**			
FULVICIN-U/F: Schering	00085-0496-03	60s	$63.83
GRISACTIN 500: Wyeth-Ayerst	00046-0444-60	60s	$69.21
GRIFULVIN V: Ortho Pharm	00062-0214-60	100s	$101.76
FULVICIN-U/F: Schering	00085-0496-06	250s	$251.75
GRIFULVIN V: Ortho Pharm	00062-0214-70	500s	$441.36

GRISEOFULVIN, ULTRAMICROCRYSTALLINE
TABLETS: 125 MG

BRAND/MANUFACTURER	NDC	SIZE	AWP
◆ **BRAND**			
FULVICIN P/G: Schering	00085-0228-03	100s	$39.05
◆ **GENERICS**			
GRIS-PEG: Allergan Herbert	00023-0763-04	100s	$43.91

TABLETS: 165 MG

AVERAGE UNIT PRICE (AVAILABLE SIZES)		GENERIC A-RATED AVERAGE PRICE (GAAP)	
BRAND	$0.56	100s	$41.33
GENERIC	$0.41		

BRAND/MANUFACTURER	NDC	SIZE	AWP
◆ **BRAND**			
FULVICIN P/G: Schering	00085-0654-03	100s	$56.36
◆ **GENERICS**			
Sidmak	50111-0415-01	100s	$35.00
Major	00904-0723-60	100s	$47.65

TABLETS: 250 MG

AVERAGE UNIT PRICE (AVAILABLE SIZES)		GENERIC A-RATED AVERAGE PRICE (GAAP)	
BRAND	$0.77	100s	$75.92
GENERIC	$0.72		

BRAND/MANUFACTURER	NDC	SIZE	AWP
◆ **BRAND**			
FULVICIN P/G: Schering	00085-0507-03	100s	$76.61
◆ **GENERICS**			
GRIS-PEG: Allergan Herbert	00023-0773-04	100s	$73.35
GRISACTIN ULTRA: Wyeth-Ayerst	00046-0435-81	100s	$78.48
GRIS-PEG: Allergan Herbert	00023-0773-50	500s	$326.29

TABLETS: 330 MG

AVERAGE UNIT PRICE (AVAILABLE SIZES)		GENERIC A-RATED AVERAGE PRICE (GAAP)	
BRAND	$0.97	100s	$83.30
GENERIC	$0.83		

BRAND/MANUFACTURER	NDC	SIZE	AWP
◆ **BRAND**			
FULVICIN P/G: Schering	00085-0352-03	100s	$97.26
◆ **GENERICS**			
Sidmak	50111-0416-01	100s	$60.00
Major	00904-0724-60	100s	$82.25
GRISACTIN ULTRA: Wyeth-Ayerst	00046-0437-81	100s	$107.64

Guaifenesin

DESCRIPTION

Each sustained-release tablet provides 600 mg Guaifenesin.

Each capsule provides 300 mg Guaifenesin in a sustained-released formulation intended for oral administration. The microencapsulated contents of a capsule may be sprinkled on a small amount of soft food immediately prior to ingestion, making the product ideal for children and other patients unable to swallow capsules or tablets. Capsules are oversized to facilitate opening but may also be swallowed whole.

Following is its chemical structure:

$$\begin{array}{c} OH \\ | \\ OCH_2CHCH_2OH \\ \hline OCH_3 \end{array}$$

CLINICAL PHARMACOLOGY

Guaifenesin is an expectorant which increases respiratory tract fluid secretions and helps to loosen phlegm and bronchial secretions. By reducing the viscosity of secretions, Guaifenesin increases the efficiency of the mucociliary mechanism in removing accumulated secretions from the upper and lower airway. Guaifenesin

---

◆ RATED THERAPEUTICALLY EQUIVALENT; ◇ THERAPEUTIC EQUIVALENCE UNCONFIRMED; ○ UNRATED

is readily absorbed from the gastrointestinal tract and is rapidly metabolized and excreted in the urine. Guaifenesin has a plasma half-life of one hour. The major urinary metabolite is β-(2-methoxyphenoxy) lactic acid.

INDICATIONS AND USAGE

Guaifenesin is indicated for the temporary relief of coughs associated with respiratory tract infections and related conditions such as sinusitis, pharyngitis, bronchitis, and asthma, when these conditions are complicated by tenacious mucus and/or mucus plugs and congestion. The drug is effective in productive as well as nonproductive cough, but is of particular value in dry, non-productive cough which tends to injure the mucous membrane of the air passages. Microencapsulated contents of capsules are particularly suitable for use in children and other patients unable to swallow tablets or capsules.

CONTRAINDICATIONS

This product is contraindicated in patients with hypersentitivity to Guaifenesin.

PRECAUTIONS

General: Before prescribing medication to suppress or modify cough, it is important to ascertain that the underlying cause of cough is identified, that modification of cough does not increase the risk of clinical or physiologic complications, and that appropriate therapy for the primary disease is instituted.

Information for Patients: Capsules may be swallowed whole or the entire contents sprinkled on a small amount of soft food (jam, etc.) immediately prior to ingestion. Capsule contents should not be subdivided, nor should they be crushed or chewed.

Drug/Laboratory Test Interactions: Guaifenesin may increase renal clearance for urate and thereby lower serum uric acid levels. Guaifenesin may produce an increase in urinary 5-hydroxyindoleacetic acid and may therefore interfere with the interpretation of this test for the diagnosis of carcinoid syndrome. It may also falsely elevate the VMA test for catechols. Administration of this drug should be discontinued 48 hours prior to the collection of urine specimens for such tests.

Carcinogenesis, Mutagenesis, Impairment of Fertility: No data are available on the long-term potential for carcinogenesis, mutagenesis, or impairment of fertility in animals or humans.

Pregnancy: Category C: Animal reproduction studies have not been conducted with Guaifenesin. It is also not known whether Guaifenesin can cause fetal harm when administered to a pregnant woman or can affect reproduction capacity. Guaifenesin should be given to a pregnant woman only if clearly needed.

Nursing Mothers: It is not known whether Guaifenesin is excreted in human milk. Because many drugs are excreted in human milk, caution should be exercised when Guaifenesin is administered to a nursing woman and a decision should be made whether to discontinue nursing or to discontinue the drug, taking into account the importance of the drug to the mother.

ADVERSE REACTIONS

No serious side effects from Guaifenesin have been reported.

OVERDOSAGE

Overdosage with Guaifenesin is unlikely to produce toxic effects since its toxicity is low. Guaifenesin, when administered by stomach tube to test animals in doses up to 5 g/kg, produced no signs of toxicity. In severe cases of overdosage, treatment should be aimed at reducing further absorption of the drug. Gastric emptying (Syrup of Ipecac) and/or lavage is recommended as soon as possible after ingestion.

DOSAGE AND ADMINISTRATION

Adults and Children Over 12 Years of Age: One or two tablets every 12 hours not to exceed 4 tablets (2400 mg) in 24 hours. *Children 6 to 12 Years:* One tablet every 12 hours not to exceed 2 tablets (1200 mg) in 24 hours. *Children 2 to 6 Years:* ½ tablet every 12 hours not to exceed 1 tablet (600 mg) in 24 hours.

Adults and Children Over 12 Years of Age: Two to four capsules every 12 hours not to exceed 8 capsules (2400 mg) in 24 hours. *Children 6 to 12 Years:* Two capsules every 12 hours not to exceed 4 capsules (1200 mg) in 24 hours. *Children 2 to 6 Years:* One capsule every 12 hours not to exceed 2 capsules (600 mg) in 24 hours.

Storage: Store at controlled room temperature between 15° C and 30° C (59° F and 86° F). Dispense in tight containers.

HOW SUPPLIED
CAPSULE, EXTENDED RELEASE: 300 MG

BRAND/MANUFACTURER	NDC	SIZE	AWP
○ BRAND			
HUMIBID PEDIATRIC: Adams	53014-0402-10	100s	$41.48

LIQUID: 100 MG/5 ML

BRAND/MANUFACTURER	NDC	SIZE	AWP
○ BRAND			
ORGANIDIN NR: Wallace	00037-4214-10	480 ml	$72.48

TABLET: 200 MG

BRAND/MANUFACTURER	NDC	SIZE	AWP
○ BRAND			
ORGANIDIN NR: Wallace	00037-4312-01	100s	$27.19

For additional alternatives, turn to the section beginning on page 2859.

Guaifenesin and Hydrocodone Bitartrate

DESCRIPTION

Guaifenesin/Hydrocodone Bitartrate expectorant syrup contains Guaifenesin, an expectorant for oral administration, and Hydrocodone (dihydrocodeinone) Bitartrate, a semi-synthetic centrally-acting narcotic antitussive.

Each teaspoonful (5 mL) contains:

Guaifenesin, USP	100 mg
Hydrocodone Bitartrate, USP	5 mg

WARNING: May be habit forming

CLINICAL PHARMACOLOGY

Clinical trials have proven Hydrocodone Bitartrate to be an effective antitussive agent which is pharmacologically 2 to 8 times as potent as codeine. At equi-effective doses, its sedative action is greater than codeine. The precise mechanism of action of Hydrocodone and other opiates is not known, however, Hydrocodone is believed to act by directly depressing the cough center. In excessive doses Hydrocodone, like other opium derivatives, can depress respiration. The effects of Hydrocodone in therapeutic doses on the cardiovascular system are insignificant. The constipation effect of Hydrocodone are much weaker than that of morphine and no stronger than that of codeine. Hydrocodone can produce miosis, euphoria, physical and psychological dependence. At therapeutic antitussive doses, it does exert analgesic effects. Following a 10 mg oral dose of Hydrocodone administered to five male human subjects, the mean peak concentration was 23.6 ± 5.2 ng/mL. Maximum serum levels were achieved at 1.3 ± 0.3 hours and half-life was determined to be 3.8 ± 0.3 hours. Hydrocodone exhibits a complex pattern of metabolism including O-demethylation, N-demethylation and 6-ketoreduction to the corresponding 6-α- and 6-β-hydroxymetabolites.

The exact mechanism of action is not established but Guaifenesin is believed to act by stimulating receptors in the gastric mucosa that initiates a reflex secretion of respiratory tract fluid, thereby increasing the volume and decreasing the viscosity of bronchial secretions. Studies with Guaifenesin indicate that it is rapidly absorbed from the gastrointestinal tract and has a half-life of one hour.

INDICATIONS AND USAGE

Guaifenesin/Hydrocodone Bitartrate experorant is indicated for the symptomatic relief of irritating nonproductive cough associated with upper and lower respiratory tract congestion.

CONTRAINDICATIONS

Guaifenesin/Hydrocodone Bitartrate expectorant is contraindicated in patients hypersensitivity to Hydrocodone or Guaifenesin. Patients known to be hypersensitive to other opioids may exhibit cross sensitivity to Guaifenesin/Hydrocodone Bitartrate expectorant. Hydrocodone is contraindicated in the presence of an intracranial lesion associated with increased intracranial pressure; and whenever ventilatory function is depressed.

WARNINGS

May be habit forming. Hydrocodone can produce drug dependence of the morphine type and therefore has the potential for being abused. Psychic dependence, physical dependence and tolerance may develop upon repeated administration of Guaifenesin/Hydrocodone Bitartrate expectorant and it should be prescribed and administered with the same degree of caution appropriate to the use of other narcotic drugs (see *"Drug Abuse and Dependence"*).

Respiratory Depression: Guaifenesin/Hydrocodone Bitartrate expectorant produces dose-related respiratory depression by directly acting on the brain stem respiratory centers. If respiratory depression occurs, it may be antagonized by the use of naloxone hydrochloride and other supportive measures when indicated.

➤ SHOWN IN PRODUCT IDENTIFICATION GUIDE

Head Injury and Increased Intracranial Pressure: The respiratory depressant properties of narcotics and their capacity to elevate cerebrospinal fluid pressure may be markedly exaggerated in the presence of head injury, other intracranial lesions or a pre-existing increase in intracranial pressure. Furthermore, narcotics produce adverse reactions which may obscure the clinical course of patients with head injuries.

Acute Abdominal Conditions: The administration of Guaifenesin/Hydrocodone Bitartrate expectorant or other opioids may obscure the diagnosis or clinical course of patients with acute abdominal conditions.

PRECAUTIONS

Before prescribing medication to suppress or modify cough, it is important to ascertain that the underlying cause of cough is identified, that modification of cough does not increase the risk of clinical or physiologic complications, and that appropriate therapy for the primary disease is provided.

Usage in Ambulatory Patients: Hydrocodone, like all narcotics, may impair the mental and/or physical abilities required for the performance of potentially hazardous tasks such as driving a car or operating machinery, and patients should be warned accordingly.

Drug Interactions: Patients receiving other narcotics, analgesics, general anesthetics, phenothiazines, other tranquilizers, sedative hypnotics or other CNS depressants (including alcohol) concomitantly with Hydrocodone may exhibit an additive CNS depression. When such combined therapy is contemplated, the dose of one or both agents should be reduced (see *"Warnings"*).

Laboratory Interactions: The metabolite of Guaifenesin has been found to produce an apparent increase in urinary 5-hydroxyindoleacetic acid, and Guaifenesin therefore may interfere with the interpretation of this test for the diagnosis of carcinoid syndrome. Guaifenesin administration should be discontinued 24 hours prior to the collection of urine specimens for the determination of 5-hydroxyindoleacetic acid.

Carcinogenesis, Mutagenesis, Impairment of Fertility: Carcinogenicity, mutagenicity and reproduction studies have not been conducted with Guaifenesin/Hydrocodone Bitartrate Expectorant.

Usage in Pregnancy: Pregnancy Category C. Animal reproduction studies have not been conducted with Guaifenesin/Hydrocodone Bitartrate Expectorant. It is also not known whether Guaifenesin/Hydrocodone Bitartrate expectorant can cause fetal harm when administered to a pregnant woman or can affect reproductive capacity. Guaifenesin/Hydrocodone Bitartrate expectorant should be given to a pregnant woman only if clearly needed.

Nonteratogenic Effects: Babies born to mothers who have been taking opioids regularly prior to delivery will be physically dependent. The withdrawal signs include irritability and excessive crying, tremors, hyperactive reflexes, increased respiratory rate, increased stools, sneezing, yawning, vomiting and fever. The intensity of the syndrome does not always correlate with the duration of maternal opioid use or dose. There is no consensus on the best method of managing withdrawal. Chlorpromazine 0.7-1.0 mg/kg q 6 h, phenobarbital 2 mg/kg q 6 h, and paregoric 2-4 drops/kg q 4 h, have been used to treat withdrawal symptoms in infants. The duration of therapy is 4 to 28 days, with the dosages decreased as tolerated.

Nursing Mothers: It is not known whether this drug is excreted in human milk. Because many drugs are excreted in human milk and because of the potential for serious adverse reactions in nursing infants from Guaifenesin/Hydrocodone Bitartrate expectorant, a decision should be made whether to discontinue nursing or discontinue the drug, taking into account the importance of the drug to the mother.

ADVERSE REACTIONS

Respiratory System: Hydrocodone produces dose-related respiratory depression by acting directly on brain stem respiratory centers.

Cardiovascular System: Hypertension, postural hypotension and palpitations.

Genitourinary System: Ureteral spasm, spasm of vesical sphincters and urinary retention have been reported with opiates.

Central Nervous System: Sedation, drowsiness, mental clouding, lethargy, impairment of mental and physical performance, anxiety, fear, dysphoria, dizziness, psychic dependence, mood changes and blurred vision.

Gastrointestinal System: Nausea and vomiting occur more frequently in ambulatory than in recumbent patients.

DRUG ABUSE AND DEPENDENCE

Special care should be exercised in prescribing Hydrocodone for emotionally unstable patients and for those with a history of drug misuse. Such patients should be closely supervised when long-term therapy is contemplated.

Guaifenesin/Hydrocodone Bitartrate expectorant is a Schedule III narcotic. Psychic dependence, physical dependence and tolerance may develop upon repeated administration of narcotics; therefore, Guaifenesin/Hydrocodone Bitartrate expectorant should always be prescribed and administered with caution. Physical dependence is the condition in which continued administration of the drug is required to prevent the appearance of a withdrawal syndrome.

Patients physically dependent on opioids will develop an abstinence syndrome upon abrupt discontinuation of the opioid or following the administration of a narcotic antagonist. The character and severity of the withdrawal symptoms are related to the degree of physical dependence. Manifestations of opioid withdrawal are similar to but milder than that of morphine and include lacrimation, rhinorrhea, yawning sweating, restlessness, dilated pupils, anorexia, goose-flesh, irritability and tremor. In more severe forms, nausea, vomiting, intestinal spasm and diarrhea, increased heart rate and blood pressure, chills, and pains in bones and muscles of the back and extremities may occur. Peak effects will usually be apparent at 48 to 72 hours.

Treatment of withdrawal is usually managed by providing sufficient quantities of an opioid to suppress *severe* withdrawal symptoms and then gradually reducing the dose of opioid over a period of several days.

OVERDOSAGE

Signs and Symptoms: Serious overdosage with Guaifenesin/Hydrocodone Bitartrate expectorant is characterized by respiratory depression (a decrease in respiratory rate and/or tidal volume, Cheyne-Stokes respiration, cyanosis), extreme somnolence progressing to stupor or coma, skeletal muscle flaccidity, cold and clammy skin, and sometimes bradycardia and hypotension. In severe overdosage apnea, circulatory collapse, cardiac arrest, and death may occur.

Treatment: Primary attention should be given to the reestablishment of adequate respiratory exchange through provision of a patent airway and the institution of assisted or controlled ventilation. The narcotic antagonist naloxone hydrochloride is a specific antidote for respiratory depression which may result from overdosage or unusual sensitivity to narcotics including Hydrocodone. Therefore, an appropriate dose of naloxone hydrochrochloride should be administered, preferably by the intravenous route, simultaneously with efforts at respiratory resuscitation. For further information, see full prescribing information for naloxone hydrochloride. An antagonist should not be administered in the absence of clinically significant respiratory depression. Oxygen, intravenous fluids, vasopressors and other supportive measures should be employed as indicated. Gastric emptying may be useful in removing unabsorbed drug. Activated charcoal may be of benefit.

DOSAGE AND ADMINISTRATION

Usual Adult Dose: One teaspoonful (5 mL) after meals and at bedtime, not less than 4 hours apart (not to exceed 6 teaspoonsful in a 24 hour period). Treatment should be initiated with one teaspoonful and subsequent doses, up to a maximum single dose of 3 teaspoonsful, adjusted if required.

Usual Children's Dose: Over 12 years: Initial dose 1 teaspoonful; maximum single dose, 2 teaspoonful.

6 to 12 years: Initial dose 1/2 teaspoonful; maximum single dose, 1 teaspoonful.

Storage: Store in a tight, light resistant container as defined in the USP. Keep tightly closed.

Store at controlled room temperature 59°-86°F (15°-30°C). A Schedule CIII Narcotic. Oral prescription where permitted by state law.

HOW SUPPLIED

LIQUID (C-III): 100 MG-5 MG/5 ML

BRAND/MANUFACTURER	NDC	SIZE	AWP
○ GENERICS			
ATUSS EX: Atley Pharm	59702-0005-16	473 ml	$22.50
CO-TUSSIN: Am Generics	58634-0032-01	480 ml	$20.95
BERTUSS SF: R&R Drugs	55419-0044-48	480 m	$20.95
VI-Q-TUSS: Qualitest	00603-1853-58	480 ml	$24.95
CODOTUSS: Major	00904-7888-16	480 ml	$30.20
FENTUSS EXP: Econolab	55053-0432-16	480 ml	$31.00
CO-TUSS V EXP: Rugby	00536-2704-85	480 ml	$31.37
PROPATUSS EXP: Norton	50732-0878-16	480 ml	$33.50
Rugby	00364-2517-16	480 ml	$37.00
HYCOSIN EXP: Barre-National	00472-0077-16	480 ml	$39.95
KWELCOF: Ascher	00225-0420-45	480 ml	$43.08

LIQUID (C-III): 300 MG-5 MG/5 ML

BRAND/MANUFACTURER	NDC	SIZE	AWP
○ BRAND			
PROLEX DH: Blansett	51674-0012-07	480 ml	$32.95

SYRUP (C-III): 100 MG-5 MG/5 ML

BRAND/MANUFACTURER	NDC	SIZE	AWP
○ BRAND			
CODICLEAR DH: Central	00131-5134-64	120 ml doz	$112.44
	00131-5134-70	480 ml	$32.80
VICODIN TUSS: Knoll	00044-0730-16	480 ml	$33.60
HYCOTUSS EXP: Dupont Multi	00056-0235-16	480 ml	$59.16
○ GENERICS			
VICOTUSS: Southwood	58016-4184-04	120 ml	$11.50
Moore, H.L.	00839-7855-69	480 ml	$20.78
HYCOCLEAR TUSS: Ethex	58177-0881-07	480 ml	$23.52
PNUMOTUSSIN HC: ECR	00095-0065-16	480 ml	$30.00
Goldline	00182-0159-40	480 ml	$30.20
COTUSS-V: Alphagen	59743-0020-16	480 ml	$32.00

◆ RATED THERAPEUTICALLY EQUIVALENT; ◇ THERAPEUTIC EQUIVALENCE UNCONFIRMED; ○ UNRATED

Aligen	00405-0095-16	480 ml	$33.98
HYDROTUSS: Rugby	00536-2660-85	480 ml	$38.25
Goldline	00182-0158-40	480 ml	$45.75

TABLET (C-III): 300 MG-5 MG

BRAND/MANUFACTURER	NDC	SIZE	AWP
○ **GENERICS**			
ENTUSS: Roberts/Hauck	59441-0141-01	100s	$38.89

Guaifenesin and Hydromorphone Hydrochloride

DESCRIPTION

Each 5 mL of cough syrup contains:

Guaifenesin 100mg
Hydromorphone Hydrochloride .... 1 mg
(WARNING: *May be habit forming)*
Alcohol 5%

Hydromorphone Hydrochloride is a hydrogenated ketone of morphine; it is a narcotic analgesic and antitussive.

CLINICAL PHARMACOLOGY

Hydromorphone HCl is a centrally acting narcotic antitussive which acts directly on the cough reflex center.

Hydromorphone HCl is also a narcotic analgesic; its principal therapeutic effect is relief of pain. The precise mechanism of action of Hydromorphone HCl and other opiates is not known, although it is believed to relate to the existence of opiate receptors in the central nervous system. There is no intrinsic limit to the analgesic effect of Hydromorphone HCl; like morphine, adequate doses will relieve even the most severe pain. Clinically, however, dosage limitations are imposed by the adverse effects, primarily respiratory depression, nausea, and vomiting, which can result from high doses.

Hydromorphone HCl has diverse additional actions. It produces drowsiness, changes in mood and mental clouding, depresses the respiratory center and the cough center, stimulates the vomiting center, produces pinpoint constriction of the pupil, enhances parasympathetic activity, elevates cerebrospinal fluid pressure, increases biliary pressure, produces transient hyperglycemia.

Generally, the analgesic action of parenterally administered Hydromorphone HCl is apparent within 15 minutes and usually remains in effect for more than five hours. The onset of action of oral Hydromorphone HCl is somewhat slower, with measurable analgesia occurring within 30 minutes.

Radioimmunoassay techniques have recently been developed for the analysis of Hydromorphone HCl in human plasma. In humans the half-life of a Hydromorphone HCl 4 mg tablet is 2.6 hours. In a random crossover study in six subjects, 4 mg of oral Hydromorphone HCl produced a mean concentration/time curve similar to that of 2 mg Hydromorphone HCl I.V., after the first hour.

Guaifenesin (glyceryl guaiacolate) reduces the viscosity of secretions, thereby increasing the efficiency of the cough reflex and of ciliary action in removing accumulated secretions from the trachea and bronchi. Unlike many other expectorants, guaifenesin rarely causes gastric irritation.

INDICATIONS AND USAGE

Guaifenesin/Hydromorphone HCl Cough Syrup is indicated for the control of persistent, exhausting cough or dry, non-productive cough.

CONTRAINDICATIONS

Guaifenesin/Hydromorphone HCl Cough Syrup is contraindicated in patients known to have a hypersensitivity to Hydromorphone; in the presence of an intracranial lesion associated with increased intracranial pressure; and whenever ventilatory function is depressed (chronic obstructive pulmonary disease, cor pulmonale, emphysema, kyphoscoliosis, status asthmaticus).

WARNINGS

Respiratory Depression: Hydromorphone HCl produces dose-related respiratory depression by acting directly on brain stem respiratory centers. Hydromorphone HCl also affects centers that control respiratory rhythm and may produce irregular and periodic breathing.

Head Injury and Increased Intracranial Pressure: The respiratory depressant effects of narcotics and their capacity to elevate cerebrospinal fluid pressure may be markedly exagerated in the presence of head injury, other intracranial lesions or a preexisting increase in intracranial pressure. Furthermore, narcotics produce adverse effects which may obscure the clinical course of patients with head injuries.

Acute Abdominal Conditions: The administration of narcotics may obscure the diagnosis or clinical course of patients with acute abdominal conditions.

PRECAUTIONS

Special Risk Patients: Guaifenesin/Hydromorphone HCl Cough Syrup should be used with caution in elderly or debilitated patients and those with impaired renal or hepatic function, hypothyroidism, Addison's disease, prostatic hypertrophy or urethral stricture. As with any narcotic analgesic agent, the usual precautions should be observed and the possibility of respiratory depression should be kept in mind.

Cough Reflex: Guaifenesin/Hydromorphone HCl Cough Syrup suppresses the cough reflex: as with all narcotics, caution should be exercised when Guaifenesin/

Hydromorphone HCl Cough Syrup is used postoperatively and in patients with pulmonary disease.

Usage in Ambulatory Patients: Narcotics may impair the mental and/or physical abilities required for the performance of potentially hazardous tasks such as driving a car or operating machinery; patients should be cautioned accordingly.

Drug Interactions: Patients receiving other narcotic analgesics, general anesthetics, phenothiazines, tranquilizers, sedative-hypnotics, tricyclic antidepressants or other CNS depressants (including alcohol) concomitantly with Guaifenesin/Hydromorphone HCl Cough Syrup may exhibit an additive CNS depression. When such combined therapy is contemplated, the dose of one or both agents should be reduced.

Usage in Pregnancy: Pregnancy Category C. Hydromorphone HCl has been shown to be teratogenic in hamsters when given in doses 600 times the human dose. There are no adequate and well-controlled studies in pregnant women. Guaifenesin/Hydromorphone HCl Cough Syrup should be used during pregnancy only if the potential benefit justifies the potential risk to the fetus.

Nonteratogenic Effects: Babies born to mothers who have been taking opioids regularly prior to delivery will be physically dependent. The withdrawal signs include irritability and excessive crying, tremors, hyperactive reflexes, increased respiratory rate, increased stools, sneezing, yawning, vomiting, and fever. The intensity of the syndrome does not always correlate with the duration of maternal opioid use or dose. There is no consensus on the best method of managing withdrawal. Chlorpromazine 0.7 to 1.0 mg/kg q6h, phenobarbital 2 mg/kg q6h, and paregoric 2 to 4 drops/kg q4h, have been used to treat withdrawal symptoms in infants. The duration of therapy is 4 to 28 days, with the dosage decreased as tolerated.

Labor and Delivery: As with all narcotics, administration of Guaifenesin/Hydromorphone HCl Cough Syrup to the mother shortly before delivery may result in some degree of respiratory depression in the newborn, especially if higher doses are used.

Nursing Mothers: It is not known whether this drug is excreted in human milk. Because many drugs are excreted in human milk and because of the potential for serious adverse reactions in nursing infants from Guaifenesin/Hydromorphone HCl Cough Syrup, a decision should be made whether to discontinue nursing or to discontinue the drug, taking into account the importance of the drug to the mother.

Pediatric Use: Safety and effectiveness in children have not been established.

FD&C Yellow No. 5: Guaifenesin/Hydomorphone HCl Cough Syrup contains FD&C Yellow No. 5 (tartrazine) dye which may cause allergic-type reactions (including bronchial asthma) in certain susceptible individuals. Although the overall incidence of FD&C Yellow No. 5 (tartrazine) dye sensitivity in the general population is low, it is frequently seen in patients who also have aspirin hypersensitivity.

ADVERSE REACTIONS

Central Nervous System: Sedation, drowsiness, mental clouding, lethargy, impairment of mental and physical performance, anxiety, fear, dysphoria, dizziness, psychic dependence, mood changes.

Gastrointestinal System: Nausea and vomiting occur more frequently in ambulatory than in recumbent patients. The antiemetic phenothiazines are useful in suppressing these effects. Prolonged administration of Hydromorphone HCl may produce constipation. Opiate agonist-induced increase in intra-luminal pressure may endanger surgical anastomosis.

Genitourinary System: Ureteral spasm, spasm of vesical sphincters and urinary retention have been reported.

Respiratory Depression: Hydromorphone HCl produces dose-related respiratory depression by acting directly on brain stem respiratory centers. Hydromorphone HCl also affects centers that control respiratory rhythm, and may produce irregular and periodic breathing. If significant respiratory depression occurs, it may be antagonized by the use of naloxone hydrochloride. The usual adult dose of 0.4 to 0.8 mg given intramuscularly or intravenously, promptly reverses the effects of morphine-like opioid agonists such as Hydromorphone HCl. In patients who are physically dependent, small doses of naloxone may be sufficient not only to antagonize respiratory depression, but also to precipitate withdrawal phenomena. The dose of naloxone should therefore be adjusted accordingly in such patients. Since the duration of action of Hydromorphone HCl may exceed that of the antagonist, the patient should be kept under continued surveillance; repeated doses of the antagonist may be required to maintain adequate respiration. Apply other supportive measures when indicated.

DRUG ABUSE AND DEPENDENCE

Hydromorphone HCl is a Schedule CII narcotic. Psychic dependence, physical dependence, and tolerance may develop upon repeated administration of narcotics; therefore, Hydromorphone HCl should be prescribed and administered with caution. However, psychic dependence is unlikely to develop when Guaifenesin/Hydromorphone HCl Cough Syrup is used for a short time as indicated. Physical dependence, the condition in which continued administration of the drug is required to prevent the appearance of a withdrawal syndrome, usually assumes clinically significant proportions only after several weeks of continued narcotic use, although some mild degree of physical dependence may develop after few days of narcotic therapy.

► SHOWN IN PRODUCT IDENTIFICATION GUIDE

OVERDOSAGE

Signs and Symptoms: Serious overdosage with Hydromorphone HCl is characterized by respiratory depression (a decrease in respiratory rate and/or tidal volume, Cheyne-Stokes respiration, cyanosis), extreme somnolence progressing to stupor or coma, skeletal muscle flaccidity, cold and clammy skin, and sometimes bradycardia and hypotension. In severe overdosage particularly by the intravenous route, apnea, circulatory collapse, cardiac arrest and death may occur.

Treatment: Primary attention should be given to the reestablishment of adequate respiratory exchange through provision of a patent airway and the institution of assisted or controlled ventilation. The narcotic antagonist naloxone hydrochloride is a specific antidote against respiratory depression which may result from overdosage or unusual sensitivity to narcotics, including Hydromorphone HCl. Therefore, naloxone hydrochloride should be administered as described under *"Adverse Reactions"* (see *"Respiratory Depression"*) in conjunction with ventilatory assistance.

Since the duration of action of Hydromorphone HCl may exceed that of the antagonist, the patient should be kept under continued surveillance; repeated doses of the antagonist may be required to maintain adequate respiration. An antagonist should not be administered in the absence of clinically significant respiratory or cardiovascular depression. Oxygen, intravenous fluids, vasopressors and other supportive measures should be employed as indicated.

In case of overdosage with oral Hydromorphone HCl, gastric lavage or induced emesis may be useful in removing unabsorbed drug from conscious patients.

DOSAGE AND ADMINISTRATION

The usual adult dose of Guaifenesin/Hydromorphone HCl Cough Syrup is one teaspoonful (5 mL) every 3 to 4 hours.

Store at 59°-86°F (15°-30°C).

HOW SUPPLIED
SYRUP (C-II): 100 MG-1 MG/5 ML

BRAND/MANUFACTURER	NDC	SIZE	AWP
○ BRAND			
DILAUDID COUGH SYRUP: Knoll	00044-1080-01	480 ml	$32.44

Guaifenesin and Phenylephrine Hydrochloride

DESCRIPTION

Each Guaifenesin and Phenylephrine Hydrochloride Capsule provides 10 mg Phenylephrine Hydrochloride and 300 mg Guaifenesin in a sustained-release formulation intended for oral administration. The microencapsulated contents of a capsule may be sprinkled on a small amount of soft food immediately prior to ingestion, making the product ideal for children and other patients unable to swallow capsules or tablets. Capsules are oversized to facilitate opening but may also be swallowed whole.

Phenylephrine Hydrochloride is an orally effective nasal decongestant. Chemically, it is (R)-3-hydroxy-α- [(methyl-amino) methyl] benzenemethanol hydrochloride, has a molecular weight of 203.67 and its molecular formula is $C_9H_{13}NO_2HCl$.

Gualfenesin is an expectorant. Chemically, it is 3-(2-methoxyphenoxy)-1,2-propanediol, and its molecular formula is $C_{10}H_{14}O_4$.

CLINICAL PHARMACOLOGY

Phenylephrine Hydrochloride effects its vasoconstrictor activity by releasing noradrenaline from sympathetic nerve endings, and from direct stimulation of α-adrenoreceptors in blood vessels. Following oral administration, constriction of blood vessels in the nasal mucosa helps relieve nasal congestion. In therapeutic doses the drug causes little, if any, central nervous system stimulation.

Gauifenesin is an expectorant which increases respiratory tract fluid secretions and helps to loosen phlegm and brochial secretions. By reducing the viscosity of secretions, Guaifenesin increases the efficiency of the mucocilary mechanism in removing accumulated secretions from the upper and lower airway. Guaifenesin is readily absorbed from the gastrointestinal tract and is rapidly metabolized and excreted in the urine. Guaifenesin has a plasma half-life of one hour. The major urinary metabolite is β-(2-methoxyphenoxy) lactic acid.

INDICATIONS AND USAGE

Guaifenesin/Phenylephrine HCl Capsules are indicated for the temporary relief of nasal congestion and cough associated with respiratory tract infections and related conditions such as sinusitis, pharyngitis, bronchitis, and asthma, when these conditions are complicated by tenacious mucus and/or mucus plugs and congestion. The product is effective in productive as well as non-productive cough, but is of particular value in dry, non-productive cough which tends to injure the mucous membrane of the air passages. Guaifenesin/Phenylephrine HCl Capsules are particularly suitable for use in children and other patients unable to swallow tablets or capsules.

CONTRAINDICATIONS

This product is contraindicated in patients with hypersensitivity to guaifenesin, or with hypersensitivity or idiosyncrasy to sympathomimetic amines which may be manifested by insomnia, dizziness, weakness, tremor or arrhythmias.

Patients known to be hypersensitive to other sympathomimetic amines may exhibit cross sensitivity with phenylephrine. Phenylephrine is contraindicated in patients with severe hypertension, severe coronary artery disease and patients on monoamine oxidase inhibitor (MAOI) therapy and for 14 days after stopping MAOI therapy. (See *"Drug Interactions"* section).

WARNINGS

Sympathomimetic amines should be used with caution in patients with hypertension, ischemic heart disease, diabetes mellitus, increased intraocular pressure, hyperthyroidism, or prostatic hypertrophy. Sympathomimetics may produce central nervous system stimulation with convulsions or cardiovascular collapse with accompanying hypotension. **Do not exceed recommended dosage**.

Hypertensive crises can occur with concurrent use of phenylephrine and MAOI, and for 14 days after stopping MAOI therapy, indomethacin or with beta-blockers and methyldopa. If a hypertensive crisis occurs, these drugs should be discontinued immediately and therapy to lower blood pressure should be instituted. Fever should be managed by means of external cooling.

PRECAUTIONS

General: Use with caution in patients with diabetes, hypertension, cardiovascular disease and intolerance to ephedrine.

Before prescribing medication to suppress or modify cough, it is important to ascertain that the underlying cause of cough is identified, that modification of cough does not increase the risk of clinical or physiologic complications, and that appropriate therapy for the primary disease is instituted.

Information for Patients: Capsules may be swallowed whole or the entire contents sprinkled on a small amount of soft food (jam, etc.) immediately prior to ingestion. Capsule contents should not be subdivided. Capsule contents should not be crushed or chewed. Patients should be instructed to check with physician if symptoms do not improve within 5 days or if fever is present.

Pediatric Use: This product is not recommended for use in children under 2 years of age.

Use in Elderly: The elderly (60 years and older) are more likely to experience adverse reactions to sympathomimetics. Overdosage of sympathomimetics in this age group may cause hallucinations, convulsions, CNS depression, and death.

Drug Interactions: Do not prescribe this product for use in patients that are now taking a prescription MAOI (certain drugs for depression, psychiatric or emotional conditions, or Parkinson's disease), or for 14 days after stopping the MAOI drug therapy. Beta-adrenergic blockers and MAOI may potentiate the pressor effect of phenylephrine (see *"Warnings"*). Concurrent use of digitalis glycosides may increase the possibility of cardiac arrhythmias. Sympathomimetics may reduce the hypotensive effects of guanethidine, mecamylamine, methyldopa, reserpine and veratrum alkaloids. Concurrent use of tricyclic antidepressants may antagonize the effect of phenylephrine.

Drug/Laboratory Test Interactions: Guaifenesin may increase renal clearance for urate and thereby lower serum uric acid levels. Guaifenesin may produce an increase in urinary 5-hydroxy-indoleacetic acid and may therefore interfere with the interpretation of this test for the diagnosis of carcinoid syndrome. It may also falsely elevate the VMA test for catechols. Administration of this drug should be discontinued 48 hours prior to the collection of urine specimens for such tests.

Carcinogenesis, Mutagenesis, Impairment of Fertility: No data are available on the long-term potential of the components of this product for carcinogenesis, mutagenesis, or impairment of fertility in animals or humans.

Pregnancy: Category C: Animal reproduction studies have not been conducted with Guaifenesin/Phenylephine HCl Capsules. It is also not known whether Guaifenesin/Phenylephine HCl Capsules can cause fetal harm when administered to a pregnant woman or can affect reproduction capacity. Accordingly, this product should be given to a pregnant woman only if clearly needed.

Nursing Mothers: Use of this product by nursing mothers is not recommended because of the higher than usual risk for infants from sympathomimetic amines.

ADVERSE REACTIONS

Hyper-reactive individuals may display ephedrine-like reactions such as tachycardia, palpitations, headache, dizziness, or nausea. Sympathomimetics have been associated with certain untoward reactions including fear, anxiety, nervousness, restlessness, tremor, weakness, pallor, respiratory difficulty, dysuria, insomnia, hallucinations, convulsions, CNS depression, arrhythmias, and cardiovascular collapse with hypotension. No serious side effects have been reported with the use of Guaifenesin.

OVERDOSAGE

Since Guaifenesin/Phenylephrine HCl SPRINKLE Capsules contain two pharmacologically different compounds, treatment of overdosage should be based upon the symptomatology of the patient as it relates to the individual ingredients. Treatment of acute overdosage would probably be based upon treating the patient for phenylephrine toxicity which may manifest itself as excessive CNS stimulation resulting in excitement, tremor, restlessness, and insomnia. Other effects may include tachycardia, hypertension, pallor, mydriasis, hyperglycemia and urinary retention. Severe overdosage may cause tachypnea or hyperpnea, hallucinations, convulsions or delirium, but in some individuals there may be CNS depression with somnolence, stupor or respiratory depression. Arrhythmias (including ventricular fibrillation) may lead to hypotension and circulatory collapse. Severe hypokalemia can occur, probably due to a compartmental shift rather than a depletion of potassium. Overdosage with Guaifenesin is unlikely to produce toxic effects since its toxicity is much lower than that of phenylephrine.

The LD$_{50}$ of Phenylephrine (single oral dose) has been reported to be 120 mg/kg in the mouse and 350 mg/kg in the rat. The toxic and lethal concentrations in human biologic fluids are not known. Guaifenesin, when administered by stomach tube to test animals in doses up to 5 grams/kg, produced no signs of toxicity.

Since the action of sustained-release products may continue for as long as 12 hours, treatment of overdosage should be directed toward reducing further absorption and supporting the patient for at least that length of time. Gastric emptying (Syrup of Ipecac) and/or lavage is recommended as soon as possible after ingestion, even if the patient has vomited spontaneously. Either isotonic or half-isotonic saline may be used for lavage. Administration of an activated charcoal slurry is beneficial after lavage and/or emesis if less than 4 hours have passed since ingestion. Saline cathartics, such as Milk of Magnesia, are useful for hastening the evacuation of unreleased medication.

Adrenergic receptor blocking agents are antidotes to phenylephrine. In practice, the most useful is the beta-blocker propranolol which is indicated when there are signs of cardiac toxicity. Theoretically, phenylephrine is dialyzable but procedures have not been clinically established.

In severe cases of overdosage, it is essential to monitor both the heart (by electrocardiograph) and plasma electrolytes, and to give intravenous potassium as indicated. Vasopressors may be used to treat hypotension. Excessive CNS stimulation may be counteracted with parenteral diazepam. Stimulants should not be used.

DOSAGE AND ADMINISTRATION

Adults and children over 12 years of age: Two to three capsules every 12 hours not to exceed 6 capsules in 24 hours.

Children 6 to 12 years: One or two capsules every 12 hours not to exceed 4 capsules in 24 hours.

Children 2 to 6 years: One capsule every 12 hours not to exceed 2 capsules in 24 hours. Capsules may be swallowed whole or the entire contents sprinkled on a small amount of soft food immediately prior to ingestion. **Subdividing the contents of a capsule is not recommended.**

Storage: Store at controlled room temperature between 15° C and 30° C (59° F and 86° F). Dispense in tight, light-resistant containers.

HOW SUPPLIED
CAPSULE:

BRAND/MANUFACTURER	NDC	SIZE	AWP
○ GENERICS			
AMIDAL: Amide	52152-0024-02	100s	$16.69
AMIDAL: Amide	52152-0024-04	500s	$73.75

CAPSULE, EXTENDED RELEASE:

BRAND/MANUFACTURER	NDC	SIZE	AWP
○ GENERICS			
SINUPAN: Ion	11808-0140-01	100s	$60.90

CAPSULE, EXTENDED RELEASE: 10 MG-300 MG

BRAND/MANUFACTURER	NDC	SIZE	AWP
○ BRAND			
DECONSAL SPRINKLE: Adams	53014-0019-10	100s	$44.02

TABLET, EXTENDED RELEASE:

BRAND/MANUFACTURER	NDC	SIZE	AWP
○ GENERICS			
ENDAL: Forest Pharm	00785-2204-01	100s	$31.56

TABLETS:

BRAND/MANUFACTURER	NDC	SIZE	AWP
○ GENERICS			
EFASIN: Major	00904-3540-60	100s	$16.45
CHEMDAL: Norton,HN	50732-0754-01	100s	$17.71
QUINDAL: Qualitest	00603-5571-21	100s	$17.88
EFASIN: Major	00904-3540-40	500s	$60.55
CHEMDAL: Norton,HN	50732-0754-05	500s	$69.87

TABLETS: 20 MG-300 MG

BRAND/MANUFACTURER	NDC	SIZE	AWP
○ GENERICS			
Goldline	00182-1206-01	100s	$16.50

Guaifenesin and Phenylpropanolamine Hydrochloride

DESCRIPTION

Each long-acting tablet for oral administration contains

Guaifenesin .... 400 mg or 600 mg
Phenylpropanolamine Hydrochloride .... 75 mg

In a special base to provide a prolonged therapeutic effect. This product contains ingredients of the following therapeutic classes: decongestant and expectorant.

Guaifenesin is an expectorant having the chemical name, 1,2-propanediol, 3-(2-methoxyphenoxy).

Phenylpropanolamine Hydrochloride is a decongestant having the chemical name, benzenemethanol, α-(1-aminoethyl)-, hydrochloride (R*, S*), (±).

CLINICAL PHARMACOLOGY

Phenylpropanolamine Hydrochloride is an α-adrenergic receptor agonist (sympathomimetic) which produces vasoconstriction by stimulating α-receptors within the mucosa of the respiratory tract. Clinically, Phenylpropanolamine shrinks swollen mucus membranes, reduces tissue hyperemia, edema, and nasal congestion, and increases nasal airway patency. Guaifenesin promotes lower respiratory tract drainage by thinning bronchial secretions, lubricates irritated respiratory tract membranes through increased mucus flow, and facilitates removal of viscous, inspissated mucus. As a result of these drugs, sinus and bronchial drainage is improved, and dry, nonproductive coughs become more productive and less frequent.

INDICATIONS AND USAGE

Guaifenesin/Phenylpropanolamine Hydrochloride is indicated for the symptomatic relief of sinusitis, bronchitis, pharyngitis, and coryza when these conditions are associated with nasal congestion and viscous mucus in the lower respiratory tract.

CONTRAINDICATIONS

Guaifenesin/Phenylpropanolamine Hydrochloride is contraindicated in individuals with known hypersensitivity to sympathomimetics, severe hypertension, or in patients receiving monoamine oxidase inhibitors.

WARNINGS

Sympathomimetic amines should be used with caution in patients with hypertension, diabetes mellitus, heart disease, peripheral vascular disease, increased intraocular pressure, hyperthyroidism, or prostatic hypertrophy.

PRECAUTIONS

Information for Patients: Do not crush or chew Guaifenesin/Phenylpropanolamine HCl long-acting tablets prior to swallowing.

Drug Interactions: Guaifenesin/Phenylpropanolamine HCl long-acting should not be used in patients taking monoamine oxidase inhibitors or other sympathomimetics.

Drug/Laboratory Test Interactions: Guaifenesin has been reported to interfere with clinical laboratory determinations of urinary 5-hydroxyindoleacetic acid (5-HIAA) and urinary vanillylmandelic acid (VMA).

Pregnancy: Pregnancy Category C. Animal reproduction studies have not been conducted with Guaifenesin/Phenylpropanolamine HCl long-acting. It is also not known whether Guaifenesin/Phenylpropanolamine HCl long-acting can cause fetal harm when administered to a pregnant woman or can affect reproduction capacity. Guaifenesin/Phenylpropanolamine HCL long-acting should be given to a pregnant woman only if clearly needed.

Nursing Mothers: It is not known whether the drugs in Guaifenesin/Phenylpropanolamine HCl long-acting are excreted in human milk. Because many drugs are excreted in human milk and because of the potential for serious adverse reactions in nursing infants, a decision should be made whether to discontinue nursing or to discontinue the product, taking into account the importance of the drug to the mother.

Pediatric Use: Safety and effectiveness of Guaifenesin/Phenylpropanolamine HCl long-acting tablets in children below the age of 6 have not been established.

ADVERSE REACTIONS

Possible adverse reactions include nervousness, insomnia, restlessness, headache, nausea, or gastric irritation. These reactions seldom, if ever, require discontinuation of therapy. Urinary retention may occur in patients with prostatic hypertrophy.

► SHOWN IN PRODUCT IDENTIFICATION GUIDE

OVERDOSAGE

The treatment of overdosage should provide symptomatic and supportive care. If the amount ingested is considered dangerous or excessive, induce vomiting with ipecac syrup unless the patient is convulsing, comatose, or has lost the gag reflex, in which case perform gastric lavage using a largebore tube. If indicated, follow with activated charcoal and a saline cathartic. Since the effects of Guaifenesin/Phenylpropanolamine HCl long-acting may last up to 12 hours, treatment should be continued for at least that length of time.

DOSAGE AND ADMINISTRATION

Adults and children 12 years of age and older: one tablet twice daily (every 12 hours).

Children 6 to under 12 years: one-half (1/2) tablet twice daily (every 12 hours). Guaifenesin/Phenylpropanolamine HCl long-acting is not recommended for children under 6 years of age.

Tablets may be broken in half for ease of administration without affecting release of medication but should not be crushed or chewed prior to swallowing.

Storage: Store at controlled room temperature, 59° to 86°F (15° to 30°C).

HOW SUPPLIED
CAPSULE, EXTENDED RELEASE: 400 MG-75 MG

BRAND/MANUFACTURER	NDC	SIZE	AWP
○ GENERICS			
NASAHIST LA: Keene	00588-3888-01	100s	$29.50
DESPEC: Intl Ethical	11584-1028-01	100s	$53.30

LIQUID: 100 MG-20 MG/5 ML

BRAND/MANUFACTURER	NDC	SIZE	AWP
○ GENERICS			
DESPEC: Intl Ethical	11584-1030-04	120 ml	$8.30

TABLET, EXTENDED RELEASE: 400 MG-75 MG

BRAND/MANUFACTURER	NDC	SIZE	AWP
○ BRAND			
➤ ENTEX LA: P&G Pharm	00149-0436-01	100s	$71.08
	00149-0436-05	500s	$344.69
○ GENERICS			
Allscrips	54569-0623-08	6s	$0.74
Allscrips	54569-0623-04	10s	$1.24
Southwood	58016-0417-10	10s	$3.04
Cheshire	55175-0165-01	10s	$3.70
Allscrips	54569-0623-03	14s	$1.74
ENOMINE LA: Major	00904-3264-54	14s	$2.35
Cheshire	55175-0165-04	14s	$4.00
Southwood	58016-0417-14	14s	$4.25
Allscrips	54569-0623-05	15s	$1.86
Cheshire	55175-0165-05	15s	$4.20
Southwood	58016-0415-15	15s	$4.56
Allscrips	54569-0623-01	20s	$2.48
ENOMINE LA: Major	00904-3264-95	20s	$2.80
Cheshire	55175-0165-00	20s	$4.70
Southwood	58016-0417-20	20s	$5.89
Allscrips	54569-0623-00	30s	$3.72
Cheshire	55175-0165-03	30s	$5.34
Southwood	58016-0417-30	30s	$7.37
Allscrips	54569-0623-02	60s	$7.44
GUAIPAX: Eon	00185-0745-01	100s	$4.95
ENOMINE LA: Major	00904-3264-60	100s	$7.75
Qualitest	00603-5214-21	100s	$8.20
AMI-TEX LA: Amide	52152-0058-02	100s	$8.25
➤ Duramed	51285-0295-02	100s	$8.25
Qualitest	00603-5215-21	100s	$8.25
GUAITEX LA: Vintage	00254-5052-28	100s	$8.31
GUAITEX LA: Vintage	00254-5051-28	100s	$8.34
ULR-LA: Geneva	00781-1503-01	100s	$8.50
Schein	00364-2138-01	100s	$8.50
URL	00677-1026-01	100s	$8.93
PHENYLFENESIN LA: Goldline	00182-1798-01	100s	$8.95
Sidmak	50111-0385-01	100s	$9.08
Sidmak	50111-0522-01	100s	$9.08
Moore,H.L.	00839-7130-06	100s	$9.11
GUIATEX L.A.: Rugby	00536-3871-01	100s	$9.30
Martec	52555-0385-01	100s	$9.35

BRAND/MANUFACTURER	NDC	SIZE	AWP
Aligen	00405-4740-01	100s	$9.56
PARTUSS-LA: Parmed	00349-8931-01	100s	$10.00
BANEX-LA: Norton,HN	50732-0788-01	100s	$11.00
Allscrips	54569-0623-06	100s	$12.40
MEDEX-LA: Med-Tek	52349-0250-10	100s	$18.80
LANTEX-LA: Bolan	44437-0111-01	100s	$19.65
RUS-DF: R&R	55419-0010-44	100s	$19.94
RYMED-TR: Edwards	00485-0045-01	100s	$19.95
STAMOIST LA: Huckaby	58407-0374-01	100s	$20.30
VANEX-LA: Abana	12463-0400-01	100s	$33.42
➤ EXGEST LA: Carnrick	00086-0063-10	100s	$34.95
MAXCOSIN LA: Johnson Labs	58118-0111-10	100s	$42.50
GUAIPAX: Eon	00185-0745-05	500s	$24.50
ENOMINE LA: Major	00904-3264-40	500s	$31.85
Moore,H.L.	00839-7130-12	500s	$35.03
Moore,H.L.	00839-7884-12	500s	$35.03
AMI-TEX LA: Amide	52152-0058-04	500s	$36.95
PHENYLFENESIN LA: Goldline	00182-1798-05	500s	$37.50
Qualitest	00603-5214-28	500s	$38.30
➤ Duramed	51285-0295-04	500s	$38.36
Qualitest	00603-5215-28	500s	$38.70
GUAITEX LA: Vintage	00254-5052-35	500s	$38.75
GUAITEX LA: Vintage	00254-5051-35	500s	$38.80
ULR-LA: Geneva	00781-1503-05	500s	$40.80
Schein	00364-2138-05	500s	$42.00
Sidmak	50111-0385-02	500s	$42.20
Sidmak	50111-0522-02	500s	$42.20
Aligen	00405-4740-02	500s	$44.42
PARTUSS-LA: Parmed	00349-8931-05	500s	$44.94
Martec	52555-0385-05	500s	$45.30
BANEX-LA: Norton,HN	50732-0788-05	500s	$52.00
➤ EXGEST LA: Carnrick	00086-0063-50	500s	$149.50
HISTACON-X:	52765-1136-05	500s	$159.95
GUAIPAX: Eon	00185-0745-10	1000s	$47.50
Major	00904-3264-80	1000s	$66.60
GUIATEX L.A.: Rugby	00536-3871-10	1000s	$85.95

TABLET, EXTENDED RELEASE: 600 MG-37.5 MG

BRAND/MANUFACTURER	NDC	SIZE	AWP
○ BRAND			
PROFEN II: Wakefield	59310-0107-10	100s	$30.00

TABLET, EXTENDED RELEASE: 600 MG-75 MG

BRAND/MANUFACTURER	NDC	SIZE	AWP
○ GENERICS			
COLDLOC-LA: Flemming Pharma	60976-0675-05	50s ud	$34.80
PROFEN LA: Wakefield	59310-0104-10	100s	$36.00
SINUVENT: WE Pharm	59196-0001-01	100s	$45.63
GUAIFENEX PPA 75: Ethex	58177-0204-04	100s	$50.33
COLDLOC-LA: Flemming Pharma	60976-0675-10	100s	$62.40
DURA-VENT: Dura	51479-0006-01	100s	$63.42
DESPEC SR: Intl Ethical	11584-0441-01	100s	$63.44
SINUVENT: WE Pharm	59196-0001-06	600s	$237.50
DURA-VENT: Dura	51479-0006-06	600s	$335.09

Guaifenesin and Pseudoephedrine Hydrochloride

DESCRIPTION

Each Guaifenesin/Pseudoephedrine Hydrochloride scored, long-acting tablet for oral administration contains:

Guaifenesin ....600 mg
Pseudoephedrine Hydrochloride ....120 mg
in a special base to provide a prolonged therapeutic effect.

Each Guaifenesin/Pseudoephedrine HCl capsule contains:

Guaifenesin ....125 mg or 250 mg
Pseudoephedrine HCl ....60 mg or 120 mg

This product contains ingredients of the following therapeutic classes: decongestant and expectorant.

Pseudoephedrine Hydrochloride is a decongestant having the chemical name, benzenemethanol, α-[1-(methylamino)ethyl]-[S(R*,R*)]-, hydrochloride. Guaifenesin is an expectorant having the chemical name, 1,2-propanediol, 3-(2-methoxyphenoxy)-,

---

◆ RATED THERAPEUTICALLY EQUIVALENT; ◇ THERAPEUTIC EQUIVALENCE UNCONFIRMED; ○ UNRATED

CLINICAL PHARMACOLOGY

Pseudoephedrine Hydrochloride is an α-adrenergic receptor agonist (sympathomimetic) which produces vasoconstriction by stimulating α-receptors within the mucosa of the respiratory tract. Clinically, Pseudoephedrine shrinks swollen mucous membranes, reduces tissue hyperemia, edema, and nasal congestion, and increases nasal airway patency. Guaifenesin promotes lower respiratory tract drainage by thinning bronchial secretions, lubricates irritated respiratory tract membranes through increased mucus flow, and facilitates removal of viscous, inspissated mucus. As a result of these drugs, sinus and bronchial drainage is improved, and dry, nonproductive coughs become more productive and less frequent.

INDICATIONS AND USAGE

Guaifenesin/Pseudoephedrine HCl tablets are indicated for the relief of nasal congestion due to the common cold, hay fever or other upper respiratory allergies, and nasal congestion associated with sinusitis. To promote nasal or sinus drainage; for the symptomatic relief of respiratory conditions characterized by dry nonproductive cough and in the presence of tenacious mucus and/or mucous plugs in the respiratory tract.

Guaifenesin/Pseudoephedrine capsules are indicated in nasal congestion, sinusitis, acute aerotitis media, bronchial asthma, serous otitis media, and symptoms of the common cold.

CONTRAINDICATIONS

Guaifenesin/Pseudoephedrine HCl tablets are contraindicated in patients with a known hypersensitivity to any of its ingredients, in nursing mothers, or in patients with severe hypertension, severe coronary artery disease, prostatic hypertrophy, or in patients on MAO inhibitor therapy.

WARNINGS

Sympathomimetic amines should be used with caution in patients with hypertension, diabetes mellitus, heart disease, peripheral vascular disease, increased intraocular pressure, hyperthyroidism, or prostatic hypertrophy. Low grade sensitivity to drugs may be experienced.

PRECAUTIONS

General: Hypertensive patients should use Guaifenesin/Pseudoephedrine HCl tablets only with medical advice, as they may experience a change in blood pressure due to added vasoconstriction.

Information for Patients: Persistent cough may indicate a serious condition. If cough persists for more than one week, tends to recur, or is accompanied by a high fever, rash, or persistent headache, consult a physician.

Drug Interactions: MAO inhibitors and beta adrenergic blockers increase effects of sympathomimetics. Sympathomimetics may reduce the antihypertensive effects of methyldopa, guanethidine, mecamylamine, reserpine and veratrum alkaloids.

Drug/Laboratory Test Interactions: Guaifenesin has been reported to interfere with clinical laboratory determinations of urinary 5-hydroxyindoleacetic acid (5-HIAA) and urinary vanillylmandelic acid (VMA).

Pregnancy: Pregnancy Category C. Animal reproduction studies have not been conducted with Guaifenesin/Pseudoephedrine HCl tablets. It is also not known whether Guaifenesin/Pseudoephedrine HCl tablets can cause fetal harm when administered to a pregnant woman or can affect reproduction capacity. Guaifenesin/Pseudoephedrine HCl tablets should be given to a pregnant woman only if clearly needed.

Nursing Mothers: Guaifenesin/Pseudoephedrine HCl tablets are contraindicated in the nursing mother because of the higher than usual risks to infants from sympathomimetic agents.

Usage in Elderly: Patients 60 years and older are more likely to experience adverse reactions to sympathomimetics. Overdose may cause hallucinations, convulsions, CNS depression and death. Demonstrate safe use of a short-acting sympathomimetic before use of a sustained action formulation in elderly patients.

Pediatric Use: Safety and effectiveness of Guaifenesin/Pseudoephedrine HCl tablets in children below the age of 6 have not been established.

ADVERSE REACTIONS

Gastrointestinal: nausea and vomiting.

Central Nervous System: nervousness, dizziness, sleeplessness, light-headedness, tremor, hallucinations, convulsions, CNS depression, fear, anxiety, headache, increased irritability or excitement.

Cardiovascular: palpitations, tachycardia, cardiovascular collapse and death.

General: weakness.

Respiratory: respiratory difficulties.

OVERDOSAGE

Symptoms: Overdosage may cause hallucinations, convulsions, CNS depression, cardiovascular collapse and death.

Treatment: Treatment of overdosage should provide symptomatic care. If the amount ingested is considered dangerous or excessive, induce vomiting with ipecac syrup unless the patient is convulsing, comatose, or has lost the gag reflex, in which case, perform gastric lavage using a large-bore tube. If indicated, follow with activated charcoal and a saline cathartic. Since the effects of Guaifenesin/Pseudoephedrine HCl tablets may last up to 12 hours, treatment should be continued for at least that length of time.

DOSAGE AND ADMINISTRATION

Adults and Children 12 Years of Age and Older: one tablet or 1 250 mg/120 mg capsule twice daily (every 12 hours).

Children under 12 years: one 125 mg/60 mg capsule as prescribed by physician.

Children 6 to under 12 years: one-half (1/2) tablet twice daily (every 12 hours). Guaifenesin/Pseudoephedrine HCl tablets are not recommended for children under 6 years of age.

Tablets may be broken in half for ease of administration without affecting release of medication but should not be crushed or chewed prior to swallowing.

Store at controlled room temperature (59°-86°F or 15°-30°C). Dispense in tight, light-resistant containers as defined in USP.

HOW SUPPLIED
CAPSULE: 250 MG-30 MG

BRAND/MANUFACTURER	NDC	SIZE	AWP
○ GENERICS			
RYMED: Edwards	00485-0043-01	100s	$18.00

CAPSULE, EXTENDED RELEASE: 125 MG-60 MG

BRAND/MANUFACTURER	NDC	SIZE	AWP
○ GENERICS			
CONGESS JR.: Fleming	00256-0174-01	100s	$25.00
CONGESS JR.: Fleming	00256-0174-02	1000s	$163.00

CAPSULE, EXTENDED RELEASE: 200 MG-60 MG

BRAND/MANUFACTURER	NDC	SIZE	AWP
○ GENERICS			
RESPAIRE-60 SR: Laser	00277-0174-01	100s	$32.52

CAPSULE, EXTENDED RELEASE: 250 MG-90 MG

BRAND/MANUFACTURER	NDC	SIZE	AWP
○ GENERICS			
NASABID: Abana	12463-0250-01	100s	$60.61

CAPSULE, EXTENDED RELEASE: 250 MG-120 MG

BRAND/MANUFACTURER	NDC	SIZE	AWP
○ BRAND			
NALEX: Blansett	51674-0001-01	100s	$42.45
○ GENERICS			
CONGESS SR.: Fleming	00256-0173-01	100s	$27.00
PSEUDOFEN: Rugby	00536-5626-01	100s	$28.20
Qualitest	00603-3776-21	100s	$29.76
Moore,H.L.	00839-7925-06	100s	$35.03
RESPAIRE-120 SR: Laser	00277-0169-01	100s	$38.46
G-PHED: Alphagen	59743-0002-01	100s	$39.00
URL	00677-1503-01	100s	$45.00
GUAIBID D: Econolab	55053-0860-01	100s	$49.95
GUAIFED: Muro	00451-4002-50	100s	$67.94
GUAIFED: Muro	00451-4002-60	500s	$322.64
CONGESS SR.: Fleming	00256-0173-02	1000s	$186.50

CAPSULE, EXTENDED RELEASE: 300 MG-60 MG

BRAND/MANUFACTURER	NDC	SIZE	AWP
○ BRAND			
NALEX JR: Blansett	51674-0003-01	100s	$32.65
○ GENERICS			
PSEUDOFEN-PD: Rugby	00536-5627-01	100s	$25.50
Qualitest	00603-3777-21	100s	$27.82
Moore,H.L.	00839-7924-06	100s	$30.80
SINUFED TIMECELLES: Roberts/Hauck	59441-0151-01	100s	$33.33
G-PHED-PD: Alphagen	59743-0003-01	100s	$35.00
VERSACAPS: Seatrace	00551-0173-01	100s	$35.70
URL	00677-1502-01	100s	$36.00
GUAIBID D PEDIATRIC: Econolab	55053-0870-01	100s	$39.50
GUAIFED-PD: Muro	00451-4003-50	100s	$54.16
GUAIFED-PD: Muro	00451-4003-60	500s	$256.71

For additional alternatives, turn to the section beginning on page 2859.

Guaifenesin and Theophylline

DESCRIPTION

Each tablet contains:
Theophylline Sodium Glycinate .....300 mg (equiv. to 150 mg Theophylline)
Guafenesin .... 100 mg

Each tablespoonful (15 mL) of elixir contains:
Theophylline Sodium Glycinate .....300 mg (equiv. to 150 mg Theophylline)
Guafenesin .... 100 mg

Each tablespoonful (15 mL) of oral liquid contains:
Theophylline Anhydrous .... 100 mg
Guafenesin .... 100 mg

The elixir supplies the active ingredients in a solution containing 15% alcohol by volume. All forms contain a bronchodilator and an expectorant.

Theophylline sodium glycinate, a methylxanthine, is a white crystalline powder that is freely soluble in water, has a slight ammoniacal odor and a bitter taste. It is an equimolar mixture of theophylline sodium and glycine buffered by an additional mole of the essential amino acid, glycine. Theophylline anhydrous has the chemical name 1H-Purine-2, 6-dione, 3, 7-dihydro-1,3-dimethyl.

The expectorant component is Guaifenesin (formerly called glyceryl guaiacolate) which helps loosen and thus clear the bronchial passageways of bothersome, thickened mucus. Guaifenesin, 3-(o-methoxyphenoxy)-1,2-propanediol, occurs as a fine, white powder having a bitter, aromatic taste and a slight odor of guaiacol. The powder tends to become lumpy on storage. It is freely soluble in alcohol and soluble in water.

CLINICAL PHARMACOLOGY

Theophylline sodium glycinate is more stable in the presence of hydrochloric acid due to the buffering action of glycine with subsequent reduction of the chance of theophylline precipitation in the stomach. This and the high solubility of the product are suggested as the reasons why this product has better gastric tolerance than aminophylline.

Theophylline, the active ingredient of Theophylline sodium glycinate, accounts for 50% of the weight of this compound. Theophylline, sodium glycinate is highly effective in relaxing the smooth muscle of the bronchioles and the pulmonary blood vessels, thus acting primarily as a bronchodilator, pulmonary vasodilator and smooth muscle relaxant. Like other xanthines, theophylline sodium glycinate is a coronary vasodilator, a diuretic, a cerebral, cardiac and skeletal muscle stimulant. It has also been demonstrated that aminophylline has a potent effect on diaphragmatic contractibility in normal persons and may then be capable of reducing fatigability and thereby improve contractibility in patients with chronic obstructive airways disease. The exact mode of action remains unsettled.

Theophylline acts by inhibiting phosphodiesterase which causes an increase in intracellular cyclic AMP. This action produces smooth muscle relaxation and inhibits the release of histamine and other bronchoconstricting mediators from mast cells. Other mechanisms proposed include an effect on translocation of intracellular calcium, prostaglandin antagonism, stimulation of catecholamines endogenously, inhibition of cyclic guanosine monophosphate metabolism and adenosine receptor antagonism. None of these mechanisms has been proven, however.

In vitro, using human white blood cells, theophylline has been shown to react synergistically with beta agonists to increase intracellular cyclic AMP. There are now available data which do demonstrate an additive effect *in vivo* with combined use. More data is required to clearly establish if theophylline and the beta agonists are synergistic or additive *in vivo*.

Guaifenesin exerts its expectorant action by reducing the viscosity of bronchial secretions, thereby increasing the efficiency of the cough reflex and of ciliary action in removing accumulated secretions from the trachea and bronchi. Unlike many other expectorants. Guaifenesin rarely causes gastric irritation.

Even after prolonged therapy, it has not been possible to demonstrate the development of tolerance to Theophylline sodium glycinate.

The half-life of Theophylline varies from individual to individual. Since effective bronchodilatation depends upon maintaining serum Theophylline levels between 10-20 mg/dl (10-20 mcg/ml), the determination of serum theophylline can be of value.

The half-life of Theophylline is prolonged in alcoholism, in patients with reduced hepatic or renal function, congestive heart failure and in patients receiving antibiotics such as triacetyloleandomycin, erythromycin, clindamycin and lincomycin. Fever can also prolong Theophylline half-life.

Newborns and neonates have extremely slow clearance rate compared to older infants and children, i.e., those over 1 year. Older children have rapid clearance rates while most non-smoking adults have clearance rates between these two extremes in premature neonates the decreased clearance is related to oxidative pathways that have yet to be established.

Cigarette smoking (1-2 packs per day) enhances Theophylline elimination. The half-life of Theophylline is shortened with cigarette smoking. This effect is probably related to the induction of enzymes and requires between three months and two years to normalize after stopping tobacco usage.

By increasing respiratory tract fluid, Guaifenesin reduces the viscosity of tenacious secretions and acts as an expectorant. The drug is effective in productive as well as nonproductive cough, but is of particular value in dry, nonproductive cough which tends to injure the mucous membranes of the air passages.

THEOPHYLLINE ELIMINATION CHARACTERISTICS

Group	Theophylline Renal Clearance Rates	Half-Life Average
1. Children	1.4 ml/kg/min	3.5 hours
2. Adults with uncomplicated asthma	1.2 ml/kg/min	7 hours
3. Older Adults with chronic obstructive pulmonary disease	0.6 ml/kg/min	up to 24 hours
4. Adults with chronic obstructive pulmonary disease and cor pulmonale or other causes of heart failure and liver pathology	0.6 ml/kg/min and less	may exceed 24 hours
5. Young smokers	Not available	4.3 hours

INDICATIONS AND USAGE

For relief and/or prevention of acute bronchial asthma and for reversible bronchospasm associated with chronic bronchitis and emphysema.

CONTRAINDICATIONS

This product is contraindicated in individuals who have shown hypersensitivity to its components. It is also contraindicated in patients with active peptic ulcer disease, and in individuals with underlying seizure disorders (unless receiving appropriate anticonvulsant medication).

WARNINGS

There is an excellent correlation between high Theophylline blood levels and the clinical manifestations of toxicity in (1) patients with lowered body plasma clearances (due to transient cardiac decomposition), (2) chronic obstructive lung disease or patients with liver dysfunction, (3) patients who are older than 55 years of age, particularly males.

There are often no early signs of Theophylline toxicity such as nausea and restlessness which may appear in up to 50% of patients. Convulsions or ventricular arrhythmias may be the first signs of toxicity.

Excessive doses of Theophylline sodium glycinate may be expected to be toxic and serum theophylline levels are recommended to monitor therapy. The incidence of toxicity increases significantly at levels greater than 20 mcg/ml. Many patients who have higher Theophylline serum levels exhibit tachycardia. Theophylline products often worsen preexisting arrhythmias.

Theophylline Guaitonesin tablets, elixir, or oral solution should never be used to treat status asthma.

PRECAUTIONS

Studies in laboratory animals (minipigs, rodents, and dogs) recorded the occurrence of cardiac arrhythmias and sudden death (with histologic evidence of myocardia necrosis) when beta-agonists and methylxanthines were administered concurrently. The significance of these findings when applied to humans is currently unknown.

PRECAUTIONS

General: Theophylline should be used with caution in patients with severe cardiovascular disease, severe hypoxemia, hypertension, hyperthyroidism, acute myocardial injury, obstructive lung disease, liver disease, in the elderly and in neonates.

Great caution should be used in giving Theophylline to patients in congestive heart failure. Such patients have markedly prolonged Theophylline blood levels which have persisted for long periods after discontinuation of the drug.

Smokers have a shorter mean half-life of Theophylline than nonsmokers and may require larger doses of Theophylline. Theophylline sodium glycinate should not be administered concurrently with other Theophylline containing products. Theophylline should be given with caution to patients with a history of peptic ulcer. Theophylline may act as a local irritant in the gastrointestinal tract.

Information for Patients: The importance of adherence to the prescribed dosage regimen should be stressed. Patients should be informed of symptoms associated with Theophylline toxicity such as nausea and restlessness.

Laboratory Tests: There is great patient-to-patient variation in the serum half-life of Theophylline. Therefore, when possible, serum Theophylline levels should be measured to assist in titration of dosage.

The serum sample should be obtained at the time of peak concentration 1 to 2 hours after administration for immediate release products it is important that the patient will not have missed or taken additional doses during the previous 48 hours and that dosing intervals will have been reasonably equally spaced. DOSAGE ADJUSTMENT BASED ON SERUM THEOPHYLLINE MEASUREMENTS WHEN THESE INSTRUCTIONS HAVE NOT BEEN FOLLOWED MAY RESULT IN RECOMMENDATIONS THAT PRESENT RISK OF TOXICITY TO THE PATIENT.

Drug Interactions: The use of Theophylline sodium glycinate with ephedrine and other sympathomimetic bronchodilators may result in a significant increase in side effects.

Drug	Effect
Aminophylline with Lithium Carbonate	Increased excretion of Lithium Carbonate
Aminophylline with Propranolol	Antagonism of Propranolol effect
Theophylline with Furosemide	Increased Diuresis
Theophylline with Hexamethonium	Decreased Hexamethonium-induced chronotropic effect
Theophylline with Reserpine	Reserpine-induced Tachycardia

◆ RATED THERAPEUTICALLY EQUIVALENT; ◇ THERAPEUTIC EQUIVALENCE UNCONFIRMED; ○ UNRATED

Drug	Effect
Theophylline with Cimetidine	Increased theophylline blood levels
Theophylline with clindamycin, troleandomycin, erythromycin, lincomycin	Increased Theophylline blood levels
Theophylline with Allopurinol (high dose)	Increased serum Theophylline levels
Theophylline with Allopurinol ciprofloxan	Increased serum Theophylline levels
Theophylline with Allopurinol oral contraceptives	Increased serum Theophylline levels
Theophylline with Phenytoin	Decreased Theophylline and phenytoin serum levels
Theophylline with Rifampin	Decreased serum Theophylline levels

Drug/Laboratory Test Interactions: Currently available analytical methods, including high pressure liquid chromatography and immunoassay techniques, for measuring serum Theophylline levels are specific Metabolites and other drugs generally do not affect the results. Other new analytic methods are also now in use. The physician should be aware of the laboratory method used and whether other drugs will interfere with the assay for Theophylline.

Theophylline has been shown to increase the urinary excretion of catecholamines. The VMA test for catechols may be falsely elevated by Guaifenesin. Theophylline may increase the apparent serum uric acid in certain manual or automated chemical procedures by being treated as if it were uric acid. Guaifenesin may increase renal clearance for urate and thereby lower the serum uric acid. It may also falsely elevate the level of urinary 5HIAA in certain serotonin metabolite chemical tests.

Carcinogenesis, Mutagenesis, Impairment of Fertility: No data are available on the long-term potential for carcinogenicity, mutagenicity or impairment of fertility in animals or humans.

Chromosome-breaking activity was detected in human cell cultures at concentrations of theophylline up to 50 times the therapeutic serum concentration in humans. Theophylline was not mutagenic in the dominant lethal assay in male mice given Theophylline intraperitoneally in doses up to 30 times the maximum daily human oral dose.

Studies to determine the effect on fertility have not been performed with Theophylline.

Pregnancy: Pregnancy Category C: Animal reproduction studies have not been conducted. Safe use in pregnancy has not been established relative to possible adverse effects in fetal development.

Therefore Theophylline should not be used in pregnant patients unless, in the judgment of the physician, the potential benefits outweigh possible hazards.

Nursing Mothers: Theophylline is distributed into breast milk and may cause irritability or other signs of toxicity in nursing infants. Because of the potential for serious adverse reactions in nursing infants, a decision should be made whether to discontinue nursing or to discontinue the drug, taking into account the importance of the drug to the mother.

Pediatric Use: Sufficient numbers of infants under the age of 1 year have not been studied in clinical trials to support use in this age group however there is evidence recorded that the use of dosage recommendations for older infants and young children (16 mg/kg/24 hours) may result in the development of toxic serum levels. Such findings very probably reflect differences in the metabolic handling of the drug related to absent or undeveloped enzyme systems. Consequently, the use of the drug in this age group should carefully consider the associated benefits and risks. If used, the maintenance dose must be conservative and in accord with the following guidelines:

INITIAL MAINTENANCE DOSAGE OF THEOPHYLLINE ANHYDROUS
Up to 24 days postnatal age - 10 mg/kg q 12h
Beyond 24 days postnatal age - 15 mg/kg q 12h

Infants 6 to 52 weeks: [(0.2 × age in weeks) + 5.0] × kg body wt = 24 hour dose in mg
Up to 26 weeks, divide into q8h dosing intervals.
From 26-52 weeks, divide into q6h dosing intervals. Final dosage should be guided by serum concentration after a steady state (no further accumulation of drug) has been achieved.

ADVERSE REACTIONS

Included in this listing which follows are adverse reactions, some of which may have been reported with Theophylline sodium glycinate. However, pharmacological similarities among the xanthine drugs require that each of the reactions be considered when Theophylline is administered. The most consistent adverse reactions are usually due to overdosage of Theophylline sodium glycinate and are:

1. Gastrointestinal: nausea, vomiting, epigastric pain, hematemesis, diarrhea.
2. Central Nervous System: headaches, irritability, restlessness, insomnia, reflex hyperexcitability, muscle twitching, clonic and tonic generalized convulsions.
3. Cardiovascular: palpitation, tachycardia, extrasystoles, flushing hypotension, circulatory failure, life-threatening ventricular arrhythmias.
4. Respiratory: tachypnea.
5. Renal: albuminuria, increased excretion of renal tubular cells and red blood cells: potentiation of diuresis.
6. Others: hyperglycemia and inappropriate ADH syndrome.

OVERDOSAGE
MANAGEMENT
A. If potential oral overdose is established and seizure has not occurred: (1) induce vomiting and resort to gastric lavage if the patient fails to vomit within 20-30 minutes; (2) administer a cathartic (this is particularly important if sustained-release preparations have been taken) and activated charcoal after successful vomiting has been induced or adequate gastric lavage performed.

B. If patient is having a seizure: (1) establish an airway; (2) administer O_2; (3) treat the seizure with intravenous diazepam 0.1 to 0.3 mg/kg up to 10 mg; (4) monitor vital signs, maintain blood pressure and provide adequate hydration.

C. Post-Seizure Coma: (1) maintain airway and oxygenation; (2) if a result of oral medication, follow above recommendations to prevent absorption of drug, but tracheal intubation and lavage will have to be performed instead of inducing emesis, and the cathartic and charcoal will need to be introduced via a large bore gastric lavage tube; (3) continue to provide full supportive care and adequate hydration while waiting for drug to be metabolized. In general, the drug is metabolized sufficiently rapidly so as to not warrant consideration of dialysis.

DOSAGE AND ADMINISTRATION
Therapeutic serum levels associated with optimal likelihood for benefit and minimal risk of toxicity are between 10-20 mcg/ml. There is great variation from patient to patient in the dosage of Theophylline needed to achieve a therapeutic blood level because of variable rates of elimination. Because of this and because of the relatively narrow therapeutic blood level range associated with optimal results, the monitoring of serum Theophylline levels is highly recommended. (See *"Laboratory Tests"*).

Effective use of Theophylline (i.e., the concentration of drug in the serum associated with optimal benefit and minimal risk of toxicity) is considered to occur when the Theophylline concentration is maintained from 10 to 20 mcg/mL. The early studies from which these levels are derived were carried out in patients immediately or shortly after recovery from acute exacerbations of their disease (some hospitalized with status asthmaticus).

Although the 20 mcg/mL level remains appropriate as a critical value (above which toxicity is more likely to occur) for safety purposes, additional data are now available which indicate that the serum Theophylline concentrations required to produce maximum physiologic benefit may, in fact, fluctuate with the degree of bronchospasm present and are variable. Therefore, the physician should individualize the range appropriate to the patient's requirements, based on both symptomatic response and improvement in pulmonary function it should be stressed that serum Theophylline concentrations maintained at the upper level of the 10 to 20 mcg/mL range may be associated with potential toxicity when factors known to reduce Theophylline clearance are operative. (See *"Warnings"*).

It it is not possible to obtain serum level determinations, restrictions of the daily dose (in otherwise healthy adults) to not greater than 13 mg/kg/day, to a maximum of 900 mg of theophylline in divided doses, will result in relatively few patients exceeding serum levels of 20 mcg/mL and the resultant greater risk of toxicity.

Caution should be exercised for younger children who cannot complain of minor side effects. Older adults those with corpulmonale congestive heart failure and/or liver disease may have unusually low dosage requirements and thus may experience toxicity at the maximal dosage recommended below.

Theophylline does not distribute into fatty tissue. Dosage should be calculated on the basis of lean (ideal) body weight where mg/kg doses are presented.

Frequency of Dosing: When immediate release products with rapid absorption are used, dosing to maintain serum levels generally requires administration every 6 hours. This is particularly true in children, but dosing intervals up to 8 hours may be satisfactory in adults since they eliminate the drug at a slower rate. Some children, and adults requiring higher than average doses (those having rapid rates of clearance, e.g., half-lives of under 6 hours) may benefit and be more effectively controlled during chronic therapy when given products with sustained-release characteristics since these provide longer dosing intervals and/or less fluctuation in serum concentration between dosing.

Dosage guidelines are approximations only and the wide range of Theophylline clearance between individuals (particularly those with concomitant disease) makes indiscriminate usage hazardous.

Usual Dosage:
Adult—1 or 2 tablets or tablespoonfuls (15-30 ml), 3 or 4 times daily.
Children 6 to 12—2 or 3 teaspoonfuls (10-15 ml), 3 or 4 times daily.
Children 3 to 6—1 to 1 ½ teaspoonfuls (5-7.5 ml), 3 or 4 times daily.
Children 1 to 3—½ to 1 teaspoonful (2.5-5 ml), 3 or 4 times daily.

Dosage Titration: A. For patients not currently receiving Theophylline products. (See related table).

B. For patients currently receiving Theophylline Products: Determine, where possible, the time, amount, route of administration and form of the patient's last dose of Theophylline.

The loading dose for Theophylline will be based on the principle that each 0.5 mg/kg of theophylline administered as a loading dose will result in a 1 mcg/ml increase in serum Theophylline concentration. Ideally, then, the loading dose should be deferred if a serum Theophylline concentration can be rapidly obtained. If this is not possible, the clinician must exercise his judgment in selecting a dose based on the potential for benefit and risk. When there is sufficient respiratory distress to warrant a small risk, 2.5 mg/kg of Theophylline is likely to increase the serum concentration when administered as a loading dose in rapidly absorbed

	Oral Loading Dose (Theophylline Sodium Glycinate)	Maintenance Dose For Next 12 Hours (Theophylline Sodium Glycinate)	Maintenance Dose Beyond 12 Hours (Theophylline Sodium Glycinate)
1. Infants	8 mg/kg *(4 mg/kg)	3-8 mg/kg q6h *(1.5-4.0 mg/kg q6h)	4-6 mg/kg q6h *(2-3 mg/kg q6h)**
2. Children 6 months to 9 years	12 mg/kg *(6 mg/kg)	8 mg/kg q4h *(4 mg/kg q4h)	8 mg/kg q6h *(4 mg/kg q6h)
3. Children age 9-16 and young adult smokers	12 mg/kg *(6 mg/kg)	6 mg/kg q4h *(3 mg/kg q4h)	6 mg/kg q8h *(3 mg/kg q8h)
4. Otherwise healthy nonsmoking adults	12 mg/kg *(6 mg/kg)	6 mg/kg q6h *(3 mg/kg q6h)	6 mg/kg q8h) *(3 mg/kg q8h)
5. Older patients and patients with Cor pulmonale	12 mg/kg *(6 mg/kg)	4 mg/kg *(2 mg/kg q6h)	4 mg/kg q8h *(2 mg/kg q8h)
6. Patients with congestive heart failure, liver failure	12 mg/kg *(6 mg/kg)	4 mg/kg q8h *(2 mg/kg q8h	2-4 mg/kg q12h *(1-2 mg/kg q12h)

Equivalent Theophylline dosage indicated in parenthesis and marked with an (*).
** Pediatrics, Vol. 55, No. 5, May 1975.

form by only about 5 mcg/ml. If the patient is not already experiencing Theophylline toxicity, this is unlikely to result in dangerous adverse effects.

Measurement of Serum Theophylline Concentration during Chronic Therapy: Blood for peak Theophylline determinations should be obtained 1-2 hours after a dose of Theophylline sodium glycinate. When determining Theophylline serum concentrations in patients who have received chronic therapy, it is essential to establish that no doses were omitted in the 48 hours prior to the determination. Missed doses could result in recommendations of future doses that would cause serious toxicity due to overdosage.

DOSAGE ADJUSTMENT BASED ON SERUM THEOPHYLLINE MEASUREMENTS WHEN THESE INSTRUCTIONS HAVE NOT BEEN FOLLOWED MAY RESULT IN RECOMMENDATIONS THAT PRESENT RISK OF TOXICITY TO THE PATIENT.

PATIENTS SHOULD NEVER BE MAINTAINED ON A DOSAGE OF THEOPHYLLINE THAT IS NOT WELL TOLERATED. Patients experiencing toxic side effects should be instructed to skip the next regular dose and to resume Theophylline therapy at a lower dosage when all side effects have disappeared.

Maximum Dose Without Measurement of Serum Concentration: Not to exceed the following: (*Warning:* DO NOT ATTEMPT TO MAINTAIN ANY DOSAGE THAT IS NOT WELL TOLERATED.)

Age	Theophylline Sodium Glycinate	Equivalent Theophylline
Under 9 years	48 mg/kg/day	24 mg/kg/day
9-12 years	40 mg/kg/day	20 mg/kg/day
12-16 years	36 mg/kg/day	18/mg/kg/day
Over 16 years	26 mg/kg/day or 1800 mg/day (WHICHEVER IS LESS)	13 mg/kg/day or 900 mg/day (WHICHEVER IS LESS)

Use ideal (lean) body weight for obese patients in computing dosage.

Dosage should always be calculated on the basis of ideal (lean) body weight when mg/kg doses are stated. Theophylline does not distribute into fatty tissue. NEVER ATTEMPT TO MAINTAIN A DOSAGE THAT IS NOT WELL TOLERATED BY THE PATIENT.

Recommended Storage: Product should be stored at controlled room temperature 15°-30° (59°-86° F)
Dispense in light containers.

HOW SUPPLIED
CAPSULE: 90 MG-150 MG

BRAND/MANUFACTURER	NDC	SIZE	AWP
○ BRAND			
QUIBRON: Roberts Pharm	54092-0067-01	100s	$35.72
	54092-0067-52	100s ud	$39.27
	54092-0067-10	1000s	$338.88
○ GENERICS			
GLYCERYL-T: Rugby	00536-3868-01	100s	$4.28
UNI-BRONCHIAL: URL	00677-0766-01	100s	$4.40
BRONCHIAL: Moore,H.L.	00839-6697-06	100s	$4.44
THEOLATE: Balan,J.J.	00304-0274-01	100s	$6.38

CAPSULE: 180 MG-300 MG

BRAND/MANUFACTURER	NDC	SIZE	AWP
○ BRAND			
QUIBRON-300: Roberts Pharm	54092-0068-01	100s	$57.14

ELIXER: 90 MG-150 MG/15 ML

BRAND/MANUFACTURER	NDC	SIZE	AWP
○ GENERICS *7NLYCERYL-T: Rugby *71 00536-0760-85	480 ml		3.50 *7NHEOCON: CMC-Cons *71 00223-6622-01

BRAND/MANUFACTURER	NDC	SIZE	AWP
	480 ml		4.50 *7N-B: Major *71 00904-0070-28
	480 ml		23.20

For additional alternatives, turn to the section beginning on page 2859.

Guaifenesin and Theophylline Sodium Glycinate

DESCRIPTION

Each tablespoonful (15 mL) of Guaifenesin/Theophylline Sodium Glycinate Elixir contains:

Guaifenesin ....100 mg
Theophylline Sodium Glycinate ....300 mg
(equivalent to 150 mg theophylline) Guaifenesin/Theophylline Sodium Glycinate contains a bronchodilator and an expectorant.

Theophylline Sodium Glycinate, a methylxanthine, is a white crystalline powder that is freely soluble in water, has a slight ammoniacal odor and a bitter taste. It is an equimolar mixture of Theophylline Sodium and glycine buffered by an additional mole of the essential amino acid, glycine.

The expectorant component is Guaifenesin (formerly called glyceryl guaiacolate) which helps loosen and thus clear the bronchial passageways of bothersome, thickened mucus. Guaifenesin, 3-(o-methoxyphenoxy)-1,2-propanediol, occurs as a fine, white powder having a bitter, aromatic taste and a slight odor of guaiacol. The powder tends to become lumpy on storage. It is freely soluble in alcohol and soluble in water.

CLINICAL PHARMACOLOGY

Theophylline Sodium Glycinate is more stable in the presence of hydrochloric acid due to the buffering action of glycine with subsequent reduction of the chance of Theophylline precipitation in the stomach. This and the high solubility of the product are suggested as the reasons why this product has better gastric tolerance than aminophylline.

Theophylline, the active ingredient of Theophylline Sodium Glycinate, accounts for 50% of the weight of this compound. Theophylline Sodium Glycinate is highly effective in relaxing the smooth muscle of the bronchioles and the pulmonary blood vessels. Thus acting primarily as a bronchodilator, pulmonary vasodilator and smooth muscle relaxant. Like other xanthines, Theophylline Sodium Glycinate is a coronary vasodilator, a diuretic, a cerebral, cardiac and skeletal muscle stimulant.

Theophylline acts by inhibiting phosphodiesterase which causes an increase in intracellular cyclic AMP. This action produces smooth muscle relaxation and inhibits the release of histamine and other bronchoconstricting mediators from mast cells.

In vitro, using human white blood cells, Theophylline has been shown to react synergistically with beta agonists to increase intracellular cyclic AMP. More data is required to clearly establish if Theophylline and the beta agonists are synergistic or additive *in vivo*. Even after prolonged therapy, it has not been possible to demonstrate the development of tolerance to Theophylline Sodium Glycinate.

The half-life of Theophylline varies from individual to individual. Since effective bronchodilatation depends upon maintaining serum Theophylline levels between 10-20 mg/dl (10-20 mcg/mL), the determination of serum Theophylline can be of value.

The half-life of Theophylline is prolonged in alcoholism, in patients with reduced hepatic or renal function, congestive heart failure and in patients receiving antibiotics such as triacetyloleandomycin, erythromycin, clindamycin and lincomycin. Fever can also prolong Theophylline half-life.

Cigarette smoking (1-2 packs per day) enhances Theophylline elimination. The half-life of Theophylline is shortened with cigarette smoking. This effect is

◆ RATED THERAPEUTICALLY EQUIVALENT; ◇ THERAPEUTIC EQUIVALENCE UNCONFIRMED; ○ UNRATED

probably related to the induction of enzymes and requires between three months and two years to normalize after stopping tobacco usage.

By increasing respiratory tract fluid, Guaifenesin reduces the viscosity of tenacious secretions and acts as an expectorant. The drug is effective in productive as well as nonproductive cough, but is of particular value in dry, nonproductive cough which tends to injure the mucous membranes of the air passages. (See Table 1).

INDICATIONS AND USAGE
For relief of acute bronchial asthma and for reversible bronchospasm associated with chronic bronchitis and emphysema.

CONTRAINDICATIONS
Guaifenesin/Theophylline Sodium Glycinate Elixir is contraindicated in individuals who have shown hypersensitivity to any of the components.

WARNINGS
There is an excellent correlation between high Theophylline blood levels and the clinical manifestations of toxicity in (1) patients with lowered body plasma clearances (due to transient cardiac decomposition), (2) chronic obstructive lung disease or patients with liver dysfunction, (3) patients who are older than 55 years of age, particularly males.

There are often no early signs of Theophylline toxicity such as nausea and restlessness which may appear in up to 50% of patients. Convulsions or ventricular arrhythmias may be the first signs of toxicity.

Excessive doses of Theophylline Sodium Glycinate may be expected to be toxic and serum Theophylline levels are recommended to monitor therapy. The incidence of toxicity increases significantly at levels greater than 20 mcg/mL. Many patients who have higher Theophylline serum levels exhibit tachycardia. Theophylline products often worsen preexisting arrhythmias.

Guaifenesin/Theophylline Sodium Glycinate Elixir and other oral Theophylline compounds should never be used to treat status asthmaticus.

PRECAUTIONS
General: Theophylline should be used with caution in patients with severe cardiovascular disease, severe hypoxemia, hypertension, hyperthyroidism, acute myocardial injury, obstructive lung disease, liver disease, in the elderly and in neonates.

Great caution should be used in giving Theophylline to patients in congestive heart failure. Such patients have markedly prolonged Theophylline blood levels which have persisted for long periods after discontinuation of the drug.

Smokers have a shorter mean half-life of Theophylline than nonsmokers and may require larger doses of Theophylline.

Theophylline Sodium Glycinate should not be administered concurrently with other Theophylline-containing products or aminophylline.

Theophylline should be given with caution to patients with a history of peptic ulcer. Theophylline may act as a local irritant in the gastrointestinal tract.

Information for Patients: The importance of adherence to the prescribed dosage regimen should be stressed. Patients should be informed of symptoms associated with Theophylline toxicity such as nausea and restlessness.

Laboratory Tests: There is a great patient-to-patient variation in the serum half-life of Theophylline. Therefore, when possible, serum Theophylline levels should be measured to assist in titration of dosage.

Drug Interactions: The use of Theophylline Sodium Glycinate with ephedrine and other sympathomimetic bronchodilators may result in a significant increase in side effects (See Table 2).

Drug/Laboratory Test Interactions: Theophylline has been shown to increase the urinary excretion of catecholamines. The VMA test for catechols may be falsely elevated by Guaifenesin. Theophylline may increase the apparent serum uric acid in certain manual or automated chemical procedures by being treated as if it were uric acid. Guaifenesin may increase renal clearance for urate and thereby lower the serum uric acid. It may also falsely elevate the level of urinary 5HIAA in certain serotonin metabolite chemical tests.

Carcinogenesis, Mutagenesis, Impairment of Fertility: No data are available on the long-term potential for carcinogenicity, mutagenicity of impairment of fertility in animals or humans.

Pregnancy: Pregnancy Category C: Animal reproduction studies have not been conducted with Guaifenesin/Theophylline Sodium Glycinate. Safe use in pregnancy has not been established relative to possible adverse effects on fetal development. Therefore, Theophylline should not be used in pregnant patients unless, in the judgment of the physician, the potential benefits outweigh possible hazards.

Nursing Mothers: It is not known whether this drug is excreted in human milk. Because many drugs are excreted in human milk, caution should be observed when Guaifenesin/Theophylline Sodium Glycinate Elixir is administered to a nursing mother.

Pediatric Use: See Dosage and Administration Section for mg/kg dosage in pediatric patients.

ADVERSE REACTIONS
Included in this listing which follows are adverse reactions, some of which may have been reported with Theophylline Sodium Glycinate. However, pharmacological similarities among the xanthine drugs require that each of the reactions be considered when Theophylline is administered. The most consistent adverse reactions are usually due to overdosage of Theophylline Sodium Glycinate and are:

1. Gastrointestinal: nausea, vomiting, epigastric pain, hematemesis, diarrhea.

2. Central Nervous System: headaches, irritability, restlessness, insomnia, reflex hyperexcitability, muscle twitching, clonic and tonic generalized convulsions.

3. Cardiovascular: palpitation, tachycardia, extrasystoles, flushing, hypotension, circulatory failure, life-threatening ventricular arrhythmias.

4. Respiratory: tachypnea.

5. Renal: albuminuria, increased excretion of renal tubular calls and red blood cells; potentiation of diuresis.

6. Others: hyperglycemia and inappropriate ADH syndrome.

OVERDOSAGE
MANAGEMENT
A. If potential oral overdose is established and seizure has not occurred: (1) induce vomiting and resort to gastric lavage if the patient fails to vomit within 20-30 minutes; (2) administer a cathartic (this is particularly important if sustained-release preparations have been taken) and activated charcoal after successful vomiting has been induced or adequate gastric lavage performed.
B. If patient is having a seizure: (1) establish an airway; (2) administer O_2; (3) treat the seizure with intravenous diazepam 0.1 to 0.3 mg/kg up to 10 mg; (4) monitor vital signs, maintain blood pressure and provide adequate hydration.
C. Post-Seizure Coma: (1) maintain airway and oxygenation; (2) if a result of oral medication, follow above recommendations to prevent absorption of drug, but tracheal intubation and lavage will have to be performed instead of inducing emesis, and the cathartic and charcoal will need to be introduced via a large bore gastric lavage tube; (3) continue to provide full supportive care and adequate hydration while waiting for drug to be metabolized. In general, the drug is metabolized sufficiently rapidly so as to not warrant consideration of dialysis.

DOSAGE AND ADMINISTRATION
Therapeutic serum levels associated with optimal likelihood for benefit and minimal risk of toxicity are between 10-20 mcg/mL. There is great variation from patient to patient in the dosage of Theophylline needed to achieve a therapeutic blood level because of variable rates of elimination. Because of this and because of the relatively narrow therapeutic blood level range associated with optimal results, the monitoring of serum Theophylline levels is highly recommended. (See Laboratory Tests).

Usual Dosage: Adults - 1 or 2 tablespoonfuls (15-30 mL), 3 or 4 times daily. Children 6 to 12 years - 2 or 3 teaspoonfuls (10-15 mL), 3 or 4 times daily. Children 3 to 6 years -1 to 1 1/2 teaspoonfuls (5-7.5 mL), 3 or 4 times daily. Children 1 to 3 years - 1/2 to 1 teaspoonful (2.5-5 mL), 3 or 4 times daily.

Dosage Titration:
A. FOR PATIENTS NOT CURRENTLY RECEIVING THEOPHYLLINE PRODUCTS: (See Table 3).
B. FOR PATIENTS CURRENTLY RECEIVING THEOPHYLLINE PRODUCTS: Determine, where possible, the time, amount, route of administration and form of the patient's last dose of Theophylline.

The loading dose of Theophylline will be based on the principle that each 0.5 mg/kg of Theophylline administered as a loading dose will result in a 1 mcg/mL increase in serum theophylline concentration. Ideally, then, the loading dose should be deferred if a serum Theophylline concentration can be rapidly obtained. If this is not possible, the clinician must exercise his judgment in selecting a dose based on the potential for benefit and risk. When there is sufficient respiratory distress to warrant a small risk, 2.5 mg/kg of Theophylline is likely to increase the serum concentration when administered as a loading dose in rapidly absorbed form by only about 5 mcg/mL. If the patient is not already experiencing Theophylline toxicity, this is unlikely to result in dangerous adverse effects.

Measurement of serum Theophylline concentration during chronic therapy: Blood for peak Theophylline determinations should be obtained 1-2 hours after a dose of Theophylline Sodium Glycinate. When determining Theophylline serum concentrations in patients who have received chronic therapy, it is essential to establish that no doses were omitted in the 48 hours prior to the determination. Missed doses could result in recommendations of future doses that would cause serious toxicity due to overdosage.

DOSAGE ADJUSTMENT BASED ON SERUM THEOPHYLLINE MEASUREMENTS WHEN THESE INSTRUCTIONS HAVE NOT BEEN FOLLOWED MAY RESULT IN RECOMMENDATIONS THAT PRESENT RISK OF TOXICITY TO THE PATIENT.

PATIENTS SHOULD NEVER BE MAINTAINED ON A DOSAGE OF THEOPHYLLINE THAT IS NOT WELL TOLERATED. Patients experiencing toxic side effects should be instructed to skip the next regular dose and to resume Theophylline therapy at a lower dosage when all side effects have disappeared.

Maximum Dose Without Measurement of Serum Concentration: Not to exceed the following (WARNING: DO NOT ATTEMPT TO MAINTAIN ANY DOSAGE THAT IS NOT WELL TOLERATED): See Table 4.

Use ideal (lean) body weight for obese patients in computing dosage.
Dosage should always be calculated on the basis of ideal (lean) body weight when mg/kg doses are stated. Theophylline does not distribute into fatty tissues. NEVER ATTEMPT TO MAINTAIN A DOSAGE THAT IS NOT WELL TOLERATED BY THE PATIENT.

Table 1
THEOPHYLLINE ELIMINATION CHARACTERISTICS

Group	Theophylline Renal Clearance Rates	Half-Life Average
1. Children	1.4 mL/kg/min	3.5 hours
2. Adults with uncomplicated asthma	1.2 mL/kg/min	7 hours
3. Older adults with chronic obstructive pulmonary disease	0.6 mL/kg/min	up to 24 hours
4. Adults with chronic obstructive pulmonary disease and cor pulmonale or other causes of heart failure and liver pathology	0.6 mL/kg/min and less	may exceed 24 hours
5. Young smokers	Not available	4.3 hours

Table 2

Drug	Effect
Aminophylline with Lithium Carbonate	Increased excretion of Lithium Carbonate
Aminophylline with Propranolol	Antagonism of Propranolol effect
Theophylline with Furosemide	Increased Diuresis
Theophylline with Hexamethonium	Decreased Hexamethonium-induced chronotropic effect
Theophylline with Reserpine	Reserpine-induced Tachycardia
Theophylline with Cimetidine	Increased theophylline blood levels
Theophylline with clindamycin, troleandomycin, erythromycin, lincomycin	Increased theophylline blood levels

Table 3

	Oral Loading Dose (Theophylline Sodium Glycinate)	Maintenance Dose For Next 12 Hours (Theophylline Sodium Glycinate)	Maintenance Dose Beyond 12 Hours (Theophylline Sodium Glycinate)
1. Infants	8 mg/kg *(4 mg/kg)	3-8 mg/kg q6h *(1.5-4.0 mg/kg q6h)	4-6 mg/kg q6h *(2-3 mg/kg q6h)**
2. Children 6 months to 9 years	12 mg/kg *(6 mg/kg)	8mg/kg q4h *(4 mg/kg q4h)	8 mg/kg q6h *(4 mg/kg q6h)
3. Children age 9-16 and young adult smokers	12 mg/kg *(6 mg/kg)	6 mg/kg q4h) *(3 mg/kg q4h)	6 mg/kg q6h *(3 mg/kg q6h)
4. Otherwise healthy nonsmoking adults	12 mg/kg *(6 mg/kg)	6 mg/kg q6h *(3 mg/kg q6h)	6 mg/kg q8h *(3 mg/kg q8h)
5. Older patients and patients with cor pulmonale	12 mg/kg *(6 mg/kg	4 mg/kg q6h *(2 mg/kg q6h)	4 mg/kg q8h *(2 mg/kg q8h)
6. Patients with congestive heart failure, liver failure	12 mg/kg *(6 mg/kg)	4 mg/kg q8h *(2 mg/kg q8h)	2-4 mg/kg q12h *(1-2 mg/kg q12h)

Equivalent Theophylline dosage indicated in parenthesis and marked with an asterisk (*).
** Pediatrics, Vol. 55, No. 5, May 1975.

Table 4

Age	Theophylline Sodium Glycinate	Equivalent Theophylline
Under 9 years	48 mg/kg/day	24 mg/kg/day
9-12 years	40 mg/kg/day	20 mg/kg/day
12-16 years	36 mg/kg/day	18 mg/kg/day
Over 16 years	26 mg/kg/day or 1800 mg/day (WHICHEVER IS LESS)	13 mg/kg/day or 900 mg/day (WHICHEVER IS LESS)

HOW SUPPLIED
Current prices are unavailable. Check wholesaler for further information.

Guaifenesin/Hydrocodone Bitartrate/Pheniramine Maleate/ Phenylephrine Hydrochloride/ Phenylpropanolamine Hydrochloride

Each 5 mL contains:

Hydrocodone Bitartrate	2.50 mg
(Warning: May be habit forming.)	
Phenylephrine HCl	5 mg
Phenylpropanolamine HCl	5 mg
Pheniramine Maleate	13.33 mg
Guaifenesin	80 mg

5% Alcohol by volume.

ACTION AND USES
This "5-action cough medicine," gives 5-action symptomatic relief of stubborn coughs and nasal congestion, due to colds or hay fever.

ADMINISTRATION AND DOSAGE
Average Adult Dosage: One teaspoonful 3 or 4 times a day as indicated, not to exceed 4 teaspoonfuls in any 24 hours.

Children: 6 to 12 years, half teaspoonful 3 or 4 times a day as indicated, not to exceed 2 teaspoonfuls in any 24 hours.

Children: 3 to 6 years, half teaspoonful; 1 to 3 years, 20 drops; 6 months to 1 year, 10 drops.

SIDE EFFECTS
The product is usually well tolerated, but if drowsiness or nausea or other side effects occur, discontinue its use immediately.
    Keep this and all medications out of children's reach.
    The product contains:
    Hydrocodone Bitartrate, a centrally acting narcotic antitussive providing cough relief for up to 6 hours.
    Phenylephrine HCl, an orally effective vasoconstrictor for relief of nasal congestion and bronchial spasm.
    Phenylpropanolamine HCl, a well known decongestant used to shrink engorged mucous membranes, caused by hay fever and allergic rhinitis.
    Pheniramine Maleate, one of the most potent antihistamines on a weight basis, Guaifenesin, an effective expectorant in the treatment of coughs.

PRECAUTIONS AND CONTRAINDICATIONS
This product contains Hydrocodone Bitartrate (7.8 dihydrocodeinone) a derivative of codeine. Warning: it may produce drug dependence and has the potential for abuse; therefore should be used with caution and only when indicated, not for a prolonged period of time. It should be used with caution in patients sensitive to antihistamines and to sympathomimetic products, or patients with arteriosclerosis, hypertension or hyperthyroidism. Patients taking this drug should not drive vehicles or operate machinery. Patients receiving narcotic analgesics, phenotiazines, other tranquilizers, sedative-hypnotics or other central nervous depressants and alcohol together with this drug may exhibit an additive CNS depression; in case of such combined therapy, the dose of one or both agents should be reduced. It is important to adopt appropriate therapy for the primary condition, before prescribing this drug to suppress or modify cough, and to make sure that the underlying cause of cough does not increase the risk of clinical or physiologic complications.

HOW SUPPLIED
LIQUID (C-III):

BRAND/MANUFACTURER	NDC	SIZE	AWP
○ **BRAND**			
S-T FORTE: Scot-Tussin	00372-0004-04	120 ml	$7.19
	00372-0005-04	120 ml	$7.19
	00372-0004-08	240 ml	$12.35
	00372-0005-08	240 ml	$12.35
	00372-0005-16	480 ml	$24.70
	00372-0004-16	480 ml	$25.27
	00372-0005-28	3840 ml	$176.82
	00372-0004-28	3840 ml	$180.83

◆ RATED THERAPEUTICALLY EQUIVALENT; ◇ THERAPEUTIC EQUIVALENCE UNCONFIRMED; ○ UNRATED

Guaifenesin/Hydrocodone Bitartrate/Phenylpropanolamine Hydrochloride/Pheniramine Maleate/Pyrilamine Maleate

DESCRIPTION

Each teaspoonful (5 ml) of Guaifenesin/Hydrocodone Bitartrate/Phenylpropanolamine Hydrochloride/Pheniramine Maleate/Pyrilamine Maleate contains: Hydrocodone Bitartrate 1.67 mg (Warning: May be habit forming), Phenylpropanolamine Hydrochloride 12.5 mg, Pheniramine Maleate 6.25 mg, Pyrilamine Maleate 6.25 mg, Guaifenesin 100 mg, and alcohol 5%.

Phenylpropanolamine Hydrochloride, a sympathomimetic drug, is structurally related to ephedrine and amphetamine. Pheniramine Maleate is an antihistamine of the alkylamine class while Pyrilamine Maleate belongs to the ethylenediamine class.

The expectorant component is Guaifenesin (3-(o-methoxyphenoxy)-1,2-propanediol) which helps loosen and thus clear the bronchial passageways of bothersome, thickened mucus. The antitussive component, Hydrocodone, is 7,8 dihydrocodeinone, a derivative of codeine.

CLINICAL PHARMACOLOGY

Phenylpropanolamine presumably acts on α-adrenergic receptors in the mucosa of the respiratory tract producing vasoconstriction which results in shrinkage of swollen mucous membranes, reduction of tissue hyperemia, edema and nasal congestion, and an increase in nasal airway patency. Antihistamines competitively act as H_1 receptor antagonists of histamine. They exhibit anticholinergic (drying) and sedative side effects. There are several classes of antihistamines which vary with respect to potency, dosage and the relative incidence of side effects. Antihistamines inhibit the effects of histamine on capillary permeability and on vascular, bronchial and many other types of smooth muscle.

By increasing respiratory tract fluid, Guaifenesin reduces the viscosity of tenacious secretions and acts as an expectorant. The drug is effective in productive as well as nonproductive cough, but is of particular value in dry, nonproductive cough which tends to injure the mucous membranes of the air passages.

Hydrocodone is a centrally acting narcotic antitussive providing cough relief for up to 6 hours.

INDICATIONS

For relief of troublesome cough, nasal congestion and postnasal drip associated with colds, nasal allergies, sinusitis, and rhinitis. Also effective for relief of severe, prolonged or refractory cough associated with other respiratory disorders. For the relief of symptoms associated with allergic rhinitis such as sneezing, rhinorrhea, pruritus and lacrimation.

CONTRAINDICATIONS

This combination is contraindicated in patients exhibiting hypersensitivity to any of the ingredients. Antihistamines are contraindicated in patients receiving monoamine oxidase inhibitors since these agents may prolong and intensify the anticholinergic effects of antihistamines (see *"Drug Interactions"*). Antihistamines *should not* be used to treat lower respiratory tract symptoms or be given to premature or newborn infants. Sympathomimetic agents such as Phenylpropanolamine are contraindicated in patients with severe hypertension, severe coronary artery disease and in those taking monoamine oxidase inhibitors. Narcotic analgesics are contraindicated in patients with acute respiratory depression. Continuous dosage over an extended period is generally contraindicated since Hydrocodone can cause addiction.

Nursing Mothers: Because of the higher risk of antihistamines for premature and newborn infants, antihistamine therapy is contraindicated in nursing mothers.

WARNINGS

This combination can produce drug dependence, and therefore has the potential for abuse.

Sympathomimetic agents should be used with caution in patients with hypertension, hyperthyroidism, diabetes mellitus and cardiovascular disease. Antihistamines should be used with caution in patients with narrow angle glaucoma, stenosing peptic ulcer, pyloroduodenal obstruction, symptomatic prostatic hypertrophy, bladder neck obstruction or chronic pulmonary disease. Narcotic analgesics should be used with caution in patients with chronic respiratory impairment, cardiac arrhythmias, history of convulsions, history of drug dependence, gallbladder disease or impaired renal or hepatic function.

Use in the Elderly (Approximately 60 Years or Older): Antihistamines are more likely to cause dizziness, sedation and hypotension in elderly patients. Overdosage of sympathomimetic agents in this age group may cause hallucinations, convulsions, CNS depression or death. Geriatric patients may be more susceptible to the effects of Hydrocodone, especially the respiratory depressant effects.

PRECAUTIONS

General: Use with caution in patients with hypertension, hyperthyroidism, diabetes mellitus, cardiovascular disease, bronchial asthma, increased intraocular pressure (see *"Warnings"*). Before prescribing medication to suppress or modify cough, it is important to ascertain that the underlying cause of cough is identified, that modification of cough does not increase the risk of clinical complications, and that appropriate therapy for the primary disease is provided.

Information for Patients: Tell patient to adhere to dosing information. Patients should be informed of the potential for sedation or drowsiness and cautioned about engaging in activities requiring mental alertness such as driving or operating machinery. The concomitant consumption of alcoholic beverages or other sedative drugs should be avoided.

Drug Interactions:

(1) Monoamine oxidase inhibitors: MAO inhibitors may prolong and intensify the anticholinergic effects of antihistamines and potentiate the pressor effects of sympathomimetics.

(2) Alcohol and CNS depressants: These agents potentiate the sedative effects of antihistamines and Hydrocodone. The CNS and respiratory depressant effects of some opioids may be exaggerated and prolonged by phenothiazines, alcohol, CNS depressants, MAO inhibitors, and tricyclic antidepressants; the mechanism of this supra-additive effect is not fully understood, but may involve alterations in the rate of metabolic transformation of the opioid or alterations in neurotransmitters involved in opioid actions.

(3) Certain antihypertensives: Sympathomimetics may reduce the antihypertensive effects of methyldopa, mecamylamine, reserpine and veratrum alkaloids.

Drug/Laboratory Test Interactions: Guaifenesin or its metabolites may cause color interference with the VMA test for catechols. It may also falsely elevate the level of urinary 5HIAA in certain serotonin metabolite chemical tests because of color interference.

Carcinogenesis, Mutagenesis, Impairment of Fertility: No data are available on the long-term potential for carcinogenicity, mutagenicity or impairment of fertility in animals or humans.

Pregnancy: Pregnancy Category C: Animal reproduction studies have not been conducted. Safe use in pregnancy has not been established relative to possible adverse effects on fetal development. Therefore, this product should not be used in pregnant patients unless, in the judgment of the physician, the potential benefits outweigh possible hazards.

Nursing Mothers: See *"Contraindications"*.

Pediatric Use: This combination is intended for administration to children 1 to 12 years of age (see *"Dosage and Administration"*). It is important to note the variability of response infants and small children exhibit to antihistamines and sympathomimetics. As in adults, the combination of an antihistamine and sympathomimetic can elicit either mild stimulation or mild sedation in children. In the young child, mild stimulation is the response most frequently seen. In infants and children, overdosage of antihistamines may cause hallucinations, convulsions or death. Pediatric patients may be more susceptible to the effects of Hydrocodone, especially the respiratory depressant effects.

ADVERSE REACTIONS

The most frequent adverse reactions are underlined.

(1) General: urticaria, drug rash, anaphylactic shock, photosensitivity, excessive perspiration, chills, dryness of mouth, nose and throat.

(2) Cardiovascular System: hypotension, headache, palpitations, tachycardia, extrasystoles.

(3) Hematologic System: hemolytic anemia, thrombocytopenia, agranulocytosis.

(4) Nervous System: sedation, sleepiness, dizziness, disturbed coordination, fatigue, confusion, restlessness, excitation, nervousness, tremor, irritability, insomnia, euphoria, paresthesias, blurred vision, diplopia, vertigo, tinnitus, acute labyrinthitis, hysteria, neuritis, convulsions, CNS depression, hallucinations.

(5) GI System: epigastric distress, anorexia, nausea, vomiting, diarrhea, constipation.

(6) GU System: urinary frequency, difficult urination, urinary retention, early menses.

(7) Respiratory System: thickening of bronchial secretions, tightness of chest and wheezing, nasal stuffiness.

Drug Abuse and Dependence: Tolerance and physical dependence may occur following prolonged administration of Hydrocodone.

OVERDOSAGE

Symptoms: The triad of coma, pinpoint pupils, and depressed respiration strongly suggest Hydrocodone poisoning. Serious overdose with this combination may be characterized by respiratory depression, extreme somnolence progressing to stupor or coma, convulsions, skeletal muscle flaccidity, cold and clammy skin, and sometimes bradycardia and hypotension. In severe overdosage, apnea, circulatory collapse, cardiac arrest and death may occur. In the presence of fever and dehydration excitation may occur in children.

Treatment of Overdose: Primary attention should be given to the reestablishment of adequate respiratory exchange through provision of patent airway and the institution of assisted or controlled ventilation. The narcotic antagonists naloxone and levallorphan are specific antidotes against respiratory depression which may result from overdosage or unusual sensitivity to narcotics, including Hydrocodone. An appropriate dose of one of these antagonists should be administered, preferably by the intravenous route, simultaneously with efforts at respiratory resuscitation. The fact that an opioid antagonist may precipitate withdrawal symptoms in patients who are physically dependent on Hydrocodone must be kept in mind and dosage titrated accordingly. Since the duration of action of Hydrocodone may exceed that of the antagonist, the patient should be kept under continued surveillance and repeated doses of the antagonist should be administered as needed to maintain adequate respiration. Oxygen, intravenous fluids, vasopressors and other supportive measures should be employed as indicated, including treatment for anticholinergic drug intoxication. Gastric emptying may be useful in removing unabsorbed drug. Activated charcoal may be of benefit.

DOSAGE AND ADMINISTRATION

Adults—2 teaspoonfuls every 4 hours; children 6 to 12—1 teaspoonful every 4 hours; children 1 to 6—½ teaspoonful every 4 hours.

Store at room temperature. This combination is a Schedule III controlled substance.

HOW SUPPLIED

LIQUID (C-III):

BRAND/MANUFACTURER	NDC	SIZE	AWP
○ **BRAND**			
TRIAMINIC-DH EXPECTORANT: Sandoz Consumer	00043-0521-16	480 ml	$38.16

Guaifenesin/Hydrocodone Bitartrate/Phenylephrine Hydrochloride

DESCRIPTION

Each 5 mL (teaspoonful) of syrup contains:

Guaifenesin ....50 mg
Hydrocodone* Bitartrate ....2.5 mg
*(Warning - May be habit forming)
Phenylephrine Hydrochloride ....7.5 mg

The syrup contains ingredients of the following therapeutic classes: antitussive, nasal decongestant and expectorant.

CLINICAL PHARMACOLOGY

Hydrocodone Bitartrate is a potent antitussive which causes suppression of the cough reflex by a direct action on the cough center. Hydrocodone is approximately three times as potent as codeine on a weight basis, but has a higher addiction potential also. Phenylephrine Hydrochloride is a sympathomimetic which acts predominantly on alpha receptors and has little action on beta receptors. It, therefore, functions as an oral nasal decongestant with minimal CNS stimulation. Guaifenesin is an expectorant which exerts its action by stimulation of reflexes from the stomach, and acts through the nauseant effect which increases the output from the secretory glands of the respiratory tract.

INDICATIONS AND USAGE

Temporary relief of cough, nasal congestion, and other symptoms associated with colds or seasonal or perennial allergic vasomotor rhinitis (hay fever).

CONTRAINDICATIONS

Patients with severe hypertension, severe coronary artery disease, and in patients on MAO inhibitor therapy. Also contraindicated in patients with urinary retention, peptic ulcer, or in patients with a hypersensitivity to any of its ingredients.

WARNINGS

Considerable caution should be exercised in patients with hypertension, diabetes mellitus, ischemic heart disease, hyperthyroidism, increased intraocular pressure and prostatic hypertrophy. The elderly (60 years or older) are more likely to exhibit adverse reactions. Hydrocodone can produce drug dependence, and, therefore, has the potential for being abused.

PRECAUTIONS

General: Caution should be exercised in patients with high blood pressure, heart disease, diabetes or thyroid disease. The Hydrocodone in this combination may exhibit additive effects with other CNS depressants, including alcohol.

Information for Patients: The Hydrocodone may cause drowsiness, and ambulatory patients who operate machinery or motor vehicles should be cautioned accordingly.

Drug Interaction: MAO inhibitors and beta adrenergic blockers increase the effects of sympathomimetics. Sympathomimetics may reduce the antihypertensive effects of methyldopa, mecamylamine, reserpine and veratrum alkaloids. Concomitant use of Hydrocodone with alcohol and other CNS depressants may have an additive effect.

Pregnancy: Pregnancy Category C: It is not known whether this combination can cause fetal harm when administered to a pregnant woman or can affect reproduction capacity. This combination should be given to a pregnant woman only if clearly needed.

Nursing Mothers: It is not known whether this drug is excreted in human milk. Because many drugs are excreted in human milk, caution should be exercised when this syrup is administered to a nursing woman.

ADVERSE REACTIONS

Adverse reactions include drowsiness, lassitude, nausea, giddiness, gastrointestinal upset, and constipation.

DRUG ABUSE AND DEPENDENCE

This syrup is a Schedule III Controlled Substance. Because of the hydrocodone content, some abuse might be expected. Psychic dependence, physical dependence, and tolerance may develop upon repeated administration. It should be prescribed and administered with the degree of caution appropriate for this type product.

OVERDOSAGE AND TREATMENT OF OVERDOSAGE

In all cases of suspected overdose, immediately call your regional poison center and/or contact a physician immediately. Symptoms of overdosage may be caused by Hydrocodone or Phenylephrine. Hydrocodone may cause the classic narcotic symptoms of coma, pinpoint pupils of the eyes, and/or depressed respiration. The treatment of choice is naloxone hydrochloride administered in small intravenous doses (consult specific product labeling before use). Symptoms of overdosage with Phenylephrine include anxiety, tenseness, respiratory difficulty, throbbing headache, and awareness of the slow forceful heartbeat. Treatment is similar to that of an overdosage of epinephrine.

DOSAGE AND ADMINISTRATION

Adults and children 12 and older, 2 teaspoonfuls. Children 6 to under 12 years of age, 1 teaspoonful. Children 3 to under 6 years of age, 1/2 teaspoonful. May be repeated every 4 to 6 hours if required for relief. Not to exceed 6 doses in 24 hours. Children under 3, at discretion of physician.

Note: Under 2 years: Narcotic antitussives are not recommended for use in children under 2 years of age. Children under 2 years may be more susceptible to the respiratory depressant effects of narcotics, including respiratory arrest, coma, and death. However, dosage based on 0.3 mg/kg/24 hours divided into four equal doses have been suggested.

Store at controlled room temperature, 15°-30° C (59°-86° F).

Dispense in a tight, light-resistant container as defined in the USP/NF with a child-resistant closure.

HOW SUPPLIED

SYRUP (C-III):

BRAND/MANUFACTURER	NDC	SIZE	AWP
○ **GENERICS**			
DONATUSSIN DC: Laser	00277-0171-34	120 ml	$7.39
DONATUSSIN DC: Laser	00277-0171-41	480 ml	$28.35

Guaifenesin/Hydrocodone Bitartrate/Pseudoephedrine Hydrochloride

DESCRIPTION

Each 5 ml (one teaspoonful) of elixir contains:

Hydrocodone* Bitartrate ....2.5 mg
* WARNING: May be habit forming
Pseudoephedrine Hydrochloride ....30 mg
Guaifenesin ....100 mg
Alcohol 5%

Hydrocodone Bitartrate is an antitussive. Chemically it is 4,5 α-epoxy-3-methoxy-17-methylmorphian-6-one-tartrate (1:1) hydrate (2:5).

Pseudoephedrine Hydrochloride is a nasal decongestant. Chemically it is [S-(R*,R*)]-α-[1-(methylamino)ethyl] benzenemethanol hydrochloride.

Guaifenesin is an expectorant. Chemically it is 3-(0-methoxy-phenoxy)-1,2 propanediol.

CLINICAL PHARMACOLOGY

Hydrocodone is a semisynthetic narcotic analgesic and antitussive with multiple actions qualitatively similar to those of codeine. Most of these involve the central nervous system and smooth muscle. Hydrocodone suppresses the cough reflex by depressing the medullary cough center. The precise mechanism of action of Hydrocodone and other opiates is not known, although it is believed to relate to the existence of opiate receptors in the central nervous system.

Pseudoephedrine Hydrochloride is an orally effective nasal decongestant that acts on alpha-adrenergic receptors in the mucosa of the respiratory tract producing vasoconstriction. Pseudoephedrine shrinks swollen nasal mucous membranes, reduces tissue hyperemia, edema and nasal congestion and increases nasal airway patency. Drainage of sinus secretions is increased and obstructed Eustachian ostia may be opened. Pseudoephedrine produces little if any rebound

---

◆ RATED THERAPEUTICALLY EQUIVALENT; ◇ THERAPEUTIC EQUIVALENCE UNCONFIRMED; ○ UNRATED

congestion. Guaifenesin is an expectorant which enhances the flow of respiratory tract secretions. The enhanced flow of less viscid secretions lubricates irritated respiratory tract membranes, promotes cilliary action and facilitates the removal of inspissated mucus. As as result, sinus and bronchial drainage is improved and nonproductive coughs become more productive and less frequent.

INDICATIONS AND USAGE

For exhausting, nonproductive cough accompanying respiratory tract congestion associated with the common cold, influenza, sinusitis, and bronchitis.

CONTRAINDICATIONS

Hydrocodone Bitartrate/Guaifenesin/Pseudoephedrine Hydrochloride Elixir (2.5 mg Hydrocodone Bitartrate [Warning: May be habit forming] 30 mg Pseudoephedrine Hydrochloride, and 100 mg Guaifenesin per teaspoonful) is contraindicated in patients with severe hypertension, severe coronary artery disease, and in patients on MAO inhibitor therapy.

Hypersensitivity: Contraindicated in patients with hypersensitivity or idiosyncracy to sympathomimetic amines, phenanthrene derivatives, or to any other formula ingredients.

Nursing Mothers: Contraindicated because of the higher than usual risk for infants for sympathomimetic amines.

WARNINGS

Hydrocodone should be prescribed and administered with the same degree of caution as all oral medications containing a narcotic analgesic. Extreme caution should be exercised in the use of Hydrocodone in patients with severe respiratory impairment or patients with impaired respiratory drive.

If sympathomimetic amines are used in patients with hypertension, diabetes mellitus, ischemic heart disease, hyperthyroidism, increased intraocular, pressure or prostatic hypertrophy, judicious caution should be exercised (see *"Contraindications"*).

Use in Elderly: The elderly (60 years and older) are more likely to have adverse reactions to sympathomimetics. Overdosage of sympathomimetics in this age group may cause hallucinations, convulsions, CNS depression and death.

PRECAUTIONS

General: Caution should be exercised if used in patients with diabetes, hypertension, cardiovascular diseases, hyperreactivity to ephedrine or decreased respiratory drive (see *"Contraindications"*).

Information for Patients: Hydrocodone may produce drowsiness. Persons who perform hazardous tasks requiring mental alertness or physical coordination should be cautioned accordingly. Concomitant use of Hydrocodone with tranquilizers, alcohol or other depressants may produce additive depressant effects. Do not exceed the prescribed dosage.

Drug Interactions: Hydrocodone may potentiate the effects of other narcotics, general anesthetics, tranquilizers, sedatives and hypnotics, tricyclic antidepressants, MAO inhibitors, alcohol, and other CNS depressants. Beta-adrenergic blockers and MAO inhibitors potentiate the sympathomimetic effects of pseudoephedrine. Sympathomimetics may reduce the antihypertensive effects of methyldopa, mecamylamine, reserpine and veratrum alkaloids.

Laboratory Test Interactions: Guaifenesin interferes with the colorimetric determination of 5-hydroxyindoleacetic acid (5-HIAA) and vanillylmandelic acid (VMA).

Pregnancy Category C: Animal reproduction studies have not been conducted with Pseudoephedrine, Guaifenesin, or Hydrocodone. It is also not known whether Pseudoephedrine, Guaifenesin or Hydrocodone can cause fetal harm when administered to a pregnant woman or can affect reproduction capacity. Pseudoephedrine, Guaifenesin or Hydrocodone may be given to a pregnant woman only if clearly needed.

Nursing Mothers: Because of the potential for serious adverse reactions in nursing infants from sympathomimetic amines, Pseudoephedrine is contraindicated in nursing mothers.

ADVERSE REACTIONS

Gastrointestinal upset, nausea, drowsiness and constipation. A slight elevation in serum transaminase levels has been noted.

Individuals hyperreactive to Pseudoephedrine may display ephedrine-like reactions such as tachycardia, palpitations, headache, dizziness or nausea. Sympathomimetic drugs have been associated with certain untoward reactions including fear, anxiety, tenseness, restlessness, tremor, weakness, pallor, respiratory difficulty, dysuria, insomnia, hallucinations, convulsions, CNS depression, arrhythmias, and cardiovascular collapse with hypotension. Patient idiosyncrasy to adrenergic agents may be manifested by insomnia, dizziness, weakness, tremor or arrhythmias.

DRUG ABUSE AND DEPENDENCE

Controlled Substance: Hydrocodone in Hydrocodone Bitartrate/Guaifenesin/Pseudoephedrine Hydrochloride Elixir is controlled by the Drug Enforcement Administration. This elixir is a Schedule III controlled substance.

Abuse: Hydrocodone is a narcotic drug related to codeine with similar abuse potential.

Dependence: Hydrocodone can produce drug dependence of the morphine type. Psychic dependence, physical dependence and tolerance may develop if dosage recommendations are greatly exceeded over a prolonged period of time.

OVERDOSAGE

Acute overdosage with Hydrocodone Bitartrate/Guaifenesin/Pseudoephedrine Hydrochloride Elixir may produce variable clinical signs as Hydrocodone produces CNS depression and cardiovascular depression while Pseudoephedrine produces CNS stimulation and variable cardiovascular effects. Hydrocodone is likely to be responsible for most of the severe reactions from overdosage. Pressor amines should be used with great caution when taking Pseudoephedrine. Patients with signs of stimulation should be treated conservatively and depressant medications should be avoided if possible because of potential drug interaction with Hydrocodone.

DOSAGE AND ADMINISTRATION

Adults: 2 teaspoonfuls (10 ml) every 4-6 hours. Children 6-12 years of age: 1 teaspoonful (5 ml) every 4-6 hours. May be given four times a day as needed. May be taken with meals.

HOW SUPPLIED

ELIXIR (C-III): 100 MG-2.5 MG-30 MG/5 ML

BRAND/MANUFACTURER	NDC	SIZE	AWP
○ GENERICS			
DURATUSS HD: Whitby	50474-0610-16	480 ml	$29.96

LIQUID (C-III):

BRAND/MANUFACTURER	NDC	SIZE	AWP
○ GENERICS			
TUSSAFIN EXPECTORANT: Rugby	00536-0542-85	480 ml	$10.88
DETUSSIN EXPECTORANT: Schein	00364-7258-16	480 ml	$12.75
DETUSSIN EXPECTORANT: Qualitest	00603-1131-58	480 ml	$12.90
DETUSSIN EXPECTORANT: Major	00904-0965-16	480 ml	$15.40
DETUSSIN EXPECTORANT: Barre	00472-0957-16	480 ml	$16.59
TUSSGEN EXPECTORANT: Goldline	00182-1164-40	480 ml	$18.00
SRC EXPECTORANT: Edwards	00485-0042-16	480 ml	$25.00
POLY-TUSSIN XP: Poly	50991-0925-16	480 ml	$30.13
NALEX EXPECTORANT: Blansett	51674-0002-07	480 ml	$31.90
DETUSSIN EXPECTORANT: Major	00904-0965-28	3840 ml	$88.10

LIQUID (C-III): 30 MG-2.5 MG-100 MG

BRAND/MANUFACTURER	NDC	SIZE	AWP
○ GENERICS			
ENTUSS-D JR.: Roberts/Hauck	59441-0439-04	120 ml	$10.00
ENTUSS-D JR.: Roberts/Hauck	59441-0439-16	480 ml	$30.56

LIQUID (C-III): 100 MG-2.5 MG-30 MG/5 ML

BRAND/MANUFACTURER	NDC	SIZE	AWP
○ GENERICS			
TUSSADUR-HD: Alphagen	59743-0056-16	480 ml	$24.50
VANEX EXPECTORANT: Abana	12463-0123-16	480 ml	$35.56

SYRUP (C-III):

BRAND/MANUFACTURER	NDC	SIZE	AWP
○ BRAND			
PANCOF XP: Pan Amer	00525-0711-16	480 ml	$30.30
○ GENERICS			
COPHENE-X-P: Dunhall	00217-2832-11	480 ml	$20.00

TABLETS (C-III): 5 MG-300 MG-30 MG

BRAND/MANUFACTURER	NDC	SIZE	AWP
○ GENERICS			
ENTUSS-D: Roberts/Hauck	59441-0142-01	100s	$41.67

Guaifenesin/Phenylephrine Hydrochloride/ Phenylpropanolamine Hydrochloride

DESCRIPTION

Each Gauifenesin/Phenylephrine Hydrochloride/Phenylpropanolamine Hydrochloride capsule for oral administration contains:

Phenylephrine HCl	.5 mg
Phenylpropanolamine HCl	.20 mg
Guaifenesin	.100 mg

Each 5 ml (one teaspoonful) of Guaifenesin/Phenylephrine/Phenylpropanolamine for oral administration contains:

Alcohol	.5%

► SHOWN IN PRODUCT IDENTIFICATION GUIDE

Phenylephrine HCl ....5 mg
Phenylpropanolamine HCl ....45 mg
Guaifenesin ....200 mg

This product contains ingredients of the following therapeutic classes: decongestant and expectorant.

Phenylephrine HCl is a decongestant having the chemical name, 3-hydroxy-α-[(methylamino)methyl]benzenemethanol hydrochloride.

Phenylpropanolamine HCl is a decongestant having the chemical name, benzenemethanol, α-(1-aminoethyl)-hydrochloride (R*, S*), (±).

Guaifenesin is an expectorant having the chemical name, 1,2-propanediol, 3-(2-methoxyphenoxy).

CLINICAL PHARMACOLOGY

Phenylephrine HCl and Phenylpropanolamine HCl are α-adrenergic receptor agonists (sympathomimetics) which produce vasoconstriction by stimulating α-receptors within the mucosa of the respiratory tract. Clinically, Phenylephrine and Phenylpropanolamine shrink swollen mucous membranes, reduce tissue hyperemia, edema, and nasal congestion, and increase nasal airway patency. Guaifenesin promotes lower respiratory tract drainage by thinning bronchial secretions, lubricates irritated respiratory tract membranes through increased mucous flow, and facilitates removal of viscous, inspissated mucus. As a result of these drugs, sinus and bronchial drainage is improved, and dry, nonproductive coughs become more productive and less frequent.

INDICATIONS AND USAGE

Guaifenesin/Phenylephrine/Phenylpropanolamine capsules and liquid are indicated for the symptomatic relief of sinusitis, bronchitis, pharyngitis, and coryza when these conditions are associated with nasal congestion and viscous mucus in the lower respiratory tract.

CONTRAINDICATIONS

Guaifenesin/Phenylephrine/Phenylpropanolamine capsules and liquid are contraindicated in individuals with known hypersensitivity to sympathomimetics, severe hypertension, or in patients receiving monoamine oxidase inhibitors.

WARNINGS

Sympathomimetic amines should be used with caution in patients with hypertension, diabetes mellitus, heart disease, peripheral vascular disease, increased intraocular pressure, hyperthyroidism, or prostatic hypertrophy.

PRECAUTIONS

Drug Interactions: Guaifenesin/Phenylephrine/Phenylpropanolamine should not be used in patients taking monoamine oxidase inhibitors or other sympathomimetics.

Drug/Laboratory Test Interactions: Guaifenesin has been reported to interfere with clinical laboratory determinations of urinary 5-hydroxyindoleacetic acid (5-HIAA) and urinary vanillylmandelic acid (VMA).

Pregnancy: Pregnancy Category C. Animal reproduction studies have not been conducted with Guaifenesin/Phenylephrine/Phenylpropanolamine. It is also not known whether Guaifenesin/Phenylephrine/Phenylpropanolamine can cause fetal harm when administered to a pregnant woman or can affect reproduction capacity. Guaifenesin/Phenylephrine/Phenylpropanolamine should be given to a pregnant woman only if clearly needed.

Nursing Mothers: It is not known whether the drugs in Guaifenesin/Phenylephrine/Phenylpropanolamine are excreted in human milk. Because many drugs are excreted in human milk and because of the potential for serious adverse reactions in nursing infants, a decision should be made whether to discontinue nursing or to discontinue the product, taking into account the importance of the drug to the mother.

Pediatric Use: Safety and effectiveness of Guaifenesin/Phenylephrine/Phenylpropanolamine capsules in children below the age of 12 and of Guaifenesin/Phenylephrine/ Phenylpropanolamine liquid in children below the age of 2, have not been established.

ADVERSE REACTIONS

Possible adverse reactions include nervousness, insomnia, restlessness, headache, nausea, or gastric irritation. These reactions seldom, if ever, require discontinuation of therapy. Urinary retention may occur in patients with prostatic hypertrophy.

OVERDOSAGE

The treatment of overdosage should provide symptomatic and supportive care. If the amount ingested is considered dangerous or excessive, induce vomiting with ipecac syrup unless the patient is convulsing, comatose, or has lost the gag reflex, in which case perform gastric lavage using a largebore tube. If indicated, follow with activated charcoal and a saline cathartic.

DOSAGE AND ADMINISTRATION

CAPSULES

Adults and children 12 years of age and older: one capsule four times daily (every 6 hours) with food or fluid. Guaifenesin/Phenylephrine/Phenylpropanolamine capsules are not recommended for children under 12 years of age.

LIQUID

All dosage should be administered four times daily (every 6 hours).

Children:

2 to under 4 years ....½ teaspoonful (2.5 ml)
4 to under 6 years ....1 teaspoonful (5 ml)
6 to under 12 years ....1 ½ teaspoonfuls (7.5 ml)

Adults and children 12 years of age and older: ....2 teaspoonfuls (10 ml)

Store below 86°F (30°C). Do not refrigerate liquid.

HOW SUPPLIED

CAPSULE:

BRAND/MANUFACTURER	NDC	SIZE	AWP
○ **BRAND**			
ENTEX: P&G Pharm	00149-0412-01	100s	$42.16
	00149-0412-05	500s	$195.29
○ **GENERICS**			
Allscrips	54569-2162-01	15s	$3.75
Southwood	58016-0492-15	15s	$4.35
Allscrips	54569-2162-03	20s	$3.65
Southwood	58016-0492-20	20s	$4.64
Allscrips	54569-2162-04	30s	$4.55
Allscrips	54569-2162-00	40s	$5.35
Allscrips	54569-2162-02	60s	$6.90
AMI-TEX: Amide	52152-0059-02	100s	$8.00
GUIATEX: Rugby	00536-4459-01	100s	$8.69
ENOMINE: Major	00904-3263-60	100s	$11.70
Moore, H.L.	00839-7201-06	100s	$17.08
BANEX: Norton,HN	50732-0789-01	100s	$19.25
DURA-GEST: Dura	51479-0005-01	100s	$37.61
AMI-TEX: Amide	52152-0059-04	500s	$39.00
ENOMINE: Major	00904-3263-40	500s	$43.50
BANEX: Norton,HN	50732-0789-05	500s	$96.25
DURA-GEST: Dura	51479-0005-05	500s	$153.09

CAPSULE: 200 MG-5 MG-45 MG

BRAND/MANUFACTURER	NDC	SIZE	AWP
○ **GENERICS**			
Allscrips	54569-3637-01	15s	$2.82
Allscrips	54569-3637-03	20s	$3.77
Allscrips	54569-3637-05	28s	$5.27
Allscrips	54569-3627-00	30s	$5.65
Allscrips	54569-3637-00	40s	$7.53
QUINTEX: Qualitest	00603-5665-21	100s	$7.65
DURATEX: Duramed	51285-0293-02	100s	$17.04
NOREL: U.S. Pharm	52747-0610-60	100s	$30.00

LIQUID:

BRAND/MANUFACTURER	NDC	SIZE	AWP
○ **BRAND**			
FENTEX: Mikart	46672-0608-16	480 ml	$11.95
ENTEX: P&G Pharm	00149-0414-16	480 ml	$31.75
○ **GENERICS**			
DESPEC: Intl Ethical	11584-1030-04	120 ml	$7.20
Southwood	58016-0475-24	120 ml	$10.73
Southwood	58016-0475-36	180 ml	$15.50
PHENYLFENESIN: Goldline	00182-6100-40	480 ml	$12.00
CRANTEX: Moore,H.L.	00839-7562-69	480 ml	$13.48
EQUI-TEX: Equipharm	57779-0112-09	480 ml	$13.75
PHENTEX: Hi-Tech	50383-0111-16	480 ml	$14.00
CRANTEX: Econolab	55053-0650-16	480 ml	$14.00
ULR: Geneva	00781-6702-16	480 ml	$14.25
BANEX: Norton,HN	50732-0833-16	480 ml	$14.28
TRI-TEX: Tri-Med	55654-0005-05	480 ml	$15.50
ALTEX LIQUID: Aligen	00405-2138-16	480 ml	$15.76
Allscrips	54569-2960-00	480 ml	$15.87
ENTAC: Barre	00472-0650-16	480 ml	$15.90
GUIATEX: Rugby	00536-2395-85	480 ml	$16.37
ENOMINE: Major	00904-3262-16	480 ml	$16.45
CONTUSS: Parmed	00349-8508-16	480 ml	$17.39
QUINTEX: Qualitest	00603-1634-58	480 ml	$17.91
P-TEX: Poly	50991-0916-01	480 ml	$21.79

LIQUID: 100 MG-5 MG-20 MG/5 ML

BRAND/MANUFACTURER	NDC	SIZE	AWP
○ **GENERICS**			
URL	00677-1354-33	480 ml	$14.80
SIL-TEX: Silarx	54838-0503-80	480 ml	$19.86
GUAIFENEX: Ethex	58177-0882-07	480 ml	$22.77
COLDLOC: Flemming Pharma	60976-0125-16	480 ml	$28.80

◆ RATED THERAPEUTICALLY EQUIVALENT; ◇ THERAPEUTIC EQUIVALENCE UNCONFIRMED; ○ UNRATED

Guaifenesin/Pseudoephedrine Hydrochloride/Theophylline

DESCRIPTION

Each Guaifenesin/Pseudoephedrine Hydrochloride/Theophylline (GG/PSE/Theo) tablet contains:

Theophylline (Anhydrous) ....100 mg.
Guaifenesin (Glyceryl Guaiacolate) ....100 mg.
Pseudoephedrine Hydrochloride ....30 mg.

ACTION AND USES

The collective effect of two widely-accepted bronchodilators, theophylline and pseudoephedrine, helps to relieve bronchospasm. The relaxation of bronchospasm counteracts the entrapment of residual air and the decrease in vital capacity, thus allaying the psychic anxiety of recurrence of asthmatic attacks. Pseudoephedrine (through its characteristic beta adrenergic action) and theophylline (as a part of the xanthine response of the smooth muscle of the bronchi) provide effective bronchodilation. Glyceryl guaiacolate helps to remove thick and tenacious mucus. GG/PSE/Theo tablets contain Pseudoephedrine which has a vasopressor effect less than that of ephedrine. GG/PSE/Theo tablets should be used as an adjunct in the overall management of the asthmatic. Severe attacks may require inhalant and/or parenteral therapy.

INDICATIONS

Indicated for the symptomatic relief of bronchial asthma, asthmatic bronchitis and related conditions associated with bronchospasm. GG/PSE/Theo tablets may be used prophylactically.

CONTRAINDICATIONS

Contraindicated in patients known to be sensitive to any of the ingredients.

PRECAUTIONS

GG/PSE/Theo tablets should be used with caution in patients with cardiovascular disease and/or severe hypertension, circulatory collapse, hyperthyroidism, prostatic hypertrophy or glaucoma. Patients with longstanding bronchial asthma and a significant degree of emphysema, who have reached the age in which degenerative heart disease is prevalent, must be given GG/PSE/Theo tablets with caution.

ADVERSE REACTIONS

Mild gastric distress, palpitation, tremulousness, ventricular arrhythmias, insomnia, difficulty of micturition and central nervous system stimulation may occur.

ADMINISTRATION AND DOSAGE

The usual adult dose is one or two tablets three or four times daily. Children eight to twelve one tablet two to three times daily. Dosage should be adjusted on an individual basis.

HOW SUPPLIED
TABLETS:

BRAND/MANUFACTURER	NDC	SIZE	AWP
○ GENERICS			
BRONCOMAR: Marlop	12939-0112-02	100s	$20.65
BRONCOMAR: Marlop	12939-0112-90	1000s	$168.50

Guaimax-D SEE GUAIFENESIN AND PSEUDOEPHEDRINE
HYDROCHLORIDE

Guanabenz Acetate

DESCRIPTION

Guanabenz Acetate, an antihypertensive agent for oral administration, is an aminoguanidine derivative, 2,6-dichlorobenzylidene-aminoguanidine acetate. It is an odorless, white to off-white, crystalline substance, sparingly soluble in water and soluble in alcohol, with a molecular weight of 291.14.

Guanabenz Acetate is available as 4 mg or 8 mg tablets for oral administration.

Following is its chemical structure:

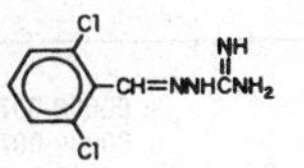

CLINICAL PHARMACOLOGY

Guanabenz Acetate is an orally active central alpha-2 adrenergic agonist. Its antihypertensive action appears to be mediated via stimulation of central alpha adrenergic receptors, resulting in a decrease of sympathetic outflow from the brain at the bulbar level to the peripheral circulatory system.

PHARMACOKINETICS

In human studies, about 75% of an orally administered dose of Guanabenz Acetate is absorbed and metabolized with less than 1% of unchanged drug recovered from the urine. Peak plasma concentrations of unchanged drug occur between two and five hours after a single oral dose. The average half-life for Guanabenz Acetate is about 6 hours. The site or sites of metabolism of Guanabenz Acetate have not been determined. The effect of meals on the absorption of Guanabenz Acetate has not been studied.

PHARMACODYNAMICS

The onset of the antihypertensive action of Guanabenz Acetate begins within 60 minutes after a single oral dose and reaches a peak effect within two to four hours. The effect of an acute single dose is reduced appreciably six to eight hours after administration, and blood pressure approaches baseline values within 12 hours of administration.

The acute antihypertensive effect of Guanabenz Acetate occurs without major changes in peripheral resistance, but its chronic effect appears to be a decrease in peripheral resistance. A decrease in blood pressure is seen in both the supine and standing positions without alterations of normal postural mechanisms, so that postural hypotension has not been observed. Guanabenz Acetate decreases pulse rate by about 5 beats per minute. Cardiac output and left ventricular ejection fraction are unchanged during long-term therapy.

In clinical trials, Guanabenz Acetate given orally to hypertensive patients, effectively controlled blood pressure without any significant effect on glomerular filtration rate, renal blood flow, body fluid volume or body weight. Guanabenz Acetate given parenterally to dogs has produced a natriuresis. Similarly, hypertensive subjects, 24 hours after salt loading, have shown a decrease in blood pressure and a natriuresis (5% to 240% increase in sodium excretion) following a single oral dose of Guanabenz Acetate. After seven consecutive days of administration and effective blood-pressure control, no significant change on glomerular filtration rate, renal blood flow, or body weight was observed. However, in clinical trials of six to thirty months duration, hypertensive patients with effective blood-pressure control by Guanabenz Acetate lost one to four pounds of body weight. The mechanism of this weight loss has not been established. Tolerance to the antihypertensive effect of Guanabenz Acetate has not been observed.

During long-term administration of Guanabenz Acetate there is a small decrease in serum cholesterol and total triglycerides without any change in the high-density lipoprotein fraction. Plasma norepinephrine, serum dopamine beta-hydroxylase and plasma renin activity are decreased during chronic administration of Guanabenz Acetate. No changes in serum electrolytes, uric acid, blood urea nitrogen, calcium, or glucose have been observed.

Guanabenz Acetate and hydrochlorothiazide have been shown to have at least partially additive effects in patients not responding adequately to either drug alone.

INDICATIONS AND USAGE

Guanabenz is indicated in the treatment of hypertension. It may be employed alone or in combination with a thiazide diuretic.

CONTRAINDICATION

Guanabenz Acetate is contraindicated in patients with a known sensitivity to the drug.

PRECAUTIONS

1. Sedation: Guanabenz Acetate causes sedation or drowsiness in a large fraction of patients. When Guanabenz Acetate is used with centrally active depressants, such as phenothiazines, barbiturates, and benzodiazepines, the potential for additive sedative effects should be considered.

2. Patients with Vascular Insufficiency: Guanabenz Acetate, like other antihypertensive agents, should be used with caution in patients with severe coronary insufficiency, recent myocardial infarction, cerebrovascular disease, or severe hepatic or renal failure.

3. Rebound: Sudden cessation of therapy with central alpha agonists like Guanabenz Acetate may rarely result in "overshoot" hypertension and more commonly produces an increase in serum catecholamines and subjective symptomatology.

4. Patients with Hepatic Impairment: The disposition of orally administered Guanabenz Acetate is altered in patients with alcohol-induced liver disease. Mean plasma concentrations of Guanabenz Acetate were higher in these patients than in healthy subjects. The clinical significance of this finding is unknown. However, careful monitoring of blood pressure is suggested when Guanabenz Acetate is administered to patients with hypertension and coexisting chronic hepatic dysfunction.

5. Patients with Renal Impairment: The disposition of orally administered Guanabenz Acetate is altered modestly in patients with renal impairment. Guanabenz Acetate's half-life is prolonged and clearance decreased, more so in patients on hemodialysis. The clinical significance of these findings is unknown. Careful monitoring of blood pressure during Guanabenz Acetate dose titration is suggested in patients with coexisting hypertension and renal impairment.

► SHOWN IN PRODUCT IDENTIFICATION GUIDE

INFORMATION FOR PATIENTS

Patients who receive Guanabenz Acetate should be advised to exercise caution when operating dangerous machinery or driving motor vehicles until it is determined that they do not become drowsy or dizzy from the medication. Patients should be warned that their tolerance for alcohol and other CNS depressants may be diminished. Patients should be advised not to discontinue therapy abruptly.

LABORATORY TESTS

In clinical trials, no clinically significant laboratory-test abnormalities were identified during either acute or chronic therapy with Guanabenz Acetate Tests carried out included CBC, urinalysis, electrolytes, SGOT, bilirubin, alkaline phosphatase, uric acid, BUN, creatinine, glucose, calcium, phosphorus, total protein, and Coombs' test. During long term administration of Guanabenz Acetate, there was a small decrease in serum cholesterol and total triglycerides without any change in the high-density lipoprotein fraction. In rare instances an occasional nonprogressive increase in liver enzymes has been observed. However, no clinical evidence of hepatic disease has been found.

DRUG INTERACTIONS

Guanabenz Acetate has not been demonstrated to cause any drug interactions when administered with other drugs, such as digitalis, diuretics, analgesics, anxiolytics, and antiinflammatory or antiinfective agents, in clinical trials. However, the potential for increased sedation when Guanabenz Acetate is administered concomitantly with CNS-depressant drugs should be noted.

DRUG/LABORATORY TEST INTERACTIONS

No laboratory test abnormalities were identified with the use of Guanabenz Acetate.

CARCINOGENESIS, MUTAGENESIS, IMPAIRMENT OF FERTILITY

No evidence of carcinogenic potential emerged in rats during a two-year oral study with Guanabenz Acetate at doses up to 9.5 mg/kg/day, i.e., about 10 times the maximum recomended human dose. In the Salmonella microsome mutagenicity (Ames) test system. Guanabenz Acetate at 200 to 500 mcg per plate or at 30 to 50 mcg/mL in suspension gave dose-related increases in the number of mutants in one (TA 1537) of five *Salmonella typhimurium* strains with or without inclusion of rat liver microsomes. No mutagenic activity was seen at doses up to those which inhibit growth in the eukaryotic microorganism, *Schizosaccharomyces pombe*, or in Chinese hamster ovary cells at doses up to those which were lethal to the cells in culture. In another eukaryotic system, *Saccharomyces cerevisiae*, Guanabenz Acetate produced no activity in an assay measuring induction of repairable DNA damage. Reproductive studies showed a decreased pregnancy rate in rats administered high oral doses (9.6 mg/kg) of Guanabenz Acetate, suggesting an impairment of fertility. The fertility of treated males (9.6 mg/kg) may also have been affected, as suggested by the decreased pregnancy rate of their mates, even though the females received Guanabenz Acetate only during the last third of pregnancy.

PREGNANCY

Pregnancy Category C

Guanabenz Acetate May Have Adverse Effects on the Fetus When Administered to Pregnant Women.

A teratology study in mice has indicated a possible increase in skeletal abnormalities when Guanabenz Acetate is given orally at doses of 3 to 6 times the maximum recommended human dose of 1.0 mg/kg. These abnormalities, principally costal and vertebral, were not noted in similar studies in rats and rabbits. However, increased fetal loss has been observed after oral Guanabenz Acetate administration to pregnant rats (14 mg/kg) and rabbits (20 mg/kg). Reproductive studies of Guanabenz Acetate in rats have shown slightly decreased live-birth indices, decreased fetal survival rate, and decreased pup body weight at oral doses of 6.4 and 9.6 mg/kg. There are no adequate, well-controlled studies in pregnant women. Guanabenz Acetate should be used during pregnancy only if the potential benefit justifies the potential risk to the fetus.

NURSING MOTHERS

Because no information is available on the excretion of Guanabenz Acetate in human milk, it should not be administered to nursing mothers.

PEDIATRIC USE

The safety and effectiveness of Guanabenz Acetate in children less than 12 years of age have not been demonstrated. Therefore, its use in this age group cannot be recommended at this time.

ADVERSE REACTIONS

The incidence of adverse effects has been ascertained from controlled clinical studies conducted in the United States and is based on data from 859 patients who received Guanabenz Acetate for up to 3 years. There is some evidence that the side effects are dose-related.

The following table shows the incidence of adverse effects occurring in at least 5% of patients in a study comparing Guanabenz Acetate to placebo, at a starting dose of 8 mg b.i.d.

Adverse Effect	Placebo (%) n=102	Guanabenz Acetate (%) n=109
Dry mouth	7	28
Drowsiness or sedation	12	39
Dizziness	7	17
Weakness	7	10
Headache	6	5

In other controlled clinical trials at the starting dose of 16 mg/day in 476 patients, the incidence of dry mouth was slightly higher (38%) and that of dizziness was slightly lower (12%), but the incidence of the most frequent adverse effects was similar to the placebo-controlled trial. Although these side effects were not serious, they led to discontinuation of treatment about 15% of the time. In more recent studies using an initial dose of 8 mg/day in 274 patients, the incidence of drowsiness or sedation was lower, about 20%.

Other adverse effects were reported during clinical trials with Guanabenz Acetate but are not clearly distinguishable from placeo effects and occurred with a frequency of 3% or less:

Cardiovascular: chest pain, edema, arrhythmias, palpitations.

Gastrointestinal: nausea, epigastric pain, diarrhea, vomiting, constipation, abdominal discomfort.

Central nervous system: anxiety, ataxia, depression, sleep disturbances.

ENT disorders: nasal congestion.

Eye disorders: blurring of vision.

Musculoskeletal: aches in extremities, muscle aches.

Respiratory: dyspnea.

Dermatologic: rash, pruritus.

Urogenital: urinary frequency, disturbances of sexual function (decreased libido, impotence).

Other: gynecomastia, taste disorders.

In very rare instances atrioventricular dysfunction, up to and including complete AV block, has been caused by Guanabenz Acetate.

DRUG ABUSE AND DEPENDENCE

No reported dependence or abuse has been associated with the administration of Guanabenz Acetate.

OVERDOSAGE

Accidental ingestion of Guanabenz Acetate caused hypotension, somnolence, lethargy, irritability, miosis, and bradycardia in two children aged one and three years. Gastric lavage and administration of pressor substances, fluids, and oral activated charcoal resulted in complete and uneventful recovery within 12 hours in both patients.

Since experience with accidental overdosage is limited, the suggested treatment is mainly supportive while the drug is being eliminated from the body and until the patient is no longer symptomatic. Vital signs and fluid balance should be carefully monitored. An adequate airway should be maintained and, if indicated, assisted respiration instituted. There are no data available on the dialyzability of Guanabenz Acetate.

DOSAGE AND ADMINISTRATION

Dosage with Guanabenz Acetate should be individualized. A starting dose of 4 mg twice a day is recommended, whether Guanabenz Acetate is used alone or with a thiazide diuretic. Dosage may be increased in increments of 4 to 8 mg per day every one to two weeks, depending on the patient's response. The maximum dose studied to date has been 32 mg twice daily, but doses as high as this are rarely needed.

Keep tightly closed.
Store at room temperature, approximately 25°C (77°F).
Dispense in light-resistant tight container.
Protect from light.

HOW SUPPLIED
TABLET: 4 MG

AVERAGE UNIT PRICE (AVAILABLE SIZES)		GENERIC A-RATED AVERAGE PRICE (GAAP)	
BRAND	$0.71	100s	$58.55
GENERIC	$0.59		

BRAND/MANUFACTURER	NDC	SIZE	AWP
◆ BRAND			
WYTENSIN: Wyeth-Ayerst	00008-0073-01	100s	$70.18
	00008-0073-05	100s	$74.78
	00008-0073-04	500s	$340.61

◆ RATED THERAPEUTICALLY EQUIVALENT; ◇ THERAPEUTIC EQUIVALENCE UNCONFIRMED; ○ UNRATED

BRAND/MANUFACTURER	NDC	SIZE	AWP
◆ **GENERICS**			
Qualitest	00603-3779-21	100s	$53.20
Martec	52555-0555-01	100s	$54.75
Moore,H.L.	00839-7932-06	100s	$59.33
Rugby	00536-5687-01	100s	$59.35
Goldline	00182-1951-01	100s	$59.35
Copley	38245-0717-10	100s	$61.92
Warner Chilcott	00047-0560-24	100s	$61.92
Copley	38245-0717-50	500s	$297.00

For additional alternatives, turn to the section beginning on page 2859.

Guanadrel Sulfate

DESCRIPTION
Guanadrel Sulfate Tablets for oral administration contain Guanadrel Sulfate, an antihypertensive agent belonging to the class of adrenergic neuron blocking drugs. Guanadrel Sulfate is (1,4-Dioxaspiro[4.5] dec-2-ylmethyl) Guanidine Sulfate with a molecular weight of 524.63. It is a white to off-white crystalline powder, which melts with decomposition at about 235°C. It is soluble in water to the extent of 76 mg/mL.

Guanadrel Sulfate Tablets are available in two strengths: 10 mg and 25 mg.

Following is its chemical structure:

$$\left[\text{} \quad O\text{—}CH_2\text{—}NHC\overset{NH}{\underset{}{\|}}NH_2 \right]_2 \cdot H_2SO_4$$

CLINICAL PHARMACOLOGY
Guanadrel Sulfate is an orally effective antihypertensive agent that lowers both systolic and diastolic arterial blood pressures. Guanadrel Sulfate inhibits sympathetic vasoconstriction by inhibiting norepinephrine release from neuronal storage sites in response to stimulation of the nerve and also causes depletion of norepinephrine from the nerve ending. This results in relaxation of vascular smooth muscle which decreases total peripheral resistance, and decreases venous return, both of which reduce the ability to maintain blood pressure in the upright position. The result is a hypotensive effect that is greater in the standing than in the supine position by about 10 mmHg systolic and 3.5 mmHg diastolic, on the average. Heart rate is also decreased usually by about 5 beats/minute. Fluid retention occurs during treatment with Guanadrel, particularly when it is not accompanied by a diuretic. The drug does not inhibit parasympathetic nerve function nor does it enter the central nervous system.

Guanadrel Sulfate is rapidly absorbed after oral administration. Plasma concentrations generally peak 1½ to 2 hours after ingestion. The half-life is about 10 hours, but individual variability is great. Approximately 85% of the drug is eliminated in the urine. Urinary excretion is approximately 85% complete within 24 hours after administration; about 40% of the dose is excreted as unchanged drug. The disposition of Guanadrel Sulfate is significantly altered in patients with impaired renal function. A study in such patients has shown that as renal function (measured as creatinine clearance) declines, apparent total body clearance, renal and apparent nonrenal clearances decrease, and the terminal elimination half-life is prolonged. Dosage adjustments may be necessary, especially in patients with creatinine clearances of less than 60 mL/min (see *"Dosage and Administration"*).

Guanadrel Sulfate begins to decrease blood pressure within two hours and produces maximal decreases in four to six hours. No significant change in cardiac output accompanies the blood pressure decline in normal individuals.

Because drugs of the adrenergic neuron blocking class are transported into the neuron by the "norepinephrine pump", drugs that compete for the pump may block their effects. Tricyclic antidepressants have been shown to block the norepinephrine-depleting effect of Guanadrel Sulfate in rats and monkeys, and the blood pressure lowering effect of Guanadrel Sulfate in monkeys. Similar effects have been seen with guanethidine and inhibition of the antihypertensive effects of Guanadrel Sulfate by tricyclic antidepressants in humans should be presumed.

Therefore caution is recommended if Guanadrel Sulfate and a tricyclic antidepressant are used concomitantly. Should patients be on both a tricyclic antidepressant and Guanadrel Sulfate, caution is advised upon discontinuation of the tricyclic antidepressant, especially if discontinued abruptly, as an enhanced effect of Guanadrel Sulfate may occur.

Chlorpromazine seems to have a similar effect on guanethidine and may affect Guanadrel as well. Indirectly acting adrenergic amines are transported into the neuron by the "norepinephrine pump" and may interfere with uptake or may displace blocking agents. Ephedrine rapidly reverses the effects of Guanadrel but other agents have not been studied. Agents of the guanethidine class cause increased sensitivity to circulating norepinephrine, probably by preventing uptake of norepinephrine by adrenergic neurons, the usual mechanism for terminating norephinephrine effects. Agents of this class are thus dangerous in the presence of excess norephinephrine, e.g., in the presence of a pheochromocytoma.

In controlled clinical studies comparing Guanadrel to guanethidine and methyldopa, involving about 2000 patients exposed to Guanadrel, patients with initial supine blood pressures averaging 160-170/105-110 mmHg had decreases in blood pressure of 20-25/15-20 mmHg in the standing position. The decreases in supine blood pressure were less than the decreases in standing blood pressure by 6-10/2-7 mmHg in different studies. Guanethidine and Guanadrel were very similar in effectiveness while methyldopa had a larger effect on supine systolic pressure. Side effects of Guanadrel and guanethidine were generally similar in type (see *"Adverse Reactions"*) while methyldopa had more central nervous system effects (depression, drowsiness) but fewer orthostatic effects and less diarrhea.

INDICATIONS AND USAGE
Guanadrel Sulfate Tablets are indicated for the treatment of hypertension in patients not responding adequately to a thiazide type diuretic. Guanadrel Sulfate should be added to a diuretic regimen for optimum blood pressure control.

UNLABELED USES
Guanadrel Sulfate is used alone or as an adjunct in the treatment of cardiovascular and neuromuscular manifestations of Graves' disease (thyrotoxicosis).

CONTRAINDICATIONS
Guanadrel Sulfate Tablets are contraindicated in known or suspected pheochromocytoma.

Guanadrel Sulfate should not be used concurrently with, or within one week of, monoamine oxidase inhibitors.

Guanadrel Sulfate should not be used in patients hypersensitive to the drug.

Guanadrel Sulfate should not be used in patients with frank congestive heart failure.

WARNINGS
A. ORTHOSTATIC HYPOTENSION
Orthostatic hypotension and its consequences (dizziness and weakness) are frequent in people treated with Guanadrel Sulfate Tablets. Rarely, fainting upon standing or exercise is seen. Careful instructions to the patient can minimize these symptoms, as can recognition by the physician that the supine blood pressure does not constitute an adequate assessment of the effects of this drug. Patients with known regional vascular disease (cerebral, coronary) are at particular risk from marked orthostatic hypotension and Guanadrel Sulfate should be avoided in them unless drugs with lesser degrees of orthostatic hypotension are ineffective or unacceptable. In such patients hypotensive episodes should be avoided, even if this requires accepting a poorer degree of blood pressure control.

Instructions to Patients: Patients should be advised about the risk of orthostatic hypotension and told to sit or lie down immediately at the onset of dizziness or weakness so that they can prevent loss of consciousness. They should be told that postural hypotension is worst in the morning and upon arising, and may be exaggerated by alcohol, fever, hot weather, prolonged standing, or exercise.

Surgery: To reduce the possibility of vascular collapse during anesthesia, Guanadrel should be discontinued 48-72 hours before elective surgery. If emergency surgery is required, the anesthesiologist should be made aware that the patient has been taking Guanadrel Sulfate and that preanesthetic and anesthetic agents should be administered cautiously in reduced dosage. If vasopressors are needed they must be used cautiously, as Guanadrel can enhance the pressor response to such agents and increase their arrhythmogenicity.

B. DRUG INTERACTIONS
As discussed above (*"Clinical Pharmacology"*), tricyclic antidepressants and indirect-acting sympathomimetics such as ephedrine or phenylpropanolamine, and possibly phenothiazines, can reverse the effects of neuronal blocking agents. IN VIEW OF THE PRESENCE OF SYMPATHOMIMETIC AMINES IN MANY NON-PRESCRIPTION DRUGS FOR THE TREATMENT OF COLDS, ALLERGY, OR ASTHMA, PATIENTS GIVEN GUANADREL SHOULD BE SPECIFICALLY WARNED NOT TO USE SUCH PREPARATIONS WITHOUT THEIR PHYSICIAN'S ADVICE.

Guanadrel enhances the activity of direct-acting sympathomimetics, like norepinephrine, by blocking neuronal uptake. Drugs that affect the adrenergic response by the same or other mechanisms would be expected to potentiate the effects of Guanadrel, causing excessive postural hypotension and bradycardia. These include alpha- or beta-adrenergic blocking agents and reserpine. There is no clinical experience with the combination of Guanadrel Sulfate with alpha-adrenergic blocking agents or reserpine.

When Guanadrel Sulfate was added to the treatment regimen in hypertensive patients inadequately controlled with a diuretic and propranolol, no significant adverse effects, including bradycardia, were reported in the 26 patients treated concomitantly with the three drugs.

The use of Guanadrel Sulfate with vasodilators has not been adequately studied and is not generally recommended because concomitant use may increase the potential for symptomatic orthostatic hypotension.

C. ASTHMATIC PATIENTS
Special care is needed in patients with bronchial asthma, as their condition may be aggravated by catecholamine depletion and sympathomimetic amines may interfere with the hypotensive effect of Guanadrel.

PRECAUTIONS
GENERAL
Salt and water retention may occur with the use of Guanadrel Sulfate Tablets. In clinical studies major problems did not arise because of concomitant diuretic use. Patients with heart failure have not been studied on Guanadrel Sulfate, but Guanadrel could interfere with the adrenergic mechanisms that maintain compensation.

In patients with a history of peptic ulcer, which could be aggravated by a relative increase in parasympathetic tone, Guanadrel Sulfate should be used cautiously.

In patients with compromised renal function, decreases in renal and nonrenal clearances and an increase in the elimination half-life of Guanadrel Sulfate have been found. This could possibly lead to an increased incidence of side effects if standard doses are used in these patients. Titration of dose based on the blood pressure response is necessary because of marked interpatient variability (see *"Dosage and Administration"*).

A transient increase in blood pressure has been observed in some patients.

INFORMATION FOR PATIENTS
See *"Warnings"* section.

DRUG INTERACTIONS
See *"Warnings"* section.

CARCINOGENESIS, MUTAGENESIS, IMPAIRMENT OF FERTILITY
No evidence of carcinogenic potential appeared in a 2-year mouse study of Guanadrel Sulfate. In a 2-year rat study, an increased number of benign testicular interstitial cell tumors was observed at dosages of 100 mg/kg/day and 400 mg/kg/day. These are common spontaneous tumors in aged rats and their significance to therapy with Guanadrel Sulfate in man is unknown. Salmonella testing (Ames test) showed no evidence of mutagenic activity.

A reproduction study was performed in male and female rats at dosages of 0, 10, 30 and 100 mg/kg/day. Suppressed libido and reduced fertility were noted at 100 mg/kg/day (12 times the maximum human dose in a 50 kg subject) and libido was suppressed to a lesser extent at 30 mg/kg/day.

PREGNANCY CATEGORY B
Teratology studies performed in rats and rabbits at doses up to 12 times the maximum recommended human dose (in a 50 kg subject) revealed no significant harm to the fetus due to Guanadrel Sulfate. There are, however, no adequate and well-controlled studies in pregnant women. Because animal reproduction studies are not always predictive, Guanadrel Sulfate should be used in pregnant women only when the potential benefit outweighs the potential risk to mother and infant.

NURSING MOTHERS
Whether Guanadrel Sulfate is excreted in human milk is not known, but because many drugs are excreted in human milk and because of the potential for serious adverse reactions in nursing infants from Guanadrel, a decision should be made whether to discontinue nursing or discontinue the drug, taking into account the importance of the drug to the mother.

PEDIATRIC USE
Safety and effectiveness in children have not been established.

ADVERSE REACTIONS
The adverse reaction data for Guanadrel is derived principally from comparative long-term (6 months to 3 years) studies with methyldopa and guanethidine in which side effects were assessed through use of periodic questionnaires, a method that tends to give high adverse reaction rates. In the tables that follow, some of the adverse effects reported may not be drug-related, but in the absence of a placebo-treated group, these cannot be readily distinguished. Comparative results with two well-known drugs, methyldopa and guanethidine, should aid in interpretation of these adverse reaction rates.

The following table displays the frequency of side effects which are believed to be related to sympathetic blocking agents: orthostatic faintness, increased bowel movements and ejaculation disturbances for peripherally acting drugs such as Guanadrel and drowsiness for centrally acting drugs such as methyldopa. The frequencies observed were generally higher during the first 8 weeks of therapy. Week 0 frequencies, which were recorded just prior to administration of the antihypertensive drugs while the patients were receiving diuretics, serve as a reference point. Frequency while on therapy are shown for the first 8 weeks and for weeks 9 to 52.

FREQUENCY OF SIDE EFFECTS

Percent of Clinic Visits in Which Side Effect Was Reported
Guanadrel

	Pre Drug		
Week	0	1-8	9-52
Number of clinic visits analyzed	470	3003	4260
SIDE EFFECT			
Morning orthostatic faintness	6.6	9.4	6.8
Orthostatic faintness during the day	7.5	10.8	8.5
Other faintness	7.8	4.8	4.5
Increased bowel movements	4.9	7.9	6.1
Drowsiness	15.3	14.4	8.7
Fatigue	25.7	26.6	23.7
Ejaculation disturbance	7.0	17.5	12.0

Methyldopa

	Pre Drug		
Week	0	1-8	9-52
Number of clinic visits analyzed	266	1610	2216
SIDE EFFECT			
Morning orthostatic faintness	6.8	8.1	7.4
Orthostatic faintness during the day	7.5	8.0	7.8
Other faintness	6.2	3.7	3.8
Increased bowel movements	4.9	5.9	3.8
Drowsiness	13.2	21.2	18.6
Fatigue	32.9	22.6	27.6
Ejaculation disturbance	10.3	13.4	11.5

Guanethidine

	Pre Drug		
Week	0	1-8	9-52
Number of clinic visits analyzed	215	1421	2009
SIDE EFFECT			
Morning orthostatic faintness	4.6	10.7	7.9
Orthostatic faintness during the day	5.6	8.9	6.3
Other faintness	5.9	2.7	2.0
Increased bowel movements	3.7	7.9	9.4
Drowsiness	10.2	10.3	6.4
Fatigue	21.4	20.5	17.5
Ejaculation disturbance	6.9	16.6	18.2

The frequency of side effects over time may be reduced by the discontinuation of drugs in patients who experience intolerable side effects. Reasons for discontinuation of therapy with Guanadrel are shown in the following table.

PERCENT OF PATIENTS WHO DISCONTINUED

	Guanadrel	Methyldopa	Guanethidine
Orthostatic faintness	0.6	0.7	6.0*
Syncope	0.4	0.3	2.0
Other faintness	1.2	0.0	0.0
Increased bowel movements	0.8	0.7	1.4
Drowsiness	0.0	1.9*	0.0
Fatigue	0.2	2.6*	0.0
Ejaculation disturbances	0.4	0.0	0.0

* *significantly greater than Guanadrel Sulfate, p < 0.003.*

The following paragraph shows the incidence of reactions often associated with adrenergic neuron blockers as the percent of patients who reported the event at least once over the treatment periods of 6 months to 3 years. For such long-term studies these incidence rates of side effects, which are found often in untreated patients, tend to be high and accumulate with time. The incidence rates for two well-known comparison drugs, methyldopa and guanethidine, should aid in interpreting the high rates. It can be seen that the serious consequences of the orthostatic effect of Guanadrel, such as syncope, were very uncommon.

1544 Guanadrel, 743 methyldopa and 330 guanethidine patients were evaluated in comparison studies. The observed incidence rates of major drug related side effects for Guanadrel, methyldopa and guanethidine, respectively, are as follows: orthostatic faintness: 49%, 41%, 48%; other faintness: 47%, 46%, 45%; increased bowel movements: 31%, 28%, 36%; ejaculation disturbances: 18%, 21%, 22%; impotence: 5.1%, 12.2%, 7.2%; syncope: 0.4%, 0.3%, 2%; urine retention: 0.2%, 0%, 0%.

Apart from these adverse effects, many others were reported. Relationship to therapy is less clear, although some (such as peripheral edema with all three drugs, depression with methyldopa) are in part drug related. All adverse effects reported in at least 1% of Guanadrel patients are listed in the following table:

Drug	Guanadrel	Methyldopa	Guanethidine
No. pts. treated	1544	743	330
Event	%	%	%
CARDIOVASCULAR RESPIRATORY			
Chest Pain	27.9	37.4	27.3
Coughing	26.9	36.2	21.5
Palpitations	29.5	35.0	24.5

Shortness of breath at rest	18.3	22.3	17.0
Shortness of breath on exertion	45.9	53.2	48.8

CENTRAL NERVOUS SYSTEM-SPECIAL SENSES

Confusion	14.8	22.6	10.9
Depression	1.9	3.9	1.8
Drowsiness	44.6	64.1	28.5
Headache	58.1	69.0	49.7
Paresthesias	25.1	35.1	16.4
Psychological problems	3.8	4.8	3.9
Sleep disorders	2.1	2.3	2.7
Visual disturbances	29.2	35.3	26.1

GASTROINTESTINAL

Abdominal distress or pain	1.7	1.9	1.5
Anorexia	18.7	23.0	17.6
Constipation	21.0	29.1	20.3
Dry mouth, dry throat	1.7	4.0	0.6
Gas pain	32.0	39.7	29.4
Glossitis	8.4	10.8	4.8
Indigestion	23.7	30.8	18.5
Nausea and/or vomiting	3.9	4.8	3.6

GENTIOURINARY

Hematuria	2.3	4.2	2.1
Nocturia	48.4	52.4	41.5
Peripheral edema	28.6	37.4	22.7
Urinary urgency or frequency	33.6	39.8	27.6

MISCELLANEOUS

Excessive weight gain	44.3	53.7	42.4
Excessive weight loss	42.2	51.1	41.5
Fatigue	63.6	76.2	57.0

MUSCULOSKELETAL

Aching limbs	42.9	51.7	33.9
Backache or neckache	1.5	1.1	1.8
Joint pain or inflammation	1.7	2.0	2.4
Leg cramps during the day	21.1	26.0	20.0
Leg cramps during the night	25.6	32.6	21.2

OVERDOSAGE

Overdosage usually produces marked dizziness and blurred vision related to postural hypotension and may progress to syncope on standing. The patient should lie down until these symptoms subside.

If excessive hypotension occurs and persists despite conservative treatment, intensive therapy may be needed to support vital functions. A vasoconstrictor such as phenylephrine will ameliorate the effect of Guanadrel Sulfate Tablets, but great care must be used because patients may be hypersensitive to such agents.

DOSAGE AND ADMINISTRATION

As with other sympathetic suppressant drugs, the dose response to Guanadrel Sulfate Tablets varies widely and must be adjusted for each patient until the therapeutic goal is achieved. With long-term therapy, some tolerance may occur and the dosage may have to be increased.

Because Guanadrel Sulfate has a substantial orthostatic effect, monitoring both supine and standing pressures is essential, especially while dosage is being adjusted.

Guanadrel Sulfate should be administered in divided doses. The usual starting dosage for treating hypertension is 10 mg per day, which can be given as 5 mg b.i.d. by breaking the 10 mg tablet. The dosage should be adjusted weekly or monthly until blood pressure is controlled. Most patients will require daily dosage in the range of 20 to 75 mg usually in twice daily doses. For larger doses 3 or 4 times daily dosing may be needed. A dosage of more than 400 mg/day is rarely required.

Dosage should be adjusted for patients with impaired renal function (see "Clinical Pharmacology" and "Precautions"). As a general guideline, it is recommended that initial therapy with Guanadrel Sulfate in patients with creatinine clearances of 30 to 60 mL/min be reduced to 5 mg every 24 hours. In patients with creatinine clearances less than 30 mL/min, the dosing interval should be increased to 48 hours. The time to achieve steady state will be increased. Dosage increases should be made cautiously at intervals not less than 7 days in patients with moderate renal insufficiency and not less than 14 days in patients with severe renal insufficiency. These recommendations are based upon human pharmacokinetic data and not clinical experience.

HOW SUPPLIED
TABLETS: 10 MG

BRAND/MANUFACTURER	NDC	SIZE	AWP
○ BRAND			
HYLOREL: Fisons Presc	00585-0787-71	100s	$71.99

TABLETS: 25 MG

BRAND/MANUFACTURER	NDC	SIZE	AWP
○ BRAND			
HYLOREL: Fisons Presc	00585-0788-71	100s	$104.20

Guanethidine Monosulfate

DESCRIPTION

Guanethidine Monosulfate USP, is an antihypertensive, available as tablets of 10 mg and 25 mg for oral administration. Each 10-mg and 25-mg tablet contains Guanethidine Monosulfate USP equivalent to 10 mg and 25 mg of Guanethidine sulfate, USP. Its chemical name is [2-(hexahydro-1(2H)-azocinyl)ethyl]guanidine sulfate 1:1.

Guanethidine Monosulfate USP is a white to off-white crystalline powder with a molecular weight of 296.38. It is very soluble in water, sparingly soluble in alcohol, and practically insoluble in chloroform.

Following is its chemical structure:

$$N-CH_2CH_2-NH-C{\overset{\displaystyle NH}{\underset{\displaystyle NH_2}{}}} \cdot H_2SO_4$$

CLINICAL PHARMACOLOGY

Guanethidine Monosulfate acts at the sympathetic neuroeffector junction by inhibiting or interfering with the release and/or distribution of the chemical mediator (presumably the catecholamine norepinephrine), rather than acting at the effector cell by inhibiting the association of the transmitter with its receptors. In contrast to ganglionic blocking agents, Guanethidine Monosulfate suppresses equally the responses mediated by alpha and beta-adrenergic receptors but does not produce parasympathetic blockade. Since sympathetic blockade results in modest decreases in peripheral resistance and cardiac output. Guanethidine Monosulfate lowers blood pressure in the supine position. It further reduces blood pressure by decreasing the degree of vasoconstriction that normally results from reflex sympathetic nervous activity upon assumption of the upright posture, thus reducing venous return and cardiac output more. The inhibition of sympathetic venoconstrictive mechanisms results in venous pooling of blood. Therefore, the effect of Guanethidine Monosulfate is especially pronounced when the patient is standing. Both the systolic and diastolic pressures are reduced.

Other actions at the sympathetic nerve terminal include depletion of norepinephrine. Once it gains access to the neuron, Guanethidine Monosulfate accumulates within the intraneuronal storage vesicles and causes depletion of norepinephrine stores within the nerve terminal. Prolonged oral administration of Guanethidine Monosulfate produces a denervation sensitivity of the neuroeffector junction, probably resulting from the chronic reduction in norepinephrine released by the sympathetic nerve endings. Systemic responses to catecholamines released from the adrenal medulla are not prevented and may even be augmented as a result of this denervation sensitivity. A paradoxical hypertensive crisis may occur if Guanethidine Monosulfate is given to patients with pheochromocytoma or if norepinephrine is given to a patient receiving the drug.

Due to its poor lipid solubility, Guanethidine Monosulfate does not readily cross the blood-brain barrier. In contrast to most neural blocking agents, Guanethidine Monosulfate does not appear to suppress plasma renin activity in many patients.

PHARMACOKINETICS
The pharmacokinetics of Guanethidine Monosulfate are complex. The amount of drug in plasma and in urine is linearly related to dose, although large differences occur between individuals because of variation in absorption and metabolism. Adrenergic blockade occurs with a minimum concentration in plasma of 8 ng/ml; this concentration is achieved in different individuals with dosages of 10-50 mg/day at steady state. Guanethidine Monosulfate is eliminated slowly because of extensive tissue binding. After chronic oral administration, the initial phase of elimination with a half-life of 1.5 days is followed by a second phase of elimination with a half-life of 4-8 days. The renal clearance of Guanethidine Monosulfate is 56 ml/min. Guanethidine Monosulfate is converted by the liver to three metabolites, which are excreted in the urine. The metabolites are pharmacologically less active than Guanethidine Monosulfate.

INDICATIONS AND USAGE

Guanethidine Monosulfate is indicated for the treatment of moderate and severe hypertension, either alone or as an adjunct, and for the treatment of renal hypertension, including that secondary to pyelonephritis, renal amyloidosis, and renal artery stenosis.

UNLABELED USES
Guanethidine Monosulfate is used alone or as an adjunct in the treatment of reflex sympathetic dystrophy including causalgia, posttraumatic painful arthrosis, Sudeck's atrophy, sympathalgia, shoulder-hand syndrome, chronic traumatic edema, posttraumatic edema, and reflex dystrophy. It is also used, when given by intravenous route, to treat Raynaud's disease.

CONTRAINDICATIONS

Known or suspected pheochromocytoma; hypersensitivity; frank congestive heart failure not due to hypertension; use of monoamine oxidase (MAO) inhibitors.

➤ SHOWN IN PRODUCT IDENTIFICATION GUIDE

WARNINGS

Guanethidine Monosulfate is a potent drug and its use can lead to disturbing and serious clinical problems. Before prescribing, physicians should familiarize themselves with the details of its use and warn patients not to deviate from instructions.

> ORTHOSTATIC HYPOTENSION CAN OCCUR FREQUENTLY, AND PATIENTS SHOULD BE PROPERLY INSTRUCTED ABOUT THIS POTENTIAL HAZARD. FAINTING SPELLS MAY OCCUR UNLESS THE PATIENT IS FOREWARNED TO SIT OR LIE DOWN WITH THE ONSET OF DIZZINESS OR WEAKNESS. POSTURAL HYPOTENSION IS MOST MARKED IN THE MORNING AND IS ACCENTUATED BY HOT WEATHER, ALCOHOL, OR EXERCISE. DIZZINESS OR WEAKNESS MAY BE PARTICULARLY BOTHERSOME DURING THE INITIAL PERIOD OF DOSAGE ADJUSTMENT AND WITH POSTURAL CHANGES, SUCH AS ARISING IN THE MORNING. THE POTENTIAL OCCURRENCE OF THESE SYMPTOMS MAY REQUIRE ALTERATION OF PREVIOUS DAILY ACTIVITY. THE PATIENT SHOULD BE CAUTIONED TO AVOID SUDDEN OR PROLONGED STANDING OR EXERCISE WHILE TAKING THE DRUG.

Inhibition of ejaculation has been reported in animals (see *"Precautions, Carcinogenesis, Mutagenesis, Impairment of Fertility"*) as well as in men given Guanethidine Monosulfate. This effect, which results from the sympathetic blockade caused by the drug's action, is reversible after Guanethidine Monosulfate has been discontinued for several weeks. The drug does not cause parasympathetic blockade, and erectile potency is usually retained during administration of Guanethidine Monosulfate. The possible occurrence of inhibition of ejaculation should be kept in mind when considering the use of Guanethidine in men of reproductive age. If possible, therapy should be withdrawn 2 weeks prior to surgery to reduce the possibility of vascular collapse and cardiac arrest during anesthesia. If emergency surgery is indicated, preanesthetic and anesthetic agents should be administered cautiously in reduced dosage. Oxygen, atropine, vasopressors, and adequate solutions for volume replacement should be ready for immediate use to counteract vascular collapse in the surgical patient. Vasopressors should be used only with extreme caution, since Guanethidine Monosulfate augments responsiveness to exogenously administered norepinephrine and vasopressors; specifically, blood pressure may rise and cardiac arrhythmias may be produced.

PRECAUTIONS

GENERAL

Dosage requirements may be reduced in the presence of fever.

Special care should be exercised when treating patients with a history of bronchial asthma; asthmatic patients are more apt to be hypersensitive to catecholamine depletion, and their condition may be aggravated.

The effects of Guanethidine Monosulfate are cumulative over long periods; initial doses should be small and increased gradually in small increments.

Guanethidine Monosulfate should be used very cautiously in hypertensive patients with renal disease and nitrogen retention or rising BUN levels, since decreased blood pressure may further compromise renal function, coronary insufficiency or recent myocardial infarction, and cerebrovascular disease, especially with encephalopathy.

Guanethidine Monosulfate should not be given to patients with severe cardiac failure except with extreme caution, since Guanethidine Monosulfate may interfere with the compensatory role of the adrenergic system in producing circulatory adjustment in patients with congestive heart failure.

Patients with incipient cardiac decompensation should be watched for weight gain or edema, which may be averted by the concomitant administration of a thiazide.

Guanethidine Monosulfate should be used cautiously in patients with a history of peptic ulcer or other chronic disorders that may be aggravated by a relative increase in parasympathetic tone.

INFORMATION FOR PATIENTS

The patient should be advised to take Guanethidine Monosulfate exactly as directed. If the patient misses a dose, he or she should be told to take only the next scheduled dose (without doubling it).

The patient should be advised to avoid sudden or prolonged standing or exercise and to arise slowly, especially in the morning, to reduce the orthostatic hypotensive effects of dizziness, lightheadedness, or fainting.

The patient should be cautioned about ingesting alcohol, since it aggravates the orthostatic hypotensive effects of Guanethidine Monosulfate.

Male patients should be advised that guanethidine may interfere with ejaculation.

DRUG INTERACTIONS

Concurrent use of Guanethidine Monosulfate and rauwolfia derivatives may cause excessive postural hypotension, bradycardia, and mental depression.

Both digitalis and Guanethidine Monosulfate slow the heart rate.

Thiazide diuretics enhance the antihypertensive action of Guanethidine Monosulfate (see *"Dosage and Administration"*).

Amphetamine-like compounds, stimulants (e.g., ephedrine, methylphenidate), tricylic antidepressants (e.g., amitriptyline, imipramine, desipramine) and other psychopharmacologic agents (e.g., phenothiazines and related compounds), as well as oral contraceptives, may reduce the hypotensive effect of Guanethidine Monosulfate.

MAO inhibitors should be discontinued for at least 1 week before starting therapy with Guanethidine Monosulfate.

CARCINOGENESIS, MUTAGENESIS, IMPAIRMENT OF FERTILITY

Long-term carcinogenicity studies in animals have not been conducted with Guanethidine Monosulfate.

While inhibition of sperm passage and accumulation of sperm debris have been reported in rats and rabbits after several weeks of administration of Guanethidine Monosulfate, 5 or 10 mg/kg per day, subcutaneously or intraperitoneally, recovery of ejaculatory function and fertility has been demonstrated in rats given Guanethidine Monosulfate intramuscularly, 25 mg/kg per day, for 8 weeks. Inhibition of ejaculation has also been reported in men (see *"Warnings"* and *"Adverse Reactions"*). This effect, which is attributable to the sympathetic blockade caused by the drug, is reversible several weeks after discontinuance of the drug.

PREGNANCY CATEGORY C

Animal reproduction studies have not been conducted with Guanethidine Monosulfate. It is also not known whether Guanethidine Monosulfate can cause fetal harm when administered to a pregnant woman or can affect reproduction capacity. Guanethidine Monosulfate should be given to a pregnant woman only if clearly needed.

NURSING MOTHERS

Guanethidine Monosulfate is excreted in breast milk in very small quantity. Caution should be exercised when Guanethidine Monosulfate is administered to a nursing woman.

PEDIATRIC USE

Safety and effectiveness in children have not been established.

ADVERSE REACTIONS

The following adverse reactions have been observed, but there are not enough data to support an estimate of their frequency. Consequently the reactions are categorized by organ system and are listed in decreasing order of severity and not frequency.

Digestive: Diarrhea, which may be severe at times and necessitate discontinuance of medication; vomiting, nausea, increased bowel movements; dry mouth, parotid tenderness.

Cardiovascular: Chest pains (angina); bradycardia; a tendency toward fluid retention and edema with occasional development of congestive heart failure.

Respiratory: Dyspnea; asthma in susceptible individuals; nasal congestion.

Neurologic: Syncope resulting from either postural or exertional hypotension; dizziness; blurred vision; muscle tremor; ptosis of the lids; mental depression; chest paresthesias; weakness; lassitude; fatigue.

Muscular: Myalgia.

Genitourinary: Rise in BUN; urinary incontinence; inhibition of ejaculation; nocturia.

Metabolic: Weight gain.

Skin and Appendages: Dermatitis; scalp hair loss.

Although a causal relationship has not been established, a few instances of blood dyscrasia (anemia, thrombocytopenia, and leukopenia) and of priapism or impotence have been reported.

OVERDOSAGE

ACUTE TOXICITY

No deaths due to acute poisoning have been reported.

Oral LD$_{50}$ in rats: 1262 mg/kg.

SIGNS AND SYMPTOMS

Postural hypotension (with dizziness, blurred vision, and possibly syncope when standing), shock, and bradycardia are most likely to occur, diarrhea (possibly severe), nausea and vomiting may also occur. Unconsciousness is unlikely if adequate blood pressure and cerebral perfusion can be maintained by placing the patient in the supine position and by administering other treatment as required.

TREATMENT

There is no specific antidote.

Treatment should consist of gastric lavage. An activated charcoal slurry should be instilled and laxatives given, if conditions permit.

In sinus bradycardia, atropine should be administered.

In previously normotensive patients, treatment has consisted essentially of restoring blood pressure and heart rate to normal by keeping the patient in the supine position. Normal homeostatic control usually returns gradually over a 72-hour period in these patients.

In previously hypertensive patients, particularly those with impaired cardiac reserve or other cardiovascular-renal disease, intensive treatment may be required to support vital functions and to control cardiac irregularities that might be present. The supine position must be maintained; if vasopressors are required, they must be used with extreme caution, since Guanethidine Monosulfate may increase responsiveness, causing a rise in blood pressure and development of cardiac arrhythmias.

◆ RATED THERAPEUTICALLY EQUIVALENT; ◇ THERAPEUTIC EQUIVALENCE UNCONFIRMED; ○ UNRATED

Diarrhea, if severe or persistent, should be treated with anticholinergic agents to reduce intestinal hypermotility; hydration and electrolyte balance should be maintained.

Since Guanethidine Monosulfate is excreted slowly, cardiovascular and renal function should be monitored for a few days.

DOSAGE AND ADMINISTRATION

Better control may be obtained, especially in the initial phases of treatment, if the patient can have his blood pressure recorded regularly at home.

AMBULATORY PATIENTS

Initial doses should be small (10 mg) and increased gradually, depending upon the patient's response. Guanethidine Monosulfate has a long duration of action; therefore, dosage increases should not be made more often than every 5-7 days, unless the patient is hospitalized.

Blood pressure should be measured in the supine position, after standing for 10 minutes, and immediately after exercise if feasible. Dosage may be increased only if there has been no decrease in the standing blood pressure from previous levels. The average daily dose is 25-50 mg; only one dose a day is usually required.

DOSAGE CHART FOR AMBULATORY PATIENTS

Visits (Intervals of 5-7 Days)	Daily Dose
Visit 1 (Patient may be started on 10-mg tablets)	10 mg
Visit 2	20 mg
Visit 3 (Patient may be changed to 25-mg tablets whenever convenient)	30 mg (three 10-mg tablets) or 37.5 mg (one and one half 25-mg tablets)
Visit 4	50 mg
Visit 5 and subsequent	Dosage may be increased by 12.5 mg or 25 mg if necessary.

The dosage should be reduced in any of the following situations: (1) normal supine pressure (2) excessive orthostatic fall in pressure (3) severe diarrhea.

HOSPITALIZED PATIENTS

Initial oral dose is 25-50 mg, increased by 25 mg or 50 mg daily or every other day, as indicated. This higher dosage is possible because hospitalized patients can be watched carefully. Unless absolutely impossible, the standing blood pressure should be measured regularly. Patients should not be discharged from the hospital until the effect of the drug on the standing blood pressure is known. Patients should be told about the possibility of orthostatic hypotension and warned not to get out of bed without help during the period of dosage adjustment.

COMBINATION THERAPY

Guanethidine Monosulfate may be added gradually to thiazides and/or hydralazine. Thiazide diuretics enhance the effectiveness of Guanethidine Monosulfate and may reduce the incidence of edema. When thiazide diuretics are added to the regimen in patients taking Guanethidine Monosulfate, it is usually necessary to reduce the dosage of Guanethidine Monosulfate. After control is established, the dosage of all drugs should be reduced to the lowest effective level.

Note: When Guanethidine Monosulfate is replacing MAO inhibitors, at least 1 week should elapse before commencing treatment with Guanethidine Monosulfate (see *"Contraindications"*). If ganglionic blockers have not been discontinued before Guanethidine Monosulfate is started, they should be gradually withdrawn to prevent a spiking blood pressure response during the transfer period.

STORAGE

Do not store above 86°F (30°C).
Dispense in tight container (USP).

HOW SUPPLIED
TABLETS: 10 MG

BRAND/MANUFACTURER	NDC	SIZE	AWP
◆ BRAND ISMELIN: Ciba Pharm	00083-0049-30	100s	$49.67

TABLETS: 25 MG

BRAND/MANUFACTURER	NDC	SIZE	AWP
◆ BRAND ISMELIN: Ciba Pharm	00083-0103-30	100s	$78.05

Guanethidine Monosulfate with Hydrochlorothiazide

WARNING

THIS FIXED-COMBINATION DRUG IS NOT INDICATED FOR INITIAL THERAPY OF HYPERTENSION. HYPERTENSION REQUIRES THERAPY TITRATED TO THE INDIVIDUAL PATIENT. IF THE FIXED COMBINATION REPRESENTS THE DOSAGE SO DETERMINED, ITS USE MAY BE MORE CONVENIENT IN PATIENT MANAGEMENT. THE TREATMENT OF HYPERTENSION IS NOT STATIC BUT MUST BE REEVALUATED AS CONDITIONS IN EACH PATIENT WARRANT.

DESCRIPTION

Guanethidine Monosulfate/Hydrochlorothiazide is an antihypertensive-diuretic combination, available as tablets for oral administration. Each tablet contains Guanethidine Monosulfate, 10 mg, and Hydrochlorothiazide 25 mg.

Guanethidine Monosulfate is [2-(hexahydro-1(2H)-azocinyl)ethyl] guanidine sulfate 1:1.

Guanethidine Monosulfate USP is a white to off-white crystalline powder with a molecular weight of 296.38. It is very soluble in water, sparingly soluble in alcohol and practically insoluble in chloroform.

Hydrochlorothiazide (HCTZ) is 6-chloro-3,4-dihydro-2H-1,2,4-benzo-thiadiazine-7-sulfonamide 1,1-dioxide.

Hydrochlorothiazide USP is a white, or practically white, practically odorless crystalline powder. It is slightly soluble in water; freely soluble in sodium hydroxide solution, in *n*-butylamine, and in dimethylformamide; sparingly soluble in methanol; and insoluble in ether, in chloroform, and in diluted mineral acids. Its molecular weight is 297.73.

CLINICAL PHARMACOLOGY
GUANETHIDINE

Guanethidine acts at the sympathetic neuroeffector junction by inhibiting or interfering with the release and/or distribution of the chemical mediator (presumably the catecholamine norepinephrine), rather than acting at the effector cell by inhibiting the association of the transmitter with its receptors. In contrast to ganglionic blocking agents, Guanethidine suppresses equally the responses mediated by alpha- and beta-adrenergic receptors but does not produce parasympathetic blockade. Since sympathetic blockade results in modest decrease in peripheral resistance and cardiac output, Guanethidine lowers blood pressure in the supine position. It further reduces blood pressure by decreasing the degree of vasoconstriction that normally results from reflex sympathetic nervous activity upon assumption of the upright posture, thus reducing venous return and cardiac output more. The inhibition of sympathetic venoconstrictive mechanisms results in venous pooling of blood. Therefore, the effect of Guanethidine is especially pronounced when the patient is standing. Both the systolic and diastolic pressures are reduced.

Other actions at the sympathetic nerve terminal include depletion of norepinephrine. Once it gains access to the neuron, Guanethidine accumulates within the intraneuronal storage vesicles and causes depletion of norepinephrine stores within the nerve terminal. Prolonged oral administration of Guanethidine produces a denervation sensitivity of the neuroeffector junction, probably resulting from the chronic reduction in norepinephrine released by the sympathetic nerve endings. Systemic responses to catecholamines released from the adrenal medulla are not prevented and may even be augmented as a result of this denervation sensitivity. A paradoxical hypertensive crisis may occur if Guanethidine is given to patients with pheochromocytoma or if norepinephrine is given to a patient receiving the drug.

Due to its poor lipid solubility, Guanethidine does not readily cross the blood-brain barrier. In contrast to most neural blocking agents, Guanethidine does not appear to suppress plasma renin activity in many patients.

PHARMACOKINETICS

The pharmacokinetics of Guanethidine are complex. The amount of drug in plasma and in urine is linearly related to dose, although large differences occur between individuals because of variation in absorption and elimination. Adrenergic blockade occurs with a minimum concentration in plasma of 8 ng/ml; this concentration is achieved in different individuals with doses of 10-50 mg per day at steady state. Guanethidine is eliminated slowly because of extensive tissue binding. After chronic oral administration, the initial phase of elimination with a half-life of 1.5 days is followed by a second phase of elimination with a half-life of 4-8 days. The renal clearance of Guanethidine is 56 ml/min. Guanethidine is converted by the liver to three metabolites, which are excreted in the urine. The metabolites are pharmacologically less active than Guanethidine.

HYDROCHLOROTHIAZIDE

Thiazides affect the renal tubular mechanism of electrolyte reabsorption. At maximal therapeutic dosage, all thiazides are approximately equal in their diuretic potency. Thiazides increase excretion of sodium and chloride in approximately equivalent amounts. Natriuresis causes a secondary loss of potassium.

The mechanism of the antihypertensive effect of thiazides is unknown. Thiazides do not affect normal blood pressure.

PHARMACOKINETICS

The onset of action of thiazides occurs in 2 hours, and the peak effect at about 4 hours. The action persists for approximately 6-12 hours. Hydrochlorothiazide is rapidly absorbed, as indicated by peak plasma concentrations 1-2.5 hours after oral administration. Plasma levels of the drug are proportional to dose; the concentration in while blood is 1.6-1.8 times higher than in plasma. Thiazides are eliminated rapidly by the kidney. After oral administration of 25- to 100-mg doses of Hydrochlorothiazide, 72-97% of the dose is excreted in the urine, indicating dose-independent absorption. Hydrochlorothiazide is eliminated from plasma in a biphasic fashion with a terminal half-life of 10-17 hours. Plasma protein binding is 67.9%. Plasma clearance is 15.9-30.0 L/hr; volume of distribution is 3.6-7.8 L/kg.

► SHOWN IN PRODUCT IDENTIFICATION GUIDE

Gastrointestinal absorption of Hydrochlorothiazide is enhanced when administered with food. Absorption is decreased in patients with congestive heart failure, and the pharmacokinetics are considerably different in these patients.

INDICATIONS AND USAGE
Guanethidine/HCTZ is indicated for the treatment of hypertension (see boxed *"Warning"*).

CONTRAINDICATIONS
GUANETHIDINE
Known or suspected pheochromocytoma: hypersensitivity; frank congestive heart failure not due to hypertension; use of monoamine oxidase (MAO) inhibitors.

HYDROCHLOROTHIAZIDE
Anuria; hypersensitivity to this or other sulfonamide-derived drugs.

WARNINGS
Guanethidine and Hydrochlorothiazide are potent drugs, and their use can lead to disturbing and serious clinical problems. Physicians should be familiar with both drugs and their combination before prescribing, and patients should be warned not to deviate from instructions.

GUANETHIDINE

> ORTHOSTATIC HYPOTENSION CAN OCCUR FREQUENTLY, AND PATIENTS SHOULD BE PROPERLY INSTRUCTED ABOUT THIS POTENTIAL HAZARD. FAINTING SPELLS MAY OCCUR UNLESS THE PATIENT IS FOREWARNED TO SIT OR LIE DOWN WITH THE ONSET OF DIZZINESS OR WEAKNESS. POSTURAL HYPOTENSION IS MOST MARKED IN THE MORNING AND IS ACCENTUATED BY HOT WEATHER, ALCOHOL, OR EXERCISE. DIZZINESS OR WEAKNESS MAY BE PARTICULARLY BOTHERSOME DURING THE INITIAL PERIOD OF DOSAGE ADJUSTMENT AND WITH POSTURAL CHANGES, SUCH AS ARISING IN THE MORNING. THE POTENTIAL OCCURRENCE OF THESE SYMPTOMS MAY REQUIRE ALTERATION OF PREVIOUS DAILY ACTIVITY. THE PATIENT SHOULD BE CAUTIONED TO AVOID SUDDEN OR PROLONGED STANDING OR EXERCISE WHILE TAKING THE DRUG.

Inhibition of ejaculation has been reported in animals (see *"Precautions, Carcinogenesis, Mutagenesis, Impairment of Fertility"*) as well as in men given Guanethidine. This effect, which results from the sympathetic blockade caused by the drug's action, is reversible after Guanethidine has been discontinued for several weeks. The drug does not cause parasympathetic blockade, and erectile potency is usually retained during administration of Guanethidine. The possible occurrence of inhibition of ejaculation should be kept in mind when considering the use of Guanethidine in men of reproductive age.

If possible, therapy should be withdrawn 2 weeks prior to surgery to reduce the possibility of vascular collapse and cardiac arrest during anesthesia. If emergency surgery is indicated, preanesthetic and anesthetic agents should be administered cautiously in reduced dosage. Oxygen, atropine, vasopressors, and adequate solutions for volume replacement should be ready for immediate use to counteract vascular collapse in the surgical patient. Vasopressors should be used only with extreme caution, since Guanethidine augments responsiveness to exogenously administered norepinephrine and vasopressors: specifically, blood pressure may rise and cardiac arrhythmias may be produced.

HYDROCHLOROTHIAZIDE
Thiazides should be used with caution in patients with severe renal disease. In patients with renal disease, thiazides may precipitate azotemia. Cumulative effects of the drug may develop in patients with impaired renal function.

Thiazides should be used with caution in patients with impaired hepatic function or progressive liver disease, since minor alterations of fluid and electrolyte imbalance may precipitate hepatic coma.

Thiazides may add to or potentiate the action of other antihypertensive drugs. Potentiation occurs with ganglionic or peripheral adrenergic blocking drugs.

Sensitivity reactions are more likely to occur in patients with a history of allergy or bronchial asthma.

The possibility of exacerbation of activation of systemic lupus erythematosus has been reported.

PRECAUTIONS
GENERAL
Guanethidine. Dosage requirements may be reduced in the presence of fever.

Special care should be exercised when treating patients with a history of bronchial asthma; asthmatic patients are more apt to be hypersensitive to catecholamine depletion, and their condition may be aggravated.

The effects of Guanethidine are cumulative over long periods; initial doses should be small and increased gradually in small increments.

Guanethidine should be used very cautiously in hypertensive patients with: renal disease and nitrogen retention or rising BUN levels, since decreased blood pressure may further compromise renal function; coronary insufficiency or recent myocardial infarction; and cerebrovascular disease, especially with encephalopathy.

Guanethidine should not be given to patients with severe cardiac failure except with extreme caution, since Guanethidine may interfere with the compensatory role of the adrenergic system in producing circulatory adjustment in patients with congestive heart failure.

Patients with incipient cardiac decompensation should be watched for weight gain or edema.

Guanethidine should be used cautiously in patients with a history of peptic ulcer or other chronic disorders that may be aggravated by a relative increase in parasympathetic tone.

Hydrochlorothiazide. All patients receiving thiazide therapy should be observed for clinical signs of fluid or electrolyte imbalance, namely hyponatremia, hypochloremic alkalosis, and hypokalemia (see *"Laboratory Tests"* and *"Drug/Drug Interactions"*). Warning signs are dryness of mouth, thirst, weakness, lethargy, drowsiness, restlessness, muscle pains or cramps, muscular fatigue, hypotension, oliguria, tachycardia, and gastrointestinal disturbance, such as nausea or vomiting.

Hypokalemia may develop, especially in cases of brisk diuresis or severe cirrhosis.

Interference with adequate oral intake of electrolytes will also contribute to hypokalemia. Hypokalemia may be avoided or treated by use of potassium supplements or foods with a high potassium content.

Any chloride deficit is generally mild and usually does not require specific treatment, except under extraordinary circumstances (as in liver disease or renal disease). Dilutional hyponatremia may occur in edematous patients in hot weather; appropriate therapy is water restriction, rather than admininistration of salt, except in rare instances when the hyponatremia is life-threatening. In cases of actual salt depletion, appropriate replacement is the therapy of choice. Hyperuricemia may occur or frank gout may be precipitated in certain patients receiving thiazide therapy.

Latent diabetes may become manifest during thiazide administration (see *"Drug/Drug Interactions"*).

The antihypertensive effects of the drug may be enhanced in the postsympathectomy patient.

If progressive renal impairment becomes evident, withholding or discontinuing diuretic therapy should be considered. Calcium excretion is decreased by thiazides. Pathological changes in the parathyroid gland with hypercalcemia and hypophosphatemia have been observed in a few patients on prolonged thiazide therapy. The common complications of hyperparathyroidism, such as renal lithiasis, bone resorption, and peptic ulceration, have not been seen.

INFORMATION FOR PATIENTS
The patient should be advised to take this medication exactly as directed. If the patient misses a dose, he or she should be told to take only the next scheduled dose (without doubling it).

The patient should be advised to avoid sudden or prolonged standing or exercise and to arise slowly, especially in the morning, to reduce the orthostatic hypotensive effects of dizziness, light-headedness, or fainting.

The patient should be cautioned about ingesting alcohol, since it aggravates the orthostatic hypotensive effects of Guanethidine.

Male patients should be advised that Guanethidine may interfere with ejaculation.

LABORATORY TESTS
Hydrochlorothiazide. Initial and periodic determinations of serum electrolytes to detect possible electrolyte imbalance should be performed at appropriate intervals.

Serum and urine electrolyte determinations are particularly important when the patient is vomiting excessively or receiving parenteral fluids.

DRUG/DRUG INTERACTIONS
Guanethidine. Concurrent use of Guanethidine and rauwolfia derivatives may cause excessive postural hypotension, bradycardia, and mental depression.

Both digitalis and Guanethidine slow the heart rate.

Amphetamine-like compounds, stimulants (e.g., ephedrine, methylphenidate), tricyclic antidepressants (e.g., amitriptyline, imipramine, desipramine) and other psychopharmacologic agents (e.g., phenothiazines and related compounds), as well as oral contraceptives, may reduce the hypotensive effect of Guanethidine.

MAO inhibitors should be discontinued for at least 1 week before starting therapy with Guanethidine.

Hydrochlorothiazide. Hypokalemia can sensitize or exaggerate the response of the heart to the toxic effects of digitalis (e.g., increased ventricular irritability).

Hypokalemia may develop during concomitant use of steroids or ACTH.

Insulin requirements in diabetic patients may be increased, decreased, or unchanged.

Thiazides may decrease arterial responsiveness to norepinephrine, but not enough to preclude effectiveness of the pressor agent for therapeutic use.

Thiazides may increase the responsiveness to tubocurarine. Lithium renal clearance is reduced by thiazides, increasing the risk of lithium toxicity.

There have been rare reports in the literature of hemolytic anemia occurring with the concomitant use of Hydrochlorothiazide and methyldopa.

Concurrent administration of some nonsteroidal anti-inflammatory agents may reduce the diuretic, natriuretic and antihypertensive effects of thiazide diuretics.

DRUG/LABORATORY TEST INTERACTIONS

Thiazides may decrease serum levels of protein-bound iodine without signs of thyroid disturbance. Guarethidine/HCTZ should be discontinued before tests for parathyroid function are made (see *"General, Hydrochlorothiazide, Calcium excretion"*).

CARCINOGENESIS, MUTAGENESIS, IMPAIRMENT OF FERTILITY

Long-term carcinogenicity studies in animals have not been conducted with Guanethidine/HCTZ.

Guanethidine: While inhibition of sperm passage and accumulation of sperm debris have been reported in rats and rabbits after several weeks of administration of Guanethidine, 5 or 10 mg/kg per day, subcutaneously or intraperitoneally, recovery of ejaculatory function and fertility has been demonstrated in rats given Guanethidine intramuscularly, 25 mg/kg per day, for 8 weeks. Inhibition of ejaculation has also been reported in men (see *"Warnings"* and *"Adverse Reactions"*). This effect, when is attributable to the sympathetic blockade caused by the drug, is reversible several weeks after discontinuance of the drug.

Hydrochlorothiazide: Two-year feeding studies in mice and rats conducted under the auspices of the National Toxicology Program (NTP) uncovered no evidence of a carcinogenic potential of Hydrochlorothiazide in female mice (at doses of up to approximately 600 mg/kg/day) or in male and female rats (at doses of up to approximately 100 mg/kg/day). The NTP, however, found equivocal evidence for hepatocarcinogenicity in male mice.

Hydrochlorothiazide was not genotoxic in *in vitro* assays using strains TA 98, TA 100, TA 1535, TA 1537, and TA 1538 of Salmonella typhimurium (Ames assay) and in the Chinese Hamster Ovary (CHO) test for chromosomal aberrations, or in in vivo assays using mouse germinal cell chromosomes, Chinese hamster bone marrow chromosomes, and the *Drosophila* sex-linked recessive lethal trait gene. Positive test results were obtained only in the in vitro CHO Sister Chromatid Exchange (clastogenicity) and in the Mouse Lymphoma Cell (mutagenicity) assays, using concentrations of Hydrochlorothiazide from 43 to 1300 μg/mL, and in *Aspergillus nidulans* nondisjunction assay at an unspecified concentration.

Hydrochlorothiazide had no adverse effects on the fertility of mice and rats of either sex in studies wherein these species were exposed, via their diet, to doses of up to 100 and 4 mg/kg/day, respectively, prior to mating and throughout gestation.

PREGNANCY: TERATOGENIC EFFECTS. PREGNANCY CATEGORY B

A reproduction study performed in rats receiving doses at least 150 times the average daily human dose of Guanethidine/HCTZ has revealed no evidence of impaired fertility or harm to the fetus due to this drug.

There are no adequate and well-controlled studies of Guanethidine/HCTZ in pregnant women. Because animal reproduction studies are not always predictive of human response, this drug should be used during pregnancy only if clearly needed.

Guanethidine. The effects of Guanethidine on teratogenesis have not been studied in animals.

Hydrochlorothiazide. Studies in which Hydrochlorothiazide was orally administered to pregnant mice and rats during their respective periods of major organogenesis at doses up to 3000 and 1000 mg/kg/day, respectively, provided no evidence of harm to the fetus.

NONTERATOGENIC EFFECTS

Hydrochlorothiazide. Thiazides cross the placental barrier and appear in cord blood, and there is a risk of fetal or neonatal jaundice, thrombocytopenia, and possibly other adverse reactions that have occurred in adults.

NURSING MOTHERS

Guanethidine is excreted in breast milk in very small quantity. Thiazides are also excreted in breast milk. Because of the potential for serious adverse reactions in nursing infants, a decision should be made whether to discontinue nursing or to discontinue Guanethidine/HCTZ, taking into account the importance of the drug to the mother.

PEDIATRIC USE

Safety and effectiveness of the combination drug in children have not been established.

ADVERSE REACTIONS

Whenever adverse reactions are moderate or severe, it may be necessary to reduce the dosage of Guanethidine/HCTZ, discontinuing the drug, or administer the individual active components, reducing the dosage of either Guanethidine or Hydrochlorothiazide.

The following adverse reactions have been observed, but there are not enough data to support an estimate of their frequency. Consequently the reactions are categorized by organ system and are listed in decreasing order of severity and not frequency.

GUANETHIDINE

Digestive: Diarrhea, which may be severe at times and necessitate discontinuance of medication; vomiting; nausea; increased bowel movements; dry mouth; parotid tenderness.

Cardiovascular: Chest pains (angina); bradycardia; a tendency toward fluid retention and edema with occasional development of congestive heart failure.

Respiratory: Dyspnea; asthma in susceptible individuals; nasal congestion.

Neurologic: Syncope resulting from either postural or exertional hypotension; dizziness; blurred vision; muscle tremor; ptosis of the lids; mental depression; chest paresthesias; weakness; lassitude; fatigue.

Muscular: Myalgia.

Genitourinary: Rise in BUN; urinary incontinence; inhibition of ejaculation; nocturia.

Metabolic: Weight gain.

Skin and Appendages: Dermatitis; scalp hair loss.

Although a causal relationship has not been established, a few instances of blood dyscrasias (anemia, thrombocytopenia, and leukopenia) and of priapism or impotence have been reported.

HYDROCHLOROTHIAZIDE

Digestive: Pancreatitis, jaundice (intrahepatic cholestatic), sialadenitis, vomiting, diarrhea, cramping, nausea, gastric irritation, constipation, anorexia.

Cardiovascular: Orthostatic hypotension (may be potentiated by alcohol, barbiturates, or narcotics).

Neurologic: Vertigo, dizziness, transient blurred vision, headache, paresthesia, xanthopsia, weakness, restlessness.

Musculoskeletal: Muscle spasm.

Hematologic: Aplastic anemia, agranulocytosis, leukopenia, thrombocytopenia.

Metabolic: Hyperglycemia, glycosuria, hyperuricemia.

Hypersensitive Reactions: Necrotizing angiitis, Stevens-Johnson syndrome, respiratory distress including pneumonitis and pulmonary edema, purpura, urticaria, rash, photosensitivity.

OVERDOSAGE

ACUTE TOXICITY

No deaths due to acute poisoning with Guanethidine/HCTZ have been reported.
Oral LD$_{50}$'s in rats (mg/kg): Guanethidine, 1262; Hydrochlorothiazide, 2750.

SIGNS AND SYMPTOMS

Guanethidine. Postural hypotension (with dizziness, blurred vision, and possibly syncope when standing), shock, and bradycardia are most likely to occur; diarrhea (possibly severe), nausea, and vomiting may also occur. Unconsciousness is unlikely if adequate blood pressure and cerebral perfusion can be maintained by placing the patient in the supine position and by administering other treatment as required.

Hydrochlorothiazide. The most prominent feature of poisoning is acute loss of fluid and electrolytes.

Cardiovascular: Tachycardia, hypotension, shock.

Neuromuscular: Weakness, confusion, dizziness, cramps of the calf muscles, paresthesia, fatigue, impairment of consciousness.

Digestive: Nausea, vomiting, thirst.

Renal: Polyuria, oliguria, or anuria (due to hemoconcentration).

Laboratory Findings: Hypokalemia, hyponatremia, hypochloremia, alkalosis, increased BUN (especially in patients with renal insufficiency).

Combined Poisoning: Signs and symptoms may be aggravated or modified by concomitant intake of antihypertensive medication, barbiturates, digitalis (hypokalemia), corticosteroids, narcotics, or alcohol.

TREATMENT

There is no specific antidote.

The stomach contents should be evacuated. An activated charcoal slurry should be instilled and laxatives given, if conditions permit.

If hypotension or shock occurs, the patient's legs should be kept raised, and lost fluid and electrolytes (potassium, sodium) should be replaced. Renal function should be monitored until conditions become normal.

In sinus bradycardia, atropine should be administered.

In previously normotensive patients, treatment has consisted essentially of restoring blood pressure and heart rate to normal by keeping the patient in the supine position. Normal homeostatic control usually returns gradually over a 72-hour period in these patients.

In previously hypertensive patients, particularly those with impaired cardiac reserve or other cardiovascular-renal disease, intensive treatment may be required to support vital functions and to control cardiac irregularities that might be present. The supine position must be maintained: if vasopressors are required, they must be used with extreme caution, since Guanethidine may increase responsiveness, causing a rise in blood pressure and development of cardiac arrhythmias.

Diarrhea, if severe or persistent, should be treated with anticholinergic agents to reduce intestinal hypermotility, and hydration and electrolyte balance should be maintained.

Since Guanethidine is excreted slowly, cardiovascular and renal function should be monitored for a few days.

DOSAGE AND ADMINISTRATION

Dosage should be determined by titration of individual components (see boxed *"Warning"*). Once the patient has successfully been given titrated doses of the individual components, Guanethidine/HCTZ may be substituted if the titrated doses are the same as those in the fixed combination.

When combined with other antihypertensive agents, doses of Hydrochlorothiazide in excess of 50 mg should be avoided. Therefore, since each Guanethidine/HCTZ tablet contains 25 mg of Hydrochlorothiazide, the daily dosage of this fixed combination should not exceed two tablets. If further blood pressure control is indicated, additional doses of Guanethidine or other nondiuretic antihypertensive agents should be considered. Before using any Guanethidine-containing product, at least 1 week should elapse after MAO inhibitors (see "Contraindications") or ganglionic blockers have been discontinued.

Do not store above 86°F (30°C)

Dispense in tight container (USP)

HOW SUPPLIED
TABLETS: 10 MG-25 MG

BRAND/MANUFACTURER	NDC	SIZE	AWP
○ BRAND			
ESIMIL: Ciba Pharm	00083-0047-30	100s	$63.90

Guanfacine Hydrochloride

DESCRIPTION
Guanfacine Hydrochloride is a centrally acting anti-hypertensive with α_2-adrenoceptor agonist properties in tablet form for oral administration.

The chemical name of Guanfacine Hydrochloride is N-amidino-2-(2,6-dichlorophenyl) acetamide hydrochloride and its molecular weight is 282.56.

Guanfacine Hydrochloride is a white to off-white powder; sparingly soluble in water and alcohol and slightly soluble in acetone.

Following is its chemical structure:

CLINICAL PHARMACOLOGY
Guanfacine Hydrochloride is an orally active antihypertensive agent whose principal mechanism of action appears to be stimulation of central α_2-adrenergic receptors. By stimulating these receptors, Guanfacine reduces sympathetic nerve impulses from the vasomotor center to the heart and blood vessels. This results in a decrease in peripheral vascular resistance and a reduction in heart rate.

The dose-response relationship for blood pressure and adverse effects of Guanfacine given once a day as monotherapy has been evaluated in patients with mild to moderate hypertension. In this study patients were randomized to placebo or to 0.5 mg, 1 mg, 2 mg, 3 mg, or 5 mg of Guanfacine Hydrochloride. Results are shown in the following table. A useful effect was not observed overall until doses of 2 mg were reached, although responses in white patients were seen at 1 mg; 24 hour effectiveness of 1 mg to 3 mg doses was documented using 24 hour ambulatory monitoring. While the 5 mg dose added an increment of effectiveness, it caused an unacceptable increase in adverse reactions. (See related table).

Controlled clinical trials in patients with mild to moderate hypertension who were receiving a thiazide-type diuretic have defined the dose-response relationship for blood pressure response and adverse reactions of Guanfacine given at bedtime and have shown that the blood pressure response to Guanfacine can persist for 24 hours after a single dose. In the 12-week, placebo-controlled dose-response study, patients were randomized to placebo or to doses of 0.5, 1, 2, and 3 mg of Guanfacine, in addition to 25 mg chlorthalidone, each given at bedtime. The observed mean changes from baseline, tabulated below, indicate the similarity of response for placebo and the 0.5 mg dose. Doses of 1, 2, and 3 mg resulted in decreased blood pressure in the sitting position with no real differences among the three doses. In the standing position there was some increase in response with dose. (See related table).

While most of the effectiveness of Guanfacine in combination (and as monotherapy in white patients) was present at 1 mg, adverse reactions at this dose were not clearly distinguishable from those associated with placebo. Adverse reactions were clearly present at 2 and 3 mg (see "Adverse Reactions").

In a second 12-week, placebo-controlled study of 1, 2 or 3 mg of Guanfacine Hydrochloride administered with 25 mg of chlorthalidone once daily, a significant decrease in blood pressure was maintained for a full 24 hours after dosing. While there was no significant difference between the 12 and 24 hour blood pressure readings, the fall in blood pressure at 24 hours was numerically smaller, suggesting possible escape of blood pressure in some patients and the need for individualization of therapy.

In a double-blind, randomized trial, either Guanfacine or clonidine was given at recommended doses with 25 mg chlorthalidone for 24 weeks and then abruptly discontinued. Results showed equal degrees of blood pressure reduction with the two drugs and there was no tendency for blood pressures to increase despite maintenance of the same daily dose of the two drugs. Signs and symptoms of rebound phenomena were infrequent upon discontinuation of either drug. Abrupt withdrawal of clonidine produced a rapid return of diastolic and especially, systolic blood pressure to approximately pretreatment levels, with occasional values significantly greater than baseline, whereas Guanfacine withdrawal produced a more gradual increase to pre-treatment levels, but also with occasional values significantly greater than baseline.

Pharmacodynamics: Hemodynamic studies in man showed that the decrease in blood pressure observed after single-dose or long-term oral treatment with Guanfacine was accompanied by a significant decrease in peripheral resistance and a slight reduction in heart rate (5 beats/min). Cardiac output under conditions of rest or exercise was not altered by Guanfacine.

Guanfacine Hydrochloride lowered elevated plasma renin activity and plasma catecholamine levels in hypertensive patients, but this does not correlate with individual blood-pressure responses.

Growth hormone secretion was stimulated with single oral doses of 2 and 4 mg of Guanfacine. Long-term use of Guanfacine Hydrochloride had no effect on growth hormone levels.

Guanfacine had no effect on plasma aldosterone. A slight but insignificant decrease in plasma volume occurred after one month of Guanfacine therapy. There were no changes in mean body weight or electrolytes.

Pharmacokinetics: Relative to an intravenous dose of 3 mg, the absolute oral bioavailability of Guanfacine is about 80%. Peak plasma concentrations occur from 1 to 4 hours with an average of 2.6 hours after single oral doses or at steady state. The area under the concentration-time curve (AUC) increases linearly with the dose.

In individuals with normal renal function, the average elimination half-life is approximately 17 hr (range 10-30 hr). Younger patients tend to have shorter elimination half-lives (13-14 hr) while older patients tend to have half-lives at the upper end of the range. Steady state blood levels were attained within 4 days in most subjects.

In individuals with normal renal function, Guanfacine and its metabolites are excreted primarily in the urine. Approximately 50% (40-75%) of the dose is eliminated in the urine as unchanged drug; the remainder is eliminated mostly as conjugates of metabolites produced by oxidative metabolism of the aromatic ring.

The Guanfacine-to-creatinine clearance ratio is greater than 1.0, which would suggest that tubular secretion of drug occurs.

The drug is approximately 70% bound to plasma proteins, independent of drug concentration.

The whole body volume of distribution is high (a mean of 6.3 L/kg), which suggests a high distribution of drug to the tissues.

The clearance of Guanfacine in patients with varying degrees of renal insufficiency is reduced, but plasma levels of drug are only slightly increased compared to patients with normal renal function. When prescribing for patients with renal impairment, the low end of the dosing range should be used. Patients on dialysis also can be given usual doses of Guanfacine Hydrochloride as the drug is poorly dialyzed.

INDICATIONS AND USAGE
Guanfacine Hydrochloride is indicated in the management of hypertension. Guanfacine Hydrochloride may be given alone or in combination with other antihypertensive agents, especially thiazide-type diuretics.

MEAN CHANGES (MM HG) FROM BASELINE IN SEATED SYSTOLIC AND DIASTOLIC BLOOD PRESSURE FOR PATIENTS COMPLETING 4 TO 8 WEEKS OF TREATMENT WITH GUANFACINE MONOTHERAPY

Mean Change S/D* Seated	n = (range)	Placebo	0.5 mg	1 mg	2 mg	3 mg	5 mg
White Patients	11-30	−1/−5	−6/−8	−8/−9	−12/−11	−15/−12	−18/−16
Black Patients	8-28	−3/−5	0/−2	−3/−5	−7/−7	−8/−9	−19/−15

*   S/D = Systolic/diastolic blood pressure.

MEAN DECREASES (MM HG) IN SEATED AND STANDING BLOOD PRESSURE FOR PATIENTS TREATED WITH GUANFACINE IN COMBINATION WITH CHLORTHALIDONE

Mean Change	n =	Placebo 63	0.5 mg 63	1 mg 64	2 mg 58	3 mg 59
S/D* Seated		−5/−7	−5/−6	−14/−13	−12/−13	−16/−13
S/D* Standing		−3/−5	−5/−4	−11/−9	−9/−10	−15/−12

*   S/D = Systolic/diastolic blood pressure

◆ RATED THERAPEUTICALLY EQUIVALENT; ◇ THERAPEUTIC EQUIVALENCE UNCONFIRMED; ○ UNRATED

UNLABELED USES
Guanfacine Hydrochloride is used alone or as an adjunct in the treatment of heroin withdrawal and hypertension associated with pregnancy.

CONTRAINDICATIONS
Guanfacine Hydrochloride is contraindicated in patients with known hypersensitivity to Guanfacine Hydrochloride.

PRECAUTIONS
General: Like other antihypertensive agents, Guanfacine Hydrochloride should be used with caution in patients with severe coronary insufficiency, recent myocardial infarction, cerebrovascular disease or chronic renal or hepatic failure.

Sedation: Guanfacine Hydrochloride, like other orally active central alpha-2-adrenergic agonists, causes sedation or drowsiness, especially when beginning therapy. These symptoms are dose-related (see *"Adverse Reactions"*). When Guanfacine Hydrochloride is used with other centrally active depressants (such as phenothiazines, barbiturates, or benzodiazepines), the potential for additive sedative effects should be considered.

Rebound: Abrupt cessation of therapy with orally active central α-2 adrenergic agonists may be associated with increases (from depressed on-therapy levels) in plasma and urinary catecholamines, symptoms of "nervousness and anxiety" and, less commonly, increases in blood pressure to levels significantly greater than those prior to therapy.

Information for Patients: Patients who receive Guanfacine Hydrochloride should be advised to exercise caution when operating dangerous machinery or driving motor vehicles until it is determined that they do not become drowsy or dizzy from the medication. Patients should be warned that their tolerance for alcohol and other CNS depressants may be diminished. Patients should be advised not to discontinue therapy abruptly.

Laboratory Tests: In clinical trials, no clinically relevant laboratory test abnormalities were identified as causally related to drug during short-term treatment with Guanfacine Hydrochloride.

Drug Interactions: The potential for increased sedation when Guanfacine Hydrochloride is given with other CNS-depressant drugs should be appreciated.

The administration of Guanfacine concomitantly with a known microsomal enzyme inducer (phenobarbital or phenytoin) to two patients with renal impairment reportedly resulted in significant reductions in elimination half-life and plasma concentration. In such cases, therefore, more frequent dosing may be required to achieve or maintain the desired hypotensive response. Further, if Guanfacine is to be discontinued in such patients, careful tapering of the dosage may be necessary in order to avoid rebound phenomena (see *Rebound* above).

Anticoagulants: Ten patients who were stabilized on oral anticoagulants were given Guanfacine, 1-2 mg/day, for 4 weeks. No changes were observed in the degree of anticoagulation.

In several well-controlled studies, Guanfacine was administered together with diuretics with no drug interactions reported. In the long-term safety studies, Guanfacine Hydrochloride was given concomitantly with many drugs without evidence of any interactions. The principal drugs given (number of patients in parentheses) were: cardiac glycosides (115), sedatives and hypnotics (103), coronary vasodilators (52), oral hypoglycemics (45), cough and cold preparations (45), NSAIDs (38), antihyperlipidemics (29), antigout drugs (24), oral contraceptives (18), bronchodilators (13), insulin (10), and beta blockers (10).

Drug/Laboratory Test Interactions: No laboratory test abnormalities related to the use of Guanfacine Hydrochloride have been identified.

Carcinogenesis, Mutagenesis, Impairment of Fertility: No carcinogenic effect was observed in studies of 78 weeks in mice at doses more than 150 times the maximum recommended human dose and 102 weeks in rats at doses more than 100 times the maximum recommended human dose. In a variety of test models, Guanfacine was not mutagenic.

No adverse effects were observed in fertility studies in male and female rats.

Pregnancy Category B: Administration of Guanfacine to rats at 70 times the maximum recommended human dose and to rabbits at 20 times the maximum recommended human dose resulted in no evidence of harm to the fetus. Higher doses (100 and 200 times the maximum recommended human dose in rabbits and rats respectively) were associated with reduced fetal survival and maternal toxicity. Rat experiments have shown that Guanfacine crosses the placenta.

There are, however, no adequate and well-controlled studies in pregnant women. Because animal reproduction studies are not always predictive of human response, this drug should be used during pregnancy only if clearly needed.

Labor and Delivery: Guanfacine Hydrochloride is not recommended in the treatment of acute hypertension associated with toxemia of pregnancy. There is no information available on the effects of Guanfacine on the course of labor and delivery.

Nursing Mothers: It is not known whether Guanfacine Hydrochloride is excreted in human milk. Because many drugs are excreted in human milk, caution should be exercised when Guanfacine Hydrochloride is administered to a nursing woman. Experiments with rats have shown that Guanfacine is excreted in the milk.

Pediatric Use: Safety and effectiveness in children under 12 years of age have not been demonstrated. Therefore, the use of Guanfacine Hydrochloride in this age group is not recommended.

ADVERSE REACTIONS
Adverse reactions noted with Guanfacine Hydrochloride are similar to those of other drugs of the central α-2 adrenoreceptor agonist class: dry mouth, sedation (somnolence), weakness (asthenia), dizziness, constipation, and impotence. While the reactions are common, most are mild and tend to disappear on continued dosing.

Skin rash with exfoliation has been reported in a few cases; although clear cause and effect relationships to Guanfacine Hydrochloride could not be established, should a rash occur, Guanfacine Hydrochloride should be discontinued and the patient monitored appropriately.

In the dose-response monotherapy study described under *"Clinical Pharmacology"*, the frequency of the most commonly observed adverse reactions showed a dose relationship from 0.5 to 3 mg as follows:

Adverse Reaction	Placebo n = 59	0.5 mg n = 60	1 mg n = 61	2 mg n = 60	3 mg n = 59
Dry Mouth	0%	10%	10%	42%	54%
Somnolence	8%	5%	10%	13%	39%
Asthenia	0%	2%	3%	7%	3%
Dizziness	8%	12%	2%	8%	15%
Headache	8%	13%	7%	5%	3%
Impotence	0%	0%	0%	7%	3%
Constipation	0%	2%	0%	5%	15%
Fatigue	2%	2%	5%	8%	10%

The percent of patients who dropped out because of adverse reactions are shown below for each dosage group.

	Placebo	0.5 mg	1 mg	2 mg	3 mg
Percent dropouts	0%	2.0%	5.0%	13%	32%

The most common reasons for dropouts among patients who received Guanfacine were dry mouth, somnolence, dizziness, fatigue, weakness, and constipation.

In the 12-week, placebo-controlled, dose-response study of Guanfacine administered with 25 mg chlorthalidone at bedtime, the frequency of the most commonly observed adverse reactions showed a clear dose relationship from 0.5 to 3 mg as follows:

Adverse Reaction	Placebo n = 73	0.5 mg n = 72	1 mg n = 72	2 mg n = 72	3 mg n = 72
Dry Mouth	5 (7%)	4 (5%)	6 (8%)	8 (11%)	20 (28%)
Somnolence	1 (1%)	3 (4%)	0 (0%)	1 (1%)	10 (14%)
Asthenia	0 (0%)	2 (3%)	0 (0%)	2 (2%)	7 (10%)
Dizziness	2 (2%)	1 (1%)	3 (4%)	6 (8%)	3 (4%)
Headache	3 (4%)	4 (3%)	3 (4%)	1 (1%)	2 (2%)
Impotence	1 (1%)	1 (0%)	0 (0%)	1 (1%)	3 (4%)
Constipation	0 (0%)	0 (0%)	0 (0%)	1 (1%)	1 (1%)
Fatigue	3 (3%)	2 (3%)	2 (3%)	5 (6%)	3 (4%)

There were 41 premature terminations because of adverse reactions in this study. The percent of patients who dropped out and the dose at which the dropout occurred were as follows:

Dose:	Placebo	0.5 mg	1 mg	2 mg	3 mg
Percent dropouts	6.9%	4.2%	3.2%	6.9%	8.3%

Reasons for dropouts among patients who received Guanfacine were: somnolence, headache, weakness, dry mouth, dizziness, impotence, insomnia, constipation, syncope, urinary incontinence, conjunctivitis, paresthesia, and dermatitis.

In a second 12-week placebo-controlled combination therapy study in which the dose could be adjusted upward to 3 mg per day in 1-mg increments at 3-week intervals, i.e., a setting more similar to ordinary clinical use, the most commonly recorded reactions were: dry mouth, 47%; constipation, 16%; fatigue, 12%; somnolence, 10%; asthenia, 6%; dizziness, 6%; headache, 4%; and insomnia, 4%.

Reasons for dropouts among patients who received Guanfacine were: somnolence, dry mouth, dizziness, impotence, constipation, confusion, depression, and palpitations.

In the clonidine/Guanfacine comparison described in *"Clinical Pharmacology"*, the most common adverse reactions noted were as follows:

Adverse Reactions	Guanfacine (n = 279)	Clonidine (n = 278)
Dry mouth	30%	37%
Somnolence	21%	35%
Dizziness	11%	8%
Constipation	10%	5%
Fatigue	9%	8%
Headache	4%	4%
Insomnia	4%	3%

Adverse reactions occurring in 3% or less of patients in the three controlled trials of Guanfacine Hydrochloride with a diuretic were:

Cardiovascular: bradycardia, palpitations, substernal pain

Gastrointestinal: abdominal pain, diarrhea, dyspepsia, dysphagia, nausea

CNS: amnesia, confusion, depression, insomnia, libido decrease

ENT disorders: rhinitis, taste perversion, tinnitus

Eye disorders: conjunctivitis, iritis, vision disturbance

Musculoskeletal: leg cramps, hypokinesia

Respiratory: dyspnea

Dermatologic: dermatitis, pruritus, purpura, sweating

Urogenital: testicular disorder, urinary incontinence

Other: malaise, paresthesia, paresis

Adverse reaction reports tend to decrease over time. In an open-label trial of one year's duration, 580 hypertensive subjects were given Guanfacine, titrated to achieve goal blood pressure, alone (51%), with diuretic (38%), with beta blocker (3%), with diuretic plus beta blocker (6%), or with diuretic plus vasodilator (2%). The mean daily dose of Guanfacine reached was 4.7 mg.

Adverse Reaction	Incidence of adverse reactions at any time during the study	Incidence of adverse reactions at the end of one year
	n = 580	n = 580
Dry mouth	60%	15%
Drowsiness	33%	6%
Dizziness	15%	1%
Constipation	14%	3%
Weakness	5%	1%
Headache	4%	0.2%
Insomnia	5%	0%

There were 52 (8.9%) dropouts due to adverse effects in this 1-year trial. The cause were: dry mouth (n = 20), weakness (n = 12), constipation (n = 7), somnolence (n = 3), nausea (n = 3), orthostatic hypotension (n = 2), insomnia (n = 1), rash (n = 1), nightmares (n = 1), headache (n = 1), and depression (n = 1).

Postmarketing Experience: An open-label postmarketing study involving 21,718 patients was conducted to assess the safety of Guanfacine Hydrochloride 1 mg/day given at bedtime for 28 days. Guanfacine Hydrochloride was administered with or without other antihypertensive agents. Adverse events reported in the postmarketing study at an incidence greater than 1% included dry mouth, dizziness, somnolence, fatigue, headache and nausea. The most commonly reported adverse events in this study were the same as those observed in controlled clinical trials.

Less frequent, possibly Guanfacine Hydrochloride related events observed in the postmarketing study and/or reported spontaneously include:

Body as a Whole: asthenia, chest pain, edema, malaise, tremor

Cardiovascular: bradycardia, palpitations, syncope, tachycardia

Central Nervous System: paresthesias, vertigo

Eye Disorders: blurred vision

Gastrointestinal System: abdominal pain, constipation, diarrhea, dyspepsia

Liver and Biliary System: abnormal liver function tests

Musculo-Skeletal System: arthralgia, leg cramps, leg pain, myalgia

Psychiatric: agitation, anxiety, confusion, depression, insomnia, nervousness

Reproductive System, Male: impotence

Respiratory System: dyspnea

Skin and Appendages: alopecia, dermatitis, exfoliative dermatitis, pruritus, rash

Special Senses: alterations in taste

Urinary System: nocturia, urinary frequency

Rare, serious disorders with no definitive cause and effect relationship to Guanfacine Hydrochloride have been reported spontaneously and/or in the postmarketing study. These events include acute renal failure, cardiac fibrillation, cerebrovascular accident, congestive heart failure, heart block, and myocardial infarction.

Drug Abuse and Dependence: No reported abuse or dependence has been associated with the administration of Guanfacine Hydrochloride.

OVERDOSAGE

Signs and Symptoms: Drowsiness, lethargy, bradycardia and hypotension have been observed following overdose with Guanfacine.

A 25-year-old female intentionally ingested 60 mg. She presented with severe drowsiness and bradycardia of 45 beats/minute. Gastric lavage was performed and an infusion of isoproterenol (0.8 mg in 12 hours) was administered. She recovered quickly and without sequelae.

A 28-year-old female who ingested 30-40 mg developed only lethargy, was treated with activated charcoal and a cathartic, was monitored for 24 hours, and was discharged in good health.

A 2-year-old male weighing 12 kg, who ingested up to 4 mg of Guanfacine, developed lethargy. Gastric lavage (followed by activated charcoal and sorbitol slurry via NG tube) removed some tablet fragments within 2 hours after ingestion, and vital signs were normal. During 24-hour observation in ICU, systolic pressure was 58 and heart rate 70 at 16 hours post-ingestion. No intervention was required, and the child was discharged fully recovered the next day.

Treatment of Overdosage: Gastric lavage and supportive therapy as appropriate. Guanfacine is not dialyzable in clinically significant amounts (2.4%).

DOSAGE AND ADMINISTRATION

The recommended initial dose of Guanfacine Hydrochloride when given alone or in combination with another antihypertensive drug is 1 mg daily given at bedtime to minimize somnolence.

If after 3 to 4 weeks of therapy, 1 mg does not give a satisfactory result, a dose of 2 mg may be given, although most of the effect of Guanfacine Hydrochloride is seen at 1 mg (see *"Clinical Pharmacology"*). Higher daily doses have been used, but adverse reactions increase significantly with doses above 3 mg/day.

The frequency of rebound hypertension is low, but it can occur. When rebound occurs, it does so after 2-4 days, which is delayed compared with clonidine hydrochloride. This is consistent with the longer half-life of Guanfacine. In most cases, after abrupt withdrawal of Guanfacine, blood pressure returns to pretreatment levels slowly (within 2-4 days) without ill effects.

Store at controlled room temperature, between 15°C and 30°C (59°F and 86°F). Dispense in tight, light-resistant container.

HOW SUPPLIED

TABLETS: 1 MG

BRAND/MANUFACTURER	NDC	SIZE	AWP
○ BRAND			
▶ TENEX: Robins Pharm	00031-8901-63	100s	$78.04
	00031-8901-64	100s ud	$84.13
	00031-8901-70	500s	$370.41

TABLETS: 2 MG

BRAND/MANUFACTURER	NDC	SIZE	AWP
○ BRAND			
▶ TENEX: Robins Pharm	00031-8903-63	100s	$107.00

Guanidine HCl *SEE* GUANIDINE HYDROCHLORIDE

Guanidine Hydrochloride

DESCRIPTION

Chemically, Guanidine (amino-methanamidide) Hydrochloride is a crystalline powder freely soluble in water and alcohol. The aqueous solution is neutral.

Each tablet contains 125 mg of Guanidine Hydrochloride.

Following is its chemical structure:

$$HN = C \underset{NH_2}{\overset{NH_2}{\diagup}} \cdot HCl$$

CLINICAL PHARMACOLOGY

Guanidine apparently acts by enhancing the release of acetylcholine following a nerve impulse. It also appears to slow the rates of depolarization and repolarization of muscle cell membranes.

INDICATIONS AND USAGE

Guanidine is indicated for the reduction of the symptoms of muscle weakness and easy fatigability associated with the myasthenic syndrome of Eaton-Lambert. It is not indicated for treating myasthenia gravis. The Eaton-Lambert syndrome is ordinarily differentiated from myasthenia gravis by the usual association of the syndrome with small cell carcinoma of the lung, but myography may be necessary to make the diagnosis.

CONTRAINDICATIONS

Guanidine is contraindicated in individuals with a history of intolerance or allergy to this drug.

WARNINGS

Fatal bone-marrow suppression, apparently dose related, can occur with Guanidine.

State use of Guanidine Hydrochloride in pregnancy has not been established. Therefore, the benefits of therapy must be weighed against the potential hazards. Because Guanidine is excreted in milk, patients on this drug should discontinue breast feeding.

Since there is inadequate experience in children who have received this drug, safety and efficacy in children have not been established.

PRECAUTIONS

Baseline blood studies should be followed by frequent red and white blood cell and differential counts. The drug should be discontinued upon appearance of bone-marrow suppression. Concurrent therapy with other drugs that may cause bone-marrow suppression should be avoided.

Renal function may be affected in some patients receiving Guanidine. Patients should therefore have regular urine examinations and serum creatinine determinations while taking this drug.

Physicians should be given adequate precautions pertaining to the gastrointestinal side effects and the possibility of induced behavior disorders.

Treatment should not be continued longer than necessary.

ADVERSE REACTIONS
Anemia, leukopenia, and thrombocytopenia resulting from bone-marrow depression attributable to Guanidine have been reported. Other adverse reactions that have been observed are:

General: sore throat, rash, fever.

Neurologic: paresthesia of lips, face, hands, feet; cold sensations in hands and feet; nervousness, light-headedness, jitteriness, increased irritability; tremor, trembling sensation; ataxia; emotional liability; psychotic state; confusion; mood changes and hallucinations.

Gastrointestinal: dry mouth; gastric irritation; anorexia; nausea; diarrhea; abdominal cramping. Gastrointestinal side effects may preclude the use of Guanidine as a desired form of therapy.

Dermatologic: rash, flushing or pink complexion; folliculitis; petechiae, purpura, ecchymoses: sweating; skin eruptions; dryness and scaling of the skin.

Renal: elevation of blood creatinine; uremia; chronic interstitial nephritis, acute interstitial nephritis, and renal tubular necrosis.

Hepatic: abnormal liver function tests.

Cardiac: palpitation, tachycardia, atrial fibrillation, hypotension.

OVERDOSAGE
Mild gastrointestinal disorders such as anorexia, increased peristalsis, or diarrhea are early warnings that tolerance is being exceeded. These symptoms may be relieved by atropine, but nevertheless note should be taken of these symptoms and dosage reductions considered. Slight numbness or tingling of the lips and fingertips shortly after taking a dose of Guanidine has been reported. This per se is not an indication to discontinue treatment and/or reduce dosage.

Severe Guanidine intoxication is characterized by nervous hyperirritability, fibrillary tremors and convulsive contractions of muscle, salivation, vomiting, diarrhea, hypoglycemia, and circulatory disturbances. Administration of intravenous calcium gluconate may control the neuromuscular and convulsive symptoms and provide some relief of other toxic manifestations.

Atropine is more effective than calcium in relieving the G.I. symptoms, circulatory disturbances, and changes in blood sugar.

DOSAGE AND ADMINISTRATION
Initial dosage is usually between 10 and 15 mg/kg (5 to 7 mg/pound) of body weight per day in 3 or 4 divided doses. This dosage may be gradually increased to a total daily dosage of 35 mg/kg (16 mg pound) of body weight per day or up to the development of side effects. As individual tolerance is highly variable, the dosage must be carefully titrated. Once a tolerable dose has been established it should be continued. Occasionally, removal of the primary neoplastic lesion may result in improvement of symptoms, permitting the discontinuance of Guanidine.

Store between 15° and 30°C (59° and 86°F).

HOW SUPPLIED
TABLETS: 125 MG

BRAND/MANUFACTURER	NDC	SIZE	AWP
○ BRAND GUANIDINE HCL: Key	00085-0492-01	100s	$18.34

Habitrol *SEE* NICOTINE

Haemophilus b Conjugate Vaccine

DESCRIPTION
Haemophilus b Conjugate Vaccine (Meningococcal Protein Conjugate), is a highly purified capsular polysaccharide (polyribosylribitol phosphate or PRP) of *Haemophilus influenzae* type b (Haemophilus b, Ross strain) that is covalently bound to an outer membrane protein complex (OMPC) of the B11 strain of *Neisseria meningitidis* sero-group B. The covalent bonding of the PRP to the OMPC which is necessary for enhanced immunogenicity of the PRP is confirmed by analysis of the conjugate's components by chemical treatment which yields a unique amino acid. This PRP-OMPC conjugate vaccine is a lyophilized preparation containing lactose as a stabilizer.

Haemophilus b Conjugate Vaccine, when reconstituted as directed, is a sterile suspension for intramuscular use formulated to contain: 15 mcg of Haemophilus b PRP, 250 mcg of *Neisseria meningitidis* OMPC.

Haemophilus b Conjugate Vaccine (Tetanus Toxoid Conjugate) is a sterile, lyophilized powder which is reconstituted at the time of use with saline diluent (0.4%) sodium chloride) or diphtheria and tetanus toxoids and pertussis vaccine adsorbed (DTP) for intramuscular use only. The vaccine consists of the

Haemophilus b polysaccharide, a high molecular weight polymer prepared from the *Haemophilus influenzae* type b strain 1482 grown in a semi-synthetic medium, covalently bound to tetanus toxoid.[1] The tetanus toxoid is prepared by extraction, ammonium sulfate purification, and formalin inactivation of the toxin from cultures of *Clostridium tetani* (Harvard strain) grown in a modified Mueller and Miller medium.[2] The toxoid is filter sterilized prior to the conjugation process. Each single dose of 0.5 ml is formulated to contain 10 µg of purified capsular polysaccharide conjugated to 24 µg of inactivated tetanus toxoid, and 8.5% of sucrose when reconstituted with saline diluent. At the time Haemophilus b Conjugate Vaccine is reconstituted with DTP vaccine, each single dose of 0.5 ml is formulated to contain 10 µg of purified capsular polysaccharide conjugated to 24 µg of inactivated tetanus toxoid, 8.5% of sucrose, 6.7 Lf of diphtheria toxoid, 5 Lf of tetanus toxoid and an estimate of 4 protective units of pertussis vaccine.

The reconstituted vaccine, using saline diluent, appears clear and colorless. The reconstituted vaccine, using DTP vaccine, appears whitish in color.

CLINICAL PHARMACOLOGY
Haemophilus influenzae type b (Haemophilus b) is the most frequent cause of bacterial meningitis and a leading cause of serious, systemic bacterial disease in young children worldwide.

Haemophilus b disease occurs primarily in children under 5 years of age and in the United States prior to the initiation of a vaccine program was estimated to account for nearly 20,000 cases of invasive infections annually, approximately 12,000 of which are meningitis. Based on its active surveillance areas, the Centers for Disease Control and Prevention (CDC) now estimate that *H influenzae* type b disease in children under the age of 5 years has been reduced by 95%.[8] Before effective vaccines were introduced, it was estimated that one in 200 children developed invasive *H influenzae* type b disease by the age of 5 years. In children less than 5 years of age, the mortality rate for invasive *H influenzae* type b disease ranged between 3% and 6%.[8] The mortality rate from Haemophilus b meningitis is about 5%. In addition, up to 35% of survivors develop neurologic sequelae including seizures, deafness, and mental retardation.[3] Other invasive diseases caused by this bacterium include cellulitis, epiglottis, sepsis, pneumonia, septic arthritis, osteomyelitis and pericarditis.

It has been estimated that 17% of all cases of Haemophilus b disease occur in infants less than 6 months of age. The peak incidence of Haemophilus b meningitis occurs between 6 to 11 months of age. Forty-seven percent of all cases occur by one year of age with the remaining 53% of cases occurring over the next four years.

Among children under 5 years of age, the risk of invasive Haemophilus b disease is further increased in certain populations including the following:

- Daycare attendees[7,8,9,10]
- Lower socio-economic groups
- Blacks (especially those who lack the Km(1) immunoglobulin allotype)
- Caucasians who lack the G2m(n or 23) immunoglobulin allotype
- Native Americans
- Household contacts of cases.[11] Adults can be colonized with *H influenzae* type b from children infected with the organism.[12]
- Individuals with asplenia, sickle cell disease, Hodgkin's disease or antibody deficiency syndromes[5,6]

An important virulence factor of the Haemophilus b bacterium is its polysaccharide capsule (PRP). Ninety-five percent of the cases of invasive *H influenzae* disease among children < 5 years of age were caused by organisms with the type b polysaccharide capsule. Approximately two-thirds of all cases of invasive *H influenzae* type b disease affected infants and children < 15 months of age, a group for which a vaccine was not available until late 1990.[4,5] Antibody to PRP (anti-PRP) has been shown to correlate with protection against Haemophilus b disease. While the anti-PRP level associated with protection using conjugated vaccines has not yet been determined, the level of anti-PRP associated with protection in studies using bacterial polysaccharide immune globulin or nonconjugated PRP vaccines ranged from ≥0.15 to ≥1.0 mcg/mL.

Nonconjugated PRP vaccines are capable of stimulating B-lymphocytes to produce antibody without the help of T-lymphocytes (T-independent). The responses to many other antigens are augmented by helper T-lymphocytes (T-dependent). Haemophilus b Conjugate Vaccine is a PRP-conjugate vaccine in which the PRP is covalently bound to the OMPC carrier producing an antigen which is postulated to convert the T-independent antigen (PRP alone) into a T-dependent antigen resulting in both an enhanced antibody response and immunologic memory.

The predominant isotype of anticapsular polysaccharide (PRP) antibody induced by Haemophilus b Conjugate Vaccine is IgG.[13] A substantial booster response has been demonstrated in children 12 months of age or older who previously received two or three doses. Bactericidal activity against *H influenzae* type b is demonstrated in serum after immunization and statistically correlates with the anti-PRP antibody response induced by Haemophilus b Conjugate Vaccine[14].

Antibody to *H influenzae* capsular polysaccharide (anti-PRP) titers of > 1.0 µg/ml following vaccination with unconjugated PRP vaccine correlated with long-term protection against invasive *H influenzae* type b disease in children older than 24 months of age.[15] Although the relevance of this threshold to clinical protection after immunization with conjugate vaccines is not known, particularly in light of the induced, immunologic memory, this level continues to be considered as indicative of long-term protection.[4] The immunogenicity and safety of Haemophilus b Conjugate Vaccine has been demonstrated in the United States and worldwide. Haemophilus b Conjugate Vaccine induced, on average anti-PRP levels $\geq$ 1.0 µg/mL in 90% of infants after the primary series and in more than 98% of infants after a booster dose.[14]

CLINICAL EVALUATION OF HAEMOPHILUS B CONJUGATE VACCINE

The protective efficacy, safety, and antibody responses to Haemophilus b Conjugate Vaccine were evaluated in 3,486 Native American (Navajo) infants who completed the primary two-dose regimen in a randomized, double-blind, placebo-controlled study (The Protective Efficacy Study). This population has a much higher incidence of Haemophilus b disease than the United States population as a whole and also has a lower antibody response to Haemophilus b Conjugate Vaccines.

Each infant in this study received two doses of either placebo or Haemophilus b Conjugate Vaccine with the first dose administered at a mean of 8 weeks of age and the second administered approximately two months later; DTP and OPV were administered concomitantly. Antibody levels were measured in a subset of each group (Table 1). (See related table).

In this study, 22 cases of invasive Haemophilus b disease occurred in the placebo group (8 cases after the first dose and 14 cases after the second dose) and only 1 case in the vaccine group (none after the first dose and 1 after the second dose). Following the recommended two-dose regimen, the protective efficacy of Haemophilus b Conjugate Vaccine was calculated to be 93% with a 95% confidence interval of 57%-98% (p = 0.001, two-tailed). In the two months between the first and second doses, the difference in number of cases of disease between placebo and vaccine recipients (8 vs 0 cases, respectively) was statistically significant (p = 0.008, two-tailed); however, a primary two-dose regimen is required for infants 2-14 months of age. A subset of 1,368 infants from this study was followed to 15 months of age with no additional cases of invasive Haemophilus b disease occurring after the primary two-dose regimen of Haemophilus b Conjugate Vaccine (see "Dosage and Administration", including "Booster Dose").

Following three doses of Haemophilus b Conjugate Vaccine at six weeks, four and six months of age, 75% of Native Americans in Alaska showed an anti-PRP antibody titer of $\geq$ 1.0 µg/mL.

Since protective efficacy with Haemophilus b Conjugate Vaccine was demonstrated in such a high risk population, it would be expected to be predictive of efficacy in other populations.

The safety and immunogenicity of Haemophilus b Conjugate Vaccine were evaluated in infants and children in other clinical studies that were conducted in various locations throughout the United States. Haemophilus b Conjugate Vaccine was highly immunogenic in all age groups studied.

Antibody responses from these clinical studies (excluding Native Americans) are shown in Table 2. These data were derived by evaluating the sera in one laboratory using a radioimmunoassay which correlated with both the Finnish National Public Health Institute assay and that recommended by the Center for Biologics Evaluation and Research of the FDA (Table 1, Table 2).

Since the magnitude of initial antibody response is lower among younger infants, a booster dose is required in infants who complete the primary two-dose regimen before 12 months of age (see Table 1 and "Dosage and Administration").

Table 2

ANTIBODY RESPONSES* TO HAEMOPHILUS B CONJUGATE VACCINE IN OTHER CLINICAL STUDIES

Age Months	Time	No. of Subjects	% Subjects Responding with >0.15 mcg/mL	% Subjects Responding with >1.0 mcg/mL	Post-Vaccination Anti-PRP GMT (mcg/mL)
2-3	Dose 1**	113	97	81	2.48
	Dose 2***	113	98	88	4.60
4-14	Dose 1**	252	98	75	2.53
	Dose 2***	252	100	92	6.04
15-17	Single Dose***	59	100	83	3.11

Table 1

ANTIBODY RESPONSES IN NAVAJO INFANTS

Vaccine	No. of Subjects	Time	% Subjects with >0.15 mcg/mL	% Subjects with >1.0 mcg/mL	Anti-PRP GMT (mcg/mL)
Haemophilus b Conjugate Vaccine*	416†	Pre-Vaccination	44	10	0.16
	416	Dose 1	88	52	0.95
	416	Dose 2	91	60	1.43
Placebo*	461†	Pre-Vaccination	44	9	0.16
	461	Dose 1	21	2	0.09
	461	Dose 2	14	1	0.08
Haemophilus b Conjugate Vaccine	27**	Prebooster	70	33	0.51
	27	Postbooster***	100	89	8.39

* Post vaccination values obtained approximately 1-3 months after each dose.
† The Protective Efficacy Study.
** Immunogenicity Trial.
*** Booster given at 12 months of age; post vaccination values obtained 1 month after administration of booster dose.

Age Months	Time	No. of Subjects	% Subjects Responding with >0.15 mcg/mL	% Subjects Responding with >1.0 mcg/mL	Post-Vaccination Anti-PRP GMT (mcg/mL)
18-23	Single	59	98	97	7.43
24-71	Dose***	52	98	92	10.55

* Only subjects with prevaccination anti-PRP ≤0.15 mcg/mL are included in this table (excluding native Americans).
** Two months post vaccination.
*** One month post vaccination.

Antibodies to the OMPC of *N. meningitidis* (see "Description") have been demonstrated in vaccinee sera but the clinical relevance of these antibodies has not been established. In a multicenter study of immunogenicity and safety in different subpopulations in the United States, antibody responses to Haemophilus b Conjugate Vaccine were evaluated in infants initially vaccinated between the ages of 2 and 3 months (Table 3).

Table 3

ANTIBODY RESPONSES* AFTER TWO DOSES OF HAEMOPHILUS B CONJUGATE VACCINE AMONG INFANTS INITIALLY VACCINATED AT 2-3 MONTHS OF AGE BY RACIAL/ETHNIC GROUP

Racial/Ethnic Groups	No. of Subjects	% With Anti-PRP >0.15 mcg/mL	% With Anti-PRP >1.0 mcg/mL	GMT (mcg/mL)
Native American†	44	95	68	2.24
Caucasian	155	99	85	4.00
Hispanic	16	100	94	4.60
Black	18	100	94	8.57

† Apache and Navajo
* One month after the second dose

Two clinical trials supported by the National Institutes of Health (NIH) have compared the anti-PRP antibody responses to three Haemophilus b conjugate vaccines in a racially mixed population of children. These studies were done in Tennessee[16] (Table 4) and in Minnesota, Missouri and Texas[17] (Table 5) in infants immunized with Haemophilus b conjugate vaccines at 2, 4 and 6 months of age. All Haemophilus b conjugate vaccines were administered concomitantly with Poliovirus Vaccine Live Oral and DTP vaccines at separate sites.

Table 4[18]

ANTI-PRP ANTIBODY RESPONSES IN 2-MONTH-OLD INFANTS NIH TRIAL IN TENNESSEE

VACCINE	N*	GEOMETRIC MEAN TITER (GMT) (µg/mL) Pre-Immunization	Post Second Immunization	Post Third Immunization	Post Third§ Immunization % ≥ 1.0 µg/mL
PRP-T†	65	0.10	0.30	3.64	83%
PRP-OMP	64	0.11	0.84	N/A	50%**
HbOC‡	61	0.07	0.13	3.08	75%

Table 5[17]c, 186
ANTI-PRP ANTIBODY RESPONSES IN 2-MONTH-OLD INFANTS NIH TRIAL IN MINNESOTA, MISSOURI AND TEXAS

		GEOMETRIC MEAN TITER (GMT) ($\mu g/mL$)			
VACCINE	N*	Pre-Immunization	Post Second Immunization	Post Third Immunization	Post Third§ Immunization % ≥ 1.0 $\mu g/mL$
PRP-T†	142	0.25	1.25	6.37	97%
PRP-OMP	149	0.18	4.00	N/A	85%**
HbOC‡	167	0.17	0.45	6.31	90%

* N = Number of Children

§ Sera were obtained after the third dose from 86 and 110 infants, in PRP-T and HbOC vaccine groups, respectively.

† Haemophilus b Conjugate Vaccine (Tetanus Toxoid Conjugate)
Haemophilus b Conjugate Vaccine (Meningococcal Protein Conjugate)

** Seroconversion after the recommended 2-dose primary immunization series is shown.

‡ Haemophilus b Conjugate Vaccine (Diphtheria CRM₁₉₇ Protein Conjugate)
N/A Not applicable in this comparison trial although third dose data have been published.[16,17]

In three U.S. trials in 12- to 15-month-old children and one trial in 17- to 24-month-old children who had not previously received Haemophilus b conjugate vaccination, a single dose of Haemophilus b Conjugate Vaccine produced an anti-PRP antibody response comparable to those seen after three doses were administered in infants (Table 6).

Table 6
ANTI-PRP ANTIBODY RESPONSES IN 12- TO 24-MONTH-OLD CHILDREN IMMUNIZED WITH A SINGLE DOSE OF HAEMOPHILUS b CONJUGATE VACCINE

AGE GROUP	N	GMT ($\mu g/mL$)		% SUBJECTS WITH ≥ 1.0 $\mu g/mL$	
		Pre	Post	Pre	Post
12 to 15 months	256	0.06	5.12	1.6	90.2
17 to 24 months	81	0.10	4.4	3.7	81.5

These trials demonstrated that Haemophilus b Conjugate Vaccine consistently conferred an anti-PRP antibody response previously shown to correlate with protection, when administered either as a regimen of three doses at least four to eight weeks apart in infants 2 to 6 months of age or as a single dose in children 12 months of age and older.

Haemophilus b Conjugate Vaccine has been found to be immunogenic in children with sickle cell anemia, a condition which may cause increased susceptibility to Haemophilus b disease. Two doses of Haemophilus b Conjugate Vaccine given at two-month intervals induced anti-PRP antibody titers of ≥ 1.0 $\mu g/mL$ in 89% of these children with a mean age of 11 months. This is comparable to anti-PRP antibody levels demonstrated in normal children of similar age following two doses of Haemophilus b Conjugate Vaccine.[18]

Comparative clinical trials demonstrated that a similar anti-PRP response was achieved in infants as young as 2 months old when one dose of whole-cell DTP vaccine was used to reconstitute one dose of lyophilized Haemophilus b Conjugate Vaccine (Table 7).[14]

Table 7
ANTI-PRP ANTIBODY RESPONSES IN 2-MONTH-OLD INFANTS FOLLOWING IMMUNIZATION WITH HAEMOPHILUS b CONJUGATE VACCINE RECONSTITUTED WITH DTP

		Geometric Mean Titer (GMT) ($\mu g/mL$)			
Study Site	N*	Pre-Immunization	Post Second Immunization	Post Third Immunization	Post Third Immunization % ≥ 1.0 $\mu g/mL$
U.S.	45	0.13	0.55	4.49	91
U.S.	135	0.12	0.43	4.46	85
Chile	94	0.09	4.31	6.94	96

* N = Number of Children

Haemophilus b Conjugate Vaccine induced antibody levels greater than 1.0 mcg/mL in children who were poor responders to nonconjugated PRP vaccines. In a study involving such a subpopulation, 34 children ranging in age from 27 to 61 months who developed invasive Haemophilus b disease despite previous vaccination with nonconjugated PRP vaccines were randomly assigned to 2 groups. One group (n = 14) was immunized with Haemophilus b Conjugate Vaccine and the other group (n = 20) with a nonconjugated PRP vaccine at a mean interval of approximately 12 months after recovery from disease. All 14 children immunized with Haemophilus b Conjugate Vaccine, but only 6 to 20 children re-immunized with a nonconjugated PRP vaccine, achieved an antibody level of > 1.0 mcg/mL. The 14 children who had not responded to revaccination with the nonconjugated PRP vaccine were then immunized with a single dose of Haemophilus b Conjugate Vaccine; following this vaccination, all achieved antibody levels of > 1.0 mcg/mL.

In addition, Haemophilus b Conjugate Vaccine has been studied in children at high risk of Haemophilus b disease because of genetically-related deficiencies [Blacks who were Km(1) allotype negative and Caucasians who were G2m(23) allotype negative] and are considered hyporesponsive to nonconjugated PRP vaccines on this basis. The hyporesponsive children had anti-PRP responses comparable to those of allotype positive children of similar age range when vaccinated with Haemophilus b Conjugate Vaccine. All children achieved anti-PRP levels of > 1.0 mcg/mL.

INDICATIONS AND USAGE
Haemophilus b Conjugate Vaccine is indicated for routine immunization against invasive disease caused by *Haemophilus influenzae* type b in infants and children 2 to 71 months of age and/or diphtheria, tetanus, and pertussis for vaccine reconstituted with DTP vaccine.

Haemophilus b Conjugate Vaccine will not protect against disease caused by *Haemophilus influenzae* other than type b or against other microorganisms that cause invasive disease such as meningitis or sepsis.

REVACCINATION
Infants completing the primary two-dose regimen before 12 months of age should receive a booster dose (see *"Dosage and Administration"*).

USE WITH OTHER VACCINES
Studies have been conducted in which Haemophilus b Conjugate Vaccine has been administered concomitantly with the primary vaccination series of DTP and OPV, or concomitantly with M-M-R II (Measles, Mumps, and Rubella Virus Vaccine Live, MSD) (using separate sites and syringes) or with a booster dose of OPV plus DTP (using separate sites and syringes for Haemophilus b Vaccine and DTP). No impairment of immune response to individual tested vaccine antigens was demonstrated. The type, frequency and severity of adverse experiences observed in these studies with Haemophilus b Conjugate Vaccine were similar to those seen when the other vaccines were given alone.

A single injection containing diphtheria, tetanus, pertussis and Haemophilus b Conjugate antigens may be more acceptable to parents and may increase compliance with vaccination programs. Therefore, in those situations where, in the judgment of the physician, it is of benefit to administer a single injection of whole-cell DTP and Haemophilus b Conjugate vaccines *only whole-cell DTP vaccine may be used for reconstitution of lyophilized Haemophilus b Conjugate Vaccine.*

Haemophilus b Conjugate Vaccine is not recommended for use in infants younger than 2 months of age.

CONTRAINDICATIONS
Hypersensitivity to any component of the vaccine or the diluent.

WARNINGS
USE ONLY THE ALUMINUM HYDROXIDE DILUENT SUPPLIED.

If Haemophilus b Conjugate Vaccine is used in persons with malignancies or those receiving immunosuppressive therapy or who are otherwise immunocompromised, the expected immune response may not be obtained. This includes patients with asymptomatic or symptomatic HIV-infection,[19] severe combined immunodeficiency, hypogammaglobulinemia, or agammaglobulinemia; altered immune states due to diseases such as leukemia, lymphoma, or generalized malignancy; or an immune system compromised by treatment with corticosteroids, alkylating drugs, antimetabolites or radiation.[20]

PRECAUTIONS
GENERAL

As for any vaccine, adequate treatment provisions, including epinephrine, should be available for immediate use should an anaphylactoid reaction occur.

Prior to an injection of any vaccine, all known precautions should be taken to prevent adverse reactions. This includes a review of the patient's history with respect to possible sensitivity and any previous adverse reactions to the vaccine or similar vaccines, previous immunization history, current health status (see *"Contraindications"; "Warnings"* sections), and a current knowledge of the literature concerning the use of the vaccine under consideration.

The health-care provider should ask the parent or guardian about the recent health status of the infant or child to be immunized including the infant's or child's previous immunization history prior to administration of Haemophilus b Conjugate Vaccine.

As with other vaccines, Haemophilus b Conjugate Vaccine may not induce protective antibody levels immediately following vaccination or even earlier than two weeks following their last recommended dose.

As with any vaccine, vaccination with Haemophilus b Conjugate Vaccine may not result in a protective antibody response in all individuals given the vaccine.

As reported with Haemophilus b Polysaccharide Vaccine and another Haemophilus b Conjugate Vaccine, cases of Haemophilus b disease may occur in the week after vaccination, prior to the onset of the protective effects of the vaccines.

There is insufficient evidence that Haemophilus b Conjugate Vaccine given immediately after exposure to natural *Haemophilus influenzae* type b will prevent illness.

Any acute infection or febrile illness is reason for delaying use of Haemophilus b Conjugate Vaccine except when in the opinion of the physician, withholding the vaccine entails a greater risk. Minor illnesses such as upper respiratory infection with or without low-grade fever are not contraindications for use of Haemophilus b Conjugate Vaccine.[21]

Antigenuria has been detected in some instances following receipt of Haemophilus b Conjugate Vaccine; therefore, urine antigen detection may not have definitive diagnostic value in suspected *H influenzae* type b disease within one week of immunization.[23]

Special care should be taken to ensure that Haemophilus b Conjugate Vaccine is not injected into a blood vessel.

Administration of Haemophilus b Conjugate Vaccine is not contraindicated in individuals with HIV infection.[20]

A separate, sterile syringe and needle or a sterile disposable unit should be used for each patient to prevent transmission of hepatitis or other infectious agents from person to person. Needles should not be recapped and should be properly disposed.

INFORMATION FOR PATIENT
The health-care provider should inform the parent or guardian of the benefits and risks of the vaccine.

Prior to administration of Haemophilus b Conjugate Vaccine, the parent or guardian should be asked about the recent health status of the infant or child to be immunized.

The physician should inform the parent or guardian about the significant adverse reactions that have been temporally associated with Haemophilus b Conjugate Vaccine reconstituted with CLI DTP vaccine administration. The parent or guardian should be instructed to report any serious adverse reactions to their health-care provider.

As part of the child's immunization record, the date, lot number and manufacturer of the vaccine administered should be recorded.[24,25,26]

The U.S. Department of Health and Human Services has established a new Vaccine Adverse Event Reporting System (VAERS) to accept all reports of suspected adverse events after the administration of any vaccine, including but not limited to the reporting of events required by the National Childhood Vaccine Injury Act of 1986.[24] The toll-free number for VAERS forms and information is 1-800-822-7967.

The National Vaccine Injury Compensation Program, established by the National Childhood Vaccine Injury Act of 1986, requires physicians and other health-care providers who administer vaccines to maintain permanent vaccination records and to report occurrences of certain adverse events to the U.S. Department of Health and Human Services. Reportable events include those listed in the Act for each vaccine and events specified in the package insert as contraindications to further doses of the vaccine.[25,26]

The health-care provider should inform the parent or guardian of the importance of completing the immunization series. The health-care provider should provide the Vaccine Information Materials (VIMs) which are required to be given with each immunization.

DRUG INTERACTIONS
When DTP vaccine is used to reconstitute Haemophilus b Conjugate Vaccine and administered to immunosuppressed persons or persons receiving immunosuppressive therapy, the expected antibody response may not be obtained.

Immunosuppressive therapies, including irradiation, antimetabolites, alkylating agents, cytotoxic drugs, and corticosteroids (used in greater than physiologic doses), may reduce the immune response to vaccines. Short-term (< 2 weeks) corticosteroid therapy or intra-articular, bursal, or tendon injections with corticosteroids should not be immunosuppressive. Although no specific studies with pertussis vaccine are available, if immunosuppressive therapy will be discontinued shortly, it is reasonable to defer vaccination until the patient has been off therapy for one month; otherwise, the patient should be vaccinated while still on therapy.[21]

If Haemophilus b Conjugate Vaccine reconstituted with DTP has been administered to persons receiving immunosuppressive therapy, a recent injection of immunoglobulin or having an immunodeficiency disorder, an adequate immunologic response may not be obtained.

As with other intramuscular injections, use with caution in patients on anticoagulant therapy.

In clinical trials, Haemophilus b Conjugate Vaccine was routinely administered, at separate sites, concomitantly with one or more of the following vaccines: DTP vaccine, Oral Poliovirus Vaccine (OPV), Measles, Mumps and Rubella vaccine (MMR), Hepatitis B vaccine and occasionally Inactivated Poliovirus Vaccine (IPV). No significant impairment of the antibody response to any antigen of DTP vaccine was observed in the three clinical trials when given either separately with Haemophilus b Conjugate Vaccine or combined with Haemophilus b Conjugate Vaccine in the same syringe. Interference with the antibody response to the pertussis component has been suggested with a DTP vaccine unlicensed in the U.S.[27] No impairment of the antibody response to the individual antigens, diphtheria, tetanus and pertussis, was demonstrated when Haemophilus b Conjugate Vaccine was given at the same time, at separate sites, with Inactivated Poliovirus Vaccine (IPV) or Measles, Mumps and Rubella vaccine (MMR). In addition, more than 47,000 infants in Finland have received a third dose of Haemophilus b Conjugate Vaccine concomitantly with MMR vaccine with no increase in serious or unexpected adverse events.

No data are available concerning the effects on immune response of OPV or Hepatitis B vaccine when given concurrently with Haemophilus b Conjugate Vaccine reconstituted with DTP.

LABORATORY TEST INTERACTIONS
Sensitive tests (e.g., Latex Agglutination Kits) may detect PRP derived from the vaccine in urine of some vaccinees for up to seven days following vaccination with Haemophilus b Conjugate Vaccine; in clinical studies with Haemophilus b Conjugate Vaccine, such children demonstrated normal immune response to the vaccine.

CARCINOGENESIS, MUTAGENESIS, AND IMPAIRMENT OF FERTILITY
Haemophilus b Conjugate Vaccine has not been evaluated for its carcinogenic or mutagenic potential, or its potential to impair fertility.

PREGNANCY
Pregnancy Category C: Animal reproduction studies have not been conducted with Haemophilus b Conjugate Vaccine. It is also not known whether Haemophilus b Conjugate Vaccine can cause fetal harm when administered to a pregnant woman or can affect reproductive capacity. Haemophilus b Conjugate Vaccine is not recommended for use in a pregnant woman.

PEDIATRIC USE
SAFETY AND EFFECTIVENESS OF HAEMOPHILUS B CONJUGATE VACCINE IN INFANTS BELOW THE AGE OF SIX WEEKS HAVE NOT BEEN ESTABLISHED. (See *"Dosage and Administration"* section.) The vaccine is not approved for use in children 5 years of age or older.

ADVERSE REACTIONS
More than 7,000 infants and young children (≤ 2 year of age) have received at least one dose of Haemophilus b Conjugate Vaccine during U.S. clinical trials. Of these, 1,064 subjects 12 to 24 months of age who received Haemophilus b Conjugate Vaccine alone reported no serious or life threatening adverse reactions.

In early clinical studies involving the administration of 8,086 doses of Haemophilus b Conjugate Vaccine alone to 5,027 healthy infants and children 2 months to 71 months of age, Haemophilus b Conjugate Vaccine was generally well tolerated. No serious adverse reactions were reported.

During a two-day period following vaccination with Haemophilus b Conjugate Vaccine in a subset of these infants and children, the most frequently reported adverse reactions, excluding those shown in Table 4, in decreasing order of frequency included irritability, sleepiness, respiratory infection/symptoms and ear infection/otitis media. Urticaria was reported in two children. Thrombocytopenia was seen in one child. A cause and effect relationship between these side effects and the vaccination has not been established.

Selected objective observations reported by parents over a 48-hour period in infants and children 2 to 71 months of age following primary vaccination with Haemophilus b Conjugate Vaccine alone are summarized in Table 8.

In The Protective Efficacy Study (see *"Clinical Pharmacology"*), 4,459 healthy Navajo infants 6 to 12 weeks of age received Haemophilus b Conjugate Vaccine or placebo. Most of these infants received DTP/OPV concomitantly. No differences were seen in the type and frequency of serious health problems expected in this Navajo population or in serious adverse experiences reported among those who received Haemophilus b Conjugate Vaccine and those who received placebo, and none was reported to be related to Haemophilus b Conjugate Vaccine. Only one serious reaction (tracheitis) was reported as possibly related to Haemophilus b Conjugate Vaccine and only one (diarrhea) as possibly related to placebo. Seizures occurred infrequently in both groups (9 occurred in vaccine recipients, 8 of whom also received DTP; 8 occurred in placebo recipients, 7 of whom also received DTP) and were not reported to be related to Haemophilus b Conjugate Vaccine. The frequencies of fever and local reactions occurring in a subset of these infants during a 48-hour period following each dose were similar to those seen in early clinical studies (Table 8). (See related table.)

Summarized in Table 9 are adverse reactions temporally associated with Haemophilus b Conjugate Vaccine immunization in 188 subjects 12 to 15 months of age.

Table 9

PERCENTAGE OF 12- TO 15-MONTH-OLD CHILDREN PRESENTING WITH LOCAL OR SYSTEMIC REACTIONS WITHIN THE FIRST 24 HOURS OF IMMUNIZATION WITH HAEMOPHILUS B CONJUGATE VACCINE (n = 188)

Reactions	Dose 1*	Dose 2*
Local		
Pain	9.0%	6.4%
Erythema (1 to 5 cm)	24.0%	18.6%
Induration	9.6%	9.0%
Systemic		
Fever (> 100.6°F)	7.4%	6.4%
Irritability	30.9%	28.2%
Lethargy	18.6%	17.0%
Anorexia	9.0%	8.5%
Rhinorrhea	24.5%	21.3%
Diarrhea	5.8%	8.5%
Vomiting	4.3%	3.7%
Cough	9.6%	4.3%

* *DTP was not administered concomitantly with Haemophilus b Conjugate Vaccine*

When Haemophilus b Conjugate Vaccine was administered to infants at 2, 4, and 6 months of age concomitantly, at separate sites, with DTP vaccine, the systemic adverse experience profile was not different from that seen when DTP vaccine was administered alone. (See related table).

Adverse reactions from a U.S. multicenter trial in 2-,4- and 6-month-old infants are summarized in Table 10. Systemic adverse reactions listed in Table 10 are more prominent than those in Table 9 because infants also received concomitant immunization with DTP.[14] (See related table).

In general, the rates of minor systemic reactions after Haemophilus b Conjugate Vaccine and DTP immunization were comparable to those usually reported after DTP vaccine alone.[28,29,30,31]

When Haemophilus b Conjugate Vaccine reconstituted with whole-cell DTP was administered in infants at 2, 4, and 6 months of age, the systemic adverse experience profile (Table 11) was comparable to that observed when the two vaccines were given separately (Table 10). An increase in the rate of local reactions was observed in some instances within the 24-hour period after immunizations. (See related table).

In a third U.S. trial where Haemophilus b Conjugated Vaccine was reconstituted with DTP, approximately 1,450 doses were administered to infants starting at 2 months of age. Adverse reactions observed at 6 and 24 hours respectively after the first immunization (n = 498) were tenderness 66.9% and 30.7%; erythema (> 1") 8.6% and 2.2%; induration 38.2% and 21.7%; irritability 77.9% and 35.7%; drowsiness 63.7% and 34.1%; anorexia 26.1% and 12.9%; diarrhea 6.8% and 9.0%; and vomiting 3.4% and 3.8%.[18] One hypotonic/hyporesponsive episode (HHE) was seen in an infant following the second dose in this trial. This is consistent with the HHE incidence rate observed with DTP vaccination alone.[4]

Adverse reactions associated with Haemophilus b Conjugated Vaccine generally subsided after 24 hours and usually do not persist beyond 48 hours after immunization.

In a randomized, double-blind U.S. clinical trial, Haemophilus b Conjugated Vaccine was given concomitantly with DTP to more than 5,000 infants and hepatitis B vaccine was given with DTP to a similar number. In this large study, deaths due to sudden infant death syndrome (SIDS) and other causes were observed but were not different in the two groups. In the first 48 hours following immunization, two definite and three possible seizures were observed after Haemophilus b Conjugated Vaccine and DTP in comparison with none after Haemophilus b Conjugated Vaccine alone.

Table 8
FEVER OR LOCAL REACTIONS IN SUBJECTS 2 TO 71 MONTHS OF AGE VACCINATED WITH HAEMOPHILUS B CONJUGATE VACCINE ALONE OTHER CLINICAL STUDIES

Age (Months)	Reaction	No. of Subjects Evaluated	Dose 1 6 hr	Dose 1 24	Dose 1 48	No. of Subjects Evaluated	Dose 2 6 hr	Dose 2 24	Dose 2 48
			Percentage						
2-14*	Fever > 38.3°C (101°F) Rectal	532	2.4	3.8	1.9	329	3.0	4.3	3.6
	Erythema > 2.5 cm diameter	1026	0.2	1.0	0.4	585	0.9	1.2	0.7
	Swelling/ Induration > 2.5 cm diameter	1026	0.6	1.5	1.6	585	0.9	2.8	3.7
15-71**	Fever > 38.3°C (101°F) Rectal	149	4.0	4.0	6.7				
	Erythema > 2.5 cm diameter	572	0.0	0.3	0.2				
	Swelling/ Induration > 2.5 cm diameter	572	0.9	2.1	1.4				

* Additional complaints reported following vaccination with the first and second dose of Haemophilus b Conjugate Vaccine, respectively, in the indicated number of subjects were: nausea, vomiting and/or diarrhea (101,41), crying for more than one-half hour (43,15), rash (16,17), and unusual high-pitched crying (4, 4).

** Additional complaints reported following vaccination with 1 dose of Haemophilus b Conjugate Vaccine in the indicated number of subjects were: nausea, vomiting and/or diarrhea (44), crying for more than one-half hour (19), rash (12), and unusual high-pitched crying (0).

Table 10[14]
PERCENTAGE OF INFANTS PRESENTING WITH LOCAL OR SYSTEMIC REACTIONS AT 6, 24, AND 48 HOURS OF IMMUNIZATION WITH HAEMOPHILUS B CONJUGATE VACCINE ADMINISTERED SIMULTANEOUSLY, AT SEPARATE SITES, WITH CLI DTP VACCINE

Reaction	2 Months (n=365) 6 Hrs	24 Hrs.	48 Hrs	4 Months (n=364) 6 Hrs.	24 Hrs.	48 Hrs.	6 Months (n=365) 6 Hrs.	24 Hrs.	48 Hrs.
Local§									
Tenderness	46.3%	11.5%	2.2%	23.4%	7.4%	1.1%	19.2%	6.0%	1.1%
Erythema	14.3%	4.1%	0.3%	8.8%	5.8%	0.6%	11.5%	6.9%	1.6%
Induration	22.5%	6.3%	1.9%	12.4%	4.7%	0.8%	9.6%	3.8%	1.1%
Systemic*									
Fever > 100.8°F†	20.1%	1.3%	0.6%	14.6%	6.6%	1.4%	15.7%	8.8%	0.8%
Irritability	72.6%	21.9%	12.6%	48.4%	25.0%	13.2%	44.1%	25.2%	10.1%
Drowsiness	57.5%	29.9%	10.4%	44.2%	18.1%	7.4%	32.6%	13.4%	2.5%
Anorexia	15.3%	5.8%	4.9%	8.0%	5.05%	3.0%	5.5%	4.9%	2.2%
Diarrhea	4.4%	6.6%	5.2%	5.0%	4.7%	4.7%	4.7%	6.3%	3.6%
Vomiting	2.7%	4.1%	2.7%	2.5%	3.3%	2.8%	2.2%	2.7%	1.9%
Persistent Crying	Percentage of infants within 72 hours after immunization was 1.6% after dose one, 0.6% after dose two, and 0.3% after dose three.								

§ Local reactions were evaluated at the Haemophilus b Conjugate Vaccine injection site.
* The adverse reaction profile is defined by the concomitant use of DTP vaccine.
† The number of individuals observed at each time point for fever varied from 357 to 363.

hepatitis B vaccine and DTP.[18] This rate of seizures following Haemophilus b Conjugated Vaccine and DTP was not greater than previously reported in infants receiving DTP alone. Other adverse reactions reported with administration of Haemophilus b Conjugate Vaccines include urticaria, seizures, hives, renal failure, early onset of Haemophilus b disease, and Guillain-Barré syndrome (GBS).[32] A cause and effect relationship among any of these events and the vaccination has not been established. When Haemophilus b Conjugated Vaccine was given with DTP and inactivated poliovirus vaccine to more than 100,000 Finnish infants, the rate and extent of serious adverse reactions was not different from those seen when other Haemophilus b Conjugate Vaccines were evaluated in Finland.

As with any vaccine, there is the possibility that broad use of Haemophilus b Conjugate Vaccine could reveal adverse reactions not observed in clinical trials.

DOSAGE AND ADMINISTRATION
FOR INTRAMUSCULAR ADMINISTRATION
DO NOT INJECT INTRAVENOUSLY
Before injection, the skin over the site to be injected should be cleansed with a suitable germicide. After insertion of the needle, aspirate to ensure that the needle has not entered a blood vessel.

HAEMOPHILUS B CONJUGATE VACCINE (MENINGOCOCCAL PROTEIN CONJUGATE)
2 to 14 Months of Age: Infants 2 to 14 months of age should receive a 0.5 mL dose of vaccine ideally beginning at 2 months of age followed by a 0.5 mL dose 2 months later (or as soon as possible thereafter). When the primary two-dose regimen is completed before 12 months of age, a booster dose is required (*see below and Table 5*).

15 Months of Age and Older: Children 15 months of age and older previously unvaccinated against Haemophilus b disease should receive a single 0.5 mL dose of vaccine.

Booster Dose: In infants completing the primary two-dose regimen before 12 months of age, a booster dose (0.5 mL) should be administered at 12 to 15 months of age but not earlier than 2 months after the second dose.

DATA ARE NOT AVAILABLE REGARDING THE INTERCHANGEABILITY OF HAEMOPHILUS b CONJUGATE VACCINES.

Vaccination regimens by age group are outlined in Table 12.

Table 12
(see circular text above for details)

Age (Months) at First Dose	Primary	Age (Months) at Booster Dose
2-10	2 doses, 2 mo. apart	12-15
11-14	2 doses, 2 mo. apart	—
15-71	1 dose	—

HAEMOPHILUS B CONJUGATE VACCINE (TETANUS TOXOID CONJUGATE)
Each dose of Haemophilus b Conjugate Vaccine is administered intramuscularly in the outer aspect of the vastus lateralis (mid-thigh) or deltoid. The vaccine should not be injected into the gluteal area or areas where there may be a nerve trunk. During the course of primary immunizations, injections should not be made more than once at the same site. When Haemophilus b Conjugate Vaccine is reconstituted with DTP vaccine, the combined vaccines are indicated for infants and children 2 months through 5 years of age for intramuscular administration in accordance with the schedule indicated in Table 13.[14]

Table 13[14]
RECOMMENDED IMMUNIZATION SCHEDULE FOR HAEMOPHILUS b CONJUGATE VACCINE AND DTP FOR PREVIOUSLY UNVACCINATED CHILDREN

Dose	Age	Immunization
First, Second and Third	At 2, 4 and 6 months	Haemophilus b Conjugate Vaccine/ reconstituted with DTP or with saline diluent (0.4% sodium chloride)
Fourth	At 15 to 18 months	Haemophilus b Conjugate Vaccine/ reconstituted with DTP or with saline diluent (0.4% sodium chloride)
Fifth	At 4 to 6 years	DTP or Acellular Pertussis (DTaP)*

* *Acellular Pertussis (DTaP) should NOT be used to reconstitute Haemophilus b Conjugate Vaccine. When administering DTaP for the fourth dose, Haemophilus influenzae type b vaccine also should be administered at this time in a separate syringe at a different site.*

For Previously Unvaccinated Children: Immunization schedules should be considered on an individual basis for children not vaccinated according to the recommended schedule. Three doses of a product containing DTP, given at approximately 2-month intervals, are required followed by a fourth dose of a product containing DTP or DTaP approximately 12 months later and a fifth dose of a product containing DTP or DTaP at 4 to 6 years of age. If the fourth dose of a pertussis-containing vaccine is not given until after the fourth birthday, no further doses of a pertussis-containing vaccine are necessary.

The number of doses of Haemophilus b Conjugate Vaccine indicated depends on the age at which immunization is begun. A child 7 to 11 months of age should receive 2 doses of Haemophilus b Conjugate Vaccine at 8-week intervals and a booster dose at 15 to 18 months of age. A child 12 to 14 months of age should receive 1 dose of Haemophilus b Conjugate Vaccine followed by a booster at 15 to 18 months of age. A child 15 to 59 months of age should receive 1 dose of Haemophilus b Conjugate Vaccine.

Preterm infants should be vaccinated according to their chronological age from birth.

Interruption of the recommended schedule with a delay between doses should not interfere with the final immunity achieved with Haemophilus b Conjugate vaccine reconstituted with DIP vaccine or saline diluent (0.4% sodium chloride). There is no need to start the series over again, regardless of the time elapsed between doses.

It is recommended that the same conjugate vaccine be used throughout each immunization schedule, consistent with the data supporting approval and licensure of the vaccine.

RECONSTITUTION
First, agitate the diluent vial, then, using sterile technique, withdraw the entire volume of diluent into the syringe to be used for reconstitution. Inject all the diluent in the syringe into the vial of lyophilized vaccine, and agitate to mix thoroughly.

Withdraw the entire contents into a new syringe and inject the total volume of reconstituted vaccine (0.5 mL) intramuscularly, preferably into the anterolateral thigh or the outer aspect of the upper arm.

It is recommended that the vaccine be used as soon as possible after reconstitution. Store reconstituted vaccine in the vaccine vial at 2-8° C (36-46° F) and discard if not used within 24 hours. Agitate prior to injection. Vaccine reconstituted with sodium chloride or DTP should be used within 30 minutes after reconstitution.

Table 11
PERCENTAGE OF INFANTS PRESENTING WITH LOCAL OR SYSTEMIC REACTIONS AT 6, 24, AND 48 HOURS OF IMMUNIZATION WITH HAEMOPHILUS b CONJUGATE VACCINE RECONSTITUTED WITH DTP VACCINE

Reaction	AGE AT IMMUNIZATION								
	2 Months (n = 204)			4 Months (n = 199)			6 Months (n = 200)		
	6 Hrs.	24 Hrs.	48 Hrs.	6 Hrs.	24 Hrs.	48 Hrs.	6 Hrs.	24 Hrs.	48 Hrs.
Local									
Tenderness	47.1%	18.6%	3.4%	33.2%	17.6%	4.0%	25.0%	17.0%	3.5%
Erythema > 1″	11.8%	2.5%	0.0%	11.6%	9.1%	2.5%	10.5%	13.5%	3.5%
Induration	31.4%	17.2%	3.9%	26.1%	20.1%	7.5%	28.5%	22.5%	10.0%
Systemic									
Fever > 100.4°F	24.6%	2.0%	0.5%	15.8%	6.1%	3.6%	13.0%	10.3%	3.1%
Irritability	70.6%	22.1%	12.8%	56.8%	31.2%	19.1%	40.5%	28.2%	15.9%
Drowsiness	60.3%	23.5%	11.3%	42.2%	20.6%	9.6%	30.3%	12.3%	5.6%
Anorexia	17.7%	6.4%	2.9%	10.1%	7.5%	5.5%	5.1%	4.6%	4.1%
Diarrhea	2.5%	5.4%	1.5%	3.5%	3.5%	2.5%	2.6%	4.1%	5.6%
Vomiting	2.9%	5.4%	2.9%	3.0%	5.0%	3.0%	3.6%	3.6%	1.5%
Persistent Crying	Percentage of infants within 72 hours after immunization was 0.0% after dose one, 0.0% after dose two, and 0.005% after dose three.								

Parenteral drug products should be inspected visually for extraneous particulate matter and discoloration prior to administration whenever solution and container permit.

Special care should be taken to ensure that the injection does not enter a blood vessel.

It is important to use a separate sterile syringe and needle for each patient to prevent transmission of hepatitis B or other infectious agents from one person to another.

After reconstitution with DTP, each 0.5 mL dose is formulated to contain 10 μg of purified capsular polysaccharide conjugated to 24 μg of inactivated tetanus toxoid, 8.5% of sucrose, 6.7 Lf of diphtheria toxoid, 5 Lf of tetanus toxoid and an estimate of 4 protective units of pertussis vaccine.

STORAGE

Before reconstitution, store the vial of lyophilized vaccine and the vial of the diluent at 2-8° C (36-46° F).

Store reconstituted vaccine in the vaccine vial at 2-8° C (36-46° F) and discard if not used within 24 hours.

DO NOT FREEZE the diluent or the reconstituted vaccine.

REFERENCES

1. Chu Cy, et al. Further studies on the immunogenicity of Haemophilus influenzae type b and pneumococcal type 6A polysaccharide-parotein conjugate. Infect immun 40: 245-246, 1983 2. Mueller JH, et al. Production of diphtheria toxin of high potency (100 Lf) on a reproducible medium. J Immunol 40: 21-32, 1941 3. Adams WG, et al. Decline of Childhood Haemophilus influenzae Type b (Hib) Disease in the Hib Vaccine Era. JAMA 269: 221-226, 1993 4. Recommendations of the Immunization Practices Advisory Committee (ACIP). Haemophilus b conjugate vaccines for prevention of Haemophilus influenzae type b disease among infants and children two months of age and older. MMWR 40: RR-I, 1991 5. Broome CV. Epidemiology of Haemophilus influenzae type b infections in the United States. Pediatr Infect Dis J 6: 779-782, 1987 6. ACIP. Polysaccharide vaccine for prevention of Haemophilus influenzae type b disease. MMWR 34: 201-205, 1985 7. Istre GR, et al. Risk factors for primary invasive Haemophilus influenzae disease: Increased risk from day care attendance and school-aged household members. J Pediatr 106: 190-195, 1985 8. Redmond SR, et al. Hemophilus influenzae type b disease. An epidemiologic study with special reference to day-care centers, JAMA 252: 2581-2584, 1984 9. Murphy TV, et al. County-wide surveillance of invasive Haemophilus influenzae infections: Risk of associated cases in Child Care Programs (CCPS). Twenty-third Interscience Conference on Antimicrobial Agents and Chemotherapy (Abstract #788) 229, 1983 10. Fleming D, et al. Haemophilus influenzae b (Hib) disease-secondary spread in day care. Twenty-fourth Interscience Conference on Antimicrobial Agents and Chemotherapy (Abstract #967) 261, 1984 11. CDC. Prevention of secondary cases of Haemophilus influenzae type b disease. MMWR 31: 672-680, 1982 12. Michaels RH, et al. Pharyngeal colonization with Haemophilus influenzae type b: A longitudinal study of families with a child with meningitis or epiglottitis due to H. influenzae type b. J Infec Dis 136: 222-227, 1977 13. Holmes SJ, et al. Immunogenicity of four Haemophilus influenzae type b conjugate vaccines in 17-to 19-month-old children J. Pediatr 118: 364-371, 1991 14. Data on file, Pasteur Mérieux Sérums à Vaccins S.A. 15. Peltola H, et al. Prevention of Haemophilus influenzae type b bacteremic infections with the capsular polysaccharide vaccine. N Engl J Med 310: 1561-1566, 1984 16. Decker MD, et al. Comparative trial in infants of four conjugate Haemophilus influenzae type b vaccines, J Pediar 120: 184-189, 1992 17. Granoff DM, et al. Differences in the immunogenicity of three Haemophilus influenzae type b conjugate vaccines in infants. J Pediatr 121: 187-194, 1992 18. Kaplan SL, et al. Immunogenicity of Haemophilus influenzae type b polysaccharide-tetanus protein conjugate vaccine in children with sickle hemoglobinopathy or malignancies, and after systemic Haemophilus influenzae type b infection. J Pediatr 120: 367-370, 1992 19. Steinhoff MC, et al. Antibody responses to Haemophilus influenzae type b vaccines in men with human immunodeficiency virus infection. N Engl J Med 325(26): 1837-1842, 1991 20. ACIP. General recommendations on immunization. MMWR 38: 205-227, 1989 21. ACIP. Diphtheria, Tetanus, and Pertussis: Recommendations for Vaccine Use and Other Preventive Measures. MMWR 40: No. RR-10, 1991 22. FDA Workshop on Haemophilus b Polysaccharide Vaccine—A Preliminary Report. MMWR 36: 529-531, 1987 23. Rothstein EP, et al. Comparison of antigenuria after immunization with three Haemophilus influenzae type b conjugate vaccines. Pediatr Infect Dis J 10: 311-314, 1991 24. Vaccine Adverse Event Reporting System—United States. MMWR 39: 730-733, 1990 25. CDC. National Childhood Vaccine Injury Act: Requirements for permanent vaccination records and for reporting of selected events after vaccination. MMWR 37: 197-200, 1988 26. National Childhood Vaccine Injury Act of 1986 (amended 1987) 27. Clemens JD, et al. Impact of Haemophilus influenzae Type b Polysaccharide-Tetanus Protein Conjugate Vaccine on responses to concurrently administered Diphtheria-Tetanus-Pertussis Vaccine. JAMA 267: 673-678, 1992 28. Cody CL, et al. Nature and rates of adverse reactions associated with DTP and DT immunizations in infants and children. Pediatr 68: 650-660, 1981 29. Barkin RM, et al. Diphtheria-tetanus-pertussis vaccine: reactogenicity of commercial products. Pediatr 63: 256-260, 1979 30. Baraff LJ, et al. DTP-associated reactions—an analysis by injection site, manufacturer, prior reactions and dose. Pediatr 73: 31-39, 1984 31. Long SS, et al. Longitudinal study of adverse reactions following diphtheria-tetanus-pertussis vaccine in infancy. Pediatr 85: 294-302, 1990 32. D'Cruz OF, et al. Acute inflammatory demyelinating polyradiculoneuropathy (Guillain-Barré Syndrome) after immunization with Haemophilus influenzae type b conjugate vaccine. J Pediatr 115: 743-746, 1989

HOW SUPPLIED

INJECTION:

BRAND/MANUFACTURER	NDC	SIZE	AWP
○ **BRAND**			
PROHIBIT: Connaught	49281-0541-05	2.5 ml	$89.81
	49281-0541-10	5 ml	$179.63
	49281-0541-01	0.5 ml 5s	$102.50
○ **GENERICS**			
HIBTITER: Lederle Labs	53124-0201-05	2.5 ml	$91.74
HIBTITER: Lederle Labs	53124-0201-10	5 ml	$194.83
HIBTITER: Lederle Labs	53124-0104-41	0.5 ml 4s	$86.36

POWDER FOR INJECTION:

BRAND/MANUFACTURER	NDC	SIZE	AWP
○ **BRAND**			
PEDVAX HIB: Merck	00006-4792-00	1s	$20.00
	00006-4797-00	5s	$100.00
OMNIHIB: SK Beecham Pharm	00007-4408-05	5s ud	$89.05
○ **GENERICS**			
ACTHIB: Connaught	49281-0549-10	1s	$323.75

Halazepam

DESCRIPTION

Halazepam is a benzodiazepine derivative having the chemical name 7-chloro-1,3-dihydro-5-phenyl-1-(2,2,2-trifluoroethyl)-2H-1,4-benzodiazepin-2-one. Each Halazepam Tablet contains 20 mg or 40 mg Halazepam. The compound is a white to light cream-colored powder with a molecular weight of 352.8.

Following is its chemical structure:

CLINICAL PHARMACOLOGY

Central nervous system agents of the 1,4-benzodiazepine class presumably exert their effects by binding at stereo specific receptors at several sites within the central nervous system. Their exact mechanism of action is unknown. Clinically, all benzodiazepines cause a dose-related central nervous system depressant activity varying from mild impairment of task performance to hypnosis.

Halazepam is rapidly and well-absorbed and primarily excreted in the urine. Maximum plasma concentration of Halazepam is achieved between one and three hours following oral administration. Studies involving 12 normal subjects indicate the median half-life of elimination of Halazepam following a 40 mg dose is approximately 14 hours. The major active plasma metabolite of Halazepam is N-desmethyldiazepam. Maximum plasma concentrations of N-desmethyldiazepam usually occur within three to six hours. This metabolite has a half-life of elimination of approximately 50 to 100 hours. Less than one percent of the dose is excreted in the urine as unchanged drug. The major metabolite of Halazepam in the urine is a conjugate, 3-hydroxyhalazepam. As with other benzodiazepines, enterohepatic recycling of Halazepam and its metabolites may occur in uremic patients.

The degree of plasma protein binding of benzodiazepines is high. Since binding is to serum albumin, the extent of binding is dependent on the albumin concentration. In chronic alcoholics, patients with cirrhosis, and newborns, reduced binding may occur. Protein binding may be greatly reduced in patients with renal insufficiency. Since hepatic biotransformation is the predominant route for the metabolism of benzodiazepines, the disposition of these drugs may be impaired in patients with chronic liver disease. Oral dosing of rats with Halazepam for a brief period induced the synthesis of hepatic microsomal drug-metabolizing enzymes. As a result, assuming similar responses in humans, the metabolism of other drugs metabolized in the liver may be increased. The transplacental transfer of Halazepam has not been studied. However, other benzodiazepines readily cross the placental barrier. Following administration of Halazepam to lactating women, Halazepam and its major metabolite, N-desmethyldiazepam, were present in the milk.

INDICATIONS AND USAGE

Halazepam Tablets are indicated for the management of anxiety disorders or the short-term relief of the symptoms of anxiety. Anxiety or tension associated with the stress of everyday life usually does not require treatment with an anxiolytic.

The effectiveness of Halazepam Tablets for long-term use, that is, more than *four* months, has not been established.

The physician should periodically reassess the usefulness of the drug for the individual patient. Except for drowsiness, the drug is well-tolerated.

CONTRAINDICATIONS

Halazepam Tablets are contraindicated in patients with known sensitivity to this drug or other benzodiazepines. It may be used in patients with open angle glaucoma who are receiving appropriate therapy, but is contraindicated in acute narrow angle glaucoma.

WARNINGS

Halazepam Tablets are not of value in the treatment of psychotic patients and should not be employed in lieu of appropriate treatment for psychosis. Halazepam Tablets are also not recommended as the primary treatment for major depressive disorders. Because of its depressant CNS effects, patients receiving Halazepam Tablets should be cautioned against engaging in hazardous occupations requiring complete mental alertness, such as operating machinery or driving a motor vehicle. For the same reason, patients should be cautioned about the simultaneous

► SHOWN IN PRODUCT IDENTIFICATION GUIDE

ingestion of alcohol and other CNS depressant drugs during treatment with Halazepam Tablets.

Benzodiazepines can potentially cause fetal harm when administered to pregnant women. If Halazepam Tablets are used during pregnancy, or if the patient becomes pregnant while taking this drug, she should be apprised of the potential hazard to the fetus. Because of experience with other members of the benzodiazepine class, Halazepam Tablets are assumed to be capable of causing an increased risk of congenital abnormalities when administered to a pregnant woman during the first trimester. Because use of these drugs is rarely a matter of urgency, their use during the first trimester should almost always be avoided. The possibility that a woman of childbearing potential may be pregnant at the time of institution of therapy should be considered. Patients should be advised that if they become pregnant during therapy or intend to become pregnant, they should communicate with their physicians about the desirability of discontinuing the drug.

PRECAUTIONS

General: If Halazepam Tablets are to be combined with other psychotropic agents or anticonvulsant drugs, careful consideration should be given to the pharmacology of the agents to be employed, particularly with compounds which might potentiate the action of benzodiazepines (see *"Drug Interactions"* section).

As with other psychotropic medications, the usual precautions with respect to administration of the drug and size of the prescription are indicated for severely depressed patients or those in whom there is reason to expect concealed suicidal ideation or plans.

In elderly and debilitated patients, it is recommended that the dosage be limited to the smallest effective amount to preclude the development of ataxia or oversedation (see *"Dosage and Administration"* section). The usual precautions in treating patients with impaired renal or hepatic function should be observed.

Information for Patients: To assure safe and effective use of benzodiazepines, the following information and instructions should be given to the patients:

1. Inform your physician about any alcohol consumption and medicine you are taking now, including drugs you buy without a prescription. Alcohol should generally not be used during treatment with benzodiazepines.

2. Inform your physician if you are planning to become pregnant, if you are pregnant, or if you become pregnant while you are taking this medication.

3. Inform your physician if you are nursing.

4. Until you experience how this medicine affects you, do not drive a car or operate potentially dangerous machinery, etc.

5. If benzodiazepines are used in large doses and/or for an extended period of time, they produce habituation, emotional and physical dependence. Therefore, do not increase the dose even if you think that the drug "does not work anymore."

6. Do not stop taking the drug abruptly without consulting your physician, since withdrawal symptoms can occur.

Laboratory Tests: Laboratory tests are not ordinarily required in otherwise healthy patients.

Drug Interactions: The benzodiazepines, including Halazepam Tablets, produce additive CNS depressant effects when co-administered with other psychotropic medications, anticonvulsants, antihistaminics, ethanol, and other drugs which themselves produce CNS depression.

Pharmacokinetic interactions with benzodiazepines have been reported. For example, cimetidine has been reported to reduce diazepam clearance. However, it is not known at this time whether a similar interaction occurs with Halazepam Tablets.

Drug/Laboratory Test Interactions: Although interactions between benzodiazepines and commonly employed clinical laboratory tests have occasionally been reported, there is no consistent pattern for a specific drug or specific test.

Carcinogenesis, Mutagenesis, Impairment of Fertility: The results of oral oncogenicity studies in rats and mice treated at doses 5 to 50 times the usual 120 mg daily human dose revealed no evidence of carcinogenicity or other significant pathology. Studies regarding mutagenesis have not been done. Reproduction studies performed in rats have revealed no evidence of impaired fertility.

Pregnancy: Teratogenic Effects: Pregnancy Category D: (See *"Warnings"* section).

Nonteratogenic Effects: The child born of a mother who is on benzodiazepines may be at some risk for withdrawal symptoms from the drug during the postnatal period. Also, neonatal flaccidity has been reported in children born of mothers who had been receiving benzodiazepines.

Labor and Delivery: Halazepam Tablets have no established use in labor or delivery.

Nursing Mothers: Halazepam and its major metabolites are excreted in the milk of lactating postpartum women. Since neonates metabolize benzodiazepines more slowly than adults, and since accumulation of the drug and its metabolites to toxic levels is possible in neonates, the drug should not be given to nursing mothers.

For example, chronic administration of the closely related benzodiazepine, diazepam, to nursing mothers has been reported to cause their infants to become lethargic and lose weight.

Pediatric Use: Safety and effectiveness in children below the age of 18 years have not been established.

ADVERSE REACTIONS

Central Nervous System: The most frequent adverse reactions to Halazepam Tablets were CNS disturbances. The most common of these was drowsiness, which occurred in approximately 29 per 100 patients. Other CNS disturbances

occurred in approximately 9 per 100 patients (e.g., headache, apathy, psychomotor retardation, disorientation, confusion, euphoria, dysarthria, depression, syncope). Less frequent CNS disturbances were: dizziness, which occurred in approximately 8 per 100 patients; ataxia which occurred in 5 per 100 patients; fatigue, which occurred in approximately 4 per 100 patients; and visual disturbances and paradoxical reaction, which occurred in 1 per 100 patients. Sleep disturbances, changes in libido, and auditory disturbances occurred in fewer than 1 per 100 patients.

Gastrointestinal: Less frequent adverse reactions were: gastrointestinal disturbances (e.g., sense of seasickness, nausea, constipation, increased salivation, difficulty in swallowing, vomiting, gastric disorder), which occurred in approximately 9 per 100 patients; change in appetite, which occurred in approximately 1 per 100 patients; and dry mouth which occurred in approximately 3 per 100 patients.

Hematologic: clinically unimportant fluctuations in the white blood and differential counts were reported in less than 5% of 761 patients.

Hepatic: small to moderate elevations of the following hepatic enzymes were reported: alkaline phosphatase in 20 (2.8%) of 705 patients; SGOT in 35 (5.4%) of 647 patients; SGPT in 3 (< 1%) of 336 patients. No serious abnormalities were seen.

The following adverse reactions were reported to occur rarely in those patients treated with Halazepam Tablets.

Cardiovascular: Cardiovascular disturbances (e.g., tachycardia, bradycardia, hypotension) were reported to occur in approximately 2 per 100 patients.

Musculoskeletal: Muscular disturbances were reported to occur in approximately 2 per 100 patients.

Other: The following adverse reactions occurred in fewer than 1 per 100 patients: allergic manifestations, genitourinary disturbance, paresthesias, and respiratory disturbance.

Adverse Reactions not reported with the use of Halazepam Tablets, but reported with the use of other benzodiazepines are: jaundice, agranulocytosis, edema, slurred speech, minor menstrual irregularities, dystonia, pruritus, incontinence, urinary retention, and diplopia.

DRUG ABUSE AND DEPENDENCE

Physical and Psychological Dependence: Withdrawal symptoms (similar in character to those noted with barbiturates and alcohol) have occurred following abrupt discontinuance of benzodiazepines. These can range from mild dysphoria and insomnia to a major syndrome which may include abdominal and muscle cramps, vomiting, sweating, tremor, and convulsions. These signs and symptoms, especially the more serious ones, are generally more common in those patients who have received excessive doses over an extended period of time. However, withdrawal symptoms have also been reported following abrupt discontinuance of benzodiazepines taken continuously, at therapeutic levels, for several months. Consequently, after extended therapy, abrupt discontinuation should generally be avoided and a gradual tapering in dosage followed.

Patients with a history of seizures or epilepsy, regardless of their concomitant anti-seizure drug therapy, should not be abruptly withdrawn from any CNS depressant agent, including Halazepam Tablets. Addiction-prone individuals (such as drug addicts or alcoholics) should be under careful surveillance when receiving Halazepam or other psychotropic agents because of the predisposition of such patients to habituation and dependence.

Controlled Substance Class: Halazepam is a controlled substance under the Controlled Substance Act and has been assigned by the Drug Enforcement Administration to Schedule IV.

OVERDOSAGE

Manifestations of Halazepam Tablets overdosage include somnolence, confusion, impaired coordination, diminished reflexes, and coma.

No delayed reactions (e.g., organ toxicity) or clinical laboratory abnormalities have been reported.

General Treatment of Overdose: Overdosage reports with Halazepam are limited. Respiration, pulse, and blood pressure should be monitored, as in all cases of drug overdosage. General supportive measures should be employed, along with immediate gastric lavage. Intravenous fluids should be administered and an adequate airway maintained. Hypotension may be combated by the use of levarterenol or metaraminol. Dialysis is of limited value. Animal experiments have suggested that forced diuresis or hemodialysis are probably of little value in treating overdosage. As with the management of intentional overdosing with any drug, it should be borne in mind that multiple agents may have been ingested.

DOSAGE AND ADMINISTRATION

Dosage should be individualized for maximum beneficial effect. While the usual daily dosages given below will meet the needs of most patients, there will be some who require higher doses. In such cases, dosage should be increased cautiously to avoid adverse effects.

Halazepam Tablets are administered orally in divided doses and the dosage should be individualized according to the severity of symptoms and response of the patient. To facilitate dosing, the tablets are scored. The usual recommended dose is 20 to 40 mg three or four times a day.

The response of the patient to several days of treatment will permit the physician to adjust the dose upward or downward. The optimal dosage usually ranges from 80 to 160 mg daily.

◆ RATED THERAPEUTICALLY EQUIVALENT; ◇ THERAPEUTIC EQUIVALENCE UNCONFIRMED; ○ UNRATED

In debilitated patients or the elderly (70 years or older), the initial recommended dosage is 20 mg once or twice a day. The dose should be adjusted as needed and tolerated.

If side effects occur with the starting dose, the dose should be lowered.

Store between 2° and 30°C (36° and 86°F). In addition, protect unit-dose packages from excessive moisture.

ANIMAL PHARMACOLOGY AND/OR ANIMAL TOXICOLOGY
In animal studies, the antianxiety activity of Halazepam was demonstrated by its ability to induce calming effects in normally aggressive species, such as the monkey, and to alleviate suppressed behavior in animals placed in a conflict situation. Halazepam was also shown to block aggressive behavior invoked by stressful stimuli. These effects occurred at substantially lower doses than those which caused motor impairment or sedation. The ratios of the doses causing these side effects to those causing antianxiety activity are greater than comparable ratios obtained with other benzodiazepines, including diazepam or chlordiazepoxide.

Halazepam has relatively little effect on autonomic function and unlike major tranquilizers such as chlorpromazine or haloperidol, it does not cause extrapyramidal side effects. As with other CNS depressants, Halazepam at relatively high doses produces transient cardiovascular depressant effects, but no EKG disturbances were seen in dogs.

A battery of tests were performed in monkeys to evaluate the abuse potential of Halazepam. Although Halazepam did cause physical dependence and positive drug-seeking behavior, these effects were judged to be weaker than those caused by diazepam or chlordiazepoxide in each case. However, the abuse potential of Halazepam in man in comparison with that of diazepam or chlordiazepoxide remains to be established.

HOW SUPPLIED
TABLETS (C-IV): 20 MG

BRAND/MANUFACTURER	NDC	SIZE	AWP
BRAND PAXIPAM: Schering	00085-0251-04	100s	$42.08

TABLETS (C-IV): 40 MG

BRAND/MANUFACTURER	NDC	SIZE	AWP
BRAND PAXIPAM: Schering	00085-0538-04	100s	$58.50

Halcinonide

DESCRIPTION
FOR DERMATOLOGIC USE ONLY. NOT FOR OPHTHALMIC USE.

The topical corticosteroids constitute a class of primarily synthetic steroids used as anti-inflammatory and antipruritic agents. The steroids in this class include Halcinonide. Halcinonide is designated chemically as 21-Chloro-9-fluoro-11β, 16α, 17-trihydroxypregn-4-ene-3,20-dione cyclic 16,17-acetal with acetone.

Each gram of 0.1% Halcinonide Cream contains 1 mg Halcinonide in a specially formulated cream. Each gram of 0.1% Halcinonide Ointment contains 1 mg Halcinonide in Plastibase ® (Plasticized Hydrocarbon Gel).

Each mL of 0.1% Halcinonide Solution contains 1 mg Halcinonide.

Each gram of 0.1% Halcinonide Cream contains 1 mg Halcinonide in a hydrophilic vanishing cream. This formulation is water-washable, greaseless, and nonstaining with moisturizing and emollient properties.

Following is its chemical structure:

CLINICAL PHARMACOLOGY
Topical corticosteroids share anti-inflammatory, antipruritic and vasoconstrictive actions.

The mechanism of anti-inflammatory activity of the topical corticosteroids is unclear. Various laboratory methods, including vasoconstrictor assays, are used to compare and predict potencies and/or clinical efficacies of the topical corticosteroids. There is some evidence to suggest that a recognizable correlation exists between vasoconstrictor potency and therapeutic efficacy in man.

PHARMACOKINETICS
The extent of percutaneous absorption of topical corticosteroids is determined by many factors including the vehicle, the integrity of the epidermal barrier, and the use of occlusive dressings.

Topical corticosteroids can be absorbed from normal intact skin. Inflammation and/or other disease processes in the skin increase percutaneous absorption. Occlusive dressings substantially increase the percutaneous absorption of topical corticosteroids. Thus, occlusive dressings may be a valuable therapeutic adjunct for treatment of resistant dermatoses (see *"Dosage and Administration"*).

Once absorbed through the skin, topical corticosteroids are handled through pharmacokinetic pathways similar to systemically administered corticosteroids. Corticosteroids are bound to plasma proteins in varying degrees. Corticosteroids are metabolized primarily in the liver and are then excreted by the kidneys. Some of the topical corticosteroids and their metabolities are also excreted into the bile.

INDICATIONS AND USAGE
Halcinonide preparations are indicated for the relief of the inflammatory and pruritic manifestations of corticosteroid-responsive dermatoses.

UNLABELED USES
Halcinonide is used as an adjunct in the treatment of cutaneous candidiasis.

CONTRAINDICATIONS
Topical corticosteroids are contraindicated in those patients with a history of hypersensitivity to any of the components of the preparations.

PRECAUTIONS
GENERAL
Systemic absorption of topical corticosteroids has produced reversible hypothalamic-pituitary-adrenal (HPA) axis suppression, manifestations of Cushing's syndrome, hyperglycemia, and glucosuria in some patients.

Conditions which augment systemic absorption include the application of the more potent steroids, use over large surface areas, prolonged use, and the addition of occlusive dressings.

Therefore, patients receiving a large dose of any potent topical steroid applied to a large surface area or under an occlusive dressing should be evaluated periodically for evidence of HPA axis suppression by using the urinary free cortisol and ACTH stimulation tests, and for impairment of thermal homeostasis. If HPA axis suppression or elevation of the body temperature occurs, an attempt should be made to withdraw the drug, to reduce the frequency of application, substitute a less potent steroid, or use a sequential approach when utilizing the occlusive technique.

Recovery of HPA axis function and thermal homeostasis are generally prompt and complete upon discontinuation of the drug. Infrequently, signs and symptoms of steroid withdrawal may occur, requiring supplemental systemic corticosteroids. Occasionally, a patient may develop a sensitivity reaction to a particular occlusive dressing material or adhesive and a substitute material may be necessary.

Children may absorb proportionally larger amounts of topical corticosteroids and thus be more susceptible to systemic toxicity (see *"Precautions, Pediatric Use"*).

If irritation develops, topical corticosteroids should be discontinued and appropriate therapy instituted.

In the presence of dermatological infections, the use of an appropriate antifungal or antibacterial agent should be instituted. If a favorable response does not occur promptly, the corticosteroid should be discontinued until the infection has been adequately controlled.

These preparations are not for ophthalmic use.

INFORMATION FOR THE PATIENT
Patients using topical corticosteroids should receive the following information and instructions:

1. These medications are to be used as directed by the physician. They are for dermatologic use only. Avoid contact with the eyes.
2. Patients should be advised not to use these medications for any disorder other than for which it was prescribed.
3. The treated skin area should not be bandaged or otherwise covered or wrapped as to be occlusive unless directed by the physician.
4. Patients should report any signs of local adverse reactions especially under occlusive dressing.
5. Parents of pediatric patients should be advised not to use tight-fitting diapers or plastic pants on a child being treated in the diaper area, as these garments may constitute occlusive dressings.

LABORATORY TESTS
A urinary free cortisol test and ACTH stimulation test may be helpful in evaluating HPA axis suppression.

CARCINOGENESIS, MUTAGENESIS, AND IMPAIRMENT OF FERTILITY
Long-term animal studies have not been performed to evaluate the carcinogenic potential or the effect on fertility of topical corticosteroids. Studies to determine mutagenicity with prednisolone and hydrocortisone showed negative results.

PREGNANCY: TERATOGENIC EFFECTS
Category C. Corticosteroids are generally teratogenic in laboratory animals when administered systemically at relatively low dosage levels. The more potent corticosteroids have been shown to be teratogenic after dermal application in laboratory animals. There are no adequate and well-controlled studies in pregnant women on teratogenic effects from topically applied corticosteroids. Therefore, topical corticosteroids should be used during pregnancy only if the potential benefit justifies the potential risk to the fetus. Drugs of this class should not be used extensively on pregnant patients, in large amounts, or for prolonged periods of time.

NURSING MOTHERS
It is not known whether topical administration of corticosteroids could result in sufficient systemic absorption to produce detectable quantities in breast milk. Systemically administered corticosteroids are secreted into breast milk in

quantities not likely to have a deleterious effect on the infant. Nevertheless, caution should be exercised when topical corticosteroids are administered to a nursing woman.

PEDIATRIC USE
Pediatric patients may demonstrate greater susceptiblity to topical corticosteroid-induced HPA axis suppression and Cushing's syndrome than mature patients because of a larger skin surface area to body weight ratio.

HPA axis suppression, Cushing's syndrome, and intracranial hypertension have been reported in children receiving topical corticosteroids. Manifestations of adrenal suppression in children include linear growth retardation, delayed weight gain, low plasma cortisol levels, and absence of response to ACTH stimulation. Manifestations of intracranial hypertension include bulging fontanelles, headaches, and bilateral papilledema.

Administration of topical corticosteroids to children should be limited to the least amount compatible with an effective therapeutic regimen. Chronic corticosteroid therapy may interfere with the growth and development of children.

ADVERSE REACTIONS
The following local adverse reactions are reported infrequently with topical corticosteroids, but may occur more frequently with the use of occlusive dressings (reactions are listed in an approximate decreasing order of occurrence): burning, itching, irritation, dryness, folliculitis, hypertrichosis, acneiform eruptions, hypopigmentation, perioral dermatitis, allergic contact dermatitis, maceration of the skin, secondary infection, skin atrophy, striae, and miliaria.

OVERDOSAGE
Topically applied corticosteroids can be absorbed in sufficient amounts to produce systemic effects (see *"Precautions, General"*).

DOSAGE AND ADMINSTRATION
Halcinonide Cream: Apply the 0.1% Halcinonide Cream to the affected area two to three times daily. Rub in gently.

Halcinonide Ointment: Apply a thin film of 0.1% Halcinonide Ointment to the affected area two to three times daily.

Halcinonide Topical Solution: Apply Halcinonide Topical Solution 0.1% to the affected area two to three times daily.

Halcinonide Cream: Apply Halcinonide Cream 0.1% to the affected area one to three times daily. Rub in gently.

OCCLUSIVE DRESSING TECHNIQUE
Occlusive dressings may be used for the management of psoriasis or other recalcitrant conditions.

Halcinonide Cream 0.1%: Gently rub a small amount of the cream into the lesion until it disappears. Reapply the preparation leaving a thin coating on the lesion, cover with a pliable nonporous film, and seal the edges. If needed, additional moisture may be provided by covering the lesion with a dampened clean cotton cloth before the nonporous film is applied or by briefly wetting the affected area with water immediately prior to applying the medication. The frequency of changing dressings is best determined on an individual basis. It may be convenient to apply Halcinonide Cream under an occlusive dressing in the evening and to remove the dressing in the morning (i.e, 12-hour occlusion). When utilizing the 12-hour occlusion regimen, additional cream should be applied, without occlusion, during the day. Reapplication is essential at each dressing change.

If an infection develops, the use of occlusive dressings should be discontinued and appropriate antimicrobial therapy instituted.

Halcinonide Ointment 0.1%: Apply a thin film of the ointment to the lesion, cover with a pliable nonporous film, and seal the edges. If needed, additional moisture may be provided by covering the lesion with a dampened clean cotton cloth before the nonporous film is applied or by briefly wetting the affected area with water immediately prior to applying the medication. The frequency of changing dressings is best determined on an individual basis. It may be convenient to apply Halcinonide Ointment under an occlusive dressing in the evening and to remove the dressing in the morning (i.e., 12-hour occlusion).

When Utilizing the 12-hour occlusion regimen, additional ointment should be applied, without occlusion, during the day. Reapplication is essential at each dressing change.

If an infection develops, the use of occlusive dressings should be discontinued and appropriate antimicrobial therapy instituted.

Halcinonide Topical Solution 0.1%: Apply the solution to the lesion, cover with a pliable nonporous film, and seal the edges. If needed, additional moisture may be provided by covering the lesion with a dampened clean cotton cloth before the nonporous film is applied or by briefly wetting the affected area with water immediately prior to applying the medication. The frequency of changing dressings is best determined on an individual basis. It may be convenient to apply Halcinonide solution under an occlusive dressing in the evening and to remove the dressing in the morning (i.e., 12-hour occlusion). When utilizing the 12-hour occlusion regimen, additional solution should be applied, without occlusion, during the day. Reapplication is essential at each dressing change.

If an infection develops, the use of occlusive dressings should be discontinued and appropriate antimicrobial therapy instituted.

STORAGE
Halcinonide Cream USP: Store at room temperature; avoid excessive heat (104 ° F); avoid freezing and refrigeration.

Halcinonide Ointment USP: Store at room temperature; avoid excessive heat (104°F).

Halcinonide Topical Solution USP: Store at room temperature; avoid freezing and temperatures above 104°F.

HOW SUPPLIED
CREAM: 0.025%

BRAND/MANUFACTURER	NDC	SIZE	AWP
○ **BRAND**			
HALOG: Westwood-Squibb	00003-0296-15	15 gm	$12.16
	00003-0296-30	60 gm	$33.21

CREAM: 0.1%

AVERAGE UNIT PRICE (AVAILABLE SIZES)		
BRAND	$0.94	

BRAND/MANUFACTURER	NDC	SIZE	AWP
◆ **BRAND**			
HALOG: Westwood-Squibb	00003-1482-15	15 gm	$17.84
HALOG-E: Westwood-Squibb	00003-1494-14	15 gm	$17.84
HALOG: Westwood-Squibb	00003-1482-20	30 gm	$28.66
HALOG-E: Westwood-Squibb	00003-1494-21	30 gm	$28.66
HALOG: Westwood-Squibb	00003-1482-30	60 gm	$48.75
HALOG-E: Westwood-Squibb	00003-1494-31	60 gm	$48.75
HALOG: Westwood-Squibb	00003-1482-40	240 gm	$155.09

OINTMENT: 0.1%

BRAND/MANUFACTURER	NDC	SIZE	AWP
○ **BRAND**			
HALOG: Westwood-Squibb	00003-0248-15	15 gm	$17.84
	00003-0248-20	30 gm	$28.66
	00003-0248-30	60 gm	$48.75
	00003-0248-40	240 gm	$155.09

SOLUTION: 0.1%

BRAND/MANUFACTURER	NDC	SIZE	AWP
○ **BRAND**			
HALOG: Westwood-Squibb	00003-0249-15	20 ml	$21.13
	00003-0249-20	60 ml	$47.33

Halcion SEE TRIAZOLAM

Haldol SEE HALOPERIDOL

Halobetasol Propionate

DESCRIPTION
Halobetasol Propionate Cream and Ointment contain the active compound Halobetasol Propionate, a synthetic corticosteroid for topical dermatological use.

Chemically, Halobetasol Propionate is 21-chloro-6α,9α-difluoro-11β,17-dihydroxy-16β-methylpregna-1,4-diene-3- 20-dione, 17-propionate, with the empirical formula $C_{25}H_{31}ClF_2O_5$, and a molecular weight of 485.

Halobetasol Propionate is a white crystalline powder insoluble in water.

Halobatasol Propionate Cream and Ointment contain Halobetasol Propionate 0.5 mg/g.

Following is its chemical structure:

CLINICAL PHARMACOLOGY
Like other topical corticosteroids, Halobetasol Propionate has anti-inflammatory, anti-pruritic and vasoconstrictive actions. The mechanism of the anti-inflammatory activity of the topical corticosteroids, in general, is unclear. However, corticosteroids are thought to act by the induction of phospholipase A_2 inhibitory proteins, collectively called lipocortins. It is postulated that these proteins control the biosynthesis of potent mediators of inflammation such as prostaglandins and

leukotrienes by inhibiting the release of their common precursor arachidonic acid. Arachidonic acid is released from membrane phospholipids by phospholipase A$_2$.

Pharmacokinetics: The extent of percutaneous absorption of topical corticosteroids is determined by many factors, including the vehicle and the integrity of the epidermal barrier. Occlusive dressings with hydrocortisone for up to 24 hours have not been demonstrated to increase penetration; however, occlusion of hydrocortisone for 96 hours markedly enhances penetration. Topical corticosteroids can be absorbed from normal intact skin while inflammation and/or other disease processes in the skin may increase percutaneous absorption.

Human and animal studies indicate that approximately 2% of the applied dose of Halobetasol Propionate enters the circulation within 96 hours following topical administration of the cream, and approximately 3% of the applied dose of Halobetasol Propionate enters the circulation within 96 hours following topical administration of the ointment.

Studies performed with Halobetasol Propionate Ointment indicate that is in the super-high range of potency as compared with other topical corticosteroids. In one of three studies conducted with Halobetasol Proprionate Cream, its potency was comparable to Halobetasol Propionate Ointment. However, in two other studies Halobetasol Proprionate Cream did not appear to be as potent as Halobetasol Propionate Ointment.

INDICATIONS AND USAGE

Halobetasol Propionate Cream 0.05% is a high to super-high potency corticosteroid (See *"Clinical Pharmacology"*) and Halobetasol Propionate Ointment 0.05% is a super-high potency corticosteroid, indicated for the relief of the inflammatory and pruritic manifestations of corticosteroid-responsive dermatoses. Treatment beyond two consecutive weeks is not recommended, and the total dosage should not exceed 50 g/week because of the potential for the drug to suppress the hypothalamic-pituitary-adrenal (HPA) axis.

CONTRAINDICATIONS

Halobetasol Propionate Cream 0.05% is contraindicated in those patients with a history of hypersensitivity to any of the components of the preparation.

PRECAUTIONS

General: Systemic absorption of topical corticosteroids can produce reversible hypothalamic-pituitary-adrenal (HPA) axis suppression with the potential for glucocorticosteroid insufficiency after withdrawal of treatment. Manifestations of Cushing's syndrome, hyperglycemia, and glucosuria can also be produced in some patients by systemic absorption of topical corticosteroids while on treatment.

Patients receiving a large dose of a higher potency topical steroid applied to a large surface area or under an occlusive dressing should be evaluated periodically for evidence of HPA axis suppression. This may be done by using the ACTH stimulation, A.M. plasma-cortisol, and urinary free-cortisol tests. Patients receiving super-potent corticosteroids should not be treated for more than 2 weeks at a time and only small areas should be treated at any one time due to the increased risk of HPA suppression.

Halobetasol Propionate Ointment produced HPA axis suppression when used in divided doses at 7 grams per day for one week in patients with psoriasis. These effects were reversible upon discontinuation of treatment.

If HPA axis suppression is noted, an attempt should be made to withdraw the drug, to reduce the frequency of application, or to substitute a less potent corticosteroid. Recovery of HPA axis function is generally prompt and complete upon discontinuation of topical corticosteroids. Infrequently, signs and symptoms of glucocorticosteroid insufficiency may occur, requiring supplemental systemic corticosteroids. For information on systemic supplementation, see prescribing information for those products.

Children may be more susceptible to systemic toxicity from equivalent doses due to their larger skin surface to body mass ratios (see *"Precautions: Pediatric Use"*).

If irritation develops Halobetasol Propionate should be discontinued and appropriate therapy instituted. Allergic contact dermatitis with corticosteroids is usually diagnosed by observing failure to heal rather than noting a clinical exacerbation as with most topical products not containing corticosteroids. Such an observation should be corroborated with appropriate diagnostic patch testing.

If concomitant skin infections are present or develop, an appropriate antifungal or antibacterial agent should be used. If a favorable response does not occur promptly, use of Halobetasol Propionate should be discontinued until the infection has been adequately controlled.

Halobetasol Propionate should not be used in the treatment of rosacea or perioral dermatitis, and it should not be used on the face, groin, or axillae.

Information for Patients: Patients using topical corticosteroids should receive the following information and instructions:

1. The medication is to be used as directed by the physician. It is for external use only. Avoid contact with the eyes.
2. The medication should not be used for any disorder other than that for which it was prescribed.
3. The treated skin area should not be bandaged or otherwise covered or wrapped so as to be occlusive unless directed by the physician.
4. Patients should report to their physician any signs of local adverse reactions.

Laboratory Tests: The following tests may be helpful in evaluating patients for HPA axis suppression: ACTH-stimulation test; A.M., plasma-cortisol test; urinary free-cortisol test.

Carcinogenesis, Mutagenesis and Impairment of Fertility: Long-term animal studies have not been performed to evaluate the carcinogenic potential of Halobetasol Propionate.

Studies in the rat following oral administration at dose levels up to 50 µg/kg/day indicated no impairment of fertility or general reproductive performance.

Positive mutagenicity effects were observed in two genotoxicity assays. Halobetasol Propionate was positive in a Chinese hamster micronucleus test, and a mouse lymphoma gene mutation assay *in vitro*.

In other genotoxicity testing Halobetasol Propionate was not found to be genotoxic in the Ames/Salmonella assay, in the sister chromatid exchange test in somatic cells of the Chinese hamster, in chromosome aberration studies of germinal and somatic cells of rodents, and in a mammalian spot test to determine point mutations.

Pregnancy, Teratogenic effects: Pregnancy Category C: Corticosteroids have been shown to be teratogenic in laboratory animals when administered systemically at relatively low dosage levels. Some corticosteroids have been shown to be teratogenic after dermal application to laboratory animals.

Halobetasol Propionate has been shown to be teratogenic in SPF rats and chinchilla-type rabbits when given systemically during gestation at doses of 0.04 to 0.1 mg/kg in rats and 0.01 mg/kg in rabbits. These doses are approximately 13, 33 and 3 times, respectively, the human topical dose of Halobetasol Propionate. Halobetasol Propionate was embryotoxic in rabbits but not in rats.

Cleft palate was observed in both rats and rabbits. Omphalocele was seen in rats, but not in rabbits.

There are no adequate and well-controlled studies of the teratogenic potential of Halobetasol Propionate in pregnant women. Therefore, Halobetasol Propionate should be used during pregnancy only if the potential benefit justifies the potential risk to the fetus.

Nursing Mothers: Systemically administered corticosteroids appear in human milk and could suppress growth, interfere with endogenous corticosteroid production, or cause other untoward effects. It is not known whether topical administration of corticosteroids could result in sufficient systemic absorption to produce detectable quantities in human milk. Because many drugs are excreted in human milk, caution should be exercised when Halobetasol Propionate is administered to a nursing woman.

Pediatric Use: Safety and effectiveness Halobetasol Propionate in children have not been established. Because of a higher ratio of skin surface area to body mass, children are at a greater risk than adults of HPA axis suppression when they are treated with topical corticosteroids. They are therefore also at greater risk of glucocorticosteroid insufficiency after withdrawal of treatment and of Cushing's syndrome while on treatment. Adverse effects including striae have been reported with inappropriate use of topical corticosteroids in infants and children. (See *"Precautions".*)

HPA axis suppression, Cushing's syndrome, and intracranial hypertension have been reported in children receiving topical corticosteroids. Manifestations of adrenal suppression in children include linear growth retardation, delayed weight gain, low plasma cortisol levels, and absence of response to ACTH stimulation. Manifestations of intracranial hypertension include bulging fontanelles, headaches, and bilateral papilledema.

ADVERSE REACTIONS

In controlled clinical trials the most frequent adverse events reported for Halobetasol Propionate Cream included stinging, burning or itching in 4.4% of the patients. Less frequently reported adverse reactions were dry skin, erythema, skin atrophy, leukoderma, vesicles and rash.

In controlled clinical trials, the most frequent adverse events reported for Halobetasol Propionate Ointment included stinging or burning in 2.4% of the patients. Less frequently reported adverse reactions were pustulation, erythema, skin atrophy, leukoderma, acne, itching, secondary infection, telangiectasia, urticaria, dry skin, miliaria, paresthesia, tingling, and rash.

The following additional local adverse reactions are reported infrequently with topical corticosteroids, but may occur more frequently with high potency corticosteroids such as Halobetasol Propionate. These reactions are listed in an approximate decreasing order of occurrence: folliculitis, hypertrichosis acneiform eruptions hypopigmentation, perioral dermatitis, allergic contact dermatitis, secondary infection, irritation, striae, and miliaria.

OVERDOSAGE

Topically applied Halobetasol Propionate can be absorbed in sufficient amounts to produce systemic effects (see *"Precautions"*).

DOSAGE AND ADMINISTRATION

Apply a thin layer of Halobetasol Propionate to the affected skin once or twice daily, as directed by your physician, and rub in gently and completely.

Halobetasol Propionate is a high potency topical corticosteroid; therefore, treatment should be limited to two consecutive weeks, and amounts greater than 50g/wk should not be used. Halobetasol Propionate should not be used with occlusive dressings.

Store between 15° and 30°C (59° and 86°F).

HOW SUPPLIED
CREAM: 0.05%

BRAND/MANUFACTURER	NDC	SIZE	AWP
○ **BRAND**			
ULTRAVATE: Westwood-Squibb	00072-1400-15	15 gm	$20.00
	00072-1400-50	50 gm	$48.98

➤ SHOWN IN PRODUCT IDENTIFICATION GUIDE

OINTMENT: 0.05%

BRAND/MANUFACTURER	NDC	SIZE	AWP
○ **BRAND**			
ULTRAVATE: Westwood-Squibb	00072-1450-15	15 gm	$20.00
	00072-1450-50	50 gm	$48.98

Halog *SEE HALCINONIDE*

Haloperidol

DESCRIPTION

Haloperidol is the first of the butyrophenone series of major tranquilizers. The chemical designation is 4-[4-(p-chlorophenyl)-4- hydroxy-piperidino]-4′-fluorobutyrophenone.

Haloperidol dosage forms include: tablets (½, 1, 2, 5, 10 and 20 mg); a concentrate with 2 mg per mL Haloperidol (as the lactate); and a sterile parenteral form for intramuscular injection. The injection provides 5 mg Haloperidol (as the lactate.)

Haloperidol Decanoate is the Decanoate ester of the butyrophenone, Haloperidol. It has a markedly extended duration of effect. It is available in sterile form for intramuscular (IM) injection. The chemical designation is 4-(4-chlorophenyl)-1-[4-(4-fluorophenyl)-4-oxobutyl]-4 piperidinyl decanoate.

Haloperidol Decanoate is almost insoluble in water (0.01 mg/mL), but is soluble in most organic solvents.

Each mL of Haloperidol Decanoate 50 for IM injection contains 50 mg Haloperidol (present as Haloperidol Decanoate 70.52 mg).

Each mL of Haloperidol Decanoate 100 for IM injection contains 100 mg Haloperidol (present as Haloperidol Decanoate 141.04 mg).

Following is its chemical structure:

Cl — HO — N—$CH_2CH_2CH_2C$ — O — F

CLINICAL PHARMACOLOGY

Haloperidol Decanoate 50 and Haloperidol Decanoate 100 are the long-acting forms of Haloperidol. The basic effects of Haloperidol Decanoate are no different from those of Haloperidol with the exception of duration of action. Haloperidol blocks the effects of dopamine and increases its turnover rate; however, the precise mechanism of action is unknown. Administration of Haloperidol Decanoate results in slow and sustained release of Haloperidol. The plasma concentrations of Haloperidol gradually rise, reaching a peak at about 6 days after the injection, and falling thereafter, with an apparent half-life of about 3 weeks. Steady state plasma concentrations are achieved after the third or fourth dose. The relationship between dose of Haloperidol Decanoate and plasma Haloperidol concentration is roughly linear for doses below 450 mg. It should be noted, however, that the pharmacokinetics of Haloperidol Decanoate following intramuscular injections can be quite variable between subjects.

INDICATIONS

Haloperidol is indicated for use in the management of manifestations of psychotic disorders.

Haloperidol is indicated for the control of tics and vocal utterances of Tourette's Disorder in children and adults.

Haloperidol is effective for the treatment of severe behavior problems in children of combative, explosive hyperexcitability (which cannot be accounted for by immediate provocation). Haloperidol is also effective in the short-term treatment of hyperactive children who show excessive motor activity with accompanying conduct disorders consisting of some or all of the following symptoms: impulsivity, difficulty sustaining attention, aggressivity, mood lability and poor frustration tolerance. Haloperidol should be reserved for these two groups of children only after failure to respond to psychotherapy or medications other than antipsychotics.

Haloperidol Decanoate 50 and Haloperidol Decanoate 100 are long-acting parenteral antipsychotic drugs intended for use in the management of patients requiring prolonged parenteral antipsychotic therapy (e.g., patients with chronic schizophrenia).

UNLABELED USES

Haloperidol is used alone or as an adjunct in the treatment of anxiety, autism, and delirium in critically ill cancer patients. It is also used in severe, treatment-resistant depression, nausea and vomiting due to cancer chemotherapy, postoperative nausea and vomiting, LSD flashback, hemiplegic episodes of migraine headache, and stuttering.

CONTRAINDICATIONS

Haloperidol is contraindicated in severe toxic central nervous system depression or comatose states from any cause and in individuals who are hypersensitive to this drug or have Parkinson's disease.

Since the pharmacologic and clinical actions of Haloperidol Decanoate 50 and Haloperidol Decanoate 100 are attributed to Haloperidol as the active medication, contraindications, warnings, and additional information are those of Haloperidol modified only to reflect the prolonged action.

WARNINGS

TARDIVE DYSKINESIA

A syndrome consisting of potentially irreversible, involuntary, dyskinetic movements may develop in patients treated with antipsychotic drugs. Although the prevalence of the syndrome appears to be highest among the elderly, especially elderly women, it is impossible to rely upon prevalence estimates to predict, at the inception of antipsychotic treatment, which patients are likely to develop the syndrome. Whether antipsychotic drug products differ in their potential to cause tardive dyskinesia is unknown.

Both the risk of developing tardive dyskinesia and the likelihood that it will become irreversible are believed to increase as the duration of treatment and the total cumulative dose of antipsychotic drugs administered to the patient increase. However, the syndrome can develop, although much less commonly, after relatively brief treatment periods at low doses.

There is no known treatment for established cases of tardive dyskinesia, although the syndrome may remit, partially or completely, if antipsychotic treatment is withdrawn. Antipsychotic treatment itself, however, may suppress (or partially suppress) the signs and symptoms of the syndrome and thereby may possibly mask the underlying process. The effect that symptomatic suppression has upon the long-term course of the syndrome is unknown.

Given these considerations, antipsychotic drugs should be prescribed in a manner that is most likely to minimize the occurrence of tardive dyskinesia. Chronic antipsychotic treatment should generally be reserved for patients who suffer from a chronic illness that, 1) is known to respond to antipsychotic drugs, and 2) for whom alternative, equally effective, but potentially less harmful treatments are not available or appropriate. In patients who do require chronic treatment, the smallest dose and the shortest duration of treatment producing a satisfactory clinical response should be sought. The need for continued treatment should be reassessed periodically.

If signs and symptoms of tardive dyskinesia appear in a patient on antipsychotics, drug discontinuation should be considered. However, some patients may require treatment despite the presence of the syndrome. (For further information about the description of tardive dyskinesia and its clinical detection, please refer to *"Adverse Reactions".*)

NEUROLEPTIC MALIGNANT SYNDROME (NMS)

A potentially fatal symptom complex sometimes referred to as Neuroleptic Malignant Syndrome (NMS) has been reported in association with antipsychotic drugs. Clinical manifestations of NMS are hyperpyrexia, muscle rigidity, altered mental status (including catatonic signs) and evidence of autonomic instability (irregular pulse or blood pressure, tachycardia, diaphoresis, and cardiac dysrhythmias). Additional signs may include elevated creatine phosphokinase, myoglobinuria (rhabdomyolysis) and acute renal failure.

The diagnostic evaluation of patients with this syndrome is complicated. In arriving at a diagnosis, it is important to identify cases where the clinical presentation includes both serious medical illness (e.g., pneumonia, systemic infection, etc.) and untreated or inadequately treated extrapyramidal signs and symptoms (EPS). Other important considerations in the differential diagnosis include central anticholinergic toxicity, heat stroke, drug fever and primary central nervous system (CNS) pathology.

The management of NMS should include 1) immediate discontinuation of antipsychotic drugs and other drugs not essential to concurrent therapy, 2) intensive symptomatic treatment and medical monitoring, and 3) treatment of any concomitant serious medical problems for which specific treatments are available. There is no general agreement about specific pharmacological treatment regimens for uncomplicated NMS.

If a patient requires antipsychotic drug treatment after recovery from NMS, the potential reintroduction of drug therapy should be carefully considered. The patient should be carefully monitored, since recurrences of NMS have been reported.

Hyperpyrexia and heat stroke, not associated with the above symptom complex, have also been reported with Haloperidol.

USAGE IN PREGNANCY

Rodents given 2 to 20 times the usual maximum human dose of Haloperidol by oral or parenteral routes showed an increase in incidence of resorption, reduced fertility, delayed delivery and pup mortality. No teratogenic effect has been reported in rats, rabbits or dogs at dosages within this range. Rodents given up to 3 times the usual maximum human dose of Baloperidol Decanoate showed an increase in incidence of restorption, fetal mortality, and pup mortality. No fetal abnormalities were observed. Cleft palate has been observed in mice given 15 times the usual maximum human dose. Cleft palate in mice appears to be a non-specific response to stress or nutritional imbalance as well as to a variety of drugs, and there is no evidence to relate this phenomenon to predictable human risk for most of these agents.

There are no adequate and well controlled studies with Haloperidol in pregnant women. There are reports, however, of cases of limb malformations observed following maternal use of Haloperidol along with other drugs which have suspected teratogenic potential during the first trimester of pregnancy. Causal relationships were not established in these cases. Since such experience does not exclude the possibility of fetal damage due to Haloperidol this drug should be used during pregnancy or in women likely to become pregnant only if the benefit clearly justifies a potential risk to the fetus. Since Haloperidol is excreted in human breast milk, infants should not be nursed during drug treatment.

◆ RATED THERAPEUTICALLY EQUIVALENT; ◇ THERAPEUTIC EQUIVALENCE UNCONFIRMED; ○ UNRATED

COMBINED USE OF HALOPERIDOL AND LITHIUM

An encephalopathic syndrome (characterized by weakness, lethargy, fever, tremulousness and confusion, extrapyramidal symptoms, leukocytosis, elevated serum enzymes, BUN, and FBS) followed by irreversible brain damage has occurred in a few patients treated with lithium plus Haloperidol. A causal relationship between these events and the concomitant administration of lithium and Haloperidol has not been established; however, patients receiving such combined therapy should be monitored closely for early evidence of neurological toxicity and treatment discontinued promptly if such signs appear.

GENERAL

A number of cases of bronchopneumonia, some fatal, have followed the use of antipsychotic drugs, including Haloperidol. It has been postulated that lethargy and decreased sensation of thirst due to central inhibition may lead to dehydration, hemoconcentration and reduced pulmonary ventilation. Therefore, if the above signs and symptoms appear, especially in the elderly, the physician should institute remedial therapy promptly.

Although not reported with Haloperidol decreased serum cholesterol and/or cutaneous and ocular changes have been reported in patients receiving chemically-related drugs.

Haloperidol may impair the mental and/or physical abilities required for the performance of hazardous tasks such as operating machinery or driving a motor vehicle. The ambulatory patient should be warned accordingly.

The use of alcohol with this drug should be avoided due to possible additive effects and hypotension.

PRECAUTIONS

Haloperidol should be administered cautiously to patients:
— with severe cardiovascular disorders, because of the possibility of transient hypotension and/or precipitation of anginal pain. Should hypotension occur and a vasopressor be required, epinephrine should not be used since Haloperidol may block its vasopressor activity and paradoxical further lowering of the blood pressure may occur. Instead, metaraminol, phenylephrine or norepinephrine should be used.
— receiving anticonvulsant medications, with a history of seizures, or with EEG abnormalities, because Haloperidol may lower the convulsive threshold. If indicated, adequate anticonvulsant therapy should be concomitantly maintained.
— with known allergies, or with a history of allergic reactions to drugs.
— receiving anticoagulants, since an isolated instance of interference occurred with the effects of one anticoagulant (phenindione).

If concomitant antiparkinson medication is required, it may have to be continued after Haloperidol is discontinued because of the difference in excretion rates or after Haloperidol Decanoate 50 or Haloperidol Decanoate 100 is discontinued because of the prolonged action of Haloperidol Decanoate. If both are discontinued simultaneously, extrapyramidal symptoms may occur. The physician should keep in mind the possible increase in intraocular pressure when anticholinergic drugs, including antiparkinson agents, are administered concomitantly with Haloperidol.

As with other antipsychotic agents, it should be noted that Haloperidol may be capable of potentiating CNS depressants such as anesthetics, opiates, and alcohol.

When Haloperidol is used to control mania in cyclic or bipolar disorders, there may be a rapid mood swing to depression.

Severe neurotoxicity (rigidity, inability to walk or talk) may occur in patients with thyrotoxicosis who are also receiving antipsychotic medication, including Haloperidol.

No mutagenic potential of Haloperidol was found in the Ames Salmonella microsomal activation assay. Negative or inconsistent positive findings have been obtained in in vitro and in vivo studies of effects of short-acting Haloperidol on chromosome structure and number. The available cytogenetic evidence is considered too inconsistent to be conclusive at this time.

Carcinogenicity studies using oral Haloperidol were conducted in Wistar rats (dosed at up to 5 mg/kg daily for 24 months) and in Albino Swiss mice (dosed at up to 5 mg/kg daily for 18 months). In the rat study survival was less than optimal in all dose groups, reducing the number of rats at risk for developing tumors. However, although a relatively greater number of rats survived to the end of the study in high dose male and female groups, these animals did not have a greater incidence of tumors than control animals. Therefore, although not optimal, this study does suggest the absence of a Haloperidol-related increase in the incidence of neoplasia in rats at doses up to 20 times the usual daily human dose for chronic or resistant patients.

In female mice at 5 and 20 times the highest initial daily dose for chronic or resistant patients, there was a statistically significant increase in mammary gland neoplasia and total tumor incidence; at 20 times the same daily dose there was a statistically significant increase in pituitary gland neoplasia. In male mice, no statistically significant differences in incidences of total tumors or specific tumor types were noted.

Antipsychotic drugs elevate prolactin levels; the elevation persists during chronic administration. Tissue culture experiments indicate that approximately one-third of human breast cancers are prolactin dependent in vitro, a factor of potential importance if the prescription of these drugs is contemplated in a patient with a previously detected breast cancer. Although disturbances such as galactorrhea, amenorrhea, gynecomastia, and impotence have been reported, the clinical significance of elevated serum prolactin levels is unknown for most patients. An increase in mammary neoplasms has been found in rodents after chronic administration of antipsychotic drugs. Neither clinical studies nor epidemiologic studies conducted to date, however, have shown an association

between chronic administration of these drugs and mammary tumorigenesis; the available evidence is considered too limited to be conclusive at this time.

ADVERSE REACTIONS
CNS EFFECTS

Extrapyramidal Symptoms (EPA): As with all injectable medications, local tissue reactions have been reported with Haloperidol Decanoate.

EPS during the adminstration of Habperidol have been reported frequently, often during the first few days of treatment. EPS can be categorized generally as Parkinson-like symptoms, akathisia, or dystonia (including opisthotonos and oculogyric crisis). While all can occur at relatively low doses, they occur more frequently and with greater severity at higher doses. The symptoms may be controlled with dose reductions or administration of antiparkinson drugs such as benztropine mesylate USP or trihexyphenidyl hydrochloride USP. It should be noted that persistent EPS have been reported; the drug may have to be discontinued in such cases.

Withdrawal Emergent Neurological Signs: Generally, patients receiving short term therapy experience no problems with abrupt discontinuation of antipsychotic drugs. However, some patients on maintenance treatment experience transient dyskinetic signs after abrupt withdrawal. In certain of these cases the dyskinetic movements are indistinguishable from the syndrome described below under "Tardive Dyskinesia" expect for duration. It is not known whether gradual withdrawal of antipsychotic drugs will reduce the rate of occurrence of withdrawal emergent neurological signs but until further evidence becomes available, it seems resonable to gradually withdraw use of Haloperidol; the long acting properties of Haloperidol Decanoate provide gradual withdrawal.

Tardive Dyskinesta: As with all antipsychotic agents Haloperidol has been associated with persistent dyskinesias. Tardive dyskinesia, a syndrome consisting of potentially irreversible, involuntary, dyskinetic movements, may appear in some patients on long-term therapy or may occur after drug therapy has been discontinued. The risk appears to be greater in elderly patients on high-dose therapy, especially females. The symptoms are persistent and in some patients appear irreversible. The syndrome is characterized by rhythmical involuntary movements of tongue, face, mouth or jaw (e.g., protrusion of tongue, puffing of cheeks, puckering of mouth, chewing movements). Sometimes these may be accompanied by involuntary movements of extremities and the trunk.

There is no known effective treatment for tardive dyskinesia: antiparkinson agents usually do not alleviate the symptoms of this syndrome. It is suggested that all antipsychotic agents be discontinued if these symptoms appear. Should it be necessary to reinstitute treatment, or increase the dosage of the agent, or switch to a different antipsychotic agent, this syndrome may be masked.

It has been reported that fine vermicular movement of the tongue may be an early sign of tardive dyskinesia and if the medication is stopped at that time the full syndrome may not develop.

Tardive Dystonia: Tardive dystonia, not associated with the above syndrome, has also been reported. Tardive dystonia is characterized by delayed onset of choreic or dystonic movements, is often persistent, and has the potential of becoming irreversible.

Other CNS Effects: Insomnia, restlessness, anxiety, euphoria, agitation, drowsiness, depression, lethargy, headache, confusion, vertigo, grand mal seizures, exacerbation of psychotic symptoms including hallucinations, and catatonic-like behavioral states which may be responsive to drug with-drawal and/or treatment with anticholinergic drugs.

Body as a Whole: Neuroleptic malignant syndrome (NMS), hyperpyrexia and heat stroke have been reported with Haloperidol. (See "Warnings" for further information concerning NMS.)

Cardiovascular Effects: Tachycardia, hypotension, hypertension and ECG changes including prolongation of the Q-T interval and ECG pattern changes compatible with the polymorphous configuration of torsades de pointes.

Hematologic Effects: Reports have appeared citing the occurrence of mild and usually transient leukopenia and leukocytosis, minimal decreases in red blood cell counts, anemia, or a tendency toward lymphomonocytosis. Agranulocytosis has rarely been reported to have occurred with the use of Haloperidol, and then only in association with other medication.

Liver Effects: Impaired liver function and/or jaundice have been reported.

Dermatologic Reactions: Maculopapular and acneiform skin reactions and isolated cases of photosensitivity and loss of hair.

Endocrine Disorders: Lactation, breast engorgement, mastalgia, menstrual irregularities, gynecomastia, impotence, increased libido, hyperglycemia, hypoglycemia and hyponatremia.

Gastrointestinal Effects: Anorexia, constipation, diarrhea, hypersalivation, dyspepsia, nausea and vomiting.

Autonomic Reactions: Dry mouth, blurred vision, urinary retention, diaphoresis and priapism.

Respiratory Effects: Laryngospasm, bronchospasm and increased depth of respiration.

Special Senses: Cataracts, retinopathy and visual disturbances.

Other: Cases of sudden and unexpected death have been reported in association with the administration of Haloperidol. The nature of the evidence makes it impossible to determine definitively what role, if any Haloperidol played in the outcome of the reported cases. The possibility that Haloperidol caused death cannot, of course, be excluded, but it is to be kept in mind that sudden and unexpected death may occur in psychotic patients when they go untreated or whey they are treated with other antipsychotic drugs.

Postmarketing Events: Hyperammonemia has been reported in a 5 ½ year old child with citrullinemia, an inherited disorder of ammonia excretion, following treatment with Haloperidol.

OVERDOSAGE

While overdosage is less likely to occur with a parenteral than with an oral medication, information pertaining to Haloperidol is presented, modified only to reflect the extended duration of action of Haloperidol Decanoate.

MANIFESTATIONS

In general, the symptoms of overdosage would be an exaggeration of known pharmacologic effects and adverse reactions, the most prominent of which would be : 1) severe extrapyramidal reactions, 2) hypotension, or 3) sedation. The patient would appear comatose with respiratory depression and hypotension which could be severe enough to produce a shock-like state. The extrapyramidal reactions would be manifested by muscular weakness or rigidity and a generalized or localized tremor as demonstrated by the akinetic or agitans types respectively. With accidental overdosage, hypertension rather than hypotension occurred in a two-year old child. The risk of ECG changes associated with torsades de pointes should be considered. (For further information regarding torsades de pointes, please refer to *"Adverse Reactions"*.)

TREATMENT

Gastric lavage or induction of emesis should be carried out immediately followed by administration of activated charcoal. Since there is no specific antidote, treatment is primarily supportive. A patent airway must be established by use of an oropharyngeal airway or endotracheal tube or, in prolonged cases of coma, by tracheostomy. Respiratory depression may be counteracted by artificial respiration and mechanical respirators. Hypotension and circulatory collapse may be counteracted by use of intravenous fluids, plasma, or concentrated albumin, and vasopressor agents such as metaraminol, phenylephrine and norepinephrine. Epinephrine should not be used. In case of severe extrapyramidal reactions, antiparkinson medication should be administered and with Haloperidol Decanoater, should be continued for several weeks, and then withdrawn and gradually as extrapyramidal symptoms may emerge. ECG and vital signs should be monitored especially for signs of Q-T prolongation or dysrhythmias and monitoring should continue until the ECG is normal. Severe arrhythmias should be treated with appropriate antiarrhythmic measures.

DOSAGE AND ADMINISTRATION

HALOPERIDOL TABLETS/CONCENTRATE/INJECTION

There is considerable variation from patient to patient in the amount of medication required for treatment. As with all antipsychotic drugs, dosage should be individualized according to the needs and response of each patient. Dosage adjustments, either upward or downward, should be carried out as rapidly as practicable to achieve optimum therapeutic control.

To determine the initial dosage, consideration should be given to the patient's age, severity of illness, previous response to other antipsychotic drugs, and any concomitant medication or disease state. Children, debilitated or geriatric patients, as well as those with a history of adverse reactions to antipsychotic drugs, may require less Haloperidol. The optimal response in such patients is usually obtained with more gradual dosage adjustments and at lower dosage levels, as recommended below.

Clinical experience suggests the following recommendations:

ORAL ADMINISTRATION

Initial Dosage Range

Adults:

Moderate Symptomatology	0.5 mg to 2.0 mg b.i.d. or t.i.d.
Severe Symptomatology	3.0 mg to 5.0 mg b.i.d. or t.i.d.

To achieve prompt control, higher doses may be required in some cases.

Geriatric or Debilitated Patients	0.5 mg to 2.0 mg b.i.d. or t.i.d.
Chronic or Resistant Patients	3.0 mg to 5.0 mg b.i.d. or t.i.d.

Patients who remain severely distributed or inadequately controlled may require dosage adjustment. Daily dosages up to 100 mg may be necessary in some cases to achieve an optimal response. Infrequently Haloperidol has been used in doses above 100 mg for severely resistant patients; however, the limited clinical usage has not demonstrated the safety of prolonged administration of such doses.

Children: The following recommendations apply to children between the ages of 3 and 12 years (weight range 15 to 40 kg). Haloperidol is not intended for children under 3 years old. Therapy should begin at the lowest dose possible (0.5 mg per day). If required, the dose should be increased by an increment of 0.5 mg at 5 to 7 day intervals until the desired therapeutic effect is obtained. (See chart below). The total dose may be divided, to be given b.i.d. or t.i.d.

Psychotic Disorders	0.05 mg/kg/day to 0.15 mg/kg/day
Nonpsychotic Behavior Disorders and Tourette's Disorder	0.05 mg/kg/day to 0.075 mg/kg/day

Severely disturbed psychotic children may require higher doses.

In severely disturbed, non-psychotic children or in hyperactive children with accompanying conduct disorders, who have failed to respond to psychotherapy or medications other than antipsychotics, it should be noted that since these behaviors may be short-lived, short-term administration of Haloperidol may suffice. There is no evidence establishing a maximum effective dosage. There is little evidence that behavior improvement is further enhanced in dosages beyond 6 mg per day.

Safety and effectiveness of Haloperidol Decanoate in children have not been established.

MAINTENANCE DOSAGE

Upon achieving a satisfactory therapeutic response, dosage should then be gradually reduced to the lowest effective maintenance level.

INTRAMUSCULAR ADMINISTRATION

Adults: Parenteral medication, administered intramuscularly in doses of 2 to 5 mg, is utilized for prompt control of the acutely agitated patient with moderately severe to very severe symptoms. Depending on the response of the patient, subsequent doses may be given, administered as often as every hour, although 4 to 8 hour intervals may be satisfactory.

Controlled trials to establish the safety and effectiveness of intramuscular administration in children have not been conducted.

Parenteral drug products should be inspected visually for particulate matter and discoloration prior to administration, whenever solution and container permit.

SWITCHOVER PROCEDURE

The oral form should supplant the injectable as soon as practicable. In the absence of bioavailability studies establishing bioequivalence between these two dosage forms the following guidelines for dosage are suggested. For an initial approximation of the total daily dose required, the parenteral dose administered in the preceding 24 hours may be used. Since this dose is only an initial estimate, it is recommended that careful monitoring of clinical signs and symptoms, including clinical efficacy, sedation, and adverse effects, be carried out periodically for the first several days following the initiation of switchover. In this way, dosage adjustments, either upward or downward, can be quickly accomplished. Depending on the patient's clinical status, the first oral dose should be given within 12-24 hours following the last parenteral dose.

HALOPERIDOL DECANOATE INJECTION

Haloperidol Decanoate 50 and Haloperidol Decanoate 100 should be administered by deep intramuscular injection. A 21 gauge needle is recommended. The maximum volume per injection site should not exceed 3 mL. DO NOT ADMINISTER INTRAVENOUSLY.

Parenteral drug products should be inspected visually for particulate matter and discoloration prior to administration, whenever solution and container permit.

Haloperidol Decanoate 50 and Haloperidol Decanoate 100 are intended for use in chronic psychotic patients who require prolonged parenteral antipsychotic therapy. These patients should be previously stabilized on antipsychotic medication before considering a conversion to Haloperidol Decanoate. Furthermore, it is recommended that patients being considered for Haloperidol Decanoate therapy have been treated with, and tolerate well, short-acting Haloperidol in order to reduce the possibility of an unexpected adverse sensitivity to Haloperidol. Close clinical supervision is required during the initial period of dose adjustment in order to minimize the risk of overdosage or reappearance of psychotic symptoms before the next injection. During dose adjustment or episodes of exacerbation of psychotic symptoms, Haloperidol Decanoate therapy can be supplemented with short-acting forms of Haloperidol.

The dose of Haloperidol Decanoate 50 or Haloperidol Decanoate 100 should be expressed in terms of its Haloperidol content. The starting dose of Haloperidol Decanoate should be based on the patient's age, clinical history, physical condition, and response to previous antipsychotic therapy. The preferred approach to determining the minimum effective dose is to begin with lower initial doses and to adjust the dose upward as needed. For patients previously maintained on low doses of antipsychotics (e.g. up to the equivalent of 10 mg/day oral Haloperidol), it is recommended that the initial dose of Haloperidol Decanoate be 10-15 times the previous daily dose in oral Haloperidol equivalents; limited clinical experience suggests that lower initial doses may be adequate.

INITIAL THERAPY

Conversion from oral Haloperidol to Haloperidol Decanoate can be achieved by using an initial dose of Haloperidol Decanoate that is 10 to 20 times the previous daily dose in oral Haloperidol equivalents.

In patients who are elderly, debilitated, or stable on low doses of oral Haloperidol (e.g. up to the equivalent of 10 mg/day oral Haloperidol), a range of 10 to 15 times the previous daily dose in oral Haloperidol equivalents is appropriate for initial conversion.

In patients previously maintained on higher doses of antipsychotics for whom a low dose approach risks recurrence of psychiatric decompensation and in patients whose long term use of Haloperidol has resulted in a tolerance to the drug, 20 times the previous daily dose in oral Haloperidol equivalents should be considered for initial conversion, with downward titration on succeeding injections.

◆ RATED THERAPEUTICALLY EQUIVALENT; ◇ THERAPEUTIC EQUIVALENCE UNCONFIRMED; ○ UNRATED

The initial dose of Haloperidol Decanoate should not exceed 100 mg regardless of previous antipsychotic dose requirements. If, therefore, conversion requires more than 100 mg of Haloperidol Decanoate as an initial dose, that dose should be administered in two injections, i.e. a maximum of 100 mg initially followed by the balance in 3 to 7 days.

MAINTENANCE THERAPY

The maintenance dosage of Haloperidol Decanoate must be individualized with titration upward or downward based on therapeutic response. The usual maintenance range is 10 to 15 times the previous daily dose in oral Haloperidol equivalents dependent on the clinical response of the patient.

HALOPERIDOL DECANOATE DOSING RECOMMENDATIONS MONTHLY

Patients	1ST Month	Maintenance
Stabilized on low daily oral doses (up to 10 mg/day)	10-15x Daily Oral Dose	10-15x Previous Daily Oral Dose
Elderly or Debilitated		
High dose		
Risk of relapse	20x Daily Oral Dose	10-15x Previous Daily Oral Dose
Tolerant to oral Haloperidol		

Close clinical supervision is required during initiation and stabilization of Haloperidol Decanoate therapy.

Haloperidol Decanoate is usually administered monthly or every 4 weeks. However, variation in patient response may dictate a need for adjustment of the dosing interval as well as the dose (see "Clinical Pharmacology").

Clinical experience with Haloperidol Decanoate at doses greater than 450 mg per month has been limited.

Dispense Haloperidol tablets and concentrate in a tight, light resistant container as defined in the official compendium.

Store Haloperidol Decanoate at controlled room temperature (15°-30°C, 59°-86°F). Do not refrigerate or freeze.

Protect from light.

J CODES

Per 50 mg IM—J1631
Up to 5 mg IM,IV—J1630

HOW SUPPLIED

HALOPERIDOL
CONCENTRATE: 2 MG/ML

AVERAGE UNIT PRICE (AVAILABLE SIZES)		GENERIC A-RATED AVERAGE PRICE (GAAP)	
GENERIC	$0.43	15 ml	$8.94
		120 ml	$31.73

BRAND/MANUFACTURER	NDC	SIZE	AWP
◆ GENERICS			
Barre	00472-0766-99	15 ml	$8.44
Roxane	00054-3350-41	15 ml	$9.43
Roxane	00054-3350-50	120 ml	$30.76
Barre	00472-0766-94	120 ml	$32.70

INJECTION: 5 MG/ML

AVERAGE UNIT PRICE (AVAILABLE SIZES)	
BRAND	$5.67

BRAND/MANUFACTURER	NDC	SIZE	AWP
◆ BRAND			
HALDOL: McNeil Pharm	00045-0255-49	10 ml	$55.93
	00045-0255-01	1 ml 10s	$57.37
◆ GENERICS			
Solo Pak	39769-0088-02	1 ml 10s	$37.50

TABLETS: 0.5 MG

AVERAGE UNIT PRICE (AVAILABLE SIZES)		GENERIC A-RATED AVERAGE PRICE (GAAP)	
BRAND	$0.24	100s	$17.05
GENERIC	$0.16	500s	$60.81
HCFA FUL (100s ea)	$0.02	1000s	$139.16

BRAND/MANUFACTURER	NDC	SIZE	AWP
◆ BRAND			
➤ HALDOL:	00045-0240-66	100s	$8.40
➤ HALDOL: McNeil Pharm	00045-0240-60	100s	$39.31
➤ HALDOL:	00045-0240-76	100s ud	$8.66
➤ HALDOL: McNeil Pharm	00045-0240-10	100s ud	$43.70
➤ HALDOL:	00045-0240-86	1000s	$84.00
➤ HALDOL: McNeil Pharm	00045-0240-80	1000s	$343.17
◆ GENERICS			
Major	00904-1730-60	100s	$11.50
Schein	00364-2204-01	100s	$12.25
Purepac	00228-2289-10	100s	$13.49

BRAND/MANUFACTURER	NDC	SIZE	AWP
Roxane	00054-4342-25	100s	$13.78
Goldline	00182-1262-01	100s	$14.50
Qualitest	00603-3782-21	100s	$14.73
Rugby	00536-3869-01	100s	$14.94
Major	00904-1830-60	100s	$14.95
URL	00677-1115-01	100s	$15.48
Mylan	00378-0351-01	100s	$17.62
Par	49884-0223-01	100s	$17.65
Parmed	00349-8944-01	100s	$17.65
Geneva	00781-1391-01	100s	$17.65
Mason Dist	11845-0242-01	100s	$17.65
Aligen	00405-4459-01	100s	$17.68
Moore,H.L.	00839-7346-06	100s	$18.56
Raway	00686-0733-20	100s ud	$5.50
U.S. Trading	56126-0335-11	100s ud	$11.01
Roxane	00054-8342-25	100s ud	$13.44
Auro	55829-0294-10	100s ud	$17.79
Major	00904-1730-61	100s ud	$24.20
Major	00904-1830-61	100s ud	$24.20
Vangard	00615-2594-13	100s ud	$24.35
UDL	51079-0733-20	100s ud	$27.80
Geneva	00781-1391-13	100s ud	$27.82
Rugby	00536-3869-05	500s	$43.43
Major	00904-1830-40	500s	$48.90
Goldline	00182-1262-05	500s	$56.00
Purepac	00228-2289-50	500s	$67.45
Par	49884-0223-05	500s	$88.25
Major	00904-1730-80	1000s	$82.30
Major	00904-1830-80	1000s	$82.30
Qualitest	00603-3782-32	1000s	$93.41
Mylan	00378-0351-10	1000s	$166.50
Geneva	00781-1391-10	1000s	$166.60
Par	49884-0223-10	1000s	$171.21
Mason Dist	11845-0242-04	1000s	$171.21
Moore,H.L.	00839-7346-16	1000s	$179.75

TABLETS: 1 MG

AVERAGE UNIT PRICE (AVAILABLE SIZES)		GENERIC A-RATED AVERAGE PRICE (GAAP)	
BRAND	$0.31	100s	$24.53
GENERIC	$0.22	500s	$85.83
HCFA FUL (100s ea)	$0.02	1000s	$181.82

BRAND/MANUFACTURER	NDC	SIZE	AWP
◆ BRAND			
➤ HALDOL:	00045-0241-66	100s	$12.00
➤ HALDOL: McNeil Pharm	00045-0241-60	100s	$58.19
➤ HALDOL:	00045-0241-76	100s ud	$12.59
➤ HALDOL: McNeil Pharm	00045-0241-10	100s ud	$59.82
➤ HALDOL:	00045-0241-86	1000s	$108.00
◆ GENERICS			
Major	00904-1731-60	100s	$18.50
Major	00904-1831-60	100s	$18.50
Par	49884-0224-01	100s	$18.55
Mason Dist	11845-0243-01	100s	$18.55
Schein	00364-2205-01	100s	$19.75
Purepac	00228-2280-10	100s	$20.15
Roxane	00054-4343-25	100s	$20.22
Goldline	00182-1263-01	100s	$21.50
Qualitest	00603-3783-21	100s	$21.82
Rugby	00536-3877-01	100s	$21.89
URL	00677-1116-01	100s	$22.87
Moore,H.L.	00839-7347-06	100s	$22.88
Aligen	00405-4460-01	100s	$23.68
Mylan	00378-0257-01	100s	$26.12
Geneva	00781-1392-01	100s	$26.15
Parmed	00349-8945-01	100s	$27.00
Raway	00686-0734-20	100s ud	$5.95
U.S. Trading	56126-0336-11	100s ud	$18.08
Roxane	00054-8343-25	100s ud	$19.13
Auro	55829-0295-10	100s ud	$26.74
Vangard	00615-2595-13	100s ud	$38.42
Major	00904-1731-61	100s ud	$38.62
Major	00904-1831-61	100s ud	$38.62
UDL	51079-0734-20	100s ud	$39.79
Geneva	00781-1392-13	100s ud	$39.80
Rugby	00536-3877-05	500s	$60.83
Goldline	00182-1263-05	500s	$89.00
Par	49884-0224-05	500s	$92.75
Purepac	00228-2280-50	500s	$100.75
Qualitest	00603-3783-32	1000s	$124.80
Major	00904-1731-80	1000s	$132.30
Major	00904-1831-80	1000s	$132.30
Par	49884-0224-10	1000s	$179.94
Mason Dist	11845-0243-04	1000s	$179.94
Parmed	00349-8643-10	1000s	$187.50
Moore,H.L.	00839-7347-16	1000s	$188.93
Roxane	00054-4343-31	1000s	$190.67
Mylan	00378-0257-10	1000s	$250.88
Geneva	00781-1392-10	1000s	$250.90

➤ SHOWN IN PRODUCT IDENTIFICATION GUIDE

TABLETS: 2 MG

AVERAGE UNIT PRICE (AVAILABLE SIZES)		GENERIC A-RATED AVERAGE PRICE (GAAP)	
BRAND	$0.47	100s	$33.67
GENERIC	$0.32	500s	$126.68
HCFA FUL (100s ea)	$0.02	1000s	$294.09

BRAND/MANUFACTURER	NDC	SIZE	AWP
◆ **BRAND**			
➤ HALDOL:	00045-0242-66	100s	$16.80
➤ HALDOL: McNeil Pharm	00045-0242-60	100s	$80.16
➤ HALDOL:	00045-0242-76	100s ud	$17.02
➤ HALDOL: McNeil Pharm	00045-0242-10	100s ud	$80.82
➤ HALDOL:	00045-0242-86	1000s	$156.00
➤ HALDOL: McNeil Pharm	00045-0242-80	1000s	$686.24
◆ **GENERICS**			
Major	00904-1732-60	100s	$22.50
Schein	00364-2206-01	100s	$25.50
Purepac	00228-2281-10	100s	$27.37
Roxane	00054-4344-25	100s	$28.08
Goldline	00182-1264-01	100s	$29.50
Qualitest	00603-3784-21	100s	$29.80
Rugby	00536-3878-01	100s	$30.63
Major	00904-1832-60	100s	$30.65
URL	00677-1117-01	100s	$32.28
Mylan	00378-0214-01	100s	$36.00
Geneva	00781-1393-01	100s	$36.05
Par	49884-0225-01	100s	$36.10
Mason Dist	11845-0244-01	100s	$36.10
Aligen	00405-4461-01	100s	$36.20
Parmed	00349-8946-01	100s	$37.00
Moore,H.L.	00839-7348-06	100s	$37.87
Raway	00686-0735-20	100s ud	$6.75
U.S. Trading	56126-0337-11	100s ud	$11.25
Roxane	00054-8344-25	100s ud	$25.82
Auro	55829-0296-10	100s ud	$35.88
Major	00904-1732-61	100s ud	$47.60
Major	00904-1832-61	100s ud	$47.60
Vangard	00615-2596-13	100s ud	$47.75
UDL	51079-0735-20	100s ud	$53.79
Geneva	00781-1393-13	100s ud	$53.80
Rugby	00536-3878-05	500s	$62.70
Purepac	00228-2281-50	500s	$136.85
Par	49884-0225-05	500s	$180.50
Major	00904-1732-80	1000s	$179.25
Major	00904-1832-80	1000s	$179.25
Qualitest	00603-3784-32	1000s	$253.40
Roxane	00054-4344-31	1000s	$267.15
Mylan	00378-0214-10	1000s	$349.88
Geneva	00781-1393-10	1000s	$349.90
Par	49884-0225-10	1000s	$350.17
Mason Dist	11845-0244-04	1000s	$350.17
Moore,H.L.	00839-7348-16	1000s	$367.61

TABLETS: 5 MG

AVERAGE UNIT PRICE (AVAILABLE SIZES)		GENERIC A-RATED AVERAGE PRICE (GAAP)	
BRAND	$0.76	100s	$55.94
GENERIC	$0.50	500s	$156.03
HCFA FUL (100s ea)	$0.03	1000s	$496.92

BRAND/MANUFACTURER	NDC	SIZE	AWP
◆ **BRAND**			
➤ HALDOL:	00045-0245-66	100s	$27.68
➤ HALDOL: McNeil Pharm	00045-0245-60	100s	$131.17
➤ HALDOL:	00045-0245-76	100s ud	$27.53
➤ HALDOL: McNeil Pharm	00045-0245-10	100s ud	$129.36
➤ HALDOL:	00045-0245-86	1000s	$259.01
➤ HALDOL: McNeil Pharm	00045-0245-80	1000s	$1125.87
◆ **GENERICS**			
Major	00904-1733-60	100s	$36.50
Qualitest	00603-3785-21	100s	$37.00
Rugby	00536-3879-01	100s	$37.75
Major	00904-1833-60	100s	$38.95
Goldline	00182-1265-01	100s	$38.95
Purepac	00228-2282-10	100s	$39.84
URL	00677-1118-01	100s	$41.70
Schein	00364-2207-01	100s	$41.75
Roxane	00054-4345-25	100s	$45.96
Mylan	00378-0327-01	100s	$58.76
Geneva	00781-1396-01	100s	$58.79
Par	49884-0226-01	100s	$59.02
Aligen	00405-4462-01	100s	$59.02
Mason Dist	11845-0245-01	100s	$59.02
Parmed	00349-8947-01	100s	$59.50
Moore,H.L.	00839-7349-06	100s	$61.97
Roxane	00054-8345-25	100s ud	$41.23
Auro	55829-0297-10	100s ud	$56.28
Vangard	00615-2597-13	100s ud	$80.41
Major	00904-1733-61	100s ud	$81.00
Major	00904-1833-61	100s ud	$81.00
UDL	51079-0736-20	100s ud	$86.06
Geneva	00781-1396-13	100s ud	$86.09
Rugby	00536-3879-05	500s	$82.28

BRAND/MANUFACTURER	NDC	SIZE	AWP
Mason Dist	11845-0245-03	500s	$98.92
Major	00904-1733-40	500s	$118.65
Major	00904-1833-40	500s	$118.65
Qualitest	00603-3785-28	500s	$140.50
Goldline	00182-1265-05	500s	$194.95
Purepac	00228-2282-50	500s	$199.20
Par	49884-0226-05	500s	$295.10
Major	00904-1833-80	1000s	$166.00
Roxane	00054-4345-31	1000s	$438.36
Mylan	00378-0327-10	1000s	$577.12
Par	49884-0226-10	1000s	$590.20
Mason Dist	11845-0245-04	1000s	$590.20
Moore,H.L.	00839-7349-16	1000s	$619.65

TABLETS: 10 MG

AVERAGE UNIT PRICE (AVAILABLE SIZES)		GENERIC A-RATED AVERAGE PRICE (GAAP)	
BRAND	$0.99	100s	$63.50
GENERIC	$0.58	500s	$208.30
HCFA FUL (100s ea)	$0.04		

BRAND/MANUFACTURER	NDC	SIZE	AWP
◆ **BRAND**			
➤ HALDOL:	00045-0246-66	100s	$42.00
➤ HALDOL: McNeil Pharm	00045-0246-60	100s	$168.29
➤ HALDOL:	00045-0246-76	100s ud	$42.67
➤ HALDOL: McNeil Pharm	00045-0246-10	100s ud	$155.94
➤ HALDOL:	00045-0246-86	1000s	$402.00
➤ HALDOL: McNeil Pharm	00045-0246-80	1000s	$1455.16
◆ **GENERICS**			
Schein	00364-2236-01	100s	$12.75
Rugby	00536-3880-01	100s	$44.87
Goldline	00182-1854-01	100s	$44.95
Major	00904-1734-60	100s	$46.40
Qualitest	00603-3786-21	100s	$46.70
URL	00677-1203-01	100s	$50.00
Parmed	00349-8948-01	100s	$64.20
Geneva	00781-1397-01	100s	$64.95
Par	49884-0227-01	100s	$65.00
Roxane	00054-4346-25	100s	$65.00
Mason Dist	11845-0246-01	100s	$65.00
Aligen	00405-4463-01	100s	$65.63
Moore,H.L.	00839-7398-06	100s	$68.24
Roxane	00054-8346-25	100s ud	$62.55
Auro	55829-0298-10	100s ud	$75.28
Geneva	00781-1397-13	100s ud	$98.98
Major	00904-1734-61	100s ud	$101.25
Major	00904-1834-61	100s ud	$101.25
Rugby	00536-3880-05	500s	$134.10
Major	00904-1734-40	500s	$165.00
Moore,H.L.	00839-7398-12	500s	$202.43
Goldline	00182-1854-05	500s	$202.45
Qualitest	00603-3786-28	500s	$220.80
Par	49884-0227-05	500s	$325.00
Roxane	00054-4346-31	1000s	$650.00

TABLETS: 20 MG

AVERAGE UNIT PRICE (AVAILABLE SIZES)		GENERIC A-RATED AVERAGE PRICE (GAAP)	
BRAND	$1.62	100s	$80.62
GENERIC	$0.77		
HCFA FUL (100s ea)	$0.12		

BRAND/MANUFACTURER	NDC	SIZE	AWP
◆ **BRAND**			
➤ HALDOL:	00045-0248-66	100s	$78.00
➤ HALDOL: McNeil Pharm	00045-0248-60	100s	$322.85
➤ HALDOL:	00045-0248-76	100s ud	$84.00
◆ **GENERICS**			
Schein	00364-2237-01	100s	$22.50
Goldline	00182-1855-01	100s	$53.20
Major	00904-1735-60	100s	$63.50
Parmed	00349-8953-01	100s	$67.73
Geneva	00781-1398-01	100s	$99.75
Roxane	00054-4347-25	100s	$115.57
Major	00904-1735-61	100s ud	$35.40
Auro	55829-0299-10	100s ud	$97.15
Roxane	00054-8347-25	100s ud	$112.50
UDL	51079-0737-20	100s ud	$138.89
Major	00904-1735-40	500s	$206.40

HALOPERIDOL DECANOATE
INJECTION: 50 MG/ML

BRAND/MANUFACTURER	NDC	SIZE	AWP
○ **BRAND**			
HALDOL DECANOATE: McNeil Pharm	00045-0253-46	5 ml	$139.76
	00045-0253-03	1 ml 3s	$83.84
	00045-0253-01	1 ml 10s	$279.44

◆ RATED THERAPEUTICALLY EQUIVALENT; ◇ THERAPEUTIC EQUIVALENCE UNCONFIRMED; ○ UNRATED

INJECTION: 100 MG/ML

BRAND/MANUFACTURER	NDC	SIZE	AWP
○ **BRAND**			
HALDOL DECANOATE: McNeil Pharm	00045-0254-46	5 ml	$256.36
	00045-0254-14	1 ml 5s	$256.36

HALOPERIDOL LACTATE
CONCENTRATE: 2 MG/ML

AVERAGE UNIT PRICE (AVAILABLE SIZES)		GENERIC A-RATED AVERAGE PRICE (GAAP)	
BRAND	$0.68	**15 ml**	$9.92
GENERIC	$0.42	**120 ml**	$32.73
HCFA FUL (15 ml)	$0.60		
HCFA FUL (120 ml)	$0.19		

BRAND/MANUFACTURER	NDC	SIZE	AWP
◆ **BRAND**			
HALDOL:	00045-0250-17	15 ml	$7.20
HALDOL: McNeil Pharm	00045-0250-15	15 ml	$21.95
HALDOL:	00045-0250-27	120 ml	$10.80
HALDOL: McNeil Pharm	00045-0250-04	120 ml	$91.73
	00045-0250-08	240 ml	$143.10
◆ **GENERICS**			
Copley	38245-0604-15	15 ml	$8.00
Silarx	54838-0501-15	15 ml	$8.86
Goldline	00182-6059-64	15 ml	$9.45
Major	00904-1729-35	15 ml	$9.60
Schein	00364-0854-72	15 ml	$10.35
Warner Chilcott	00047-2913-35	15 ml	$12.22
Rugby	00536-1011-97	120 ml	$26.75
Copley	38245-0604-14	120 ml	$27.00
Warner Chilcott	00047-2913-36	120 ml	$30.48
Geneva	00781-6205-04	120 ml	$32.70
Qualitest	00603-1290-54	120 ml	$32.75
Aligen	00405-2850-76	120 ml	$32.80
Major	00904-1729-20	120 ml	$32.95
Goldline	00182-6059-71	120 ml	$33.00
Silarx	54838-0501-40	120 ml	$34.40
Schein	00364-0854-77	120 ml	$37.10
Lemmon	00093-0553-12	120 ml	$41.86

Haloprogin

DESCRIPTION
Haloprogin Cream/Solution for topical use. Each gram of the cream contains 10 mg Haloprogin in a water-dispersible base.

Each mL of the solution contains 10 mg Haloprogin in a clear, colorless vehicle.

The chemical name for Haloprogin is 1,2,4-trichloro-5[(3-iodo-2-propynyl)oxy]benzene.

Following is its chemical structure:

CLINICAL PHARMACOLOGY
The mechanism of antifungal activity for Haloprogin in yeast cells is believed to be inhibition of respiration and disruption of the yeast cell membrane. The mechanism of antifungal activity in dermatophytes is unknown. *Dermal penetration* studies utilizing single applications of ^{14}C ring-labeled Haloprogin formulated as creams, or dissolved in acetone or alcoholic solutions, were performed in 18 male subjects. Urinary recovery from 3 subjects ranged from 9.47% (0.25% cream) to 14.89% (1% cream) over 5 days. The 0.25% and 1% alcoholic solutions were associated with lesser recoveries of 3% and 6%, respectively. Subtotal inunction studies have been conducted with both the cream and the solution. Fifteen grams of Haloprogin Cream (n = 8) and 15 mL of Haloprogin Solution (n = 14) were administered to the entire body for 10 consecutive days. Physical examinations and clinical laboratory tests conducted throughout the study showed no abnormalities. Repeat patch testing for contact sensitization and photosensitivity also were negative.

The following *in vitro* data on Haloprogin are available, but their clinical significance is not known.

Organism (# Strains Tested)	MIC^1 ($\mu g/ml$) Range Found	
Microsporum audouini (2)	< 0.0470 -	0.390
M. canis (2)	< 0.0470 -	0.390
M. gypsum (2)	0.0950 -	0.190
Other *Microsporum* spp (3)	0.0030 -	0.190
Trichophyton mentagrophytes (5)	0.0950 -	0.780
T. rubrum (4)	0.0120 -	0.780
Other *Trichophyton* spp (9)	0.0015 -	0.095
Candida albicans (3)	0.0500 -	0.400
Other *Candida* spp (2)	0.4000 -	0.800
Other Yeasts/yeast-like fungi (8)	0.0500 -	0.400
Staphylococus aureus (5)	1.5600 -	3.120
Streptococcus pyrogenes (3)	0.7800 -	50.000
Other gram pos. organisms (6)	25.00 -	> 100.000
Gram neg. organisms		> 100

^{1} *Minimal Inhibitory Concentration*

INDICATIONS AND USAGE
Haloprogin Cream and Solution are indicated for the treatment of superficial mycotic infections including tinea pedis, tinea cruris, tinea corporis and tinea manulum due to infection with *Tricophyton rubrum, T. tonsurans, T. mentagrophytes, Microsporum canis* and *Epidermophyton flocossum*. Haloprogin also is indicated for the treatment of tinea versicolor caused by *Malassezia furfur*.

CONTRAINDICATIONS
Haloprogin Cream and Solution should not be used by patients known to have hypersensitivity to any of the listed ingredients.

WARNINGS
See *"Contraindications"* and *"Precautions"*.

PRECAUTIONS
General: Treatment with Haloprogin Cream or Solution should be discontinued in case of sensitization or persistent irritation and appropriate therapy instituted. The diagnosis in patients showing no improvement after four weeks of treatment with Haloprogin should be reconsidered.

In mixed infections, where bacteria or nonsusceptible fungi are present, supplementary anti-infective therapy may be indicated.

Information for Patients: Haloprogin is for topical use only.

Contact of this drug with the eyes should be avoided.

Use of Haloprogin should be discontinued and a physician contacted in the event of increased irritation.

In order to minimize the risk of recurrence, use the prescribed medication for the full duration even if symptoms have abated.

Laboratory Tests: KOH preparations of the afflicted areas may be useful to verify the diagnosis of fungal infection prior to treatment. Periodic repeat KOH preparations at 2-week intervals during treatment and at 2-4 weeks after treatment will document the response to the drug. Cultures of specimens from any area which does not respond to treatment for bacteria or fungi may help to elucidate the lack of response.

In the event of a suspected irritation or sensitization, patch testing with components of the formulation used may help verify the reaction and identify its cause.

Carcinogenesis, Mutagenesis, Impairment of Fertility: The carcinogenic potential of Haloprogin in laboratory animals has not been evaluated. Haloprogin was shown to be nonmutagenic in The Ames Salmonella/Microsome Plate Assay.

Pregnancy: Pregnancy Category B: Reproduction studies have been performed in rats and rabbits, each group being given 10 daily topical applications, representing up to 5 times the estimated total human dose needed for a 30-day course of therapy. No evidence of impaired fertility or harm to the fetus due to Haloprogin was revealed. There are, however, no adequate and well-controlled studies in pregnant women. Because animal reproduction studies are not always predictive of human response, this drug should be used during pregnancy only if clearly needed.

Nursing Mothers: It is not known whether this drug is excreted in human milk. Because many drugs are excreted in human milk, caution should be exercised when Haloprogin formulations are applied to a nursing mother.

Pediatric Use: Safety and efficacy studies in children have not been performed.

ADVERSE REACTIONS
In clinical studies with the cream and the solution 26 adverse reactions were noted out of a total 1796 patients treated. These reactions are tabulated below for each formulation.

Reaction	Formulation	
	Cream (n = 977)	Solution (n = 819)
Burning and/or irritation on application	8	14
Erythema and Scaling	1	—
Erythema and Itching	1	—
Folliculitis	1	—
Pruritus and Vesicle Formation	—	1

Reactions noted did not always require interruption of treatment.

▶ SHOWN IN PRODUCT IDENTIFICATION GUIDE

OVERDOSAGE

The oral LD$_{50}$ of Haloprogin is $\geq$ 3000 mg/kg in mice, rats, dogs and rabbits. The maximum Haloprogin in any single package is 300 mg total. There is no experience to allow extrapolation of acute toxicity and expected symptoms in man.

DOSAGE AND ADMINISTRATION

Haloprogin Cream and Solution should be applied liberally to the affected areas twice daily for 2-3 weeks. Intertriginous areas may require 4 weeks of treatment.

HOW SUPPLIED
CREAM:

BRAND/MANUFACTURER	NDC	SIZE	AWP
○ BRAND			
HALOTEX: Westwood-Squibb	00072-7130-15	15 gm	$12.24
	00072-7130-02	30 gm	$21.49

SOLUTION:

BRAND/MANUFACTURER	NDC	SIZE	AWP
○ BRAND			
HALOTEX: Westwood-Squibb	00072-7200-10	10 ml	$11.44
	00072-7200-30	30 ml	$22.98

Halotestin SEE FLUOXYMESTERONE

Halotex SEE HALOPROGIN

Halothane

DESCRIPTION

Halothane, is supplied as a liquid and is vaporized for use as an inhalation anesthetic. It is 2-bromo-2-chloro-1, 1, 1-trifluoro-ethane. Its molecular formula is $C_2HBrClF_3$ The molecular weight is 197.38. The drug substance halothane molecule has an asymmetric carbon atom: the commercial product is a racemic mixture. Resolution of the mixture has not been reported.*

Halothane is miscible with alcohol, chloroform, ether, and other fat solvents.

The specific gravity is 1.872-1.877 at 20°C, and the boiling point (range) is 49°C-51°C at 760 mm Hg. The vapor pressure is 243 mm Hg at 20°C. The blood/gas coefficient is 2.5 at 37°C, and the olive oil/water coefficient is 220 at 37°C. Vapor concentrations within anesthetic range are nonirritating and have a pleasant odor.

Halothane is nonflammable, and its vapors mixed with oxygen in proportions from 0.5 to 50% (v/v) are not explosive.

Halothane does not decompose in contact with warm soda lime. When moisture is present, the vapor attacks aluminum, brass, and lead, but not copper. Rubber, some plastics and similar materials are soluble in Halothane; such materials will deteriorate rapidly in contact with Halothane vapor or liquid. Stability of Halothane is maintained by the addition of 0.01% thymol (w/w), up to 0.00025% ammonia (w/w).

Following is its chemical structure:

$$\begin{array}{c} Br \quad F \\ | \quad\quad | \\ H-C-C-F \\ | \quad\quad | \\ Cl \quad F \end{array}$$

CLINICAL PHARMACOLOGY

Halothane is an inhalation anesthetic. Induction and recovery are rapid, and depth of anesthesia can be rapidly altered.

Halothane progressively depresses respiration. There may be tachypnea with reduced tidal volume and alveolar ventilation. Halothane is not an irritant to the respiratory tract, and no increase in salivary or bronchial secretions ordinarily occurs. Pharyngeal and laryngeal reflexes are rapidly obtunded. It causes bronchodilation. Hypoxia, acidosis, or apnea, may develop during deep anesthesia.

Halothane reduces the blood pressure and frequently decreases the pulse rate. The greater the concentration of the drug, the more evident these changes become. Atropine may reverse the bradycardia. Halothane does not cause the release of catecholamines from adrenergic stores.

Halothane also causes dilation of the vessels of the skin and skeletal muscles.

Cardiac arrhythmias may occur during Halothane anesthesia. These include nodal rhythm, AV dissociation, ventricular extrasystoles and asystole. Halothane sensitizes the myocardial conduction system to the action of epinephrine and norepinephrine, and the combination may cause serious cardiac arrhythmias. Halothane increases cerebrospinal-fluid pressure. Halothane produces moderate muscular relaxation. Muscle relaxants are used as adjuncts in order to maintain

---

* Klaus Florey, editor, Analytical Profiles of Drug Substances, Vol. 1, page 127, (1972).

lighter levels of anesthesia. Halothane augments the action of nondeplorizing relaxants and ganglionic blocking agents. Halothane is a potent uterine relaxant.

The mechanism(s) whereby Halothane and other subtances induce general anesthesia is unknown. Halothane is a very potent anesthetic in humans, with a minimum alveolar concentration (MAC) determined to be 0.64%. The MAC has been found to decrease with age (see MAC table in "Dosage and Administration").

INDICATIONS AND USAGE

Halothane is indicated for the induction and maintenance of general anesthesia.

CONTRAINDICATIONS

Halothane is not recommended for obstetrical anesthesia except when uterine relaxation is required.

WARNINGS

When previous exposure to Halothane was followed by unexplained hepatic dysfunction and/or jaundice, consideration should be given to the use of other agents.

PRECAUTIONS
GENERAL

Halothane should be used in vaporizers that permit a reasonable approximation of output, and preferably of the calibrated type. The vaporizer should be placed out of circuit in closed-circuit rebreathing systems; otherwise, overdosage is difficult to avoid. The patient should be closely observed for signs of overdosage, i.e., depression of blood pressure, pulse rate, and ventilation, particularly during assisted or controlled ventilation.

Halothane increases cerebrospinal-fluid pressure. Therefore, in patients with markedly raised intracranial pressure, if Halothane is indicated, administration should be preceded by measures ordinarily used to reduce cerebrospinal-fluid pressure. Ventilation should be carefully assessed, and it may be necessary to assist or control ventilation to ensure adequate oxygenation and carbon dioxide removal.

In susceptible individuals, Halothane anesthesia may trigger a skeletal-muscle hypermetabolic state leading to a high oxygen demand and the clinical syndrome known as malignant hyperthermia. The syndrome includes nonspecific features such as muscle rigidity, tachycardia, tachypnea, cyanosis, arrhythmias, and unstable blood pressure. (It should also be noted that many of these nonspecific signs may appear with light anesthesia, acute hypoxia, etc.) An increase in overall metabolism may be reflected in an elevated temperature (which may rise rapidly, early or late in the case, but usually is not the first sign of augmented metabolism) and an increased usage of the CO_2 absorption system (hot canister). PaO$_2$ and pH may decrease, and hyperkalemia and a base deficit may appear. Treatment includes discontinuance of triggering agents (e.g., Halothane), administration of intravenous dantrolene, and application of supportive therapy. Such therapy includes vigorous efforts to restore body temperature to normal, respiratory and circulatory support as indicated, and management of electrolyte-fluid-acid-base derangements. Renal failure may appear later, and urine flow should be sustained if possible. It should be noted that the syndrome of malignant hyperthermia secondary to Halothane appears to be rare.

INFORMATION FOR PATIENTS

When appropriate, as in some cases where discharge is anticipated soon after general anesthesia, patients should be cautioned not to drive automobiles, operate hazardous machinery, or engage in hazardous sports for 24 hours or more (depending on the total dose of Halothane condition of the patient, and consideration given to other drugs administered after anesthesia).

DRUG INTERACTIONS

Epinephrine or norepinephrine should be employed cautiously, if at all, during Halothane anesthesia since their simultaneous use may induce ventricular tachycardia or fibrillation.

Nondepolarizing relaxants and ganglionic-blocking agents should be administered cautiously, since their actions are augmented by Halothane.

Clinical experience and animal experiments suggest that pancuronium should be given with caution to patients receiving chronic tricyclic antidepressant therapy who are anesthetized with Halothane because severe ventricular arrhythmias may result from such usage.

CARCINOGENESIS, MUTAGENESIS, IMPAIRMENT OF FERTILITY

An 18-month inhalational carcinogenicity study of Halothane at 0.05% in the mouse revealed no evidence of anesthetic-related carcinogenicity. This concentration is equivalent to 24 hours of 1% Halothane.

Mutagenesis testing of Halothane revealed both positive and negative results. In the rat, one-year exposure to trace concentrations of Halothane (1 and 10 ppm) and nitrous oxide produced chromosomal damage to spermatogonia cells and bone marrow cells. Negative mutagenesis tests included: Ames bacterial assay, Chinese hamster lung fibroblast assay, sister chromatid exchange in Chinese hamster ovary cells, and human leukocyte culture assay.

Reproduction studies of Halothane (10 ppm) and nitrous oxide in the rat caused decreased fertility. This trace concentration corresponds to 1/1000 the human maintenance dose.

PREGNANCY

Teratogenic Effects: Pregnancy Category C. Some studies have shown Halothane to be teratogenic, embryotoxic, and fetotoxic in the mouse, rat, hamster, and rabbit at subanesthetic and/or anesthetic concentrations. There are no adequate

---

and well-controlled studies in pregnant women. Halothane should be used during pregnancy only if the potential benefit justifies the potential risk to the fetus.

LABOR AND DELIVERY
The uterine relaxation obtained with Halothane, unless carefully controlled, may fail to respond to ergot derivatives and oxytocic posterior pituitary extract.

NURSING MOTHERS
It is not known whether this drug is excreted in human milk. Because many drugs are excreted in human milk, caution should be exercised when Halothane is administered to a nursing woman.

PEDIATRIC USE
Extensive clinical experience reveals that maintenance concentrations of Halothane are generally higher in infants and children, and that maintenance requirements decrease with age. (See MAC table, based upon age, in *"Dosage And Administration"*.)

ADVERSE REACTIONS
The following adverse reactions have been reported: mild, moderate, and severe hepatic dysfunction (including hepatic necrosis): cardiac arrest; hypotension; respiratory arrest; cardiac arrhythmias; hyperpyrexia; shivering; nausea; and emesis.

OVERDOSAGE
In the event of overdosage, or what may appear to be overdosage, drug administration should be stopped, and assisted or controlled ventilation with pure oxygen initiated.

DOSAGE AND ADMINISTRATION
Halothane may be administered by the nonrebreathing technique, partial rebreathing, or closed technique. The induction dose varies from patient to patient but is usually within the range of 0.5% to 3%. The maintenance dose varies from 0.5% to 1.5%.

Halothane may be administered with either oxygen or a mixture of oxygen and nitrous oxide.

Halothane should not be kept indefinitely in vaporizer bottles not specifically designed for its use. Thymol does not volatilize along with Halothane and, therefore, accumulates in the vaporizer and may, in time, impart a yellow color to the remaining liquid or to wicks in vaporizers. The development of such discoloration may be used as an indicator that the vaporizer should be drained and cleaned and the discolored Halothane discarded. Accumulation of thymol may be removed by washing with diethyl ether. After cleaning a wick or vaporizer, make certain all the diethyl ether has been removed before reusing the equipment to avoid introducing ether into the system.

Because of the more rapid uptake of Halothane and the increased blood concentration required for anesthesia in younger patients, the minimum alveolar concentration (MAC)[1] values will decrease with age as follows:

Age	MAC %
Infants	1.08
3 yrs.	0.91
10 yrs.	0.87
15 yrs.	0.92
24 yrs.	0.84
42 yrs.	0.76
81 yrs.	0.64

Store at room temperature (approximately 25°C) in a tight, closed container. Protect from light.

HOW SUPPLIED
LIQUID:
AVERAGE UNIT PRICE (AVAILABLE SIZES)

BRAND			$0.34
BRAND/MANUFACTURER	NDC	SIZE	AWP
◆ BRAND			
FLUOTHANE: Wyeth-Ayerst	00046-3125-81	125 ml	$43.55
	00046-3125-82	250 ml	$84.29
◆ GENERICS			
Abbott Hosp	00074-4894-02	250 ml 12s	$1338.79

Harmonyl *SEE* DESERPIDINE

H-BIG *SEE* HEPATITIS B IMMUNE GLOBULIN (HUMAN)

Healon *SEE* SODIUM HYALURONATE

Helixate *SEE* ANTIHEMOPHILIC FACTOR

Hemabate *SEE* CARBOPROST TROMETHAMINE

Hemin

> HEMIN SHOULD ONLY BE USED BY PHYSICIANS EXPERIENCED IN THE MANAGEMENT OF PORPHYRIAS IN HOSPITALS WHERE THE RECOMMENDED CLINICAL AND LABORATORY DIAGNOSTIC AND MONITORING TECHNIQUES ARE AVAILABLE.
>
> HEMIN THERAPY SHOULD BE CONSIDERED AFTER AN APPROPRIATE PERIOD OF ALTERNATE THERAPY (I.E., 400 G GLUCOSE/DAY FOR 1 TO 2 DAYS). (SEE *"WARNINGS"*, *"PRECAUTIONS"* AND *"DOSAGE AND ADMINISTRATION"* SECTION).

DESCRIPTION
Hemin is an enzyme inhibitor derived from processed red blood cells. Hemin for injection was known previously as hematin. The term hematin has been used to describe the chemical reaction product of Hemin and sodium carbonate solution. Hemin is an iron containing metalloporphyrin. Chemically, Hemin is represented as chloro[7,12-diethenyl-3,8,13,17-tetramethyl-21H,23H-porphine-2, 18-dipropanoato (2-)-N^{21},N^{22},N^{23},N^{24}] iron.

Hemin is a sterile, lyophilized powder suitable for intravenous administration after reconstitution. Each dispensing vial of Hemin contains the equivalent of 313 mg Hemin, 215 mg sodium carbonate and 300 mg of sorbitol. The pH may have been adjusted with hydrochloric acid. When mixed as directed with Sterile Water for Injection, USP, each 43 mL provides the equivalent of approximately 301 mg Hemin (7 mg/mL).

Following is its chemical structure:

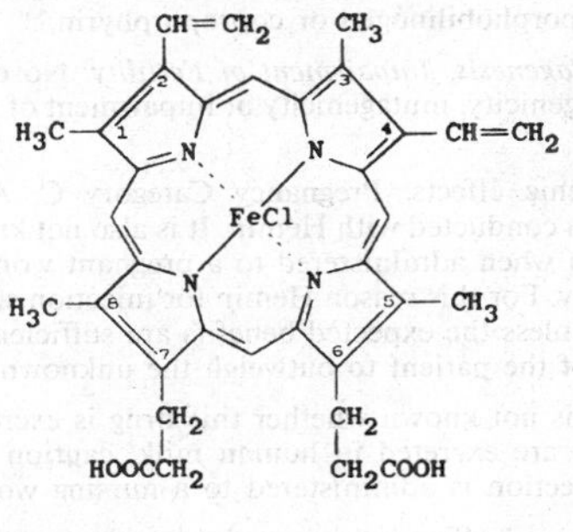

CLINICAL PHARMACOLOGY
Hemin acts to limit the hepatic and/or marrow synthesis of porphyrin. This action is likely due to the inhibition of delta-aminolevulinic acid synthetase, the enzyme which limits the rate of the porphyrin/heme biosynthetic pathway. The exact mechanism by which Hemin produces symptomatic improvement in patients with acute episodes of the hepatic porphyrias has not been elucidated.[1,9]

Following intravenous administration of Hemin in nonjaundiced human patients, an increase in fecal urobilinogen can be observed which is roughly proportional to the amount of Hemin administered. This suggests an enterohepatic pathway as at least one route of elimination. Bilirubin metabolites are also excreted in the urine following Hemin injections.[2]

Hemin therapy for the acute porphyrias is not curative. After discontinuation Hemin treatment, symptoms generally return although in some cases remission is prolonged. Some neurological symptoms have improved weeks to months after therapy although little or no response was noted at the time of treatment.

Other aspects of human pharmacokinetics have not been defined.

INDICATIONS AND USAGE
Hemin is indicated for the amelioration of recurrent attacks of acute intermittent porphyria temporarily related to the menstrual cycle in susceptible women.

Manifestations such as pain, hypertension, tachycardia, abnormal mental status and mild to progressive neurologic signs may be controlled in selected patients with this disorder.

Similar findings have been reported in other patients with acute intermittent porphyria, porphyria variegata and hereditary coproporphyria. Hemin is not indicated in porphyria cutanea tarda.

UNLABELED USES
Hemin is used alone or as an adjunct in the treatment of hepatic porphyria.

CONTRAINDICATIONS
Hemin for injection is contraindicated in patients with known hypersensitivity to this drug.

➤ SHOWN IN PRODUCT IDENTIFICATION GUIDE

WARNINGS

Hemin therapy is intended to limit the rate of porphyria/heme biosynthesis possibly by inhibiting the enzyme delta-aminolevulinic acid synthetase. For this reason, drugs such as estrogens, barbituric acid derivatives and steroid metabolites which increase the activity of delta-aminolevulinic acid synthetase should be avoided.

Also, because Hemin has exhibited transient, mild anticoagulant effects during clinical studies, concurrent anticoagulant therapy should be avoided.[9] The extent and duration of the hypocoagulable state induced by Hemin has not been established.

PRECAUTIONS

General: Clinical benefit from Hemin depends on prompt administration. Attacks of porphyria may progress to a point where irreversible neuronal damage has occurred. Hemin therapy is intended to prevent an attack from reaching the critical stage of neuronal degeneration. Hemin is not effective in repairing neuronal damage.[9]

Recommended dosage guidelines should be strictly followed. Reversible renal shutdown has been observed in a case where an excessive Hemin dose (12.2 mg/kg) was administered in a single infusion. Oliguria and increased nitrogen retention occurred although the patient remained asymptomatic.[4] No worsening of renal function has been seen with administration of recommended dosages of Hemin.[9]

A large arm vein or a central venous catheter should be utilized for the administration of Hemin for injection to avoid the possibility of phlebitis.

Since reconstituted Hemin is not transparent, any undissolved particulate matter is difficult to see when inspected visually. Therefore, terminal filtration through a sterile 0.45 micron or smaller filter is recommended.

Tests for Diagnosis and Monitoring of Therapy: Before Hemin therapy is begun, the presence of acute porphyria must be diagnosed using the following criteria:[9]
 a. Presence of clinical symptoms.
 b. Positive Watson-Schwartz or Hoesch test. (A negative Watson-Schwartz or Hoesch test indicates a porphyric attack is highly unlikely. When in doubt quantitative measures of delta-aminolevulinic acid and porphobilinogen in serum or urine may aid in diagnosis.)

Urinary concentrations of the following compounds may be *monitored* during Hemin therapy. Drug effect will be demonstrated by a decrease in one or more of the following compounds.[3-6] ALA—delta-aminolevulinic acid, UPG —uroporphyrinogen, PBG—porphobilinogen or coproporphyrin.

Carcinogenesis, Mutagenesis, Impairment of Fertility: No data are available on potential for carcinogenicity, mutagenicity or impairment of fertility in animals or humans.

Pregnancy: Teratogenic effects: Pregnancy Category C. Animal reproduction studies have not been conducted with Hemin. It is also not known whether Hemin can cause fetal harm when administered to a pregnant woman unless the affect reproduction capacity. For this reason Hemin for injection should not be given to a pregnant woman unless the expected benefits are sufficiently important to the health and welfare of the patient to outweigh the unknown hazard to the fetus.

Nursing Mothers: It is not known whether this drug is excreted in human milk. Because many drugs are excreted in human milk, caution should be exercised when Hemin for Injection is administered to a nursing woman.

Pediatric Use: Safety and effectiveness in children have not been established.

ADVERSE REACTIONS

Reversible renal shutdown has occurred with administration of excessive doses (see "*Precautions*" section).

Phlebitis with or without leucocytosis and with or without mild pyrexia has occurred after administration of Hemin through small arm veins.

There has been one report in the literature[8] of coagulopathy occurring in a patient receiving Hemin therapy. This patient exhibited prolonged prothrombin time and partial thromboplastin time, thrombocytopenia, mild hypofibrinogenemia, mild elevation of fibrin split products and a 10% fall in hematocrit.

OVERDOSAGE

Reversible renal shutdown has been observed in a case where an excessive Hemin dose (12.2 mg/kg) was administered in a single infusion. Treatment of this case consisted of ethacrynic acid and mannitol.[7]

DOSAGE AND ADMINISTRATION

Before administering Hemin for injection, an appropriate period of alternate therapy (i.e., 400 g glucose/day for 1 or 2 days) must be considered. If improvement is unsatisfactory for the treatment of acute attacks of porphyria, an intravenous infusion of Hemin containing a dose of 1 to 4 mg/kg/day of Hemin should be given over a period of 10 to 15 minutes for 3 to 14 days based on the clinical signs. In more severe cases this dose may be repeated no earlier than every 12 hours. No more than 6 mg/kg of Hemin should be given in any 24-hour period.

After reconstitution each mL of Hemin contains the equivalent of approximately 7 mg of Hemin. The drug may be administered directly from the vial.

DOSAGE CALCULATION TABLE

1 mg Hematin equivalent	= 0.14 mL Hemin
2 mg Hematin equivalent	= 0.28 mL Hemin
3 mg Hematin equivalent	= 0.42 ml Hemin
4 mg Hematin equivalent	= 0.56 mL Hemin

Since reconstitute Hemin is not transparent, any undissolved particulate matter is difficult to see when inspected visually. Therefore, terminal filtration through a sterile 0.45 micron or smaller filter is recommended.

Preparation of Solution: Reconstitute Hemin by aseptically adding 43 mL of Sterile Water for Injection, USP, to the dispensing vial. Immediately after adding diluent, the product should be shaken well for a period of 2 to 3 minutes to aid dissolution. *Note:* **Because Hemin contains no preservative and because Hemin undergoes rapid chemical decomposition in solution, it should not be reconstituted until immediately before use. After the first withdrawal from the vial, any solution remaining must be discarded.**

No drug or chemical agent should be added to a Hemin fluid admixture unless its effect on the chemical and physical stability has first been determined.

REFERENCES

1. Bickers, D., Treatment of the Porphyrias: Mechanisms of Action, *J Invest Dermatol* 77(1):107-113, 1981. 2. Watson, C.J., Hematin and Porphyria, editorial, *N Engl J Med* 293(12):605-607, September 18, 1975. 3. Lamon, J. M., Hematin Therapy for Acute Porphyria, *Medicine* 58(3):252-269, 1979. 4. Dhar, G.J., et al., Effects of Hematin in Hepatic Porphyria, *Ann Intern Med* 83:20-30,1975. 5. Watson, C.J., et al., Use of Hematin in the Acute Attack of the "Inducible" Hepatic Porphyrias, *Adv Intern Med* 23:265-286, 1978. 6. McColl, K.E., et al., Treatment with Hematin in Acute Hepatic Porphyria, *Q J Med*, New Series L (198):161-174, Spring, 1981. 7. Dhar, G.J., et al., Transitory Renal Failure Following Rapid Administration of a Relatively Large Amount of Hematin in a Patient with Acute International Porphyria in Clinical Remission, *Acta Med Scand* 203:437 443, 1978. 8. Morris, D.L., et al., Coagulopathy Associated with Hematin Treatment for Acute Intermittent Porphyria, *Ann Intern Med* 95:700-701, 1981. 9. Pierach, C.A., Hematin Therapy for the Porphyric Attack, *Semin Liver Dis* 2(2):125-131 May, 1982.

HOW SUPPLIED
POWDER FOR INJECTION: 313 MG

BRAND/MANUFACTURER	NDC	SIZE	AWP
BRAND			
PANHEMATIN: Abbott Pharm	00074-2000-43	1s	$255.53

Hemo-Pad *SEE* COLLAGEN HEMOSTAT

Hemophilus b Conjugate Vaccine (Tetanus Toxoid Conjugate)

DESCRIPTION

Hemophilus b Conjugate Vaccine (Tetanus Toxoid Conjugate), produced by Pasteur Mérieux Sérums & Vaccins S.A., for intramuscular use, is a sterile, lyophilized powder which is reconstituted at the time of use with saline diluent (0.4% Sodium Chloride). The vaccine consists of the Hemophilus b polysaccharide, a high molecular weight polymer prepared from the *Hemophilus influenzae* type b strain 1482 grown in a semi-synthetic medium, covalently bound to tetanus toxoid.[1] The lyophilized powder and saline diluent contain no preservatives. Each single dose of 0.5 mL is formulated to contain 10 μg of purified capsular polysaccharide, 24 μg of tetanus toxoid and 8.5% of sucrose. The tetanus toxoid is prepared by extraction, ammonium sulfate purification, and formalin inactivation of the toxin from cultures of *Clostridium tetani* (Harvard strain) grown in a modified Mueller and Miller medium.[2] The toxoid is filter sterilized prior to the conjugation process. Potency of Hemophilus b Conjugate Vaccine (Tetanus Toxoid Conjugate) is specified on each lot by limits on the content of PRP polysaccharide and protein in each dose and the proportion of polysaccharide and protein in the vaccine which is characterized as high molecular weight conjugate. The reconstituted vaccine is clear and colorless.

CLINICAL PHARMACOLOGY

H influenzae type b was the leading cause of invasive bacterial disease among children in the United States prior licensing of Hemophilus b Conjugate Vaccines. Based on its active surveillance areas, the Centers for Disease Control and Prevention (CDC) now estimate that *H influenzae* type b disease in children under the age of 5 years has been reduced by 95%.[3] Before effective vaccines were introduced, it was estimated that one in 200 children developed invasive *H influenzae* type b disease by the age of 5 years. In children less than 5 years of age, the mortality rate for invasive *H influenzae* type b disease ranged between 3% and 6%.[3] In more than 60% of these children, meningitis was the clinical syndrome and permanent sequelae ranging from mild hearing loss to mental retardation affecting 20% to 30% of all survivors.[3] Ninety-five percent of the cases of invasive *H influenzae* disease among children < 5 years of age were caused by organisms with the type b polysaccharide capsule. Approximately two-thirds of all cases of invasive *H influenzae* type b disease affected infants and children < 15 months of age, a group for which a vaccine was not available until late 1990.[4,5]

Incidence rates of invasive *H influenzae* type b disease have been shown to be increased in certain high-risk groups, such as native Americans (both American Indians and Eskimos), blacks, individuals of lower socioeconomic status, and patients with asplenia, sickle cell disease, Hodgkin's disease, and antibody deficiency syndromes.[5,6] Studies also have suggested that the risk of acquiring primary invasive *H influenzae* type b disease for children under 5 years of age appears to be greater for those who attend day-care facilities.[7,8,9,10]

◆ RATED THERAPEUTICALLY EQUIVALENT; ◇ THERAPEUTIC EQUIVALENCE UNCONFIRMED; ○ UNRATED

The potential for person to person transmission of the organism among susceptible individuals has been recognized. Studies of secondary spread of disease in household contacts of index patients have shown a substantially increased risk among exposed household contacts under 4 years of age.[11] Adults can be colonized with *H influenzae* type b from children infected with the organisms.[12]

The response to Hemophilus b Conjugate Vaccine (Tetanus Toxoid Conjugate) is typical of a T-dependent immune response to antigen. The predominant isotype of anticapsular polysaccharide (polyribosyl-ribitol-phosphate or PRP) antibody induced by Hemophilus b Conjugate Vaccine (Tetanus Toxoid Conjugate) is IgG.[13] A substantial booster response has been demonstrated in children 12 months of age or older who previously received two or three doses. Bactericidal activity against *H influenzae* type b is demonstrated in serum after immunization and statistically correlates with the anti-PRP antibody response induced by Hemophilus b Conjugate Vaccine (Tetanus Toxoid Conjugate).[14]

Antibody to *H influenzae* capsular polysaccharide (anti-PRP) titers of > 1.0 µg/mL following vaccination with unconjugated PRP vaccine correlated with long-term protection against invasive *H influenzae* type b disease in children older than 24 months of age.[15] Although the relevance of this threshold to clinical protection after immunization with conjugate vaccines is not known, particularly in light of the induced, immunologic memory, this level continues to be considered as indicative of long-term protection.[4] The immunogenicity and safety of Hemophilus b Conjugate Vaccine (Tetanus Toxoid Conjugate) has been demonstrated in the United States and worldwide. Hemophilus b Conjugate Vaccine (Tetanus Toxoid Conjugate) induced, on average anti-PRP levels ≥ 1.0 µg/mL in 90% of infants after a booster dose.[14]

Two clinical trials supported by the National Institute of Health (NIH) have compared the anti-PRP antibody responses to three Hemophilus b Conjugate Vaccines in a racially mixed population of children. These studies were done in Tennessee[16] (Table 1) and in Minnesota, Missouri and Texas[17] (Table 2) in infants immunized with Hemophilus b Conjugate Vaccine (Tetanus Toxoid Conjugate) and other Hemophilus b Conjugate vaccines at 2, 4 and 6 months of age. All Hemophilus b Conjugate vaccines were administered concomitantly with Poliovirus Vaccine Live Oral and DTP vaccines at separate sites. (See related tables).

N/A Not applicable in this comparison trial although third dose data have been published.[16,17]

Native American populations have high rates of *H influenzae* type b disease and have been observed to have low immune responses to Hemophilus b Conjugate Vaccines. Following three doses of Hemophilus b Conjugate Vaccine (Tetanus Toxoid Conjugate) at six weeks, four and six months of age, 75% of Native Americans in Alaska showed an anti-PRP antibody titer of ≥ 1.0 µg/mL.[18]

In three U.S. trials in 12- to 15-month-old children and one trial in 17- to 24-month-old children who had not previously received Hemophilus b Conjugate vaccination, a single dose of Hemophilus b Conjugate Vaccine (Tetanus Toxoid Conjugate) produced an anti-PRP antibody response comparable to those seen after three doses were administered in infants (Table 3).[18]

Table 3[18]

ANTI-PRP ANTIBODY RESPONSES IN 12- TO 24-MONTH-OLD CHILDREN IMMUNIZED WITH A SINGLE DOSE OF HEMOPHILUS B CONJUGATE VACCINE (TETANUS TOXOID CONJUGATE)

Age Group	N	GMT (µg/mL)		% Subjects Responding with ≥ 1.0 µg/mL	
		Pre	Post	Pre	Post
12 to 15 months	256	0.06	5.12	1.6	90.2
17 to 24 months	81	0.10	4.4	3.7	18.5

These trials demonstrated that Hemophilus b Conjugate Vaccine (Tetanus Toxoid Conjugate) consistently conferred an anti-PRP antibody response previously shown to correlate with protection, when administered either as a regimen of three doses at least four to eight weeks apart in infants 2 to 6 months of age or as a single dose in children 12 months of age and older.[18]

Hemophilus b Conjugate Vaccine (Tetanus Toxoid Conjugate) has been found to be immunogenic in children with sickle cell anemia, a condition which may cause increased susceptibility to Hemophilus b disease. Two doses of Hemophilus b Conjugate Vaccine (Tetanus Toxoid Conjugate) given at two month intervals induced anti-PRP antibody titers of > 1.0 µg/mL in 89% of these children with a mean age of 11 months. This is comparable to anti-PRP antibody levels demonstrated in normal children of similar age following two doses of Hemophilus b Conjugate Vaccine (Tetanus Toxoid Conjugate).[19]

Although Hemophilus b Conjugate Vaccine (Tetanus Toxoid Conjugate) produces an antibody response to tetanus toxoid, data do not exist to substantiate the correlation of this response with protection against tetanus. IMMUNIZATION WITH HEMOPHILUS B CONJUGATE VACCINE (TETANUS TOXOID CONJUGATE) ALONE DOES NOT SUBSTITUTE FOR ROUTINE TETANUS IMMUNIZATION.

INDICATIONS AND USAGE

Hemophilus b Conjugate Vaccine (Tetanus Toxoid Conjugate) is indicated for the active immunization of infants and children 2 months through 5 years of age for the prevention of invasive disease caused by *H influenzae* type b.

Antibody levels associated with protection may not be achieved earlier than two weeks following the last recommended dose.

As with any vaccine, vaccination with Hemophilus b Conjugate Vaccine (Tetanus Toxoid Conjugate) may not protect 100% of susceptible individuals.

CONTRAINDICATIONS

HEMOPHILUS B CONJUGATE VACCINE (TETANUS TOXOID CONJUGATE) IS CONTRAINDICATED IN CHILDREN WITH A HISTORY OF HYPERSENSITIVITY TO ANY COMPONENT OF THIS VACCINE, INCLUDING TETANUS TOXOID.

Table 1[16]
ANTI-PRP ANTIBODY RESPONSES IN 2-MONTH-OLD INFANTS NIH TRIAL IN TENNESSEE

Vaccine	N*	GEOMETRIC MEAN TITER (GMT) (µg/mL)			POST THIRD IMMUNIZATION
		Pre-Immunization	Post Second Immunization	Post Third Immunization	% ≥ 1.0 µg/mL
PRP-T†	65	0.10	0.30	3.64	83%
PRP-OMP△	64	0.11	0.84	N/A	50%**
HbOC‡	61	0.07	0.13	3.08	75%

Table 2[17]
ANTI-PRP ANTIBODY RESPONSES IN 2-MONTH-OLD INFANTS NIH TRIAL IN MINNESOTA, MISSOURI AND TEXAS

Vaccine	N*	GEOMETRIC MEAN TITER (GMT) (µg/mL)			POST THIRD § IMMUNIZATION
		Pre-Immunization	Post Second Immunization	Post Third§ Immunization	% ≥ 1.0 µg/mL
PRP-T†	142	0.25	1.25	6.37	97%
PRP-OMP△	149	0.18	4.00	N/A	85%**
HbOC§	167	0.17	0.45	6.31	90%

* N = Number of Children
§ Sera were obtained after the third dose from 86 and 110 infants, in PRP-T and HbOC vaccine groups, respectively.
† Hemophilus b Conjugate Vaccine (Tetanus Toxoid Conjugate)
△ Hemophilus b Conjugate Vaccine (Meningococcal Protein Conjugate)
** Seroconversion after the recommended 2-dose primary immunization series is shown.
‡ Hemophilus b Conjugate Vaccine (Diptheria CRM$_{197}$ Protein Conjugate)

➤ SHOWN IN PRODUCT IDENTIFICATION GUIDE

WARNINGS

If Hemophilus b Conjugate Vaccine (Tetanus Toxoid Conjugate) is administered to immunosuppressed persons or persons receiving immunosuppressive therapy, the expected antibody response may not be obtained. This includes patients with asymptomatic or symptomatic HIV-infection,[20] severe combined immunodeficiency, hypogammaglobulinemia, or agammaglobulinemia; altered immune states due to diseases such as leukemia, lymphoma, or generalized malignancy; or an immune system compromised by treatment with corticosteroids, alkylating drugs, antimetabolites or radiation.[21]

IMMUNIZATION WITH HEMOPHILUS B CONJUGATE VACCINE (TETANUS TOXOID CONJUGATE) ALONE DOES NOT SUBSTITUTE FOR ROUTINE TETANUS IMMUNIZATION.

PRECAUTIONS

GENERAL

Epinephrine Injection (1:0000) Must Be Immediately Available Should An Anaphylactic Or Other Allergic Reaction Occur Due To Any Component Of The Vaccine.

Prior to an injection of any vaccine, all known precautions should be taken to prevent adverse reactions. This includes a review of the patient's history with respect to possible hypersensitivity to this vaccine or similar vaccines. The healthcare provider should ask the parent or guardian about the recent health status of the infant or child to be immunized including the infant's or child's previous immunization history prior to administration of Hemophilus b Conjugate Vaccine (Tetanus Toxoid Conjugate).

Any acute infection or febrile illness is reason for delaying use of Hemophilus b Conjugate Vaccine (Tetanus Toxoid Conjugate) except when in the opinion of the physician, withholding the vaccine entails a greater risk.

As reported with Hemophilus b polysaccharide vaccines,[22] cases of *H influenzae* type b disease may occur subsequent to vaccination and prior to the onset of protective effects of the vaccine.[18] (See *"Indications and Usage"* section).

Antigenuria has been detected in some instances following receipt of Hemophilus b Conjugate Vaccine (Tetanus Toxoid Conjugate); therefore, urine antigen detection may not have definitive diagnostic value in suspected *H influenzae* type b disease within one week of immunization.[23]

Special care should be taken to ensure that Hemophilus b Conjugate Vaccine (Tetanus Toxoid Conjugate) is not injected into a blood vessel.

Administration of Hemophilus b Conjugate Vaccine (Tetanus Toxoid Conjugate) is not contraindicated in individuals with an HIV infection.[21]

A separate, sterile syringe and needle or a sterile disposable unit should be used for each patient to prevent transmission of hepatitis or other infectious agents from person to person. Needles should not be recapped and should be properly disposed.

INFORMATION FOR PATIENT

The health-care provider should inform the parent or guardian of the benefits and risks of the vaccine.

The physician should inform the parent or guardian about the significant adverse reactions that have been temporally associated with Hemophilus b Conjugate Vaccine (Tetanus Toxoid Conjugate) administration. The parent or guardian should be instructed to report any serious adverse reactions to the health-care provider.

As part of the child's immunization record, the date, lot number and manufacturer of the vaccine administered should be recorded.[24,25,26]

The U.S. Department of Health and Human Services has established a new Vaccine Adverse Event Reporting System (VAERS) to accept all reports of suspected adverse events after the administration of any vaccine, including but not limited to the reporting of events required by the National Childhood Vaccine Injury Act of 1986.[24] The toll-free number for VAERS forms and information is 1-800-822-7967.

The National Vaccine Injury Compensation Program, established by the National Childhood Vaccine Injury Act of 1986, requires physicians and other health-care providers who administer vaccines to maintain permanent vaccination records and to report occurrences of certain adverse events to the U.S. Department of Health and Human Services. Reportable events include those listed in the Act for each vaccine and events specified in the package insert as contraindications to further doses of the vaccine.[25,26]

The health-care provider should inform the parent or guardian of the importance of completing the immunization series. The health-care provider should provide the Vaccine Information Materials (VIMs) which are required to be given with each immunization.

DRUG INTERACTIONS

There are no known interactions of Hemophilus b Conjugate Vaccine (Tetanus Toxoid Conjugate) with drugs or foods.

In clinical trials, Hemophilus b Conjugate Vaccine (Tetanus Toxoid Conjugate) was routinely administered, at separate sites, concomitantly with one or more of the following vaccines: DTP vaccine, Poliovirus Vaccine Live Oral, Measles, Mumps and Rubella vaccine (MMR), Hepatitis B vaccine and occasionally Inactivated Polio Vaccine (IPV). No significant impairment of the antibody response to any antigen was observed in three clinical trials when Connaught Laboratories, Inc. (CLI) DTP vaccine was given concurrently with Hemophilus b Conjugate Vaccine (Tetanus Toxoid Conjugate) at separate sites.[18] Interference with the antibody response to the pertussis component has been suggested with a DTP vaccine unlicensed in the U.S.[27] No impairment of the antibody response to the individual antigens was demonstrated when Hemophilus b Conjugate Vaccine (Tetanus Toxoid Conjugate) was given at the same time, at separate sites, with

Inactivated Polio Vaccine (IPV) or Measles, Mumps and Rubella vaccine (MMR).[18] In addition, more than 47,000 infants in Finland have received a third dose of Hemophilus b Conjugate Vaccine (Tetanus Toxoid Conjugate) concomitantly with MMR vaccine.[18] No data are available on the antibody response to OPV or Hepatitis B vaccines when given concurrently with Hemophilus b Conjugate Vaccine (Tetanus Toxoid Conjugate).

CARCINOGENESIS, MUTAGENESIS, IMPAIRMENT OF FERTILITY

Hemophilus b Conjugate Vaccine (Tetanus Toxoid Conjugate) has not been evaluated for its carcinogenic, mutagenic potential or impairment of fertility.

PREGNANCY

Reproductive Studies: Pregnancy Category C: Animal reproduction studies have not been conducted with Hemophilus b Conjugate Vaccine (Tetanus Toxoid Conjugate). It is also not known whether Hemophilus b Conjugate Vaccine (Tetanus Toxoid Conjugate) can cause fetal harm when administered to a pregnant woman or can affect reproduction capacity. Hemophilus b Conjugate Vaccine (Tetanus Toxoid Conjugate) is NOT recommended for use in a pregnant woman.

PEDIATRIC USE

Safety And Effectiveness Of Hemophilus B Conjugate Vaccine (Tetanus Toxoid Conjugate) In Infants Below The Age Of Six Weeks Have Not Been Established. (See *"Dosage and Administration"* section.)

ADVERSE REACTIONS

More than 7,000 infants and young children ($\leq$ 2 years of age) have received at least one dose of Hemophilus b Conjugate Vaccine (Tetanus Toxoid Conjugate) during U.S. clinical trials. Of these, 1,064 subjects 12 to 24 months of age who received Hemophilus b Conjugate Vaccine (Tetanus Toxoid Conjugate) alone reported no serious or life threatening adverse reactions.

Summarized in Table 4 are adverse reactions temporally associated with Hemophilus b Conjugate Vaccine (Tetanus Toxoid Conjugate) immunizations in 188 subjects 12 to 15 months of age.[18]

Table 4[18]

PERCENTAGE OF 12- TO 15-MONTH-OLD CHILDREN PRESENTING WITH LOCAL OR SYSTEMIC REACTIONS WITHIN THE FIRST 24 HOURS OF IMMUNIZATION WITH HEMOPHILUS B CONJUGATE VACCINE (TETANUS TOXOID CONJUGATE) (N = 188)

Reactions	Dose 1*	Dose 2*
Local		
Pain	9.0%	6.4%
Erythema (1 to 5 cm)	24.0%	18.6%
Induration	9.6%	9.0%
Systemic:		
Fever (> 100.6°F)	7.4%	6.4%
Irritability	30.9%	28.2%
Lethargy	18.6%	17.0%
Anorexia	9.0%	8.5%
Rhinorrhea	24.5%	21.3%
Diarrhea	5.8%	8.5%
Vomiting	4.3%	3.7%
Cough	9.6%	4.3%

DTP was not administered concomitantly with Hemophilus b Conjugate Vaccine (Tetanus Toxoid Conjugate).

When Hemophilus b Conjugate Vaccine (Tetanus Toxoid Conjugate) was administered to infants at 2, 4, and 6 months of age concomitantly, at separate sites, with CLI DTP vaccine, the systemic adverse experience profile was not different from that seen when CLI DTP vaccine was administered alone.[18] *Refer to product insert for CLI whole-cell DTP.*

Adverse reactions from a U.S. multicenter trial in 2-, 4- and 6-month-old infants are summarized in Table 5. Systemic adverse reactions listed in Table 5 are more prominent than those in Table 4 because infants also received concomitant immunization with DTP.[14,18] (See related table.)

In general, the rates of minor systemic reactions after Hemophilus b Conjugate Vaccines (Tetanus Toxoid Conjugate) and DTP immunization were comparable to those usually reported after DTP vaccine alone.[28,29,30,31]

Adverse reactions associated with Hemophilus b Conjugate Vaccine (Tetanus Toxoid Conjugate) generally subsided after 24 hours and usually do not persist beyond 48 hours after immunization.

In a randomized, double-blind U.S. clinical trial, Hemophilus b Conjugate Vaccine (Tetanus Toxoid Conjugate) was given concomitantly with DTP to more than 5,000 infants and hepatitis B vaccine was given with DTP to a similar number. In this large study, deaths due to sudden infant death syndrome (SIDS) and other causes were observed but were not different in the two groups. In the first 48 hours following immunization, two definite and three possible seizures were observed after Hemophilus b Conjugate Vaccine (Tetanus Toxoid Conjugate) and DTP in comparison with none after hepatitis B vaccine and DTP.[18] This rate of seizures following Hemophilus b Conjugate Vaccine (Tetanus Toxoid Conjugate) and DTP was not greater than previously reported in infants receiving DTP alone. Other adverse reactions reported with administration of other Hemophilus b Conjugate Vaccines include urticaria, seizures, hives, renal failure and Guillain-Barre syndrome (GBS).[18,32] A cause and effect relationship among any of these events and the vaccination has not been established.

◆ RATED THERAPEUTICALLY EQUIVALENT; ◇ THERAPEUTIC EQUIVALENCE UNCONFIRMED; ○ UNRATED

When Hemophilus b Conjugate Vaccine (Tetanus Toxoid Conjugate) was given with DTP and inactivated poliovirus vaccine to more than 100,000 Finnish infants, the rate and extent of serious adverse reactions were not different from those seen when other Hemophilus b Conjugate Vaccines were evaluated in Finland.

REPORTING OF ADVERSE EVENTS

Reporting by the parent or guardian of all adverse events occurring after vaccine administration should be encouraged. Adverse events following immunization with vaccine should be reported by the health-care provider to the U.S. Department of Health and Human Services (DHHS) Vaccine Adverse Event Reporting System (VAERS). Reporting forms and information about reporting requirements or completion of the form can be obtained from VAERS through a tollfree number:
1-800-822-7967.[24,25,26]

DOSAGE AND ADMINISTRATION

Parenteral drug products should be inspected visually for particulate matter and/or discoloration prior to administration, whenever solution and container permit. If these conditions exist, the vaccine should not be administered.

RECONSTITUTION

With Diluent Supplied: Prior to reconstitution, cleanse the vaccine vial rubber barrier with a suitable germicide and inject the entire volume of diluent contained in the syringe into the vial of lyophilized vaccine. Thorough agitation is advised to ensure complete rehydration. The entire volume of reconstituted vaccine is then drawn back into a new syringe before injection of one 0.5 mL dose. The vaccine will appear clear and colorless.

Administer Hemophilus b Conjugate Vaccine (Tetanus Toxoid Conjugate) intramuscularly after reconstitution with diluent supplied. (In the event of coagulation disorders, Hemophilus b Conjugate Vaccine (Tetanus Toxoid Conjugate) may be given subcutaneously in the mid-lateral aspect of the thigh.[14]) *Vaccine should be used immediately after reconstitution.*

Each 0.5 mL dose is formulated to contain 10 μg of purified capsular polysaccharide conjugated to 24 μg of inactivated tetanus toxoid and 8.5% of sucrose.

Before injection, the skin over the site to be injected should be cleansed with a suitable germicide. After insertion of the needle, aspirate to ensure that the needle has not entered a blood vessel.

DO NOT INJECT INTRAVENOUSLY

Each dose of Hemophilus b Vaccine Conjugate (Tetanus Toxoid Conjugate) is administered intramuscularly in the outer aspect of the vastus lateralis (mid-thigh) or deltoid. The vaccine should not be injected into the gluteal area or areas where there may be a nerve trunk. During the course of primary immunizations, injections should not be made more than once at the same site.

Hemophilus b Vaccine Conjugate (Tetanus Toxoid Conjugate) is indicated for infants and children 2 months through 5 years of age for intramuscular administration in accordance with the schedule indicated in Table 6.[14,16]

Infants between 2 and 6 months of age should receive three 0.5 mL doses at eight week intervals, followed by a booster dose at 15 to 18 months of age. Infants 7 to 11 months of age who have not been previously immunized should receive two 0.5 mL doses at eight week intervals, followed by a booster dose at 15 to 18 months of age; children 12 to 14 months of age who have not been previously immunized should receive one 0.5 mL dose, followed by a booster dose at 15 to 18 months of age; and children 15 to 60 months of age who have not been previously immunized should receive a single 0.5 mL dose.

Table 6[14,16,33]
IMMUNIZATION SCHEDULE

Age at First Dose	Primary Series	Booster
2 to 6 months	3 Doses, 8 weeks apart	1 Dose, 15 to 18 months
7 to 11 months	2 Doses, 8 weeks apart	1 Dose, 15 to 18 months
12 to 14 months	1 Dose	1 Dose, 15 to 18 months*
15 to 60 months	1 Dose	None

* *Administer vaccine not earlier than 2 months after the previous dose.*

Preterm infants should be vaccinated according to their chronological age from birth.[33]

Interruption of the recommended schedule with a delay between doses should not interfere with the final immunity achieved with Hemophilus b Vaccine Conjugate (Tetanus Toxoid Conjugate). There is no need to start the series over again, regardless of the time elapsed between doses. No data are available to support the interchangeability of Hemophilus b Vaccine Conjugate (Tetanus Toxoid Conjugate) with other Hemophilus b Conjugate Vaccines. Therefore, it is recommended that the same Conjugate Vaccine be used throughout each immunization schedule, consistent with the data supporting approval and licensure of the vaccine. *Administer vaccine immediately after reconstitution.*

STORAGE
Store lyophilized vaccine and prefilled syringe containing diluent between 2°-8°C (35°-46°F). DO NOT FREEZE.

REFERENCES
1. Chu CY, et al. Further studies on the immunogenicity of *Haemophilus influenzae* type b and pneumococcal type 6A polysaccharide-protein conjugate. Infect Immun 40: 245-246, 1983. 2. Mueller JH, et al. Production of diphtheria toxin of high potency (100 Lf) on a reproducible medium. J Immunol 40:21-32, 1941. 3. Adams WG, et al. Decline of Childhood *Haemophilus influenzae* Type b (Hib) Disease in the Hib Vaccine Era. JAMA 269: 221-226, 1993. 4. Recommendations of the Immunization Practices Advisory Committee (ACIP). Haemophilus b conjugate vaccines for prevention of *Haemophilus influenzae* type b disease among infants and children two months of age and older. MMWR 40: No. RR-1, 1991 5. Broome CV. Epidemiology of *Haemophilus influenzae* type b infections in the United States. Pediatr Infect Dis J 6: 779-782, 1987 6. ACIP. Polysaccharide vaccine for prevention of *Haemophilus influenzae* type b disease. MMWR 34:201-205, 1985 7. Istre GR, et al. Risk factors for primary invasive *Haemophilus influenzae* disease: Increased risk from day care attendance and school-aged household members. J Pediatr 106:190-195, 1985 8. Redmond SR, et al. *Haemophilus influenzae* type b disease. An epidemiologic study with special reference to day-care centers. JAMA 252: 2581-2584, 1984 9. Murphy TV, et al. County-wide surveillance of invasive Haemophilus infections: Risk of associated cases in Child Care Programs (CCPs). Twenty-third Interscience Conference on Antimicrobial Agents and Chemotherapy (Abstract #788) 229, 1983 10. Fleming D, et al. *Haemophilus influenzae* b (Hib) disease-secondary spread in day care. Twenty-fourth Interscience Conference on Antimicrobial Agents and Chemotherapy (Abstract #967) 261, 1984 11. CDC. Prevention of secondary cases of *Haemophilus influenzae* type b disease. MMWR 31: 672-680, 1982 12. Michaels RH, et al. Pharyngeal colonization with *Haemophilus influenzae* type b: A longitudinal study of families with a child with meningitis or epiglottitis due to *H. influenzae* type b. J Infec Dis 136: 222-227, 1977 13. Holmes SJ, et al. Immunogenicity of four *Haemophilus influenzae* type b conjugate vaccines in 17- to 19-month-old children. J Pediatr 118: 364-371, 1991 14. Data on file, Pasteur Mérieux Sérums & Vaccins S.A. 15. Peltola H, et al. Prevention of *Haemophilus influenzae* type b bacteremic infections with the capsular polysaccharide vaccine. N Engl J Med 310: 1561-1566, 1984 16. Decker MD, et al. Comparative trial in infants of four conjugate *Haemophilus influenzae* type b vaccines. J Pediatr 120:184-189, 1992 17.

Table 5[14]
PERCENTAGE OF INFANTS PRESENTING WITH LOCAL OR SYSTEMIC REACTIONS AT 6, 24 AND 48 HOURS OF IMMUNIZATION WITH HEMOPHILUS B CONJUGATE VACCINE (TETANUS TOXOID CONJUGATE) ADMINISTERED SIMULTANEOUSLY, AT SEPARATE SITES, WITH CLI DTP VACCINE

Reaction	2 Months (n = 365)			4 Months (n = 364)			6 Months (n = 365)		
	6 Hrs.	24 Hrs.	48 Hrs.	6 Hrs.	24 Hrs.	48 Hrs.	6 Hrs.	24 Hrs.	48 Hrs.
Locals									
Tenderness	46.3%	11.5%	2.2%	23.4%	7.4%	1.1%	19.2%	6.0%	1.1%
Erythema	14.3%	4.1%	0.3%	8.8%	5.8%	0.6%	11.5%	6.9%	1.6%
Induration	22.5%	6.3%	1.9%	12.4%	4.7%	0.8%	9.6%	3.8%	1.1%
Systemic*									
Fever > 100.8°F†	20.1%	1.3%	0.6%	14.6%	6.6%	1.4%	15.7%	8.8%	0.8%
Irritability	72.6%	21.9%	12.6%	48.4%	25.0%	13.2%	44.1%	25.2%	10.1%
Drowsiness	57.5%	29.9%	10.4%	44.2%	18.1%	7.4%	32.6%	13.4%	2.5%
Anorexia	15.3%	5.8%	4.9%	8.0%	5.0%	3.0%	5.5%	4.9%	2.2%
Diarrhea	4.4%	6.6%	5.2%	5.0%	4.7%	4.7%	4.7%	6.3%	3.6%
Vomiting	2.7%	4.1%	2.7%	2.5%	3.3%	2.8%	2.2%	2.7%	1.9%
Persistent Crying	Percentage of infants within 72 hours after immunization was 1.6% after dose one, 0.6% after dose two, and 0.3% after dose three.								

§ *Local reactions were evaluated at the Hemophilus b Conjugate Vaccine (Tetanus Toxoid Conjugate) injection site.*
* *The adverse reaction profile is defined by the concomitant use of CLI DTP vaccine.*
† *The number of individuals observed at each time point for fever varied from 357 to 363.*

➤ SHOWN IN PRODUCT IDENTIFICATION GUIDE

Granoff DM, et al. Differences in the immunogenicity of three *Haemophilus influenzae* type b conjugate vaccines in infants. J Pediatr 121:187-194, 1992 18. Data on file, Connaught Laboratories, Inc. 19. Kaplan SL, et al. Immunogenicity of *Haemophilus influenzae* type b, polysaccharide tetanus protein conjugate vaccine in children with sickle hemoglobinopathy or malignancies, and after systemic *Haemophilus influenzae* type b infection. J Pediatr 120:367-370, 1992 20. Steinhoff MC, et al. Antibody responses to *Haemophilus influenzae* type b vaccines in men with human immunodeficiency virus infection. N Engl J Med 325 (26): 1837-1842, 1991 21. ACIP. General recommendations on immunization. MMWR 38: 205-227, 1989 22. FDA Workshop on Haemophilus b Polysaccharide Vaccine-A Preliminary Report. MMWR 36: 529-531, 1987 23. Rothstein EP, et al. Comparison of antigenuria after immunization with three *Haemophilus influenzae* type b conjugate vaccines. Pediatr Infect Dis J 10: 311-314, 1991 24. Vaccine Adverse Event Reporting System-United States. MMWR 39: 730-733, 1990 25. CDC. National Childhood Vaccine Injury Act: Requirements for permanent vaccination records and for reporting of selected events after vaccination. MMWR 37: 197-200, 1988 26. National Childhood Vaccine Injury Act of 1986 (Amended 1987) 27. Clemens JD, et al. Impact of *Haemophilus influenzae* Type b Polysaccharide-Tetanus Protein Conjugate Vaccine on responses to concurrently administered Diphtheria-Tetanus-Pertussis Vaccine. JAMA 267: 673-678, 1992 28. Cody CL, et al. Nature and rates of adverse reactions associated with DTP and DT immunizations in infants and children. Pediatr 68: 650-660, 1981 29. Barkin RM, et al. Diphtheria-tetanus-pertussis vaccine: reactogenicity of commercial products. Pediatr 63: 256-260, 1979 30. Baraff LJ, et al. DTP associated reactions: an analysis by injection site, manufacturer, prior reactions and dose. Pediatr 73: 31-39, 1984 31. Long SS, et al. Longitudinal study of adverse reactions following diphtheria-tetanus-pertussis vaccine in infancy. Pediatr 85: 294-302, 1990 32. D'Cruz OF, et al. Acute inflammatory demyelinating polyradiculoneuropathy (Guillain-Barre Syndrome) after immunization with *Haemophilus influenzae* type b conjugate vaccine. J Pediatr 115: 743-746, 1989 33. Report on the Committee on Infectious Diseases. American Academy of Pediatrics. Twenty-second Edition, 1991

HOW SUPPLIED
INJECTION:

BRAND/MANUFACTURER	NDC	SIZE	AWP
○ **BRAND**			
PROHIBIT: Connaught	49281-0541-05	2.5 ml	$89.81
	49281-0541-10	5 ml	$179.63
	49281-0541-01	0.5 ml 5s	$102.50
○ **GENERICS**			
HIBTITER: Lederle Labs	53124-0201-05	2.5 ml	$91.74
HIBTITER: Lederle Labs	53124-0201-10	5 ml	$194.83
HIBTITER: Lederle Labs	53124-0104-41	0.5 ml 4s	$86.36

POWDER FOR INJECTION:

BRAND/MANUFACTURER	NDC	SIZE	AWP
○ **BRAND**			
PEDVAX HIB: Merck	00006-4792-00	1s	$20.00
	00006-4797-00	5s	$100.00
OMNIHIB: SK Beecham Pharm	00007-4408-05	5s ud	$89.05
○ **GENERICS**			
ACTHIB: Connaught	49281-0549-10	1s	$323.75

Hemotene *SEE* COLLAGEN HEMOSTAT

Hep-B-Gammagee *SEE* HEPATITIS B IMMUNE
GLOBULIN (HUMAN)

Hep-Pak *SEE* HEPARIN

Heparin

DESCRIPTION
Heparin is a heterogenous group of straight-chain anionic mucopolysaccharides, called glycosaminoglycans, having anticoagulant properties. Although others may be present, the main sugars in Heparin are: (1) α-L-iduronic acid 2-sulfate, (2) 2-deoxy-2-sulfamino-α-D-glucose 6-sulfate, (3) β-D-glucuronic acid, (4) 2-acetamido-2-deoxy-α-D-glucose, and (5) α-L-iduronic acid. These sugars are present in decreasing amounts, usually in the order (2) > (1) > (4) > (3) > (5), and are joined by glycosidic linkages, forming polymers of varying sizes. Heparin is strongly acidic because of its covalently linked sulfate and carboxylic acid groups. In Heparin sodium, the acidic protons of the sulfate units are partially replaced by sodium ions.

Heparin sodium injection is a sterile solution of Heparin sodium derived from porcine intestinal mucosa or bovine lung tissue, which is standardized for anticoagulant activity. It is to be administered by intravenous or deep subcutaneous routes. The potency is determined by a biological assay using a USP reference standard based on units of Heparin activity per milligram.

Each ml of solution for injection contains:

Heparin ....10,000 units
or
Heparin sodium ....1,000, 2,500, 5,000, 7,500, 10,000, 15,000, or 20,000 units

Each ml of lock flush solution contains:

Heparin sodium ....10 or 100 units

CLINICAL PHARMACOLOGY
Heparin inhibits reactions that lead to the clotting of blood and the formation of fibrin clots both *in vitro* and *in vivo*. Heparin acts at multiple sites in the normal coagulation system. Small amounts of Heparin in combination with antithrombin III (Heparin cofactor) can inhibit thrombosis by inactivating activated Factor X and inhibiting the conversion of prothrombin to thrombin. Once active thrombosis has developed, larger amounts of Heparin can inhibit further coagulation by inactivating thrombin and preventing the conversion of fibrinogen to fibrin. Heparin also prevents the formation of a stable fibrin clot by inhibiting the activation of the fibrin stabilizing factor.

Bleeding time is usually unaffected by Heparin. Clotting time is prolonged by full therapeutic doses of Heparin; in most cases, it is not measurably affected by low doses of Heparin.

Peak plasma levels of Heparin are achieved 2 to 4 hours following subcutaneous administration, although there are considerable individual variations. Log linear plots of Heparin plasma concentrations with time for a wide range of dose levels are linear, which suggests the absence of zero order processes. The liver and the reticuloendothelial system are the sites of biotransformation. The biphasic elimination curve, a rapidly declining α phase ($t_{1/2}$ = 10 minutes) and, after the age of 40, a slower β phase, indicate uptake in organs. The absence of a relationship between anticoagulant half-life and concentration half-life may reflect factors such as protein binding of Heparin.

Heparin does not have fibrinolytic activity; therefore, it will not lyse existing clots.

INDICATIONS AND USAGE
Heparin sodium is indicated for:

Anticoagulant therapy in prophylaxis and treatment of venous thrombosis and its extension.

Prevention (in a low-dose regimen) of postoperative deep venous thrombosis and pulmonary embolism in patients undergoing major abdominothoracic surgery or who, for other reasons, are at risk of developing thromboembolic disease (see *"Dosage and Administration"*)

Prophylaxis and treatment of pulmonary embolism

Atrial fibrillation with embolization

Diagnosis and treatment of acute and chronic consumption coagulopathies (eg, disseminated intravascular coagulation)

Prevention of clotting in arterial and heart surgery

Prophylaxis and treatment of peripheral arterial embolism

As an anticoagulant in blood transfusions, extracorporeal circulation, and dialysis procedures and in blood samples for laboratory purposes

Heparin lock flush solution is intended to maintain patency of an indwelling venipuncture device designed for intermittent injection or infusion therapy, or blood sampling. Heparin lock flush solution may be used following initial placement of the device in the vein, after each injection of a medication, or after withdrawal of blood for laboratory tests.

Heparin lock flush sodium is not to be used for anticoagulant therapy.

CONTRAINDICATIONS
Heparin sodium should not be used in patients with severe thrombocytopenia or patients in whom suitable blood coagulation tests (eg, tests for whole-blood clotting time and partial thromboplastin time) cannot be performed at appropriate intervals. (This restriction refers to full-dose administration of Heparin; it is usually unnecessary to monitor coagulation parameters in patients receiving low-dose Heparin). In addition, Heparin sodium should not be administered to patients in an uncontrollable active bleeding state (see *"Warnings"*), except when this condition is the result of disseminated intravascular coagulation.

WARNINGS
Heparin is not intended for intramuscular use.

Hypersensitivity: Patients with documented hypersensitivity to Heparin should be given the drug only in clearly life-threatening situations.

Hemorrhage: Hemorrhage can occur at virtually any site in patients receiving Heparin. An unexplained fall in hematocrit, a fall in blood pressure, or any other unexplained symptom warrants consideration of a hemorrhagic event.

Heparin sodium should be used with extreme caution in disease states in which there is increased danger of hemorrhage. Some of the conditions in which this danger exists are as follows:

Cardiovascular: Subacute bacterial endocarditis. Severe hypertension.

Surgical: During and immediately following (a) a spinal tap or spinal anesthesia or (b) major surgery, especially involving the brain, spinal cord, or eye.

Hematologic: Conditions associated with increased bleeding tendencies, such as hemophilia, thrombocytopenia, and some vascular purpuras.

Gastrointestinal: Ulcerative lesions and continuous tube drainage of the stomach or small intestine.

Other: Menstruation and liver disease with impaired hemostasis.

Coagulation Testing: When Heparin sodium is administered in therapeutic amounts, its dosage should be regulated by frequent blood coagulation tests. If the

---

◆ RATED THERAPEUTICALLY EQUIVALENT; ◇ THERAPEUTIC EQUIVALENCE UNCONFIRMED; ○ UNRATED

coagulation test is unduly prolonged or if hemorrhage occurs, Heparin sodium should be discontinued promptly (see *"Overdosage"*).

Thrombocytopenia: Thrombocytopenia occurs in patients receiving Heparin with a reported incidence of 0% to 30%. Mild thrombocytopenia (count greater than 100,000/mm^3) may remain stable or reverse, even if Heparin is continued. However, thrombocytopenia of any degree should be monitored closely. If the count falls below 100,000/mm^3 or if recurrent thrombosis develops (see *"Precautions, White-Clot Syndrome"*), the Heparin product should be discontinued. If continued Heparin therapy is essential, utilize Heparin from a different organ source and reinstitute therapy with caution.

Miscellaneous: Some brands contain benzyl alcohol as a preservative. Benzyl alcohol has been reported to be associated with a fatal "gasping syndrome" in premature infants.

PRECAUTIONS

General: White-Clot Syndrome: It has been reported that patients taking Heparin may develop new thrombus formation in association with thrombocytopenia. This development is the result of the irreversible aggregation of platelets induced by Heparin, ie, the so-called "white-clot syndrome." The process may lead to severe thromboembolic complications such as skin necrosis, gangrene of the extremities that may lead to amputation, myocardial infarction, pulmonary embolism, stroke, and possibly death. Therefore, Heparin administration should be promptly discontinued if a patient develops new thrombosis in association with thrombocytopenia.

Heparin Resistance: Increased resistance to Heparin is frequently encountered in cases involving fever, thrombosis, thrombophlebitis, infections with thrombosing tendencies, myocardial infarction, and cancer. Increased resistance can also occur in postsurgical patients.

Increased Risk in Older Women: A higher incidence of bleeding has been reported in women over 60 years of age.

Laboratory Tests: Periodic platelet counts, hematocrit determinations, and tests for occult blood in the stool are recommended during the entire course of Heparin therapy, regardless of the route of administration (see *"Dosage and Administration"*).

Drug Interactions: Oral anticoagulants: Heparin sodium may prolong the one-stage prothrombin time. Therefore, if a valid prothrombin time is to be obtained when Heparin sodium is given with dicumarol or warfarin sodium, a period of at least 5 hours after the last intravenous dose or 24 hours after the last subcutaneous dose should elapse before blood is drawn.

Platelet inhibitors: Drugs such as acetylsalicylic acid, dextran, phenylbutazone, ibuprofen, indomethacin, dipyridamole, hydroxychloroquine, and others that interfere with platelet-aggregation reactions (the main hemostatic defense of heparinized patients) may induce bleeding and should be used with caution in patients receiving Heparin sodium.

Other interactions: Digitalis, tetracyclines, nicotine, or antihistamines may partially counteract the anticoagulant action of Heparin sodium.

Intravenous nitroglycerin administered to heparinized patients may result in a decrease of the partial thromboplastin time with subsequent rebound effect upon discontinuation of nitroglycerin. Careful monitoring of partial thromboplastin time and adjustment of Heparin dosage are recommended during coadministration of Heparin and intravenous nitroglycerin.

When clinical circumstances require reversal heparinization, consult the labeling of protamine sulfate injection, USP.

Drug/Laboratory Test Interaction: Hyperaminotransferasemia. Significant elevations of aminotransferase (SGOT and SGPT) levels have occurred in a high percentage of patients (and healthy subjects) who have received Heparin. Since aminotransferase determinations are important in the differential diagnosis of myocardial infarction, liver disease, and pulmonary emboli, increases that might be caused by drugs (eg, Heparin) should be interpreted with caution.

Carcinogenesis, Mutagenesis, Impairment of Fertility: No long-term studies in animals have been performed to evaluate the carcinogenic potential of Heparin. Also, no reproduction studies in animals have been performed concerning mutagenesis or impairment of fertility.

Pregnancy-Teratogenic Effect: Pregnancy Category C: Animal reproduction studies have not been conducted with Heparin sodium. It is also not known whether Heparin sodium can cause fetal harm when administered to a pregnant woman or can affect reproduction capacity. Heparin sodium should be given to a pregnant woman only if clearly needed.

Nonteratogenic Effects: Heparin does not cross the placental barrier.

Nursing Mothers: Heparin is not excreted in human milk.

Pediatric Use: See *"Dosage and Administration."*

ADVERSE REACTIONS

Hemorrhage: Hemorrhage is the chief complication that may result from Heparin therapy (see *"Warnings"*). An overly prolonged clotting time or minor bleeding during therapy can usually be controlled by withdrawing the drug (see *"Overdosage"*). *Gastrointestinal or urinary tract bleeding during anticoagulant therapy may indicate the presence of an underlying occult lesion.* Bleeding can occur at any site, but certain specific hemorrhagic complications may be difficult to detect:

Adrenal hemorrhage, with resultant acute adrenal insufficiency, has occurred during anticoagulant therapy. Therefore, such treatment should be discontinued in patients who develop signs and symptoms of acute adrenal hemorrhage and

insufficiency. Initiation of corrective therapy should not be delayed for laboratory confirmation of the diagnosis, since any delay in an acute situation may result in the patient's death.

Ovarian (corpus luteum) hemorrhage developed in a number of women of reproductive age receiving short- or long-term anticoagulant therapy. If unrecognized, this complication may be fatal.

Retroperitoneal hemorrhage has occurred.

Local Irritation: Local irritation, erythema, mild pain, hematoma, or ulceration may follow deep subcutaneous (intrafat) injection of Heparin sodium. These complications are much more common after intramuscular use; therefore, such use is not recommended.

Hypersensitivity: Generalized hypersensitivity reactions have been reported, with chills, fever, and urticaria as the most common manifestations; asthma, rhinitis, lacrimation, headache, nausea and vomiting, and anaphylactoid reactions (including shock) have occurred more rarely. Itching and burning, especially on the plantar site of the feet, may occur.

The occurrence of thrombocytopenia has been reported in patients receiving Heparin, with an incidence of 0% to 30%. Although often mild and of no obvious clinical significance, thromboembolic complications, such as skin necrosis, gangrene of the extremities that may lead to amputation, myocardial infarction, pulmonary embolism, stroke, and possibly death (see *"Warnings"* and *"Precautions"*).

Certain episodes of painful, ischemic, and cyanosed limbs have, in the past, been attributed to allergic vasospastic reactions. Whether these are, in fact, identical to the thrombocytopenia-associated complications remains to be determined.

Miscellaneous: Osteoporosis following long-term administration of high doses of Heparin, cutaneous necrosis after systemic administration, suppression of aldosterone synthesis, delayed transient alopecia, priapism, and rebound hyperlipemia occurring after discontinuation of Heparin sodium have also been reported.

Significant elevations of aminotransferase (SGOT and SGPT) levels have occurred in a high percentage of patients (and healthy subjects) who have received Heparin.

OVERDOSAGE

Signs and Symptoms: Overdose of Heparin may follow parenteral administration, but oral Heparin has little systemic effect. Bleeding is the chief sign of Heparin overdosage. Nosebleeds, blood in urine or tarry stools may be noted as the first sign of bleeding. Easy bruising or petechial formations may precede frank bleeding. Excessive Heparin effect also increases whole-blood clotting time and activated partial thromboplastin time (APTT). The half-life of Heparin ranges from 0.5 to 2.5 hours and may vary widely in cases involving an overdose.

The intravenous median lethal dose in mice is 1,500 mg/kg.

Treatment: To obtain up-to-date information about the treatment of overdose, a good resource is your certified Regional Poison Control Center. Telephone numbers of certified poison control centers are listed in the *Physicians' Desk Reference (PDR)*. In managing overdosage, consider the possibility of multiple drug overdoses, interaction among drugs, and unusual drug kinetics in your patient.

Minor bleeding occurring during therapy with Heparin can often be treated by reducing the dose or increasing the dosing interval.

For major bleeding episodes, Heparin may be neutralized by slow infusion of protamine; no more than 50 mg should be administered, very slowly, in any 10-minute period. Each mg of protamine will neutralize approximately 100 or 115 units of Heparin.

Protamine dosage may be guided by determining the amount of time by which clotting is shortened *in vitro* or by the results of other hematologic tests. The amount of protamine required decreases over time as Heparin is metabolized. Although the metabolism of Heparin is complex, it may, for the purpose of choosing a protamine dose, be assumed to have a half-life of about ½ hour after intravenous injection. Note that protamine may cause severe hypotensive and anaphylactoid reactions that may be life threatening. Because fatal reactions often resembling anaphylaxis have been reported, the drug should be given only when resuscitation techniques and treatment of anaphylactoid shock are readily available. (See the protamine label for additional information.) The administration for whole blood or fresh frozen plasma should be considered for patients with significant blood losses. Vitamin K will not reverse the activity of Heparin.

DOSAGE AND ADMINISTRATION

Parenteral drug products should be inspected visually for particulate matter and discoloration prior to administration if solution and container permit. Slight discoloration does not alter potency.

When Heparin is added to an infusion solution for continuous intravenous administration, the container should be inverted at least 6 times to ensure adequate mixing and prevent pooling of the Heparin in the solution.

Heparin sodium is not effective by oral administration and should be given by intermittent intravenous injection, intravenous infusion, or deep subcutaneous (intrafat, ie, above the iliac crest or abdominal fat layer) injection. *The intramuscular route of administration should be avoided because of frequent occurrence of hematoma at the injection site.*

The dosage of Heparin sodium should be adjusted according to the patient's coagulation test results. When Heparin is given by continuous intravenous infusion, the coagulation time should be determined approximately every 4 hours in the early stages of treatment. When the drug is administered intermittently by intravenous injection, coagulation tests should be performed before each injection during the early stages of treatment and at appropriate intervals thereafter. Dosage is considered adequate when the activated partial thromboplastin time (APTT) is 1.5 to 2 times normal or when the whole-blood clotting time is elevated approximately 2.5 to 3 times the control value. After deep subcutaneous (intrafat) injections, tests for adequacy of dosage are best performed on samples drawn 4 to 6 hours after the injections.

Periodic platelet counts, hematocrit determinations, and tests for occult blood in the stool are recommended during the entire course of Heparin therapy, regardless of the route of administration.

Heparin sodium injection should not be mixed with doxorubicin or droperidol since it has been reported that these drugs are incompatible with Heparin and a precipitate may form.

Converting to Oral Anticoagulant: When an oral anticoagulant of the coumarin (or similar) type is to be administered in patients receiving Heparin sodium, baseline and subsequent tests of prothrombin activity must be determined at times during which Heparin activity is too low to affect the prothrombin time. Such a time usually occurs about 5 hours after the last IV bolus and 24 hours after the last subcutaneous dose. If Heparin is continuously infused by IV, prothrombin time can usually be measured at any time. In converting from Heparin to an oral anticoagulant, the oral anticoagulant should be given in the usual initial amount; thereafter, prothrombin time should be determined at the usual intervals. To ensure continuous anticoagulation, it is advisable to continue full Heparin therapy for several days after the prothrombin time has reached the limit of the therapeutic range. Heparin therapy may then be discontinued without tapering.

Therapeutic Anticoagulant Effect With Full-Dose Heparin: Although dosage must be adjusted for the individual patient according to the results of appropriate laboratory tests, the following dosage schedule may be used as a guideline. (See related table).

Pediatric Use: Follow recommendations of appropriate pediatric reference texts.
In general, the following dosage schedule may be used as a guideline:

Initial Dose: 50 units/kg (IV, drip)

Maintenance Dose: 100 units/kg (IV, drip) every 4 hours, or 20,000 units/m^2/24 hours, infused continuously.

Surgery of the Heart and Blood Vessels: Patients undergoing total body perfusion for open heart surgery should receive an initial dose of not less than 150 units of Heparin sodium per kg of body weight. Frequently, a dose of 300 units/kg is used for procedures estimated to last less than 60 minutes; a dose of 400 units/kg is often used for those procedures likely to last longer than 60 minutes.

Low-Dose Prophylaxis of Postoperative Thromboembolism: A number of well-controlled clinical trials have demonstrated that low-dose Heparin prophylaxis, given just prior to and after surgery, will reduce the incidence of postoperative deep-vein thrombosis in the legs (as measured by the I-125 fibrinogen technique and venography) and of clinical pulmonary embolism. The most widely used dosage is 5,000 units given 2 hours before surgery and 5,000 units given every 8 to 12 hours thereafter for 7 days or until the patient is fully ambulatory, whichever is longer. The Heparin is given by deep subcutaneous (intrafat, ie, above the iliac crest or abdominal fat layer, arm, or thigh) injection with a fine (25- to 26-gauge) needle to minimize tissue trauma. A concentrated solution of Heparin sodium is recommended. Such prophylaxis should be reserved for patients over the age of 40 who are undergoing major surgery. Patients with bleeding disorders and those having brain or spinal-cord surgery, spinal anesthesia, eye surgery, or potentially sanguineous operations should be excluded from this treatment, as should patients receiving oral anticoagulants or platelet-active drugs (see *"Warnings"*). The value of such prophylaxis in hip surgery has not been established. The possibility of increased bleeding during surgery or postoperatively should be borne in mind. If such bleeding occurs, discontinuance of Heparin and neutralization with protamine sulfate are advisable. If clinical evidence of thromboembolism develops despite low-dose prophylaxis, full therapeutic doses of anticoagulants should be given unless contraindicated. Prior to initiating heparinization, the physician should rule out the probability of bleeding disorders by taking a thorough history and performing the appropriate laboratory tests. Appropriate coagulation tests should be repeated, just prior to surgery. Coagulation test values should be normal or only slightly elevated at these times. There is

usually no need for daily monitoring of the effect of low-dose Heparin in patients with normal coagulation parameters.

Extracorporeal Dialysis: Follow equipment manufacturers' operating directions carefully.

Blood Transfusion: The addition of 400 to 600 USP units to each 100 ml of whole blood for transfusion is usually employed to prevent coagulation. Usually, 7,500 USP units of Heparin sodium are mixed with 100 ml of 0.9% sodium chloride injection, usp (or 75,000 usp units/1,000 ml of 0.9% sodium chloride injection, usp); 6 to 8 ml of this sterile solution is then added to each 100 ml of whole blood used.

Laboratory Samples: 70 to 150 units of Heparin sodium are usually added per 10 to 20-ml sample of whole blood to prevent coagulation of the sample. Leukocyte counts should be performed on heparinized blood within 2 hours after the addition of the Heparin. Heparinized blood should not be used for isoagglutinin, complement, or erythrocyte fragility tests or for taking platelet counts.

Withdrawal of Blood Samples: Heparin lock flush solution may also be used after each withdrawal of blood for laboratory tests. When Heparin (or sodium chloride) would interfere with or alter the results of blood tests, the Heparin solution should be cleared from the device by aspirating and discarding it before withdrawing the blood sample.

Clearing Intermittent Infusion (Heparin Lock) Sets: To prevent clot formation in a Heparin lock set or central venous catheter following its proper insertion, Heparin lock flush solution should be injected via the injection hub in a quantity sufficient to fill the entire device to the needle tip. This solution should be replaced each time the device is used. Aspirate before administering any solution via the device in order to confirm the patency and location of the needle or catheter tip. If the drug to be administered is incompatible with Heparin, the entire device lock should be flushed with sterile water or normal saline before and after the medication is administered; following the second cleansing flush, Heparin lock flush solution may be reinstilled in the device. The device manufacturer's instructions should be consulted for specifics concerning its use. Usually this dilute Heparin solution will maintain anti-coagulation within the device for up to 4 hours.

Note: Since repeated injections of small doses of Heparin can alter tests for activated partial thromboplastin time (APTT), a baseline value for APTT should be obtained prior to insertion of an intravenous device.

Storage: Protect from light. Store at controlled room temperature, 59° to 86° F (15° to 30° C). Do not freeze. Do not use if solution is discolored or contains a precipitate.

J CODES
30 ml IV,SC—J1640

HOW SUPPLIED

HEPARIN LOCK FLUSH
INJECTION: 10 U/ML

GENERIC A-RATED AVERAGE PRICE (GAAP)	
1 ml 25s	$32.71
2 ml 25s	$13.07
10 ml 25s	$28.83
30 ml 25s	$52.83
1 ml 50s	$44.31
2 ml 50s	$55.59
2.5 ml 50s	$54.07
1 ml 120s	$181.50
3 ml 120s	$264.00
5 ml 120s	$304.50

AVERAGE UNIT PRICE (AVAILABLE SIZES)	
BRAND	$13.99
GENERIC	$0.65

BRAND/MANUFACTURER	NDC	SIZE	AWP
◆ BRAND			
HEP-PAK: Sanofi Winthrop	00024-0741-12	1 ml	$72.78
	00024-0725-02	2 ml 30s	$88.15
	00024-0725-03	1 ml 50s	$114.76

Method of Administration	Frequency	Recommended Dose*
Deep Subcutaneous (Intrafat) Injection (A different site should be used for each injection to prevent the development of massive hematoma)	Initial dose	5,000 units by IV injection, followed by 10,000-20,000 units of a concentrated solution, subcutaneously
	Every 8 hours or	8,000-10,000 units of a concentrated solution
	Every 12 hours	15,000-20,000 units of a concentrated solution
Intermittent Intravenous Injection	Initial dose	10,000 units, either undiluted or in 50-100 ml of 0.9% sodium chloride injection USP.
	Every 4 to 6 hours	5,000-10,000 units, either undiluted or in 50-100 ml of 0.9% sodium chloride injection USP
Continuous Intravenous Infusion	Initial dose	5,000 units by IV injection
	Continuous Infusion	20,000-40,000 units/24 hours in 1,000 ml of 0.9% sodium chloride injection USP (or in any compatible solution) for infusion

*Based on 150-lb (68-kg) patient.

◆ RATED THERAPEUTICALLY EQUIVALENT; ◇ THERAPEUTIC EQUIVALENCE UNCONFIRMED; ○ UNRATED

BRAND/MANUFACTURER	NDC	SIZE	AWP
LOK-PAK-N KIT: Solo Pak Medical	59747-0117-71	1 ml 200s	$833.25
	59747-0117-73	3 ml 200s	$1005.00
	59747-0117-75	5 ml 200s	$1542.50
◆ GENERICS			
Fujisawa	00469-3001-15	1 ml	$0.84
HEP FLUSH-10: Fujisawa	00469-1700-30	10 ml	$3.35
Elkins-Sinn	00641-0392-25	1 ml 25s	$9.65
Elkins-Sinn	00641-0414-25	1 ml 25s	$10.98
Solo Pak	39769-0018-01	1 ml 25s	$13.13
Abbott Hosp	00074-4822-01	1 ml 25s	$97.08
Elkins-Sinn	00641-0393-25	2 ml 25s	$11.14
Solo Pak	39769-0018-02	2 ml 25s	$15.00
Solo Pak	39769-0018-05	5 ml 25s	$18.13
Elkins-Sinn	00641-2438-45	10 ml 25s	$15.91
Abbott Hosp	00074-1151-70	10 ml 25s	$30.28
Solo Pak	39769-0035-10	10 ml 25s	$40.31
Elkins-Sinn	00641-2442-45	30 ml 25s	$40.64
Solo Pak	39769-0035-30	30 ml 25s	$47.50
Abbott Hosp	00074-1151-78	30 ml 25s	$70.36
Elkins-Sinn	00641-3260-09	1 ml 50s	$33.94
Wyeth-Ayerst	00008-0523-01	1 ml 50s	$34.50
Sanofi Winthrop	00024-0721-12	1 ml 50s	$37.49
Wyeth-Ayerst	00008-0523-50	1 ml 50s	$53.25
Sanofi Winthrop	00024-0721-16	1 ml 50s	$62.35
Sanofi Winthrop	00024-0721-13	2 ml 50s	$48.82
Sanofi Winthrop	00024-0721-17	2 ml 50s	$62.35
Elkins-Sinn	00641-3261-09	2.5 ml 50s	$53.64
Wyeth-Ayerst	00008-0523-02	2.5 ml 50s	$54.49
Solo Pak Medical	59747-0106-71	1 ml 120s	$181.50
Solo Pak Medical	59747-0106-81	1 ml 120s	$181.50
Solo Pak Medical	59747-0106-73	3 ml 120s	$264.00
Solo Pak Medical	59747-0106-83	3 ml 120s	$264.00
Solo Pak Medical	59747-0106-75	5 ml 120s	$304.50
Solo Pak Medical	59747-0106-85	5 ml 120s	$304.50

INJECTION: 20 U/ML

BRAND/MANUFACTURER	NDC	SIZE	AWP
◆ GENERICS			
Sanofi Winthrop	00024-0722-13	2 ml 50s	$48.82

INJECTION: 25 U/2.5 ML

BRAND/MANUFACTURER	NDC	SIZE	AWP
◆ GENERICS			
Wyeth-Ayerst	00008-0523-51	2.5 ml 50s	$73.24

INJECTION: 100 U/ML

AVERAGE UNIT PRICE (AVAILABLE SIZES)		GENERIC A-RATED AVERAGE PRICE (GAAP)	
BRAND	$13.99	1 ml 25s	$11.25
GENERIC	$1.009	2 ml 25s	$13.07
		10 ml 25s	$30.77
		30 ml 25s	$57.83
		1 ml 50s	$44.31
		1 ml 120s	$181.50
		3 ml 120s	$264.00
		5 ml 120s	$304.50

BRAND/MANUFACTURER	NDC	SIZE	AWP
◆ BRAND			
HEP-PAK: Sanofi Winthrop	00024-0742-12	1 ml	$72.78
	00024-0736-02	2 ml 30s	$88.15
	00024-0736-03	1 ml 50s	$114.76
LOK-PAK-N KIT: Solo Pak Medical	59747-0118-71	1 ml 200s	$833.25
	59747-0118-73	3 ml 200s	$1005.00
	59747-0118-75	5 ml 200s	$1542.50
◆ GENERICS			
Fujisawa	00469-3101-15	1 ml	$1.01
Sanofi Winthrop	00024-0722-33	3 ml	$40.15
Fujisawa	00469-3105-20	5 ml	$1.28
Elkins-Sinn	00641-0389-25	1 ml 25s	$9.65
Elkins-Sinn	00641-0411-25	1 ml 25s	$10.98
Solo Pak	39769-0011-01	1 ml 25s	$13.13
Elkins-Sinn	00641-0387-25	2 ml 25s	$11.14
Solo Pak	39769-0011-02	2 ml 25s	$15.00
Solo Pak	39769-0011-05	5 ml 25s	$18.13
Elkins-Sinn	00641-2436-45	10 ml 25s	$17.56
Abbott Hosp	00074-1152-70	10 ml 25s	$34.44
Solo Pak	39769-0036-10	10 ml 25s	$40.31
Elkins-Sinn	00641-2443-45	30 ml 25s	$46.13
Solo Pak	39769-0036-30	30 ml 25s	$47.50
Abbott Hosp	00074-1152-78	30 ml 25s	$79.86
Elkins-Sinn	00641-3262-09	1 ml 50s	$33.94
Wyeth-Ayerst	00008-0487-01	1 ml 50s	$34.50
Sanofi Winthrop	00024-0722-12	1 ml 50s	$37.49
Wyeth-Ayerst	00008-0487-50	1 ml 50s	$53.25
Sanofi Winthrop	00024-0722-16	1 ml 50s	$62.35
Sanofi Winthrop	00024-0722-17	2 ml 50s	$62.35
Wyeth-Ayerst	00008-0487-03	2.5 ml 50s	$54.49
Solo Pak Medical	59747-0107-71	1 ml 120s	$181.50
Solo Pak Medical	59747-0107-81	1 ml 120s	$181.50

BRAND/MANUFACTURER	NDC	SIZE	AWP
Solo Pak Medical	59747-0107-73	3 ml 120s	$264.00
Solo Pak Medical	59747-0107-83	3 ml 120s	$264.00
Solo Pak Medical	59747-0107-75	5 ml 120s	$304.50
Solo Pak Medical	59747-0107-85	5 ml 120s	$304.50

INJECTION: 250 U/ML

BRAND/MANUFACTURER	NDC	SIZE	AWP
◆ GENERICS			
Elkins-Sinn	00641-3263-09	2.5 ml 50s	$53.64

INJECTION: 250 U/2.5 ML

BRAND/MANUFACTURER	NDC	SIZE	AWP
◆ GENERICS			
Wyeth-Ayerst	00008-0487-51	2.5 ml 50s	$73.24

KIT: 10 U/ML

AVERAGE UNIT PRICE (AVAILABLE SIZES)	
BRAND	$2.80

BRAND/MANUFACTURER	NDC	SIZE	AWP
◆ BRAND			
HEPARIN FLUSH: Wyeth-Ayerst	00008-2528-51	30s	$114.78
	00008-2528-01	50s	$103.98
	00008-2528-03	50s	$103.98
	00008-2528-50	50s	$160.23

KIT: 25 U

BRAND/MANUFACTURER	NDC	SIZE	AWP
◆ BRAND			
CVC HEPARIN FLUSH: Wyeth-Ayerst	00008-2528-02	30s	$81.03

KIT: 100 U/ML

AVERAGE UNIT PRICE (AVAILABLE SIZES)	
BRAND	$2.64

BRAND/MANUFACTURER	NDC	SIZE	AWP
◆ BRAND			
HEPARIN FLUSH: Wyeth-Ayerst	00008-2529-01	50s	$103.98
	00008-2529-03	50s	$103.98
	00008-2529-50	50s	$160.23
	00008-2529-52	50s	$160.23

KIT: 250 U

BRAND/MANUFACTURER	NDC	SIZE	AWP
◆ BRAND			
CVC HEPARIN FLUSH: Wyeth-Ayerst	00008-2529-02	30s	$81.03

HEPARIN SODIUM

INJECTION: 2 U/ML

AVERAGE UNIT PRICE (AVAILABLE SIZES)	
GENERIC	$0.01

BRAND/MANUFACTURER	NDC	SIZE	AWP
◆ GENERICS			
Baxter	00338-0433-04	1000 ml 12s	$87.84
Baxter	00338-0431-03	500 ml 18s	$123.66

INJECTION: 10,000 U/ML

AVERAGE UNIT PRICE (AVAILABLE SIZES)		GENERIC A-RATED AVERAGE PRICE (GAAP)	
GENERIC	$1.93	1 ml	$2.50
		4 ml	$9.82
		10 ml	$10.92
		1 ml 10s	$20.04
		1 ml 25s	$46.43
		4 ml 25s	$161.50
		2 ml 50s	$68.44

BRAND/MANUFACTURER	NDC	SIZE	AWP
◆ GENERICS			
Fujisawa	00469-2152-15	1 ml	$1.88
Fujisawa	00469-0833-00	1 ml	$2.73
Upjohn	00009-0317-01	1 ml	$2.90
Fujisawa	00469-0833-70	4 ml	$8.84
Upjohn	00009-0317-02	4 ml	$10.79
Lilly	00002-7217-01	5 ml	$24.58
Schein	00364-6539-54	10 ml	$7.75
Steris	00402-0049-10	10 ml	$7.75
Rugby	00536-4925-70	10 ml	$17.25

BRAND/MANUFACTURER	NDC	SIZE	AWP
Elkins-Sinn	00641-2470-41	4 ml	$7.94
Wyeth-Ayerst	00008-0277-02	0.5 ml 10s	$15.98
Sanofi Winthrop	00024-0733-02	1 ml 10s	$17.12
Elkins-Sinn	00641-3268-03	1 ml 10s	$20.95
Wyeth-Ayerst	00008-0277-01	1 ml 10s	$22.05
Sanofi Winthrop	00024-0733-05	2 ml 10s	$10.25
Elkins-Sinn	00641-0410-25	1 ml 25s	$20.36
Upjohn	00009-0317-08	1 ml 25s	$72.50
Elkins-Sinn	00641-2470-45	4 ml 25s	$53.31
Upjohn	00009-0317-09	4 ml 25s	$269.69
Abbott Hosp	00074-2581-02	5 ml 25s	$67.98
Wyeth-Ayerst	00008-0277-03	0.5 ml 50s	$78.05
Sanofi Winthrop	00024-0733-15	2 ml 50s	$51.29
Sanofi Winthrop	00024-0733-12	2 ml 50s	$85.59

INJECTION: 10,000 U

BRAND/MANUFACTURER	NDC	SIZE	AWP
◆ GENERICS			
Abbott Hosp	00074-6286-11	150 ml 12s	$207.48

INJECTION: 12,500 U/ML

BRAND/MANUFACTURER	NDC	SIZE	AWP
◆ GENERICS			
Abbott Hosp	00074-2582-02	5 ml 25s	$81.94

INJECTION: 12,500 U

AVERAGE UNIT PRICE (AVAILABLE SIZES)	
GENERIC	$0.06

BRAND/MANUFACTURER	NDC	SIZE	AWP
◆ GENERICS			
Abbott Hosp	00074-6287-02	250 ml 12s	$220.59
Abbott Hosp	00074-7651-62	250 ml 24s	$229.14

INJECTION: 20,000 U/ML

AVERAGE UNIT PRICE (AVAILABLE SIZES)		GENERIC A-RATED AVERAGE PRICE (GAAP)	
GENERIC	$3.03	5 ml	$15.85

BRAND/MANUFACTURER	NDC	SIZE	AWP
◆ GENERICS			
Schein	00364-6540-53	5 ml	$15.83
Steris	00402-0050-05	5 ml	$15.83
Rugby	00536-4950-65	5 ml	$15.90
Wyeth-Ayerst	00008-0276-01	1 ml 10s	$41.30
Schein	00364-6540-46	1 ml 25s	$93.75
Schein	00364-6540-48	2 ml 25s	$166.65
Abbott Hosp	00074-2583-02	10 ml 25s	$121.42

INJECTION: 20,000 U

BRAND/MANUFACTURER	NDC	SIZE	AWP
◆ GENERICS			
McGaw	00264-9567-10	500 ml	$21.30

INJECTION: 20 MILLION U/ML

BRAND/MANUFACTURER	NDC	SIZE	AWP
◆ GENERICS			
Fujisawa	00469-1155-15	1 ml	$3.84

INJECTION: 25,000 U/ML

BRAND/MANUFACTURER	NDC	SIZE	AWP
◆ GENERICS			
Abbott Hosp	00074-2584-02	10 ml 25s	$157.64

INJECTION: 25,000 U

AVERAGE UNIT PRICE (AVAILABLE SIZES)	
GENERIC	$0.05

BRAND/MANUFACTURER	NDC	SIZE	AWP
◆ GENERICS			
McGaw	00264-9587-20	250 ml	$22.15
McGaw	00264-9577-10	500 ml	$21.38
McGaw	00264-5577-10	500 ml 10s	$205.20
Abbott Hosp	00074-6286-02	250 ml 12s	$264.77
Abbott Hosp	00074-6287-03	500 ml 12s	$264.77
Abbott Hosp	00074-7650-62	250 ml 24s	$243.11
Abbott Hosp	00074-7651-03	500 ml 24s	$243.11

INJECTION: 40 U/ML

BRAND/MANUFACTURER	NDC	SIZE	AWP
◆ GENERICS			
Baxter	00338-0449-03	500 ml 12s	$110.45

INJECTION: 40,000 U/ML

AVERAGE UNIT PRICE (AVAILABLE SIZES)		GENERIC A-RATED AVERAGE PRICE (GAAP)	
GENERIC	$5.19	5 ml	$16.50

BRAND/MANUFACTURER	NDC	SIZE	AWP
◆ GENERICS			
Schein	00364-2364-53	5 ml	$16.50
Steris	00402-0519-05	5 ml	$16.50
Schein	00364-2364-46	1 ml 25s	$187.50
Schein	00364-2364-48	2 ml 25s	$333.38

INJECTION: 50 U/ML

BRAND/MANUFACTURER	NDC	SIZE	AWP
◆ GENERICS			
Baxter	00338-0450-03	500 ml 12s	$119.23

INJECTION: 100 U/ML

BRAND/MANUFACTURER	NDC	SIZE	AWP
◆ GENERICS			
Baxter	00338-0451-02	250 ml 18s	$178.92

INJECTION: 1000 U/ML

AVERAGE UNIT PRICE (AVAILABLE SIZES)		GENERIC A-RATED AVERAGE PRICE (GAAP)	
GENERIC	$0.47	10 ml	$3.01
		30 ml	$7.59
		1 ml 10s	$7.19
		10 ml 25s	$44.43
		30 ml 25s	$45.68

BRAND/MANUFACTURER	NDC	SIZE	AWP
◆ GENERICS			
Fujisawa	00469-1033-15	1 ml	$1.10
Fujisawa	00469-2760-10	2 ml	$5.03
Elkins-Sinn	00641-2440-41	10 ml	$2.55
Fujisawa	00469-0813-30	10 ml	$2.79
Upjohn	00009-0268-01	10 ml	$2.90
Schein	00364-6669-54	10 ml	$3.10
Steris	00402-0463-10	10 ml	$3.10
Fujisawa	00469-0033-25	10 ml	$3.60
Fujisawa	00469-0813-50	30 ml	$6.45
Elkins-Sinn	00641-2450-41	30 ml	$8.06
Upjohn	00009-0268-02	30 ml	$8.25
Elkins-Sinn	00641-3264-03	1 ml 10s	$6.94
Wyeth-Ayerst	00008-0275-01	1 ml 10s	$7.44
Elkins-Sinn	00641-0391-25	1 ml 25s	$10.94
Apothecon	00003-2963-20	5 ml 25s	$87.30
Elkins-Sinn	00641-2440-45	10 ml 25s	$21.74
Solo Pak	39769-0019-10	10 ml 25s	$39.06
Upjohn	00009-0268-07	10 ml 25s	$72.50
Elkins-Sinn	00641-2450-45	30 ml 25s	$38.23
Solo Pak	39769-0019-30	30 ml 25s	$53.13

INJECTION: 1000 U

AVERAGE UNIT PRICE (AVAILABLE SIZES)	
GENERIC	$0.02

BRAND/MANUFACTURER	NDC	SIZE	AWP
◆ GENERICS			
McGaw	00264-9872-10	500 ml	$13.85
McGaw	00264-8872-10	500 ml 10s	$93.72
Abbott Hosp	00074-7620-03	500 ml 24s	$228.57

INJECTION: 2000 U

BRAND/MANUFACTURER	NDC	SIZE	AWP
◆ GENERICS			
Abbott Hosp	00074-7620-59	1000 ml 12s	$114.29

INJECTION: 2500 U/ML

BRAND/MANUFACTURER	NDC	SIZE	AWP
◆ GENERICS			
Wyeth-Ayerst	00008-0482-01	1 ml 10s	$13.46

◆ RATED THERAPEUTICALLY EQUIVALENT; ◇ THERAPEUTIC EQUIVALENCE UNCONFIRMED; ○ UNRATED

INJECTION: 5000 U/ML

AVERAGE UNIT PRICE (AVAILABLE SIZES)		GENERIC A-RATED AVERAGE PRICE (GAAP)	
GENERIC	$0.97	10 ml	$8.75
		1 ml 10s	$13.79

BRAND/MANUFACTURER	NDC	SIZE	AWP
◆ GENERICS			
Fujisawa	00469-1262-15	1 ml	$1.44
Fujisawa	00469-0923-30	10 ml	$6.48
URL	00677-0275-21	10 ml	$7.50
Schein	00364-6538-54	10 ml	$7.50
Steris	00402-0418-10	10 ml	$7.50
Rugby	00536-4900-70	10 ml	$10.08
Upjohn	00009-0291-01	10 ml	$13.45
Elkins-Sinn	00641-2460-41	10 ml	$8.63
Sanofi Winthrop	00024-0793-02	1 ml 10s	$10.25
Elkins-Sinn	00641-3267-03	1 ml 10s	$15.15
Wyeth-Ayerst	00008-0278-02	1 ml 10s	$15.98
Elkins-Sinn	00641-0400-25	1 ml 25s	$15.09
Elkins-Sinn	00641-2460-45	10 ml 25s	$56.88
Sanofi Winthrop	00024-0793-12	1 ml 50s	$51.29

INJECTION: 5000 U/0.5 ML

BRAND/MANUFACTURER	NDC	SIZE	AWP
◆ GENERICS			
Elkins-Sinn	00641-3266-03	0.5 ml 10s	$15.15

INJECTION: 7500 U/ML

BRAND/MANUFACTURER	NDC	SIZE	AWP
◆ GENERICS			
Wyeth-Ayerst	00008-0293-01	1 ml 10s	$18.30

Heparin Flush *SEE* HEPARIN

Hepatitis b Immune Globulin (Human)

DESCRIPTION

Hepatitis B Immune Globulin (Human) is a sterile solution of human immuno-globulin 10%-18% protein) which is prepared by cold alcohol fractionation from pooled plasma of individuals with high titers of antibody to the hepatitis B surface antigen (anti-HBs). The product is stabilized with M glycine and is preserved with thimerosal (a mercury derivative). The solution has a pH of 6.4-7.2.

Each vial contains anti-HBs antibody equivalent to or exceeding the potency of anti-HBs in a U.S. reference hepatitis B immune globulin (Center for Biologics Evaluation and Research, FDA). The U.S. reference has been tested against the World Health Organization standard Hepatitis B Immune Globulin and found to be equal to 217 international units (IU) per mL. Hepatitis B Immune Globulin must be administered intramuscularly.

There is no evidence to suggest that the causative virus of AIDS (HIV) has been transmitted by Hepatitis B Immune Globulin prepared by the cold ethanol process.

CLINICAL PHARMACOLOGY

Hepatitis B Immune Globulin (Human) provides passive immunization for individuals exposed to the hepatitis B virus (HBV) as evidenced by a reduction in the attack rate of hepatitis B following its use.[1-6] The administration of the usual recommended dose of this immune globulin generally results in a detectable level of circulating anti-HBs which persists for approximately 2 months or longer. The highest antibody (IgG) serum levels were seen in the following distribution of subjects studied:

Day	% Of Subjects
3	38.9%
7	41.7%
14	11.1%
21	8.3%

Mean values for half-life were between 17.5 and 25 days, with the shortest being 5.9 days and the longest 35 days.[7]

Cases of type B hepatitis are rarely seen following exposure to HBV in persons with pre-existing anti-HBs. No confirmed instance of transmission of hepatitis B has been associated with this product.

INDICATIONS AND USAGE

Hepatitis B Immune Globulin (Human) is indicated for postexposure prophylaxis following either sexual exposure, parenteral exposure, e.g., by accidental "needle-stick," direct mucous membrane contact (accidental splash), or oral ingestion (pipetting accident) involving HBsAg-positive materials such as blood, plasma or serum.

Hepatitis B Immune Globulin also indicated for prophylaxis of infants born to HBsAg-positive mothers. Such infants are at risk of being infected with hepatitis B virus and becoming chronic carriers.[5,8-10] The risk is especially great if the mother is HBeAg-positive.[11,12] For perinatal exposure to an HBsAg-positive, HBeAg-positive mother, a regimen combining one dose of Hepatitis B Immune Globulin (Human) at birth with the Hepatitis B Vaccine series started soon after birth is 94% effective in preventing development of the HB carrier state.[13] Regimens involving either multiple doses of Hepatitis B Immune Globulin (Human) alone, or Hepatitis B Vaccine series alone, have a 70%-75% efficacy, while a single dose of Hepatitis B Immune Globulin (Human) alone has only 50% efficacy.

Administration of Hepatitis B Immune Globulin (Human) either preceding or concomitant with the commencement of active immunization with Hepatitis B Vaccine provides for more rapid achievement of protective levels of hepatitis B antibody, than when the vaccine alone is administered.[15] Rapid achievement of protective levels of antibody to hepatitis B virus may be desirable in certain clinical situations, as in cases of accidental inoculations with contaminated medical instruments.[15] Administration of Hepatitis B Immune Globulin (Human) either 1 month preceding or at the time of commencement of a program of active vaccination with Hepatitis B Vaccine has been shown not to interfere with the active immune response to the vaccine.[15]

CONTRAINDICATIONS

Hypersensitivity to any component of the product.

WARNINGS

Persons with isolated immunoglobulin A deficiency have the potential for developing antibodies to immunoglobulin A and could have anaphylactic reactions to subsequent administration of blood products that contain immuno-globulin A. Therefore, as with any immunoglobulin preparation, Hepatitis B Immune Globulin (Human) should be given to such persons only if the expected benefits outweigh the potential risks.

Hepatitis B Immune Globulin should be given with caution to patients with a history of prior systemic allergic reactions following the administration of human immune globulin preparations or in patients who are known to have had an allergic response to thimerosal. Epinephrine should be available.

In patients who have severe thrombocytopenia or any coagulation disorder that would contraindicate intramuscular injections, Hepatitis B Immune Globulin (Human) should be given only if the expected benefits outweigh the risks.

PRECAUTIONS

GENERAL

Hepatitis B Immune Globulin (Human) should **not** be administered intravenously because of the potential for serious reactions. Injections should be made intramuscularly, and care should be taken to draw back on the plunger of the syringe before injection in order to be certain that the needle is not in a blood vessel.

Intramuscular injections are preferably administered in the anterolateral aspects of the upper thigh and the deltoid muscle of the upper arm. The gluteal region should not be used routinely as an injection site because of the risk of injury to the sciatic nerve. An individual decision as to which muscle is injected must be made for each patient based on the volume of material to be administered. If the gluteal region is used when very large volumes are to be injected or multiple doses are necessary, the central region MUST be avoided; only the upper, outer quadrant should be used.[16]

There is no evidence that the causative virus of AIDS (HIV-1) is transmitted by Hepatitis B Immune Globulin which is prepared by a cold alcohol process.

Some investigational intravenous immunoglobulin products have been linked to transmission of non-A, non-B hepatitis; however, there have been no reports of this in association with Hepatitis B Immune Globulin.

LABORATORY TESTS

None required.

DRUG INTERACTIONS

Although administration of Hepatitis B Immune Globulin (Human) did not interfere with measles vaccination,[17] it is not known whether Hepatitis B Immune Globulin (Human) may interfere with other live virus vaccines. Therefore, use of such vaccines should be deferred until approximately three months after Hepatitis B Immune Globulin (Human) administration. Hepatitis B Vaccine may be administered at the same time, but at a different injection site, without interfering with the immune response.[15] It may be necessary to revaccinate persons who received Hepatitis B Immune Globulin (Human) shortly after live virus vaccination. No interactions with other products are known.

PREGNANCY CATEGORY C

Animal reproduction studies have not been conducted with Hepatitis B Immune Globulin. It is also not known whether Hepatitis B Immune Globulin can cause fetal harm when administered to a pregnant woman or can affect reproduction capacity. Hepatitis B Immune Globulin should be given to a pregnant woman only if clearly needed.

NURSING MOTHERS

It is not known whether this drug is excreted in human milk. Because many drugs are excreted in human milk, caution should be exercised when Hepatitis B Immune Globulin is administered to a nursing woman.

RECOMMENDATIONS FOR HEPATITIS B PROPHYLAXIS FOLLOWING PRECUTANEOUS EXPOSURE

Source	Exposed Person	
	Unvaccinated	Vaccinated
HBsAg-Positive	1. Hepatitis B Immune Globulin (Human)×1 immediately* 2. Initiate HB Vaccine series†	1. Test exposed person for anti-HBs. 2. If inadequate antibody,‡ Hepatitis B Immune Globulin (Human) (×1) immediately plus HB Vaccine booster dose at two different sites.
Known Source (High Risk)	1. Initiate HB Vaccine series 2. Test source for HBsAg. If positive, Hepatitis B Immune Globulin (Human)×1	1. Test Source for HBsAg only if exposed is vaccine nonresponder; if source is HBsAg-positive, give Hepatitis B Immune Globulin (Human)×1 immediately plus HB Vaccine booster dose.
Low Risk HBsAg-Positive	Initiate HB Vaccine series.	Nothing required.
Unknown Source	Initiate HB Vaccine series.	Nothing required.

* *Hepatitis B Immune Globulin (Human), dose 0.06 mL/kg IM.*
† *HB Vaccine dose 20 µg IM for adults; 10 µg IM for infants for children under 10 years of age. First dose within 1 week; second and third doses, 1 and 6 months later.*
‡ *Less than 10 sample ratio units (SRU) by radioimmunoassay (RIA), negative by enzyme immunoassay (EIA).*

ADVERSE REACTIONS
Local pain and tenderness at the injection site, urticaria and angioedema may occur; anaphylactic reactions, although rare, have been reported following the injection of human immune globulin preparations.[18] Anapylaxis is more likely to occur if Hepatitis B Immune Globulin (Human) is given intravenously; therefore, Hepatitis B Immune Globulin (Human) must be administered *only* intramuscularly. In highly allergic individuals, repeated injections may lead to anaphylactic shock.

OVERDOSAGE
Although no data are available, clinical experience with other immunoglobulin preparations suggests that the only manifestations would be pain and tenderness at the injection site.

DOSAGE AND ADMINISTRATION
ACUTE EXPOSURE TO BLOOD CONTAINING HBSAG[14]
The following table summarizes prophylaxis for percutaneous (needlestick or bite), ocular, or mucous-membrane exposure to blood according to the source of exposure and vaccination status of the exposed person. For greatest effectiveness, passive prophylaxis with Hepatitis B Immune Globulin (Human) should be given as soon as possible after exposure (its value beyond 7 days of exposure is unclear). If Hepatitis B Immune Globulin (Human) is indicated (see table below), an injection of 0.06 mL/kg of body weight should be administered intramuscularly (see *"Precautions"*). Consult Hepatitis B Vaccine package insert for dosage information regarding that product. (See related table).

For persons who refuse Hepatitis B Vaccine, a second dose of Hepatitis B Immune Globulin should be given 1 month after the first dose.

PROPHYLAXIS OF INFANTS BORN TO HBs:UCAG
AND HBe:UCAG POSITIVE MOTHERS
Infants born to HBsAg positive mothers are at high risk of becoming chronic carriers of hepatitis B virus and of developing the chronic sequelae of hepatitis B virus infection.

Efficacy of prophylactic Hepatitis B Immune Globulin (Human) in infants at risk depends on administering Hepatitis B Immune Globulin (Human) on the day of birth. It is therefore vital that HBsAg-positive mothers are identified before delivery.

Hepatitis B Immune Globulin (Human) (0.5 mL) should be administered intramuscularly (IM) to the newborn infant after physiologic stabilization of the infant and preferably within 12 hours of birth. Hepatitis B Immune Globulin (Human) efficacy decreases markedly if treatment is delayed beyond 48 hours. Hepatitis B Vaccine should be administered IM in three doses of 0.5 mL of vaccine (10 µg) each. The first dose should be given within 7 days of birth and may be given concurrently with Hepatitis B Immune Globulin (Human) but in the opposite anterolateral thigh. The second and third doses of vaccine should be given 1 month and 6 months, respectively, after the first. If administration of the first dose of Hepatitis B Vaccine is delayed for as long as 3 months, then a 0.5 mL dose of Hepatitis B Immune Globulin (Human) should be repeated at 3 months. If Hepatitis B Vaccine is refused, the 0.5 mL dose of Hepatitis B Immune Globulin (Human) should be repeated at 3 and 6 months. Hepatitis B Immune Globulin (Human) administered at birth should not interfere with oral polio and diphtheria-tetanus-pertussis vaccines administered at 2 months of age.[14]

Hepatitis B Immune Globulin (Human) may be administered at the same time (but at a different site), or up to 1 month preceding Hepatitis B Vaccination without impairing the active immune response from Hepatitis B Vaccination.[15]

Testing for HBsAg and anti-HBs is recommended at 12-15 months of age. If HBsAg is not detectable, and anti-HBs is present, the child has been protected.

Parenteral drug products should be inspected visually for particulate matter and discoloration prior to administration, whenever solution and container permit.

Administer intramuscularly. Do not inject intravenously.

It is important to use a separate sterile syringe and needle for each individual patient to prevent transmission of hepatitis B and other infectious agents from one person to another.

STORAGE
Store at 2°-8°C (35°-46°F). Do not freeze. Do not use after expiration date.

REFERENCES
1. Grady GF, Lee VA: Hepatitis B immune globulin—prevention of hepatitis from accidental exposure among medical personnel. *N Engl J Med* 293(21): 1067-70, 1975. 2. Seeff LB, Zimmerman HJ, Wright EC, et al: Efficacy of hepatitis B immune serum globulin after accidental exposure. *Lancet* 2(7942):939-41, 1975. 3. Krugman S, Giles JP: Viral hepatitis, type B (MS-2-strain). Further observations on natural history and prevention. *N Engl J Med* 288(15):755-60, 1973. 4. Current trends: Health status of Indochinese refugees: malaria and hepatitis B. *MMWR* 28(39):463-4; 469-70, 1979. 5. Jhaveri R, Rosenfeld W, Salazar JD, et al: High titer multiple dose therapy with HBIG in newborn infants of HBsAg positive mothers. *J Pediatr* 97(2):305-8, 1980. 6. Hoofnagle JH, Seeff LB, Bales ZB, et al: Passive-active immunity from hepatitis B immune globulin. *Ann Intern Med* 91(6):813-8, 1979. 7. Scheiermann N, Kuwert EK: Uptake and elimination of hepatitis B immunoglobulins after intramuscular application in man. *Dev Biol Stand* 54:347-55, 1983. 8. Stevens CE, Beasley RP, Tsui J, et al: Vertical transmission of hepatitis B antigen in Taiwan. *N Engl J Med* 292(15):771-4, 1975. 9. Shiraki K, Yoshihara N, Kawana T, et al: Hepatitis B surface antigen and chronic hepatitis in infants born to asymptomatic carrier mothers. *Am J Dis Child* 131(6):644-7, 1977. 10. Recommendation of the Immunization Practices Advisory Committee (ACIP): Immune globulins for protection against viral hepatitis. *MMWR* 30(34):423-8; 433-5, 1981. 11. Okada K, Kamiyama I, Inomata M, et al: e antigen and anti-e in the serum of asymptomatic carrier mothers as indicators of positive and negative transmission of hepatitis B virus to their infants. *N Engl J Med* 294(14):746-9, 1976. 12. Beasley RP, Trepo C, Stevens CE, et al: The e antigen and vertical transmission of hepatitis B surface antigen. *Am J Epidemiol* 105(2):94-8, 1977. 13. Beasley RP, Hwang LY, Lee GCY, et al: Prevention of perinatally transmitted hepatitis B virus infections with hepatitis B immune globulin and hepatitis B vaccine. *Lancet* 2(8359):1099-102, 1983. 14. Recommendation of the Immunization Practices Advisory Committee (ACIP): Recommendations for protection against viral hepatitis. *MMWR* 34(22):313-35, 1985. 15. Szmuness W, Stevens CE, Olesko WR, et al: Passive-active immunisation against hepatitis B: Immunogenicity studies in adult Americans. *Lancet* 1:575-77, 1981. 16. Recommendations of the Immunization Practices Advisory Committee (ACIP): General recommendations on immunization. *MMWR* 38(13):205-14; 219-27, 1989. 17. Beasley RP, Hwang LY: Measles vaccination not interfered with by hepatitis B immune globulin. *Lancet* 1:161, 1982. 18. Ellis EF, Henney CS: Adverse reactions following administration of human gamma globulin. *J Allerg* 43(1):45-54, 1969.

HOW SUPPLIED
INJECTION:

BRAND/MANUFACTURER	NDC	SIZE	AWP
BRAND			
HYPERHEP: Miles Biol	00192-0616-00	0.5 ml	$35.41
H-BIG:	00074-8399-11	0.5 ml	$56.25
	00074-8399-01	1 ml	$53.44
HYPERHEP: Miles Biol	00192-0616-01	1 ml	$71.75
H-BIG:	00074-8399-04	4 ml	$156.75
	00074-8399-05	5 ml	$182.88
HYPERHEP: Miles Biol	00192-0616-05	5 ml	$240.19
HEP-B-GAMMAGEE: Merck	00006-4692-00	5 ml	$393.84
H-BIG: Nabi	05973-0399-11	0.5 ml	$45.00
	05973-0399-01	1 ml	$45.00
	05973-0399-05	5 ml	$146.00

Hepatitis B Vaccine, Recombinant

DESCRIPTION
Hepatitis B Vaccine-Recombinant is a noninfectious subunit viral vaccine derived from Hepatitis B surface antigen (HBsAg) produced in yeast cells. A

portion of the hepatitis B virus gene, coding for HBsAg, is cloned into yeast, and the vaccine for hepatitis B is produced from cultures of this recombinant yeast strain.

The antigen is harvested and purified from fermentation cultures of a recombinant strain of the yeast *Saccharomyces cerevisiae* containing the gene for the *adw* subtype of HBsAg. The HBsAg protein is released from the yeast cells by cell disruption and purified by a series of physical and chemical methods. The vaccine contains no detectable yeast DNA but may contain 1% to 5% yeast protein. The vaccine has been shown to be comparable to the plasma-derived vaccine in terms of animal potency (mouse, monkey, and chimpanzee) and protective efficacy (chimpanzee and human).

Some vaccines against hepatitis B, prepared from recombinant yeast cultures, are free of association with human blood or blood products. No substances of human origin are used in the manufacture of others.

Each lot of Hepatitis B Vaccine is tested for safety, in mice and guinea pigs, and for sterility.

Hepatitis B Vaccine-Recombinant is a sterile suspension for intramuscular injection. However, for persons at risk of hemorrhage following intramuscular injection, the vaccine may be administered subcutaneously. (See *"Dosage And Administration".*) The vaccine is ready for use without reconstitution; it must be shaken before administration since a fine white deposit with a clear colorless supernatant may form on storage.

Hepatitis B Vaccine-Recombinant is supplied in formulations.

Pediatric Formulation, 5 or 20 mcg/mL: each 0.5 mL dose contains 2.5 or 10 mcg of hepatitis B surface antigen.

Adolescent/High-Risk Infant, 10 mcg/mL: each 0.5 mL dose contains 5 mcg of hepatitis B surface antigen.

Adult Formulation, 10 or 20 mcg/mL each 1 mL dose contains 10 or 20 mcg of hepatitis B surface antigen.

Dialysis Formulation, 40 mcg/mL: each 1 mL dose contains 40 mcg of hepatitis B surface antigen.

The vaccine is of the *adw* subtype. Hepatitis B Vaccine-Recombinant is indicated for vaccination of persons at risk of infection from hepatitis B virus including all known subtypes. Hepatitis B Vaccine-Recombinant Dialysis Formulation is indicated for vaccination of adult predialysis and dialysis patients against infection caused by all known subtypes of hepatitis B virus.

CLINICAL PHARMACOLOGY

Hepatitis B virus is one of at least three hepatitis viruses that cause a systemic infection, with a major pathology in the liver. The others include hepatitis A virus, and non-A, non-B hepatitis viruses. The estimated lifetime risk of HBV infection in the United States varies from almost 100% for the highest-risk groups to approximately 5% for the population as a whole.[1]

Hepatitis B virus is an important cause of viral hepatitis. There is no specific treatment for this disease. The incubation period for hepatitis B is relatively long; six weeks to six months may elapse between exposure and the onset of clinical symptoms. The prognosis following infection with hepatitis B virus is variable and dependent on at least three factors: (1) Age—Infants and younger children usually experience milder initial disease than older persons; (2) Dose of virus—The higher the dose, the more likely acute icteric hepatitis B will result; and, (3) Severity of associated underlying disease—underlying malignancy or pre-existing hepatic disease predisposes to increased mortality and morbidity.

Persistence of viral infection (the chronic hepatitis B virus carrier state) occurs in 5-10% of persons following acute hepatitis B, and occurs more frequently after initial anicteric hepatitis B than after initial icteric disease. Consequently, carriers of hepatitis B surface antigen (HBsAg) frequently give no history of having had recognized acute hepatitis. Sixty to 80% of neonates and 6 to 10% of adults who are infected in the United States will become hepatitis B virus carriers.[1] It has been estimated that more than 170 million people in the world today are persistently infected with hepatitis B virus. The Centers for Disease Control (CDC) estimates that there are approximately 0.75 to 1 million chronic carriers of hepatitis B virus in the USA. Chronic carriers represent the largest human reservoir of hepatitis B virus.

The serious complications and sequelae of hepatitis B virus infection include massive hepatic necrosis, cirrhosis of the liver, chronic active hepatitis, and hepatocellular carcinoma. Chroninc carriers of HBsAg can infect others and appear to be at increased risk of developing primary hepatocellular carcinoma. Although a number of etiologic factors are associated with development of hepatocellular carcinoma, the single most important etiologic factor appears to be active infection with the hepatitis B virus.[1,3] Considering the serious consequences of infection, immunization should be considered for all persons at potential risk of exposure to the hepatitis B virus.

There is also evidence that several diseases other than hepatitis have been associated with hepatitis B virus infection through an immunologic mechanism involving antigen-antibody complexes. Such diseases include a syndrome with rash, urticaria, and arthralgia resembling serum sickness; periarteritis nodosa; membranous glomerulonephritis; and infantile papular acrodermatitis.

Although the vehicles for transmission of the virus are often blood and blood products, viral antigen has also been found in tears, saliva, breast milk, urine, semen and vaginal secretions. Hepatitis B virus is capable of surviving for days on environmental surfaces exposed to body fluids containing hepatitis B virus. Infection may occur when hepatitis B virus, transmitted by infected body fluids, is implanted via mucous surfaces or percutaneously introduced through accidental or deliberate breaks in the skin.

Transmission of hepatitis B virus infection is often associated with close interpersonal contact with an infected individual and with crowded living conditions. In such circumstances, transmission by inoculation via routes other than overt percutaneous ones may be quite common. Perinatal transmission of hepatitis B infection from infected mother to child, at or shortly after birth, can occur if the mother is a hepatitis B surface antigen (HBsAg) carrier or if the mother has an acute hepatitis B infection in the third trimester. Infection in infancy by the hepatitis B virus usually leads to the chronic carrier state. Among infants born to women whose sera are positive for both the hepatitis B surface antigen and the e antigen, 85-90% are infected and become chronic carriers. Therefore, screening of pregnant women for hepatitis B is recommended. Well-controlled studies have shown that administration of three 0.5 mL doses of Hepatitis B Immune Globulin (Human) starting at birth is 75% effective in preventing establishment of the chronic carrier state in these infants during the first year of life. However, the protective effect of Hepatitis B Immune Globulin (Human) is transient. Hepatitis B is endemic throughout the world and is a serious medical problem in population groups at increased risk. Because vaccination limited to high-risk individuals has failed to substantially lower the overall incidence of hepatitis B infection, both the immunization Practices Advisory Committee (ACIP) and the Committee on Infectious Diseases of the American Academy of Pediatrics (AAP) have also endorsed universal infant immunization as part of a comprehensive strategy for the control of hepatitis B infection. These advisory groups further recommended broad-based vaccination of adolescents. The ACIP encourages universal hepatitis B vaccination of adolescents in communities where use of illicit injectable drugs, pregnancy among teenagers, and/or sexually transmitted diseases are common. Similarly, the AAP recommends that universal immunization of all adolescents should be implemented when resources permit with emphasis on those individuals in high-risk settings. (Refer to *"Indications and Usage".*)

Numerous epidemiological studies have shown that persons who develop anti-HBs following active infection with the hepatitis B virus are protected against the disease on reexposure to the virus.

Clinical studies have shown that Hepatitis B Vaccine-Recombinant when injected into the deltoid muscle induced protective levels of antibody in 96% of 1213 healthy adults who received the recommended 3-dose regimen. Antibody responses varied with age; a protective level of antibody was induced in 98% of 787 young adults 20-29 years of age, 94% of 249 adults 30-39 years of age and in 89% of 177 adults $\geq$ 40 years of age. Studies with hepatitis B vaccine derived from plasma have shown that a lower response rate (81%) to vaccine may be obtained if the vaccine is administered as a buttock injection. Seroconversion rates and geometric mean antibody titers were measured 1 to 2 months after the 3rd dose. Multiple clinical studies have defined a protective antibody (anti-HBs) level as 1) 10 or more sample ratio units (SRU) as determined by radioimmunoassay or 2) a positive result as determined by enzyme immunoassay. Note: 10 SRU is comparable to 10 mIU/mL of antibody. Seroconversion is defined as antibody titers $\geq$ 1 mIU/mL.

Other clinical trials in healthy adult and adolescent subjects have shown that following a course of three dosesof 20 mcg Hepatitis B Vaccine-Recombinant given according to the Immunization Practices Advisory Committee (ACIP) recommended schedule of injections at months 0, 1 and 6, the seroprotection (antibody titers $\geq$ 10 mIU/mL) rate for all individuals was 79% at month 6 and 96% at month 7; the geometric mean antibody titer (GMT) for seroconverters at month 7 was 2,204 mIU/mL. On an alternate schedule (injections at months 0, 1 and 2) designed for certain populations (e.g., neonates born of hepatitis B infected mothers, individuals who have or might have been recently exposed to the virus, and certain travelers to high-risk areas. See *"Indications and Usage."* 99% of all individuals were seroprotected at month 3 and remained protected through month 12. On the alternate schedule, an additional dose at 12 months produced a GMT for seroconverters at month 13 of 9,163 mIU/mL.

Hepatitis B Vaccine-Recombinant is highly immunogenic in younger individuals In clinical studies, 99% of 94 infants under 1 year of age born of non-carrier mothers, 96% of 48 children 1-10 years of age, and 99% of 112 children and adolescents 11-19 years of age developed a protective level of antibody following the recommended 3-dose regimen of vaccine (see *"Dosage and Administrtion"*).

The protective efficacy of three 5 mcg doses of Hepatitis B Vaccine-Recombinant has been demonstrated in neonates born of mothers positive for both HBsAg and HBeAg (a core-associated antigenic complex which correlates with high infectivity). In a clinical study of infants who received one dose of Hepatitis B Immune Globulin at birth followed by the recommended three dose regimen of Hepatitis B Vaccine-Recombinant, chronic infection had not occurred in 96% of 130 infants after nine months of follow-up. The estimated efficacy in prevention of chronic hepatitis B infection was 95% as compared to the infection rate in untreated historical controls. Significantly fewer neonates became chronically infected when given one dose of Hepatitis B Immune Globulin at birth followed by the recommended three dose regimen of Hepatitis B Vaccine-Recombinant, when compared to historical controls who received only a single dose of Hepatitis B Immune Globulin. Testing for HBsAg and anti-HBs is recommended at 12-15 months of age. If HBsAg is not detectable and anti-HBs is present, the child has been protected.

As demonstrated in the above study, Hepatitis B Immune Globulin, when administered simultaneously with Hepatitis B Vaccine-Recombinant at separate body sites, did not interfere with the induction of protective antibodies against hepatitis B virus elicited by the vaccine.

Immunogenicity in Neonates: Immunization with 10 mcg at 0, 1 and 2 months of age produced a seroprotection rate of 96% infants by month 4, with a GMT among seroconverters of 210 mlU/mL (N = 311); an additional dose at month 12 produced a GMT among seroconverters of 2,941 mlU/mL at month 13 (N = 126).

Immunization with 10 meg at 0. 1 and 6 months of age produced seroconversion in 100% of infants by month 7 with a GMT of 713 mlU/mL (N = 52), and the seroprotection rate was 97%.

Clinical trials indicate that administration of hepatitis B immune globulin at birth does not alter the response to Hepatitis B Vaccine-Recombinant.

In clinical trials with 242 children ages 6 months to, and including, 10 years given 10 meg at months 0.1 and 6, the seroprotection rate was 98% one to two months after the third dose; the GMT of seroconverters was 4,023 mlU/mL.

Immunogenicity in Older Subjects: Among older subjects given 20 meg at months 0.1 and 6, the seroprotection rate one month after the third dose was 88%. However, as with other hepatitis B vaccines, in adults over 40 years of age. Hepatitis B Vaccine-Recombinant produced anti-HBs titers that were lower than those in younger adults (GMT among seroconverters one month after the third 20 meg dose with a 0,1, 6-month schedule: 610 mlU/mL for individuals over 40 years of age, N = 50).

The duration of the protective effect of Hepatitis B Vaccine-Recombinant in healthy vaccines is unknown at present and the need for booster doses is not yet defined. However, long-term follow-up (5 to 9 years) of approximately 3000 high-risk vaccinees (infants of carrier mothers, male homosexuals, Alaskan Natives) who developed an anti-HBs titer of ≥ 10 mlU/mL when given a similar plasma-derived vaccine of intervals of 0, 1, and 6 months showed that no subjects developed clinically apparent hepatitis B infection and that 5 subjects developed antigenemia, even though up to half of the subjects failed to maintain a titer at this level. Persistence of immunologic memory was demonstrated by an anamnestic antibody response to a booster dose of Hepatitis B Vaccine-Recombinant in healthy adults given plasma-derived vaccine 5 to 7 years earlier at intervals of 0, 1, and 6 months.

Protective efficacy with Hepatitis B Vaccine-Recombinant has been demonstrated in a clinical trial in neonates at high risk of hepatitis B infection.[6,7] Fifty-eight neonates born of mothers who were both HBsAg and HBeAg positive were given Hepatitis B Vaccine-Recombinant (10 meg at 0, 1 and 2 months) without concomitant hepatitis B immune globulin. Two infants became chronic carriers in the 12-month follow-up period after initial inoculation. Assuming an expected carrier rate of 70%,[1] the protective efficacy rate against the chronic carrier state during the first 12 months of life was 95%.

Other Clinical Studies: In one study,[8] four of 244 (1.6%) adults (homosexual men) at high risk of contracting hepatitis B virus became infected during the period prior to completion of three doses of Hepatitis B Vaccine-Recombinant (20 mcg at 0, 1, 6 months). No additional patients became infected during the 18-month follow-up period after completion of the immunization course.

Predialysis and Dialysis Patients: Hemodialysis patients given hepatis B vaccines respond with lower titers,[5] which remain at protective levels for shorter durations than in normal subjects. In a study in which patients on chronic hemodialysis (mean time on dialysis was 24 months: N = 562) received 40 mcg of the plasma-derived vaccine at months 0, 1, and 6, approximately 50% of patients achieved antibody titers ≥ 10 mlU/mL.[5]

Since a fourth dose of Hepatitis B Vaccine-Recombinant given to healthy adults at month 12 following the 0, 1, 2-month schedule resulted in a substantial increase in the GMT (see above), a four-dose regimen was studied in hemodialysis patients. In a clinical trial of adults who had been on hemodialysis for a mean of 56 months (N = 43), 67% of patients were seroprotected two months after the last dose of 40 mcg of Hepatitis B Vaccine-Recombinant (two × 20 mcg) given on a 0, 1, 2, 6-month schedule; the GMT among seroconverters was 93 mlU/mL.

In addition, the responses to these vaccines may be lower if the vaccine is administered as a buttock injection. When 40 mcg of Hepatitis B Vaccine-Recombinant was administered in the deltoid muscle, 89% of 28 participants developed anti-HBs with 86% achieving levels ≥ 10 mlU/mL. However, when the same dosage of this vaccine was administered inappropriately either in the buttock or a combination of buttock and deltoid, 62% of 47 participants developed anti-HBs with 55% achieving levels ≥ 10 mlU/mL.

Revaccination with Hepatitis B Vaccine-Recombinant Dialysis Formulation may be considered in predialysis/dialysis patients if the anti-HBs level is less than 10 mlU/mL.

Reports in the literature describe a more virulent form of hepatitis B associated with superinfections or coinfections by delta virus, an imcomplete RNA virus. Delta virus can only infect and cause illness in persons infected with hepatitis B virus since the delta agent requires a coat of HBsAg in order to become infectious. Therefore, persons immune to hepatitis B virus infection should also be immune to delta virus infection.

Interchangeability of Plasma-Derived and Recombinant Hepatitis B Vaccines: Recombinant DNA vaccines are produced in yeast by expression of a hepatitis B virus gene sequence that codes for the hepatitis B surface antigen. Like plasma-derived vaccine, the yeast-derived vaccines are protein particles visible by electron microscopy and have hepatitis B surface antigen epitopes as determined by monoclonal antibody analyses.

Yeast-derived vaccines have been shown by *in vitro* analyses to induce antibodies (anti-HBs) which are immunologically comparable by epitope specificity and binding affinity to antibodies induced by plasma-derived vaccine.[9] In cross absorption studies, no differences were detected in the spectra of antibodies induced in man to plasma-derived or to yeast-derived hepatitis B vaccines.[9]

Additionally, patients immunized approximately three years previously with plasma-derived vaccine and whose antibody titers were < 100 mlU/mL (GMT: 35

mlU/mL; range: 9-94) were given a 20 mcg dose of Hepatitis B Vaccine-Recombinant. All patients, including two who had not responded to the plasma-derived vaccine, showed a response to Hepatitis B Vaccine-Recombinant (GMT: 5,069 mlU/mL; range: 624-15,019).

There have been no clinical studies in which a three-dose vaccine series was initiated with a plasma-derived hepatitis B vaccine and completed with Hepatitis B Vaccine-Recombinant, or vice versa. However, because the *in vitro* and *in vivo* studies described above indicate the comparability of the antibody produced in response to plasma-derived vaccine and Hepatitis B Vaccine-Recombinant it should be possible to interchange the use of Hepatitis B Vaccine-Recombinant and plasma-derived vaccines (but see *"Contraindications"*).

A controlled study (N = 48) demonstrated that completion of a course of immunization with one dose of Hepatitis B Vaccine-Recombinant (20 mcg, month 6) following two doses of Plasma-derived Hepatitis B Vaccine (10 mcg, months 0 and 1) produced a similar GMT (4,077 mlU/mL) to immunization with three doses of Plasma-derived Hepatitis B Vaccine (10 mcg, months 0, 1 and 6; 2,654 mlU/mL). Thus, Hepatitis B Vaccine-Recombinant can be used to complete a vaccination course initiated with Plasma-derived Hepatitis B Vaccine.

INDICATIONS AND USAGE

Hepatitis B Vaccine-Recombinant is indicated for vaccination against infection caused by all known subtypes of hepatitis B virus. As hepatitis D (caused by the delta virus) does not occur in the absence of hepatitis B infection, it can be expected that hepatitis D will also be prevented by Hepatitis B Vaccine-Recombinant vaccination. Vaccination with Hepatitis B Vaccine-Recombinant is recommended for:

1) Infants including those born to HBsAg positive mothers (high-risk infants) whether HBeAg positive or negative.
2) Adolescents (see *"Clinical Pharmacology"*).
3) Other persons of all ages in areas of high prevalence or those who are or may be at increased risk of infection with hepatitis B virus, such as:

■ *Health Care Personnel*
   Dentists and oral surgeons.
   Physicians, surgeons and pediatrists.
   Nurses.
   Paramedical and ambulance personnel and custodial staff who may be exposed to the virus via blood or other patient specimens.
   Dental hygienists and dental nurses.
   Laboratory personnel handling blood, blood products, and other patient specimens.
   Dental, medical and nursing students.
   Hospital cleaning staff who handle waste.
■ *Selected Patients and Patient Contacts*
   Patients and staff in hemodialysis units and hematology/oncology units.
   Patients requiring frequent and/or large volume blood transfusions or clotting factor concentrates (e.g., persons with hemophilia, thalassemia, sickle-cell anemia, cirrhosis).
   Clients (residents) and staff of institutions for the mentally handicapped.
   Classroom contacts of deinstitutionalized mentally handicapped persons who have persistent hepatitis B surface antigenemia and who show aggressive behavior.
   Household and other intimate contacts of persons with persistent hepatitis B surface antigenemia.
■ *Sub-populations with a known high incidence of the disease,* such as:
   Alaskan Natives.
   Pacific Islanders.
   Refugees from areas where hepatitis B virus infection is endemic.
   All infants of women born in areas where the infection is highly endemic.
■ *Persons who may be exposed to the hepatitis B virus by travel to high risk areas (See ACIP Guidelines, 1985.)*
■ *Military Personnel identified as being at increased risk*
■ *Morticians and Embalmers*
■ *Blood bank and plasma fractionation workers*
■ *Persons at increased risk of the disease due to their sexual practices, such as:*
   Persons who have heterosexual activity with multiple partners.
   Persons who have contracted or repeatedly contract sexually transmitted diseases.
   Homosexually active males.
   Female prostitutes.
■ *Prisoners*
■ *Users of illicit injectable drugs*
■ *Others*
   Police and fire department personnel who render first aid or medical assistance, and any others who, through their work or personal life-style, may be exposed to the hepatitis B virus.

Neither dosage strength will prevent hepatitis caused by other agents, such as hepatitis A virus, non-A, non-B hepatitis viruses, or other viruses known to infect the liver.

Revaccination: (See *"Clinical Pharmacology."*)

Use with Other Vaccines: Specific data are not yet available for the simultaneous administration of Hepatitis B Vaccine-Recombinant with other vaccines. However, the Immunization Practices Advisory Committee states that, in general, simultaneous administration of certain live and inactivated pediatric vaccines has not resulted in impaired antibody responses or increased rates of adverse reactions.[12] Separate sites and syringes should be used for simultaneous administration of injectable vaccines.

CONTRAINDICATIONS
Hypersensitivity to yeast or any component of the vaccine.

WARNINGS
Patients who develop symptoms suggestive of hypersensitivity after an injection should not receive further injections of the vaccine (see "Contraindications").

Because of the long incubation period for hepatitis B, it is possible for unrecognized infection to be present at the time the vaccine is given. The vaccine may not prevent hepatitis B in such patients. Additionally, it may not prevent infection in individuals who do not achieve protective antibody titers.

PRECAUTIONS
GENERAL
As with any percutaneous vaccine, epinephrine should be available for immediate use should an anaphylactoid reaction occur.

Any febrile illness or serious active infection is reason for delaying use of the vaccine except when in the opinion of the physician, withholding the vaccine entails a greater risk.

Caution and appropriate care should be exercised in administering the vaccine to individuals with severely compromised cardiopulmonary status or to others in whom a febrile or systemic reaction could pose a significant risk.

PREGNANCY
Pregnancy Category C: Animal reproduction studies have not been conducted with the vaccine. It is also not known whether the vaccine can cause fetal harm when administered to a pregnant woman or can affect reproduction capacity. The vaccine should be given to a pregnant woman only if clearly needed.

NURSING MOTHERS
It is not known whether the vaccine is excreted in human milk. Because many drugs are excreted in human milk, cautions should be exercised when the vaccine is administered to a nursing woman.

PEDIATRIC USE
Hepatitis B Vaccine-Recombinant has been shown to be usually well-tolerated and highly immunogenic in infants and children of all ages. Newborns also respond well; maternally transferred antibodies do not interfere with the active immune response to the vaccine. (See "Clinical Pharmacology" for seroconversion rates and titers in neonates and children. See "Dosage and Administration" for recommended pediatric dosage and for recommended dosage for infants born to HBsAg positive mothers.)

The safety and effectiveness of Hepatitis B Vaccine-Recombinant Dialysis Formulation in children have not been established.

ADVERSE REACTIONS
Hepatitis B Vaccine-Recombinant is generally well-tolerated. No serious adverse reactions attributable to the vaccine have been reported during the course of clinical trials. No adverse experiences were reported during clinical trials which could be related to changes in the titers of antibodies to yeast. As with any vaccine, there is the possibility that broad use of the vaccine could reveal adverse reactions not observed in clinical trials.

In a group of studies, 1636 doses of Hepatitis B Vaccine-Recombinant were administered to 653 healthy infants and children (up to 10 years of age) who were monitored for 5 days after each dose.

Injection site reactions (including erythema and swelling) and systemic complaints were reported following 8% and 17% of the injections, respectively. The most frequently reported systemic adverse reactions (> 1% injections), in decreasing order of frequency, were irritability, tiredness, fever (> 101°F oral equivalent), crying, diarrhea, vomiting diminished appetite, and insomnia.

In a group of studies, 3258 doses of Hepatitis B Vaccine-Recombinant were administered to 1252 healthy adults who were monitored for 5 days after each dose. Injection site and systemic complaints were reported following 17% and 15% of the injections, respectively. The following adverse reactions were reported:

Ten double-blind studies involving 2,252 subjects showed no significant difference in the frequency or severity of adverse experiences between Hepatitis B Vaccine-Recombinant and plasma-derived vaccines. In 36 clinical studies a total of 13,495 doses of Hepatitis B Vaccine-Recombinant were administered to 5,071 healthy adults and children who were initially seronegative for hepatitis B markers, and healthy neonates. All subjects were monitored for 4 days post-administration. Frequency of adverse experiences tended to decrease with successive doses of Hepatitis B Vaccine-Recombinant. Using a symptom checklist, the most frequently reported adverse reactions were injection site soreness (22%) and fatigue (14%). Other reactions are listed below.

INCIDENCE EQUAL TO OR GREATER THAN 1% OF INJECTIONS
Local Reaction (Injection Site): Injection site reactions consisting principally of soreness, and including pain, tenderness, pruritus, erythema, induration, ecchymosis, swelling, warmth, and nodule formation.

Body as a Whole: The most frequent systemic complaints include fatigue/weakness; headache; fever (≥ 100°F or > 37.5°C); and malaise.

Digestive System: Nausea; and diarrhea

Respiratory System: Pharyngitis; and upper respiratory infection

INCIDENCE LESS THAN 1% OF INFECTIONS
Body as a Whole: Sweating; achiness; sensation of warmth; light-headedness; malaise; tingling; chills; and flushing

Digestive System: Vomiting; abdominal pains/cramps; dyspepsia; and diminished appetite

Respiratory System: Rhinitis; influenza, and cough

Nervous System: Vertigo/dizziness: somnolence; insomnia; irritability; agitation; and paresthesia

Integumentary System: Pruritus; rash (non-specified); angioedema; and urticaria.

Musculoskeletal System: Arthralgia including monoarticular; myalgia; back pain, neck pain; arm and shoulder pain: and neck stiffness

Hemic/Lymphatic System: Lymphadenopathy

Psychiatric/Behavioral: Insomnia/Disturbed sleep

Special Senses: Earache

Urogenital System: Dysuria

Cardiovascular System: Hypotension

The following additional adverse reactions have been reported with use of the marketed vaccine. In many instances, the relationship to the vaccine was unclear.

HYPERSENSITIVITY
Anaphylaxis and symptoms of immediate hypersensitivity reactions including rash, pruritus, urticaria, edema, angioedema, dyspnea, chest discomfort, bronchial spasm, palpitation, or symptoms consistent with a hypotensive episode have been reported within the first few hours after vaccination. An apparent hypersensitivity syndrome (serum-sickness-like) of delayed onset has been reported days to weeks after vaccination, including: arthralgia/arthritis (usually transient), fever, and dermatologic reactions such as urticaria, erythema multiforme including Stevens Johnson syndrome, ecchymoses and erythema nodosum (see "Warnings and Precautions").

Digestive System: Elevation of liver enzymes and abnormal liver function tests; constipation.

Nervous System: Peripheral neuropathy including Bell's Palsy; muscle weakness; Guillain-Barre syndrome; radiculopathy; herpes zoster; hypesthesia; migraine; syncope; paresis; multiple sclerosis; myelitis including transverse myelitis.

Integumentary System: Stevens-Johnson Syndrome; petechiae; eczema; purpura; herpes zoster; erythema nodosum.

Hematologic: Increased erythrocyte sedimentation rate; thrombocytopenia.

Psychiatric/Behavioral: Irritability; agitation; somnolence.

Special Senses: Optic neuritis; tinnitus; conjunctivitis; visual disturbances;

Cardiovascular System: Syncope; tachycardia; palpitations.

Respiratory System: Bronchospasm, including asthma-like symptoms

The following adverse reaction has been reported with a Hepatitis B Vaccine-Recombinant but not with with Recombivax Hb: keratitis.

DOSAGE AND ADMINISTRATION
DO NOT INJECT INTRAVENOUSLY OR INTRADERMALLY
Hepatitis B Vaccine-Recombinant Dialysis Formulation (40 mcg/mL) is intended only for adult predialysis/dialysis patients.

Hepatitis B Vaccine-Recombinant Pediatric, adolescent/high-risk infant, and adult formulations are not intended for use in predialysis/dialysis patients.

Table 1 summarizes the dose and formulation of Hepatitis B Vaccine-Recombinant for specific populations. The vaccination regimen for each population EXCEPT Infants of HBsAg Positive Mothers (see Table 2) consists of 3 doses of vaccine given according to the following schedule:
- 1st dose: at elected date
- 2nd dose: 1 month later
- 3rd dose: 6 months after the first dose

There is an alternate schedule with injections at 0, 1 and 2 months designed for certain populations (e.g., neonates born of hepatitis B infected mothers, others who have or might have been recently exposed to the virus, certain travelers to high-risk areas. See "Indications and Usage".) On this alternate schedule, an additional dose at 12 months is recommended for infants born of infected mothers and for others for whom prolonged maintenance of protective titers is desired.

In infants born of mothers who are not hepatitis B infected, Hepatitis B Vaccine-Recombinant may be administered at birth, 1 month of age and 6 months of age.

Table 1

Group	Dose*
Infants born of:	
HBsAg Negative	2.5 mcg
Mothers	(0.5 mL)
HBsAg Positive	5 mcg
Mothers†	(0.5 mL)
1-10 years of age	2.5 or 10 mcg (0.5 mL)
11-19 years of age	5 or 20 mcg (0.5 mL)

Group	Dose*
≥ 20 years of age	10 or 20 mcg (1.0 mL)
	40 mcg/1.0 mL at 0, 1, 2 and 6
Predialysis and Dialysis Patients**	months.

† See Table 2

* If the suggested formulation is not available, the appropriate dosage can be achieved from another formulation provided that the total volume of vaccine administered does not exceed 1 mL. However, the Dialysis Formulation may be used only for adult predialysis/dialysis patients.

** See also recommendations for revaccination of "Predialysis and Dialysis Patients" under "Revaccination, Dosage and Administration".

Hepatitis B Vaccine-Recombinant is for intramuscular injection. The *deltoid muscle* is the preferred site for intramuscular injection in adults. Data suggests that injections given in the buttocks frequently are given into fatty tissue instead of into muscle. Such injections have resulted in a lower seroconversion rate than was expected. The *anterolateral thigh* is the recommended site for intramuscular injection in infants and young children.

For persons at risk of hemorrhage following intramuscular injection, Hepatitis B Vaccine-Recombinant may be administered subcutaneously. However, Hepatitis B Vaccines administered subcutaneously are known to result in lower GMTs. Additionally, when other aluminum-adsorbed vaccines have been administered subcutaneously, an increased incidence of local reactions including subcutaneous nodules has been observed. Therefore, subcutaneous administration should be used only in persons (e.g., hemophiliacs) who are at risk of hemorrhage following intramuscular injections.

The vaccine should be used as supplied; no dilution or reconstitution is necessary. The full recommended dose of the vaccine should be used.

It is important to use a separate sterile syringe and needle for each individual patient to prevent transmission of hepatitis and other infectious agents from one person to another.

Shake well before withdrawal and use: Thorough agitation at the time of administration is necessary to maintain suspension of the vaccine.

Parenteral drug products should be inspected visually for particulate matter and discoloration prior to administration. After thorough agitation, the vaccine is a slightly opaque, white suspension. Discard if it appears otherwise.

For Syringe Use Only: Withdraw the recommended dose from the vial using a sterile needle and syringe free of preservatives, antiseptics, and detergents.

Injection must be accomplished with a needle long enough to ensure intramuscular deposition of the vaccine.

The Immunization Practices Advisory Committee has recommended that "for an intramuscular injection, the needle and syringe should be of sufficient length and bore to reach the muscle mass itself and prevent vaccine from seeping into subcutaneous tissue. For children, a 20- or 22-gauge needle 1 to 1 ¼ inches long is recommended. For small infants, a 25-gauge ⅝-inch-long needle may be adequate. For adults, the suggested needle length is 1 ½ inches."

Dosage for Infants Born of HBsAg Positive Mothers (High-Risk Infants) or Mothers of Unknown HBsAg Status: The recommended regimen for infants born of HBsAg positive mothers is as follows:

Table 2

Birth*	Within 7 days	1 month	6 months
Hepatitis B Vaccine-Recombinant Adolescent/High-Risk Infant yellow color code	5 mcg** (0.5 mL)	5 mcg (0.5 mL)	5 mcg (0.5 mL)
Hepatitis B Immune Globulin 0.5 mL	—	—	—

* The first 5 mcg/0.5 mL dose of Hepatitis B Vaccine-Recombinant is given preferably within the first 12 hours of birth but may be given within the first 7 days.

** The first 5 mcg/0.5 mL dose of Hepatitis B Vaccine-Recombinant may be given at birth at the same time as Hepatitis B Immune Globulin, but should be administered in the opposite anterolateral thigh.

Recommendations from the Immunization Practices Advisory Committee for infants born of mothers of unknown HBsAg status are summarized as follows: In the event that a mother's HBsAg status is unknown, vaccination should be initiated as soon as possible with a 5 mcg/0.5 mL dose of vaccine (Adolescent/High-Risk Infant, yellow color code). If within 7 days of delivery the mother is determined to be HBsAg positive, the infant should also be given a dose of Hepatitis B Immune Globulin immediately; the vaccination series should then be completed with 5 mcg/0.5 mL dosages. If the mother's HBsAg antigen test is negative, then complete the vaccination series with 2.5 mcg/0.5 mL dosages (Pediatric Formulation, brown color code).

REVACCINATION

The duration of the protective effect of Hepatitis B Vaccine-Recombinant in healthy vaccinees is unknown at present and the need for booster doses is not yet defined.

For hemodialysis patients, in whom vaccine-induced protection is less complete and may persist only as long as antibody levels remain above 10 mIU/mL, the need for booster doses should be assessed by annual antibody testing, 40 mcg (two × 20 mcg) booster doses with Hepatitis B Vaccine-Recombinant should be given when antibody levels decline below 10 mIU/mL.[1] Data show individuals given a booster with Hepatitis B Vaccine-Recombinant achieve high antibody titers. (See "Clinical Pharmacology".)

KNOWN OR PRESUMED EXPOSURE TO HBSAG

There are no prospective studies directly testing the efficacy of a combination of Hepatitis B Immune Globulin (Human) and Hepatitis B Vaccine-Recombinant preventing clinical hepatitis B following percutaneous, ocular or mucous membrane exposure to hepatitis B virus. However, since most persons with such exposures (e.g., health-care workers) are candidates for Hepatitis B Vaccine-Recombinant and since combined Hepatitis B Immune Globulin (Human) plus vaccine is more efficacious than Hepatitis B Immune Globulin (Human) alone in perinatal exposures, the following guidelines are recommended for neonates born of infected mothers and persons who have been exposed to hepatitis B virus such as through (1) percutaneous (needlestick), ocular, mucous membrane exposure to blood known or presumed to contain HBsAg, (2) human bites by known or presumed HBsAg carriers that penetrate the skin, or (3) following intimate sexual contact with known or presumed HBsAg carriers:

Hepatitis B Immune Globulin (Human) (0.06 mL/kg) should be given intramuscularly as soon as possible after exposure and within 24 hours if possible. Hepatitis B Vaccine-Recombinant (see "Dosage Recommendation") should be given intramuscularly at a separate site within 7 days of exposure and second and third doses given one and six months, respectively, after the first dose.

BOOSTER VACCINATIONS

Whenever administration of a booster dose is appropriate, the dose of Hepatitis B Vaccine-Recombinant is 10 mcg for children 10 years of age and under; 20 mcg for other children and adults. Studies have demonstrated a substantial increase in antibody titers after Hepatitis B Vaccine-Recombinant booster vaccination following an initial course with both plasma- and yeast-derived vaccines. (See "Clinical Pharmacology".)

STORAGE

Store vials at 2-8°C (36°-46°F). Storage above or below the recommended temperature may reduce potency.

Do not freeze since freezing destroys potency.

REFERENCES

1. Centers for Disease Control: Protection against viral hepatitis; recommendations of the Immunization Practices Advisory Committee (ACIP), *MMWR.* 39(No. RR-2), 1990. 2. Robinson, W.S.: Hepatitis B virus and the delta virus. In Mandell, G.L., Douglas, R.G., Bennett, J.E. (eds); *Principles and practice of infectious diseases*, vol. 3, New York, John Wiley & Sons, 1990, pp. 1204-1231. 3. Beasley, R.P., et al.: Efficacy of hepatitis B immune globulin for prevention of perinatal transmission of hepatitis B virus carrier state: final report of a randomized double-blind, placebo-controlled trial. *Hepatology* 3:135-141, 1983. 4. Centers for Disease Control: Hepatitis B virus: a comprehensive strategy for eliminating transmission in the United States through universal childhood vaccination: recommendations of the Immunization Practices Advisory Committee (ACIP). *MMWR.* 40(No. RR-13):1-25, 1991. 5. Committee on Infectious Diseases: Universal hepatitis immunization. *Pediatrics*, 89(4):795-800, 1992. 6. Ambrosch, F.: Persistence of vaccine-induced antibodies to hepatitis B surface antigen-the need for booster vaccination in adult subjects. *Postgrad. Med. J.* 63(Suppl. 2):129-135, 1987. 7. Stevens, C.E., et al.: Hepatitis B vaccine in patients receiving hemodialysis, *N. Engl. J. Med.* 311:496-501, 1984. 8. Andre, F.E., and Safary, A.: Clinical experience with a yeast-derived hepatitis B vaccine. In Zuckerman, A.J.(ed): *Viral hepatitis and liver disease*, Alan R. Liss, Inc. 1988, pp. 1025-1030. 9. Poovorawan, Y., et al.: Protective efficacy of a recombinant DNA hepatitis B vaccine in neonates of HBe antigen-positive mothers. *JAMA.* 261(22):3278-3281, June 9, 1989. 10. Goilav, C., et al.: Immunization of homosexual men with a recombinant DNA vaccine against hepatitis B; immunogenicity and protection. In Zuckerman, A.J.(ed): *Viral hepatitis and liver disease*, Alan R. Liss, Inc., 1988, pp. 1057-1058. 11. Hauser, P. et al.: Immunological properties of recombinant HBsAg produced in yeast. *Postgrad. Med. J.* 63(Suppl. 2):83-91, 1987. 12. Centers for Disease Control: Recommendations on the Immunization Practices Advisory Committee (ACIP): General Recommendations on Immunization. *MMWR* 38(13):April 7, 1989.

HOW SUPPLIED

INJECTION: 2.5 MCG/0.5 ML

BRAND/MANUFACTURER	NDC	SIZE	AWP
○ **BRAND**			
RECOMBIVAX-HB: Merck	00006-4799-00	0.5 ml	$22.50
	00006-4761-00	3 ml	$121.25

INJECTION: 5 MCG/0.5 ML

BRAND/MANUFACTURER	NDC	SIZE	AWP
○ **BRAND**			
RECOMBIVAX-HB: Merck	00006-4769-00	0.5 ml	$37.50

INJECTION: 10 MCG/ML

BRAND/MANUFACTURER	NDC	SIZE	AWP
○ **BRAND**			
RECOMBIVAX-HB: Merck	00006-4775-00	1 ml	$55.78
	00006-4773-00	3 ml	$167.35

INJECTION: 10 MCG/0.5 ML

BRAND/MANUFACTURER	NDC	SIZE	AWP
○ **BRAND**			
ENGERIX-B PEDIATRIC: SK Beecham Pharm	58160-0859-01	0.5 ml	$23.45

INJECTION: 20 MCG/ML

BRAND/MANUFACTURER	NDC	SIZE	AWP
○ **BRAND**			
ENGERIX-B: SK Beecham Pharm	58160-0860-01	1 ml	$54.35
	58160-0860-16	1 ml 25s	$1359.10

INJECTION: 40 MCG/ML

BRAND/MANUFACTURER	NDC	SIZE	AWP
○ **BRAND**			
RECOMBIVAX-HB: Merck	00006-4776-00	1 ml	$156.30

Hespan *SEE* HETASTARCH

Hetastarch

DESCRIPTION

Hetastarch (6% Hetastarch in 0.9% sodium chloride injection) is a sterile, nonpyrogenic solution.

Each 100 mL contains:

Hetastarch	6.0 g
Sodium Chloride, USP	0.9 g
Water for Injection, USP	qs

pH adjusted with sodium hydroxide
Concentration of Electrolytes (mEq/liter): Sodium 154, Chloride 154
pH: 3.5-7.0; Calc. Osmolarity: 310 mOsM/liter

Hetastarch is an artificial colloid derived from a waxy starch composed almost entirely of amylopectin. Hydroxyethyl ether groups are introduced into the glucose units of the starch and the resultant material is hydrolyzed to yield a product with a molecular weight suitable for use as a plasma volume expander and erythrocyte sedimenting agent. Hetastarch is characterized by its molar substitution, and also by its molecular weight. The molar substitution is 0.7 which means Hetastarch has 7 hydroxyethyl groups for every 10 glucose units. The weight average molecular weight is approximately 480,000 with a range of 400,000 to 550,000 and with 80% of the polymers falling between the range of 30,000 and 2,400,000. Hydroxyethyl groups are attached by ether linkage primarily at C-2 of the glucose unit and to a lesser extent at C-3 and C-6. The polymerized glucose units are joined primarily by 1-4 linkages with occasional 1-6 branching linkages. The degree of branching is approximately 1:20 which means that there is one 1-6 branch for every 20 glucose monomer units.

The chemical name for Hetastarch is hydroxyethyl starch.

Amylopectin derivative in which R_2, R_3, and R_6 are H or CH_2CH_2OH, or R_6 is a branching point in the starch polymer connected through a 1-6 linkage to additional *a*-D-glucopyranosyl units.

Hetastarch is a clear, pale yellow to amber solution. Exposure to prolonged adverse storage conditions may result in a change to a turbid deep brown or the formation of a crystalline precipitate. Do not use the solution if these conditions are evident.

Following is its chemical structure:

Amylose derivative:

in which either **R** or **R'** may be either H or CH_2CH_2OH

Amylopectin derivative: Similar to the above, except that the sequence is frequently interrupted by a similar unit that differs in that **R'** is the residue of an additional O-hydroxy-ethylated α-D-glucopyranosyl moiety that constitutes the first unit in a branch or sub-branch of the polymer.

CLINICAL PHARMACOLOGY

The plasma volume expansion produced by Hetastarch approximate those of 5% human albumin. Intravenous infusion of Hetastarch results in expansion of plasma volume that decreases over the succeeding 24 to 36 hours. The degree of plasma volume expansion and improvement in hemodynamic state depend upon the patient's intravascular status. Hetastarch molecules below 50,000 molecular weight are rapidly eliminated by renal excretion. A single dose of approximately 500 mL of Hetastarch (approximately 30 g) results in elimination in the urine of approximately 33% of the dose within 24 hours. This is a variable process but generally results in an intravascular Hetastarch concentration of less than 10% of the total dose injected by two weeks. The hydroxyethyl group is not cleaved by the body, but remains intact and attached to glucose units when excreted. Significant

quantities of glucose are not produced as hydroxyethylation prevents complete metabolism of the smaller polymers.

The addition of Hetastarch to whole blood increases the erythrocyte sedimentation rate. Therefore, Hetastarch is used to improve the efficiency of granulocyte collection by centrifugal means.

INDICATIONS AND USAGE

Hetastarch is indicated in the treatment of hypovolemia when plasma volume expansion is desired. It is not a substitute for blood or plasma.

The adjunctive use of Hetastarch in leukapheresis has also been shown to be safe and efficacious in improving the harvesting and increasing the yield of granulocytes by centrifugal means.

CONTRAINDICATIONS

Hetastarch is contraindicated in patients with known hypersensitivity to hydroxyethyl starch, or with bleeding disorders, or with congestive heart failure where volume overload is a potential problem. Hetastarch should not be used in renal disease with oliguria or anuria not related to hypovolemia.

WARNINGS

USAGE IN PLASMA VOLUME EXPANSION

Large volumes may alter the coagulation mechanism. Thus, administration of Hetastarch may result in transient prolongation of prothrombin, partial thromboplastin and clotting times. With administration of large doses, the physician should also be alert to the possibility of transient prolongation of bleeding time.

Hematocrit may be decreased and plasma proteins diluted excessively by administration of large volumes of Hetastarch (6% Hetastarch in 0.9% sodium chloride injection). Administration of packed red cells, platelets, and fresh frozen plasma should be considered if excessive dilution occurs.

Use over extended periods Hetastarch has not been adequately evaluated to establish its safety in situations other than leukapheresis that require frequent use of colloidal solutions over extended periods. Certain conditions may affect the safe use of Hetastarch on a chronic basis. For example, in patients with subarachnoid hemorrhage where Hetastarch is used repeatedly over a period of days for the prevention of cerebral vasospasm, significant clinical bleeding may occur.

USAGE IN LEUKAPHERESIS

Slight declines in platelet counts and hemoglobin levels have been observed in donors undergoing repeated leukapheresis procedures using Hetastarch due to the volume expanding effects of Hetastarch and to the collection of platelets and erythrocytes. Hemoglobin levels usually return to normal within 24 hours. Hemodilution by Hetastarch and saline may also result in 24 hour declines of total protein, albumin, calcium and fibrinogen values. None of these decreases are to a degree recognized to be clinically significant risks to healthy donors.

PRECAUTIONS

GENERAL

Regular and frequent clinical evaluation and complete blood counts (CBC) are necessary for proper monitoring of Hetastarch use during leukapheresis. If the frequency of leukapheresis is to exceed the guidelines for whole blood donation, you may wish to consider the following additional studies: total leukocyte and platelet counts, leukocyte differential count, hemoglobin and hematocrit, prothrombin time (PT), and partial thromboplastin time (PTT) tests.

The possibility of circulatory overload should be kept in mind. Caution should be used when the risk of pulmonary edema and/or congestive heart failure is increased. Special care should be exercised in patients who have impaired renal clearance since this is the principal way in which Hetastarch is eliminated.

Indirect bilirubin levels of 8.3 mg/L (normal 0.0-7.0 mg/L) have been reported in 2 out of 20 normal subjects who received multiple Hetastarch infusions. Total bilirubin was within normal limits at all times; indirect bilirubin returned to normal by 96 hours following the final infusion. The significance, if any, of these elevations is not known; however, caution should be observed before administering Hetastarch to patients with a history of liver disease.

Hetastarch has been reported to produce hypersensitivity reactions such as wheezing and urticaria. However, Hetastarch has not been observed to stimulate antibody formation. If hypersensitivity effects occur, they are readily controlled by discontinuation of the drug and, if necessary, administration of an antihistaminic agent.

Elevated serum amylase levels may be observed temporarily following administration of Hetastarch, although no association with pancreatitis has been demonstrated.

If administration is by pressure infusion, all air should be withdrawn or expelled from the bag through the medication port prior to infusion.

CARCINOGENESIS, MUTAGENESIS, IMPAIRMENT OF FERTILITY

Long-term studies of animals have not been performed to evaluate the carcinogenic potential of Hetastarch.

TERATOGENIC EFFECTS

Pregnancy Category C. Animal reproduction studies have not been conducted with Hetastarch. It is also not known whether Hetastarch can cause fetal harm when administered to a pregnant woman or can affect reproduction capacity. Hetastarch should be given to a pregnant woman only if clearly needed.

➤ SHOWN IN PRODUCT IDENTIFICATION GUIDE

NURSING MOTHERS

It is not known whether Hetastarch is excreted in human milk. Because many drugs are excreted in human milk, caution should be exercised when Hetastarch is administered to a nursing woman.

PEDIATRIC USE

The safety and effectiveness of Hetastarch in children have not been established.

ADVERSE REACTIONS

The following have been reported: vomiting, fever, chills, pruritus, submaxillary and parotid glandular enlargement, mild influenza-like symptoms, headaches, muscle pains, peripheral edema of the lower extremities, anaphylactoid reactions (periorbital edema, urticaria, wheezing), bleeding due to hemodilution (see *"Warnings"*), and circulatory overload and pulmonary edema (see *"Precautions"*).

DOSAGE AND ADMINISTRATION

DOSAGE FOR ACUTE USE IN PLASMA VOLUME EXPANSION

Hetastarch is administered by intravenous infusion only. Total dosage and rate of infusion depend upon the amount of blood or plasma lost and the resultant hemoconcentration.

In adults, the amount usually administered is 500 to 1000 mL. Doses of more than 1500 mL per day for the typical 70 kg patient (approximately 20 mL per kg of body weight) are usually not required, although higher doses have been reported in postoperative and trauma patients where severe blood loss has occurred.

DOSAGE IN LEUKAPHERESIS

250 to 700 mL of Hetastarch to which citrate anticoagulant has been added is typically administered by aseptic addition to the input line of the centrifugation apparatus at a ratio of 1:8 to 1:13 to venous whole blood. The Hetastarch and citrate should be thoroughly mixed to assure effective anticoagulation of blood as it flows through the leukapheresis machine.

Do not use plastic container in series connection.

If administration is controlled by a pumping device, care must be taken to discontinue pumping action before the container runs dry or air embolism may result.

This solution is intended for intravenous administration using sterile equipment. It is recommended that intravenous administration apparatus be replaced at least once every 24 hours.

Use only if solution is clear and container and seals are intact.

Parenteral drug products should be inspected for particulate matter and discoloration prior to administration whenever solution and container permit.

The safety and compatibility of other additives have not been established.

If administration is by pressure infusion, all air should be withdrawn or expelled from the bag through the medication port prior to infusion.

Exposure of pharmaceutical products to heat should be minimized. Avoid excessive heat. Protect from freezing. It is recommended that the product be stored at room temperature (25°C); however, brief exposure up to 40°C does not adversely affect the product.

DIRECTIONS FOR USE (PLASTIC CONTAINER)
Caution: Before administering to the patient, review these directions:

VISUAL CHECKING
1. Do not remove the plastic infusion container from its overwrap until immediately before use.
2. While the overwrap is intact, identify the solution— Hetastarch (6% Hetastarch in 0.9% sodium chloride injection), lot number, and expiration date.
3. Check that the solution is clear.
4. Inspect the intact unit for signs of obvious damage. If present, the unit should not be used.

REMOVAL OF OVERWRAP
To open overwrap, tear at any notch located at either end of unit. After removing overwrap, check for minute leaks by squeezing container firmly. If leaks are found, discard unit as sterility may be impaired.

PREPARATION FOR ADMINISTRATION (USE ASEPTIC TECHNIQUE)
1. Close flow control clamp of administration set.
   Twist off plug from port designated "Infusion Set Port".
3. Insert spike of infusion set into port with a twisting motion until the set is firmly seated.
4. Suspend container from hanger.
5. Follow manufacturer's recommended procedures for the administration set.
6. Discontinue administration and notify physician immediately if patient exhibits signs of adverse reactions.

HOW SUPPLIED
INJECTION:

BRAND/MANUFACTURER	NDC	SIZE	AWP
○ **BRAND**			
HESPAN: Du Pont Pharma	00056-0037-44	500 ml	$69.60

Hexabrix *SEE* IOXAGLATE MEGLUMINE AND IOXAGLATE SODIUM

Hexachlorophene

DESCRIPTION

Hexachlorophene detergent cleanser, is an antibacterial sudsing emulsion for topical administration. Hexachlorophene contains a colloidal dispersion of Hexachlorophene 3% (w/w) in a stable emulsion.

Chemically, Hexachlorophene is Phenol, 2,2'-methylenebis[3,4,6-trichloro-].

Following is its chemical structure:

CLINICAL PHARMACOLOGY

Hexachlorophene is a bacteriostatic cleansing agent. It cleanses the skin thoroughly and has bacteriostatic action against staphylococci and other gram-positive bacteria. Cumulative antibacterial action develops with repeated use. Cleansing with alcohol or soaps containing alcohol removes the antibacterial residue.

Detectable blood levels of Hexachlorophene following absorption through intact skin have been found in subjects who regularly scrubbed with Hexachlorophene emulsion 3%. (See *"Warnings"* for additional information.)

Hexachlorophene has the same slight acidity as normal skin (pH value 5.0 to 6.0).

INDICATIONS AND USAGE

Hexachlorophene is indicated for use as a surgical scrub and a bacteriostatic skin cleanser. It may also be used to control an outbreak of gram-positive infection where other infection control procedures have been unsuccessful. Use only as long as necessary for infection control.

CONTRAINDICATIONS

Hexachlorophene should not be used on burned or denuded skin. It should not be used as an occlusive dressing, wet pack, or lotion.

It should not be used routinely for prophylactic total body bathing.

It should not be used as a vaginal pack or tampon, or on any mucous membranes.

Hexachlorophene should not be used on persons with sensitivity to any of its components. It should not be used on persons who have demonstrated primary light sensitivity to halogenated phenol derivatives because of the possibility of cross-sensitivity to Hexachlorophene.

WARNINGS

Rinse thoroughly after each use: Patients should be closely monitored and use should be immediately discontinued at the first sign of any of the symptoms described below.

Rapid absorption of Hexachlorophene may occur with resultant toxic blood levels when preparations containing Hexachlorophene are applied to skin lesions such as ichthyosis congenita, the dermatitis of Letterer-Siwe's syndrome, or other generalized dermatological conditions. Application to burns has also produced neurotoxicity and death.

Hexachlorophene Should be Discontinued Promptly if Signs or Symptoms of Cerebral Irritability Occur.

Infants, especially premature infants or those with dermatoses, are particularly susceptible to Hexachlorophene absorption. Systemic toxicity may be manifested by signs of stimulation (irritation) of the central nervous system, sometimes with convulsions.

Infants have developed dermatitis, irritability, generalized clonic muscular contractions and decerebrate rigidity following application of a 6 percent Hexachlorophene powder. Examination of brainstems of those infants revealed vacuolization like that which can be produced in newborn experimental animals following repeated topical application of 3 percent Hexachlorophene. Moreover, a study of histologic sections of premature infants who died of unrelated causes has shown a positive correlation between Hexachlorophene baths and lesions in white matter of brains.

PRECAUTIONS
GENERAL
Avoid accidental contact of Hexachlorophene with the eyes.

If contact occurs, promptly rinse thoroughly with water. To assist in the detection of ocular irritation, applications to the head and periorbital skin areas should be performed only in responsive patients with unanesthetized eyes.

Rinse thoroughly after use: especially from sensitive areas such as the scrotum and perineum.

Hexachlorophene is intended for external use only. If swallowed, Hexachlorophene is harmful, especially to infants and children. *Hexachlorophene should not be poured into measuring cups, medicine bottles, or similar containers since it may be mistaken for baby formula or other medications.*

◆ RATED THERAPEUTICALLY EQUIVALENT; ◇ THERAPEUTIC EQUIVALENCE UNCONFIRMED; ○ UNRATED

CARCINOGENESIS, MUTAGENESIS, IMPAIRMENT OF FERTILITY
Carcinogenicity Studies in Animals: Hexachlorophene was tested in one experiment in rats by oral administration; it had no carcinogenic effect.

Hexachlorophene was not mutagenic in *Salmonella typhimurium* and was negative in a dominant lethal assay in male mice. Cytogenetic tests with cultured human lymphocytes were also negative.

Human Data: No case reports or epidemiological studies were available.

Impairment of Fertility: Topical exposure of neonatal rats to 3% Hexachlorophene solution caused reduced fertility in 7-month-old males, due to inability to ejaculate.

EMBRYOTOXICITY AND TERATOGENICITY
Placental transfer of Hexachlorophene has been demonstrated in rats.

Hexachlorophene is embroytoxic and produces some teratogenic effects.

PREGNANCY CATEGORY C
There are no adequate and well-controlled studies in pregnant women. Hexachlorophene should be used during pregnancy only if the potential benefit justifies potential risk to the fetus.

Hexachlorophene has been shown to be teratogenic and embryotoxic in rats when given by mouth, or instilled into the vagina in large doses.

Administration of 500 mg/kg diet or 20 to 30 mg/kg bw/day by gavage to rats caused some malformations (angulated ribs, cleft palate, micro- and anophthalmia) and reduction in litter size.

Placental transfer and excretion in milk of Hexachlorophene has been demonstrated in rats.

In another study, doses of up to 50 mg/kg diet failed to produce any effects in 3 generations of rats. Hexachlorophene did not interfere with reproduction in hamsters.

NURSING MOTHERS
It is not known whether this drug is excreted in human milk. Because many drugs are excreted in human milk and because of the potential for serious adverse reactions in nursing infants from Hexachlorophene, a decision should be made whether to discontinue nursing or to discontinue the drug taking into account the importance of the drug to the mother.

PEDIATRIC USE
Hexachlorophene detergent cleanser, should not be used routinely for bathing infants. See *"Warnings"*. For premature infants: see *"Warnings"*.

ADVERSE REACTIONS
Adverse reactions to Hexachlorophene may include dermatitis and photosensitivity. Sensitivity to Hexachlorophene is rare; however, persons who have developed photoallergy to similar compounds also may become sensitive to Hexachlorophene.

In persons with highly sensitive skin the use of Hexachlorophene may at times produce a reaction characterized by redness and/or mild scaling or dryness, especially when it is combined with such mechanical factors as excessive rubbing or exposure to heat or cold.

OVERDOSAGE
The accidental ingestion of Hexachlorophene amounts from 1 oz to 4 oz has caused anorexia, vomiting, abdominal cramps, diarrhea, dehydration, convulsions, hypotension, and shock, and in several reported instances, fatalities.

If patients are seen early, the stomach should be evacuated by emesis or gastric lavage. Olive oil or vegetable oil (60 mL or 2 fl oz) may then be given to delay absorption of Hexachlorophene, followed by a saline cathartic to hasten removal.

Treatment is symptomatic and supportive; intravenous fluids (5 percent dextrose in physiologic saline solution) may be given for dehydration. Any other electrolyte derangement should be corrected. If marked hypotension occurs, vasopressor therapy is indicated. Use of opiates may be considered if gastrointestinal symptoms (cramping, diarrhea) are severe. Scheduled medical or surgical procedures should be postponed until the patient's condition has been evaluated and stabilized.

DOSAGE AND ADMINISTRATION
SURGICAL HAND SCRUB
1. Wet hands and forearms with water. Apply approximately 5 mL of Hexachlorophene over the hands and rub into a copious lather by adding small amounts of water. Spread suds over hands and forearms and scrub well with a wet brush for 3 minutes. Pay particular attention to the nails and interdigital spaces. A separate nail cleaner may be used. *Rinse thoroughly* under running water.

2. Apply 5 mL of Hexachlorophene to hands again and scrub as above for another 3 minutes. *Rinse thoroughly* with running water and dry.

3. For repeat surgical scrubs during the day, scrub thoroughly with the same amount of Hexachlorophene for 3 minutes only. *Rinse thoroughly* with water and dry.

BACTERIOSTATIC CLEANSING
Wet hands with water. Dispense approximately 5 mL of Hexachlorophene into the palm, work up a lather with water and apply to area to be cleansed.

RINSE THOROUGHLY AFTER EACH WASHING

Infant Care: Hexachlorophene should not be used routinely for bathing infants. See *"Warnings"*.

Premature Infants: see *"Warnings"*.
Use of baby skin products containing alcohol may decrease the antibacterial action Hexachlorophene detergent cleanser.

HEXACHLOROPHENE SHOULD NOT BE DISPENSED FROM, OR STORED IN, CONTAINERS WITH ORDINARY METAL PARTS. A SPECIAL TYPE OF STAINLESS STEEL MUST BE USED OR UNDESIRABLE DISCOLORATION OF THE PRODUCT OR OXIDATION OF METAL MAY OCCUR. SPECIALLY DESIGNED DISPENSERS FOR HOSPITAL OR OFFICE USE MAY BE OBTAINED THROUGH YOUR LOCAL DEALER.

Directions for Cleaning Dispensers: Before initial installation and use, run an antiseptic, such as an aqueous solution of benzalkonium chloride, NF, 1:500 to 1:750, or alcohol, through the working parts: rinse with sterile water. At weekly intervals thereafter, remove dispenser and pour off remainder of Hexachlorophene emulsion. Rinse empty dispenser with water. Run water through the working parts by operating the dispenser. Sanitize as described above. Rinse thoroughly with sterile water.

ANIMAL TOXICITY
The oral LD$_{50}$ of Hexachlorophene in male rats is 66 mg/kg bw, in females 56 mg/kg bw, and in weanling rats 120 mg/kg bw.

In suckling rats (10-days old), it is 9 mg/kg bw.

HOW SUPPLIED
FOAM:

BRAND/MANUFACTURER	NDC	SIZE	AWP
○ BRAND			
SEPTISOL: Calgon Vestal	00519-6288-56	180 gm	$5.48
	00519-6288-72	600 gm	$11.52

LIQUID:

BRAND/MANUFACTURER	NDC	SIZE	AWP
○ BRAND			
PHISOHEX: Sanofi Winthrop	00024-1535-05	50s	$29.40

LIQUID: 3%

BRAND/MANUFACTURER	NDC	SIZE	AWP
○ BRAND			
PHISOHEX: Sanofi Winthrop	00024-1535-02	150 ml	$12.14
	00024-1535-06	480 ml	$23.42
	00024-1535-08	3840 ml	$116.04

Hexadrol *SEE* DEXAMETHASONE, ORAL

Hexalen *SEE* ALTRETAMINE

Hiprex *SEE* METHENAMINE HIPPURATE

Hismanal *SEE* ASTEMIZOLE

Histalet *SEE* CHLORPHENIRAMINE MALEATE AND PSEUDOEPHEDRINE HYDROCHLORIDE, CHLORPHENIRAMINE MALEATE/PHENYLEPHRINE HYDROCHLORIDE/ PHENYLPROPANOLAMINE HYDROCHLORIDE/PYRILAMINE MALEATE *AND* GUAIFENESIN AND PSEUDOEPHEDRINE HYDROCHLORIDE

Histamine Phosphate

DESCRIPTION
The chemical formula for Histamine Phosphate is $C_5H_9N_3 \cdot 2H_3PO_4$; its molecular weight is 307.14. For prick, puncture or scratch testing, the product contains 1 mg/mL Histamine base (2.75 mg/mL Histamine Phosphate) in Water for Injection.

Following is its chemical structure:

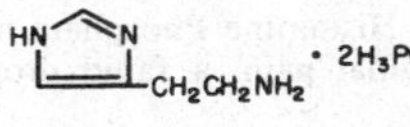

➤ SHOWN IN PRODUCT IDENTIFICATION GUIDE

CLINICAL PHARMACOLOGY

Histamine acts as a potent vasodilator when released from mast cells during an allergic reaction. It is largely responsible for the immediate skin test reaction of a sensitive patient when challenged with an offending allergen.

The effect of added glycerin (50% v/v) to 1 mg/mL Histamine base was studied by puncture testing using a bifurcated needle in twelve volunteer subjects. The mean sum of cross diameters of the wheals was 13.25mm for the non-glycerinated, and 12.54mm for the glycerinated formulation. Sum of cross-diameters of erythema was 52.88mm for the nonglycerinated, and 54.42mm for the glycerinated formulation. These differences are not statistically significant.

INDICATIONS AND USAGE

For use as a positive control in evaluation of allergenic (immediate hypersensitivity or "Type I") skin testing.

CONTRAINDICATIONS

Histamine should not be injected into individuals with hypotension, severe hypertension, severe cardiac, pulmonary, or renal disease. Not to be used for diagnosis of pheochromocytoma or to test the ability of the gastric mucosa to secrete hydrochloric acid.

WARNINGS

Care must be taken in intracutaneous testing to avoid injection into a venule or capillary. Pull back gently on the syringe plunger and note if blood is drawn. If blood is drawn, withdraw needle and inject into another skin site.

Small doses by any route of administration may precipitate asthma in patients with bronchial hyperactivity. This product is not intended for inhalation, intracutaneous or subcutaneous injection. The utmost caution is advised in using Histamine in such patients and in those with a history of bronchial asthma.

PRECAUTIONS

GENERAL

A separate sterile needle or other percutaneous testing device should be used for each individual patient to prevent transmission of hepatitis and other infectious agents from one person to another.

Epinephrine injection (1:1,000) and injectable antihistamines should be available for immediate use in the event the patient exhibits a severe response. A tourniquet can be applied above the test site to slow absorption if a severe response occurs.

DRUG INTERACTIONS

Drugs can interfere with the performance of skin tests in general, and specifically with Histamine.[1]

Antihistamines: Response to Histamine is suppressed by antihistamines. The length of suppression varies, and is dependent on individual patient, type of antihistamine and length of time the patient has been on antihistamines. The duration of this suppression may be as little as 24 hours (chlorpheniramine), and can be as long as 40 days (astemizole).

Tricyclic Antidepressants: These exert a potent and sustained decrease of skin reactivity to Histamine, which may last for a few weeks.

Beta$_2$ Agonists: Oral terbutaline and parenteral ephedrine, in general, have been shown to decrease allergen induced wheal. Theoretically, this may also reduce whealing capacity to Histamine.

Dopamine: Intravenous infusion of dopamine has been shown to inhibit skin test responses to Histamine.

Beta Blocking Agents: Propranolol can significantly increase skin test reactivity, including Histamine.

Other Drugs: Short acting steroids, inhaled beta$_2$ agonists, theophylline and cromolyn do not seem to affect skin test response.

PREGNANCY CATEGORY C

There are no adequate and well-controlled studies in pregnant women. However, based on Histamine's known ability to contract uterine muscle, exposure or repeated doses should be avoided. Histamine Phosphate should be used during pregnancy only if the potential benefit justifies the potential risk to the fetus or mother.

PEDIATRIC USE

Histamine solutions for percutaneous testing have been given safely in infants and young children.[2,3,4,5] Neonates and infants have lower skin test reactivity to Histamines as well as common allergens.[3,4,5,6] About 20% of infants less than six months of age have been observed to have a negative reaction to Histamine hydrochloride (1 mg/mL of salt).[4] Skin test reactivity gradually increases to age six and plateaus to age sixty.[2,3] Therefore, small skin test reactions should be anticipated in children under age six.

ADVERSE REACTIONS

Following the injection of large doses of Histamine, systemic reactions may include flushing, dizziness, headache, bronchial constriction, urticaria, asthma, marked hypertension or hypotension, abdominal cramps, vomiting, metallic taste, and local or generalized allergic manifestations.

OVERDOSAGE

A large subcutaneous dose of Histamine Phosphate may cause severe occipital headache, blurred vision, anginal pain, a rapid drop in blood pressure, and cyanosis of the face.

Overdosage may cause severe symptoms including vasomotor collapse, shock, and even death.

Epinephrine injection given subcutaneously or intramuscularly should be used in case of emergency due to severe reactions (see *"Precautions"*). An antihistamine preparation may be given intramuscularly to ameliorate systemic reaction to overdose.

DOSAGE AND ADMINISTRATION

FOR PRICK, PUNCTURE AND SCRATCH TESTING

Histamine base 1 mg/mL (Histamine Phosphate 2.75 mg/mL) should be used to give a reaction. (Refer to *"Interpretation"* section below.)

PRICK, PUNCTURE OR SCRATCH TEST TECHNIQUES

1. The skin in the test area should be cleansed with alcohol and air dried.
2. The Histamine control skin test solution should be placed at the same site with the other skin test antigens, either on the patient's back or on the volar surface of the forearm. The patient should be placed in a comfortable position before the testing is begun.
3. For the prick test, a sharp needle is used to puncture the skin, but not to draw blood. If the scratch test is used, carefully break or scratch the skin with a sterile scarifier. Do not draw blood. Each scratch should be about 2 mm - 4 mm in length.
4. A small drop of the Histamine base 1 mg/mL (Histamine Phosphate 2.75 mg/mL) is placed on the abraded skin site no closer than 4 or 5 cm from an adjacent test site. Some physicians prefer to place the solution on the test area and then prick through the drop with a sharp needle.
5. Use a separate sterile scarifier or needle for each patient.
6. The test should be read in 15-20 minutes; if a large wheal reaction occurs before that time, the test site should be wiped free of Histamine.

INTERPRETATION

The patient's response is based on the size of: erythema (degree of redness) and/or size of wheal (smooth, slightly elevated area) which appear after 15-20 minutes.

For prick, puncture and scratch testing Histamine base 1 mg/mL (Histamine Phosphate 2.75 mg/mL) should be used to give a positive reaction. In a large population, the NHANES II survey reports a mean diameter (average of length and width) wheal of 4.4 mm ± 1.65 mm (± standard deviation) and a mean erythema of 18.4 mm ± 8.55 mm (± standard deviation) when using 25 gauge B-D needle by prick puncture (Pepys) technique.[7] All positive reactions should be interpreted against an appropriate negative control.

FOR INTRADERMAL SKIN TESTING

Histamine base 0.1 mg/mL (Histamine Phosphate 0.275 mg/mL) or 0.01 mg/mL should be used to give a reaction. (Refer to *"Interpretation"* section above.)

INTRACUTANEOUSLY (INTRADERMAL) TEST TECHNIQUES

1. The skin should be cleansed with alcohol and air dried.
2. A sterile one milliliter tuberculin syringe with 26 or 27 gauge needle should be used. A single sterile syringe should be used for each solution to assure sterility. Only the Histamine base 0.1 mg/mL (Histamine Phosphate, 0.275 mg/mL) or greater dilution solution should be used.
3. The Histamine base skin test solution should be injected at the same site with the other skin test allergens, either on the patient's back or on the arm. The patient should be placed in a comfortable position before the testing is begun.
4. The skin is held tense and the needle is inserted almost parallel to the skin, bevel side up, far enough to cover the beveled portion. Slowly inject 0.01 mL or 0.02 mL, making a small bleb approximately 3 mm - 5 mm in diameter.
5. The test should be read in 15-20 minutes.

INTERPRETATION

The patient's response is based on the size of: erythema (degree of redness) and/or size of wheal (smooth, slightly elevated area) which appear after 15-20 minutes.

For intradermal skin testing, Histamine base 0.1 mg/mL (Histamine Phosphate 0.275 mg/mL) or 0.01 mg/mL should be used to give a positive reaction. The available 0.1 mg/mL concentration must be diluted ten-fold to achieve this dose. All positive reactions should be interpreted against an appropriate negative control. In two successive years of testing, the Committee on Standardization of the American College of Allergy reported positive reactions at Histamine base doses of 0.01 mg/mL and higher.[7] Mean sum of wheal diameters was approximately 14 mm ± 4.8 mm and sum of erythema diameters was approximately 52 mm ± 21.6 mm following 0.01 mL intradermal doses of 0.01 mg/mL Histamine base. When 0.01 mL of 0.1 mg/mL Histamine base was injected, the sum of crossed diameters of wheal ranged from 15 - 20 mm and the sum of crossed diameters of erythema ranged from 60 - 80 mm.[8]

STORAGE

Store at 2°-8°C.

REFERENCES

1. Bousquet, J.: In vivo methods for the study of allergy: skin test, techniques, and interpretation. In Allergy Principles and Practice, 3rd Edition, Middleton, et al eds., C.V. Mosby, St. Louis, MO, 1988. 2. Skassa-Brociek, W., et al.: Skin test reactivity to histamine from infancy to old age. J. Allergy Clin. Immunol. 80:711, 1987. 3. Menardo, J.L. et al.: Skin test reactivity in infancy, J. Allergy Clin. Immunol. 75:646, 1985. 4. Van Asperen, P.P., et al.: Skin test reactivity and clinical allergen sensitivity in infancy. J. Allergy Clin. Immunol. 73:381, 1984. 5. Matheson, A., et al.: Reactivity of the skin of the newborn infant. Pediatrics 10:181, 1952. 6. Stevenson, D.D., et al.: Development of IgE in newborn human infants. J. Allergy 48:61, 1971. 7. Committee on Standardization. Report of the Committee on Standardization: 1. A method of evaluating skin test response. Ann. Allergy 29:30-34, 1971. 8. National Center for Health Statistics, P.J.

Gergen and P.C. Turkeltaub: Percutaneous immediate hypersensitivity to eight allergens. United States, 1976-80. *Vital and Health Statistics.* Series 11, No. 235, DHHS Pub. No. (PHS) 86-1685. Public Health Service, Washington. U.S. Government Printing Office, July 1986.

HOW SUPPLIED
Current prices are unavailable. Check wholesaler for further information.

Histrelin Acetate

DESCRIPTION
Histrelin Acetate Injection contains a synthetic nonapeptide agonist of the naturally occuring gonadotropin releasing hormone (GnRH or LHRH). The analog possesses a greater potency than the natural sequence hormone. The amino acid sequence and chemical name of Histrelin Acetate is:

5-oxo-L-prolyl-L-histidyl-L-tryptophyl-L-seryl-L-tyrosyl-N^t- benzyl-D-histidyl-L-leucyl-L-arginyl-N-ethyl-L-prolinamide acetate (salt) $[C_{66}H_{86}N_{18}O$ (1.7-2.8 moles) CH_3COOH. (0.6-7.0 moles) $H_2O]$.

The molecular weight of the peptide base is 1323.52

Histrelin Acetate Injection is a sterile, aqueous solution for subcutaneous administration available in single-use vials of 0.6 mL. It contains histrelin equivalent to either 200 mcg/mL, 500 mcg/mL, or 1000 mcg/mL peptide base with 0.9% sodium chloride and 10% mannitol. The pH of the 200 mcg/mL solution is 4.5-6.5 and the pH of the 500 mcg/mL and 1000 mcg/mL solutions is 4.5-6.0.

Following is its chemical structure:

H-5-oxoPro-His-Trp-Ser-Tyr-D-His(N^T-PhCH$_2$-)-Leu-Arg-Pro-NHEt
  1   2   3   4   5   6   7   8   9

CLINICAL PHARMACOLOGY
Histrelin Acetate Injection, a GnRH agonist, is a potent inhibitor of gonadotropin secretion when administered daily in therapeutic doses. Both animal and human studies indicate that following an initial stimulatory phase, chronic, subcutaneous administration of histrelin acetate desensitizes responsiveness of the pituitary gonadotropin which, in turn, causes a reduction in ovarian and testicular steroidogenesis. Although animal studies have shown that *acute* administration of Histrelin Acetate Injection results in stimulation of the reproductive system, *chronic* Histrelin Acetate Injection administration in the rat delays sexual development, inhibits estrous cyclicity and pregnancy, reduces reproductive organ weight, and inhibits ovarian and testicular steroidogenesis in a reversible fashion. In the rabbit, chronic administration of Histrelin Acetate Injection resulted in decreased reproductive organ weights.

In human studies, chronic administration of Histrelin Acetate Injection controls the secretion of pituitary gonadotropins resulting in decreased sex steroid levels and in the regression of secondary sexual characteristics in children with precocious puberty. In girls, menses cease, serum estradiol levels are decreased to prepubertal levels, linear growth velocities decrease, skeletal maturation is slowed, and adult height predictions increase. In boys, testicular steroidogenesis is inhibited and testicular volume is reduced.

Continuous Histrelin Acetate Injection administration to patients with central precocious puberty can be monitored by standard GnRH testing and by serial determinations of sex steroid levels. The decreases in LH, FSH, and sex steroid levels are evident within three months of the initiation of therapy. These effects have been demonstrated in the 10 female patients who were studied for periods up to eighteen months. The metabolism, distribution, and excretion of Histrelin Acetate Injection in humans have not been determined.

INDICATIONS AND USAGE
Histrelin Acetate Injection is indicated for the control of the biochemical and clinical manifestations of central precocious puberty.

Selection of Patients:
1. Only patients with centrally mediated precocious puberty (either idiopathic or neurogenic and occurring before age 8 years in girls or 9.5 years in boys) should receive Histrelin Acetate Injection treatment.
2. Before treatment with Histrelin Acetate Injection is instituted, a thorough physical and endocrinologic evaluation should be performed. This should include:
    a. Height and weight as baseline for serial monitoring.
    b. Hand and wrist x-ray for bone age determination, to document advanced skeletal age and as baseline for serially monitoring predicted height.
    c. Total sex steroid level (estradiol or testosterone).
    d. Adrenal steroid level, to exclude congenital adrenal hyperplasia.
    e. Beta-Human Chorionic Gonadotropin level, to rule out a chorionic gonadotropin-secreting tumor.
    f. GnRH stimulation test, to demonstrate activation of the Hypothalamic-Pituitary-Gonadal (HPG) axis.
    g. Pelvic/adrenal/testicular ultrasound, to rule out a steroid-secreting tumor and to document gonadal size for serial monitoring.
    h. Computerized tomography of the head, to rule out previously undiagnosed intracranial tumor.
3. Patients must be able to maintain compliance with a *daily* regimen of injections.

UNLABELED USES
Histrelin Acetate is used alone or as an adjunct in the treatment of acute intermittent porphyria, endometriosis, and premenstrual syndrome. It is also used in the treatment of uterine leiomyomata.

CONTRAINDICATIONS
Histrelin Acetate Injection should not be administered to patients known to be hypersensitive to any of its components.

Histrelin Acetate Injection is contraindicated in women who are or may become pregnant while receiving the drug and in nursing mothers. There was increased fetal size and mortality in rats and increased fetal mortality in rabbits but not in mice after Histrelin Acetate Injection administration. Other responses to Histrelin Acetate Injection included dystocia, a greater incidence of unilateral hydroureter, and incomplete ossification in rat fetuses in all treated groups. When administered to rabbits on days 6-18 of pregnancy at doses of 20 to 80 mcg/kg/day (2 to 8 times the human dose), Histrelin Acetate Injection produced early termination of pregnancy and increased fetal death. In rats administered Histrelin Acetate Injection on days 7-20 of pregnancy at doses of 1 to 15 mcg/kg/day (0.1 to 1.5 times the human dose) there was an increase in fetal resorptions. In mice treated on days 6-15 of pregnancy at 10 to 100 times the human dose, Supprelin Injection had no adverse effects. The effects on fetal mortality are expected consequences of the alterations in hormonal levels brought about by the drug. If this drug is inadvertently used during pregnancy or in the rare event that a patient becomes pregnant while taking this drug, she should be apprised of the potential hazard to the fetus.

It is not known if this drugs are excreted in human milk, but because many drugs are excreted in human milk and because of the potential for serious adverse reactions in nursing infants from Histrelin Acetate, the drug should not be given to nursing mothers.

WARNINGS
Noncompliance with drug regimen or inadequate dosing may result in inadequate control of the pubertal process. The consequences of poor control include the return of pubertal signs such as menses, breast development, and testicular growth. The long-term consequences of inadequate control of gonadal steroid secretion are unknown, but may include a further compromise of adult stature.

Serious hypersensitivity reactions (angioedema, urticaria) have been reported following Histrelin Acetate Injection administration. Clinical manifestations may include: cardiovascular collapse, hypotension, tachycardia, loss of consciousness, angioedema, bronchospasm, dyspnea, urticaria, flushing and pruritus. If any allergic reaction occurs, therapy with Histrelin Acetate should be discontinued. Serious acute hypersensitivity reactions may require emergency medical treatment.

PRECAUTIONS
General: Studies in rats and monkeys have indicated that all of the known biochemical and antifertility effects of Histrelin Acetate Injection are reversible. Because animal studies are not always predictive of human response, and because children who have received Histrelin Acetate Injection have not been followed sufficiently long to ensure reactivation of the HPG axis following long-term therapy, this drug should be used only when the benefits to the patient outweigh the potential risks. In addition, the patient (and/or guardian) should be advised that hypogonadism may result if the HPG axis fails to reactivate after the drug is discontinued.

Information to Patient: Prior to Histrelin Acetate Injection therapy, patients and their families should be informed of the importance of complying with the schedule of single, daily injections, given at approximately the same time each day. If injections are not given daily, the pubertal process may be reactivated. Histrelin Acetate Injection contains no preservative. Patients should be informed that vials are to be used once and any unused solution is to be discarded. Medication should be allowed to reach room temperature before injecting. Daily injections should be rotated through different body sites (upper arms, thighs, abdomen).

Patients should be made aware of the required monitoring of their condition and of the potential risks of therapy. Within the first month of therapy, girls being treated with Histrelin Acetate Injection may experience a light menstrual flow. This menstrual flow is common and likely is related to the lower estrogen levels brought about by treatment, and the withdrawal of estrogen support from the endometrium.

Irritation, redness, or swelling at the injection sites may occur. If these reactions are severe, or do not go away, the patient's doctor should be notified.

The patients and their families should be advised to discontinue the drug and seek medical attention at the first sign of skin rash, urticaria, rapid heartbeat, difficulty in swallowing and breathing, or any swelling which may suggest angioedema. (See *"Warnings"* and *"Adverse Reactions"*).

Clinical Evaluations/Laboratory Tests: An initial pelvic ultrasound should be performed to exclude other conditions before treating with Histrelin Acetate Injection. The patient should be monitored carefully after 3 months and every 6 to 12 months thereafter by serial clinical evaluations, repeated height measurements, bone age determinations (yearly), and serial GnRH testing to document that gonadotropin responsiveness of the pituitary remains prepubertal while on therapy. During the initial agonistic phase of treatment, the patient may demonstrate transient increases in breast tissue, moodiness, vaginal secretions, or testicular volume. After this initial agonistic phase (usually one to three weeks), control of the biochemical and physical manifestations of puberty should remain as long as chronic therapy is in effect. Treatment should be discontinued when the onset of puberty is desired. Following the discontinuation of Histrelin Acetate Injection treatment, the onset of normal puberty should be documented. In addition, patients should be monitored to assess menstrual cyclicity, reproductive function, and ultimate adult height.

Carcinogenesis, Mutagenesis, and Impairment of Fertility: Carcinogenicity studies were conducted in rats for 2 years at doses of 5, 25 or 150 mcg/kg/day (up to 15 times the human dose) and in mice for 18 months at doses of 20, 200, or 2000 mcg/kg/day (up to 200 times the human dose). As seen with other GnRH agonists, Histrelin Acetate Injection administration was associated with an increase in tumors of hormonally responsive tissues. There was a significant increase in pituitary adenomas in rats. There was an increase in pancreatic islet-cell adenomas in treated female rats and a non-dose-related increase in testicular Leydig-cell tumors (highest incidence in the low-dose group). In mice, there was a significant increase in mammary-gland adenocarcinomas in all treated females. In addition, there were increases in stomach papillomas in male rats given high doses, and an increase in histiocytic sarcomas in female mice at the highest dose.

Mutagenicity studies have not been performed. Fertility studies have been conducted in rats and monkeys given subcutaneous daily doses of Histrelin Acetate Injection up to 180 mcg/kg for 6 months and full reversibility of fertility suppression was demonstrated. The development and reproductive performance of offspring from parents treated with Histrelin Acetate Injection has not been investigated.

Pregnancy, Teratogenic Effects: Pregnancy Category X. See *"Contraindications"* section.

Nursing Mothers: See *"Contraindications"* section.

Pediatric Use: Safety and effectiveness in children below the age of two years have not been established.

ADVERSE REACTIONS

At least one adverse experience was reported for 139 of the 183 (76%) children in clinical studies of central precocious puberty. Three of the 183 children (2%) stopped therapy due to a hypersensitivity reaction.

Adverse experience considered related or probably related to drug therapy included:

Skin reactions at the medication site (redness, swelling, and itching)	45%
Vaginal bleeding (usually only one episode within 1 to 3 weeks of starting therapy lasting several days)	22%
Urticaria	4%
Purpura	2%
Convulsions (increased frequency)	2%
Visual disturbances	2%
Hot flashes/flushes	2%
Edema (other than at medication site)	2%
Mood changes	2%
Erythema (other than at medication site)	1%
Conduct disorder	1%

Other adverse experiences considered possibly related to drug therapy and reported in at least 1% of patients are as follows:

Cardiovascular: (1-3%)—palpitations, tachycardia, epistaxis, hypertension, migraine headache, pallor.

Endocrine: (6%)—leukorrhea; (1%)—goiter, hyperlipidemia, anemia, breast edema, breast pain, breast discharge, glycosuria.

Gastrointestinal: (3-10%)—gastrointestinal pain, abdominal pain, nausea, vomiting, diarrhea; (1-3%)—GI cramps, GI distress, constipation, appetite decreased, thirsty.

Miscellaneous: (14%)—pyrexia; (6%)—extremity pain: (1-3%)—fatigue, chills, malaise, neck, chest or trunk pain, viral infection.

Musculoskeletal: (4%)—arthralgia; (1%)—pain, hypotonia.

Nervous System: (22%)—headache; 1-3%)—somnolence, lethergy, dizziness impared consciousness, syncope, tremor, hyperkinesia, nervousness, anxiety, depression.

Respiratory: (3-10%)—cough, pharyngitis; (1-3%)—hyperventilation, upper respiratory infection.

Skin: (7%)—rash; (1-3%)—pruritus, dyschromia, keratoderma, alopecia, sweating.

Special Senses: (1-3%)—abnormal pupillary function, otalgia, hearing loss, polyopia, photophobia.

Urogenital: (1-3%)—irritation or odor or pruritus or infections of the female genitalia, polyuria, dysuria, urinary frequency, incontinence, hematuria, nocturia.

Acute generalized (angioedema, urticaria) hypersensitivity reactions have been reported (See *"Warnings"* and *"Precautions"*).

OTHER PATIENTS

Histrelin Acetate Injection has been studied in other patients for various indications (N = 196). Adverse experiences occurring in 2% or more of the study population are:

Cardiovascular: (35%)—vasodilation; (3%)—edema, migraine headache, hypertension

Endocrine: (12%)—vaginal dryness; (3-10%)—metrorrhagia, breast pain, breast edema; (2-3%)—leukorrhea, breast discharge, decreased breast size, tenderness of female genitalia

Gastrointestinal: (3-10%)—nausea, GI pain, flatulence, decreased appetite, dyspepsia; (2-3%)—vomiting, constipation, diarrhea, GI cramps, gastritis

Miscellaneous: (12%)—abdominal pain; (3-10%)—pain in trunk, body, or extremities, fatigue, pyrexia, weight gain, chest pain, viral infection; (2-3%)—chills, malaise, head/face pain, neck pain, purpura

Musculoskeletal: (3-10%)—arthralgia, joint stiffness, muscle cramps (2-3%)—muscle stiffness, myalgia

Nervous System: (22%)—headache; (3-10%)—mood changes, nervousness, dizziness, depression, libido changes, insomnia, anxiety; (2-3%)—paresthesia, cognitive changes, syncope

Respiratory: (3-10%)—upper respiratory infection, pharyngitis, respiratory congestion; (2-3%)—cough, asthma, breathing disorder, rhinorrhea, bronchitis, sinusitis

Skin: (12%)—skin reaction at the medication site; (3-10%)—acne, rash, sweating; (2-3%)—keratoderma, pruritus, pain

Special Senses: (6%)—visual disturbances; (2-3%)—ear congestion, otalgia

Urogenital: (3-10%)—pain of female genitalia, vaginitis, dysmenorrhea; (2-3%)—dyspareunia, dysuria, hypertrophy of female genitalia, pruritus of external female genitalia Urticaria which was reported by less than 2% of the population, may be clinically significant.

DRUG ABUSE AND DEPENDENCE

No instances of drug abuse or dependence have been reported.

OVERDOSAGE

Histrelin Acetate Injection of up to 200 mcg/kg (rats, rabbits), or 2000 mcg/kg (mice) resulted in no systemic toxicity. This represents 20 to 200 times the maximal recommended human dose of 10 mcg/kg/day.

DOSAGE AND ADMINISTRATION

The dose of Histrelin Acetate Injection that is recommended for the treatment of central precocious puberty is 10 mcg/kg of body weight administered as a single, daily subcutaneous injection. If prepubertal levels of sex steroids and/or a prepubertal gonadotropin response to GnRH testing are not achieved within the first 3 months of treatment, the patient should be reevaluated. Doses greater than 10 mcg/kg/day have not been evaluated in clinical trials. The injection site should be varied daily.

Note: Parenteral drug products should be inspected visually for discoloration and particulate matter before use. Histrelin Acetate contains no preservative. Vials are to be used once. Any unused solution is to be discarded.

Store refrigerated at 2-8°C (36-46°F) and protect from light. Remove vial from packaging only at time of use. Allow vial to reach room temperature before injecting contents. Discard unused portion of the vial after administration.

HOW SUPPLIED
KIT: 200 MCG/ML

BRAND/MANUFACTURER	NDC	SIZE	AWP
○ **BRAND** SUPPRELIN: Roberts Pharm	54092-0637-75	1s	$269.09

KIT: 500 MCG/5 ML

BRAND/MANUFACTURER	NDC	SIZE	AWP
○ **BRAND** SUPPRELIN: Roberts Pharm	54092-0638-75	1s	$413.99

KIT: 1000 MCG/ML

BRAND/MANUFACTURER	NDC	SIZE	AWP
○ **BRAND** SUPPRELIN: Roberts Pharm	54092-0639-75	1s	$600.27

Hivid *SEE* ZALCITABINE

HMS *SEE* MEDRYSONE

◆ RATED THERAPEUTICALLY EQUIVALENT; ◇ THERAPEUTIC EQUIVALENCE UNCONFIRMED; ○ UNRATED

Homatropine Hydrobromide

DESCRIPTION

Homatropine Hydrobromide is an anticholinergic prepared as a sterile topical ophthalmic solution supplied in two strengths.

The chemical name is benzeneacetic acid, α-hydroxy-, 8-methyl-8-azabicyclo[3,2.1]-oct-3-yl ester, hydrobromide, endo-(±).

Each ml contains: Homatropine Hydrobromide 2.0% or 5.0%.

Following is its chemical structure:

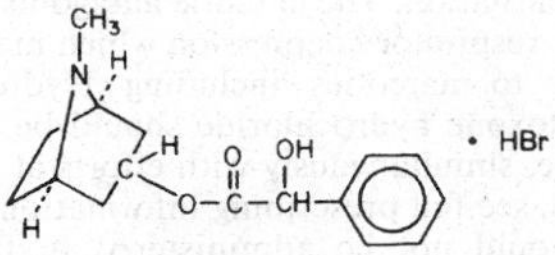

CLINICAL PHARMACOLOGY

This anticholinergic preparation blocks the responses of the sphincter muscle of the iris and the accommodative muscle of the ciliary body to cholinergic stimulation, producing pupilary dilation (mydriasis) and paralysis of accommodation (cycloplegia).

INDICATIONS AND USAGE

A moderately long-acting mydriatic and cycloplegic for cycloplegic refraction and in the treatment of inflammatory conditions of the uveal tract. For pre- and postoperative states when mydriasis is required. Use as an ontical aid in some cases of axial lens opacities.

CONTRAINDICATIONS

Contraindicated in persons with primary glaucoma or a tendency toward glaucoma, e.g., narrow anterior chamber angle, and in those persons showing hypersensitivity to any component of the preparation.

WARNING

For topical use only—not for injection. Risk-benefit should be considered when the following medical problems exist: keratoconus (Homatropine may produce fixed dilated pupil); Down's syndrome, children with brain damage and the elderly (increased susceptibility). In infants and small children, use with extreme caution.

PRECAUTIONS

General: To avoid excessive systemic absorption, the lacrimal sac should be compressed by digital pressure for two to three minutes after instillation. To avoid inducing angle closure glaucoma, an estimation of the depth of the angle of the anterior chamber should be made. Excessive topical use of this drug can potentially lead to a confusional state characterized by delirium, agitation, and, rarely, coma. This state is more apt to occur in the pediatric and geriatric age groups. The specific antidote for this systemic anticholinergic syndrome is injectable physostigmine salicylate.

Information for Patients: Patient should be advised not to drive or engage in other hazardous activities while pupils are dilated. Patient may experience sensitivity to light and should protect eyes in bright illumination during dilation. Parents should be warned not to get this preparation in their child's mouth and to wash their own hands and the child's hands following administration. Do not touch dropper tip to any surface, as this may contaminate the solution.

Carcinogenesis, Mutagenesis, Impairment of Fertility: There have been no long-term studies done using Homatropine HBr in animals to evaluate carcinogenic potential.

Pregnancy: Pregnancy Category C. Animal reproduction studies have not been conducted with Homatropine HBr. It is also not known whether Homatropine HBr can cause fetal harm when administered to a pregnant woman or can affect reproduction capacity. Homatropine HBr should be given to a pregnant woman only if clearly needed.

Nursing Mothers: It is not known whether this drug is excreted in human milk. Because many drugs are excreted in human milk, caution should be exercised when Homatropine HBr is administered to a nursing woman.

ADVERSE REACTIONS

Transient symptoms of stinging and burning may occur. Prolonged use may produce local irritation characterized by follicular conjunctivitis, vascular congestion, edema, exudate, and an eczematoid dermatitis. Thirst or dryness of mouth, eye irritation not present before therapy, or increased sensitivity of eyes to light may occur.

DOSAGE AND ADMINISTRATION

For refraction, instill one or two drops topically in the eye(s). May be repeated in five to ten minutes if necessary. For uveitis, instill one or two drops topically up to every three to four hours. Individuals with heavily pigmented irides may require larger doses. Only the 2% strength should be used in pediatric patients.

Store at 8°-24°C (46°-75°F).

HOW SUPPLIED
DROP: 2%

BRAND/MANUFACTURER	NDC	SIZE	AWP
○ **BRAND**			
ISOPTO HOMATROPINE: Alcon Labs	00998-0311-05	5 ml	$10.94
	00998-0311-15	15 ml	$15.13
○ **GENERICS**			
Southwood	58016-6324-01	1 ml 12s	$33.44

DROP: 5%

BRAND/MANUFACTURER	NDC	SIZE	AWP
○ **BRAND**			
ISOPTO HOMATROPINE: Alcon Labs	00998-0315-05	5 ml	$12.25
	00998-0315-15	15 ml	$16.38
○ **GENERICS**			
Paco	52967-0536-35	5 ml	$1.65
Iolab	00058-2467-05	5 ml	$9.72
Allscrips	54569-1750-01	5 ml	$9.72
Paco	52967-0536-45	15 ml	$1.95
Iolab	00058-7778-12	1 ml 12s	$24.96
Alcon Surg	00065-0712-12	2 ml 12s	$37.80

Homatropine Methylbromide and Hydrocodone Bitartrate

DESCRIPTION

Homatropine Methylbromide/Hydrocodone Bitartrate contains Hydrocodone (dihydrocodeinone) Bitartrate, a semisynthetic centrally-acting narcotic antitussive. Homatropine Methylbromide is included in a subtherapeutic amount to discourage deliberate overdosage.

Each tablet or teaspoonful (5 mL) contains:

Hydrocodone Bitartrate, USP ....5 mg
WARNING: May be habit forming.
Homatropine Methylbromide, USP ....1.5 mg

The Hydrocodone component is 4,5α-epoxy-3-methoxy-17-methylmorphinan-6-one tartrate (1:1) hydrate (2:5), a fine white crystal or crystalline powder, which is derived from the opium alkaloid, thebaine, has a molecular weight of (494.50).

Homatropine Methylbromide is 8-Azoniabicyclo-[3.2.1] octane, 3-[(hydroxyphenylacetyl) oxy]-8, 8-dimethylbromide, endo-; a white crystal or fine white crystalline powder, with a molecular weight of (370.29).

CLINICAL PHARMACOLOGY

Hydrocodone is a semisynthetic narcotic antitussive and analgesic with multiple actions qualitatively similar to those of codeine. The precise mechanism of action of Hydrocodone and other opiates is not known; however, Hydrocodone is believed to act directly on the cough center. In excessive doses, Hydrocodone, like other opium derivatives, will depress respiration. The effects of Hydrocodone in therapeutic doses on the cardiovascular system are insignificant. Hydrocodone can produce miosis, euphoria, physical and physiological dependence.

Following a 10 mg oral dose of Hydrocodone administered to five adult male subjects, the mean peak concentration was 23.6 ± 5.2 ng/mL. Maximum serum levels were achieved at 1.3 ± 0.3 hours and the half-life was determined to be 3.8 ± 0.3 hours. Hydrocodone exhibits a complex pattern of metabolism including O-demethylation, N-demethylation and 6-keto reduction to the corresponding 6-α- and 6-β-hydroxymetabolites.

INDICATIONS AND USAGE

Homatropine/Hydrocodone is indicated for the symptomatic relief of cough.

CONTRAINDICATIONS

Homatropine/Hydrocodone should not be administered to patients who are hypersensitive to Hydrocodone or Homatropine Methylbromide.

WARNINGS

May be habit forming. Hydrocodone can produce drug dependence of the morphine type and, therefore, has the potential for being abused. Psychic dependence, physical dependence and tolerance may develop upon repeated administration of Homatropine/Hydrocodone and it should be prescribed and administered with the same degree of caution appropriate to the use of other narcotic drugs (see "Drug Abuse and Dependence").

Respiratory Depression: Homatropine/Hydrocodone produces dose-related respiratory depression by directly acting on brain stem respiratory centers. If respiratory depression occurs, it may be antagonized by the use of naloxone hydrochloride and other supportive measures when indicated.

Head Injury and Increased Intracranial Pressure: The respiratory depression properties of narcotics and their capacity to elevate cerebrospinal fluid pressure may be markedly exaggerated in the presence of head injury, other intracranial lesions or a pre-existing increase in intracranial pressure. Furthermore, narcotics produce adverse reactions which may obscure the clinical course of patients with head injuries.

➤ SHOWN IN PRODUCT IDENTIFICATION GUIDE

Acute Abdominal Conditions: The administration of Homatropine/Hydrocodone or other narcotics may obscure the diagnosis or clinical course of patients with acute abdominal conditions.

Pediatric Use: In young children, as well as adults, the respiratory center is sensitive to the depressant action of narcotic cough suppressants in a dose-dependent manner. Benefit to risk ratio should be carefully considered especially in children with respiratory embarrassment (e.g., croup).

PRECAUTIONS

General: Before prescribing medication to suppress or modify cough, it is important to ascertain that the underlying cause of cough is identified, that modification of cough does not increase the risk of clinical or physiological complications, and that appropriate therapy for the primary disease is provided.

Special Risk Patients: Homatropine/Hydrocodone should be given with caution to certain patients such as the elderly or debilitated, and those with severe impairment of hepatic or renal functions, hypothyroidism, Addison's disease, prostatic hypertrophy or urethral stricture, asthma, and narrow angle glaucoma.

Information For Patients: Hydrocodone may impair the mental and/or physical abilities required for the performance of potentially hazardous tasks such as driving a car or operating machinery. The patient using Homatropine/Hydrocodone should be cautioned accordingly.

Drug Interactions: Patients receiving narcotics, antihistamines, antipsychotics, antianxiety agents or other CNS depressants (including alcohol) concomitantly with Homatropine/Hydrocodone may exhibit an additive CNS depression. When combined therapy is contemplated, the dose of one or both agents should be reduced. The use of MAO inhibitors or tricyclic antidepressants with hydrocodone preparations may increase the effect of either the antidepressant or Hydrocodone.

Carcinogenesis, Mutagenesis, Impairment of Fertility: Studies of Homatropine/Hydrocodone in animals to evaluate the carcinogenic and mutagenic potential and the effect on fertility have not been conducted.

PREGNANCY

Teratogenic Effects: Pregnancy Category C: Animal reproduction studies have not been conducted with Homatropine/Hydrocodone (hydrocodone bitartrate and homatropine methylbromide). It is also not known whether Homatropine/Hydrocodone can cause fetal harm when administered to a pregnant woman or can affect reproduction capacity. Homatropine/Hydrocodone should be given to a pregnant woman only if clearly needed.

Nonteratogenic Effects: Babies born to mothers who have been taking opioids regularly prior to delivery will be physically dependent. The withdrawal signs include irritability and excessive crying, tremors, hyperactive reflexes, increased respiratory rate, increased stools, sneezing, yawning, vomiting and fever. The intensity of the syndrome does not always correlate with the duration of maternal opioid use or dose.

Labor and Delivery: As with all narcotics, administration of Homatropine/Hydrocodone to the mother shortly before delivery may result in some degree of respiratory depression in the newborn, especially if higher doses are used.

Nursing Mothers: It is not known whether this drug is excreted in human milk. Because many drugs are excreted in human milk and because of the potential for serious adverse reactions in nursing infants from Homatropine/Hydrocodone a decision should be made whether to discontinue nursing or to discontinue the drug, taking into account the importance of the drug to the mother.

Pediatric Use: Safety and effectiveness of Homatropine/Hydrocodone in children under six have not been established.

ADVERSE REACTIONS

Central Nervous System: Sedation, drowsiness, mental clouding, lethargy, impairment of mental and physical performance, anxiety, fear, dysphoria, dizziness, psychic dependence, mood changes.

Gastrointestinal System: Nausea and vomiting may occur; they are more frequent in ambulatory than in recumbent patients. Prolonged administration of Homatropine/Hydrocodone may produce constipation.

Genitourinary System: Ureteral spasm, spasm of vesicle sphincters and urinary retention have been reported with opiates.

Respiratory Depression: Homatropine/Hydrocodone may produce dose-related respiratory depression by acting directly on brain stem respiratory centers (see "Overdosage").

Dermatological: Skin rash, pruritus.

DRUG ABUSE AND DEPENDENCE

Homatropine/Hydrocodone is a Schedule III narcotic. Psychic dependence, physical dependence and tolerance may develop upon repeated administration of narcotics; therefore, Homatropine/Hydrocodone should be prescribed and administered with caution. However, psychic dependence is unlikely to develop when Homatropine/Hydrocodone is used for a short time for the treatment of cough. Physical dependence, the condition in which continued administration of the drug is required to prevent the appearance of a withdrawal syndrome, assumes clinically significant proportions only after several weeks of continued oral narcotic use, although some mild degree of physical dependence may develop after a few days of narcotic therapy.

OVERDOSAGE

Signs and Symptoms: Serious overdosage with Hydrocodone is characterized by respiratory depression (a decrease in respiratory rate and/or tidal volume, Cheyne-Stokes respiration, cyanosis), extreme somnolence progressing to stupor or coma, skeletal muscle flaccidity, cold and clammy skin, and sometimes bradycardia and hypotension. In severe overdosage apnea, circulatory collapse, cardiac arrest and death may occur. The ingestion of very large amounts of Homatropine/Hydrocodone may, in addition, result in acute Homatropine intoxication.

Treatment: Primary attention should be given to the reestablishment of adequate respiratory exchange through provision of a patent airway and the institution of assisted or controlled ventilation. The narcotic antagonist naloxone hydrochloride is a specific antidote for respiratory depression which may result from overdosage or unusual sensitivity to narcotics including Hydrocodone. Therefore, an appropriate dose of naloxone hydrochloride should be administered, preferably by the intravenous route, simultaneously with efforts at respiratory resuscitation. For further information, see full prescribing information for naloxone hydrochloride. An antagonist should not be administered in the absence of clinically significant respiratory depression. Oxygen, intravenous fluids, vasopressors and other supportive measures should be employed as indicated. Gastric emptying may be useful in removing unabsorbed drug.

DOSAGE AND ADMINISTRATION

Adults: One (1) tablet or one (1) teaspoonful (5 mL) of the syrup every 4 to 6 hours as needed: do not exceed six (6) tablets or six (6) teaspoonfuls in 24 hours.

Children 6 to 12 years of age: One-half (½) tablet or one-half (½) teaspoonful (2.5 mL) of the syrup every 4 to 6 hours as needed: do not exceed three (3) tablets or three (3) teaspoonfuls in 24 hours.

Storage: Store at controlled room temperature (59°-86° F, 15°-30° C).

HOW SUPPLIED
SYRUP (C-III): 1.5 MG-5 MG/5 ML

AVERAGE UNIT PRICE (AVAILABLE SIZES)		GENERIC A-RATED AVERAGE PRICE (GAAP)	
BRAND	$0.13	480 ml	$11.95
GENERIC	$0.02	3840 ml	$81.06
HCFA FUL (480 ml)	$0.02		

BRAND/MANUFACTURER	NDC	SIZE	AWP
◆ **BRAND**			
HYCODAN: Du Pont Multi	00056-0234-16	480 ml	$60.36
◆ **GENERICS**			
HYDROTROPINE: Rugby	00536-0920-85	480 ml	$9.88
Qualitest	00603-1296-58	480 ml	$10.71
Goldline	00182-1155-40	480 ml	$10.95
Geneva	00781-6526-16	480 ml	$11.50
Pennex	00426-8455-16	480 ml	$12.32
Pennex	00832-8455-16	480 ml	$12.32
HYDROMIDE: Major	00904-0956-16	480 ml	$12.50
HYDROPANE: Aligen	00405-0098-16	480 ml	$13.10
Halsey Pharm	00879-0455-16	480 ml	$13.10
HYDROMET: Barre	00472-1030-16	480 ml	$13.13
Schein	00364-2487-16	480 ml	$13.50
HYDROTROPINE: Rugby	00536-0920-90	3840 ml	$65.44
HYDROMIDE: Major	00904-0956-28	3840 ml	$75.25
Halsey Pharm	00879-0455-28	3840 ml	$91.65
HYDROMET: Barre	00472-1030-28	3840 ml	$91.88

TABLETS (C-III): 1.5 MG-5 MG

AVERAGE UNIT PRICE (AVAILABLE SIZES)	
BRAND	$0.50
GENERIC	$0.25

BRAND/MANUFACTURER	NDC	SIZE	AWP
◆ **BRAND**			
HYCODAN: Du Pont Multi	00056-0042-70	100s	$51.90
	00056-0042-85	500s	$235.74
◆ **GENERICS**			
TUSSIGON: Daniels	00689-0082-01	100s	$25.60
TUSSIGON: Daniels	00689-0082-05	500s	$116.71

House Dust Treatment Set *SEE*
ALLERGENIC EXTRACTS

Humate-P *SEE* **ANTIHEMOPHILIC FACTOR, HUMAN**

Humatin *SEE* **PAROMOMYCIN SULFATE**

Humatrope *SEE* **SOMATROPIN**

◆ RATED THERAPEUTICALLY EQUIVALENT; ◇ THERAPEUTIC EQUIVALENCE UNCONFIRMED; ○ UNRATED

Humibid DM *SEE* DEXTROMETHORPHAN
HYDROBROMIDE AND GUAIFENESIN

Humibid L.A. *SEE* GUAIFENESIN

Humorsol Ocumeter *SEE* DEMECARIUM
BROMIDE

Hyaluronidase

DESCRIPTION

Hyaluronidase, a protein enzyme, is a preparation of highly purified bovine testicular Hyaluronidase. The exact chemical structure of this enzyme is unknown. Hyaluronidase is available in two dosage forms:

HYALURONIDASE LYOPHILIZED

Hyaluronidase, dehydrated in the frozen state under high vacuum, is supplied as a sterile, white, odorless, amorphous solid and is to be reconstituted before use, usually in the proportion of one mL of diluent per 150 USP units of Hyaluronidase Lyophilized.

HYALURONIDASE STABILIZED SOLUTION

A Hyaluronidase injection solution ready for use, colorless and odorless, containing 150 USP units of Hyaluronidase per mL.

The USP and the NF Hyaluronidase units are equivalent to the turbidity-reducing (TR) unit and to the International Unit.

CLINICAL PHARMACOLOGY

Hyaluronidase is a spreading or diffusing substance which modifies the permeability of connective tissue through the hydrolysis of hyaluronic acid, a polysaccharide found in the intercellular ground substance of connective tissue, and of certain specialized tissues, such as the umbilical cord and vitreous humor. Hyaluronic acid is also present in the capsules of type A and C hemolytic streptococci. Hyaluronidase hydrolyzes hyaluronic acid by splitting the glucosaminidic bond between C_1 of the glucosamine moiety and C_4 of glucuronic acid. This temporarily decreases the viscosity of the cellular cement and promotes diffusion of injected fluids or of localized transudates or exudates, thus facilitating their absorption.

When no spreading factor is present, material injected subcutaneously spreads very slowly, but Hyaluronidase causes rapid spreading, provided local interstitial pressure is adequate to furnish the necessary mechanical impulse. Such an impulse is normally initiated by injected solutions. The rate of diffusion is proportionate to the amount of enzyme, and the extent is proportionate to the volume of solution.

Animal studies indicated that in dogs, given 160,000 U/kg Hyaluronidase intravenously, peak protein excretion in the urine occurred in the first hour and accounted for most of the 82 mg of protein recovered from the urine. The recovery represents 5% of the total amount of protein injected. One hour after the intravenous administration of 160,000 U/kg of Hyaluronidase to rabbits, the agent could no longer be detected in the blood (mucin clot assay). It was also noted that the sojourn of Hyaluronidase in the blood, as measured by the spreading technique, is considerably longer than the sojourn determined by the mucin clot assay. Rabbits and dogs were given 80,000 to 160,000 U/kg Hyaluronidase intravenously, plasma and urine samples were collected and were injected into the shaven skin of another rabbit. The spreading activity (trypan blue as indicator) of the plasma reached a maximum within 5 minutes, remained constant for the first hour, and then declined slowly over 5 hours. The spreading activity of the urine reached a maximum within the first hour and paralleled that of the plasma thereafter.

A study in rats, sacrificed 3 hours after 2,400—3,000 U of radio-labeled Hyaluronidase was administered intraperitoneally, indicated that all organs and tissues investigated displayed radioactivity, and that particularly high radioactivity was observed in the thymus, pancreas, kidneys, and ovaries.

Knowledge of the mechanisms involved in the disappearance of injected Hyaluronidase is limited. It is known, however, that the blood of a number of mammalian species brings about the inactivation of Hyaluronidase. Studies have demonstrated that Hyaluronidase is antigenic; repeated injections of relatively large amounts of this enzyme may result in the formation of neutralizing antibodies. The reconstitution of the dermal barrier removed by intradermal injection of Hyaluronidase (20, 2, 0.2, 0.02, and 0.002 U/mL) to adult humans indicated that at 24 hours the restoration of the barrier is incomplete and inversely related to the dosage of enzyme; at 48 hours the barrier is completely restored in all treated areas.

Results from an experimental study, in humans, on the influence of Hyaluronidase in bone repair support the conclusion that this enzyme alone, in the usual clinical dosage, does not deter bone healing.

INDICATIONS AND USAGE

Hyaluronidase is indicated as an adjuvant to increase the absorption and dispersion of other injected drugs; for hypodermoclysis; and as an adjunct in subcutaneous urography for improving resorption of radiopaque agents.

CONTRAINDICATIONS

Hypersensitivity to Hyaluronidase. A preliminary test for sensitivity should be conducted. (See *"Precautions—Laboratory Tests"*.)

Because of the danger of spreading a localized infection, Hyaluronidase should not be injected into or around an infected or acutely inflamed area. Similarly, Hyaluronidase should not be injected into an area that is known or suspected to be cancerous.

PRECAUTIONS

GENERAL

When considering the administration of any other drug with Hyaluronidase, it is recommended that appropriate references first be consulted to determine the usual precautions for the use of the other drug; e.g., when epinephrine is injected along with Hyaluronidase, the precautions for the use of epinephrine in cardiovascular disease, thyroid disease, diabetes, digital nerve block, ischemia of the fingers and toes, etc., should be observed.

LABORATORY TESTS

A preliminary skin test for sensitivity to Hyaluronidase should be performed with an intradermal injection of approximately 0.02 mL of the solution. A positive reaction consists of a wheal with pseudopods appearing within five minutes and persisting for 20 to 30 minutes and accompanied by localized itching. Transient vasodilation at the site of the test, i.e., erythema, is not a positive reaction.

DRUG INTERACTIONS

When Hyaluronidase is added to a local anesthetic agent, it hastens the onset of analgesia and tends to reduce the swelling caused by local infiltration, but the wider spread of the local anesthetic solution increases its absorption; this shortens its duration of action and tends to increase the incidence of systemic reaction.

CARCINOGENESIS, MUTAGENESIS, IMPAIRMENT OF FERTILITY

Long-term animal studies have not been performed to assess the carcinogenic or mutagenic potential of Hyaluronidase. It has been observed that intravenous administration of as much as 75,000 U (500 times the therapeutic dose) of Hyaluronidase in animals caused no changes in the tissues.

Long-term animal studies have not been performed to assess whether Hyaluronidase impaired fertility; however, it has been reported that testicular degeneration may occur with the production of organ-specific antibodies against this enzyme following repeated injections. Human studies on the effect of intravaginal Hyaluronidase in sterility due to oligospermia indicated that Hyaluronidase may have aided conception. Thus, it appears that Hyaluronidase may not adversely affect fertility in females.

PREGNANCY

Teratogenic Effects—Pregnancy Category C: Animal reproductive studies have not been conducted with Hyaluronidase. It is also not known whether Hyaluronidase can cause fetal harm when administered to a pregnant woman. Hyaluronidase should be given to a pregnant woman only if clearly needed.

LABOR AND DELIVERY

Administration of Hyaluronidase during labor was reported to cause no complications: no increase in blood loss or differences in cervical trauma were observed. It is not known whether Hyaluronidase has an effect on the fetus if used during labor; the effect of Hyaluronidase on the later growth, development, and functional maturation of the infant is unknown.

NURSING MOTHERS

It is not known whether Hyaluronidase is excreted in human milk. Because many drugs are excreted in human milk, caution should be exercised when Hyaluronidase is administered to a nursing woman.

PEDIATRIC USE

Hyaluronidase may be added to small volumes of solution (up to 200 mL), such as a small clysis for infants or solutions of drugs for subcutaneous injection. The potential for chemical or physical incompatibilities should be kept in mind. (See *"Dosage and Administration"*.)

ADVERSE REACTIONS

The subcutaneous administration of Hyaluronidase has been associated with very few adverse reactions. Allergic reactions (urticaria) are rare. Anaphylactic-like reactions following retrobulbar block or intravenous injections have occurred in isolated cases. Cardiac fibrillation has been encountered once.

OVERDOSAGE

Symptoms of toxicity consist of local edema or urticaria, erythema, chills, nausea, vomiting, dizziness, tachycardia, and hypotension. The enzyme should be discontinued and supportive measures initiated immediately. Agents such as epinephrine, corticosteroids, and antihistamines should always be available for emergency treatment.

DOSAGE AND ADMINISTRATION

Hyaluronidase should be administered only as discussed below, since its effects relative to absorption and dispersion of other drugs are not produced when it is administered intravenously.

➤ SHOWN IN PRODUCT IDENTIFICATION GUIDE

RECONSTITUTION

If the lyophilized powder for injection is used, 1 mL of diluent should be added to a vial containing 150 U of Hyaluronidase, and 10 mL of diluent to a vial containing 1,500 U of Hyaluronidase, respectively, to provide a solution containing approximately 150 U/mL.

ABSORPTION AND DISPERSION OF INJECTED DRUGS

Absorption and dispersion of other injected drugs may be enhanced by adding 150 U Hyaluronidase to the injection solution. In order to prepare a solution containing epinephrine, add 0.5 mL epinephrine to the above solution.

Before adding Hyaluronidase to a solution containing another drug, it is recommended that appropriate references be consulted regarding physical or chemical incompatibilities.

HYPODERMOCLYSIS

Insert needle with aseptic precautions. With tip lying free and movable between skin and muscle, begin clysis; fluid should start in readily without pain or lump. Then inject solution Hyaluronidase into rubber tubing close to needle.

An alternate method is to inject Hyaluronidase under skin prior to clysis. 150 U will facilitate absorption of 1,000 mL or more of solution. As with all parenteral fluid therapy, observe the effect closely, with the same precautions for restoring fluid and electrolyte balance as in intravenous injections. The dose, the rate of injection, and the type of solution (saline, glucose, Ringer's, etc.) must be adjusted carefully to the individual patient. When solutions devoid of inorganic electrolytes are given by hypodermoclysis, hypovolemia may occur. This may be prevented by using solutions containing adequate amounts of inorganic electrolytes and/or controlling the volume and speed of administration.

Hyaluronidase may be added to small volumes of solution (up to 200 mL), such as small clysis for infants or solutions of drugs for subcutaneous injection. For children less than 3 years old, the volume of a single clysis should be limited to 200 mL; and in premature infants or during the neonatal period, the daily dosage should not exceed 25 mL/kg of body weight; the rate of administration should not be greater than 2 mL per minute. For older patients, the rate and volume of administration should not exceed those employed for intravenous infusion.

SUBCUTANEOUS UROGRAPHY

The subcutaneous route of administration of urographic contrast media is indicated when intravenous administration cannot be successfully accomplished, particularly in infants and small children. With the patient prone, 75 U of Hyaluronidase is injected subcutaneously over each scapula, followed by injection of the contrast medium at the same sites.

Parenteral drug products should be inspected visually for particulate matter and discoloration prior to administration, whenever solution and container permit.

STORAGE

Store Hyaluronidase lyophilized at controlled room temperature in a dry place. Store sterile reconstituted solution below 30° C (86° F). Use within 14 days. Following reconstitution, store vial in upright position.

Store Hyaluronidase stable solution in a refrigerator. Do not use if solution is discolored or contains a precipitate.

J CODES
Up to 150 units SC,IV—J3470

HOW SUPPLIED
INJECTION: 150 U/ML

BRAND/MANUFACTURER	NDC	SIZE	AWP
○ BRAND			
WYDASE: Wyeth-Ayerst	00008-0170-01	1 ml	$7.03
	00008-0170-02	10 ml	$19.89

POWDER FOR INJECTION: 150 U/ML

BRAND/MANUFACTURER	NDC	SIZE	AWP
○ BRAND			
WYDASE: Wyeth-Ayerst	00008-0121-01	1s	$6.60
	00008-0149-01	1s	$19.48

Hyate:C SEE ANTIHEMOPHILIC FACTOR, PORCINE

Hycodan SEE HOMATROPINE METHYLBROMIDE AND HYDROCODONE BITARTRATE

Hycomine SEE HYDROCODONE BITARTRATE WITH PHENYLPROPANOLAMINE HYDROCHLORIDE

Hycomine Compound SEE ACETAMINOPHEN/ CAFFEINE/CHLORPHENIRAMINE/HYDROCODONE/PHENYLEPHRINE

Hycotuss Expectorant SEE GUAIFENESIN AND HYDROCODONE BITARTRATE

Hydeltra-T.B.A. SEE PREDNISOLONE TEBUTATE

Hydeltrasol SEE PREDNISOLONE, SYSTEMIC

Hydergine SEE ERGOLOID MESYLATES

Hydralazine Hydrochloride

DESCRIPTION
Hydralazine Hydrochloride is an antihypertensive. Its chemical name is 1-hydrazinophthalazine monohydrochloride. It is available as tablets for oral administration and injection for intravenous or intramuscular administration.

Each tablet contains:	
Hydralazine HCl	.......10, 25, 50, or 100 mg

Each ml of solution for injection contains:
Hydralazine HCl ....20 mg.

Hydralazine Hydrochloride USP is a white to off-white, odorless crystalline powder. It is soluble in water, slightly soluble in alcohol, and very slightly soluble in ether. It melts at about 275°C, with decomposition, and has a molecular weight of 196.64.

Following is its chemical structure:

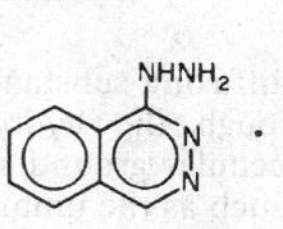

CLINICAL PHARMACOLOGY
Although the precise mechanism of action of Hydralazine is not fully understood, the major effects are on the cardiovascular system. Hydralazine apparently lowers blood pressure by exerting a peripheral vasodilating effect through a direct relaxation of vascular smooth muscle. Hydralazine, by altering cellular calcium metabolism, interferes with the calcium movements within the vascular smooth muscle that are responsible for initiating or maintaining the contractile state. The peripheral vasodilating effect of Hydralazine results in decreased arterial blood pressure (diastolic more than systolic); decreased peripheral vascular resistance; and an increased heart rate, stroke volume, and cardiac output. The preferential dilatation of arterioles, as compared to veins, minimizes postural hypotension and promotes the increase in cardiac output. Hydralazine usually increases renin activity in plasma, presumably as a result of increased secretion of renin by the renal juxtaglomerular cells in response to reflex sympathetic discharge. This increase in renin activity leads to the production of angiotensin II, which then causes stimulation of aldosterone and consequent sodium reabsorption. Hydralazine also maintains or increases renal and cerebral blood flow.

Hydralazine is rapidly absorbed after oral administration, and peak plasma levels are reached at 1-2 hours. Plasma levels of apparent Hydralazine decline with a half-life of 3-7 hours. Binding to human plasma protein is 87%. Plasma levels of Hydralazine vary widely among individuals. Hydralazine is subject to polymorphic acetylation; slow acetylators generally have higher plasma levels of Hydralazine and require lower doses to maintain control of blood pressure. Hydralazine undergoes extensive hepatic metabolism; it is excreted mainly in the form of metabolites in the urine.

The average maximal decrease in blood pressure usually occurs 10-80 minutes after administration of parenteral Hydralazine. No other pharmacokinetic data on parenteral Hydralazine are available.

INDICATION AND USAGE
Essential hypertension, alone or as adjunct. Hydralazine injection is indicated for severe essential hypertension when the drug cannot be given orally or when there is an urgent need to lower blood pressure.

UNLABELED USES
Hydralazine Hydrochloride is used alone or as an adjunct in the treatment of anorexia and cachexia in patients with advanced cancer, to improve cardiac performance and reduce regurgitant flow acutely and chronically in patients with severe aortic insufficiency, and congestive heart failure. It is also used to treat hypertension in pregnancy, and pulmonary hypertension.

CONTRAINDICATIONS
Hypersensitivity to Hydralazine; coronary artery disease; mitral valvular rheumatic heart disease.

◆ RATED THERAPEUTICALLY EQUIVALENT; ◇ THERAPEUTIC EQUIVALENCE UNCONFIRMED; ○ UNRATED

WARNINGS

In a few patients Hydralazine may produce a clinical picture simulating systemic lupus erythematosus including glomerulonephritis. In such patients Hydralazine should be discontinued unless the benefit-to-risk determination requires continued antihypertensive therapy with this drug. Symptoms and signs usually regress when the drug is discontinued but residua have been detected many years later. Long-term treatment with steroids may be necessary. (See *"Precautions, Laboratory Tests".*)

PRECAUTIONS

General: Myocardial stimulation produced by Hydralazine HCl can cause anginal attacks and ECG changes of myocardial ischemia. The drug has been implicated in the production of myocardial infarction. It must, therefore, be used with caution in patients with suspected coronary artery disease.

The "hyperdynamic" circulation caused by Hydralazine HCl may accentuate specific cardiovascular inadequacies. For example, Hydralazine HCl may increase pulmonary artery pressure in patients with mitral valvular disease. The drug may reduce the pressor responses to epinephrine. Postural hypotension may result from Hydralazine HCl but is less common than with ganglionic blocking agents. It should be used with caution in patients with cerebral vascular accidents.

In hypertensive patients with normal kidneys who are treated with Hydralazine HCl, there is evidence of increased renal blood flow and a maintenance of glomerular filtration rate. In some instances where control values were below normal, improved renal function has been noted after administration of Hydralazine HCl. However, as with any antihypertensive agent, Hydralazine HCl should be used with caution in patients with advanced renal damage.

Peripheral neuritis, evidenced by paresthesia, numbness, and tingling, has been observed. Published evidence suggests an antipyridoxine effect, and that pyridoxine should be added to the regimen if symptoms develop.

Certain brands of Hydralazine contain FD&C Yellow No. 5 (tartrazine), which may cause allergic-type reactions (including bronchial asthma) in certain susceptible individuals. Although the overall incidence of sensitivity in the general population is low, it is frequently seen in patients who are also hypersensitive to aspirin.

Information for Patients: Patients should be informed of possible side effects and advised to take the tablets regularly and continuously as directed.

Laboratory Tests: Complete blood counts and antinuclear antibody titer determinations are indicated before and periodically during prolonged therapy with Hydralazine even though the patient is asymptomatic. These studies are also indicated if the patient develops arthralgia, fever, chest pain, continued malaise, or other unexplained signs or symptoms. A positive antinuclear antibody titer requires that the physician carefully weigh the implications of the test results against the benefits to be derived from antihypertensive therapy with Hydralazine.

Blood dyscrasias, consisting of reduction in hemoglobin and red cell count, leukopenia, agranulocytosis, and purpura, have been reported. If such abnormalities develop, therapy should be discontinued.

Drug/Drug Interactions: MAO inhibitors should be used with caution in patients receiving Hydralazine.

When other potent parenteral antihypertensive drugs, such as diazoxide, are used in combination with Hydralazine, patients should be continuously observed for several hours for any excessive fall in blood pressure. Profound hypotensive episodes may occur when diazoxide injection and Hydralazine HCl are used concomitantly.

Drug/Food Interactions: Administration of Hydralazine tablets with food results in higher plasma levels.

Carcinogenesis, Mutagenesis, Impairment of Fertility: In a lifetime study in Swiss albino mice, there was a statistically significant increase in the incidence of lung tumors (adenomas and adenocarcinomas) of both male and female mice given Hydralazine continuously in their drinking water at a dosage of about 250 mg/kg per day (about 80 times the maximum recommended human dose). In a 2-year carcinogenicity study of rats given Hydralazine by gavage at dose levels of 15, 30, and 60 mg/kg/day (approximately 5 to 20 times the recommended human daily dosage), microscopic examination of the liver revealed a small, but statistically significant, increase in benign neoplastic nodules in male and female rats from the high-dose group and in female rats from the intermediate-dose group. Benign interstitial cell tumors of the testes were also significantly increased in male rats from the high-dose group. The tumors observed are common in aged rats and a significantly increased incidence was not observed until 18 months of treatment. Hydralazine was shown to be mutagenic in bacterial systems (Gene Mutation and DNA Repair) and in one of two rat and one rabbit hepatocyte *in vitro* DNA repair studies. Additional *in vivo* and *in vitro* studies using lymphoma cells, germinal cells, and fibroblasts from mice, bone marrow cells from Chinese hamsters and fibroblasts from human cell lines did not demonstrate any mutagenic potential for Hydralazine.

The extent to which these findings indicate a risk to man is uncertain. While long-term clinical observation has not suggested that human cancer is associated with Hydralazine use, epidemiologic studies have so far been insufficient to arrive at any conclusions.

Pregnancy Category C: Animal studies indicate that Hydralazine is teratogenic in mice at 20-30 times the maximum daily human dose of 200-300 mg and possibly in rabbits at 10-15 times the maximum daily human dose, but that it is nonteratogenic in rats. Teratogenic effects observed were cleft palate and malformations of facial and cranial bones. There are no adequate and well-controlled studies in pregnant women. Although clinical experience does not include any positive evidence of adverse effects on the human fetus, Hydralazine should be used during pregnancy only if the expected benefit justifies the potential risk to the fetus.

Nursing Mothers: It is not known whether this drug is excreted in human milk. Because many drugs are excreted in human milk, caution should be exercised when Hydralazine HCl is administered to a nursing woman.

Pediatric Use: Safety and effectiveness in children have not been established in controlled clinical trials, although there is experience with the use of Hydralazine HCl in children. The usual recommended oral starting dosage is 0.75 mg/kg of body weight daily in four divided doses. Dosage may be increased gradually over the next 3-4 weeks to a maximum of 7.5 mg/kg or 200 mg daily. The usual recommended parenteral dosage, administered intramuscularly or intravenously, is 1.7-3.5 mg/kg of body weight daily, divided into four to six doses.

ADVERSE REACTIONS

Adverse reactions with Hydralazine HCl are usually reversible when dosage is reduced. However, in some cases it may be necessary to discontinue the drug.

The following adverse reactions have been observed, but there has not been enough systematic collection of data to support an estimate of their frequency.

Common: Headache, anorexia, nausea, vomiting, diarrhea, palpitations, tachycardia, angina pectoris.

Less Frequent: Digestive: constipation, paralytic ileus.

Cardiovascular: hypotension, paradoxical pressor response, edema.

Respiratory: dyspnea.

Neurologic: peripheral neuritis, evidenced by paresthesia, numbness, and tingling; dizziness; tremors; muscle cramps; psychotic reactions characterized by depression, disorientation, or anxiety.

Genitourinary: difficulty in urination.

Hematologic: blood dyscrasias, consisting of reduction in hemoglobin and red cell count, leukopenia, agranulocytosis, purpura; lymphadenopathy; splenomegaly.

Hypersensitive Reactions: rash, urticaria, pruritus, fever, chills, arthralgia, eosinophilia, and, rarely, hepatitis.

Other: nasal congestion, flushing, lacrimation, conjunctivitis.

OVERDOSAGE

Acute Toxicity: No deaths due to acute poisoning have been reported.

Highest known dose survived: adults, 10 g orally.

Oral LD_{50} in rats: 173 and 187 mg/kg.

Signs and Symptoms: Signs and symptoms of overdosage include hypotension, tachycardia, headache, and generalized skin flushing.

Complications can include myocardial ischemia and subsequent myocardial infarction, cardiac arrhythmia, and profound shock.

Treatment: There is no specific antidote.

After oral ingestion, the gastric contents should be evacuated, taking adequate precautions against aspiration and for protection of the airway. An activated charcoal slurry may be instilled if conditions permit. These manipulations may have to be omitted or carried out after cardiovascular status has been stabilized, since they might precipitate cardiac arrhythmias or increase the depth of shock.

Support of the cardiovascular system is of primary importance. Shock should be treated with plasma expanders. If possible, vasopressors should not be given, but if a vasopressor is required, care should be taken not to precipitate or aggravate cardiac arrhythmia. Tachycardia responds to beta blockers. Digitalization may be necessary, and renal function should be monitored and supported as required.

No experience has been reported with extracorporeal or peritoneal dialysis.

DOSAGE AND ADMINISTRATION

Tablets: Initiate therapy in gradually increasing dosages; adjust according to individual response. Start with 10 mg four times daily for the first 2-4 days, increase to 25 mg four times daily for the balance of the first week. For the second and subsequent weeks, increase dosage to 50 mg four times daily. For maintenance, adjust dosage to the lowest effective levels.

The incidence of toxic reactions, particularly the L.E. cell syndrome, is high in the group of patients receiving large doses of Hydralazine HCl.

In a few resistant patients, up to 300 mg of Hydralazine HCl daily may be required for a significant antihypertensive effect. In such cases, a lower dosage of Hydralazine HCl combined with a thiazide and/or reserpine or a beta blocker may be considered. However, when combining therapy, individual titration is essential to ensure the lowest possible therapeutic dose of each drug.

When there is urgent need, therapy in the hospitalized patient may be initiated intramuscularly or as a rapid intravenous bolus injection directly into the vein. Parenteral Hydralazine HCl should be used only when the drug cannot be given orally. The usual dose is 20-40 mg, repeated as necessary. Certain patients (especially those with marked renal damage) may require a lower dose. Blood pressure should be checked frequently. It may begin to fall within a few minutes after injection, with the average maximal decrease occurring in 10-80 minutes. In cases where there has been increased intracranial pressure, lowering the blood pressure may increase cerebral ischemia. Most patients can be transferred to oral Hydralazine HCl within 24-48 hours.

The product should be used immediately after the container is opened. It should not be added to infusion solutions. Hydralazine HCl parenteral may discolor upon contact with metal; discolored solutions should be discarded.

Parenteral drug products should be inspected visually for particulate matter and discoloration prior to administration, whenever solution and container permit.

Do not store tablets above 86°F (30°C).

Dispense in tight, light-resistant container (USP).

Store solution for injection between 59° and 86°F (15°-30°C).

J CODES
Up to 20 mg IV,IM—J0360

HOW SUPPLIED
INJECTION: 20 MG/ML

BRAND/MANUFACTURER	NDC	SIZE	AWP
◆ GENERICS			
Solo Pak	39769-0021-01	1 ml 25s	$140.63

TABLETS: 10 MG

AVERAGE UNIT PRICE (AVAILABLE SIZES)		GENERIC A-RATED AVERAGE PRICE (GAAP)	
BRAND	$0.20	100s	$4.43
GENERIC	$0.04	1000s	$18.06
HCFA FUL (100s ea)	$0.02		

BRAND/MANUFACTURER	NDC	SIZE	AWP
◆ BRAND			
APRESOLINE: Ciba Pharm	00083-0037-30	100s	$19.81
◆ GENERICS			
Schein	00364-0647-01	100s	$2.00
Rugby	00536-3890-01	100s	$2.16
Goldline	00182-0905-01	100s	$2.25
Moore,H.L.	00839-6114-06	100s	$2.63
URL	00677-0650-01	100s	$2.65
Mutual	53489-0123-01	100s	$2.65
UDL	51079-0074-40	100s	$2.70
Major	00904-2338-60	100s	$3.00
Camall	00147-0255-10	100s	$3.08
Qualitest	00603-3830-21	100s	$3.40
Par	49884-0029-01	100s	$3.50
Aligen	00405-4469-01	100s	$3.50
Sidmak	50111-0398-01	100s	$3.50
Martec	52555-0029-01	100s	$3.57
Major	00904-2338-61	100s ud	$4.58
Raway	00686-0074-20	100s ud	$4.95
Goldline	00182-0905-89	100s ud	$6.20
Vangard	00615-0516-13	100s ud	$6.86
Auro	55829-0300-10	100s ud	$7.31
Medirex	57480-0331-01	100s ud	$11.30
UDL	51079-0074-20	100s ud	$11.32
Camall	00147-0255-20	1000s	$9.90
Rugby	00536-3890-10	1000s	$12.09
Major	00904-2338-80	1000s	$12.50
Sidmak	50111-0398-03	1000s	$15.05
Moore,H.L.	00839-6114-16	1000s	$15.11
Martec	52555-0029-10	1000s	$16.27
Mutual	53489-0123-10	1000s	$16.50
URL	00677-0650-10	1000s	$16.79
Qualitest	00603-3830-32	1000s	$16.84
Schein	00364-0647-02	1000s	$17.80
Par	49884-0029-10	1000s	$33.95
Aligen	00405-4469-03	1000s	$33.95

TABLETS: 25 MG

AVERAGE UNIT PRICE (AVAILABLE SIZES)		GENERIC A-RATED AVERAGE PRICE (GAAP)	
BRAND	$0.28	100s	$5.54
GENERIC	$0.04	1000s	$25.97
HCFA FUL (100s ea)	$0.02		

BRAND/MANUFACTURER	NDC	SIZE	AWP
◆ BRAND			
APRESOLINE: Ciba Pharm	00083-0039-30	100s	$28.31
◆ GENERICS			
Richlyn	00115-3660-01	100s	$2.69
Rugby	00536-3862-01	100s	$2.79
Moore,H.L.	00839-1361-06	100s	$2.90
URL	00677-0447-01	100s	$3.50
Schein	00364-0144-01	100s	$3.50
Goldline	00182-0554-01	100s	$3.50
Qualitest	00603-3831-21	100s	$3.51
Mutual	53489-0124-01	100s	$3.65
Major	00904-2339-60	100s	$3.95
Sidmak	50111-0327-01	100s	$4.20
Par	49884-0027-01	100s	$4.25
Aligen	00405-4470-01	100s	$4.32
Martec	52555-0027-01	100s	$4.34
U.S. Trading	56126-0027-11	100s ud	$3.78
Raway	00686-0075-20	100s ud	$5.00

BRAND/MANUFACTURER	NDC	SIZE	AWP
Major	00904-2339-61	100s ud	$6.21
Goldline	00182-0554-89	100s ud	$8.10
Auro	55829-0301-10	100s ud	$8.76
Vangard	00615-0531-13	100s ud	$8.96
UDL	51079-0075-20	100s ud	$14.25
Medirex	57480-0332-01	100s ud	$14.25
Camall	00147-0256-20	1000s	$16.04
Sidmak	50111-0327-03	1000s	$17.25
Goldline	00182-0554-10	1000s	$17.25
Richlyn	00115-3660-03	1000s	$20.70
Qualitest	00603-3831-32	1000s	$20.70
Rugby	00536-3862-10	1000s	$20.93
Major	00904-2339-80	1000s	$20.95
Moore,H.L.	00839-1361-16	1000s	$23.36
URL	00677-0447-10	1000s	$24.65
Mutual	53489-0124-10	1000s	$24.65
Schein	00364-0144-02	1000s	$24.75
Lederle Std Prod	00005-3564-34	1000s	$33.84
Par	49884-0027-10	1000s	$41.23
Aligen	00405-4470-03	1000s	$41.23
Martec	52555-0027-10	1000s	$42.05

TABLETS: 50 MG

AVERAGE UNIT PRICE (AVAILABLE SIZES)		GENERIC A-RATED AVERAGE PRICE (GAAP)	
BRAND	$0.42	100s	$6.42
GENERIC	$0.05	1000s	$31.66
HCFA FUL (100s ea)	$0.03		

BRAND/MANUFACTURER	NDC	SIZE	AWP
◆ BRAND			
APRESOLINE: Ciba Pharm	00083-0073-30	100s	$42.21
◆ GENERICS			
Rugby	00536-3863-01	100s	$2.93
Schein	00364-0145-01	100s	$3.70
URL	00677-0451-01	100s	$3.75
Qualitest	00603-3832-21	100s	$3.78
Goldline	00182-0555-01	100s	$3.80
Sidmak	50111-0328-01	100s	$4.00
Richlyn	00115-3662-01	100s	$4.50
Mutual	53489-0125-01	100s	$4.60
Moore,H.L.	00839-1363-06	100s	$4.66
Par	49884-0028-01	100s	$4.75
Aligen	00405-4471-01	100s	$4.75
Martec	52555-0028-01	100s	$4.85
Major	00904-2340-60	100s	$5.00
U.S. Trading	56126-0028-11	100s ud	$3.50
Raway	00686-0076-20	100s ud	$5.75
Major	00904-2340-61	100s ud	$7.45
Goldline	00182-0555-89	100s ud	$8.60
Auro	55829-0302-10	100s ud	$9.73
Vangard	00615-0532-13	100s ud	$9.79
UDL	51079-0076-20	100s ud	$17.46
Medirex	57480-0333-01	100s ud	$17.50
Rugby	00536-3863-10	1000s	$20.93
Goldline	00182-0555-10	1000s	$22.50
Schein	00364-0145-02	1000s	$24.75
Sidmak	50111-0328-03	1000s	$24.75
Qualitest	00603-3832-32	1000s	$25.46
Major	00904-2340-80	1000s	$26.25
Camall	00147-0257-20	1000s	$27.32
URL	00677-0451-10	1000s	$27.75
Mutual	53489-0125-10	1000s	$27.75
Moore,H.L.	00839-1363-16	1000s	$33.28
Richlyn	00115-3662-03	1000s	$34.65
Lederle Std Prod	00005-3565-34	1000s	$40.29
Par	49884-0028-10	1000s	$46.08
Aligen	00405-4471-03	1000s	$46.08
Martec	52555-0028-10	1000s	$47.00

TABLETS: 100 MG

AVERAGE UNIT PRICE (AVAILABLE SIZES)		GENERIC A-RATED AVERAGE PRICE (GAAP)	
BRAND	$0.59	100s	$8.30
GENERIC	$0.08	1000s	$49.62
HCFA FUL (100s ea)	$0.04		

BRAND/MANUFACTURER	NDC	SIZE	AWP
◆ BRAND			
APRESOLINE: Ciba Pharm	00083-0101-30	100s	$59.38
◆ GENERICS			
Schein	00364-0696-01	100s	$4.80
Rugby	00536-3891-01	100s	$4.94
Camall	00147-0258-01	100s	$5.16
Qualitest	00603-3833-21	100s	$5.51
URL	00677-0922-01	100s	$5.95
Goldline	00182-1553-01	100s	$6.00
Major	00904-2341-60	100s	$6.90
UDL	51079-0183-40	100s	$7.20
Par	49884-0121-01	100s	$7.70
Sidmak	50111-0397-01	100s	$7.75
Martec	52555-0026-01	100s	$7.85
Moore,H.L.	00839-6761-06	100s	$8.09

◆ RATED THERAPEUTICALLY EQUIVALENT; ◇ THERAPEUTIC EQUIVALENCE UNCONFIRMED; ○ UNRATED

BRAND/MANUFACTURER	NDC	SIZE	AWP
Raway	00686-0183-20	100s ud	$8.75
UDL	51079-0183-20	100s ud	$18.76
Auro	55829-0303-10	100s ud	$19.12
Sidmak	50111-0397-03	1000s	$34.38
Rugby	00536-3891-10	1000s	$41.19
Camall	00147-0258-20	1000s	$48.22
Par	49884-0121-10	1000s	$74.69

Hydralazine Hydrochloride with Hydrochlorothiazide

WARNING

THIS FIXED-COMBINATION DRUG IS NOT INDICATED FOR INITIAL THERAPY OF HYPERTENSION. HYPERTENSION REQUIRES THERAPY TITRATED TO THE INDIVIDUAL PATIENT. IF THE FIXED COMBINATION REPRESENTS THE DOSAGE SO DETERMINED, ITS USE MAY BE MORE CONVENIENT IN PATIENT MANAGEMENT. THE TREATMENT OF HYPERTENSION IS NOT STATIC BUT MUST BE REEVALUATED AS CONDITIONS IN EACH PATIENT WARRANT.

DESCRIPTION

Hydralazine Hydrochloride/Hydrochlorothiazide (Hydralazine/HCTZ) is an antihypertensive-diuretic combination available as capsules for oral administration. Hydralazine/HCTZ capsules of 25/25 contain 25 mg of Hydralazine Hydrochloride USP and 25 mg of Hydrochlorothiazide USP; capsules of 50/50 contain 50 mg of Hydralazine Hydrochloride USP and 50 mg of Hydrochlorothiazide USP; and capsules of 100/50 contain 100 mg of Hydralazine Hydrochloride USP and 50 mg of Hydrochlorothiazide USP.

Hydralazine Hydrochloride is 1-hydrazinophthalazine monohydrochloride.

Hydralazine Hydrochloride USP is a white to off-white, odorless crystalline powder. It is soluble in water, slightly soluble in alcohol, and very slightly soluble in ether. It melts at about 275°C, with decomposition, and has a molecular weight of 196.64.

Hydrochlorothiazide is 6-chloro-3,4-dihydro-$2H$-1,2,4-benzo-thiadiazine-7-sulfonamide 1,1-dioxide.

Hydrochlorothiazide USP is a white, or practically white, practically odorless crystalline powder. It is freely soluble in sodium hydroxide solution, in *n*-butylamine, and in dimethylformamide; sparingly soluble in methanol; slightly soluble in water; and insoluble in ether, in chloroform, and in dilute mineral acids. Its molecular weight is 297.73.

CLINICAL PHARMACOLOGY

HYDRALAZINE

Although the precise mechanism of action of Hydralazine is not fully understood, the major effects are on the cardiovascular system. Hydralazine apparently lowers blood pressure by exerting a peripheral vasodilating effect through a direct relaxation of vascular smooth muscle. Hydralazine, by altering cellular calcium metabolism, interferes with the calcium movements within the vascular smooth muscle that are responsible for initiating or maintaining the contractile state. The peripheral vasodilating effect of Hydralazine results in decreased arterial blood pressure (diastolic more than systolic); decreased peripheral vascular resistance; and an increased heart rate, stroke volume, and cardiac output. The preferential dilatation of arterioles, as compared to veins, minimizes postural hypotension and promotes the increase in cardiac output. Hydralazine usually increases renin activity in plasma, presumably as a result of increased secretion of renin by the renal juxtaglomerular cells in response to reflex sympathetic discharge. This increase in renin activity leads to the production of angiotension II, which then causes stimulation of aldosterone and consequent sodium reabsorption. Hydralazine also maintains or increases renal and cerebral blood flow.

HYDROCHLOROTHIAZIDE

Thiazides affect the renal tubular mechanism of electrolyte reabsorption. At maximal therapeutic dosage, all thiazides are approximately equal in their diuretic potency. Thiazides increase excretion of sodium and chloride in approximately equivalent amounts. Natriuresis causes a secondary loss of potassium.

The mechanism of the antihypertensive effect of thiazides is unknown. Thiazides do not affect normal blood pressure.

PHARMACOKINETICS

Hydralazine. Hydralazine is rapidly absorbed after oral administration, and peak plasma levels are reached at 1-2 hours. Plasma levels decline with a half-life of 3-7 hours. Binding to human plasma protein is 87%. Plasma levels of Hydralazine vary widely among individuals. Hydralazine is subject to polymorphic acetylation; slow acetylators generally have higher plasma levels of Hydralazine and require lower doses to maintain control of blood pressure. Hydralazine undergoes extensive hepatic metabolism; it is excreted mainly in the form of metabolites in the urine.

Administration of Hydralazine with food results in higher levels of the drug in plasma.

Hydrochlorothiazide. Onset of action of thiazides occurs in 2 hours and the peak effect at about 4 hours. The action persists for approximately 6-12 hours. Hydrochlorothiazide is rapidly absorbed, as indicated by peak concentrations 1-2.5 hours after oral administration. Plasma levels of the drug are proportional to dose; the concentration in whole blood is 1.6-1.8 times higher than in plasma. Thiazides are eliminated rapidly by the kidney. After oral administration of 25- to 100-mg doses, 72-97% of the dose is excreted in the urine, indicating dose-independent absorption. Hydrochlorothiazide is eliminated from plasma in a biphasic fashion with a terminal half-life of 10-17 hours. Plasma protein binding is 67.9%. Plasma clearance is 15.9-30.0 L/hr; volume of distribution is 3.6-7.8 L/kg.

Gastrointestinal absorption of Hydrochlorothiazide is enhanced when administered with food. Absorption is decreased in patients with congestive heart failure, and the pharmacokinetics are considerably different in these patients.

INDICATIONS AND USAGE

Hypertension (see boxed *"Warnings"*).

CONTRAINDICATIONS

HYDRALAZINE

Hypersensitivity to Hydralazine; coronary artery disease; mitral valvular rheumatic heart disease.

HYDROCHLOROTHIAZIDE

Anuria; hypersensitivity to this or other sulfonamide-derived drugs.

WARNINGS

HYDRALAZINE

In a few patients Hydralazine may produce a clinical picture simulating systemic lupus erythematosus including glomerulonephritis. In such patients Hydralazine should be discontinued unless the benefit-to-risk determination requires continued antihypertensive therapy with this drug. Signs and symptoms usually regress when the drug is discontinued, but residua have been detected many years later. Long-term treatment with steroids may be necessary. (See *"Precautions: Laboratory Tests."*)

HYDROCHLOROTHIAZIDE

Thiazides should be used with caution in patients with severe renal disease. In patients with renal disease, thiazides may precipitate azotemia. Cumulative effects of the drug may develop in patients with impaired renal function.

Thiazides should be used with caution in patients with impaired hepatic function or progressive liver disease, since minor alterations of fluid and electrolyte imbalance may precipitate hepatic coma.

Thiazides may add to or potentiate the action of other antihypertensive drugs. Potentiation occurs with ganglionic or peripheral adrenergic blocking drugs.

Sensitivity reactions are more likely to occur in patients with a history of allergy or bronchial asthma.

The possibility of exacerbation or activation of systemic lupus erythematosus has been reported.

PRECAUTIONS

GENERAL

Hydralazine: Myocardial stimulation produced by Hydralazine can cause anginal attacks and ECG changes indicative of myocardial ischemia. The drug has been implicated in the production of myocardial infarction. It must, therefore, be used with caution in patients with suspected coronary artery disease.

The "hyperdynamic" circulation caused by Hydralazine may accentuate specific cardiovascular inadequacies. For example, Hydralazine may increase pulmonary artery pressure in patients with mitral valvular disease. The drug may reduce the pressor responses to epinephrine. Postural hypotension may result from Hydralazine but is less common than with ganglionic blocking agents. It should be used with caution in patients with cerebral vascular accidents.

In hypertensive patients with normal kidneys who are treated with Hydralazine, there is evidence of increased renal blood flow and a maintenance of glomerular filtration rate. In some instances where control values were below normal, improved renal function has been noted after administration of Hydralazine. However, as with any antihypertensive agent, Hydralazine should be used with caution in patients with advanced renal damage.

Peripheral neuritis, evidenced by paresthesia, numbness, and tingling, has been observed. Published evidence suggests that Hydralazine has an antipyridoxine effect and that pyridoxine should be added to the regimen if symptoms develop.

Hydrochlorothiazide: All patients receiving thiazide therapy should be observed for clinical signs of fluid or electrolyte imbalance, namely hyponatremia, hypochloremic alkalosis, and hypokalemia (see *"Laboratory Tests"* and *"Drug/Drug Interactions"*). Warning signs are dryness of mouth, thirst, weakness, lethargy, drowsiness, restlessness, muscle pains or cramps, muscular fatigue, hypotension, oliguria, tachycardia, and gastrointestinal disturbance, such as nausea or vomiting.

Hypokalemia may develop, especially in cases of brisk diuresis or severe cirrhosis.

Interference with adequate oral intake of electrolytes will also contribute to hypokalemia. Hypokalemia may be avoided or treated by the use of potassium supplements or foods with a high potassium content.

Any chloride deficit is generally mild and usually does not require specific treatment, except under extraordinary circumstances (as in liver disease or renal disease). Dilutional hyponatremia may occur in edematous patients in hot weather; appropriate therapy is water restriction, rather than administration of salt, except in rare instances when the hyponatremia is life-threatening. In cases of actual salt depletion, appropriate replacement is the therapy of choice. Hyperuricemia may occur or frank gout may be precipitated in certain patients receiving thiazide therapy.

Latent diabetes may become manifest during thiazide administration (see *"Drug/Drug Interactions"*).

The antihypertensive effects of the drug may be enhanced in the postsympathectomy patient.

If progressive renal impairment becomes evident, withholding or discontinuing diuretic therapy should be considered. Calcium excretion is decreased by thiazides. Pathological changes in the parathyroid gland with hypercalcemia and hypophosphatemia have been observed in a few patients on prolonged thiazide therapy. The common complications of hyperparathyroidism, such as renal lithiasis, bone resorption, and peptic ulceration, have not been seen.

Thiazide diuretics have been shown to increase the urinary excretion of magnesium; this may result in hypomagnesemia.

INFORMATION FOR PATIENTS
Patients should be informed of possible side effects and advised to take the medication regularly and continuously as directed.

LABORATORY TESTS
Hydralazine: Complete blood counts and antinuclear antibody titer determinations are indicated before and periodically during prolonged therapy with Hydralazine even though the patient is asymptomatic. These studies are also indicated if the patient develops arthralgia, fever, chest pain, continued malaise, or other unexplained signs or symptoms. A positive antinuclear antibody titer requires that the physician carefully weigh the implications of the test results against the benefits to be derived from antihypertensive therapy with a combination drug containing Hydralazine. Blood dyscrasias, consisting of reduction in hemoglobin and red cell count, leukopenia, agranulocytosis, and purpura, have been reported. If such abnormalities develop, therapy should be discontinued.

Hydrochlorothiazide: Initial and periodic determinations of serum electrolytes to detect possible electrolyte imbalance should be performed at appropriate intervals.

Serum and urine electrolyte determinations are particularly important when the patient is vomiting excessively or receiving parenteral fluids.

DRUG/DRUG INTERACTIONS
Hydralazine: MAO inhibitors should be used with caution in patients receiving Hydralazine.

When other potent parenteral antihypertensive drugs, such as diazoxide, are used in combination with Hydralazine, patients should be continuously observed for several hours for any excessive fall in blood pressure. Profound hypotensive episodes may occur when diazoxide injections and Hydralazine are used concomitantly.

Hydrochlorothiazide: Hypokalemia can sensitize or exaggerate the response of the heart to the toxic effects of digitalis (e.g., increased ventricular irritability).

Hypokalemia may develop during concomitant use of steroids or ACTH.

Insulin requirements in diabetic patients may be increased, decreased, or unchanged.

Thiazides may decrease arterial responsiveness to norepinephrine, but not enough to preclude effectiveness of the pressor agent for therapeutic use.

Thiazides may increase the responsiveness to tubocurarine. Lithium renal clearance is reduced by thiazides, increasing the risk of lithium toxicity.

There have been rare reports in the literature of hemolytic anemia occurring with the concomitant use of Hydrochlorothiazide and methyldopa.

Concurrent administration of some nonsteroidal anti-inflammatory agents may reduce the diuretic, natriuretic and antihypertensive effects of thiazide diuretics.

DRUG/LABORATORY TEST INTERACTIONS
Thiazides may decrease serum levels of protein-bound iodine without signs of thyroid disturbance. Hydralazine/HCTZ should be discontinued before tests for parathyroid function are made (See *"Precautions: General, Hydrochlorothiazide, Calcium Excretion"*).

CARCINOGENESIS, MUTAGENESIS, IMPAIRMENT OF FERTILITY
Carcinogenicity, mutagenicity, and fertility studies in animals have not been conducted with Hydralazine/HCTZ.

Hydralazine: In a lifetime study in Swiss albino mice, there was a statistically significant increase in the incidence of lung tumors (adenomas and adenocarcinomas) of both male and female mice given Hydralazine continuously in their drinking water at a dosage of about 250 mg/kg per day (about 80 times the maximum recommended human dose). In a 2-year carcinogenicity study of rats given Hydralazine by gavage at dosages of 15, 30, and 60 mg/kg per day (approximately 5 to 20 times the recommended human daily dose), microscopic examination of the liver revealed a small, but statistically significant, increase in benign neoplastic nodules in male and female rats from the high-dose group and in female rats from the intermediate-dose group. Benign interstitial cell tumors of the testes were also significantly increased in male rats from the high-dose group. The tumors observed are common in aged rats, and a significantly increased incidence was not observed until 18 months of treatment. Hydralazine was shown

to be mutagenic in bacterial systems (Gene Mutation and DNA Repair) and in one of two rat and one rabbit hepatocyte in vitro DNA repair studies. Additional in vivo and in vitro studies using lymphoma cells, germinal cells, and fibroblasts from mice, bone marrow cells from Chinese hamsters, and fibroblasts from human cell lines did not demonstrate any mutagenic potential for Hydralazine.

The extent to which these findings indicate a risk to man is uncertain. While long-term clinical observation has not suggested that human cancer is associated with Hydralazine use, epidemiologic studies have so far been insufficient to arrive at any conclusions.

Fertility studies in animals have not been conducted with Hydralazine.

Hydrochlorothiazide. Two-year feeding studies in mice and rats conducted under the auspices of the National Toxicology Program (NTP) uncovered no evidence of a carcinogenic potential of Hydrochlorothiazide in female mice (at doses of up to approximately 600 mg/kg/day) or in male and female rats (at doses of up to approximately 100 mg/kg/day). The NTP, however, found equivocal evidence for hepatocarcinogenicity in male mice.

Hydrochlorothiazide was not genotoxic in in vitro assays using strains TA 98, TA 100, TA 1535, TA 1537, and TA 1538 of *Salmonella typhimurium* (Ames assay) and in the Chinese Hamster Ovary (CHO) test for chromosomal aberrations, or in in vivo assays using mouse germinal cell chromosomes, Chinese hamster bone marrow chromosomes, and the *Drosophila* sex-linked recessive lethal trait gene. Positive test results were obtained only in the in vitro CHO Sister Chromatid Exchange (clastogenicity) and in the Mouse Lymphoma Cell (mutagenicity) assays, using concentrations of Hydrochlorothiazide from 43 to 1300 µg/mL, and in the *Aspergillus nidulans* nondisjunction assay at an unspecified concentration.

Hydrochlorothiazide had no adverse effects on the fertility of mice and rats of either sex in studies wherein these species were exposed, via their diet, to doses of up to 100 and 4 mg/kg/day, respectively, prior to mating, and throughout gestation.

PREGNANCY: TERATOGENIC EFFECTS. PREGNANCY CATEGORY C
Animal reproduction studies have not been conducted with Hydrazaline/HCTZ.

Hydralazine. Animal studies indicate that Hydralazine is teratogenic in mice at 20-30 times the maximum daily human dose of 200-300 mg and possibly in rabbits at 10-15 times the maximum daily human dose, but that it is non-teratogenic in rats. Teratogenic effects observed were cleft palate and malformations of facial and cranial bones.

Hydrochlorothiazide. Studies in which Hydrochlorothiazide was orally administered to pregnant mice and rats during their respective periods of major organogenesis at doses up to 3000 and 1000 mg/kg/day, respectively, provided no evidence of harm to the fetus. There are, however, no adequate and well-controlled studies of Hydrazaline/HCTZ in pregnant women. Because animal reproduction studies are not always predictive of human response, this combination drug should be used during pregnancy only if clearly needed.

Nonteratogenic Effects. Hydrochlorothiazide. There are no adequate and well-controlled studies of Hydrazaline/HCTZ in pregnant women. However, thiazides cross the placental barrier and appear in cord blood, and there is a risk of fetal or neonatal jaundice, thrombocytopenia, and possibly other adverse reactions that have occurred in adults.

NURSING MOTHERS
It is not known whether Hydralazine is excreted in human milk. Thiazides are excreted in human milk. Because of the potential for serious adverse reactions in nursing infants, a decision should be made whether to discontinue nursing or to discontinue the drug, taking into account the importance of the drug to the mother.

PEDIATRIC USE
Safety and effectiveness of the combination drug in children have not been established.

ADVERSE REACTIONS
Adverse reactions are usually reversible upon reduction of dosage or discontinuation of Hydralazine/HCTZ. Whenever adverse reactions are moderate or severe, it may be necessary to discontinue the drug.

HYDRALAZINE
The following adverse reactions have been observed, but there has not been enough systematic collection of data to support an estimate of their frequency.

COMMON
Headache, anorexia, nausea, vomiting, diarrhea, palpitations, tachycardia, angina pectoris.

LESS FREQUENT
Digestive: Constipation, paralytic ileus.

Cardiovascular: Hypotension, paradoxical pressor response, edema.

Respiratory: Dyspenea.

Neurologic: Peripheral neuritis, evidenced by paresthesia, numbness and tingling; dizziness; tremors; muscle cramps; psychotic reactions characterized by depression, disorientation, or anxiety.

Genitourinary: Difficulty in urination.

Hematologic: Blood dyscrasias, consisting of reduction in hemoglobin and red cell count, leukopenia, agranulocytosis, purpura; lymphadenopathy; splenomegaly.

◆ RATED THERAPEUTICALLY EQUIVALENT; ◇ THERAPEUTIC EQUIVALENCE UNCONFIRMED; ○ UNRATED

Hypersensitive Reactions: Rash, urticaria, pruritus, fever, chills, arthralgia, eosinophilia, and, rarely, hepatitis.

Other: Nasal congestion, flushing, lacrimation, conjunctivitis.

HYDROCHLOROTHIAZIDE

The following adverse reactions have been observed, but there has not been enough systematic collection of data to support an estimate of their frequency. Consequently the reactions are categorized by organ systems and are listed in decreasing order of severity and not frequency.

Digestive: Pancreatitis, jaundice (intrahepatic cholestatic), sialadenitis, vomiting, diarrhea, cramping, nausea, gastric irritation, constipation, anorexia.

Cardiovascular: Orthostatic hypotension (may be potentiated by alcohol, barbiturates, or narcotics).

Neurologic: Vertigo, dizziness, transient blurred vision, headache, paresthesia, xanthopsia, weakness, restlessness.

Musculoskeletal: Muscle spasm.

Hematologic: Aplastic anemia, agranulocytosis, leukopenia, thrombocytopenia.

Metabolic: Hyperglycemia, glycosuria, hyperuricemia.

Hypersensitive Reactions: Necrotizing angiitis, Stevens-Johnson syndrome, respiratory distress including pneumonitis and pulmonary edema, purpura, urticaria, rash, photosensitivity.

OVERDOSAGE

ACUTE TOXICITY
Oral LD_{50}'s in rats (mg/kg): Hydralazine, 173 and 187; Hydrochlorothiazide, 2750.

SIGNS AND SYMPTOMS
Hydralazine: Signs and symptoms of overdosage include hypotension, tachycardia, headache, and generalized skin flushing.

Complications can include myocardial ischemia and subsequent myocardial infarction, cardiac arrhythmia, and profound shock.

Hydrochlorothiazide: The most prominent feature of poisoning is acute loss of fluid and electrolytes.

Cardiovascular: Tachycardia, hypotension, shock.

Neuromuscular: Weakness, confusion, dizziness, cramps of the calf muscles, paresthesia, fatigue, impairment of consciousness.

Digestive: Nausea, vomiting, thirst.

Renal: Polyuria, oliguria, or anuria (due to hemoconcentration).

Laboratory Findings: Hypokalemia, hyponatremia, hypochloremia, alkalosis; increased BUN (especially in patients with renal insufficiency).

Combined Poisoning: Signs and symptoms may be aggravated or modified by concomitant intake of antihypertensive medication, barbiturates, curare, digitalis (hypokalemia), corticosteroids, narcotics, or alcohol.

TREATMENT
There is no specific antidote.

The gastric contents should be evacuated, taking adequate precautions against aspiration and for protection of the airway. An activated charcoal slurry may be instilled if conditions permit. Dialysis may not be effective for elimination of Hydralazine/HCTZ because of its plasma protein binding (see *"Clinical Pharmacology"*).

These manipulations may have to be omitted or carried out after cardiovascular status has been stabilized, since they might precipitate cardiac arrhythmias or increase the depth of shock.

Support of the cardiovascular system is of primary importance in suspected Hydralazine overdosage. Shock should be treated with plasma expanders. The patient's legs should be kept raised and lost fluid and electrolytes (potassium, sodium) should be replaced. If possible, vasopressors should not be given, but if a vasopressor is required, care should be taken not to precipitate or aggravate cardiac arrhythmia. Tachycardia responds to beta blockers. Digitalization may be necessary, and renal function should be monitored and supported as required.

DOSAGE AND ADMINISTRATION
Dosage should be determined by individual titration (see boxed *"Warning"*).

The usual dosage is one Hydralazine/HCTZ capsule twice daily, the strength depending upon individual requirement following titration. For maintenance, the dosage should be adjusted to the lowest effective level.

When necessary, other antihypertensive agents such as sympathetic inhibitors may be added gradually in reduced dosages, and the effects should be watched carefully.

Do not store above 86°F (30°C).

Dispense in tight, light-resistant container (USP).

HOW SUPPLIED
CAPSULE: 25 MG-25 MG

AVERAGE UNIT PRICE (AVAILABLE SIZES)		GENERIC A-RATED AVERAGE PRICE (GAAP)	
BRAND	$0.38	100s	$13.53
GENERIC	$0.13	500s	$62.32
HCFA FUL (100s ea)	$0.07		

BRAND/MANUFACTURER	NDC	SIZE	AWP
◆ BRAND			
APRESAZIDE: Ciba Pharm	00083-0139-30	100s	$37.64
◆ GENERICS			
Qualitest	00603-3834-21	100s	$13.30
Rugby	00536-3885-01	100s	$13.43
URL	00677-0773-01	100s	$13.45
Par	49884-0143-01	100s	$13.45
Major	00904-2852-60	100s	$13.45
Goldline	00182-1509-01	100s	$13.45
Goldline	00182-1483-01	100s	$13.45
Martec	52555-0143-01	100s	$13.72
Moore,H.L.	00839-6582-06	100s	$14.11
Rugby	00536-3885-05	500s	$59.40
Par	49884-0143-05	500s	$65.23
Moore,H.L.	00839-6582-16	1000s	$102.20

CAPSULE: 50 MG-50 MG

AVERAGE UNIT PRICE (AVAILABLE SIZES)		GENERIC A-RATED AVERAGE PRICE (GAAP)	
BRAND	$0.56	100s	$20.32
GENERIC	$0.20		
HCFA FUL (100s ea)	$0.09		

BRAND/MANUFACTURER	NDC	SIZE	AWP
◆ BRAND			
APRESAZIDE: Ciba Pharm	00083-0149-30	100s	$56.25
◆ GENERICS			
Qualitest	00603-3835-21	100s	$19.90
URL	00677-0774-01	100s	$20.10
Rugby	00536-3886-01	100s	$20.15
Major	00904-2853-60	100s	$20.20
Goldline	00182-1510-01	100s	$20.20
Goldline	00182-1484-01	100s	$20.20
Par	49884-0144-01	100s	$20.25
Martec	52555-0144-01	100s	$20.66
Moore,H.L.	00839-6583-06	100s	$21.26
Par	49884-0144-05	500s	$98.21

CAPSULE: 100 MG-50 MG

AVERAGE UNIT PRICE (AVAILABLE SIZES)		GENERIC A-RATED AVERAGE PRICE (GAAP)	
BRAND	$0.69	100s	$30.02
GENERIC	$0.30		
HCFA FUL (100s ea)	$0.19		

BRAND/MANUFACTURER	NDC	SIZE	AWP
◆ BRAND			
APRESAZIDE: Ciba Pharm	00083-0159-30	100s	$68.54
◆ GENERICS			
Qualitest	00603-3836-21	100s	$28.71
Par	49884-0145-01	100s	$31.32
Par	49884-0145-05	500s	$151.90

Hydralazine Hydrochloride/ Hydrochlorothiazide/Reserpine

> **WARNING**
> THIS FIXED-COMBINATION DRUG IS NOT INDICATED FOR INITIAL THERAPY OF HYPERTENSION. HYPERTENSION REQUIRES THERAPY TITRATED TO THE INDIVIDUAL PATIENT. IF THE FIXED COMBINATION REPRESENTS THE DOSAGE SO DETERMINED, ITS USE MAY BE MORE CONVENIENT IN PATIENT MANAGEMENT. THE TREATMENT OF HYPERTENSION IS NOT STATIC BUT MUST BE REEVALUATED AS CONDITIONS IN EACH PATIENT WARRANT.

DESCRIPTION

Hydralazine Hydrochloride/Hydrochlorothiazide/Reserpine is an antihypertensive-diuretic combination, available as tablets for oral administration. Each tablet contains Reserpine USP, 0.1 mg; Hydralazine Hydrochloride USP, 25 mg; and Hydrochlorothiazide USP, 15 mg.

Reserpine is methyl 18β-hydroxy-11, 17α-dimethoxy-3β, 20α-yohimban-16β-carboxylate 3,4,5-trimethoxybenzoate (ester).

Reserpine USP, a pure crystalline alkaloid of rauwolfia, is a white or pale buff to slightly yellowish, odorless crystalline powder. It darkens slowly on exposure to light, but more rapidly when in solution. It is insoluble in water, freely soluble in acetic acid and in chloroform, slightly soluble in benzene, and very slightly soluble in alcohol and in ether. Its molecular weight is 608.69.

Hydralazine Hydrochloride is 1-hydrazinophthalazine mono-hydrochloride.

Hydralazine Hydrochloride USP is a white to off-white, odorless crystalline powder. It is soluble in water, slightly soluble in alcohol, and very slightly soluble in ether. It melts at about 275°C, with decomposition, and has a molecular weight of 196.64.

Hydrochlorothiazide is 6-chloro-3,4-dihydro-2 *H*-1,2,4-benzothiadiazine- 7-sulfonamide-1, 1-dioxide.

Hydrochlorothiazide USP is a white, or practically white, practically odorless crystalline powder. It is slightly soluble in water; freely soluble in sodium hydroxide solution, in *n*-butylamine, and in dimethylformamide; sparingly soluble in methanol; and insoluble in ether, in chloroform, and in dilute mineral acids. Its molecular weight is 297.73.

CLINICAL PHARMACOLOGY

Reserpine: Reserpine depletes stores of catecholamines and 5-hydroxytryptamine in many organs, including the brain and adrenal medulla. Most of its pharmacological effects have been attributed to this action. Depletion is slower and less complete in the adrenal medulla than in other tissues. The depression of sympathetic nerve function results in a decreased heart rate and a lowering of arterial blood pressure. The sedative and tranquilizing properties of Reserpine are thought to be related to depletion of catecholamines and 5-hydroxytryptamine from the brain.

Reserpine, like other rauwolfia compounds, is characterized by slow onset of action and sustained effects. Both cardiovascular and central nervous system effects may persist for a period of time following withdrawal of the drug.

Mean maximum plasma levels of 1.54 ng/ml were attained after a median of 3.5 hours in six normal subjects receiving a single oral dose of four 0.25-mg Serpasil tablets. Bioavailability was approximately 50% of that of a corresponding intravenous dose. Plasma levels of Reserpine after intravenous administration declined with a mean half-life of 33 hours. Reserpine is extensively bound (96%) to plasma proteins. No definitive studies on the human metabolism of Reserpine have been made.

Hydralazine: Although the precise mechanism of action of Hydralazine is not fully understood, the major effects are on the cardiovascular system. Hydralazine apparently lowers blood pressure by exerting a peripheral vasodilating effect through a direct relaxation of vascular smooth muscle. Hydralazine, by altering cellular calcium metabolism, interferes with the calcium movements within the vascular smooth muscle that are responsible for initiating or maintaining the contractile state.

The peripheral vasodilating effect of Hydralazine results in decreased arterial blood pressure (diastolic more than systolic); decreased peripheral vascular resistance; and in increased heart rate, stroke volume, and cardiac output. The preferential dilatation of arterioles, as compared to veins, minimizes postural hypotension and promotes the increase in cardiac output. Hydralazine usually increases renin activity in plasma, presumably as a result of increased secretion of renin by the renal juxtaglomerular cells in response to reflex sympathetic discharge. This increase in renin activity leads to the production of angiotensin II, which then causes stimulation of aldosterone and consequent sodium reabsorption. Hydralazine also maintains or increases renal and cerebral blood flow.

Hydralazine is rapidly absorbed after oral administration, and peak plasma levels are reached at 1-2 hours. Plasma levels decline with a half-life of 3-7 hours. Binding to human plasma protein is 87%. Plasma levels of Hydralazine vary widely among individuals. Hydralazine is subject to polymorphic acetylation; slow acetylators generally have higher plasma levels of Hydralazine and require lower doses to maintain control of blood pressure. Hydralazine undergoes extensive hepatic metabolism; it is excreted mainly in the form of metabolites in the urine.

Administration of Hydralazine with food results in higher levels of the drug in plasma.

Hydrochlorothiazide: Thiazides affect the renal tubular mechanism of electrolyte reabsorption. At maximal therapeutic dosage, all thiazides are approximately equal in their diuretic potency. Thiazides increase excretion of sodium and chloride in approximately equivalent amounts. Natriuresis causes a secondary loss of potassium.

The mechanism of the antihypertensive effect of thiazides is unknown. Thiazides do not affect normal blood pressure. The onset of action of thiazides occurs in 2 hours, and the peak effect at about 4 hours. The action persists for approximately 6-12 hours. Hydrochlorothiazide is rapidly absorbed, as indicated by peak plasma concentrations 1-2.5 hours after oral administration. Plasma levels of the drug are proportional to dose; the concentration in whole blood is 1.6-1.8 times higher than in plasma. Thiazides are eliminated rapidly by the kidney. After oral administration of 25- to 100-mg doses of Hydrochlorothiazide, 72-97% of the dose is excreted in the urine, indicating dose-independent absorption. Hydrochlorothiazide is eliminated from plasma in a biphasic fashion with a terminal half-life of 10-17 hours. Plasma protein binding is 67.9%. Plasma clearance is 15.9-30.0 L/hr; volume of distribution is 3.6-7.8 L/kg.

Gastrointestinal absorption of Hydrochlorothiazide is enhanced when administered with food. Absorption is decreased in patients with congestive heart failure, and the pharmacokinetics are considerably different in these patients.

INDICATIONS AND USAGE

Hypertension (see boxed "Warning").

CONTRAINDICATIONS

Reserpine: Hypersensitivity to Reserpine; mental depression or history of mental depression (especially with suicidal tendencies); active peptic ulcer, ulcerative colitis; patients receiving electroconvulsive therapy.

Hydralazine: Hypersensitivity to Hydralazine; coronary artery disease; mitral valvular rheumatic heart disease.

Hydrochlorothiazide: Anuria; hypersensitivity to this or other sulfonamide-derived drugs.

WARNINGS

Reserpine: Reserpine may cause mental depression. Recognition of depression may be difficult because this condition may often be disguised by somatic complaints. The drug should be discontinued at first signs of depression such as despondency, early morning insomnia, loss of appetite, impotence, or self-deprecation. Drug-induced depression may persist for several months after drug withdrawal and may be severe enough to result in suicide.

Hydralazine: In a few patients Hydralazine may produce a clinical picture simulating systemic lupus erythematosus including glomerulonephritis. In such patients Hydralazine should be discontinued unless the benefit-to-risk determination requires continued antihypertensive therapy with this drug. Signs and symptoms usually regress when the drug is discontinued, but residua have been detected many years later. Long-term treatment with steroids may be necessary. (See "Precautions", Laboratory Tests.)

Hydrochlorothiazide: Thiazides should be used with caution in patients with severe renal disease. In patients with renal disease, thiazides may precipitate azotemia. Cumulative effects of the drug may develop in patients with impaired renal function.

Thiazides should be used with caution in patients with impaired hepatic function or progressive liver disease, since minor alterations of fluid and electrolyte imbalance may precipitate hepatic coma.

Thiazides may add to or potentiate the action of other antihypertensive drugs. Potentiation occurs with ganglionic or peripheral adrenergic blocking drugs.

Sensitivity reactions are more likely to occur in patients with a history of allergy or bronchial asthma.

The possibility of exacerbation or activation of systemic lupus erythematosus has been reported.

PRECAUTIONS

GENERAL

Reserpine: Since Reserpine increases gastrointestinal motility and secretion, it should be used cautiously in patients with a history of peptic ulcer, ulcerative colitis, or gallstones (biliary colic may be precipitated).

Caution should be exercised when treating hypertensive patients with renal insufficiency, since they adjust poorly to lowered blood pressure levels.

Preoperative withdrawal of Reserpine does not assure that circulatory instability will not occur. It is important that the anesthesiologist be aware of the patient's drug intake and consider this in the overall management, since hypotension has occurred in patients receiving rauwolfia preparations. Anticholinergic and adrenergic drugs (e.g., metaraminol, norepinephrine) have been employed to treat adverse vagocirculatory effects.

Hydralazine: Myocardial stimulation produced by Hydralazine can cause anginal attacks and ECG changes indicative of myocardial ischemia. The drug has been implicated in the production of myocardial infarction. It must, therefore, be used with caution in patients with suspected coronary artery disease.

The "hyperdynamic" circulation caused by Hydralazine may accentuate specific cardiovascular inadequacies. For example, Hydralazine may increase pulmonary artery pressure in patients with mitral valvular disease. The drug may reduce the pressor responses to epinephrine. Postural hypotension may result from Hydralazine but is less common than with ganglionic blocking agents. It should be used with caution in patients with cerebral vascular accidents.

In hypertensive patients with normal kidneys who are treated with Hydralazine, there is evidence of increased renal blood flow and a maintenance of glomerular filtration rate. In some instances where control values were below normal, improved renal function have been noted after administration of Hydralazine. However, as with any antihypertensive agent, Hydralazine should be used with caution in patients with advanced renal damage.

Peripheral neuritis, evidenced by paresthesia, numbness, and tingling, has been observed. Published evidence suggests that Hydralazine has an antipyridoxine effect and that pyridoxine should be added to the regimen if symptoms develop.

Hydrochlorothiazide: All patients receiving thiazide therapy should be observed for clinical signs of fluid or electrolyte imbalance, namely hyponatremia, hypochloremic alkalosis, and hypokalemia (see "Laboratory Tests" and "Drug/Drug Interactions"). Warning signs are dryness of mouth, thirst, weakness, lethargy, drowsiness, restlessness, muscle pains or cramps, muscular fatigue, hypotension, oliguria, tachycardia, and gastrointestinal disturbance, such as nausea or vomiting.

Hypokalemia may develop, especially in cases of brisk diuresis or severe cirrhosis.

Interference with adequate oral intake of electrolytes will also contribute to hypokalemia. Hypokalemia may be avoided or treated by use of potassium supplements or foods with a high potassium content.

Any chloride deficit is generally mild and usually does not require specific treatment, except under extraordinary circumstances (as in liver disease or renal disease). Dilutional hyponatremia may occur in edematous patients in hot

---

weather; appropriate therapy is water restriction, rather than administration of salt, except in rare instances when the hyponatremia is life-threatening. In cases of actual salt depletion, appropriate replacement is the therapy of choice. Hyperuricemia may occur or frank gout may be precipitated in certain patients receiving thiazide therapy.

Latent diabetes may become manifest during thiazide administration (see "Drug/Drug Interactions").

The antihypertensive effects of the drug may be enhanced in the postsympathectomy patient.

If progressive renal impairment becomes evident, withholding or discontinuing diuretic therapy should be considered.

Calcium excretion is decreased by thiazides. Pathological changes in the parathyroid gland with hypercalcemia and hypophosphatemia have been observed in a few patients on prolonged thiazide therapy. The common complications of hyperparathyroidism, such as renal lithiasis, bone resorption, and peptic ulceration, have not been seen.

Thiazide diuretics have been shown to increase the urinary excretion of magnesium; this may result in hypomagnesemia.

Information for Patients: Patients should be informed of possible side effects and advised to take the medication regularly and continuously as directed.

LABORATORY TESTS
Hydralazine: Complete blood counts and antinuclear antibody titer determinations are indicated before and periodically during prolonged therapy with Hydralazine even though the patient is asymptomatic. These studies are also indicated if the patient develops arthralgia, fever, chest pain, continued malaise, or other unexplained signs or symptoms. A positive antinuclear antibody titer requires that the physician carefully weigh the implications of the test results against the benefits to be derived from antihypertensive therapy with a combination drug containing Hydralazine.

Blood dyscrasias, consisting of reduction in hemoglobin and red cell count, leukopenia, agranulocytosis, and purpura, have been reported. If such abnormalities develop, therapy should be discontinued.

Hydrochlorothiazide: Initial and periodic determinations of serum electrolytes to detect possible electrolyte imbalance should be performed at appropriate intervals.

Serum and urine electrolyte determinations are particularly important when the patient is vomiting excessively or receiving parenteral fluids.

DRUG/DRUG INTERACTIONS
Reserpine: MAO inhibitors should be avoided or used with extreme caution.

Reserpine should be used cautiously with digitalis and quinidine, since cardiac arrhythmias have occurred with rauwolfia preparations.

Concurrent use of tricyclic antidepressants may decrease the antihypertensive effect of Reserpine (see "Contraindications").

Concurrent use of Reserpine and direct or indirect-acting sympathomimetics should be closely monitored. The action of direct-acting amines (epinephrine, isoproterenol, phenylephrine, metaraminol) may be prolonged when given to patients taking Reserpine. The action of indirect-acting amines (ephedrine, tyramine, amphetamines) is inhibited.

Hydralazine: MAO inhibitors should be used with caution in patients receiving Hydralazine.

When other potent parenteral antihypertensive drugs, such as diazoxide, are used in combination with Hydralazine, patients should be continuously observed for several hours for any excessive fall in blood pressure. Profound hypotensive episodes may occur when diazoxide injections and Hydralazine are used concomitantly.

Hydrochlorothiazide: Hypokalemia can sensitize or exaggerate the response of the heart to the toxic effects of digitalis (e.g., increased ventricular irritability).

Hypokalemia may develop during concomitant use of steroids or ACTH.

Insulin requirements in diabetic patients may be increased, decreased, or unchanged.

Thiazides may decrease arterial responsiveness to norepinephrine, but not enough to preclude effectiveness of the pressor agent for therapeutic use.

Thiazides may increase the responsiveness to tubocurarine. Lithium renal clearance is reduced by thiazides, increasing the risk of lithium toxicity.

There have been rare reports in the literature of hemolytic anemia occurring with the concomitant use of hydrochlorothiazide and methyldopa.

Concurrent administration of some nonsteroidal anti-inflammatory agents may reduce the diuretic, natriuretic and antihypertensive effects of thiazide diuretics.

Drug/Laboratory Test Interactions: Thiazides may decrease serum levels of protein-bound iodine without signs of thyroid disturbance. Hydralazine/HCTZ/Reserpine should be discontinued before tests for parathyroid function are made (see "Precautions, General, Hydrochlorothiazide, Calcium Excecretion").

Carcinogenesis, Mutagenesis, Impairment of Fertility: Carcinogenicity, mutagenicity, and fertility studies in animals have not been conducted with Hydralazine/HCTZ/Reserpine.

Reserpine. Animal Tumorigenicity: Rodent studies have shown that Reserpine is an animal tumorigen, causing an increased incidence of mammary fibroadenomas in female mice, malignant tumors of the seminal vesicles in male mice, and malignant adrenal medullary tumors in male rats. These findings arose in 2-year studies in which the drug was administered in the feed at concentrations of 5 and 10 ppm—about 100 to 300 times the usual human dose. The breast neoplasms are

thought to be related to Reserpine's prolactin-elevating effect. Several other prolactin-elevating drugs have also been associated with an increased incidence of mammary neoplasia in rodents.

The extent to which these findings indicate a risk to humans is uncertain. Tissue culture experiments show that about one third of human breast tumors are prolactin-dependent in vitro, a factor of considerable importance if the use of the drug is contemplated in a patient with previously detected breast cancer. The possibility of an increased risk of breast cancer in Reserpine users has been studied extensively; however, no firm conclusion has emerged. Although a few epidemiologic studies have suggested a slightly increased risk (less than twofold in all studies except one) in women who have used Reserpine, other studies of generally similar design have not confirmed this. Epidemiologic studies conducted using other drugs (neuroleptic agents) that, like Reserpine, increase prolactin levels and therefore would be considered rodent mammary carcinogens have not shown an association between chronic administration of the drug and human mammary tumorigenesis. While long-term clinical observation has not suggested such an association, the available evidence is considered too limited to be conclusive at this time. An association of Reserpine intake with pheochromocytoma or tumors of the seminal vesicles has not been explored.

Hydralazine: In a lifetime study in Swiss albino mice, there was a statistically significant increase in the incidence of lung tumors (adenomas and adenocarcinomas) of both male and female mice given Hydralazine continuously in their drinking water at a dosage of about 250 mg/kg/day (about 80 times the maximum recommended human dose). In a 2-year carcinogenicity study of rats given Hydralazine by gavage at dose levels of 15, 30, and 60 mg/kg/day (approximately 5 to 20 times the recommended human daily dosage), microscopic examination of the liver revealed a small, but statistically significant, increase in benign neoplastic nodules in male and female rats from the high-dose group and in female rats from the intermediate-dose group. Benign interstitial cell tumors of the testes were also significantly increased in male rats from the high-dose group. The tumors observed are common in aged rats and a significantly increased incidence was not observed until 18 months of treatment. Hydralazine was shown to be mutagenic in bacterial systems (Gene Mutation and DNA Repair) and in one of two rat and one rabbit hepatocyte in vitro DNA repair studies. Additional in vivo and in vitro studies using lymphoma cells, germinal cells, and fibroblasts from mice, bone marrow cells from Chinese hamsters and fibroblasts from human cell lines did not demonstrate any mutagenic potential for Hydralazine.

The extent to which these findings indicate a risk to man is uncertain. While long-term clinical observation has not suggested that human cancer is associated with Hydralazine use, epidemiologic studies have so far been insufficient to arrive at any conclusions.

Fertility studies in animals have not been conducted with Hydralazine.

Hydrochlorothiazide: Two-year feeding studies in mice and rats conducted under the auspices of the National Toxicology Program (NTP) uncovered no evidence of a carcinogenic potential of Hydrochlorothiazide in female mice (at doses of up to approximately 600 mg/kg/day) or in male and female rats (at doses of up to approximately 100 mg/kg/day). The NTP, however, found equivocal evidence for hepatocarcinogenicity in male mice.

Hydrochlorothiazide was not genotoxic in in vitro assays using strains TA 98, TA 100, TA 1535, TA 1537, and TA 1538 of *Salmonella typhimurium* (Ames assay) and in the Chinese Hamster Ovary (CHO) test for chromosomal aberrations, or in in vivo assays using mouse germinal cell chromosomes, Chinese hamster bone marrow chromosomes, and the *Drosophila* sex-linked recessive lethal trait gene. Positive test results were obtained only in the *in vitro* CHO Sister Chromatid Exchange (clastogenicity) and in the Mouse Lymphoma Cell (mutagenicity) assays, using concentrations of Hydrochlorothiazide from 43 to 1300 μg/mL, and in the *Aspergillus nidulans* nondisjunction assay at an unspecified concentration.

Hydrochlorothiazide had no adverse effects on the fertility of mice and rats of either sex in studies wherein these species were exposed, via their diet, to doses of up to 100 and 4 mg/kg/day, respectively, prior to mating, and throughout gestation.

Pregnancy Category C: Pregnancy: Teratogenic Effects: Animal reproduction studies have not been conducted with Hydralazine/HCTZ/Reserpine.

Reserpine. Reserpine administered parenterally has been shown to be teratogenic in rats at doses up to 2 mg/kg and to have an embryocidal effect in guinea pigs given dosages of 0.5 mg daily.

Hydralazine. Animal studies indicate that Hydralazine is teteratogenic in mice at 20-30 times the maximum daily human dose of 200-300 mg and possibly in rabbits at 10-15 times the maximum daily human dose, but that it is nonteratogenic in rats. Teratogenic effects observed were cleft palate and malformations of facial and cranial bones.

Hydrochlorothiazide. Studies in which Hydrochlorothiazide was orally administered to pregnant mice and rats during their respective periods of major organogenesis at doses up to 3000 and 1000 mg/kg/day, respectively, provided no evidence of harm to the fetus. There are, however, no adequate and well-controlled studies of Hydralazine/HCTZ/Reserpine in pregnant women. Because animal reproduction studies are not always predictive of human response, this combination drug should be used during pregnancy only if clearly needed.

Nonteratogenic Effects. Reserpine. Reserpine crosses the placental barrier and increased respiratory tract secretions, nasal congestion, cyanosis, and anorexia may occur in neonates of mothers treated with Reserpine.

Hydrochlorothiazide. Thiazides also cross the placental barrier and appear in cord blood, and there is a risk of fetal or neonatal jaundice, fibrocytopenia, and possibly other adverse reactions that have occurred in adults.

Nursing Mothers: Reserpine is excreted in maternal breast milk, and increased respiratory tract secretions, nasal congestion, cyanosis, and anorexia may occur in breast-fed infants. Thiazides are also excreted in breast milk. Because of the potential for serious adverse reactions in nursing infants and the potential for tumorigenicity shown for Reserpine in animal studies, a decision should be made whether to discontinue nursing or to discontinue Hydralazine/HCTZ/Reserpine, taking into account the importance of the drug to the mother.

Pediatric Use: Safety and effectiveness of the combination drug in children have not been established.

ADVERSE REACTIONS

Adverse reactions are usually reversible upon reduction of dosage or discontinuation of Hydralazine/HCTZ/Reserpine. Whenever adverse reactions are moderate or severe, it may be necessary to discontinue the drug.

The following adverse reactions have been observed, but there has not been enough systematic collection of data to support an estimate of their frequency. Consequently the reactions are categorized by organ system and are listed in decreasing order of severity and not frequency.

Reserpine: The following have been observed with rauwolfia preparations:

Digestive: Vomiting, diarrhea, nausea, anorexia, dryness of mouth, hypersecretion.

Cardiovascular: Arrhythmia (particularly when used concurrently with digitalis or quinidine), syncope, angina-like symptoms, bradycardia, edema.

Respiratory: Dyspnea, epistaxis, nasal congestion.

Neurologic: Rare parkinsonian syndrome and other extra-pyramidal tract symptoms; dizziness; headache; paradoxical anxiety; depression; nervousness; nightmares; dull sensorium; drowsiness.

Musculoskeletal: Muscular aches.

Genitourinary: Pseudolactation, impotence, dysuria, gynecomastia, decreased libido, breast engorgement.

Metabolic: Weight gain.

Special Senses: Deafness, optic atrophy, glaucoma, uveitis, conjunctival injection.

Hypersensitive Reactions: Purpura, rash, pruritus.

Hydralazine:

Digestive: Hepatitis, paralytic ileus, vomiting, diarrhea, nausea, constipation, anorexia.

Cardiovascular: Angina pectoris, hypotension, paradoxical pressor response, tachycardia, palpitations, edema, flushing.

Respiratory: Dyspnea, nasal congestion.

Neurologic: Psychotic reactions characterized by depression, disorientation, or anxiety; peripheral neuritis, evidenced by paresthesia, numbness, and tingling; tremors; dizziness; headache.

Musculoskeletal: Muscle cramps, arthralgia.

Genitourinary: Difficulty in urination.

Hematologic: Blood dyscrasias, consisting of reduction in hemoglobin and red cell count, leukopenia, agranulocytosis; lymphadenopathy; splenomegaly; eosinophilia.

Special Senses: Conjunctivitis, lacrimation.

Hypersensitive Reactions: Purpura, fever, urticaria, rash, pruritus, chills.

Hydrochlorothiazide:

Digestive: Pancreatitis, jaundice (intrahepatic cholestatic), sialadenitis, vomiting, diarrhea, cramping, nausea, gastric irritation, constipation, anorexia.

Cardiovascular: Orthostatic hypotension (may be potentiated by alcohol, barbiturates, or narcotics).

Neurologic: Vertigo, dizziness, transient blurred vision, headache, paresthesia, xanthopsia, weakness, restlessness.

Musculoskeletal: Muscle spasm.

Hematologic: Aplastic anemia, agranulocytosis, leukopenia, thrombocytopenia.

Metabolic: Hyperglycemia, glycosuria, hyperuricemia.

Hypersensitive Reactions: Necrotizing angitis, Stevens-Johnson syndrome, respiratory distress including pneumonitis and pulmonary edema, purpura, urticaria, rash, photosensitivity.

OVERDOSAGE

Acute Toxicity: No deaths due to acute poisoning with Hydralazine/HCTZ/Reserpine have been reported.

Oral LD$_{50}$'s in animals (mg/kg): rats, 397; mice 272.

SIGNS AND SYMPTOMS

Reserpine. The clinical picture of acute poisoning is characterized chiefly by signs and symptoms due to the reflex parasympathomimetic effect of reserpine.

Impairment of consciousness may occur and may range from drowsiness to coma, depending upon the severity of overdosage. Flushing of the skin, conjunctival injection, and pupillary constriction are to be expected. Hypotension, hypothermia, central respiratory depression, and bradycardia may develop in cases of severe overdosage. Increased salivary and gastric secretion and diarrhea may also occur.

Hydralazine. Signs and symptoms of overdosage include hypotension, tachycardia, headache, and generalized skin flushing.

Complications can include myocardial ischemia and subsequent myocardial infarction, cardiac arrhythmia, and profound shock.

Hydrochlorothiazide. The most prominent feature of poisoning is acute loss of fluid and electrolytes.

Cardiovascular: Trachycardia, hypotension, shock.

Neuromuscular: Weakness, confusion, dizziness, cramps of the calf muscles, paresthesia, fatigue, impairment of consciousness.

Digestive: Nausea, vomiting, thirst.

Renal: Polyuria, oliguria, or anuria (due to hemoconcentration).

Laboratory Findings: Hypokalemia, hyponatremia, hypochloremia, alkalosis; increased BUN (especially in patients with renal insufficiency).

Combined Poisoning: Signs and symptoms may be aggravated or modified by concomitant intake of antihypertensive medication, barbiturates, digitalis (hypokalemia), corticosteroids, narcotics, or alcohol.

Treatment: There is no specific antidote.

The gastric contents should be evacuated, taking adequate precautions against aspiration and for protection of the airway. An activated charcoal slurry may be instilled if conditions permit. Dialysis may not be effective for elimination of Hydralazine Hydrochloride/HCTZ/Reserpine because of its plasma protein binding (see *"Clinical Pharmacology"*).

These manipulations may have to be omitted or carried out after cardiovascular status has been stabilized, since they might precipitate cardiac arrhythmias or increase the depth of shock.

If hypotension or shock occurs, the patient's legs should be kept raised and lost fluid and electrolytes (potassium, sodium) should be replaced.

Support of the cardiovascular system is of primary importance in suspected hydralazine overdosage. If possible, vasopressors should not be given, but if a vasopressor is required, care should be taken not to precipitate or aggravate cardiac arrhythmia. Tachycardia responds to beta blockers. Digitalization may be necessary.

If hypotension is severe enough to require treatment with a vasopressor, one having a direct action upon vascular smooth muscle (e.g., phenylephrine, levarterenol, metaraminol) should be used to treat the symptomatic effects of Reserpine overdosage.

Fluid and electrolyte balance (especially serum potassium) and renal function should be monitored until conditions become normal. Since Reserpine is long-acting, the patient should be observed carefully for at least 72 hours.

DOSAGE AND ADMINISTRATION

Dosage should be determined by individual titration (see boxed *"Warning"*). Dosage regimens that exceed 0.25 mg of Reserpine per day are not recommended.

Do not store above 86°F (30°C).

Dispense in tight, light-resistant container (USP).

HOW SUPPLIED
TABLETS:

BRAND/MANUFACTURER	NDC	SIZE	AWP
◇ **GENERICS**			
SERPAZIDE: Major	00904-2334-60	100s	$5.25
TRI-HYDROSERPINE: Rugby	00536-4909-01	100s	$6.75
SERPAZIDE: Major	00904-2334-80	1000s	$35.95
TRI-HYDROSERPINE: Rugby	00536-4909-10	1000s	$39.30

TABLETS: 25 MG-15 MG-0.1 MG

BRAND/MANUFACTURER	NDC	SIZE	AWP
◇ **BRAND**			
SER-AP-ES: Ciba Pharm	00083-0071-30	100s	$47.59
	00083-0071-40	1000s	$471.00
◇ **GENERICS**			
Schein	00364-0361-01	100s	$3.90
Aligen	00405-4484-01	100s	$4.91
DIURETIC AP-ES: Moore,H.L.	00839-1282-06	100s	$5.33
UNI SERP: URL	00677-0415-01	100s	$6.40
Goldline	00182-1820-01	100s	$6.45
Qualitest	00603-3807-21	100s	$8.07
Camall	00147-0124-10	100s	$8.31
MARPRES: Marnel	00682-1800-01	100s	$15.20
UNIPRES: Solvay	00032-1132-01	100s	$40.88
Schein	00364-0361-02	1000s	$25.50
UNI SERP: URL	00677-0415-10	1000s	$35.90
Aligen	00405-4484-03	1000s	$38.51
DIURETIC AP-ES: Moore,H.L.	00839-1282-16	1000s	$39.02
Goldline	00182-1820-10	1000s	$42.00
Qualitest	00603-3807-32	1000s	$48.06

◆ RATED THERAPEUTICALLY EQUIVALENT; ◇ THERAPEUTIC EQUIVALENCE UNCONFIRMED; ○ UNRATED

BRAND/MANUFACTURER	NDC	SIZE	AWP
Camall	00147-0124-20	1000s	$49.50
HYDRAP-ES: Parmed	00349-2076-10	1000s	$62.00

Hydrea *SEE* HYDROXYUREA

Hydrochlorothiazide

DESCRIPTION
Hydrochlorothiazide is a diuretic and antihypertensive. It is the 3,4-dihydro derivative of chlorothiazide. Its chemical name is 6-chloro-3,4-dihydro-$2H$-1,2,4-benzothiadiazine-7-sulfonamide 1,1-dioxide. Its empirical formula is $C_7H_8ClN_3O_4S_2$.

It is a white, or practically white, crystalline powder with a molecular weight of 297.72, which is slightly soluble in water, but freely soluble in sodium hydroxide solution.

Hydrochlorothiazide is supplied as 25 mg, 50 mg and 100 mg tablets for oral use.

Following is its chemical structure:

CLINICAL PHARMACOLOGY
The mechanism of the antihypertensive effect of thiazides is unknown. Hydrochlorothiazide does not usually affect normal blood pressure.

Hydrochlorothiazide affects the distal renal tubular mechanism of electrolyte reabsorption. At maximal therapeutic dosage all thiazides are approximately equal in their diuretic efficacy. Hydrochlorothiazide increases excretion of sodium and chloride in approximately equivalent amounts. Natriuresis may be accompanied by some loss of potassium and bicarbonate.

After oral use diuresis begins within 2 hours, peaks in about 4 hours and lasts about 6 to 12 hours.

PHARMACOKINETICS AND METABOLISM
Hydrochlorothiazide is not metabolized but is eliminated rapidly by the kidney. When plasma levels have been followed for at least 24 hours, the plasma half-life has been observed to vary between 5.6 and 14.8 hours. At least 61 percent of the oral dose is eliminated unchanged within 24 hours. Hydrochlorothiazide crosses the placental but not the blood-brain barrier and is excreted in breast milk.

INDICATIONS AND USAGE
Hydrochlorothiazide is indicated as adjunctive therapy in edema associated with congestive heart failure, hepatic cirrhosis, and corticosteroid and estrogen therapy.

Hydrochlorothiazide has also been found useful in edema due to various forms of renal dysfunction such as nephrotic syndrome, acute glomerulonephritis, and chronic renal failure. Hydrochlorothiazide is indicated in the management of hypertension either as the sole therapeutic agent or to enhance the effectiveness of other antihypertensive drugs in the more severe forms of hypertension.

Use in Pregnancy. Routine use of diuretics during normal pregnancy is inappropriate and exposes mother and fetus to unnecessary hazard. Diuretics do not prevent development of toxemia of pregnancy and there is no satisfactory evidence that they are useful in the treatment of toxemia.

Edema during pregnancy may arise from pathologic causes or from the physiologic and mechanical consequences of pregnancy. Thiazides are indicated in pregnancy when edema is due to pathologic causes, just as they are in the absence of pregnancy (see *"Precautions, Pregnancy"*). Dependent edema in pregnancy, resulting from restriction of venous return by the gravid uterus, is properly treated through elevation of the lower extremities and use of support stockings. Use of diuretics to lower intravascular volume in this instance is illogical and unnecessary. During normal pregnancy there is hypervolemia which is not harmful to the fetus or the mother in the absence of cardiovascular disease. However, it may be associated with edema, rarely generalized edema. If such edema causes discomfort, increased recumbency will often provide relief. Rarely this edema may cause extreme discomfort which is not relieved by rest. In these instances, a short course of diuretic therapy may provide relief and be appropriate.

CONTRAINDICATIONS
Anuria.

Hypersensitivity to this product or to other sulfonamide-derived drugs.

WARNINGS
Use with caution in severe renal disease. In patients with renal disease, thiazides may precipitate azotemia. Cumulative effects of the drug may develop in patients with impaired renal function.

Thiazides should be used with caution in patients with impaired hepatic function or progressive liver disease, since minor alterations of fluid and electrolyte balance may precipitate hepatic coma.

Thiazides may add to or potentiate the action of other anti-hypertensive drugs. Sensitivity reactions may occur in patients with or without a history of allergy or bronchial asthma.

The possibility of exacerbation or activation of systemic lupus erythematosus has been reported.

Lithium generally should not be given with diuretics (see *"Precautions, Drug Interactions"*).

PRECAUTIONS
GENERAL
All patients receiving diuretic therapy should be observed for evidence of fluid or electrolyte imbalance; namely, hyponatremia, hypochloremic alkalosis, and hypokalemia. Serum and urine electrolyte determinations are particularly important when the patient is vomiting excessively or receiving parenteral fluids. Warning signs or symptoms of fluid and electrolyte imbalance, irrespective of cause, include dryness of mouth, thirst, weakness, lethargy, drowsiness, restlessness, confusion, seizures, muscle pains or cramps, muscular fatigue, hypotension, oliguria, tachycardia, and gastrointestinal disturbances such as nausea and vomiting.

Hypokalemia may develop, especially with brisk diuresis, when severe cirrhosis is present or after prolonged therapy. Interference with adequate oral electrolyte intake will also contribute to hypokalemia. Hypokalemia may cause cardiac arrhythmia and may also sensitize or exaggerate the response of the heart to the toxic effects of digitalis (e.g., increased ventricular irritability). Hypokalemia may be avoided or treated by use of potassium sparing diuretics or potassium supplements such as foods with a high potassium content.

Although any chloride deficit is generally mild and usually does not require specific treatment except under extraordinary circumstances (as in liver disease or renal disease), chloride replacement may be required in the treatment of metabolic alkalosis.

Dilutional hyponatremia may occur in edematous patients in hot weather; appropriate therapy is water restriction, rather than administration of salt, except in rare instances when the hyponatremia is life threatening. In actual salt depletion, appropriate replacement is the therapy of choice. Hyperuricemia may occur or acute gout may be precipitated in certain patients receiving thiazides.

In diabetic patients dosage adjustments of insulin or oral hypoglycemic agents may be required. Hyperglycemia may occur with thiazide diuretics. Thus latent diabetes mellitus may become manifest during thiazide therapy.

The antihypertensive effects of the drug may be enhanced in the post-sympathectomy patient.

If progressive renal impairment becomes evident, consider withholding or discontinuing diuretic therapy.

Thiazides have been shown to increase the urinary excretion of magnesium; this may result in hypomagnesemia.

Thiazides may decrease urinary calcium excretion. Thiazides may cause intermittent and slight elevation of serum calcium in the absence of known disorders of calcium metabolism. Marked hypercalcemia may be evidence of hidden hyperparathyroidism. Thiazides should be discontinued before carrying out tests for parathyroid function.

Increases in cholesterol and triglyceride levels may be associated with thiazide diuretic therapy.

LABORATORY TESTS
Periodic determination of serum electrolytes to detect possible electrolyte imbalance should be done at appropriate intervals.

DRUG INTERACTIONS
When given concurrently the following drugs may interact with thiazide diuretics.

Alcohol, Barbiturates, or Narcotics: potentiation of orthostatic hypotension may occur.

Antidiabetic Drugs: (oral agents and insulin): dosage adjustment of the antidiabetic drug may be required.

Other Antihypertensive Drugs: additive effect or potentiation.

Cholestyramine and Colestipol Resins: Absorption of Hydrochlorothiazide is impaired in the presence of anionic exchange resins. Single doses of either cholestyramine or colestipol resins bind the Hydrochlorothiazide and reduce its absorption from the gastrointestinal tract by up to 85 and 43 percent, respectively.

Corticosteroids, ACTH: intensified electrolyte depletion, particularly hypokalemia.

Pressor Amines (e.g., norepinephrine): possible decreased response to pressor amines but not sufficient to preclude their use.

Skeletal Muscle Relaxants, Nondepolarizing (e.g., Tubocurarine): possible increased responsiveness to the muscle relaxant.

Lithium: generally should not be given with diuretics. Diuretic agents reduce the renal clearance of lithium and add a high risk of lithium toxicity. Refer to the package insert for lithium preparations before use of such preparations with Hydrochlorothiazide.

Nonsteroidal Anti-inflammatory Drugs: In some patients, the administration of a non-steroidal anti-inflammatory agent can reduce the diuretic, natriuretic, and antihypertensive effects of loop, potassium-sparing and thiazide diuretics. Therefore, when Hydrochlorothiazide and nonsteroidal anti-inflammatory agents are used concomitantly, the patient should be observed closely to determine if the desired effect of the diuretic is obtained.

➤ SHOWN IN PRODUCT IDENTIFICATION GUIDE

DRUG/LABORATORY TEST INTERACTIONS

Thiazides should be discontinued before carrying out tests for parathyroid function (see "Precautions, General").

Carcinogenesis, Mutagenesis, Impairment of Fertility: Two-year feeding studies in mice and rats conducted under the auspices of the National Toxicology Program (NTP) uncovered no evidence of a carcinogenic potential of Hydrochlorothiazide in female mice (at doses of up to approximately 600 mg/kg/day) or in male and female rats (at doses of up to approximately 100 mg/kg/day). The NTP, however, found equivocal evidence for hepatocarcinogenicity in male mice. Hydrochlorothiazide was not genotoxic *in vitro* in the Ames mutagenicity assay of *Salmonella typhimurium* strains TA 98, TA 100, TA 1535, TA 1537, and TA 1538 and in the Chinese Hamster Ovary (CHO) test for chromosomal aberrations, or *in vivo* in assays using mouse germinal cell chromosomes, Chinese hamster bone marrow chromosomes, and the *Drosophilia* sex-linked recessive lethal trait gene. Positive test results were obtained only in the *in vitro* CHO Sister Chromatid Exchange (clastogenicity) and in the Mouse Lymphoma Cell (mutagenicity) assays, using concentrations of Hydrochlorothiazide from 43 to 1300 μg/mL, and in the *Aspergillus nidulans* nondisjunction assay at an unspecified concentration.

Hydrochlorothiazide had no adverse effects on the fertility of mice and rats of either sex in studies wherein these species were exposed, via their diet, to doses of up to 100 and 4 mg/kg, respectively, prior to conception and throughout gestation.

PREGNANCY

Teratogenic Effects—Pregnancy Category B: Studies in which Hydrochlorothiazide was orally administered to pregnant mice and rats during their respective periods of major organogenesis at doses up to 3000 and 1000 mg Hydrochlorothiazide/kg, respectively, provided no evidence of harm to the fetus.

There are, however, no adequate and well-controlled studies in pregnant women. Because animal reproduction studies are not always predictive of human response, this drug should be used during pregnancy only if clearly needed.

Nonteratogenic Effects: Thiazides cross the placental barrier and appear in cord blood. There is a risk of fetal or neonatal jaundice, thrombocytopenia, and possibly other adverse reactions that have occurred in adults.

NURSING MOTHERS

Thiazides are excreted in breast milk. Because of the potential for serious adverse reactions in nursing infants, a decision should be made whether to discontinue nursing or to discontinue Hydrochlorothiazide, taking into account the importance of the drug to the mother.

PEDIATRIC USE

Safety and effectiveness in children have not been established.

ADVERSE REACTIONS

The following adverse reactions have been reported and, within each category, are listed in order of decreasing severity.

Body as a Whole: Weakness.

Cardiovascular: Hypotension including orthostatic hypotension (may be aggravated by alcohol, barbiturates, narcotics or antihypertensive drugs).

Digestive: Pancreatitis, jaundice (intrahepatic cholestatic jaundice), diarrhea, vomiting, sialadenitis, cramping, constipation, gastric irritation, nausea, anorexia.

Hematologic: Aplastic anemia, agranulocytosis, leukopenia, hemolytic anemia, thrombocytopenia.

Hypersensitivity: Anaphylactic reactions, necrotizing angiitis (vasculitis and cutaneous vasculitis), respiratory distress including pneumonitis and pulmonary edema, photosensitivity, fever, urticaria, rash, purpura.

Metabolic: Electrolyte imbalance (see "Precautions"), hyperglycemia, glycosuria, hyperuricemia.

Musculoskeletal: Muscle spasm.

Nervous System/Psychiatric: Vertigo, paresthesias, dizziness, headache, restlessness.

Renal: Renal failure, renal dysfunction, interstitial nephritis. (See "Warnings.")

Skin: Erythema multiforme including Stevens-Johnson syndrome, exfoliative dermatitis including toxic epidermal necrolysis, alopecia.

Special Senses: Transient blurred vision, xanthopsia.

Urogenital: Impotence.

Whenever adverse reactions are moderate or severe, thiazide dosage should be reduced or therapy withdrawn.

OVERDOSAGE

The most common signs and symptoms observed are those caused by electrolyte depletion (hypokalemia, hypochloremia, hyponatremia) and dehydration resulting from excessive diuresis. If digitalis has also been administered, hypokalemia may accentuate cardiac arrhythmias.

In the event of overdosage, symptomatic and supportive measures should be employed. Emesis should be induced or gastric lavage performed. Correct dehydration, electrolyte imbalance, hepatic coma and hypotension by established procedures. If required, give oxygen or artificial respiration for respiratory impairment. The degree to which Hydrochlorothiazide is removed by hemodialysis has not been established.

The oral LD_{50} of Hydrochlorothiazide is greater than 10 g/kg in the mouse and rat.

DOSAGE AND ADMINISTRATION

Therapy should be individualized according to patient response. Use the smallest dosage necessary to achieve the required response.

ADULTS

For Edema: The usual adult dosage is 25 to 100 mg daily as a single or divided dose. Many patients with edema respond to intermittent therapy, i.e., administration on alternate days or on three to five days each week. With an intermittent schedule, excessive response and the resulting undesirable electrolyte imbalance are less likely to occur.

For Control of Hypertension: The usual initial dose in adults is 25 mg daily given as a single dose. The dose may be increased to 50 mg daily, given as a single or two divided doses. Doses above 50 mg are often associated with marked reductions in serum potassium (see also "Precautions").

Patients usually do not require doses in excess of 50 mg of Hydrochlorothiazide daily when used concomitantly with other antihypertensive agents.

INFANTS AND CHILDREN

The usual pediatric dosage is based on 1.0 mg of Hydrochlorothiazide per pound of body weight per day in two doses. Infants under 6 months of age may require up to 1.5 mg per pound per day in two doses.

On this basis, infants up to 2 years of age may be given 12.5 to 37.5 mg daily in two doses. Children from 2 to 12 years of age may be given 37.5 to 100 mg daily in two doses. Dosage in both age groups should be based on body weight. However, pediatric patients with hypertension only rarely will benefit from doses larger than 50 mg daily.

STORAGE

Keep container tightly closed. Protect from light, moisture, freezing [−20°C (−4°F)] and store at room temperature, 15-30°C (59-86°F).

HOW SUPPLIED
SOLUTION: 50 MG/5 ML

BRAND/MANUFACTURER	NDC	SIZE	AWP
◆ **GENERICS**			
Roxane	00054-3383-63	500 ml	$15.37

TABLETS: 25 MG

AVERAGE UNIT PRICE (AVAILABLE SIZES)		GENERIC A-RATED AVERAGE PRICE (GAAP)	
BRAND	$0.12	30s	$2.69
GENERIC	$0.03	90s	$4.26
HCFA FUL (100s ea)	$0.02	100s	$4.43
		1000s	$12.98

BRAND/MANUFACTURER	NDC	SIZE	AWP
◆ **BRAND**			
➤ ESIDRIX: Ciba Pharm	00083-0022-30	100s	$11.56
➤ HYDRODIURIL: Merck	00006-0042-68	100s	$13.06
	00006-0042-82	1000s	$125.65
◆ **GENERICS**			
Major	00904-2083-46	30s	$2.25
Medirex	57480-0334-06	30s	$3.12
Vangard	00615-1561-06	60s	$1.14
Allscrips	54569-8540-00	90s	$3.11
Major	00904-2083-89	90s	$5.40
Richlyn	00115-3670-01	100s	$1.40
Schein	00364-0322-01	100s	$2.50
➤ Rugby	00536-3922-01	100s	$2.69
URL	00677-0346-01	100s	$2.86
Qualitest	00603-3858-21	100s	$2.86
Major	00904-2083-60	100s	$2.95
Moore,H.L.	00839-5135-06	100s	$2.96
Camall	00147-0116-10	100s	$3.15
➤ Geneva	00781-1480-01	100s	$3.45
ORETIC: Abbott Pharm	00074-6978-01	100s	$4.19
➤ Geneva	00781-1480-13	100s ud	$4.65
Goldline	00182-0556-89	100s ud	$4.75
Vangard	00615-1561-13	100s ud	$4.78
Auro	55829-0290-10	100s ud	$4.87
Raway	00686-0049-20	100s ud	$5.00
Major	00904-2083-61	100s ud	$5.11
ORETIC: Abbott Pharm	00074-6978-05	100s ud	$5.66
UDL	51079-0049-20	100s ud	$10.20
Medirex	57480-0334-01	100s ud	$10.20
Qualitest	00603-3858-32	1000s	$8.33
Schein	00364-0322-02	1000s	$9.54
Camall	00147-0116-20	1000s	$10.22
Major	00904-2083-80	1000s	$10.50
Goldline	00182-0556-10	1000s	$10.50
Richlyn	00115-3670-03	1000s	$10.80
➤ Zenith	00172-2083-80	1000s	$11.70
Moore,H.L.	00839-5135-16	1000s	$11.87
Martec	52555-0297-10	1000s	$12.05
Lederle Std Prod	00005-3752-34	1000s	$15.13
URL	00677-0346-10	1000s	$15.20
➤ Geneva	00781-1480-10	1000s	$15.25
HYDRO PAR: Parmed	00349-2070-10	1000s	$15.85
➤ Rugby	00536-3922-10	1000s	$15.95
➤ Purepac	00228-2221-96	1000s	$17.21

◆ RATED THERAPEUTICALLY EQUIVALENT; ◇ THERAPEUTIC EQUIVALENCE UNCONFIRMED; ○ UNRATED

BRAND/MANUFACTURER	NDC	SIZE	AWP
ORETIC: Abbott Pharm	00074-6978-02	1000s	$17.59
HYDRO PAR: Parmed	00349-2070-51	5000s	$60.46

TABLETS: 50 MG

AVERAGE UNIT PRICE (AVAILABLE SIZES)		GENERIC A-RATED AVERAGE PRICE (GAAP)	
BRAND	$0.19	30s	$3.29
GENERIC	$0.04	100s	$5.32
HCFA FUL (100s ea)	$0.02	1000s	$18.11
		5000s	$55.12

BRAND/MANUFACTURER	NDC	SIZE	AWP
◆ BRAND			
➤ ESIDRIX: Ciba Pharm	00083-0046-30	100s	$18.32
➤ HYDRODIURIL: Merck	00006-0105-68	100s	$20.70
➤ ESIDRIX: Ciba Pharm	00083-0046-73	720s	$136.96
➤ HYDRODIURIL: Merck	00006-0105-82	1000s	$196.29
	00006-0105-86	5000s	$923.55
◆ GENERICS			
Major	00904-2089-46	30s	$1.70
Medirex	57480-0335-06	30s	$4.87
Allscrips	54569-8587-00	90s	$3.56
Richlyn	00115-3675-01	100s	$1.66
➤ Schein	00364-0328-01	100s	$2.50
Major	00904-2205-60	100s	$2.60
West-Ward	00143-1257-01	100s	$2.75
Major	00904-2089-60	100s	$3.40
Camall	00147-0108-10	100s	$3.46
➤ Rugby	00536-3921-01	100s	$3.55
➤ Geneva	00781-1481-01	100s	$3.60
URL	00677-0347-01	100s	$3.66
➤ Rugby	00536-3919-01	100s	$3.70
Qualitest	00603-3859-21	100s	$3.70
Moore,H.L.	00839-5136-06	100s	$3.71
Goldline	00182-0557-01	100s	$3.75
Parmed	00349-2071-01	100s	$3.90
EZIDE: EconoMed	38130-0020-01	100s	$3.94
Camall	00147-0123-10	100s	$4.45
ORETIC: Abbott Pharm	00074-6985-01	100s	$6.64
CAROZIDE: Seneca	47028-0003-01	100s	$9.80
➤ Schein	00364-0328-90	100s ud	$5.25
Major	00904-2089-61	100s ud	$5.26
Goldline	00182-0557-89	100s ud	$5.40
Raway	00686-0111-20	100s ud	$5.50
➤ Geneva	00781-1481-13	100s ud	$5.65
Vangard	00615-1562-13	100s ud	$6.31
ORETIC: Abbott Pharm	00074-6985-06	100s ud	$8.24
Auro	55829-0291-10	100s ud	$8.38
West-Ward	00143-1257-25	100s ud	$9.00
Medirex	57480-0335-01	100s ud	$12.30
UDL	51079-0111-20	100s ud	$12.33
West-Ward	00143-1257-10	1000s	$8.24
Major	00904-2205-80	1000s	$9.24
Camall	00147-0108-20	1000s	$11.91
Richlyn	00115-3675-03	1000s	$12.75
➤ Schein	00364-0328-02	1000s	$13.02
Qualitest	00603-3859-32	1000s	$14.05
➤ Zenith	00172-2089-80	1000s	$14.10
Martec	52555-0298-10	1000s	$14.80
➤ Rugby	00536-3919-10	1000s	$16.25
Major	00904-2089-80	1000s	$16.50
Moore,H.L.	00839-5136-16	1000s	$16.59
➤ Rugby	00536-3921-10	1000s	$16.60
HYDRO PAR: Parmed	00349-2071-10	1000s	$17.50
Camall	00147-0123-20	1000s	$18.48
Goldline	00182-0557-10	1000s	$20.00
Lederle Std Prod	00005-3753-34	1000s	$21.09
ORETIC: Abbott Pharm	00074-6985-02	1000s	$23.60
URL	00677-0347-10	1000s	$23.92
Purepac	00228-2222-96	1000s	$23.98
➤ Geneva	00781-1481-10	1000s	$24.25
Aligen	00405-4490-03	1000s	$26.62
EZIDE: EconoMed	38130-0020-10	1000s	$34.90
Major	00904-2089-90	5000s	$38.85
➤ Rugby	00536-3919-50	5000s	$43.50
➤ Geneva	00781-1481-51	5000s	$45.50
Camall	00147-0108-30	5000s	$53.23
Moore,H.L.	00839-5136-20	5000s	$53.39
URL	00677-0347-50	5000s	$54.05
➤ Schein	00364-0328-03	5000s	$54.10
Goldline	00182-0557-50	5000s	$60.00
➤ Zenith	00172-2089-85	5000s	$67.65
HYDRO PAR: Parmed	00349-2071-51	5000s	$80.95

TABLETS: 100 MG

AVERAGE UNIT PRICE (AVAILABLE SIZES)		GENERIC A-RATED AVERAGE PRICE (GAAP)	
BRAND	$0.37	100s	$5.14
GENERIC	$0.05	1000s	$27.38
HCFA FUL (100s ea)	$0.04		

BRAND/MANUFACTURER	NDC	SIZE	AWP
◆ BRAND			
➤ HYDRODIURIL: Merck	00006-0410-68	100s	$37.15

BRAND/MANUFACTURER	NDC	SIZE	AWP
◆ GENERICS			
Richlyn	00115-3677-01	100s	$2.89
Rugby	00536-3923-01	100s	$4.25
Schein	00364-0421-01	100s	$4.51
Major	00904-2478-60	100s	$5.25
➤ Zenith	00172-2485-60	100s	$6.00
Martec	52555-0299-01	100s	$6.20
URL	00677-0764-01	100s	$6.30
Moore,H.L.	00839-6013-06	100s	$6.87
Major	00904-2478-61	100s ud	$4.00
Major	00904-2478-80	1000s	$14.95
Richlyn	00115-3677-03	1000s	$22.20
➤ Zenith	00172-2485-80	1000s	$45.00

Hydrochlorothiazide and Triamterene

DESCRIPTION

Hydrochlorothiazide/Triamterene is available in the following combinations: Hydrochlorothiazide 50 mg and Triamterene 75 mg or Hydrochlorothiazide 25 mg and Triamterene 37.5 mg. Hydrochlorothiazide is a diuretic/antihypertensive agent and Triamterene is an antikaliuretic agent.

Hydrochlorothiazide is slightly soluble in water. It is soluble in dilute ammonia, n-butylamine, dilute aqueous sodium hydroxide and dimethylformamide. It is sparingly soluble in methanol and insoluble in ether, chloroform, and dilute mineral acids. Hydrochlorothiazide is 6-chloro-3,4-dihydro-2H-1,2,4-benzothiadiazine-7-sulfonamide 1,1-dioxide. Its molecular weight is 297.73.

At 50°C, Triamterene is practically insoluble in water (less than 0.1%), benzene, chloroform, ether, and dilute alkali hydrozites. It is soluble in formic acid, sparingly soluble in methoxyethanol and very slightly soluble in alcohol, acetic acid, and dilute mineral acids. Triamterene is 2,4,7-triamino-6-phenylteridine. Its molecular weight is 253.27.

CLINICAL PHARMACOLOGY

Hydrochlorothiazide/Triamterene is a diuretic/antihypertensive drug product that combines natriuretic and antikaliuretic effects. Each component complements the action of the other. The Hydrochlorothiazide component blocks the reabsorption of sodium and chloride ions, and thereby increases the quantity of sodium traversing the distal tubule and the volume of water excreted. A portion of the additional sodium presented to the distal tubule is exchanged there for potassium and hydrogen ions. With continued use of Hydrochlorothiazide and depletion of sodium, compensatory mechanisms tend to increase this exchange and may produce excessive loss of potassium, hydrogen and chloride ions. Hydrochlorothiazide also decreases the excretion of calcium and uric acid, may increase the excretion of iodide and may reduce glomerular filtration rate. Onset of Hydrochlorothiazide's diuretic effect occurs within 2 hours and the peak action takes place in 4 hours. Diuretic activity persists for approximately 6 to 12 hours. The exact mechanism of the antihypertensive effect of Hydrochlorothiazide is not known, although it may relate to the excretion and redistribution of body sodium. Hydrochlorothiazide does not affect normal blood pressure.

Following oral administration, peak Hydrochlorothiazide plasma levels are attained in approximately 2 hours. It is excreted rapidly and unchanged in the urine.

Well-controlled studies have demonstrated that doses of Hydrochlorothiazide as low as 25 mg given once daily are effective in treating hypertension, but the dose response has not been clearly established.

The Triamterene component of Hydrochlorothiazide/Triamterene exerts its diuretic effect on the distal renal tubule to inhibit the reabsorption of sodium in exchange for potassium and hydrogen ions. Its natriuretic activity is limited by the amount of sodium reaching its site of action. Although it blocks the increase in this exchange that is stimulated by mineralocorticoids (chiefly aldosterone), it is not a competitive antagonist of aldosterone and its activity can be demonstrated in adrenalectomized rats and patients with Addison's disease. As a result, the dose of Triamterene required is not proportionally related to the level of mineralocorticoid activity, but is dictated by the response of the individual patients, and the kaliuretic effect of concomitantly administered drugs. By inhibiting the distal tubular exchange mechanism, Triamterene maintains or increases the sodium excretion and reduces the excess loss of potassium, hydrogen, and chloride ions induced by Hydrochlorothiazide. As with Hydrochlorothiazide, Triamterene may reduce glomerular filtration and renal plasma flow. Via this mechanism it may reduce uric acid excretion although it has no tubular effect on uric acid reabsorption or secretion. Triamterene does not affect calcium excretion. No predictable antihypertensive effect has been demonstrated for Triamterene.

Triamterene is rapidly absorbed following oral administration. Peak plasma levels are achieved within 1 hour after dosing. Triamterene is primarily metabolized to the sulfate conjugate of hydroxytriamterene. Both the plasma and urine levels of this metabolite greatly exceed Triamterene levels.

The amount of Triamterene added to 50 mg of Hydrochlorothiazide/Triamterene was determined from steady-state dose response evaluations in which various doses of liquid preparations of Triamterene were administered to hypertensive persons who developed hypokalemia with Hydrochlorothiazide/Triamterene (50 mg given once daily). Single daily doses of 75 mg Triamterene resulted in greater increases in serum potassium than lower doses (25 mg and 50 mg), while doses greater than 75 mg of Triamterene resulted in no additional elevations in serum potassium levels. The amount of Triamterene added to 25 mg of Hydrochlorothiazide/Triamterene was also determined from steady-state dose response evaluations in which various doses of liquid preparations of Triamterene were administered to hypertensive persons who developed hypokalemia with Hydrochlorothiazide/Triamterene (25 mg given once daily). Single daily doses of 37.5 mg Triamterene resulted in greater increases in serum potassium than a lower dose (25 mg), while doses greater than 37.5 mg of Triamterene, i.e., 75 mg and 100 mg, resulted in no additional elevations in serum potassium levels. The dose response relationship of Triamterene was also evaluated in patients rendered hypokalemic by Hydrochlorothiazide/Triamterene given 25 mg twice daily. Triamterene given twice daily increased serum potassium levels in a dose-related fashion. However, the combination of Triamterene and Hydrochlorothiazide/Triamterene given twice daily also appeared to produce an increased frequency of elevation in serum BUN and creatinine levels. The largest increases in serum potassium, BUN and creatinine in this study were observed with 50 mg of Triamterene given twice daily, the largest dose tested. Ordinarily, Triamterene does not entirely compensate for the kaliuretic effect of Hydrochlorothiazide/Triamterene and some patients may remain hypokalemic while receiving Triamterene and Hydrochlorothiazide/Triamterene. In some individuals, however, it may induce hyperkalemia (see *"Warnings"*).

Duration of diuretic activity and effective dosage range of the Hydrochlorothiazide and Triamterene components of Hydrochlorothiazide/Triamterene are similar. Onset of diuresis with Hydrochlorothiazide/Triamterene takes place within one hour, peaks at two to three hours and tapers off during the subsequent seven to nine hours.

The bioavailability of the Hydrochlorothiazide and the Triamterene components of Hydrochlorothiazide/Triamterene is, in each case, about 50% of that observed with an aqueous suspension of the components. (See *"Precautions, Bioavailability".)*

The Triamterene and Hydrochlorothiazide components of Hydrochlorothiazide/Triamterene are well absorbed and are bioequivalent to liquid preparations of the individual components administered orally. Food does not influence the absorption of Triamterene or Hydrochlorothiazide/Triamterene. The Hydrochlorothiazide component of Hydrochlorothiazide/Triamterene is bioequivalent to single-entity Hydrochlorothiazide tablet formulations.

Upon administration of a single oral dose to fasted normal male volunteers, the following mean pharmacokinetic parameters were determined: (See related table). where AUC(0-48), Cmax, Tmax and Ae represent area under the plasma concentration versus time plot, maximum plasma concentration, time to reach Cmax and amount excreted in urine over 48 hours.

Hydrochlorothiazide/Triamterene capsule is bioequivalent to a single-entity 25 mg Hydrochlorothiazide tablet and 37.5 mg Triamterene capsule used in the double-blind clinical trial below. (See *"Clinical Trials."*)

CLINICAL TRIALS

A placebo-controlled, double-blind trial was conducted to evaluate the efficacy of Hydrochlorothiazide/Triamterene capsules. This trial demonstrated that Hydrochlorothiazide/Triamterene (25 mg Hydrochlorothiazide/37.5 mg Triamterene) was effective in controlling blood pressure while reducing the incidence of Hydrochlorothiazide induced hypokalemia. This trial involved 636 patients with mild to moderate hypertension controlled by Hydrochlorothiazide 25 mg daily and who had hypokalemia (serum potassium < 3.5 mEq/L) secondary to the Hydrochlorothiazide. Patients were randomly assigned to 4 weeks treatment with once-daily regimens of 25 mg Hydrochlorothiazide plus placebo, or 25 mg Hydrochlorothiazide combined with one of the following doses of Triamterene: 25 mg, 37.5 mg, 50 mg or 75 mg.

Blood pressure and serum potassium were monitored at baseline and throughout the trial. All five treatment groups had similar mean blood pressure and serum potassium concentrations at baseline (mean systolic blood pressure range: 137 ± 14 mmHg to 140 ± 16 mmHg: mean diastolic blood pressure range: 86 ± 9 mmHg to 88 ± 8 mmHg: mean serum potassium range: 2.3 to 3.4 mEq/L with the majority of patients having values between 3.1 and 3.4 mEq/L).

While all Triamterene regimens reversed hypokalemia, at week 4 the 37.5 mg regimen proved optimal compared with the other tested regimens. On this regimen, 81% of the patients had a significant ($p < 0.05$) reversal of hypokalemia vs. 59% of patients on the placebo/Hydrochlorothiazide regimen. The mean serum potassium concentration on 37.5 mg Triamterene went from 3.2 ± 0.2 mEq/L at baseline to 3.7 ± 0.3 mEq/L at week 4, a significantly greater ($p < 0.05$) improvement than that achieved with placebo/Hydrochlorothiazide (i.e., 3.2 ± 0.2 mEq/L at baseline and 3.5 ± 0.4 mEq/L at week 4). Also, 51% of patients in the 37.5 mg Triamterene group had an increase in serum potassium of ≥ 0.5 mEq/L at week 4 vs. 33% in the placebo group. The 37.5 mg Triamterene/25 mg Hydrochlorothiazide regimen also maintained control of blood pressure; mean supine systolic blood pressure at week 4 was 138 ± 21 mmHg while mean supine diastolic blood pressure was 87 ± 13 mmHg.

INDICATIONS AND USAGE

This fixed combination drug is not indicated for the initial therapy of edema or hypertension except in individuals in whom the development of hypokalemia cannot be risked.

Hydrochlorothiazide/Triamterene is indicated for the treatment of hypertension or edema in patients who develop hypokalemia on Hydrochlorothiazide alone.

Hydrochlorothiazide/Triamterene is also indicated for those patients who require a thiazide diuretic and in whom the development of hypokalemia cannot be risked, (eg, patients on concomitant digitalis preparations, or with a history of cardiac arrhythmias, etc.).

Hydrochlorothiazide/Triamterene may be used alone or as an adjunct to other antihypertensive drugs, such as beta-blockers. Since Hydrochlorothiazide/Triamterene may enhance the action of these agents, dosage adjustments may be necessary.

Usage in Pregnancy: The routine use of diuretics in an otherwise healthy woman is inappropriate and exposes mother and fetus to unnecessary hazard. Diuretics do not prevent development of toxemia of pregnancy, and there is no satisfactory evidence that they are useful in the treatment of developed toxemia.

Edema during pregnancy may arise from pathological causes or from the physiologic and mechanical consequences of pregnancy. Diuretics are indicated in pregnancy when edema is due to pathologic causes, just as they are in the absence of pregnancy. Dependent edema in pregnancy resulting from restriction of venous return by the expanded uterus is properly treated through elevation of the lower extremities and use of support hose; use of diuretics to lower intravascular volume in this case is illogical and unnecessary. There is hypervolemia during normal pregnancy which is harmful to neither the fetus nor the mother (in the absence of cardiovascular disease), but which is associated with edema, including generalized edema, in the majority of pregnant women. If this edema produces discomfort, increased recumbency will often provide relief. In rare instances this edema may cause extreme discomfort which is not relieved by rest. In these cases a short course of diuretics may provide relief and may be appropriate.

CONTRAINDICATIONS

ANTIKALIURETIC THERAPY AND POTASSIUM SUPPLEMENTATION
Hydrochlorothiazide/Triamterene should not be given to patients receiving other potassium-conserving agents such as spironolactone, amiloride or other formulations containing Triamterene. Concomitant potassium-containing salt substitutes should also not be used.

Potassium supplementation in the form of medication or potassium-enriched diets should not be used with Hydrochlorothiazide/Triamterene except in severe cases of hypokalemia. Such concomitant therapy can be associated with rapid increases in serum potassium levels. If potassium supplementation is used, careful monitoring of the serum potassium level is necessary.

IMPAIRED RENAL FUNCTION
Hydrochlorothiazide/Triamterene is contraindicated in patients with anuria, acute and chronic renal insufficiency or significant renal impairment.

HYPERSENSITIVITY
Hypersensitivity to either drug in the preparation or to other sulfonamide-derived drugs is a contraindication.

HYPERKALEMIA
Hydrochlorothiazide/Triamterene should not be used in the presence of elevated serum potassium levels (greater than or equal to 5.5 mEq/L). If hyperkalemia develops, this drug should be discontinued and a thiazide alone should be substituted.

WARNINGS
HYPERKALEMIA

ABNORMAL ELEVATION OF SERUM POTASSIUM LEVELS (GREATER THAN OR EQUAL TO 5.5 MEQ/L) CAN OCCUR WITH ALL POTASSIUM-CONSERVING DIURETIC COMBINATIONS, INCLUDING HYDROCHLORO-THIAZIDE/TRIAMTERENE. HYPERKALEMIA IS MORE LIKELY TO OCCUR IN PATIENTS WITH RENAL IMPAIRMENT AND DIABETES (EVEN WITHOUT EVIDENCE OF RENAL IMPAIRMENT), AND IN THE ELDERLY OR SEVERELY ILL. SINCE UNCORRECTED HYPERKALEMIA MAY BE FATAL, SERUM POTASSIUM LEVELS MUST BE MONITORED AT FREQUENT INTERVALS ESPECIALLY IN PATIENTS FIRST RECEIVING HYDROCHLOROTHIAZIDE/TRIAMTERENE, WHEN DOSAGES ARE CHANGED OR WITH ANY ILLNESS THAT MAY INFLUENCE RENAL FUNCTION.

If hyperkalemia is suspected (warning signs include paresthesias, muscular weakness, fatigue, flaccid paralysis of the extremities, bradycardia and shock), an electrocardiogram (ECG) should be obtained. However, it is important to monitor

	AUC(0-48) ng*hrs/mL (±SD)	Cmax ng/mL (±SD)	Median Tmax hrs	Ae mg (±SD)
Triamterene	148.7 (87.9)	46.4 (29.4)	1.1	2.7 (1.4)
hydroxytriamterene sulfate	1865 (471)	720 (364)	1.3	19.7 (6.1)
Hydrochlorothiazide	834 (177	135.1 (35.7)	2.0	14.3 (3.8)

◆ RATED THERAPEUTICALLY EQUIVALENT; ◇ THERAPEUTIC EQUIVALENCE UNCONFIRMED; ○ UNRATED

serum potassium levels because mild hyperkalemia may not be associated with ECG changes.

If hyperkalemia is present, Hydrochlorothiazide/Triamterene should be discontinued immediately and a thiazide alone should be substituted. If the serum potassium exceeds 6.5 mEq/liter more vigorous therapy is required. The clinical situation dictates the procedures to be employed. These include the intravenous administration of calcium chloride solution, sodium bicarbonate solution and/or the oral or parenteral administration of glucose with a rapid-acting insulin preparation. Cationic exchange resins such as sodium polystyrene sulfonate may be orally or rectally administered. Persistent hyperkalemia may require dialysis.

The development of hyperkalemia associated with potassium-sparing diuretics is accentuated in the presence of renal impairment (see *"Contraindications"* section). Patients with mild renal functional impairment should not receive this drug without frequent and continuing monitoring of serum electrolytes. Cumulative drug effects may be observed in patients with impaired renal function. The renal clearances of Hydrochlorothiazide and the pharmacologically active metabolite of Triamterene, the sulfate ester of hydroxytriamterene, have been shown to be reduced and the plasma levels increased following Hydrochlorothiazide/Triamterene administration to elderly patients and patients with impaired renal function. Hyperkalemia has been reported in diabetic patients with the use of potassium-conserving agents even in the absence of apparent renal impairment. Accordingly, Hydrochlorothiazide/Triamterene should be avoided in diabetic patients. If it is employed, serum electrolytes must be frequently monitored.

Because of the potassium-sparing properties of angiotensin-converting enzyme (ACE) inhibitors, Hydrochlorothiazide/Triamterene should be used cautiously, if at all, with these agents (see *"Precautions, Drug Interactions"*).

METABOLIC OR RESPIRATORY ACIDOSIS
Potassium-conserving therapy should also be avoided in severely ill patients in whom respiratory or metabolic acidosis may occur. Acidosis may be associated with rapid elevations in serum potassium levels. If Hydrochlorothiazide/Triamterene is employed, frequent evaluations of acid/base balance and serum electrolytes are necessary.

PRECAUTIONS
GENERAL
Bioavailability: The bioavailability of the Hydrochlorothiazide and Triamterene components of Hydrochlorothiazide/Triamterene is about 50% of the maximum obtainable with oral therapy. A patient transferred from therapy with Hydrochlorothiazide with or without Triamterene might show an increase in blood pressure, fluid retention, or change in serum potassium. Extensive clinical experience with Hydrochlorothiazide/Triamterene, however, suggests that these conditions have not been commonly observed in clinical practice. (See *"Clinical Pharmacology"*.)

IMPAIRED HEPATIC FUNCTION
Thiazides should be used with caution in patients with impaired hepatic function or progressive liver disease. Minor alterations of fluid and electrolyte balance can precipitate hepatic coma in patients with severe liver disease. Potassium depletion induced by the thiazide may be important in this connection.

Administer Hydrochlorothiazide/Triamterene cautiously and be alert for such early signs of impending coma as confusion, drowsiness and tremor; if mental confusion increases, discontinue Hydrochlorothiazide/Triamterene for a few days. Attention must be given to other factors that may precipitate hepatic coma, such as blood in the gastrointestinal tract or preexisting potassium depletion.

HYPOKALEMIA
Hypokalemia may develop with thiazide therapy, especially with brisk diuresis, when severe cirrhosis is present, or during concomitant use of corticosteroids, ACTH, amphotericin B or after prolonged thiazide therapy. However, hypokalemia of this type is usually prevented by the Triamterene component of Hydrochlorothiazide/Triamterene.

Interference with adequate oral electrolyte intake will also contribute to hypokalemia. Hypokalemia can sensitize or exaggerate the response of the heart to the toxic effects of digitalis (eg, increased ventricular irritability).

Hypokalemia is uncommon with Hydrochlorothiazide/Triamterene but, should it develop, corrective measures should be taken such as potassium supplementation or increased intake of potassium-rich foods. Institute such measures cautiously with frequent determinations of serum potassium levels, especially in patients receiving digitalis or with a history of cardiac arrhythmias. If serious hypokalemia (serum potassium less than 3.0 mEq/L) is demonstrated by repeat serum potassium determinations, Hydrochlorothiazide/Triamterene should be discontinued and potassium chloride supplementation initiated. Less serious hypokalemia should be evaluated with regard to other coexisting conditions and treated accordingly.

ELECTROLYTE IMBALANCE
Electrolyte imbalance, often encountered in such conditions as heart failure, renal disease or cirrhosis of the liver, may also be aggravated by diuretics and should be considered during Hydrochlorothiazide/Triamterene therapy when using high doses for prolonged periods or in patients on a salt-restricted diet. Serum determinations of electrolytes should be performed, and are particularly important if the patient is vomiting excessively or receiving fluids parenterally. Possible fluid and electrolyte imbalance may be indicated by such warning signs as: dry mouth, thirst, weakness, lethargy, drowsiness, restlessness, muscle pain or cramps, muscular fatigue, hypotension, oliguria, tachycardia and gastrointestinal symptoms such as nausea and vomiting.

HYPOCHLOREMIA
Although any chloride deficit during thiazide therapy is generally mild and usually does not require specific treatment except under extraordinary circumstances (as in liver disease or renal disease), chloride replacement may be required in the treatment of metabolic alkalosis. Dilutional hyponatremia may occur in edematous patients in hot weather; appropriate therapy is water restriction, rather than administration of salt, except in rare instances when the hyponatremia is life threatening. In actual salt depletion, appropriate replacement is the therapy of choice.

RENAL STONES
Triamterene has been found in renal stones in association with the other usual calculus components. Hydrochlorothiazide/Triamterene should be used with caution in patients with a history of renal stones.

FOLIC ACID DEFICIENCY
Triamterene is a weak folic acid antagonist and may contribute to the appearance of megaloblastosis in instances where folic acid stores are decreased. In such patients, periodic blood evaluations are recommended.

HYPERURICEMIA
Hyperuricemia may occur or acute gout may be precipitated in certain patients receiving thiazide therapy.

Insulin requirements in diabetic patients may be increased, decreased or unchanged. Diabetes mellitus which has been latent may become manifest during thiazide administration.

HYPERSENSITIVITY
Sensitivity reactions to thiazides may occur in patients with or without a history of allergy or bronchial asthma.

Possible exacerbation or activation of systemic lupus erythematosus by thiazides has been reported.

LABORATORY TESTS
Serum Potassium: The normal adult range of serum potassium is 3.5 to 5.0 mEq per liter with 4.5 mEq often being used for a reference point. If hypokalemia should develop, corrective measures should be taken such as potassium supplementation or increased dietary intake of potassium-rich foods. Institute such measures cautiously with frequent determinations of serum potassium levels. Potassium levels persistently above 6 mEq per liter require careful observation and treatment. Serum potassium levels do not necessarily indicate true body potassium concentration. A rise in plasma pH may cause a decrease in plasma potassium concentration and an increase in the intracellular potassium concentration. Discontinue corrective measures for hypokalemia immediately if laboratory determinations reveal an abnormal elevation of serum potassium. Discontinue Hydrochlorothiazide/Triamterene and substitute a thiazide diuretic alone until potassium levels return to normal.

Serum Creatinine and BUN: Hydrochlorothiazide/Triamterene may produce an elevated blood urea nitrogen level, creatinine level or both. This apparently is secondary to a reversible reduction of glomerular filtration rate or a depletion of intravascular fluid volume (prerenal azotemia) rather than renal toxicity; levels usually return to normal when Hydrochlorothiazide/Triamterene is discontinued. Elevations in BUN and creatinine levels may be more frequent in patients receiving divided dose diuretic therapy. If azotemia increases, discontinue Hydrochlorothiazide/Triamterene. Periodic BUN and serum creatinine determinations should be made, especially in elderly patients and in patients with suspected or confirmed hepatic disease or renal insufficiency.

Serum PBI: Thiazide may decrease serum PBI levels without sign of thyroid disturbance.

Parathyroid Function: Thiazides should be discontinued before carrying out tests for parathyroid function. Calcium excretion is decreased by thiazides. Pathologic changes in the parathyroid glands with hypercalcemia and hypophosphatemia have been observed in a few patients on prolonged thiazide therapy. The common complications of hyperparathyroidism such as renal lithiasis, bone resorption and peptic ulceration have not been seen.

DRUG INTERACTIONS
Angiotensin-converting Enzyme Inhibitors: Potassium-sparing agents should be used with caution in conjunction with angiotensin-converting enzyme (ACE) inhibitors due to an increased risk of hyperkalemia. Serum potassium should be monitored frequently.

Oral Hypoglycemic Drugs: Concurrent use with chlorpropamide may increase the risk of severe hyponatremia.

Nonsteroidal Anti-inflammatory Drugs: A possible interaction resulting in acute renal failure has been reported in a few patients on Hydrochlorothiazide/Triamterene when treated with indomethacin, a nonsteroidal anti-inflammatory agent. Caution is advised in administering nonsteroidal anti-inflammatory agents with Hydrochlorothiazide/Triamterene.

Lithium: Lithium generally should not be given with diuretics because they reduce its renal clearance and increase the risk of lithium toxicity. Read circulars for lithium preparations before use of such concomitant therapy with Hydrochlorothiazide/Triamterene.

Surgical considerations: Thiazides have been shown to decrease arterial responsiveness to norepinephrine (an effect attributed to loss of sodium). This diminution is not sufficient to preclude effectiveness of the pressor agent for therapeutic use. Thiazides have also been shown to increase the paralyzing effect of nondepolarizing muscle relaxants such as tubocurarine (an effect attributed to potassium loss); consequently, caution should be observed in patients undergoing surgery.

Other Considerations: Concurrent use of Hydrochlorothiazide with amphotericin B or corticosteroids or corticotropin (ACTH) may intensify electrolyte imbalance, particularly hypokalemia, although the presence of Triamterene minimizes the hypokalemic effect.

Thiazides may add to or potentiate the action of other antihypertensive drugs. See *"Indications and Usage"* for concomitant use with other antihypertensive drugs.

The effect of oral anticoagulants may be decreased when used concurrently with Hydrochlorothiazide; dosage adjustments may be necessary.

Hydrochlorothiazide/Triamterene may raise the level of blood uric acid; dosage adjustments of antigout medication may be necessary to control hyperuricemia and gout.

The following agents given together with Triamterene may promote serum potassium accumulation and possibly result in hyperkalemia because of the potassium-sparing nature of Triamterene, especially in patients with renal insufficiency: blood from blood bank (may contain up to 30 mEq of potassium per liter of plasma or up to 65 mEq per liter of whole blood when stored for more than 10 days); low-salt milk (may contain up to 60 mEq of potassium per liter); potassium-containing medications (such as parenteral penicillin G potassium); salt substitutes (most contain substantial amounts of potassium).

Exchange resins, such as sodium polystyrene sulfonate, whether administered orally or rectally, reduce serum potassium levels by sodium replacement of the potassium; fluid retention may occur in some patients because of the increased sodium intake.

Chronic or overuse of laxatives may reduce serum potassium levels by promoting excessive potassium loss from the intestinal tract; laxatives may interfere with the potassium-retaining effects of Triamterene.

The effectiveness of methenamine may be decreased when used concurrently with Hydrochlorothiazide because of alkalinization of the urine.

DRUG/LABORATORY TEST INTERACTIONS

Triamterene and quinidine have similar fluorescence spectra; thus, Hydrochlorothiazide/Triamterene will interfere with the fluorescent measurement of quinidine.

CARCINOGENESIS, MUTAGENESIS, IMPAIRMENT OF FERTILITY

Studies have not been performed to evaluate the mutagenic or carcinogenic potential of Hydrochlorothiazide/Triamterene.

Hydrochlorothiazide: Two-year feeding studies in mice and rats conducted under the auspices of the National Toxicology Program (NTP) uncovered no evidence of a carcinogenic potential of Hydrochlorothiazide in female mice (at doses of up to approximately 600 mg/kg day) or in male and female rats (at doeses of up to approximately 100 mg/kg/day). The NTP, however, found equivocal evidence for hepatocarcinogenicity in male mice. Hydrochlorothiazide was not genotoxic in *in vitro* assays using strains TA 98, TA 100, TA 1535, TA 1537 and TA 1538 of *Salmonella typhimurium* (Ames assay) and in the Chinese Hamster Ovary (CHO) test for chromosomal aberrations, or in *in vivo* assays using mouse germinal cell chromosomes, Chinese hamster bone marrow chromosomes, and the *Drosophila* sex-linked recessive lethal trait gene. Positive test results were obtained only in the *in vitro* CHO Sister Chromatid Exchange (clastogenicity) and in the Mouse Lymphoma Cell (mutagenicity) assays, using concentrations of Hydrochlorothiazide from 43 to 1300 μg/mL, and in the *Aspergillus nidulans* non-disjunction assay at an unspecified concentration of Hydrochlorothiazide.

Hydrochlorothiazide had no adverse effects on the fertility of mice and rats of either sex in studies wherein these species were exposed, via their diet, to doses of up to 100 and 4 mg/kg, respectively, prior to conception and throughout gestation.

Corresponding multiples of the MRHD are 100 (mice) and 4 (rats) on the basis of body-weight and 9.4 (mice) and 0.8 (rats) on the basis of body-surface area.

Triamterene: Reproductive studies have been performed in rats at doses up to 30 times the human dose and have revealed no evidence of impaired fertility.

PREGNANCY: CATEGORY C

Hydrochlorothiazide/Triamterene: Animal reproduction studies to determine the potential for fetal harm by Hydrochlorothiazide/Triamterene have not been conducted. However, a One Generation Study in the rat approximated Hydrochlorothiazide/Triamterene composition by using a 1:1 ratio of Triamterene to Hydrochlorothiazide (30:30 mg/kg/day); there was no evidence of teratogenicity at those doses which were, on a body-weight basis, 15 and 30 times, respectively, the MRHD, and on the basis of body-surface area, 3.1 and 6.2 times, respectively, the MRHD.

The safe use of Hydrochlorothiazide/Triamterene in pregnancy has not been established since there are no adequate and well-controlled studies with Hydrochlorothiazide/Triamterene pregnant women. Hydrochlorothiazide/Triamterene should be used during pregnancy only if the potential benefit justifies the risk to the fetus.

Triamterene: Reproduction studies have been performed in rats at doses as high as 20 times the MRHD on the basis of body-weight, and 6 times the human dose on the basis of body-surface area without evidence of harm to the fetus due to Triamterene.

Because animal reproduction studies are not always predictive of human response, this drug should be used during pregnancy only if clearly needed.

Hydrochlorothiazide: Hydrochlorothiazide was orally administered to pregnant mice and rats during respective periods of major organogenesis at doses up to 3000 and 1000 mg/kg/day, respectively. At these doses, which are multiples of the MRHD equal to 3000 for mice and 1000 for rats, based on body-weight, and equal to 282 for mice and 206 for rats, based on body-surface area, there was no evidence of harm to the fetus.

There are, however, no adequate and well-controlled studies in pregnant women. Because animal reproduction studies are not always predictive of human response, this drug should be used during pregnancy only if clearly needed.

Nonteratogenic Effects: Thiazides and Triamterene have been shown to cross the placental barrier and appear in cord blood. The use of thiazides and Triamterene in pregnant women requires that the anticipated benefit be weighed against possible hazards to the fetus. These hazards include fetal or neonatal jaundice, pancreatitis, thrombocytopenia, and possible other adverse reactions which have occurred in the adult.

Nursing Mothers: Thiazides and Triamterene in combination have not been studied in nursing mothers. Triamterene appears in animal milk; this may occur in humans. Thiazides are excreted in human breast milk. If use of the combination drug product is deemed essential, the patient should stop nursing.

Pediatric Use: Safety and effectiveness in children have not been established.

ADVERSE REACTIONS

Side effects observed in association with the use of Hydrochlorothiazide/Triamterene and products containing Triamterene or Hydrochlorothiazide include the following:

Gastrointestinal: jaundice (intrahepatic cholestatic jaundice) and/or liver enzyme abnormalities, pancreatitis, nausea, appetite disturbance, taste alteration, vomiting, diarrhea, constipation, anorexia, gastric irritation, abdominal pain and cramping.

Central Nervous System: drowsiness and fatigue, insomnia, headache, dizziness, dry mouth, depression, anxiety, vertigo, restlessness, paresthesias, weakness.

Cardiovascular: tachycardia and other arrhythmias, shortness of breath and chest pain, orthostatic or postural hypotension (may be aggravated by alcohol, barbiturates or narcotics).

Renal: acute renal failure (one case of irreversible renal failure has been reported), acute interstitial nephritis, renal stones composed of Triamterene in association with other calculus materials, urine discoloration, elevated BUN and serum creatinine, abnormal urinary sediment.

Metabolic: diabetes melitus, hyperglycemia, glycosuria, hyperuricemia, acidosis.

Hematologic: leukopenia, agranulocytosis, thrombocytopenia, aplastic anemia, hemolytic anemia and megaloblastosis.

Ophthalmic: xanthopsia, transient blurred vision.

Hypersensitivity: anaphylaxis, photosensitivity, rash, urticaria, purpura, necrotizing angiitis (vasculitis, cutaneous vasculitis), fever, respiratory distress including pneumonitis.

Other: muscle cramps and weakness, decreased sexual performance, sialadenitis necrotizing vasculitis, exacerbation of lupus.

Neonate and Infancy: thrombocytopenia and pancreatitis—rarely, in newborns whose mothers have received thiazides during pregnancy. Whenever adverse reactions are moderate to severe, therapy should be reduced or withdrawn.

Altered Laboratory Findings: Serum Electrolytes: hyperkalemia, hypokalemia, hyponatremia, hypomagnesemia, hypochloremia (see *"Warnings," "Precautions"*).

Creatinine, Blood Urea Nitrogen: Reversible elevations in BUN and serum creatinine have been observed in hypertensive patients treated with Hydrochlorothiazide/Triamterene.

Glucose: hyperglycemia, glycosuria and diabetes mellitus (see *"Precautions"*).

Serum Uric Acid, PBI and Calcium: (see *"Precautions"*).

Other: Elevated liver enzymes have been reported in patients receiving Hydrochlorothiazide/Triamterene.

OVERDOSAGE

No specific data are available regarding Hydrochlorothiazide/Triamterene overdosage in humans and no specific antidote is available.

Fluid and electrolyte imbalances are the most important concern. Excessive doses of the Triamterene component may elicit hyperkalemia, dehydration, nausea, vomiting and weakness and possibly hypotension. Overdosing with hydrochlorothiazide has been associated with hypokalemia, hypochloremia, hyponatremia, dehydration, lethargy (may progress to coma) and gastrointestinal irritation.

Other symptoms reported include: polyuria, lassitude, fever, flushed face, and hyperactive deep tendon reflexes. Treatment is symptomatic and supportive. Therapy with Hydrochlorothiazide/Triamterene should be discontinued. If hypotension occurs, it may be treated with pressor agents such as levarterenol to maintain blood pressure. Carefully evaluate the electrolyte pattern and fluid balance. Induce immediate evacuation of the stomach through emesis or gastric lavage. Institute supportive measures as required to maintain hydration, electrolyte balance, respiratory, cardiovascular and renal function. There is no specific antidote.

◆ RATED THERAPEUTICALLY EQUIVALENT; ◇ THERAPEUTIC EQUIVALENCE UNCONFIRMED; ○ UNRATED

Reversible acute renal failure following ingestion of 50 tablets of a product containing a combination of 50 mg Triamterene and 25 mg Hydrochlorothiazide has been reported. Although Triamterene is largely protein-bound (approximately 67%), there may be some benefit to dialysis in cases of overdosage.

DOSAGE AND ADMINISTRATION

The usual dose of Hydrochlorothiazide/Triamterene is one or two capsules or tablets given once daily, with appropriate monitoring of serum potassium and of the clinical effect. (See *"Warnings, Hyperkalemia"*).

There is no experience with the use of more than one 50-mg Hydrochlorothiazide combination tablet daily or more than two 25-mg Hydrochlorothiazide combination tablets or capsules daily. Clinical experience with the administration of two 25-mg Hydrochlorothiazide combination tablets or capsules daily in divided doses (rather than as a single dose) suggests an increased risk of electrolyte imbalance and renal dysfunction.

Patients receiving 50 mg of Hydrochlorothiazide who become hypokalemic may be transferred to Hydrochlorothiazide 50 mg/Triamterene 75 mg directly. Patients receiving 25 mg Hydrochlorothiazide who become hypokalemic may be transferred to Hydrochlorothiazide 25 mg/Triamterene 37.5 mg directly.

In patients requiring Hydrochlorothiazide therapy and in whom hypokalemia cannot be risked, therapy may be initiated with Hydrochlorothiazide 25 mg/Triamterene 37.5 mg. If an optimal blood pressure response is not obtained with Hydrochlorothiazide 25 mg/Triamterene 37.5 mg, the dose should be increased to two Hydrochlorothiazide 25 mg/Triamterene 37.5 mg tablets daily as a single dose, or one Hydrochlorothiazide 50 mg/Triamterene 75 mg tablet daily. If blood pressure still is not controlled, another antihypertensive agent may be added (see *"Precautions, Drug Interactions"*).

Clinical studies have shown that patients taking less bioavailable formulations of Triamterene and Hydrochlorothiazide in daily doses of 25 to 50 mg Hydrochlorothiazide and 50 to 100 mg Triamterene may be safely changed to one Hydrochlorothiazide 25 mg/Triamterene 37.5 mg tablet daily. All patients changed from less bioavailable formulations to Hydrochlorothiazide 50 mg/ Triamterene 75 mg should be monitored clinically and for serum potassium after the transfer.

Store at controlled room temperature, (15°-30°C [59°-86°F]). Protect from light. Dispense in a tight, light-resistant container.

HOW SUPPLIED
CAPSULE: 25 MG-37.5 MG

BRAND/MANUFACTURER	NDC	SIZE	AWP
○ **BRAND**			
DYAZIDE: SK Beecham Pharm	00007-3650-22	100s	$38.25
	00007-3650-21	100s ud	$40.35
	00007-3650-30	1000s	$367.35
○ **GENERICS**			
Geneva	00781-2056-01	100s	$34.43
Geneva	00781-2056-10	1000s	$330.62

CAPSULE: 25 MG-50 MG

AVERAGE UNIT PRICE (AVAILABLE SIZES)		GENERIC A-RATED AVERAGE PRICE (GAAP)	
GENERIC	$0.28	90s	$25.41
		100s	$29.39
		1000s	$266.46

BRAND/MANUFACTURER	NDC	SIZE	AWP
◆ **GENERICS**			
Allscrips	54569-0543-04	3s	$0.85
Allscrips	54569-0543-05	6s	$1.69
Allscrips	54569-0543-01	30s	$8.47
Allscrips	54569-0543-02	60s	$16.94
Allscrips	54569-8015-00	90s	$25.41
Allscrips	54569-8502-00	90s	$25.41
➤ Geneva	00781-2540-01	100s	$27.95
➤ Geneva	00781-2715-01	100s	$27.95
Qualitest	00603-6181-21	100s	$27.95
Alligen	00405-5047-01	100s	$28.00
Sidmak	50111-0850-01	100s	$28.00
Goldline	00182-1750-01	100s	$28.00
Allscrips	54569-0543-00	100s	$28.23
Allscrips	54569-8015-01	100s	$28.23
Major	00904-1936-60	100s	$29.95
➤ Geneva	00781-2715-13	100s ud	$32.00
Raway	00686-0432-20	100s ud	$37.00
Allscrips	54569-8502-01	180s	$50.81
Major	00904-1936-80	1000s	$255.70
Qualitest	00603-6181-32	1000s	$267.50
Alligen	00405-5047-03	1000s	$268.00
Sidmak	50111-0850-10	1000s	$268.00
Goldline	00182-1750-10	1000s	$268.00
➤ Geneva	00781-2540-10	1000s	$269.00
➤ Geneva	00781-2715-10	1000s	$269.00

TABLET: 25 MG-37.5 MG

AVERAGE UNIT PRICE (AVAILABLE SIZES)		GENERIC A-RATED AVERAGE PRICE (GAAP)	
BRAND	$0.42	100s	$32.66
GENERIC	$0.32	500s	$157.91

BRAND/MANUFACTURER	NDC	SIZE	AWP
◆ **BRAND**			
➤ MAXZIDE: Lederle Labs	00005-4464-43	100s	$39.30
	00005-4464-60	100s ud	$43.61
◆ **GENERICS**			
Allscrips	54569-8596-00	90s	$28.94
Qualitest	00603-6180-21	100s	$29.90
Watson	52544-0424-01	100s	$30.86
Alligen	00405-5049-01	100s	$32.48
Rugby	00536-5665-01	100s	$32.67
Caremark	00339-5837-12	100s	$33.16
Major	00904-7873-60	100s	$33.65
Geneva	00781-1123-01	100s	$33.65
Goldline	00182-1903-01	100s	$33.65
Moore,H.L.	00839-7950-06	100s	$33.95
Watson	52544-0424-05	500s	$146.59
Alligen	00405-5049-02	500s	$154.31
Rugby	00536-5665-05	500s	$155.18
Geneva	00781-1123-05	500s	$155.40
Major	00904-7873-40	500s	$167.95
Goldline	00182-1903-05	500s	$168.00

TABLET: 50 MG-75 MG

AVERAGE UNIT PRICE (AVAILABLE SIZES)		GENERIC A-RATED AVERAGE PRICE (GAAP)	
BRAND	$0.81	100s	$38.01
GENERIC	$0.34	500s	$152.56
HCFA FUL (100s ea)	$0.06	1000s	$300.70

BRAND/MANUFACTURER	NDC	SIZE	AWP
◆ **BRAND**			
➤ MAXZIDE: Lederle Labs	00005-4460-43	100s	$79.49
	00005-4460-60	100s ud	$85.15
	00005-4460-31	500s	$397.44
◆ **GENERICS**			
Vangard	00615-0567-35	15s	$2.66
Vangard	00615-0567-30	30s	$3.46
Allscrips	54569-8526-00	90s	$29.55
➤ Schein	00364-2242-01	100s	$28.42
Qualitest	00603-6182-21	100s	$28.46
➤ Rugby	00536-4956-01	100s	$28.50
Major	00904-1965-60	100s	$28.50
Barr	00555-0444-02	100s	$28.78
Alligen	00405-5048-01	100s	$28.90
Geneva	00781-1008-01	100s	$28.90
Martec	52555-0974-01	100s	$28.90
URL	00677-1212-01	100s	$28.94
Moore,H.L.	00839-7422-06	100s	$28.96
Caremark	00339-5625-12	100s	$32.83
Parmed	00349-8749-01	100s	$33.71
Par	49884-0279-01	100s	$49.98
Watson	52544-0348-01	100s	$49.98
Goldline	00182-1872-01	100s	$49.98
Warner Chilcott	00047-0833-24	100s	$52.17
U.S. Trading	56126-0394-11	100s ud	$8.39
Vangard	00615-0567-13	100s ud	$38.02
Geneva	00781-1008-13	100s ud	$38.10
Major	00904-1965-61	100s ud	$39.76
➤ Schein	00364-2242-90	100s ud	$43.10
Goldline	00182-1872-89	100s ud	$51.00
Medirex	57480-0373-01	100s ud	$69.00
UDL	51079-0433-20	100s ud	$69.03
Qualitest	00603-6182-28	500s	$101.84
➤ Rugby	00536-4956-05	500s	$101.90
Barr	00555-0444-04	500s	$101.96
Major	00904-1965-40	500s	$102.20
Alligen	00405-5048-02	500s	$102.22
➤ Schein	00364-2242-05	500s	$125.50
Martec	52555-0974-05	500s	$127.50
Geneva	00781-1008-05	500s	$129.80
URL	00677-1212-05	500s	$130.00
Moore,H.L.	00839-7422-12	500s	$132.23
Parmed	00349-8749-05	500s	$157.50
Par	49884-0279-05	500s	$241.95
Watson	52544-0348-05	500s	$241.95
Goldline	00182-1872-05	500s	$241.95
Warner Chilcott	00047-0833-30	500s	$249.83
Major	00904-1965-80	1000s	$173.40
Martec	52555-0974-10	1000s	$252.75
Parmed	00349-8749-10	1000s	$316.95
Watson	52544-0348-10	1000s	$459.71

Hydrochlorothiazide and Lisinopril

DESCRIPTION

Hydrochlorothiazide/Lisinopril combines an angiotensin converting enzyme inhibitor, Lisinopril, and a diuretic, Hydrochlorothiazide.

Lisinopril, a synthetic peptide derivative, is an oral long-acting angiotensin converting enzyme inhibitor. It is chemically described as (S)-1-[N^2-(1-carboxy-3-phenylpropyl)-L-lysyl]-L-proline dihydrate. Its empirical formula is $C_{21}H_{31}N_3O_5 \cdot 2H_2O$.

Lisinopril is a white to off-white, crystalline powder, with a molecular weight of 441.53. It is soluble in water, sparingly soluble in methanol, and practically insoluble in ethanol.

Hydrochlorothiazide is 6-chloro-3,4-dihydro-2H-1,2,4-benzothiadiazine-7-sulfonamide 1,1-dioxide. Its empirical formula is $C_7H_8ClN_3O_4S_2$ and its structural formula is:

Hydrochlorothiazide is a white, or practically white, crystalline powder with a molecular weight of 297.72, which is slightly soluble in water, but freely soluble in sodium hydroxide solution.

Hydrochlorothiazide/Lisinopril is available for oral use in two tablet combinations of Lisinopril with Hydrochlorothiazide. Hydrochlorothiazide/Lisinopril 20-12.5 containing 20 mg Lisinopril and 12.5 mg Hydrochlorothiazide; and, Hydrochlorothiazide/Lisinopril 20-25 containing 20 mg Lisinopril and 25 mg Hydrochlorothiazide.

As a result of its diuretic effects, Hydrochlorothiazide increases plasma renin activity, increases aldosterone secretion, and decreases serum potassium. Administration of Lisinopril blocks the renin-angiotensin aldosterone axis and tends to reverse the potassium loss associated with the diuretic.

In clinical studies, the extent of blood pressure reduction seen with the combination of Lisinopril and Hydrochlorothiazide was approximately additive. The combination appeared somewhat less effective in black patients, but relatively few black patients were studied. In most patients, the antihypertensive effect of Hydrochlorothiazide/Lisinopril was sustained for at least 24 hours.

In a randomized, controlled comparison, the mean antihypertensive effects of Hydrochlorothiazide/Lisinopril 20-12.5 and Hydrochlorothiazide/Lisinopril 20-25 were similar, suggesting that many patients who respond adequately to the latter combination may be controlled with Hydrochlorothiazide/Lisinopril 20-12.5 (See *"Dosage and Administration"*.)

Concomitant administration of Lisinopril and Hydrochlorothiazide has little or no effect on the bioavailability of either drug. The combination tablet is bioequivalent to concomitant administration of the separate entities.

LISINOPRIL

Mechanism of Action: Lisinopril inhibits angiotensin-converting enzyme (ACE) in human subjects and animals. ACE is a peptidyl dipeptidase that catalyzes the conversion of angiotensin I to the vasoconstrictor substance, angiotensin II. Angiotensin II also stimulates aldosterone secretion by the adrenal cortex. Inhibition of ACE results in decreased plasma angiotensin II which leads to decreased vasopressor activity and to decreased aldosterone secretion. The latter decrease may result in a small increase of serum potassium. Removal of angiotensin II negative feedback on renin secretion leads to increased plasma renin activity. In hypertensive patients with normal renal function treated with Lisinopril alone for up to 24 weeks, the mean increase in serum potassium was less than 0.1 mEq/L; however, approximately 15 percent of patients had increases greater than 0.5 mEq/L and approximately six percent had a decrease greater than 0.5 mEq/L. In the same study, patients treated with Lisinopril plus a thiazide diuretic showed essentially no change in serum potassium. (See *"Precautions"*.)

ACE is identical to kininase, an enzyme that degrades bradykinin. Whether increased levels of bradykinin, a potent vasodepressor peptide, play a role in the therapeutic effects of Lisinopril remains to be elucidated.

While the mechanism through which Lisinopril lowers blood pressure is believed to be primarily suppression of the renin-angiotensin-aldosterone system, Lisinopril is antihypertensive even in patients with low-renin hypertension. Although Lisinopril was antihypertensive in all races studied, black hypertensive patients (usually a low-renin hypertensive population) had a smaller average response to Lisinopril monotherapy than nonblack patients.

Pharmacokinetics and Metabolism: Following oral administration of Lisinopril, peak serum concentrations occur within about 7 hours. Declining serum concentrations exhibit a prolonged terminal phase which does not contribute to drug accumulation. This terminal phase probably represents saturable binding to ACE and is not proportional to dose. Lisinopril does not appear to be bound to other serum proteins.

Lisinopril does not undergo metabolism and is excreted unchanged entirely in the urine. Based on urinary recovery, the mean extent of absorption of Lisinopril is approximately 25 percent, with large intersubject variability (6%-60%) at all doses tested (5-80 mg). Lisinopril absorption is not influenced by the presence of food in the gastrointestinal tract. Upon multiple dosing, Lisinopril exhibits an effective half-life of accumulation of 12 hours.

Impaired renal function decreases elimination of Lisinopril, which is excreted principally through the kidneys, but this decrease becomes clinically important only when the glomerular filtration rate is below 30 mL/min. Above this glomerular filtration rate, the elimination half-life is little changed. With greater impairment, however, peak and trough Lisinopril levels increase, time to peak concentration increases and time to attain steady state is prolonged. Older patients, on average, have (approximately doubled) higher blood levels and area under the plasma concentration time curve (AUC) than younger patients. (See *"Dosage and Administration"*.) Lisinopril can be removed by hemodialysis.

Studies in rats indicate that Lisinopril crosses the blood-brain barrier poorly. Multiple doses of Lisinopril in rats do not result in accumulation in any tissues. However, milk of lactating rats contains radioactivity following administration of ^{14}C Lisinopril. By whole body autoradiography, radioactivity was found in the placenta following administration of labeled drug to pregnant rats, but none was found in the fetuses.

Pharmacodynamics: Administration of Lisinopril to patients with hypertension results in a reduction of supine and standing blood pressure to about the same extent with no compensatory tachycardia. Symptomatic postural hypotension is usually not observed although it can occur and should be anticipated in volume and/or salt-depleted patients. (See *"Warnings"*.)

In most patients studied, onset of antihypertensive activity was seen at one hour after oral administration of an individual dose of Lisinopril, with peak reduction of blood pressure achieved by six hours.

In some patients achievement of optimal blood pressure reduction may require two to four weeks of therapy.

At recommended single daily doses, antihypertensive effects have been maintained for at least 24 hours, after dosing, although the effect at 24 hours was substantially smaller than the effect six hours after dosing.

The antihypertensive effects of Lisinopril have continued during long term therapy. Abrupt withdrawal of Lisinopril has not been associated with a rapid increase in blood pressure; nor with a significant overshoot of pretreatment blood pressure.

In hemodynamic studies in patients with essential hypertension, blood pressure reduction was accompanied by a reduction in peripheral arterial resistance with little or no change in cardiac output and in heart rate. In a study in nine hypertensive patients, following administration of Lisinopril, there was an increase in mean renal blood flow that was not significant. Data from several small studies are inconsistent with respect to the effect of Lisinopril on glomerular filtration rate in hypertensive patients with normal renal function, but suggest that changes, if any, are not large.

In patients with renovascular hypertension Lisinopril has been shown to be well tolerated and effective in controlling blood pressure. (See *"Precautions"*.)

HYDROCHLOROTHIAZIDE

The mechanism of the antihypertensive effect of thiazides is unknown. Thiazides do not usually affect normal blood pressure.

Hydrochlorothiazide is a diuretic and antihypertensive. It affects the distal renal tubular mechanism of electrolyte reabsorption. Hydrochlorothiazide increases excretion of sodium and chloride in approximately equivalent amounts. Natriuresis may be accompanied by some loss of potassium and bicarbonate.

After oral use diuresis begins within two hours, peaks in about four hours and lasts about 6 to 12 hours.

Hydrochlorothiazide is not metabolized but is eliminated rapidly by the kidney. When plasma levels have been followed for at least 24 hours, the plasma half-life has been observed to vary between 5.6 and 14.8 hours. At least 61 percent of the oral dose is eliminated unchanged within 24 hours. Hydrochlorothiazide crosses the placental but not the blood-brain barrier.

INDICATIONS AND USAGE

Hydrochlorothiazide/Lisinopril is indicated for the treatment of hypertension in patients for whom combination therapy is appropriate.

This fixed dose combination is not indicated for initial therapy. Patients already receiving a diuretic when Lisinopril is initiated, or given a diuretic and Lisinopril simultaneously, can develop symptomatic hypotension. In the initial titration of the individual entities, it is important, if possible, to stop the diuretic for several days before starting Lisinopril or, if this is not possible, begin Lisinopril at a low initial dose. (See *"Dosage and Administration"*.)

In using Hydrochlorothiazide/Lisinopril, consideration should be given to the fact that an angiotensin converting enzyme inhibitor, captopril, has caused agranulocytosis, particularly in patients with renal impairment or collagen vascular disease, and that available data are insufficient to show that Lisinopril does not have a similar risk. (See *"Warnings"*.)

CONTRAINDICATIONS

Hydrochlorothiazide/Lisinopril is contraindicated in patients who are hypersensitive to any component of this product and in patients with a history of angioedema related to previous treatment with an angiotensin converting enzyme inhibitor. Because of the hydrochlorothiazide component, this product is contraindicated in patients with anuria or hypersensitivity to other sulfonamide-derived drugs.

WARNINGS
LISINOPRIL
Angioedema: Angioedema of the face, extremities, lips, tongue, glottis and/or larynx has been reported rarely in patients treated with angiotensin converting enzyme inhibitors, including Lisinopril. In such cases Hydrochlorothiazide/Lisinopril should be promptly discontinued and the appropriate therapy and monitoring should be provided until complete and sustained resolution of signs and symptoms has occurred. In instances where swelling has been confined to the face and lips the condition has generally resolved without treatment, although antihistamines have been useful in relieving symptoms. Angioedema associated with laryngeal edema may be fatal. **Where there is involvement of the tongue, glottis or larynx, likely to cause airway obstruction, subcutaneous epinephrine solution 1:1000 (0.3 mL to 0.5 mL) and/or measures necessary to ensure a patient airway should be promptly provided. (See** *"Adverse Reactions".***)**

Hypotension and Related Effects: Excessive hypotension was rarely seen in uncomplicated hypertensive patients but is a possible consequence of Lisinopril use in salt/volume-depleted persons such as those treated vigorously with diuretics or patients on dialysis. (See *"Precautions, Drug Interactions"* and *"Adverse Reactions".*)

Syncope has been reported in 0.8 percent of patients receiving Hydrochlorothiazide/Lisinopril. In patients with hypertension receiving Lisinopril alone, the incidence of syncope was 0.1 percent. The overall incidence of syncope may be reduced by proper titration of the individual components. (See *"Precautions, Drug Interactions", "Adverse Reactions"* and *"Dosage and Administration".*)

In patients with severe congestive heart failure, with or without associated renal insufficiency, excessive hypotension has been observed and may be associated with oliguria and/or progressive azotemia, and rarely with acute renal failure and/or death. Because of the potential fall in blood pressure in these patients, therapy should be started under very close medical supervision. Such patients should be followed closely for the first two weeks of treatment and whenever the dose of Lisinopril and/or diuretic is increased. Similar considerations apply to patients with ischemic heart or cerebrovascular disease in whom an excessive fall in blood pressure could result in a myocardial infarction or cerebrovascular accident.

If hypotension occurs, the patient should be placed in supine position and, if necessary, receive an intravenous infusion of normal saline. A transient hypotensive response is not a contraindication to further doses which usually can be given without difficulty once the blood pressure has increased after volume expansion.

Neutropenia/Agranulocytosis: Another angiotensin converting enzyme inhibitor, captopril, has been shown to cause agranulocytosis and bone marrow depression, rarely in uncomplicated patients but more frequently in patients with renal impairment, especially if they also have a collagen vascular disease. Available data from clinical trials of Lisinopril are insufficient to show that Lisinopril does not cause agranulocytosis at similar rates. Marketing experience has revealed rare cases of neutropenia and bone marrow depression in which a causal relationship to Lisinopril cannot be excluded. Periodic monitoring of white blood cell counts in patients with collagen vascular disease and renal disease should be considered.

PREGNANCY
Lisinopril and Hydrochlorothiazide: Teratogenicity studies were conducted in mice and rats with up to 90 mg/kg/day of Lisinopril (56 times the maximum recommended human dose) in combination with 10 mg/kg/day of Hydrochlorothiazide (2.5 times the maximum recommended human dose). Maternal or fetotoxic effects were not seen in mice with the combination. In rats decreased maternal weight gain and decreased fetal weight occurred down to 3/10 mg/kg/day (the lowest dose tested). Associated with the decreased fetal weight was a delay in fetal ossification. The decreased fetal weight and delay in fetal ossification were not seen in saline-supplemented animals given 90/10 mg/kg/day.

When used in pregnancy during the second and third trimesters, ACE inhibitors can cause injury and even death to the developing fetus. When pregnancy is detected Hydrochlorothiazide/Lisinopril should be discontinued as soon as possible. (See *"Lisinopril, Fetal/Neonatal Morbidity and Mortality"* below.)

LISINOPRIL
Fetal/Neonatal Morbidity and Mortality: ACE inhibitors can cause fetal and neonatal morbidity and death when administered to pregnant women. Several dozen cases have been reported in the world literature. When pregnancy is detected, ACE inhibitor therapy should be discontinued as soon as possible.

The use of ACE inhibitors during the second and third trimesters of pregnancy has been associated with fetal and neonatal injury, including hypotension, neonatal skull hypoplasia, anuria, reversible or irreversible renal failure, and death. Oligohydramnios has also been reported, presumably resulting from decreased fetal renal function; oligohydramnios in this setting has been associated with fetal limb contractures, craniofacial deformation, and hypoplastic lung development. Prematurity, intrauterine growth retardation, and patent ductus arteriosus have also been reported, although it is not clear whether these occurrences were due to the ACE-inhibitor exposure.

These adverse effects do not appear to have resulted from intrauterine ACE-inhibitor exposure that has been limited to the first trimester. Mothers whose embryos and fetuses are exposed to ACE inhibitors only during the first trimester should be so informed. Nonetheless, when patients become pregnant, physicians should make every effort to discontinue the use of Hydrochlorothiazide/Lisinopril as soon as possible.

Rarely (probably less often than once in every thousand pregnancies), no alternative to ACE inhibitors will be found. In these rare cases, the mothers should be apprised of the potential hazards to their fetuses, and serial ultrasound examinations should be performed to assess the intraamniotic environment.

If oligohydramnios is observed, Hydrochlorothiazide/Lisinopril should be discontinued unless it is considered lifesaving for the mother. Contraction stress testing (CST), a nonstress test (NST), or biophysical profiling (BPP) may be appropriate, depending upon the week of pregnancy. Patients and physicians should be aware, however, that oligohydramnios may not appear until after the fetus has sustained irreversible injury.

Infants with histories of in utero exposure to ACE inhibitors should be closely observed for hypotension, oliguria, and hyperkalemia. If oliguria occurs, attention should be directed toward support of blood pressure and renal perfusion. Exchange transfusion or dialysis may be required as means of reversing hypotension and/or substituting for disordered renal function. Lisinopril, which crosses the placenta, has been removed from neonatal circulation by peritoneal dialysis with some clinical benefit, and theoretically may be removed by exchange transfusion, although there is no experience with the latter procedure.

No teratogenic effects of Lisinopril were seen in studies of pregnant rats, mice, and rabbits. On a mg/kg basis, the doses used were up to 625 times (in mice), 188 times (in rats), 0.6 times (in rabbits) the maximum recommended human dose.

HYDROCHLOROTHIAZIDE
Teratogenic Effects: Reproduction studies in the rabbit, the mouse and the rat at doses up to 100 mg/kg/day (50 times the human dose) showed no evidence of external abnormalities of the fetus due to Hydrochlorothiazide. Hydrochlorothiazide given in a two-litter study in rats at doses of 4-5.6 mg/kg/day (approximately 1-2 times the usual daily human dose) did not impair fertility or produce birth abnormalities in the offspring. Thiazides cross the placental barrier and appear in cord blood.

Nonteratogenic Effects: These may include fetal or neonatal jaundice, thrombocytopenia, and possibly other adverse reactions have occurred in the adult.

HYDROCHLOROTHIAZIDE
Thiazides should be used with caution in severe renal disease. In patients with renal disease, thiazides may precipitate azotemia. Cumulative effects of the drug may develop in patients with impaired renal function.

Thiazides should be used with caution in patients with impaired hepatic function or progressive liver disease, since minor alterations of fluid and electrolyte balance may precipitate hepatic coma.

Sensitivity reactions may occur in patients with or without a history of allergy or bronchial asthma.

The possibility of exacerbation or activation of systemic lupus erythematosus has been reported.

Lithium generally should not be given with thiazides. (See *"Precautions, Drug Interactions, Lisinopril* and *Hydrochlorothiazide".*)

PRECAUTIONS
GENERAL
LISINOPRIL
Impaired Renal Function: As a consequence of inhibiting the renin-angiotensin-aldosterone system, changes in renal function may be anticipated in susceptible individuals. In patients with severe congestive heart failure whose renal function may depend on the activity of the renin-angiotensin-aldosterone system, treatment with angiotensin converting enzyme inhibitors, including Lisinopril, may be associated with oliguria and/or progressive azotemia and rarely with acute renal failure and/or death.

In hypertensive patients with unilateral or bilateral renal artery stenosis, increases in blood urea nitrogen and serum creatinine may occur. Experience with another angiotensin coverting enzyme inhibitor suggest that these increases are usually reversible upon discontinuation of Lisinopril and/or diuretic therapy. In such patients renal function should be monitored during the first few weeks of therapy. Some hypertensive patients with no apparent pre-existing renal vascular disease have developed increases in blood urea and serum creatinine, usually minor and transient, especially when Lisinopril has been given concomitantly with a diuretic. This is more likely to occur in patients with pre-existing renal impairment. Dosage reduction of Lisinopril and/or discontinuation of the diuretic may be required.

Evaluation of the hypertensive patient should always include assessment of renal function. (See *"Dosage and Administration".***)**

Hemodialysis Patients: Thiazide-containing combination products, such as Hydrochlorothiazide/Lisinopril are not recommended in patients with severe renal dysfunction. In patients treated with an ACE inhibitor, sudden and potentially life-threatening anaphylactoid reactions have been reported in some patients dialyzed with high-flux membranes (eg. AN69).

In such patients, dialysis must be stopped immediately, and aggressive therapy for anaphylactoid reactions be initiated. Symptoms have not responded to antihistamines in these situations. In these patients consideration should be given to using a different type of dialysis membrane or a different class of antihypertensive agent.

Hyperkalemia: In clinical trials hyperkalemia (serum potassium greater than 5.7 mEq/L) occurred in approximately 1.4 percent of hypertensive patients treated with Lisinopril plus Hydrochlorothiazide. In most cases these were isolated values which resolved despite continued therapy. Hyperkalemia was not a cause of discontinuation of therapy. Risk factors for the development of hyperkalemia include renal insufficiency, diabetes mellitus, and the concomitant use of potassium-sparing diuretics, potassium supplements and/or potassium-containing salt substitutes, which should be used cautiously if at all with Hydrochlorothiazide/Lisinopril. (See *"Drug Interactions".*)

Cough: Cough has been reported with the use of ACE inhibitors. Characteristically, the cough is nonproductive, persistent and resolves after discontinuation of therapy. ACE inhibitor-induced cough should be considered as part of the differential diagnosis of cough.

Surgery/Anesthesia: In patients undergoing major surgery or during anesthesia with agents that produce hypotension, Lisinopril may block angiotensin II formation secondary to compensatory renin release. If hypotension occurs and is considered to be due to this mechanism, it can be corrected by volume expansion.

HYDROCHLOROTHIAZIDE
Periodic determination of serum electrolytes to detect possible electrolyte imbalance should be performed at appropriate intervals.

All patients receiving thiazide therapy should be observed for clinical signs of fluid or electrolyte imbalance: namely, hyponatremia, hypochloremic alkalosis, and hypokalemia. Serum and urine electrolyte determinations are particularly important when the patient is vomiting excessively or receiving parenteral fluids. Warning signs or symptoms of fluid and electrolyte imbalance, irrespective of cause, include dryness of mouth, thirst, weakness, lethargy, drowsiness, restlessness, confusion, seizures, muscle pains or cramps, muscular fatigue hypotension, oliguria, tachycardia, and gastrointestinal disturbances such as nausea and vomiting.

Hypokalemia may develop, especially with brisk diuresis, when severe cirrhosis is present, or after prolonged therapy. Interference with adequate oral electrolyte intake will also contribute to hypokalemia. Hypokalemia may cause cardiac arrhythmia and may also sensitize or exaggerate the response of the heart to the toxic effects of digitalis (eg, increased ventricular irritability). Because Lisinopril reduces the production of aldosterone, concomitant therapy with Lisinopril attenuates the diuretic-induced potassium loss. (See *"Drug Interactions, Agents Increasing Serum Potassium".*)

Although any chloride deficit is generally, mild and usually does not require specific treatment, except under extraordinary circumstances (as in liver disease or renal disease), chloride replacement may be required in the treatment of metabolic alkalosis.

Dilutional hyponatremia may occur in edematous patients in hot weather; appropriate therapy is water restriction, rather than administration of salt except in rare instances when the hyponatremia is life-threatening. In actual salt depletion, appropriate replacement is the therapy of choice.

Hyperuricemia may occur or frank gout may be precipitated in certain patients receiving thiazide therapy.

In diabetic patients dosage adjustments of insulin or oral hypoglycemic agents may be required. Hyperglycemia may occur with thiazide diuretics. Thus latent diabetes mellitus may become manifest during thiazide therapy.

The antihypertensive effects of the drug may be enhanced in the postsympathectomy patient.

If progressive renal impairment becomes evident consider withholding or discontinuing diuretic therapy.

Thiazides have been shown to increase the urinary excretion of magnesium: this may result in hypomagnesemia.

Thiazides may decrease urinary calcium excretion. Thiazides may cause intermittent and slight elevation of serum calcium in the absence of known disorders of calcium metabolism. Marked hypercalcemia may be evidence of hidden hyperparathyroidism. Thiazides should be discontinued before carrying out tests for parathyroid function.

Increases in cholesterol and triglyceride levels may be associated with thiazide diuretic therapy.

INFORMATION FOR PATIENTS
Angioedema: Angioedema, including laryngeal edema, may occur especially following the first dose of Lisinopril. Patients should be so advised and told to report immediately any signs or symptoms suggesting angioedema (swelling of face, extremities, eyes, lips, tongue, difficulty in swallowing or breathing) and to take no more drug until they have consulted with the prescribing physician.

Symptomatic Hypotension: Patients should be cautioned to report light-headedness especially during the first few days of therapy. If actual syncope occurs, the patients should be told to discontinue the drug until they have consulted with the prescribing physician.

All patients should be cautioned that excessive perspiration and dehydration may lead to an excessive fall in blood pressure because of reduction in fluid volume. Other causes of volume depletion such as vomiting or diarrhea may also lead to a fall in blood pressure; patients should be advised to consult with their physician.

Hyperkalemia: Patients should be told not to use salt substitutes containing potassium without consulting their physician.

Neutropenia: Patients should be told to report promptly any indication of infection (eg, sore throat, fever) which may be a sign of neutropenia.

Pregnancy: Female patients of childbearing age should be told about the consequences of second- and third-trimester exposure to ACE inhibitors, and they should also be told that these consequences do not appear to have resulted from

intrauterine ACE-inhibitor exposure that has been limited to the first trimester. These patients should be asked to report pregnancies to their physicians as soon as possible.

Note: As with many other drugs, certain advise to patients being treated with Hydrochlorothiazide/Lisinopril is warranted. This information is intended to aid in the safe and effective use of this medication. It is not a disclosure of all possible adverse or intended effects.

DRUG INTERACTIONS
LISINOPRIL
Hypotension—Patients of Diuretic Therapy: Patients on diuretics and especially those in whom diuretic therapy was recently instituted, may occasionally experience an excessive reduction of blood pressure after initiation of therapy with Lisinopril. The possibility of hypotensive effects with Lisinopril can be minimized by either discontinuing the diuretic or increasing the salt intake prior to initiation of treatment with Lisinopril at a dose of 5 mg daily, and provide close medical supervision after the initial dose for at least two hours and until blood pressure has stabilized for at least an additional hour. (See *"Warnings"* and *"Dosage and Administration".*) When a diuretic is added to the therapy of a patient receiving Lisinopril, an additional antihypertensive effect is usually observed. (See *"Dosage and Administration".*)

Indomethacin: In a study in 36 patients with mild to moderate hypertension where the antihypertensive effects of Lisinopril alone were compared to Lisinopril given concomitantly with indomethacin, the use of indomethacin was associated with a reduced effect, although the difference between the two regimens was not significant.

Other Agents: Lisinopril has been used concomitantly with nitrates and/or digoxin without evidence of clinically significant adverse interactions. No meaningful clinically important pharmacokinetic interactions occurred when Lisinopril was used concomitantly with propranolol, digoxin, or Hydrochlorothiazide. The presence of food in the stomach does not alter the bioavailability of Lisinopril.

Agents Increasing Serum Potassium: Lisinopril attenuates potassium loss caused by thiazide-type diuretics. Use of Lisinopril with potassium-sparing diuretics (eg, spironolactone, triamterene, or amiloride), potassium supplements, or potassium-containing salt substitutes may lead to significant increases in serum potassium. Therefore, if concomitant use of these agents is indicated, because of demonstrated hypokalemia, they should be used with caution and with frequent monitoring of serum potassium.

Lithium: Lithium toxicity has been reported in patients receiving lithium concomitantly with drugs which cause elimination of sodium, including ACE inhibitors. Lithium toxicity was usually reversible upon discontinuation of lithium and the ACE inhibitor. It is recommended that serum lithium levels be monitored frequently if Lisinopril is administered concomitantly with lithium.

HYDROCHLOROTHIAZIDE
When administered concurrently the following drugs may interact with thiazide diuretics:

Alcohol, barbiturates, or narcotics: potentiation of orthostatic hypotension may occur.

Antidiabetic drugs (oral agents and insulin): dosage adjustment of the antidiabetic drug may be required.

Other antihypertensive drugs: additive effect or potentiation.

Cholestyramine and colestipol resins: Cholestyramine and colestipol resins bind the Hydrochlorothiazide and reduce its absorption from the gastrointestinal tract by up to 85 and 43 percent, respectively. Thiazides may be administered two to four hours before the resin when the two drugs are used concomitantly.

Corticosteroids, ACTH: intensified electrolyte depletion, particularly hypokalemia.

Pressor amines (eg, norepinephrine): possible decreased response to pressor amines but not sufficient to preclude their use.

Skeletal muscle relaxants, nondepolarizing (eg, tubocurarine): possible increased responsiveness to the muscle relaxant.

Lithium: should not generally be given with diuretics. Diuretic agents reduce the renal clearance of lithium and add a high risk of lithium toxicity. Refer to the package insert for lithium preparations before use of such preparations with Hydrochlorothiazide/Lisinopril.

Nonsteroidal Anti-inflammatory Drugs: In some patients, the administration of a nonsteroidal anti-inflammatory agent can reduce the diuretic, natriuretic, and antihypertensive effects of loop, potassium-sparing and thiazide diuretics. Therefore, when Hydrochlorothiazide/Lisinopril and nonsteroidal anti-inflammatory agents are used concomitantly, the patient should be observed closely to determine if the desired effect of Hydrochlorothiazide/Lisinopril is obtained.

CARCINOGENESIS, MUTAGENESIS, IMPAIRMENT OF FERTILITY
Lisinopril and Hydrochlorothiazide: Lisinopril in combination with Hydrochlorothiazide was not mutagenic in a microbial mutagen test using *Salmonella typhimurium* (Ames test) or *Escherichia coli* with or without metabolic activation or in a forward mutation assay using Chinese hamster lung cells. Lisinopril and Hydrochlorothiazide did not produce DNA single strand breaks in an *in vitro* alkaline elution rat hepatocyte assay. In addition, it did not produce increases in

---

chromosomal aberrations in an *in vitro* test in Chinese hamster ovary cells or in an *in vivo* study in mouse bone marrow.

Lisinopril: There was no evidence of a tumorigenic effect when Lisinopril was administered for 105 weeks to male and female rats at doses up to 90 mg/kg/day (about 56 or 9 times* the maximum daily human dose, based on body weight and body surface area respectively). There was no evidence of carcinogenicity when Lisinopril was administered for 92 weeks to (male and female) mice at doses up to 135 mg/kg/day (about 84 times* the maximum recommended daily human dose). This dose was 6.8 times the maximum human dose based on body surface area in mice.

* Calculations assume a human weight of 50 kg and human body surface area of 1.62 m^2.

Lisinopril was not mutagenic in the Ames microbial mutagen test with or without metabolic activation. It was also negative in a forward mutation assay using Chinese hamster lung cells. Lisinopril did not produce single strand DNA breaks in an *in vitro* alkaline elution rat hepatocyte assay. In addition, Lisinopril did not produce increase in chromosomal aberrations in an *in vitro* test in Chinese hamster ovary cells or in an *in vivo* study in mouse bone marrow.

There were no adverse effects on reproductive performance in male and female rats treated with up to 300 mg/kg/day of Lisinopril. This dose is 188 times and 30 times the maximum daily human dose based on mg/kg and mg/m^2, respectively.

Hydrochlorothiazide: Two-year feeding studies in mice and rats conducted under the auspices of the National Toxicology Program (NTP) uncovered no evidence of a carcinogenic potential of Hydrochlorothiazide in female mice (at doses of up to approximately 600 mg/kg/day) or in male and female rats (at doses of up to approximately 100 mg/kg/day). These doses are 150 times and 12 times for mice and 25 times and 4 times for rats the maximum human daily dose based on mg/kg and mg/m^2, respectively. The NTP, however, found equivocal evidence for hepatocarcinogenicity in male mice.

Hydrochlorothiazide was not genotoxic *in vitro* in the Ames mutagenicity assay of *Salmonella typhimurium* strains TA 98, TA 100, TA 1535, TA 1537, and TA 1538 and in the Chinese Hamster Ovary (CHO) test for chromosomal aberrations, or *in vivo* in assays using mouse germinal cell chromosomes. Chinese hamster bone marrow chromosomes, and the *Drosophilia* sex-linked recessive lethal trait gene. Positive test results were obtained only in the *in vitro* CHO Sister Chromatid Exchange (clastogenicity) and in the Mouse Lymphoma Cell (mutagenicity) assays, using concentrations of Hydrochlorothiazide from 43 to 1300 μg/mL, and in the *Aspergillus nidulans* nondisjunction assay at an unspecified concentration.

Hydrochlorothiazide had no adverse effect on the fertility of mice and rats of either sex in studies in wherein these species were exposed via their diet, to doses of up to 100 and 4 mg/kg/day, respectively, prior to conception and throughout gestation. In mice this dose is 25 times and 2 times the maximum daily human dose based on mg/kg and mg/m^2, respectively. In rats this dose is 1 times and 0.2 times the maximum daily human dose based on mg/kg and mg/m^2, respectively.

PREGNANCY
Pregnancy Categories C (first trimester) and D (second and third trimesters): See *"Warnings, Pregnancy, Lisinopril, Fetal/Neonatal Morbidity and Mortality".)*

NURSING MOTHERS
It is not known whether Lisinopril is excreted in human milk. However, milk of lactating rats contains radioactivity following administration of ^{14}C Lisinopril. In another study, Lisinopril was present in rat milk at levels similar to plasma levels in the dams. Thiazides do appear in human milk. Because of the potential for serious adverse reactions in nursing infants from ACE inhibitors and Hydrochlorothiazide, a decision should be made whether to discontinue nursing and/or discontinue Hydrochlorothiazide/Lisinopril, taking into account the importance of the drug to the mother.

PEDIATRIC USE
Safety and effectiveness in children have not been established.

ADVERSE REACTIONS
Hydrochlorothiazide/Lisinopril has been evaluated for safety in 930 patients including 100 patients treated for 50 weeks or more.

In clinical trials with Hydrochlorothiazide/Lisinopril no adverse experiences peculiar to this combination drug have been observed. Adverse experiences that have occurred have been limited to those that have been previously reported with Lisinopril or Hydrochlorothiazide.

The most frequent clinical adverse experiences in controlled trials (including open label extensions) with any combination of Lisinopril and Hydrochlorothiazide were: dizziness (7.5%), headache (5.2%), cough (3.9%), fatigue (3.7%) and orthostatic effects (3.2%) all of which were more common than in placebo-treated patients. Generally, adverse experiences were mild and transient in nature, but see *"Warnings"* regarding angioedema and excessive hypotension or syncope. Discontinuation of therapy due to adverse effects was required in 4.4% of patients principally because of dizziness, cough, fatigue and muscle cramps.

Adverse experiences occurring in greater than one percent of patients treated with Lisinopril plus Hydrochlorothiazide in controlled clinical trials are shown below.

PERCENT OF PATIENTS IN CONTROLLED STUDIES

	Lisinopril and Hydrochlorothiazide (n=930) Incidence (discontinuation)		Placebo (n=207) Incidence
Dizziness	7.5	(0.8)	1.9
Headache	5.2	(0.3)	1.9
Cough	3.9	(0.6)	1.0
Fatigue	3.7	(0.4)	1.0
Orthostatic Effects	3.2	(0.1)	1.0
Diarrhea	2.5	(0.2)	2.4
Nausea	2.2	(0.1)	2.4
Upper Respiratory Infection	2.2	(0.0)	0.0
Muscle Cramps	2.0	(0.4)	0.5
Asthenia	1.8	(0.2)	1.0
Paresthesia	1.5	(0.1)	0.0
Hypotension	1.4	(0.3)	0.5
Vomiting	1.4	(0.1)	0.5
Dyspepsia	1.3	(0.0)	0.0
Rash	1.2	(0.1)	0.5
Impotence	1.2	(0.3)	0.0

Clinical adverse experiences occurring in 0.3% to 1.0% of patients in controlled trails included:

Body as a Whole: Chest pain, abdominal pain, syncope, chest discomfort, fever, trauma, virus infection.

Cardiovascular: Palpitation, orthostatic hypotension.

Digestive: Gastrointestinal cramps, dry mouth, constipation, heartburn.

Musculoskeletal: Back pain, shoulder pain, knee pain, back strain, myalgia, foot pain.

Nervous/Psychiatric: Decreased libido, vertigo, depression, somnolence.

Respiratory: Common cold, nasal congestion, influenza, bronchitis, pharyngeal pain, dyspnea, pulmonary congestion, chronic sinusitis, allergic rhinitis, pharyngeal discomfort.

Skin: Flushing, pruritus, skin inflammation, diaphoresis.

Special Senses: Blurred vision, tinnitus, otalgia.

Urogenital: Urinary tract infection.

Angioedema: Angioedema of the face, extremities, lips, tongue, glottis and/or larynx has been reported rarely. (See *"Warnings".*)

Hypotension: In clinical trials, adverse effects relating to hypotension occurred as follows: hypotension (1.4%), orthostatic hypotension (0.5%), other orthostatic effects (3.2%). In addition syncope occurred in 0.8% of patients. (See *"Warnings".*)

Cough: See *"Precautions, Cough".*

CLINICAL LABORATORY TEST FINDINGS
Serum Electrolytes: (See *"Precautions".*)

Creatinine, Blood Urea Nitrogen: Minor reversible increases in blood urea nitrogen and serum creatinine were observed in patients with essential hypertension treated with Hydrochlorothiazide/Lisinopril. More marked increases have also been reported and were more likely to occur in patients with renal artery stenosis. (See *"Precautions".*)

Serum Uric Acid, Glucose, Magnesium, Cholesterol, Triglycerides and Calcium: (See *"Precautions".*)

Hemoglobin and Hematocrit: Small decreases in hemoglobin and hematocrit (mean decreases of approximately 0.5 g% and 1.5 vol%, respectively) occurred frequently in hypertensive patients treated with Hydrochlorothiazide/Lisinopril but were rarely of clinical importance unless another cause of anemia coexisted. In clinical trials. 0.4% of patients discontinued therapy due to anemia.

Liver Function Tests: Rarely, elevations of liver enzymes and/or serum bilirubin have occurred.

Other adverse reactions that have been reported with the individual components are listed below:

Lisinopril: Lisinopril has been evaluated for safety in 2003 patients. In clinical trials adverse reactions which occurred with Lisinopril were also seen with Hydrochlorothiazide/Lisinopril. In addition and since Lisinopril has been marketed, the following adverse reactions have been reported.

Body as a Whole: Malaise, anaphylactoid reactions (See *"Precautions-Hemodialysis Patients"*);

Cardiovascular: Myocardial infarction or cerebrovascular accident, possibly secondary to excessive hypotension in high risk patients (see *"Warnings, Hypotension"*); angina pectoris, rhythm disturbances, tachycardia, peripheral edema, vasculitis;

Digestive: Pancreatitis, hepatitis (hepatocellular or cholestatic jaundice), anorexia, flatulence;

Hematologic: Rare cases of neutropenia, thrombocytopenia and bone marrow depression have been reported in which a causal relationship to Lisinopril cannot be excluded;

Metabolic: Gout;

Musculoskeletal: Joint pain;

Nervous System/Psychiatric: Insomnia, stroke, nervousness, confusion;

Skin: Urticaria, photosensitivity;

Urogenital: Oliguria, progressive azotemia, acute renal failure.

Miscellaneous: A symptom complex has been reported which may include a positive ANA, an elevated erythrocyte sedimentation rate, arthralgia/arthritis, myalgia, fever, vasculitis, eosinophilia and leukocytosis. Rash, photosensitivity or other dermatological manifestations may occur alone or in combination with these symptoms.

FETAL/NEONATAL MORBIDITY AND MORTALITY
See *"Warnings—Pregnancy, Lisinopril, Fetal/Neonatal Morbidity and Mortality"*.

Hydrochlorothiazide: Body as a Whole: Weakness;

Digestive: Anorexia, gastric irritation, cramping, jaundice (intrahepatic cholestatic jaundice), pancreatitis, sialoadenitis, constipation;

Hematologic: Leukopenia, agranulocytosis, thrombocytopenia, aplastic anemia, hemolytic anemia;

Musculoskeletal: Muscle spasm;

Nervous System/Psychiatric: Restlessness;

Renal: Renal failure, renal dysfunction, interstitial nephritis (see *"Warnings"*);

Skin: Erythema multiforme including Stevens-Johnson syndrome, exfoliative dermatitis including toxic epidermal necrolysis, alopecia;

Special Senses: Xanthopsia;

Hypersensitivity: Purpura, photo-sensitivity, urticaria, necrotizing angitis (vasculitis and cutaneous vasculitis, respiratory distress including pneumonitis and pulmonary edema, anaphylactic reactions.

OVERDOSAGE
No specific information is available on the treatment of overdosage with Hydrochlorothiazide/Lisinopril. Treatment is symptomatic and supportive. Therapy with Hydrochlorothiazide/Lisinopril should be discontinued and the patient observed closely. Suggested measures include induction of emesis and/or gastric lavage, and correction of dehydration, electrolyte imbalance and hypotension by established procedures.

Lisinopril: Following a single oral dose of 20g/kg no lethality occurred in rats and death occurred in one of 20 mice receiving the same dose. The most likely manifestation of overdosage would be hypotension, for which the usual treatment would be intravenous infusion of normal saline solution.

Lisinopril can be removed by hemodialysis.

Hydrochlorothiazide: Oral administration of a single oral dose of 10g/kg mice and rats was not lethal. The most common signs and symptoms observed are those caused by electrolyte depletion (hypokalemia, hypochloremia, hyponatremia) and dehydration resulting from excessive diuresis. If digitalis has also been administered, hypokalemia may accentuate cardiac arrhythmias.

DOSAGE AND ADMINISTRATION
DOSAGE MUST BE INDIVIDUALIZED. THE FIXED COMBINATION IS NOT FOR INITIAL THERAPY. IT MAY BE SUBSTITUTED FOR THE TITRATED INDIVIDUAL COMPONENTS. ALTERNATIVELY, PATIENTS WHO HAVE RECEIVED LISINOPRIL MONOTHERAPY 20 OR 40 MG MAY BE GIVEN HYDROCHLOROTHIAZIDE/LISINOPRIL (20-12.5), THEN HYDROCHLOROTHIAZIDE/LISINOPRIL (20-25), THUS TITRATING THE HYDROCHLOROTHIAZIDE COMPONENT USING THE COMBINATION.

The usual dose is one or two tablets of Hydrochlorothiazide/Lisinopril or Hydrochlorothiazide/Lisinopril 20-25 once daily. The recommended dose of Hydrochlorothiazide/Lisinopril 10-12.5 is one tablet daily. (See *"Indications and Usage"* and *"Warnings"*.) However, because data from a clinical trial suggest that the mean group antihypertensive response is similar when Lisinopril 20 mg is combined with Hydrochlorothiazide 12.5 mg or 25 mg, patients whose blood pressure is controlled with Lisinopril 20 mg plus Hydrochlorothiazide 25 mg ordinarily should be given a trial of Hydrochlorothiazide/Lisinopril 20-12.5 before Hydrochlorothiazide/Lisinopril 20-25 is used. (See *"Description, Lisinopril and Hydrochlorothiazide."*)

Patients usually do not require doses in excess of 50 mg of Hydrochlorothiazide daily, particularly when it is combined with other antihypertensive agents.

For Lisinopril monotherapy the recommended initial dose in patients not on diuretics is 10 mg of Lisinopril once a day. Dosage should be adjusted according to blood pressure response. The usual dosage range of Lisinopril is 20 to 40 mg administered in a single daily dose; the maximum recommended dose is 80 mg in a single daily dose. Blood pressure should be measured at the interdosing interval to ensure that there is an adequate antihypertensive response at that time. If blood pressure is not controlled with Lisinopril alone, a diuretic may be added. Hydrochlorothiazide 12.5 mg has been shown to provide an additive effect. After addition of the diuretic it may be possible to reduce the dose of Lisinopril. In patients who are currently being treated with a diuretic, symptomatic hypotension occasionally may occur following the initial dose of Lisinopril. The diuretic should, if possible, be discontinued for two to three days before beginning therapy with Lisinopril to reduce the likelihood of hypotension. (See *"Warnings"*.) If the patient's blood pressure is not controlled with Lisinopril alone, diuretic therapy may be resumed.

If the diuretic cannot be discontinued, an initial dose of 5 mg of Lisinopril should be used under medical supervision for at least two hours and until blood pressure has stabilized for at least an additional hour. (See *"Warnings"* and *"Precautions, Drug Interactions"*.)

Concomitant administration of Hydrochlorothiazide/Lisinopril with potassium supplements, potassium salt substitutes or potassium-sparing diuretics may lead to increases of serum potassium. (See *"Precautions"*.)

Dosage Adjustment in Renal Impairment: The usual dose of Hydrochlorothiazide/Lisinopril is recommended for patients with a creatinine clearance > 30 mL/min (serum creatinine of up to approximately 3 mg/dL).

When concomitant diuretic therapy is required in patients with severe renal impairment, a loop diuretic, rather than a thiazide diuretic is preferred for use with Lisinopril; therefore, for patients with severe renal dysfunction the Lisinopril and Hydrochlorothiazide combination tablet is not recommended.

Use in Elderly: In general, blood pressure response and adverse experiences were similar in younger and older patients given Hydrochlorothiazide/Lisinopril. However, in a multiple dose pharmacokinetic study in elderly versus young patients using the Lisinopril/Hydrochlorothiazide combination, area under the plasma concentration time curve (AUC) increased approximately 120% for Lisinopril and approximately 80% for Hydrochlorothiazide in older patients. Therefore, dosage adjustments in elderly patients should be made with particular caution.

Storage: Store at controlled room temperature, 15-30°C (59-86°F).
Protect from excessive light and humidity.
Dispense in a well-closed container, if product package is subdivided.

HOW SUPPLIED
TABLETS: 10 MG-12.5 MG

AVERAGE UNIT PRICE (AVAILABLE SIZES)			
BRAND	$0.88		

BRAND/MANUFACTURER	NDC	SIZE	AWP
◆ BRAND			
► PRINZIDE: Merck	00006-0145-31	30s	$26.45
	00006-0145-58	100s	$88.18

TABLETS: 20 MG-12.5 MG

AVERAGE UNIT PRICE (AVAILABLE SIZES)			
BRAND	$0.94		

BRAND/MANUFACTURER	NDC	SIZE	AWP
◆ BRAND			
► PRINZIDE: Merck	00006-0140-31	30s	$28.32
► ZESTORETIC: Stuart	00038-0142-10	100s	$94.22
► PRINZIDE: Merck	00006-0140-58	100s	$94.40

TABLETS: 20 MG-25 MG

AVERAGE UNIT PRICE (AVAILABLE SIZES)			
BRAND	$0.96		

BRAND/MANUFACTURER	NDC	SIZE	AWP
◆ BRAND			
► PRINZIDE: Merck	00006-0142-31	30s	$28.66
► ZESTORETIC: Stuart	00038-0145-10	100s	$95.39
► PRINZIDE: Merck	00006-0142-58	100s	$95.57

Hydrochlorothiazide and Methyldopa

WARNING

THIS FIXED COMBINATION DRUG IS NOT INDICATED FOR INITIAL THERAPY OF HYPERTENSION. HYPERTENSION REQUIRES THERAPY TITRATED TO THE INDIVIDUAL PATIENT. IF THE FIXED COMBINATION REPRESENTS THE DOSAGE SO DETERMINED, ITS USE MAY BE MORE CONVENIENT IN PATIENT MANAGEMENT. THE TREATMENT OF HYPERTENSION IS NOT STATIC, BUT MUST BE RE-EVALUATED AS CONDITIONS IN EACH PATIENT WARRANT.

DESCRIPTION
Hydrochlorothiazide/Methyldopa (HCTZ/Methyldopa) combines two antihypertensives: Methyldopa and Hydrochlorothiazide.

Each tablet contains:

Methyldopa	250 mg
Hydrochlorothiazide	15 mg
Methyldopa	250 mg
Hydrochlorothiazide	25 mg
Methyldopa	500 mg
Hydrochlorothiazide	30 mg
Methyldopa	500 mg
Hydrochlorothiazide	50 mg

◆ RATED THERAPEUTICALLY EQUIVALENT; ◇ THERAPEUTIC EQUIVALENCE UNCONFIRMED; ○ UNRATED

METHYLDOPA

Methyldopa is an antihypertensive and is the *L*-isomer of alphamethyldopa. It is levo-3-(3,4-dihydroxyphenyl)-2-methylalanine. Its empirical formula is $C_{10}H_{13}NO_4$, with a molecular weight of 211.22.

Methyldopa is a white to yellowish white, odorless fine powder, and is soluble in water.

HYDROCHLOROTHIAZIDE

Hydrochlorothiazide is a diuretic and antihypertensive. It is the 3,4-dihydro derivative of chlorothiazide. Its chemical name is 6-chloro-3,4-dihydro-2*H*-1,2,4-benzothiadiazine-7-sulfonamide 1,1-dioxide. Its empirical formula is $C_7H_8ClN_3O_4S_2$.

Hydrochlorothiazide is a white, or practically white, crystalline powder with a molecular weight of 297.72, which is slightly soluble in water, but freely soluble in sodium hydroxide solution.

CLINICAL PHARMACOLOGY

METHYLDOPA

Methyldopa is an aromatic-amino-acid decarboxylase inhibitor in animals and in man. Although the mechanism of action has yet to be conclusively demonstrated, the antihypertensive effect of Methyldopa probably is due to its metabolism to alpha-methylnorepinephrine, which then lowers arterial pressure by stimulation of central inhibitory alpha-adrenergic receptors, false neurotransmission, and/or reduction of plasma renin activity. Methyldopa has been shown to cause a net reduction in the tissue concentration of serotonin, dopamine, norepinephrine, and epinephrine.

Only Methyldopa, the *L*-isomer of alpha-Methyldopa, has the ability to inhibit dopa decarboxylase and to deplete animal tissues of norepinephrine. In man, the antihypertensive activity appears to be due solely to the *L*-isomer. About twice the dose of the racemate (*DL*-alpha-methyldopa) is required for equal antihypertensive effect.

Methyldopa has no direct effect on cardiac function and usually does not reduce glomerular filtration rate, renal blood flow, or filtration fraction. Cardiac output usually is maintained without cardiac acceleration. In some patients the heart rate is slowed.

Normal or elevated plasma renin activity may decrease in the course of Methyldopa therapy.

Methyldopa reduces both supine and standing blood pressure. It usually produces highly effective lowering of the supine pressure with infrequent symptomatic postural hypotension. Exercise hypotension and diurnal blood pressure variations rarely occur.

HYDROCHLOROTHIAZIDE

The mechanism of the antihypertensive effect of thiazides is unknown. Hydrochlorothiazide does not usually affect normal blood pressure.

Hydrochlorothiazide affects the distal renal tubular mechanism of electrolyte reabsorption. At maximal therapeutic dosage all thiazides are approximately equal in their diuretic efficacy.

Hydrochlorothiazide increases excretion of sodium and chloride in approximately equivalent amounts. Natriuresis may be accompanied by some loss of potassium and bicarbonate. After oral use diuresis begins within 2 hours, peaks in about 4 hours and lasts about 6 to 12 hours.

PHARMACOKINETICS AND METABOLISM

Methyldopa: The maximum decrease in blood pressure occurs four to six hours after oral dosage. Once an effective dosage level is attained, a smooth blood pressure response occurs in most patients in 12 to 24 hours. After withdrawal, blood pressure usually returns to pretreatment levels within 24-48 hours. Methyldopa is extensively metabolized. The known urinary metabolites are: α-methyldopa mono-0-sulfate; 3-0-methyl-α-methyldopa; 3,4-dihydroxyphenylacetone; α-methyldopamine; 3-0-methyl-α-methyldopamine and their conjugates. Approximately 70 percent of the drug which is absorbed is excreted in the urine as Methyldopa and its mono-0-sulfate conjugate. The renal clearance is about 130 mL/min in normal subjects and is diminished in renal insufficiency. The plasma half-life of methyldopa is 105 minutes. After oral doses, excretion is essentially complete in 36 hours.

Methyldopa crosses the placental barrier, appears in cord blood, and appears in breast milk.

Hydrochlorothiazide: Hydrochlorothiazide is not metabolized but is eliminated rapidly by the kidney. When plasma levels have been followed for at least 24 hours, the plasma half-life has been observed to vary between 5.6 and 14.8 hours. At least 61 percent of the oral dose is eliminated unchanged within 24 hours. Hydrochlorothiazide crosses the placental but not the blood-brain barrier and is excreted in breast milk.

INDICATION AND USAGE

Hypertension (see box *"Warning"*).

CONTRAINDICATIONS

Active hepatic disease, such as acute hepatitis and active cirrhosis.

If previous Methyldopa therapy has been associated with liver disorders (see *"Warnings"*).

Anuria.

Hypersensitivity to Methyldopa, or to Hydrochlorothiazide or other sulfonamide-derived drugs.

WARNINGS

METHYLDOPA

It is important to recognize that a positive Coombs test, hemolytic anemia, and liver disorders may occur with methyldopa therapy. The rare occurrences of hemolytic anemia or liver disorders could lead to potentially fatal complications unless properly recognized and managed. Read this section carefully to understand these reactions.

With prolonged Methyldopa therapy, 10 to 20 percent of patients develop a positive direct Coombs test which usually occurs between 6 and 12 months of Methyldopa therapy. Lowest incidence is at daily dosage of 1 g or less. This on rare occasions may be associated with hemolytic anemia, which could lead to potentially fatal complications. One cannot predict which patients with a positive direct Coombs test may develop hemolytic anemia.

Prior existence or development of a positive direct Coombs test is not in itself a contraindication to use of Methyldopa. If a positive Coombs test develops during Methyldopa therapy, the physician should determine whether hemolytic anemia exists and whether the positive Coombs test may be a problem. For example, in addition to a positive direct Coombs test there is less often a positive indirect Coombs test which may interfere with cross matching of blood.

Before treatment is started it is desirable to do a blood count (hematocrit, hemoglobin, or red cell count) for a baseline or to establish whether there is anemia. Periodic blood counts should be done during therapy to detect hemolytic anemia. It may be useful to do a direct Coombs test before therapy and at 6 and 12 months after the start of therapy.

If Coombs-positive hemolytic anemia occurs, the cause may be Methyldopa and the drug should be discontinued. Usually the anemia remits promptly. If not, corticosteroids may be given and other causes of anemia should be considered. If the hemolytic anemia is related to Methyldopa, the drug should not be reinstituted.

When Methyldopa causes Coombs positivity alone or with hemolytic anemia, the red cells is usually coated with gamma globulin of the IgG (gamma G) class only. The positive Coombs test may not revert to normal until weeks to months after Methyldopa is stopped.

Should the need for transfusion arise in a patient receiving Methyldopa, both a direct and an indirect Coombs test should be performed. In the absence of hemolytic anemia, usually only the direct Coombs test will be positive. A positive direct Coombs test alone will not interfere with typing or cross matching. If the indirect Coombs test is also positive, problems may arise in the major cross match and the assistance of a hemotologist or transfusion expert will be needed. Occasionally, fever has occurred within the first three weeks of Methyldopa therapy, associated in some cases with eosinophilia or abnormalities in one or more liver function tests, such as serum alkaline phosphatase, serum transaminases (SGOT, SGPT), bilirubin, and prothrombin time. Jaundice, with or without fever, may occur with onset usually within the first two to three months of therapy. In some patients the findings are consistent with those of cholestasis. In others the findings are consistent with hepatitis and hepatocellular injury.

Rarely fatal hepatic necrosis has been reported after use of methyldopa. These hepatic changes may represent hypersensitivity reactions. Periodic determination of hepatic function should be done particularly during the first 6 to 12 weeks of therapy or whenever an unexplained fever occurs. If fever, abnormalities in liver function tests, or jaundice appear, stop therapy with Methyldopa. If caused by methyldopa, the temperature and abnormalities in liver function characteristically have reverted to normal when the drug was discontinued. Methyldopa should not be reinstituted in such patients.

Rarely, a reversible reduction of the white blood cell count with a primary effect on the granulocytes has been seen. The granulocyte count returned promptly to normal on discontinuance of the drug. Rare cases of granulocytopenia have been reported. In each instance, upon stopping the drug, the white cell count returned to normal. Reversible thrombocytopenia has occurred rarely.

HYDROCHLOROTHIAZIDE

Use with caution in severe renal disease. In patients with renal disease, thiazides may precipitate azotemia. Cumulative effects of the drug may develop in patients with impaired renal function.

Thiazides should be used with caution in patients with impaired hepatic function or progressive liver disease, since minor alterations of fluid and electrolyte balance may precipitate hepatic coma.

Thiazides may add to or potentiate the action of other antihypertensive drugs. Sensitivity reactions may occur in patients with or without a history of allergy or bronchial asthma.

The possibility of exacerbation or activation of systemic lupus erythematosus has been reported.

Lithium generally should not be given with diuretics (see *"Precautions, Drug Interactions"*).

PRECAUTIONS

GENERAL

METHYLDOPA

Methyldopa should be used with caution in patients with a history of previous liver disease or dysfunction (see *"Warnings"*).

Some patients taking Methyldopa experience clinical edema or weight gain which may be controlled by use of a diuretic. Methyldopa should not be continued if edema progresses or signs of heart failure appear.

Hypertension has recurred occassionally after dialysis in patients given Methyldopa because the drug is removed by this procedure.

Rarely involuntary choreoathetotic movements have been observed during therapy with methyldopa in patients with severe bilateral cerebrovascular disease. Should these movements occur, stop therapy.

HYDROCHLOROTHIAZIDE

All patients receiving diuretic therapy should be observed for evidence of fluid or electrolyte imbalance: namely: hyponatremia, hypochloremic alkalosis, and hypokalemia. Serum and urine electrolyte determinations are particularly important when the patient is vomiting excessively or receiving pareternal fluids. Warning signs or symptoms of fluid and electrolyte imbalance, irrespective of cause, include dryness of mouth, thirst, weakness, lethargy, drowsiness, restlessness, confusion, seizures, muscle pains or cramps, muscular fatigue, hypotension, oliguria, tachycardia, and gastrointestinal disturbances such as nausea and vomiting.

Hypokalemia may develop especially after prolonged therapy or when severe cirrhosis is present (see "Contraindications" and "Warnings").

Interference with adequate oral electrolyte intake will also contribute to hypokalemia. Hypokalemia may cause cardiac arrhythmia and may also sensitize or exaggerate the response of the heart to the toxic effects of digitalis (e.g., increased ventricular irritability). Hypokalemia may be avoided or treated by use of potassium sparing diuretics or potassium supplements such as foods with a high potassium content.

Although any chloride deficit is generally mild and usually does not require specific treatment except under extraordinary circumstances (as in liver disease or renal disease), chloride replacement may be required in the treatment of metabolic alkalosis.

Dilutional hyponatremia may occur in edematous patients in hot weather: appropriate therapy is water restriction, rather than administration of salt, except in rare instances when the hyponatremia is life threatening. In actual salt depletion, appropriate replacement is the therapy of choice. Hyperuricemia may occur or acute gout may be precipitated in certain patients receiving thiazides.

In diabetic patients dosage adjustment of insulin or oral hypoglycemic agents may be required. Hyperglycemia may occur with thiazide diuretics. Thus latent diabetes mellitus may become manifest during thiazide therapy.

The antihypertensive effects of the drug may be enhanced in the postsympathectomy patient.

If progressive renal impairment becomes evident, consider withholding or discontinuing diuretic therapy.

Thiazides have been shown to increase the urinary excretion of magnesium; this may result in hypomagnesemia.

Thiazides may decrease urinary calcium excretion. Thiazides may cause intermittent and slight elevation of serum calcium in the absence of known disorders of calcium metabolism. Marked hypercalcemia may be evidence of hidden hyperparathyroidism. Thiazides should be discontinued before carrying out tests for parathyroid function.

Increases in cholesterol and triglyceride levels may be associated with thiazide diuretic therapy.

LABORATORY TESTS

METHYLDOPA

Blood count. Coombs test and liver function test, are recommended before initiating therapy and at periodic intervals (see "Warnings").

HYDROCHLOROTHIAZIDE

Periodic determination of serum electrolytes to detect possible electrolyte imbalance should be done at appropriate intervals.

DRUG INTERACTIONS

METHYLDOPA

When Methyldopa is used with other antihypertensive drugs, potentiation of antihypertensive effect may occur. Patients should be followed carefully to detect side reactions or unusual manifestations of drug idiosyncrasy.

Patients may require reduced doses of anesthetics when on Methyldopa. If hypotension does occur during anesthesia, it usually can be controlled by vasopressors. The adrenergic receptors remain sensitive during treatment with Methyldopa.

HYDROCHLOROTHIAZIDE

When given concurrently the following drugs may interact with thiazide diuretics.

Alcohol, Barbiturates, or Narcotics: potentiation of orthostatic hypotension may occur.

Antidiabetic Drugs: (Oral Agents and Insulin)—dosage adjustment of the antidiabetic drug may be required.

Other Antihypertensive Drugs: additive effect or potentiation.

Cholestyramine and Colestipol Resins: Absorption of hydrochlorothiazide is impaired in the presence of anionic exchange resins. Single doses of either Cholestyramine or Colestipol resins bind the Hydrochlorothiazide and reduce its absorption from the gastrointestinal tract by up to 85 and 43 percent, respectively.

Corticosteriods, ACTH: intensified electrolyte depletion, particularly hypokalemia.

Pressor Amines (e.g., norepinephrine): possible decreased response to pressor amines but not sufficient to preclude their use.

Skeletal Muscle Relaxants, Nondepolarizing (e.g., Tubocurarine): possible increased responsiveness to the muscle relaxant.

Lithium: genrally should not be given with diuretics. Diuretic agents reduce the renal clearance of lithium and add a high risk of lithium toxicity. Refer to the package insert for lithium preparations before use of such preparations with HCTZ/Methyldopa.

Nonsteroidal Anti-inflammatory Drugs: In some patients, the administration of a nonsteroidal anti-inflammatory agent can reduce the diuretic, natriuretic, and antihypertensive effects of loop, potassium-sparing and thiazide diuretics. Therefore, when HCTZ/Methyldopa and non-steroidal anti-inflammatory agents are used concomitantly, the patients should be observed closely to determine if the desired effect of the diuretic is obtained.

DRUG/LABORATORY TEST INTERACTIONS

METHYLDOPA

Methyldopa may interfere with measurement of: urinary uric acid by the phosphotungstate method, serum creatinine by the alkaline picrate method, and SGOT by colorimetric methods. Interference with spectrophotometric methods for SGOT analysis has not been reported.

Since Methyldopa causes fluorescence in urine samples at the same wave lengths as catecholamines, falsely high levels of urinary catecholamines may be reported. This will interfere with the diagnosis of pheochromocytoma. It is important to recognize this phenomenon before a patient with a possible pheochromocytoma is subjected to surgery. Methyldopa does not interfere with measurement of VMA (vanillylmandelic acid), a test for pheochromocytoma, by those methods which convert VMA to vanillin. Methyldopa is not recommended for the treatment of patients with pheochromocytoma. Rarely, when urine is exposed to air after voiding, it may darken because of breakdown of Methyldopa or its metabolites.

HYDROCHLOROTHIAZIDE

Thiazides should be discontinued before carrying out tests for parathyroid function (see "Precautions, General").

CARCINOGENESIS, MUTAGENESIS, IMPAIRMENT OF FERTILITY

Long-term studies in animals have not been performed to evaluate the effects upon fertility, mutagenic or carcinogenic potential of the combination.

METHYLDOPA

No evidence of a tumorigenic effect was seen when Methyldopa was given for two years to mice at doses up to 1800 mg/kg/day or to rats at doses up to 240 mg/kg/day (30 and 4 times the maximum recommended human dose in mice and rats, respectively, when compared on the basis of body weight: 2.5 and 0.6 times the maximum recommended human dose in mice and rats, respectively, when compared on the basis of body surface area; calculations assume a patient weight of 50 kg).

Methyldopa was not mutagenic in the Ames Test and did not increase chromosomal aberration or sister chromatid exchanges in Chinese hamster ovary cells. These in vitro studies were carried out both with and without exogenous metabolic activation.

Fertility was unaffected when Methyldopa was given to male and female rats at 100 mg/kg/day (1.7 times the maximum daily human dose when compared on the basis of body weight: 0.2 times the maximum daily human dose when compared on the basis of body surface area). Methyldopa decreased sperm count, sperm motility, the number of late spermatids and the male fertility index when given to male rats at 200 and 400 mg/kg/day (3.3 and 6.7 times the maximum daily human dose when compared on the basis of body weight: 0.5 and 1 times the maximum daily human dose when compared on the basis of body surface area).

HYDROCHLOROTHIAZIDE

Two-year feeding studies in mice and rats conducted under the auspices of the National Toxicology Program (NTP) uncovered no evidence of a carcinogenic potential of Hydrochlorothiazide in female mice (at doses of up to approximately 600 mg/kg/day) or in male and female rats (at doses of up to approximately 100 mg/kg/day). The NTP, however, found equivocal evidence for hepatocarcinogenicity in male mice. Hydrochlorothiazide was not genotoxic in vitro in the Ames mutagenicity assay of *Salmonella typhimurium* strains TA 98, TA 100, TA 1535, TA 1537, and TA 1538 and in the Chinese Hamster Ovary (CHO) test for chromosomal aberrations, or in vivo in assays using mouse germinal cell chromosomes, Chinese hamster bone marrow chromosomes, and the *Drosophila* sex-linked recessive lethal trait gene. Positive test results were obtained only in the in vitro CHO Sister Chromatid Exchange (clastogenicity) and in the Mouse Lymphoma Cell (mutagenicity) assays, using concentrations of Hydrochlorothiazide from 43 to 1300 μg/mL, and in the *Aspergillus nidulans* non-disjunction assay at an unspecified concentration.

Hydrochlorothiazide had no adverse effects on the fertility of mice and rats of either sex in studies wherein these species were exposed, via their diet, to doses of up to 100 and 4 mg/kg, respectively, prior to conception and throughout gestation.

PREGNANCY

Use of diuretics during normal pregnancy is inappropriate and exposes mother and fetus to unnecessary hazard. Diuretics do not prevent development of toxemia of pregnancy and there is no satisfactory evidence that they are useful in the treatment of toxemia.

Teratogenic Effects—Pregnancy Category C: Animal reproduction studies have not been conducted with HCTZ/Methyldopa. It is also not known whether HCTZ/Methyldopa can affect reproduction capacity or can cause fetal harm when given to a pregnant woman. HCTZ/Methyldopa should be given to a pregnant woman only if clearly needed.

◆ RATED THERAPEUTICALLY EQUIVALENT; ◇ THERAPEUTIC EQUIVALENCE UNCONFIRMED; ○ UNRATED

Hydrochlorothiazide: Studies in which Hydrochlorothiazide was orally administered to pregnant mice and rats during their respective periods of major organogenesis at doses up to 3000 and 1000 mg Hydrochlorothiazide/kg, respectively, provided no evidence of harm to the fetus. There are, however, no adequate and well-controlled studies in pregnant women.

Methyldopa: Reproduction studies performed with Methyldopa at oral doses up to 1000 mg/kg in mice, 200 mg/kg in rabbits and 100 mg/kg in rats revealed no evidence of harm to the fetus. These doses are 16.6 times, 3.3 times and 1.7 times, respectively, the maximum daily human dose when compared on the basis of body weight: 1.4 times, 1.1 times and 0.2 times, respectively, when compared on the basis of body surface area: calculations assume a patient weight of 50 kg. There are, however, no adequate and well-controlled studies in pregnant women in the first trimester of pregnancy. Because animal reproduction studies are not always predictive of human response, Methyldopa should be used during pregnancy only if clearly needed.

Published reports of the use of Methyldopa during all trimesters indicate that if this drug is used during pregnancy the possibility of fetal harm appears remote. In five studies, three of which were controlled, involving 332 pregnant hypertensive women, treatment with Methyldopa was associated with an improved fetal outcome. The majority of these women were in the third trimester when Methyldopa therapy was begun.

In one study, women who had begun Methyldopa treatment between weeks 16 and 20 of pregnancy gave birth to infants whose average head circumference was reduced by a small amount (34.2 ± 1.7 cm vs. 34.6 ± 1.3 cm [mean ± 1 S.D.]). Long term follow-up of 195 (97.5%) of the children born to Methyldopa-treated pregnant women (including those who began treatment between weeks 16 and 20) failed to uncover any significant adverse effect on the children. At four years of age, the developmental delay commonly seen in children born to hypertensive mothers was less evident in those whose mothers were treated with Methyldopa during pregnancy than those whose mothers were untreated. The children of the treated group scored consistently higher than the children of the untreated group on five major indices of intellectual and motor development. At age 7 and one-half developmental scores and intelligence indices showed no significant differences in children of treated or untreated hypertensive women.

Nonteratogenic Effects: Thiazides cross the placental barrier and appear in cord blood. There is a risk of fetal or neonatal jaundice, thrombocytopenia, and possibly other adverse reactions that have occurred in adults.

NURSING MOTHERS
Methyldopa and thiazides appear in breast milk. Therefore, because of the potential for serious adverse reactions in nursing infants from Hydrochlorothiazide, a decision should be made whether to discontinue nursing or to discontinue the drug, taking into account the importance of the drug to the mother.

PEDIATRIC USE
Safety and effectiveness of HCTZ/Methyldopa in children have not been established.

ADVERSE REACTIONS
The following adverse reactions have been reported and, within each category, are listed in order of decreasing severity.

METHYLDOPA
Sedation, usually transient, may occur during the initial period of therapy or whenever the dose is increased. Headache, asthenia, or weakness may be noted as early and transient symptoms. However, significant adverse effects due to methyldopa have been infrequent and this agent usually is well tolerated.

Cardiovascular: Aggravation of angina pectoris, congestive heart failure, prolonged carotid sinus hypersensitivity, orthostatic hypotension (decrease daily dosage), edema or weight gain, bradycardia.

Digestive: Pancreatitis, colitis, vomiting, diarrhea, sialadenitis, sore or "black" tongue, nausea, constipation, distension, flatus, dryness of mouth.

Endocrine: Hyperprolactinemia.

Hematologic: Bone marrow depression, leukopenia, granulocytopenia, thrombocytopenia, hemolytic anemia: positive tests for antinuclear antibody, LE cells, and rheumatoid factor, positive Coombs test.

Hepatic: Liver disorders including hepatitis, jaundice, abnormal liver function tests (see *"Warnings"*).

Hypersensitivity: Myocarditis, pericarditis, vasculitis, lupus-like syndrome, drug-related fever.

Nervous System/Psychiatric: Parkinsonism, Bell's palsy, decreased mental acuity, involuntary choreoathetotic movements, symptoms of cerebrovascular insufficiency, psychic disturbances including nightmares and reversible mild psychoses or depression, headache, sedation, asthenia or weakness, dizziness, lightheadedness, paresthesias.

Metabolic: Rise in BUN.

Musculoskeletal: Arthralgia, with or without joint swelling; myalgia.

Respiratory: Nasal stuffiness.

Skin: Toxic epidermal necrolysis, rash.

Urogenital: Amenorrhea, breast enlargement, gynecomastia, lactation, impotence, decreased libido.

HYDROCHLOROTHIAZIDE
Body as a Whole: Weakness.

Cardiovascular: Hypotension including orthostatic hypotension (may be aggravated by alcohol, barbiturates, narcotics or antihypertensive drugs).

Digestive: Pancreatitis, jaundice (intrahepatic cholestatic jaundice), diarrhea, vomiting, sialadenitis, cramping, constipation, gastric irritation, nausea, anorexia.

Hematologic: Aplastic anemia, agranulocytosis, leukopenia, hemolytic anemia, thrombocytopenia.

Hypersensitivity: Anaphylactic reactions, necrotizing angiitis (vasculitis and cutaneous vasculitis), respiratory distress including pneumonitis and pulmonary edema photosensitivity, fever, urticaria, rash, purpura.

Metabolic: Electrolyte imbalance (see *"Precautions"*), hyperglycemia, glycosuria, hyperuricemia.

Musculoskeletal: Muscle spasm.

Nervous System/Psychiatric: Vertigo, paresthesias, dizziness, headache, restlessness.

Renal: Renal failure, renal dysfunction, interstitial nephritis. (See *"Warnings."*)

Skin: Erythema multiforme including Stevens-Johnson syndrome, exfoliative dermatitis including toxic epidermal necrolysis, alopecia.

Special Senses: Transient blurred vision, xanthopsia.

Urogenital: Impotence.

OVERDOSAGE
Acute overdosage may produce acute hypotension with other responses attributable to brain and gastrointestinal malfunction (excessive sedation, weakness, bradycardia, dizziness, lightheadedness, constipation, distention, flatus, diarrhea, nausea, vomiting).

In the event of overdosage, symptomatic and supportive measures should be employed. When ingestion is recent, gastric lavage or emesis may reduce absorption. When ingestion has been earlier, infusions may be helpful to promote urinary excretion. Otherwise, management includes special attention to cardiac rate and output, blood volume, electrolyte balance, paralytic ileus, urinary function and cerebral activity.

Sympathomimetic drugs (e.g., levarterenol, epinephrine, metaraminol bitartrate) may be indicated. Methyldopa is dialyzable. The degree to which Hydrochlorothiazide is removed by hemodialysis has not been established.

The oral LD_{50} of Methyldopa is greater than 1.5 g/kg in both the mouse and the rat. The oral LD_{50} of Hydrochlorothiazide is greater than 10 g/kg in the mouse and rat.

DOSAGE AND ADMINISTRATION
DOSAGE MUST BE INDIVIDUALIZED, AS DETERMINED BY TITRATION OF THE INDIVIDUAL COMPONENTS (see *"Warning"*). Once the patient has been successfully titrated. HCTZ/Methyldopa may be substituted if the previously determined titrated doses are the same as in the combination. The usual starting dosage is one tablet of HCTZ 15 mg/Methyldopa 250 mg two or three times a day or one tablet of HCTZ 25 mg/Methyldopa 250 mg two times a day. For those patients requiring higher doses, one tablet of HCTZ 30 mg/Methyldopa 500 mg or HCTZ 50 mg/Methyldopa 500 mg two times a day may be used.

Patients usually do not require doses of Hydrochlorothiazide in excess of 50 mg daily when combined with other antihypertensive agents. The usual daily dosage of Methyldopa is 500 mg to 2 g. To minimize the sedation associated with Methyldopa, start dosage increases in the evening.

Occasionally tolerance to Methyldopa may occur, usually between the second and third month of therapy. Additional separate doses of Methyldopa or replacement of HCTZ/Methyldopa with single entity agents is necessary until the new effective dose ratio is re-established by titration. The maximum recommended daily dose Methyldopa is 3 g and of Hydrochlorothiazide is 200 mg.

If HCTZ/Methyldopa does not adequately control blood pressure, additional does of other agents may be given. When HCTZ/Methyldopa is given with antihypertensives other than thiazides, the initial dosage of Methyldopa should be limited to 500 mg daily in divided doses and the dose of these other agents may need to be adjusted to effect a smooth transition.

Since both components of HCTZ/Methyldopa have a relatively short duration of action, withdrawal is followed by return of hypertension usually within 48 hours. This is not complicated by an overshoot of blood pressure.

Since Methyldopa is largely excreted by the kidney, patients with impaired renal function may respond to smaller doses. Syncope in older patients may be related to an increased sensitivity and advanced arteriosclerotic vascular disease. This may be avoided by lower doses.

Keep container tightly closed. Protect from light, moisture, freezing. −20°C (−4°F) and store at controlled room temperature, 15-30°C (59-86°F).

HOW SUPPLIED
CAPSULE: 15 MG-250 MG

BRAND/MANUFACTURER	NDC	SIZE	AWP
◆ GENERICS			
Major	00904-2403-61	100s ud	$28.07

TABLETS: 15 MG-250 MG

AVERAGE UNIT PRICE (AVAILABLE SIZES)		GENERIC A-RATED AVERAGE PRICE (GAAP)	
BRAND	$0.44	100s	$23.68
GENERIC	$0.23	500s	$111.17
HCFA FUL (100s ea)	$0.10	1000s	$198.50

BRAND/MANUFACTURER	NDC	SIZE	AWP
◆ BRAND			
ALDORIL-15: Merck	00006-0423-68	100s	$44.48
	00006-0423-82	1000s	$431.69
◆ GENERICS			
Watson	52544-0357-01	100s	$18.52
Warner Chilcott	00047-0030-24	100s	$20.80
Goldline	00182-1830-01	100s	$21.00
Rugby	00536-4887-01	100s	$21.56
Rugby	00536-5651-01	100s	$21.56
Major	00904-2403-60	100s	$21.95
Major	00904-7813-60	100s	$21.95
Qualitest	00603-4543-21	100s	$22.70
Lederle Std Prod	00005-3852-23	100s	$23.30
Invamed	52189-0205-24	100s	$24.14
Schein	00364-0827-01	100s	$25.23
URL	00677-1051-01	100s	$25.94
Moore,H.L.	00839-7141-06	100s	$25.99
Par	49884-0186-01	100s	$26.00
Aligen	00405-4658-01	100s	$26.54
Geneva	00781-1809-01	100s	$27.50
Mylan	00378-0507-01	100s	$27.95
Watson	52544-0357-05	500s	$87.97
Invamed	52189-0205-29	500s	$119.45
Par	49884-0186-05	500s	$126.10
Major	00904-2403-80	1000s	$170.55
Major	00904-7813-80	1000s	$170.55
Watson	52544-0357-10	1000s	$175.94
Qualitest	00603-4543-32	1000s	$200.30
Lederle Std Prod	00005-3852-34	1000s	$221.43
Par	49884-0186-10	1000s	$252.20

TABLETS: 25 MG-250 MG

AVERAGE UNIT PRICE (AVAILABLE SIZES)		GENERIC A-RATED AVERAGE PRICE (GAAP)	
BRAND	$0.53	100s	$28.31
GENERIC	$0.27	500s	$126.50
HCFA FUL (100s ea)	$0.10	1000s	$236.04

BRAND/MANUFACTURER	NDC	SIZE	AWP
◆ BRAND			
ALDORIL-25: Merck	00006-0456-68	100s	$52.39
	00006-0456-28	100s ud	$56.70
	00006-0456-82	1000s	$508.76
◆ GENERICS			
Watson	52544-0358-01	100s	$19.42
Warner Chilcott	00047-0031-24	100s	$23.53
Qualitest	00603-4544-21	100s	$23.68
Rugby	00536-4888-01	100s	$23.69
Rugby	00536-5652-01	100s	$23.69
Goldline	00182-1310-01	100s	$24.00
Goldline	00182-1831-01	100s	$24.00
Major	00904-2404-60	100s	$24.70
Major	00904-7814-60	100s	$24.70
Lederle Std Prod	00005-3853-23	100s	$25.79
Invamed	52189-0206-24	100s	$27.34
Schein	00364-0828-01	100s	$29.40
URL	00677-1052-01	100s	$31.08
Moore,H.L.	00839-7142-06	100s	$31.12
Geneva	00781-1819-01	100s	$31.25
Par	49884-0187-01	100s	$31.30
Mylan	00378-0711-01	100s	$31.95
Aligen	00405-4659-01	100s	$33.19
Major	00904-2404-61	100s ud	$31.48
Geneva	00781-1819-13	100s ud	$36.65
UDL	51079-0647-20	100s ud	$42.50
Watson	52544-0358-05	500s	$92.25
Invamed	52189-0206-29	500s	$135.45
Par	49884-0187-05	500s	$151.80
Major	00904-2404-80	1000s	$180.35
Major	00904-7814-80	1000s	$180.35
Watson	52544-0358-10	1000s	$184.49
Schein	00364-0828-02	1000s	$205.50
Qualitest	00603-4544-32	1000s	$208.16
Warner Chilcott	00047-0031-32	1000s	$222.24
Lederle Std Prod	00005-3853-34	1000s	$244.93
Geneva	00781-1819-10	1000s	$281.25
Mylan	00378-0711-10	1000s	$281.95
Par	49884-0187-10	1000s	$303.61
Aligen	00405-4659-03	1000s	$303.61

TABLETS: 30 MG-500 MG

AVERAGE UNIT PRICE (AVAILABLE SIZES)		GENERIC A-RATED AVERAGE PRICE (GAAP)	
BRAND	$0.83	100s	$45.00
GENERIC	$0.44		
HCFA FUL (100s ea)	$0.37		

BRAND/MANUFACTURER	NDC	SIZE	AWP
◆ BRAND			
ALDORIL D30: Merck	00006-0694-68	100s	$83.30
◆ GENERICS			
Watson	52544-0359-01	100s	$38.44
Warner Chilcott	00047-0032-24	100s	$40.18
Major	00904-2423-60	100s	$41.95
Rugby	00536-5653-01	100s	$44.78
Schein	00364-2400-01	100s	$45.43
Par	49884-0188-01	100s	$49.00
Aligen	00405-4660-01	100s	$49.00
Geneva	00781-1843-01	100s	$49.95
Major	00904-2423-61	100s ud	$46.26
Watson	52544-0359-05	500s	$182.59

TABLETS: 50 MG-500 MG

AVERAGE UNIT PRICE (AVAILABLE SIZES)		GENERIC A-RATED AVERAGE PRICE (GAAP)	
BRAND	$0.90	100s	$48.02
GENERIC	$0.47		
HCFA FUL (100s ea)	$0.37		

BRAND/MANUFACTURER	NDC	SIZE	AWP
◆ BRAND			
ALDORIL D50: Merck	00006-0935-68	100s	$89.56
◆ GENERICS			
Watson	52544-0360-01	100s	$39.46
Warner Chilcott	00047-0033-24	100s	$43.21
Major	00904-2424-60	100s	$44.95
Schein	00364-2401-01	100s	$45.67
Rugby	00536-4890-01	100s	$49.13
Rugby	00536-5654-01	100s	$49.13
Par	49884-0189-01	100s	$51.00
Aligen	00405-4661-01	100s	$51.00
Geneva	00781-1853-01	100s	$53.40
Major	00904-2424-61	100 ud	$53.28
Watson	52544-0360-05	500s	$187.44

Hydrochlorothiazide and Propranolol Hydrochloride

Each Hydrochlorothiazide/Propranolol Hydrochloride Long Acting 80/50 Capsule contains:

Propranolol HCl ....80 mg
Hydrochlorothiazide ....50 mg

Each Hydrochlorothiazide/Propranolol Hydrochloride Long Acting 120/50 Capsule contains:
Propranolol HCl ....120 mg
Hydrochlorothiazide ....50 mg

Each Hydrochlorothiazide/Propranolol Hydrochloride Long Acting 160/50 Capsule contains:
Propanolol HCl ....160 mg
Hydrochlorothiazide ....50 mg

Each Hydrochlorothiazide/ Propranolol Hydrochloride 40/25 Tablet contains:
Hydrochlorothiazide ....25 mg
Propranolol HCl ....40 mg

Each Hydrochlorothiazide/Propranolol Hydrochloride 80/25 Tablet contains:
Hydrochlorothiazide ....25 mg
Propranolol HCl ....80 mg

DESCRIPTION

Long-acting Hydrochlorothiazide/Propranolol capsules are indicated in the once-daily management of hypertension; Hydrochlorothiazide/Propranolol HCl tablets for oral administration are indicated for twice-daily management of hypertension.

Hydrochlorothiazide/Propranolol HCl combines two antihypertensive agents: Propranolol HCl, a beta-adrenergic receptor-blocking agent, and Hydrochlorothiazide, a thiazide diuretic-antihypertensive.

Propranolol HCl is a synthetic beta-adrenergic receptor-blocking agent chemically described as 1-(Isopropylamino)-3-(1-naphthyloxy)-2-propanol hydrochloride.

Propranolol HCl is a stable, white, crystalline solid which is readily soluble in water and ethanol. Its molecular weight is 295.81.

Hydrochlorothiazide is a white, or practically white, practically odorless, crystalline powder. It is slightly soluble in water; freely soluble in sodium hydroxide solution; sparingly soluble in methanol; insoluble in ether, chloroform,

◆ RATED THERAPEUTICALLY EQUIVALENT; ◇ THERAPEUTIC EQUIVALENCE UNCONFIRMED; ○ UNRATED

benzene, and dilute mineral acids. Its chemical name is 6-Chloro-3,4-dihydro-2H-1,2,4-benzothiadiazine-7-sulfonamide 1,1-dioxide.

CLINICAL PHARMACOLOGY

PROPRANOLOL HYDROCHLORIDE

Propranolol is a nonselective, beta-adrenergic receptor-blocking agent possessing no other autonomic nervous system activity. It specifically competes with beta-adrenergic receptor-stimulating agents for available receptor sites. When access to beta-receptor sites is blocked by Propranolol, the chronotropic, inotropic, and vasodilator responses to beta-adrenergic stimulation are decreased proportionately.

Propranolol is almost completely absorbed from the gastrointestinal tract, but a portion is immediately metabolized by the liver on its first pass through the portal circulation.

Peak effect occurs in one to one-and-one-half hours. The biologic half-life is approximately four hours. Propranolol is not significantly dialyzable. There is no simple correlation between dose or plasma level and therapeutic effect, and the dose-sensitivity range, as observed in clinical practice, is wide. The principal reason for this is that sympathetic tone varies widely between individuals. Since there is no reliable test to estimate sympathetic tone or to determine whether total beta blockade has been achieved, proper dosage requires titration.

Hydrochlorothiazide/Propranolol HCl Long Acting Capsules (80/50, 120/50, and 160/50 mg) release Propranolol HCl at a controlled and predictable rate. Peak Propranolol blood levels following dosing with Hydrochlorothiazide/Propranolol HCl Long Acting occur at about 6 hours, and the apparent plasma half-life is about 10 hours. Over a 24-hour period, Propranolol blood levels are fairly constant for about 12 hours, then decline exponentially. When measured at steady state over a 24-hour period, the areas under the Propranolol plasma concentration-time curve (AUCs) for the capsules are approximately 60% to 65% of the AUCs for a comparable divided daily dose of Propranolol HCl tablets. The lower AUCs for the capsules are due to greater hepatic metabolism of Propranolol resulting from the slower rate of absorption of Propranolol. Hydrochlorothiazide/Propranolol HCl Long Acting should not be considered a simple mg-for-mg substitute for conventional Hydrochlorothiazide/Propranolol HCl tablets, and the Propranolol blood levels achieved do not match (are lower than) those of twice-daily dosing of Hydrochlorothiazide/Propranolol HCl tablets with the same dose. When changing to Hydrochlorothiazide/Propranolol Hydrochloride Long Acting from conventional Hydrochlorothiazide/Propranolol HCl tablets, a possible need for retitration upwards should be considered.

The mechanism of the antihypertensive effect of Propranolol has not been established. Among the factors that may be involved in contributing to the antihypertensive action are: (1) decreased cardiac output, (2) inhibition of renin release by the kidneys, and (3) diminution of tonic sympathetic nerve outflow from vasomotor centers in the brain.

Propranolol HCl decreases heart rate, cardiac output, and blood pressure. Although total peripheral vascular resistance may increase initially, it readjusts to or below the pretreatment level with chronic usage. Effects on plasma volume appear to be minor and somewhat variable. Propranolol has been shown to cause a small increase in serum potassium concentration when used in the treatment of hypertensive patients.

Beta-receptor blockade is useful in conditions in which, because of pathologic or functional changes, sympathetic activity is excessive or inappropriate, and detrimental to the patient. But there are also situations in which sympathetic stimulation is vital. For example, in patients with severely damaged hearts, adequate ventricular function is maintained by virtue of sympathetic drive, which should be preserved. In the presence of AV block greater than first degree, beta blockade may prevent the necessary facilitating effect of sympathetic activity on conduction. Beta blockade results in bronchial constriction by interfering with adrenergic bronchodilator activity, which should be preserved in patients subject to bronchospasm.

The proper objective of beta-blockade therapy is to decrease adverse sympathetic stimulation, but not to the degree that may impair necessary sympathetic support.

HYDROCHLOROTHIAZIDE

Hydrochlorothiazide is a benzothiadiazine (thiazide) diuretic closely related to chlorothiazide. The mechanism of the antihypertensive effect of the thiazides is unknown. Thiazides usually do not affect normal blood pressure.

Thiazides affect the renal tubular mechanism of electrolyte reabsorption. At maximal therapeutic dosage, all thiazides are approximately equal in their diuretic efficacy.

Thiazides increase excretion of sodium and chloride in approximately equivalent amounts. Natriuresis causes a secondary loss of potassium and bicarbonate.

Onset of diuretic action of thiazides occurs in 2 hours, and the peak effect in about 4 hours. Its action persists for approximately 6 to 12 hours. Thiazides are eliminated rapidly by the kidney. The Hydrochlorothiazide in Hydrochlorothiazide/Propranolol HCl Long Acting is a conventional (not sustained-release) formulation.

INDICATIONS AND USAGE

Hydrochlorothiazide/Propranolol HCl is indicated in the management of hypertension.

This fixed-combination drug is not indicated for initial therapy of hypertension. Hypertension requires therapy titrated to the individual patient. If the fixed combination represents the dosage so determined, its use may be more convenient in patient management. The treatment of hypertension is not static, but must be reevaluated as conditions in each patient warrant.

CONTRAINDICATIONS

PROPRANOLOL HCL

Propranolol is contraindicated in: 1) cardiogenic shock; 2) sinus bradycardia and greater than first-degree block; 3) bronchial asthma; 4) congestive heart failure (see "Warnings"), unless the failure is secondary to a tachyarrhythmia treatable with Propranolol.

HYDROCHLOROTHIAZIDE

Hydrochlorothiazide is contraindicated in patients with anuria or hypersensitivity to this or other sulfonamide-derived drugs.

WARNINGS

PROPRANOLOL HCL

Cardiac Failure: Sympathetic stimulation may be a vital component supporting circulatory function in patients with congestive heart failure, and its inhibition by beta blockade may further depress myocardial contractility and precipitate more severe failure. Although beta blockers should be avoided in overt congestive heart failure, if necessary, they can be used with close follow-up in patients with a history of failure who are well compensated and are receiving digitalis and diuretics. Propranolol acts selectively without abolishing the inotropic action of digitalis on the heart muscle (i.e., that of supporting the strength of myocardial contractions). In patients already receiving digitalis, the positive inotropic action of digitalis may be reduced by Propranolol's negative inotropic effect. The effects of Propranolol and digitalis are additive in depressing AV conduction.

In Patients Without a History of Heart Failure, continued use of beta blockers, i.e., continued depression of the myocardium over a period of time, can, in some cases, lead to cardiac failure. In rare instances, this has been observed during Propranolol therapy. Therefore, at the first sign or symptom of impending heart failure, the patient should be digitalized and/or treated with diuretics, and the response observed closely: a) if cardiac failure continues, despite adequate digitalization and diuretic therapy, Propranolol therapy should be withdrawn (gradually, if possible); b) if tachyarrhythmia is being controlled, patients should be maintained on combined therapy and the patient closely followed until threat of cardiac failure is over.

IN PATIENTS WITH ANGINA PECTORIS: THERE HAVE BEEN REPORTS OF EXACERBATION OF ANGINA AND, IN SOME CASES, MYOCARDIAL INFARCTION, FOLLOWING *ABRUPT* DISCONTINUANCE OF PROPRANOLOL THERAPY. THEREFORE, WHEN DISCONTINUANCE OF PROPRANOLOL IS PLANNED, THE DOSAGE SHOULD BE GRADUALLY REDUCED AND THE PATIENT CAREFULLY MONITORED. IN ADDITION, WHEN PROPRANOLOL IS PRESCRIBED FOR ANGINA PECTORIS, THE PATIENT SHOULD BE CAUTIONED AGAINST INTERRUPTION OR CESSATION OF THERAPY WITHOUT THE PHYSICIAN'S ADVICE. IF PROPRANOLOL THERAPY IS INTERRUPTED AND EXACERBATION OF ANGINA OCCURS, IT USUALLY IS ADVISABLE TO REINSTITUTE PROPRANOLOL THERAPY AND TAKE OTHER MEASURES APPROPRIATE FOR THE MANAGEMENT OF UNSTABLE ANGINA PECTORIS. SINCE CORONARY ARTERY DISEASE MAY BE UNRECOGNIZED, IT MAY BE PRUDENT TO FOLLOW THE ABOVE ADVICE IN PATIENTS CONSIDERED AT RISK OF HAVING OCCULT ATHEROSCLEROTIC HEART DISEASE WHO ARE GIVEN PROPRANOLOL FOR OTHER INDICATIONS.

Thyrotoxicosis: Beta blockade may mask certain clinical signs of hyperthyroidism. Therefore, abrupt withdrawal of Propranolol may be followed by an exacerbation of symptoms of hyperthyroidism, including thyroid storm.

In Patients With Wolff-Parkinson-White Syndrome: several cases have been reported in which, after Propranolol, the tachycardia was replaced by a severe bradycardia requiring a demand pacemaker. In one case this resulted after an initial dose of 5 mg Propranolol.

Major Surgery: The necessity or desirability of withdrawal of beta-blocking therapy prior to major surgery is controversial. It should be noted, however, that the impaired ability of the heart to respond to reflex adrenergic stimuli may augment the risk of general anesthesia and surgical procedures.

Propranolol, like other beta blockers, is a competitive inhibitor of beta-receptor agonists, and its effects can be reversed by administration of such agents, e.g., dobutamine or isoproterenol. However, such patients may be subject to protracted severe hypotension. Difficulty in starting and maintaining the heartbeat has also been reported with beta blockers.

Nonallergic Bronchospasm (e.g., chronic bronchitis, emphysema): Patients with bronchospastic diseases should, in general, not receive beta blockers: Propranolol should be administered with caution since it may block bronchodilation produced by endogenous and exogenous catecholamine stimulation of beta receptors.

Diabetes and Hypoglycemia: Beta blockers should be used with caution in diabetic patients if a beta-blocking agent is required. Beta-adrenergic blockade may prevent the appearance of certain premonitory signs and symptoms (pulse rate and pressure changes) of acute hypoglycemia in labile insulin-dependent diabetes. In these patients, it may be more difficult to adjust the dosage of insulin. Beta blockers may mask tachycardia occurring with hypoglycemia, but other manifestations such as dizziness and sweating may not be significantly affected. Following insulin-induced hypoglycemia, Propranolol may cause a delay in the recovery of blood glucose to normal levels. Hypoglycemic attacks may be accompanied by a precipitous elevation of blood pressure.

HYDROCHLOROTHIAZIDE
Thiazides should be used with caution in severe renal disease. In patients with renal disease, thiazides may precipitate azotemia. In patients with impaired renal function, cumulative effects of the drug may develop.

Thiazides should also be used with caution in patients with impaired hepatic function or progressive liver disease, since minor alterations of fluid and electrolyte balance may precipitate hepatic coma.

Thiazides may add to or potentiate the action of other antihypertensive drugs. Potentiation occurs with ganglionic or peripheral adrenergic-blocking drugs.

Sensitivity reactions may occur in patients with a history of allergy or bronchial asthma. The possibility of exacerbation or activation of systemic lupus erythematosus has been reported.

PRECAUTIONS
PROPRANOLOL HCL
General: Propranolol should be used with caution in patients with impaired hepatic or renal function. Propranolol is not indicated for the treatment of hypertensive emergencies.

Beta-adrenoreceptor blockade can cause reduction of intraocular pressure. Patients should be told that Propranolol may interfere with the glaucoma screening test. Withdrawal may lead to a return of increased intraocular pressure.

Clinical Laboratory Tests: Elevated blood urea levels in patients with severe heart disease, elevated serum transaminase, alkaline phosphatase, lactate dehydrogenase.

Drug Interactions: Patients receiving catecholamine-depleting drugs, such as reserpine, should be closely observed if Propranolol is administered. The added catecholamine-blocking action may produce an excessive reduction of resting sympathetic nervous activity, which may result in hypotension, marked bradycardia, vertigo, syncopal attacks, or orthostatic hypotension.

Caution should be exercised when patients receiving a beta blocker are administered a calcium-channel blocking drug, especially intravenous verapamil, for both agents may depress myocardial contractility or atrioventricular conduction. On rare occasions, the concomitant intravenous use of a beta blocker and verapamil has resulted in serious adverse reactions, especially in patients with severe cardiomyopathy, congestive heart failure, or recent myocardial infarction.

Blunting of the antihypertensive effect of beta-adrenoceptor blocking agents by nonsteroidal anti-inflammatory drugs has been reported.

Hypotension and coronary arrest have been reported with the concomitant use of Propranolol and haloperidol.

Aluminum hydroxide gel greatly reduces intestinal absorption of Propranolol.

Ethanol slows the rate of absorption of Propranolol.

Phenytoin, phenobarbitone, and rifampin accelerate Propranolol clearance.

Chlorpromazine when used concomitantly with Propranolol, results in increased plasma levels of both drugs.

Antipyrine and lidocaine have reduced clearance when used concomitantly with Propranolol.

Thyroxine may result in a lower than expected T_3 concentration when used concomitantly with Propranolol.

Cimetidine decreases the hepatic metabolism of Propranolol, delaying elimination and increasing blood levels.

Theophylline clearance is reduced when used concomitantly with Propranolol.

Carcinogenesis, Mutagenesis, Impairment of Fertility: Long-term studies in animals have been conducted to evaluate toxic effects and carcinogenic potential. In 18-month studies, in both rats and mice, employing doses up to 150 mg/kg/day there was no evidence of significant drug-induced toxicity. There were no drug-related tumorigenic effects at any of the dosage levels. Reproductive studies in animals did not show any impairment of fertility that was attributable to the drug.

Long-term studies in animals have not been conducted to evaluate the toxic effects and carcinogenic potential of Hydrochlorothiazide/Propranolol HCl.

Pregnancy: Pregnancy Category C. Propranolol has been shown to be embryotoxic in animal studies at doses about 10 times greater than the maximum recommended human dose. There are no adequate and well-controlled studies in pregnant women. Propranolol should be used during pregnancy only if the potential benefit justifies the potential risk to the fetus.

Nursing Mothers: Propranolol is excreted in human milk. Caution should be exercised when Propranolol is administered to a nursing mother.

Pediatric Use: Safety and effectiveness in children have not been established.

HYDROCHLOROTHIAZIDE
General: Periodic determination of serum electrolytes to detect possible electrolyte imbalance should be performed at appropriate intervals.

All patients receiving thiazide therapy should be observed for clinical signs of fluid or electrolyte imbalance, namely: Hyponatremia, hypochloremic alkalosis, and hypokalemia. Serum and urine electrolyte determinations are particularly important when the patient is vomiting excessively or receiving parenteral fluids. Medication such as digitalis may also influence serum electrolytes. Warning signs irrespective of cause are: Dryness of mouth, thirst, weakness, lethargy, drowsiness,

restlessness, muscle pains or cramps, muscular fatigue, hypotension, oliguria, tachycardia, and gastrointestinal disturbances such as nausea and vomiting.

Hypokalemia may develop, especially with brisk diuresis, when severe cirrhosis is present or during concomitant use of corticosteroids or ACTH.

Interference with adequate oral electrolyte intake will also contribute to hypokalemia. Hypokalemia can sensitize or exaggerate the response of the heart to the toxic effect of digitalis (e.g., increased ventricular irritability). Hypokalemia may be avoided or treated by use of potassium supplements, such as foods with a high potassium content.

Any chloride deficit is generally mild and usually does not require specific treatment, except under extraordinary circumstances (as in liver or renal disease). Dilutional hyponatremia may occur in edematous patients in hot weather; appropriate therapy is water restriction, rather than administration of salt, except in rare instances when the hyponatremia is life-threatening. In actual salt depletion, appropriate replacement is the therapy of choice.

Hyperuricemia may occur or frank gout may be precipitated in certain patients receiving thiazide therapy.

Insulin requirements in diabetic patients may be increased, decreased, or unchanged. Diabetes mellitus which has been latent may become manifest during thiazide administration. If progressive renal impairment becomes evident, consider withholding or discontinuing diuretic therapy.

Thiazides may decrease serum PBI levels without signs of thyroid disturbance. Calcium excretion is decreased by thiazides. Pathologic changes in the parathyroid gland with hypercalcemia and hypophosphatemia have been observed in a few patients on prolonged thiazide therapy. The common complications of hyperparathyroidism, such as renal lithiasis, bone resorption, and peptic ulceration have not been seen. Thiazides should be discontinued before carrying out tests for parathyroid function.

Drug Interactions: Thiazide drugs may increase the responsiveness to tubocurarine.

The antihypertensive effects of thiazides may be enhanced in the postsympathectomy patient. Thiazides may decrease arterial responsiveness to norepinephrine. This diminution is not sufficient to preclude effectiveness of the pressor agent for therapeutic use.

Carcinogenesis, Mutagenesis, Impairment of Fertility: Hydrochlorothiazide is presently under study for carcinogenesis in rats and mice in the National Toxicology Research and Testing Program.

Hydrochlorothiazide was not mutagenic in *in vitro* Ames mutagenicity assays of *Salmonella typhimurium* strains TA 98, TA 100, TA 1535, TA 1537, and TA 1538 or in *in vivo* mutagenicity assays of mouse germinal-cell chromosomes and Chinese hamster bone-marrow-cell chromosomes. It was, however, mutagenic in inducing nondisjunction (96% frequency) in diploid strains of *Aspergillus nidulans*. Hydrochlorothiazide had no adverse effects on fertility in rats at a dose equivalent to the recommended maximum human dose and in mice at a dose equivalent to 25 times the recommended maximum human dose (4 mg/kg. assumed body weight of 50 kg).

Pregnancy: Pregnancy Category C. Thiazides cross the placental barrier and appear in cord blood. The use of thiazides in pregnancy requires that the anticipated benefit be weighed against possible hazards to the fetus. These hazards include fetal or neonatal jaundice, thrombocytopenia, and possibly other adverse reactions which have occurred in the adult.

Available information indicates that Hydrochlorothiazide at doses as high as 330 times the recommended maximum human dose was not teratogenic in pregnant rats.

Nursing Mothers: Thiazides appear in human milk. If use of the drug is deemed essential, the patient should stop nursing.

Pediatric Use: Safety and effectiveness in children have not been established.

ADVERSE REACTIONS
The following adverse reations have been observed, but there is not enough systematic collection of data to support an estimate of their frequency. Although many side effects are mild and transient, some require discontinuation of therapy.

PROPRANOLOL HCL
Most adverse effects have been mild and transient and have rarely required the withdrawal of therapy.

Cardiovascular: Bradycardia; congestive heart failure; intensification of AV block; hypotension; paresthesia of hands; thrombocytopenic purpura; arterial insufficiency, usually of the Raynaud type.

Central Nervous System: Light-headedness; mental depression manifested by insomnia, lassitude, weakness, fatigue; reversible mental depression progressing to catatonia; visual disturbances; vivid dreams; hallucinations; an acute reversible syndrome characterized by disorientation for time and place, short-term memory loss, emotional lability, slightly clouded sensorium, and decreased performance on neuropsychometrics.

Total daily doses above 160 mg (when administered as divided doses of greater than 80 mg each) may be associated with an increased incidence of fatigue, lethargy, and vivid dreams.

Gastrointestinal: Nausea, vomiting, epigastric distress, abdominal cramping, diarrhea, constipation, mesenteric arterial thrombosis, ischemic colitis.

Allergic: Pharyngitis and agranulocytosis; erythematous rash; fever combined with aching and sore throat; laryngospasm and respiratory distress.

Respiratory: Bronchospasm.

◆ RATED THERAPEUTICALLY EQUIVALENT; ◇ THERAPEUTIC EQUIVALENCE UNCONFIRMED; ○ UNRATED

Hematologic: Agranulocytosis; nonthrombocytopenic purpura, thrombocytopenic purpura.

Autoimmune: In extremely rare instances, systemic lupus erythematosus has been reported.

Miscellaneous: Alopecia, LE-like reactions; psoriasiform rashes; dry eyes; male impotence; and Peyronie's disease have been reported rarely. Oculomucocutaneous reactions involving the skin, serous membranes, and conjunctivae reported for a beta blocker (practolol) have not been associated with Propranolol.

HYDROCHLOROTHIAZIDE
Gastrointestinal: Anorexia, gastric irriation, nausea, vomiting, cramping; diarrhea; constipation; jaundice (intrahepatic cholestatic jaundice); pancreatitis; sialadenitis.

Central Nervous System: Dizziness, vertigo; paresthesias; headache; xanthopsia.

Hematologic: Leukopenia; agranulocytosis; thrombocytopenia; aplastic anemia.

Cardiovascular: Orthostatic hypotension (may be aggravated by alcohol, barbiturates, or narcotics).

Hypersensitivity: Purpura; photosensitivity; rash; urticaria; necrotizing angiitis (vasculitis, cutaneous vasculitis); fever; respiratory distress, including pneumonitis; anaphylactic reactions.

Other: Hyperglycemia; glycosuria; hyperuricemia; muscle spasm; weakness; restlessness; transient blurred vision. Whenever adverse reactions are moderate or severe, thiazide dosage should be reduced or therapy withdrawn.

DOSAGE AND ADMINISTRATION
The dosage must be determined by individual titration.

Hydrochlorothiazide can be given at doses of 25 to 100 mg per day when used alone, but in most patients, 50 mg exerts a maximal effect. The initial dose of Propranolol is 80 mg daily, and it may be increased gradually until optimal blood pressure control is achieved. The usual effective dose, when used alone is 160 to 480 mg per day.

One Hydrochlorothiazide/Propranolol HCl Long Acting capsule once a day can be used to administer up to 160 mg of Propranolol and 50 mg of Hydrochlorothiazide. One Hydrochlorothiazide/Propranolol HCl tablet twice daily can be used to administer up to 160 mg of Propranolol and 50 mg of Hydrochlorothiazide. For doses of Propranolol greater than 160 mg, the combination products are not appropriate because their use would lead to an excessive dose of the thiazide component.

Hydrochlorothiazide/Propranolol HCl Long Acting provides Propranolol HCl in a sustained-release form and Hydrochlorothiazide in conventional formulation, for once-daily administration. If patients are switched from Hydrochlorothiazide/Propranolol HCl tablets (or Propranolol plus Hydrochlorothiazide to Hydrochlorothiazide/Propranolol HCl Long Acting, care should be taken to ensure that the desired therapeutic effect is maintained. Hydrochlorothiazide/Propranolol HCl Long Acting should not be considered a mg-for-mg substitute for Hydrochlorothiazide/Propranolol HCl or Propranolol plus Hydrochlorothiazide. Hydrochlorothiazide/Propranolol HCl Long Acting has different kinetics and produces lower blood levels. Retitration may be necessary, especially to maintain effectiveness at the end of the 24-hour dosing interval.

When necessary, another antihypertensive agent may be added gradually, beginning with 50% of the usual recommended starting dose, to avoid an excessive fall in blood pressure.

OVERDOSAGE OR EXAGGERATED RESPONSE
The Propranolol Hydrochloride component may cause bradycardia, cardiac failure, hypotension, or bronchospasm. Propranolol is not significantly dialyzable.

The Hydrochlorothiazide component can be expected to cause diuresis. Lethargy of varying degree may appear and may progress to coma within a few hours, with minimal depression of respiration and cardiovascular function, and in the absence of significant serum electrolyte changes or dehydration. The mechanism of central nervous system depression with thiazide overdosage is unknown. Gastrointestinal irritation and hypermotility can occur; temporary elevation of BUN has been reported and serum electrolyte changes could occur, especially in patients with impairment of renal function.

The oral LD$_{50}$ dosages in rats and mice for Propranolol, Hydrochlorothiazide, and combined Propranolol/Hydrochlorothiazide (40/25, 80/25) are 364 to 533 mg/kg, greater than 2,750 to 5,000 mg/kg, and 538 to 845 mg/kg, respectively.

TREATMENT
The following measures should be employed:

General: If ingestion is, or may have been, recent, evacuate gastric contents, taking care to prevent pulmonary aspiration.

Bradycardia: Administer atropine (0.25 to 1.0 mg). If there is no response to vagal blockade, administer isoproterenol cautiously.

Cardiac Failure: Digitalization and diuretics.

Hypotension: Vasopressors, e.g., levarterenol or epinephrine.

Bronchospasm: Administer isoproterenol and aminophylline.

Stupor or Coma: Administer supportive therapy as clinically warranted.

Gastrointestinal Effects: Though usually of short duration, these may require symptomatic treatment.

Abnormalities in BUN and/or Serum Electrolytes: Monitor serum electrolyte levels and renal function; institute supportive measures, as required individually, to maintain hydration, electrolyte balance, respiration, and cardiovascular-renal function.

Store at room temperature (approximately 25° C).

Protect from light, moisture, freezing, and excessive heat. Dispense in a tight, light-resistant container as defined in the USP.

HOW SUPPLIED
CAPSULE: 50 MG-80 MG

BRAND/MANUFACTURER	NDC	SIZE	AWP
○ BRAND			
➤ INDERIDE LA: Wyeth-Ayerst	00046-0455-81	100s	$125.83

CAPSULE: 50 MG-120 MG

BRAND/MANUFACTURER	NDC	SIZE	AWP
○ BRAND			
➤ INDERIDE LA: Wyeth-Ayerst	00046-0457-81	100s	$149.50

CAPSULE: 50 MG-160 MG

BRAND/MANUFACTURER	NDC	SIZE	AWP
○ BRAND			
➤ INDERIDE LA: Wyeth-Ayerst	00046-0459-81	100s	$167.63

TABLETS: 25 MG-40 MG

AVERAGE UNIT PRICE (AVAILABLE SIZES)		GENERIC A-RATED AVERAGE PRICE (GAAP)	
BRAND	$0.86	100s	$30.65
GENERIC	$0.29	500s	$116.62
HCFA FUL (100s ea)	$0.08	1000s	$255.73

BRAND/MANUFACTURER	NDC	SIZE	AWP
◆ BRAND			
➤ INDERIDE-40/25: Wyeth-Ayerst	00046-0484-81	100s	$87.95
	00046-0484-91	1000s	$844.09
◆ GENERICS			
Sidmak	50111-0473-01	100s	$16.78
Barr	00555-0427-02	100s	$21.04
Mylan	00378-0731-01	100s	$23.72
Qualitest	00603-5503-21	100s	$24.08
Rugby	00536-4402-01	100s	$24.69
Goldline	00182-1833-01	100s	$24.90
Purepac	00228-2358-10	100s	$25.75
Geneva	00781-1431-01	100s	$26.07
Major	00904-0434-60	100s	$26.50
Schein	00364-0838-01	100s	$26.50
URL	00677-1106-01	100s	$26.90
Moore,H.L.	00839-7197-06	100s	$31.12
Aligen	00405-4894-01	100s	$35.58
Major	00904-0434-80	100s	$96.85
Major	00904-0434-61	100s ud	$29.24
Sidmak	50111-0473-02	500s	$80.58
Qualitest	00603-5503-28	500s	$110.45
Rugby	00536-4402-05	500s	$112.38
Purepac	00228-2358-50	500s	$128.75
Parmed	00349-8509-05	500s	$150.95
Barr	00555-0427-05	1000s	$173.24
Purepac	00228-2358-96	1000s	$338.22

TABLETS: 25 MG-80 MG

AVERAGE UNIT PRICE (AVAILABLE SIZES)		GENERIC A-RATED AVERAGE PRICE (GAAP)	
BRAND	$1.18	100s	$34.81
GENERIC	$0.34		
HCFA FUL (100s ea)	$0.09		

BRAND/MANUFACTURER	NDC	SIZE	AWP
◆ BRAND			
➤ INDERIDE-80/25: Wyeth-Ayerst	00046-0488-81	100s	$118.10
◆ GENERICS			
Sidmak	50111-0474-01	100s	$23.43
Barr	00555-0428-02	100s	$29.60
Mylan	00378-0347-01	100s	$32.86
Goldline	00182-1834-01	100s	$34.10
Rugby	00536-4403-01	100s	$34.25
Qualitest	00603-5504-21	100s	$34.44
Purepac	00228-2360-10	100s	$35.99
Geneva	00781-1432-01	100s	$36.20
Major	00904-0438-60	100s	$37.90
Schein	00364-0839-01	100s	$37.90
URL	00677-1107-01	100s	$38.47
Moore,H.L.	00839-7198-06	100s	$38.48
Aligen	00405-4895-01	100s	$38.95
Sidmak	50111-0474-02	500s	$112.64
Purepac	00228-2360-96	1000s	$349.43

➤ SHOWN IN PRODUCT IDENTIFICATION GUIDE

Hydrochlorothiazide and Timolol Maleate

DESCRIPTION

Hydrochlorothiazide/Timolol Maleate is for the treatment of hypertension. It combines the antihypertensive activity of two agents: a non-selective beta-adrenergic receptor blocking agent (Timolol Maleate) and a diuretic (Hydrochlorothiazide).

Timolol Maleate is (S)-1-[(1,1-dimethylethyl)amino]-3-[[4-(4-morpholinyl)-1,2,5-thiadiazol-3-yl]oxy]-2-propanol (Z)-2-butenedioate (1:1) salt. Its empirical formula is $C_{13}H_{24}N_4O_3S \cdot C_4H_4O_4$.

Hydrochlorothiazide is 6-chloro-3,4-dihydro-2H-1,2,4-benzothiadiazine-7-sulfonamide 1, 1-dioxide. Its empirical formula is $C_7H_8ClN_3O_4S_2$.

Hydrochlorothiazide has a molecular weight of 297.72. It is a white, or practically white, crystalline powder which is slightly soluble in water, but freely soluble in sodium hydroxide solution.

Hydrochlorothiazide/Timolol Maleate is supplied as tablets containing 10 mg of Timolol Maleate and 25 mg of Hydrochlorothiazide for oral administration.

CLINICAL PHARMACOLOGY

HYDROCHLOROTHIAZIDE/TIMOLOL MALEATE

Timolol Maleate and Hydrochlorothiazide have been used singly and concomitantly for the treatment of hypertension. The antihypertensive effects of these agents are additive. The two components of Hydrochlorothiazide/Timolol Maleate have similar dosage schedules, and studies have shown that there is no interference with bioavailability when these agents are given together in the single combination tablet. Therefore, this combination provides a convenient formulation for the concomitant administration of these two entities.

In controlled clinical trials with Hydrochlorothiazide/Timolol Maleate in selected patients with mild to moderate essential hypertension, about 90 percent had a good to excellent response. In patients with more severe hypertension, Hydrochlorothiazide/Timolol Maleate may be administered with other antihypertensives such as methyldopa or a vasodilator.

Although the mechanisms of action of Timolol Maleate and Hydrochlorothiazide in the treatment of hypertension have not been established, they are thought to be different; for example, Hydrochlorothiazide increases plasma renin activity while Timolol Maleate reduces plasma renin activity.

TIMOLOL MALEATE

Timolol Maleate is a beta$_1$ and beta$_2$ (non-selective) adrenergic receptor blocking agent that does not have significant intrinsic sympathomimetic, direct myocardial depressant, or local anesthetic activity.

PHARMACODYNAMICS

Clinical pharmacology studies have confirmed the beta-adrenergic blocking activity as shown by (1) changes in resting heart rate and response of heart rate to changes in posture; (2) inhibition of isoproterenol-induced tachycardia; (3) alteration of the response to the Valsalva maneuver and amyl nitrite administration; and (4) reduction of heart rate and blood pressure changes on exercise.

Timolol Maleate decreases the positive chronotropic, positive inotropic, bronchodilator, and vasodilator responses caused by beta-adrenergic receptor agonists. The magnitude of this decreased response is proportional to the existing sympathetic tone and the concentration of Timolol Maleate at receptor sites.

In normal volunteers, the reduction in heart rate response to a standard exercise was dose dependent over the test range of 0.5 to 20 mg, with a peak reduction at 2 hours of approximately 30% at higher doses.

Beta-adrenergic receptor blockade reduces cardiac output in both healthy subjects and patients with heart disease. In patients with severe impairment of myocardial function beta-adrenergic receptor blockade may inhibit the stimulatory effect of the sympathetic nervous system necessary to maintain adequate cardiac function.

Beta-adrenergic receptor blockade in the bronchi and bronchioles results in increased airway resistance from unopposed parasympathetic activity. Such an effect in patients with asthma or other bronchospastic conditions is potentially dangerous.

Clinical studies indicate that Timolol Maleate at a dosage of 20-60 mg/day reduces blood pressure without causing postural hypotension in most patients with essential hypertension. Administration of Timolol Maleate to patients with hypertension results initially in a decrease in cardiac output, little immediate change in blood pressure, and an increase in calculated peripheral resistance. With continued administration of Timolol Maleate blood pressure decreases within a few days, cardiac output usually remains reduced, and peripheral resistance falls toward pretreatment levels. Plasma volume may decrease or remain unchanged during therapy with Timolol Maleate. In the majority of patients with hypertension, Timolol Maleate also decreases plasma renin activity. Dosage adjustment to achieve optimal antihypertensive effect may require a few weeks. When therapy with Timolol Maleate is discontinued, the blood pressure tends to return to pretreatment levels gradually. In most patients the antihypertensive activity of Timolol Maleate is maintained with long-term therapy and is well tolerated.

The mechanism of the antihypertensive effects of beta-adrenergic receptor blocking agents is not established at this time. Possible mechanisms of action include reduction in cardiac output, reduction in plasma renin activity, and a central nervous system sympatholytic action.

PHARMACOKINETICS AND METABOLISM

Timolol Maleate is rapidly and nearly completely absorbed (about 90%) following oral ingestion. Detectable plasma levels of Timolol occur within one-half hour and peak plasma levels occur in about one to two hours. The drug half-life in plasma is approximately 4 hours and this is essentially unchanged in patients with moderate renal insufficiency. Timolol is partially metabolized by the liver and Timolol and its metabolites are excreted by the kidney. Timolol is not extensively bound to plasma proteins; i.e., < 10% by equilibrium dialysis and approximately 60% by ultrafiltration. An *in vitro* hemodialysis study, using ^{14}C Timolol added to human plasma or whole blood, showed that Timolol was readily dialyzed from these fluids; however, a study of patients with renal failure showed that Timolol did not dialyze readily. Plasma levels following oral administration are about half those following intravenous administration indicating approximately 50% first pass metabolism. The level of beta sympathetic activity varies widely among individuals, and no simple correlation exists between the dose or plasma level of Timolol Maleate and its therapeutic activity. Therefore, objective clinical measurements such as reduction of heart rate and/or blood pressure should be used as guides in determining the optimal dosage for each patient.

HYDROCHLOROTHIAZIDE

Hydrochlorothiazide is a diuretic and antihypertensive agent. It affects the renal tubular mechanism of electrolyte reabsorption. Hydrochlorothiazide increases excretion of sodium and chloride in approximately equivalent amounts. Natriuresis may be accompanied by some loss of potassium and bicarbonate. The mechanism of the antihypertensive effect of thiazides may be related to the excretion and redistribution of body sodium. Hydrochlorothiazide usually does not cause clinically important changes in normal blood pressure.

INDICATIONS AND USAGE

Hydrochlorothiazide/Timolol Maleate is indicated for the treatment of hypertension. This fixed combination drug is not indicated for initial therapy of hypertension. If the fixed combination represents the dose titrated to an individual patient's needs, it may be more convenient than the separate components.

CONTRAINDICATIONS

Hydrochlorothiazide/Timolol Maleate is contraindicated in patients with bronchial asthma or with a history of bronchial asthma, or severe chronic obstructive pulmonary disease (see *"Warnings"*); sinus bradycardia; second and third degree atrioventricular block; overt cardiac failure (see *"Warnings"*); cardiogenic shock; anuria; hypersensitivity to this product or to sulfonamide-derived drugs.

WARNINGS

CARDIAC FAILURE

Sympathetic stimulation may be essential for support of the circulation in individuals with diminished myocardial contractility, and its inhibition by beta-adrenergic receptor blockade may precipitate more severe failure. Although beta blockers should be avoided in overt congestive heart failure, they can be used, if necessary, with caution in patients with a history of failure who are well-compensated, usually with digitalis and diuretics. Both digitalis and Timolol Maleate slow AV conduction. If cardiac failure persists, therapy with Hydrochlorothiazide/Timolol Maleate should be withdrawn.

In Patients Without a History of Cardiac Failure: continued depression of the myocardium with beta-blocking agents over a period of time can, in some cases, lead to cardiac failure. At the first sign or symptom of cardiac failure, patients receiving Hydrochlorothiazide/Timolol Maleate should be digitalized and/or be given additional diuretic therapy. Observe the patient closely. If cardiac failure continues, despite adequate digitalization and diuretic therapy, Hydrochlorothiazide/Timolol Maleate should be withdrawn.

RENAL AND HEPATIC DISEASE AND ELECTROLYTE DISTURBANCES

Since Timolol Maleate is partially metabolized in the liver and excreted mainly by the kidneys, dosage reductions may be necessary when hepatic and/or renal insufficiency is present.

Although the pharmacokinetics of Timolol Maleate are not greatly altered by renal impairment, marked hypotensive responses have been seen in patients with marked renal impairment undergoing dialysis after 20 mg doses. Dosing in such patients should therefore be especially cautious.

In patients with renal disease, thiazides may precipitate azotemia, and cumulative effects may develop in the presence of impaired renal function. If progressive renal impairment becomes evident, Hydrochlorothiazide/Timolol Maleate should be discontinued. In patients with impaired hepatic function or progressive liver disease, even minor alterations in fluid and electrolyte balance may precipitate hepatic coma. Hepatic encephalopathy, manifested by tremors, confusion, and coma, has been reported in association with diuretic therapy including Hydrochlorothiazide.

EXACERBATION OF ISCHEMIC HEART DISEASE FOLLOWING ABRUPT WITHDRAWAL: HYPERSENSITIVITY TO CATECHOLAMINES HAS BEEN OBSERVED IN PATIENTS WITHDRAWN FROM BETA BLOCKER THERAPY; EXACERBATION OF ANGINA AND, IN SOME CASES, MYOCARDIAL INFARCTION HAVE OCCURRED AFTER *ABRUPT* DISCONTINUATION OF SUCH THERAPY. WHEN DISCONTINUING CHRONICALLY ADMINISTERED TIMOLOL MALEATE, PARTICULARLY IN PATIENTS WITH ISCHEMIC HEART DISEASE, THE DOSAGE SHOULD BE GRADUALLY REDUCED OVER

◆ RATED THERAPEUTICALLY EQUIVALENT; ◇ THERAPEUTIC EQUIVALENCE UNCONFIRMED; ○ UNRATED

A PERIOD OF ONE TO TWO WEEKS AND THE PATIENT SHOULD BE CAREFULLY MONITORED. IF ANGINA MARKEDLY WORSENS OR ACUTE CORONARY INSUFFICIENCY DEVELOPS, TIMOLOL MALEATE ADMINISTRATION SHOULD BE REINSTITUTED PROMPTLY, AT LEAST TEMPORARILY, AND OTHER MEASURES APPROPRIATE FOR THE MANAGEMENT OF UNSTABLE ANGINA SHOULD BE TAKEN. PATIENTS SHOULD BE WARNED AGAINST INTERRUPTION OR DISCONTINUATION OF THERAPY WITHOUT THE PHYSICIAN'S ADVICE. BECAUSE CORONARY ARTERY DISEASE IS COMMON AND MAY BE UNRECOGNIZED, IT MAY BE PRUDENT NOT TO DISCONTINUE TIMOLOL MALEATE THERAPY ABRUPTLY EVEN IN PATIENTS TREATED ONLY FOR HYPERTENSION.

OBSTRUCTIVE PULMONARY DISEASE
Patients with chronic obstructive pulmonary disease (e.g., chronic bronchitis, emphysema) of mild or moderate severity, bronchospastic disease (other than bronchial asthma or a history of bronchial asthma in which Hydrochlorothiazide/Timolol Maleate is contraindicated (see "Contraindications"), should in general not receive beta blockers, including Hydrochlorothiazide/Timolol Maleate. However, if Hydrochlorothiazide/Timolol Maleate is necessary in such patients, then the drug should be administered with caution since it may block bronchodilation produced by endogenous and exogenous catecholamine stimulation of beta$_2$ receptors.

MAJOR SURGERY
The necessity or desirability of withdrawal of beta-blocking therapy prior to major surgery is controversial. Beta-adrenergic receptor blockade impairs the ability of the heart to respond to beta-adrenergically mediated reflex stimuli. This may augment the risk of general anesthesia in surgical procedures. Some patients receiving beta-adrenergic receptor blocking agents have been subject to protracted severe hypotension during anesthesia. Difficulty in restarting and maintaining the heartbeat has also been reported. For these reasons, in patients undergoing elective surgery, some authorities recommend gradual withdrawal of beta-adrenergic receptor blocking agents.

If necessary during surgery, the effects of beta-adrenergic blocking agents may be reversed by sufficient doses of such agonists as isoproterenol, dopamine, dobutamine or levarterenol (see *"Overdosage"*).

METABOLIC AND ENDOCRINE EFFECTS
Beta-adrenergic blockade may mask certain clinical signs (e.g., tachycardia) of hyperthyroidism. Patients suspected of developing thyrotoxicosis should be managed carefully to avoid abrupt withdrawal of beta blockade which might precipitate a thyroid storm. Thiazides may decrease serum PBI levels without signs of thyroid disturbance.

Beta-adrenergic receptor blocking agents may mask the signs and symptoms of acute hypoglycemia. Therefore, Hydrochlorothiazide/Timolol Maleate should be administered with caution to patients subject to spontaneous hypoglycemia, or to diabetic patients (especially those with labile diabetes) who are receiving insulin or oral hypoglycemic agents. Insulin requirements in diabetic patients may be increased, decreased, or unchanged by thiazides. Diabetes mellitus which has been latent may become manifest during administration of thiazide diuretics. Because calcium excretion is decreased by thiazides Hydrochlorothiazide/Timolol Maleate should be discontinued before carrying out tests for parathyroid function. Pathologic changes in the parathyroid glands, with hypercalcemia and hypophosphatemia, have been observed in a few patients on prolonged thiazide therapy; however, the common complications of hyperparathyroidism such as renal lithiasis, bone resorption, and peptic ulceration have not been seen.

Hyperuricemia may occur or acute gout may be precipitated in certain patients receiving thiazide therapy.

PRECAUTIONS
GENERAL
Electrolyte and Fluid Balance Status: Periodic determination of serum electrolytes to detect possible electrolyte imbalance should be performed at appropriate intervals.

Patients should be observed for clinical signs of fluid or electrolyte imbalance, i.e., hyponatremia, hypochloremic alkalosis, and hypokalemia. Serum and urine electrolyte determinations are particularly important when the patient is vomiting excessively or receiving parenteral fluids. Warning signs or symptoms of fluid and electrolyte imbalance, irrespective of cause, include dryness of the mouth, thirst, weakness, lethargy, drowsiness, restlessness, confusion, seizures, muscle pains or cramps, muscular fatigue, hypotension, oliguria, tachycardia, and gastrointestinal disturbances such as nausea and vomiting.

Hypokalemia may develop, especially with brisk diuresis, when severe cirrhosis is present, or during concomitant use of corticosteroids or ACTH.

Interference with adequate oral electrolyte intake will also contribute to hypokalemia. Hypokalemia may cause cardiac arrhythmia and may also sensitize or exaggerate the response of the heart to the toxic effects of digitalis (e.g., increased ventricular irritability). Hypokalemia may be avoided or treated by use of potassium sparing diuretics or potassium supplements such as foods with a high potassium content.

Any chloride deficit during thiazide therapy is generally mild and usually does not require specific treatment except under extraordinary circumstances (as in liver disease or renal disease). Dilutional hyponatremia may occur in edematous patients in hot weather; appropriate therapy is water restriction rather than

administration of salt except in rare instances when the hyponatremia is life threatening. In actual salt depletion, appropriate replacement is the therapy of choice.

Thiazides have been shown to increase urinary excretion of magnesium, which may result in hypomagnesemia.

Effects on Cholesterol and Triglyceride Levels: Increases in cholesterol and triglyceride levels may, be associated with thiazide diuretic therapy.

Muscle Weakness: Beta-adrenergic blockade has been reported to potentiate muscle weakness consistent with certain myasthenic symptoms (e.g., diplopia, ptosis, and generalized weakness). Timolol has been reported rarely to increase muscle weakness in some patients with myasthenia gravis or myasthenic symptoms.

Cerebrovascular Insufficiency: Because of potential effects of beta-adrenergic blocking agents relative to blood pressure and pulse, these agents should be used with caution in patients with cerebrovascular insufficiency. If signs or symptoms suggesting reduced cerebral blood flow are observed, consideration should be given to discontinuation these agents.

DRUG INTERACTIONS
Hydrochlorothiazide/Timolol Maleate may potentiate the action of other antihypertensive agents used concomitantly. Close observation of the patient is recommended when Hydrochlorothiazide/Timolol Maleate is administered to patients receiving catecholamine-depleting drugs such as reserpine, because of possible additive effects and the production of hypotension and/or marked bradycardia, which may produce vertigo, syncope, or postural hypotension.

Blunting of the antihypertensive effect of beta-adrenoceptor blocking agents by non-steroidal anti-inflammatory drugs has been reported. In some patients, the administration of a non-steroidal anti-inflammatory agent can reduce the diuretic, natriuretic, and antihypertensive effects of loop, potassium-spring and thiazide diuretics. Therefore, when Hydrochlorothiazide/Timolol Maleate and non-steroidal anti-inflammatory agents are used concomitantly, the patient should be observed closely to determine if the desired therapeutic effect has been obtained.

Literature reports suggest that oral calcium antagonists may be used in combination with beta-adrenergic blocking agents when heart function is normal, but should be avoided in patients with impaired cardiac function. Hypotension, AV conduction disturbances, and left ventricular failure have been reported in some patients receiving beta-adrenergic blocking agents when an oral calcium antagonist was added to the treatment regimen. Hypotension was more likely to occur if the calcium antagonist were a dihydropyridine derivative, e.g., nifedipine, while left ventricular failure and AV conduction disturbances were more likely to occur with either verapamil or diltiazem.

Intravenous calcium antagonists should be used with caution in patients receiving beta-adrenergic blocking agents. The concomitant use of beta-adrenergic blocking agents with digitalis and either diltiazem or verapamil may have additive effects in prolonging AV conduction time.

Absorption of Hydrochlorothiazide is impaired in the presence of anionic exchange resins. Single doses of either cholestyramine or colestipol resins bind the Hydrochlorothiazide and reduce its absorption from the gastrointestinal tract by up to 85 and 43 percent, respectively.

Risk from Anaphylactic Reaction: While taking beta-blockers, patients with a history of atopy or a history of severe anaphylactic reaction to a variety of allergens may be more reactive to repeated accidental, diagnostic, or therapeutic challenge with such allergens. Such patients may be unresponsive to the usual doses of epinephrine used to treat anaphylactic reactions.

In patients receiving thiazides, sensitivity reactions may occur with or without a history of allergy or bronchial asthma. The possible exacerbation or activation of systemic lupus erythematosus has been reported. The antihypertensive effects of thiazides may be enhanced in the post-sympathectomy patient.

Thiazides may decrease arterial responsiveness to norepinephrine. This diminution is not sufficient to preclude the therapeutic effectiveness of norepinephrine. Thiazides may increase the responsiveness to tubocurarine.

Lithium generally should not be given with diuretics because they reduce its renal clearance and add a high risk of lithium toxicity. Read circulars for lithium preparations before use of such preparations with Hydrochlorothiazide/Timolol Maleate.

CARCINOGENESIS, MUTAGENESIS, IMPAIRMENT OF FERTILITY
Carcinogenicity, mutagenicity, and fertility studies have not been conducted in animals with Hydrochlorothiazide/Timolol Maleate.

Timolol Maleate: In a two-year study of Timolol Maleate in rats, there was a statistically significant increase in the incidence of adrenal pheochromocytomas in male rats administered 300 mg/kg/day (250 times* the maximum recommended daily human dose). Similar differences were not observed in rats administered doses equivalent to approximately 20 or 80 times* the maximum recommended daily human dose.

In a lifetime study in mice, there were statistically significant increases in the incidence of benign and malignant pulmonary tumors, benign uterine polyps and mammary adenocarcinoma in female mice at 500 mg/kg/day (approximately 400 times* the maximum recommended daily human dose), but not at 5 or 50 mg/kg/day. In a subsequent study in female mice, in which post-mortem examinations were limited to uterus and lungs, a statistically significant increase in the incidence of pulmonary tumors was again observed at 500 mg/kg/day.

---
* Based on patient weight of 50 kg

The increased occurrence of mammary adenocarcinoma was associated with elevations of serum prolactin that occurred in female mice administered Timolol at 500 mg/kg/day, but not at doses of 5 or 50 mg/kg/day. An increase incidence of mammary adenocarcinomas in rodents has been associated with administration of several other therapeutic agents which elevate serum prolactin, but no correlation between serum prolactin levels and mammary tumors has been established in man. Furthermore, in adult human female subjects who received oral dosages of up to 60 mg of Timolol Maleate, the maximum recommended daily human oral dosage, there were no clinically meaningful changes in serum prolactin.

Timolol Maleate was devoid of mutagenic potential when evaluated *in vivo* (mouse) in the micronucleus test and cytogenetic assay (doses up to 800 mg/kg) and *in vitro* in a neoplastic cell transformation assay (up to 100 μg/mL). In Ames tests the highest concentrations of Timolol employed, 5000 or 10,000 μg/plate, were associated with statistically significant elevations of revertants observed with tester strain TA100 (in seven replicate assays), but not in the remaining three strains. In the assays with tester strain TA100, no consistent dose response relationship was observed, nor did the ratio of test to control revertants reach 2. A ratio of 2 is usually considered the criterion for a positive Ames test.

Reproduction and fertility studies in rats showed no adverse effect on male or female fertility at doses up to 125 times* the maximum recommended daily dose.

Hydrochlorothiazide: Two-year feeding studies in mice and rats conducted under the auspices of the National Toxicology Program (NTP) uncovered no evidence of a carcinogenic potential of Hydrochlorothiazide in female mice (at doses of up to approximately 600 mg/kg/day) or in male and female rats (at doses of up to approximately 100 mg/kg/day). The NTP, however, found equivocal evidence for hepatocarcinogenicity in male mice.

Hydrochlorothiazide was not genotoxic *in vitro* in the Ames mutagenicity assay of *Salmonella typhimurium* strains TA 98, TA 100, TA 1535, TA 1537, and TA 1538 and in the Chinese Hamster Ovary (CHO) test for chromosomal aberrations, or *in vivo* in assays using mouse germinal cell chromosomes, Chinese hamster bone marrow chromosomes, and the *Drosophila* sex-linked recessive lethal trait gene. Positive test results were obtained only in the *in vitro* CHO Sister Chromatid Exchange (clastogenicity) and in the Mouse Lymphoma Cell (mutagenicity) assay, using concentrations of Hydrochlorothiazide from 43 to 1300 μg/ mL, and in the *Aspergillus nidulans* nondisjunction assay at an unspecified concentration.

Hydrochlorothiazide had no adverse effects on the fertility of mice and rats of either sex in studies wherein these species were exposed, via their diet, to doses of up to 100 and 4 mg/kg, respectively, prior to conception and throughout gestation.

PREGNANCY
Teratogenic Effects

Pregnancy Category C: Combinations of Timolol Maleate and Hydrochlorothiazide were studied for teratogenic potential in the mouse and rabbit. The Timolol Maleate/Hydrochlorothiazide combinations were administered orally to pregnant mice and pregnant rabbits at dosage levels of 1/2.5, 4/10, or 8/10 mg/kg/day. No teratogenic, embryotoxic, fetotoxic, or maternotoxic effects attributable to treatment were observed in either species. There are no adequate and well-controlled studies in pregnant women with Hydrochlorothiazide/Timolol Maleate. Because of the data listed below with the individual components, Hydrochlorothiazide/Timolol Maleate should be used during pregnancy only if the potential benefit justifies the potential risk to the fetus.

Timolol Maleate: Teratogenicity studies with Timolol Maleate in mice, rats and rabbits at doses up to 50 mg/kg/day (approximately 40 times* the maximum recommended daily human dose) showed no evidence of fetal malformations. Although delayed fetal ossification was observed at this dose in rats, there were no adverse effects on postnatal development of offspring. Doses of 1000 mg/kg/day (approximately 830 times* the maximum recommended daily human dose) were maternotoxic in mice and resulted in an increased number of fetal resorptions. Increased fetal resorptions were also seen in rabbits at doses of approximately 40 times the maximum recommended daily human dose, in this case without apparent maternotoxicity.

Hydrochlorothiazide: Studies in which Hydrochlorothiazide was orally administered to pregnant mice and rats during their respective periods of major organogenesis at doses up to 3000 and 1000 Hydrochlorothiazide/kg, respectively, provided no evidence of harm to the fetus.

Nonteratogenic Effects

Hydrochlorothiazide: Hydrochlorothiazide/Timolol Maleate contains Hydrochlorothiazide. Thiazides cross the placental barrier and appear in cord blood. The possible hazards to the fetus include fetal or neonatal jaundice, thrombocytopenia, and possibly other adverse reactions which have occurred in the adult.

NURSING MOTHERS
Timolol Maleate and thiazides have been detected in human milk. Because of the potential for serious adverse reactions from Timolol and Hydrochlorothiazide in nursing infants, a decision should be made whether to discontinue nursing or to discontinue the drug, taking into account the importance of the drug to the mother.

PEDIATRIC USE
Safety and effectiveness in children have not been established.

* Based on patient weight of 50 kg

ADVERSE REACTIONS
Hydrochlorothiazide/Timolol Maleate is usually well tolerated in properly selected patients. Most adverse effects have been mild and transient. The adverse reactions listed in the following table were spontaneously reported and have been arranged into two groups: (1) incidence greater than 1%; and (2) incidence less than 1%. The incidence was obtained from clinical studies conducted in the United States (257 patients treated with Hydrochlorothiazide/Timolol Maleate.

Incidence Greater Than 1%	Incidence Less Than 1%
Body as a Whole	
fatigue/tiredness (1.9%)	chest pain
asthenia (1.9%)	headache
Cardiovascular	
hypotension (1.6%)	arrhythmia
bradycardia (1.2%)	syncope
	cardiac failure
Digestive System	
none	diarrhea
	dyspepsia
	nausea
	gastrointestinal pain
	constipation
Integumentary	
none	rash
	increased pigmentation
	dry mucous membranes
Musculoskeletal	
none	myalgia
Nervous System	
dizziness (1.2%)	none
Psychiatric	
none	insomnia
	decreased libido
	nervousness
	confusion
	trouble concentrating
	somnolence
Respiratory	
bronchial spasm (1.6%)	rales
dyspnea (1.2%)	
Urogenital	
none	renal colic

The following additional adverse effects have been reported in clinical experience with the drug: cerebral ischemia, cerebral vascular accident, gout, muscle cramps, oculogyric crisis, worsening of chronic obstructive pulmonary disease, earache, and impotence.

Other Adverse Reactions that have been reported with the individual components are listed below:

TIMOLOL MALEATE
Body as a Whole: extremity pain, decreased exercise tolerance, weight loss, fever;

Cardiovascular: cardiac arrest, cerebral vascular accident, worsening of angina pectoris, sinoatrial block, AV block, worsening of arterial insufficiency, Raynaud's phenomenon, claudication, palpitations, vasodilatation, cold hands and feet, edema;

Digestive: hepatomegaly, elevated liver function tests, vomiting;

Hematologic: nonthrombocytopenic purpura;

Endocrine: hyperglycemia, hypoglycemia;

Skin: skin irritation, pruritus, sweating, alopecia;

Musculoskeletal: arthralgia;

Nervous System: local weakness, vertigo, paresthesia, increase in signs and symptoms of myasthenia gravis;

Psychiatric: depression, nightmares, hallucinations;

Respiratory: cough;

Special Senses: visual disturbances, diplopia, ptosis, eye irritation, dry eyes, tinnitus;

Urogenital: urination difficulties.

There have been reports of retroperitoneal fibrosis in patients receiving Timolol Maleate and in patients receiving other beta-adrenergic blocking agents. A causal relationship between this condition and therapy with beta-adrenergic blocking agents has not been established.

HYDROCHLOROTHIAZIDE
Body as a Whole: weakness;

Digestive: anorexia, gastric irritation, vomiting, cramping, jaundice (intrahepatic cholestatic jaundice), pancreatitis, sialadenitis;

Nervous System/Psychiatric: vertigo, paresthesias, restlessness;

Hematologic: leukopenia, agranulocytosis, thrombocytopenia, aplastic anemia, hemolytic anemia;

Cardiovascular: hypotension including orthostatic hypotension (may be aggravated by alcohol, barbiturates, narcotics or antihypertensive drugs);

Hypersensitivity: purpura, photosensitivity, urticaria, necrotizing angiitis (vasculitis, cutaneous vasculitis) fever, respiratory distress including pneumonitis and pulmonary edema, anaphylactic reactions;

Metabolic: hyperglycemia; glycosuria, hyperuricemia, electrolyte imbalance (see "*Precautions*");

Musculoskeletal: muscle spasm;

Renal: renal failure, renal dysfunction, interstitial nephritis (see "*Warnings*");

Skin: erythema multiforme including Stevens-Johnson syndrome, exfoliative dermatitis including toxic epidermal necrolysis, alopecia;

Special Senses: transient blurred vision, xanthopsia.

Potential Adverse Effects: In addition, a variety of adverse effects not observed in clinical trials with Timolol Maleate, but reported with other beta-adrenergic blocking agents, should be considered potential adverse effects of Timolol Maleate:

Nervous System: reversible mental depression progressing to catatonia; an acute reversible syndrome characterized by disorientation for time and place, short-term memory loss, emotional lability, slightly clouded sensorium, and decreased performance on neuropsychometrics;

Cardiovascular: intensification of AV block (see "*Contraindications*");

Digestive: mesenteric arterial thrombosis, ischemic colitis;

Hematologic: agranulocytosis, thrombocytopenic purpura;

Allergic: erythematous rash, fever combined with aching and sore throat, laryngospasm with respiratory distress;

Miscellaneous: Peyronie's disease.

There have been reports of a syndrome comprising psoriasiform skin rash, conjunctivitis sicca, otitis, and sclerosing serositis attributed to the beta-adrenergic receptor blocking agent, practolol. This syndrome has not been reported with Hydrochlorothiazide/Timolol Maleate or Timolol Maleate.

Clinical Laboratory Test Findings: Clinically important changes in standard laboratory parameters were rarely associated with the administration of Hydrochlorothiazide/Timolol Maleate. The changes in laboratory parameters were not progressive and usually were not associated with clinical manifestations. The most common changes were increases in serum triglycerides and uric acid and decreases in serum potassium and chloride. Decreases in HDL cholesterol have been reported.

OVERDOSAGE

Overdosage has been reported with Timolol Maleate Tablets. A 30-year-old female ingested 650 mg of Timolol Maleate (maximum recommended daily dose—60 mg) and experienced second and third degree heart block. She recovered without treatment but approximately two months later developed irregular heart beat, hypertension, dizziness, tinnitus, faintness, increased pulse rate and borderline first degree heart block. Pretreatment of mice with Hydrochlorothiazide (5 mg/kg) did not alter the LD_{50} of Timolol (1320 mg/kg compared to 1300 mg/kg without pretreatment).

No specific information is available on the treatment of overdosage with Hydrochlorothiazide/Timolol Maleate and no specific antidote is available. Treatment is symptomatic and supportive. Therapy with Hydrochlorothiazide/Timolol Maleate should be discontinued and the patient observed closely. Suggested measures include induction of emesis and/or gastric lavage, and correction of dehydration, electrolyte imbalance, and hypotension by established procedures.

TIMOLOL MALEATE
No data are available in regard to overdosage in humans. The oral LD_{50} of the drug is 1190 and 900 mg/kg in female mice and female rats, respectively.

An *in vitro* hemodialysis study, using [14]C Timolol added to human plasma and whole blood, showed that Timolol was readily dialyzed from these fluids; however, a study of patients with renal failure showed that Timolol did not dialyze readily.

The most common signs and symptoms to be expected with overdosage with a beta-adrenergic receptor blocking agent are symptomatic bradycardia, hypotension, bronchospasm, and acute cardiac failure. If overdosage occurs the following therapeutic measures should be considered.

(1) Gastric lavage:

(2) Symptomatic bradycardia: Use atropine sulfate intravenously in a dosage of 0.25 mg to 2 mg to induce vagal blockade. If bradycardia persists, intravenous isoproterenol hydrochloride should be administered cautiously. In refractory cases the use of a transvenous cardiac pacemaker may be considered.

(3) Hypotension: Use sympathomimetic pressor drug therapy, such as dopamine, dobutamine or levarterenol. In refractory cases the use of glucagon hydrochloride has been reported to be useful.

(4) Bronchospasm: Use isoproterenol hydrochloride. Additional therapy with aminophylline may be considered.

(5) Acute cardiac failure: Conventional therapy with digitalis, diuretics, and oxygen should be instituted immediately. In refractory cases the use of intravenous aminophylline is suggested. This may be followed, if necessary, by glucagon hydrochloride which has been reported to be useful

(6) Heart block (second or third degree): Use isoproterenol hydrochloride or a transvenous cardiac pacemaker.

HYDROCHLOROTHIAZIDE
The most common signs and symptoms observed with Hydrochlorothiazide overdosage are those caused by electrolyte depletion (hypokalemia, hypochloremia, hyponatremia) and dehydration resulting from excessive diuresis. if digitalis has also been administered, hypokalemia may accentuate cardiac arrhythmias.

DOSAGE AND ADMINISTRATION
The recommended starting and maintenance dosage is 1 tablet twice a day or 2 tablets once a day. Patients usually do not require doses in excess of 50 mg of Hydrochlorothiazide daily when combined with other antihypertensive agents. If the antihypertensive response is not satisfactory, another nondiuretic antihypertensive agent may be added.

Store in a well-closed container, protected from light.

HOW SUPPLIED
TABLETS:

BRAND/MANUFACTURER	NDC	SIZE	AWP
○ BRAND			
TIMOLIDE 10-25: Merck	00006-0067-68	100s	$61.80

Hydrochlorothiazide with Metoprolol Tartrate

DESCRIPTION
Hydrochlorothiazide/Metoprolol Tartrate (HCTZ/Metoprolol) has the antihypertensive effect of Metoprolol Tartrate, a selective beta$_1$-adrenoreceptor blocking agent, and the antihypertensive and diuretic actions of Hydrochlorothiazide. It is available as tablets for oral administration. The 50/25 tablets contain 50 mg of Metoprolol Tartrate USP and 25 mg of Hydrochlorothiazide USP; the 100/25 tablets contain 100 mg of Metoprolol Tartrate USP and 25 mg of Hydrochlorothiazide USP; and the 100/50 tablets contain 100 mg of Metoprolol Tartrate USP and 50 mg of Hydrochlorothiazide USP.

Metoprolol Tartrate USP is ($\pm$)-1-Isopropylamino-3-[*p*-(2-methoxyethyl)phenoxyl]-2-propanol 2:1 *dextro*-Tartrate salt. Metoprolol Tartrate USP is a white, crystalline powder with a molecular weight of 684.82. It is very soluble in water; freely soluble in methylene chloride, in chloroform, and in alcohol; slightly soluble in acetone; and insoluble in either. Hydrochlorothiazide is 6-chloro-3,4-dihydro-2*H*-1,2,4-benzothiadiazine-7-sulfonamide, 1,1-dioxide.

Hydrochlorothiazide USP is a white, or practically white, practically odorless, crystalline powder. It is freely soluble in sodium hydroxide solution, in *n*-butylamine, and in dimethylformamide; sparingly soluble in methanol; slightly soluble in water; and insoluble in either, in chloroform, and in dilute mineral acids. Its molecular weight is 297.73.

CLINICAL PHARMACOLOGY
METOPROLOL
Metoprolol is a beta-adrenergic receptor blocking agent. *In vitro* and *in vivo* animal studies have shown that it has a preferential effect on beta$_1$ adrenoreceptors, chiefly located in cardiac muscle. This preferential effect is not absolute, however, and at higher doses, Metoprolol also inhibits beta$_2$ adrenoreceptors, chiefly located in the bronchial and vascular musculature.

Clinical pharmacology studies have confirmed the beta-blocking activity of Metoprolol in man, as shown by (1) reduction in heart rate and cardiac output at rest and upon exercise, (2) reduction of systolic blood pressure upon exercise, (3) inhibition of isoproterenol-induced tachycardia, and (4) reduction of reflex orthostatic tachycardia.

Relative beta$_1$ selectivity has been confirmed by the following: (1) in normal subjects, Metoprolol is unable to reverse the beta$_2$-mediated vasodilating effects of epinephrine. This contrasts with the effect of nonselective (beta$_1$ plus beta$_2$) beta blockers, which completely reverse the vasodilating effects of epinephrine. (2) In asthmatic patients, Metoprolol reduces FEV_1 and FVC significantly less than a nonselective beta blocker, propranolol at equivalent beta$_1$-receptor blocking doses.

Metoprolol has no intrinsic sympathomimetic activity and only weak membrane-stabilizing activity. Metoprolol crosses the blood-brain barrier and has been reported in the CSF in a concentration 78% of the simultaneous plasma concentration. Animal and human experiments indicate that Metoprolol slows the sinus rate and decreases AV nodal conduction. In controlled clinical studies, Metoprolol has been shown to be an effective antihypertensive agent when used alone or as concomitant therapy with thiazide-type diuretics, at dosages of 100-450 mg daily. In controlled, comparative, clinical studies, Metoprolol has been shown to be as effective an antihypertensive agent as propranolol, methyldopa, and thiazide-type diuretics, and to be equally effective in supine and standing positions.

The mechanism of the antihypertensive effects of beta-blocking agents has not been elucidated. However, several possible mechanisms have been proposed: (1) competitive antagonism of catecholamines at peripheral (especially cardiac) adrenergic neuron sites, leading to decreased cardiac output; (2) a central effect leading to reduced sympathetic outflow to the periphery; and (3) suppression of renin activity.

In man, absorption of Metoprolol is rapid and complete. Plasma levels following oral administration, however, approximate 50% of levels following intravenous administration, indicating about 50% first-pass metabolism. Plasma levels achieved are highly variable after oral administration. Only a small fraction of the drug (about 12%) is bound to human serum albumin. Elimination is mainly by biotransformation in the liver, and the plasma half-life ranges from approximately 3 to 7 hours. Less than 5% of an oral dose of Metoprolol is recovered unchanged in the urine; the rest is excreted by the kidneys as metabolites that appear to have no clinical significance. The systemic availability and half-life of Metoprolol in patients with renal failure do not differ to a clinically significant degree from those in normal subjects. Consequently, no reduction in dosage is usually needed in patients with chronic renal failure.

Significant beta-blocking effect (as measured by reduction of exercise heart rate) occurs within 1 hour after oral administration, and its duration is dose-related. For example, a 50% reduction of the maximum registered effect after single oral doses of 20, 50, and 100 mg occurred at 3.3, 5.0, and 6.4 hours, respectively, in normal subjects. After repeated oral dosages of 100 mg twice daily, a significant reduction in exercise systolic blood pressure was evident at 12 hours.

There is a linear relationship between the log of plasma levels and reduction of exercise heart rate. However, antihypertensive activity does not appear to be related to plasma levels. Because of variable plasma levels attained with a given dose and lack of a consistent relationship of antihypertensive activity to dose, selection of proper dosage requires individual titration.

HYDROCHLOROTHIAZIDE

Thiazides affect the renal tubular mechanism of electrolyte reabsorption. At maximal therapeutic dosage, all thiazides are approximately equal in their diuretic potency. Thiazides increase excretion of sodium and chloride in approximately equivalent amounts. Natriuresis causes a secondary loss of potassium.

The mechanism of the antihypertensive effect of thiazides is unknown. Thiazides do not affect normal blood pressure. The onset of action of thiazides occurs in 2 hours and the peak effect at about 4 hours. The action persists for approximately 6-12 hours. Hydrochlorothiazide is rapidly absorbed, as indicated by peak plasma concentrations 1-2.5 hours after oral administration. Plasma levels of the drug are proportional to dose; the concentration in whole blood is 1.6-1.8 times higher than in plasma. Thiazides are eliminated rapidly by the kidney. After oral administration of 25- to 100-mg doses, 72-97% of the dose is excreted in the urine, indicating dose-independent absorption. Hydrochlorothiazide is eliminated from plasma in a biphasic fashion with a terminal half-life of 10-17 hours. Plasma protein binding is 67.9%. Plasma clearance is 15.9-30.0 L/hr; volume of distribution is 3.6-7.8 L/kg.

Gastrointestinal absorption of Hydrochlorothiazide is enhanced when administered with food. Absorption is decreased in patients with congestive heart failure, and the pharmacokinetics are considerably different in these patients.

INDICATIONS AND USAGE

HCTZ/Metoprolol is indicated for the management of hypertension.

This fixed-combination drug is not indicated for initial therapy of hypertension. If the fixed combination represents the dose titrated to the individual patient's needs, therapy with the fixed combination may be more convenient than with the separate components.

CONTRAINDICATIONS

METOPROLOL

Metoprolol is contraindicated in sinus bradycardia, heart block greater than first degree, cardiogenic shock, and overt cardiac failure (see "Warnings").

HYDROCHLOROTHIAZIDE

Hydrochlorothiazide is contraindicated in patients with anuria or hypersensitivity to this or other sulfonamide-derived drugs (see "Warnings").

WARNINGS

METOPROLOL

Cardiac Failure: Sympathetic stimulation is a vital component supporting circulatory function in congestive heart failure, and beta blockade carries the potential hazard of further depressing myocardial contractility and precipitating more severe failure. In hypertensive patients who have congestive heart failure controlled by digitalis and diuretics, Metoprolol should be administered cautiously. Both digitalis and Metoprolol slow AV conduction.

In Patients Without a History of Cardiac Failure: Continued depression of the myocardium with beta-blocking agents over a period of time can, in some cases, lead to cardiac failure. At the first sign of symptom of impending cardiac failure, patients should be fully digitalized and/or given a diuretic. The response should be observed closely. If cardiac failure continues, despite adequate digitalization and diuretic therapy, Metoprolol should be withdrawn.

Ischemic Heart Disease: Following abrupt cessation of therapy with certain beta-blocking agents, exacerbations of angina pectoris and, in some cases, myocardial infarction have been reported. Even in the absence of overt angina pectoris, when discontinuing therapy, Metoprolol should not be withdrawn abruptly, and patients should be cautioned against interruption of therapy without the physician's advice (see "Precautions, Information for Patients").

Bronchospastic Diseases: **PATIENTS WITH BRONCHOSPASTIC DISEASES SHOULD, IN GENERAL, NOT RECEIVE BETA BLOCKERS.** Because of its relative $beta_1$ selectivity, however, Metoprolol may be used with caution in patients with bronchospastic disease who do not respond to, or cannot tolerate, other antihypertensive treatment. Since $beta_1$ selectivity is not absolute, a $beta_2$-stimulating agent should be administered concomitantly, and the lowest possible dose of Metoprolol should be used. In these circumstances it would be prudent initially to administer Metoprolol in smaller doses three times daily, instead of larger doses two times daily, to avoid the higher plasma levels associated with the longer dosing interval. (see "Dosage and Administration").

Major Surgery: The necessity or desirability of withdrawing beta-blocking therapy prior to major surgery is controversial; the impaired ability of the heart to respond to reflex adrenergic stimuli may augment the risks of general anesthesia and surgical procedures.

Metoprolol, like other beta blockers, is a competitive inhibitor of beta-receptor agonists, and its effects can be reversed by administration of such agents, e.g., dobutamine or isoproterenol. However, such patients may be subject to protracted severe hypotension. Difficulty in restarting and maintaining the heart beat has also been reported with beta blockers.

Diabetes and Hypoglycemia: Metoprolol should be used with caution in diabetic patients if a beta-blocking agent is required. Beta blockers may mask tachycardia occurring with hypoglycemia, but other manifestations such as dizziness and sweating may not be significantly affected. Selective beta blockers do not potentiate insulin-induced hypoglycemia and, unlike nonselective beta blockers, do not delay recovery of blood glucose to normal levels.

Thyrotoxicosis: Beta-adrenergic blockade may mask certain clinical signs (e.g., tachycardia) or hyperthyroidism. Patients suspected of developing thyrotoxicosis should be managed carefully to avoid abrupt withdrawal of beta blockade, which might precipitate a thyroid storm.

HYDROCHLOROTHIAZIDE

Thiazides should be used with caution in patients with severe renal disease. In patients with renal disease, thiazides may precipitate azotemia. Cumulative effects of the drug may develop in patients with impaired renal function.

Thiazides should be used with caution in patients with impaired hepatic function or progressive liver disease, since minor alterations of fluid and electrolyte imbalance may precipitate hepatic coma.

Thiazides may add to or potentiate the action of other antihypertensive drugs. Potentiation occurs with ganglionic or peripheral adrenergic blocking drugs.

Sensitivity reactions are more likely to occur in patients with a history of allergy or bronchial asthma.

The possibility of exacerbation or activation of systemic lupus erythematosus has been reported.

PRECAUTIONS

GENERAL

Metoprolol: Metoprolol should be used with caution in patients with impaired hepatic function.

Hydrochlorothiazide: All patients receiving thiazide therapy should be observed for clinical signs of fluid or electrolyte imbalance, namely hyponatremia, hypochloremic alkalosis, and hypokalemia (see "Laboratory Tests" and "Drug/Drug Interactions"). Warning signs are dryness of mouth, thirst, weakness, lethargy, drowsiness, restlessness, muscle pains or cramps, muscular fatigue, hypotension, oliguria, tachycardia, and gastrointestinal disturbance, such as nausea or vomiting.

Hypokalemia may develop, especially in cases of brisk diuresis or severe cirrhosis.

Interference with adequate oral intake of electrolytes will also contribute to hypokalemia. Hypokalemia may be avoided or treated by the use of potassium supplements or foods with a high potassium content.

Any chloride deficit is generally mild and usually does not require specific treatment, except under extraordinary circumstances (as in liver disease or renal disease). Dilutional hyponatremia may occur in edematous patients in hot weather; appropriate therapy is water restriction, rather than administration of salt, except in rare instances when the hyponatremia is life-threatening. In cases of actual salt depletion, appropriate replacement is the therapy of choice. Hyperuricemia may occur or frank gout may be precipitated in certain patients receiving thiazide therapy.

Latent diabetes may become manifest during thiazide administration (see "Drug/Drug Interactions").

The antihypertensive effects of the drug may be enhanced in the postsympathectomy patient.

If progressive renal impairment becomes evident, withholding or discontinuing diuretic therapy should be considered. Calcium excretion is decreased by thiazides. Pathological changes in the parathyroid gland with hypercalcemia and hypophosphatemia have been observed in a few patients on prolonged thiazide therapy. The common complications of hyperparathyroidism, such as renal lithiasis, bone resorption, and peptic ulceration, have not been seen.

INFORMATION FOR PATIENTS

Patients should be advised to take HCTZ/Metoprolol regularly and continuously, as directed, with or immediately following meals. If a dose should be missed, the patient should take only the next scheduled dose (without doubling it). Patients should not discontinue HCTZ/Metoprolol without consulting the physician.

Patients should be advised (1) to avoid operating automobiles and machinery or engaging in other tasks requiring alertness until the patient's response to therapy with Metoprolol has been determined; (2) to contact the physician if any difficulty in breathing occurs; (3) to inform the physician or dentist before any type of surgery that he or she is taking HCTZ/Metoprolol.

LABORATORY TESTS

Metoprolol: Clinical laboratory findings may include elevated levels of serum transaminase, alkaline phosphatase, and lactate dehydrogenase.

Hydrochlorothiazide: Initial and periodic determinations of serum electrolytes to detect possible electrolyte imbalance should be performed at appropriate intervals.

Serum and urine electrolyte determinations are particularly important when the patient is vomiting excessively or receiving parenteral fluids.

DRUG/DRUG INTERACTIONS

Metoprolol: Catecholamine-depleting drugs (e.g., reserpine) may have an additive effect when given with beta-blocking agents. Patients treated with Metoprolol plus a catecholamine depletor should therefore be closely observed for evidence of hypotension or marked bradycardia, which may produce vertigo, syncope, or postural hypotension.

Risk of Anaphylactic Reaction: While taking beta-blockers, patients with a history of severe anaphylactic reaction to a variety of allergens may be more reactive to repeated challenge, either accidental, diagnostic, or therapeutic. Such patients may be unresponsive to the usual doses of epinephrine used to treat allergic reaction.

Hydrochlorothiazide: Hypokalemia can sensitize or exaggerate the response of the heart to the toxic effects of digitalis (e.g., increased ventricular irritability).

Hypokalemia may develop during concomitant use of steroids or ACTH.

Insulin requirements in diabetic patients may be increased, decreased, or unchanged.

Thiazides may decrease arterial responsiveness to norepinephrine, but not enough to preclude effectiveness of the pressor agent for therapeutic use.

Thiazides may increase the responsiveness to tubocurarine. Lithium renal clearance is reduced by thiazides, increasing the risk of lithium toxicity.

There have been rare reports in the literature of hemolytic anemia occurring with the concomitant use of Hydrochlorothiazide and methyldopa.

Concurrent administration of some nonsteroidal anti-inflammatory agents may reduce the diuretic, natriuretic and antihypertensive effects of thiazide diuretics.

DRUG/LABORATORY TEST INTERACTIONS

Hydrochlorothiazide: Thiazides may decrease serum levels of protein-bound iodine without signs of thyroid disturbance. Thiazides should be discontinued before tests for parathyroid function are made. (See *"General, Hydrochlorothiazide, Calcium excretion"*).

CARCINOGENESIS, MUTAGENESIS, IMPAIRMENT OF FERTILITY

Metoprolol: Long-term studies in animals have been conducted to evaluate carcinogenic potential. In a 2-year study in rats at three oral dosage levels of up to 800 mg/kg per day, there was no increase in the development of spontaneously occurring benign or malignant neoplasms of any type. The only histologic changes that appeared to be drug related were an increased incidence of generally mild focal accumulation of foamy macrophages in pulmonary alveoli and a slight increase in biliary hyperplasia. In a 21-month study in Swiss albino mice at three oral dosage levels of up to 750 mg/kg per day, benign lung tumors (small adenomas) occurred more frequently in female mice receiving the highest dose than in untreated control animals. There was no increase in malignant or total (benign plus malignant) lung tumors, nor in the overall incidence of tumors or malignant tumors. This 21-month study was repeated in CD-1 mice, and no statistically or biologically significant differences were observed between treated and control mice of either sex for any type of tumor.

All mutagenicity tests performed (a dominant lethal study in mice, chromosome studies in somatic cells, a *Salmonella*/mammalian-microsome mutagenicity test, and a nucleus anomaly test in somatic interphase nuclei) were negative. No evidence of impaired fertility due to Metoprolol was observed in a study performed in rats at doses up to 55.5 times the maximum daily human dose of 450 mg.

Hydrochlorothiazide: Long-term carcinogenicity studies in animals have not been conducted. Hydrochlorothiazide was not mutagenic in in vitro Ames mutagenicity assay of *Salmonella typhimurium* strains TA 98, TA 100, TA 1535, TA 1537, and TA 1538 or in in vivo mutagenicity assays of mouse germinal cell chromosomes and chinese hamster bone marrow cell chromosomes. It was however, mutagenic in inducing nondisjunction (96% frequency) in diploid strains of *Aspergillus nidulans.*

Hydrochlorothiazide had no adverse effect on fertility of male or females mice or rats in studies in which these species were exposed to doses up to 4 and 100 mg/kg, respectively.

PREGNANCY CATEGORY C

Metoprolol has been shown to increase postimplantation loss and decrease neonatal survival in rats at doses up to 55.5 times the maximum daily human dose of 450 mg. Distribution studies in mice confirm exposure of the fetus when Metoprolol is administered to the pregnant animal. These studies have revealed no evidence of impaired fertility or teratogenicity.

There are no adequate and well-controlled studies in pregnant women with HCTZ/Metoprolol. Because animal reproduction studies are not always predictive of human response, this drug should be used during pregnancy only if clearly needed.

Nonteratogenic Effects: Thiazides cross the placental barrier and appear in cord blood, and there is a risk of fetal or neonatal jaundice, thrombocytopenia, and possibly other adverse reactions that have occurred in adults.

NURSING MOTHERS

Metoprolol is excreted in breast milk in very small quantity. An infant consuming 1 liter of breast milk daily would receive a dose of Metoprolol of less than 1 mg. Thiazides are also excreted in breast milk. If the use of HCTZ/Metoprolol is deemed essential, the patient should stop nursing.

PEDIATRIC USE

Safety and effectiveness in children have not been established.

ADVERSE REACTIONS

HCTZ/METOPROLOL

The following adverse reactions were reported in controlled clinical studies of the combination of Metoprolol and Hydrochlorothiazide.

Body as a Whole: Fatigue or lethargy and flu syndrome have each been reported in about 10 in 100 patients.

Nervous System: Dizziness or vertigo, drowsiness or somnolence, and headache have each occurred in about 10 in 100 patients. Nightmare has occurred in 1 in 100 patients.

Cardiovascular: Bradycardia has occurred in about 6 in 100 patients. Decreased exercise tolerance and dyspnea have each occurred in about 1 of 100 patients.

Digestive: Diarrhea, digestive disorder, dry mouth, nausea or vomiting, and constipation have each occurred in about 1 in 100 patients.

Metabolic and Nutritional: Hypokalemia has occurred in fewer than 10 in 100 patients. Edema, gout, and anorexia have each occurred in 1 in 100 patients.

Special Senses: Blurred vision, tinnitus, and earache have each been reported in 1 in 100 patients.

Skin: Sweating and purpura have each occurred in 1 in 100 patients.

Urogenital: Impotence has occurred in 1 in 100 patients.

Musculoskeletal: Muscle pain has occurred in 1 in 100 patients.

METOPROLOL

Most adverse effects have been mild and transient.

Central Nervous System: Tiredness and dizziness have occurred in about 10 of 100 patients. Depression has been reported in about 5 of 100 patients. Mental confusion and short-term memory loss have been reported. Headache, nightmares, and insomnia have also been reported, but a drug relationship is not clear.

Cardiovascular: Shortness of breath and bradycardia have occurred in approximately 3 of 100 patients. Cold extremities; arterial insufficiency, usually of the Raynaud type; palpitations; and congestive heart failure have been reported. (See *"Contraindications," "Warnings,"* and *"Precautions"*).

Respiratory: Wheezing (bronchospasm) has been reported in fewer than 1 of 100 patients (see *"Warnings"*).

Gastrointestinal: Diarrhea has occurred in about 5 of 100 patients. Nausea, gastric pain, constipation, flatulence, and heartburn have been reported in 1 of 100, or fewer, patients.

Hypersensitive Reactions: Pruritus has occurred in fewer than 1 of 100 patients. Rash has been reported.

Miscellaneous: Peyronie's disease has been reported in fewer than 1 of 100,000 patients. Alopecia has been reported. The oculomucocutaneous syndrome associated with the beta blocker practolol has not been reported with Metoprolol.

POTENTIAL ADVERSE REACTIONS

A variety of adverse reactions not listed above have been reported with other beta-adrenergic blocking agents and should be considered potential adverse reactions to Metoprolol.

Central Nervous System: Reversible mental depression progressing to catatonia; visual disturbances; hallucinations; an acute reversible syndrome characterized by disorientation for time and place, short-term memory loss, emotional lability, slightly clouded sensorium, and decreased performance on neuropsychometrics.

Cardiovascular: Intensification of AV block. (see *"Contraindications"*).

Hematologic: Agranulocytosis, nonthrombocytopenic purpura, thrombocytopenic purpura.

Hypersensitive Reactions: Fever combined with aching and sore throat, laryngospasm, and respiratory distress.

HYDROCHLOROTHIAZIDE

The following adverse reactions have been observed, but there has not been enough systematic collection of data to support an estimate of their frequency. Consequently the reactions are categorized by organ systems and are listed in decreasing order of severity and not frequency.

Digestive: Pancreatitis, jaundice (intrahepatic cholestatic), sialadenitis, vomiting, diarrhea, cramping, nausea, gastric irritation, constipation, anorexia.

Cardiovascular: Orthostatic hypotension (may be potentiated by alcohol, barbiturates, or narcotics).

Neurologic: Vertigo, dizziness, transient blurred vision, headache, paresthesia, xanthopsia, weakness, restlessness.

Musculoskeletal: Muscle spasm.

Hematologic: Aplastic anemia, agranulocytosis, leukopenia, thrombocytopenia.

Metabolic: Hyperglycemia, glycosuria, hyperuricemia.

Hypersensitive Reactions: Necrotizing angiitis, Stevens-Johnson syndrome, respiratory distress including pneumonitis and pulmonary edema, purpura, urticaria, rash, photosensitivity.

OVERDOSAGE
ACUTE TOXICITY
Several cases of overdosage with Metoprolol have been reported, some leading to death. No deaths have been reported with Hydrochlorothiazide.

Oral LD_{50}'s (mg/kg); mice, 1158 (Metoprolol); rats, 3090 (Metoprolol), 2750 (Hydrochlorothiazide).

SIGNS AND SYMPTOMS
Metoprolol: Potential signs and symptoms associated with overdosage with Metoprolol are bradycardia, hypotension, bronchospasm, and cardiac failure.

Hydrochlorothiazide: The most prominent feature of poisoning is acute loss of fluid and electrolytes.

Cardiovascular: Tachycardia, hypotension, shock.

Neuromuscular: Weakness, confusion, dizziness, cramps of the calf muscles, paresthesia, fatigue, impairment of consciousness.

Digestive: Nausea, vomiting, thirst.

Renal: Polyuria, oliguria, or anuria (due to hemoconcentration).

Laboratory Findings: Hypokalemia, hyponatremia, hypochloremia, alkalosis: increased BUN (especially in patients with renal insufficiency).

Combined Poisoning: Signs and symptoms may be aggravated or modified by concomitant intake of antihypertensive medication, barbiturates, curare, digitalis (hypokalemia), corticosteroids, narcotics, or alcohol.

TREATMENT
There is no specific antidote.

On the basis of the pharmacologic actions of Metoprolol and Hydrochlorothiazide, the following general measures should be employed:

Elimination of the Drug: Inducement of vomiting, gastric lavage, and activated charcoal.

Bradycardia: Atropine should be administered. If there is no response to vagal blockade, isoproterenol should be administered cautiously.

Hypotension: The patient's legs should be elevated, and lost fluid and electrolytes (potassium, sodium) should be replaced. A vasopressor should be administered, e.g., levarterenol or dopamine.

Bronchospasm: A $beta_2$-stimulating agent and/or a theophylline derivative should be administered.

Cardiac Failure: A digitalis glycoside and diuretic should be administered. In shock resulting from inadequate cardiac contractility, administration of dobutamine, isoproterenol, or glucagon may be considered.

Surveillance: Fluid and electrolyte balance (especially serum potassium) and renal function should be monitored until conditions become normal.

DOSAGE AND ADMINISTRATION
Dosage should be determined by individual titration (see *"Indications and Usage"*).

Hydrochlorothiazide is usually given at a dosage of 25 to 100 mg per day. The usual initial dosage of Metoprolol is 100 mg daily in single or divided doses. Dosage may be increased gradually until optimum blood pressure control is achieved. The effective dosage range is 100 to 450 mg per day. While once-daily dosing is effective and can maintain a reduction in blood pressure throughout the day, lower doses (especially 100 mg) may not maintain a full effect at the end of the 24-hour period, and larger or more frequent daily doses may be required. This can be evaluated by measuring blood pressure near the end of the dosing interval to determine whether satisfactory control is being maintained throughout the day. $Beta_1$ selectivity diminishes as dosage of Metoprolol is increased.

The following dosage schedule may be used to administer from 100 to 200 mg of Metoprolol per day and from 25 to 50 mg of Hydrochlorothiazide per day:

HCTZ/ Metoprolol	Dosage
Tablets of 50/25	2 tablets per day in single or divided doses
Tablets of 100/25	1 to 2 tablets per day in single or divided doses
Tablets of 100/50	1 tablet per day in single or divided doses

Dosing regimens that exceed 50 mg of Hydrochlorothiazide per day are not recommended. When necessary, another antihypertensive agent may be added gradually, beginning with 50% of the usual recommended starting dose to avoid an excessive fall in blood pressure.

Store between 59°-86°F (15°-30°C). Protect from moisture.

Dispense in tight, light-resistant container (USP).

HOW SUPPLIED
TABLETS: 25 MG-50 MG

BRAND/MANUFACTURER	NDC	SIZE	AWP
○ BRAND			
➤ LOPRESSOR HCT: Geigy	00028-0035-01	100s	$56.88

TABLETS: 25 MG-100 MG

BRAND/MANUFACTURER	NDC	SIZE	AWP
○ BRAND			
➤ LOPRESSOR HCT: Geigy	00028-0053-01	100s	$88.88

TABLETS: 50 MG-100 MG

BRAND/MANUFACTURER	NDC	SIZE	AWP
○ BRAND			
➤ LOPRESSOR HCT: Geigy	00028-0073-01	100s	$94.27

Hydrochlorothiazide with Reserpine

> **WARNING**
> THIS FIXED COMBINATION DRUG IS NOT INDICATED FOR INITIAL THERAPY OF HYPERTENSION. HYPERTENSION REQUIRES THERAPY TITRATED TO THE INDIVIDUAL PATIENT. IF THE FIXED COMBINATION REPRESENTS THE DOSAGE SO DETERMINED, ITS USE MAY BE MORE CONVENIENT IN PATIENT MANAGEMENT. THE TREATMENT OF HYPERTENSION IS NOT STATIC, BUT MUST BE RE-EVALUATED AS CONDITIONS IN EACH PATIENT WARRANT.

DESCRIPTION
HYDROCHLOROTHIAZIDE
Hydrochlorothiazide is a diuretic and antihypertensive. It is the 3,4-dihydro derivative of chlorothiazide. Its chemical name is 6-chloro-3,4-dihydro-2H-1,2,4-benzothiadiazine-7-sulfonamide 1,1-dioxide. Its empirical formula is $C_7H_8ClN_3O_4S_2$.

Hydrochlorothiazide is a white, or practically white, crystalline powder with a molecular weight of 297.72, which is slightly soluble in water, but freely soluble in sodium hydroxide solution.

RESERPINE
The chemical name for Reserpine is (11,17α-dimethoxy-18β-[(3,4,5-trimethoxy-benzoyl) oxy]-3β, 20α-yohimban-16β-carboxylic acid methyl ester). It is a crystalline alkaloid derived from Rauwolfia serpentina. Its empirical formula is $C_{33}H_{40}N_2O_9$.

Reserpine is a white or pale buff to slightly yellowish, odorless, crystalline powder with a molecular weight of 608.69, is insoluble in water, and freely soluble in glacial acetic acid. Hydrochlorothiazide/Reserpine is supplied as tablets in two strengths for oral use:

One, contains 25 mg of Hydrochlorothiazide and 0.125 mg of Reserpine.

The other contains 50 mg of Hydrochlorothiazide and 0.125 mg of Reserpine.

CLINICAL PHARMACOLOGY
HYDROCHLOROTHIAZIDE
The mechanism of the antihypertensive effect of thiazides is unknown. Hydrochlorothiazide does not usually affect normal blood pressure.

Hydrochlorothiazide affects the distal renal tubular mechanism of electrolyte reabsorption. At maximal therapeutic dosage all thiazides are approximately equal in their diuretic efficacy.

Hydrochlorothiazide increases excretion of sodium and chloride in approximately equivalent amounts. Natriuresis may be accompanied by some loss of potassium and bicarbonate. After oral use, diuresis begins within 2 hours, peaks in about 4 hours and lasts about 6 to 12 hours.

RESERPINE
Reserpine has antihypertensive, bradycardic, and tranquilizing properties. It lowers arterial blood pressure by depletion of catecholamines. Reserpine is

---

◆ RATED THERAPEUTICALLY EQUIVALENT; ◇ THERAPEUTIC EQUIVALENCE UNCONFIRMED; ○ UNRATED

beneficial in relieving anxiety, tension, and headache in the hypertensive patient. It acts at the hypothalamic level of the central nervous system to promote relaxation without hypnosis or analgesia. The sleep pattern shown by the electroencephalogram following barbiturates does not occur with this drug. In laboratory animals spontaneous activity and response to external stimuli are decreased, but confusion or difficulty of movement is not evident.

The bradycardic action of Reserpine promotes relaxation and may eliminate sinus tachycardia. It is most pronounced in subjects with sinus tachycardia and usually is not prominent in persons with a normal pulse rate.

Miosis, relaxation of the nictitating membrane, ptosis, hypothermia, and increased gastrointestinal activity are noted in animals given Reserpine, sometimes in subclinical doses. None of these effects, except increased gastrointestinal activity, has been found to be clinically significant in man with therapeutic doses.

PHARMACOKINETICS AND METABOLISM
Hydrochlorothiazide: Hydrochlorothiazide is not metabolized but is eliminated rapidly by the kidney. When plasma levels have been followed for at least 24 hours, the plasma half-life has been observed to vary between 5.6 and 14.8 hours. At least 61 percent of the oral dose is eliminated unchanged within 24 hours. Hydrochlorothiazide crosses the placental but not the blood-brain barrier and is excreted in breast milk.

Reserpine: Oral Reserpine is rapidly absorbed from the gastrointestinal tract. Methylreserpate and trimethoxybenzoic acid are the primary metabolites which result from the hydrolytic cleavage of Reserpine. Maximal blood levels are achieved approximately 2 hours after the oral dosage of ^{3}H-Reserpine to six normal volunteers; within 96 hours approximately 8 percent was excreted in urine and 62 percent in feces. Reserpine appears in human breast milk. Reserpine crosses the placental barrier in guinea pigs.

INDICATION AND USAGE
Hypertension (see box *"Warning"*).

CONTRAINDICATIONS
Hydrochlorothiazide is contraindicated in anuria.

Hydrochlorothiazide/Reserpine is contraindicated in hypersensitivity to Hydrochlorothiazide or other sulfonamide-derived drugs or to Reserpine.

Electroshock therapy should not be given to patients while on Reserpine, as severe and even fatal reactions have been reported with minimal convulsive electroshock dosage. After discontinuing Reserpine, allow at least seven days before starting electroshock therapy.

Active peptic ulcer, ulcerative colitis, and active or a history of mental depression, especially suicidal tendencies, are contraindications to Reserpine therapy.

WARNINGS
HYDROCHLOROTHIAZIDE
Use with caution in severe renal disease. In patients with renal disease, thiazides may precipitate azotemia. Cumulative effects of the drug may develop in patients with impaired renal function.

Thiazides should be used with caution in patients with impaired hepatic function or progressive liver disease, since minor alterations of fluid and electrolyte balance may precipitate hepatic coma.

Thiazides may add to or potentiate the action of other antihypertensive drugs.

Sensitivity reactions may occur in patients with or without a history of allergy or bronchial asthma.

The possibility of exacerbation or activation of systemic lupus erythematosus has been reported.

Lithium generally should not be given with diuretics (see *"Precautions, Drug Interactions"*).

RESERPINE
Reserpine may cause mental depression. Recognition of depression may be difficult because this condition may often be disguised by somatic complaints (masked depression). The drug should be discontinued at first signs of depression such as despondency, early morning insomnia, loss of appetite, impotence or self deprecation. Drug induced depression may persist for several months after drug withdrawal and may be severe enough to result in suicide.

The occurrence of mental depression due to Reserpine in doses of 0.25 mg daily or less is unusual. In any event, Hydrochlorothiazide/Reserpine should be discontinued at the first sign of depression.

PRECAUTIONS
GENERAL
Hydrochlorothiazide: All patients receiving diuretic therapy should be observed for evidence of fluid or electrolyte imbalance; namely, hyponatremia, hypochloremic alkalosis, and hypokalemia. Serum and urine electrolyte determinations are particularly important when the patient is vomiting excessively or receiving parenteral fluids. Warning signs or symptoms of fluid and electrolyte imbalance irrespective of cause, include dryness of mouth, thirst, weakness, lethargy, drowsiness, restlessness, confusion, seizures, muscle pains or cramps, muscular fatigue, hypotension, oliguria, tachycardia, and gastrointestinal disturbances such as nausea and vomiting. Hypokalemia may develop, especially with brisk diuresis, when severe cirrhosis is present or after prolonged therapy. Interference with adequate oral electrolyte intake will contribute to hypokalemia. Hypokalemia may cause cardiac arrhythmia and may also sensitize or exaggerate the response of the heart to the toxic effects of digitals (e.g., increased ventricular irritability).

Hypokalemia may be avoided or treated by use of potassium sparing diuretic or potassium supplements such as foods with a high potassium content.

Although any chloride deficit is generally mild and usually does not require specific treatment except under extraordinary circumstances (as in liver disease or renal disease), chloride replacement may be required in the treatment of metabolic alkalosis.

Dilutional hyponatremia may occur in edematous patients in hot weather. Appropriate therapy is water restriction, rather than administration of salt, except in rare instances when the hyponatremia is life threatening. In actual salt depletion, appropriate replacement is the therapy of choice. Hyperuricemia may occur or acute gout may be precipitated in certain patients receiving thiazides.

In diabetic patients dosage adjustment of insulin or oral hypoglycemic agents may be required. Hyperglycemia may occur with thiazide diuretics. Thus latent diabetes mellitus may become manifest during thiazide therapy.

The antihypertensive effect of the drug may be enhanced in the postsympathectomy patient.

If progressive renal impairment becomes evident, consider withholding or discontinuing diuretic therapy.

Thiazides have been shown to increase the urinary excretion of magnesium; this may result in hypomagnesemia.

Thiazides may decrease urinary calcium excretion. Thiazides may cause intermittent and slight elevation of serum calcium in the absence of known disorders of calcium metabolism. Marked hypercalcemia may be evidence of hidden hyperparathyroidism. Thiazides should be discontinued before carrying out tests for parathyroid function.

Increases in cholesterol and triglyceride levels may be associated with thiazide diuretic therapy.

Reserpine: Since Reserpine may increase gastric secretion and motility, it should be used cautiously in patients with a history of peptic ulcer, ulcerative colitis, or other gastrointestinal disorder. This compound may precipitate biliary colic in patients with gallstones, or bronchial asthma in susceptible persons. Reserpine may cause hypotension including orthostatic hypotension.

Anxiety or depression, as well as psychosis, may develop during Reserpine therapy. If depression is present when therapy is begun, it may be aggravated. Mental depression is unusual with Reserpine doses of 0.25 mg daily or less. In any case, Hydrochlorothiazide/Reserpine should be discontinued at the first sign of depression. Extreme caution should be used in treating patients with a history of mental depression, and the possibility of suicide should be kept in mind.

As with most antihypertensive therapy, caution should be exercised when treating hypertensive patients with renal insufficiency, since they adjust poorly to lowered blood pressure.

When two or more antihypertensives are given, the individual dosages may have to be reduced to prevent excessive drop in blood pressure. In hypertensive patients with coronary artery disease, it is important to avoid a precipitous drop in blood pressure.

LABORATORY TESTS
Periodic determination of serum electrolytes to detect possible electrolyte imbalance should be done at appropriate intervals.

DRUG INTERACTIONS
Hydrochlorothiazide: When given concurrently the following drugs may interact with thiazide diuretics.

Alcohol, Barbiturates, or Narcotics: potentiation of orthostatic hypotension may occur.

Antidiabetic Drugs (Oral Agents and Insulin): dosage adjustment of the antidiabetic drug may be required.

Other Antihypertensive Drugs: additive effect or potentiation.

Cholestyramine and Colestipol Resins: Absorption of Hydrochlorothiazide is impaired in the presence of anionic exchange resins. Single doses of either cholestyramine or colestipol resins bind the Hydrochlorothiazide and reduce its absorption from the gastrointestinal tract by up to 85 and 43 percent, respectively.

Corticosteroids, ACTH: intensified electrolyte depletion, particularly hypokalemia.

Pressor Amines (e.g., norepinephrine): possible decreased response to pressor amines but not sufficient to preclude their use.

Skeletal muscle relaxants, nondepolarizing (e.g., tubocurarine): possible increased responsiveness to the muscle relaxant.

Lithium: generally should not be given with diuretics. Diuretic agents reduce the renal clearance of lithium and add a high risk of lithium toxicity. Refer to the package insert for lithium preparations before use of such preparations with Hydrochlorothiazide/Reserpine.

Nonsteroidal Anti-inflammatory Drugs: In some patients, the administration of a non-steroidal anti-inflammatory agent can reduce the diuretic, natriuretic, and antihypertensive effects of loop, potassium-sparing and thiazide diuretics. Therefore, when Hydrochlorothiazide/Reserpine and non-steroidal anti-inflammatory agents are used concomitantly, the patient should be observed closely to determine if the desired effect of the diuretic is obtained.

Reserpine: In hypertensive patients on Reserpine therapy significant hypotension and bradycardia may develop during surgical anesthesia. The anesthesiologist should be aware that Reserpine has been taken, since it may be necessary to give vagal blocking agents parenterally to prevent or reverse hypotension and/or bradycardia.

Use Reserpine cautiously with digitalis and quinidine; cardiac arrhythmias have occurred with Reserpine preparations.

Barbiturates enhance the central nervous system depressant effects of Reserpine.

DRUG/LABORATORY TEST INTERACTIONS
Thiazides should be discontinued before carrying out tests for parathyroid function (see *"Precautions"*, General).

CARCINOGENESIS, MUTAGENESIS, IMPAIRMENT OF FERTILITY
Long-term carcinogenic or mutagenic studies have not been done with Hydrochlorothiazide/Reserpine.

In a two-litter study in the rat at an oral dose of 5.0/0.25 mg/kg, the combination of Hydrochlorothiazide/Reserpine did not impair fertility or produce abnormalities in the fetus.

Hydrochlorothiazide: Two-year feeding studies in mice and rats conducted under the auspices of the National Toxicology Program (NTP) uncovered no evidence of a carcinogenic potential of Hydrochlorothiazide in female mice (at doses of up to approximately 600 mg/kg/day) or in male and female rats (at doses of up to approximately 100 mg/kg/day). The NTP, however, found equivocal evidence for hepatocarcinogenicity in male mice. Hydrochlorothiazide was not genotoxic *in vitro* in the Ames mutagenicity assay of *Salmonella typhimurium* strains TA 98, TA 100, TA 1535, TA 1537, and TA 1538 and in the Chinese Hamster Ovary (CHO) test for chromosomal aberrations, or *in vivo* in assays using mouse germinal cell chromosomes, Chinese hamster bone marrow chromosomes, and the *Drosophila* sex-linked recessive lethal trait gene. Positive test results were obtained only in the *in vitro* CHO Sister Chromatid Exchange (clastogenicity) and in the Mouse Lymphoma Cell (mutagenicity) assays, using concentrations of Hydrochlorothiazide from 43 to 1300 µg/mL, and in the *Aspergillus nidulans* nondisjunction assay at an unspecified concentration.

Hydrochlorothiazide had no adverse effects on the fertility of mice and rats of either sex in studies wherein this species were exposed, via their diet, to doses of up to 100 and 4 mg/kg, respectively, prior to conception and throughout gestation.

Reserpine: Reserpine at a concentration of 1 to 5000 mcg/plate had no mutagenic activity against four strains of *S. typhimurium in vitro* in the Ames microbial mutagen test with or without metabolic activation. Reserpine did not induce malignant transformation of mouse fibroblasts *in vitro* at concentrations of 0.3 to 10 mcg/mL.

A few chromosomal aberrations were induced by Reserpine *in vitro* in cultured mouse mammary carcinoma cells but were considered negative in this study. The drug did not produce chromosomal aberrations in human peripheral leucocyte cultures although an increase in mitotic figures occurred. One study reported chromosomal aberrations and dominant lethal mutations in mice at doses up to 10 mg/kg of Reserpine in the form of a pharmaceutical preparation. Another study did not show dominant lethal mutations in mice at IP doses of 0.92 and 4.6 mg/kg of Reserpine.

Reserpine did not impair fertility in a two-litter study in the rat at an oral dose of 0.25 mg/kg (35 times the maximum recommended human dose).

Rodent studies have shown that Reserpine is an animal tumorigen, causing an increased incidence of mammary fibroadenomas in female mice, malignant tumors of the seminal vesicles in male mice, and malignant adrenal medullary tumors in male rats. These findings arose in 2 year studies in which the drug was administered in the feed at concentrations of 5 and 10 ppm—about 100 to 300 times the usual human dose. The breast neoplasms are thought to be related to Reserpine's prolactin-elevating effect. Several other prolactin-elevating drugs have also been associated with an increased incidence of mammary neoplasia in rodents.

The extent to which these findings indicate a risk to humans is uncertain. Tissue culture experiments show that about one-third of human breast tumors are prolactin-dependent *in vitro*, a factor of considerable importance if the use of the drug is contemplated in a patient with previously detected breast cancer. The possibility of an increased risk of breast cancer in Reserpine users has been studied extensively; however, no firm conclusion has emerged. Although a few epidemiologic studies have suggested a slightly increased risk (less than twofold in all studies except one) in women who have used Reserpine, other studies of generally similar design have not confirmed this. Epidemiologic studies conducted using other drugs (neuroleptic agents) that, like Reserpine, increase prolactin levels and therefore would be considered rodent mammary carcinogens, have not shown an association between chronic administration of the drug and human mammary tumorigenesis. While long-term clinical observation has not suggested such an association, the available evidence is considered too limited to be conclusive at this time. An association of Reserpine intake with pheochromocytoma or tumors of the seminal vesicles has not been explored.

PREGNANCY
Use of diuretics during normal pregnancy is inappropriate and exposes mother and fetus to unnecessary hazard. Diuretics do not prevent development of toxemia of pregnancy and there is no satisfactory evidence that they are useful in the treatment of toxemia.

TERATOGENIC EFFECTS
Pregnancy Category C: Hydrochlorothiazide/Reserpine may cause fetal harm when given to a pregnant woman. There are no adequate and well-controlled studies with Hydrochlorothiazide/Reserpine in pregnant women. Hydrochlorothiazide/Reserpine should be used during pregnancy only if the potential benefit justifies the potential risk to the fetus.

Reserpine: Reproduction studies in rats have shown that Reserpine is teratogenic at doses of 1-2 mg/kg (125 to 250 times the maximum recommended human dose) IM or IP given early in pregnancy. A variety of abnormalities was produced including anophthalmia, absence of the axial skeleton, hydronephrosis, etc. Pregnancy in rabbits was interrupted when doses as low as 0.04 mg/kg (10 times the maximum recommended human dose) were given early or late in pregnancy.

Hydrochlorothiazide: Studies in which Hydrochlorothiazide was orally administered to pregnant mice and rats during their respective periods of major organogenesis at doses up to 3000 and 1000 mg Hydrochlorothiazide/kg, respectively, provided no evidence of harm to the fetus.

NONTERATOGENIC EFFECTS
Reserpine: Reserpine has been demonstrated to cross the placental barrier in guinea pigs with depression of adrenal catecholamine stores in the newborn. There is some evidence that side effects such as nasal congestion, lethargy, depressed Moro reflex, and bradycardia may appear in infants born of Reserpine-treated mothers.

Hydrochlorothiazide: Thiazides cross the placental barrier and appear in cord blood. There is a risk of fetal or neonatal jaundice, thrombocytopenia, and possibly other adverse reactions that have occurred in adults.

NURSING MOTHERS
Thiazides and Reserpine appear in breast milk. Because of the potential for serious adverse reactions in nursing infants from Hydrochlorothiazide/Reserpine, a decision should be made whether to discontinue nursing or to discontinue the drug, taking into account the importance of the drug to the mother.

PEDIATRIC USE
Safety and effectiveness of Hydrochlorothiazide/Reserpine in children has not been established.

ADVERSE REACTIONS
The following adverse reactions have been reported and, within each category, are listed in order of decreasing severity.

HYDROCHLOROTHIAZIDE
Body as a Whole: Weakness.

Cardiovascular: Hypotension including orthostatic hypotension (may be aggravated by alcohol, barbiturates, narcotics or antihypertensive drugs).

Digestive: Pancreatitis, jaundice (intrahepatic cholestatic jaundice), diarrhea, vomiting, sialadenitis, cramping, constipation, gastric irritation, nausea, anorexia.

Hematologic: Aplastic anemia, agranulocytosis, leukopenia, hemolytic anemia, thrombocytopenia.

Hypersensitivity: Anaphylactic reactions, necrotizing angiitis (vasculitis and cutaneous vasculitis), respiratory distress including pneumonitis and pulmonary edema, photosensitivity, fever, urticaria, rash, purpura.

Metabolic: Electrolyte imbalance (see *"Precautions"*), hyperglycemia, glycosuria, hyperuricemia.

Musculoskeletal: Muscle spasm.

Nervous System/Psychiatric: Vertigo, paresthesias, dizziness, headache, restlessness.

Renal: Renal failure, renal dysfunction, interstitial nephritis. (See *"Warnings."*)

Skin: Erythema multiforme including Stevens-Johnson syndrome, exfoliative dermatitis including toxic epidermal necrolysis, alopecia.

Special Senses: Transient blurred vision, xanthopsia.

Urogenital: Impotence.

RESERPINE
Cardiovascular: Angina pectoris, arrhythmia, premature ventricular contractions, other direct cardiac effects (e.g., fluid retention, congestive heart failure), bradycardia.

Digestive: Vomiting, diarrhea, nausea, hypersecretion and increased motility, anorexia, dryness of mouth, increased salivation.

Hematologic: Thrombocytopenic purpura, excessive bleeding following prostatic surgery.

Hypersensitivity: Pruritus, rash, flushing of skin.

Metabolic: Weight gain.

Musculoskeletal: Muscular aches.

Nervous System/Psychiatric: Mental depression, dull sensorium, syncope, paradoxical anxiety, excessive sedation, nightmares, headache, dizziness, nervousness, parkinsonism (usually reversible with decreased dosage or discontinuance of therapy).

Respiratory: Dyspnea, epistaxis, nasal congestion, enhanced susceptibility to colds.

Special Senses: Optic atrophy, uveitis, deafness, glaucoma, conjunctival injection, blurred vision.

◆ RATED THERAPEUTICALLY EQUIVALENT; ◇ THERAPEUTIC EQUIVALENCE UNCONFIRMED; ○ UNRATED

Urogenital: Dysuria, impotence, decreased libido, nonpuerperal lactation.

OVERDOSAGE

Overdosage may lead to excessive sedation, mental depression, severe hypotension, extrapyramidal reactions.

There is no specific antidote. In the event of overdosage, symptomatic and supportive measures should be employed.

Emesis should be induced or gastric lavage performed. Correct dehydration, electrolyte imbalance, hepatic coma and hypotension by established procedures. If required, give oxygen or artificial respiration for respiratory impairment. In the event of severe hypotension from the Reserpine component, intravenous use of a vasopressor is indicated (Metaraminol bitartrate, levarerenol, phenylephrine). Anticholinergics may be needed to relieve gastrointestinal distress from Reserpine. Because the effects of the rauwolfia alkaloids are prolonged, the patient should be closely observed for at least 72 hours.

Reserpine is not dialyzable. The degree to which Hydrochlorothiazide is removed by hemodialysis has not been established.

The oral LD_{50} of Hydrochlorothiazide is greater than 10 g/kg in the mouse and rat. The oral LD_{50} of Reserpine in the mouse is 390 mg/kg.

DOSAGE AND ADMINISTRATION

The initial dosage of Hydrochlorothiazide/Reserpine should conform to the dosages of the individual components established during titration (see *"Box Warning"*).

The usual adult dosage of Hydrochlorothiazide/Reserpine 25 is 1 or 2 tablets once a day; that of Hydrochlorothiazide/Reserpine 50 is 1 tablet once a day.

Patients usually do not require doses in excess of 50 mg of Hydrochlorothiazide daily when combined with other antihypertensive agents. Dosage may require adjustment according to the blood pressure response of the patient. For maintenance, dosage should be adjusted to the lowest requirements of the individual patient. Doses higher than 0.25 mg daily of Reserpine should be used cautiously, because occurrence of serious mental depression and other side effects may increase considerably (see *"Warnings"*).

Keep container tightly closed. Protect from light, moisture, freezing, −20°C (−4°F) and store at room temperature, 15-30°C (59-86°F).

HOW SUPPLIED
TABLETS: 25 MG-0.125 MG

BRAND/MANUFACTURER	NDC	SIZE	AWP
◇ **BRAND**			
HYDROPRES-25: Merck	00006-0053-68	100s	$27.26
	00006-0053-82	1000s	$252.40
◇ **GENERICS**			
HYDROSERPINE: Major	00904-2169-60	100s	$3.55
HYDROSERPINE: Schein	00364-0354-01	100s	$3.70
HYDROSERPINE: Moore,H.L.	00839-5137-06	100s	$3.77
Aligen	00405-4495-01	100s	$3.95
HYDROSERPINE #1: Rugby	00536-3915-01	100s	$4.79
HYDROSERPINE: Major	00904-2169-70	250s	$4.15
HYDROSERPINE: Schein	00364-0354-02	1000s	$20.40
HYDROSERPINE: Major	00904-2169-80	1000s	$27.75

TABLETS: 50 MG-0.125 MG

BRAND/MANUFACTURER	NDC	SIZE	AWP
◇ **BRAND**			
HYDROPRES-50: Merck	00006-0127-68	100s	$42.51
	00006-0127-82	1000s	$391.06
◇ **GENERICS**			
Aligen	00405-4496-01	100s	$3.97
HYDROSERPINE: Moore,H.L.	00839-5138-06	100s	$3.98
HYDROSERPINE: Major	00904-2168-60	100s	$4.15
HYDROSERPINE: Schein	00364-0355-01	100s	$4.16
HYDROSERPINE #2: Rugby	00536-3916-01	100s	$5.94
HYDROSERPINE: Major	00904-2168-70	250s	$4.80
HYDROSERPINE: Moore,H.L.	00839-5138-16	1000s	$22.28
HYDROSERPINE: Schein	00364-0355-02	1000s	$25.95
HYDROSERPINE: Major	00904-2168-80	1000s	$32.80

Hydrochlorothiazide with Spironolactone

WARNING

SPIRONOLACTONE HAS BEEN SHOWN TO BE A TUMORIGEN IN CHRONIC TOXICITY STUDIES IN RATS (SEE *"WARNINGS"*). HYDROCHLOROTHIAZIDE/SPIRONOLACTONE SHOULD BE USED ONLY IN THOSE CONDITIONS DESCRIBED UNDER *INDICATIONS AND USAGE.* UNNECESSARY USE OF THIS DRUG SHOULD BE AVOIDED.

FIXED-DOSE COMBINATION DRUGS ARE NOT INDICATED FOR INITIAL THERAPY OF EDEMA OR HYPERTENSION. EDEMA OR HYPERTENSION REQUIRES THERAPY TITRATED TO THE INDIVIDUAL PATIENT. IF THE FIXED COMBINATION REPRESENTS THE DOSAGE SO DETERMINED, ITS USE MAY BE MORE CONVENIENT IN PATIENT MANAGEMENT. THE TREATMENT OF HYPERTENSION AND EDEMA IS NOT STATIC BUT MUST BE REEVALUATED AS CONDITIONS IN EACH PATIENT WARRANT.

DESCRIPTION

Hydrochlorothiazide/Spironolactone oral tablets contain:

Hydrochlorothiazide ....25 mg
Spironolactone ....25 mg
or
Hydrochlorothiazide ....50 mg
Spironolactone ....50 mg

Hydrochlorothiazide, a diuretic and antihypertensive, is 6-chloro-3, 4-dihydro-2H-1,2,4-benzothiadiadiazine-7-sulfonamide 1,1-dioxide.

Hydrochlorothiazide is slightly soluble in water and freely soluble in sodium hydroxide solution.

Spironolactone, an aldosterone antagonist, is 17-hydroxy-7α-mercapto-3-oxo-17α-pregn-4-ene-21-carboxylic acid γ-lactone acetate.

Spironolactone is practically insoluble in water, soluble in alcohol, and freely soluble in benzene and in chloroform.

CLINICAL PHARMACOLOGY

Mechanism of Action: Hydrochlorothiazide/Spironolactone is a combination of two diuretic agents with different but complementary mechanisms and sites of action, thereby providing additive diuretic and antihypertensive effects. Additionally, the Spironolactone component helps to minimize the potassium loss characteristically induced by the thiazide component.

Hydrochlorothiazide promotes the excretion of sodium and water primarily by inhibiting their reabsorption in the cortical diluting segment of the distal renal tubule.

The diuretic effect of Spironolactone is mediated through its action as a specific pharmacologic antagonist of aldosterone, primarily by competitive binding of receptors at the aldosterone-dependent sodium-potassium exchange site in the distal convoluted renal tubule.

Hydrochlorothiazide/Spironolactone is effective in significantly lowering the systolic and diastolic blood pressure in many patients with essential hypertension, even when aldosterone secretion is within normal limits.

Both Hydrochlorothiazide and Spironolactone reduce exchangeable sodium, plasma volume, body weight, and blood pressure. The diuretic and antihypertensive effects of the individual components are potentiated when Hydrochlorothiazide and Spironolactone are given concurrently.

Hydrochlorothiazide is rapidly absorbed following oral administration. Onset of action of Hydrochlorothiazide is observed within one hour and persists for 6 to 12 hours. Hydrochlorothiazide plasma concentrations attain peak levels at one to two hours and decline with a half-life of four to five hours. Hydrochlorothiazide undergoes only slight metabolic alteration and is excreted in urine. It is distributed throughout the extracellular space, with essentially no tissue accumulation except in the kidney.

Pharmacokinetics: Spironlactone is rapidly and extensively metabolized. Sulfur-containing products are the predominant metabolites and are thought to be primarily responsible, together with Spironolactone, for the therapeutic effects of the drug. The following pharmacokinetic data were obtained from 12 healthy volunteers following the administration of 100 mg of Spironolactone daily for 15 days. On the 15th day, Spironolactone was given immediately after a low-fat breakfast and blood was drawn thereafter. (See related table).

The pharmacological activity of Spironolactone metabolites in man is not known. However, in the adrenalectomized rat the antimineralocorticoid activities of the metabolites C. TMS, and HTMS, relative to Spironolactone, were 1.10 1.28, and 0.32, respectively. Relative to Spironolactone, their binding affinities to the aldosterone receptors in rat kidney slices were 0.19, 0.86, and 0.06, respectively.

In humans the potencies of TMS and 7-α-thiospirolactone in reversing the effects of the synthetic mineralocorticoid, fludrocortisone, on urinary electrolyte composition were 0.33 and 0.26, respectively, relative to Spironolactone. However, since the serum concentrations of these steroids were not determined, their incomplete absorption and/or first-pass metabolism could not be ruled out as a reason for their reduced *in vivo* activities.

Both Spironolactone and canrenone are more than 90% bound to plasma proteins. The metabolites are excreted primarily in the urine and secondarily in bile.

The effect of food on Spironolactone absorption was assessed in a single dose study of 9 healthy, drug-free volunteers. Food increased the bioavailability of unmetabolized Spironolactone by almost 100%. The clinical importance of this finding is not known.

INDICATIONS AND USAGE

Spironolactone, an ingredient of Hydrochlorothiazide/Spironolactone, has been shown to be a tumorigen in chronic toxicity studies in rats (see *Warnings* section). Hydrochlorothiazide/Spironolactone, should be used only in those conditions described below. Unnecessary use of this drug should be avoided.

Hydrochlorothiazide/Spironolactone is indicated for:

EDEMATOUS CONDITIONS FOR PATIENTS WITH
Congestive Heart Failure: For the management of edema and sodium retention when the patient is only partially responsive to, or is intolerant of, other therapeutic measures. The treatment of diuretic-induced hypokalemia in patients

with congestive heart failure when other measures are considered inappropriate. The treatment of patients with congestive heart failure taking digitalis when other therapies are considered inadequate or inappropriate.

Cirrhosis of the Liver accompanied by Edema and/or Ascites: Aldosterone levels may be exceptionally high in this condition. Hydrochlorothiazide/Spironolactone is indicated for maintenance therapy together with bed rest and the restriction of fluid and sodium.

The Nephrotic Syndrome: For nephrotic patients when treatment of the underlying disease, restriction of fluid and sodium intake, and the use of other diuretics do not provide an adequate response.

ESSENTIAL HYPERTENSION
For patients with essential hypertension in whom other measures are considered inadequate or inappropriate. In hypertensive patients for the treatment of a diuretic-induced hypokalemia when other measures are considered inappropriate.

Usage in Pregnancy: The routine use of diuretics in an otherwise healthy woman is inappropriate and exposes mother and fetus to unnecessary hazard. Diuretics do not prevent development of toxemia of pregnancy, and there is no satisfactory evidence that they are useful in the treatment of developing toxemia.

Edema during pregnancy may arise from pathologic causes or from the physiologic and mechanical consequences of pregnancy. Hydrochlorothiazide/Spironolactone is indicated in pregnancy when edema is due to pathologic causes just as it is in the absence of pregnancy (however, see *"Warnings"* section). Dependent edema in pregnancy, resulting from restriction of venous return by the expanded uterus, is properly treated through elevation of the lower extremities and use of support hose; use of diuretics to lower intravascular volume in this case is unsupported and unnecessary. There is hypervolemia during normal pregnancy which is not harmful to either the fetus or the mother (in the absence of cardiovascular disease), but which is associated with edema, including generalized edema, in the majority of pregnant women. If this edema produces discomfort, increased recumbency will often provide relief. In rare instances, this edema may cause extreme discomfort which is not relieved by rest. In these cases, a short course of diuretics may provide relief and may be appropriate.

CONTRAINDICATIONS
Hydrochlorothiazide/Spironolactone is contraindicated in patients with anuria, acute renal insufficiency, significant impairment of renal excretory function, or hyperkalemia, and in patients who are allergic to thiazide diuretics or to other sulfonamide-derived drugs. Hydrochlorothiazide/Spironolactone may also be contraindicated in acute or severe hepatic failure.

WARNINGS
Potassium supplementation, either in the form of medication or as a diet rich in potassium, should not ordinarily be given in association with Hydrochlorothiazide/Spironolactone therapy. Excessive potassium intake may cause hyperkalemia in patients receiving Hydrochlorothiazide/Spironolactone (see *"Precautions"* section). Hydrochlorothiazide/Spironolactone should not be administered concurrently with other potassium-sparing diuretics. Spironolactone, when used with ACE inhibitors, even in the presence of a diuretic, has been associated with severe hyperkalemia. Extreme caution should be exercised when Hydrochlorothiazide/Spironolactone is given concomitantly with ACE inhibitors (see *"Precautions"*).

Sulfonamide derivatives, including thiazides, have been reported to exacerbate or activate systemic lupus erythematosus.

Spironolactone has been shown to be a tumorigen in chronic toxicity studies performed in rats, with its proliferative effects manifested on endocrine organs and the liver. In one study using 25, 75, and 250 times the usual daily human dose (2 mg/kg) there was a statistically significant dose-related increase in benign adenomas of the thyroid and testes. In female rats there was a statistically significant increase in malignant mammary tumors at the mid-dose only. In male rats there was a dose-related increase in proliferative changes in the liver. At the highest dosage level (500 mg/kg), the range of effects included hepatocytomegaly, hyperplastic nodules, and hepatocellular carcinoma; the last was not statistically significant at a value of p = 0.05. A dose-related (above 20 mg/kg/day) incidence of myelocytic leukemia was observed in rats fed daily doses of potassium canrenoate for a period of one year. In long-term (two-year) oral carcinogenicity studies of potassium canrenoate in the rat, myelocytic leukemia and hepatic, thyroid, testicular, and mammary tumors were observed. Potassium canrenoate did not produce a mutagenic effect in tests using bacteria or yeast. It did produce a positive mutagenic effect in several *in vitro* tests in mammalian cells following metabolic activation. In an *in vivo* mammalian system potassium canrenoate was not mutagenic. Canrenone and canrenoic acid are the major metabolites of potassium canrenoate. Spironolactone is also metabolized to canrenone. An increased incidence of leukemia was not observed in chronic rat toxicity studies conducted with Spironolactone at doses up to 500 mg/kg/day.

PRECAUTIONS
Patients receiving Hydrochlorothiazide/Spironolactone therapy should be carefully evaluated for possible disturbances of fluid and electrolyte balance. Hyperkalemia may occur in patients with impaired renal function or excessive potassium intake and can cause cardiac irregularities, which may be fatal. Consequently, no potassium supplement should ordinarily be given with Hydrochlorothiazide/Spironolactone. Hyperkalemia can be treated promptly by the rapid intravenous administration of glucose (20% to 50%) and regular insulin, using 0.25 to 0.5 units of insulin per gram of glucose. This is a temporary measure to be repeated as required. Hydrochlorothiazide/Spironolactone use should be discontinued and potassium intake (including dietary potassium) restricted.

Hypokalemia may develop as a result of profound diuresis, particularly when Hydrochlorothiazide/Spironolactone is used concomitantly with loop diuretics, glucocorticoids, or ACTH. Hypokalemia may exaggerate the effects of digitalis therapy. Potassium depletion may induce signs of digitalis intoxication at previously tolerated dosage levels.

Concomitant administration of potassium-sparing diuretics and ACE inhibitors or indomethacin has been associated with severe hyperkalemia.

Warning signs of possible fluid and electrolyte imbalance include dryness of the mouth, thirst, weakness, lethargy, drowsiness, restlessness, muscle pains or cramps, muscular fatigue, hypotension, oliguria, tachycardia, and gastrointestinal symptoms.

Hydrochlorothiazide/Spironolactone therapy may cause a transient elevation of BUN. This appears to represent a concentration phenomenon rather than renal toxicity, since the BUN level returns to normal after use of Hydrochlorothiazide/Spironolactone is discontinued. Progressive elevation of BUN is suggestive of the presence of preexisting renal impairment.

Reversible hyperchloremic metabolic acidosis, usually in association with hyperkalemia, has been reported to occur in some patients with decompensated hepatic cirrhosis, even in the presence of normal renal function.

Dilutional hyponatremia, manifested by dryness of the mouth, thirst, lethargy, and drowsiness, and confirmed by a low serum sodium level, may be induced, especially when Hydrochlorothiazide/Spironolactone is administered in combination with other diuretics. A true low-salt syndrome may rarely develop with Hydrochlorothiazide/Spironolactone therapy and may be manifested by increasing mental confusion similar to that observed with hepatic coma. This syndrome is differentiated from dilutional hyponatremia in that it does not occur with obvious fluid retention. Its treatment requires that diuretic therapy be discontinued and sodium administered.

Thiazides have been demonstrated to alter the metabolism of uric acid and carbohydrates, with possible development of hyperuricemia, gout, and decreased glucose tolerance. Thiazides may temporarily exaggerate abnormalities of glucose metabolism in diabetic patients or cause abnormalities to appear in patients with latent diabetes.

The antihypertensive effects of Hydrochlorothiazide may be enhanced in patients who have undergone sympathectomy.

Pathologic changes in the parathyroid gland with hypercalcemia and hypophosphatemia have been observed in patients on prolonged thiazide therapy. Thiazides may also decrease serum PBI levels without evidence of alteration of thyroid function.

Gynecomastia may develop in association with the use of Spironolactone; physicians should be alert to its possible onset. The development of gynecomastia appears to be related to both dosage level and duration of therapy and is normally reversible when Hydrochlorothiazide/Spironolactone is discontinued. In rare instances some breast enlargement may persist when Hydrochlorothiazide/Spironolactone is discontinued.

A determination of serum electrolytes to detect possible electrolyte imbalance should be performed at periodic intervals.

Both Hydrochlorothiazide and Spironolactone reduce the vascular responsiveness to norepinephrine. Therefore, caution should be exercised in the management of patients subjected to regional or general anesthesia while they are being treated with Hydrochlorothiazide/Spironolactone. Thiazides may also increase the responsiveness to tubocurarine.

Hydrochlorothiazide may raise the concentration of blood uric acid. Dosage adjustment of antigout medications may be necessary. Hydrochlorothiazide may also raise blood glucose concentrations. Dosage adjustments of insulin or hypoglycemic medications may be necessary. Concurrent use of diuretics with lithium is not recommended as it may produce lithium toxicity.

Spironolactone has been shown to increase the half-life of digoxin. This may result in increased serum digoxin levels and subsequent digitalis toxicity. It may be necessary to reduce the maintenance and digitalization doses when Spironolactone is administered, and the patient should be carefully monitored to avoid over- or underdigitalization.

Several reports of possible interference with digoxin radio-immunoassays by Spironolactone, or its metabolites, have appeared in the literature. Neither the

	Accumulation Factor: AUC (0-24 hr, day 15)/ AUC (0-24 hr, day 1)	Mean Peak Serum Concentration	Mean (SD) Post-Steady State Half-life
7-α-(thiomethyl) spirolactone (TMS)	1.25	391 ng/mL at 3.2 hr	13.8 hr (6.4) (terminal)
6-β-hydroxy-7-a-(thiomethyl) spirolactone (HTMS)	1.50	125 ng/mL at 5.1 hr	15.0 hr (4.0) (terminal)
Canrenone (C)	1.41	181 ng/mL at 4.3 hr	16.5 hr (6.3) (terminal)
Spironolactone	1.30	80 ng/mL at 2.6 hr	Approximately 1.4 hr (0.5) (β half-life)

◆ RATED THERAPEUTICALLY EQUIVALENT; ◇ THERAPEUTIC EQUIVALENCE UNCONFIRMED; ○ UNRATED

extent nor the potential clinical significance of its interference (which may be assay-specific) has been fully established.

Usage in Pregnancy. Hydrochlorothiazide does, and Spironolactone or its metabolites may, cross the placental barrier. Therefore, the use of Hydrochlorothiazide/Spironolactone in pregnant women requires that the anticipated benefit be weighed against possible hazards to the fetus. These hazards include fetal or neonatal jaundice, thrombocytopenia, and possible other adverse reactions which have been reported in the adult.

Nursing Mothers. Hydrochlorothiazide and canrenone, a metabolite of Spironolactone appear in breast milk. If use of these drugs is deemed essential, an alternative method of infant feeding should be instituted.

ADVERSE REACTIONS

Adverse reactions reported in association with the use of thiazides include: gastrointestinal symptoms (anorexia, nausea, vomiting, diarrhea, abdominal cramps), purpura, thrombocytopenia, leukopenia, agranulocytosis, dermatologic symptoms (cutaneous eruptions, pruritus, erythema multiforme), paresthesia, acute pancreatitis, jaundice, dizziness, vertigo, headache, xanthopsia, photosensitivity, necrotizing angiitis, aplastic anemia, orthostatic hypotension, muscle spasm, weakness, restlessness, and hypokalemia.

Gynecomastia is observed not infrequently. A few cases of agranulocytosis have been reported in patients taking Spironolactone. Other adverse reactions that have been reported in association with the use of Spironolactone are: gastrointestinal symptoms including cramping and diarrhea, drowsiness, lethargy, headache, maculopapular or erythematous cutaneous eruptions, urticaria, mental confusion, drug fever, ataxia, inability to achieve or maintain erection, irregular menses or amenorrhea, postmenopausal bleeding, hirsutism, deepening of the voice, gastric bleeding, ulceration, gastritis, and vomiting. Carcinoma of the breast has been reported in patients taking Spironolactone, but a cause and effect relationship has not been established.

Adverse reactions are usually reversible upon discontinuation of Hydrochlorothiazide/Spironolactone.

DOSAGE AND ADMINISTRATION

Optimal dosage should be established by individual titration of the components (see box *"Warning"*).

Edema in adults: (Congestive Heart Failure, Hepatic Cirrhosis, or Nephrotic Syndrome). The usual maintenance dose of Hydrochlorothiazide/Spironolactone is 100 mg each of Hydrochlorothiazide and Spironolactone daily, administered in a single dose or in divided doses, but may range from 25 mg to 200 mg of each component daily depending on the response to the initial titration. In some instances it may be desirable to administer separate tablets of either Spironolactone or Hydrochlorothiazide in addition to Hydrochlorothiazide/Spironolactone in order to provide optimal individual therapy.

The onset of diuresis with Hydrochlorothiazide/Spironolactone occurs promptly and, due to prolonged effect of the Spironolactone component, persists for two to three days after Hydrochlorothiazide/Spironolactone is discontinued.

Edema in Children: The usual daily maintenance dose of Hydrochlorothiazide/Spironolactone should be that which provides 0.75 to 1.5 mg of Spironolactone per pound of body weight (1.65 to 3.3 mg/kg).

Essential Hypertension. Although the dosage will vary depending on the results of titration of the individual ingredients, many patients will be found to have an optimal response to 50 mg to 100 mg each of Hydrochlorothiazide and Spironolactone daily, given in a single dose or in divided doses.

Concurrent potassium supplementation is not recommended when Hydrochlorothiazide/Spironolactone is used in the long-term management of hypertension or in the treatment of most edematous conditions, since the Spironolactone content of Hydrochlorothiazide/Spironolactone is usually sufficient to minimize loss induced by the Hydrochlorothiazide component.

Storage: Store below 86°F (30°C).

HOW SUPPLIED
TABLETS: 25 MG

BRAND/MANUFACTURER	NDC	SIZE	AWP
◆ GENERICS			
U.S. Trading	56126-0305-11	100s ud	$9.87

TABLETS: 25 MG-25 MG

AVERAGE UNIT PRICE (AVAILABLE SIZES)		GENERIC A-RATED AVERAGE PRICE (GAAP)	
BRAND	$0.38	100s	$8.85
GENERIC	$0.07	500s	$29.66
HCFA FUL (100s ea)	$0.05	1000s	$57.57

BRAND/MANUFACTURER	NDC	SIZE	AWP
◆ BRAND			
▶ ALDACTAZIDE 25/25: Searle	00025-1011-31	100s	$40.10
	00025-1011-52	1000s	$368.94
	00025-1011-55	2500s	$896.30
◆ GENERICS			
Major	00904-0344-60	100s	$5.65
Geneva	00781-1149-01	100s	$7.08
Mylan	00378-0141-01	100s	$7.10

BRAND/MANUFACTURER	NDC	SIZE	AWP
Caremark	00339-5357-12	100s	$7.16
SPIROZIDE: Rugby	00536-4576-01	100s	$7.25
Qualitest	00603-5767-21	100s	$7.30
Mutual	53489-0144-01	100s	$7.50
Goldline	00182-1158-01	100s	$7.50
Moore,H.L.	00839-6322-06	100s	$7.63
URL	00677-0624-01	100s	$7.74
Schein	00364-0513-01	100s	$7.75
Aligen	00405-4946-01	100s	$8.18
Parmed	00349-2306-01	100s	$8.60
Raway	00686-0104-20	100s ud	$8.00
Major	00904-0344-61	100s ud	$11.10
UDL	51079-0104-20	100s ud	$17.45
Auro	55829-0472-10	100s ud	$11.95
Major	00904-0344-70	250s	$11.95
Major	00904-0344-40	500s	$24.40
Mylan	00378-0141-05	500s	$27.12
Qualitest	00603-5767-28	500s	$31.66
Mutual	53489-0144-05	500s	$32.50
SPIROZIDE: Rugby	00536-4576-05	500s	$32.60
Major	00904-0344-80	1000s	$39.75
Schein	00364-0513-02	1000s	$40.80
URL	00677-0624-10	1000s	$53.26
Moore,H.L.	00839-6322-16	1000s	$53.26
Geneva	00781-1149-10	1000s	$59.95
Mutual	53489-0144-10	1000s	$64.20
SPIROZIDE: Rugby	00536-4576-10	1000s	$65.50
Parmed	00349-2306-10	1000s	$67.95
Aligen	00405-4946-03	1000s	$73.49

TABLETS: 50 MG-50 MG

BRAND/MANUFACTURER	NDC	SIZE	AWP
○ BRAND			
▶ ALDACTAZIDE 50/50: Searle	00025-1021-31	100s	$70.43

Hydrocodone Bitartrate with Phenylephrine Hydrochloride

DESCRIPTION

Each teaspoonful (5 ml) contains:

Hydrocodone bitartrate ....1.67 mg
(Warning: May be habit forming.)
Phenylephrine hydrochloride ....5 mg
Alcohol 5%

CLINICAL PHARMACOLOGY

Hydrocodone Bitartrate is a potent antitussive which causes suppression of the cough reflex by direct action on the cough center. Hydrocodone is approximately 3 times as potent as codeine on a weight basis and has a higher addiction potential also.

Phenylephrine Hydrochloride is a sympathomimetic which acts predominately on alpha receptors and has little action on beta receptors. It therefore functions on an oral nasel decongestant with minimal CNS stimulation.

INDICATIONS

For the temporary relief of cough due to the common cold or other upper respiratory infections or irritations.

CONTRAINDICATIONS

Contraindicated in individuals with known hypersensitivity to any of the ingredients. Also contraindicated in patients with severe hypertension and patients on *MAO* inhibitor therapy.

WARNINGS

Hydrocodone can produce drug dependence and therefore has the potential for being abused. This product should be prescribed and administered with the degree of caution appropriate for this type product. Considerable caution should also be exercised in patients with hypertension, diabetes mellitus, ischemic heart disease, hyperthyroidism, increased intraocular pressure and prostatic hypertrophy. The elderly (60 years or older) are more likely to exhibit adverse reactions.

PRECAUTIONS

General: The Hydrocodone in this product may exhibit additive effects with other CNS depressants, including alcohol. Respiratory depression can be a real hazard so caution should be used, especially in patients with chronic obstructive pulmonary disease. Caution should be exercised in patients with high blood pressure, heart disease, diabetes or thyroid disease.

Drug Interactions: MAO inhibitors and beta adrenergic blockers increase the effects of sympathomimetics. Sympathomimetics may reduce the antihypertensive effects of methyldopa, mecamylamine, reserpine and veretrum alkaloids. Concomitant use of Hydrocodone with alcohol and/or other CNS depressants may have an additive effect.

▶ **SHOWN IN PRODUCT IDENTIFICATION GUIDE**

Usage in Pregnancy: Pregnancy Category C. Hydrocodone has been shown to be teratogenic in hamsters when given in doses 700 times the human dose. There are no adequate and well-controlled studies in pregnant women. This product should be used during pregnancy only if the potential benefit justifies the potential risk to the fetus.

Nursing Mothers: Due to the possible passage of the ingredients into breast milk, this product should not be given to nursing mothers.

ADVERSE REACTIONS

Adverse reactions include drowsiness, lassitude, nausea, giddiness, constipation, respiratory depression and addiction, nervousness, insomnia, restlessness, or headache. These reactions seldom, if ever, require discontinuation of therapy. Urinary retention may occur in patients with prostatic hypertrophy.

DOSAGE AND ADMINISTRATION

Adults, orally 2 teaspoonfuls every 4 to 6 hours. Children 6 to 12 years, 1 teaspoonful every 4 to 6 hours. Children 2 to 6 years, 1/2 to 1 teaspoonful every 4 to 6 hours, according to age. Dosage for children should not be repeated more than 4 times in any 24 hour period.

Store and dispense in tight containers as defined in USP/NF.

Store at controlled room temperature 15°-30°C (59°-86°F).

Dispense in child-resistant container.

HOW SUPPLIED
LIQUID (C-III):

BRAND/MANUFACTURER	NDC	SIZE	AWP
○ BRAND NALEX DH: Blansett	51674-0005-07	480 ml	$27.95

Hydrocodone Bitartrate with Phenylpropanolamine Hydrochloride

DESCRIPTION

Hydrocodone/Phenylpropanolamine contains Hydrocodone (dihydrocodeinone) Bitartrate, a semi-synthetic centrally-acting narcotic antitussive and Phenylpropanolamine Hydrochloride, a sympathomimetic amine decongestant for oral administration.

	Pediatric Syrup	Syrup
Each teaspoonful (5 mL) contains:		
Hydrocodone Bitartrate, USP	2.5 mg	5 mg
WARNING: May Be habit forming		
Phenylpropanolamine Hydrochloride, USP	12.5 mg	25 mg

CLINICAL PHARMACOLOGY

Hydrocodone is a semisynthetic narcotic antitussive and analgesic with multiple actions qualitatively similar to those of codeine. The precise mechanism of action of Hydrocodone and other opiates is not known; however, Hydrocodone is believed to act directly on the cough center. In excessive doses, Hydrocodone, like other opium derivatives, will depress respiration. The effects of Hydrocodone in therapeutic doses on the cardiovascular system are insignificant. Hydrocodone can produce miosis, euphoria, physical and physiological dependence.

Following a 10 mg oral dose of Hydrocodone administered to five adult male subjects, the mean peak concentration was 23.6 ± 5.2 ng/mL. Maximum serum levels were achieved at 1.3 ± 0.3 hours and the half-life was determined to be 3.8 ± 0.3 hours. Hydrocodone exhibits a complex pattern of metabolism including O-demethylation, N-demethylation and 6-keto reduction to the corresponding 6-α- and 6-β-hydroxymetabolites.

Phenylpropanolamine effects its vasoconstrictor activity by releasing noradrenaline from sympathetic nerve endings, and from direct stimulation of α-adrenoceptors of blood vessels.

INDICATIONS AND USAGE

Hydrocodone/Phenylpropanolamine is indicated for the symptomatic relief of cough and nasal congestion.

CONTRAINDICATIONS

Hydrocodone/Phenylpropanolamine is contraindicated in patients hypersensitive to Hydrocodone or Phenylpropanolamine, and in patients on concurrent MAO inhibitor therapy. Patients known to be hypersensitive to other opioids or sympathomimetic amines may exhibit cross sensitivity to Hydrocodone/Phenylpropanolamine Phenylpropanolamine is contraindicated in patients with heart disease, hypertension, diabetes or hyperthyroidism. Hydrocodone is contraindicated in the presence of an intracranial lesion associated with increased intracranial pressure; and whenever ventilatory function is depressed.

WARNINGS

May be habit forming. Hydrocodone can produce drug dependence of the morphine type and, therefore, has the potential for being abused. Psychic dependence, physical dependence and tolerance may develop upon repeated administration of Hydrocodone/Phenylpropanolamine and it should be prescribed and administered with the same degree of caution appropriate to the use of other narcotic drugs (see *"Drug Abuse and Dependence"*).

Respiratory Depression: Hydrocodone/Phenylpropanolamine produces dose-related respiratory depression by directly acting on brain stem respiratory centers. If respiratory depression occurs, it may be antagonized by the use of naloxone hydrochloride and other supportive measures when indicated.

Head Injury and Increased Intracranial Pressure: The respiratory depression properties of narcotics and their capacity to elevate cerebrospinal fluid pressure may be markedly exaggerated in the presence of head injury, other intracranial lesions or a preexisting increase in intracranial pressure. Furthermore, narcotics produce adverse reactions which may obscure the clinical course of patients with head injuries.

Acute Abdominal Conditions: The administration of Hydrocodone/Phenylpropanolamine or other narcotics may obscure the diagnosis or clinical course of patients with acute abdominal conditions.

Pediatric Use: In young children, as well as adults, the respiratory center is sensitive to the depressant action of narcotic cough suppressants in a dose-dependent manner. Benefit to risk ratio should be carefully considered especially in children with respiratory embarrassment (e.g., croup).

Phenylpropanolamine: Hypertensive crises can occur with concurrent use of Phenylpropanolamine and monoamine oxidase (MAO) inhibitors, indomethacin or with beta-blockers and methyldopa.

If a hypertensive crisis occurs, these drugs should be discontinued immediately and therapy to lower blood pressure should be instituted immediately. Fever should be managed by means of external cooling.

PRECAUTIONS

General: Before prescribing medication to suppress or modify cough, it is important to ascertain that the underlying cause of cough is identified, that modification of cough does not increase the risk of clinical or physiologic complications, and that appropriate therapy for the primary disease is provided.

Special Risk Patients: Hydrocodone/Phenylpropanolamine should be given with caution to certain patients such as the elderly or debilitated, and those with severe impairment of hepatic or renal functions, hypothyroidism, Addison's disease, prostatic hypertrophy or urethral stricture, asthma, narrow-angle glaucoma, and uncontrolled hypertension.

Information for Patients: Hydrocodone may impair the mental and/or physical abilities required for the performance of potentially hazardous tasks such as driving a car or operating machinery; phenylpropanolamine may produce a rapid pulse, dizziness or palpitations. The patient using Hydrocodone/Phenylpropanolamine should be cautioned accordingly.

Drug Interactions: Patients receiving other narcotic analgesics, general anesthetics, phenothiazines, other tranquilizers, sedative-hypnotics or other CNS depressants (including alcohol) concomitantly with Hydrocodone may exhibit an additive CNS depression. When such combined therapy is contemplated, the dose of one or both agents should be reduced. The use of Phenylpropanolamine with other sympathomimetic amines and MAO inhibitors may produce an additive elevation of blood pressure (see *"Warnings"*).

Carcinogenesis, Mutagenesis, Impairment of Fertility: Carcinogenicity, mutagenicity and reproduction studies have not been conducted with Hydrocodone/Phenylpropanolamine.

Pregnancy: Teratogenic Effects: Pregnancy Category C: Animal reproduction studies have not been conducted with Hydrocodone/Phenylpropanolamine. It is also not known whether Hydrocodone/Phenylpropanolamine can cause fetal harm when administered to a pregnant woman or can affect reproductive capacity. Hydrocodone/Phenylpropanolamine should be given to a pregnant woman only if clearly needed.

Nonteratogenic Effects: Babies born to mothers who have been taking opioids regularly prior to delivery will be physically dependent. The withdrawal signs include irritability and excessive crying, tremors, hyperactive reflexes, increased respiratory rate, increased stools, sneezing, yawning, vomiting and fever. The intensity of the syndrome does not always correlate with the duration of maternal opioid use or dose.

Labor and Delivery: As with all narcotics, administration of Hydrocodone/Phenylpropanolamine to the mother shortly before delivery may result in some degree of respiratory depression in the newborn, especially if higher doses are used.

Nursing Mothers: It is not known whether this drug is excreted in human milk. Because many drugs are excreted in human milk and because of the potential for serious adverse reactions in nursing infants from Hydrocodone/Phenylpropanolamine a decision should be made whether to discontinue nursing or discontinue the drug, taking into account the importance of the drug to the mother.

Pediatric Use: Safety and effectiveness of Hydrocodone/Phenylpropanolamine in children under six have not been established.

◆ RATED THERAPEUTICALLY EQUIVALENT; ◇ THERAPEUTIC EQUIVALENCE UNCONFIRMED; ○ UNRATED

ADVERSE REACTIONS

Respiratory System: Hydrocodone produces dose-related respiratory depression by acting directly on brain stem respiratory centers. (See *"Overdosage"*).

Cardiovascular System: Hypertension, postural hypotension, tachycardia and palpitations.

Genitourinary System: Ureteral spasm, spasm of vesical sphincters and urinary retention have been reported with opiates.

Central Nervous System: Sedation, drowsiness, mental clouding, lethargy, impairment of mental and physical performance, anxiety, fear, dysphoria, dizziness, psychic dependence, mood changes and blurred vision.

Gastrointestinal System: Nausea and vomiting occur more frequently in ambulatory than in recumbent patients. Prolonged administration of Hydrocodone/Phenylpropanolamine may produce constipation.

Dermatological: Skin rash, pruritus.

DRUG ABUSE AND DEPENDENCE

Hydrocodone/Phenylpropanolamine is a Schedule III narcotic. Psychic dependence, physical dependence, and tolerance may develop upon repeated administration of narcotics; therefore, Hydrocodone/Phenylpropanolamine should be prescribed and administered with caution. However, psychic dependence is unlikely to develop when Hydrocodone/Phenylpropanolamine is used for a short time for the treatment of cough. Physical dependence, the condition in which continued administration of the drug is required to prevent the appearance of a withdrawal syndrome, assumes clinically significant proportions only after several weeks of continued oral narcotic use, although some mild degree of physical dependence may develop after a few days of narcotic therapy.

OVERDOSAGE

Signs and Symptoms: Serious overdosage with Hydrocodone/Phenylpropanolamine is characterized by respiratory depression (a decrease in respiratory rate and/or tidal volume, Cheyne-Stokes respiration, cyanosis), extreme somnolence progressing to stupor or coma, skeletal muscle flaccidity, cold and clammy skin, and sometimes bradycardia and hypotension. In severe overdosage apnea, circulatory collapse, cardiac arrest, and death may occur.

The signs and symptoms of overdosage of the individual components of Hydrocodone/Phenylpropanolamine may be modified in varying degrees by the presence of other active ingredients. Overdosage with Phenylpropanolamine alone may result in tremor, restlessness, increased motor activity, agitation and hallucinations.

Treatment: Primary attention should be given to the reestablishment of adequate respiratory exchange through provision of a patent airway and the institution of assisted or controlled ventilation. The narcotic antagonist naloxone hydrochloride is a specific antidote for respiratory depression which may result from overdosage or unusual sensitivity to narcotics including Hydrocodone. Therefore, an appropriate dose of naloxone hydrochloride should be administered preferably by the intravenous route, simultaneously with efforts at respiratory resuscitation.

For further information, see full prescribing information for naloxone hydrochloride. An antagonist should not be administered in the absence of clinically significant respiratory depression. Oxygen, intravenous fluids, vasopressors, and other supportive measures should be employed as indicated. Gastric emptying may be useful in removing unabsorbed drug.

DOSAGE AND ADMINISTRATION

Adults: The usual dose for adults is one teaspoonful Hydrocodone/Phenylpropanolamine every four hours as needed, not to exceed six teaspoonfuls in a 24 hour period. Children 6 to 12 years of age: The usual dose for children 6 to 12 years of age is one teaspoonful Hydrocodone/Phenylpropanolamine Pediatric Syrup (Hydrocodone Bitartrate 2.5 mg and Phenylpropanolamine Hydrochloride 12.5 mg/5 cc) every four hours as needed, not to exceed six teaspoonfuls in a 24 hour period.

Store at controlled room temperature (59°-86°F, 15°-30°C). Oral prescription where permitted by state law.

HOW SUPPLIED
SYRUP (C-III): 2.5 MG-12.5 MG/5 ML

BRAND/MANUFACTURER	NDC	SIZE	AWP
○ BRAND			
HYCOMINE PEDIATRIC: Du Pont Multi	00056-0247-16	480 ml	$52.26

For additional alternatives, turn to the section beginning on page 2859.

Hydrocodone Bitartrate with Pseudoephedrine Hydrochloride

DESCRIPTION

Each 5 mL (one teaspoonful) of Hydrocodone Bitartrate/Pseudoephedrine Hydrochloride Liquid for oral use contains Hydrocodone Bitartrate, 5 mg (Warning: May be habit forming), and Pseudoephedrine Hydrochloride 60 mg.

Hydrocodone Bitartrate is an antitussive. Chemically it is 4,5α-epoxy-3-methoxy-17-methylmorphinan-6-one tartrate (1:1) hydrate (2:5).

Pseudoephedrine Hydrochloride is a nasal decongestant. Chemically it is benzenemethanol, α-[1-(methylamino)ethyl],[S-(R^*,R^*)]-, hydrochloride.

CLINICAL PHARMACOLOGY

Hydrocodone is a narcotic-analgesic chemically and pharmacologically related to codeine. Hydrocodone suppresses the cough reflex by depressing the medullary cough center. The duration of antitussive action of hydrocodone in man after oral administration is 4 to 8 hours. Hydrocodone is approximately three times more potent than codeine on a weight basis.

Pseudoephedrine is an orally active sympathomimetic amine and exerts a decongestant action on the nasal mucosa. Pseudoephedrine produces peripheral effects similar to those of ephedrine and central effects similar to, but less intense than amphetamines. It has the potential for excitatory side effects. At the recommended oral dosages it has little or no pressor effect in normotensive adults.

The serum half-life (T-1/2) of Pseudoephedrine is approximately 4 to 8 hours. T-1/2 is decreased with increased excretion of drug at a urine pH lower than 6 and may be increased with decreased excretion at urine pH higher than 8.

INDICATIONS

For exhausting cough spasms accompanying upper respiratory tract congestion associated with the common cold, influenza, bronchitis and sinusitis.

CONTRAINDICATIONS

Patients with severe hypertension, severe coronary artery disease, and in patients on MAO inhibitor therapy.

Hypersensitivity: Contraindicated in patients with hypersensitivity or Idiosyncrasy to sympathomimetic amines, phenanthrene derivatives or to any other formula ingredients.

Nursing Mothers: Contraindicated because of the higher than usual risk for infants from sympathomimetic amines.

WARNINGS

Hydrocodone should be prescribed and administered with the same degree of caution as all oral medications containing a narcotic analgesic. Extreme caution should be exercised in the use of hydrocodone in patients with severe respiratory impairment or patients with impaired respiratory drive.

If sympathomimetic amines are used in patients with hypertension, diabetes mellitus, ischemic heart disease, hyperthyroidism, increased intraocular pressure or prostatic hypertrophy, judicious caution should be exercised (see *"Contraindications"*).

Use in Elderly: The elderly (60 years and older) are more likely to have adverse reactions to sympathomimetics. Overdosage of sympathomimetics in the age group may cause hallucinations, convulsions, CNS depressions and death.

PRECAUTIONS

General: Caution should be exercised if used in patients with diabetes, hypertension, cardiovascular disease, hyperreactivity to ephedrine, or decreased respiratory drive (see *"Contraindications"*). Information for Patients: Hydrocodone may produce drowsiness. Persons who perform hazardous tasks requiring mental alertness or physical coordination should be cautioned accordingly. Concomitant use of hydrocodone with tranquilizers, alcohol or other depressants may produce additive depressant effects. Do not exceed the prescribed dosage.

Drug Interactions: Hydrocodone may potentiate the effects of other narcotics, general anesthetics, tranquilizers, sedatives and hypnotics, tricyclic antidepressants, MAO inhibitors, alcohol, and other CNS depressants. Beta adrenergic blockers and MAO inhibitors potentiate the sympathomimetic effects of pseudoephedrine. Sympathomimetics may reduce the antihypertensive effects of methyldopa, mecamylamine, reserpine and veratrum alkaloids.

Pregnancy Category C: Animal reproduction studies have not been conducted with Pseudoephedrine or Hydrocodone. It is also not known whether Pseudoephedrine or Hydrocodone can cause fetal harm when administered to a pregnant woman or can affect reproduction capacity. Pseudoephedrine or Hydrocodone may be given to a pregnant woman only if clearly needed.

Nursing Mothers: Because of the potential for serious adverse reactions in nursing infants from sympathomimetic amines, Pseudoephedrine is contraindicated in nursing mothers.

ADVERSE REACTIONS

Gastrointestinal upset, nausea, drowsiness and constipation.

A slight elevation in serum transaminase levels has been noted.

Individuals hyperreactive to Pseudoephedrine may display ephedrine-like reactions such as tachycardia, palpitations, headache, dizziness or nausea. Sympathomimetic drugs have been associated with certain untoward reactions including fear, anxiety, tenseness, restlessness, tremor, weakness, pallor, respiratory difficulty, dysuria, insomnia, hallucinations, convulsions, CNS depression, arrhythmias and cardiovascular collapse with hypotension.

Patient idiosyncrasy to adrenergic agents may be manifested by insomnia, dizziness, weakness, tremor or arrhythmias.

DRUG ABUSE AND DEPENDENCE

Controlled Substance: Hydrocodone is controlled by the Drug Enforcement Administration. Hydrocodone Bitartrate/Pseudoephedrine Hydrochloride Liquid is a Schedule III controlled substance.

Abuse: Human experience indicates that abuse of this product is uncommon. However, Hydrocodone is a narcotic drug related to codeine with roughly three times the abuse potential of codeine on a weight basis.

Dependence: Hydrocodone can produce drug dependence of the morphine type. Psychic dependence, physical dependence and tolerance may develop if dosage recommendations are greatly exceeded over a prolonged period of time.

OVERDOSAGE

Acute overdosage may produce variable clinical signs as Hydrocodone produces CNS depression and cardiovascular depression while Pseudoephedrine produces CNS stimulation and variable cardiovascular effects. Hydrocodone is likely to be responsible for most of the severe reactions from overdosage. Pressor amines should be used with great caution when taking Pseudoephedrine. Patients with signs of stimulation should be treated conservatively and depressant medications should be avoided if possible because of potential drug interaction with Hydrocodone.

DOSAGE AND ADMINISTRATION

Adults and children over 90 lbs, 1 teaspoonful; children 50 to 90 lbs, ½ teaspoonful; children 25 to 50 lbs, 1/4 teaspoonful.
   May be given four times a day as needed. May be taken with meals.
   Store at controlled room temperature 15°-30°C (59°-86°F).
   Dispense in a tight, light-resistant container as defined in the USP.

HOW SUPPLIED
ELIXIR (C-III)

BRAND/MANUFACTURER	NDC	SIZE	AWP
○ GENERICS			
TUSSAFIN: Rugby	00536-0532-85	480 ml	$9.13
DETUSSIN: Qualitest	00603-1130-58	480 ml	$12.20

LIQUID (C-III):

BRAND/MANUFACTURER	NDC	SIZE	AWP
○ GENERICS			
DETUSSIN: Schein	00364-7257-16	480 ml	$12.79
DETUSSIN: Major	00904-0967-16	480 ml	$13.00
DETUSSIN: Barre	00472-0958-16	480 ml	$13.65
TUSSGEN: Goldline	00182-1163-40	480 ml	$14.55
HYDROPHED: Norton,HN	50732-0834-16	480 ml	$28.94
HYDROPHED: Norton,HN	50732-0835-16	480 ml	$29.17
DETUSSIN: Major	00904-0967-28	3840 ml	$62.00

LIQUID (C-III): 5 MG-300 MG-30 MG

BRAND/MANUFACTURER	NDC	SIZE	AWP
○ GENERICS			
ENTUSS-D: Roberts/Hauck	59441-0438-16	480 ml	$41.67

TABLETS (C-III): 5 MG-60 MG

BRAND/MANUFACTURER	NDC	SIZE	AWP
○ BRAND			
P-V-TUSSIN: Solvay	00032-1091-01	100s	$59.03

Hydrocodone Bitartrate/ Pheniramine Maleate/ Phenylephrine Hydrochloride/ Phenylpropanolamine Hydrochloride/Pyrilamine Maleate

DESCRIPTION

Each 5 mL (one teaspoonful) contains:

Hydrocodone bitartrate ....1.7 mg
(Warning: May be habit forming)
Phenylephrine HCl ....5.0 mg
Phenylpropanolamine HCl ....3.3 mg
Pyrilamine Maleate ....3.3 mg
Pheniramine Maleate ....3.3 mg
Alcohol 5%

CLINICAL PHARMACOLOGY

Hydrocodone Bitartrate is a potent antitussive which causes suppression of the cough reflex by direct action on the cough center. Hydrocodone is approximately three times as potent as codeine on a weight basis and has a higher addiction potential also.

   Pheniramine Maleate and Pyrilamine Maleate are antihistamines which act by competing with histamine for receptor sites on effector cells. They thereby prevent, but do not reverse, responses mediated by histamine alone. The antimuscarinic actions provide a drying effect on the nasal mucosa.

   Phenylephrine Hydrochloride and Phenylpropanolamine Hydrochloride are sympathomimetics which act predominantly on alpha receptors and have little action on beta receptors. They therefore function as oral nasal decongestants with minimal CNS stimulation.

INDICATIONS

For the temporary relief of cough and other symptoms of the common cold, pertussis, or influenza.

CONTRAINDICATIONS

Hypersensitivity to any of the ingredients. Also contraindicated in patients with severe hypertension, severe coronary artery disease, patients on MAO inhibitor therapy, patients with narrow-angle glaucoma, urinary retention, peptic ulcer, and during an asthmatic attack.

WARNINGS

Hydrocodone can produce drug dependence and therefore has the potential for being abused. This product should be prescribed and administered with the appropriate degree of caution.

   Considerable caution should be exercised in patients with hypertension, diabetes mellitus, ischemic heart disease, hyperthyroidism, increased intraocular pressure and prostatic hypertrophy. The elderly (60 years and older) are more likely to exhibit adverse reactions. Antihistamines may cause excitability, especially in children. At dosages higher than the recommended dose, nervousness, dizziness, or sleeplessness may occur.

PRECAUTIONS

General: Caution should be exercised in patients with high blood pressure, heart disease, diabetes or thyroid disease. The Hydrocodone and antihistamine in this product may exhibit additive effects with other CNS depressants, including alcohol. Respiratory depression can be a real hazard so caution should be used, especially in patients with chronic obstructive pulmonary disease.

Information For Patients: Hydrocodone and antihistamines may cause drowsiness and ambulatory patients who operate machinery or motor vehicles should be cautioned accordingly.

Drug Interactions: MAO inhibitors and beta adrenergic blockers increase the effects of sympathomimetics. Sympathomimetics may reduce the antihypertensive effects of methyldopa, mecamylamine, reserpine and veratrum alkaloids. Concomitant use of narcotics and antihistamines with alcohol and other CNS depressants may have an additive effect.

Pregnancy: Pregnancy Category C: Animal reproduction studies have not been conducted with this product. It is also not known whether it can cause fetal harm when administered to a pregnant woman or can affect reproduction capacity. This product should be given to a pregnant woman only if clearly needed.

Nursing Mothers: Due to the possible passage of the ingredients into breast milk this product should not be given to nursing mothers.

ADVERSE REACTIONS

Adverse reactions include drowsiness, lassitude, nausea, giddiness, constipation, respiratory depression, addiction, dryness of mouth, blurred vision, cardiac palpitations, flushing, increased irritability or excitement (especially in children).

DRUG ABUSE AND DEPENDENCE

This product is a Schedule III Controlled Substance. Because of the Hydrocodone Bitartrate content, some abuse might be expected. Psychic dependence, physical dependence and tolerance may develop upon repeated administration. It should be prescribed and administered with appropriate caution.

OVERDOSAGE

Symptoms of overdosage include respiratory depression, extreme somnolence progressing to stupor or coma, skeletal muscle flaccidity, cold and clammy skin and other symptoms common with narcotic overdosage.

   Primary treatment consists of insuring adequate respiration through provision of a patent airway and the institution of assisted or controlled ventilation. Naloxone hydrochloride should be administered in small intravenous doses (consult specific product labeling before use). In addition, oxygen, intravenous fluids, vasopressors and other supportive measures should be employed as indicated. Gastric emptying may be useful in removing unabsorbed drug. Activated charcoal may also be of benefit.

DOSAGE AND ADMINISTRATION

Adults and children over 12 years: 2 teaspoonfuls.
   Children 6 to 12 years of age: 1 teaspoonful.
   Children 2 to 6 years of age: 1/2 teaspoonful.
   These doses may be given four times daily as needed. Not recommended for children under 2 years of age.
   Store at controlled room temperature 15°-30°C (59°-86°F).
   Dispense in a tight, light-resistant container as described in the USP/NF.

◆ RATED THERAPEUTICALLY EQUIVALENT; ◇ THERAPEUTIC EQUIVALENCE UNCONFIRMED; ○ UNRATED

HOW SUPPLIED
LIQUID (C-III):

BRAND/MANUFACTURER	NDC	SIZE	AWP
○ GENERICS			
ROLATUSS W/HYDROCODONE: Major	00904-1201-16	480 ml	$14.25
BAN-TUSS HC: Norton,HN	50732-0607-16	480 ml	$18.67
STATUSS GREEN: Huckaby	58407-0372-16	480 ml	$22.29
BAN-TUSS HC: Norton,HN	50732-0607-28	3840 ml	$124.73

SYRUP (C-III):

BRAND/MANUFACTURER	NDC	SIZE	AWP
○ GENERICS			
QRP TUSSIN SYRUP:	52765-0602-04	120 ml	$8.50

Hydrocodone Bitartrate/ Phenylephrine Hydrochloride/ Pyrilamine Maleate

DESCRIPTION
Each teaspoonful (5 mL) contains:

Hydrocodone Bitartrate ....1.66 mg
(Warning — May be habit forming)
Phenylephrine Hydrochloride ....5 mg
Pyrilamine Maleate ....8.33 mg

This product contains ingredients of the following therapeutic classes: antitussive, nasal decongestant and antihistamine.

CLINICAL PHARMACOLOGY
Hydrocodone Bitartrate is a potent antitussive which causes suppression of the cough reflex by a direct action on the cough center. Hydrocodone is approximately three times as potent as codeine on a weight basis, and has a higher addiction potential also. Phenylephrine Hydrochloride is a sympathonimetic which acts predominantly on alpha receptors and has little action on beta receptors. It therefore functions as an oral nasal decongestant with minimal CNS stimulation. Pyrilamine Maleate is an antihistamine used in suppressing symptoms of allergic rhinitis. However, it is more prone to cause drowsiness than some other antihistamines.

INDICATIONS
Temporary relief of cough, nasal congestion, and other symptoms associated with colds, or seasonal or perennial allergic vasomotor rhinitis (hay fever).

CONTRAINDICATIONS
Patients with severe hypertension, severe coronary artery disease, in patients on MAO inhibitor therapy and in nursing mothers. Also contraindicated in patients with narrow-angle glaucoma, urinary retention, peptic ulcer or in patients with a hypersensitivity to any of its ingredients.

WARNINGS
Considerable caution should be exercised in patients with hypertension, diabetes mellitus, ischemic heart disease, hyperthyroidism, increased intraocular pressure and prostatic hypertrophy. The elderly (60 years or older) are more likely to exhibit adverse reactions. Antihistamines may cause excitability, especially in children. At dosages higher than the recommended dose, nervousness, dizziness or sleeplessness may occur. Hydrocodone can produce drug dependence and therefore has the potential for being abused.

PRECAUTIONS
General: Caution should be exercised in patients with high blood pressure, heart disease, diabetes or thyroid disease. The Antihistamines and Hydrocodone in this product may exhibit additive effects with other CNS depressants, including alcohol.

Information for Patients: The Hydrocodone and Antihistamines may cause drowsiness and ambulatory patients who operate machinery or motor vehicles should be cautioned accordingly.

Drug Interactions: MAO inhibitors and beta adrenergic blockers may increase the effects of sympathomimetics. Sympathomimetics may reduce the antihypertensive effects of methyldopa, mecamylamine, reserpine and veratrum alkaloids. Concomitant use of Hydrocodone and Antihistamines with alcohol and other CNS depressants may have an additive effect.

Pregnancy: Pregnancy Category C: Hydrocodone has been shown to be teratogenic in hamsters when given doses 700 times the human dose. There are no adequate and well-controlled studies in pregnant women. Hydrocodone/Phenylephrine/Pyrilamine should be used during pregnancy only if the potential benefit justifies the potential risk to the fetus.

ADVERSE REACTIONS
Adverse reactions include drowsiness, lassitude, nausea, giddiness, dryness of mouth, blurred vision, cardiac palpitations, flushing, increased irritability or excitement (especially in children).

DRUG ABUSE AND DEPENDENCE
This product is a Schedule III controlled substance. Because of the Hydrocodone content, some abuse may be expected. Psychic dependence, physical dependence, and tolerance may develop upon repeated administration. It should be prescribed and administered with the degree of caution appropriate for this type product.

DOSAGE AND ADMINISTRATION
Adults and older children: 1 to 2 teaspoonfuls every 4 hours.

Children, 6 to 12 years of age: 1 teaspoonful every 4 hours.

Children, 2 to 6 years of age: ½ teaspoonful every 4 hours.

Under 2 years: Narcotic antitussives are not recommended for use in children under 2 years of age. Children under 2 years may be more susceptible to the respiratory depressant effects of narcotics, including respiratory arrest, coma, and death. However, dosages based on hydrocodone, 0.3 mg/kg/24 hours, divided into four equal doses have been suggested.

Dispense syrup in a tight container as defined in usp/nf with a child-resistant closure.

Store at controlled room temperature 15°-30°C (59°-86°F).

HOW SUPPLIED
SYRUP (C-III): 1.66 MG-5 MG-8.33MG/5ML

BRAND/MANUFACTURER	NDC	SIZE	AWP
○ BRAND			
CODIMAL DH: Central	00131-5129-64	120 ml doz	$77.88
	00131-5129-70	480 ml	$21.15
	00131-5129-72	3840 ml	$147.55
○ GENERICS			
DICOMAL-DH: Econolab	55053-0900-04	118 ml	$5.52
DICOMAL-DH: Econolab	55053-0900-16	480 ml	$17.95

Hydrocodone Bitartrate with Potassium Guaiacolsulfonate

DESCRIPTION
Each teaspoonful (5 ml.) contains:

Hydrocodone Bitartrate ....5 mg
(Warning-May be habit forming)
Potassium Guaiacolsulfonate ....300 mg

This product contains ingredients of the following therapeutic classes: antitussive and expectorant.

CLINICAL PHARMACOLOGY
Hydrocodone Bitartrate is a potent antitussive which causes suppression of the cough reflex by direct action on the cough center. Hydrocodone is approximately three times as potent as codeine on a weight basis and has a higher addiction potential also. Potassium Guaiacolsulfonate has been used empirically for many decades as an expectorant.

INDICATIONS
For the temporary relief of dry, nonproductive cough due to colds, pertussis or influenza.

CONTRAINDICATIONS
Hypersensitivity to any of the ingredients.

WARNINGS
Hydrocodone can produce drug dependence and therefore has the potential for being abused. Hydrocodone Bitartrate/Potassium Guaiacolsulfonate should be prescribed and administered with the degree of caution appropriate for this type product.

PRECAUTIONS
General: The Hydrocodone in this product may exhibit additive effects with other CNS depressants, including alcohol. Respiratory depression can be a real hazard so caution should be used, especially in patients with chronic obstructive pulmonary disease.

Information for Patients: The Hydrocodone may cause drowsiness and ambulatory patients who operate machinery or motor vehicles should be cautioned accordingly.

Drug Interactions: Concomitant use of Hydrocodone with alcohol and/or other CNS depressants may have an addictive effect.

Pregnancy: The safety of use of the product in pregnancy has not been established.

ADVERSE REACTIONS
Adverse reactions include drowsiness, lassitude, nausea, giddiness, constipation, respiratory depression and addiction.

➤ SHOWN IN PRODUCT IDENTIFICATION GUIDE

DRUG ABUSE AND DEPENDENCE

This product is a Schedule III Controlled Substance. Because of the Hydrocodone content, some abuse might be expected. Psychic dependence, physical dependence and tolerance may develop upon repeated administration. It should be prescribed and administered with the degree of caution appropriate for this type product.

OVERDOSAGE

Symptoms of overdosage include respiratory depression, extreme somnolence progressing to stupor or coma, skeletal muscle flaccidity, cold and clammy skin and other symptoms common with narcotic overdosage.

Primary treatment consists of insuring adequate respiration through provision of a patent airway and the institution of assisted or controlled ventilation. Naloxone hydrochloride should be administered in small intravenous doses (consult specific product labeling before use). In addition, oxygen, intravenous fluids, vasopressors and other supportive measures should be employed as indicated. Gastric emptying may be useful in removing unabsorbed drug. Activated charcoal may also be of benefit.

DOSAGE AND ADMINISTRATION

Adults and older children: 1 to 1 ½ teaspoonfuls

Children, 6 to 12 years of age: ½ to 1 teaspoonful

Children, 3 to 6 years of age: ¼ to ½ teaspoonful. These doses may be given four times daily as needed. Not recommended for children under 3 years of age.

Store and dispense syrup in tight containers as defined in USP/NF. Store between 15°-30°C (50°-86°F).

Dispense in child-resistant containers.

HOW SUPPLIED
LIQUID (C-III): 5 MG-300 MG/5 ML

BRAND/MANUFACTURER	NDC	SIZE	AWP
○ GENERICS			
PROTUSS: Horizon Pharm	59630-0100-04	120 ml	$10.50
PROTUSS: Horizon Pharm	59630-0100-16	480 ml	$36.25

LIQUID (C-V):

BRAND/MANUFACTURER	NDC	SIZE	AWP
○ GENERICS			
MARCOF EXPECTORANT: Marnel	00682-0445-16	480 ml	$22.30

Hydrocodone/Pheniramine/ Phenylephrine/ Phenylpropanolamine/Pyrilamine

DESCRIPTION

Each 5 mL (one teaspoonful) contains:

Hydrocodone Bitartrate	1.7 mg
(WARNING: MAY BE HABIT FORMING)	
Phenylephrine Hydrochloride	5.0 mg
Phenylpropanolamine Hydrochloride	3.3 mg
Pheniramine Maleate	3.3 mg
Pyrilamine Maleate	3.3 mg
Alcohol	5%

This combination is an oral antitussive, antihistaminic and nasal decongestant preparation.

INDICATIONS AND USAGE

This combination is indicated for the temporary relief of symptoms associated with hay fever, allergies, nasal congestion and cough due to the common cold.

CONTRAINDICATIONS

Hypersensitivity to antihistamines. Concomitant use of antihypertensive or antidepressant drugs containing a monoamine oxidase inhibitor is contraindicated.

This combination is contraindicated in patients with glaucoma, bronchial asthma and in women who are pregnant.

WARNINGS

Patients should be warned of the potential that this combination may be habit forming.

This combination may cause drowsiness.

Patients should be warned of the possible additive effects caused by taking antihistamines with alcohol, hypnotics, sedatives and tranquilizers.

PRECAUTIONS

Patients taking this combination should avoid driving a motor vehicle or operating dangerous machinery (See *"Warnings"*).

Caution should be taken with patients having hypertension and cardiovascular disease.

ADVERSE REACTIONS

Gastrointestinal: nausea, vomiting, diarrhea, constipation, epigastric distress.

Genitourinary System: urinary frequency and dysuria.

Central Nervous System: drowsiness, giddiness, dizziness, headache, incoordination, faintness, hyperirritability, nervousness and insomnia, mydriasis.

Special Senses: tinnitus, visual disturbances, blurred vision.

Metabolic/Endocrine: anorexia, lassitude.

Cardiovascular: tightness of the chest, palpitations, tachycardia, hypotension/ hypertension.

Miscellaneous: dryness of mucous membranes, xerostomia.

Respiratory: thickening of bronchial secretions.

OVERDOSAGE

Overdosing may cause restlessness, excitation, delirium, tremors, euphoria, stupor, tachycardia and even convulsions.

DOSAGE AND ADMINISTRATION

Adults and children 12 years and older: 2 teaspoonfuls every 4 to 6 hours.
Children 6 to under 12 years of age: 1 teaspoonful every 4 to 6 hours.
Children 2 to under 6 years of age: ½ to 1 teaspoonful every 4 to 6 hours, according to age.

Note: Doses for children should not be repeated more than 4 times in any 24 hour period.

Store at controlled room temperature 15°-30°C (59°-86°F)

HOW SUPPLIED
LIQUID (C-III):

BRAND/MANUFACTURER	NDC	SIZE	AWP
○ GENERICS			
Q-TUSS HC: Qualitest	00603-1596-58	480 ml	$16.80
TRI-PHEN-PYRL HC: Goldline	00182-0157-40	480 ml	$20.00
RU-TUSS W/HYDROCODONE: Boots Pharm	00048-1007-16	480 ml	$40.00

Hydrocortisone 1% In Absorbase *SEE*
HYDROCORTISONE, TOPICAL

Hydrocortisone Acetate and Pramoxine Hydrochloride

DESCRIPTION

Hydrocortisone Pramoxine Cream contains:

Hydrocortisone Acetate	0.5%, 1%, or 2.5%
Pramoxine Hydrochloride in a hydrophilic cream base	1%

Hydrocortisone/Pramoxine Lotion contains:

Hydrocortisone Acetate	0.5%, 1%, or 2.5%
Pramoxine Hydrochloride	1%

Hydrocortisone/Pramoxine Ointment contains:

Hydrocortisone Acetate	1% or 2.5%
Pramoxine Hydrochloride in an emollient ointment base	1%

Hydrocortisone/Pramoxine Topical Aerosol contains:

Hydrocortisone Acetate	1%
Pramoxine Hydrochloride	1%

Topical corticosteroids are anti-inflammatory and antipruritic agents. The chemical structural formulae for the active ingredients are presented below.

Hydrocortisone Acetate
(Pregn-4-ene-3,20-dione, 21-(acetyloxy)-11,17-dihydroxy-, (11β). $C_{23}H_{23}O_6$:mol wt:404.50.

Pramoxine Hydrochloride
(4-(3-p-butoxyphenoxy)propyl)morpholine hydrochloride) $C_{17}H_{27}$ NO_3 HCl:mol wt:329.87.

CLINICAL PHARMACOLOGY

Topical corticosteroids share anti-inflammatory, antipruritic and vasoconstrictive actions.

The mechanism of anti-inflammatory activity of the topical corticosteroids is unclear. Various laboratory methods, including vasoconstrictor assays, are used to compare and predict potencies and/or clinical efficacies of the topical corticosteroids. There is some evidence to suggest that a recognizable correlation exists between vasoconstrictor potency and therapeutic efficacy in man.

Pramoxine Hydrochloride is a topical anesthetic agent which provides temporary relief from itching and pain. It acts by stabilizing the neuronal membrane of nerve endings with which it comes into contact. It is not chemically related to the "caine" types of local anesthetics. Its unique chemical structure is

---

◆ RATED THERAPEUTICALLY EQUIVALENT; ◇ THERAPEUTIC EQUIVALENCE UNCONFIRMED; ○ UNRATED

likely to minimize the danger of cross-sensitivity reactions in patients allergic to other local anesthetics.

PHARMACOKINETICS

The extent of percutaneous absorption of topical corticosteroids is determined by many factors including the vehicle, the integrity of the epidermal barrier, and the use of occlusive dressings.

Topical corticosteroids can be absorbed from normal intact skin. Inflammation and/or other disease processes in the skin increase the percutaneous absorption. Occlusive dressings substantially increase the percutaneous absorption of topical corticosteroids. Thus, occlusive dressings may be a valuable therapeutic adjunct for treatment of resistant dermatoses. (See "Dosage and Administration").

Once absorbed through the skin, topical corticosteroids are handled through pharmacokinetic pathways similar to systemically administered corticosteroids. Corticosteroids are bound to plasma proteins in varying degrees. Corticosteroids are metabolized primarily in the liver and are then excreted by the kidneys. Some of the topical corticosteroids and their metabolites are also excreted into the bile.

INDICATIONS AND USAGE

Topical corticosteroids are indicated for the relief of the inflammatory and pruritic manifestations of corticosteroid-responsive dermatoses.

HYDROCORTISONE/PRAMOXINE TOPICAL AEROSOL

Topical corticosteroids are indicated for the relief of the inflammatory and pruritic manifestations of corticosteroid-responsive dermatoses of the anal region.

CONTRAINDICATIONS

Topical corticosteroids are contraindicated in those patients with a history of hypersensitivity to any of the components of the preparation.

WARNINGS

Do not insert any part of the aerosol container into the anus. Contents of the container are under pressure. Do not burn or puncture the aerosol container. *Store at temperatures below 120°F.* If there is no evidence of clinical or proctologic improvement within two or three weeks after therapy, or if the patient's condition worsens, discontinue the drug. Keep this and all medicines out of the reach of children.

PRECAUTIONS

General: Systemic absorption of topical corticosteroids has produced reversible hypothalamic-pituitary-adrenal (HPA) axis suppression, manifestations of Cushing's syndrome, hyperglycemia, and glucosuria in some patients.

Conditions which augment systemic absorption include the application of the more potent steroids, use over large surface areas, prolonged use, and the addition of occlusive dressings.

Therefore, patients receiving a large dose of a potent topical steroid applied to a large surface area and/or under an occlusive dressing should be evaluated periodically for evidence of HPA axis suppression by using the urinary free cortisol and ACTH stimulation tests. If HPA axis suppression is noted, an attempt should be made to withdraw the drug, to reduce the frequency of application, or to substitute a less potent steroid.

Recovery of HPA axis function is generally prompt and complete upon discontinuation of the drug. Infrequently, signs and symptoms of steroid withdrawal may occur, requiring supplemental systemic corticosteroids.

Children may absorb proportionally larger amounts of topical corticosteroids and, thus, be more susceptible to systemic toxicity. (See *Precautions—Pediatric Use.*")

If irritation develops, topical corticosteroids should be discontinued and appropriate therapy instituted.

In the presence of dermatological infections, the use of an appropriate antifungal or antibacterial agent should be instituted. If a favorable response does not occur promptly, the corticosteroid should be discontinued until the infection has been adequately controlled.

Information for the Patient: Patients using topical corticosteroids should receive the following information and instructions.

1. The medication is to be used as directed by the physician. It is for external use only; some brands are for anal or perianal use only. Avoid contact with the eyes.

2. Patients should be advised not to use this medication for any disorder other than for which it was prescribed.

3. The treated skin area should not be bandaged or otherwise covered or wrapped as to be occlusive unless directed by the physician.

4. Patients should report any signs of local adverse reactions especially under occlusive dressing.

5. Parents of pediatric patients should be advised not to use tight-fitting diapers or plastic pants on a child being treated in the diaper area, as these garments may constitute occlusive dressings.

Laboratory Tests: The following tests may be helpful in evaluating the HPA axis suppression:
Urinary free cortisol test
ACTH stimulation test

Carcinogenesis, Mutagenesis, and Impairment of Fertility: Long-term animal studies have not been performed to evaluate the carcinogenic potential or the effect on fertility of topical corticosteroids.

Studies to determine mutagenicity with prednisolone and hydrocortisone have revealed negative results.

Pregnancy Category C: Corticosteroids are generally teratogenic in laboratory animals when administered systemically at relatively low dosage levels. The more potent corticosteroids have been shown to be teratogenic after dermal application in laboratory animals. There are no adequate and well-controlled studies in pregnant women on teratogenic effects from topically applied corticosteroids. Therefore, topical corticosteroids should be used during pregnancy only if the potential benefit justifies the potential risk to the fetus. Drugs of this class should not be used extensively on pregnant patients, in large amounts, or for prolonged periods of time.

Nursing Mothers: It is not known whether topical administration of corticosteroids could result in sufficient systemic absorption to produce detectable amounts in breast milk. Systemically administered corticosteroids are secreted into breast milk in quantities NOT likely to have a deleterious effect on the infant. Nevertheless, caution should be exercised when topical corticosteroids are administered to a nursing woman.

Pediatric Use: PEDIATRIC PATIENTS MAY DEMONSTRATE GREATER SUSCEPTIBILITY TO TOPICAL CORTICOSTEROID-INDUCED HPA AXIS SUPPRESSION AND CUSHING'S SYNDROME THAN MATURE PATIENTS BECAUSE OF A LARGER SKIN SURFACE AREA TO BODY WEIGHT RATIO.

Hypothalamic-pituitary-adrenal (HPA) axis suppression, Cushing's syndrome, and intracranial hypertension have been reported in children receiving topical corticosteroids. Manifestations of adrenal suppression in children include linear growth retardation, delayed weight gain, low plasma cortisol levels, and absence of response to ACTH stimulation. Manifestations of intracranial hypertension include bulging fontanelles, headaches, and bilateral papilledema.

Administration of topical corticosteroids to children should be limited to the least amount compatible with an effective therapeutic regimen. Chronic corticosteroid therapy may interfere with the growth and development of children.

ADVERSE REACTIONS

The following local adverse reactions are reported infrequently with topical corticosteroids, but may occur more frequently with the use of occlusive dressings. These reactions are listed in an approximate decreasing order of occurrence:
Burning
Itching
Irritation
Dryness
Folliculitis
Hypertrichosis
Acneiform eruptions
Hypopigmentation
Perioral dermatitis
Allergic contact dermatitis
Maceration of the skin
Secondary infection
Skin atrophy
Striae
Miliaria

OVERDOSAGE

Topically applied corticosteroids can be absorbed in sufficient amounts to produce systemic effects (see *"Precautions"*).

DOSAGE AND ADMINISTRATION

Topical corticosteroids are generally applied to the affected area as a thin film three or four times daily depending on the severity of the condition.

Occlusive dressings may be used for the management of psoriasis or recalcitrant conditions.

If an infection develops, the use of occlusive dressings should be discontinued and appropriate antimicrobial therapy instituted.

DIRECTIONS FOR USE
Topical Aerosol
1. Shake foam container vigorously before use.
2. Hold container upright and apply only a small amount directly to affected areas. Alternatively, dispense a small amount onto a pad and apply to affected areas.
3. The container and cap should be disassembled and rinsed with warm water after use.

Note: The aerosol container should never be inserted into the vagina or anus.

TOPICAL AEROSOL FOR ANAL CONDITIONS
Apply to affected areas 3 or 4 times daily. Use the applicator supplied for anal administration. For perianal use, transfer a small quantity to a tissue and rub in gently.
1. Shake foam container vigorously before use. Hold container upright and insert into opening of the tip of the applicator. Be sure applicator plunger is drawn all the way out. **CONTAINER MUST BE HELD UPRIGHT TO OBTAIN PROPER FLOW OF MEDICATION.**
2. To fill, press down slowly on container cap. Repeat until foam reaches fill line in the applicator. *Caution.* The aerosol container should never be inserted directly into the anus.
3. Remove applicator from container. Allow some foam to remain on the applicator tip. Hold applicator by barrel and gently insert tip into the anus. With applicator in place, push plunger in order to expel foam, then withdraw

applicator. (Applicator parts should be pulled apart for thorough cleaning with warm water.)

Store at controlled room temperature 15°-30°C (59°-86°F).

Store aerosol containers upright.

HOW SUPPLIED
AEROSOL SOLID INGREDIENTS: 1%-1%

BRAND/MANUFACTURER	NDC	SIZE	AWP
◇ GENERICS			
Copley	38245-0624-05	10 gm	$11.70

CREAM: 1%-1%

BRAND/MANUFACTURER	NDC	SIZE	AWP
◇ GENERICS			
ANALPRAM-HC: Ferndale	00496-0778-04	30 gm	$13.95
PROCTOCREAM HC: Reed & Carnrick	00021-4260-10	30 gm	$17.75

CREAM: 2.5%-1%

BRAND/MANUFACTURER	NDC	SIZE	AWP
◇ GENERICS			
ANALPRAM-HC: Ferndale	00496-0800-04	30 gm	$19.55

CREAM: 2.5%-1%

BRAND/MANUFACTURER	NDC	SIZE	AWP
○ BRAND			
PRAMOSONE: Ferndale	00496-0717-04	30 gm	$15.90
	00496-0717-03	60 gm	$25.45

CREAM: 1%-1%

BRAND/MANUFACTURER	NDC	SIZE	AWP
○ BRAND			
PRAMOSONE: Ferndale	00496-0716-04	30 gm	$8.00
	00496-0716-03	60 gm	$12.80

CREAM: 0.5%

BRAND/MANUFACTURER	NDC	SIZE	AWP
○ BRAND			
PRAMOSONE: Ferndale	00496-0715-04	30 gm	$6.75

CREAM: 2.5%

BRAND/MANUFACTURER	NDC	SIZE	AWP
◇ GENERICS			
PROCTOCREAM HC: Reed & Carnrick	00021-4640-24	30 gm	$18.86

FOAM: 1%-1%

BRAND/MANUFACTURER	NDC	SIZE	AWP
◇ BRAND			
EPIFOAM: Reed & Carnrick	00021-0740-10	10 gm	$11.57
PROCTOFOAM HC: Reed & Carnrick	00021-0690-10	10 gm	$21.05
◇ GENERICS			
Rugby	00536-2145-19	10 gm	$15.03

LOTION: 1%-1%

BRAND/MANUFACTURER	NDC	SIZE	AWP
○ BRAND			
PRAMOSONE: Ferndale	00496-0729-06	60 ml	$13.35
	00496-0729-04	120 ml	$21.35
	00496-0729-03	240 ml	$34.15

LOTION: 2.5%-1%

BRAND/MANUFACTURER	NDC	SIZE	AWP
○ BRAND			
PRAMOSONE: Ferndale	00496-0726-06	60 ml	$23.75
	00496-0726-04	120 ml	$38.00

OINTMENT: 1%-1%

BRAND/MANUFACTURER	NDC	SIZE	AWP
○ BRAND			
PRAMOSONE: Ferndale	00496-0763-04	30 gm	$9.35

OINTMENT: 2.5%-1%

BRAND/MANUFACTURER	NDC	SIZE	AWP
○ BRAND			
PRAMOSONE: Ferndale	00496-0777-04	30 gm	$17.15

Hydrocortisone Acetate with Lidocaine

DESCRIPTION
Hydrocortisone Acetate/Lidocaine Creme contains 3% Lidocaine and 1/2% micro-dispersed Hydrocortisone Acetate.

Lidocaine is a local anesthetic. Chemically, it is [2-(diethylamino)-N-(2, 6-dimethyl-phenyl) acetamide].

Hydrocortisone Acetate is a corticosteroid. Chemically, Hydrocortisone Acetate is pregn-4-ene-3, 20-dione, 21-(acetyloxy)-11, 17-dihydroxy-, (11β).

CLINICAL PHARMACOLOGY
Lidocaine is not absorbed from the intact skin. It can be absorbed from the abraded skin and mucous membrane. When absorbed, Lidocaine is metabolized in the liver by microsomal mixed-function oxidases by dealkylation to monoethyl-glycine and xylidide. Xylidide retains significant local anesthetic and toxic activity of Lidocaine. In man about 75% of the xylidide is excreted in the urine as the further metabolite. 4-hydroxy-2, 6-dimethyl-aniline.

Hydrocortisone is a vasoconstrictive agent. Studies have shown that Hydrocortisone is not retained in the dermis to any significant extent in most subjects. The barrier to penetration of Hydrocortisone is in the epidermis. Relative to the epidermis, the dermis presents little hindrance to the penetration. Hydrocortisone does not accumulate in the dermis as it is rapidly removed from the area by cutaneous blood supply. Quantitative absorption of Hydrocortisone in this concentration from the skin is not known. Topical steroids are primarily effective because of their anti-inflammatory, antipruritic and vasoconstrictive actions.

INDICATIONS AND USAGE
Hydrocortisone Acetate/Lidocaine Creme is used for relief of pruritus, pain, soreness, and discomfort due to pruritus vulva, pruritic eczemas, abrasions, hemorrhoids, anal fissures, minor burns, and similar conditions of the skin and mucous membranes.

CONTRAINDICATIONS
Hydrocortisone Acetate/Lidocaine Creme is contraindicated in those patients with a history of hypersensitivity to any of the components. It should not be applied on traumatized mucosa and lesions with secondary bacterial infection.

WARNINGS
As with any local anesthetic, adverse reactions may result from high plasma levels of Lidocaine due to excessive dosage or rapid absorption. Caution should be exercised in persistent, severe or extensive skin disorders or bleeding hemorrhoids. Advise patients to use only as directed. In case of rectal bleeding, advise patient to consult physician promptly. Keep out of reach of children.

PRECAUTIONS
If irritation develops, the product should be discontinued and appropriate therapy instituted.

If favorable response does not occur promptly, or new infection appears, the product should be discontinued and the use of an appropriate antifungal or antibacterial agent should be instituted.

Hydrocortisone Acetate/Lidocaine Creme should be used with caution in patients with severely traumatized mucosa and sepsis in the region of proposed application.

No long term studies in animals have been performed to evaluate the carcinogenic potential of topical steroids and Lidocaine.

Pregnancy Category C: In laboratory animals, topical steroids have been associated with an increase in the incidence of fetal abnormalities when gestating females have been exposed to rather low dosage levels. There are no adequate and well controlled studies in pregnant women. Hydrocortisone Acetate/Lidocaine Creme should only be used during pregnancy if the potential benefit justifies the risk to the fetus. Drugs of this class should not be used extensively on pregnant patients, in large amounts, or for prolonged periods of time.

Teratogenic effect of Lidocaine when applied topically has not been studied in animals.

It is not known whether this drug is excreted in human milk. Because many drugs are excreted in human milk and because of the potential for serious adverse reactions in nursing infants from Hydrocortisone Acetate/Lidocaine Creme, a decision should be made whether to discontinue nursing or to discontinue the drug, taking into account the importance of the drug to the mother.

If extensive areas are treated or if the occlusive technique is used there will be increased systemic absorption of the corticosteroid and Lidocaine and suitable precautions should be taken, particularly in children and infants.

ADVERSE REACTIONS
The following local adverse reactions have been reported with topical corticosteroids, especially under occlusive dressings.

1. Burning
2. Itching

◆ RATED THERAPEUTICALLY EQUIVALENT; ◇ THERAPEUTIC EQUIVALENCE UNCONFIRMED; ○ UNRATED

3. Irritation
4. Dryness
5. Folliculitis
6. Hypertrichosis
7. Acneiform eruptions
8. Hypopigmentation
9. Perioral dermatitis
10. Allergic Contact Dermatitis
11. Maceration of the skin
12. Secondary infection
13. Skin atrophy
14. Striae
15. Miliaria

DRUG ABUSE AND DEPENDENCE
Drug abuse and dependence has not been reported in patients treated with Hydrocortisone Acetate/Lidocaine Creme.

OVERDOSAGE
Systemic adverse reactions have not been reported with Hydrocortisone Acetate/Lidocaine Creme. However, as with any local anesthetic, adverse reactions may result from high plasma levels due to excessive dosage or rapid absorption. Systemic reactions due to overdosage (high plasma levels) involve the central nervous system (CNS) and/or the cardiovascular system (CVS).

CNS reactions are excitory and/or depressant, and may be characterized by nervousness, dizziness, blurred vision, and tremors followed by drowsiness, convulsions, unconsciousness, and possibly respiratory arrest. The excitory reaction may be very brief or may not occur at all, in which case the first manifestations of toxicity may be drowsiness, merging into unconsciousness and respiratory arrest.

Cardiovascular reactions are depressant, and may be characterized by hypotension, myocardial depression, bradycardia, and possibly cardiac arrest.

Treatment of a patient with toxic manifestations consist of assuring and maintaining a patent airway and supporting ventilation using oxygen and assisted or controlled respiration as required. This usually will be sufficient in the management of most reactions. If circulatory depression occurs vasopressors such as (ephedrine or metaraminol), and intravenous fluids may be used. If convulsions persist in spite of oxygen therapy ultra-short acting barbiturates (thiopental or thiamytal) may be used.

DOSAGE AND ADMINISTRATION
Apply to the affected areas two or three times daily.
Store below 86°F (30°C), avoid freezing.

HOW SUPPLIED
CREAM:

BRAND/MANUFACTURER	NDC	SIZE	AWP
○ BRAND			
LIDA-MANTLE-HC: Miles Pharm	00026-1508-81	30 gm	$35.13

Hydrocortisone Acetate with Neomycin Sulfate

DESCRIPTION
Hydrocortisone Acetate/Neomycin Sulfate Ointment contains the anti-inflammatory agent Hydrocortisone Acetate 1% and the broad-spectrum antibiotic Neomycin Sulfate equivalent to 3.5 mg Neomycin.

CLINICAL PHARMACOLOGY
Topical steroids are primarily effective because of their anti-inflammatory, antipruritic and vasoconstrictive actions.

Hydrocortisone exerts a marked anti-inflammatory effect through its controlling influence on the vascular and connective tissue components. In inhibiting the inflammatory reaction, Hydrocortisone does not appear to interfere with antibody formation or with antigen-antibody union.

Applied topically on the skin, Hydrocortisone inhibits more markedly than cortisone, similarly employed, the various aspects of inflammation (particularly of the allergic type) including edema, hyperemia, cellular infiltration and pruritus. In acute allergic dermatitis topical application has been found to be rapidly effective. In many instances objective signs of improvement, subsidence of erythema and edema with symptomatic relief, occur within a few hours of the first application. Following discontinuance of the application no "rebound" activation of the lesions has been observed. Even in acute exudative lesions the application of Hydrocortisone/Neomycin Ointment is effective. The results are questionable in dermatitic lesions in which there is considerable thickening or scaling of the skin.

Neomycin is an antibacterial substance derived from cultures of the soil organism *Streptomyces fradiae*. It exhibits a wider spectrum of antibacterial activity than either bacitracin, streptomycin, or *penicillin* and is active against a variety of gram-positive and gram-negative organisms including staphylococci, *Escherichia coli*, and *Hemophilus influenzae*. It is not active against fungi. Neomycin rarely causes resistant strains of microorganisms to develop; in addition, it is unusually nontoxic for human epithelial cells in tissue culture and is nonirritating topically in therapeutic concentrations.

INDICATIONS AND USAGE
For the treatment of corticosteroid-responsive dermatoses with secondary infection. It has not been demonstrated that this steroid-antibiotic combination provides greater benefit than the steroid component alone after seven days of treatment. (See "Warnings" section.)

CONTRAINDICATIONS
This preparation is contraindicated in cutaneous tuberculosis, fungus infections and certain virus infections (herpes simplex, vaccinia and varicella) for which an effective antibiotic or chemotherapeutic agent is not available for simultaneous application, and in those patients with a history of hypersensitivity to any of its components.

WARNINGS
Because of the potential hazard of nephrotoxicity and ototoxicity, prolonged use or use of large amounts of this product should be avoided in the treatment of skin infections following extensive burns, trophic ulceration and other conditions where absorption of Neomycin is possible.

Because of the concern of nephrotoxicity and ototoxicity associated with Neomycin, this combination product should not be used over a wide area or for extended periods of time.

PRECAUTIONS
This preparation is usually well tolerated. However, Neomycin may occasionally induce sensitivity reactions. If signs of irritation or sensitivity should develop, application should be discontinued.

If extensive areas are treated or if the occlusive technique is used, the possibility exists of increased absorption of the corticoid and suitable precautions should be taken.

The safety of the use of topical steroid preparations during pregnancy has not been fully established. Therefore, they should not be used unnecessarily during pregnancy, on extended areas, in large amounts, or for prolonged periods of time.

This product should not be put in the eyes or, if the ear drum is perforated, in the external ear canal.

Note: The prolonged use of antibiotic-containing preparations may result in overgrowth of nonsusceptible organisms, particularly fungi. If new infections appear during treatment, appropriate therapy should be instituted.

ADVERSE REACTIONS
When steroid preparations are used for long periods in intertriginous areas or under occlusive dressing, localized atrophy and striae may occur.

Other local adverse reactions associated with topically applied corticoids either with or without occlusive dressings include: burning sensations, itching, irritation, dryness, folliculitis, secondary infection, atrophy of the skin, acneiform eruption and hypopigmentation.

Ototoxicity and nephrotoxicity have been reported following absorption of topically applied Neomycin.

According to current medical literature there has been an increase in the prevalence of Neomycin hypersensitivity.

DOSAGE AND ADMINISTRATION
After thorough cleansing of the affected skin, a small amount of the ointment is applied and rubbed gently into the involved areas. Application may be made one to three times daily. In many instances the amount of the ointment required is small and applications at intervals as long as two or three days may be sufficient.

HOW SUPPLIED
HYDROCORTISONE/NEOMYCIN SULFATE
CREAM: 1%-0.5%

AVERAGE UNIT PRICE (AVAILABLE SIZES)			
GENERIC	$0.11		

BRAND/MANUFACTURER	NDC	SIZE	AWP
◆ GENERICS			
Clay-Park	45802-0062-02	20 gm	$2.70
Clay-Park	45802-0062-05	454 gm	$34.56

OINTMENT: 1%-0.5%

BRAND/MANUFACTURER	NDC	SIZE	AWP
◆ GENERICS			
Rugby	00536-0601-99	20 gm	$2.85

HYDROCORTISONE ACETATE/NEOMYCIN SULFATE
OINTMENT:

BRAND/MANUFACTURER	NDC	SIZE	AWP
○ BRAND			
NEO-CORTEF: Upjohn	00009-0622-02	20 gm	$21.33
○ GENERICS			
Major	00904-2786-29	20 gm	$3.15

➤ SHOWN IN PRODUCT IDENTIFICATION GUIDE

Hydrocortisone Acetate with Oxytetracycline Hydrochloride

DESCRIPTION

Hydrocortisone Acetate/Oxytetracycline Hydrochloride suspension combines the antibiotic, Oxytetracycline HCl ($C_{22}H_{24}N_2O_9 \cdot HCl$) and the adrenocorticoid, Hydrocortisone Acetate ($C_{23}H_{32}O_6$).

Each mL of Hydrocortisone Acetate/Oxytetracycline Hydrochloride contains Oxytetracycline Hydrochloride equivalent to 5 mg of Oxytetracycline, and 15 mg of Hydrocortisone Acetate incorporated in mineral oil with aluminum tristearate.

For ophthalmic use only.

CLINICAL PHARMACOLOGY

Corticosteroids suppress the inflammatory response to a variety of agents and they probably delay or slow healing. Since corticoids may inhibit the body's defense mechanism against infection, a concomitant antimicrobial drug may be used when this inhibition is considered to be clinically significant in a particular case.

The anti-infective component in the combination is included to provide action against specific organisms susceptible to it. Hydrocortisone Acetate/Oxytetracycline Hydrochloride is considered active against the following microorganisms:

Rickettsiae (Rocky Mountain spotted fever, typhus fever and the typhus group, Q fever, rickettsialpox and tick fevers),
Mycoplasma pneumoniae (PPLO, Eaton Agent),
Agents of psittacosis and ornithosis,
Agents of lymphogranuloma venereum and granuloma inguinale,
The spirochetal agent of relapsing fever (*Borrelia recurrentis*).
The following gram-negative microorganisms:
Haemophilus ducreyi (chancroid),
Pasteurella pestis and *Pasteurella tularensis*,
Bartonella bacilliformis,
Bacteroides species,
Vibrio comma and *Vibrio fetus*,
Brucella species (in conjunction with streptomycin).

Because many strains of the following groups of microorganisms have been shown to be resistant to tetracyclines, culture and susceptibility testing are recommended.

Oxytetracycline is indicated for treatment of infections caused by the following gram-negative microorganisms, when bacteriologic testing indicates appropriate susceptibility to the drug:

Escherichia coli,
Enterobacter aerogenes (formerly *Aerobacter aerogenes*),
Shigella species,
Mima species and *Herellea* species,
Haemophilus influenzae (respiratory infections),
Klebsiella species (respiratory and urinary infections).

Oxytetracycline is indicated for treatment of infections caused by the following gram-positive microorganisms when bacteriologic testing indicates appropriate susceptibility to the drug:

Streptococcus species:
Up to 44 percent of strains of *Streptococcus pyogenes* and 74 percent of *Streptococcus faecalis* have been found to be resistant to tetracycline drugs. Therefore, tetracyclines should not be used for streptococcal disease unless the organism has been demonstrated to be sensitive.

For upper respiratory infections due to Group A beta-hemolytic streptococci, penicillin is the usual drug of choice, including prophylaxis of rheumatic fever.
Diplococcus pneumoniae,
Staphylococcus cureus, skin and soft tissue infections. Oxytetracycline is not the drug of choice in the treatment of any type of staphylococcus infections.

When penicillin is contraindicated, tetracyclines are alternative drugs in the treatment of infections due to:

Neisseria gonorrhoeae,
Treponema pallidum and *Treponema pertenue* (syphilis and yaws),
Listeria monocytogenes,
Clostridium species,
Bacillus anthracis,
Fusobacterium fusiforme (Vincent's infection),
Actinomyces species:
Tetracyclines are indicated in the treatment of trachoma, although the infectious agent is not always eliminated, as judged by immunofluorescence.

Inclusion conjunctivitis may be treated with oral tetracyclines or with a combination of oral and topical agents.

When a decision to administer both a corticoid and an antimicrobial is made, the administration of such drugs in combination has the advantage of greater patient compliance and convenience, with the added assurance that the appropriate dosage of both drugs is administered, plus assured compatibility of ingredients when both types of drug are in the same formulation and, particularly, that the correct volume of drug is delivered and retained.

The relative potency of corticosteroids depends on the molecular structure, concentration, and release from the vehicle.

INDICATIONS AND USAGE

For steroid-responsive inflammatory ocular conditions for which a corticosteroid is indicated and where bacterial infection or risk of bacterial ocular infection exists.

Ocular steroids are indicated in inflammatory conditions of the palpebral and bulbar conjunctiva, cornea, and anterior segment of the globe where the inherent risk of steroid use in certain infective conjunctivitides is accepted to obtain a diminution in edema and inflammation. They are also indicated in chronic anterior uveitis and corneal injury from chemical radiation, thermal burns, or penetration of foreign bodies The use of a combination drug with an anti-infective component is indicated where the risk of infection is high or where there is an expectation that potentially dangerous numbers of bacteria will be present in the eye.

The particular anti-infective drug in this product is active against the following common bacterial eye pathogens:
Staphylococcus aureus
Streptococci, including *Streptococcus pneumoniae*
Escherichia coli
Neisseria species
The product does not provide adequate coverage against:
Haemophilus influenzae
Klebsiella/Enterobacter species
Pseudomonas aeruginosa
Serratia marcescens

CONTRAINDICATIONS

Epithelial herpes simplex keratitis (dendritic keratitis), vaccinia, varicella, and many other viral diseases of the cornea and conjunctiva. Mycobacterial infection of the eye. Fungal diseases of ocular structures. Hypersensitivity to a component of the medication. (Hypersensitivity to the antibiotic component occurs at a higher rate than for other components.)

The use of these combinations is always contraindicated after uncomplicated removal of a corneal foreign body.

WARNINGS

Prolonged use may result in glaucoma, with damage to the optic nerve, defects in visual acuity and fields of vision, and posterior subcapsular cataract formation. Prolonged use may suppress the host response and thus increase the hazard of secondary ocular infections. In those diseases causing thinning of the cornea or sclera, perforations have been known to occur with the use of topical steroids. In acute purulent conditions of the eye, steroids may mask infection or enhance existing infection. If these products are used for 10 days or longer, intraocular pressure should be routinely monitored even though it may be difficult in children and uncooperative patients.

Employment of steroid medication in the treatment of herpes simplex requires great caution.

PRECAUTIONS

The initial prescription and renewal of the medication order beyond 20 milliliters should be made by a physician only after examination of the patient with the aid of magnification, such as slit lamp biomicroscopy and, where appropriate, fluorescein staining.

The possibility of persistent fungal infections of the cornea should be considered after prolonged steroid dosing.

ADVERSE REACTIONS

Adverse reactions have occurred with steroid/anti-infective combination drugs which can be attributed to the steroid component, the anti-infective component, or the combination. Exact incidence figures are not available since no denominator of treated patients is available.

Reactions occurring most often from the presence of the anti-infective ingredient are allergic sensitizations. The reactions due to the steroid component in decreasing order of frequency are: elevation of intraocular pressure (IOP) with possible development of glaucoma, and infrequent optic nerve damage; posterior subcapsular cataract formation; and delayed would healing.

Secondary Infection: The development of secondary infection has occurred after use of combinations containing steroids and antimicrobials. Fungal infections of the cornea are particularly prone to develop coincidentally with long-term applications of steroid. The possibility of fungal invasion must be considered in any persistent corneal ulceration where steroid treatment has been used.

Secondary bacterial ocular infection following suppression of host responses also occurs.

DOSAGE AND ADMINISTRATION

Instill 1 or 2 drops of Hydrocortisone/Oxytetracycline Ophthalmic Suspension into the affected eye three times daily.

Not more than 20 milliliters should be prescribed initially and the prescription should not be refilled without further evaluation as outlined in *"Precautions"* above.

◆ RATED THERAPEUTICALLY EQUIVALENT; ◇ THERAPEUTIC EQUIVALENCE UNCONFIRMED; ○ UNRATED

HOW SUPPLIED

DROP:

BRAND/MANUFACTURER	NDC	SIZE	AWP
○ **BRAND**			
TERRA-CORTIL: Roerig,J.B.	00049-0670-48	5 ml	$20.33

Hydrocortisone Cypionate

DESCRIPTION

Hydrocortisone Cypionate oral suspension contains Hydrocortisone Cypionate which is a glucocorticoid. Glucocorticoids are adrenocortical steroids, both naturally occurring and synthetic, which are readily absorbed from the gastrointestinal tract. Hydrocortisone Cypionate is the water-insoluble Cypionate ester of Hydrocortisone. It is both tasteless and odorless, and by the oral route and in equimolar doses, is equivalent to Hydrocortisone free alcohol in biologic activity (rat liver-glycogen assay). Determinations of plasma and urinary 17-hydroxycorticoid levels in man following oral administration indicate that this ester is as efficiently absorbed and metabolized as the free alcohol.

The chemical name for Hydrocortisone Cypionate is pregn-4-ene-3,20-dione, 21-(3-cyclopentyl-1-oxopropoxy)-11,17-dihydroxy-,(11β)-and the molecular weight is 486.65.

Hydrocortisone Cypionate, a preparation for oral use, contains 13.4 mg Hydrocortisone Cypionate (equivalent to 10 mg Hydrocortisone) in each 5 mL.

Hydrocortisone Cypionate is stable at room temperature. The pH is within the USP specified range of 2.8 to 3.2.

ACTIONS

Naturally occurring glucocorticoids (Hydrocortisone and cortisone), which also have salt-retaining properties, are used as replacement therapy in adrenocortical deficiency states. Their synthetic analogs are primarily used for their potent anti-inflammatory effects in disorders of many organ systems.

Glucocorticoids cause profound and varied metabolic effects. In addition, they modify the body's immune responses to diverse stimuli.

INDICATIONS

Hydrocortisone Cypionate oral suspension is indicated in the following conditions:

1. Endocrine Disorders: Primary or secondary adrenocortical insufficiency (hydrocortisone or cortisone is the first choice; synthetic analogs may be used in conjunction with mineralocorticoids where applicable; in infancy mineralocorticoid supplementation is of particular importance); Congenital adrenal hyperplasia; Hypercalcemia associated with cancer; Nonsuppurative thyroiditis

2. Rheumatic Disorders: As adjunctive therapy for short-term administration (to tide the patient over an acute episode or exacerbation) in: Psoriatic arthritis; Rheumatoid arthritis, including juvenile rheumatoid arthritis (selected cases may require low-dose maintenance therapy); Ankylosing spondylitis; Acute and subacute bursitis; Acute nonspecific tenosynovitis; Acute gouty arthritis; Post-traumatic osteoarthritis; Synovitis of osteoarthritis; Epicondylitis

3. Collagen Diseases: During an exacerbation or as maintenance therapy in selected cases of: Systemic lupus erythematosus; Systemic dermatomyositis (polymyositis); Acute rheumatic carditis

4. Dermatologic Diseases: Pemphigus Bullous dermatitis herpetiformis; Severe erythema multiforme; (Stevens-Johnson syndrome); Exfoliative dermatitis; Mycosis fungoides; Severe psoriasis; Severe seborrheic dermatitis

5. Allergic States: Control of severe or incapacitating allergic conditions intractable to adequate trials of conventional treatment: Seasonal or perennial allergic rhinitis; Serum sickness; Bronchial asthma; Atopic dermatitis; Contact dermatitis; Drug hypersensitivity reactions

6. Ophthalmic Diseases: Severe acute and chronic allergic and inflammatory processes involving the eye and its adnexa such as: Allergic corneal marginal ulcers; Herpes zoster ophthalmicus; Anterior segment inflammation; Diffuse posterior uveitis and choroiditis; Sympathetic ophthalmia; Allergic conjunctivitis; Keratitis; Chorioretinitis; Optic neuritis; Iritis and iridocyclitis

7. Respiratory Diseases: Symptomatic sarcoidosis Loeffler's syndrome not manageable by other means Berylliosis Fulminating or disseminated pulmonary tuberculosis when used concurrently with appropriate antituberculous chemotherapy; Aspiration pneumonitis

8. Hematologic Disorders: Idiopathic thrombocytopenic purpura in adults; Secondary thrombocytopenia in adults; Acquired (autoimmune) hemolytic anemia; Erythroblastopenia (RBC anemia); Congenital (erythroid) hypoplastic anemia

9. Neoplastic Diseases: For palliative management of: Leukemias and lymphomas in adults; Acute leukemia of childhood

10. Edematous States: To induce a diuresis or remission of proteinuria in the nephrotic syndrome, without uremia, of the idiopathic type or that due to lupus erythematosus

11. Gastrointestinal Diseases: To tide the patient over a critical period of the disease in: Ulcerative colitis; Regional enteritis

12. Miscellaneous: Tuberculous meningitis with subarachnoid block or impending block when used concurrently with appropriate antituberculous chemotherapy; Trichinosis with neurologic or myocardial involvement

UNLABELED USES

Hydrocortisone Cypionate is used alone or as an adjunct in the treatment of breast carcinoma.

CONTRAINDICATIONS

Systemic fungal infections and known hypersensitivity to components.

WARNINGS

In patients on corticosteroid therapy subjected to unusual stress, increased dosage of rapidly acting corticosteroids before, during, and after the stressful situation is indicated.

Corticosteroids may mask some signs of infection, and new infections may appear during their use. There may be decreased resistance and inability to localize infection when corticosteroids are used.

Prolonged use of corticosteroids may produce posterior subcapsular cataracts, glaucoma with possible damage to the optic nerves, and may enhance the establishment of secondary ocular infections due to fungi or viruses.

Usage in Pregnancy: Since adequate human reproduction studies have not not been done with corticosteroids, the use of these drugs in pregnancy, nursing mothers or women of childbearing potential requires that the possible benefits of the drug be weighed against the potential hazards to the mother and embryo or fetus. Infants born of mothers who have received substantial doses of corticosteroids during pregnancy, should be carefully observed for signs of hypoadrenalism.

Average and large doses of Hydrocortisone or cortisone can cause elevation of blood pressure, salt and water retention, and increased excretion of potassium. These effects are less likely to occur with the synthetic derivatives except when used in large doses. Dietary salt restriction and potassium supplementation may be necessary. All corticosteroids increase calcium excretion.

While on corticosteroid therapy patients should not be vaccinated against small-pox. Other immunization procedures should not be undertaken in patients who are on corticosteroids, especially on high dose, because of possible hazards of neurological complications and a lack of antibody response.

The use of Hydrocortisone Cypionate Oral Suspension in active tuberculosis should be restricted to those cases of fulminating or disseminated tuberculosis in which the corticosteroid is used for the management of the disease in conjunction with an appropriate antituberculous regimen.

If corticosteroids are indicated in patients with latent tuberculosis or tuberculin reactivity, close observation is necessary as reactivation of the disease may occur. During prolonged corticosteroid therapy, these patients should receive chemoprophylaxis.

Persons who are on drugs which suppress the immune system are more susceptible to infections than healthy individuals. Chicken pox and measles, for example, can have a more serious or even fatal course in nonimmune children or adults on corticosteroids. In such children or adults who have not had these diseases, particular care should be taken to avoid exposure. How the dose, route and duration of corticosteroid administration affects the risk of developing a disseminated infection is not known. The contribution of the underlying disease and/or prior corticosteroid treatment to the risk is also not known. If exposed to chicken pox, prophylaxis with varicella zoster immune globulin (VZIG) may be indicated. If exposed to measles, prophylaxis with pooled intramuscular immunoglobulin (IG) may be indicated. (See the respective package inserts for complete VZIG and IG prescribing information.) If chickenpox develops, treatment with antiviral agents may be considered.

PRECAUTIONS

GENERAL PRECAUTIONS

Drug-induced secondary adrenocortical insufficiency may be minimized by gradual reduction of dosage. This type of relative insufficiency may persist for months after discontinuation of therapy; therefore, in any situation of stress occurring during that period, hormone therapy should be reinstituted. Since mineralocorticoid secretion may be impaired, salt and/or a mineralocorticoid should be administered concurrently.

There is an enhanced effect of corticosteroids on patients with hypothyroidism and in those with cirrhosis.

Corticosteroids should be used cautiously in patients with ocular herpes simplex because of possible corneal perforation.

The lowest possible dose of corticosteroid should be used to control the condition under treatment, and when reduction in dosage is possible, the reduction should be gradual.

Psychic derangements may appear when corticosteroids are used, ranging from euphoria, insomnia, mood swings, personality changes, and severe depression, to frank psychotic manifestations. Also, existing emotional instability or psychotic tendencies may be aggravated by corticosteroids.

Steroids should be used with caution in nonspecific ulcerative colitis, if there is a probability of impending perforation, abscess or other pyogenic infection; diverticulitis; fresh intestinal anastomoses; active or latent peptic ulcer; renal insufficiency; hypertension; osteoporosis; and myasthenia gravis.

Growth and development of infants and children on prolonged corticosteroid therapy should be carefully observed.

DRUG INTERACTIONS

The pharmacokinetic interactions listed below are potentially clinically important. Drugs that induce hepatic enzymes such as phenobarbital, phenytoin and rifampin may increase the clearance of corticosteroids and may require increases in corticosteroid dose to achieve the desired response. Drugs such as troleandomycin and ketoconazole may inhibit the metabolism of corticosteroids and thus decrease their clearance. Therefore, the dose of corticosteroid should be titrated to avoid steroid toxicity. Corticosteroids may increase the clearance of chronic high dose aspirin. This could lead to decreased salicylate serum levels or increase the risk of salicylate toxicity when corticosteroid is withdrawn. Aspirin should be used cautiously in conjunction with corticosteroids in patients suffering from hypoprothrombinemia. The effect of corticosteroids on oral anticoagulants is variable. There are reports of enhanced as well as diminished effects of anticoagulants when given concurrently with corticosteroids. Therefore, coagulation indices should be monitored to maintain the desired anticoagulant effect.

INFORMATION FOR THE PATIENT
Persons who are on immunosuppressant doses of corticosteroids should be warned to avoid exposure to chicken pox or measles. Patients should also be advised that if they are exposed, medical advice should be sought without delay.

ADVERSE REACTIONS
Fluid and Electrolyte Disturbances
  Sodium retention
  Fluid retention
  Congestive heart failure in susceptible patients
  Potassium loss
  Hypokalemic alkalosis
  Hypertension
Musculoskeletal
  Muscle weakness
  Steroid myopathy
  Loss of muscle mass
  Osteoporosis
  Vertebral compression fractures
  Aseptic necrosis of femoral and humeral heads
  Pathologic fracture of long bones
Gastrointestinal
  Peptic ulcer with possible perforation and hemorrhage
  Pancreatitis
  Abdominal distention
  Ulcerative esophagitis
  Increases in alanine transaminase
  (ALT, SGPT), aspartate transaminase
  (AST, SGOT) and alkaline
  Phosphatase have been observed following corticosteroid treatment.
  These changes are usually small, not associated with any clinical syndrome and are reversible upon discontinuation.
Dermatologic
  Impaired wound healing
  Thin fragile skin
  Petechiae and ecchymoses
  Facial erythema
  Increased sweating
  May suppress reactions to skin tests
Metabolic
  Negative nitrogen balance due to protein catabolism
Neurological
  Increased intracranial pressure with papilledema (pseudotumor cerebri) usually after treatment
  Convulsions
  Vertigo
  Headache
Endocrine
  Menstrual irregularities
  Development of Cushingoid state
  Secondary adrenocortical and pituitary unresponsiveness, particularly in times of stress, as in trauma, surgery or illness
  Suppression of growth in children
  Decreased carbohydrate tolerance
  Manifestations of latent diabetes mellitus
  Increased requirements for insulin or oral hypoglycemic agents in diabetics
Ophthalmic
  Posterior subcapsular cataracts
  Increased intraocular pressure
  Glaucoma
  Exophthalmos

DOSAGE AND ADMINISTRATION
The initial dosage Hydrocortisone Cypionate Oral Suspension may vary from 2 to 24 teaspoonsful (10-120 mL) per day depending on the specific disease entity being treated. This provides a daily dosage of 26.8 mg to 321.6 mg of Hydrocortisone Cypionate, equivalent in activity to 20 to 240 mg of hydrocortisone. In situations of less severity lower doses will generally suffice while in selected patients higher initial doses may be required. The initial dosage should be maintained or adjusted until a satisfactory response is noted. If after a reasonable period of time there is a lack of satisfactory clinical response, Hydrocortisone Cypionate should be discontinued and the patient transferred to other appropriate therapy. **IT SHOULD BE EMPHASIZED THAT DOSAGE REQUIREMENTS ARE VARIABLE AND**

MUST BE INDIVIDUALIZED ON THE BASIS OF THE DISEASE UNDER TREATMENT AND THE RESPONSE OF THE PATIENT. After a favorable response is noted, the proper maintenance dosage should be determined by decreasing the initial drug dosage in small decrements at appropriate time intervals until the lowest dosage which will maintain an adequate clinical response is reached. It should be kept in mind that constant monitoring is needed in regard to drug dosage. Included in the situations which may make dosage adjustments necessary are changes in clinical status secondary to remissions or exacerbations in the disease process, the patient's individual drug responsiveness, and the effect of patient exposure to stressful situations not directly related to the disease entity under treatment; in this latter situation it may be necessary to increase the dosage of Hydrocortisone Cypionate for a period of time consistent with the patient's condition. If after long-term therapy the drug is to be stopped, it is recommended that it be withdrawn gradually rather than abruptly.

HOW SUPPLIED
SUSPENSION: 10 MG/5 ML

BRAND/MANUFACTURER	NDC	SIZE	AWP
○ BRAND			
CORTEF: Upjohn	00009-0142-01	120 ml	$15.69

Hydrocortisone with Iodoquinol

DESCRIPTION
Each gram of Hydrocortisone/Iodoquinol Cream 0.5% and 1% contains 5 mg or 10 mg of Hydrocortisone, respectively, and 10 mg of Iodoquinol.
  Chemically Hydrocortisone is 11, 17, 21-trihydroxypregn-4-ene-3, 20-dione $(C_{21}H_{30}O_5)$.
  Iodoquinol is 5,7-diiodo-8-quinolinol $(C_9H_5I_2NO)$.
  Hydrocortisone is an anti-inflammatory and antipruritic agent, while Iodoquinol is an antifungal and antibacterial agent.

CLINICAL PHARMACOLOGY
Hydrocortisone has anti-inflammatory, antipruritic and vasoconstrictor properties. The mechanism of anti-inflammatory activity is unclear. There is some evidence to suggest that a recognizable correlation exists between vasoconstrictor potency and therapeutic efficacy in man.
  Iodoquinol has both antifungal and antibacterial properties.

PHARMACOKINETICS
The extent of percutaneous absorption of topical corticosteroids is determined by many factors including vehicle, the integrity of the epidermal barrier, and the use of occlusive dressings.
  Hydrocortisone can be absorbed from normal intact skin. Inflammation and/or other inflammatory disease processes in the skin increase percutaneous absorption. Occlusive dressings substantially increase the percutaneous absorption of topical corticosteroids.
  Once absorbed through the skin Hydrocortisone is metabolized in the liver and most body tissues to hydrogenated and degraded forms such as tetrahydrocortisone and tetrahydrocortisol. These are excreted in the urine, mainly conjugated as glucuronides, together with a very small porportion of unchanged Hydrocortisone.
  There are no data available regarding the percutaneous absorption of Iodoquinol; however, following oral administration, 3-5% of the dose was recovered in the urine as a glucuronide.

INDICATIONS AND USAGE

BASED ON A REVIEW OF A RELATED DRUG BY THE NATIONAL RESEARCH COUNCIL AND SUBSEQUENT FDA CLASSIFICATION FOR THAT DRUG, THE INDICATIONS ARE AS FOLLOWS:
  "POSSIBLY" EFFECTIVE; CONTACT OR ATOPIC DERMATITIS; IMPETIGINIZED ECZEMA; NUMMULAR ECZEMA; INFANTILE ECZEMA; ENDOGENOUS CHRONIC INFECTIOUS DERMATITIS; STATIS DERMATITIS; PYODERMIA; NUCHAL EZCEMA AND CHRONIC EZCEMATOID OTITIS EXTERNA; ACNETURTICATA; LOCALIZED OR DISSEMINATED NEURODERMATITIS; LICHEN SIMPLEX CHRONICUS; ANOGENITAL PRURITUS (VULVAE, SCROTI, ANI); FOLLICULITIS; BACTERIAL DERMATOSES; MYCOTIC DERMATOSES SUCH AS TINEA (CAPITIS, CRURIS, CORPORIS, PEDIS); MONILIASIS, INTERTRIGO. FINAL CLASSIFICATION OF THE LESS-THAN-EFFECTIVE INDICATIONS REQUIRES FURTHER INVESTIGATION.

CONTRAINDICATIONS
Hydrocortisone/Iodoquinol Cream is contraindicated in those patients with a history of hypersensitivity to Hydrocortisone Iodoquinol or any other components of the preparation.

WARNINGS AND PRECAUTIONS
For external use only. Keep away from eyes. If irritation develops, the use of Hydrocortisone/Iodoquinol Cream should be discontinued and appropriate therapy instituted. Staining of the skin and fabrics may occur. If extensive areas are treated or if the occlusive technique is used, the possibility exists of increased systemic absorption of the corticosteroid, and suitable precautions should be

taken. Children may absorb proportionally larger amounts of topical corticosteroids and thus be more susceptible to systemic toxicity. Parents of pediatric patients should be advised not to use tight-fitting diapers or plastic pants on a child being treated in the diaper area, as these garments may constitute occlusive dressings. Iodoquinol may be absorbed through the skin and interfere with thyroid function tests. If such tests are contemplated, wait at least one month after discontinuance of therapy to perform these tests. The ferric chloride test for phenylketonuria (PKU) can yield a false positive result if Iodoquinol is present in the diaper or urine.

Prolonged use may result in overgrowth of non-susceptible organisms requiring appropriate therapy. Keep out of reach of children.

Carcinogenesis, Mutagenesis and Impairment of Fertility: Long term animal studies have not been performed to evaluate the carcinogenic potential or the effect on fertility of Hydrocortisone or Iodoquinol.

In vitro studies to determine mutagenicity with Hydrocortisone have revealed negative results. Mutagenicity studies have not been conducted with Iodoquinol.

Pregnancy Category C: Animal reproductive studies have not been conducted with Hydrocortisone/Iodoquinol Cream. It is not known whether Hydrocortisone/Iodoquinol Cream can cause fetal harm when administered to a pregnant woman or can affect reproductive capacity, Hydrocortisone/Iodoquinol Cream should be given to a pregnant woman only if clearly needed.

Nursing Mothers: It is not known whether this drug is excreted in human milk. Because many drugs are excreted in human milk, caution should be exercised when Hydrocortisone/Iodoquinol Cream is administered to a nursing woman.

Pediatric Use: Safety and effectiveness in children under the age of 12 have not been established.

ADVERSE REACTIONS

The following local adverse reactions are reported infrequently with topical corticosteroids. These reactions are listed in an approximate decreasing order of occurrence.

Burning	Perioral dermatitis
Itching	Allergic contact dermatitis
Irritation	Maceration of the skin
Dryness	Secondary infection
Folliculitis	Skin atrophy
Hypertrichosis	Striae
Acneiform eruptions	Miliaria
Hypopigmentation	

DOSAGE AND ADMINISTRATION

Apply to affected area 3 to 4 times daily in accordance with physician's directions.

HOW SUPPLIED
CREAM: 1%

BRAND/MANUFACTURER	NDC	SIZE	AWP
○ BRAND			
VYTONE: Dermik	00066-0051-01	30 gm	$21.71

Hydrocortisone, Rectal

DESCRIPTION

Each Hydrocortisone, 25-mg Suppository contains 25 mg Hydrocortisone Acetate in a hydrogenated cocoglyceride base. Hydrocortisone Acetate is a corticosteroid. Chemically, Hydrocortisone Acetate is pregn-4-ene-3,20-dione, 21-(acetyloxy)-11,17-dihydroxy-,(11β)-.

Hydrocortisone Rectal Enema is a convenient disposable single-dose Hydrocortisone enema designed for ease of self-administration. Hydrocortisone is a naturally occurring glucocorticoid (adrenal corticosteroid) which, similarly as its acetate and sodium hemisuccinate derivatives, is partially absorbed following rectal administration. Absorption studies in ulcerative colitis patients have shown up to 50% absorption of Hydrocortisone administered as Hydrocortisone Rectal Enema and up to 30% of Hydrocortisone Acetate administered in an identical vehicle.

Hydrocortisone Rectal Foam contains Hydrocortisone Acetate 10% as the sole active ingredients in 20 g of a foam.

Each application delivers approximately 900 mg of foam containing 80 mg of Hydrocortisone (90 mg of Hydrocortisone Acetate).

Following is its chemical structure:

CLINICAL PHARMACOLOGY

In normal subjects, about 26 percent of Hydrocortisone Acetate is absorbed when the Hydrocortisone Acetate suppository is applied to the rectum. Absorption of Hydrocortisone Acetate may vary across abraded or inflamed surfaces.

Topical steroids are primarily effective because of their anti-inflammatory, antipruritic and vasoconstrictive action.

Hydrocortisone Rectal Enema provides the potent anti-inflammatory effect of Hydrocortisone. Because this drug is absorbed from the colon, it acts both topically and systemically. Although rectal Hydrocortisone, used as recommended for Hydrocortisone Rectal Enema, has a low incidence of reported adverse reactions, prolonged use presumably may cause systemic reactions associated with oral dosage forms.

Hydrocortisone Rectal Foam provides effective topical administration of an anti-inflammatory corticosteroid as adjunctive therapy of ulcerative proctitis.

INDICATIONS AND USAGE

Hydrocortisone Rectal suppositories are for use in inflamed hemorrhoids, post irradiation (factitial) proctitis, as an adjunct in the treatment of chronic ulcerative colitis, cryptitis, other inflammatory conditions of the anorectum, and pruritus ani.

Hydrocortisone Rectal Enema is indicated as adjunctive therapy in the treatment of ulcerative colitis, especially distal forms, including ulcerative proctitis, ulcerative protosigmoiditis, and left-sided ulcerative colitis. It has proved useful also in some cases involving the transverse and ascending colons.

Hydrocortisone Rectal Foam is indicated as adjunctive therapy in the topical treatment of ulcerative proctitis of the distal portion of the rectum in patients who cannot retain Hydrocortisone or other corticosteroid enemas. Direct observations of methylene blue-containing foam have shown staining about 10 centimeters into the rectum.

CONTRAINDICATIONS

Hydrocortisone Rectal Suppositories are contraindicated in those patients with a history of hypersensitivity to any of the components.

Hydrocortisone Rectal Enema is contraindicated in systemic fungal infections; and ileocolostomy during the immediate or early post-operative period.

Hydrocortisone Rectal Foam: Local contraindications to the use of intrarectal steroids include obstruction, abscess, perforation, peritonitis, fresh intestinal anastomoses, extensive fistulas and sinus tracts. Tuberculosis (active, latent or questionably healed), ocular herpes simplex and acute psychosis are usually considered absolute contraindications to the use of corticosteroids. Relative contraindications include active peptic ulcer, acute glomerulonephritis, myasthenia gravis, osteoporosis, diverticulitis, thrombophlebitis, psychic disturbances, pregnancy, diabetes, hyperthyroidism, acute coronary disease, hypertension, limited cardiac reserve, and local or systemic infections, including fungal or exanthematous diseases. Where these conditions exist, the expected benefits from steroid therapy must be weighed against the risks involved in its use. Pregnancy is a relative contraindication to corticosteroids, particularly during third trimester. If corticosteroids must be administered in pregnancy, watch newborn infant closely for signs of hypoadrenalism, and administer appropriate therapy if needed.

WARNINGS

In severe ulcerative colitis, it is hazardous to delay needed surgery while awaiting response to medical treatment.

Damage to the rectal wall can result from careless or improper insertion of an enema tip.

In patients on corticosteroid therapy subjected to unusual stress, increased dosage of rapidly acting corticosteroids before, during, and after the stressful situation is indicated. Corticosteroids may mask some signs of infection, and new infections may appear during their use. There may be decreased resistance and inability to localize infection when corticosteroids are used.

Prolonged use of corticosteroids may produce posterior subcapsular cataracts, glaucoma with possible damage to the optic nerves, and may enhance the establishment of secondary ocular infections due to fungi or viruses.

Do not insert any part of aerosol container into the anus. Contents of the container are under pressure, but not flammable. Do not burn or puncture the aerosol container. Store at room temperature and not over 120° F. Because Hydrocortisone Rectal Foam is not expelled, systemic hydrocortisone absorption may be greater from Hydrocortisone Rectal Foam than from corticosteroid enema formulations. If there is not evidence of clinical or proctologic improvement within two or three weeks after starting Hydrocortisone Rectal Foam therapy, or if the patient's condition worsens, discontinue the drug.

Children who are on immunosuppressant drugs are more susceptible to infections than healthy children. Chickenpox and measles, for example, can have a more serious or even fatal course in children on immunosuppressant corticosteroids. In such children, or in adults who have not had these diseases, particular care should be taken to avoid exposure. If exposed, therapy with varicella zoster immune globulin (VZIG) or pooled intravenous immunoglobulin (IVIG), as appropriate, may be indicated. If chickenpox develops, treatment with antiviral agents may be considered.

Average and large doses of Hydrocortisone or cortisone can cause elevation of blood pressure, salt and water retention, and increased excretion of potassium. These effects are less likely to occur with the synthetic derivatives except when used in large doses. Dietary salt restriction and potassium supplementation may be necessary. All corticosteroids increase calcium excretion.

While on corticosteroid therapy patients should not be vaccinated against smallpox. Other immunization procedures should not be undertaken in patients who are on corticosteroids, especially on high dose, because of possible hazards of neurological complications and a lack of antibody response.

If corticosteroids are indicated in patients with latent tuberculosis or tuberculin reactivity, close observation is necessary as reactivation of the disease may occur. During prolonged corticosteroid therapy, these patients should receive chemoprophylaxis.

PRECAUTIONS

Do not use unless adequate proctologic examination is made. If irritation develops, the product should be discontinued and appropriate therapy instituted.

In the presence of an infection, the use of an appropriate antifungal or antibacterial agent should be instituted. If a favorable response does not occur promptly, the corticosteroid should be discontinued until the infection has been adequately controlled.

No long-term studies in animals have been performed to evaluate the carcinogenic potential of corticosteroid suppositories.

Steroid therapy should be administered with caution in patients with severe ulcerative disease because these patients are predisposed to perforation of the bowel wall. Where surgery is imminent, it is hazardous to wait more than a few days for a satisfactory response to medical treatment. General precautions common to all corticosteroid therapy should be observed during treatment with Hydrocortisone Rectal Foam. These include gradual withdrawal of therapy to allow for possible adrenal insufficiency and awareness to possible growth suppression in children. Patients should be kept under close observation, for, as with all drugs, rare individuals may react unfavorably under certain conditions. If severe reactions or idiosyncrasies occur, steroids should be discontinued immediately and appropriate measures instituted. Do not employ in immediate or early postoperative period following ileorectostomy.

Hydrocortisone Rectal Enema should be used with caution where there is a probability of impending perforation, abscess or other pyogenic infection; fresh intestinal anastomoses; obstruction; or extensive fistulas and sinus tracts. Use with caution in presence of active or latent peptic ulcer; diverticulitis; renal insufficiency; hypertension; osteoporosis; and myasthenia gravis.

Steroid therapy might impair prognosis in surgery by increasing the hazard of infection. If infection is suspected, appropriate antibiotic therapy must be administered, usually in larger than ordinary doses.

Drug-induced secondary adrenocortical insufficiency may occur with prolonged Hydrocortison Rectal Enema therapy. This is minimized by gradual reduction of dosage. This type of relative insufficiency may persist for months after discontinuation of therapy; therefore, in any situation of stress occurring during that period, hormone therapy should be reinstituted. Since mineralocorticoid secretion may be impaired, salt and/or a mineralocorticoid should be administered concurrently. There is an enhanced effect of corticosteroids on patients with hypothyroidism and in those with cirrhosis.

Corticosteroid should be used cautiously in patients with ocular herpes simplex because of possible corneal perforation.

The lowest possible dose of corticosteroid should be used to control the conditions under treatment, and when reduction in dosage is possible, the reduction should be gradual.

Psychic derangement may appear when corticosteroids are used, ranging from euphoria, insomnia, mood swings, personality changes, and severe depression, to frank psychotic manifestations. Also, existing emotional instability or psychotic tendencies may be aggravated by corticosteroids.

Aspirin should be used cautiously in conjunction with corticosteroids in hypoprothrombinemia.

Growth and development of infants and children on prolonged corticosteroid therapy should be carefully observed.

INFORMATION FOR PATIENTS

Staining of fabric may occur with use of the suppository. Precautionary measures are recommended.

Patients who are on immunosuppressant doses of corticosteroids should be warned to avoid exposure to chickenpox or measles and, if exposed, to obtain medical advice.

PREGNANCY CATEGORY C

In laboratory animals, topical steroids have been associated with an increase in the incidence of fetal abnormalities when gestating females have been exposed to rather low dosage levels. There are no adequate and well-controlled studies in pregnant women. Hydrocortisone Rectal suppositories should only be used during pregnancy if the potential benefit justifies the risk to the fetus. Drugs of this class should not be used extensively on pregnant patients, in large amounts, or for prolonged periods of time. Infants born of mothers who have received substantial doses of corticosteroids during pregnancy should be carefully observed for signs of hypoadrenalism.

It is not known whether this drug is excreted in human milk, and because many drugs are excreted in human milk and because of the potential for serious adverse reactions in nursing infants from Hydrocortisone Rectal suppositories, a decision should be made whether to discontinue nursing or to discontinue the drug, taking into account the importance of the drug to the mother.

ADVERSE REACTIONS

The following local adverse reactions have been reported with corticosteroid suppositories:

1. Burning
2. Itching
3. Irritation
4. Dryness
5. Folliculitis
6. Hypopigmentation
7. Allergic Contact Dermatitis
8. Secondary infection

Local pain or burning and rectal bleeding attributed to Hydrocortisone Rectal Enema have been reported rarely. Apparent exacerbations or sensitivity reactions also occur rarely. The following adverse reactions should be kept in mind whenever corticosteroids are given by rectal administration.

Fluid and Electrolyte Disturbances: Sodium retention; fluid retention; congestive heart failure in susceptible -patients; potassium loss; hypokalemic alkalosis; hypertension.

Musculoskeletal: Muscle weakness; steroid myopathy; loss of muscle mass; osteoporosis; vertebral compression fractures; aseptic necrosis of femoral and humeral heads; pathologic fracture of long bones.

Gastrointestinal: Peptic ulcer with possible perforation and hemorrhage; pancreatitis; abdominal distention; ulcerative esophagitis.

Dermatologic: Impaired wound healing; thin fragile skin; petechiae and ecchymoses; facial erythema; increased sweating; may suppress reactions to skin tests.

Neurological: Convulsions; increased intracranial pressure with papilledema (pseudo-tumor cerebri) usually after treatment; vertigo; headache.

Endocrine: Menstrual irregularities; development of Cushingoid state; suppression of growth in children; secondary adrenocortical and pituitary unresponsiveness, particularly in times of stress, as in trauma, surgery or illness; decreased carbohydrate or glucose tolerance; manifestations of latent diabetes mellitus; increased requirements for insulin or oral hypoglycemic agents in diabetics.

Ophthalmic: Posterior subcapsular cataracts; increased intraocular pressure; glaucoma; exophthalmos.

Metabolic: Negative nitrogen balance due to protein catabolism, with delayed bone and wound healing.

Corticosteroid therapy may also produce these side effects: excessive appetite and weight gain, abnormal fat deposits, mental symptoms, hypertrichosis, acne, pigmentation, dry scaly skin, thinning scalp hair, thrombophlebitis, decreased resistance to infection, neuropathy, adrenal insufficiency, necrotizing angiitis, and hypertension. Long-term use of all corticosteroids results in catabolic effects characterized by negative protein and calcium balance. Osteoporosis, spontaneous fractures and aseptic necrosis of the hip and humerus may occur as part of this catabolic phenomenon. Where hypopotassemia and other symptoms associated with fluid and electrolyte imbalance call for potassium supplementation and salt poor or salt-free diets, these may be instituted and are compatible with diet requirements for ulcerative proctitis.

DRUG ABUSE AND DEPENDENCE

Drug abuse and dependence have not been reported in patients treated with Hydrocortisone Rectal suppositories.

OVERDOSAGE

If signs and symptoms of systemic overdosage occur discontinue use.

DOSAGE AND ADMINISTRATION

HYDROCORTISONE RECTAL SUPPOSITORIES

Usual dosage: One suppository in the rectum morning and night for two weeks, in nonspecific proctitis. In more severe cases, one suppository three times daily; or two suppositories twice daily. In factitial proctitis, recommended therapy is six to eight weeks or less, according to response.

HYDROCORTISONE RECTAL ENEMA

The use of Hydrocortisone Rectal Enema is predicated upon the concomitant use of modern supportive measures such as rational dietary control, sedatives, antidiarrheal agents, antibacterial therapy, blood replacement if necessary, etc.

The usual course of therapy is one Hydrocortisone, Rectal, Enema nightly for 21 days, or until the patient comes into remission both clinically and proctologically. Clinical symptoms usually subside promptly within 3 to 5 days. Improvement in the appearance of the mucosa, as seen by sigmoidoscopic examination, may lag somewhat behind clinical improvement. Difficult cases may require as long as 2 or 3 months of Hydrocortisone Rectal Enema treatment. Where the course of therapy extends beyond 21 days, Hydrocortisone Rectal Enema should be discontinued gradually by reducing administration to every other night for 2 or 3 weeks.

If clinical or proctologic improvement fail to occur within 2 or 3 weeks after starting Hydrocortisone Rectal Enema, discontinue its use.

Symptomatic improvement, evidenced by decreased diarrhea and bleeding; weight gain; improved appetite; lessened fever; and decreased leukocytosis, may be misleading and should not be used as the sole criterion in judging efficacy. Sigmoidoscopic examination and X-ray visualization are essential for adequate monitoring of ulcerative colitis. Biopsy is useful for differential diagnosis.

Patient instructions for administering Hydrocortisone Rectal Enema are enclosed in each box of seven units. We recommend that the patient lie on his left side during administration and for 30 minutes thereafter, so that the fluid will distribute throughout the left colon. Every effort should be made to retain the enema for at least an hour and, preferably, all night. This may be facilitated by prior sedation and/or antidiarrheal medication, especially early in therapy, when the urge to evacuate is great.

HYDROCORTISONE RECTAL FOAM:

NOTE: SEE INNER PACKAGE FOR FULL DIRECTIONS FOR USE.

Usual dose is one applicatorful once or twice daily for two or three weeks, and every second day thereafter, administered rectally. The patient direction package

◆ RATED THERAPEUTICALLY EQUIVALENT; ◇ THERAPEUTIC EQUIVALENCE UNCONFIRMED; ○ UNRATED

with the applicator describes how to use the aerosol container and applicator. Satisfactory response usually occurs within five to seven days marked by a decrease in symptoms. Symptomatic improvement in ulcerative proctitis should not be used as the sole criterion for evaluating efficacy. Sigmoidoscopy is also recommended to judge dosage adjustment, duration of therapy and rate of improvement.

Directions for Use: 1) Shake foam container vigorously before use. Hold container upright and insert into the opening of the tip of the applicator. **Be sure applicator plunger is drawn all the way out.** Container must be held upright to obtain proper flow of medication. 2) To fill, press down slowly on container cap. When foam reaches <u>fill line</u> in the applicator, it is ready for use.

Caution: The aerosol container should never be inserted directly into the anus. 3) Remove applicator from container. Allow some foam to remain on the applicator tip. Hold applicator by barrel and gently insert tip into the anus. With applicator in place, push plunger in order to expel foam, then withdraw applicator. (Applicator parts should be pulled apart for thorough cleaning with warm water.)

STORAGE

Store suppositories below 30°C (86°F). Protect from freezing.

Store enemas at controlled room temperature, 15°-30°C (59°-86°F).

Store foam upright at controlled room temperature, 15°-30°C (59°-86°F).

HOW SUPPLIED

HYDROCORTISONE
CREAM: 1%

AVERAGE UNIT PRICE (AVAILABLE SIZES)	
BRAND	$0.40
HCFA FUL (15 gm)	$0.15
HCFA FUL (20 gm)	$0.12
HCFA FUL (30 gm)	$0.05
HCFA FUL (60 gm)	$0.07
HCFA FUL (120 gm)	$0.06
HCFA FUL (454 gm)	$0.05

BRAND/MANUFACTURER	NDC	SIZE	AWP
◆ BRAND			
PROCTO-KIT 1%: Amer Generics	58634-0024-01	30 gm	$10.95
PROCTOCORT: Solvay	00032-1920-61	30 gm	$18.72

CREAM: 2.5%

AVERAGE UNIT PRICE (AVAILABLE SIZES)		GENERIC A-RATED AVERAGE PRICE (GAAP)	
BRAND	$0.65	30 gm	$9.49
GENERIC	$0.32		
HCFA FUL (20 gm)	$0.21		
HCFA FUL (30 gm)	$0.16		

BRAND/MANUFACTURER	NDC	SIZE	AWP
◆ BRAND			
ANUSOL-HC: Parke-Davis	00071-3131-13	30 gm	$20.65
PROCTO-KIT 2.5%: Amer Generics	58634-0028-01	30 gm	$26.95
◆ GENERICS			
Clay-Park	45802-0287-03	30 gm	$7.02
PROCTOSOL-HC: Amer Generics	58634-0025-01	30 gm	$11.95

SOLUTION: 100 MG/60 ML

BRAND/MANUFACTURER	NDC	SIZE	AWP
○ BRAND			
CORTENEMA: Solvay	00032-1904-73	60 ml	$7.68
	00032-1904-82	60 ml 7s	$44.72

HYDROCORTISONE ACETATE
AEROSOL SOLID INGREDIENTS:

BRAND/MANUFACTURER	NDC	SIZE	AWP
○ BRAND			
CORTIFOAM: Reed & Carnrick	00021-0695-20	20 gm	$43.73

SUPPOSITORY: 25 MG

BRAND/MANUFACTURER	NDC	SIZE	AWP
○ BRAND			
ANUSOL-HC: Parke-Davis	00071-1726-07	12s	$22.97
CORT-DOME HIGH POTENCY: Miles Pharm	00026-5005-12	12s	$35.90
ANUSOL-HC: Parke-Davis	00071-1726-13	24s	$40.24

Hydrocortisone, Systemic

DESCRIPTION

Hydrocortisone, Systemic, is available as an injection and as tablets for oral administration.

Each ml of suspension for injection contains:
Hydrocortisone Acetate ....25 or 50 mg

Each ml of solution for injection contains:
Hydrocortisone Sodium Phosphate equivalent to ....50 mg Hydrocortisone

Each ml of reconstituted solution for injection contains:
Hydrocortisone Sodium Succinate
equivalent to ....50 or 125 mg Hydrocortisone

Each tablet contains:
Hydrocortisone ....10 or 20 mg

Glucocorticoids are adrenocortical steroids, both naturally occurring and synthetic, which are readily absorbed from the gastrointestinal tract. Hydrocortisone is believed to be the principal hormone secreted by the adrenal cortex.

Hydrocortisone is a white to practically white, odorless, crystalline powder, very slightly soluble in water. The molecular weight is 362.47. It is designated chemically as 11β,17,21-trihydroxypregn-4-ene-3,20-dione. The empirical formula is $C_{12}H_{30}O_5$.

Hydrocortisone acetate, a synthetic adrenocortical steroid, is a white to practically white, odorless, crystalline powder. It is insoluble in water and slightly in alcohol and chloroform. The molecular weight is 404.50. It is designated chemically as 21-(acetyloxy)-11β,17-dihydroxypregn-4-ene-3,20-dione. The empirical formula is $C_{23}H_{32}O_6$.

Hydrocortisone sodium phosphate, a synthetic adrenocortical steroid, is a white to light yellow, odorless or practically odorless powder. It is freely soluble in water and is exceedingly hygroscopic. The molecular weight is 486.41. It is designated chemically as 11β,17-dihydroxy-21-(phosphonooxyl)-pregn-4-ene-3,20-dione disodium salt. The empirical formula is $C_{21}H_{29}Na_2O_8P$.

Hydrocortisone sodium succinate is a white or nearly white, odorless, hygroscopic amorphous solid. It is very soluble in water and in alcohol, very slightly soluble in acetone and insoluble in chloroform. The chemical name is pregn-4-ene-3,20-dione,21-(3-carboxy-1-oxopropoxy)-11,17-dihydroxy-, monosodium salt, (11β)-and its molecular weight is 484.52.

ACTIONS

Naturally occurring glucocorticoids (Hydrocortisone and cortisone), which also have salt-retaining properties, are used as replacement therapy in adrenocortical deficiency states. They are also used for their potent anti-inflammatory effect in disorders of many organ systems.

Glucocorticoids cause profound and varied metabolic effects. In addition, they modify the body's immune responses to diverse stimuli.

Hydrocortisone acetate sterile suspension has a slow onset but long duration of action when compared with more soluble preparations. Because of its insolubility, it is suitable for intra-articular, intralesional, and soft tissue injection where its anti-inflammatory effects are confined mainly to the area in which it has been injected, although it is capable of producing systemic hormonal effects.

Hydrocortisone phosphate injection has a rapid onset but short duration of action when compared with less soluble preparations. Because of this, it is suitable for the treatment of acute disorders responsive to adrenocortical steroid therapy.

Hydrocortisone sodium succinate has the same metabolic and anti-inflammatory actions as hydrocortisone. When given parenterally and in equimolar quantities, the two compounds are equivalent in biologic activity. Following the intravenous injection of Hydrocortisone sodium succinate, demonstrable effects are evident within one hour and persist for a variable period. Excretion of the administered dose is nearly complete within 12 hours. Thus, if constantly high blood levels are required, injections should be made every 4 to 6 hours. This preparation is also rapidly absorbed when administered intramuscularly and is excreted in a pattern similar to that observed after intravenous injection.

INDICATIONS

HYDROCORTISONE ACETATE SUSPENSION
1. By intra-articular or soft tissue injection

As adjunctive therapy for short-term administration (to tide the patient over an acute episode or exacerbation) in:

Synovitis of osteoarthritis
Rheumatoid arthritis
Acute and subacute bursitis
Acute gouty arthritis
Epicondylitis
Acute nonspecific tenosynovitis
Post-traumatic osteoarthritis

2. By intralesional injection:

Keloids
Localized hypertrophic, infiltrated, inflammatory lesions of: lichen planus, psoriatic plaques, granuloma annulare, and lichen simplex chronicus (neurodermatitis)
Discoid lupus erythematosus
Necrobiosis lipoidica diabeticorum
Alopecia areata
May also be useful in cystic tumors of an aponeurosis or tendon (ganglia).

HYDROCORTISONE TABLETS, HYDROCORTISONE SODIUM PHOSPHATE SOLUTION, HYDROCORTISONE SODIUM SUCCINATE
The parenteral forms are indicated when oral therapy is not feasible.

1. Endocrine Disorders

Primary or secondary adrenocortical insufficiency (hydrocortisone or cortisone is the first choice; synthetic analogs may be used in conjunction with mineralocorticoids where applicable; in infancy mineralocorticoid supplementation is of particular importance)

Congenital adrenal hyperplasia
Nonsuppurative thyroiditis
Hypercalcemia associated with cancer

The parenteral forms are additionally indicated in:

Acute adrenocortical insufficiency (Hydrocortisone or cortisone is the drug of choice; mineralocorticoid supplementation may be necessary, particularly when synthetic analogs are used)

Preoperatively, and in the event of serious trauma or illness, in patients with known adrenal insufficiency or when adrenocortical reserve is doubtful

Shock unresponsive to conventional therapy if adrenocortical insufficiency exists or is suspected

2. *Rheumatic Disorders*

As adjunctive therapy for short-term administration (to tide the patient over an acute episode or exacerbation) in:

Psoriatic arthritis
Rheumatoid arthritis, including juvenile rheumatoid arthritis (selected cases may require low-dose maintenance therapy)
Ankylosing spondylitis
Acute and subacute bursitis
Acute nonspecific tenosynovitis
Acute gouty arthritis
Post-traumatic osteoarthritis
Synovitis of osteoarthritis
Epicondylitis

3. *Collagen Diseases*

During an exacerbation or as maintenance therapy in selected cases of:

Systemic lupus erythematosus
Acute rheumatic carditis
Systemic dermatomyositis (polymyositis)

4. *Dermatologic Diseases*

Pemphigus
Bullous dermatitis herpetiformis
Severe erythema multiforme (Stevens-Johnson syndrome)
Exfoliative dermatitis
Mycosis fungoides
Severe psoriasis
Severe seborrheic dermatitis

5. *Allergic States*

Control of severe or incapacitating allergic conditions intractable to adequate trials of conventional treatment:

Seasonal or perennial allergic rhinitis
Bronchial asthma
Contact dermatitis
Atopic dermatitis
Serum sickness
Drug hypersensitivity reactions

The parenteral forms are additionally indicated in:

Urticarial transfusion reactions
Acute noninfectious laryngeal edema (epinephrine is the drug of first choice)

6. *Ophthalmic Diseases*

Severe acute and chronic allergic and inflammatory processes involving the eye and its adnexa, such as:

Allergic conjunctivitis
Keratitis
Allergic corneal marginal ulcers
Herpes zoster ophthalmicus
Iritis and iridocyclitis
Chorioretinitis
Anterior segment inflammation
Diffuse posterior uveitis and choroiditis
Optic neuritis
Sympathetic ophthalmia

7. *Respiratory Diseases*

Symptomatic sarcoidosis
Loeffler's syndrome not manageable by other means
Berylliosis
Fulminating or disseminated pulmonary tuberculosis when used concurrently with appropriate antituberculous chemotherapy
Aspiration pneumonitis

8. *Hematologic Disorders*

Idiopathic thrombocytopenic purpura in adults (IM administration is contraindicated)
Secondary thrombocytopenia in adults
Acquired (autoimmune) hemolytic anemia
Erythroblastopenia (RBC anemia)
Congenital (erythroid) hypoplastic anemia

9. *Neoplastic Diseases*

For palliative management of:
Leukemias and lymphomas in adults
Acute leukemia of childhood

10. *Edematous States*

To induce diuresis or remission of proteinuria in the nephrotic syndrome, without uremia, of the idiopathic type or that due to lupus erythematosus

11. *Gastrointestinal Diseases*

To tide the patient over a critical period of the disease in:
Ulcerative colitis
Regional enteritis

12. *Miscellaneous*

Tuberculous meningitis with subarachnoid block or impending block when used concurrently with appropriate antituberculous chemotherapy
Trichinosis with neurologic or myocardial involvement

Hydrocortisone sodium succinate is additionally indicated in:

13. *Nervous System:* Acute exacerbations of multiple sclerosis

UNLABELED USES

Hydrocortisone is used alone or as an adjunct in the diagnosis of leukopenia to differentiate idiopathic from drug-induced leukopenia. It is also used as an adjunct in the treatment of disseminated breast cancer, is used to induce labor, and is prescribed to reduce the risk of hyaline membrane disease in premature labor.

CONTRAINDICATIONS

Systemic fungal infections.

Hypersensitivity to any component of this product.

Some brands and/or formulations are contraindicated in premature infants because they contain benzyl alcohol. Benzyl alcohol has been reported to be associated with a fatal "Gasping Syndrome" in premature infants.

WARNINGS

Because rare instances of anaphylactoid reactions have occurred in patients receiving parenteral corticosteroid therapy, appropriate precautionary measures should be taken prior to administration, especially when the patient has a history of allergy to any drug. Anaphylactoid and hypersensitivity reactions have been reported for Hydrocortisone phosphate injection.

Some brands contain sodium bisulfite, a sulfite that may cause allergic-type reactions including anaphylactic symptoms and life-threatening or less severe asthmatic episodes in certain susceptible people. The overall prevalence of sulfite sensitivity in the general population is unknown and probably low. Sulfite sensitivity is seen more frequently in asthmatic than in nonasthmatic people.

Corticosteroids may exacerbate systemic fungal infections and therefore should not be used in the presence of such infections unless they are needed to control drug reactions due to amphotericin B. Moreover, there have been cases reported in which concomitant use of amphotericin B and Hydrocortisone was followed by cardiac enlargement and congestive failure.

In patients on corticosteroid therapy subjected to any unusual stress, increased dosage of rapidly acting corticosteroids before, during, and after the stressful situation is indicated.

Drug-induced secondary adrenocortical insufficiency may result from too rapid withdrawal of corticosteroids and may be minimized by gradual reduction of dosage. This type of relative insufficiency may persist for months after discontinuation of therapy; therefore, in any situation of stress occurring during that period, hormone therapy should be reinstituted. If the patient is receiving steroids already, dosage may have to be increased. Since mineralocorticoid secretion may be impaired, salt and/or a mineralocorticoid should be administered concurrently.

Corticosteroids may mask some signs of infection, and new infections may appear during their use. There may be decreased resistance and inability to localize infection when corticosteroids are used. Moreover, corticosteroids may affect the nitroblue-tetrazolium test for bacterial infection and produce false negative results.

In cerebral malaria, a double-blind trial has shown that the use of corticosteroids is associated with prolongation of coma and a higher incidence of pneumonia and gastrointestinal bleeding.

Corticosteroids may activate latent amebiasis. Therefore, it is recommended that latent or active amebiasis be ruled out before initiating corticosteroid therapy in any patient who has spent time in the tropics or any patient with unexplained diarrhea.

Prolonged use of corticosteroids may produce posterior subcapsular cataracts, glaucoma with possible damage to the optic nerves, and may enhance the establishment of secondary ocular infections due to fungi or viruses.

Usage in Pregnancy: Since adequate human reproduction studies have not been done with corticosteroids, use of these drugs in pregnancy or in women of childbearing potential requires that the anticipated benefits be weighed against the possible hazards to the mother and embryo or fetus. Infants born of mothers who have received substantial doses of corticosteroids during pregnancy should be carefully observed for signs of hypoadrenalism.

Corticosteroids appear in breast milk and could suppress growth, interfere with endogenous corticosteroid production, or cause other unwanted effects. Mothers taking pharmacologic doses of corticosteroids should be advised not to nurse. Average and large doses of cortisone or Hydrocortisone can cause elevation of blood pressure, salt and water retention, and increased excretion of potassium. These effects are less likely to occur with the synthetic derivatives except when used in large doses. Dietary salt restriction and potassium supplementation may be necessary. All corticosteroids increase calcium excretion.

◆ **RATED THERAPEUTICALLY EQUIVALENT;** ◇ **THERAPEUTIC EQUIVALENCE UNCONFIRMED;** ○ **UNRATED**

Administration of live virus vaccines, including smallpox, is contraindicated in individuals receiving immunosuppressive doses of corticosteroids. If inactivated viral or bacterial vaccines are administered to individuals receiving immunosuppressive doses of corticosteroids, there is a risk of neurological complications and the expected serum antibody response may not be obtained. However, immunization procedures may be undertaken in patients who are receiving corticosteroids as replacement therapy, e.g., for Addison's disease.

Patients who are on drugs which suppress the immune system are more susceptible to infections than healthy individuals. Chickenpox and measles, for example, can have a more serious or even fatal course in non-immune children or adults on corticosteroids. In such children or adults who have not had these diseases, particular care should be taken to avoid exposure. The risk of developing a disseminated infection varies among individuals and can be related to the dose, route and duration of corticosteroid administration as well as to the underlying disease. If exposed to chickenpox, prophylaxis with varicella zoster immune globulin (VZIG) may be indicated. If chickenpox develops, treatment with antiviral agents may be considered. If exposed to measles, prophylaxis with immune globulin (IG) may be indicated. (See the respective package inserts for VZIG and IG for complete prescribing information.)

The use of Hydrocortisone tablets, Hydrocortisone phosphate injection, or Hydrocortisone sodium succinate injection in active tuberculosis should be restricted to those cases of fulminating or disseminated tuberculosis in which the corticosteroid is used for the management of the disease in conjunction with an appropriate antituberculous regimen.

If corticosteroids are indicated in patients with latent tuberculosis or tuberculin reactivity, close observation is necessary as reactivation of the disease may occur. During prolonged corticosteroid therapy, these patients should receive chemoprophylaxis.

Literature reports suggest an apparent association between use of corticosteroids and left ventricular free wall rupture after a recent myocardial infarction; therefore, therapy with corticosteroids should be used with great caution in these patients.

PRECAUTIONS
This product, like many other steroid formulations, is sensitive to heat. Therefore, it should not be autoclaved when it is desirable to sterilize the exterior of the container vial.

Following prolonged therapy, withdrawal of corticosteroids may result in symptoms of the corticosteroid withdrawal syndrome including fever, myalgia, arthralgia, and malaise. This may occur in patients even without evidence of adrenal insufficiency.

There is an enhanced effect of corticosteroids in patients with hypothyroidism and in those with cirrhosis.

Corticosteroids should be used cautiously in patients with ocular herpes simplex for fear of corneal perforation.

The lowest possible dose of corticosteroid should be used to control the condition under treatment, and when reduction in dosage is possible, the reduction should be gradual.

Psychic derangements may appear when corticosteroids are used, ranging from euphoria, insomnia, mood swings, personality changes, and severe depression to frank psychotic manifestations. Also, existing emotional instability or psychotic tendencies may be aggravated by corticosteroids.

Corticosteroids may increase the clearance of chronic high dose aspirin. This could lead to decreased salicylate serum levels or increase the risk of salicylate toxicity when corticosteroid is withdrawn.

Aspirin should be used cautiously in conjunction with corticosteroids in hypoprothrombinemia.

Steroids should be used with caution in nonspecific ulcerative colitis, if there is a probability of impending perforation, abscess, or other pyogenic infection, also in diverticulitis, fresh intestinal anastomoses, active or latent peptic ulcer, renal insufficiency, hypertension, osteoporosis, and myasthenia gravis. Signs of peritoneal irritation following gastrointestinal perforation in patients receiving large doses of corticosteroids may be minimal or absent. Fat embolism has been reported as a possible complication of hypercortisonism.

When large doses are given, some authorities advise that oral corticosteroids be taken with meals and antacids administered between meals to help to prevent peptic ulcer.

Growth and development of infants and children on prolonged corticosteroid therapy should be carefully followed.

Steroids may increase or decrease motility and number of spermatozoa in some patients.

Drugs that induce hepatic enzymes such as phenytoin, phenobarbital, ephedrine, and rifampin may enhance the metabolic clearance of corticosteroids, resulting in decreased blood levels and lessened physiologic activity, thus requiring adjustment in corticosteroid dosage.

Drugs such as troleandomycin and ketoconazole may inhibit the metabolism of corticosteroids and thus decrease their clearance. Therefore, the dose of corticosteroid should be titrated to avoid steroid toxicity.

The prothrombin time should be checked frequently in patients who are receiving corticosteroids and coumarin anticoagulants at the same time because of reports that corticosteroids have altered the response to these anticoagulants. Studies have shown that the usual effect produced by adding corticosteroids is inhibition of response to coumarins, although there have been some conflicting reports of potentiation not substantiated by studies.

When corticosteroids are administered concomitantly with potassium-depleting diuretics, patients should be observed closely for development of hypokalemia.

Intra-articular injection of a corticosteroid may produce systemic as well as local effects.

Appropriate examination of any joint fluid present is necessary to exclude a septic process.

A marked increase in pain accompanied by local swelling, further restriction of joint motion, fever, and malaise is suggestive of septic arthritis. If this complication occurs and the diagnosis of sepsis is confirmed, appropriate antimicrobial therapy should be instituted.

Injection of a steroid into an infected site is to be avoided.

The slower rate of absorption by intramuscular administration should be recognized.

Corticosteroids should not be injected into unstable joints. Patients should be impressed strongly with the importance of not overusing joints in which symptomatic benefit has been obtained as long as the inflammatory process remains active.

Frequent intra-articular injection may result in damage to joint tissues.

Although controlled clinical trials have shown corticosteroids to be effective in speeding the resolution of acute exacerbations of multiple sclerosis, they do not show that corticosteroids affect the ultimate outcome or natural history of the disease. The studies do show that relatively high doses of corticosteroids are necessary to demonstrate a significant effect. (See "Administration and Dosage".)

Since complications of treatment with glucocorticoids are dependent on the size of the dose and the duration of treatment, a risk/benefit decision must be made in each individual case as to dose and duration of treatment and as to whether daily or intermittent therapy should be used.

Information for Patients: Susceptible patients who are on immunosuppressant doses of corticosteroids should be warned to avoid exposure to chickenpox or measles. Patients should also be advised that if they are exposed, medical advice should be sought without delay.

ADVERSE REACTIONS
Fluid and electrolyte disturbances
Sodium retention
Fluid retention
Congestive heart failure in susceptible patients
Potassium loss
Hypokalemic alkalosis
Hypertension

Musculoskeletal
Muscle weakness
Steroid myopathy
Loss of muscle mass
Osteoporosis
Vertebral compression fractures
Aseptic necrosis of femoral and humeral heads
Pathologic fracture of long bones
Tendon rupture

Gastrointestinal
Peptic ulcer with possible subsequent perforation and hemorrhage
Perforation of the small and large bowel, particularly in patients with inflammatory bowel disease
Pancreatitis
Abdominal distention
Ulcerative esophagitis
Increases in alanine transaminase (ALT, SGPT), aspartate transaminase (AST, SGOT) and alkaline phosphatase have been observed following corticosteroid treatment. These changes are usually small, not associated with any clinical syndrome and are reversible upon discontinuation.

Dermatologic:
Impaired wound healing
Thin fragile skin
Petechiae and ecchymoses
Erythema
Increased sweating
May suppress reactions to skin tests
Burning or tingling, especially in the perineal area (after IV injection)
Other cutaneous reactions, such as allergic dermatitis, urticaria, angioneurotic edema

Neurologic
Convulsions
Increased intracranial pressure with papilledema (pseudotumor cerebri) usually after treatment
Vertigo
Headache
Psychic disturbances

Endocrine
Menstrual irregularities
Development of cushingoid state
Suppression of growth in children
Secondary adrenocortical and pituitary unresponsiveness, particularly in times of stress, as in trauma, surgery, or illness

Decreased carbohydrate tolerance
Manifestations of latent diabetes mellitus
Increased requirements for insulin or oral hypoglycemic agents in diabetics
Hirsutism

Ophthalmic
Posterior subcapsular cataracts
Increased intraocular pressure
Glaucoma
Exophthalmos

Metabolic
Negative nitrogen balance due to protein catabolism

Cardiovascular
Myocardial rupture following recent myocardial infarction (see *"Warnings"*).

Other
Anaphylactoid or hypersensitivity reactions
Thromboembolism
Weight gain
Increased appetite
Nausea
Malaise

The following *additional* adverse reactions are related to injection of corticosteroids:
Rare instances of blindness associated with intralesional therapy around the face and head
Hyperpigmentation or hypopigmentation
Subcutaneous and cutaneous atrophy
Sterile abscess
Postinjection flare (following intra-articular use)
Charcot-like arthropathy.

OVERDOSAGE

Reports of acute toxicity and/or death following overdosage of glucocorticoids are rare. In the event of overdosage, no specific antidote is available; treatment is supportive and symptomatic.

The intraperitoneal LD_{50} of Hydrocortisone in female mice was 1740 mg/kg.

DOSAGE AND ADMINISTRATION

HYDROCORTISONE ACETATE SUSPENSION
For intra-articular, intralesional, and soft tissue injection only

NOT FOR INTRAVENOUS USE
Dosage and frequency of injection are variable and must be individualized on the basis of the disease and the response of the patient.

The initial dose varies from 5 to 75 mg depending on the disease being treated and the size of the area to be injected. Frequency of injection depends on symptomatic response, and usually is once every two or three weeks. Severe conditions may require injection once a week. Frequent intra-articular injection may result in damage to joint tissues. If satisfactory clinical response does not occur after a reasonable period of time, discontinue Hydrocortisone acetate sterile suspension and transfer the patient to other therapy.

Patients should be observed closely for signs that might require dosage adjustment, including changes in clinical status resulting from remissions or exacerbations of the disease, and individual drug responsiveness.

Some of the usual single doses are:

Large Joints (e.g., Knee)	25 mg, occasionally 37.5 mg. Doses over 50 mg not recommended
Small Joints (e.g, Interphalangeal, Temporomandibular)	10 to 25 mg
Bursae	25 to 37.5 mg
Tendon Sheaths	5 to 12.5 mg
Soft Tissue Infiltration	25 to 50 mg, occasionally 75 mg
Ganglia	12.5 to 25 mg

For rapid onset of action, a soluble adrenocortical hormone preparation, such as dexamethasone sodium phosphate injection or prednisolone sodium phosphate injection, may be given with Hydrocortisone acetate sterile suspension.

If desired, a local anesthetic may be used, and may be injected before Hydrocortisone acetate sterile suspension or mixed in a syringe with Hydrocortisone acetate sterile suspension and given simultaneously.

If used prior to intra-articular injection of the steroid, inject most of the anesthetic into the soft tissues of the surrounding area and instill a small amount into the joint.

If given together, mixing should be done in the injection syringe by drawing the steroid in *first*, then the anesthetic. In this way, the anesthetic will not be introduced inadvertently into the vial of steroid. *The mixture must be used immediately and any unused portion discarded.*

HYDROCORTISONE SODIUM PHOSPHATE SOLUTION
For intravenous, intramuscular, and subcutaneous injection. Hydrocortisone sodium phosphate injection can be given directly or it can be added to sodium chloride injection or dextrose injection and administered by intravenous drip.

Benzyl alcohol as a preservative has been associated with toxicity in premature infants. Solutions used for intravenous administration or further dilution of this product should be preservative-free when used in the neonate, especially the premature infant.

When it is mixed with an infusion solution, sterile precautions should be observed. Since infusion solutions generally do not contain preservatives, mixtures should be used within 24 hours.

Dosage requirements are variable and must be individualized on the basis of the disease and the response of the patient.

The initial dosage varies from 15 to 240 mg a day depending on the disease being treated. In less severe diseases doses lower than 15 mg may suffice, while in severe diseases doses higher than 240 mg may be required. Usually the parenteral dosage ranges are one-third to one-half the oral dose given every 12 hours. However, in certain overwhelming, acute, life-threatening situations, administration in dosages exceeding the usual dosages may be justified and may be in multiples of the oral dosages.

The initial dosage should be maintained or adjusted until the patient's response is satisfactory. If a satisfactory clinical response does not occur after a reasonable period of time, discontinue Hydrocortisone sodium phosphate injection and transfer the patient to other therapy.

After a favorable initial response, the proper maintenance dosage should be determined by decreasing the initial dosage in small amounts to the lowest dosage that maintains an adequate clinical response.

Patients should be observed closely for signs that might require dosage adjustment, including changes in clinical status resulting from remissions or exacerbations of the disease, individual drug responsiveness, and the effect of stress (e.g., surgery, infection, trauma). During stress it may be necessary to increase dosage temporarily.

If the drug is to be stopped after more than a few days of treatment, it usually should be withdrawn gradually.

HYDROCORTISONE SODIUM SUCCINATE POWDER FOR RECONSTITUTION

This preparation may be administered by intravenous injection, by intravenous infusion, or by intramuscular injection, the preferred method for initial emergency use being intravenous injection. Following the initial emergency period, consideration should be given to employing a longer acting injectable preparation or an oral preparation.

Therapy is initiated by administering Hydrocortisone sodium succinate sterile intravenously over a period of 30 seconds (eg, 100 mg) to 10 minutes (eg, 500 mg or more). In general, high-dose corticosteroid therapy should be continued only until the patient's condition has stabilized—usually not beyond 48 to 72 hours. Although adverse effects associated with high dose, short-term corticoid therapy are uncommon, peptic ulceration may occur. Prophylactic antacid therapy may be indicated.

When high dose Hydrocortisone therapy must be continued beyond 48-72 hours, hypernatremia may occur. Under such circumstances it may be desirable to replace Hydrocortisone sodium succinate with a corticoid such as methylprednisolone sodium succinate, which causes little or no sodium retention.

The initial dose of Hydrocortisone sodium succinate sterile powder is 100 mg to 500 mg, depending on the severity of the condition. This dose may be repeated at intervals of 2, 4 or 6 hours as indicated by the patient's response and clinical condition. While the dose may be reduced for infants and children, it is governed more by the severity of the condition and response of the patient than by age or body weight but should not be less than 25 mg daily.

Patients subjected to severe stress following corticosteroid therapy should be observed closely for signs and symptoms of adrenocortical insufficiency.

Corticoid therapy is an adjunct to, and not a replacement for, conventional therapy.

Multiple Sclerosis: In the treatment of acute exacerbations of multiple sclerosis daily doses of 200 mg of prednisolone for a week followed by 80 mg every other day for one month have been shown to be effective (20 mg of Hydrocortisone is equivalent to 5 mg of prednisolone).

Preparation of Solutions: For intravenous or intramuscular injection, prepare solution by aseptically adding 2.1 ml, 2 ml, 4 ml, or 8 ml bacteriostatic water for injection or bacteriostatic sodium chloride injection to 100, 250, 500 or 1,000 mg Hydrocortisone sodium succinate powder. *For intravenous infusion,* first prepare solution by adding *not more than 2 ml* of bacteriostatic water for injection to the 100, 250, 500, or 1,000 mg powder; this solution may then be added to 100 to 1000 ml (but not less than 100 ml) of the following: 5% dextrose in water (or isotonic saline solution or 5% dextrose in isotonic saline solution if patient is not on sodium restriction).

Further dilution is not necessary for intravenous or intramuscular injection. For intravenous infusion, first prepare solution as just described. The *100 mg* solution may then be added to 100 to 1000 ml of 5% dextrose in water (or isotonic saline solution or 5% dextrose in isotonic saline solution if patient is not on sodium restriction). The *250 mg* solution may be added to 250 to 1000 ml, the *500 mg* solution may be added to 500 to 1000 ml and the *1000 mg* solution to 1000 ml of the same diluents. In cases where administration of a small volume of fluid is desirable, 100 mg to 3000 mg of Hydrocortisone sodium succinate sterile powder may be added to 50 ml of the above diluents. The resulting solutions are stable for at least 4 hours and may be administered either directly or by IV piggyback.

◆ RATED THERAPEUTICALLY EQUIVALENT; ◇ THERAPEUTIC EQUIVALENCE UNCONFIRMED; ○ UNRATED

HYDROCORTISONE TABLETS
For oral administration

Dosage requirements are available and must be individualized on the basis of the disease and the response of the patient.

The initial dosage varies from 20 to 240 mg a day depending on the disease being treated. In less severe diseases doses lower than 20 mg may suffice, while in severe diseases doses higher than 240 mg may be required. The initial dosage should be maintained or adjusted until the patient's response is satisfactory. If satisfactory clinical response does not occur after a reasonable period of time, discontinue Hydrocortisone tablets and transfer the patient to other therapy.

After a favorable initial response, the proper maintenance dosage should be determined by decreasing the initial dosage in small amounts to the lowest dosage that maintains an adequate clinical response.

Patients should be observed closely for signs that might require dosage adjustment, including changes in clinical status resulting from remissions or exacerbations of the disease, individual drug responsiveness, and the effect of stress (e.g., surgery, infection, trauma). During stress it may be necessary to increase dosage temporarily.

If the drug is to be stopped after more than a few days of treatment, it usually should be withdrawn gradually.

STORAGE
Hydrocortisone acetate suspension, Hydrocortisone sodium phosphate solution:
Sensitive to heat. Do not autoclave. Protect from freezing.
Hydrocortisone sodium succinate:
Parenteral drug products should be inspected visually for particulate matter and discoloration prior to administration, whenever solution and container permit. Use only if solution is clear.

J CODES
Up to 100 mg IV,IM,SC—J1720
Up to 50 mg IV,IM,SC—J1710
Up to 25 mg IV,IM,SC—J1700

HOW SUPPLIED

HYDROCORTISONE SODIUM PHOSPHATE
INJECTION: 50 MG/ML

AVERAGE UNIT PRICE (AVAILABLE SIZES)			
BRAND	$4.98		

BRAND/MANUFACTURER	NDC	SIZE	AWP
◆ BRAND			
HYDROCORTONE PHOSPHATE: Merck	00006-7633-04	2 ml	$10.11
	00006-7633-10	10 ml	$48.96

HYDROCORTISONE
TABLETS: 5 MG

BRAND/MANUFACTURER	NDC	SIZE	AWP
◇ BRAND			
CORTEF: Upjohn	00009-0012-01	50s	$5.33

TABLETS: 10 MG

BRAND/MANUFACTURER	NDC	SIZE	AWP
◇ BRAND			
CORTEF: Upjohn	00009-0031-01	100s	$18.83
HYDROCORTONE: Merck	00006-0619-68	100s	$19.48

TABLETS: 20 MG

BRAND/MANUFACTURER	NDC	SIZE	AWP
◇ BRAND			
CORTEF: Upjohn	00009-0044-01	100s	$35.71
HYDROCORTONE: Merck	00006-0625-68	100s	$37.16
◇ GENERICS			
Moore,H.L.	00839-1365-06	100s	$7.14
West-Ward	00143-1254-01	100s	$8.00
URL	00677-0076-01	100s	$8.10
Major	00904-2674-60	100s	$8.65
Richlyn	00115-3685-01	100s	$8.93
Rugby	00536-3913-01	100s	$11.55
West-Ward	00143-1254-25	100s ud	$8.25
Richlyn	00115-3685-03	1000s	$68.70

HYDROCORTISONE ACETATE
INJECTION: 25 MG/ML

BRAND/MANUFACTURER	NDC	SIZE	AWP
◇ GENERICS			
Schein	00364-6624-54	10 ml	$3.75
Steris	00402-0051-10	10 ml	$3.75
Major	00904-0855-10	10 ml	$4.45
Rugby	00536-1200-70	10 ml	$4.58

INJECTION: 50 MG/ML

BRAND/MANUFACTURER	NDC	SIZE	AWP
◇ BRAND			
HYDROCORTONE ACETATE: Merck	00006-7519-03	5 ml	$26.14

HYDROCORTISONE SODIUM SUCCINATE
POWDER FOR INJECTION: 100 MG

AVERAGE UNIT PRICE (AVAILABLE SIZES)			
BRAND	$3.10		

BRAND/MANUFACTURER	NDC	SIZE	AWP
◆ BRAND			
SOLU-CORTEF: Upjohn	00009-0825-01	1s	$3.26
	00009-0900-13	1s	$3.34
	00009-0900-15	1s	$3.34
A-HYDROCORT: Abbott Hosp	00074-5671-02	10s	$24.58

POWDER FOR INJECTION: 250 MG

AVERAGE UNIT PRICE (AVAILABLE SIZES)			
BRAND	$6.89		

BRAND/MANUFACTURER	NDC	SIZE	AWP
◆ BRAND			
SOLU-CORTEF: Upjohn	00009-0909-08	1s	$7.56
	00009-0909-09	1s	$7.56
A-HYDROCORT: Abbott Hosp	00074-5672-02	10s	$55.58

POWDER FOR INJECTION: 500 MG

AVERAGE UNIT PRICE (AVAILABLE SIZES)			
BRAND	$12.77		

BRAND/MANUFACTURER	NDC	SIZE	AWP
◆ BRAND			
SOLU-CORTEF: Upjohn	00009-0912-05	1s	$14.71
A-HYDROCORT: Abbott Hosp	00074-5673-04	25s	$270.75

POWDER FOR INJECTION: 1 GM

AVERAGE UNIT PRICE (AVAILABLE SIZES)			
BRAND	$25.66		

BRAND/MANUFACTURER	NDC	SIZE	AWP
◆ BRAND			
SOLU-CORTEF: Upjohn	00009-0920-03	1s	$29.29
A-HYDROCORT: Abbott Hosp	00074-5674-08	25s	$550.70

Hydrocortisone, Topical

DESCRIPTION
Hydrocortisone, Topical, is available as a cream, ointment, topical solution, lotion, and oral paste.

Each gm of cream contains:

Hydrocortisone . . . . .10 or 25 mg
or
Hydrocortisone Butyrate . . . . .1 mg
or
Hydrocortisone Valerate . . . . .2 mg

Each gm of ointment contains:
Hydrocortisone . . . . .10 or 25 mg
or
Hydrocortisone Butyrate 1mg
or
Hydrocortisone Valerate . . . . .2 mg

Each ml of topical solution contains:
Hydrocortisone Butyrate . . . . .1 mg

Each ml of lotion contains:
Hydrocortisone . . . . .10 or 25 mg

Each gm of oral paste contains:
Hydrocortisone Acetate . . . . .5 mg

The topical corticosteroids, including Hydrocortisone, Hydrocortisone Acetate, Hydrocortisone Butyrate, and Hydrocortisone Valerate, constitute a class of primarily synthetic steroids used as anti-inflammatory and antipruritic agents. Hydrocortisone Acetate is a natural corticosteroid. Hydrocortisone is known chemically as 11, 17, 21-trihydroxypregn-4-ene, 3, 20-dione.

Hydrocortisone Acetate, an adrenocorticoid topical dental paste for application to the oral mucosa, is Pregn-4-ene, 20-dione, 21-(acetyloxy)-11, 17 dihydroxy-, (11β)-. It is also known as cortisol acetate.

Hydrocortisone Butyrate, a non-fluorinated hydrocortisone ester, has the chemical name: pregn-4-ene-3,20-dione, 11,21-dihydroxy-17-[(1-oxobutyl)oxy]-, 11β); the molecular formula: $C_{25}H_{36}O_6$; and the molecular weight: 432.54.

Hydrocortisone valerate, a non-fluorinated steroid, has the chemical name Pregn-4-ene-3, 20-dione, 11, 21-dihydroxy-17-[(1-oxo-pentyl) oxy]-, (11β)-; the empirical formula is $C_{26}H_{38}O_6$ and the molecular weight is 44.58.

CLINICAL PHARMACOLOGY

Topical corticosteroids share anti-inflammatory, anti-pruritic and vasoconstrictive actions.

The mechanism of anti-inflammatory activity of the topical corticosteroids is unclear. Various laboratory methods, including vasoconstrictor assays, are used to compare and predict potencies and/or clinical efficacies of the topical corticosteroids. There is some evidence to suggest that a recognizable correlation exists between vasoconstrictor potency and therapeutic efficacy in man.

PHARMACOKINETICS

The extent of percutaneous absorption of topical corticosteroids is determined by many factors including the vehicle, the integrity of the epidermal barrier, and the use of occlusive dressings.

Topical corticosteroids can be absorbed from normal intact skin. Inflammation and/or other disease processes in the skin increase percutaneous absorption. Occlusive dressings substantially increase the percutaneous absorption of topical corticosteroids. Thus, occlusive dressings may be a valuable therapeutic adjunct for treatment of resistant dermatoses. (See *"Dosage and Administration"*.)

Once absorbed, topical corticosteroids are handled through pharmacokinetic pathways similar to systemically administered corticosteroids. Corticosteroids are bound to plasma proteins in varying degrees. Corticosteroids are metabolized primarily in the liver and are then excreted by the kidneys. Some of the topical corticosteroids and their metabolites are also excreted into the bile.

The oral paste acts as an adhesive vehicle for applying the active medication to oral tissues. The protective action of the adhesive vehicle may serve to reduce oral irritation.

INDICATIONS AND USAGE

Topical corticosteroids are indicated for the relief of the inflammatory and pruritic manifestations of corticosteroid-responsive dermatoses.

Hydrocortisone Butyrate topical solution is also indicated for the relief of the inflammatory and pruritic manifestations of seborrheic dermatitis.

Indicated for adjunctive treatment and for temporary relief of symptoms associated with oral inflammatory lesions and ulcerative lesions resulting from trauma.

CONTRAINDICATIONS

Topical corticosteroids are contraindicated in those patients with a history of hypersensitivity to any of the components of the preparation. Because it contains a corticosteroid, contraindicated in the presence of fungal, viral, or bacterial infections of the mouth or throat.

PRECAUTIONS

General: Systemic absorption of topical corticosteroids has produced reversible hypothalamic-pituitary-adrenal (HPA) axis suppression, manifestations of Cushing's syndrome, hyperglycemia, and glucosuria in some patients. Conditions which augment systemic absorption include the application of the more potent steroid, use over large surface areas, prolonged use, and the addition of occlusive dressings.

Therefore, patients receiving a large dose of a potent topical steroid applied to a large surface area or under an occlusive dressing should be evaluated periodically for evidence of HPA axis suppression by using the urinary free cortisol and ACTH stimulation tests. If HPA axis suppression is noted, an attempt should be made to withdraw the drug, to reduce the frequency of application, or to substitute a less potent steroid.

Recovery of HPA axis function is generally prompt and complete upon discontinuation of the drug. Infrequently, signs and symptoms of steroid withdrawal may occur, requiring supplemental systemic corticosteroids.

Children may absorb proportionally larger amounts of topical corticosteroids and thus be more susceptible to systemic toxicity (see *"Precautions—Pediatric Use"*.)

If irritation develops, topical corticosteroids should be discontinued and appropriate therapy instituted. In the presence of dermatological or oral infections, the use of an appropriate antifungal or antibacterial agent should be instituted. If a favorable response does not occur promptly, the corticosteroid should be discontinued until the infection has been adequately controlled.

INFORMATION FOR THE PATIENT

Patients using topical corticosteroids should receive the following information and instructions:

1. This medication is to be used as directed by the dentist or physician. It is for external or oral, when appropriate, use only. Avoid contact with the eyes.

2. Patients should be advised not to use this medication for any disorder other than for which it was prescribed.

3. The treated area should not be bandaged or otherwise covered or wrapped as to be occlusive unless directed by the dentist or physician.

4. Patients should report any signs of local adverse reactions especially under occlusive dressing.

5. Parents of pediatric patients should be advised not to use tight-fitting diapers or plastic pants on a child being treated in the diaper area, as these garments may constitute occlusive dressings.

LABORATORY TESTS

The following tests may be helpful in evaluating the HPA axis suppression:
   Urinary free cortisol test
   ACTH stimulation test.

CARCINOGENESIS, MUTAGENESIS, AND IMPAIRMENT OF FERTILITY

Long-term animal studies have not been performed to evaluate the carcinogenic potential or the effect on fertility of topical corticosteroids.

Studies to determine mutagenicity with prednisolone and hydrocortisone have revealed negative results.

PREGNANCY CATEGORY C

Corticosteroids are generally teratogenic in laboratory animals when administered systemically at relatively low dosage levels. The more potent corticosteroids have been shown to be teratogenic after dermal application in laboratory animals. There are no adequate and well-controlled studies in pregnant women on teratogenic effects from topically applied corticosteroids. Therefore, topical corticosteroids should be used during pregnancy only if the potential benefit justifies the potential risk to the fetus. Drugs of this class should not be used extensively on pregnant patients, in large amounts, or for prolonged periods of time.

NURSING MOTHERS

It is not known whether topical administration of corticosteroids could result in sufficient systemic absorption to produce detectable quantities in breast milk. Systemically administered corticosteroids are secreted into breast milk, in quantities not likely to have a deleterious effect on the infant. Nevertheless, caution should be exercised when topical corticosteroids are administered to a nursing woman.

PEDIATRIC USE

Pediatric patients may demonstrate greater susceptibility to topical corticosteroid-induced HPA axis suppression and Cushing's syndrome than mature patients because of a larger skin surface area to body weight ratio.

Hypothalamic-pituitary-adrenal (HPA) axis suppression, Cushing's syndrome, and intracranal hypertension have been reported in children receiving topical corticosteroids. Manifestations of adrenal suppression in children include linear growth retardation, delayed weight gain, low plasma cortisol levels, and absence of response to ACTH stimulation. Manifestations of intracranial hypertension include bulging fontanelles, headaches, and bilateral papilledema.

Administration of topical corticosteroids to children should be limited to the least amount compatible with an effective therapeutic regimen. Chronic corticosteroid therapy may interfere with the growth and development of children.

ADVERSE REACTIONS

The following local adverse reactions are reported infrequently with topical corticosteroids, but may occur more frequently with the use of occlusive dressings. These reactions are listed in an approximate decreasing order of occurrence: burning, itching, irritation, dryness, folliculitis, hypertrichosis, acneiform eruptions, hypopigmentation, perioral dermatitis, allergic contact dermatitis, maceration of the skin, secondary infection, skin atrophy, striae, miliaria.

OVERDOSAGE

Topically applied corticosteroids can be absorbed in sufficient amounts to produce systemic effects. (See *"Precautions"*.)

DOSAGE AND ADMINISTRATION

Hydrocortisone preparations should be applied to the affected area as a thin film two to four times daily depending on the severity of the condition.

Occlusive dressings may be used for the management of psoriasis or recalcitrant conditions.

If an infection develops, the use of occlusive dressings should be discontinued and appropriate antimicrobial therapy instituted.

Hydrocortisone Acetate oral paste: Dab, **do not rub**, on the lesion until the paste adheres. (Rubbing this preparation on lesions may result in a granular, gritty sensation.) After application, a smooth, slippery film develops.

Usual adult dose: Topical, to the oral mucous membrane, 2 or 3 times a day following meals and at bedtime.

Usual pediatric dose: Dosage has not been established.

STORAGE

Hydrocortisone Butyrate cream: Store between 46° and 77°F (8° and 25°C).

Hydrocortisone Butyrate ointment: Store between 36° and 86°F (2° and 30°C).

Hydrocortisone Butyrate solution: Store between 41° and 77°F (5° and 25°C).

Hydrocortisone Valerate cream and ointment: Store below 78°F (26°C).

HOW SUPPLIED

HYDROCORTISONE VALERATE
CREAM: 0.2%

BRAND/MANUFACTURER	NDC	SIZE	AWP
○ **BRAND**			
WESTCORT: Westwood-Squibb	00072-8100-15	15 gm	$11.95
	00072-8100-45	45 gm	$24.79
	00072-8100-60	60 gm	$29.82

◆ RATED THERAPEUTICALLY EQUIVALENT; ◇ THERAPEUTIC EQUIVALENCE UNCONFIRMED; ○ UNRATED

BRAND/MANUFACTURER	NDC	SIZE	AWP
	00072-8100-12	120 gm	$41.12

OINTMENT: 0.2%

BRAND/MANUFACTURER	NDC	SIZE	AWP
○ BRAND			
WESTCORT: Westwood-Squibb	00072-7800-15	15 gm	$11.95
	00072-7800-45	45 gm	$24.79
	00072-7800-60	60 gm	$29.82

HYDROCORTISONE

CREAM: 0.5%

BRAND/MANUFACTURER	NDC	SIZE	AWP
◆ BRAND			
CORT-DOME: Miles Pharm	00026-1631-81	30 gm	$12.31

CREAM: 1%

AVERAGE UNIT PRICE (AVAILABLE SIZES)		GENERIC A-RATED AVERAGE PRICE (GAAP)	
BRAND	$0.40	20 gm	$2.63
GENERIC	$0.10	30 gm	$3.36
HCFA FUL (15 gm)	$0.15	60 gm	$6.44
HCFA FUL (20 gm)	$0.12	120 gm	$8.56
HCFA FUL (30 gm)	$0.05	454 gm	$28.05
HCFA FUL (60 gm)	$0.07	480 gm	$24.58
HCFA FUL (120 gm)	$0.06		
HCFA FUL (454 gm)	$0.05		

BRAND/MANUFACTURER	NDC	SIZE	AWP
◆ BRAND			
HYTONE: Dermik	00066-0083-01	30 gm	$8.41
CORT-DOME: Miles Pharm	00026-1641-81	30 gm	$20.41
DERMACORT: Solvay	00032-6002-68	454 gm	$25.95
◆ GENERICS			
Thames	49158-0101-07	20 gm	$1.90
Moore,H.L.	00839-5207-45	20 gm	$2.15
Rugby	00536-0501-99	20 gm	$2.90
LEMODERM: Seneca	47028-0024-20	20 gm	$3.58
Thames	49158-0101-08	30 gm	$2.00
HYDROCORT CREAM: Geneva	00781-7018-24	30 gm	$2.13
NMC	23317-0321-28	30 gm	$2.36
Moore,H.L.	00839-5207-49	30 gm	$2.42
Moore,H.L.	00839-7721-49	30 gm	$2.42
Schein	00364-7087-56	30 gm	$2.60
Med-Derm	45565-0500-09	30 gm	$2.90
Major	00904-0749-31	30 gm	$2.95
Rugby	00536-0501-95	30 gm	$2.97
Parmed	00349-8758-48	30 gm	$3.00
Fougera	00168-0015-31	30 gm	$3.10
Goldline	00182-5060-34	30 gm	$3.15
HYDRO-TEX: Syosset	47854-0567-05	30 gm	$3.95
HI-COR 1.0: C & M	00398-0100-01	30 gm	$4.86
ALA-CORT: Del-Ray	00316-0126-01	30 gm	$5.85
PENECORT: Allergan Inc	00023-0510-30	30 gm	$7.11
NMC	23317-0321-57	60 gm	$4.70
Goldline	00182-5060-43	60 gm	$5.25
HYDRO-TEX: Syosset	47854-0567-07	60 gm	$6.50
HI-COR 1.0: C & M	00398-0100-02	60 gm	$9.30
ALA-CORT: Del-Ray	00316-0126-03	90 gm	$9.74
Major	00904-0749-22	120 gm	$7.50
Thames	49158-0101-12	120 gm	$7.50
Med-Derm	45565-0500-13	120 gm	$7.90
HYDRO-TEX: Syosset	47854-0567-09	120 gm	$8.50
Rugby	00536-0501-97	120 gm	$11.39
Thames	49158-0101-16	454 gm	$21.60
Clay-Park	45802-0003-05	454 gm	$21.60
Syosset	47854-0567-13	454 gm	$22.50
NMC	23317-0321-16	454 gm	$27.52
Moore,H.L.	00839-5207-60	454 gm	$27.52
Fougera	00168-0015-16	454 gm	$27.84
Goldline	00182-5060-45	454 gm	$29.25
Rugby	00536-0501-98	454 gm	$32.67
HI-COR 1.0: C & M	00398-0100-16	454 gm	$41.94
Major	00904-0749-27	480 gm	$24.35
HYDROCORT CREAM: Geneva	00781-7018-16	480 gm	$24.81
Goldline	00182-5060-30	0.9 gm 144s ud	$15.00

CREAM: 2.5%

AVERAGE UNIT PRICE (AVAILABLE SIZES)		GENERIC A-RATED AVERAGE PRICE (GAAP)	
BRAND	$0.48	20 gm	$4.72
GENERIC	$0.16	30 gm	$6.94
HCFA FUL (20 gm)	$0.21	454 gm	$61.09
HCFA FUL (30 gm)	$0.16		

BRAND/MANUFACTURER	NDC	SIZE	AWP
◆ BRAND			
HYTONE: Dermik	00066-0095-01	30 gm	$16.70
	00066-0095-02	60 gm	$26.71

BRAND/MANUFACTURER	NDC	SIZE	AWP
◆ GENERICS			
Moore,H.L.	00839-6376-45	20 gm	$3.71
Thames	49158-0200-07	20 gm	$3.80
Clay-Park	45802-0004-02	20 gm	$4.10
Major	00904-0756-29	20 gm	$4.65
NMC	23317-0322-20	20 gm	$4.70
HYDROCORT CREAM: Geneva	00781-7011-22	20 gm	$4.89
URL	00677-0718-38	20 gm	$5.20
Goldline	00182-5005-48	20 gm	$5.55
Rugby	00536-0611-99	20 gm	$5.88
Moore,H.L.	00839-6376-49	30 gm	$4.98
Thames	49158-0200-08	30 gm	$5.80
Qualitest	00603-7781-78	30 gm	$5.85
Clay-Park	45802-0004-03	30 gm	$5.94
NMC	23317-0322-30	30 gm	$6.24
Major	00904-0756-30	30 gm	$6.75
Major	00904-0756-31	30 gm	$6.75
HYDROCORT CREAM: Geneva	00781-7011-24	30 gm	$7.26
Fougera	00168-0080-31	30 gm	$8.06
HI-COR 2.5: C & M	00398-0019-01	30 gm	$8.34
Rugby	00536-0611-95	30 gm	$10.32
HI-COR 2.5: C & M	00398-0019-02	60 gm	$13.68
Thames	49158-0200-16	454 gm	$56.70
Clay-Park	45802-0004-05	454 gm	$58.32
NMC	23317-0322-16	454 gm	$68.24
HI-COR 2.5: C & M	00398-0019-16	454 gm	$74.88

LOTION: 0.25%

BRAND/MANUFACTURER	NDC	SIZE	AWP
○ BRAND			
CETACORT: Galderma	00299-3947-04	120 ml	$13.86
CORT-DOME: Miles Pharm	00026-1622-04	120 ml	$16.29

LOTION: 0.5%

HCFA FUL (60 ml)	$0.04
HCFA FUL (120 ml)	$0.04

BRAND/MANUFACTURER	NDC	SIZE	AWP
◆ BRAND			
CETACORT: Galderma	00299-3948-02	60 ml	$13.86
◆ GENERICS			
COTACORT: Truxton	00463-8010-04	120 ml	$7.20

LOTION: 1%

AVERAGE UNIT PRICE (AVAILABLE SIZES)		GENERIC A-RATED AVERAGE PRICE (GAAP)	
BRAND	$0.19	120 ml	$11.15
GENERIC	$0.10		
HCFA FUL (60 ml)	$0.07		
HCFA FUL (120 ml)	$0.05		

BRAND/MANUFACTURER	NDC	SIZE	AWP
◆ BRAND			
NUTRACORT: Galderma	00299-5830-01	60 ml	$14.44
CETACORT: Galderma	00299-3949-02	60 ml	$15.72
DERMACORT: Solvay	00032-6008-74	120 ml	$9.31
NUTRACORT: Galderma	00299-5830-02	120 ml	$21.63
HYTONE: Dermik	00066-0090-04	120 ml	$22.40
◆ GENERICS			
LACTICARE-HC: Stiefel	00145-2537-04	118 ml	$14.40
Thames	49158-0203-12	120 ml	$7.00
Moore,H.L.	00839-6233-53	120 ml	$8.22
ALA-CORT: Del-Ray	00316-0131-04	120 ml	$12.09
Glades	59366-2707-04	120 ml	$14.21
Qualitest	00603-7783-54	120 ml	$14.24

LOTION: 2.5%

AVERAGE UNIT PRICE (AVAILABLE SIZES)		GENERIC A-RATED AVERAGE PRICE (GAAP)	
BRAND	$0.32	15.70	$60 ML
GENERIC	$0.27		
HCFA FUL (60 ml)	$0.26		

BRAND/MANUFACTURER	NDC	SIZE	AWP
◆ BRAND			
NUTRACORT: Galderma	00299-5825-01	60 ml	$18.38
HYTONE: Dermik	00066-0098-02	60 ml	$24.92
NUTRACORT: Galderma	00299-5825-02	120 ml	$28.88
◆ GENERICS			
LACTICARE-HC: Stiefel	00145-2538-02	59 ml	$16.69
Qualitest	00603-7785-52	60 ml	$15.69
Glades	59366-2708-02	60 ml	$15.70

➤ SHOWN IN PRODUCT IDENTIFICATION GUIDE

OINTMENT: 1%

AVERAGE UNIT PRICE (AVAILABLE SIZES)		GENERIC A-RATED AVERAGE PRICE (GAAP)	
BRAND	$0.17	20 gm	$2.13
GENERIC	$0.09	30 gm	$2.89
HCFA FUL (20 gm)	$0.13	454 gm	$28.49
HCFA FUL (30 gm)	$0.09		
HCFA FUL (120 gm)	$0.06		
HCFA FUL (454 gm)	$0.05		

BRAND/MANUFACTURER	NDC	SIZE	AWP
◆ BRAND			
HYTONE: Dermik	00066-0087-01	30 gm	$9.83
HYDROCORTISONE 1% IN ABSORBASE: Carolina	46287-0003-16	454 gm	$29.82
	46287-0003-01	25 gm 12s	$56.25
	46287-0003-04	110 gm 12s	$106.65
◆ GENERICS			
Thames	49158-0103-07	20 gm	$1.90
Moore,H.L.	00839-5208-45	20 gm	$2.36
Thames	49158-0103-08	30 gm	$2.00
Major	00904-0751-31	30 gm	$2.25
Schein	00364-0785-56	30 gm	$2.25
NMC	23317-0326-28	30 gm	$2.36
Moore,H.L.	00839-5208-49	30 gm	$2.69
Moore,H.L.	00839-7722-49	30 gm	$2.69
Goldline	00182-0845-34	30 gm	$2.85
Fougera	00168-0020-31	30 gm	$2.92
Rugby	00536-0515-95	30 gm	$2.97
Goldline	00182-5061-34	30 gm	$3.15
C & M	00398-0050-01	30 gm	$5.70
Goldline	00182-5061-43	60 gm	$5.25
Moore,H.L.	00839-5208-53	120 gm	$7.14
Thames	49158-0103-16	454 gm	$21.60
Moore,H.L.	00839-5208-60	454 gm	$21.72
Rugby	00536-2570-98	454 gm	$23.27
Clay-Park	45802-0013-05	454 gm	$23.76
NMC	23317-0326-16	454 gm	$27.90
Fougera	00168-0020-16	454 gm	$27.97
C & M	00398-0050-16	454 gm	$53.22

OINTMENT: 2.5%

AVERAGE UNIT PRICE (AVAILABLE SIZES)		GENERIC A-RATED AVERAGE PRICE (GAAP)	
BRAND	$0.60	20 gm	$5.12
GENERIC	$0.24		
HCFA FUL (20 gm)	$0.27		

BRAND/MANUFACTURER	NDC	SIZE	AWP
◆ BRAND			
HYTONE: Dermik	00066-0085-01	30 gm	$17.99
◆ GENERICS			
Clay-Park	45802-0014-02	20 gm	$4.32
Schein	00364-7088-55	20 gm	$4.75
URL	00677-0724-38	20 gm	$4.90
Moore,H.L.	00839-5209-45	20 gm	$4.93
Rugby	00536-0620-99	20 gm	$5.88
Major	00904-0757-29	20 gm	$5.95
Clay-Park	45802-0014-05	454 gm	$58.32

SOLUTION: 1%

BRAND/MANUFACTURER	NDC	SIZE	AWP
◆ BRAND			
TEXACORT: Genderm	52761-0247-01	30 ml	$7.48

SOLUTION: 2.5%

BRAND/MANUFACTURER	NDC	SIZE	AWP
◆ BRAND			
TEXACORT: Genderm	52761-0293-01	30 ml	$14.40

HYDROCORTISONE BUTYRATE
CREAM: 0.1%

BRAND/MANUFACTURER	NDC	SIZE	AWP
○ BRAND			
LOCOID: Ferndale	00496-0802-15	15 gm	$11.95
	00496-0802-45	45 gm	$24.85

OINTMENT: 0.1%

BRAND/MANUFACTURER	NDC	SIZE	AWP
○ BRAND			
LOCOID: Ferndale	00496-0803-15	15 gm	$11.95
	00496-0803-45	45 gm	$24.85

SOLUTION: 0.1%

BRAND/MANUFACTURER	NDC	SIZE	AWP
○ BRAND			
LOCOID: Ferndale	00496-0804-20	20 ml	$17.65
	00496-0804-60	60 ml	$35.30

HYDROCORTISONE ACETATE
CREAM: 1%

AVERAGE UNIT PRICE (AVAILABLE SIZES)	
GENERIC	$0.18

BRAND/MANUFACTURER	NDC	SIZE	AWP
◆ GENERICS			
Thames	49158-0227-08	30 gm	$7.00
Thames	49158-0227-12	120 gm	$15.50

PASTE: 0.5%

Hydrocortisone/Neomycin Sulfate/Polymyxin B Sulfate

DESCRIPTION

Hydrocortisone/Neomycin Sulfate/Polymyxin B Sulfate is available as a sterile antimicrobial and anti-inflammatory suspension for ophthalmic use, suspension and solution for otic use, and a topical antibacterial cream.

Each ml of the ophthalmic suspension contains: Hydrocortisone 10 mg (1%), Neomycin Sulfate equivalent to 3.5 mg Neomycin buse, and Polymyxin B Sulfate 10,000 units.

Each gram of the cream contains: Hydrocortisone Acetate 5 mg (0.5%), Neomycin Sulfate equivalent to 3.5 mg Neomycin buse, and Polymyxin B Sulfate 10,000 units.

Each ml of the otic suspension contains hydrocortisone 10 mg (1%), Neomycin Sulfate equivalent to 3.5 mg Neomycin base, and Polymyxin B Sulfate equivalent ro 10,000 Polymyxin B units.

Hydrocortisone, 11β, 17, 21-trihydroxypregn-4-ene-3,20-dione, is an anti-inflammatory hormone. Hydrocortisone acetate is the acetate ester of Hydrocortisone, an anti-inflammatory hormone. Its chemical name is 21-(acetyloxy)-11β,17-dihydroxypregn-4-ene-3,20-dione.

Neomycin sulfate is the sulfate salt of neomycin B and C, which are produced by the growth of *Streptomyces fradiae* Waksman (Fam. Streptomycetaceae). It has a potency equivalent of not less than 600 μg of Neomycin standard per mg, calculated on an anhydrous basis.

Polymyxin B Sulfate is the sulfate salt of Polymyxin B_1 and B_2, which are produced by the growth of *Bacillus polymyxa* (Prazmowski) Migula (Fam. Bacillaceae). It has a potency of not less than 6,000 Polymyxin B units per mg, calculated on an anhydrous basis.

CLINICAL PHARMACOLOGY

Corticoids suppress the inflammatory response to a variety of agents and they may delay healing. Since corticoids may inhibit the body's defense mechanism against infection, a concomitant antimicrobial drug may be used when this inhibition is considered to be clinically significant in a particular case.

The anti-infective components in the combination are included to provide action against specific organisms susceptible to them. Polymyxin B Sulfate and Neomycin Sulfate together are considered active against the following microorganisms: *Staphylococcus aureus, Escherichia coli, Haemophilus influenzae, Klebsiella-Enterobacter* species, *Neisseria* species and *Pseudomonas aeruginosa.*

When used topically, Neomycin and Polymyxin B are rarely irritating, and absorption from the intact skin or mucous membrane is insignificant. The incidence of skin sensitization to this combination has been shown to be low on normal skin.[1,2] Since these antibiotics are seldom used systemically, the patient is spared sensitization to those antibiotics which might later be required systemically.

When a decision to administer both a corticoid and antimicrobials is made, the administration of such drugs in combination has the advantage of greater patient compliance and convenience, with the added assurance that the intended dosage of both drugs is administered, plus assured compatibility of ingredients when both types of drug are in the same formulation and, particularly that the intended volume of each drug is delivered simultaneously, thereby avoiding dilution of either medication by successive instillations.

The relative potency of corticosteroids depends on the molecular structure, concentration, and release from the vehicle.

The acid pH of the cream helps restore normal cutaneous acidity. Owing to its excellent spreading and penetrating properties, the cream facilitates treatment of hairy and intertriginous areas. It may also be of value in selective cases where the lesions are moist.

INDICATIONS AND USAGE

The ophthalmic suspension is indicated for steroid-responsive inflammatory ocular conditions for which a corticosteroid is indicated and where bacterial infection or a risk of bacterial ocular infection exists.

◆ RATED THERAPEUTICALLY EQUIVALENT; ◇ THERAPEUTIC EQUIVALENCE UNCONFIRMED; ○ UNRATED

Ocular steroids are indicated in inflammatory conditions of the palpebral and bulbar conjunctiva, cornea and anterior segment of the globe where the inherent risk of steroid use in certain infective conjunctivitides is accepted to obtain a diminution in edema and inflammation. They are also indicated in chronic anterior uveitis and corneal injury from chemical, radiation, or thermal burns, or penetration of foreign bodies. The use of a combination drug with an anti-infective component is indicated where the risk of infection is high or where there is an expectation that potentially dangerous numbers of bacteria will be present in the eye.

The particular anti-infective drugs in this product are active against the following common bacterial eye pathogens: *Staphylococcus aureus, Escherichia coli, Haemophilus influenzae, Klebsiella-Enterobacter* species, *Neisseria* species, and *Pseudomonas aeruginosa*.

The otic suspension and solution are indicated for the treatment of superficial bacterial infections of the external auditory canal caused by organisms susceptible to the action of the antibiotics. The otic suspension is also indicated for the treatment of infections of mastoidectomy and fenestration cavities caused by organisms susceptible to the antibiotics.

The cream is indicated for the treatment of corticosteroid-responsive dermatoses with secondary infection. It has not been demonstrated that this steroid-antibiotic combination provides greater benefit than the steroid component alone after 7 days of treatment (see *"Warnings"* section).

None of these formulations provides adequate coverage against *Serratia marcescens* and streptococci, including *Streptococcus pneumoniae*.

CONTRAINDICATIONS

The ophthalmic suspension is contraindicated in epithelial herpes simplex keratitis (dendritic keratitis), vaccinia, varicella, and many other viral diseases of the cornea and conjunctiva. Mycobacterial infection of the eye. Fungal diseases of ocular structures. The otic suspension and solution are contraindicated in herpes simplex, vaccinia, and varicella infections. The cream is contraindicated in tuberculous, fungal, or viral lesions of the skin (herpes simplex, vaccinia, and varicella). All formulations are contraindicated when there is hypersensitivity to a component of the medication. (Hypersensitivity to the antibiotic component occurs at a higher rate than for other components.)

The use of these combinations in the ophthalmic suspension is always contraindicated after uncomplicated removal of a corneal foreign body.

The cream is not for use in the eyes or in the external ear canal if the eardrum is perforated.

WARNINGS

Prolonged use may result in glaucoma, with damage to the optic nerve, defects in visual acuity and fields of vision, and posterior subcapsular cataract formation. Prolonged use may suppress the host response and thus increase the hazard of secondary ocular infections. In those diseases causing thinning of the cornea or sclera, perforations have been known to occur with the use of topical steroids. In acute purulent conditions of the eye, steroids may mask infection or enhance existing infection. If these products are used for 10 days or longer, intraocular pressure should be routinely monitored even though it may be difficult in children and uncooperative patients.

Employment of steroid medication in the treatment of herpes simplex requires great caution.

Neomycin Sulfate may cause cutaneous sensitization. A precise incidence of hypersensitivity reactions (primarily skin rash) due to topical Neomycin is not known.

When using Neomycin-containing products to control secondary infection in the chronic dermatoses, such as chronic otitis externa or stasis dermatitis, it should be borne in mind that the skin in these conditions is more liable than normal skin to become sensitized to many substances, including Neomycin. The manifestations of sensitization to neomycin are usually itching, reddening, dry scaling, and swelling. It may be manifest simply as a failure to heal. During long-term use of Neomycin-containing products, periodic examination for such signs is advisable, and the patient should be told to discontinue the product if they are observed. These symptoms subside quickly on withdrawing the medication.

Neomycin-containing applications should be avoided for the patient thereafter.

The otic suspension and solution should be used with care in cases of perforated eardrum or when the integrity of the tympanic membrane is in question and in longstanding cases of chronic otitis media because of the possibility of ototoxicity, and because stinging and burning may occur when this product gains access to the middle ear.

Some brands contain potassium metabisulfite, a sulfite that may cause allergic-type reactions including anaphylactic symptoms and life-threatening or less severe asthmatic episodes in certain susceptible people. The overall prevalence of sulfite sensitivity in the general population is unknown and probably low. Sulfite sensitivity is seen more frequently in asthmatic than in nonasthmatic people.

Because of the concern of nephrotoxicity and ototoxicity associated with Neomycin, this combination as a cream should not be used over a wide area or for extended periods of time.

PRECAUTIONS

General: The initial prescription and renewal of the ophthalmic suspension order beyond 20 milliliters should be made by a physician only after examination of the patient with the aid of magnification, such as slit lamp biomicroscopy and, where appropriate, fluorescein staining.

The possibility of persistent fungal infections of the cornea should be considered after prolonged steroid dosing.

As with other antibiotic preparations, prolonged use may result in overgrowth of nonsusceptible organisms, including fungi.

If the ear infection is not improved after one week, cultures and susceptibility tests should be repeated to verify the identity of the organism and to determine whether therapy should be changed. Treatment should not be continued for longer than ten days.

Appropriate measures should be taken if such infection occurs while using the cream. Use of steroids on infected areas should be supervised with care as anti-inflammatory steroids may encourage spread of infection. If this occurs, steroid therapy should be stopped and appropriate antibacterial drugs used. Generalized dermatological conditions may require systemic corticosteroid therapy.

Signs and symptoms of exogenous hyperadrenocorticism can occur with the use of topical corticosteroids, including adrenal suppression. Systemic absorption of topically applied steroids will be increased if extensive body surface areas are treated or if occlusive dressings are used. Under these circumstances, suitable precautions should be taken when long-term use is anticipated.

Allergic cross-reactions may occur which could prevent the use of any or all of the following antibiotics for the treatment of future infections: kanamycin, paromomycin, streptomycin, and possibly gentamicin.

Information for Patients: Avoid contaminating the otic suspension or solution dropper with material from the ear, fingers, or other source. This caution is necessary if the sterility of the drops is to be preserved. If sensitization or irritation occurs, discontinue use immediately and contact your physician.

Do not use the otic suspension or solution in the eyes.

If redness, irritation, swelling or pain persists or increases with use of the cream, discontinue use and notify physician. Do not use in the eyes.

Laboratory Tests: Systemic effects of excessive levels of Hydrocortisone may include a reduction in the number of circulating eosinophils and a decrease in urinary excretion of 17-hydroxycorticosteroids.

Carcinogenesis, Mutagenesis, Impairment of Fertility: Long-term studies in animals (rats, rabbits, mice) showed no evidence of carcinogenicity attributable to oral administration of corticosteroids.

Pregnancy: Teratogenic Effects: Pregnancy Category C. Corticosteroids have been shown to be teratogenic in rabbits when applied topically at concentrations of 0.5% on days 6-18 of gestation and in mice when applied topically at a concentration of 15% on days 10-13 of gestation. There are no adequate and well-controlled studies in pregnant women. Corticosteroids should be used during pregnancy only if the potential benefit justifies the potential risk to the fetus.

Nursing Mothers: Hydrocortisone appears in human milk following oral administration of the drug. Since systemic absorption of Hydrocortisone may occur when applied topically, caution should be exercised when Hydrocortisone/Neomycin Sulfate/Polymyxin B Sulfate ophthalmic suspension, otic suspension/solution, or cream is used by a nursing woman.

Pediatric Use: (See *"Dosage and Administration"*.)

Sufficient percutaneous absorption of Hydrocortisone can occur in infants and children during prolonged use to cause cessation of growth, as well as other systemic signs and symptoms of hyperadrenocorticism.

ADVERSE REACTIONS

Ophthalmic Suspension: Adverse reactions have occurred with steroid/anti-infective combination drugs which can be attributed to the steroid component, the anti-infective component, or the combination. Reactions occurring most often from the presence of the anti-infective ingredient are localized hypersensitivity, including itching, swelling and conjunctival erythema. Local irritation on instillation has also been reported. Exact incidence figures are not available since no denominator of treated patients is available.

The reactions due to the steroid component in decreasing order of frequency are: elevation of intraocular pressure (IOP) with possible development of glaucoma, and infrequent optic nerve damage; posterior subcapsular cataract formation; and delayed wound healing.

Secondary Infection: The development of secondary infection has occurred after use of combinations containing steroids and antimicrobials. Fungal infections of the cornea are particularly prone to develop coincidentally with long-term applications of steroid. The possibility of fungal invasion must be considered in any persistent corneal ulceration where steroid treatment has been used.

Secondary bacterial ocular infection following suppression of host responses also occurs.

Otic Suspension and Solution, Cream: Neomycin occasionally causes skin sensitization. Ototoxicity and nephrotoxicity have also been reported (see *"Warnings"* section.) Adverse reactions have occurred with topical use of antibiotic combinations including Neomycin and Polymyxin B. Exact incidence figures are not available since no denominator of treated patients is available. The reaction occurring most often is allergic sensitization. In one clinical study, using a 20% Neomycin patch, Neomycin-induced allergic skin reactions occurred in two of 2,175 (0.09%) individuals in the general population.[1] In another study, the incidence was found to be approximately 1%.[2]

The following local adverse reactions have been reported with topical corticosteroids, especially under occlusive dressings: burning, itching, irritation, dryness, folliculitis, hypertrichosis, acneiform eruptions, hypopigmentation, peri-oral dermatitis, allergic contact dermatitis, maceration of the skin, secondary infection, skin atrophy, striae and miliaria. Stinging and burning have been reported when this drug has gained access to the middle ear. When topical steroid preparations are used for long periods of time in intertriginous areas or over extensive body areas, with or without occlusive non-permeable dressings, striae may occur; also there exists the possibility of systemic side effects when steroid preparations are used over large areas or for a long period of time.

DOSAGE AND ADMINISTRATION

Ophthalmic Suspension: One or two drops in the affected eye every 3 or 4 hours, depending on the severity of the condition. The suspension may be used more frequently if necessary.

Not more than 20 milliliters should be prescribed initially and the prescription should not be refilled without further evaluation as outlined in *"Precautions"* above.

The Otic Suspension and Solution: The external auditory canal should be thoroughly cleansed and dried with a sterile cotton applicator.

For adults, 4 drops of the suspension or solution should be instilled into the affected ear 3 or 4 times daily.

For infants and children, 3 drops are suggested because of the smaller capacity of the ear canal.

The patient should lie with the affected ear upward and then the drops should be instilled. This position should be maintained for 5 minutes to facilitate penetration of the drops into the ear canal. Repeat, if necessary, for the opposite ear. If preferred, a cotton wick may be inserted into the canal and then the cotton may be saturated with the suspension. This wick should be kept moist by adding further suspension or solution every four hours. The wick should be replaced at least once every 24 hours.

SHAKE THE OPHTHALMIC AND OTIC SUSPENSIONS WELL BEFORE USING.

Cream: A small quantity of the cream should be applied 2 to 4 times daily, as required. The cream should, if conditions permit, be gently rubbed into the affected areas.

Storage: Store all formulations at 15°-25°C (59°-77°F).

REFERENCES

1. Leyden JJ and Kligman AM. Contact Dermatitis to Neomycin Sulfate. *JAMA 242 (12):* 1276-1278, 1979. 2. Prystowsky SD, Allen AM, Smith RW, Nonomura JH, Odom RB and Akers WA. Allergic Contact Hypersensitivity to Nickel, Neomycin, Ethylenediamine, and Benzocaine. *Arch Dermatol 115:* 959-962, 1979.

HOW SUPPLIED
CREAM:

BRAND/MANUFACTURER	NDC	SIZE	AWP
○ BRAND			
CORTISPORIN: Burr Wellcome	00081-0185-98	7.5 gm	$15.18

DROP:

AVERAGE UNIT PRICE (AVAILABLE SIZES)			
BRAND			$0.80

BRAND/MANUFACTURER	NDC	SIZE	AWP
◆ BRAND			
DROTIC: Ascher	00225-0340-55	10 ml	$7.50
EAR-EZE: Hyrex	00314-0020-10	10 ml	$8.40

DROP: 1%-0.35%-10,000 U/ML

AVERAGE UNIT PRICE (AVAILABLE SIZES)		GENERIC A-RATED AVERAGE PRICE (GAAP)	
BRAND	$1.94	7.5 ml	$10.02
GENERIC	$0.87	10 ml	$7.80
HCFA FUL (10 ml)	$0.45		

BRAND/MANUFACTURER	NDC	SIZE	AWP
◆ BRAND			
CORTISPORIN: Burr Wellcome	00081-0193-02	7.5 ml	$15.72
	00081-0198-92	10 ml	$18.65
	00081-0199-92	10 ml	$18.65
◆ GENERICS			
PHN-OTIC: Major	00904-7668-32	7.5 ml	$7.45
OTITRICIN: Bausch&Lomb Pharm	24208-0556-61	7.5 ml	$7.68
TRIPLE-GEN: Goldline	00182-7076-83	7.5 ml	$8.40
CORTOMYCIN: Major	00904-2994-32	7.5 ml	$8.95
AK-SPORE HC: Akorn	17478-0231-09	7.5 ml	$9.38
Steris	00402-0774-07	7.5 ml	$10.50
PEDIOTIC: Burr Wellcome	00081-0910-02	7.5 ml	$13.67
Aligen	00405-6130-07	7.5 ml	$14.21
MASPORIN OTIC: Mason Dist	11845-7080-02	10 ml	$3.12
CORTATRIGEN MODIFIED: Goldline	00182-1388-63	10 ml	$4.15
OCTICAIR: Bausch&Lomb Pharm	24208-0630-04	10 ml	$4.16
OCTICAIR: Bausch&Lomb Pharm	24208-0635-62	10 ml	$4.41
URL	00677-0680-21	10 ml	$4.50
MASPORIN OTIC: Mason Dist	11845-8950-02	10 ml	$6.00
Moore,H.L.	00839-6490-30	10 ml	$7.02
Steris	00402-0708-10	10 ml	$7.25
Schein	00364-7300-54	10 ml	$7.25
URL	00677-0874-21	10 ml	$7.35
OTIMAR: Marlop	12939-0205-05	10 ml	$7.45
OTOCORT: Lemmon	00093-0047-43	10 ml	$7.50
Moore,H.L.	00839-6664-90	10 ml	$7.55

BRAND/MANUFACTURER	NDC	SIZE	AWP
Geneva	00781-7409-70	10 ml	$7.70
Aligen	00405-6160-10	10 ml	$7.70
AK-SPORE HC: Akorn	17478-0236-11	10 ml	$7.81
Rugby	00536-4071-70	10 ml	$7.85
CORTOMYCIN: Major	00904-3017-10	10 ml	$7.90
CORTOMYCIN: Major	00904-3141-10	10 ml	$7.90
OTIMAR: Marlop	12939-0204-10	10 ml	$7.95
AK-SPORE HC: Akorn	17478-0237-11	10 ml	$8.13
Steris	00402-0736-10	10 ml	$8.75
Schein	00364-7374-54	10 ml	$8.75
OTIC CARE: Parmed	00349-8202-70	10 ml	$8.95
OTIC CARE EAR: Parmed	00349-8895-70	10 ml	$8.95
OTOCORT: Lemmon	00093-0363-43	10 ml	$9.00
Aligen	00405-6161-10	10 ml	$9.21
CORTATRIGEN: Goldline	00182-1563-63	10 ml	$9.90
OTIC EAR CARE: Parmed	00349-8894-70	10 ml	$10.99
Rugby	00536-4050-70	10 ml	$12.38
UAD OTIC: Forest Pharm	00785-9069-10	10 ml	$14.35

DROP: 1%-3.5 MG-10,000 U/ML

AVERAGE UNIT PRICE (AVAILABLE SIZES)		GENERIC A-RATED AVERAGE PRICE (GAAP)	
GENERIC	$1.29	7.5 ml	$9.08

BRAND/MANUFACTURER	NDC	SIZE	AWP
◆ GENERICS			
OCUTRICIN HC: Raway	00686-0526-61	7.5 ml	$6.70
Rugby	00536-2590-77	7.5 ml	$10.89
OCUTRICIN HC: Moore,H.L.	00839-7175-28	7.5 ml	$11.46

DROP: 3.5 MG-10,000 U-1%

BRAND/MANUFACTURER	NDC	SIZE	AWP
◆ GENERICS			
Schein	00364-0842-71	7.5 ml	$10.50

Hydrocortone *SEE* HYDROCORTISONE, SYSTEMIC

HydroDIURIL *SEE* HYDROCHLOROTHIAZIDE

Hydroflumethiazide

DESCRIPTION

Hydroflumethiazide is an oral thiazide (benzothiadiazide) diuretic-antihypertensive agent.

Hydroflumethiazide is available as 50 mg tablets for oral administration.

Chemical Name: 3,4-Dihydro-6-(trifluoromethyl)-2H-1,2,4-benzothiadiazine-7-sulfonamide 1,1-dioxide.

Hydroflumethiazide is an odorless white to cream-colored, finely divided, crystalline powder. It has a melting point between 270° and 275°C. Hydroflumethiazide is freely soluble in acetone, soluble in alcohol, and very slightly soluble in water.

Following is its chemical structure:

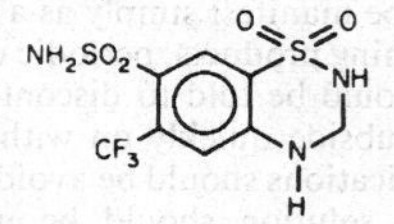

CLINICAL PHARMACOLOGY

Hydroflumethiazide is incompletely but fairly rapidly absorbed from the gastrointestinal tract. It appears to have a biphasic biological half-life with an estimated alpha-phase of about 2 hours and an estimated beta-phase of about 17 hours; it has a metabolite with a longer half-life, which is extensively bound to the red blood cells. Hydroflumethiazide is excreted in the urine; its metabolite has also been detected in the urine.

The mechanism of action results in an interference with the renal tubular mechanism of electrolyte reabsorption. At maximal therapeutic dosage, all thiazides are approximately equal in their diuretic potency. The mechanism whereby thiazides function in the control of hypertension is unknown.

INDICATIONS AND USAGE

Hydroflumethiazide is indicated as adjunctive therapy in edema associated with congestive heart failure, hepatic cirrhosis, and corticosteroid and estrogen therapy.

Hydroflumethiazide has also been found useful in edema due to various forms of renal dysfunction such as: nephrotic syndrome; acute glomerulonephritis; and chronic renal failure.

◆ RATED THERAPEUTICALLY EQUIVALENT; ◇ THERAPEUTIC EQUIVALENCE UNCONFIRMED; ○ UNRATED

Hydroflumethiazide is indicated in the management of hypertension either as the sole therapeutic agent or to enhance the effectiveness of other antihypertensive drugs in the more severe forms of hypertension.

USAGE IN PREGNANCY

The routine use of diuretics in an otherwise healthy woman is inappropriate and exposes mother and fetus to unnecessary hazard. Diuretics do not prevent development of toxemia of pregnancy, and there is no satisfactory evidence that they are useful in the treatment of developed toxemia.

Edema during pregnancy may arise from pathological causes or from the physiologic and mechanical consequences of pregnancy. Thiazides are indicated in pregnancy when edema is due to pathologic causes just as they are in the absence of pregnancy (however, see *"Precautions—Pregnancy"* below). Dependent edema in pregnancy, resulting from restriction of venous return by the expanded uterus, is properly treated through elevation of the lower extremities and use of support hose. Use of diuretics to lower intravascular volume in this case is illogical and unnecessary. There is hypervolemia during normal pregnancy which is harmful to neither the fetus nor the mother (in the absence of cardiovascular disease), but which is associated with edema, including generalized edema, in the majority of pregnant women. If this edema produces discomfort, increased recumbency will often provide relief. In rare instances, this edema may cause extreme discomfort which is not relieved by rest. In these cases, a short course of diuretics may provide relief and may be appropriate.

UNLABELED USES
Hydroflumethiazide is used as an adjunct in the treatment of diabetes insipidus.

CONTRAINDICATIONS
Anuria.
Hypersensitivity to this or other sulfonamide-derived drugs.

WARNINGS
Hydroflumethiazide should be used with caution in severe renal disease. In patients with renal disease, thiazides may precipitate azotemia. Cumulative effects of the drug may develop in patients with impaired renal function.

Thiazides should be used with caution in patients with impaired hepatic function or progressive liver disease, since minor alterations of fluid and electrolyte balance may precipitate hepatic coma.

Thiazides may add to or potentiate the action of other antihypertensive drugs. Potentiation occurs with ganglionic or peripheral adrenergic blocking drugs.

Sensitivity reactions may occur in patients with a history of allergy or bronchial asthma.

The possibility of exacerbation or activation of systemic lupus erythematosus has been reported.

PRECAUTIONS
GENERAL
All patients receiving thiazide therapy should be observed for clinical signs of fluid or electrolyte imbalance; namely, hyponatremia, hypochloremic alkalosis, and hypokalemia. Serum and urine electrolyte determinations are particularly important when the patient is vomiting excessively or receiving parenteral fluids. Medication such as digitalis may also influence serum electrolytes. Warning signs, irrespective of cause, are: dryness of mouth, thirst, weakness, lethargy, drowsiness, restlessness, muscle pains or cramps, muscular fatigue, hypotension, oliguria, tachycardia, and gastrointestinal disturbances such as nausea and vomiting.

Hypokalemia may develop with thiazides as with any other potent diuretic, especially with brisk diuresis, when severe cirrhosis is present, or during concomitant use of corticosteroids or ACTH.

Interference with adequate oral electrolyte intake will also contribute to hypokalemia. Digitalis therapy may exaggerate metabolic effects of hypokalemia, especially with reference to myocardial activity.

Any chloride deficit is generally mild and usually does not require specific treatment except under extraordinary circumstances (as in liver disease or renal disease). Dilutional hyponatremia may occur in edematous patients in hot weather; appropriate therapy is water restriction, rather than administration of salt, except in rare instances when the hyponatremia is life-threatening. In actual salt depletion, appropriate replacement is the therapy of choice.

Hyperuricemia may occur or frank gout may be precipitated in certain patients receiving thiazide therapy.

Insulin requirements in diabetic patients may be increased, decreased, or unchanged. Latent diabetes mellitus may become manifested during thiazide administration.

The antihypertensive effects of the drug may be enhanced in the postsympathectomy patient.

If progressive renal impairment becomes evident, as indicated by a rising creatinine or blood urea nitrogen, a careful reappraisal of therapy is necessary with consideration given to withholding or discontinuing diuretic therapy.

Thiazides may decrease serum PBI levels without signs of thyroid disturbance.

Lithium generally should not be given with diuretics because they reduce its renal clearance and increase the risk of lithium toxicity. Read circulars for lithium preparations before use of such concomitant therapy with Hydroflumethiazide.

Thiazides have been shown to increase the urinary excretion of magnesium; this may result in hypomagnesemia.

Calcium excretion is decreased by thiazides. Pathological changes in the parathyroid gland with hypercalcemia and hypophosphatemia have been observed in a few patients on prolonged thiazide therapy. The common complica-

tions of hyperparathyroidism, such as renal lithiasis, bone resorption, and peptic ulceration, have not been seen.

INFORMATION FOR PATIENTS
This medicine may cause a loss of potassium from your body. To help prevent this, your doctor may want you to:
■ eat or drink foods that have a high potassium content (for example, orange or other citrus fruit juices), or
■ take a potassium supplement, or
■ take another medicine to help prevent the loss of the potassium in the first place.
It is very important to follow these directions. Also, it is important not to change your diet on your own. This is more important if you are already on a special diet (as for diabetes), or if you are taking a potassium supplement or a medicine to reduce potassium loss. Extra potassium may not be necessary and, in some cases, too much potassium could be harmful.

Check with your doctor if you become sick and have severe or continuing vomiting or diarrhea. These problems may cause you to lose additional water and potassium.

Caution Diabetics: Thiazide diuretics may raise blood sugar levels. While you are using this medicine, be especially careful in testing for sugar in your urine. If you have any questions about this, check with your doctor.

A few people who take this medicine may become more sensitive to sunlight than they are normally. When you begin to take this medicine, avoid too much sun or use of a sunlamp until you see how you react, especially if you tend to burn easily. If you have a severe reaction, check with your doctor.

For patients taking this medicine for high blood pressure:
■ *Do not take other medicines unless they have been discussed with your doctor.* This especially includes over-the-counter (nonprescription) medicines for appetite control, asthma, colds, cough, hay fever, or sinus.
Abstracted from USP DI "Advice for the Patient" ©1984 USP Convention.

LABORATORY TESTS
Periodic determination of serum electrolytes to detect possible electrolyte imbalance should be performed at appropriate intervals.

DRUG INTERACTIONS
Anticoagulants, oral (Effects may be decreased when used concurrently with thiazide diuretics; dosage adjustments may be necessary.)

Antigout medications (Thiazide diuretics may raise the level of blood uric acid; dosage adjustment of antigout medications may be necessary to control hyperuricemia and gout.)

Antihypertensive medications, other, especially diazoxide, or preanes- thetic and anesthetic agents used in surgery or skeletal muscle relaxants, nondepolarizing, used in surgery (Effects may be potentiated when used concurrently with thiazide diuretics; dosage adjustments may be necessary.)

Amphotericin B or Corticosteroids or Corticotropin (ACTH) (Concurrent use with thiazide diuretics may intensify electrolyte imbalance, particularly hypokalemia.)

Cardiac glycosides (Concurrent use with thiazide diuretics may enhance the possibility of digitalis toxicity associated with hypokalemia.)

Colestipol (May inhibit gastrointestinal absorption of the thiazide diuretics; administration 1 hour before or 4 hours after colestipol is recommended.)

Hypoglycemics (Thiazide diuretics may raise blood glucose levels; for adult-onset diabetics, dosage adjustment of hypoglycemic medications may be necessary during and after thiazide diuretic therapy; insulin requirements may be increased, decreased, or unchanged.)

Lithium salts (Concurrent use with thiazide diuretics is not recommended, as they may provoke lithium toxicity because of reduced renal clearance.)

Methenamine (Effectiveness may be decreased when used concurrently with thiazide diuretics because of alkalinization of the urine.)

Nonsteroidal anti-inflammatory agents (In some patients, the steroidal anti-inflammatory agent can reduce the diuretic, natriuretic, and antihypertensive effects of loop, potassium sparing, and thiazide diuretics. Therefore, when hydroflumethiazide and nonsteroidal anti-inflammatory agents are used concomitantly, the patient should be observed closely to determine if the desired effect of the diuretic is obtained.)

Norepinephrine (Thiazides may decrease arterial responsiveness to norepinephrine. This diminution is not sufficient to preclude effectiveness of the pressor agent for therapeutic use.)

Tubocurarine (Thiazide drugs may increase the responsiveness to tubocurarine.)

DIAGNOSTIC INTERFERENCE
With expected physiologic effects:

Blood and urine glucose levels (usually only in patients with a predisposition for glucose imbalance) and
Serum bilirubin levels (by displacement from albumin binding) and
Serum calcium levels (thiazide diuretics should be discontinued before parathyroid-function tests are carried out) and
Serum uric acid levels (may be increased)

Serum magnesium, potassium, and sodium levels (may be decreased; serum magnesium levels may increase in uremic patients)
Serum protein-bound iodine (PBI) levels (may be decreased)
Thiazides should be discontinued before carrying out tests for parathyroid function (see *"Precautions—General, Calcium Excretion"*).

CARCINOGENESIS, MUTAGENESIS, IMPAIRMENT OF FERTILITY

No studies have been performed to evaluate carcinogenic or mutagenic potential of Hydroflumethiazide or the potential of Hydroflumethiazide to impair fertility.

PREGNANCY

Teratogenic Effects—Pregnancy Category C: Animal reproduction studies have not been conducted with Hydroflumethiazide. It is also not known whether Hydroflumethiazide can cause fetal harm when administered to a pregnant woman or can affect reproduction capacity. Hydroflumethiazide should be given to a pregnant woman only if clearly needed.

Nonteratogenic Effects: Fetal or neonatal jaundice, thrombocytopenia, and possibly other adverse reactions which have occurred in the adult.

NURSING MOTHERS

Thiazides appear in breast milk. If use of the drug is deemed essential, the patient may consider stopping nursing.

PEDIATRIC USE

Safety and effectiveness in children have not been established.

ADVERSE REACTIONS

The following adverse reactions have been observed, but there is not enough systematic collection of data to support an estimate of their frequency.

GASTROINTESTINAL SYSTEM

Anorexia, gastric irritation, nausea, vomiting, cramping, diarrhea, constipation, jaundice (intrahepatic cholestatic jaundice), pancreatitis, sialadenitis.

CENTRAL NERVOUS SYSTEM

Dizziness, vertigo, paresthesias, headache, xanthopsia.

HEMATOLOGIC

Leukopenia, agranulocytosis, thrombocytopenia, aplastic anemia, hemolytic anemia.

CARDIOVASCULAR

Orthostatic hypotension (may be aggravated by alcohol, barbiturates, or narcotics).

DERMATOLOGIC—HYPERSENSITIVITY

Purpura, photosensitivity, rash, urticaria, necrotizing angiitis (vasculitis, cutaneous vasculitis), fever, respiratory distress including pneumonitis, anaphylactic reactions.

OTHER

Hyperglycemia, glycosuria, hyperuricemia, muscle spasm, weakness, restlessness, transient blurred vision.

Whenever adverse reactions are moderate or severe, thiazide dosage should be reduced or therapy withdrawn.

OVERDOSAGE

SIGNS AND SYMPTOMS

Diuresis, lethargy progressing to coma, with minimal cardiorespiratory depression and with or without significant serum electrolyte changes or dehydration; GI irritation; hypermotility; transient elevation in BUN level.

TREATMENT

Empty stomach by gastric lavage, taking care to avoid aspiration. Monitor serum electrolyte levels and renal function, and institute supportive measures, as required to maintain hydration, electrolyte balance, respiration, and cardiovascular and renal function. Treat GI effects symptomatically.

DOSAGE AND ADMINISTRATION

The average adult diuretic dose is 25 to 200 mg per day. The average adult antihypertensive dose is 50 to 100 mg per day.

Therapy should be individualized according to patient response. This therapy should be titrated to gain maximal response as well as the minimal dose possible to maintain that therapeutic response.

Store at room temperature (approximately 25° C)

HOW SUPPLIED
TABLETS: 50 MG

AVERAGE UNIT PRICE (AVAILABLE SIZES)

BRAND		$0.48		
BRAND/MANUFACTURER		NDC	SIZE	AWP
◆ BRAND				
DIUCARDIN: Wyeth-Ayerst		00046-0702-81	100s	$42.88
SALURON: Roberts Pharm		00015-5410-60	100s	$53.04

Hydroflumethiazide with Reserpine

> **WARNING**
>
> THIS FIXED COMBINATION DRUG IS NOT INDICATED FOR INITIAL THERAPY OF HYPERTENSION. HYPERTENSION REQUIRES THERAPY TITRATED TO THE INDIVIDUAL PATIENT. IF THE FIXED COMBINATION REPRESENTS THE DOSAGE SO DETERMINED, ITS USE MAY BE MORE CONVENIENT IN PATIENT MANAGEMENT. THE TREATMENT OF HYPERTENSION IS NOT STATIC, BUT MUST BE REEVALUATED AS CONDITIONS IN EACH PATIENT WARRANT.

DESCRIPTION

Hydroflumethiazide/Reserpine is a combination of two antihypertensive agents. The chemical name for Hydroflumethiazide is 3,4-dihydro-7-sulfamyl-6-trifluoro-methyl-2H-1,2,4-benzothiadiazine-1,1-dioxide. Hydroflumethiazide is very slightly soluble in water, soluble in methanol and freely soluble in acetone.

Reserpine (3,4,5-trimethoxybenzoyl methyl reserpate) is a crystalline alkaloid derived from rauwolfia serpentina. It is very slightly soluble in water, slightly soluble in acetone, methanol and ethanol and freely soluble in chloroform and methylene chloride.

Two available combinations contain the following:

Hydroflumethiazide	50 mg
Reserpine	0.125 mg
Hydroflumethiazide	25 mg
Reserpine	0.125 mg

CLINICAL PHARMACOLOGY

Hydroflumethiazide is incompletely but fairly rapidly absorbed from the gastrointestinal tract. It appears to have a biphasic biological half-life with an estimated alpha-phase of about 2 hours and an estimated beta-phase of about 17 hours; it has a metabolite with a longer half-life, which is extensively bound to the red blood cells. Hydroflumethiazide is excreted in the urine; its metabolite has also been detected in the urine.

Hydroflumethiazide is an oral diuretic-antihypertensive agent. It exerts its effect by inhibiting renal tubular reabsorption, including increased excretion of sodium and chloride and water with variable concomitant loss of potassium and bicarbonate as well. When used alone as an antihypertensive agent, Hydroflumethiazide usually induces a gradual but sustained decrease in abnormally elevated blood-pressure—both systolic and diastolic. Hypertensive patients who have been maintained on chlorothiazide or hydrochlorothiazide may also be maintained on Hydroflumethiazide.

Reserpine is absorbed from the gastrointestinal tract. About 6% has been reported to be excreted in the urine in the first 24 hours and about 8% in the first 4 days, mainly as the metabolite trimethyoxybenzoic acid. Over 60% is excreted in the faeces in the first 4 days, mainly unchanged. Reserpine crosses the placental barrier and also appears in breast milk.

The component, reserpine, probably produces its antihypertensive effects through depletion of tissue stores of catecholamines (epinephrine and norepinephrine) from peripheral sites. By contrast, its sedative and tranquilizing properties are thought to be related to depletion of 5-hydroxytryptamine from the brain.

Reserpine is characterized by slow onset of action and sustained effect. Both its cardiovascular and central nervous system effects may persist following withdrawal of the drug.

Careful observation for changes in blood pressure must be made when Hydroflumethiazide/Reserpine is used with other antihypertensive drugs.

INDICATIONS AND USAGE

Hypertension (see box *"Warning"*).

CONTRAINDICATIONS

Hydroflumethiazide/Reserpine is contraindicated in patients with a history of mental depression because of the possibility that it will potentiate depression and increase the possibility of suicide or in patients who have previously demonstrated hypersensitivity to its components. Patients with anuria or oliguria should not be given this medication. The presence of an active peptic ulcer, ulcerative colitis or depression contraindicates the use of reserpine. If electroshock therapy

---

◆ RATED THERAPEUTICALLY EQUIVALENT; ◇ THERAPEUTIC EQUIVALENCE UNCONFIRMED; ○ UNRATED

is necessary, treatment with Hydroflumethiazide/Reserpine should be discontinued at least seven (7) days prior to this therapy.

WARNINGS

Azotemia may be precipitated or increased by Hydroflumethiazide. Special caution is necessary in patients with impaired renal function to avoid cumulative or toxic effects.

Since in hepatic cirrhosis, minor alterations of fluid and electrolyte balance may precipitate coma, Hydroflurmethiazide should be given with caution.

The possibility of sensitivity reactions should be considered in patients with a history of allergy or bronchial asthma.

Hydroflumethiazide potentiates the action of other antihypertensive drugs. Therefore, the dosage of these agents, especially the ganglion blockers, must be reduced by at least 50 percent as soon as Hydroflumethiazide is added to the regimen.

The possibility of exacerbation or activation of systemic lupus erythematosus has been reported for sulfonamide derivatives (including thiazides) and reserpine.

Reserpine may cause mental depression. Recognition of depression may be difficult because depression may often be disguised by somatic complaints (Masked Depression). The drug should be discontinued at first signs of depression such as despondency, early morning insomnia, loss of appetite, impotence, or self-deprecation. Drug-induced depression may persist for several months after drug withdrawal and may be severe enough to result in suicide.

PRECAUTIONS

GENERAL

Hydroflumethiazide/Reserpine is a combination of these individual components. Precautions to be observed are associated with each component and are listed below.

HYDROFLUMETHIAZIDE

Careful check should be kept for signs of fluid and electrolyte imbalance. Serum and urine electrolyte determinations are particularly important when the patient is vomiting excessively or receiving parenteral fluids. Warning signs, irrespective of cause, are: dryness of mouth, thirst, weakness, lethargy, drowsiness, restlessness, muscle pains or cramps, muscular fatigue, hypotension, oliguria, tachycardia, and gastrointestinal disturbances.

Potassium excretion is usually minimal. However, hypokalemia may develop with Hydroflumethiazide as with any other potent diuretic, especially with brisk diuresis, when severe cirrhosis is present, or during concomitant use of steroids of ACTH. Interference with adequate electrolyte intake will contribute to hypokalemia. Digitalis therapy may exaggerate metabolic effects of hypokalemia especially with reference to myocardial activity. If dietary salt is unduly restricted, especially during hot weather, in severely edematous patients with congestive failure or renal disease, a low salt syndrome may complicate therapy with thiazides.

Hypokalemia may be avoided or treated by use of potassium chloride or giving foods with a high potassium content. Any chloride deficit may similarly be corrected by use of ammonium chloride (excepting patients with hepatic disease) and largely prevented by a near normal salt intake.

Thiazide drugs may increase the responsiveness to tubocurarine. The antihypertensive effect of the drug may be enhanced in the postsympathectomy patient. Hydroflumethiazide decreases arterial responsiveness to norepinephrine, as do other thiazoles, necessitating due care in surgical patients. It is recommended that thiazides be discontinued 48 hours before elective surgery. Orthostatic hypotension may occur and may be potentiated by alcohol, barbiturates, or narcotics.

Pathological changes in the parathyroid glands with hypercalcemia and hypophosphatemia have been observed in a few patients on prolonged thiazide therapy. The common complications of hyperparathyroidism such as renal lithiasis, bone resorption, and peptic ulceration have not been seen. The effect of discontinuance of thiazide therapy on serum calcium and phosphorus levels may be helpful in assessing the need for parathyroid surgery in such patients. Parathyroidectomy has been followed by subjective clinical improvement in most patients, but is without effect on the hypertension. Following surgery, thiazide therapy may be resumed.

Caution is necessary in patients with hyperuricemia or a history of gout, since gout may be precipitated. Insulin requirements in diabetic patients may be increased, decreased, or unchanged. In latent diabetics, Hydroflumethiazide, in common with other benzothiadiazines, may cause hyperglycemia and glycosuria.

RESERPINE

Since Reserpine may increase gastric secretion and motility, it should be used cautiously in patients with a history of peptic ulcer, ulcerative colitis, or other gastrointestinal disorders. This compound may precipitate biliary colic in patients with gallstones, or bronchial asthma in susceptible persons.

Reserpine may cause hypotension including orthostatic hypotension. In hypertensive patients on Reserpine therapy significant hypotension and bradycardia may develop during surgical anesthesia. Therefore, the drug should be discontinued two weeks before giving anesthesia. For emergency surgical procedures, it may be necessary to give vagal blocking agents parenterally to prevent or reverse hypotension and/or bradycardia.

Anxiety or depression, as well as psychosis, may develop during Reserpine therapy. If depression is present when therapy is begun, it may be aggravated. Mental depression is unusual with Reserpine doses of 0.25 mg daily or less. In any case, Hydroflumethiazide/Reserpine should be discontinued at the first sign of depression.

As with most antihypertensive therapy, caution should be exercised when treating hypertensive patients with renal insufficiency, since they adjust poorly to lowered blood pressure levels. Use Reserpine cautiously with digitalis and quinione: cardiac arrhythmias have occurred with Reserpine preparations. Thiazides may decrease serum P.B.I. levels without signs of thyroid disturbance.

LABORATORY TESTS

Determination of serum electrolytes to detect possible electrolyte imbalance should be performed at appropriate intervals.

DRUG INTERACTIONS

RESERPINE

Alcohol or CNS depressants (concurrent use may enhance the CNS depressant effects of either these medications or rauwolfia alkaloids).

Antihypertensives, other, or diuretics (antihypertensive effects may be potentiated when used concurrently with rauwolfia alkaloids: although some combinations are frequently used for therapeutic advantage, when used concurrently, dosage adjustments may be necessary)

Beta-blockers (concurrent administration with beta-blockers may result in additive and possible excessive beta-adrenergic blockade. Although this effect is largely theoretical, close observation is recommended)

Digitalis glycosides or quinidine (concurrent use may result in cardiac arrhythmias; although this interaction is controversial and does not appear to be significant with usual doses, caution is recommended, especially when large doses of rauwolfia alkaloids are used in digitalized patients)

Levodopa (since rauwolfia alkaloids may cause dopamine depletion and parkinsonism effects, concurrent use is not recommended)

Methotrimeprazine (concurrent use may result in additive hypotension)

Monoamine oxidase (MAO) inhibitors (concurrent use with rauwolfia alkaloids may result in moderate to sudden and severe hypertension and hyperpyrexia which can reach crisis levels)

Sympathomimetics, indirect-acting amines such as amphetamines, ephedrine, methylphenidate, phenylpropanolamine, pseudoephedrine, tyramine (rauwolfia alkaloids inhibit the action of indirect-acting sympathomimetics by depleting catecholamine stores)

Direct-acting amines such as epinephrine, isoproterenol, and norepinephrine (levarterenol). Included are metaraminol and phenylephrine which are thought to act both directly and indirectly (rauwolfia alkaloids may theoretically prolong the action of direct-acting sympathomimetics by preventing uptake into storage granules: a "denervation supersensitivity" response is also possible; although concurrent use with rauwolfia alkaloids is not known to produce severe adverse effects, a significant increase in blood pressure has been documented when phenylephrine ophthalmic drops have been administered to patients taking Reserpine, and caution and close observation are recommended)

Tricyclic antidepressants (concurrent use may decrease the hypotensive effects of rauwolfia alkaloids and interfere with the antidepressant effects of these medications)

HYDROFLUMETHIAZIDE

Other antihypertensive medications, especially diazoxide, or
Preanesthetic and anesthetic agents used in surgery or
Skeletal muscle relaxants, nondepolarizing, used in surgery (effects may be potentiated when used concurrently with thiazide diuretics: dosage adjustments may be necessary)

Amphotericin B or
Corticosteroids or
Corticotropin (ACTH) (concurrent use with thiazide diuretics may intensify electrolyte imbalance, particularly hypokalemia)

Cardiac glycosides (concurrent use with thiazide diuretics may enhance the possibility of digitalis toxicity associated with hypokalemia)

Colestipol (may inhibit gastrointestinal absorption of the thiazide diuretics; administration 1 hour before or 4 hours after colestipol is recommended)

Hypoglycemics (thiazide diuretics may raise blood glucose levels; for adult onset diabetics, dosage adjustment of hypoglycemic medications may be necessary during and after thiazide diuretic therapy; insulin requirements may be increased, decreased, or unchanged)

Lithium salts (concurrent use with thiazide diuretics is not recommended, as they may provoke lithium toxicity because of reduced renal clearance)

Methenamine (effectiveness may be decreased when used concurrently with thiazide diuretics because of alkalinization of the urine)

Nonsteroidal anti-inflammatories (in some patients, the administration of a nonsteroidal anti-inflammatory agent can reduce the diuretic, natriuretic and antihypertensive effects of loop, potassium-sparing and thiazide diuretics. Therefore, when Hydroflurethiazide/Reserpine and nonsteroidal anti-inflammatory agents are used concomitantly, the patient should be observed closely to determine if the desired effect of the diuretic is obtained.)

DIAGNOSTIC INTERFERENCE

RESERPINE

With diagnostic test results

Urinary steroid colorimetric determinations by modified Glenn-Nelson technique or Holtorff Koch modification of Zimmerman reaction (falsely low because rauwolfia alkaloids slightly decrease absorbance)

With expected physiologic effects

Serum prolactin levels (may be increased)

Urinary catecholamine excretion (large parenteral doses of reserpine may cause an initial increase, although an overall decrease is usually noted with chronic administration of rauwolfia alkaloids)

Urinary vanilmandelic acid (VMA) excretion (intramuscular administration of reserpine causes an initial increase of about 40%, followed by a decrease by the end of the second day; chronic or parenteral administration of rauwolfia alkaloids results in an overall decrease)

HYDROFLUMETHIAZIDE
With expected physiologic effects

Blood and urine glucose levels (usually only in patients with a predisposition to glucose intolerance) and

Serum bilirubin levels (by displacement from albumin binding) and

Serum calcium levels (thiazide diuretics should be discontinued before parathyroid function tests are carried out) and

Serum uric acid levels (may be increased)

Serum magnesium, potassium, and sodium levels (may be decreased; serum magnesium levels may increase in uremic patients)

Serum protein-bound iodine (PBI) levels (may be decreased)

ANIMAL TUMORIGENICITY
Rodent studies have shown that Reserpine is an animal tumorigen, causing an increased incidence of mammary fibroadenomas in female mice, malignant tumors of the seminal vesicals in male mice, and malignant adrenal medullary tumors in male rats. These findings arose in 2 year studies in which the drug was administered in the feed at concentrations of 5 and 10 ppm — about 100 to 300 times the usual human dose. The breast neoplasms are thought to be related to Reserpine's prolactin-elevating effect. Several other prolactin-elevating drugs have also been associated with an increased incidence of mammary neoplasma in rodents.

The extent to which these findings indicate a risk to humans is uncertain. Tissue culture experiments show that about one-third of human breast tumors are prolactin-dependent *in vitro*, a factor of considerable importance if the use of the drug is contemplated in a patient with previously detected breast cancer. The possibility of an increased risk of breast cancer in Reserpine users has been studied extensively; however, no firm conclusion has emerged. Although a few epidemiologic studies have suggested a slightly increased risk (less than two-fold in all studies except one) in women who have used Reserpine, other studies of generally similar design have not confirmed this. Epidemiologic studies conducted using other drugs (neuroleptic agents) that, like Reserpine, increase prolactin levels and therefore would be considered rodent mammary carcinogens, have not shown an association between chronic administration of the drug and human mammary tumorigenesis. While long term clinical observation has not suggested such an association, the available evidence is considered too limited to be conclusive at this time. An association of Reserpine intake with pheochromocytoma or tumors of the seminal vesicles has not been explored.

PREGNANCY
Teratogenic Effects: Pregnancy Category C—Animal reproduction studies have not been conducted with Hydroflumethiazide/Reserpine. It is also not known whether Hydroflumethiazide/Reserpine can cause fetal harm when administered to a pregnant woman or can affect reproduction capacity. Hydroflumethiazide/Reserpine should be given to a pregnant woman only if clearly indicated.

Nonteratogenic Effects: There is some evidence that side effects such as nasal congestion, lethargy, depressed Moro reflex, and bradycardia may appear in infants born of Reserpine treated mothers. Thiazides cross the placental barrier and appear in cord blood. When Hydroflumethiazide/Reserpine is used in women of childbearing age, the potential benefits of the drug should be weighed against the possible hazards to the fetus. These hazards included fetal or neonatal jaundice, thrombocytopenia, and possibly other adverse reactions which have occurred in the adult.

NURSING MOTHERS
Thiazides and Reserpine appear in breast milk. If use of the drug is deemed essential, the mother may consider stopping nursing.

PEDIATRIC USE
Safety and effectiveness in children have not been established.

ADVERSE REACTIONS
The following adverse reactions have been observed, but there is not enough systematic collection of data to support an estimate of their frequency.

HYDROFLUMETHIAZIDE
A. *Gastrointestinal System Reactions:* anorexia, gastric irritation, nausea, vomiting, cramping, diarrhea, constipation, jaundice (intrahepatic cholestatic jaundice), pancreatitis, hyperglycemia, and glycosuria.

B. *Central Nervous System Reactions:* dizziness, vertigo, paresthesias, headache, and xanthopsia.

C. *Hematologic Reactions:* leukopenia, thrombocytopenia, agranulocytosis, and aplastic anemia.

D. *Dermatologic-Hypersensitivity Reactions:* purpura, photosensitivity, rash, urticaria, and necrotizing angiitis (vasculitis) (cutaneous vasculitus).

E. *Cardiovascular Reaction:* orthostatic hypotension may occur and may be aggravated by alcohol, barbiturates or narcotics.

F. *Miscellaneous:* muscle spasm, weakness, restlessness, fever, respiratory distress including pneumonitis, pulmonary edema and anaphylactic reactions.

Whenever adverse reactions are moderate or severe, thiazole dosage should be reduced or therapy withdrawn.

RESERPINE
A. *Gastrointestinal System Reactions:* anorena, nausea, increased intestinal motility, diarrhea, dryness of the mouth, increased salivation, vomiting.

B. *Central Nervous System Reactions:* excessive sedation, nightmares, headaches, dizziness, blurred vision, syncope, impotence or decreased libido, mental depression, nervousness, paradoxical anxiety, dull sensorium, deafness, glaucoma, uveitis, optic atrophy, Parkinsonian-like syndrome.

C. *Hematologic Reactions:* epistaxis, purpura due to thrombocytopenia.

D. *Dermatological Reactions:* conjunctival injection, flushing of the skin, pruritus, rash.

E. *Cardiovascular Reactions:* bradycardia, dyspnea, angina pectoris and other direct cardiac effects (e.g. premature ventricular contractions, fluid retention, congestive failure).

F. *Miscellaneous:* nasal congestion, weight gain, muscular aches, enhanced susceptibility to colds, dysuria, non-puerperal lactation.

OVERDOSAGE
SIGNS AND SYMPTOMS
Hydroflumethiazide-related Effects: diuresis, lethargy progressing to coma with minimal cardiorespiratory depression, GI irritation, hypermotility, elevated BUN, serum electrolyte changes.

Reserpine-related Effects: impairment of consciousness ranging from drowsiness to coma, flushing, conjunctival injection, miosis, hypotension, hypothermia, respiratory depression, bradycardia, diarrhea.

TREATMENT
Induce emesis or use gastric lavage, followed by activated charcoal, to empty stomach. Treat hypotension by volume expansion, if possible. If a vasopressor is needed, use phenylephrine, levarterenol, or metarminol. Treat significant bradycardia with vagal blocking agents, along with other appropriate measures. Monitor serum electrolytes and renal function, and institute supportive measures, as required. Treat GI effects symptomatically. Observe patient for at least 72 hours.

DIALYZABILITY
There is no information available on the dialyzability of Reserpine and Hydroflumethiazide.

DOSAGE AND ADMINISTRATION
As determined by individual titration (see box warning)

The usual adult dose of Hydroflumethiazide 50 mg/Reserpine 0.125 mg is one tablet once or twice daily if a smaller amount of thiazide diuretic is desired. Hydroflumethiazide 25 mg/Reserpine 0.125 mg, one tablet once or twice daily, can be given. Most patients will respond to this dosage level. In cases where a patient has been previously titrated to a higher dose of Reserpine than that contained in 1 or 2 tablets of Hydroflumethiazide 50mg/Reserpine 0.125mg, Reserpine should be added as the single entity alone. Doses of Hydroflumethiazide greater than 100 mg a day can significantly increase the incidence of hypokalemia and other adverse effects without any evidence that such doses increase the antihypertensive efficacy of the combination.

Store below 86°F (30°C).

HOW SUPPLIED
TABLETS: 25 MG-0.125 MG

BRAND/MANUFACTURER	NDC	SIZE	AWP
◇ BRAND			
SALUTENSIN-DEMI: Roberts Pharm	00015-5455-60	100s	$72.39

TABLETS: 50 MG-0.125 MG

BRAND/MANUFACTURER	NDC	SIZE	AWP
◇ BRAND			
SALUTENSIN: Roberts Pharm	00015-5436-60	100s	$93.05
	00015-5436-90	1000s	$902.99

Hydromorphone Hydrochloride

DESCRIPTION
Hydromorphone Hydrochloride (*"Warning"*: May be habit forming), a hydrogenated ketone of morphine, is a narcotic analgesic.

Each ampule (for parenteral administration) contains:

Hydromorphone Hydrochloride	1 mg per mL
	2 mg per mL
	4 mg per mL

Each multiple dose vial (for parenteral administration) contains:

Hydromorphone Hydrochloride	2 mg per mL

Each suppository (for rectal administration) contains:

Hydromorphone Hydrochloride	3 mg

Each 5 mL (1 teaspoon) Oral Liquid contains:

Hydromorphone Hydrochloride	5 mg

◆ RATED THERAPEUTICALLY EQUIVALENT; ◇ THERAPEUTIC EQUIVALENCE UNCONFIRMED; ○ UNRATED

Each Tablet contains:
Hydromorphone Hydrochloride ....2 mg
4 mg
8 mg

Each High-Potency ampule or single-dose vial (for intravenous, subcutaneous, or intramuscular administration) contains:
Hydromorphone Hydrochloride ....10 mg

Non-Sterile Powder (for prescription compounding) contains:
Hydromorphone Hydrochloride

Following is its chemical structure:

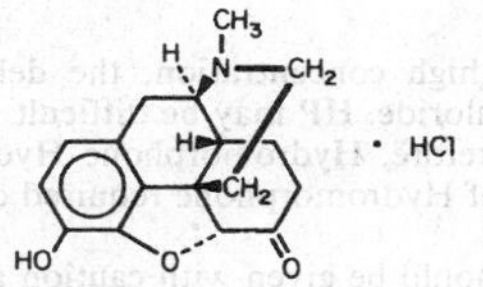

CLINICAL PHARMACOLOGY

Many of the effects described below are common to the class of narcotic analgesics. In some instances, data may not exist to demonstrate that Hydromorphone Hydrochloride possesses similar or different effects than those observed with other narcotic analgesics. However, in the absence of data to the contrary, it is assumed that Hydromorphone Hydrochloride would possess these effects.

Central Nervous System: Narcotic analgesics have multiple actions but exert their primary effects on the central nervous system and organs containing smooth muscle. The principal actions of therapeutic value are analgesia and sedation. A distinctive feature of the analgesia is that it occurs without loss of consciousness. Narcotic analgesics also suppress the cough reflex and cause respiratory depression, mood changes, mental clouding, euphoria, dysphoria, nausea, vomiting and electroencephalographic changes. The precise mode of analgesic action of narcotic analgesics is unknown. However, specific CNS opiate receptors have been identified. Narcotics are believed to express their pharmacological effects by combining with these receptors.

There is no intrinsic limit to the analgesic effect of Hydromorphone Hydrochloride; like morphine, adequate doses will relieve even the most severe pain. Clinically, however, dosage limitations are imposed by the adverse effects, primarily respiratory depression, nausea, and vomiting, which can result from high doses.

Narcotics depress the cough reflex by direct effect on the cough center in the medulla.

Narcotics produce respiratory depression by direct effect on brain stem respiratory centers. The mechanism of respiratory depression also involves a reduction in the responsiveness of the brain stem respiratory centers to increases in carbon dioxide tension.

Narcotics cause miosis. Pinpoint pupils are a common sign of narcotic overdose but are not pathognomonic (e.g., pontine lesions of hemorrhagic or ischemic origin may produce similar findings) and marked mydriasis occurs when asphyxia intervenes.

Gastrointestinal Tract and Other Smooth Muscle: Gastric, biliary and pancreatic secretions are decreased by narcotics. Narcotics cause a reduction in motility associated with an increase in tone in the antrum portion of the stomach and duodenum. Digestion of food in the small intestine is delayed and propulsive contractions are decreased. Propulsive peristaltic waves in the colon are decreased, and tone may be increased to the point of spasm. The end result is constipation. Narcotics can cause a marked increase in biliary tract pressure as a result of spasm of the sphincter of Oddi.

Cardiovascular System: Certain narcotics produce peripheral vasodilation which may result in orthostatic hypotension. Release of histamine may occur with narcotics and may contribute to narcotic-induced hypotension. Other manifestations of histamine release and/or peripheral vasodilation may include pruritus, flushing, and red eyes.

Effects on the myocardium after i.v. administration of narcotics are not significant in normal persons, vary with different narcotic analgesic agents and vary with the hemodynamic state of the patient, state of hydration and sympathetic drive.

Pharmacokinetics: In normal human volunteers Hydromorphone is metabolized primarily in the liver. It is excreted primarily as the glucuronidated conjugate, with small amounts of parent drug and minor amounts of 6-hydroxy reduction metabolites.

Following intravenous administration of Hydromorphone Hydrochloride to normal volunteers, the mean half-life of elimination was 2.64 ± 0.88 hours. The mean volume of distribution was 91.5 liters, suggesting extensive tissue uptake. Hydromorphone Hydrochloride is rapidly removed from the blood stream and distributed to skeletal muscle, kidneys, liver, intestinal tract, lungs, spleen and brain. Hydromorphone Hydrochloride also crosses the placental membranes.

In terms of area under the analgesic time-effect curve, Hydromorphone is approximately 8 times more potent than morphine (i.e., 1.3 mg of Hydromorphone produces analgesia equal to that produced by 10 mg of morphine). After intramuscular administration, Hydromorphone has a slightly more rapid onset and slightly shorter duration of action than morphine. The duration of Hydromorphone Hydrochloride analgesia in the non-tolerant patient with usual doses may be up to 4-5 hours. However, in tolerant subjects, duration will vary substantially depending on tolerance and dose. Dose should be adjusted so that 3-4 hours of pain relief may be achieved.

Generally, the analgesic action of parenterally administered Hydromorphone Hydrochloride is apparent within 15 minutes and usually remains in effect for more than five hours. The onset of action of oral Hydromorphone Hydrochloride is somewhat slower, with measurable analgesia occurring within 30 minutes.

In human plasma the half-life of a Hydromorphone Hydrochloride 4 mg tablet is 2.6 hours. In a random crossover study in six subjects, 4 mg of *oral* Hydromorphone Hydrochloride produced a mean concentration/time curve similar to that of 2 mg Hydromorphone Hydrochloride I.V., after the first hours.

In a single-dose crossover study in 27 normal subjects the pharmacokinetics of Hydromorphone Hydrochloride 8 mg tablets was compared to that of 8 mL of Hydromorphone Hydrochloride Oral Liquid (1 mg/mL). Plasma Hydromorphone concentration was determined using a sensitive and specific assay. The pharmacokinetic parameters from this study are outlined below.

Parameter Mean & (CV)	8 mg Tablet		8 mg Oral Liquid (1 mg/mL)	
C_{max} (ng/mL)	5.5	(33%)	5.7	(31%)
T_{max} (hr)	0.74	(34%)	0.73	(71%)
$AUC_{0-\infty}$ (ng*hr/mL)	23.7	(28%)	24.6	(29%)
$T\frac{1}{2}$ (hr)	2.6	(18%)	2.8	(20%)

Dose proportionality between the 8 mg Hydromorphone Hydrochloride tablets and other strengths of Hydromorphone Hydrochloride tablets has not been established. In normal human volunteers Hydromorphone is metabolized primarily in the liver. It is excreted in the urine primarily as the glucuronidated conjugate, with small amounts of parent drug and minor amounts of 6-hydroxy reduction metabolites. The effects of renal disease on the clearance of Hydromorphone are unknown, but caution should be taken to guard against unanticipated accumulation if renal and/or hepatic functions are seriously impaired. Hydromorphone has been shown to cross placental membranes.

CLINICAL TRIALS

Analgesic effects of single doses of Hydromorphone Hydrochloride oral liquid administered to patients with post-surgical pain have been studied in double-blind controlled trials. In one study with 61 patients, both 5 mg and 10 mg of Hydromorphone Hydrochloride provided significantly more analgesia than placebo. In another trial with 80 patients, 5 mg and 10 mg of Hydromorphone Hydrochloride Oral Liquid were compared to 30 mg and 60 mg of morphine sulfate oral liquid. The pain relief provided by 5 mg and 10 mg Hydromorphone Hydrochloride was comparable to 30 mg and 60 mg oral morphine sulfate, respectively.

In patients receiving opioids, both the dose and duration of analgesia will vary substantially depending on the patient's opioid tolerance. The dose should be selected and adjusted so that at least 3-4 hours of pain relief may be achieved. In patients taking opioid analgesics, the starting dose of Hydromorphone Hydrochloride should be based on the prior opioid usage. This should be done by converting the total daily usage of the previous opioid to an equivalent total daily dosage of oral Hydromorphone Hydrochloride using an equianalgesic table (see below). For opioids not in the table, first estimate the equivalent total daily usage of oral morphine, then use the table to find the equivalent total daily dosage of Hydromorphone Hydrochloride.

Once the total daily dosage of Hydromorphone Hydrochloride has been estimated, it should be divided into the desired number of doses. Since there is individual variation in response to different opioid drugs, only ½ to ⅔ of the estimated dose of Hydromorphone Hydrochloride calculated from equivalence tables should be given for the first few doses, then increased as needed according to the patient's response.

In chronic pain, doses should be administered around-the-clock. A supplemental dose of 5-15% of the total daily usage may be administered every two hours on an "as-needed" basis.

Periodic reassessment after the initial dosing is always required. If pain management is not satisfactory and in the absence of significant opioid-induced adverse events, the Hydromorphone dose may be increased gradually. If excessive opioid side effects are observed early in the dosing interval, the Hydromorphone dose should be reduced. If this results in breakthrough pain at the end of the dosing interval, the dosing interval may need to be shortened. Dose titration should be guided more by the need for analgesia than the absolute dose of opioid employed.

OPIOID ANALGESIC EQUIVALENTS WITH APPROXIMATELY EQUIANALGESIC POTENCY*

Nonproprietary (Trade) Name	IM or SC Dose	Oral Dose
Morphine Sulfate	10 mg	40-60 mg
Hydromorphone HCl	1.3-2.0 mg	6.5-7.5 mg
Oxymorphone	1.0-1.1 mg	6.6 mg
Levorphanol	2-2.3 mg	4 mg
Meperidine	75-100 mg	300-400 mg
Methadone	10 mg	10-20 mg

Dosages, and ranges of dosages represented, are a compilation of estimated equipotent dosages from published references comparing opioid analgesics in cancer and severe pain.

INDICATIONS AND USAGE

Hydromorphone Hydrochloride Oral Liquid and 8 mg Tablets are indicated for the management of pain in patients where an opioid analgesic is appropriate.

Parenteral Hydromorphone Hydrochloride is indicated for the relief of moderate to severe pain such as that due to:
- Surgery
- Cancer
- Trauma (soft tissue & bone)
- Biliary Colic
- Myocardial Infarction
- Burns
- Renal Colic

Hydromorphone Hydrochloride, HP is indicated for the relief of moderate-to-severe pain in narcotic-tolerant patients who require larger than usual doses of narcotics to provide adequate pain relief. Because Hydromorphone Hydrochloride, HP contains 10 mg of Hydromorphone per mL, a smaller injection volume can be used than with other parenteral narcotic formulations. Discomfort associated with the intramuscular or subcutaneous injection of an unusually large volume of solution can therefore be avoided.

CONTRAINDICATIONS:

Hydromorphone Hydrochloride, HP is contraindicated in: patients who are not already receiving large amounts of parenteral narcotics; all forms of Hydromorphone Hydrochloride are contraindicated in patients with known hypersensitivity to the drug; Hydromorphone Hydrochloride Oral Liquid, Tablets, and HP are contraindicated in patients with respiratory depression in the absence of resuscitative equipment, and in patients with status asthmaticus and for use in obstetrical analgesia. Parenteral Hydromorphone Hydrochloride is contraindicated in the presence of an intracranial lesion associated with increased intracranial pressure; and whenever ventilatory function is depressed (chronic obstructive pulmonary disease, cor pulmonale, emphysema, kyphoscoliosis, status asthmaticus).

WARNINGS

Drug Dependence: Hydromorphone Hydrochloride is a Schedule II narcotic. Hydromorphone Hydrochloride can produce drug dependence of the morphine type and therefore has the potential for being abused. Psychic dependence, physical dependence and tolerance may develop upon repeated administration of Hydromorphone Hydrochloride, and it should be prescribed and administered with the same degree of caution appropriate for the use of morphine. Abrupt discontinuance in the administration of Hydromorphone Hydrochloride is likely to result in a withdrawal syndrome. (See *"Drug Abuse and Dependence."*)

Infants born to mothers physically dependent on Hydromorphone Hydrochloride will also be physically dependent and may exhibit respiratory difficulties and withdrawal symptoms (see *"Drug Abuse and Dependence"*). The withdrawal signs include irritability and excessive crying, tremors, hyperactive reflexes, increased respiratory rate, increased stools, sneezing, yawning, vomiting, and fever. The intensity of the syndrome does not always correlate with the duration of maternal opioid use or dose. There is no consensus on the best method of managing withdrawal. Chlorpromazine 0.7 to 1.0 mg/kg q6h, phenobarbital 2 mg/kg q6h, and paregoric 2 to 4 drops/kg q4h, have been used to treat withdrawal symptoms in infants. The duration of therapy is 4 to 28 days, with the dosages decreased as tolerated.

Impaired Respiration: Respiratory depression is the chief hazard of Hydromorphone Hydrochloride. Hydromorphone Hydrochloride produces dose-related respiratory depression by acting directly on brain stem respiratory centers. Hydromorphone Hydrochloride also affects centers that control respiratory rhythm, and may produce irregular and periodic breathing. Respiratory depression occurs most frequently in overdose situations, in the elderly, in the debilitated, and in those suffering from conditions accompanied by hypoxia or hypercapnia when even moderate therapeutic doses may dangerously decrease pulmonary ventilation.

Hydromorphone Hydrochloride should be used with extreme caution in patients with chronic obstructive pulmonary disease or cor pulmonale, patients having a substantially decreased respiratory reserve, hypoxia, hypercapnia, or preexisting respiratory depression. In such patients even usual therapeutic doses of narcotic analgesics may decrease respiratory drive while simultaneously increasing airway resistance to the point of apnea.

Head Injury and Increased Intracranial Pressure: The respiratory depressant effects of Hydromorphone Hydrochloride with carbon dioxide retention and secondary elevation of cerebrospinal fluid pressure may be markedly exaggerated in the presence of head injury, other intracranial lesions, or preexisting increase in intracranial pressure. Narcotic analgesics including Hydromorphone Hydrochloride may produce effects which can obscure the clinical course and neurologic signs of further increase in pressure in patients with head injuries.

Acute Abdominal Conditions: The administration of narcotics may obscure the diagnosis or clinical course of patients with acute abdominal conditions and may aggravate preexisting convulsions in patients with convulsive disorders.

Hypotensive Effect: Narcotic analgesics, including Hydromorphone Hydrochloride may cause severe hypotension in an individual whose ability to maintain his blood pressure has already been compromised by a depleted blood volume, or a concurrent administration of drugs such as phenothiazines or general anesthetics (see also *"Precautions — Drug Interactions"*). Hydromorphone Hydrochloride may produce orthostatic hypotension in ambulatory patients.

Hydromorphone Hydrochloride should be administered with caution to patients in circulatory shock, since vasodilation produced by the drug may further reduce cardiac output and blood pressure.

Sulfites: Some brands of Hydromorphone Hydrochloride Oral Liquid and Tablets may contain sodium bisulfite, a sulfite that may cause allergic-type reactions including anaphylactic symptoms and life-threatening or less severe asthmatic episodes in certain susceptible people. The overall prevalence of sulfite sensitivity in the general population is unknown and probably low. Sulfite sensitivity is seen more frequently in asthmatic than in nonasthmatic people.

PRECAUTIONS

General: Because of its high concentration, the delivery of precise doses of Hydromorphone Hydrochloride, HP may be difficult if low doses of Hydromorphone are required. Therefore, Hydromorphone Hydrochloride, HP should be used only if the amount of Hydromorphone required can be delivered accurately with this formulation.

In general, narcotics should be given with caution and the initial dose should be reduced in the elderly or debilitated and those with severe impairment of hepatic, pulmonary or renal function; myxedema or hypothyroidism; adrenocortical insufficiency (e.g., Addison's Disease); CNS depression or coma; toxic psychoses; prostatic hypertrophy or urethral stricture; gallbladder disease; acute alcoholism; delirium tremens; kyphoscoliosis; or following gastrointestinal surgery.

In the case of Hydromorphone Hydrochloride, HP, however, the patient is presumed to be receiving a narcotic to which he or she exhibits tolerance and the initial dose of Hydromorphone Hydrochloride, HP selected should be estimated based on the relative potency of Hydromorphone and the narcotic previously used by the patient. See *"Dosage and Administration"* section.

Narcotic analgesics including Hydromorphone Hydrochloride should also be used with caution in patients about to undergo surgery of the biliary tract since it may cause spasm of the sphincter of Oddi.

Cough Reflex: Hydromorphone Hydrochloride suppresses the cough reflex; as with all narcotics, caution should be exercised when Hydromorphone Hydrochloride is used postoperatively and in patients with pulmonary disease.

Usage in Ambulatory Patients: Narcotics may impair the mental and/or physical abilities required for the performance of potentially hazardous tasks such as driving a car or operating machinery; patients should be cautioned accordingly.

Parenteral Administration: The parenteral form of Hydromorphone Hydrochloride may be given intravenously, but the injection should be given very slowly. Rapid intravenous injection of narcotic analgesics increases the possibility of side effects such as hypotension and respiratory depression.

Drug Interactions: The concomitant use of other central nervous system depressants including sedatives or hypnotics, general anesthetics, phenothiazines, tranquilizers and alcohol may produce additive depressant effects. Respiratory depression, hypotension and profound sedation or coma may occur. When such combined therapy is contemplated, the dose of one or both agents should be reduced. Hydromorphone Hydrochloride should not be taken with alcohol. Narcotic analgesics, including Hydromorphone Hydrochloride, may enhance the action of neuromuscular blocking agents and produce an increased degree of respiratory depression.

Use in Drug and Alcohol Dependent Patients: Hydromorphone Hydrochloride should be used with caution in patients with alcoholism and other drug dependencies due to the increased frequency of narcotic tolerance, dependence, and the risk of addiction observed in these patient populations. Abuse of Hydromorphone Hydrochloride in combination with other CNS depressant drugs can result in serious risk to the patient.

Carcinogenesis, Mutagenesis, Impairment of Fertility: Studies in animals to evaluate the drug's carcinogenic and mutagenic potential or the effect on fertility, have not been conducted.

PREGNANCY—CATEGORY C:

Human: Adequate animal studies on reproduction have not been performed to determine whether Hydromorphone affects fertility in males or females. There are no well-controlled studies in women. Hydromorphone is known to cross placental membranes. Reports based on marketing experience do not identify any specific teratogenic risks following routine (short-term) clinical use. Although there is no clearly defined risk, such reports do not exclude the possibility of infrequent or subtle damage to the human fetus. Hydromorphone Hydrochloride, should be used in pregnant women only when clearly needed or if the potential benefit justifies the potential risk to the fetus (see *"Labor and Delivery"* and *"Drug Abuse and Dependence"*).

Animal: Literature reports of Hydromorphone Hydrochloride administration to pregnant Syrian hamsters show that Hydromorphone Hydrochloride is teratogenic at a dose of 20 mg/kg which is 600 times the human dose. A maximal teratogenic effect (50% of fetuses affected) in the Syrian hamster was observed at a dose of 125 mg/kg (738 mg/m^2).

Labor and Delivery: Hydromorphone Hydrochloride, HP, Oral Liquid, and Tablets are contraindicated in Labor and Delivery (see *"Contraindications"* section).

As with all narcotics, administration of parenteral Hydromorphone Hydrochloride to the mother shortly before delivery may result in some degree of respiratory depression in the newborn, especially if higher doses are used.

Nursing Mothers: Low levels of narcotic analgesics have been detected in human milk. As a general rule, nursing should not be undertaken while a patient is receiving Hydromorphone Hydrochloride since it, and other drugs in this class, may be excreted in the milk.

Pediatric Use: Safety and effectiveness in children have not been established.

Geriatric Use: Hydromorphone Hydrochloride has not been studied in geriatric patients. Elderly subjects have been shown to have at least twice the sensitivity (as measured by EEG changes) of young adults to some opioids. When administering Hydromorphone Hydrochloride to the elderly, the initial dose should be reduced.

ADVERSE REACTIONS
The adverse effects of Hydromorphone Hydrochloride are similar to those of other narcotic analgesics, and represent established pharmacological effects of the drug class. The major hazards include respiratory depression and apnea. To a lesser degree, circulatory depression, respiratory arrest, shock and cardiac arrest have occurred.

The most frequently observed adverse effects are lightheadedness, dizziness, sedation, nausea, vomiting, and sweating. These effects seem to be more prominent in ambulatory patients and in those not experiencing severe pain. Some adverse reactions in ambulatory patients may be alleviated if the patient lies down.

Nausea and vomiting are more frequent in ambulatory than in recumbent patients. The antiemetic phenothiazines are useful in suppressing these effects; however, some phenothiazine derivatives seem to be antianalgesic and to increase the amount of narcotic required to produce pain relief, while other phenothiazines reduce the amount of narcotic required to produce a given level of analgesia. Opiate agonist-induced increase in intraluminal pressure may endanger surgical anastomosis.

Respiratory Depression: Hydromorphone Hydrochloride produces dose-related respiratory depression by acting directly on brain stem respiratory centers. Hydromorphone Hydrochloride also affects centers that control respiratory rhythm, and may produce irregular and periodic breathing. If significant respiratory depression occurs, it may be antagonized by the use of naloxone hydrochloride. The usual adult dose of 0.4 to 0.8 mg given *intramuscularly* or *intravenously*, promptly reverses the effects of morphine-like opioid agonists such as Hydromorphone Hydrochloride. In patients who are physically dependent, small doses of naloxone may be sufficient not only to antagonize respiratory depression, but also to precipitate withdrawal phenomena. The dose of naloxone should therefore be adjusted accordingly in such patients. Since the duration of action of Hydromorphone Hydrochloride may exceed that of the antagonist, the patient should be kept under continued surveillance; repeated doses of the antagonist may be required to maintain adequate respiration. Apply other supportive measures when indicated.

LESS FREQUENTLY OBSERVED WITH NARCOTIC ANALGESICS
General and CNS: Dysphoria, euphoria, weakness, headache, agitation, tremor, uncoordinated muscle movements, alterations of mood (nervousness, apprehension, depression, floating feelings, dreams), muscle rigidity, paresthesia, muscle tremor, blurred vision, nystagmus, diplopia and miosis, transient hallucinations* and disorientation, visual disturbances, insomnia and increased intracranial pressure may occur. Also occurring with some forms of the drug: drowsiness, mental clouding, lethargy, impairment of mental and physical performance, anxiety, fear, psychic dependence, and mood changes.

Cardiovascular: Flushing of the face, chills, tachycardia, bradycardia, palpitation, faintness, syncope, hypotension and hypertension have been reported.

Circulatory depression, peripheral circulatory collapse and cardiac arrest have occurred after rapid intravenous injection. Orthostatic hypotension and fainting may occur if a patient stands up suddenly after receiving an injection of Hydromorphone Hydrochloride.

Respiratory: Bronchospasm and laryngospasm have been known to occur.

Gastrointestinal: Dry mouth, constipation, biliary tract spasm, ileus, anorexia, diarrhea, cramps and taste alterations have been reported.

Genitourinary: Urinary retention or hesitancy, ureteral spasm, spasm of vesical sphincters, and antidiuretic effects have been reported.

Dermatologic: Pruritus, urticaria, other skin rashes, wheal and flare over the vein with intravenous injection, and diaphoresis have been reported with narcotic analgesics.

Other: In clinical trials, neither local tissue irritation nor induration was observed at the site of subcutaneous injection of Hydromorphone Hydrochloride; pain at the injection site was rarely observed. However, local irritation and induration have been seen following parenteral injection of other narcotic drug products.

DRUG ABUSE AND DEPENDENCE
Hydromorphone Hydrochloride is a Schedule II narcotic, similar to morphine. Narcotic analgesics may cause psychological and physical dependence (see

---

* Hallucinations, although unusual with pure agonist narcotics, have been observed in one patient following both a 6 mg and a 4 mg Hydromorphone Hydrochloride, HP dose. However, the patient was receiving several concomitant medications during the second episode and a causal relationship cannot be established.

"Warnings"). Psychic dependence is unlikely to develop when Hydromorphone Hydrochloride is used for a short time for the treatment of pain. Physical dependence results in withdrawal symptoms in patients who abruptly discontinue the drug. Withdrawal symptoms also may be precipitated in the patient with physical dependence by the administration of a drug with narcotic antagonist activity, e.g., naloxone (see also *"Overdosage"*). Physical dependence usually does not occur to a clinically significant degree until after several weeks of continued narcotic usage. Tolerance, in which increasingly large doses are required in order to produce the same degree of analgesia, is initially manifested by a shortened duration of analgesic effect, and subsequently, by decreases in the intensity of analgesia. In chronic pain patients, and in narcotic-tolerant cancer patients, the dose of Hydromorphone Hydrochloride should be guided by the degree of tolerance manifested.

In chronic pain patients in whom narcotic analgesics including Hydromorphone Hydrochloride are abruptly discontinued, a severe abstinence syndrome should be anticipated. This may be similar to the abstinence syndrome noted in patients who withdraw from heroin. The latter abstinence syndrome may be characterized by restlessness, lacrimation, rhinorrhea, yawning, perspiration, gooseflesh, restless sleep or "yen" and mydriasis during the first 24 hours. These symptoms may increase in severity and over the next 72 hours may be accompanied by increasing irritability, anxiety, weakness, twitching and spasms of muscles, kicking movements, severe backache, abdominal and leg pains, abdominal and muscle cramps, hot and cold flashes, insomnia, nausea, anorexia, vomiting, intestinal spasm, diarrhea, coryza and repetitive sneezing, increase in body temperature, blood pressure, respiratory rate and heart rate.

Because of excessive loss of fluids through sweating, or vomiting and diarrhea, there is usually marked weight loss, dehydration, ketosis, and disturbances in acid-base balance. Cardiovascular collapse can occur. Without treatment most observable symptoms disappear in 5-14 days; however, there appears to be a phase of secondary or chronic abstinence which may last for 2-6 months characterized by insomnia, irritability, muscular aches, and autonomic instability.

In the treatment of physical dependence on Hydromorphone Hydrochloride, the patient may be detoxified by gradual reduction of the dosage, although this is unlikely to be necessary in the terminal cancer patient. If abstinence symptoms become severe, the patient may be given methadone. Temporary administration of tranquilizers and sedatives may aid in reducing patient anxiety. Gastrointestinal disturbances or dehydration should be treated accordingly.

OVERDOSAGE
Serious overdosage with Hydromorphone Hydrochloride is characterized by respiratory depression (a decrease in respiratory rate and/or tidal volume, Cheyne-Stokes respiration, cyanosis), somnolence progressing to stupor or coma, skeletal muscle flaccidity, cold and clammy skin, constricted pupils, and sometimes bradycardia and hypotension. In serious overdosage, particularly following intravenous injection, apnea, circulatory collapse, cardiac arrest and death may occur.

In the treatment of overdosage primary attention should be given to the reestablishment of adequate respiratory exchange through provision of a patent airway and institution of assisted or controlled ventilation. A potentially serious oral ingestion, if recent, should be managed with gut decontamination. In unconscious patients with a secure airway, instill activated charcoal (30-100 g in adults, 1-2 g/kg in infants) via a nasogastric tube. A saline cathartic or sorbitol may be added to the first dose of activated charcoal. Gastric lavage or induced emesis may be useful in removing unabsorbed drug from conscious patients.

Narcotic-Tolerant Patient: Since tolerance to the respiratory and CNS depressant effects of narcotics develops concomitantly with tolerance to their analgesic effects, serious respiratory depression due to an acute overdose is unlikely to be seen in narcotic-tolerant patients receiving the usual therapeutic dosage of Hydromorphone Hydrochloride for chronic pain.

Note: In such an individual who is physically dependent on narcotics, administration of the usual dose of an opioid antagonist will precipitate an acute withdrawal syndrome. The severity will depend on the degree of physical dependence and the dose of the antagonist administered. Use of a narcotic antagonist in such a person should be avoided. If necessary to treat serious respiratory depression in the physically-dependent patient, the antagonist should be administered with extreme care and by titration with smaller than usual, or fractional (one fifth to one tenth), doses of the antagonist.

Nontolerant Patient: The narcotic antagonist, naloxone, is a specific antidote against respiratory depression which may result from overdosage, or unusual sensitivity to Hydromorphone Hydrochloride. A dose of naloxone (usually given as a test dose of 0.4 mg, followed by up to 2.0 mg if needed) should be administered intravenously, if possible, simultaneously with respiratory resuscitation. The dose can be repeated in 3 minutes. Naloxone should not be administered in the absence of clinically significant respiratory or circulatory depression. Naloxone should be administered cautiously to persons who are known, or suspected to be physically dependent on Hydromorphone Hydrochloride. In such cases, an abrupt or complete reversal of narcotic effects may precipitate an acute abstinence syndrome.

Since the duration of action of Hydromorphone Hydrochloride may exceed that of the antagonist, the patient should be kept under continued surveillance; repeated doses of the antagonist may be required to maintain adequate respiration. Apply other supportive measures when indicated.

Supportive measures (including oxygen, vasopressors) should be employed in the management of circulatory shock and pulmonary edema accompanying overdose as indicated. Cardiac arrest or arrhythmias may require cardiac massage or defibrillation.

DOSAGE AND ADMINISTRATION

Parenteral: The usual starting dose is 1-2 mg *subcutaneously* or *intramuscularly* every 4 to 6 hours as necessary for pain control. The dose should be adjusted according to the severity of pain, as well as the patient's underlying disease, age, and size. Patients with terminal cancer may be tolerant to narcotic analgesics and may, therefore, require higher doses for adequate pain relief. Intravenous or subcutaneous administration is usually not painful. Should intravenous administration be necessary, the injection should be given *slowly*, over at least 2 to 3 minutes, depending on the dose. A gradual increase in dose may be required if analgesia is inadequate, tolerance occurs, or if pain severity increases. The first sign of tolerance is usually a reduced duration of effect.

Oral Tablets: The usual oral dose is 2 mg to 4 mg every 4 to 6 hours as necessary. Appropriate use of the 8 mg tablet must be decided by careful evaluation of each clinical situation. The dose must be individually adjusted according to severity of pain, patient response and patient size. More severe pain may require 4 mg or more every 4 to 6 hours. If the pain increases in severity, analgesia is not adequate or tolerance occurs, a gradual increase in dosage may be required. If pain is exceedingly severe, or if prompt response is desired, parenteral Hydromorphone Hydrochloride should be used initially in adequate amounts to control the pain.

Rectal: Hydromorphone Hydrochloride suppositories (3 mg) may provide longer duration of relief which could obviate additional medication during the sleeping hours. The usual adult dose is one (1) suppository inserted rectally every 6 to 8 hours or as directed by physician.

Oral Liquid: The usual adult oral dosage of Hydromorphone Hydrochloride oral liquid is one-half (2.5 mL) to two teaspoonfuls (10 mL) (2.5 mg-10 mg) every 3 to 6 hours as directed by the clinical situation. Oral dosages higher than the usual dosages may be required in some patients.

SAFETY AND HANDLING INSTRUCTIONS

Hydromorphone Hydrochloride oral liquid and 8 mg tablets pose little risk of direct exposure to health care personnel and should be handled and disposed of prudently in accordance with hospital or institutional policy. Significant absorption from dermal exposure is unlikely; accidental dermal exposure to Hydromorphone Hydrochloride oral liquid should be treated by removal of any contaminated clothing and rinsing the affected area with cool water. Patients and their families should be instructed to flush any Hydromorphone Hydrochloride oral liquid and 8 mg tablets that are no longer needed.

Access to abusable drugs such as Hydromorphone Hydrochloride oral liquid and Hydromorphone Hydrochloride Tablets presents an occupational hazard for addiction in the health care industry. Routine procedures for handling controlled substances developed to protect the public may not be adequate to protect health care workers. Implementation of more effective accounting procedures and measures to restrict access to drugs of this class (appropriate to the practice setting) may minimize the risk of self-administration by health care providers.

Parenteral: HYDROMORPHONE HYDROCHLORIDE, HP SHOULD BE GIVEN ONLY TO PATIENTS WHO ARE ALREADY RECEIVING LARGE DOSES OF NARCOTICS. Hydromorphone Hydrochloride, HP is indicated for relief of moderate-to-severe pain in narcotic-tolerant patients. Thus, these patients will already have been treated with other narcotic analgesics. If the patient is being changed from regular Hydromorphone Hydrochloride to Hydromorphone Hydrochloride, HP, similar doses should be used, depending on the patient's clinical response to the drug. If Hydromorphone Hydrochloride, HP is substituted for a different narcotic analgesic, the following equivalency table should be used as a guide to determine the appropriate starting dose of Hydromorphone Hydrochloride, HP.

STRONG ANALGESICS AND STRUCTURALLY RELATED DRUGS USED IN THE TREATMENT OF CANCER PAIN*

	IM or SC Administration	
Nonproprietary Names	*Dose, mg Equianalgesic to 10 mg of IM Morphine†*	*Duration Compared With Morphine*
Morphine sulfate	10	Same
Papaveretum	20	Same
Hydromorphone Hydrochloride	1.3	Slightly shorter
Oxymorphone hydrochloride	1.1	Slightly shorter
Nalbuphine hydrochloride	12	Same
Heroin, diamorphine hydrochloride	4-5	Slightly shorter
Levorphanol tartrate	2.3	Same
Butorphanol tartrate	1.5-2.5	Same
Pentazocine lactate or hydrochloride	60	Shorter
Meperidine, pethidine hydrochloride	80	Shorter
Methadone hydrochloride	10	Same

* *From Beaver WT. Management of cancer pain with parenteral medication. J. Am. Med. Assoc. 244:2653-2657 (1980).*

† *(In terms of the area under the analgesic time-effect curve.)*

In open clinical trials with Hydromorphone Hydrochloride, HP in patients with terminal cancer, doses ranged from 1-14 mg subcutaneously or intramuscularly; one patient received 30 mg subcutaneously on two occasions. In these trials, both subcutaneous and intramuscular injections of Hydromorphone Hydrochloride,

HP were well-tolerated, with minimal pain and/or burning at the injection site. Mild erythema was rarely noted after intramuscular injection. There was no induration after either intramuscular or subcutaneous administration of Hydromorphone Hydrochloride, HP. Subcutaneous injections of Hydromorphone Hydrochloride, HP were particularly well accepted when administered with a short, 30-gauge needle.

Experience with administration of Hydromorphone Hydrochloride, HP by the intravenous route is limited. Should intravenous administration be necessary, the injection should be given slowly, over at least 2 to 3 minutes. The intravenous route is usually painless.

A gradual increase in dose may be required if analgesia is inadequate, tolerance occurs, or if pain severity increases. The first sign of tolerance is usually a reduced duration of effect.

Note: Parenteral drug products should be inspected visually for particulate matter and discoloration prior to administration, whenever solution and container permit. A slight yellowish discoloration may develop in Hydromorphone Hydrochloride ampules and multiple-dose vials. No loss of potency has been demonstrated. Hydromorphone Hydrochloride injection is physically compatible and chemically stable for at least 24 hours at 25°C protected from light in most common large volume parenteral solutions.

500mg/50mL Vial: To use this single dose presentation, do not penetrate the stopper with a syringe. Instead, remove both the aluminum flipseal and rubber stopper in a suitable work area such as under a laminar flow hood (or equivalent clean air compounding area). The contents may then be withdrawn for preparation of a single, large volume parenteral solution. Any unused portion should be discarded in an appropriate manner.

Storage: Parenteral and oral forms of Hydromorphone Hydrochloride should be stored at 59°-77° or 86°F, (15°-25° or 30°C). Protect from light.

Hydromorphone Hydrochloride suppositories should be stored in a refrigerator.

J CODES
Up to 4 mg SC,IM,IV—J1170

HOW SUPPLIED
INJECTION (C-II): 1 MG/ML

BRAND/MANUFACTURER	NDC	SIZE	AWP
○ **BRAND**			
DILAUDID: Knoll	00044-1011-01	1 ml 10s	$10.29
○ **GENERICS**			
Wyeth-Ayerst	00008-0387-03	1 ml 10s	$9.63
Wyeth-Ayerst	00008-0387-50	1 ml 10s	$13.38
Sanofi Winthrop	00024-0726-02	2 ml 10s	$9.07

INJECTION (C-II): 2 MG/ML

BRAND/MANUFACTURER	NDC	SIZE	AWP
○ **BRAND**			
DILAUDID: Knoll	00044-1062-05	20 ml	$17.49
	00044-1012-01	1 ml 10s	$11.34
	00044-1012-09	1 ml 25s	$27.00
○ **GENERICS**			
Elkins-Sinn	00641-2341-41	20 ml	$10.63
Astra	00186-1309-01	20 ml	$11.56
Schein	00364-2422-55	20 ml	$12.50
Steris	00402-0918-20	20 ml	$12.50
Wyeth-Ayerst	00008-0295-02	1 ml 10s	$9.46
Wyeth-Ayerst	00008-0295-01	1 ml 10s	$9.94
Wyeth-Ayerst	00008-0295-50	1 ml 10s	$13.69
Sanofi Winthrop	00024-0728-02	2 ml 10s	$9.39
Elkins-Sinn	00641-0121-25	1 ml 25s	$15.63
Elkins-Sinn	00641-0121-26	1 ml 100s	$63.44

INJECTION (C-II): 3 MG/ML

BRAND/MANUFACTURER	NDC	SIZE	AWP
○ **GENERICS**			
Wyeth-Ayerst	00008-0388-01	1 ml 10s	$10.34

INJECTION (C-II): 4 MG/ML

BRAND/MANUFACTURER	NDC	SIZE	AWP
○ **BRAND**			
DILAUDID: Knoll	00044-1014-01	1 ml 10s	$13.74
○ **GENERICS**			
Wyeth-Ayerst	00008-0296-01	1 ml 10s	$10.69
Wyeth-Ayerst	00008-0296-50	1 ml 10s	$14.44
Sanofi Winthrop	00024-0727-02	2 ml 10s	$10.09

◆ RATED THERAPEUTICALLY EQUIVALENT; ◇ THERAPEUTIC EQUIVALENCE UNCONFIRMED; ○ UNRATED

INJECTION (C-II): 10 MG/ML

BRAND/MANUFACTURER	NDC	SIZE	AWP
○ **BRAND**			
DILAUDID-HP: Knoll	00044-1017-10	1 ml 10s	$30.48
DILAUDID-HP: Knoll	00044-1017-06	50 ml	$137.53
DILAUDID-HP: Knoll	00044-1017-25	5 ml 10s	$144.75

LIQUID (C-II): 1 MG/ML

BRAND/MANUFACTURER	NDC	SIZE	AWP
○ **BRAND**			
DILAUDID-5: Knoll	00044-1085-01	480 ml	$81.11

POWDER (C-II):

BRAND/MANUFACTURER	NDC	SIZE	AWP
○ **BRAND**			
DILAUDID: Knoll	00044-1040-01	1 gm	$165.18
○ **GENERICS**			
Mallinckrodt-II	00406-3245-52	1 gm	$162.50

SUPPOSITORY (C-II): 3 MG

BRAND/MANUFACTURER	NDC	SIZE	AWP
○ **BRAND**			
DILAUDID: Knoll	00044-1053-01	6s	$17.96

TABLETS (C-II): 1 MG

BRAND/MANUFACTURER	NDC	SIZE	AWP
○ **GENERICS**			
HYDROSTAT IR: Richwood	58521-0001-01	100s	$22.00

TABLETS (C-II): 2 MG

BRAND/MANUFACTURER	NDC	SIZE	AWP
○ **BRAND**			
➤ DILAUDID: Knoll	00044-1022-02	100s	$36.88
	00044-1022-45	100s ud	$46.78
	00044-1022-03	500s	$175.15
○ **GENERICS**			
Halsey Pharm	00879-0715-50	50s	$13.20
Halsey Pharm	00879-0715-01	100s	$22.15
Rexar	00478-5402-01	100s	$23.33
➤ Roxane	00054-4392-25	100s	$25.44
Qualitest	00603-3925-21	100s	$28.12
HYDROSTAT IR: Richwood	58521-0002-01	100s	$32.20
Roxane	00054-8392-24	100s ud	$28.27

TABLETS (C-II): 3 MG

BRAND/MANUFACTURER	NDC	SIZE	AWP
○ **BRAND**			
DILAUDID: Knoll	00044-1023-01	100s	$45.33
○ **GENERICS**			
HYDROSTAT IR: Richwood	58521-0003-01	100s	$42.50

TABLETS (C-II): 4 MG

BRAND/MANUFACTURER	NDC	SIZE	AWP
○ **BRAND**			
➤ DILAUDID: Knoll	00044-1024-02	100s	$60.40
	00044-1024-45	100s ud	$71.13
	00044-1024-03	500s	$287.63
○ **GENERICS**			
Halsey Pharm	00879-0717-50	50s	$21.50
Halsey Pharm	00879-0717-01	100s	$39.00
Rexar	00478-5404-01	100s	$39.17
Goldline	00182-9173-01	100s	$40.00
➤ Roxane	00054-4394-25	100s	$41.95
Qualitest	00603-3926-21	100s	$45.45
HYDROSTAT IR: Richwood	58521-0004-01	100s	$52.30
Goldline	00182-9178-01	100s	$52.75
Roxane	00054-8394-24	100s ud	$43.31

TABLETS (C-II): 8 MG

BRAND/MANUFACTURER	NDC	SIZE	AWP
○ **BRAND**			
DILAUDID: Knoll	00044-1028-02	100s	$114.85

Hydropres *SEE* HYDROCHLOROTHIAZIDE WITH RESERPINE

Hydroquinone

DESCRIPTION

Hydroquinone Cream, Cream with Sunblack, Cream with Sunscreens, and Gel with Sunscreens contain: Hydroquinone 40 mg/gm. Hydroquinone Topical Solution contains: Hydroquinone 30 mg/ml

Each package of Topical Solution includes a cap with a plastic rod applicator (for small, more precise application) and a sponge top applicator cator for larger areas of skin involvement. If neither applicator is specified on prescription, install the sponge top unit.

Following is its chemical structure:

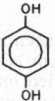

CLINICAL PHARMACOLOGY

Topical application of Hydroquinone produces a reversible depigmentation of the skin by inhibition of the enzymatic oxidation of tyrosine to 3, 4-dihydroxyphenylalanine (dopa) and suppression of other melanocyte metabolic processes. The selective inhibition of the enzyme affects melanogenesis in the melanocytes resulting in cessation of melanin formation and subsequent reduction in pigmentation. Additional studies indicate Hydroquinone acts on the essential subcellular metabolic processes of melanocytes with resultant cytolysis, i.e., nonenzymediated depigmentation. Exposure to sunlight or ultraviolet light will cause repigmentation of the bleached areas, which may be prevented by the sunblocking agents or broad spectrum sunscreen agents contained in Hydroquinone Creams or Gel.

INDICATIONS AND USAGE

Hydroquinone Cream is indicated for the gradual bleaching of hyperpigmented skin conditions such as chloasma, melasma, freckles, senile lentigines, and other unwanted areas of melanin hyperpigmentation.

Hydroquinone Topical Solution is indicated in the temporary bleaching of these skin conditions. Hydroquinone Cream is intended for night-time use only since it contains no sunblocking agents.

CONTRAINDICATIONS

Prior history of sensitivity or allergic reaction to this product or any of its ingredients. The safety of topical Hydroquinone use during pregnancy or in children (12 years and under) has not been established.

WARNINGS

A. *Caution:* Hydroquinone is a skin bleaching agent which may produce unwanted cosmetic effects if not used as directed. The physician should be familiar with the contents of this insert before prescribing or dispensing this medication.

B. Test for skin sensitivity before using Hydroquinone Cream or Gel by applying a small amount to an unbroken patch of skin and check in 24 hours. Minor redness is not a contraindication, but where there is itching or vesicle formation or excessive inflammatory response, further treatment is not advised. If rash or irritation occurs with use of Hydroquinone Topical Solution, discontinue use. Close patient supervision is recommended.

Contact with the eyes should be avoided. In case of accidental contact, patient should rinse eyes thoroughly with water and contact physician. A bitter taste and anesthetic effect may occur if applied to lips. Keep out of reach of children. Use of Hydroquinone Topical Solution in paranasal and infraorbital areas increases the chance of irritation (see *"Adverse Reactions"*). If no bleaching or lightening effect is noted after 2 months of treatment use, Hydroquinone Cream Topical Solution or Gel should be discontinued. Hydroquinone Cream and Gel are formulated for use as a skin bleaching agent and should not be used for the prevention of sunburn.

C. Sunscreen use is an essential aspect of Hydroquinone therapy because even minimal sunlight exposure sustains melanocytic activity. The sunscreens in Hydroquinone Cream and Gel provide the necessary sun protection during skin bleaching therapy. After clearing and during maintenance therapy, sun exposure should be avoided on bleached skin by application of a sunscreen or sunblock agent, or protective clothing to prevent repigmentation.

There are no sunblocking or sunscreening agents in some Hydroquinone Creams and since minimal sunlight exposure may reverse the bleaching effect of this preparation, it should be used only at night or on areas of the body covered by protective clothing. During the daytime, sunblocking or broad spectrum sunscreen preparations or protective clothing should be used to prevent the bleached areas from repigmentation.

➤ SHOWN IN PRODUCT IDENTIFICATION GUIDE

D. Keep this and all medications out of the reach of children. In case of accidental ingestion, call a physician or a poison control center immediately.

E. *Warning:* Some brands contain sodium metabisulfite, a sulfite that may cause serious allergic type reactions (e.g. hives, itching, wheezing, anaphylaxis, severe asthma attacks) in certain susceptible persons.

PRECAUTIONS
See *"Warnings".*

A. Pregnancy Category C. Animal reproduction studies have not been conducted with topical Hydroquinone. It is also not known whether Hydroquinone can cause fetal harm when used topically on a pregnant woman or affect reproductive capacity. It is not known to what degree, if any, topical Hydroquinone is absorbed systemically. Topical Hydroquinone should be used in women only when clearly indicated.

B. Nursing mothers. It is not known whether topical Hydroquinone is absorbed or excreted in human milk. Caution is advised when topical Hydroquinone is used by a nursing mother.

C. Pediatric usage. Safety and effectiveness in children below the age of 12 years have not been established.

Concurrent use of Hydroquinone Topical Solution with peroxide products may result in transient dark staining of skin areas so treated. This is due to the oxidation of Hydroquinone by the peroxide. This transient staining can be removed by discontinuing concurrent usage and normal soap cleansing.

ADVERSE REACTIONS
No systemic adverse reactions have been reported. Occasional hypersensitivity (localized contact dermatitis) may occur in which case the medication should be discontinued and the physician notified immediately.

The following have been reported with Hydroquinone Topical Solution: dryness and fissuring of the paranasal and infraorbital areas, erythema, and stinging. Hydroquinone has been known to produce irritation and sensitization in susceptible individuals.

OVERDOSAGE
There have been no systemic reactions from the use of topical Hydroquinone or the sunblockers in Hydroquinone Creams or Gel. However, treatment should be limited to relatively small areas of the body at one time since some patients experience a transient skin reddening and a mild burning sensation which does not preclude treatment.

DRUG DOSAGE AND ADMINISTRATION
A thin application of Hydroquinone Cream or Gel should be applied to the affected area twice daily or as directed by a physician. Consult product label for instructions on whether to rub in or not. There is no recommendation for children under 12 years of age except under the advice and supervision of a physician.

Apply Hydroquinone Topical Solution to affected areas twice daily, in the morning and before bedtime. During the day, an effective broad spectrum sunscreen like Sunblock SPF 15 or SPF 30 should be used and unnecessary solar exposure avoided, or protective clothing should be worn to cover bleached skin in order to prevent repigmentation from occurring.

Hydroquinone Creams and Gel should be stored at controlled room temperature (15-30°C) (59-86°F). Store Topical Solution at room temperature or below; avoid excessive heat.

REFERENCES
1. Denton, C., A.B. Lerner and T.B. Fitzpatrick, "Inhibition of Melanin Formation by Chemical Agents", *Journal of Investigative Dermatology*, 18:119-135, 1952. 2. Jimbow, K., H. Obata, M. Pathak, and T.B. Fitzpatrick, "Mechanism of Depigmentation by Hydroquinone", *Journal of Investigative Dermatology*, 62:436-449, 1974. 3. Parrish, J.A., R.R. Anderson, F. Urbach, D. Pitts, *UVA, Biological Effects of Ultraviolet Radiation with Emphasis on Human Responses to Longwave Ultraviolet.* Plenum Press, New York and London, 1978, p. 151.

HOW SUPPLIED
CREAM: 4%

BRAND/MANUFACTURER	NDC	SIZE	AWP
○ **BRAND**			
ELDOQUIN FORTE: ICN	00187-0394-31	30 gm	$30.84
SOLAQUIN FORTE: ICN	00187-0396-31	30 gm	$30.84
ELDOPAQUE FORTE: ICN	00187-0395-31	30 gm	$30.84
○ **GENERICS**			
NUQUIN HP: Stratus	58980-0574-05	15 gm	$11.25
MELQUIN HP: Stratus	58980-0472-05	15 gm	$11.25
NUQUIN HP: Stratus	58980-0574-10	30 gm	$17.90
MELQUIN HP: Stratus	58980-0472-10	30 gm	$17.90
CMC-Cons	00223-4330-02	60 gm	$3.00
NUQUIN HP: Stratus	58980-0574-20	60 gm	$30.30
CMC-Cons	00223-4330-04	120 gm	$4.00

GEL: 4%

BRAND/MANUFACTURER	NDC	SIZE	AWP
○ **BRAND**			
SOLAQUIN FORTE: ICN	00187-0523-31	30 gm	$30.84
○ **GENERICS**			
NUQUIN HP: Stratus	58980-0475-05	15 gm	$11.25
NUQUIN HP: Stratus	58980-0575-10	30 gm	$17.90
NUQUIN HP: Stratus	58980-0475-20	60 gm	$30.30

SOLUTION: 3%

BRAND/MANUFACTURER	NDC	SIZE	AWP
○ **BRAND**			
MELQUIN-3: Stratus	58980-0476-10	30 ml	$8.70
MELANEX: Neutrogena	10812-9300-01	30 ml	$11.94

Hydroxyamphetamine Hydrobromide with Tropicamide

DESCRIPTION
Hydroxyamphetamine Hydrobromide/Tropicamide sterile ophthalmic solution is a topical mydriatic combination product for ophthalmic use.

Chemical Name: Hydroxyamphetamine Hydrobromide: Phenol, 4-(2-amino-propyl)-, Hydrobromide. Tropicamide: Benzeneacetamide, N-ethyl-α-(hydroxymethyl)-N-(4-pyridinylmethyl)-, troperamide.

Contains: Hydroxyamphetamine Hydrobromide, USP 1.0%. Tropicamide, USP 0.25%. pH of Hydroxyamphetamine Hydrobromide/Tropicamide can range from 4.2 to 5.8 during its shelf life. The osmolality of Hydroxyamphetamine Hydrobromide/Tropicamide is approximately 307 mOsm/l.

CLINICAL PHARMACOLOGY
Hydroxyamphetamine Hydrodromide/Tropicamide Solution combines the effects of the adrenergic agent, Hydroxyamphetamine Hydrobromide, and the anticholinergic agent, Tropicamide. Hydroxyamphetamine Hydrobromide is an indirectly-acting sympathomimetic agent which, when applied topically to the eye, causes the release of endogenous norepinephrine from intact adrenergic nerve terminals, resulting in mydriasis. Since Hydroxyamphetamine Hydrobromide has little or no direct activity on the receptor site, dilation does not usually occur if there is damage to the presynaptic nerve terminal, e.g., Horner's Syndrome. However, it is not known whether damage to the presynaptic nerve terminal will influence the extent of mydriasis produced by Hydroxyamphetamine Hydrobromide/Tropicamide. Hydroxyamphetamine Hydrobromide has minimal cycloplegic action. Tropicamide is a parasympatholytic agent which, when applied topically to the eye, blocks the responses of the sphincter muscle of the iris and ciliary muscle to cholinergic stimulation, producing dilation of the pupil and paralysis of the ciliary muscle. Tropicamide produces short-duration mydriasis. Although cycloplegia occurs with higher doses of Tropicamide, there is evidence with 0.25% Tropicamide that full cycloplegia does not occur. Since both these agents act on different effector sites, their simultaneous use produces an additive mydriatic effect. Hydroxyamphetamine Hydrobromide/Tropicamide provides diminished pupil responsiveness to light, facilitating ophthalmoscopy. The onset of action with Hydroxyamphetamine Hydrobromide/Tropicamide occurs within 15 minutes, followed by maximum effect within 60 minutes after instillation of one drop. Clinically significant dilation, inhibition of pupillary light response, and partial cycloplegia last 3 hours, with recovery beginning at approximately 90 minutes and with complete recovery occurring in most patients in 6 to 8 hours. However, in some cases, complete recovery may take up to 24 hours. Effectiveness may differ slightly in patients with light and dark irides, with those patients with light irides experiencing a slightly greater mydriasis.

INDICATIONS
Hydroxyamphetamine Hydrobromide/Tropicamide Solution is indicated for mydriasis in routine diagnostic procedures and in conditions where short-term pupil dilation is desired Hydroxyamphetamine Hydrobromide/Tropicamide provides clinically significant mydriasis with partial cycloplegia.

CONTRAINDICATIONS
Hydroxyamphetamine Hydrobromide/Tropicamide Solution should not be used in patients with angle-closure glaucoma or in those with narrow angles in whom dilation of the pupil may precipitate an attack of angle-closure glaucoma. This product is also contraindicated in patients who are hypersensitive to any of its components.

WARNINGS
For topical ophthalmic use only, not for injection. There is evidence that mydriatics may produce a transient elevation of intraocular pressure in patients with open-angle glaucoma. This preparation rarely may cause CNS disturbances which may be particularly dangerous in infants, children or the aged. Psychotic reactions, behavioral disturbances and vasomotor or cardio-respiratory collapse in children have been reported with the use of anticholinergic drugs.

PRECAUTIONS
General: Patients with hypertension, hyperthyroidism, diabetes or cardiac disease (i.e., arrhythmias or chronic ischemic heart disease) should be monitored after instillation. The elderly and others in whom glaucoma or increased intraocular pressure may be encountered following administration of Hydroxyamphetamine Hydrobromide/Tropicamide Solution should also be monitored closely. To avoid inducing angle-closure glaucoma, an estimation of the depth of the angle of the anterior chamber should be made.

◆ RATED THERAPEUTICALLY EQUIVALENT; ◇ THERAPEUTIC EQUIVALENCE UNCONFIRMED; ○ UNRATED

Information for Patients: Patients should be advised not to touch the dropper tip to any surface since this may contaminate the solution. Patients should be advised to use caution when driving or engaging in other hazardous activities while pupils are dilated. Patients may experience photophobia and/or blurred vision and should protect their eyes in bright illumination when pupils are dilated. Parents should be warned not to get this preparation in their child's mouth and to wash their own hands and the child's hands following administration.

Carcinogenesis, Mutagenesis, Impairment of Fertility: No studies have been performed to evaluate the carcinogenic, mutagenic or impairment of fertility, potential of Hydroxyamphetamine Hydrobromide/Tropicamide.

Pregnancy: Pregnancy Category C: Animal reproduction studies have not been conducted with Hydroxyamphetamine Hydrobromide/Tropicamide. It is also not known whether Hydroxyamphetamine Hydrobromide/Tropicamide can cause fetal harm when administered to a pregnant woman or can affect reproduction capability. Hydroxyamphetamine Hydrobromide/Tropicamide should be given to a pregnant woman only if clearly needed.

Nursing Mothers: It is not known whether this drug is excreted in human milk. Because many drugs are excreted in human milk, caution should be exercised when Hydroxyamphetamine Hydrobromide/Tropicamide is administered to a nursing woman.

Pediatric Use: Safety and effectiveness in children have not been established, Hydroxyamphetamine Hydrobromide/Tropicamide may rarely cause CNS disturbances which may be dangerous in infants and children. Psychotic reactions, behavioral disturbances and vasomotor or cardio-respiratory collapse in children have been reported with the use of anticholinergic drugs. (See *"Warnings"*.) Keep this and all medications out of the reach of children.

ADVERSE REACTIONS

Increased intraocular pressure has been reported following use of mydriatics. Transient stringing, dryness of the mouth, blurred vision, photophobia with or without corneal staining, tachycardia, headache, allergic reactions, nausea, vomiting, pallor, and muscle rigidity have been reported with the use of Tropicamide and/or Hydroxyamphetamine Hydrobromide, and thus may occur with Hydroxyamphetamine Hydrobromide/Tropicamide Solution. Central nervous system disturbances have also been reported. Psychotic reactions, behavioral disturbances, and vasomotor or cardiorespiratory collapse in children have been reported with the use of anticholinergic drugs.

OVERDOSAGE

Ocular overdosage will cause dilation of the pupils. Systemic overdosage or ingestion of large doses may result in hypertension, cardiac arrhythmias, substernal discomfort, headache, sweating, nausea, vomiting and gastrointestinal irritation. Patients with systemic overdosage should be carefully monitored and treated symptomatically.

DOSAGE AND ADMINISTRATION

One to two drops in the conjunctival sac. The onset of action with Hydroxyamphetamine Hydrobromide/Tropicamide Solution occurs within 15 minutes, followed by maximum effect within 60 minutes. Clinically significant dilation, inhibition of pupillary light response, and partial cycloplegia last 3 hours. Mydriasis will reverse spontaneously with time, typically in 6 to 8 hours. However, in some cases, complete recovery may take up to 24 hours.

Note: Protect from light. Store between 15 °C to 25 °C (59 °F to 77 °F).

HOW SUPPLIED
DROP: 1%-0.25%

BRAND/MANUFACTURER	NDC	SIZE	AWP
○ BRAND			
PAREMYD: Allergan Pharm	11980-0289-15	15 ml	$7.81

Hydroxychloroquine Sulfate

> **WARNING**
> PHYSICIANS SHOULD COMPLETELY FAMILIARIZE THEMSELVES WITH THE COMPLETE CONTENTS OF THIS LEAFLET BEFORE PRESCRIBING HYDROXYCHLOROQUINE.

DESCRIPTION

The compound is a colorless crystalline solid, soluble in water to at least 20 percent; chemically the drug is 2-[[4-[(7-Chloro-4- quinolyl) amino, pentyl] ethylamino] ethanol sulfate (1:1).

The following is its chemical structure:

Following is its chemical structure:

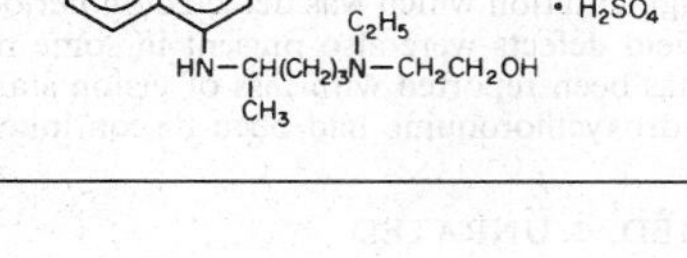

ACTIONS

The drug possesses antimalarial actions and also exerts a beneficial effect in lupus erythematosus (chronic discoid or systemic) and acute or chronic rheumatoid arthritis. The precise mechanism of action is not known.

INDICATIONS

Hydroxychloroquine Sulfate is indicated for the suppressive treatment and treatment of acute attacks of malaria due to *Plasmodium vivax, P. malariae, P. ovale,* and susceptible strains of *P. falciparum.* It is also indicated for the treatment of discoid and systemic lupus erythematosus, and rheumatoid arthritis.

UNLABELED USES

Hydroxychloroquine is used alone or as an adjunct in the treatment of asthma, noninsulin-dependent diabetes mellitus, and porphyria cutanea tarda. It is also used in pulmonary embolism and to diminish autoantibody titers in patients with primary Sjogren's syndrome.

CONTRAINDICATIONS

Use of this drug is contraindicated (1) in the presence of retinal or visual field changes attributable to any 4-aminoquinoline compound, (2) in patients with known hypersensitivity to 4-aminoquinoline compounds, and (3) for long-term therapy in children.

WARNINGS
GENERAL

Hydroxychloroquine Sulfate is not effective against chloroquine-resistant strains of *P. falciparum.*

Children are especially sensitive to the 4-aminoquinoline compounds. A number of fatalities have been reported following the accidental ingestion of chloroquine, sometimes in relatively small doses (0.75 g or 1 g in one 3-year-old child). Patients should be strongly warned to keep these drugs out of the reach of children.

Use of Hydroxychloroquine Sulfate in patients with psoriasis may precipitate a severe attack of psoriasis. When used in patients with porphyria the condition may be exacerbated. The preparation should not be used in these conditions unless in the judgment of the physician the benefit to the patient outweighs the possible hazard.

Usage in Pregnancy: Usage of this drug during pregnancy should be avoided except in the suppression or treatment of malaria when in the judgment of the physician the benefit outweighs the possible hazard. It should be noted that radioactively-tagged chloroquine administered intravenously to pregnant, pigmented CBA mice passed rapidly across the placenta. It accumulated selectively in the melanin structures of the fetal eyes and was retained in the ocular tissues for five months after the drug had been eliminated from the rest of the body.

PRECAUTIONS

General: Antimalarial compound should be used with caution in patients with hepatic disease or alcoholism or in conjunction with known hepatotoxic drugs.

Periodic blood cell counts should be made if patients are given prolonged therapy. If any severe blood disorder appears which is not attributable to the disease under treatment, discontinuation of the drug should be considered. The drug should be administered with caution in patients having G-6-PD (glucose-6-phosphate dehydrogenase) deficiency.

OVERDOSAGE

The 4-aminoquinoline compounds are very rapidly and completely absorbed after ingestion, and in accidental overdosage, or rarely with lower doses in hypersensitive patients, toxic symptoms may occur within 30 minutes. These consist of headache, drowsiness, visual disturbances, cardiovascular collapse, and convulsions, followed by sudden and early respiratory and cardiac arrest. The electrocardiogram may reveal atrial standstill, nodal rhythm, prolonged intraventricular conduction time, and progressive bradycardia leading to ventricular fibrillation and/or arrest. Treatment is symptomatic and must be prompt with immediate evacuation of the stomach by emesis (at home, before transportation to the hospital) or gastric lavage until the stomach is completely emptied. If finely powdered, activated charcoal is introduced by the stomach tube, after lavage, and within 30 minutes after ingestion of the tablets, it may inhibit further intestinal absorption of the drug. To be effective, the dose of activated charcoal should be at least five times the estimated dose of Hydroxychloroquine ingested. Convulsions, if present, should be controlled before attempting gastric lavage. If due to cerebral stimulation, cautious administration of an ultrashort-acting barbiturate may be tried but, if due to anoxia, it should be corrected by oxygen administration, artificial respiration or, in shock with hypotension, by vasopressor therapy. Because of the importance of supporting respiration, tracheal intubation or tracheostomy, followed by gastric lavage, may also be necessary. Exchange transfusions have been used to reduce the level of 4-aminoquinoline drug in the blood.

A patient who survives the acute phase and is asymptomatic should be closely observed for at least six hours. Fluids may be forced, and sufficient ammonium chloride (8 g daily in divided doses for adults) may be administered for a few days to acidify the urine to help promote urinary excretion in cases of both overdosage and sensitivity.

MALARIA

ACTIONS

Like chloroquine phosphate, USP, Hydroxychloroquine Sulfate is highly active against the erythrocytic forms of *P. vivax* and *malariae* and most strains of *P. falciparum* (but not the gametocytes of *P. falciparum*).

Hydroxychloroquine Sulfate does not prevent relapses in patients with *vivax* or *malariae* malaria because it is not effective against exo-erythrocytic forms of the parasite, nor will it prevent *vivax* or *malariae* infection when administered as a prophylactic. It is highly effective as a suppressive agent in patients with *vivax* or *malariae* malaria, in terminating acute attacks, and significantly lengthening the interval between treatment and relapse. In patients with *falciparum* malaria, it abolishes the acute attack and effects complete cure of the infection, unless due to a resistant strain of *P. falciparum*.

INDICATIONS

Hydroxychloroquine Sulfate is indicated for the treatment of acute attacks and suppression of malaria.

WARNING

In recent years, it has been found that certain strains of *P. falciparum* have become resistant to 4-aminoquinoline compounds (including Hydroxychloroquine) as shown by the fact that normally adequate doses have failed to prevent or cure clinical malaria or parasitemia. Treatment with quinine or other specific forms of therapy is therefore advised for patients infected with a resistant strain of parasites.

ADVERSE REACTIONS

Following the administration in doses adequate for the treatment of an acute malarial attack, mild and transient headache, dizziness, and gastrointestinal complaints (diarrhea, anorexia, nausea, abdominal cramps and, on rare occasions, vomiting) may occur.

DOSAGE AND ADMINISTRATION

One tablet of 200 mg of Hydroxychloroquine Sulfate is equivalent to 155 mg base.

Malaria: Suppression—*In adults,* 400 mg (= 310 mg base) on exactly the same day of each week. *In infants and children,* the weekly suppressive dosage is 5 mg, calculated as base, per kg of body weight, but should not exceed the adult dose regardless of weight.

If circumstances permit, suppressive therapy should begin two weeks prior to exposure. However, failing this, in adults an initial double (loading) dose of 800 mg (= 620 mg base), or in children 10 mg base/kg may be taken in two divided doses, six hours apart. The suppressive therapy should be continued for eight weeks after leaving the endemic area.

Treatment of the acute attack—*In adults,* an initial dose of 800 mg (= 620 mg base) followed by 400 mg (= 310 mg base) in six to eight hours and 400 mg (310 mg base) on each of two consecutive days (total 2 g hydroxychloroquine sulfate or 1.55 g base). An alternative method, employing a single dose of 800 mg (= 620 mg base), has also proved effective.

The dosage for adults may also be calculated on the basis of body weight; this method is preferred for infants and children. A total dose representing 25 mg of base per kg of body weight is administered in three days, as follows:

First dose: 10 mg base per kg (but not exceeding a single dose of 620 mg base).
Second dose: 5 mg base per kg (but not exceeding a single dose of 310 mg base) 6 hours after first dose.
Third dose: 5 mg base per kg 18 hours after second dose.
Fourth dose: 5 mg base per kg 24 hours after third dose.

For radical cure of *vivax* and *malariae* malaria concomitant therapy with an 8-aminoquinoline compound is necessary.

LUPUS ERYTHEMATOSUS AND RHEUMATOID ARTHRITIS

INDICATIONS

Hydroxychloroquine Sulfate is useful in patients with the following disorders who have not responded satisfactorily to drugs with less potential for serious side effects: lupus erythematosus (chronic discoid and systemic) and acute or chronic rheumatoid arthritis.

WARNINGS

PHYSICIANS SHOULD COMPLETELY FAMILIARIZE THEMSELVES WITH THE COMPLETE CONTENTS OF THIS LEAFLET BEFORE PRESCRIBING HYDROXYCHLOROQUINE SULFATE.

Irreversible retinal damage has been observed in some patients who had received long-term or high-dosage 4-amino-quinoline therapy for discoid and systemic lupus erythematosus, or rheumatoid arthritis. Retinopathy has been reported to be dose related.

When prolonged therapy with any antimalarial compound is contemplated, initial (base line) and periodic (every three months) ophthalmologic examinations (including visual acuity, expert slit-lamp, funduscopic, and visual field tests) should be performed.

If there is any indication of abnormality in the visual acuity, visual field, or retinal macular areas (such as pigmentary changes, loss of foveal reflex), or any visual symptoms (such as light flashes and streaks) which are not fully explainable by difficulties of accommodation or corneal opacities, the drug should be discontinued immediately and the patient closely observed for possible progression. Retinal changes (and visual disturbances) may progress even after cessation of therapy.

All patients on long-term therapy with this preparation should be questioned and examined periodically, including the testing of knee and ankle reflexes, to detect any evidence of muscular weakness. If weakness occurs, discontinue the drug.

In the treatment of rheumatoid arthritis, if objective improvement (such as reduced joint swelling, increased mobility) does not occur within six months, the drug should be discontinued. Safe use of the drug in the treatment of juvenile arthritis has not been established.

PRECAUTIONS

Dermatologic reactions to Hydroxychloroquine Sulfate tablets may occur and, therefore, proper care should be exercised when it is administered to any patient receiving a drug with a significant tendency to produce dermatitis.

The methods recommended for early diagnosis of "chloroquine retinopathy" consist of (1) funduscopic examination of the macula for fine pigmentary disturbances or loss of the foveal reflex and (2) examination of the central visual field with a small red test object for pericentral or paracentral scotoma or determination of retinal thresholds to red. Any unexplained visual symptoms, such as light flashes or streaks should also be regarded with suspicion as possible manifestations of retinopathy.

If serious toxic symptoms occur from overdosage or sensitivity, it has been suggested that ammonium chloride (8 g daily in divided doses for adults) be administered orally three or four days a week for several months after therapy has been stopped, as acidification of the urine increases renal excretion of the 4-aminoquinoline compounds by 20 to 90 percent. However, caution must be exercised in patients with impaired renal function and/or metabolic acidosis.

ADVERSE REACTIONS

Not all of the following reactions have been observed with every 4-aminoquinoline compound during long-term therapy, but they have been reported with one or more and should be borne in mind when drugs of this class are administered. Adverse effects with different compounds vary in type and frequency.

CNS REACTIONS

Irritability, nervousness, emotional changes, nightmares, psychosis, headache, dizziness, vertigo, tinnitus, nystagmus, nerve deafness, convulsions, ataxia.

NEUROMUSCULAR REACTIONS

Extraocular muscle palsies, skeletal, muscle weakness, absent or hypoactive deep tendon reflexes.

OCULAR REACTIONS

A. Ciliary Body: Disturbance of accommodation with symptoms of blurred vision. This reaction is dose related and reversible with cessation of therapy.

B. Cornea: Transient edema, punctate to lineal opacities, decreased corneal sensitivity. The corneal changes, with or without accompanying symptoms (blurred vision, halos around lights, photophobia), are fairly common, but reversible. Corneal deposits may appear as early as three weeks following initiation of therapy.

The incidence of corneal changes and visual side effects appears to be considerably lower with Hydroxychloroquine than with chloroquine.

C. Retina:
Macula: Edema, atrophy, abnormal pigmentation (mild pigment stippling to a "bull's-eye" appearance), loss of foveal reflex, increased macular recovery time following exposure to a bright light (photo-stress test), elevated retinal threshold to red light in macular, paramacular and peripheral retinal areas.

Other fundus changes: Include optic disc pallor and atrophy, attenuation of retinal arterioles, fine granular pigmentary disturbances in the peripheral retina and prominent choroidal patterns in advanced stage.

D. Visual Field Defects: Pericentral or paracentral scotoma, central scotoma with decreased visual acuity, rarely field constriction.

The most common visual symptoms attributed to the retinopathy are: reading and seeing difficulties (words, letters, or parts of objects missing), photophobia, blurred distance vision, missing or blacked out areas in the central or peripheral visual field, light flashes and streaks.

Retinopathy appears to be dose related and has occurred within several months (rarely) to several years of daily therapy; a small number of cases have been reported several years after antimalarial drug therapy was discontinued. It has not been noted during prolonged use of weekly doses of the 4-aminoquinoline compounds for suppression of malaria. Patients with retinal changes may have visual symptoms or may be asymptomatic (with or without visual field changes). Rarely, scotomatous vision or field defects may occur without obvious retinal change.

Retinopathy may progress even after the drug is discontinued. In a number of patients, early retinopathy (macular pigmentation sometimes with central field defects) diminished or regressed completely after therapy was discontinued. Paracentral scotoma to red targets (sometimes called "premaculopathy") is indicative of early retinal dysfunction which is usually reversible with cessation of therapy.

A small number of cases of retinal changes have been reported as occurring in patients who received only Hydroxychloroquine. These usually consisted of alteration in retinal pigmentation which was detected on periodic ophthalmologic examination; visual field defects were also present in some instances. A case of delayed retinopathy has been reported with loss of vision starting one year after administration of Hydroxychloroquine had been discontinued.

DERMATOLOGIC REACTIONS

Bleaching of hair, alopecia, pruritus, skin and mucosal pigmentation, skin eruptions (urticarial, morbilliform, lichenoid, maculopapular, purpuric, erythema annulare centrifugum and exfoliative dermatitis.

HEMATOLOGIC REACTIONS

Various blood dyscrasias such as aplastic anemia, agranulocytosis, leukopenia, thrombocytopenia (hemolysis in individuals with glucose-6-phosphate dehydrogenase (G-6-PD) deficiency).

GASTROINTESTINAL REACTIONS

Anorexia, nausea, vomiting, diarrhea, and abdominal cramps.

MISCELLANEOUS REACTIONS

Weight loss, lassitude, exacerbation or precipitation of porphyria and nonlight-sensitive psoriasis.

Cardiomyopathy has been rarely reported and the relationship to Hydroxychloroquine is unclear.

DOSAGE AND ADMINISTRATION

One tablet of Hydroxychloroquine Sulfate, 200 mg, is equivalent to 155 mg base.

Lupus Erythematosus: Initially, the average *adult* dose is 400 mg (= 310 mg base) once or twice daily. This may be continued for several weeks or months depending on the response of the patient. For prolonged maintenance therapy, a smaller dose, from 200 mg to 400 mg (= 155 mg to 310 mg base) daily will frequently suffice.

The incidence of retinopathy has been reported to be higher when this maintenance dose is exceeded.

Rheumatoid Arthritis: The compound is cumulative in action and will require several weeks to exert its beneficial therapeutic effects, whereas minor side effects may occur relatively early. Several months of therapy may be required before maximum effects can be obtained. If objective improvement (such as reduced joint swelling, increased mobility) does not occur within six months, the drug should be discontinued. Safe use of the drug in the treatment of juvenile rheumatoid arthritis has not been established.

Initial Dosage: In *adults,* from 400 mg to 600 mg (= 310 mg to 465 mg base) daily, each dose to be taken with a meal or a glass of milk. In a small percentage of patients, troublesome side effects may require temporary reduction of the initial dosage. Later (usually from five to ten days), the dose may gradually be increased to the optimum response level, often without return of side effects.

Maintenance Dosage: When a good response is obtained (usually in four to twelve weeks), the dosage is reduced by 50 percent and continued at a usual maintenance level of 200 mg to 400 mg (= 155 mg to 310 mg base) daily, each dose to be taken with a meal or a glass of milk. The incidence of retinopathy has been reported to be higher when this maintenance dose is exceeded.

Should a relapse occur after medication is withdrawn, therapy may be resumed or continued on an intermittent schedule if there are no ocular contraindications.

Corticosteroids and Salicylates: may be used in conjunction with this compound, and they can generally be decreased gradually in dosage or eliminated after the drug has been used for several weeks. When gradual reduction of steroid dosage is indicated, it may be done by reducing every four to five days the dose of cortisone by no more than from 5 mg to 15 mg; of hydrocortisone from 5 mg to 10 mg; of prednisolone and prednisone from 1 mg to 2.5 mg; of methylprednisolone and triamcinolone from 1 mg to 2 mg; and of dexamethasone from 0.25 mg to 0.5 mg.

HOW SUPPLIED

TABLETS: 200 MG

BRAND/MANUFACTURER	NDC	SIZE	AWP
○ **BRAND**			
► PLAQUENIL SULFATE: Sanofi Winthrop	00024-1562-10	100s	$110.42

Hydroxyprogesterone Caproate

WARNING

THE USE OF HYDROXYPROGESTERONE CAPROATE DURING THE FIRST FOUR MONTHS OF PREGNANCY IS NOT RECOMMENDED.

PROGESTATIONAL AGENTS HAVE BEEN USED BEGINNING WITH THE FIRST TRIMESTER OF PREGNANCY IN AN ATTEMPT TO PREVENT HABITUAL ABORTION OR TREAT THREATENED ABORTION. THERE IS NO ADEQUATE EVIDENCE THAT SUCH USE IS EFFECTIVE AND THERE IS EVIDENCE OF POTENTIAL HARM TO THE FETUS WHEN SUCH DRUGS ARE GIVEN DURING THE FIRST 4 MONTHS OF PREGNANCY. FURTHERMORE, IN THE VAST MAJORITY OF WOMEN, THE CAUSE OF ABORTION IS A DEFECTIVE OVUM, WHICH PROGESTATIONAL AGENTS COULD NOT BE EXPECTED TO INFLUENCE. IN ADDITION, THE USE OF PROGESTATIONAL AGENTS, WITH THEIR UTERINE-RELAXANT PROPERTIES, IN PATIENTS WITH FERTILIZED DEFECTIVE OVA MAY CAUSE A DELAY IN SPONTANEOUS ABORTION. THEREFORE, THE USE OF SUCH DRUGS DURING THE FIRST 4 MONTHS OF PREGNANCY IS NOT RECOMMENDED.

SEVERAL REPORTS SUGGEST AN ASSOCIATION BETWEEN INTRAUTERINE EXPOSURE TO PROGESTATIONAL DRUGS IN THE FIRST TRIMESTER OF PREGNANCY AND GENITAL ABNORMALITIES IN MALE AND FEMALE FETUSES. THE RISK OF HYPOSPADIAS, 5 TO 8 PER 1,000 MALE BIRTHS IN THE GENERAL POPULATION, MAY BE APPROXIMATELY DOUBLED WITH EXPOSURE TO THESE DRUGS. THERE ARE INSUFFICIENT DATA TO QUANTIFY THE RISK TO EXPOSED FEMALE FETUSES, BUT INSOFAR AS SOME OF THESE DRUGS INDUCE MILD VIRILIZATION OF THE EXTERNAL GENITALIA OF THE FEMALE FETUS, AND BECAUSE OF THE INCREASED ASSOCIATION OF HYPOSPADIAS IN THE MALE FETUS, IT IS PRUDENT TO AVOID THE USE OF THESE DRUGS DURING THE FIRST TRIMESTER OF PREGNANCY.

SEVERAL REPORTS SUGGEST AN ASSOCIATION BETWEEN INTRAUTERINE EXPOSURE TO FEMALE SEX HORMONES AND CONGENITAL ANOMALIES, INCLUDING CONGENITAL HEART DEFECTS AND LIMB REDUCTION DEFECTS (REFS. 1-5). ONE STUDY (REF. 4) ESTIMATED A 4.7-FOLD INCREASED RISK OF LIMB REDUCTION DEFECTS IN INFANTS EXPOSED *IN UTERO* TO SEX HORMONES (ORAL CONTRACEPTIVES, HORMONE WITHDRAWAL TESTS FOR PREGNANCY, OR ATTEMPTED TREATMENT FOR THREATENED ABORTION). SOME OF THESE EXPOSURES WERE VERY SHORT AND INVOLVED ONLY A FEW DAYS OF TREATMENT. THE DATA SUGGEST THAT THE RISK OF LIMB REDUCTION DEFECTS IN EXPOSED FETUSES IS SOMEWHAT LESS THAN 1 IN 1,000.

IF THE PATIENT IS EXPOSED TO HYDROXYPROGESTERONE CAPROATE DURING THE FIRST FOUR MONTHS OF PREGNANCY OR IF SHE BECOMES PREGNANT WHILE TAKING THIS DRUG, SHE SHOULD BE APPRISED OF THE POTENTIAL RISKS TO THE FETUS.

DESCRIPTION

Hydroxyprogesterone Caproate injection is a sterile solution of Hydroxyprogesterone Caproate. *Each mL contains*: Hydroxyprogesterone Caproate 125 or 250 mg.

Hydroxyprogesterone Caproate 17-Hydroxypregn-4-ene-3, 20-dione hexanoate is a white or off white crystalline powder. The empirical fromula is $C_{27}H_{40}O_4$ and the molecular weight 428.62.

Hydroxyprogesterone Caproate is classed as a progestogen for intramuscular injection.

Following is its chemical structure:

CLINICAL PHARMACOLOGY

Hydroxyprogesterone Caproate transforms proliferative endometrium into secretory endometrium.

Inhibits (at the usual dose range) the secretion of pituitary gonadotropins, which in turn prevents follicular maturation and ovulation.

May also demonstrate some estrogenic, anabolic, androgenic or corticoid activity but should not be relied upon for these effects.

INDICATIONS AND USAGE

This drug is indicated in amenorrhea, abnormal uterine bleeding due to hormonal imbalance in the absence of organic pathology, such as submucous fibriods or uterine cancer; for production of secretory endometrium and desquamation; as a test for endogenous estrogen production ("Medical D and C").

UNLABELED USES

Hydroxyprogesterone Caproate is used alone or as an adjunct in the treatment of androgenetic alopecia, benign prostatic hyperplasia, ureteral calculi, and preterm labor.

CONTRAINDICATIONS

1. Thrombophlebitis, thromboembolic disorders, cerebral apoplexy or patients with a past history of these conditions.
2. Known or suspected carcinoma of the breast.
3. Undiagnosed vaginal bleeding.
4. Missed abortion.
5. As a diagnostic test for pregnancy.

WARNINGS

Hydroxyprogesterone Caproate may cause fetal harm when administered to a pregnant woman.

If this drug is used during pregnancy, or if the patient becomes pregnant while taking this drug, the patient should be apprised of the potential hazard to the fetus.

There is an increased risk of birth defects in children whose mothers take this drug during the first four months of pregnancy.

Hydroxyprogesterone is similar to the progesterone hormones naturally produced by the body. Hydroxyprogesterone and progesterone-like drugs are used to treat menstrual disorders, to test if the body is producing certain hormones, and to treat some forms of cancer in women.

They have been used as a test for pregnancy but such use is no longer considered safe because of possible damage to a developing baby. Also, more rapid methods for testing for pregnancy are now available.

These drugs have also been used to prevent miscarriage in the first few months of pregnancy. No adequate evidence is available to show that they are effective for this purpose and there is evidence of an increased risk of birth defects, such as heart or limb defects, if these drugs are taken during the first four months of pregnancy. Furthermore, most cases of early miscarriage are due to causes which could not be helped by these drugs.

The exact risk of taking this drug early in pregnancy and having a baby with a birth defect is not known. However, one study found that babies born to women who had taken sex hormones (such as progesterone-like drugs) during the first three months of pregnancy were 4 to 5 times more likely to have abnormalities of the arms or legs than if their mothers had not taken such drugs. Some of these women had taken these drugs for only a few days. The chance that an infant whose mother had taken this drug will have this type of defect is about 1 in 1,000.

Masculinization of the female fetus has occurred when progestogens have been used in pregnant women.

Discontinue medication pending examination if there is a sudden partial or complete loss of vision, or if there is sudden onset of proptosis, diplopia or migraine. If examination reveals papilledema or retinal vascular lesions, medication should be withdrawn.

Because of the occasional occurrence of thrombophlebitis and pulmonary embolism in patients taking progestogens, the physician should be alert to the earliest manifestation of the disease. If these occur or are suspected the drug should be discontinued immediately.

PRECAUTIONS

General: The pretreatment physical examination should include special reference to breast and pelvic organs, as well as Papanicolaou smear.

Because this drug may cause some degree of fluid retention, conditions which might be influenced by this factor, such as epilepsy, migraine, asthma, cardiac or renal dysfunction, require careful observation.

In cases of breakthrough bleeding, as in all cases of irregular bleeding per vaginam, nonfunctional causes should be borne in mind. In cases of undiagnosed vaginal bleeding, adequate diagnostic measures are indicated.

Patients who have a history of psychic depression should be carefully observed and the drug discontinued if the depression recurs to a serious degree.

Any possible influence of prolonged progestin therapy on pituitary, ovarian, adrenal, hepatic or uterine functions awaits further study.

A decrease in glucose tolerance has been observed in a small percentage of patients on estrogen-progestin combination drugs. The mechanism of this decrease is obscure. For this reason, diabetic patients should be carefully observed while receiving progestin therapy.

The age of the patient constitutes no absolute limiting factor although treatment with progestins may mask the onset of the climacteric.

The pathologist should be advised of progestin therapy when relevant specimens are submitted.

Studies of the addition of a progestin product to an estrogen replacement regimen for seven or more days of a cycle of estrogen administration have reported a lowered incidence of endometrial hyperplasia. Morphological and biochemical studies of endometrium suggest that 10 to 13 days of a progestin are needed to provide maximal maturation of the endometrium and to eliminate any hyperplastic changes. Whether this will provide protection from endometrial carcinoma has not been clearly established. There are possible additional risks which may be associated with the inclusion of progestin in estrogen replacement regimens. The potential risks include adverse effects on carbohydrate and lipid metabolism. The dosage used may be important in minimizing these adverse effects.

PATIENT LABELING FOR PROGESTATIONAL DRUG PRODUCTS WARNING FOR WOMEN

Progesterone is similar to the progesterone hormones naturally produced by the body. Progesterone and progesterone-like drugs are used to treat menstrual disorders, to test if the body is producing certain hormones, and to treat some forms of cancer in women.

Progesterone or progesteron-like drugs have been used to prevent miscarriage in the first few months of pregnancy. No adequate evidence is available to show that they are effective for this purpose and there is evidence of an increased risk of birth defects, such as heart or limb defects, if these drugs are taken during the first four months of pregnancy. Furthermore, most cases of early miscarriage are due to causes which could not be helped by these drugs.

There is an increased risk of minor birth defects in children whose mothers take this drug during the first 4 months of pregnancy. Several reports suggest an association between mothers who take these drugs in the first trimester of pregnancy and genital abnormalities in male and female babies. The risk to the male baby is the possibility of being born with a condition in which the opening of the penis is on the underside rather than the tip of the penis (hypospadias). Hypospadias occurs in about 5 to 8 per 1,000 male births and is about doubled with exposure to these drugs. There is not enough information to quantify the risk to exposed female fetuses, but enlargement of the clitoris and fusion of the labia may occur, although rarely.

Therefore, since drugs of this type may induce mild masculinization of the external genitalia of the female fetus, as well as hypospadias in the male fetus, it is wise to avoid using the drug during the first trimester of pregnancy.

The exact risk of taking this drug early in pregnancy and having a baby with a birth defect is not known. However, one study found that babies born to women who had taken sex hormones (such as progesterone-like drugs) during the first three months of pregnancy were 4 to 5 times more likely to have abnormalities of the arms or legs than if their mothers had not taken such drugs. Some of these women had taken these drugs for only a few days. The chance that an infant whose mother had taken this drug will have this type of defect is about 1 in 1,000.

These drugs have been used as a test for pregnancy but such use is no longer considered safe because of possible damage to a developing baby. Also, more rapid methods for testing for pregnancy are now available.

If you take progesterone or a progesterone-like drug and later find you were pregnant when you took it, be sure to discuss this with your doctor as soon as possible.

Drug/Laboratory Test Interactions: The following laboratory result may be altered by the use of progestogens: Pregnanediol determination.

In addition, the following laboratory results may be altered by the concomitant use of estrogens with progestogens:

1. Hepatic function.
2. Coagulation tests: increase in prothrombin, Factors VII, VIII, IX and X.
3. Increase in PBI, BEI and a decrease in T uptake.
4. Metyrapone test.

Carcinogenesis, Mutagenesis, Impairment of Fertility: Beagle dogs treated with medroxyprogesterone acetate (MPA) injection (a progestin closely related to Hydroxyprogesterone Caproate) developed mammary nodules, some of which were malignant.

Although nodules occasionally appeared in control animals, they were intermittent in nature, whereas the nodules in the drug-treated animals were larger, more numerous, persistent, and there were some breast malignancies with metastases. Their significance with respect to humans has not been established.

Pregnancy Category D: See "Warnings" section.

Nursing Mothers: Caution should be exercised when Hydroxyprogesterone Caproate is administered to a nursing woman.

Detectable amounts of progestogens have been identified in the milk of mothers receiving them. The effect of this on the nursing infant has not been determined.

Pediatric Use: Hydroxyprogesterone Caproate is not indicated for pediatric use; therefore safety and effectiveness in children have not been established.

ADVERSE REACTIONS

The following adverse reactions have been observed in women taking progestogens:

Breakthrough bleeding, spotting, change in menstrual flow, amenorrhea, edema, changes in weight (increase or decrease), changes in cervical erosion and cervical secretions, cholestatic jaundice, rash (allergic) with and without pruritus, melasma or chloasma, and mental depression.

A statistically significant association has been demonstrated between use of estrogen-progestin combination drugs and the following serious adverse reactions: thrombophlebitis; pulmonary embolism and cerebral thrombosis and embolism. For this reason patients on progestin therapy should be carefully observed.

Although available evidence is suggestive of an association, such a relationship has been neither confirmed nor refuted for the following serious, adverse reactions:

Neuro-ocular lesions, e.g., retinal thrombosis and optic neuritis.

The following adverse reactions have been observed in patients receiving estrogen-progestin combination drugs:

Rise in blood pressure in susceptible individuals, premenstrual-like syndrome, changes in libido, changes in appetite, cystitis-like syndrome, headache, nervousness, dizziness, fatigue, backache, hirsutism, loss of scalp hair, erythema multiforme, erythema nodosum, hemorrhagic eruption and itching.

In view of these observations, patients on progestin therapy should be carefully observed for their occurrence.

DOSAGE AND ADMINISTRATION

Route of administration: Intramuscular.

Hydroxyprogesterone Caproate is effective for the following conditions:
1. Amenorrhea—Usual adult dose: 375 mg.
2. Dysfunctional uterine bleeding, metrorrhagia—Usual adult dose. 375 mg.
3. Production of secretory endometrium and desquamation. Test for continous endogenous estrogen production (Medical D and C)—Usual

Adult Dose: 125 to 250 mg given on 10th day of cycle; repeat every 7 days until suppression is no longer desired.

Parenteral drug products should be inspected visually for particulate matter and discoloration prior to administration whenever the solution and container permit.

REFERENCES

1. Gal, I., B. Kirman, and J. Stern, "Hormone Pregnancy Tests and Congenital Malformation," *Nature*, 216:83, 1967. 2. Levy, E.P., A. Cohen, and F.C. Fraser, "Hormone Treatment During Pregnancy and Congenital Heart Defects," *Lancet*, 1:611, 1973. 3. Nora, J. and A. Nora, "Birth Defects and Oral Contraceptives," *Lancet*, 1:941-942, 1973. 4. Janerich, D.T., J.M. Piper, and D.M. Glebatis, "Oral Contraceptives and Congenital Limb-Reduction Defects," *New England Journal of Medicine*, 291:697-700, 1974. 5. Heinonen, O.P., D. Slone, R.R. Monson, E.B. Hook and S. Shapiro, "Cardiovascular Birth Defects and Antenatal Exposure to Female Sex Hormones," *New England Journal of Medicine*, 296:67-70, 1977.

J CODES
250 mg/ml IM—J1741
125 mg/ml IM—J1739

HOW SUPPLIED
INJECTION: 125 MG/ML

BRAND/MANUFACTURER	NDC	SIZE	AWP
◆ GENERICS			
Schein	00364-2184-54	10 ml	$11.25

INJECTION: 250 MG/ML

AVERAGE UNIT PRICE (AVAILABLE SIZES)		GENERIC A-RATED AVERAGE PRICE (GAAP)	
GENERIC	$2.61	5 ml	$13.04

BRAND/MANUFACTURER	NDC	SIZE	AWP
◆ GENERICS			
Schein	00364-6690-53	5 ml	$10.80
Steris	00402-0598-05	5 ml	$10.80
Major	00904-0852-05	5 ml	$13.15
HYLUTIN: Hyrex	00314-0891-75	5 ml	$13.30
Moore,H.L.	00839-6279-25	5 ml	$14.43
Rugby	00536-1695-65	5 ml	$15.75

Hydroxypropyl Cellulose

DESCRIPTION
Hydroxypropyl Cellulose is a sterile, translucent, rod-shaped, water soluble, ophthalmic insert made of Hydroxypropyl Cellulose for administration into the inferior cul-de-sac of the eye.

The chemical name for Hydroxypropyl Cellulose is Cellulose, 2-Hydroxypropyl ether. It is an ether of Cellulose in which Hydroxypropyl groups (-$CH_2CHOHCH_3$) are attached to the Hydroxyls present in the anhydroglucose rings of Cellulose by ether linkages.

The molecular weight is typically 1×10^6.

Hydroxypropyl Cellulose is an off-white, odorless, tasteless powder. It is soluble in water below 38°C, and in many polar organic solvents such as ethanol, propylene glycol, dioxane, methanol, isopropyl alcohol (95%), dimethyl sulfoxide, and dimethyl formamide.

Each Hydroxypropyl Cellulose sterile opthalmic insert consists of 5 mg of Hydroxypropyl Cellulose. It contains no preservatives or other ingredients. It is about 1.27 mm in diameter by about 3.5 mm long.

Inserts are supplied in packages of 60 units, together with illustrated instructions and a special applicator for removing the insert from the unit dose blister and inserting it into the eye. A spare applicator is included in each package.

CLINICAL PHARMACOLOGY
PHARMACODYNAMICS
Hydroxypropyl Cellulose acts to stabilize and thicken the precorneal tear film and prolong the tear film breakup time which is usually accelerated in patients with dry eye states. Hydroxypropyl Cellulose also acts to lubricate and protect the eye. Hydroxypropyl Cellulose usually reduces the signs and symptoms resulting from moderate to severe dry eye syndromes, such as conjunctival hyperemia, corneal and conjunctival staining with rose bengal, exudation, itching, burning, foreign body sensation, smarting, photophobia, dryness and blurred or cloudy vision. Progressive visual deterioration which occurs in some patients may be retarded, halted, or sometimes reversed. In a multicenter crossover study the 5 mg Hydroxypropyl Cellulose administered once a day during the waking hours was compared to artificial tears used four or more times daily. There was a prolongation of tear film breakup time and a decrease in foreign body sensation associated with dry eye syndrome in patients during treatment with inserts as compared to artificial tears; these findings were statistically significantly different between the treatment groups. Improvement, as measured by amelioration of symptoms, by slit-lamp examination and by rose bengal staining of the cornea and conjunctiva, was greater in most patients with moderate to severe symptoms during treatment with Hydroxypropyl Cellulose. Patient comfort was usually better with Hydroxypropyl Cellulose than with artificial tears solution, and most patients preferred Hydroxypropyl Cellulose.

In most patients treated with Hydroxypropyl Cellulose for over one year, improvement was observed as evidenced by amelioration of symptoms generally associated with keratoconjunctivitis sicca such as burning, tearing, foreign body sensation, itching, photophobia and blurred or cloudy vision.

During studies in healthy volunteers, a thickened precorneal tear film was usually observed through the slit-lamp while Hydroxypropyl Cellulose was present in the conjunctival sac.

PHARMACOKINETICS AND METABOLISM
Hydroxypropyl Cellulose is a physiologically inert substance. In a study of rats fed Hydroxypropyl Cellulose or unmodified Cellulose at levels up to 5% of their diet, it was found that the two were biologically equivalent in that neither was metabolized.

Studies conducted in rats fed ^{14}C-labeled Hydroxypropyl Cellulose demonstrated that when orally administered, Hydroxypropyl Cellulose is not absorbed from the gastrointestinal tract and is quantitatively excreted in the feces.

Dissolution studies in rabbits showed that Hydroxypropyl Cellulose inserts became softer within 1 hour after they were placed in the conjunctival sac. Most of the inserts dissolved completely in 14 to 18 hours; with a single exception, all had disappeared by 24 hours after insertion. Similar dissolution of the inserts was observed during prolonged administration (up to 54 weeks).

INDICATIONS AND USAGE
Hydroxypropyl Cellulose is indicated in patients with moderate to severe dry eye syndromes, including keratoconjunctivitis sicca. Hydroxypropyl Cellulose is indicated especially in patients who remain symptomatic after an adequate trial of therapy with artificial tear solutions.

Hydroxypropyl Cellulose is also indicated for patients with:

Exposure keratitis
Decreased corneal sensitivity
Recurrent corneal erosions

CONTRAINDICATIONS
Hydroxypropyl Cellulose is contraindicated in patients who are hypersensitive to Hydroxypropyl Cellulose.

WARNINGS
Instructions for inserting and removing Hydroxypropyl Cellulose should be carefully followed.

PRECAUTIONS
GENERAL
If improperly placed, Hydroxypropyl Cellulose may result in corneal abrasion (see "Dosage and Administration").

INFORMATION FOR PATIENTS
Patients should be advised to follow the instructions for using Hydroxypropyl Cellulose which accompany the package.

Because this product may produce transient blurring of vision, patients should be instructed to exercise caution when operating hazardous machinery or driving a motor vehicle.

DRUG INTERACTIONS
Application of Hydroxypropyl Cellulose inserts to the eyes of unanesthetized rabbits immediately prior to or two hours before instilling pilocarpine, proparacaine HCl (0.5%), or phenylephrine (5%) did not markedly alter the magnitude and/or duration of the miotic, local corneal anesthetic, or mydriatic activity, respectively, of these agents.

Under various treatment schedules, the anti-inflammatory effect of ocularly instilled dexamethasone (0.1%) in unanesthetized rabbits with primary uveitis was not affected by the presence of Hydroxypropyl Cellulose inserts.

CARCINOGENESIS, MUTAGENESIS, IMPAIRMENT OF FERTILITY
Feeding of Hydroxypropyl Cellulose to rats at levels up to 5% of their diet produced no gross or histopathologic changes or other deleterious effects.

ADVERSE REACTIONS
The following adverse reactions have been reported in patients treated with Hydroxypropyl Cellulose, but were in most instances mild and transient:

Transient blurring of vision (see "Precautions")
Ocular discomfort or irritation
Matting or stickiness of eyelashes
Photophobia
Hypersensitivity
Edema of the eyelids
Hyperemia

DOSAGE AND ADMINISTRATION
One Hydroxypropyl Cellulose ophthalmic insert in each eye once daily is usually sufficient to relieve the symptoms associated with moderate to severe dry eye syndromes. Individual patients may require more flexibility in the use of Hydroxypropyl Cellulose; some patients may require twice daily use for optimal results.

Clinical experience with Hydroxypropyl Cellulose indicates that in some patients several weeks may be required before satisfactory improvement of symptoms is achieved.

Hydroxypropyl Cellulose is inserted into the inferior cul-de-sac of the eye beneath the base of the tarsus, not in apposition to the cornea, nor beneath the eyelid at the level of the tarsal plate. If not properly positioned, it will be expelled into the interpalpebral fissure, and may cause symptoms of a foreign body. Illustrated instructions are included in each package. While in the licensed practitioner's office, the patient should read the instructions, then practice insertion and removal of Hydroxypropyl Cellulose until proficiency is achieved.

Note: Occasionally Hydroxypropyl Cellulose is inadvertently expelled from the eye, especially in patients with shallow conjunctival fornices. The patient should be cautioned against rubbing the eye(s) containing Hydroxypropyl Cellulose especially upon awakening, so as not to dislodge or expel the insert. If required, another Hydroxypropyl Cellulose ophthalmic insert may be inserted. If experience indicates that transient blurred vision develops in an individual patient, the patient may want to remove Hydroxypropyl Cellulose a few hours after insertion to avoid this. Another Hydroxypropyl Cellulose ophthalmic insert may be inserted if needed.

➤ SHOWN IN PRODUCT IDENTIFICATION GUIDE

If Hydroxypropyl Cellulose causes worsening of symptoms, the patient should be instructed to inspect the conjunctival sac to make certain Hydroxypropyl Cellulose is in the proper location, deep in the inferior cul-de-sac of the eye beneath the base of the tarsus. If these symptoms persist, Hydroxypropyl Cellulose should be removed and the patient should contact the practitioner.

Store below 30°C (86°F).

HOW SUPPLIED
DEVICE: 5 MG

BRAND/MANUFACTURER	NDC	SIZE	AWP
○ BRAND LACRISERT: Merck	00006-3380-60	60s	$49.29

Hydroxypropylmethylcellulose

DESCRIPTION
Hydroxypropylmethylcellulose is a sterile, isotonic, nonpyrogenic viscoelastic solution. It is a 2% solution which is highly purified, noninflammatory, and has a high molecular weight greater than 80,000 daltons. Hydroxypropylmethylcellulose is supplied in 1 mL syringes. Each mL provides 20 mg/mL of Hydroxypropylmethylcellulose dissolved in a physiological balanced salt solution containing 0.49% sodium chloride, 0.075% potassium chloride, 0.048% calcium chloride, 0.03% magnesium chloride, 0.39% sodium acetate, 0.17% sodium citrate and water for injection. The osmolarity of Hydroxypropylmethylcellulose is 285±32 mOsM; the viscosity is 4000±1500 cst; and the pH is 7.2±0.4.

CHARACTERISTICS
Hydroxypropylmethylcellulose is an ophthalmic surgical aid for use in anterior segment surgery.
Hydroxypropylmethylcellulose:
1. Is a space occupying, tissue protective substance
2. Exhibits excellent flow properties
3. Is completely transparent
4. Is nonantigenic
5. Is easily removed from the anterior chamber
6. Contains no proteins which may cause inflammation or foreign body reactions
7. Requires no refrigeration or restrictive storage conditions
8. Does not interfere with normal wound healing process
9. Clears the trabecular meshwork in 24 hours (98% clearance rate).

INDICATIONS
Hydroxypropylmethylcellulose is indicated for use as an ophthalmic surgical aid in anterior segment surgical procedures including cataract extraction and intraocular lens implantation. Hydroxypropylmethylcellulose maintains a deep chamber during anterior segment surgery and thereby allows for more efficient manipulation with less trauma to the corneal endothelium and other ocular tissues. The viscoelasticity of Hydroxypropylmethylcellulose helps the vitreous face to be pushed back, thus preventing formation of a postoperative flat chamber.

CONTRAINDICATIONS
At present, there are no known contraindications to the use of Hydroxypropylmethylcellulose when used as recommended.

PRECAUTIONS
Precautions are limited to those normally associated with the ophthalmic surgical procedure being performed. There may be transient increased intraocular pressure following surgery because of pre-existing glaucoma or due to the surgery itself. For these reasons, the following precautions should be considered:
- Hydroxypropylmethylcellulose should be removed from the anterior chamber at the end of surgery.
- If the postoperative intraocular pressure increases above expected values, appropriate therapy should be administered.

ADVERSE REACTIONS
Clinical testing of Hydroxypropylmethylcellulose showed it to be extremely well tolerated after injection into the human eye. A transient rise in intraocular pressure postoperatively has been reported in some cases.

Rarely, postoperative inflammatory reactions (iritis, hypopyon) as well as incidents of corneal edema and corneal decompensation have been reported with viscoelastic agents. Their relationship to Hydroxypropylmethylcellulose has not been established.

CLINICAL APPLICATIONS
In anterior segment surgery, Hydroxypropylmethylcellulose should be carefully introduced into the anterior chamber using a 20 gauge or smaller cannula. Hydroxypropylmethylcellulose may be injected into the chamber prior to or following delivery of the crystalline lens. Injection of Hydroxypropylmethylcellulose prior to lens delivery will provide additional protection to the corneal endothelium and other ocular tissues. Injection of the material at this point is significant in that a coating of Hydroxypropylmethylcellulose may protect the corneal endothelium from possible damage arising from surgical instrumentation during the cataract extraction surgery.

Hydroxypropylmethylcellulose 2% may also be used to coat an intraocular lens as well as tips of surgical instruments prior to implantation surgery. Additional Hydroxypropylmethylcellulose may be injected during anterior segment surgery to fully maintain the chamber, or to replace fluid lost during the surgical procedure. Hydroxypropylmethylcellulose should be removed from the anterior chamber at the end of surgery. Rather than aspirate Hydroxypropylmethylcellulose from the eye with the Hydroxypropylmethylcellulose syringe, it is recommended that Hydroxypropylmethylcellulose be aspirated using an automated I/A device or irrigated using an irrigation syringe or a BSS squeeze bottle.

Store at room temperature; avoid excessive heat (60°C). Protect from light. For intraocular use.

REFERENCES
1. Fechner, PU, Fechner, MU. Methylcellulose and lens implantation. *Br J Ophthalmol.* 1983:67. 2. Aron-Rosa, D. et al. Methylcellulose instead of Hyaluronidase in extracapsular surgery with intraocular lens implantation. *Ophthalmology.* 1983:90:10. 3. Smith, SG, et al. Safety and efficacy of 2% methylcellulose in cat and monkey cataract-implant surgery. *Am Intraocular Implant Soc J.* 1984:10. 4. Liesegang, TJ, et al. The use of hydroxypropyl methylcellulose in extracapsular cataract extraction with intraocular lens implantation. *Am J Ophthalmol.* 1986:102.

HOW SUPPLIED
DROP: 2.5%

BRAND/MANUFACTURER	NDC	SIZE	AWP
○ GENERICS GONIOSOFT: Ocusoft	54799-0503-15	15 ml	$10.30

Hydroxyurea

DESCRIPTION
Hydroxyurea is an antineoplastic agent, available for oral use as capsules providing 500 mg Hydroxyurea.

Hydroxyurea occurs as an essentially tasteless, white crystalline powder.

Following is its chemical structure:

$$H_2NCONHOH$$

ACTIONS
MECHANISM OF ACTION
The precise mechanism by which Hydroxyurea produces its cytotoxic effects cannot, at present, be described. However, the reports of various studies in tissue culture in rats and man lend support to the hypothesis that Hydroxyurea causes an immediate inhibition of DNA synthesis without interfering with the synthesis of ribonucleic acid or of protein. This hypothesis explains why, under certain conditions, Hydroxyurea may induce teratogenic effects.

Three mechanisms of action have been postulated for the increased effectiveness of concomitant use of Hydroxyurea therapy with irradiation on squamous cell (epidermoid) carcinomas of the head and neck. *In vitro* studies utilizing Chinese hamster cells suggest that Hydroxyurea (1) is lethal to normally radioresistant S-stage cells, and (2) holds other cells of the cell cycle in the G1 or pre-DNA synthesis stage where they are most susceptible to the effects of irradiation. The third mechanism of action has been theorized on the basis of *in vitro* studies of HeLa cells: it appears that Hydroxyurea, by inhibition of DNA synthesis, hinders the normal repair process of cells damaged but not killed by irradiation, thereby decreasing their survival rate; RNA and protein syntheses have shown no alteration.

ABSORPTION, METABOLISM, FATE AND EXCRETION
After oral administration in man, Hydroxyurea is readily absorbed from the gastrointestinal tract. The drug reaches peak serum concentrations within 2 hours; by 24 hours the concentration in the serum is essentially zero. Approximately 80% of an oral or intravenous dose of 7 to 30 mg/kg may be recovered in the urine within 12 hours.

ANIMAL PHARMACOLOGY AND TOXICOLOGY
The oral LD_{50} of Hydroxyurea is 7330 mg/kg in mice and 5780 mg/kg in rats, given as a single dose.

In subacute and chronic toxicity studies in the rat, the most consistent pathological findings were an apparent dose-related mild to moderate bone marrow hypoplasia as well as pulmonary congestion and mottling of the lungs. At the highest dosage levels (1260 mg/kg/day for 37 days then 2520 mg/kg/day for 40 days), testicular atrophy with absence of spermatogenesis occurred; in several animals, hepatic cell damage with fatty metamorphosis was noted. In the dog, mild to marked bone marrow depression was a consistent finding except at the lower dosage levels. Additionally, at the higher dose levels (140 to 420 mg or 140 to 1260 mg/kg/week given 3 or 7 days weekly for 12 weeks), growth retardation, slightly increased blood glucose values, and hemosiderosis of the liver or spleen were found; reversible spermatogenic arrest was noted. In the monkey, bone marrow depression, lymphoid atrophy of the spleen, and degenerative changes in the epithelium of the small and large intestines were found. At the higher, often lethal, doses (400 to 800 mg/kg/day for 7 to 15 days), hemorrhage and congestion were found in the lungs, brain and urinary tract. Cardiovascular effects (changes in heart rate, blood pressure, orthostatic hypotension, EKG changes) and hematological changes (slight hemolysis, slight methemoglobinemia) were observed in some species of laboratory animals at doses exceeding clinical levels.

◆ RATED THERAPEUTICALLY EQUIVALENT; ◇ THERAPEUTIC EQUIVALENCE UNCONFIRMED; ○ UNRATED

INDICATIONS AND USAGE

Significant tumor response to Hydroxyurea has been demonstrated in melanoma, resistant chronic myelocytic leukemia, and recurrent, metastatic, or inoperable carcinoma of the ovary.

Hydroxyurea used concomitantly with irradiation therapy is intended for use in the local control of primary squamous cell (epidermoid) carcinomas of the head and neck, excluding the lip.

UNLABELED USES
Hydroxyurea is used alone or as an adjunct in the treatment of sickle cell anemia, hypereosinophilic syndrome, and recalcitrant psoriasis. It is also used with appropriate antibiotics as adjunctive therapy for chronic urinary tract infections (renal calculi).

CONTRAINDICATIONS

Hydroxyurea is contraindicated in patients with marked bone marrow depression, ie, leukopenia (< 2500 WBC) or thrombocytopenia (< 100,000), or severe anemia.

WARNINGS

Treatment with Hydroxyurea should not be initiated if bone marrow function is markedly depressed (see *"Contraindications"*). Bone marrow suppression may occur, and leukopenia is generally its first and most common manifestation. Thrombocytopenia and anemia occur less often, and are seldom seen without a preceding leukopenia. However, the recovery from myelosuppression is rapid when therapy is interrupted. It should be borne in mind that bone marrow depression is more likely in patients who have previously received radiotherapy or cytotoxic cancer chemotherapeutic agents; Hydroxyurea should be used cautiously in such patients.

Patients who have received irradiation therapy in the past may have an exacerbation of postirradiation erythema.

Severe anemia must be corrected with whole blood replacement before initiating therapy with Hydroxyurea.

Erythrocytic abnormalities: megaloblastic erythropoiesis, which is self-limiting, is often seen early in the course of Hydroxyurea therapy. The morphologic change resembles pernicious anemia, but is not related to vitamin B_{12} or folic acid deficiency. Hydroxyurea may also delay plasma iron clearance and reduce the rate of iron utilization by erythrocytes, but it does not appear to alter the red blood cell survival time.

Hydroxyurea should be used with caution in patients with marked renal dysfunction.

Elderly patients may be more sensitive to the effects of Hydroxyurea, and may require a lower dose regimen.

USAGE IN PREGNANCY

Drugs which affect DNA synthesis, such as Hydroxyurea, may be potential mutagenic agents. The physician should carefully consider this possibility before administering this drug to male or female patients who may contemplate conception.

Hydroxyurea is a known teratogenic agent in animals. Therefore Hydroxyurea should not be used in women who are or may become pregnant unless in the judgment of the physician the potential benefits outweigh the possible hazards.

PRECAUTIONS

Therapy with Hydroxyurea requires close supervision. The complete status of the blood, including bone marrow examination, if indicated, as well as kidney function and liver function should be determined prior to, and repeatedly during, treatment. The determination of the hemoglobin level, total leukocyte counts, and platelet counts should be performed at least once a week throughout the course of Hydroxyurea therapy. If the white blood cell count decreases to less than 2500/ mm^3, or the platelet count to less than 100,000/mm^3, therapy should be interrupted until the values rise significantly toward normal levels. Anemia, if it occurs, should be managed with whole blood replacement, without interrupting Hydroxyurea therapy.

ADVERSE REACTIONS

Adverse reactions have been primarily bone marrow depression (leukopenia, anemia, and occasionally thrombocytopenia), and less frequently gastrointestinal symptoms (stomatitis, anorexia, nausea, vomiting, diarrhea, and constipation), and dermatological reactions such as maculopapular rash and facial erythema. Dysuria and alopecia occur very rarely. Large doses may produce moderate drowsiness. Neurological disturbances have occurred extremely rarely and were limited to headache, dizziness, disorientation, hallucinations, and convulsions. Hydroxyurea occasionally may cause temporary impairment of renal tubular function accompanied by elevations in serum uric acid, BUN, and creatinine levels. Abnormal BSP retention has been reported. Fever, chills, malaise, and elevation of hepatic enzymes have also been reported.

Adverse reactions observed with combined Hydroxyurea and irradiation therapy are similar to those reported with the use of Hydroxyurea alone. These effects primarily include bone marrow depression (anemia and leukopenia), and gastric irritation. Almost all patients receiving an adequate course of combined Hydroxyurea and irradiation therapy will demonstrate concurrent leukopenia. Platelet depression (less than 100,000 cells/mm^3) has occurred rarely and only in the presence of marked leukopenia. Gastric distress has also been reported with irradiation alone and in combination with Hydroxyurea therapy.

It should be borne in mind that therapeutic doses of irradiation alone produce the same adverse reactions as Hydroxyurea; combined therapy may cause an increase in the incidence and severity of these side effects.

Although inflammation of the mucous membranes at the irradiated site (mucositis) is attributed to irradiation alone, some investigators believe that the more severe cases are due to combination therapy.

DOSAGE AND ADMINISTRATION

Procedures for proper handling and disposal of antineoplastic drugs should be considered. Several guidelines on this subject have been published.[1-7] There is no general agreement that all of the procedures recommended in the guidelines are necessary or appropriate.

Because of the rarity of melanoma, resistant chronic myelocytic leukemia, carcinoma of the ovary, and carcinomas of the head and neck in children, dosage regimens have not been established.

All dosage should be based on the patient's actual or ideal weight, whichever is less.

Note: If the patient prefers, or is unable to swallow capsules, the contents of the capsules may be emptied into a glass of water and taken immediately. Some inert material used as a vehicle in the capsule may not dissolve, and may float on the surface.

SOLID TUMORS

Intermittent Therapy: 80 mg/kg administered orally as a *single* dose every *third* day.

Continuous Therapy: 20 to 30 mg/kg administered orally as a *single* dose *daily*. The intermittent dosage schedule offers the advantage of reduced toxicity since patients on this dosage regimen have rarely required complete discontinuation of therapy because of toxicity.

Concomitant Therapy with Irradiation: (*Carcinoma of the head and neck*) 80 mg/kg administered orally as a *single* dose every *third* day.

Administration of Hydroxyurea should be begun at least 7 days before initiation of irradiation and continued during radiotherapy as well as indefinitely afterwards provided that the patient may be kept under adequate observation and evidences no unusual or severe reactions.

Irradiation should be given at the maximum dose considered appropriate for the particular therapeutic situation: adjustment of irradiation dosage is not usually necessary when hydroxurea is used concomitantly.

RESISTANT CHRONIC MYELOCYTIC LEUKEMIA

Until the intermittent therapy regimen has been evaluated, CONTINUOUS therapy (20 to 30 mg/kg adminsterd orally as a *single* dose *daily*) is recommended.

An adequate trial period for determining the antineoplastic effectiveness of Hydroxyurea is 6 weeks of therapy. When there is regression in tumor size or arrest in tumor growth, therapy should be continued indefinitely. Thereapy should be interrupted if the white blood cell count drops below 2500/mm^3, or the platelet count below 100,000/mm^3. In these cases, the counts should be rechecked after 3 days, and therapy resumed when the counts rise significantly toward normal values. Since the hematopoietic rebound is prompt, it is usually necessary to omit only a few doses. If prompt rebound has not occurred during combined Hydroxyurea and irradiation therapy, irradiation may also be interrupted. However, the need for postponement of irradiation has been rare; radiotherapy has usually been continued using the recommended dosage and technique. Anemia, if it occurs, should be corrected with whole blood replacement, without interrupting Hydroxyurea therapy. Because hematopoiesis may be compromised by extensive irradiation or by other antineoplastic agents, it is recommended that Hydroxyurea be administered cautiously to patients who have recently received extensive radiation therapy or chemotherapy with other cytotoxic drugs.

Pain or discomfort from inflammation of the mucous membranes at the irradiated site (mucositis) is usually controlled by measures such as topical anesthetics and orally administered analgesics. If the reaction is severe Hydroxyurea therapy may be temporarily interrupted; if it is extremely severe, irradiation dosage may, in addition, be temporarily postponed. However, it has rarely been necessary to terminate these therapies.

Severe gastric distress, such as nausea, vomiting, and anorexia, resulting from combined therapy may usually be controlled by temporary interruption of Hydroxyurea administration; rarely has the additional interruption of irradiation been necessary.

STORAGE

Store at room temperature; avoid excessive heat.

REFERENCES

1. Recommendations for the Safe Handling of Parenteral Antineoplastic Drugs. NIH Publication No. 83-2621. Available from Superintendent of Documents, US Government Printing Office, Washington, DC 20402.   2. AMA Council Report: Guidelines for Handling Parenteral Antineoplastics. *JAMA.* 1985; 253:1590-1592.   3. National Study Commission on Cytotoxic Exposure: Recommendations for Handling Cytotoxic Agents. Available from Louis P. Jeffrey, ScD, Director of Pharmacy Services, Rhode Island Hospital, 593 Eddy Street, Providence, RI 02902.   4. Clinical Oncological Society of Australia: Guidelines and Recommendations for Safe Handling of Antineoplastic Agents. *Med J Australia.* 1983; 1:426-428.   5. Jones RB, et al: Safe handling of chemotherapeutic agents: A report from the Mount Sinai Medical Center, CA—*A Cancer J for Clinicians.* 1983; 133:258-263.   6. American Society of Hospital Pharmacists Technical Assistance Bulletin on Handling Cytotoxic and Hazardous Drugs in Hospitals. *Am J Hosp Pharm.* 1990; 47:1033-1049.   7. OSHA Work-Practice Guidelines for Personnel Dealing with Cytotoxic (Antineoplastic) Drugs. *Am J Hosp Pharm.* 1986; 43:1193-1204.

➤ SHOWN IN PRODUCT IDENTIFICATION GUIDE

HOW SUPPLIED
CAPSULE: 500 MG

BRAND/MANUFACTURER

	NDC	SIZE	AWP
○ **BRAND**			
HYDREA: Bristol-Myer Onc/Hiv	00003-0830-50	100s	$136.46

Hydroxyzine

DESCRIPTION

Hydroxyzine Pamoate is designed chemically as 1-(p-chlorobenzhydryl)4-[2-(2-hydroxyethoxy)ethyl] diethylenediamine, salt of 1,1'-methylone-bis-(2-hydroxy-3-naphthalone (carboxylic acid).

Hyroxyzine Hydrochloride is designated chemically as 1-(p-chlorobenzhydryl)4-[2-(2-hydroxyethoxy)ethyl]piperazine dihydrochloride.

Following is its chemical structure:

$$CH_2CH_2OCH_2CH_2OH$$

· 2HCl

CLINICAL PHARMACOLOGY

Hydroxyzine is unrelated chemically to the phenothiazines, reserpine, meprobamate, or the benzodiazepines.

Hydroxyzine HCl Intramascular (IM) has demonstrated its clinical effectiveness in the chemotherapeutic aspect of the total management of neuroses and emotional disturbances manifested by anxiety, tension, agitation, apprehension or confusion.

Hydroxyzine HCl IM has been shown clinically to be a rapid-acting true ataraxic with a wide margin of safety. It induces a calming effect in anxious, tense, psychoneurotic adults and also in anxious, hyperkinetic children without impairing mental alertness. It is not a cortical depressant but its action may be due to a suppression of activity in certain key regions of the subcortical area of the central nervous system.

Hydroxyzine is not a cortical depressant, but its action may be due to a suppression of activity in certain key regions of the subcortical area of the central nervous system. Primary skeletal muscle relaxation has been demonstrated experimentally.

Hydroxyzine HCl IM has been shown experimentally to have antispasmodic properties, apparently mediated through interference with the mechanism that responds to spasmogenic agents such as serotonin, acetylcholine, and histamine.

Bronchodilator activity, and antihistaminic and analgesic effects have been demonstrated experimentally and confirmed clinically. An antiemetic effect, both by the apomorphine test and the veriloid test, has been demonstrated. Pharmacological and clinical studies indicate that Hydroxyzine in therapeutic dosage does not increase gastric secretion or acidity and in most cases has mild antisecretory activity. Hydroxyzine is rapidly absorbed from the gastrointestinal tract and Hydroxyzine's clinical effects are usually noted within 15 to 30 minutes after oral administration.

INDICATIONS
CAPSULES, ORAL SUSPENSION, TABLETS, AND SYRUP

For symptomatic relief of anxiety and tension associated with psychoneurosis and as an adjunct in organic disease states in which anxiety is manifested.

Useful in the management of pruritus due to allergic conditions such as chronic urticaria and atopic and contact dermatoses, and in histamine-mediated pruritus.

As a sedative when used as premedication and following general anesthesia, *Hydroxyzine may potentiate meperidine and barbiturates:* so their use in preanesthetic adjunctive therapy should be modified on an individual basis. Atropine and other belladonna alkaloids are not affected by the drug.

INTRAMUSCULAR

The total management of anxiety, tension, and psychomotor agitation in conditions of emotional stress requires in most instances a combined approach of psychotherapy and chemotherapy. Hydroxyzine IM has been found to be particularly useful for this latter phase of therapy in its ability to render the disturbed patient more amenable to psychotherapy in long term treatment of the psychoneurotic and psychotic, although it should not be used as the sole treatment of psychosis or of clearly demonstrated cases of depression.

Hydroxyzine IM is also useful in alleviating the manifestations of anxiety and tension as in the preparation for dental procedures and in acute emotional problems. It has also been recommended for the management of anxiety associated with organic disturbances and as adjunctive therapy in alcoholism and allergic conditions with strong emotional overlay, such as in asthma, chronic urticaria, and pruritus.

Hydroxyzine Intramuscular Solution is useful in treating the following types of patients when intramuscular administration is indicated:

1. The acutely disturbed or hysterical patient.
2. The acute or chronic alcoholic with anxiety withdrawal symptoms or delirium tremens.
3. As pre- and postoperative and pre- and postpartum adjunctive medication to permit reduction in narcotic dosage, allay anxiety and control emesis.

Hydroxyzine has also demonstrated effectiveness in controlling nausea and vomiting, excluding nausea and vomiting of pregnancy. (See *"Contraindications."*)

In prepartum states, the reduction in narcotic requirement effected by Hydroxyzine is of particular benefit to both mother and neonate.

Hydroxyzine benefits the cardiac patient by its ability to allay the associated anxiety and apprehension attendant to certain types of heart disease.

Hydroxyzine is not known to interfere with the action of digitalis in any way and may be used concurrently with this agent.

The effectiveness of Hydroxyzine as an antianxiety agent for long term use, that is more than 4 months, has not been assessed by systematic clinical studies. The physician should reassess periodically the usefulness of the drug for the individual patient.

UNLABELED USES

Hydroxyzine is used alone or as an adjunct in the treatment of atopic dermatitis and bronchial asthma.

CONTRAINDICATIONS

Hydroxyzine, when administered to the pregnant mouse, rat, and rabbit, induced fetal abnormalities in the rat and mouse at doses substantially above the human therapeutic range. Clinical data in human beings are inadequate to establish safety in early pregnancy. Until such data are available, Hydroxyzine is contraindicated in early pregnancy.

Hydroxyzine is contraindicated for patients who have shown a previous hypersensitivity to it.

Hydroxyzine Intramuscular Solution is intended only for intramuscular administration and should not, under any circumstances, be injected subcutaneously, intra-arterially, or intravenously.

WARNINGS

Nursing Mothers: It is not known whether this drug is excreted in human milk. Since many drugs are so excreted, Hydroxyzine should not be given to nursing mothers.

For Tablets Only: Some brands are manufactured with 1,1,1-trichloroethane, a substance which harms public health and the environment by destroying ozone in the upper atmosphere.

PRECAUTIONS

The Potentiating Action Of Hydroxyzine Must Be Considered When The Drug Is Used In Conjunction With Central Nervous System Depressants Such As Narcotics, Non-Narcotic Analgesics And Barbiturates. Therefore, when central nervous system depressants are administered concomitantly with Hydroxyzine their dosage should be reduced. Since drowsiness may occur with use of the drug, patients should be warned of this possibility and cautioned against driving a car or operating dangerous machinery while taking Hydroxyzine. Patients should be advised against the simultaneous use of other CNS depressant drugs, and cautioned that the effect of alcohol may be increased.

Rarely, cardiac arrests and death have been reported in association with the combined use of Hydroxyzine HCl IM and other CNS depressants. Therefore, when central nervous system depressants are administered concomitantly with Hydroxyzine HCl IM their dosage should be reduced up to 50 per cent. The efficacy of Hydroxyzine as adjunctive pre- and postoperative sedative medication has also been well established, especially as regards its ability to allay anxiety, control emesis, and reduce the amount of narcotic required.

Hydroxyzine May Potentiate Narcotics And Barbiturates so their use in preanesthetic adjunctive therapy should be modified on an individual basis. Atropine and other belladonna alkaloids are not affected by the drug. When Hydroxyzine is used preoperatively or prepartum, narcotic requirements may be reduced as much as 50 per cent. Thus, when 50 mg of Hydroxyzine HCl IM Solution is employed, meperidine dosage may be reduced from 100 mg to 50 mg. The administration of meperidine may result in severe hypotension in the postoperative patient or any individual whose ability to maintain blood pressure has been compromised by a depleted blood volume. Meperidine should be used with great caution and in reduced dosage in patients who are receiving other pre- and/or postoperative medications and in whom there is a risk of respiratory depression, hypotension, and profound sedation or coma occurring. Before using any medications concomitant with Hydroxyzine, the manufacturer's prescribing information should be read carefully.

As with all intramuscular preparations Hydroxyzine Intramuscular Solution should be injected well within the body of a relatively large muscle. Inadvertent subcutaneous injection may result in significant tissue damage.

Adults: The preferred site is the upper outer quadrant of the buttock, (i.e., gluteus maximus), or the mid-lateral thigh.

Children: It is recommended that intramuscular injections be given preferably in the mid-lateral muscles of the thigh. In infants and small children the periphery of the upper outer quadrant of the gluteal region should be used only when necessary, such as in burn patients, in order to minimize the possibility of damage to the sciatic nerve.

The deltoid area should be used only if well developed such as in certain adults and older children, and then only with caution to avoid radial nerve injury. Intramuscular injections should not be made into the lower and mid-third of the upper arm. As with all intramuscular injections, aspiration is necessary to help avoid inadvertent injection into a blood vessel.

ADVERSE REACTIONS

Side effects reported with the administration of Hydroxyzine are usually mild and transitory in nature.

Anticholinergic: Dry mouth.

Central Nervous System: Drowsiness is usually transitory and may disappear in a few days of continued therapy or upon reduction of the dose. Involuntary motor activity including rare instances of tremor and convulsions has been reported, usually with doses considerably higher than those recommended. Clinically significant respiratory depression has not been reported at recommended doses.

Extensive clinical use has substantiated the absence of toxic effects on the liver or bone marrow when Hydroxyzine HCl IM is administered in the recommended doses for over four years of uninterrupted therapy. The absence of adverse effects has been further demonstrated in experimental studies in which excessively high doses were administered.

Involuntary motor activity, including rare instances of tremor and convulsions, has been reported with Hydroxyzine HCl IM, usually with doses considerably higher than those recommended. Continuous therapy with over one gram per day has been employed in some patients without these effects having been encountered.

OVERDOSAGE

The most common manifestation of overdosage of Hydroxyzine is hypersedation. As in the management of overdosage with any drug, it should be borne in mind that multiple agents may have been taken.

If vomiting has not occurred spontaneously, it should be induced. Immediate gastric lavage is also recommended. General supportive care, including frequent monitoring of the vital signs and close observation of the patient, is indicated. Hypotension, though unlikely, may be controlled with intravenous fluids and Levarterenol or Metaraminol. Do not use epinephrine as Hydroxyzine counteracts its pressor action. Caffeine and Sodium Benzoate Injection, U.S.P., may be used to counteract central nervous system depressant effects.

There is no specific antidote. It is doubtful that hemodialysis would be of any value in the treatment of overdosage with Hydroxyzine. However, if other agents such as barbiturates have been ingested concomitantly, hemodialysis may be indicated. There is no practical method to quantitate Hydroxyzine in body fluids or tissue after its ingestion or administration.

DOSAGE

For symptomatic relief of anxiety and tension associated with psychoneurosis and as an adjunct in organic disease states in which anxiety is manifested: in adults, 50-100 mg q.i.d.; children under 6 years, 50 mg daily in divided doses and over 6 years, 50-100 mg daily in divided doses.

For use in the management of pruritus due to allergic conditions such as chronic urticaria and atopic and contact dermatoses, and in histamine-mediated pruritus; in adults, 25 mg t.i.d. or q.i.d.; children under 6 years, 50 mg daily in divided doses and over 6 years, 50-100 mg daily in divided doses.

As a sedative when used as a premedication and following general anesthesia: 50-100 mg in adults, and 0.6 mg/kg in children.

The recommended dosages for Hydroxyzine HCl IM Solution are:

For adult psychiatric and emotional emergencies, including acute alcoholism. I.M.: 50-100 mg stat., and q. 4-6h., p.r.n.

Nausea and vomiting excluding nausea and vomiting of pregnancy. Adults: 25-100 mg I.M. Children: 0.5 mg/lb. body weight I.M.

Pre- and postoperative adjunctive medication. Adults: 25-100 mg I.M. Children: 0.5 mg/lb. body weight I.M.

Pre- and postpartum adjunctive therapy. 25-100 mg I.M.

As with all patients medications, the dosage should be adjusted according to the patient's response to therapy.

For Additional Information On The Administration And Site Of Selection See Precautions Section Note: Hydroxyzine HCl IM Solution may be administered without further dilution.

When treatment is initiated by the intramuscular route of administration, subsequent doses may be administered orally. Patients should be maintained on oral therapy whenever this route is practicable.

As with all medications, the dosage should be adjusted according to the patient's response to therapy.

J CODES

Up to 25 mg IM—J3410

HOW SUPPLIED

HYDROXYZINE HYDROCHLORIDE
INJECTION: 25 MG/ML

AVERAGE UNIT PRICE (AVAILABLE SIZES)		GENERIC A-RATED AVERAGE PRICE (GAAP)	
BRAND	$1.14	10 ml	$3.57
GENERIC	$0.47	1 ml 25s	$14.96

BRAND/MANUFACTURER	NDC	SIZE	AWP
◆ BRAND			
VISTARIL IM: Roerig	00049-5450-74	10 ml	$11.44

BRAND/MANUFACTURER	NDC	SIZE	AWP
◆ GENERICS			
Fujisawa	00469-2100-00	1 ml	$0.65
Moore, H.L.	00839-6337-30	10 ml	$2.03
Schein	00364-6718-54	10 ml	$2.93
Steris	00402-0170-10	10 ml	$2.93
Rugby	00536-5050-70	10 ml	$6.38
Sanofi Winthrop	00024-0711-02	2 ml 10s	$6.23
Elkins-Sinn	00641-0432-25	1 ml 25s	$12.05
Solo Pak	39769-0023-02	1 ml 25s	$14.38
Amer Regent	00517-4201-25	1 ml 25s	$18.44

INJECTION: 50 MG/ML

AVERAGE UNIT PRICE (AVAILABLE SIZES)		GENERIC A-RATED AVERAGE PRICE (GAAP)	
BRAND	$1.83	10 ml	$5.23
GENERIC	$0.52	2 ml 10s	$7.67
		1 ml 25s	$16.21
		2 ml 25s	$23.29

BRAND/MANUFACTURER	NDC	SIZE	AWP
◆ BRAND			
VISTARIL IM: Roerig	00049-5460-74	10 ml	$18.25
◆ GENERICS			
Fujisawa	00469-5100-00	1 ml	$0.78
Fujisawa	00469-5100-10	2 ml	$0.92
Moore, H.L.	00839-6338-30	10 ml	$2.63
Elkins-Sinn	00641-2518-41	10 ml	$3.03
Insource	58441-1107-01	10 ml	$3.19
Schein	00364-6719-54	10 ml	$3.38
Steris	00402-0171-10	10 ml	$3.38
Goldline	00182-1182-63	10 ml	$3.90
Major	00904-0365-10	10 ml	$4.35
Fujisawa	00469-0350-25	10 ml	$4.79
HYZINE: Hyrex	00314-1400-70	10 ml	$7.00
Rugby	00536-5060-70	10 ml	$7.13
VISTAJECT-50: Mayrand	00259-0340-10	10 ml	$14.80
Sanofi Winthrop	00024-0712-02	2 ml 10s	$7.19
Sanofi Winthrop	00024-0713-02	2 ml 10s	$8.14
Elkins-Sinn	00641-0433-25	1 ml 25s	$12.05
Solo Pak	39769-0024-02	1 ml 25s	$14.38
Amer Regent	00517-5601-25	1 ml 25s	$22.19
Solo Pak	39769-0024-06	2 ml 25s	$14.38
Amer Regent	00517-5602-25	2 ml 25s	$32.19
Amer Regent	00517-5610-25	10 ml 25s	$78.44

INJECTION: 100 MG/ML

BRAND/MANUFACTURER	NDC	SIZE	AWP
◆ GENERICS			
Elkins-Sinn	00641-0434-25	2 ml 25s	$12.05

SYRUP: 2 MG/ML

BRAND/MANUFACTURER	NDC	SIZE	AWP
◆ GENERICS			
Geneva	00781-6570-16	480 ml	$11.25

SYRUP: 10 MG/5 ML

AVERAGE UNIT PRICE (AVAILABLE SIZES)		GENERIC A-RATED AVERAGE PRICE (GAAP)	
BRAND	$0.11	120 ml	$3.85
GENERIC	$0.02	480 ml	$11.21
HCFA FUL (480 ml)	$0.02	3840 ml	$71.14

BRAND/MANUFACTURER	NDC	SIZE	AWP
◆ BRAND			
ATARAX: Roerig	00049-5590-93	480 ml	$51.49
◆ GENERICS			
Pennex	00832-8150-04	120 ml	$3.40
Pennex	00426-8150-04	120 ml	$4.30
Pennex	00426-8150-16	480 ml	$10.00
Qualitest	00603-1310-58	480 ml	$10.44
Pennex	00832-8150-16	480 ml	$10.56
Warner Chilcott	00047-2902-23	480 ml	$10.56
Schein	00364-7273-16	480 ml	$11.00
Moore, H.L.	00839-6476-69	480 ml	$11.00
URL	00677-1421-33	480 ml	$11.20
Mason Dist	11845-0431-13	480 ml	$11.37
Major	00904-0379-16	480 ml	$11.55
Goldline	00182-1376-40	480 ml	$12.00
Rugby	00536-1002-85	480 ml	$12.79
Barre	00472-0771-16	480 ml	$12.81
Major	00904-0379-28	3840 ml	$56.70
Barre	00472-0771-28	3840 ml	$85.57

SYRUP: 10 MG

AVERAGE UNIT PRICE (AVAILABLE SIZES)

GENERIC	$0.05

BRAND/MANUFACTURER	NDC	SIZE	AWP
◆ **GENERICS**			
Aligen	00405-2900-16	480 ml	$12.20
UDL	51079-0533-10	5 ml 50s ud	$20.00

SYRUP: 25 MG

BRAND/MANUFACTURER	NDC	SIZE	AWP
◆ **GENERICS**			
UDL	51079-0534-10	12.5 ml 50s ud	$25.10

SYRUP: 50 MG

BRAND/MANUFACTURER	NDC	SIZE	AWP
◆ **GENERICS**			
UDL	51079-0535-10	25 ml 50s ud	$39.60

TABLETS: 10 MG

AVERAGE UNIT PRICE (AVAILABLE SIZES)

		GENERIC A-RATED AVERAGE PRICE (GAAP)	
BRAND	$0.53	100s	$11.60
GENERIC	$0.09	500s	$30.48
HCFA FUL (100s ea)	$0.03	1000s	$55.25

BRAND/MANUFACTURER	NDC	SIZE	AWP
◆ **BRAND**			
➤ ATARAX: Roerig	00049-5600-66	100s	$54.42
	00049-5600-73	500s	$258.68
◆ **GENERICS**			
Medirex	57480-0415-06	30s	$10.79
➤ Rugby	00536-4567-01	100s	$6.33
Goldline	00182-1492-01	100s	$6.40
Moore,H.L.	00839-7437-06	100s	$6.47
Schein	00364-0494-01	100s	$6.50
Major	00904-0357-60	100s	$6.75
URL	00677-0604-01	100s	$6.79
Qualitest	00603-3970-21	100s	$6.80
Geneva	00781-1332-01	100s	$6.85
Mutual	53489-0126-01	100s	$7.00
Sidmak	50111-0307-01	100s	$7.20
Martec	52555-0159-01	100s	$7.42
Royce	51875-0345-01	100s	$7.55
Aligen	00405-4511-01	100s	$7.58
REZINE: Stewart Jackson	45565-0403-01	100s	$14.90
REZINE: Marnel	00682-9403-01	100s	$15.20
U.S. Trading	56126-0012-11	100s ud	$4.25
Major	00904-0357-61	100s ud	$11.81
Schein	00364-0494-90	100s ud	$12.50
Goldline	00182-1492-89	100s ud	$15.10
Vangard	00615-1525-13	100s ud	$15.55
Auro	55829-0306-10	100s ud	$15.99
Medirex	57480-0415-01	100s ud	$35.95
UDL	51079-0530-20	100s ud	$35.97
Major	00904-0357-70	250s	$15.20
Moore,H.L.	00839-7437-12	500s	$26.99
➤ Rugby	00536-4567-05	500s	$29.48
Goldline	00182-1492-05	500s	$29.55
URL	00677-0604-05	500s	$29.79
Qualitest	00603-3970-28	500s	$29.80
Schein	00364-0494-05	500s	$29.90
Geneva	00781-1332-05	500s	$29.95
Aligen	00405-4511-05	500s	$30.08
Sidmak	50111-0307-02	500s	$30.50
Martec	52555-0159-05	500s	$31.10
Mutual	53489-0126-05	500s	$32.70
Royce	51875-0345-02	500s	$35.88
Schein	00364-0494-02	1000s	$47.00
Goldline	00182-1492-10	1000s	$47.00
Martec	52555-0159-10	1000s	$50.60
URL	00677-0604-10	1000s	$55.10
Rugby	00536-4567-10	1000s	$55.13
Major	00904-0357-80	1000s	$55.25
Geneva	00781-1332-10	1000s	$55.25
Mutual	53489-0126-10	1000s	$57.95
Sidmak	50111-0307-03	1000s	$58.25
Aligen	00405-4511-03	1000s	$61.32
Royce	51875-0345-04	1000s	$64.88

TABLETS: 25 MG

AVERAGE UNIT PRICE (AVAILABLE SIZES)

		GENERIC A-RATED AVERAGE PRICE (GAAP)	
BRAND	$0.78	100s	$15.98
GENERIC	$0.13	500s	$43.88
HCFA FUL (100s ea)	$0.03	1000s	$80.49

BRAND/MANUFACTURER	NDC	SIZE	AWP
◆ **BRAND**			
➤ ATARAX: Roerig	00049-5610-66	100s	$79.83
	00049-5610-73	500s	$380.74

BRAND/MANUFACTURER	NDC	SIZE	AWP
◆ **GENERICS**			
Medirex	57480-0429-06	30s	$12.72
➤ Rugby	00536-4568-01	100s	$8.48
Qualitest	00603-3971-21	100s	$8.50
Goldline	00182-1493-01	100s	$8.55
Moore,H.L.	00839-7438-06	100s	$9.17
URL	00677-0605-01	100s	$9.49
Major	00904-0358-60	100s	$9.50
Schein	00364-0495-01	100s	$9.50
Sidmak	50111-0308-01	100s	$9.85
Geneva	00781-1334-01	100s	$9.95
Mutual	53489-0127-01	100s	$9.95
Martec	52555-0558-01	100s	$10.34
Aligen	00405-4512-01	100s	$10.37
ANX: EconoMed	38130-0044-01	100s	$10.98
Royce	51875-0346-01	100s	$11.07
REZINE: Stewart Jackson	45565-0404-01	100s	$19.50
REZINE: Marnel	00682-9404-01	100s	$21.90
U.S. Trading	56126-0013-11	100s ud	$5.43
Major	00904-0358-61	100s ud	$13.72
Schein	00364-0495-90	100s ud	$15.00
Goldline	00182-1493-89	100s ud	$19.50
Auro	55829-0307-10	100s ud	$20.95
Vangard	00615-1526-13	100s ud	$31.12
Geneva	00781-1334-13	100s ud	$32.00
UDL	51079-0531-20	100s ud	$42.40
Medirex	57480-0429-01	100s ud	$42.40
Major	00904-0358-70	250s	$21.40
➤ Rugby	00536-4568-05	500s	$40.49
Goldline	00182-1493-05	500s	$40.55
Qualitest	00603-3971-28	500s	$40.55
URL	00677-0605-05	500s	$40.94
Schein	00364-0495-05	500s	$40.95
Major	00904-0358-40	500s	$42.75
Martec	52555-0558-05	500s	$42.75
Geneva	00781-1334-05	500s	$44.95
Sidmak	50111-0308-02	500s	$45.50
Mutual	53489-0127-05	500s	$46.20
Aligen	00405-4512-02	500s	$48.32
Royce	51875-0346-02	500s	$52.58
Moore,H.L.	00839-7438-16	1000s	$73.91
Schein	00364-0495-02	1000s	$76.25
Qualitest	00603-3971-32	1000s	$76.77
➤ Rugby	00536-4568-10	1000s	$76.80
URL	00677-0605-10	1000s	$76.82
Goldline	00182-1493-10	1000s	$76.85
Major	00904-0358-80	1000s	$76.95
Martec	52555-0160-10	1000s	$79.20
Geneva	00781-1334-10	1000s	$79.95
Mutual	53489-0127-10	1000s	$82.95
Sidmak	50111-0308-03	1000s	$87.45
Aligen	00405-4512-03	1000s	$87.82
Royce	51875-0346-04	1000s	$94.64

TABLETS: 50 MG

AVERAGE UNIT PRICE (AVAILABLE SIZES)

		GENERIC A-RATED AVERAGE PRICE (GAAP)	
BRAND	$0.95	100s	$16.53
GENERIC	$0.14	500s	$49.38
HCFA FUL (100s ea)	$0.04	1000s	$95.42

BRAND/MANUFACTURER	NDC	SIZE	AWP
◆ **BRAND**			
➤ ATARAX: Roerig	00049-5620-66	100s	$97.29
	00049-5620-73	500s	$464.18
◆ **GENERICS**			
Medirex	57480-0430-06	30s	$6.95
Moore,H.L.	00839-7439-06	100s	$7.63
Qualitest	00603-3972-21	100s	$10.60
➤ Rugby	00536-4569-01	100s	$10.62
Major	00904-0359-60	100s	$10.70
Sidmak	50111-0309-01	100s	$10.95
URL	00677-0606-01	100s	$11.24
Schein	00364-0496-01	100s	$11.25
Martec	52555-0559-01	100s	$11.50
Mutual	53489-0128-01	100s	$12.00
Geneva	00781-1336-01	100s	$12.10
Aligen	00405-4513-01	100s	$12.11
Royce	51875-0347-01	100s	$12.59
U.S. Trading	56126-0014-11	100s ud	$7.20
Major	00904-0359-61	100s ud	$16.87
Schein	00364-0496-90	100s ud	$20.00
Goldline	00182-1494-89	100s ud	$22.00
Auro	55829-0308-10	100s ud	$25.15
Vangard	00615-1527-13	100s ud	$34.44
UDL	51079-0532-20	100s ud	$35.49
Medirex	57480-0430-01	100s ud	$36.10
Major	00904-0359-70	250s	$19.90
Major	00904-0359-40	500s	$36.20
Qualitest	00603-3972-28	500s	$46.40
➤ Rugby	00536-4569-05	500s	$46.88
Goldline	00182-1494-05	500s	$46.95
Martec	52555-0161-05	500s	$49.40

◆ RATED THERAPEUTICALLY EQUIVALENT; ◇ THERAPEUTIC EQUIVALENCE UNCONFIRMED; ○ UNRATED

BRAND/MANUFACTURER	NDC	SIZE	AWP
Mutual	53489-0128-05	500s	$49.95
Sidmak	50111-0309-02	500s	$52.25
URL	00677-0606-05	500s	$52.50
Geneva	00781-1336-05	500s	$52.50
Schein	00364-0496-05	500s	$53.50
Royce	51875-0347-02	500s	$56.65
Martec	52555-0559-10	1000s	$87.45
➤ Rugby	00536-4569-10	1000s	$89.55
URL	00677-0606-10	1000s	$96.75
Sidmak	50111-0309-03	1000s	$96.80
Mutual	53489-0128-10	1000s	$100.00
Royce	51875-0347-04	1000s	$101.97

TABLETS: 100 MG

BRAND/MANUFACTURER	NDC	SIZE	AWP
◆ BRAND			
➤ ATARAX: Roerig	00049-5630-66	100s	$119.56

HYDROXYZINE PAMOATE
CAPSULE: 25 MG

AVERAGE UNIT PRICE (AVAILABLE SIZES)		GENERIC A-RATED AVERAGE PRICE (GAAP)	
BRAND	$0.82	100s	$19.34
GENERIC	$0.18	500s	$72.39
HCFA FUL (100s ea)	$0.12	1000s	$126.83

BRAND/MANUFACTURER	NDC	SIZE	AWP
◆ BRAND			
VISTARIL: Pfizer Labs	00069-5410-66	100s	$79.82
	00069-5410-41	100s ud	$90.68
	00069-5410-73	500s	$380.73
◆ GENERICS			
Medirex	57480-0395-06	30s	$13.29
Eon	00185-0613-01	100s	$10.00
Rugby	00536-3893-01	100s	$13.73
Moore,H.L.	00839-6270-06	100s	$14.38
Geneva	00781-2252-01	100s	$15.00
Goldline	00182-1098-01	100s	$15.00
URL	00677-0596-01	100s	$15.10
Major	00904-0362-60	100s	$15.15
Qualitest	00603-3994-21	100s	$15.40
Schein	00364-0483-01	100s	$15.49
Barr	00555-0323-02	100s	$17.38
Martec	52555-0326-01	100s	$17.82
Raway	00686-0077-20	100s	$18.00
Zenith	00172-2911-60	100s	$18.75
Aligen	00405-4518-01	100s	$20.46
Parmed	00349-8919-01	100s	$20.95
U.S. Trading	56126-0069-11	100s ud	$5.97
Vangard	00615-0331-13	100s ud	$19.92
Goldline	00182-1098-89	100s ud	$20.00
Auro	55829-0665-10	100s ud	$23.14
Major	00904-0362-61	100s ud	$23.17
Medirex	57480-0395-01	100s ud	$44.30
UDL	51079-0077-20	100s ud	$44.31
Eon	00185-0613-05	500s	$44.65
Rugby	00536-3893-05	500s	$60.87
Moore,H.L.	00839-6270-12	500s	$64.79
Qualitest	00603-3994-28	500s	$70.12
URL	00677-0596-05	500s	$70.48
Geneva	00781-2252-05	500s	$70.50
Major	00904-0362-40	500s	$70.80
Goldline	00182-1098-05	500s	$72.00
Schein	00364-0483-05	500s	$73.23
Barr	00555-0323-04	500s	$82.38
Martec	52555-0326-05	500s	$82.52
Zenith	00172-2911-70	500s	$86.80
Aligen	00405-4518-02	500s	$101.87
Rugby	00536-3893-10	1000s	$115.65
Goldline	00182-1098-10	1000s	$138.00

CAPSULE: 50 MG

AVERAGE UNIT PRICE (AVAILABLE SIZES)		GENERIC A-RATED AVERAGE PRICE (GAAP)	
BRAND	$1.001	100s	$20.96
GENERIC	$0.20	500s	$77.82
HCFA FUL (100s ea)	$0.13		

BRAND/MANUFACTURER	NDC	SIZE	AWP
◆ BRAND			
VISTARIL: Pfizer Labs	00069-5420-66	100s	$97.29
	00069-5420-41	100s ud	$110.10
	00069-5420-73	500s	$464.18
◆ GENERICS			
Medirex	57480-0396-06	30s	$18.83
Eon	00185-0615-01	100s	$12.55
Rugby	00536-3894-01	100s	$13.86
Moore,H.L.	00839-6271-06	100s	$15.26
Schein	00364-0484-01	100s	$15.75
Major	00904-0363-60	100s	$16.50

BRAND/MANUFACTURER	NDC	SIZE	AWP
URL	00677-0597-01	100s	$18.00
Goldline	00182-1099-01	100s	$18.00
Qualitest	00603-3995-21	100s	$18.01
Geneva	00781-2254-01	100s	$18.25
Martec	52555-0327-01	100s	$18.83
Zenith	00172-2909-60	100s	$20.00
Aligen	00405-4519-01	100s	$21.24
Parmed	00349-8920-01	100s	$22.00
U.S. Trading	56126-0070-11	100s ud	$6.42
Raway	00686-0078-20	100s ud	$19.00
Vangard	00615-0332-13	100s ud	$24.13
Goldline	00182-1099-89	100s ud	$24.15
Auro	55829-0666-10	100s ud	$26.31
Major	00904-0363-61	100s ud	$28.18
UDL	51079-0078-20	100s ud	$62.72
Eon	00185-0615-05	500s	$50.00
Rugby	00536-3894-05	500s	$60.81
Moore,H.L.	00839-6271-12	500s	$68.30
Schein	00364-0484-05	500s	$75.00
Major	00904-0363-40	500s	$76.50
URL	00677-0597-05	500s	$78.37
Qualitest	00603-3995-28	500s	$78.38
Goldline	00182-1099-05	500s	$81.00
Zenith	00172-2909-70	500s	$95.00
Aligen	00405-4519-02	500s	$95.00
Martec	52555-0327-05	500s	$97.61
Rugby	00536-3894-10	1000s	$115.55

CAPSULE: 100 MG

AVERAGE UNIT PRICE (AVAILABLE SIZES)		GENERIC A-RATED AVERAGE PRICE (GAAP)	
BRAND	$1.23	100s	$37.34
GENERIC	$0.36		
HCFA FUL (100s ea)	$0.21		

BRAND/MANUFACTURER	NDC	SIZE	AWP
◆ BRAND			
VISTARIL: Pfizer Labs	00069-5430-66	100s	$119.56
	00069-5430-41	100s ud	$132.85
	00069-5430-73	50s	$585.78
◆ GENERICS			
Moore,H.L.	00839-6272-06	100s	$29.50
Rugby	00536-3896-01	100s	$31.43
Goldline	00182-1991-01	100s	$32.38
Qualitest	00603-3996-21	100s	$34.10
Major	00904-0360-60	100s	$39.75
Major	00904-0364-60	100s	$39.75
Aligen	00405-4520-01	100s	$41.71
Major	00904-0364-61	100s ud	$18.50
Raway	00686-0058-20	100s ud	$24.00
UDL	51079-0528-20	100s ud	$82.24
Major	00904-0364-40	500s	$93.85

SUSPENSION: 25 MG/5 ML

AVERAGE UNIT PRICE (AVAILABLE SIZES)	
BRAND	$0.25

BRAND/MANUFACTURER	NDC	SIZE	AWP
◆ BRAND			
VISTARIL: Pfizer Labs	00069-5440-93	480 ml	$121.79
	00069-5440-97	120 ml 4s	$121.78

Hygroton SEE CHLORTHALIDONE

Hylorel SEE GUANADREL SULFATE

Hyoscyamine Sulfate

DESCRIPTION

Hyoscyamine Sulfate is one of the principal anticholinergic/antispasmodic components of belladonna alkaloids. The empirical formula is $(C_{17}H_{23}NO_3)_2 \cdot H_2SO_4 \cdot 2H_2O$ and the molecular weight is 712.85. Chemically, it is benzeneacetic acid, α-(hydroxymethyl)-,8-methyl-8-azabicyclo [3.2.1.] oct-3-yl ester, [3(S)-endol-, sulfate (2:1), dihydrate.

Hyoscyamine Sulfate/SL Tablets contain 0.125 mg and are formulated for sublingual administration. However, the tablets may also be chewed or taken orally.

Hyoscyamine Sulfate Tablets contain 0.125 mg formulated for oral administration.

Hyoscyamine Sulfate Elixir contains 0.125 mg per 5 mL (teaspoonful) with 20% alcohol for oral use.

Hyoscyamine Sulfate Drops, oral solution, contain 0.125 mg per mL with 5% alcohol.

➤ SHOWN IN PRODUCT IDENTIFICATION GUIDE

Hyoscyamine Sulfate Injection is a sterile solution containing 0.5 mg per mL.

Hyoscyamine Sulfate Timed-Release Capsules contain 0.375 mg and are designed for oral b.i.d. dosage.

Following is its chemical structure:

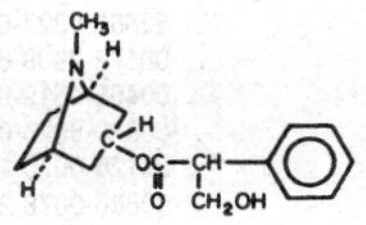

CLINICAL PHARMACOLOGY

Hyoscyamine Sulfate inhibits specifically the actions of acetylcholine on structures innervated by postganglionic cholinergic nerves and on smooth muscles that respond to acetylcholine but lack cholinergic innervation. These peripheral cholinergic receptors are present in the autonomic effector cells of the smooth muscle, cardiac muscle, the sinoatrial node, the atrioventricular node, and the exocrine glands. It is completely devoid of any action in the autonomic ganglia. Hyoscyamine Sulfate inhibits gastrointestinal propulsive motility and decreases gastric acid secretion. Hyoscyamine Sulfate also controls excessive pharyngeal, tracheal and bronchial secretions.

Hyoscyamine Sulfate is absorbed totally and completely by sublingual administration as well as oral administration. Once absorbed, Hyoscyamine Sulfate disappears rapidly from the blood and is distributed throughout the entire body. The half-life of Hyoscyamine Sulfate is 3 ½ hours. Hyoscyamine Sulfate is partly hydrolyzed to tropic acid and tropine but the majority of the drug is excreted in the urine unchanged within the first 12 hours. Only traces of this drug are found in breast milk. Hyoscyamine Sulfate passes the blood brain barrier and the placental barrier.

The Timed-Release Capsules release 0.375 mg Hyoscyamine Sulfate at a controlled and predictable rate for 12 hours. Peak blood levels occur in 2 ½ hours and the apparent plasma half-life is approximately 7 hours. The relative bioavailability of the timed-release dosage form is approximately 81% that of the immediate-release dosage form. The urinary excretion from both the immediate-release dosage form and the timed-release dosage form is equal and uniform over a 24 hour period.

INDICATIONS AND USAGE

Hyoscyamine Sulfate is effective as adjunctive therapy in the treatment of peptic ulcer. It can also be used to control gastric secretion, visceral spasm, and hypermotility in spastic colitis, spastic bladder, cystitis, pylorospasm, and associated abdominal cramps. May be used in functional intestinal disorders to reduce symptoms such as those seen in mild dysenteries, diverticulitis, and acute enterocolitis. For use as adjunctive therapy in the treatment of irritable bowel syndrome (irritable colon, spastic colon, mucous colitis) and functional gastrointestinal disorders. Also as adjunctive therapy in the treatment of neurogenic bladder and neurogenic bowel disturbances including the splenic flexure syndrome and neurogenic colon. Also used in the treatment of infant colic (elixir and drops). Hyoscyamine Sulfate is indicated along with morphine or other narcotics in symptomatic relief of biliary and renal colic; as a "drying agent" in the relief of symptoms of acute rhinitis; in the therapy of parkinsonism to reduce rigidity and tremors and to control associated sialorrhea and hyperhidrosis. May be used in the therapy of poisoning by anticholinesterase agents.

Parenterally administered Hyoscyamine Sulfate is also effective in reducing duodenal motility to facilitate the diagnostic radiologic procedure, hypotonic duodenography. Hyoscyamine Sulfate may be used to reduce pain and hypersecretion in pancreatitis. Hyoscyamine Sulfate may also be used in certain cases of partial heart block associated with vagal activity.

IN ANESTHESIA

Hyoscyamine Sulfate Injection is indicated as a pre-operative antimuscarinic to reduce salivary, tracheobronchial, and pharyngeal secretions; to reduce the volume and acidity of gastric secretions, and to block cardiac vagal inhibitory reflexes during induction of anesthesia and intubation. Hyoscyamine Sulfate protects against the peripheral muscarinic effects such as bradycardia and excessive secretions produced by halogenated hydrocarbons and cholinergic agents such as physostigmine, neostigmine and pyridostigmine given to reverse the actions of curariform agents.

IN UROLOGY

Hyoscyamine Sulfate Injection may also be used intravenously to improve radiologic visibility of the kidneys.

CONTRAINDICATIONS

Glaucoma; obstructive uropathy (for example, bladder neck obstruction due to prostatic hypertrophy); obstructive disease of the gastrointestinal tract (as in achalasia, pyloroduodenal stenosis); paralytic ileus, intestinal atony of elderly or debitated patients; unstable cardiovascular status in acute hemorrhage; severe ulcerative colitis; toxic megacolon complicating ulcerative colitis; myasthenia gravis.

WARNINGS

In the presence of high environmental temperature, heat prostration can occur with drug use (fever and heat stroke due to decreased sweating). Diarrhea may be an early symptom of incomplete intestinal obstruction, especially in patients with ileostomy or colostomy. In this instance, treatment with this drug would be inappropriate and possibly harmful. Like other anticholinergic agents. Hyoscya-

mine Sulfate may produce drowsiness or blurred vision. In this event, the patient should be warned not to engage in activities requiring mental alertness such as operating a motor vehicle or other machinery or to perform hazardous work while taking this drug.

Psychosis has been reported in sensitive individuals given anticholinergic drugs. CNS signs and symptoms inlude confusion, disorientation, short term memory loss, hallucinations, dysarthria, ataxia, coma, euphoria, decreased anxiety, fatigue, insomnia, agitation and mannerisms, and inappropriate affect. These CNS signs and symptoms usually resolve within 12-48 hours after discontinuation of the drug.

The 10 mL multiple-dose vial of Hyoscyamine Sulfate Injection contains sodium metabisulfite, a sulfite that may cause allergic-type reactions including anaphylactic symptoms and life-threatening or less severe asthmatic episodes in certain susceptible people. The overall prevalence of sulfite sensitivity in the general population is unknown and probably low. Sulfite sensitivity is seen more frequently in asthmatic than in nonasthmatic people.

PRECAUTIONS

GENERAL

Use with caution in patients with: autonomic neuropathy, hyperthyroidism, coronary heart disease, congestive heart failure, cardiac arrhythmias, hypertension and renal disease. Investigate any tachycardia before giving any anticholinergic drug since they may increase the heart rate. Use with caution in patients with hiatal hernia associated with reflux esophagitis.

INFORMATION FOR PATIENTS

Hyoscyamine Sulfate may cause drowsiness, dizziness or blurred vision; patients should observe caution before driving, using machinery or performing other tasks requiring mental alertness.

Use of Hyoscyamine Sulfate may decrease sweating resulting in heat prostration, fever or heat stroke; febrile patients or those who may be exposed to elevated environmental temperatures should use caution.

DRUG INTERACTIONS

Additive adverse effects resulting from cholinergic blockade may occur when Hyoscyamine Sulfate is administered concomitantly with other antimuscarinics, amantadine, haloperidol, phenothiazines, monoamine oxidase (MAO) inhibitors, tricyclic antidepressants or some antihistamines.

Antacids may interfere with the absorption of Hyoscyamine Sulfate; take Hyoscyamine Sulfate before meals and antacids after meals.

CARCINOGENESIS, MUTAGENESIS, IMPAIRMENT OF FERTILITY

No long term studies in animals have been performed to determine the carcinogenic, mutagenic or impairment of fertility potential of Hyoscyamine Sulfate; however, over 30 years of marketing experience shows no demonstrable evidence of a problem.

PREGNANCY—PREGNANCY CATEGORY C

Animal reproduction studies have not been conducted with Hyoscyamine Sulfate. It is also not known whether Hyoscyamine Sulfate can cause fetal harm when administered to a pregnant woman or can affect reproduction capacity. Hyoscyamine Sulfate should be given to a pregnant woman only if clearly needed.

NURSING MOTHERS

Hyoscyamine Sulfate is excreted in human milk. Caution should be exercised when Hyoscyamine Sulfate is administered to a nursing woman.

ADVERSE REACTIONS

Not all of the following adverse reactions have been reported with Hyoscyamine Sulfate. The following adverse reactions have been reported for pharmacologically similar drugs with anticholinergic/antispasmodic action. Adverse reactions may include dryness of the mouth; urinary hesitancy and retention; blurred vision; tachycardia; palpitations; mydriasis; cycloplegia; increased ocular tension; loss of taste; headache; nervousness; drowsiness; weakness; dizziness; insomnia; nausea; vomiting; impotence; suppression of lactation; constipation; bloated feeling; allergic reactions or drug idiosyncrasies; urticaria and other dermal manifestations; ataxia; speech disturbance; some degree of mental confusion and/or excitement (especially in elderly persons); and decreased sweating.

OVERDOSAGE

The signs and symptoms of overdose are headache, nausea, vomiting, blurred vision, dilated pupils, hot dry skin, dizziness, dryness of the mouth, difficulty in swallowing and CNS stimulation.

Measures to be taken are immediate lavage of the stomach and injection of physostigmine 0.5 to 2 mg intravenously and repeated as necessary up to a total of 5 mg. Fever may be treated symptomatically (tepid water sponge baths, hypothermic blanket). Excitement to a degree which demands attention may be managed with sodium thiopental 2% solution given slowly intravenously or chloral hydrate (100-200 mL of a 2% solution) by rectal infusion. In the event of progression of the curare-like effect to paralysis of the respiratory muscles, artificial respiration should be instituted and maintained until effective respiratory action returns.

In rats, the LD_{50} for Hyoscyamine Sulfate is 375 mg/kg. Hyoscyamine Sulfate is dialyzable.

DOSAGE AND ADMINISTRATION

Dosage may be adjusted according to the conditions and severity of symptoms.

HYOSCYAMINE SULFATE/SL TABLETS
The tablets may be taken sublingually, orally or chewed.

Adults and children 12 years of age and older: 1 to 2 tablets every four hours or as needed. Do not exceed 12 tablets in 24 hours.

Children 2 to under 12 years of age: ½ to 1 tablet every four hours or as needed. Do not exceed 6 tablets in 24 hours.

HYOSCYAMINE SULFATE TABLETS
The tablets may be taken orally or sublingually.

Adults and children 12 years of age and older: 1 to 2 tablets every four hours or as needed. Do not exceed 12 tablets in 24 hours.

Children 2 to under 12 years of age: ½ to 1 tablet every four hours or as needed. Do not exceed 6 tablets in 24 hours.

HYOSCYAMINE SULFATE ELIXIR
Adults and children 12 years of age and older: 1 to 2 teaspoonfuls every four hours or as needed. Do not exceed 12 teaspoonfuls in 24 hours.

Children 2 to under 12 years of age: ¼ to 1 teaspoonful every four hours or as needed. Do not exceed 6 teaspoonfuls in 24 hours.
    The following dosage guide is based upon body weight. The doses may be repeated every four hours or as needed.

Body Weight	Usual Dose
10 kg (22 lb)	¼ tsp
20 kg (44 lb)	½ tsp
40 kg (88 lb)	¾ tsp
50 kg (110 lb)	1 tsp

HYOSCYAMINE SULFATE DROPS
Adults and children 12 years of age and older: 1 to 2 mL every four hours or as needed. Do not exceed 12 mL in 24 hours.

Children 2 to under 12 years of age: ¼ to 1 mL every four hours or as needed. Do not exceed 6 mL in 24 hours.

Children under 2 years of age: The following dosage guide is based upon body weight. The doses may be repeated every four hours or as needed.

Body Weight	Usual Dose	Do Not Exceed in 24 Hours
2.3 kg (5 lb)	3 drops	18 drops
3.4 kg (7.5 lb)	4 drops	24 drops
5 kg (11 lb)	5 drops	30 drops
7 kg (15 lb)	6 drops	36 drops
10 kg (22 lb)	8 drops	48 drops
15 kg (33 lb)	11 drops	66 drops

HYOSCYAMINE SULFATE INJECTION
The dose may be administered subcutaneously, intramuscularly, or intravenously without dilution.

Gastrointestinal Disorders: The usual adult recommended dose is 0.5 to 1.0 mL (0.25 to 0.5 mg). Some patients may need only a single dose; others may require administration two, three, or four times a day at four hour intervals.

Hypotonic Duodenography: The usual adult recommended dose is 0.5 to 1.0 mL (0.25 to 0.5 mg) administered 5 to 10 minutes prior to the diagnostic procedure.

Anesthesia: Adults and children over 2 years of age: As a pre-anesthetic medication, the recommended dose is 5 µg (0.005 mg) per kg of body weight. This dose is usually given 30 to 60 minutes prior to the anticipated time of induction of anesthesia or at the time the pre-anesthetic narcotic or sedative is administered.
    Hyoscyamine Sulfate Injection may be used during surgery to reduce drug-induced bradycardia. It should be administered intravenously in increments of 0.25 mL and repeated as needed. To achieve reversal of neuromuscular blockade, the recommended dose is 0.2 mg (0.4 mL) Hyoscyamine Sulfate Injection for every 1 mg neostigmine or the equivalent dose of physotigmine or pyridostigmine.
    Parenteral drug products should be inspected visually for particulate matter and discoloration prior to administration, whenever solution and container permit.

HYOSCYAMINE SULFATE TIME/RELEASE CAPSULES
Adults and children 12 years of age and older: 1 to 2 capsules every 12 hours. Dosage may be adjusted to 1 capsule every 8 hours if needed. Do not exceed 4 capsules in 24 hours.

Children 2 to under 12 years of age: 1 capsule every 12 hours. Do not exceed 2 capsules in 24 hours.
    Store at controlled room temperature 15°-30°C (59°-86°F).

J CODES
Up to 0.25 mg SC,IM,IV—J1980

HOW SUPPLIED
CAPSULE: 0.375 MG

BRAND/MANUFACTURER	NDC	SIZE	AWP
○ **BRAND**			
CYSTOSPAZ-M: Polymedica	00998-2260-10	100s	$58.13

CAPSULE, EXTENDED RELEASE: 0.375 MG

BRAND/MANUFACTURER	NDC	SIZE	AWP
○ **BRAND**			
► LEVSINEX: Schwarz	00091-3537-01	100s	$55.78
○ **GENERICS**			
Ethex	58177-0017-04	100s	$42.70
Econolab	55053-0310-01	100s	$43.45
Qualitest	00603-4004-21	100s	$44.06
Major	00904-7833-60	100s	$45.95
URL	00677-1507-01	100s	$47.30
Rugby	00536-5592-01	100s	$48.04
Aligen	00405-4522-01	100s	$48.20
Moore,H.L.	00839-7910-06	100s	$51.00
Pecos	59879-0109-01	100s	$51.00

DROP:

BRAND/MANUFACTURER	NDC	SIZE	AWP
○ **BRAND**			
LEVSIN: Schwarz	00091-4538-15	15 ml	$14.30
○ **GENERICS**			
SPASDEL: Marlop	12939-0774-15	15 ml	$6.05
GASTROSED: Roberts/Hauck	59441-0447-15	15 ml	$11.11

DROP: 0.125 MG

BRAND/MANUFACTURER	NDC	SIZE	AWP
○ **GENERICS**			
Rugby	00536-2680-72	15 ml	$8.40
Marlop	12939-0345-15	15 ml	$8.40

ELIXIR:

BRAND/MANUFACTURER	NDC	SIZE	AWP
○ **BRAND**			
LEVSIN: Schwarz	00091-4532-16	480 ml	$36.44
○ **GENERICS**			
URL	00677-0511-33	480 ml	$7.35
Goldline	00182-6136-40	480 ml	$12.00
SPASDEL: Marlop	12939-0775-16	480 ml	$12.50
HYCO ELIXIR: Hi-Tech	50383-0290-16	480 ml	$20.00
LIQUI-SOOTH: Liquipharm	54198-0147-16	480 ml	$25.00
SPASDEL: Marlop	12939-0775-28	3840 ml	$90.00

ELIXIR: 0.125 MG

BRAND/MANUFACTURER	NDC	SIZE	AWP
○ **GENERICS**			
Marlop	12939-0346-16	480 ml	$10.30

INJECTION: 0.5 MG/ML

BRAND/MANUFACTURER	NDC	SIZE	AWP
○ **BRAND**			
LEVSIN: Schwarz	00091-1536-05	1 ml 5s	$31.81

LIQUID:

BRAND/MANUFACTURER	NDC	SIZE	AWP
○ **GENERICS**			
LIQUI-SOOTH: Liquipharm	54198-0146-15	15 ml	$9.30

SOLUTION: 0.125 MG

BRAND/MANUFACTURER	NDC	SIZE	AWP
○ **GENERICS**			
Econolab	55053-0380-15	15 ml	$10.25

TABLETS:

BRAND/MANUFACTURER	NDC	SIZE	AWP
○ **BRAND**			
ESPASMOTEX: Kramer Dist	52083-0835-60	60s	$8.00
ANASPAZ: Ascher	00225-0295-15	100s	$18.24
► LEVSIN SL: Schwarz	00091-3532-01	100s	$27.00
ANASPAZ: Ascher	00225-0295-20	500s	$88.74
► LEVSIN SL: Schwarz	00091-3532-05	500s	$130.00
○ **GENERICS**			
DONNAMAR: Marnel	00682-0106-01	100s	$11.30
Breckenridge	51991-0130-01	100s	$13.50
MEDISPAZ: Med-Tek	52349-0240-10	100s	$20.89
SETAMINE:	52765-1377-00	1000s	$12.95

► SHOWN IN PRODUCT IDENTIFICATION GUIDE

TABLETS: 0.125 MG

BRAND/MANUFACTURER	NDC	SIZE	AWP
○ **BRAND**			
▶ LEVSIN: Schwarz	00091-3531-01	100s	$27.00
	00091-3531-05	500s	$130.00
○ **GENERICS**			
Alphagen	59743-0026-01	100s	$11.25
Qualitest	00603-4003-21	100s	$11.61
SPASDEL: Marlop	12939-0773-60	100s	$11.80
Major	00904-2496-60	100s	$11.95
Equipharm	57779-0101-04	100s	$12.37
Aligen	00405-4521-01	100s	$13.50
Econolab	55053-0130-01	100s	$13.50
URL	00677-1419-01	100s	$13.75
Goldline	00182-1607-01	100s	$13.80
GASTROSED: Roberts/Hauck	59441-0143-01	100s	$15.00
Marlop	12939-0347-10	100s	$15.50
Rugby	00536-3918-01	100s	$15.68
ED SPAZ: Edwards	00485-0056-01	100s	$18.00
HYOSOL/SL: Econolab	55053-0717-01	100s	$18.95
Moore,H.L.	00839-7818-06	100s	$19.78
Moore,H.L.	00839-7521-06	100s	$19.78
Rugby	00536-5575-01	100s	$21.65
Moore,H.L.	00839-7806-06	100s	$21.80
URL	00677-1536-01	100s	$22.90

TABLETS: 0.15 MG

BRAND/MANUFACTURER	NDC	SIZE	AWP
○ **BRAND**			
CYSTOSPAZ: Polymedica	00998-2225-10	100s	$41.25
○ **GENERICS**			
HYOSPAZ: Econolab	55053-0111-01	100s	$21.25

Hyoscyamine Sulfate and Phenobarbital

Each tablet contains:

Hyoscyamine Sulfate ....0.125 mg
Phenobarbital ....15 mg
(WARNING: May be habit-forming)

Each ml of oral solution contains:

Hyoscyamine Sulfate ....0.125 mg
Phenobarbital ....15 mg
(WARNING: May be habit-forming)

Each 5 ml of elixir contains:

Hyoscyamine Sulfate ....0.125 mg
Phenobarbital ....15 mg
(WARNING: May be habit-forming)

CLINICAL PHARMACOLOGY

Hyoscyamine Sulfate is one of the principal anticholinergic/antispasmodic components of belladonna alkaloids. Hyoscyamine Sulfate also inhibits the action of acetylcholine at the postganglionic nerve endings of the parasympathetic nervous system. A fixed ratio combination with Phenobarbital provides mild sedation to protect patients against the physical and emotional stresses often present in conditions causing vagotonia or parasympathotonia.

INDICATIONS AND USAGE

BASED ON A REVIEW OF THESE DRUGS BY THE NATIONAL ACADEMY OF SCIENCES-NATIONAL RESEARCH COUNCIL AND/OR OTHER INFORMATION, FDA HAS CLASSIFIED THE INDICATION AS FOLLOWS: "POSSIBLY" EFFECTIVE:

FOR USE AS ADJUNCTIVE THERAPY IN THE TREATMENT OF PEPTIC ULCER.

IT SHOULD BE NOTED AT THIS POINT IN TIME THAT THERE IS A LACK OF CONCURRENCE AS TO THE VALUE OF ANTICHOLINERGICS/ANTISPASMODICS IN THE TREATMENT OF GASTRIC ULCER. IT HAS NOT BEEN SHOWN CONCLUSIVELY WHETHER ANTICHOLINERGIC/ANTISPASMODIC DRUGS AND IN THE HEALING OF A PEPTIC ULCER, DECREASE THE RATE OF RECURRENCES, OR PREVENT COMPLICATION.

MAY ALSO BE USEFUL IN THE IRRITABLE BOWEL SYNDROME (IRRITABLE COLON, SPASTIC COLON, MUCOUS COLITIS), AND ACUTE ENTEROCOLITIS.

FINAL CLASSIFICATION OF THE LESS-THAN-EFFECTIVE INDICATIONS REQUIRES FURTHER INVESTIGATION.

CONTRAINDICATIONS

Glaucoma, obstructive uropathy (for example, bladder neck obstruction due to prostatic hypertrophy); obstructive disease of the gastrointestinal tract (as in achalasia, pyloroduodenal stenosis, etc.); paralytic ileus, intestinal atony of the elderly or debilitated patient; unstable cardiovascular status in acute hemorrhage; severe ulcerative colitis especially if complicated by toxic megacolon; myasthenia gravis; hiatal hernia associated with reflux esophagitis.

Phenobarbital is contraindicated in acute intermittent porphyria. A sensitivity to phenobarbital contraindicates the use of Hyoscyamine Sulfate/Phenobarbital and in patients in whom Phenobarbital produces restlessness and/or excitement.

WARNINGS

Belladonna alkaloids with Phenobarbital should be used in pregnancy, lactation, or in women of childbearing age only when, in the judgment of the physician, the expected benefits outweigh the potential hazards to the mother and child.

In the presence of high environmental temperature, heat prostration can occur with the drug use (fever and heatstroke due to decreased sweating).

Diarrhea may be an early symptom of incomplete intestinal obstruction, especially in patients with ileostomy or colostomy. In this instance, treatment with this drug would be inappropriate and possibly harmful.

Hyoscyamine Sulfate/Phenobarbital may produce drowsiness or blurred vision. In this event, the patient should be warned not to engage in activities requiring mental alertness such as operating a motor vehicle or other machinery, or perform hazardous work while taking this drug.

Phenobarbital in patients taking anticoagulants may decrease the effect of the anticoagulant and thus require larger doses of the anticoagulant for optimal effect. When the phenobarbital is discontinued, the dose of the anticoagulant may have to be decreased. Barbiturates may thus decrease the action of anticoagulant drugs.

Phenobarbital may be habit forming and should not be administered to individuals known to be addiction prone or to those with a history of physical and/or psychological dependence upon habit-forming drugs. Since barbiturates are metabolized in the liver, use with initial small doses and caution in patients with hepatic dysfunction.

PRECAUTIONS

General: Use with caution in patients with: autonomic neuropathy, hepatic or renal disease, hyperthyroidism, coronary heart disease, congestive heart failure, cardiac arrhythmias, and hypertension.

It should be noted that the use of anticholinergic/antispasmodic drugs in the treatment of gastric ulcer may produce a delay in gastric emptying time and may complicate such therapy (antral stasis).

Do not rely on the use of the drug in the presence of complication of biliary tract disease.

Investigate any tachycardia before giving anticholinergic (atropine-like) drugs since they may increase the heart rate.

With overdosage, a curare-like action may occur.

ADVERSE REACTIONS

Adverse reactions may include dryness of the mouth; urinary hesitancy and retention; blurred vision; tachycardia; palpitation; mydriasis; cycloplegia; increased ocular tension; loss of taste; headache; nervousness; drowsiness; weakness; dizziness; insomnia; nausea; vomiting, impotence; suppression of lactation; constipation; bloated feeling; severe allergic reaction or drug idiosyncrasies including anaphylaxis; urticaria and other dermal manifestations; and decreased sweating. Elderly patients may react with symptoms of excitement, agitation, drowsiness, and other untoward manifestations to even small doses of the drug.

Phenobarbital may produce excitement in some patients rather than a sedative effect. An occasional patient may experience musculoskeletal pain. Some patients may acquire a sensitivity to barbiturates and experience allergic phenomena and/or dermatologic response.

In patients habituated to barbiturates, abrupt withdrawal may produce delirium or convulsions.

OVERDOSAGE

The signs and symptoms of overdose are headache, nausea, vomiting, blurred vision, dilated pupils, hot dry skin, dizziness, dryness of the mouth, difficulty in swallowing, and CNS stimulation. Treatment should consist of gastric lavage, emetics, and activated charcoal. If indicated, parenteral cholinergic agents such as bethanechol chloride USP should be used.

DOSAGE AND ADMINISTRATION

The dosage may be adjusted to the needs of the individual patient to assure symptomatic control with a minimum of adverse effects.

TABLETS ORAL SOLUTION

Adults: 1 or 2 tablets three or four times a day according to conditions and severity of symptoms.

1-2 ml every four hours or as needed.

Children: 1-10 *years*: ½ to 1 ml every four hours or as needed.

Infants: The following dosage guide is based on body weight. The doses may be repeated every four hours or as needed.

Body Weight	Starting Dose
5 lb	3 drops
7.5 lb	4 drops
10 lb	6 drops

◆ RATED THERAPEUTICALLY EQUIVALENT; ◇ THERAPEUTIC EQUIVALENCE UNCONFIRMED; ○ UNRATED

Body Weight	Starting Dose
15 lb	7 drops
20 lb	9 drops

STORAGE
Store at controlled room temperature, 15°-30°C (59°-86°F).

HOW SUPPLIED
DROP:

BRAND/MANUFACTURER	NDC	SIZE	AWP
○ **BRAND**			
LEVSIN W/PHENOBARBITAL: Schwarz	00091-4536-15	15 ml	$19.66

LIQUID:

BRAND/MANUFACTURER	NDC	SIZE	AWP
○ **GENERICS**			
ELIXIRAL: Vita Elixir	00181-0626-00	480 ml	$9.50
ELIXIRAL: Vita Elixir	00181-0627-00	3840 ml	$52.00

TABLETS: 0.125 MG-15 MG

BRAND/MANUFACTURER	NDC	SIZE	AWP
○ **BRAND**			
LEVSIN W/PHENOBARBITAL: Schwarz	00091-3534-01	100s	$41.63

Hypaque SEE DIATRIZOATE MEGLUMINE

Hypaque SEE DIATRIZOATE SODIUM

Hyper-Tet SEE TETANUS IMMUNE GLOBULIN

Hyperab SEE RABIES IMMUNE GLOBULIN (HUMAN)

HyperHep SEE HEPATITIS B IMMUNE GLOBULIN (HUMAN)

Hyperlyte SEE DEXTROSE AND ELECTROLYTES *AND* ELECTROLYTES, INJECTABLE

Hyperstat SEE DIAZOXIDE, INJECTABLE

Hyprho-D Mini-Dose SEE GLOBULIN, IMMUNE RHO₀(D) *AND* RH₀(D) IMMUNE GLOBULIN

Hyskon SEE DEXTRAN-70 IN DEXTROSE

Hytakerol SEE DIHYDROTACHYSTEROL

Hytone SEE HYDROCORTISONE, TOPICAL

Hytrin SEE TERAZOSIN HYDROCHLORIDE

Iberet-Folic-500 SEE FERROUS SULFATE/FOLIC ACID/VITAMINS, MULTI

Ibuprofen

DESCRIPTION
The active ingredient in Ibuprofen is chemically designated as (±)-2-(p-isobutyl-phenyl) propionic acid. Ibuprofen is a white powder with a melting point of 74-77°C and is very slightly soluble in water (< 1 mg/ml) and readily soluble in organic solvents such as ethanol and acetone.

Ibuprofen, a nonsteroidal anti-inflammatory agent, is available in 300 mg, 400 mg, 600 mg, and 800 mg tablets for oral administration. Ibuprofen is also available as a suspension for oral administration containing 100 mg per 5 ml.

Following is its chemical structure:

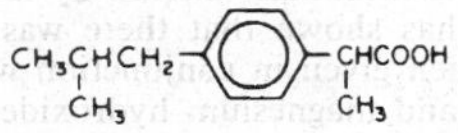

$$CH_3CHCH_2 \underset{CH_3}{\overset{}{\bigcirc}} CHCOOH \, CH_3$$

CLINICAL PHARMACOLOGY
Ibuprofen possesses analgesic and antipyretic activities. Its mode of action, like that of other nonsteroidal anti-inflammatory agents, is not completely understood, but may be related to prostaglandin synthetase inhibition.

In clinical studies in adult patients with rheumatoid arthritis and osteoarthritis Ibuprofen has been shown to be comparable to aspirin in controlling pain and inflammation and to be associated with a statistically significant reduction in the milder gastrointestinal side effects (see *"Adverse Reactions"*). Ibuprofen may be well tolerated in some patients who have had gastrointestinal side effects with aspirin, but these patients when treated with Ibuprofen should be carefully followed for signs and symptoms of gastrointestinal ulceration and bleeding. Although it is not definitely known whether Ibuprofen causes less peptic ulceration than aspirin, in one study involving 885 adult patients with rheumatoid arthritis treated for up to one year, there were no reports of gastric ulceration with Ibuprofen whereas frank ulceration was reported in 13 patients in the aspirin group (statistically significant p < .001).

Gastroscopic studies at varying doses show an increased tendency toward gastric irritation at higher doses. However, at comparable doses, gastric irritation is approximately half that seen with aspirin. Studies using ^{51}Cr-tagged red cells indicate that fecal blood loss associated with Ibuprofen in doses up to 2400 mg daily did not exceed the normal range, and was significantly less than that seen in aspirin-treated patients.

In clinical studies in patients with rheumatoid arthritis, Ibuprofen has been shown to be comparable to indomethacin in controlling the signs and symptoms of disease activity and to be associated with a statistically significant reduction of the milder gastrointestinal (see *"Adverse Reactions"*) and CNS side effects.

Ibuprofen may be used in combination with gold salts and/or corticosteroids.

Controlled studies in adults have demonstrated that Ibuprofen is a more effective analgesic than propoxyphene for the relief of episiotomy pain, pain following dental extraction procedures, and for the relief of the symptoms of primary dysmenorrhea.

In clinical studies in patients aged 2 to 15 with juvenile arthritis, Ibuprofen Suspension in doses of 20 to 50 mg/kg/day divided into 3 or 4 daily doses, has been shown to be similar to aspirin in controlling the signs and symptoms of their disease. In these trials, there was a significantly lower incidence of liver test abnormalities associated with Ibuprofen Suspension than with aspirin. Although Ibuprofen may be better tolerated in terms of liver test abnormalities in children treated with Ibuprofen Suspension, they should be carefully followed for signs and symptoms suggesting liver dysfunction particularly with doses above 30mg/kg/day, or if abnormal liver tests have occurred with previous NSAID treatment (see *"Precautions"*).

Controlled clinical trials comparing doses of 5 and 10mg/kg Ibuprofen and 10-15 mg/kg of acetaminophen have been conducted in children 6 months to 12 years of age with fever primarily due to viral illnesses. In these studies there were no differences between treatments in fever reduction for the first hour and maximum fever reduction occurred between 2 and 4 hours. Response after 1 hour was dependent on both the level of temperature elevation as well as the treatment. In children with baseline temperatures at or below 102.5°F, both Ibuprofen doses and acetaminophen were equally effective in their maximum effect. In those children with temperatures above 102.5°F, the Ibuprofen 10mg/kg dose was more effective. By 6 hours children treated with Ibuprofen 5mg/kg tended to have recurrence of fever, whereas children treated with Ibuprofen 10 mg/kg still had significant fever reduction at 8 hours. In control groups treated with 10mg/kg acetaminophen, fever reduction resembled that seen in children treated with 5 mg/kg of Ibuprofen, with the exception that temperature elevation tended to return 1-2 hours earlier. In other trials, the antipyretic effect of Ibuprofen Suspension at 10 mg/kg was similar to that of acetaminophen at 15 mg/kg.

In patients with primary dysmenorrhea, Ibuprofen has been shown to reduce elevated levels of prostaglandin activity in the menstrual fluid and to reduce resting and active intra-uterine pressure, as well as the frequency of uterine contractions. The probable mechanism of action is to inhibit prostaglandin synthesis rather than simply to provide analgesia. Ibuprofen is rapidly absorbed when administered orally. As is true with most tablet and suspension formulations, Ibuprofen Suspension is absorbed somewhat faster than the tablet with a time to peak serum level generally within one hour. Peak serum Ibuprofen levels are generally attained one to two hours after administration of Ibuprofen tablets and within about 1 hour after the suspension. With single, oral, solid doses up to 800 mg adults, a linear relationship exists between amount of drug administered and the integrated area under the serum drug concentration vs time curve. Above 800 mg, however, the area under the curve increases less than proportionally to increases in dose. There is no evidence of drug accumulation or enzyme induction. There is no evidence of age-dependent kinetics in patients 2 to 11 years old. With single doses of Ibuprofen Suspension ranging up to 10mg/kg, a dose/response relationship exists between the amount of drug administered to febrile children and the serum concentration vs. time curve. There is also a correlation between reduction of fever and drug concentration over time, although the peak reduction in fever occurs 2-4 hours after dosing.

The administration of Ibuprofen either under fasting conditions or immediately before meals yields quite similar serum Ibuprofen concentration-time profiles. When Ibuprofen is administered immediately after a meal, there is a reduction in the rate of absorption but no appreciable decrease in the extent of absorption. The bioavailability of the drug is minimally altered by the presence of food.

A bioavailability study has shown that there was no interference with the absorption of Ibuprofen when given in conjunction with an antacid containing both aluminum hydroxide and magnesium hydroxide.

Ibuprofen is rapidly metabolized and eliminated in the urine. The excretion of Ibuprofen is virtually complete 24 hours after the last dose. The serum half-life is 1.8 to 2.0 hours.

Studies have shown that following ingestion of the drug, 45% to 79% of the dose was recovered in the urine within 24 hours as metabolite A (25%), (+)-2-[p-(2hydroxymethylpropyl)-phenyl] propionic acid and metabolite B (37%), (+)-2-[p-(2carboxypropyl)-phenyl] propionic acid; the percentages of free and conjugated Ibuprofen were approximately 1% and 14%, respectively.

INDICATIONS AND USAGE

Ibuprofen Tables are indicated for relief of the signs and symptoms of rheumatoid arthritis and osteoarthritis. The suspension is indicated for juvenile arthritis, rheumatoid arthritis and osteoarthritis. It is also indicated for the relief of mild to moderate pain and of primary dysmenorrhea, and for the reduction of fever in patients ages 6 months and older.

Ibuprofen is indicated for relief of mild to moderate pain.

Ibuprofen is also indicated for the treatment of primary dysmenorrhea.

Since there have been no controlled clinical trials to demonstrate whether or not there is any beneficial effect or harmful interaction with the use of Ibuprofen in conjunction with aspirin, the combination cannot be recommended (see "Drug Interactions").

Safety and efficacy of Ibuprofen Suspension in children below the age of 6 months has not been established.

UNLABELED USES

Ibuprofen is used alone or as an adjunct in the treatment of Barouer's syndrome and chronic uveitis, both anterior and posterior. It is also used in IUD-associated uterine bleeding, and prophylactically to reduce the severity of nausea and prevent radiation-induced vomiting in patients receiving pelvic irradiation. Ibuprofen is also prescribed for diabetic neuropathy and acute migraine headache, and is used in hemophilic arthropathy.

CONTRAINDICATIONS

Ibuprofen should not be used in patients who have previously exhibited hypersensitivity to the drug, or in individuals with the syndrome of nasal polyps, angioedema and bronchospastic reactivity to aspirin or other nonsteroidal anti-inflammatory agents. Anaphylactoid reactions have occurred in such patients.

WARNINGS

Risk of GI Ulceration, Bleeding and Perforation with Nonsteroidal Anti-inflammatory Therapy: Serious gastrointestinal toxicity such as bleeding, ulceration, and perforation, can occur at any time, with or without warning symptoms, in patients treated chronically with nonsteroidal anti-inflammatory drugs. Although minor upper gastrointestinal problems, such as dyspepsia, are common, usually developing early in therapy, physicians should remain alert for ulceration and bleeding in patients treated chronically with nonsteroidal anti-inflammatory drugs even in the absence of previous GI tract symptoms. In patients observed in clinical trials of several months to two years duration, symptomatic upper GI ulcers, gross bleeding or perforation appear to occur in approximately 1% of patients treated for 3-6 months, and in about 2-4% of patients treated for one year. Physicians should inform patients about the signs and/or symptoms of serious GI toxicity and what steps to take if they occur.

Studies to date have not identified any subset of patients not at risk of developing peptic ulceration and bleeding. Except for a prior history of serious GI events and other risk factors known to be associated with peptic ulcer disease, such as alcoholism, smoking, etc., no risk factors (e.g., age, sex) have been associated with increased risk. Elderly or debilitated patients seem to tolerate ulceration or bleeding less well than other individuals and most spontaneous reports of fatal GI events are in this population. Studies to date are inconclusive concerning the relative risk of various nonsteroidal anti-inflammatory agents in causing such reactions. High doses of any such agents probably carry a greater risk of these reactions, although controlled clinical trials showing this do not exist in most cases. In considering the use of relatively large doses (within the recommended dosage range), sufficient benefit should be anticipated to offset the potential increased risk of GI toxicity.

PRECAUTIONS

Blurred and/or diminished vision, scotomata, and/or changes in color vision have been reported. If a patient develops such complaints while receiving Ibuprofen, the drug should be discontinued and the patient should have an ophthalmologic examination which includes central visual fields and color vision testing.

Fluid retention and edema have been reported in association with Ibuprofen; therefore, the drug should be used with caution in patients with a history of cardiac decompensation or hypertension.

Ibuprofen, like other nonsteroidal anti-inflammatory agents, can inhibit platelet aggregation but the effect is quantitatively less and of shorter duration than that seen with aspirin. Ibuprofen has been shown to prolong bleeding time (but within the normal range) in normal subjects. Because this prolonged bleeding effect may be exaggerated in patients with underlying hemostatic defects, Ibuprofen should be used with caution in persons with intrinsic coagulation defects and those on anticoagulant therapy.

Patients on Ibuprofen should report to their physicians signs or symptoms of gastrointestinal ulceration or bleeding, blurred vision or other eye symptoms, skin rash, weight gain, or edema.

In order to avoid exacerbation of disease or adrenal insufficiency, patients who have been on prolonged corticosteroid therapy should have their therapy tapered slowly rather than discontinued abruptly when Ibuprofen is added to the treatment program.

The antipyretic and anti-inflammatory activity of Ibuprofen may reduce fever and inflammation, thus diminishing their utility as diagnostic signs in detecting complications of presumed noninfectious noninflammatory painful conditions. As with other nonsteroidal anti-inflammatory drugs, border-line elevations of one or more liver function tests may occur in up to 15% of patients. These abnormalities may progress, may remain essentially unchanged, or may be transient with continued therapy. The SGPT (ALT) test is probably the most sensitive indicator of liver dysfunction. Meaningful (3 times the upper limit of normal) elevations of SGPT or SGOT (AST) occurred in controlled clinical trials in less than 1% of patients. A patient with symptoms and/or signs suggesting liver dysfunction, or in whom an abnormal liver test has occurred, should be evaluated for evidence of the development of more severe hepatic reactions while on therapy with Ibuprofen. Severe hepatic reactions, including jaundice and cases of fatal hepatitis, have been reported with Ibuprofen as with other nonsteroidal anti-inflammatory drugs. Although such reactions are rare, if abnormal liver tests persist or worsen, if clinical signs and symptoms consistent with liver disease develop, or if systemic manifestations occur (e.g., eosinophilia, rash, etc.), Ibuprofen should be discontinued.

In cross-study comparisons with doses ranging from 1200 mg to 3200 mg daily for several weeks, a slight dose-response decrease in hemoglobin/hematocrit was noted. This has been observed with other nonsteroidal anti-inflammatory drugs; the mechanism is unknown. With daily doses of 3200 mg, the total decrease in hemoglobin may exceed 1 gram; if there are no signs of bleeding, it is probably not clinically important. In two postmarketing clinical studies the incidence of a decreased hemoglobin level was greater than previously reported. Decrease in hemoglobin of 1 gram or more was observed in 17.1% of 193 patients on 1600 mg Ibuprofen daily (osteoarthritis), and in 22.8% of 189 patients taking 2400 mg of Ibuprofen daily (rheumatoid arthritis). Positive stool occult blood tests and elevated serum creatinine levels were also observed in these studies.

Aseptic Meningitis: Aseptic meningitis with fever and coma has been observed on rare occasions in patients on Ibuprofen therapy. Although it is probably more likely to occur in patients with systemic lupus erythematosus and related connective tissue diseases, it has been reported in patients who do not have an underlying chronic disease. If signs or symptoms of meningitis develop in a patient on Ibuprofen, the possibility of its being related to Ibuprofen should be considered.

Renal Effects: As with other nonsteroidal anti-inflammatory drugs, long term administration of Ibuprofen to animals has resulted in renal papillary necrosis and other abnormal renal pathology. In humans, there have been reports of acute interstitial nephritis with hematuria, proteinuria, and occasionally nephrotic syndrome.

A second form of renal toxicity has been seen in patients with prerenal conditions leading to a reduction in renal blood flow or blood volume, where the renal prostaglandins have a supportive role in the maintenance of renal perfusion. In these patients administration of a nonsteroidal anti-inflammatory drug may cause a dose dependent reduction in prostaglandin formation and may precipitate overt renal decompensation. Patients at greatest risk of this reaction are those with impaired renal function, heart failure, liver dysfunction, those taking diuretics and the elderly. Discontinuation of nonsteroidal anti-inflammatory drug therapy is typically followed by recovery to the pretreatment state. Those patients at high risk who chronically take Ibuprofen should have renal function monitored if they have signs or symptoms which may be consistent with mild azotemia, such as malaise, fatigue, loss of appetite, etc. Occasional patients may develop some elevation of serum creatinine and BUN levels without signs or symptoms.

Since Ibuprofen is eliminated primarily by the kidneys, patients with significantly impaired renal function should be closely monitored; and a reduction in dosage should be anticipated to avoid drug accumulation. Prospective studies on the safety of Ibuprofen in patients with chronic renal failure have not been conducted.

INFORMATION FOR PATIENTS

Ibuprofen, like other drugs of its class, is not free of side effects. The side effects of these drugs can cause discomfort and, rarely, there are more serious side effects, such as gastrointestinal bleeding, which may result in hospitalization and even fatal outcomes.

Nonsteroidal anti-inflammatory drugs are often essential agents in the management of arthritis and have a major role in the treatment of pain, but they also may be commonly employed for conditions which are less serious.

Physicians may wish to discuss with their patients the potential risks (see *"Warnings"*, *"Precautions"*, and *"Adverse Reactions"*) and likely benefits of nonsteroidal anti-inflammatory drug treatment, particularly when the drugs are used for less serious conditions where treatment without such agents may represent an acceptable alternative to both the patient and physician.

LABORATORY TESTS
Because serious GI tract ulcerations and bleeding can occur without warning symptoms, physicians should follow chronically treated patients for the signs and symptoms of ulcerations and bleeding and should inform them of the importance of this follow-up (see Risk of GI Ulceration, Bleeding and Perforation with Nonsteroidal Anti-inflammatory therapy).

Drug Interactions: Coumarin-type anticoagulants: Several short-term controlled studies failed to show that Ibuprofen significantly affected prothrombin times or a variety of other clotting factors when administered to individuals on coumarin-type anticoagulants. However, because bleeding has been reported when Ibuprofen and other nonsteroidal anti-inflammatory agents have been administered to patients on coumarin-type anticoagulants, the physician should be cautious when administering Ibuprofen to patients on anticoagulants.

Aspirin: Animal studies show that aspirin given with nonsteroidal anti-inflammatory agents, including Ibuprofen, yields a net decrease in anti-inflammatory activity with lowered blood levels of the non-aspirin drug. Single dose bioavailability studies in normal volunteers have failed to show an effect of aspirin on Ibuprofen blood levels. Correlative clinical studies have not been done.

Methotrexate: Ibuprofen, as well as other nonsteroidal anti-inflammatory drugs, probably reduces the tubular secretion of methotrexate based on *in-vitro* studies in rabbit kidney slices. This may indicate that Ibuprofen could enhance the toxicity of methotrexate. Caution should be used if Ibuprofen is administered concomitantly with methotrexate.

H-2 Antagonists: In studies with human volunteers, co-administration of cimetidine or ranitidine with Ibuprofen had no substantive effect on Ibuprofen serum concentrations.

Furosemide: Clinical studies, as well as random observations, have shown that Ibuprofen can reduce the natriuretic effect of furosemide and thiazides in some patients. This response has been attributed to inhibition of renal prostaglandin synthesis. During concomitant therapy with Ibuprofen, the patient should be observed closely for signs of renal failure (See *"Precautions, Renal Effects"*) as well as to assure diuretic efficacy.

Lithium: Ibuprofen produced an elevation of plasma lithium levels and a reduction in renal lithium clearance in a study of eleven normal volunteers. The mean minimum lithium concentration increased 15% and the renal clearance of lithium was decreased by 19% during this period of concomitant drug administration. This effect has been attributed to inhibition of renal prostaglandin synthesis by Ibuprofen. Thus, when Ibuprofen and lithium are administered concurrently, subjects should be observed carefully for signs of lithium toxicity. (Read circulars for lithium preparation before use of such concurrent therapy.)

Diabetes: Each 5 mL of Ibuprofen suspension contains approximately 1.5 or 2.5 grams of sucrose, which should be taken into consideration when treating patients with impaired glucose tolerance. Some brands also contain 350mg of sorbitol per 5mL. Although in clinical trials Ibuprofen Suspension was not associated with more diarrhea than control treatments, should a patient develop diarrhea, the physician may wish to review the patient's dietary intake of sorbitol from other sources.

Pregnancy: Reproductive studies conducted in rats and rabbits at doses somewhat less than the maximal adult clinical dose did not demonstrate evidence of developmental abnormalities. However, animal reproduction studies are not always predictive of human response. As there are no adequate and well-controlled studies in pregnant women, this drug should be used during pregnancy only if clearly needed. Because of the known effects of nonsteroidal anti-inflammatory drugs on the fetal cardiovascular system (closure of ductus arteriosus), use during late pregnancy should be avoided. As with other drugs known to inhibit prostaglandin synthesis, an increased incidence of dystocia and delayed parturition occurred in rats. Administration of Ibuprofen is not recommended during pregnancy.

Nursing Mothers: In limited studies, an assay capable of detecting 1 mcg/ml did not demonstrate Ibuprofen in the milk of lactating mothers. However, because of the limited nature of the studies, and the possible adverse effects of prostaglandin-inhibiting drugs on neonates, Ibuprofen is not recommended for use in nursing mothers.

ADVERSE REACTIONS
The most frequent type of adverse reaction occurring with Ibuprofen is gastrointestinal. In controlled clinical trials the percentage of adult patients reporting one or more gastrointestinal complaints ranged from 4% to 16%.

In controlled studies in adults when Ibuprofen was compared to aspirin and indomethacin in equally effective doses, the overall incidence of gastrointestinal complaints was about half that seen in either the aspirin- or indomethacin-treated patients. In a 12-week comparison of Ibuprofen Suspension (n = 45) and aspirin (n = 47) in children with juvenile arthritis, the most common adverse experiences were also gastrointestinal in nature, usually of mild severity. Abdominal pain of possible drug relationship was reported in about 25% of patients on Ibuprofen and/or aspirin; other possibly drug-related effects associated with the digestive system were reported in 42% of the children taking Ibuprofen and in 70% of those taking aspirin.

Adverse reactions observed during controlled clinical trials in adults at an incidence greater than 1% are listed in the table. Those reactions listed in Column One encompass observations in approximately 3,000 adult patients. More than 500 of these patients were treated for periods of at least 54 weeks.

Still other reactions occurring less frequently than 1 in 100 were reported in controlled clinical trials and from marketing experience. These reactions have been divided into two categories: Column Two of the following table lists reactions with therapy with Ibuprofen where the probability of a causal relationship exists: for the reactions in Column Three, a causal relationship with Ibuprofen has not been established. Reported side effects were higher at doses of 3200 mg/day than at doses of 2400 mg or less per day in clinical trials of adult patients with rheumatoid arthritis. The increases in incidence were slight and still within the ranges reported in the following table. (See related table).

OVERDOSAGE
Approximately 1 1/2 hours after the reported ingestion of from 7 to 10 Ibuprofen tablets (400 mg), a 19-month old child weighing 12 kg was seen in the hospital emergency room, apneic and cyanotic, responding only to painful stimuli. This type of stimulus, however, was sufficient to induce respiration. Oxygen and parenteral fluids were given; a greenish-yellow fluid was aspirated from the stomach with no evidence to indicate the presence of Ibuprofen. Two hours after ingestion the child's condition seemed stable; she still responded only to painful stimuli and continued to have periods of apnea lasting from 5 to 10 seconds. She was admitted to intensive care and sodium bicarbonate was administered as well as infusions of dextrose and normal saline. By four hours post-ingestion she could be aroused easily, sit by herself and respond to spoken commands. Blood level of Ibuprofen, was 102.9 μg/ml approximately 8 1/2 hours after accidental ingestion. At 12 hours she appeared to be completely recovered.

In two other reported cases where children (each weighing approximately 10 kg) accidentally, acutely ingested approximately 120 mg/kg, there were no signs of acute intoxication or late sequelae. Blood level in one child 90 minutes after ingestion was 700 μg/ml—about 10 times the peak levels seen in absorption-excretion studies.

A 19-year old male who had taken 8,000 mg of Ibuprofen over a period of a few hours complained of dizziness, and nystagmus was noted. After hospitalization, parenteral hydration and three days' bed rest, he recovered with no reported sequelae.

In cases of acute overdosage, the stomach should be emptied by vomiting or lavage, though little drug will likely be recovered if more than an hour has elapsed since ingestion. Because the drug is acidic and is excreted in the urine, it is theoretically beneficial to administer alkali and induce diuresis. In addition to supportive measures the use of oral activated charcoal may help to reduce the absorption and reabsorption of Ibuprofen.

DOSAGE AND ADMINISTRATION
Do not exceed 3200 mg total daily dose. If gastrointestinal complaints occur, administer Ibuprofen with meals or milk. Shake the suspension well prior to administration.

RHEUMATOID ARTHRITIS AND OSTEOARTHRITIS, INCLUDING FLARE-UPS OF CHRONIC DISEASE
Suggested Adult Dosage: 1200 mg-3200 mg daily (300 mg qid; 400 mg, 600 mg or 800 mg tid or qid). Individual patients may show a better response to 3200 mg daily, as compared with 2400 mg, although in well-controlled clinical trials patients on 3200 mg did not show a better mean response in terms of efficacy. Therefore, when treating patients with 3200 mg/day, the physician should observe sufficient increased clinical benefits to offset potential increased risk.

The dose should be tailored to each patient, and may be lowered or raised depending on the severity of symptoms either at the time of initiating drug therapy or as the patient responds or fails to respond.

In general, patients with rheumatoid arthritis seem to require higher doses of Ibuprofen than do patients with osteoarthritis.

The smallest dose of Ibuprofen that yields acceptable control should be employed. A linear blood level dose-response relationship exists with single doses up to 800 mg (see *"Clinical Pharmacology"* for effects of food on rate of absorption).

The availability of four tablet strengths facilitates dosage adjustment.

In chronic conditions, a therapeutic response to therapy with Ibuprofen is sometimes seen in a few days to a week but most often is observed by two weeks. After a satisfactory response has been achieved, the patient's dose should be reviewed and adjusted as required.

JUVENILE ARTHRITIS
The usual dose is 30 to 40mg/kg/day divided into 3 or 4 doses. Patients with milder disease may be adequately treated with 20mg/kg/day.

Doses above 50mg/kg/day are not recommended because they have not been studied and because side effects appear to be dose related.

Therapeutic response may require from a few days to several weeks to be achieved. Once a clinical response is obtained, dosage can be lowered to the smallest dose of Ibuprofen suspension needed to maintain adequate control of disease.

MILD TO MODERATE PAIN
400 mg every 4 to 6 hours as necessary for relief of pain in adults. In controlled analgesic clinical trials, doses of Ibuprofen greater than 400 mg were no more effective than the 400 mg dose.

➤ SHOWN IN PRODUCT IDENTIFICATION GUIDE

DYSMENORRHEA

For the treatment of dysmenorrhea, beginning with the earliest onset of such pain, Ibuprofen should be given in a dose of 400 mg every 4 hours as necessary for the relief of pain.

FEVER REDUCTION IN CHILDREN 6 MONTHS TO 12 YEARS OF AGE

Dosage should be adjusted on the basis of the initial temperature level (see "Clinical Pharmacology" for a description of the controlled clinical trial results). The recommended dose is 5mg/kg if the baseline temperature is 102.5°F or below or 10mg/kg if the baseline temperature is greater than 102.5°F. The duration of fever reduction is generally 6-8 hours and is longer with the higher dose. The recommended maximum daily dose is 40mg/kg.

Age	Weight (lb)	5mg/kg (Fever < 102.5°F) (mg)	(tsp)	10mg/kg (Fever > 102.5°F) (mg)	(tsp)
6-11 mos	13-17	25	1/4	50	1/2
12-23 mos	18-23	50	1/2	100	1
2-3 yrs	24-35	75	3/4	150	1 1/2
4-5 yrs	36-47	100	1	200	2
6-8 yrs	48-59	125	1 1/4	250	2 1/2
9-10 yrs	60-71	150	1 1/2	300	3
11-12 yrs	72-95	200	2	400	4

FEVER REDUCTION IN ADULTS

400mg every 4-6 hours as necessary.

STORAGE

Ibuprofen suspension should be stored at room temperature, 15°C to 30°C (59°F to 86°F).

Shake well before use, Keep container tightly closed.

HOW SUPPLIED

SUSPENSION: 100 MG/5 ML

BRAND/MANUFACTURER	NDC	SIZE	AWP
◇ **BRAND**			
MOTRIN CHILDREN'S: McNeil Cons	00045-0801-04	10 ml	$6.18
CHILDREN'S ADVIL: Wyeth-Ayerst	00008-0800-01	120 ml	$6.44
MOTRIN CHILDREN'S:	00045-0469-17	480 ml	$16.40
MOTRIN CHILDREN'S: McNeil Cons	00045-0801-16	480 ml	$20.66
CHILDREN'S ADVIL: Wyeth-Ayerst	00008-0800-03	480 ml	$21.53

TABLETS: 200 MG

BRAND/MANUFACTURER	NDC	SIZE	AWP
◆ **GENERICS**			
UDL	51079-0731-20	100s ud	$6.86

TABLETS: 300 MG

AVERAGE UNIT PRICE (AVAILABLE SIZES)		GENERIC A-RATED AVERAGE PRICE (GAAP)	
BRAND	$0.18	100s	$7.80
GENERIC	$0.07	500s	$29.30

BRAND/MANUFACTURER	NDC	SIZE	AWP
◆ **BRAND**			
MOTRIN: Upjohn	00009-0733-01	60s	$11.91
	00009-0733-02	500s	$76.05
◆ **GENERICS**			
Major	00904-1638-51	50s	$5.20
Major	00904-1638-60	100s	$6.00
URL	00677-1091-01	100s	$8.30
Mutual	53489-0130-01	100s	$8.30
U.S. Trading	56126-0161-11	100s ud	$8.58
U.S. Trading	56126-0161-05	500s	$13.50
Major	00904-1638-40	500s	$26.00
URL	00677-1091-05	500s	$35.50
Mutual	53489-0130-05	500s	$35.50
Goldline	00182-1770-05	500s	$36.00

IBUPROFEN

Incidence Greater than 1% (but less than 3%) Probable Causal Relationship	Precise Incidence Unknown (but less than 1%) Probable Causal Relationship**	Precise Incidence Unknown (but less than 1%) Causal Relationship Unknown**
Gastrointestinal		
Nausea*, epigastric pain*, heartburn*, diarrhea, abdominal distress, nausea and vomiting, indigestion, constipation, abdominal cramps or pain, fullness of GI tract (bloating and flatulence)	Gastric or duodenal ulcer with bleeding and/or perforation, gastrointestinal hemorrhage, melena, gastritis, hepatitis, jaundice, abnormal liver function tests; pancreatis	
Central Nervous System		
Dizziness*, headache, nervousness	Depression, insomnia, confusion, emotional lability, somnolence, aseptic meningitis with fever and coma	Paresthesias, hallucinations, dream abnormalities, pseudotumor cerebri
Dermatologic		
Rash* (including maculopapular type), pruritus	Vesiculobullous eruptions, urticaria, erythema multiforme, Stevens-Johnson syndrome, alopecia	Toxic epidermal necrolysis, photoallergic skin reactions
Special Senses		
Tinnitus	Hearing loss, amblyopia (blurred and/or diminished vision, scotomata and/or changes in color vision) (see "Precautions")	Conjunctivitis, diplopia, optic neuritis, cataracts
Hematologic		
	Neutropenia, agranulocytosis, aplastic anemia, hemolytic anemia (sometimes Coombs positive), thrombocytopenia with or without purpura, eosinophilia, decreases in hemoglobin and hematocrit (see "Precautions")	Bleeding episodes (e.g., epistaxis, menorrhagia)
Metabolic/Endocrine		
Decreased appetite		Gynecomastia, hypoglycemic reaction, acidosis
Cardiovascular		
Edema, fluid retention (generally responds promptly to drug discontinuation; see "Precautions")	Congestive heart failure in patients with marginal cardiac function, elevated blood pressure, palpitations	Arrhythmias (sinus tachycardia, sinus bradycardia)
Allergic		
	Syndrome of abdominal pain, fever, chills, nausea and vomiting; anaphylaxis; bronchospasm (see "Contraindications") in patients with pre-existing significantly impaired renal function	Serum sickness, lupus erythematosus syndrome, Henoch-Schönlein vasculitis, angioedema
Renal		
	Acute renal failure (see "Precautions"), decreased creatinine clearance, polyuria, azotemia, cystitis, hematuria	Renal papillary necrosis
Miscellaneous		
	Dry eyes and mouth, gingival ulcer, rhinitis	

* Reactions occurring in 3% to 9% of adult patients treated with Ibuprofen. (Those reactions occurring in less than 3% of the patients are unmarked).

** Reactions are classified under "Probable Causal Relationship (PCR)" if there has been one positive rechallenge or if three or more cases occur which might be causally related. Reactions are classified under "Causal Relationship Unknown" if seven or more events have been reported but the criteria for PCR have not been met.

◆ RATED THERAPEUTICALLY EQUIVALENT; ◇ THERAPEUTIC EQUIVALENCE UNCONFIRMED; ○ UNRATED

TABLETS: 400 MG

AVERAGE UNIT PRICE (AVAILABLE SIZES)		GENERIC A-RATED AVERAGE PRICE (GAAP)	
BRAND	$0.17	50s	$5.75
GENERIC	$0.13	60s	$34.23
HCFA FUL (100s ea)	$0.04	90s	$10.23
		100s	$13.33
		500s	$50.89
		1000s	$81.28

BRAND/MANUFACTURER	NDC	SIZE	AWP
◆ BRAND			
➤ MOTRIN: Upjohn	00009-0750-25	100s	$19.83
	00009-0750-06	100s ud	$21.55
	00009-0750-26	120s	$23.79
	00009-0750-02	500s	$82.20
	00009-0750-40	10000s	$803.45
◆ GENERICS			
Vangard	00615-2525-35	15s	$2.29
Vangard	00615-2525-19	20s	$2.45
Vangard	00615-2525-30	30s	$3.80
OHM	51660-0440-51	50s	$5.75
OHM	51660-0446-51	50s	$5.75
Vangard	00615-2525-06	60s	$8.45
UDL	51079-0281-98	60s	$60.00
Vangard	00615-2525-90	90s	$10.09
Allscrips	54569-3820-00	90s	$10.37
Medirex	57480-0336-06	100s	$6.63
Interpharm	53746-0131-01	100s	$8.77
OHM	51660-0440-01	100s	$9.90
OHM	51660-0446-01	100s	$9.90
Sidmak	50111-0387-01	100s	$10.01
Warner Chilcott	00047-0516-24	100s	$10.47
Lemmon	00093-0491-01	100s	$10.50
Qualitest	00603-4018-21	100s	$10.90
Goldline	00182-1809-01	100s	$11.00
Norton,HN	50732-0744-01	100s	$11.00
Caremark	00339-5915-12	100s	$11.30
Geneva	00781-1352-01	100s	$11.52
URL	00677-1031-01	100s	$11.60
Major	00904-1648-60	100s	$11.60
Major	00904-1748-60	100s	$11.60
Mutual	53489-0131-01	100s	$11.60
Purepac	00228-2124-10	100s	$11.69
➤ Rugby	00536-4604-01	100s	$11.94
Schein	00364-0765-01	100s	$12.00
Winsor	59004-0140-50	100s	$12.00
Invamed	52189-0223-24	100s	$12.12
IBU: Boots Labs	00524-0165-01	100s	$12.35
Aligen	00405-4527-01	100s	$12.38
➤ Par	49884-0162-01	100s	$12.39
Moore,H.L.	00839-7112-06	100s	$12.96
IBU-TAB: Alra	51641-0214-01	100s	$15.41
Vangard	00615-2525-01	100s	$15.41
Parmed	00349-8282-01	100s	$15.95
➤ RUFEN: Boots Pharm	00048-0039-01	100s	$18.40
U.S. Trading	56126-0162-11	100s ud	$4.67
Raway	00686-0281-20	100s ud	$8.00
Schein	00364-0765-90	100s ud	$15.05
Winsor	59004-0140-55	100s ud	$16.00
Major	00904-1748-61	100s ud	$16.01
Goldline	00182-1809-89	100s ud	$16.05
West-Ward	00143-1300-25	100s ud	$17.00
Auro	55829-0312-10	100s ud	$17.43
Vangard	00615-2525-13	100s ud	$17.88
UDL	51079-0281-20	100s ud	$22.10
Medirex	57480-0336-01	100s ud	$22.10
IBU-TAB: Alra	51641-0214-11	100s ud	$33.29
Vangard	00615-2525-12	120s	$9.04
Schein	00364-0765-05	500s	$37.25
Warner Chilcott	00047-0516-30	500s	$41.04
OHM	51660-0440-05	500s	$44.00
OHM	51660-0446-05	500s	$44.00
Mason Dist	11845-0116-03	500s	$45.72
Lemmon	00093-0491-05	500s	$46.90
Geneva	00781-1352-05	500s	$46.90
Interpharm	53746-0131-05	500s	$47.00
Purepac	00228-2124-50	500s	$47.86
Qualitest	00603-4018-28	500s	$48.05
Goldline	00182-1809-05	500s	$48.20
Major	00904-1648-40	500s	$48.70
Major	00904-1748-40	500s	$48.70
Martec	52555-0162-05	500s	$48.90
Winsor	59004-0140-80	500s	$49.00
IBU: Boots Labs	00524-0165-05	500s	$49.35
Aligen	00405-4527-02	500s	$49.42
Sidmak	50111-0387-05	500s	$49.50
IBU-TAB: Alra	51641-0214-05	500s	$49.59
Norton,HN	50732-0744-05	500s	$49.95
Invamed	52189-0223-29	500s	$50.26
URL	00677-1031-05	500s	$50.50
Mutual	53489-0131-05	500s	$50.50
Goldline	00182-1771-05	500s	$52.50
Vangard	00615-2525-05	500s	$53.37
➤ Rugby	00536-4604-05	500s	$53.95
Parmed	00349-8282-05	500s	$54.25

BRAND/MANUFACTURER	NDC	SIZE	AWP
Mylan	00378-1401-05	500s	$54.74
Moore,H.L.	00839-7699-12	500s	$54.74
➤ Par	49884-0162-05	500s	$58.00
Moore,H.L.	00839-7112-12	500s	$60.89
DOLGESIC: Marlop	12939-0814-05	500s	$64.55
➤ RUFEN: Boots Pharm	00048-0039-05	500s	$81.20
OHM	51660-0440-10	1000s	$73.90
OHM	51660-0446-10	1000s	$73.90
IBU-TAB: Alra	51641-0214-10	1000s	$96.03

TABLETS: 600 MG

AVERAGE UNIT PRICE (AVAILABLE SIZES)		GENERIC A-RATED AVERAGE PRICE (GAAP)	
BRAND	$0.25	30s	$5.90
GENERIC	$0.18	60s	$32.30
HCFA FUL (100s ea)	$0.05	100s	$18.91
		500s	$71.12
		1000s	$128.65

BRAND/MANUFACTURER	NDC	SIZE	AWP
◆ BRAND			
➤ MOTRIN: Upjohn	00009-0742-08	90s	$25.33
	00009-0742-03	100s	$28.11
	00009-0742-09	100s ud	$31.49
	00009-0742-02	500s	$116.39
	00009-0742-25	8000s	$1030.50
◆ GENERICS			
Major	00904-1758-46	30s	$2.95
Medirex	57480-0337-06	30s	$8.85
Major	00904-1758-52	60s	$4.60
UDL	51079-0282-98	60s	$60.00
Vangard	00615-2526-90	90s	$9.71
Warner Chilcott	00047-0922-24	100s	$13.56
Lemmon	00093-0492-01	100s	$13.95
Interpharm	53746-0132-01	100s	$14.50
Norton,HN	50732-0747-01	100s	$14.75
Qualitest	00603-4019-21	100s	$14.80
Goldline	00182-1810-01	100s	$15.00
Mutual	53489-0132-01	100s	$15.10
Sidmak	50111-0388-01	100s	$15.13
Martec	52555-0163-01	100s	$15.58
Caremark	00339-5917-12	100s	$15.60
Purepac	00228-2125-10	100s	$15.61
Winsor	59004-0160-50	100s	$16.50
IBU: Boots Labs	00524-0162-01	100s	$16.70
➤ Par	49884-0163-01	100s	$16.75
Rugby	00536-4605-01	100s	$16.75
Major	00904-1658-60	100s	$16.75
Major	00904-1758-60	100s	$16.75
Aligen	00405-4528-01	100s	$16.83
URL	00677-1032-01	100s	$16.85
Schein	00364-0766-01	100s	$16.85
Geneva	00781-1362-01	100s	$16.85
Invamed	52189-0224-24	100s	$17.19
Moore,H.L.	00839-7113-06	100s	$17.55
IBU-TAB: Alra	51641-0213-01	100s	$18.50
Vangard	00615-2526-01	100s	$22.05
Parmed	00349-8425-01	100s	$24.25
➤ RUFEN: Boots Pharm	00048-0062-01	100s	$25.65
U.S. Trading	56126-0163-11	100s ud	$6.08
Raway	00686-0282-20	100s ud	$10.00
Schein	00364-0766-90	100s ud	$22.00
Winsor	59004-0160-55	100s ud	$22.00
Major	00904-1758-61	100s ud	$23.38
Auro	55829-0313-10	100s ud	$23.91
Goldline	00182-1810-89	100s ud	$24.70
Vangard	00615-2526-13	100s ud	$24.94
West-Ward	00143-1302-25	100s ud	$25.00
Medirex	57480-0337-01	100s ud	$29.50
UDL	51079-0282-20	100s ud	$29.60
IBU-TAB: Alra	51641-0213-11	100s ud	$40.00
Major	00904-1758-18	120s	$7.70
Schein	00364-0766-05	500s	$41.15
Warner Chilcott	00047-0922-30	500s	$56.06
Mason Dist	11845-0117-03	500s	$65.25
Purepac	00228-2125-50	500s	$65.32
Lemmon	00093-0492-05	500s	$65.65
Norton,HN	50732-0747-05	500s	$65.95
Qualitest	00603-4019-28	500s	$67.91
Interpharm	53746-0132-05	500s	$68.35
Vangard	00615-2526-05	500s	$68.51
Rugby	00536-4605-05	500s	$68.69
Geneva	00781-1362-05	500s	$68.69
Major	00904-1658-40	500s	$68.75
Major	00904-1758-40	500s	$68.75
Goldline	00182-1810-05	500s	$68.75
URL	00677-1032-05	500s	$68.90
Martec	52555-0163-05	500s	$68.90
Mutual	53489-0132-05	500s	$68.90
Sidmak	50111-0388-02	500s	$68.97
Invamed	52189-0224-29	500s	$71.16
Winsor	59004-0160-80	500s	$72.00
IBU: Boots Labs	00524-0162-05	500s	$72.15

BRAND/MANUFACTURER	NDC	SIZE	AWP
Aligen	00405-4528-02	500s	$72.20
IBU-TAB: Alra	51641-0213-05	500s	$72.26
Moore,H.L.	00839-7700-12	500s	$75.05
Mylan	00378-1601-05	500s	$79.35
Parmed	00349-8425-05	500s	$79.35
➤ Par	49884-0163-05	500s	$83.75
Moore,H.L.	00839-7113-12	500s	$87.95
➤ RUFEN: Boots Pharm	00048-0062-05	500s	$113.70
Parmed	00349-8425-10	1000s	$120.00
IBU-TAB: Alra	51641-0213-10	1000s	$137.29

TABLETS: 800 MG

AVERAGE UNIT PRICE (AVAILABLE SIZES)		GENERIC A-RATED AVERAGE PRICE (GAAP)	
BRAND	$0.32	30s	$6.72
GENERIC	$0.24	90s	$10.62
HCFA FUL (100s ea)	$0.07	100s	$24.57
		500s	$105.17
		1000s	$190.93

BRAND/MANUFACTURER	NDC	SIZE	AWP
◆ BRAND			
➤ MOTRIN: Upjohn	00009-0725-08	90s	$33.23
	00009-0725-01	100s	$36.90
	00009-0725-02	100s ud	$39.89
	00009-0725-03	500s	$147.61
	00009-0725-13	8000s	$1396.66
◆ GENERICS			
Major	00904-1760-46	30s	$3.95
Medirex	57480-0338-06	30s	$9.49
UDL	51079-0596-98	60s ud	$60.00
Major	00904-1760-89	90s	$9.20
Vangard	00615-2528-90	90s	$12.04
Vangard	00615-2528-01	100s	$14.67
Warner Chilcott	00047-0914-24	100s	$19.33
Lemmon	00093-0498-01	100s	$20.63
Sidmak	50111-0451-01	100s	$21.45
Caremark	00339-5919-12	100s	$21.73
➤ Schein	00364-2137-01	100s	$21.75
➤ Rugby	00536-4606-01	100s	$21.88
Qualitest	00603-4020-21	100s	$21.90
Major	00904-1760-60	100s	$21.95
Goldline	00182-1297-01	100s	$21.95
Purepac	00228-2111-10	100s	$22.07
IBU-TAB: Alra	51641-0212-01	100s	$22.51
Invamed	52189-0225-24	100s	$22.57
Geneva	00781-1363-01	100s	$23.00
Winsor	59004-0180-50	100s	$23.00
Norton,HN	50732-0781-01	100s	$23.00
IBU: Boots Labs	00524-0173-01	100s	$23.05
Aligen	00405-4529-01	100s	$23.18
URL	00677-1119-01	100s	$23.25
Mutual	53489-0137-01	100s	$23.25
Par	49884-0216-01	100s	$23.89
Parmed	00349-8609-01	100s	$24.95
Interpharm	53746-0137-01	100s	$25.00
Moore,H.L.	00839-7236-06	100s	$25.04
➤ RUFEN: Boots Pharm	00048-0073-01	100s	$34.40
U.S. Trading	56126-0359-11	100s ud	$8.79
Winsor	59004-0180-55	100s ud	$27.00
Goldline	00182-1297-89	100s ud	$27.75
Auro	55829-0314-10	100s ud	$27.77
➤ Schein	00364-2137-90	100s ud	$27.85
Vangard	00615-2528-13	100s ud	$29.52
West-Ward	00143-1304-25	100s ud	$30.00
Medirex	57480-0338-01	100s ud	$31.50
UDL	51079-0596-20	100s ud	$31.60
IBU-TAB: Alra	51641-0021-11	100s ud	$48.78
Warner Chilcott	00047-0914-30	500s	$83.13
Invamed	52189-0225-29	500s	$90.25
Purepac	00228-2111-50	500s	$91.57
Moore,H.L.	00839-7239-12	500s	$96.24
Mason Dist	11845-0118-03	500s	$99.64
Sidmak	50111-0451-05	500s	$101.75
Martec	52555-0216-05	500s	$102.75
Lemmon	00093-0498-05	500s	$103.15
Geneva	00781-1363-05	500s	$103.15
Qualitest	00603-4020-28	500s	$103.15
URL	00677-1119-05	500s	$104.00
Mutual	53489-0137-05	500s	$104.00
Winsor	59004-0180-80	500s	$104.00
IBU: Boots Labs	00524-0173-05	500s	$104.10
Aligen	00405-4529-05	500s	$104.20
➤ Rugby	00536-4606-05	500s	$104.88
Major	00904-1760-40	500s	$104.90
➤ Schein	00364-2137-05	500s	$104.95
Goldline	00182-1297-05	500s	$104.95
Interpharm	53746-0137-05	500s	$105.00
IBU-TAB: Alra	51641-0021-05	500s	$105.04
Norton,HN	50732-0781-05	500s	$108.00
Parmed	00349-8609-05	500s	$110.00
Mylan	00378-1801-05	500s	$114.50
Par	49884-0216-05	500s	$119.45
Moore,H.L.	00839-7236-12	500s	$125.42

BRAND/MANUFACTURER	NDC	SIZE	AWP
➤ RUFEN: Boots Pharm	00048-0073-05	500s	$137.30
Parmed	00349-8609-10	1000s	$181.90
IBU-TAB: Alra	51641-0212-10	1000s	$199.95

Idamycin SEE IDARUBICIN HYDROCHLORIDE

Idarubicin Hydrochloride

WARNINGS

1. IDARUBICIN HYDROCHLORIDE SHOULD BE GIVEN SLOWLY INTO A FREELY FLOWING INTRAVENOUS INFUSION. IT MUST *NEVER* BE GIVEN INTRAMUSCULARLY OR SUBCUTANEOUSLY. SEVERE LOCAL TISSUE NECROSIS CAN OCCUR IF THERE IS EXTRAVASATION DURING ADMINISTRATION.

2. AS IN THE CASE WITH OTHER ANTHRACYCLINES THE USE OF IDARUBICIN HYDROCHLORIDE CAN CAUSE MYOCARDIAL TOXICITY LEADING TO CONGESTIVE HEART FAILURE. CARDIAC TOXICITY IS MORE COMMON IN PATIENTS WHO HAVE RECEIVED PRIOR ANTHRACYCLINES OR WHO HAVE PRE-EXISTING CARDIAC DISEASE.

3. AS IS USUAL WITH ANTILEUKEMIC AGENTS, SEVERE MYELO-SUPPRESSION OCCURS WHEN IDARUBICIN HYDROCHLORIDE IS USED AT EFFECTIVE THERAPEUTIC DOSES.

4. IT IS RECOMMENDED THAT IDARUBICIN HYDROCHLORIDE BE ADMINISTERED ONLY UNDER THE SUPERVISION OF A PHYSICIAN WHO IS EXPERIENCED IN LEUKEMIA CHEMOTHERAPY AND IN FACILITIES WITH LABORATORY AND SUPPORTIVE RESOURCES ADEQUATE TO MONITOR DRUG TOLERANCE AND PROTECT AND MAINTAIN A PATIENT COMPROMISED BY DRUG TOXICITY. THE PHYSICIAN AND INSTITUTION MUST BE CAPABLE OF RESPONDING RAPIDLY AND COMPLETELY TO SEVERE HEMORRHAGIC CONDITIONS AND/OR OVERWHELMING INFECTION.

5. DOSAGE SHOULD BE REDUCED IN PATIENTS WITH IMPAIRED HEPATIC OR RENAL FUNCTION. (SEE "DOSAGE AND ADMINISTRATION".)

DESCRIPTION

Idarubicin Hydrochloride is a sterile, synthetic antineoplastic anthracycline for intravenous use. Chemically, Idarubicin Hydrochloride is 5,12-Naphthacene-dione, 9-acetyl-7-[(3-amino-2,3,6-trideoxy -α-L-*lyxo*-hexopyranosyl)oxy]-7,8,9,10-tetrahydro-6,9,11-trihydroxy-hydrochlo- ride,(7S-*cis*). Its molecular formula is $C_{26}H_{27}NO_9 \cdot HCl$ and molecular weight is 533.96.

Idarubicin Hydrochloride, a sterile parenteral, is available in 5 mg and 10 mg single use only vials.

Each 5 mg vial contains 5 mg Idarubicin Hydrochloride and 50 mg of Lactose NF(hydrous) as an orange-red, lyophilized powder.

Each 10 mg vial contains 10 mg Idarubicin Hydrochloride and 100 mg of Lactose NF(hydrous) as an orange-red, lyophilized powder.

Following is its chemical structure:

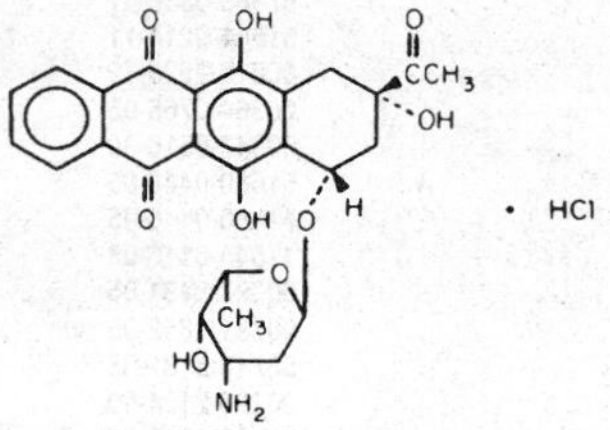

CLINICAL PHARMACOLOGY

Idarubicin Hydrochloride is a DNA-intercalating analog of daunorubicin which has an inhibitory effect on nucleic acid synthesis and interacts with the enzyme topoisomerase II. The absence of a methoxy group at position 4 of the anthracycline structure gives the compound a high lipophilicity which results in an increased rate of cellular uptake compared with other anthracyclines.

Pharmacokinetic studies have been performed in adult leukemia patients with normal renal and hepatic function following intravenous administration of 10-12 mg/m^2 of Idarubicin Hydrochloride daily for 3 to 4 days, as a single agent or combined with cytarabine (Ara-C). The plasma concentrations of Idarubicin Hydrochloride are best described by a two or three compartment open model. The disposition profile shows a rapid distributive phase with a very high volume of distribution presumably reflecting extensive issue binding. The plasma clearance is twice the expected hepatic plasma flow indicating extensive extrahepatic metabolism. The drug is eliminated predominately by biliary and to a lesser

---

◆ RATED THERAPEUTICALLY EQUIVALENT; ◇ THERAPEUTIC EQUIVALENCE UNCONFIRMED; ○ UNRATED

extent by renal excretion, mostly in the form of the primary metabolite, 13-dihydroidarubicin (idarubicinol).

The elimination rate of Idarubicin Hydrochloride from plasma is slow with an estimated mean terminal half-life of 22 hours (range: 4 to 46 hours) when used as a single agent and 20 hours (range: 7 to 38 hours) when used in combination with cytarabine. The elimination of idarubicinol is considerably slower than that of the parent drug, with an estimated mean terminal half-life that exceeds 45 hours; hence its plasma levels are sustained for a period greater than 8 days. As Idarubicinol has cytotoxic activity it presumably contributes to the effects of Idarubicin Hydrochloride.

The extent of drug and metabolite accumulation predicted in leukemia patients for Day 2 and 3 of dosing, based on the mean plasma levels and half-life obtained after the first dose, is 1.7-and 2.3-fold, respectively, and suggests no change in kinetics following a daily $\times$ 3 regimen.

The pharmacokinetics of Idarubicin Hydrochloride have not been evaluated in leukemia patients with hepatic impairment. It is expected that in patients with moderate or severe hepatic dysfunction, the metabolism of Idarubicin Hydrochloride may be impaired and lead to higher systemic drug levels.

Studies of cellular (nucleated blood and bone marrow cells) drug concentrations in leukemia patients have shown that peak cellular Idarubicin Hydrochloride concentrations are reached a few minutes after injection Idarubicin Hydrochloride and Idarubicinol concentrations in nucleated blood and bone marrow cells are more than a hundred times the plasma concentrations. Idarubicin Hydrochloride disappearance rates in plasma and cells were comparable with a terminal half-life of about 15 hours. The terminal half-life of Idarubicinol in cells was about 72 hours.

Protein binding was studied *in vitro* by equilibrium dialysis at concentrations of Idarubicin Hydrochloride and Idarubicinol similar to the maximum plasma level obtained in the pharmacokinetic studies. The percentages of Idarubicin Hydrochloride and idarubicinol bound to human plasma proteins averaged 97% and 94%, respectively. The binding is concentration independent.

Idarubicin Hydrochloride studies in pediatric leukemia patients, at doses of 4.2 to 13.3 mg/m^2/day $\times$ 3, suggest dose independent kinetics. There is no difference between the half-lives of the drug following daily $\times$ 3 or weekly $\times$ 3 administration.

Cerebrospinal fluid (CSF) levels of Idarubicin Hydrochloride and its active metabolite, idarubicinol, were measured in pediatric leukemia patients treated intravenously. Idarubicin was detected in 2 of 21 CSF samples (0.14 and 1.57 ng/mL), while idarubicinol was detected in 20 of these 21 CSF samples obtained 18-30 hours after dosing (mean = 0.51 ng/mL, range 0.22 − 1.05 ng/mL). The clinical relevance of these findings is currently being evaluated.

CLINICAL STUDIES

Four prospective randomized studies, three U.S. and one Italian, have been conducted to compare the efficacy and safety of Idarubicin Hydrochloride (IDR) to that of daunorubicin (DNR), each in combination with cytarabine (Ara-C) as induction therapy in previously untreated adult patients with acute myeloid leukemia (AML). These data are summarized in the following table and demonstrate significantly greater complete remission rates for the IDR regimen in two of the three U.S. studies and significantly longer overall survival for the IDR regimen in two of the three U.S. studies. (See related table).

There is no consensus regarding optional regimens to be used for consolidation; however, the following consolidation regimens were used in U.S. controlled trials. Patients received the same anthracycline for consolidation as was used for induction.

Studies 1 and 3 utilized 2 courses of consolidation therapy consisting of Idarubicin Hydrochloride 12 or 13 mg/m^2 daily for 2 days, respectively (or DNR 50 or 45 mg/m^2 daily for 2 days), and Ara-C, either 25 mg/m^2 daily by IV bolus followed by 200 mg/m^2 daily by continuous infusion for 4 days (Study 1), or 100 mg/m^2 daily for 5 days by continuous infusion (Study 3). A rest period of 4 to 6 weeks is recommended prior to initiation of consolidation and between the courses. Hematologic recovery is mandatory prior to initiation of each consolidation course.

Study 2 utilized 3 consolidation courses, administered at intervals of 21 days or upon hematologic recovery. Each course consisted of Idarubicin Hydrochloride 15 mg/m^2 IV for 1 dose (or DNR 50 mg/m^2 IV for 1 dose), Ara-C 100 mg/m^2 every 12 hours for 10 doses and 6-thioguanine 100 mg/m^2 po for 10 doses. If severe myelosuppression occurred, subsequent courses were given with 25% reduction in the doses of all drugs. In addition, this study included 4 courses of maintenance therapy (2 days of the same anthracycline as was used in induction and 5 days of Ara-C).

Toxicities and duration of aplasia were similar during induction on the 2 arms in the U.S. studies except for an increase in mucositis on the IDR arm in one study. During consolidation, duration of aplasia on the IDR arm was longer in all three studies and mucositis was more frequent in two studies. During consolidation, transfusion requirements were higher on the IDR arm in the two studies in which they were tabulated, and patients on the IDR arm in Study 3 spent more days on IV antibiotics (Study 3 used a higher dose of Idarubicin Hydrochloride).

The benefit of consolidation and maintenance therapy in prolonging the duration of remission and survival is not proven.

Intensive maintenance with Idarubicin Hydrochloride is not recommended in view of the considerable toxicity (including deaths in remission) experienced by patients during the maintenance phase of Study 2.

A higher induction death rate was noted in patients on the IDR arm in the Italian trial. Since this was not noted in patients of similar age in the U.S. trials, one may speculate that it was due to a difference in the level of supportive care.

INDICATIONS AND USAGE

Idarubicin Hydrochloride in combination with other approved antileukemic drugs is indicated for the treatment of acute myeloid leukemia (AML) in adults. This includes French-American-British (FAB) classifications M1 through M7.

UNLABELED USES

Idarubicin Hydrochloride is used alone or as an adjunct in the treatment of breast cancer.

WARNINGS

Idarubicin Hydrochloride is intended for administration under the supervision of a physician who is experienced in leukemia chemotherapy.

Idarubicin Hydrochloride is a potent bone marrow suppressant. Idarubicin Hydrochloride should not be given to patients with pre-existing bone marrow suppression induced by previous drug therapy or radiotherapy unless the benefit warrants the risk.

Severe myelosuppression will occur in all patients given a therapeutic dose of this agent for induction, consolidation or maintenance. Careful hematologic monitoring is required. Deaths due to infection and/or bleeding have been reported during the period of severe myelosuppression. Facilities with laboratory and supportive resources adequate to monitor drug tolerability and protect and maintain a patient compromised by drug toxicity should be available. It must be possible to treat rapidly and completely a severe hemorrhagic condition and/or a severe infection.

	Induction[a] Regimen Dose in mg/m^2- Daily $\times$ 3 Days		Complete Remission Rate, All Pts Randomized		Median Survival (Days) All Pts Randomized	
	IDR	DNR	IDR	DNR	IDR	DNR
U.S. (IND Studies)						
1. MSKCC* (Age $\leq$ 60 years)	12[b]	50[b]	51/65+ (78%)	38/65 (58%)	508+	435
2. SEG** (Age $\geq$ 15 years)	12[c]	45[c]	76/111+ (69%)	65/119 (55%)	328	277
3. U.S. Multicenter (Age $\geq$ 18 years)	13[c]	45[c]	68/101 (67%)	66/113 (58%)	393+	281
Foreign (non-IND study) GIMEMA*** (Age $\geq$ 55 years)	12[c]	45[c]	49/124 (40%)	49/125 (39%)	87	169

* Memorial Sloan Kettering Cancer Center
** Southeastern Cancer Study Group
*** Gruppo Italiano Malattie Ematologiche Maligne dell' Adulto
+ *Overall p < 0.05, unadjusted for prognostic factors or multiple endpoints.*
[a] *Patients who had persistent leukemia after the first induction course received a second course.*
[b] *Ara-C 25 mg/m^2 bolus IV followed by 200 mg/m^2 daily $\times$ 5 days by continuous infusion.*
[c] *Ara-C 100 mg/m^2 daily $\times$ 7 days by continuous infusion.*

Pre-existing heart disease and previous therapy with anthracyclines at high cumulative doses or other potentially cardiotoxic agents are co-factors for increased risk of Idarubicin Hydrochloride-induced cardiac toxicity and the benefit to risk ratio of Idarubicin Hydrochloride therapy in such patients should be weighed before starting treatment with Idarubicin Hydrochloride.

Myocardial toxicity as manifested by potentially fatal congestive heart failure, acute life-threatening arrhythmias or other cardiomyopathies may occur following therapy with Idarubicin Hydrochloride. Appropriate therapeutic measures for the management of congestive heart failure and/or arrhythmias are indicated.

Cardiac function should be carefully monitored during treatment in order to minimize the risk of cardiac toxicity of the type described for other anthracycline compounds. The risk of such myocardial toxicity may be higher following concomitant or previous radiation to the mediastinal-pericardial area or in patients with anemia, bone marrow depression, infections, leukemic pericarditis and/or myocarditis. While there are no reliable means for predicting congestive heart failure, cardiomyopathy induced by anthracyclines is usually associated with a decrease of the left ventricular ejection fraction (LVEF) from pretreatment baseline values.

Since hepatic and/or renal function impairment can affect the disposition of Idarubicin Hydrochloride, liver and kidney function should be evaluated with conventional clinical laboratory tests (using serum bilirubin and serum creatinine as indicators) prior to and during treatment. In a number of Phase III clinical trials, treatment was not given if bilirubin and/or creatinine serum levels exceeded 2 mg%. However, in one Phase III trial, patients with bilirubin levels between 2.6 and 5 mg% received the anthracycline with a 50% reduction in dose. Dose reduction of Idarubicin Hydrochloride should be considered if the bilirubin and/or creatinine levels are above normal range (see *"Dosage and Administration"*).

Pregnancy Category D: Idarubicin Hydrochloride was embryotoxic and teratogenic in the rat at a dose of 1.2 mg/m^2/day or one tenth the human dose, which was nontoxic to dams. Idarubicin Hydrochloride was embryotoxic but not teratogenic in the rabbit even at a dose of 2.4 mg/m^2/day or two tenths the human dose, which was toxic to dams. There is no conclusive information about Idarubicin Hydrochloride adversely affecting human fertility or causing teratogenesis.

There are no adequate and well-controlled studies in pregnant women. If Idarubicin Hydrochloride is to be used during pregnancy, or if the patient becomes pregnant during therapy, the patient should be apprised of the potential hazard to the fetus. Women of childbearing potential should be advised to avoid pregnancy.

PRECAUTIONS

GENERAL
Therapy with Idarubicin Hydrochloride requires close observation of the patient and careful laboratory monitoring. Hyperuricemia secondary to rapid lysis of leukemic cells may be induced. Appropriate measures must be taken to prevent hyperuricemia and to control any systemic infection before beginning therapy.

Extravasation of Idarubicin Hydrochloride can cause severe local tissue necrosis. Extravasation may occur with or without an accompanying stinging or burning sensation even if blood returns well on aspiration of the infusion needle. If signs or symptoms of extravasation occur the injection or infusion should be terminated immediately and restarted in another vein. (See *"Dosage and Administration"*).

LABORATORY TESTS
Frequent complete blood counts and monitoring of hepatic and renal function tests are recommended.

CARCINOGENESIS, MUTAGENESIS, IMPAIRMENT OF FERTILITY
Formal long-term carcinogenicity studies have not been conducted with Idarubicin Hydrochloride. Idarubicin Hydrochloride and related compounds have been shown to have mutagenic and carcinogenic properties when tested in experimental models (including bacterial systems, mammalian cells in culture and female Sprague-Dawley rats).

In male dogs given 1.8 mg/m^2/day or more Idarubicin (3 times/wk for 13 weeks), testicular atrophy was observed with inhibition of spermiogenesis and sperm maturation, and few or no mature sperm. Effects were not readily reversible after an eight week recovery period.

PREGNANCY
Category I: (See *"Warnings"*.)

NURSING MOTHERS
It is not known whether this drug is excreted in human milk. Because many drugs are excreted in human milk and because of the potential for serious adverse reactions in nursing infants from Idarubicin Hydrochloride, mothers should discontinue nursing prior to taking this drug.

PEDIATRIC USE
Safety and effectiveness in children have not been established.

ADVERSE REACTIONS
Approximately 550 patients with AML have received Idarubicin Hydrochloride in combination with Ara-C in controlled clinical trials worldwide. In addition, over 550 patients with acute leukemia have been treated in uncontrolled trials utilizing Idarubicin Hydrochloride as a single agent or in combination. The table below lists the adverse experiences reported in U.S. Study 2 (see *"Clinical Studies"*) and is representative of the experience in other studies. These adverse experiences constitute all reported or observed experiences, including those not considered to be drug related. Patients undergoing induction therapy for AML are seriously ill due to their disease, are receiving multiple transfusions, and concomitant medications including potentially toxic antibiotics and antifungal agents. The contribution of the study drug to the adverse experience profile is difficult to establish.

Induction Phase	Percentage of Patients	
Adverse Experiences	IDR (N = 110)	DNR (N = 118)
Infection	95%	97%
Nausea & Vomiting	82%	80%
Hair Loss	77%	72%
Abdominal Cramps/Diarrhea	73%	68%
Hemorrhage	63%	65%
Mucositis	50%	55%
Dermatologic	46%	40%
Mental Status	41%	34%
Pulmonary-Clinical	39%	39%
Fever (not elsewhere classified)	26%	28%
Headache	20%	24%
Cardiac-Clinical	16%	24%
Neurologic-Peripheral Nerves	7%	9%
Pulmonary Allergy	2%	5%
Seizure	4%	5%
Cerebellar	4%	4%

The duration of aplasia and incidence of mucositis were greater on the IDR arm than the DNR arm, especially during consolidation in some U.S. controlled trials (see *"Clinical Studies"*).

The following information reflects experience based on U.S. controlled clinical trials.

MYELOSUPPRESSION
Severe myelosuppression is the major toxicity associated with Idarubicin Hydrochloride therapy, but this effect of the drug is required in order to eradicate the leukemic clone. During the period of myelosuppression, patients are at risk of developing infection and bleeding which may be life-threatening or fatal.

GASTROINTESTINAL
Nausea and/or vomiting, mucositis, abdominal pain and diarrhea were reported frequently, but were severe (equivalent to WHO Grade 4) in less than 5% of patients. Severe enterocolitis with perforation has been reported rarely. The risk of perforation may be increased by instrumental intervention. The possibility of perforation should be considered in patients who develop severe abdominal pain and appropriate steps for diagnosis and management should be taken.

DERMATOLOGIC
Alopecia was reported frequently and dermatologic reactions including generalized rash, urticaria and a bullous erythrodermatous rash of the palms and soles have occurred. The dermatologic reactions were usually attributed to concomitant antibiotic therapy. Local reactions including hives at the injection site have been reported.

HEPATIC AND RENAL
Changes in hepatic and renal function tests have been observed. These changes were usually transient and occurred in the setting of sepsis and while patients were receiving potentially hepatotoxic and nephrotoxic antibiotics and antifungal agents. Severe changes in renal function (equivalent to WHO Grade 4) occurred in no more than 1% of patients, while severe changes in hepatic function (equivalent to WHO Grade 4) occurred in less than 5% of patients.

CARDIAC
Congestive heart failure (frequently attributed to fluid overload), serious arrhythmias including atrial fibrillation, chest pain, myocardial infarction and asymptomatic declines in LVEF have been reported in patients undergoing induction therapy for AML. Myocardial insufficiency and arrhythmias were usually reversible and occurred in the setting of sepsis, anemia and aggressive intravenous fluid administration. The events were reported more frequently in patients over age 60 years and in those with pe-existing cardiac disease.

OVERDOSAGE
There is no known antidote to Idarubicin Hydrochloride. Two cases of fatal overdosage in patients receiving therapy for AML have been reported. The doses were 135 mg/m^2 over 3 days and 45 mg/m^2 of Idarubicin Hydrochloride and 90 mg/m^2 of daunorubicin over a three day period.

It is anticipated that overdosage with Idarubicin Hydrochloride will result in severe and prolonged myelosuppression and possibly in increased severity of gastrointestinal toxicity. Adequate supportive care including platelet transfusions, antibiotics and symptomatic treatment of mucositis is required. The effect of acute overdose on cardiac function is not fully known, but severe arrhythmia occurred in 1 of the 2 patients exposed. It is anticipated that very high doses of Idarubicin Hydrochloride may cause acute cardiac toxicity and may be associated with a higher incidence of delayed cardiac failure.

Disposition studies with Idarubicin Hydrochloride in patients undergoing dialysis have not been carried out. The profound multicompartment behavior, extensive extravascular distribution and tissue binding, coupled with the low

---

unbound fraction available in the plasma pool make it unlikely that therapeutic efficacy or toxicity would be altered by conventional peritoneal or hemodialysis.

DOSAGE AND ADMINISTRATION
(See "Warnings.")

For induction therapy in adult patients with AML the following dose schedule is recommended:

Idarubicin Hydrochloride 12 mg/m^2 daily for 3 days by slow (10 to 15 min) intravenous injection in combination with Ara-C. The Ara-C may be given as 100 mg/m^2 daily by continuous infusion for 7 days or as Ara-C 25 mg/m^2 intravenous bolus followed by Ara-C 200 mg/m^2 daily for 5 days continuous infusion. In patients with unequivocal evidence of leukemia after the first induction course, a second course may be administered. Administration of the second course should be delayed in patients who experience severe mucositis, until recovery from this toxicity has occurred, and a dose reduction of 25% is recommended. In patients with hepatic and/or renal impairment, a dose reduction of Idarubicin Hydrochloride should be considered. Idarubicin Hydrochloride should not be administered if the bilirubin level exceeds 5 mg%. (See "Warnings").

The benefit of consolidation in prolonging the duration of remissions and survival is not proven. There is no consensus regarding optional regimens to be used for consolidation. (See "Clinical Studies" for doses used in U.S. clinical studies).

PREPARATION OF SOLUTION
Caution in handling of the powder and preparation of the solution must be exercised as skin reactions associated with Idarubicin Hydrochloride should be washed thoroughly with soap and water, and if the eyes are involved, standard irrigation techniques should be used immediately. The use of goggles, gloves, and protective gowns is recommended during preparation and administration of the drug.

Idarubicin Hydrochloride 5 mg and 10 mg vials should be reconstituted with 5 mL and 10 mL, respectively, of Sodium Chloride Injection USP (0.9%) to give a final concentration of 1 mg/mL of Idarubicin Hydrochloride. Bacteriostatic diluents are not recommended.

The vial contents are under a negative pressure to minimize aerosol formation during reconstitution; therefore, particular care should be taken when the needle is inserted. Inhalation of any aerosol produced during reconstitution must be avoided.

Reconstituted solutions are physically and chemically stable for at least 168 hours (7 days) under refrigeration (2°-8°C, 36°-46°F) and 72 hours (3 days) at controlled room temperature, (15°-30°C, 59°-86°F). Discard unused solutions in an appropriate manner (see "Handling and Disposal").

Care in the administration of Idarubicin Hydrochloride will reduce the chance of perivenous infiltration. It may also decrease the chance of local reactions such as urticaria and erythematous streaking. During intravenous administration of Idarubicin Hydrochloride extravasation may occur with or without an accompanying stinging or burning sensation even if blood returns well on aspiration of the infusion needle. If any signs or symptoms of extravasation have occurred, the injection or infusion should be immediately terminated and restarted in another vein. If it is known or suspected that subcutaneous extravasation has occurred it is recommended that intermittent ice packs (1/2 hour immediately, then 1/2 hour 4 times per day for 3 days) be placed over the area of extravasation and that the affected extremity be elevated. Because of the progressive nature of extravasation reactions, the area of injection should be frequently examined and plastic surgery consultation obtained early if there is any sign of a local reaction such as pain, erythema, edema or vesication. If ulceration begins or there is severe persistent pain at the site of extravasation, early wide excision of the involved area should be considered.[1]

Idarubicin Hydrochloride should be administered slowly (over 10 to 15 minutes) into the tubing of a freely running intravenous infusion of Sodium Chloride Injection USP (0.9%) or 5% Dextrose Injection USP. The tubing should be attached to a Butterfly needle or other suitable device and inserted preferably into a large vein.

INCOMPATIBILITY
Unless specific compatibility data are available, Idarubicin Hydrochloride should not be mixed with other drugs. Precipitation occurs with heparin. Prolonged contact with any solution of an alkaline pH will result in degradation of the drug. Parenteral drug products should be inspected visually for particulate matter and discoloration prior to administration whenever solution and containers permit.

Handling and Disposal: Procedures for handling and disposal of anticancer drugs should be considered. Several guidelines on this subject have been published.[2-8] There is no general agreement that all of the procedures recommended in the guidelines are necessary or appropriate.

Store at controlled room temperature, 15°-30°C (59°-86°F), and protect from light.

REFERENCES
1. Rudolph R, Larson DL: Etiology and Treatment of Chemotherapeutic Agent Extravasation Injuries: A Review. J. Clin Oncol 5: 1116-1126, 1987. 2. Recommendations for the Safe Handling of Parenteral Antineoplastic Drugs. NIH Publication No. 83-2621, US Government Printing Office, Washington, DC 20402. 3. Council on Scientific Affairs: Guidelines for Handling Parenteral Antineoplastics. JAMA 1985; 253:1590. 4. National Study Commission on Cytotoxic Agents. Available from Louis P. Jeffrey, ScD., Director of Pharmacy Services, Rhode Island Hospital, 593 Eddy Street, Providence, Rhode Island 02902. 5. Clinical Oncological Society of Australia: Guidelines and Recommendations for Safe Handling of Antineoplastic Agents. Med J Aust 1983; 1:426. 6. Jones RB, et al.: Safe Handling of Chemotherapeutic Agents: A Report from the Mount Sinai Medical Center. CA 33:258; Sept/Oct 1983. 7. American Society of Hospital Pharmacists: Technical Assistance Bulletin on Handling Cytotoxic Drugs in Hospitals. Am J Hosp Pharm 1990; 47:1033-1049. 8. OSHA Work-Practice Guidelines for Personnel Dealing with Cytotoxic (Antineoplastic) Drugs. Am J Hosp Pharm 1986; 43:1193-1204.

J CODES
5 mg IV—J9211

HOW SUPPLIED
POWDER FOR INJECTION: 5 MG

BRAND/MANUFACTURER	NDC	SIZE	AWP
◆ BRAND			
IDAMYCIN: Pharmacia	00013-2506-94	1s	$254.15

POWDER FOR INJECTION: 10 MG

BRAND/MANUFACTURER	NDC	SIZE	AWP
◆ BRAND			
IDAMYCIN: Pharmacia	00013-2516-86	1s	$508.30

Idoxuridine

DESCRIPTION
Idoxuridine sterile ophthalmic solution is a topical ophthalmic antiviral chemotherapeutic preparation.

Chemical Name: 2'-Deoxy-5-iodouridine.

Following is its chemical structure:

CLINICAL PHARMACOLOGY
In chemical structure Idoxuridine closely approximates the configuration of thymidine, one of the four building blocks of DNA—the genetic material of the herpes virus. As a result, Idoxuridine is able to replace thymidine in the enzymatic step of viral replication or "growth". The consequent production of faulty DNA results in a pseudostructure which cannot infect or destroy tissue. In short, by preempting a vital building block in the genetic material of the herpes simplex virus, Idoxuridine destroys the infective and destructive capacity of the viral material.

INDICATIONS AND USAGE
Idoxuridine is indicated for the treatment of keratitis caused by the herpes simplex virus.

CONTRAINDICATIONS
Idoxuridine is contraindicated for those who have a hypersensitivity to the active ingredient or other components of this medication.

WARNINGS
Recurrence may occur if medication is not continued 5 to 7 days after lesion is apparently healed (does not stain).

PRECAUTIONS
General: Some strains of herpes simplex virus appear resistant to the action of Idoxuridine. If there is no lessening of fluorescein staining in 14 days, another form of therapy should be undertaken.

Drug Interactions: Boric acid should not be administered during the course of therapy. The potential exists for interaction between boric acid and ingredients in Idoxuridine which may result in precipitate formation.

Carcinogenesis, Mutagenesis, Impairment of Fertility: The studies performed to date on Idoxuridine are inadequate for assessment of carcinogenicity. This cytotoxic drug should be regarded as being potentially carcinogenic. It can inhibit DNA synthesis or function and is incorporated into the DNA of mammalian cells as well as into the genome of DNA viruses. Idoxuridine has been reported to induce RNA tumor virus (type C particles) production from virus-negative mouse cells. The degree of oncogenic activity of Idoxuridine-induced oncornaviruses has not been documented. However, several Idoxuridine-activated oncornaviruses have caused *in vitro* cell transformation and induction of specific neoplasms (lymphatic leukemias and carcinomas) upon inoculation into syngeneic mice.

Idoxuridine has been reported to cause chromosome aberrations in mice and to be mutagenic in mammalian cells in culture (e.g., diploid human lymphoblasts and mouse lymphoma cells), drosophila melanogaster and in host-mediated assay system utilizing mammalian cells.

Pregnancy Category C: Idoxuridine has been reported to cross the placental barrier and to produce fetal malformations in rabbits when administered topically to the eyes of pregnant females in doses similar to those used clinically.

Idoxuridine has also been reported to produce fetal malformations in the rat after intraperitoneal and oral administration and in the mouse after subcutaneous administration. There are no adequate and well-controlled studies in pregnant women. Idoxuridine should be used during pregnancy only if the potential benefit justifies the potential risk to the fetus.

Nursing Mothers: It is not known whether this drug is excreted in human milk. Because of the potential for tumorigenicity shown for Idoxuridine in animal studies, a decision should be made whether to discontinue nursing or to discontinue the drug, taking into account the importance of the drug to the mother.

Pediatric Use: Safety and effectiveness in children have not been established.

ADVERSE REACTIONS
Exact incidence figures are not available since no denominator of treated patients is available.

Adverse reactions associated with topical Idoxuridine administration include occasional irritation, pain, pruritus, inflammation, edema of the eyes or lids, allergic reactions, photophobia, occasional corneal clouding, stippling, and punctate defects of the epithelium.

OVERDOSAGE
Overdosage will not ordinarily cause acute problems. Should accidental overdosage in the eye(s) occur, flush the eye(s) with water or normal saline. If accidentally ingested, drink fluids to dilute.

DOSAGE AND ADMINISTRATION
For optimal results, the infected tissues should be kept "saturated" with Idoxuridine. Under practical, clinical conditions, one of the following "high frequency" dosage schedules is recommended.

1. Instill one drop in the infected eye(s) every hour during the day. At night the dosage may be reduced to one drop every other hour.
2. Instill one drop every minute for 5 minutes. This schedule should be repeated every four hours—night and day.

Store at controlled room temperature (59°-86°F). Protect from light.

HOW SUPPLIED
DROP: 0.1%

BRAND/MANUFACTURER	NDC	SIZE	AWP
◆ GENERICS			
HERPLEX: Allergan Optical	00023-0033-15	15 ml	$13.21

Ifex *SEE* IFOSFAMIDE

Ifex/Mesnex *SEE* MESNA

Ifosfamide

WARNING

IFOSFAMIDE SHOULD BE ADMINISTERED UNDER THE SUPERVISION OF A QUALIFIED PHYSICIAN EXPERIENCED IN THE USE OF CANCER CHEMOTHERAPEUTIC AGENTS. UROTOXIC SIDE EFFECTS, ESPECIALLY HEMORRHAGIC CYSTITIS, AS WELL AS CNS TOXICITIES SUCH AS CONFUSION AND COMA HAVE BEEN ASSOCIATED WITH THE USE OF IFOSFAMIDE. WHEN THEY OCCUR, THEY MAY REQUIRE CESSATION OF IFOSFAMIDE THERAPY. SEVERE MYELOSUPPRESSION HAS BEEN REPORTED. (SEE *"ADVERSE REACTIONS"* SECTION.)

DESCRIPTION
Ifosfamide sterile single-dose vials for constitution and administration by intravenous infusion each contain 1 gram or 3 grams. Ifosfamide is a chemotherapeutic agent chemically related to the nitrogen mustards and a synthetic analog of cyclophosphamide. Ifosfamide is 3-(2-chloroethyl)-2-[(2-chloroethyl)amino]-tetrahydro-2H-1,3, 2-oxazaphosphorine 2-oxide. The molecular formula is $C_7H_{15}Cl_2N_2O_2P$ and its molecular weight is 261.1.

Ifosfamide is a white crystalline powder that is soluble in water.

Following is its chemical structure:

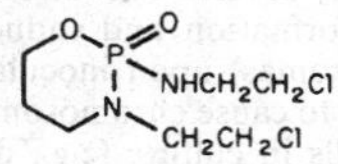

CLINICAL PHARMACOLOGY
Ifosfamide has been shown to require metabolic activation by microsomal liver enzymes to produce biologically active metabolites. Activation occurs by hydroxylation at the ring carbon atom 4 to form the unstable intermediate 4-hydroxyifos-

famide. This metabolite rapidly degrades to the stable urinary metabolite 4-ketoifosfamide. Opening of the ring results in formation of the stable urinary metabolite, 4-carboxyifosfamide. These urinary metabolites have not been found to be cytotoxic. N, N-*bis*(2-chloroethyl)-phosphoric acid diamide (Ifosphoramide) and acrolein are also found. Enzymatic oxidation of the chloroethyl side chains and subsequent dealkylation produces the major urinary metabolites, dechloroethyl Ifosfamide and dechloroethyl cyclophosphamide. The alkylated metabolites of Ifosfamide have been shown to interact with DNA.

In vitro incubation of DNA with activated Ifosfamide has produced phosphotriesters. The treatment of intact cell nuclei may also result in the formation of DNA-DNA crosslinks. DNA repair most likely occurs in G-1 and G-2 stage cells.

PHARMACOKINETICS
Ifosfamide exhibits dose-dependent pharmacokinetics in humans. At single doses of 3.8-5.0 g/m², the plasma concentrations decay biphasically and the mean terminal elimination half-life is about 15 hours. At doses of 1.6-2.4 g/m²/day, the plasma decay is monoexponential and the terminal elimination half-life is about 7 hours. Ifosfamide is extensively metabolized in humans and the metabolic pathways appear to be saturated at high doses.

After administration of doses of 5 g/m² of ¹⁴C-labeled Ifosfamide, from 70% to 86% of the dosed radioactivity was recovered in the urine, with about 61% of the dose excreted as parent compound. At doses of 1.6-2.4 g/m² only 12% to 18% of the dose was excreted in the urine as unchanged drug within 72 hours.

Two different dechloroethylated derivatives of Ifosfamide, 4-carboxyifosfamide, thiodiacetic acid and cysteine conjugates of chloroacetic acid have been identified as the major urinary metabolites of Ifosfamide in humans and only small amounts of 4-hydroxyifosfamide and acrolein are present. Small quantities (nmole/mL) of Ifosfamide mustard and 4-hydroxyifosfamide are detectable in human plasma. Metabolism of Ifosfamide is required for the generation of the biologically active species and while metabolism is extensive, it is also quite variable among patients.

In a study at Indiana University, 50 fully evaluable patients with germ cell testicular cancer were treated with Ifosfamide in combination with cisplatin and either vinblastine or etoposide after failing (47 of 50 patients) at least two prior chemotherapy regimens consisting of cisplatin/vinblastine/bleomycin, (PVB), cisplatin/vinblastine/actinomycin D/bleomycin/cyclophosphamide, (VAB6), or the combination of cisplatin and etoposide. Patients were selected for remaining cisplatin sensitivity because they had previously responded to a cisplatin containing regimen and had not progressed while on the cisplatin containing regimen or within 3 weeks of stopping it. Patients served as their own control based on the premise that long term complete responses could not be achieved by retreatment with a regimen to which they had previously responded and subsequently relapsed.

Ten of 50 fully evaluable patients were still alive 2 to 5 years after treatment. Four of the 10 long term survivors were rendered free of cancer by surgical resection after treatment with the Ifosfamide regimen; median survival for the entire group of 50 fully evaluable patients was 53 weeks.

INDICATION AND USAGE
Ifosfamide, used in combination with certain other approved antineoplastic agents, is indicated for third line chemotherapy of germ cell testicular cancer. It should ordinarily be used in combination with a prophylactic agent for hemorrhagic cystitis, such as mesna.

UNLABELED USES
Ifosfamide is used alone or as an adjunct in the treatment of bronchogenic carcinoma, pancreatic carcinoma, renal cell carcinoma, and osteosarcoma.

CONTRAINDICATIONS
Continued use of Ifosfamide is contraindicated in patients with severely depressed bone marrow function (see *"Warnings"* and *"Precautions"* sections). Ifosfamide is also contraindicated in patients who have demonstrated a previous hypersensitivity to it.

WARNINGS
URINARY SYSTEM
Urotoxic side effects, especially hemorrhagic cystitis, have been frequently associated with the use of Ifosfamide. It is recommended that a urinalysis should be obtained prior to each dose of Ifosfamide. If microscopic hematuria (greater than 10 RBCs per high power field) is present, then subsequent administration should be withheld until complete resolution. Further administration of Ifosfamide should be given with vigorous oral or parenteral hydration.

HEMATOPOIETIC SYSTEM
When Ifosfamide is given in combination with other chemotherapeutic agents, severe myelosuppression is frequently observed. Close hematologic monitoring is recommended. White blood cell (WBC) count, platelet count and hemoglobin should be obtained prior to each administration and at appropriate intervals. Unless clinically essential, Ifosfamide should not be given to patients with a WBC count below 2000/µL and/or a platelet count below 50,000/µL.

CENTRAL NERVOUS SYSTEM
Neurologic manifestations consisting of somnolence, confusion, hallucinations and in some instances, coma, have been reported following Ifosfamide therapy. The occurrence of these symptoms requires discontinuing Ifosfamide therapy. The symptoms have usually been reversible and supportive therapy should be maintained until their complete resolution.

◆ RATED THERAPEUTICALLY EQUIVALENT; ◇ THERAPEUTIC EQUIVALENCE UNCONFIRMED; ○ UNRATED

PREGNANCY

Animal studies indicate that the drug is capable of causing gene mutations and chromosomal damage *in vivo*. Embryotoxic and teratogenic effects have been observed in mice, rats and rabbits at doses 0.05-0.075 times the human dose. Ifosfamide can cause fetal damage when administered to a pregnant woman. If Ifosfamide is used during pregnancy, or if the patient becomes pregnant while taking this drug, the patient should be apprised of the potential hazard to the fetus.

PRECAUTIONS

GENERAL

Ifosfamide should be given cautiously to patients with impaired renal function as well as to those with compromised bone marrow reserve, as indicated by: leukopenia, granulocytopenia, extensive bone marrow metastases, prior radiation therapy, or prior therapy with other cytotoxic agents.

LABORATORY TESTS

During treatment, the patient's hematologic profile (particularly neutrophils and platelets) should be monitored regularly to determine the degree of hematopoietic suppression. Urine should also be examined regularly for red cells which may precede hemorrhagic cystitis.

DRUG INTERACTIONS

The physician should be alert for possible combined drug actions, desirable or undesirable, involving Ifosfamide even though Ifosfamide has been used successfully concurrently with other drugs, including other cytotoxic drugs.

WOUND HEALING

Ifosfamide may interfere with normal wound healing.

PREGNANCY

Pregnancy "Category D." (See *"Warnings"* section.)

NURSING MOTHERS

Ifosfamide is excreted in breast milk. Because of the potential for serious adverse events and the tumorigenicity shown for Ifosfamide in animal studies, a decision should be made whether to discontinue nursing or to discontinue the drug, taking into account the importance of the drug to the mother.

CARCINOGENESIS, MUTAGENESIS, IMPAIRMENT OF FERTILITY

Ifosfamide has been shown to be carcinogenic in rats, with female rats showing a significant incidence of leiomyosarcomas and mammary fibroadenomas.

The mutagenic potential of Ifosfamide has been documented in bacterial systems *in vitro* and mammalian cells *in vivo*. In *vivo*, Ifosfamide has induced mutagenic effects in mice and *Drosophila melanogaster* germ cells, and has induced a significant increase in dominant lethal mutations in male mice as well as recessive sex-linked lethal mutations in Drosophila. In pregnant mice, resorptions increased and anomalies were present at day 19 after 30 mg/m^2 dose of Ifosfamide was administered on day 11 of gestation. Embryolethal effects were observed in rats following the administration of 54 mg/m^2 doses of Ifosfamide from the 6th through the 15th day of gestation and embryotoxic effects were apparent after dams received 18 mg/m^2 doses over the same dosing period. Ifosfamide is embryotoxic to rabbits receiving 88 mg/m^2/day doses from the 6th through the 18th day after mating. The number of anomalies was also significantly increased over the control group.

PEDIATRIC USE

Safety and effectiveness in children have not been established.

ADVERSE REACTIONS

In patients receiving Ifosfamide as a single agent, the dose-limiting toxicities are myelosuppression and urotoxicity. Dose fractionation, vigorous hydration, and a protector such as mesna can significantly reduce the incidence of hematuria, especially gross hematuria, associated with hemorrhagic cystitis. At a dose of 1.2 g/m^2 daily for 5 consecutive days, leukopenia, when it occurs, is usually mild to moderate. Other significant side effects include alopecia, nausea, vomiting, and central nervous system toxicities.

Adverse Reaction	*Incidence %
Alopecia	83
Nausea-Vomiting	58
Hematuria	46
Gross Hematuria	12
CNS Toxicity	12
Infection	8
Renal Impairment	6
Liver Dysfunction	3
Phlebitis	2
Fever	1
Allergic Reaction	< 1
Anorexia	< 1
Cardiotoxicity	< 1
Coagulopathy	< 1
Constipation	< 1
Dermatitis	< 1
Diarrhea	< 1
Fatigue	< 1

Adverse Reaction	*Incidence %
Hypertension	< 1
Hypotension	< 1
Malaise	< 1
Polyneuropathy	< 1
Pulmonary Symptoms	< 1
Salivation	< 1
Stomatitis	< 1

* *Based upon 2,070 patients from the published literature in 30 single agent studies.*

HEMATOLOGIC TOXICITY

Myelosuppression was dose related and dose limiting. It consisted mainly of leukopenia and, to a lesser extent, thrombocytopenia. A WBC count < 3000/μL is expected in 50% of the patients treated with Ifosfamide single agent at doses of 1.2 g/m^2 per day for 5 consecutive days. At this dose level, thrombocytopenia (platelets < 100,000/μL) occurred in about 20% of the patients. At higher dosages, leukopenia was almost universal, and at total dosages of 10 to 12 g/m^2/cycle, one half of the patients had a WBC count below 1000/μL and 8% of patients had platelet counts less than 50,000/μL. Myelosuppression was usually reversible and treatment can be given every 3 to 4 weeks. When Ifosfamide is used in combination with other myelosuppressive agents, adjustments in dosing may be necessary. Patients who experience severe myelosuppression are potentially at increased risk for infection.

DIGESTIVE SYSTEM

Nausea and vomiting occurred in 58% of the patients who received Ifosfamide. They were usually controlled by standard antiemetic therapy. Other gastrointestinal side effects include anorexia, diarrhea, and in some cases, constipation.

URINARY SYSTEM

Urotoxicity consisted of hemorrhagic cystitis, dysuria, urinary frequency and other symptoms of bladder irritation. Hematuria occurred in 6% to 92% of patients treated with Ifosfamide. The incidence and severity of hematuria can be significantly reduced by using vigorous hydration, a fractionated dose schedule and a protector such as mesna. At daily doses of 1.2 g/m^2 for 5 consecutive days without a protector, microscopic hematuria is expected in about one half of the patients and gross hematuria in about 8% of patients.

Renal toxicity occurred in 6% of the patients treated with Ifosfamide as a single agent. Clinical signs, such as elevation in BUN or serum creatinine or decrease in creatinine clearance, were usually transient. They were most likely to be related to tubular damage. One episode of renal tubular acidosis which progressed into chronic renal failure was reported. Proteinuria and acidosis also occurred in rare instances. Metabolic acidosis was reported in 31% of patients in one study when Ifosfamide was administered at doses of 2.0 to 2.5 g/m^2/day for 4 days. Renal tubular acidosis, Fanconi syndrome and renal rickets have been reported. Close clinical monitoring of serum and urine chemistries including phosphorus, potassium, alkaline phosphatase and other appropriate laboratory studies is recommended. Appropriate replacement therapy should be administered as indicated.

CENTRAL NERVOUS SYSTEM

CNS side effects were observed in 12% of patients treated with Ifosfamide. Those most commonly seen were somnolence, confusion, depressive psychosis, and hallucinations. Other less frequent symptoms include dizziness, disorientation, and cranial nerve dysfunction. Seizures and coma were occasionally reported. The incidence of CNS toxicity may be higher in patients with altered renal function.

OTHER

Alopecia occurred in approximately 83% of the patients treated with Ifosfamide as a single agent. In combination, this incidence may be as high as 100%, depending on the other agents included in the chemotherapy regimen. Increases in liver enzymes and/or bilirubin were noted in 3% of the patients. Other less frequent side effects included phlebitis, pulmonary symptoms, fever of unknown origin, allergic reactions, stomatitis, cardiotoxicity, and polyneuropathy.

OVERDOSAGE

No specific antidote for Ifosfamide is known. Management of overdosage would include general supportive measures to sustain the patient through any period of toxicity that might occur.

DOSAGE AND ADMINISTRATION

Ifosfamide should be administered intravenously at a dose of 1.2 g/m^2 per day for 5 consecutive days. Treatment is repeated every 3 weeks or after recovery from hematologic toxicity (Platelets $\geq$ 100,000/μL, WBC $\geq$ 4,000/μL). In order to prevent bladder toxicity, Ifosfamide should be given with extensive hydration consisting of at least two liters of oral or intravenous fluid per day. A protector, such as mesna, should also be used to prevent hemorrhagic cystitis. Ifosfamide should be administered as a slow intravenous infusion lasting a minimum of 30 minutes. Although Ifosfamide has been administered to a small number of patients with compromised hepatic and/or renal function, studies to establish optimal dose schedules of Ifosfamide in such patients have not been conducted.

PREPARATION FOR INTRAVENOUS ADMINISTRATION/STABILITY

Injections are prepared for parenteral use by adding *Sterile Water for Injection* USP, or *Bacteriostatic Water for Injection USP* (benzyl alcohol or parabens preserved) to the vial and shaking to dissolve. Use the quantity of diluent shown below to reconstitute the product:

Dosage Strength	Quantity of Diluent	Final Concentration
1 gram	20 mL	50 mg/mL
3 grams	60 mL	50 mg/mL

Reconstituted solutions are chemically and physically stable for 1 week at 30°C or 3 weeks at 5°C.

Solutions of Ifosfamide may be diluted further to achieve concentrations of 0.6 to 20 mg/mL in the following fluids:

5% Dextrose Injection, USP
0.9% Sodium Chloride Injection, USP
Lactated Ringer's Injection, USP
Sterile Water for Injection, USP

Such admixtures, when stored in large volume parenteral glass bottles, Viaflex bags, or PAB® bags, are physically and chemically stable for at least 1 week at 30°C or 6 weeks at 5°C.

Because essentially identical stability results were obtained for Sterile Water admixtures as for the other admixtures (5% Dextrose Injection, 0.9% Sodium Chloride Injection, and Lactated Ringer's Injection), the use of large volume parenteral glass bottles, Viaflex bags or PAB® bags that contain intermediate concentrations or mixtures of excipients (eg, 2.5% Dextrose Injection, 0.45% Sodium Chloride Injection, or 5% Dextrose and 0.9% Sodium Chloride Injection) is also acceptable.

The microbiological qualities of the constituted products or prepared admixtures should be considered, particularly where unpreserved vehicles are used.

Dilutions of Ifosfamide not prepared by constitution with Bacteriostatic Water for Injection, USP (benzyl alcohol or parabens preserved), should be refrigerated and used within 6 hours. Parenteral drug products should be inspected visually for particulate matter and discoloration prior to administration.

Store at controlled room temperature 15°C to 30°C.

Procedures for proper handling and disposal of anticancer drugs should be considered. Skin reactions associated with accidental exposure to Ifosfamide may occur. The use of gloves is recommended. If Ifosfamide solution contacts the skin or mucosa, immediately wash the skin thoroughly with soap and water or rinse the mucosa with copious amounts of water. Several guidelines on this subject have been published.[1-7] There is no general agreement that all of the procedures recommended in the guidelines are necessary or appropriate.

REFERENCES
1. Recommendations for the Safe Handling of Parenteral Antineoplastic Drugs. NIH Publication No. 83-2621. For sale by the Superintendent of Documents, U.S. Government Printing Office, Washington, DC 20402. 2. AMA Council Report, Guidelines for Handling Parenteral Antineoplastics, *JAMA*. 1985; 253 (11): 1590-1592. 3. National Study Commission on Cytotoxic Exposure—Recommendations for Handling Cytotoxic Agents. Available from Louis P. Jeffrey, Sc.D., Chairman, National Study Commission on Cytotoxic Exposure, Massachusetts College of Pharmacy and Allied Health Sciences, 179 Longwood Avenue, Boston Massachusetts 02115. 4. Clinical Oncological Society of Australia: Guidelines and Recommendations for Safe Handling of Antineoplastic Agents. *Med J Australia*. 1983; 1:426-428. 5. Jones, RB, et al: Safe Handling of Chemotherapeutic Agents: A Report from the Mount Sinai Medical Center, *CA—A Cancer J for Clinicians*. 1983; Sept/Oct. 258-263. 6. American Society of Hospital Pharmacists Technical Assistance Bulletin on Handling Cytotoxic and Hazardous Drugs. *Am J Hosp Pharm*. 1990; 47:1033-1049. 7. OSHA Work-Practice Guidelines for Personnel Dealing with Cytotoxic (Antineoplastic) Drugs. *Am J Hosp Pharm*. 1986; 43:1193-1204.

J CODES
Per 1 g IV—J9208

HOW SUPPLIED
POWDER FOR INJECTION:

BRAND/MANUFACTURER	NDC	SIZE	AWP
○ **BRAND**			
IFEX: Bristol-Myer Onc/Hiv	00015-0556-41	1s	$101.94
	00015-0557-41	1s	$305.81

Iletin II Reg. Pork SEE INSULIN-PORK, CONCENTRATED

Ilopan SEE DEXPANTHENOL

Ilopan-Choline SEE CHOLINE BITARTRATE AND DEXPANTHENOL

Ilosone SEE ERYTHROMYCIN, ORAL

Ilotycin SEE ERYTHROMYCIN, INJECTABLE AND ERYTHROMYCIN, OPHTHALMIC

Imdur SEE ISOSORBIDE MONONITRATE

Imiglucerase

DESCRIPTION
Imiglucerase for injection is an analogue of the human enzyme β-glucocerebrosidase produced by recombinant DNA technology. β-Glucocerebrosidase (β-D-glucosyl-N-acylsphingosine glucohydrolase, E.C. 3.2.1.45) is a lysosomal glycoprotein enzyme which catalyzes the hydrolysis of the glycolipid glucocerebroside to glucose and ceramide.

Imiglucerase is produced by recombinant DNA technology using mammalian cell culture (Chinese hamster ovary). Purified Imiglucerase is a monomeric glycoprotein of 497 amino acids, containing 4 N-linked glycosylation sites (Mr = 60,430). Imiglucerase differs from placental glucocerebrosidase by one amino acid at position 495 where histidine is substituted for arginine. The oligosaccharide chains at the glycosylation sites have been modified to terminate in mannose sugars.

The modified carbohydrate structures on Imiglucerase are somewhat different from those on placental glucocerebrosidase. These mannose-terminated oligosaccharide chains of Imiglucerase are specifically recognized by endocytic carbohydrate recognized by endocytic carbohydrate receptors on macrophages, the cells that accumulate lipid in Gaucher disease.

Imiglucerase is supplied as a sterile, non-pyrogenic, white to off-white lyophilized product. The quantitative composition of the lyophilized drug per vial is:

Imiglucerase 212 units (total amount)

This provides a withdrawal dose of 200 units of Imiglucerase.

An enzyme unit (U) is defined as the amount of enzyme that catalyzes the hydrolysis of one micromole of the synthetic substrate para-nitrophenyl β-D-glucopyranoside (pNP-Glc) per minute at 37°C. The product is stored at 2-8°C (36-46°F.). After reconstitution with 5.1 mL of Sterile Water for Injection, USP, the Imiglucerase concentration is 40 U/mL in a final volume of 5.3 mL which provides a withdrawal volume of 5.0 mL (200 enzyme units). Reconstituted solutions have a pH of approximately 6.1.

In addition, cross-linked gelatin polypeptides, which are used as a stabilizing agent during the manufacturing process, may also be present in very small amounts in the final product.

CLINICAL PHARMACOLOGY
MECHANISM OF ACTION/PHARMACODYNAMICS
Gaucher disease is characterized by a deficiency of β-glucocerebrosidase activity, resulting in accumulation of glucocerebroside in tissue macrophages which become engorged and are typically found in the liver, spleen, and bone marrow and occasionally in lung, kidney, and intestine. Secondary hematologic sequelae include severe anemia and thrombocytopenia in addition to the characteristic progressive hepatosplenomegaly, skeletal complications, including osteonecrosis and osteopenia with secondary pathological fractures.

Imiglucerase for injection catalyzes the hydrolysis of glucocerebroside to glucose and ceramide. In clinical trials, Imiglucerase improved anemia and thrombocytopenia, reduced spleen and liver size, and decreased cachexia to a degree similar to that observed with alglucerase.

PHARMACOKINETICS
During one hour intravenous infusions of four doses (7.5, 15, 30, 60 U/Kg) of Imiglucerase for injection steady-state enzymatic activity was achieved by 30 minutes. Following infusion, plasma enzymatic activity declined rapidly with a half-life ranging from 3.6 to 10.4 minutes. Plasma clearance ranged from 9.8 to 20.3 mL/min/Kg (mean ± S.D. 14.5 ± 4.0 mL/min/Kg). The volume of distribution corrected for weight ranged from 0.09 to 0.15 L/Kg (0.12 ± 0.02 L/kg).

These variables do not appear to be influenced by dose or duration of infusion. However, only one or two patients were studied at each dose level and infusion rate. The pharmacokinetics of Imiglucerase do not appear to be different from placental-derived alglucerase Imiglucerase.

In patients who developed IgG antibody to Imiglucerase, an apparent effect on serum enzyme levels resulted in diminished volume of distribution and clearance and increased elimination half-life compared to patients without antibody (see "Warnings").

INDICATIONS AND USAGE
Imiglucerase for injection is indicated for long-term enzyme replacement therapy for patients with a confirmed diagnosis of Type 1 Gaucher disease that results in one or more of the following conditions:
   a. anemia
   b. thrombocytopenia
   c. bone disease
   d. hepatomegaly or splenomegaly

◆ RATED THERAPEUTICALLY EQUIVALENT; ◇ THERAPEUTIC EQUIVALENCE UNCONFIRMED; ○ UNRATED

CONTRAINDICATIONS

There are no known contraindications to the use of Imiglucerase for injection. Treatment with Imiglucerase should be carefully re-evaluated if there is significant clinical evidence of hypersensitivity to the product.

WARNINGS

During the clinical trials (duration 9 months), 4 of 25 patients (16%) treated with Imiglucerase for injection developed IgG antibodies reactive with Imiglucerase. During the same clinical trial, 6 to 15 patients (40%) treated with placental-derived alglucerase developed IgG antibodies to alglucerase, and one of these patients had clinical allergic signs and symptoms resulting in withdrawal from the study.

Of those patients treated with Imiglucerase, only one patient developed a transient rash. No patients treated with Imiglucerase, either initially or after changing over from alglucerase, have exhibited serious symptoms of immediate hypersensitivity, although a risk for such reactions may be present.

Treatment with Imiglucerase should be approached with caution in patients who have exhibited symptoms of hypersensitivity to the product.

PRECAUTIONS

GENERAL

Therapy with Imiglucerase for injection should be directed by physicians knowledgeable in the management of patients with Gaucher disease.

Caution may be advisable in administration of Imiglucerase to patients previously treated with alglucerase and who have developed antibody to alglucerase or who have exhibited symptoms of hypersensitivity to alglucerase.

CARCINOGENESIS, MUTAGENESIS, IMPAIRMENT OF FERTILITY

Studies have not been conducted in either animals or humans to assess the potential effects of Imiglucerase for injection on carcinogenesis, mutagenesis, or impairment of fertility.

TERATOGENIC EFFECTS: PREGNANCY CATEGORY C

Animal reproduction studies have not been conducted with Imiglucerase for injection. It is also not known whether Imiglucerase can cause fetal harm when administered to a pregnant woman, or can affect reproductive capacity. Imiglucerase should not be administered during pregnancy except when the indication and need are clear and the potential benefit is judged by the physician to substantially justify the risk.

NURSING MOTHERS

It is not known whether this drug is excreted in human milk. Because many drugs are excreted in human milk, caution should be exercised when Imiglucerase for injection is administered to a nursing woman.

ADVERSE REACTIONS

During clinical trials with Imiglucerase involving 25 patients with Gaucher disease, the following adverse events were noted that were possibly related to Imiglucerase.

Headache was noted in three patients. Nausea, abdominal discomfort, dizziness, pruritus, and rash occurred in one patient each. One patient was noted to have a mild decrease in blood pressure and another a decrease in urinary frequency. None of these events was judged to be serious or to warrant medical intervention or interruption of therapy. All proved transient and did not recur frequently.

Symptoms suggestive of allergic hypersensitivity have been noted in a number of patients treated with alglucerase (see *"Warnings"*).

OVERDOSAGE

Effects of dosages exceeding 120 U/kg per four weeks have not been studied and therefore dosages above 120 U/kg are not recommended.

DOSAGE AND ADMINISTRATION

Imiglucerase for injection is administered by intravenous infusion over 1-2 hours. Dosage should be individualized to each patient. Initial dosage may be as little as 2.5 units/kg of body weight 3 times a week up to as much as 60 U/kg administered as frequently as once a week or as infrequently as every 4 weeks. 60 units/kg every 2 weeks is the dosage for which the most data are available. Disease severity may dictate that treatment be initiated at a relatively high dose or relatively frequent administration. After patient response is well established, a reduction in dosage may be attempted for maintenance therapy. Progressive reductions can be made at intervals of 3-6 months while carefully monitoring response parameters.

Imiglucerase should be stored at 2-8° C (36-46° F). Each vial, after reconstitution with 5.1 mL Sterile Water for Injection, USP, should be inspected visually for particulate matter and discoloration before use. Any vials exhibiting particulate matter or discoloration should not be used. *Do not use* Imiglucerase after the expiration date on the vial.

On the day of use, after the correct amount of Imiglucerase to be administered to the patient has been determined, the appropriate number of vials are each reconstituted with 5.1 mL of Sterile Water for Injection. USP, to give a reconstituted volume of 5.3 mL. A nominal 5.0 mL volume is then withdrawn from each vial and pooled with 0.9% Sodium Chloride Injection, USP, to a final volume of 100 to 200 mL. Imiglucerase is administered by intravenous infusion over 1 to 2 hours. Alternatively, the appropriate dose of Imiglucerase may be administered such that a rate of no greater than 1 unit per kg body weight per minute is infused. Aseptic techniques should be used when diluting the dose. Since Imiglucerase does not contain any preservative, after reconstitution, vials should be promptly diluted and not stored for subsequent use. Imiglucerase, when

diluted to 50 mL has been shown to be stable for up to 24 hours when stored at 2-8° C (36-46° F).

Relatively low toxicity, combined with the extended time course of response, allows small dosage adjustments to be made occasionally to avoid discarding partially used bottles. Thus, the dosage administered in individual infusions may be slightly increased or decreased to utilize fully each vial as long as the monthly administered dosage remains substantially unaltered.

HOW SUPPLIED

POWDER FOR INJECTION: 200 U

BRAND/MANUFACTURER	NDC	SIZE	AWP
○ **BRAND**			
CEREZYME: Genzyme	58468-1983-01	1s	$740.00

Imipramine

DESCRIPTION

Imipramine, the original tricyclic antidepressant, is a member of the dibenzazepine group of compounds. It is designated 5-[3-(Dimethylamino)propyl]-10, 11-dihydro-5H-dibenz[b,f] azepine Monohydrochloride. Imipramine Hydrochloride USP is a white to off-white, odorless, or practically odorless crystalline powder. It is freely soluble in water and in alcohol, soluble in acetone, and insoluble in ether and in benzene. Its molecular weight is 316.87.

Imipramine Pamoate is a tricyclic antidepressant, available as capsules for oral administration. The 75-, 100-, 125-, and 150-mg capsules contain Imipramine Pamoate equivalent to 75, 100, 125, and 150 mg of Imipramine Hydrochloride.

Imipramine Pamoate is 5-(3-[dimethylamino)propyl]-10,11-dihydro-5H-dibenz[b,f]azepine 4,4'-methylenebis-(3-hydroxy-2-naphthoate) (2:1).

Imipramine Pamoate is a fine, yellow, tasteless and odorless powder. It is soluble in ethanol, in acetone, in ether, in chloroform, and in carbon tetrachloride, and is insoluble in water. Its molecular weight is 949.21.

CLINICAL PHARMACOLOGY

The mechanism of action of Imipramine is not definitely known. However, it does not act primarily by stimulation of the central nervous system. The clinical effect is hypothesized as being due to potentiation of adrenergic synapses by blocking uptake of norepinephrine at nerve endings. The mode of action of the drug in controlling childhood enuresis is thought to be apart from its antidepressant effect.

INDICATIONS

Depression: For the relief of symptoms of depression. Endogenous depression is more likely to be alleviated than other depressive states. One to three weeks of treatment may be needed before optimal therapeutic effects are evident.

Childhood Enuresis: Imipramine Hydrochloride, oral, may be useful as temporary adjunctive therapy in reducing enuresis in children aged 6 years and older, after possible organic causes have been excluded by appropriate tests. In patients having daytime symptoms of frequency and urgency, examination should include voiding cystourethrography and cystoscopy, as necessary. The effectiveness of treatment may decrease with continued drug administration.

UNLABELED USES

Imipramine is used alone or as an adjunct in the treatment of agoraphobia, attention deficit disorder, refractory depression, and diabetic neuropathy. It is also used in the treatment of pathological crying or laughing (emotionalism), drug-induced extrapyramidal symptoms, and cardiac arrhythmias, and is prescribed for posttraumatic stress disorder, retrograde ejaculation, sleep apnea syndrome, and premenstrual syndrome.

CONTRAINDICATIONS

The concomitant use of monoamine oxidase inhibiting compounds is contraindicated. Hyperpyretic crises or severe convulsive seizures may occur in patients receiving such combinations. The potentiation of adverse effects can be serious, or even fatal. When it is desired to substitute Imipramine in patients receiving a monoamine oxidase inhibitor, as long an interval should elapse as the clinical situation will allow, with a minimum of 14 days. Initial dosage should be low and increases should be gradual and cautiously prescribed.

The drug is contraindicated during the acute recovery period after a myocardial infarction. Patients with a known hypersensitivity to this compound should not be given the drug. The possibility of cross-sensitivity to other dibenzazepine compounds should be kept in mind.

WARNINGS

Children: A dose of 2.5 mg/kg/day of Imipramine should not be exceeded in childhood. ECG changes of unknown significance have been reported in pediatric patients with doses twice this amount.

Imipramine Pamoate should not be used in children of any age because of the increased potential for acute overdosage due to the high unit potency (75 mg, 100 mg, 125 mg and 150 mg). Each capsule contains Imipramine Pamoate equivalent to 75 mg, 100 mg, 125 mg or 150 mg Imipramine Hydrochloride.

Extreme caution should be used when this drug is given to: patients with cardiovascular disease because of the possibility of conduction defects, arrhythmias, congestive heart failure, myocardial infarction, strokes and tachycardia. These patients require cardiac surveillance at all dosage levels of the drug:

▶ SHOWN IN PRODUCT IDENTIFICATION GUIDE

patients with increased intraocular pressure, history of urinary retention, or history of narrow-angle glaucoma because of the drug's anticholinergic properties;

hyperthyroid patients or those on thyroid medication because of the possibility of cardiovascular toxicity;

patients with a history of seizure disorder because this drug has been shown to lower the seizure threshold;

patients receiving guanethidine, clonidine, or similar agents, since Imipramine may block the pharmacologic effects of these drugs;

patients receiving methylphenidate hydrochloride. Since methylphenidate hydrochloride may inhibit the metabolism of Imipramine, downward dosage adjustment of Imipramine may be required when given concomitantly with methylphenidate hydrochloride.

Imipramine may enhance the CNS depressant effects of alcohol. Therefore, it should be borne in mind that the dangers inherent in a suicide attempt or accidental overdosage with the drug may be increased for the patient who uses excessive amounts of alcohol. (See "Precautions".)

Since Imipramine may impair the mental and/or physical abilities required for the performance of potentially hazardous tasks, such as operating an automobile or machinery, the patient should be cautioned accordingly.

Some brands of Imipramine contain sodium sulfite and sodium bisulfite, that may cause allergic-type reactions including anaphylactic symptoms and life-threatening or less severe asthmatic episodes in certain susceptible people. The overall prevalence of sulfite sensitivity in the general population is unknown and probably low. Sulfite sensitivity is seen more frequently in asthmatic than in nonasthmatic people.

PRECAUTIONS

An ECG recording should be taken prior to the initiation of larger-than-usual doses of Imipramine and at appropriate intervals thereafter until steady state is achieved. (Patients with any evidence of cardiovascular disease require cardiac surveillance at all dosage levels of the drug. See "Warnings".)

Elderly patients and patients with cardiac disease or a prior history of cardiac disease are at special risk of developing the cardiac abnormalities associated with the use of Imipramine. It should be kept in mind that the possibility of suicide in seriously depressed patients is inherent in the illness and may persist until significant remission occurs. Such patients should be carefully supervised during the early phase of treatment with Imipramine and may require hospitalization. Prescriptions should be written for the smallest amount feasible.

Hypomanic or manic episodes may occur, particularly in patients with cyclic disorders. Such reactions may necessitate discontinuation of the drug. If needed, Imipramine may be resumed in lower dosage when these episodes are relieved. Administration of a tranquilizer may be useful in controlling such episodes.

An activation of the psychosis may occasionally be observed in schizophrenic patients and may require reduction of dosage and the addition of a phenothiazine.

Concurrent administration of Imipramine with electroshock therapy may increase the hazards; such treatment should be limited to those patients for whom it is essential, since there is limited clinical experience.

Usage During Pregnancy and Lactation: Animal reproduction studies have yielded inconclusive results. (See also "Animal Pharmacology and Toxicology".)

There have been no well-controlled studies conducted with pregnant women to determine the effect of Imipramine on the fetus. However, there have been clinical reports of congenital malformations associated with the use of the drug. Although a causal relationship between these effects and the drug could not be established, the possibility of fetal risk from the maternal ingestion of Imipramine cannot be excluded. Therefore, Imipramine should be used in women who are or might become pregnant only if the clinical condition clearly justifies potential risk to the fetus.

Limited data suggest that Imipramine is likely to be excreted in human breast milk. As a general rule, a woman taking a drug should not nurse since the possibility exists that the drug may be excreted in breast milk and be harmful to the child.

Usage in Children: The effectiveness of the drug (given orally) in children for conditions other than nocturnal enuresis, has not been established.

The safety and effectiveness of the oral drug as temporary adjunctive therapy for nocturnal enuresis in children less than 6 years of age has not been established.

The safety of the oral drug for long-term, chronic use as adjunctive therapy for nocturnal enuresis in children 6 years of age or older has not been established; consideration should be given to instituting a drug-free period following an adequate therapeutic trial with a favorable response.

A dose of 2.5 mg/kg/day, orally, should not be exceeded in childhood. ECG changes of unknown significance have been reported in pediatric patients with doses twice this amount.

Patients should be warned that Imipramine may enhance the CNS depressant effects of alcohol. (See "Warnings".)

Imipramine should be used with caution in patients with significantly impaired renal or hepatic function.

Patients who develop a fever and a sore throat during therapy with Imipramine should have leukocyte and differential blood counts performed. Imipramine should be discontinued if there is evidence of pathological neutrophil depression.

Prior to elective surgery, Imipramine should be discontinued for as long as the clinical situation will allow.

In occasional susceptible patients or in those receiving anticholinergic drugs (including antiparkinsonism agents) in addition, the atropine-like effects may become more pronounced (e.g., paralytic ileus).

Close supervision and careful adjustment of dosage is required when Imipramine is administered concomitantly with anticholinergic drugs.

Avoid the use of preparations, such as decongestants and local anesthetics, which contain any sympathomimetic amine (e.g., epinephrine, norepinephrine), since it has been reported that tricyclic antidepressants can potentiate the effects of catecholamines.

Caution should be exercised when Imipramine is used with agents that lower blood pressure.

Imipramine may potentiate the effects of CNS depressant drugs. The plasma concentration of Imipramine may increase when the drug is given concomitantly with hepatic enzyme inhibitors (e.g., cimetidine, fluoxetine) and decrease by concomitant administration of hepatic enzyme inducers (e.g., barbiturates, phenytoin), and adjustment of the dosage of Imipramine may therefore be necessary.

Patients taking Imipramine should avoid excessive exposure to sunlight since there have been reports of photosensitization. Both elevation and lowering of blood sugar levels have been reported with Imipramine use.

ADVERSE REACTIONS

Note: Although the listing which follows includes a few adverse reactions which have not been reported with this specific drug, the pharmacological similarities among the tricyclic antidepressant drugs require that each of the reactions be considered when Imipramine is administered.

Cardiovascular: Orthostatic hypotension, hypertension, tachycardia, palpitation, myocardial infarction, arrhythmias, heart block, ECG changes, precipitation of congestive heart failure, stroke.

Psychiatric: Confusional states (especially in the elderly) with hallucinations, disorientation, delusions; anxiety, restlessness, agitation; insomnia and nightmares; hypomania; exacerbation of psychosis.

Neurological: Numbness, tingling, paresthesias of extremities; incoordination, ataxia, tremors; peripheral neuropathy; extrapyramidal symptoms; seizures, alterations in EEG patterns; tinnitus.

Anticholinergic: Dry mouth, and, rarely, associated sublingual adenitis; blurred vision, disturbances of accommodation, mydriasis; constipation, paralytic ileus; urinary retention, delayed micturition, dilation of the urinary tract.

Allergic: Skin rash, petechiae, urticaria, itching, photosensitization; edema (general or of face and tongue); drug fever; cross-sensitivity with desipramine.

Hematologic: Bone marrow depression including agranulocytosis; eosinophilia; purpura; thrombocytopenia.

Gastrointestinal: Nausea and vomiting, anorexia, epigastric distress, diarrhea; peculiar taste, stomatitis, abdominal cramps, black tongue.

Endocrine: Gynecomastia in the male; breast enlargement and galactorrhea in the female; increased or decreased libido, impotence; testicular swelling; elevation or depression of blood sugar levels; inappropriate antidiuretic hormone (ADH) secretion syndrome.

Other: Jaundice (simulating obstructive); altered liver function; weight gain or loss; perspiration; flushing; urinary frequency; drowsiness; dizziness, weakness and fatigue; headache; parotid swelling; alopecia; proneness to falling.

Withdrawal Symptoms: Though not indicative of addiction, abrupt cessation of treatment after prolonged therapy may produce nausea, headache and malaise.

Note: In enuretic children treated with oral Imipramine, the most common adverse reactions have been nervousness, sleep disorders, tiredness, and mild gastrointestinal disturbances. These usually disappear during continued drug administration or when dosage is decreased. Other reactions which have been reported include constipation, convulsions, anxiety, emotional instability, syncope, and collapse. All of the adverse reactions reported with adult use should be considered.

DOSAGE AND ADMINISTRATION

Depression: Lower dosages are recommended for elderly patients and adolescents. Lower dosages are also recommended for outpatients as compared to hospitalized patients who will be under close supervision. Dosage should be initiated at a low level and increased gradually, noting carefully the clinical response and any evidence of intolerance. Following remission, maintenance medication may be required for a longer period of time, at the lowest dose that will maintain remission.

IMIPRAMINE HYDROCHLORIDE, ORAL
USUAL ADULT DOSE:
Hospitalized Patients: Initially, 100 mg/day in divided doses gradually increased to 200 mg/day as required. If no response after two weeks, increase to 250-300 mg/day.

Outpatients: Initially, 75 mg/day increased to 150 mg/day. Dosages over 200 mg/day are not recommended. Maintenance, 50-150 mg/day.

Adolescent and geriatric patients: Initially, 30-40 mg/day; it is generally not necessary to exceed 100 mg/day.

Childhood Enuresis: Initially, an oral dose of 25 mg/day should be tried in children aged 6 and older. Medication should be given one hour before bedtime. If a satisfactory response does not occur within one week, increase the dose to 50 mg nightly in children under 12 years; children over 12 may receive up to 75 mg nightly. A daily dose greater than 75 mg does not enhance efficacy and tends to increase side effects. Evidence suggests that in early night bedwetters, the drug is more effective given earlier and in divided amounts, i.e., 25 mg in midafternoon, repeated at bedtime. Consideration should be given to instituting a drug-free period following an adequate therapeutic trial with a favorable response. Dosage should be tapered off gradually rather than abruptly discontinued; this may reduce the tendency to relapse. Children who relapse when the drug is discontinued do not always respond to a subsequent course of treatment.

A dose of 2.5 mg/kg/day should not be exceeded. ECG changes of unknown significance have been reported in pediatric patients with doses twice this amount.

The safety and effectiveness of Imipramine as temporary adjunctive therapy for nocturnal enuresis in children less than 6 years of age has not been established.

IMIPRAMINE HYDROCHLORIDE, INTRAMUSCULAR
Initially, up to 100 mg/day intramuscularly in divided doses. Parenteral administration should be used only for starting therapy in patients unable or unwilling to use oral medication. The oral form should supplant the injectable as soon as possible.

IMIPRAMINE PAMOATE
The following recommended dosages for Imipramine Pamoate should be modified as necessary by the clinical response and any evidence of intolerance.

INITIAL ADULT DOSAGE
Outpatients: Therapy should be initiated at 75 mg/day. Dosage may be increased to 150 mg/day which is the dose level at which optimum response is usually obtained. If necessary, dosage may be increased to 200 mg/day.

Dosage higher than 75 mg/day may also be administered on a once-a-day basis after the optimum dosage and tolerance have been determined. The daily dosage may be given at bedtime. In some patients it may be necessary to employ a divided-dose schedule.

As with all tricyclics, the antidepressant effect of Imipramine may not be evident for one to three weeks in some patients.

Hospitalized Patients: Therapy should be initiated at 100-150 mg/day and may be increased to 200 mg/day. If there is no response after two weeks, dosage should be increased to 250-300 mg/day.

Dosage higher than 150 mg/day may also be administered on a once-a-day basis after the optimum dosage and tolerance have been determined. The daily dosage may be given at bedtime. In some patients it may be necessary to employ a divided-dose schedule.

As with all tricyclics, the antidepressant effect of Imipramine may not be evident for one to three weeks in some patients.

Adult Maintenance Dosage: Following remission, maintenance medication may be required for a longer period of time at the lowest dose that will maintain remission after which the dosage should gradually be decreased.

The usual maintenance dosage is 75-150 mg/day. The total daily dosage can be administered on a once-a-day basis, preferably at bedtime. In some patients it may be necessary to employ a divided-dose schedule.

In cases of relapse due to premature withdrawal of the drug, the effective dosage of Imipramine should be reinstituted.

Adolescent and Geriatic Patients: Therapy in these age groups should be initiated with Imipramine Hydrochloride tablets at a total daily dosage of 25-50 mg, since Imipramine Pamoate capsules are not available in these strengths. Dosage may be increased according to response and tolerance, but it is generally unnecessary to exceed 100 mg/day in these patients. Imipramine Pamoate capsules may be used when total daily dosage is established at 75 mg or higher. The total daily dosage can be administered on a once-a-day basis, preferably at bedtime. In some patients it may be necessary to employ a divided-dose schedule.

As with all tricyclics, the antidepressant effect of Imipramine may not be evident for one to three weeks in some patients.

Adolescent and geriatric patients can usually be maintained at lower dosage. Following remission, maintenance medication may be required for a longer period of time at the lowest dose that will maintain remission after which the dosage should gradually be decreased.

The total daily maintenance dosage can be administered on a once-a-day basis, preferably at bedtime. In some patients it may be necessary to employ a divided-dose schedule.

In cases of relapse due to premature withdrawal of the drug, the effective dosage of Imipramine should be reinstituted.

OVERDOSAGE
Children have been reported to be more sensitive than adults to an acute overdosage of Imipramine. An acute overdose of any amount in infants or young children, especially, must be considered serious and potentially fatal.

Signs and Symptoms: These may vary in severity depending upon factors such as the amount of drug absorbed, the age of the patient, and the interval between drug ingestion and the start of treatment. Blood and urine levels of Imipramine may not reflect the severity of poisoning; they have chiefly a qualitative rather than quantitative value, and are unreliable indicators in the clinical management of the patient.

CNS abnormalities may include drowsiness, stupor, coma, ataxia, restlessness, agitation, hyperactive reflexes, muscle rigidity, athetoid and choreiform movements and convulsions.

Cardiac abnormalities may include arrhythmia, tachycardia, ECG evidence of impaired conduction, and signs of congestive failure.

Respiratory depression, cyanosis, hypotension, shock, vomiting, hyperpyrexia, mydriasis, and diaphoresis may also be present.

Treatment: The recommended treatment for overdosage with tricyclic antidepressants may change periodically. Therefore, it is recommended that the physician contact a poison control center for current information on treatment. Because CNS involvement, respiratory depression and cardiac arrhythmia can occur suddenly, hospitalization and close observation may be necessary, even when the amount ingested is thought to be small or the initial degree of intoxication appears slight or moderate. All patients with ECG abnormalities should have continuous cardiac monitoring and be closely observed until well after cardiac status has returned to normal; relapses may occur after apparent recovery.

In the alert patient, empty the stomach promptly by lavage. In the obtunded patient, secure the airway with a cuffed endotracheal tube before beginning lavage (do not induce emesis). Instillation of activated charcoal slurry may help reduce absorption of Imipramine.

Minimize external stimulation to reduce the tendency to convulsions. If anticonvulsants are necessary, diazepam, and phenytoin may be useful.

Maintain adequate respiratory exchange. Do not use respiratory stimulants.

Shock should be treated with supportive measures, such as appropriate position, intravenous fluids, and, if necessary, a vasopressor agent. The use of corticosteroids in shock is controversial and may be contraindicated in cases of overdosage with tricyclic antidepressants. Digitalis may increase conduction abnormalities and further irritate an already sensitized myocardium. If congestive heart failure necessitates rapid digitalization, particular care must be exercised.

Hyperpyrexia should be controlled by whatever external means are available, inclding ice packs and cooling sponge baths, if necessary.

Hemodialysis, peritoneal dialysis, exchange transfusions and forced diuresis have been generally reported as ineffective because of the rapid fixation of Imipramine in tissues. Blood and urine levels of Imipramine may not correlate with the degree of intoxication, and are unreliable indicators in the clinical management of the patient.

The slow intravenous administration of physostigmine salicylate has been used as a last resort to reverse severe CNS anticholinergic manifestations of overdosage with tricyclic antidepressants; however, it should not be used routinely, since it may induce seizures and cholinergic crises.

Store between 59°-86° (15°-30°C)
Dispense in tight container (USP).

Note: Upon storage, minute crystals may form in some ampuls. This has no influence on the therapeutic efficacy of the preparation, and the crystals redissolve when the affected ampuls are immersed in hot tap water for 1 minute.

ANIMAL PHARMACOLOGY AND TOXICOLOGY
IMIPRAMINE HYDROCHLORIDE
A. Acute: Oral LD_{50} ranges are as follows:
Rat   355 to 682 mg/kg
Dog   100 to 215 mg/kg

Depending on the dosage in both species, toxic signs proceeded progressively from depression, irregular respiration and ataxia to convulsions and death.

B. Reproduction/Teratogenic: The overall evaluation may be summed up in the following manner:

Oral: Independent studies in three species (rat, mouse and rabbit) revealed that when Imipramine is administered orally in doses up to approximately 2½ times the maximum human dose in the first 2 species and up to 25 times the maximum human dose in the third species, the drug is essentially free from teratogenic potential. In the three species studied, only one instance of fetal abnormality occurred (in the rabbit), and in that study there was likewise an abnormality in the control group. However, evidence does exist from the rat studies that some systemic and embryotoxic potential is demonstrable. This is manifested by reduced litter size, a slight increase in the stillborn rate and a reduction in the mean birth weight.

Parenteral: In contradistinction to the oral data, Impiramine does exhibit a slight but definite teratogenic potential when administered by the subcutaneous route. Drug effects on both the mother and fetus in the rabbit are manifested in higher resorption rates and decrease in mean fetal birth weights, while teratogenic findings occurred at a level of 5 times the maximum human dose. In the mouse, teratogenicity occurred in 1½ and 6½ times the maximum human dose, but no teratogenic effects were seen at levels 3 times the maximum human dose. Thus, in the mouse, the findings are equivocal.

IMIPRAMINE PAMOATE

A. Acute: Oral LD$_{50}$:

Mouse   2185 mg/kg
Rat (F)   1142 mg/kg
     (M)   1807 mg/kg
Rabbit   1016 mg/kg
Dog   693 mg/kg (Emesis ED$_{50}$)

B. Subacute: Two three-month studies in dogs gave evidence of an adverse drug effect on the testes, but only at the highest dose level employed. i.e., 90 mg/kg (10 times the maximum human dose). Depending on the histological section of the testes examined, the findings consisted of a range of degenerative changes up to and including complete atrophy of the seminiferous tubules, with spermatogenesis usually arrested.

Human studies show no definitive effect on sperm count, sperm motility, sperm morphology or volume of ejaculate.

Rat: One three-month study was done in rats at dosage levels comparable to those of the dog studies. No adverse drug effect on the testes was noted in this study, as confirmed by histological examination.

C. Reproduction/Teratogenic:

Oral: Imipramine Pamoate was fed to male and female albino rats for 28 weeks through two breeding cycles at dose levels of 15 mg/kg/day and 40 mg/kg/day (equivalent to 2½ and 7 times the maximum human dose). No abnormalities which could be related to drug administration were noted in gross inspection. Autopsies performed on pups from the second breeding likewise revealed no pathological changes in organs or tissues; however, a decrease in mean litter size from both matings was noted in the drug-treated groups and significant growth suppression occurred in the nursing pups of both sexes in the high group as well as in the females of the low-level group. Finally, the lactation index (pups weaned divided by number left to nurse) was significantly lower in the second litter of the high-level group.

J CODES
Up to 25 mg IM—J3270

HOW SUPPLIED

IMIPRAMINE HYDROCHLORIDE
INJECTION: 12.5 MG/ML

BRAND/MANUFACTURER	NDC	SIZE	AWP
○ **BRAND**			
TOFRANIL: Geigy	00028-0065-23	2 ml 10s	$22.52

TABLET: 10 MG

AVERAGE UNIT PRICE (AVAILABLE SIZES)		GENERIC A-RATED AVERAGE PRICE (GAAP)	
BRAND	$0.26	100s	$4.86
GENERIC	$0.04	750s	$49.58
HCFA FUL (100s ea)	$0.02	1000s	$24.06

BRAND/MANUFACTURER	NDC	SIZE	AWP
◆ **BRAND**			
➤ TOFRANIL: Geigy	00028-0032-01	100s	$26.09
◆ **GENERICS**			
Medirex	57480-0403-06	30s	$2.40
Rugby	00536-3929-01	100s	$2.85
Biocraft	00332-2111-09	100s	$3.07
Moore,H.L.	00839-1370-06	100s	$3.09
Qualitest	00603-4043-21	100s	$3.12
Mutual	53489-0330-01	100s	$3.90
URL	00677-0421-01	100s	$4.32
Purepac	00228-2231-10	100s	$4.40
Schein	00364-0443-01	100s	$4.45
Geneva	00781-1762-01	100s	$4.47
Par	49884-0054-01	100s	$4.50
Goldline	00182-0826-01	100s	$4.50
Martec	52555-0254-01	100s	$4.60
Aligen	00405-4534-01	100s	$4.62
Parmed	00349-2079-01	100s	$4.95
U.S. Trading	56126-0054-11	100s ud	$3.15
Raway	00686-0079-20	100s ud	$5.95
Vangard	00615-0528-13	100s ud	$6.61
UDL	51079-0079-20	100s ud	$7.98
TIPRAMINE: Major	00904-0925-61	100s ud	$11.89
TIPRAMINE: Major	00904-0925-70	250s	$6.70
Glasgow	60809-0104-55	750s ud	$49.58
Glasgow	60809-0104-72	750s ud	$49.58
TIPRAMINE: Major	00904-0925-80	1000s	$17.10
Moore,H.L.	00839-1370-16	1000s	$19.83
Rugby	00536-3929-10	1000s	$20.25
URL	00677-0421-10	1000s	$21.38
Qualitest	00603-4043-32	1000s	$21.40
Mutual	53489-0330-10	1000s	$21.60
Biocraft	00332-2111-15	1000s	$21.85
Par	49884-0054-10	1000s	$31.15
Martec	52555-0254-10	1000s	$31.80
Parmed	00349-2079-10	1000s	$34.26

TABLET: 25 MG

AVERAGE UNIT PRICE (AVAILABLE SIZES)		GENERIC A-RATED AVERAGE PRICE (GAAP)	
BRAND	$0.44	100s	$6.69
GENERIC	$0.06	750s	$60.15
HCFA FUL (100s ea)	$0.02	1000s	$40.88

BRAND/MANUFACTURER	NDC	SIZE	AWP
◆ **BRAND**			
➤ TOFRANIL: Geigy	00028-0140-01	100s	$43.63
◆ **GENERICS**			
Medirex	57480-0404-06	30s	$3.05
Qualitest	00603-4044-21	100s	$3.15
Biocraft	00332-2113-09	100s	$3.42
Moore,H.L.	00839-1371-06	100s	$3.77
Rugby	00536-3930-01	100s	$3.83
URL	00677-0422-01	100s	$4.59
Schein	00364-0406-01	100s	$4.60
➤ Geneva	00781-1764-01	100s	$4.62
Mutual	53489-0331-01	100s	$4.70
Par	49884-0055-01	100s	$6.05
Goldline	00182-0827-01	100s	$6.05
Aligen	00405-4535-01	100s	$6.10
Martec	52555-0255-01	100s	$6.17
Parmed	00349-2080-01	100s	$6.25
U.S. Trading	56126-0055-11	100s ud	$4.31
Raway	00686-0080-20	100s ud	$6.50
Vangard	00615-0529-13	100s ud	$8.02
UDL	51079-0080-20	100s ud	$10.14
➤ Geneva	00781-1764-13	100s ud	$10.15
Goldline	00182-0827-89	100s ud	$10.30
Roxane	00054-8419-25	100s ud	$10.54
TIPRAMINE: Major	00904-0927-61	100s ud	$17.23
TIPRAMINE: Major	00904-0927-70	250s	$7.65
Glasgow	60809-0105-55	750s	$60.15
Glasgow	60809-0105-72	750s ud	$60.15
Qualitest	00603-4044-32	1000s	$22.30
Schein	00364-0406-02	1000s	$23.70
Moore,H.L.	00839-1371-16	1000s	$26.31
Rugby	00536-3930-10	1000s	$26.70
TIPRAMINE: Major	00904-0927-80	1000s	$29.25
Mutual	53489-0331-10	1000s	$29.75
URL	00677-0422-10	1000s	$30.13
Biocraft	00332-2113-15	1000s	$33.16
➤ Geneva	00781-1764-10	1000s	$43.89
Purepac	00228-2232-96	1000s	$48.64
Par	49884-0055-10	1000s	$52.63
Goldline	00182-0827-10	1000s	$52.63
Aligen	00405-4535-03	1000s	$52.82
Martec	52555-0255-10	1000s	$53.68
Parmed	00349-2080-10	1000s	$57.95
Roxane	00054-4419-31	1000s	$70.53

For additional alternatives, turn to the section beginning on page 2859.

Imitrex *SEE* SUMATRIPTAN SUCCINATE

Imodium *SEE* LOPERAMIDE HYDROCHLORIDE

Imogam Rabies *SEE* RABIES IMMUNE GLOBULIN (HUMAN)

Imovax Rabies *SEE* RABIES VACCINE *AND* RABIES VACCINE ADSORBED

Imuran *SEE* AZATHIOPRINE

Inapsine *SEE* DROPERIDOL

◆ RATED THERAPEUTICALLY EQUIVALENT; ◇ THERAPEUTIC EQUIVALENCE UNCONFIRMED; ○ UNRATED

Indapamide

DESCRIPTION

Indapamide is an oral antihypertensive/diuretic. Its molecule contains both a polar sulfamoyl chlorobenzamide moiety and a lipid-soluble methylindoline moiety. It differs chemically from the thiazides in that it does not possess the thiazide ring system and contains only one sulfonamide group. The chemical name of Indapamide is 1-(4-chloro-3-sulfamoylbenzamido)-2-methylindoline, and its molecular weight is 365.84. The compound is a weak acid, $pK_a = 8.8$, and is soluble in aqueous solutions of strong bases. It is a white to yellow-white crystalline (tetragonal) powder.

Following is its chemical structure:

CLINICAL PHARMACOLOGY

Indapamide is the first of a new class of antihypertensive/diuretics, the indolines. The oral administration of 2.5 mg (two 1.25 mg tablets) of Indapamide to male subjects produced peak concentrations of approximately 115 ng/mL of the drug in blood within two hours. The oral administration of 5 mg (two 2.5-mg tablets) of Indapamide to healthy male subjects produced peak concentrations of approximately 260 ng/mL of the drug in the blood within two hours. A minimum of 70% of a single oral dose is eliminated by the kidneys and an additional 23% by the gastrointestinal tract, probably including the biliary route. The half-life of Indapamide in whole blood is approximately 14 hours.

Indapamide is preferentially and reversibly taken up by the erythrocytes in the peripheral blood. The whole blood/plasma ratio is approximately 6:1 at the time of peak concentration and decreases to 3.5:1 at eight hours. From 71 to 79% of the Indapamide in plasma is reversibly bound to plasma proteins.

Indapamide is an extensively metabolized drug, with only about 7% of the total dose administered, recovered in the urine as unchanged drug during the first 48 hours after administration. The urinary elimination of ^{14}C-labeled Indapamide and metabolites is biphasic with a terminal half-life of excretion of total radioactivity of 26 hours.

In a parallel design double-blind, placebo controlled trial in hypertension, daily doses of Indapamide between 1.25 mg and 10.0 mg produced dose-related antihypertensive effects. Doses of 5.0 and 10.0 mg were not distinguishable from each other although each was differentiated from placebo and 1.25 mg Indapamide. At daily doses of 1.25 mg, 5.0 mg and 10.0 mg, a mean decrease of serum potassium of 0.28, 0.61 and 0.76 mEq/L, respectively, was observed and uric acid increased by about 0.69 mg/100 mL.

In other parallel design, dose-ranging clinical trials in hypertension and edema, daily doses of Indapamide between 0.5 and 5.0 mg produced dose-related effects. Generally, doses of 2.5 and 5.0 mg were not distinguishable from each other although each was differentiated from placebo and from 0.5 or 1.0 mg Indapamide. At daily doses of 2.5 and 5.0 mg a mean decrease of serum potassium of 0.5 and 0.6 mEq/Liter, respectively, was observed and uric acid increased by about 1.0 mg/100 mL.

At these doses, the effects of Indapamide on blood pressure and edema are approximately equal to those obtained with conventional doses of other antihypertensive/diuretics.

In hypertensive patients, daily doses of 1.25, 2.5 and 5.0 mg of Indapamide have no appreciable cardiac inotropic or chronotropic effect. The drug decreases peripheral resistance, with little or no effect on cardiac output, rate or rhythm. Chronic administration of Indapamide to hypertensive patients has little or no effect on glomerular filtration rate or renal plasma flow.

Indapamide had an antihypertensive effect in patients with varying degrees of renal impairment, although in general, diuretic effects declined as renal function decreased.

In a small number of controlled studies, Indapamide taken with other antihypertensive drugs such as hydralazine, propranolol, guanethidine, and methyldopa, appeared to have the additive effect typical of thiazide-type diuretics.

INDICATIONS

Indapamide is indicated for the treatment of hypertension, alone or in combination with other antihypertensive drugs.

Indapamide is also indicated for the treatment of salt and fluid retention associated with congestive heart failure.

Usage in Pregnancy: The routine use of diuretics in an otherwise healthy woman is inappropriate and exposes mother and fetus to unnecessary hazard (see *"Precautions"* below).

Diuretics do not prevent development of toxemia of pregnancy, and there is no satisfactory evidence that they are useful in the treatment of developed toxemia. Edema during pregnancy may arise from pathological causes or from the physiologic and mechanical consequences of pregnancy. Indapamide is indicated in pregnancy when edema is due to pathologic causes, just as it is in the absence of pregnancy (however, see *"Precautions"* below). Dependent edema in pregnancy, resulting from restriction of venous return by the expanded uterus, is properly treated through elevation of the lower extremities and use of support hose; use of diuretics to lower intravascular volume in this case is illogical and unnecessary. There is hypervolemia during normal pregnancy which is not harmful to either the fetus or the mother (in the absence of cardiovascular disease), but which is associated with edema, including generalized edema in the majority of pregnant women. If this edema produces discomfort, increased recumbency will often provide relief. In rare instances, this edema may cause extreme discomfort which is not relieved by rest. In these cases, a short course of diuretics may provide relief and may be appropriate.

CONTRAINDICATIONS

Anuria. Known hypersensitivity to Indapamide or to other sulfonamide-derived drugs.

WARNINGS

Infrequent cases of severe hyponatremia, accompanied by hypokalemia, have been reported with 2.5 mg and 5.0 mg Indapamide primarily in elderly females. Symptoms were reversed by electrolyte replenishment. Hyponatremia considered possibly clinically significant (< 125 mEq/L) has not been observed in clinical trials with the 1.25 mg dosage (see *"Precautions"*).

Hypokalemia occurs commonly with diuretics (see *"Adverse Reactions, Hypokalemia"*), and electrolyte monitoring is essential, particularly in patients who would be at increased risk from hypokalemia, such as those with cardiac arrhythmias or who are receiving concomitant cardiac glycosides.

In general, diuretics should not be given concomitantly with lithium because they reduce its renal clearance and add a high risk of lithium toxicity. Read prescribing information for lithium preparations before use of such concomitant therapy.

PRECAUTIONS

GENERAL

1. Hypokalemia, Hyponatremia, and Other Fluid and Electrolyte Imbalances: Periodic determinations of serum electrolytes should be performed at appropriate intervals. In addition, patients should be observed for clinical signs of fluid or electrolyte imbalance, such as hyponatremia, hypochloremic alkalosis, or hypokalemia. Warning signs include dry mouth, thirst, weakness, fatigue, lethargy, drowsiness, restlessness, muscle pains or cramps, hypotension, oliguria, tachycardia, and gastrointestinal disturbance. Electrolyte determinations are particularly important in patients who are vomiting excessively or receiving parenteral fluids, in patients subject to electrolyte imbalance (including those with heart failure, kidney disease, and cirrhosis), and in patients on a salt-restricted diet.

The risk of hypokalemia secondary to diuresis and natriuresis is increased when larger doses are used, when the diuresis is brisk, when severe cirrhosis is present and during concomitant use of corticosteroids or ACTH. Interference with adequate oral intake of electrolytes will also contribute to hypokalemia. Hypokalemia can sensitize or exaggerate the response of the heart to the toxic effects of digitalis, such as increased ventricular irritability.

Dilutional hyponatremia may occur in edematous patients; the appropriate treatment is restriction of water rather than administration of salt, except in rare instances when the hyponatremia is life threatening. However, in actual salt depletion, appropriate replacement is the treatment of choice. Any chloride deficit that may occur during treatment is generally mild and usually does not require specific treatment except in extraordinary circumstances as in liver or renal disease. Thiazide-like diuretics have been shown to increase the urinary excretion of magnesium; this may result in hypomagnesemia.

2. Hyperuricemia and Gout: Serum concentrations of uric acid increased by an average of 0.69 mg/100 mL in patients treated with Indapamide 1.25 mg, and by an average of 1.0 mg/100 mL in patients treated with Indapamide 2.5 mg and 5.0 mg and frank gout may be precipitated in certain patients receiving Indapamide (see *"Adverse Reactions"* below). Serum concentrations of uric acid should, therefore, be monitored periodically during treatment.

3. Renal Impairment: Indapamide, like the thiazides, should be used with caution in patients with severe renal disease, as reduced plasma volume may exacerbate or precipitate azotemia. If progressive renal impairment is observed in a patient receiving Indapamide, withholding or discontinuing diuretic therapy should be considered. Renal function tests should be performed periodically during treatment with Indapamide.

4. Impaired Hepatic Function: Indapamide, like the thiazides, should be used with caution in patients with impaired hepatic function or progressive liver disease, since minor alterations of fluid and electrolyte balance may precipitate hepatic coma.

5. Glucose Tolerance: Latent diabetes may become manifest and insulin requirements in diabetic patients may be altered during thiazide administration. A mean increase in glucose of 6.47 mg/dL was observed in patients treated with Indapamide 1.25 mg, which was not considered clinically significant in these trials. Serum concentrations of glucose should be monitored routinely during treatment with Indapamide.

6. Calcium Excretion: Calcium excretion is decreased by diuretics pharmacologically related to Indapamide. After six to eight weeks of Indapamide 1.25 mg treatment and in long-term studies of hypertensive patients with higher doses of Indapamide, however, serum concentrations of calcium increased only slightly with Indapamide. Prolonged treatment with drugs pharmacologically related to Indapamide may in rare instances be associated with hypercalcemia and hypophosphatemia secondary to physiologic changes in the parathyroid gland;

however, the common complications of hyperparathyroidism, such as renal lithiasis, bone resorption, and peptic ulcer, have not been seen. Treatment should be discontinued before tests for parathyroid function are performed. Like the thiazides, Indapamide may decrease serum PBI levels without signs of thyroid disturbance.

7. *Interaction With Systemic Lupus Erthematosus:* Thiazides have exacerbated or activated systemic lupus erythematosus and this possibility should be considered with Indapamide as well.

DRUG INTERACTIONS
1. *Other Antihypertensives:* Indapamide may add to or potentiate the action of other antihypertensive drugs. In limited controlled trials that compared the effect of Indapamide combined with other antihypertensive drugs with the effect of the other drugs administered alone, there was no notable change in the nature or frequency of adverse reactions associated with the combined therapy.

2. *Lithium:* See *"Warnings"*.

3. *Post-Sympathectomy Patient:* The antihypertensive effect of the drug may be enhanced in the postsympathectomized patient.

4. *Norepinephrine:* Indapamide, like the thiazides, may decrease arterial responsiveness to norepinephrine, but this diminution is not sufficient to preclude effectiveness of the pressor agent for therapeutic use.

Carcinogenesis, Mutagenesis, Impairment of Fertility: Both mouse and rat lifetime carcinogenicity studies were conducted. There was no significant difference in the incidence of tumors between the Indapamide-treated animals and the control groups.

Pregnancy/Teratogenic Effects: Pregnancy Category B. Reproduction studies have been performed in rats, mice, and rabbits at doses up to 6,250 times the therapeutic human dose and have revealed no evidence of impaired fertility or harm to the fetus due to Indapamide. Postnatal development in rats and mice was unaffected by pretreatment of parent animals during gestation. There are, however, no adequate and well-controlled studies in pregnant women. Moreover, diuretics are known to cross the placental barrier and appear in cord blood. Because animal reproduction studies are not always predictive of human response, this drug should be used during pregnancy only if clearly needed. There may be hazards associated with this use such as fetal or neonatal jaundice, thrombocytopenia, and possibly other adverse reactions that have occurred in the adult.

Nursing Mothers: It is not known whether this drug is excreted in human milk. Because most drugs are excreted in human milk, if use of this drug is deemed essential, the patient should stop nursing.

ADVERSE REACTIONS
Most adverse effects have been mild and transient.

The clinical adverse reactions listed in table 1 represent data from Phase II/III placebo-controlled studies (306 patients given Indapamide 1.25 mg). The clinical adverse reactions listed in table 2 represent data from Phase II placebo-controlled studies and long-term controlled clinical trials (426 patients given Indapamide 2.5 mg or 5.0 mg). The reactions are arranged into two groups: 1) a cumulative incidence equal to or greater than 5%; 2) a cumulative incidence less than 5%. Reactions are counted regardless of reaction to drug.

Table 1
ADVERSE REACTIONS FROM STUDIES OF 1.25 MG

Incidence ≥ 5%	*Incidence* < 5%*
Body as a Whole	
Headache	Asthenia
Infection	Flu Syndrome
Pain	Abdominal Pain
Back Pain	Chest Pain
Gastrointestinal System	Constipation
	Diarrhea
	Dyspepsia
	Nausea
Metabolic System	Peripheral Edema
Central Nervous System	Nervousness
Dizziness	Hypertonia
Respiratory System	Cough
Rhinitis	Pharyngitis
	Sinusitis
Special Senses	Conjunctivitis

* *Other*

All other clinical adverse reactions occurred at an incidence of < 1%.

Approximately 4% of patients given Indapamide 1.25 mg compared to 5% of the patients given placebo discontinued treatment in the trials of up to eight weeks because of adverse reactions.

In controlled clinical trials of six to eight weeks in duration, 20% of patients receiving Indapamide 1.25 mg, 61% of patients receiving Indapamide 5.0 mg, and 80% of patients receiving Indapamide 10.0 mg had at least one potassium value below 3.4 mEq/L. In the Indapamide 1.25 mg group, about 40% of those patients who reported hypokalemia as a laboratory adverse event returned to normal serum potassium values without intervention. Hypokalemia with concomitant

clinical signs or symptoms occurred in 2% of patients receiving Indapamide 1.25 mg.

Table 2
ADVERSE REACTIONS FROM STUDIES OF 2.5 MG AND 5.0 MG

Incidence ≥ 5%	*Incidence* < 5%
Central Nervous System/ Neuromuscular	
Headache	Light-headedness
Dizziness	Drowsiness
Fatigue, weakness, loss of energy, lethargy, tiredness, or malaise	Vertigo
	Insomnia
	Depression
Muscle cramps or spasm, or numbness of the extremities	Blurred Vision
Nervousness, tension, anxiety, irritability, or agitation	
Gastrointestinal System	Constipation
	Nausea
	Vomiting
	Diarrhea
	Gastric irritation
	Abdominal pain or cramps
	Anorexia
Cardiovascular System	Orthostatic hypotension
	Premature ventricular contractions
	Irregular heart beat
	Palpitations
Genitourinary System	Frequency of urination
	Nocturia Polyuria
Dermatologic/Hypersensitivity	Rash
	Hives
	Pruritus
	Vasculitis
Other	Impotence or reduced libido
	Rhinorrhea
	Flushing
	Hyperuricemia
	Hyperglycemia
	Hyponatremia
	Hypochloremia
	Increase in serum urea nitrogen (BUN) or creatinine
	Glycosuria
	Weight loss
	Dry mouth
	Tingling of extremities

Because most of these data are from long-term studies (up to 40 weeks of treatment), it is probable that many of the adverse experiences reported are due to causes other than the drug. Approximately 10% of patients given Indapamide discontinued treatment in long-term trials because of reactions either related or unrelated to the drug.

Hypokalemia with concomitant clinical signs or symptoms occurred in 3% of patients receiving Indapamide 2.5 mg q.d. and 7% of patients receiving Indapamide 5 mg q.d. In long-term controlled clinical trials comparing the hypokalemic effects of daily doses of Indapamide and hydrochlorothiazide, however, 47% of patients receiving Indapamide 2.5 mg, 72% of patients receiving Indapamide 5 mg, and 44% of patients receiving hydrochlorothiazide 50 mg had at least one potassium value (out of a total of 11 taken during the study) below 3.5 mEq/L. In the Indapamide 2.5 mg group, over 50% of those patients returned to normal serum potassium values without intervention.

In clinical trials of six to eight weeks, the mean changes in selected values were as shown in the tables below.

MEAN CHANGES FROM BASELINE AFTER 8 WEEKS OF TREATMENT —1.25 MG

	Serum Electrolytes (mEq/L) Potassium Sodium Chloride			Serum Uric Acid (mg/dL)	BUN (mg/ dL)
Indapamide 1.25 mg (n = 255-257)	− 0.28	− 0.63	− 2.60	0.69	1.46
Placebo (n = 263-266)	0.00	− 0.11	− 0.21	0.06	0.06

No patients receiving Indapamide 1.25 mg experienced hyponatremia considered possibly clinically significant (< 125 mEq/L).

Indapamide had no adverse effects on lipids.

◆ RATED THERAPEUTICALLY EQUIVALENT; ◇ THERAPEUTIC EQUIVALENCE UNCONFIRMED; ○ UNRATED

MEAN CHANGES FROM BASELINE AFTER 40 WEEKS OF TREATMENT — 2.5 MG AND 5.0 MG

	Serum Electrolytes (mEq/L) Potassium Sodium Chloride			Serum Uric Acid (mg/dL)	BUN (mg/dL)
Indapamide 2.5 mg (n = 76)	− 0.4	− 0.6	− 3.6	0.7	− 0.1
Indapamide 5.0 mg (n = 81)	− 0.6	− 0.7	− 5.1	1.1	1.4

Other adverse reactions reported with antihypertensive/diuretics are jaundice (intrahepatic cholestatic jaundice), sialadenitis, xanthopsia, photosensitivity, purpura, bullous eruptions, Stevens-Johnson Syndrome, necrotizing angiitis, fever, respiratory distress (including pneumonitis), and anaphylactic reactions; also, agranulocytosis, leukopenia, thrombocytopenia, and aplastic anemia. These reactions should be considered as possible occurrence with clinical usage of Indapamide.

OVERDOSAGE

Symptoms of overdosage include nausea, vomiting, weakness, gastrointestinal disorders and disturbances of electrolyte balance. In severe instances, hypotension and depressed respiration may be observed. If this occurs, support of respiration and cardiac circulation should be instituted. There is no specific antidote. An evacuation of the stomach is recommended by emesis and gastric lavage after which the electrolyte and fluid balance should be evaluated carefully.

DOSAGE AND ADMINISTRATION

Hypertension: The adult starting Indapamide dose for hypertension is 1.25 mg as a single daily dose taken in the morning. If the response to 1.25 mg is not satisfactory after four weeks, the daily dose may be increased to 2.5 mg taken once daily. If the response to 2.5 mg is not satisfactory after four weeks, the daily dose may be increased to 5.0 mg taken once daily, but adding another antihypertensive should be considered.

Edema of Congestive Heart Failure: The adult starting Indapamide dose for edema of congestive heart failure is 2.5 mg as a single daily dose taken in the morning. If the response to 2.5 mg is not satisfactory after one week, the daily dose may be increased to 5.0 mg taken once daily.

If the antihypertensive response to Indapamide is insufficient, Indapamide may be combined with other antithypertensive drugs, with careful monitoring of blood pressure. It is recommended that the usual dose of other agents be reduced by 50% during initial combination therapy. As the blood pressure response becomes evident, further dosage adjustments may be necessary.

In general, doses of 5.0 mg and larger have not appeared to provide additional effects on blood pressure or heart failure, but are associated with a greater degree of hypokalemia. There is minimal clinical trial experience in patients with doses greater than 5.0 mg once a day.

Keep tightly closed. Store at controlled room temperature, 15°-30°C (59°-86°F). Avoid excessive heat. Dispense in tight containers as defined in USP.

HOW SUPPLIED
TABLETS: 1.25 MG

BRAND/MANUFACTURER	NDC	SIZE	AWP
○ BRAND			
▶ LOZOL: RPR	00075-0700-00	100s	$63.04

TABLETS: 2.5 MG

BRAND/MANUFACTURER	NDC	SIZE	AWP
○ BRAND			
▶ LOZOL: RPR	00075-0082-00	100s	$79.93
	00075-0082-62	100s ud	$79.93
	00075-0082-99	1000s	$789.00
	00075-0082-23	20000s	$14704.85
○ GENERICS			
Aligen	00405-4538-01	100s	$65.98
Arcola	00070-3000-00	100s	$65.98
Arcola	00070-3000-99	1000s	$651.30

Inderal *SEE* PROPRANOLOL HYDROCHLORIDE

Inderide *SEE* HYDROCHLOROTHIAZIDE AND PROPRANOLOL HYDROCHLORIDE

Indigotindisulfonate Sodium

DESCRIPTION

Each 5 mL contains: 40 mg of Indigotindisulfonate Sodium, in Water for Injection, q.s. pH adjusted, when necessary, with Citric Acid and/or Sodium Citrate. Sterile, nonpyrogenic.

Sufficient Indigotindisulfonate Sodium is contained in each 5 mL ampule to permit accurate withdrawal and administration of the full dose. It gives a deep blue solution when dissolved in water. Its molecular formula is $C_{16}H_8N_2Na_2O_8S_2$ and molecular weight is 466.35.

Following is its chemical structure:

CLINICAL PHARMACOLOGY

Indigotindisulfonate Sodium is excreted largely by the kidneys, retaining its blue color during passage through the body.

Elimination of the dye begins soon after injection, appearing in the urine within 10 minutes in average cases. The biological half-life is 4 to 5 minutes following intravenous injection. Larger quantities are necessary when intramuscular injection is employed. Appearance time and elimination are delayed following intramuscular injection.

INDICATIONS

Originally employed as a kidney function test, the chief application of Indigotindisulfonate Sodium at present is localizing ureteral orifices during cystoscopy and ureteral catheterization.

CONTRAINDICATIONS

Indigotindisulfonate Sodium is contraindicated in patients who have previously experienced an adverse reaction following its use.

WARNINGS

An occasional idiosyncratic drug reaction may occur. A mild pressor effect may be encountered in some patients.

Since precipitation of Indigotindisulfonate Sodium may occur, Indigotindisulfonate Sodium Solution must **not** be diluted prior to injection or injected with infusion assemblies which were used with other solutions.

PRECAUTIONS

Indigotindisulfonate Sodium should be stored in the dark, away from direct light, preferably in the original package.

Pregnancy Category C: Animal Reproduction studies have not been conducted with Indigotindisulfonate Sodium injection. It is also not known whether Indigotindisulfonate Sodium injection can cause fetal harm when administered to a pregnant woman or can affect reproduction capacity. Indigotindisulfonate Sodium injection should be given to a pregnant woman only if clearly needed.

It is not known whether this drug is excreted in human milk. Because many drugs are excreted in human milk, caution should be exercised when Indigotindisulfonate Sodium is administered to a nursing woman.

ADVERSE REACTIONS

See *"Warning"* section.

DRUG ABUSE AND DEPENDENCE

Indigotindisulfonate Sodium is not a controlled substance listed in any of the Drug Enforcement Administration Schedules. Its use is not known to lead to dependence or abuse.

OVERDOSAGE

There are no data available describing the signs, symptoms or laboratory findings accompanying overdosage.

No discernible symptoms of toxicity have been observed in mice with an intravenous dose of 200 mg/kg. After intravenous administration the LD_{80} was established at 300 mg/kg in mice.

DOSAGE AND ADMINISTRATION

Indigotindisulfonate Sodium solution is injected either by the intravenous or intramuscular route, and its appearance at the ureteral orifices is watched with the cystoscope in place. The intravenous method is preferred because a 5 mL injection is sufficient. A lesser dosage in infants, children and underweight patients will prevent skin coloration.

Parenteral drug products should be inspected visually for particulate matter and discoloration prior to administration, whenever solution and container permit.

Protect from light
Store at controlled room temperature 15°-30°C (59°-86°F).

HOW SUPPLIED
INJECTION: 0.8%

BRAND/MANUFACTURER	NDC	SIZE	AWP
○ GENERICS			
Amer Regent	00517-0375-10	5 ml 10s	$90.00
Pasadena	00418-2501-31	5 ml 10s	$130.90
CMC-Cons	00223-7902-05	5 ml 10s	$150.00

INJECTION: 8 MG/ML

BRAND/MANUFACTURER	NDC	SIZE	AWP
○ GENERICS			
BD Microbiology	00011-8366-09	5 ml 10s	$102.00
Raway	00686-0375-10	5 ml 10s	$120.00

Indium In-111 Pentetreotide

DESCRIPTION
Indium In-111 Pentetreotide is a diagnostic radiopharmaceutical consisting of two components:

—10 μg Pentetreotide [N-(diethylenetriamine-N,N,N′,N″-tetraacetic acid-N″-acetyl)-D-phenyl-alanyl-L-hemicystyl-L-phenyl-alanyl-D-tryptophyl-L -lysyl-L-threonyl-L-hemicystyl-L-threoninol cyclic (2→7) disulfide], (also known as octreotide DTPA).

—Indium In-111 chloride sterile solution contains: 1.1 mL of 111 MBq/mL (3.0 mCi/mL) Indium In-111 chloride in 0.02N HCl at time of calibration. The contents are sterile and nonpyrogenic.

Indium In-111 Pentetreotide is prepared by combining the two components (see *"Instructions for the Preparation of Indium In-111 Pentetreotide"*). Indium In-111 reacts with the diethylenetriaminetetraacetic acid portion of the Pentetreotide molecule to form Indium In-111 Pentetreotide. The pH of the resultant Indium In-111 Pentetreotide solution is between 3.8 and 4.3.

The Indium In-111 Pentetreotide solution is suitable for intravenous administration as is, or it may be diluted to a maximum volume of 3.0 mL with 0.9% sodium chloride injection immediately before intravenous administration. In either case, the labeling yield of Indium In-111 Pentetreotide should be determined before administration to the patient. A method recommended for determining the labeling yield is presented at the end of this material.

PHYSICAL CHARACTERISTICS
Indium In-111 decays by electron capture to cadmium-111 (stable) and has a physical half-life of 2.805 days (67.32 hours).[1] The principal photons that are useful for detection and imaging are listed in Table 1.

Table 1
PRINCIPAL RADIATION EMISSION DATA[2]

Radiation	Mean Percent Per Disintegration	Energy (keV)
Gamma-2	90.2	171.3
Gamma-3	94.0	245.4

The specific gamma ray constant for In-111 is 3.21 R/hr-mCi at 1 cm[1]. The first half-value thickness of lead (Pb) for In-111 is 0.023 cm. Selected coefficients of attenuation are listed in Table 2 as a function of lead shield thickness. For example, the use of 0.834 cm of lead will attenuate the external radiation by a factor of about 1000.

Table 2
RADIATION ATTENUATION BY LEAD SHIELDING[1]

Shield Thickness (Pb) cm	Coefficient of Attenuation
0.023	0.5
0.203	0.1
0.513	0.01
0.834	0.001
1.12	0.0001

Table 3 lists fractions remaining at selected time intervals before and after calibration. This information may be used to correct for physical decay of the radionuclide.

Table 3
PHYSICAL DECAY CHART: INDIUM IN-111, HALF-LIFE 2.805 DAYS (67.32 HOURS)

Hours	Fraction Remaining	Hours	Fraction Remaining
−72	2.100	0*	1.000
−60	1.854	3	0.970
−48	1.639	6	0.940
−36	1.448	12	0.885
−24	1.280	24	0.781
−12	1.131	36	0.690
−6	1.064	48	0.610

* Calibration time

CLINICAL PHARMACOLOGY
General: Pentetreotide is a DTPA conjugate of octreotide, which is a long-acting analog of the human hormone, somatostatin. Indium In-111 Pentetreotide binds to somatostatin receptors on cell surfaces throughout the body. Within an hour of injection, most of the dose of Indium In-111 Pentetreotide distributes from plasma to extravascular body tissues and concentrates in tumors containing a high density of somatostatin receptors. After background clearance, visualization of somatostatin receptor-rich tissue is achieved. In addition to somatostatin receptor-rich tumors, the normal pituitary gland, thyroid gland, liver, spleen and urinary bladder also are visualized in most patients, as is the bowel, to a lesser extent. Excretion is almost exclusively via the kidneys.

Pharmacokinetics: Radioactivity leaves the plasma rapidly; one-third of the radioactive injected dose remains in the blood pool at 10 minutes after administration. Plasma levels continue to decline so that by 20 hours post-injection, about 1% of the radioactive dose is found in the blood pool. The biological half-life of Indium In-111 Pentetreotide is 6 hours.

Half of the injected dose is recoverable in urine within six hours after injection, 85% is recovered in the first 24 hours, and over 90% is recovered in urine by two days.

Hepatobiliary excretion represents a minor route of elimination, and less than 2% of the injected dose is recovered in feces within three days after injection.

Metabolism: For several hours after administration, plasma radioactivity is predominantly in parent form. Ten percent of the radioactivity excreted is nonpeptide-bound.

Pharmacodynamics: Indium In-111 Pentetreotide binds to cell surface receptors for somatostatin. In nonclinical pharmacologic studies, the hormonal effect of Indium In-111 Pentetreotide *in vitro* is one-tenth that of octreotide. Since diagnostic imaging doses of Indium In-111 Pentetreotide are lower than the therapeutic doses of octreotide, Indium In-111 Pentetreotide is not expected to exert clinically significant somatostatin effects.

Indium In-111 Pentetreotide is cleared from the body primarily by renal excretion. Indium In-111 Pentetreotide elimination has not been studied in anephric patients or in those with poorly functioning kidneys. It is not known whether Indium In-111 Pentetreotide can be removed by dialysis. Dosage adjustments in patients with decreased renal function have not been studied.

CLINICAL TRIALS
Indium In-111 Pentetreotide was studied in nine unblinded clinical studies in a total of 365 patients. Of these patients, 174 were male and 191 were female. Their mean age was 54.0 years (range 1.8 to 86 years). One patient was under the age of 2 and 2 patients were between the ages of 2 and 12; 223 patients (61.1%) were between 18 and 60 years; and 136 patients (37.3%) were older than 60 years. A racial distribution is not available.

Eligible patients had a demonstrated or high clinical suspicion of a neuroendocrine tumor. The most common tumors were carcinoids (132 of 309 evaluable patients). Scintigraphic results were compared to results of conventional localization procedures (CT, ultrasound, MRI, angiography, surgery and/or biopsy). The mean dose of radioactivity administered was 173.4 MBq (4.7 mCi).

Indium In-111 Pentetreotide results were consistent with the final diagnosis (success) in 267 of 309 evaluable patients (86.4%). Compared with carcinoids and gastrinomas, lower success rates were noted for localization of insulinomas, neuroblastomas, pituitary adenomas and medullary thyroid carcinomas. Indium In-111 Pentetreotide success was observed in 27 of 32 patients (84.4%) with clinically nonfunctioning neuroendocrine tumors (i.e., no symptom of a clinical syndrome mediated by abnormally elevated hormones). Indium In-111 Pentetreotide localized previously unidentified tumors in 57/204 patients. In 55/195 patients, Indium In-111 Pentetreotide uptake occurred in lesions not thought to have somatostatin receptors. In a small subgroup of 39 patients who had tissue confirmation, the sensitivity rate for Indium In-111 Pentetreotide scintigraphy was 85.7%; for CT/MRI the rate was 68%. The specificity rate for Indium In-111 Pentetreotide scintigraphy was 50%, the rate for CT/MRI was 12%. Larger studies are needed to confirm these comparisons. Overall, including all tumor types with or without the presence of somatostatin receptors, there were 3/508 false positives and 104/508 false negatives.

Of the 309 patients, 87 had received octreotide for therapeutic purposes within 72 hours of Indium In-111 Pentetreotide administration. These patients had an overall 95% success rate. The effect of different dose levels of octreotide on success rates has not been evaluated.

INDICATIONS AND USAGE
Indium In-111 Pentetreotide is an agent for the scintigraphic localization of primary and metastatic neuroendocrine tumors bearing somatostatin receptors.

CONTRAINDICATIONS
None known.

WARNINGS
DO NOT ADMINISTER IN TOTAL PARENTERAL NUTRITION (TPN) ADMIXTURES OR INJECT INTO TPN INTRAVENOUS ADMINISTRATION LINES; IN THESE SOLUTIONS, A COMPLEX GLYCOSYL OCTREOTIDE CONJUGATE MAY FORM.

The sensitivity of scintigraphy with Indium In-111 Pentetreotide may be reduced in patients concurrently receiving therapeutic doses of octreotide acetate. Consideration should be given to temporarily suspending octreotide acetate therapy before the administration of Indium In-111 Pentetreotide and to monitoring the patient for any signs of withdrawal.

PRECAUTIONS
GENERAL
1. Therapy with octreotide acetate can produce severe hypoglycemia in patients with insulinomas. Since Pentetreotide is an analog of octreotide, an intravenous line is recommended in any patient suspected of having an insulinoma. An intravenous solution containing glucose should be administered just before and during administration of Indium In-111 Pentetreotide.
2. The two components of Indium In-111 Pentetreotide are NOT to be administered separately to the patient.
3. Since Indium In-111 Pentetreotide is eliminated primarily by renal excretion, use in patients with impaired renal function should be carefully considered.
4. To help reduce the radiation dose to the thyroid, kidneys, bladder, and other target organs, patients should be well hydrated before the administration of Indium In-111 Pentetreotide. They should increase fluid intake and void frequently for one day after administration of this drug. In addition, it is recommended that patients be given a mild laxative (e.g., bisacodyl or lactulose) before and after administration of Indium In-111 Pentetreotide (see *"Dosage and Administration"* section).
5. Indium In-111 Pentetreotide should be tested for labeling yield of radioactivity prior to administration. The product must be used within six hours of preparation.
6. To maintain sterility, it is essential that directions are followed carefully. Aseptic technique must be used during the preparation and administration of Indium In-111 Pentetreotide.
7. Octreotide acetate and the natural somatostatin hormone may be associated with cholelithiasis, presumably by altering fat absorption and possibly by decreasing motility of the gallbladder. A single dose of Indium In-111 Pentetreotide is not expected to cause cholelithiasis.
8. As with any other radioactive material, appropriate shielding should be used to avoid unnecessary radiation exposure to the patient, occupational workers, and other persons.
9. Radiopharmaceuticals should be used only by physicians who are qualified by specific training in the safe use and handling of radionuclides.

CARCINOGENESIS, MUTAGENESIS, IMPAIRMENT OF FERTILITY
Studies have not been performed with Indium In-111 Pentetreotide to evaluate carcinogenic potential or effects on fertility. Pentetreotide was evaluated for mutagenic potential in an *in vitro* mouse lymphoma forward mutation assay and an *in vivo* mouse micronucleus assay; evidence of mutagenicity was not found.

PREGNANCY CATEGORY C
Animal reproduction studies have not been conducted with Indium In-111 Pentetreotide. It is not known whether Indium In-111 Pentetreotide can cause fetal harm when administered to a pregnant woman or can affect reproduction capacity. Therefore, Indium In-111 Pentetreotide should not be administered to a pregnant woman unless the potential benefit justifies the potential risk to the fetus.

NURSING MOTHERS
It is not known whether this drug is excreted in human milk. Because many drugs are excreted in human milk, caution should be exercised when Indium In-111 Pentetreotide is administered to a nursing woman.

PEDIATRIC USE
Safety and effectiveness in children have not been established.

ADVERSE REACTIONS
The following adverse effects were observed in clinical trials at a frequency of less than 1% of 538 patients: dizziness, fever, flush, headache, hypotension, changes in liver enzymes, joint pain, nausea, sweating, and weakness. These adverse effects were transient. Also in clinical trials, there was one reported case of bradycardia and one case of decreased hematocrit and hemoglobin.

Pentetreotide is derived from octreotide which is used as a therapeutic agent to control symptoms from certain tumors. The usual dose for Indium In-111 Pentetreotide is approximately 5 to 20 times less than for octreotide and is subtherapeutic. The following adverse reactions have been associated with octreotide in 3% to 10% of patients: nausea, injection site pain, diarrhea, abdominal pain/discomfort, loose stools, and vomiting. Hypertension and hyper- and hypoglycemia have also been reported with the use of octreotide.

DOSAGE AND ADMINISTRATION
Before administration, a patient should be well hydrated. After administration, the patient must be encouraged to drink fluids liberally. Elimination of extra fluid intake will help reduce the radiation dose by flushing out unbound, labeled Pentetreotide by glomerular filtration. It is also recommended that a mild laxative (e.g., bisacodyl or lactulose) be given to the patient starting the evening before the radioactive drug is administered, and continuing for 48 hours. Ample fluid uptake is necessary during this period as a support both to renal elimination and the bowel-cleansing process. In a patient with an insulinoma, bowel-cleansing should be undertaken only after consultation with an endocrinologist.

The recommended intravenous dose for *planar* imaging is 111 MBq (3.0 mCi) of Indium In-111 Pentetreotide. The recommended intravenous for *SPECT* imaging is 222 MBq (6.0 mCi) of Indium In-111 Pentetreotide.

The dose should be confirmed by a suitably calibrated radioactivity ionization chamber immediately before administration.

As with all intravenously administered products, Indium In-111 Pentetreotide should be inspected visually for particulate matter and discoloration prior to administration, whenever solution and container permit. Preparations containing particulate matter of discoloration should not be administered. They should be disposed of in a safe manner, in compliance with applicable regulations.

Aseptic techniques and effective shielding should be employed in withdrawing doses for administration to patients. Waterproof gloves should be worn during the administration procedure.

Do not administer Indium In-111 Pentetreotide in TPN solutions or through the same intravenous line.

RADIATION DOSIMETRY
The estimated radiation doses* to the average adult (70 kg) from intravenous administration of 111 MBq (3 mCi) and 222 MBq (6 mCi) are presented in Table 4. These estimates were calculated by Oak Ridge Associated Universities using the data published by Krenning, et al.[3]

Table 4.

ESTIMATED ABSORBED RADIATION DOSES AFTER INTRAVENOUS ADMINISTRATION OF INDIUM IN-111 PENTETREOTIDE[a] TO A 70 KG PATIENT

Organ	Planar		Spect	
	mGy/111 MBq	rads/3 mCi	mGy/222 MBq	rads/6 mCi
Kidneys	54.16	5.42	108.32	10.83
Liver	12.15	1.22	24.31	2.43
Spleen	73.86	7.39	147.73	14.77
Uterus	6.34	0.63	12.67	1.27
Ovaries	4.89	0.49	9.79	0.98
Testes	2.90	0.29	5.80	0.58
Red Marrow	3.46	0.35	6.91	0.69
Urinary Bladder Wall	30.24	3.02	60.48	6.05
GI Tract				
Stomach Wall	5.67	0.57	11.34	1.13
Small Intestine	4.78	0.48	9.56	0.96
Upper Large Intestine	5.80	0.58	11.59	1.16
Lower Large Intestine	7.73	0.77	15.46	1.55
Adrenals	7.55	0.76	15.11	1.51
Thyroid	7.43	0.74	14.86	1.49
	mSv/111 MBq	rem/3 mCi	mSv/222 MBq	rem/6 mCi
Effective Dose[b] Equivalent	13.03	1.30	26.06	2.61

a   Assumes 4.8 hour voiding interval and International Commission on Radiological Protection (ICRP) 30 model for the gastrointestinal tract calculations.
b   Estimated according to ICRP Publication 53.

STORAGE
Indium In-111 Pentetreotide should be stored at 2°C to 8°C (36°F to 46°F). After reconstitution, store at or below 25°C (77°F). Indium In-111 Pentetreotide must be used within six hours of preparation.

INSTRUCTIONS FOR THE PREPARATION OF INDIUM IN-111 PENTETREOTIDE
Note: Read complete directions thoroughly before starting preparation.

Procedure Precautions and Notes

1. All transfers and penetrations of the vial stoppers by a needle must use aseptic technique.
2. Wear waterproof gloves during the entire procedure and while withdrawing the patient-dose of Pentetreotide.

---

* Values listed include a correction for a maximum of 0.1% Indium In-114m radiocontaminant at calibration.

3. Transfer Indium In-111 chloride sterile solution with an adequately shielded, sterile syringe.
4. Adequate shielding should be maintained at all times until the preparation is administered to the patient, disposed of in an approved manner, or allowed to decay to safe levels of radioactivity. A shielded, sterile syringe should be used for withdrawing and injecting the preparation.
5. Do not inject into TPN administration bags or their intravenous lines.

Procedure for the Preparation of Indium In-111 Pentetreotide

1. Place the Pentetreotide in a lead dispensing shield (of minimum wall thickness 1/4 inch) fitted with a lid.
2. Aseptically remove the Indium In-111 chloride sterile solution using the needle provided and a shielded, sterile syringe.
3. Inject the Indium In-111 chloride sterile solution into the Pentetreotide.
4. Gently swirl the Pentetreotide until the lyophilized pellet is completely dissolved.
5. Incubate the Indium In-111 Pentetreotide solution at or below 25°C (77°F) for a minimum of 30 minutes. Note: A 30 minute incubation time is required. Shorter incubation periods may result in inadequate labeling.
6. Using proper shielding, visually inspect the vial contents. The solution should be clear, colorless, and free of particulate matter. If not, the solution should not be used. It should be disposed in a safe and approved manner.
7. Assay the Indium In-111 Pentetreotide solution using a suitably calibrated ionization chamber. Record the date, time, total activity, and patient identifier (e.g., patient name and number) on the radioassay information label and affix the label to the lead dispensing shield.
8. The labeling yield of the reconstituted solution should be checked before administration to the patient. If the radiochemical purity is less than 90%, the product should not be used.
9. Store the reaction vial containing the Indium In-111 Pentetreotide solution at or below 25°C (77°F) until use. The Indium In-111 Pentetreotide must be used within six hours of preparation.
10. If desired, the preparation can be diluted to a maximum volume of 3 mL with 0.9% sodium chloride injection immediately prior to injection. The sample should be drawn into a shielded, sterile syringe and administered to the patient.

REFERENCES
1. From Radiopharmaceutical Internal Dosimetry Information Center, Oak Ridge Associated Universities, Oak Ridge, TN 37831-0117, February 1985. 2. Kocher, David C., "Radioactive Decay Data Tables," DOE/TIC-11026,115 (1981). 3. E.P. Krenning, W.H. Bakker, P.P.M. Kooij, W.A.P. Breeman, H.Y. Oei, M. de Jong, J.C. Reubi, T.J. Visser, C. Bruns, D.J. Kwekkeboom, A.E.M. Reijs, P.M. van Hagen, J.W. Koper, and S.W.J. Lamberts, "Somatostatin Receptor Scintigraphy with Indium-111-DTPA-D-Phe-1-Octreotide in Man: Metabolism, Dosimetry and Comparison with Iodine-123-Try-3-Octreotide." The Journal of Nuclear Medicine, Vol. 33, No. 5, May 1992, pp. 652-658.

HOW SUPPLIED
KIT:

BRAND/MANUFACTURER	NDC	SIZE	AWP
○ **BRAND** OCTREOSCAN: Mallinckrodt Med	00019-9050-40	1s	$800.00

Indocin *SEE* INDOMETHACIN

Indocyanine Green

DESCRIPTION
Indocyanine Green is a sterile, water soluble, tricarbocyanine dye with a peak spectral absorption at 800-810 nm in blood plasma or blood. Indocyanine Green contains not more than 5.0% sodium iodide. Indocyanine Green is to be administered intravenously.

The Aqueous Solvent provided with this product, pH of 5.5 to 6.5, is a prepared Sterile Water for injection used to dissolve Indocyanine Green.

Following is its chemical structure:

CLINICAL PHARMACOLOGY
Following intravenous injection, Indocyanine Green is rapidly bound to plasma protein, of which albumin is the principle carrier (95%). Indocyanine Green undergoes no significant extrahepatic or enterohepatic circulation; simultaneous arterial and venous blood estimations have shown negligible renal, peripheral, lung or cerebro-spinal uptake of the dye. Indocyanine Green is taken up from the plasma almost exclusively by the hepatic parenchymal cells and is secreted entirely into the bile. After biliary obstruction, the dye appears in the hepatic lymph, independently of the bile, suggesting that the biliary mucosa is sufficiently intact to prevent diffusion of the dye, though allowing diffusion of bilirubin. These characteristics make Indocyanine Green a helpful index of hepatic function.

INDICATIONS
For determining cardiac output, hepatic function and liver blood flow, and for ophthalmic angiography.

CONTRAINDICATIONS
Indocyanine Green contains sodium iodide and should be used with caution in patients who have a history of allergy to iodides.

WARNINGS
Two anaphylactic deaths have been reported following Indocyanine Green administration during cardiac catheterization. One of these was in a patient with a history of sensitivity to penicillin and sulfa drugs.

The Aqueous Solvent provided with this product, pH 5.5 to 6.5, which is especially prepared Sterile Water for injection, should be used to dissolve Indocyanine Green because there have been reports of incompatibility with some commercially available Water for injection.

PRECAUTIONS
General: Indocyanine Green Powder and Solution: Indocyanine Green is unstable in aqueous solution and must be used within 10 hours. However, the dye is stable in plasma and whole blood so that samples obtained in discontinuous sampling techniques may be read hours later. Sterile techniques should be used in handling the dye solution as well as in the performance of the dilution curves.

Indocyanine Green, USP powder may cling to the vial or lump together because it is freeze-dried in the vials. *This is not due to the presence of water*—the moisture content is carefully controlled.

Heparin preparations containing sodium bisulfite reduce the absorption peak of Indocyanine Green, USP in blood and, therefore, should not be used as an anticoagulant for the collection of samples for analysis.

The plasma fractional disappearance rate at the recommended 0.5 mg/kg dose has been reported to be significantly greater in women than in men, although there was no significant difference in the calculated value for clearance.

Radio-active iodine uptake studies should not be performed for at least a week following the use of Indocyanine Green, USP.

Pregnancy Category C: Animal Reproduction studies have not been conducted with Indocyanine Green, USP. It is also not known whether Indocyanine Green, USP can cause fetal harm when administered to a pregnant woman or can affect reproduction capacity. Indocyanine Green, USP should be given to a pregnant woman only if clearly indicated.

Nursing Mothers: It is not known whether this drug is excreted in human milk. Because many drugs are excreted in human milk, caution should be exercised when Indocyanine Green, USP is administered to a nursing woman.

ADVERSE REACTIONS
Anaphylactic or urticarial reactions have been reported in patients with or without history of allergy to iodides. If such reactions occur, treatment with the appropriate agents, e.g., epinephrine, antihistamines, and corticosteroids should be administered.

DRUG ABUSE AND DEPENDENCE
Indocyanine Green, USP is not a controlled substance listed in any of the Drug Enforcement Administration schedules. Its use is not known to lead to dependence or abuse.

OVERDOSAGE
There are no data available describing the signs, symptoms, or laboratory findings accompanying overdosage. The LD$_{50}$ after IV administration ranges between 60 and 80 mg/kg in mice, 50 and 70 mg/kg in rats and 50 and 80 mg/kg in rabbits.

DOSAGE AND ADMINISTRATION
Indicator-Dilution Studies: Indocyanine Green, USP permits recording of the indicator-dilution curves for both diagnostic and research purposes independently of fluctuations in oxygen saturation. In the performance of dye dilution curves, a known amount of dye is usually injected as a single bolus as rapidly as possible via a cardiac catheter into selected sites in the vascular system. A recording instrument (oximeter or densitometer) is attached to a needle or catheter for sampling of the dye-blood mixture from a systemic arterial sampling site.

Under sterile conditions, the Indocyanine Green, USP powder should be dissolved with the Aqueous Solvent furnished, and the solution used within 10 hours after it is prepared. The amount of solvent to be used can be calculated from the dosage form which follows. It is recommended that the syringe used for injection of the dye be rinsed with this diluent. Isotonic saline should be used to flush the residual dye from the cardiac catheter into the circulation so as to avoid hemolysis. With the exception of the rinsing of the dye injection syringe, saline is used in all other parts of the catheterization procedure.

This matter of rinsing the dye syringe with distilled water may not be critical, since it is known that an amount of sodium chloride sufficient to make an isotonic solution may be added to dye *that has first been dissolved in distilled water*. This procedure has been used for constant-rate injection techniques without precipitation of the dye.

The usual doses of Indocyanine Green, USP which have been used for dilution curves are as follows:
Adults-5 mg
Children-2.5 mg
Infants-1.25 mg

These doses of the dye are usually injected in a ml volume. An average of five dilution curves are required in the performance of a diagnostic cardiac catheterization. The total dose of dye injected should be kept below 2 mg/kg.

Calibrating Dye Curves: To quantitate the dilution curves, standard dilutions of Indocyanine Green, USP in whole blood are made as follows. It is strongly recommended that the same dye that was used for the injections be used in the preparation of these standard dilutions. The most concentrated dye solution is made by accurately diluting 1 ml of the 5 mg/ml dye with 7 ml of distilled water. This concentration is then successfully halved by diluting 4 ml of the previous concentration with 4 ml of distilled water. (If a 2.5 mg/ml concentration was used for the dilution curves, 1 ml of the 2.5 mg/ml dye is added to 3 ml of distilled water to make the most concentrated "standard" solution. This concentration is then successively halved by diluting 2 ml of the previous concentration with 2 ml of distilled water.) Then 0.2 ml portions (accurately measured from a calibrated syringe) of these dye solutions are added to 5 ml aliquots of the subject's blood, giving final concentrations of the dye in blood beginning with 24.0 mg/liter, approximately (actual concentration depends on the exact volume of dye added). This concentration is, of course, successively halved in the succeeding aliquots of the subject's blood. These aliquots of blood containing known amounts of dye, as well as a blank sample of which 0.2 ml of saline containing no dye has been added, are then passed through the detecting instrument and a calibration curve is constructed from the deflections recorded.

Hepatic Function Studies: Due to its absorption spectrum, changing concentrations of Indocyanine Green, USP in the blood can be monitored by ear densitometry or by obtaining blood specimens at timed intervals. The technique for both methods is as follows.

The patient should be studied in a fasting, basal state. The patient should be weighed and the dosage calculated on the basis of 0.5 mg/kg of body weight.

Under sterile conditions, the Indocyanine Green, USP powder should be dissolved with the Aqueous Solvent furnished. Exactly 5 ml of aqueous solvent should be added to the 25 mg vial or exactly 10 ml of aqueous solvent should be added to the 50 mg vial, giving 5 mg of dye per ml of solution.

Inject the correct amount of dye into the lumen of an arm vein as rapidly as possible, without allowing the dye to escape outside the vein. (*If the photometric method is used, prior to injecting Indocyanine Green, USP, withdraw 6 ml of venous blood from the patient's arm for serum blank and standard curve construction, and through the same needle, inject the correct amount of dye.*)

Ear Densitometry: Ear oximetry has also been used and makes it possible to monitor the appearance and disappearance of Indocyanine Green, USP without the necessity of withdrawal and spectrophotometric analysis of blood samples for calibration. An ear densitometer which has a compensatory photo-electric cell to correct for changes in blood volume and hematocrit, and a detection photocell which registers Indocyanine Green, USP levels has been described. This device permits simultaneous measurement of cardiac output, blood volume and hepatic clearance of Indocyanine Green, USP and was found to provide a reliable index of plasma removal kinetics after single injections or continuous intrusions of Indocyanine Green, USP. This technique was employed in newborn infants, healthy adults and in children and adults with liver disease. The normal subject has a removal rate of 18-24% per minute. Due to the absence of extra-hepatic removal, Indocyanine Green, USP was found to be ideally suited for serial study of severe chronic liver disease and to provide a stable measurement of hepatic blood flow. In larger doses, Indocyanine Green, USP has proven to be particularly valuable in detecting drug-induced alterations of hepatic function and in the detection of mild liver injury.

Using the ear densitometer, a dosage of 0.5 mg/kg in normal subjects gives the following clearance pattern.

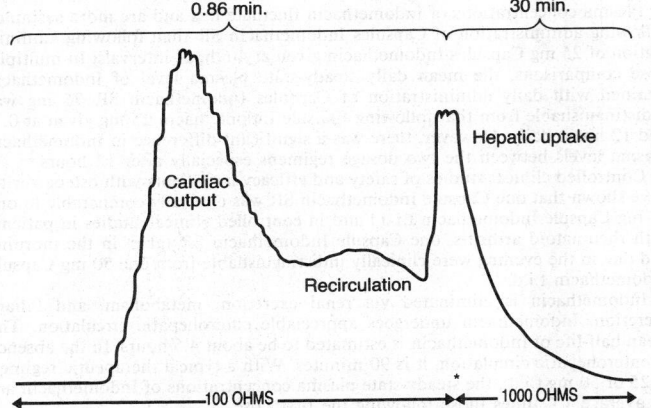

* cross-over indicating a manual gain change in densitometer system.

PHOTOMETRIC METHOD
Determination Using Percentage Retention of Dye: A typical curve obtained by plotting dye concentration versus optical density is shown nearby. Percent retention can be read from this plot.

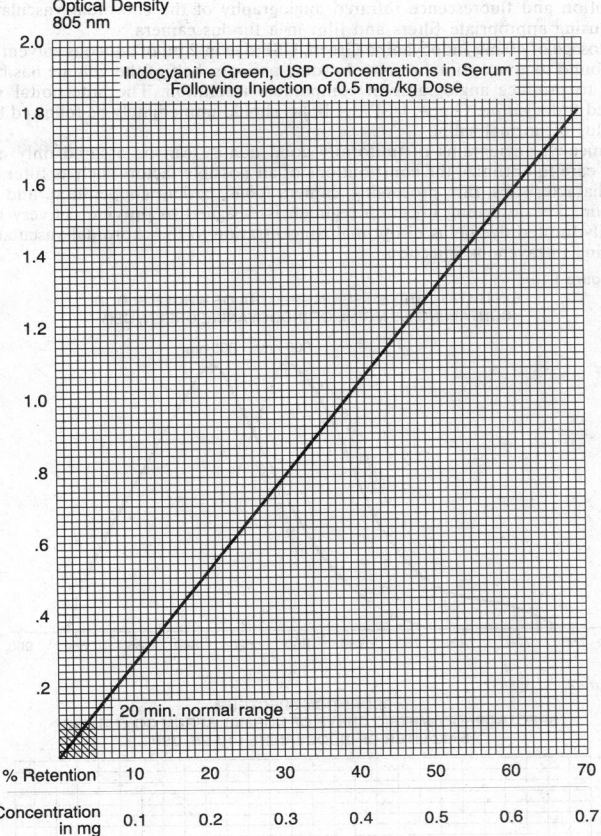

If more accurate results are desired, a curve using the patient's blood and the vial of Indocyanine Green, USP being used in the determination can be constructed as follows:

1. Take 6 ml of non-dye-containing venous blood from the patient's arm. Place in a test tube and allow the blood to clot. The serum is separated by centrifugation.
2. Pipette 1 ml of the serum into a microcuvette.
3. Add 1 lambda (λ) of the 5 mg/ml aqueous Indocyanine Green, USP solution to the serum, giving a dilution of 5 mg/liter, the standard for 50% retention. (The addition of 2 lambda (λ) of the 5 mg/ml Indocyanine Green, USP solution would give 100% retention; however, this concentration cannot be read on the spectrophotometer.)
4. The optical density of this solution is read at 805 nm, using normal serum as the blank.
5. Using graph paper similar to that used in the illustration, plot the 50% figure obtained in Step 4, and draw a line connecting this point with the zero coordinates.

Percentage Retention: A single 20-minute sample (withdrawn from a vein in the opposite arm to that injected) is allowed to clot, centrifuged and its optical density is determined at 805 nm using the patient's normal serum as the blank. Dye concentration is read from the curve above. A single 20-minute sample of serum in healthy subjects should contain no more than 4% of the initial concentration of the dye. The use of percentage retention is less accurate than percentage disappearance rate, but provides reproducible results. Hemolysis does not interfere with a reading.

Determination Using Disappearance Rate of Dye: To calculate the percentage disappearance rate, obtain samples at 5, 10, 15 and 20 minutes after injecting the dye. Prepare the samples as in the previous section and measure the optical densities at 805 nm, using the patient's normal serum as the blank. The Indocyanine Green, USP in each timed specimen can be determined by using the concentration curve illustrated. Plot values on semilogarithmic paper.

Specimens containing Indocyanine Green, USP should be read at the same temperature since its optical density is influenced by temperature variations.

Normal Values: Percentage disappearance rate in healthy subjects is 18-24% per minute. Normal biological half-time is 2.5-3.0 minutes.

Ophthalmic Angiography Studies: The excitation and emission spectra (Figure 1) and the absorption spectra (Figure 2) of Indocyanine Green, USP make it useful in ophthalmic angiography. The peak absorption and emission of Indocyanine Green, USP lie in a region (800-850 nm) where transmission of energy by the pigment epithelium is more efficient than in the region of visible light energy. Indocyanine Green, USP also has the property of being nearly 98% bound to blood protein, and therefore, excessive dye extravasation does not take place in the highly fenestrated choroidal vasculature. It is, therefore, useful in both absorption and fluorescence infrared angiography of the choroidal vasculature when using appropriate filters and film in a fundus camera.

A dosage of 40 mg Indocyanine Green, USP dye in 2 ml of aqueous solvent has been found to give optimal results. In some patients, half of the volume has been found to produce angiograms of comparable resolution. The antecubital vein injected Indocyanine Green, USP dye bolus should immediately be followed by 5 ml bolus of normal saline.

Clinically, angiograms of uniformly good quality can be assured only after taking care to optimize the contributions of all possible factors such as filter and film characteristics, film processing, camera focus, patient cooperation, and dye injection. The foregoing injection regimen is designed to provide delivery of a spatially limited dye bolus of optimal concentration to the choroidal vasculature following intravenous injection.

Figure 1

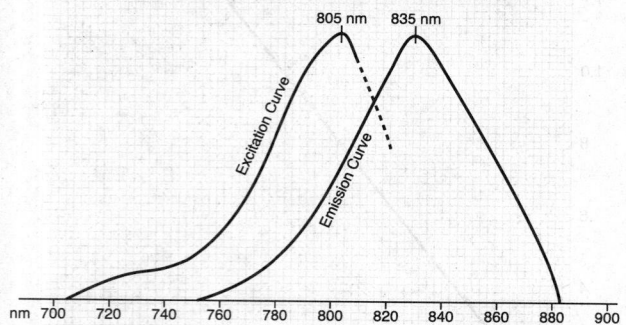

EXCITATION AND EMISSION SPECTRA OF WHOLE BLOOD CONTAINING .05 MG/ML OF INDOCYANINE GREEN, USP

Figure 2

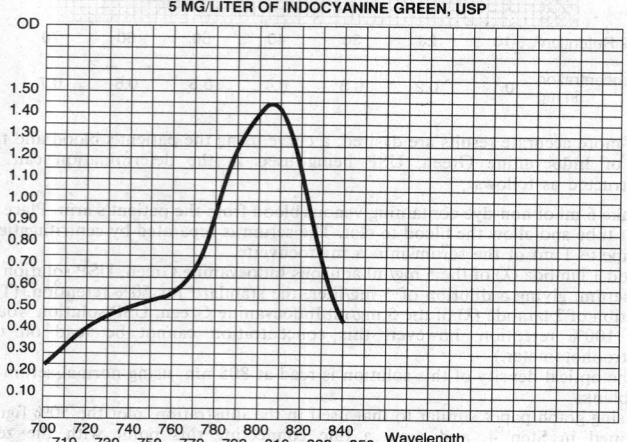

ABSORPTION SPECTRUM
SPECTROPHOTOMETRIC CURVE OF NORMAL SERUM CONTAINING
5 MG/LITER OF INDOCYANINE GREEN, USP

HOW SUPPLIED
POWDER FOR INJECTION: 25 MG

BRAND/MANUFACTURER	NDC	SIZE	AWP
○ BRAND			
CARDIO-GREEN: BD Microbiology	00011-8361-20	2s	$22.65

POWDER FOR INJECTION: 50 MG

BRAND/MANUFACTURER	NDC	SIZE	AWP
○ BRAND			
CARDIO-GREEN: BD Microbiology	00011-8362-55	10 ml 2s	$30.60

Indomethacin

DESCRIPTION

Indomethacin cannot be considered a simple analgesic and should not be used in conditions other than those recommended under *"Indications."*

Indomethacin is supplied in four dosage forms. Capsules Indomethacin for oral administration contain either 25 mg or 50 mg of Indomethacin. Capsules Indomethacin SR for sustained release oral administration contain 75 mg of Indomethacin. Capsules Indomethacin SR conform to the requirements of the USP Drug Release Test for Indomethacin Extended-release Capsules. Suspension Indomethacin for oral use contains 25 mg of Indomethacin per 5 mL. Supposito-

ries Indomethacin for rectal use contain 50 mg of Indomethacin. Indomethacin is a non-steroidal anti-inflammatory indole derivative designated chemically as 1-(4-chlorobenzoyl)-5-methoxy-2-methyl-1H-indole-3-acetic acid. Indomethacin is practically insoluble in water and sparingly soluble in alcohol. It has a pKa of 4.5 and is stable in neutral or slightly acidic media and decomposes in strong alkali. The suspension has a pH of 4.0-5.0.

Following is its chemical structure:

CLINICAL PHARMACOLOGY

Indomethacin is a nonsteroidal drug with anti-inflammatory, antipyretic and analgesic properties. Its mode of action, like that of other anti-inflammatory drugs, is not known. However, its therapeutic action is not due to pituitary-adrenal stimulation.

Indomethacin is a potent inhibitor of prostaglandin synthesis *in vitro*. Concentrations are reached during therapy which have been demonstrated to have an effect *in vivo* as well. Prostaglandins sensitize afferent nerves and potentiate the action of bradykinin in inducing pain in animal models. Moreover, prostaglandins are known to be among the mediators of inflammation. Since Indomethacin is an inhibitor of prostaglandin synthesis, its mode of action may be due to a decrease of prostaglandins in peripheral tissues.

Indomethacin has been shown to be an effective anti-inflammatory agent, appropriate for long-term use in rheumatoid arthritis, ankylosing spondylitis, and osteoarthritis.

Indomethacin affords relief of symptoms; it does not alter the progressive course of the underlying disease.

Indomethacin suppresses inflammation in rheumatoid arthritis as demonstrated by relief of pain, and reduction of fever, swelling and tenderness. Improvement in patients treated with Indomethacin for rheumatoid arthritis has been demonstrated by a reduction in joint swelling, average number of joints involved, and morning stiffness; by increased mobility as demonstrated by a decrease in walking time; and by improved functional capability as demonstrated by an increase in grip strength.

Indomethacin has been reported to diminish basal and CO_2 stimulated cerebral blood flow in healthy volunteers following acute oral and intravenous administration. In one study after one week of treatment with orally administered Indomethacin, this effect on basal cerebral blood flow had disappeared. The clinical significance of this effect has not been established.

Capsules Indomethacin have been found effective in relieving the pain, reducing the fever, swelling, redness, and tenderness of acute gouty arthritis. Capsules Indomethacin rather than Capsules Indomethacin SR are recommended for treatment of acute gouty arthritis—see Indications.

Following single oral doses of Capsules Indomethacin 25 mg or 50 mg, Indomethacin is readily absorbed, attaining peak plasma concentrations of about 1 and 2 mcg/mL, respectively, at about 2 hours. Orally administered Capsules Indomethacin are virtually 100% bioavailable, with 90% of the dose absorbed within 4 hours. A single 50 mg dose of Oral Suspension Indomethacin was found to be bioequivalent to a 50 mg Indomethacin capsule when each was administered with food.

Capsules Indomethacin SR 75 mg are designed to release 25 mg of the drug initially and the remaining 50 mg over approximately 12 hours (90% of dose absorbed by 12 hours). When measured over a 24-hour period, the cumulative amount and time-course of Indomethacin absorption from a single Capsule Indomethacin SR are comparable to those of 3 doses of 25 mg Capsules Indomethacin given at 4-6 hour intervals.

Plasma concentrations of Indomethacin fluctuate less and are more sustained following administration of Capsules Indomethacin SR than following administration of 25 mg Capsules Indomethacin given at 4-6 hour intervals. In multiple-dose comparisons, the mean daily steady-state plasma level of Indomethacin attained with daily administration of Capsules Indomethacin SR 75 mg was indistinguishable from that following Capsule Indomethacin 25 mg given at 0, 6 and 12 hours daily. However, there was a significant difference in Indomethacin plasma levels between the two dosage regimens especially after 12 hours.

Controlled clinical studies of safety and efficacy in patients with osteoarthritis have shown that one Capsule Indomethacin SR was clinically comparable to one 25 mg Capsule Indomethacin t.i.d.; and in controlled clinical studies in patients with rheumatoid arthritis, one Capsule Indomethacin SR taken in the morning and one in the evening were clinically indistinguishable from one 50 mg Capsule Indomethacin t.i.d.

Indomethacin is eliminated via renal excretion, metabolism, and biliary excretion. Indomethacin undergoes appreciable enterohepatic circulation. The mean half-life of Indomethacin is estimated to be about 4.5 hours. In the absence of enterohepatic circulation, it is 90 minutes. With a typical therapeutic regimen of 25 or 50 mg t.i.d., the steady-state plasma concentrations of Indomethacin are an average 1.4 times those following the first dose.

The rate of absorption is more rapid from the rectal suppository than from Capsules Indomethacin. Ordinarily, therefore, the total amount absorbed from the suppository would be expected to be at least equivalent to the capsule. In controlled clinical trials, however, the amount of Indomethacin absorbed was found to be somewhat less (80-90%) than that absorbed from Capsules Indomethacin. This is probably because some subjects did not retain the material from the suppository for the one hour necessary to assure complete absorption. Since

---

the suppository dissolves rather quickly rather than melting slowly, it is seldom recovered in recognizable form if the patient retains the suppository for more than a few minutes.

Indomethacin exists in the plasma as the parent drug and its desmethyl, desbenzoyl, and desmethyl-desbenzoyl metabolites, all in the unconjugated form. About 60 percent of an oral dosage is recovered in urine as drug and metabolites (26 percent as Indomethacin and its glucuronide), and 33 percent is recovered in feces (1.5 percent as Indomethacin).

In adults, about 99% of Indomethacin is bound to protein in plasma over the expected range of therapeutic plasma concentrations. The percent bound in neonates has not been studied. In controlled trials in premature infants, however, no evidence of bilirubin displacement has been observed as evidenced by increased incidence of bilirubin encephalopathy (kernicterus).

In a gastroscopic study in 45 healthy subjects, the number of gastric mucosal abnormalities was significantly higher in the group receiving Capsules Indomethacin than in the group taking Suppositories Indomethacin or placebo.

In a double-blind comparative clinical study involving 175 patients with rheumatoid arthritis, however, the incidence of upper gastrointestinal adverse effects with Suppositories or Capsules Indomethacin was comparable. The incidence of lower gastrointestinal adverse effect was greater in the suppository group.

Although the exact mechanism of action through which Indomethacin causes closure of a patent ductus arteriosus is not known, it is believed to be through inhibition of prostaglandin synthesis. In human newborns with certain congenital heart malformations, PGE 1 dilates the ductus arteriosus. In fetal and newborn lambs, E type prostaglandins have also been shown to maintain the patency of the ductus, and as in human newborns, Indomethacin causes its constriction.

Studies in healthy young animals and in premature infants with patent ductus arteriosus indicated that, after the first dose of intravenous Indomethacin, there was a transient reduction in cerebral blood flow velocity and cerebral blood flow. The clinical significance of this effect has not been established.

In double-blind placebo-controlled studies of Indomethacin IV in 460 small pre-term infants, weighing 1750 g or less, the infants treated with placebo had a ductus closure rate after 48 hours of 25 to 30 percent, whereas those treated with Indomethacin IV had a 75 to 80 percent closure rate. In one of these studies, a multicenter study, involving 405 pre-term infants, later re-opening of the ductus arteriosus occurred in 26 percent of infants treated with Indomethacin IV, however, 70 percent of these closed subsequently without the need for surgery or additional Indomethacin.

PHARMACOKINETICS AND METABOLISM
The disposition of Indomethacin following intravenous administration (0.2 mg/kg) in pre-term neonates with patent ductus arteriosus has not been extensively evaluated. Even though the plasma half-life of Indomethacin was variable among premature infants, it was shown to vary inversely with postnatal age and weight. In one study, of 28 infants who could be evaluated, the plasma half-life in those infants less than 7 days old averaged 20 hours (range: 3-60 hours, n = 18). In infants older than 7 days, the mean plasma half-life of Indomethacin was 12 hours (range: 4-38 hours, n = 10). Grouping the infants by weight, mean plasma half-life in those weighing less than 1000 g was 21 hours (range: 9-60 hours, n = 10); in those infants weighing more than 1000 g, the mean plasma half-life was 15 hours (range: 3-52 hours, n = 18).

INDICATIONS
Indomethacin has been found effective in active stages of the following:

1. Moderate to severe rheumatoid arthritis including acute flares of chronic disease.
2. Moderate to severe ankylosing spondylitis.
3. Moderate to severe osteoarthritis.
4. Acute painful shoulder (bursitis and/or tendinitis).
5. Acute gouty arthritis.

Capsules Indomethacin SR are recommended for all of the indications for Capsules Indomethacin except acute gouty arthritis. Indomethacin may enable the reduction of steroid dosage in patients receiving steroids for the more severe forms of rheumatoid arthritis. In such instances the steroid dosage should be reduced slowly and the patients followed very closely for any possible adverse effects.

The use of Indomethacin in conjunction with aspirin or other salicylates is not recommended. Controlled clinical studies have shown that the combined use of Indomethacin and aspirin does not produce any greater therapeutic effect than the use of Indomethacin alone. Furthermore, in one of these clinical studies, the incidence of gastrointestinal side effects was significantly increased with combined therapy (see "Drug Interactions").

UNLABELED USES
Indomethacin is used alone or as an adjunct in the treatment of biliary, acute renal, and ureteral colic. It is also used in the treatment of Bartter's syndrome and primary dysmenorrhea, to reduce miosis during cataract surgery, and to provide symptomatic relief in cholecystitis and pericarditis. Indomethacin is used in the treatment of fever due to various causes, benign exertional headache, hypercalcemia of malignancy, and pain due to acute pancreatitis. It is also used in Reiter's syndrome, polyhydramnios, and Posner and Sclossman's syndrome, and is prescribed for prevention of heteroptic ossification.

Indomethacin IV is indicated to close a hemodynamically significant patent ductus arteriosus in premature infants weighing between 500 and 1750 g when after 48 hours usual medical management (e.g., fluid restriction, diuretics,

digitalis, respiratory support, etc.) is ineffective. Clear-cut clinical evidence of a hemodynamically significant patent ductus arteriosus should be present, such as respiratory distress, a continuous murmur, a hyperactive precordium, cardiomegaly and pulmonary plethora on chest x-ray.

CONTRAINDICATIONS
Indomethacin should not be used in:

Patients who are hypersensitive to this product.
Patients in whom acute asthmatic attacks, urticaria, or rhinitis are precipitated by aspirin or other non-steroidal anti-inflammatory agents.
Suppositories Indomethacin are contraindicated in patients with a history of proctitis or recent rectal bleeding.

Indomethacin IV is contraindicated in: infants with proven or suspected infection that is untreated; infants who are bleeding, especially those with active intracranial hemorrhage or gastrointestinal bleeding; infants with thrombocytopenia; infants with coagulation defects; infants with or who are suspected of having necrotizing enterocolitis; infants with significant impairment of renal function; infants with congenital heart disease in whom patency of the ductus arteriosus is necessary for satisfactory pulmonary or systemic blood flow (e.g., pulmonary atresia, severe tetralogy of Fallot, severe coarctation of the aorta).

WARNINGS
GENERAL
Because of the variability of the potential of Indomethacin to cause adverse reactions in the individual patient, the following are strongly recommended:

1. The lowest possible effective dose for the individual patient should be prescribed. Increased dosage tends to increase adverse effects, particularly in doses over 150-200 mg/day, without corresponding increase in clinical benefits.
2. Careful instructions to, and observations of, the individual patient are essential to the prevention of serious adverse reactions. As advancing years appear to increase the possibility of adverse reactions, Indomethacin should be used with greater care in the aged.
3. Effectiveness of Indomethacin Capsules and Suppositories in children has not been established. Indomethacin should not be prescribed for children 14 years of age and younger unless toxicity or lack of efficacy associated with other drugs warrants the risk.
In experience with more than 900 children who were treated with Capsules Indomethacin, side effects in children were comparable to those reported in adults. Experience in children has been confined to the use of Capsules Indomethacin. If a decision is made to use Indomethacin for children two years of age or older, such patients should be monitored closely and periodic assessment of liver function is recommended. There have been cases of hepatotoxicity reported in children with juvenile rheumatoid arthritis, including fatalities.
If Indomethacin treatment is instituted, a suggested starting dose is 2 mg/kg/day given in divided doses. Maximum daily dosage should not exceed 4 mg/kg/day or 150-200 mg/day, whichever is less. As symptoms subside, the total daily dosage should be reduced to the lowest level required to control symptoms, or the drug should be discontinued.
4. If Capsules Indomethacin SR are used for initial therapy or during dosage adjustment, observe the patient closely (see "Dosage and Administration").

GASTROINTESTINAL EFFECTS
Capsules and Suppositories: Single or multiple ulcerations, including perforation and hemorrhage of the esophagus, stomach, duodenum or small and large intestine, have been reported to occur with Indomethacin. Fatalities have been reported in some instances. Rarely, intestinal ulceration has been associated with stenosis and obstruction.

Gastrointestinal bleeding without obvious ulcer formation and perforation of pre-existing sigmoid lesions (diverticulum, carcinoma, etc.) have occurred. Increased abdominal pain in ulcerative colitis patients or the development of ulcerative colitis and regional ileitis have been reported to occur rarely.

Because of the occurrence, and at times severity, of gastrointestinal reactions to Indomethacin, the prescribing physician must be continuously alert for any sign or symptom signaling a possible gastrointestinal reaction. The risks of continuing therapy with Indomethacin in the face of such symptoms must be weighed against the possible benefits to the individual patient.

Indomethacin should not be given to patients with active gastrointestinal lesions or with a history of recurrent gastrointestinal lesions except under circumstances which warrant the very high risk and where patients can be monitored very closely.

The gastrointestinal effects may be reduced by giving Capsules Indomethacin or Capsules Indomethacin SR immediately after meals, with food, or with antacids.

Intravenous: In the collaborative study, major gastrointestinal bleeding was no more common in those infants receiving Indomethacin than in those infants on placebo. However, minor gastrointestinal bleeding (i.e., chemical detection of blood in the stool) was more commonly noted in those infants treated with Indomethacin. Severe gastrointestinal effects have been reported in adults with various arthritic disorders treated chronically with oral Indomethacin.

RISK OF GI ULCERATIONS, BLEEDING AND PERFORATION WITH NSAID THERAPY
Serious gastrointestinal toxicity such as bleeding, ulceration, and perforation, can occur at any time, with or without warning symptoms, in patients treated chronically with NSAID therapy. Although minor upper gastrointestinal problems, such as dyspepsia, are common, usually developing early in therapy,

➤ SHOWN IN PRODUCT IDENTIFICATION GUIDE

physicians should remain alert for ulceration and bleeding in patients treated chronically with NSAIDs even in the absence of previous GI tract symptoms. In patients observed in clinical trials of several months to two years duration, symptomatic upper GI ulcers, gross bleeding or perforation appear to occur in approximately 1% of patients treated for 3-6 months, and in about 2-4% of patients treated for one year. Physicians should inform patients about the signs and/or symptoms of serious GI toxicity and what steps to take if they occur.

Studies to date have not identified any subset of patients not at risk of developing peptic ulceration and bleeding. Except for a prior history of serious GI events and other risk factors known to be associated with peptic ulcer disease, such as alcoholism, smoking, etc., no risk factors (e.g., age, sex) have been associated with increased risk. Elderly or debilitated patients seem to tolerate ulceration or bleeding less well than other individuals and most spontaneous reports of fatal GI events are in this population. Studies to date are inconclusive concerning the relative risk of various NSAIDs in causing such reactions. High doses of any NSAID probably carry a greater risk of these reactions, although controlled clinical trials showing this do not exist in most cases. In considering the use of relatively large doses (within the recommended dosage range), sufficient benefit should be anticipated to offset the potential increased risk of GI toxicity.

RENAL EFFECTS

Capsules and Suppositories: As with other nonsteroidal anti-inflammatory drugs, long term administration of Indomethacin to animals has resulted in renal papillary necrosis and other abnormal renal pathology. In humans, there have been reports of acute interstitial nephritis with hematuria, proteinuria, and occasionally nephrotic syndrome.

A second form of renal toxicity has been seen in patients with prerenal and renal conditions leading to a reduction in renal blood flow or blood volume, where the renal prostaglandins have a supportive role in the maintenance of renal perfusion. In these patients administration of an NSAID may cause a dose dependent reduction in prostaglandin formation and may precipitate overt renal decompensation. Patients at greatest risk of this reaction are those with conditions such as renal or hepatic dysfunction, diabetes mellitus, advanced age, extracellular volume depletion from any cause, congestive heart failure, septicemia, pyelonephritis, or concomitant use of any nephrotoxic drug. Indomethacin or other NSAIDs should be given with caution and renal function should be monitored in any patient who may have reduced renal reserve. Discontinuation of NSAID therapy is typically followed by recovery to the pretreatment state.

Increases in serum potassium concentration, including hyperkalemia, have been reported, even in some patients without renal impairment. In patients with normal renal function, these effects have been attributed to a hyporeninemic-hypoaldosteronism state (see "Precautions, Drug Interactions").

Since Indomethacin is eliminated primarily by the kidneys, patients with significantly impaired renal function should be closely monitored; a lower daily dosage should be anticipated to avoid excessive drug accumulation.

Indomethacin IV may cause significant reduction in urine output (50 percent or more) with concomitant elevations of blood urea nitrogen and creatinine, and reductions in glomerular filtration rate and creatinine clearance. These effects in most infants are transient, disappearing with cessation of therapy with Indomethacin IV. However, because adequate renal function can depend upon renal prostaglandin synthesis, Indomethacin IV may precipitate renal insufficiency, including acute renal failure, especially in infants with other conditions that may adversely affect renal function (e.g., extracellular volume depletion from any cause, congestive heart failure, sepsis, concomitant use of any nephrotoxic drug, hepatic dysfunction). When significant suppression of urine volume occurs after a dose of Indomethacin IV, no additional dose should be given until the urine output returns to normal levels.

Indomethacin IV in pre-term infants may suppress water excretion to a greater extent than sodium excretion. When this occurs, a significant reduction in serum sodium values (i.e., hyponatremia) may result. Infants should have serum electrolyte determinations done during therapy with Indomethacin IV Renal function and serum electrolytes should be monitored (see "Precautions, Drug Interactions" and "Dosage and Administration").

OCULAR EFFECTS

Capsules and Suppositories: Corneal deposits and retinal disturbances, including those of the macula, have been observed in some patients who had received prolonged therapy with Indomethacin. The prescribing physician should be alert to the possible association between the changes noted and Indomethacin. It is advisable to discontinue therapy if such changes are observed. Blurred vision may be a significant symptom and warrants a thorough ophthalmological examination. Since these changes may be asymptomatic, ophthalmologic examination at periodic intervals is desirable in patients where therapy is prolonged.

CENTRAL NERVOUS SYSTEM EFFECTS

Capsules and Suppositories: Indomethacin may aggravate depression or other psychiatric disturbances, epilepsy, and parkinsonism, and should be used with considerable caution in patients with these conditions. If severe CNS adverse reactions develop, Indomethacin should be discontinued.

Indomethacin may cause drowsiness; therefore, patients should be cautioned about engaging in activities requiring mental alertness and motor coordination, such as driving a car. Indomethacin may also cause headache. Headache which persists despite dosage reduction requires cessation of therapy with Indomethacin.

USE IN PREGNANCY AND THE NEONATAL PERIOD

Intravenous: Prematurity per se, is associated with an increased incidence of spontaneous intraventricular hemorrhage. Because Indomethacin may inhibit

platelet aggregation, the potential for intraventricular bleeding may be increased. However, in the large multi-center study of Indomethacin IV (see "Clinical Pharmacology"), the incidence of intraventricular hemorrhage in babies treated with Indomethacin IV was not significantly higher than in the control infants.

Capsules and Suppositories: Indomethacin is not recommended for use in pregnant women, since safety for use has not been established, and because of the known effect of drugs of this class on the human fetus (closure of the ductus arteriosus, platelet dysfunction with resultant bleeding, renal dysfunction or failure with oligohydramnios, gastrointestinal bleeding or perforation, and myocardial degenerative changes) during the third trimester of pregnancy).

Teratogenic studies were conducted in mice and rats at dosages of 0.5, 1.0, 2.0, and 4.0 mg/kg/day. Except for retarded fetal ossification at 4 mg/kg/day considered secondary to the decreased average fetal weights, no increase in fetal malformations was observed as compared with control groups. Pregnant rats, given 2.0 mg/kg/day and 4.0 mg/kg/day during the last trimester of gestation, delivered offspring whose pulmonary blood vessels were both reduced in number and excessively muscularized. These findings are similar to those observed in the syndrome of persistent pulmonary hypertension of the newborn.

Other studies in mice reported in the literature using higher doses (5 to 15 mg/kg/day) have described maternal toxicity and death, increased fetal resorptions, and fetal malformations. Comparable studies in rodents using high doses of aspirin have shown similar maternal and fetal effects.

As with other non-steroidal anti-inflammatory agents which inhibit prostaglandin synthesis, Indomethacin has been found to delay parturition in rats.

In rats and mice, 4.0 mg/kg/day given during the last three days of gestation caused a decrease in maternal weight gain and some maternal and fetal deaths. An increased incidence of neuronal necrosis in the diencephalon in the live-born fetuses was observed. At 2.0 mg/kg/day, no increase in neuronal necrosis was observed as compared to the control groups. Administration of 0.5 or 4.0 mg/kg/day during the first three days of life did not cause an increase in neuronal necrosis at either dose level.

USE IN NURSING MOTHERS

Indomethacin is excreted in the milk of lactating mothers. Indomethacin is not recommended for use in nursing mothers.

PRECAUTIONS

GENERAL

Nonsteroidal anti-inflammatory drugs, including Indomethacin, may mask the usual signs and symptoms of infection. Therefore, the physician must be continually on the alert for this and should use the drug with extra care in the presence of existing infection.

Fluid retention and peripheral edema have been observed in some patients taking Indomethacin. Therefore, as with other nonsteroidal anti-inflammatory drugs, Indomethacin should be used with caution in patients with cardiac dysfunction, hypertension, or other conditions predisposing to fluid retention.

In a study of patients with severe heart failure and hyponatremia, Indomethacin was associated with significant deterioration of circulatory hemodynamics, presumably due to inhibition of prostaglandin dependent compensatory mechanisms. Indomethacin, like other nonsteroidal anti-inflammatory agents, can inhibit platelet aggregation. This effect is of shorter duration than that seen with aspirin and usually disappears within 24 hours after discontinuation of Indomethacin. In one small study, platelet aggregation was grossly abnormal after Indomethacin therapy (given orally to premature infants to close the ductus arteriosus). Platelet aggregation returned to normal by the tenth day. Premature infants should be observed for signs of bleeding. Indomethacin has been shown to prolong bleeding time (but within the normal range) in normal subjects. Because this effect may be exaggerated in patients with underlying hemostatic defects Indomethacin should be used with caution in persons with coagulation defects.

As with other nonsteroidal anti-inflammatory drugs, borderline elevations of one or more liver tests may occur in up to 15% of patients. These abnormalities may progress, may remain essentially unchanged, or may be transient with continued therapy. The SGPT (ALT) test is probably the most sensitive indicator of liver dysfunction. Meaningful (3 times the upper limit of normal) elevations of SGPT or SGOT (AST) occurred in controlled clinical trials in less than 1% of patients. A patient with symptoms and/or signs suggesting liver dysfunction, or in whom an abnormal liver test has occurred, should be evaluated for evidence of the development of more severe hepatic reaction while on therapy with Indomethacin. Severe hepatic reactions, including jaundice and cases of fatal hepatitis, have been reported with Indomethacin as with other nonsteroidal anti-inflammatory drugs. Although such reactions are rare, if abnormal liver tests persist or worsen, if clinical signs and symptoms consistent with liver disease develop, or if systemic manifestations occur (e.g., eosinophilia, rash, etc.), Indomethacin should be discontinued. If clinical signs and symptoms consistent with liver disease develop in the neonate on Indomethacin IV or if systemic manifestations occur, Indomethacin IV should be discontinued.

Indomethacin IV should be administered carefully to avoid extravascular injection or leakage as the solution may be irritating to tissue.

INFORMATION FOR PATIENTS

Indomethacin, like other drugs of its class, is not free of side effects. The side effects of these drugs can cause discomfort and, rarely, there are more serious side effects such as gastrointestinal bleeding, which may result in hospitalization and even fatal outcomes.

NSAIDs (Nonsteroidal Anti-inflammatory Drugs) are often essential agents in the management of arthritis; but they also may be commonly employed for conditions which are less serious.

◆ RATED THERAPEUTICALLY EQUIVALENT; ◇ THERAPEUTIC EQUIVALENCE UNCONFIRMED; ○ UNRATED

Physicians may wish to discuss with their patients the potential risks (see *"Warnings"*, *"Precautions"* and *"Adverse Reactions"*) and likely benefits of NSAID treatment, particularly when the drugs are used for less serious conditions where treatment without NSAIDs may represent an acceptable alternative to both the patient and physician.

LABORATORY TESTS

Because serious GI tract ulceration and bleeding can occur without warning symptoms, physicians should follow chronically treated patients for the signs and symptoms of ulceration and bleeding and should inform them of the importance of this follow-up (see *"Warnings, Risk of GI Ulcerations, Bleeding and Perforation with NSAID Therapy"*).

CARCINOGENESIS, MUTAGENESIS, IMPAIRMENT OF FERTILITY

In an 81-week chronic oral toxicity study in the rat at doses up to 1 mg/kg/day, Indomethacin had no tumorigenic effect. Indomethacin produced no neoplastic or hyperplastic changes related to treatment in carcinogenic studies in the rat (dosing period 73-110 weeks) and the mouse (dosing period 62-88 weeks) at doses up to 1.5 mg/kg/day.

Indomethacin did not have any mutagenic effect in *in vitro* bacterial tests (Ames test and *E. coli* with or without metabolic activation) and a series of *in vivo* tests including the host-mediated assay, sex-linked recessive lethals in *Drosophila*, and the micronucleus test in mice.

Indomethacin at dosage levels up to 0.5 mg/kg/day had no effect on fertility in mice in a two generation reproduction study or a two litter reproduction study in rats.

DRUG INTERACTIONS

In normal volunteers receiving Indomethacin, the administration of diflunisal decreased the renal clearance and significantly increased the plasma levels of Indomethacin. In some patients, combined use of Indomethacin and diflunisal has been associated with fatal gastrointestinal hemorrhage. Therefore, diflunisal and Indomethacin should not be used concomitantly.

In a study in normal volunteers, it was found that chronic concurrent administration of 3.6 g of aspirin per day decreases Indomethacin blood levels approximately 20%.

Clinical studies have shown that Indomethacin does not influence the hypoprothrombinemia produced by anticoagulants. However, when any additional drug, including Indomethacin is added to the treatment of patients on anticoagulant therapy, the patients should be observed for alterations of the prothrombin time.

When Indomethacin is given to patients receiving probenecid, the plasma levels of Indomethacin are likely to be increased. Therefore, a lower total daily dosage of Indomethacin may produce a satisfactory therapeutic effect. When increases in the dose of Indomethacin are made, they should be made carefully and in small increments.

Caution should be used if Indomethacin is administered simultaneously with methotrexate. Indomethacin has been reported to decrease the tubular secretion of methotrexate and to potentiate its toxicity.

Administration of nonsteroidal anti-inflammatory drugs concomitantly with cyclosporine has been associated with an increase in cyclosporine-induced toxicity, possibly due to decreased synthesis of renal prostacyclin. NSAIDs should be used with caution in patients taking cyclosporine, and renal function should be monitored.

Capsules Indomethacin 50 mg t.i.d. produced a clinically relevant elevation of plasma lithium and reduction in renal lithium clearance in psychiatric patients and normal subjects with steady state plasma lithium concentrations. This effect has been attributed to inhibition of prostaglandin synthesis. As a consequence, when Indomethacin and lithium are given concomitantly, the patient should be carefully observed for signs of lithium toxicity. (Read circulars for lithium preparations before use of such concomitant therapy.) In addition, the frequency of monitoring serum lithium concentration should be increased at the outset of such combination drug treatment.

Indomethacin given concomitantly with digoxin has been reported to increase the serum concentration and prolong the half-life of digoxin. Therefore, when Indomethacin and digoxin are used concomitantly, serum digoxin levels should be closely monitored.

In some patients, the administration of Indomethacin can reduce the diuretic, natriuretic, and, antihypertensive effects of loop, potassium-sparing, and thiazide diuretics. Therefore, when Indomethacin and diuretics are used concomitantly, the patient should be observed closely to determine if the desired effect of the diuretic is obtained.

Indomethacin reduces basal plasma renin activity (PRA), as well as those elevations of PRA induced by furosemide administration, or salt or volume depletion. These facts should be considered when evaluating plasma renin activity in hypertensive patients. Therapy with Indomethacin may blunt the natriuretic effect of furosemide. This response has been attributed to inhibition of prostaglandin synthesis by nonsteroidal anti-inflammatory drugs. In a study of 19 premature infants with patent ductus arteriosus treated with either Indomethacin I.V. alone or a combination of Indomethacin I.V. and furosemide, results showed that infants receiving both Indomethacin I.V. and furosemide had significantly higher urinary output, higher levels of sodium and chloride excretion, and higher glomerular filtration rates than did those infants receiving Indomethacin I.V. alone. In this study, the data suggested that therapy with furosemide helped to maintain renal function in the premature infant when Indomethacin I.V. was added to the treatment of patent ductus arteriosus.

It has been reported that the addition of triamterene to a maintenance schedule of Indomethacin resulted in reversible acute renal failure in two of four healthy volunteers. Indomethacin and triamterene should not be administered together. Indomethacin and potassium-sparing diuretics each may be associated with increased serum potassium levels. The potential effects of Indomethacin and potassium-sparing diuretics on potassium kinetics and renal function should be considered when these agents are administered concurrently.

Most of the above effects concerning diuretics have been attributed, at least in part, to mechanisms involving inhibition of prostaglandin synthesis by Indomethacin.

Blunting of the antihypertensive effect of beta-adrenoceptor blocking agents by non-steroidal anti-inflammatory drugs including Indomethacin has been reported. Therefore, when using these blocking agents to treat hypertension, patients should be observed carefully in order to confirm that the desired therapeutic effect has been obtained. There are reports that Indomethacin can reduce the antihypertensive effect of captopril in some patients.

False-negative results in the dexamethasone suppression test (DST) in patients being treated with Indomethacin have been reported. Thus, results of the DST should be interpreted with caution in these patients.

Since renal function may be reduced by Indomethacin IV consideration should be given to reduction in dosage of those medications that rely on adequate renal function for their elimination. Because the half-life of digitalis (given frequently to pre-term infants with patent ductus arteriosus and associated cardiac failure) may be prolonged when given concomitantly with Indomethacin, the infant should be observed closely; frequent ECGs and serum digitalis levels may be required to prevent or detect digitalis toxicity early. Furthermore, in one study of premature infants treated with Indomethacin IV and also receiving either gentamicin or amikacin, both peak and trough levels of these aminoglycosides were significantly elevated.

PEDIATRIC USE

Effectiveness of Indomethacin Capsules and Suppositories in children 14 years of age and younger has not been established (see *"Warnings"*).

ADVERSE REACTIONS

Capsules and Suppositories: The adverse reactions for Capsules Indomethacin listed in the following table have been arranged into two groups: (1) incidence greater than 1%; and (2) incidence less than 1%. The incidence for group (1) was obtained from 33 double-blind controlled clinical trials reported in the literature (1,092 patients). The incidence for group (2) was based on reports in clinical trials, in the literature, and on voluntary reports since marketing. The probability of a causal relationship exists between Indomethacin and these adverse reactions, some of which have been reported only rarely.

In controlled clinical trials, the incidence of adverse reactions to Capsules Indomethacin SR and equal 24-hour doses of Capsules Indomethacin were similar.

The adverse reactions reported with Capsules Indomethacin may occur with use of the suppositories. In addition, rectal irritation and tenesmus have been reported in patients who have received the suppositories.

The adverse reactions reported with Capsules Indomethacin may also occur with use of the suspension.

Incidence greater than 1%	Incidence less than 1%	
Gastrointestinal		
nausea* with or without vomiting	anorexia	gastrointestinal bleeding without obvious ulcer
dyspepsia* (including indigestion, heartburn and epigastric pain)	bloating (includes distention)	formation and perforation of pre-existing
	flatulence	
	peptic ulcer	
	gastroenteritis	sigmoid lesions
diarrhea	rectal bleeding	(diverticulum,
abdominal distress or pain	proctitis	carcinoma, etc.)
constipation	single or multiple ulcerations including perforation and hemorrhage of the esophagus, stomach, duodenum or small and large intestines intestinal ulceration associated with stenosis and obstruction	development of ulcerative colitis and regional ileitis ulcerative stomatitis toxic hepatitis and jaundice (some fatal cases have been reported)
Central Nervous System		
headache (11.7%)	anxiety (includes nervousness)	light-headedness
dizziness*	muscle weakness	syncope
vertigo	involuntary muscle movements	paresthesia
somnolence	insomnia	aggravation of epilepsy and parkinsonism
depression and fatigue (including malaise and listlessness)	muzziness	depersonalization
	psychic distur-	coma

Incidence greater than 1%	Incidence less than 1%	
	bances including psychotic episodes mental confusion drowsiness	peripheral neuropathy convulsions dysarthria
Special Senses		
tinnitus	ocular—corneal deposits and retinal distur- bances, including those of the macula, have been reported in some patients on pro- longed therapy with Indomethacin	blurred vision diplopia hearing disturbances deafness
Cardiovascular		
none	hypertension hypotension tachycardia chest pain	congestive heart failure arrhythmia; palpitations
Metabolic		
none	edema weight gain fluid retention flushing or sweating	hyperglycemia glycosuria hyperkalemia
Integumentary		
none	pruritus rash; urticaria petechiae or ecchymosis	exfoliative dermatitis erythema nodosum loss of hair Stevens-Johnson syndrome erythema multiforme toxic epidermal necrolysis
Hematologic		
none	leukopenia bone marrow depression anemia secondary to obvious or occult gastrointestinal bleeding	aplastic anemia hemolytic anemia agranulocytosis thrombocytopenic purpura disseminated intravascular coagulation
Hypersensitivity		
none	acute anaphylaxis acute repiratory distress rapid fall in blood pressure resembling a shock-like-state angioedema	dyspnea asthma purpura angiitis pulmonary edema fever
Genitourinary		
none	hematuria vaginal bleeding proteinuria nephrotic syndrome interstitial nephritis	BUN elevation renal sufficiency, including renal failure
Miscellaneous		
none	epistaxis breast changes, including enlargement and tenderness, or gynecomastia	

* *Reactions occurring in 3% to 9% of patients treated with Indomethacin. (Those reactions occurring in less than 3% of the patients are unmarked.)*

Causal Relationship Unknown: Other reactions have been reported but occurred under circumstances where a causal relationship could not be established. However, in these rarely reported events, the possibility cannot be excluded. Therefore, these observations are being listed to serve as alerting information to physicians:

Cardiovascular: Thrombophlebitis

Hematologic: Although there have been several reports of leukemia, the supporting information is weak.

Genitourinary: Urinary frequency.

A rare occurrence of fulminant necrotizing fasciitis, particularly in association with Group A β-hemolytic streptococcus, has been described in persons treated with nonsteroidal anti-inflammatory agents, including Indomethacin, sometimes with fatal outcome (see also *"Precautions, General"*).

Intravenous: In a double-blind placebo-controlled trial of 405 premature infants weighing less than or equal to 1750 g with evidence of large ductal shunting, in those infants treated with Indomethacin (n = 206), there was a statistically significantly greater incidence of bleeding problems, including gross or microscopic bleeding into the gastrointestinal tract, oozing from the skin after needle stick, pulmonary hemorrhage, and disseminated intravascular coagulopathy. There was no statistically significant difference between treatment groups with reference to intracranial hemorrhage.

The infants treated with Indomethacin sodium trihydrate also had a significantly higher incidence of transient oliguria and elevations of serum creatinine (greater than or equal to 1.8 mg/dL) than did the infants treated with placebo.

The incidences of retrolental fibroplasia (grades III and IV) and pneumothorax in infants treated with Indomethacin IV were no greater than in placebo controls and were statistically significantly lower than in surgically-treated infants. The following additional adverse reactions in infants have been reported from the collaborative study, anecdotal case reports, and from other studies using rectal, oral, or intravenous Indomethacin for treatment of patent ductus arteriosus. The rates are based on the experience of 849 Indomethacin-treated infants reported in the medical literature, regardless of the route of administration. One year follow-up is available on 175 infants and shows no long-term sequelae which could be attributed to Indomethacin. In controlled clinical studies, only electrolyte imbalance and renal dysfunction (of the reactions listed below) occurred statistically significantly more frequently after Indomethacin I.V. than after placebo.

Renal: renal dysfunction in 41 percent of infants, including one or more of the following: reduced urinary output; reduced urine sodium, chloride, or potassium, urine osmolality, free water clearance, or glomerular filtration rate; elevated serum creatinine or BUN; uremia.

Cardiovascular: intracranial bleeding**, pulmonary hypertension.

Gastrointestinal: gastrointestinal bleeding*, vomiting, abdominal distention, transient ileus, localized perforation(s) of the small and/or large intestine.

Metabolic: hyponatremia*, elevated serum potassium*, reduction in blood sugar, including hypoglycemia, increased weight gain (fluid retention).

Coagulation: decreased platelet aggregation (see *"Precautions"*).

The following adverse reactions have also been reported in infants treated with Indomethacin, however, a causal relationship to therapy with Indomethacin I.V. has not been established:

Cardiovascular: bradycardia.

Respiratory: apnea, exacerbation of pre-existing pulmonary infection.

Metabolic: acidosis/alkalosis.

Hematologic: disseminated intravascular coagulation.

Gastrointestinal: necrotizing enterocolitis.

Ophthalmic: retrolental fibroplasia.**

OVERDOSAGE

The following symptoms may be observed following overdosage; nausea, vomiting, intense headache, dizziness, mental confusion, disorientation, or lethargy. There have been reports of parethesias, numbness, and convulsions.

Treatment is symptomatic and supportive. The stomach should be emptied as quickly as possible if the ingestion is recent. If vomiting has not occurred spontaneously, the patient should be induced to vomit with syrup of ipecac. If the patient is unable to vomit, gastric lavage should be performed. Once the stomach has been emptied, 25 or 50 g of activated charcoal may be given. Depending on the condition of the patient, close medical observation and nursing care may be required. The patient should be followed for several days because gastrointestinal ulceration and hemorrhage have been reported as adverse reactions of Indomethacin. Use of antacids may be helpful.

The oral LD_{50} of Indomethacin in mice and rats (based on 14 day mortality response) was 50 and 12 mg/kg, respectively.

DOSAGE AND ADMINISTRATION

Capsules and Suppositories: Indomethacin is available as 25 and 50 mg Capsules Indomethacin, 75 mg Capsules Indomethacin SR for oral use, Oral Suspension Indomethacin, containing 25 mg of Indomethacin per 5 mL, and 50 mg Suppositories Indomethacin for rectal use. Capsules Indomethacin SR 75 mg once a day can be substituted for Capsules Indomethacin 25 mg t.i.d. However, there will be significant differences between the two dosage regimens in Indomethacin blood levels, especially after 12 hours (see *"Clinical Pharmacology"*). In addition, Capsules Indomethacin SR 75 mg b.i.d. can be substituted for Capsules Indomethacin 50 mg t.i.d. Capsules Indomethacin SR may be substituted for all the indications for Capsules Indomethacin except acute gouty arthritis. Adverse reactions appear to correlate with the size of the dose of Indomethacin in most patients but not all. Therefore, every effort should be made to determine the smallest effective dosage for the individual patient.

* Incidence 3-9 percent. Those reactions which are unmarked occurred in 1-3 percent of patients.
** Incidence in both Indomethacin and placebo-treated infants 3-9 percent. Those reactions which are unmarked occurred in less than 3 percent.

◆ RATED THERAPEUTICALLY EQUIVALENT; ◇ THERAPEUTIC EQUIVALENCE UNCONFIRMED; ○ UNRATED

Always give Capsules Indomethacin, Capsules Indomethacin SR, or Oral Suspension Indomethacin with food, immediately after meals, or with antacids to reduce gastric irritation.

PEDIATRIC USE
Indomethacin ordinarily should not be prescribed for children 14 years of age and under (see *"Warnings"*).

ADULT USE
Dosage Recommendations for Active Stages of the Following:

1. Moderate to severe rheumatoid arthritis including acute flares of chronic disease: moderate to severe ankylosing spondylitis; and moderate to severe osteoarthritis.
Suggested Dosage:
Capsules Indomethacin 25 mg b.i.d. or t.i.d. If this is well tolerated, increase the daily dosage by 25 or by 50 mg, if required by continuing symptoms, at weekly intervals until a satisfactory response is obtained or until a total daily dose of 150-200 mg is reached. *DOSES ABOVE THIS AMOUNT GENERALLY DO NOT INCREASE THE EFFECTIVENESS OF THE DRUG.*
In patients who have persistent night pain and/or morning stiffness, the giving of a large portion, up to a maximum of 100 mg, of the total daily dose at bedtime, either orally or by rectal suppositories, may be helpful in affording relief. The total daily dose should not exceed 200 mg. In acute flares of chronic rheumatoid arthritis, it may be necessary to increase the dosage by 25 mg or, if required, by 50 mg daily.
If Capsules Indomethacin SR 75 mg are used for initiating Indomethacin treatment, one capsule daily should be the usual starting dose in order to observe patient tolerance since 75 mg per day is the maximum recommended starting dose for Indomethacin (see above). If Capsules Indomethacin SR are used to increase the daily dose, patients should be observed for possible signs and symptoms of intolerance since the daily increment will exceed the daily increment recommended for the other dosage forms. For patients who require 150 mg of Indomethacin per day and have demonstrated acceptable tolerance, Indomethacin SR may be prescribed as one capsule twice daily.
If minor adverse effects develop as the dosage is increased, reduce the dosage rapidly to a tolerated dose and *OBSERVE THE PATIENT CLOSELY.*
If severe adverse reactions occur, *STOP THE DRUG.* After the acute phase of the disease is under control, an attempt to reduce the daily dose should be made repeatedly until the patient is receiving the smallest effective dose or the drug is discontinued.
Careful instructions to, and observations of, the individual patient are essential to the prevention of serious, irreversible, including fatal, adverse reactions.
As advancing years appear to increase the possibility of adverse reactions, Indomethacin should be used with greater care in the aged.
2. Acute painful shoulder (bursitis and/or tendinitis).
Initial Dose:
75-150 mg daily in 3 or 4 divided doses.
   The drug should be discontinued after the signs and symptoms of inflammation have been controlled for several days. The usual course of therapy is 7-14 days.
3. Acute gouty arthritis.
Suggested Dosage:
Capsules Indomethacin 50 mg t.i.d. until pain is tolerable. The dose should then be rapidly reduced to complete cessation of the drug. Definite relief of pain has been reported within 2 to 4 hours. Tenderness and heat usually subside in 24 to 36 hours, and swelling gradually disappears in 3 to 5 days.

INTRAVENOUS: FOR INTRAVENOUS ADMINISTRATION ONLY.
Dosage recommendations for closure of the ductus arteriosus depends on the age of the infant at the time of therapy. A course of therapy is defined as three intravenous doses of Indomethacin I.V. given at 12-24 hour intervals, with careful attention to urinary output. If anuria or marked oliguria (urinary output < 0.6 mL/kg/hr) is evident at the scheduled time of the second or third dose of Indomethacin I.V., no additional doses should be given until laboratory studies indicate that renal function has returned to normal (see *"Warnings, Renal Effects"*).
   Dosage according to age is as follows:

Age at 1st dose	Dosage (mg/kg)		
	1st	*2nd*	*3rd*
Less than 48 hours	0.2	0.1	0.1
2-7 days	0.2	0.2	0.2
over 7 days	0.2	0.25	0.25

If the ductus arteriosus closes or is significantly reduced in size after an interval of 48 hours or more from completion of the first course of Indomethacin IV no further doses are necessary. If the ductus arteriosus re-opens, a second course of 1-3 doses may be given, each dose separated by a 12-24 hour interval as described above.
   If the infant remains unresponsive to therapy with Indomethacin IV after 2 courses, surgery may be necessary for closure of the ductus arteriosus. If severe adverse reactions occur, STOP THE DRUG.

DIRECTIONS FOR USE
Parenteral drug products should be inspected visually for particulate matter and discoloration prior to administration whenever solution and container permit.

The solution should be prepared only with 1 to 2 mL of preservative-free sterile Sodium Chloride Injection, 0.9 percent or preservative-free Sterile Water for Injection. Benzyl alcohol as a preservative has been associated with toxicity in newborns. Therefore, all diluents should be preservative-free. If 1 mL of diluent is used, the concentration of Indomethacin in the solution will equal approximately 0.1 mg/0.1 mL; if 2 mL of diluent are used, the concentration of the solution will equal approximately 0.05 mg/0.1 mL. Any unused portion of the solution should be discarded because there is no preservative contained in the vial. A fresh solution should be prepared just prior to each administration. Once reconstituted, the Indomethacin solution may be injected intravenously over 5-10 seconds.
   Further dilution with intravenous infusion solutions is not recommended. Indomethacin I.V. is not buffered, and reconstitution with solutions at pH values below 6.0 may result in precipitation of the insoluble Indomethacin free acid moiety.

STORAGE
Store Oral Suspension Indomethacin below 30°C (86°F). Avoid temperatures above 50°C (122°F). Protect from freezing.
   Store Suppositories Indomethacin below 30°C (86°F). Avoid transient temperatures above 40°C (104°F).

HOW SUPPLIED
CAPSULE: 25 MG

AVERAGE UNIT PRICE (AVAILABLE SIZES)		GENERIC A-RATED AVERAGE PRICE (GAAP)	
BRAND	$0.53	100s	$16.13
GENERIC	$0.14	500s	$51.46
HCFA FUL (100s ea)	$0.03	1000s	$111.39

BRAND/MANUFACTURER	NDC	SIZE	AWP
◆ BRAND			
➤ INDOCIN: Merck	00006-0025-68	100s	$52.21
	00006-0025-28	100s ud	$56.08
	00006-0025-82	1000s	$506.54
◆ GENERICS			
Medirex	57480-0406-06	30s	$8.40
Major	00904-1175-89	90s	$4.15
Novopharm	55953-0420-40	100s	$6.15
Watson	52544-0303-01	100s	$8.45
Raway	00686-0190-20	100s	$9.00
Rugby	00536-3981-01	100s	$10.62
Major	00904-1175-60	100s	$10.70
Geneva	00781-2325-01	100s	$10.75
➤ West Point	59591-0172-68	100s	$10.85
Warner Chilcott	00047-0887-24	100s	$11.45
Moore,H.L.	00839-6762-06	100s	$11.46
Schein	00364-0691-01	100s	$11.95
Martec	52555-0474-01	100s	$12.05
Zenith	00172-4029-60	100s	$12.10
Goldline	00182-1681-01	100s	$12.10
Qualitest	00603-4067-21	100s	$13.94
Par	49884-0067-01	100s	$14.90
URL	00677-0872-01	100s	$15.90
Mutual	53489-0133-01	100s	$15.90
Sidmak	50111-0406-01	100s	$15.95
Aligen	00405-4541-01	100s	$15.99
➤ Mylan	00378-0143-01	100s	$17.75
Lederle Std Prod	00005-3761-23	100s	$20.90
Parmed	00349-8341-01	100s	$24.56
U.S. Trading	56126-0067-11	100s ud	$4.61
Novopharm	55953-0420-01	100s ud	$9.33
Vangard	00615-2516-13	100s ud	$31.71
UDL	51079-0190-20	100s ud	$31.81
Medirex	57480-0406-01	100s ud	$32.00
Goldline	00182-1681-89	100s ud	$32.30
Geneva	00781-2325-13	100s ud	$32.50
Novopharm	55953-0420-70	500s	$27.12
Parmed	00349-8341-05	500s	$44.54
Rugby	00536-3981-05	500s	$47.19
Goldline	00182-1681-05	500s	$47.25
Zenith	00172-4029-70	500s	$57.48
Mutual	53489-0133-05	500s	$59.00
URL	00677-0872-05	500s	$64.30
Par	49884-0067-05	500s	$64.83
Novopharm	55953-0420-80	1000s	$48.17
Qualitest	00603-4067-32	1000s	$63.91
Major	00904-1175-80	1000s	$64.00
Geneva	00781-2325-10	1000s	$65.00
Watson	52544-0303-10	1000s	$65.95
Rugby	00536-3981-10	1000s	$76.68
➤ West Point	59591-0172-82	1000s	$81.80
Schein	00364-0691-02	1000s	$81.95
Moore,H.L.	00839-6762-16	1000s	$83.36
URL	00677-0872-10	1000s	$114.00
Mutual	53489-0133-10	1000s	$114.00
Warner Chilcott	00047-0887-32	1000s	$114.50
Zenith	00172-4029-80	1000s	$114.95
Goldline	00182-1681-10	1000s	$114.95
Par	49884-0067-10	1000s	$129.63
Parmed	00349-8341-10	1000s	$159.90
➤ Mylan	00378-0143-10	1000s	$159.95
Aligen	00405-4541-03	1000s	$187.55
Sidmak	50111-0406-03	1000s	$187.55
Lederle Std Prod	00005-3761-34	1000s	$200.00

➤ SHOWN IN PRODUCT IDENTIFICATION GUIDE

CAPSULE: 50 MG

AVERAGE UNIT PRICE (AVAILABLE SIZES)		GENERIC A-RATED AVERAGE PRICE (GAAP)	
BRAND	$0.87	100s	$25.01
GENERIC	$0.22	500s	$97.52
HCFA FUL (100s ea)	$0.04	1000s	$149.52

BRAND/MANUFACTURER	NDC	SIZE	AWP
◆ **BRAND**			
➤ INDOCIN: Merck	00006-0050-68	100s	$85.20
	00006-0050-28	100s ud	$89.09
◆ **GENERICS**			
Raway	00686-0191-20	100s	$11.00
Novopharm	55953-0439-40	100s	$11.54
Watson	52544-0304-01	100s	$14.07
Geneva	00781-2350-01	100s	$16.25
➤ West Point	59591-0159-68	100s	$17.70
Warner Chilcott	00047-0888-24	100s	$19.15
Moore,H.L.	00839-6763-06	100s	$19.24
Qualitest	00603-4068-21	100s	$19.40
Rugby	00536-3982-01	100s	$19.50
Major	00904-1176-60	100s	$19.55
Schein	00364-0692-01	100s	$19.55
Martec	52555-0475-01	100s	$19.65
Zenith	00172-4030-60	100s	$20.58
Goldline	00182-1682-01	100s	$20.58
Par	49884-0068-01	100s	$22.40
URL	00677-0873-01	100s	$30.00
Mutual	53489-0134-01	100s	$30.00
Aligen	00405-4542-01	100s	$30.25
Sidmak	50111-0407-01	100s	$30.25
Mylan	00378-0147-01	100s	$30.50
Parmed	00349-8342-01	100s	$35.26
Lederle Std Prod	00005-3762-23	100s	$37.65
U.S. Trading	56126-0068-11	100s ud	$6.92
Novopharm	55953-0439-01	100s ud	$14.04
UDL	51079-0191-20	100s ud	$52.98
Geneva	00781-2350-13	100s ud	$53.50
Goldline	00182-1682-89	100s ud	$53.70
Novopharm	55953-0439-70	500s	$45.10
Geneva	00781-2350-05	500s	$62.50
Major	00904-1176-40	500s	$64.00
Watson	52544-0304-05	500s	$65.95
Rugby	00536-3982-05	500s	$76.68
Moore,H.L.	00839-6763-12	500s	$80.93
Mutual	53489-0134-05	500s	$89.00
Schein	00364-0692-05	500s	$89.50
URL	00677-0873-05	500s	$89.65
Qualitest	00603-4068-28	500s	$89.70
Parmed	00349-8342-05	500s	$96.25
Zenith	00172-4030-70	500s	$97.76
Goldline	00182-1682-05	500s	$97.76
Par	49884-0068-05	500s	$112.80
Aligen	00405-4542-02	500s	$134.70
Sidmak	50111-0407-05	500s	$134.75
Mylan	00378-0147-05	500s	$144.85
Lederle Std Prod	00005-3762-31	500s	$183.54
Novopharm	55953-0439-80	1000s	$85.69
Mutual	53489-0134-10	1000s	$168.00
Par	49884-0068-10	1000s	$194.88

For additional alternatives, turn to the section beginning on page 2859.

Inflamase *SEE* PREDNISOLONE, SYSTEMIC

Influenza Virus Vaccine

DESCRIPTION

Influenza Virus Vaccine Types A and B (Surface Antigen or Purified Subviron) is a sterile parenteral for intramuscular use only.

The purified-surface-antigen vaccine is prepared from the extraembryonic fluid of embryonated chicken eggs inoculated with a specific type of influenza virus containing neomycin and polymyxin. The fluid containing the virus is harvested and clarified by centrifugation and filtration prior to inactivation with betapropiolactone. The inactivated virus is concentrated and purified by zonal centrifugation.

The surface antigens, hemagglutinin and neuraminidase, are obtained from the influenza virus particle by further centrifugation in the presence of Triton®[†] N101, a process which removes most of the internal proteins. The Triton N101 is removed from the surface antigen preparation and the antigens are suspended in 0.01M phosphate buffered saline. The purified-subvirion vaccine is prepared from the allantoic fluid of chick embryos innoculated with a specific type of influenza virus. During processing, not more than 5 μg of gentamicin sulfate per mL is added. The harvested virus is inactivated with formaldehyde and is concentrated and purified by a column-chromatographic procedure. At the same time, addition of tri(n)butylphosphate and Polysorbate 80, USP, to the column-eluting fluids effects disruption and inactivation of a significant proportion of the

virus to smaller subunit particles. The recovered subvirion (split-virus) suspension is freed of substantial portions of the disrupting agents by dialysis and of other undesirable materials by selective filtration through membranes of controlled pore size.

The hemagglutinin content is standardized according to current United States Public Health Service requirements. Each dose (0.5 mL) contains the recommended ratio of not less than 15 μg of hemagglutinin of each strain similar to: A/Texas/36/91-(H$_1$N$_1$), A/Beijing/32/92-(H$_3$N$_2$), and B/Panama/45/90 viruses.[1]

Thimerosal (mercury derivative) 0.01% is added as a preservative. Polymyxin, neomycin, betapropiolactone, and gentamicin sulfate cannot be detected in the final product by current assay procedures.

CLINICAL PHARMACOLOGY

The administration of inactivated influenza vaccine to high-risk persons each year before the influenza season is the single most important influenza-control measure. The injection of antigens prepared from inactivated influenza virus stimulates the production of specific antibodies.

Influenza A viruses are classified into subtypes on the basis of two surface antigens: hemagglutinin (H) and neuraminidase (N). Three subtypes of hemagglutinin (H$_1$, H$_2$, and H$_3$) and two subtypes of neuraminidase (N$_1$, N$_2$) are recognized among influenza A viruses that have caused widespread human disease. Immunity to these antigens, especially the hemagglutinin, reduces the likelihood of infection and lessens the severity of the disease if infection occurs. Infection with a virus of one subtype confers little or no protection against viruses of other subtypes. Furthermore, over time, antigenic variation (antigenic drift) within a subtype may be so marked that infection or immunization with one strain may not induce immunity to distantly related strains of the same subtype. Although influenza B viruses have shown more antigenic stability than influenza A viruses, antigenic variation does occur. For these reasons major epidemics of respiratory disease caused by new variants of influenza continue to occur. The antigenic characteristics of strains currently circulating provide the basis for selecting virus strains to include in each year's vaccine.[2]

Typical influenza illness is characterized by abrupt onset of fever, myalgia, sore throat, and nonproductive cough. Unlike other common respiratory infections, influenza can cause severe malaise lasting several days. More severe illness can result if primary influenza pneumonia or secondary bacterial pneumonia occurs. During influenza epidemics, high attack rates of acute illness result in increased numbers of visits to physicians' offices, walk-in clinics, and emergency rooms and increased hospitalization for management of lower respiratory tract complications.[2]

Elderly persons and persons with underlying health problems are at increased risk of complications from influenza infection. If infected, such high-risk persons or groups (listed as "groups at increased risk for influenza-related complications" under Target Groups for Special Vaccination Programs) are more likely than the general population to require hospitalization. During major epidemics, hospitalization rates for high-risk persons may increase two to fivefold, depending on the age group. Previously healthy children and young adults may also require hospitalization for influenza-related complications, but the relative increase in their hospitalization rates is less than for persons who belong to high-risk groups.[2]

An increase in mortality further indicates the impact of influenza epidemics. Increased mortality results not only from influenza and pneumonia, but also from cardiopulmonary and other chronic diseases that can be exacerbated by influenza infection. It is estimated that more than 10,000 excess deaths occurred during each of 7 different US epidemics in the period 1977 to 1988, and more than 40,000 excess deaths occurred during each of two of these epidemics. Approximately 80% to 90% of the excess deaths attributed to pneumonia and influenza were among persons 65 years of age or older.[2] However, during major epidemics, influenza-associated deaths also occur among children and previously healthy adults under 65 years of age.

Because the proportion of elderly persons in the United States population is increasing and because age and its associated chronic diseases are risk factors for severe influenza illness, the toll from influenza can be expected to increase unless control measures are used more vigorously. The number of younger persons at increased risk for influenza-related complications is also increasing for various reasons, such as the success of neonatal intensive care units, better management of diseases such as cystic fibrosis, acquired immunodeficiency syndrome (AIDS), and better survival rates for organ transplant recipients.[2]

Reye syndrome has been associated primarily with influenza B, but also with influenza A infection.[3]

The effectiveness of influenza vaccine in preventing or attenuating illness varies, depending primarily upon the age and immunocompetence of the vaccine recipient and the degree of similarity between the virus strains included in the vaccine and those that circulate during the influenza season. When there is a good match between vaccine and circulating viruses, influenza vaccine has been shown to prevent illness in approximately 70% of healthy children and younger adults. Under these circumstances, studies have also shown influenza vaccine to be approximately 70% effective in preventing hospitalization for pneumonia and influenza among elderly persons living in the community. Among elderly persons residing in nursing homes, the vaccine is most effective in preventing severe illness, secondary complications, and death. Studies of this population have shown influenza vaccine to be 50% to 60% effective in preventing hospitalization and pneumonia and up to 80% effective in preventing death, even though efficacy in preventing influenza illness may often be in the range of 30% to 40%. Achieving high rates of vaccination among nursing home residents has been shown to reduce the spread of infection when it is introduced into a facility, thus preventing infection through herd immunity.[2] The Public Health Service (PHS) regularly reviews the antigenic characteristics of current strains in order to select those to be included in the contemporary vaccine. Based upon epidemiological studies of circulating influenza virus strains, the PHS has recommended that the 1993-1994 vaccine will be trivalent and contain 15 µg of hemagglutinin of each strain similar to: A/Texas/36/91-(H$_1$N$_1$), A/Beijing/32/92-(H$_3$N$_2$), and B/Panama/45/90 viruses.[1]

INDICATIONS AND USAGE
Influenza Virus Vaccine, Types A and B, is indicated for immunization against influenza viruses containing antigens related to those in the vaccine.

Influenza vaccine is strongly recommended for persons 6 months of age or older who, by virtue of age or underlying medical condition, are at increased risk of complications from influenza. Health care workers and others (including household members) in close contact with high-risk persons should also be immunized. In addition, influenza vaccine may be given to children and teenagers receiving long-term aspirin therapy who, therefore, may be at increased risk of developing Rye's Sydrome after an influenza virus infection and to any person who wishes to reduce the chances of becoming infected with influenza. Guidelines for the use of vaccine among different groups follow.[2]

Although the current Influenza Virus Vaccine can contain one or more antigens used in previous years, annual immunization using the current vaccine is necessary because immunity declines in the year following immunization.[2] *Because the 1993-1994 vaccine differs from the 1992-1993 vaccine, supplies of 1992-1993 vaccine should not be used to provide protection for the 1993-1994 influenza season.*[2]

Two doses given at least one month apart may be required for a satisfactory response among previously unvaccinated children less than 9 years of age; however, studies with vaccines similar to those in current use have shown little or no improvement in antibody responses when a second dose is given to adults during the same season.[2]

TARGET GROUPS FOR SPECIAL IMMUNIZATION PROGRAMS
To maximize protection of high-risk persons, they and their close contacts should be targeted for organized immunization programs.

GROUPS AT INCREASED MEDICAL RISK OF INFLUENZA-RELATED COMPLICATIONS
1. Persons 65 years of age or older[2] (regardless of health status).
2. Residents of nursing homes and other chronic-care facilities housing persons of any age with chronic medical conditions.[2]
3. Adults and children with chronic disorders of the pulmonary or cardiovascular systems requiring regular medical follow-up or hospitalization during the preceding year, including children with asthma.[2]
4. Adults and children who have required regular medical follow-up or hospitalization during the preceding year because of chronic metabolic diseases (including diabetes mellitus), renal dysfunction, hemoglobinopathies, or immunosuppression (including immunosuppression caused by medication).[2]
5. Children and teenagers (6 months through 18 years of age) who are receiving long-term aspirin therapy and, therefore, may be at risk of developing Reye syndrome following influenza infection.[2]

Elderly persons and persons with certain chronic diseases may develop lower postvaccination antibody titers than healthy young adults and thus may remain susceptible to influenza upper-respiratory-tract infections. Nevertheless, even if such persons develop influenza illness, the vaccine has been shown to be effective in preventing lower-respiratory-tract involvement or other complications, thereby reducing the risk of hospitalization and death.

GROUPS THAT CAN TRANSMIT INFLUENZA TO HIGH-RISK PERSONS
Persons who are clinically or subclinically infected or are themselves incubating infection and who attend or live with high-risk persons can transmit influenza virus to them. Some high-risk persons (eg, the elderly, transplant recipients, or persons with acquired immunodeficiency syndrome [AIDS]) can have low antibody responses to influenza vaccine. Efforts to protect these high-risk persons against influenza may be improved by reducing the chances of exposure to influenza from their care providers. Therefore, the following groups should be immunized:[2]
1. Physicians, nurses, and other personnel in both hospital and outpatient care settings who have contact with high-risk persons among all age groups, including infants.[2]
2. Employees of nursing homes and chronic-care facilities who have contact with patients or residents.[2]
3. Providers of home care to high-risk persons (eg, visiting nurses and/or volunteer workers).[2]
4. Household members (including children) of high-risk persons.[2]

IMMUNIZATION OF OTHER GROUPS
General Population: Physicians should administer influenza vaccine to any person who wishes to reduce the chances of acquiring influenza infection. Persons who provide essential community services may be considered for immunization to minimize disruption of essential activities during influenza outbreaks. Similarly, students or other persons in institutional settings such as those who reside in dormitories should be considered for immunization to minimize the disruption of routine activities during epidemics.[2]

Pregnant Women: Influenza-associated excess mortality among pregnant women has not been documented, except in the pandemics of 1918-1919 and 1957-1958. However, the Immunization Practices Advisory Committee (ACIP) of the United

States Public Health Service recommends that pregnant women who have other medical conditions that increase their risk of complications from influenza should be immunized, as the vaccine is considered safe for pregnant women. The ACIP has stated that administering the vaccine after the first trimester is a reasonable precaution to minimize any concern over the theoretical possibility of teratogenicity. The ACIP has also stated however that it may be *undesirable* to delay immunization of pregnant women with high-risk conditions who will still be in the first trimester of pregnancy when the influenza season begins.[2] **The clinical judgment of the attending physician should prevail at all times in determining whether to administer the vaccine to a pregnant woman (see "Precautions, Use in Pregnancy").**

Persons Infected with Human Immunodeficiency Virus (HIV): Little information exists regarding the frequency and severity of influenza illness in human immunodeficiency virus (HIV)-infected persons, but recent reports suggest that symptoms of influenza may be prolonged and the risk of complications increased in this high-risk group.[2]

Because influenza may result in serious illness and complications in some HIV-infected persons, immunization is a prudent precaution and will result in protective antibody levels in many recipients.[2] However, the antibody response to vaccine may be low in persons with advanced HIV-related illnesses; a booster dose of vaccine has not improved the immune response in these individuals.[2]

Foreign Travelers: Increasingly, the elderly and persons with high-risk medical conditions are embarking on international travel. The risk of exposure to influenza during foreign travel varies, depending on, among other factors, the season and destination. Influenza can occur throughout the year in the tropics; the season of greatest influenza activity in the southern hemisphere is April through September. Because of the short incubation period for influenza, exposure to the virus during travel can result in clinical illness that also begins during travel, an inconvenient or potentially dangerous situation, especially for those at increased risk for complications. Persons preparing to travel to the tropics at any time of year or to the southern hemisphere during April through September should review their influenza immunization histories. If they were not immunized the previous fall/winter, they should be considered for influenza immunization prior to travel. The most current available vaccine should be used. High-risk persons given the previous season's vaccine prior to travel should be reimmunized in the fall/winter with current vaccine.[2]

TIMING OF IMMUNIZATION
Beginning each September, when vaccine for the upcoming influenza season becomes available, high-risk persons who are seen by health care providers for routine care or as a result of hospitalization should be offered influenza vaccine. Opportunities to vaccinate persons at high-risk for complications of influenza should not be missed.

The optimal time for organized vaccination campaigns for high-risk persons usually is the period between mid-October and mid-November. In the United States influenza activity generally peaks between late December and early March, and high levels of influenza activity infrequently occur in the contiguous 48 states before December. It is particularly important to avoid administering vaccine too far in advance of the influenza season in facilities such as nursing homes because antibody levels may begin to decline within a few months of vaccination. Vaccination programs may be undertaken as soon as current vaccine is available if regional influenza activity is expected to begin earlier than December.[2] Children under 9 years of age who have not been immunized previously require two doses with at least one month between doses. The second dose should be given before December, if possible. Vaccine can be given to both children and adults up to the time influenza virus activity is documented in a region, and even thereafter, which may be as late as April in some areas.[2]

If this product is to be used in an immunization program sponsored by an organization *where a traditional physician/patient relationship does not exist*, each participant (or legal guardian) should be made aware of the possible risks that have been associated with the use of influenza virus vaccines, including the possible risk of a form of paralysis sometimes known as Guillain-Barré syndrome. Information about possible side effects and adverse reactions is presented below, and consent, preferably written, should be obtained from the intended recipient (or legal guardian) before vaccine administration.

Simultaneous Administration of Pnuemococcal or Pediatric Vaccines: Pnuemococcal vaccine and influenza vaccine can be given at the same time at different sites without increased side effects. However, it should be emphasized that whereas influenza vaccine is given annually, pneumococcal vaccine is generally given only once to all but those at highest risk of fatal pneumococcal disease.

It may be desirable to simultaneously administer influenza vaccine, if indicated, with routine pediatric vaccine but at different sites. Although studies have not been done, no diminution of immunogenicity or enhancement of adverse reactions should be expected. Influenza vaccine should not be given within 3 days of vaccination with pertussis vaccine.

CONTRAINDICATIONS
INFLUENZA VIRUS IS PROPAGATED IN EGGS FOR THE PREPARATION OF INFLUENZA VIRUS VACCINE. THUS, THIS VACCINE SHOULD NOT BE ADMINISTERED TO ANYONE WITH A HISTORY OF HYPERSENSITIVITY (ALLERGY) TO CHICKEN EGGS.[2] THE VACCINE IS ALSO CONTRAINDICATED IN INDIVIDUALS HYPERSENSITIVE TO ANY COMPONENT OF THE VACCINE INCLUDING THIMEROSAL (A MERCURY DERIVATIVE) (SEE *"ADVERSE REACTIONS"*). EPINEPHRINE INJECTION (1:1000) MUST BE IMMEDIATELY AVAILABLE SHOULD AN ACUTE ANAPHYLACTIC REACTION OCCUR DUE TO ANY COMPONENT OF THE VACCINE. BEFORE BEING VACCINATED, PERSONS KNOWN TO BE

HYPERSENSITIVE TO EGG PROTEIN OR OTHER COMPONENTS SHOULD BE GIVEN A SKIN TEST OR OTHER ALLERGY-EVALUATING TEST, USING THE INFLUENZA VIRUS VACCINE AS THE ANTIGEN. PERSONS WITH ADVERSE REACTIONS TO SUCH TESTING SHOULD NOT BE VACCINATED. CHEMOPROPHYLAXIS MAY BE INDICATED FOR PREVENTION OF INFLUENZA IN SUCH PERSONS. HOWEVER, PERSONS WITH A HISTORY OF ANAPHYLACTIC HYPERSENSITIVITY TO VACCINE COMPONENTS BUT WHO ARE ALSO AT HIGHEST RISK FOR COMPLICATIONS OF INFLUENZA INFECTIONS MAY BENEFIT FROM VACCINE AFTER APPROPRIATE EVALUATION AND DESENSITIZATION.

IMMUNIZATION SHOULD BE DELAYED IN PERSONS WITH AN ACTIVE NEUROLOGICAL DISORDER CHARACTERIZED BY CHANGING NEUROLOGICAL FINDINGS, BUT SHOULD BE CONSIDERED WHEN THE DISEASE PROCESS HAS BEEN STABILIZED.

THE OCCURRENCE OF ANY NEUROLOGICAL SYMPTOMS OR SIGNS FOLLOWING ADMINISTRATION OF THIS PRODUCT IS A CONTRAINDICATION TO FURTHER USE.

PERSONS WITH A PAST HISTORY OF GUILLAIN-BARRÉ SYNDROME (GBS) SHOULD NOT BE GIVEN INFLUENZA VIRUS VACCINE.

THE VACCINE SHOULD NOT BE ADMINISTERED TO PERSONS WITH ACUTE FEBRILE ILLNESSES UNTIL THEIR TEMPORARY SYMPTOMS HAVE ABATED. HOWEVER, MINOR ILLNESSES, WITH OR WITHOUT FEVER, SHOULD NOT CONTRAINDICATE THE USE OF INFLUENZA VACCINE PARTICULARLY AMONG CHILDREN WITH A MILD UPPER RESPIRATORY TRACT INFECTION OR ALLERGIC RHINITIS.[2,3]

ALTHOUGH GENTAMICIN SULFATE IS NOT DETECTABLE IN FORMS OF INFLUENZA VIRUS VACCINE CONTAINING IT BY CURRENT ASSAY PROCEDURES, THE VACCINE SHOULD NOT BE ADMINISTERED TO PERSONS WITH KNOWN SENSITIVITY TO GENTAMICIN OR OTHER AMINOGLYCOSIDES.

The clinical judgment of the attending physician should prevail at all times.

WARNINGS

Influenza Virus Vaccine should not be given to individuals with thrombocytopenia or any coagulation disorder that would contraindicate intramuscular injection unless, in the judgment of the physician, the potential benefits clearly outweigh the risk of administration.

Patients with impaired immune responsiveness, whether due to the use of immunosuppressive therapy (including irradiation, corticosteroids, antimetabolites, alkylating agents, and cytotoxic agents), a genetic defect, human immunodeficiency virus (HIV) infection, leukemia, lymphoma, generalized malignancy, or other causes, may have a reduced antibody response to active immunization procedures. Short-term (less than 2 weeks) corticosteroid therapy or intra-articular, bursal, or tendon injections with corticosteroids should not be immunosuppressive. Inactivated vaccines are not a risk to immunocompromised individuals, although their efficacy may be substantially reduced. Because patients with immunodeficiencies may not have an adequate response to immunizing agents, they may remain susceptible despite having received an appropriate vaccine. If feasible, specific serum antibody titers or other immunologic responses may be determined after immunization to assess immunity. Chemoprophylaxis may be indicated for high-risk persons who are expected to have a poor antibody response to influenza vaccine.

Because of the lower potential for causing febrile reactions, only split-virus vaccines should be used for children. These vaccines may be labeled as "split," "subvirion," or "purified-surface-antigen" vaccine. For adults, immunogenicity and side effects of split- and whole-virus vaccines are comparable when the vaccines are used at the recommended dosage.[2]

Since the likelihood of febrile convulsions from any cause is greater in children between 6 and 35 months, special care should be taken in weighing the relative risks and benefits of immunization in this age group.

As with any vaccine, immunization with Influenza Virus Vaccine may not result in seroconversion of all individuals given the vaccine.

PRECAUTIONS

GENERAL:
1. PRIOR TO ADMINISTRATION OF ANY DOSE OF INFLUENZA VIRUS VACCINE, THE PARENT, GUARDIAN, OR ADULT PATIENT SHOULD BE ASKED ABOUT THE RECENT HEALTH STATUS, MEDICAL AND IMMUNIZATION HISTORY OF THE PATIENT TO BE IMMUNIZED IN ORDER TO DETERMINE THE EXISTENCE OF ANY CONTRAINDICATION TO IMMUNIZATION WITH INFLUENZA VIRUS VACCINE (SEE "CONTRAINDICATIONS", "WARNINGS").

2. BEFORE ADMINISTRATION OF ANY BIOLOGICAL, THE PHYSICIAN SHOULD TAKE ALL PRECAUTIONS KNOWN FOR PREVENTION OF ALLERGIC OR ANY OTHER SIDE REACTIONS. This should include: a review of the patient's history regarding possible sensitivity, the ready availability of epinephrine 1:1000 and other appropriate agents used for control of immediate allergic reactions, and a knowledge of the recent literature pertaining to use of the biological concerned, including the nature of side effects and adverse reactions that may follow its use.

3. A separate sterile syringe and needle or a sterile disposable unit should be used for each individual patient to prevent transmission of hepatitis B or other infectious agents from one person to another. Reusable glass syringes and needles should be heat-sterilized.

4. Special care should be taken to prevent injection into a blood vessel.

Influenza virus is remarkably capricious antigenically, and significant changes may occur from time to time. It is known definitely that Influenza Virus Vaccine is not effective against all possible strains of influenza virus. Protection is afforded most people only against those strains of virus from which the vaccine is prepared or against closely related strains.

Influenza vaccine often contains one or more antigens used in previous years. However, immunity declines during the year following immunization. Therefore, revaccination on a yearly basis is necessary to provide optimal protection for the current season. REMAINING 1992-1993 VACCINE SHOULD NOT BE USED.

Information for the Patient: PRIOR TO ADMINISTRATION OF THIS VACCINE, HEALTH CARE PERSONNEL SHOULD INFORM THE PARENT, GUARDIAN, OR ADULT PATIENT OF THE BENEFITS AND RISKS OF IMMUNIZATION AGAINST INFLUENZA.

Drug Interactions: Although influenza immunization can inhibit the clearance of warfarin and theophylline, studies have failed to show any adverse clinical effects attributable to these drugs in patients receiving influenza vaccine.[2] Nevertheless, observation for possible enhanced drug effect or toxicity is indicated for those persons taking theophylline preparations or warfarin sodium.

Individuals receiving immunosuppressive therapy (including irradiation, corticosteroids, antimetabolites, alkylating agents, and cytotoxic agents) may have a reduced antibody response to immunization with Influenza Virus Vaccine.

There have been conflicting reports on the effects of Influenza Virus Vaccine on the elimination of some drugs metabolized by the hepatic cytochrome P-450 system.

Use in Pregnancy: Pregnancy Category C: Animal reproduction studies have not been conducted with Influenza Virus Vaccine. It is also not known whether Influenza Virus Vaccine can cause fetal harm when administered to a pregnant woman or can affect reproductive capacity. Influenza Virus Vaccine should therefore be given to a pregnant woman ONLY if clearly needed. The ACIP has clearly stated that administering the vaccine after the first trimester is a reasonable precaution to minimize any concern over the theoretical possibility of teratogenicity. The ACIP has also stated however that it may be undesirable to delay immunization of pregnant women with high-risk conditions who will still be in the first trimester of pregnancy when the influenza season begins[2] (see "Indications and Usage, Pregnant Women").

The clinical judgment of the attending physician should prevail at all times in determining whether to administer Influenza Virus Vaccine to a pregnant woman.

ADVERSE REACTIONS

Side effects of influenza vaccination are generally inconsequential in adults and occur at low frequency, but at younger ages side effects may be more common.

Because influenza vaccine contains only noninfectious purified viral proteins, it cannot cause influenza. Occasional cases of respiratory disease following immunization represent coincidental illnesses unrelated to influenza immunization.[2]

Vaccine Adverse Event Reporting System: The US Department of Health and Human Services has established a new Vaccine Adverse Event Reporting System (VAERS) to accept all reports of suspected adverse events after the administration of any vaccine, including, but not limited to the reporting of events required by the National Childhood Vaccine Injury Act of 1986.[4] The VAERS toll-free number for VAERS forms and information is 1-800-822-7967.[5]

Local Symptoms: Slight tenderness, redness or induration at the site of injection lasting for 1 or 2 days may occur in less than one third of recipients.[2]

Systemic Symptoms: Fever, malaise, myalgia, and other systemic symptoms occur infrequently and most often affect persons who have had no exposure to the influenza virus antigens in the vaccine (eg, young children). These reactions begin 6 to 12 hours after immunization and can persist for 1 or 2 days.[2]

Immediate, presumably allergic, reactions such as hives, angioedema, allergic asthma, or systemic anaphylaxis occur rarely after influenza immunization. These reactions probably result from hypersensitivity to some vaccine component—most likely residual egg protein. Although current influenza vaccines contain only a small quantity of egg protein, this protein is presumed capable of inducing immediate hypersensitivity reactions in persons with severe egg allergy, and such persons should not be given influenza vaccine. This includes persons who develop hives, have swelling of the lips or tongue, or experience acute respiratory distress or collapse after eating eggs. Persons with a documented immunoglobulin E (IgE)-mediated hypersensitivity to eggs, including those who have experienced occupational asthma or other allergic responses from occupational exposure to egg protein, may also be at increased risk of reactions from influenza vaccine[2] (see "Contraindications"). The protocol for influenza vaccination developed by Murphy and Strunk may be considered for patients who have egg allergies and medical conditions that place them at increased risk for influenza infection or its complications. The potential exists for hypersensitivity reactions to any vaccine components. Although exposure to vaccines containing thimerosal can lead to induction of hypersensitivity, most patients do not develop reactions to thimerosal administered as a component of vaccines even when patch or intradermal tests for thimerosal indicate hypersensitivity. When it has been reported, hypersensitivity to thimerosal has usually consisted of local delayed type hypersensitivity reactions.

Guillain-Barré Syndrome (GBS) is an uncommon illness characterized by ascending paralysis which is usually self-limited and reversible. Though most persons with GBS recover without residual weakness, approximately 5% of cases are fatal. Before 1976, no association of GBS with influenza vaccine use was recognized. Unlike the 1976-77 swine influenza vaccine, subsequent vaccines prepared from other virus strains have not been clearly associated with an increased frequency of GBS.[2,3,6-9] However, it is difficult to make a precise estimate of risk for a rare condition such as GBS. In 1990-91, although there was no overall increase in frequency of GBS among vaccine recipients, there may have been a small increase in GBS cases in vaccinated persons 18-64 years of age, but not in those aged ≥ 65 years. In contrast to the swine influenza vaccine, the epidemiologic features of the possible association of the 1990-91 vaccine with GBS were not as convincing. Even if GBS were a true side effect, the very low estimated risk of GBS is less than that of severe influenza that could be prevented by vaccine. Candidates for Influenza Virus Vaccine should be made aware of the benefits and possible risks of vaccine administration. Other neurological disorders, including encephalopathies not defined as GBS, have been temporally associated with influenza immunization, but no causal link has been established.[10,11]

DOSAGE AND ADMINISTRATION

For Intramuscular Use Only: Shake well before withdrawing each dose. DO NOT INJECT INTRAVENOUSLY.

Parenteral drug products should be inspected visually for particulate matter and discoloration prior to administration whenever solution and container permit (see *"Description"*).

Remaining 1992-1993 influenza vaccine should not be used.

Although Influenza Virus Vaccine often contains one or more antigens used in previous years, immunity declines during the year following immunization. Therefore, a history of immunization in any previous year with a vaccine containing one or more antigens included in the current vaccine does NOT preclude the need for reimmunization for the 1993-1994 influenza season in order to provide optimal protection.

See *"Indications and Usage"* section for information regarding the optimal time of administration of this vaccine. During the past decade, data on influenza vaccine immunogenicity and side effects have generally been obtained when vaccine has been administered intramuscularly. Because there has been no adequate evaluation of recent influenza vaccines administered by other routes, the intramuscular route should be used. Adults and older children should be immunized in the deltoid muscle; infants and young children in the anterolateral aspect of the thigh.

Before immunization, the skin over the site to be injected should be cleansed with a suitable germicide. After insertion of the needle, aspirate to help avoid inadvertent injection into a blood vessel.

Because of the lower potential for causing febrile reactions, only split-virus vaccines should be used for children under age 13. These vaccines may be labeled as "split," "subvirion," or "purified-surface-antigen" vaccine. For adults, immunogenicity and side effects of split- and whole-virus vaccines are comparable when vaccines are used at the recommended dosage.[2]

INFLUENZA VACCINE DOSAGE, BY AGE GROUP, 1993-1994 SEASON

Age Group	Product	Dose	No. of Doses (see below for details)
6-35 months	Split-virus only	0.25 mL	1 or 2 Doses
3-8 years	Split-virus only	0.50 mL	1 or 2 Doses
9-12 years	Split-virus only	0.50 mL	1 Dose
13 years and older	Whole or Split virus	0.50 mL	1 Dose

A single dose is considered sufficient for those under 9 years who have received at least 1 dose of Influenza Virus Vaccine. Two doses given at least one month apart are recommended for children under 9 years of age who are receiving influenza vaccine for the first time. With the two-dose regimen, allow four weeks or more between doses.[2,3]

SIMULTANEOUS ADMINISTRATION WITH OTHER VACCINES

The target groups for influenza and pneumococcal immunization overlap considerably. Both vaccines may be given at the same time at different sites without increasing side effects. However, influenza vaccine is given annually, while it is currently recommended that, with few exceptions, pneumococcal vaccine be given only once. Detailed immunization records should be provided to each patient to record the date when pneumococcal vaccine was administered.[2,12]

The ACIP states that children at high-risk of influenza complications may receive influenza vaccine at the same time as Measles-Mumps-Rubella, Haemophilus b Conjugate Vaccine, Pneumococcal and Oral Polio Vaccine, Diphtheria and Tetanus Toxoids, and Pertussis Adsorbed and Acellular Pertussis Vaccines. Vaccines should be given at different sites.[2] The American Academy of Pediatrics suggests that since influenza vaccine and pertussis-containing vaccine may produce febrile reactions in children, it may be prudent not to administer these vaccines simultaneously.[2,3]

IMPORTANT INFORMATION for Group Immunization Programs:

If this vaccine is to be used in an immunization program sponsored by any organization *WHERE A TRADITIONAL PHYSICIAN/PATIENT RELATIONSHIP DOES NOT EXIST,* each recipient (or legal guardian) must be made aware of the benefits and risks of immunization. These are summarized in the current labeling and informed consent should be obtained from the recipient (or legal guardian) before immunization. Copies of the Centers for Disease Control and Prevention Important Information about Influenza and Influenza Consent Form are available.

Do not freeze. Store refrigerated, away from freezer compartment, at 2°C to 8°C (36°F to 46°F).

REFERENCES

1. Composition of the 1993-1994 influenza vaccine. *MMWR.* 1993;42(10):177-180. 2. Prevention and control of influenza. Recommendations of the Immunization Practices Advisory Committee (ACIP). *MMWR.* 1993;42 RR-6:1-15. 3. American Academy of Pediatrics: *Report of the Committee on Infectious Diseases,* ed. 22. Elk Grove Village, IL: American Academy of Pediatrics; 1991. 4. National Childhood Vaccine Injury Act: Requirements for permanent vaccination records and for reporting of selected events after vaccination. *MMWR.* 1988; 37(13):197-200. 5. CDC. Vaccine Adverse Event Reporting System—United States. *MMWR.* 1990;39(41):730-733. 6. Schonberger LB, Hurwitz ES, Katona P, *et al:* Guilllain-Barré syndrome: Its epidemiology and associations with influenza vaccination. *Ann Neurol.* 1981;9 (Suppl 31). 7. Hurwitz ES, Schonberger LB, Nelson DB, *et al*: Guillain-Barré syndrome and the 1978-1979 influenza vaccine. *New Eng J Med.* 1981;304:1557-1561. 8. Kaplan J, Katona P, Hurwitz ES, *et al*: Guillain-Barré syndrome in the United States, 1979-1980 and 1980-1981. Lack of association with influenza vaccination. *JAMA.* 1982;248:689-700. 9. Safranek TJ, Lawrence DN, Kurland LT, *et al*: Reassessment of the association between Guillain-Barré syndrome and receipt of swine influenza vaccine in 1976-1977: results of a two-state study. *Am J Epidemiol.* 1991;133(9):940-951. 10. Centers for Disease Control: December 1986; Adverse events following immunization: Report No. 2, 1982-1984. 11. Retailliou H, Curtis AC, Storr G *et al*: Illness after influenza vaccination reported through a nation-wide surveillance system, 1976-1977. *Am J Epidemiol.* 1980;111:270-278. 12. Recommendations of the Immunization Practices Advisory Committee. Pneumococcal polysaccharide vaccine. *MMWR.* 1989;38(5):64-8, 73-6.

HOW SUPPLIED
INJECTION:

BRAND/MANUFACTURER	NDC	SIZE	AWP
○ **BRAND**			
FLUOGEN: Parke-Davis	00071-4094-40	0.5 ml	$48.95
FLUSHIELD: Wyeth-Ayerst	00008-0840-01	5 ml	$35.16
FLUVIRIN: Adams	53014-0100-10	5 ml	$42.15
FLUOGEN: Parke-Davis	00071-4094-08	5 ml	$44.44
FLUZONE: Connaught	49281-0347-10	0.5 ml 10s	$39.88
	49281-0348-15	0.5 ml 10s	$39.88
FLUSHIELD: Wyeth-Ayerst	00008-0840-02	0.5 ml 10s	$45.59
FLUZONE: Connaught	49281-0348-11	0.5 ml 10s	$48.94
○ **GENERICS**			
Wyeth-Ayerst	00008-0835-02	0.5 ml	$43.75
Wyeth-Ayerst	00008-0815-01	5 ml	$33.75
Wyeth-Ayerst	00008-0835-01	5 ml	$33.75
Wyeth-Ayerst	00008-0815-02	0.5 ml 10s	$43.75

Infumorph *SEE* MORPHINE SULFATE

Innovar *SEE* DROPERIDOL AND FENTANYL CITRATE

Inocor I.V. *SEE* AMRINONE LACTATE

Inpersol *SEE* DEXTROSE AND ELECTROLYTES *AND* DEXTROSE AND ELECTROLYTES, INTRAPERITONEAL

Insulin-Pork, Concentrated

WARNINGS

ANY CHANGE OF INSULIN SHOULD BE MADE CAUTIOUSLY AND ONLY UNDER MEDICAL SUPERVISION. CHANGES IN PURITY, STRENGTH (U-100), BRAND (MANUFACTURER), TYPE (LENTE®, NPH, REGULAR, ETC.), AND/OR SPECIES SOURCE (BEEF, PORK, BEEF-PORK, OR HUMAN) MAY RESULT IN THE NEED FOR A CHANGE IN DOSAGE. SEE BELOW.

IT IS NOT POSSIBLE TO IDENTIFY WHICH PATIENTS WILL REQUIRE A *REDUCTION* IN DOSE TO AVOID HYPOGLYCEMIA WHEN USING THIS INSULIN. HOWEVER, IT IS KNOWN THAT A SMALL NUMBER OF PATIENTS MAY REQUIRE A SIGNIFICANT CHANGE.

ADJUSTMENT MAY BE NEEDED WITH THE FIRST DOSE OR OCCUR OVER A PERIOD OF SEVERAL WEEKS. BE AWARE OF THE POSSIBILITY OF SYMPTOMS OF EITHER HYPOGLYCEMIA OR HYPERGLYCEMIA.

This insulin is prepared from Pork pancreas only. The dose of Pork Insulin for patients with Insulin resistance due to antibodies to beef Insulin may be only a fraction of that of beef Insulin

This Insulin preparation contains 500 units of Insulin in each milliliter. Extreme caution must be observed in the measurement of dosage because inadvertent overdose may result in irreversible insulin shock. Serious consequences may result if it is used other than under constant medical supervision.

DESCRIPTION

The Lilly Pork Insulin product differs from previous Pork Insulin preparations because it has undergone additional steps of chromatographic purification.

Insulin—Pork, Concentrated is an aqueous solution made from the antidiabetic principle of Pork pancreas as stated on the label. Each milliliter contains 500 units of regular (unmodified) Insulin and approximately 1.6% glycerin (w/v), with approximately 0.25% m-cresol (w/v) as a preservative. Sodium hydroxide and hydrochloric acid are added during manufacture to adjust the pH. All preparations of Insulin—Pork, Concentrated are made from zinc-insulin crystals.

CLINICAL PHARMACOLOGY

Adequate Insulin dosage permits the diabetic patient to utilize carbohydrates and fats in a comparatively satisfactory manner. Regardless of concentration, the action of Insulin is basically the same: to enable carbohydrate metabolism to occur and thus to prevent the production of ketone bodies by the liver. Although, under usual circumstances, diabetes can be controlled with doses in the vicinity of 40 to 60 units or less, an occasional patient develops such resistance or becomes so unresponsive to the effect of Insulin that daily doses of several hundred, or even several thousand, units are required. Patients who require doses in excess of 300 to 500 units daily usually have impaired receptor function. Occasionally, a cause of the Insulin resistance can be found (such as hemochromatosis, cirrhosis of the liver, some complicating disease of the endocrine glands other than the pancreas, allergy, or infection), but in other cases, no cause of the high Insulin requirement can be determined.

Insulin—Pork, Concentrated is unmodified by any agent that might prolong its action; however, clinical experience has shown that it frequently has a time action similar to a repository Insulin preparation and that a single dose may show activity over a 24-hour period. This effect has been credited to the high concentration of the preparation.

INDICATIONS AND USAGE

Insulin—Pork, Concentrated, is especially useful for the treatment of diabetic patients with marked Insulin resistance (daily requirements more than 200 units), since a large dose may be administered subcutaneously in a reasonable volume.

CONTRAINDICATIONS

Patients with a history of systemic allergic reactions to Pork or mixed beef/Pork Insulin should not receive the Insulin formulation unless they have been successfully desensitized.

PRECAUTIONS

General: Every patient exhibiting Insulin resistance who requires Insulin—Pork, Concentrated, for control of diabetes should be under close observation until dosage is established. The response will vary among patients. Some can be controlled with a single dose daily: others may require 2 or 3 injections per day. Most patients will show a "tolerance" to Insulin, so that minor variations in dosage can occur without the development of untoward symptoms of Insulin shock.

Insulin resistance is frequently self-limited; after several weeks or months during which high dosage is required, responsiveness to the pharmacologic effect of Insulin may be regained and dosage can be reduced.

Patients with immunologic Insulin resistance to Beef Insulin (this diagnosis is usually confirmed by the finding of increased serum antibody titers) may require an immediate dosage reduction of 20 to 50% when treated with Pork Insulin.

Information for Patients: Patients should be instructed regarding their dosage and should be reminded that this formulation requires the administration of a smaller volume of solution than is the case with less concentrated formulations.

Laboratory Tests: Blood and urine glucose, glycohemoglobin, and urine ketones should be monitored frequently.

Drug Interactions: The concurrent use of oral hypoglycemic agents with Insulin-Pork, Concentrated, is not recommended since there are no data to support such use.

Pregnancy—Teratogenic Effects: No reproduction studies have been conducted in animals, and there are no adequate and well-controlled studies in pregnant women. It would be anticipated that the benefits of this Insulin preparation would outweigh any risk to the developing fetus.

Nonteratogenic Effects: Insulin does not cross the placenta as does glucose.

Labor and Delivery: Careful monitoring of the patient is required, since the Insulin requirement may decrease following delivery.

Nursing Mothers: It is not known whether Insulin is excreted in significant amounts in human milk. Because many drugs are excreted in human milk, caution should be exercised when Insulin—Pork, Concentrated injection is administered to a nursing woman.

Pediatric Use: There are no special precautions relating to the use of this Insulin formulation in the pediatric age group.

ADVERSE REACTIONS

As with other Insulin preparations, hypoglycemic reactions may be associated with the administration of Insulin—Pork, Concentrated. However, deep secondary hypoglycemic reactions may develop 18 to 24 hours after the original injection of Insulin—Pork, Concentrated. Consequently, patients should be carefully observed, and prompt treatment of such reactions should be initiated with glucagon injections and/or with glucose by intravenous injection or gavage.

ALLERGIC REACTIONS

Erythema, swelling, or pruritus may occur at injection sites. Such localized allergic manifestations usually resolve within a few days to a few weeks.

Less common, but potentially more serious, is systemic allergy to Insulin, manifested by generalized urticaria, dyspnea, and wheezing, which may progress to anaphylaxis. If a severe allergic reaction occurs, the drug should be discontinued and the patient treated with the usual agents (eg, epinephrine, antihistamines, or corticosteroids). Patients who have experienced severe systemic allergic reactions to insulin (eg, generalized urticaria, angioedema, anaphylaxis) should be skin-tested with each new preparation to be used before starting therapy with that

preparation. Desensitization procedures may permit resumption of Insulin administration.

DOSAGE AND ADMINISTRATION

Insulin—Pork, Concentrated can be administered by both the subcutaneous and the intramuscular routes. It is inadvisable to inject Insulin—Pork, Concentrated, intravenously because of the possible development of allergic or anaphylactoid reactions.

It is recommended that a tuberculin type of syringe be utilized for the measurement of dosage. Variations in dosage are frequently possible in the Insulin-resistant patient, since the individual is unresponsive to the pharmacologic effect of the Insulin. Nevertheless, accuracy of measurement is to be encouraged because of the potential danger of the preparation.

Insulin should be kept in a cold place, preferably in a refrigerator, but must not be frozen.

Do not inject Insulin that is not water-clear. Discoloration, turbidity, or unusual viscosity indicates deterioration or contamination.

Use of a package of Insulin should not be started after the expiration date stamped on it.

J CODES

Up to 100 units SC—J1820

HOW SUPPLIED
INJECTION: 500 U/ML

BRAND/MANUFACTURER	NDC	SIZE	AWP
○ **BRAND**			
ILETIN II REG. PORK: Lilly	00002-8500-01	20 ml	$121.27

Intal *SEE* CROMOLYN SODIUM

Interferon Alfa-2A

DESCRIPTION

Interferon Alfa-2A is a sterile protein product for use by injection. Interferon Alfa-2A is manufactured by recombinant DNA technology that employs a genetically engineered *E. coli* bacterium containing DNA that codes for the human protein. Interferon Alfa-2A is a highly purified protein containing 165 amino acids, and it has an approximate molecular weight of 19,000 daltons. The purification procedure includes affinity chromatography using a murine monoclonal antibody. Fermentation is carried out in a defined nutrient medium containing the antibiotic tetracycline hydrochloride, 5 mg/L. However, the presence of the antibiotic is not detectable in the final product. Interferon Alfa-2A is supplied as an injectable solution or as a sterile powder for injection with its accompanying diluent.

The specific activity of Interferon Alfa-2A, is 2×10^8 IU/mg protein. The route of administration is subcutaneous or intramuscular.

Following is its chemical structure:

```
H— Cys-Asp-Leu-Pro-Gln-Thr-His-Ser-Leu-Gly-Ser-Arg-Arg-Thr-Leu-Met-Leu-Leu-Ala-Gln-
     1   2   3   4   5   6   7   8   9  10  11  12  13  14  15  16  17  18  19  20

Met-Arg-Lys-Ile-Ser-Leu-Phe-Ser-Cys-Leu-Lys-Asp-Arg-His-Asp-Phe-Gly-Phe-Pro-Gln-
 21  22  23  24  25  26  27  28  29  30  31  32  33  34  35  36  37  38  39  40

Glu-Glu-Phe-Gly-Asn-Gln-Phe-Gln-Lys-Ala-Glu-Thr-Ile-Pro-Val-Leu-His-Glu-Met-Ile-
 41  42  43  44  45  46  47  48  49  50  51  52  53  54  55  56  57  58  59  60

Gln-Gln-Ile-Phe-Asn-Leu-Phe-Ser-Thr-Lys-Asp-Ser-Ser-Ala-Ala-Trp-Asp-Glu-Thr-Leu-
 61  62  63  64  65  66  67  68  69  70  71  72  73  74  75  76  77  78  79  80

Leu-Asp-Lys-Phe-Tyr-Thr-Glu-Leu-Tyr-Gln-Gln-Leu-Asn-Asp-Leu-Glu-Ala-Cys-Val-Ile-
 81  82  83  84  85  86  87  88  89  90  91  92  93  94  95  96  97  98  99 100

Gln-Gly-Val-Gly-Val-Thr-Glu-Thr-Pro-Leu-Met-Lys-Glu-Asp-Ser-Ile-Leu-Ala-Val-Arg-
101 102 103 104 105 106 107 108 109 110 111 112 113 114 115 116 117 118 119 120

Lys-Tyr-Phe-Gln-Arg-Ile-Thr-Leu-Tyr-Leu-Lys-Glu-Lys-Lys-Tyr-Ser-Pro-Cys-Ala-Trp-
121 122 123 124 125 126 127 128 129 130 131 132 133 134 135 136 137 138 139 140

Glu-Val-Val-Arg-Ala-Glu-Ile-Met-Arg-Ser-Phe-Ser-Leu-Ser-Thr-Asn-Leu-Gln-Glu-Ser-
141 142 143 144 145 146 147 148 149 150 151 152 153 154 155 156 157 158 159 160

Leu-Arg-Ser-Lys-Glu —OH
161 162 163 164 165
```

CLINICAL PHARMACOLOGY

The mechanism by which Interferon Alfa-2A or any other interferon, exerts antitumor activity is not clearly understood. However, it is believed that direct antiproliferative action against tumor cells and modulation of the host immune response play important roles in the antitumor activity.

The biological activities of Interferon Alfa-2A are species-restricted, *i.e.*, they are expressed in a very limited number of species other than humans. As a consequence, preclinical evaluation of Interferon Alfa-2A has involved *in vitro* experiments with human cells and some *in vivo* experiments.[1] Using human cells in culture, Interferon Alfa-2A has been shown to have antiproliferative and immunomodulatory activities that are very similar to those of the mixture of Interferon Alfa subtypes produced by human leukocytes. *In vivo*, Interferon Alfa-2A has been shown to inhibit the growth of several human tumors growing in immunocompromised (nude) mice. Because of its species-restricted activity, it has

---

◆ RATED THERAPEUTICALLY EQUIVALENT; ◇ THERAPEUTIC EQUIVALENCE UNCONFIRMED; ○ UNRATED

not been possible to demonstrate antitumor activity in immunologically intact syngeneic tumor model systems, where effects on the host immune system would be observable. However, such antitumor activity has been repeatedly demonstrated with, for example, mouse interferon-Alfa in transplantable mouse tumor systems. The clinical significance of these findings is unknown.

The metabolism of Interferon Alfa-2A, is consistent with that of alfa interferons in general. Alfa interferons are totally filtered through the glomeruli and undergo rapid proteolytic degradation during tubular reabsorption, rendering a negligible reappearance of intact alfa interferon in the systemic circulation. Small amounts of radiolabeled Interferon Alfa-2A, appear in the urine of isolated rat kidneys, suggesting near complete reabsorption of Interferon Alfa-2A catabolites. Liver metabolism and subsequent biliary excretion are considered minor pathways of elimination for alfa interferons.

The serum concentrations of Interferon Alfa-2A reflected a large intersubject variation in both healthy volunteers and patients with disseminated cancer. In healthy people, Interferon Alfa-2A exhibited an elimination half-life of 3.7 to 8.5 hours (mean 5.1 hours), volume of distribution at steady-state of 0.223 to 0.748 L/kg (mean 0.400 L/kg) and a total body clearance of 2.14 to 3.62 mL/min/kg (mean 2.79 mL/min/kg) after a 36 million IU (2.2×10^8 pg) intravenous infusion. After intramuscular and subcutaneous administrations of 36 million IU, peak serum concentrations ranged from 1500 to 2580 pg/mL (mean 2020 pg/mL) at a mean time to peak of 3.8 hours and from 1250 to 2320 pg/mL (mean 1730 pg/mL) at a mean time to peak of 7.3 hours, respectively. The apparent fraction of the dose absorbed after intramuscular injection was greater than 80%.

The pharmacokinetics of Interferon Alfa-2A after single intramuscular doses to patients with disseminated cancer were similar to those found in healthy volunteers. Dose proportional increases in serum concentrations were observed after single doses up to 198 million IU. There were no changes in the distribution or elimination of Interferon Alfa-2A during twice daily (0.5 to 36 million IU), once daily (1 to 54 million IU), or three times weekly (1 to 136 million IU) dosing regimens up to 28 days of dosing. Multiple intramuscular doses of Interferon Alfa-2A resulted in an accumulation of 2 to 4 times the single dose serum concentrations. Pharmacokinetic information in patients with hairy cell leukemia or AIDS-related Kaposi's sarcoma is presently unknown.

Serum neutralizing activity, determined by a highly sensitive enzyme immunoassay and a neutralization bioassay, was detected in approximately 25% of all patients who received Interferon-Alfa-2A.[2] Antibodies to human leukocyte interferon may occur spontaneously in certain clinical conditions (cancer, systemic lupus erythematosus, herpes zoster) in patients who have never received exogenous interferon.[3] The significance of the appearance of serum neutralizing activity is not known.

The acute parenteral toxicity of Interferon Alfa-2A has been studied in mice, rats, rabbits and ferrets at doses up to 30 million IU/kg intravenously, and 500 million IU/kg intramuscularly. No treatment-related mortality was noted in any species given Interferon Alfa-2A by any of the routes of administration.

Effects on Hairy Cell Leukemia: During the first one to two months of treatment of patients with hairy cell leukemia, significant depression of hematopoiesis was likely to occur. Subsequently, there was improvement in circulating blood cell counts.

Of the 75 patients who were evaluable for efficacy following at least 16 weeks of therapy, 46 (61%) achieved complete or partial response. Twenty-one patients (28%) had a minor remission, eight (11%) remained stable, and none had worsening of disease. All patients who achieved either a complete or partial response had complete or partial normalization of all peripheral blood elements including hemoglobin level, white blood cell, neutrophil, monocyte and platelet counts with a concomitant decrease in peripheral blood and bone marrow hairy cells. Responding patients also exhibited a marked reduction in red blood cell and platelet transfusion requirements, a decrease in infectious episodes and improvement in performance status. The probability of survival for two years in patients receiving Interferon Alfa-2A (94%) was statistically increased compared to a historical control group (75%).

Effects on AIDS-related Kaposi's sarcoma: In six studies with Interferon Alfa-2A, doses of 3 to 54 million IU daily were evaluated for the treatment of AIDS-related Kaposi's sarcoma in more than 350 patients. Four dosage regimens of Interferon Alfa-2A were evaluated for initial induction. Thirty-nine patients received 3 million IU daily; 99 patients received an escalating regimen of 3 million, 9 million and 18 million IU each daily for 3 days, followed by 36 million IU daily; 119 patients received 36 million IU daily; and 16 patients received doses greater than 36 million IU to a maximum of 54 million IU daily. An additional 81 patients received Interferon Alfa-2A in combination with vinblastine. The best response rate associated with acceptable toxicity was observed when Interferon Alfa-2A was administered as a single agent at a dose of 36 million IU daily. The escalating regimen of 3 to 36 million IU daily provided equivalent therapeutic benefit with some amelioration of acute toxicity in some patients. In AIDS-related Kaposi's sarcoma, lower doses were less effective in inducing tumor regression and doses higher than 36 million IU daily were associated with unacceptable toxicity.

As summarized in Table 1, the likelihood of response to Interferon Alfa-2A varied with the clinical manifestations of human immunodeficiency virus (HIV) infection. Patients with prior opportunistic infection or B symptoms are unlikely to respond to treatment with Interferon Alfa-2A.

Table 1

LIKELIHOOD OF RESPONSE TO INTERFERON ALPHA-2A IN PATIENTS WITH AIDS-RELATED KAPOSI'S SARCOMA

No. Pts.*	$CD_4(T_4)$ Lymphocyte Count (cells/mm^3)	Objective Response Rate (%)		
		CR	PR	Total
83	0-200	3.6	3.6	7.2
51	> 200-400	15.7	11.8	27.5
33	> 400	24.2	21.2	45.4

In the 28 patients evaluated who had prior opportunistic infection or B symptoms, the response rate was 3.6%.

* Patients had no prior opportunistic infection or B symptoms. B symptoms include night sweats, weight loss of greater than 10% of body weight or 15 lbs., or fever greater than 100°F without an identifiable source of infection.

Patients who were otherwise asymptomatic, with no prior opportunistic infection and near-normal levels of CD_4 lymphocytes, experienced higher response rates. Responding patients with a baseline CD_4 lymphocyte count greater than 200 cells/mm^3 had a distinct survival advantage over both responding patients with a baseline CD_4 lymphocyte count of 200 cells/mm^3 or less and nonresponding patients regardless of their baseline CD_4 lymphocyte count. Median survival for responding patients with CD_4 lymphocyte counts of greater than 200 to 400 cells/mm^3 had not been reached but was greater than 32.7 months from the initiation of therapy. For responding patients with CD_4 lymphocyte counts of greater than 400 cells/mm^3, the median survival had not been reached but was greater than 29.5 months.

A classification system for staging AIDS-related Kaposi's sarcoma has been described based on location and extent of disease. In studies of Interferon Alfa-2A no difference was noted in response rates for patients with different stages of Kaposi's sarcoma. Likelihood of response was related to manifestations of HIV Infection (baseline CD_4 lymphocyte count, prior opportunistic infection or B symptoms) and not to extent of tumor involvement. The median time to response was 2.7 months. The median duration of response for patients achieving a partial or complete response was 6.3 and 20.7 months, respectively. Complete and partial responses lasting in excess of three years have been observed. Therapy was discontinued because of progression of Kaposi's sarcoma, development of severe opportunistic infection or severe adverse effects. The median time to discontinuation of treatment was 12.5 months for responding patients and 2.3 months for patients who did not respond.

INDICATIONS AND USAGE
Interferon Alfa-2A is indicated for use in the treatment of hairy cell leukemia and AIDS-related Kaposi's sarcoma in select patients 18 years of age or older. Studies have shown that Interferon Alfa-2A can produce clinically meaningful tumor regression or disease stabilization in patients with hairy cell leukemia or in patients with AIDS-related Kaposi's sarcoma.[4-6]

For Patients with Hairy Cell Leukemia: Prior to initiation of therapy, tests should be performed to quantitate peripheral blood hemoglobin, platelets, granulocytes and hairy cells and bone marrow hairy cells. These parameters should be monitored periodically (e.g., monthly) during treatment to determine whether response to treatment has occurred. If a patient does not respond within six months, treatment should be discontinued. If a response to treatment does occur, treatment should be continued until no further improvement is observed and these laboratory parameters have been stable for about three months. It is not known whether continued treatment after that time is beneficial. Studies are in progress to evaluate this question.

For Patients with AIDS-related Kaposi's Sarcoma: Interferon Alfa-2A is useful for the treatment of AIDS-related Kaposi's sarcoma in a select group of patients. In determining whether a patient should be treated, the physician should assess the likelihood of response based on the clinical manifestations of HIV infection and the manifestations of Kaposi's sarcoma requiring treatment. See *"Clinical Pharmacology".*

Indicator lesion measurements and total lesion count should be performed before initiation of therapy. These parameters should be monitored periodically (e.g., monthly) during treatment to determine whether response to treatment or disease stabilization has occurred. When disease stabilization or a response to treatment occurs, treatment should continue until there is no further evidence of tumor or until discontinuation is required because of a severe opportunistic infection or adverse effects.

UNLABELED USES
Interferon Alfa-2A is used alone or as an adjunct in the treatment of cryoglobulinemia, genital herpes infections, chronic hepatitis C (non-a, non-b hepatitis), and in patients who are Philadelphia-chromosome-positive with chronic myelogenous leukemia. It is also used in cutaneous T-cell lymphomas including mycosis fungoides, the Sezary syndrome, and non-Hodgkin's lymphomas, multiple myeloma, and squamous cell skin cancer.

CONTRAINDICATIONS
Interferon Alfa-2A is contraindicated in patients with known hypersensitivity to alfa interferon, mouse immunoglobulin or any component of the product.

➤ SHOWN IN PRODUCT IDENTIFICATION GUIDE

WARNINGS

Interferon Alfa-2A should be administered under the guidance of a qualified physician. (See *"Dosage and Administration."*) Appropriate management of the therapy and its complications is possible only when adequate diagnostic and treatment facilities are readily available.

Interferon Alfa-2A should not be used for the treatment of visceral AIDS-related Kaposi's sarcoma associated with rapidly progressive or life-threatening disease.

Interferon Alfa-2A should be used with caution in patients with severe preexisting cardiac disease, severe renal or hepatic disease, seizure disorders and/or compromised central nervous system function.

Because of the possibility of severe or even fatal adverse reactions, patients should be informed not only of the benefits of therapy but also of the risks involved.

Interferon Alfa-2A should be administered with caution to patients with cardiac disease or with any history of cardiac illness. No direct cardiotoxic effect has been demonstrated, but it is likely that acute, self-limited toxicities (*i.e.*, fever, chills) frequently associated with Interferon Alfa-2A administration may exacerbate preexisting cardiac conditions. Rarely, myocardial infarction has occurred in patients receiving Interferon Alfa-2A. Cases of cardiomyopathy have been observed on rare occasions in patients treated with alfa-interferons.

Caution should be exercised when administering Interferon Alfa-2A to patients with myelosuppression or when Interferon Alfa-2A is used in combination with other agents that are known to cause myelosuppression. Synergistic toxicity has been observed when Interferon Alfa-2A is administered in combination with Zidovudine (AZT).[7] The effects of Interferon Alfa-2A when combined with other drugs used in the treatment of AIDS-related disease are not known.

Central nervous system adverse reactions have been reported in a number of patients. These reactions included decreased mental status, exaggerated central nervous system function, and dizziness. More severe obtundation and coma have been rarely observed. Most of these abnormalities are mild and reversible within a few days to three weeks upon dose reduction or discontinuation of Interferon Alfa-2A therapy. Careful periodic neuropsychiatric monitoring of all patients is recommended.

Leukopenia and elevation of hepatic enzymes occurred frequently but were rarely dose-limiting. Thrombocytopenia occurred less frequently. Proteinuria and increased cells in urinary sediment were also seen infrequently. Rarely, significant hepatic, renal and myelosuppressive toxicities were noted.

PRECAUTIONS

General: In all instances where the use of Interferon Alfa-2A is considered for chemotherapy, the physician must evaluate the need and usefulness of the drug against the risk of adverse reactions. Most adverse reactions are reversible if detected early. If severe reactions occur, the drug should be reduced in dosage or discontinued and appropriate corrective measures should be taken according to the clinical judgment of the physician. Reinstitution of Interferon Alfa-2A therapy should be carried out with caution and with adequate consideration of the further need for the drug and alertness as to possible recurrence of toxicity.

The minimum effective doses of Interferon Alfa-2A for treatment of hairy cell leukemia and AIDS-related Kaposi's sarcoma have not been established. Variations in dosage and adverse reactions exist among different brands of Interferon. Therefore, do not use different brands of Interferon in a single treatment regimen.

Information for Patient: Patients should be cautioned not to change brands of Interferon without medical consultation, as a change in dosage may result. Patients should be informed regarding the potential benefits and risks attendant to the use of Interferon Alfa-2A. If home use is determined to be desirable by the physician, instructions on appropriate use should be given, including review of the contents of the enclosed Patient Information Sheet. Patients should be well hydrated, especially during the initial stages of treatment.

Patients should be thoroughly instructed in the importance of proper disposal procedures and cautioned against reusing syringes and needles. If home use is prescribed, a puncture resistant container for the disposal of used syringes and needles should be supplied to the patient. The full container should be disposed of according to directions provided by the physician.

Patients receiving high dose Alfa-Interferon should be cautioned against performing tasks that require complete mental alertness such as operating machinery or driving a motor vehicle.

Laboratory Tests: Complete blood counts and clinical chemistry tests should be performed before initiation of Interferon Alfa-2A therapy and at appropriate periods during therapy. Since responses of hairy cell leukemia and AIDS-related Kaposi's sarcoma are not generally observed for one to three months after initiation of treatment, very careful monitoring for severe depression of blood cell counts is warranted during the initial phase of treatment.

Those patients who have preexisting cardiac abnormalities and/or are in advanced stages of cancer should have electrocardiograms taken before and during the course of treatment.

Carcinogenesis, Mutagenesis and Impairment of Fertility:

Carcinogenesis: Interferon Alfa-2A has not been tested for its carcinogenic potential.

Mutagenesis: A. Internal studies—Ames tests using six different tester strains, with and without metabolic activation, were performed with Interferon Alfa-2A to a concentration of 1920 µg/plate. There was no evidence of mutagenicity.

Human lymphocyte cultures were treated *in vitro* with Interferon Alfa-2A at noncytotoxic concentrations. No increase in the incidence of chromosomal damage was noted.

B. Published studies—There are no published studies on the mutagenic potential of Interferon Alfa-2A. However, a number of studies on the genotoxicity of human leukocyte interferon have been reported.

A chromosomal defect following the addition of human leukocyte interferon to lymphocyte cultures from a patient suffering from a lymphoproliferative disorder has been reported.

In contrast, other studies have failed to detect chromosomal abnormalities following treatment of lymphocyte cultures from healthy volunteers with human leukocyte interferon. It has also been shown that human leukocyte interferon protects primary chick embryo fibroblasts from chromosomal aberrations produced by gamma rays.

Impairment of Fertility: Interferon Alfa-2A has been studied for its effect on fertility in Macaca mulatta (rhesus monkeys). Non-pregnant rhesus females treated with Interferon Alfa-2A at doses of 5 and 25 million IU/kg day have shown menstrual cycle irregularities, including prolonged or shortened menstrual periods and erratic bleeding; these cycles were considered to be anovulatory on the basis that reduced progesterone levels were noted and that expected increases in preovulatory estrogen and luteinizing hormones were not observed. These monkeys returned to a normal menstrual rhythm following discontinuation of treatment.

Drug Interactions: Interferon Alfa-2A, apparently through an unknown effect on certain microsomal enzyme systems, has been reported to reduce the clearance of theophylline.[8,9] The clinical relevance of this interaction is presently unknown.

Interactions between Interferon Alfa-2A and other drugs have not been fully evaluated. Caution should be exercised when administering Interferon Alfa-2A in combination with other potentially myelosuppressive agents. See *"Warnings"*.

PREGNANCY

Teratogenic Effects: Pregnancy Category C. Interferon Alfa-2A has been shown to demonstrate a statistically significant increase in abortifacient activity in rhesus monkeys when given at approximately 20 to 500 times the human dose. A study in pregnant rhesus monkeys treated with 1, 5 or 25 million IU/kg/day of Interferon Alfa-2A in their early to midfetal period (days 22 to 70 of gestation) has failed to demonstrate teratogenic activity for Interferon Alfa-2A.

There are no adequate and well-controlled studies in pregnant women.

Nonteratogenic Effects: Dose-related abortifacient activity was observed in pregnant rhesus monkeys treated with 1, 5 or 25 million IU/kg/day of Interferon Alfa-2A in their early to mid-fetal period (days 22 to 70 of gestation). A late-fetal period study (days 79 to 100 of gestation) is in progress and as yet there have been no reports of any increased rate of abortion.

Usage in Pregnancy: Safe use in human pregnancy has not been established. Therefore, Interferon Alfa-2A should be used during pregnancy only if the potential benefit justifies the potential risk to the fetus. Information from primate studies showed dose-related menstrual irregularities and an increased incidence of spontaneous abortions. Decreases in serum estradiol and progesterone concentrations have been reported in women treated with human leukocyte interferon.[10] Therefore, fertile women should not receive Interferon Alfa-2A unless they are using effective contraception during the therapy period.

Male fertility and teratologic evaluations have yielded no significant adverse effects to date.

Nursing Mothers: It is not known whether this drug is excreted in human milk. Because many drugs are excreted in human milk and because of the potential for serious adverse reactions in nursing infants from Interferon Alfa-2A, a decision should be made whether to discontinue nursing or to discontinue the drug, taking into account the importance of the drug to the mother.

Pediatric Use: Safety and effectiveness in children under 18 years of age have not been established.

ADVERSE REACTIONS

The following data on adverse reactions are based on the subcutaneous or intramuscular administration of Interferon Alfa-2A as a single agent. Most of the adverse reactions reported were mild to moderate and diminished in severity and number with continued therapy. More severe adverse reactions were observed at higher doses and may require dose reduction.
For Patients with Hairy Cell Leukemia:

Flu-like Symptoms: Fever (98%), fatigue (89%), myalgia (73%), headache (71%), chills (64%) and arthralgia (5%).

Gastrointestinal: Anorexia (46%), nausea (32%), diarrhea (29%) and emesis (10%).

Central and Peripheral Nervous System: Dizziness (21%), paresthesia (6%), numbness (6%) and transient impotence (6%).

Skin: Rash (18%), dry skin or pruritus (13%) and partial alopecia (8%).

Other: Dryness or inflammation of the oropharynx (16%), weight loss (14%), change in taste (13%), diaphoresis (8%) and reactivation of herpes liabialis (8%).

Rarely (< 3%), central nervous system effects including decreased mental status, depression, visual disturbances, sleep disturbances and nervousness, as well as cardiac adverse events, including hypertension, chest pain, arrhythmias and palpitations, were reported. Adverse experiences that occurred rarely, and may have been related to underlying disease, included epistaxis, bleeding gums, ecchymosis and petechiae. Miscellaneous adverse events, such as night sweats, urticaria, conjunctivitis and inflammation at the site of injection, were also rarely observed.

For Patients with AIDS-related Kaposi's Sarcoma:

Flu-like Symptoms: Fatigue (95%), fever (74%), myalgia (69%), headache (66%), chills (41%) and arthralgia (24%).

Gastrointestinal: Anorexia (65%), nausea (51%), diarrhea (42%), emesis (17%) and abdominal pain (15%).

Central and Peripheral Nervous System: Dizziness (40%), decreased mental status (17%), depression (16%), paresthesia (8%), confusion (8%), diaphoresis (7%), visual disturbances (5%), sleep disturbances (5%) and numbness (3%).

Pulmonary and Cardiovascular: Coughing (27%), dyspnea (11%), edema (9%), chest pain (4%) and hypotension (4%).

Skin: Partial alopecia (22%), rash (11%) and dry skin or pruritus (5%).

Other: Weight loss (25%), change in taste (25%), dryness or inflammation of the oropharynx (14%), night sweats (8%) and rhinorrhea (4%).

Occasionally (<3%) nervous system effects including anxiety, nervousness, emotional lability, vertigo and forgetfulness, as well as cardiac adverse events, including palpitations and arrhythmia, were reported. Other adverse experiences that occurred occasionally (<3%) and may have been related to underlying disease, included sinusitis, constipation, chest congestion, urticaria, and flatulence. Adverse experiences which occurred rarely (<1%) included ataxia, seizures, cyanosis, gastric distress, bronchospasm, pain at injection site, earache, eye irritation and rhinitis. Miscellaneous adverse experiences such as poor coordination, lethargy, muscle contractions, neuropathy, tremor, involuntary movement, syncope, aphasia, aphonia, dysarthria, amnesia, weakness, and flushing of skin were observed in less than 0.5% of patients. Cases of cardiomyopathy have been observed on rare occasions in patients treated with alfa-interferons.

In other investigational studies of Interferon Alpha-2A in addition to the adverse experiences noted above, other adverse experiences that occurred included: abdominal fullness, hypermotility, hepatitis, gait disturbance, hallucinations, encephalopathy, psychomotor retardation, coma, stroke, transient ischemic attacks, dysphasia, sedation, apathy, irritability, hyperactivity, claustrophobia, loss of libido, congestive heart failure, myocardial infarction, Raynaud's phenomenon, hot flashes, tachypnea, and excessive salivation. These adverse experiences occurred rarely (<1%).

Abnormal Laboratory Test Values: The percentage of patients with hairy cell leukemia or AIDS-related Kaposi's sarcoma who experienced a significant abnormal laboratory test value (NCI grades III or IV) at least once during their treatment with Interferon Alfa-2A is shown in the following table:

ABNORMAL LABORATORY TEST VALUES

	Hairy Cell Leukemia (n = 63)	AIDS-Related Kaposi's Sarcoma (n = 241)
Leukopenia	NA*	49%
Neutropenia	NA	52%
Thrombocytopenia	NA	35%
Decreased Hemoglobin	NA	27%
SGOT	42%	46%
Alkaline Phosphatase	8%	11%
LDH	13%	10%
Bilirubin	2%	<1%
BUN	4%	0%
Serum Creatinine	2%	<1%
Proteinuria	0%	<1%

* *Not applicable—Patient's initial hematologic laboratory test values were abnormal due to their underlying disease.*

Increases in fasting serum glucose, serum phosphorus and serum uric acid levels and decreases in serum calcium levels were also observed in less than 5% of patients.

DOSAGE AND ADMINISTRATION

The recommended dosages of Interferon Alfa-2A differ for hairy cell leukemia and AIDS-related Kaposi's sarcoma. See indication-specific dosages below.

Hairy Cell Leukemia: The induction dose of Interferon Alfa-2A is 3 million IU daily for 16 to 24 weeks, administered as a subcutaneous or intramuscular injection. Subcutaneous administration is particularly suggested for, but not limited to, thrombocytopenia patients (platelet count <50,000) or for patients at risk for bleeding. The recommended maintenance dose is 3 million IU, three times per week. Dose reduction by one-half or withholding of individual doses may be needed when severe adverse reactions occur. The use of doses higher than 3 million IU is not recommended in hairy cell leukemia. The 9 and 36 million IU dosage forms should not be used for the treatment of hairy cell leukemia.

Patients should be treated for approximately six months before the physician determines whether to continue therapy in patients who respond or discontinue therapy in patients who did not respond. Patients with hairy cell leukemia have been treated for up to 24 consecutive months. The optimal duration of treatment for this disease has not been determined.

AIDS-Related Kaposi's sarcoma: The recommended induction dose of Interferon Alfa-2A is 36 million IU daily for 10 to 12 weeks, administered as an intramuscular or subcutaneous injection. Subcutaneous administration is particu-

larly suggested for, but not limited to, patients who are thrombocytopenic (platelet count <50,000) or who are at risk for bleeding. The recommended maintenance dose is 36 million IU, three times per week. Dose reductions by one-half or withholding of individual doses may be required when severe adverse reactions occur. An escalating schedule of 3 million IU, 9 million IU and 18 million IU each daily for 3 days followed by 36 million IU daily for the remainder of the 10 to 12 week induction period has also produced equivalent therapeutic benefit with some amelioration of the acute toxicity in some patients.

When disease stabilization or a response to treatment occurs, treatment should continue until there is no further evidence of tumor or until discontinuation is required because of a severe opportunistic infection or adverse effects. The optimal duration of treatment for this disease has not been determined.

If severe reactions occur, the dose should be modified (50% reduction) or therapy should be temporarily discontinued until the adverse reactions abate. The need for dose reduction should take into account the effects of prior x-ray therapy or chemotherapy that may have compromised bone marrow reserve. The minimum effective doses of Interferon Alfa-2A for the treatment of hairy cell leukemia and AIDS-related Kaposi's sarcoma have not been established.

Parenteral drug products should be inspected visually for particulate matter and discoloration before administration, whenever solution and container permit.

Storage: The sterile powder and its accompanying diluent, the reconstituted solution and the injectable solution should be stored in the refrigerator at 36° to 46°F (2° to 8°C). Do *not* freeze or shake.

REFERENCES

1. Trown PW *et al: Cancer* 57 (Suppl.): 1648-1656, 1986. 2. Itri LM *et al: Cancer* 59: 668-674, 1987. 3. Jones GJ, Itri LM: *Cancer* 57 (Suppl.): 1709-1715, 1986. 4. Foon KA *et al: Blood* 64 (Suppl. 1): 164a, 1984. 5. Quesada JR *et al: Cancer* 57 (Suppl.): 1678-1680, 1986. 6. Krown SE *et al: N Eng. J Med* 308: 1071-1076, 1983. 7. Krown SE *et al: Proc Am Soc Clin Oncol* 7: 1, 1988, 8. Williams SJ *et al: Lancet* 2:939-941, 1987. 9. Jonkman JHG *et al: Br J Clin Pharmacol* 2(27) 795-802, 1989. 10. Kauppila A *et al: Int J Cancer* 29:291-294, 1982. Revised: August 1992.

J CODES
3 million units SC,IM—J9213

HOW SUPPLIED
INJECTION: 3 MILLION U

BRAND/MANUFACTURER	NDC	SIZE	AWP
○ BRAND ROFERON-A: Roche Labs	00004-1987-09	1 ml	$29.87

INJECTION: 9 MILLION U

BRAND/MANUFACTURER	NDC	SIZE	AWP
○ BRAND ROFERON-A: Roche Labs	00004-6900-09	0.9 ml	$84.14

INJECTION: 18 MILLION U

BRAND/MANUFACTURER	NDC	SIZE	AWP
○ BRAND ROFERON-A: Roche Labs	00004-1993-09	1s	$179.20
	00004-1988-09	3 ml	$179.20

INJECTION: 36 MILLION U

BRAND/MANUFACTURER	NDC	SIZE	AWP
○ BRAND ROFERON-A: Roche Labs	00004-2005-09	1 ml	$358.38

Interferon Alfa-2B

DESCRIPTION
Interferon Alfa-2B, recombinant for intramuscular, subcutaneous or intralesional injection, is a purified sterile recombinant interferon product.

Powder for Injection: The 3 million, 5 million, 18 million multidose, 25 million, and 50 million IU packages are for use by intramuscular or subcutaneous injection. The 10 million IU package is for intramuscular, subcutaneous, or intralesional injection. (See *"Warnings"* and *"Precautions"*.)

Solution for Injection: The 10 million and 25 million IU packages are for use by intramuscular or subcutaneous injection, and not for intralesional use. (See *"Warnings"*and *"Precautions"*.)

Interferon Alfa-2B recombinant for injection has been classified as an alpha Interferon and is a water soluble protein with a molecular weight of 19,271 daltons produced by recombinant DNA techniques. It is obtained from the bacterial fermentation of a strain of *Escherichia coli* bearing a genetically engineered plasmid containing an Interferon Alfa-2B gene from human leukocytes. The fermentation is carried out in a defined nutrient medium containing the antibiotic tetracycline hydrochloride at a concentration of 5 to 10 mg/L; the presence of this antibiotic is not detectable in the final product. The specific activity of Interferon Alfa-2B, recombinant is approximately 2×10^8 IU/mg protein.

Powder for Injection: After reconstitution, the 3 million, 5 million, 10 million (1 mL), 18 million, 25 million, and 50 million IU vials contain, respectively, per mL either 3 million, 5 million, 10 million, 6 million, 5 million, or 50 million IU of Interferon Alfa-2B, recombinant, 20 mg glycine, 2.3 mg sodium phosphate dibasic, 0.55 mg sodium phosphate monobasic, and 1.0 mg human albumin are also present. Based on the specific activity of approximately 2×10^8 IU/mg protein, the corresponding quantities of Interferon Alfa-2B, recombinant in the vials described above are approximately 0.015 mg, 0.025 mg, 0.05 mg, 0.09 mg, 0.125 mg, and 0.25 mg protein, respectively. Prior to administration, the Interferon Alfa-2B, a powder for injection, is to be reconstituted with the provided diluent for Interferon Alfa-2B, recombinant for injection (bacteriostatic water for injection) containing 0.9% benzyl alcohol as a preservative. (See *"Dosage and Administration"*.) Interferon Alfa-2B powder for injection is a white to cream colored powder.

Solution for Injection: Each Interferon Alfa-2B vial contains either 10 million IU of Interferon Alfa-2B, recombinant per 2 mL or 25 million IU of Interferon Alfa-2B, recombinant per 5 mL. Each mL also contains 20 mg glycine, 2.3 mg sodium phosphate dibasic, 0.55 mg sodium phosphate monobasic, 1.0 mg human albumin, and 1.2 mg methylparaben and 0.12 mg propylparaben as preservatives. Based on the specific activity of approximately 2×10^8 IU/mg protein, the corresponding quantities of Interferon Alfa-2B, recombinant in the vials described above are approximately 0.05 mg and 0.125 mg protein, respectively. These packages do not require reconstitution prior to administration. Interferon Alfa-2B solution for injection is a colorless to light yellow solution.

Following is its chemical structure:

CLINICAL PHARMACOLOGY

General: The interferons are a family of naturally occurring small proteins and glycoproteins with molecular weights of approximately 15,000 to 27,600 daltons produced and secreted by cells in response to viral infections and to synthetic or biological inducers.

Preclinical Pharmacology: Interferons exert their cellular activities by binding to specific membrane receptors on the cell surface. Once bound to the cell membrane, interferons initiate a complex sequence of intracellular events. *In vitro* studies demonstrated that these include the induction of certain enzymes, suppression of cell proliferation, immunomodulating activities such as enhancement of the phagocytic activity of macrophages and augmentation of the specific cytotoxicity of lymphocytes for target cells, and inhibition of virus replication in virus-infected cells.

In a study using human hepatoblastoma cell line, HB 611, the *in vitro* antiviral activity of alpha interferon was demonstrated by its inhibition of hepatitis B virus (HBV) replication.

The correlation between these *in vitro* data and the clinical results is unknown. Any of these activities might contribute to interferon's therapeutic effects.

Pharmacokinetics: The pharmacokinetics of Interferon Alfa-2B, recombinant for injection were studied in 12 healthy male volunteers following single doses of 5 million IU/m² administered intramuscularly, subcutaneously and as a 30-minute intravenous infusion in a crossover design. Interferon Alfa-2B concentrations were determined using a radioimmunoassay (RIA) with a detection limit equal to 10 IU/mL.

The mean serum Interferon Alfa-2B concentrations following intramuscular and subcutaneous injections were comparable. The maximum serum concentrations obtained via these routes were approximately 18 to 116 IU/mL and occurred 3 to 12 hours after administration. The elimination half-life of Interferon Alfa-2B, recombinant for injection following both intramuscular and subcutaneous injections was approximately two to three hours. Serum concentrations were below the detection limit by 16 hours after the injections.

After intravenous administration, serum Interferon Alfa-2B concentrations peaked (135 to 273 IU/mL) by the end of the 30-minutes infusion, then declined at a slightly more rapid rate than after intramuscular or subcutaneous drug administration, becoming undetectable four hours after the infusion. The elimination half-life was approximately two hours.

Urine Interferon Alfa-2B concentrations following a single dose (5 million IU/m²) were not detectable after any of the parenteral routes of administration. This result was expected since preliminary studies with isolated and perfused rabbit kidneys have shown that the kidney may be the main site of interferon catabolism.

There are no pharmacokinetic data available for the intralesional route of administration.

Serum Neutralizing Antibodies: In Interferon Alfa-2B treated patients tested for antibody activity in clinical trials, serum anti-interferon neutralizing antibodies

were detected in 0% (0/90) of patients with hairy cell leukemia, 0.8% (2/260) of patients treated intralesionally for condylomata acuminata, and 4% (1/24) of patients with AIDS-Related Kaposi's Sarcoma. Serum neutralizing antibodies have been detected in < 3% of patients treated with higher Interferon Alfa-2B doses in malignancies other than hairy cell leukemia or AIDS-Related Kaposi's Sarcoma. The clinical significance of the appearance of serum anti-interferon neutralizing activity in these indications is not known.

Serum anti-interferon neutralizing antibodies were detected in 15% (7/46) of patients with chronic hepatitis NANB/C and in 13% (6/48) of patients who received Interferon Alfa-2B therapy for chronic hepatitis B at 5 million IU, QD for 4 months, and in 3% (1/33) of patients treated at 10 million IU, TIW. In patients with chronic hepatitis the titers detected were low ($\leq 1:40$) and the appearance of serum anti-interferon neutralizing activity did not appear to affect safety or efficacy.

Hairy Cell Leukemia: In clinical trials in patients with hairy cell leukemia, there was depression of hematopoiesis during the first 1 to 2 months of Interferon Alfa-2B treatment, resulting in reduced numbers of circulating red and white blood cells, and platelets. Subsequently, both splenectomized and non-splenectomized patients achieved substantial and sustained improvements in granulocytes, platelets, and hemoglobin levels in 75% of treated patients and at least some improvement (minor responses) occurred in 90%. Interferon Alfa-2B treatment resulted in a decrease in bone marrow hypercellularity and hairy cell infiltrates. The hairy cell index (HCI), which represents the percent of bone marrow cellularity times the percent of hairy cell infiltrate, was greater than or equal to 50% at the beginning of the study in 87% of patients. The percentage of patients with such an HCI decreased to 25% after six months and to 14% after one year. These results indicate that even though hematologic improvement had occurred earlier, prolonged Interferon Alfa-2B treatment may be required to obtain maximal reduction in tumor cell infiltrates in the bone marrow.

The percentage of patients with hairy cell leukemia who required red blood cell or platelet transfusions decreased significantly during treatment and the percentage of patients with confirmed and serious infections declined as granulocyte counts improved. Reversal of splenomegaly and of clinically significant hypersplenism was demonstrated in some patients.

A study was conducted to assess the effects of extended Interferon Alfa-2B treatment on duration of response for patients who responded to initial therapy. In this study, 126 responding patients were randomized to receive additional Interferon Alfa-2B treatment for 6 months or observation for a comparable period, after 12 months of initial Interferon Alfa-2B. During this 6-month period, 3% (2/66) of Interferon Alfa-2B treated patients relapsed compared with 18% (11/60) who were not treated. This represents a significant difference in time to relapse in favor of continued Interferon Alfa-2B treatment (p = 0.006/0.01, Logrank/Wilcoxon). Since a small proportion of the total population had relapsed, median time to relapse could not be estimated in either group. A similar pattern in relapses was seen when all randomized treatment, including that beyond 6 months, and available follow-up data were assessed. The 15% (10/66) relapses among Interferon Alfa-2B patients occurred over a significantly longer period of time than the 40% (24/60) with observation (p = 0.0002/0.0001, Logrank/Wilcoxon). Median time to relapse was estimated, using the Kaplan-Meier method, to be 6.8 months in the observation group but could not be estimated in the Interferon Alfa-2B group.

Subsequent follow-up with a median time of approximately 40 months demonstrated an overall survival of 87.8%. In a comparable historical control group followed for 24 months, overall median survival was approximately 40%.

Condylomata Acuminata: Condylomata acuminata (venereal or genital warts) are associated with infections of the human papilloma virus (HPV). The safety and efficacy of Interferon Alfa-2B, recombinant for injection in the treatment of condylomata acuminata were evaluated in three controlled double-blind clinical trials. In these studies Interferon Alfa-2B doses of 1 million IU per lesion were administered intralesionally three times a week (TIW), in ≤ 5 lesions per patient for 3 weeks. The patients were observed for up to 16 weeks after completion of the full treatment course.

Interferon Alfa-2B treatment of condylomata was significantly more effective than placebo, as measured by disappearance of lesions, decreases in lesion size, and by an overall change in disease status. Of 192 Interferon Alfa-2B treated patients and 206 placebo treated patients who were evaluable for efficacy at the time of best response during the course of the study, 42% of Interferon Alfa-2B patients *versus* 17% of placebo patients experienced complete clearing of all treated lesions. Likewise 24% of Interferon Alfa-2B patients *versus* 8% of placebo patients experienced marked ($\geq 75\%$ to < 100%) reduction in lesion size, 18% *versus* 9% experienced moderate ($\geq 50\%$ to $\leq 75\%$) reduction in lesion size, 10% *versus* 42% had a slight (< 50%) reduction in lesion size, 5% *versus* 24% had no change in lesion size and 0% *versus* 1% experienced exacerbation (p < 0.001).

In one of these studies, 43% (54/125) of patients in whom multiple (≥ 3) lesions were treated, experienced complete clearing of all treated lesions during the course of the study. Of these patients, 81% remained cleared 16 weeks after treatment was initiated.

Patients who did not achieve total clearing of all their treated lesions had these same lesions treated with a second course of therapy. During this second course of treatment, 38% to 67% of patients had clearing of all treated lesions. The overall percentage of patients who had cleared all their treated lesions after 2 courses of treatment ranged from 57% to 85%.

Interferon Alfa-2B treated lesions showed improvement within 2 to 4 weeks after the start of treatment in the above study; maximal response to Interferon Alfa-2B therapy was noted 4 to 8 weeks after initiation of treatment.

◆ RATED THERAPEUTICALLY EQUIVALENT; ◇ THERAPEUTIC EQUIVALENCE UNCONFIRMED; ○ UNRATED

The response to Interferon Alfa-2B therapy was better in patients who had condylomata for shorter durations than in patients with lesions for a longer duration.

Another study involved 97 patients in whom three lesions were treated with either an intralesional injection of 1.5 million IU of Interferon Alfa-2B, recombinant for injection per lesion followed by a topical application of 25% podophyllin, or a topical application of 25% podophyllin alone. Treatment was given once a week for 3 weeks. The combined treatment of Interferon Alfa-2B, recombinant for injection and podophyllin was shown to be significantly more effective than podophyllin alone, as determined by the number of patients whose lesions cleared. This significant difference in response was evident after the second treatment (week 3) and continued through 8 weeks posttreatment. At the time of the patient's best response, 67% (33/49) of the Interferon Alfa-2B, recombinant for injection and podophyllin treated patients had all three treated lesions clear while 42% (20/48) of the podophyllin treated patients had all three clear (p = 0.003).

AIDS-Related Kaposi's Sarcoma: The safety and efficacy of Interferon Alfa-2B, recombinant for injection in the treatment of Kaposi's Sarcoma (KS), a common manifestation of the Acquired Immune Deficiency Syndrome (AIDS), were evaluated in clinical trials in 144 patients.

In one study, Interferon Alfa-2B doses of 30 million IU/m^2 were administered subcutaneously three times per week (TIW), to patients with AIDS-Related KS. Doses were adjusted for patient tolerance. The average weekly dose delivered in the first 4 weeks was 150 million IU; at the end of 12 weeks this averaged 110 million IU/week; and by 24 weeks averaged 75 million IU/week.

Forty-four percent of asymptomatic patients responded *versus* 7% of symptomatic patients. The median time to response was approximately 2 months and 1 month, respectively, for asymptomatic and symptomatic patients. The median duration of response was approximately 3 months and 1 month, respectively, for the asymptomatic and symptomatic patients. Baseline T4/T8 ratios were 0.46 for responders *versus* 0.33 for nonresponders.

In another study, Interferon Alfa-2B doses of 35 million IU were administered subcutaneously, daily (QD), for 12 weeks. Maintenance treatment, with every other day dosing (QOD), was continued for up to 1 year in patients achieving antitumor and antiviral responses. The median time to response was 2 months and the median duration of response was 5 months in the asymptomatic patients.

In all studies, the likelihood of response was greatest in patients with relatively intact immune systems as assessed by baseline CD4 counts. Results at doses of 30 million IU/m^2 TIW and 35 million IU/QD, subcutaneously were similar and are provided together in Table 1. This table demonstrates the relationship of response to baseline CD4 count in both asymptomatic and symptomatic patients in the 30 million IU/m^2 TIW and the 35 million IU/QD treatment groups.

In the 30 million IU study group, 7% (5/72) of patients were complete responders and 22% (16/72) of the patients were partial responders. The 35 million IU study had 13% (3/23) patients complete responders and 17% (4/23) partial responders.

For patients who received 30 million IU, TIW, the median survival time was longer in patients with CD4 greater than 200 (30.7 months) than in patients with CD4 less than or equal to 200 (8.9 months). Among responders, the median survival time was 22.6 months *versus* 9.7 months in nonresponders.

Table 1
RESPONSE BY BASELINE CD4 COUNT*
IN AIDS-RELATED KS PATIENTS

	30 million IU/m^2 TIW, SC and 35 million IU QD, SC	
	Asymptomatic	Symptomatic
CD4 < 200	4/14 (29%)	0/19 (0%)
200 ≤ CD4 ≤ 400	6/12 (50%)	0/5 (0%)
	58%	
CD4 > 400	5/7 (71%)	0/0 (0%)

* Data for CD4, and asymptomatic and symptomatic classification were not available for all patients.

Chronic Hepatitis Non-A, Non-B/C (NANB/C): The safety and efficacy of Interferon Alfa-2B, recombinant for injection in the treatment of chronic hepatitis NANB/C were evaluated in 4 randomized controlled clinical studies in which Interferon Alfa-2B doses of 1, 2, or 3 million IU three times a week (TIW), were administered subcutaneously for 6 months (23 or 24 weeks). The patients were 18 years of age or older and had compensated liver disease. Of the 332 patients evaluable for efficacy, 81% had a history of blood or blood product exposure, 8% had a history of intravenous drug abuse, 2% had a history of surgery without blood products, and the remainder had other exposure. Retrospectively, 86% (172/199) of the patients with blood or blood product exposure who were tested were found to be positive for antibody to hepatitis C virus (HCV).

In each of 3 clinical studies, Interferon Alfa-2B therapy at 3 million IU, TIW, resulted in a reduction in serum alanine aminotransferase (ALT) in a statistically significantly greater proportion of patients *versus* control patients (see Table 2). Of the 54% of patients responding to Interferon Alfa-2B therapy at a dose of 3 million IU, 70% achieved reductions in ALT levels to normal, 18% achieved reductions to near normal levels, and 12% achieved partial responses.

Histological improvement was evaluated by comparison of pre- and post-treatment liver biopsies using the semi-quantitative Knodell Histology Activity Index (HAI).[4]

In one of the three studies there was histological improvement in a statistically significantly greater proportion of Interferon Alfa-2B treated patients compared to controls (see Table 3). A similar, but not statistically significant trend for improvement was observed in the other two studies.

Subsequent combined analysis of results for the 3 studies showed histological improvement in a statistically significantly greater proportion of patients treated with Interferon Alfa-2B doses of 3 million IU than in control patients (p = 0.04). The improvement was due primarily to decreases in severity of necrosis and degeneration in the lobular and periportal regions (Knodell HAI Categories I + II), which were observed in 65% (52/80) of patients treated at 3 million IU compared to 46% (32/70) of controls. Diminution of disease activity in these regions of the liver was accompanied by a reduction or normalization of serum ALT in many patients. Disease activity increased in these regions in only 3% of all Interferon Alfa-2B treated patients, whereas an increase was observed in 16% of the controls. No patient achieving an ALT response with 3 million IU Interferon Alfa-2B therapy showed increased periportal or lobular necrosis and degeneration.

Patients were followed for 6 months after the end of Interferon Alfa-2B therapy. During this period the ALT response was maintained in 51% (26/51) of patients who responded at the 3 million IU TIW dose. Of patients who relapsed during the follow-up period and were retreated at this dose, 83% (15/18) responded to retreatment.

Table 2
ALT RESPONSES† IN CHRONIC HEPATITIS NANB/C PATIENTS

	Treatment Group			
	Number of Patients (%)			
Study Number	Interferon Alfa-2B 3 million IU		Controls‡	P § Value
1[1]	29/55	(53%)	5/55 (9%)	< 0.001
2[2]	10/23	(43%)	3/25 (12%)	0.02
3[3]	12/17	(71%)	3/17 (18%)	0.005
All Studies	**51/95**	**(54%)**	**11/97 (11%)**	**< 0.001**

† Includes reduction in serum ALT to: normal, near normal (≤ 1.5 times the upper limit of normal), or partial response (> 50% decrease in serum ALT).
‡ Untreated or Placebo
§ Interferon Alfa-2B 3 million IU, TIW, 6 months versus control.

Table 3
HISTOLOGICAL IMPROVEMENT£ IN CHRONIC HEPATITIS NANB/C PATIENTS

	Treatment Group			
	Number of Patients (%)			
Study Number	Interferon Alfa-2B 3 million IU		Controls**	P†† Value
1	29/45	(64%)	18/36 (50%)	0.26
2	12/19	(63%)	10/18 (56%)	0.75
3	14/16	(88%)	8/15 (53%)	0.054
All Studies	**55/80**	**(69%)**	**36/69 (52%)**	**0.04**

£ Assessed by the Knodell Histology Activity Index which includes:
Category I—Periportal necrosis
Category II—Intralobular degeneration and necrosis
Category III—Portal inflammation
Category IV—Fibrosis
** Untreated or Placebo
†† Interferon Alfa-2B 3 million IU, TIW, 6 months compared to control for improvement versus no improvement.

Chronic Hepatitis B: The safety and efficacy of Interferon Alfa-2B, recombinant for injection in the treatment of chronic hepatitis B were evaluated in three clinical trials in which Interferon Alfa-2B doses of 30 to 35 million IU per week were administered subcutaneously (SC), as either 5 million IU daily (QD), or 10 million IU three times a week (TIW) for 16 weeks *versus* no treatment. All patients were 18 years of age or older with compensated liver disease, and had chronic hepatitis B virus (HBV) infection (serum HBsAg positive for at least 6 months) and HBV replication (serum HBeAg positive). Patients were also serum HBV-DNA positive, an additional indicator of HBV replication, as measured by a research assay.[5,6] All patients had elevated serum alanine aminotransferase (ALT), and liver biopsy findings compatible with the diagnosis of chronic hepatitis. Patients with the presence of antibody to human immunodeficiency virus (anti-HIV) or antibody to hepatitis delta virus (anti-HDV) in the serum were excluded from the studies.

Virologic response to treatment was defined in these studies as a loss of serum markers of HBV replication (HBeAg and HBV-DNA). Secondary parameters of response included loss of serum HBsAg, decreases in serum ALT, and improvement in liver histology.

In each of two randomized controlled studies, a significantly greater proportion of Interferon Alfa - 2B treated patients exhibited a virologic response compared with untreated control patients (see Table 4). In a third study without a concurrent control group, a similar response rate to Interferon Alfa - 2B therapy was observed. Pretreatment with prednisone, evaluated in two of the studies, did not improve the response rate and provided no additional benefit.

The response to Interferon Alfa - 2B therapy was durable. No patient responding to Interferon Alfa - 2B therapy at a dose of 5 million IU, QD or 10 million IU, TIW, relapsed during the follow-up period which ranged from 2 to 6 months after treatment ended. The loss of serum HBeAg and HBV-DNA was maintained in 100% of 19 responding patients followed for 3.5 to 36 months after the end of therapy.

In a proportion of responding patients, loss of HBeAg was followed by the loss of HBsAg. HBsAg was lost in 27% (4/15) of patients who responded to Interferon Alfa-2B therapy at a dose of 5 million IU, QD, and 35 (8/23) of patients who responded to 10 million IU, TIW. No untreated control patient lost HBsAg in these studies.

In a pilot study, 12 patients responding to Interferon Alfa-2B therapy were followed for 3.8 to 6.6 years after treatment; 100% (12/12) remained serum HBeAg negative and 58% (7/12) lost serum HBsAg.

Interferon Alfa-2B therapy resulted in normalization of serum ALT in a significantly greater proportion of treated patients compared to untreated patients in each of two controlled studies (see Table 5). In a third study without a concurrent control group, normalization of serum ALT was observed in 50% (12/24) of patients receiving Interferon Alfa-2B therapy.

Virologic response was associated with a reduction in serum ALT to normal or near normal (≥ 1.5 times the upper limit of normal) in 87% (13/15) of patients responding to Interferon Alfa-2B therapy at 5 million IU, QD, and 100% (23/23) of patients responding to 10 million IU, TIW.

Improvement in liver histology was evaluated in Studies 1 and 3, by comparison of pre- and 6 month posttreatment liver biopsies using the semi-quantitative Knodell Histology Activity Index. No statistically significant difference in liver histology was observed in treated patients compared to control patients in Study 1. Although statistically significant histological improvement from baseline was observed in treated patients in Study 3 ($p \geq 0.01$), there was no control group for comparison. Of those patients exhibiting a virologic response following treatment with 5 million IU, QD or 10 million IU, TIW histological improvement was observed in 85% (17/20) compared to 36% (9/25) of patients who were not virologic responders. The histological improvement was due primarily to decreases in severity of necrosis, degeneration, and inflammation in the periportal, lobular, and portal regions of the liver (Knodell Categories I + II + III). Continued histological improvement was observed in four responding patients who lost serum HBsAg and were followed 2 to 4 years after the end of Interferon Alfa-2B therapy.[7]

Table 4
VIROLOGIC RESPONSE* IN CHRONIC HEPATITIS B PATIENTS

	Treatment Group £ Number of Patients (%)				
Study Number	Interferon Alfa-2B 5 million IU, QD	Interferon Alfa-2B 10 million, IU, TIW	Untreated Controls		P** Value
1[5]	15/38 (39%)	—	3/42	(7%)	0.0009
2	—	10/24 (42%)	1/22	(5%)	0.005
3[6]	—	13/24‡ (54%)	2/27	(7%)‡	NA‡
All Studies	15/38 (39%)	23/48 (48%)	6/91	(7%)	—

* Loss of HBeAg and HBV-DNA by 6 months posttherapy.
£ Patients pretreated with prednisone not shown.
** Interferon Alfa-2B treatment group versus untreated control.
‡ Untreated control patients evaluated after 24 weeks observation period. A subgroup subsequently received Interferon Alfa-2B therapy. A direct comparison is not applicable (NA).

Table 5
ALT RESPONSES* IN CHRONIC HEPATITIS B PATIENTS

	Treatment Group Number of Patients (%)				
Study Number	Interferon Alfa-2B 5 million IU,QD	Interferon Alfa-2B 10 million IU, TIW	Untreated Controls		P** Value
1	16/38 (42%)	—	8/42	(19%)	0.03
2	—	10/24 (42%)	1/22	(5%)	0.0034
3	—	12/24† (50%)	2/27	(7%)†	NA†
All Studies	16/38 (42%)	22/48 (46%)	11/91	(12%)	—

* Reduction in serum ALT to normal by 6 months posttherapy.
** Interferon Alfa-2B treatment group versus untreated control.
† Untreated control patients evaluated after 24 week observation period. A subgroup subsequently received Interferon Alfa-2B therapy. A direct comparison is not applicable (NA).

INDICATIONS AND USAGE

General: Interferon Alfa-2B, recombinant for injection is indicated in patients 18 years of age or older for the treatment of hairy cell leukemia, selected cases of condylomata acuminata involving external surfaces of the genital and perianal areas, selected patients with AIDS-Related Kaposi's Sarcoma, chronic hepatitis Non-A, Non-B/C (NANB/C) in patients with compensated liver disease who have a history of blood or blood product exposure and/or are HCV antibody positive, and chronic hepatitis B in patients with compensated liver disease and HBV replication (serum HBeAg positive).

Hairy Cell Leukemia: Interferon Alfa-2B, recombinant for injection is indicated for the treatment of patients 18 years of age or older with hairy cell leukemia. Studies have shown that Interferon Alfa-2B therapy can produce clinically meaningful regression or stabilization of this disease, both in previously splenectomized and non-splenectomized patients. Prior to initiation of therapy, tests should be performed to quantitate peripheral blood hemoglobin, platelets, granulocytes and hairy cells and bone marrow hairy cells. These parameters should be monitored periodically during treatment to determine whether response to treatment has occurred. If a patient does not respond within 6 months, treatment should be discontinued. If a response to treatment does occur, treatment usually should be continued until no further improvement is observed and these laboratory parameters have been stable for about 3 months (see *"Dosage and Administration"*). Responding patients may benefit from continued treatment after that time point with fewer relapses and a longer relapse-free interval. If treatment with Interferon Alfa-2B therapy has been interrupted, it should be noted that re-treatment with Interferon Alfa-2B therapy has led to response in greater than 90% of patients.

Condylomata Acuminata: Interferon Alfa-2B, recombinant for injection is indicated for intralesional treatment of selected patients 18 years of age or older with condylomata acuminata involving external surfaces of the genital and perianal areas (see *"Dosage and Administration"*).

In selecting patients for Interferon Alfa-2B treatment, the physician should consider the nature of the patient's lesion and the patient's past treatment history, in addition to the patient's ability to comply with the treatment regimen. Interferon Alfa-2B therapy offers an additional approach to treatment in condylomata and is particularly useful for those patients who do not respond satisfactorily to other treatment modalities (eg, podophyllin resin, surgery, cryotherapy, chemotherapy, and laser therapy), or whose lesions are more readily treatable by Interferon Alfa-2B, recombinant for injection than by other treatments.

The use of this product in adolescents has not been studied. Interferon alpha has been shown to affect the menstrual cycle in non-human primates and to decrease serum estradiol and progesterone levels in women. Consideration should be given as to whether the adolescent patient should be treated.

AIDS-Related Kaposi's Sarcoma: Interferon Alfa-2B, recombinant for injection is indicated for the treatment of selected patients 18 years of age or older with AIDS-Related Kaposi's Sarcoma. Studies have demonstrated a greater likelihood of response to Interferon Alfa-2B therapy in patients who are without systemic symptoms, who have limited lymphadenopathy and who have a relatively intact immune system.

Lesion measurements and blood counts should be performed prior to initiation of therapy and should be monitored periodically during treatment to determine whether response to treatment or disease stabilization has occurred.

When disease stabilization or a response to treatment occurs, treatment should continue until there is no further evidence of tumor or until discontinuation is required by evidence of a severe opportunistic infection or adverse effect (see *"Dosage and Administration"*).

Chronic Hepatitis Non-A, Non-B/C (NANB/C): Interferon Alfa-2B, recombinant for injection is indicated for the treatment of chronic hepatitis Non-A, Non-B/C (NANB/C) in patients 18 years of age or older with compensated liver disease who have a history of blood or blood product exposure and/or are HCV antibody positive. Studies in these patients demonstrated that Interferon Alfa-2B therapy can produce clinically meaningful effects on this disease, manifested by normalization of serum alanine aminotransferase (ALT) and reduction in liver necrosis and degeneration.

A liver biopsy should be performed to establish the diagnosis of chronic hepatitis. Patients should be tested for the presence of antibody to HCV. Patients with other causes of chronic hepatitis, including autoimmune hepatitis, should be excluded. Prior to initiation of Interferon Alfa-2B therapy, the physician should establish that the patient has compensated liver disease. The following patient entrance criteria for compensated liver disease were used in the clinical studies and should be considered before Interferon Alfa-2B treatment of patients with chronic hepatitis NANB/C.

- No history of hepatic encephalopathy, variceal bleeding, ascites, or other clinical signs of decompensation
- Bilirubin ≤ 2 mg/dL
- Albumin Stable and within normal limits
- Prothrombin Time < 3 seconds prolonged
- WBC ≥ 3000/mm³
- Platelets ≥ 70,000/mm³

Serum creatinine should be normal or near normal. Prior to initiation of Interferon Alfa-2B therapy, CBC and platelet counts should be evaluated in order to establish baselines for monitoring potential toxicity. These tests should be repeated at weeks 1 and 2 following initiation of Interferon Alfa-2B therapy, and monthly thereafter. Serum ALT should be evaluated after 2, 16, and 24 weeks of therapy to assess response to treatment (see *"Dosage and Administration"*).

Patients with preexisting thyroid abnormalities may be treated if thyroid stimulating hormone (TSH) levels can be maintained in the normal range by medication. TSH levels must be within normal limits upon initiation of Interferon

Alfa-2B treatment and TSH testing should be repeated at 3 and 6 months (see *"Precautions—Laboratory Tests"*).

Chronic Hepatitis B Interferon Alfa-2B, recombinant for injection is indicated for the treatment of chronic hepatitis B in patients 18 years of age or older with compensated liver disease and HBV replication. Patients must be serum HBsAg positive for at least 6 months and have HBV replication (serum HBeAg positive) with elevated serum ALT. Studies in these patients demonstrated that Interferon Alfa-2B therapy can produce virologic remission of this disease (loss of serum HBeAg), and normalization of serum amino-transferases. Interferon-Alfa-2B therapy resulted in the loss of serum HBsAg in some responding patients.

Prior to initiation of Interferon Alfa-2B therapy, it is recommended that a liver biopsy be performed to establish the presence of chronic hepatitis and the extent of liver damage. The physician should establish that the patient has compensated liver disease. The following patient entrance criteria for compensated liver disease were used in the clinical studies and should be considered before Interferon Alfa-2B treatment of patients with chronic hepatitis B:
- No history of hepatic encephalopathy, variceal bleeding, ascites, or other signs of clinical decompensation

■ Bilirubin	Normal
■ Albumin	Stable and within normal limits
■ Prothrombin Time	< 3 seconds prolonged
■ WBC	$\geq 4000/mm^3$
■ Platelets	$\geq 100,000/mm^3$

Patients with causes of chronic hepatitis other than chronic hepatitis B or chronic hepatitis NANB/C should not be treated with Interferon Alfa-2B, recombinant for injection. CBC and platelet counts should be evaluated prior to initiation of Interferon Alfa-2B therapy in order to establish baselines for monitoring potential toxicity. These tests should be repeated at treatment weeks 1, 2, 4, 8, 12, and 16. Liver function tests, including serum ALT, albumin and bilirubin, should be evaluated at treatment weeks 1, 2, 4, 8, 12, and 16. HBeAg, HBsAg, and ALT should be evaluated at the end of therapy, as well as 3 and 6 months posttherapy, since patients may become virologic responders during the 6 month period following the end of treatment. In clinical studies, 39% (15/38) of responding patients lost HBeAg 1 to 6 months following the end of Interferon Alfa-2B therapy. Of responding patients who lost HBsAg, 58% (7/12) did so 1 to 6 months posttreatment.

A transient increase in ALT ≥ 2 times baseline value (flare) can occur during Interferon Alfa-2B therapy for chronic hepatitis B. In clinical trials, this flare generally occurred 8 to 12 weeks after initiation of therapy and was more frequent in responders (63%, 24/38) than in nonresponders (27%, 13/48). However, elevations in bilirubin ≥ 3 mg/dL occurred infrequently (2%, 2/86) during therapy. When ALT flare occurs, in general, Interferon Alfa-2B therapy should be continued unless signs and symptoms of liver failure are observed. During ALT flare, clinical symptomatology and liver function tests including ALT, prothrombin time, alkaline phosphatase, albumin, and bilirubin, should be monitored at approximately 2 week intervals (see *"Warnings"*).

UNLABELED USES
Interferon Alfa-2B is used alone or as an adjunct in the treatment of chronic myelogenous leukemia (CML), acute hepatitis B, cervical cancer, and to slow the progression of HIV disease. It is also used in the treatment of chronic hepatitis D infection, mycosis fungoides, non-Hodgkin's lymphoma, malignant melanoma, and multiple myeloma. In addition, Interferon Alfa-2B is also used as prophylaxis against rhinovirus infections, in the treatment of essential thrombocythemia, and to alleviate vulvar pain in women with vulvar vestibulitis syndrome.

CONTRAINDICATIONS
Interferon-Alfa-2B, recombinant for injection is contraindicated in patients with a history of hypersensitivity to Interferon Alfa or any component of the injection.

WARNINGS
General: Moderate to severe adverse experiences may require modification of the patient's dosage regimen, or in some cases termination of Interferon Alfa-2B therapy. Because of the fever and other "flu-like" symptoms associated with Interferon Alfa-2B administration, it should be used cautiously in patients with debilitating medical conditions, such as those with a history of pulmonary disease (eg, chronic obstructive pulmonary disease), or diabetes mellitus prone to ketoacidosis. Caution should also be observed in patients with coagulation disorders (eg, thrombophlebitis, pulmonary embolism) or severe myelosuppression.

Patients with platelet counts of less than 50,000/mm³ should not be administered Interferon Alfa-2B, recombinant for injection intramuscularly, but instead by subcutaneous administration.

Interferon Alfa-2B therapy should be used cautiously in patients with a history of cardiovascular disease such as unstable angina or uncontrolled congestive heart failure. Those patients with a recent history of myocardial infarction and/or previous or current arrhythmic disorder who require Interferon Alfa-2B therapy should be closely monitored (see *"Laboratory Tests"*). Cardiovascular adverse experiences, which include hypotension, arrhythmia, or tachycardia of 150 beats per minute or greater, and transient reversible cardiomyopathy have been observed in some Interferon Alfa-2B treated patients. Transient reversible cardiomyopathy was reported in approximately 2% of the AIDS-Related Kaposi's Sarcoma patients treated with Interferon Alfa-2B, recombinant for injection. The incidence of these complications in patients with preexisting heart disease is unknown. Hypotension may occur during Interferon Alfa-2B administration, or up to two days posttherapy, and may require supportive therapy including fluid replacement to maintain intravascular volume. Supraventricular arrhythmias

occurred rarely and appeared to be correlated with preexisting conditions and prior therapy with cardiotoxic agents. These adverse experiences were controlled by modifying the dose or discontinuing treatment, but may require specific additional therapy.

Patients with a preexisting psychiatric condition, especially depression, or a history of severe psychiatric disorder should not be treated with Interferon Alfa-2B, recombinant for injection.[8] Interferon Alfa-2B therapy should be discontinued for any patient developing severe depression or other psychiatric disorder during treatment. Central nervous system effects manifested by depression, confusion and other alterations of mental status have been observed in some Interferon Alfa-2B treated patients, and suicidal ideation and attempted suicide have been observed rarely. These adverse effects have occurred in patients treated with recommended doses as well as in patients treated with higher Interferon Alfa-2B doses. More significant obtundation and coma have also been observed in some patients, usually elderly, treated at higher doses. While these effects are usually rapidly reversible upon discontinuation of therapy, full resolution of symptoms has taken up to three weeks in a few severe episodes. Narcotics, hypnotics, or sedatives may be used concurrently with caution and patients should be closely monitored until the adverse effects have resolved.

Patients with preexisting thyroid abnormalities whose thyroid function cannot be maintained in the normal range by medication should not be treated with Interferon Alfa-2B, recombinant for Injection. Therapy should be discontinued for patients developing thyroid abnormalities during treatment whose thyroid function cannot be normalized by medication.

Hepatotoxicity, including fatality, has been observed rarely in Interferon Alfa-2B treated patients. Any patient developing liver function abnormalities during treatment should be monitored closely and, if appropriate, treatment should be discontinued.

Pulmonary infiltrates, pneumonitis and pneumonia, including fatality, have been observed rarely in Interferon Alfa treated patients including those treated with Interferon Alfa-2B, recombinant for injection. The etiologic explanation for these pulmonary findings has yet to be established. Any patient developing fever, cough, dyspnea, or other respiratory symptoms should have a chest x-ray taken. If the chest x-ray shows pulmonary infiltrates or there is evidence of pulmonary function impairment, the patient should be closely monitored, and, if appropriate, Interferon Alfa treatment should be discontinued. While this has been reported more often in patients with chronic hepatitis NANB/C treated with Interferon Alfa, it has also been reported in patients with oncologic diseases treated with Interferon Alfa.

Retinal hemorrhages, cotton-wool spots, and retinal artery or vein obstruction have been observed rarely in patients treated with Interferon Alfa, including those treated with Interferon Alfa-2B, recombinant for Injection. The etiologic explanation for these findings has not yet been established. These events appear to occur after use of the drug for several months, but also have been reported after shorter treatment periods. Diabetes mellitus or hypertension have been present in some patients. Any patient complaining of changes in visual acuity or visual fields, or reporting other ophthalmologic symptoms during treatment with Interferon Alfa-2B, recombinant; should have an eye examination. Because the retinal events may have to be differentiated from those seen with diabetic or hypertensive retinopathy, a baseline ocular examination is recommended prior to treatment with Interferon in patients with diabetes mellitus or hypertension.

The 50 million IU strength of the Interferon Alfa-2B powder for injection is *not* to be used for the treatment of hairy cell leukemia, condylomata acuminata, chronic hepatitis NANB/C, or chronic hepatitis B. The 3 million, 5 million, 18 million multidose, and 25 million IU strengths of the Interferon Alfa-2B powder for injection are *not* to be used for the intralesional treatment of condylomata acuminata since the dilution required for the intralesional use would result in a hypertonic solution.

The 10 million and 25 million IU strengths of the Interferon Alfa-2B solution for injection are *not* to be used for the treatment of condylomata acuminata or AIDS-Related Kaposi's Sarcoma.

AIDS-Related Kaposi's Sarcoma: Interferon Alfa-2B therapy should not be used for patients with rapidly progressive visceral disease (see *"Clinical Pharmacology"*). Also of note, there may be synergistic adverse effects between Interferon Alfa-2B, recombinant for injection and zidovudine. Patients receiving concomitant zidovudine have had a higher incidence of neutropenia than that expected with zidovudine alone. Careful monitoring of the WBC count is indicated in all patients who are myelosuppressed and in all patients receiving other myelosuppressive medications. The effects of Interferon Alfa-2B, recombinant for injection when combined with other drugs used in the treatment of AIDS-Related disease are unknown.

Chronic Hepatitis Non-A, Non-B/C (NANB/C) and Chronic Hepatitis B: Patients with decompensated liver disease, autoimmune hepatitis or a history of autoimmune disease, and patients who are immunosuppressed transplant recipients should not be treated with Interferon Alfa-2B recombinant for injection. There are reports of worsening liver disease, including jaundice, hepatic encephalopathy, hepatic failure and death following Interferon Alfa-2B therapy in such patients. Therapy should be discontinued for any patient developing signs and symptoms of liver failure.

Chronic hepatitis B patients with evidence of decreasing hepatic synthetic functions, such as decreasing albumin levels or prolongation of prothrombin time, who nevertheless meet the entry criteria to start therapy, may be at increased risk of clinical decompensation if a flare of aminotransferases occurs during Interferon Alfa-2B treatment. In such patients, if increases in ALT occur during Interferon Alfa-2B therapy for chronic hepatitis B, they should be followed carefully including close monitoring of clinical symptomatology and liver function tests, including ALT, prothrombin time, alkaline phosphatase, albumin, and bilirubin.

In considering these patients for Interferon Alfa-2B therapy, the potential risks must be evaluated against the potential benefits of treatment.

PRECAUTIONS

General: Acute serious hypersensitivity reactions (eg, urticaria, angioedema, bronchoconstriction, anaphylaxis) have been observed rarely in Interferon Alfa-2B treated patients; if such an acute reaction develops, the drug should be discontinued immediately and appropriate medical therapy instituted. Transient rashes have occurred in some patients following injection, but have not necessitated treatment interruption. While fever may be related to the flu-like syndrome reported commonly in patients treated with interferon, other causes of persistent fever should be ruled out.

There have been reports of interferon exacerbating preexisting psoriasis; therefore, Interferon Alfa-2B therapy should be used in these patients only if the potential benefit justifies the potential risk.

Variations in dosage, routes of administration, and adverse reactions exist among different brands of interferon. Therefore, do not use different brands of interferon in any single treatment regimen.

Drug Interactions: Interactions between Interferon Alfa-2B, recombinant for injection and other drugs have not been fully evaluated. Caution should be exercised when administering Interferon Alfa-2B therapy in combination with other potentially myelosuppressive agents such as zidovudine.

Information for Patients: Patients receiving Interferon Alfa-2B treatment should be directed in its appropriate use, informed of benefits and risks associated with treatment, and referred to the *"Patient Information Sheet".* This information is intended to aid in the safe and effective use of this medication. It is not a disclosure of all possible adverse or intended effects.

If home use is prescribed, a puncture-resistant container for the disposal of used syringes and needles should be supplied to the patient. Patients should be thoroughly instructed in the importance of proper disposal and cautioned against any reuse of needles and syringes. The full container should be disposed of according to the directions provided by the physician (see *"Patient Information Sheet").*

Patients should be cautioned not to change brands of Interferon without medical consultation as a change in dosage may result.

Patients receiving high Interferon Alfa-2B doses should be cautioned against performing tasks that would require complete mental alertness, such as operating machinery or driving a motor vehicle.

The most common adverse experiences occurring with Interferon Alfa-2B therapy are "flu-like" symptoms, such as fever, headache, fatigue, anorexia, nausea, or vomiting (see *"Adverse Reactions"* section) and appear to decrease in severity as treatment continues. Some of these "flu-like" symptoms may be minimized by bedtime administration. Acetaminophen may be used to prevent or partially alleviate the fever and headache. Another common adverse experience is thinning of the hair.

It is advised that patients be well hydrated especially during the initial stages of treatment.

Laboratory Tests: In addition to those tests normally required for monitoring patients, the following laboratory tests are recommended for all patients on Interferon Alfa-2B therapy, prior to beginning treatment and then periodically thereafter.

■ Standard hematologic tests—including hemoglobin, complete and differential white blood cell counts and platelet count.

■ Blood chemistries—electrolytes, liver function tests, and TSH.

Those patients who have preexisting cardiac abnormalities and/or are in advanced stages of cancer, should have electrocardiograms taken prior to and during the course of treatment.

Mild to moderate leukopenia and elevated serum liver enzyme (SGOT) levels have been reported with intralesional administration of Interferon Alfa-2B, recombinant for injection (see *"Adverse Reactions"* section); therefore, the monitoring of these laboratory parameters should be considered.

Baseline chest X-rays are suggested and should be repeated if clinically indicated.

For specific recommendations in chronic hepatitis NANB/C and chronic hepatitis B, see *"Indications and Usage"* section.

Carcinogenesis, Mutagenesis, Impairment of Fertility: Studies with Interferon Alfa-2B, recombinant for injection have not been performed to determine carcinogenicity.

Interferon may impair fertility. In studies of interferon administration in non-human primates, menstrual cycle abnormalities have been observed. Decreases in serum estradiol and progesterone concentrations have been reported in women treated with human leukocyte interferon.[9] Therefore, fertile women should not receive Interferon Alfa-2B therapy unless they are using effective contraception during the therapy period. Interferon Alfa-2B therapy should be used with caution in fertile men.

Mutagenicity studies have demonstrated that Interferon Alfa-2B, recombinant for injection is not mutagenic.

Studies in mice (0.1, 1.0 million IU/day), rats (4, 20, 100 million IU/kg/day), and cynomolgus monkeys (1.1 million IU/kg/day; 0.25, 0.75, 2.5 million IU/kg/day) injected with Interferon Alfa-2B, recombinant for injection for up to 9 days, 3 months, and 1 month, respectively, have revealed no evidence of toxicity. However, in cynomolgus monkeys (4, 20, 100 million IU/kg/day) injected daily for 3 months with Interferon Alfa-2B, recombinant for injection toxicity was observed at the mid- and high-doses and mortality was observed at the high dose.

However, due to the known species-specificity of interferon, the effects in animals are unlikely to be predictive of those in man.

Pregnancy Category C: Interferon Alfa-2B, recombinant for injection has been shown to have abortificient effects in *Macaca mulatta* (rhesus monkeys) at 7.5, 15, and 30 million IU/kg (90, 180, and 360 times the intramuscular or subcutaneous dose of 2 million IU/m^2). Although abortion was observed in all dose groups, it was only statistically significant at the mid- and high-dose groups. There are no adequate and well-controlled studies in pregnant women. Interferon Alfa-2B therapy should be used during pregnancy only if the potential benefit justifies the potential risk to the fetus.

Nursing Mothers: It is not known whether this drug is excreted in human milk. However, studies in mice have shown that mouse interferons are excreted into the milk. Because of the potential for serious adverse reactions from the drug in nursing infants, a decision should be made whether to discontinue nursing or to discontinue Interferon Alfa-2B therapy, taking into account the importance of the drug to the mother.

Pediatric Use: Safety and effectiveness have not been established in patients below the age of 18 years.

ADVERSE REACTIONS

General: The adverse experiences listed below were reported to be possibly or probably related to Interferon Alfa-2B therapy during clinical trials. Most of these adverse reactions were mild to moderate in severity and were manageable. Some were transient and most diminished with continued therapy.

The most frequently reported adverse reactions were flu-like symptoms, particularly fever, headache, chills, myalgia, and fatigue. More severe toxicities are observed generally at higher doses and may be difficult for patients to tolerate. (See related table).

Hairy Cell Leukemia: The adverse reactions most frequently reported during clinical trials in 145 patients with hairy cell leukemia were the flu-like symptoms of fever (68%), fatigue (61%), and chills (46%).

Condylomata Acuminata: Eighty-eight percent (311/352) of patients treated with Interferon Alfa-2B, recombinant for injection for condylomata acuminata who were evaluable for safety, reported an adverse reaction during treatment. The incidence of the adverse reactions reported increased when the number of treated lesions increased from 1 to 5. All 40 patients who had 5 warts treated, reported some type of adverse reaction during treatment.

Adverse reactions and abnormal laboratory test values reported by patients who were retreated were qualitatively and quantitatively similar to those reported during the initial Interferon Alfa-2B treatment period.

AIDS-Related Kaposi's Sarcoma: In patients with AIDS-Related Kaposi's Sarcoma, some type of adverse reaction occurred in 100% of the 74 patients treated with 30 million IU/m^2 three times a week and in 97% of the 29 patients treated with 35 million IU per day.

Of these adverse reactions, those classified as severe (World Health Organization grade 3 or 4) were reported in 27% to 55% of patients. Severe adverse reactions in the 30 million IU/m^2 TIW study included: fatigue (20%), influenza-like symptoms (15%), anorexia (12%), dry mouth (4%), headache (4%), confusion (3%), fever (3%), myalgia (3%), and nausea and vomiting (1% each). Severe adverse reactions for patients who received the 35 million IU QD included: fever (24%), fatigue (17%), influenza-like symptoms (14%), dyspnea (14%), headache (10%), pharyngitis (7%), and ataxia, confusion, dysphagia, GI hemorrhage, abnormal hepatic function, increased SGOT, myalgia, cardiomyopathy, face edema, depression, emotional lability, suicide attempt, chest pain, and coughing (1 patient each). Overall, the incidence of severe toxicity was higher among patients who received the 35 million IU per day dose.

Chronic Hepatitis Non-A, Non-B/C (NANB/C): In patients with chronic hepatitis NANB/C, alopecia, injection site reactions, rash, depression, and irritability apparently increased in incidence with continued treatment; residual mild alopecia persisted posttreatment.

Infrequently, patients receiving Interferon Alfa-2B therapy for chronic hepatitis NANB/C developed thyroid abnormalities, either hypothyroid or hyperthyroid. In clinical trials < 1% (4/426) developed thyroid abnormalities. The abnormalities were controlled by conventional therapy for thyroid dysfunction. The mechanism by which Interferon Alfa-2B, recombinant for injection may alter thyroid status is unknown. Prior to initiation of Interferon Alfa-2B therapy for the treatment of chronic hepatitis NANB/C, serum TSH should be evaluated. Patients developing symptoms consistent with possible thyroid dysfunction during the course of Interferon Alfa-2B therapy should have their thyroid function evaluated and appropriate treatment instituted. Interferon Alfa-2B treatment may be continued if TSH levels can be maintained in the normal range by medication. Discontinuation of Interferon Alfa-2B therapy has not always reversed thyroid dysfunction occurring during treatment.

Chronic Hepatitis B: In patients with chronic hepatitis B, some type of adverse reaction occurred in 98% of the 101 patients treated at 5 million IU, QD and 90% of the 78 patients treated at 10 million IU, TIW. Most of these adverse reactions were mild to moderate in severity, were manageable, and were reversible following the end of therapy.

Adverse reactions classified as severe (causing a significant interference with normal daily activities or clinical state) were reported in 21% to 44% of patients. The severe adverse reactions reported most frequently were the flu-like symptoms of fever (28%), fatigue (15%), headache (5%), myalgia (4%), and rigors (4%), and

TREATMENT-RELATED ADVERSE EXPERIENCES BY INDICATION

Adverse Experience	Hairy Cell Leukemia 2 million IU/m² TIW/SC N = 145	Condylomata Acuminata 1 million IU/lesion N = 352	Dosing Regimens Percentage (%) of Patients* AIDS-Related Kaposi's Sarcoma 30 million IU/m² TIW/SC N = 74	35 million IU/QD/SC N = 29	Chronic Hepatitis NANB/C 3 million IU TIW N = 159	5 million IU QD N = 101	Chronic Hepatitis B 10 million IU TIW N = 78
Application-Site Disorders	20						
injection site inflammation					7	3	—
other (< 5%)	burning, injection site bleeding, injection site pain, injection site reaction, itching						
Blood Disorders (< 5%)	anemia, granulocytopenia, hemolytic anemia, leukopenia, thrombocytopenia						
Body as a Whole							
facial edema	—	< 1	—	10	1	3	1
weight decrease	< 1	< 1	5	—	< 1	2	5
other (< 5%)	cachexia, dehydration, earache, hypercalcemia, lymphadenopathy, periorbital edema, peripheral edema, thirst, weakness						
Cardiovascular System Disorders (< 5%)	arrhythmia, atrial fibrillation, bradycardia, cardiac failure, cardiomyopathy, extrasystoles, hypertension, hypotension, palpitations, postural hypotension, tachycardia						
Endocrine System Disorders (< 5%)	aggravation of diabetes mellitus, gynecomastia, thyroid disorder, virilism						
Flu-like Symptoms							
fever	68	56	47	55	43	66	86
headache	39	47	36	21	43	61	44
chills	46	45					
myalgia	39	44	34	28	42	59	40
fatigue	61	18	84	48	19	75	69
increased sweating	8	2	4	21	3	1	1
asthenia	7	—	11	—	24	5	15
rigors	—	—	30	14	27	38	42
arthralgia	8	9	—	3	19	19	8
dizziness	12	9	7	24	9	13	10
influenza-like symptoms	37	—	45	79	9	5	—
back pain	19	6	1	3	3	—	—
dry mouth	19	—	22	28	4	6	5
chest pain	< 1	< 1	1	28	1	4	—
malaise	—	14	5	—	3	9	6
pain (unspecified)	18	3	3	3			
other (< 5%)	chest pain substernal, rhinitis, rhinorrhea						
Gastrointestinal System Disorders							
diarrhea	18	2	18	45	13	19	8
anorexia	19	1	38	41	13	43	53
nausea	21	17	28	21	23	50	33
taste alteration	13	< 1	5	7	1	10	—
abdominal pain	< 5	1	5	21	6	5	4
loose stools	—	< 1	—	10	3	2	—
vomiting	6	2	11	14	3	7	10
constipation	< 1	—	—	10	< 1	5	—
gingivitis				14			
dyspepsia	—	2	4	—	3	3	8
other (< 5%)	abdominal distention, dysphagia, eructation, esophagitis, flatulence, gastric ulcer, gastrointestinal hemorrhage, gastrointestinal mucosal discoloration, gingival bleeding, gum hyperplasia, increased appetite, increased saliva, melena, oral leukoplakia, bleeding after stool, rectal hemorrhage, stomatitis, stomatitis ulcerative, taste loss						
Liver and Biliary System Disorders (< 5%)	abnormal hepatic function tests, bilirubinemia, increased transaminases, jaundice, right upper quadrant pain and very rarely hepatic encephalopathy, hepatic failure, and death						
Musculoskeletal System Disorders							
musculoskeletal pain	—	—	—	—	—	9	1
other (< 5%)	arthritis, arthrosis, bone pain, leg cramps, muscle weakness						
Nervous System and Psychiatric Disorders							
depression	6	3	9	28	8	17	6
paresthesia	6	1	3	21	1	6	3
impaired concentration	—	< 1	3	14	4	8	5
amnesia	< 5	—	—	14	—	—	—
confusion	< 5	4	12	10	—	—	—
hypoesthesia	< 5	1	—	10			12
irritability	—	—	—	—	4	16	12
somnolence	< 5	3	3	—	1	14	9
anxiety	5	< 1	1	3	1	2	—
insomnia	—	< 1	3	3	4	11	6

➤ SHOWN IN PRODUCT IDENTIFICATION GUIDE

Adverse Experience	Hairy Cell Leukemia 2 million IU/m² TIW/SC N = 145	Condylomata Acuminata 1 million IU/ lesion N = 352	Dosing Regimens Percentage (%) of Patients* AIDS-Related Kaposi's Sarcoma 30 million IU/m² TIW/SC N = 74	35 million IU/QD/SC N = 29	Chronic Hepatitis NANB/C 3 million IU TIW N = 159	5 million IU QD N = 101	Chronic Hepatitis B 10 million IU TIW N = 78
nervousness	—	1	—	3	—	3	—
decreased libido		< 5			1	5	1
other (< 5%)							

other (< 5%): abnormal coordination, abnormal dreaming, abnormal gait, abnormal thinking, aggravated depression, aggressive reaction agitation, apathy, aphasia, ataxia, CNS dysfunction, coma, convulsions, dysphoria, emotional lability, extrapyramidal disorder, feeling of ebriety, flushing, hearing disorder, hot flashes, hyperesthesia, hyperkinesia, hypertonia, hypokinesia, impaired consciousness, migraine, neuropathy, neurosis, paresis, paroniria, parosmia, personality disorder, polyneuropathy, speech disorder, suicide attempt, syncope, tinnitus, tremor, vertigo

Reproduction System Disorders (< 5%)
amenorrhea, impotence, leukorrhea, menorrhagia, uterine bleeding

Resistance Mechanism Disorders

Adverse Experience	Hairy Cell	Condylomata	AIDS 30m	AIDS 35m	Hep 3m	Hep 5m	Hep B
moniliasis	—	< 1	17	—	—	—	—
herpes simplex	—	1	3	—	—	5	—

other (< 5%): abscess, conjunctivitis, sepsis, stye

Respiratory System Disorders

Adverse Experience	Hairy Cell	Condylomata	AIDS 30m	AIDS 35m	Hep 3m	Hep 5m	Hep B
dyspnea	< 1	1	34		< 1	5	
coughing	< 1		31		< 1	4	
pharyngitis	< 5	1	31		1	7	1
sinusitis			21				
nonproductive coughing			14				
nasal congestion		1	10			4	

other (< 5%): bronchospasm, cyanosis, epistaxis, pleural pain, pneumonia, sneezing, wheezing

Skin and Appendages Disorders

Adverse Experience	Hairy Cell	Condylomata	AIDS 30m	AIDS 35m	Hep 3m	Hep 5m	Hep B
dermatitis	8	—	—	—	—	1	—
alopecia	8	—	12	31	17	26	38
pruritus	11	1	7	—	6	6	4
rash	25	—	9	10	6	8	1
dry skin	9	—	9	10	< 1	3	—

other (< 5%): abnormal hair texture, acne, cyanosis of the hand, cold and clammy skin, dermatitis lichenoides, epidermal necrolysis, erythema furunculosis, increased hair growth, lacrimal gland disorder, melanosis, nail disorders, nonherpetic cold sores, peripheral ischemia, photosensitivity, purpura, skin depigmentation, skin discoloration, urticaria, vitiligo

Urinary System Disorders (< 5%)
increased BUN, hematuria, micturition disorder, micturition frequency, nocturia, polyuria

Vision Disorders (< 5%)
abnormal vision, blurred vision, diplopia, dry eyes, eye pain, photophobia

* Dash (—) indicates not reported

other severe flu-like symptoms which occurred in 1% to 3% of patients. Other severe adverse reactions occurring in more than one patient were alopecia (8%), anorexia (6%), depression (3%), nausea (3%), and vomiting (2%).

To manage side effects, the dose was reduced, or Interferon Alfa-2B therapy was interrupted in 25% to 38% of patients. Five percent of patients discontinued treatment due to adverse experiences. (See related table).

DOSAGE AND ADMINISTRATION

Important: Interferon Alfa-2B, recombinant for injection dosing regimens are different for each of the following indications described in this section of the product information sheet.

Hairy Cell Leukemia: The recommended dosage of Interferon Alfa-2B, recombinant for injection for the treatment of hairy cell leukemia is 2 million IU/m² administered intramuscularly (see *"Warnings"*) or subcutaneously 3 times a week. The 50 million IU strength of the Interferon Alfa-2B powder for injection is not to be used for the treatment of hairy cell leukemia. Higher doses are not recommended. The normalization of one or more hematologic variables usually begins within 2 months of initiation of therapy. Improvement in all three hematologic variables may require 6 months or more of therapy.

This dosage regimen should be maintained unless the disease progresses rapidly, or severe intolerance is manifested. If severe adverse reactions develop, the dosage should be modified (50% reduction) or therapy should be temporarily discontinued until the adverse reactions abate. If persistent or recurrent intolerance develops following adequate dosage adjustment, or disease progresses, Interferon Alfa-2B treatment should be discontinued. The minimum effective Interferon Alfa-2B dose has not been established.

Condylomata Acuminata: The 10 million IU vial of Interferon Alfa-2B powder for injection must be reconstituted with *1 mL of diluent for Interferon Alfa-2B recombinant for injection* (bacteriostatic water for injection). Do *not* reconstitute the 10 million IU vial of Interferon Alfa-2B powder for injection with more than 1 mL of diluent since the injection would be subpotent. Do *not* use the 3 million, 5 million, 18 million multidose, 25 million, or 50 million IU vials of Interferon Alfa-2B powder for injection for the treatment of condylomata acuminata since the resulting reconstituted solution would be either hypertonic or an inappropriate concentration. Do *not* use the 10 million or 25 million IU vials of Interferon

Alfa-2B solution for injection for the intralesional treatment of condylomata acuminata since the concentrations are inappropriate for such use.

Inject 1.0 million IU of Interferon Alfa-2B, recombinant for injection (0.1 mL of reconstituted Interferon Alfa-2B solution) into each lesion three times per week on alternate days, for three weeks. The injection should be administered intralesionally using a Tuberculin or similar syringe and a 25-30 gauge needle. The needle should be directed at the center of the base of the wart and at an angle almost parallel to the plane of the skin (approximating that in the commonly used PPD test). This will deliver the interferon to the dermal core of the lesion, infiltrating the lesion and causing a small wheal. Care should be taken *not* to go beneath the lesion too deeply; subcutaneous injection should be avoided, since this area is below the base of the lesion. Do not inject too superficially since this will result in possible leakage, infiltrating only the keratinized layer, and not the dermal core. As many as 5 lesions can be treated at one time. To reduce side effects, Interferon Alfa-2B injections may be administered in the evening, when possible. Additionally, acetaminophen may be administered at the time of injection to alleviate some of the potential side effects.

The maximum response usually occurs four to eight weeks after initiation of the first treatment course. If results at 12 to 16 weeks after the initial treatment course has concluded are not satisfactory, a second course of treatment using the above dosage schedule may be instituted providing that clinical symptoms and signs, or changes in laboratory parameters (liver function tests, WBC and platelets) do not preclude such a course of action.

Patients with six to ten condylomata may receive a second (sequential) course of treatment at the above dosage schedule, to treat up to five additional condylomata per course of treatment. Patients with greater than ten condylomata may receive additional sequences depending on how large a number of condylomata are present.

AIDS-Related Kaposi's Sarcoma: The recommended Interferon Alfa-2B dosage is 30 million IU/m² three times a week administered subcutaneously or intramuscularly. The 10 million and 25 million IU vials of the Interferon Alfa-2B solution for injection are *not* to be used for the treatment of condylomata acuminata or AIDS-Related Kaposi's Sarcoma.

The selected dosage regimen should be maintained unless the disease progresses rapidly or severe intolerance is manifested. If severe adverse reactions develop, the dosage should be modified (50% reduction) or therapy should be

ABNORMAL LABORATORY TEST VALUES BY INDICATION

Laboratory Tests	Hairy Cell Leukemia 2 million IU/m² TIW/SC N = 145	Condylomata Acuminata 1 million IU/ lesion N = 352	AIDS-Related Kaposi's Sarcoma 30 million IU/m² TIW/SC N = 69-73	AIDS-Related Kaposi's Sarcoma 35 million IU/QD/SC N = 26-28	Chronic Hepatitis NANB/C 3 million IU TIW N = 87-158	Chronic Hepatitis NANB/C 5 million IU QD N = 96-101	Chronic Hepatitis B 10 million TIW N = 75
Hemoglobin	NA	—	1%	15%	15%	32%*	23%
White Blood Cell Count	NA	17%	10%	22%	18%	68%†	34%
Platelet Count	NA	0%	0%	8%	9%	12%‡	5%
Serum Creatinine	0%	—	—	—	2%	3%	0%
Alkaline Phosphatase	4%	—	—	—	3%	8%	4%
Lactate Dehydrogenase	0%	—	—	—	—	—	—
Serum Urea Nitrogen	0%	—	—	—	1%	2%	0%
SGOT	4%	12%	11%	41%	—	—	—
SGPT	13%		10%	15%	—	—	—
Granulocyte Count							
• Total	NA		31%	39%	37%§	75%§	61%
• 1000- <1500/mm³	—	—	—	—	—	30%	32%
• 750 - < 1000/mm³	—	—	—	—	—	24%	18%
• 500 - < 750/mm³	—	—	—	—	—	17%	9%
• < 500/mm³	—	—	—	—	—	4%	2%

NA—Not Applicable—Patients' initial hematologic laboratory test values were abnormal due to their conditions.
* Decrease of ≥ 2 g/dL
† Decrease to < 3000/mm³
‡ Decrease to < 70,000/mm³
§ Neutrophils plus bands

temporarily discontinued until the adverse reactions abate. When patients initiate therapy at 30 million IU/m² TIW, the average dose tolerated at the end of 12 weeks of therapy is 110 million IU/week and 75 million IU/week at the end of 24 weeks of therapy.

When disease stabilization or a response to treatment occurs, treatment should continue until there is no further evidence of tumor or until discontinuation is required by evidence of a severe opportunistic infection or adverse effect.

Chronic Hepatitis Non-A, Non-B/C (NANB/C): The recommended dosage of Interferon Alfa-2B, recombinant for injection for the treatment of chronic hepatitis NANB/C is 3 million IU three times a week (TIW) administered subcutaneously or intramuscularly.

Normalization of serum alanine aminotransferase (ALT) may occur in some patients as early as two weeks after initiation of treatment; however, current experience suggests that patients responding to Interferon Alfa-2B therapy with a reduction in serum ALT should complete 6 months (24 weeks) of treatment. The optimal dose and duration of therapy are currently under investigation.

In clinical trials, 54% (51/95) of the patients at a dose of 3 million IU TIW responded with a reduction in serum ALT after 6 months of Interferon Alfa-2B therapy. Since most of these patients (49/51) responded within the first 16 weeks of treatment, consideration could be given to discontinuing Interferon Alfa-2B therapy in patients who fail to respond after 16 weeks. The effect of dose escalation in these patients is under investigation.

If severe adverse reactions develop during Interferon Alfa-2B treatment, the dose should be modified (50% reduction) or therapy should be temporarily discontinued until the adverse reactions abate. If intolerance persists after dose adjustment, Interferon Alfa-2B therapy should be discontinued.

Patients who relapse following Interferon Alfa-2B therapy may be retreated with the same dosage regimen to which they had previously responded.

Chronic Hepatitis B: The recommended dosage of Interferon Alfa-2B, recombinant for injection for the treatment of chronic hepatitis B is 30 to 35 million IU per week, administered subcutaneously or intramuscularly either as 5 million IU daily (QD), or as 10 million IU three times a week (TIW), for 16 weeks.

If severe adverse reactions or laboratory abnormalities develop during Interferon Alfa-2B therapy, the dose should be modified (50% reduction), or discontinued if appropriate, until the adverse reactions abate. If intolerance persists after dose adjustment, Interferon Alfa-2B therapy should be discontinued.

For patients with decreases in granulocyte or platelet counts, the following guidelines for dose modification were used in the clinical trials:

Interferon Alfa-2B Dose	Granulocyte Count	Platelet Count
Reduce 50%	< 750/mm³	< 50,000/mm³
Interrupt	< 500/m³	< 30,000/m³

Interferon Alfa-2B therapy was resumed at up to 100% of the initial dose when granulocyte and/or platelet counts returned to normal or baseline values.

At the discretion of the physician, the patient may self-administer the medication. (See illustrated *"Patient Information Sheet"* for instructions.)

PREPARATION AND ADMINISTRATION OF INTERFERON ALFA-2B, RECOMBINANT POWDER FOR INJECTION

Reconstitution of Interferon Alfa-2B powder for injection: Inject the amount of diluent for Interferon Alfa-2B, recombinant (bacteriostatic water for injection) stated in the appropriate chart below into the Interferon Alfa-2B vial. Swirl gently to hasten complete dissolution of the powder. The appropriate Interferon Alfa-2B dose should then be withdrawn and injected intramuscularly, subcutaneously, or intralesionally. (See *"Patient Information Sheet"* for detailed instructions.)

After preparation and administration of the Interferon Alfa-2B injection, it is essential to follow the procedure for proper disposal of syringes and needles. (See *"Patient Information Sheet"* for detailed instructions.)

HAIRY CELL LEUKEMIA

Vial Strength	mL Diluent	Final Concentration
3 million IU	1	3 million IU/mL
5 million IU	1	5 million IU/mL
10 million IU	2	5 million IU/mL
18 million IU multidose‡	3.8	6 million IU/mL
25 million IU	5	5 million IU/mL

‡ This is a multidose vial to deliver 18 million IU of Interferon Alfa-2B, recombinant for injection when reconstituted with 3.8 mL of the diluent provided.

CONDYLOMATA ACUMINATA

Vial Strength	mL Diluent	Final Concentration
*10 million IU	1	10 million IU/mL

* Important: For patients with condylomata acuminata, reconstitute the 10 million IU vial with only 1 mL of the diluent provided to reach a final concentration of 10 million IU/mL to be administered intralesionally. (See "Dosage and Administration, Condylomata Acuminata.")

AIDS-RELATED KAPOSI'S SARCOMA

Vial Strength	mL Diluent	Final Concentration
50 million IU	1	50 million IU/mL

IMPORTANT: This vial size is to be used *only* for treatment of patients with AIDS-Related Kaposi's Sarcoma (see *"Dosage and Administration, AIDS-Related Kaposi's Sarcoma"*).

► SHOWN IN PRODUCT IDENTIFICATION GUIDE

CHRONIC HEPATITIS NON-A, NON-B/C

Vial Strength	mL Diluent	Final Concentration
3 million IU	1	3 million IU/mL
18 million IU multidose†	3.8	6 million IU/mL

† *This is a multidose vial to deliver 18 million IU of Interferon Alfa-2B, recombinant for injection when reconstituted with 3.8 mL of the diluent provided..*

CHRONIC HEPATITIS B

Vial Strength	mL Diluent	Final Concentration
5 million IU	1	5 million IU/mL
10 million IU	1	10 million IU/mL

Stability: Interferon Alfa-2B, recombinant powder for injection provided in vials ranging from 3 to 50 million IU per vial, is stable at 45°C (113°F) for up to 7 days. After reconstitution with diluent for Interferon Alfa-2B, recombinant for injection (bacteriostatic water for injection) the solution is stable for 1 month at 2° to 8°C (36° to 46°F). The reconstituted solution is clear and colorless to light yellow.

PREPARATION AND ADMINISTRATION OF INTERFERON ALFA-2B, RECOMBINANT SOLUTION FOR INJECTION
The 10 million and 25 million IU vials of Interferon Alfa-2B solution for injection are supplied in 2 mL vials and 5 mL vials, respectively. The solution is colorless to light yellow. These packages do not require reconstitution prior to administration. The appropriate Interferon Alfa-2B dose should be withdrawn from the vial and injected intramuscularly or subcutaneously. (See *"Patient Information Sheet"* for detailed instructions.) After administration of Interferon Alfa-2B solution for injection, it is essential to follow the procedure for proper disposal of syringes and needles. (See *"Patient Information Sheet"* for detailed instructions.)

HAIRY CELL LEUKEMIA

Vial Strength	mL Solution	Final Concentration
10 million IU	2 mL	5 million IU/mL
25 million IU	5 mL	5 million IU/mL

CHRONIC HEPATITIS NON-A, NON-B/C

Vial Strength	mL Solution	Final Concentration
10 million IU	2 mL	5 million IU/mL
25 million IU	5 mL	5 million IU/mL

CHRONIC HEPATITIS B

Vial Strength	mL Solution	Final Concentration
10 million IU	2 mL	5 million IU/mL
25 million IU	5mL	5 million IU/mL

Important: The 10 million and 25 million IU strengths of Interferon Alfa-2B a solution for injection are *not* to be used for condylomata acuminata or for AIDS-Related Kaposi's Sarcoma. (See *"Dosage and Administration, Condylomata Acuminata,"* *"Dosage and Administration, AIDS-Related Kaposi's Sarcoma"*.)

Parenteral drug products should be inspected visually for particulate matter and discoloration prior to administration, whenever solution and container permit.

Interferon Alfa-2B, recombinant for injection may be administered using either sterilized glass or plastic disposable syringes.

Storage: Store Interferon Alfa-2B, recombinant solution for injection between 2° and 8°C (36° and 46°F).

REFERENCES
1. Davis G, et al. *N Engl J Med.* 1989;321:1501-1506. 2. Cause X, et al. *Gastroenterology.* 1991;101:497-502. 3. Marcellin P, et al. *Hepatology.* 1991;13:393-397. 4. Knodell R, et al. *Hepatology.* 1981;1:431-435. 5. Perrillo R, et al. *N Engl J Med.* 1990;323:295-301. 6. Perez V, et al. *J Hepatol.* 1990; 11PS,113-S117. 7. Perrillo R, et al. *Ann Intern Med.* 1991;115:113-115. 8. Renault P, et al. *Arch Intern Med.* 1987;147:1577-1580. 9. Kauppila A, et al. *Int J Cancer.* 1982;29:291-294.

J CODES
1 million units SC,IM—J9214

HOW SUPPLIED
POWDER FOR INJECTION: 3 MILLION IU

BRAND/MANUFACTURER	NDC	SIZE	AWP
○ **BRAND**			
INTRON-A: Schering	00085-0647-03	1s	$29.87
	00085-0647-04	1s	$29.87
	00085-0647-05	6s	$179.18

POWDER FOR INJECTION: 5 MILLION IU

BRAND/MANUFACTURER	NDC	SIZE	AWP
○ **BRAND**			
INTRON-A: Schering	00085-0120-02	1s	$49.78
	00085-0120-03	1s	$49.78
	00085-0120-04	14s	$696.86

POWDER FOR INJECTION: 10 MILLION U

BRAND/MANUFACTURER	NDC	SIZE	AWP
◇ **BRAND**			
INTRON-A: Schering	00085-0923-01	1s	$99.55

POWDER FOR INJECTION: 10 MILLION IU

BRAND/MANUFACTURER	NDC	SIZE	AWP
◇ **BRAND**			
INTRON-A: Schering	00085-0571-02	1s	$99.55
	00085-0571-06	6s	$597.30

POWDER FOR INJECTION: 18 MILLION IU

BRAND/MANUFACTURER	NDC	SIZE	AWP
◇ **BRAND**			
INTRON-A: Schering	00085-0689-01	1s	$179.18

POWDER FOR INJECTION: 25 MILLION IU

BRAND/MANUFACTURER	NDC	SIZE	AWP
◇ **BRAND**			
INTRON-A: Schering	00085-0285-02	1s	$248.88
	00085-0769-01	1s	$248.88

POWDER FOR INJECTION: 50 MILLION IU

BRAND/MANUFACTURER	NDC	SIZE	AWP
◇ **BRAND**			
INTRON-A: Schering	00085-0539-01	1s	$497.75

Interferon Alfa-N3

DESCRIPTION
Interferon alfa-n3 (Human Leukocyte Derived) is a sterile aqueous formulation of purified, natural, human Interferon alpha proteins for use by injection. Interferon alfa-n3 Injection consists of Interferon alpha proteins comprising approximately 166 amino acids ranging in molecular weights from 16,000 to 27,000 daltons. The specific activity of Interferon alfa-n3 is approximately equal to, or greater than, 2×10^8 IU/mg of protein.

Interferon alfa-n3 is manufactured from pooled units of human leukocytes which have been induced by incomplete infection with an avian virus (Sendai virus) to produce Interferon alfa-n3. The manufacturing process includes immunoaffinity chromatography with a murine monoclonal antibody, acidification (pH 2) for 5 days at 4°C, and gel filtration chromatography.

Since Interferon alfa-n3 is manufactured using source leukocytes, human, donor screening is performed to minimize the risk that the leukocytes could contain infectious agents. In addition, the manufacturing process contains steps which have been shown to inactivate viruses, and there has been no evidence of infection transmission to recipients in clinical trials. The laboratory and clinical data obtained support the conclusion that Interferon alfa-n3 is equivalent to other products derived from human blood or plasma which are free of risk of transmission of infectious agents, such as immunoglobulin and albumin.

The Interferon alfa-n3 manufacturing process was evaluated for quantitative removal or inactivation of model pathogenic viruses. The viruses were deliberately added to the leukocytes in amounts far exceeding those present in contaminated blood, i.e., $\geq 10^9$ infectious units per milliliter. The manufacturing process yielded a cumulative reduction of $\geq 10^{14}$ of infectious HIV-1, i.e., $\geq 10^{6,5}$ removal by acid inactivation and $\geq 10^{7,9}$ removal by the purification process. In the validation studies, there was 10^8 reduction in the titer of hepatitis B virus as determined by HBsAg assay, and a 10^9 reduction in the infectious titer of herpes simplex virus-1 (HSV-1). Cultivation of Interferon alfa-n3 with human indicator cells, i.e., MRC-5 cells, peripheral blood leukocytes in the presence of Cyclosporin A, and fetal cord blood cells, did not detect the presence of infectious viruses.

As part of a validation study, Interferon alfa-n3 was examined for the presence of the following viruses: Sendai virus (SV), HIV-1, HTLV-1, HBV, HSV-1, CMV, and EBV Interferon alfa-n3 contained no detectable quantities of these viruses. In addition other studies, i.e., Polymerase Chain Reaction (PCR) and Dot Blot Hybridization (DBH), have shown no detectable genetic material from these viruses in Interferon alfa-n3. The sensitivity of the PCR was 10 copies for HIV-1 (env gene probe) and 10 copies for HBV (S/P gene probe). The sensitivity of the DBH was 1 pg for EBV, < 10 pg for CMV, < 10 pg for HSV-1, and < 2 pg for SV. Furthermore, sera from 105 patients treated with Interferon alfa-n3 (95 with condylomata acuminata and 10 with cancer) were tested for antibody HIV-1 and HIV p24 antigen. There was no evidence to suggest transmission of HIV-1 by Interferon alfa-n3. Sera from 135 patients with condylomata acuminata treated with Interferon alfa-n3 were tested to determine abnormal SGOT laboratory values. There was no evidence to suggest transmission of hepatitis by Interferon alfa-n3 based on both SGOT results and patient data collected during clinical trials.

Interferon alfa-n3 has been extensively purified using immunoaffinity chromatography with a murine monoclonal antibody, acidification (pH 2) for 5 days at 4°C, and gel filtration chromatography. Interferon alfa-n3 has been subjected to the acid treatment for five days during its manufacture in order to reduce the risk of viral transmission. Subsequent analyses of the Interferon alfa-n3 Purified Drug

◆ RATED THERAPEUTICALLY EQUIVALENT; ◇ THERAPEUTIC EQUIVALENCE UNCONFIRMED; ○ UNRATED

Concentrate confirm the absence of detectable infectious or non-infectious viral particles.

The leukocyte nutrient medium contains the antibiotic neomycin sulfate at a concentration of 35 mg/L; however, neomycin sulfate is not detectable in the final product, i.e., < 0.64 µg/ml.

Murine immunoglobulin (IgG) is detected in the Interferon alfa-n3 Purified Drug Concentrate at levels below 0.15% of the Interferon alfa-n3 protein. This equates to levels less than 8 ng of murine IgG per million IU Interferon alfa-n3 (range of 0.9 to 5.6 ng typically found).

Interferon alfa-n3 is available in an injectable solution containing 5 million IU Interferon alfa-n3 per vial for intralesional injection. The solution is clear and colorless. Each milliliter (ml) contains five million IU of Interferon alfa-n3 in phosphate buffered saline (8.0 mg sodium chloride, 1.74 mg sodium phosphate dibasic, 0.20 mg potassium phosphate monobasic, and 0.20 mg potassium chloride) containing 3.3 mg phenol as a preservative and 1 mg Albumin (Human) as a stabilizer.

CLINICAL PHARMACOLOGY

General: Interferons are naturally occurring proteins with both antiviral and antiproliferative properties. They are produced and secreted in response to viral infections and to a variety of other synthetic and biological inducers. Three major families of interferons have been identified; alpha, beta, and gamma. The interferon alpha family contains at least 15 different molecular species. Their molecular weights range from 16,000 to 27,000 daltons.

Interferons bind to specific membrane receptors on cell surfaces. Interferon alfa-n3 has been shown to bind to the same receptors as Interferon alfa-2b. The receptors have a high degree of selectivity for the binding of human but not mouse Interferon. This correlates with the high species specificity found in laboratory studies.

Binding of Interferon to membrane receptors initiates a series of events including induction of protein synthesis. These actions are followed by a variety of cellular responses, including inhibition of virus replication and suppression of cell proliferation Immunomodulation, including enhancement of phagocytosis by macrophages, augmentation of the cytotoxicity of lymphocytes and enhancement of human leukocyte antigen expression occurs in response to exposure to Interferons. One or more of these activities may contribute to the therapeutic effect of Interferon.

Pharmacokinetics: In a study of intralesional use of Interferon alfa-n3 (Human Leukocyte Derived) for the treatment of condylomata acuminata, plasma concentrations of Interferon were below the detection limit of the assay, i.e., ≤ 3 IU/ml. Minor systemic effects (e.g., myalgias, fever, and headaches) were noted, indicating that some of the injected Interferon entered the systemic circulation (see *"Adverse Reactions"*).

Condylomata Acuminata: Condylomata acuminata (venereal or genital warts) are associated with infections of human papilloma virus (HPV), especially HPV type-6 and possibly type-11. Given the antiviral and antiproliferative activities of Interferons and the viral etiology of condylomata, a placebo-controlled clinical trial was conducted to evaluate the safety and efficacy of intralesional injection of Interferon alfa-n3 in the treatment of condylomata acuminata.

In a multicenter randomized double-blind, placebo-controlled clinical trial, intralesional administration of Interferon alfa-n3 was an effective treatment for condylomata acuminata.[1-4] One hundred fifty-six patients were evaluable for efficacy (81 Interferon alfa-n3 patients and 75 placebo patients). Patients had a mean of five warts (range was 2-14) and all warts were treated. Patients were injected intralesionally with a mean of 225,000 IU of Interferon alfa-n3 per wart 2 times a week for up to 8 weeks. Overall, 80% (65/81) of patients treated with Interferon alfa-n3 had a complete or partial resolution of warts compared with 44% (33/75) of placebo-treated patients (p < 0.001). Interferon alfa-n3 was significantly more effective than placebo in producing a complete resolution of warts (p < 0.001), as shown by the following table: (See related table).

Of the patients who had a complete resolution of warts, approximately half (21/44) the patients had complete resolution of warts by the end of treatment, and half (23/44) had complete resolution of warts during the three months after the cessation of treatment. Patients with complete resolution of warts were followed for a median of 48 weeks. Overall, 76% (31/41) of Interferon alfa-n3 treated patients who achieved complete resolution of warts remained clear of all treated lesions during follow-up, while 79% (11/14) of the placebo-treated patients remained clear of all treated lesions during follow-up. A total of 762 evaluable warts were injected in this trial. Of the 407 Interferon alfa-n3-treated warts, 73% (297/407) completely resolved, as compared to 35% (125/355) of the placebo-treated warts (p < 0.0001). Interferon alfa-n3 was effective in treating lesions of all sizes, and there was no difference in resolution for perianal, penile, or vulvar lesions.

There was no difference in resolution for patients who had received prior treatment of their warts and for those who had not. Among patients with recalcitrant warts (i.e., warts that were refractory to previous treatment or recurring), 82% (58/71) of the evaluable patients had complete or partial resolution of warts due to intralesional administration of Interferon alfa-n3 as compared to 43% (29/67) of placebo patients (p < 0.001). Fifty-four percent (38/71) of the evaluable Interferon alfa-n3 patients had complete resolution of warts as compared to 18% (12/67) of placebo patients (p < 0.001). Patients with primary occurrence of genital warts (i.e., no prior treatment of warts) had a similar resolution rate compared to the patients with recalcitrant warts: 70% (7/10) had complete or partial resolution of warts due to Interferon alfa-n3 treatment and 60% (6/10) had complete resolution of warts, as compared to 50% (4/8) of placebo recipients who had complete or partial resolution of warts and 38% (3/8) who had complete resolution. Overall, 83% (5/6) of Interferon alfa-n3-treated patients with primary occurrence, who achieved complete resolution of warts, remained clear of all treated lesions during a median follow-up of 52 weeks. Because the number of patients with primary occurrence of warts was small (10 Interferon alfa-n3 recipients and 8 placebo recipients), the difference between Interferon alfa-n3 and placebo treatment was not statistically significant. However, when the resolution of primary warts was examined, 75% (33/44) of the Interferon alfa-n3-treated primary warts resolved completely as compared to 39% (11/28) of the placebo-treated primary warts (p = 0.003).

In an open clinical trial using a once a week treatment schedule for up to 16 weeks, 28 patients were evaluable for efficacy. Eighty-nine percent (25/28) of patients had a complete or partial resolution of warts following treatment with Interferon alfa-n3. The condylomata acuminata resolved completely in 46% (13/28) of the patients. Of the 154 warts treated, 77% (118/154) resolved completely.

After injections of Interferon alfa-n3 side effects were minor and transient. After 4 weeks of treatment, the frequency of adverse reactions was similar in Interferon alfa-n3 and placebo treatment groups. The most frequent side effects were myalgias, fever, and headache (see *"Adverse Reactions"*).

ANTIGENICITY

1. Interferon alfa-n3

One hundred and five (105) patients treated with Interferon alfa-n3 during clinical trials were tested for the presence of anti-Interferon antibodies using three different antibody assays: Immunoradiometric Assay (IRMA), Enzyme Linked Immunosorbent Assay (ELISA), and neutralization by the Cytopathic Effect Assay (CPE). To date, no antibodies to Interferon alfa-n3 have been detected in any of the patients.

2. Mouse Proteins

No hypersensitivity reactions to the components in Interferon alfa-n3 have been observed. Interferon alfa-n3 uses a murine monoclonal antibody in one of the purification procedures. A possibility exists that patients treated with Interferon alfa-n3 may develop hypersensitivity to the mouse proteins. However, none of the patients receiving Interferon alfa-n3 during clinical trials developed antibodies or hypersensitivity to mouse proteins (see *"Contraindications"*).

3. Egg Protein

The initial stage in the manufacture of Interferon alfa-n3 uses Sendai virus which was grown in chicken eggs as the specific Interferon alfa-n3 inducer. Although no egg protein (ovalbumin) has been detected in the initial stage of Interferon manufacture using an ELISA (sensitivity of 16 ng/ml), a possibility exists that patients treated with Interferon alfa-n3 may develop hypersensitivity to egg protein (see *"Contraindications"*).

INDICATIONS AND USAGE

Interferon alfa-n3 is indicated for the intralesional treatment of refractory or recurring external condylomata acuminata in patients 18 years of age or older (see *"Dosage and Administration"*).

The physician should select patients for treatment with Interferon alfa-n3 after consideration of a number of factors: the locations and sizes of the lesions, past treatment and response thereto, and the patient's ability to comply with the treatment regimen. Interferon alfa-n3 is particularly useful for patients who have not responded satisfactorily to other treatment modalities, e.g., podophyllin resin, surgery, laser or cryotherapy.

There have been no studies with this product in adolescents. This product is not recommended for use in patients less than 18 years of age.

UNLABELED USES

Interferon alfa-n3 is used alone or as an adjunct in the treatment of breast cancer and chickenpox.

CONTRAINDICATIONS

Interferon alfa-n3 is contraindicated in patients with known hypersensitivity to human Interferon alpha or any component of the product. The product also is

Table 1
DEGREE OF RESOLUTION AS MEASURED BY TOTAL WART VOLUME PER PATIENT

	Percent of Patients with:			
	Complete Resolution	Partial Resolution (≥ 50% resolution)	Minor Resolution (< 50% resolution)	Progression/ No change
Interferon alfa-n3 (n = 81)	54%	26%	15%	5%
Placebo (n = 75)	20%	24%	13%	43%

contraindicated in patients who have anaphylactic sensitivity to mouse immuno-globulin (IgG), egg protein or neomycin.

WARNINGS

Because of the fever and other "flu-like" symptoms associated with Interferon alfa-n3 (see "*Adverse Reactions*"), it should be used cautiously in patients with debilitating medical conditions such as cardiovascular disease (e.g., unstable angina and uncontrolled congestive heart failure), severe pulmonary disease (e.g., chronic obstructive pulmonary disease), or diabetes mellitus with ketoacidosis. Interferon alfa-n3 should be used cautiously in patients with coagulation disorders (e.g., thrombophlebitis, pulmonary embolism and hemophilia), severe myelosup-pression, or seizure disorders. Acute, serious hypersensitivity reactions (e.g., urticaria, angioedema, bronchoconstriction, and anaphylaxis) have not been observed in patients receiving Interferon alfa-n3. However, if such reactions develop, drug administration should be discontinued immediately and appropri-ate medical therapy should be instituted.

PRECAUTIONS

General: Patients being treated with Interferon alfa-n3 should be informed of the benefits and risks associated with the treatment. Because the manufacturing process, strength, and type of Interferon (e.g., natural, human leukocyte Interferon versus single-subspecies recombinant Interferon) may vary for different Interferon formulations, changing brands may require a change in dosage. Therefore, physicians are cautioned not to change from one Interferon product to another without considering these factors.

Information for Patients: Patients should be informed of the early signs of hypersensitivity reactions including hives, generalized urticaria, tightness of the chest, wheezing, hypotension, and anaphylaxis, and should be advised to contact their physician if these symptoms occur.

Patients being treated with Interferon alfa-n3 should be informed of benefits and risks associated with treatment. Patients should be cautioned not to change brands of Interferon without medical consultation, as a change in dosage may occur.

Carcinogenesis, Mutagenesis, Impairment of Fertility: Studies with Interferon alfa-n3 have not been performed to determine carcinogenicity, mutagenicity, or the effect on fertility. In studies with adult females, Interferon alpha has been shown to affect the menstrual cycle and decrease serum estradiol and progesterone levels[5].

Interferon alfa-n3 should be used with caution in fertile men. Fertile women should be cautioned to use effective contraception while being treated with Interferon alfa-n3. Changes in the menstrual cycle and abortions have been reported to occur in non-human primates given extremely high doses of recombinant Interferon alfa-n3. In these studies, Macaca mulatta (rhesus monkeys) were given Interferon daily by intramuscular injection. When given at daily intramuscular doses 326 times the average intralesional dose of Interferon alfa-n3 (120 times the maximum recommended dose), this recombinant Interfer-on formulation produced menstrual cycle changes in the monkeys.

In human clinical trials with Interferon alfa-n3 menstrual cycle data were reported by 51 patients (36 Interferon alfa-n3 and 15 placebo). There was no significant difference between Interferon alfa-n3 and placebo treatment groups with regard to menstrual cycle changes.

Pregnancy—Pregnancy Category C: Animal reproduction studies have not been conducted with Interferon alfa-n3. It is also not known whether Interferon alfa-n3 can cause fetal harm when administered to a pregnant woman or can affect reproductive capacity. Interferon alfa-n3 should be given to a pregnant woman only if clearly needed. Changes in the menstrual cycle and abortions have been reported to occur in non-human primates given extremely high doses of recombinant Interferon alpha. In these studies, Macaca mulatta (rhesus monkeys) were given Interferon alfa-n3 daily by intramuscular injection. Abortifacient effects were noted when the recombinant Interferon alpha was given daily during early to mid-gestation at intramuscular doses of 978 times the average intralesion-al dose of Interferon alfa-n3 (360 times the maximum recommended dose).

Nursing Mothers: It is not known whether Interferon alfa-n3 is excreted in human milk. Studies in mice have shown that mouse Interferons are excreted in milk[7]. Because many drugs are excreted in human milk and because of the potential for serious adverse reactions in nursing infants, a decision should be made whether to discontinue nursing or to not initiate drug treatment, taking into account the importance of the drug to the mother and the potential risk to the infant.

Pediatric Use: Safety and effectiveness have not been established in patients below the age of 18 years.

ADVERSE REACTIONS

Adverse reactions were evaluated in 202 patients with condylomata acuminata receiving Interferon alfa-n3 by intralesional administration and in 31 patients with cancer receiving Interferon alfa-n3 by systemic administration. In the double-blind efficacy trial for the treatment of condylomata acuminata, 104 patients were treated with doses of Interferon alfa-n3 of 0.05 million to 2.5 million IU per treatment session (average dose = 0.92 million IU per treatment session) by intralesional injection. In open trials, an additional 98 patients received a dose range of 0.05 to 4.6 million IU of Interferon alfa-n3 per treatment session (average dose = 1.12 million IU per treatment session). Patients with cancer were given doses of Interferon alfa-n3 of 3 million, 9 million, or 15 million IU per day for ten days by intramuscular injection.

Adverse Reactions in Patients with Condylomata Acuminata: A total of 104 patients with condylomata acuminata was treated with Interferon alfa-n3 during the double-blind clinical trial. Adverse reactions were reported to be likely, unlikely, or not known to be related to Interferon alfa-n3. Adverse reactions consisted primarily of "flu-like" symptoms (myalgias, fever, and/or headache) which were in most cases mild or moderate, and transient, and did not interfere with treatment.

The "flu-like" adverse reactions, consisting of fever myalgias, and/or headache, occurred primarily after the first treatment session and were reported by 30% of the patients. The frequency of "flu-like" adverse reactions abated with repeated dosing of Interferon alfa-n3 so that the incidences due to Interferon alfa-n3 and placebo were similar after three to four weeks of treatment (after six to eight treatment sessions). "Flu-like" symptoms were relieved by administration of acetaminophen.

Adverse reactions were reported at least once during the course of treatment in the following percentages of patients in each treatment group.

Table 2
PERCENT OF PATIENTS WITH ADVERSE REACTIONS

Adverse Reactions	Interferon alfa-n3 (n = 104)	Placebo (n = 85)
Autonomic Nervous System		
Sweating	2%	1%
Vasovagal Reaction	2%	0%
Body as a Whole		
Fever	40%	19%
Chills	14%	2%
Fatigue	14%	6%
Malaise	9%	9%
Skin		
Generalized Pruritus	2%	0%
Central & Peripheral Nervous System		
Dizziness	9%	4%
Insomnia	2%	1%
Gastrointestinal System		
Nausea	4%	7%
Vomiting	3%	0%
Dyspepsia/Heartburn	3%	1%
Diarrhea	2%	2%
Musculoskeletal System		
Arthralgia	5%	1%
Back Pain	4%	1%
Myalgias	45%	15%
Headache	31%	15%
Psychiatric Disorders		
Depression	2%	1%
Nasopharyngeal		
Nose/sinus drainage	2%	2%

Most of the systemic adverse reactions were mild or moderate. Severe systemic adverse reactions were reported by 18% of Interferon alfa-n3- treated patients and 13% of placebo-treated patients (not a statistically significant difference). Most of the severe systemic adverse reactions reported were "flu-like". Other severe systemic adverse reactions included back pain, insomnia, and sensitivity to allergens. Those adverse reactions which were reported by 1% of patients treated with Interferon alfa-n3 in the double-blind trial include left groin lymph node swelling, tongue hyperaesthesia, thirst, tingling of legs/feet, hot sensation on bottom of feet, strange taste in mouth, increased salivation, heat intolerance, visual disturbances, pharyngitis, sensitivity to allergens, muscle cramps, nose bleed, throat tightness, and papular rash on neck. Additional adverse reactions which were reported by 1% of patients treated with placebo include: pharyngitis, oral pain, penile discharge, cold, knuckle stiffness, herpes outbreak, cough, disorientation, and weight/appetite loss.

Additional adverse reactions which occurred only in open clinical trials of intralesional use of Interferon alfa-n3 for treatment of condylomata acuminata were herpes labialis, hot flashes, nervousness, decrease in concentration, dysuria, photosensitivity, and swollen lymph nodes. These reactions occurred in 1% of the patients. One patient with a history of epilepsy, who was not taking anticonvul-sant medication, had a grand mal seizure while being treated with Interferon alfa-n3; this seizure was judged to be unrelated to Interferon alfa-n3 administration.

Application Site Disorders: The frequency of application site disorders (such as itching and pain) for patients treated with Interferon alfa-n3 was significantly less than that reported with placebo (12% versus 26%). No severe application site disorders were reported by patients treated with Interferon alfa-n3, while 7% of placebo-treated patients reported severe disorders.

Laboratory Test Values: Abnormalities were seen with statistically equivalent frequencies in both the Interferon alfa-n3 and placebo groups. None of the laboratory abnormalities were considered clinically significant. The abnormalities in the Interferon alfa-n3-treated patients consisted primarily of decreased WBC (11%). Decreases also occurred in 4% of the placebo patients (not a statistically significant difference). The abnormalities in Interferon alfa-n3-treated patients involved increases of only one WHO grade.

◆ RATED THERAPEUTICALLY EQUIVALENT; ◇ THERAPEUTIC EQUIVALENCE UNCONFIRMED; ○ UNRATED

Adverse Reactions in Patients with Cancer: Thirty-one patients with cancer were treated with a maximum of ten intramuscular injections of Interferon alfa-n3 in doses of 3 million IU, 9 million IU, or 15 million IU per treatment session. The occurrence of adverse reactions was judged to be unrelated to the dose of Interferon alfa-n3. The following adverse reactions were reported at least once (the percentage of patients experiencing the reaction is indicated in parentheses): chills (87%), fever (81%), anorexia (68%), malaise (65%), nausea (48%), vomiting (29%), myalgias (16%), arthralgia (10%), chest pains (10%), soreness at injection site (10%), sleepiness (10%), headache (10%), diarrhea (6%), fatigue (6%), low blood pressure (6%), sore mouth/stomatitis (6%), and blurred vision (6%). Those adverse reactions which were each reported by only one patient treated with Interferon alfa-n3 include: stiff shoulders, face flushed, edema, dry mouth, mucositis, coughing, numbness, numbness in hands, numbness in fingers, pain on ocular rotation, shakes/shivers, ringing in ears, cramps, constipation, muscle soreness, confusion, light-headedness, depression, upset stomach, and sweating. The following adverse reactions were reported as severe by at least one patient (the percentage of patients experiencing the reaction is indicated in parentheses): fever (55%), malaise (54%), anorexia (45%), chills (45%), nausea (16%), myalgias (13%), vomiting (10%), fatigue (6%), low blood pressure (6%), chest pains (6%), sore mouth/stomatitis (6%), headache (3%), diarrhea (3%), sleepiness (3%), arthralgia (3%), blurred vision (3%), stiff shoulders (3%), numbness (3%), pain on ocular rotation (3%), muscle soreness (3%), and sweating (3%).

The number and percentage of patients with cancer who experienced a significant abnormal laboratory test value (values that changed from WHO Grades 0, 1, or 2 at baseline to WHO Grades 3 or 4 during or after treatment) at least once during the trials are shown in the following table:

Table 3
ABNORMAL LABORATORY TEST VALUES

	Cancer (n = 31)
Hemoglobin Level	2 (7%)
White Blood Cell Count	1 (3%)
Platelet Count	1 (3%)
GGT	1 (6%)
SGOT	1 (3%)
Alkaline Phosphatase	2 (8%)
Total Bilirubin	1 (4%)

DOSAGE AND ADMINISTRATION

The recommended dose of Interferon alfa-n3 for the treatment of condylomata acuminata is 0.05 ml (250,000 IU) per wart. Interferon alfa-n3 should be administered twice weekly for up to 8 weeks. The maximum recommended dose per treatment session is 0.5 ml (2.5 million IU). Interferon alfa-n3 should be injected into the base of each wart, preferably using a 30 gauge needle. For large warts, Interferon alfa-n3 may be injected at several points around the periphery of the wart, using a total dose of 0.05 ml per wart. The minimum effective dose of Interferon alfa-n3 for the treatment of condylomata acuminata has not been established. Moderate to severe adverse experiences may require modification of the dosage regimen or, in some cases, termination of therapy with Interferon alfa-n3.

Genital warts usually begin to disappear after several weeks of treatment with Interferon alfa-n3. Treatment should continue for a maximum of 8 weeks. In clinical trials with Interferon alfa-n3 many patients who had partial resolution of warts during treatment experienced further resolution of their warts after cessation of treatment. Of the patients who had complete resolution of warts due to treatment, half the patients had complete resolution of warts by the end of the treatment and half had complete resolution of warts during the 3 months after cessation of treatment. Thus, it is recommended that no further therapy (Interferon alfa-n3 or conventional therapy) be administered for 3 months after the initial 8-week course of treatment unless the warts enlarge or new warts appear. Studies to determine the safety and efficacy of a second course of treatment with Interferon alfa-n3 have not been conducted.

Parenteral drug products should be inspected visually for particulate matter and discoloration prior to administration, whenever solution and container permit.

Interferon alfa-n3 should be stored at 2° to 8°C (36° to 46°F). Do not freeze. Do not shake.

REFERENCES
1. Friedman-Kien, AE, Eron, LJ, Conant, M. et al., *JAMA,* 259:533-538, 1988. 2. Kirby, P. (editorial comment), *JAMA,* 259:570-572, 1988. 3. Friedman-Kien, AE, Plasse, TF, et al., *Papilloma Viruses: Molecular and Clinical Aspects* [Howley, PM, Broker, TR (eds)], New York, Alan R. Liss, Inc., 1986, pp. 217-233. 4. Geffen, JR, Klein, RJ, Friedman-Kien, AE, *J Infect. Dis.,* 150:612-615, 1984. 5. Kauppila, A, et al., *Int. J. Cancer,* 29:291-294, 1982. 6. Trown, PW, et al., *Cancer, 57 (Suppl):* 1648-1656, 1986. 7. Schafer, TW, et al., *Science,* 176:1326-1327, 1972.

J CODES
250,000 IU IM—J9215

HOW SUPPLIED
INJECTION: 5 MILLION IU

BRAND/MANUFACTURER	NDC	SIZE	AWP
○ **BRAND**			
ALFERON N: Purdue Frederick	00034-1019-01	1 ml	$132.35

Interferon Beta-1B

DESCRIPTION
Interferon Beta-1B is a purified, sterile, lyophilized protein product produced by recombinant DNA techniques and formulated for use by injection. Interferon Beta-1B is manufactured by bacterial fermentation of a strain of *Escherichia coli* that bears a genetically engineered plasmid containing the gene for human Interferon Beta$_{ser17}$. The native gene was obtained from human fibroblasts and altered in a way that substitutes serine for the cysteine residue found at position 17. Interferon Beta-1B is a highly purified protein that has 165 amino acids and an approximate molecular weight of 18,500 daltons. It does not include the carbohydrate side chains found in the natural material.

The specific activity of Interferon Beta-1B is approximately 32 million international units (IU)/mg Interferon Beta-1B. Each vial contains 0.3 mg (9.6 million IU) of Interferon Beta-1B. The unit measurement is derived by comparing the antiviral activity of the product to the World Health Organization (WHO) reference standard of recombinant human Interferon Beta. Dextrose and Albumin Human, USP (15 mg each/vial) are added as stabilizers. Prior to 1993, a different analytical standard was used to determine potency. It assigned 54 million IU to 0.3 mg Interferon Beta-1B.

Lyophilized Interferon Beta-1B is a sterile, white to off-white powder intended for subcutaneous injection after reconstitution with the diluent supplied (sodium chloride, 0.54% solution).

CLINICAL PHARMACOLOGY
General: Interferons are a family of naturally occurring proteins, which have molecular weights ranging from 15,000 to 21,000 daltons. Three major classes of interferons have been identified: alfa, beta, and gamma. Interferon Beta-1B, interferon alfa, and interferon gamma have overlapping yet distinct biologic activities.[1-5] The activities of Interferon Beta-1B are species-restricted and, therefore, the most pertinent pharmacologic information on Interferon Beta-1B is derived from studies of human cells in culture and in humans.

Biologic Activities: Interferon Beta-1B has been shown to possess both antiviral and immunoregulatory activities. The mechanisms by which Interferon Beta-1B exerts its actions in multiple sclerosis (MS) are not clearly understood. However, it is known that the biologic response-modifying properties of Interferon Beta-1B are mediated through its interactions with specific cell receptors found on the surface of human cells. The binding of Interferon Beta-1B to these receptors induces the expression of a number of interferon-induced gene products (e.g., 2',5'-oligoadenylate synthetase, protein kinase, and indoleamine 2,3-dioxygenase) that are believed to be the mediators of the biological actions of Interferon Beta-1B.[1,3,6-10] A number of these Interferon-induced products have been readily reassured in the serum and cellular fractions of blood collected from patients treated with Interferon Beta-1B.[11,12]

Pharmacokinetics: Because serum concentrations of Interferon Beta-1B are low or not detectable following subcutaneous administration of 0.25 mg (8 million IU) or less of Interferon Beta-1B, pharmacokinetic information in patients with MS receiving the recommended dose of Interferon Beta-1B is not available. Following single and multiple daily subcutaneous administrations of 0.5 mg (16 million IU) Interferon Beta-1B to healthy volunteers (N = 12), serum Interferon Beta-1B concentrations were generally below 100 IU/mL. Peak serum Interferon Beta-1B concentrations occurred between 1 to 8 hours, with a mean peak serum interferon concentration of 40 IU/mL. Bioavailability, based on a total dose of 0.5 mg (16 million IU) Interferon Beta-1B given as two subcutaneous injections at different sites, was approximately 50%.

After intravenous administration of Interferon Beta-1B (0.006 mg [0.2 million IU] to 2.0 mg [64 million IU]), similar pharmacokinetic profiles were obtained from healthy volunteers (N = 12) and from patients with diseases other than MS (N = 142). In patients receiving single intravenous doses up to 2.0 mg (64 million IU), increases in serum concentrations were dose proportional.

Mean serum clearance values ranged from 9.4 mL/min.kg^{-1} to 28.9 mL/min.kg^{-1} and were independent of dose. Mean terminal elimination half-life values ranged from 8.0 minutes to 4.3 hours and mean steady-state volume of distribution values ranged from 0.25 L/kg to 2.88 L/kg. Three-times-a-week intravenous dosing for 2 weeks resulted in no accumulation of Interferon Beta-1B in the serum of patients. Pharmacokinetic parameters after single and multiple intravenous doses of Interferon Beta-1B were comparable.

Clinical Trials: The effectiveness of Interferon Beta-1B in relapsing-remitting MS was evaluated in a double-blind, multiclinic (11 sites: 4 Canadian and 7 United States), randomized, parallel, placebo-controlled clinical investigation of 2 years duration. The study enrolled MS patients, aged 18 to 50, who were ambulatory (Kurtzke expanded disability status scale [EDSS] of ≤ 5.5), exhibited a relapsing-remitting clinical course, met Poser's criteria[13] for clinically definite and/or laboratory supported definite MS and had experienced at least two exacerbations over 2 years preceding the trial without exacerbation in the preceding month. Patients who had received prior immunosuppressant therapy were excluded. An exacerbation was defined, per protocol, as the appearance of a new clinical sign/symptom or the clinical worsening of a previous sign/symptom (one that had been stable for at least 30 days) that persisted for a minimum of 24 hours. Patients selected for study were randomized to treatment with either placebo (N = 123), 0.05 mg (1.6 million IU) of Interferon Beta-1B (N = 125), or 0.25 mg (8 million IU) of Interferon Beta-1B (N = 124) self-administered subcutaneously every other day. Outcome based on the 372 randomized patients was evaluated after 2 years.

interferons are thought to act through the same receptor. Patients who experience these symptoms should be closely monitored and cessation of therapy considered.

Additional common adverse clinical and laboratory events associated with the use of Interferon Beta-1B are listed in the following paragraphs. These events occurred at an incidence of 5% or more in the 124 MS patients treated with 0.25 mg (8 million IU) of Interferon Beta-1B every other day for periods of up to 3 years in the controlled trial, and at an incidence that was at least twice that observed in the 123 placebo patients. Common adverse clinical and laboratory events associated with the use of Interferon Beta-1B were: injection site reaction (85%), injection site necrosis (5%), flu-like symptoms (53%), palpitation (8%), hypertension (7%), tachycardia (6%), peripheral vascular disorders (5%), gastrointestinal disorders (6%), absolute neutrophil count < 1500/mm³ (18%), WBC < 3000/mm³ (16%), SGPT > 5 times baseline value (19%), total bilirubin > 2.5 times baseline value (6%), somnolence (6%), dyspnea (8%), laryngitis (6%), menstrual disorder (17%), cystitis (8%), breast pain (7%), pelvic pain (6%), and menorrhagia (6%).

A total of 277 MS patients have been treated with Interferon Beta-1B in doses ranging from 0.025 mg (0.8 million IU) to 0.5 mg (16 million IU). During the first 3 years of treatment, withdrawals due to clinical adverse events or laboratory abnormalities not mentioned above included: fatigue (2%, 6 patients), cardiac arrhythmia (< 1%, 1 patient), allergic urticarial skin reaction to injections (< 1%, 1 patient), headache (< 1%, 1 patient), unspecified adverse events (< 1%, 1 patient) and "felt sick" (< 1%, 1 patient).

The table that follows enumerates adverse events and laboratory abnormalities that occurred at an incidence of 2% or more among the 124 MS patients treated with 0.25 mg (8 million IU) Interferon Beta-1B every other day for periods of up to 3 years in the controlled trial and at an incidence that was at least 2% more than that observed in the 123 placebo patients. Reported adverse events have been reclassified using the standard COSTART glossary to reduce the total number of terms employed in the table. In the following table, terms so general as to be uninformative, and those events where a drug cause was remote have been excluded.

Table 2

ADVERSE REACTIONS AND LABORATORY ABNORMALITIES

Adverse Reaction	Placebo N = 123	0.25 mg (8 mIU) N = 124
Body as a Whole		
Injection site reaction*	37%	85%
Headache	77%	84%
Fever*	41%	59%
Flu-like symptom complex*	56%	76%
Pain	48%	52%
Asthenia*	35%	49%
Chills*	19%	46%
Abdominal pain	24%	32%
Malaise*	3%	15%
Generalized edema	6%	8%
Pelvic pain	3%	6%
Injection site necrosis*	0%	5%
Cyst	2%	4%
Necrosis	0%	2%
Suicide attempt	0%	2%
Cardiovascular System		
Migraine	7%	12%
Palpitation*	2%	8%
Hypertension	2%	7%
Tachycardia	3%	6%
Peripheral vascular disorder	2%	5%
Hemorrhage	1%	3%
Digestive System		
Diarrhea	29%	35%
Constipation	18%	24%
Vomiting	19%	21%
Gastrointestinal disorder	3%	6%
Endocrine System		
Goiter	0%	2%
Hemic and Lymphatic System		
Lymphocytes less than 1500/mm²	67%	82%
ANC < 1500/mm³*	6%	18%
WBC < 3000/mm³*	5%	16%
Lymphadenopathy	11%	14%
Metabolic and Nutritional Disorders		
SGPT < 5 times baseline*	6%	19%
Glucose > 55 mg/dL	13%	15%
Total bilirubin ≥ 2.5 times baseline	2%	6%
Urine protein < 1 +	3%	5%
SGOT > 5 times baseline*	0%	4%
Weight gain	0%	4%
Weight loss	2%	4%

Adverse Reaction	Placebo N = 123	0.25 mg (8 mIU) N = 124
Musculoskeletal System		
Myalgie*	28%	44%
Myasthenia	10%	13%
Nervous System		
Dizziness	28%	35%
Hypertonia	24%	26%
Anxiety	13%	15%
Nervousness	5%	8%
Somnolence	3%	6%
Confusion	2%	4%
Speech Disorder	0%	2%
Hyperkinesia	0%	2%
Amnesia	20%	2%
Respiratory System		
Sinusitis	26%	36%
Dyspnea*	2%	6%
Laryngitis	2%	6%
Skin and Appendages		
Sweating*	11%	23%
Alopecia	2%	4%
Special Senses		
Conjunctivitis	10%	12%
Abnormal vision	4%	7%
Urogenital System		
Dysmenorrhea	11%	18%
Menstrual disorder*	8%	17%
Metrorrhagia	8%	15%
Cystitis	4%	8%
Breast pain	3%	7%
Menorrhagia	3%	6%
Urinary Urgency	2%	4%
Fibrocystic breast	1%	3%
Breast neoplasm	0%	2%

* - *Significantly associated with Interferon Beta-1B treatment*

It should be noted that the figures cited in the table cannot be used to predict the incidence of side effects in the course of usual medical practice where patient characteristics and other factors differ from those that prevailed in the clinical trials. The cited figures do provide the prescribing physician with some basis for estimating the relative contribution of drug and nondrug factors to the side effect incidence rate in the population studied.

Other events observed during parmarketing evaluation of various doses of Interferon Beta-1B in 1440 patients are listed in the paragraph that follows. Because most of the events were observed in open and uncontrolled studies, the role of Interferon Beta-1B in their causation cannot be reliably determined.

Body as a Whole: abscess, adenoma, anaphylactoic reaction, ascites, cellulitis, hernia, hydrocephalus, hypothermia, infection, peritonitis, photosensitivity, sarcoma, sepsis, and shock;

Cardiovascular System: angina pectoris, arrhythmia, atrial fibrillation, cardiomegaly, cardiac arrest, cerebral, hemorrhage, cerebral ischemia, endocarditis, heart failure, hypotension, myocardial infarct, pericardial effusion, postural hypotension, pulmonalry embolus, spider angioma, subarachnoid hemorrhage, syncope, thrombophlebitis, thrombosis, varicose vein, vasospasm, syncope, thrombophlebitis, thrombosis, varicose vein, vasospasm, venous pressure increased, ventricular extrasystoles, and ventricular fibrillation;

Digestive System: aphthous stomatitis, cardiospasm, chelitis, cholecystitis, choleithiasis, duodenal ulcer, dry mouth, enteritis, esophagitis, fecal impaction, fecal incontinence, flatulence, gastritis, gastrointestinal hemorrhage, gingivitis, glossitis, hematemesis, hepatic neoplasia, hepatitis, hepatomegaly, ileus, increased salivation, intestinal obstruction, melena, nausea, oral leukoplakia, oral moniliasis, pancreatitis, periodontal abscess proctitis, rectal hemorrhage, salivary gland enlargement, stomach ulcer, and tenesmus;

Endocrine System: Cushing's Syndrome, diabetes insipidus, diabetes mellitus, hypothyroidism, and inappropriate ADH;

Hemic and Lymphatic System: chronic lymphocytic leukemia, hemoglobin less than 9.4 g/100 mL, petechia, platelets less than 75,000/mm³, and splenomegaly;

Metabolic and Nutritional Disorders: alcohol intolerance, alkaline phosphatase greater than 5 times baseline value, BUN greater than 40 mg/dL, calcium greater than 11.5 mg/dL, cyanosis, edema, glucose greater than 160 mg/dL, glycosuria, hypoglycemic reaction, hypoxia, ketosis, and thirst;

Musculoskeletal System: arthritis, arthrosis, bursitis, leg cramps, muscle atrophy, myopathy, myositis, ptosis, and tenosynovitis;

Nervous System: abnormal gait, acute brain syndrome, agitation, apathy, aphasia, ataxia, brain edema, chronic brain syndrome, coma, delirium, delusions, dementia, depersonalization, diplopia, dystonia, encephalopathy, euphoria, facial paral-

---

ysis, foot drop, hallucinations, hemiplegia, hypalgesia, hyperesthesia, incoordination, intracranial hypertension, libido decreased, manic reaction, meningitis, neuralgia, neuropathy, neurosis, nystagmus, oculogyric crisis, ophthalmoplegia, papilledema, paralysis, paranoid reaction, psychosis, reflexes decreased, stupor, subdural hematoma, torticollis, tremor, and urinary retention.

Respiratory System: apnea, asthma, atelectasis, carcinoma of lung, hemoptysis, hiccup, hyperventilation, hypoventilation, interstitial pneumonia, lung edema, pleural effusion, pneumonia, and pneumothorax.

Skin and Appendages: contact dermatitis, erythema nodosum, exfoliative dermatitis, furunculosis, hirsutism, leukoderma, lichenoid dermatitis, maculopapular rash, psoriasis, seborrhea, skin benign neoplasm, skin carcinoma, skin hypertrophy skin necrosis, skin ulcer, urticaria, and vesiculobullous rash.

Special Senses: blepharitis, blindness, deafness, dry eyes, ear pain, iritis, keratoconjunctivitis, mydriasis, otitis externa, otitis media, parosmia, photophobia, retinitis, taste loss, taste perversion, and visual field defect.

Urogenital system: anuria, balanitis, breast engorgement, cervicitis, epididymitis, gynecomastia, hematuria, impotence, kidney calculus, kidney failure, kidney tabular disorder, leukorrhea; nephritis, nocturia, oliguria, polyuria, salpingitis, urethritis, urinary incontinence, uterine fibroids enlarged, uterine neoplasm, and vaginal hemorrhage.

DRUG ABUSE AND DEPENDENCE
No evidence or experience suggests that abuse or dependence occurs with Interferon Beta-1B therapy; however, the risk of dependence has not been systematically evaluated.

DOSAGE AND ADMINISTRATION
The recommended dose of Interferon Beta-1B for the treatment of ambulatory relapsing-remitting MS is 0.25 mg (8 million IU) injected subcutaneously every other day. Limited data regarding the activity of a lower dose are presented above (see *"Clinical Pharmacology, Clinical Trials"*).

Evidence of efficacy beyond 2 years is not known since the primary evidence of efficacy derives from a 2-year, double-blind, placebo-controlled clinical trial (see *"Clinical Pharmacology, Clinical Trials"*). Safety data are not available beyond the third year. Patients were discontinued from this trial due to unremitting disease progression of 6 months or greater.

To reconstitute lyophilized Interferon Beta-1B for injection, use a sterile syringe and needle to inject 1.2 mL of the diluent supplied, sodium chloride, 0.54% solution, into the Interferon Beta-1B vial. Gently swirl the vial of Interferon Beta-1B to dissolve the drug completely; do not shake. Inspect the reconstituted product visually and discard the product before use if it contains particulate matter or is discolored. After reconstitution with accompanying diluent, Interferon Beta-1B vials contain 0.25 mg (8 million IU) Interferon Beta-1B/mL of solution.

Withdraw 1 mL of reconstituted solution from the vial into a sterile syringe fitted with a 27-gauge needle and inject the solution subcutaneously. Sites for self-injection include arms, abdomen, hips, and thighs. A vial is suitable for single use only; unused portions should be discarded. (See *"Interferon Beta-1B Patient Information sheet for Self-Injection Procedure."*)

Stability: The reconstituted product contains no preservative. Before and after reconstitution with diluent, store 2° to 8°C (36° to 46°F). Product should be used within 3 hours of reconstitution.

REFERENCES
1. Ruzicka FJ, et al. J Biol Chem, 1987; 262: 16142-16149. 2. Uze G, et al. Cell, 1990; 60: 225-234. 3. DeMaeyer E, et al. In: Interferons and other regulatory cytokines, NY, Wiley 1988. 4. Colby CB, et al. J Immunol 1984; 133: 3091-3095. 5. Pestka S, et al. Annu Rev Biochem 1987; 56; 727-777. 6. Lengyel P, Annu Rev Biochem 1982; 51: 251-282. 7. Witt PL, et al. J Interferon Res 1990; 10: 393-402. 8. Schiller JH, et al. J Biol Resp Mod 1990; 9: 377-386. 9. Rosenblum MG, et al. J Interferon Res 1990; 10: 141-151. 10. Carlin JM, et al. J Immuno 1987; 130(7): 2414-2418. 11. Witt PL, et al. J Immunotherapy 1993; 13: 191-200. 12. Goldstein D, et al. J Natl Cancer Inst 1989; 81: 1061-1068. 13. Poser CM, et al. Ann Neurol 1983; 13(3): 227-231. 14. Blaschke TF, et al. Clinical Research 1985; 33(1): 19A, Part Number L 1147

INTERFERON BETA-1B PATIENT INFORMATION
(Interferon Beta-1B) is intended for use under the guidance and supervision of a physician. Your physician or his/her delegate should instruct you in the preparation of Betaseron for administration and in the technique of self injection. Do not attempt self-administration until you are sure that you understand the requirements for mixing the product and giving an injection to yourself.

Interferon Beta-1B should be used as prescribed by your physician. However, if you miss a dose, take it as soon as you remember. Your next injection, however, should be scheduled about 48 hours later. While using Interferon Beta-1B, please keep in mind the following facts:

■ Interferon Beta-1B must be kept cold. Be sure to store it in a refrigerator before and after reconstitution. Do not freeze.
■ Keep syringes and needles away from children. Do not reuse needles or syringes. Discard used syringes and needles in a syringe disposal unit as instructed by your physician.
■ Women: Interferon Beta-1B should not be used during pregnancy or if you are trying to become pregnant. If you wish to become pregnant while using Interferon Beta-1B, discuss the matter with your doctor. While using Interferon Beta-1B, women of childbearing age should use birth control measures. If you do become pregnant you should discontinue treatment and contact your doctor immediately.

■ Injection site reactions are common. They include redness, pain and swelling, and discoloration. To minimize the chances for a reaction, ask your doctor to suggest a series of injection sites so that you will not have to use the same one repeatedly. Do not make an injection into skin that is tender, red, or hard.
■ Flu-like symptoms are also common. They include fever, chills, sweating, fatigue, and muscle aches. Taking Interferon Beta-1B at night may help lessen the impact of flu-like symptoms.
■ Depression, including suicide attempts, has been reported by patients. If you experience such symptoms, contact your physician promptly.
■ As with any prescription medication, side effects related to therapy can occur. Consult with your physician if you have any problems, whether or not you think they may be related to Interferon Beta-1B.

SELF-INJECTION PROCEDURE TO MIX
THE CONTENTS OF ONE VIAL
Only the vial of diluent (liquid) that comes inside your prescription package should be used to dissolve the white cake of drug in the Interferon Beta-1B vial.

1. *Wash* your hands thoroughly with soap and water.
2. *Collect* all your equipment before you begin the process.
You'll need:

■ vial of Diluent for Interferon Beta-1B (Sodium Chloride 0.54%)
■ vial of Interferon Beta-1B
■ 3-mL syringe with 21-gauge needle (1)
■ 1-mL syringe with 27-gauge needle (1)
■ alcohol wipes
■ disposal unit (an opaque, puncture-resistant, sealable container for used syringes/needles)

Note: Be sure needle guards are on the needles tightly.
3. *Remove* the protective caps from both vials.
4. Use alcohol wipes to *clean* the tops of the vials—move in one direction and use one wipe per vial.

Note: Leave an alcohol wipe on top of each vial until you are ready to use it.
5. Resting your hands on a stable surface, *remove* the needle cover on the 3-mL syringe by pulling the cover straight off the needle.
6. *Pull back* the plunger (on the 3-mL syringe) to the 1.2 mL mark.

Note: Read the labels on the vials—find the Diluent for Interferon Beta-1B vial and throw away the alcohol wipe on top of it.
7. Holding the vial of Diluent for Interferon Beta-1B on a stable surface, slowly *insert* the needle straight through the stopper, into the top of the vial.

Note: When inserting and removing needles from vials, *be sure* not to touch the needles or the rubber stoppers on the vials with your hands.

If you do touch a stopper, clean it with a fresh alcohol wipe. If you touch a needle, throw away the entire syringe into the disposal unit and start over with a new syringe.

If the needle touches any surface, throw away the entire syringe into the disposal unit and start over with a new syringe.

8. *Push* in the plunger all the way to gently inject air into the vial (*leave* the needle *in* the vial of Diluent for Interferon Beta-1B).
9. Turn the vial of Diluent for Interferon Beta-1B *upside down*.

Note: Keep the needle tip in the liquid.

10. Resting your hands on a stable surface, hold the vial and syringe in one hand and slowly *pull back* the plunger on the syringe to the 1.2 mL mark (to draw up that amount of liquid) with your other hand.
11. Keeping the vial upside down, gently *tap* the syringe until any air bubbles that formed rise to the top of the barrel of the syringe.
12. Carefully *push in* the plunger to eject ONLY THE AIR through the needle.
13. *Remove* the needle/syringe from the vial of Diluent for Interferon Beta-1B.

Note: Find the Interferon Beta-1B vial and *throw away* the alcohol wipe on top of it.

14. Holding the Interferon Beta-1B vial on a stable surface, slowly *insert* the needle of the syringe (containing 1.2 mL of liquid) all the way through the stopper of the vial.
15. *Push* the plunger down slowly, *directing* the needle toward the side of the vial to allow the liquid to run down the inside wall (injecting Diluent for Interferon Beta-1B directly onto the cake of drug will cause excess foaming).
16. Remove the needle/syringe from the Interferon Beta-1B vial.
17. *Throw away* the 3 mL syringe into the diposal unit.

Note: Double-check that you are throwing away the correct syringe into the disposal unit.

18. *Roll* the vial between your hands gently to completely dissolve the white cake of Interferon Beta-1B (DO NOT SHAKE).
19. *Look* closely at the solution (it should be clear).

Note: If the mixture contains particles or is discolored, discard it and start again.

PREPARING THE INJECTION
1. *Remove* the needle guard of the 1 mL syringe and *pull back* the plunger to the 1 mL mark.
2. *Insert* the needle of the 1 mL syringe through the stopper of the vial of Interferon Beta-1B solution.

3. Gently *push* the plunger all the way down to inject air into the vial (leave the needle in the vial).

4. Turn the vial of Interferon Beta-1B solution *upside down*.

Note: Keep the needle tip in the liquid.

5. *Pull back* the plunger to withdraw 1 mL of liquid into the syringe.

6. *Hold* the syringe with the needle pointing upward.

7. *Tap* the syringe gently until any air bubbles that formed rise to the top of the barrel of the syringe.

8. Carefully *push in* the plunger to eject ONLY THE AIR through the needle.

9. *Remove* the needle/syringe from the vial.

10. *Recap* the needle on the syringe.

Note: The injection should be administered immediately after mixing (if the injection is delayed, refrigerate the solution and inject it within 3 hours).
Do not freeze.

11. *Throw away* unused portion of the solution remaining in the vial.

GIVING THE INJECTION
Subcutaneous (under the skin) self-administration

1. *Choose* an injection site (see *"Injection Sites"* diagram); you may want to hold the syringe like a pencil or dart. Use a different site each day you inject:

- Arms (upper back portion)
- Abdomen (except around navel and waistline)
- Hips (upper, outer rear quadrant)
- Thighs (front and sides except at groin and knee)

Note: Do not use any areas in which you feel lumps, firm knots, depressions, pain, or discoloration; talk to your doctor or healthcare professional about anything you find.

2. Use an alcohol wipe to *clean* the skin at the injection site; let it air dry.

3. *Throw away* the wipe.

4. *Uncap* the needle.

5. Gently *pinch* the skin together around the site (to lift it up a bit).

6. Resting your wrist on the skin near the site, *stick* the needle straight into the skin at a 90° angle with a quick, firm motion.

7. *Inject* the drug by using a slow, steady push (push the plunger all the way in until the syringe is empty).

8. *Hold* a swab on the injection site.
Remove the needle from the skin.

9. Gently *massage* the injection site with a dry cotton ball or gauze.

10. *Throw away* the 1 mL syringe in the disposal unit.

INJECTION SITE
Picking an injection site: Interferon Beta-1B therapy should be injected into subcutaneous tissue (between the fat layer just under the skin and the muscles beneath). The best areas for injection are loose and soft (flabby), away from joints and nerves. Each therapy day you can choose an injection site. It's a good idea to know where your injection will be given *before* you prepare your syringe.

If there are any sites that are difficult for you to reach, you can ask your support person (or someone who has been trained to give injections) to help you.

Rotating injection sites: Changing sites each time helps prevent injection reactions; it gives the site time to "bounce back" from the last injection. Today's injection should not be given in the same areas as the last one. Keep a record of where and when you last gave yourself an injection. One way to do that is to note the injection site on a calendar.

You may use a site again after waiting 1 week. If all areas become tender, talk to the doctor about choosing other injection sites.

HOW SUPPLIED
POWDER FOR INJECTION: 0.3 MG

BRAND/MANUFACTURER	NDC	SIZE	AWP
○ **BRAND**			
BETASERON: Berlex Labs	50419-0521-15	5s	$360.00

Interferon Gamma-1B

DESCRIPTION
Interferon Gamma-1B a biologic response modifier, is a single-chain polypeptide containing 140 amino acids. Production of Interferon Gamma-1B is achieved by fermentation of a genetically engineered *Escherichia coli* bacterium containing the DNA which encodes for the human protein. Purification of the product is achieved by conventional column chromatography. Interferon Gamma-1B is a highly purified sterile solution consisting of non-covalent dimers of two identical 16,465 dalton monomers; with a specific activity of 30 million U/mg.

Interferon Gamma-1B is a sterile, clear, colorless solution filled in a single-dose vial for subcutaneous injection. Each 0.5 mL contains 100 mcg (3 million U) of Gamma-1B formulated in 20 mg mannitol, 0.36 mg sodium succinate, 0.05 mg polysorbate 20 and Sterile Water for Injection.

CLINICAL PHARMACOLOGY
GENERAL
Interferons are a family of functionally related, species-specific proteins synthesized by eukaryotic cells in response to viruses and a variety of natural and synthetic stimuli. The most striking differences between interferon-gamma and other classes of interferon concern the immunomodulatory properties of this molecule. While gamma, alpha and beta interferons share certain properties, interferon-gamma has potent phagocyte-activating effects not seen with other interferon preparations. These effects include the generation of toxic oxygen metabolites within phagocytes, which are capable of mediating the killing of microorganisms such as *Staphyloccus aureus, Toxoplasma gondii, Leishmania donovani, Listeria monocytogenes, and Mycobacterium avium intracellulare.*

Clinical studies in patients using interferon-gamma have revealed a broad range of biological activities including the enhancement of the oxidative metabolism of tissue macrophages, enhancement of antibody-dependent cellular cytotoxicity (ADCC) and natural killer (NK) cell activity. Additionally, effects on Fc receptor expression on monocytes and major histocompatibility antigen expression have been noted.[1,2]

To the extent that interferon-gamma is produced by antigen-stimulated T lymphocytes and regulates the activity of immune cells, it is appropriate to characterize interferon-gamma as a lymphokine of the interleukin type. There is growing evidence that interferon-gamma interacts functionally with other interleukin molecules such as interleukin-2 and that all of the interleukins form part of a complex, lymphokine regulatory network.[3] For example, interferon-gamma and interleukin-4 appear to reciprocally interact to regulate murine IgE levels: interferon-gamma can suppress IgE levels in humans.[4,5] Interferon-gamma also inhibits the production of collagen at the transcription level in human systems.[6]

More specifically, with respect to Chronic Granulomatous Disease (an inherited disorder characterized by deficient phagocyte oxidative metabolism), pilot clinical trials of the systemic administration of Interferon Gamma-1B in patients with Chronic Granulomatous Disease were initiated which provided evidence for a treatment-related enhancement of phagocyte function including elevation of superoxide levels and improved killing of *Staphylococcus aureus.*[7,8] Based on this evidence, a randomized, double-blind, placebo-controlled clinical study was initiated to further delineate the effects of Interferon Gamma-1B in Chronic Granulomatous Disease.

PHARMACOKINETICS
The intravenous, intramuscular, and subcutaneous pharmacokinetics of Interferon Gamma-1B have been investigated in 24 healthy male subjects following single-dose administration of 100 mcg/m^2. Interferon Gamma-1B is rapidly cleared after intravenous administration (1.4 liters/minute) and slowly absorbed after intramuscular or subcutaneous injection. After intramuscular or subcutaneous injection, the apparent fraction of dose absorbed was greater than 89%. The mean elimination half-life after intravenous administration of 100 mcg/m^2 in healthy male subjects was 38 minutes. The mean elimination half-lives for intramuscular and subcutaneous dosing with 100 mcg/m^2 were 2.9 and 5.9 hours, respectively. Peak plasma concentrations, determined by ELISA, occurred approximately 4 hours (1.5 ng/mL) after intramuscular dosing and 7 hours (0.6 ng/mL) after subcutaneous dosing. Multiple dose subcutaneous pharmacokinetic studies were conducted in 38 healthy male subjects. There was no accumulation of Interferon Gamma-1B after 12 consecutive daily injections of 100 mcg/m^2. Pharmacokinetic studies in patients with Chronic Granulomatous Disease have not been performed.

Excretion studies of Interferon Gamma-1B have been performed. Trace amounts of interferon-gamma were detected in the urine of squirrel monkeys following intravenous administration of 500 mcg/kg. Interferon-gamma was not detected in the urine of healthy human volunteers following administration of 100 mcg/m^2 of Interferon Gamma-1B by the intravenous, intramuscular and subcutaneous routes. *In vitro* perfusion studies utilizing rabbit livers and kidneys demonstrate that these organs are capable of clearing interferon-gamma from perfusate. Studies of the administration of interferon-gamma to nephrectomized mice and squirrel monkeys demonstrate a reduction in clearance of interferon-gamma from blood; however, prior nephrectomy did not prevent elimination.

EFFECTS OF CHRONIC GRANULOMATOUS DISEASE
A randomized, double-blind, placebo-controlled study of Interferon Gamma-1B in patients with Chronic Granulomatous Disease, was performed to determine whether Interferon Gamma-1B administered subcutaneously on a three times weekly schedule could decrease the incidence of serious infectious episodes and improve existing infectious and inflammatory conditions in patients with Chronic Granulomatous Disease. One hundred twenty-eight eligible patients were enrolled on this study including patients with different patterns of inheritance. Most patients received prophylactic antibiotics. Patients ranged in age from 1 to 44 years with the mean age being 14.6 years. The study was terminated early following demonstration of a highly statistically significant benefit of Interferon Gamma-1B therapy compared to placebo with respect to time to serious infection (p=0.0036), the primary endpoint of the investigation. Serious infection was defined as a clinical event requiring hospitalization and the use of parenteral antibiotics. The final analysis provided further support for the primary end-point (p=0.0006). There was a 67 percent reduction in relative risk of serious infection in patients receiving Interferon Gamma-1B (n=63) compared to placebo (n=65). Additional supportive evidence of treatment benefit included a twofold reduction in the number of primary serious infections in the Interferon Gamma-1B group (30 on placebo versus 14 on Interferon Gamma-1B (p=0.002) and the total number and rate of serious infections including recurrent events (56 on placebo

versus 20 on Interferon Gamma-1B (p = < 0.0001). Moreover, the length of hospitalization for the treatment of all clinical events provided evidence highly supportive of an Interferon Gamma-1B treatment benefit. Placebo patients required three times as many inpatient hospitalization days for treatment of clinical events compared to patients receiving Interferon Gamma-1B (1493 versus 497 total days, p=0.02). An Interferon Gamma-1B treatment benefit with respect to time to serious infection was consistently demonstrated in all subgroup analyses according to stratification factors, including pattern of inheritance, use of prophylactic antibiotics, as well as age. There was a 67 percent reduction in relative risk of serious infection in patients receiving Interferon Gamma-1B compared to placebo across all groups. The beneficial effect of Interferon Gamma-1B therapy was observed throughout the entire study, in which the mean duration of Interferon Gamma-1B administration was 8.9 months/patient.

INDICATIONS AND USAGE

Interferon Gamma-1B is indicated for reducing the frequency and severity of serious infections associated with Chronic Granulomatous Disease. The safety and effectiveness in children under the age of 1 year has not been established.

UNLABELED USES

Interferon Gamma-1B is used alone or as an adjunct in the treatment of basal cell carcinoma, atopic dermatitis, bowenoid papulosis, and visceral leishmaniasis. It is also used in non-small cell lung cancer, rheumatoid arthritis, acquired immunodeficiency syndrome and leukemia, including chronic myelogenous leukemia.

CONTRAINDICATIONS

Interferon Gamma-1B is contraindicated in patients who develop or have known hypersensitivity to interferon-gamma, *E. coli* derived products, or any component of the product.

WARNINGS

Interferon Gamma-1B should be used with caution in patients with pre-existing cardiac disease, including symptoms of ischemia, congestive heart failure or arrhythemia. No direct cardiotoxic effect has been demonstrated but it is possible that acute and transient 'flu-like' or constitutional symptoms such as fever and chills frequently associated with Interferon Gamma-1B administration at doses of 250 mcg/m^2/day or higher may exacerbate pre-existing cardiac conditions.

Caution should be exercised when treating patients with known seizure disorders and or compromised central nervous system function. Central nervous system adverse reactions including decreased mental status, gait disturbance and dizziness have been observed, particularly in patients receiving doses greater than 250 mcg/mg^2/day. Most of these abnormalities were mild and reversible within a few days upon dose reduction or discontinuation of therapy.

Caution should be exercised when administering Interferon Gamma-1B to patients with myelosuppression. Reversible neutropenia and elevation of hepatic enzymes can be dose limiting above 250mcg/m^2/day. Thrombocytopenia and proteinuria have also been seen rarely.

PRECAUTIONS

GENERAL

Acute serious hypersensitivity reactions have not been observed in patients receiving Interferon Gamma-1B; however, if such an acute reaction develops the drug should be discontinued immediately and appropriate medical therapy instituted. Transient cutaneous rashes have occurred in some patients following injection but have rarely necessitated treatment interruption.

INFORMATION FOR PATIENTS

Patients being treated with Interferon Gamma-1B and/or their parents should be informed regarding the potential benefits and risks associated with treatment. If home use is determined to be desirable by the physician, instructions on appropriate use should be given, including review of the contents of the Patient Information Insert. This information is intended to aid in the safe and effective use of the medication. It is not a disclosure of all possible adverse or intended effects.

If home use is prescribed, a puncture resistant container for the disposal of used syringes and needles should be supplied to the patient. Patients should be thoroughly instructed in the importance of proper disposal and cautioned against any reuse of needles and syringes. The full container should be disposed of according to the directions provided by the physician (see *"Patient Information Insert"*).

The most common adverse experiences occurring with Interferon Gamma-1B therapy are 'flu-like' or constitutional symptoms such as fever, headache, chills, myalgia or fatigue (see *"Adverse Reactions"* section) which may decrease in severity as treatment continues. Some of the 'flu-like' symptoms may be minimized by bedtime administration. Acetaminophen may be used to prevent or partially alleviate the fever and headache.

The long-term effects of Interferon Gamma-1B therapy on growth, development or other parameters, are not known.

LABORATORY TESTS

In addition to those tests normally required for monitoring patients with Chronic Granulomatous Disease, the following laboratory tests are recommended for all patients on Interferon Gamma-1B therapy prior to the beginning of and at three month intervals during treatment.

- Hematologic tests — including complete blood counts, differential and platelet counts.
- Blood chemistries — including renal and liver function tests.
- Urinalysis.

DRUG INTERACTIONS

Interactions between Interferon Gamma-1B and other drugs have not been fully evaluated. Caution should be exercised when administering Interferon Gamma-1B in combination with other potentially myelosuppressive agents (see *"Warnings"*).

Preclinical studies in rodents using species-specific inteferon-gamma have demonstrated a decrease in hepatic microsomal cytochrome P-450 concentrations. This could potentially lead to a depression of the hepatic metabolism of certain drugs that utilize this degradative pathway.

CARINOGENESIS, MUTAGENESIS, AND IMPAIRMENT OF FERTILITY

Carcinogenesis: Interferon Gamma-1B has not been tested for its carcinogenic potential.

Mutagenesis: Ames tests using five different tester strains of bacteria with and without metabolic activation revealed no evidence of mutagenic potential. Interferon Gamma-1B was tested in a micronucleus assay for its ability to induce chromosomal damage in bone marrow cells of mice following two intravenous doses of 20 mg/kg. No evidence of chromosomal damage was noted.

Impairment of Fertility: Female cynomolgus monkeys treated with daily subcutaneous doses of 150 mcg/kg Interferon Gamma-1B approximately 100 times the human dose) exhibited irregular menstrual cycles or absence of cyclicity during treatment. Similar findings were not observed in aninals treated with 3 or 30 mcg/kg Interferon Gamma - 1B. No studies have been performed assessing any potential effects of Interferon Gamma-1B on male fertility.

PREGNANCY

Teratogenic Effects: Pregnancy Category C. Interferon Gamma-1B has shown an increased incidence of abortions in primates when given in doses approximately 100 × the human dose. A study in pregnant primates treated with intravenous doses 2-100× the human dose failed to demonstrate teratogenic activity for Interferon Gamma-1B. There are no adequate and well-controlled studies in pregnant women. Interferon Gamma-1B should be used during pregnancy only if the potential benefit justifies the potential risk to the fetus. In addition, studies evaluating recombinant murine interferon-gamma in pregnant mice, revealed increased incidences of uterine bleeding and abortifacient activity and decreased neonatal viability at maternally toxic doses. The clinical significance of this latter observation with recombinant murine interferon-gamma tested in a homologus system is uncertain.

NURSING MOTHERS

It is not known whether Interferon Gamma-1B is excreted in human milk. Because many drugs are excreted in human milk and because of the potential for serious adverse reactions in nursing infants from Interferon Gamma-1B a decision should be made whether to discontinue nursing or to discontinue the drug dependent upon the importance of the drug to the mother.

PEDIATRIC USE

Safety and effectiveness in children under the age of 1 year has not been established.

ADVERSE REACTIONS

The following data on adverse reactions are based on the subcutaneous administration of Interferon Gamma-1B at a dose of 50 mcg/m^2, three times weekly, in 63 patients with Chronic Granulomatous Disease during an investigational trial in the United States and Europe. Sixty-five additional patients with Chronic Granulomatous Disease received placebo on this study. The following table represents the percentage of patients experiencing common adverse reactions observed on this study.

Clinical Toxicity	Percent of Patients Interferon Gamma-1B	Placebo
Fever	52	28
Headache	33	9
Rash	17	6
Chills	14	0
Injection site erythema or tenderness	14	2
Fatigue	14	11
Diarrhea	14	12
Vomiting	13	5
Nausea	10	2
Weight loss	6	6
Myalgia	6	0
Anorexia	3	5
Arthralgia	2	0
Injection site pain	0	2

Miscellaneous adverse events which occurred infrequently and may have been related to underlying diseases included back pain (2 percent versus 0 percent), abdominal pain (8 percent versus 3 percent) and depression (3 percent versus 0 percent) for Interferon Gamma-1B and placebo treated patients, respectively.

Interferon Gamma-1B has also been evaluated in additional disease states in studies in which patients have generally received higher doses (>100 mcg/m^2/day) administered by intramuscular injection or intravenous infusion. All of the previously described adverse reactions which occurred in patients with Chronic

► SHOWN IN PRODUCT IDENTIFICATION GUIDE

Granulomatous Disease have also been observed in patients receiving higher doses. Adverse reactions not observed in patients with Chronic Granulomatous Disease receiving doses less than 100 mcg/m^2/day but seen rarely in patients receiving Interferon Gamma-1B in other studies include:

Cardiovascular: hypotension, syncope, tachyarrhythmia, heart block, heart failure, and myocardial infarction

Central Nervous System: confusion, disorientation, gait disturbance, Parkinsonian symptoms, seizure, hallucinations, and transient ischemic attacks.

Gastrointestinal: hepatic insufficiency, gastrointestinal bleeding, and pancreatitis.

Renal: reversible renal insufficiency.

Hematologic: deep venous thrombosis and pulmonary embolism.

Pulmonary: tachypnea, bronchospasm, and interstitial pneumonitis.

Metabolic: hyponatremia and hyperglycemia.

Other: exacerbation of dermatomyositis.

Abnormal Laboratory Test Values: No statistically significant differences between the Interferon Gamma-1B and placebo treatment groups were observed with regard to effect of treatment on hematologic, coagulation, hepatic and renal laboratory studies.

No neutralizing antibodies to Interferon Gamma-1B have been detected in any Chronic Granulomatous Disease patient receiving Interferon Gamma-1B.

DOSAGE AND ADMINISTRATION

The recommended dosage of Interferon Gamma-1B for the treatment of patients with Chronic Granulomatous Disease is 50 mcg/m^2 (1.5 million U/m^2) for patients whose body surface area is greater than 0.5m^2 and 1.5 mcg/kg/dose for patients whose body surface area is equal to or less than 0.5 m^2. Injections should be administered subcutaneously three times weekly (for example, Monday, Wednesday, Friday). The optimum sites of injection are the right and left deltoid and anterior thigh. Interferon Gamma-1B can be administered by a physician, nurse, family member or patient when trained in the administration of subcutaneous injections. Parenteral drug products should be inspected visually for particulate matter and discoloration prior to administration, whenever solution and container permit.

The formulation does not contain a preservative. A vial of Interferon Gamma-1B is suitable for a single dose only. The unused portion of any vial should be discarded.

Higher doses are not recommended. Safety and efficacy has not been established for Interferon Gamma-1B given in doses greater or less than the recommended dose of 50 mcg/m^2. The minimum effective dose of Interferon Gamma-1B has not been established.

If severe reactions occur, the dosage should be modified (50 percent reduction) or therapy should be discontinued until the adverse reaction abates.

Interferon Gamma-1B may be administered using either sterilized glass or plastic disposable syringes.

Vials of Interferon Gamma-1B must be placed in a 2-8°C (36-46°F) refrigerator immediately upon receipt to insure optimal retention of physical and biochemical integrity. DO NOT FREEZE. Avoid excessive or vigorous agitation. DO NOT SHAKE. An unentered vial of Interferon Gamma-1B should not be left at room temperature for a total time exceeding 12 hours prior to use. Vials exceeding this time period should not be returned to the refrigerator; such vials should be discarded.

Do not use beyond the expiration date stamped on the vial.

REFERENCES

1. Maluish AE, Urba WJ, Longo DL, *et al:* The determination of an immunologically active dose of interferon gamma in patients with melanoma J Clin Onc *6:* 434-445, 1988. 2. Nathan CF, Kaplan G. Levis W, *et al:* Local and systemic effects of intradermal recombinant interferon gamma in patients with lepromatous leprosy, NEJM *315:* 6-11, 1986. 3. Facui AS, Rosenberg SA, Sherwin SA, *et al:* Immunomodulators in clinical medicine. Ann Internal Med. *106:* 421-433, 1987. 4. Snapper CM, Paul WE: Interferon-gamma and B cell stimulatory factor-1 reciprocally regulate Ig isotype production. Science *236:* 944-947, 1987. 5. King CL, Gallin JI, Malech HL, *et al:* Regulation of immunoglobulin production in hyperimmunoglobulin E recurrent-infection syndrome by interferon gamma. PNAS USA *86:* 10085-10089, 1989. 6. Rosenbloom J. Feldman G. Freundlich B, Jimenez SA: Inhibition of excessive scleroderma fibroblast collagen production by recombinant gamma-interferon. Arth Rheum *29:* 851-856, 1986. 7. Ezekowitz RAB, Dinauer MC, Jaffe HS, *et al:* Partial correction of the phagocyte defect in patients with X-linked chronic granulomatous disease by subcutaneous interferon gamma. NEJM *319:* 146-151, 1988. 8. Sechler JMG, Malech HL, White CJ, Gallin JI: Recombinant human interferon-gamma reconstitutes defective phagocyte function in patients with chronic granulomatous disease of childhood. PNAS USA *85:* 4874-4878, 1988.

J CODES
3 million units SC—J9216

HOW SUPPLIED
INJECTION: 3 MILLION U

BRAND/MANUFACTURER	NDC	SIZE	AWP
○ BRAND			
ACTIMMUNE: Genentech	50242-0052-23	0.5 ml doz	$1526.00
	50242-0052-14	0.5 ml	$140.00

Intralipid *SEE* FAT EMULSION

Intron-A *SEE* INTERFERON ALFA-2B

Inversine *SEE* MECAMYLAMINE HYDROCHLORIDE

Iodamide Meglumine

DESCRIPTION

Iodamide Meglumine is a radiopaque contrast agent supplied as a sterile, non-pyrogenic, aqueous, intravenous solution. Each ml provides 240 mg Iodamide Meglumine and 0.0368 mg edetate disodium as a sequestering stabilizing agent; the pH has been adjusted to 6.5 to 7.7 with Iodamide. *Each ml of solution contains approximately 0.0046 mg (0.0002 mEq) sodium* and approximately 111 mg organically bound iodine. The clear, colorless to pale yellow solution has a viscosity of 1.8 cps at 37°C and 2.0 cps at 25°C. The solution has an osmolarity of approximately 0.5 mOsm per ml at 37°C. At the time of manufacture, the air in the container is replaced with nitrogen.

Chemically, Iodamide Meglumine is 3-(acetylamino)-5[(acetylamino)methyl]-2,4,6-triiodo-benzoic acid, N-methylglucamine salt.

Following is its chemical structure:

CLINICAL PHARMACOLOGY

Following intravenous infusion, Iodamide Meglumine is rapidly transported through the bloodstream to the kidneys and is excreted essentially unchanged in the urine, principally by glomerular filtration. However, at least one-third of the intravenous dose is secreted by the renal tubules.

DRIP INFUSION PYELOGRAPHY

After infusion, the contrast agent permits visualization of the kidneys and urinary passages through the natural physiologic mechanism of excretion.

Renal accumulation is sufficiently rapid so that the period of maximal opacification of the renal passages may begin within five minutes after start of infusion. Normal kidneys rapidly eliminate the contrast medium. In nephropathic conditions, particularly when excretory capacity has been altered, the rate of excretion varies unpredictably, and opacification may be delayed for 60 minutes or more after start of infusion; with severe renal impairment, opacification may not occur. Generally the medium is concentrated sufficiently and promptly enough to permit satisfactory visualization of the urinary tract.

COMPUTED TOMOGRAPHY

Iodamide Meglumine enhances computed tomographic brain imaging through augmentation of radiographic efficiency. The degree of enhancement of visualization of tissue density is directly related to the iodine content in an administered dose; peak iodine blood levels occur immediately following rapid infusion of the dose. These levels fall rapidly within five to ten minutes. This can be accounted for by the dilution in the vascular and extracellular fluid compartments which causes an initial sharp fall in plasma concentration. Equilibration with the extracellular compartments is reached in about ten minutes; thereafter, the fall becomes exponential. Maximum contrast enhancement frequently occurs after peak blood iodine levels are reached. The delay in maximum contrast enhancement can range from five to forty minutes, depending on the peak iodine levels achieved and the cell type of the lesion. This lag suggests that radiographic contrast enhancement is at least in part dependent on the accumulation of iodine within the lesion and outside the blood pool, although the mechanism by which this occurs is not clear. The radiographic enhancement of nontumoral lesions, such as arteriovenous malformations and aneurysms is probably dependent on the iodine content of the circulating blood pool.

INDICATIONS AND USAGE

Iodamide Meglumine is an intravenous diagnostic agent for excretion urography and radiographic contrast enhancement in computed tomography (CT) of the brain.

CONTRAST ENHANCEMENT OF COMPUTED TOMOGRAPHIC (CT) BRAIN IMAGING

Contrast enhancement is advantageous in delineating or ruling out disease in suspicious areas which may otherwise not have been satisfactorily visualized.

TUMORS

Iodamide Meglumine may be useful to demonstrate the presence and extent of certain malignancies such as: gliomas including malignant gliomas, glioblastomas, astrocytomas, oligodendrogliomas and gangliomas; ependymomas; medulloblastomas; meningiomas; neuromas; pinealomas; pituitary adenomas; cranio-pharyngiomas; germinomas; and metastatic lesions.

The usefulness of contrast enhancement for the investigation of the retrobulbar space and in cases of low grade or infiltrative gliomas has not been demonstrated. In cases where lesions have calcified, there is less likelihood of enhancement. Following therapy, tumors may show decreased or no enhancement.

NON-NEOPLASTIC CONDITIONS
The use of an iodinated contrast agent may be beneficial in the enhancement of images of lesions not due to neoplasms. Cerebral infarctions of recent onset may be better visualized with the contrast enhancement, while some infarctions are obscured if a contrast medium is used. The use of Iodamide Meglumine improved the contrast enhancement in approximately 60 percent of cerebral infarctions studied from one week to four weeks from the onset of symptoms.

Imaging of sites of active infection may also be enhanced following contrast medium administration.

Arteriovenous malformations and aneurysms will show contrast enhancement. In the case of these vascular lesions, the enhancement is probably dependent on the iodine content of the circulating blood pool.

Hematomas and intraparenchymal bleeders seldom demonstrate any contrast enhancement. However, in cases of intraparenchymal clot, for which there is no obvious clinical explanation, contrast medium administration may be helpful in ruling out the possibility of associated arteriovenous malformation.

The opacification of the inferior vermis following contrast medium administration has resulted in false-positive diagnoses in a number of normal studies.

CONTRAINDICATIONS
There are no absolute contraindications to the use of Iodamide Meglumine (see "Warnings").

WARNINGS
A definite risk exists in the performance of excretion urography in patients who are known to have multiple myeloma, because of the great possibility of producing transient to fatal renal failure. The risk of excretion urography in myelomatous patients is not a contraindication to the procedure; however, dehydration in the preparation of these patients should be avoided, since this may predispose to the precipitation of protein in the renal tubules.

Administration of radiopaque materials to patients known or suspected to have pheochromocytoma should be performed only if the physician deems that the possible benefits outweigh the considered risks; the procedure should then be performed with extreme caution and the volume of radiopaque medium injected should be kept to an absolute minimum. The blood pressure should be assessed throughout the procedure and measures for treatment of a hypertensive crisis should be available.

Contrast media administered intravenously have been shown to promote the phenomenon of sickling in individuals who are homozygous for sickle cell disease.

Urography should be performed with extreme caution in patients with severe concomitant hepatic and renal disease, or anuria.

A history of sensitivity to iodine *per se* or to any contrast agent is not an absolute contraindication to the use of iodamide meglumin, but calls for extreme caution in administration.

PRECAUTIONS
General: All procedures utilizing contrast media carry a definite risk of producing adverse reactions. While most reactions may be minor, life-threatening and fatal reactions may occur without warning. The risk-benefit factor should always be carefully evaluated before such a procedure is undertaken. At all times a fully equipped emergency cart, or equivalent supplies and equipment, and personnel competent in recognizing and treating adverse reactions of all severity (or situations which may arise as a result of the procedure) should be immediately available. If a serious reaction should occur, administration should be discontinued immediately.

Since severe delayed reactions have been known to occur, emergency facilities and competent personnel should be available for at least 30 to 60 minutes after administration.

Renal toxicity has been reported in a few patients with liver dysfunction who were given oral cholecystographic agents followed by urographic agents. Administration of Iodamide Meglumine should therefore be postponed in any patient with a known or suspected hepatic or biliary disorder who has recently taken a cholecystographic contrast agent.

Caution should be exercised with the use of radiopaque media in severely debilitated patients and in those with marked hypertension. The increased osmotic load associated with drip infusion pyelography should also be considered in patients with congestive heart failure.

Consideration must be given to the functional ability of the kidneys before infusing this preparation.

The diuretic effect of the drip infusion pyelography procedure may hinder assessment of residual urine in the bladder.

When any intravenous infusion technique is employed, the possibility of thrombosis or of other complications due to the mechanical trauma of the procedure should be borne in mind.

The recommended rate of infusion should not be exceeded.

Contrast agents may interfere with some chemical determinations made on urine specimens; therefore, urine should be collected before administration of the contrast medium or two or more days afterwards.

Recent reports of thyroid storm occurring following the intravascular use of iodinated radiopaque agents in patients with hyperthyroidism or with an autonomously functioning thyroid nodule suggest that this additional risk be evaluated in such patients before use of this drug.

Since iodine-containing contrast agents may alter the results of thyroid function tests which depend on iodine estimations (e.g., PBI and radioactive iodine uptake studies), such tests, if indicated, should be performed prior to administration of this preparation. However, measurements of serum thyroxine concentration involving use of tests such as the Resin Triiodothyronine Uptake test, "RT$_3$U," or the Thyroxine (Displacement) assay, "T$_4$(D)," are not affected.

Premedication with antihistamines to avoid or minimize possible allergic reactions, or their use in the management of adverse reactions, may be considered; however, admixture of an antihistamine with a contrast agent may result in a precipitate (see "Dosage and Administration"). A separate syringe should be used for this injection.

Use of a diuretic prior to the examination in order to increase the urinary concentration of the contrast medium is not desirable (see "Dosage and Administration"); dehydration may predispose to a greater incidence of, or more severe, reactions.

Sensitivity Testing: Severe, life-threatening reactions to radiopaque agents often resemble hypersensitivity phenomena. This has prompted the use of several pretesting methods, none of which can be relied on to predict severe reactions. Many authorities question the value of any pretest. A history of bronchial asthma or allergy, a family history of allergy, or a previous reaction to a contrast agent warrant special attention. Such a history, by suggesting histamine sensitivity and a consequent proneness to reactions, may be more accurate than pretesting in predicting the likelihood of a reaction, although it will not necessarily indicate the severity or type of reaction in the individual case.

The sensitivity test most often performed is the slow intravenous injection of 0.5 to 1.0 ml of the radiopaque medium prior to infusion of the full diagnostic dose. It should be noted that the absence of a reaction to the test dose does not preclude the possibility of a reaction to the full diagnostic dose. If the test dose causes an untoward response of any kind, the necessity for continuing with the examination should be carefully reevaluated and, if it is deemed essential, the examination should be conducted with all possible caution. In rare instances reactions to the test dose itself may be extremely severe; therefore, close observation of the patient, and facilities for emergency treatment are essential.

Pregnancy Category B: No teratogenic effects attributable to Iodamide Meglumine have been observed in reproduction studies performed in mice, rats, and rabbits.

Safety for use during pregnancy in humans has not been established. Although there is no clearly defined risk, the possibility of infrequent or subtle damage to the fetus cannot be excluded. Iodamide Meglumine should be used in pregnant women only when clearly needed.

Nursing Mothers: Iodamide Meglumine is excreted unchanged in human milk. Although it has not been established that serious adverse reactions have occurred in nursing infants, caution should be exercised when iodamide meglumine is administered to a nursing woman because of the potential for adverse reactions.

Pediatric Use: Administration of Iodamide Meglumine by infusion has not been evaluated in pediatric patients; however, Iodamide Meglumine, the less dilute formulation, is available for use in infants and children. See the package insert accompanying that product for complete information.

ADVERSE REACTIONS
In clinical studies with iodamide meglumine, adverse reactions occurred in approximately 9.5 to 13 percent of patients. The most frequently seen adverse reactions were nausea and/or vomiting, urticaria, pruritus, and a rise or fall in blood pressure, individually occurring at a frequency of approximately one to five percent. Reactions were usually mild. Reactions occurring less frequently are generalized flushing, retching, nasal congestion, sneezing, flank tenderness, chills, syncope, pulse rate increase, hyperpnea, shortness of breath, chest pain, tachycardia, and hemiparesis.

Other reactions to iodinated contrast media may occur including fever; dizziness; headache; lacrimation; sweating and weakness; light-headedness; restlessness; pallor; coughing; choking; hoarseness; laryngeal or pulmonary edema; dysphagia; malaise; edema of the eyelids; bitter or metallic taste; pharyngeal burning sensation; facial or conjunctival petechiae; rash and other eruptions; itching; perianal burning sensation; wheezing; asthmatic reaction; cramps; tremors; anxiety; pain, erythema, hematomas, ecchymoses, and tissue necrosis around injection site due to faulty technique; warmth or burning sensation; venospasm or venous pain; partial collapse of the injected vein; thrombophlebitis and cellulitis following injection; red blood cell clumping and agglutination; crenation and interference in clot formation; neutropenia; transient proteinuria; hysterical reaction and numbness of head and neck; bradycardia; shock; and convulsions. "Iodism" (salivary gland swelling) has been reported infrequently; immediate or delayed rigors sometimes with hyperpyrexia has occurred rarely.

Antihistaminic agents may be of benefit in the event of adverse reactions. Adverse reactions may be severe enough to require discontinuation of infusion.

Severe reactions to contrast agents which may require emergency measures (see "Precautions"), may take the form of a cardiovascular reaction characterized by peripheral vasodilatation with resultant hypotension and reflex tachycardia, dyspnea, agitation, confusion, and cyanosis progressing to unconsciousness.

Rare cases of cardiac arrest, ventricular fibrillation, cardiac arrhythmias, and hypertension may occur. The histamine-liberating effect of these compounds may induce an allergic-like reaction which may range in severity from rhinitis or angioneurotic edema to laryngeal or bronchial spasm and, rarely, anaphylactoid shock.

Rarely, temporary renal shutdown or other nephropathy may occur.

DOSAGE AND ADMINISTRATION

Iodamide Meglumine should be at body temperature when infused, and may need to be warmed before use.

DRIP INFUSION PYELOGRAPHY

Appropriate preparation of the patient is desirable for optimal results. A laxative the night before the examination and a low residue diet the day before the procedure may be used to clear the gastrointestinal tract. However, a normal liquid intake during this time is desirable.

The recommended adult dose is 4.5 ml per kg of body weight, administered intravenously by continuous infusion, with a maximum total dose of 300 ml; the appropriate volume should be infused in approximately 10 minutes (about 30 ml per minute for a 147 lb or heavier patient), through a large-bore (usually 17- or 18-gauge) needle. In older patients and in patients with known or suspected cardiac decompensation, a slower rate of infusion is probably wise. If flushing or nausea occurs during administration, infusion should be slowed or briefly interrupted until the side effects have disappeared. If a serious reaction should occur, administration should be discontinued immediately.

The admixture of diphenhydramine hydrochloride Injection with Iodamide Meglumine may cause a precipitate to form in the tubing. If antihistamines are administered concomitantly (see *"Precautions"*), they should *not* be mixed with the contrast agent and should be administered at another site.

ROENTGENOGRAPHIC PROCEDURE

A scout film should be made before the contrast medium is administered. Several films should be exposed after infusion to allow for individual variation and to insure visualization of the desired sites of the urinary tract. Times at which optimal opacification may be first observed in the majority of patients are as follows: renal parenchyma at 10 minutes after start of infusion, calyces and pelves at 20 minutes, and ureters and bladder at 30 minutes. In patients with renal dysfunction, optimal visualization may be delayed until 60 minutes or more after the start of infusion.

COMPUTED TOMOGRAPHY

The suggested dose is 4.5 ml of Iodamide Meglumine per kg of body weight, administered by intravenous drip infusion. The first 200 ml of Iodamide Meglumine should be infused in about five minutes, at which time imaging should commence. The balance of the dose should be infused during imaging. A maximum total dose of 300 ml should not be exceeded.

PATIENT PREPARATION

No special patient preparation is required for contrast enhancement of CT brain imaging. However, it is advisable to insure that patients are well hydrated prior to examination.

STORAGE

The preparation should be stored at room temperature, protected from light and excessive heat. If precipitation or solidification has occurred due to storage in the cold, immerse the container in hot water and shake intermittently to dissolve any solids.

HOW SUPPLIED
INJECTION: 24%

BRAND/MANUFACTURER	NDC	SIZE	AWP
○ BRAND			
RENOVUE-DIP: Bracco Diag	00003-1407-10	300 ml 10s	$265.28
	00003-1407-15	300 ml 10s	$523.99

INJECTION: 65%

BRAND/MANUFACTURER	NDC	SIZE	AWP
○ BRAND			
RENOVUE-65: Bracco Diag	00003-1406-40	50 ml 25s	$448.91

Iodipamide Meglumine

DESCRIPTION

Iodipamide Meglumine is a radiopaque contrast agent for slow intravenous cholangiography and cholecystography supplied as a sterile, aqueous solution. Each ml provides 103 mg Iodipamide Meglumine; agent. The pH has been adjusted between 6.5 and 7.7 with Meglumine. *Each ml of solution also contains*: 51 mg organically bound iodine (5.1 g 100 ml).

The appearance of the solution may vary from essentially colorless to pale yellow. Solutions which have become substantially darker, however, should not be used.

Following is its chemical structure:

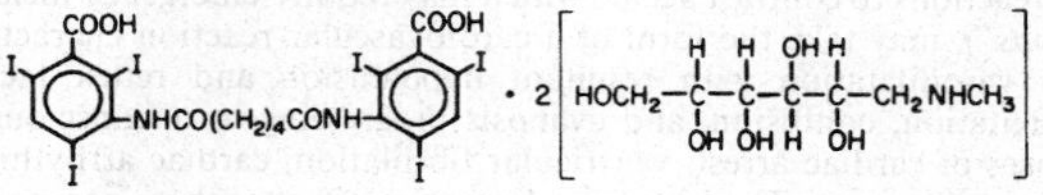

CLINICAL PHARMACOLOGY

Following intravenous administration of Iodipamide Meglumine, Iodipamide is carried to the liver where it is rapidly excreted. The contrast medium appears in the bile, thus permitting visualization of the hepatic and common bile ducts, even in cholecystectomized patients. The biliary ducts are readily visualized after administration, except in patients with impaired liver function; visualization may be apparent from 20 to 40 minutes after the infusion is started, with optimum visualization usually occurring after 40 to 80 minutes. The gallbladder begins to fill within an hour after the infusion is completed; maximum filling is reached after three hours. The contrast medium is finally eliminated in the feces without passing through the enterohepatic circulation, except for approximately 10 percent of the intravenously administered dose which is excreted through the kidneys.

INDICATIONS AND USAGE

Iodipamide Meglumine is indicated for intravenous cholangiography and cholecystography as follows: (a) visualization of the gallbladder and biliary ducts in the differential diagnosis of acute abdominal conditions. (b) visualization of the biliary ducts, especially in patients with symptoms after cholecystectomy, and (c) visualization of the gallbladder in patients unable to take oral contrast media or to absorb contrast media from the gastrointestinal tract.

CONTRAINDICATIONS

Iodipamide Meglumine is contraindicated in patients with a hypersensitivity to salts of Iodipamide or who exhibit sensitivity reactions to the test dose. It is also contraindicated in patients with concomitant severe impairment of renal and liver function.

WARNINGS

Administration of radiopaque materials to patients known or suspected to have pheochromocytoma should be performed with extreme caution. If, in the opinion of the physician, the possible benefits of such procedures outweigh the considered risks, the procedures may be performed; however, the amount of radiopaque medium injected should be kept to an absolute minimum. The blood pressure should be assessed throughout the procedure and measures for treatment of a hypertensive crisis should be available.

Contrast media have been shown to promote the phenomenon of sickling in individuals who are homozygous for sickle cell disease when the material is injected intravenously or intra-arterially.

Since iodine-containing contrast agents may alter the results of thyroid function tests, such tests, if indicated, should be performed prior to the administration of this preparation.

A history of sensitivity to iodine *per se* or to other contrast agents is not an absolute contraindication to the use of Iodipamide Meglumine, but calls for extreme caution in administration.

PRECAUTIONS

Diagnostic procedures which involve the use of radiopaque contrast agents should be carried out under the direction of personnel with the prerequisite training and with a thorough knowledge of the particular procedure to be performed. Appropriate facilities should be available for coping with situations which may arise as a result of the procedure, as well as for emergency treatment of severe reactions to the contrast agent itself.

After intravascular administration of a radiopaque agent, competent personnel and emergency facilities should be available for at least 30 to 60 minutes, since severe delayed reactions have been known to occur.

These severe, life-threatening reactions suggest hypersensitivity to the radiopaque agent, which has prompted the use of several pretesting methods, none of which can be relied upon to predict severe reactions. Many authorities question the value of any pretest. A history of bronchial asthma or allergy, a family history of allergy, or a previous reaction to a contrast agent warrant special attention. Such a history, by suggesting histamine sensitivity and a consequent proneness to reactions, may be more accurate than pretesting in predicting the likelihood of a reaction, although not necessarily the severity or type of reaction in the individual case.

The sensitivity test most often performed is the slow injection of 0.5 to 1.0 ml of the radiopaque medium, administered intravenously, prior to infusion of the full diagnostic dose. It should be noted that the absence of a reaction to the test dose does not preclude the possibility of a reaction to the full diagnostic dose. If the test dose causes an untoward response of any kind, the necessity for continuing with the examination should be carefully reevaluated and, if it is deemed essential, the examination should be conducted with all possible caution. In rare instances reactions to the test dose itself may be extremely severe; therefore, close observation of the patient, and facilities for emergency treatment, appear indicated.

Caution should be exercised with the use of radiopaque media in severely debilitated patients and in those with marked hypertension. The possibility of thrombosis should be borne in mind when intravenous techniques are employed.

Contrast agents may interfere with some chemical determinations made on urine specimens; therefore, urine should be collected before administration of the contrast medium or two or three days afterwards.

The admixture of Diphenhydramine Hydrochloride Injection with Iodipamide Meglumine may cause a precipitate which may form in the syringe or tubing. If antihistamines are administered concomitantly, they should not be mixed with the contrast agent but administered at another site.

USAGE IN PREGNANCY

The safety of Iodipamide Meglumine for use during pregnancy has not been established; therefore, it should be used in pregnant patients, only when, in the judgment of the physician, its use is deemed essential to the welfare of the patient.

◆ RATED THERAPEUTICALLY EQUIVALENT; ◇ THERAPEUTIC EQUIVALENCE UNCONFIRMED; ○ UNRATED

ADVERSE REACTIONS

Local reactions at the site of infusion are not observed, unless excessive amounts are extravasated during infusion. After too rapid administration, mild transient symptoms such as restlessness, sensations of warmth, sneezing, perspiration, salivation, flushing, pressure in the upper abdomen, dizziness, nausea, vomiting, chills, fever, headache, pallor and tremors may occur. These symptoms disappear when the infusion has been completed. Rarely, swollen eyelids, laryngospasm, respiratory difficulties, hypotension, cardiac reactions and cyanosis have been reported. Hypersensitivity reactions may occur. In rare instances, despite the most careful sensitivity testing, anaphylactoid reactions may occur.

Renal function tests may be altered and renal failure may occur.

DOSAGE AND ADMINISTRATION

Iodipamide Meglumine is for intravenous use only.

DIRECTIONS FOR USE

Preparation of the Patient: For best results, the usual preliminary measures for cholecystography are recommended, particularly in cholecystectomized patients, i.e., a low residue diet on the day before examination and administration of castor oil the night before or neostigmine at the time of examination to dispel excess intestinal gas. Cholecystography is preferably carried out in the morning with the patient fasting.

Dose: The usual adult dose is 100 ml.

Note: The dose should not be repeated for 24 hours.

Administration: After warming to body temperature, Iodipamide Meglumine should be given by slow intravenous infusion, following the usual precautions of intravenous administration. *It is preferable that the preparation be infused slowly over a period of 30 to 45 minutes.* During the infusion, the patient should be watched for untoward reactions such as a feeling of warmth, flushing and occasionally nausea. Nausea indicates that the infusion rate is too rapid.

Radiography: A scout film should be exposed routinely before the intravenous infusion is made.

Position of the Patient: With the patient prone and the right side elevated, radiographs are made in the posterior-anterior projection. Some radiologists prefer the supine position with the left side elevated. Serial exposures should begin 20 minutes after the infusion is started and be continued every 20 minutes until optimal visualization of the *biliary ducts* is obtained. Wet films should be examined immediately by the radiologist. In some cases a 15-degree rotation or the upright position may prove helpful. Depending on the situation revealed by the roentgenograms in which the duct is first seen, the position of the subject should be changed to displace the shadow of the common bile duct from that of the spine. Tomography is a useful technique for enhancing bile duct visualization after administration of the radiopaque medium.

Examination of the *gallbladder* should be started about two hours after the infusion is completed. The standard positions in routine examination of the gallbladder should be used unless otherwise indicated. There is no need for the patient to remain quiet awaiting the time for the gallbladder film to be exposed. If the contrast medium should stratify in the gallbladder, decubitus as well as upright films should be obtained. Additional exposures may be made after the ingestion of a fatty meal.

If visualization is not achieved after two and one-half hours, the patient should be returned for a 24-hour film, whenever possible. Occasionally, delayed opacification of the gallbladder will occur in 24 hours.

Note: In the presence of liver disease (BSP retention greater than 30% to 40%), the contrast medium is not excreted efficiently by the liver and visualization is usually not achieved. Visualization is rarely achieved in the presence of a serum bilirubin of 3.0 mg per 100 ml if the elevated bilirubin level is due to mechanical obstruction or hepatocellular damage. In the presence of severe liver damage, the contrast agent is excreted by the kidneys.

Interpretation: When intravenous cholecystography and cholangiography are used as an aid in the differential diagnosis of acute abdominal conditions, visualization of the gallbladder is considered strong evidence against a diagnosis of acute cholecystitis, while nonvisualization of the gallbladder two and one-half hours after administration *with* visualization of the bile ducts is considered strong evidence in favor of a diagnosis of acute cholecystitis (if the bile ducts are only faintly visualized, gallbladder films four hours after administration may occasionally show visualization of the gallbladder). When neither the bile ducts nor the gallbladder is visualized, the study provides no definite information with regard to determining the presence or absence of acute cholecystitis.

STORAGE

Protect from light. Store at room temperature; avoid excessive heat.

HOW SUPPLIED
INJECTION: 10.3%

BRAND/MANUFACTURER	NDC	SIZE	AWP
○ **BRAND**			
CHOLOGRAFIN MEGLUMINE: Bracco Diag	00003-0393-30	100 ml 10s	$608.81

INJECTION: 52%

BRAND/MANUFACTURER	NDC	SIZE	AWP
○ **BRAND**			
CHOLOGRAFIN MEGLUMINE: Bracco Diag	00003-0265-20	20 ml	$52.11
	00003-0265-25	20 ml 25s	$1218.89

Iodopen *SEE* SODIUM IODIDE

Iodoquinol

DESCRIPTION

Iodoquinol is of a light yellowish to tan color, nearly odorless and stable in air. The compound is practically insoluble in water, and sparingly soluble in most other solvents. It contains 64 per cent organically bound iodine.

Following is its chemical structure:

ACTION

Iodoquinol is amebicidal against Entamoeba histolytica and is considered effective against the trophozoite and cyst forms.

INDICATIONS

Iodoquinol is used in the treatment of intestinal amebiasis. Iodoquinol is not recommended for the treatment of non-specific diarrhea.

UNLABELED USES

Iodoquinol is used alone or as an adjunct in the treatment of monilial and nonspecific vulvovaginitis.

CONTRAINDICATIONS

Known hypersensitivity to iodine and 8-hydroxyquinolines. Contraindicated in patients with hepatic damage.

WARNINGS

Optic neuritis, optic atrophy, and peripheral neuropathy have been reported following prolonged high dosage therapy with halogenated 8-hydroxyquinolines. Long term use of this drug should be avoided.

USE IN PREGNANCY

Safety for use in pregnancy or during lactation has not been established.

PRECAUTIONS

Iodoquinol should be used with caution in patients with thyroid disease.

Protein-bound serum iodine levels may be increased during treatment with Iodoquinol and therefore interfere with certain thyroid function tests. These effects may persist for as long as six months after discontinuation of therapy. Discontinue the drug if hypersensitivity reactions occur.

ADVERSE REACTIONS

Skin: various forms of skin eruptions (acneiform papular and pustular; bullae; vegetating of tuberous iododerma), urticaria and pruritus.

Gastrointestinal: nausea, vomiting, abdominal cramps, diarrhea, and pruritus ani.

Fever, chills, headache, vertigo and enlargement of thyroid have been reported. Optic neuritis, optic atrophy and peripheral neuropathy have been reported in association with prolonged high-dosage 8-hydroxyquinoline therapy.

DOSAGE AND ADMINISTRATION

Usual adult dose: (210 mg each) 3 tablets three times daily, after meals for 20 days. Children 6 to 12 years: (210 mg each) 2 tablets, t.i.d. Children under 6: (210 mg each) one tablet per 15 pounds of body weight. Usual adult dose: (650 mg each) one tablet three times a day for twenty days, to be taken after meals. Children (650 mg each): For twenty days, 40 mg per Kg of body weight daily divided into 3 doses, not to exceed 1.95 grams in 24 hours, for 20 days.

Storage: Store at controlled room temperature, 15-30°C. (59-86°F).

HOW SUPPLIED
POWDER:

BRAND/MANUFACTURER	NDC	SIZE	AWP
○ **GENERICS**			
YODOXIN: Glenwood	00516-0091-26	25 gm	$27.18

TABLETS: 210 MG

BRAND/MANUFACTURER	NDC	SIZE	AWP
○ **GENERICS**			
YODOXIN: Glenwood	00516-0092-01	100s	$31.83
YODOXIN: Glenwood	00516-0092-10	1000s	$226.47

➤ SHOWN IN PRODUCT IDENTIFICATION GUIDE

TABLETS: 650 MG

BRAND/MANUFACTURER	NDC	SIZE	AWP
○ **GENERICS**			
YODOQUINOL: Liquipharm	54198-0500-01	100s	$18.20
DIQUINOL: CMC-Cons	00223-0850-01	100s	$30.00
CMC-Cons	00223-0851-01	100s	$30.00
YODOXIN: Glenwood	00516-0093-01	100s	$39.11
DIQUINOL: CMC-Cons	00223-0850-05	500s	$145.00
CMC-Cons	00223-0851-05	500s	$145.00
YODOXIN: Glenwood	00516-0093-10	1000s	$304.31

Iohexol

DESCRIPTION

Iohexol, N,N'-Bis(2,3-dihydroxypropyl)-5-[N-(2, 3-dihydroxypropyl)-acetamido]-2,4,6-triiodoisophthalamide, is a nonionic, water-soluble radiographic contrast medium with a molecular weight of 821.14 (iodine content 46.36%). In aqueous solution each triiodinated molecule remains undissociated.

Iohexol is a sterile, pyrogen-free, colorless to pale yellow solution, in the following iodine concentrations: 140, 180, 210, 240, 300, and 350 mgI/mL. Iohexol 140 contains 302 mg of Iohexol equivalent to 140 mg of organic iodine per mL; Iohexol 180 contains 388 mg of Iohexol equivalent to 180 mg of organic iodine per mL; Iohexol 210 contains 453 mg of Iohexol equivalent to 210 mg of organic iodine per mL; Iohexol 240 contains 518 mg of Iohexol equivalent to 240 mg of organic iodine per mL; Iohexol 300 contains 647 mg of Iohexol equivalent to 300 mg of organic iodine per mL; and Iohexol 350 contains 755 mg of Iohexol equivalent to 350 mg of organic iodine per mL. Each milliliter of Iohexol solution contains 1.21 mg tromethamine and 0.1 mg edetate calcium disodium with the pH adjusted between 6.8 and 7.7 with hydrochloric acid or sodium hydroxide. All solutions are sterilized by autoclaving and contain no preservatives. Unused portions must be discarded. Iohexol solution is sensitive to light and therefore should be protected from exposure.

The available concentrations have the following physical properties: (See related table).

Iohexol has an osmolality from approximately 1.1 to 3.0 times that of plasma (285 mOsm/kg water) or cerebrospinal fluid (301 mOsm/kg water) as shown in the above table and is hypertonic under conditions of use.

Following is its chemical structure:

SECTION I
CLINICAL PHARMACOLOGY
INTRATHECAL

Iohexol is absorbed from cerebrospinal fluid (CSF) into the bloodstream and is eliminated by renal excretion. No significant metabolism, deiodination, or biotransformation occurs. In five adult patients receiving 16 to 18 milliliters of Iohexol (180 mgI/mL) by lumbar intrathecal injection, approximately 88 (73.1-98.2) percent of the injected dose was excreted in the urine within the first 24 hours after administration. The renal and body clearances were 99 (47-137) milliliters per minute and 109 (52-138) milliliters per minute. The mean maximal plasma concentration was 119 (72-177) micrograms of Iohexol per milliliter and occurred after 3.8 (2-6) hours. The volume of distribution was 557 (350-849) milliliters per kilogram. In one patient with a large spinal cord tumor, excretion was delayed (67 percent of the dose appeared in the urine within the first 24 hours) with no difference in the total overall recovery in the urine after 48 hours. The delay in excretion appeared to be related to a decrease in the rate of transfer of Iohexol from the cerebrospinal fluid to the blood (plasma maximal concentration was approximately 30 micrograms/mL).

The initial concentration and volume of the medium, in conjunction with appropriate patient manipulation and the volume of CSF into which the medium is placed, will determine the extent of the diagnostic contrast that can be achieved.

Following intrathecal injection in conventional radiography, Iohexol 180, Iohexol 210, Iohexol 240, and Iohexol 300 will continue to provide good

diagnostic contrast for at least 30 minutes. Slow diffusion of Iohexol takes place throughout the CSF with subsequent absorption into the bloodstream. Once in the systemic circulation, Iohexol displays little tendency to bind to serum or plasma proteins. At approximately 1 hour following injection, contrast of diagnostic quality will no longer be available for conventional myelography. If computerized tomographic (CT) myelography is to follow, consideration should be given to a delay of several hours to allow the degree of contrast to decrease.

After administration into the lumbar subarachnoid space, computerized tomography shows the presence of contrast medium in the thoracic region in about 1 hour, in the cervical region in about 2 hours, and in the basal cisterns in 3 to 4 hours.

In patients with renal impairment, depending on the degree of impairment, prolonged plasma Iohexol levels may be anticipated due to decreased renal elimination.

INDICATIONS AND USAGE
INTRATHECAL

Iohexol 180, Iohexol 240, and Iohexol 300 are indicated for intrathecal administration in adults including myelography (lumbar, thoracic, cervical, total columnar) and in contrast enhancement for computerized tomography (myelography, cisternography, ventriculography).

Iohexol 180 and Iohexol 210 are indicated for intrathecal administration in children including myelography (lumbar, thoracic, cervical, total columnar) and in contrast enhancement for computerized tomography (myelography, cisternography).

CONTRAINDICATIONS
INTRATHECAL

Iohexol should not be administered to patients with a known hypersensitivity to Iohexol.

Myelography should not be performed in the presence of significant local or systemic infection where bacteremia is likely.

Intrathecal administration of corticosteroids with Iohexol is contraindicated.

Because of the possibility of overdosage, immediate repeat myelography in the event of technical failure is contraindicated (see "Dosage and Administration").

WARNINGS
GENERAL

If grossly bloody CSF is encountered, the possible benefits of a myelographic procedure should be considered in terms of the risk to the patient.

Caution is advised in patients with a history of epilepsy, severe cardiovascular disease, chronic alcoholism, or multiple sclerosis.

Elderly patients may present a greater risk following myelography. The need for the procedure in these patients should be evaluated carefully. Special attention must be paid to dose and concentration of the medium, hydration, and technique used.

Patients who are receiving anticonvulsants should be maintained on this therapy. Should a seizure occur, intravenous diazepam or phenobarbital sodium is recommended. In patients with a history of seizure activity who are not on anticonvulsant therapy, premedication with barbiturates should be considered.

Prophylactic anticonvulsant treatment with barbiturates should be considered in patients with evidence of inadvertent intracranial entry of a large or concentrated bolus of the contrast medium since there may be an increased risk of seizure in such cases.

Drugs which lower the seizure threshold, especially phenothiazine derivatives, including those used for their antihistamine properties, are not recommended for use with Iohexol. Others include MAO inhibitors, tricyclic antidepressants, CNS stimulants, and psychoactive drugs described as analeptics, major tranquilizers, or antipsychotic drugs. While the contributory role of these medications has not been established, the use of such drugs should be based on physician evaluation of potential benefits and potential risks. Physicans have discontinued these agents at least 48 hours before and for at least 24 hours postprocedure. Care is required in patient management to prevent inadvertent intracranial entry of a large dose or concentrated bolus of the medium. Also, effort should be directed to avoid rapid dispersion of the medium causing inadvertent rise to intracranial levels (e.g., by active patient movement). Direct intracisternal or ventricular administration for standard radiography (not CT) is not recommended.

In most reported cases of major motor seizures with nonionic myelographic media, one or more of the following factors were present. Therefore avoid:

- Deviations from recommended procedure or in myelographic management.
- Use in patients with a history of epilepsy.

Concentration (mgI/mL)	Osmolality* (mOsm/kg water)	Osmolarity (mOsm/L)	Absolute Viscosity (cp)		Specific Gravity 37°C
			20°C	37°C	
140	322	273	2.3	1.5	1.164
180	408	331	3.1	2.0	1.209
210	460	362	4.2	2.5	1.244
240	520	391	5.8	3.4	1.280
300	672	465	11.8	6.3	1.349
350	844	541	20.4	10.4	1.406

* By vapor-pressure osmometry.

◆ RATED THERAPEUTICALLY EQUIVALENT; ◇ THERAPEUTIC EQUIVALENCE UNCONFIRMED; ○ UNRATED

- Overdosage.
- Intracranial entry of a bolus or premature diffusion of a high concentration of the medium.
- Medication with neuroleptic drugs or phenothiazine antinauseants.
- Failure to maintain elevation of the head during the procedure, on the stretcher, or in bed.
- Excessive and particularly active patient movement or straining.

PRECAUTIONS

GENERAL

Diagnostic procedures which involve the use of radiopaque diagnostic agents should be carried out under the direction of personnel with the prerequisite training and with a thorough knowledge of the particular procedure to be performed. Appropriate facilities should be available for coping with any complication of the procedure, as well as for emergency treatment of severe reactions to the contrast agent itself. After parenteral administration of a radiopaque agent, competent personnel and emergency facilities should be available for at least 30 to 60 minutes since severe delayed reactions have occurred. (See *"Adverse Reactions"*.)

Preparatory dehydration is dangerous and may contribute to acute renal failure in patients with advanced vascular disease, diabetic patients, and in susceptible nondiabetic patients (often elderly with preexisting renal disease). Dehydration in these patients seems to be enhanced by the osmotic diuretic action of contrast agents. *Patients should be well hydrated prior to and following administration of any contrast medium, including Iohexol.*

The possibility of a reaction, including serious, life-threatening, fatal, anaphylactoid, cardiovascular or central nervous system reactions, should always be considered (see *"Adverse Reactions"*). Therefore, it is of utmost importance that a course of action be carefully planned in advance for the immediate treatment of serious reactions, and that adequate and appropriate facilities and personnel be readily available in case of any reaction.

The possibility of an idiosyncratic reaction in susceptible patients should always be considered (see *"Adverse Reactions"*). The susceptible population includes, but is not limited to, patients with a history of a previous reaction to contrast media, patients with a known sensitivity to iodine per se, and patients with a known clinical hypersensitivity: bronchial asthma, hay fever, and food allergies.

The occurrence of severe idiosyncratic reactions has prompted the use of several pretesting methods. However, pretesting cannot be relied upon to predict severe reactions and may itself be hazardous for the patient. It is suggested that a thorough medical history with emphasis on allergy and hypersensitivity, prior to the injection of any contrast media, may be more accurate than pretesting in predicting potential adverse reactions.

A positive history of allergies or hypersensitivity does not arbitrarily contraindicate the use of a contrast agent where a diagnostic procedure is thought essential, but caution should be exercised (see *"Adverse Reactions"*). Premedication with antihistamines or corticosteroids to avoid or minimize possible allergic reactions in such patients should be considered. Recent reports indicate that such pretreatment does not prevent serious life-threatening reactions, but may reduce both their incidence and severity.

In patients with severe renal insufficiency or failure, compensatory biliary excretion of the drug is anticipated to occur, with a slow clearance into the bile. Patients with hepatorenal insufficiency should not be examined unless the possibility of benefit clearly outweighs the additional risk.

Administration of contrast media should be performed by qualified personnel familiar with the procedure and appropriate patient management (see *"Patient Management"*). Sterile technique must be used with any spinal puncture.

When Iohexol is to be injected using plastic disposable syringes, the contrast medium should be drawn into the syringe and used immediately.

If nondisposable equipment is used, scrupulous care should be taken to prevent residual contamination with traces of cleansing agents.

Parenteral products should be inspected visually for particulate matter and discoloration prior to administration. If particulate matter or discoloration is present, do not use.

Repeat Procedures: If in the clinical judgment of the physician sequential or repeat examinations are required, a suitable interval of time between administrations should be observed to allow for normal clearance of the drug from the body (see *"Dosage and Administration"* and *"Clinical Pharmacology"*).

Information for Patients (or if applicable, children): Patients receiving injectable radiopaque diagnostic agents should be instructed to:

1. Inform your physician if you are pregnant (see *"Clinical Pharmacology"*).
2. Inform your physician if you are diabetic or if you have multiple myeloma, pheochromocytoma, homozygous sickle cell disease or known thyroid disorder (see *"Warnings"*).
3. Inform your physician if you are allergic to any drugs, food, or if you had any reactions to previous injections of dyes used for x-ray procedures (see *"Precautions—General"*).
4. Inform your physician about any other medications you are currently taking, including nonprescription drugs, before you are administered this drug.

Drug Interactions: Drugs which lower seizure threshold, especially phenothiazine derivatives including those used for their antihistaminic or antinauseant properties, are not recommended for use with Iohexol. Others include monoamine oxidase (MAO) inhibitors, tricyclic antidepressants, CNS stimulants, psychoactive drugs described as analeptics, major tranquilizers, or antipsychotic drugs.

Such medications should be discontinued at least 48 hours before myelography, should not be used for the control of nausea or vomiting during or after myelography, and should not be resumed for at least 24 hours postprocedure. In nonelective procedures in patients on these drugs, consider prophylactic use of anticonvulsants.

Carcinogenesis, Mutagenesis, Impairment of Fertility: No long-term animal studies have been performed to evaluate carcinogenic potential, mutagenesis, or whether Iohexol can affect fertility in men or women.

Pregnancy Category B: Reproduction studies have been performed in rats and rabbits with up to 100 times the recommended human dose. No evidence of impaired fertility or harm to the fetus has been demonstrated due to Iohexol. There are, however, no studies in pregnant women. Because animal reproduction studies are not always predictive of human response, this drug should be used during pregnancy only if clearly needed.

Nursing Mothers: It is not known to what extent Iohexol is excreted in human milk. However, many injectable contrast agents are excreted unchanged in human milk. Although it has not been established that serious adverse reactions occur in nursing infants, caution should be exercised when intravascular contrast media are administered to nursing women. Bottle feedings may be substituted for breast feedings for 24 hours following administration of Iohexol.

Pediatric Use: Pediatric patients at higher risk of experiencing adverse events during contrast medium administration may include those having asthma, a sensitivity to medication and/or allergens, congestive heart failure, a serum creatinine greater than 1.5 mg/dL or those less than 12 months of age.

ADVERSE REACTIONS

INTRATHECAL

The most frequently reported adverse reactions with Iohexol are headache, mild to moderate pain including backache, neckache and stiffness, nausea, and vomitting. These reactions usually occur 1 to 10 hours after injection, and almost all occur within 24 hours. They are usually mild to moderate in degree, lasting for a few hours, and usually disappearing within 24 hours. Rarely, headaches may be severe or persist for days. Headache is often accompanied by nausea and vomiting and tends to be more frequent and persistent in patients not optimally hydrated.

Transient alterations in vital signs may occur and their significance must be assessed on an individual basis. Those reactions reported in clinical studies with Iohexol are listed below in decreasing order of occurrence, based on clinical studies of 1531 patients.

Headaches: The most frequently occurring adverse reaction following myelography has been headache, with an incidence of approximately 18%. Headache may be caused by either a direct effect of the contrast medium or by CSF leakage at the dural puncture site. However, in managing the patient, it is considered more important to minimize intracranial entry of contrast medium by postural management than attempting to control possible CSF leakage (see *"Patient Management"*).

Pain: Mild to moderate pain including backache, neckache and stiffness, and neuralgia occurred following injection with an incidence of about 8%.

Nausea and Vomiting: Nausea was reported with an incidence of about 6%, and vomiting about 3% (see *"Patient Management"*). Maintaining normal hydration is very important. The use of phenothiazine antinauseants is not recommended. (See *"Warnings—General."*) Reassurance to the patient that the nausea will clear usually is all that is required.

Dizziness: Transient dizziness was reported in about 2% of the patients.

Other Reactions: Other reactions occurring with an individual incidence of less than 0.1% included: feeling of heaviness, hypotension, hypertonia, sensation of heat, sweating, vertigo, loss of appetite, drowsiness, hypertension, photophobia, tinnitus, neuralgia, paresthesia, difficulty in micturition, and neurological changes. All were transient and mild with no clinical sequelae.

Pediatrics: In controlled clinical trials involving 152 patients for pediatric myelography by lumbar puncture, adverse events following the use of Iohexol 180 and Iohexol 210 were generally less frequent than with adults.

Headache: 9%

Vomiting: 6%

Backache: 1.3%

Other Reactions: Other reactions occurring with an individual incidence of less than 0.7% included: fever, hives, stomachache, visual hallucination, and neurological changes. All were transient and mild with no clinical sequelae.

General Adverse Reactions to Contrast Media: Physicians should remain alert for the occurrence of adverse effects in addition to those discussed above, particularly the following reactions which have been reported in the literature for other nonionic, water-soluble myelographic media, and rarely with Iohexol. These have included, but are not limited to, convulsion, aseptic and bacterial meningitis, and CNS and other neurological disturbances.

An aseptic meningitis syndrome has been reported rarely (less than 0.01%). It was usually preceded by pronounced headaches, nausea and vomiting. Onset usually occurred about 12 to 18 hours postprocedure. Prominent features were meningismus, fever, sometimes with oculomotor signs and mental confusion. Lumbar puncture revealed a high white cell count, high protein content often with a low glucose level and with absence of organisms. The condition usually started to clear spontaneously about 10 hours after onset, with complete recovery over 2 to 3 days.

Allergy or Idiosyncrasy: Chills, fever, profuse diaphoresis, pruritus, urticaria, nasal congestion, dyspnea, and a case of Guillain-Barré syndrome.

CNS Irritation: Mild and transitory perceptual aberrations such as hallucinations, depersonalization, amnesia, hostility, amblyopia, diplopia, photophobia, psychosis, insomnia, anxiety, depression, hyperesthesia, visual or auditory or speech disturbances, confusion and disorientation. In addition, malaise, weakness, convulsion, EEG changes, meningismus, hyperreflexia or areflexia, hypertonia or flaccidity, hemiplegia, paralysis, quadriplegia, restlessness, tremor, echoacousia, echolalia, asterixis, cerebral hemorrhage, and dysphasia have occurred.

Profound mental disturbances have also rarely been reported. They have usually consisted of various forms and degrees of aphasia, mental confusion, or disorientation. The onset is usually at 8 to 10 hours and lasts for about 24 hours, without aftereffects. However, occasionally they have been manifest as apprehension, agitation, or progressive withdrawal in several instances to the point of somnolence, stupor, and coma. In a few cases these have been accompanied by transitory hearing loss or other auditory symptoms and visual disturbances (believed subjective or delusional), including unilateral or bilateral loss of vision which may last for hours. In one case, persistent cortical loss of vision has been reported in association with convulsions. Ventricular block has been reported; amnesia of varying degrees may be present for the reaction event.

Rarely, persistent though transitory weakness in the leg or ocular muscles has been reported.

Peripheral neuropathies have been rare and transitory. They include sensory and/or motor or nerve root disturbances, myelitis, persistent leg muscle pain or weakness, 6th nerve palsy, or cauda equina syndrome. Muscle cramps, fasciculation or myoclonia, spinal convulsion, or spasticity is unusual and has responded promptly to a small intravenous dose of diazepam.

In general, the reactions which are known to occur upon parenteral administration of iodinated contrast agents are possible with any nonionic agent. Approximately 95 percent of adverse reactions accompanying the use of water-soluble contrast agents are mild to moderate in degree. However, severe, life-threatening, anaphylactoid and fatal reactions, mostly of cardiovascular origin and central nervous system origin, have occurred.

Adverse reactions to injectable contrast media fall into two categories: chemotoxic reactions and idiosyncratic reactions. Chemotoxic reactions result from the physicochemical properties of the contrast media, the dose, and speed of injection. All hemodynamic disturbances and injuries to organs or vessels perfused by the contrast medium are included in this category.

Idiosyncratic reactions include all other reactions. They occur more frequently in patients 20 to 40 years old. Idiosyncratic reactions may or may not be dependent on the amount of dose injected, the speed of injection, and the radiographic procedure. Idiosyncratic reactions are subdivided into minor, intermediate, and severe. The minor reactions are self-limited and of short duration; the severe reactions are life-threatening and treatment is urgent and mandatory.

The reported incidence of adverse reactions to contrast media in patients with a history of allergy is twice that of the general population. Patients with a history of previous reactions to a contrast medium are three times more susceptible than other patients. However, sensitivity to contrast media does not appear to increase with repeated examinations.

Most adverse reactions to injectable contrast media appear within 1 to 3 minutes after the start of injection, but delayed reactions may occur.

OVERDOSAGE

Clinical consequences of overdosage with Iohexol have not been reported. However, based on experience with other nonionic myelographic media, physicians should be alert to a potential increase in frequency and severity of CNS-mediated reactions. Even use of a recommended dose can produce effects tantamount to overdosage, if incorrect management of the patient during or immediately following the procedure permits inadvertent early intracranial entry of a large portion of the medium.

The intracisternal LD_{50} value of Iohexol (in grams of iodine per kilogram body weight) is greater than 2.0 in mice.

DOSAGE AND ADMINISTRATION

INTRATHECAL

The volume and concentration of Iohexol 180, Iohexol 210, Iohexol 240, or Iohexol 800 to be administered will depend on the degree and extent of contrast required in the area(s) under examination and on the equipment and technique employed.

Iohexol 180 at a concentration of 180 mgI/mL, Iohexol 240 at a concentration of 240 mgI/mL, or Iohexol 300 at a concentration of 300 mgI/mL is recommended for the examination of the lumbar, thoracic, and cervical regions in adults by lumbar or direct cervical injection and is slightly hypertonic to CSF.

Iohexol 180 at a concentration of 180 mgI/mL or Iohexol 210 at a concentration of 210 mgI/mL is recommended for the examination of the lumbar, thoracic, and cervical regions in children by lumbar injection and is slightly hypertonic to CSF.

A total dose of 3060 mg iodine or a concentration of 300 mgI/mL should not be exceeded in adults and a total dose of 2940 mg iodine or a concentration of 210 mgI/mL should not be exceeded in children in a single myleographic examination. This is based on clinical trial evaluation to date. As in all diagnostic procedures, the minimum volume and dose to produce adequate visualization should be used. Most procedures do not require either maximum dose or concentration.

Anesthesia is not necessary. Premedication sedatives or tranquilizers are usually not needed (see *"Precautions"*). Patients should be well hydrated prior to and following contrast administration. Seizure-prone patients should be maintained on anticonvulsant medication.

Many radiopaque contrast agents are incompatible *in vitro* with some antihistamines and many other drugs; therefore, concurrent drugs should not be physically admixed with contrast agents.

Rate of Injection: To avoid excessive mixing with CSF and consequent dilution of contrast, injection should be made slowly over 1 to 2 minutes.

Depending on the estimated volume of contrast medium which may be required for the procedure a small amount of CSF may be removed to minimize distention of the subarachnoid spaces.

The lumbar or cervical puncture needle may be removed immediately following injection since it is not necessary to remove Iohexol after injection into the subarachnoid space.

Adults: The usual recommended total doses for use in lumbar, thoracic, cervical, and total columnar myelography in adults are 1.2 gI to 3.06 gI as follows: (See related table).

Pediatrics: The usual recommended total doses for lumbar, thoracic, cervical, and/or total columnar myelography by lumbar puncture in children are 0.36 gI to 2.94 gI (see table below). Actual volumes administered depend largely on patient age and the following guidelines are recommended.

Age	Conc. (mgI/mL)	Volume (mL)	Dose (gI)
0 to < 3 mos.	180	2— 4	0.36—0.72
	210	2— 3	0.42—0.63
3 to < 36 mos.	180	4— 8	0.72—1.44
	210	3— 6	0.63—1.26
3 to < 7 yrs.	180	5—10	0.9 —1.8
	210	5— 8	1.05—1.68
7 to < 13 yrs.	180	5—12	0.9 —2.16
	210	5—10	1.05—2.1
13 to 18 yrs.	180	6—15	1.08—2.7
	210	6—14	1.26—2.94

Withdrawal of contrast agents from their containers should be accomplished under aseptic conditions with sterile syringes. Spinal puncture must always be performed under sterile conditions.

Parenteral products should be inspected visually for particulate matter or discoloration prior to administration. If particulate matter or discoloration is present, do not use.

Repeat Procedures: If in the clinical judgment of the physician sequential or repeat examinations are required, a suitable interval of time between administrations should be observed to allow for normal clearance of the drug from the body. An interval of at least 48 hours should be allowed before repeat examination; however, whenever possible, 5 to 7 days is recommended.

PATIENT MANAGEMENT

INTRATHECAL

Suggestions for Usual Patient Management

Good patient management should be exercised at all times to minimize the potential for procedurally related complications.

Preprocedure:
- Discontinuance of neuroleptic drugs (including phenothiazines, e.g., chlorpromazine, prochlorperazine, and promethazine) at least 48 hours beforehand should be considered.
- Maintain normal diet up to 2 hours before procedure.
- Ensure hydration—fluids up to procedure.

During Procedure:
- Use minimum dose and concentration required for satisfactory contrast (see *"Dosage and Administration"*).
- In all positioning techniques keep the patient's head elevated above highest level of spine.
- Do not lower head of table more than 15° in moving contrast medium cranially.
- In patients with excessive lordosis, consider lateral position for injection and movement of the medium cephalad.
- Inject slowly (over 1 to 2 minutes) to avoid excessive mixing.
- To maintain as a bolus, move medium to distal area *very slowly*. Use fluoroscopic monitoring.
- Avoid intracranial entry of a bolus.
- Avoid early and high cephalad dispersion of the medium.
- Avoid abrupt or active patient movement to minimize excessive mixing of medium with CSF. Instruct patient to remain *passive*. Move patient *slowly* and only as necessary.

Postprocedure:
- Raise head of stretcher to at least 30° before moving patient onto it.
- Movement onto and off the stretcher should be done slowly with the patient completely passive, maintaining *head-up* position.
- Before moving patient onto bed, raise head of bed 30° to 45°.
- Advise patient to remain still in bed, in a sitting or semisitting position, especially in the first few hours.
- Maintain close observation for at least 12 hours after myelogram.

◆ RATED THERAPEUTICALLY EQUIVALENT; ◇ THERAPEUTIC EQUIVALENCE UNCONFIRMED; ○ UNRATED

- Obtain vistors' cooperation in keeping the patient quiet and in *head-up* position, especially in first few hours.
- Encourage oral fluids. Diet as tolerated.
- *If nausea or vomiting occurs*, do not use phenothiazine antinauseants. Persistent nausea and vomiting will result in dehydration. Therefore, prompt consideration of replacement by intravenous fluids is recommended.

Alternative Postprocedure Method:
- Recent evidence with nonionic, water-soluble contrast media suggests that maintaining the patient postmyelography in an upright position (via wheelchair or ambulation) may help minimize adverse effects. The upright position may help to delay upward dispersion of the medium and to maximize the spinal arachnoid absorption.

Storage: Protect vials of Iohexol from strong daylight and direct exposure to sunlight. Do not freeze. Store at 59°F to 86°F (15°C to 30°C).

SECTION II
CLINICAL PHARMACOLOGY
INTRAVASCULAR
Following intravascular injection, Iohexol is distributed in the extracellular fluid compartment and is excreted unchanged by glomerular filtration. It will opacify those vessels in the path of flow of the contrast medium permitting radiographic visualization of the internal structures until significant hemodilution occurs.

Approximately 90% or more of the injected dose is excreted within the first 24 hours, with the peak urine concentrations occurring in the first hour after administration. Plasma and urine Iohexol levels indicate that the Iohexol body clearance is due primarily to renal clearance. An increase in the dose from 500 mgI/kg to 1500 mgI/kg does not significantly alter the clearance of the drug. The following pharmacokinetic values were observed following the intravenous administration of Iohexol (between 500 mgI/kg to 1500 mgI/kg) to 16 adult human subjects: renal clearance—120 (86-162) mL/min; total body clearance—131 (98-165) mL/min; and volume of distribution—165 (108-219) mL/kg.

Renal accumulation is sufficiently rapid that the period of maximal opacification of the renal passages may begin as early as 1 minute after intravenous injection. Urograms become apparent in about 1 to 3 minutes with optimal contrast occurring between 5 to 15 minutes. In nephropathic conditions, particularly when excretory capacity has been altered, the rate of excretion may vary unpredictably, and opacification may be delayed after injection. Severe renal impairment may result in a lack of diagnostic opacification of the collecting system and, depending on the degree of renal impairment, prolonged plasma Iohexol levels may be anticipated. In these patients, as well as in infants with immature kidneys, the route of excretion through the gallbladder and into the small intestine may increase.

Iohexol displays a low affinity for serum or plasma proteins and is poorly bound to serum albumin. No significant metabolism deiodination or biotransformation occurs.

Iohexol probably crosses the placental barrier in humans by simple diffusion. It is not known to what extent Iohexol is excreted in human milk.

Animal studies indicate that Iohexol does not cross an intact blood-brain barrier to any significant extent following intravascular administration.

Iohexol enhances computed tomographic imaging through augmentation of radiographic efficiency. The degree of density enhancement is directly related to the iodine content in an administered dose; peak iodine blood levels occur immediately following rapid intravenous injection. Blood levels fall rapidly within 5 to 10 minutes and the vascular compartment half-life is approximately 20 minutes. This can be accounted for by the dilution in the vascular and extravascular fluid compartments which causes an initial sharp fall in plasma concentration. Equilibration with the extracellular compartments is reached in about ten minutes; thereafter, the fall becomes exponential.

The pharmacokinetics of Iohexol in both normal and abnormal tissue have been shown to be variable. Contrast enhancement appears to be greatest immediately after bolus administration (15 seconds to 120 seconds). Thus, greatest enhancement may be detected by a series of consecutive two-to-three second scans performed within 30 to 90 seconds after injection (i.e., dynamic computed tomographic imaging). Utilization of a continuous scanning technique (i.e., dynamic CT scanning) may improve enhancement and diagnostic assessment of tumor and other lesions such as abscess, occasionally revealing unsuspected or more extensive disease. For example, a cyst may be distinguished from a vascularized solid lesion when precontrast and enhanced scans are compared; the nonperfused mass shows unchanged x-ray absorption (CT number). A vascularized lesion is characterized by an increase in CT number in the few minutes after a bolus of intravascular contrast agent; it may be malignant, benign, or normal tissue, but would probably not be a cyst, hematoma, or other nonvascular lesion.

Because unenhanced scanning may provide adequate diagnostic information in the individual patient, the decision to employ contrast enhancement, which may be associated with risk and increased radiation exposure, should be based upon a careful evaluation of clinical, other radiological, and unenhanced CT findings.

CT SCANNING OF THE HEAD
In contrast enhanced computed tomographic head imaging, Iohexol does not accumulate in normal brain tissue due to the presence of the normal blood-brain barrier. The increase in x-ray absorption in normal brain is due to the presence of contrast agent within the blood pool. A break in the blood-brain barrier such as occurs in malignant tumors of the brain allows for the accumulation of contrast medium within the interstitial tissue of the tumor. Adjacent normal brain tissue does not contain the contrast medium.

Maximum contrast enhancement in tissue frequently occurs after peak blood iodine levels are reached. A delay in maximum contrast enhancement can occur. Diagnostic contrast enhanced images of the brain have been obtained up to 1 hour after intravenous bolus administration. This delay suggests that radiographic contrast enhancement is at least in part dependent on the accumulation of iodine containing medium within the lesion and outside the blood pool, although the mechanism by which this occurs is not clear. The radiographic enhancement of nontumoral lesions, such as arteriovenous malformations and aneurysms, is probably dependent on the iodine content of the circulating blood pool. In patients where the blood-brain barrier is known or suspected to be disrupted, the use of any radiographic contrast medium must be assessed on an individual risk to benefit basis. However, compared to ionic media, nonionic media are less toxic to the central nervous system.

CT SCANNING OF THE BODY
In contrast enhanced computed tomographic body imaging (nonneural tissue), Iohexol diffuses rapidly from the vascular into the extravascular space. Increase in x-ray absorption is related to blood flow, concentration of the contrast medium, and extraction of the contrast medium by interstitial tissue of tumors since no barrier exists. Contrast enhancement is thus due to the relative differences in extravascular diffusion between normal and abnormal tissue, quite different from that in the brain.

INDICATIONS AND USAGE
INTRAVASCULAR
General: Iohexol 350 is indicated in adults for angiocardiography (ventriculography, selective coronary arteriography), aortography including studies of the aortic root, aortic arch, ascending aorta, abdominal aorta and its branches, contrast enhancement for computed tomographic head and body imaging, intravenous digital subtraction angiography of the head, neck, abdominal, renal and peripheral vessels, peripheral arteriography, and excretory urography.

Iohexol 350 is indicated in children for angiocardiography (ventriculography, pulmonary arteriography, and venography; studies of the collateral arteries and aortography, including the aortic root, aortic arch, ascending and descending aorta).

Iohexol 300 is indicated in adults for aortography including studies of the aortic arch, abdominal aorta and its branches, contrast enhancement for computed tomographic head and body imaging, cerebral arteriography, peripheral venography (phlebography), and excretory urography.

Iohexol 300 is indicated in children for angiocardiography (ventriculography), excretory urography, and contrast enhancement for computed tomographic head imaging.

Iohexol 240 is indicated in adults for contrast enhancement for computed tomographic head imaging and peripheral venography (phlebography).

Iohexol 140 is indicated in adults for intra-arterial digital subtraction angiography of the head, neck, abdominal, renal and peripheral vessels.

Iohexol 240 is indicated in children for contrast enhancement for computed tomographic head imaging.

Procedure	Formulations	Concentration (mgI/mL)	Volume (mL)	Dose (gI)
Lumbar Myelography (via lumbar injection)	Iohexol 180	180	10—17	1.8—3.06
	Iohexol 240	240	7—12.5	1.7—3.0
Thoracic Myelography (via lumbar or cervical injection)	Iohexol 240	240	6—12.5	1.7—3.0
	Iohexol 300	300	6—10	1.8—3.0
Cervical Myelography (via lumbar injection)	Iohexol 240	240	6—12.5	1.4—3.0
	Iohexol 300	300	6—10	1.8—3.0
Cervical Myelography (via C1-2 injection)	Iohexol 180	180	7—10	1.3—1.8
	Iohexol 240	240	6—12.5	1.4—3.0
	Iohexol 300	300	4—10	1.2—3.0
Total Columnar Myelography (via lumbar injection)	Iohexol 240	240	6—12.5	1.4—3.0
	Iohexol 300	300	6—10	1.8—3.0

➤ SHOWN IN PRODUCT IDENTIFICATION GUIDE

CONTRAINDICATIONS

Iohexol should not be administered to patients with a known hypersensitivity to Iohexol.

WARNINGS

General: Nonionic iodinated contrast media inhibit blood coagulation, *in vitro,* less than ionic contrast media. Clotting has been reported when blood remains in contact with syringes containing nonionic contrast media.

Serious, rarely fatal, thromboembolic events causing myocardial infarction and stroke have been reported during angiographic procedures with both ionic and nonionic contrast media. Therefore, meticulous intravascular administration technique is necessary, particularly during angiographic procedures, to minimize thromboembolic events. Numerous factors, including length of procedure, catheter and syringe material, underlying disease state, and concomitant medications may contribute to the development of thromboembolic events. For these reasons, meticulous angiographic techniques are recommended including close attention to guidewire and catheter manipulation, use of manifold systems and/or three-way stopcocks, frequent catheter flushing with heparinized saline solutions and minimizing the length of the procedure. The use of plastic syringes in place of glass syringes has been reported to decrease but not eliminate the likelihood of *in vitro* clotting.

Iohexol should be used with extreme care in patients with severe functional disturbances of the liver and kidneys, severe thyrotoxicosis, or myelomatosis. Diabetics with a serum creatinine level above 3 mg/dL should not be examined unless the possible benefits of the examination clearly outweigh the additional risk. Iohexol is not recommended for use in patients with anuria.

Radiopaque contrast agents are potentially hazardous in patients with multiple myeloma or other paraproteinemia, particularly in those with therapeutically resistant anuria. Although neither the contrast agent nor dehydration has separately proven to be the cause of anuria in myeloma, it has been speculated that the combination of both may be causative factors. The risk in myelomatous patients is not a contraindication; however, special precautions are necessary. Partial dehydration in the preparation of these patients prior to injection is not recommended since this may predispose the patient to precipitation of the myeloma protein in the renal tubules. No form of therapy, including dialysis, has been successful in reversing the effect. Myeloma, which occurs most commonly in persons over age 40, should be considered before instituting intravascular administration of contrast agents.

Ionic contrast media, when injected intravenously or intraarterially, may promote sickling in individuals who are homozygous for sickle cell disease.

Administration of radiopaque materials to patients known or suspected of having pheochromocytoma should be performed with extreme caution. If, in the opinion of the physician, the possible benefits of such procedures outweigh the considered risks, the procedures may be performed; however, the amount of radiopaque medium injected should be kept to an absolute minimum. The patient's blood pressure should be assessed throughout the procedure and measures for the treatment of hypertensive crisis should be readily available.

Reports of thyroid storm following the use of iodinated, ionic radiopaque contrast media in patients with hyperthyroidism or with an autonomously functioning thyroid nodule suggest that this additional risk be evaluated in such patients before use of any contrast medium.

Urography should be performed with caution in patients with severely impaired renal function and patients with combined renal and hepatic disease.

PRECAUTIONS

General: Diagnostic procedures which involve the use of radiopaque diagnostic agents should be carried out under the direction of personnel with the prerequisite training and with a thorough knowledge of the particular procedure to be performed. Appropriate facilities should be available for coping with any complication of the procedure, as well as for emergency treatment of severe reactions to the contrast agent itself. After parenteral administration of a radiopaque agent, competent personnel and emergency facilities should be available for at least 30 to 60 minutes since severe delayed reactions have occurred (see *"Adverse Reactions: Intravascular—General"*).

Preparatory dehydration is dangerous and may contribute to acute renal failure in patients with advanced vascular disease, diabetic patients, and in susceptible nondiabetic patients (often elderly with preexisting renal disease), infants and small children. Dehydration in these patients seems to be enhanced by the osmotic diuretic action of urographic agents. It is believed that overnight fluid restriction prior to excretory urography generally does not provide better visualization in normal patients. *Patients should be well hydrated prior to and following administration of any contrast medium, including Iohexol.*

Acute renal failure has been reported in diabetic patients with diabetic nephropathy and in susceptible nondiabetic patients (often elderly with preexisting renal disease) following excretory urography. Therefore, careful consideration of the potential risks should be given before performing this radiographic procedure in these patients.

Immediately following surgery, excretory urography should be used with caution in renal transplant recipients.

The possibility of a reaction, including serious, life-threatening, fatal, anaphylactoid or cardiovascular reactions should always be considered (see *"Adverse Reactions: Intravascular—General"*). It is of utmost importance that a course of action be carefully planned in advance for immediate treatment of serious reactions, and that adequate and appropriate personnel be readily available in case of any reaction.

The possibility of an idiosyncratic reaction in susceptible patients should always be considered (see *"Adverse Reactions: Intravascular—General"*). The

susceptible population includes, but is not limited to, patients with a history of a previous reaction to contrast media, patients with a known sensitivity to iodine per se, and patients with a known clinical hypersensitivity; bronchial asthma, hay fever, and food allergies.

The occurrence of severe idiosyncratic reactions has prompted the use of several pretesting methods. However, pretesting cannot be relied upon to predict severe reactions and may itself be hazardous for the patient. It is suggested that a thorough medical history with emphasis on allergy and hypersensitivity, prior to the injection of any contrast media, may be more accurate than pretesting in predicting potential adverse reactions.

A positive history of allergies or hypersensitivity does not arbitrarily contraindicate the use of a contrast agent where a diagnostic procedure is thought essential, but caution should be exercised (see *"Adverse Reactions: Intravascular—General"*). Premedication with antihistamines or corticosteroids to avoid or minimize possible allergic reactions in such patients should be considered and administered using separate syringes. Recent reports indicate that such pretreatment does not prevent serious life-threatening reactions, but may reduce both their incidence and severity.

Even though the osmolality of Iohexol is low compared to diatrizoate- or iothalamate-based ionic agents of comparable iodine concentration, the potential transitory increase in the circulatory osmotic load in patients with congestive heart failure requires caution during injection. These patients should be observed for several hours following the procedure to detect delayed hemodynamic disturbances.

General anesthesia may be indicated in the performance of some procedures in selected adult patients; however, a higher incidence of adverse reactions has been reported in these patients, and may be attributable to the inability of the patient to identify untoward symptoms, or to the hypotensive effect of anesthesia which can reduce cardiac output and increase the duration of exposure to the contrast agent.

Angiography should be avoided whenever possible in patients with homocystinuria, because of the risk of inducing thrombosis and embolism.

In angiographic procedures, the possibility of dislodging plaques or damaging or perforating the vessel wall should be borne in mind during the catheter manipulations and contrast medium injection. Test injections to ensure proper catheter placement are recommended.

Selective coronary arteriography should be performed only in those patients in whom the expected benefits outweigh the potential risk. The inherent risks of angiocardiography in patients with chronic pulmonary emphysema must be weighed against the necessity for performing this procedure. When Iohexol is to be injected using plastic disposable syringes, the contrast medium should be drawn into the syringe and used immediately.

If nondisposable equipment is used, scrupulous care should be taken to prevent residual contamination with traces of cleansing agents.

Parenteral products should be inspected visually for particulate matter and discoloration prior to administration. If particulate matter or discoloration is present, do not use.

Information for Patients: Patients receiving injectable radiopaque diagnostic agents should be instructed to:

1. Inform your physician if you are pregnant (see *"Clinical Pharmacology—Intravascular"*).
2. Inform your physician if you are diabetic or if you have multiple myeloma, pheochromocytoma, homozygous sickle cell disease, or known thyroid disorder (see *"Warnings"*).
3. Inform your physician if you are allergic to any drugs, food, or if you had any reactions to previous injections of dyes used for x-ray procedures (see *"Precautions—General"*).
4. Inform your physician about any other medications you are currently taking, including nonprescription drugs, before you are administered this drug.

Drug/Laboratory Test Interaction: If iodine-containing isotopes are to be administered for the diagnosis of thyroid disease, the iodine-binding capacity of thyroid tissue may be reduced for up to 2 weeks after contrast medium administration. Thyroid function tests which do not depend on iodine estimation, e.g., T_3 resin uptake or direct thyroxine assays, are not affected.

Many radiopaque contrast agents are incompatible *in vitro* with some antihistamines and many other drugs; therefore, no other pharmaceuticals should be admixed with contrast agents.

Carcinogenesis, Mutagenesis, Impairment of Fertility: No long-term animal studies have been performed to evaluate carcinogenic potential, mutagenesis, or whether Iohexol can affect fertility in men or women.

Pregnancy Category B: Reproduction studies have been performed in rats and rabbits with up to 100 times the recommended human dose. No evidence of impaired fertility or harm to the fetus has been demonstrated due to Iohexol. There are, however, no studies in pregnant women. Because animal reproduction studies are not always predictive of human response, this drug should be used during pregnancy only if clearly needed.

Nursing Mothers: It is not known to what extent Iohexol is excreted in human milk. However, many injectable contrast agents are excreted unchanged in human milk. Although it has not been established that serious adverse reactions occur in nursing infants, caution should be exercised when intravascular contrast media are administered to nursing women. Bottle feedings may be substituted for breast feedings for 24 hours following administration of Iohexol.

Pediatric Use: Pediatric patients at higher risk of experiencing adverse events during contrast medium administration may include those having asthma, a sensitivity to medication and/or allergens, congestive heart failure, a serum creatinine greater than 1.5 mg/dL or those less than 12 months of age.

ADVERSE REACTIONS

INTRAVASCULAR

General: Adverse reactions following the use of Iohexol 140, Iohexol 240, Iohexol 300, and Iohexol 350 are usually of mild to moderate severity. However, serious, life-threatening and fatal reactions, mostly of cardiovascular origin, have been associated with the administration of iodine-containing contrast media, including Iohexol. The injection of contrast media is frequently associated with the sensation of warmth and pain, especially in peripheral angiography; pain and warmth are less frequent and less severe with Iohexol than with many contrast media.

Cardiovascular System: Arrhythmias including PVCs and PACs (2%), angina/chest pain (1%), and hypotension (0.7%). Others including cardiac failure, asystole, bradycardia, tachycardia, and vasovagal reaction were reported with an individual incidence of 0.3% or less. In controlled clinical trials involving 1485 patients, one fatality occurred. A cause and effect relationship between this death and Iohexol has not been established.

Nervous System: Vertigo (including dizziness and light-headedness) (0.5%), pain (3%), vision abnormalities (including blurred vision and photomas) (2%), headache (2%), and taste perversion (1%). Others including anxiety, fever, motor and speech dysfunction, convulsion, paresthesia, somnolence, stiff neck, hemiparesis, syncope, shivering, transient ischemic attack, cerebral infarction, and nystagmus were reported, with an individual incidence of 0.3% or less.

Respiratory System: Dyspnea, rhinitis, coughing, and laryngitis, with an individual incidence of 0.2% or less.

Gastrointestinal System: Nausea (2%) and vomiting (0.7%). Others including diarrhea, dyspepsia, cramp, and dry mouth were reported, with an individual incidence of less than 0.1%.

Skin and Appendages: Urticaria (0.3%), purpura (0.1%), abscess (0.1%), and pruritus (0.1%).

Individual adverse reactions which occurred to a significantly greater extent for a specific procedure are listed under that indication.

Pediatrics: In controlled clinical trials involving 391 patients for pediatric angiocardiography, urography, and contrast enhanced computed tomographic head imaging, adverse reactions following the use of Iohexol 240, Iohexol 300, and Iohexol 350 were generally less frequent than with adults.

Cardiovascular System: Ventricular tachycardia (0.5%), 2:1 heart block (0.5%), hypertension (0.3%), and anemia (0.3%).

Nervous System: Pain (0.8%), fever (0.5%), taste abnormality (0.5%), and convulsion (0.3%).

Respiratory System: Congestion (0.3%) and apnea (0.3%).

Gastrointestinal System: Nausea (1%), hypoglycemia (0.3%), and vomiting (2%).

Skin and Appendages: Rash (0.3%).

General Adverse Reactions to Contrast Media: Physicians should remain alert for the occurrence of adverse effects in addition to those discussed above.

The following reactions have been reported after administration of other intravascular iodinated contrast media, and rarely with Iohexol.

Reactions Due to Technique: hematomas and ecchymoses.

Hemodynamic reactions: vein cramp and thrombophlebitis following intravenous injection.

Cardiovascular Reactions: rare cases of cardiac arrhythmias, reflex tachycardia, chest pain, cyanosis, hypertension, hypotension, peripheral vasodilatation, shock, and cardiac arrest.

Renal Reactions: occasionally, transient proteinuria, and rarely, oliguria or anuria.

Allergic Reactions: asthmatic attacks, nasal and conjunctival symptoms, dermal reactions such as urticaria with or without pruritus, as well as pleomorphic rashes, sneezing and lacrimation and, rarely, anaphylactic reactions. Rare fatalities have occurred, due to this or unknown causes.

Signs and Symptoms related to the respiratory system: pulmonary or laryngeal edema, bronchospasm, dyspnea: *or to the nervous system:* restlessness, tremors, convulsions.

Other Reactions: flushing, pain, warmth, metallic taste, nausea, vomiting, anxiety, headache, confusion, pallor, weakness, sweating, localized areas of edema, especially facial cramps, neutropenia, and dizziness.

Rarely, immediate or delayed rigors can occur, sometimes accompanied by hyperpyrexia. Infrequently, "iodism" (salivary gland swelling) from organic iodinated compounds, appears two days after exposure and subsides by the sixth day.

In general, the reactions which are known to occur upon parenteral administration of iodinated contrast agents are possible with any nonionic agent. Approximately 95 percent of adverse reactions accompanying the use of water-soluble intravascularly administered contrast agents are mild to moderate in degree. However, severe, life-threatening anaphylactoid reactions, mostly of cardiovascular origin, have occurred. Reported incidences of death range from 6.6 per 1 million (0.00066 percent) to 1 in 10,000 (0.01 percent). Most deaths occur during injection or 5 to 10 minutes later; the main feature being cardiac arrest with

cardiovascular disease as the main aggravating factor. Isolated reports of hypotensive collapse and shock are found in the literature. The incidence of shock is estimated to be 1 out of 20,000 (0.005 percent) patients.

Adverse reactions to injectable contrast media fall into two categories: chemotoxic reactions and idiosyncratic reactions. Chemotoxic reactions result from the physicochemical properties of the contrast media, the dose, and speed of injection. All hemodynamic disturbances and injuries to organs or vessels perfused by the contrast medium are included in this category.

Idiosyncratic reactions include all other reactions. They occur more frequently in patients 20 to 40 years old. Idiosyncratic reactions may or may not be dependent on the amount of dose injected, the speed of injection, and the radiographic procedure. Idiosyncratic reactions are subdivided into minor, intermediate, and severe. The minor reactions are self-limited and of short duration; the severe reactions are life-threatening and treatment is urgent and mandatory.

The reported incidence of adverse reactions to contrast media in patients with a history of allergy are twice that of the general population. Patients with a history of previous reactions to a contrast medium are three times more susceptible than other patients. However, sensitivity to contrast media does not appear to increase with repeated examinations.

Most adverse reactions to injectable contrast media appear within 1 to 3 minutes after the start of injection, but delayed reactions may occur.

Regardless of the contrast agent employed, the overall estimated incidence of serious adverse reactions is higher with angiocardiography than with other procedures. Cardiac decompensation, serious arrhythmias, angina pectoris, or myocardial ischemia or infarction may occur during angiocardiography and left ventriculography. Electrocardiographic and hemodynamic abnormalities occur less frequently with Iohexol than with diatrizoate meglumine and diatrizoate sodium injection.

OVERDOSAGE

Overdosage may occur. The adverse effects of overdosage are life-threatening and affect mainly the pulmonary and cardiovascular systems. The symptoms included: cyanosis, bradycardia, acidosis, pulmonary hemorrhage, convulsions, coma, and cardiac arrest. Treatment of an overdosage is directed toward the support of all vital functions, and prompt institution of symptomatic therapy.

The intravenous LD_{50} values of Iohexol (in grams of iodine per kilogram body weight) are 24.2 in mice and 15.0 in rats.

DOSAGE AND ADMINISTRATION

General: As with all radiopaque contrast agents, the lowest dose of Iohexol necessary to obtain adequate visualization should be used. A lower dose may reduce the possibility of an adverse reaction. Most procedures do not require use of either the maximum volume or the highest concentration of Iohexol. The combination of volume and concentration of Iohexol to be used should be carefully individualized accounting for factors such as age, body weight, size of the vessel and the rate of blood flow within the vessel. Other factors such as anticipated pathology, degree and extent of opacification required, structure(s) or area to be examined, disease processes affecting the patient, and equipment and technique to be employed should be considered.

Sterile technique must be used in all vascular injections involving contrast media.

Withdrawal of contrast agents from their containers should be accomplished under aseptic conditions with sterile equipment. Sterile techniques must be used with any invasive procedure.

If nondisposable equipment is used, scrupulous care should be taken to prevent residual contamination with traces of cleansing agents.

It may be desirable that solutions of radiopaque diagnostic agents be used at body temperature when injected.

Parenteral products should be inspected visually for particulate matter and discoloration prior to administration whenever solution and container permit. Solutions of Iohexol should be used only if clear and within the normal colorless to pale yellow range. If particulate matter or discoloration is present, do not use.

INDIVIDUAL INDICATIONS AND USAGE

ANGIOCARDIOGRAPHY

Pharmacology—Hemodynamic Changes: Iohexol 350 at a concentration of 35 mgI/mL is indicated in adults for angiocardiography (ventriculography, aortic root injections, and selective coronary arteriography). Iohexol 350 at a concentration of 350 mgI/mL is indicated in children for angiocardiography (ventriculography, pulmonary arteriography, and venography, and studies of the collateral arteries).

Iohexol 300 at a concentration of 300 mgI/mL is indicated in children for angiocardiography (ventriculography). After both ventricular and coronary injection, decreases in systolic pressure were less pronounced and returned to baseline values earlier with Iohexol 350 than with diatrizoate meglumine and diatrizoate sodium injection.

Iohexol 350 produced less Q-T interval prolongation than seen with diatrizoate meglumine and diatrizoate sodium injection.

In children, after injection of all sites, but particularly following ventricular and pulmonary artery injections, decreases in both systolic and diastolic intravascular pressure were significantly less pronounced with Iohexol 350 than with diatrizoate meglumine and diatrizoate sodium injection. In children, Iohexol 350 produced significantly less shortening of the R-R interval than seen with diatrizoate meglumine and diatrizoate sodium injection.

If repeat injections are made in rapid succession, all these changes are likely to be more pronounced. (See *"Dosage and Administration".*)

Precautions: During administration of large doses of Iohexol 350, continuous monitoring of vital signs is desirable. Caution is advised in the administration of large volumes to patients with incipient heart failure because of the possibility of aggravating the preexisting condition. Hypotension should be corrected promptly since it may induce serious arrhythmias.

Special care regarding dosage should be observed in patients with right ventricular failure, pulmonary hypertension, or stenotic pulmonary vascular beds because of the hemodynamic changes which may occur after injection into the right heart outflow tract. (See *"Precautions—General."*) Pediatric patients at higher risk of experiencing adverse events during contrast medium administration may include those having asthma, a sensitivity to medication and/or allergens, congestive heart failure, a serum creatinine greater than 1.5 mg/dL or those less than 12 months of age.

Adverse Reactions: Cardiovascular system reactions in angiocardiography included angina (8%), hypotension (2.5%), bradycardia (1.0%), and tachycardia (1.0%). (See *"Adverse Reactions: Intravascular—General."*)

Dosage and Administration: The individual dose or volume is determined by the size of the structure to be visualized, the anticipated degree of hemodilution, and valvular competence. Weight is a minor consideration in adults, but must be considered in infants and young children. The volume of each individual injection is a more important consideration than the total dosage used. When large individual volumes are administered, as in ventriculography and aortography, it has been suggested that several minutes be permitted to elapse between each injection to allow for subsidence of possible hemodynamic disturbances.

The recommended single injection volume of Iohexol 350 for angiocardiographic procedures in adults and the recommended single injection volumes of Iohexol 350 and Iohexol 300 for angiographic procedures in children are as follows:

Ventriculography:

Adults: The usual adult volume for a single injection is 40 mL with a range of 30 mL to 60 mL. This may be repeated as necessary. When combined with selective coronary arteriography, the total administered volume should not exceed 250 mL (87.5 gI).

Pediatrics: The usual single injection dose of Iohexol 350 is 1.25 mL/kg of body weight with a range of 1.0 mL/kg to 1.5 mL/kg. For Iohexol 300 the usual single injection dose is 1.75 mL/kg with a range of 1.5 mL/kg to 2.0 mL/kg. When multiple injections are given, the total administered dose should not exceed 5 mL/kg up to a total volume of 250 mL of Iohexol 350 or up to a total volume of 291 mL of Iohexol 300.

Selective Coronary Arteriography: The usual adult volume for right or left coronary arteriography is 5 mL (range 3 mL to 14 mL) per injection.

Aortic Root and Arch Study When Used Alone: The usual adult single injection volume is 50 mL, with a range of 20 mL to 75 mL.

Pulmonary Angiography:

Pediatrics: The usual single injection dose is 1.0 mL/kg of Iohexol 350.

Combined Angiocardiographic Procedures

Multiple Procedures:

Adults: The visualization of multiple vascular systems and target organs is possible during a single radiographic examination of the patient.

Large doses of Iohexol 350 were well tolerated in angiographic procedures requiring multiple injections.

The maximum total volume for multiple procedures should not exceed 250 mL of 350 mgI/mL (87.5 gI).

Pediatrics: Visualization of multiple vascular systems and target organs is possible during a single radiographic examination of the patient.

The maximum total dose for multiple injection procedures should not exceed 5.0 mL/kg up to a total volume of 250 mL of Iohexol 350 or 6.0 mL/kg up to a total volume of 291 mL of Iohexol 300.

AORTOGRAPHY AND SELECTIVE VISCERAL ARTERIOGRAPHY

Iohexol 300 at a concentration of 300 mgI/mL and Iohexol 350 at a concentration of 350 mgI/mL are indicated in adults for use in aortography and selective visceral arteriography including studies of the aortic arch, ascending aorta, and abdominal aorta and its branches (celiac, mesenteric, renal, hepatic and splenic arteries).

Iohexol 350 at a concentration of 350 mgI/mL is indicated in children for use in aortography including studies of the aortic root, aortic arch, ascending and descending aorta.

Precautions: Under conditions of slowed aortic circulation there is an increased likelihood for aortography to cause muscle spasm. Occasional serious neurologic complications, including paraplegia, have also been reported in patients with aortoiliac obstruction, femoral artery obstruction, abdominal compression, hypotension, hypertension, spinal anesthesia, and injection of vasopressors to increase contrast. In these patients the concentration, volume, and number of repeat injections of the medium should be maintained at a minimum with appropriate intervals between injections. The position of the patient and catheter tip should be carefully monitored.

Entry of a large aortic dose into the renal artery may cause, even in the absence of symptoms, albuminuria, hematuria, and an elevated creatinine and urea nitrogen. Rapid and complete return of function usually follows. (See *"Precautions—General."*)

Adverse Reactions: See *"Adverse Reactions: Intravascular—General"* and *"Adverse Reactions—Angiocardiography."*

Dosage and Administration:

Adults: The usual adult volume as a single injection is 50 mL to 80 mL for the aorta, 30 mL to 60 mL for major branches including celiac and mesenteric arteries, and 5 mL to 15 mL for renal arteries. Repeated injections may be performed if indicated, but the total volume should not exceed 291 mL of Iohexol 300 or 250 mL of Iohexol 350 (87.5 gI/mL).

Pediatrics: The usual single injection dose is 1.0 mL/kg of Iohexol 350 and should not exceed 5.0 mL/kg up to a total volume of 250 mL of Iohexol 350.

CEREBRAL ARTERIOGRAPHY

Iohexol 300 at a concentration of 300 mgI/mL is indicated in adults for use in cerebral arteriography.

The degree of pain and flushing as the result of the use of Iohexol 300 in cerebral arteriography is less than that seen with comparable injections of many contrast media.

In cerebral arteriography, patients should be appropriately prepared consistent with existing or suspected disease states.

Precautions: Cerebral arteriography should be undertaken with extreme care with special caution in elderly patients, patients in poor clinical condition, advanced arteriosclerosis, severe arterial hypertension, recent cerebral embolism or thrombosis, and cardiac decompensation.

Since the contrast medium is given by rapid injection, the patient should be monitored for possible untoward reactions. (See *"Precautions—General."*)

Adverse Reactions: Cerebral arteriography with water-soluble contrast media has been associated with temporary neurologic complications including seizures, drowsiness, transient paresis, and mild disturbances in vision such as photomas of 1-second or less duration.

Central nervous system reactions in cerebral arteriography included photomas (15%), headache (5.5%), and pain (4.5%). (See *"Adverse Reactions: Intravascular—General."*)

Dosage and Administration: Iohexol 300 is recommended for cerebral arteriography at the following volumes: common carotid artery (6 mL to 12 mL), internal carotid artery (8 mL to 10 mL), external carotid artery (6 mL to 9 mL), and vertebral artery (6 mL to 10 mL).

CONTRAST ENHANCED COMPUTED TOMOGRAPHY

Iohexol 240 at a concentration of 240 mgI/mL, Iohexol 300 at a concentration of 300 mgI/mL, and Iohexol 350 at a concentration of 350 mgI/mL are indicated in adults for use in intravenous contrast enhanced computed tomographic head and body imaging by rapid injection or infusion technique.

Iohexol 240 at a concentration of 240 mgI/mL and Iohexol 300 at a concentration of 300 mgI/mL are indicated in children for use in intravenous contrast enhanced computed tomographic head imaging by rapid bolus injection.

CT SCANNING OF THE HEAD

Iohexol may be used to redefine diagnostic precision in areas of the brain which may not otherwise have been satisfactorily visualized.

Tumors: Iohexol may be useful to investigate the presence and extent of certain malignancies such as: gliomas including malignant gliomas, glioblastomas, astrocytomas, oligodendrogliomas and gangliomas, ependymomas, medull-oblastomas, meningiomas, neuromas, pinealomas, pituitary adenomas, carniopharyngiomas, germinomas, and metastatic lesions. The usefulness of contrast enhancement for the investigation of the retrobulbar space and in cases of low grade or infiltrative glioma has not been demonstrated. In calcified lesions, there is less likelihood of enhancement. Following therapy, tumors may show decreased or no enhancement. The opacification of the inferior vermis following contrast media administration has resulted in false positive diagnosis in a number of otherwise normal studies.

Nonneoplastic Conditions: Iohexol may be beneficial in the image enhancement of nonneoplastic lesions. Cerebral infarctions of recent onset may be better visualized with contrast enhancement, while some infarctions are obscured if contrast medium is used. The use of iodinated contrast media results in enhancement in about 60 percent of cerebral infarctions studied from one to four weeks from the onset of symptoms.

Sites of active infection may also be enhanced following contrast medium administration.

Arteriovenous malformations and aneurysms will show contrast enhancement. For these vascular lesions the enhancement is probably dependent on the iodine content of the circulating blood pool. Hematomas and intraparenchymal bleeders seldom demonstrate contrast enhancement. However, in cases of intraparenchymal clot, for which there is no obvious clinical explanation, contrast media administration may be helpful in ruling out the possibility of associated arteriovenous malformation.

CT SCANNING OF THE BODY

Iohexol may be useful for enhancement of computed tomographic images for detection and evaluation of lesions in the liver, pancreas, kidneys, aorta, mediastinum, pelvis, abdominal cavity, and retroperitoneal space.

Enhancement of computed tomography with Iohexol may be of benefit in establishing diagnoses of certain lesions in these sites with greater assurance than is possible with CT alone. In other cases, the contrast agent may allow visualization of lesions not seen with CT alone (i.e., tumor extension) or may help to define suspicious lesions seen with unenhanced CT (i.e., pancreatic cyst).

For information regarding the use of dilute oral plus intravenous Iohexol in CT of the abdomen, see "Individual Indications and Usage—Oral Use."

Precautions: See "Precautions—General".

Adverse Reactions: Immediately following intravascular injection of contrast medium, a transient sensation of mild warmth is not unusual. Warmth is less frequent with Iohexol than with ionic media. (See "Adverse Reactions: Intravascular—General".)

Dosage and Administration: The concentration and volume required will depend on the equipment and imaging technique used.

Iohexol Injection:

The dosage recommended for use in adults for contrast enhanced computed tomography is as follows:

Head Imaging by Injection:	70 mL to 150 mL (21 gI to 45 gI) of Iohexol 300 (300 mgI/mL) 80 mL (28 gI) of Iohexol 350 (350 mgI/mL)
Head Imaging by Infusion:	120 mL to 250 mL (29 gI to 60 gI) of Iohexol 240 (240 mgI/mL)
Body Imaging by Injection	50 mL to 200 mL (15 gI to 60 gI) of Iohexol 300 (300 mgI/mL) 60 mL to 100 mL (21 gI to 35 gI) of Iohexol 350 (350 mgI/mL)

The dosage recommended for use in children for contrast enhanced computed tomographic head imaging is 1.0 mL/kg to 2.0 mL/kg for Iohexol 240 or Iohexol 300. It should not be necessary to exceed a maximum dose of 28 gI with Iohexol 240 or 35 gI with Iohexol 300.

DIGITAL SUBTRACTION ANGIOGRAPHY
Intravenous Administration: Iohexol 350 at a concentration of 350 mgI/mL is indicated in adults for use in intravenous digital subtraction angiography (I.V. DSA) of the vessels of the head, neck, and abdominal, renal and peripheral vessels.

Arteriograms of diagnostic quality can be obtained following the intravenous administration of contrast media employing digital subtraction and computer imaging enhancement techniques. The intravenous route of administration using these techniques has the advantage of being less invasive than the corresponding selective catheter placement of medium. The dose is administered into a peripheral vein, the superior vena cava or right atrium, usually by mechanical injection although sometimes by rapid manual injection. The technique has been used to visualize the ventricles, aorta and most of its larger branches, including the carotids, cerebrals, vertebrals, renal, celiac, mesenterics, and the major peripheral vessels of the limbs. Radiographic visualization of these structures is possible until significant hemodilution occurs.

Iohexol 350 can be injected intravenously as a rapid bolus to provide arterial visualization using digital subtraction radiography. Preprocedural medications are not considered necessary. Iohexol 350 has provided diagnostic arterial radiographs in about 95% of patients. In some cases, poor arterial visualization has been attributed to patient movement. Iohexol 350 is very well tolerated in the vascular system. Patient discomfort (general sensation of heat and/or pain) following injection is less than with various other contrast media.

Precautions: Since the contrast medium is usually administered mechanically under high pressure, rupture of smaller peripheral veins can occur. It has been suggested that this can be avoided by using an intravenous catheter threaded proximally beyond larger tributaries or, in the case of the antecubital vein, into the superior vena cava. Sometimes the femoral vein is used. (See "Precautions—General".)

Adverse Reactions: Cardiovascular system reactions in digital arteriography included transient PVCs (16%) and PACs (6.5%). (See "Adverse Reactions: Intravascular—General.")

Dosage and Administration: The usual injection volume of Iohexol 350 for the intravenous digital technique is 30 mL to 50 mL of a 350 mgI/mL solution. This is administered as a bolus at 7.5 to 30 mL/second using a pressure injector. The volume and rate of injection will depend primarily on the type of equipment and technique used.

Frequently three or more injections may be required, up to a total volume not to exceed 250 mL (87.5 gI).

Intra-arterial Administration: Iohexol 140 at a concentration of 140 mgI/mL is indicated for use in intra-arterial digital subtraction angiography of head, neck, abdominal, renal and peripheral vessels. The intra-arterial route of administration has the advantages of allowing a lower total dose of contrast agent since there is less hemodilution than with the intravenous route of administration. Patients with poor cardiac output would be expected to have better contrast enhancement following intra-arterial administration as compared with intravenous administration. A higher concentration of contrast agent may be needed to facilitate catheter placement under fluoroscopic control.

Precautions: High pressure intra-arterial injections may cause the rupture of smaller peripheral arteries. (See "Precautions—General.")

Adverse Reactions: Central nervous system reactions in intra-arterial digital angiography include transient ischemia attacks (1.6%) and cerebral infarctions (1.6%). These occurred in high risk patients having a cerebral examination and the relationship to the contrast medium was uncertain. (See "Adverse Reactions—General.") Headache occurred in 6.3% of the patients, all of whom were having cerebral examinations.

Dosage and Administration: Mechanical or hand injection can be used to administer one or more bolus intra-arterial injections of Iohexol 140. The volume and rate of injection will depend on the type of equipment, technique used, and the vascular area to be visualized. The following volumes and rates of injection have been used with Iohexol 140.

Arteries	Injection/ Volume (mL)	Rate of Injection (mL/sec)
Aorta	20-45	8-20
Carotid	5-10	3-6
Femoral	9-20	3-6
Vertebral	4-10	2-8
Renal	6-12	3-6
Other Branches of the Aorta (includes subclavian, axillary, innominate and iliac)	8-25	3-10

PERIPHERAL ANGIOGRAPHY
Iohexol 300 at a concentration of 300 mgI/mL or Iohexol 350 at a concentration of 350 mgI/mL is indicated in adults for use in peripheral arteriography. Iohexol 240 at a concentration of 240 mgI/mL or Iohexol 300 at a concentration of 300 mgI/mL is indicated in adults for use in peripheral venography.

Sedative medication may be employed prior to use. Anesthesia is not considered necessary.

Patient discomfort during and immediately following injection is substantially less than that following injection of various other contrast media. Moderate to severe discomfort is very unusual.

Precautions: Pulsation should be present in the artery to be injected. In thromboangiitis obliterans, or ascending infection associated with severe ischemia, angiography should be performed with extreme caution, if at all. (See "Precautions—General.")

Adverse Reactions: A transient sensation of mild warmth is usual, immediately following injection. This has not interfered with the procedure.

In phlebography the incidence of leg pain was 21%. This usually was mild and lasted a short time after injection. (See "Adverse Reactions: Intravascular—General.")

Dosage and Administration: The volume required will depend on the size, flow rate, and disease state of the injected vessel and on the size and condition of the patient, as well as the imaging technique used.

The dosage recommended for use in peripheral angiography is as follows:

Aortofemoral runoffs: 20 mL to 70 mL of Iohexol 350 (350 mgI/mL) 30 mL to 90 mL of Iohexol 300 (300 mgI/mL)

Selective arteriograms (femoral/iliac): 10 mL to 30 mL of Iohexol 350 (350 mgI/mL) 10 mL to 60 mL of Iohexol 300 (300 mgI/mL)

Venography (per leg): 20 mL to 150 mL of Iohexol 240 (240 mgI/mL) 40 mL to 100 mL of Iohexol 300 (300 mgI/mL)

EXCRETORY UROGRAPHY
Iohexol 300 at a concentration of 300 mgI/mL or Iohexol 350 at a concentration of 350 mgI/mL is indicated for use in adults in excretory urography to provide diagnostic contrast of the urinary tract.

Iohexol 300 at a concentration of 300 mgI/mL is indicated in children for excretory urography. (See "Section III" for information on "Voiding Cystourethrography.")

For pharmacokinetics of excretion in adults, see "Clinical Pharmacology—Intravascular."

Precautions: Preparatory dehydration is not recommended in the elderly, infants, young children, diabetic or azotemic patients, or in patients with suspected myelomatosis.

Pediatric patients at higher risk of experiencing adverse events during contrast medium administration may include those having asthma, a sensitivity to medication and/or allergens, congestive heart failure, a serum creatinine greater than 1.5 mg/dL or those less than 12 months of age.

Since there is a possibility of temporary suppression of urine formation, it is recommended that a suitable interval elapse before excretory urography is repeated, especially in patients with unilateral or bilateral reduction in renal function. (See "Precautions—General.")

Adverse Reactions: See "Adverse Reactions: Intravascular—General."

Dosage and Administration: Adults: Iohexol 300 and Iohexol 350 at dosages from 200 mgI/kg body weight to 350 mgI/kg body weight have produced diagnostic opacification of the excretory system in patients with normal renal function.

Pediatrics: Excretory Urography: Iohexol 300 at doses of 0.5 mL/kg to 3.0 mL/kg of body weight has produced diagnostic opacification of the excretory tract. The usual dose for children is 1.0 mL/kg to 1.5 mL/kg. Dosage for infants and children should be administered in proportion to age and body weight. The total administered dose should not exceed 3 mL/kg.

SECTION III
CLINICAL PHARMACOLOGY
ORAL/BODY CAVITY USE

For most body cavities, the injected Iohexol is absorbed into the surrounding tissue and eliminated by the kidneys and bowel as previously described in *"Section II, Clinical Pharmacology—Intravascular."* Examinations of the uterus (hysterosalpingography) and bladder (voiding cystourethrography) involve the almost immediate drainage of contrast medium from the cavity upon conclusion of the radiographic procedure.

Orally administered Iohexol is very poorly absorbed from the normal gastrointestinal tract. Only 0.1 to 0.5 percent of the oral dose was excreted by the kidneys. This amount may increase in the presence of bowel perforation or bowel obstruction. Iohexol is well tolerated and readily absorbed if leakage into the peritoneal cavity occurs.

Visualization of the joint spaces, uterus, fallopian tubes, peritoneal herniations, pancreatic and bile ducts, and bladder can be accomplished by direct injection of contrast medium into the region to be studied. The use of appropriate iodine concentrations assures diagnostic density.

Orally administered Iohexol produces good visualization of the gastrointestinal tract. Iohexol is particularly useful when barium sulfate is contraindicated as in patients with suspected bowel perforation or those where aspiration of contrast medium is a possibility.

INDICATIONS AND USAGE
ORAL/BODY CAVITY USE

General: Iohexol 210, Iohexol 240, Iohexol 300, and Iohexol 350 have osmolalities from approximately 1.6 to 3.0 times that of plasma (285 mOsm/kg water) and are hypertonic under conditions of use.

Adults: Iohexol 350 is indicated in adults for arthrography and oral pass-thru examination of the gastrointestinal tract.

Iohexol 300 is indicated in adults for arthrography and hysterosalpingography.

Iohexol 240 is indicated in adults for arthrography, endoscopic retrograde pancreatography and cholangiopancreatography, herniography, and hysterosalpingography.

Iohexol 210 is indicated in adults for arthrography.

Iohexol diluted to concentrations from 6 mgI/mL to 9 mgI/mL administered orally in conjunction with Iohexol 300 at a concentration of 300 mgI/mL administered intravenously is indicated in adults for contrast enhanced computed tomography of the abdomen.

Children: Iohexol diluted to concentrations from 50 mgI/mL to 100 mgI/mL is indicated in children for voiding cystourethrography.

Iohexol diluted to concentrations from 9 mgI/mL to 21 mgI/mL administered orally in conjunction with Iohexol 240 at a concentration of 240 mgI/mL or Iohexol 300 at a concentration of 300 mgI/mL administered intravenously are indicated in children for use in contrast enhanced computed tomography of the abdomen.

CONTRAINDICATIONS

Iohexol should not be administered to patients with a known hypersensitivity to Iohexol.

WARNINGS

General: See *"Section II, Warnings—General."*

PRECAUTIONS

General: See *"Section II, Precautions—General."*

Orally administered hypertonic contrast media draw fluid into the intestines which, if severe enough, could result in hypovolemia. Plasma fluid loss in elderly cachectic patients may be sufficient to cause a shocklike state which, if untreated, could be dangerous. It is advisable to correct any electrolyte disturbances before using hypertonic contrast media and promptly correct any hypovolemic episodes caused by the media.

Bronchial entry of hypertonic contrast medium causes osmotic effusion and should be avoided.

ADVERSE REACTIONS
ORAL/BODY CAVITY USE
General:

Body Cavities: In controlled clinical trials involving 285 adult patients for various body cavity examinations using Iohexol 210, 240, 300 and 350, the following adverse reactions were reported.

Cardiovascular System
  Incidence > 1%: None
  Incidence ≤ 1%: Hypertension

Nervous System
  Incidence > 1%: Pain (26%)
  Incidence ≤ 1%: Headache, somnolence, fever, muscle weakness, burning, unwell feeling, tremors, lightheadedness, syncope.

Respiratory System
  None

Gastrointestinal System
  Incidence > 1%: None
  Incidence ≤ 1%: Flatulence, diarrhea, nausea, vomiting, abdominal pressure.

Skin and Appendages
  Incidence > 1%: Swelling (22%), heat (7%)
  Incidence ≤ 1%: Hematoma at injection site

The most frequent reactions, pain and swelling, were almost exclusively reported after arthrography and were generally related to the procedure rather than the contrast medium. Gastrointestinal reactions were almost exclusively reported after oral pass-thru examinations. For additional information on adverse reactions that may be expected with specific procedures, see *"Individual Indications and Usage."* For information on general adverse reactions to contrast media, see *"Section II, Adverse Reactions: Intravascular—General."*

No adverse reactions associated with the use of Iohexol for VCU procedures were reported in 51 pediatric patients studied.

Oral Use: See *"Individual Indications and Usage", "Oral Use—Adverse Reactions."*

OVERDOSAGE

See also *"Section II, Overdosage."*

The recommended dose of Iohexol 350 at a concentration of 350 mgI/mL for adult oral pass-thru examination of the gastrointestinal tract is 50 mL to 100 mL. In a Phase I study, 150 mL of Iohexol 350 was administered orally to 11 healthy male subjects. The incidence of diarrhea was 91% (10 of 11) and abdominal cramping was 27% (3 of 11). Despite all of these events being mild and transient the occurrences were more than double that seen at the recommended doses. It is apparent from this finding that larger volumes of hypertonic contrast media, like Iohexol increase the osmotic load in the bowel which may result in greater fluid shifts.

DOSAGE AND ADMINISTRATION
GENERAL

See *"Section II, Dosage and Administration—General."*

INDIVIDUAL INDICATIONS AND USAGE
Oral Use:

Adults: Iohexol 350 at a concentration of 350 mgI/mL is indicated in adults for use in oral pass-thru examination of the gastrointestinal tract.

Iohexol diluted to concentrations from 6 mgI/mL to 9 mgI/mL administered orally in conjunction with Iohexol 300 at a concentration of 300 mgI/mL administered intravenously are indicated in adults for use in contrast enhanced computed tomography of the abdomen. Dilute oral plus intravenous Iohexol may be useful when unenhanced imaging does not provide sufficient delineation between normal loops of the bowel and adjacent organs or areas of suspected pathology.

Children: Iohexol diluted to concentrations from 9 mgI/mL to 21 mgI/mL administered orally in conjunction with Iohexol 240 at a concentration of 240 mgI/mL or Iohexol 300 at a concentration of 300 mgI/mL administered intravenously are indicated in children for use in contrast enhanced computed tomography of the abdomen.

Precautions: See *"Precautions—General."*

Adverse Reactions: Oral administration of Iohexol is most often associated with mild, transient diarrhea especially when high concentrations and large volumes are administered. Nausea, vomiting, and moderate diarrhea have also been reported following orally administered Iohexol but much less frequently. For CT examinations using dilute oral plus intravenous contrast medium, adverse events are more likely to be associated with the intravenous injection than the hypotonic oral solution. It should be noted that serious or anaphylactoid reactions that may occur with intravascular iodinated media are possible following administration by other routes.

In controlled clinical trials involving 54 adult patients for oral pass-thru examination of the gastrointestinal tract using Iohexol 350, the following adverse reactions were reported: diarrhea (42%), nausea (15%), vomiting (11%), abdominal pain (7%), flatulence (2%), and headache (2%). In controlled clinical studies involving 44 adult patients for dilute oral plus intravenous CT examination of the gastrointestinal tract using Iohexol 300, adverse reactions were limited to a single report of vomiting (2%).

In controlled clinical studies involving 69 pediatric patients for dilute oral plus intravenous CT examination of the gastrointestinal tract using Iohexol 240 and Iohexol 300, adverse reactions were limited to a single report of vomiting (1.4%).

Dosage and Administration:

Adults: The recommended dosage of Iohexol 350 at a concentration of 350 mgI/mL for oral pass-thru examination of the gastrointestinal tract in adults is 50 mL to 100 mL depending on the nature of the examination and the size of the patient.

The recommended oral dosage of Iohexol diluted to concentrations of 6 mgI/mL to 9 mgI/mL for contrast enhanced computed tomography of the abdomen in adults is 500 mL to 1000 mL. Smaller administered volumes are needed as the concentration of the final solution is increased (see Table below). In conjunction with dilute oral administration, the recommended dosage of Iohexol 300 administered intravenously is 100 mL to 150 mL. The oral dose is administered about 20 to 40 minutes prior to the intravenous dose and image acquisition.

Children: The recommended oral dosage of Iohexol diluted to concentrations of 9 mgI/mL to 21 mgI/mL for contrast enhanced computed tomography of the abdomen in children is 180 mL to 750 mL. Smaller administered volumes are needed as the concentration of the final solution is increased (see Table below). The total oral dose in grams of iodine should generally not exceed 5 gI for children under 3 years of age and 10 gI for children from 3 to 18 years of age. The oral dosage may be given all at once or over a period of 30 to 45 minutes if there is difficulty in consuming the required volume.

In conjunction with dilute oral administration the recommended dosage of Iohexol 240 and Iohexol 300 is 2.0 mL/kg when administered intravenously with a range of 1.0 mL/kg to 2.0 mL/kg. Dosage for infants and children should be administered in proportion to age and body weight. The total intravenously administered dose should not exceed 3 mL/kg. The oral dose is administered about 30 to 60 minutes prior to the intravenous dose and image acquisition.

Iohexol may be diluted with water or beverage as follows:

To Achieve	Add		To
One Liter of Contrast Medium at A Final Concentration (mgI/mL) of	Stock Concentration of Iohexol (mgI/mL)	Volume (mL)	Water, Carbonated Beverage, Milk, or Juice (mL)
6	240	25	975
	300	20	980
	350	17	983
9	240	38	962
	300	30	970
	350	26	974
12	240	50	950
	300	40	960
	350	35	965
15	240	63	937
	300	50	950
	350	43	957
18	240	75	925
	300	60	940
	350	52	948
21	240	88	912
	300	70	930
	350	60	940

Dilutions of Iohexol should be prepared just prior to use and any unused portion discarded after the procedure.

VOIDING CYSTOURETHROGRAPHY (VCU)
Iohexol diluted to concentrations from 50 mgI/mL to 100 mgI/mL is indicated in children for voiding cystourethrography. VCUs are often performed in conjunction with excretory urography.

Precautions: See "Precautions—General."
Since the VCU procedure requires instrumentation, special precautions should be observed in those patients known to have an acute urinary tract infection. Filling of the bladder should be done at a steady rate, exercising caution to avoid excessive pressure. Sterile procedures are essential.

Adverse Reactions: See "Adverse Reactions—General."

Dosage and Administration: Iohexol may be diluted, utilizing aseptic technique, with Sterile Water for Injection to a concentration of 50 mgI/mL to 100 mgI/mL for voiding cystourethrography. The concentration may vary depending upon the patient's size and age and also with the technique and equipment used. Sufficient volume of contrast medium should be administered to adequately fill the bladder. The usual volume ranges from 50 mL to 300 mL of Iohexol at a concentration of 100 mgI/mL and 50 mL to 600 mL of Iohexol at a concentration of 50 mgI/mL. Iohexol may be diluted with Sterile Water for Injection as indicated in the table below:

To Achieve	Add to		
A Final Concentration	Each 100 mL of Iohexol Sterile Water for Injection, USP (mL)		
(mgI/mL) of	Iohexol 240	Iohexol 300	Iohexol 350
100	140	200	250
90	167	233	289
80	200	275	338
70	243	330	400
60	300	400	483
50	380	500	600

Dilutions of Iohexol should be prepared just prior to use and any unused portion discarded after the procedure.

ARTHROGRAPHY
Iohexol 240 at a concentration of 240 mgI/mL or Iohexol 300 at a concentration of 300 mgI/mL or Iohexol 350 at a concentration of 350 mgI/mL is indicated in radiography of the knee joint in adults, and Iohexol 210 at a concentration of 210 mgI/mL or Iohexol 240 at a concentration of 240 mgI/mL or Iohexol 300 at a concentration of 300 mgI/mL is indicated in radiography of the shoulder joint in adults, and Iohexol 300 at a concentration of 300 mgI/mL is indicated in

radiography of the temporomandibular joint in adults. Arthrography may be helpful in the diagnosis of posttraumatic or degenerative joint diseases, synovial rupture, the visualization of communicating bursae or cysts, and in meniscography.

Precautions: See "Precautions—General."
Strict aseptic technique is required to prevent infection. Fluoroscopic control should be used to ensure proper needle placement, prevent extracapsular injection, and prevent dilution of contrast medium. Undue pressure should not be exerted during injection.

Adverse Reactions: Injection of Iohexol into the joint is associated with transient discomfort, i.e., pain, swelling. However, delayed, severe or persistent discomfort may occur occasionally. Severe pain may often result from undue use of pressure or the injection of large volumes. Joint swelling after injection is less with Iohexol than with high osmolar ionic contrast medium. These types of reactions are generally procedurally dependent and of greater frequency when double-contrast technique is employed.

Nervous System: Swelling sensation (42%), pain (29%), heat sensation (13%), and muscle weakness (0.7%).

Skin and Appendages: Hematoma at injection site (0.7%).

Dosage and Administration: Arthrography is usually performed under local anesthesia. The amount of Iohexol injected is dependent on the size of the joint to be examined and the technique employed. Lower volumes of contrast medium are usually injected for knee and shoulder arthrography when double-contrast examinations using 15 mL to 100 mL of air are performed.

The following concentrations and volumes are recommended for normal adult knee, shoulder, and temporomandibular joints but should serve as guidelines since joints may require more or less contrast medium for optimal visualization.

KNEE
Iohexol 240	5 mL to 15 mL
Iohexol 300	5 mL to 15 mL
Iohexol 350	5 mL to 10 mL

SHOULDER
Iohexol 300	10 mL
Iohexol 240	3 mL
Iohexol 210	3 mL

TEMPOROMANDIBULAR
Iohexol 300	0.5 mL to 1.0 mL

Lower volumes recommended for double-contrast examinations; higher volumes recommended for single-contrast examinations.
Passive or active manipulation is used to disperse the medium throughout the joint space.

ENDOSCOPIC RETROGRADE PANCREATOGRAPHY (ERP)/ ENDOSCOPIC RETROGRADE CHOLANGIOPANCREATOGRAPHY (ERCP)
Iohexol 240 at a concentration of 240 mgI/mL is indicated in adults for use in ERP/ERCP.

Precautions: See "Precautions—General."

Adverse Reactions: Injection of Iohexol in ERP/ERCP is associated with transient pain. However, delayed, severe or persistent pain may occur and can persist for 24 hours. The cause of the pain may be due as much to the procedure itself as to the contrast medium injected, therefore, attention should be paid to the injection pressure and total volume injected to minimize disruptive distention of the ducts examined.

Cardiovascular system: Hypertension (1%).

Nervous system: Pain (17%), somnolence (1%), and burning (1%).

Gastrointestinal system: Vomiting, diarrhea, and pressure, each with an individual incidence of 1%.

Dosage and Administration: The recommended dose of Iohexol 240 at a concentration of 240 mgI/mL is 10 mL to 50 mL but may vary depending on individual anatomy and/or disease state.

HYSTEROSALPINGOGRAPHY
Iohexol 240 at a concentration of 240 mgI/mL or Iohexol 300 at a concentration of 300 mgI/mL is indicated in radiography of the internal group of adult female reproductive organs; ovaries, fallopian tubes, uterus, and vagina. Hysterosalpingography is utilized as a diagnostic and therapeutic modality in the treatment of infertility and other abnormal gynecological conditions.

Contraindications: The procedure should not be performed during the menstrual period or when menstrual flow is imminent, nor should it be performed when infection is present in any portion of the genital tract, including the external genitalia. The procedure is also contraindicated for pregnant women or for those in whom pregnancy is suspected. Its use is not advised for 6 months after termination of pregnancy or 30 days after conization or curettage.

Precautions: In patients with carcinoma or in those in whom the condition is suspected, caution should be exercised to avoid possible spreading of the lesion by the procedure.

Adverse Reactions: Injection of Iohexol in hysterosalpingography is associated with immediate but transient pain. The cause of the pain may be due as much to the procedure itself as to the contrast medium injected, therefore attention should be paid to the injection pressure and volume instilled to avoid disruptive distention of the uterus and fallopian tubes. Fluoroscopic monitoring is recommended.

Nervous system: Pain (49%), somnolence and fever each with an individual incidence of 3%.

Gastrointestinal system: Nausea (3%).

Dosage and Administration: The recommended dosage of Iohexol 240 is 15 mL to 20 mL and of Iohexol 300 is 15 mL to 20 mL but will vary depending on individual anatomy and/or disease state.

HERNIOGRAPHY
Iohexol 240 at a concentration of 240 mgI/mL is indicated in adults for use in herniography.

Precautions: See "Precautions—General."

Adverse Reactions:

Nervous System: Pain (7%), headache (3%), and unwell feeling (3%).

Gastrointestinal System: Diarrhea (3%) and flatulence (10%).

Dosage and Administration: The recommended dosage of Iohexol 240 is 50 mL but may vary depending on individual anatomy and/or disease state.
DO NOT USE FLEXIBLE CONTAINER IN SERIES CONNECTIONS.

Storage: Protect vials, bottles, and flexible containers of Iohexol from strong daylight and direct exposure to sunlight. Do not freeze. Store at controlled room temperature 15°C to 30°C (59°F to 86°F).

HOW SUPPLIED
INJECTION: 140 MG

BRAND/MANUFACTURER	NDC	SIZE	AWP
○ **BRAND**			
OMNIPAQUE: Sanofi Winthrop	00024-1401-50	50 ml 10s	$389.41
OMNIPAQUE 140: Sanofi Winthrop	00024-1401-51	50 ml 10s	$389.41

INJECTION: 180 MG

BRAND/MANUFACTURER	NDC	SIZE	AWP
○ **BRAND**			
OMNIPAQUE 180 REDI-UNIT: Sanofi Winthrop	00024-1411-07	10 ml 5s	$246.17
MYELO-KIT: Sanofi Winthrop	00024-1415-05	10 ml 5s	$310.93
OMNIPAQUE 180 REDI-UNIT: Sanofi Winthrop	00024-1411-08	20 ml 5s	$274.32
MYELO-KIT: Sanofi Winthrop	00024-1415-06	20 ml 5s	$338.96
OMNIPAQUE 180: Sanofi Winthrop	00024-1411-10	10 ml 10s	$480.54
	00024-1411-20	20 ml 10s	$536.95

INJECTION: 210 MG

BRAND/MANUFACTURER	NDC	SIZE	AWP
○ **BRAND**			
OMNIPAQUE 210: Sanofi Winthrop	00024-1402-15	15 ml 10s	$529.18

INJECTION: 240 MG

BRAND/MANUFACTURER	NDC	SIZE	AWP
○ **BRAND**			
OMNIPAQUE 240 REDI-UNIT: Sanofi Winthrop	00024-1412-07	10 ml 5s	$267.08
MYELO-KIT: Sanofi Winthrop	00024-1416-05	10 ml 5s	$331.85
OMNIPAQUE 240: Sanofi Winthrop	00024-1412-10	10 ml 10s	$522.47
	00024-1412-20	20 ml 10s	$552.19
	00024-1412-50	50 ml 10s	$456.47
	00024-1412-51	50 ml 10s	$456.47
	00024-1412-52	75 ml 10s	$670.59
OMNIPAQUE 'FLEXIPAK': Sanofi Winthrop	00024-1412-70	100 ml 10s	$782.30
OMNIPAQUE 240: Sanofi Winthrop	00024-1412-60	100 ml 10s	$888.41
	00024-1412-53	125 ml 10s	$1088.23
OMNIPAQUE 'FLEXIPAK': Sanofi Winthrop	00024-1412-75	150 ml 10s	$1052.20
OMNIPAQUE 240: Sanofi Winthrop	00024-1412-49	150 ml 10s	$1207.06
OMNIPAQUE 'FLEXIPAK': Sanofi Winthrop	00024-1412-72	200 ml 10s	$1428.50
OMNIPAQUE 240: Sanofi Winthrop	00024-1412-17	200 ml 10s	$1646.35

INJECTION: 300 MG

BRAND/MANUFACTURER	NDC	SIZE	AWP
○ **BRAND**			
OMNIPAQUE: Sanofi Winthrop	00024-1413-10	10 ml 10s	$482.40
OMNIPAQUE 300: Sanofi Winthrop	00024-1413-30	30 ml 10s	$485.18
	00024-1413-50	50 ml 10s	$540.00
	00024-1413-51	50 ml 10s	$540.00
	00024-1413-52	75 ml 10s	$811.76
OMNIPAQUE 'FLEXIPAK': Sanofi Winthrop	00024-1413-80	100 ml 10s	$932.50
OMNIPAQUE 300: Sanofi Winthrop	00024-1413-60	100 ml 10s	$1058.12
	00024-1413-53	125 ml 10s	$1308.82
OMNIPAQUE 'FLEXIPAK': Sanofi Winthrop	00024-1413-85	150 ml 10s	$1342.10
OMNIPAQUE 300: Sanofi Winthrop	00024-1413-90	150 ml 10s	$1543.29

INJECTION: 350 MG

BRAND/MANUFACTURER	NDC	SIZE	AWP
○ **BRAND**			
OMNIPAQUE 350: Sanofi Winthrop	00024-1414-75	75 ml	$880.12
	00024-1414-76	125 ml	$1389.65
OMNIPAQUE: Sanofi Winthrop	00024-1414-77	200 ml	$1801.41
OMNIPAQUE 350: Sanofi Winthrop	00024-1414-50	50 ml 10s	$588.12
	00024-1414-51	50 ml 10s	$588.12
OMNIPAQUE 'FLEXIPAK': Sanofi Winthrop	00024-1414-61	100 ml 10s	$1019.70
OMNIPAQUE 350: Sanofi Winthrop	00024-1414-60	100 ml 10s	$1175.76
OMNIPAQUE 'FLEXIPAK': Sanofi Winthrop	00024-1414-65	150 ml 10s	$1424.90
OMNIPAQUE 'FLEXIPAK': Sanofi Winthrop	00024-1414-03	200 ml 10s	$1623.18
OMNIPAQUE 'FLEXIPAK': Sanofi Winthrop	00024-1414-62	200 ml 10s	$1765.20
OMNIPAQUE 350: Sanofi Winthrop	00024-1414-04	200 ml 10s	$1999.53
OMNIPAQUE: Sanofi Winthrop	00024-1414-80	250 ml 10s	$2411.76

Ionamin *SEE* PHENTERMINE

Iopamidol

DESCRIPTION
Iopamidol formulations are stable, aqueous, sterile, and nonpyrogenic solutions for intravascular, intrathecal, or intra-arterial administration.

Each mL of Iopamidol for intravascular administration contains:

Iopamidol	408 mg/iodine 200 mg
Iopamidol	510 mg/iodine 250 mg
Iopamidol	612 mg/iodine 300 mg
Iopamidol	755 mg/iodine 370 mg

Each mL of Iopamidol for intrathecal administration contains:

Iopamidol	408 mg/iodine 200 mg
Iopamidol	612 mg/iodine 300 mg

Each mL of Iopamidol for intra-arterial administration contains:

Iopamidol	261 mg/iodine 128 mg

The pH of Iopamidol contrast media is 6.5-7.5. Pertinent physiochemical data are noted below. Iopamidol is hypertonic as compared to plasma and cerebrospinal fluid (approximately 285 and 301 mOsm/kg water, respectively).

IOPAMIDOL

Parameter	26%	41%	51%	61%	76%
Concentration (mgI/mL)	128	200	250	300	370
Osmolality @ 37° C (mOsm/kg water)	290	413	524	616	796
Viscosity (cP)					
@ 37° C	1.4	2.0	3.0	4.7	9.4
@ 20° C	2.1	3.3	5.1	8.8	20.9
Specific Gravity @ 37° C	1.143	1.216	1.281	1.328	1.405

Iopamidol is designated chemically as (S)-N,N'-bis[2-hydroxy-1-(hydroxymethyl)-ethyl]-2,4,6-triiodo-5- lactamidoisophthalamide.

Following is its chemical structure:

CLINICAL PHARMACOLOGY
Intravascular injection of a radiopaque diagnostic agent opacifies those vessels in the path of flow of the contrast medium, permitting radiographic visualization of the internal structures of the human body until significant hemodilution occurs.

Following intravascular injection, radiopaque diagnostic agents are immediately diluted in the circulating plasma. Calculations of apparent volume of distribution at steady-state indicate that Iopamidol is distributed between the circulating blood volume and other extracellular fluid; there appears to be no significant deposition of Iopamidol in tissues. Uniform distribution of Iopamidol in extracellular fluid is reflected by its demonstrated utility in contrast enhancement of computed tomographic imaging of the head and body following intravenous administration.

The pharmacokinetics of intravenously administered Iopamidol in normal subjects conform to an open two-compartment model with first order elimination (a rapid alpha phase for drug distribution and a slow beta phase for drug

---

◆ RATED THERAPEUTICALLY EQUIVALENT; ◇ THERAPEUTIC EQUIVALENCE UNCONFIRMED; ○ UNRATED

elimination). The elimination serum or plasma half-life is approximately two hours; the half-life is not dose dependent. No significant metabolism, deiodination, or biotransformation occurs.

Iopamidol is rapidly absorbed into the bloodstream from cerebrospinal fluid (CSF); following intrathecal administration, iopamidol appears in plasma within one hour and virtually all of the drug reaches the systemic circulation within 24 hours.

Iopamidol is excreted mainly through the kidneys following intravascular, intrathecal, or intra-arterial administration and the drug is essentially undetectable in the plasma 48 hours later. In patients with impaired renal function, the elimination half-life is prolonged dependent upon the degree of impairment. In the absence of renal dysfunction, the cumulative urinary excretion for Iopamidol, expressed as a percentage of administered intravenous dose, is approximately 35 to 40 percent at 60 minutes, 80 to 90 percent at 8 hours, and 90 percent or more in the 72- to 96-hour period after administration. In normal subjects, approximately one percent or less of the administered dose appears in cumulative 72- to 96-hour fecal specimens.

Iopamidol may be visualized in the renal parenchyma within 30-60 seconds following rapid intravenous administration. Opacification of the calyces and pelves in patients with normal renal function becomes apparent within 1 to 3 minutes, with optimum contrast occurring between 5 and 15 minutes. In patients with renal impairment, contrast visualization may be delayed.

Iopamidol displays little tendency to bind to serum or plasma proteins.

No evidence of *in vivo* complement activation has been found in normal subjects.

Animal studies indicate that Iopamidol does not cross the blood-brain barrier to any significant extent following intravascular administration.

Iopamidol enhances computed tomographic brain imaging through augmentation of radiographic efficiency. The degree of enhancement of visualization of tissue density is directly related to the iodine content in an administered dose; peak iodine blood levels occur immediately following rapid injection of the dose. These levels fall rapidly within five to ten minutes. This can be accounted for by the dilution in the vascular and extracellular fluid compartments which causes an initial sharp fall in plasma concentration. Equilibration with the extracellular compartments is reached in about ten minutes; thereafter, the fall becomes exponential. Maximum contrast enhancement frequently occurs after peak blood iodine levels are reached. The delay in maximum contrast enhancement can range from five to forty minutes depending on the peak iodine levels achieved and the cell type of the lesion. This lag suggests that radiographic contrast enhancement is at least in part dependent on the accumulation of iodine within the lesion and outside the blood pool, although the mechanism by which this occurs is not clear. The radiographic enhancement of nontumoral lesions, such as arteriovenous malformations and aneurysms, is probably dependent on the iodine content of the circulating blood pool.

In CECT head imaging, Iopamidol does not accumulate in normal brain tissue due to the presence of the "blood-brain" barrier. The increase in x-ray absorption in normal brain is due to the presence of contrast agent within the blood pool. A break in the blood-brain barrier such as occurs in malignant tumors of the brain allows the accumulation of the contrast medium within the interstitial tissue of the tumor. Adjacent normal brain tissue does not contain the contrast medium.

In nonneural tissues (during computed tomography of the body), Iopamidol diffuses rapidly from the vascular into the extravascular space. Increase in x-ray absorption is related to blood flow, concentration of the contrast medium, and extraction of the contrast medium by interstitial tissue of tumors since no barrier exists. Contrast enhancement is thus due to the relative differences in extravascular diffusion between normal and abnormal tissue, quite different from that in the brain.

The pharmacokinetics of Iopamidol in both normal and abnormal tissue have been shown to be variable. Contrast enhancement appears to be greatest soon after administration of the contrast medium, and following intraarterial rather than intravenous administration. Thus, greatest enhancement can be detected by a series of consecutive two- to three-second scans performed just after injection (within 30 to 90 seconds), i.e., dynamic computed tomographic imaging.

INDICATIONS AND USAGE

Iopamidol for intravascular injection is indicated for angiography throughout the cardiovascular system, including cerebral and peripheral arteriography, coronary arteriography and ventriculography, pediatric angiocardiography, selective visceral arteriography and aortography, peripheral venography (phlebography), and adult and pediatric intravenous excretory urography and intravenous adult and pediatric contrast enhancement of computed tomographic (CECT) head and body imaging (see below).

CECT HEAD IMAGING

Iopamidol (intravascular) may be used to refine diagnostic precision in areas of the brain which may not otherwise have been satisfactorily visualized.

TUMORS

Iopamidol (intravascular) may be useful to investigate the presence and extent of certain malignancies such as: gliomas including malignant gliomas, glioblastomas, astrocytomas, oligodendrogliomas and gangliomas, ependymomas, medulloblastomas, meningiomas, neuromas, pinealomas, pituitary adenomas, craniopharyngiomas, germinomas, and metastatic lesions. The usefulness of contrast enhancement for the investigation of the retrobulbar space and in cases of low grade or infiltrative glioma has not been demonstrated.

In calcified lesions, there is less likelihood of enhancement. Following therapy, tumors may show decreased or no enhancement.

The opacification of the inferior vermis following contrast media administration has resulted in false-positive diagnosis in a number of otherwise normal studies.

NONNEOPLASTIC CONDITIONS

Iopamidol (intravascular) may be beneficial in the image enhancement of nonneoplastic lesions. Cerebral infarctions of recent onset may be better visualized with contrast enhancement, while some infarctions are obscured if contrast media are used. The use of iodinated contrast media results in contrast enhancement in about 60 percent of cerebral infarction studied from one to four weeks from the onset of symptoms.

Sites of active infection may also be enhanced following contrast media administration.

Arteriovenous malformations and aneurysms will show contrast enhancement. For these vascular lesions, the enhancement is probably dependent on the iodine content of the circulating blood pool.

Hematomas and intraparenchymal bleeders seldom demonstrate any contrast enhancement. However, in cases of intraparenchymal clot, for which there is no obvious clinical explanation, contrast media administration may be helpful in ruling out the possibility of associated arteriovenous malformation.

CECT BODY IMAGING

Iopamidol (intravascular) may be used for enhancement of computed tomographic images for detection and evaluation of lesions in the liver, pancreas, kidneys, aorta, mediastinum, abdominal cavity, pelvis and retroperitoneal space.

Enhancement of computed tomography with Iopamidol (intravascular) may be of benefit in establishing diagnoses of certain lesions in these sites with greater assurance than is possible with CT alone, and in supplying additional features of the lesions (e.g., hepatic abscess delineation prior to percutaneous drainage). In other cases, the contrast agent may allow visualization of lesions not seen with CT alone (e.g., tumor extension), or may help to define suspicious lesions seen with unenhanced CT (e.g., pancreatic cyst).

Contrast enhancement appears to be greatest within 60 to 90 seconds after bolus administration of contrast agent. Therefore, utilization of a continuous scanning technique ("dynamic CT scanning") may improve enhancement and diagnostic assessment of tumor and other lesions such as an abscess, occasionally revealing unsuspected or more extensive disease. For example, a cyst may be distinguished from a vascularized solid lesion when precontrast and enhanced scans are compared; the nonperfused mass shows unchanged x-ray absorption (CT number). A vascularized lesion is characterized by an increase in CT number in the few minutes after a bolus of intravascular contrast agent; it may be malignant, benign, or normal tissue, but would probably not be a cyst, hematoma, or other nonvascular lesion.

Because unenhanced scanning may provide adequate diagnostic information in the individual patient, the decision to employ contrast enhancement, which may be associated with risk and increased radiation exposure, should be based upon a careful evaluation of clinical, other radiological, and unenhanced CT findings.

Iopamidol for intrathecal administration is indicated in adult neuroradiology including myelography (lumbar, thoracic, cervical, total columnar), and for contrast enhancement of computed tomographic (CECT) cisternography and ventriculography. Iopamidol for intrathecal administration is indicated for thoraco-lumbar myelography in children over the age of two years.

Iopamidol for intra-arterial administration is indicated for intra-arterial digital subtraction angiography (DSA) of the cerebral and abdominal vasculature.

CONTRAINDICATIONS

None.

Intrathecal administration of corticosteroids with Iopamidol is contraindicated. Because of overdosage considerations, immediate repeat myelography in the event of technical failure is contraindicated (see interval recommendation under *"Dosage and Administration"*). Myelography should not be performed in the presence of significant local or systemic infection where bacteremia is likely.

There are no known contraindications to the use of Iopamidol for intravascular or intra-arterial administration.

WARNINGS

IOPAMIDOL FOR INTRAVASCULAR AND INTRA-ARTERIAL ADMINISTRATION

Nonionic iodinated contrast media inhibit blood coagulation, *in vitro*, less than ionic contrast media. Clotting has been reported when blood remains in contact with syringes containing nonionic contrast media.

Serious, rarely fatal, thromboembolic events causing myocardial infarction and stroke have been reported during angiographic procedures with both ionic and nonionic contrast media. Therefore, meticulous intravascular administration technique is necessary, particularly during angiographic procedures, to minimize thromboembolic events. Numerous factors, including length of procedure, catheter and syringe material, underlying disease state, and concomitant medications may contribute to the development of thromboembolic events. For these reasons, meticulous angiographic techniques are recommended including close attention to guidewire and catheter manipulation, use of manifold systems and/or three way stopcocks, frequent catheter flushing with heparinized saline solutions, and minimizing the length of the procedure. The use of plastic syringes in place of glass syringes has been reported to decrease but not eliminate the likelihood of *in vitro* clotting.

Caution must be exercised in patients with severely impaired renal function, those with combined renal and hepatic disease, or anuria, particularly when larger doses are administered.

Radiopaque diagnostic contrast agents are potentially hazardous in patients with multiple myeloma or other paraproteinemia, particularly in those with therapeutically resistant anuria. Myeloma occurs most commonly in persons over age 40. Although neither the contrast agent nor dehydration has been proved separately to be the cause of anuria in myelomatous patients, it has been speculated that the combination of both may be causative. The risk in myelomatous patients is not a contraindication; however, special precautions are required.

Contrast media may promote sickling in individuals who are homozygous for sickle cell disease when injected intravenously or intra-arterially.

Administration of radiopaque materials to patients known or suspected of having pheochromocytoma should be performed with extreme caution. If, in the opinion of the physician, the possible benefits of such procedures outweigh the considered risks, the procedures may be performed; however, the amount of radiopaque medium injected should be kept to an absolute minimum. The blood pressure should be assessed throughout the procedure and measures for treatment of a hypertensive crisis should be available. These patients should be monitored very closely during contrast enhanced procedures.

Reports of thyroid storm following the use of iodinated radiopaque diagnostic agents in patients with hyperthyroidism or with an autonomously functioning thyroid nodule suggest that this additional risk be evaluated in such patients before use of any contrast medium.

IOPAMIDOL FOR INTRATHECAL ADMINISTRATION
The need for myelographic examination should be carefully evaluated. Iopamidol should be administered with caution in patients with increased intracranial pressure or suspicion of intracranial tumor, abscess or hematoma, those with a history of convulsive disorder, severe cardiovascular disease, chronic alcoholism, or multiple sclerosis, and elderly patients. Particular attention must be given to state of hydration, concentration of medium, dose, and technique used in these patients.

If frankly bloody cerebrospinal fluid is observed, the possible benefits of a myelographic examination should be considered in terms of risk to the patient.

Patients on anticonvulsant medication should be maintained on this therapy.

Direct intracisternal or ventricular administration for standard radiography (without computerized tomographic enhancement) is not recommended. Inadvertent intracranial entry of a large or concentrated bolus of the contrast medium, which increases the risk of neurotoxicity, can be prevented by careful patient management. Also, effort should be directed to avoid rapid dispersion of the medium causing inadvertent rise to intracranial levels (e.g., by active patient movement). If such intracranial entry of the medium occurs, prophylactic anticonvulsant treatment with diazepam or barbiturates orally for 24 to 48 hours should be considered.

Use of medications that may lower the seizure threshold (phenothiazine derivatives, including those used for their antihistaminic properties; tricyclic antidepressants; MAO inhibitors; CNS stimulants; analeptics; antipsychotic agents) should be carefully evaluated. While the contributory role of such medications has not been established, some physicians have discontinued these agents at least 48 hours before and for at least 24 hours following intrathecal use.

Focal and generalized motor seizures have been reported after intrathecal use of water-soluble contrast agents including Iopamidol. In several of those cases reported with Iopamidol, higher than recommended doses were employed. Therefore *avoid*:

■ Deviations from recommended neuroradiologic procedure or patient management.
■ Use in patients with a history of epilepsy unless medically justified.
■ Overdosage.
■ Intracranial entry of a bolus or premature diffusion of a high concentration of the medium.
■ Failure to maintain elevation of the head during the procedure, on the stretcher, and in bed.
■ Excessive and particularly active patient movement or straining.

PRECAUTIONS
GENERAL
Diagnostic procedures which involve the use of any radiopaque agent should be carried out under the direction of personnel with the prerequisite training and with a thorough knowledge of the particular procedure to be performed. Appropriate facilities should be available for coping with any complication of the procedure, as well as for emergency treatment of severe reaction to the contrast agent itself. After parenteral administration of a radiopaque agent, competent personnel and emergency facilities should be available for at least 30 to 60 minutes since severe delayed reactions may occur.

Preparatory dehydration is dangerous and may contribute to acute renal failure in patients with advanced vascular disease, diabetic patients, and in susceptible nondiabetic patients (often elderly with preexisting renal disease). *Patients should be well hydrated prior to and following Iopamidol administration.*

The possibility of a reaction, including serious, life-threatening, fatal, anaphylactoid or cardiovascular reactions, should always be considered (see *"Adverse Reactions"*). Patients at increased risk include those with a history of previous reaction to a contrast medium, patients with a known sensitivity to iodine *per se*, and patients with a known clinical hypersensitivity (bronchial asthma, hay fever, and food allergies). The occurrence of severe idiosyncratic reactions has prompted the use of several pretesting methods. However, pretesting cannot be relied upon to predict severe reactions and may itself be hazardous for the patient. It is suggested that a thorough medical history with emphasis on allergy and

hypersensitivity, prior to the injection of any contrast medium, may be more accurate than pretesting in predicting potential adverse reactions. A positive history of allergies or hypersensitivity does not arbitrarily contraindicate the use of a contrast agent where a diagnostic procedure is thought essential, but caution should be exercised. Premedication with antihistamines or corticosteroids to avoid or minimize possible allergic reactions in such patients should be considered. Recent reports indicate that such pretreatment does not prevent serious life-threatening reactions, but may reduce both their incidence and severity.

General anesthesia may be indicated in the performance of some procedures in selected patients; however, a higher incidence of adverse reactions has been reported with intravascularly or intra-arterially administered radiopaque media in anesthetized patients, which may be attributable to the inability of the patient to identify untoward symptoms, or to the hypotensive effect of anesthesia which can reduce cardiac output and increase the duration of exposure to the contrast agent.

Even though the osmolality of intravascularly administered Iopamidol is low compared to diatrizoate or iothalamate based ionic agents of comparable iodine concentration and of intra-arterially administered Iopamidol comparable to that of plasma, the potential transitory increase in the circulatory osmotic load in patients with congestive heart failure requires caution during injection. These patients should be observed for several hours following the procedure to detect delayed hemodynamic disturbances.

In angiographic procedures, the possibility of dislodging plaques or damaging or perforating the vessel wall should be borne in mind during catheter manipulations and contrast medium injection. Test injections to ensure proper catheter placement are suggested.

Selective coronary arteriography should be performed only in selected patients and those in whom the expected benefits outweigh the procedural risk. The inherent risks of *angiocardiography* in patients with chronic pulmonary emphysema must be weighed against the necessity for performing this procedure. Following arteriographic procedures with intra-arterially administered Iopamidol, gentle pressure hemostasis is required, followed by observation and immobilization of the limb for several hours to prevent hemorrhage from the site of arterial puncture. *Angiography* should be avoided whenever possible in patients with homocystinuria, because of the risk of inducing thrombosis and embolism. See also Pediatric Use.

In addition to the general precautions previously described, special care is required when intravascular venography is performed in patients with suspected thrombosis, phlebitis, severe ischemic disease, local infection or a totally obstructed venous system.

Extreme caution during intravascular injection of contrast media is necessary to avoid extravasation and fluoroscopy is recommended. This is especially important in patients with severe arterial or venous disease.

The possibility of inducing bacterial meningitis in patients during intrathecal procedures should always be considered. To avoid bacterial contamination during spinal puncture, a sterile field should be maintained at all times.

If nondisposable equipment is used, scrupulous care should be taken to prevent residual contamination with traces of cleansing agents.

INFORMATION FOR PATIENTS
Patients receiving injectable radiopaque diagnostic agents should be instructed to:

1. Inform your physician if you are pregnant.
2. Inform your physician if you are a diabetic or if you have multiple myeloma, pheochromocytoma, homozygous sickle cell disease, or known thyroid disorder (see *"Warnings"*).
3. Inform your physician if you are allergic to any drugs, food, or if you had any reactions to previous injections of substances used for x-ray procedures (see *"Precautions, General"*).
4. Inform your physician about any other medications you are currently taking, including nonprescription drugs, before you have this procedure.

DRUG INTERACTIONS
Renal toxicity has been reported in a few patients with liver dysfunction who were given oral cholecystographic agents followed by intravascular contrast agents. Administration of intravascular agents should therefore be postponed in any patient with a known or suspected hepatic or biliary disorder who has recently received a cholecystographic contrast agent.

Other drugs should not be admixed with Iopamidol.

DRUG/LABORATORY TEST INTERACTIONS
The results of PBI and radioactive iodine uptake studies, which depend on iodine estimations, will not accurately reflect thyroid function for up to 16 days following administration of iodinated contrast media. However, thyroid function tests not depending on iodine estimations, e.g., T3 resin uptake and total or free thyroxine (T4) assays are not affected.

Any test which might be affected by contrast media should be performed prior to administration of the contrast medium.

LABORATORY TEST FINDINGS
In vitro studies with animal blood showed that many radiopaque contrast agents, including Iopamidol, produced a slight depression of plasma coagulation factors including prothrombin time, partial thromboplastin time, and fibrinogen, as well as a slight tendency to cause platelet and/or red blood cell aggregation (see *"Precautions, General"*).

Transitory changes may occur in red cell and leucocyte counts, serum calcium, serum creatinine, serum glutamic oxalacetic transaminase (SGOT), and uric acid in urine; transient albuminuria may occur.

◆ RATED THERAPEUTICALLY EQUIVALENT; ◇ THERAPEUTIC EQUIVALENCE UNCONFIRMED; ○ UNRATED

These findings have not been associated with clinical manifestations.

CARCINOGENESIS, MUTAGENESIS, IMPAIRMENT OF FERTILITY
Long-term studies in animals have not been performed to evaluate carcinogenic potential. No evidence of genetic toxicity was obtained in *in vitro* tests.

In animal reproduction studies performed on rats, intravenously administered Iopamidol did not induce adverse effects on fertility or general reproductive performance.

In studies to determine mutagenic activity, Iopamidol did not cause any increase in mutation rates.

PREGNANCY
Teratogenic Effects: Pregnancy Category B Reproduction studies have been performed in rats and rabbits at doses up to 2.7 and 1.4 times the maximum recommended human dose (1.48 gI/kg in a 50 kg individual), respectively, and have revealed no evidence of impaired fertility or harm to the fetus due to Iopamidol. There are, however, no adequate and well-controlled studies in pregnant women. It is not known whether Iopamidol crosses the placental barrier or reaches fetal tissues. However, many injectable contrast agents cross the placental barrier in humans and appear to enter fetal tissues passively. Because animal reproduction studies are not always predictive of human response, this drug should be used during pregnancy only if clearly needed.

Radiologic procedures involve a certain risk related to the exposure of the fetus to ionizing radiation.

LABOR AND DELIVERY
It is not known whether use of contrast agents during labor or delivery has immediate or delayed adverse effects on the fetus, prolongs the duration of labor or increases the likelihood that forceps delivery or other obstetrical intervention or resuscitation of the newborn will be necessary.

NURSING MOTHERS
It is not known whether this drug is excreted in human milk. However, many injectable contrast agents are excreted unchanged in human milk. Although it has not been established that serious adverse reactions occur in nursing infants, caution should be exercised when intravascular contrast media are administered to nursing women because of potential adverse reactions, and consideration should be given to temporarily discontinuing nursing.

PEDIATRIC USE
Safety and effectiveness in children have been established in intravascularly administered pediatric angiocardiography, computed tomography (head and body) and excretory urography. Pediatric patients at higher risk of experiencing adverse events during contrast medium administration may include those having asthma, a sensitivity to medication and/or allergens, cyanotic heart disease, congestive heart failure, a serum creatinine greater than 1.5 mg/dL or those less than 12 months of age.

See "*Dosage and Administration*" for pediatric use of intrathecally administered Iopamidol. Safety and effectiveness for intra-arterially administered Iopamidol in children have not been established.

ADVERSE REACTIONS
INTRAVASCULARLY AND INTRA-ARTERIALLY ADMINISTERED IOPAMIDOL
Adverse reactions following the use of Iopamidol are usually mild to moderate, self-limited, and transient.

In angiocardiography (597 patients), the adverse reactions with an estimated incidence of one percent or higher are: hot flashes 3.4%; angina pectoris 3.0%; flushing 1.8%; bradycardia 1.3%; hypotension 1.0%; hives 1.0%.

In a clinical trial with 76 pediatric patients undergoing angiocardiography, 2 adverse reactions (2.6%) both remotely attributed to the contrast media were reported. Both patients were less than 2 years of age, both had cyanotic heart disease with underlying right ventricular abnormalities and abnormal pulmonary circulation. In one patient pre-existing cyanosis was transiently intensified following contrast media administration. In the second patient pre-existing decreased peripheral perfusion was intensified for 24 hours following the examination (see "*Precautions*" section for information on high risk nature of these patients).

Intravascular injection of contrast media is frequently associated with the sensation of warmth and pain, especially in peripheral arteriography and venography; pain and warmth are less frequent and less severe with Iopamidol than with diatrizoate meglumine and diatrizoate sodium injection.

In a clinical trial with 100 patients, adverse reactions possibly attributed to Iopamidol (intra-arterial) administration were nausea (2%), headache (1%) and vomiting (1%). One patient with preexisting renal impairment and severe bilateral renal vascular disease experienced renal failure, possibly secondary to a subsequent acute episode of congestive heart failure and/or drug administration (see "*Warnings*").

The following table of incidence of reactions is based on clinical studies with Iopamidol (intravascular) in about 2246 to 2191 patients. These reactions may or may not occur with Iopamidol (intra-arterial) with the same frequency.

ADVERSE REACTIONS

| System | Estimated Overall Incidence | |
	> 1%	≤ 1%
Cardiovascular	none	tachycardia

| System | Estimated Overall Incidence | |
	> 1%	≤ 1%
		hypotension
		hypertension
		myocardial ischemia
		circulatory collapse
		S-T segment
		depression
		bigeminy
		extrasystoles
		ventricular fibrillation
		angina pectoris
		bradycardia
		transient ischemia
		attack
		thrombophlebitis
Nervous	pain (2.8%)	vasovagal reaction
	burning sensation (1.4%)	tingling in arms
		grimace
		faintness
Digestive	nausea (1.2%)	vomiting
		anorexia
Respiratory	none	throat constriction
		dyspnea
		pulmonary edema
Skin and Appendages	none	rash
		urticaria
		pruritus
		flushing
Body as a Whole	hot flashes (1.5%)	headache
		fever
		chills
		excessive sweating
		back spasm
Special Senses	warmth (1.1%)	taste alterations
		nasal congestion
		visual disturbances
Urogenital	none	urinary retention

Regardless of the contrast agent employed, the overall estimated incidence of serious adverse reactions is higher with *coronary arteriography* than with other procedures. Cardiac decompensation, serious arrhythmias, or myocardial ischemia or infarction may occur during *coronary arteriography and left ventriculography*. Following coronary and ventricular injections, certain electrocardiographic changes (increased QTc, increased R-R, T-wave amplitude) and certain hemodynamic changes (decreased systolic pressure) occurred less frequently with Iopamidol than with diatrizoate meglumine and diatrizoate sodium injection; increased LVEDP occurred less frequently after ventricular Iopamidol injections.

In *aortography*, the risks of procedures also include injury to the aorta and neighboring organs, pleural puncture, renal damage including infarction and acute tubular necrosis with oliguria and anuria, accidental selective filling of the right renal artery during the translumbar procedure in the presence of preexisting renal disease, retroperitoneal hemorrhage from the translumbar approach, and spinal cord injury and pathology associated with the syndrome of transverse myelitis.

Adverse effects reported in clinical literature for Iopamidol include arrhythmia, arterial spasms, hematuria, periorbital edema, involuntary leg movement, malaise, and triggering of deglutition; some of these may occur as a consequence of the procedure. Other reactions may also occur with the use of any contrast agent as a consequence of the procedural hazard; these include hemorrhage or pseudoaneurysms at the puncture site, brachial plexus palsy following axillary artery injections, chest pain, myocardial infarction, and transient changes in hepatorenal chemistry tests. Arterial thrombosis, displacement of arterial plaques, venous thrombosis, dissection of the coronary vessels and transient sinus arrest are rare complications.

INTRATHECALLY ADMINISTERED IOPAMIDOL
The most frequently reported adverse reactions following intrathecal administration of Iopamidol are headache, nausea, vomiting, and musculoskeletal pain. These reactions usually occur 1 to 10 hours after injection, almost all occurring within 24 hours. They are usually mild to moderate in degree, lasting for a few hours and usually disappearing within 24 hours. Rarely, headaches may be severe or persist for days. Headache is often accompanied by nausea and vomiting, and tends to be more frequent and persistent in patients not optimally hydrated. Backache, neck stiffness, numbness and paresthesias, leg or sciatic-type pain occurred less frequently, often in the form of a transient exacerbation of preexisting symptomatology. Transient alterations in vital signs may occur and their significance must be assessed on an individual basis.

The following table of incidence of reactions is based on clinical studies with Iopamidol (intrathecal) in about 686 patients.

ADVERSE REACTIONS

| System | Estimated Overall Incidence | |
	> 1%	≤ 1%
Body as a Whole	headache (16.4%)	pyrexia

System	Estimated Overall Incidence	
	> 1%	≤ 1%
		muscle weakness
		hot flashes
		malaise
		fatigue
		weakness
Digestive	nausea (7.3%)	diarrhea
	vomiting (3.6%)	heartburn
Musculoskeletal	back pain (2.2%)	leg cramps
	leg pain (1.4%)	sciatica
	neck pain (1.1%)	cervicobrachial
		irritation
		meningeal irritation
		radicular irritation,
		lumbosacral
		other musculoskeletal
		pain
		involuntary movement
		burning sensation
Cardiovascular	hypotension (1.1%)	tachycardia
		hypertension
		chest pain
Nervous	none	emotional stress
		dizziness
		paresthesia
		confusion
		hallucinations
		lightheadedness
		syncope
		numbness
		cold extremities
		ataxia
		irritability
Urogenital	none	urinary retention
Respiratory	none	dyspnea
Skin and Appendages	none	rash
Miscellaneous	none	injection site pain

Other adverse effects reported in clinical literature for Iopamidol include facial neuralgia, tinnitus, and sweating.

Major motor seizures have been reported in the clinical literature and since market introduction in the United States. Early onset of seizures (less than two hours) is indicative of early substantial intracranial entry. Transitory EEG changes occur and usually take the form of slow wave activity.

While not observed in controlled clinical studies with Iopamidol (intrathecal), the following adverse reactions may occur because they have been reported with Iopamidol (intrathecal) and other nonionic water soluble contrast agents

Cardiovascular: (arrhythmias)

Pulmonary: (apnea):

Bacterial meningitis and aseptic meningitis syndrome

Allergy or idiosyncrasy: (chills, pruritus, nasal congestion, Guillain-Barre syndrome)

CNS irritation: (psycho-organic syndrome: mild and transitory perceptual aberrations such as depersonalization, anxiety, depression, hyperesthesia, disturbances in speech, sight, or hearing, and disorientation; in addition, hyperreflexia or areflexia, hypertonia or flaccidity, restlessness, tremor, echoacousia, echolalia, asterixis or dysphasia have occurred).

Profound mental disturbances have rarely been reported (various forms and degrees of aphasia, mental confusion or disorientation); the onset is usually at 8 to 10 hours and lasts for about 24 hours without aftereffects. However, occasionally they have been manifest as apprehension, agitation, or progressive withdrawal to the point of stupor or coma. In a few cases, these have been accompanied by transitory hearing loss or other auditory symptoms and visual disturbances (believed subjective or delusional). Persistent cortical loss of vision in association with convulsions, and ventricular block have been reported. Rarely, persistent though transitory weakness in the leg or ocular muscles has been reported. *Peripheral neuropathies* have been rare and transitory. They include sensory and/or motor or nerve root disturbances, myelitis, persistent leg muscle pain or weakness, or sixth nerve palsy, or cauda equina syndrome. Muscle cramps, fasciculation or myoclonia, spinal convulsion, paralysis, or spasticity are unusual.

GENERAL ADVERSE REACTIONS TO CONTRAST MEDIA
Reactions known to occur with parenteral administration of iodinated ionic contrast agents (see the listing below) are possible with any nonionic agent. Approximately 95 percent of adverse reactions accompanying the use of other water-soluble intravascularly administered contrast agents are mild to moderate in degree. However, life-threatening reactions and fatalities, mostly of cardiovascular origin, have occurred. Reported incidences of death from the administration of other iodinated contrast media range from 6.6 per 1 million (0.00066 percent) to 1 in 10,000 patients (0.01 percent). Most deaths occur during injection or 5 to 10 minutes later, the main feature being cardiac arrest with cardiovascular disease as the main aggravating factor. Isolated reports of hypotensive collapse and shock

are found in the literature. The incidence of shock is estimated to be 1 out of 20,000 (0.005 percent) patients.

Adverse reactions to injectable contrast media fall into two categories: chemotoxic reactions and idiosyncratic reactions. Chemotoxic reactions result from the physicochemical properties of the contrast medium, the dose, and the speed of injection. All hemodynamic disturbances and injuries to organs or vessels perfused by the contrast medium are included in this category. Experience with Iopamidol suggests there is much less discomfort (e.g., pain and/or warmth) with peripheral arteriography. Fewer changes are noted in ventricular function after ventriculography and coronary arteriography. During intrathecal use, there is a lower incidence of electroencephalographic changes as well as neurotoxicity by virtue of the intrinsic properties of the Iopamidol molecule.

Idiosyncratic reactions include all other reactions. They occur more frequently in patients 20 to 40 years old. Idiosyncratic reactions may or may not be dependent on the amount of drug injected, the speed of injection, the mode of injection, and the radiographic procedure. Idiosyncratic reactions are subdivided into minor, intermediate, and severe. The minor reactions are self-limited and of short duration; the severe reactions are life-threatening and treatment is urgent and mandatory.

The reported incidence of adverse reactions to contrast media in patients with a history of allergy is twice that for the general population. Patients with a history of previous reactions to a contrast medium are three times more susceptible than other patients. However, sensitivity to contrast media does not appear to increase with repeated examinations. Most adverse reactions to intravascular contrast agents appear within one to three minutes after the start of injection, but delayed reactions may occur (see *"Precautions, General"*).

In addition to the adverse drug reactions reported for Iopamidol, the following additional adverse reactions have been reported with the use of other intravascular contrast agents and are possible with the use of any water-soluble iodinated contrast agent. Because measurable plasma levels are attained following the intrathecal administration of iopamidol, adverse reactions reported with the use of intravascular contrast agents are theoretically possible.

Cardiovascular: vasodilation, cerebral hematomas, petechiae, hemodynamic disturbances, sinus bradycardia, transient electrocardiographic abnormalities, ventricular fibrillation.

Digestive: nausea, vomiting, severe unilateral or bilateral swelling of the parotid and submaxillary glands.

Nervous: paresthesia, dizziness, convulsions, paralysis, coma.

Respiratory: Increased cough, asthma, laryngeal edema, pulmonary edema, bronchospasm, rhinitis dyspnea.

Skin and Appendages: Injection site pain usually due to extravasation and/or erythematous swelling, skin necrosis urticaria.

Urogenital: osmotic nephrosis of proximal tubular cells, renal failure, pain.

Special Senses: bilateral ocular irritation, lacrimation, conjunctival chemosis, infection, and conjunctivitis, preversion of taste, itching.

The following reactions may also occur: neutropenia, thrombophlebitis, flushing, pallor, weakness, severe retching and choking, wheezing, cramps, tremors, and sneezing.

OVERDOSAGE
A dose of 3000 mgI in adults and 2400 mgI in children is sufficient for most myelographic procedures. Doses above these levels may result in an increased frequency and severity of adverse reactions including seizures. However, in myelography, even use of a recommended dose can produce mental aberrations tantamount to overdosage, if incorrect management of the patient during or immediately following the procedure permits inadvertent early intracranial entry of a large portion of the medium.

Treatment of an overdose of an injectable radiopaque contrast medium is directed toward the support of all vital functions, and prompt institution of symptomatic therapy.

Intravenous LD$_{50}$ values (gI/kg) for Iopamidol in animals: 21.8 (mice), 13.8 (rats), 9.6 (rabbits), 17.0 (dogs).

DOSAGE AND ADMINISTRATION
GENERAL
It is desirable that solutions of radiopaque diagnostic agents for intravascular or intrathecal use be at body temperature when injected. In the event that crystallization of the medium has occurred, place the vial in hot (60°-100°C) water for about five minutes, then shake gently to obtain a clear solution. Cool to body temperature before use. Discard vial without use if solids persist.

Withdrawal of contrast agents from their containers should be accomplished under aseptic conditions with sterile syringes. Sterile techniques must be used with any intravascular injection, and with catheters and guidewires.

Parenteral drug products should be inspected visually for particulate matter and discoloration prior to administration, whenever solution and container permit. Iopamidol solutions should be used only if clear and within the normal colorless to pale yellow range.

Patients should be well hydrated prior to and following Iopamidol administration.

As with all radiopaque contrast agents, only the lowest dose of Iopamidol necessary to obtain adequate visualization should be used. A lower dose reduces the possibility of an adverse reaction. Most procedures do not require use of either a maximum dose or the highest available concentration of Iopamidol the combination of dose and Iopamidol concentration to be used should be carefully

---

◆ RATED THERAPEUTICALLY EQUIVALENT; ◇ THERAPEUTIC EQUIVALENCE UNCONFIRMED; ○ UNRATED

individualized, and factors such as age, body size, size of the vessel and its blood flow rate, anticipated pathology and degree and extent of opacification required, structure(s) or area to be examined, disease processes affecting the patient, and equipment and technique to be employed should be considered.

Intravasularly administered Iopamidol:

CEREBRAL ARTERIOGRAPHY

Iopamidol injection, 300 mgI/mL should be used. The usual individual injection by carotid puncture or transfemoral catheterization is 8 to 12 mL, with total multiple doses ranging to 90 mL.

PERIPHERAL ARTERIOGRAPHY

Iopamidol 300 mgI/mL usually provides adequate visualization. For injection into the femoral artery or subclavian artery, 5 to 40 mL may be used; for injection into the aorta for a distal runoff, 25 to 50 mL may be used. Doses up to a total of 250 mL of Iopamidol 300 mgI/mL have been administered during peripheral arteriography.

PERIPHERAL VENOGRAPHY (PHLEBOGRAPHY)

Iopamidol injection, 200 mgI/mL should be used. The usual dose is 25 to 150 mL per lower extremity. The combined total dose for multiple injections has not exceeded 350 mL.

SELECTIVE VISCERAL ARTERIOGRAPHY AND AORTOGRAPHY

Iopamidol injection, 370 mgI/mL should be used. Doses up to 50 mL may be required for injection into the larger vessels such as the aorta or celiac artery; doses up to 10 mL may be required for injection into the renal arteries. Often, lower doses will be sufficient. The combined total dose for multiple injections has not exceeded 225 mL.

PEDIATRIC ANGIOCARDIOGRAPHY

Iopamidol injection, 370 mgI/mL should be used. Pediatric angiocardiography may be performed by injection into a large peripheral vein or by direct catheterization of the heart.

The usual dose range for single injections is provided in the following table:

SINGLE INJECTION USUAL DOSAGE RANGE

Age	mL
< 2 years	10-15
2-9 years	15-30
10-18 years	20-50

The usual dose for cumulative injections is provided in the following table:

CUMULATIVE INJECTIONS USUAL DOSE RANGE

Age	mL
< 2 years	40
2-4 years	50
5-9 years	100
10-18 years	125

CORONARY ARTERIOGRAPHY AND VENTRICULOGRAPHY

Iopamidol 370 mgI/mL should be used. The usual dose for selective coronary artery injections is 2 to 10 mL. The usual dose for ventriculography, or for nonselective opacification of multiple coronary arteries following injection at the aortic root, is 25 to 50 mL. The total dose for combined procedures has not exceeded 200 mL. EKG monitoring is essential.

EXCRETORY UROGRAPHY

Iopamidol 250 mgI/mL or Iopamidol 300 mgI/mL may be used. The usual adult dose for Iopamidol 250 mgI/mL is 50 to 100 mL and for Iopamidol 300 mgI/mL is 50 mL administered by rapid intravenous injection; doses up to 100mL of Iopamidol 300 mgI/mL have been administered.

PEDIATRIC EXCRETORY UROGRAPHY

Iopamidol 250 mgI/mL or Iopamidol 300 mgI/mL may be used. The dosage recommended for use in children for excretory urography is 1.2 mL/kg to 3.6 mL/kg for Iopamidol 250 mgI/mL and 1.0 mL/kg to 3.0 mL/kg for Iopamidol 300 mgI/mL. It should not be necessary to exceed a total dose of 30 gI.

COMPUTED TOMOGRAPHY

Iopamidol 250 mgI/mL or Iopamidol 300 mgI/mL may be used *Head Imaging*: The suggested dose range for Iopamidol 250 mgI/mL is 100 to 150 mL and for Iopamidol 300 mgI/mL is 50 to 100 mL by intravenous administration; imaging may be performed immediately after completion of administration.

Body Imaging: The usual adult dose for Iopamidol 250 mgI/mL is 130 mL and for Iopamidol 300 mgI/mL is 100 mL administered by rapid intravenous infusion or bolus injection. Imaging is performed immediately after injection.

Equivalent doses of Iopamidol 370 mgI/mL, based on organically bound iodine content, may also be used.

PEDIATRIC COMPUTED TOMOGRAPHY

Iopamidol 250 mgI/mL or Iopamidol 300 mgI/mL may be used. The dosage recommended for use in children for contrast enhanced computed tomography is 1.2 mL/kg to 3.6 mL/kg for Iopamidol 250 mgI/mL and 10 mL/kg to 3.0 mL/kg for Iopamidol 300 mgI/mL. It should not be necessary to exceed a total dose of 30 gI.

INTRATHECALLY ADMINISTERED IOPAMIDOL

In adults a solution that is approximately isotonic Iopamidol 200 mgI/mL is recommended for examination of the lumbar region. For movement of the contrast medium to distant target areas, the more concentrated Iopamidol 300 mgI/mL preparation should be used to compensate for dilution of Iopamidol (intrathecal) with cerebrospinal fluid.

The usual recommended adult dose range for Iopamidol is 2000-3000 mg iodine. Iopamidol formulated to contain more than 300 mgI/mL should not be used intrathecally in adults. The minimum dose needed to perform a procedure should always be used.

In pediatric patients, a solution that is approximately isotonic Iopamidol 200 mgI/mL is recommended for all intrathecal procedures. In children, loss of contrast due to mixing on movement of the medium is less apt to occur because of their shorter spinal cord.

The usual recommended pediatric dose range for Iopamidol is 1400-2400 mg iodine. Iopamidol formulated to contain more than 200 mgI/mL should not be used intrathecally in children. The minimum dose needed to perform a procedure should always be used. See pediatric dosage table for recommended dosage.

Anesthesia is not necessary. However, young children may require general anesthesia for technical reasons. Premedication with sedatives or tranquilizers is usually not needed. In patients with a history of seizure activity who are not on anticonvulsant therapy, premedication with barbiturates or phenytoin should be considered.

Lumbar puncture is usually made between L3 and L4; if pathology is suspected at this level, the interspace immediately above or below may be selected. A lateral cervical puncture may also be used.

Rate of Injection: To avoid excessive mixing with cerebrospinal fluid and consequent loss of contrast as well as premature cephalad dispersion, injection must be made slowly over one to two minutes; the needle may then be removed.

An interval of at least 48 hours should be allowed before repeat examination; however, whenever possible five to seven days is recommended.

As with all radiopaque contrast agents, only the lowest dose of Iopamidol (intrathecal) necessary to obtain adequate visualization should be used. A lower dose reduces the possibility of an adverse reaction. Most procedures do not require use of either a maximum dose or the highest available concentration of Iopamidol (intrathecal); the combination of dose and Iopamidol (intrathecal) concentration to be used should be carefully individualized, and factors such as age, body size, anticipated pathology and degree and extent of opacification required, structure(s) or area to be examined, disease processes affecting the patient, and equipment and technique to be employed should be considered. **Following are the usual recommended pediatric and adult doses of Iopamidol (intrathecal).**

The pediatric doses listed below, intended as a guideline, are based on age rather than weight because the brain and CSF capacity is independent of weight. Variations will depend on such factors as height, suspected pathology, the patient's condition, technique used, etc., (e.g., CT or standard radiology or movement of the contrast media directed distal to the site of injection).

PEDIATRIC DOSAGE TABLE
IOPAMIDOL (INTRATHECAL) (200 MGI/ML)

Procedure	Age Years	Usual Recommended Dose (mL)
Lumbar, thoracic myelogram	2- 7	7- 9
	8-12	8-11
	13-18	10-12

ADULT DOSAGE TABLE

Procedure	Concentration of Solution (mgI/mL)	Usual Recommended Dose (mL)
Lumbar myelogram	200	10 to 15
Thoracic myelogram	200	10 to 15
Cervical myelogram	200	10 to 15
(via lumbar injection)	300	10
Cervical myelogram	200	10
(via lateral cervical injection)		
Total columnar myelography	300	10
CT cisternography (via lumbar injection)	200	4 to 6

Following subarachnoid injection, conventional radiography will continue to provide good diagnostic contrast for at least 30 minutes. At about one hour, diagnostic degree of contrast will not usually be available. However, sufficient contrast for CT myelography will be available for several hours. CT myelography following conventional myelography should be deferred for at least four hours to reduce the degree of contrast.

Aspiration of Iopamidol is unnecessary following intrathecal administration (see "Clinical Pharmacology").

SUGGESTIONS FOR USUAL PATIENT MANAGEMENT
Preprocedure:

- See *"Warnings"* regarding discontinuation of neuroleptic agents.
- Maintain normal diet up to 2 hours before procedure.
- Ensure hydration — fluids up to time of procedure.

➤ SHOWN IN PRODUCT IDENTIFICATION GUIDE

During Procedure:

- Use minimum dose and concentration required for satisfactory contrast.
- Injection slowly over 1 to 2 minutes to avoid excessive mixing.
- Abrupt or active patient movement causes excessive mixing with CSF.
- Instruct patient to remain *passive*. Move patient *slowly* and only as necessary.
- To maintain as a bolus, move medium to distal area *very slowly* under fluoroscopic control.
- In all positioning techniques keep the patient's head elevated above highest level of spine.
- Do not lower head of table more than 15° during thoraco-cervical procedures.
- In patients with excessive lordosis, consider lateral position for injection and movement of the medium cephalad.
- Avoid intracranial entry of a bolus.
- Avoid early and high cephalad dispersion of the medium.
- At completion of direct cervical or lumbo-cervical procedures, raise head of table steeply (45°) for about 2 minutes to restore medium to lower levels.

Postprocedure:

- Raise head of stretcher to at least 30° before moving patient onto it.
- Movement onto stretcher, and off the stretcher to bed, should be done slowly with patient completely passive, maintaining *head up* position.
- Before moving patient onto bed, raise head of bed 30° to 45° and maintain the patient in this position under close observation for 12 to 24 hours.
- Advise patient to remain still in bed, in *head up* position for the first 24 hours.
- Obtain visitors cooperation in keeping the patient quiet and in *head up* position, especially in first few hours.
- Encourage oral fluids and diet as tolerated.
- Antinauseants of the phenothiazine class should not be administered to treat postprocedural nausea or vomiting (see *"Warnings"*). Since persistent nausea and vomiting may result in dehydration, prompt consideration of volume replacement by intravenous fluids is recommended.

INTRA-ARTERIALLY ADMINISTERED IOPAMIDOL

The following dosing schedule should serve as a guide only, since the volume and rate of contrast administration will depend on the vessel size and on the technical specifications of the imaging equipment being used. As a general rule, the volume and flow rates used for intra-arterial DSA are less than that used for conventional film arteriography.

    Carotid or Vertebral arteries 6-12 mL
    Aortic Arch 25-60 mL
    Renal arteries 6-15 mL
    Branches of the aorta 12-50 mL
    Abdominal Aorta 25-60 mL
    The combined total dose for multiple injections should not exceed 350 mL.

DRUG INCOMPATIBILITIES

Many radiopaque contrast agents are incompatible *in vitro* with some antihistamines and many other drugs; therefore, no other pharmaceuticals should be admixed with contrast agents.

STORAGE

Store at room temperature not exceeding 30°C (86°F). Protect from light.

HOW SUPPLIED
INJECTION: 26%

BRAND/MANUFACTURER	NDC	SIZE	AWP
○ **BRAND**			
ISOVUE-128: Bracco Diag	00003-2153-10	50 ml 10s	$468.75

INJECTION: 41%

BRAND/MANUFACTURER	NDC	SIZE	AWP
○ **BRAND**			
ISOVUE-M-200: Bracco Diag	00003-1411-11	10 ml 10s	$538.24
	00003-1411-25	20 ml 10s	$737.25
ISOVUE-200: Bracco Diag	00003-1314-30	50 ml 10s	$537.50
	00003-1314-34	100 ml 10s	$875.00
	00003-1314-40	200 ml 10s	$1575.00

INJECTION: 51%

BRAND/MANUFACTURER	NDC	SIZE	AWP
○ **BRAND**			
ISOVUE-250: Bracco Diag	00003-1317-05	50 ml 10s	$553.13
	00003-1317-02	100 ml 10s	$981.50
	00003-1317-03	150 ml 10s	$1286.63
	00003-1317-01	200 ml 10s	$1839.00

INJECTION: 61%

BRAND/MANUFACTURER	NDC	SIZE	AWP
○ **BRAND**			
ISOVUE-M-300: Bracco Diag	00003-1412-15	15 ml 10s	$714.74
ISOVUE-300: Bracco Diag	00003-1315-25	30 ml 10s	$515.00
	00003-1315-30	50 ml 10s	$574.88
	00003-1315-47	75 ml 10s	$887.50
	00003-1315-35	100 ml 10s	$1123.50
	00003-1315-50	150 ml 10s	$1637.50
	00003-1315-37	150 ml 10s	$1650.00

INJECTION: 76%

BRAND/MANUFACTURER	NDC	SIZE	AWP
○ **BRAND**			
ISOVUE-370: Bracco Diag	00003-1316-07	20 ml 10s	$350.00
	00003-1316-47	30 ml 10s	$544.63
	00003-1316-01	50 ml 10s	$625.00
	00003-1316-30	50 ml 10s	$625.00
	00003-1316-52	75 ml 10s	$937.50
	00003-1316-35	100 ml 10s	$1246.88
	00003-1316-04	125 ml 10s	$1473.63
	00003-1316-37	150 ml 10s	$1725.00
	00003-1316-44	175 ml 10s	$1913.75
	00003-1316-40	200 ml 10s	$2200.00

Iopanoic Acid

DESCRIPTION

Iopanoic Acid is a diagnostic enteral cholecystographic radiopaque agent used for radiographic visualization of the gallbladder and biliary tract. Iopanoic Acid is an oral radiopaque medium for cholecystography and cholangiography. Each tablet contains 500 mg Iopanoic Acid.

Iopanoic Acid is a cream-colored solid which is insoluble in water. It contains 66.68 percent organically bound iodine. The molecular weight is 570.93.

Iopanoic Acid is a substituted, triiodinated, benzoic acid derivative, and is chemically 3-amino-α-ethyl-2,4,6-triiodohydrocinnamic acid ($C_{11}H_{12}I_3NO_2$)

Following is its chemical structure:

CLINICAL PHARMACOLOGY

The most important characteristic of contrast media is the iodine content. The relatively high atomic weight of iodine contributes sufficient radiodensity for radiographic contrast with surrounding tissues.

Diagnostic enteral radiopaque agents have few known pharmacological effects. They are moderately uricosuric. Iopanoic Acid when absorbed systemically may have iodine-mediated thyrotropic effects described under *"Precautions"*.

PHARMACOKINETICS

Iopanoic Acid is absorbed by passive diffusion across the gastrointestinal mucosa. Absorption of the agent can be improved by increasing the gastrointestinal pH, drug solubility, and availability of bile salts.

Controversy exists regarding the effects of food on the absorption and clinical efficacy of the cholecystographic agents. In one study, the number of satisfactory cholecystograms obtained with Iopanoic Acid administered with a high-fat meal was greater than with a nonfat meal. However, the fat content of the meal had no significant effect on the number of satisfactory cholecystograms obtained with Iopanoic Acid. Therefore, recommendations regarding the size or content of the evening meal on the day prior to oral cholecystography are made at the discretion of the physician.

Once absorbed, oral cholecystographic agents enter the systemic circulation via the portal venous system. They are then transported to the liver and bound to plasma albumin. The affinity for albumin may determine the primary route of elimination, biliary or renal, with the more extensively bound agents, primarily excreted by the hepatobiliary system.

In the liver Iopanoic Acid is metabolized to glucuronide esters which are then actively excreted into the hepatic ducts and concentrated by the gallbladder. The time of peak opacification of the gallbladder is approximately 14 to 19 hours for Iopanoic Acid. However, diagnostically adequate visualization of gallbladder may occur within 5 to 6 hours.

Iopanoic Acid is removed from the body by two pathways: excretion into the duodenum via the common bile duct and renal elimination. The ratio of renal to fecal elimination for Iopanoic Acid is 35:65 respectively in normal subjects. It appears that the bulk of an administered dose is eliminated from the body within a week. However, effects on thyroid function tests may persist for longer periods.

Oral cholecystographic agents are excreted in breast milk. (See *"Precautions—Nursing Mothers"*.)

Oral cholecystographic agents may produce changes in thyroid studies attributable to changes in circulating iodide. Thyroid function tests may not accurately reflect thyroid status for up to 1 year following cholecystography. Additionally, oral cholecystographic agents tend to elevate BSP (sulfobromophthalein) determinations. (See *"Precautions—Drug/Laboratory Test Interactions"*.)

INDICATIONS AND USAGE

Iopanoic Acid is indicated for use in oral cholecystography. It may also be used for oral cholangiography, although it is not considered the method of choice.

CONTRAINDICATIONS

Administration of Iopanoic Acid is contraindicated in severe impairment of renal function and particularly in advanced hepatorenal disease. It is also contraindicated in severe gastrointestinal disorders that prevent absorption, and in those patients who are allergic to iodinated compounds.

◆ RATED THERAPEUTICALLY EQUIVALENT; ◇ THERAPEUTIC EQUIVALENCE UNCONFIRMED; ○ UNRATED

PRECAUTIONS
GENERAL
Cholecystography in severely ill or debilitated patients or in those with severe hepatic or renal disease could result in partial or total renal shutdown.

Renal Effect: Acute renal insufficiency has followed the use of oral cholecystographic agents. Most reported cases were attributed to the use of large doses or multiple agents, to preexisting dehydration, or hepatic disease.

Patients with preexisting renal disease should not receive high doses of cholecystographic media. Possible renal irritation in susceptible individuals could result in reflex vascular spasm with partial or complete renal shutdown.

Liver Disease: Iopanoic Acid is generally well tolerated by patients with moderately impaired liver function, and adequate gallbladder visualization can often be achieved in the presence of hepatic disease. However, severe, advanced liver disease (e.g., bilirubin exceeding 5 mg per 100 mL) very frequently results in nonvisualization of the gallbladder.

Severe, advanced liver disease may interfere with metabolism of the radiopaque medium, and therefore, a greater amount of unchanged Iopanoic Acid will be diverted for renal excretion, increasing the load on the kidneys. Although renal difficulty has rarely been attributed to Iopanoic Acid, renal function in patients with severe, advanced liver disease should be assessed before cholecystography, and renal output and hepatic function should be observed for a few days after the procedure.

Dehydration: All patients, especially those with renal or hepatic diseases, should not be dehydrated beforehand and should drink liberal amounts of fluids with the tablets.

Uricosuric Effect: It has been shown that Iopanoic Acid has uricosuric activity. Therefore, patients with hyperuricemia should be well hydrated to maintain adequate urinary output to prevent uric acid crystal formation.

Coronary Disease: Caution is advised in patients with coronary disorders, especially those with recent symptoms of coronary artery disease. Blood pressure should be observed after administration of cholecystographic media to these patients.

Thyroid Disease: Caution should be exercised when administering cholecystographic agents to hyperthyroid and euthyroid goiterous patients (see "*Adverse Reactions*").

Elderly Patients: For elderly patients, see "*Dosage and Administration*".

INFORMATION FOR THE PATIENT
Patients receiving oral cholecystographic agents should be given the following information and instructions.

This drug has been prescribed to perform an x-ray study of the gallbladder. All the medication must be taken with water following dinner the evening prior to the test. Thereafter, nothing except water should be taken until the test has been completed.

Patients should be questioned regarding medicines, including nonprescription drugs, currently being used. Allergies to iodine, any foods, or x-ray dyes should also be disclosed.

Patients should inform the physician of any liver or kidney disease or pregnancy before taking this drug.

Patients should consult the physician if, at some future date, any thyroid tests are planned. The iodine in this agent may interfere with later thyroid tests.

This drug may cause abdominal cramping, nausea, vomiting, diarrhea, skin rashes, itching, heartburn, dizziness or headache in some patients but most reactions are mild and pass quickly.

DRUG INTERACTIONS
Concurrent administration of cholestyramine and Iopanoic Acid reportedly resulted in abnormal cholecystography. *In vitro* studies indicate that cholestyramine has an apparent high affinity for Iopanoic Acid. To avoid nonvisualization or poor visualization, oral cholecystography should be performed after cholestyramine has been discontinued long enough for complete evacuation from at least the small bowel.

The administration of both oral cholecystographic agents and intravenous iodipamide meglumine within 24 hours is not recommended. The prior administration of an oral cholecystographic agent seems to block the hepatic excretion of the intravenously administered iodipamide meglumine.

Renal toxicity has been reported in a few patients with liver dysfunction who were given oral cholecystographic agents followed by urographic agents. Administration of urographic agents should therefore be postponed in any patient with a known or suspected hepatic or biliary disorder who has recently taken a cholecystographic contrast agent.

DRUG/LABORATORY TEST INTERACTIONS
Thyroid Function Tests: The results of PBI and RAI uptake studies, which depend on iodine estimations, will not reflect thyroid function for several months following administration of cholecystographic media. However, function tests not depending on iodine estimations, eg, T_3 resin uptake or free thyroxine assays, are not affected.

Liver Function Tests: Bilirubin, thymol turbidity, cephalin flocculation, and serum enzyme values are unaffected but Iopanoic Acid may delay BSP clearance values for up to two days.

Urine Tests: Pseudoalbuminuria may be present for three days in response to certain chemical protein precipitation tests. Positive reactions should be verified by the heat-and-acetic acid or colorimetric dip-strip methods.

Uricosuric Effect: Iopanoic Acid may increase the rate of excretion of uric acid, lowering blood levels and raising urinary excretion values for a few days.

CARCINOGENESIS, MUTAGENESIS, IMPAIRMENT OF FERTILITY
Long-term studies in animals have not been performed in order to evaluate the carcinogenic potential, mutagenesis, or whether Iopanoic Acid can affect fertility in males or females.

PREGNANCY CATEGORY C
Animal reproduction studies have not been conducted with Iopanoic Acid. It is also not known whether Iopanoic Acid can cause fetal harm when administered to a pregnant woman or can affect reproduction capacity. Iopanoic Acid should be given to a pregnant woman only if clearly needed.

NURSING MOTHERS
Iopanoic Acid is excreted in the milk of nursing mothers. Therefore, caution should be exercised when Iopanoic Acid is administered.

ADVERSE REACTIONS
Most reactions following the oral administration of Iopanoic Acid have been mild and transitory. Moderately severe reactions are unusual and severe reactions or morbidity is extremely rare.

Gastrointestinal: By far the most frequent adverse response to Iopanoic Acid is gastrointestinal, mostly affecting the lower bowel (20%). Thus a few loose stools are common, frank diarrhea or abdominal cramps unusual and severe diarrhea with prostration is rare.

Mild nausea (10%) with vomiting (1%) is also frequent.

Allergic: (0.5%)—Skin, mucous membrane, and systemic hypersensitivity reactions are unusual and include urticaria with or without pruritus, erythema, morbilliform rash, and localized areas of edema. Rarely a systemic serum sickness-type reaction with fever, rash, and arthralgia. A few cases of transitory thrombocytopenia with petechiae have been reported.

Urinary: A mild stinging sensation during urination may occur (3%).

Hepatorenal and Cardiovascular: Very rare disturbances in function have been reported, usually occurring in patients with preexisting disease (see "*Precautions—General*").

Goiter: Cases of hyperthyroidism have been reported with the use of oral contrast media. Some of these patients reportedly had multinodular goiters which may have been responsible for the increased hormone synthesis in response to excess iodine. Thyroid storm has occurred in these patients.

OVERDOSAGE
A few cases of large overdoses of Iopanoic Acid have been reported, involving ingestion of 30 g, 36 g, and 75 g of the drug. Mild transient renal dysfunction was reported. All patients experienced extreme nausea, diarrhea, and vomiting, but survived without permanent adverse effects.

Based upon the clinical pharmacology of Iopanoic Acid, the following treatment measures are recommended. While specific recommendations for other enteral radiopaque agents are unavailable, the following measures may be beneficial:
- Lavage the stomach and administer enemas to remove remaining potentially absorbable contrast material.
- Force fluids to avoid concentration and possible precipitation or crystallization of the contrast material or uric acid in the kidneys.
- Alkalinize the urine to increase the solubility of the drug-glucuronide complex and of uric acid.
- Administer cholestyramine to chelate and reduce absorption of the drug.
- Monitor blood pressure.

The acute oral LD_{50} of Iopanoic Acid in the mouse is 6.6 ± 0.7 to 15.8 ± 1.1 g/kg $\pm$ Standard Error.

DOSAGE AND ADMINISTRATION
The standard adult dose of 3 g (six tablets) administered individually is usually ingested with water in the evening after a fat-free dinner, about 14 hours before the cholecystography. In some instances, double doses of 6 g (12 tablets) may be ingested, eg, for duct visualization or for some repeat examinations made over 7 days later. Many radiologists prefer that the patient take a laxative (eg, castor oil) about four to six hours before ingesting Iopanoic Acid. (See also "*Nonvisualization—Repeat Examination*".) Preparatory dehydration is unnecessary and undesirable, especially in elderly patients.

The use of large or repeated doses over a number of days to force visualization of a poorly functioning gallbladder *in elderly patients* is not recommended.

DIET BEFORE CHOLECYSTOGRAPHY
Patients presenting for a cholecystogram are frequently on various types of diet, eg, weight reducing diet, gallbladder diet. In these diets the fat content is low or absent. The resulting gallbladder stasis often results in a viscous inspissated bile content in a distended bladder, making entry of Iopanoic Acid opacified bile difficult. It is recommended, therefore, that these patients be placed on a normal (fat containing) diet for several days before Iopanoic Acid cholecystography.

THE EVENING MEAL—FAT CONTENT

There is not a consensus as to whether or not the evening meal immediately prior to Iopanoic Acid cholecystography should contain fat. This is based on the following two considerations:

■ Fat is a prolonged cholecystagogue causing intermittent gallbladder emptying for up to eight hours. This renders accumulation and concentration by the healthy gallbladder difficult and may account for spurious nonvisualization on the first examination in some patients.

■ A normal fat containing diet, including fat in the evening meal, promotes increased opacified bile flow facilitating gallbladder accumulation and concentration.

Both views are based on animal and clinical observation. The radiologist should choose which regimen for the patient to follow in preparation for the cholecystogram.

During the interval between ingestion of Iopanoic Acid and the morning of cholecystographic examination the patient should take *nothing by mouth* except water, and should not smoke or chew gum. In the morning, before the radiologic examination, the patient may take an enema in order to remove accumulated gas which might interfere with visualization.

FATTY MEAL AFTER CHOLECYSTOGRAPHY

After the gallbladder has been visualized the patient may be given a fat-containing meal or a commercially available cholecystagogue, for determining the extent and duration of gallbladder contractility (thus, the degree of function), to help identify small radiolucent stones or to visualize the bile ducts. In recent years most radiologists consider the value of the fat meal in this manner mostly unrewarding and have dispensed with its routine use.

DUCT VISUALIZATION

Occasionally, the bile ducts may be visualized on the original film during cholecystography. However, in a substantial percentage of patients, administration of a fat is necessary. The more frequent the roentgenographic exposures, the greater the probability of visualization of the ducts; however, the best time intervals are usually 20 and 30 minutes after the fatty meal. Some investigators believe contrast in the ducts is enhanced by an increased dose of Iopanoic Acid (up to 6 g).

NONVISUALIZATION—REPEAT EXAMINATION

Nonvisualization (or nondiagnostic faint visualization) following a primary examination can occur in up to 15% to 20% of cholecystographic examinations, irrespective of the medium used. This is only "indicative" evidence of gallbladder disease. There are, however, also a large number of extrabiliary diseases and situations which can result in nonvisualization. Following nonvisualization on the first examination, a repeat cholecystogram using a single dose is therefore indicated to exclude extrabiliary causes. The radiologic diagnosis is based on the results of the repeat examination. If nonvisualization also occurs following the second examination, gallbladder disease may be inferred with reasonable certainty (98% to 100%).

For repeat examination on the same day as the initial cholecystographic procedure, an additional 3 g (six tablets) may be given. However, if repeat cholecystography is to be performed with a double dose, a period of at least five to seven days should intervene between the first and the repeat examinations. No more than a total of 6 g (12 tablets) should be ingested during a 24-hour period.

STORAGE

Protect tablets from light.

HOW SUPPLIED
TABLETS: 500 MG

BRAND/MANUFACTURER	NDC	SIZE	AWP
○ BRAND TELEPAQUE: Sanofi Winthrop	00024-1931-03	150s	$99.47

Iopidine *SEE* APRACLONIDINE HYDROCHLORIDE

Iothalamate

DESCRIPTION

Iothalamate is a sterile aqueous solution intended for use as a diagnostic radiopaque medium. Iothalamate contains 60% w/v Iothalamate Meglumine which is 1-deoxy-1-(methylamino)-D-glucitol 5-acetamido-2,4,6 triiodo-N-methylisophthalamate (salt) 54.3% or 66.8% w/v of iothalamate sodium which is monosodium 5-acetamido-2,4,6-triiodo-N-methylisophthalamate.

Each ml contains:
Iothalamate Meglumine ....600 mg
or
Iothalamate Sodium ....543 or 668 mg.

Iothalamate Meglumine solution provides 282 mg/ml organically bound iodine; Iothalamate Sodium provides 325 or 400 mg/ml. Iothalamate Meglumine has an osmolarity of approximately 1000 mOsmol per liter, an osmolality of approximately 1400 mOsmol per kilogram and is, therefore, hypertonic under conditions

of use. The viscosity (cps) is approximately 6 at 25°C and 4 at 37°C. The pH is 6.5-7.7.

Iothalamate Sodium has an osmolarity of approximately 1400 or 1700 mOsmol per liter, an osmolality of approximately 1700 or 2300 mOsmol per kilogram and is, therefore, hypertonic under conditions of use. The viscosity (cps) is approximately 4 or 7 at 25°C and 3 or 4.5 at 37°C. The pH is 7.0-7.6 or 6.5-7.7. Iothalamate is a clear solution containing no undissolved solids. Crystallization does not occur at normal room temperatures. It is supplied in containers from which the air has been displaced by nitrogen.

Following is its chemical structure:

CLINICAL PHARMACOLOGY

Following intravascular injection, Iothalamate is rapidly transported through the circulatory system to the kidneys and is excreted unchanged in the urine by glomerular filtration. The pharmacokinetics of intravascularly administered radiopaque contrast media are usually best described by a two compartment model with a rapid alpha phase for drug distribution and a slower beta phase for drug elimination. In patients with normal renal function, the alpha and beta half-lives of Iothalamate were approximately 10 and 90 minutes.

Angiography may be performed following intravascular injection which will permit visualization until significant hemodilution occurs.

Renal accumulation is sufficiently rapid that maximum radiographic density in the calyces and pelves occurs in most instances about 3-8 minutes after injection. In patients with impaired renal function, diagnostic opacification frequently is achieved only after prolonged periods.

Injectable iodinated contrast agents are excreted either through the kidneys or through the liver. These two excretory pathways are not mutually exclusive, but the main route of excretion seems to be related to the affinity of the contrast medium for serum albumin. Iothalamate salts are poorly bound to serum albumin, and are excreted mainly through the kidneys.

The liver and small intestine provide the major alternate route of excretion. In patients with severe renal impairment, the excretion of this contrast medium through the gallbladder and into the small intestine sharply increases.

Iothalamate salts cross the placental barrier in humans and are excreted unchanged in human milk.

The biliary system, pancreatic duct or joint spaces may be visualized by the direct injection of Iothalamate Meglumine contrast medium into the region to be studied.

CT SCANNING OF THE HEAD

When used for contrast enhancement in computed tomographic brain scanning, the degree of enhancement is directly related to the amount of iodine administered. Rapid injection of the entire dose yields peak blood iodine concentrations immediately following the injection, which fall rapidly over the next five to ten minutes. This can be accounted for by the dilution in the vascular and extracellular fluid compartments which causes an initial sharp fall in plasma concentration. Equilibration with the extracellular compartments is reached by about ten minutes; thereafter the fall becomes exponential. Maximum contrast enhancement frequently occurs after peak blood iodine levels are reached. The delay in maximum contrast enhancement can range from five to forty minutes, depending on the peak iodine levels achieved and the cell type of the lesion. This lag suggests that the contrast enhancement of the image is at least in part dependent on the accumulation of iodine within the lesion and outside the blood pool.

In brain scanning, the contrast medium (Iothalamate) does not accumulate in normal brain tissue due to the presence of the "blood brain barrier". The increase in x-ray absorption in the normal brain is due to the presence of the contrast agent within the blood pool. A break in the blood brain barrier, such as occurs in malignant tumors of the brain, allows accumulation of contrast medium within the interstitial tumor tissue; adjacent normal brain tissue does not contain the contrast medium.

The image enhancement of non-tumoral lesions, such as arteriovenous malformations and aneurysms, is dependent on the iodine content of the circulating blood pool.

When Iothalamate Meglumine is used for cranial computerized angiotomography, rapid bolus injection and/or infusion combined with rapid CT scanning will provide clear delineation of the cerebral vessels.

CT SCANNING OF THE BODY[1]

In non-neural tissues (during CT of the body), Iothalamate diffuses rapidly from the vascular to the extra-vascular space. Increase in x-ray absorption is related to blood flow, concentration of the contrast medium and extraction of the contrast medium by interstitial tissue since no barrier exists; contrast enhancement is thus due to the relative differences in extravascular diffusion between normal and abnormal tissue, a situation quite different than that in the brain.

The pharmacokinetics of Iothalamate in normal and abnormal tissues has been shown to be variable.

Enhancement of CT with Iothalamate may be of benefit in establishing diagnoses of certain lesions in some sites with greater assurance than is possible with unenhanced CT and in supplying additional features of the lesions. In other

---

◆ RATED THERAPEUTICALLY EQUIVALENT; ◇ THERAPEUTIC EQUIVALENCE UNCONFIRMED; ○ UNRATED

cases, the contrast medium may allow visualization of lesions not seen with CT alone or may help to define suspicious lesions seen with unenhanced CT.

Contrast enhancement appears to be greatest within the 30-90 seconds after bolus administration of the contrast agent, and after intra-arterial rather than intravenous administration. Therefore, the use of a continuous scanning technique (a series of 2-3 second scans beginning at the injection—dynamic CT scanning) may improve enhancement and diagnostic assessment of tumors and other lesions such as an abscess, occasionally revealing more extensive disease. A cyst, or similar non-vascularized lesion may be distinguished from vascularized solid lesions by comparing enhanced and unenhanced scans; the non-vascularized lesions show no change in CT number, the vascularized lesions would show an increase. The latter might be benign, malignant or normal, but it is unlikely that it would be a cyst, hematoma, or other nonvascularized lesion.

Because *unenhanced* scanning may provide adequate information in the individual patient, the decision to employ contrast enhancement, which is associated with additional risk and increased radiation exposure, should be based upon a careful evaluation of clinical, other radiological, and unenhanced CT findings.

INDICATIONS AND USAGE

Iothalamate Meglumine is indicated for use in excretory urography, cerebral angiography, peripheral arteriography, venography, arthrography, direct cholangiography, endoscopic retrograde cholangiopancreatography, contrast enhancement of computed tomographic brain images, cranial computerized angiotomography, intravenous digital subtraction angiography and arterial digital subtraction angiography.

Iothalamate Sodium with 325 mg/ml iodine is indicated for use in intravenous excretory urography. Iothalamate Sodium with 400 mg/ml iodine is indicated for use in excretory urography, angiocardiography, aortography and for contrast enhancement of computed tomographic brain images.

Iothalamate Meglumine and Iothalamate Sodium with 400 mg/ml iodine may also be used for enhancement of computed tomographic scans performed for detection and evaluation of lesions in the liver, pancreas, kidneys, abdominal aorta, mediastinum, abdominal cavity and retroperitoneal space. Continuous or multiple scans separated by intervals of 1-3 seconds during the first 30-90 seconds post-injection of the contrast medium (dynamic CT scanning) may provide enhancement of diagnostic significance, and may be of benefit in establishing diagnoses of certain lesions in these sites with greater assurance than is possible with CT alone, and in supplying additional features of the lesions. In other cases, the contrast agent may allow visualization of lesions not seen with CT alone, or may help to define suspicious lesions seen with unenhanced CT. (See "Clinical Pharmacology"). Subsets of patients in whom delayed body CT scans might be helpful have not been identified. Inconsistent results have been reported and abnormal and normal tissues may be isodense during the time frame used for delayed CT scanning. The risks of such indiscriminate use of contrast media are well known and such use is not recommended. At present, consistent results have been documented using dynamic CT techniques only.

CONTRAINDICATIONS

Refer to "Precautions, General", concerning hypersensitivity. Iothalamate should not be used for myelography. Arthrography should not be performed if infection is present in or near the joint. Percutaneous transhepatic cholangiography is contraindicated in patients with coagulation defects and prolonged prothrombin times. Endoscopic retrograde cholangiopancreatography is contraindicated during an acute attack of pancreatitis or during severe clinically evident cholangitis and in patients in whom endoscopy is prohibited.

Iothalamate Sodium with 400 mg/ml iodine should not be used for cerebral angiography by direct injection into the carotid or vertebral arteries due to the high concentration of the solution. (See "Warnings".)

WARNINGS

Ionic iodinated contrast media inhibit blood coagulation, *in vitro,* more than nonionic contrast media. Nonetheless, it is prudent to avoid prolonged contact of blood with syringes containing ionic contrast media.

Serious, rarely fatal, thromboembolic events causing myocardial infarction and stroke have been reported during angiographic procedures with both ionic and nonionic contrast media. Therefore, meticulous intravascular administration technique is necessary, particularly during angiographic procedures, to minimize thromboembolic events. Numerous factors, including length of procedure, catheter and syringe material, underlying disease state and concomitant medications may contribute to the development of thromboembolic events. For these reasons, meticulous angiographic techniques are recommended including close attention to guidewire and catheter manipulation, use of manifold systems and/or three-way stopcocks, frequent catheter flushing with heparinized saline solutions and minimizing the length of the procedure. The use of plastic syringes in place of glass syringes has been reported to decrease but not eliminate the likelihood of *in vitro* clotting.

Serious or fatal reactions have been associated with the administration of iodine containing radiopaque media. It is of utmost importance to be completely prepared to treat any contrast medium reaction.

Serious neurologic sequelae, including permanent paralysis, have been reported following cerebral arteriography, selective spinal arteriography and arteriography of vessels supplying the spinal cord following inadvertent injections of excessive amounts of concentrated contrast media into arteries supplying the spinal cord. The intravascular injection of a contrast medium should never be made following the administration of vasopressors since they strongly potentiate neurologic effects.

In patients with subarachnoid hemorrhage, a rare association between contrast administration and clinical deterioration, including convulsions and death, has been reported. Therefore, administration of intravascular iodinated ionic contrast media in these patients should be undertaken with caution.

A definite risk exists in the use of intravascular contrast agents in patients who are known to have multiple myeloma. In such instances anuria has developed resulting in progressive uremia, renal failure and eventually death. Although neither the contrast agent nor dehydration has separately proved to be the cause of anuria in myeloma, it has been speculated that the combination of both may be causative factors. The risk in myelomatous patients is not a contraindication to the procedure; however, partial dehydration in the preparation of these patients for the examination is not recommended since this may pre-dispose to precipitation of myeloma protein in the renal tubules. No form of therapy, including dialysis, has been successful in reversing the effect. Myeloma, which occurs most commonly in persons over 40, should be considered before instituting intravascular administration of contrast agents.

Administration of radiopaque materials to patients known or suspected to have pheochromocytoma should be performed with extreme caution. If, in the opinion of the physician, the possible benefits of such procedures outweigh the considered risks, the procedures may be performed; however, the amount of radiopaque medium injected should be kept to an absolute minimum. The blood pressure should be assessed throughout the procedure, and measures for treatment of a hypertensive crisis should be available.

Contrast media have been shown to promote the phenomenon of sickling in individuals who are homozygous for sickle cell disease when the material is injected intravenously or intra-arterially.

Convulsions have occurred in patients with primary or metastatic cerebral lesions following the administration of iodine-containing radiopaque media for the contrast enhancement of CT brain images.

In patients with advanced renal disease, iodinated contrast media should be used with caution, and only when the need for the examination dictates, since excretion of the medium may be impaired. Patients with combined renal and hepatic disease, those with severe hypertension or congestive heart failure, and recent renal transplant recipients may present an additional risk.

Renal failure has been reported in patients with liver dysfunction who were given an oral cholecystographic agent followed by an intravascular iodinated radiopaque agent and also in patients with occult renal disease, notably diabetics and hypertensives. In these classes of patients there should be no fluid restriction and every attempt should be made to maintain normal hydration, prior to contrast medium administration, since dehydration is the single most important factor influencing further renal impairment.

Acute renal failure has been reported in diabetic patients with diabetic nephropathy and in susceptible non-diabetic patients (often elderly with pre-existing renal disease) following the administration of iodinated contrast agents. Therefore, careful consideration of the potential risks should be given before performing this radiographic procedure in these patients.

Caution should be exercised in performing contrast medium studies in patients with endotoxemia and/or those with elevated body temperatures.

Reports of thyroid storm occurring following the intravascular use of iodinated radiopaque agents in patients with hyperthyroidism or with an autonomously functioning thyroid nodule, suggest that this additional risk be evaluated in such patients before use of this drug. Iodine containing contrast agents may alter the results of thyroid function tests which depend on iodine estimation, e.g. PBI and radioactive iodine uptake studies. Such tests, if indicated, should be performed prior to the administration of this preparation.

PRECAUTIONS

GENERAL

Diagnostic procedures which involve the use of iodinated intra-vascular contrast agents should be carried out under the direction of personnel skilled and experienced in the particular procedure to be performed. All procedures utilizing contrast media carry a definite risk of producing adverse reactions. While most reactions may be minor, life threatening and fatal reactions may occur without warning. The risk-benefit factor should always be carefully evaluated before such a procedure is undertaken. At all times a fully equipped emergency cart, or equivalent supplies and equipment, and personnel competent in recognizing and treating adverse reactions of all severity, or situations which may arise as a result of the procedure, should be immediately available. If a serious reaction should occur, immediately discontinue administration. Since severe delayed reactions have been known to occur, emergency facilities and competent personnel should be available for at least 30 to 60 minutes after administration (See "Adverse Reactions").

Preparatory dehydration is dangerous and may contribute to acute renal failure in infants, young children, the elderly, patients with pre-existing renal insufficiency, patients with advanced vascular disease and diabetic patients.

Severe reactions to contrast media often resemble allergic responses. This has prompted the use of several provocative pretesting methods, none of which can be relied on to predict severe reactions. No conclusive relationship between severe reactions and antigen-antibody reactions or other manifestations of allergy has been established. The possibility of an idiosyncratic reaction in patients who have previously received a contrast medium without ill effect should always be considered. Prior to the injection of any contrast medium, the patient should be questioned to obtain a medical history with emphasis on allergy and hypersensitivity. A positive history of bronchial asthma or allergy, including food, a family history of allergy, or a previous reaction or hypersensitivity to a contrast agent may imply a greater than usual risk. Such a history, by suggesting histamine sensitivity and consequently proneness to reactions, may be more accurate than pre-testing in predicting the potential for reaction, although not necessarily the severity or type of reaction in the individual case. A positive history of this type does not arbitrarily contraindicate the use of a contrast agent when a diagnostic procedure is thought essential, but does call for caution. (See *"Adverse Reactions"*.)

Prophylactic therapy including corticosteroids and antihistamines should be considered for patients who present with a strong allergic history, a previous reaction to a contrast medium, or a positive pretest since in these patients the incidence of reaction is two to three times that of the general population. Adequate doses of corticosteroids should be started early enough prior to contrast medium injection to be effective and should continue through the time of injection and for 24 hours after injection. Antihistamines should be administered within 30 minutes of the contrast medium injection. Recent reports indicate that such pre-treatment does not prevent serious early life-threatening reactions, but may reduce both their incidence and severity. A separate syringe should be used for these injections.

General anesthesia may be indicated in the performance of some procedures in young or uncooperative children and in selected adult patients; however, a higher incidence of adverse reactions has been reported in these patients, and may be attributable to the inability of the patient to identify untoward symptoms or to the hypotensive effect of anesthesia which can prolong the circulation time and increase the duration of contact of the contrast agent.

Angiography should be avoided whenever possible in patients with hemocystinuria because of the risk of inducing thrombosis and embolism.

Information for Patients: Patients receiving iodinated intravascular contrast agents should be instructed to:
1. Inform your physician if you are pregnant.
2. Inform your physician if you are diabetic or if you have multiple myeloma, pheochromocytoma, homozygous sickle cell disease or known thyroid disease. (See *"Warnings"*).
3. Inform your physician if you are allergic to any drugs, food or if you had any reactions to previous injections of dyes used for x-ray procedures. (See *"Precautions, General"*).
4. Inform your physician about any other medications you are currently taking including non-prescription drugs.

Carcinogenesis, Mutagenesis, Impairment of Fertility: No long-term animal studies have been performed to evaluate carcinogenic potential. However, animal studies suggest that this drug is not mutagenic and does not affect fertility in males or females.

Pregnancy Category B: Reproduction studies have been performed in mice, rats, and rabbits at doses up to 6.6 times the human dose and have revealed no evidence of impaired fertility or harm to the fetus due to Iothalamate. There are, however, no adequate and well controlled studies in pregnant women. Because animal reproduction studies are not always predictive of human response, this drug should be used during pregnancy only if clearly needed.

Nursing Mothers: Iothalamate salts are excreted unchanged in human milk. Because of the potential for adverse effects in nursing infants, bottle feedings should be substituted for breast feedings for 24 hours following the administration of this drug.
(Precautions for specific procedures receive comment under that procedure.)

ADVERSE REACTIONS
Adverse reactions to injectable contrast media fall into two categories: chemotoxic reactions and idiosyncratic reactions.

Chemotoxic reactions result from the physio-chemical properties of the contrast media, the dose and speed of injection. All hemodynamic disturbances and injuries to organs or vessels perfused by the contrast medium are included in this category.

Idiosyncratic reactions include all other reactions. They occur more frequently in patients 20 to 40 years old. Idiosyncratic reactions may or may not be dependent on the amount of dose injected, the speed of injection, the mode of injection and the radiographic procedure. Idiosyncratic reactions are subdivided into minor, intermediate and severe. The minor reactions are self-limited and of short duration; the severe reactions are life-threatening and treatment is urgent and mandatory.

Fatalities have been reported following the administration of iodine-containing contrast agents. Based upon clinical literature, the incidence of death is reported to range from one in 10,000 (0.01 percent) to less than one in 100,000 (0.001 percent).

The following adverse reactions have been observed in conjunction with the use of iodine-containing contrast agents.

The most frequent adverse reactions are nausea, vomiting, facial flush and a feeling of body warmth. These are usually of brief duration. Other reactions include the following:

Hypersensitivity Reactions: Dermal manifestations of urticaria with or without pruritus, erythema and maculopapular rash. Dry mouth. Sweating. Conjunctival symptoms. Facial, peripheral and angioneurotic edema. Symptoms related to the respiratory system include sneezing, nasal stuffiness, coughing, choking, dyspnea, chest tightness and wheezing, which may be initial manifestations of more severe and infrequent reactions including asthmatic attack, laryngospasm and bronchospasm with or without edema, pulmonary edema, apnea and cyanosis. Rarely, these allergic-type reactions can progress into anaphylaxis with loss of consciousness and coma and severe cardiovascular disturbances.

Cardiovascular Reactions: Generalized vasodilation, flushing and venospasm. Occasionally, thrombosis or rarely, thrombophlebitis. Red blood cell clumping and agglutination, crenation and interference in clot formation. Extremely rare cases of disseminated intravascular coagulation resulting in death have been reported. Severe cardiovascular responses include rare cases of hypotensive shock, coronary insufficiency, cardiac arrhythmia, fibrillation and arrest. These severe reactions are usually reversible with prompt and appropriate management; however, fatalities have occurred.

Technique Reactions: Extravasation with burning pain, hematomas, ecchymosis and tissue necrosis, paresthesia or numbness, vascular constriction due to injection rate, thrombosis and thrombophlebitis.

Neurological Reactions: Spasm, convulsions, aphasia, syncope, paresis, paralysis resulting from spinal cord injury and pathology associated with syndrome of transverse myelitis, visual field losses which are usually transient but may be permanent, coma and death.

Other Reactions: Headache, trembling, shaking, chills without fever and light-headedness. Temporary renal shutdown or other nephropathy.
(Adverse reactions to specific procedures receive comment under that procedure.)

OVERDOSAGE
Overdosage may occur. The adverse effects of overdosage are life-threatening and affect mainly the pulmonary and cardiovascular systems. The symptoms may include cyanosis, bradycardia, acidosis, pulmonary hemorrhage, convulsions, coma and cardiac arrest. Treatment of an overdose is directed toward the support of all vital functions and prompt institution of symptomatic therapy.

Iothalamate salts are dialyzable.

The intravenous LD_{50} value of various concentrations of Iothalamate Meglumine (in grams of iodine/kilogram body weight) varied from 5.7 to 8.9 g/kg in mice and 9.8 to 11.2 g/kg in rats. The intravenous LD_{50} value of various concentrations of Iothalamate Sodium (in grams of iodine/kilogram body weight) varied from 6.4 to 13.5 g/kg in mice, 6.9 to 9.5 g/kg in rats and 8.3 to 11.1 g/kg in rabbits. The LD_{50} values decrease as the rate of injection increases.

DOSAGE AND ADMINISTRATION
It is advisable that Iothalamate be at or close to body temperature when injected.

The patient should be instructed to omit the meal that precedes the examination. Appropriate premedication, which may include a barbiturate, tranquilizer or analgesic drug, may be administered prior to the examination.

A preliminary film is recommended to check the position of the patient and the x-ray exposure factors.

If during administration a minor reaction occurs the injection should be slowed or stopped until the reaction has subsided. If a major reaction occurs the injection should be discontinued immediately.

Under no circumstances should either corticosteroids or antihistamines, or other drugs, be mixed in the same syringe or IV administration set with the contrast medium because of a potential for chemical incompatibility.

Parenteral drug products should be inspected visually for particulate matter and discoloration prior to administration.

EXCRETORY UROGRAPHY
Following intravenous injection, Iothalamate is rapidly excreted by the kidneys. Iothalamate may be visualized in the renal parenchyma 30 seconds following bolus injection. Maximum radiographic density in the calyces and pelves occurs in most instances within 3-8 minutes after injection. In patients with severe renal impairment contrast visualization may be substantially delayed.

PATIENT PREPARATION
Appropriate preparation of the patient is important for optimal visualization. A low residue diet is recommended for the day preceding the examination and a laxative is given the evening before the examination, unless contraindicated.

PRECAUTIONS
Infants and small children should not have any fluid restrictions prior to excretory urography. Injections of Iothalamate represent an osmotic load which, if superimposed on increased serum osmolality due to partial dehydration, may magnify hypertonic dehydration. (See *"Warnings"* and *"Precautions, General"* concerning preparatory dehydration).

ADVERSE REACTIONS
See section on general *"Adverse Reactions"*.

USUAL DOSAGE
Adults: The usual dose of Iothalamate Meglumine and Iothalamate Sodium/325 mg iodine is 30-60 ml, of Iothalamate Sodium/400 mg iodine 25-50 ml. Children 14 years of age and over, of average weight, may receive the adult dose. The total dose is normally injected within 30-90 seconds. Higher dosage may be indicated to achieve optimum results in instances where poor visualization may be anticipated (e.g., elderly patients or patients with impaired renal function). When nephrograms and/or sequential urograms are desired, the total dose should be rapidly injected, normally within 15-30 seconds.

The dosage for children is reduced in proportion to age and body weight. The following approximate schedule is recommended for infants and children based on a dosage of about 0.5 mL/kg of body weight:

Under 6 months of age	5 mL
6-12 months	8 mL

1-2 years	10 mL
2-5 years	12 mL
5-8 years	15 mL
8-12 years	18 mL
12-14 years	20-30 mL

CEREBRAL ANGIOGRAPHY
Iothalamate Meglumine may be used to visualize the cerebral vasculature by any of the accepted techniques.

PATIENT PREPARATION
Cerebral angiography is normally performed with local or general anesthesia. (See *"Precautions, General"*). Premedication may be employed as indicated.

A preliminary radiograph is usually made prior to injection of the contrast agent.

PRECAUTIONS
In addition to the general precautions previously described, cerebral angiography should be performed with special caution in patients with advanced arteriosclerosis, severe hypertension, cardiac decompensation, senility, recent cerebral thrombosis or embolism, and migraine.

ADVERSE REACTIONS
The major sources of cerebral arteriographic adverse reactions appear to be related to repeated injections of the contrast material, administration of doses higher than those recommended, the presence of occlusive atherosclerotic vascular disease and the method and technique of injection.

Adverse reactions are normally mild and transient. A feeling of warmth in the face and neck is frequently experienced. Infrequently, a more severe burning discomfort is observed.

Serious neurological reactions that have been associated with cerebral angiography and not listed under the general Adverse Reactions include stroke, amnesia and respiratory difficulties.

Cardiovascular reactions that may occur with some frequency are bradycardia and decrease in systemic blood pressure. The blood pressure change is transient and usually requires no treatment.

USUAL DOSAGE
The usual dosage employed varies with the site and method of injection and the age, condition and weight of the patient. In adults, carotid and vertebral angiography, by either the percutaneous needle or catheter methods is usually performed with a single rapid injection of 6-10 mL. Additional injections are made as indicated. Retrograde brachial cerebral angiography, in adults, is usually performed with a single rapid injection of 35-50 mL into the right brachial artery. Other dosages may be employed depending upon the vessel injected and the procedure followed. The dose for children is reduced in approximate proportion to age and body weight.

PERIPHERAL ARTERIOGRAPHY AND VENOGRAPHY
Iothalamate Meglumine may be injected to visualize the arterial and venous peripheral circulation. Arteriograms of the upper and lower extremities may be obtained by any of the established techniques. Most frequently a percutaneous injection is made into the brachial artery in the arm or the femoral artery in the leg. Venograms are obtained by injection into an appropriate vein in the upper and lower extremity.

PATIENT PREPARATION
The procedure is normally performed with local or general anesthesia. (See *"Precautions, General."*) Premedication may be employed as indicated.

A preliminary radiograph is usually made prior to the injection of the contrast agent.

PRECAUTIONS
In addition to the general precautions previously described, moderate decreases in blood pressure occur frequently with intra-arterial (brachial) injections. This change is usually transient and requires no treatment; however, the blood pressure should be monitored for approximately ten minutes following injection. Special care is required when venography is performed in patients with suspected thrombosis, phlebitis, severe ischemic disease, local infection or a totally obstructed venous system. In the presence of venous stasis, vein irrigation with normal saline should be considered following the procedure. Venography is optimally performed with a more dilute solution such as Iothalamate Meglumine injection 43%.

Extreme caution during injection of the contrast agent is necessary to avoid extravasation and fluoroscopy is recommended. This is especially important in patients with severe arterial or venous disease.

ADVERSE REACTIONS
In addition to the general adverse reactions previously described, hemorrhage and thrombosis have occurred at the puncture site of the percutaneous injection. Brachial plexus injury has been reported following axillary artery injection. Thrombophlebitis, syncope and very rare cases of gangrene have been reported following venography.

USUAL DOSAGE
Peripheral Arteriography: In adults a single rapid injection of 20-40 mL is normally sufficient to visualize the entire extremity. The dose for children is reduced in proportion to body weight. Venography: The usual dose for adults is a single rapid injection of 20-40 mL. The dose for children is reduced in proportion to body weight. Following the procedure, the venous system should be flushed with either 5% dextrose in water (D5W) or normal saline (Sodium Chloride Injection) or the contrast medium should be removed by leg massage and/or leg elevation.

ARTHOGRAPHY
PRECAUTIONS
In addition to the general precautions previously described, strict aseptic technique in administering Iothalamate Meglumine is required to prevent the introduction of infection. Fluoroscopic control should be used to insure proper introduction of the needle into the synovial space and prevent extracapsular injection. Aspiration of excessive synovial fluid will reduce the pain on injection and prevent the rapid dilution of the contrast agent. It is important that undue pressure not be exerted during the injection.

ADVERSE REACTIONS
In addition to the general adverse reactions previously described arthrography may induce joint pain or discomfort which is usually mild and transient but occasionally may be severe and persist for 24 to 48 hours following the procedure. Effusion requiring aspiration may occur in patients with rheumatoid arthritis.

USUAL DOSAGE
Arthrography is usually performed under local anesthesia. The amount of Iothalamate Meglumine required is solely dependent on the size of the joint to be injected and the technique employed.

The following dosage schedule for normal adult joints should serve only as a guide since joints may require more or less contrast medium for optimal visualization. Dosage should be reduced for children in proportion to body weight.

Knee, hip	5-15 mL
Shoulder, ankle	5-10 mL
Other	1- 4 mL

Passive or active manipulation is used to disperse the medium throughout the joint space.

The lower volumes of contrast medium are usually employed for double contrast examinations. Following the injection of the contrast medium 50-100 cc of either filtered room air or carbon dioxide is introduced for examination of the knee and lesser volumes for other joints. The concomitant use of epinephrine 1:1000 will reduce the rate of contrast medium absorption as well as the production of synovial fluids and consequent dilution of the medium.

DIRECT CHOLANGIOGRAPHY
PRECAUTIONS
In addition to the general precautions previously described, in the presence of acute pancreatitis, direct cholangiography, if necessary, should be employed with caution, injecting no more than 5 to 10 mL of Iothalamate Meglumine without undue pressure. Percutaneous transhepatic cholangiography should only be attempted when compatible blood for potential transfusions is in readiness and emergency surgical facilities are available. The patient should be carefully monitored for at least 24 hours to insure prompt detection of bile leakage and hemorrhage. Appropriate premedication of the patient is recommended and drugs which are cholespastic, such as morphine, should be avoided. Respiratory movements should be controlled during introduction of the needle.

ADVERSE REACTIONS
Adverse reactions may often be attributed to injection pressure or excessive volume of the medium resulting in over-distention of the ducts and producing local pain.

Some of the medium may enter the pancreatic duct which may result in pancreatic irritation. Occasionally, nausea, vomiting, fever, and tachycardia have been observed. Pancholangitis resulting in liver abscess or septicemia has been reported.

In percutaneous transhepatic cholangiography, some discomfort is common, but severe pain is unusual. Complications of the procedure are often serious and have been reported in 4 to 6 percent of patients. These reactions have included bile leakage and biliary peritonitis, gall bladder perforation, internal bleeding (sometimes massive), blood-bile fistula resulting in septicemia involving gramnegative organisms, and tension pneumothorax from inadvertent puncture of the diaphragm or lung. Bile leakage is more likely to occur in patients with obstructions that cause unrelieved high biliary pressure.

DOSAGE AND ADMINISTRATION
It is advisable that Iothalamate Meglumine be at or close to body temperature when injected. The injection is made slowly without undue pressure, taking the necessary precautions to avoid the introduction of bubbles.

Operative: The usual dose is 10 mL but as much as 25 mL may be needed depending upon the caliber of the ducts. If desired, the contrast agent may be diluted 1:1 with Sodium Chloride Injection U.S.P. using strict aseptic procedures. Following surgical exploration of the ductal system, repeat studies may be performed before closure of the abdomen, using the same dose as before.

Postoperative: Postoperatively, the ductal system may be examined by injection of the contrast agent through an in-place T-tube. These delayed cholangiograms are usually made from the fifth to the tenth postoperative day prior to removal of the T-tube. The usual dose is the same as for operative cholangiography.

Percutaneous Transhepatic Cholangiography: This procedure is recommended for carefully selected patients for the differential diagnosis of jaundice due to extrahepatic biliary obstruction or parenchymal disease. The procedure is only employed where oral or intravenous cholangiography and other procedures have failed to provide the necessary information. In obstructed cases, percutaneous transhepatic cholangiography is used to determine the cause and site of obstruction to help plan surgery. The technique may also be of value in avoiding laparotomy in poor risk jaundice patients since failure to enter a duct suggests hepatocellular disease. Careful attention to technique is essential for the success and safety of the procedure. The procedure is usually performed under local anesthesia following analgesic premedication.

Depending upon the caliber of the biliary tree, a dose of 20 to 40 mL is generally sufficient to opacify the entire ductal system. If desired, the contrast agent may be diluted 1:1 with Sodium Chloride Injection U.S.P. using strict aseptic procedures.

As the needle is advanced or withdrawn, a bile duct may be located by frequent aspiration for bile or mucus. Before the dose is administered, as much bile as possible is aspirated. The injection may be repeated for exposures in different planes and repositioning of the patient, if necessary, should be done with care. If a duct is not readily located by aspiration, successive small doses of 1 to 2 mL of the medium are injected into the liver as the needle is gradually withdrawn, until a duct is visualized by x-ray.

If no duct can be located after 3 or 4 attempts, the procedure should be terminated. Inability to enter a duct by a person experienced in the technique is generally considered to be strongly suggestive of hepatocellular disease.

ENDOSCOPIC RETROGRADE CHOLANGIOPANCREATOGRAPHY

Endoscopic retrograde cholangiopancreatography (ERCP), using Iothalamate Meglumine, is indicated in carefully selected patients with known or suspected pancreatic or biliary tract disease when other diagnostic procedures have failed to provide the necessary diagnostic information. Prior to the development of ERCP, x-ray examination of the pancreatic ducts could only be obtained at laparotomy.

PRECAUTIONS

Endoscopic retrograde cholangiopancreatography should only be performed by personnel skilled and experienced with the procedure, and careful attention to technique is essential for the success and safety of the procedure. Fluoroscopy is mandatory during injection to prevent overdistention of the duct systems.

ADVERSE REACTIONS

Adverse reactions that have occurred which are attributable to either the procedure or contrast agent include nausea, vomiting, fever, severe abdominal pain, duodenal wall intravasation, septicemia, pancreatitis and perforation of the common bile duct associated with pathology.

DOSAGE AND ADMINISTRATION

The procedure is usually performed following pharyngeal anesthesia and analgesic or sedative premedication. Duodenal motility may be controlled in patients with active duodenal peristalsis with an appropriate antiperistaltic agent.

Iothalamate Meglumine should be injected slowly under fluoroscopic control employing the minimal dose that is adequate to visualize the common bile duct, the pancreatic duct, or both duct systems. The dosage will vary greatly depending on the pathological findings and can range from 10-100 mL for visualization of the common bile duct and from 2-10 mL for visualization of the pancreatic duct.

Following the procedure, the patient should be kept under close observation for 24 hours.

CONTRAST ENHANCEMENT OF COMPUTED TOMOGRAPHIC (CT) BRAIN IMAGING
TUMORS

Iothalamate Meglumine and Iothalamate Sodium/400 mg/ml Iodine may be useful to enhance the demonstration of the presence and extent of certain malignancies such as: gliomas including malignant gliomas, glioblastomas, astrocytomas, oligodendrogliomas and gangliomas; ependymomas; medulloblastomas; meningiomas; neuromas; pinealomas; pituitary adenomas; craniopharyngiomas; germinomas; and metastatic lesions.

The usefulness of contrast enhancement for the investigation of the retrobulbar space and in cases of low grade or infiltrative glioma has not been demonstrated.

In cases where lesions have calcified, there is less likelihood of enhancement. Following therapy, tumors may show decreased or no enhancement.

NON-NEOPLASTIC CONDITIONS

The use of Iothalamate Meglumine and Iothalamate Sodium/400 mg/ml Iodine may be beneficial in the image enhancement of non-neoplastic lesions. General (Iothalamate Meglumine) or cerebral (Iothalamate Sodium) infarctions of recent onset may be better visualized with the contrast enhancement, while some infarctions are obscured if contrast media are used. The use of iodinated contrast media results in contrast enhancement in about 60% of cerebral infarctions studied from one to four weeks from the onset of symptoms.

Sites of active infection may also be enhanced following contrast medium administration.

Arteriovenous malformations and aneurysms will show contrast enhancement. In the case of these vascular lesions, the enhancement is probably dependent on the iodine content of the circulating blood pool.

The opacification of the inferior vermis following contrast medium administration has resulted in false positive diagnoses in a number of normal studies.

PATIENT PREPARATION

No special patient preparation is required for contrast enhancement of CT brain scanning. However, it is advisable to insure that patients are well hydrated prior to examination.

USUAL DOSAGE

The usual dosage of Iothalamate Meglumine in adults and children is 2 mL/kg (1 mL/lb) by intravenous administration, not to exceed a total dose of 150 mL. The usual dose of Iothalamate Sodium/400 mg/ml iodine in adults and children is 1.5 mL/kg (0.7 mL/lb) by rapid intravenous administration, not to exceed a total dose of 100 mL. In most cases, scanning may be performed immediately after completion of administration; however, when fast scanning equipment (less than 1 minute) is used consideration should be given to waiting approximately 5 minutes to allow for maximum contrast enhancement.

CRANIAL COMPUTERIZED ANGIOTOMOGRAPHY

Iothalamate Meglumine may be administered for cranial computerized angiotomography when necessary to visualize the cerebral vessels to detect cerebrovascular lesions and to evaluate the anatomical relationship between the cerebral blood vessels and other parenchymal or space occupying lesions.

USUAL DOSAGE

Iothalamate Meglumine may be administered by intravenous bolus injection, or by bolus injection followed by rapid infusion.

For bolus injection, the usual dose in adults and children is 0.5 to 1.0 mL/kg at an injection rate of 2 mL/second with scanning begun immediately after administration. This dose may be repeated as necessary. The total dose per procedure should not exceed 200 mL, and in children the total dose is reduced in approximate proportion to age and body weight.

In adults, when the combination bolus and infusion technique is used, a 50 mL bolus injection followed by a rapid infusion of 150 mL may be given or a 100 mL bolus injection followed by a rapid infusion of 100 mL may be used. Scanning is begun immediately after the bolus administration. In children, the dose is reduced in approximate proportion to age and body weight.

CONTRAST ENHANCEMENT IN BODY COMPUTED TOMOGRAPHY[1]

Iothalamate Meglumine and Iothalamate Sodium/400 mg/ml iodine may be administered when necessary to visualize vessels and organs in patients undergoing CT of the chest, abdomen and pelvis.

PATIENT PREPARATION

No special patient preparation is required for contrast enhancement in body CT. In patients undergoing abdominal or pelvic examination, opacification of the bowel may be valuable in scan interpretation.

PRECAUTIONS

In addition to the general precautions previously described, it is advisable to insure that patients are adequately hydrated prior to examination. Patient motion, including respiration, can markedly affect image quality, therefore, patient cooperation is essential. The use of an intravascular contrast medium can obscure tumors in patients undergoing CT evaluation of the liver resulting in a false negative diagnosis. Dynamic CT scanning is the procedure of choice for malignant tumor enhancement. (See *"Clinical Pharmacology".*)

USUAL DOSAGE

Iothalamate Meglumine may be administered by bolus injection, by rapid infusion or by a combination of both.

For vascular opacification, a bolus injection of 25-50 mL may be used, repeated as necessary. When prolonged arterial or venous phase enhancement is required and for the enhancement of specific lesions, a rapid infusion of 150 mL may be used. In some instances, a 100-150 mL infusion may be employed to define the area of interest followed by bolus injections of 20-50 mL to clarify selected scans.

The usual adult dose of Iothalamate Sodium/400 mg/ml iodine is 25 to 60 mL administered by rapid intravenous bolus injection. Scanning is performed immediately or within 30 to 90 seconds after injection.

INTRAVENOUS DIGITAL SUBTRACTION ANGIOGRAPHY

Intravenous digital subtraction angiography (IV DSA) is a radiographic modality which allows dynamic imaging of the arterial system following intravenous injection of Iothalamate Meglumine through the use of image intensification, enhancement of the iodine signal and digital processing of the image data. Temporal subtraction of the images obtained during the "first arterial pass" of the injected contrast medium injection yield images which are devoid of bone and soft tissue.

Areas that have been most frequently examined by intravenous DSA are the heart, including coronary by-pass grafts; the pulmonary arteries; the arteries of the brachiocephalic circulation; the aortic arch; the abdominal aorta and its major branches including the celiac, mesenterics and renal arteries; the iliac arteries; and the arteries of the extremities.

PATIENT PREPARATION

No special patient preparation is required for intravenous digital subtraction angiography. However, it is advisable to insure that patients are well hydrated prior to examination.

PRECAUTIONS

In addition to the general precautions previously described, the risks associated with IV DSA are those usually attendant with catheter procedures and include

---

◆ RATED THERAPEUTICALLY EQUIVALENT; ◇ THERAPEUTIC EQUIVALENCE UNCONFIRMED; ○ UNRATED

intramural injections, vessel dissection and tissue extravasation. Small test injections of Iothalamate Meglumine made under fluoroscopic observation to insure the catheter tip is properly positioned, and in the case of peripheral placement that the vein is of adequate size, will reduce this potential.

Patient motion, including respiration and swallowing, can result in marked image degradation yielding non-diagnostic studies. Therefore, patient cooperation is essential.

ADVERSE REACTIONS
See section on general *"Adverse Reactions"*.

USUAL DOSAGE
Iothalamate Meglumine may be injected either centrally, into the superior or inferior vena cava, or peripherally into an appropriate arm vein. For central injections, catheters may be introduced at the antecubital fossa into either the basilic or cephalic vein or at the leg into the femoral vein and advanced to the distal segment of the corresponding vena cava. For peripheral injections, the catheter is introduced at the antecubital fossa into the appropriate size arm vein. In order to reduce the potential for extravastation during peripheral injection, a catheter of approximately 20 cm in length should be employed.

Depending on the area to be imaged, the usual dose range is 20-40 mL. Injections may be repeated as necessary.

Central catheter injections are usually made with a power injector with an injection rate of between 10 and 30 ml/second. When making peripheral injections, rates of 12 to 20 ml/second should be used, depending on the size of the vein. Also, since contrast medium may remain in the arm vein for an extended period following injection, it may be advisable to flush the vein, immediately following injection with an appropriate volume (20-25 mL) of 5% Dextrose in water or normal saline.

ARTERIAL DIGITAL SUBTRACTION ANGIOGRAPHY
Arterial digital subtraction angiography, using Iothalamate Meglumine, provides images similar in quality to conventional film-screen systems. The advantages of arterial DSA when compared to standard film angiography include: the use of less contrast medium; the use of lower concentrations for some procedures; a decreased need for selective arterial catherization reducing the possibility of dislodging atheromatous plaques or significantly reducing the blood flow in the artery; and a shortened examination time. The limitations of arterial DSA include: reduced spatial resolution; limited field size; and the inability to conduct simultaneous biplane examinations.

PATIENT PREPARATION
No special patient preparation is required for arterial DSA. However, it is advisable to insure that patients are well hydrated prior to examination.

PRECAUTIONS
In addition to the general precautions described, the risks associated with arterial DSA are those usually attendant with catheter procedures. Following the procedure, gentle pressure hemostasis is required, followed by observation and immobilization of the limb for several hours to prevent hemorrhage from the site of arterial puncture.

USUAL DOSAGE
The following dosage schedule for adults should serve only as a guide since the volume administered, the concentration selected and the flow rate will be determined by the resolution of the equipment being used. As a general rule, the volume used and the flow rates for arterial DSA are 50% or less than that used for conventional film arteriography. Diagnostic studies have been obtained using Iothalamate Meglumine undiluted (28.2% iodine), diluted 1:1 (14.1% iodine) and diluted 1:2 (9.4% iodine). Sodium Chloride Injection U.S.P. or Water for Injection U.S.P. may be used for dilution.

The following doses, equivalent in iodine content to undiluted Iothalamate Meglumine, have been used.

Carotid or vertebral arteries:	3-8 mL
Aortic Arch:	15-25 mL
Subclavian and brachial arteries:	5-15 mL
Major branches of the aorta:	5-20 mL
Lumbar aorta (bifurcation):	10-25 mL

ANGIOCARDIOGRAPHY
Iothalamate Sodium/400 mg/ml iodine may be administered by injection into an appropriate peripheral vein, or by means of a catheter, directed to the chambers of the heart or associated large blood vessels to be visualized. Injection through a catheter usually provides adequate opacity with a lower dosage because less dilution of the medium takes place. Regardless of the mode of administration, rapid injection is essential. Satisfactory results usually require injection of the total dosage in 1-2 seconds. In most cases, this may be accomplished by manual injection. If indicated, shorter injection times may be obtained with a mechanical injector.

PRECAUTIONS
In addition to the general precautions previously described, continuous monitoring of ECG and vital signs is recommended during the procedure. When large individual doses are administered, a minimum of 15 minutes between injections is recommended to permit subsidence of any hemodynamic disturbances.

Adult: Caution should be used when injection of this agent is made into the right ventricle or pulmonary artery in patients with pulmonary hypertension or right ventricular failure, since this may result in increased right atrial, right ventricular and pulmonary artery pressure with subsequent bradycardia and systemic hypotension. Patients with chronic pulmonary emphysema present additional risks.

Pediatric: Particular caution is advised in cyanotic infants since apnea, bradycardia, other arrhythmias and a tendency to acidosis are more likely to occur. Infants are more likely to respond with convulsions than are adults. The amount of total dosage in infants is of particular importance. Repeated injections are particularly hazardous in infants weighing less than 7 kg and the risk is significantly increased if these infants have pre-existing compromised right heart function or obliterated pulmonary vascular beds.

ADVERSE REACTIONS
In addition to the adverse reactions previously listed, this procedure has been complicated by intramural injection with marked adverse effects on cardiac function. Hemodynamic changes which occur on injection into the heart chambers can aggravate incipient heart failure and serious arrhythmias, and cardiac arrest may be precipitated.

USUAL DOSAGE
The volume of individual doses should be determined by the size of the structure to be visualized, and in adults, the weight of the patient is only a minor consideration. The anticipated degree of hemodilution at the site of injection and valvular competence should also be taken into consideration.

Adults: Catheter angiocardiography usually requires single doses of 40-50 mL of Iothalamate Sodium/400 mg/ml iodine. Intravenous angiocardiography requires 50-100 mL.

Children: Usual dose is 0.5-1.0 mL/kg for subjects with normal heart size. Minimum dosage should be applied to patients with stenotic lesions or questionable valvular competence.

Infants (2 months old or less): Dosages are the same as those described for children; however, the total dosage administered in any one procedure should be kept below 3 mL/kg.

AORTOGRAPHY
To visualize the aorta and its major branches, Iothalamate Sodium/400 mg/ml iodine may be administered by the arterial or intravenous methods. Renal arteriograms may be obtained by any accepted technique which provides for delivery of the medium above the level of the renal arteries. Nephrograms or nephrotomograms may also be obtained by these methods of administration.

PRECAUTIONS
In addition to the general precautions previously described, the hazards of aortography include those associated with the particular technique employed, the contrast medium and the underlying pathology which warrants the procedure. There is, therefore, a definite risk.

In order to prevent the inadvertent injection of a large dose into a branch of the aorta or intramurally the position of the catheter tip or needle should be carefully evaluated. A small dose of 1-2 ml should be administered to locate the exact site of the needle or catheter tip. Inadvertent direct injection of contrast medium into brachiocephalic vessels may result in significant slowing of heart rate, peripheral hypotension and severe CNS reactions, including convulsions. Toxic effects may also be produced if large quantities of contrast medium are injected directly into aortic branches such as the renal artery, and repetitive injection of the recommended clinical dosage may be hazardous.

Occasional serious neurologic complications, including paraplegia and quadriplegia have been reported and may be attributable to excess doses injected into arterial trunks supplying the spinal arteries or to prolonged contact time of the concentrated contrast medium on the CNS tissue. Conditions which can contribute to prolonged contact time include decreased circulation, aortic occlusions distal to the site of injection, abdominal compression, hypotension, general anesthesia or the administration of vasopressors. When these conditions exist or occur, the necessity of performing or continuing the procedure should be carefully evaluated and the dose and number of repeat injections should be maintained at a minimum with appropriate intervals between injections.

Severe pain, paresthesia, or peripheral muscle spasm during injection may require discontinuance of the procedure and a reevaluation of the placement of the catheter tip or needle. When employing the translumbar technique, extreme caution is advised to avoid inadvertent intrathecal injection.

Following catheter procedures, gentle pressure hemostasis is advised, followed by observation and immobilization of the limb for several hours to prevent hemorrhage from the site of arterial puncture.

ADVERSE REACTIONS
In addition to the general adverse reactions previously listed, adverse reactions following aortography include injury to the aorta and to neighboring organs, renal damage including infarction and acute tubular necrosis, spinal cord damage resembling transverse myelitis, retroperitoneal hemorrhage, arterial thrombosis, intestinal necrosis and diffuse cutaneous petechiae.

USUAL DOSAGE
Retrograde or antegrade catheter aortography: The usual dose for adults and children over 14 years of age and of average weight is 20-50 mL. The dose for younger children is reduced in proportion to body weight.

Intravenous aortography: For adults and children, the usual dose is 1 mL/kg to a maximum of 80-100 mL per injection. The dose may be divided equally for simultaneous bilateral injection.

Percutaneous translumbar aortography: For adults and children over 14 years of age and of average weight, the usual dose is 20 mL. The dose for younger children is reduced in proportion to body weight and size.

Renal arteriograms by aortography: For adults and children over 14 years of age and of average weight, the usual dose is 10-25 mL. The dose for younger children is reduced in proportion to body weight.

STORAGE

Store below 30°C (86°F). Exposing these products to very cold temperatures may result in crystallization of the salt. If this occurs the container should be brought to room temperature. Shake vigorously to assure complete dissolution of any crystals. The speed of dissolution may be increased by heating with circulating warm air. Submersion of syringes in water is not recommended. Before use, examine the product to assure that all solids are redissolved and that the container and closure have not been damaged.

These preparations are sensitive to light and must be protected from strong daylight or direct exposure to the sun.

Do not reautoclave plastic container because of possible damage to syringe.

As with all contrast media, glass and plastic containers should be inspected prior to use to ensure that breakage or other damage has not occurred during shipping and handling. All containers should be inspected for closure integrity. Damaged containers should not be used.

REFERENCE

1. Young, S. W., Turner, R.J., Castellino, R.A.: 'A strategy for the contrast enhancement of malignant tumors using dynamic computed tomography and intravascular pharmacokinetics,' *Radiology*, 137:137-147, October 1980.

HOW SUPPLIED
INJECTION: 66.8%

BRAND/MANUFACTURER	NDC	SIZE	AWP
○ **BRAND**			
CONRAY-400: Mallinckrodt Med	00019-0954-15	50 ml	$11.70

Iothalamate Meglumine

DESCRIPTION

Iothalamate Meglumine is a sterile aqueous solution intended for use as a diagnostic radiopaque medium. Some solutions are injected intravascularly and some are instilled by sterile catheter. The solutions contain 30% or 43% (injection) or 17.2% or 43% (instillation) w/v Iothalamate Meglumine, which is 1-deoxy-1-(methylamino)-D-glucitol 5-acetamido-2,4,6 triiodo-N-methylisophthalamate (salt).

Each ml (injection) contains:
Iodine (organically bound) ....141 or 202 mg (14.1% or 20.2%)
Iothalamate Meglumine ....300 or 430 mg

Each ml (instillation) contains:
Iodine (organically bound) ....81 or 202 mg (8.1% or 20.2%)
Iothalamate Meglumine ....172 or 430 mg
Iothalamate Meglumine is hypertonic under conditions of use.

Iothalamate Meglomine is a clear solution containing no undissolved solids. Crystallization does not occur at normal room temperatures.

Following is its chemical structure:

CLINICAL PHARMACOLOGY

The most important characteristic of contrast media is the iodine content. The relatively high atomic weight of iodine contributes sufficient radiodensity for radiographic contrast.

Following intravascular injection, Iothalamate Meglumine is rapidly transported through the circulatory system to the kidneys and is excreted unchanged in the urine by glomerular filtration. The pharmacokinetics of intravascularly administered radiopaque contrast media are usually best described by a two compartment model with a rapid alpha phase for drug distribution and a slower beta phase for drug elimination. In patients with normal renal function, the alpha and beta half-

lives of Iothalamate Meglumine were approximately 10 and 90 minutes, respectively.

Arteriography and venography (43%), or angiography (30%), may be performed following injection into an appropriate vessel and will permit visualization until significant hemodilution occurs.

Following infusion of Iothalamate Meglumine the upper and lower urinary tract is opacified. Renal accumulation is sufficiently rapid that maximum radiographic density in the calyces and pelves occurs by the time the infusion is complete. In patients with impaired renal function, diagnostic opacification frequently is achieved only after prolonged periods.

Injectable iodinated contrast agents are excreted either through the kidneys or through the liver. These two excretory pathways are not mutually exclusive, but the main route of excretion seems to be related to the affinity of the contrast medium for serum albumin. Iothalamate salts are poorly bound to serum albumin, and are excreted mainly through the kidneys.

The liver and small intestine provide the major alternate route of excretion. In patients with severe renal impairment, the excretion of this contrast medium through the gallbladder and into the small intestine sharply increases.

Iothalamate salts cross the placental barrier in humans and are excreted unchanged in human milk.

Following instillation by sterile catheter, Iothalamate Meglumine provides for visualization of the lower urinary tract. Clinical literature reports indicate that routinely less than 1% of a retrograde urographic radiopaque is absorbed systemically, however, as much as 12% absorption was observed with pyelorenal back flow and may produce iodine medicated thyrotropic effects described under *"Precautions"*.

CT SCANNING OF THE HEAD INJECTION

When used for contrast enhancement in computed tomographic brain scanning, the degree of enhancement is directly related to the amount of iodine administered. Rapid injection of the entire dose yields peak blood iodine concentrations immediately following the injection, which fall rapidly over the next five to ten minutes. This can be accounted for by the dilution in the vascular and extracellular fluid compartments which causes an initial sharp fall in plasma concentration. Equilibration with the extracellular compartments is reached by about ten minutes; thereafter, the fall becomes exponential. Maximum contrast enhancement frequently occurs after peak blood iodine levels are reached. The delay in maximum contrast enhancement can range from five to forty minutes, depending on the peak iodine levels achieved and the cell type of the lesion. This lag suggests that the contrast enhancement of the image is at least in part dependent on the accumulation of iodine within the lesion and outside the blood pool.

In brain scanning, the contrast medium Iothalamate Meglumine does not accumulate in normal brain tissue due to the presence of the "blood brain barrier". The increase in x-ray absorption in the normal brain is due to the presence of the contrast agent within the blood pool. A break in the blood brain barrier, such as occurs in malignant tumors of the brain, allows accumulation of contrast medium within the interstitial tumor tissue; adjacent normal brain tissue does not contain the contrast medium.

The image enhancement of non-tumoral lesions, such as arteriovenous malformations and aneurysms, is dependent on the iodine content of the circulating blood pool.

CT SCANNING OF THE BODY (INJECTION)

Iothalamate Meglumine 43% may also be used for enhancement of computed tomographic scans performed for detection and evaluation of lesions in the liver, pancreas, kidneys, abdominal aorta, mediastinum, abdominal cavity and retroperitoneal space.

In non-neural tissues (during computed tomography of the body), Iothalamate Meglumine diffuses rapidly from the vascular to the extravascular space. Increase in x-ray absorption is related to blood flow, concentration of the contrast medium and extraction of the contrast medium by interstitial tissue since no barrier exists; contrast enhancement is thus due to the relative differences in extravascular diffusion between normal and abnormal tissue, a situation quite different from that in the brain.

The pharmacokinetics of Iothalamate Meglumine in normal and abnormal tissues has been shown to be variable.

Enhancement of CT with Iothalamate Meglumine may be of benefit in establishing diagnoses of certain lesions in some sites with greater assurance than is possible with unenhanced CT and in supplying additional features of the lesions. In other cases, the contrast medium may allow visualization of lesions not seen with CT alone or may help to define suspicious lesions seen with unenhanced CT.

Contrast enhancement appears to be greatest within the 30-90 seconds after bolus administration of the contrast agent, and after intra-arterial rather than intravenous administration. Therefore, the use of a continuous scanning technique (a series of two to three second scans beginning at the injection—dynamic CT scanning) may improve enhancement and diagnostic assessment of tumors and other lesions such as an abscess, occasionally revealing more extensive disease.

A cyst or similar non-vascularized lesion may be distinguished from vascularized solid lesions by comparing enhanced and unenhanced scans; the nonvascularized lesions show no change in CT number, the vascularized lesions would show an increase. The latter might be benign, malignant or normal, but it is unlikely that it would be a cyst, hematoma, or other non-vascularized lesion.

Because *unenhanced* scanning may provide adequate information in the individual patient, the decision to employ contrast enhancement, which is

---

◆ RATED THERAPEUTICALLY EQUIVALENT;   ◇ THERAPEUTIC EQUIVALENCE UNCONFIRMED;   ○ UNRATED

associated with additional risk and increased radiation exposure, should be based upon a careful evaluation of clinical, other radiological, and unenhanced CT findings.

INDICATIONS AND USAGE

Injection: Iothalamate Meglumine 30% and 43% are indicated for use in intravenous infusion urography, contrast enhancement of computed tomographic brain images and arterial digital subtraction angiography. Iothalamate Meglumine 43% is indicated for use in lower extremity venography.

Iothalamate Meglumine 43% may also be used for enhancement of computed tomographic scans performed for detection and evaluation of lesions in the liver, pancreas, kidneys, abdominal aorta, mediastinum, abdominal cavity and retroperitoneal space. Continuous or multiple scans separated by intervals of 1-3 seconds during the first 30-90 seconds post-injection of the contrast medium (dynamic CT scanning) may provide enhancement of diagnostic significance, and may be of benefit in establishing diagnoses of certain lesions in these sites with greater assurance than is possible with CT alone and in supplying additional features of the lesions. In other cases, the contrast agent may allow visualization of lesions not seen with CT alone, or may help to define suspicious lesions seen with unenhanced CT. (See *"Clinical Pharmacology."*) Subsets of patients in whom delayed body CT scans might be helpful have not been identified. Inconsistent results have been reported and abnormal and normal tissues may be isodense during the same time frame used for delayed CT scanning. The risks of such indiscriminate use of contrast media are well known and such use is not recommended. At present, consistent results have been documented using dynamic CT techniques only.

Instillation: Iothalamate Meglumine 17.2% and 43% are indicated for use in retrograde cystography and cystourethrography. Iothalamate Meglumine 43% is also indicated for use in retrograde pyelography.

CONTRAINDICATIONS

Injection: Iothalamate Meglumine should not be used for myelography.

Refer to *"Precautions, General",*) concerning hypersensitivity.

Catheter: Contraindications to the procedure of retrograde pyelography include obstruction to endoscopy or catherization of the ureters, severe systemic disease which contraindicates instrumentation and acute infection of the upper urinary tract.

WARNINGS

Injection: Ionic iodinated contrast media inhibit blood coagulation, *in vitro*, more than nonionic contrast media. Nonetheless, it is prudent to avoid prolonged contact of blood with syringes containing ionic contrast media.

Serious, rarely fatal, thromboembolic events causing myocardial infarction and stroke have been reported during angiographic procedures with both ionic and nonionic contrast media. Therefore, meticulous intravascular administration technique is necessary, particularly during angiographic procedures, to minimize thromboembolic events. Numerous factors, including length of procedure, catheter and syringe material, underlying disease state and concomitant medications may contribute to the development of thromboembolic events. For these reasons, meticulous angiographic techniques are recommended including close attention to guidewire and catheter manipulation, use of manifold systems and/or three-way stopcocks, frequent catheter flushing with heparinized saline solutions and minimizing the length of the procedure. The use of plastic syringes in place of glass syringes has been reported to decrease but not eliminate the likelihood of *in vitro* clotting.

Serious or fatal reactions have been associated with the administration of iodine containing radiopaque media. It is of utmost importance to be completely prepared to treat any contrast medium reaction.

Serious neurologic sequelae, including permanent paralysis, have been reported following cerebral arteriography, selective spinal arteriography and arteriography of vessels supplying the spinal cord. The intravascular injection of a contrast medium should never be made following the administration of vasopressors since they strongly potentiate neurologic effects.

In patients with subarachnoid hemorrhage, a rare association between contrast administration and clinical deterioration, including convulsions and death, has been reported. Therefore, administration of intravascular iodinated ionic contrast media in these patients should be undertaken with caution.

A definite risk exists in the use of intravascular contrast agents in patients who are known to have multiple myeloma. In such instances anuria has developed resulting in progressive uremia, renal failure and eventually death. Although neither the contrast agent nor dehydration has separately proved to be the cause of anuria in myeloma, it has been speculated that the combination of both may be causative factors. The risk in myelomatous patients is not a contraindication to the procedure; however, partial dehydration in the preparation of these patients for the examination is not recommended since this may predispose to precipitation of myeloma protein in the renal tubules. No form of therapy, including dialysis, has been successful in reversing the effect. Myeloma, which occurs most commonly in persons over 40, should be considered before instituting intravascular administration of contrast agents.

Administration of radiopaque materials to patients known or suspected to have pheochromocytoma should be performed with extreme caution. If, in the opinion of the physician, the possible benefits of such procedures outweigh the considered risks, the procedures may be performed; however, the amount of radiopaque medium injected should be kept to an absolute minimum. The blood pressure

should be assessed throughout the procedure, and measures for treatment of a hypertensive crisis should be available.

Contrast media have been shown to promote the phenomenon of sickling in individuals who are homozygous for sickle cell disease when the material is injected intravenously or intra-arterially. Convulsions have occurred in patients with primary or metastatic cerebral lesions following the administration of iodine-containing radiopaque media for the contrast enhancement of CT brain images.

In patients with advanced renal disease, iodinated contrast media should be used with caution, and only when the need for the examination dictates, since excretion of the medium may be impaired. Patients with combined renal and hepatic disease, those with severe hypertension or congestive heart failure, and recent renal transplant recipients may present an additional risk.

Renal failure has been reported in patients with liver dysfunction who were given an oral cholecystographic agent followed by an intravascular iodinated radiopaque agent and also in patients with occult renal disease, notably diabetics and hypertensives. In these classes of patients there should be no fluid restriction and every attempt made to maintain normal hydration, prior to contrast medium administration, since dehydration is the single most important factor influencing further renal impairment.

Acute renal failure has been reported in diabetic patients with diabetic nephropathy and in susceptible non-diabetic patients (often elderly with pre-existing renal disease) following the administration of iodinated contrast agents. Therefore, careful consideration of the potential risks should be given before performing this radiographic procedure in these patients.

Caution should be exercised in performing contrast medium studies in patients with endotoxemia and/or those with elevated body temperatures.

Reports of thyroid storm occurring following the intravascular use of iodinated radiopaque agents in patients with hyperthyroidism or with an autonomously functioning thyroid nodule, suggest that this additional risk be evaluated in such patients before use of this drug. Iodine containing contrast agents may alter the results of thyroid function tests which depend on iodine estimation, e.g. PBI and radioactive iodine uptake studies. Such tests, if indicated, should be performed prior to the administration of this preparation.

Instillation: There are no known warnings with regard to use of these contrast media.

PRECAUTIONS

GENERAL

Diagnostic procedures which involve the use of radiopaque diagnostic agents should be carried out under the direction of personnel with the prerequisite training in and with a thorough knowledge of the particular procedure to be performed. All procedures utilizing contrast media carry a definite risk of producing adverse reactions. While most reactions may be minor, life threatening and fatal reactions may occur without warning. The risk-benefit factor should always be carefully evaluated before such a procedure is undertaken. At all times a fully equipped emergency cart, or equivalent supplies and equipment, and personnel competent in recognizing and treating adverse reactions of all severity, or situations which may arise as a result of the procedure, should be immediately available. If a serious reaction should occur, immediately discontinue administration. Since severe delayed reactions have been known to occur, emergency facilities and competent personnel should be available for at least 30 to 60 minutes after administration. (See *"Adverse Reactions."*)

Preparatory dehydration is dangerous and may contribute to acute renal failure in infants, young children, the elderly, patients with pre-existing renal insufficiency, patients with advanced vascular disease and diabetic patients.

Severe reactions to contrast media often resemble allergic responses. This has prompted the use of several provocative pretesting methods, none of which can be relied on to predict severe reactions. No conclusive relationship between severe reactions and antigen-antibody reactions or other manifestations of allergy has been established. The possibility of an idiosyncratic reaction in patients who have previously received a contrast medium without ill effect or in susceptible patients should always be considered. Prior to the injection of any contrast medium, the patient should be questioned to obtain a medical history with emphasis on allergy and hypersensitivity. A positive history of bronchial asthma, hay fever, or allergy, including food, a family history of allergy, a known sensitivity to iodine per se, or a previous reaction or hypersensitivity to a contrast agent may imply a greater than usual risk. Such a history, by suggesting histamine sensitivity and consequently proneness to reactions, may be more accurate than pre-testing in predicting the potential for reaction, although not necessarily the severity or type of reaction in the individual case. A positive history of this type does not arbitrarily contraindicate the use of a contrast agent, when a diagnostic procedure is thought essential, but does call for caution. (See *"Adverse Reactions."*)

Prophylactic therapy including corticosteroids and antihistamines should be considered for patients who present with a strong allergic history, a previous reaction to a contrast medium, or a positive pre-test since in these patients the incidence of reaction is two to three times that of the general population. Adequate doses of corticosteroids should be started early enough prior to contrast medium injection to be effective and should continue through the time of injection and for 24 hours after injection. Antihistamines should be administered within 30 minutes of the contrast medium injection. Recent reports indicate that such pretreatment does not prevent life-threatening reactions, but may reduce both their incidence and severity. A separate syringe should be used for these injections.

Since these procedures require instrumentation, special precautions should be observed in those patients known to have an acute urinary tract infection.

Filling of the bladder should be done at a steady rate, exercising caution to avoid excessive pressure. Sterile procedures should be employed in administration.

Angiography should be avoided whenever possible in patients with homocystinuria because of the risk of inducing thrombosis and embolism.

Information for Patients: Patients receiving iodinated intravascular contrast agents or diagnostic agents for instillation urography should be instructed to:

1. Inform your physician if you are pregnant.
2. Inform your physician if you are diabetic or if you have multiple myeloma, pheochromocytoma, homozygous sickle cell disease or known thyroid disease. (See *"Warnings."*)
3. Inform your physician if you are allergic to any drugs, food or if you had any reactions to previous injections of dyes used for x-ray procedures. (See *"Precautions, General."*)
4. Inform your physican about any other medications you are currently taking including non-prescription drugs.
5. Consult with your physician if, at some future date, any thyroid tests are planned. The iodine in this agent may interfere with later thyroid tests.

Carcinogenesis, Mutagenesis, Impairment of Fertility: No long-term animal studies have been performed to evaluate carcinogenic potential or, with Iothalamate Meglumine (catheter), mutagenic potential or whether this drug affects fertility. However, animal studies suggest that Iothalamate Meglumine (injection) is not mutagenic and does not affect fertility in males or females.

Use in Pregnancy:

Injection: Pregnancy Category B: Reproduction studies have been performed in mice, rats, and rabbits at doses up to 6.6 times the human dose and have revealed no evidence of impaired fertility or harm to the fetus due to Iothalamate Meglumine. There are, however, no adequate and well controlled studies in pregnant woman. Because animal reproduction studies are not always predictive of human response, this drug should be used during pregnancy only if clearly needed.

Instillation: Pregnancy Category C: Animal reproduction studies have not been conducted with Iothalamate Meglumine for catheter instillation. It is also not known whether this drug can cause fetal harm when administered to a pregnant woman or can affect reproduction capacity. Iothalamate Meglumine for catheter instillation should be used in pregnant women only if clearly needed.

Nursing Mothers: Iothalamate salts are excreted unchanged in human milk. Because of the potential for adverse effects in nursing infants, bottle feedings should be substituted for breast feedings for 24 hours following the administration of this drug.

(Precautions for specific procedures receive comment under that procedure).

Use In Children: Safety and effectiveness of Iothalamate Meglumine 30% for infusion urography have not been established in children under 12 years of age.

DRUG/LABORATORY TEST INTERACTION
Thyroid Function Tests: If indicated, these tests generally should be performed prior to the administration of any iodinated agent. However, thyroid function can be evaluated after use of these agents by using T_3 resin uptake or free thyroxine assays.

ADVERSE REACTIONS
INJECTION
Adverse reactions to injectable contrast media fall into two categories: chemotoxic reactions and idiosyncratic reactions.

Chemotoxic reactions result from the physio-chemical properties of the contrast media, the dose and speed of injection. All hemodynamic disturbances and injuries to organs or vessels perfused by the contrast medium are included in this category.

Idiosyncratic reactions include all other reactions. They occur more frequently in patients 20 to 40 years old. Idiosyncratic reactions may or may not be dependent on the amount of dose injected, the speed of injection, the mode of injection and the radiographic procedure. Idiosyncratic reactions are subdivided into minor, intermediate and severe. The minor reactions are self-limited and of short duration; the severe reactions are life-threatening and treatment is urgent and mandatory.

Fatalities have been reported following the administration of iodine-containing contrast agents. Based upon clinical literature, the incidence of death is reported to range from one in 10,000 (0.01%) to less than one in 100,000 (0.001%).

The following adverse reactions have been observed in conjunction with the use of iodine-containing contrast agents.

The most frequent adverse reactions are nausea, vomiting, facial flush and a feeling of body warmth. These are usually of brief duration. Other reactions include the following:

Hypersensitivity Reactions: Dermal manifestations of urticaria with or without pruritus, erythema and maculopapular rash. Dry mouth. Sweating. Conjunctival symptoms. Facial, peripheral and angioneurotic edema. Symptoms related to the respiratory system include sneezing, nasal stuffiness, coughing, choking, dyspnea, chest tightness and wheezing, which may be initial manifestations of more severe and infrequent reactions including asthmatic attack, laryngospasm and bronchospasm with or without edema, pulmonary edema, apnea and cyanosis. Rarely, these allergic-type reactions can progress into anaphylaxis with loss of consciousness and coma and severe cardiovascular disturbances.

Cardiovascular Reactions: Generalized vasodilation, flushing and venospasm. Occasionally, thrombosis or rarely, thrombophlebitis. Red blood cell clumping and agglutination, crenation and interference in clot formation. Extremely rare cases of disseminated intravascular coagulation resulting in death have been reported. Severe cardiovascular responses include rare cases of hypotensive shock, coronary insufficiency, cardiac arrhythmia, fibrillation and arrest. These severe reactions are usually reversible with prompt and appropriate management; however, fatalities have occurred.

Technique Reactions: Extravasation with burning pain, hematomas, ecchymosis and tissue necrosis, paresthesia or numbness, vascular constriction due to injection rate, thrombosis and thrombophlebitis.

Neurological Reactions: Spasm, convulsions, aphasia, syncope, paresis, paralysis resulting from spinal cord injury and pathology associated with syndrome of transverse myelitis, visual field losses which are usually transient but may be permanent, coma and death.

Other Reactions: Headache, trembling, shaking, chills without fever and light-headedness. Temporary renal shutdown or other nephropathy.

(Adverse reactions to specific procedures receive comment under that procedure).

INSTILLATION
Irritation of the bladder or ureter, common to some degree to all contrast media administered for retrograde urographic procedures, may occasionally occur.

As with all contrast media, intravasation may lead to hypersensitivity reactions such as a sense of warmth, flushing, sneezing, sweating, chills, fever, urticaria, laryngeal edema, bronchospasm, hypertension, hypotension, cardiac arrhythmias and cardiac arrest.

Oliguria or anuria may occur following retrograde pyelography, especially in patients with severe pre-existing renal disease.

Adverse reactions associated with procedural technique include injury to the urethra, bladder, ureter, and introduction of infection.

In the event of serious or anaphylactoid reactions, it should be kept in mind that the reactions known to occur with intravenous administration of radiopaque contrast materials are possible.

OVERDOSAGE
Overdosage may occur. The adverse effects of overdosage are life-threatening and affect mainly the pulmonary and cardiovascular system. The symptoms may include cyanosis, bradycardia, acidosis, pulmonary hemorrhage, convulsions, coma and cardiac arrest. Treatment of an overdose is directed toward the support of all vital functions and prompt institution of symptomatic therapy.

Iothalamate salts are dialyzable.

The intravenous LD_{50} value of various concentrations of Iothalamate Meglumine (in grams of iodine/kilogram body weight) varied from 5.7 to 8.9 g/kg in mice and 9.8 to 11.2 g/kg in rats. The LD_{50} values decrease as the rate of injection increases.

DOSAGE AND ADMINISTRATION
INJECTION
It is advisable that Iothalamate Meglumine be at or close to body temperature when injected.

The patient should be instructed to omit the meal that precedes the examination. Appropriate premedication, which may include a barbiturate, tranquilizer or analgesic drug, may be administered prior to the examination.

A preliminary film is recommended to check the position of the patient and the x-ray exposure factors.

If during administration a minor reaction occurs, the injection should be slowed or stopped until the reaction has subsided. If a major reaction occurs the injection should be discontinued immediately.

Under no circumstances should either corticosteroids or antihistamines be mixed in the same syringe with the contrast medium because of a potential for chemical incompatibility.

Parenteral drug products should be inspected visually for particulate matter and discoloration prior to administration.

LOWER EXTREMITY VENOGRAPHY
Precautions: All patients should be well hydrated prior to the procedure. In addition to the general precautions previously described, special care is required when venography is performed in patients with suspected thrombosis, phlebitis, severe ischemic disease, local infection or a totally obstructed venous system. Extreme caution during injection of the contrast agent is necessary to avoid extravasation and fluoroscopy is recommended. This is especially important in patients with severe arterial or venous disease.

Adverse Reactions: In addition to the general adverse reactions previously described, thrombophlebitis, syncope and very rare cases of gangrene have been reported following venography.

Usual Dosage: The usual dose for adults is 30-125 mL of Iothalamate Meglumine 43% per lower extremity. The dose for children is reduced in proportion to body weight. Following the procedure, the venous system should be flushed with either 5% dextrose in water (D5W) or normal saline (Sodium Chloride Injection U.S.P.) or the contrast medium should be removed by leg massage and/or leg elevation.

INTRAVENOUS INFUSION UROGRAPHY
Intravenous infusion urography enhances the potential for more diagnostic information in those patients in whom the usual excretory urographic technique

---

either has not provided or is not expected to provide satisfactory visualization. The entire urinary tract, including nephrogram and cystogram, may be visualized in the unobstructed patient with normal renal function.

Patient Preparation: Appropriate preparation of the patient is important for optimal visualization. A low residue diet is recommended for the day preceding the examination and a laxative is given the evening before the examination, unless contraindicated.

Dehydration is not indicated for the performance of infusion urography. Patients should be maintained in an optimal state of hydration prior to the procedure.

Usual Dosage: The usual dose of Iothalamate Meglumine 43% in adults and children is 3 mL/kg (1.5 mL/lb) by intravenous administration, not to exceed a total dose of 200 mL.

The recommended adult dose is 200-300 mL of Iothalamate Meglumine 30% (4 mL/kg) with a maximum of 300 mL.

Safety and effectiveness for infusion urography in children below the age of 12 have not been established.

The solution is infused through an appropriate I.V. needle at a rate of approximately 40-50 mL per minute for Iothalamate Meglumine 43% or 50 mL per minute for Iothalamate Meglumine 30%. Any appropriate intravenous administration set may be used observing the usual precautions for maintaining sterility and safety in administration. Films are usually taken at 5 minute intervals following the initiation of the infusion for a total of 20 minutes.

In patients with impaired renal function, diagnostic opacification frequently is achieved only after prolonged periods. In these individuals, periodic films obtained up to 24 hours after infusion might yield useful information.

CONTRAST ENHANCEMENT OF COMPUTED TOMOGRAPHIC (CT) HEAD (BRAIN) IMAGING

Tumors: Iothalamate Meglumine may be useful to enhance the demonstration of the presence and extent of certain malignancies such as: gliomas including malignant gliomas, glioblastomas, astrocytomas, oligodendrogliomas and gangliomas; ependymomas; medulloblastomas; meningiomas; neuromas; pinealomas; pituitary adenomas; craniopharyngiomas; germinomas; and metastatic lesions.

The usefulness of contrast enhancement for the investigation of the retrobulbar space and in cases of low grade or infiltrative glioma has not been demonstrated.

In cases where lesions have calcified, there is less likelihood of enhancement. Following therapy, tumors may show decreased or no enhancement.

Non-Neoplastic Conditions: The use of Iothalamate Meglumine may be beneficial in the image enhancement of non-neoplastic lesions. Cerebral infarctions of recent onset may be better visualized with the contrast enhancement, while some infarctions are obscured if contrast media are used. The use of iodinated contrast media results in contrast enhancement in about 60% of cerebral infarctions studied from one to four weeks from the onset of symptoms.

Sites of active infection may also be enhanced following contrast medium administration.

Arteriovenous malformations and aneurysms will show contrast enhancement. In the case of these vascular lesions, the enhancement is probably dependent on the iodine content of the circulating blood pool.

The opacification of the inferior vermis following contrast medium administration has resulted in false positive diagnoses in a number of normal studies.

Patient Preparation: No special patient preparation is required for contrast enhancement of CT head (brain) scanning. However, it is advisable to insure that patients are well hydrated prior to examination.

Usage Dosage: The usual dose of Iothalamate Meglumine 43% in adults and children is 3 mL/kg (1.5 mL/lb) by intravenous administration, not to exceed a total dose of 200 mL. The recommended adult dose is 200-300 mL of Iothalamate Meglumine 30%. For children under 12 years of age and patients weighing less than 100 pounds, a dose of 4 mL/kg (2 mL/lb) is recommended. The dose should be infused as rapidly as possible through any well vented intravenous administration set and needle, observing the usual precautions for maintaining sterility. In most cases, scanning may be performed immediately after completion of administration; however, when fast scanning equipment (less than 1 minute) is used, consideration should be given to waiting approximately 5 minutes to allow for maximum contrast enhancement.

CONTRAST ENHANCEMENT IN BODY COMPUTED TOMOGRAPHY

Patient Preparation: No special patient preparation is required. However, it is advisable to insure that patients are well hydrated. In patients undergoing abdominal or pelvic examination, opacification of the bowel may be valuable in scan interpretation.

Precautions: In addition to the general precautions previously described, patient cooperation is essential since patient motion, including respiration, can markedly affect image quality. The use of an intravascular contrast medium can obscure tumors in patients undergoing CT evaluation of the liver resulting in a false negative diagnosis. Dynamic CT scanning is the procedure of choice for malignant tumor enhancement. (See *"Clinical Pharmacology."*)

Usage Dosage: The usual adult dose is 200 to 250 mL of Iothalamate Meglumine 43% administered by bolus injection, by rapid infusion or by a combination of both.

In adults, when the combination bolus and infusion technique is used, a 50 to 100 mL bolus injection followed by a rapid infusion of 100 to 150 mL may be used. In children, the dose is reduced in proportion to body weight.

ARTERIAL DIGITAL SUBTRACTION ANGIOGRAPHY

Arterial digital subtraction angiography provides images similar in quality to conventional film-screen systems. The advantages of arterial DSA when compared to standard film angiography include the use of less contrast medium; the use of a lower concentration of contrast medium as provided by Iothalamate Meglumine; a decreased need for selective arterial catheterization and a shortened examination time. The limitations of arterial DSA include: reduced spatial resolution and limited field size.

Patient Preparation: No special patient preparation is required for arterial DSA. However, it is advisable to insure that patients are well hydrated prior to examination.

Precautions: In addition to the general precautions described, the risks associated with arterial DSA are those usually attendant with catheter procedures. Following the procedure, gentle pressure hemostasis is required, followed by observation and immobilization of the limb for several hours to prevent hemorrhage from the site of arterial puncture.

Usual Dosage: It is advisable to inject at rates approximately equal to the flow rate of the vessel being injected. The following volumes per injection, have been used, and may be repeated as necessary:

Carotid or Vertebral Arteries	3-10 mL
Aortic Arch	15-30 mL
Subclavian and Brachial Arteries	5-15 mL
Major branches of the Aorta	5-30 mL
Abdominal Aorta	10-30 mL

A total dose of 200 mL (representing 40.4 gm of iodine) of Iothalamate Meglumine 43% or 250 mL (representing 35.2 g of iodine) of Iothalamate Meglumine 30% should not be exceeded. Consideration should be given to the patient's clinical condition and whether large volumes of fluids may be detrimental to patient care.

CYSTOGRAPHY, CYSTOURETHROGRAPHY, AND RETROGRADE PYELOGRAPHY

Patient Preparation: Unless contraindicated, an appropriate laxative is given the night before the examination.

Radiographic Technique: The radiographic procedure normally employed for cystography, cystourethrography and retrograde pyelography should be employed. A preliminary radiograph is recommended before the contrast agent is administered.

Administration: Sterile catheterization is essential. Iothalamate Meglumine may be introduced by gravity flow using an appropriate venoclysis set or by syringe. Excessive pressure should be avoided with any method of administration.

Usual Dosage: Retrograde Pyelography: Ordinarily about 25 mL of Iothalamate Meglumine 43% are required for bilateral and 15 mL for unilateral pyelograms. About 5-6 mL are usually administered for each exposure. Children usually require a volume reduced in proportion to their body size.

Cystography and Cystourethrography: Either Iothalamate Meglumine supplied at 43% w/v concentration or Iothalamate Meglumine supplied at a 17.2% w/v concentration may be used for these procedures. The desired concentration will vary depending upon the patient's size and age and also with the technique and equipment used. Sufficient volume of contrast medium is administered to adequately fill the urinary bladder. The volume of solution required will vary depending upon the individual patient. Adults usually require a volume in the range of 200-400 mL. Children require a volume in proportion to their body size. The usual dose ranges from 30 to 300 mL.

STORAGE

Store below 30°C (86°F). Exposing this product to very cold temperatures may result in crystallization of the salt. If this occurs, the container should be brought to room temperature. Shake vigorously to assure complete dissolution of any crystals. The speed of dissolution may be increased by heating with circulating warm air. Submersion of syringes in water is not recommended. Before use, examine the product to assure that all solids are redissolved and that the container and closure have not been damaged. This preparation is sensitive to light and must be protected from strong daylight or direct exposure to the sun.

Do not reautoclave plastic container because of possible damage to syringe.

As with all contrast media, glass and plastic containers should be inspected prior to use to ensure that breakage or other damage has not occurred during shipping and handling. All containers should be inspected for closure integrity. Damaged containers should not be used.

HOW SUPPLIED
INJECTION: 17.2%

BRAND/MANUFACTURER	NDC	SIZE	AWP
○ **BRAND**			
CYSTO-CONRAY II: Mallinckrodt Med	00019-0862-07	250 ml	$13.80
	00019-0862-09	500 ml	$20.00

➤ SHOWN IN PRODUCT IDENTIFICATION GUIDE

INJECTION: 30%

BRAND/MANUFACTURER	NDC	SIZE	AWP
○ **BRAND**			
CONRAY-30: Mallinckrodt Med	00019-0952-15	50 ml	$4.15
	00019-0952-11	150 ml	$12.45
	00019-0952-01	300 ml	$24.84

INJECTION: 43%

BRAND/MANUFACTURER	NDC	SIZE	AWP
○ **BRAND**			
CONRAY-43: Mallinckrodt Med	00019-3183-75	50 ml	$159.60
CYSTO-CONRAY: Mallinckrodt Med	00019-7649-15	50 ml	$7.50
CYSTO-CONRAY: Mallinckrodt Med	00019-3183-07	1000 ml	$13.12
CONRAY-43: Mallinckrodt Med	00019-3183-08	150 ml	$13.91
	00019-3183-11	200 ml	$18.58
	00019-3183-09	250 ml	$20.05
CYSTO-CONRAY: Mallinckrodt Med	00019-7649-03	250 ml	$22.84
CONRAY-43: Mallinckrodt Med	00019-3183-15	50 ml	$6.88
CYSTO-CONRAY: Mallinckrodt Med			

INJECTION: 60%

BRAND/MANUFACTURER	NDC	SIZE	AWP
○ **BRAND**			
CONRAY: Mallinckrodt Med	00019-0953-13	30 ml	$5.77
	00019-0953-73	30 ml	$6.99
	00019-0953-15	50 ml	$8.75
	00019-0953-75	50 ml	$9.74
	00019-0953-03	100 ml	$17.22
	00019-0953-09	100 ml	$18.95
	00019-0953-81	125 ml	$23.00
	00019-0953-11	150 ml	$24.62
	00019-0953-12	200 ml	$30.30

Iothalamate Meglumine and Iothalamate Sodium

DESCRIPTION

Iothalamate Meglumine/Iothalamate Sodium is a sterile aqueous solution intended for intravascular administration as a diagnostic radiopaque medium. Iothalamate Meglumine/Iothalamate Sodium (Iothalamate Salts) contains 52% w/v 1-Deoxy-1-(methylamino)-D-glucitol 5-acetamido-2, 4, 6-triiodo-N-methylisophthalate (salt) and 26% w/v monosodium 5-acetamido-2, 4, 6-triiodo-N-methylisophthalate.

Each milliliter contains 520 mg of Iothalamate Meglumine, 260 mg of Iothalamate Sodium.

The solution contains approximately 9.4 mg (0.408 mEq) sodium in each milliliter of solution and provides 40% (400 mg/mL) organically bound iodine.

Iothalamate Salts has an osmolarity of approximately 1600 mOsmol per liter, an osmolality of approximately 2400 mOsmol per kilogram and is, therefore, hypertonic under conditions of use. The viscosity (cps) is approximately 17 at 25° C and 9 at 37° C. The pH is 6.5-7.7.

Iothalamate Salts is a clear solution containing no undissolved solids. Crystallization does not occur at normal room temperatures. It is supplied in containers from which the air has been displaced by nitrogen.

CLINICAL PHARMACOLOGY

Following intravascular injection, Iothalamate Salts is rapidly transported through the circulatory system to the kidneys and is excreted unchanged in the urine by glomerular filtration. The pharmacokinetics of intravascularly administered radiopaque contrast media are usually best described by a two compartment model with a rapid alpha phase for drug distribution and a slower beta phase for drug elimination. In patients with normal renal function, the alpha and beta half-lives of Iothalamate Salts were approximately 10 and 90 minutes, respectively.

Angiography may be performed following intravascular injection which will permit visualization until significant hemodilution occurs.

Renal accumulation is sufficiently rapid that maximum radiographic density in the calyces and pelves occurs in most instances about 3-8 minutes after injection. In patients with impaired renal function, diagnostic opacification frequently is achieved only after prolonged periods.

Injectable iodinated contrast agents are excreted either through the kidneys or through the liver. These two excretory pathways are not mutually exclusive, but the main route of excretion seems to be related to the affinity of the contrast medium for serum albumin. Iothalamate salts are poorly bound to serum albumin, and are excreted mainly through the kidneys.

The liver and small intestine provide the major alternate route of excretion. In patients with severe renal impairment, the excretion of this contrast medium through the gallbladder and into the small intestine sharply increases.

Iothalamate Salts cross the placental barrier in humans and are excreted unchanged in human milk.

CT SCANNING OF THE HEAD

When used for contrast enhancement in computed tomographic brain scanning, the degree of enhancement is directly related to the amount of iodine administered. Rapid injection of the entire dose yields peak blood iodine concentrations immediately following the injection, which fall rapidly over the next five to ten minutes. This can be accounted for by the dilution in the vascular and extracellular fluid compartments which causes an initial sharp fall in plasma concentration. Equilibration with the extracellular compartments is reached by about ten minutes; thereafter the fall becomes exponential. Maximum contrast enhancement frequently occurs after peak blood iodine levels are reached. The delay in maximum contrast enhancement can range from five to forty minutes, depending on the peak iodine levels achieved and the cell type of the lesion. This lag suggests that the contrast enhancement of the image is at least in part dependent on the accumulation of iodine within the lesion and outside the blood pool.

In brain scanning, the contrast medium, Iothalamate Salts, does not accumulate in normal brain tissue due to the presence of the "blood brain barrier". The increase in x-ray absorption in the normal brain is due to the presence of the contrast agent within the blood pool. A break in the blood brain barrier, such as occurs in malignant tumors of the brain, allows accumulation of contrast medium within the interstitial tumor tissue; adjacent normal brain tissue does not contain the contrast medium.

The image enhancement of non-tumoral lesions, such as arteriovenous malformations and aneurysms, is dependent on the iodine content of the circulating blood pool.

INDICATIONS AND USAGE

Iothalamate Salts is indicated for use in excretory urography, angiocardiography, aortography, selective renal arteriography, selective coronary arteriography, intravenous digital subtraction angiography, and for contrast enhancement of computed tomographic brain images.

CONTRAINDICATIONS

Iothalamate Salts should not be used for myelography.

This product should not be used for cerebral angiography by direct injection into the carotid or vertebral arteries due to the high concentration of the solution. (Refer to *"Warnings".*)

Refer to *"Precautions, General"* concerning hypersensitivity.

WARNINGS

Ionic iodinated contrast media inhibit blood coagulation, *in vitro*, more than nonionic contrast media. Nonetheless, it is prudent to avoid prolonged contact of blood with syringes containing ionic contrast media.

Serious, rarely fatal, thromboembolic events causing myocardial infarction and stroke have been reported during angiographic procedures with both ionic and nonionic contrast media. Therefore, meticulous intravascular administration technique is necessary, particularly during angiographic procedures, to minimize thromboembolic events. Numerous factors, including length of procedure, catheter and syringe material, underlying disease state and concomitant medications may contribute to the development of thromboembolic events. For these reasons, meticulous angiographic techniques are recommended including close attention to guidewire and catheter manipulation, use of manifold systems and/or three-way stopcocks, frequent catheter flushing with heparinized saline solutions and minimizing the length of the procedure. The use of plastic syringes in place of glass syringes has been reported to decrease but not eliminate the likelihood of *in vitro* clotting.

Serious or fatal reactions have been associated with the administration of iodine-containing radiopaque media. It is of utmost importance to be completely prepared to treat any contrast medium reaction.

Serious neurologic sequelae, including permanent paralysis, have been reported following inadvertent injections of excessive amounts of concentrated contrast media into arteries supplying the spinal cord. The injection of a contrast medium should never be made following the administration of vasopressors since they strongly potentiate neurologic effects. (See *"Precautions"* pertaining to Aortography.)

In patients with subarachnoid hemorrhage, a rare association between contrast administration and clinical deterioration, including convulsions and death, has been reported. Therefore, administration of intravascular iodinated ionic contrast media in these patients should be undertaken with caution.

A definite risk exists in the use of intravascular contrast agents in patients who are known to have multiple myeloma. In such instances anuria has developed resulting in progressive uremia, renal failure and eventually death. Although neither the contrast agent nor dehydration has separately proved to be the cause of anuria in myeloma, it has been speculated that the combination of both may be causative factors. The risk in myelomatous patients is not a contraindication to the procedure; however, partial dehydration in the preparation of these patients for the examination is not recommended since this may predispose to precipitation of myeloma protein in the renal tubules. No form of therapy, including dialysis, has been successful in reversing the effect. Myeloma, which occurs most commonly in persons over 40, should be considered before instituting intravascular administration of contrast agents.

Administration of radiopaque materials to patients known or suspected to have pheochromocytoma should be performed with extreme caution. If, in the opinion of the physician, the possible benefits of such procedures outweigh the considered risks, the procedures may be performed; however, the amount of radiopaque medium injected should be kept to an absolute minimum. The blood pressure should be assessed throughout the procedure, and measures for treatment of a hypertensive crisis should be available. *Contrast media have been shown to promote the phenomenon of sickling in individuals who are homozygous for sickle cell disease when the material is injected intravenously or intraarterially.*

Convulsions have occurred in patients with primary or metastatic cerebral lesions following the administration of iodine-containing radiopaque media for the contrast enhancement of CT brain images.

In patients with advanced renal disease, iodinated contrast media should be used with caution, and only when the need for the examination dictates, since excretion of the medium may be impaired. Patients with combined renal and hepatic disease, those with severe hypertension or congestive heart failure and recent renal transplant recipients present an additional risk.

Renal failure has been reported in patients with liver dysfunction who were given an oral cholecystographic agent followed by an intravascular iodinated radiopaque agent and also in patients with occult renal disease, notably diabetics and hypertensives. In these classes of patients there should be no fluid restriction and every attempt should be made to maintain normal hydration, prior to contrast medium administration, since dehydration is the single most important factor influencing further renal impairment.

Acute renal failure has been reported in diabetic patients with diabetic nephropathy and in susceptible nondiabetic patients (often elderly with pre-existing renal disease) following the administration of iodinated contrast agents. Therefore, careful consideration of the potential risks should be given before performing this radiographic procedure in these patients.

Caution should be exercised in performing contrast medium studies in patients with endotoxemia and/or those with elevated body temperatures.

Reports of thyroid storm occurring following the intravascular use of iodinated radiopaque agents in patients with hyperthyroidism or with an autonomously functioning thyroid nodule suggest that this additional risk be evaluated in such patients before use of this drug. Iodine-containing contrast agents may alter the results of thyroid function tests which depend on iodine estimation, e.g. PBI and radioactive iodine uptake studies. Such tests, if indicated, should be performed prior to the administration of this preparation.

PRECAUTIONS

General: Diagnostic procedures which involve the use of iodinated intravascular contrast agents should be carried out under the direction of personnel skilled and experienced in the particular procedure to be performed. All procedures utilizing contrast media carry a definite risk of producing adverse reactions. While most reactions may be minor, life-threatening and fatal reactions may occur without warning. The risk-benefit factor should always be carefully evaluated before such a procedure is undertaken. A fully equipped emergency cart, or equivalent supplies and equipment, and personnel competent in recognizing and treating adverse reactions of all types should always be available. If a serious reaction should occur, immediately discontinue administration. Since severe delayed reactions have been known to occur, emergency facilities and competent personnel should be available for at least 30 to 60 minutes after administration. (See *"Adverse Reactions"*).

Preparatory dehydration is dangerous and may contribute to acute renal failure in infants, young children, the elderly, patients with pre-existing renal insufficiency, patients with advanced vascular disease and diabetic patients.

Severe reactions to contrast media often resemble allergic responses. This has prompted the use of several provocative pretesting methods, none of which can be relied on to predict severe reactions. No conclusive relationship between severe reactions and antigen-antibody reactions or other manifestations of allergy has been established. The possibility of an idiosyncratic reaction in patients who have previously received a contrast medium without ill effect should always be considered. Prior to the injection of any contrast medium, the patient should be questioned to obtain a medical history with emphasis on allergy and hypersensitivity. A positive history of bronchial asthma or allergy, a family history of allergy (including food), or a previous reaction or hypersensitivity to a contrast agent may imply a greater than usual risk. Such a history, by suggesting histamine sensitivity and consequently proneness to reactions, may be more accurate than pretesting in predicting the potential for reaction, although not necessarily the severity or type of reaction in the individual case. A positive history of this type does not arbitrarily contraindicate the use of a contrast agent when a diagnostic procedure is thought essential, but does call for caution. (See *"Adverse Reactions"*.)

Prophylactic therapy including corticosteroids and antihistamines should be considered for patients who present with a strong allergic history, a previous reaction to a contrast medium, or a positive pretest, since in these patients the incidence of reaction is two to three times that of the general population. Adequate doses of corticosteroids should be started early enough prior to contrast medium injection to be effective and should continue through the time of injection and for 24 hours after injection. Antihistamines should be administered within 30 minutes of the contrast medium injection. Recent reports indicate that such pretreatment does not prevent serious life-threatening reactions, but may reduce both their incidence and severity. A separate syringe should be used for these injections.

Clinical trials have not been conducted using Iothalamate Salts for routine angiography of the extremities.

General anesthesia may be indicated in the performance of some procedures in young or uncooperative children and in selected adult patients; however, a higher incidence of adverse reactions has been reported in these patients, and may be attributable to the inability of the patient to identify untoward symptoms or to the hypotensive effect of anesthesia which can prolong the circulation time and increase the duration of contact of the contrast agent.

Angiography should be avoided whenever possible in patients with hemocystinuria, because of the risk of inducing thrombosis and embolism.

Information for Patients: Patients receiving iodinated intravascular contrast agents should be instructed to:
1. Inform your physician if you are pregnant.
2. Inform your physician if you are diabetic or if you have multiple myeloma, pheochromocytoma, homozygous sickle cell disease or known thyroid disease. (See *"Warnings"*.)
3. Inform your physician if you are allergic to any drugs, food or if you had any reactions to previous injections of dyes used for x-ray procedures. (See *"Precautions, General"*.)
4. Inform your physician about any other medications you are currently taking, including non-prescription drugs.

Carcinogenesis, Mutagenesis, Impairment of Fertility: No long-term animal studies have been performed to evaluate carcinogenic potential. However, animal studies suggest that this drug is not mutagenic and does not affect fertility in males or females.

Pregnancy Category B: Reproduction studies have been performed in mice, rats and rabbits at doses up to 6.6 times the human dose and have revealed no evidence of impaired fertility or harm to the fetus due to Iothalamate Salts. There are however no adequate and well controlled studies in pregnant women. Because animal reproduction studies are not always predictive of human response, this drug should be used during pregnancy only if clearly needed.

Nursing Mothers: Iothalamate salts are excreted unchanged in human milk. Because of the potential for adverse effects in nursing infants, bottle feedings should be substituted for breast feedings for 24 hours following the administration of this drug.

(Precautions for specific procedures receive comment under that procedure.)

ADVERSE REACTIONS

General: Adverse reactions to injectable contrast media fall into two categories: chemotoxic reactions and idiosyncratic reactions.

Chemotoxic reactions result from the physio-chemical properties of the contrast media, the dose and speed of injection. All hemodynamic disturbances and injuries to organs or vessels perfused by the contrast medium are included in this category.

Idiosyncratic reactions include all other reactions. They occur more frequently in patients 20 to 40 years old. Idiosyncratic reactions may or may not be dependent on the amount of dose injected, the speed of injection, the mode of injection and the radiographic procedure. Idiosyncratic reactions are subdivided into minor, intermediate and severe. The minor reactions are self-limited and of short duration; the severe reactions are life-threatening and treatment is urgent and mandatory.

Fatalities have been reported following the administration of iodine-containing agents. Based upon clinical literature, the incidence of death is reported to range from one in 10,000 (0.01 percent) to less than one in 100,000 (0.001 percent).

The following adverse reactions have been observed in conjunction with the use of iodine-containing contrast agents.

The most frequent adverse reactions are nausea, vomiting, facial flush and feeling of body warmth. These are usually of brief duration. Other reactions include the following:

Hypersensitivity Reactions: Dermal manifestations of urticaria with or without pruritus, erythema and maculopapular rash. Dry mouth. Sweating. Conjunctival symptoms. Facial, peripheral and angioneurotic edema. Symptoms related to the respiratory system include sneezing, nasal stuffiness, coughing, choking, dyspnea, chest tightness and wheezing, which may be initial manifestations of more severe and infrequent reactions including asthmatic attack, laryngospasm and bronchospasm with or without edema, pulmonary edema, apnea and cyanosis. Rarely, these allergic-type reactions can progress into anaphylaxis with loss of consciousness and coma and severe cardiovascular disturbances.

Cardiovascular Reactions: Generalized vasodilation, flushing and venospasm. Occasionally, thrombosis or rarely, thrombophlebitis. Red blood cell clumping and agglutination, crenation and interference in clot formation. Extremely rare cases of disseminated intravascular coagulation resulting in death have been reported. Severe cardiovascular responses include rare cases of hypotensive shock, coronary insufficiency; cardiac arrhythmia, fibrillation and arrest. These severe reactions are usually reversible with prompt and appropriate management; however, fatalities have occurred.

Technique Reactions: Extravasation with burning pain, hematomas ecchymosis and tissue necrosis, paresthesia or numbness, vascular constriction due to injection rate, thrombosis and thrombophlebitis.

Neurological Reactions: Spasm, convulsions, aphasia, syncope, paresis, paralysis resulting from spinal cord injury and pathology associated with the syndrome of transverse myelitis, visual field losses which are usually transient but may be permanent, coma and death.

Other Reactions: Headache, trembling, shaking, chills without fever and lightheadness. Temporary renal shutdown or other nephropathy.

(Adverse reactions to specific procedures receive comment under that procedure.)

OVERDOSAGE

Overdosage may occur. The adverse effects of overdosage are life-threatening and affect mainly the pulmonary and cardiovascular systems. The symptoms may include cyanosis, bradycardia, acidosis, pulmonary hemorrhage, convulsions, coma and cardiac arrest. Treatment of an overdose is directed toward the support of all vital functions and prompt institution of symptomatic therapy.

Iothalamate salts are dialyzable.

The intravenous LD$_{50}$ value of Iothalamate Salts (in grams of iodine/kilogram body weight) varied from 8.4 to 12.0 g/kg in mice. The LD$_{50}$ values decrease as the rate of injection increases.

DOSAGE AND ADMINISTRATION

It is advisable that Iothalamate Salts be at or close to body temperature when injected.

The patient should be instructed to omit the meal that precedes the examination. Appropriate premedication, which may include a barbiturate, tranquilizer or analgesic drug, may be administered prior to the examination.

A preliminary film is recommended to check the position of the patient and the x-ray exposure factors.

If during the administration a minor reaction occurs the injection should be slowed or stopped until the reaction has subsided. If a major reaction occurs the injection should be discontinued immediately.

Under no circumstances should either corticosteroids or antihistamines be mixed in the same syringe with the contrast medium because of a potential for chemical incompatibility.

Parenteral drug products should be inspected visually for particulate matter and discoloration prior to administration.

EXCRETORY UROGRAPHY

Following intravenous injection, Iothalamate Salts is rapidly excreted by the kidneys. Iothalamate Salts may be visualized in the renal parenchyma 30 seconds following bolus injection. Maximum radiographic density in the calyces and pelves occurs in most instances within 3-8 minutes after injection. In patients with severe renal impairment contrast visualization may be substantially delayed.

Patient Preparation: Appropriate preparation of the patient is important for optimal visualization. A low residue diet is recommended for the day preceding the examination and a laxative is given the evening before the examination, unless contraindicated.

Precautions: In addition to the general precautions previously described, infants and small children should not have any fluid restrictions prior to excretory urography. Injections of Iothalamate Salts represent an osmotic load which, if superimposed on increased serum osmolality due to partial dehydration, may magnify hypertonic dehydration. (See *"Warnings"* and *"Precautions, General"* concerning preparatory dehydration).

Adverse Reactions: See section on *"Adverse Reactions, General"*.

Usual Dosage: Adults—The usual dose is 25-50 mL. Children 14 years of age and over, of average weight, may receive the adult dose. The total dose is normally injected within 30-90 seconds. Higher dosage may be indicated to achieve optimum results in instances where poor visualization may be anticipated (e.g., elderly patients or patients with impaired renal function). When nephrograms and/or sequential urograms are desired, the total dose should be rapidly injected, normally within 15-30 seconds.

The dosage for children is reduced in proportion to age and body weight. The following approximate schedule is recommended for infants and children based on a dosage of about 0.5 mL/kg of body weight:

Under 6 months of age	5 mL
6-12 months	8 mL
1-2 years	10 mL
2-5 years	12 mL
5-8 years	15 mL
8-12 years	18 mL
12-14 years	20-30 mL

ANGIOCARDIOGRAPHY

Iothalamate Salts may be administered by injection into an appropriate peripheral vein, or by means of a catheter, directed to the chambers of the heart or associated large blood vessel to be visualized. Injection through a catheter usually provides adequate opacity with a lower dosage because less dilution of the medium takes place. Regardless of the mode of administration, rapid injection is essential. Satisfactory results usually require injection of the total dosage in 1-2 seconds. In most cases, this may be accomplished by manual injection. If indicated, shorter injection times may be obtained with a mechanical injector.

Precautions: In addition to the general precautions previously described, continuous monitoring of ECG and vital signs is recommended during the procedure. When large individual doses are administered, a minimum of 15 minutes between injections is recommended to permit subsidence of any hemodynamic disturbances.

Adult: Caution should be used when injection of this agent is made into the right ventricle or pulmonary artery in patients with pulmonary hypertension or right ventricular failure, since this may result in increased right atrial, right ventricular and pulmonary artery pressure with subsequent bradycardia and systemic hypotension. Patients with chronic pulmonary emphysema present additional risks.

Pediatric: Particular caution is advised in cyanotic infants since apnea, bradycardia, other arrhythmias and a tendency to acidosis are more likely to occur. Infants are more likely to respond with convulsions than are adults. The amount of total dosage in infants is of particular importance. Repeated injections are particularly

hazardous in infants weighing less than 7 kg and the risk is significantly increased if these infants have pre-existing compromised right heart function or obliterated pulmonary vascular beds.

Adverse Reactions: In addition to the adverse reactions previously listed, this procedure has been complicated by intramural injection with marked adverse effects on cardiac function. Hemodynamic changes which occur on injection into the heart chambers can aggravate incipient heart failure and serious arrhythmias, and cardiac arrest may be precipitated.

Usual Dosage: The volume of individual doses should be determined by the size of the structure to be visualized, and in adults, the weight of the patient is only a minor consideration. The anticipated degree of hemodilution at the site of injection and valvular competence should also be taken into consideration.

Adults: Catheter angiocardiography usually requires single doses of 40-50 mL of Iothalamate Salts. Intravenous angiocardiography requires 50-100 mL.

Children: Usual dose is 0.5-1.0 mL/kg for subjects with normal heart size. Minimum dosage should be applied to patients with stenotic lesions or questionable valvular competence.

Infants (2 months old or less): Dosages are the same as those described for children, however, the total dosage administered in any one procedure should be kept below 3 mL/kg.

ARTERIOGRAPHY AORTOGRAPHY

To visualize the aorta and its major branches, Iothalamate Salts may be administered by the arterial or intravenous methods. Iothalamate Salts may be utilized to visualize the aorta and its major branches by any commonly accepted technique. Nephrograms and nephrotomograms may also be obtained subsequent to these procedures when the medium is injected above the level of the renal arteries.

Precautions: In addition to the general precautions previously described, the hazards of aortography include those associated with the particular technique employed, the contrast medium and the underlying pathology which warrants the procedure. There is, therefore, a definite risk. In order to prevent the inadvertent injection of a large dose into a branch of the aorta or intramurally the position of the catheter tip or needle should be carefully evaluated. A small dose of 1-2 mL should be administered to locate the exact site of the needle or catheter tip. Inadvertent direct injection of contrast medium into branchiocephalic vessels may result in significant slowing of heart rate, peripheral hypotension and severe CNS reactions, including convulsions. Toxic effects may also be produced if large quantities of contrast medium are injected directly into aortic branches such as the renal artery, and repetitive injection of the recommended clinical dosage may be hazardous.

Occasional serious neurologic complications, including paraplegia and quadriplegia have been reported and may be attributable to excess doses injected into arterial trunks supplying the spinal arteries or to prolonged contact time of the concentrated contrast medium on the CNS tissue.

Conditions which can contribute to prolonged contact time include decreased circulation, aortic occlusions distal to the site of injection, abdominal compression, hypotension, general anesthesia or the administration of vasopressors. When these conditions exist or occur, the necessity of performing or continuing the procedure should be carefully evaluated and the dose and number of repeat injections should be maintained at a minimum with appropriate intervals between injections.

Severe pain, paresthesia, or peripheral muscle spasm during injection may require discontinuation of the procedure and a re-evaluation of the placement of the catheter tip or needle. When employing the translumbar technique, extreme caution is advised to avoid inadvertent intrathecal injection.

Following catheter procedures, gentle pressure hemostasis is advised, followed by observation and immobilization of the limb for several hours to prevent hemorrhage from the site of arterial puncture.

Adverse Reactions: In addition to the general adverse reactions previously listed, adverse reactions following aortography include injury to the aorta and to neighboring organs, renal damage including infarction and acute tubular necrosis, spinal cord damage resembling transverse myelitis, retroperitoneal hemorrhage, arterial thrombosis, intestinal necrosis and diffuse cutaneous petechiae.

Usual Dosage: Retrograde or antegrade catheter aortography. The usual dose for adults and children over 14 years of age and of average weight is 20-50 mL. The dose for younger children is reduced in proportion to body weight.

Intravenous aortography: For adults and children, the usual dose is 1 mL/kg to a maximum of 80-100 mL per injection. The dose may be divided equally for simultaneous bilateral injection.

Percutaneous translumbar aortography: For adults and children over 14 years of age and of average weight, the usual dose is 15-30 mL. The dose for younger children is reduced in proportion to body weight and size.

CORONARY ARTERIOGRAPHY

Contraindications: In addition to the previously listed contraindications, coronary arteriography should be deferred for a period of four weeks in patients with clinically evident myocardial infarction.

Precautions: In addition to the general precautions previously described, coronary arteriography should only be performed in carefully selected patients when the value of the anticipated information outweighs the risk involved. Mandatory prerequisites to the procedure are experienced personnel, ECG monitoring apparatus, and adequate facilities for immediate resuscitation and cardioversion.

◆ RATED THERAPEUTICALLY EQUIVALENT; ◇ THERAPEUTIC EQUIVALENCE UNCONFIRMED; ○ UNRATED

Adverse Reactions: Most patients will have transient ECG changes during the procedure. Serious cardiac arrhythmias, including bradycardia, ventricular tachycardia, ventricular fibrillation and cardiac arrest have occurred. Other adverse effects include hypotension, shock, anginal pain and myocardial infarction.

Fatalities have been reported. Complications due to the procedure include dissection of coronary arteries, dislodgement of atheromatous plaques, perforation, hemorrhage and thrombosis.

Usual Dosage: Nonselective coronary arteriography: The usual dose for adults is 30-50 mL delivered immediately cephalad to the root of the aorta. One-half the usual dose (15-25 mL) may be injected at the sinus of Valsalva on either side.

Selective coronary arteriography: The usual dose is 4-7 mL injected into either coronary artery. This dose may be injected alternately and repeated.

RENAL ARTERIOGRAPHY
Renal arteriography may be undertaken by aortography or by selective catherization of either renal artery.

Precautions: See "Precautions, General" and "Precautions", specific for "Aortography".

Adverse Reactions: See "Adverse Reactions, General" and "Adverse Reactions", specific for "Aortography".

Usual Dosage: Aortography: For adults and children over 14 years of age and of average weight the usual dose is 10-25 mL delivered above the level of the renal arteries. The dose for younger children is reduced in proportion to body size and weight.

Selective procedures: The usual dose is 4-8 mL injected into either renal artery. The dose may be repeated as indicated.

INTRAVENOUS DIGITAL SUBTRACTION ANGIOGRAPHY
Digital subtraction angiography (DSA) is a radiographic modality which allows dynamic imaging of the arterial system following intravenous injection of iodinated x-ray contrast media through the use of image intensification, enhancement of the iodine signal and digital processing of the image data. Temporal subtraction of the images obtained during the "first arterial pass" of the injected contrast medium from images obtained before and after contrast medium injection yield images which are devoid of bone and soft tissue.

Areas that have been most frequently examined by intravenous DSA are the heart, including coronary by-pass grafts; the pulmonary arteries; the arteries of the brachiocephalic circulation; the aortic arch; the abdominal aorta and its major branches including the celiac, mesenterics and renal arteries; the iliac arteries; and the arteries of the extremities.

Patient Preparation: No special patient preparation is required for DSA. However, it is advisable to insure that patients are well hydrated prior to examination.

Precautions: In addition to the general precautions described, the risks associated with DSA are those usually attendent with catheter procedures and include intramural injections, vessel dissection and tissue extravasation. Small test injections of contrast medium should be made under fluoroscopic observation. This insures that the catheter tip is properly positioned, and in the case of peripheral placement that the vein is of adequate size.

Patient motion, including respiration and swallowing, can result in marked image degradation yielding non-diagnostic studies. Therefore, patient cooperation is essential.

Adverse Reactions: See section on "Adverse Reactions, General".

Usual Dosage: Iothalamate Salts may be injected either centrally, into the superior or inferior vena cava, or peripherally into an appropriate arm vein. For central injections, catheters may be introduced at the antecubital fossa into either the basilic or cephalic vein or at the leg into the femoral vein and advanced to the distal segment of the corresponding vena cava. For peripheral injections, the catheter is introduced at the antecubital fossa into an appropriate size arm vein. In order to reduce the potential for extravasation during peripheral injection, a catheter of approximately 20 cm in length should be employed.

Depending on the area to be imaged, the usual dose range is 20-60 mL. Injections may be repeated as necessary.

Central catheter injections are usually made with a power injector with an injection rate of between 10 and 30 mL/second. When making peripheral injections, rates of 12 to 20 mL/second should be used, depending on the size of the vein. Also, since contrast medium may remain in the arm vein for an extended period following injection, it may be advisable to flush the vein, immediately following injection with an appropriate volume (20-25 mL) of 5% Dextrose in water or normal saline.

CONTRAST ENHANCEMENT OF COMPUTED TOMOGRAPHIC (CT) BRAIN IMAGING
Tumors: Iothalamate Salts may be useful to enhance the demonstration of the presence and extent of certain malignancies such as: gliomas including malignant gliomas, glioblastomas, astrocytomas, oligodendrogliomas and gangliomas; ependymomas; medulloblastomas; meningiomas; neuromas; pinealomas; pituitary adenomas; craniopharyngiomas; germinomas; and metastatic lesions.

The usefulness of contrast enhancement for the investigation of the retrobulbar space and in cases of low grade or infiltrative glioma has not been demonstrated.

In cases where lesions have calcified, there is less likelihood of enhancement. Following therapy, tumors may show decreased or no enhancement.

Non-Neoplastic Conditions: The use of Iothalamate Salts may be beneficial in the image enhancement of non-neoplastic lesions. Cerebral infarctions of recent onset may be better visualized with the contrast enhancement, while some infarctions are obscured if contrast media are used. The use of iodinated contrast media results in contrast enhancement in about 60% of cerebral infarctions studied from one to four weeks from the onset of symptoms.

Sites of active infection may also be enhanced following contrast medium administration.

Arteriovenous malformations and aneurysms will show contrast enhancement. In the case of these vascular lesions, the enhancement is probably dependent on the iodine content of the circulating blood pool.

The opacification of the inferior vermis following contrast medium administration has resulted in false positive diagnoses in a number of normal studies.

Patient Preparation: No special patient preparation is required for contrast enhancement of CT brain scanning. However, it is advisable to insure that patients are well hydrated prior to examination.

Usual Dosage: The usual dose in adults and children is 1.5 mL/kg (0.7 mL/lb) by rapid intravenous administration, not to exceed a total dose of 100 mL. In most cases, scanning may be performed immediately after completion of administration, however, when fast scanning equipment (less than 1 minute) is used consideration should be given to waiting approximately 5 minutes to allow for maximum contrast enhancement.

Storage: Store vials below 30°C (86° F). Exposing this product to very cold temperatures may result in crystallization of the salt. If this occurs the vial should be brought to room temperature. Intermittent shaking may be necessary to completely redissolve the crystals. Before use, examine the product to assure that all solids are redissolved and that the container and closure have not been damaged.

This preparation is sensitive to light and must be protected from strong daylight or direct exposure to the sun.

HOW SUPPLIED
Current prices are unavailable. Check wholesaler for further information.

Ioversol

DESCRIPTION
Ioversol formulations are sterile, nonpyrogenic, aqueous solutions intended for intravascular administration as diagnostic radiopaque media. Ioversol is designated chemically as N,N'-bis (2,3-dihydroxypropyl)-5-[N-(2-hydroxyethyl)-glycolamido]-2,4,6-triiodoisophthalamide.

The molecular weight of Ioversol is 807.13 and the organically bound iodine content is 47.2%. Ioversol is nonionic and does not dissociate in solution.

The pH of the Ioversol formulations has been adjusted to 6.0 to 7.4 with hydrochloric acid or sodium hydroxide. All solutions are sterilized by autoclaving and contain no preservatives. Unused portions should be discarded. Ioversol solutions are sensitive to light and therefore should be protected from exposure.

Some physical and chemical properties of these formulations are listed below:

	Ioversol 160	Ioversol 240	Ioversol 300	Ioversol 320	Ioversol 350
Ioversol content (mg/mL)	339	509	636	678	741
Iodine content (mg I/mL)	160	240	300	320	350
Osmolality (mOsm/kg water)	355	502	651	702	792
Viscosity (cps)					
at 25°C	2.7	4.6	8.2	9.9	14.3
at 37°C	1.9	3.0	5.5	5.8	9.0
Specific Gravity at 37°C	1.188	1.281	1.352	1.371	1.405

The Ioversol formulations are clear, colorless to pale yellow solutions containing no undissolved solids. Crystallization does not occur at room temperature. The products are supplied in containers from which the air has been displaced by nitrogen. Ioversol solutions have osmolalities 1.2 to 2.8 times that of plasma (285 mOsm/kg water) as shown in the above table and are hypertonic under conditions of use.

Following is its chemical structure:

CLINICAL PHARMACOLOGY

The pharmacokinetics of Ioversol intravascularly administered in normal subjects conform to an open two compartment model with first order elimination (a rapid alpha phase for drug distribution and a slower beta phase for drug elimination). Based on the blood clearance curves for 12 healthy volunteers (6 receiving 50 mL and 6 receiving 150 mL of Ioversol 320), the biological half-life was 1.5 hours for both dose levels and there was no evidence of any dose related difference in the rate of elimination.

Ioversol is excreted mainly through the kidneys following intravascular administration. In patients with impaired renal function, the elimination half-life is prolonged. In the absence of renal dysfunction, the mean half-life for urinary excretion following a 50 mL dose was 118 minutes (105-156) and following a 150 mL dose was 105 minutes (74-141). Greater than 95% of the administered dose was excreted within the first 24 hours, with the peak urine concentration occurring in the first 2 hours after administration. Fecal elimination was negligible.

Ioversol does not bind to serum or plasma proteins to any extent and no significant metabolism, deiodination or biotransformation occurs.

Ioversol probably crosses the placental barrier in humans by simple diffusion. It is not known to what extent Ioversol is excreted in human milk.

Intravascular injection of Ioversol opacifies those vessels in the path of the flow of the contrast medium, permitting radiographic visualization of the internal structures until significant hemodilution occurs.

Ioversol may be visualized in the renal parenchyma within 30-60 seconds following rapid intravenous injection. Opacification of the calyces and pelves in patients with normal renal function becomes apparent within 1-3 minutes, with optimum contrast occurring within 5-15 minutes.

Animal studies indicate that Ioversol does not cross the blood-brain barrier or cause endothelial damage to any significant extent.

Ioversol enhances computed tomographic imaging through augmentation of radiographic efficiency. The degree of density enhancement is directly related to the iodine content in an administered dose; peak iodine blood levels occur immediately following rapid intravenous injection. Blood levels fall rapidly within 5 to 10 minutes and the vascular compartment half-life is approximately 20 minutes. This can be accounted for by the dilution in the vascular and extravascular fluid compartments which causes an initial sharp fall in plasma concentration. Equilibrium with the extracellular compartments is reached in about 10 minutes; thereafter, the fall becomes exponential.

The pharmacokinetics of Ioversol in both normal and abnormal tissue have been shown to be variable. Contrast enhancement appears to be greatest immediately after bolus administration (15 seconds to 120 seconds). Thus, greatest enhancement may be detected by a series of consecutive two-to-three second scans performed within 30 to 90 seconds after injection (i.e. dynamic computed tomographic imaging). Utilization of a continuous scanning technique (i.e., dynamic CT scanning) may improve enhancement and diagnostic assessment of tumor and other lesions such as abscess, occasionally revealing unsuspected or more extensive disease. For example, a cyst may be distinguished from a vascularized solid lesion when precontrast and enhanced scans are compared; the nonperfused mass shows unchanged x-ray absorption (CT number). A vascularized lesion is characterized by an increase in CT number in the few minutes after a bolus of intravascular contrast agent; it may be malignant, benign, or normal tissue, but would probably not be a cyst, hematoma, or other nonvascular lesion.

Because unenhanced scanning may provide adequate diagnostic information in the individual patient, the decision to employ contrast enhancement, which may be associated with risk and increased radiation exposure, should be based upon a careful evaluation of clinical, other radiological, and unenhanced CT findings.

CT SCANNING OF THE HEAD

In contrast enhanced computed tomographic head imaging, Ioversol does not accumulate in normal brain tissue due to the presence of the normal blood-brain barrier. The increase in x-ray absorption in normal brain is due to the presence of contrast agent within the blood pool. A break in the blood-brain barrier such as occurs in malignant tumors of the brain allows for the accumulation of contrast medium within the interstitial tissue of the tumor. Adjacent normal brain tissue does not contain the contrast medium.

Maximum contrast enhancement in tissue frequently occurs after peak blood iodine levels are reached. A delay in maximum contrast enhancement can occur. Diagnostic contrast enhanced images of the brain have been obtained up to 1 hour after intravenous bolus administration. This delay suggests that radiographic contrast enhancement is at least in part dependent on the accumulation of iodine containing medium within the lesion and outside the blood pool, although the mechanism by which this occurs is not clear. The radiographic enhancement of nontumoral lesions, such as arteriovenous malformations and aneurysms, is probably dependent on the iodine content of the circulating blood pool.

In patients where the blood-brain barrier is known or suspected to be disrupted, the use of any radiographic contrast medium must be assessed on an individual risk to benefit basis. However, compared to ionic media, nonionic media are less toxic to the central nervous system.

CT SCANNING OF THE BODY

In contrast enhanced computed tomographic body imaging (nonneural tissue), Ioversol diffuses rapidly from the vascular into the extravascular space. Increase in x-ray absorption is related to blood flow, concentration of the contrast medium, and extraction of the contrast medium by interstitial tissue of tumors since no barrier exists. Contrast enhancement is thus due to the relative differences in extravascular diffusion between normal and abnormal tissue, quite different from that in the brain.

INDICATIONS AND USAGE

Ioversal 350 is indicated in adults for coronary arteriography and left ventriculography. Ioversal 350 is also indicated for contrast enhanced computed tomographic imaging of the body, intravenous excretory urography, intravenous digital subtraction angiography and venography. Ioversal 350 is indicated in children for angiocardiography.

Ioversal 320 is indicated in adults for angiography throughout the cardiovascular system. The uses include cerebral, coronary, peripheral, visceral and renal arteriography, aortography, and left ventriculography. Ioversal 320 is also indicated for contrast enhanced computed tomographic imaging of the head and body, and intravenous excretory urography.

Ioversal 320 is indicated in children for angiocardiography, contrast enhanced computed tomographic imaging of the head and body, and intravenous excretory urography.

Ioversal 300 is indicated for cerebral angiography and peripheral arteriography. Ioversal 300 is also indicated for contrast enhanced computed tomographic imaging of the head and body and intravenous excretory urography.

Ioversal 240 is indicated for cerebral angiography and venography. Ioversal 240 is also indicated for contrast enhanced computed tomographic imaging of the head and body and intravenous excretory urography.

Ioversal 160 is indicated for intra-arterial digital subtraction angiography (IA-DSA).

CONTRAINDICATIONS

None.

WARNINGS

Nonionic iodinated contrast media inhibit blood coagulation, in vitro, less than ionic contrast media. Clotting has been reported when blood remains in contact with syringes containing nonionic contrast media.

Serious, rarely fatal, thromboembolic events causing myocardial infarction and stroke have been reported during angiographic procedures with both ionic and non-ionic contrast media. Therefore, meticulous intravascular administration technique is necessary, particularly during angiographic procedures, to minimize thromboembolic events. Numerous factors, including length of procedure, catheter and syringe material, underlying disease state, and concomitant medications may contribute to the development of thromboembolic events. For these reasons, meticulous angiographic techniques are recommended including close attention to guidewire and catheter manipulation, use of manifold systems and/or three-way stopcocks, frequent catheter flushing with heparinized saline solutions and minimizing the length of the procedure. The use of plastic syringes in place of glass syringes has been reported to decrease but not eliminate the likelihood of in vitro clotting.

Serious or fatal reactions have been associated with the administration of iodine-containing radiopaque media. It is of utmost importance to be completely prepared to treat any contrast medium reaction.

As with any contrast medium, serious neurologic sequelae, including permanent paralysis, can occur following cerebral arteriography, selective spinal arteriography and arteriography of vessels supplying the spinal cord. A cause-effect relationship to the contrast medium has not been established since the patients' pre-existing condition and procedural technique are causative factors in themselves. The arterial injection of a contrast medium should never be made following the administration of vasopressors since they strongly potentiate neurologic effects.

Caution must be exercised in patients with severely impaired renal function, combined renal and hepatic disease, severe thyrotoxicosis, myelomatosis, or anuria, particularly when large doses are administered.

Intravascularly administered iodine-containing radiopaque media are potentially hazardous in patients with multiple myeloma or other paraproteinemia, particularly in those with therapeutically resistant anuria. Myeloma occurs most commonly in persons over age 40. Although neither the contrast agent nor dehydration has been proved separately to be the cause of anuria in myelomatous patients, it has been speculated that the combination of both may be causative. The risk in myelomatous patients is not a contraindication to the procedure; however, special precautions, including maintenance of normal hydration and close monitoring, are required. Partial dehydration in the preparation of these patients prior to injection is not recommended since this may predispose the patient to precipitation of the myeloma protein.

Administration of radiopaque materials to patients known or suspected of having pheochromocytoma should be performed with extreme caution. If, in the opinion of the physician, the possible benefits of such procedures outweigh the

---

considered risks, the procedures may be performed; however, the amount of radiopaque medium injected should be kept to an absolute minimum. The blood pressure should be assessed throughout the procedure, and measures for treatment of a hypertensive crisis should be available.

Contrast media may promote sickling in individuals who are homozygous for sickle cell disease when administered intravascularly.

Reports of thyroid storm following the intravascular use of iodinated radiopaque agents in patients with hyperthyroidism or with an autonomously functioning thyroid nodule, suggest that this additional risk be evaluated in such patients before use of any contrast medium.

PRECAUTIONS

GENERAL

Diagnostic procedures which involve the use of iodinated intravascular contrast agents should be carried out under the direction of personnel skilled and experienced in the particular procedure to be performed. A fully equipped emergency cart, or equivalent supplies and equipment, and personnel competent in recognizing and treating adverse reactions of all types should always be available. Since severe delayed reactions have been known to occur, emergency facilities and competent personnel should be available for at least 30 to 60 minutes after administration.

Preparatory dehydration is dangerous and may contribute to acute renal failure in patients with advanced vascular disease, diabetic patients, and in susceptible non-diabetic patients (often elderly with pre-existing renal disease). **Patients should be well hydrated prior to and following the administration of Ioversol.**

The possibility of a reaction, including serious, life-threatening, fatal, anaphylactoid or cardiovascular reactions, should always be considered (See *"Adverse Reactions"*). Increased risk is associated with a history of previous reaction to a contrast medium, a known sensitivity to iodine and known allergies (i.e., bronchial asthma, hay fever and food allergies) or hypersensitivities.

The occurrence of severe idiosyncratic reactions has prompted the use of several pretesting methods. However, pretesting cannot be relied upon to predict severe reactions and may itself be hazardous to the patient. It is suggested that a thorough medical history with emphasis on allergy and hypersensitivity, prior to the injection of any contrast medium, may be more accurate than pretesting in predicting potential adverse reactions. A positive history of allergies or hypersensitivity does not arbitrarily contraindicate the use of a contrast agent when a diagnostic procedure is thought essential, but caution should be exercised. Premedication with antihistamines or corticosteroids to avoid or minimize possible allergic reactions in such patients should be considered. Reports indicate that such pretreatment does not prevent serious life-threatening reactions, but may reduce both their incidence and severity.

General anesthesia may be indicated in the performance of some procedures in selected patients; however, a higher incidence of adverse reactions has been reported in these patients, and may be attributable to the inability of the patient to identify untoward symptoms or to the hypotensive effect of anesthesia which can prolong the circulation time and increase the duration of exposure to the contrast agent.

In angiographic procedures, the possibility of dislodging plaques or damaging or perforating the vessel wall should be considered during catheter manipulations and contrast medium injection. Test injections to insure proper catheter placement are suggested.

Angiography should be avoided whenever possible in patients with homocystinuria because of the risk of inducing thrombosis and embolism.

Patients with congestive heart failure should be observed for several hours following the procedure to detect delayed hemodynamic disturbances which may be associated with a transitory increase in the circulating osmotic load.

Selective coronary arteriography should be performed only in selected patients and those in whom the expected benefits outweigh the procedural risk. The inherent risks of angiocardiography in patients with chronic pulmonary emphysema must be weighed against the necessity for performing this procedure.

Extreme caution during injection of a contrast medium is necessary to avoid extravasation. This is especially important in patients with severe arterial or venous disease.

Information for Patients: Patients receiving iodinated intravascular contrast agents should be instructed to:

1. Inform your physician if you are pregnant.
2. Inform your physician if you are diabetic or if you have multiple myeloma, pheochromocytoma, homozygous sickle cell disease or known thyroid disorder. (See *"Warnings"*).
3. Inform your physician if you are allergic to any drugs or food, or if you had any reactions to previous injections of dyes used for x-ray procedures. (See *"Precautions, General"*).
4. Inform your physician about any other medications you are currently taking including non-prescription drugs.

DRUG INTERACTIONS

Renal toxicity has been reported in a few patients with liver dysfunction who were given oral cholecystographic agents followed by intravascular contrast agents. Administration of any intravascular contrast agent should therefore be postponed in patients who have recently received a cholecystographic contrast agent.

Other drugs should not be mixed with Ioversol injection.

DRUG LABORATORY TEST INTERACTIONS

The results of PBI and radioactive iodine uptake studies, which depend on iodine estimation, will not accurately reflect thyroid function for up to 16 days following administration of iodinated contrast media. However, thyroid function tests not depending on iodine estimations, e.g., T3 resin uptake and total or free thyroxine (T4) assays are not affected.

Carcinogenesis, Mutagenesis, Impairment of Fertility: No long term animal studies have been performed to evaluate carcinogenic potential. However, animal studies suggest that this drug is not mutagenic and does not affect fertility.

Pregnancy Category B: No teratogenic effects attributable to Ioversol have been observed in teratology studies performed in animals. There are, however, no adequate and well controlled studies in pregnant women. It is not known whether Ioversol crosses the placental barrier or reaches fetal tissues. However, many injectable contrast agents cross the placental barrier in humans and appear to enter fetal tissue passively. Because animal teratology studies are not always predictive of human response, this drug should be used during pregnancy only if clearly needed. X-ray procedures involve a certain risk related to the exposure of the fetus.

Nursing Mothers: It is not known whether Ioversol is excreted in human milk. However, many injectable contrast agents are excreted unchanged in human milk. Although it has not been established that serious adverse reactions occur in nursing infants, caution should be exercised when intravascular contrast media are administered to nursing women because of potential adverse reactions, and consideration should be given to temporarily discontinuing nursing.

PEDIATRIC USE

Safety and effectiveness in children have been established for the use of Ioversol 350 and Ioversol 320 in angiocardiography, and for Ioversol 320 in contrast enhanced computed tomographic imaging of the head and body, and intravenous excretory urography.

Safety and effectiveness in newborns have not been established.

ADVERSE REACTIONS

Adverse reactions following the use of Ioversol formulations are usually mild to moderate, of short duration and resolve spontaneously (without treatment). However, serious, life-threatening and fatal reactions, mostly of cardiovascular origin, have been associated with the administration of iodine-containing contrast media.

Injections of contrast media are often associated with sensations of warmth and pain. In controlled double-blind clinical studies, significantly less warmth and pain were associated with the injection of Ioversol than with iothalamate meglumine, diatrizoate meglumine, and diatrizoate meglumine and diatrizoate sodium.

When Ioversol was used for coronary arteriography and ventriculography in double-blind clinical trials, electrocardiographic and hemodynamic changes occurred with less frequency and severity with Ioversol injection than with diatrizoate meglumine and diatrizoate sodium.

Following coronary artery and left ventricular injection, electrocardiographic parameters were affected less with Ioversol Injection than with diatrizoate meglumine and diatrizoate sodium injection. These parameters included the following: bradycardia, tachycardia, T-wave amplitude, ST depression and ST elevation.

Ioversol has also been shown to cause fewer changes in cardiac function and systemic blood pressure than conventional ionic media. These include cardiac output, left ventricular systolic and end-diastolic pressure, right ventricular systolic and pulmonary artery systolic pressures and decreases in systolic and diastolic blood pressures.

The following table of incidence of reactions is based upon clinical trials with Ioversol formulations in 1,954 patients. This listing includes all adverse reactions which were coincidental to the administration of Ioversol regardless of their direct attributability to the drug or the procedure. Adverse reactions are listed by organ system and in decreasing order of occurrence. Significantly more severe reactions are listed before others in a system regardless of frequency.

ADVERSE REACTIONS

System	>1%	≤1%
Cardiovascular	none	angina pectoris
		hypotension
		blood pressure fluctuation
		arterial spasm
		bradycardia
		conduction defect
		false aneurysm
		hypertension
		transient arrhythmia
		vascular trauma
Digestive	none	nausea
		vomiting
Nervous	none	cerebral infarct
		headache
		blurred vision
		vertigo
		light-headedness
		visual hallucination
		vasovagal reaction
		disorientation
		paresthesia
		dysphasia

System	>1%	≤1%
Respiratory	none	muscle spasm syncope laryngeal edema pulmonary edema sneezing nasal congestion coughing shortness of breath hypoxia
Skin	none	periorbital edema urticaria pruritus facial edema flush erythema
Miscellaneous	none	extravasation hematoma shaking chills bad taste general pain renal colic

Regardless of the contrast medium employed, the overall incidence of serious adverse reaction is higher with coronary arteriography than with other procedures. Cardiac decompensation, serious arrhythmias, myocardial ischemia or myocardial infarction may occur during coronary arteriography and left ventriculography.

Pediatrics: In controlled clinical trials involving 159 patients for pediatric angiocardiography, contrast enhanced computed tomographic imaging of the head and body, and intravenous excretory urography, adverse reactions reported were as follows: fever (1.3%), nausea (0.6%), muscle spasm (0.6%), LV pressure changes (0.6%).

GENERAL ADVERSE REACTIONS TO CONTRAST MEDIA
The following adverse reactions are possible with any parenterally administered iodinated contrast medium. Severe life-threatening reactions and fatalities, mostly of cardiovascular origin, have occurred. Most deaths occur during injection or 5 to 10 minutes later; the main feature being cardiac arrest with cardiovascular disease as the main aggravating factor. Isolated reports of hypotensive collapse and shock are found in the literature. Based upon clinical literature, reported deaths from the administration of conventional iodinated contrast agents range from 6.6 per 1 million (0.00066 percent) to 1 in 10,000 patients (0.01 percent).

The reported incidence of adverse reactions to contrast media in patients with a history of allergy is twice that of the general population. Patients with a history of previous reactions to a contrast medium are three times more susceptible than other patients. However, sensitivity to contrast media does not appear to increase with repeated examinations.

Adverse reactions to injectable contrast media fall into two categories: chemotoxic reactions and idiosyncratic reactions.

Chemotoxic reactions result from the physicochemical properties of the contrast medium, the dose and the speed of injection. All hemodynamic disturbances and injuries to organs or vessels perfused by the contrast medium are included in this category.

Idiosyncratic reactions include all other reactions. They occur more frequently in patients 20 to 40 years old. Idiosyncratic reactions may or may not be dependent on the dose injected, the speed of injection, the mode of injection and the radiographic procedure. Idiosyncratic reactions are subdivided into minor, intermediate and severe. The minor reactions are self-limited and of short duration; the severe reactions are life-threatening and treatment is urgent and mandatory.

In addition to the adverse reactions reported for Ioversol, the following additional adverse reactions have been reported with the use of other contrast agents and are possible with any water soluble, iodinated contrast agent.

Nervous: convulsions, aphasia, paralysis, visual field losses which are usually transient but may be permanent, coma and death.

Cardiovascular: angioneurotic edema, peripheral edema, vasodilation, thrombosis and rarely thrombophlebitis, disseminated intravascular coagulation and shock.

Skin: maculopapular rash, erythema, conjunctival symptoms, ecchymosis and tissue necrosis.

Respiratory: choking, dyspnea, wheezing which may be an initial manifestation of more severe and infrequent reactions including asthmatic attack, laryngospasm and bronchospasm, apnea and cyanosis. Rarely these allergic-type reactions can progress into anaphylaxis with loss of consciousness, coma, severe cardiovascular disturbances and death.

Miscellaneous: hyperthermia, temporary anuria or other nephropathy.

Other reactions may also occur with the use of any contrast agent as a consequence of the procedural hazard; these include hemorrhage or pseudoaneurysms at the puncture site, brachial plexus palsy following axillary artery injections, chest pain, myocardial infarction, and transient changes in hepatorenal chemistry tests. Arterial thrombosis, displacement of arterial plaques, venous

thrombosis, dissection of the coronary vessels and transient sinus arrest are rare complications.

(Adverse reactions for specific procedures receive comment in the *"Individual Usage and Procedural Information"* section.)

OVERDOSAGE
The adverse effects of overdosage are life-threatening and effect mainly the pulmonary and cardiovascular system. Treatment of an overdosage is directed toward the support of all vital functions and prompt institution of symptomatic therapy.

Ioversol does not bind to plasma or serum protein and is therefore, dialyzable.

The intravenous LD_{50} values (gI/kg) for Ioversol in animals were: 17 (mice), and 15 (rats).

DOSAGE AND ADMINISTRATION
GENERAL
As with all radiopaque contrast agents, only the lowest dose necessary to obtain adequate visualization should be used. A lower dose may reduce the possibility of an adverse reaction. Most procedures do not require use of either the maximum volume or the highest concentration of Ioversol. The combination of volume and concentration of Ioversol to be used should be carefully individualized accounting for factors such as age, body weight, size of the vessel and the rate of blood flow within the vessel. Other factors such as anticipated pathology, degree and extent of opacification required, structure(s) or area to be examined, disease processes affecting the patient, and equipment and technique to be employed should be considered.

It is desirable that intravascularly administered iodinated contrast agents be at or close to body temperature when injected.

If during administration a reaction occurs, the injection should be stopped until the reaction has subsided.

Patients should be well hydrated prior to and following Ioversol administration.

As with all contrast media, other drugs should not be mixed with Ioversol solutions because of the potential for chemical incompatibility.

Sterile technique must be used in all vascular injections involving contrast media.

If nondisposable equipment is used, scrupulous care should be taken to prevent residual contamination with traces of cleansing agents.

Withdrawal of contrast agents from their containers should be accomplished under strict aseptic conditions using only sterile syringes and transfer devices. Contrast agents which have been transferred into other delivery systems should be used immediately.

Parenteral drug products should be inspected visually for particulate matter and discoloration prior to administration and should not be used if particulates are observed or marked discoloration has occurred.

The Ioversol formulations are supplied in single dose containers. Discard unused portion.

INDIVIDUAL INDICATIONS, USAGE AND PROCEDURAL INFORMATION
GENERAL ANGIOGRAPHY
Visualization of the cardiovascular system may be accomplished by any accepted radiological technique. Since intra-arterial digital subtraction angiography (IA-DSA) requires adjustments in the method of administration, this procedure is described separately.

CEREBRAL ARTERIOGRAPHY
Additional Precautions and Adverse Reactions: Extreme caution is advised in patients with advanced arteriosclerosis, severe hypertension, cardiac decompensation, senility, recent cerebral thrombosis or embolism, and migraine. Cardiovascular reactions that may occur with some frequency are bradycardia and either an increase or decrease in systemic blood pressure. Neurological reactions that may occur are: seizures, drowsiness, transient paresis, and mild disturbances in vision.

Central nervous system reactions with Ioversol in controlled clinical studies in cerebral arteriography that were considered drug-related and occurred with frequencies greater than 1% were: headache, bradycardia, blood pressure fluctuation, disorientation, nausea and vertigo.

Dosage and Administration: Ioversol 240, Ioversol 300 or Ioversol 320 is recommended for this procedure. The usual individual injection for visualization of the carotid or vertebral arteries is 2-12 mL, repeated as necessary. Aortic arch injection for a simultaneous four vessel study requires 20-50 mL. Total procedural doses should not usually exceed 200 mL.

PERIPHERAL ARTERIOGRAPHY
Additional Precautions: Pulsation should be present in the artery to be injected. In thromboangiitis obliterans, or ascending infection associated with severe ischemia, angiography should be performed with extreme caution, if at all.

Dosage and Administration: Ioversol 300 or Ioversol 320 is recommended for this procedure. The usual individual injection volumes for visualization of various peripheral arteries are as follows:

aorto-iliac runoff—60 mL (range 20-90 mL)
common iliac, femoral—40 mL (range 10-50 mL)
subclavian, brachial—20 mL (range 15-30 mL)
These doses may be repeated as necessary. Total procedural doses should not usually exceed 250 mL.

VISCERAL AND RENAL ARTERIOGRAPHY AND AORTOGRAPHY
Additional Precautions and Adverse Effects: In aortography, depending on the technique employed, the risks of this procedure also include the following: injury

to the aorta and neighboring organs, pleural puncture, renal damage including infarction and acute tubular necrosis with oliguria and anuria, retroperitoneal hemorrhage from the translumbar approach and spinal cord injury and pathology associated with the syndrome of transverse myelitis.

Under conditions of slowed aortic circulation there is an increased likelihood for aortography to cause muscle spasm. Occasional serious neurologic complications, including paraplegia, have also been reported in patients with aortoiliac obstruction, femoral artery obstruction, abdominal compression, hypotension, hypertension, spinal anesthesia, and injection of vasopressors to increase contrast. In these patients the concentration, volume, and number of repeat injections of the medium should be maintained at a minimum with appropriate intervals between injections. The position of the patient and catheter tip should be carefully monitored.

Entry of a large aortic dose into the renal artery may cause, even in the absence of symptoms, albuminuria, hematuria, and an elevated creatinine and urea nitrogen. Rapid and complete return of function usually follows.

Dosage and Administration: Ioversol 320 is recommended for this procedure. The usual individual injection volumes for visualization for the aorta and various visceral arteries are as follows:

aorta—45 mL (range 10-80 mL)
celiac—45 mL (range 15-60 mL)
superior mesenteric—45 mL (range 15-60 mL)
renal or inferior mesenteric—9 mL (range 6-15 mL)

These doses may be repeated as necessary. Total procedural doses should not usually exceed 250 mL.

CORONARY ARTERIOGRAPHY AND LEFT VENTRICULOGRAPHY

Additional Precautions: Mandatory prerequisites to the procedure are specialized personnel, ECG monitoring apparatus and adequate facilities for immediate resuscitation and cardioversion. Electrocardiograms and vital signs should be routinely monitored throughout the procedure.

Adverse Reactions: There were no cardiovascular system reactions with Ioversol in controlled clinical studies in coronary arteriography with left ventriculography that were considered drug-related and occurred with a frequency greater than 1%.

Dosage and Administration: Ioversol 320 or Ioversol 350 is recommended for this procedure. The usual individual injection volumes for visualization of the coronary arteries and left ventricle are:

left coronary—8 mL (range 2-10 mL)
right coronary—6 mL (range 1-10 mL)
left ventricle—40 mL (range 30-50 mL)

These doses may be repeated as necessary. Total procedural dose for the combined procedures should not usually exceed 250 mL. When large individual volumes are administered, as in ventriculography and aortography, it has been suggested that several minutes be permitted to elapse between each injection to allow for subsidence of possible hemodynamic disturbances.

PEDIATRIC ANGIOCARDIOGRAPHY

Additional Precautions: Mandatory prerequisites to the procedure are specialized personnel, ECG monitoring apparatus and adequate facilities for immediate resuscitation and cardioversion. Electrocardiograms and vital signs should be routinely monitored throughout the procedure. Pediatric patients at higher risk of experiencing adverse events during contrast medium administration may include those having asthma, a sensitivity to medication and/or allergens, congestive heart failure, a serum creatinine greater than 1.5 mg/dL, or those less than 12 months of age.

Dosage and Administration: Ioversol 350 or Ioversol 320 is recommended for this procedure. The usual single ventricular injection of Ioversol 350 or Ioversol 320 is 1.25 mL/kg of body weight with a range of 1 mL/kg to 1.5 mL/kg. When multiple injections are given, the total administered dose should not exceed 5 mL/kg up to a total volume of 250 mL.

INTRA-ARTERIAL DIGITAL SUBTRACTION ANGIOGRAPHY (IA-DSA)

All of the arteriographic procedures described above can be performed using digital subtraction techniques.

Dosage and Administration: Ioversol 160 is recommended for this procedure. As a general rule, the volume and concentration used for IA-DSA are about 50% or less, of that used for conventional procedures. The actual dosage and flow rate will vary depending on the selectivity of the injection site and the area being examined.

The following suggested volumes per injection are intended only as a guide.

Injections may be repeated as necessary. It is advisable to inject at rates approximately equal to the flow of the vessel being injected.

Carotid Arteries	6-10 mL
Vertebral Arteries	4-8 mL
Aorta	25-50 mL
Subclavian or Brachial Arteries	2-10 mL
Major Branches of the Abdominal Aorta	2-20 mL
Dosage should not usually exceed 250 mL.	

VENOGRAPHY

Additional Precautions: Special care is required when venography is performed in patients with suspected thrombosis, phlebitis, severe ischemic disease, local infection or a totally obstructed venous system. In order to minimize extravasation during injection, fluoroscopy is recommended.

Dosage and Administration: Ioversol 240 or Ioversol 350 is recommended for this procedure. The usual dose is 50-100 mL per extremity with smaller or larger volumes indicated in some cases. Dosage should not usually exceed 250 mL.

Following the procedure, the venous system should be flushed with Sodium Chloride Injection U.S.P. or 5% Dextrose in Water (D5W). Massage and elevation are also helpful for clearing the contrast medium from the extremity.

COMPUTED TOMOGRAPHY

Ioversol 320, Ioversol 300 or Ioversol 240 is recommended for head imaging.

Ioversol 350, Ioversol 320, Iversol 300 or Ioversol 240 is recommended for body imaging.

HEAD IMAGING

Tumors: Ioversol may be useful to investigate the presence and extent of certain malignancies such as: gliomas including malignant gliomas, glioblastomas, astrocytomas, oligodendrogliomas and gangliomas, ependymomas, medulloblastomas, meningiomas, neuromas, pinealomas, pituitary adenomas, craniopharyngiomas, germinomas, and metastatic lesions. The usefulness of contrast enhancement for the investigation of the retrobulbar space and in cases of low grade or infiltrative glioma has not been demonstrated. In calcified lesions, there is less likelihood of enhancement. Following therapy, tumors may show decreased or no enhancement. The opacification of the inferior vermis following contrast media administration has resulted in false-positive diagnosis in a number of otherwise normal studies.

Nonneoplastic Conditions: Ioversol may be beneficial in the image enhancement of nonneoplastic lesions. Cerebral infarctions of recent onset may be better visualized with contrast enhancement, while some infarctions are obscured if contrast medium is used. The use of iodinated contrast media results in enhancement in about 60% of cerebral infarctions studied from one to four weeks from the onset of symptoms.

Sites of active infection may also be enhanced following contrast medium administration.

Arteriovenous malformations and aneurysms will show contrast enhancement. For these vascular lesions the enhancement is probably dependent on the iodine content of the circulating blood pool. Hematomas and intraparenchymal bleeders seldom demonstrate contrast enhancement. However, in cases of intraparenchymal clot, for which there is no obvious clinical explanation, contrast media administration may be helpful in ruling out the possibility of associated arteriovenous malformation.

Dosage and Administration: Adults: For adults, the usual dosage is 50 to 150 mL of Ioversol 320 or Ioversol 300 or 100 to 250 mL of Ioversol 240. Scanning may be performed immediately after completion of the intravenous administration. Dosage should not usually exceed 150 mL of Ioversol 320 or Ioversol 300 or 250 mL of Ioversol 240.

Children: The dosage recommended for use in children is 1 mL/kg to 3 mL/kg of Ioversol 320.

BODY IMAGING

Ioversol may be useful for enhancement of computed tomographic images for detection and evaluation of lesions in the liver, pancreas, kidneys, aorta, mediastinum, pelvis, abdominal cavity, and retroperitoneal space.

Enhancement of computed tomography with Ioversol may be of benefit in establishing diagnoses of certain lesions in these sites with greater assurance than is possible with CT alone. In other cases, the contrast agent may allow visualization of lesions not seen with CT alone (i.e., tumor extension) or may help to define suspicious lesions seen with unenhanced CT (i.e., pancreatic cyst).

Dosage and Administration: Adults: Ioversol 350, Ioversol 320, Ioversol 300 or Ioversol 240 may be administered by bolus injection, by rapid infusion, or by a combination of both. The usual doses are summarized below:

	bolus injection	infusion
Ioversol 350	25-75 mL	50-150 mL
Ioversol 320	25-75 mL	50-150 mL
Ioversol 300	25-75 mL	50-150 mL
Ioversol 240	35-100 mL	70-200 mL

Dosage should not usually exceed 150 mL of Ioversol 350, Ioversol 320 or Ioversol 300 or 250 mL of Ioversol 240.

Children: The dosage recommended for use in children is 1 mL/kg to 3 mL/kg of Ioversol 320, with a usual dose of 2 mL/kg.

INTRAVENOUS DIGITAL SUBTRACTION ANGIOGRAPHY

Intravenous digital subtraction angiography (IV DSA) is a radiographic modality which allows dynamic imaging of the arterial system following intravenous injection of iodinated x-ray contrast media through the use of image intensification, enhancement of the iodine signal and digital processing of the image data. Temporal subtraction of the images obtained prior to and during the "first arterial pass" of the injected contrast medium yields images which are devoid of bone and soft tissue.

IV DSA is most frequently used to examine the heart, including coronary bypass grafts; the pulmonary arteries; arteries of the brachiocephalic circulation; the aortic arch; the abdominal aorta and its major branches; the iliac arteries; and the arteries of the extremities.

PATIENT PREPARATION

No special patient preparation is required for IV DSA. However, it is advisable to insure that patients are well hydrated prior to examination.

PRECAUTIONS

In addition to the general precautions previously described, the risks associated with IV DSA include those usually attendant with catheter procedures and include intramural injections, vessel dissection and tissue extravasation. The potential risk is reduced when small test injections of contrast medium are made under fluoroscopic observation to insure that the catheter tip is properly positioned and, in the case of peripheral placement, that the vein is of adequate size.

Patient motion, including respiration and swallowing, can result in misregistration leading to image degradation and non-diagnostic studies.

USUAL DOSAGE

Ioversol 350 may be injected centrally, in either the superior or inferior vena cava or right artium; or peripherally into an appropriate arm vein. For central injections, catheters may be introduced at the antecubital fossa into either the basilic or cephalic vein or at the leg into the femoral vein and advanced to the distal segment of the corresponding vena cava. For peripheral injections, the catheter is introduced at the antecubital fossa into an appropriate size arm vein. In order to reduce the potential for extravasation during peripheral injection, a catheter of approximately 20 cm in length should be employed.

Depending on the area to be imaged, the usual dose range per injection is 30-50 mL. Injections may be repeated as necessary. The total procedureal dose should not exceed 250 mL.

Injection rates will vary depending on the site of catheter placement and vessel size. Central catheter injections are usually made at a rate of between 10 and 30 mL/second. Peripheral injections are usually made at a rate of between 12 and 20 mL/second. Since the injected medium can sometimes remain in the arm vein for an extended period, it is advisable to flush the vein, immediately following injection with an appropriate volume (20-25 mL) of Sodium Chloride Injection U.S.P. or 5% Dextrose in Water (D5W).

INTRAVENOUS UROGRAPHY

Dosage and Administration: Ioversol 350, Ioversol 320, Ioversol 300 or Ioversol 240 is recommended for routine and high dose excretory urography. Preparatory dehydration is dangerous and may contribute to acute renal failure (see "Precautions, General").

Adults: The usual dose for routine excretory urography in adults is 50-75 mL of Ioversol 350, Ioversol 320 or Ioversol 300 or 75-100 mL of Ioversol 240. Higher dosages may be indicated to achieve optimum results where poor visualization is anticipated (e.g., elderly patients or patients with impaired renal function). In these patients, high dose urography may be preferred, using Ioversol 350 at a dose of 1.4 mL/kg (maximum 140 mL), Ioversol 320 at a dose of 1.5-2 mL/kg (maximum 150 mL), Ioversol 300 at a dose of 1.6 mL/kg (maximum 150 mL) or Ioversol 240 at a dose of 2 mL/kg (maximum 200 mL).

Children: Ioversol 320 at doses of 0.5 mL/kg to 3 mL/kg of body weight has produced diagnostic opacification of the excretory tract. The usual dose for children is 1 mL/kg to 1.5 mL/kg. Dosage for infants and children should be administered in proportion to age and body weight. The total administered dose should not exceed 3 mL/kg.

Storage: Store below 30°C (86°F). These products are sensitive to light and must be protected from strong daylight or direct exposure to the sun. If product is frozen or if crystallization occurs, examine the container for physical damage. If no damage has occurred, the container should be brought to room temperature. Shake vigorously to assure complete dissolution of any crystals. The speed of dissolution may be increased by heating with circulating warm air. Submersion of syringes in water is not recommended. Ioversol may be stored at 37°C for up to one month in a contrast media warmer utilizing circulating warm air. For periods longer than one month, store below 30°C (86°F). Before use, examine the product to assure that all solids are redissolved. Do not reautoclave plastic container because of possible damage to syringe.

As with all contrast media, glass and plastic containers should be inspected prior to use to ensure that breakage or other damage has not occurred during shipping and handling. All containers should be inspected for closure integrity. Damaged containers should not be used.

HOW SUPPLIED
INJECTION: 160 MG/ML

BRAND/MANUFACTURER	NDC	SIZE	AWP
○ **BRAND**			
OPTIRAY-160: Mallinckrodt Med	00019-1325-06	50 ml	$33.00
	00019-1325-11	100 ml	$59.00

INJECTION: 240 MG/ML

BRAND/MANUFACTURER	NDC	SIZE	AWP
○ **BRAND**			
OPTIRAY-240: Mallinckrodt Med	00019-1324-06	50 ml	$38.75
	00019-1324-75	50 ml	$41.00
	00019-1324-11	100 ml	$69.50
	00019-1324-81	125 ml	$98.00
	00019-1324-21	200 ml	$133.00

INJECTION: 300 MG/ML

BRAND/MANUFACTURER	NDC	SIZE	AWP
○ **BRAND**			
OPTIRAY-300: Mallinckrodt Med	00019-1332-83	100 ml 20s	$1920.00

INJECTION: 320 MG/ML

BRAND/MANUFACTURER	NDC	SIZE	AWP
○ **BRAND**			
OPTIRAY-320: Mallinckrodt Med	00019-1323-02	20 ml	$26.25
	00019-1323-04	30 ml	$39.25
	00019-1323-06	50 ml	$43.75
	00019-1323-75	50 ml	$48.00
	00019-1323-77	50 ml	$51.00
	00019-1323-11	100 ml	$87.00
	00019-1323-83	125 ml	$119.50
	00019-1323-16	150 ml	$125.25
	00019-1323-21	200 ml	$165.75

INJECTION: 350 MG/ML

BRAND/MANUFACTURER	NDC	SIZE	AWP
○ **GENERICS**			
OPTIRAY-350: Mallinckrodt Med	00019-1333-40	30 ml	$42.50
OPTIRAY-350: Mallinckrodt Med	00019-1333-73	30 ml	$44.00
OPTIRAY-350: Mallinckrodt Med	00019-1333-06	50 ml	$47.50
OPTIRAY-350: Mallinckrodt Med	00019-1333-75	50 ml	$51.00
OPTIRAY-350: Mallinckrodt Med	00019-1333-77	50 ml	$54.00
OPTIRAY-350: Mallinckrodt Med	00019-1333-41	75 ml	$72.50
OPTIRAY-350: Mallinckrodt Med	00019-1333-11	100 ml	$95.00
OPTIRAY-350: Mallinckrodt Med	00019-1333-83	100 ml	$103.00
OPTIRAY-350: Mallinckrodt Med	00019-1333-81	125 ml	$123.00
OPTIRAY-350: Mallinckrodt Med	00019-1333-16	150 ml	$133.00
OPTIRAY-350: Mallinckrodt Med	00019-1333-21	200 ml	$168.75

Ioxaglate Meglumine and Ioxaglate Sodium

DESCRIPTION

Ioxaglate Meglumine/Ioxaglate Sodium is a sterile, non-pyrogenic, aqueous solution intended for use as a diagnostic radiopaque medium. Ioxaglate Meglumine/Ioxaglate Sodium contains 39.3% w/v N-(2-hydroxyethyl)-2,4,6-triiodo-5-[2-(2,4,6-triiodo-3-(N-methylacetamido)-5-(methylcarbamoyl) benzamido acetamido)-isophthalamic acid, compounded with 1-deoxy-1-(methylamino-D-glucitol (1:1) and 19.6% w/v sodium N-(2-hydroxyethyl)-2,4,6 triiodo-5-[2-(2,4,6-triiodo-3-(N-methylacetamido)-5-(methylcarbamoyl) benzamido acetamido)-isophthalamate.

Each milliliter contains 393 mg of Ioxaglate Meglumine, 196 mg of Ioxaglate Sodium and 0.10 mg edetate calcium disodium as a stabilizer.

Solutions of Ioxaglate Meglumine/Ioxaglate Sodium provide six iodine atoms for each two dissociated ions. Ioxaglate Meglumine/Ioxaglate Sodium is an ionic contrast agent. Ioxaglate Meglumine/Ioxaglate Sodium has an osmolarity of approximately 460 mOsmol/L, an osmolality of approximately 600 mOsmol/kg of water and is, therefore, hypertonic under conditions of use.

Ioxaglate Meglumine/Ioxaglate Sodium has a viscosity (cps) of 15.7 at 20°C and 7.5 at 37°C. The pH has been adjusted to 6.0—7.6 with Meglumine, sodium hydroxide or Ioxaglic acid.

Ioxaglate Meglumine/Ioxaglate Sodium is a clear, colorless to pale yellow solution containing no undissolved solids. Crystallization does not occur at normal room temperatures. It is supplied in containers from which the air has been displaced by nitrogen.

CLINICAL PHARMACOLOGY

Intravascular injection of a radiopaque diagnostic agent opacifies those vessels in the path of the flow of the contrast medium, permitting radiographic visualization of the internal structures of the human body until significant hemodilution occurs.

Following intravascular injection, Ioxaglate Meglumine/Ioxaglate Sodium is rapidly transported through the circulatory system to the kidneys and is excreted unchanged in the urine. The pharmacokinetics of intravascularly administered radiopaque contrast media are usually best described by a two compartment model with a rapid alpha phase for drug distribution and a slower beta phase for drug elimination. In 10 patients with normal renal function, the alpha and beta half-lives of Ioxaglate Meglumine/Ioxaglate Sodium were 12 (4-17) and 92 (61-140) minutes, respectively. Following the intravenous administration of 50 mL of Ioxaglate Meglumine/Ioxaglate Sodium in 10 normal volunteers, the mean peak plasma concentration occurred at two (1-3) minutes, reaching a concentration of 2.1 (1.8-2.8) mg/mL. Approximately 50 (42-67) percent of the intravenously administered dose was recovered in the urine at two hours, and 90 (68-105) percent was recovered at 24 hours.

The joint spaces as well as the uterus and fallopian tubes may be visualized by the direct injection of the contrast medium into the region to be studied.

Injectable iodinated contrast agents are excreted either through the kidneys or through the liver. These two excretory pathways are not mutually exclusive, but the main route of excretion seems to be related to the affinity of the contrast medium for serum albumin. Ioxaglate salts are poorly bound to serum albumin, and are excreted mainly through the kidneys.

The liver and small intestine provide the major alternate route of excretion. In patients with severe renal impairment, the excretion of this contrast medium through the gallbladder and into the small intestine sharply increases.

Ioxaglate salts cross the placental barrier in humans and are excreted unchanged in human milk.

CT SCANNING OF THE HEAD
When used for contrast enhancement in computed tomographic (CT) head imaging, the degree of enhancement is directly related to the amount of iodine administered. Rapid injection of the entire dose yields peak blood iodine concentrations immediately following the injection, which falls rapidly over the next five to ten minutes as a result of dilution in the vascular and extravascular fluid compartments. Equilibration is reached in about ten minutes and thereafter the fall in iodine plasma concentration becomes exponential.

In brain scanning, contrast media do not accumulate in normal brain tissue due to the blood brain barrier (BBB). The increase in x-ray attenuation usually seen in normal tissue following contrast medium injection is due to the presence of the contrast medium in the blood pool. Disruption in the BBB, such as occurs in malignant tumors of the brain, allows accumulation of contrast medium within the interstitial tumor tissue; adjacent normal brain tissue does not contain the contrast medium. Maximum contrast enhancement frequently occurs after peak blood iodine levels are reached. A delay in maximum contrast enhancement can occur depending on the peak iodine level achieved and the cell type of the lesion. This lag in enhancement is probably associated with the accumulation of the contrast medium within the lesion and outside the blood pool.

The image enhancement of non-tumor lesions, such as arteriovenous malformations and aneurysms, is dependent on the iodine content of the circulating blood pool.

CT SCANNING OF THE BODY
Ioxaglate Meglumine/Ioxaglate Sodium may also be used for enhancement of computed tomographic scans performed for detection and evaluation of lesions in the liver, pancreas, kidneys, abdominal aorta, mediastinum, abdominal cavity and retroperitoneal space.

In non-neural tissues (during computed tomography of the body), Ioxaglate Meglumine/Ioxaglate Sodium diffuses rapidly from the vascular to the extravasular space. Increase in x-ray absorption is related to blood flow, concentration of the contrast medium and extraction of the contrast medium by interstitial tissue since no barrier exists; contrast enhancement is thus due to the relative differences in extra-vascular diffusion between normal and abnormal tissue, a situation quite different than that in the brain.

The pharmacokinetics of Ioxaglate Meglumine/Ioxaglate Sodium in normal and abnormal tissues has been shown to be variable.

Enhancement of CT with Ioxaglate Meglumine/Ioxaglate Sodium may be of benefit in establishing diagnoses of certain lesions in some sites with greater assurance than is possible with unenhanced CT and in supplying additional features of the lesions. In other cases, the contrast medium may allow visualization of lesions not seen with CT alone or may help to define suspicious lesions seen with unenhanced CT.

Contrast enhancement appears to be greatest within the 30-90 seconds after bolus administration of the contrast agent, and after intra-arterial rather than intravenous administration. Therefore, the use of a continuous scanning technique (a series of two to three second scans beginning at the injection—dynamic CT scanning) may improve enhancement and diagnostic assessment of tumors and other lesions such as an abscess, occasionally revealing more extensive disease.

Because *unenhanced* scanning may provide adequate information in the individual patient, the decision to employ contrast enhancement, which is associated with additional risk and increased radiation exposure, should be based upon a careful evaluation of clinical, other radiological, and unenhanced CT findings.

INDICATIONS AND USAGE
Ioxaglate Meglumine/Ioxaglate Sodium is indicated for use in pediatric angiocardiography, selective coronary arteriography with or without left ventriculography, peripheral arteriography, aortography, selective visceral arteriography, cerebral angiography, intra-arterial digital subtraction angiography, intravenous digital subtraction angiography, peripheral venography (phlebography), excretory urography, contrast enhancement of computed tomographic head imaging and body imaging, arthrography and hysterosalpingography.

CONTRAINDICATIONS
Ioxaglate Meglumine/Ioxaglate Sodium is contraindicated for use in myelography. Refer to *"Precautions, General,"* concerning hypersensitivity. Hysterosalpingography should not be performed during the menstrual period; in pregnant patients; in patients with known infection in any portion of the genital tract; or in patients in whom cervical conization or curettage has been performed within 30 days. Arthrography should not be performed if infection is present in or near the joint.

WARNINGS
Ionic iodinated contrast media inhibit blood coagulation, *in vitro*, more than nonionic contrast media. Nonetheless, it is prudent to avoid prolonged contact of blood with syringes containing ionic contrast media.

Serious, rarely fatal, thromboembolic events causing myocardial infarction and stroke have been reported during angiographic procedures with both ionic and nonionic contrast media. Therefore, meticulous intravascular administration technique is necessary, particularly during angiographic procedures, to minimize thromboembolic events. Numerous factors, including length of procedure, catheter and syringe material, underlying disease state and concomitant medications may contribute to the development of thromboembolic events. For these reasons, meticulous angiographic techniques are recommended including close attention to guidewire and catheter manipulation, use of manifold systems and/or three-way stopcocks, frequent catheter flushing with heparinized saline solutions and minimizing the length of the procedure. The use of plastic syringes in place of glass syringes has been reported to decrease but not eliminate the likelihood of *in vitro* clotting.

Serious or fatal reactions have been associated with the administration of iodine containing radiopaque media. It is of utmost importance to be completely prepared to treat any contrast medium reaction.

As with any contrast medium, serious neurologic sequelae, including permanent paralysis, can occur following cerebral arteriography, selective spinal arteriography and arteriography of vessels supplying the spinal cord. The injection of a contrast medium should never be made following the administration of vasopressors since they strongly potentiate neurologic effects.

In patients with subarachnoid hemorrhage, a rare association between contrast administration and clinical deterioration, including convulsions and death, has been reported. Therefore, administration of intravascular iodinated contrast media in these patients should be undertaken with caution.

A definite risk exists in the use of intravascular contrast agents in patients who are known to have multiple myeloma. In such instances anuria has developed resulting in progressive uremia, renal failure and eventually death. Although neither the contrast agent nor dehydration has separately proved to be the cause of anuria in myeloma, it has been speculated that the combination of both may be causative factors. The risk in myelomatous patients is not a contraindication to the procedure; however, partial dehydration in the preparation of these patients for the examination is not recommended since this may predispose to precipitation of myeloma protein in the renal tubules. No form of therapy, including dialysis, has been successful in reversing the effect. Myeloma, which occurs most commonly in persons over 40, should be considered before instituting intravascular administration of contrast agents.

Administration of radiopaque materials to patients known or suspected to have pheochromocytoma should be performed with extreme caution. If, in the opinion of the physician, the possible benefits of such procedures outweigh the considered risks, the procedures may be performed; however, the amount of radiopaque medium injected should be kept to an absolute minimum. The blood pressure should be assessed throughout the procedure and measures for treatment of a hypertensive crisis should be available.

Since intravascular administration of contrast media may promote sickling in individuals who are homozygous for sickle cell disease, fluid restriction is not advised.

In patients with advanced renal disease, iodinated contrast media should be used with caution and only when the need for the examination dictates, since excretion of the medium may be impaired. Patients with combined renal and hepatic disease, those with severe hypertension or congestive heart failure and recent renal transplant recipients present an additional risk.

Renal failure has been reported in patients with liver dysfunction who were given an oral cholecystographic agent followed by an intravascular iodinated radiopaque agent and also in patients with occult renal disease, notably diabetics and hypertensives. In these classes of patients there should be no fluid restriction and every attempt made to maintain normal hydration, prior to contrast medium administration, since dehydration is the single most important factor influencing further renal impairment.

Caution should be exercised in performing contrast medium studies in patients with endotoxemia and/or those with elevated body temperatures.

Reports of thyroid storm occurring following the intravascular use of iodinated radiopaque agents in patients with hyperthyroidism or with an autonomously functioning thyroid nodule, suggest that this additional risk be evaluated in such patients before use of this drug. Iodine containing contrast agents may alter the results of thyroid function tests which depend on iodine estimation, e.g., PBI, and may also affect results of radioactive iodine uptake studies. Such tests, if indicated, should be performed prior to the administration of this preparation.

PRECAUTIONS
General: Diagnostic procedures which involve the use of iodinated intravascular contrast agents should be carried out under the direction of personnel skilled and experienced in the particular procedure to be performed. All procedures utilizing contrast media carry a definite risk of producing adverse reactions. While most reactions are minor, life-threatening and fatal reactions may occur without warning, and this risk must be weighed against the benefit of the procedure. A fully equipped emergency cart, or equivalent supplies and equipment, and personnel competent in recognizing and treating adverse reactions of all types should always be available. If a serious reaction should occur, immediately discontinue administration. Since severe delayed reactions have been known to occur, emergency facilities and competent personnel should be available for at least 30 to 60 minutes after administration. (See *"Adverse Reactions, General"*.)

Preparatory dehydration is dangerous and may contribute to acute renal failure in infants, young children, the elderly, patients with pre-existing renal insufficiency, patients with multiple myeloma, patients with advanced vascular disease and diabetic patients.

Acute renal failure has been reported in diabetic patients with diabetic nephropathy and in susceptible nondiabetic patients (often elderly with preexisting renal disease) following the administration of iodinated contrast agents. Therefore, careful consideration of the potential risks should be given before performing this radiographic procedure in these patients.

Severe reactions to contrast media often resemble allergic responses. This has prompted the use of several provocative pretesting methods, none of which can be relied on to predict severe reactions. No conclusive relationship between severe reactions and antigen-antibody reactions or other manifestations of allergy has been established. The possibility of an idiosyncratic reaction in patients who have previously received a contrast medium without ill effect should always be considered. Prior to the injection of any contrast medium, the patient should be questioned to obtain a medical history with emphasis on allergy and hypersensitivity. A positive history of bronchial asthma or allergy (including food), a family history of allergy, or a previous reaction or hypersensitivity to a contrast agent may imply a greater than usual risk. Such a history may be more accurate than pre-testing in predicting the potential for reaction, although not necessarily the severity or type of reaction in the individual case. A positive history of this type does not arbitrarily contraindicate the use of a contrast agent, when a diagnostic procedure is though essential, but does call for caution. (See *"Adverse Reactions, General".*)

Prophylactic therapy including corticosteroids and antihistamines should be considered for patients who present with a strong allergic history, a previous reaction to a contrast medium, or a positive pre-test since in these patients the incidence of reaction is two to three times that of the general population. Adequate doses of corticosteroids should be started early enough prior to contrast medium injection to be effective and should continue through the time of injection and for 24 hours after injection. Antihistamines should be administered within 30 minutes of the contrast medium injection. Recent reports indicate that such pre-treatment does not prevent serious life-threatening reactions, but may reduce both their incidence and severity. A separate syringe should be used for these injections.

General anesthesia may be indicated in the performance of some procedures in selected patients; however, a higher incidence of adverse reactions has been reported in these patients, and may be attributable to the inability of the patient to identify untoward symptoms or to the hypotensive effect of anethesia which can prolong the circulation time and increase the duration of contact of the contrast agent.

Angiography should be avoided whenever possible in patients with homocystinuria because of the risk of inducing thrombosis and embolism.

Information for Patients: Patients receiving iodinated intravascular contrast agents should be instructed to:
1. Inform your physician if you are pregnant.
2. Inform your physician if you are diabetic or if you have multiple myeloma, pheochromocytoma, homozygous sickle cell disease or known thyroid disease. (See *"Warnings"*.)
3. Inform your physician if you are allergic to any drugs, food or if you had any reactions to previous injections of dyes used for x-ray procedures. (See *"Precautions, General".*)
4. Inform your physician about any other medications you are currently taking including nonprescription drugs.

Carcinogenesis, Mutagenesis, Impairment of Fertility: No long-term animal studies have been performed to evaluate carcinogenic potential. However, animal studies suggest that this drug is not mutagenic and does not affect fertility in males or females.

Pregnancy Category B: Reproduction studies have been performed in rats and rabbits at doses up to two times the maximum adult human dose and have revealed no evidence of impaired fertility or harm to the fetus due to Ioxaglate Meglumine/Ioxaglate Sodium. There are, however, no adequate and well controlled studies in pregnant women. Because animal reproduction studies are not always predictive of human response, this drug should be used during pregnancy only if clearly needed.

Nursing Mothers: Ioxaglate salts are excreted unchanged in human milk. Because of the potential for adverse effects in nursing infants, bottle feedings should be substituted for breast feedings for 24 hours following the administration of this drug.

Pediatric Use: Safety and effectiveness in children have been established in pediatric angiocardiography and intravenous excretory urography. Data have not been submitted to support the safety and effectiveness of Ioxaglate Meglumine/ Ioxaglate Sodium in any other indication.

(Precautions for specific procedures receive comment under that procedure.)

ADVERSE REACTIONS

General: Adverse reactions to injectable contrast media fall into two categories: chemotoxic reactions and idiosyncratic reactions.

Chemotoxic reactions result from the physio-chemical properties of the contrast media, the dose and the speed of injection. All hemodynamic disturbances and injuries to organs or vessels perfused by the contrast medium are included in this category.

Idiosyncratic reactions include all other reactions. They occur more frequently in patients 20 to 40 years old. Idiosyncratic reactions may or may not be dependent on the dose injected, the speed of injection, the mode of injection and the radiographic procedure. Idiosyncratic reactions are subdivided into minor, intermediate and severe. The minor reactions are self-limited and of short duration; the severe reactions are life-threatening and treatment is urgent and mandatory.

Note: Not all of the following adverse reactions have been reported with Ioxaglate Meglumine/Ioxaglate Sodium. Because Ioxaglate Meglumine/Ioxaglate Sodium is an iodinated intravascular contrast agent, all of the side effects and toxicity associated with agents of this class are theoretically possible, and this should be borne in mind when Ioxaglate Meglumine/Ioxaglate Sodium is administered.

Severe, life-threatening anaphylactoid reactions, mostly of cardiovascular origin, have occurred following the administration of Ioxaglate Meglumine/ Ioxaglate Sodium as well as other iodine-containing contrast agents. Most deaths occur during injection or 5 to 10 minutes later; the main feature being cardiac arrest with cardiovascular disease as the main aggravating factor. Isolated reports of hypotensive collapse and shock are found in the literature. Based upon clinical literature, reported deaths from the administration of conventional iodinated contrast agents range from 6.6 per 1 million (0.00066 percent) to 1 in 10,000 patients (0.01 percent).

Regardless of the contrast agent employed, the overall estimated incidence of serious adverse reactions is higher with coronary arteriography than with other procedures. Cardiac decompensation, serious arrhythmias, or myocardial ischemia or infarction may occur during coronary arteriography and left ventriculography.

The most frequent adverse reactions are nausea, vomiting, facial flush and a feeling of body warmth. These are usually of brief duration. In double-blind clinical trials, Ioxaglate Meglumine/Ioxaglate Sodium produced less discomfort upon injection (pain and heat) when compared to various other contrast agents. Other reactions include the following:

Hypersensitivity Reactions: Dermal manifestations of urticaria with or without pruritus, erythema and maculopapular rash. Dry mouth. Sweating. Conjunctival symptoms. Facial, peripheral and angioneurotic edema. Symptoms related to the respiratory system include sneezing, nasal stuffiness, coughing, choking, dyspnea, chest tightness and wheezing, which may be initial manifestations of more severe and infrequent reactions including asthmatic attack, laryngospasm and bronchospasm with or without edema, pulmonary edema, apnea and cyanosis. Rarely, these allergic-type reactions can progress into anaphylaxis with loss of consciousness, coma, severe cardiovascular disturbances, and death.

Cardiovascular Reactions: Generalized vasodilation, flushing and venospasm. Occasionally, thrombosis or rarely, thrombophlebitis. Extremely rare cases of disseminated intravascular coagulation resulting in death have been reported. Severe cardiovascular responses include rare cases of hypotensive shock, coronary insufficiency, cardiac arrhythmia, fibrillation and arrest. These severe reactions are usually reversible with prompt and appropriate management; however, fatalities have occurred.

Technique Reactions: Extravasation with burning pain, hematomas, ecchymosis and tissue necrosis, vascular constriction due to injection rate, thrombosis and thrombophlebitis.

Neurological Reactions: Spasm, convulsions, aphasia, syncope, paresis, paralysis resulting from spinal cord injury and pathology associated with the syndrome of transverse myelitis, visual field losses which are usually transient but may be permanent, coma and death.

Other Reactions: Headache, trembling, shaking, chills without fever, hyperthermia and light-headedness. Temporary renal shutdown or other nephropathy.

(Adverse reactions to specific procedures receive comment under that procedure.)

OVERDOSAGE

Overdosage may occur. The adverse effects of overdosage are life-threatening and affect mainly the pulmonary and cardiovascular systems. The symptoms may include cyanosis, bradycardia, acidosis, pulmonary hemorrhage, convulsions, coma and cardiac arrest. Treatment of an overdose is directed toward the support of all vital functions and prompt institution of symptomatic therapy.

Ioxaglate salts are dialyzable.

The intravenous LD_{50} values of Ioxaglate Meglumine/Ioxaglate Sodium (in grams of iodine/kilogram body weight) were 11.2 g/kg in mice, > 8 g/kg in rats, > 6.4 g/kg in rabbits and > 10.2 g/kg in dogs.

DOSAGE AND ADMINISTRATION

It is advisable that Ioxaglate Meglumine/Ioxaglate Sodium be at or close to body temperature when injected.

The patient should be instructed to omit the meal that precedes the examination. Appropriate premedication, which may include a barbiturate, tranquilizer or analgesic drug, may be administered prior to the examination.

A preliminary film is recommended to check the position of the patient and the x-ray exposure factors prior to the injection of the contrast medium.

If during administration a minor reaction occurs, the injection should be slowed or stopped until the reaction has subsided. If a major reaction occurs, the injection should be discontinued immediately.

Under no circumstances should other drugs be administered concomitantly in the same syringe or IV administration set because of a potential for chemical incompatibility.

Parenteral drug products should be inspected visually for particulate matter and discoloration prior to administration.

PEDIATRIC ANGIOCARDIOGRAPHY

Ioxaglate Meglumine/Ioxaglate Sodium may be administered by catheter injection into the chambers of the heart or associated large blood vessels. Rapid injection is essential and satisfactory results usually require injection of the total dosage in 1-2 seconds.

◆ RATED THERAPEUTICALLY EQUIVALENT; ◇ THERAPEUTIC EQUIVALENCE UNCONFIRMED; ○ UNRATED

PRECAUTIONS

In addition to the general precautions previously described, it is advisable to monitor for ECG and vital signs changes throughout the procedure.

When large individual doses are administered sufficient time should be allowed for any observed changes to return to or near baseline prior to making the next injection.

Caution should be used when making right heart injections in patients with pulmonary hypertension or incipient heart failure since this may lead to increased right side pressures with subsequent bradycardia and systemic hypotension. Patients with pulmonary disease present additional risks.

Caution is advised in cyanotic infants since apnea, bradycardia, other arrhythmias and a tendency to acidosis are more likely to occur.

Since infants are more likely to respond with convulsions than are adults, the amount of total dosage is of particular importance. Repeated injections are hazardous in infants weighing less than 7 kg, particularly when these infants have pre-existing compromised right heart function or obliterated pulmonary vascular beds.

ADVERSE REACTIONS

In addition to the adverse reactions previously listed, this procedure has been complicated by intramural injection with marked adverse effects on cardiac function.

USUAL DOSAGE

The volume of individual doses should be determined by the size of the structure to be visualized and the anticipated degree of hemodilution at the site of injection. Valvular competence should also be taken into consideration.

Older Children: Catheter angiocardiography usually requires single doses of 30-45 mL of Ioxaglate Meglumine/Ioxaglate Sodium.

Infants and Young Children: The recommended single dose of Ioxaglate Meglumine/Ioxaglate Sodium is about 1.5 mL/kg (range 1 mL/kg to 2 mL/kg). In addition, small test volumes of about 2 mL may be used for catheter placement.

The usual total dose of Ioxaglate Meglumine/Ioxaglate Sodium per procedure, which includes diagnostic and test doses is about 4 mL/kg. This dosage may be as small as 1.5 mL/kg and should not normally exceed 5 mL/kg.

SELECTIVE CORONARY ARTERIOGRAPHY WITH OR WITHOUT LEFT VENTRICULOGRAPHY

PRECAUTIONS

During the administration of large doses of Ioxaglate Meglumine/Ioxaglate Sodium continuous monitoring of vital signs is desirable. Caution is advised in the administration of large volumes to patients with incipient heart failure because of the possibility of aggravating the pre-existing condition. Hypotension should be corrected promptly since it may result in serious arrhythmias.

Special care regarding dosage should be observed in patients with right ventricular failure, pulmonary hypertension, or stenotic pulmonary vascular beds because of hemodynamic changes which may occur after injection into the right heart outflow tract.

ADVERSE REACTION

Patients may have clinically insignificant ECG changes during the procedure. The following adverse effects have occurred in conjunction with the administration of iodinated intravascular contrast agents for this procedure: hypotension, shock, anginal pain, myocardial infarction, cardiac arrhythmias (bradycardia, ventricular tachycardia, ventricular fibrillation) and cardiac arrest. Fatalities have been reported.

Complications to the procedure include dissection of coronary arteries, dislodgement of atheromatous plaques, perforation, hemorrhage and thrombosis.

USUAL DOSAGE

The usual adult dose for left coronary arteriography is 8 mL (range 2-14 mL) and for right coronary arteriography is 5 mL (range 1-10 mL). The doses may be repeated as necessary; doses up to a total of 150 mL have been given. For left ventriculography, the usual adult dose in a single injection is 45 mL (range 35-45 mL) and repeated as necessary. The total dose for combined selective coronary arteriography and left ventriculography should not exceed 250 mL.

PERIPHERAL ARTERIOGRAPHY

Ioxaglate Meglumine/Ioxaglate Sodium may be injected to visualize the peripheral arterial circulation. Arteriograms of the upper and lower extremities may be obtained by any of the established techniques.

PATIENT PREPARATION

The procedure is normally performed with local anesthesia. Rarely, general anesthesia may be required. (See *"Precautions, General."*)

A preliminary radiograph is usually made prior to the injection of the contrast agent.

PRECAUTIONS

In addition to the general precautions previously described, moderate decreases in blood pressure occur frequently with intra-arterial (brachial) injections. This change is usually transient and requires no treatment; however, the blood pressure should be monitored for approximately ten minutes following injection.

Extreme caution during injection of the contrast agent is necessary to avoid extravasation and fluoroscopy is recommended. This is especially important in patients with severe arterial disease.

ADVERSE REACTIONS

In addition to the general adverse reactions previously described, hemorrhage and thrombosis have occurred at the puncture site of the percutaneous injection. Brachial plexus injury has been reported following axillary artery injection.

USUAL DOSAGE

The single adult dose for aorto-iliac runoff studies is 45 mL (range 20-80 mL). The single adult dose for the common iliac, the external iliac and the femoral arteries is 30 mL (range 10-50 mL). These doses may be repeated as necessary. For the upper limb, the usual single adult dose is 20 mL (range 15-30 mL), repeated as necessary. The total procedural dose should not exceed 250 mL.

AORTOGRAPHY AND SELECTIVE VISCERAL ARTERIOGRAPHY

Ioxaglate Meglumine/Ioxaglate Sodium may be used to visualize the aorta and its major abdominal branches.

USUAL DOSAGE

The usual dose for injections into the aorta is 25 to 50 mL; the celiac artery is 40 mL; the superior mesenteric artery is 20 to 40 mL; the inferior mesenteric artery is 8 to 15 mL. These doses may be repeated as necessary. The total dose should not exceed 250 mL.

CEREBRAL ANGIOGRAPHY

Ioxaglate Meglumine/Ioxaglate Sodium may be used to visualize the cerebral vasculature by any of the accepted techniques.

PATIENT PREPARATION

Cerebral angiography is normally performed with local or general anesthesia. (See *"Precautions, General."*)

PRECAUTIONS

In addition to the general precautions previously described, cerebral angiography should be performed with special caution in patients with advanced arteriosclerosis, severe hypertension, cardiac decompensation, senility, recent cerebral thrombosis or embolism, and migraine.

ADVERSE REACTIONS

The major causes of cerebral arteriographic adverse reactions appear to be repeated injections of the contrast material, administration of doses higher than those recommended, the presence of occlusive atherosclerotic vascular disease and the method and technique of injection.

Adverse reactions are normally mild and transient. A feeling of warmth in the face and neck is frequently experienced. Infrequently, a more severe buring discomfort is observed. Transient visual hallucinations have been reported.

Serious neurological reactions that have been associated with cerebral angiography and not listed under *"Adverse Reactions, General,"* including stroke, amnesia and respiratory difficulties.

Visual field defects with anopsia and reversible neurological deficit lasting from 24 hours to 48 hours have been reported. Confusion, disorientation with hallucination, and absence of vision sometimes lasting for one week have also been reported.

Cardiovascular reactions that may occur with some frequency are bradycardia and either an increase or decrease in systemic blood pressure. The blood pressure change is transient and usually requires no treatment.

USUAL DOSAGE

The usual dosage employed varies with the site and method of injection and the age and condition of the patient. In adults, cerebral angiography is usually performed by a selective injection of 9 mL (range 6-12 mL) for the common carotid arteries and 8 mL (range 5-12 mL) for the vertebral arteries. Additional injections may be made as indicated. When aortic arch injections (four vessel studies) are performed in conjunction with cerebral angiography, the usual dose is 40 mL (range 30-50 mL). Other dosages may be employed for more selective injections, depending upon the vessel injected. The total dose per procedure should not exceed 150 mL.

INTRA-ARTERIAL DIGITAL SUBTRACTION ANGIOGRAPHY (IA-DSA)

Intra-arterial digital subtraction angiography (IA-DSA) is a radiographic modality which produces arterial images similar to conventional film-screen systems following arterial injection. The advantages include: the use of less contrast medium; the use of lower iodine concentrations; a decreased need for selective arterial catheterization; and a shortened examination time.

PATIENT PREPARATION

No special patient preparation is required for IA-DSA. However, it is advisable to insure that patients are well hydrated prior to examination.

PRECAUTIONS

In addition to the general precautions described, the risks associated with IA-DSA are those usually attendant with catheter procedures. Following the procedure, gentle pressure hemostasis is required, followed by observation and immobilization of the limb for several hours to prevent hemorrhage from the site of arterial puncture.

Patient motion, including respiration and swallowing, can result in misregistration leading to image degradation and non-diagnostic studies.

USUAL DOSAGE

As a general rule, the volume and concentration used for IA-DSA are about 50%, or less, of that used for conventional procedures. The actual dosage and flow rate will vary depending on the selectivity of the injection site and the area being examined.

The most versatile concentration of Ioxaglate Meglumine/Ioxaglate Sodium is a 1:1 dilution with Sterile Water for Injection, U.S.P. This dilution provides 16% iodine and is isotonic.

The following suggested volumes per injection are intended only as a guide. Injections may be repeated as necessary. It is advisable to inject at rates approximately equal to the flow rate of the vessel being injected.

Carotid Arteries	6-10 mL
Vertebral Arteries	4-8 mL
Aorta	25-50 mL
Subclavian or Brachial Arteries	2-10 mL
Major Branches of the Abdominal Aorta	2-20 mL

INTRAVENOUS DIGITAL SUBTRACTION ANGIOGRAPHY
Intravenous digital subtraction angiography (IV DSA) is a radiographic modality which allows dynamic imaging of the arterial system following intravenous injection of iodinated x-ray contrast media through the use of image intensification, enhancement of the iodine signal and digital processing of the image data. Temporal subtraction of the images obtained prior to and during the "first arterial pass" of the injected contrast medium yields images which are devoid of bone and soft tissue.

IV DSA is most frequently used to examine the heart, including coronary by-pass grafts; the pulmonary arteries; arteries of the brachiocephalic circulation; the aortic arch; the thoracic aorta and its major branches; the iliac arteries; and the arteries of the extremities.

PATIENT PREPARATION
No special patient preparation is required for IV DSA. However, it is advisable to insure that patients are well hydrated prior to examination.

PRECAUTIONS
In addition to the general precautions previously described, the risks associated with IV DSA include those usually attendant with catheter procedures and include intramural injections, vessel dissection and tissue extravasation. The potential risk is reduced when small test injections of contrast medium are made under fluoroscopic observation to insure that the catheter tip is properly positioned and, in the case of peripheral placement, that the vein is of adequate size.

Patient motion, including respiration and swallowing, can result in misregistration leading to image degradation and non-diagnostic studies.

USUAL DOSAGE
Ioxaglate Meglumine/Ioxaglate Sodium may be injected centrally, in either the superior or inferior vena cava or right atrium; or peripherally into an appropriate arm vein. For central injections, catheters may be introduced at the antecubital fossa into either the basilic or cephalic vein or at the leg into the femoral vein and advanced to the distal segment of the corresponding vena cava. For peripheral injections, the catheter is introduced at the antecubital fossa into an appropriate size arm vein. In order to reduce the potential for extravasation during peripheral injection, a catheter of approximately 20 cm in length should be employed.

Depending on the area to be imaged, the usual dose range per injection is 30-50 mL. Injections may be repeated as necessary. The total procedural dose should not exceed 250 mL.

Injection rates will vary depending on the site of catheter placement and vessel size. Central catheter injections are usually made at a rate of between 10 and 30 mL/second. Peripheral injections are usually made at a rate of between 12 and 20 mL/second. Since the injected medium can sometimes remain in the arm vein for an extended period, it may be advisable to flush the vein, immediately following injection with an appropriate volume (20-25 mL) of 5% Dextrose in water or normal saline.

PERIPHERAL VENOGRAPHY (PHLEBOGRAPHY)
Ioxaglate Meglumine/Ioxaglate Sodium may be injected to visualize the peripheral venous circulation. Venograms are obtained by injection or infusion into an appropriate vein in the upper or lower extremity. Post-venography thrombophlebitis, as detected by fibrinogen I-125 uptake studies, is significantly less in patients receiving Ioxaglate Meglumine/Ioxaglate Sodium when compared to conventional contrast agents.

PRECAUTIONS
In addition to the general precautions previously described, special care is required when venography is performed in patients with suspected thrombosis, phlebitis, severe ischemic disease, local infection or a totally obstructed venous system.

Extreme caution during injection of contrast media is necessary to avoid extravasation and fluoroscopy is recommended. This is especially important in patients with severe arterial or venous disease.

USUAL DOSAGE
The dose for adults will usually range from 50-100 mL per extremity of full strength (32% iodine) Ioxaglate Meglumine/Ioxaglate Sodium as a single rapid injection. The dosage will vary according to the patient's size and condition and

the technique employed. Smaller or larger volumes may be indicated in some cases.

Reduced concentrations to as low as 20% w/v iodine may be effectively employed. These dilute solutions may be prepared by addition of normal saline (Sodium Chloride Injection, U.S.P.), 5% Dextrose in water (D5W) or Water for Injection, U.S.P. To prepare a 20% w/v solution, dilute each milliliter of Ioxaglate Meglumine/Ioxaglate Sodium with 0.6 milliliters of the diluent selected (e.g., 50 mL Ioxaglate Meglumine/Ioxaglate Sodium plus 30 mL of diluent equals 80 mL of a 20% iodine concentration). The usual dose of dilute medium will range from 75-150 mL per extremity.

Following the procedure, the venous system should be flushed with any one of the diluents listed above. Massage and elevation are also helpful for clearing the contrast medium from the extremity.

EXCRETORY UROGRAPHY
Following intravenous injection, Ioxaglate Meglumine/Ioxaglate Sodium is rapidly excreted by the kidneys. Ioxaglate Meglumine/Ioxaglate Sodium may be visualized in the renal parenchyma one minute following bolus injection. Maximum radiographic density in the calyces and pelves occurs in most instances within 7 to 12 minutes after injection. In patients with severe renal impairment, contrast visualization may be substantially delayed.

PATIENT PREPARATION
A low residue diet the day preceding the examination and a laxative the evening before the examination may be given, unless contraindicated.

PRECAUTIONS
Infants and small children should not have any fluid restrictions prior to excretory urography. (See "Warnings" and "Precautions, General" concerning preparatory dehydration.)

USUAL DOSAGE
Adults—The usual adult dose is 50 to 75 mL (0.7 to 1.0 mL/kg). The total dose is normally injected within 30 to 90 seconds. A higher dosage may be indicated where poor visualization is anticipated (e.g., elderly patients, obese patients, patients with impaired renal function or patients in whom dense opacification of the pelvo-calyceal system and ureters is desired). In these patients, a dose of 100 to 150 mL (1.5 to 2.0 mL/kg) may be used.

Children—The following schedule is recommended for infants and children.

Under 6 months of age	3 mL/kg
Over 6 months of age	2 mL/kg

The total dosage in children should not exceed 5 mL/kg.

CONTRAST ENHANCEMENT OF COMPUTED TOMOGRAPHIC (CT)
HEAD IMAGING
Ioxaglate Meglumine/Ioxaglate Sodium may be useful to enhance the presence and better define the extent of primary and metastatic malignancies of the head. In cases where lesions have calcified, there is less likelihood of enhancement. Following therapy, tumors may show decreased or no enhancement.

The use of Ioxaglate Meglumine/Ioxaglate Sodium may also be beneficial in the image enhancement of non-neoplastic lesions, such as cerebral infarcts, sites of active infection, arteriovenous malformations and aneurysms.

The opacification of the inferior vermis occurs occasionally in normal studies.

PATIENT PREPARATION
No special preparation is required; however, it is advisable to insure that patients are well hydrated prior to examination.

USUAL DOSAGE
For adults weighing up to 150 pounds, the usual dosage is 0.9 mL/lb. Patients weighing more than 150 pounds can usually undergo satisfactory examination with a dose of 135 mL not to exceed 150 mL.

CONTRAST ENHANCEMENT IN BODY COMPUTED TOMOGRAPHY
PATIENT PREPARATION
No special patient preparation is required. However, it is advisable to insure that patients are well hydrated. In patients undergoing abdominal or pelvic examination, opacification of the bowel may be valuable in scan interpretation.

PRECAUTIONS
In addition to the general precautions described, patient cooperation is essential since patient motion, including respiration, can markedly affect image quality. The use of an intravascular contrast medium can obscure tumors in patients undergoing CT evaluation of the liver resulting in a false negative diagnosis. Dynamic CT scanning is the procedure of choice for malignant tumor enhancement. (See "Clinical Pharmacology.")

USUAL DOSAGE
Ioxaglate Meglumine/Ioxaglate Sodium may be administered by bolus injection, rapid infusion or by a combination of both. Depending on the area to be examined, doses of 30-150 mL (0.4-0.9 mL/lb) may be administered. When prolonged enhancement is required up to 150 mL can be used, usually with 25-50 mL as a rapid bolus and the remainder as an infusion.

ARTHROGRAPHY
Due to the low osmolality of Ioxaglate Meglumine/Ioxaglate Sodium the concomitant use of epinephrine is not necessary since the rate of contrast medium

---

◆ RATED THERAPEUTICALLY EQUIVALENT; ◇ THERAPEUTIC EQUIVALENCE UNCONFIRMED; ○ UNRATED

absorption as well as the production of synovial fluid and consequent dilution of the medium are reduced.

PRECAUTIONS
In addition to the general precautions previously described, strict aseptic technique is required to prevent the introduction of infection. Fluoroscopic control should be used to insure proper introduction of the needle into the synovial space and prevent extracapsular injection. Aspiration of excessive synovial fluid will reduce the pain on injection and prevent the dilution of the contrast agent. It is important that undue pressure not be exerted during the injection.

ADVERSE REACTIONS
In addition to the general adverse reactions previously described, arthrography may induce joint pain or discomfort which is usually mild and transient but occasionally may be severe and persist for 24 to 48 hours following the procedure. Effusion requiring aspiration may occur in patients with rheumatoid arthritis.

USUAL DOSAGE
Arthrography is usually performed under local anesthesia. The amount of contrast agent required is solely dependent on the size of the joint to be injected and the technique employed.

The following dosage schedule for normal adult joints should serve only as a guide since joints may require more or less contrast medium for optimal visualization.

Knee, hip	5-15 mL
Shoulder, ankle	5-20 mL
Temporomandibular	0.5-0.7 mL

Passive or active manipulation is used to disperse the medium throughout the joint space.

The lower volumes of contrast medium are usually employed for double contrast examinations in which 30-100 cc of either filtered room air or carbon dioxide may be introduced for examination of the knee and lesser volumes for other joints.

HYSTEROSALPINGOGRAPHY

PATIENT PREPARATION
It is preferable to perform the procedure approximately eight to ten days after the onset of menses. The patient should empty the bladder before the examination.

PRECAUTIONS
Caution should be exercised in patients suspected of having cervical or tubal carcinoma to avoid possible spread of the lesion by the procedure. Delayed onset of pain and fever (1-2 days) may be indicative of pelvic infection.

ADVERSE REACTIONS
In addition to the general adverse reactions described previously, fever and pain, cramping and tenderness of the abdomen have been reported.

USUAL DOSAGE
The total volume administered will vary depending upon anatomical variations and/or disease processes. The usual dose varies from 5 to 15 mL, administered slowly under fluoroscopic control, without undue pressure.

Storage: Store below 30°C (86°F). Do not freeze. If product is frozen or if crystallization of the salt has occurred, examine the container for physical damage. If no damage has occurred, the container should be brought to room temperature. Shake vigorously to assure complete dissolution of any crystals. The speed of dissolution may be increased by heating with circulating warm air. Submersion of syringes in water is not recommended. Before use, examine the product to assure that all solids are redissolved and that the container and closure have not been damaged.

This preparation is sensitive to light and must be protected from strong daylight or direct exposure to the sun.

Do not reautoclave plastic container because of possible damage to syringe.

As with all contrast media, glass and plastic containers should be inspected prior to use to ensure that breakage or other damage has not occurred during shipping and handling. All containers should be inspected for closure integrity. Damaged containers should not be used.

HOW SUPPLIED
INJECTION:

BRAND/MANUFACTURER	NDC	SIZE	AWP
○ **BRAND**			
HEXABRIX: Mallinckrodt Med	00019-5505-04	30 ml	$36.50
	00019-5505-06	50 ml	$53.50
	00019-5505-41	75 ml	$79.95
	00019-5505-08	100 ml	$105.60
	00019-5505-81	125 ml	$123.00
	00019-5505-10	150 ml	$149.50
	00019-5505-21	200 ml	$197.95

Ipodate

DESCRIPTION
Ipodate Calcium and Ipodate Sodium are oral radiopaque media for cholangiography and cholecystography.

Ipodate Calcium is available in foil packets providing 3 g Ipodate calcium.

Ipodate Sodium is available in capsules providing 500 mg iopodate sodium per capsule.

The organically bound iodine content of Ipodate Calcium and Ipodate Sodium is 61.7% (approximately 1.85 g/packet) and 61.4% (approximately 307 mg/capsule), respectively.

Following is its chemical structure:

CLINICAL PHARMACOLOGY
Ipodate Calcium and Ipodate Sodium are absorbed from the gastrointestinal tract, excreted by the liver into the bile, and stored and concentrated in the gallbladder. The calcium salt, which is absorbed somewhat faster than the sodium salt, appears in the ducts as early as 30 minutes after ingestion. Optimal concentration of either salt in the hepatic and biliary ducts occurs within one to three hours after ingestion in nearly all cases; rarely, maximal opacification may be delayed for as much as five hours. Adequate opacification of the ducts usually persists for about 45 minutes. The ducts may be visualized in patients who have undergone cholecystectomy.

The gallbladder is optimally opacified approximately 10 hours after ingestion of either salt. Diagnostically adequate filling, however, often takes place within five hours or less after ingestion, particularly with the calcium salt. Thus, studies of ducts and gallbladder may be carried out in as little as five hours when necessary or desirable. In this connection, it should be pointed out that both salts have been administered to unprepared patients as well as to previously prepared patients, with no significant difference in results.

INDICATIONS AND USAGE
Ipodate Calcium and Ipodate Sodium are indicated for cholecystography. They may also be used for cholangiography, although they are not considered the drugs of choice.

CONTRAINDICATIONS
Both preparations are contraindicated in patients who are hypersensitive to Ipodate salts.

WARNINGS
A history of sensitivity to iodine *per se* or to other iodinated compounds is not an absolute contraindication to the use of these preparations, but calls for extreme caution in administration.

USAGE IN PREGNANCY
The safety of these preparations for use during pregnancy has not been established; therefore, they should be used in pregnant patients only when, in the judgment of the physician, their use is deemed essential to the welfare of the patient.

PRECAUTIONS
Increasing the dosage above that recommended increases the possibility of hypotension.

Anuria may result when these preparations are administered to patients with combined renal and hepatic disease or severe renal impairment.

Renal toxicity has been reported in a few patients with liver dysfunction who were given oral cholecystographic agents followed by urographic agents. Administration of urographic agents should therefore be postponed in any patient with a known or suspected hepatic or biliary disorder who has recently taken a cholecystographic contrast agent.

Gastrointestinal disorders which interfere with absorption, liver disorders which interfere with excretion, or obstruction of the biliary duct may result in nonvisualization of the hepatic and biliary ducts and the gallbladder.

Contrast agents may interfere with some chemical determinations made on urine specimens; therefore, urine should be collected before administration of the contrast media or two or more days afterwards.

Thyroid function tests, if indicated, should be performed prior to the administration of these preparations since iodine-containing contrast agents may alter the results of these tests.

Ipodate Sodium contains FD&C Yellow No. 5 (tartrazine) which may cause allergic-type reactions (including bronchial asthma) in certain susceptible individuals. Although the overall incidence of FD&C Yellow No. 5 (tartrazine) sensitivity in the general population is low, it is frequently seen in patients who also have aspirin hypersensitivity.

ADVERSE REACTIONS
Ipodate Calcium and Ipodate Sodium are usually well tolerated. Unwanted effects such as mild and transient nausea, vomiting, or diarrhea sometimes occur but the incidence can be reduced by restricting the dosage to 3 g and administering only

► SHOWN IN PRODUCT IDENTIFICATION GUIDE

the granules to patients who may be prone to gastrointestinal reactions. Headache, dysuria, or abdominal pains may occur infrequently as transient disturbances.

Hypersensitivity reactions may include urticaria, serum sickness-like reactions (fever, rash, arthralgia), other skin rashes, and, rarely, anaphylactoid shock. They are more likely to occur in individuals with a history of allergy, asthma, hay fever, or urticaria, and in those who have previously demonstrated hypersensitivity to iodine compounds. The following adverse reactions have been reported: thrombocytopenia, disseminated intravascular coagulation, cardiogenic shock, cardiac arrest and death.

DOSAGE AND ADMINISTRATION

The capsules should be taken with as little water as possible. They may be swallowed in rapid succession or slowly over the course of ½ hour or more, depending on patient preference.

The granules should be stirred vigorously into a small amount of water (¼ glass or less) and swallowed immediately. If lukewarm rather than cold water is used, the patient will find the suspension quite palatable and there will be less likelihood of nausea.

A total dose of 6 g (12 capsules or two packets of granules) per 24 hour period should not be exceeded.

When an upper gastrointestinal barium study is scheduled, prior administration of either salt will not interfere. Either salt may also be used in conjunction with an intravenous cholangiographic agent.

The recommended dosage and patient preparation for cholangiography and/or cholecystography are as follows:

ROUTINE CHOLECYSTOGRAPHY

On the day before the examination, the patient may, if feasible, eat a high-fat lunch so that the gallbladder will evacuate and refill with opacified bile. The evening meal should be eaten two hours before the contrast medium is taken; there is no need to change the patient's customary diet, whether low-fat or routine. The contrast agent should be administered 10 to 12 hours before the roentgenologic examination. The usual dose is six capsules (providing 3 g ipodate sodium), although up to 12 capsules may be given; one to two packets of granules may be used instead. No other food or drink except small amounts of water should be taken before the examination. A mild laxative or other cathartic may be given, but is not generally necessary.

Roentgenologic examination of the gallbladder is performed the next morning in the usual manner, employing the standard positions. An immediate study of the wet films will determine any need for repositioning of the patient. Administration of a fat meal or other cholecystokinetic agent provides good dynamic studies of gallbladder function. If a barium meal examination is also to be performed, the fat meal may be given simultaneously with or following the barium meal. Gallbladder function studies are then made after the barium meal examination is completed.

REPEAT EXAMINATION

To minimize the possibility of diagnostic error, it may be desirable to repeat the study when the initial examination results in nonvisualization or is non-diagnostic. If the repeat examination also results in nonvisualization, gallbladder disease may be inferred although it should be recognized that nonvisualization may be due to other factors (see *"Precautions"*); also, a small proportion of normal gallbladders may fail to visualize.

Reexamination can be performed on the same day if the usual dose (3 g) was administered initially; administer 3 g (one packet) of the granules or, alternatively, 3 g ipodate sodium (six capsules).

At least five days should intervene between the initial and repeat examinations when the total dose will exceed 6 g.

A total dose of 6 g per 24 hour period should not be exceeded.

CHOLANGIOGRAPHY

No prior preparation of the patient is necessary. For this procedure, the granules should be used. They are administered one hour before cholangiography. Although only one packet (providing 3 g ipodate calcium) may suffice, two packets (6 g) are usually necessary for visualization of the ducts.

Beginning one hour after ingestion of the granules, and at 15-minute intervals thereafter, films should be taken, preferably with the aid of tomography or laminography. With proper positioning of the patient, residual contrast medium gastrointestinal tract is not likely to be a problem, particularly with the more rapidly absorbed calcium salt. Optimal visualization of the ducts is generally achieved between 1 ½ and 2 ½ hours after ingestion of the medium.

COMBINED CHOLANGIOGRAPHY AND CHOLECYSTOGRAPHY

Preparation of the patient and administration of dosage should be as outlined under *"Routine Cholecystography"*, with a dose of six capsules or, if preferred, one packet of granules taken on the evening before examination. On the following morning, one hour before the examination, one additional packet of granulues should be administered.

Beginning one hour after the morning dose, and at 15-minute intervals thereafter, films should be made, preferably with the use of tomography or laminography. While the gallbladder will have concentrated the evening dose of the medium, the additional morning dose will provide opacification of the ducts, and simultaneous visualization may be achieved. When satisfactory films have been obtained, a fat meal may be administered to provide gallbladder function studies.

RAPID COMBINED CHOLANGIOGRAPHY AND CHOLECYSTOGRAPHY

No prior preparation of the patient is necessary. On the day of examination, the patient should be given two packets of granules. Beginning one hour later, examination of the ducts should be performed as described above under *"Cholangiography"*. If the gallbladder has not opacified sufficiently by the time the cholangiographic examination is completed, further cholecystograms may be taken after two or three hours. Dynamic studies of gallbladder function may be carried out in the usual manner.

STORAGE

Store the capsules and granules at room temperature. The capsules should also be protected from exposure to excessive heat.

HOW SUPPLIED

IPODATE CALCIUM

GRANULE FOR RECONSTITUTION: 3 GM

BRAND/MANUFACTURER	NDC	SIZE	AWP
○ BRAND			
ORAGRAFIN CALCIUM: Bracco Diag	00003-0454-70	8 gm 25s	$208.54

IPODATE SODIUM

CAPSULE: 500 MG

AVERAGE UNIT PRICE (AVAILABLE SIZES)			
BRAND	$1.02		

BRAND/MANUFACTURER	NDC	SIZE	AWP
◆ BRAND			
ORAGRAFIN SODIUM: Bracco Diag	00003-0455-50	100s	$97.01
	00003-0455-51	100s ud	$99.36
	00003-0455-20	144s	$157.95

IPOL *SEE* POLIO VACCINE

Ipratropium Bromide

DESCRIPTION

Ipratropium Bromide is an anticholinergic bronchodilator chemically described as 8-azoniabicyclo(3.2.1)-octane, 3-(3-hydroxy-1-oxo-2-phenyl propoxy)-8-methyl-8-(1-methylethyl)-, bromide, monohydrate (*endo, syn*), (±)-; a synthetic quaternary ammonium compound, chemically related to atropine. The molecular weight of Ipratropium Bromide is 430.4; the empirical formula is $C_{20}H_{30}BrNO_3 \cdot H_2O$.

Ipratropium Bromide is a white crystalline substance, freely soluble in water and lower alcohols but insoluble in lipophilic solvents such as ether, chloroform, and fluorocarbons. It is a quaternary ammonium compound and thus exists in an ionized state in aqueous solutions. It is relatively insoluble in nonpolar media. Ipratropium Bromide is available as an inhalation aerosol for oral administration and as an inhalation solution for oral inhalation with the aid of a nebulizer. The aerosol yields 200 inhalations. Each actuation of the valve delivers 18 mcg of Ipratropium Bromide from the mouthpiece. The inhalation solution contains Ipratropium Bromide 0.02% (anhydrous basis); each vial contains 500 mcg of drug.

Following is its chemical structure:

CLINICAL PHARMACOLOGY

Ipratropium Bromide is an anticholinergic (parasympatholytic) agent which, based on animal studies, appears to inhibit vagally mediated reflexes by antagonizing the action of acetylcholine, the transmitter agent released from the vagus nerve. Anticholinergics prevent the increases in intracellular concentration of cyclic guanosine monophosphate (cyclic GMP) which are caused by interaction of acetylcholine with the muscarinic receptor on bronchial smooth muscle.

The bronchodilation following inhalation of Ipratropium Bromide is primarily a local, site-specific effect, not a systemic one. Much of an inhaled dose is swallowed but not absorbed, as shown by fecal excretion studies. Ipratropium Bromide is not readily absorbed into the systemic circulation either from the surface of the lung or from the gastrointestinal tract as confirmed by blood level and renal excretion studies. Following nebulization of a 2 mg dose of inhalation solution, a mean 7% of the dose was absorbed into the systemic circulation either from the surface of the lung or from the gastrointestinal tract.

The half-life of elimination is about 2 hours after inhalation or intravenous administration. Ipratropium Bromide is minimally (0 to 9% *in vitro*) bound to plasma albumin and α₁-acid glycoproteins. It is partially metabolized. Autoradiographic studies in rats have shown that Ipratropium Bromide does not penetrate the blood-brain barrier.

Ipratropium Bromide has not been studied in patients with hepatic or renal insufficiency. It should be used with caution in those patient populations.

In controlled 90-day studies of Ipratropium Bromide aerosol in patients with bronchospasm associated with chronic obstructive pulmonary disease (chronic bronchitis and emphysema) significant improvements in pulmonary function (FEV_1 and FEF_{25-75}% increases of 15% or more) occurred within 15 minutes, reached a peak in 1–2 hours, and persisted for periods of 3 to 4 hours in the majority of patients and up to 6 hours in some patients. In addition, significant increases in Forced Vital Capacity (FVC) have been demonstrated.

In controlled 12-week studies of Ipratropium Bromide inhalation solution in patients with bronchospasm associated with chronic obstructive pulmonary disease (chronic bronchitis and emphysema) significant improvements in pulmonary function (FEV_1 increases of 15% or more) occurred within 15 to 30 minutes, reached a peak in 1–2 hours, and persisted for periods of 4–5 hours in the majority of patients, with about 25–38% of the patients demonstrating increases of 15% or more for at least 7–8 hours. Continued effectiveness of Ipratropium Bromide inhalation solution was demonstrated throughout the 12-week period. In addition, significant increases in forced vital capacity (FVC) have been demonstrated. However, Ipratropium Bromide did not consistently produce significant improvement in subjective symptom scores nor in quality of life scores over the 12-week duration of study.

Additional controlled 12-week studies were conducted to evaluate the safety and effectiveness of Ipratropium Bromide inhalation solution administered concomitantly with the beta adrenergic bronchodilator solutions metaproterenol and albuterol compared with the administration of each of the beta agonists alone. Combined therapy produced significant additional improvement in FEV_1 and FVC. On combined therapy, the median duration of 15% improvement in FEV_1 was 5–7 hours, compared with 3–4 hours in patients receiving a beta agonist alone.

Controlled clinical studies have demonstrated that Ipratropium Bromide does not alter either mucociliary clearance or the volume or viscosity of respiratory secretions. In studies without a positive control Ipratropium Bromide did not alter pupil size, accommodation or visual acuity (see *"Adverse Reactions"*).

Ventilation/perfusion studies have shown no clinically significant effects on pulmonary gas exchange or arterial oxygen tension. Ipratropium Bromide does not produce clinically significant changes in pulse rate or blood pressure.

INDICATIONS AND USAGE

Ipratropium Bromide is indicated as a bronchodilator for maintenance treatment of bronchospasm associated with chronic obstructive pulmonary disease, including chronic bronchitis and emphysema. The inhalation solution can be administered either alone or with other bronchodilators, especially beta adrenergics.

UNLABELED USES

Ipratropium Bromide is used alone or as an adjunct in the treatment of allergic rhinitis, rhinorrhea, and airway obstruction secondary to tuberculosis.

CONTRAINDICATIONS

Hypersensitivity to atropine or its derivatives or to Ipratropium Bromide.

Ipratropium Bromide is not indicated for the initial treatment of acute episodes of bronchospasm where rapid response is required.

WARNINGS

The use of Ipratropium Bromide inhalation solution as a single agent for the relief of bronchospasm in acute COPD exacerbation has not been adequately studied. Drugs with faster onset of action may be preferable as initial therapy in this situation. Combination of Ipratropium Bromide and beta agonists has not been shown to be more effective than either drug alone in reversing the bronchospasm associated with acute COPD exacerbation.

PRECAUTIONS

General: Ipratropium Bromide should be used with caution in patients with narrow-angle glaucoma, prostatic hypertrophy or bladder-neck obstruction.

Information for Patients: Patients should be advised that temporary blurring of vision may result if the aerosol is sprayed into the eyes or if the solution comes into direct contact with the eyes; additional dangers with the solution are precipitation or worsening of narrow-angle glaucoma and eye pain. Use of a nebulizer with mouthpiece rather than face mask may be preferable, to reduce the likelihood of the nebulizer solution reaching the eyes. Patients should be advised that Ipratropium Bromide inhalation solution can be mixed in the nebulizer with albuterol if used within one hour. Compatibility data are not currently available with other drugs.

Patients should be reminded that Ipratropium Bromide is not intended for occasional use, but rather, in order to be maximally effective, must be used consistently as prescribed throughout the course of therapy.

Drug Interactions: Ipratropium Bromide has been used concomitantly with other drugs, including sympathomimetic bronchodilators, methylxanthines, steroids and cromolyn sodium, commonly used in the treatment of chronic obstructive pulmonary disease, without adverse drug reactions. There are no formal studies fully evaluating the interactive effects of Ipratropium Bromide and these drugs with respect to effectiveness.

Carcinogenesis, Mutagenesis, Impairment of Fertility: Two-year oral carcinogenicity studies in rats and mice have revealed no carcinogenic potential at doses up to

1,250 times the maximum recommended human daily dose for Ipratropium Bromide aerosol (up to 6 mg/kg/day of inhalation solution). Results of various mutagenicity studies (Ames test, mouse dominant lethal test, mouse micronucleus test and chromosome aberration of bone marrow in Chinese hamsters) were negative.

Fertility of male or female rats at oral doses up to approximately 10,000 times the maximum recommended human daily dose of aerosol (up to 50 mg/kg/day of inhalation solution) was unaffected by Ipratropium Bromide administration. At doses above 18,000 times the maximum recommended human daily dose of aerosol (above 90 mg/kg of inhalation solution), increased resorption and decreased conception rates were observed.

Pregnancy/Teratogenic Effects: Pregnancy Category B: Oral reproduction studies performed in mice, rats and rabbits (at doses approximately 2,000, 200,000 and 26,000 times the maximum recommended human daily dose, respectively) of aerosol (10, 100, and 125 mg/kg, respectively, of inhalation solution), and inhalation reproduction studies in rats and rabbits (at doses approximately 312 and 375 times the maximum recommended human daily dose, of aerosol and 38 and 45 times the recommended human daily dose—1.5 and 1.8 mg/kg—of inhalation solution respectively) have demonstrated no evidence of teratogenic effects as a result of Ipratropium Bromide. However, no adequate or well controlled studies have been conducted in pregnant women. Because animal reproduction studies are not always predictive of human response, Ipratropium Bromide should be used during pregnancy only if clearly needed.

Nursing Mothers: It is not known whether Ipratropium Bromide is excreted in human milk. Although lipid-insoluble quaternary bases pass into breast milk, it is unlikely that Ipratropium Bromide would reach the infant to an important extent, especially when taken by aerosol or inhalation; Ipratropium Bromide is not well absorbed systemically after inhalation or oral administration. However, because many drugs are excreted in human milk, caution should be exercised when Ipratropium Bromide is administered to a nursing woman.

Pediatric Use: Safety and effectiveness in children below the age of 12 have not been established.

ADVERSE REACTIONS

Adverse reaction information concerning Ipratropium Bromide is derived from 90 day controlled clinical trials (N = 254) with the aerosol, other controlled clinical trials using recommended doses of Ipratropium Bromide aerosol (N = 377) and an uncontrolled study (N = 1924), and from 12-week active-controlled clinical trials of inhalation solution. Additional information is derived from the foreign post-marketing experience and the published literature.

Ipratropium Bromide aerosol: Adverse reactions occurring in greater than one percent of patients in the 90 day controlled clinical trials appear in the following table:

Reaction	Percent of Patients	
	Ipratropium Bromide N = 254	Metaproterenol sulfate N = 249
Cardiovascular		
Palpitations	1.8	1.6
Central Nervous System		
Nervousness	3.1	6.8
Dizziness	2.4	2.8
Headache	2.4	2.0
Dermatological		
Rash	1.2	0.4
Gastrointestinal		
Nausea	2.8	1.2
Gastrointestinal distress	2.4	2.8
Vomiting	0	1.2
Musculoskeletal		
Tremor	0	2.4
Ophthalmological		
Blurred vision	1.2	0.8
Oro-Otolaryngeal		
Dry mouth	2.4	0.8
Irritation from aerosol	1.6	1.6
Respiratory		
Cough	5.9	1.2
Exacerbation of symptoms	2.4	3.6

Additional adverse reactions reported in less than one percent of the patients considered possibly due to Ipratropium Bromide aerosol include urinary difficulty, fatigue, insomnia and hoarseness.

The large uncontrolled, open-label study included seriously ill patients. About 7% of patients treated discontinued the program because of adverse events.

Of the 2301 patients treated in the large uncontrolled study and in clinical trials other than the 90-day studies, the most common adverse reactions reported were: dryness of the oropharynx, about 5 in 100; cough, exacerbation of symptoms and irritation from aerosol, each about 3 in 100; headache, about 2 in 100; nausea, dizziness, blurred vision/difficulty in accommodation, and drying of secretions, each about 1 in 100. Less frequently reported adverse reactions that were possibly due to Ipratropium Bromide aerosol include tachycardia, paresthe-

ALL ADVERSE EVENTS, FROM A DOUBLE BLIND, PARALLEL 12-WEEK STUDY OF PATIENTS WITH COPD*

	Percent of Patients				
	Ipratropium Bromide (500 mcg t.i.d) n = 219	Metaproterenol Sulfate (15 mg t.i.d.) n = 212	Ipratropium Bromide/Metaproterenol Sulfate (500 mcg t.i.d/15 mg t.i.d) n = 108	Albuterol (2.5 mg t.i.d) n = 205	Ipratropium Bromide/Albuterol (500 mcg t.i.d/2.5 mg t.i.d) n = 100
Body as a Whole–General Disorders					
Headache	6.4	5.2	6.5	6.3	9.0
Pain	4.1	3.3	0.9	2.9	5.0
Influenza-like symptoms	3.7	4.7	6.5	0.5	1.0
Back pain	3.2	1.9	1.9	2.4	0.0
Chest pain	3.2	4.2	5.6	2.0	1.0
Cardiovascular Disorders					
Hypertension/Hypertension Aggravated	0.9	1.9	0.9	1.5	4.0
Central & Peripheral Nervous System					
Dizziness	2.3	3.3	1.9	3.9	4.0
Insomnia	0.9	0.5	4.6	1.0	1.0
Tremor	0.9	7.1	8.3	1.0	1.0
Nervousness	0.5	4.7	6.5	1.0	1.0
Gastrointestinal System Disorders					
Mouth Dryness	3.2	0.0	1.9	2.0	3.0
Nausea	4.1	3.8	1.9	2.9	2.0
Constipation	0.9	0.0	3.7	1.0	1.0
Musculo-skeletal System Disorders					
Arthritis	0.9	1.4	0.9	0.5	3.0
Respiratory System Disorders (Lower)					
Coughing	4.6	8.0	6.5	5.4	6.0
Dyspnea	9.6	13.2	16.7	12.7	9.0
Bronchitis	14.6	24.5	15.7	16.6	20.0
Bronchospasm	2.3	2.8	4.6	5.4	5.0
Sputum Increased	1.4	1.4	4.6	3.4	4.0
Respiratory Disorder	0.0	6.1	6.5	2.0	4.0
Respiratory System Disorders (Upper)					
Upper Respiratory Tract Infection	13.2	11.3	9.3	12.2	16.0
Pharyngitis	3.7	4.2	5.6	2.9	4.0
Rhinitis	2.3	4.2	1.9	2.4	0.0
Sinusitis	2.3	2.8	0.9	5.4	4.0

* All adverse events, regardless of drug relationship, reported by three percent or more patients in the 12-week controlled clinical trials.

sias, drowsiness, coordination difficulty, itching, hives, flushing, alopecia, constipation, tremor, mucosal ulcers.

Cases of precipitation or worsening of narrow-angle glaucoma, acute eye pain and hypotension have been reported. A case of giant urticaria with positive rechallenge has been reported from the foreign marketing experience. (See "Contraindications".)

Ipratropium Bromide inhalation solution: All adverse events, regardless of drug relationship, reported by three percent or more patients in the 12-week controlled clinical trials appear in the table below: (See related table).

Additional adverse reactions reported in less than three percent of the patients treated with Ipratropium Bromide include tachycardia, palpitations, eye pain, urinary retention, urinary tract infection and urticaria. A single case of anaphylaxis thought to be possibly related to Ipratropium Bromide has been reported. Cases of precipitation or worsening of narrow-angle glaucoma and acute eye pain have been reported.

Lower respiratory adverse reactions (bronchitis, dyspnea and bronchospasm) were the most common events leading to discontinuation of Ipratropium Bromide therapy in the 12-week trials.

Headache, mouth dryness and aggravation of COPD symptoms are more common when the total daily dose of Ipratropium Bromide equals or exceeds 2,000 mcg.

OVERDOSAGE

Acute overdosage by inhalation is unlikely since Ipratropium Bromide is not well absorbed systemically after aerosol administration, inhalation at up to four-fold the recommended dose, or after oral administration at up to forty-fold the recommended dose. The oral LD$_{50}$ of Ipratropium Bromide ranged between 1001 and 2010 mg/kg in mice; between 1667 and more than 4000 mg/kg in rats; and between 400 and 1300 mg/kg in dogs.

DOSAGE AND ADMINISTRATION

The usual starting dose of Ipratropium Bromide aerosol is two inhalations (36 mcg) four times a day. Patients may take additional inhalations as required; however, the total number of inhalations should not exceed 12 in 24 hours.

The usual dosage of Ipratropium Bromide inhalation solution is 500 mcg, administered three to four times a day by oral nebulization, with doses 6 to 8 hours apart. Ipratropium Bromide inhalation solution can be mixed in the nebulizer with albuterol if used within one hour. Compatibility data are not currently available with other drugs.

Store between 59°F (15°C) and 86°F (30°C). Avoid excessive humidity. Protect from light.

HOW SUPPLIED
AEROSOL SOLID W/ADAPTER:

BRAND/MANUFACTURER	NDC	SIZE	AWP
○ **BRAND**			
ATROVENT: Boehr Ingelheim	00597-0082-18	14 gm	$24.71
	00597-0082-14	14 gm	$27.00

SOLUTION: 0.02%

BRAND/MANUFACTURER	NDC	SIZE	AWP
○ **BRAND**			
ATROVENT: Boehr Ingelheim	00597-0080-62	2.5 ml 25s ud	$46.69

Iron Dextran

WARNING
THE PARENTERAL USE OF COMPLEXES OF IRON AND CARBOHYDRATES HAS RESULTED IN FATAL ANAPHYLACTIC-TYPE REACTIONS. DEATHS

ASSOCIATED WITH SUCH ADMINISTRATION HAVE BEEN REPORTED. THEREFORE, IRON DEXTRAN SHOULD BE USED ONLY IN THOSE PATIENTS IN WHOM THE INDICATIONS HAVE BEEN CLEARLY ESTABLISHED AND LABORATORY INVESTIGATIONS CONFIRM AN IRON DEFICIENT STATE NOT AMENABLE TO ORAL IRON THERAPY.

DESCRIPTION
Iron Dextran, a hematinic agent, is a dark brown, slightly viscous liquid complex of ferric hydroxide and Dextran for intramuscular or intravenous use.

Each mL contains the equivalent of 50 mg of iron as an Iron Dextran complex.

CLINICAL PHARMACOLOGY
The Iron Dextran complex is dissociated by the reticuloendothelial system, and the ferric iron is transported by transferrin and incorporated into hemoglobin and storage sites.

INDICATIONS AND USAGE
Intravenous or intramuscular injections of Iron Dextran are indicated for treatment of patients with documented iron deficiency in whom oral administration is unsatisfactory or impossible.

CONTRAINDICATIONS
Hypersensitivity to the product. All anemias not associated with iron deficiency.

WARNINGS
Two mL of undiluted Iron Dextran is the maximum recommended daily dose.

The following pattern of signs/symptoms has been reported as a delayed (1-2 days) reaction at recommended doses: modest-high fever, chills, backache, headache, myalgia, malaise, nausea, vomiting, and dizziness. These reactions have been reported in an unexpectedly high incidence with certain batches. Therefore, in estimating the benefit/risk of treatment for an individual patient, it must be assumed that there is a real possibility that such a delayed reaction may occur.

This preparation should be used with extreme care in the presence of serious impairment of liver function.

A risk of carcinogenesis may attend the intramuscular injection of iron carbohydrate complexes. Such complexes have been found under experimental conditions to produce sarcoma when large doses are injected in rats, mice, and rabbits, and possibly in hamsters.

The long latent period between the injection of a potential carcinogen and the appearance of a tumor makes it impossible to measure the risk in man accurately. There have, however, been several reports in the literature describing tumors at the injection site in humans who had previously received intramuscular injections of iron-carbohydrate complexes.

Use in Pregnancy: Animal studies have shown that administration of Iron Dextran during pregnancy caused an increase in the number of stillbirths and fetal anomalies, fetal edema, and a decrease in neonatal survival. In addition, these studies show that the fetus can obtain from 80 to 90% of the iron administered to the pregnant dam during the third trimester of pregnancy. Whether this represents a danger to the fetus and whether the drug is effective in treating maternal iron deficiency under these circumstances is not known.

For these reasons, Iron Dextran should not be used in pregnancy or in women of child-bearing potential unless, in the judgment of the physician, the potential benefits outweigh the possible hazards.

PRECAUTIONS
Unwarranted therapy with parenteral iron will cause excess storage of iron with the consequent possibility of exogenous hemosiderosis. Such iron overload is particularly apt to occur in patients with hemoglobinopathies and other refractory anemias which might be erroneously diagnosed as iron deficiency anemia.

Iron Dextran should be used with caution in individuals with histories of significant allergies and/or asthma. Epinephrine should be immediately available in the event of acute hypersensitivity reactions. (Usual adult dose: 0.5 mL of a 1:1000 solution, by subcutaneous or intramuscular injection.)

Patients with iron deficiency anemia and rheumatoid arthritis may have an acute exacerbation of joint pain and swelling following the intravenous administration of Iron Dextran.

ADVERSE REACTIONS
Anaphylactic reactions including fatal anaphylaxis; other hypersensitivity reactions including dyspnea, urticaria, other rashes and itching, arthralgia and myalgia, and febrile episodes; variable degree of soreness and inflammation at or near injection site, including sterile abscesses (IM injection); brown skin discoloration at injection site (IM injection); lymphadenopathy; local phlebitis at injection site (IV injection); peripheral vascular flushing with overly rapid IV administration; hypotensive reaction; possible arthritic reactivation in patients with quiescent rheumatoid arthritis; leucocytosis, frequently with fever; headache, backache, dizziness, malaise, transitory paresthesias, nausea and shivering.

DOSAGE AND ADMINISTRATION
A. IRON DEFICIENCY ANEMIA—DOSAGE
Periodic hematologic determinations should be used as a guide in therapy. It should be recognized that iron storage may lag behind the appearance of normal blood morphology. Although there are significant variations in body build and weight distribution among males and females, the accompanying table and formula represent a simple and convenient means for estimating the total iron

required. This total iron requirement reflects the amount of iron needed to restore hemoglobin to normal or near normal levels plus an additional 50% allowance to provide adequate replenishment of iron stores in most individuals with moderately or severely reduced levels of hemoglobin. Factors contributing to the formula are shown below.

The formula should not be used for patients weighing 30 pounds or less. (Adjustments have been made in the table values to account for the lower normal hemoglobins for those weighing 30 pounds or less.)

Note: The table and accompanying formula are applicable for dosage determinations only in patients with *iron deficiency anemia;* they are not to be used for dosage determinations in patients requiring *iron replacement for blood loss.* (See related tables).

TOTAL AMOUNT OF IRON DEXTRAN REQUIRED (TO THE NEAREST ML) FOR RESTORATION OF HEMOGLOBIN AND REPLACEMENT OF DEPLETED IRON STORES, BASED ON OBSERVED HEMOGLOBIN AND BODY WEIGHT

Patient Weight		Milliliter Requirement Based on Observed Hemoglobin of			
lb	kg	4.0 (g/dl)	6.0 (g/dl)	8.0 (g/dl)	10.0 (g/dl)
10	4.5	3 mL	3 mL	2 mL	2 mL
20	9.1	7	6	4	3
30	13.6	10	8	7	5
40	18.1	18	14	11	8
50	22.7	22	18	14	10
60	27.2	26	21	17	12
70	31.8	31	25	19	14
80	36.3	35	28	22	16
90	40.8	39	32	25	18
100	45.4	44	35	28	20
110	49.9	48	39	30	21
120	54.4	53	42	33	23
130	59.0	57	46	36	25
140	63.5	61	50	39	27
150	68.1	66	53	41	29
160	72.6	70	57	44	31
170	77.1	74	60	47	33
180	81.7	79	64	50	35

The total amount of iron (in mg) required to restore hemoglobin to normal levels and to replenish iron stores may be approximated from the formula: (See related table).

Administration:
1. Intravenous Injection: The total amount of Iron Dextran required for the treatment of iron deficiency anemia is determined from the formula or table (see "Dosage" section above).

Test Dose: Prior to receiving their first Iron Dextran therapeutic dose, all patients should be given an intravenous test dose of 0.5 mL. Although anaphylactic reactions known to occur following Iron Dextran administration are usually evident within a few minutes, or sooner, it is recommended that a period of an hour or longer elapse before the remainder of the initial therapeutic dose is given. Individual doses of 2 mL or less may be given on a daily basis until the calculated total amount required has been reached. Iron Dextran is given undiluted and *slowly* (1 mL or less per minute).

2. *Intramuscular Injection:* The total amount of Iron Dextran required for the treatment of iron deficiency anemia is determined from the formula or table. (See "Dosage" section above.)

Test Dose: Prior to receiving their first Iron Dextran therapeutic dose, all patients should be given an intramuscular test dose of 0.5 mL, administered in the same recommended test site and by the same technique as described in the last paragraph of this section. Although anaphylactic reactions known to occur following Iron Dextran administration are usually evident within a few minutes or sooner, it is recommended that a period of an hour or longer elapse before the remainder of the initial therapeutic dose is given.

If no adverse reactions are observed, the injection can be given according to the following schedule until the calculated total amount required has been reached. Each day's dose should ordinarily not exceed 0.5 mL (25 mg of iron) for infants under 10 lb, 1.0 mL (50 mg of iron) for children under 20 lb, 2.0 mL (100 mg of iron) for other users.

Iron Dextran should be injected only into the muscle mass of the upper outer quadrant of the buttock—never into the arm or other exposed areas—and should be injected deeply, with a 2-inch or 3-inch 19 or 20 gauge needle. If the patient is standing, he should be bearing his weight on the leg opposite the injection site, or if in bed, he should be in the lateral position with injection site upper-most. To avoid injection or leakage into the subcutaneous tissue, a Z-track technique (displacement of the skin laterally prior to injection) is recommended.

B. IRON REPLACEMENT FOR BLOOD LOSS
Some individuals sustain blood losses on an intermittent or repetitive basis. Such blood losses may occur periodically in patients with hemorrhagic diatheses

$$\frac{mg\ blood\ iron}{lb\ body\ weight} = \frac{mL\ blood}{lb\ body\ weight} \times \frac{g\ hemoglobin}{mL\ blood} \times \frac{mg\ iron}{g\ hemoglobin}$$

a) Blood volume .... 8.5% body weight
b) Normal hemoglobin (males and females)
 over 30 pounds .... 14.8 g/dl
 30 pounds or less .... 12.0 g/dl
c) Iron content of hemoglobin 0.34%
d) Hemoglobin deficit
e) Weight
Based on the above factors, individuals with normal hemoglobin levels will have approximately 20 mg of blood iron per pound of
 body weight.

$$0.3 \times \text{Body Weight in Pounds} \times 100 - \frac{hemoglobin\ in\ g/dl \times 100}{14.8}$$

(To calculate dose in mL of Iron Dextran divide this result by 50.)

(familial telangiectasia; hemophilia; gastro-intestinal bleeding) and on a repetitive basis from procedures such as renal hemodialysis.

Iron therapy in these patients should be directed toward replacement of the equivalent amount of iron represented in the blood loss. The table and formula described under "A. Iron Deficiency Anemia" are *not* applicable for simple iron replacement values.

Quantitative estimates of the individual's periodic blood loss and hematocrit during the bleeding episode provide a convenient method for the calculation of the required iron dose. The formula shown below is based on the approximation that 1 mL of normocytic, normochromic red cells contains 1 mg of elemental iron:

Replacement iron (in mg) = Blood loss (in mL) × hematocrit Example: Blood loss of 500 mL with 20% hematocrit
Replacement Iron = 500 × 0.20 = 100 mg
Iron Dextran dose = $\frac{100\ mg}{50}$ = 2 mL

Parenteral drug products should be inspected visually for particulate matter and discoloration prior to administration, whenever the solution and container permit.

STORAGE
Store at controlled room temperature 15°-30° C (59°-86° F).

J CODES
10 cc IV,IM—J1780
5 cc IV,IM—J1770
2 cc IV,IM—J1760

HOW SUPPLIED
INJECTION: 50 MG/ML

BRAND/MANUFACTURER	NDC	SIZE	AWP
◇ GENERICS			
INFED: Schein	00364-3012-47	2 ml 10s	$349.59

Irrigating Solution G SEE CITRIC ACID/
MAGNESIUM OXIDE/SODIUM CARBONATE

Ismelin SEE GUANETHIDINE MONOSULFATE

ISMO SEE ISOSORBIDE MONONITRATE

Ismotic SEE ISOSORBIDE

Isoetharine Hydrochloride

DESCRIPTION
Isoetharine Inhalation Solution, USP (sulfite-free) is a sterile solution for oral inhalation packaged in plastic vials for single use. Each vial contains Isoetharine Hydrochloride 0.062%, 0.125%, 0.167%, 0.2% or 0.25% in a sterile aqueous solution. The solution is for use in aerosol bronchodilator therapy employing oxygen aerosolization or intermittent positive pressure breathing (IPPB). It is also available as a pocket nebulizer containing Isoetharine mesylate 0.61% (w/w) delivering approximately 20 metered doses per ml of solution. Each average 56 mg delivery contains 340 µg of Isoetharine. Isoetharine Hydrochloride is a sympathomimetic amine and is chemically 3,4-dihydroxy-α-[1-(isopropylamino)propyl] benzyl alcohol hydrochloride.

Following is its chemical structure:

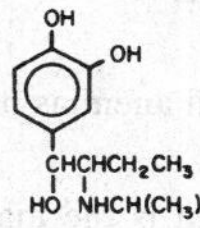

CLINICAL PHARMACOLOGY
Isoetharine is a sympathomimetic amine with preferential affinity for $Beta_2$ adrenergic receptor sites of bronchial and certain arteriolar musculature and a lower order of affinity for $Beta_1$ adrenergic receptors. Its activity in symptomatic relief of bronchospasm is rapid and of relatively long duration. By relieving bronchospasm, Isoetharine helps give prompt relief and significantly increases FVC, FEV_1, and FEF 25%-75%.

Recent studies in laboratory animals (minipigs, rodents and dogs) recorded the occurrence of cardiac arrhythmias and sudden death (with histologic evidence of myocardial necrosis) when beta agonists and methylxanthines were administered concurrently. The significance of these findings when applied to human usage is currently unknown.

INDICATIONS AND USAGE
Isoetharine Hydrochloride is indicated for use as a bronchodilator for bronchial asthma and for reversible bronchospasm that may occur in association with bronchitis and emphysema.

CONTRAINDICATIONS
Isoetharine inhalation solution should not be administered to patients who are hypersensitive to any of its components.

WARNINGS
Not for injection.

Excessive use of an adrenergic aerosol should be discouraged as it may lose its effectiveness. Occasional patients have been reported to develop severe paradoxical airway resistance with repeated excessive use of an aerosol adrenergic inhalation preparation. The cause of this refractory state is unknown. It is advisable that in such instances the use of the aerosol adrenergic be discontinued immediately and alternative therapy instituted, since in the reported cases the patients did not respond to other forms of therapy until the drug was withdrawn. Cardiac arrest has been noted in several instances.

Isoetharine should not be administered along with epinephrine or other sympathomimetic amines, since these drugs are direct cardiac stimulants and may cause excessive tachycardia. They may, however, be alternated if desired.

Some forms of Isoetharine contain acetone sodium bisulfite, a sulfite that may cause allergic-type reactions including anaphyactic Symptoms and life-threatening or less severe asthmatic episodes in certain susceptible people. The overall prevalence of sulfite sensitivity in the general population is unknown and probably low. Sulfite sensitivity is seen more frequently in asthmatic than in nonasthmatic people.

PRECAUTIONS
General: Dosage must be carefully adjusted in patients with hyperthyroidism, hypertension, acute coronary disease, cardiac asthma, limited cardiac reserve and in individuals sensitive to sympathomimetic amines since overdosage may result in tachycardia, palpitations, nausea, headache or epinephrine-like side effects.

Drug Interactions: Isoetharine should not be administered along with epinephrine or other sympathomimetic amines, since these drugs are direct cardiac stimulants and may cause excessive tachycardia. They may, however, be alternated if desired.

Carcinogenesis, Mutagenesis, Impairment of Fertility: Chronic toxicity studies up to twelve months in dogs with doses up to 20 mg/kg/day (equivalent to approximately 200 times the human dose based on a 70 kg individual) and chronic toxicity studies in rats with the doses up to 45 mg/kg/day (equivalent to approximately 450 times the human dose, based on a 70 kg individual) revealed no evidence of carcinogenicity due to isoetharine.

◆ RATED THERAPEUTICALLY EQUIVALENT; ◇ THERAPEUTIC EQUIVALENCE UNCONFIRMED; ○ UNRATED

Pregnancy—Category C: Animal reproduction studies have not been conducted with Isoetharine hydrochloride. It is also not known whether Isoetharine hydrochloride can cause fetal harm when administered to a pregnant woman or can affect reproduction capacity, although there is no evidence of such harm or effects. Isoetharine hydrochloride should be given to a pregnant woman only if in the physician's judgment the potential benefit to the pregnant woman outweighs the risk to the fetus.

Nursing Mothers: It is not known whether this drug is excreted in human milk. Because many drugs are excreted in human milk, caution should be exercised when isoetharine hydrochloride is administered to a nursing woman.

Pediatric Use: The safety and efficacy of this product in children under the age of 12 have not been established.

ADVERSE REACTIONS

Although Isoetharine Hydrochloride is relatively free of toxic side effects, too frequent use may cause the following effects, as is the case with other sympathomimetic amines:

CNS Effects: headache, anxiety, tension, restlessness, insomnia, weakness, dizziness, excitement.

Cardiovascular Effects: tachycardia, palpitations, changes in blood pressure.

Gastrointestinal Effects: nausea.

Other: tremor, weakness.

OVERDOSAGE

Overdosage of Isoetharine Hydrochloride may produce signs and symptoms typical of excessive sympathomimetic effects, including tachycardia, palpitations, nausea, headache, blood pressure changes, anxiety, restlessness, insomnia, tremor, weakness, dizziness, and excitation. Excessive use of adrenergic aerosols may result in loss of effectiveness or severe paradoxical airway resistance. Cardiac arrest has been noted in several instances. In all cases of overdosage, the drug should be discontinued immediately and vital functions supported until the patient is stabilized. It is not known whether Isoetharine Hydrochloride is dialyzable.

The single dose amount of drug that may be toxic or life threatening is highly variable according to patient characteristics and drug history. The acute oral LD_{50} in mice is 1630 mg/kg of pure drug (Isoetharine Hydrochloride).

DOSAGE AND ADMINISTRATION

Isoetharine Hydrochloride is for oral inhalation only and can be administered by hand nebulizer, oxygen aerosolization, or intermittent positive pressure breathing devices (IPPB). Usually, treatment need not be repeated more than every four hours, although in severe cases more frequent administration may be necessary.

The average adult dose of Isoetharine pocket nebulizer is one or two inhalations, occasionally, more maybe required. It is important, however, to wait one full minute after the initial one or two inhalations in order to be certain whether another is necessary.

Method of Administration	Usual Dose (1% Solution)*	Range
Hand nebulizer	4 inhalations	3-7 inhalations
Oxygen aerosolization**	0.5 mL	0.25 to 0.5 mL
IPPB†	0.5 mL	0.25 to 1 mL

The doses given are for the 1% solution which must be suitably diluted prior to administration. Below are the dose equivalents for the entire prediluted and ready-to-use product line:

Product Strength (%)	Volume (mL)	Equivalent to _mL of Isoetharine HCl 1%
0.062%	4 mL	0.25 mL
0.125%	4 mL	0.5 mL
0.167%	3 mL	0.5 mL
0.2%	2.5 mL	0.5 mL
0.25%	2 mL	0.5 mL

** *Administered with oxygen flow adjusted to 4 to 6 liters/minute over a period of 15 to 20 minutes.*
† *Usually an inspiratory flow rate of 15 liters/minute at a cycling pressure of 15 cm H$_2$O is recommended. It may be necessary, according to patient and type of IPPB apparatus, to adjust flow rate to 6 to 30 liters per minute, cycling pressure to 10-15 cm H$_2$O and further dilution according to needs of patient.*

Store at controlled room temperature, 15°-30°C (59°-86°F). PROTECT FROM LIGHT. Store vial in pouch until time of use. Do not use solution if its color is pinkish or darker than slightly yellow or if it contains a precipitate.

J CODES

1.0% per ml INH—J7655
0.25% per ml INH—J7654
0.2% per ml INH—J7653
0.167% per ml INH—J7652
0.125% per ml INH—J7651
0.1% per ml INH—J7650

HOW SUPPLIED

SOLUTION: 0.062%

BRAND/MANUFACTURER		NDC	SIZE	AWP
◆ GENERICS				
Astra		00186-4110-01	4 ml 100s	$57.38

SOLUTION: 0.08%

BRAND/MANUFACTURER		NDC	SIZE	AWP
◆ GENERICS				
Dey		49502-0661-03	3 ml 25s	$19.90

SOLUTION: 0.1%

AVERAGE UNIT PRICE (AVAILABLE SIZES)				
GENERIC	$0.28			

BRAND/MANUFACTURER		NDC	SIZE	AWP
◆ GENERICS				
Dey		49502-0664-05	5 ml 25s	$19.90
Roxane		00054-8429-25	2.5 ml 100s ud	$99.35

SOLUTION: 0.125%

AVERAGE UNIT PRICE (AVAILABLE SIZES)		GENERIC A-RATED AVERAGE PRICE (GAAP)	
GENERIC	$0.20	4 ml 100s	$78.37

BRAND/MANUFACTURER		NDC	SIZE	AWP
◆ GENERICS				
Astra		00186-4112-01	4 ml 100s	$57.38
Roxane		00054-8430-25	4 ml 100s ud	$99.35

SOLUTION: 0.167%

AVERAGE UNIT PRICE (AVAILABLE SIZES)		GENERIC A-RATED AVERAGE PRICE (GAAP)	
GENERIC	$0.26	3 ml 100s	$78.37

BRAND/MANUFACTURER		NDC	SIZE	AWP
◆ GENERICS				
Astra		00186-4111-01	3 ml 100s	$57.38
Roxane		00054-8432-25	3 ml 100s ud	$99.35

SOLUTION: 0.17%

BRAND/MANUFACTURER		NDC	SIZE	AWP
◆ GENERICS				
Dey		49502-0660-03	3 ml 100s	$19.90

SOLUTION: 0.2%

AVERAGE UNIT PRICE (AVAILABLE SIZES)		GENERIC A-RATED AVERAGE PRICE (GAAP)	
GENERIC	$0.31	2.5 ml 100s	$78.37

BRAND/MANUFACTURER		NDC	SIZE	AWP
◆ GENERICS				
Astra		00186-4113-01	2.5 ml 100s	$57.38
Roxane		00054-8431-25	2.5 ml 100s ud	$99.35

SOLUTION: 0.25%

AVERAGE UNIT PRICE (AVAILABLE SIZES)		GENERIC A-RATED AVERAGE PRICE (GAAP)	
GENERIC	$0.39	2 ml 100s	$78.37

BRAND/MANUFACTURER		NDC	SIZE	AWP
◆ GENERICS				
Dey		49502-0659-02	2 ml 25s	$19.90
Astra		00186-4115-01	2 ml 100s	$57.38
Roxane		00054-8434-25	2 ml 100s ud	$99.35

SOLUTION: 1%

AVERAGE UNIT PRICE (AVAILABLE SIZES)		GENERIC A-RATED AVERAGE PRICE (GAAP)	
BRAND	$1.63	10 ml	$5.97
GENERIC	$0.60	30 ml	$17.97
HCFA FUL (10 ml)	$0.75		
HCFA FUL (30 ml)	$0.50		

BRAND/MANUFACTURER		NDC	SIZE	AWP
◆ BRAND				
BRONKOSOL: Sanofi Winthrop		00024-1071-10	10 ml	$16.99
		00024-1071-30	30 ml	$46.56
◆ GENERICS				
BETA-2: Nephron		00487-7601-00	10 ml	$5.60
Roxane		00054-3408-40	10 ml	$5.81
Major		00904-2353-10	10 ml	$6.50

► SHOWN IN PRODUCT IDENTIFICATION GUIDE

BRAND/MANUFACTURER	NDC	SIZE	AWP
BETA-2: Nephron	00487-7601-01	30 ml	$14.00
Roxane	00054-3408-44	30 ml	$16.81
Major	00904-2353-30	30 ml	$23.10

Isoetharine Mesylate

DESCRIPTION

Isoetharine Mesylate inhalation aerosol is a nebulizer containing Isoetharine Mesylate 0.61% (w/w).

Isoetharine Mesylate is 1,2-Benzenediol, 4-[l-hydroxy-2-[(l-methylethyl)-amino]-butyl]-, methanesulfonate (salt). Each average 56 mg delivery contains 340 µg Isoetharine.

Following is its chemical structure:

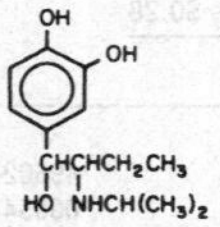

CLINICAL PHARMACOLOGY

Isoetharine is a sympathomimetic amine with preferential affinity for beta$_2$ adrenergic receptor sites of bronchial and certain arteriolar musculature, and a lower order of affinity for beta, adrenergic receptors. Its activity in symptomatic relief of bronchospasm is rapid and of relatively long duration. By relieving bronchospasm, Isoetharine Mesylate inhalation aerosol helps give prompt relief and significantly increases vital capacity.

INDICATIONS AND USAGE

Isoetharine Mesylate inhalation aerosol is indicated for use as a bronchodilator for bronchial asthma and for reversible bronchospasm that may occur in association with bronchitis and emphysema.

CONTRAINDICATION

Isoetharine Mesylate inhalation aerosol should not be administered to patients who are hypersensitive to any of its ingredients.

WARNINGS

Excessive use of an adrenergic aerosol should be discouraged as it may lose its effectiveness. Occasional patients have been reported to develop severe paradoxical airway resistance with repeated excessive use of an aerosol adrenergic inhalation preparation. The cause of this refractory state is unknown. It is advisable that in such instances the use of the aerosol adrenergic be discontinued immediately and alternative therapy instituted, since in the reported cases the patients did not respond to other forms of therapy until the drug was withdrawn. Cardiac arrest has been noted in several instances.

Isoetharine Mesylate inhalation aerosol should not be administered along with epinephrine or other sympathomimetic amines, since these drugs are direct cardiac stimulants and may cause excessive tachycardia. They may, however, be alternated if desired.

Usage in Pregnancy: Although there has been no evidence of teratogenic effects with this drug, use of any drug in pregnancy, lactation, or in women of childbearing potential requires that the potential benefit of the drug be weighed against its possible hazard to the mother or child.

PRECAUTIONS

Dosage must be carefully adjusted in patients with hyperthyroidism, hypertension, acute coronary disease, cardiac asthma, limited cardiac reserve, and in individuals sensitive to sympathomimetic amines, since overdosage may result in tachycardia, palpitation, nausea, headache, or epinephrine-like side effects.

ADVERSE REACTIONS

Although Isoetharine Mesylate inhalation aerosol is relatively free of toxic side effects, too frequent use may cause tachycardia, palpitation, nausea, headache, changes in blood pressure, anxiety, tension, restlessness, insomnia, tremor, weakness, dizziness, and excitement, as is the case with other sympathomimetic amines.

DOSAGE AND ADMINISTRATION

The average adult dose is one or two inhalations. Occasionally, more may be required. It is important, however, to wait one full minute after the initial one or two inhalations in order to be certain whether another is necessary. In most cases, inhalations need not be repeated more often than every four hours, although more frequent administration may be necessary in severe cases.

HOW SUPPLIED
AEROSOL LIQUID:

BRAND/MANUFACTURER	NDC	SIZE	AWP
◇ BRAND			
BRONKOMETER: Sanofi Winthrop	00024-1041-01	10 ml	$21.12
	00024-1041-03	15 ml	$27.26

AEROSOL LIQUID W/ADAPTER:

BRAND/MANUFACTURER	NDC	SIZE	AWP
◇ BRAND			
BRONKOMETER: Sanofi Winthrop	00024-1040-01	10 ml	$22.53
	00024-1040-03	15 ml	$29.94

Isoflurane

DESCRIPTION

Isoflurane, a nonflammable liquid administered by vaporizing, is a general inhalation anesthetic drug. It is 1-chloro-2,2,2-trifluoroethyl difluoromethyl ether.

Some physical constants are:

Molecular weight	184.5
Boiling point at 760 mm Hg	48.5°C (uncorr.)
Refractive index n$_D^{20}$	1.2990-1.3005
Specific gravity 25°/25°C	1.496
Vapor pressure in mm Hg**	

20°C	238
25°C	295
30°C	367
35°C	450

Equation for vapor pressure calculation:

$$\log_{10}P_{vap} = A + \frac{B}{T} \text{ where:}$$

$A = 8.058$
$B = -1664.58$
$T = °C + 273.16 \text{ (Kelvin)}$

Partition coefficients at 37°C

Water/gas	0.61
Blood/gas	1.43
Oil/gas	90.8

Partition coefficients at 25°C — rubber and plastic

Conductive rubber/gas	62.0
Butyl rubber/gas	75.0
Polyvinyl chloride/gas	110.0
Polyethylene/gas	~2.0
Polyurethane/gas	~1.4
Polyolefin/gas	~1.1
Butylacetate/gas	~2.5
Purity by gas chromatography	> 99.9%

Lower limit of flammability in oxygen or nitrous oxide at 9 joules/sec. and 23°C	None
Lower limit of flammability in oxygen or nitrous oxide at 900 joules/sec. and 23°C	Greater than useful concentration in anesthesia.

Isoflurane is a clear, colorless, stable liquid containing no additives or chemical stabilizers. Isoflurane has a mildly pungent, musty, ethereal odor. Samples stored in indirect sunlight in clear, colorless glass for five years, as well as samples directly exposed for 30 hours to a 2 amp, 115 volt, 60 cycle long wave U.V. light were unchanged in composition as determined by gas chromatography. Isoflurane in one normal sodium methoxide-methanol solution, a strong base, for over six months consumed essentially no alkali, indicative of strong base stability. Isoflurane does not decompose in the presence of soda lime (at normal operating temperatures), and does not attack aluminum, tin, brass, iron or copper.

Following is its chemical structure:

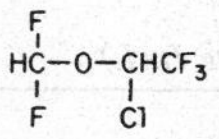

CLINICAL PHARMACOLOGY

Isoflurane is an inhalation anesthetic. The MAC (minimum alveolar concentration) in man is as follows:

Age	100% Oxygen	70% N$_2$O
26 ± 4	1.28	0.56
44 ± 7	1.15	0.50
64 ± 5	1.05	0.37

Induction of and recovery from Isoflurane anesthesia are rapid. Isoflurane has a mild pungency which limits the rate of induction, although excessive salivation or tracheobronchial secretions do not appear to be stimulated. Pharyngeal and laryngeal reflexes are readily obtunded. The level of anesthesia may be changed rapidly with Isoflurane. Isoflurane is a profound respiratory depressant. RESPIRATION MUST BE MONITORED CLOSELY AND SUPPORTED WHEN NECESSARY. As anesthetic dose is increased, tidal volume decreases and respiratory rate is unchanged. This depression is partially reversed by surgical stimulation, even at deeper levels of anesthesia. Isoflurane evokes a sigh response reminiscent of that seen with diethyl ether and enflurane, although the frequency is less than with enflurane.

◆ RATED THERAPEUTICALLY EQUIVALENT; ◇ THERAPEUTIC EQUIVALENCE UNCONFIRMED; ○ UNRATED

Blood pressure decreases with induction of anesthesia but returns toward normal with surgical stimulation. Progressive increases in depth of anesthesia produce corresponding decreases in blood pressure. Nitrous oxide diminishes the inspiratory concentration of Isoflurane required to reach a desired level of anesthesia and may reduce the arterial hypotension seen with Isoflurane alone. Heart rhythm is remarkably stable. With controlled ventilation and normal $PaCO_2$, cardiac output is maintained despite increasing depth of anesthesia, primarily through an increase in heart rate which compensates for a reduction in stroke volume. The hypercapnia which attends spontaneous ventilation during Isoflurane anesthesia further increases heart rate and raises cardiac output above awake levels. Isoflurane does not sensitize the myocardium to exogenously administered epinephrine in the dog. Limited data indicate that subcutaneous injection of 0.25 mg of epinephrine (50 mL of 1:200,000 solution) does not produce an increase in ventricular arrhythmias in patients anesthetized with Isoflurane.

Muscle relaxation is often adequate for intra-abdominal operations at normal levels of anesthesia. Complete muscle paralysis can be attained with small doses of muscle relaxants. ALL COMMONLY USED MUSCLE RELAXANTS ARE MARKEDLY POTENTIATED WITH ISOFLURANE, THE EFFECT BEING MOST PROFOUND WITH THE NONDEPOLARIZING TYPE. Neostigmine reverses the effect of nondepolarizing muscle relaxants in the presence of Isoflurane. All commonly used muscle relaxants are compatible with Isoflurane.

Isoflurane can produce coronary vasodilation at the arteriolar level in selected animal models[1,2]; the drug is probably also a coronary dilator in humans. Isoflurane, like some other coronary arteriolar dilators, has been shown to divert blood from collateral dependent myocardium to normally perfused areas in an animal model ("coronary steal")[3]. Clinical studies to date evaluating myocardial ischemia, infarction and death as outcome parameters have not established that the coronary arteriolar dilation property of Isoflurane is associated with coronary steal or myocardial ischemia in patients with coronary artery disease[4,5,6,7].

Pharmacokinetics: Isoflurane undergoes minimal biotransformation in man. In the postanesthesia period, only 0.17% of the Isoflurane taken up can be recovered as urinary metabolites.

INDICATIONS AND USAGE
Isoflurane may be used for induction and maintenance of general anesthesia. Adequate data have not been developed to establish its application in obstetrical anesthesia.

UNLABELED USES
Isoflurane is used alone or as an adjunct for the treatment of obstetrical pain.

CONTRAINDICATIONS
Known sensitivity to Isoflurane or to other halogenated agents.
  Known or suspected genetic susceptibility to malignant hyperthermia.

WARNINGS
Since levels of anesthesia may be altered easily and rapidly, only vaporizers producing predictable concentrations should be used. Hypotension and respiratory depression increase as anesthesia is deepened.
  Increased blood loss comparable to that seen with halothane has been observed in patients undergoing abortions.
  Isoflurane markedly increases cerebral blood flow at deeper levels of anesthesia. There may be a transient rise in cerebral spinal fluid pressure which is fully reversible with hyperventilation.

PRECAUTIONS
General: As with any potent general anesthetic, Isoflurane should only be administered in an adequately equipped anesthetizing environment by those who are familiar with the pharmacology of the drug and qualified by training and experience to manage the anesthetized patient.
  Regardless of the anesthetics employed, maintenance of normal hemodynamics is important to the avoidance of myocardial ischemia in patients with coronary artery disease[4,5,6,7].

Information to Patients: Isoflurane, as well as other general anesthetics, may cause a slight decrease in intellectual function for 2 or 3 days following anesthesia. As with other anesthetics, small changes in moods and symptoms may persist for up to 6 days after administration.

Laboratory Tests: Transient increases in BSP retention, blood glucose and serum creatinine with decrease in BUN, serum cholesterol and alkaline phosphatase have been observed.

Drug Interactions: Isoflurane potentiates the muscle relaxant effect of all muscle relaxants, most notably nondepolarizing muscle relaxants, and MAC (minimum alveolar concentration) is reduced by concomitant administration of N_2O. See "Clinical Pharmacology".

Carcinogenesis: Swiss ICR mice were given Isoflurane to determine whether such exposure might induce neoplasia. Isoflurane was given at 1/2, 1/8 and 1/32 MAC for four in-utero exposures and for 24 exposures to the pups during the first nine weeks of life. The mice were killed at 15 months of age. The incidence of tumors in these mice was the same as in untreated control mice which were given the same background gases, but not the anesthetic.

Pregnancy Category C: Isoflurane has been shown to have a possible anesthetic-related fetotoxic effect in mice when given in doses 6 times the human dose. There are no adequate and well-controlled studies in pregnant women. Isoflurane

should be used during pregnancy only if the potential benefit justifies the potential risk to the fetus.

Nursing Mothers: It is not known whether this drug is excreted in human milk. Because many drugs are excreted in human milk, caution should be exercised when Isoflurane is administered to a nursing woman.

Malignant Hyperthermia: In susceptible individuals, Isoflurane anesthesia may trigger a skeletal muscle hypermetabolic state leading to high oxygen demand and the clinical syndrome known as malignant hyperthermia. The syndrome includes nonspecific features such as muscle rigidity, tachycardia, tachypnea, cyanosis, arrhythmias, and unstable blood pressure. (It should also be noted that many of these nonspecific signs may appear with light anesthesia, acute hypoxia, etc.) An increase in overall metabolism may be reflected in an elevated temperature, (which may rise rapidly early or late in the case, but usually is not the first sign of augmented metabolism) and an increased usage of the CO_2 absorption system (hot canister). PaO_2 and pH may decrease, and hyperkalemia and a base deficit may appear. Treatment includes discontinuance of triggering agents (e.g., Isoflurane), administration of intravenous dantrolene sodium, and application of supportive therapy. Such therapy includes vigorous efforts to restore body temperature to normal, respiratory and circulatory support as indicated, and management of electrolyte-fluid-acid-base derangements. (Consult prescribing information for dantrolene sodium intravenous for additional information on patient management.) Renal failure may appear later, and urine flow should be sustained if possible.

ADVERSE REACTIONS
Adverse reactions encountered in the administration of Isoflurane are in general dose dependent extensions of pharmacophysiologic effects and include respiratory depression, hypotension and arrhythmias.
  Shivering, nausea, vomiting and ileus have been observed in the postoperative period.
  As with all other general anesthetics, transient elevations in white blood count have been observed even in the absence of surgical stress. See "Precautions" for information regarding malignant hyperthemia.
  During marketing, there have been rare reports of mild, moderate and severe (some fatal) postoperative hepatic dysfunction. The causal relationship is unknown.

OVERDOSAGE
In the event of overdosage, or what may appear to be overdosage, the following action should be taken:
  Stop drug administration, establish a clear airway, and initiate assisted or controlled ventilation with pure oxygen.

DOSAGE AND ADMINISTRATION
Premedication: Premedication should be selected according to the need of the individual patient, taking into account that secretions are weakly stimulated by Isoflurane and the heart rate tends to be increased. The use of anticholinergic drugs is a matter of choice.

Inspired Concentration: The concentration of Isoflurane being delivered from a vaporizer during anesthesia should be known. This may be accomplished by using:
  a) vaporizers calibrated specifically for Isoflurane:
  b) vaporizers from which delivered flows can be calculated, such as vaporizers delivering a saturated vapor which is then diluted. The delivered concentration from such a vaporizer may be calculated using the formula:

$$\% \text{ Isoflurane} = \frac{100 \, P_V \, F_V}{F_T \, (P_A - P_V)}$$

where:
  P_A = Pressure of atmosphere
  P_V = Vapor pressure of Isoflurane
  F_V = Flow of gas through vaporizer (mL/min)
  F_T = Total gas flow (mL/min)

Isoflurane contains no stabilizer. Nothing in the agent alters calibration or operation of these vaporizers.

Induction: Induction with Isoflurance in oxygen or in combination with oxygen-nitrous oxide mixtures may produce coughing, breath holding, or laryngospasm. These difficulties may be avoided by the use of a hypnotic dose of an ultra-short-acting barbiturate. Inspired concentrations of 1.5 to 3.0% Isoflurance usually produce surgical anesthesia in 7 to 10 minutes.

Maintenance: Surgical levels of anesthesia may be sustained with a 1.0 to 2.5% concentration when nitrous oxide is used concomitantly. An additional 0.5 to 1.0% may be required when Isoflurane is given using oxygen alone. If added relaxation is required, supplemental doses of muscle relaxants may be used.
  The level of blood pressure during maintenance is an inverse function of Isoflurane concentration in the absence of other complicating problems. Excessive decreases may be due to depth of anesthesia and in such instances may be corrected by lightening anesthesia.

Storage: Store at room temperature 15° - 30°C (59° - 86°F). Isoflurane contains no additives and has been demonstrated to be stable at room temperature for periods in excess of five years.

REFERENCES
1. JC Sill, et al, Anesthesiology 66:273-279, 1987. 2. RF Hickey, et al, Anesthesiology 68:21-30, 1988. 3. CW Buffington, et al, Anesthesiology 66:280-292, 1987. 4. S Reis, et al, Anesthesiology 59:91-97, 1983 5. S Slogoff and AS Keats, Anesthesiology 70:179-

188, 1989. 6. KJ Tuman, et al, Anesthesiology 70:189-198, 1989. 7. DT Mangano, Editorial Views, Anesthesiology 70:175-178, 1989.

HOW SUPPLIED
LIQUID:

BRAND/MANUFACTURER	NDC	SIZE	AWP
○ **BRAND**			
FORANE: Ohmeda	10019-0360-40	100 ml	$96.00
○ **GENERICS**			
Abbott Hosp	00074-3292-01	100 ml	$123.29

Isoflurophate

DESCRIPTION
Isoflurophate is available as 0.025% sterile ophthalmic ointment. Isoflurophate has a molecular weight of 184.15 and is known chemically as bis (1-methylethyl) phosphorofluoridate. Its empirical formula is $C_6H_{14}FO_3P$.

Following is its chemical structure:

$$(CH_3)_2CHO-\overset{\overset{\displaystyle F}{|}}{\underset{\underset{\displaystyle O}{||}}{P}}-OCH(CH_3)_2$$

CLINICAL PHARMACOLOGY
Isoflurophate is a cholinesterase inhibitor with sustained activity. Application to the eye produces intense miosis and ciliary muscle contraction due to inhibition of cholinesterase, allowing acetylcholine to accumulate at sites of cholinergic transmission.

Isoflurophate *irreversibly* inactivates cholinesterase. Thus, following use of Isoflurophate in the eye, cholinesterase must be either regenerated or supplied from depots elsewhere in the body before ophthalmic action dependent on cholinesterase returns.

If given systemically in sufficient amounts, Isoflurophate reduces plasma cholinesterase to zero. However, when applied locally to the eye, plasma cholinesterase is usually reduced only slightly.

INDICATIONS AND USAGE
Open-angle glaucoma (Isoflurophate should be used in glaucoma only when shorter-acting miotics have proven inadequate.)
Conditions obstructing aqueous outflow, such as synechial formation, that are amenable to miotic therapy
Following iridectomy
Accommodative esotropia (accommodative convergent strabismus)

CONTRAINDICATIONS
Hypersensitivity to any component of this product.

Because of the toxicity of cholinesterase inhibitors in general, Isoflurophate is contraindicated in women who are or who may become pregnant. If this drug is used during pregnancy, or if the patient becomes pregnant while taking this drug, the patient should be apprised of the potential hazard to the fetus.

Because miotics may aggravate inflammation, Isoflurophate should not be used in active uveal inflammation and/or glaucoma associated with iridocyclitis.

WARNINGS
In patients receiving cholinesterase inhibitors such as Isoflurophate, succinylcholine should be administered with extreme caution before and during general anesthesia because of possible respiratory and cardiovascular collapse.

Because of possible adverse additive effects, Isoflurophate should be administered only with extreme caution to patients with myasthenia gravis who are receiving systemic anticholinesterase therapy; conversely, extreme caution should be exercised in the use of an anticholinesterase drug for the treatment of myasthenia gravis patients who are already undergoing topical therapy with cholinesterase inhibitors.

PRECAUTIONS
GENERAL
Isoflurophate should be used with caution in patients with chronic angle-closure (narrow-angle) glaucoma or in patients with narrow angles, because of the possibility of producing pupillary block and increasing angle blockage.

Gonioscopy is recommended prior to medication with Isoflurophate.

When an intraocular inflammatory process is present, the intensity and persistence of miosis and ciliary muscle contraction that result from anticholinesterase therapy require abstention from, or cautious use of Isoflurophate.

Systemic effects are infrequent when Isoflurophate is applied carefully. The hands should be washed immediately following application.

Discontinue Isoflurophate if salivation, urinary incontinence, diarrhea, profuse sweating, muscle weakness, respiratory difficulties, shock, or cardiac irregularities occur.

Persons receiving cholinesterase inhibitors who are exposed to organophosphate-type insecticides and pesticides (gardeners, organophosphate plant or warehouse workers, farmers, residents of communities which are undergoing insecticide spraying or dusting, etc.) should be warned of the added systemic effects possible from absorption through the respiratory tract or skin. Wearing of respiratory masks, frequent washing, and clothing changes may be advisable.

Anticholinesterase drugs should be used with extreme caution, if at all, in patients with marked vagotonia, bronchial asthma, spastic gastrointestinal disturbances, peptic ulcer, pronounced bradycardia and hypotension, recent myocardial infarction, epilepsy, parkinsonism, and other disorders that may respond adversely to vagotonic effects.

After long-term use of Isoflurophate, dilation of blood vessels and resulting greater permeability increase the possibility of hyphema during ophthalmic surgery. Therefore, this drug should be discontinued before surgery.

Despite observance of all precautions and the use of only the recommended dose, there is some evidence that repeated administration may cause depression of the concentration of cholinesterase in the serum and erythrocytes, with resultant systemic effects.

There have been reports of bacterial keratitis associated with the use of multiple dose containers of topical ophthalmic products. These containers had been inadvertently contaminated by patients who, in most cases, had a concurrent corneal disease or a disruption of the ocular epithelial surface. (See *"Precautions, Information for Patients"*.)

INFORMATION FOR PATIENTS
Patients should be instructed to avoid allowing the tip of the dispensing container to contact the eye or surrounding structures.

Patients should also be instructed that ocular preparations, if handled improperly, can become contaminated by common bacteria known to cause ocular infections. Serious damage to the eye and subsequent loss of vision may result from using contaminated preparations. (See *"Precautions, General."*) Patients should also be advised that if they develop an intercurrent ocular condition (e.g., trauma, ocular surgery or infection), they should immediately seek their physician's advice concerning the continued use of the present multidose container.

DRUG INTERACTIONS
See *"Warnings"* regarding possible drug interactions of Isoflurophate with succinylcholine or with other anticholinesterase agents.

CARCINOGENESIS, MUTAGENESIS, IMPAIRMENT OF FERTILITY
Long-term studies in animals have not been performed to evaluate the effects of Isoflurophate on fertility or carcinogenic potential.

PREGNANCY
Pregnancy Category X: See *"Contraindications."*

NURSING MOTHERS
It is not known whether this drug is excreted in human milk. Because of the potential for serious adverse reactions in nursing infants from Isoflurophate, a decision should be made whether to discontinue nursing or to discontinue the drug, taking into account the importance of the drug to the mother.

PEDIATRIC USE
The occurrence of iris cysts is more frequent in children. (See *"Adverse Reactions"* and *"Dosage and Administration."*)

Extreme caution should be exercised in children receiving Isofluro- phate who may require general anesthesia (see *"Warnings"*).

Since Isoflurophate is a potent cholinesterase inhibitor it should be kept out of the reach of children.

ADVERSE REACTIONS
Stinging, burning, lacrimation, lid muscle twitching, conjunctival and ciliary redness, brow ache, headache, and induced myopia with visual blurring may occur.

As with all miotic therapy, retinal detachment has been reported occasionally.
Activation of latent iritis or uveitis may occur.

Iris cysts may form, enlarge, and obscure vision. Occurrence is more frequent in children. The iris cyst usually shrinks upon discontinuance of the miotic. Rarely, the cyst may rupture or break free into the aqueous. Frequent examination for this occurrence is advised.

Prolonged use may cause conjunctival thickening and obstruction of nasolacrimal canals.

Systemic effects, which occur rarely, are suggestive of increased cholinergic activity. Such effects may include nausea, vomiting, abdominal cramps, diarrhea, urinary incontinence, salivation, sweating, difficulty in breathing, bradycardia, or cardiac irregularities. Medical management of systemic effects may be indicated (see *"Treatment of Adverse Effects"*).

Lens opacities have been reported in patients on miotic therapy. Routine slit-lamp examinations, including the lens, should accompany prolonged use.

Paradoxical increase in intraocular pressure may follow anticholinesterase application. This may be alleviated by pupil-dilating medication.

TREATMENT OF ADVERSE EFFECTS
If Isoflurophate is taken systemically by accident, or if systemic effects occur after topical application in the eye or from accidental skin contact, atropine sulfate in a dose (for adults) of 0.4 to 0.6 mg or more should be given parenterally (intravenously if necessary). The recommended dosage of atropine in infants and children up to 12 years of age is 0.01 mg/kg repeated every two hours as needed until the desired effect is obtained, or adverse effects of atropine preclude further usage. The maximum single dose should not exceed 0.4 mg.

The use of much larger doses of atropine in treating anticholinesterase intoxication in adults has been reported in the literature. Initially 2 to 6 mg may be given followed by 2 mg every hour or more often, as long as muscarinic effects

---

continue. The greater possibility of atropinization with large doses, particularly in sensitive individuals, should be borne in mind.

Pralidoxime chloride has been reported to be useful in treatment of systemic effects due to cholinesterase inhibitors. However, its use is recommended in addition to and not as a substitute for atropine.

A short-acting barbiturate is indicated if convulsions occur that are not entirely relieved by atropine. Barbiturate dosage should be carefully adjusted to avoid central respiratory depression. Marked weakness or paralysis of muscles of respiration should be treated promptly by artificial respiration and maintenance of a clear airway.

The oral LD_{50} of Isoflurophate is 37 mg/kg in the mouse, 5—10 mg/kg in the rat, and 4—10 mg/kg in the rabbit.

DOSAGE AND ADMINISTRATION

Isoflurophate *is intended solely for topical use in the conjunctival sac.*

Isoflurophate hydrolyzes in the presence of water to form hydrofluoric acid. To prevent absorption of moisture and loss of potency, the ointment tube should be kept tightly closed; the tip of the tube should not be washed or allowed to touch the eyelid or other moist surface.

Whenever possible, Isoflurophate should be applied at night before retiring to lessen blurring of vision. As it is an extremely potent drug, it should be used with great care and only by those familiar with its use and thoroughly indoctrinated in the technic of application.

The required dose is applied in the conjunctival sac, with the patient supine, care being taken not to touch the cornea with the tip of the tube. *Wash the hands immediately after administration.*

Isoflurophate *should not be used more often than directed. Caution is necessary to avoid overdosage.*

Keep frequency of use to a minimum in all patients, but especially in children, to reduce the chance of iris cyst development (see *"Adverse Reactions"*). If tolerance develops, another miotic should be used. Isoflurophate may be resumed later.

GLAUCOMA

For initial therapy 1/4 inch strip of ophthalmic ointment Isoflurophate 0.025 per cent is placed in the glaucomatous eye every 8 to 72 hours. A decrease in intraocular pressure should occur within a few hours. During this period, keep the patient under supervision and make tonometric examinations at least hourly for 3 or 4 hours to be sure that no immediate rise in pressure occurs (see *"Adverse Reactions"*).

STRABISMUS

Essentially equal visual acuity of both eyes is a prerequisite to successful treatment. For initial evaluation Isoflurophate may be used as a diagnostic aid to determine if an accommodative factor exists. This is especially useful preoperatively in young children and in patients with normal hypermetropic refractive errors. Not more than 1/4 inch strip of ointment is administered every night for 2 weeks. If the eyes become straighter, an accommodative factor is demonstrated. This technic may supplement or complement standard testing with atropine and trial with glasses for the accommodative factor.

In esotropia uncomplicated by amblyopia or anisometropia, ophthalmic ointment Isoflurophate may be used in both eyes, not more than 1/4 inch strip at a time every night for 2 weeks, as too severe a degree of miosis may interfere with vision. The dosage is then reduced from 1/4 inch strip every other day to 1/4 inch strip once a week for 2 months, after which the patient's status should be reevaluated.

If benefit can not be maintained with a dosage interval of at least 48 hours, therapy with Isoflurophate should be stopped. Frequency of administration and duration of maintenance therapy depend on how long the eyes remain straight without medication. Intervals between administration should be gradually increased to the greatest length compatible with good results. Therapy may need to be continued for many years in some patients; in others, it has been possible to discontinue therapy after several months.

STORAGE

Protect from moisture, freezing and excessive heat.

HOW SUPPLIED
OINTMENT: 0.025%

BRAND/MANUFACTURER	NDC	SIZE	AWP
○ **BRAND**			
FLOROPRYL: Merck	00006-7742-04	3.5 gm	$8.14

Isolyte *SEE DEXTROSE AND ELECTROLYTES AND ELECTROLYTES, INJECTABLE*

Isoniazid

MANY MONTHS OF TREATMENT. THIS RISK OF DEVELOPING HEPATITIS IS AGE RELATED. APPROXIMATE CASE RATES BY AGE ARE: 0 PER 1,000 FOR PERSONS UNDER 20 YEARS OF AGE, 3 PER 1,000 FOR PERSONS IN THE 20 TO 34 YEAR AGE GROUP, 12 PER 1,000 FOR PERSONS IN THE 35 TO 49 YEAR AGE GROUP, 23 PER 1,000 FOR PERSONS IN THE 50 TO 64 YEAR AGE GROUP, AND 8 PER 1,000 FOR PERSONS OVER 65 YEARS OF AGE. THIS RISK OF HEPATITIS IS INCREASED WITH DAILY CONSUMPTION OF ALCOHOL. PRECISE DATA TO PROVIDE A FATALITY RATE FOR ISONIAZID-RELATED HEPATITIS IS NOT AVAILABLE; HOWEVER, IN A US PUBLIC HEALTH SERVICE SURVEILLANCE STUDY OF 13,838 PERSONS TAKING ISONIAZID, THERE WERE 8 DEATHS AMONG 174 CASES OF HEPATITIS.

THEREFORE, PATIENTS GIVEN ISONIAZID SHOULD BE CAREFULLY MONITORED AND INTERVIEWED AT MONTHLY INTERVALS. SERUM TRANSAMINASE CONCENTRATION BECOMES ELEVATED IN ABOUT 10 TO 20 PERCENT OF PATIENTS, USUALLY DURING THE FIRST FEW MONTHS OF THERAPY BUT IT CAN OCCUR AT ANY TIME. USUALLY ENZYME LEVELS RETURN TO NORMAL DESPITE CONTINUANCE OF DRUG BUT IN SOME CASES PROGRESSIVE LIVER DYSFUNCTION OCCURS. PATIENTS SHOULD BE INSTRUCTED TO REPORT IMMEDIATELY ANY OF THE PRODROMAL SYMPTOMS OF HEPATITIS, SUCH AS FATIGUE, WEAKNESS, MALAISE, ANOREXIA, NAUSEA, OR VOMITING. IF THESE SYMPTOMS APPEAR OR IF SIGNS SUGGESTIVE OF HEPATIC DAMAGE ARE DETECTED, ISONIAZID SHOULD BE DISCONTINUED PROMPTLY, SINCE CONTINUED USE OF THE DRUG IN THESE CASES HAS BEEN REPORTED TO CAUSE A MORE SEVERE FORM OF LIVER DAMAGE.

PATIENTS WITH TUBERCULOSIS SHOULD BE GIVEN APPROPRIATE TREATMENT WITH ALTERNATIVE DRUGS. IF ISONIAZID MUST BE REINSTITUTED, IT SHOULD BE REINSTITUTED ONLY AFTER SYMPTOMS AND LABORATORY ABNORMALITIES HAVE CLEARED. THE DRUG SHOULD BE RESTARTED IN VERY SMALL AND GRADUALLY INCREASING DOSES AND SHOULD BE WITHDRAWN IMMEDIATELY IF THERE IS ANY INDICATION OF RECURRENT LIVER INVOLVEMENT. PREVENTIVE TREATMENT SHOULD BE DEFERRED IN PERSONS WITH ACUTE HEPATIC DISEASES.

DESCRIPTION

Isoniazid is the hydrazide of isonicotinic acid available as tablets or injection. Each tablet contains 50, 100, or 300 mg Isoniazid. Isoniazid injection provides 100 mg Isoniazid per ml.

Ioniazid 4-Pyridinecarboxylic acid, hydrazide, is colorless or white crystals or white crystalline powder. It is odorless and slowly affected by exposure to air and light. It is freely soluble in water, sparingly soluble in alcohol, and slightly soluble in chloroform and in ether. Its molecular formular is $C_6H_7N_3O$ and its molecular weight 137.14.

Following is its chemical structure:

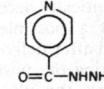

CLINICAL PHARMACOLOGY

Isoniazid acts against actively growing tubercle bacilli.

Within one to two hours after oral administration, Isoniazid produces peak blood levels which decline to 50 percent or less within six hours. It diffuses readily into all body fluids (cerebrospinal, pleural, and ascitic), tissues, organs, and excreta (saliva, sputum, and feces). The drug also passes through the placental barrier and into maternal breast milk in concentrations comparable to those in the plasma. From 50 to 70 percent of a dose of Isoniazid is excreted in the urine in 24 hours.

Isoniazid is metabolized primarily by acetylation and dehydrazination. The rate of acetylation is genetically determined. Approximately 50 percent of Blacks and Caucasians are "slow acetylators" and the rest are "rapid acetylators": the majority of Eskimos and Orientals are "rapid acetylators".

The rate of acetylation does not significantly alter the effectiveness of Isoniazid therapy when dosage is administered daily. However, slow acetylation may lead to higher blood levels of the drug and thus an increase in toxic reactions.

Pyridoxine (vitamin B_6) deficiency is sometimes observed in adults with high doses of Isoniazid and is considered probably due to its competition with pyridoxal phosphate for the enzyme apotryptophanase.

INDICATIONS AND USAGE

Isoniazid is recommended for all forms of tuberculosis in which organisms are susceptible.

Intramuscular administration is intended for use whenever administration by the oral route is not possible.

Isoniazid is recommended for preventive therapy for the following groups, in order to priority:

1. Household members and other close associates of persons with recently diagnosed tuberculous disease.

2. Positive tuberculin skin test reactors with findings on the chest roentgenogram consistent with nonprogressive tuberculous disease, in whom there are neither positive bacteriologic findings nor a history of adequate chemotherapy.

3. Newly infected person.

4. Positive tuberculin skin test reactors in the special clinical situations as follows: prolonged therapy with adrenocorticosteroids; immunosuppressive therapy; some hematologic and reticuloendothelial diseases, such as leukemia or Hodgkin's disease; diabetes mellitus; silicosis; after gastrectomy.

5. Other positive tuberculin reactors under 35 years of age. The risk of hepatitis must be weighed against the risk of tuberculosis in positive tuberculin reactors over the age of 35. However, the use of Isoniazid is recommended for those with the additional risk factors listed above (1 to 4) and on an individual basis in situations where there is likelihood of serious consequences to contacts who may become infected.

UNLABELED USES

Isoniazid is used alone or as an adjunct in the treatment of Huntington's chorea, and cerebellar tremor. It is also used in the determination of a patient's acetylator status.

CONTRAINDICATIONS

Isoniazid is contraindicated in patients who develop severe hypersensitivity reactions, including drug-induced hepatitis. Previous Isoniazid-associated hepatic injury: severe adverse reactions to Isoniazid, such as drug fever, chills, and arthritis; acute liver disease of any etiology.

WARNINGS

See the boxed *"Warnings"*.

PRECAUTIONS

All drugs should be stopped and an evaluation made at the first sign of a hypersensitivity reaction. If Isoniazid therapy must be reinstituted, the drug should be given only after symptoms have cleared. The drug should be restarted in very small and gradually increasing doses and should be withdrawn immediately if there is any indication of recurrent hypersensitivity reaction.

Use of Isoniazid should be carefully monitored in the following:

1. Patients who are receiving phenytoin concurrently. Isoniazid may decrease the excretion of phenytoin or may enhance its effects. To avoid phenytoin intoxication, appropriate dosage adjustment of the anticonvulsant should be made.

2. Daily users of alcohol. Daily ingestion of alcohol may be associated with a higher incidence of Isoniazid related hepatitis.

3. Those patients with current chronic liver disease or severe renal dysfunction.

Ophthalmologic examinations (including ophthalmoscopy) should be done *before* INH is started and periodically there-after, even without occurrence of visual symptoms.

USAGE IN PREGNANCY AND LACTATION

It has been reported that in both rats and rabbits, Isoniazid may exert an embryocidal effect when administered orally during pregnancy, although no Isoniazid-related congenital anomalies have been found in reproduction studies in mammalian species (mice, rats and rabbits). Isoniazid should be prescribed during pregnancy only when therapeutically necessary. The benefit of preventive therapy should be weighed against a possible risk to the fetus. Preventive treatment generally should be started after delivery because of the increased risk of tuberculosis for new mothers during the postpartum period.

Since Isoniazid is known to cross the placental barrier and to pass into maternal breast milk, neonates and breast-fed infants of Isoniazid-treated mothers should be carefully observed for any evidence of adverse effects.

CARCINOGENESIS

Isoniazid has been reported to induce pulmonary tumors in a number of strains of mice.

ADVERSE REACTIONS

The most frequent reactions are those affecting the nervous system and the liver.

Nervous system: Peripheral neuropathy is the most common toxic effect. It is dose related, occurs most often in the malnourished and in those predisposed to neuritis (e.g., alcoholics and diabetics), and is usually preceded by paresthesias of the feet and hands. The incidence is higher in "slow acetylators."

Other neurotoxic effects which are uncommon with conventional doses are convulsions, toxic encephalopathy, optic neuritis and atrophy, memory impairment, and toxic psychosis.

Gastrointestinal: Nausea, vomiting, and epigastric distress.

Hepatic: Elevated serum transaminases (SGOT, SGPT), bilirubinemia, bilirubinuria, jaundice, and occasionally severe and sometimes fatal hepatitis. The common prodromal symptoms are anorexia, nausea, vomiting, fatigue, malaise, and weakness. Mild and transient elevation of serum transaminase levels occurs in 10 to 20 percent of persons taking Isoniazid. The abnormality usually occurs in the first four to six months of treatment but can occur at any time during therapy. In most instances, enzyme levels return to normal without need to discontinue medication. In occasional instances, progressive liver damage occurs with accompanying symptoms. In these cases, the drug should be discontinued immediately. The frequency of progressive liver damage increases with age. It is rare in individuals under 20, but occurs in up to 2.3 percent of those over 50 years of age.

Hematologic: Agranulocytosis; hemolytic, sideroblastic, or aplastic anemia; thrombocytopenia; and eosinophila.

Hypersensitivity: Fever, skin eruptions (morbilliform, maculopapular, purpuric, or exfoliative), lymphadenopathy, and vasculitis.

Metabolic and Endocrine: Pyridoxine deficiency, pellagra, hyperglycemia, metabolic acidosis, and gynecomastia.

Miscellaneous: Rheumatic syndrome and systemic lupus erythematosus-like syndrome. Local irritation has been observed at the site of intramuscular injection.

OVERDOSAGE

SIGNS AND SYMPTOMS

Isoniazid overdosage produces signs and symptoms within 30 minutes to three hours after ingestion. Nausea, vomiting, dizziness, slurring of speech, blurring of vision, and visual hallucinations (including bright colors and strange designs) are among the early manifestations. With marked overdosage, respiratory distress and CNS depression, progressing rapidly from stupor to profound coma, are to be expected, along with severe, intractable seizures. Severe metabolic acidosis, acetonuria, and hyperglycemia are typical laboratory findings.

TREATMENT

Untreated or inadequately treated cases of gross Isoniazid overdosage can terminate fatally, but good response has been reported in most patients brought under adequate treatment within the first few hours after drug ingestion. Secure the airway and establish adequate respiratory exchange. Gastric lavage within the first 2 to 3 hours is advised, but should not be attempted until convulsions are under control. To control convulsions, administer I.V. short-acting barbiturates and I.V. pyridoxine (usually 1 mg/mg Isoniazid ingested).

Obtain blood samples for immediate determination of gases, electrolytes, BUN, glucose, etc.; type and crossmatch blood in preparation for possible hemodialysis.

Rapid control of metabolic acidosis is fundamental to management. Give I.V. sodium bicarbonate at once and repeat as needed, adjusting subsequent dosage on the basis of laboratory findings (i.e., serum sodium, pH, etc.).

Forced osmotic diuresis must be started early and should be continued for some hours after clinical improvement to hasten renal clearance of the drug and help prevent relapse. Fluid intake and output should be monitored.

Hemodialysis is advised for severe cases; if this is not available, peritoneal dialysis can be used along with forced diuresis.

Along with measures based on initial and repeated determination of blood gases and other laboratory tests as needed, meticulous respiratory and other intensive care should be utilized to protect against hypoxia, hypotension, aspiration pneumonitis, etc.

DOSAGE AND ADMINISTRATION

Note: For preventive therapy of tuberculous infection it is recommended that physicians be familiar with the joint recommendations of the American Thoracic Society, American Lung Association, and the Centers for Disease Control, as published in the American Review of Respiratory Disease, Vol. 110, No. 3, September, 1974, or CDC's Morbidity and Mortality Weekly Report, Vol. 24, No. 8, February 22, 1975.

FOR TREATMENT OF ACTIVE TUBERCULOSIS

Isoniazid is used in conjunction with other effective antituberculous agents. If the bacilli become resistant, therapy must be changed to agents to which the bacilli are susceptible.

USUAL DOSAGE

Adults: 5 mg/kg up to 300 mg daily in a single dose.

Infants and Children: 10 to 20 mg/kg depending on severity of infection (up to 300 to 500 mg daily) in a single dose.

FOR PREVENTIVE THERAPY

Adults: 300 mg per day in a single dose.

Infants and Children: 10 mg/kg (up to 300 mg daily) in a single dose.

Continuous administration of Isoniazid for a sufficient period of time is an essential part of the regimen because relapse rates are higher if chemotherapy is stopped prematurely. In the treatment of tuberculosis, resistant organisms may multiply and their emergence during the treatment may necessitate a change in the regimen.

Concomitant administration of pyridoxine (vitamin B_6) is recommended in the malnourished and in those predisposed to neuropathy (e.g., alcoholics and diabetics).

STORAGE

Store tablets at controlled room temperature, 15°-30°C (59°-86°F).

Store injection at room temperature. Protect from light and moisture. Isoniazid injection may crystallize at low temperatures. If this occurs, warm the vial to room temperature before use to redissolve the crystals.

HOW SUPPLIED

INJECTION: 100 MG/ML

BRAND/MANUFACTURER	NDC	SIZE	AWP
○ BRAND			
NYDRAZID: Apothecon	00003-0643-50	10 ml	$15.22

◆ RATED THERAPEUTICALLY EQUIVALENT; ◇ THERAPEUTIC EQUIVALENCE UNCONFIRMED; ○ UNRATED

SYRUP:

BRAND/MANUFACTURER	NDC	SIZE	AWP
◆ GENERICS			
Carolina	46287-0009-01	480 ml	$16.90

TABLETS: 100 MG

AVERAGE UNIT PRICE (AVAILABLE SIZES)		GENERIC A-RATED AVERAGE PRICE (GAAP)	
GENERIC	$0.05	100s	$5.63
HCFA FUL (100s ea)	$0.05	1000s	$32.20

BRAND/MANUFACTURER	NDC	SIZE	AWP
◆ GENERICS			
Eon	00185-4351-30	30s	$1.95
Richlyn	00115-3706-01	100s	$2.14
West-Ward	00143-1260-01	100s	$2.50
	00574-0100-01	100s	$3.90
Eon	00185-4351-01	100s	$4.00
▶ Barr	00555-0066-02	100s	$5.16
Rugby	00536-3948-01	100s	$5.61
Major	00904-2095-60	100s	$5.70
Goldline	00182-0559-01	100s	$5.85
Aligen	00405-4552-01	100s	$5.92
Dixon-Shane	17236-0180-01	100s	$6.60
Halsey Pharm	00879-0113-01	100s	$6.60
U.S. Trading	56126-0264-11	100s ud	$6.45
UDL	51079-0082-20	100s ud	$9.39
Raway	00686-0082-20	100s ud	$9.95
West-Ward	00143-1260-10	1000s	$11.00
Richlyn	00115-3706-03	1000s	$16.50
Qualitest	00603-4093-32	1000s	$22.10
Eon	00185-4351-10	1000s	$23.50
Barr	00555-0066-05	1000s	$28.73
Rugby	00536-3948-10	1000s	$30.83
Major	00904-2095-80	1000s	$32.20
Halsey Pharm	00879-0113-10	1000s	$57.65
Schein	00364-0150-02	1000s	$67.30

TABLETS: 300 MG

AVERAGE UNIT PRICE (AVAILABLE SIZES)		GENERIC A-RATED AVERAGE PRICE (GAAP)	
GENERIC	$0.09	30s	$3.91
HCFA FUL (100s ea)	$0.06	35s	$4.33
		100s	$8.23
		1000s	$60.36

BRAND/MANUFACTURER	NDC	SIZE	AWP
◆ GENERICS			
Major	00904-2096-46	30s	$1.95
Dixon-Shane	17236-0182-30	30s	$2.90
Eon	00185-4350-30	30s	$2.95
Medirex	57480-0495-06	30s	$3.44
	00574-0300-03	30s	$3.50
Duramed	51285-0277-30	30s	$5.20
Barr	00555-0071-01	30s	$7.45
Dixon-Shane	17236-0182-35	35s	$3.10
Halsey Pharm	00879-0341-35	35s	$5.55
West-Ward	00143-1261-01	100s	$3.50
Eon	00185-4350-01	100s	$5.75
Dixon-Shane	17236-0182-01	100s	$7.00
Halsey Pharm	00879-0341-01	100s	$8.00
Duramed	51285-0277-02	100s	$8.02
Aligen	00405-4553-01	100s	$8.43
Barr	00555-0071-02	100s	$8.55
Rugby	00536-3941-01	100s	$8.58
Major	00904-2096-60	100s	$8.70
Goldline	00182-1356-01	100s	$9.00
Schein	00364-0151-01	100s	$10.46
UDL	51079-0083-40	100s	$10.49
Major	00904-2096-61	100s ud	$4.66
U.S. Trading	56126-0265-11	100s ud	$5.21
Raway	00686-0083-20	100s ud	$11.00
UDL	51079-0083-20	100s ud	$11.19
Medirex	57480-0495-01	100s ud	$11.45
Schein	00364-0151-05	500s	$40.40
West-Ward	00143-1261-10	1000s	$21.00
Eon	00185-4350-10	1000s	$49.95
Goldline	00182-1356-10	1000s	$68.00
Rugby	00536-3941-10	1000s	$68.07
Halsey Pharm	00879-0341-10	1000s	$68.55
Barr	00555-0071-05	1000s	$68.65
Duramed	51285-0277-05	1000s	$68.72
Major	00904-2096-80	1000s	$69.90

Isoniazid and Rifampin

WARNING

SEVERE AND SOMETIMES FATAL HEPATITIS ASSOCIATED WITH ISONIAZID THERAPY MAY OCCUR AND MAY DEVELOP EVEN AFTER MANY MONTHS OF TREATMENT. THE RISK OF DEVELOPING HEPATITIS IS AGE RELATED. APPROXIMATE CASE RATES BY AGE ARE: 0 PER 1,000 FOR PERSONS UNDER 20 YEARS OF AGE, 3 PER 1,000 FOR PERSONS IN THE 20-34 YEAR AGE GROUP, 12 PER 1,000 FOR PERSONS IN THE 35-49 YEAR AGE GROUP, 23 PER 1,000 FOR PERSONS IN THE 50-64 YEAR AGE GROUP, AND 8 PER 1,000 FOR PERSONS OVER 65 YEARS OF AGE. THE RISK OF HEPATITIS IS INCREASED WITH DAILY CONSUMPTION OF ALCOHOL. PRECISE DATA TO PROVIDE A FATALITY RATE FOR ISONIAZID-RELATED HEPATITIS IS NOT AVAILABLE; HOWEVER, IN A U.S. PUBLIC HEALTH SERVICE SURVEILLANCE STUDY OF 13,838 PERSONS TAKING ISONIAZID, THERE WERE 8 DEATHS AMONG 174 CASES OF HEPATITIS. THEREFORE, PATIENTS GIVEN ISONIAZID SHOULD BE CAREFULLY MONITORED AND INTERVIEWED AT MONTHLY INTERVALS. SERUM TRANSAMINASE CONCENTRATION BECOMES ELEVATED IN ABOUT 10-20 PERCENT OF PATIENTS, USUALLY DURING THE FIRST FEW MONTHS OF THERAPY, BUT IT CAN OCCUR AT ANY TIME. USUALLY ENZYME LEVELS RETURN TO NORMAL DESPITE CONTINUANCE OF DRUG BUT IN SOME CASES PROGRESSIVE LIVER DYSFUNCTION OCCURS. PATIENTS SHOULD BE INSTRUCTED TO REPORT IMMEDIATELY ANY OF THE PRODROMAL SYMPTOMS OF HEPATITIS, SUCH AS FATIGUE, WEAKNESS, MALAISE, ANOREXIA, NAUSEA, OR VOMITING. IF THESE SYMPTOMS APPEAR OR IF SIGNS SUGGESTIVE OF HEPATIC DAMAGE ARE DETECTED, ISONIAZID SHOULD BE DISCONTINUED PROMPTLY, SINCE CONTINUED USE OF THE DRUG IN THESE CASES HAS BEEN REPORTED TO CAUSE A MORE SEVERE FORM OF LIVER DAMAGE.

PATIENTS WITH TUBERCULOSIS SHOULD BE GIVEN APPROPRIATE TREATMENT WITH ALTERNATIVE DRUGS. IF ISONIAZID MUST BE REINSTITUTED, IT SHOULD BE REINSTITUTED ONLY AFTER SYMPTOMS AND LABORATORY ABNORMALITIES HAVE CLEARED. THE DRUG SHOULD BE RESTARTED IN VERY SMALL AND GRADUALLY INCREASING DOSES AND SHOULD BE WITHDRAWN IMMEDIATELY IF THERE IS ANY INDICATION OF RECURRENT LIVER INVOLVEMENT. TREATMENT SHOULD BE DEFERRED IN PERSONS WITH ACUTE HEPATIC DISEASES.

DESCRIPTION

Each capsule contains 300 mg Rifampin and 150 mg Isoniazid.

Rifampin is a semisynthetic antibiotic derivative of rifamycin B. The chemical name for Rifampin is 3-(4-methyl-1-piperazinyl-iminomethyl) rifamycin SV.

Isoniazid is the hydrazide of isonicotinic acid. It exists as colorless or white crystals or as a white, crystalline powder that is water soluble, odorless, and slowly affected by exposure to air and light.

ACTIONS

RIFAMPIN

Rifampin inhibits DNA-dependent RNA polymerase activity in susceptible cells. Specifically, it interacts with bacterial RNA polymerase but does not inhibit the mammalian enzyme. This is the mechanism of action by which Rifampin exerts its therapeutic effect. Rifampin cross resistance has only been shown with other rifamycins.

In a study of 14 normal human adult males, peak blood levels of Rifampin occurred 1½ to 3 hours following oral administration of two Isoniazid/Rifampin capsules. The peaks ranged from 6.9 to 14 mcg/ml with an average of 10 mcg/mL.

In normal subjects the T½ (biological half-life) of Rifampin in blood is approximately 3 hours. Elimination occurs mainly through the bile and, to a much lesser extent, the urine.

ISONIAZID

Isoniazid acts against actively growing tubercle bacilli.

After oral administration Isoniazid produces peak blood levels within 1 to 2 hours which decline to 50% or less within 6 hours. It diffuses readily into all body fluids (cerebrospinal, pleural, and ascitic fluids), tissues, organs and excreta (saliva, sputum, and feces). The drug also passes through the placental barrier and into milk in concentrations comparable to those in the plasma. From 50 to 70% of a dose of Isoniazid is excreted in the urine in 24 hours.

Isoniazid is metabolized primarily by acetylation and dehydrazination. The rate of acetylation is genetically determined. Approximately 50% of Blacks and Caucasians are "slow inactivators"; the majority of Eskimos and Orientals are "rapid inactivators."

The rate of acetylation does not significantly alter the effectiveness of Isoniazid. However, slow acetylation may lead to higher blood levels of the drug, and thus an increase in toxic reactions.

Pyridoxine deficiency (B_6) is sometimes observed in adults with high doses of Isoniazid and is considered probably due to its competition with pyridoxal phosphate for the enzyme apotryptophanase.

INDICATIONS

For pulmonary tuberculosis in which organisms are susceptible, and when the patient has been titrated on the individual components and it has therefore been established that this fixed dosage is therapeutically effective.

This fixed-dosage combination drug is not recommended for initial therapy of tuberculosis or for preventive therapy.

▶ SHOWN IN PRODUCT IDENTIFICATION GUIDE

In the treatment of tuberculosis, small numbers of resistant cells, present within large populations of susceptible cells, can rapidly become the predominating type. Since rapid emergence of resistance can occur, culture and susceptibility tests should be performed in the event of persistent positive cultures.

This drug is *not* indicated for the treatment of meningococcal infections or asymptomatic carriers of *N. meningitidis* to eliminate meningococci from the nasopharynx.

CONTRAINDICATIONS

Previous Isoniazid-associated hepatic injury; severe adverse reactions to Isoniazid, such as drug fever, chills, and arthritis; acute liver disease of any etiology.

A history of previous hypersensitivity reaction to any of the rifamycins or to Isoniazid, including drug-induced hepatitis.

WARNINGS

Isoniazid and Rifampin have each been associated with liver dysfunction. Liver function tests should be performed prior to therapy with Isoniazid/Rifampin and periodically during treatment.

RIFAMPIN

Rifampin has been shown to produce liver dysfunction. There have been fatalities associated with jaundice in patients with liver disease or receiving Rifampin concomitantly with other hepatotoxic agents. Since an increased risk may exist for individuals with liver disease, benefits must be weighed carefully against the risk of further liver damage.

Several studies of tumorigenicity potential have been done in rodents. In one strain of mice known to be particularly susceptible to the spontaneous development of hepatomas, Rifampin given at a level 2-10 times the maximum dosage used clinically, resulted in a significant increase in the occurrence of hepatomas in female mice of this strain after one year of administration. There was no evidence of tumorigenicity in the males of this strain, in males or females of another mouse strain, or in rats.

ISONIAZID
See the boxed *"Warning"*.

PRECAUTIONS

RIFAMPIN

Rifampin is not recommended for intermittent therapy; the patient should be cautioned against intentional or accidental interruption of the daily dosage regimen since rare renal hypersensitivity reactions have been reported when therapy was resumed in such cases.

Rifampin has been observed to increase the requirements for anticoagulant drugs of the coumarin type. The cause of the phenomenon is unknown. In patients receiving anticoagulants and Rifampin concurrently, it is recommended that the prothrombin time be performed daily or as frequently as necessary to establish and maintain the required dose of anticoagulant.

Urine, feces, saliva, sputum, sweat and tears may be colored red-orange by Rifampin and its metabolites. Soft contact lenses may be permanently stained. Individuals to be treated should be made aware of these possibilities.

It has been reported that the reliability of oral contraceptives may be affected in some patients being treated for tuberculosis with Rifampin in combination with at least one other antituberculosis drug. In such cases, alternative contraceptive measures may need to be considered.

It has also been reported that Rifampin given in combination with other antituberculosis drugs may decrease the pharmacologic activity of methadone, oral hypoglycemics, digitoxin, quinidine, disopyramide, dapsone and corticosteroids. In these cases, dosage adjustment of the interacting drugs is recommended.

Therapeutic levels of Rifampin have been shown to inhibit standard microbiological assays for serum folate and vitamin B_{12}. Alternative methods must be considered when determining folate and vitamin B_{12} concentrations in the presence of Rifampin.

Since Rifampin has been reported to cross the placental barrier and appear in cord blood and in maternal milk, neonates and newborns of Rifampin treated mothers should be carefully observed for any evidence of untoward effects.

ISONIAZID

All drugs should be stopped and an evaluation of the patient should be made at the first sign of a hypersensitivity reaction.

Use of Isoniazid should be carefully monitored in the following:

1. Patients who are receiving phenytoin (diphenylhydantoin) concurrently. Isoniazid may decrease the excretion of phenytoin or may enhance its effects. To avoid phenytoin intoxication, appropriate adjustment of the anticonvulsant dose should be made.

2. Daily users of alcohol. Daily ingestion of alcohol may be associated with a higher incidence of Isoniazid hepatitis.

3. Patients with current chronic liver disease or severe renal dysfunction.

Periodic ophthalmoscopic examination during Isoniazid therapy is recommended when visual symptoms occur.

USAGE IN PREGNANCY AND LACTATION

RIFAMPIN

Although Rifampin has been reported to cross the placental barrier and appear in cord blood, the effect of Rifampin, alone or in combination with other antituberculosis drugs, on the human fetus is not known. An increase in congenital malformations, primarily spina bifida and cleft palate, has been reported in the offspring of rodents given oral doses of 150-250 mg/kg/day of Rifampin during pregnancy.

The possible teratogenic potential in women capable of bearing children should be carefully weighed against the benefits of therapy.

ISONIAZID

It has been reported that in both rats and rabbits, Isoniazid may exert an embryocidal effect when administered orally during pregnancy, although no Isoniazid-related congenital anomalies have been found in reproduction studies in mammalian species (mice, rats, and rabbits). Isoniazid should be prescribed during pregnancy only when therapeutically necessary. The benefit of preventive therapy should be weighed against a possible risk to the fetus. Preventive treatment generally should be started after delivery because of the increased risk of tuberculosis for new mothers.

Since Isoniazid is known to cross the placental barrier and to pass into maternal breast milk, neonates and breast-fed infants of Isoniazid treated mothers should be carefully observed for any evidence of adverse effects.

Carcinogenesis: Isoniazid has been reported to induce pulmonary tumors in a number of strains of mice.

ADVERSE REACTIONS

RIFAMPIN

Nervous System Reactions: headache, drowsiness, fatigue, ataxia, dizziness, inability to concentrate, mental confusion, visual disturbances, muscular weakness, pain in extremities and generalized numbness.

Gastrointestinal Disturbances: in some patients heartburn, epigastric distress, anorexia, nausea, vomiting, gas, cramps, and diarrhea.

Hepatic Reactions: transient abnormalities in liver function tests (e.g., elevations in serum bilirubin, BSP, alkaline phosphatase, serum transaminase) have been observed. Rarely, hepatitis or a shocklike syndrome with hepatic involvement and abnormal liver function tests.

Renal Reactions: Elevations in BUN and serum uric acid have been reported. Rarely, hemolysis, hemoglobinuria, hematuria, interstitial nephritis, renal insufficiency and acute renal failure have been noted. These are generally considered to be hypersensitivity reactions. They usually occur during intermittent therapy or when treatment is resumed following intentional or accidental interruption of a daily dosage regimen, and are reversible when Rifampin is discontinued and appropriate therapy instituted.

Hematologic Reactions: thrombocytopenia, transient leukopenia, hemolytic anemia, eosinophilia and decreased hemoglobin have been observed. Thrombocytopenia has occurred when Rifampin and ethambutol were administered concomitantly according to an intermittent dose schedule twice weekly and in high doses.

Allergic and Immunological Reactions: occasionally pruritus, urticaria, rash, pemphigoid reaction, eosinophilia, sore mouth, sore tongue and exudative conjunctivitis. Rarely, hemolysis, hemoglobinuria, hematuria, renal insufficiency or acute renal failure have been reported which are generally considered to be hypersensitivity reactions. These have usually occurred during intermittent therapy or when treatment was resumed following intentional or accidental interruption of a daily dosage regimen and were reversible when Rifampin was discontinued and appropriate therapy instituted.

Although Rifampin has been reported to have an immuno-suppressive effect in some animal experiments, available human data indicate that this has no clinical significance.

Metabolic Reactions: elevations in BUN and serum uric acid have occurred.

Miscellaneous Reactions: fever and menstrual disturbances have been noted.

ISONIAZID

The most frequent reactions are those affecting the nervous system and the liver.

Nervous System Reactions: Peripheral neuropathy is the most common toxic effect. It is dose-related, occurs most often in the malnourished and in those predisposed to neuritis (e.g., alcholics and diabetics), and is usually preceded by paresthesias of the feet and hands. The incidence is higher in "slow inactivators."

Other neurotoxic effects, which are uncommon with conventional doses, are convulsions, toxic encephalopathy, optic neuritis and atrophy, memory impairment, and toxic psychosis.

Gastrointestinal Reactions: Nausea, vomiting, and epigastric distress.

Hepatic Reactions: Elevated serum transaminases (SGOT; SGPT), bilirubinemia, bilirubinuria, jaundice, and occasionally severe and sometimes fatal hepatitis. The common prodromal symptoms are anorexia, nausea, vomiting, fatigue, malaise, and weakness. Mild and transient elevation of serum transaminase levels occurs in 10 to 20 percent of persons taking Isoniazid. The abnormality usually occurs in the first 4 to 6 months of treatment but can occur at any time during therapy. In most instances, enzyme levels return to normal with no necessity to discontinue medication. In occasional instances, progressive liver damage occurs, with accompanying symptoms. In these cases, the drug should be discontinued immediately. The frequency of progressive liver damage increases with age. It is rare in persons under 20, but occurs in up to 2.3 percent of those over 50 years of age.

Hematologic Reactions: agranulocytosis, hemolytic sideroblastic or aplastic anemia, thrombocytopenia and eosinophilia.

Hypersensitivity Reactions: fever, skin eruptions (morbilliform, maculopapular, purpuric, or exfoliative), lymphadenopathy and vasculitis.

Metabolic and Endocrine Reactions: pyridoxine deficiency, pellagra, hyperglycemia, metabolic acidosis, and gynecomastia.

Miscellaneous Reactions: rheumatic syndrome and systemic lupus erythematosus-like syndrome.

OVERDOSAGE

RIFAMPIN

SIGNS AND SYMPTOMS

Nausea, vomiting, and increasing lethargy will probably occur within a short time after ingestion; actual unconsciousness may occur with severe hepatic involvement. Brownish-red or orange discoloration of the skin, urine, sweat, saliva, tears, and feces is proportional to amount ingested.

Liver enlargement, possibly with tenderness, can develop within a few hours after severe overdosage and jaundice may develop rapidly. Hepatic involvement may be more marked in patients with prior impairment of hepatic function. Other physical findings remain essentially normal.

Direct and total bilirubin levels may increase rapidly with severe overdosage; hepatic enzyme levels may be affected, especially with prior impairment of hepatic function. A direct effect upon hemopoietic system, electrolyte levels or acid-base balance is unlikely.

ISONIAZID

SIGNS AND SYMPTOMS

Isoniazid overdosage produces signs and symptoms within 30 minutes to 3 hours. Nausea, vomiting, dizziness, slurring of speech, blurring of vision, visual hallucinations (including bright colors and strange designs), are among the early manifestations. With marked overdosage, respiratory distress and CNS depression, progressing rapidly from stupor to profound coma, are to be expected, along with severe, intractable seizures. Severe metabolic acidosis, acetonuria, and hyperglycemia are typical laboratory findings.

ISONIAZID RIFAMPIN CAPSULES

TREATMENT

The airway should be secured and adequate respiratory exchange established. Only then should gastric emptying (lavage-aspiration) be attempted; this may be difficult because of seizures. Since nausea and vomiting are likely to be present, gastric lavage is probably preferable to induction of emesis.

Activated charcoal slurry instilled into the stomach following evacuation of gastric contents can help absorb any remaining drug in the GI tract. Antiemetic medication may be required to control severe nausea and vomiting.

Blood samples should be obtained for immediate determination of gases, electrolytes, BUN, glucose, etc. Blood should be typed and crossmatched in preparation for possible hemodialysis.

Rapid control of metabolic acidosis is fundamental to management. Intravenous sodium bicarbonate should be given at once and repeated as needed, adjusting subsequent dosage on the basis of laboratory findings (i.e. serum sodium, pH, etc.). At the same time, anticonvulsants should be given intravenously (i.e., barbiturates, diphenylhydantoin, diazepam) as required, and large doses of intravenous pyridoxine. Forced osmotic diuresis must be started early and should be continued for some hours after clinical improvement to hasten renal clearance of drug and help prevent relapse. Fluid intake and output should be monitored.

Bile drainage may be indicated in presence of serious impairment of hepatic function lasting more than 24-48 hours. Under these circumstances, and for severe cases, extracorporeal hemodialysis may be required; if this is not available, peritoneal dialysis can be used along with forced diuresis. Along with measures based on initial and repeated determination of blood gases and other laboratory tests as needed, meticulous respiratory and other intensive care should be utilized to protect against hypoxia, hypotension, aspiration, pneumonitis, etc.

In patients with previously adequate hepatic function, reversal of liver enlargement and impaired hepatic excretory function probably will be noted within 72 hours, with rapid return toward normal thereafter.

Untreated or inadequately treated cases of gross Isoniazid overdosage can terminate fatally, but good response has been reported in most patients brought under adequate treatment within the first few hours after drug ingestion.

DOSAGE AND ADMINISTRATION

In general, therapy should be continued until bacterial conversion and maximal improvement have occurred.

Adults: Two Isoniazid/Rifampin capsules (600 mg Rifampin, 300 mg Isoniazid) once daily, administered one hour before or two hours after a meal.

Concomitant administration of pyridoxine (B$_6$) is recommended in the malnourished, in those predisposed to neuropathy (e.g., diabetics) and in adolescents.

SUSCEPTIBILITY TESTING

RIFAMPIN

Rifampin susceptibility powders are available for both direct and indirect methods of determining the susceptibility of strains of mycobacteria. The MIC's (minimal inhibitory concentrations) of susceptible clinical isolates when determined in 7H10 or other non-egg-containing media have ranged from 0.1 to 2 mcg/ml.

Quantitative methods that require measurement of zone diameters give the most precise estimates of antibiotic susceptibility. One such procedure has been recommended for use with discs for testing susceptibility to Rifampin. Interpretations correlate zone diameters from the disc test with MIC values for Rifampin.

HOW SUPPLIED
CAPSULE: 300 MG-150 MG

BRAND/MANUFACTURER	NDC	SIZE	AWP
○ **BRAND**			
RIFAMATE: Marion Merrell Dow	00068-0509-60	60s	$145.92

Isoniazid/Pyrazinamide/Rifampin

> **WARNING**
>
> SEVERE AND SOMETIMES FATAL HEPATITIS ASSOCIATED WITH ISONIAZID THERAPY MAY OCCUR AND MAY DEVELOP EVEN AFTER MANY MONTHS OF TREATMENT. THE RISK OF DEVELOPING HEPATITIS IS AGE RELATED. APPROXIMATE CASE RATES BY AGE ARE: 0 PER 1,000 FOR PERSONS UNDER 20 YEARS OF AGE, 3 PER 1,000 FOR PERSONS IN THE 20 TO 34 YEAR AGE GROUP, 12 PER 1,000 FOR PERSONS IN THE 35 TO 49 YEAR AGE GROUP, 23 PER 1,000 FOR PERSONS IN THE 50 TO 64 YEAR AGE GROUP, AND 8 PER 1,000 FOR PERSONS OVER 65 YEARS OF AGE. THE RISK OF HEPATITIS IS INCREASED WITH DAILY CONSUMPTION OF ALCOHOL. PRECISE DATA TO PROVIDE A FATALITY RATE FOR ISONIAZID-RELATED HEPATITIS IS NOT AVAILABLE; HOWEVER, IN A U.S. PUBLIC HEALTH SERVICE SURVEILLANCE STUDY OF 13,838 PERSONS TAKING ISONIAZID, THERE WERE 8 DEATHS AMONG 174 CASES OF HEPATITIS.
>
> THEREFORE, PATIENTS GIVEN ISONIAZID SHOULD BE CAREFULLY MONITORED AND INTERVIEWED AT MONTHLY INTERVALS. SERUM TRANSAMINASE CONCENTRATION BECOMES ELEVATED IN ABOUT 10% TO 20% OF PATIENTS, USUALLY DURING THE FIRST FEW MONTHS OF THERAPY, BUT IT CAN OCCUR AT ANY TIME. USUALLY ENZYME LEVELS RETURN TO NORMAL DESPITE CONTINUANCE OF DRUG, BUT IN SOME CASES PROGRESSIVE LIVER DYSFUNCTION OCCURS. PATIENTS SHOULD BE INSTRUCTED TO REPORT IMMEDIATELY ANY OF THE PRODROMAL SYMPTOMS OF HEPATITIS, SUCH AS FATIGUE, WEAKNESS, MALAISE, ANOREXIA, NAUSEA, OR VOMITING. IF THESE SYMPTOMS APPEAR OR IF SIGNS SUGGESTIVE OF HEPATIC DAMAGE ARE DETECTED, ISONIAZID SHOULD BE DISCONTINUED PROMPTLY SINCE CONTINUED USE OF THE DRUG IN THESE CASES HAS BEEN REPORTED TO CAUSE A MORE SEVERE FORM OF LIVER DAMAGE.
>
> PATIENTS WITH TUBERCULOSIS SHOULD BE GIVEN APPROPRIATE TREATMENT WITH ALTERNATIVE DRUGS. IF ISONIAZID MUST BE REINSTITUTED, IT SHOULD BE REINSTITUTED ONLY AFTER SYMPTOMS AND LABORATORY ABNORMALITIES HAVE CLEARED. THE DRUG SHOULD BE RESTARTED IN VERY SMALL AND GRADUALLY INCREASING DOSES AND SHOULD BE WITHDRAWN IMMEDIATELY IF THERE IS ANY INDICATION OF RECURRENT LIVER INVOLVEMENT. TREATMENT SHOULD BE DEFERRED IN PERSONS WITH ACUTE HEPATIC DISEASES.

DESCRIPTION

Isoniazid/Pyrazinamide/Rifampin tablets are combination tablets for use in antibacterial therapy.

Each tablet contains:

Isoniazid	50 mg
Pyrazinamide	300 mg
Rifampin	120 mg

The Isoniazid/Pyrazinamide/Rifampin triple therapy combination was developed for dosing convenience.

Rifampin is a semisynthetic antibiotic derivative of rifamycin B. Rifampin is a red-brown crystalline powder very slightly soluble in water at neutral pH, freely soluble in chloroform, soluble in ethyl acetate and methanol. Its molecular weight is 822.95 and its chemical formula is $C_{43}H_{58}N_4O_{12}$. The chemical name for Rifampin is either:

3-[[(4-methyl-1-piperazinyl) imino]-methyl]-rifamycin; or 5,6,9,17,19,21-hexahydroxy-23methoxy-2,4,12,16,18,20,22 heptamethyl-8-[N-(4-methyl-1-piperazinyl) formimidoyl]-2,7-(epoxypentadeca [1,11,13]trienimino)naphthol-[2,1-b] furan-1, 11(2H)-dione 21-acetate.

Isoniazid is the hydroxide of isonicotinic acid. It is a colorless or white crystalline powder or white crystals. It is odorless and slowly affected by exposure to air and light. It is freely soluble in water, sparingly soluble in alcohol and slightly soluble in chloroform and in ether. Its molecular weight is 137.14 and its chemical formula is $C_6H_7N_3O$. The chemical name for Isoniazid is 4-pyridine-carboxylic acid, hydrazide.

Pyrazinamide, the pyrazine analogue of nicotinamide, is a white, crystalline powder, stable at room temperature, and sparingly soluble in water. The chemical name for Pyrazinamide is pyrazinecarboxamide and its molecular weight is 123.11. Its chemical formula is $C_5H_5N_3O$.

▶ SHOWN IN PRODUCT IDENTIFICATION GUIDE

Parameter	C_{max} (µg/mL)		Half-life (hr)		Apparent Oral Clearance (L/hr)		Bioavailability (%)
Treatment	A	B	A	B	A	B	A
Isoniazid	3.09 ± 0.88	3.14 ± 0.92	2.80 ± 1.02	2.80 ± 1.11	24.02 ± 15.29	25.72 ± 18.38	100.6 ± 16.6
Pyrazinamide	28.02 ± 4.52	29.21 ± 4.35	10.04 ± 1.54	10.08 ± 1.29	3.82 ± 0.65	3.70 ± 0.59	96.8 ± 7.6
Rifampin	11.04 ± 3.08	13.61 ± 3.96	3.19 ± 0.63	3.41 ± 0.86	9.62 ± 3.00	8.30 ± 2.50	88.8 ± 16.5

The effect of food on the pharmacokinetics of Isoniazid/Pyrazinamide/Rifampin tablets was not studied.

CLINICAL PHARMACOLOGY
GENERAL
Isoniazid. After oral administration, Isoniazid is readily absorbed from the GI tract and produces peak blood levels within 1 to 2 hours. It diffuses readily into all body fluids (cerebrospinal, pleural, and ascitic fluids), tissues, organs, and excreta (saliva, sputum, and feces). Isoniazid is not substantially bound to plasma proteins. The drug also passes through the placental barrier and into milk in concentrations comparable to those in the plasma. The plasma half-life of Isoniazid in patients with normal renal and hepatic function ranges from 1-4 hours, depending on the rate of metabolism. From 50% to 70% of a dose of Isoniazid is excreted in the urine within 24 hours, mostly as metabolites.

Isoniazid is metabolized in the liver mainly by acetylation and dehydrazination. The rate of acetylation is genetically determined. Approximately 50% of African American and Caucasians are "slow inactivators" and the rest are "rapid inactivators"; the majority of Eskimos and Asians are "rapid inactivators." The rate of acetylation does not significantly alter the effectiveness of Isoniazid. However, slow acetylation may lead to higher blood levels of the drug, and thus, an increase in toxic reactions.

Pyridoxine (B_6) deficiency is sometimes observed in adults with high doses of Isoniazid and is probably due to its competition with pyridoxal phosphate for the enzyme apotryptophanase.

Pyrazinamide. Pyrazinamide is well absorbed from the gastrointestinal tract and attains peak plasma concentrations within 2 hours. Plasma concentrations generally range from 30 to 50 µg/mL with doses of 20 to 25 mg/kg. It is widely distributed in body tissues and fluids including the liver, lungs, and cerebrospinal fluid (CSF). The CSF concentration is approximately equal to concurrent steady-state plasma concentrations in patients with inflamed meninges. Pyrazinamide is approximately 10% bound to plasma proteins. The plasma half-life of Pyrazinamide is 9 to 10 hours in patients with normal renal and hepatic function. The half-life of the drug may be prolonged in patients with impaired renal or hepatic function. Pyrazinamide is hydrolyzed in the liver to its major active metabolite, pyrazinoic acid. Pyrazinoic acid is hydroxylated to the main excretory product, 5-hydroxypyrazinoic acid.

Within 24 hours, approximately 70% of an oral dose of Pyrazinamide is excreted in urine, mainly by glomerular filtration. About 4% to 14% of the dose is excreted as unchanged drug; the remainder is excreted as metabolites.

Rifampin: Rifampin is readily absorbed from the gastrointestinal tract. Peak serum levels in normal adults and children vary widely from individual to individual. Following a single 600 mg oral dose of Rifampin in healthy adults, the peak serum level averages 7 µg/mL but may vary from 4 to 32 µg/mL. Absorption of Rifampin is reduced when the drug is ingested with food.

In normal subjects, the biological half-life of Rifampin in serum averages about 3 hours after a 600-mg oral dose, with increases up to 5.1 hours reported after a 900-mg dose. With repeated administration, the half-life decreases and reaches average values of approximately 2 to 3 hours. The half-life does not differ in patients with renal failure at doses not exceeding 600 mg daily and, consequently, no dosage adjustment is required. The half-life of Rifampin at a dose of 720 mg daily has not been established in patients with renal failure. Following a single 900 mg oral dose of Rifampin in patients with varying degrees of renal insufficiency, the half-life increased from 3.6 hours in normal subjects to 5.0, 7.3 and 11.0 hours in patients with glomerular filtration rates of 30-50 mL/min, less than 30 mL/min, and in anuric patients, respectively. Refer to *"Warnings"* section for information regarding patients with hepatic insufficiency.

After absorption, Rifampin in rapdily eliminated in the bile, and an enterohepatic circulation ensues. During this process, Rifampin undergoes progressive deacetylation so that nearly all the drug in the bile is in this form in about 6 hours. This metabolite has antibacterial activity. Intestinal reabsorption is reduced by deacetylation, and elimination is facilitated. Up to 30% of a dose is excreted in the urine, with about half as unchanged drug. Rifampin is widely distributed throughout the body. It is present in effective concentrations in many organs and body fluids, including cerebrospinal fluid. Rifampin is about 80% protein bound. Most of the unbound fraction is not ionized and therefore is diffused freely in tissues.

ISONIAZID/PYRAZINAMIDE/RIFAMPIN
In a single-dose bioavailability study of five Isoniazid/Pyrazinamide/Rifampin tablets (Treatment A, n = 23) versus Isoniazid 250 mg, Pyrazinamide 1500 mg, and Rifampin 600 mg (Treatment B, n = 24) administered concurrently in normal subjects, there was no difference in extent of absorption, as measured by the area under the plasma concentration versus time curve (AUC), of all three components. However, the mean peak plasma concentration of Rifampin was approximately 18% lower following the single-dose administration of Isoniazid/Pyrazinamide/Rifampin tablets as compared to Rifampin administered in combination with Pyrazinamide and Isoniazid. Mean (± SD) pharmacokinetic parameters are summarized in the following table.

MICROBIOLOGY
Isoniazid, Pyrazinamide, and Rifampin at the therapeutic levels have demonstrated bactericidal activity against both intracellular and extracellular *Mycobacterium tuberculosis* organisms.

MECHANISM OF ACTION
Isoniazid. Isoniazid kills actively growing tubercle bacilli by inhibiting the biosynthesis of mycolic acids which are major components of the cell wall of *Mycobacterium tuberculosis.*

Pyrazinamide. The exact mechanism of action by which Pyrazinamide inhibits the growth of *Mycobacterium tuberculosis* organisms is unknown. *In vitro* and *in vivo* studies have demonstrated that Pyrazinamide is only active at a slightly acidic pH (pH 5.5).

Rifampin: Rifampin inhibits DNA-dependent RNA polymerase activity in susceptible *Mycobacterium tuberculosis* organisms. Specifically, it interacts with bacterial RNA polymerase, but does not inhibit the mammalian enzyme. Organisms resistant to Rifampin are likely to be resistant to other rifamycins.

SUSCEPTIBILITY TESTING
Prior to initiation of therapy, appropriate specimens should be collected for identification of the infecting organism and *in vitro* susceptibility tests. (See related table).

Two standardized *in vitro* susceptibility methods are available for testing Isoniazid, Pyrazinamide, and Rifampin against *Mycobacterium tuberculosis* organisms. The agar proportion method (CDC or NCCLS M24-P) utilizes Middlebrook 7H10 medium impregnated with Isoniazid at 0.2 and 1.0 µg/mL and Rifampin at 1.0 µg/mL for the final concentrations of drug. The final concentration for Pyrazinamide is 25.0 µg/mL at pH 5.5. After 3 weeks of incubation MIC_{99} values are calculated by comparing the quantity of organisms growing in the medium containing drug to the control cultures. Mycobacterial growth in the presence of drug ≥ 1% of the control indicates resistance.

The radiometric broth method employs the BACTEC 460 machine to compare the growth index from untreated control cultures to cultures grown in the presence of 0.2 and 1.0 µg/mL of Isoniazid and 2.0 µg/mL of Rifampin. Strict adherence to the manufacturer's instructions for sample processing and data interpretation is required for this assay. The radiometric broth method has not been approved for the testing of Pyrazinamide.

Susceptibility test results obtained by the two different methods can only be compared if the appropriate Rifampin or Isoniazid concentrations are used for each test method as indicated above. Both test procedures require the use of *Mycobacterium tuberculosis* H37Rv, ATCC 27294, as a control organism.

The clinical relevance of *in vitro* susceptibility test results for mycobacterial species other than *Mycobacterium tuberculosis* using either the radiometric broth method or the proportion method has not been determined.

CLINICAL TRIALS
A total of 250 patients were enrolled in an open label, prospective, randomized, parallel group, active controlled trial, for the treatment of pulmonary tuberculosis. There were 241 patients evaluable for efficacy, 123 patients received Isoniazid, Pyrazinamide, and Rifampin as separate tablets and capsules for 56 days, and 118 patients received 4 to 6 Isoniazid/Pyrazinamide/Rifampin tablets based on body weight for 56 days. Isoniazid/Pyrazinamide/Rifampin tablets and the drugs dosed as separate tablets and capsules were administered based on body weight during the intensive phase of treatment according to the following table.

DOSE OF ISONIAZID, PYRAZINAMIDE, AND RIFAMPIN ADMINISTERED AS SEPARATE DRUGS

Patient Weight	Isoniazid (mg)	Pyrazinamide (mg)	Rifampin (mg)
< 50 kg	300	1500	450
≥ 50 kg	300	2000	600

DOSE OF ISONIAZID, PYRAZINAMIDE, AND RIFAMPIN ADMINISTERED AS ISONIAZID/PYRAZINAMIDE/RIFAMPIN

Patient Weight	Number of Tablets	Isoniazid (mg)	Pyrazinamide (mg)	Rifampin (mg)
≤ 44 kg	4	200	1200	480
45 to 54 kg	5	250	1500	600
≥ 55 kg	6	300	1800	720

During the continuation phase, both treatment groups received 450 mg of Rifampin and 300 mg of Isoniazid per day for 4 months if the patient weighed < 50 kg or 600 mg of Rifampin and 300 mg of Isoniazid per day for 4 months if the

---

◆ RATED THERAPEUTICALLY EQUIVALENT; ◇ THERAPEUTIC EQUIVALENCE UNCONFIRMED; ○ UNRATED

patient weighed ≥ 50 kg. Patients were followed for occurrence of relapses for up to 30 months after the end of therapy.

There were no significant differences in the negative bacteriological sputum results (available in a subset of patients) between the two treatments at 2 and 6 months during the trial and during the follow-up period. See table below.

Treatment	Negative Sputums/No. of Patients (Percent Negative)		
	2 Months	6 Months	Follow-up Period*
Isoniazid/ Pyrazinamide/ Rifampin	91/96 (95%)	100/104 (96%)	99/101 (98%)
Separate†	99/108 (92%)	95/96 (99%)	105/106 (99%)

* *The median follow-up time for all the Isoniazid/Pyrazinamide/Rifampin patients was 756 days with a range of 42 to 1325 days and 745 days with a range of 50 to 1427 days for the patients dosed with separate tablets and capsules.*

† *Isoniazid, Pyrazinamide, and Rifampin dosed as separate tablets and capsules.*

For adverse events, see "Adverse Reactions" section.

INDICATIONS AND USAGE

Isoniazid/Pyrazinamide/Rifampin is indicated in the initial phase of the short-course treatment of pulmonary tuberculosis. During this phase, which should last 2 months, Isoniazid/Pyrazinamide/Rifampin should be administered on a daily, continous basis (see "Dosage and Administration" section).

Following the initial phase and treatment with Isoniazid/Pyrazinamide/Rifampin, treatment should be continued with Rifampin and Isoniazid for at least 4 months. Treatment should be continued for a longer period of time if the patient is still sputum or culture positive, if resistant organisms are present, or if the patient is HIV positive.

In the treatment of tuberculosis, the small number of resistant cells present within large populations of susceptible cells can rapidly become the predominant type. Since resistance can emerge rapidly, susceptibility tests should be performed in the event of persistent positive cultures during the course of treatment. Bacteriologic smears or cultures should be obtained before the start of therapy to confirm the susceptibility of the organism to Isoniazid, Pyrazinamide, and Rifampin and they should be repeated throughout therapy to monitor response to the treatment. If test results show resistance to any of the components of Isoniazid/Pyrazinamide/Rifampin and the patient is not responding to therapy, the drug regimen should be modified.

CONTRAINDICATIONS

Isoniazid/Pyrazinamide/Rifampin is contraindicated in patients with a history of hypersensitivity to Isoniazid, Pyrazinamide, Rifampin, or any of the components. Other contraindications include patients with severe hepatic damage; severe adverse reactions to Isoniazid, such as drug fever, chills, and arthritis; patients with acute liver disease of any etiology; and patients with acute gout.

WARNINGS

Each of the individual drugs in Isoniazid/Pyrazinamide/Rifampin has been associated with liver dysfunction.

Isoniazid: See the boxed "Warning".

Since Isoniazid/Pyrazinamide/Rifampin contains Isoniazid, ophthalmologic examinations (including ophthalmoscopy) should be done before treatment is started and periodically thereafter, even without occurrence of visual symptoms.

Pyrazinamide: Since Isoniazid/Pyrazinamide/Rifampin contains Pyrazinamide, patients started on Isoniazid/Pyrazinamide/Rifampin should have baseline serum uric acid and liver function determinations. Patients with preexisting liver disease or those patients at increased risk for drug related hepatitis (eg, alcohol abusers) should be followed closely.

Because it contains Pyrazinamide, Isoniazid/Pyrazinamide/Rifampin should be discontinued and not be resumed if signs of hepatocellular damage or hyperuricemia accompanied by an acute gouty arthritis appear. If hyperuricemia accompanied by an acute gouty arthritis occurs without liver dysfunction, the patient should be transferred to a regimen not containing Pyrazinamide.

Rifampin: Rifampin has been shown to produce liver dysfunction. Fatalities associated with jaundice have occurred in patients with liver disease and in patients taking Rifampin with other hepatotoxic agents. Because Isoniazid/Pyrazinamide/Rifampin contains both Rifampin and Isoniazid, it should only be given with caution and under strict medical supervision to patients with impaired liver function. In these patients, careful monitoring of liver function, especially serum glutamic pyruvic transaminase (SGPT) and serum glutamic oxaloacetic transaminase (SGOT) should be carried out prior to therapy and then every 2 to 4 weeks during therapy. If signs of hepatocellular damage occur, Isoniazid/Pyrazinamide/Rifampin should be withdrawn.

In some cases, hyperbilirubinemia resulting from competition between Rifampin and bilirubin for excretory pathways of the liver at the cell level can occur in the early days of treatment. An isolated report showing a moderate rise in bilirubin and/or transaminase level is not in itself an indication for interrupting treatment; rather, the decision should be made after repeating the tests, noting trends in the levels, and considering them in conjunction with the patient's clinical condition.

Rifampin has enzyme-inducing properties, including induction of delta amino levulinic acid synthetase. Isolated reports have associated porphyria exacerbation with Rifampin administration.

PRECAUTIONS

GENERAL

Isoniazid/Pyrazinamide/Rifampin should be used with caution in patients with a history of diabetes mellitus, as diabetes management may be more difficult.

Isoniazid: All drugs should be stopped and an evaluation of the patient should be made at the first sign of a hypersensitivity reaction.

Use of Isoniazid/Pyrazinamide/Rifampin, because it contains Isoniazid, should be carefully monitored in the following:

1. Patients who are receiving phenytoin (diphenylhydantoin) concurrently. Isoniazid may decrease the excretion of phenytoin or may enhance its effects. To avoid phenytoin intoxication, appropriate adjustment of the anticonvulsant dose should be made.

2. Daily users of alcohol. Daily ingestion of alcohol may be associated with a higher incidence of Isoniazid hepatitis.

3. Patients with current chronic liver disease or severe renal dysfunction.

Pyrazinamide: Pyrazinamide inhibits renal excretion of urates, frequently resulting in hyperuricemia which is usually asymptomatic. If hyperuricemia is accompanied by acute gouty arthritis, Isoniazid/Pyrazinamide/Rifampin, because it contains Pyrazinamide, should be discontinued.

Rifampin: For treatment of tuberculosis, Rifampin is usually administered on a daily basis. Doses of Rifampin (> 600 mg) given once or twice weekly have resulted in a higher incidence of adverse reactions, including the "flu syndrome" (fever, chills and malaise); hematopoietic reactions (leukopenia, thrombocytopenia, or acute hemolytic anemia); cutaneous, gastrointestinal, and hepatic reactions; shortness of breath; shock and renal failure.

The patient should be advised that the reliability of oral contraceptives may be affected; consideration should be given to using alternative contraceptive measures.

INFORMATION FOR PATIENTS

Food Interactions: Because Isoniazid has some monoamine oxidase inhibiting activity, an interaction with tyramine-containing foods (cheese, red wine) may occur. Diamine oxidase may also be inhibited, causing exaggerated response, (e.g., headache, sweating, palpitations, flushing, hypotension) to foods containing histamine (e.g., skipjack, tuna, other tropical fish). Tyramine- and histamine-containing foods should be avoided in patients receiving Isoniazid/Pyrazinamide/Rifampin.

Isoniazid/Pyrazinamide/Rifampin, because it contains Rifampin, may produce a reddish coloration of the urine, sweat, sputum, and tears, and the patient should be forewarned of this. Soft contact lenses may be permanently stained.

Patients should be instructed to take Isoniazid/Pyrazinamide/Rifampin either 1 hour before or 2 hours after a meal.

Patients should be instructed to notify their physicians promptly if they experience any of the following: fever, loss of appetite, malaise, nausea and vomiting, darkened urine, yellowish discoloration of the skin and eyes, pain or swelling of the joints.

Compliance with the full course of therapy must be emphasized, and the importance of not missing any doses must be stressed.

LABORATORY TESTS

A complete blood count (CBC), liver function tests, and blood uric acid determinations should be obtained prior to instituting therapy and periodically throughout the course of therapy. Because of a possible transient rise in transaminase and bilirubin values, blood for baseline clinical chemistries should be obtained before Isoniazid/Pyrazinamide/Rifampin dosing.

DRUG INTERACTIONS

Isoniazid: Enzyme Inhibition: Isoniazid is known to inhibit certain cytochrome P-450 enzymes. Coadministration of Isoniazid with drugs that undergo biotransformation through these metabolic pathways may decrease elimination. Consequently, dosages of drugs metabolized by these enzymes may require adjustment when starting or stopping concomitantly administered Isoniazid/Pyrazinamide/Rifampin, because it contains Isoniazid, to maintain optimum therapeutic blood levels.

Isoniazid has been reported to inhibit the metabolism of the following drugs: anticonvulsants (eg, carbamazepine, phenytoin, primidone, valproic acid), benzodiazepines (eg, diazepam), haloperidol, ketoconazole, theophylline, and warfarin. It may be necessary to adjust the dosages of these drugs if they are given concurrently with Isoniazid/Pyrazinamide/Rifampin because it contains Isoniazid. The impact of the competing effects of Rifampin and Isoniazid on the metabolism of these drugs is unknown.

Other Interactions: Concomitant antacid administration may reduce the absorption of Isoniazid. Ingestion with food may also reduce the absorption of Isoniazid. Daily doses of Isoniazid/Pyrazinamide/Rifampin, because it contains Isoniazid, should be given on an empty stomach at least 1 hour before the ingestion of antacids or food.

Corticosteroids (eg, prednisolone) may decrease the serum concentration of Isoniazid by increasing acetylation rate and/or renal clearance. Para-aminosalicylic acid may increase the plasma concentration and elimination half-life of Isoniazid by competition of acetylating enzymes.

Pharmacodynamic Interactions: Daily ingestion of alcohol may be associated with a higher incidence of Isoniazid hepatitis. Isoniazid when given concomitantly with Rifampin, has been reported to increase the hepatotoxicity of both drugs. Patients receiving both Rifampin and Isoniazid as in Isoniazid/Pyrazinamide/Rifampin should be monitored closely for hepatotoxicity.

The CNS effects of meperidine (drowsiness), cycloserine (dizziness, drowsiness), and disulfiram (acute behavioral and coordination changes) may be exaggerated when concomitant Isoniazid/Pyrazinamide/Rifampin, because it contains Isoniazid, is given. Concurrent Isoniazid/Pyrazinamide/Rifampin, because it contains Isoniazid, and levodopa administration may produce symptoms of excess catecholamine stimulation (agitation, flushing, palpitations) or lack of levodopa effect.

Isoniazid may produce hyperglycemia and lead to loss of glucose control in patients on oral hypoglycemics.

Fast acetylation of Isoniazid may produce high concentrations of hydrazine which facilitate deflorination of enflurane. Renal function should be monitored in patients receiving both Isoniazid/Pyrazinamide/Rifampin and enflurane.

Food Interactions: Because Isoniazid has some monoamine oxidase inhibiting activity, an interaction with tyramine-containing foods (cheese, red wine) may occur. Diamine oxidase may also be inhibited, causing exaggerated response (e.g., headache, sweating, palpitations, flushing, hypotension) to foods containing histamine (eg, skipjack, tuna, other tropical fish). Tyramine- and histamine-containing foods should be avoided by patients receiving Isoniazid/Pyrazinamide/Rifampin.

Rifampin: Enzyme Introduction: Rifampin is known to induce certain cytochrome P-450 enzymes. Coadministration of Isoniazid/Pyrazinamide/Rifampin, because it contains Rifampin, with drugs that undergo biotransformation through these metabolic pathways may accelerate elimination. To maintain optimum therapeutic blood levels, dosages of drugs metabolized by these enzymes may require adjustment when starting or stopping concomitantly administered Rifampin.

Rifampin has been reported to accelerate the metabolism of the following drugs: anticonvulsants (eg, phenytoin), antiarrhythmics (eg, disopyramide, mexiletine, quinidine, tocainide), anticoagulants, antifungals (eg, fluconazole, itraconazole, ketoconazole), barbiturates, beta-blockers, calcium channel blockers (eg, diltiazem, nifedipine, verapamil), chloramphenicol, ciprofloxacin, corticosteroids, cyclosporine, cardiac glycoside preparations, clofibrate, oral contraceptives, dapsone, diazepam, haloperidol, oral hypoglycemic agents (sulfonylureas), methadone, narcotic analgesics, nortriptyline, progestins, and theophylline. If may be necessary to adjust dosages of these drugs if they are given concurrently with Isoniazid/Pyrazinamide/Rifampin since it contains Rifampin.

Rifampin has been observed to increase the requirements for anticoagulant drugs of the coumarin type. In patients receiving anticoagulants and Isoniazid/Pyrazinamide/Rifampin concurrently, it is recommended that the prothrombin time be performed daily or as frequently as necessary to establish and maintain the required dose of anticoagulant.

Concurrent use of ketoconazole and Rifampin has resulted in decreased serum concentration of both drugs. Concurrent use of Rifampin and enalapril has resulted in decreased concentrations of enalaprilat, the active metabolite of enalapril. Since Isoniazid/Pyrazinamide/Rifampin contains Rifampin, dosage adjustments should be made if Isoniazid/Pyrazinamide/Rifampin is concurrently administered with ketoconazole or enalapril if indicated by the patient's clinical condition.

Other Interactions: Concomitant anticid administration may reduce the absorption of Rifampin. Daily doses of Isoniazid/Pyrazinamide/Rifampin, because it contains Rifampin, should be given at least 1 hour before the ingestion of antacids.

Probenecid and cotrimoxazole have been reported to increase the blood level of Rifampin.

When Rifampin is given concomitantly with either halothane or Isoniazid the potential for hepatotoxicity is increased. The concomitant use of Isoniazid/Pyrazinamide/Rifampin, because it contains both Rifampin and Isoniazid, and halothane should be avoided. Patients receiving both Rifampin and Isoniazid as in Isoniazid/Pyrazinamide/Rifampin should be monitored closely for hepatotoxicity. See the boxed *"Warning".*

Plasma concentrations of sulfapyridine may be reduced following the concomitant administration of sulfasalazine and Isoniazid/Pyrazinamide/Rifampin, because it contains Rifampin. This finding may be the result of alteration in the colonic bacteria responsible for the reduction of sulfasalazine to sulfapyridine and mesalamine.

DRUG/LABORATORY TESTS INTERACTION
Pyrazinamide: Pyrazinamide has been reported to interfere with ACETEST® and KETOSTIX® urine tests to produce a pink-brown color.

Rifampin: Therapeutic levels of Rifampin have been shown to inhibit standard microbiological assays for serum folate and vitamin B_{12}. Therefore, alternative assay methods should be considered. Transient abnormalities in liver function tests (eg, elevation in serum bilirubin, abnormal bromsulphalein [BSP] excretion, alkaline phosphatase and serum transaminases), and reduced biliary excretion of contrast media used for visualization of the gallbladder have also been observed. Therefore, tests should be performed before the morning dose of Isoniazid/Pyrazinamide/Rifampin.

Rifampin and Isoniazid have been reported to alter vitamin D metabolism. In some cases, reduced levels of circulating 25-hydroxy vitamin D and 1,25-dihydroxy vitamin D have been accompanied by reduced serum calcium and phosphate and elevated parathyroid hormone.

CARCINOGENESIS, MUTAGENESIS, IMPAIRMENT OF FERTILITY
Increased frequency of chromosomal aberrations was observed *in vitro* in lymphocytes obtained from patients treated with combinations of Isoniazid, Pyrazinamide and Rifampin and combinations of streptomycin, Isoniazid, Pyrazinamide and Rifampin.

Isoniazid: Isoniazid has been reported to induce pulmonary tumors in a number of strains of mice.

Pyrazinamide: In lifetime bioassays in rats and mice, Pyrazinamide was administered in the diet at concentrations of up to 10,000 ppm. This resulted in estimated daily doses of 2 g/kg for the mouse, or 40 times the maximum human dose, and 0.5 g/kg for the rat, or 10 times the maximum human dose. Pyrazinamide was not carcinogenic in rats or male mice and no conclusion was possible for female mice.

Pyrazinamide was not mutagenic in the Ames bacterial test, but induced chromosomal aberrations in human lymphocyte cell cultures.

Rifampin: There are no known human data on long-term potential for carcinogenicity, mutagenicity, or impairment of fertility. A few cases of accelerated growth of lung carcinoma have been reported in man, but a causal relationship with the drug has not been established. An increase in the incidence of hepatomas in female mice (of a strain known to be particularly susceptible to the spontaneous development of hepatomas) was observed when Rifampicin was administered in doses two to ten times the average daily human dose for 60 weeks followed by an observation period of 46 weeks. No evidence of carcinogenicity was found in male mice of the same strain, mice of a different strain, or rats under similar experimental conditions.

Rifampin has been reported to possess immunosuppressive potential in rabbits, mice, rats, guinea pigs, human lymphocytes *in vitro*, and humans. Antitumor activity *in vitro* has also been shown with Rifampin.

There was no evidence of mutagenicity in bacteria, *Drosophilia melanogaster*, or mice. An increase in chromatid breaks was noted when whole blood cell cultures were treated with Rifampin.

PREGNANCY—TERATOGENIC EFFECTS
Category C. Animal reproduction studies have not been conducted with Isoniazid/Pyrazinamide/Rifampin. It is also not known whether Isoniazid/Pyrazinamide/Rifampin can cause fetal harm when administered to a pregnant woman. Isoniazid/Pyrazinamide/Rifampin should be given to a pregnant woman only if clearly needed.

Isoniazid: It has been reported that in both rats and rabbits, Isoniazid may exert an embryocidal effect when administered orally during pregnancy, although no Isoniazid-related congenital anomalies have been found in reproduction studies in mammalian species (mice, rats, and rabbits). Isoniazid/Pyrazinamide/Rifampin, because it contains Isoniazid, should be prescribed during pregnancy only when therapeutically necessary. The benefit of preventive therapy should be weighed against a possible risk to the fetus. Preventive treatment generally should be started after delivery because of the increased risk of tuberculosis for new mothers.

Pyrazinamide: Animal reproductive studies have not been conducted with Pyrazinamide. It is also not known whether Pyrazinamide can cause fetal harm when administered to a pregnant woman. Isoniazid/Pyrazinamide/Rifampin, because it contains Pyrazinamide, should be given to a pregnant woman only if clearly needed.

Rifampin: Although Rifampin has been reported to cross the placental barrier and appear in cord blood, the effect of Rifampin, alone or in combination with other antituberculosis drugs, on the human fetus is not known. An increase in congenital malformations, primarily spina bifida and cleft palate, has been reported in the offspring of rodents given oral doses of 150 to 250 mg/kg/day of Rifampin during pregnancy. The possible teratogenic potential in women capable of bearing children should be carefully weighed against the benefits of Isoniazid/Pyrazinamide/Rifampin therapy.

PREGNANCY—NON-TERATOGENIC EFFECTS
It is not known whether Isoniazid/Pyrazinamide/Rifampin can affect reproduction capacity.

Rifampin: When administered during the last few weeks of pregnancy, Rifampin can cause postnatal hemorrhages in the mother and infant. In this case, treatment with vitamin K may be indicated for postnatal hemorrhage.

NURSING MOTHERS
Since Isoniazid, Pyrazinamide, and Rifampin are known to pass into maternal breast milk, a decision should be made whether to discontinue nursing or to discontinue Isoniazid/Pyrazinamide/Rifampin taking into account the importance of the drug to the mother.

PEDIATRIC USE
Safety and effectiveness in children or adolescents under the age of 15 have not been established.

◆ RATED THERAPEUTICALLY EQUIVALENT; ◇ THERAPEUTIC EQUIVALENCE UNCONFIRMED; ○ UNRATED

ADVERSE REACTIONS

ADVERSE EXPERIENCES DURING THE CLINICAL TRIAL

Adverse event data reported for the Isoniazid/Pyrazinamide/Rifampin and the separate drug treatment groups during the first 2 months of the trial are shown in the table below.

ADVERSE EVENTS REPORTED DURING THE CLINICAL STUDY

Adverse Events by Body Systems During First 2 Months of Trial	Number of Patients With Adverse Events*	
	Isoniazid/ Pyrazinamide/ Rifampin n = 122‡	Separate† n = 123‡
Cutaneous (rash, erythroderma, erythema, exfoliative dermatitis, Lyell syndrome, urticaria, localized skin rash, diffuse skin rash, pruritus, generalized hypersensitivity)	8 (7%)	21 (17%)
Gastrointestinal (nausea, vomiting, digestive pain, diarrhea)	8 (7%)	14 (11%)
Musculoskeletal (arthralgia, long bone pain, phlebitis localized joint pain, diffuse joint pain, edema of the legs)	5 (4%)	8 (7%)
Hearing and Vestibular (tinnitus, vertigo, vertigo with loss of equilibrium)	3 (2%)	6 (5%)
Liver and Biliary (hepatitis with conjunctival jaundice, hepatitis with deep jaundice)	0 (0%)	2 (2%)
Central and Peripheral Nervous System (sweating, headache, insomnia, diffuse paresthesia of the legs, anxiety, diabetic coma)	5 (4%)	4 (3%)
Total Body (spiking fever, persistent fever)	2 (2%)	4 (3%)
Cardiorespiratory (tightness in chest, coughing, diffuse chest pain, hemoptysis, angina, palpitation, total pneumothorax)	8 (7%)	3 (2%)
Total number of patients with one or more adverse events	29	43

*   A given patient may have experienced ≥ 1 adverse event.
†   Isoniazid, Pyrazinamide, and Rifampin dosed as separate tablets and capsules.
‡   A total of 250 patients (124 Isoniazid/Pyrazinamide/Rifampin; 126 separate) were originally enrolled in the study. Five patients (2 Isoniazid/Pyrazinamide/Rifampin; 3 separate) were excluded due to admission errors.

No serious adverse events were reported in the patients receiving Isoniazid/Pyrazinamide/Rifampin tablets. Three serious adverse events were reported in the patients given Isoniazid, Pyrazinamide, and Rifampin as separate tablets and capsules. The three serious adverse events were two general hypersensitivity reactions and one jaundice reaction. There were no significant differences between the two treatment groups in standard liver function, renal function and hematological laboratory test values measured at baseline and after 8 weeks of treatment. As would be expected for these drugs, there were alterations in liver enzymes (SGOT, SGPT) and serum uric acid levels. The adverse reactions reported during therapy with Isoniazid/Pyrazinamide/Rifampin are consistent with those described below for the individual components.

ADVERSE REACTIONS REPORTED FOR INDIVIDUAL COMPONENTS

Isoniazid: The most frequent reactions are those affecting the nervous system and the liver. See the boxed *"Warning"*.

Nervous System: Peripheral neuropathy is the most common toxic effect. It is dose-related, occurs most often in the malnourished and in those predisposed to neuritis (eg, alcoholics and diabetics), and is usually preceded by paresthesias of the feet and hands. The incidence is higher in "slow inactivators."

Other neurotoxic effects, which are uncommon with conventional doses, are convulsions, toxic encephalopathy, optic neuritis and atrophy, memory impairment, and toxic psychosis.

Gastrointestinal: Nausea, vomiting, and epigastric distress.

Hepatic: Elevated serum transaminases (SGOT, SGPT), bilirubinemia, bilirubinuria, jaundice, and occasionally severe and sometimes fatal hepatitis. The common prodromal symptoms are anorexia, nausea, vomiting, fatigue, malaise, and weakness. Mild and transient elevation of serum transaminase levels occurs in 10 to 20% of persons taking Isoniazid. The abnormality usually occurs in the first 4 to 6 months of treatment but can occur at any time during therapy. In most instances, enzyme levels return to normal with no necessity to discontinue medication. In occasional instances, progressive liver damage occurs, with accompanying symptoms. In these cases, the drug should be discontinued immediately. The frequency of progressive liver damage increases with age. It is rare in persons under 20, but occurs in up to 2.3% of those over 50 years of age.

Hematologic: Agranulocytosis; hemolytic, sideroblastic, or aplastic anemia, thrombocytopenia; and eosinophilia.

Hypersensitivity Reactions: Fever, skin eruptions (morbilliform, maculopapular, purpuric, or exfoliative), lymphadenopathy, and vasculitis.

Metabolic and Endocrine: Pyridoxine deficiency, pellagra, hyperglycemia, metabolic acidosis, and gynecomastia.

Miscellaneous: Rheumatic syndrome and systemic lupus erythematosus-like syndrome.

Pyrazinamide: The principal adverse effect is a hepatic reaction (see *"Warnings"*). Hepatotoxicity appears to be dose related and may appear at any time during therapy. Pyrazinamide can cause hyperuricemia and gout (see *"Precautions"*).

Gastrointestinal: GI disturbances including nausea, vomiting, and anorexia have also been reported.

Hematologic and Lymphatic: Thrombocytopenia and sideroblastic anemia with erythroid hyperplasia, vacuolation of erythrocytes and increased serum concentration have occurred rarely with this drug. Adverse effects on blood clotting mechanisms have also been rarely reported.

Other: Mild arthralgia and myalgia have been reported frequently. Hypersensitivity reactions including rashes, urticaria, and pruritus have been reported. Fever, acne, photosensitivity, porphyria, dysuria, and interstitial nephritis have been reported rarely.

Rifampin:

Gastrointestinal: Heartburn, epigastric distress, anorexia, nausea, vomiting, jaundice, flatulence, cramps, and diarrhea have been noted in some patients. Although *Clostridium difficile* has been shown *in vitro* to be sensitive to Rifampin, pseudomembranous colitis has been reported with the use of Rifampin (and other broad-spectrum antibiotics). Therefore, it is important to consider this diagnosis in patients who develop diarrhea in association with antibiotic use. Rarely, hepatitis or a shocklike syndrome with hepatic involvement and abnormal liver function tests has been reported.

Hematologic: Thrombocytopenia has occurred primarily with high dose intermittent therapy, but has also been noted after resumption of interrupted treatment. It rarely occurs during well-supervised daily therapy. This effect is reversible if the drug is discontinued as soon as purpura occurs. Cerebral hemorrhage and fatalities have been reported when Rifampin administration has been continued or resumed after the appearance of purpura.

Transient leukopenia, hemolytic anemia, and decreased hemoglobin have been observed.

Central Nervous System: Headache, fever, drowsiness, fatigue, ataxia, dizziness, inability to concentrate, mental confusion, behavioral changes, muscular weakness, pains in extremities, and generalized numbness have been observed.

Rare reports of myopathy have also been observed.

Ocular: Visual disturbances have been observed.

Endocrine: Menstrual disturbances have been observed.

Renal: Elevations in BUN and serum uric acid have been reported. Rarely, hemolysis, hemoglobinuria, hematuria, interstitial nephritis, renal insufficiency, and acute renal failure have been noted. These are generally considered to be hypersensitivity reactions. They usually occur during intermittent therapy or when treatment is resumed following intentional or accidental interruption of a daily dosage regimen, and are reversible when Rifampin is discontinued and appropriate therapy instituted.

Dermatologic: Cutaneous reactions are mild and self-limiting and do not appear to be hypersensitivity reactions. Typically, they consist of flushing and itching with or without a rash. More serious cutaneous reactions which may be due to hypersensitivity occur but are uncommon.

Hypersensitivity Reactions: Occasionally pruritus, urticaria, rash, pemphigoid reaction, eosinophilia, sore mouth, sore tongue and conjunctivitis have been observed.

Miscellaneous: Edema of the face and extremities have been reported. Other reactions which have occurred with intermittent dosage regimens include "flu" syndrome (such as episodes of fever, chills, headache, dizziness, and bone pain), shortness of breath, wheezing, decrease in blood pressure and shock. The "flu" syndrome may also appear if Rifampin is taken irregularly by the patient or if daily administration is resumed after a drug free interval.

OVERDOSAGE

There is no human experience with Isoniazid/Pyrazinamide/Rifampin overdosage.

Isoniazid: Untreated or inadequately treated cases of gross Isoniazid overdosage can be fatal, but good response has been reported in most patients treated within the first few hours after drug ingestion.

Ingested acutely, as little as 1.5 gm Isoniazid may cause toxicity in adults. Doses of 35 to 40 mg/kg have resulted in seizures. Ingestion of 80 to 150 mg/kg Isoniazid has been associated with severe toxicity and, if untreated, significant mortality.

Pyrazinamide: Overdosage experience with Pyrazinamide is limited.

Rifampin: Nonfatal overdoses with as high as 12 gm of Rifampin have been reported. One case of fatal overdose is known: A 26-year old man died after self-administering 60 gm of Rifampin.

SIGNS AND SYMPTOMS

The following signs and symptoms have been seen with each individual component in an overdosage situation.

Isoniazid: Isoniazid overdosage produces signs and symptoms within 30 minutes to 3 hours. Nausea, vomiting, dizziness, slurring of speech, blurring of vision, and visual hallucinations (including bright colors and strange designs) are among the early manifestations. With marked overdosage, respiratory distress and CNS depression, progressing rapidly from stupor to profound coma, are to be expected along with severe, intractable seizures. Severe metabolic acidosis, acetonuria, and hyperglycemia are typical laboratory findings.

Pyrazinamide: In one case of Pyrazinamide overdosage, abnormal liver function tests developed. These spontaneously reverted to normal when the drug was stopped.

Rifampin: Nausea, vomiting, and increasing lethargy will probably occur within a short time after Rifampin overdosage; unconsciousness may occur when there is severe hepatic disease. Brownish red or orange discoloration of the skin, urine, sweat, saliva, tears, and feces will occur, and its intensity is proportional to the amount ingested.

Liver enlargement, possibly with tenderness, can develop within a few hours after severe overdosage; bilirubin levels may increase and jaundice may develop rapidly. Hepatic involvement may be more marked in patients with prior impairment of hepatic function. Other physical findings remain essentially normal. A direct effect upon the hematopoietic system, electrolyte levels, or acid-base balance is unlikely.

TREATMENT

The airway should be secured and adequate respiratory exchange should be established in cases of overdosage with Isoniazid/Pyrazinamide/Rifampin.

Obtain blood samples for immediate determination of gases, electrolytes, BUN, glucose, etc. type and cross-match blood in preparation for possible hemodialysis.

Gastric lavage within the first 2 to 3 hours after ingestion is advised, but it should not be attempted until convulsions are under control. To treat convulsions, administer IV diazepam or short-acting barbiturates, and IV pyridoxine (usually 1 mg/1 mg Isoniazid ingested). Following evacuation of gastric contents, the instillation of activated charcoal slurry into the stomach may help absorb any remaining drug from the gastrointestinal tract. Antiemetic medication may be required to control severe nausea and vomiting.

Rapid Control of Metabolic Acidosis is Fundamental to Management: Give IV sodium bicarbonate at once and repeat as needed, adjusting subsequent dosage on the basis of laboratory findings (ie, serum sodium, pH, etc.)

Forced osmotic diuresis must be started early and should be continued for some hours after clinical improvement to hasten renal clearance of drug and help prevent relapse; monitor fluid intake and output.

Hemodialysis is advised for severe cases; if this is not available, peritoneal dialysis can be used along with forced diuresis.

Along with measures based on initial and repeated determination of blood gases and other laboratory tests as needed, utilize meticulous respiratory and other intensive care to protect against hypoxia, hypotension, aspiration pneumonitis, etc.

DOSAGE AND ADMINISTRATION

Adults: Patients should be given the following single daily dose of Isoniazid/Pyrazinamide/Rifampin either 1 hour before or 2 hours after a meal with a full glass of water.

Patients weighing ≤ 44 kg—4 tablets
Patients weighing between 45-54 kg—5 tablets
Patients weighing ≥ 55 kg—6 tablets

Children: The ratio of the drugs in Isoniazid/Pyrazinamide/Rifampin may not be appropriate in children or adolescents under the age of 15 (eg, higher mg/kg doses of Isoniazid are usually given in children than adults).

Isoniazid/Pyrazinamide/Rifampin is recommended in the initial phase of short-course therapy which is usually continued for 2 months. The Advisory Council for the Elimination of Tuberculosis, the American Thoracic Society, and the Centers for Disease Control and Prevention recommend that either streptomycin or ethambutol be added as a fourth drug in a regimen containing Isoniazid (INH), Pyrazinamide, and Rifampin for initial treatment of tuberculosis unless the likelihood of INH or Rifampin resistance is very low. The need for a fourth drug should be reassessed when the results of susceptibility testing are known. If community rates of INH resistance are currently less than 4%, an initial treatment regimen with less than four drugs may be considered.

Following the initial phase, treatment should be continued with Rifampin and Isoniazid for at least 4 months. Treatment should be continued for longer if the patient is still sputum or culture positive, if resistant organisms are present, or if the patient is HIV positive.

Concomitant administration of pyridoxine (B_6) is recommended in the malnourished, in those predisposed to neuropathy (e.g., alcoholics and diabetics), and in adolescents.

See *"Clinical Pharmacology, General"* for dosing information in patients with renal failure.

Storage Conditions: Store at controlled room temperature, 59-86°F (15-30°C). Protect from excessive humidity.

REFERENCE

1. National Committee for Clinical Laboratory Standards. 1990. Antimycobacterial Susceptibility Testing (Proposed Standard). Document M24-P.

HOW SUPPLIED
TABLETS: 50 MG-300 MG-120 MG

BRAND/MANUFACTURER	NDC	SIZE	AWP
○ **BRAND**			
▶ RIFATER: Marion Merrell Dow	00088-0576-41	60s	$108.00

Isoproterenol

DESCRIPTION

Isoproterenol is a beta agonist sympathomimetic bronchodilator. Isoproterenol inhalation solution contains Isoproterenol hydrochloride 5 mg/mL or 10 mg/mL.

Each metered dose of Isoproterenol inhalation aerosol delivers 0.08 mg Isoproterenol Sulfate of appropriate particle size (the majority less than 5μ or 131 μg of Isoproterenol Hydrochloride).

Each milliliter of the sterile 1:5000 solution contains Isoproterenol HCl Injection, USP, 0.2 mg.

The sterile 1:5000 solution can be administered by the intravenous, intramuscular, subcutaneous, or intracardiac routes.

Isoproterenol HCl is soluble in water (1 g Isoproterenol HCl dissolves in 3 mL H_2O). The solution and injection have a pH range of 3 to 4.5.

Isoproterenol HCl is a racemic compound with a molecular weight of 247.72 and the molecular formula $C_{11}H_{17}NO_3 \cdot HCl$.

Chemically, Isoproterenol HCl is 3,4-Dihydroxy-α-[(isopropylamino)methyl]benzyl alcohol hydrochloride, a synthetic sympathomimetic amine that is structurally related to epinephrine.

Chemically, Isoproterenol sulfate is 4-[1-hydroxy-2-[(1-methylethyl)amino]ethyl]-1,2-benzenediol sulfate.

CLINICAL PHARMACOLOGY

Isoproterenol relaxes bronchial spasm and facilitates expectoration of pulmonary secretions by acting almost exclusively on beta receptors. It is frequently effective when epinephrine and other drugs fail, and it has a wide margin of safety.

Isoproterenol acts directly on beta-adrenergic receptors of tissues supplied by sympathetic nerves. The beta-adrenergic effects stem from the release of cyclic AMP following the activation of the enzyme adenyl cyclase. Therapeutic doses of Isoproterenol result in relaxation of the smooth muscle of the bronchial tree and decrease in peripheral vascular resistance; increased cardiac output and stroke volume may occur due to its positive inotropic and chronotropic action. The coronary arteries may be dilated, increasing the blood flow. Isoproterenol also inhibits uterine motility and causes decreased tone and motility of intestinal musculature even when epinephrine causes contraction.

In patients with bronchial constriction, Isoproterenol relieves bronchospasm, increases pulmonary function, decreases residual air, and facilitates lung clearance by increasing ciliary motility and mucous transport. Bronchodilatation occurs quickly after oral inhalation and lasts up to one hour. It is one of the most potent bronchodilators known and can be used in patients who do not respond to the bronchodilating action of epinephrine. The drug will prevent or overcome histamine-induced asthma in both experimental animals and man, and is effective when used prophylactically.

Isoproterenol has a cardio-accelerating effect, but its vasoconstricting action is less pronounced than that of epinephrine. Therapeutic doses may produce a slight increase in systolic blood pressure but a slight decrease in diastolic. Larger doses may cause peripheral vasodilation in the renal, mesenteric, and femoral beds; some patients respond with a decrease in diastolic but no change in systolic pressure. Such effects are usually of very short duration.

Pharmacokinetics: The average plasma half-life for Isoproterenol given intravenously in seven healthy volunteers was four minutes while the average half-life of the drug administered by aerosol to five patients was five minutes. In children, the decline in plasma concentration was biphasic, with a half-life during the first phase of two to five minutes and of three to seven hours during the second phase. A plasma concentration of 0.03 ng/ml was found within minutes following an aerosol inhalation dose of 500 mcg.

Isoproterenol is readily absorbed when given as an aerosol. Excretion following inhalation administration is primarily renal and the major metabolite is the sulfate conjugate of Isoproterenol. When the drug is administered directly into the bronchial tree, it is inactivated by the enzyme catechol-o-methyl transferase, and the predominant metabolite is 3-o-methylisoproterenol sulfate. The explanation for this difference is supported by the observation that most (90%) of an aerosol dose is deposited in the mouth and pharynx and is swallowed. The swallowed Isoproterenol is converted to its sulfate conjugate in the gut wall, and to a lesser extent in the liver. The remaining Isoproterenol is excreted as follows: 1% to 2% unchanged, 1% to 2% free methylated metabolite, and small amounts of metabolites in the bile.

Recent studies in laboratory animals (minipigs, rodents, and dogs) recorded the occurrence of cardiac arrhythmias and sudden death (with histologic evidence of myocardial necrosis) when beta agonists and methylxanthines were concomitantly administered. The significance of these findings when applied to human usage is currently unknown.

Isoproterenol HCl injection acts primarily on the heart and on smooth muscle of bronchi, skeletal muscle vasculature, and alimentary tract. The positive

---

◆ RATED THERAPEUTICALLY EQUIVALENT; ◇ THERAPEUTIC EQUIVALENCE UNCONFIRMED; ○ UNRATED

inotropic and chronotropic actions of the drug result in an increase in minute blood flow. There is an increase in heart rate, an approximately unchanged stroke volume, and an increase in ejection velocity. The rate of discharge of cardiac pacemakers is increased with Isoproterenol HCl injection. Venous return to the heart is increased through a decreased compliance of the venous bed. Systemic resistance and pulmonary vascular resistance are decreased, and there is an increase in coronary and renal blood flow. Systolic blood pressure may increase and diastolic blood pressure may decrease. Mean arterial blood pressure is usually unchanged or reduced. The peripheral and coronary vasodilating effects of the drug may aid tissue perfusion.

Isoproterenol HCl injection relaxes most smooth muscle, the most pronounced effect being on bronchial and gastrointestinal smooth muscle. It produces marked relaxation in the smaller bronchi and may even dilate the trachea and main bronchi past the resting diameter.

Isoproterenol HCl injection is metabolized primarily in the liver by COMT. The duration of action of Isoproterenol HCl injection may be longer than epinephrine, but it is still brief.

INDICATIONS AND USAGE

Isoproterenol is indicated for the relief of bronchospasm associated with acute and chronic asthma and reversible bronchospasm which may be associated with chronic bronchitis or emphysema.

Isoproterenol HCl injection is indicated:

- For mild or transient episodes of heart block that do not require electric shock or pacemaker therapy.
- For serious episodes of heart block and Adams-Stokes attacks (except when caused by ventricular tachycardia or fibrillation). (See *"Contraindications"*.)
- For use in cardiac arrest until electric shock or pacemaker therapy, the treatments of choice, is available. (See *"Contraindications"*.)
- For bronchospasm occurring during anesthesia.
- As an adjunct to fluid and electrolyte replacement therapy and the use of other drugs and procedures in the treatment of hypovolemic and septic shock, low cardiac output (hypoperfusion) states, congestive heart failure, and cardiogenic shock. (See *"Warnings"*.)

UNLABELED USES

Isoproterenol is used alone or as an adjunct in the treatment of philmonary hypertension, cerebral vasospasm, and bronchopulmonary dysplasia.

CONTRAINDICATION

Use of Isoproterenol in patients with preexisting cardiac arrhythmias associated with tachycardia is generally considered contraindicated because the cardiac stimulant effect of the drug may aggravate such disorders. The use of this medication is contraindicated in those patients who have a known hypersensitivity to Isoproterenol or other sympathomimetic amines or to any of the other components of this drug.

Use of Isoproterenol HCl injection is contraindicated in patients with tachyarrhythmias; tachycardia or heartblock caused by digitalis intoxication; ventricular arrhythmias which require inotropic therapy; and angina pectoris.

WARNINGS

Excessive use of an adrenergic aerosol should be discouraged as it may lose its effectiveness.

Isoproterenol administration as a solution for nebulization has been associated with a decrease in arterial pO₂ in asthmatic patients as a result of ventilation-perfusion abnormalities despite improvement in airway obstruction. The clinical significance of this relative hypoxemia is unclear.

In patients with status asthmaticus and abnormal blood gas tensions, improvement in vital capacity and in blood gas tensions may not accompany apparent relief of bronchospasm. Facilities for administering oxygen mixtures and ventilatory assistance are necessary to such patients.

Occasional patients have been reported to develop severe paradoxical airway resistance with repeated, excessive use of isoproterenol inhalation preparations. The cause of this refractory state is unknown. It is advisable that in such instances the use of this preparation be discontinued immediately and alternative therapy instituted, since in the reported cases the patients did not respond to other forms of therapy until the drug was withdrawn.

Deaths have been reported following excessive use of Isoproterenol inhalation preparations and the exact cause is unknown. Cardiac arrest was noted in several instances. It is therefore essential that the physician instruct the patient in the need for further evaluation if his/her asthma worsens.

Isoproterenol HCl injection, by increasing myocardial oxygen requirements while decreasing effective coronary perfusion, may have a deleterious effect on the injured or failing heart. Most experts discourage its use as the initial agent in treating cardiogenic shock following myocardial infarction. However, when a low arterial pressure has been elevated by other means, Isoproterenol HCl injection may produce beneficial hemodynamic and metabolic effects.

In a few patients, presumably with organic disease of the AV node and its branches, Isoproterenol HCl injection has paradoxically been reported to worsen heart block or to precipitate Adams-Stokes attacks during normal sinus rhythm or transient heart block.

Some brands of Isoproterenol contain sodium metabisulfite, a sulfite that may cause allergic-type reactions including anaphylactic symptoms and life-threatening or less severe asthmatic episodes in certain susceptible people. The overall prevalence of sulfite sensitivity in the general population is unknown and probably low. Sulfite sensitivity is seen more frequently in asthmatic than in nonasthmatic people.

PRECAUTIONS

Isoproterenol, as with all sympathomimetic amines, should be used with caution in patients with cardiovascular disorders, especially coronary insufficiency, cardiac arrhythmias, and hypertension; in patients with convulsive disorders, hyperthyroidism, or diabetes mellitus; and in patients who are unusually responsive to sympathomimetic amines. Clinically significant changes in systolic and diastolic blood pressure have been seen in some patients after use of any beta adrenergic bronchodilator.

Any patient who requires more than three aerosol treatments within a 24-hour period should be under the close supervision of his physician. Further therapy with the bronchodilator aerosol alone is inadvisable when three to five treatments within six to twelve hours produce minimal or no relief.

When compressed oxygen is employed as the aerosol propellant, the percentage of oxygen used should be determined by the patient's individual requirements to avoid depression of respiratory drive.

Isoproterenol and epinephrine may be used interchangeably if the patient becomes unresponsive to one or the other, but should not be used concurrently. If desired, these drugs may be alternated, provided an interval of at least four hours has elapsed.

Information for Patients: Patients who are being treated with Isoproterenol inhalation aerosol should be informed adequately of the dangers of overusage, tolerance, and rebound bronchospasm (see *"Warnings, Adverse Reactions"*). They should be instructed to take no more than two inhalations at any one time, nor more than six in any one hour during a 24-hour period, unless advised by the physician (see *"Dosage and Administration"*; Patient Instructions for Use).

Isoproterenol may cause the patient's saliva to turn pinkish to red in color. Proper use of Isoproterenol oral inhaler should be demonstrated and discussed. Patient Instructions for Use are available with the package insert and should be provided when the medication is dispensed.

As with any drug, patients should be advised against the ingestion of alcohol during treatment.

GENERAL

Isoproterenol HCl injection should generally be started at the lowest recommended dose. This may be gradually increased, if necessary, while carefully monitoring the patient. Doses sufficient to increase the heart rate to more than 130 beats per minute may increase the likelihood of inducing ventricular arrhythmias. Such increases in heart rate will also tend to increase cardiac work and oxygen requirements which may adversely affect the failing heart or the heart with a significant degree of arteriosclerosis.

Adequate filling of the intravascular compartment by suitable volume expanders is of primary importance in most cases of shock, and should precede the administration of vasoactive drugs. In patients with normal cardiac function, determination of central venous pressure is a reliable guide during volume replacement. If evidence of hypoperfusion persists after adequate volume replacement, Isoproterenol HCl injection may be given.

In addition to the routine monitoring of systemic blood pressure, heart rate, urine flow, and the electrocardiograph, the response to therapy should also be monitored by frequent determination of the central venous pressure and blood gases. Patients in shock should be closely observed during Isoproterenol HCl injection administration. If the heart rate exceeds 110 beats per minute, it may be advisable to decrease the infusion rate or temporarily discontinue the infusion. Determinations of cardiac output and circulation time may also be helpful. Appropriate measures should be taken to ensure adequate ventilation. Careful attention should be paid to acid-base balance and to the correction of electrolyte disturbances. In cases of shock associated with bacteremia, suitable antimicrobial therapy is, of course, imperative.

Drug Interactions: Other sympathomimetic aerosol bronchodilators or epinephrine should not be used concomitantly with Isoproterenol. If additional adrenergic drugs are to be administered by any route to the patient using Isoproterenol, they should be used with caution to avoid deleterious cardiovascular effects.

Beta adrenergic agonists should be administered with caution to patients being treated with MAO inhibitors or tricyclic antidepressants since the action of the beta adrenergic agonists on the vascular system may be potentiated. No adverse cardiovascular effects were observed in normal volunteers given Isoproterenol by inhalation along with a monoamine oxidase inhibitor or a tricyclic antidepressant.

Beta receptor blocking agents and Isoproterenol inhibit the effects of each other.

Corticosteroids may be used to restore responsiveness to Isoproterenol if necessary. This may come about by increasing the sensitivity of the beta-adrenergic receptors to isoproterenol.

Concomitant administration of ergot alkaloids and Isoproterenol may result in additive peripheral vasoconstriction. Arrhythmias may result from the administration of Isoproterenol to patients who are receiving digitalis, epinephrine, cyclopropane, or halogenated hydrocarbon anesthetics. Beta-adrenergic blocking drugs such as propranolol antagonize the cardiac, bronchodilating, and vasodilating effects of isoproterenol.

Isoproterenol should be used with caution, if at all, when potent inhalational anesthetics such as halothane are employed because of potential to sensitize the myocardium to effects of sympathomimetic amines.

Drug/Laboratory Test Interactions: Isoproterenol causes false elevations of bilirubin as measured *in vitro* by a sequential multiple analyzer. An effect on serum bilirubin determinations in patients receiving the drug has not been determined. Isoproterenol inhalation may result in enough absorption of the drug

▶ **SHOWN IN PRODUCT IDENTIFICATION GUIDE**

to produce elevated values for urinary epinephrine. This effect is probably small with standard inhalation doses, but is likely to increase with larger doses.

Carcinogenesis, Mutagenesis, Impairment of Fertility: Long-term chronic toxicity studies in animals have not been done to evaluate Isoproterenol in these areas.

Pregnancy Category C: Animal reproduction studies have not been conducted with Isoproterenol HCl. It is also not known whether Isoproterenol HCl can cause fetal harm when administered to a pregnant woman or can effect reproduction capacity. Isoproterenol HCl should be given to a pregnant woman only if clearly needed.

Pregnancy Category B: Reproduction studies of Isoproterenol Sulfate have been performed in rats and rabbits at aerosol doses (30 minutes per day for 12 days) up to 15 times the human dose and have revealed no evidence of impaired fertility or harm to the fetus due to Isoproterenol. There are, however, no adequate and well-controlled studies in pregnant women. Because animal reproduction studies are not always predictive of human response, this drug should be used during pregnancy only if clearly needed.

Labor and Delivery: Isoproterenol has no recognized use during labor and delivery, and its effect during these processes is unknown.

Nursing Mothers: It is not known whether this drug is excreted in human milk. Because many drugs are excreted in human milk, caution should be exercised when Isoproterenol is administered to a nursing woman.

Pediatric Use: In general, the technique of Isoproterenol Hydrochloride solution in administration to children is similar to that of adults, since children's smaller ventilatory exchange capacity automatically provides proportionally smaller aerosol intake. However, it is generally recommended that the 1:200 solution (rather than the 1:100) be used for an acute attack of bronchospasm, and no more than 0.25 mL of the 1:200 solution should be used for each 10 to 15 minute programmed treatment in chronic bronchospastic disease.

Safe and effective use of Isoproterenol Sulfate aerosol in children below the age of 12 has not been established.

Geriatric Use: Lower doses in elderly patients may be required due to increased sympathomimetic sensitivity (see *"Dosage and Administration"*).

ADVERSE REACTIONS

The mist from some brands of Isoproterenol HCl inhalation aerosol contains alcohol but is generally very well tolerated. An occasional patient may experience some transient throat irritation which has been attributed to the alcohol content.

Serious reactions to Isoproterenol are infrequent. The following reactions, however, have been reported:

CNS: Nervousness, headache, dizziness, weakness, vertigo, central excitation, insomnia.

Gastrointestinal: Nausea, vomiting.

Cardiovascular: Tachycardia, palpitations, precordial distress, anginal-type pain, coronary insufficiency, flushing of the skin, blood pressure changes, cardiac arrhythmias, cardiac arrest.

Pulmonary: Paradoxical airway resistance (see *"Warnings"*), rebound bronchospasm.

Other: Flushing of the skin, tremor, and sweating.

The inhalation route is usually accompanied by a minimum of side effects. These untoward reactions disappear quickly and do not as a rule, inconvenience the patient to the extent that the drug must be discontinued. No cumulative effects have been reported.

DRUG ABUSE AND DEPENDENCE

Drug abuse and dependence have not been reported with Isoproterenol Sulfate inhalation aerosol.

In a few patients, presumably with organic disease of the AV node and its branches, Isoproterenol HCl injection has been reported to precipitate Adams-Stokes seizures during normal sinus rhythm or transient heart block.

OVERDOSAGE

The acute toxicity of Isoproterenol HCl in animals is much less than that of epinephrine. Excessive doses in animals or man can cause a striking drop in blood pressure, and repeated large doses in animals may result in cardiac enlargement and focal myocarditis.

Overdosage of Isoproterenol HCl may produce signs and symptoms typical of excessive sympathomimetic effects, including tachycardia, palpitations, angina, hypotension, hypertension, nervousness, nausea, and vomiting. Excessive use of adrenergic aerosols may result in loss of effectiveness or severe paradoxical airway resistance. Cardiac arrest has been noted in several instances. In all cases of overdose or excessive use of Isoproterenol HCl, the drug should be discontinued immediately or the rate of injection reduced and vital functions supported until the patient is stabilized. It is not known whether Isoproterenol HCl is dialyzable.

The acute oral LD_{50} in mice is 3,850 mg/kg $\pm$ 1.190 mg/kg of pure drug in solution (Isoproterenol HCl). In dogs, the toxic dose is 1,000 times the therapeutic dose. Converted to the amount used clinically in man, this would be about 2,500 times the therapeutic dose.

The oral LD_{50} values for Isoproterenol Sulfate are as follows: mouse, 1260 mg/kg: rabbit, 3070 mg/kg; male rat, 2230 mg/kg; female rat, 2840 mg/kg; and dog, 600 mg/kg. The intravenous LD^{50} values are as follows: mouse, 126 mg/kg; rabbit, 27 mg/kg; male rat, 96 mg/kg; female rat, 112 mg/kg; and dog, 50 mg/kg. Overdosage effects may occur at doses equal to the therapeutic dose.

Symptoms: Manifestations of acute overdosage include chest pain, dizziness, headache, irregular heartbeat, fast or pounding heartbeat, nausea or vomiting, restlessness, weakness, flushing, or decreased diastolic pressure.

Treatment: Discontinued dosing allows rapid reversal of adverse effects. Blood pressure and ECG may be monitored and the following treatment used, as appropriate: tachycardia in asthmatic patients may be treated with cardio-selective beta-blockers (metoprolol or atenolol, but used cautiously since cardio-selectivity may not be absolute) and in nonasthmatics with propranolol; blood pressure may be regulated with rapid-acting vasodilators (nitrites, sodium nitroprusside) or alpha-blocking agents (quinidine, phentolamine).

It is not known if Isoproterenol Sulfate dialyzable; however, its rapid elimination should preclude the need for dialysis.

DOSAGE AND ADMINISTRATION

Isoproterenol HCl solutions can be administered as an aerosol mist by hand-bulb nebulizer, compressed air or oxygen operated nebulizer, or by intermittent positive pressure breathing (IPPB) devices. The method of delivery, and the treatment regimen employed in the management of the reversible bronchospastic element accompanying bronchial asthma, chronic bronchitis, and chronic obstructive lung diseases, will depend on such factors as the severity of the bronchospasm, patient age, tolerance to the medication, complicating cardiopulmonary conditions, and whether therapy is for an intermittent acute attack of bronchospasm or is part of a programmed treatment regimen for constant bronchospasm.

Acute Bronchial Asthma. Hand-Bulb Nebulizer: Depending on the frequency of treatment and the type of nebulizer used, a volume of solution Isoproterenol HCl, sufficient for not more than one day's treatment, should be placed in the nebulizer using the dropper provided. In time, the patient can learn to adjust the volume required. For adults and children, the 1:200 solution is administered by hand-bulb nebulization in a dosage of 5 to 15 deep inhalations (using an all glass or plastic nebulizer). In adults, the 1:100 solution may be used if a stronger solution seems to be indicated. The dose is 3 to 7 deep inhalations. If after about 5 to 10 minutes inadequate relief is observed, these doses may be repeated one more time. If the acute attack recurs, treatments may be repeated up to 5 times daily if necessary. (See *"Precautions"*.)

Bronchospasm in Chronic Obstructive Lung Disease. Hand-Bulb Nebulizer: A solution of 1:200 or 1:100 of Isoproterenol HCl may be administered daily at not less than 3 to 4 hour intervals for subacute bronchospastic attacks or as part of a programmed treatment regimen in patients with chronic obstructive lung disease with a reversible bronchospastic component. An adequate dose is usually 5 to 15 deep inhalations, using the 1:200 solution. Some patients with severe attacks of bronchospasm may require 3 to 7 deep inhalations using the 1:100 solution of Isoproterenol HCl.

Nebulization by Compressed Air or Oxygen: A method often used in patients with severe chronic obstructive lung disease is to deliver the Isoproterenol mist *in more dilute form over a longer period of time.* The purpose is, not so much to increase the dose supplied, as to achieve progressively deeper bronchodilatation and thus insure that the mist achieves maximum penetration of the finer bronchioles. In this method, 0.5 mL of a 1:200 solution of Isoproterenol HCl is diluted to 2 mL to 2.5 mL with water or isotonic saline to achieve a use concentration of 1:800 to 1:1000. If desired, 0.25 mL of the 1:100 solution may be similarly diluted to achieve the same use concentration. The diluted solution is placed in a nebulizer connected to either a source of compressed air or oxygen. The flow rate is regulated to suit the particular nebulizer so that the diluted solution of Isoproterenol HCl will be delivered over approximately 10 to 20 minutes. A treatment may be repeated up to 5 times daily if necessary. Although the total delivered dose of Isoproterenol is somewhat higher than with the treatment regimen employing the hand-bulb nebulizer, patients usually tolerate it well because of the greater dilution and longer application-time factors.

Intermittent Positive Pressure Breathing (IPPB): Diluted solutions of 1:200 or 1:100 of Isoproterenol HCl are used in a programmed regimen for the treatment of reversible bronchospasm in patients with chronic obstructive lung disease who require intermittent positive pressure breathing therapy. These devices generally have a small nebulizer, usually of 3 mL to 5 mL capacity, on a patient-operated side arm. The effectiveness of IPPB therapy is greatly enhanced by the simultaneous use of aerosolized bronchodilators. As with compressed air or oxygen operated nebulizers, the usual regimen is to place 0.5 mL of 1:200 solution of Isoproterenol HCl diluted to 2 mL to 2.5 mL with water or isotonic saline in the nebulizer cup and follow the IPPB manufacturer's operating instructions. IPPB-bronchodilator treatments are usually administered over 15 to 20 minutes, up to 5 times daily if necessary.

Children's Dosage: In general, the technique of Isoproterenol HCl solution in administration to children is similar to that of adults, since children's smaller ventilatory exchange capacity automatically provides proportionally smaller aerosol intake. However, it is generally recommended that the 1:200 solution (rather than the 1:100) be used for an acute attack of bronchospasm, and no more than 0.25 mL of the 1:200 solution should be used for each 10 to 15 minute programmed treatment in chronic bronchospastic disease.

Adults: The usual dose of Isoproterenol Sulfate aerosol inhalation for the relief of dyspnea in the acute episode is one or two inhalations. Start with a single inhalation. If no relief is evident after two to five minutes, a second inhalation may be taken. For daily maintenance, use one or two inhalations four to six times daily or as directed by the physician. The physician should be careful to instruct

---

♦ RATED THERAPEUTICALLY EQUIVALENT; ◇ THERAPEUTIC EQUIVALENCE UNCONFIRMED; ○ UNRATED

the patient in the proper technique of administration so that the number of inhalations per treatment and the frequency of retreatment may be titrated to the patient's response.

No more than two inhalations should be taken at any one time, nor more than six inhalations in any one hour during a 24-hour period, unless advised by the physician. Lower doses in elderly patients may be required due to increased sympathomimetic sensitivity.

Each depression of the valve delivers through the oral adapter 0.08 mg Isoproterenol Sulfate.

Children: Safety and effectiveness for children under 12 years have not been established (see *"Pediatric Use"*).

DIRECTIONS FOR USE
Before each use, remove dust cap and inspect mouthpiece for foreign objects. Shake Isoproterenol Sulfate inhalation aerosol unit.

1. Breathe out fully and place mouthpiece well into the mouth aimed at the back of the throat.
2. As you begin to breathe in deeply, press the vial firmly down into the adapter with the index finger. This releases one dose.
3. Release pressure on vial and remove unit from mouth. Hold your breath as long as possible, then breathe out slowly.

Replace dust cap after each use.

Isoproterenol HCl injection 1:5000 should generally be started at the lowest recommended dose and the rate of administration gradually increased if necessary while carefully monitoring the patient. The usual route of administration is by intravenous infusion or bolus intravenous injection. In dire emergencies, the drug may be administered by intracardiac injection. If time is not of the utmost importance, initial therapy by intramuscular or subcutaneous injection is preferred. (See related table).

There are no well-controlled studies in children to establish appropriate dosing; however, the American Heart Association recommends an initial infusion rate of 0.1 µg/kg/min, with the usual range being 0.1 µg/kg/min to 1.0 µg/kg/min.

RECOMMENDED DOSAGE FOR ADULTS WITH SHOCK AND HYPOPERFUSION STATES

Route of Administration	Preparation of Dilution†	Infusion Rate††
Intravenous infusion	Dilute 5 mL (1 mg) in 500 mL of 5% Dextrose Injection, USP	0.5 µg to 5 µg per minute (0.25 mL to 2.5 mL of diluted solution)

† Concentrations up to 10 times greater have been used when limitation of volume is essential.
†† Rates over 30 µg per minute have been used in advanced stages of shock. The rate of infusion should be adjusted on the basis of heart rate, central venous pressure, systemic blood pressure, and urine flow. If the heart rate exceeds 110 beats per minute, it may be advisable to decrease or temporarily discontinue the infusion.

RECOMMENDED DOSAGE FOR ADULTS WITH BRONCHOSPASM OCCURRING DURING ANESTHESIA

Route of Administration	Preparation of Dilution	Initial Dose	Subsequent Dose
Bolus intravenous injection	Dilute 1 mL (0.2 mg) to 10 mL with Sodium Chloride Injection, USP, or 5% Dextrose Injection, USP	0.01 mg to 0.02 mg (0.5 mL to 1 mL of diluted solution)	The initial dose may be repeated when necessary

Parenteral drug products should be inspected visually for particulate matter and discoloration prior to administration, whenever solution and container permit. Such solution should not be used.

Storage: Store at controlled room temperature, 15°C to 30°C (59°F to 86°F).
Contents of aerosol container under pressure. Do not puncture or incinerate container. Keep out of the reach of children.

Store Isoproterenol HCl injection in a cool place between 8°C to 15°C (46°F to 59°F). Do not use if the injection is pinkish to brownish in color or contains a precipitate.

J CODES
1.0% per ml INH—J7665
0.5% per ml INH—J7660

HOW SUPPLIED

ISOPROTERENOL HYDROCHLORIDE
AEROSOL LIQUID: 1:400

BRAND/MANUFACTURER	NDC	SIZE	AWP
○ BRAND			
ISUPREL MISTOMETER: Sanofi Winthrop	00024-0879-01	15 ml	$26.33

AEROSOL LIQUID W/ADAPTER: 1:400

BRAND/MANUFACTURER	NDC	SIZE	AWP
○ BRAND			
ISUPREL MISTOMETER: Sanofi Winthrop	00024-0878-05	10 ml	$22.53
	00024-0878-01	15 ml	$29.71

INJECTION: 1:50,000

BRAND/MANUFACTURER	NDC	SIZE	AWP
◆ GENERICS			
Abbott Hosp	00074-4905-01	10 ml 10s	$127.30

INJECTION: 1:5,000

AVERAGE UNIT PRICE (AVAILABLE SIZES)			
GENERIC	$2.09		

BRAND/MANUFACTURER	NDC	SIZE	AWP
◆ GENERICS			
Abbott Hosp	00074-4978-01	5 ml 10s	$124.93
Abbott Hosp	00074-4977-01	10 ml 10s	$168.74

INJECTION: 0.2 MG/ML

AVERAGE UNIT PRICE (AVAILABLE SIZES)			
BRAND	$4.27		

BRAND/MANUFACTURER	NDC	SIZE	AWP
◆ BRAND			
ISUPREL HCL: Sanofi Winthrop	00024-0866-02	5 ml 10s	$179.12
	00024-0866-25	1 ml 25s	$123.82
◆ GENERICS			
Elkins-Sinn	00641-1438-35	5 ml 25s	$89.43

SOLUTION: 1:200

AVERAGE UNIT PRICE (AVAILABLE SIZES)			
BRAND	$1.86		

BRAND/MANUFACTURER	NDC	SIZE	AWP
◆ BRAND			
ISUPREL HCL: Sanofi Winthrop	00024-0871-01	10 ml	$22.04
	00024-0871-03	60 ml	$90.49

SOLUTION: 1:100

BRAND/MANUFACTURER	NDC	SIZE	AWP
◆ BRAND			
ISUPREL HCL: Sanofi Winthrop	00024-0873-01	10 ml	$23.28

RECOMMENDED DOSAGE FOR ADULTS WITH HEART BLOCK, ADAMS-STOKES ATTACKS, AND CARDIAC ARREST

Route of Administration	Preparation of Dilution	Initial Dose	Subsequent Dose Range*
Bolus intravenous injection	Dilute 1 mL (0.2 mg) to 10 mL with Sodium Chloride Injection, USP, or 5% Dextrose Injection, USP	0.02 mg to 0.06 mg (1 mL to 3 mL of diluted solution)	0.01 mg to 0.2 mg (0.5 mL to 10 mL of diluted solution)
Intravenous infusion	Dilute 10 mL (2 mg) in 500 mL of 5% Dextrose Injection, USP	5 µg/min. (1.25 mL of diluted solution per minute)	
Intramuscular	Use Solution 1:5000 undiluted	0.2 mg (1 mL)	0.02 mg to 1 mg (0.1 mL to 5 mL)
Subcutaneous	Use Solution 1:5000 undiluted	0.2 mg (1 mL)	0.15 to 0.2 mg (0.75 mL to 1 mL)
Intracardiac	Use Solution 1:5000 undiluted	0.02 mg (0.1 mL)	

* Subsequent dosage and method of administration depend on the ventricular rate and the rapidity with which the cardiac pacemaker can take over when the drug is gradually withdrawn.

► SHOWN IN PRODUCT IDENTIFICATION GUIDE

TABLETS: 10 MG

BRAND/MANUFACTURER	NDC	SIZE	AWP
◆ **BRAND**			
ISUPREL HCL GLOSSETS: Sanofi Winthrop	00024-0875-02	50s	$31.98

ISOPROTERENOL SULFATE
AEROSOL LIQUID: 1:500

BRAND/MANUFACTURER	NDC	SIZE	AWP
○ **BRAND**			
MEDIHALER-ISO: 3M Pharm	00089-0785-11	15 ml	$20.52

AEROSOL LIQUID W/ADAPTER: 1:500

BRAND/MANUFACTURER	NDC	SIZE	AWP
○ **BRAND**			
MEDIHALER-ISO: 3M Pharm	00089-0785-21	15 ml	$23.16

Isoproterenol Hydrochloride with Phenylephrine Bitartrate

DESCRIPTION
Isoproterenol Hydrochloride/Phenylephrine Bitartrate is a combination of two sympathomimetics administered by oral inhalation for the treatment of broncho-constriction. Each metered dose of the aerosol delivers through the oral adapter 0.16 mg Isoproterenol Hydrochloride and 0.24 mg Phenylephrine Bitartrate of appropriate particle size (the majority less than 5 μ).

CLINICAL PHARMACOLOGY
Isoproterenol acts directly on beta-adrenergic receptors and Phenylephrine acts directly on alpha-adrenergic receptors. The beta-adrenergic effects stem from the release of cyclic AMP following activation of the enzyme adenyl cyclase. Alpha-adrenergic effects probably result from inhibition of adenyl cyclase. Isoproterenol produces bronchodilatation, systemic vasodilation, mild hypotension, and tachy-cardia. Phenylephrine produces mild bronchodilatation, systemic vasoconstric-tion, mild hypertension, and bradycardia. These two drugs appear to act synergistically to allow the expression of each product's ability to relax bronchial smooth muscle. The vasoconstrictor effect of Phenylephrine reduces bronchiolar blood flow thereby producing a decongestant effect promotes retention of the drug in the bronchial mucosa, and blocks the tachycardia of isoproterenol. After oral inhalation of the combination, the pulmonary effects occur within a few minutes and persist up to three hours.

Studies demonstrate that the ventilatory effects of Isoproterenol/ Phenyleph-rine are superior to those obtained with the administration of Isoproterenol alone. Because Isoproterenol is a potent vasodilator that lowers blood pressure and acts upon the heart to increase cardiac output and pulse rate, its combination with Phenylephrine results in a product with fewer cardiovascular effects. Studies have shown the absence of tachycardia and hypotension.

Isoproterenol alone often lowers arterial blood oxygen (PO₂). Several studies have shown that the combination of Isoproterenol and Phenylephrine rarely produces a significant drop in arterial oxygen tension while usually producing an increase in P_aO_2 in asthmatic patients.

Pharmacokinetics: The average half-life for Isoproterenol administered by aerosol was five minutes. A plasma concentration of 0.03 ng/ml was found within minutes following an inhalation dose of 500 mcg Isoproterenol.

Isoproterenol excretion following oral or inhalation administration is primarily renal. When given by inhalation, the major metabolite is the sulfate conjugate of the drug. When the drug is administered directly into the bronchial tree, it is inactivated by the enzyme catechol-o-methyl transferase, and the predominant metabolite is 3-o-methylisoproterenol sulfate. The explanation for this difference is supported by the observation that most (90%) of an aerosol dose is deposited in the mouth, swallowed, and converted to its sulfate conjugate in the gut wall, and to a lesser extent in the liver. The remaining Isoproterenol is excreted as follows: 1% to 2% unchanged, 1% to 2% free methylated metabolite, and small amounts of metabolites in the bile.

Plasma levels following inhalation of Phenylephrine have not been reported. Following oral and intravenous administrations, the average half-life was about 2.5 hours. Phenylephrine is metabolized in the liver and intestine by the enzyme monoamine oxidase. About 30% of a dose is recovered in the urine, primarily as phenolic conjugates and *m*-hydroxymandelic acid. About 16% of a dose is excreted as unchanged drug following intravenous administration and, due to first pass metabolism, less than 3% is excreted unchanged following oral dosing.

Recent studies in laboratory animals (minipigs, rodents, and dogs) recorded the occurrence of cardiac arrhythmias and sudden death (with histologic evidence of myocardial necrosis) when beta agonists and methylxanthines were concomitantly administered. The significance of these findings when applied to human usage is currently unknown.

INDICATIONS AND USAGE
Isoproterenol HCl/Phenylephrine Bitartrate is indicated for the treatment of bronchospasm associated with acute and chronic asthma and reversible broncho-spasm which may be associated with chronic bronchitis or emphysema.

CONTRAINDICATIONS
Isoproterenol HCl/Phenylephrine Bitartrate must not be used by patients with known hypersensitivity to sympathomimetics. The use of Isoproterenol in patients with pre-existing cardiac arrhythmias associated with tachycardia is contraindicated because the cardiac stimulant effects of the drug may aggravate such disorders.

WARNINGS
Excessive use of an adrenergic aerosol should be discouraged, as it may lose effectiveness. Occasional patients have been reported to develop severe paradoxi-cal airway resistance with repeated, excessive use of Isoproterenol inhalation preparations (see "Adverse Reactions"). The cause of this is unknown. It is advisable that in such instances the use of this preparation be discontinued immediately and alternative therapy instituted, since in the reported cases the patients did not respond to other forms of therapy until the drug was withdrawn. Deaths have been reported following excessive use of Isoproterenol inhalation preparations, and the exact cause is unknown. Cardiac arrest was noted in several instances (see "Adverse Reactions").

PRECAUTIONS
General: As with all sympathomimetic drugs, Isoproterenol HCl/Phenylephrine Bitartrate should be used with great caution in the presence of coronary insufficiency, hypertension, hyperthyroidism, and diabetes.

Information for Patients: Patients who are being treated with Isoproterenol HCl/ Phenylephrine Bitartrate should be informed adequately of the dangers of overusage, tolerance and rebound bronchospasm (see "Warnings" and "Adverse Reactions" sections). They should be instructed to take no more than two inhalations at any one time, nor more than six in any one hour during a 24-hour period, unless advised by the physician (see "Dosage and Administration" and "Patient Instructions for Use" sections).

Isoproterenol HCl may cause the patient's saliva to turn pinkish to red in color. Proper use of Isoproterenol HCl/Phenylephrine Bitartrate oral inhaler should be demonstrated and discussed. Patient Instructions for Use are available with the package insert and should be provided when the medication is dispensed.

As with any drug, patients should be advised against the ingestion of alcohol during treatment.

Drug Interactions: A monoamine oxidase (MAO) inhibitor, a tricyclic antidepres-sant, or guanethidine may increase the cardiac and pressor effects of Phenyleph-rine and Isoproterenol, however, normal volunteers given Isoproterenol by inhalation along with an MAO inhibitor or a tricyclic antidepressant had no adverse cardiovascular effects.

Arrhythmias may result from the concurrent administration of Isoproterenol or Phenylephrine to patients who are receiving digitalis, epinephrine, cyclopropane, or halogenated hydrocarbon anesthetics.

Beta-adrenergic blocking drugs such as propranolol antagonize the cardiac, bronchodilating, and vasodilating effects of Isoproterenol and the stimulating effects of Phenylephrine.

Ergot alkaloids may increase blood pressure in patients receiving Isoproterenol or Phenylephrine. Phentolamine mesylate, an alpha-adrenergic blocker, may decrease the pressor response to Phenylephrine.

Phenothiazine drugs have some alpha-adrenergic blocking activity and may reduce the pressor effects and duration of action of Phenylephrine.

Drug/Laboratory Test Interactions: Isoproterenol causes false elevations of bilirubin as measured *in vitro* by sequential multiple analyzer. An effect on serum bilirubin determinations in patients receiving the drug has not been determined. One case of surreptitious self-administration of a 500 mg subcutaneous dose of Isoproterenol resulted in increased urinary excretion of epinephrine, norepineph-rine, and vanilmandelic acid. Isoproterenol inhalation may result in enough absorption of the drug to produce increased values for urinary epinephrine. This effect is probably small with standard doses, but is likely to increase with larger doses.

Carcinogenesis, Mutagenesis and Impairment of Fertility: Isoproterenol HCl and Phenylephrine Bitartrate have not been evaluated for carcinogenicity, mutagenici-ty or impairment of fertility.

Pregnancy: Teratogenic Effects - Pregnancy Category C: Reproduction studies have not been done with the Isoproterenol HCl/Phenylephrine Bitartrate combi-nation or with phenylephrine alone. Reproduction studies with Isoproterenol have been performed in rats and rabbits with aerosol doses (30 minutes per day for 12 days) up to 15 times the human dose and have revealed no evidence of impaired fertility or harm to the fetus. It is also not known whether Isoproterenol HCl/Phenylephrine Bitartrate can cause fetal harm when administered to a pregnant woman or can affect reproduction capacity. Isoproterenol HCl/Phenyl-ephrine Bitartrate should be given to a pregnant woman only if clearly needed.

Labor and Delivery: Isoproterenol HCl/Phenylephrine Bitartrate has no recog-nized use during labor and delivery. Phenylephrine Bitartrate administration during late pregnancy or labor may cause fetal anoxia and bradycardia by increasing uterine contractility and decreasing uterine blood flow.

Nursing Mothers: It is not known whether Isoproterenol HCl or Phenylephrine Bitartrate is excreted in human milk. Because many drugs are excreted in human milk, caution should be exercised when Isoproterenol HCl/Phenylephrine Bitar-trate Inhaler is administered to a nursing woman.

Pediatric Use: Safe and effective use of Isoproterenol HCl/Phenylephrine Bitar-trate Inhaler in children below the age of 12 has not been established.

◆ RATED THERAPEUTICALLY EQUIVALENT; ◇ THERAPEUTIC EQUIVALENCE UNCONFIRMED; ○ UNRATED

Geriatric Use: Lower doses in elderly patients may be required due to increased sympathomimetic sensitivity (see *"Dosage and Administration"*).

ADVERSE REACTIONS

The following adverse effects, listed by organ system in decreasing frequency have been associated with the use of Isoproterenol HCl/Phenylephrine Bitartrate Inhaler and are similar to those produced by other sympathomimetic agents:

	Isoproterenol	Phenylephrine
Cardiovascular:	palpitation	bradycardia
	tachycardia	decreased cardiac
	coronary	output
	insufficiency	blanching of skin
	flushing of skin	peripheral and
	blood pressure changes	visceral vasoconstriction
	cardiac arrhythmias	cardiac
	cardiac arrest	irregularities
	anginal pain	anginal pain
Pulmonary:	paradoxical airway	respiratory
	resistance	distress
	rebound bronchospasm	
Central Nervous System:	headache	tremor
	tremor	dizziness
	vertigo	central excitation
	central excitation	pilomotor
	insomnia	response
Gastrointestinal:	nausea	

DRUG ABUSE AND DEPENDENCE

Drug abuse and dependence have not been reported with Isoproterenol HCl/Phenylephrine Bitartrate Inhaler.

OVERDOSAGE

Isoproterenol: The oral LD$_{50}$ values are as follows: mouse, 1260 mg/kg; rabbit, 3070 mg/kg; male rat, 2230 mg/kg; female rat, 2840 mg/kg; and dog, 600 mg/kg. The intravenous LD$_{50}$ values are as follows: mouse, 126 mg/kg; rabbit, 27 mg/kg; male rat, 96 mg/kg; female rat, 112 mg/kg; and dog, 50 mg/kg.

Phenylephrine: The oral LD$_{50}$ values are as follows: rat, 350 mg/kg; and mouse, 120 mg/kg. The intravenous LD$_{50}$ values are as follows: rat, 6.8 mg/kg; and mouse, 21 mg/kg.

Symptoms: The individual patient's sensitivity to either drug will dictate the overdosage signs. There is reason to believe, however, that the overdosage effects of either drug are antagonized by the other drug in the combination. Severe symptoms of overdosage are more likely to result from parenteral administration of Isoproterenol HCl rather than from oral inhalation of Isoproterenol and Phenylephrine HCl in an aerosol.

Manifestations of acute overdosage include chest pain, dizziness, headache, irregular heartbeat, fast or pounding heartbeat, bradycardia, nausea or vomiting, restlessness, weakness, flushing, decreased diastolic pressure, convulsions, cerebral hemorrhage, or hypertension.

Treatment: Discontinued dosing allows rapid reversal of adverse effects. Blood pressure and ECG may be monitored and the following treatment used, as appropriate: Tachycardia in asthmatic patients may be treated with cardioselective beta-blockers (metoprolol or atenolol, but use cautiously since cardioselectivity may not be absolute) and in nonasthmatics with propranolol; bradycardia may be treated with atropine; blood pressure may be regulated with rapid-acting vasodilators (nitrites, sodium nitroprusside) or alpha-blocking agents (quinidine, phentolamine). It is not known if Isoproterenol or Phenylephrine are dialyzable.

DOSAGE AND ADMINISTRATION

Adults: The usual dose for the relief of dyspnea caused by acute bronchospasm is one or two inhalations. Start with a single inhalation. If no relief is evident after two to five minutes, a second inhalation may be taken. For daily maintenance, use one or two inhalations four to six times daily or as directed by the physician. The physician should be careful to instruct the patient in the proper technique of administration so that the number of inhalations per treatment and the frequency of retreatment may be titrated to the patient's response.

No more than two inhalations should be taken at any one time, nor more than six inhalations in any one hour during a 24-hour period, unless advised by the physician. Lower doses in elderly patients may be required due to increased sympathomimetic sensitivity. Each depression of the valve delivers through the oral adapter 0.16 mg Isoproterenol Hydrochloride and 0.24 mg Phenylephrine Bitartrate.

Children: Safety and effectiveness for children under 12 years have not yet been established (see *"Pediatric Use"*).

DIRECTIONS FOR USE

Before each use, remove dust cap and inspect mouthpiece for foreign objects. Shake Isoproterenol HCl/Prenylephrine Bitartrate Inhaler.

1. Breathe out fully and place mouthpiece well into the mouth aimed at the back of the throat.
2. As you begin to breathe in deeply, press the vial firmly down into the adapter with the index finger. This releases one dose.

3. Release pressure on vial and remove unit from mouth. Hold your breath as long as possible, then breathe out slowly.

Replace dust cap after each use.

Warning: Contains trichloromonofluoromethane, dichlorodifluoromethane, and dichlorotetrafluoroethane, substances which harm public health and environment by destroying ozone in the upper atmosphere.

Storage: CONTENTS UNDER PRESSURE. Do not puncture or incinerate container. Store at controlled room temperature between 15°C and 30°C (59°F and 86°F). KEEP OUT OF THE REACH OF CHILDREN.

HOW SUPPLIED
AEROSOL LIQUID:

BRAND/MANUFACTURER	NDC	SIZE	AWP
○ **BRAND**			
DUO-MEDIHALER: 3M Pharm	00089-0735-11	15 ml	$23.34

AEROSOL LIQUID W/ADAPTER:

BRAND/MANUFACTURER	NDC	SIZE	AWP
○ **BRAND**			
DUO-MEDIHALER: 3M Pharm	00089-0735-21	15 ml	$26.34

Isoptin *SEE* VERAPAMIL HYDROCHLORIDE

Isopto Atropine *SEE* ATROPINE SULFATE, OPHTHALMIC

Isopto Carbachol *SEE* CARBACHOL

Isopto Carpine *SEE* PILOCARPINE, OPHTHALMIC

Isopto Cetamide *SEE* SULFACETAMIDE SODIUM, OPHTHALMIC

Isopto Cetapred *SEE* PREDNISOLONE AND SULFACETAMIDE SODIUM

Isopto Homatropine *SEE* HOMATROPINE HYDROBROMIDE

Isopto Hyoscine *SEE* SCOPOLAMINE HYDROBROMIDE, OPHTHALMIC

Isordil *SEE* ISOSORBIDE DINITRATE

Isosorbide

DESCRIPTION

Each mL contains: Isosorbide 45% w/v (Isosorbide concentrate 60.6%), water.

Typical Analysis of Electrolyte Content: 4.6 mEq. of sodium, 220 mL Isosorbide solution 0.9 meq. of potassium/220 mL Isosorbide solution.

Isosorbide, an osmotic agent, is Isosorbide, is a dihydric alcohol with the formula $C_6H_{10}O_4$.

Established name: Isosorbide

Chemical name: 1,4:3,6-dianhydro-D-glucitol.

Following is its chemical structure:

$$\begin{array}{c} CH_2\text{---} \\ HCOH \\ CH \\ HC \\ HCOH \\ CH_2\text{---} \end{array}$$

CLINICAL PHARMACOLOGY

Isosorbide is rapidly absorbed after oral administration. It is essentially non-metabolized, and in the circulation, it contributes to the tonicity of the blood until it is eliminated by the kidney unchanged. While in the blood, Isosorbide acts as an osmotic agent to promote redistribution of water toward the circulation with ultimate elimination in the urine. The physical action of Isosorbide is similar to that of other osmotic drugs.

INDICATIONS AND USAGE

For the short-term reduction of intraocular pressure. May be used prior to and after intraocular surgery. May be used to interrupt an acute attack of glaucoma. Use where less risk of nausea and vomiting than that posed by other oral hyperosmotic agents is needed.

CONTRAINDICATIONS

1. Well-established anuria.
2. Severe dehydration.
3. Frank or impending acute pulmonary edema.
4. Severe cardiac decompensation.
5. Hypersensitivity to any component of this preparation.

WARNINGS

1. With repeated doses, consideration should be given to maintenance of adequate fluid and electrolyte balance.

2. If urinary output continues to decrease, the patient's clinical status should be closely reviewed. Accumulation of Isosorbide may result in over-expansion of the extracellular fluid.

As with all medications, keep out of the reach of children.

PRECAUTIONS

For oral use only—not for injection. Repetitive doses should be used with caution particularly in patients with diseases associated with salt retention. Ensure that patient's bladder has been emptied prior to surgery.

Usage in Pregnancy: Pregnancy Category B: Reproduction studies have been performed in rats and rabbits and there was no evidence of impaired fertility or harm to the animal fetus due to Isosorbide. There are no adequate or well controlled studies on whether this drug may affect fertility in human males or females or have a teratogenic potential or other adverse effect on the fetus. Because animal reproduction studies are not always predictive of human responses, this drug should be used during pregnancy only if clearly needed.

ADVERSE REACTIONS

Nausea, vomiting, headache, confusion and disorientation may occur. Occurrences of syncope, gastric discomfort, lethargy, vertigo, thirst, dizziness, hiccups, hypernatremia, hyperosmolarity, irritability, rash, and light-headedness have been reported.

DOSAGE AND ADMINISTRATION

The recommended initial dose 1.5 gm/kg body weight of Isosorbide (equivalent to 1.5 mL/lb of body weight). The onset of action is usually within 30 minutes while the maximum effect is expected at 1 to 1 ½ hours. The useful dose range is 1 to 3 gm/kg body weight and the drug effect will persist up to 5 to 6 hours. Use two to four times a day as indicated. Palatability may be improved if the medication is poured over cracked ice and sipped.

RECOMMENDED DOSAGES

Pounds	Milliliters	Pounds	Milliliters
100	150	155	235
105	155	160	240
110	165	165	250
115	170	170	255
120	180	175	265
125	190	180	270
130	195	185	280
135	205	190	285
140	210	195	295
145	220	200	300
150	225		

Store at room temperature.

HOW SUPPLIED
SOLUTION:

BRAND/MANUFACTURER	NDC	SIZE	AWP
○ **BRAND** ISMOTIC: Alcon Surg	00065-0034-08	220 ml 12s	$237.60

Isosorbide Dinitrate

DESCRIPTION

Isosorbide Dinitrate, an organic nitrate, is a vasodilator with effects on both arteries and veins. Isosorbide Dinitrate is available as 2.5 mg, 5 mg, and 10 mg sublingual tablets; 5 mg, 10 mg, 20 mg, 30 mg, and 40 mg standard oral tablets; 40 mg controlled-release oral capsules and tablets and 40 mg sustained release capsules.

The chemical name for Isosorbide Dinitrate is 1,4,3,6-dianhydro-sorbitol-2,5-dinitrate. The molecular weight is 236.14.

Isosorbide Dinitrate is a white, crystalline, odorless compound which is stable in air and in solution, has a melting point of 70° C and has an optical rotation of + 134° (c = 1.0, alcohol, 20° C). Isosorbide Dinitrate is freely soluble in organic solvents such as acetone, alcohol, and ether, but is only sparingly soluble in water.

Following is its chemical structure:

$$\begin{array}{c} CH_2\text{---} \\ HCONO_2 \\ CH \\ HC \\ HCONO_2 \\ CH_2\text{---} \end{array}$$

CLINICAL PHARMACOLOGY

The principal pharmacological action of Isosorbide Dinitrate is relaxation of vascular smooth muscle, producing a vasodilatory effect on both peripheral arteries and veins, with predominant effects on the latter. Dilation of the postcapillary vessels, including large veins, promotes peripheral pooling of blood and decreases venous return to the heart, thereby reducing left-ventricular end-diastolic pressure (preload). Arteriolar relaxation reduces systemic vascular resistance and arterial pressure (afterload).

The mechanism by which Isosorbide Dinitrate relieves angina pectoris is not fully understood. Myocardial oxygen consumption or demand (as measured by the pressure-rate product, tension-time index, and stroke-work index) is decreased by both the arterial and venous effects of Isosorbide Dinitrate and, presumably, a more favorable supply-demand ratio is achieved. While the large epicardial coronary arteries are also dilated by Isosorbide Dinitrate, the extent to which this contributes to relief of exertional angina is unclear.

Therapeutic doses of Isosorbide Dinitrate may reduce systolic, diastolic, and mean arterial blood pressures, especially in the upright posture. Effective coronary perfusion is usually maintained. The decrease in systemic blood pressure may result in reflex tachycardia, an effect which could unfavorably influence myocardial oxygen demand. Hemodynamic studies indicate that Isosorbide Dinitrate may reduce the abnormally elevated left ventricular end-diastolic and pulmonary capillary wedge pressures that occur during an acute episode of angina pectoris.

Isosorbide Dinitrate is metabolized by enzymatic denitration to the intermediate products, Isosorbide-2-mononitrate and Isosorbide-5-mononitrate. Both metabolites have biological activity, especially the 5-mononitrate which is also the principal metabolite. The liver is a principal site of metabolism, and oral Isosorbide Dinitrate is subject to a large first pass effect. The systemic clearance of the drug following intravenous infusion is about 3.4 liters/min. Since the clearance exceeds hepatic blood flow, considerable extrahepatic metabolism must also occur.

The average bioavailability of Isosorbide Dinitrate is 59 and 22 percent following sublingual and oral administration, respectively. The terminal half-life is about 20 minutes, 60 minutes, and 4 hours following IV, sublingual, and oral administration, respectively. The dependence of half-life on the route of administration is not understood. Over limited ranges of IV dosing, the pharmacokinetics of Isosorbide Dinitrate appear linear. However, both the 2- and 5-mononitrate metabolites have been shown to decrease the rate of disappearance of the dinitrate from the blood. The half-lives of Isosorbide-5-mononitrate and Isosorbide-2-mononitrate range from 4.0 to 5.6 and 1.5 to 3.1 hours, respectively.

The pharmacokinetics and/or bioavailability of Isosorbide Dinitrate during multiple dosing have not been well studied. Because the metabolites influence the clearance of Isosorbide Dinitrate, prediction of blood levels of parent compound or metabolites from single-dose studies is uncertain.

INDICATIONS AND USAGE

Isosorbide Dinitrate is indicated for the treatment and prevention of angina pectoris. Controlled clinical trials have demonstrated that the sublingual, chewable, immediate release, and controlled-release oral dosage forms of Isosorbide Dinitrate are effective in improving exercise tolerance in patients with angina pectoris. When single sublingual or chewable doses (5 mg) of Isosorbide Dinitrate were administered prophylactically to patients with angina pectoris in various clinical studies, duration of exercise until chest pain or fatigue was significantly improved for at least 45 minutes (and as long as 2 hours in some studies) following dosing. Similar studies after single oral (15 to 120 mg) and oral controlled-release (40 to 80 mg) doses of Isosorbide Dinitrate have shown significant improvement in exercise tolerance for up to 8 hours following dosing. The exercise electrocardiographic evidence suggests that improved exercise tolerance with Isosorbide Dinitrate is not at the expense of greater myocardial ischemia. All dosage forms of Isosorbide Dinitrate may therefore be used prophylactically to decrease frequency and severity of anginal attacks and can be expected to decrease the need for sublingual nitroglycerin.

The sublingual and chewable forms of the drug are indicated for acute prophylaxis of angina pectoris when taken a few minutes before situations likely to provoke anginal attacks. Because of a slower onset of effect, the oral forms of Isosorbide Dinitrate are not indicated for acute prophylaxis.

In controlled clinical trials chewable and sublingual Isosorbide Dinitrate were effective in relieving an acute attack of angina pectoris. Relief occurred with a mean time of 2.9 and 3.4 minutes (chewable and sublingual, respectively) compared to relief of angina with a mean time of 1.9 minutes following sublingual nitroglycerin. Because of the more rapid relief of chest pain with sublingual nitroglycerin, the use of sublingual or chewable Isosorbide Dinitrate for aborting an acute anginal attack should be limited to patients intolerant or unresponsive to sublingual nitroglycerin.

UNLABELED USES
Isosorbide Dinitrate is used alone or as an adjunct in the treatment of congestive heart failure and complications from esophageal varices.

CONTRAINDICATIONS
Isosorbide Dinitrate is contraindicated in patients who have shown purported hypersensitivity or idiosyncrasy to it or other nitrates or nitrites.

WARNINGS
The benefits of Isosorbide Dinitrate during the early days of an acute myocardial infarction have not been established. If one elects to use organic nitrates in early infarction, hemodynamic monitoring and frequent clinical assessment should be used because of the potential deleterious effects of hypotension.

PRECAUTIONS
GENERAL
Severe hypotensive response, particularly with upright posture, may occur with even small doses of Isosorbide Dinitrate. The drug should therefore be used with caution in subjects who may have blood volume depletion from diuretic therapy or in subjects who have low systolic blood pressure (e.g., below 90 mm Hg). Paradoxical bradycardia and increased angina pectoris may accompany nitrate-induced hypotension. Nitrate therapy may aggravate the angina caused by hypertrophic cardiomyopathy. Tolerance to this drug and cross-tolerance to other nitrates and nitrites may occur.

Marked symptomatic, orthostatic hypotension has been reported when calcium channel blockers and organic nitrates were used in combination. Dose adjustment of either class of agents may be necessary.

Tolerance to the vascular and antianginal effects of Isosorbide Dinitrate or nitroglycerin has been demonstrated in clinical trials, experience through occupational exposure, and in isolated tissue experiments in the laboratory. The importance of tolerance to the appropriate use of Isosorbide Dinitrate in the management of patients with angina pectoris has not been determined. However, one clinical trial using treadmill exercise tolerance (as an endpoint) found an 8 hour duration of action of oral Isosorbide Dinitrate following the first dose (after a 2-week placebo washout) and only a 2-hour duration of effect of the same dose after 1 week of repetitive dosing at conventional dosing intervals. On the other hand, several trials have been able to differentiate Isosorbide Dinitrate from placebo after 4 weeks of therapy, and in open trials an effect seems detectable for as long as several months.

Tolerance clearly occurs in industrial workers continuously exposed to nitroglycerin. Moreover, physical dependence also occurs, since chest pain, acute myocardial infarction, and even sudden death have occurred during temporary withdrawal of nitroglycerin from the workers. In clinical trials in angina patients, there are reports of anginal attacks being more easily provoked and of rebound in the hemodynamic effects soon after nitrate withdrawal. The relative importance of these observations to the routine, clinical use of Isosorbide Dinitrate is not known. However, it seems prudent to gradually withdraw patients from Isosorbide Dinitrate when the therapy is being terminated, rather than stopping the drug abruptly.

INFORMATION FOR PATIENTS
Headache may occur during initial therapy with Isosorbide Dinitrate. Headache is usually relieved by the use of standard headache remedies, or by lowering the dose, and tends to disappear after the first week or two of use.

DRUG INTERACTIONS
Alcohol may enhance any marked sensitivity to the hypotensive effect of nitrates.

Isosorbide Dinitrate acts directly on vascular smooth muscle; therefore, any other agent that depends on vascular smooth muscle as the final common path can be expected to have decreased or increased effect, depending on the agent.

CARCINOGENESIS, MUTAGENESIS, IMPAIRMENT OF FERTILITY
No long-term studies in animals have been performed to evaluate the carcinogenic potential of this drug. A modified two-litter reproduction study in rats fed Isosorbide Dinitrate at 25 or 100 mg/kg/day did not reveal any effects on fertility or gestation or any remarkable growth pathology in any parent or offspring fed Isosorbide Dinitrate as compared with rats fed a basal-controlled diet.

PREGNANCY CATEGORY C
Isosorbide Dinitrate has been shown to cause a dose-related increase in embryotoxicity (increase in mummified pups) in rabbits at oral doses 35 and 150 times the maximum recommended human daily dose. There are no adequate and well-controlled studies in pregnant women. Isosorbide Dinitrate should be used during pregnancy only if the potential benefit justifies the potential risk to the fetus.

NURSING MOTHERS
It is not known whether this drug is excreted in human milk. Because many drugs are excreted in human milk, caution should be exercised when Isosorbide Dinitrate is administered to a nursing woman.

PEDIATRIC USE
The safety and effectiveness of Isosorbide Dinitrate in children have not been established.

ADVERSE REACTIONS
Adverse reactions, particularly headache and hypotension, are dose-related. In clinical trials at various doses, the following have been observed:

Headache is the most common adverse reaction and may be severe and persistent; reported incidence varies widely, apparently being dose-related, with an average occurrence of about 25%.

Cutaneous vasodilation with flushing may occur.

Transient episodes of dizziness and weakness, as well as other signs of cerebral ischemia associated with postural hypotension, may occasionally develop (the incidence of reported symptomatic hypotension ranges from 2% to 36%). An occasional individual will exhibit marked sensitivity to the hypotensive effects of nitrates, and severe responses (nausea, vomiting, weakness, restlessness, pallor, perspiration, and collapse) may occur even with the usual therapeutic dose. Drug rash and/or exfoliative dermatitis may occasionally occur. Nausea and vomiting appear to be uncommon.

OVERDOSAGE
SIGNS AND SYMPTOMS
These may include the following: a prompt fall in blood pressure, persistent and throbbing headache, vertigo, palpitation, visual disturbances, flushed and perspiring skin (later becoming cold and cyanotic), nausea and vomiting (possibly with colic and even bloody diarrhea), syncope (especially in the upright position), methemoglobinemia with cyanosis and anoxia, initial hyperpnea, dyspnea and slow breathing, slow pulse (dicrotic and intermittent), heart block, increased intracranial pressure with cerebral symptoms of confusion and moderate fever, paralysis and coma followed by clonic convulsions and possibly death due to circulatory collapse.

It is not known what dose of the drug is associated with symptoms of overdosing or what dose of the drug would be life-threatening. The acute oral LD50 of Isosorbide Dinitrate in rats was found to be approximately 1100 mg/kg of body weight. These animal experiments indicate that approximately 500 times the usual therapeutic dose would be required to produce such toxic symptoms in humans. It is not known whether the drug is dialyzable.

TREATMENT OF OVERDOSAGE
Prompt removal of the ingested material by gastric lavage is reasonable but not documented to be useful. Keep the patient recumbent in a shock position and comfortably warm. Passive movements of the extremities may aid venous return. Administer oxygen and artificial respiration if necessary. If methemoglobinemia is present, administer methylene blue (1% solution), 1 to 2 mg/kg intravenously.

METHEMOGLOBIN
Case reports of clinically significant methemoglobinemia are rare at conventional doses of organic nitrates. The formation of methemoglobin is dose-related, and in the case of genetic abnormalities of hemoglobin that favor methemoglobin formation, even conventional doses of organic nitrate could produce harmful concentrations of methemoglobin.

WARNING
Epinephrine is ineffective in reversing the severe hypotensive events associated with overdose. It and related compounds are contraindicated in this situation.

DOSAGE AND ADMINISTRATION
For the treatment of angina pectoris, the usual starting dose of sublingual Isosorbide Dinitrate is 2.5 to 5 mg.

Isosorbide Dinitrate should be titrated upward until angina is relieved or side effects limit the dose. In ambulatory patients, the magnitude of the incremental dose increase should be guided by measurements of standing blood pressure.

The initial dosage of sublingual Isosorbide Dinitrate for acute prophylactic therapy in angina pectoris patients is generally 5 or 10 mg every 2 to 3 hours. Adequate, controlled clinical studies demonstrating the effectiveness of chronic maintenance therapy with these dosage forms have not been reported.

Because of a slower onset of effect, the oral forms of Isosorbide Dinitrate are not indicated for acute prophylaxis or for the treatment of acute anginal attacks.

For the treatment of chronic stable angina pectoris, the usual starting dose for immediate-release (swallowed) tablets is 5 to 20 mg; and for controlled release forms, 40 mg. For maintenance therapy, oral doses of 10 to 40 mg given every 6 hours or oral controlled-release doses of 40 to 80 mg given every 8 to 12 hours are generally recommended. The extent to which development of tolerance should modify the dosage program has not been defined. The oral controlled-release forms of Isosorbide Dinitrate should not be chewed.

Protect from light and moisture.

Store at room temperature, approximately 25 ° C (77°F). Keep tightly closed. Dispense in a tight, light-resistant container.

HOW SUPPLIED
CAPSULE, EXTENDED RELEASE: 40 MG

BRAND/MANUFACTURER	NDC	SIZE	AWP
◇ **BRAND**			
ISORDIL TEMBIDS: Wyeth-Ayerst	00008-4140-01	100s	$49.35
	00008-4140-02	500s	$234.54
◇ **GENERICS**			
DILATRATE-SR: Reed & Carnrick	00021-0920-02	60s	$30.44
DILATRATE-SR: Reed & Carnrick	00021-0920-01	100s	$48.28

CHEW TABLET: 5 MG

AVERAGE UNIT PRICE (AVAILABLE SIZES)			
BRAND	$0.19		

BRAND/MANUFACTURER	NDC	SIZE	AWP
◆ **BRAND**			
SORBITRATE CHEWABLE: Zeneca	00310-0810-10	100s	$19.22
	00310-0810-50	500s	$93.19

CHEW TABLET: 10 MG

BRAND/MANUFACTURER	NDC	SIZE	AWP
◆ **BRAND**			
SORBITRATE CHEWABLE: Zeneca	00310-0815-10	100s	$22.07

TABLET, EXTENDED RELEASE: 40 MG

AVERAGE UNIT PRICE (AVAILABLE SIZES)		GENERIC A-RATED AVERAGE PRICE (GAAP)	
GENERIC	$0.08	100s	$8.79
		1000s	$78.26

BRAND/MANUFACTURER	NDC	SIZE	AWP
◆ **GENERICS**			
Parmed	00349-2083-01	100s	$5.83
Goldline	00182-0879-01	100s	$10.05
Schein	00364-0401-01	100s	$10.50
Parmed	00349-2083-10	1000s	$66.02
Goldline	00182-0879-10	1000s	$76.50
Schein	00364-0401-02	1000s	$92.25

TABLET, EXTENDED RELEASE: 40 MG

BRAND/MANUFACTURER	NDC	SIZE	AWP
○ **BRAND**			
➤ ISORDIL TEMBIDS: Wyeth-Ayerst	00008-4125-01	100s	$49.35
	00008-4125-02	500s	$234.54
	00008-4125-03	1000s	$461.70

TABLETS: 2.5 MG

AVERAGE UNIT PRICE (AVAILABLE SIZES)		GENERIC A-RATED AVERAGE PRICE (GAAP)	
BRAND	$0.21	100s	$4.69
GENERIC	$0.02	1000s	$17.90
GENERIC	$0.04		
HCFA FUL (100s ea)	$0.03		

BRAND/MANUFACTURER	NDC	SIZE	AWP
◆ **BRAND**			
➤ SORBITRATE SUBLINGUAL: Zeneca	00310-0853-10	100s	$17.90
➤ ISORDIL: Wyeth-Ayerst	00008-4139-01	100s	$21.54
	00008-4139-05	100s ud	$23.21
	00008-4139-03	500s	$102.15
◆ **GENERICS**			
Schein	00364-0367-01	100s	$2.85
West-Ward	00143-1765-01	100s	$3.50
Caremark	00339-5655-12	100s	$4.07
Major	00904-2342-60	100s	$4.15
Moore,H.L.	00839-5044-06	100s	$4.17
Qualitest	00603-4122-21	100s	$4.25
➤ ISDN: Geneva	00781-1515-01	100s	$4.35
Rugby	00536-3928-01	100s	$4.45
Aligen	00405-4569-01	100s	$5.92
➤ ISDN: Geneva	00781-1515-13	100s ud	$8.00
West-Ward	00143-1765-10	1000s	$13.50
Schein	00364-0367-02	1000s	$14.20
Major	00904-2342-80	1000s	$15.10
Qualitest	00603-4122-32	1000s	$18.30
Moore,H.L.	00839-5044-16	1000s	$18.56
➤ ISDN: Geneva	00781-1515-10	1000s	$20.50
Rugby	00536-3928-10	1000s	$20.75

TABLETS: 5 MG

AVERAGE UNIT PRICE (AVAILABLE SIZES)		GENERIC A-RATED AVERAGE PRICE (GAAP)	
BRAND	$0.22	100s	$5.23
GENERIC	$0.05	1000s	$17.56
GENERIC	$0.04		
HCFA FUL (100s ea)	$0.03		

BRAND/MANUFACTURER	NDC	SIZE	AWP
◆ **BRAND**			
➤ SORBITRATE ORAL: Zeneca	00310-0770-10	100s	$19.22
➤ SORBITRATE SUBLINGUAL: Zeneca	00310-0760-10	100s	$19.22
➤ ISORDIL: Wyeth-Ayerst	00008-4126-01	100s	$23.01
➤ ISORDIL TITRADOSE: Wyeth-Ayerst	00008-4152-01	100s	$23.11
➤ SORBITRATE ORAL: Zeneca	00310-0770-39	100s ud	$22.07
➤ ISORDIL: Wyeth-Ayerst	00008-4126-07	100s ud	$24.83
➤ ISORDIL TITRADOSE: Wyeth-Ayerst	00008-4152-05	100s ud	$24.94
➤ SORBITRATE ORAL: Zeneca	00310-0770-50	500s	$93.19
➤ ISORDIL: Wyeth-Ayerst	00008-4126-03	500s	$109.65
➤ ISORDIL TITRADOSE: Wyeth-Ayerst	00008-4152-02	500s	$110.18
	00008-4152-03	1000s	$216.83
◆ **GENERICS**			
Medirex	57480-0339-06	30s	$4.49
West-Ward	00143-1769-01	100s	$2.64
Schein	00364-0340-01	100s	$2.75
Rugby	00536-3967-01	100s	$2.90
Moore,H.L.	00839-1378-06	100s	$2.96
URL	00677-0572-01	100s	$3.00
Caraco	57664-0102-08	100s	$3.00
Goldline	00182-0550-01	100s	$3.00
Major	00904-2150-60	100s	$3.10
Qualitest	00603-4116-21	100s	$3.15
Caremark	00339-5572-12	100s	$3.24
Schein	00364-0368-01	100s	$3.25
West-Ward	00143-1767-01	100s	$3.60
Rugby	00536-3944-01	100s	$4.13
➤ ISDN: Geneva	00781-1635-01	100s	$4.35
Par	49884-0020-01	100s	$4.35
Aligen	00405-4558-01	100s	$4.35
Major	00904-2343-60	100s	$4.45
Caremark	00339-5657-12	100s	$4.46
Qualitest	00603-4123-21	100s	$4.50
URL	00677-0409-01	100s	$4.60
➤ ISDN: Geneva	00781-1565-01	100s	$4.66
Moore,H.L.	00839-5043-06	100s	$5.06
Aligen	00405-4570-01	100s	$5.92
Major	00904-2343-61	100s ud	$4.85
Raway	00686-0084-20	100s ud	$5.50
Major	00904-2150-61	100s ud	$6.04
Auro	55829-0323-10	100s ud	$6.52
➤ ISDN: Geneva	00781-1565-13	100s ud	$6.65
Vangard	00615-1564-13	100s ud	$7.88
West-Ward	00143-1769-25	100s ud	$8.00
➤ ISDN: Geneva	00781-1635-13	100s ud	$9.85
UDL	51079-0084-20	100s ud	$14.95
Medirex	57480-0339-01	100s ud	$14.95
West-Ward	00143-1769-10	1000s	$10.68
Rugby	00536-3967-10	1000s	$11.72
Moore,H.L.	00839-1378-16	1000s	$12.14
Major	00904-2150-80	1000s	$12.50
West-Ward	00143-1767-10	1000s	$13.75
Schein	00364-0368-02	1000s	$15.00
Schein	00364-0340-02	1000s	$15.90
URL	00677-0572-10	1000s	$16.00
Goldline	00182-0550-10	1000s	$16.00
Qualitest	00603-4116-32	1000s	$16.85
Rugby	00536-3944-10	1000s	$16.87
➤ ISDN: Geneva	00781-1635-10	1000s	$16.95
Major	00904-2343-80	1000s	$17.10
Moore,H.L.	00839-5043-16	1000s	$18.56
Qualitest	00603-4123-32	1000s	$19.86
➤ ISDN: Geneva	00781-1565-10	1000s	$21.50
Par	49884-0020-10	1000s	$27.84
Aligen	00405-4558-03	1000s	$27.84

TABLETS: 10 MG

AVERAGE UNIT PRICE (AVAILABLE SIZES)		GENERIC A-RATED AVERAGE PRICE (GAAP)	
BRAND	$0.25	100s	$6.53
GENERIC	$0.05	500s	$12.40
HCFA FUL (100s ea)	$0.02	1000s	$20.09

BRAND/MANUFACTURER	NDC	SIZE	AWP
◆ **BRAND**			
➤ SORBITRATE ORAL: Zeneca	00310-0780-10	100s	$22.07
➤ SORBITRATE SUBLINGUAL: Zeneca	00310-0761-10	100s	$22.07
➤ ISORDIL TITRADOSE: Wyeth-Ayerst	00008-4153-01	100s	$25.84
➤ ISORDIL: Wyeth-Ayerst	00008-4161-01	100s	$26.86
➤ SORBITRATE ORAL: Zeneca	00310-0780-39	100s ud	$25.39
➤ ISORDIL TITRADOSE: Wyeth-Ayerst	00008-4153-05	100s ud	$28.18
➤ SORBITRATE ORAL: Zeneca	00310-0780-50	500s	$107.06
➤ ISORDIL TITRADOSE: Wyeth-Ayerst	00008-4153-02	500s	$122.83
	00008-4153-03	1000s	$242.99

◆ RATED THERAPEUTICALLY EQUIVALENT; ◇ THERAPEUTIC EQUIVALENCE UNCONFIRMED; ○ UNRATED

BRAND/MANUFACTURER	NDC	SIZE	AWP
◆ GENERICS			
Medirex	57480-0340-06	30s	$5.46
Qualitest	00603-4117-21	100s	$2.75
West-Ward	00143-1771-01	100s	$2.82
Schein	00364-0341-01	100s	$2.93
➤ Rugby	00536-3943-01	100s	$3.14
Caraco	57664-0106-08	100s	$3.15
Goldline	00182-0514-01	100s	$3.15
Parmed	00349-2327-01	100s	$3.45
Caremark	00339-5573-12	100s	$3.54
URL	00677-0348-01	100s	$4.15
Moore,H.L.	00839-1381-06	100s	$4.17
Major	00904-2151-60	100s	$4.40
➤ ISDN: Geneva	00781-1556-01	100s	$4.62
Par	49884-0021-01	100s	$4.85
Aligen	00405-4559-01	100s	$4.85
Raway	00686-0029-20	100s ud	$5.95
Major	00904-2151-61	100s ud	$6.14
Auro	55829-0324-10	100s ud	$8.01
West-Ward	00143-1771-25	100s ud	$9.50
Vangard	00615-1560-13	100s ud	$9.62
Goldline	00182-0514-89	100s ud	$10.80
➤ ISDN: Geneva	00781-1556-13	100s ud	$11.85
UDL	51079-0029-20	100s ud	$18.20
Medirex	57480-0340-01	100s ud	$18.20
West-Ward	00143-1771-05	500s	$8.58
➤ ISDN: Geneva	00781-1556-05	500s	$16.22
West-Ward	00143-1771-10	1000s	$11.03
➤ Rugby	00536-3943-10	1000s	$13.13
Schein	00364-0341-02	1000s	$16.90
Caraco	57664-0106-18	1000s	$17.00
Moore,H.L.	00839-1381-16	1000s	$18.21
URL	00677-0348-10	1000s	$18.99
Goldline	00182-0514-10	1000s	$19.00
Qualitest	00603-4117-32	1000s	$19.20
➤ ISDN: Geneva	00781-1556-10	1000s	$19.25
Parmed	00349-2327-10	1000s	$22.00
Major	00904-2151-80	1000s	$22.10
Par	49884-0021-10	1000s	$32.19
Aligen	00405-4559-03	1000s	$32.19

TABLETS: 20 MG

AVERAGE UNIT PRICE (AVAILABLE SIZES)		GENERIC A-RATED AVERAGE PRICE (GAAP)	
BRAND	$0.40	100s	$7.54
GENERIC	$0.05	1000s	$23.72
HCFA FUL (100s ea)	$0.02		

BRAND/MANUFACTURER	NDC	SIZE	AWP
◆ BRAND			
➤ SORBITRATE ORAL: Zeneca	00310-0820-10	100s	$35.09
➤ ISORDIL TITRADOSE: Wyeth-Ayerst	00008-4154-01	100s	$41.69
➤ SORBITRATE ORAL: Zeneca	00310-0820-39	100s ud	$40.42
➤ ISORDIL TITRADOSE: Wyeth-Ayerst	00008-4154-05	100s ud	$45.01
	00008-4154-02	500s	$198.18
◆ GENERICS			
Major	00904-2154-89	90s	$3.05
West-Ward	00143-1772-01	100s	$2.91
Qualitest	00603-4118-21	100s	$3.16
Schein	00364-0509-01	100s	$3.20
Parmed	00349-2348-01	100s	$3.24
Caraco	57664-0107-08	100s	$3.70
Caremark	00339-5574-12	100s	$3.87
Goldline	00182-0868-01	100s	$3.90
URL	00677-0689-01	100s	$4.30
Moore,H.L.	00839-6017-06	100s	$4.31
➤ Rugby	00536-3927-01	100s	$4.55
Major	00904-2154-60	100s	$4.60
➤ ISDN: Geneva	00781-1695-01	100s	$5.25
Par	49884-0022-01	100s	$5.50
Aligen	00405-4560-01	100s	$5.50
Auro	55829-0325-10	100s ud	$9.03
West-Ward	00143-1772-25	100s ud	$17.00
Major	00904-2154-61	100s ud	$17.53
➤ ISDN: Geneva	00781-1695-13	100s ud	$19.63
UDL	51079-0085-20	100s ud	$22.10
Major	00904-2154-18	120s	$3.60
Major	00904-2154-93	180s	$4.65
Major	00904-2154-34	240s	$5.75
Major	00904-2154-53	360s	$8.00
West-Ward	00143-1772-10	1000s	$12.80
Schein	00364-0509-02	1000s	$18.50
Goldline	00182-0868-10	1000s	$19.50
Qualitest	00603-4118-32	1000s	$20.80
URL	00677-0689-10	1000s	$21.19
Caraco	57664-0107-18	1000s	$21.25
➤ ISDN: Geneva	00781-1695-10	1000s	$21.73
➤ Rugby	00536-3927-10	1000s	$22.25
Major	00904-2154-80	1000s	$23.25
Moore,H.L.	00839-6017-16	1000s	$23.34
Parmed	00349-2348-10	1000s	$28.00
Par	49884-0022-10	1000s	$37.85
Aligen	00405-4560-03	1000s	$37.88

TABLETS: 30 MG

AVERAGE UNIT PRICE (AVAILABLE SIZES)		GENERIC A-RATED AVERAGE PRICE (GAAP)	
BRAND	$0.45	100s	$7.15
GENERIC	$0.06	1000s	$37.95
HCFA FUL (100s ea)	$0.03		

BRAND/MANUFACTURER	NDC	SIZE	AWP
◆ BRAND			
➤ SORBITRATE ORAL: Zeneca	00310-0773-10	100s	$39.04
➤ ISORDIL TITRADOSE: Wyeth-Ayerst	00008-4159-01	100s	$46.91
➤ SORBITRATE ORAL: Zeneca	00310-0773-39	100s ud	$44.84
➤ ISORDIL TITRADOSE: Wyeth-Ayerst	00008-4159-04	100s ud	$50.61
	00008-4159-02	500s	$222.69
◆ GENERICS			
Major	00904-2682-60	100s	$4.15
Rugby	00536-3938-01	100s	$4.43
URL	00677-0786-01	100s	$4.60
Caremark	00339-5653-12	100s	$4.78
Qualitest	00603-4119-21	100s	$4.81
Par	49884-0009-01	100s	$6.45
Aligen	00405-4561-01	100s	$6.48
Moore,H.L.	00839-6618-06	100s	$6.75
Auro	55829-0326-10	100s ud	$11.09
Major	00904-2682-61	100s ud	$17.97
URL	00677-0786-10	1000s	$28.38
Rugby	00536-3938-10	1000s	$28.43
Major	00904-2682-80	1000s	$30.25
Par	49884-0009-10	1000s	$46.11
Aligen	00405-4561-03	1000s	$46.11
Moore,H.L.	00839-6618-16	1000s	$48.40

TABLETS: 40 MG

AVERAGE UNIT PRICE (AVAILABLE SIZES)	
BRAND	$0.49

BRAND/MANUFACTURER	NDC	SIZE	AWP
◆ BRAND			
➤ SORBITRATE ORAL: Zeneca	00310-0774-10	100s	$41.08
➤ ISORDIL TITRADOSE: Wyeth-Ayerst	00008-4192-01	100s	$50.93
➤ SORBITRATE ORAL: Zeneca	00310-0774-39	100s ud	$47.22
➤ ISORDIL TITRADOSE: Wyeth-Ayerst	00008-4192-04	100s ud	$54.90

Isosorbide Mononitrate

DESCRIPTION

Isosorbide Mononitrate (ISMN), an organic nitrate and the major biologically active metabolite of isosorbide dinitrate (ISDN), is a vasodilator with effects on both arteries and veins. The empirical formula is $C_6H_9NO_6$ and the molecular weight is 191.14.

The chemical name for ISMN is 1,4:3,6-dianhydro-, D-glucitol 5-nitrate.

ISMN immediate release tablets contain 10 or 20 mg of the drug; ISMN extended release tablets contain 60 mg.

ISMN is a white, crystalline, odorless compound which is stable in air and in solution, has a melting point of about 90°C, and an optical rotation of +144° (2% in water, 20°C).

ISMN is freely soluble in water, ethanol, methanol, chloroform, ethyl acetate, and dichloromethane.

Following is its chemical structure:

$$
\begin{array}{c}
CH_2 \\
| \\
HCOH \\
| \\
O \\
| \\
O - CH \\
| \\
HC \\
| \\
HC \\
| \\
HCONO_2 \\
| \\
CH_2
\end{array}
$$

CLINICAL PHARMACOLOGY

Mechanism of Action: ISMN is the major active metabolite of isosorbide dinitrate; most of the clinical activity of the dinitrate is attributable to the mononitrate.

The principal pharmacological action of ISMN and all organic nitrates in general is relaxation of vascular smooth muscle, producing dilatation of peripheral arteries and veins, especially the latter. Dilatation of the veins promotes peripheral pooling of blood, decreases venous return to the heart, thereby reducing left ventricular end-diastolic pressure and pulmonary capillary wedge pressure (preload). Arteriolar relaxation reduces systemic vascular resistance, and systolic arterial pressure and mean arterial pressure (afterload). Dilatation of the coronary arteries also occurs. The relative importance of preload reduction, afterload reduction, and coronary dilatation remains undefined.

Pharmacodynamics: Dosing regimens for most chronically used drugs are designed to provide plasma concentrations that are continuously greater than a minimally effective concentration. This strategy is inappropriate for organic nitrates. Several well-controlled clinical trials have used exercise testing to assess

➤ SHOWN IN PRODUCT IDENTIFICATION GUIDE

the antianginal efficacy of continuously delivered nitrates. In the large majority of these trials, active agents were indistinguishable from placebo after 24 hours (or less) of continuous therapy. Attempts to overcome tolerance by dose escalation, even to doses far in excess of those used acutely, have consistently failed. Only after nitrates have been absent from the body for several hours has their antianginal efficacy been restored. The drug-free interval sufficient to avoid tolerance to ISMN has not been completely defined. In the only regimen of twice-daily ISMN that has been shown to avoid development of tolerance, the two doses of ISMN tablets are given 7 hours apart, so there is a gap of 17 hours between the second dose of each day and the first dose of the next day. Taking account of the relatively long half-life of ISMN this result is consistent with those obtained for other organic nitrates.

The asymmetric twice daily regimen of ISMN tablets successfully avoided significant rebound/withdrawal effects. The incidence and magnitude of such phenomena have appeared, in studies of other nitrates, to be highly dependent upon the schedule of nitrate administration.

ISMN extended-release tablets during long-term use over 42 days dosed at 120 mg once daily continued to improve exercise performance at 4 hours and at 12 hours after dosing but its effects (although better than placebo) are less than or at best equal to the effects of the first dose of 60 mg.

Pharmacokinetics and Metabolism: ISMN is rapidly and completely absorbed from the gastrointestinal tract. After oral administration of ISMN as a solution or immediate-release tablets, maximum plasma concentrations of ISMN are achieved in 30 to 60 minutes, with an absolute bioavailability of approximately 100%. After intravenous administration, ISMN is distributed into total body water in about 9 minutes with a volume of distribution of approximately 0.6-0.7 L/kg; volume of distribution for immediate-release tablets is approximately 0.6 L/kg. ISMN is approximately 4% to 5% bound to human plasma proteins and is distributed into blood cells and saliva. ISMN is primarily metabolized by the liver, but unlike oral ISDN it is not subject to first-pass metabolism. ISMN is cleared by denitration to isosorbide and glucuronidation as the mononitrate, with 93% of the dose excreted in the urine within 48 hours, 96% excreted in the urine within 5 days, and only about 1% eliminated in the feces. At least six different compounds have been detected in urine, with about 1% to 2% of the dose excreted as the unchanged drug and at least five metabolites. The metabolites are not pharmacologically active. Renal clearance accounts for only about 4% of total body clearance. The mean plasma elimination half-life of ISMN is approximately 5 hours.

ISMN has no known effect on renal and hepatic function. The disposition of ISMN in patients with various degrees of renal insufficiency, liver cirrhosis, or cardiac dysfunction and in elderly patients was evaluated and found to be similar to that observed in healthy subjects. The elimination half-life of ISMN was not prolonged, and there was no drug accumulation in patients with chronic renal failure after multiple oral dosing.

The pharmacokinetics and/or bioavailability of ISMN tablets have been studied in both normal volunteers and patients following single- and multiple-dose administration. Data from these studies suggest that the pharmacokinetics of ISMN tablets are similar between normal healthy volunteers and patients with angina pectoris. In single- and multiple-dose studies, the pharmacokinetics of ISMN were dose proportional between 20 mg and 240 mg.

In a multiple-dose study, the effect of age on the pharmacokinetic profile of ISMN extended release 60 mg and 120 mg (2 × 60 mg) tablets was evaluated in subjects ≥45 years. The results of that study indicate that there are no significant differences in any of the pharmacokinetic variables of ISMN between elderly (≥65 years) and younger individuals (45-64 years) for the ISMN extended release 60 mg dose. The administration of ISMN extended release tablets 120 mg (2 × 60 mg tablets every 24 hours for 7 days) produced a dose-proportional increase in C_{max} and AUC, without changes in T_{max} or the terminal half-life. The older group (65-74 years) showed 30% lower apparent oral clearance (Cl/F) following the higher dose, ie, 120 mg, compared to the younger group (45-64 years); Cl/F was not different between the two groups following the 60 mg regimen. While Cl/F was independent of dose in the younger group, the older group showed slightly lower Cl/F following the 120 mg regimen compared to the 60 mg regimen. Differences between the two age groups, however, were not statistically significant. In the same study, females showed a slight (15%) reduction in clearance when the dose was increased. Females showed higher AUCs and C_{max} compared to males, but these differences were accounted for by differences in body weight between the two groups. When the data were analyzed using age as a variable, the results indicated that there were no significant differences in any of the pharmacokinetic variables of ISMN between older (≥65 years) and younger individuals (45-64 years). The results of this study, however, should be viewed with caution due to the small numbers of subjects in each age subgroup and consequently the lack of sufficient statistical power.

The following table summarizes key pharmacokinetic parameters of ISMN after single- and multiple-dose administration of ISMN as an oral solution or ISMN extended release tablets. (See related table).

Food Effects: The influence of food on the bioavailability of ISMN after single-dose administration of ISMN extended release tablets 60 mg was evaluated in three different studies involving either a "light" breakfast or a high-calorie, high-fat breakfast. Results of these and other studies indicate that concomitant food intake may decrease the rate (increase in T_{max}) but not the extent (AUC) of absorption or bioavailability of ISMN immediate release or extended release.

ISMN is significantly removed from the blood during hemodialysis; however, an additional dose to compensate for drug lost is not necessary. In patients undergoing continuous ambulatory peritoneal dialysis, blood levels are similar to patients not on dialysis.

CLINICAL TRIALS

The acute and chronic antianginal efficacy of ISMN immediate release has been confirmed in clinical trials. The clinical efficacy of ISMN immediate release was studied in 21 stable angina pectoris patients. After single dose administration of ISMN immediate release, 20 mg, the exercise capacity was increased by 42.7% after one hour, 29.6% after 6 hours and by 25% after eight hours when compared to placebo. Controlled trials of single doses of ISMN immediate release tablets have demonstrated that antianginal activity is present about 1 hour after dosing, with peak effect seen from 1-4 hours after dosing.

In one multicenter placebo controlled trial ISMN immediate release was found to be safe and effective during acute and chronic (3 weeks) treatment of angina pectoris. Two hundred fourteen (214) patients were enrolled in the trial; 54 patients were randomized to receive placebo and 106 patients were randomized to receive 10 or 20 mg of ISMN immediate release twice daily seven hours apart. The largest effect of ISMN immediate release compared to placebo, was on day one–dose one. Although 14 hours after the first dose of day 14, the increase in exercise tolerance due to ISMN immediate release was statistically significant, the increase was about half of that seen 2 hours after the first dose of day one. On day 21, two hours after the first dose the effect of ISMN was 60 to 70% of that seen on day one.

Controlled trials of single doses of ISMN immediate release tablets have demonstrated that antianginal activity is present about 1 hour after dosing, with peak effect seen from 1-4 hours after dosing. In other placebo-controlled trials lasting 2-3 weeks, ISMN immediate release tablets were administered twice daily, in asymmetric regimens (with interdosing intervals of 7 and 17 hours) designed to avoid tolerance. One trial tested doses of 10 mg and 20 mg; one trial tested doses of 20 mg, 40 mg, and 60 mg; and three trials tested only doses of 20 mg. In each trial, the subjects were persons with known chronic stable angina, and the primary measure of efficacy was exercise tolerance on a standardized treadmill test. After initial dosing and for at least three weeks, exercise tolerance in patients treated with ISMN immediate release 20 mg tablets was significantly greater than that seen in patients treated with placebo, although there was some attenuation of effect with time. Treatment with ISMN immediate release tablets was superior to placebo for at least 12 hours after the first dose (i.e., 5 hours after the second dose) of each day. Significant tolerance and rebound phenomena were not observed. The 10 mg dose was not unequivocally superior to placebo, while the effect of the 40 mg dose was similar to that of the 20 mg dose. The 60 mg dose appeared to be less effective, and it was associated with a rebound phenomenon (early-morning worsening). Administration of ISMN extended release tablets once daily, taken early in the morning on arising, provided at least 12 hours of antianginal activity.

In a placebo control parallel study, 30, 60, 120, and 240 mg of ISMN extended release tablets were administered once daily for up to 6 weeks. Prior to randomization, all patients completed a 1- to 3-week single-blind placebo phase to demonstrate nitrate responsiveness and total exercise treadmill time reproducibility. Exercise tolerance tests using the Bruce Protocol were conducted prior to and at 4 and 12 hours after the morning dose on days 1, 7, 14, 28, and 42 of the double-blind period. ISMN extended release tablets 30 and 60 mg (only doses evaluated acutely) demonstrated a significant increase from baseline in total treadmill time relative to placebo at 4 and 12 hours after the administration of the first dose. At day 42, the 120 and 240 mg dose of ISMN extended release tablets demonstrated a significant increase in total treadmill time at 4 and 12 hours post dosing, but by day 42 the 30 and 60 mg doses no longer were differentiable from placebo. Throughout chronic dosing rebound was not observed in any ISMN extended release treatment group.

Pooled data from two other trials, comparing ISMN extended release tablets 60 mg once daily, ISDN 30 mg qid, and placebo qid in patients with chronic stable angina using a randomized, double-blind, three-way crossover design found statistically significant increases in exercise tolerance times for ISMN extended release tablets compared to placebo at hours 4, 8, and 12 and to ISDN at hour 4. The increases in exercise tolerance on day 14, although statistically significant compared to placebo, were about half of that seen on day 1 of the trial.

INDICATIONS AND USAGE

ISMN tablets are indicated for the prevention and treatment of angina pectoris due to coronary artery disease. The onset of action of oral ISMN is not sufficiently rapid for this product to be useful in aborting an acute anginal episode.

UNLABELED USES

Isosorbide Mononitrate is used alone or as an adjunct in the treatment of acute myocardial infarction, acute pulmonary edema, and congestive heart failure.

CONTRAINDICATIONS

Allergic reactions to organic nitrates are extremely rare, but they do occur. ISMN is contraindicated in patients who have shown hypersensitivity or idiosyncratic reactions to it or to other nitrates or nitrites.

WARNINGS

The benefits of ISMN in patients with acute myocardial infarction or congestive heart failure have not been established; because the effects of ISMN are difficult to terminate rapidly, this drug is not recommended in these settings.

If ISMN is used in these conditions, careful clinical or hemodynamic monitoring must be used to avoid the hazards of hypotension and tachycardia.

PRECAUTIONS

General: Severe hypotension, particularly with upright posture, may occur with even small doses of ISMN. This drug should therefore be used with caution in patients who may be volume depleted or who, for whatever reason, are already

---

Parameter	Single-Dose Studies		Multiple-Dose Studies	
	ISMN 60 mg	ISMN extended release 60 mg	ISMN extended release 60 mg	ISMN extended release 120 mg
C_{max} (ng/mL)	1242-1534	424-541	557-572	1151-1180
T_{max} (hr)	0.6-0.7	3.1-4.5	2.9-4.2	3.1-3.2
AUC (ng•hr/mL)	8189-8313	5990-7452	6625-7555	14241-16800
$t_{1/2}$ (hr)	4.8-5.1	6.3-6.6	6.2-6.3	6.2-6.4
Cl/F (mL/min)	120-122	151-187	132-151	119-140

hypotensive. Hypotension induced by ISMN may be accompanied by paradoxical bradycardia and increased angina pectoris.

Nitrate therapy may aggravate the angina caused by hypertrophic cardiomyopathy.

In industrial workers who have had long-term exposure to unknown (presumably high) doses of organic nitrates, tolerance clearly occurs. Chest pain, acute myocardial infarction, and even sudden death have occurred during temporary withdrawal of nitrates from these workers, demonstrating the existence of true physical dependence. The importance of these observations to the routine, clinical use of oral ISMN is not known.

Information for Patients: Patients should be told that the antianginal efficacy of ISMN tablets can be maintained by carefully following the prescribed schedule of dosing. For most patients, this can be accomplished by taking the first dose on awakening and the second dose 7 hours later or, with single dosage, the dose on arising.

As with other nitrates, daily headaches sometimes accompany treatment with Isosorbide Mononitrate. In patients who get these headaches, the headaches are a marker of the activity of the drug. Patients should resist the temptation to avoid headaches by altering the schedule of their treatment with ISMN, since loss of headache may be associated with simultaneous loss of antianginal efficacy. Aspirin or acetaminophen often successfully relieves ISMN-induced headaches with no deleterious effect on ISMN's antianginal efficacy.

Treatment with ISMN may be associated with light-headedness on standing, especially just after rising from a recumbent or seated position. This effect may be more frequent in patients who have also consumed alcohol.

Drug Interactions: The vasodilating effects of ISMN may be additive with those of other vasodilators. Alcohol, in particular, has been found to exhibit additive effects of this variety.

Marked symptomatic orthostatic hypotension has been reported when calcium channel blockers and organic nitrates were used in combination. Dose adjustments of either class of agents may be necessary.

Metoprolol coadministration did not change the pharmacokinetics of ISMN.

Drug/Laboratory Test Interactions: Nitrates and nitrites may interfere with the Zlatkis-Zak color reaction, causing falsely low readings in serum cholesterol determinations.

Carcinogenesis, Mutagenesis, Impairment of Fertility: No carcinogenic effects were observed in mice exposed to oral Isosorbide Mononitrate for 104 weeks at doses of up to 900 mg/kg/day (102 × the human exposure comparing body surface area).

No evidence of carcinogenicity was observed in rats exposed to ISMN in their diets at doses of up to 900 mg/kg/day for the first six months and 500 mg/kg/day for the remaining duration of a study in which males were dosed for up to 121 weeks and females were dosed for up to 137 weeks. No evidence of mutagenicity was *in vitro* in the Salmonella test (Ames test), in human peripheral lymphocytes, in Chinese hamster cells (V79) or, *in vivo* in the rat micronucleus test. In a study on the fertility and breeding capacity of two generations of rats, ISMN had no adverse effects on fertility or general reproductive performance with oral doses up to 120 mg/kg/day. A dose of 360 mg/kg/day was associated with increased mortality in treated males and females and a reduced fertility index. (See table in "Pregnancy" section for animal-to-human dosage comparisons.) In another study, no adverse effects on fertility were observed when ISMN was administered to male and female rats at doses up to 500 mg/kg/day (125 × the human exposure comparing body surface area).

ISMN is a metabolite of ISDN. Plasma levels of ISMN achieved from a therapeutic dose of ISMN extended release tablets do not significantly exceed the levels of ISMN achieved from a therapeutic dose of ISDN.

No effects on fertility were observed in a study in which male and female rats were administered doses of up to 750 mg/kg/day beginning, in males, 9 weeks prior to mating, and in females, 2 weeks prior to mating.

PREGNANCY

In studies designed to detect effects of ISMN on embryo-fetal development, doses of up to 240 or 248 mg/kg/day, administered to pregnant rats and rabbits, were unassociated with evidence of such effects. These animal doses are about 100 times the maximum recommended human dose (120 mg in a 50 kg woman) when comparison is based on body weight; when comparison is based on body surface area, the rat dose is about 17 times the human dose and the rabbit dose is about 38 times the human dose. Reproduction studies performed in rats and rabbits at doses of up to 540 and 810 mg/kg/day, respectively, have also revealed no evidence of harm to the fetus due to ISMN. There are, however, no adequate and well-controlled studies in pregnant women. Because animal reproduction studies are not always predictive of human response, ISMN tablets should be used during pregnancy only if clearly needed.

Nonteratogenic Effects: Neonatal survival and development, birth weights, and incidence of stillbirths were adversely affected when pregnant rats were administered oral doses of 540 (but not 270) or 750 (but not 300) mg ISMN/kg/day during late gestation and lactation. These doses (the latter about 312 times the human dose when comparison is based on body weight and 54 times the human dose when comparison is based on body surface area) were associated with decreases in maternal weight gain and motor activity and evidence of impaired lactation.

Species	Daily Dose (mg/kg)	Multiple of MRHD* Based on:	
		Body Weight	Body Surface
Rabbit	810	1013	375
Rat	900	1125	195
	540	675	117
	500	625	108
	360	450	78
	270	338	59

* Maximum recommended human dose (MRHD) is 20 mg bid.

Calculations assume a human weight of 50 kg and human body surface area of 1.46 m², a rabbit weight of 2 kg and rabbit body surface area of 0.163 m², and a rat weight of 150 g and rat body surface area of 0.025 m².

For some brands, ISMN has been shown to be associated with stillbirths and neonatal death in rats receiving 500 mg/kg/day of ISMN (125 × the human exposure comparing body surface area). At 250 mg/kg/day, no adverse effects on reproduction and development were reported.

In rats and rabbits receiving ISMN at up to 250 mg/kg/day, no developmental abnormalities, fetal malformations, or other effects upon reproductive performance were detected; these doses are larger than the maximum recommended human dose by factors between 70 (body-surface-area basis in rabbits) and 310 (body-weight basis, either species). In rats receiving 500 mg/kg/day, there were small but statistically significant increases in the rates of prolonged gestation, prolonged parturition, stillbirth, and neonatal death; and there were small but statistically significant decreases in birth weight, live litter size, and pup survival.

Nursing Mothers: It is not known whether this drug is excreted in human milk. Because many drugs are excreted in human milk, caution should be exercised when ISMN is administered to a nursing mother.

Pediatric Use: The safety and effectiveness of ISMN in children have not been established.

ADVERSE REACTIONS

Immediate Release Tablets: Headache is the most frequent side effect and was the cause of 2% of all dropouts from controlled-clinical trials. Headache decreased in incidence after the first few days of therapy.

The following table shows the frequency of adverse reactions observed in 1% or more of subjects in 6 placebo-controlled trials, conducted in the United States and abroad. The same table shows the frequency of withdrawal for these adverse reactions. In many cases the adverse reactions were of uncertain relation to drug treatment. (See related table).

Other adverse reactions, each reported by fewer than 1% of exposed patients, and in many cases of uncertain relation to drug treatment, were:

Cardiovascular: acute myocardial infarction, apoplexy, arrhythmias, bradycardia, edema, hypertension, hypotension, pallor, palpitations, susurrus aurium, tachycardia.

Dermatologic: sweating.

Gastrointestinal: anorexia, dry mouth, dyspepsia, thirst, vomiting, decreased weight.

Genitourinary: prostatic disorder.

Miscellaneous: amblyopia, back pain, bitter taste, muscle cramps, neck pain, paresthesia.

Neurologic: anxiety, impaired concentration, depression, insomnia, nervousness, nightmares, restlessness, tremor, vertigo.

Respiratory: asthma, dyspnea, sinusitis.

Extremely rarely, ordinary doses of organic nitrates have caused methemoglobinemia in normal-seeming patients; for further discussion of its diagnosis and treatment see under "Overdosage."

The table below shows the frequencies of the adverse reactions observed in more than 1% of the subjects (a) in 6 placebo-controlled domestic studies in which patients in the active-treatment arm received 20 mg ISMN twice daily, and (b) in all studies in which patients received ISMN in a variety of regimens. In parentheses, the same table shows the frequencies with which these adverse reactions led to discontinuation of treatment. Overall, eleven percent of the patients who received ISMN in the six controlled U.S. studies discontinued treatment because of adverse reactions. Most of these discontinued because of headache.

"Dizziness" and nausea were also frequently associated with withdrawal from these studies. (See related table.)

Other adverse reactions, each reported by fewer than 1% of exposed patients, and in many cases of uncertain relation to drug treatment, were:
Cardiovascular: angina pectoris, arrhythmias, atrial fibrillation, hypotension, palpitations, postural hypotension, premature ventricular contractions, supraventricular tachycardia, syncope.
Dermatologic: pruritus, rash.
Gastrointestinal: abdominal pain, diarrhea, dyspepsia, tenesmus, tooth disorder, vomiting.
Genitourinary: dysuria, impotence, urinary frequency.
Miscellaneous: asthenia, blurred vision, cold sweat, diplopia, edema, malaise, neck stiffness, rigors.
Musculoskeletal: arthralgia.
Neurologic: agitation, anxiety, confusion, dyscoordination, hypoesthesia, hypokinesia, increased appetite, insomnia, nervousness, nightmares.
Respiratory: bronchitis, pneumonia, upper respiratory tract infection.

Extended Release Tablets: The table below shows the frequencies of the adverse events that occurred in > 5% of the subjects in three placebo-controlled North American studies, in which patients in the active treatment arm received 30 mg, 60 mg, 120 mg, or 240 mg of ISMN extended release tablets once daily. In parentheses, the same table shows the frequencies with which these adverse events were associated with the discontinuation of treatment. Overall, 8% of the patients who received 30 mg, 60 mg, 120 mg, or 240 mg of ISMN extended release in the three placebo-controlled North American studies discontinued treatment because of adverse events. Most of these discontinued because of headache. Dizziness was rarely associated with withdrawal from these studies. Since headache appears to be a dose-related adverse effect and tends to disappear with continued treatment, it is recommended that ISMN extended release treatment be initiated at low doses for several days before being increased to desired levels.

FREQUENCY AND ADVERSE EVENTS (DISCONTINUED)*

Three Controlled North American Studies

Dose	Placebo	30 mg	60 mg	120 mg**	240 mg**
Patients	96	60	102	65	65
Headache	15%	38%	51%	42%	57%
	(0%)	(5%)	(8%)	(5%)	(8%)
Dizziness	4%	8%	11%	9%	9%
	(0%)	(0%)	(1%)	(2%)	(2%)

* *Some individuals discontinued for multiple reasons.*
** *Patients were started on 60 mg and titrated to their final dose.*

FREQUENCY OF ADVERSE REACTIONS (DISCONTINUATIONS)*

			6 Placebo Controlled Studies	
Dose	Placebo	5 mg	10 mg	20 mg
Patients	160	54	52	159
Headache	6% (0%)	17% (0%)	13% (0%)	35% (5%)
Fatigue	2% (0%)	0% (0%)	4% (0%)	1% (0%)
Upper Respiratory Infection	< 1% (0%)	0% (0%)	4% (0%)	1% (0%)
Pain	< 1% (0%)	4% (0%)	0% (0%)	< 1% (0%)
Dizziness	1% (0%)	0% (0%)	0% (0%)	4% (0%)
Nausea	< 1% (0%)	0% (0%)	0% (0%)	3% (2%)
Increased Cough	< 1% (0%)	0% (0%)	2% (0%)	1% (0%)
Rash	0% (0%)	2% (2%)	2% (0%)	< 1% (0%)
Abdominal Pain	< 1% (0%)	0% (0%)	2% (0%)	0% (0%)
Allergic Reaction	0% (0%)	0% (0%)	2% (0%)	0% (0%)
Cardiovascular Disorder	0% (0%)	2% (0%)	0% (0%)	0% (0%)
Chest Pain	< 1% (0%)	0% (0%)	2% (0%)	< 0% (0%)
Diarrhea	0% (0%)	0% (0%)	2% (0%)	0% (0%)
Flushing	0% (0%)	0% (0%)	2% (0%)	0% (0%)
Emotional Lability	0% (0%)	2% (0%)	0% (0%)	0% (0%)
Pruritus	1% (0%)	2% (2%)	0% (0%)	0% (0%)

* *Some individuals discontinued for multiple reasons.*

FREQUENTLY AND ADVERSE REACTIONS (DISCONTINUATIONS)*

			6 Controlled Studies		*92 Clinical Studies*
Dose	Placebo		20 mg		(varied)
Patients	204		219		3344
Headache	9%	(0%)	38%	(9%)	19% (4.3%)
Dizziness	1%	(0%)	5%	(1%)	3% (0.2%)
Nausea, Vomiting	< 1%	(0%)	4%	(3%)	2% (0.2%)

* *Some individuals discontinued for multiple reasons.*

In addition, the three North American trials were pooled with 11 controlled trials conducted in Europe. Among the 14 controlled trials, a total of 711 patients were randomized to ISMN extended release tablets. When the pooled data were reviewed, headache and dizziness were the only adverse events that were reported by > 5% of patients. Other adverse events, each reported by ≤ 5% of exposed patients, and in many cases of uncertain relation to drug treatment, were:

Autonomic Nervous System Disorders: Dry mouth, hot flushes.

Body as a Whole: Asthenia, back pain, chest pain, edema, fatigue, fever, flu-like symptoms, malaise, rigors.

Cardiovascular Disorders, General: Cardiac failure, hypertension, hypotension.

Central and Peripheral Nervous System Disorders: Dizziness, headache, hypoesthesia, migraine, neuritis, paresis, paresthesia, ptosis, tremor, vertigo.

Gastrointestinal System Disorders: Abdominal pain, constipation, diarrhea, dyspepsia, flatulence, gastric ulcer, gastritis, glossitis, hemorrhagic gastric ulcer, hemorrhoids, loose stools, melena, nausea, vomiting.

Hearing and Vestibular Disorders: Earache, tinnitus, tympanic membrane perforation.

Heart Rate and Rhythm Disorders: Arrhythmia, arrhythmia atrial, atrial fibrillation, bradycardia, bundle branch block, extrasystole, palpitation, tachycardia, ventricular tachycardia.

Liver and Biliary System Disorders: SGOT increase, SGPT increase.

Metabolic and Nutritional Disorders: Hyperuricemia, hypokalemia.

Musculoskeletal System Disorders: Arthralgia, frozen shoulder, muscle weakness, musculoskeletal pain, myalgia, myositis, tendon disorder, torticollis.

Myo-, Endo-, Pericardial and Valve Disorders: Angina pectoris aggravated, heart murmur, heart sound abnormal, myocardial infarction, Q-Wave abnormality.

Platelet, Bleeding, and Clotting Disorders: Purpura, thrombocytopenia.

Psychiatric Disorders: Anxiety, concentration impaired, confusion, decreased libido, depression, impotence, insomnia, nervousness, paroniria, somnolence.

Red Blood Cell Disorder: Hypochromic anemia.

Reproductive Disorders, Female: Atrophic vaginitis, breast pain.

Resistance Mechanism Disorders: Bacterial infection, moniliasis, viral infection.

Respiratory System Disorders: Bronchitis, bronchospasm, coughing, dyspnea, increased sputum, nasal congestion, pharyngitis, pneumonia, pulmonary infiltration, rales, rhinitis, sinusitis.

Skin and Appendages Disorders: Acne, hair texture abnormal, increased sweating, pruritus, rash, skin nodule.

◆ RATED THERAPEUTICALLY EQUIVALENT; ◇ THERAPEUTIC EQUIVALENCE UNCONFIRMED; ○ UNRATED

Urinary System Disorders: Polyuria, renal calculus, urinary tract infection.

Vascular (Extracardiac) Disorders: Flushing, intermittent claudication, leg ulcer, varicose vein.

Vision Disorders: Conjunctivitis, photophobia, vision abnormal.

OVERDOSAGE

Hemodynamic Effects: The ill effects of ISMN overdose are generally the results of ISMN's capacity to induce vasodilatation, venous pooling, reduced cardiac output, and hypotension. These hemodynamic changes may have protean manifestations, including increased intracranial pressure, with any or all of persistent throbbing headache, confusion, and moderate fever; vertigo; palpitations; visual disturbances; nausea and vomiting (possibly with colic and even bloody diarrhea); syncope (especially in the upright posture); air hunger and dyspnea, later followed by reduced ventilatory effort; diaphoresis, with the skin either flushed or cold and clammy; heart block and bradycardia; paralysis; coma; seizures and death.

Laboratory determinations of serum levels of ISMN and its metabolites are not widely available, and such determinations have, in any event, no established role in the management of ISMN overdose.

There are no data suggesting what dose of ISMN is likely to be life threatening in humans. In rats and mice, there is significant lethality at doses of 1965 to 2000 mg/kg and 2581 to 3000 mg/kg, respectively.

No data are available to suggest physiological maneuvers (e.g., maneuvers to change the pH of the urine) that might accelerate elimination of ISMN. In particular, dialysis is known to be ineffective in removing ISMN from the body.

No specific antagonist to the vasodilator effects of ISMN is known, and no intervention has been subject to controlled study as a therapy of ISMN overdose. Because the hypotension associated with ISMN overdose is the result of venodilatation and arterial hypovolemia, prudent therapy in this situation should be directed toward an increase in central fluid volume. Passive elevation of the patient's legs may be sufficient, but intravenous infusion of normal saline or similar fluid may also be necessary.

The use of epinephrine or other arterial vasoconstrictors in this setting is likely to do more harm than good.

In patients with renal disease or congestive heart failure, therapy resulting in central volume expansion is not without hazard. Treatment of ISMN overdose in these patients may be subtle and difficult, and invasive monitoring may be required.

Methemoglobinemia: Methemoglobinemia has been reported in patients receiving other organic nitrates, and it probably could also occur as a side effect of ISMN. Certainly nitrate ions liberated during metabolism of ISMN can oxidize hemoglobin into methemoglobin. Even in patients totally without cytochrome b_5 reductase activity, however, and even assuming that the nitrate moiety of ISMN is quantitatively applied to oxidation of hemoglobin, about 2 mg/kg of ISMN should be required before any of these patients manifest clinically significant ($\geq$ 10%) methemoglobinemia. In patients with normal reductase function, significant production of methemoglobin should require even larger doses of ISMN. In one study in which 36 patients received 2-4 weeks of continuous nitroglycerin therapy at 3.1 to 4.4 mg/hr (equivalent, in total administered dose of nitrate ions, to 7.8-11.1 mg of ISMN per hour), the average methemoglobin level measured was 0.2%; this was comparable to that observed in parallel patients who received placebo.

Notwithstanding these observations, there are case reports of significant methemoglobinemia in association with moderate overdoses of organic nitrates. None of the affected patients had been thought to be unusually susceptible.

Methemoglobin levels are available from most clinical laboratories. The diagnosis should be suspected in patients who exhibit signs of impaired oxygen delivery despite adequate cardiac output and adequate arterial pO$_2$. Classically, methemoglobinemic blood is described as chocolate brown, without color change on exposure to air.

When methemoglobinemia is diagnosed, the treatment of choice is methylene blue, 1-2 mg/kg intravenously.

DOSAGE AND ADMINISTRATION

The recommended regimen of ISMN immediate release tablets is 20 mg twice daily, with the doses seven hours apart. For most patients, this can be accomplished by taking the first dose on awakening and the second dose 7 hours later. A starting dose of 5 mg (1/2 tablet of the 10 mg dosing strength) might be appropriate for persons of particularly small stature but should be increased to at least 10 mg by the second or third day of therapy. Dosage adjustments are not necessary for elderly patients or patients with altered hepatic or renal function.

As noted above ("Clinical Pharmacology"), multiple studies of organic nitrates have shown that maintenance of continuous 24-hour plasma levels results in refractory tolerance. The asymmetric (2 doses, 7 hours apart) dosing regimen for ISMN tablets provides a daily nitrate-free interval to minimize the development of tolerance.

As also noted under *"Clinical Pharmacology"*, well-controlled studies have shown that tolerance to ISMN tablets occurs to some extent or may be avoided when using the twice daily regimen in which the two doses are given seven hours apart. This regimen has been shown to have antianginal efficacy beginning one hour after the first dose and lasting at least five to seven hours after the second dose. The duration (if any) of antianginal activity beyond twelve to fourteen hours has not been studied; large controlled studies with other nitrates suggest that no dosing regimen should be expected to provide more than about twelve hours of continuous antianginal efficacy per day.

In clinical trials, ISMN has been administered in a variety of regimens and doses. Single doses less than 20 mg have not been adequately studied, while single doses greater than 20 mg have demonstrated no greater efficacy than doses of 20 mg. Doses above 20 mg twice a day (with the doses seven hours apart) have not been adequately studied. Doses of 5 mg twice a day are clearly effective (effectiveness based on exercise tolerance) for only the first day of a twice-a-day (with doses 7 hours apart) regimen. The recommended starting dose of ISMN extended release tablets is 30 mg (given as 1/2 of a 60 mg tablet) or 60 mg (given as a single tablet) once daily. After several days the dosage may be increased to 120 mg (given as two 60 mg tablets) once daily. Rarely, 240 mg may be required. The daily dose of ISMN extended release tablets should be taken in the morning on arising. ISMN extended release tablets should not be chewed or crushed and should be swallowed together with a half-glassful of fluid.

Store immediate release tablets at controlled room temperature 15°-30°C (59°-86°F). Keep tightly closed.

Store extended release tablets between 2° and 30°C (36° and 86°F). Protect unit dose from excessive moisture.

HOW SUPPLIED
TABLET, EXTENDED RELEASE: 60 MG

BRAND/MANUFACTURER	NDC	SIZE	AWP
○ BRAND			
► IMDUR: Schering	00085-4110-03	100s	$75.62
	00085-4110-01	100s ud	$83.18

TABLETS: 10 MG

BRAND/MANUFACTURER	NDC	SIZE	AWP
○ BRAND			
► MONOKET: Schwarz	00091-3610-60	60s	$30.00
	00091-3610-01	100s	$50.00
	00091-3610-11	100s ud	$55.00
	00091-3610-18	180s	$90.00

TABLETS: 20 MG

AVERAGE UNIT PRICE (AVAILABLE SIZES)	
BRAND	$0.54

BRAND/MANUFACTURER	NDC	SIZE	AWP
◆ BRAND			
MONOKET: Schwarz	00091-3620-60	60s	$31.59
	00091-3620-01	100s	$52.65
	00091-3620-11	100s ud	$57.90
	00091-3620-18	180s	$94.78

TABLETS: 20 MG

BRAND/MANUFACTURER	NDC	SIZE	AWP
○ BRAND			
► ISMO: Wyeth-Ayerst	00008-0771-01	100s	$65.81
	00008-0771-02	100s ud	$72.38

Isosulfan Blue

DESCRIPTION

The chemical name for Isosulfan Blue is N-[4-[[4-(diethylamino)phenyl](2,5-disulfophenyl) methylene]-2,5-cyclohexadien-1-ylidene]-N-ethylethanaminium hydroxide, inner salt, sodium salt.

Isosulfan Blue is a sterile aqueous solution for subcutaneous administration. Each ml of solution contains 10 mg Isosulfan Blue.

Isosulfan Blue 1% is a contrast agent for the delineation of lymphatic vessels.

CLINICAL PHARMACOLOGY

Isosulfan Blue 1% has no known pharmacologic action. Following subcutaneous administration, Isosulfan Blue is selectively picked up by the lymphatic vessels. Thus, the lymphatic vessels are delineated by a bright blue color making them discernible from surrounding tissue.

There is some evidence that 50% of Isosulfan Blue, from aqueous solution, is weakly bound to serum protein (albumin). Since interstitial protein is presumed to be carried almost exclusively by lymphatics, and in view of evidence of binding of dyes to proteins, visualization may be due to protein binding phenomenon.

ABSORPTION

Following a single 1 ml subcutaneous injection of a 1% solution by triphenylmethane dye in the rat, 34% is absorbed in 30 minutes from the injection site. Absorption of 69% and 100% occurs at 1 and 24 hours respectively.

EXCRETION

Up to 10% of the subcutaneously administered dose of Isosulfan Blue 1% is excreted unchanged in the urine in 24 hours in man. Presumably, 90% is excreted through the biliary route.

► SHOWN IN PRODUCT IDENTIFICATION GUIDE

INDICATIONS

Isosulfan Blue 1% upon subcutaneous administration, delineates the lymphatic vessels. It is an adjunct to lymphography (in primary and secondary lymphedema of the extremities; chyluria, chylous ascites or chylothorax; lymph node involvement by primary or secondary neoplasm; and lymph node response to therapeutic modalities) for visualization of the lymphatic system draining the region of injection.

CONTRAINDICATIONS

Isosulfan Blue 1% is contraindicated in those individuals with known hypersensitivity to triphenylmethane or related compounds.

WARNINGS

The lymphographic procedure which involves the use of Isosulfan Blue 1% should be carried out under the direction of personnel with the prerequisite training and with a thorough knowledge of the procedure to be performed. Appropriate facilities should be available for coping with situations which may arise as a result of the procedure, as well as for emergency treatment of severe reactions to the drug.

After subcutaneous administration of Isosulfan Blue 1%, competent personnel and emergency facilities should be available for at least 30 to 60 minutes, since severe delayed reactions have been known to occur with similar compounds.

The admixture of Isosulfan Blue 1% with local anesthetics (i.e., lidocaine) in the same syringe prior to administration results in an immediate precipitation of 4-9% drug complex. This technique is not recommended. If it is in the best interest of the patient to give a local anesthetic, it is suggested that administration be made via a separate syringe.

PRECAUTIONS

INFORMATION FOR PATIENTS

Since up to 10% of Isosulfan Blue 1% is excreted unchanged in the urine, the patient should be advised that urine color may be blue for 24 hours following its administration.

CARCINOGENESIS, MUTAGENESIS, IMPAIRMENT OF FERTILITY

Long-term studies in animals have not been performed to evaluate the carcinogenic potential of Isosulfan Blue 1% and are, therefore, unknown. Similarly, reproduction studies in animals have not been conducted and, therefore, it is unknown if a problem concerning mutagenesis or impairment of fertility in either males or females exists.

TERATOGENIC EFFECTS

Pregnancy Category C: Animal reproduction studies have not been conducted with Isosulfan Blue 1%. It is also not known whether Isosulfan Blue 1% can cause fetal harm when administered to a pregnant woman or can affect reproduction capacity. Isosulfan Blue 1% should be given to a pregnant woman only if clearly needed.

NURSING MOTHERS

It is not known whether this drug is excreted in human milk. Because many drugs are excreted in human milk, caution should be exercised when Isosulfan Blue 1% is administered to a nursing mother.

PEDIATRIC USE

Safety and effectiveness of Isosulfan Blue 1% in children have not been established.

ADVERSE REACTIONS

Isosulfan Blue 1% has demonstrated a 1.5% incidence of adverse reactions. All the reactions were of an allergic type. Localized swelling at the site of administration and mild pruritus of hands, abdomen and neck have been reported within several minutes following administration of the drug.

Reports of mild to severe reactions have appeared in the literature for compounds similar to Isosulfan Blue. A death has been reported following the intravenous administration of a similar compound employed to estimate depth of a severe burn. Severe reactions may be manifested by edema of the face and glottis, respiratory distress or shock; such reactions may prove fatal unless promptly controlled by such emergency measures as maintenance of a clear airway and immediate use of oxygen and resuscitative drugs. Like other sensitivity phenomena, severe reactions are more likely to occur in patients with a personal or family history of bronchial asthma, significant allergies, drug reactions or previous reactions to triphenylmethane dyes.

DOSAGE AND ADMINISTRATION

Isosulfan Blue 1% is to be administered subcutaneously, one-half (1/2) ml into three (3) interdigital spaces of each extremity per study. A maximum dose of 3 ml (30 mg) Isosulfan Blue is, therefore, injected.

Store at room temperature. Avoid excessive heat.

HOW SUPPLIED

INJECTION: 10 MG/ML

BRAND/MANUFACTURER	NDC	SIZE	AWP
○ **BRAND**			
LYMPHAZURIN: Hirsch	50673-0250-21	5 ml 6s	$195.00

Isotretinoin

CONTRAINDICATION AND WARNING

ISOTRETINOIN MUST NOT BE USED BY FEMALES WHO ARE PREGNANT OR WHO MAY BECOME PREGNANT WHILE UNDERGOING TREATMENT. THERE IS AN EXTREMELY HIGH RISK THAT A DEFORMED INFANT WILL RESULT IF PREGNANCY OCCURS WHILE TAKING ISOTRETINOIN IN ANY AMOUNT EVEN FOR SHORT PERIODS. POTENTIALLY ALL EXPOSED FETUSES CAN BE AFFECTED.

ISOTRETINOIN IS CONTRAINDICATED IN WOMEN OF CHILDBEARING POTENTIAL UNLESS THE *PATIENT MEETS ALL OF THE FOLLOWING CONDITIONS*:

- HAS SEVERE DISFIGURING CYSTIC ACNE THAT IS RECALCITRANT TO STANDARD THERAPIES
- IS RELIABLE IN UNDERSTANDING AND CARRYING OUT INSTRUCTIONS
- IS CAPABLE OF COMPLYING WITH THE MANDATORY CONTRACEPTIVE MEASURES
- HAS RECEIVED BOTH ORAL AND WRITTEN WARNINGS OF THE HAZARDS OF TAKING ISOTRETINOIN DURING PREGNANCY AND THE RISK OF POSSIBLE CONTRACEPTION FAILURE AND HAS ACKNOWLEDGED HER UNDERSTANDING OF THESE WARNINGS IN WRITING
- HAS HAD A NEGATIVE SERUM PREGNANCY TEST WITHIN TWO WEEKS PRIOR TO BEGINNING THERAPY (IT IS ALSO RECOMMENDED THAT PREGNANCY TESTING AND CONTRACEPTION COUNSELING BE REPEATED ON A MONTHLY BASIS. TO ENCOURAGE COMPLIANCE WITH THIS RECOMMENDATION, THE PHYSICIAN SHOULD PRESCRIBE NO MORE THAN A ONE MONTH SUPPLY OF THE DRUG.)
- WILL BEGIN THERAPY ONLY ON THE SECOND OR THIRD DAY OF THE NEXT NORMAL MENSTRUAL PERIOD

MAJOR HUMAN FETAL ABNORMALITIES RELATED TO ISOTRETINOIN ADMINISTRATION HAVE BEEN DOCUMENTED: CNS ABNORMALITIES (INCLUDING CEREBRAL ABNORMALITIES, CEREBELLAR MALFORMATION, HYDROCEPHALUS, MICROCEPHALY, CRANIAL NERVE DEFICIT); SKULL ABNORMALITY; EXTERNAL EAR ABNORMALITIES (INCLUDING ANOTIA, MICROPINNA, SMALL OR ABSENT EXTERNAL AUDITORY CANALS); EYE ABNORMALITIES (INCLUDING MICROPHTHALMIA); CARDIOVASCULAR ABNORMALITIES; FACIAL DYSMORPHIA; THYMUS GLAND ABNORMALITY; PARATHYROID HORMONE DEFICIENCY. IN SOME CASES DEATH HAS OCCURRED WITH CERTAIN OF THE ABNORMALITIES PREVIOUSLY NOTED. CASES OF IQ SCORES LESS THAN 85 WITH OR WITHOUT OBVIOUS CNS ABNORMALITIES HAVE ALSO BEEN REPORTED. THERE IS AN INCREASED RISK OF SPONTANEOUS ABORTION. IN ADDITION, PREMATURE BIRTHS HAVE BEEN REPORTED.

EFFECTIVE CONTRACEPTION MUST BE USED FOR AT LEAST ONE MONTH BEFORE BEGINNING ISOTRETINOIN THERAPY, DURING THERAPY AND FOR ONE MONTH FOLLOWING DISCONTINUATION OF THERAPY EVEN WHERE THERE HAS BEEN A HISTORY OF INFERTILITY, UNLESS DUE TO HYSTERECTOMY. IT IS RECOMMENDED THAT TWO RELIABLE FORMS OF CONTRACEPTION BE USED SIMULTANEOUSLY UNLESS ABSTINENCE IS THE CHOSEN METHOD.

IF PREGNANCY DOES OCCUR DURING TREATMENT, THE PHYSICIAN AND PATIENT SHOULD DISCUSS THE DESIRABILITY TO CONTINUING THE PREGNANCY.

ISOTRETINOIN SHOULD BE PRESCRIBED ONLY BY PHYSICIANS WHO HAVE SPECIAL COMPETENCE IN THE DIAGNOSIS AND TREATMENT OF SEVERE RECALCITRANT CYSTIC ACNE, ARE EXPERIENCED IN THE USE OF SYSTEMIC RETINOIDS AND UNDERSTAND THE RISK OF TERATOGENICITY IF ISOTRETINOIN IS USED DURING PREGNANCY.

DESCRIPTION

Isotretinoin, a retinoid which inhibits sebaceous gland function and keratinization, is available in 10-mg, 20-mg and 40-mg soft gelatin capsules for oral administration.

Chemically, Isotretinoin is 13-*cis*-retinoic acid and is related to both retinoic acid and retinol (vitamin A). It is a yellow-orange to orange crystalline powder with a molecular weight of 300.44.

Following is its chemical structure:

CLINICAL PHARMACOLOGY

The exact mechanism of action of Isotretinoin is unknown.

Cystic Acne: Clinical improvement in cystic acne patients occurs in association with a reduction in sebum secretion. The decrease in sebum secretion is temporary and is related to the dose and duration of treatment with Isotretinoin, and reflects a reduction in sebaceous gland size and an inhibition of sebaceous gland differentiation.[1]

Clinical Pharmacokinetics: The pharmacokinetic profile of Isotretinoin is predictable and can be described using linear pharmacokinetic theory.

After oral administration of 80 mg (two 40-mg capsules), peak blood concentrations ranged from 167 to 459 ng/mL (mean 256 ng/mL) and mean time to peak was 3.2 hours in normal volunteers, while in acne patients peak concentrations ranged from 98 to 535 ng/mL (mean 262 ng/mL) with a mean time to peak of 2.9 hours. The drug is 99.9% bound in human plamsa almost exclusively to albumin. The terminal elimination half-life of Isotretinoin ranged from 10 to 20 hours in volunteers and patients. Following an 80-mg liquid suspension oral dose of ^{14}C-Isotretinoin, ^{14}C-activity in blood declined with a half-life of 90 hours. Relatively equal amounts of radioactivity were recovered in the urine and feces with 65% to 83% of the dose recovered.

The major identified metabolite in blood is 4-*oxo*-isotretinoin. The mean elimination half-life of this metabolite is 25 hours (range 17-50 hours). Tretinoin and 4-oxo-tretinoin were also observed. After two 40-mg capsules of Isotretinoin, maximum concentrations of the metabolite of 87 to 399 ng/mL occurred at 6 to 20 hours. The blood concentration of the major metabolite generally exceeded that of Isotretinoin after six hours.

When taken with food or milk, the oral absorption of Isotretinoin is increased.

The mean ± SD minimum steady-state blood concentration of Isotretinoin was 160 ± 19 ng/mL in ten patients receiving 40-mg *b.i.d.* doses. After single and multiple doses the mean ratio of areas under the blood concentration time curves of 4-*oxo*-isotretinoin to Isotretinoin was 3 to 3.5.

Tissue Distribution in Animals: Tissue distribution of ^{14}C-Isotretinoin in rats after oral dosing revealed high concentrations of radioactivity in many tissues after 15 minutes, with a maximum in one hour, and declining to nondetectable levels by 24 hours in most tissues. After seven days, however, low levels of radioactivity were detected in the liver, ureter, adrenal, ovary and lacrimal gland.

INDICATIONS AND USAGE

Cystic Acne: Isotretinoin is indicated for the treatment of severe recalcitrant cystic acne, and a single course of therapy has been shown to result in complete and prolonged remission of disease in many patients.[1-3] If a second course of therapy is needed, it should not be initiated until at least eight weeks after completion of the first course, since experience has shown that patients may continue to improve while off drug.

Because of significant adverse effects associated with its use, Isotretinoin should be reserved for patients with severe cystic acne who are unresponsive to conventional therapy, including systemic antibiotics.

UNLABELED USES

Isotretinoin is used alone or as an adjunct in the treatment of basal cell carcinoma, cervical cancer, and mycosis fungoides (cutaneous T-cell lymphoma). It is also used in Darier's disease, lamellar ichthyosis, and pityriasis rubra pilaris, and is prescribed for the treatment of herpes simplex infections, Grover's disease, lichen planus, refractory rosacea, keratosis palmaris et plantaris, leukoplakia, squamous cell skin cancer, and xeroderma pigmentosum.

CONTRAINDICATIONS

Pregnancy: Category X: (see boxed "*Contraindication and Warning.*")

Isotretinion should not be given to patients who are sensitive to parabens, which are used as preservatives in the gelatin capsule.

WARNINGS

PSEUDOTUMOR CEREBRI: ISOTRETINOIN USE HAS BEEN ASSOCIATED WITH A NUMBER OF CASES OF PSEUDOTUMOR CEREBRI (BENIGN INTRACRANIAL HYPERTENSION). EARLY SIGNS AND SYMPTOMS OF PSEUDOTUMOR CEREBRI INCLUDE PAPILLEDEMA, HEADACHE, NAUSEA AND VOMITING, AND VISUAL DISTURBANCES. PATIENTS WITH THESE SYMPTOMS SHOULD BE SCREENED FOR PAPILLEDEMA AND, IF PRESENT, THEY SHOULD BE TOLD TO DISCONTINUE ISOTRETINOIN IMMEDIATELY AND BE REFERRED TO A NEUROLOGIST FOR FURTHER DIAGNOSIS AND CARE.

Decreased Night Vision: A number of cases of decreased night vision have occurred during Isotretinoin therapy. Because the onset in some patients was sudden, patients should be advised of this potential problem and warned to be cautious when driving or operating any vehicle at night. Visual problems should be carefully monitored.

Corneal opacities: Corneal opacities have occurred in patients receiving Isotretinoin for acne and more frequently when higher drug dosages were used in patients with disorders of keratinization. All Isotretinoin patients experiencing visual difficulties should discontinue the drug and have an ophthalmological examination. The corneal opacities that have been observed in patients treated with Isotretinoin have either completely resolved or were resolving at follow-up six to seven weeks after discontinuation of the drug. See "*Adverse Reactions.*"

Inflammatory Bowel Disease: Isotretinoin has been temporally associated with inflammatory bowel disease (including regional ileitis) in patients without a prior history of intestinal disorders. Patients experiencing abdominal pain, rectal bleeding or severe diarrhea should discontinue Isotretinoin immediately.

Lipids: Blood lipid determinations should be performed before Isotretinoin is given and then at intervals until the lipid response to Isotretinoin is established, which usually occurs within four weeks. See "*Precautions.*"

Approximately 25% of patients receiving Isotretinoin experienced an elevation in plasma triglycerides. Approximately 15% developed a decrease in high density lipoproteins and about 7% showed an increase in cholesterol levels. These effects on triglycerides, HDL and cholesterol were reversible upon cessation of Isotretinoin therapy.

Patients with increased tendency to develop hypertriglyceridemia include those with diabetes mellitus, obesity, increased alcohol intake and familial history.

The cardiovascular consequences of hypertriglyceridemia are not well understood, but may increase the patient's risk status. In addition, elevation of serum triglycerides in excess of 800 mg/dL has been associated with acute pancreatitis, Therefore, every attempt should be made to control significant triglyceride elevation.

Some patients have been able to reverse triglyceride elevation by reduction in weight, restriction of dietary fat and alcohol, and reduction in dose while continuing Isotretinoin.[4] An obese male patient with Darier's disease developed elevated triglycerides and subsequent eruptive xanthomas.[5]

Hyperostosis: In clinical trials of disorders of keratinization with a mean dose of 2.24 mg/kg/day, a high prevalence of skeletal hyperostosis was noted. Two children showed x-ray findings suggestive of premature closure of the epiphysis. Additionally, skeletal hyperostosis was noted in six of eight patients in a prospective study of disorders of keratinization.[6] Minimal skeletal hyperostosis has also been observed by x-rays in prospective studies of cystic acne patients treated with a single course of therapy at recommended doses.

Hepatotoxicity: Several cases of clinical hepatitis have been noted which are considered to be possibly or probably related to Isotretinoin therapy. Additionally, mild to moderate elevations of liver enzymes have been observed in approximately 15% of individuals treated during clinical trials, some of which normalized with dosage reduction or continued administration of the drug. If normalization does not readily occur or if hepatitis is suspected during treatment with Isotretinoin, the drug should be discontinued and the etiology further investigated.

Animal Studies: In rats given 32 or 8 mg/kg/day of Isotretinoin for 18 months or longer, the incidences of focal calcification, fibrosis and inflammation of the myocardium, calcification of coronary, pulmonary and mesenteric arteries and metastatic calcification of the gastric mucosa were greater than in control rats of similar age. Focal endocardial and myocardial calcifications associated with calcification of the coronary arteries were observed in two dogs after approximately six to seven months of treatment with Isotretinoin at a dosage of 60 to 120 mg/kg/day.

In dogs given Isotretinoin chronically at a dosage of 60 mg/kg/day, corneal ulcers and corneal opacities were encountered at a higher incidence than in control dogs. In general, these ocular changes tended to revert toward normal when treatment with Isotretinoin was stopped, but did not completely clear during the observation period.

In rats given Isotretinoin at a dosage of 32 mg/kg/day for approximately 15 weeks, long bone fracture has been observed.

PRECAUTIONS

Information for Patients: Women of childbearing potential should be instructed that they must not be pregnant when Isotretinoin therapy is initiated, and that they should use effective contraception while taking Isotretinoin and for one month after Isotretinoin has been stopped. They should also sign a consent form prior to beginning Isotretinoin therapy. See boxed "*Contraindication and Warning.*"

Because of the relationship of Isotretinoin to vitamin A, patients should be advised against taking vitamin supplements containing vitamin A to avoid additive toxic effects.

Patients should be informed that transient exacerbation of acne has been seen, generally during the initial period of therapy.

Patients should be informed that they may experience decreased tolerance to contact lenses during and after therapy. It is recommended that patients not donate blood during therapy and for at least one month following discontinuance of the drug.

Laboratory Tests: The incidence of hypertriglyceridemia is 1 patient in 4 on Isotretinoin therapy. Pretreatment and follow-up blood lipids should be obtained under fasting conditions. After consumption of alcohol at least 36 hours should elapse before these determinations are made. It is recommended that these tests be performed at weekly or biweekly intervals until the lipid response to Isotretinoin is established. Since elevations of liver enzymes have been observed during clinical trials, pretreatment and follow-up liver function tests should be performed at weekly or biweekly intervals until the response to Isotretinoin has been established.

Certain patients receiving Isotretinoin have experienced problems in the control of their blood sugar. In addition, new cases of diabetes have been diagnosed during Isotretinoin therapy, although no causal relationship has been established. Some patients undergoing vigorous physical activity while on Isotretinoin therapy have experienced elevated CPK levels; however, the clinical significance is unknown.

Carcinogenesis, Mutagenesis, Impairment of Fertility: In Fischer 344 rats given Isotretinoin at dosages of 32 or 8 mg/kg/day for greater than 18 months, there was an increased incidence of pheochromocytoma. The incidence of adrenal medullary hyperplasia was also increased at the higher dosage. The relatively high level of spontaneous pheochromocytomas occurring in the Fischer 344 rat makes it a poor model for study of this tumor, since the increase in adrenal medullary proliferative lesions following chronic treatment with relatively high dosages of Isotretinoin may be an accentuation of a genetic predisposition in the Fischer 344 rat, and its relevance to the human population is not clear. In addition, a decreased incidence of liver adenomas, liver angiomas and leukemia was noted at the dose levels of 8 and 32 mg/kg/day.

The Ames test was conducted in two laboratories. The results of the tests in one laboratory were negative while in the second laboratory a weekly-positive response (less than $1.6 \times$ background) was noted in S. typhimurium TA100 when the assay was conducted with metabolic activation. No dose-response effect was seen and all other strains were negative. Additionally, other tests designed to assess genotoxicity (Chinese hamster cell assay, mouse micronucleus test, S. cerevisiae D7 assay, *in vitro* clastogenesis assay in human-derived lymphocytes and unscheduled DNA synthesis assay) were all negative.

No adverse effects on gonadal function, fertility, conception rate, gestation or parturition were observed at dose levels of 2, 8 or 32 mg/kg/day in male and female rats.

In dogs, testicular atrophy was noted after treatment with Isotretinoin for approximately 30 weeks at dosages of 60 or 20 mg/kg/day. In general, there was microscopic evidence for appreciable depression of spermatogenesis but some sperm were observed in all testes examined and in no instance were completely atrophic tubules seen. In studies in 66 human males, 30 of whom were patients with cystic acne, no significant changes were noted in the count or motility of spermatozoa in the ejaculate. In a study of 50 men (ages 17-32 years) receiving Isotretinoin therapy for cystic acne, no significant effects were seen on ejaculate volume, sperm count, total sperm motility, morphology or seminal plasma fructose.

Pregnancy: Category X.: See boxed *"Contraindication and Warnings."*

Nursing Mothers: It is not known whether this drug is excreted in human milk. Because of the potential for adverse effects, nursing mothers should not receive Isotretinoin.

ADVERSE REACTIONS

Clinical: Many of the side effects and adverse reactions seen or expected in patients receiving Isotretinoin are similar to those described in patients taking high doses of vitamin A. The percentages of adverse reactions listed below reflect the total experience in Isotretinoin studies, including investigational studies of disorders of keratinization, with the exception of those pertaining to dry skin and mucous membranes. These latter reflect the experience only in patients with cystic acne because reactions relating to dryness are more commonly recognized as adverse reactions in this disease. Included in this category are dry skin, skin fragility, pruritus, epistaxis, dry nose and dry mouth, which may be seen in up to 80% of cystic acne patients.

The most frequent adverse reaction to Isotretinoin is cheilitis, which occurs in over 90% of patients. A less frequent reaction was conjunctivitis (about two patients in five).

Skeletal hyperostosis has been observed on x-rays of patients treated with Isotretinoin. See *"Warnings."* Other types of bone abnormalities have also been reported; however, no causal relationship has been established.

Approximately 16% of patients treated with Isotretinoin developed musculo-skeletal symptoms (including arthralgia) during treatment. In general, these were mild to moderate and have occasionally required discontinuation of drug. Less frequently, transient pain in the chest has also been reported. These symptoms generally cleared rapidly after discontinuation of Isotretinoin but in rare cases have persisted. In less than one patient in ten—rash (including erythema, seborrhea and eczema); thinning of hair, which in rare cases has persisted.

In approximately one patient in twenty—peeling of palms and soles, skin infections, nonspecific urogenital findings, nonspecific gastrointestinal symptoms, fatigue, headache and increased susceptibility to sunburn.

Isotretinoin has been associated with a number of cases of pseudotumor cerebri, some of which involved concomitant use of tetracyclines. See *"Warnings."*

The following CNS reactions have been reported and may bear no relationship to therapy—seizures, emotional instability, dizziness, nervousness, drowsiness, malaise, weakness, insomnia, lethargy and paresthesias.

Depression has been reported in some patients on Isotretinoin therapy. In some of these patients, this has subsided with discontinuation of therapy and recurred with reinstitution of therapy.

The following reactions have been reported in less than 1% of patients and may bear no relationship to therapy—changes in skin pigment (hypo- and hyperpigmentation), flushing, urticaria, bruising, disseminated herpes simplex, edema, hair problems (other than thinning), hirsutism, respiratory infections, weight loss, erythema nodosum, paronychia, nail dystrophy, bleeding and inflammation of the gums, abnormal menses, optic neuritis, photophobia, eye lid inflammation, arthritis, anemia, palpitation, tachycardia, lymphadenopathy, sweating, tinnitus and voice alteration. A few isolated reports of vasculitis, including Wegener's granulomatosis, have been received, but no causal relationship to Isotretinoin therapy has been established.

In Isotretinoin studies to date, of 72 patients who had normal pretreatment ophthalmological examinations, five developed corneal opacities while on Isotretinoin (all five patients had a disorder of keratinization). Corneal opacities have also been reported in cystic acne patients treated with Isotretinoin. See *"Warnings."* Dry eyes and decrease in night vision have been reported and in rare instances have persisted. See *"Warnings."* Cataracts and visual disturbances have also been reported.

Isotretinoin has been temporally associated with inflammatory bowel disease. See *"Warnings."*

As may be seen with healing cystic acne lesions, an occasional exaggerated healing response, manifested by exuberant granulation tissue with crusting, has also been reported in patients receiving therapy with Isotretinoin. Pyogenic granuloma has also been diagnosed in a number of cases.

Laboratory: Isotretinoin therapy induces change in serum lipids in a significant number of treated subjects. Approximately 25% of patients had elevation of plasma triglycerides. Five out of 135 patients treated for cystic acne and 32 out of 298 total subjects treated for all diagnoses showed an elevation of triglycerides above 500 mg percent. About 16% of patients showed a mild to moderate decrease in serum high density lipoprotein (HDL) levels while receiving treatment with Isotretinoin and about 7% of patients experienced minimal elevations of serum cholesterol during treatment. Abnormalities of serum triglycerides, HDL and cholesterol were reversible upon cessation of Isotretinoin therapy.

Approximately 40% of patients receiving Isotretinoin developed elevated sedimentation rates, often from elevated baseline values.

From one in ten to one in five patients showed decreases in red blood cell parameters and white blood cell counts, elevated platelet counts, white cells in the urine, increased alkaline phosphatase, SGOT, SGPT, GGTP or LDH. See *"Warnings: Hepatotoxicity."*

Less than one in ten patients showed proteinuria, microscopic or gross hematuria, elevated fasting blood sugar, elevated CPK, hyperuricemia or thrombocytopenia.

Dose Relationship and Duration: Cheilitis and hypertriglyceridemia are usually dose-related.

Most adverse reactions were reversible when therapy was discontinued; however, some have persisted after cessation of therapy. (See *"Warnings"* and *"Adverse Reactions."*)

Overdosage: The oral LD_{50} of Isotretinoin is greater than 4000 mg/kg in rats and mice and is approximately 1960 mg/kg in rabbits. Overdose has been associated with transient headache, vomiting, facial flushing, cheilosis, abdominal pain, headache, dizziness and ataxia. All symptoms quickly resolved without apparent residual effects.

DOSAGE AND ADMINISTRATION

The recommended dosage range for Isotretinoin is 0.5 to 2 mg/kg given in two divided doses daily for 15 to 20 weeks. In studies comparing 0.1, 0.5 and 1 mg/kg/day,[7] it was found that all doses provided initial clearing of disease but there was a greater need for retreatment with the lower dose(s). It is recommended that for most patients the initial dose of Isotretinoin be 0.5 to 1 mg/kg/day. Patients whose disease is very severe or is primarily manifest on the body may require up to the maximum recommended dose, 2 mg/kg/day. During treatment, the dose may be adjusted according to response of the disease and/or the appearance of clinical side effects—some of which may be dose-related.

If the total cyst count has been reduced by more than 70 percent prior to completing 15 to 20 weeks of treatment, the drug may be discontinued. After a period of two months or more off therapy, and if warranted by persistent or recurring severe cystic acne, a second course of therapy may be initiated. Contraceptive measures must be followed for any subsequent course of therapy.

Isotretinoin should be administered with food.

ISOTRETINOIN DOSING BY BODY WEIGHT

Body Weight		Total Mg/Day		
kilograms	*pounds*	*0.5 mg/kg*	*1 mg/kg*	*2 mg/kg*
40	88	20	40	80
50	110	25	50	100
60	132	30	60	120
70	154	35	70	140
80	176	40	80	160
90	198	45	90	180
100	220	50	100	200

Store at 59° to 86°F; 15° to 30°C. Protect from light.

REFERENCES

1. Peck GL, Olsen TG, Yoder FW, Strauss JS, Downing DT, Pandya M, Butkus D, Arnaud-Battandier J: Prolonged remissions of cystic and conglobate acne with 13-*cis*-retinoic acid. *N Engl J Med* 300:329-333, 1979. 2. Farrell LN, Strauss JS, Stranieri AM: The treatment of severe cystic acne with 13-*cis*-retinoic acid. Evaluation of sebum production and the clinical response in a multiple-dose trial. *J Am Acad Dermatol* 3:602-611, 1980. 3. Jones H, Blanc D, Cunliffe WJ: 13-*cis*-retinoic acid and acne. *Lancet* 2:1048-1049, 1980. 4. Katz RA, Jorgensen H, Nigra TP: Elevation of serum triglyceride levels from oral isotretinoin in disorders of keratinization. *Arch Dermatol* 116:1369-1372, 1980. 5. Dicken CH, Connolly SM: Eruptive xanthomas associated with isotretinoin (13-*cis*-retinoic acid). *Arch Dermatol* 116:951-952, 1980. 6. Ellis CN, Madison KC, Pennes DR, Martel W, Voorhees JJ: Isotretinoin therapy is associated with early skeletal radiographic changes. *J Am Acad Dermatol* 10:1024-1029, 1984. 7. Strauss JS, Rapini RP, Shalita AR, Konecky E, Pochi PE, Comite H, Exner JH: Isotretinoin therapy for acne: Results of a multicenter dose-response study. *J Am Acad Dermatol* 10:490-496, 1984.

◆ RATED THERAPEUTICALLY EQUIVALENT; ◇ THERAPEUTIC EQUIVALENCE UNCONFIRMED; ○ UNRATED

HOW SUPPLIED
CAPSULE: 10 MG

BRAND/MANUFACTURER	NDC	SIZE	AWP
○ BRAND			
➤ ACCUTANE: Roche Labs	00004-0155-49	100s	$297.45

CAPSULE: 20 MG

BRAND/MANUFACTURER	NDC	SIZE	AWP
○ BRAND			
➤ ACCUTANE: Roche Labs	00004-0169-49	100s	$352.76

CAPSULE: 40 MG

BRAND/MANUFACTURER	NDC	SIZE	AWP
○ BRAND			
➤ ACCUTANE: Roche Labs	00004-0156-49	100s	$409.83

Isovue SEE IOPAMIDOL

Isoxsuprine Hydrochloride

DESCRIPTION
Isoxsuprine Hydrochloride tablets, USP, contain 10 mg and 20 mg of Isoxsuprine Hydrochloride.

Following is its chemical structure:

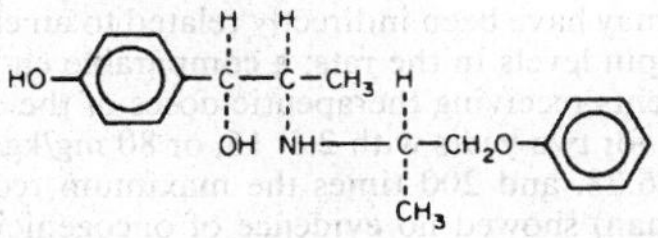

INDICATIONS

BASED ON A REVIEW OF THIS DRUG BY THE NATIONAL ACADEMY OF SCIENCES-NATIONAL RESEARCH COUNCIL AND/OR OTHER INFORMATION, THE FDA HAS CLASSIFIED THE INDICATIONS AS FOLLOWS:
POSSIBLY EFFECTIVE:
1. FOR THE RELIEF OF SYMPTOMS ASSOCIATED WITH CEREBROVASCULAR INSUFFICIENCY.
2. IN PERIPHERAL VASCULAR DISEASE OF ARTERIOSCLEROSIS OBLITERANS, THROMBOANGIITIS OBLITERANS (BUERGER'S DISEASE), AND RAYNAUD'S DISEASE.
FINAL CLASSIFICATION OF THE LESS-THAN-EFFECTIVE INDICATIONS REQUIRES FURTHER INVESTIGATION.

CONTRAINDICATIONS
Oral: There are no known contraindications to oral use when administered in recommended doses. Should not be given immediately postpartum or in the presence of arterial bleeding.

ADVERSE REACTIONS
On rare occasions oral administration of the drug has been associated, in time, with the occurrence of hypotension, tachycardia, chest pain, nausea, vomiting, dizziness, abdominal distress, and severe rash. If rash appears, the drug should be discontinued.

Although available evidence suggests a temporal association of these reactions with Isoxsuprine Hydrochloride, a causal relationship can be neither confirmed nor refuted.

β-Adrenergic receptor stimulants such as Isoxsuprine Hydrochloride have been used to inhibit preterm labor. Maternal and fetal tachycardia may occur under such use. Hypocalcemia, hypoglycemia, hypotension, and ileus have been reported to occur in infants whose mothers received Isoxsuprine Hydrochloride. Pulmonary edema has been reported in mothers treated with β-stimulants. Isoxsuprine Hydrochloride is neither approved nor recommended for use in the treatment of premature labor.

DOSAGE AND ADMINISTRATION
Oral: 10 to 20 mg three or four times daily.

HOW SUPPLIED
TABLET: 10 MG

BRAND/MANUFACTURER	NDC	SIZE	AWP
○ BRAND			
VASODILAN: Apothecon	00087-0543-01	100s	$28.82
	00087-0543-05	100s ud	$34.99
	00087-0543-02	1000s	$274.07

BRAND/MANUFACTURER	NDC	SIZE	AWP
○ GENERICS			
Amide	52152-0009-02	100s	$3.95
Eon	00185-0530-01	100s	$4.30
Geneva	00781-1840-01	100s	$4.95
Pharmacist's Choice	54979-0152-01	100s	$5.25
Goldline	00182-1055-01	100s	$5.55
Rugby	00536-3935-01	100s	$5.78
Qualitest	00603-4146-21	100s	$5.79
Major	00904-0635-60	100s	$5.80
Moore,H.L.	00839-1382-06	100s	$5.81
Aligen	00405-4575-01	100s	$5.83
Rugby	00536-3935-10	1000s	$23.94
Amide	52152-0009-05	1000s	$26.00
Major	00904-0635-80	1000s	$31.30
Pharmacist's Choice	54979-0152-10	1000s	$34.35
Eon	00185-0530-10	1000s	$34.45
Goldline	00182-1055-10	1000s	$34.95
Moore,H.L.	00839-1382-16	1000s	$39.81
Geneva	00781-1840-10	1000s	$79.60

For additional alternatives, turn to the section beginning on page 2859.

Isradipine

DESCRIPTION
Isradipine is a calcium antagonist available for oral administration in capsules containing 2.5 mg or 5 mg.

Chemically, Isradipine is 3.5-Pyridinedicarboxylic acid, 4-(4-benzofurazanyl)-1,4-dihydro-2,6-dimethyl-, methyl 1-methylethyl ester. It has a molecular weight of 371.39. Isradipine is a yellow, fine crystalline powder which is odorless or has a faint characteristic odor. Isradipine is practically insoluble in water (< 10 mg/L at 37°C), but is soluble in ethanol and freely soluble in acetone, chloroform, and methylene chloride.

Following is its chemical structure:

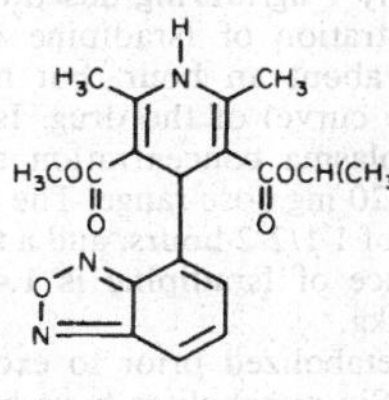

CLINICAL PHARMACOLOGY
MECHANISM OF ACTION
Isradipine is a dihydropyridine calcium channel blocker. It binds to calcium channels with high affinity and specificity and inhibits calcium flux into cardiac and smooth muscle. The effects observed in mechanistic experiments *in vitro* and studied in intact animals and man are compatible with this mechanism of action and are typical of the class.

Except for diuretic activity, the mechanism of which is not clearly understood, the pharmacodynamic effects of Isradipine observed in whole animals can also be explained by calcium channel blocking activity, especially dilating effects in arterioles which reduce systemic resistance and lower blood pressure, with a small increase in resting heart rate. Although like other dihydropyridine calcium channel blockers, Isradipine has negative inotropic effects *in vitro*, studies conducted in intact anesthetized animals have shown that the vasodilating effect occurs at doses lower than those which affect contractility. In patients with normal ventricular function, Isradipine's afterload reducing properties lead to some increase in cardiac output.

Effects in patients with impaired ventricular function have not been fully studied.

CLINICAL EFFECTS
Dose-related reductions in supine and standing blood pressure are achieved within 2-3 hours following single oral doses of 2.5 mg, 5 mg, 10 mg, and 20 mg Isradipine, with a duration of action (at least 50% of peak response) of more than 12 hours following administration of the highest dose.

Isradipine has been shown in controlled, double-blind clinical trials to be an effective antihypertensive agent when used as monotherapy, or when added to therapy with thiazide-type diuretics. During chronic administration, divided doses (b.i.d.) in the range of 5 mg-20 mg daily have been shown to be effective, with response at trough (prior to next dose) over 50% of the peak blood pressure effect. The response is dose-related between 5-10 mg daily. Isradipine is equally effective in reducing supine, sitting, and standing blood pressure.

On chronic administration, increases in resting pulse rate averaged about 3-5 beats/min. These increases were not dose-related.

HEMODYNAMICS
In man, peripheral vasodilation produced by Isradipine is reflected by decreased systemic vascular resistance and increased cardiac output. Hemodynamic studies conducted in patients with normal left ventricular function produced, following intravenous Isradipine administration, increases in cardiac index, stroke volume index, coronary sinus blood flow, heart rate, and peak positive left ventricular dP/dt. Systemic, coronary, and pulmonary vascular resistance were decreased. These

studies were conducted with doses of Isradipine which produced clinically significant decreases in blood pressure. The clinical consequences of these hemodynamic effects, if any, have not been evaluated.

Effects on heart rate are variable, dependent upon rate of administration and presence of underlying cardiac condition. While increases in both peak positive dP/dt and LV ejection fraction are seen when intravenous Isradipine is given, it is impossible to conclude that these represent a positive inotropic effect due to simultaneous changes in preload and afterload. In patients with coronary artery disease undergoing atrial pacing during cardiac catheterization, intravenous Isradipine diminished abnormalities of systolic performance. In patients with moderate left ventricular dysfunction, oral and intravenous Isradipine in doses which reduce blood pressure by 12-30%, resulted in improvement in cardiac index without increase in heart rate, and with no change or reduction in pulmonary capillary wedge pressure. Combination of Isradipine and propranolol did not significantly affect left ventricular dP/dt max. The clinical consequences of these effects have not been evaluated.

ELECTROPHYSIOLOGIC EFFECTS
In general, no detrimental effects on the cardiac conduction system were seen with the use of Isradipine. Electrophysiologic studies were conducted on patients with normal sinus and atrioventricular node function. Intravenous Isradipine in doses which reduce systolic blood pressure did not affect PR, QRS, AH* or HV* intervals.

No changes were seen in Wenckebach cycle length, atrial, and ventricular refractory periods. Slight prolongation of QTc interval of 3% was seen in one study. Effects on sinus node recovery time (CSNRT) were mild or not seen.

In patients with sick sinus syndrome, at doses which significantly reduced blood pressure, intravenous Isradipine resulted in no depressant effect on sinus and atrioventricular node function.

PHARMACOKINETICS AND METABOLISM
Isradipine is 90-95% absorbed and is subject to extensive first-pass metabolism, resulting in a bioavailability of about 15-24%. Isradipine is detectable in plasma within 20 minutes after administration of single oral doses of 2.5-20 mg, and peak concentrations of approximately 1 ng/mL/mg dosed occur about 1.5 hours after drug administration. Administration of Isradipine with food significantly increases the time to peak by about an hour, but has no effect on the total bioavailability (area under the curve) of the drug. Isradipine is 95% bound to plasma proteins. Both peak plasma concentration and AUC exhibit a linear relationship to dose over the 0-20 mg dose range. The elimination of Isradipine is biphasic with an early half-life of 1 1/2-2 hours, and a terminal half-life of about 8 hours. The total body clearance of Isradipine is 1.4 L/min and the apparent volume of distribution is 3 L/kg.

Isradipine is completely metabolized prior to excretion, and no unchanged drug is detected in the urine. Six metabolites have been characterized in blood and urine, with the mono acids of the pyridine derivative and a cyclic lactone product accounting for > 75% of the material identified. Approximately 60-65% of an administered dose is excreted in the urine and 25-30% in the feces. Mild renal impairment (creatinine clearance 30-80 mL/min) increases the bioavailability (AUC) of Isradipine by 45%. Progressive deterioration reverses this trend, and patients with severe renal failure (creatinine clearance < 10 mL/min) who have been on hemodialysis show a 20-50% lower AUC than healthy volunteers. No pharmacokinetic information is available on drug therapy during hemodialysis. In elderly patients, C_{max} and AUC are increased by 13% and 40%, respectively; in patients with hepatic impairment, C_{max} and AUC are increased by 32% and 52%, respectively (see *"Dosage and Administration"*).

INDICATIONS AND USAGE
HYPERTENSION
Isradipine is indicated in the management of hypertension. It may be used alone or concurrently with thiazide-type diuretics.

UNLABELED USES
Isradipine is used alone or as an adjunct in the treatment of angina pectoris and in the management of preterm labor.

CONTRAINDICATIONS
Isradipine is contraindicated in individuals who have shown hypersensitivity to any of the ingredients in the formulation.

WARNINGS
None.

PRECAUTIONS
GENERAL
Blood Pressure: Because Isradipine decreases peripheral resistance, like other calcium blockers Isradipine may occasionally produce symptomatic hypotension. However, symptoms like syncope and severe dizziness have rarely been reported in hypertensive patients administered Isradipine, particularly at the initial recommended doses (see *"Dosage and Administration"*).

Use in Patients with Congestive Heart Failure: Although acute hemodynamic studies in patients with congestive heart failure have shown that Isradipine reduced afterload without impairing myocardial contractility, it has a negative

inotropic effect at high doses *in vitro*, and possibly in some patients. Caution should be exercised when using the drug in congestive heart failure patients, particularly in combination with a beta-blocker.

DRUG INTERACTIONS
Nitroglycerin: Isradipine has been safely coadministered with nitroglycerin.

Hydrochlorothiazide: A study in normal healthy volunteers has shown that concomitant administration of Isradipine and hydrochlorothiazide does not result in altered pharmacokinetics of either drug. In a study in hypertensive patients, addition of Isradipine to existing hydrochlorothiazide therapy did not result in any unexpected adverse effects, and Isradipine had an additional antihypertensive effect.

Propranolol: In a single dose study in normal volunteers, coadministration of propranolol had a small effect on the rate but no effect on the extent of Isradipine bioavailability. Coadministration of Isradipine resulted in significant increases in AUC (27%) and C_{max} (58%) and decreases in t_{max} (23%) of propranolol.

Digoxin: The concomitant administration of Isradipine and digoxin in a single-dose pharmacokinetic study did not affect renal, non-renal, and total body clearance of digoxin.

Fentanyl Anesthesia: Severe hypotension has been reported during fentanyl anesthesia with concomitant use of a beta blocker and a calcium channel blocker. Even though such interactions have not been seen in clinical studies with Isradipine, an increased volume of circulating fluids might be required if such an interaction were to occur.

CARCINOGENESIS, MUTAGENESIS, IMPAIRMENT OF FERTILITY
Treatment of male rats for 2 years with 2.5, 12.5, or 62.5 mg/kg/day Isradipine admixed with the diet (approximately 6, 31, and 156 times the maximum recommended daily dose based on a 50 kg man) resulted in dose dependent increases in the incidence of benign Leydig cell tumors and testicular hyperplasia relative to untreated control animals. These findings, which were replicated in a subsequent experiment, may have been indirectly related to an effect of Isradipine on circulating gonadotropin levels in the rats; a comparable endocrine effect was not evident in male patients receiving therapeutic doses of the drug on a chronic basis. Treatment of mice for two years with 2.5, 15, or 80 mg/kg/day Isradipine in the diet (approximately 6.38, and 200 times the maximum recommended daily dose based on a 50 kg man) showed no evidence of oncogenicity. There was no evidence of mutagenic potential based on the results of a battery of mutagenicity tests. No effect on fertility was observed in male and female rats treated with up to 60 mg/kg/day Isradipine.

PREGNANCY
Pregnancy Category C: Isradipine was administered orally to rats and rabbits during organogenesis. Treatment of pregnant rats with doses of 6, 20, or 60 mg/kg/day produced a significant reduction in maternal weight gain during treatment with the highest dose (150 times the maximum recommended human daily dose) but with no lasting effect on the mother or the offspring. Treatment of pregnant rabbits with doses of 1, 3, or 10 mg/kg/day (2.5, 7.5, and 25 times the maximum recommended human daily dose) produced decrements in maternal body weight gain and increased fetal resorptions at the two higher doses. There was no evidence of embryotoxicity at doses which were not maternotoxic and no evidence of teratogenicity at any dose tested. In a peri/postnatal administration study in rats, reduced maternal body weight gain during late pregnancy at oral doses of 20 and 60 mg/kg/day Isradipine was associated with reduced birth weights and decreased peri and postnatal pup survival.

NURSING MOTHERS
It is not known whether Isradipine is excreted in human milk. Because many drugs are excreted in human milk, and because of the potential for adverse effects of Isradipine on nursing infants, a decision should be made as to whether to discontinue nursing or discontinue the drug, taking into account the importance of the drug to the mother.

PEDIATRIC USE
Safety and effectiveness have not been established in children.

ADVERSE REACTIONS
In multiple dose U.S. studies in hypertension, 1228 patients received Isradipine alone or in combination with other agents, principally a thiazide diuretic, 934 of them in controlled comparisons with placebo or active agents. An additional 652 patients (which includes 374 normal volunteers) received Isradipine in U.S. studies of conditions other than hypertension, and 1321 patients received Isradipine in non-U.S. studies. About 500 patients received Isradipine in long-term hypertension studies, 410 of them for at least 6 months. The adverse reaction rates given below are principally based on controlled hypertension studies, but rarer serious events are derived from all exposures to Isradipine including foreign marketing experience.

Most adverse reactions were mild and related to the vasodilatory effects of Isradipine (dizziness, edema, palpitations, flushing, tachycardia), and many were transient. About 5% of Isradipine patients left studies prematurely because of adverse reactions (vs. 3% of placebo patients and 6% of active control patients), principally due to headache, edema, dizziness, palpitations, and gastrointestinal disturbances.

The table below shows the most common adverse reactions, volunteered or elicited, considered by the investigator to be at least possibly drug related. The results for the Isradipine treated patients are presented for all doses pooled

---

* AH = conduction time from low right atrium to His bundle deflection, or AV nodal conduction time; HV = conduction time through the His bundle and the bundle branch-Purkinje system.

together (reported by 1% or greater of patients receiving any dose of Isradipine), and also for the two treatment regimens most applicable to the treatment of hypertension with Isradipine: (1) initial and maintenance dose of 2.5 mg b.i.d., and (2) initial dose of 2.5 mg b.i.d. followed by maintenance dose of 5.0 mg b.i.d. (See related table).

Except for headache, which is not clearly drug-related (see table above), the more frequent adverse reactions listed above show little change, or increase slightly, in frequency over time, as shown in the following table: (See related table).

Edema, palpitations, fatigue, and flushing appear to be dose-related, especially at the higher doses of 15-20 mg/day.

In open-label, long-term studies of up to two years in duration, the adverse events reported were generally the same as those reported in the short-term controlled trials. The overall frequencies of these adverse events were slightly higher in the long-term than in the controlled studies, but as in the controlled trials most adverse reactions were mild and transient.

The following adverse events were reported in 0.5-1.0% of the Isradipine-treated patients in hypertension studies, or are rare. More serious events from this and other data sources, including postmarketing exposure, are shown in italics. The relationship of these adverse events to Isradipine administration is uncertain.

SKIN
Pruritus, *urticaria*

MUSCULOSKELETAL
Cramps of legs/feet

RESPIRATORY
Cough

CARDIOVASCULAR
Shortness of breath, hypotension, *atrial fibrillation, ventricular fibrillation, myocardial infarction, heart failure.*

GASTROINTESTINAL
Abdominal discomfort, constipation, diarrhea.

UROGENITAL
Nocturia

NERVOUS SYSTEM
Drowsiness, insomnia, lethargy, nervousness, impotence, decreased libido, depression, *syncope, paresthesia* (which includes numbness and tingling), *transient ischemic attack, stroke.*

AUTONOMIC
Hyperhidrosis, visual disturbance, dry mouth, numbness.

MISCELLANEOUS
Throat discomfort, *leukopenia, elevated liver function tests.*

OVERDOSAGE
Although there is no well documented experience with Isradipine overdosage, available data suggest that, as with other dihydropyridines, gross overdosage would result in excessive peripheral vasodilation with subsequent marked and probably prolonged systemic hypotension. Clinically significant hypotension overdosage calls for active cardiovascular support including monitoring of cardiac and respiratory function, elevation of lower extremities, and attention to circulating fluid volume and urine output. A vasoconstrictor (such as epinephrine, norepinephrine, or levarterenol) may be helpful in restoring vascular tone and blood pressure, provided that there is no contraindication to its use. Since Isradipine is highly protein-bound, dialysis is not likely to be of benefit.

Significant lethality was observed in mice given oral doses of over 200 mg/kg and rabbits given about 50 mg/kg of Isradipine. Rats tolerated doses of over 2000 mg/kg without effects on survival.

	Isradipine					
N = Adverse Experience	All Doses 934 %	2.5 mg b.i.d. 199 %	5 mg b.i.d.† 150 %	10 mg b.i.d.†† 59 %	Placebo 297 %	Active Controls* 414 %
Headache	13.7	12.6	10.7	22.0	14.1	9.4
Dizziness	7.3	8.0	5.3	3.4	4.4	8.2
Edema	7.2	3.5	8.7	8.5	3.0	2.9
Palpitations	4.0	1.0	4.7	5.1	1.4	1.5
Fatigue	3.9	2.5	2.0	8.5	0.3	6.3
Flushing	2.6	3.0	2.0	5.1	0.0	1.2
Chest Pain	2.4	2.5	2.7	1.7	2.4	2.9
Nausea	1.8	1.0	2.7	5.1	1.7	3.1
Dyspnea	1.8	0.5	2.7	3.4	1.0	2.2
Abdominal Discomfort	1.7	0.0	3.3	1.7	1.7	3.9
Tachycardia	1.5	1.0	1.3	3.4	0.3	0.5
Rash	1.5	1.5	2.0	1.7	0.3	0.7
Pollakiuria	1.5	2.0	1.3	3.4	0.0	< 1.0
Weakness	1.2	0.0	0.7	0.0	0.0	1.2
Vomiting	1.1	1.0	1.3	0.0	0.3	0.2
Diarrhea	1.1	0.0	2.7	3.4	2.0	1.9

† Initial dose of 2.5 mg b.i.d. followed by maintenance dose of 5.0 mg b.i.d.
†† Initial dose of 2.5 mg b.i.d. followed by sequential titration to 5.0 mg b.i.d., 7.5 mg b.i.d., and maintenance dose of 10.0 mg b.i.d.
* Propranolol, prazosin, hydrochlorothiazide, enalapril, captopril.

INCIDENCE RATES FOR ISRADIPINE (ALL DOSES) BY WEEK (%)

Week N=	1 694	2 906	3 649	4 847	5 432	6 494
Adverse Reaction						
Headache	6.5	6.1	5.2	5.2	5.8	4.5
Dizziness	1.6	1.9	1.7	2.2	2.3	2.0
Edema	1.2	2.5	3.2	3.2	5.3	5.5
Palpitations	1.2	1.3	1.4	1.9	2.1	1.4
Fatigue	0.4	1.0	1.4	1.2	1.2	1.6
Flushing	1.2	1.3	2.0	1.4	2.1	1.4

Week N=	7 153	8 377	9 261	10 362	11 107	12 105
Adverse Reaction						
Headache	2.0	2.7	1.9	2.8	2.8	3.8
Dizziness	2.0	1.9	2.3	3.9	4.7	3.8
Edema	5.9	5.0	4.6	4.7	3.8	3.8
Palpitations	1.3	0.8	0.8	1.7	1.9	2.9
Fatigue	2.0	2.7	1.5	1.4	0.9	1.9
Flushing	3.3	1.3	1.1	0.8	0.0	0.0

DOSAGE AND ADMINISTRATION

The dosage of Isradipine should be individualized. The recommended initial dose of Isradipine is 2.5 mg b.i.d. alone or in combination with a thiazide diuretic. An antihypertensive response usually occurs within 2-3 hours. Maximal response may require 2-4 weeks. If a satisfactory reduction in blood pressure does not occur after this period, the dose may be adjusted in increments of 5 mg/day at 2-4 week intervals up to a maximum of 20 mg/day. Most patients, however, show no additional response to doses above 10 mg/day, and adverse effects are increased in frequency above 10 mg/day.

The bioavailability of Isradipine (increased AUC) is increased in elderly patients (above 65 years of age), patients with hepatic functional impairment, and patients with mild renal impairment. Ordinarily, the starting dose should still be 2.5 mg b.i.d. in these patients.

Store and Dispense: Below 86°F (30°C) in a tight container. Protect from light.

HOW SUPPLIED
CAPSULE: 2.5 MG

BRAND/MANUFACTURER	NDC	SIZE	AWP
○ BRAND			
▶ DYNACIRC: Sandoz Pharm	00078-0226-44	60s	$31.20
	00078-0226-05	100s	$50.88
▶ DYNACIRC: Sandocare	00078-0226-65	640s ud	$346.92

CAPSULE: 5 MG

BRAND/MANUFACTURER	NDC	SIZE	AWP
○ BRAND			
▶ DYNACIRC: Sandoz Pharm	00078-0227-44	60s	$45.48
	00078-0227-05	100s	$74.58
▶ DYNACIRC: Sandocare	00078-0227-65	640s ud	$498.66

Isuprel *SEE* ISOPROTERENOL

Itraconazole

> ## WARNING
> COADMINISTRATION OF TERFENADINE WITH ITRACONAZOLE IS CONTRAINDICATED. RARE CASES OF SERIOUS CARDIOVASCULAR ADVERSE EVENTS, INCLUDING DEATH, VENTRICULAR TACHYCARDIA AND TORSADES DE POINTES HAVE BEEN OBSERVED IN PATIENTS TAKING ITRACONAZOLE CONCOMITANTLY WITH TERFENADINE, DUE TO INCREASED TERFENADINE CONCENTRATIONS INDUCED BY ITRACONAZOLE. SEE ''CONTRAINDICATIONS,'' ''WARNINGS'' AND ''PRECAUTIONS'' SECTIONS.
>
> PHARMACOKINETIC DATA INDICATE THAT ANOTHER ORAL ANTIFUNGAL, KETOCONAZOLE, INHIBITS THE METABOLISM OF ASTEMIZOLE, RESULTING IN ELEVATED PLASMA LEVELS OF ASTEMIZOLE AND ITS ACTIVE METABOLITE DESMETHYLASTEMIZOLE WHICH MAY PROLONG QT INTERVALS. *IN VITRO* DATA SUGGEST THAT ITRACONAZOLE, WHEN COMPARED TO KETOCONAZOLE, HAS A LESS PRONOUNCED EFFECT ON THE BIOTRANSFORMATION SYSTEM RESPONSIBLE FOR THE METABOLISM OF ASTEMIZOLE. BASED ON THE CHEMICAL RESEMBLANCE OF ITRACONAZOLE AND KETOCONAZOLE, COADMINISTRATION OF ASTEMIZOLE WITH ITRACONAZOLE IS CONTRAINDICATED. SEE ''CONTRAINDICATIONS,'' ''WARNINGS'' AND ''PRECAUTIONS'' SECTIONS.

DESCRIPTION

Itraconazole is a synthetic triazole antifungal agent. Itraconazole is a 1:1:1:1 racemic mixture of four diastereomers (two enantiomeric pairs), each possessing three chiral centers.

(±)-1-[(R*)-sec-Butyl]-4-[p-[4-[p-[[2R*,4S*]-2-(2,4-dichlorophenyl)-2-(1H-1,2,4-triazol-1-ylmethyl)-1,3-dioxolan-4-yl] methoxy]phenyl]-1-piperazinyl]phenyl]-Δ²-1,2,4-triazolin-5-one mixture with (±)-1-[(R*)-sec-butyl]-4-[p-[4-[p-[[2S*4R*]-2-(2,4-dichlorophenyl)-2-(1H-1,2,4-triazol-1-ylmethyl)-1,3-dioxolan-4-yl]methoxyl]phenyl]-1-piperazinyl]phenyl]-Δ²-1,2,4-triazolin-5-one or (±)-1-[(RS)-sec-Butyl]-4-[p-[4-[p-[[(2R,4S)-2-(2,4-dichlorophenyl)-2-(1H-1,2,4-triazol-1-ylmethyl)-1,3-dioxolan-4-yl] methoxy]phenyl]-1-piperazinyl]phenyl]-Δ²-1,2,4-triazolin-5-one

Itraconazole has a molecular formula of $C_{35}H_{28}Cl_2N_8O_4$ and a molecular weight of 705.64. It is a white to slightly yellowish powder. It is insoluble in water at pH 1-12, very slightly soluble in alcohols, and freely soluble in dichloromethane. It has a pKa of 3.70 (based on extrapolation of values obtained from methanolic solutions) and a log (n-octanol/water partition coefficient) of 5.66 at pH 8.1.

Following is its chemical structure:

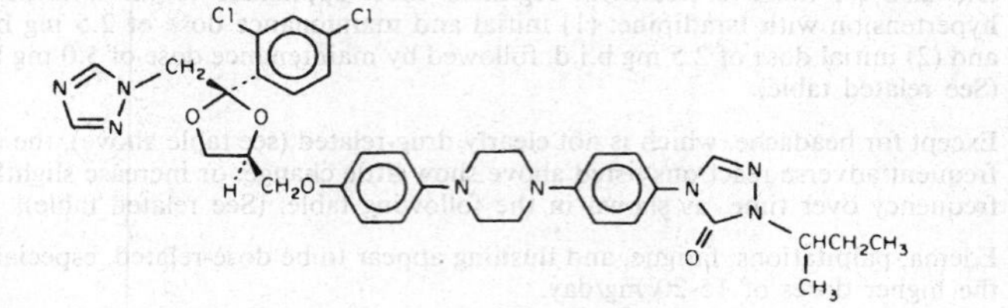

CLINICAL PHARMACOLOGY

Mode of Action: In vitro studies have demonstrated that Itraconazole inhibits the cytochrome P-450-dependent synthesis of ergosterol, which is a vital component of fungal cell membranes.

Pharmacokinetics and Metabolism: Note: The plasma concentrations reported below were measured by high performance liquid chromatography (HPLC) specific for Itraconazole. When Itraconazole in plasma is measured by a bioassay, values reported are approximately 3.3 times higher than those obtained by HPLC due to the presence of the bioactive metabolite, hydroxyitraconazole. (See "Microbiology" section.)

The pharmacokinetics of Itraconazole after intravenous administration and its absolute oral bioavailability from an oral solution were studied in a randomized cross-over study using six healthy male volunteers. The total plasma clearance averaged 381 ± 95 mL/min and the apparent volume of distribution averaged 796 ± 185 L. The observed absolute oral bioavailability of Itraconazole was 55%.

The oral bioavailability of Itraconazole Capsules is maximal when taken with food. The pharmacokinetics of Itraconazole were studied using six healthy male volunteers who received, in a cross-over design, single 100 mg doses of Itraconazole as a polyethylene glycol capsule, with or without food. The same six volunteers also received 50 mg or 200 mg with food in a cross-over design. In this study, only Itraconazole plasma concentrations were measured. Presented in the table below are the respective pharmacokinetic parameters for Itraconazole:

	50 mg (fed)	100 mg (fed)	100 mg (fasted)	200 mg (fed)
C_{max} (ng/mL)	45 ± 16	132 ± 67	38 ± 20	289 ± 100
T_{max} (hours)	3.2 ± 1.3	4.0 ± 1.1	3.3 ± 1.0	4.7 ± 1.4
$AUC_{0-\infty}$ (ng.h/mL)	567 ± 264	1899 ± 838	722 ± 289	5211 ± 2116

Values are means ± standard deviation

Doubling the Itraconazole dose results in approximately a three-fold increase in the Itraconazole plasma concentrations.

Values given in the table below represent data from a cross-over pharmacokinetics study in which 27 healthy male volunteers each took a single 200 mg dose of Itraconazole with or without food:

	Itraconazole		Hydroxyitraconazole	
	Fed	Fasted	Fed	Fasted
C_{max} (ng/mL)	239 ± 85	140 ± 65	397 ± 103	286 ± 101
T_{max} (hours)	4.5 ± 1.1	3.9 ± 1.0	5.1 ± 1.6	4.5 ± 1.1
$AUC_{0-\infty}$ (ng.h/mL)	3423 ± 1154	2094 ± 905	7978 ± 2648	5191 ± 2489
$t_{1/2}$ (hours)	21 ± 5	21 ± 7	12 ± 3	12 ± 3

Values are means ± standard deviation

Steady-state concentrations were reached within 15 days following oral doses of 50-400 mg daily. Values given in the table below are data at steady-state from a pharmacokinetics study in which 27 healthy male volunteers took 200 mg Itraconazole b.i.d. (with food) for 15 days:

	Itraconazole	Hydroxyitraconazole
C^{max} (ng/mL)	2282 ± 514	3488 ± 742
C^{min} (ng/mL)	1855 ± 535	3349 ± 761
T^{max} (hours)	4.6 ± 1.8	3.4 ± 3.4
AUC^{0-12h} (ng.h/mL)	22569 ± 5375	38572 ± 8450
$t^{1/2}$ (hours)	64 ± 32	56 ± 24

Values are means ± standard deviation

◆ RATED THERAPEUTICALLY EQUIVALENT; ◇ THERAPEUTIC EQUIVALENCE UNCONFIRMED; ○ UNRATED

Results of the pharmacokinetics study suggest that Itraconazole may undergo saturation metabolism with multiple dosing.

Itraconazole is extensively metabolized by the liver into a large number of metabolites including hydroxyitraconazole, the major metabolite. Fecal excretion of the parent drug varies between 3-18% of the dose. Renal excretion of the parent drug is less than 0.03% of the dose. About 40% of the dose is excreted as inactive metabolites in the urine. No excreted single metabolite represents more than 5% of a dose. The main metabolic pathways are oxidative scission of the dioxolane ring, aliphatic oxidation at the 1-methylpropyl substituent. *N*-dealkylation of this 1-methylpropyl substituent, oxidative degradation of the piperazine ring and triazolone scission.

Plasma concentrations of Itraconazole in subjects with renal insufficiency were comparable to those obtained in healthy subjects. The effect of hepatic impairment on the plasma concentration of Itraconazole is unknown. It is recommended that plasma concentrations of Itraconazole in patients with hepatic impairment be carefully monitored.

The plasma protein binding of Itraconazole is 99.8% and that of hydroxyitraconazole is 99.5%. Itraconazole is not removed by hemodialysis.

In animal studies, Itraconazole is extensively distributed into lipophilic tissues. Concentrations of Itraconazole in fatty tissues, omentum, liver, kidney and skin tissues are 2-20 times the corresponding plasma concentrations. Aqueous fluids such as cerebrospinal fluid and saliva contain negligible amounts of the drug.

Microbiology: Itraconazole exhibits *in vitro* activity against *Blastomyces dermatitidis, Histoplasma capsulatum, Histoplasma duboisii, Aspergillus flavus, Aspergillus fumigatus* and *Cryptococcus neoformans.* Itraconazole also exhibits varying *in vitro* activity against *Sporothrix schenckii*, Trichophyton spp., *Candida albicans* and Candida spp. In addition, the bioactive metabolite, hydroxyItraconazole, was evaluated *in vitro.* Although the activity has not been evaluated against *Histoplasma capsulatum* and *Blastomyces dermatitidis*, the *in vitro* antifungal activity of hydroxyitraconazole against eleven other fungal species was shown to be comparable to that of Itraconazole. Correlation between *in vitro* minimum inhibitory concentration (MIC) results and clinical outcome has yet to be established for azole antifungal agents.

Itraconazole administered orally was active in a variety of animal models of fungal infection using standard laboratory strains of fungi. Fungistatic activity has been demonstrated against disseminated fungal infections caused by *Blastomyces dermatitidis, Histoplasma duboisii, Aspergillus fumigatus, Coccidioides immitis, Cryptococcus neoformans, Paracoccidioides brasiliensis, Sporothrix schenckii* and *Trichophyton mentagrophytes.* In immunocompromised mice infected with *Aspergillus fumigatus* via the intravenous route, Itraconazole was effective in reducing the organism load in tissue. However, when infected with *Aspergillus fumigatus* via the intranasal route, animals were non-responsive to Itraconazole treatment. Itraconazole has demonstrated antifungal activity in a variety of animal models infected with *Candida albicans* and other Candida species.

INDICATIONS AND USAGE

Itraconazole is indicated for the treatment of the following fungal infections in immunocompromised and non-immunocompromised patients. (For HIV-infected subjects, see *"Histoplasmosis in HIV-infected Patients"* under *"Precautions."*)

1. Blastomycosis, pulmonary and extrapulmonary.
2. Histoplasmosis, including chronic cavitary pulmonary disease and disseminated, non-meningeal histoplasmosis.

Specimens for fungal cultures and other relevant laboratory studies (wet mount, histopathology, serology) should be obtained prior to therapy to isolate and identify causative organisms. Therapy may be instituted before the results of the cultures and other laboratory studies are known; however, once these results become available, anti-infective therapy should be adjusted accordingly.

UNLABELED USES

Itraconazole is used alone or as an adjunct in the treatment of oral candidiasis, including chronic mucocutaneous candidiasis and in the treatment of vaginal candidiasis, onychomycosis, and coccidioidomycosis. This drug is also used in the treatment of systemic mycoses, including chromoblastomycosis, cryptococcosis, sporotrichosis, aspergillosis, cryptococcal meningitis, histoplasmosis, systemic candidiasis, paracoccidioidomycosis, phaeohyphomycosis, and blastomycosis.

CONTRAINDICATIONS

Coadministration of terfenadine or astemizole with Itraconazole is contraindicated. (See *"Box Warning," "Warnings,"* and *"Precautions"* sections.)

Itraconazole is contraindicated in patients who have shown hypersensitivity to the drug or its excipients. There is no information regarding cross hypersensitivity between Itraconazole and other azole antifungal agents. Caution should be used in prescribing Itraconazole to patients with hypersensitivity to other azoles.

WARNINGS

In U.S. clinical trials prior to marketing, there have been three cases of reversible idiosyncratic hepatitis reported among more than 2500 patients taking Itraconazole. One patient outside the U.S. developed fulminant hepatitis and died during Itraconazole administration. Since this patient was on multiple medications, the causal association with Itraconazole is uncertain. If clinical signs and symptoms consistent with liver disease develop that may be attributable to Itraconazole, should be discontinued.

Prior to U.S. marketing, there have been three cases of life-threatening cardiac dysrhythmias and one death reported in patients receiving terfenadine and Itraconazole. (See *"Box Warning," "Contraindications,"* and *"Precautions"* sections.)

Coadministration of astemizole with Itraconazole is contraindicated. (See *"Box Warning," "Contraindications,"* and *"Precautions"* sections.)

PRECAUTIONS

General: Hepatic enzyme test values should be monitored in patients with preexisting hepatic function abnormalities.

Information for Patients: Patients should be instructed to take Itraconazole with food.

Patients should be instructed to report any signs and symptoms that may suggest liver dysfunction so that the appropriate laboratory testing can be done. Such signs and symptoms may include unusual fatigue, anorexia, nausea and/or vomiting, jaundice, dark urine or pale stool.

Drug Interactions: Coadministration of terfenadine with Itraconazole has led to elevated plasma concentrations of terfenadine, resulting in rare instances of life-threatening cardiac dysrhythmias and one death. (See *"Box Warning," "Contraindications,"* and *"Warnings"* sections.)

Pharmacokinetic data indicate that another oral antifungal, ketoconazole, inhibits the metabolism of astemizole, resulting in elevated plasma levels of astemizole and its active metabolite desmethylastemizole which may prolong QT intervals. *In vitro* data suggest that Itraconazole, when compared to ketoconazole, has a less pronounced effect on the biotransformation system responsible for the metabolism of astemizole. Based on the chemical resemblance of Itraconazole and ketoconazole, coadministration of astemizole with Itraconazole is contraindicated. (See *"Box Warning," "Contraindications,"* and *"Warnings"* sections.)

Coadministration of Itraconazole and cyclosporine or digoxin has led to increased plasma concentrations of the latter two drugs. When digoxin is given concurrently with Itraconazole the physician is advised to monitor digoxin concentrations and reduce the dosage as needed. Although no studies have been conducted, literature case reports suggest that the dose of cyclosporine should be reduced by 50% when Itraconazole doses greater than 100 mg daily are given. Cyclosporine concentrations should be monitored frequently and the dose adjusted appropriately.

When Itraconazole was coadministered with phenytoin, rifampin, or H$_2$ antagonists, reduced plasma concentrations of Itraconazole were reported. The physician is advised to monitor the plasma concentrations of Itraconazole when any of these drugs is taken concurrently, and to increase the dose of Itraconazole if necessary. Although no studies have been conducted, concomitant administration of Itraconazole and phenytoin may alter the metabolism of phenytoin; therefore, plasma concentrations of phenytoin should also be monitored with it is given concurrently with Itraconazole. It has been reported that Itraconazole enhances the anticoagulant effect of coumarin-like drugs. Therefore, prothrombin time should be carefully monitored in patients receiving Itraconazole and coumarin-like drugs simultaneously.

Plasma concentrations of azole antifungal agents are reduced when given concurrently with isoniazid. Itraconazole plasma concentrations should be monitored when Itraconazole and isoniazid are coadministered.

Severe hypoglycemia has been reported in patients concomitantly receiving azole antifungal agents and oral hypoglycemic agents. Blood glucose concentrations should be carefully monitored when Itraconazole and oral hypoglycemic agents are coadministered.

Carcinogenesis, Mutagenesis and Impairment of Fertility: Itraconazole showed no evidence of carcinogenicity potential in mice treated orally for 23 months at dosage levels up to 80 mg/kg/day [approximately 10 × the maximum recommended human dose (MRHD)]. Male rats treated with 25 mg/kg/day (3.1 × MRHD) had a slightly increased incidence of soft tissue sarcoma. These sarcomas may have been a consequence of hypercholesterolemia, which is a response of rats, but not dogs or humans, to chronic Itraconazole administration. Female rats treated with 50 mg/kg/day (6.25 × MRHD) had an increased incidence of squamous cell carcinoma of the lung (2/50) as compared to the untreated group. Although the occurrence of squamous cell carcinoma in the lung is extremely uncommon in untreated rats, the increase in this study was not statistically significant.

Itraconazole produced no mutagenic effects when assayed in appropriate bacterial, non-mammalian and mammalian test systems.

Itraconazole did not affect the fertility of male or female rats treated orally with dosage levels of up to 40 mg/kg/day (5 × MRHD) even though parental toxicity was present at this dosage level. More severe signs of parental toxicity, including death, were present in the next higher dosage level, 160 mg/kg/day (20 × MRHD).

Pregnancy: Teratogenic Effects. Pregnancy Category C: Itraconazole was found to cause a dose-related increase in maternal toxicity, embryotoxicity and teratogenicity in rats at dosage levels of approximately 40-160 mg/kg/day (5-20 × MRHD) and in mice at dosage levels of approximately 80 mg/kg/day (10 × MRHD). In rats, the teratogenicity consisted of major skeletal defects; in mice it consisted of encephaloceles and/or macroglossia.

There are no studies in pregnant women. Itraconazole should be used in pregnancy only if the benefit outweighs the potential risk.

Nursing Mothers: Itraconazole is excreted in human milk; therefore, Itraconazole should not be administered to a nursing woman.

Pediatric Use: The efficacy and safety of Itraconazole have not been established in children. No pharmacokinetic data are available in children. A small number of patients from age 3 to 16 years have been treated with 100 mg/day of Itraconazole for systemic fungal infections and no serious adverse effects have been reported.

Toxicological studies have shown that Itraconazole, when administered to rats, can produce bone toxicity. While no such toxicity has been reported in adult patients, the long term effect of Itraconazole in children is unknown. (See "Animal Toxicology" section.)

Histoplasmosis in HIV-infected Patients: Data from a small number of HIV-infected patients suggested that the response rate of histoplasmosis in HIV-infected patients is similar to non-HIV-infected patients. The clinical course of histoplasmosis in HIV-infected patients is more severe and usually requires maintenance therapy to prevent relapse. The optimal dosage regimen for treatment and maintenance therapy are unknown. Studies to investigate the efficacy and safety of Itraconazole including optimal dosage and duration in HIV-infected patients, are ongoing.

Because hypochlorhydria has been reported in HIV-infected individuals, the absorption of Itraconazole in these patients may be decreased.

The results from a study in which eight HIV-infected individuals were treated with zidovudine, 8 ± 0.4 mg/kg/day, with or without Itraconazole 100 mg b.i.d., showed that the pharmacokinetics of zidovudine were not affected during concomitant administration of Itraconazole.

ADVERSE REACTIONS

In U.S. clinical trials prior to marketing, there have been three cases of reversible idiosyncratic hepatitis reported among more than 2500 patients. One patient outside the U.S. developed fulminant hepatitis and died during Itraconazole administration. Because this patient was on multiple medications, the causal association with Itraconazole is uncertain. (See *"Warnings."*)

U.S. adverse experience data are derived from 602 patients with systemic fungal disease, who were immunocompromised or receiving multiple concomitant medications. Of these patients, treatment was discontinued in 10.5% of patients due to adverse events. The median duration before discontinuation of therapy was 81 days, with a range of 2-776 days. The worldwide experience data are derived from 5751 patients treated for at least seven days in clinical trials primarily of nonsystemic fungal infections. Of these patients, treatment was discontinued in 3% of patients due to adverse events. The table below lists adverse events reported by at least 1% of patients treated with Itraconazole in U.S. clinical trials. The worldwide experience data are included for comparison.

	United States	Worldwide
Total number of patients	602	5751
Body System/Adverse Event (Incidence ≤ 1%)		*Incidence (1%)*
Gastrointestinal Disorders		
Nausea	10.6	2.4
Vomiting	5.1	0.8
Diarrhea	3.3	0.6
Abdominal Pain	1.5	1.4
Anorexia	1.2	0.3
Body as a Whole		
Edema	3.5	0.4
Fatigue	2.8	0.5
Fever	2.5	0.3
Malaise	1.2	0.1
Skin and Appendages		
Rash	8.6*	1.1
Pruritus	2.5	0.7
Central and Peripheral Nervouse System		
Headache	3.8	1.5
Dizziness	1.7	0.7
Psychiatric Disorders		
Libido decreased	1.2	0.2
Somnolence	1.2	0.3
Cardiovascular Disorders		
Hypertension	3.2	0.3
Metabolic and Nutritional Disorders		
Hypokalemia	2.0	0.2
Urinary System Disorders		
Albuminuria	1.2	0.1
Liver and Biliary System Disorders		
Hepatic function abnormal	2.7	0.3
Reproductive Disorders		
Male Impotence	1.2	0.2

* *Rash tends to occur more frequently in immunocompromised patients receiving immunosuppressive medications.*

Adverse events reported by less than 1% of patients in U.S. clinical trials included: flatulence, depression, insomnia, tinnitus, adrenal insufficiency, gynecomastia and male breast pain.

OVERDOSAGE

Itraconazole is not removed by dialysis. In the event of accidental overdosage, supportive measures, including gastric lavage with sodium bicarbonate, should be employed.

No significant lethality was observed when Itraconazole was administered orally to mice and rats at dosage levels of 320 mg/kg or to dogs at 200 mg/kg.

DOSAGE AND ADMINISTRATION

Itraconazole should be taken with food to ensure maximal absorption.

The recommended dose is 200 mg once daily (2 capsules). If there is no obvious improvement or there is evidence of progressive fungal disease, the dose should be increased in 100 mg increments to a maximum of 400 mg daily. Doses above 200 mg per day should be given in two divided doses. In life-threatening situations: Although these studies did not provide for a loading dose, it is recommended, based on pharmacokinetic data, that a loading dose of 200 mg (2 capsules) t.i.d. (600 mg/day) be given for the first three days. Treatment should be continued for a minimum of three months and until clinical parameters and laboratory tests indicate that the active fungal infection has subsided. An inadequate period of treatment may lead to recurrence of active infection.

Store at controlled room temperature, 15°-30°C (59°-86°F). Protect from light and moisture.

ANIMAL TOXICOLOGY

In three toxicology studies using rats, Itraconazole induced bone defects at dosage levels as low as 20 mg/kg/day (2.5 × MRHD). The induced defects included reduced bone plate activity, thinning of the zona compacta of the large bones and increased bone fragility. At a dosage level of 80 mg/kg/day (10 × MRHD) over one year or 160 mg/kg/day (20 × MRHD) for six months, Itraconazole induced small tooth pulp with hypocellular appearance in some rats.

HOW SUPPLIED
CAPSULE: 100 MG

BRAND/MANUFACTURER	NDC	SIZE	AWP
○ **BRAND**			
▶ SPORANOX: Janssen	50458-0290-04	30s	$154.84
	50458-0290-01	30s ud	$154.84

Japanese Encephalitis Virus Vaccine

DESCRIPTION

Japanese Encephalitis Virus Vaccine Inactivated, is a sterile, lyophilized vaccine for subcutaneous use, prepared by inoculating mice intracerebrally with Japanese Encephalitis (JE) Virus. "Nakayama-NIH" strain. Infected brains are harvested and homogenized in phosphate buffered saline, pH 8.0. The homogenate is centrifuged and the supernatant inactivated with formaldehyde, then processed to yield a partially purified, inactivated virus suspension. This is further purified by ultra centrifugation through 40 w/v% sucrose. The suspension is then lyophilized in final containers and sealed under dry nitrogen atmosphere. Thimerosal (mercury derivative) is added as a preservative to a final concentration of 0.007%. The diluent, Sterile Water for Injection, contains no preservative. Each 1.0 mL dose contains approximately 500 μg of gelatin, less than 100 μg of formaldehyde, and less than 50 ng of mouse serum protein. No myelin basic protein can be detected at the detection threshold of the assay (< 2 ng/mL). Prior to reconstitution, the vaccine is a white caked powder, and after reconstitution the vaccine is a colorless transparent liquid. The potency of JE Vaccine is determined by immunizing mice with either the test vaccine or the JE reference vaccine. Neutralizing antibodies are measured in a plaque neutralization assay performed on sera from the immunized mice. The potency of the test vaccine must be no less than that of the reference vaccine.

CLINICAL PHARMACOLOGY

Japanese Encephalitis (JE), a mosquito-borne arboviral Flavivirus infection, is the leading cause of viral encephalitis in Asia. Infection leads to overt encephalitis in 1 of 20 to 1000 cases. Encephalitis usually is severe, resulting in a fatal outcome in 25% of cases and residual neuropsychiatric sequelae in 50% of cases. JE acquired during the first or second trimesters of pregnancy may cause intrauterine infection and miscarriage. Infections that occur during the third trimester of pregnancy have not been associated with adverse outcomes in newborns.[1]

The virus is transmitted in an enzootic cycle among mosquitoes and vertebrate amplifying hosts, chiefly domestic pigs and, in some areas, wild Ardeid (wading) birds. Viral infection rates in mosquitoes range from < 1% to 3%. These species are prolific in rural areas where their larvae breed in ground pools and flooded rice fields. Thus all elements of the transmission cycle are prevalent in rural areas of Asia and human infections occur principally in this setting. Because vertebrate amplifying hosts and agricultural activities may be situated within and at the periphery of cities, human cases occasionally are reported from urban locations.[1]

JE Virus is transmitted seasonally in most areas of Asia. The seasonal patterns of viral transmission are correlated with the abundance of vector mosquitoes and of vertebrate amplifying hosts. Although the abundance of vector mosquitoes fluctuates with the amount of rainfall, and with the impact of the rainy season in some tropical locations, irrigation associated with agricultural practices is a more important factor affecting vector abundance, and transmission may occur year-round. Thus the periods of greatest risk for JE viral transmission vary regionally and within countries, and from year to year.[1]

In areas where JE is endemic, annual incidence ranges from 1 to 10 per 10,000 people. Cases occur primarily in children under 10 years of age. Seroprevalence studies in these endemic areas indicate nearly universal exposure by adulthood (calculating from a ratio of asymptomatic to symptomatic infections of 200 to 1, approximately 10% of the susceptible population is infected per year). In addition

---

to children < 10 years, an increase in JE incidence has been observed in the elderly.[1]

Challenge experiments in passively protected mice have defined the levels of neutralizing antibody that may be protective for humans.[2]

Mice passively immunized to achieve a neutralizing antibody titer of $\geq 1:10$ were protected from a JE virus challenge of $10^5 LD_{50}$, a viral dose thought to be transmitted by an infected mosquito.[2]

The efficacy of the BIKEN Nakayama-NIH strain Japanese Encephalitis Virus Vaccine Inactivated was demonstrated in a placebo-controlled, randomized clinical trial in Thai children, sponsored by the U.S. Army.[3] In this trial, children between 1 and 14 years of age received BIKEN monovalent Nakayama-NIH strain (n = 21,628) or a bivalent vaccine containing the Nakayama-NIH and Beijing JE Virus strains (n = 22,080) or tetanus toxoid as a placebo (n = 21,516). Immunization consisted of two (2) subcutaneous 1.0 mL doses of vaccine, except in children under 3 years of age who received two 0.5 mL doses. One case (5 cases/100,000) of JE occurred in the monovalent vaccine group, one case (5 cases/100,000) in the bivalent vaccine group, and 11 cases (51 cases/100,000) in the placebo group. The observed efficacy of both monovalent and bivalent vaccines was 91% (95% confidence interval, 54% to 98%). Side effects of vaccination, including headache, sore arm, rash, and swelling were reported at rates similar to those in the placebo group, usually less than 1%. Symptoms did not increase after the second dose. It should be noted that a schedule of two doses, separated by seven days, as employed in this trial, may be appropriate for use in residents of endemic or epidemic areas, where pre-existing exposure to Flaviviruses may contribute to the immune response.[3]

A three-dose vaccination schedule is recommended for U.S. travelers and military personnel, based on the Centers for Disease Control and Prevention (CDC) experience and on a controlled immunogenicity trial perfomed in U.S.military personnel.[4,5] The CDC experience demonstrated that neutralizing antibody was produced in fewer than 80% of vaccinees following two doses of vaccine in U.S. travelers and antibody levels declined substantially in most vaccinees within six months. The U.S. Army studies the immunogenicity of Japanese Encephalitis Virus Vaccine in 538 volunteers. Two three-dose regimens were evaluated (Day 0, 7, and 14 or Day 0, 7, and 30). All vaccine recipients demonstrated neutralizing antibodies at 2 months and 6 months after initiation of vaccination. The schedule of Day 0, 7, and 30 produced higher antibody responses than the Day 0, 7, and 14 schedule. Two hundred and seventy-three of the original study participants were tested at 12 months post-vaccination and there was no longer a statistical difference in antibody titers between the two vaccination regimens.[5]

The full duration of protection is unknown. Of U.S. Army volunteers completing a three-dose regimen, 252 agreed to receive a booster dose of vaccine one year after the primary series. All boosted participants still had antibody 12 months after the booster. Protective levels of neutralizing antibody persisted for 24 months (2 years) in all 21 persons who had not received a booster.[5] Definitive recommendations cannot be given on the timing of booster doses at this time.

INDICATIONS AND USAGE
Japanese Encephalitis Virus Vaccine is indicated for active immunization against JE for persons one year of age and older. For recommended primary immunization series see *"Dosage And Administration"* section.

Japanese Encephalitis Virus Vaccine should be considered for use in person who plan to reside in or travel to areas where JE is endemic or epidemic during a transmission season. *Japanese Encephalitis Virus Vaccine is NOT recommended for all persons traveling to or residing in Asia.* The incidence of JE in the location of intended stay, the conditions of housing, nature of activities, duration of stay, and the possibility of unexpected travel to high-risk areas are factors that should be considered in the decision to administer vaccine. In general, vaccine should be considered for use in persons spending a month or longer in epidemic or endemic areas during the transmission season, especially if travel will include rural areas. Depending on the epidemic circumstances, vaccine should be considered for persons spending less than 30 days whose activites, such as extensive outdoor activities in rural areas, place them at particularly high risk for exposure.[1]

In all instances, travelers are advised to take personal precautions to reduce exposure to mosquito bites. (See *"Information for Patients"* section.)

Current CDC advisories should be consulted with regard to JE epidemicity in specific locales.[1]

The decision to use Japanese Encephalitis Virus Vaccine should balance the risk for exposure to the virus and for developing illness, the availability and acceptability of repellents and other alternative measures, and the side effects of vaccination. Assessments should be interpreted cautiously because risk can vary within areas and from year to year and available data are incomplete. Estimates suggest that risk of JE in highly endemic areas during the transmission season can reach 1 per 5000 per month of exposure; risk for most short-term travelers may be 1 per million or less. Although JE vaccine is reactogenic, rates of serious allergic reactions (generalized urticaria and/or angioedema) are low (approximately 1-104 per 10,000).[1]

Advanced age may be a risk factor for developing symptomic illness after infection. JE acquired during pregnancy carries the potential for intrauterine infection and fetal death. These factors should be considered when advising elderly persons and pregnant women who plan visits to JE endemic areas.

There are no data on the safety and efficacy of JE Vaccine in infants under one year of age. Whenever possible, immunization of infants should be deferred until they are one year of age or order.[1]

Research Laboratory Workers: Laboratory acquired JE has been reported in 22 cases. JE Virus may be transmitted in a laboratory setting through needle sticks and other accidental exposures Vaccine-derived immunity presumably protects against exposure through these percutaneous routes. Exposure to aerosolized JE Virus, and particular to high concentrations of virus, such as may occur during viral purification potentially could lead to infection through mucous membranes and possibly directly into the central nervous system through the olfactory mucosa. It is unknown whether vaccine-derived immunity protects against such exposures, but immunization is recommended for all laboratory workers with a potential for exposure to infectious JE Virus.[1]

As with any vaccine, vaccination with Japanese Encephalitis Virus Vaccine may not result in protection in all individuals Long-term protection, as demonstrated by persistence of neutralizing antibody for more than two years, has not yet been shown.

UNLABELED USES
Japanese Encephalitis Virus Vaccine is used alone or as an adjunct in the treatment of dengue and dengue hemorrhagic fever.

CONTRAINDICATIONS
Adverse reactions to a prior dose of JE Vaccine manifesting as generalized urticaria and angioedema are considered to be contraindications to further vaccination.

Patients who develop allergic or unusual adverse events after vaccination should be reported through the Vaccine Adverse Event Reporting System (VAERS) 1-800-822-7967.[1]

JE Vaccine is produced in mouse brains and should not be administered to persons with a proven or suspected hypersensitivity to proteins or rodent or neural origin. *Hypersensitivity to thimerosal is a contraindication to vaccination.*[1]

WARNINGS
Adverse reactions to JE Vaccine manifesting as generalized urticaria or angioedema may occur within minutes following vaccination. A possibly related reaction has occurred as late as 17 days after vaccination. Most reactions occur within 10 days with the majority occurring within 48 hours. (See *"Adverse Reactions"* section)

Vaccinees should be observed for 30 minutes after vaccination and warned about the possibility of delayed generalized urticaria, often in a generalized distribution or angioedema of the extremities, face and oropharynx, especially of the lips.[1]

Vaccinees should be advised to remain in areas where they have ready access to medical care for 10 days after receiving a dose of JE Vaccine. Vaccinees should be instructed to seek medical attention immediately upon onset of any reaction.[1]

Persons should not embark on international travel within 10 days of Japanese Encephalitis Virus Vaccine immunization because of the possibility of delayed allergic reactions.[1]

Persons with a past history of urticaria after hymenoptera envenomation, drugs, physical or other provocations, or of idiopathic cause appear to have a greater risk of developing reactions to JE Vaccine (relative risk 9.1, 95% confidence interval 1.8 to 50.9).[6] This history should be considered when weighing risks and benefits of the vaccine for an individual patient. When patients with such a history are offered JE Vaccine, they should be alerted to their increased risk for reaction and monitored appropriately. There are no data supporting the efficacy of prophylactic antihistamines or steroids in preventing JE Vaccine-related allergic reactions.[1]

Epinephrine and other medications and equipment to treat anaphylaxis should be available at vaccine administration centers.

PRECAUTIONS
GENERAL
Epinephrine Injection (1:1000) must be immediately available should an acute anaphylactic reaction occur due to any component of the vaccine.

Prior to injection of any vaccine, all known precautions should be taken to prevent adverse reactions. This includes a review of the patient's history with respect to possible sensitivity to this vaccine, a similar vaccine or allergic disorders in general (see *"Contraindications"* section).

A separate, sterile syringe and needle or a disposable unit should be used for each patient to prevent transmission of infectious agents from person to person. Needles should not be recapped and should be disposed of properly.

Although substantial neutralizing antibody titers are elicited by Japanese Encephalitis Virus Vaccine in more than 90% of U.S. travelers without history of prior JE immunization or of prior exposure to JE, the precise relationship between antibody level and efficacy has not been established even though these titers persisted for at least two years after immunization.[7]

The decision to administer JE Vaccine should balance the risks for exposure to the virus and for developing illness, the availability and acceptability of repellents and other alternative protective measures, and the side effects of vaccination.

INFORMATION FOR PATIENTS
Patients should be advised of the following:
- Japanese Encephalitis Virus Vaccine is given to provide immunization against Japanese Encephalitis Virus.
- A three-dose immunizing series should be completed, except in unusual circumstances. (See *"Contraindications"* and *"Dosage and Administration"* sections.)
- Japanese Encephalitis Virus Vaccine should be given to a pregnant woman only if, in the opinion of a physician, withholding the vaccine entails even greater risk.

■ Any adverse events following Japanese Encephalitis Virus Vaccine should be reported through the Vaccine Adverse Event Reporting System (VAERS) 1-800-822-7967 after contacting the physician immediately.

■ If the patient has a past history of urticaria (hives) (following hymenoptera envenomation, drugs, physical or other provocation or of idiopathic origin), adverse effects are more likely.

■ Adverse events consisting of arm soreness and local redness can occur shortly after vaccination.

■ Adverse events consisting of headache, rash, edema and generalized urticaria or angioedema may occur shortly after vaccination or up to 17 days (usually within 10 days) following vaccination.

■ International travel should not be initiated within 10 days of Japanese Encephalitis Virus Vaccine vaccination because of the possibility of delayed adverse reactions. Patients should be instructed to seek medical attention immediately upon onset of any adverse reaction.

■ Personal precautions should be taken to avoid exposure to mosquito bites by the use of insect repellents, and protective clothing. Avoiding outdoor activity, especially during twilight periods and in the evening, will reduce risk even further.

DRUG INTERACTIONS
There are no data on the effect of concurrent administration of other vaccines, drugs (e.g. chloroquine, mefloquine) or biologicals on the safety and immunogenicity of JE vaccine.

CARCINOGENESIS, MUTAGENESIS, IMPAIRMENT OF FERTILITY
No studies have been performed to evaluate carcinogenicity, mutagenic potential, or impact on fertility.

PREGNANCY
Reproductive Studies: Pregnancy Category C: Animal reproduction studies have not been conducted with Japanese Encephalitis Virus Vaccine. It is not not known whether Japanese Encephalitis Virus Vaccine can cause fetal harm when administered to a pregnant woman or can affect reproductive capacity. Pregnant women who must travel to an area where risk of JE is high should be immunized when the theoretical risks of immunization are outweighed by the risk of infection to the mother and developing fetus. Japanese Encephalitis Virus Vaccine should be given to a pregnant woman only if clearly needed.

NURSING MOTHERS
It is not known whether Japanese Encephalitis Virus Vaccine is excreted in human milk. Because many drugs are excreted in human milk, caution should be exercised when Japanese Encephalitis Virus Vaccine is administered to a nursing woman.

PEDIATRIC USE
Safety and efficacy of JE Vaccine in infants under one year of age have not been established.

ADVERSE REACTIONS
JE Vaccine is associated with a moderate frequency of local and mild systemic adverse effects.[3,4,5,8,9,10,11] Tenderness, redness, swelling and other local effects have been reported in about 20% of vaccines (< 1% to 31%). Systemic side effects, principally fever, headache, malaise, rash, and other reactions, such as chills, dizziness, myalgia, nausea, vomiting and abdominal pain have been reported in approximately 10% of vaccinees.

In a study conducted by the CDC less than 5% of the 1,756 U.S. travelers immunized with a three-dose regimen of the vaccine reported headache, flu-like symptoms, fever, and other systemic complaints. Hives and facial swelling were reported in 0.2% and 0.1% of vaccines, respectively. Local soreness occurred in 5.9% and local redness in 2.9%. There was no increase in the number or severity of reactions with increasing numbers of doses.[7]

The U.S. Army studied 4,034 personnel from 1987 to 1989.[10] Using a two- or three-dose regimen of JE Vaccine, arm soreness was described in 22.7%, local redness in 4.8%, headache in 15.2%, and a febrile episode in 5.5%. In another trial evaluating the safety and immunogenicity of a three-dose immunizing series (Day 0, 7, and 30 or Day 0, 7, and 14), performed in 538 adult volunteers in 1990, the Army determined that local soreness and redness occurred in 21% of vaccinees after the first dose, then decreased with subsequent injections (p < 0.0001, Chi-square for downward trend). Systemic symptoms including feverishness, headache and rash occurred in 5% of vaccinees after the first dose, then decreased with subsequent injections (p < 0.001, Chi-square for downward trend).[5] Participants who received the third dose on Day 14 reported more side effects than those who received the injection on Day 30. Among these volunteers, 252 received a booster injection of vaccine one year after receiving the first dose of the primary series. Side effects reported after the booster injection included local symptoms of soreness (24.5%) and redness (6.1%) at the injection site and systemic complaints of headache (4.9%), fever (1.6%), and rash (0.8%). Less than 1% of all reported symptoms was graded as severe. No generalized urticaria or anaphylaxis was reported.

Since 1989, an apparently new pattern of adverse reactions has been reported among vaccinees in Europe, North America, and Australia.[11,12,13] The reactions have been characterized by urticaria, often in a generalized distribution, or angioedema of the extremities and face, especially of the lips and oropharynx. Three vaccine recipients developed respiratory distress. Distress or collapse due to hypotension or other causes led to hospitalization in several cases. Most reactions were treated successfully with antihistamines or oral steroids; however some patients were hospitalized for parenteral steroid therapy. Three patients developed an erythema multiforme or erythema nodosum and some patients have

had joint swelling. Some vaccinees complained of generalized itching without objective evidence of a rash.

An important feature of the reactions has been the interval between vaccination and onset of symptoms. Reactions after a first vaccine dose occurred after a median of 12 hours after immunization (88% of reactions occurred within 3 days). The interval between administration of a second dose and onset of symptoms generally was longer, (median 3 days and possibly as long as 2 weeks). Reactions have occurred after a second or third dose, when preceding doses were received uneventfully.

Between November 1991 and May 1992, the U.S. Navy immunized 35,253 U.S. personnel (marines, other military and dependents) with Japanese Encephalitis Virus Vaccine on Okinawa. The overall reaction rate, 62.4 per 10,000 vaccinees (95% confidence interval 54.2 to 70.6) includes persons reporting urticaria, angioedema, generalized itching and wheezing. The reaction rate per 10,000 vaccinees was 26.7 (95% confidence interval 21.3 to 32.1), 30.8 (95% confidence interval 24.6 to 37.0) or 12.2 (95% confidence interval 7.9 to 16.5) after the first, second or third dose, respectively.[6] These reactions were generally mild to moderate in severity. Nine out of 35,253 persons immunized were hospitalized (2.6 per 10,000 vaccinees) primarily to allow administration of intravenous steroids for refractory urticaria. None of these reactions were considered life-threatening.

A case-control study conducted as part of the JE immunization campaign in Okinawa found that persons developing these reactions after JE vaccination were more likely to have had a past history of urticaria after hymenoptera envenomation, drugs, physical or other provocations or of idiopathic origins (relative risk 9.1, 95% confidence interval 1.8 to 50.9).[6] The vaccine constituents responsible for these adverse reactions have not been identified.

Other serious adverse events reported following vaccination include (1) one case of Guillain-Barre syndrome after JE vaccination has been reported in the United States since 1984, however, this patient was diagnosed as having mononucleosis three weeks before the onset of weakness; (2) one case of urticaria, hepatitis and respiratory failure one week after dose 2 (this person showed effusion and infiltrate on chest x-ray and eosinophilia); and (3) one case of respiratory and renal failure one week after a dose (this 26-month-old male had infiltrate on chest x-ray and acid fast bacilli in sputum); and (4) one case of newly diagnosed hypertension in a young adult male presenting with a headache several hours after receiving dose one. The etiology of these adverse events is unknown.

Sudden death occurred approximately 60 hours after receiving the first dose of JE Vaccine in a 21-year-old U.S. military person with a history of recurrent hypersensitivity and an episode of possible anaphylaxis. This person also received the third dose of plague vaccine approximately 12-15 hours prior to the death. There was no evidence of urticaria or angioedema. Cause of death was not established at autopsy.

Surveillance of JE Vaccine related complications in Japan from 1965 to 1973 disclosed neurologic events (primarily encephalitis, encephalopathy, seizures, and peripheral neuropathy) in 1 to 2.3 per million vaccines.[14,15] Very rarely, deaths occurred with vaccine-associated encephalitis. Between 1987 and 1989, two cases of neurologic dysfunction were reported from Japan; one of these was a transverse myelitis, while the second included seizures, cranial nerve paresis, cerebellar ataxia, and behavior disorder.[15] In 1992, two cases of acute disseminated encephalomyelitis were reported from Japan; one occurred 14 days after the second dose and the second occurred 17 days after a booster dose of JE Vaccine. Both cases recovered.[16] One case of Bell's Palsy was reported from Thailand.

REPORTING OF ADVERSE EVENTS
Reporting by parents and patients of all adverse events occurring after antigen administration should be encouraged. Adverse events following immunization with vaccine should be reported by the health-care provider to the U.S. Department of Health and Human Services (DHHS) Vaccine Adverse Event Reporting System (VAERS). Reporting forms and information about reporting requirements or completion of the form can be obtained from VAERS through a toll-free number 1-800-822-7967.[17]

Health-care providers also should report these events to Director of Medical Affairs, Connaught Laboratories, Inc., Route 611, P.O. Box 187, Swiftwater, PA 18370 or call 1-800-822-2463.

DOSAGE AND ADMINISTRATION
Parenteral drug products should be inspected visually for extraneous particulate matter and/or discoloration prior to administration whenever solution and container permit. If either of these conditions exist, the vaccine should not be administered.

For persons 3 years of age and older, a single dose is 1.0 mL of vaccine. *For children 1 year to 3 years of age, a single dose is 0.5 mL of vaccine.* (See "Primary Immunization Schedule" below.)

Single-Dose vial of lyophilized vaccine: Remove plastic tab of flip-off cap. DO NOT REMOVE RUBBER STOPPER. Cleanse stopper with a suitable disinfectant. Reconstitute only with the supplied 1.3 mL of diluent (Sterile Water for Injection). Shake vial thoroughly. After reconstitution the vaccine should be stored between 2° — 8°C (35° — 46° F) and used within 8 hours. DO NOT FREEZE RECONSTITUTED VACCINE.

10-Dose vial of lyophilized vaccine: Remove plastic tab of flip-off cap. DO NOT REMOVE RUBBER STOPPER. Cleanse stopper with a suitable disinfectant. Reconstitute only with the supplied 11 mL of diluent (Sterile Water for Injection). Shake vial thoroughly. After reconstitution the vaccine should be stored between 2° — 8°C (35° — 46° F) and used within 8 hours. DO NOT FREEZE RECONSTITUTED VACCINE.

A separate, sterile syringe and needle or a sterile disposable unit should be used for each patient to prevent transmission of infectious agents from person to person. Needles should not be recapped and should be disposed of properly.

SHAKE VIAL WELL.

PRIMARY IMMUNIZATION SCHEDULE

The recommended primary immunization series is three doses of 1.0 mL each for individuals > 3 years of age given subcutaneously on days 0, 7, and 30. *For children 1 to 3 years of age a series of three doses of 0.5 mL each should be given subcutaneously on days 0, 7, and 30.* An abbreviated schedule of days 0, 7, and 14 can be used when the longer schedule is impractical because of time constraints. (When it is impossible to follow one of the above recommended schedules, two doses given a week apart will induce antibodies in approximately 80% of vaccinees; however, this two-dose regimen should not be used except under unusual circumstances). The last dose should be given at least 10 days before the commencement of international travel to ensure an adequate immune response and access to medical care in the event of delayed adverse reactions.

A booster dose of 1.0 mL *(0.5 mL for children from 1 to 3 years of age)* may be given after two years. In the absence of firm data on the persistence of antibody after primary immunization, a definite recommendation cannot be made on the spacing of boosters beyond two years.

There are no data on the safety and efficacy of JE Vaccine in infants under one year of age. Whenever possible, immunization of infants should be deferred until they are one year of age or older.[1]

The skin at the site of injection first should be cleansed and disinfected. Shake vial thoroughly before each use. Cleanse top of rubber stopper of the vial with a suitable antiseptic and wipe away all excess before withdrawing vaccine.

When Japanese Encephalitis Virus Vaccine and any other vaccines are given concurrently, separate syringes and separate sites should be used.

For persons 3 years of age and older, a single dose is 1.0 mL of vaccine. *For children 1 year to 3 years of age, a single dose is 0.5 mL of vaccine.* (See *"Primary Immunization Schedule"* above.)

STORAGE

The vaccine should be stored between 2° — 8°C (35° — 46°F). DO NOT FREEZE. After reconstitution the vaccine should be stored between 2° — 8°C (35° — 46°F) and used within 8 hours. DO NOT FREEZE RECONSTITUTED VACCINE.

REFERENCES

1. Recommendations of the Advisory Committee on Immunization Practices (ACIP). Inactivated Japanese Encephalitis Virus Vaccine. MMWR (In Press) 2. Oya A. Japanese Encephalitis Vaccine. Acta Paediatr Jpn 30: 175-184, 1988 3. Hoke CH, et al. Protection Against Japanese Encephalitis by Inactivated Vaccines. N Eng J Med 319; 608-614, 1988 4. Poland JD, et al. Evaluation of the Potency and Safety of Inactivated Japanese Encephalitis Vaccine in US Inhabitants. J Infect Dis 161: 878-882, 1990 5. DeFraites RF. Immunogenicity and Safety of Japanese Encephalitis Vaccine (Inactivated: Nakayama/BIKEN) in U.S. Army Soldiers; Evaluation of Three Consecutively Manufactured Lots of Vaccine Administered in Two Dosing Regimens. April 30, 1991, and November 12, 1992. Unpublished Data, on file with BIKEN and with Walter Reed Army Institute of Research, Washington, DC 6. Berg WS. Navy Environmental Health Center, Norfolk, VA June 16, 1992 (unpublished) 7. Unpublished data on file with "BIKEN" and CDC 8. Rojanasuphot S, et al. A field trial of Japanese encephalitis vaccine produced in Thailand. Southeast Asian J Trop Med Publ Health 20: 653-654, 1989 9. Rao Bhau LN, et al. Safety and efficacy of Japanese encephalitis vaccine produced in India. Indian J Med Res 88: 301-307, 1988 10. Sanchez JL, et al. Further Experience with Japanese Encephalitis Vaccine. Lancet 335: 972-973, 1990 11. Japanese Encephalitis Vaccine and Adverse Effects among Travelers. Canada Diseases Weekly Report. Vol. 17-32; 173-177, 1991 12. Anderson MM, et al. Side-Effects with Japanese Encephalitis Vaccine. Lancet 337: 1044, 1991 13. Ruff TA, et al. Adverse Reactions to Japanese Encephalitis Vaccine. Lancet 338: 881-882, 1991 14. Kitaoka M. Follow-up on use of vaccine in children in Japan, in McDHammon W, Kitaoka M, Downs WG eds. Immunization for Japanese encephalitis. Excerpta Medica, Amsterdam 275-277, 1972 15. Unpublished data on file with "BIKEN" 16. Ohtaki E, et al. Acute disseminated encephalomyelitis after Japanese B Encephalitis Vaccination. Pediatric Neurology Vol. 8 No. 2: 137-139, 1992 17. CDC. Vaccine Adverse Event Reporting System-United States. MMWR 39: 730-733, 1990

HOW SUPPLIED
POWDER FOR INJECTION:

BRAND/MANUFACTURER	NDC	SIZE	AWP
○ **BRAND**			
JE-VAX/Connaught	49281-0680-30	3	$145.06

JE-VAX *SEE* **JAPANESE ENCEPHALITIS VIRUS VACCINE**

Jenest-28 *SEE* **ETHINYL ESTRADIOL AND NORETHINDRONE**

K-Dur *SEE* **POTASSIUM CHLORIDE, ORAL**

K-Lor *SEE* **POTASSIUM CHLORIDE, ORAL**

K-Lyte Cl *SEE* **POTASSIUM CHLORIDE, ORAL**

K-Lyte DS *SEE* **CITRIC ACID AND POTASSIUM BICARBONATE**

K-Norm *SEE* **POTASSIUM CHLORIDE, ORAL**

K-Phos *SEE* **POTASSIUM ACID PHOSPHATE, POTASSIUM ACID PHOSPHATE AND SODIUM ACID PHOSPHATE** *AND* **POTASSIUM PHOSPHATE, MONOBASIC AND SODIUM PHOSPHATE, DIBASIC**

K-Tab *SEE* **POTASSIUM CHLORIDE, ORAL**

Kabikinase *SEE* **STREPTOKINASE**

Kanamycin Sulfate

WARNING

PATIENTS TREATED WITH AMINOGLYCOSIDES BY ANY ROUTE SHOULD BE UNDER CLOSE CLINICAL OBSERVATION BECAUSE OF THE POTENTIAL TOXICITY ASSOCIATED WITH THEIR USE. AS WITH OTHER AMINOGLYCOSIDES, THE MAJOR TOXIC EFFECTS OF KANAMYCIN SULFATE ARE ITS ACTION ON THE AUDITORY AND VESTIBULAR BRANCHES OF THE EIGHTH NERVE AND THE RENAL TUBULES. NEUROTOXICITY IS MANIFESTED BY BILATERAL AUDITORY TOXICITY WHICH OFTEN IS PERMANENT AND, SOMETIMES, BY VESTIBULAR OTOTOXICITY. LOSS OF HIGH FREQUENCY PERCEPTION USUALLY OCCURS BEFORE THERE IS NOTICEABLE CLINICAL HEARING LOSS AND CAN BE DETECTED BY AUDIOMETRIC TESTING. THERE MAY NOT BE CLINICAL SYMPTOMS TO WARN OF DEVELOPING COCHLEAR DAMAGE. VERTIGO MAY OCCUR AND MAY BE EVIDENCE OF VESTIBULAR INJURY. OTHER MANIFESTATIONS OF NEUROTOXICITY MAY INCLUDE NUMBNESS, SKIN TINGLING, MUSCLE TWITCHING, AND CONVULSIONS. THE RISK OF HEARING LOSS INCREASES WITH THE DEGREE OF EXPOSURE TO EITHER HIGH PEAK OR HIGH TROUGH SERUM CONCENTRATIONS AND CONTINUES TO PROGRESS AFTER DRUG WITHDRAWAL.

RENAL IMPAIRMENT MAY BE CHARACTERIZED BY DECREASED CREATININE CLEARANCE, THE PRESENCE OF CELLS OR CASTS, OLIGURIA, PROTEINURIA, DECREASED URINE SPECIFIC GRAVITY, OR EVIDENCE OF INCREASING NITROGEN RETENTION (INCREASING BUN, NPN, OR SERUM CREATININE).

THE RISKS OF SEVERE OTOTOXIC AND NEPHROTOXIC REACTIONS ARE SHARPLY INCREASED IN PATIENTS WITH IMPAIRED RENAL FUNCTION AND IN THOSE WITH NORMAL RENAL FUNCTION WHO RECEIVED HIGH DOSES OR PROLONGED THERAPY.

RENAL AND EIGHTH NERVE FUNCTION SHOULD BE CLOSELY MONITORED, ESPECIALLY IN PATIENTS WITH KNOWN OR SUSPECTED REDUCED RENAL FUNCTION AT THE ONSET OF THERAPY, AND ALSO IN THOSE WHOSE RENAL FUNCTION IS INITIALLY NORMAL BUT WHO DEVELOP SIGNS OF RENAL DYSFUNCTION DURING THERAPY. SERUM CONCENTRATIONS OF PARENTERALLY ADMINISTERED AMINO-GLYCOSIDES SHOULD BE MONITORED WHEN FEASIBLE TO ASSURE ADEQUATE LEVELS AND TO AVOID POTENTIALLY TOXIC LEVELS. URINE SHOULD BE EXAMINED FOR DECREASED SPECIFIC GRAVITY, INCREASED EXCRETION OF PROTEIN, AND THE PRESENCE OF CELLS OR CASTS. BLOOD UREA NITROGEN, SERUM CREATININE, OR CREATININE CLEARANCE SHOULD BE MEASURED PERIODICALLY. SERIAL AUDIOGRAMS SHOULD BE OBTAINED WHEN FEASIBLE IN PATIENTS OLD ENOUGH TO BE TESTED, PARTICULARLY HIGH RISK PATIENTS. EVIDENCE OF OTOTOXICITY (DIZZINESS, VERTIGO, TINNITUS, ROARING IN THE EARS, AND HEARING LOSS) OR NEPHROTOXICITY REQUIRES DOSAGE ADJUSTMENT OR DISCONTINUANCE OF THE DRUG.

NEUROMUSCULAR BLOCKADE WITH RESPIRATORY PARALYSIS MAY OCCUR WHEN KANAMYCIN SULFATE IS INSTILLED INTRA-PERITONEALLY CONCOMITANTLY WITH ANESTHESIA AND MUSCLE-RELAXING DRUGS. NEUROMUSCULAR BLOCKADE HAS BEEN REPORTED FOLLOWING PARENTERAL INJECTION AND THE ORAL USE OF AMINOGLYCOSIDES. THE POSSIBILITY OF THE OCCURRENCE OF

➤ SHOWN IN PRODUCT IDENTIFICATION GUIDE

NEUROMUSCULAR BLOCKADE AND RESPIRATORY PARALYSIS SHOULD BE CONSIDERED IF AMINOGLYCOSIDES ARE ADMINISTERED BY ANY ROUTE, ESPECIALLY IN PATIENTS RECEIVING ANESTHETICS, NEUROMUSCULAR-BLOCKING AGENTS SUCH AS TUBOCURARINE, SUCCINYLCHOLINE, DECAMETHONIUM, OR IN PATIENTS RECEIVING MASSIVE TRANSFUSIONS OF CITRATE-ANTICOAGULATED BLOOD. IF BLOCKAGE OCCURS, CALCIUM SALTS MAY REDUCE THESE PHENOMENA BUT MECHANICAL RESPIRATORY ASSISTANCE MAY BE NECESSARY.

THE CONCURRENT AND/OR SEQUENTIAL SYSTEMIC, ORAL, OR TOPICAL USE OF KANAMYCIN AND OTHER POTENTIALLY NEPHROTOXIC, AND/OR NEUROTOXIC DRUGS, PARTICULARLY POLYMYXIN B, BACITRACIN, STREPTOMYCIN, NEOMYCIN, VIOMYCIN, GENTAMICIN, CEPHALORIDINE, COLISTIN, OTOTOXIC, AMPHOTERICIN B, CISPLATIN, VANCOMYCIN, AND ALL OTHER AMINOGLYCOSIDES (INCLUDING PAROMOMYCIN) SHOULD BE AVOIDED BECAUSE THE TOXICITY MAY BE ADDITIVE. OTHER FACTORS WHICH MAY INCREASE PATIENT RISK OF TOXICITY ARE ADVANCED AGE AND DEHYDRATION.

KANAMYCIN SULFATE SHOULD NOT BE GIVEN CONCURRENTLY WITH POTENT DIURETICS (ETHACRYNIC ACID, FUROSEMIDE, MERALLURIDE SODIUM, SODIUM MERCAPTOMERIN, OR MANNITOL). THEY MAY CAUSE CUMULATIVE ADVERSE EFFECTS OR THE KANAMYCIN ON THE KIDNEY AND AUDITORY NERVE. SOME DIURETICS THEMSELVES CAUSE OTOTOXICITY, AND INTRAVENOUSLY ADMINISTERED DIURETICS MAY ENHANCE AMINOGLYCOSIDE TOXICITY BY ALTERING ANTIBIOTIC CONCENTRATIONS IN SERUM AND TISSUE.

DESCRIPTION

Kanamycin Sulfate is an aminoglycoside antibiotic produced by *Streptomyces kanamyceticus*. Kanamycin Sulfate is available as an injection for intramuscular or intravenous use and as capsules for oral administration. It is supplied in oral formulation for topical effect within the gastrointestinal tract, because it is absorbed only very slightly when administered orally, and is excreted unchanged in the feces.

Each 2 ml of solution for injection contains:
Kanamycin Sulfate equivalent to ....75 mg (pediatric) or 500 mg Kanamycin

Each 3 ml of solution for injection contains:
Kanamycin Sulfate equivalent to ....1 gm Kanamycin

Each capsule contains:
Kanamycin Sulfate equivalent to ....500 mg Kanamycin

It is $C_{18}H_{36}N_4O_{11} \cdot 2H_2SO_4$. D-Streptamine, 0-3-amino-3-deoxy-α-D-glucopyranosyl - (1 → 6) -0- [6-amino-6-deoxy-α-D-glucopyranosyl- (1 → 4)]-2-deoxy, sulfate 1:2 (salt). It consists of two amino sugars glycosidically linked to deoxystreptamine.

Following is its chemical structure:

CLINICAL PHARMACOLOGY

The drug is rapidly absorbed after intramuscular injection and peak serum levels are generally reached within approximately one hour. Doses of 7.5 mg/kg give mean peak levels of 22 μg/mL. At 8 hours following a 7.5 mg/kg dose, mean serum levels are 3.2 μg/mL. The serum half-life is 2 ½ hours. Intravenous administration of Kanamycin over a period of one hour resulted in serum concentrations similar to those obtained by intramuscular administration.

Kanamycin diffuses rapidly into most body fluids including synovial and peritoneal fluids and bile. Significant levels of the drug appear in cord blood and amniotic fluid following intramuscular administration to pregnant patients. Spinal fluid concentrations in normal infants are approximately 10 to 20% of serum levels and may reach 50% when the meninges are inflamed.

Studies in normal adult patients have shown only trace levels of Kanamycin in spinal fluid. No data are available on adults with meningitis.

The drug is excreted almost entirely by glomerular filtration and is not reabsorbed by the renal tubules. Hence, high concentrations are attained in the nephron, and the urine may contain levels 10 to 20 times higher than those in serum. Little, if any, metabolic transformation occurs. Renal excretion is extremely rapid. In patients with normal renal function, approximately one-half of the administered dose is cleared within 4 hours and excretion is complete within 24 to 48 hours. Patients with impaired renal function or with diminished glomerular filtration pressure excrete Kanamycin more slowly. Such patients may build up excessively high blood levels which greatly increase the risk of ototocic reactions. In severely burned patients the half-life may be significantly decreased and resulting serum concentrations may be lower than anticipated from the mg per kg dose.

Oral administered Kanamycin is poorly absorbed from the normal gastrointestinal tract. The small absorbed fraction is rapidly excreted with normal kidney function. The unabsorbed portion of the drug is eliminated unchanged in the feces.

Microbiology: Kanamycin Sulfate is a bactericidal antibiotic which acts by inhibiting the synthesis of protein in susceptible microorganisms. Parenteral Kanamycin Sulfate is active *in vitro* against many strains of *Staphylococcus aureus* (including penicillinase and nonpenicillinase-producing strains), *Staphylococcus epidermidis, N. gonorrhoeae, H. Influenzae, E. coli, Enterobacter aerogenes, Shigella* and *Salmonella* species, *K, pneumoniae, Serratia marcescens, Providencia* species, *Acinetobacter* species and *Citrobacter freundii* and *Citrobacter* species, and many strains of both indole-positive and indole-negative *Proteus* strains that are frequently resistant to other antibiotics.

Aminoglycosides have a low order of activity against most gram-positive organisms including *Streptococcus pyogenes, Streptococcus pneumoniae* and *enterococci. In vitro* studies have demonstrated that an aminoglycoside combined with an antibiotic which interferes with cell wall synthesis (ie, Pencillin G or ampicillin) affects some Group D streptococcal strains synergistically. Bacteriological testing and tests for antibiotic synergism are necessary.

Enzymatic inactivation of deoxystreptamine is the principal mechanism of resistance.

Most intestinal bacteria are eliminated rapidly following oral administration of Kanamycin, with bacterial suppression persisting for 48 to 72 hours.

Susceptibility Testing: Quantitative methods for susceptibility testing that require measurement of zone diameters give the most precise estimates of antibiotic susceptibility. One such procedure has been recommended for use with discs to test susceptibility to Kanamycin. Interpretation involves correlation of the diameters obtained in the disc test with minimal inhibitory concentration (MIC) values for Kanamycin.

Reports from the laboratory give results of the standardized single disc susceptibility test (Bauer, et al., Am. J. Clin. Path. 1966; 45:493 and Federal Register 37:20525-20529, 1972), using a 30-μg Kanamycin disc should be interpreted according to the following criteria:

Organisms producing zones of 18 mm or greater, or MIC's of 16 μg or less are considered susceptible, indicating that the test organism is likely to respond to therapy.

Resistant organisms produce zones of 14 mm or less or MIC's of 16μg or greater. A report of 'resistant' from the laboratory indicates that the infecting organism is not likely to respond to therapy.

Zones greater than 14 mm and less than 18 mm, or MIC's of greater than 16 μg and less than 65 μg, indicate intermediate susceptibility. A report of "intermediate" susceptibility suggests that the organism would be susceptible if the infection is confined to tissues and fluids (eg, urine), in which high antibiotic levels are attained.

Control organisms are recommended for susceptibility testing. Each time the test is performed one or more of the following organisms should be included: *Escherichi coli* ATCC 15922, *Staphylococcus aureus* ATCC 25923 and *Pseudomonas aeruginosa* ATCC 27853. The control organisms should produce zones of inhibition within the following ranges:

Escherichia coli (ATCC 15922)	22-30 mm
Staphylococcus aureus (ATCC 25923)	22-31 mm
Pseudomonas aeruginosa (ATCC 27853)	17-23 mm

INDICATIONS AND USAGE

PARENTERAL

Kanamycin is indicated in the short-term treatment of serious infections caused by susceptible strains of the designated microorganisms below. Bacteriological studies to identify the causative organisms and to determine their susceptibility to Kanamycin should be performed. Therapy may be instituted prior to obtaining the results of susceptibility testing.

Kanamycin may be considered as initial therapy in the treatment of infections where one or more of the following are the known or suspected pathogens: *E. coli, Proteus* species (both indole-positive and indole-negative), *Enterobacter aerogenes, Klebsiella pneumoniae, Serratia marcescens, Acinetobacter* species. The decision to continue therapy with the drug should be based on results of the susceptibility tests, the response of the infection to therapy, and the important additional concepts contained in the "*Warnings*" box above.

In serious infections when the causative organisms are unknown, Kanamycin Sulfate may be administered as initial therapy in conjunction with a penicillin- or cephalosporin-type drug before obtaining results of susceptibility testing.

If anaerobic organisms are suspected, consideration should be given to using other suitable antimicrobial therapy in conjunction with Kanamycin.

Although Kanamycin is not the drug of choice for staphylococcal infections, it may be indicated under certain conditions for the treatment of known or suspected staphylococcal disease. These situations include the initial therapy of severe infections where the organism is thought to be either a Gram-negative bacterium or a staphylococcus, infections due to susceptible strains of staphylococci in patients allergic to other antibiotics, and mixed staphylococcal/Gram-negative infections.

◆ RATED THERAPEUTICALLY EQUIVALENT; ◇ THERAPEUTIC EQUIVALENCE UNCONFIRMED; ○ UNRATED

ORAL

Suppression of intestinal bacteria: Kanamycin is indicated when suppression of the normal bacterial flora of the bowel is desirable for short-term adjunctive therapy.

Hepatic Coma: Prolonged administration has been shown to be effective adjunctive therapy in *Hepatic Coma* by reduction of the ammonia-formin bacteria in the intestinal tract. The subsequent reduction in blood ammonia has resulted in neurologic improvement.

UNLABELED USES

Kanamycin Sulfate is used alone or as an adjunct in the treatment of endocarditis, gonococcal ophthalmia neonatorum, gonorrhea, and gram-negative septicemia. It is also used in severe gram-negative infections, including acute pyelonephritis, acute prostatitis, clolangeohepatitis, and appendix abscess. In addition, Kanamycin is also used in neonatal necrotizing enterocolitis, urinary tract infections, and to prevent wound infections.

CONTRAINDICATIONS

A history of hypersensitivity or toxic reaction to one aminoglycoside may also contraindicate the use of any other aminoglycoside, because of the known cross-sensitivity and cumulative effects of drugs in this category.

This drug is not indicated in long-term therapy (eg Tuberculosis) because of the toxic hazard associated with extended administration.

Oral Kanamycin Sulfate is contraindicated in the presence of intestinal obstruction.

WARNING

See *"Warning"* box above.

Aminoglycosides can cause fetal harm when administered to pregnant women. Aminoglycoside antibiotics cross the placenta and there have been several reports of total, irreversible, bilateral congenital deafness in children whose mothers received streptomycin during pregnancy. Although serious side effects to fetus or newborn have not been reported in treatment of pregnant women with other aminoglycosides, the potential for harm exists.

Reproductive studies have been performed in rats and rabbits and have revealed no evidence of impaired fertility or teratogenic effects. Dosages of 200 mg/kg/day in pregnant rats and pregnant guinea pigs led to hearing impairment in the off-spring. There are no well-controlled studies in pregnant women but clinical experience does not include any positive evidence of adverse effects on the fetus. However, if the drug is used during pregnancy, or if the patient becomes pregnant while taking this drug, the patient should be apprized of the potential hazard on the fetus.

Some brands contains sodium bisulfite, a sulfite that may cause allergic-type reactions including anaphylactic symptoms and life-threatening or less severe asthmatic episodes in certain susceptible people. The overall prevalence of sulfite sensitivity in the general population is unknown and probably low. Sulfite sensitivity is seen more frequently in asthmatic than in nonasthmatic people.

Although negligible amounts of orally administered Kanamycin are absorbed through intact intestinal mucosa (approximately 1 percent), the possibility of increased absorption from ulcerated or denuded areas should be considered. If renal insufficiency develops during treatment, the dosage should be reduced or the antibiotic discontinued. Urine and blood examinations and audiometric tests should be given prior to and during extended therapy in individuals with hepatic and/or renal disease.

PRECAUTIONS

GENERAL

Neurotoxic and nephrotoxic antibiotics may be almost completely absorbed from body surfaces (except the urinary bladder) after local irrigation and after topical application during surgical procedures. The potential toxic effects of antibiotics administered in this fashion (oto- and nephrotoxicity, neuromuscular blockade, respiratory paralysis) should be considered. (See *"Warning"* box).

Increased nephrotoxicity has been reported following concomitant administration of aminoglycoside antibiotics with some cephalosporins.

Aminoglycosides should be used with caution in patients with neuromuscular disorders such as myasthenia gravis, parkinsonism, or infant botulism, since these drugs may aggravate muscle weakness because of their potential curare-like effect on neuromuscular junction.

Elderly patients may have a decrease in renal function which may not be evident in the results of routine screening tests, such as BUN or serum creatinine levels. Measurement of creatinine clearance or an estimate based on published nomograms or equations may be more useful. Monitoring of renal function during treatment with Kanamycin, as with other aminoglycosides, is particularly important in such patients.

Because of high concentrations of Kanamycin Sulfate in the urinary excretory system, patients should be well hydrated before treatment to prevent irritation of the renal tubules.

Note: The risk of toxic reactions is low in well-hydrated patients with normal kidney function, who receive a total dose of 15 g of Kanamycin or less.

Treatment with Kanamycin may result in overgrowth of nonsusceptible organisms. If this occurs, Kanamycin should be discontinued and appropriate therapy initiated.

LABORATORY TESTS

Tests of eighth cranial nerve functions: Serial audiometric tests are suggested, particularly when renal function is impaired and/or prolonged aminoglycoside therapy is required; such tests should also be repeated periodically after treatment

if there is evidence of a hearing deficit or vestibular abnormalities before or during therapy; or when consecutive or concomitant use of other potentially ototoxic drug is unavoidable.

Test of renal function: It should be emphasized that since renal function may alter appreciably during therapy, renal function should be tested daily or more frequently. Urine should be examined for increased excretion of protein and for presence of cells and casts, keeping in mind the effects of the primary illness on these tests. One or more of the following laboratory measurements should be obtained at the onset of therapy, frequently during therapy, and at, or shortly after, the end of therapy:

Creatinine clearance rate (either carefully measured or estimated from published nomograms or equations based on patient's age, sex, body weight, and serial creatinine concentrations) (preferred over BUN).

Serum creatinine concentration (preferred over BUN).

Blood urea nitrogen (BUN).

More frequent testing is desirable if renal function is changing. If signs of renal irritation appear, such as casts, white or red cells, and albumin hydration should be increased and a reduction in dosage may be desirable (see *"Dosage and Administration"*). These signs usually disappear when treatment is completed. However, if azotemia or a progressive decrease of urine output occurs, treatment should be stopped.

Drug Interactions: In vitro mixing of an aminoglycoside with beta-lactam-type antibiotics (penicillins or cephalosporins) may result in a significant mutual inactivation. Even when an aminoglycoside and a penicillin-type drug are administered separately by different routes, a reduction in aminoglycoside serum half-life or serum levels has been reported in patients with impaired renal function and in some patients with normal renal function. Usually, such inactivation of the aminoglycoside is clinically significant only in patients with severely impaired renal function. (See also *"Laboratory Test Interactions"*).

See *"Warnings"* box regarding concurrent use of potent diuretics, concurrent and/or sequential use of other neurotoxic and/or nephrotoxic antibiotics, and for other essential information.

Laboratory Test Interactions: Concomitant cephalosporin therapy may spuriously elevate creatinine determinations.

The inactivation between aminoglycosides and beta-lactam antibiotics described in *"Drug Interactions"* may continue in specimens of body fluids collected for assay, resulting in inaccurate, false low aminoglycoside readings. Such specimens should be properly handled, ie, assayed promptly, frozen, or treated with beta-lactamase.

Carcinogenesis, Mutagenesis, Impairment of Fertility: Studies have not been performed with Kanamycin to determine its effect in carcinogenesis, mutagenesis, or impairment of fertility.

Pregnancy Category D: (See *"Warnings"* section.)

Nursing Mothers: Kanamycin Sulfate is excreted in minute amounts in human milk. Because of the potential for serious adverse reactions from aminoglycosides in nursing infants, a decision should be made whether to discontinue nursing or to discontinue the drug taking into account the importance of the drug to the mother.

Pediatric Use: Aminoglycosides should be used with caution in prematures and neonates because of the renal immaturity of these patients and the resulting prolongation of serum half-life of these drugs.

ADVERSE REACTIONS

Kanamycin has the potential to induce auditory and sometimes vestibular toxicity, renal toxicity, and neuromuscular blockade. The risks are higher for patients with a present or past history of renal impairment (especially if hemodialysis is required), for those receiving concomitant or sequential treatment with other ototoxic or nephrotoxic drugs or rapid acting diuretic agents given intravenously (ethacrynic acid, furosemide, and mannitol), and for patients treated for longer periods and/or with higher doses than recommended.

Ototoxicity: Toxic effects of Kanamycin on the eighth cranial nerve can result in partially reversible or irreversible bilateral loss of hearing, loss of balance, or both. Tinnitus or vertigo may or may not be experienced. Cochlear damage is usually manifested initially by small changes in audiometric test results at the high frequencies and may not be associated with subjective hearing loss. Vestibular dysfunction is usually manifested by nystagmus, vertigo, nausea, vomiting, or acute Meniere's syndrome.

Nephrotoxicity: Albuminuria, presence of red-and-white cells, and granular casts; azotemia and oliguria have been reported. Renal function changes are usually reversible when the drug is discontinued. Renal impairment may be characterized by a rise in serum creatinine and may be accompanied by oliguria, presence of casts, cells, and protein in the urine, by rising levels of BUN or by decrease in creatinine clearance.

Neuromuscular Blockade: Acute muscular paralysis and apnea can occur following treatment with aminoglycoside antibiotics. Neurotoxicity can occur after intrapleural and interperitoneal instillation of large doses of an aminoglycoside; however, the reaction has followed intravenous, intramuscular, and even the oral administration of these agents.

Other: Some local irritation or pain may follow the intramuscular injection of Kanamycin. Other adverse reactions of the drug reported on rare occasions are skin rash, drug fever, headache, paresthesia, nausea, vomiting, and diarrhea. The "malabsorption syndrome" characterized by an increase in fecal fat, decrease in serum carotene, and fall in xylose absorption, reportedly has occurred with prolonged parenteral or oral therapy. Nephrotoxicity and ototoxicity have been reported following prolonged and high dosage therapy in hepatic coma.

OVERDOSAGE
In the event of overdosage or toxic reaction, hemodialysis or peritoneal dialysis will aid in the removal of Kanamycin from the blood. In the newborn infant, exchange transfusion may also be considered.

DOSAGE AND ADMINISTRATION
PARENTERAL
Kanamycin Sulfate injection may be given intramuscularly or intravenously. The patient's pretreatment body weight should be obtained for calculation of the correct dosage. The dosage of an aminoglycoside in obese patients should be based on an estimate of the lean body mass. The status of renal function should be determined by measurement of serum creatinine concentration or calculation of the endogenous creatinine clearance rate. The blood urea nitrogen (BUN) level is much less reliable for this purpose. Renal function should be reassessed frequently during therapy.

It is desirable to measure both peak and trough serum concentrations intermittently during therapy since both concentrations are used to determine the adequacy and safety of the dose and to adjust the dosage during treatment. Peak serum concentrations (30 to 90 minutes after injection) above 35 µg per mL and trough concentrations (just prior to the next dose) above 10 µg per mL should be avoided.

Intramuscular Route: Inject deeply into the upper outer quadrant of the gluteal muscle. The recommended dose for adults or children is 15 mg/kg/day in two equally divided dosages administered at equally divided intervals; ie, 7.5 mg/kg q 12h. If continuously high blood levels are desired, the daily dose of 15 mg/kg may be given in equally divided doses every 6 or 8 hours.

Treatment of patients in the heavier weight classes, ie, 100 kg, should not exceed 1.5 g/day.

In patients with impaired renal function, it is desirable to follow therapy by appropriate serum assays. If this is not feasible, a suggested method is to reduce the frequency of administration in patients with renal dysfunction.

The interval between doses may be calculated with the following formula:
Serum creatinine (mg/100 ml) × 9 = Dosage interval (in hours); eg, if the serum creatinine is 2 mg, the recommended dose (7.5 mg/kg) should be administered every 18 hours. Changes in creatinine concentration during therapy would, of course, necessitate changes in the dosage frequency.

It is desirable to limit the duration of treatment with Kanamycin to short term. The usual duration of treatment is 7 to 10 days. Total daily dose by all routes of administration should not exceed 1.5 g/day. If longer therapy is required, measurement of Kanamycin peak and trough serum concentrations is particularly important as a basis for determining the adequacy and safety of the dose. These patients should be carefully monitored for changes in renal, auditory, and vestibular function. Dosage should be adjusted as needed. The risks of toxicity multiply as the length of treatment increases.

At the recommended dosage level, uncomplicated infections due to Kanamycin-susceptible organisms should respond to therapy in 24 to 48 hours. If definite clinical response does not occur within 3 to 5 days, therapy should be stopped and the antibiotic susceptibility pattern of the invading organism should be rechecked. Failure of the infection to respond may be due to resistance of the organism or to the presence of septic foci requiring surgical drainage.

Intravenous Administration: The dose should not exceed 15 mg/kg per day and must be administered slowly. The solution for intravenous use is prepared by adding the contents of a 500-mg vial to 100 to 200 ml of sterile diluent such as normal saline or 5% Dextrose in water, or the contents of a 1.0-g vial to 200 to 400 ml of sterile diluent. The appropriate dose is administered over a 30- to 60-minute period. The total daily dose should be divided into 2 or 3 equally divided doses.

In pediatric patients the amount of diluent used should be sufficient to infuse the Kanamycin Sulfate over a 30- to 60-minute period.

Kanamycin Sulfate injections should not be physically mixed with other antibacterial agents but each should be administered separately in accordance with its recommended route of administration and dosage schedule.

Intraperitoneal Use: (Following exploration for established peritonitis or after peritoneal contamination due to fecal spill during surgery.)

Adults: 500 mg diluted in 20 ml sterile distilled water may be instilled through a polyethylene catheter sutured into the wound at closure. If possible, instillation should be postponed until the patient has fully recovered from the effects of anesthesia and muscle-relaxing drugs (see duration of treatment statement above and ''Warning'' box). Serum levels should be carefully monitored during treatment.

Aerosol Treatment: 250 mg 2 to 4 times a day. Withdraw 250 mg (1.0 ml) and dilute it with 3 ml Physiological saline and nebulize.
Serum levels should be carefully monitored during treatment.

Other Routes of Administration: Kanamycin Sulfate injection in concentrations of 0.25% (2.5 mg/ml) has been used as an irrigating solution in abscess cavities, pleural space, peritoneal and ventricular cavities. Possible absorption of Kanamycin Sulfate by such routes must be taken into account and dosage adjustments should be arranged so that a maximum total dose of 1.5 g/day by all routes of administration is not exceeded. Serum levels should be carefully monitored during treatment.

PEDIATRIC DOSAGE GUIDE FOR KANAMYCIN SULFATE PEDIATRIC INJECTION, 75 MG/2 ML — AMOUNT PER 24 HOURS TO BE GIVEN IN DIVIDED DOSES

Weight in lb	Weight in kg	Daily Dosage in Milligrams	Daily Dosage in Milliliters
2.2	1.00	15.0	0.4
2.8	1.25	18.8	0.5
3.3	1.50	22.5	0.6
3.9	1.75	26.2	0.7
4.4	2.00	30.0	0.8
5.0	2.25	33.8	0.9
5.5	2.50	37.5	1.0
6.0	2.75	41.2	1.1
6.6	3.00	45.0	1.2
7.7	3.50	52.5	1.4
8.8	4.00	60.0	1.6
9.9	4.50	67.5	1.8
11.0	5.00	75.0	2.0

STABILITY
Occasionally, some vials may darken during the shelf life of the product, but this does not indicate a loss of potency.
Parenteral drug products should be inspected visually for particulate matter and discoloration prior to administration, whenever container and solution permit.

ORAL
Suppression of Intestinal Bacteria: 1. As an adjunct in therapy of hepatic coma for extended therapy: 8 to 12 g per day in divided doses.
2. As an adjunct to mechanical cleansing of the large bowel in short-term therapy: 1 g (2 capsules) every hour for 4 hours followed by 1 g (2 capsules) every 6 hours for 36 to 72 hours.
Duration of therapy within this range depends on the condition of the patient, the type and amount of concurrent mechanical cleansing (catharsis and enemas), and the customary medical routine.

J CODES
Up to 75 mg IM,IV—J1850
Up to 500 mg IM,IV—J1840

HOW SUPPLIED
CAPSULE: 500 MG

BRAND/MANUFACTURER	NDC	SIZE	AWP
○ **BRAND**			
KANTREX: Apothecon	00015-3506-25	20s	$41.29
	00015-3506-60	100s	$198.25

INJECTION: 75 MG/2 ML

BRAND/MANUFACTURER	NDC	SIZE	AWP
◆ **GENERICS**			
Solo Pak	39769-0065-02	2 ml 10s	$50.63

INJECTION: 75 MG

BRAND/MANUFACTURER	NDC	SIZE	AWP
◆ **BRAND**			
KANTREX: Apothecon	00015-3512-20	2 ml	$3.04

INJECTION: 500 MG/2 ML

BRAND/MANUFACTURER	NDC	SIZE	AWP
◆ **GENERICS**			
Solo Pak	39769-0064-02	2 ml 10s	$111.25

INJECTION: 500 MG

BRAND/MANUFACTURER	NDC	SIZE	AWP
◆ **BRAND**			
KANTREX: Apothecon	00015-3502-20	2 ml	$6.85

INJECTION: 1 GM

BRAND/MANUFACTURER	NDC	SIZE	AWP
◆ **BRAND**			
KANTREX: Apothecon	00015-3503-20	3 ml	$13.56

INJECTION: 1 GM/3 ML

BRAND/MANUFACTURER	NDC	SIZE	AWP
◆ **GENERICS**			
Solo Pak	39769-0063-05	3 ml 10s	$238.13

Kantrex *SEE* **KANAMYCIN SULFATE**

◆ RATED THERAPEUTICALLY EQUIVALENT; ◇ THERAPEUTIC EQUIVALENCE UNCONFIRMED; ○ UNRATED

Kaochlor SEE POTASSIUM CHLORIDE, ORAL

Kaon SEE POTASSIUM CHLORIDE AND POTASSIUM GLUCONATE

Kaon-Cl SEE POTASSIUM CHLORIDE, ORAL

Karidium SEE SODIUM FLUORIDE

Kato SEE POTASSIUM CHLORIDE, ORAL

Kay Ciel SEE POTASSIUM CHLORIDE, ORAL

Kayexalate SEE SODIUM POLYSTYRENE SULFONATE

Keflex SEE CEPHALEXIN

Keflin SEE CEPHALOTHIN SODIUM

Keftab SEE CEPHALEXIN

Kefurox SEE CEFUROXIME SODIUM

Kefzol SEE CEFAZOLIN SODIUM

Kemadrin SEE PROCYCLIDINE HYDROCHLORIDE

Kenalog SEE TRIAMCINOLONE ACETONIDE, INJECTABLE AND TRIAMCINOLONE ACETONIDE, TOPICAL

Kerlone SEE BETAXOLOL HYDROCHLORIDE, ORAL

Ketalar SEE KETAMINE HYDROCHLORIDE

Ketamine Hydrochloride

SPECIAL NOTE

EMERGENCE REACTIONS HAVE OCCURRED IN APPROXIMATELY 12 PERCENT OF PATIENTS

THE PSYCHOLOGICAL MANIFESTATIONS VARY IN SEVERITY BETWEEN PLEASANT, DREAM-LIKE STATES, VIVID IMAGERY, HALLUCINATIONS, AND EMERGENCE DELIRIUM. IN SOME CASES, THESE STATES HAVE BEEN ACCOMPANIED BY CONFUSION, EXCITEMENT, AND IRRATIONAL BEHAVIOR WHICH A FEW PATIENTS RECALL AS AN UNPLEASANT EXPERIENCE. THE DURATION ORDINARILY IS NO MORE THAN A FEW HOURS; IN A FEW CASES, HOWEVER, RECURRENCES HAVE TAKEN PLACE UP TO 24 HOURS POST-OPERATIVELY. NO RESIDUAL PSYCHOLOGICAL EFFECTS ARE KNOWN TO HAVE RESULTED FROM USE OF KETAMINE HYDROCHLORIDE.

THE INCIDENCE OF THESE EMERGENCE PHENOMENA IS LEAST IN THE YOUNG (15 YEARS OF AGE OR LESS) AND ELDERLY (OVER 65 YEARS OF AGE) PATIENT. ALSO, THEY ARE LESS FREQUENT WHEN THE DRUG IS GIVEN INTRAMUSCULARLY AND THE INCIDENCE IS REDUCED AS EXPERIENCE WITH THE DRUG IS GAINED.

THE INCIDENCE OF PSYCHOLOGICAL MANIFESTATIONS DURING EMERGENCE, PARTICULARLY DREAM-LIKE OBSERVATIONS AND EMERGENCE DELIRIUM, MAY BE REDUCED BY USING LOWER RECOMMENDED DOSAGES OF KETAMINE HYDROCHLORIDE IN CONJUNCTION WITH INTRAVENOUS DIAZEPAM DURING INDUCTION AND MAINTENANCE OF ANESTHESIA. (SEE *"DOSAGE AND ADMINISTRATION."*) ALSO, THESE REACTIONS MAY BE REDUCED IF VERBAL, TACTILE AND VISUAL STIMULATION OF THE PATIENT IS MINIMIZED DURING THE RECOVERY PERIOD. THIS DOES NOT PRECLUDE THE MONITORING OF VITAL SIGNS.

IN ORDER TO TERMINATE A SEVERE EMERGENCE REACTION, THE USE OF A SMALL HYPNOTIC DOSE OF A SHORT-ACTING OR ULTRASHORT-ACTING BARBITURATE MAY BE REQUIRED.

WHEN KETAMINE HYDROCHLORIDE IS USED ON AN OUTPATIENT BASIS, THE PATIENT SHOULD NOT BE RELEASED UNTIL RECOVERY FROM ANESTHESIA IS COMPLETE AND THEN SHOULD BE ACCOMPANIED BY A RESPONSIBLE ADULT.

DESCRIPTION

Ketamine Hydrochloride is a nonbarbiturate anesthetic chemically designated *dl* 2-(0-chlorophenyl)-2-(methylamino) cyclohexanone hydrochloride. It is formulated as a slightly acid (pH 3.5-5.5) sterile solution for intravenous or intramuscular injection in concentrations containing the equivalent of either 10, 50 or 100 mg Ketamine base per milliliter and contains not more than 0.1 mg/mL benzethonium chloride added as a preservative. The 10 mg/mL solution has been made isotonic with sodium chloride.

Following is its chemical structure:

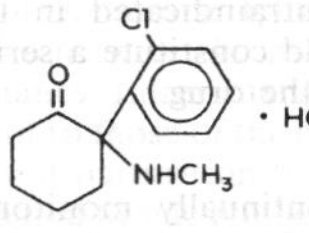

CLINICAL PHARMACOLOGY

Ketamine HCl is a rapid-acting general anesthetic producing an anesthetic state characterized by profound analgesia, normal pharyngeal-laryngeal reflexes, normal or slightly enhanced skeletal muscle tone, cardiovascular and respiratory stimulation, and occasionally a transient and minimal respiratory depression.

A patent airway is maintained partly by virtue of unimpaired pharyngeal and laryngeal reflexes. (See Warnings and Precautions.)

The biotransformation of Ketamine HCl includes N-dealkylation (metabolite I), hydroxylation of the cyclohexone ring (metabolites III and IV), conjugation with glucuronic acid and dehydration of the hydroxylated metabolites to form the cyclohexene derivative (metabolite II).

Following intravenous administration, the Ketamine concentration has an initial slope (alpha phase) lasting about 45 minutes with a half-life of 10 to 15 minutes. This first phase corresponds clinically to the anesthetic effect of the drug. The anesthetic action is terminated by a combination of redistribution from the CNS to slower equilibrating peripheral tissues and by hepatic biotransformation to metabolite I. This metabolite is about 1/3 as active as Ketamine in reducing halothane requirements (MAC) of the rat. The later half-life of Ketamine (beta phase) is 2.5 hours.

The anesthetic state produced by Ketamine has been termed "dissociative anesthesia" in that it appears to selectively interrupt association pathways of the brain before producing somesthetic sensory blockade. It may selectively depress the thalamoneocortical system before significantly obtunding the more ancient cerebral centers and pathways (reticular-activating and limbic systems).

Elevation of blood pressure begins shortly after injection, reaches a maximum within a few minutes and usually returns to preanesthetic values within 15 minutes after injection. In the majority of cases, the systolic and diastolic blood pressure peaks from 10% to 50% above preanesthetic levels shortly after induction of anesthesia, but the elevation can be higher or longer in individual cases (see Contraindications).

Ketamine has a wide margin of safety; several instances of unintentional administration of overdoses of Ketamine HCl (up to ten times that usually required) have been followed by prolonged but complete recovery.

Ketamine HCl has been studied in over 12,000 operative and diagnostic procedures, involving over 10,000 patients from 105 separate studies. During the course of these studies, Ketamine HCl was administered as the sole agent, as induction for other general agents, or to supplement low-potency agents.

Specific areas of application have included the following:

1. debridement, painful dressings, and skin grafting in burn patients, as well as other superficial surgical procedures;

2. neurodiagnostic procedures such as pneumonencephalograms, ventriculograms, myelograms, and lumbar punctures. See also Precaution concerning increased intracranial pressure.

3. diagnostic and operative procedures of the eye, ear, nose, and mouth, including dental extractions.

4. diagnostic and operative procedures of the pharynx, larynx, or bronchial tree. NOTE: Muscle relaxants, with proper attention to respiration, may be required (see Precautions).

5. sigmoidoscopy and minor surgery of the anus and rectum, and circumcision.

IS THEREFORE CONTRAINDICATED. SEE "CONTRAINDICATIONS", "WARNINGS," AND "PRECAUTIONS" SECTIONS.

DESCRIPTION

Ketoconazole is a synthetic, broad-spectrum, antifungal agent available for oral administration.

Ketoconazole is cis-1-acetyl-4-[4-[[2-(2,4-dichlorophenyl) -2-(1H-imidazol-1-yl-methyl)-1,3-dioxolan-4-yl] methoxyl]phenyl] piperazine.

Ketoconazole is a white to slightly beige, odorless powder, soluble in acids, with a molecular weight of 531.44.

Following is its chemical structure:

CLINICAL PHARMACOLOGY

Mean peak plasma levels of approximately 3.5 µg/mL are reached within 1 to 2 hours, following oral administration of a single 200 mg dose taken with a meal. Subsequent plasma elimination is biphasic with a half-life of 2 hours during the first 10 hours and 8 hours thereafter. Following absorption from the gastrointestinal tract, Ketoconazole is converted into several inactive metabolites. The major identified metabolic pathways are oxidation and degradation of the imidazole and piperazine rings, oxidative O-dealkylation and aromatic hydroxylation. About 13% of the dose is excreted in the urine, of which 2 to 4% is unchanged drug. The major route of excretion is through the bile into the intestinal tract. In vitro, the plasma protein binding is about 99% mainly to the albumin fraction. Only a negligible proportion of Ketoconazole reaches the cerebral-spinal fluid. Ketoconazole is a weak dibasic agent and thus requires acidity for dissolution and absorption.

Ketoconazole tablets are active against clinical infections with Blastomyces dermatitidis, Candida spp, Coccidioides immitis, Histoplasma capsulatum, Paracoccidioides brasiliensis, and Phialophora spp. Ketoconazole tablets are also active against Trichophyton spp, Epidermophyton spp., and Microsporum spp. Ketoconazole is also active in vitro against a variety of fungi and yeast. In animal models, activity has been demonstrated against Candida spp., Blastomyces dermatitidis, Histoplasma capsulatum, Malassezia furfur, Coccidioides immitis, and Cryptococcus neoformans.

Mode of Action: In vitro studies suggest that Ketoconazole impairs the synthesis of ergosterol, which is a vital component of fungal cell membranes.

INDICATIONS AND USAGE

Ketoconazole tablets are indicated for the treatment of the following systemic fungal infections: candidiasis, chronic mucocutaneous candidiasis, oral thrush, candiduria, blastomycosis, coccidioidomycosis, histoplasmosis, chromomycosis, and paracoccidioidomycosis Ketoconazole tablets should not be used for fungal meningitis because it penetrates poorly into the cerebral-spinal fluid.

Ketoconazole tablets are also indicated for the treatment of patients with severe recalcitrant cutaneous dermatophyte infections who have not responded to topical therapy or oral griseofulvin, or who are unable to take griseofulvin.

UNLABELED USES

Ketoconazole is used alone or as an adjunct in the treatment of fungal urinary infections caused by candida species, vulvovaginal candidiasis, and leishmaniasis, including Panamanian cutaneous leishmaniasis and visceral leishmaniasis. It is used in onychomycosis, ovarian hyperandrogenism, and precocious puberty unresponsive to LHRH-analogue therapy, as well as in the treatment and palliation of advanced prostatic cancer. Ketoconazole is prescribed in the treatment of pseudallsecheriasis caused by Petriellidium boydii infections and recalcitrant Tinea cruris, and is used in the long-term systemic treatment of chronic symptomatic Tinea pedis. It is also used to diminish the nephrotoxicity induced by cyclosporine in organ transplantation and to control hypercorticoidism associated with Cushing's disease.

CONTRAINDICATIONS

Coadministration of terfenadine or astemizole with ketoconazole tablets is contraindicated. (See box "Warning", "Warnings" and "Precautions" section.)

Ketoconazole is contraindicated in patients who have shown hypersensitivity to the drug.

WARNINGS

Hepatotoxicity, primarily of the hepatocellular type, has been associated with the use of Ketoconazole tablets, including rare fatalities. The reported incidence of hepatotoxicity has been about 1:10,000 exposed patients, but this probably represents some degree of under-reporting, as is the case for most reported adverse reactions to drugs. The median duration of Ketoconazole tablet therapy in patients who developed symptomatic hepatotoxicity was about 28 days, although the range extended to as low as 3 days. The hepatic injury has usually, but not always, been reversible upon discontinuation of Ketoconazole tablet treatment. Several cases of hepatitis have been reported in children.

Prompt recognition of liver injury is essential. Liver function tests (such as SGGT, alkaline phosphatase, SGPT, SGOT and bilirubin) should be measured before starting treatment and at frequent intervals during treatment. Patients receiving Ketoconazole tablets concurrently with other potentially hepatotoxic drugs should be carefully monitored, particularly those patients requiring prolonged therapy or those who have had a history of liver disease.

Most of the reported cases of hepatic toxicity have to date been in patients treated for onychomycosis. Of 180 patients worldwide developing idiosyncratic liver dysfunction during Ketoconazole tablet therapy, 61.3% had onychomycosis and 16.8% had chronic recalcitrant dermatophytoses.

Transient minor elevations in liver enzymes have occurred during treatment with Ketoconazole tablets. The drug should be discontinued if these persist, if the abnormalities worsen, or if the abnormalities become accompanied by symptoms of possible liver injury.

In rare cases anaphylaxis has been reported after the first dose: Several cases of hypersensitivity reactions including urticaria have also been reported.

Coadministration of Ketoconazole tablets and terfenadine has led to elevated plasma concentrations of terfenadine which may prolong QT intervals, sometimes resulting in life-threatening cardiac dysrhythmias. Cases of torsades de pointes and other serious ventricular dysrhythmias, in rare cases leading to fatality, have been reported among patients taking terfenadine concurrently with Ketoconazole tablets. Coadministration of Ketoconazole tablets and terfenadine is contraindicated.

Coadministration of astemizole with Ketoconazole tablets is contraindicated. (See "Box Warning, Contraindications, and Precautions" sections).

In European clinical trials involving 350 patients with metastatic prostatic cancer, eleven deaths were reported within two weeks of starting treatment with high doses of Ketoconazole tablets (1200 mg/day). It is not possible to ascertain from the information available whether death was related to Ketoconazole therapy in these patients with serious underlying disease. However, high doses of Ketoconazole tablets are known to suppress adrenal corticosteroid secretion.

In female rats treated three to six months with Ketoconazole at dose levels of 80 mg/kg and higher, increased fragility of long bones, in some cases leading to fracture, was seen. The maximum "no-effect" dose level in these studies was 20 mg/kg (2.5 times the maximum recommended human dose). The mechanism responsible for this phenomenon is obscure. Limited studies in dogs failed to demonstrate such an effect on the metacarpals and ribs.

PRECAUTIONS

General: Ketoconazole tablets have been demonstrated to lower serum testosterone. Once therapy with Ketoconazole has been discontinued, serum testosterone levels return to baseline values. Testosterone levels are impaired with doses of 800 mg per day and abolished by 1600 mg per day. Ketoconazole tablets also decrease ACTH-induced corticosteroid serum levels at similar high doses. The recommended dose of 200 mg-400 mg daily should be followed closely.

In four subjects with drug-induced achlorhydria, a marked reduction in Ketoconazole absorption was observed. Ketoconazole tablets require acidity for dissolution. If concomitant antacids, anti-cholinergics, and H_2-blockers are needed, they should be given at least two hours after administration of Ketoconazole tablets. In cases of achlorhydria, the patients should be instructed to dissolve each tablet in 4 mL aqueous solution of 0.2 N HCl. For ingesting the resulting mixture, they should use a drinking straw so as to avoid contact with the teeth. This administration should be followed with a cup of tap water.

Information for patients: Patients should be instructed to report any signs and symptoms which may suggest liver dysfunction so that appropriate biochemical testing can be done. Such signs and symptoms may include unusual fatigue, anorexia, nausea and/or vomiting, jaundice, dark urine or pale stools (see "Warnings").

Drug Interactions: When taken orally, imidazole compounds like Ketoconazole may enhance the anticoagulant effect of coumarin-like drugs. In simultaneous treatment with imidazole drugs and coumarin drugs, the anticoagulant effect should be carefully titrated and monitored.

Concomitant administration of rifampin with Ketoconazole tablets reduces the blood levels of the latter. INH (Isoniazid) is also reported to affect Ketoconazole concentrations adversely. These drugs should not be given concomitantly.

Ketoconazole tablets may alter the metabolism of cyclosporine and methylprednisolone, resulting in elevated plasma concentrations of the latter drugs. Dosage adjustment may be required if cyclosporine or methylprednisolone are given concomitantly with ketoconazole tablets.

Concomitant administration of Ketoconazole tablets with phenytoin may alter the metabolism of one or both of the drugs. It is suggested to monitor both Ketoconazole and phenytoin.

Because severe hypoglycemia has been reported in patients concomitantly receiving oral miconazole (an imidazole) and oral hypoglycemic agents, such a potential interaction involving the latter agents when used concomitantly with Ketoconazole tablets (an imidazole) can not be ruled out.

Ketoconazole tablets inhibit the metabolism of terfenadine, resulting in an increased plasma concentration of terfenadine and a delay in the elimination of its acid metabolite. The increased plasma concentration of terfenadine or its metabolite may result in prolonged QT intervals. (See box "Warning," "Contraindications", and "Warnings" sections.)

Pharmacokinetic data indicate that oral Ketoconazole inhibits the metabolism of astemizole, resulting in elevated plasma levels of astemizole and its active metabolite desmethylastemizole which may prolong QT intervals. Coadministration of astemizole and Ketoconazole tablets is therefore contraindicated. (See box "Warning", "Contraindications", and "Warnings" sections.)

After the coadministration of 200 mg oral Ketoconazole twice daily and one 20 mg of loratadine to 11 subjects, the AUC and C_{max} of loratadine averaged 302% ($\pm$ 142 S.D.) and 251% ($\pm$ 68 S.D.), respectively, of those obtained after cotreatment with placebo. The AUC and C_{max} of descarboethoxyloratadine, an active metabolite, averaged 155% ($\pm$ 27 S.D.) and 141% ($\pm$ 35 S.D.), respectively. However, no related changes were noted in the QT_c on ECG taken at 2, 6, and 24 hours after the coadministration. Also, there were no clinically significant differences in adverse events when loratadine was administered with or without Ketoconazole. Rare cases of a disulfiram-like reaction to alcohol have been reported. These experiences have been characterized by flushing, rash, peripheral edema, nausea, and headache. Symptoms resolved within a few hours.

Carcinogenesis, Mutagenesis, Impairment of Fertility: The dominant lethal mutation test in male and female mice revealed that single oral doses of Ketoconazole as high as 80 mg/kg produced no mutation in any stage of germ cell development. The *Ames Salmonella* microsomal activator assay was also negative. A long term feeding study in Swiss Albino mice and in Wistar rats showed no evidence of oncogenic activity.

Pregnancy: Teratogenic effects: Pregnancy Category C: Ketoconazole has been shown to be teratogenic (syndactylia and oligodactylia) in the rat when given in the diet at 80 mg/kg/day (10 times the maximum recommended human dose). However, these effects may be related to maternal toxicity, evidence of which also was seen at this and higher dose levels.

There are no adequate and well-controlled studies in pregnant women. Ketoconazole should be used during pregnancy only if the potential benefit justifies the potential risk to the fetus.

Nonteratogenic Effects: Ketoconazole has also been found to be embryotoxic in the rat when given in the diet at doses higher than 80 mg/kg during the first trimester of gestation. In addition, dystocia (difficult labor) was noted in rats administered oral Ketoconazole during the third trimester of gestation. This occurred when Ketoconazole was administered at doses higher than 10 mg/kg (higher than 1.25 times the maximum human dose).

It is likely that both the malformations and the embryotoxicity resulting from the administration of oral Ketoconazole during gestation are a reflection of the particular sensitivity of the female rat to this drug. For example, the oral LD_{50} of Ketoconazole given by gavage to the female rat is 166 mg/kg whereas in the male rat the oral LD_{50} is 287 mg/kg.

Nursing Mothers: Since Ketoconazole is probably excreted in the milk, mothers who are under treatment should not breast feed.

Pediatric Use: Ketoconazole tablets have not been systematically studied in children of any age, and essentially no information is available on children under 2 years. Ketoconazole should not be used in pediatric patients unless the potential benefit outweighs the risks.

ADVERSE REACTIONS

In rare cases, anaphylaxis has been reported after the first dose: Several cases of hypersensitivity reactions including urticaria have also been reported. However, the most frequent adverse reactions were nausea and/or vomiting in approximately 3%, abdominal pain in 1.2%, pruritus in 1.5%, and the following in less than 1% of the patients: headache, dizziness, somnolence, fever and chills, photophobia, diarrhea, gynecomastia, impotence, thrombocytopenia, leukopenia, hemolytic anemia, and bulging fontanelles. Oligospermia has been reported in investigational studies with the drug at dosages above those currently approved. Oligospermia has not been reported at dosages up to 400 mg daily, however sperm counts have been obtained infrequently in patients treated with these dosages. Most of these reactions were mild and transient and rarely required discontinuation of Ketoconazole tablets. In contrast, the rare occurrences of hepatic dysfunction require special attention (see "Warnings").

Neuropsychiatric disturbances, including suicidal tendencies and severe depression, have occurred rarely in patients using Ketoconazole tablets.

Ventricular dysrhythmias (prolonged QT intervals) have occurred with the concomitant use of terfenadine with Ketoconazole tablets. (See "Box Warning, Contraindications, and Warnings" sections.)

OVERDOSAGE

In the event of accidental overdosage, supportive measures, including gastric lavage with sodium bicarbonate, should be employed.

DOSAGE AND ADMINISTRATION

Adults: The recommended starting dose of Ketoconazole tablets is a single daily administration of 200 mg (one tablet). In very serious infections or if clinical responsiveness is insufficient within the expected time, the dose of Ketoconazole may be increased to 400 mg (two tablets) once daily.

Children: In small numbers of children over 2 years of age, a single daily dose of 3.3 to 6.6 mg/kg has been used. Ketoconazole tablets have not been studied in children under 2 years of age.

There should be laboratory as well as clinical documentation of infection prior to starting ketoconazole therapy. Treatment should be continued until tests indicate that active fungal infection has subsided. Inadequate periods of treatment may yield poor response and lead to early recurrence of clinical symptoms. Minimum treatment for candidiasis is one or two weeks. Patients with chronic mucocutaneous candidiasis usually require maintenance therapy. Minimum treatment for the other indicated systemic mycoses is six months.

Minimum treatment for recalcitrant dermatophyte infections is four weeks in cases involving glabrous skin. Palmar and plantar infections may respond more slowly. Apparent cures may subsequently recur after discontinuation of therapy in some cases.

Storage: Store at room temperature, 15°-30°C (59°-86°F).

HOW SUPPLIED
TABLETS: 200 MG

BRAND/MANUFACTURER	NDC	SIZE	AWP
BRAND			
NIZORAL: Janssen	50458-0220-10	100s	$258.26
	50458-0220-01	100s ud	$283.99

Ketoconazole, Topical

DESCRIPTION

Ketoconazole is a broad-spectrum synthetic antifungal agent, Ketoconazole, Topical, is available as a cream and a shampoo in 2% potency.

Ketoconazole is *cis*-1-acetyl-4-[4-[[2-(2,4-dichlorophenyl)-2- (1 *H*-imidazol-1-ylmethyl) 1,3-dioxolan-4-yl] methoxy] phenyl]piperazine.

Following is its chemical structure:

CLINICAL PHARMACOLOGY

When Ketoconazole cream was applied dermally to intact or abraded skin of beagle dogs for 28 consecutive days at a dose of 80 mg, there were no detectable plasma levels using an assay method having a lower detection limit of 2 ng/ml.

After a single topical application to the chest, back and arms of normal volunteers, systemic absorption of Ketoconazole was not detected at the 5 ng/ml level in blood over a 72-hour period.

Two dermal irritancy studies, a human sensitization test, a phototoxicity study and a photoallergy study conducted in 38 male and 62 female volunteers showed no contact sensitization of the delayed hypersensitivity type, no irritation, no phototoxicity and no photoallergenic potential due to Ketoconazole cream.

When Ketoconazole shampoo was applied dermally to intact or abraded skin of rabbits for 28 days at doses up to 50 mg/kg and allowed to remain one hour before being washed away, there were no detectable plasma Ketoconazole levels using an assay method having a lower detection limit of 5 ng/ml Ketoconazole was not detected in plasma in 39 patients who shampooed 4-10 times per week for 6 months or in 33 patients who shampooed 2-3 times per week for 3-26 months (mean: 16 months).

Twelve hours after a single shampoo, hair samples taken from six patients showed that high amounts of Ketoconazole were present on the hair but only about 5% had penetrated into the hair keratin. Chronic shampooing (twice weekly for two months) increased the Ketoconazole levels in the hair keratin to 20%, but did not increase levels on the hair. There were no detectable plasma levels.

An exaggerated use washing test on the sensitive antecubital skin of 10 subjects twice daily for five consecutive days showed that the irritancy potential of Ketoconazole shampoo was significantly less than that of 2.5% selenium sulfide shampoo.

A human sensitization test, a phototoxicity study, and a photallergy study conducted in 38 male and 22 female volunteers showed no contact sensitization of the delayed hypersensitivity type, no phototoxicity and no photoallergenic potential due to Ketoconazole shampoo.

Microbiology: Ketoconazole is a broad spectrum synthetic antifungal agent which inhibits the *in vitro* growth of the following common dermatophytes and yeasts by altering the permeability of the cell membrane: dermatophytes: *Trichophyton* rubrum, T. mentagrophytes, T. tonsurans, Microsporum canis, M. audouini, M. gypseum and Epidermophyton floccosum: yeasts: Candida albicans, Malassezia ovale (Pityrosporum ovale) and C. tropicalis; and the organism responsible for tinea versicolor, Malassezia furfur (Pityrosporum orbiculare). Only those organisms listed in the Section have been proven to be clinically affected. Development of resistance to Ketoconazole has not been reported.

Mode of Action: In vitro studies suggest that Ketoconazole impairs the synthesis of ergosterol, which is a vital component of fungal cell membranes. It is postulated that the therapeutic effect of Ketoconazole in seborrheic dermatitis and dandruff is due to the reduction of M. ovale, but this has not been proven.

Support for the latter hypothesis comes from a 4-week double-blind, placebo-controlled clinical trial, in which the decrease in *P. ovale* on the scalp was significantly greater with Ketoconazole (36 patients) than with placebo (20 patients) and was comparable to that with selenium sulfide (42 patients). In the same study, Ketoconazole and selenium sulfide reduced the severity of adherent dandruff significantly more than the placebo did. Ketoconazole produced significantly higher proportions of patients with at least 50% reductions in adherent dandruff (50% vs. 15%) and in loose dandruff (67% vs. 15%) than did the placebo.

INDICATIONS AND USAGE

Ketoconazole cream is indicated for the topical treatment of tinea corporis and tinea cruris and tinea pedis caused by *Trichophyton rubrum, T. mentagrophytes* and *Epidermophyton floccosum*: in the treatment of tinea (pityriasis) versicolor caused by *Malassezia furfur (Pityrosporum orbiculare)*; in the treatment of cutaneous candidiasis caused by *Candida spp* and in the treatment of seborrheic dermatitis.

Ketoconazole shampoo is indicated for the reduction of scaling due to dandruff.

UNLABELED USES

Ketoconazole is used alone or as an adjunct in the treatment of blepharitis.

CONTRAINDICATIONS

Ketoconazole cream and shampoo are contraindicated in persons who have shown hypersensitivity to the active or excipient ingredients of this formulation.

WARNINGS

Ketoconazole 2% cream is not for ophthalmic use.

Ketoconazole 2% cream contains sodium sulfite anhydrous, a sulfite that may cause allergic-type reactions including anaphylactic symptoms and life-threatening or less severe asthamatic episodes in certain susceptible people. The overall prevalence of sulfite sensitivity in the general population is unknown and probably low. Sulfite sensitivity is seen more frequently in asthmatic than in nonasthmatic people.

PRECAUTIONS

General: If a reaction suggesting sensitivity or chemical irritation should occur, use of the medication should be discontinued. Hepatitis (1:10,000 reported incidence) and, at high doses, lowered testosterone and ACTH induced corticosteroid serum levels have been seen with orally administered Ketoconazole; these effects have not been seen with topical Ketoconazole.

Information for Patients: May be irritating to mucous membranes of the eyes and contact with this area should be avoided.

There have been reports that use of the shampoo resulted in removal of the curl from permanently waved hair.

Carcinogenesis, Mutagenesis, Impairment of Fertility: A long-term feeding study in Swiss Albino mice and in Wistar rats showed no evidence of oncogenic activity. The dominant lethal mutation test in male and female mice revealed that single oral doses of Ketoconazole as high as 80 mg/kg produced no mutation in any stage of germ cell development. The Ames' *Salmonella* microsomal activator assay was also negative.

Pregnancy: Teratogenic effects: Pregnancy Category C: Ketoconazole is not detected in plasma after chronic shampooing. Ketoconazole has been shown to be teratogenic (syndactylia and oligodactylia) in the rat when given orally in the diet at 80 mg/kg/day (10 times the maximum recommended human oral dose). However, these effects may be related to maternal toxicity, which was seen at this and higher dose levels.

There are no adequate and well-controlled studies in pregnant women. Ketoconazole should be used during pregnancy only if the potential benefit justifies the potential risk to the fetus.

Nursing Mothers: It is not known whether Ketoconazole cream administered topically could result in sufficient systemic absorption to produce detectable quantities in breast milk. Nevertheless, a decision should be made whether to discontinue nursing or discontinue the drug, taking into account the importance of the drug to the mother. Ketoconazole is not detected in plasma after chronic shampooing. Nevertheless, caution should be exercised when Ketoconazole shampoo is administered to a nursing woman.

Pediatric Use: Safety and effectiveness in children have not been established.

ADVERSE REACTIONS

During clinical trials 45 (5.0%) of 905 patients treated with Ketoconazole cream and 5 (2.4%) of 208 patients treated with placebo reported side effects consisting mainly of severe irritation, pruritus and stinging. One of the patients treated with Ketoconazole cream developed a painful allergic reaction.

In 11 double-blind trials in 264 patients using Ketoconazole shampoo, an increase in normal hair loss and irritation occurred in less than 1% of patients. In three open-label safety trials in which 41 patients shampooed 4-10 times weekly for six months, the following adverse experiences each occurred once: abnormal hair texture, scalp pustules, mild dryness of the skin, and itching. As with other shampoos, oilness and dryness of hair and scalp have been reported.

OVERDOSAGE

Ketoconazole shampoo is intended for external use only. In the event of ingestion, supportive measures, including gastric lavage with sodium bicarbonate, should be employed.

DOSAGE AND ADMINISTRATION

KETOCONAZOLE CREAM

Cutaneous candidiasis, tinea corporis, tinea cruris, and tinea (pityriasis) versicolor: It is recommended that Ketoconazole cream be applied once daily to cover the affected and immediate surrounding area. Clinical improvement may be seen fairly soon after treatment is begun; however, candidal infections and tinea cruris and corporis should be treated for two weeks in order to reduce the possibility of recurrence. Patients with tinea versicolor usually require two weeks of treatment. Patients with tinea pedis require six weeks of treatment.

Seborrheic dermatitis: Ketoconazole cream should be applied to the affected area twice daily for four weeks or until clinical clearing.

If a patient shows no clinical improvement after the treatment period, the diagnosis should be redetermined.

KETOCONAZOLE SHAMPOO

1. Moisten hair and scalp thoroughly with water.
2. Apply sufficient shampoo to produce enough lather to wash the scalp and hair and gently massage it over the entire scalp area for approximately 1 minute.
3. Rinse the hair thoroughly with warm water.
4. Repeat, leaving the shampoo on the scalp for an additional 3 minutes.
5. After the second thorough rinse, dry the hair with a towel or warm air flow.

Shampoo twice a week for four weeks with at least three days between each shampooing, then intermittently as needed to maintain control.

Storage conditions: Store shampoo at a temperature not above 25° C (77°F). Protect from light.

HOW SUPPLIED

CREAM: 2%

BRAND/MANUFACTURER	NDC	SIZE	AWP
○ **BRAND**			
NIZORAL: Janssen	50458-0221-15	15 gm	$12.89
	50458-0221-30	30 gm	$21.66
	50458-0221-60	60 gm	$32.92

SHAMPOO: 2%

BRAND/MANUFACTURER	NDC	SIZE	AWP
○ **BRAND**			
NIZORAL: Janssen	50458-0223-04	120 ml	$15.92

Ketoprofen

DESCRIPTION

Ketoprofen is a nonsteroidal anti-inflammatory drug. The chemical name for Ketoprofen is 2-(3-benzoylphenyl)-propionic acid.

Its empirical formula is $C_{16}H_{14}O_3$, with a molecular weight of 254.29. It has a pKa of 5.94 in methanol:water (3:1) and an n-octanol:water partition coefficient of 0.97 (buffer pH 7.4). Ketoprofen is a white or off-white, odorless, nonhygroscopic, fine to granular powder, melting at about 95°C. It is freely soluble in ethanol, chloroform, acetone, ether and soluble in benzene and strong alkali, but practically insoluble in water at 20°C.

Ketoprofen capsules contain 25 mg, 50 mg, or 75 mg of Ketoprofen for oral administration. Each Ketoprofen extended release capsule contain 200 mg of Ketoprofen in the form of hundreds of coated pellets. The dissolution of the pellets is pH dependent with optimum dissolution occurring at pH 6.5-7.5. There is no dissolution at pH 1.

Following is its chemical structure:

CLINICAL PHARMACOLOGY

Ketoprofen is a nonsteroidal anti-inflammatory drug with analgesic and antipyretic properties.

The anti-inflammatory, analgesic, and antipyretic properties of Ketoprofen have been demonstrated in classical animal and *in vitro* test systems. In anti-inflammatory models Ketoprofen has been shown to have inhibitory effects on prostaglandin and leukotriene synthesis, to have antibradykinin activity, as well as to have lysosomal membrane-stabilizing action. However, its mode of action, like that of other nonsteroidal anti-inflammatory drugs, is not fully understood.

PHARMACODYNAMICS

Ketoprofen is a racemate with only the S enantiomer possessing pharmacological activity. The enantiomers have similar concentration time curves and do not appear to interact with one another.

An analgesic effect-concentration relationship for Ketoprofen was established in an oral surgery pain study with Ketoprofen. The effect-site rate constant (k_{e0}) was estimated to be 0.9 hour^{-1} (95% confidence limits: 0 to 2.1), and the concentration (Ce_{50}) of Ketoprofen that produced one-half the maximum PID (pain intensity difference) was 0.3 µg/mL (95% confidence limits: 0.1 to 0.5). Thirty-three (33) to 68% of patients had an onset of action (as measured by reporting some pain relief) within 30 minutes following a single oral dose in postoperative pain and dysmenorrhea studies. Pain relief (as measured by remedication) persisted for up to 6 hours in 26 to 72% of patients in these studies.

PHARMACOKINETICS

GENERAL

Ketoprofen and Ketoprofen extended release capsules both contain Ketoprofen. They differ only in their release characteristics Ketoprofen capsules release drug in the stomach whereas the pellets in Ketoprofen extended release capsules are designed to resist dissolution in the low pH of gastric fluid but release drug at a controlled rate in the higher pH environment of the small intestine (see "Description").

Irrespective of the pattern of release, the systemic availability (F_s) when either oral formulation is compared with IV administration is approximately 90% in humans. For 75 to 200 mg single doses, the area under the curve has been shown to be dose proportional. The figure depicts the plasma time curves associated with both products.

Ketoprofen is > 99% bound to plasma proteins, mainly to albumin.

Separate sections follow which dellheate differences between Ketoprofen and Ketoprofen extended release capsules.

ABSORPTION

Ketoprofen capsules—Ketoprofen is rapidly and well-absorbed, with peak plasma levels occurring within 0.5 to 2 hours.

Ketoprofen extended release capsules—Ketoprofen is also well-absorbed from this dosage form, although an observable increase in plasma levels does not occur until approximately 2 to 3 hours after taking the formulation. Peak plasma levels are usually reached 6 to 7 hours after dosing. (See Table, below).

When Ketoprofen is administered with food, its total bioavailability (AUC) is not altered; however, the rate of absorption from either dosage form is slowed.

Ketoprofen capsules—Food intake reduces C_{max} by approximately one-half and increases the mean time to peak concentration (t_{max}) from 1.2 hours for fasting subjects (range, 0.5 to 3 hours) to 2.0 hours for fed subjects (range, 0.75 to 3 hours). The fluctuation of plasma peaks may also be influenced by circadian changes in the absorption process.

Concomitant administration of magnesium hydroxide and aluminum hydroxide does not interfere with absorption of Ketoprofen from Ketoprofen capsules

Ketoprofen extended release capsules—Administration of Ketoprofen with a high-fat meal causes a delay of about 2 hours in reaching the C_{max}: neither the total bioavailability (AUC) nor the C_{max} is affected. Circardian changes in the absorption process have not been studied.

The administration of antacids or other drugs which may raise stomach pH would not be expected to change the rate or extent of absorption of Ketoprofen from Ketoprofen extended release capsules.

MULTIPLE DOSING

Steady-state concentrations of Ketoprofen are attained within 24 hours after commencing treatment with Ketoprofen or Ketoprofen extended release capsules. In studies with healthy male volunteers, trough levels at 24 hours following administration of Ketoprofen capsules were 0.4 mg/L compared with 0.07 mg/L at 24 hours following administration of Ketoprofen 50 mg capsules QID (12 hours) or 0.13 mg/L following administration of Ketoprofen 75 mg capsules TID for 12 hours. Thus, relative to the peak plasma concentration, the accumulation of Ketoprofen after multiple doses of Ketoprofen extended release or Ketoprofen capsules is minimal.

A reduction in peak concentration and its duration occurs after the second 50 mg dose. This is probably due to a combination of food effects, circadian effects, and plasma sampling times. It is unclear to what extent each factor contributes to the loss.

COMPARISON OF PHARMACOKINETIC PARAMETERS FOR KETOPROFEN AND KETOPROFEN EXTENDED RELEASE

Kinetic Parameters	Ketoprofen (4 × 50 mg)	Ketoprofen extended release (1 × 200 mg)
Extent of oral absorption (bioavailability) F_s (%)	~90	~90

Kinetic Parameters	Ketoprofen (4 × 50 mg)	Ketoprofen extended release (1 × 200 mg)
Peak plasma levels C_{max} (mg/L)		
Fasted	3.9±1.3	3.1±1.2
Fed	2.4±1.0	3.4±1.3
Time to peak concentration t_{max} (h)		
Fasted	1.2±0.6	6.8±2.1
Fed	2.0±0.8	9.2±2.6
Area under plasma concentration-time curve AUC_{0-24h} (mg h/L)		
Fasted	32.1±7.2	30.1±7.9
Fed	36.6±8.1	31.3±8.1
Oral-dose clearance CL/F (L/h)	6.9±0.8	6.8±1.8
Half-life $t_{1/2}$ (h) [See footnote 1]	2.1±1.2 +t3	5.4±2.2

\# Values expressed are mean ± standard deviation
[1] In the case of Ketoprofen extended release absorption is slowed, intrinsic clearance is unchanged, but because the rate of elimination is dependent on absorption, the half-time is prolonged.

METABOLISM

The metabolic fate of Ketoprofen is glucuronide conjugation to form an unstable acyl-glucuronide. The glucuronic acid moiety can be converted back to the parent compound. Thus, the metabolite serves as a potential reservoir for parent drug and this may be important in persons with renal insufficiency, whereby the conjugate may accumulate in the serum and undergo deconjugation back to the parent drug (see "Special Populations: Renally impaired"). The conjugates are reported to appear only in trace amounts in plasma in healthy adults, but are higher in elderly subjects—presumably because of reduced renal clearance. It has been demonstrated that in elderly subjects following multiple doses (50 mg every 6 h), the ratio of conjugated to parent Ketoprofen AUC was 30% and 3%, respectively for the S & R enantiomers.

There are no known active metabolites of Ketoprofen. Ketoprofen has been shown not to induce drug-metabolizing enzymes.

ELIMINATION

The plasma clearance of Ketoprofen is approximately 0.08 L/kg/h with a V_d of 0.1 L/kg after IV administration. The elimination half-life of Ketoprofen has been reported to be 2.05±0.58 h (Mean ± S.D.) following IV administration, from 2 to 4 h following administration of Ketoprofen extended release capsules, and 5.4±2.2 h after administration of Ketoprofen extended release capsules, in cases of slow drug absorption, the elimination rate is dependent on the absorption rate and thus $t_{1/2}$ relative to an IV dose appears prolonged.

After a single 200 mg dose of Ketoprofen extended release, the plasma levels decline slowly, and average 0.4 mg/L after 24 hours (see Figure above).

In a 24-hour period, approximately 80% of an administered dose of Ketoprofen is excreted in the urine, primarily as the glucuronide metabolite.

Enterohepatic recirculation of the drug has been postulated, although biliary levels have never been measured to confirm this.

SPECIAL POPULATIONS

ELDERLY: CLEARANCE AND UNBOUND FRACTION

The plasma and renal clearance of Ketoprofen is reduced in the elderly (mean age, 73 years) compared to a younger normal population (mean age, 27 years). Hence, Ketoprofen peak concentration and AUC increase with increasing age. In addition, there is a corresponding increase in unbound fraction with increasing age. Data from one trial suggest that the increase is greater in women than in men. It has not been determined whether age-related changes in absorption among the elderly contribute to the changes in bioavailability of Ketoprofen.

Ketoprofen capsules—In a study conducted with young and elderly men and women, results for subjects older than 75 years of age showed that free drug AUC increased by 40% and C_{max} increased by 60% as compared with estimates of the same parameters in young subjects (those younger than 35 years of age; see "Individualization of Dosage").

Also in the elderly, the ratio of intrinsic clearance/availability decreased by 35% and plasma half-life was prolonged by 26%. This reduction is thought to be due to a decrease in hepatic extraction associated with aging.

Ketoprofen extended release capsules—The effects of age and gender on Ketoprofen disposition were investigated in 2 small studies in which elderly male and female subjects received Ketoprofen extended release capsules. The results were compared with those from another study conducted in healthy young men.

Compared to the younger subject group, the elimination half-life in the elderly was prolonged by 54% and total drug C_{max} and AUC were 40% and 70% higher, respectively. Plasma concentrations in the elderly after single doses and at steady state were essentially the same. Thus, no drug accumulation occurs.

In comparison to younger subjects taking the immediate-release formulation of Ketoprofen there was a decrease of 16% and 25% in total drug C_{max} and AUC,

► SHOWN IN PRODUCT IDENTIFICATION GUIDE

respectively, among the elderly. Free drug data are not available for Ketoprofen extended release.

RENALLY IMPAIRED
Studies of the effects of renal-function impairment have been small. They indicate a decrease in clearance in patients with impaired renal function. In 23 patients with renal impairment, free Ketoprofen peak concentration was not significantly elevated, but free Ketoprofen clearance was reduced from 15 L/h/kg for normal subjects to 7 L/h/kg in patients with mildly impaired renal function, and to 4 L/h/kg in patients with moderately to severely impaired renal function. The elimination $t_{1/2}$ was prolonged form 1.6 hours in normal subjects to approximately 3 hours in patients with mild renal impairment, and to approximately 5 to 9 hours in patients with moderately to severely impaired renal function. No studies have been conducted in patients with renal impairment taking Ketoprofen extended release capsules. It is recommended that only the immediate-release formulation of Ketoprofen be used to treat patients with significant renal impairment (see "Individualization of Dosage").

HEPATICALLY IMPAIRED
For patients with alcoholic cirrhosis, no significant changes in the kinetic disposition of Ketoprofen capsules were observed relative to age-matched normal subjects: the plasma clearance of drug was 0.07 L/h/kg in 26 hepatically impaired patients. The elimination half-time was comparable to that observed for normal subjects. However, the unbound (biologically active) fraction was approximately doubled, probably due to hypoalbuminemia and high variability which was observed in the pharmacokinetics for cirrhotic patients. Therefore, these patients should be carefully monitored and daily doses of Ketoprofen kept at the minimum providing the desired therapeutic effect.

No studies have been conducted in patients with heptic impairment taking Ketoprofen extended release capsules. It is recommended that only the immediate-release formulation of Ketoprofen be used to treat patients who have hepatic impairment and serum albumin levels below 3.5 g/dL. (See "Individualization of Dosage".)

CLINICAL TRIALS
RHEUMATOID ARTHRITIS AND OSTEOARTHRITIS
The efficacy of Ketoprofen has been demonstrated in patients with rheumatoid arthritis and osteoarthritis. Using standard assessments of therapeutic response, there were no detectable differences in effectiveness or in the incidence of adverse events in crossover comparison of Ketoprofen and Ketoprofen extended release In other trials, Ketoprofen demonstrated effectiveness comparable to aspirin, ibuprofen, naproxen, piroxicam, diclofenac and indomethacin. In some of these studies there were more dropouts due to gastrointestinal side effects among patients on Ketoprofen than among patients on other NSAIDs.

In studies with patients with rheumatoid arthritis, Ketoprofen was administered in combination with gold salts, antimalarials, low-dose methotrexate, d-pencillamine, and/or corticosteroids with results comparable to those seen with control nonsteroidal drugs.

MANAGEMENT OF PAIN
The effectiveness of Ketoprofen as a general-purpose analgesic has been studied in standard pain models which have shown the effectiveness of doses of 25 to 150 mg. Doses of 25 mg were superior to placebo. Doses larger than 25 mg generally could not be shown to be significantly more effective, but there was a tendency toward faster onset and greater duration of action with 50 mg, and, in the case of dysmenorrhea, a significantly greater effect overall with 75 mg. Doses greater than 50 to 75 mg did not have increased analgesic effect. Studies in postoperative pain have shown that Ketoprofen in doses of 25 to 100 mg was comparable to 650 mg of acetaminophen with 60 mg of codeine, or 650 mg of acetaminophen with 10 mg of oxycodone. Ketoprofen tended to be somewhat slower in onset; peak pain relief was about the same and the duration of the effect tended to be 1 to 2 hours longer, particularly with the higher doses of Ketoprofen.

The use of Ketoprofen extended release in patients with acute pain is not recommended, since, in comparison to Ketoprofen, Ketoprofen extended release would be expected to have a delayed analgesic response due to its controlled-release characteristics.

INDIVIDULIZATION OF DOSAGE
In patients with significant renal impairment Ketoprofen rather than Ketoprofen extended release should be used.

The initial dosage should be reduced to 25 to 50 mg TID in patients with mildly impaired renal function and to 25 to 50 mg twice daily (BID) in patients with a more severe renal impairment (GFR less than 25 mL/min/1.73m^2 or end-stage renal impairment). In elderly patients, renal function may be reduced with apparently normal serum creatinine and/or BUN levels.

Therefore, Ketoprofen is the recommended formulation of Ketoprofen and the initial dosage for patients over 75 years of age should be reduced to 75 to 150 mg/day.

It is recommended that for patients with impaired liver function and serum albumin concentration less than 3.5 g/dL, Ketoprofen rather than Ketoprofen should be used and the initial dosage reduced to 75 to 150 mg/day. All patients with metabolic impairment, particularly those with both hypoalbuminemia and reduced renal function, may have increased levels of free (biologically active) Ketoprofen and should be closely monitored. The dosage may be increased to the range recommended for the general population, if necessary, only after good individual tolerance has been ascertained.

Because hypoalbuminemia and reduced renal function both increase the fraction of free drug (biologically active form), patients who have both conditions may be at greater risk of adverse effects. Therefore, it is recommended that such patients also be started on lower doses of Ketoprofen and closely monitored.

As with other nonsteroidal anti-inflammatory drugs, the predominant adverse effects of Ketoprofen are gastrointestinal. To attempt to minimize these effect, physicians may wish to prescribe that either Ketoprofen formulation be taken with antacids, food, or milk. Although food delays the absorption of both formulations (see "Clinical Pharmacology"), in most of the clinical trials Ketoprofen was taken with food or milk.

Physicians may want to make specific recommendations to patients about when they should take Ketoprofen or Ketoprofen extended release in relation to food and/or what patients should do if they experience minor GI symptoms associated with either formulation.

INDICATIONS AND USAGE
Ketoprofen or Ketoprofen extended release are indicated for the management of the signs and symptoms of rheumatoid arthritis and osteoarthritis. Ketoprofen extended release is not recommended for treatment of acute pain because of its controlled-release characteristics (see "Pharmacokinetics").

Ketoprofen is indicated for the management of pain Ketoprofen is also indicated for treatment of primary dysmenorrhea.

CONTRAINDICATIONS
Ketoprofen is contraindicated in patients who have shown hypersensitivity to it. Ketoprofen should not be given to patients in whom aspirin or other nonsteroidal anti-inflammatory drugs induce asthma, urticaria, or other allergic-type reactions, because severe, rarely fatal, anaphylactic reactions to Ketoprofen have been reported in such patients.

WARNINGS
RISK OF GI ULCERATION, BLEEDING, AND PERFORATION WITH NSAID THERAPY
Serious gastrointestinal toxicity, such as bleeding, ulceration, and perforation, can occur at any time with or without warning symptoms, in patients treated chronically with NSAID therapy. Although minor upper-gastrointestinal problems, such as dyspepsia, are common, usually developing early in therapy, physicians should remain alert for ulceration and bleeding in patients treated chronically with NSAIDs even in the absence of previous GI-tract symptoms. In patients observed in clinical trials of several months to two years' duration, symptomatic upper-GI ulcers, gross bleeding, or perforation appear to occur in approximately 1% of patients treated for 3 to 6 months, and in about 2-4% of patients treated for one year. Physicians should inform patients about the signs and/or symptoms of serious GI toxicity and what steps to take if they occur.

Studies to date have not identified any subset of patients not at risk of developing peptic ulceration and bleeding. Except for a prior history of serious GI events and other risk factors known to be associated with peptic ulcer disease, such as alcoholism, smoking, etc., no other risk factors (e.g., age, sex) have been associated with increased risk. Elderly or debilitated patients seem to tolerate ulceration or bleeding less well than other individuals, and most spontaneous reports of fatal GI events are in this population. Studies to date are inconclusive concerning the relative risk of various NSAIDs in causing such reactions. High doses of any NSAID probably carry a greater risk of these reactions, although controlled clinical trials showing this do not exist in most cases. In considering the use of relatively large doses (within the recommended dosage range), sufficient benefit should be anticipated to offset the potential increased risk of GI toxicity.

GENERAL PRECAUTIONS
Ketoprofen and other nonsteroidal anti-inflammatory drugs cause nephritis in mice and rats associated with chronic administration. Rare cases of interstitial nephritis or nephrotic syndrome have been reported in humans with Ketoprofen since it has been marketed.

A second form of renal toxicity has been seen in patients with conditions leading to a reduction in renal blood flow or blood volume, where renal prostaglandins have a supportive role in the maintenance of renal blood flow. In these patients, administration of a nonsteroidal anti-inflammatory drug results in a dose-dependent decrease in prostaglandin synthesis and, secondarily, in renal blood flow which may precipitate overt renal failure. Patients at greatest risk of this reaction are those with impaired renal function, heart failure, liver dysfunction, those taking diuretics, and the elderly. Discontinuation of nonsteroidal anti-inflammatory drug therapy is typically followed by recovery to the pretreatment state.

Since Ketoprofen is primarily eliminated by the kidneys and its pharmacokinetics are altered by renal failure (see "Clinical Pharmacology"), patients with significantly impaired renal function should be closely monitored, and a reduction of dosage should be anticipated to avoid accumulation of Ketoprofen and/or its metabolites (see "Individualization of Dosage").

As with other nonsteroidal anti-inflammatory drugs, borderline elevations of one or more liver function tests may occur in up to 15% of patients. These abnormalities may progress, may remain essentially unchanged, or may disappear with continued therapy. The ALT (SGPT) test is probably the most sensitive indicator of liver dysfunction. Meaningful (3 times the upper limit of normal) elevations of ALT or AST (SGOT) occurred in controlled clinical trials in less than 1% of patients. A patient with symptoms and/or signs suggesting liver dysfunction, or in whom an abnormal liver test has occurred, should be evaluated for evidence of the development of a more severe hepatic reaction while on therapy with Ketoprofen. Serious hepatic reactions, including jaundice, have been

---

reported from post-marketing experience with Ketoprofen as well as with other nonsteroidal anti-inflammatory drugs.

In patients with chronic liver disease with reduced serum albumin levels, Ketoprofen's pharmacokinetics are altered (see *"Clinical Pharmacology"*). Such patients should be closely monitored, and a reduction of dosage should be anticipated to avoid high blood levels of Ketoprofen and/or its metabolites (see *"Individualization of Dosage"*).

If steroid dosage is reduced or eliminated during therapy, it should be reduced slowly and the patients observed closely for any evidence of adverse effects, including adrenal insufficiency and exacerbation of symptoms of arthritis.

Anemia is commonly observed in rheumatoid arthritis and is sometimes aggravated by nonsteroidal anti-inflammatory drugs, which may produce fluid retention or significant gastrointestinal blood loss in some patients. Patients on long-term treatment with NSAIDs, including Ketoprofen or Ketoprofen extended release should have their hemoglobin or hematocrit checked if they develop signs or symptoms of anemia.

Peripheral edema has been observed in approximately 2% of patients taking Ketoprofen. Therefore, as with other nonsteroidal anti-inflammatory drugs, Ketoprofen should be used with caution in patients with fluid retention, hypertension, or heart failure.

INFORMATION FOR PATIENTS
Ketoprofen or Ketoprofen extended release contain Ketoprofen. Like other drugs of its class, Ketoprofen is not free of side effects. The side effects of these drugs can cause discomfort and, rarely, there are more serious side effects, such as gastrointestinal bleeding, which may result in hospitalization and even fatal outcomes.

NSAIDs are often essential agents in the management of arthritis and have a major role in the treatment of pain, but they also may be commonly employed for conditions which are less serious. Physicians may wish to discuss with their patients the potential risks (see *"Warnings"*, *"General Precautions"*, and *"Adverse Reactions"* sections) and likely benefits of NSAID treatment, particularly when the drugs are used for less serious conditions where treatment without NSAIDs may represent an acceptable alternative to both the patient and physician.

Because aspirin causes an increase in the level of unbound Ketoprofen, patients should be advised not to take aspirin while taking Ketoprofen (see *"Drug Interactions"*). It is possible that minor adverse symptoms of gastric intolerance may be prevented by administering Ketoprofen with antacids, food, or milk. Ketoprofen extended release has not been studied with antacids. Because food and milk do alter the rate but not the extent of absorption (see *"Clinical Pharmacology"*) physicians may want to make specific recommendations to patients about when they should take Ketoprofen in relation to food and/or what patients should do if they experience minor GI symptoms associated with Ketoprofen therapy.

LABORATORY TESTS
Because serious GI-tract ulceration and bleeding can occur without warning symptoms, physicians should follow chronically treated patients for the signs and symptoms of ulceration and bleeding and should inform them of the importance of this follow-up (see *"Warnings—Risk of GI Ulceration, Bleeding, and Perforation with Nsaid Therapy"*).

DRUG INTERACTIONS
The following drug interactions were studied with Ketoprofen doses of 200 mg/day. The possibility of increased interaction should be kept in mind when Ketoprofen does greater than 50 mg as a single dose or 200 mg of Ketoprofen per day are used concomitantly with highly bound drugs.

1. ANTACIDS
Concomitant administration of magnesium hydroxide and aluminum hydroxide does not interfere with the rate or extent of the absorption of Ketoprofen administered as Orudis.

2. ASPIRIN
Ketoprofen does not alter aspirin absorption; however, in a study of 12 normal subjects, concurrent administration of aspirin decreased Ketoprofen protein binding and increased Ketoprofen plasma clearance from 0.07 L/h/kg without aspirin to 0.11 L/h/kg with aspirin. The clinical significance of these changes has not been adequately studied. Therefore, concurrent use of aspirin and Ketoprofen is not recommended.

3. DIURETIC
Hydrochlorothiazide, given concomitantly with Ketoprofen, produces a reduction in urinary potassium and chloride excretion compared to hydrochlorothiazide alone. Patients taking diuretics are at greater risk of developing renal failure secondary to a decrease in renal blood flow caused by prostaglandin inhibition (see *"General Precautions"*).

4. DIGOXIN
In a study in 12 patients with congestive heart failure where Ketoprofen and digoxin were concomitantly administered, Ketoprofen did not alter the serum levels of digoxin.

5. WARFARIN
In a short-term controlled study in 14 normal volunteers, Ketoprofen did not significantly interfere with the effect of warfarin on prothrombin time. Bleeding from a number of sites may be a complication of warfarin treatment and GI bleeding a complication of Ketoprofen treatment. Because prostaglandins play an

important role in hemostasis and Ketoprofen has an effect on platelet function as well (see *"Drug/Laboratory Test Interactions: Effect On Blood Coagulation"*), concurrent therapy with Ketoprofen and warfarin requires close monitoring of patients on both drugs.

6. PROBENECID
Probenecid increases both free and bound Ketoprofen by reducing the plasma clearance of Ketoprofen to about one-third, as well as decreasing its protein-binding. Therefore, the combination of Ketoprofen and probenecid is not recommended.

7. METHOTREXATE
Ketoprofen, like other NSAIDs, may cause changes in the elimination of methotrexate leading to elevated serum levels of the drug and increased toxicity.

8. LITHIUM
Nonsteroidal anti-inflammatory agents have been reported to increase steady-state plasma lithium levels. It is recommended that plasma lithium levels be monitored when Ketoprofen is co-administered with lithium.

DRUG/LABORATORY TEST INTERACTIONS: EFFECT ON BLOOD COAGULATION
Ketoprofen decreases platelet adhesion and aggregation. Therefore, it can prolong bleeding time by approximately 3 to 4 minutes from baseline values. There is no significant change in platelet count, prothrombin time, partial thromboplastin time, or thrombin time.

CARCINOGENESIS, MUTAGENESIS, IMPAIRMENT OF FERTILITY
Chronic oral toxicity studies in mice (up to 32 mg/kg/day; 96 mg/m^2/day) did not indicate a carcinogenic potential for Ketoprofen. The maximum recommended human therapeutic dose is 300 mg/day for a 60 kg patient with a body surface area of 1.6 m^2, which is 5 mg/kg/day or 185 mg/m^2/day. Thus the mice were treated at 0.5 times the maximum human daily dose based on surface area.

A 2-year carcinogenicity study in rats, using doses up to 6.0 mg/kg/day (36 mg/m^2/day), showed no evidence of tumorigenic potential. All groups were treated for 104 weeks except the females receiving 6.0 mg/kg/day (36 mg/m^2/day) where the drug treatment was terminated in week 81 because of low survival; the remaining rats were sacrificed after week 87. Their survival in the groups treated for 104 weeks was within 6% of the control group. An earlier 2-year study with doses up to 12.5 mg/kg/day (75 mg/m^2/day) also showed no evidence of tumorigenicity, but the survival rate was low and the study was therefore judged inconclusive. Ketoprofen did not show mutagenic potential in the Ames Test. Ketoprofen administered to male rats (up to 9 mg/kg/day; or 54 mg/m^2/day) had no significant effect on reproductive performance or fertility. In female rats administered 6 or 9 mg/kg/day (36 or 54 mg/m^2/day), a decrease in the number of implantation sites has been noted. The dosages of 36 mg/m^2/day in rats represent 0.2 times the maximum recommended human dose of 185 mg/m^2/day (see above).

Abnormal spermatogenesis or inhibition of spermatogenesis developed in rats and dogs at high doses, and a decrease in the weight of the testes occurred in dogs and baboons at high doses.

TERATOGENIC EFFECTS: PREGNANCY CATEGORY B
In teratology studies Ketoprofen administered to mice at doses up to 12 mg/kg/day (36 mg/m^2/day) and rats at doses up to 9 mg/kg/day (54 mg/m^2/day), the approximate equivalent of 0.2 times the maximum recommended therapeutic dose of 185 mg/m^2/day, showed no teratogenic or embryotoxic effects. In separate studies in rabbits, maternally toxic doses were associated with embryotoxicity but not teratogenicity.

There are no adequate and well-controlled studies in pregnant women. Because animal teratology studies are not always predictive of the human response, Ketoprofen should be used during pregnancy only if the potential benefit justifies the risk.

LABOR AND DELIVERY
The effects of Ketoprofen on labor and delivery in pregnant women are unknown. Studies in rats have shown Ketoprofen at doses of 6 mg/kg (36 mg/m^2/day, approximately equal to 0.2 times the maximum recommended human dose) prolongs pregnancy when given before the onset of labor. Because of the known effects of prostaglandin-inhibiting drugs on the fetal cardiovascular system (closure of ductus arteriosus), use of Ketoprofen during late pregnancy should be avoided.

NURSING MOTHERS
Data on secretion in human milk after ingestion of Ketoprofen do not exist. In rats, Ketoprofen at doses of 9 mg/kg (54 mg/m^2/day; approximately 0.3 times the maximum human therapeutic dose) did not affect perinatal development. Upon administration to lactating dogs, the milk concentration of Ketoprofen was found to be 4 to 5% of the plasma drug level. As with other drugs that are excreted in milk, Ketoprofen is not recommended for use in nursing mothers.

PEDIATRIC USE
Ketoprofen is not recommended for use in children, because its safety and effectiveness have not been studied in children.

ADVERSE REACTIONS
The incidence of common adverse reactions (above 1%) was obtained from a population of 835 Ketoprofen treated patients in double-blind trials lasting from 4 to 54 weeks and in 622 Ketoprofen extended release treated patients in trials

➤ **SHOWN IN PRODUCT IDENTIFICATION GUIDE**

lasting from 4 to 16 weeks. Minor gastrointestinal side effects predominated; upper gastrointestinal symptoms were more common than lower gastrointestinal symptoms. In crossover trials in 321 patients with rheumatoid arthritis or osteoarthritis, there was no difference in either upper or lower gastrointestinal symptoms between patients treated with 200 mg of Ketoprofen extended release once a day or 75 mg of Ketoprofen TID (225 mg/day). Peptic ulcer or GI bleeding occurred in controlled clinical trials in less than 1% of 1,076 patients; however, in open label continuation studies in 1,292 patients the rate was greater than 2%.

The incidence of peptic ulceration in patients on NSAIDs is dependent on many risk factors including age, sex, smoking, alcohol use, diet, stress, concomitant drugs such as aspirin and corticosteroids, as well as the dose and duration of treatment with NSAIDs (see *"Warnings"*).

Gastrointestinal reactions were followed in frequency by central nervous system side effects, such as headache, dizziness, or drowsiness. The incidence of some adverse reactions appears to be dose-related (see *"Dosage and Administration"*). Rare adverse reactions (incidence less than 1%) were collected from foreign reports to manufacturers and regulatory agencies, publications, and U.S. clinical trials. Reactions are listed below under body system, then by incidence or number of cases in decreasing incidence.

INCIDENCE GREATER THAN 1%
(PROBABLE CAUSAL RELATIONSHIP)
Digestive: Dyspepsia (11%), nausea*, abdominal pain*, diarrhea*, constipation*, flatulence*, anorexia, vomiting, stomatitis.

Nervous System: Headache*, dizziness, CNS inhibition (i.e., pooled reports of somnolence, malaise, depression, etc.) or excitation (i.e., insomnia, nervousness, dreams, etc.)*.

Special Senses: Tinnitus, visual disturbance.

Skin and Appendages: Rash.

Urogenital: Impairment of renal function (edema, increased BUN)*, signs or symptoms of urinary-tract irritation.

INCIDENCE LESS THAN 1%
(PROBABLE CAUSAL RELATIONSHIP)
Body as a Whole: Chills, facial edema, infection, pain, allergic reaction, anaphylaxis.

Cardiovascular: Hypertension, palpitation, tachycardia, congestive heart failure, peripheral vascular disease, vasodilation.

Digestive: Appetite increased, dry mouth, eructation, gastritis, rectal hemorrhage, melena, fecal occult blood, salivation, peptic ulcer, gastrointestinal perforation, hematemesis, intestinal ulceration.

Hemic: Hypocoagulability, agranulocytosis, anemia, hemolysis, purpura, thrombocytopenia.

Metabolic and Nutritional: Thirst, weight gain, weight loss, hepatic dysfunction, hyponatremia.

Musculoskeletal: Myalgia.

Nervous System: Amnesia, confusion, impotence, migraine, paresthesia, vertigo.

Respiratory: Dyspnea, hemoptysis, epistaxis, pharyngitis, rhinitis, bronchospasm, laryngeal edema.

Skin and Appendages: Alopecia, eczema, pruritus, purpuric rash, sweating, urticaria, bullous rash, exfoliative dermatitis, photosensitivity, skin discoloration, onycholysis.

Special Senses: Conjunctivitis, conjunctivitis sicca, eye pain, hearing impairment, retinal hemorrhage and pigmentation change, taste perversion.

Urogenital: Menometrorrhagia, hematuria, renal failure, interstitial nephritis, nephrotic syndrome.

INCIDENCE LESS THAN 1%
(CAUSAL RELATIONSHIP UNKNOWN)
The following rare adverse reactions, whose causal relationship to Ketoprofen is uncertain, are being listed to serve as alerting information to the physician.

Body as a Whole: Septicemia, shock.

Cardiovascular: Arrhythmias, myocardial infarction.

Digestive: Buccal necrosis, ulcerative colitis, microvesicular steatosis, jaundice, pancreatitis.

Endocrine: Diabetes mellitus (aggravated).

Nervous System: Dysphoria, hallucination, libido disturbance, nightmares, personality disorder.

Urogenital: Acute tubulopathy, gynecomastia.

OVERDOSAGE
Signs and symptoms following acute NSAID overdose are usually limited to lethargy, drowsiness, nausea, vomiting, and epigastric pain, which are generally reversible with supportive care. Respiratory depression, coma, or convulsions have occurred following large Ketoprofen overdoses. Gastrointestinal bleeding, hypotension, hypertension, or acute renal failure may occur, but are rare.

---

* Adverse events occurring in 3 to 9% of patients.

Patients should be managed by symptomatic and supportive care following an NSAID overdose. There are no specific antidotes. Gut decontamination may be indicated in patients with symptoms seen within 4 hours (longer for sustained-release products) or following a large overdose (5 to 10 times the usual dose). This should be accomplished via emesis and/or activated charcoal (60 to 100 g in adults, 1 to 2g/kg in children) with a saline cathartic or sorbitol added to the first dose. Forced diuresis, alkalinization of the urine, hemodialysis or hemoperfusion would probably not be useful due to Ketoprofen's high protein binding.

Case reports include twenty-six overdoses: 6 were in children, 16 in adolescents, and 4 in adults. Five of these patients had minor symptoms (vomiting in 4, drowsiness in 1 child). A 12-year-old girl had tonic-clonic convulsions 1-2 hours after ingesting an unknown quantity of Ketoprofen and 1 or 2 tablets of acetaminophen with hydrocodone. Her Ketoprofen level was 1128 mg/L (56 times the upper therapeutic level of 20 mg/L) 3-4 hours post ingestion. Full recovery ensued 18 hours after ingestion following management with intubation, diazepam, and activated charcoal. A 45-year-old woman ingested twelve 200 mg Ketoprofen extended release and 375 mL vodka, was treated with emesis and supportive measures 2 hours after ingestion, and recovered completely with her only complaint being mild epigastric pain.

DOSAGE AND ADMINISTRATION
RHEUMATOID ARTHRITIS AND OSTEOARTHRITIS
The recommended starting dose of Ketoprofen in otherwise healthy patients is for Ketoprofen 75 mg three times or 50 mg four times a day or for Ketoprofen extended release 200 mg administered once a day. A smaller dose should be utilized initially in small individuals, in debilitated or elderly patients Ketoprofen is recommended for such initial dosage titration and Ketoprofen extended release is recommended for chronic treatment of those patients whose optimum dose is 200 mg/day. The recommended maximum daily dose of Ketoprofen is 300 mg/day (see *"Individualization of Dosage"*).

During titration with Ketoprofen, if minor side effects appear they may disappear at a lower dose which may still have an adequate therapeutic effect. If well tolerated but not optimally effective, the dosage may be increased. Individual patients may show a better response to 300 mg daily as compared to 200 mg, although in well-controlled clinical trials patients on 300 mg did not show greater mean effectiveness. They did, however, show an increased frequency of upper-and lower-GI distress and headaches. It is of interest that women also had an increased frequency of these adverse effects compared to men. When treating patients with 300 mg/day, the physician should observe sufficient increased clinical benefit to offset potential increased risk. Dosages higher than 300 mg/day are not recommended because they have not been adequately studied. Relatively smaller people may need smaller doses (see *"Individualization of Dosage"*).

MANAGEMENT OF PAIN AND DYSMENORRHEA
The usual dose of Ketoprofen recommended for mild-to-moderate pain and dysmenorrhea is 25 to 50 mg every 6 to 8 hours as necessary. A smaller dose should be utilized initially in small individuals, in debilitated or elderly patients, or in patients with renal or liver disease (see *"General Precautions"*). A larger dose may be tried if the patient's response to a previous dose was less than satisfactory, but doses above 75 mg have not been shown to give added analgesia. Daily doses above 300 mg are not recommended because they have not been adequately studied. Because of its typical nonsteroidal anti-inflammatory drug-side-effect profile, including as its principal adverse effect GI side effects (see *"Warnings"* and *"Adverse Reactions"*), higher doses of Ketoprofen should be used with caution and patients receiving them observed carefully (see *"Individualization of Dosage"*).

Ketoprofen extended release is not recommended for use in treating acute pain because of its controlled-release characteristics.

STORAGE
Keep tightly closed.
Store at room temperature, approximately 25°C (177°F).
Dispense in a tight container.

HOW SUPPLIED
CAPSULE: 25 MG

AVERAGE UNIT PRICE (AVAILABLE SIZES)

BRAND	$0.81	GENERIC A-RATED AVERAGE PRICE (GAAP)	
GENERIC	$0.72	100s	$71.53

BRAND/MANUFACTURER		NDC	SIZE	AWP
◆ **BRAND**				
➤ ORUDIS: Wyeth-Ayerst		00008-4186-01	100s	$80.66
◆ **GENERICS**				
Biocraft		00332-3191-09	100s	$65.68
Goldline		00182-1958-01	100s	$67.50
Geneva		00781-2409-01	100s	$70.98
West Point		59591-0001-68	100s	$72.15
Lederle Std Prod		00005-3284-43	100s	$74.35
Aligen		00405-4578-01	100s	$78.50

◆ RATED THERAPEUTICALLY EQUIVALENT; ◇ THERAPEUTIC EQUIVALENCE UNCONFIRMED; ○ UNRATED

CAPSULE: 50 MG

AVERAGE UNIT PRICE (AVAILABLE SIZES)		GENERIC A-RATED AVERAGE PRICE (GAAP)	
BRAND	$0.99	100s	$87.95
GENERIC	$0.88		

BRAND/MANUFACTURER	NDC	SIZE	AWP
◆ BRAND			
➤ ORUDIS: Wyeth-Ayerst	00008-4181-01	100s	$99.01
◆ GENERICS			
Biocraft	00332-3193-09	100s	$80.62
Qualitest	00603-4177-21	100s	$80.62
Geneva	00781-2410-01	100s	$87.13
Goldline	00182-1959-01	100s	$88.00
Warner Chilcott	00047-0528-24	100s	$89.10
URL	00677-1463-01	100s	$89.11
Rugby	00536-5564-01	100s	$89.11
West Point	59591-0002-68	100s	$89.15
Schein	00364-2571-01	100s	$89.11
Major	00904-7711-60	100s	$89.25
Lederle Std Prod	00005-3285-43	100s	$91.91
Aligen	00405-4579-01	100s	$92.20

CAPSULE: 75 MG

AVERAGE UNIT PRICE (AVAILABLE SIZES)		GENERIC A-RATED AVERAGE PRICE (GAAP)	
BRAND	$1.10	100s	$98.32
GENERIC	$0.95	500s	$455.12

BRAND/MANUFACTURER	NDC	SIZE	AWP
◆ BRAND			
➤ ORUDIS: Wyeth-Ayerst	00008-4187-01	100s	$110.13
	00008-4187-04	100s ud	$114.41
	00008-4187-02	500s	$524.60
◆ GENERICS			
Biocraft	00332-3195-09	100s	$89.67
Geneva	00781-2411-01	100s	$96.91
Goldline	00182-1960-01	100s	$98.00
Qualitest	00603-4178-21	100s	$98.90
Rugby	00536-5565-01	100s	$99.00
Warner Chilcott	00047-0566-24	100s	$99.00
URL	00677-1464-01	100s	$99.11
West Point	59591-0003-68	100s	$99.15
Aligen	00405-4580-01	100s	$99.29
Major	00904-7712-60	100s	$99.30
Schein	00364-2572-01	100s	$99.32
Lederle Std Prod	00005-3286-43	100s	$102.21
Aligen	00405-4580-02	500s	$427.12
Biocraft	00332-3195-13	500s	$427.12
Qualitest	00603-4178-28	500s	$427.12
Geneva	00781-2411-05	500s	$461.65
Goldline	00182-1960-05	500s	$464.00
Rugby	00536-5565-05	500s	$472.14
Warner Chilcott	00047-0566-30	500s	$472.14
Schein	00364-2572-05	500s	$472.36
Major	00904-7712-40	500s	$472.40

CAPSULE, EXTENDED RELEASE: 200 MG

BRAND/MANUFACTURER	NDC	SIZE	AWP
○ BRAND			
➤ ORUVAIL: Wyeth-Ayerst	00008-0690-01	100s	$206.89
	00008-0690-02	100s	$206.89

Ketorolac Tromethamine, Ophthalmic

DESCRIPTION
Ketorolac Tromethamine is a member of the pyrrolo-pyrolle group of nonsteroidal anti-inflammatory drugs (NSAIDs) for ophthalmic use. Its chemical name is (±)-5-benzoyl-2,3-dihydro-1-*H*-pyrrolizine-1-carboxylic acid compound with 2-amino-2-(hydroxymethyl)-1,3-propanediol (1:1).

Ketorolac Tromethamine is supplied as a sterile isotonic aqueous 0.5% solution, with a pH of 7.4. Ketorolac Tromethamine is a racemic mixture of R-(+)- and S-(−)- Ketorolac Tromethamine. Ketorolac Tromethamine may exist in three crystal forms. All forms are equally soluble in water. The pKa of Ketorolac is 3.5. This white to off-white crystalline substance discolors on prolonged exposure to light. The molecular weight of Ketorolac Tromethamine is 376.41. Each mL of Ketorolac Tromethamine ophthalmic solution contains Ketorolac Tromethamine 0.5%, benzalkonium chloride 0.01%, edetate disodium 0.1%, octoxynol 40, sodium chloride, hydrochloric acid and/or sodium hydroxide to adjust the pH, and purified water. The osmolality of Ketorolac Tromethamine is 290 mOsmol/kg.

Following is its chemical structure:

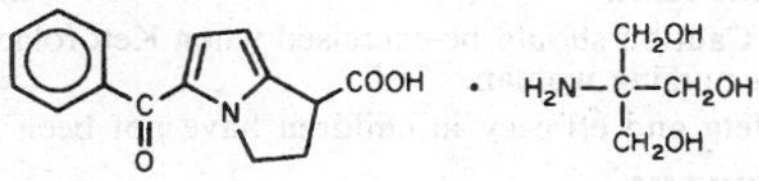

ANIMAL PHARMACOLOGY
Ketorolac Tromethamine prevented the development of increased intraocular pressure induced in rabbits with topically applied arachidonic acid. Ketorolac did not inhibit rabbit lens aldose reductase *in vitro*.

Ketorolac Tromethamine ophthalmic solution did not enhance the spread of ocular infections induced in rabbits with *Candida albicans, Herpes simplex* virus type one, or *Pseudomonas aeruginosa*.

CLINICAL PHARMACOLOGY
Ketorolac Tromethamine is a nonsteroidal anti-inflammatory drug which, when administered systemically, has demonstrated analgesic, anti-inflammatory and antipyretic activity. The mechanism of its action is thought to be due, in part, to its ability to inhibit prostaglandin biosynthesis. Ocular administration of Ketorolac Tromethamine reduces prostaglandin E_2 levels in aqueous humor. The mean concentration of PGE_2 was 80 pg/mL in the aqueous humor of eyes receiving vehicle and 28 pg/mL in the eyes receiving 0.5% Ketorolac Tromethamine ophthalmic solution. Ketorolac Tromethamine given systemically does not cause pupil constriction.

Results from clinical studies indicate that Ketorolac Tromethamine ophthalmic solution has no significant effect upon intraocular pressure.

Two controlled clinical studies showed that Ketorolac Tromethamine ophthalmic solution was significantly more effective than its vehicle in relieving ocular itching caused by seasonal allergic conjunctivitis. Two drops (0.1 mL) of 0.5% Ketorolac Tromethamine ophthalmic solution instilled into the eyes of patients 12 hours and 1 hour prior to cataract extraction achieved measurable levels in 8 of 9 patients' eyes (mean Ketorolac concentration 95 ng/mL aqueous humor, range 40 to 170 ng/mL). One drop (0.05 mL) of 0.5% Ketorolac Tromethamine ophthalmic solution was instilled into one eye and one drop of vehicle into the other eye tid in 26 normal subjects. Only 5 of 26 subjects had a detectable amount of Ketorolac in their plasma (range 10.7 to 22.5 ng/mL) at Day 10 during topical ocular treatment. When Ketorolac Tromethamine 10 mg is administered systemically every 6 hours, peak plasma levels at steady state are around 960 ng/mL. Ketorolac Tromethamine ophthalmic solution has been safely administered in conjunction with other ophthalmic medications, such as antibiotics, beta blockers, carbonic anhydrase inhibitors, cycloplegics, and mydriatics.

INDICATIONS AND USAGE
Ketorolac Tromethamine ophthalmic solution is indicated for the relief of ocular itching due to seasonal allergic conjunctivitis.

CONTRAINDICATIONS
Ketorolac Tromethamine ophthalmic solution is contraindicated in patients while wearing soft contact lenses and in patients with previously demonstrated hypersensitivity to any of the ingredients in the formulation.

WARNINGS
There is the potential for cross-sensitivity to acetylsalicylic acid, phenylacetic acid derivatives, and other nonsteroidal anti-inflammatory agents. Therefore, caution should be used when treating individuals who have previously exhibited sensitivities to these drugs.

With some nonsteroidal anti-inflammatory drugs, there exists the potential for increased bleeding time due to interference with thrombocyte aggregation. There have been reports that ocularly applied nonsteroidal anti-inflammatory drugs may cause increased bleeding of ocular tissues (including hyphemas) in conjunction with ocular surgery.

PRECAUTIONS
General: It is recommended that Ketorolac Tromethamine ophthalmic solution be used with caution in patients with known bleeding tendencies or who are receiving other medications which may prolong bleeding time.

Carcinogenesis, Mutagenesis, and Impairment of Fertility: An 18-month study in mice at oral doses of Ketorolac Tromethamine equal to the parenteral MRHD (Maximum Recommended Human Dose) and a 24-month study in rats at oral doses 2.5 times the parenteral MRHD, showed no evidence of tumorigenicity.

Ketorolac Tromethamine was not mutagenic in Ames test, unscheduled DNA synthesis and repair, and in forward mutation assays. Ketorolac did not cause chromosome breakage in the *in vivo* mouse micronucleus assay. At 1590 ug/mL (approximately 1000 times the average human plasma levels) and at higher concentrations, Ketorolac Tromethamine increased the incidence of chromosomal aberrations in Chinese hamster ovarian cells.

Impairment of fertility did not occur in male or female rats at oral doses of 9 mg/kg (53.1 mg/m^2) and 16 mg/kg (94.4 mg/m^2) respectively.

Pregnancy: Pregnancy Category C: Reproduction studies have been performed in rabbits, using daily oral doses at 3.6 mg/kg (42.35 mg/m^2) and in rats at 10 mg/kg (59 mg/m^2) during organogenesis. Results of these studies did not reveal evidence of teratogenicity to the fetus. Oral doses of Ketorolac Tromethamine at 1.5 mg/kg (8.8 mg/m^2), which was half of the human oral exposure, administered after gestation day 17 caused dystocia and higher pup mortality in rats. There are no adequate and well-controlled studies in pregnant women. Ketorolac Tromethamine should be used during pregnancy only if the potential benefit justifies the potential risk to the fetus.

Nursing Mothers: Caution should be exercised when Ketorolac Tromethamine is administered to a nursing woman.

Pediatric Use: Safety and efficacy in children have not been established.

ADVERSE REACTIONS

In patients with allergic conjunctivitis, the most frequent adverse events reported with the use of Ketorolac Tromethamine ophthalmic solution have been transient stinging and burning on instillation. These events were reported by approximately 40% of patients treated with Ketorolac Tromethamine ophthalmic solution. In all development studies conducted, other adverse events reported during treatment with Ketorolac Tromethamine include ocular irritation (3%), allergic reactions (3%), superficial ocular infections (0.5%) and superficial keratitis (1%).

DOSAGE AND ADMINISTRATION

The recommended dose of Ketorolac Tromethamine ophthalmic solution is one drop (0.25 mg) four times a day for relief of ocular itching due to seasonal allergic conjunctivitis. The efficacy of Ketorolac Tromethamine ophthalmic solution has not been established beyond one week of therapy.

Store at controlled room temperature 15-30°C (59-86°F) with protection from light.

HOW SUPPLIED
DROP: 0.5%

BRAND/MANUFACTURER	NDC	SIZE	AWP
○ **BRAND**			
ACULAR: Allergan Optical	00023-2181-05	5 ml	$26.60

Ketorolac Tromethamine, Systemic

DESCRIPTION

Ketorolac Tromethamine is a member of the pyrrolo-pyrrole group of nonsteroidal anti-inflammatory drugs (NSAIDs). The chemical name for Ketorolac Tromethamine is (±)-5-benzoyl-2,3-dihydro-1H-pyrrolizine-1-carboxylic acid, 2-amino-2-(hydroxymethyl)-1,3-propanediol.

Ketorolac Tromethamine, Systemic is a racemic mixture of R-(+)- and S-(−)-Ketorolac Tromethamine. Ketorolac Tromethamine may exist in three crystal forms. All forms are equally soluble in water. Ketorolac Tromethamine has a pKa of 3.5 and an n-octanol/water partition coefficient of 0.26. The molecular weight of Ketorolac Tromethamine is 376.41.

Ketorolac Tromethamine is available for intramuscular (IM) administration as 15 mg in 1 mL (1.5%), 30 mg in 1 mL (35), or 60 mg in 2 mL (35) of Ketorolac Tromethamine in sterile solution.

Ketorolac Tromethamine oral tablet contains 10 mg of Ketorolac Tromethamine.

Following is its chemical structure:

CLINICAL PHARMACOLOGY
PHARMACODYNAMICS

Ketorolac is a nonsteroidal anti-inflammatory drug (NSAID) that exhibits analgesic, anti-inflammatory, and antipyretic activity. Ketorolac inhibits synthesis of prostaglandins and may be considered a peripherally acting analgesic. As with other NSAIDs, the biological activity of Ketorolac is associated with the S form. Ketorolac does not have any known effects on opiate receptors.

Pain relief, following extraction of impacted third molars, is clinically evident when steady state plasma levels average approximately 0.3 µg/mL, while side effects are frequent above concentrations of 5 µg/mL. Pain relief is comparable following IM or oral administration. Pain relief is statistically different from that following placebo at 1/2 hour (the first time point at which it was measured) following the largest recommended doses of Ketorolac and by 1 hour following the smallest recommended dose. The peak analgesic effect occurs at 2 to 3 hours and is not statistically significantly different over the recommended dosage range of Ketorolac. The greatest difference between large and small doses of Ketorolac Tromethamine by either route is in the duration of analgesia. In controlled clinical trials 75% of patients receiving 90 mg of Ketorolac Tromethamine IM or 100 mg Ketorolac Tromethamine Oral did not request remedication at 6 hours as compared to 56% of those patients receiving 10 mg of Ketorolac Tromethamine IM or 10 to 12.5 mg Ketorolac Tromethamine Oral.

TABLE OF ESTIMATED PHARMACODYNAMIC PARAMETERS FOLLOWING ORAL OR INTRAMUSCULAR DOSES OF KETOROLAC TROMETHAMINE

$C_{50}est^1$	0.3 µg/mL
$C_{toxic}est^2$	5 µg/mL

[1] *Estimated concentration required to obtain 50% decreases in pain intensity scores in dental surgery pain*
[2] *Estimated concentration above which side effects are frequent.*

PHARMACOKINETICS (SEE *"TABLES"* AND *"GRAPH"*)

The pharmacokinetics of Ketorolac in humans, following single or multiple intramuscular or oral doses, are apparently linear, i.e., plasma levels are approximately proportional to dosage. Steady state plasma levels are achieved after dosing every 6 hours for one day. No changes in clearance occur with chronic dosing. More than 99% of the Ketorolac in plasma is protein bound over a wide concentration range.

The pharmacokinetic profiles of IM and oral doses are very similar. Following IM administration, some individuals have slower absorption which is reflected below in the two tables showing results of studies of 15, 30, and 60 mg of Ketorolac Tromethamine IM and 10 mg of Ketorolac Tromethamine Oral. Note that the studies used different but comparable subject populations. The tables show slightly longer times to peak plasma levels and slightly longer apparent half-lives following IM administration.

Ketorolac Tromethamine IM is completely absorbed following intramuscular administration with mean peak plasma concentrations of 2.2-3.0 µg/mL occurring an average of 50 minutes after a single 30 mg dose. The terminal plasma half-life is 3.5-9.2 hours in young adults and 4.7-8.6 hours in elderly subjects (mean age 72).

Ketorolac Tromethamine Oral is completely absorbed following oral administration with a mean peak plasma concentration of 0.7-1.1 µg/mL occurring an average of 44 minutes after a single 10 mg dose in fasted subjects. The terminal plasma half-life is 2.4-9.0 hours in young adults and 4.3-7.6 hours in elderly subjects (mean age 72).

A high fat meal decreased the peak and delayed the time to peak concentration, but did not affect the extent of absorption, while antacid had no effect upon absorption of Ketorolac Tromethamine Oral.

Ketorolac, following intravenous, intramuscular and oral administration, displays characteristics of a two-compartment model. In order to minimize the time delay in achieving adequate analgesic effect, an IM or oral loading dose equal to twice the maintenance dose is recommended. This is based upon the pharmacokinetic principle that when the dosing interval is near the drug's half-life, the target steady-state plasma level is achieved faster if the first dose is twice the maintenance dose. Due to the two-compartment characteristics of Ketorolac, the loading dose results in plasma levels during the first dosing interval that are higher than in subsequent intervals (see graph of IM dosing which illustrates this).

METABOLISM AND EXCRETION

The primary route of excretion of Ketorolac and its metabolites (conjugates and a para-hydroxy metabolite) is in the urine (mean 91.4%) and the remainder (mean 6.1%) is excreted in the feces. In patients with serum creatinine values ranging from 1.9 to 5.0 mg/dL, the rate of Ketorolac clearance was reduced to approximately two-thirds of normal. Decreases in serum albumin, such as encountered in liver cirrhosis, would be expected to change Ketorolac clearance. However, in a study of 7 patients with liver cirrhosis, no correlation was found between serum albumin concentration and ketorolac clearance.

Hemodynamics of anesthetized patients were not altered by parenteral administration of Ketorolac. Unlike opiate analgesics such as morphine, Ketorolac does not cause respiratory depression.

Ketorolac poorly penetrates the blood-brain barrier (levels in the cerebrospinal fluid were found to be 0.002 times or less than those in plasma).

TABLE OF APPROXIMATE AVERAGE PHARMACOKINETIC PARAMETERS FOLLOWING INTRAMUSCULAR AND ORAL DOSES OF KETOROLAC TROMETHAMINE

Pharmacokinetic Parameter (units)	Oral†		Intramuscular†	
	10 mg	15 mg	30 mg	60 mg
Bioavailability (extent)	100%	100%	100%	100%
T_{max}^1 (min)	20-60	30-60	30-60	30-60
C_{max}^2 (µg/mL)				
[single dose]	0.7-1.1	1.0-1.4	2.2-3.0	4.0-4.5
C_{max} (µg/mL)				
[steady state qid]	0.7-1.2	1.1-1.7	2.3-3.5	N/A‡
C_{min}^3 (µg/mL)				
[steady state qid]	0.2-0.3	0.2-0.3	0.3-0.7	N/A
C_{ave}^4 (µg/mL)				
[steady state qid]	0.3-0.6	0.6-0.8	1.3-1.5	N/A
$Vd(\beta)^5$ (L/kg)	0.15-0.33			

% Dose metabolized = <50	% Dose excreted in feces = 6
% dose excreted in urine = 91	% Plasma protein binding = 99

* *Derived from IM pharmacokinetic studies in 32 normal volunteers.*
† *Derived from PO pharmacokinetic studies in 23 normal fasted volunteers.*
†† *Not applicable because 60 mg is only recommended as a loading dose.*
[1] *Time to peak plasma concentration*
[2] *Peak plasma concentration*
[3] *Trough plasma concentration*
[4] *Average plasma concentration*
[5] *Volume of distribution (calculated from mean clearance and terminal half-life)*

◆ RATED THERAPEUTICALLY EQUIVALENT; ◇ THERAPEUTIC EQUIVALENCE UNCONFIRMED; ○ UNRATED

Plasma Levels After Recommended Ketorolac Tromethamine I.M. Dosing Schedules

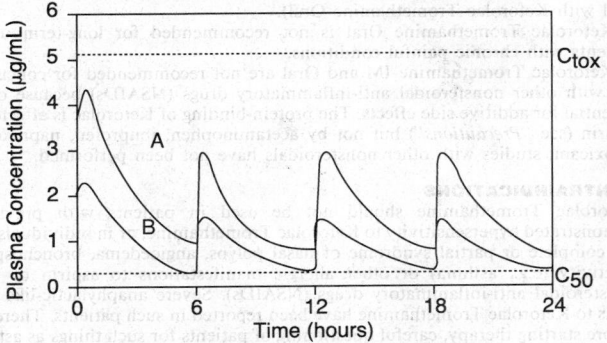

A=Ketorolac tromethamine 60 mg followed by 30 mg doses (q6h)
B=Ketorolac tromethamine 30 mg followed by 15 mg doses (q6h)
C_{tox}=Estimated concentration above which side effects are frequent
C_{50}=Estimated concentration required to obtain 50% decreases in
 pain intensity scores in dental surgery pain

(See related table).

CLINICAL STUDIES
The analgesic efficacy of intramuscularly and orally administered Ketorolac was investigated in two postoperative pain models; general surgery (orthopedic, gynecologic and abdominal) and oral surgery (removal of impacted third molars). The studies were primarily double-blind, single dose, parallel trial designs in patients with moderate to severe pain at baseline. Ketorolac Tromethamine IM was compared to meperidine or morphine administered intramuscularly. Ketorolac Tromethamine Oral was compared to naproxen, ibuprofen, aspirin, acetaminophen and aspirin or acetaminophen with codeine.

SHORT TERM USE (UP TO 5 DAYS)
In the comparisons of intramuscular administration during the first hour, the onset of analgesic action was similar between Ketorolac Tromethamine and the narcotics. Ketorolac Tromethamine 30 or 90 mg intramuscularly gave pain relief comparable to meperidine 100 mg or morphine 12 mg. Ketorolac Tromethamine 10 mg was comparable to 50 mg of meperidine or 6 mg morphine. The duration of analgesia was longer with all three doses of Ketorolac Tromethamine. The percentage of patients who did not remedicate by 6 hours, i.e., by the end of the studies, was roughly 70%, 60% and 50% for Ketorolac Tromethamine 90, 30 and 10 mg respectively, as compared to 30% and 20% for the high and low doses of the two narcotics. In a multi-dose, postoperative (general surgery) double-blind trial of Ketorolac Tromethamine 30 mg versus morphine 6 and 12 mg, each drug given on an "as needed" basis for up to 5 days, the overall analgesic effect of Ketorolac Tromethamine 30 mg was in between that of morphine 6 and 12 mg. Ketorolac Tromethamine 30 mg caused less drowsiness, nausea and vomiting than morphine 12 mg. The majority of patients treated with either Ketorolac Tromethamine or morphine were dosed for up to 3 days; a small percentage of patients received 5 days of dosing.

In the first hour, the comparisons of Ketorolac Tromethamine Oral in dental surgery studies, 10 or 20 mg of Ketorolac Tromethamine Oral gave comparable pain relief to ibuprofen 400 mg, aspirin 650 mg, acetaminophen 600 mg and acetaminophen 600 mg combined with codeine 60 mg. The peak effects of the 2 Ketorolac Tromethamine Oral doses and ibuprofen were comparable and beyond

2 to 3 hours, the patients who received those 3 treatments had statistically significantly better pain relief than patients who received the other 3 treatments. The percentage of patients who required remediation after 3 hours were as follows:

Treatment	4 hr	5 hr	6 hr
Ketorolac 10 mg	20%	35%	46%
Ketorolac 20 mg	23%	41%	54%
Ibuprofen 400 mg	35%	41%	65%
Aspirin 650 mg	38%	62%	76%
Acetaminophen 600 mg	50%	69%	78%
Acetaminophen 600 mg with codeine 60 mg	46%	69%	74%

In the comparisons of Ketorolac Tromethamine Oral in postoperative patients following other surgical procedures, 10 mg of Ketorolac Tromethamine Oral resulted in comparable pain relief to aspirin 650 mg combined with codeine 60 mg and naproxen sodium 550 mg in onset, duration and peak effect. The percentages of patients who required remediation after 3 hours were as follows:

Treatment	4 hour	5 hour	6 hour
Ketorolac 10 mg	24%	37%	43%
Aspirin 650 mg	27%	39%	51%
Aspirin 650 mg with codeine 60 mg	20%	27%	38%
Naproxen 500 mg or naproxen sodium 550 mg	13%	16%	19%

LIMITED DURATION USE OF KETOROLAC TROMETHAMINE IM FOLLOWED BY KETOROLAC TROMETHAMINE ORAL PRN FOR ACUTE POST-SURGICAL PAIN.
The use of Ketorolac Tromethamine Oral (10 mg) following Ketorolac Tromethamine IM (30 mg) therapy after surgery was evaluated in 210 patients in a double-blind trial compared to IM meperidine 100 mg followed by oral acetaminophen 600 mg with codeine 60 mg. The use of both IM and oral treatment in this study was prn. Patients received Ketorolac Tromethamine IM for a median duration of 2 days (median dose 60 mg/day) followed by Ketorolac Tromethamine Oral for a median duration of 8 days (median dose 25 mg/day). The efficacy of the Ketorolac was comparable to the meperidine/acetaminophen plus codeine regimen. The adverse events are shown in the following table:

TABLE OF DIFFERENCES IN ADVERSE EVENTS

Body System and Term	Meperidine IM followed by Acetaminophen + Codeine (n=104)	Ketorolac IM followed by Ketorolac Oral (n=106)
Gastrointestinal		
Nausea	66%	39%
Constipation	24%	8%
Diarrhea	3%	9%
Nervous System		
Dizziness	28%	8%
Somnolence	28%	8%
Dry Mouth	20%	9%
Insomnia	9%	14%
Nervousness	2%	6%
Tremor	5%	0%

THE INFLUENCE OF AGE, LIVER AND KIDNEY FUNCTION ON THE CLEARANCE AND TERMINAL HALF-LIFE OF KETOROLAC TROMETHAMINE IM[1] AND ORAL[2]

Type of Subjects	Total Clearance (in L/h/kg)[3]		Terminal Half-life (in hours)	
	IM mean (range)	Oral mean (range)	IM mean (range)	Oral mean (range)
Normal subjects IM (n=54), Oral (n=77)	0.023 (0.010-0.046)	0.025 (0.013-0.050)	5.3 (3.5-9.2)	5.3 (2.4-9.0)
Healthy elderly subjects IM (n=13), Oral (n=12) (mean age=72, range=65-78)	0.019 (0.013-0.034)	0.024 (0.018-0.034)	7.0 (4.7-8.6)	6.1 (4.3-7.6)
Patients with Hepatic Dysfunction IM and Oral (n=7)	0.029 (0.013-0.066)	0.033 (0.019-0.051)	5.4 (2.2-6.9)	4.5 (1.6-7.6)
Patients with Renal Impairment IM and Oral (n=9) (serum creatinine 1.9-5.0 mg/dL)	0.014 (0.007-0.043)	0.016 (0.007-0.052)	10.3 (8.1-15.7)	10.8 (3.4-18.9)
Renal Dialysis Patients IM (n=9)	0.016 (0.003-0.036)	—	13.6 (8.0-39.1)	—

1. *Estimated from 30 mg single IM doses of Ketorolac Tromethamine*
2. *Estimated from 10 mg single oral doses of Ketorolac Tromethamine*
3. *Liters/hour/kilogram*

Body System and Term	Meperidine IM followed by Acetaminophen + Codeine (n=104)	Ketorolac IM followed by Ketorolac Oral (n=106)
Skin		
Pruritus	10%	4%
Rash	6%	3%
Urogenital		
Urinary Retention	8%	0%

There were no serious adverse reactions reported during this study or in other studies of 490 additional patients who received Ketorolac Tromethamine IM 10 or 30 mg single dose or qid prn followed by Ketorolac Tromethamine Oral 10 mg qid prn for 3-10 days.

LONG TERM USE OF KETOROLAC TROMETHAMINE
Ketorolac Tromethamine IM is not recommended for use beyond 5 days at recommended doses because of the increase in side effects which may occur.

In a clinical trial in 823 patients with chronic pain states comparing Ketorolac Tromethamine Oral 10 mg qid (553 patients) with aspirin 650 mg qid (270 patients), during the first week there was a 2.4% dropout rate because of upper GI complaints in the Ketorolac Tromethamine Oral treated patients as compared with a 0.4% rate in the aspirin treated group. After the first 2 weeks, the dropout rates due to GI pain or discomfort were comparable in both treatment groups. The time-adjusted percentages of patients who developed ulcers or upper GI bleeding are as follows:

CUMULATIVE OCCURRENCE

Interval	Ketorolac	Aspirin
≤ 3 month	0.69	0
≤ 6 months	1.59	0.73

PHYSICIANS SHOULD CAREFULLY WEIGH THE POTENTIAL RISKS AND BENEFITS OF KETORO-LAC TROMETHAMINE ORAL USE ON A LONG-TERM BASIS. PATIENTS SHOULD BE INSTRUCTED TO WATCH FOR SIGNS OF SERIOUS GI ADVERSE EVENTS AND THEY SHOULD BE MONITORED MORE CLOSELY THAN IF THEY WERE ON ANOTHER NSAID.

INDIVIDUALIZATION OF DOSAGE
Suggestions for using Ketorolac Tromethamine IM on a PRN schedule.
Since the half-life of Ketorolac Tromethamine is approximately 6 hours, an assessment of the size of a repeat dose can be based on the duration of pain relief from the previous dose. For example, if pain returns within 3 to 5 hours of a maintenance dose (15 or 30 mg), the next dose could be increased by up to 50% [Note: The recommended maximum total daily dose is 120 mg (150 mg on the first day); an alternative would be to use morphine or meperidine concomitantly (see *"Indications"* and *"Drug Interactions"*). Alternatively, if pain does not return for 8 to 12 hours, the next dose could be decreased by as much as 50%, or the dosage interval could be increased to 8 to 12 hours.

Note: The initial intramuscular loading dose (30 or 60 mg) should be given only once, unless therapy has been interrupted for 3 half-lives (15-40 hours, see half-life of Ketorolac Tromethamine IM in Table in *"Clinical Pharmacology"*).

Ketorolac Tromethamine IM is only recommended for short-term therapy (not over 5 days), because adverse reactions may increase with longer use at recommended doses (see *"Warnings"* and *"Precautions"*).

The lower end of the dosage range is recommended for patients under 50 kg (110 pounds) of body weight, for patients over 65 years of age, and for patients with reduced renal function (see *"Clinical Pharmacology"* and *"Precautions"*).

If management by regular scheduled doses is elected, see *"Dosage and Administration"* for dosing recommendations.

The most logical use of Ketorolac Tromethamine Oral is in patients who have benefited from Ketorolac Tromethamine IM without limiting side effects. They can be continued on analgesic treatment with Ketorolac Tromethamine Oral (see *"Dosage and Administration—Transition from Ketorolac Tromethamine IM to Ketorolac Tromethamine Oral"*). It is recommended to use the lowest effective dose of Ketorolac Tromethamine IM at the transition to Ketorolac Tromethamine Oral and to continue treatment with Ketorolac Tromethamine Oral for as short a time as possible (see *"Warnings"* and *"Adverse Reactions"*).

INDICATIONS AND USAGE
Ketorolac Tromethamine IM is indicated for the short-term management (up to 5 days) of pain (see *"Clinical Studies"* in *"Clinical Pharmacology"*) Ketorolac Tromethamine IM is not recommended for longer use (more than 5 days) because of the possibility of increased frequency and severity of adverse reactions associated with the recommended doses (see *"Warnings"*, *"Dosage and Adminis-tration"* and *"Adverse Reactions"*).

Ketorolac Tromethamine IM is not recommended as a pre-operative medication for support of anesthesia, because it inhibits platelet aggregation and may prolong bleeding time (see *"Precautions—Hematologic Effects"*) and because it possesses no sedative or anxiolytic properties.

Ketorolac Tromethamine IM is not recommended in obstetric analgesia because it has not been adequately studied for such use and because of the known effects of drugs that inhibit prostaglandin synthesis on uterine contraction and fetal circulation.

Ketorolac Tromethamine IM has been used concomitantly with morphine and meperidine without apparent adverse effects.

Ketorolac Tromethamine Oral is indicated for limited duration prn use in the management of pain (see *"Warnings,"* *"Adverse Reactions"* and *"Clinical Pharmacology—Clinical Studies"* sections for details about relative risks associated with Ketorolac Tromethamine Oral).

Ketorolac Tromethamine Oral is not recommended for long-term use in patients with chronic painful conditions.

Ketorolac Tromethamine IM and Oral are not recommended for concurrent use with other nonsteroidal anti-inflammatory drugs (NSAIDs) because of the potential for additive side effects. The protein-binding of Ketorolac is affected by aspirin (see *"Precautions"*) but not by acetaminophen, ibuprofen, naproxen or piroxicam; studies with other nonsteroidals have not been performed.

CONTRAINDICATIONS
Ketorolac Tromethamine should not be used in patients with previously demonstrated hypersensitivity to Ketorolac Tromethamine, or in individuals with the complete or partial syndrome of nasal polyps, angioedema, bronchospastic reactivity (e.g., asthma) or other allergic manifestations to aspirin or other nonsteroidal anti-inflammatory drugs (NSAIDs). Severe anaphylactic-like reactions to Ketorolac Tromethamine have been reported in such patients. Therefore, before starting therapy, careful questioning of patients for such things as asthma, nasal polyps, urticaria, and hypotension associated with nonsteroidal anti-inflammatory drugs is important. In addition, if such symptoms occur during therapy, treatment should be discontinued.

WARNINGS
The most serious risks associated with Ketorolac Tromethamine are: *gastrointestinal* ulcerations, bleeding and perforation (see *"Precautions"*), *renal* events ranging from interstitial nephritis to acute renal failure (see *"Precautions"*), especially in patients with pre-existing kidney problems; *hemorrhage*, especially in patients where strict hemostasis is critical (see *"Precautions"*); *hypersensitivity reactions* such as anaphylaxis, bronchospasm, vascular collapse, urticaria, angioedema, Stevens-Johnson syndrome and vesicular bullous rash. Anaphylactoid reactions may occur in patients with a history of hypersensitivity to aspirin, other nonsteroidal anti-inflammatory drugs, or Ketorolac Tromethamine. They may, however, also occur in patients without a known previous exposure or hypersensitivity to these agents. Both types of reactions may be fatal.

The use of Ketorolac Tromethamine IM at recommended doses for more than 5 days is associated with an increased frequency and severity of adverse events.

The use of Ketorolac Tromethamine Oral 10 mg on a long-term basis is associated with more GI tract adverse effects than aspirin 650 mg qid (see *"Clinical Pharmacology—Clinical Studies"*). Long-term treatment is not recommended (see *"Indications and Usage"*).

High oral doses (e.g., 80 or 120 mg/day) are not recommended because risks of serious adverse events are greater with daily doses exceeding the recommended 40 mg oral per day (see *"Adverse Reactions"*).

PRECAUTIONS
Physicians should be alert to the pharmacologic similarity of Ketorolac Tromethamine to other nonsteroidal anti-inflammatory drugs (NSAIDs) that inhibit cyclo-oxygenase.

GENERAL PRECAUTIONS
Risk of Gastrointestinal Ulcerations, Bleeding and Perforation: Serious gastrointestinal toxicity, such as bleeding, ulceration, and perforation, can occur at any time, with or without warning symptoms, in patients treated with NSAIDs.

Studies to date with NSAIDs have not identified any subset of patients not at risk of developing peptic ulceration and bleeding. Except for a prior history of serious GI events and other risk factors known to be associated with peptic ulcer disease, such as alcoholism, smoking, etc., no other factors have been associated with increased risk. Elderly or debilitated patients seem to tolerate ulceration or bleeding less well than other individuals, and most spontaneous reports of fatal GI events are in this population. Postmarketing experience with Ketorolac Tromethamine IM suggests that there may be a greater risk of gastrointestinal ulcerations, bleeding and perforation in the elderly.

Studies so far are inconclusive concerning the relative risk of various nonsteroidal anti-inflammatory drugs (NSAIDs) in causing such reactions. High doses of any such agent probably carry a greater risk of these reactions, although this is rarely established in controlled clinical trials. In considering the intramuscular use of relatively large doses (within the recommended dosage range), or treatment with Ketorolac Tromethamine IM for a duration longer than 5 days, sufficient benefit should be anticipated to offset the potential increased risk of GI toxicity.

The risks of gastrointestinal side effects associated with long-term use of Ketorolac Tromethamine Oral are described under *"Clinical Pharmacology—Clinical Studies (Long-Term Use of Ketorolac Tromethamine"*).

Impaired Renal or Hepatic Function: As with other nonsteroidal anti-inflammatory drugs (NSAIDs), Ketorolac Tromethamine should be used with caution in patients with impaired renal or hepatic function, or a history of kidney or liver disease.

Renal Effects: As with other nonsteroidal anti-inflammatory drugs (NSAIDs), administration of Ketorolac Tromethamine to animals resulted in renal papillary necrosis and other abnormal renal pathology. In humans, there have been reports of hematuria, proteinuria, glomerular nephritis, interstitial nephritis, renal papillary necrosis, nephrotic syndrome, and acute renal failure.

Another, equally important, renal toxicity has been seen in patients with conditions leading to a reduction in blood volume and/or renal blood flow, where renal prostaglandins have a supportive role in the maintenance of renal perfusion. In these patients, administration of a nonsteroidal anti-inflammatory drug (NSAID) may cause a dose-dependent reduction in renal prostaglandin formation and may precipitate acute renal failure. Patients at greatest risk of this reaction are those with impaired renal function, heart failure, or liver dysfunction, those taking diuretics and the elderly. Discontinuation of NSAID therapy is usually followed by recovery to the pretreatment state.

Ketorolac Tromethamine and its metabolites are eliminated primarily by the kidneys which, in patients with reduced creatinine clearance, will result in diminished clearance of the drug (see "Clinical Pharmacology"). Therefore, Ketorolac Tromethamine should be used with caution in patients with impaired renal function (see "Warnings" and "Dosage and Administration") and such patients should be followed closely.

Fluid Retention and Edema: As with other nonsteroidal anti-inflammatory drugs (NSAIDs) that inhibit prostaglandin biosynthesis, fluid retention, edema, retention of NaCl, oliguria, elevations of serum urea nitrogen and creatinine have been reported in clinical trials with Ketorolac Tromethamine. Therefore Ketorolac Tromethamine should be used with caution in patients with acute renal failure, cardiac decompensation, hypertension, or similar conditions.

Hepatic Effects: As with other nonsteroidal anti-inflammatory drugs (NSAIDs) treatment with Ketorolac Tromethamine may cause elevations of liver enzymes, and in patients with pre-existing liver dysfunction, it may lead to the development of a more severe hepatic reaction. The ALT (SGPT) test is probably the most sensitive indicator of liver injury. In patients with symptoms and signs suggesting liver dysfunction, or in whom an abnormal liver test has occurred as a result of Ketorolac Tromethamine therapy, the administration of the drug should be discontinued.

Hematologic Effects: Ketorolac Tromethamine inhibits platelet aggregation and may prolong bleeding time. Unlike aspirin, the inhibition of platelet function by Ketorolac Tromethamine disappears within 24 to 48 hours after the drug is discontinued. Ketorolac Tromethamine does not appear to affect platelet count, prothrombin time (PT) or partial thromboplastin time (PTT). In controlled clinical studies where Ketorolac Tromethamine was administered intramuscularly or intravenously postoperatively, the incidence of clinically significant postoperative bleeding was 0.4% for Ketorolac Tromethamine compared to 0.2% in the control groups receiving narcotic analgesics.

Because prostaglandins play an important role on hemostasis, NSAIDs affect platelet aggregation as well, use of Ketorolac Tromethamine in patients who have coagulation disorders should be undertaken with caution, and those patients should be carefully monitored. Patients on therapeutic doses of anticoagulants (e.g., heparin or dicumarol derivatives) have an increased risk of bleeding complications if given Ketorolac Tromethamine concurrently; physicians should administer such concomitant therapy with extreme caution. The concurrent use of Ketorolac Tromethamine and prophylatic, low-dose heparin (2500-5000 units q12h) has not been studied extensively, but may also be associated with an increased risk of bleeding. Physicians should weigh the benefits against the risk, and exercise caution in using such concomitant therapy in these patients. In patients who receive anticoagulants for any reason, there is an increased risk of intramuscular hematoma formation from Ketorolac Tromethamine IM injections (see "Precautions—Drug Interactions").

In postmarketing experience, postoperative hematomas and other signs of wound bleeding have been reported in association with the perioperative use of Ketorolac Tromethamine IM. Caution should be used, therefore, when Ketorolac Tromethamine is administered pre- or intra-operatively. Perioperative use of Ketorolac Tromethamine should be undertaken with caution when strict hemostasis is critical.

INFORMATION FOR PATIENTS
Ketorolac Tromethamine like other drugs of its class, is not free of side effects. The side effects of these drugs can cause discomfort and, rarely, there are more serious side effects, such as gastrointestinal bleeding, which may result in hospitalization and even fatal outcomes.

Physicians may wish to discuss with their patients the potential risks (see "Warnings," "Precautions," and "Adverse Reactions" sections) and likely benefits of Ketorolac Tromethamine treatment, particularly when it is used for less serious conditions when lengthy treatment is anticipated and when acceptable alternatives to both the patient and physician may be available.

LABORATORY TESTS
Because serious GI tract ulceration and bleeding can occur without warning symptoms, physicians should follow patients for the signs and symptoms of ulceration and bleeding and should inform them of the importance of this follow-up (see "Precautions—Risk of GI Ulceration, Bleeding and Perforation").

DRUG INTERACTIONS
Ketorolac Tromethamine is highly bound to human plasma protein (mean 99.2%) and binding is independent of concentration.

The *in vitro* binding of *warfarin* to plasma proteins is only slightly reduced by Ketorolac Tromethamine (99.5% control vs 99.3%) with Ketorolac Tromethamine plasma concentrations of 5 to 10 µg/mL. Ketorolac Tromethamine does not alter *digoxin* protein binding.

In vitro studies indicate that, at therapeutic plasma concentrations of *salicylate* (300 µg/mL), the binding of Ketorolac Tromethamine was reduced from approximately 99.2% to 97.5%, representing a potential two-fold increase in unbound Ketorolac Tromethamine plasma levels; hence Ketorolac Tromethamine should be used with caution (or at a reduced dosage) in patients being treated with

high-dose salicylate regimens. Therapeutic concentrations of *digoxin, warfarin, ibuprofen, naproxen, piroxicam, acetaminophen, phenytoin,* and *tolbutamide* did not alter Ketorolac Tromethamine protein binding.

In a study involving 12 volunteers, oral Ketorolac Tromethamine was co-administered with a single dose of 25 mg *warfarin*, causing no significant changes in pharmacokinetics or pharmacodynamics of warfarin. In another study, intramuscular Ketorolac Tromethamine (following oral dosing) was given with two doses of 5000 U of *heparin* to 11 healthy volunteers, resulting in a mean template bleeding time of 6.4 minutes (3.2-11.4 min) compared to a mean of 6.0 minutes (3.4-7.5 min) for heparin alone and 5.1 minutes (3.5-8.5 min) for placebo. Although these results do not indicate significant interaction between Ketorolac Tromethamine and warfarin or heparin, the administration of Ketorolac Tromethamine, or other NSAIDs, to patients taking anticoagulants should be done with caution and patients should be closely monitored (see "Precautions—Hematologic Effects").

Intramuscular Ketorolac Tromethamine reduced the diuretic response to *furosemide* in normovolemic healthy subjects by approximately 20% (mean sodium and urinary output decreased 17%).

Concomitant administration of oral Ketorolac Tromethamine and *probenecid* resulted in decreased clearance of ketorolac and significant increases in Ketorolac plasma levels (total AUC increased approximately 3-fold from 5.4 to 17.8 µg.h/mL) and terminal half-life (increased approximately 2-fold from 6.6 to 15.1 hours).

Inhibition of renal *lithium* clearance, leading to an increase in plasma lithium concentration, has been reported with some prostaglandin synthesis inhibiting drugs. The effect of Ketorolac Tromethamine on plasma lithium has not been studied.

Concomitant administration of *methotrexate* and some NSAIDs has been reported to reduce the clearance of methotrexate, enhancing the toxicity of methotrexate. The effect of Ketorolac Tromethamine on methotrexate clearance has not been studied. In post-marketing experience, there have been three reports of a possible interaction between Ketorolac Tromethamine IM and *non-depolarizing muscle relaxants*, appearing to enhance the effect of the muscle relaxant. The concurrent use of Ketorolac Tromethamine with muscle relaxants has not been formally studied. Intramuscular Ketorolac Tromethamine has been administered concurrently with *morphine* in several clinical trials of postoperative pain without evidence of adverse interactions.

There is no evidence, in animal or human studies, that Ketorolac Tromethamine induces or inhibits hepatic enzymes capable of metabolizing itself or other drugs.

CARCINOGENESIS, MUTAGENESIS, AND IMPAIRMENT OF FERTILITY
An 18-month study in mice at oral doses of Ketorolac Tromethamine equal to the parenteral MRHD (Maximum Recommended Human Dose) and a 24-month study in rats at oral doses 2.5 times the parenteral MRHD, showed no evidence of tumorigenicity.

Ketorolac Tromethamine was not mutagenic in Ames test, unscheduled DNA synthesis and repair, and in forward mutation assays. Ketorolac did not cause chromosome breakage in the *in vivo* mouse micronucleus assay. At 1590 µg/mL (approximately 1000 times the average human plasma levels) and at higher concentrations, Ketorolac Tromethamine increased the incidence of chromosomal aberrations in Chinese hamster ovarian cells.

Impairment of fertility did not occur in male or female rats at oral doses of 9 mg/kg (53.1 mg/m^2) and 16 mg/kg (94.4 mg/m^2), respectively.

PREGNANCY:
PREGNANCY CATEGORY C
Reproduction studies have been performed in rabbits, using daily oral doses at 3.6 mg/kg (42.35 mg/m^2) and in rats at 10 mg/kg (59 mg/m^2) during organogenesis. Results of these studies did not reveal evidence of teratogenicity to the fetus. Oral doses of Ketorolac Tromethamine at 1.5 mg/kg (8.8 mg/m^2), which was half of the human oral exposure, administered after gestation day 17 caused dystocia and higher pup mortality in rats. There are no adequate and well-controlled studies in pregnant women. Ketorolac Tromethamine should be used during pregnancy only if the potential benefit justifies the potential risk to the fetus.

LABOR AND DELIVERY
Ketorolac Tromethamine is not recommended for use during labor and delivery (see "Indications").

LACTATION AND NURSING
After a single oral administration of 10 mg of Ketorolac Tromethamine Oral to humans, the maximum milk concentration observed was 7.3 ng/mL and the maximum milk-to-plasma ratio was 0.037. After one day of dosing (qid), the maximum milk concentration was 7.9 ng/mL and the maximum milk-to-plasma ratio was 0.025. Caution should be exercised when Ketorolac Tromethamine IM or Oral is administered to a nursing woman.

PEDIATRIC USE
Safety and efficacy in children have not been established. Therefore, Ketorolac Tromethamine is not recommended for use in children.

USE IN THE ELDERLY
Because Ketorolac Tromethamine is cleared somewhat more slowly by the elderly (see "Clinical Pharmacology") who are also more sensitive to the renal effects of NSAIDs (see "Precautions—Renal Effects"), extra caution and reduced dosages

(see *"Dosage and Administration"*) should be used when treating the elderly with Ketorolac Tromethamine.

ADVERSE REACTIONS
Adverse reaction rates from short-term use of NSAIDs are generally from $1/10$ to $1/2$ the rates associated with long-term use. This is also true for Ketorolac Tromethamine. Adverse reaction rates also may increase with higher doses of Ketorolac Tromethamine (see *"Warnings"* and *"Dosage and Administration"*).

Ketorolac Tromethamine IM is indicated for short-term use. Physicians using Ketorolac Tromethamine IM should be alert for the usual complications of NSAID treatment, and should be aware that with longer use (exceeding 5 days) of Ketorolac Tromethamine IM, the frequency and severity of adverse reactions may increase.

Physicians using Ketorolac Tromethamine Oral should be alert to the relative risks associated with dose and dose duration as described in *"Clinical Pharmacology—Clinical Studies"*.

Physicians using Ketorolac Tromethamine should be alert for the usual complications of NSAID treatment.

The adverse reactions listed below were reported in clinical trials with Ketorolac Tromethamine in which patients received up to 20 doses, in 5 days, of Ketorolac Tromethamine IM 30 mg or up to 4 doses a day from long-term studies of Ketorolac Tromethamine Oral 10 mg qid. In addition, adverse reactions that were reported from Ketorolac Tromethamine IM post-marketing surveillance are included in "Incidence 1% or Less."

INCIDENCE GREATER THAN 1% (PROBABLY CAUSALLY RELATED)
Body as a Whole: EDEMA*

Cardiovascular: HYPERTENSION

Dermatologic: RASH, pruritus*

Gastrointestinal: NAUSEA (12%), DYSPEPSIA (12%), GASTROINTESTINAL PAIN (13%), constipation, diarrhea* flatulence, gastrointestinal fullness, vomiting, STOMATITIS

Hemic and Lymphatic: purpura

Nervous System: drowsiness*, dizziness*, HEADACHE (17%), sweating

Injection site pain was reported by 2% of patients in multidose studies (vs. 5% for morphine control group).

INCIDENCE 1% OR LESS (PROBABLY CAUSALLY RELATED)
Body as a Whole: hypersensitivity reactions such as *anaphylaxis*[1], *bronchospasm, laryngeal edema, tongue edema, hypotension,* and *flushing,* weight gain, fever

Cardiovascular: flushing, palpitation, pallor, *hypotension, syncope*

Dermatologic: Lyell's syndrome, Stevens-Johnson syndrome, exfoliative dermatitis, muculo-papular rash, urticaria

Gastrointestinal: peptic ulceration, GI hemorrhage, GI perforation (see *"Warnings"* and *"Precautions"*), *melena,* rectal bleeding, gastritis, eructation, anorexia, increased appetite

Hemic and Lymphatic: postoperative wound hemorrhage, rarely requiring blood transfusion (see *"Warnings"* and *"Precautions"*), thrombocytopenia, epistaxis, anemia

Nervous System: convulsions, vertigo, tremors, abnormal dreams, hallucinations, euphoria

Respiratory: dyspnea, *asthma,* pulmonary edema

Urogenital: acute renal failure (see *"Warnings"* and *"Precautions"*), *flank pain with or without hematuria and/or azotemia,* oliguria, nephritis

OTHER ADVERSE EVENTS (CAUSAL RELATIONSHIP UNKNOWN)[2]
Body as a Whole: asthenia

Gastrointestinal: pancreatitis

Hemic and Lymphatic: leukopenia, EOSINOPHILIA

Nervous System: paresthesia, depression, insomnia, nervousness, excessive thirst, dry mouth, abnormal thinking, inability to concentrate, hyperkinesia, stupor

Respiratory: RHINITIS, COUGH, dyspnea

Special Senses: abnormal taste, abnormal vision, blurred vision, tinnitus, HEARING LOSS

Urogenital: polyuria, increased urinary frequency

DRUG ABUSE AND PHYSICAL DEPENDENCE
Ketorolac Tromethamine is not a narcotic agonist or antagonist. Subjects did not show any subjective symptoms or objective signs of drug withdrawal upon abrupt discontinuation of intravenous or intramuscular dosing. Patients receiving Ketorolac Tromethamine Oral for long-term therapy have not developed tolerance to the drug and there is no pharmacologic basis to expect addiction.

---

* Incidence of reported reaction between 3% and 9%. Those reactions occurring in less than 3% of the patients are unmarked. Reactions reported predominantly from long-term Ketorolac Tromethamine Oral studies are CAPITALIZED.
1 *Italics* denote reactions reported from *postmarketing experience.*
2 Reactions occurred under circumstances where causal relationship to Ketorolac Tromethamine treatment has not been clearly established; they are presented as alerting information for physicians. Reactions reported predominantly from long-term Ketorolac Tromethamine Oral studies are CAPITALIZED.

Ketorolac did not exhibit activity in classical animal studies which are reasonable predictors of opiate analgesic action. *In vitro,* Ketorolac does not bind to opiate receptors. These studies demonstrate that Ketorolac does not have central opiate-like activity.

OVERDOSAGE
The absence of experience with acute overdosage precludes characterization of sequelae and assessment of antidotal efficacy at this time. At single oral doses greater than 100 mg/kg in rats, mice and monkeys, symptoms such as decreased activity, diarrhea, pallor, labored breathing, rales, and vomiting were observed.

DOSAGE AND ADMINISTRATION
Ketorolac Tromethamine IM may be used on a regular schedule or prn ("as needed"), based on the return of pain. For the short-term management of pain on a regular schedule (see *"Clinical Pharmacology"* for details of clinical trials), the recommended initial dose is 30 or 60 mg IM, as a loading dose, followed by half of the loading dose, i.e., 15 or 30 mg, every 6 hours. The maximum recommended daily dose is 150 mg for the first day and 120 mg/day thereafter. It is recommended that intramuscular Ketorolac Tromethamine be limited to short-term therapy (not over 5 days) because the frequency and severity of adverse events may increase with longer use at recommended doses (see *"Warnings"* and *"Precautions"*).

Note: The initial intramuscular loading dose should be given only once, unless therapy has been interrupted for 3 half-lives (15-40 hours, see half-life of Ketorolac Tromethamine IM in Table in "Clinical Pharmacology").

The lower end of the dosage range is recommended for patients under 50 kg (110 pounds) of body weight, for patients over 65 years of age, and for patients with reduced renal function (see *"Clinical Pharmacology"* and *"Precautions"*).

If prn management is elected, see *"Individualization of Dosage"* in *"Clinical Pharmacology"* for suggestions. Parenteral drug products should be inspected visually for particulate matter and discoloration prior to administration, whenever solution and container permit.

PHARMACEUTICAL COMPATIBILITY OF KETOROLAC TROMETHAMINE IM
Ketorolac Tromethamine IM should not be mixed in small volume (e.g., in a syringe) with morphine sulfate, meperidine hydrochloride, promethazine hydrochloride or hydrolyzine hydrochloride; this will result in precipitation of Ketorolac from solution.

Ketorolac Tromethamine Oral is indicated for the management of pain. The recommended oral dose is 10 mg prn every 4 to 6 hours for limited duration. Doses of 10 mg qid chronically are not recommended (see *"Warnings"*, *"Adverse Reactions"* and *"Clinical Pharmacology—Clinical Studies"* sections for details about relative risks associated with Ketorolac Tromethamine Oral).

TRANSITION FROM KETOROLAC TROMETHAMINE IM TO KETOROLAC TROMETHAMINE ORAL
When Ketorolac Tromethamine Oral is used as follow-on therapy to Ketorolac Tromethamine IM the total combined dose should not exceed 120 mg on the day of transition, including a maximum of 40 mg orally. Subsequent oral dosing should not exceed the recommended daily maximum of 40 mg.

STORAGE
Injection: Store at controlled room temperature 15-30°C (59°-86°F) with protection from light.

Tablets: Store bottles at controlled room temperature, 15°-30°C (59°-86°F). Store blister packages at controlled room temperature, 15°-30°C (59°-86°F). Protect from excessive humidity and light.

J CODES
Per 15 mg IM,IV—J1885

HOW SUPPLIED
INJECTION: 15 MG/ML

BRAND/MANUFACTURER	NDC	SIZE	AWP
○ BRAND			
TORADOL: Syntex	00033-2443-50	1 ml 10s	$73.27

INJECTION: 30 MG/ML

BRAND/MANUFACTURER	NDC	SIZE	AWP
○ BRAND			
TORADOL: Syntex	00033-2434-50	1 ml 10s	$76.75

INJECTION: 60 MG/2 ML

BRAND/MANUFACTURER	NDC	SIZE	AWP
○ BRAND			
TORADOL: Syntex	00033-2444-50	2 ml 10s	$80.48

TABLETS: 10 MG

BRAND/MANUFACTURER	NDC	SIZE	AWP
○ BRAND			
▶ TORADOL: Syntex	00033-2435-42	100s	$114.30
	00033-2435-53	100s ud	$114.30

◆ RATED THERAPEUTICALLY EQUIVALENT; ◇ THERAPEUTIC EQUIVALENCE UNCONFIRMED; ○ UNRATED

Kinesed SEE BELLADONNA AND PHENOBARBITAL

Kinevac SEE SINCALIDE

Klonopin SEE CLONAZEPAM

Klorvess SEE POTASSIUM CHLORIDE, ORAL

Klorvess Effervescent SEE LYSINE HYDROCHLORIDE/POTASSIUM BICARBONATE/POTASSIUM CHLORIDE

Klotrix SEE POTASSIUM CHLORIDE, ORAL

KoGENate SEE ANTIHEMOPHILIC FACTOR

Konakion SEE PHYTONADIONE

Ku-Zyme SEE AMYLASE/CELLULASE/LIPASE/PROTEASE

Kutapressin SEE LIVER DERIVATIVE COMPLEX

Kutrase SEE DIGESTIVE ENZYMES/HYOSCYAMINE SULFATE/ PHENYLTOLOXAMINE CITRATE

Kytril SEE GRANISETRON HYDROCHLORIDE

L-Cysteine Hydrochloride

DESCRIPTION

L-Cysteine Hydrochloride Injection, USP, is a sterile nonpyrogenic solution. Each mL contains: 50 mg of L-Cysteine Hydrochloride (Monohydrate).

L-Cysteine is a sulfur containing amino acid. In premixed solutions of crystalline amino acids, Cysteine is relatively unstable over time, eventually converting to insoluble cystine. To avoid such precipitation, L-Cysteine Hydrochloride Injection, USP is intended to be used as an additive with Crystalline Amino Acid Injection immediately prior to administration to the patient.

Its molecular formula is $C_3H_7NO_2S \cdot HCl \cdot H_2O$ and molecular weight is 175.63.

Following is its chemical structure:

$$HSCH_2 - \overset{\overset{\displaystyle H}{|}}{\underset{\underset{\displaystyle NH_2}{|}}{C}} - COOH \cdot HCl \cdot H_2O$$

CLINICAL PHARMACOLOGY

L-Cysteine is synthesized from methionine via the trans-sulfuration pathway in the adult, but newborn infants lack the enzyme necessary to effect this conversion. Therefore, L-Cysteine is generally considered to be an essential amino acid in infants.

INDICATIONS AND USAGE

L-Cysteine Hydrochloride Injection, USP is indicated for use only after dilution as an additive to Crystalline Amino Acid Injection to meet the intravenous amino acid nutritional requirements of infants receiving total parenteral nutrition.

CONTRAINDICATIONS

This preparation should not be used in patients with hepatic coma or metabolic disorders involving impaired nitrogen utilization.

WARNINGS

Peripheral intravenous infusion of amino acids may induce a rise in blood urea nitrogen (BUN) especially in patients with impaired hepatic or renal function. Appropriate laboratory tests should be performed periodically and infusion discontinued if BUN levels exceed normal postprandial limits and continue to rise. It should be noted that a modest rise in BUN normally occurs as a result of increased protein intake.

Administration of amino acid solutions to a patient with hepatic insufficiency may result in serum amino acid imbalances, metabolic alkalosis, prerenal azotemia, hyperammonemia, stupor and coma.

Administration of amino acid solutions in the presence of impaired renal function may augment an increasing BUN, as does any protein dietary component.

Solutions containing sodium ion should be used with great care, if at all, in patients with congestive heart failure, severe renal insufficiency, and in clinical states in which there exists edema with sodium retention.

Solutions which contain potassium ion should be used with great care, if at all, in patients with hyperkalemia, severe renal failure and in conditions in which potassium retention is present.

Solutions containing acetate ion should be used with great care in patients with metabolic or respiratory alkalosis. Acetate should be administered with great care in those conditions in which there is an increased level or an impaired utilization of this ion such as severe hepatic insufficiency.

Hyperammonemia is of special significance in infants, as it can result in mental retardation. Therefore it is essential that blood ammonia levels be measured frequently in infants.

Instances of asymptomatic hyperammonemia have been reported in patients without overt liver dysfunction. The mechanisms of this reaction are not clearly defined but may involve genetic defects and immature or subclinically impaired liver function.

Frequent Clinical Evaluations and Laboratory Determinations are Necessary for Proper Monitoring During Administration: Blood studies should include glucose, urea nitrogen, serum electrolytes, ammonia, cholesterol, acid-base balance, serum proteins, kidney and liver function tests, osmolality and hemogram. White blood count and blood cultures are to be determined if indicated. Urinary osmolality and glucose should be determined frequently.

PREGNANCY

Safe use during pregnancy has not been established, therefore, infusion of amino acids should be undertaken during pregnancy only when this is deemed essential to the patients' welfare, as judged by the physician.

PRECAUTIONS

Special care must be taken when administering hypertonic glucose to provide calories in diabetic or prediabetic patients.

Because of its antianabolic activity, concurrent administration of tetracycline may reduce the nitrogen sparing effects of infused amino acids.

Do not withdraw venous blood chemistries through the peripheral infusion site, as interference with estimations of nitrogen containing substances may occur.

Intravenous feeding regiments which include amino acids should be used with caution in patients with a history of renal disease, pulmonary disease, or with cardiac insufficiency so as to avoid excessive fluid accumulation.

The effect of infusion of amino acids, without dextrose, upon carbohydrate metabolism of children is not known at this time.

Nitrogen intake should be carefully monitored in patients with impaired renal function. For long-term total nutrition, or if a patient has inadequate fat stores, it is essential to provide adequate exogenous calories concurrently with the amino acids. Concentrated dextrose solutions are an effective source of such calories. Such strongly hypertonic nutrient solutions should be administered through an indwelling intravenous catheter with the tip located in the superior vena cava.

ADVERSE REACTIONS

Local reactions consisting of a warm sensation, erythema, phlebitis and thrombosis at the infusion site have occurred with peripheral intravenous infusion of amino acids, particularly if other substances, such as antibiotics, are also administered through the same site. In such cases the infusion site should be changed promptly to another vein. Use of large peripheral veins, inline filters, and slowing the rate of infusion may reduce the incidence of local venous irritation. Electrolyte additives should be spread throughout the day. Irritating additive medications may need to be injected at another venous site.

Generalized flushing, fever and nausea also have been reported during peripheral infusions of amino acid solutions.

DRUG ABUSE AND DEPENDENCE

None known.

DOSAGE AND ADMINISTRATION

L-Cysteine Hydrochloride Injection, USP is intended for use only after dilution in Crystalline Amino Acid Injection. Each 0.5 gram of L-Cysteine Hydrochloride Monohydrate should be combined aseptically with 12.5 grams of Crystalline Amino Acid Injection, such as that present in 250 mL of 5% Crystalline Amino Acid Injection. The admixture is then diluted with 250 mL of dextrose 50% or such lesser volume as indicated. Equal volumes of 5% Crystalline Amino Acid and dextrose 50% produce a final solution which contains Crystalline Amino Acid Injection 2.5% in dextrose 25%, which is suitable for administration by central venous infusion. Administration of the final admixture should begin within one hour of mixing. Otherwise, the admixture should be refrigerated immediately and used within 24 hours of the time of mixing. For the recommended rate of administration, see the Crystalline Amino Acid Injection package insert.

Parenteral drug products should be inspected visually for particulate matter and discoloration prior to administration, whenever solution and container permit.

Store at controlled room temperature 15-30°C (59°-86°F). Do not freeze.

HOW SUPPLIED
INJECTION: 50 MG/ML

BRAND/MANUFACTURER	NDC	SIZE	AWP
○ GENERICS			
Amer Regent	00517-2064-05	10 ml 5s	$44.38
Gensia	00703-5324-03	10 ml 10s	$106.25

Labetalol Hydrochloride

DESCRIPTION

Labetalol Hydrochloride Tablets and Labetalol Hydrochloride Injection are adrenergic receptor blocking agents that have both selective alpha$_1$-adrenergic and nonselective beta-adrenergic receptor blocking actions in a single substance.

Labetalol Hydrochloride is a racemate chemically designated as 2-hydroxy-5-[1-hydroxy-2-[(1-methyl-3-phenylpropyl)amino]ethyl] benzamide monohydrochloride. Labetalol HCl has the empirical formula $C_{19}H_{24}N_2O_3 \cdot HCl$ and a molecular weight of 364.9. It has two asymmetric centers and therefore exists as a molecular complex of two diastereoisomeric pairs. Dilevalol, the R,R' stereoisomer, makes up 25% of racemic Labetalol.

Labetalol Hydrochloride is a white or off-white crystalline powder, soluble in water.

Labetalol Hydrochloride is available as 100, 200, 300 mg tablets for oral use.

Labetalol Injection is a clear, colorless to light yellow, aqueous, sterile, isotonic solution for intravenous (IV) injection. It has a pH range of 3-4. Each milliliter contains 5 mg of Labetalol Hydrochloride.

Following is its chemical structure:

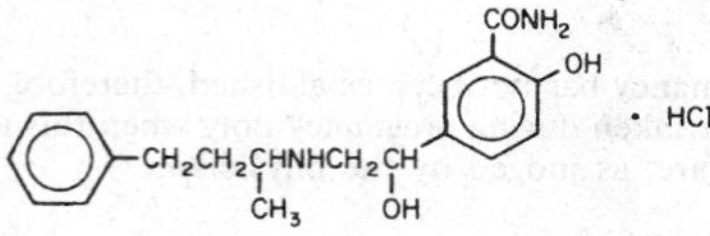

CLINICAL PHARMACOLOGY

Labetalol Hydrochloride combines both selective, competitive, alpha$_1$-adrenergic blocking and nonselective, competitive, beta-adrenergic blocking activity in a single substance. In man, the ratios of alpha-to beta-blockade have been estimated to be approximately 1:3 and 1:7 following oral and IV administration, respectively. Beta$_2$-agonist activity has been demonstrated in animals with minimal beta$_1$-agonist (ISA) activity detected. In animals, at doses greater than those required for alpha- or beta-adrenergic blockade, a membrane stabilizing effect has been demonstrated.

Pharmacodynamics: The capacity of Labetalol Hydrochloride to block alpha receptors in man has been demonstrated by attenuation of the pressor effect of phenylephrine and by a significant reduction of the pressor response caused by immersing the hand in ice-cold water ("cold-pressor test"). Labetalol Hydrochloride beta$_1$-receptor blockade in man was demonstrated by a small decrease in the resting heart rate, attenuation of tachycardia produced by isoproterenol or exercise, and by attenuation of the reflex tachycardia to the hypotension produced by amyl nitrite. Beta$_2$-receptor blockade was demonstrated by inhibition of the isoproterenol-induced fall in diastolic blood pressure. Both the alpha- and beta-blocking actions of orally administered Labetalol Hydrochloride contribute to a decrease in blood pressure in hypertensive patients. Labetalol HCl consistently, in dose-related fashion, blunted increases in exercise-induced blood pressure and heart rate, and in their double product. The pulmonary circulation during exercise was not affected by Labetalol Hydrochloride dosing.

Single oral doses of Labetalol Hydrochloride administered to patients with coronary artery disease had no significant effect on sinus rate, intraventricular conduction, or QRS duration. The atrioventricular (A-V) conduction time was modestly prolonged in two of seven patients. In another study, IV Labetalol Hydrochloride slightly prolonged A-V nodal conduction time and atrial effective refractory period with only small changes in heart rate. The effects on A-V nodal refractoriness were inconsistent.

Labetalol Hydrochloride produces dose-related falls in blood pressure without reflex tachycardia and without significant reduction in heart rate, presumably through a mixture of its alpha- and beta-blocking effects. Hemodynamic effects are variable, with small, nonsignificant changes in cardiac output seen in some studies, but not others, and small decreases in total peripheral resistance. Elevated plasma renins are reduced. Doses of Labetalol Hydrochloride that controlled hypertension did not affect renal function in mildly to severely hypertensive patients with normal renal function.

Due to the alpha$_1$-receptor blocking activity of Labetalol Hydrochloride, blood pressure is lowered more in the standing than in the supine position, and symptoms of postural hypotension (2%), including rare instances of syncope, can occur. Following oral administration, when postural hypotension has occurred, it

has been transient and is uncommon when the recommended starting dose and titration increments are closely followed (see "Dosage and Administration"). Symptomatic postural hypotension is most likely to occur 2-4 hours after a dose, especially following the use of large initial doses or upon large changes in dose. During dosing with IV Labetalol Hydrochloride, the contribution of the postural component should be considered when positioning the patient for treatment, and the patient should not be allowed to move to an erect position unmonitored until his ability to do so is established.

The peak effects of single oral doses of Labetalol Hydrochloride occur within 2-4 hours. The duration of effect depends upon dose, lasting at least 8 hours following single oral doses of 100 mg and more than 12 hours following single oral doses of 300 mg. The maximum, steady-state blood pressure response upon oral, twice-a-day dosing occurs within 24-72 hours.

The antihypertensive effect of Labetalol has a linear correlation with the logarithm of Labetalol plasma concentration, and there is also a linear correlation between the reduction in exercise-induced tachycardia occurring at 2 hours after oral administration of Labetalol Hydrochloride and the logarithm of the plasma concentration.

About 70% of the maximum beta-blocking effect is present for 5 hours after the administration of a single oral dose of 400 mg with suggestion that about 40% remains at 8 hours. The antianginal efficacy of Labetalol Hydrochloride has not been studied. In 37 patients with hypertension and coronary artery disease, Labetalol Hydrochloride did not increase the incidence or severity of angina attacks.

In a clinical pharmacologic study in severe-hypertensives, an initial 0.25-mg/kg injection of Labetalol Hydrochloride administered to patients in the supine position decreased blood pressure by an average of 11/7 mmHg. Additional injections of 0.5 mg/kg at 15-minute intervals up to a total cumulative dose of 1.75 mg/kg of Labetalol Hydrochloride caused further dose-related decreases in blood pressure. Some patients required cumulative doses of up to 3.25 mg/kg. The maximal effect of each dose level occurred within 5 minutes. Following discontinuation of IV treatment with Labetalol Hydrochloride, the blood pressure rose gradually and progressively, approaching pretreatment baseline values within an average of 16-18 hours in the majority of patients.

Similar results were obtained in the treatment of patients with severe hypertension who required urgent blood pressure reduction with an initial dose of 20 mg (which corresponds to 0.25 mg/kg for an 80-kg patient) followed by additional doses of either 40 or 80 mg at 10-minute intervals to achieve the desired effect, or up to a cumulative dose of 300 mg.

Labetalol Hydrochloride administered as a continuous IV infusion, with a mean dose of 136 mg (27-300 mg) over a period of 2-3 hours (mean of 2 hours and 39 minutes), lowered the blood pressure by an average of 60/35 mmHg.

Exacerbation of angina and, in some cases, myocardial infarction and ventricular dysrhythmias have been reported after abrupt discontinuation of therapy with beta-adrenergic blocking agents in patients with coronary artery disease. Abrupt withdrawal of these agents in patients without coronary artery disease has resulted in transient symptoms, including tremulousness, sweating, palpitation, headache, and malaise. Several mechanisms have been proposed to explain these phenomena, among them increased sensitivity to catecholamines because of increased numbers of beta receptors. Although beta-adrenergic receptor blockade is useful in the treatment of angina and hypertension, there are also situations in which sympathetic stimulation is vital. For example, in patients with severely damaged hearts, adequate ventricular function may depend on sympathetic drive. Beta-adrenergic blockade may worsen A-V block by preventing the necessary facilitating effects of sympathetic activity on conduction. Beta$_2$-adrenergic blockade results in passive bronchial constriction by interfering with endogenous adrenergic bronchodilator activity in patients subject to bronchospasm, and it may also interfere with exogenous bronchodilators in such patients.

Pharmacokinetics and Metabolism: Labetalol Hydrochloride is completely absorbed from the gastrointestinal tract with peak plasma levels occurring 1-2 hours after oral administration. The relative bioavailability of Labetalol Hydrochloride tablets compared to an oral solution is 100%. The absolute bioavailability (fraction of drug reaching systemic circulation) of Labetalol when compared to an IV infusion is 25%; this is due to extensive "first-pass" metabolism. Despite "first-pass" metabolism, there is a linear relationship between oral doses of 100-3,000 mg and peak plasma levels. The absolute bioavailability of Labetalol is increased when administered with food. Following IV infusion of Labetalol, the elimination half-life is about 5.5 hours and the total body clearance is approximately 33 mL/min/kg. The plasma half-life of Labetalol following oral administration is about 6-8 hours. Steady-state plasma levels of Labetalol during repetitive dosing are reached by about the third day of dosing. In patients with decreased hepatic or renal function, the elimination half-life of Labetalol is not altered; however, the relative bioavailability in hepatically impaired patients is increased due to decreased "first-pass" metabolism.

The metabolism of Labetalol is mainly through conjugation to glucuronide metabolites. These metabolites are present in plasma and are excreted in the urine and, via the bile, into the feces. Approximately 55%-60% of a dose appears in the urine as conjugates or unchanged Labetalol within the first 24 hours of dosing.

Labetalol has been shown to cross the placental barrier in humans. Only negligible amounts of the drug crossed the blood-brain barrier in animal studies. Labetalol is approximately 50% protein bound. Neither hemodialysis nor peritoneal dialysis removes a significant amount of Labetalol Hydrochloride from the general circulation (< 1%).

◆ RATED THERAPEUTICALLY EQUIVALENT; ◇ THERAPEUTIC EQUIVALENCE UNCONFIRMED; ○ UNRATED

INDICATIONS AND USAGE

Labetalol Hydrochloride Tablets are indicated in the management of hypertension. Labetalol Hydrochloride Tablets may be used alone or in combination with other antihypertensive agents, especially thiazide and loop diuretics.

Labetalol Hydrochloride Injection is indicated for control of blood pressure in severe hypertension.

UNLABELED USES

Labetalol is used alone or as an adjunct in the treatment of angina. It is used in myocardial infarction patients with associated hypertension and in cases of malignant hypertension. It is also used in Raynaud's disease and pheochromocytoma, and to manage the sympathetic overactivity observed in severe tetanus.

CONTRAINDICATIONS

Labetalol Hydrochloride Tablets and Labetalol Hydrochloride Injection are contraindicated in bronchial asthma, overt cardiac failure, greater-than-first-degree heart block, cardiogenic shock, severe bradycardia, other conditions associated with severe and prolonged hypotension, and in patients with a history of hypersensitivity to any component of the product (see "Warnings").

WARNINGS

Hepatic Injury: Severe hepatocellular injury, confirmed by rechallenge in at least one case, occurs rarely with Labetalol therapy. The hepatic injury is usually reversible, but hepatic necrosis and death have been reported. Injury has occurred after both short- and long-term treatment and may be slowly progressive despite minimal symptomatology. Similar hepatic events have been reported with a related research compound, dilevalol Hydrochloride, including two deaths. Dilevalol Hydrochloride is one of the four isomers of Labetalol Hydrochloride. Thus, for patients taking Labetalol, periodic determination of suitable hepatic laboratory tests would be appropriate. Appropriate laboratory testing should be done at the first symptom/sign of liver dysfunction (e.g., pruritus, dark urine, persistent anorexia, jaundice, right upper quadrant tenderness, or unexplained "flu-like" symptoms). If the patient has laboratory evidence of liver injury or jaundice, Labetalol should be stopped and not restarted.

Cardiac Failure: Sympathetic stimulation is a vital component supporting circulatory function in congestive heart failure. Beta-blockade carries a potential hazard of further depressing myocardial contractility and precipitating more severe failure. Although beta-blockers should be avoided in overt congestive heart failure, if necessary, Labetalol Hydrochloride can be used with caution in patients with a history of heart failure who are well compensated. Congestive heart failure has been observed in patients receiving Labetalol Hydrochloride. Labetalol Hydrochloride does not abolish the inotropic action of digitalis on heart muscle.

In Patients Without a History of Cardiac Failure: In patients with latent cardiac insufficiency, continued depression of the myocardium with beta-blocking agents over a period of time can, in some cases, lead to cardiac failure. At the first sign or symptom of impending cardiac failure, patients should be fully digitalized and/or be given a diuretic, and the response should be observed closely. If cardiac failure continues despite adequate digitalization and diuretic, Labetalol Hydrochloride Tablets and Labetalol Hydrochloride Injection therapy should be withdrawn (gradually, if possible).

Exacerbation of Ischemic Heart Disease Following Abrupt Withdrawal: Labetalol Hydrochloride Tablets: Angina pectoris has not been reported upon Labetalol Hydrochloride discontinuation. However, hypersensitivity to catecholamines has been observed in patients withdrawn from beta-blocker therapy; exacerbation of angina and, in some cases, myocardial infarction have occurred after *abrupt* discontinuation of such therapy. When discontinuing chronically administered Labetalol Hydrochloride Tablets, particularly in patients with ischemic heart disease, the dosage should be gradually reduced over a period of 1-2 weeks and the patient should be carefully monitored. If angina markedly worsens or acute coronary insufficiency develops, Labetalol Hydrochloride Tablets therapy should be reinstituted promptly, at least temporarily, and other measures appropriate for the management of unstable angina should be taken. Patients should be warned against interruption or discontinuation of therapy without the physician's advice. Because coronary artery disease is common and may be unrecognized, it may be prudent not to discontinue Labetalol Hydrochloride Tablets therapy abruptly in patients being treated for hypertension.

Ischemic Heart Disease: Labetalol Hydrochloride Injection: Angina pectoris has not been reported upon Labetalol Hydrochloride discontinuation. However, following abrupt cessation of therapy with some beta-blocking agents in patients with coronary artery disease, exacerbations of angina pectoris and, in some cases, myocardial infarction have been reported. Therefore, such patients should be cautioned against interruption of therapy without the physician's advice. Even in the absence of overt angina pectoris, when discontinuation of Labetalol Hydrochloride Injection is planned, the patient should be carefully observed and should be advised to limit physical activity. If angina markedly worsens or acute coronary insufficiency develops, Labetalol Hydrochloride Injection administration should be reinstituted promptly, at least temporarily, and other measures appropriate for the management of unstable angina should be taken.

Nonallergic Bronchospasm (e.g., Chronic Bronchitis and Emphysema): Patients with bronchospastic disease should, in general, not receive beta-blockers. Labetalol Hydrochloride Tablets may be used with caution, however, in patients who do not respond to, or cannot tolerate, other antihypertensive agents. It is prudent, if Labetalol Hydrochloride Tablets are used, to use the smallest effective dose, so that inhibition of endogenous or exogenous beta-agonists is minimized. Since Labetalol Hydrochloride Injection at the usual IV therapeutic doses has not been studied in patients with nonallergic bronchospastic disease, it should not be used in such patients.

Pheochromocytoma: Labetalol Hydrochloride has been shown to be effective in lowering blood pressure and relieving symptoms in patients with pheochromocytoma; higher than usual IV doses may be required. However, paradoxical hypertensive responses have been reported in a few patients with this tumor; therefore, use caution when administering Labetalol Hydrochloride to patients with pheochromocytoma.

Diabetes Mellitus and Hypoglycemia: Beta-adrenergic blockade may prevent the appearance of premonitory signs and symptoms (e.g., tachycardia) of acute hypoglycemia. This is especially important in patients with labile diabetics. Beta-blockade also reduces the release of insulin in response to hyperglycemia; it may therefore be necessary to adjust the dose of antidiabetic drugs.

Major Surgery: The necessity or desirability of withdrawing beta-blocking therapy before major surgery is controversial. Protracted severe hypotension and difficulty in restarting or maintaining a heartbeat have been reported with beta-blockers. The effect of Labetalol Hydrochloride alpha-adrenergic activity has not been evaluated in this setting.

A synergism between Labetalol Hydrochloride and halothane anesthesia has been shown (see *"Precautions: Drug Interactions"*).

Rapid Decreases of Blood Pressure: Caution must be observed when reducing severely elevated blood pressure. Although such findings have not been reported with IV Labetalol Hydrochloride, a number of adverse reactions, including cerebral infarction, optic nerve infarction, angina, and ischemic changes in the electrocardiogram, have been reported with other agents when severely elevated blood pressure was reduced over time courses of several hours to as long as 1 or 2 days. The desired blood pressure lowering should therefore be achieved over as long a period of time as is compatible with the patient's status.

PRECAUTIONS

General: Labetalol Hydrochloride Tablets: Impaired Hepatic Function: Labetalol Hydrochloride Tablets should be used with caution in patients with impaired hepatic function since metabolism of the drug may be diminished.

Jaundice or Hepatic Dysfunction: (see *"Warnings"*).

Labetalol Hydrochloride Injection: Impaired Hepatic Function: Labetalol Hydrochloride Injection should be used with caution in patients with impaired hepatic function since metabolism of the drug may be diminished.

Hypotension: Symptomatic postural hypotension (incidence, 58%) is likely to occur if patients are tilted or allowed to assume the upright position within 3 hours of receiving Labetalol Hydrochloride Injection. Therefore, the patient's ability to tolerate an upright position should be established before permitting any ambulation.

Following Coronary Artery Bypass Surgery: In one uncontrolled study, patients with low cardiac indices and elevated systemic vascular resistance following intravenous Labetalol Hydrochloride experienced significant declines in cardiac output with little change in systemic vascular resistance. One of these patients developed hypotension following Labetalol treatment. Therefore, use of Labetalol Hydrochloride should be avoided in such patients.

High Dose Labetalol: Administration of up to 3 g per day as an infusion for up to 2-3 days has been anecdotally reported: several patients have experienced hypotension or bradycardia.

Jaundice or Hepatic Dysfunction: (see *"Warnings"*).

Information for Patients: As with all drugs with beta-blocking activity, certain advice to patients being treated with Labetalol Hydrochloride is warranted. This information is intended to aid in the safe and effective use of this medication. It is not a disclosure of all possible adverse or intended effects. While no incident of the abrupt withdrawal phenomenon (exacerbation of angina pectoris) has been reported with Labetalol Hydrochloride, dosing with Labetalol Hydrochloride Tablets should not be interrupted or discontinued without a physician's advice. Patients being treated with Labetalol Hydrochloride Tablets should consult a physician at any signs or symptoms of impending cardiac failure or hepatic dysfunction (see *"Warnings"*). Also, transient scalp tingling may occur, usually when treatment with Labetalol Hydrochloride Tablets is initiated (see *"Adverse Reactions"*).

During and immediately following (for up to 3 hours) Labetalol Hydrochloride Injection, the patient should remain supine. Subsequently, the patient should be advised on how to proceed gradually to become ambulatory and should be observed at the time of first ambulation.

When the patient is started on Labetalol Hydrochloride Tablets following adequate control of blood pressure with Labetalol Hydrochloride Injection, appropriate directions for titration of dosage should be provided (see *"Dosage and Administration"*).

Laboratory Tests: As with any new drug given over prolonged periods, laboratory parameters should be observed over regular intervals. In patients with concomitant illnesses, such as impaired renal function, appropriate tests should be done to monitor these conditions.

Routine laboratory tests are ordinarily not required before or after IV Labetalol Hydrochloride.

Drug Interactions: Since Labetalol Hydrochloride Injection may be administered to patients already being treated with other medications, including other antihypertensive agents, careful monitoring of these patients is necessary to detect and treat promptly any undesired effect from concomitant administration.

In one survey, 2.3% of patients taking Labetalol Hydrochloride orally in combination with tricyclic antidepressants experienced tremor, as compared to 0.7% reported to occur with Labetalol Hydrochloride alone. The contribution of each of the treatments to this adverse reaction is unknown, but the possibility of a drug interaction cannot be excluded.

Drugs possessing beta-blocking properties can blunt the bronchodilator effect of beta-receptor agonist drugs in patients with bronchospasm; therefore, doses greater than the normal antiasthmatic dose of beta-agonist bronchodilator drugs may be required.

Cimetidine has been shown to increase the bioavailability of Labetalol Hydrocholine administered orally. Since this could be explained either by enhanced absorption or by an alteration of hepatic metabolism of Labetalol Hydrochloride, special care should be used in establishing the dose required for blood pressure control in such patients.

Synergism has been shown between halothane anesthesia and intravenously administered Labetalol Hydrochloride. During controlled hypotensive anesthesia using Labetalol Hydrochloride in association with halothane, high concentrations (3% or above) of halothane should not be used because the degree of hypotension will be increased and because of the possibility of a large reduction in cardiac output and an increase in central venous pressure. The anesthesiologist should be informed when a patient is receiving Labetalol Hydrochloride.

Labetalol Hydrochloride blunts the reflex tachycardia produced by nitroglycerin without preventing its hypotensive effect. If Labetalol Hydrochloride is used with nitroglycerin in patients with angina pectoris, additional antihypertensive effects may occur. Care should be taken if Labetalol is used concomitantly with calcium antagonists of the verapamil type.

Risk of Anaphylactic Reaction: While taking beta-blockers, patients with a history of severe anaphylactic reaction to a variety of allergens may be more reactive to repeated challenge, either accidental, diagnostic, or therapeutic. Such patients may be unresponsive to the usual doses of epinephrine used to treat allergic reaction.

Drug/Laboratory Test Interactions: The presence of Labetalol metabolites in the urine may result in falsely elevated levels of urinary catecholamines, metanephrine, normetanephrine, and vanillylmandelic acid when measured by fluorimetric or photometric methods. In screening patients suspected of having a pheochromocytoma and being treated with Labetalol Hydrochloride, a specific method, such as a high performance liquid chromatographic assay with solid phase extraction (e.g., *J Chromatog* 385:241, 1987) should be employed in determining levels of catecholamines.

Labetalol Hydrochloride has also been reported to produce a false-positive test for amphetamine when screening urine for the presence of drugs using the commercially available assay methods Toxi-Lab A® (thin-layer chromatographic assay) and Emit-d.a.u.® (radioenzymatic assay). When patients being treated with Labetalol have a positive urine test for amphetamine using these techniques, confirmation should be made by using more specific methods, such as a gas chromatographic-mass spectrometer technique.

Carcinogenesis, Mutagenesis, Impairment of Fertility: Long-term oral dosing studies with Labetalol Hydrochloride for 18 months in mice and for 2 years in rats showed no evidence of carcinogenesis. Studies with Labetalol Hydrochloride using dominant lethal assays in rats and mice and exposing microorganisms according to modified Ames tests showed no evidence of mutagenesis.

Pregnancy: Teratogenic Effects: Pregnancy Category C: Teratogenic studies were performed with Labetalol in rats and rabbits at oral doses up to approximately six and four times the maximum recommended human dose (MRHD), respectively. No reproducible evidence of fetal malformations was observed. Increased fetal resorptions were seen in both species at doses approximating the MRHD. A teratology study performed with Labetalol in rabbits at IV doses up to 1.7 times the MRHD revealed no evidence of drug-related harm to the fetus. There are no adequate and well-controlled studies in pregnant women. Labetalol should be used during pregnancy only if the potential benefit justifies the potential risk to the fetus.

Nonteratogenic Effects: Hypotension, bradycardia, hypoglycemia, and respiratory depression have been reported in infants of mothers who were treated with Labetalol Hydrochloride for hypertension during pregnancy. Oral administration of Labetalol to rats during late gestation through weaning at doses of two to four times the MRHD caused a decrease in neonatal survival.

Labor and Delivery: Labetalol Hydrochloride given to pregnant women with hypertension did not appear to affect the usual course of labor and delivery.

Nursing Mothers: Small amounts of Labetalol (approximately 0.004% of the maternal dose) are excreted in human milk. Caution should be exercised when Labetalol Hydrochloride is administered to a nursing woman.

Pediatric Use: Safety and effectiveness in children have not been established.

ADVERSE REACTIONS

Labetalol Hydrochloride Tablets: Most adverse effects are mild and transient and occur early in the course of treatment. In controlled clinical trials of 3-4 months' duration, discontinuation of Labetalol Hydrochloride Tablets due to one or more adverse effects was required in 7% of all patients. In these same trials, other agents with solely beta-blocking activity used in the control groups led to discontinuation in 8%-10% of patients, and a centrally acting alpha-agonist led to discontinuation in 30% of patients.

The incidence rates of adverse reactions listed in the following table were derived from multicenter, controlled clinical trials comparing Labetalol Hydrochloride, placebo, metoprolol, and propranolol over treatment periods of 3 and 4 months. Where the frequency of adverse effects for Labetalol Hydrochloride and placebo is similar, causal relationship is uncertain. The rates are based on adverse reactions considered probably drug related by the investigator. If all reports are considered, the rates are somewhat higher (e.g., dizziness, 20%; nausea, 14%; fatigue, 11%), but the overall conclusions are unchanged. (See related table).

The adverse effects were reported spontaneously and are representative of the incidence of adverse effects that may be observed in a properly selected hypertensive patient population, i.e., a group excluding patients with bronchospastic disease, overt congestive heart failure, or other contraindications to beta-blocker therapy.

Clinical trials also included studies utilizing daily doses up to 2,400 mg in more severely hypertensive patients. Certain of the side effects increased with

	Labetalol HCl (n = 227) %	Placebo (n = 98) %	Propranolol (n = 84) %	Metoprolol (n = 49) %
Body as a Whole				
Fatigue	5	0	12	12
asthenia	1	1	1	0
headache	2	1	0	2
Gastrointestinal				
nausea	6	1	1	2
vomiting	< 1	0	0	0
dyspepsia	3	1	0	0
abdominal pain	0	0	0	2
diarrhea	< 1	0	2	0
taste distortion	1	0	0	0
Central and Peripheral Nervous Systems				
dizziness	11	3	4	4
paresthesia	< 1	0	0	0
drowsiness	< 1	2	2	2
Autonomic nervous system				
nasal stuffiness	3	0	0	0
ejaculation failure	2	0	0	0
impotence	1	0	1	0
increased sweating	< 1	0	0	0
Cardiovascular				
edema	1	0	0	0
postural hypotension	1	0	0	0
bradycardia	0	0	5	12
Respiratory				
dyspnea	2	0	1	0
Skin				
rash	1	0	0	0
Special senses				
vision abnormality	1	0	0	0
vertigo	2	1	0	0

increasing dose, as shown in the following table that depicts the entire US therapeutic trials data base for adverse reactions that are clearly or possibly dose related. (See related table).

In addition, a number of other less common adverse events have been reported:

Body as a Whole: Fever.

Cardiovascular: Hypotension, and rarely, syncope, bradycardia, heart block.

Central and Peripheral Nervous Systems: Paresthesia, most frequently described as scalp tingling. In most cases, it was mild and transient and usually occurred at the beginning of treatment.

Collagen Disorders: Systemic lupus erythematosus, positive antinuclear factor.

Eyes: Dry eyes.

Immunological System: Antimitochondrial antibodies.

Liver and Biliary System: Hepatic necrosis, hepatitis, cholestatic jaundice, elevated liver function tests.

Musculoskeletal System: Muscle cramps, toxic myopathy.

Respiratory System: Bronchospasm.

Skin and Appendages: Rashes of various types, such as generalized maculopapular, lichenoid, urticarial, bullous lichen planus, psoriaform, and facial erythema; Peyronie's disease; reversible alopecia.

Urinary System: Difficulty in micturition, including acute urinary bladder retention.

Hypersensitivity: Rare reports of hypersensitivity (e.g., rash, urticaria, pruritus, angioedema, dyspnea) and anaphylactoid reactions.

Following approval for marketing in the United Kingdom, a monitored release survey involving approximately 6,800 patients was conducted for further safety and efficacy evaluation of this product. Results of this survey indicate that the type, severity, and incidence of adverse effects were comparable to those cited above.

Potential Adverse Effects: In addition, other adverse effects not listed above have been reported with other beta-adrenergic blocking agents.

Central Nervous System: Reversible mental depression progressing to catatonia, an acute reversible syndrome characterized by disorientation for time and place, short-term memory loss, emotional lability, slightly clouded sensorium, and decreased performance on psychometrics.

Cardiovascular: Intensification of A-V block (see "Contraindications").

Allergic: Fever combined with aching and sore throat, laryngospasm, respiratory distress.

Hematologic: Agranulocytosis, thrombocytopenic or nonthrombocytopenic purpura.

Gastrointestinal: Mesenteric artery thrombosis, ischemic colitis.

Labetalol Hydrochloride Injection: Labetalol Hydrochloride Injection is usually well tolerated. Most adverse effects have been mild and transient and, in controlled trials involving 92 patients, did not require Labetalol Hydrochloride withdrawal. Symptomatic postural hypotension (incidence, 58%) is likely to occur if patients are tilted or allowed to assume the upright position within 3 hours of receiving Labetalol Hydrochloride Injection. Moderate hypotension occurred in 1 of 100 patients while supine. Increased sweating was noted in 4 of 100 patients, and flushing occurred in 1 of 100 patients.

The following also were reported with Labetalol Hydrochloride Injection with the incidence per 100 patients as noted:

Cardiovascular System: Ventricular arrhythmia in 1.

Central and Peripheral Nervous Systems: Dizziness in 9, tingling of the scalp/skin in 7, hypoesthesia (numbness) and vertigo in 1 each.

Gastrointestinal System: Nausea in 13, vomiting in 4, dyspepsia and taste distortion in 1 each.

Metabolic Disorders: Transient increases in blood urea nitrogen and serum creatinine levels occurred in 8 of 100 patients; these were associated with drops in blood pressure, generally in patients with prior renal insufficiency.

Psychiatric Disorders: Somnolence/yawning in 3.

Respiratory System: Wheezing in 1.

Skin: Pruritus in 1.

The incidence of adverse reactions depends upon the dose of Labetalol Hydrochloride. The largest experience is with oral Labetalol Hydrochloride (see above for details). Certain of the side effects increased with increasing oral dose, as shown in the above table that depicts the entire US therapeutic trials data base for adverse reactions that are clearly or possibly dose related. In addition, a number of other less common adverse events have been reported:

Cardiovascular: Hypotension, and rarely, syncope, bradycardia, heart block.

Liver and Biliary System: Hepatic necrosis, hepatitis, cholestatic jaundice, elevated liver function tests.

Hypersensitivity: Rare reports of hypersensitivity (e.g., rash, urticaria, pruritus, angioedema, dyspnea) and anaphylactoid reactions.

The oculomucocutaneous syndrome associated with the beta-blocker practolol has not been reported with Labetalol Hydrochloride.

Clinical Laboratory Tests: Among patients dosed with Labetalol HCl Tablets, there have been reversible increases of serum transaminases in 4% of patients tested and, more rarely, reversible increases in blood urea.

OVERDOSAGE

Overdosage with Labetalol Hydrochloride causes excessive hypotension that is posture sensitive and, sometimes, excessive bradycardia. Patients should be placed supine and their legs raised if necessary to improve the blood supply to the brain. If overdosage with Labetalol Hydrochloride follows oral ingestion, gastric lavage or pharmacologically induced emesis (using syrup of ipecac) may be useful for removal of the drug shortly after ingestion. The following additional measures should be employed if necessary:

Excessive Bradycardia: Administer atropine or epinephrine.

Cardiac Failure: administer a digitalis glycoside and a diuretic. Dopamine or dobutamine may also be useful.

Hypotension: administer vasopressors, e.g., norepinephrine. There is pharmacologic evidence that norepinephrine may be the drug of choice.

Bronchospasm: administer epinephrine and/or an aerosolized beta$_2$-agonist.

Seizures: administer diazepam.

In severe beta-blocker overdose resulting in hypotension and/or bradycardia, glucagon has been shown to be effective when administered in large doses (5-10 mg rapidly over 30 seconds, followed by continuous infusion of 5 mg per hour that can be reduced as the patient improves).

Neither hemodialysis nor peritoneal dialysis removes a significant amount of Labetalol Hydrochloride from the general circulation (< 1%).

The oral LD$_{50}$ value of Labetalol Hydrochloride in the mouse is approximately 600 mg/kg and in the rat is greater than 2 g/kg. The IV LD$_{50}$ in these species is 50-60 mg/kg.

DOSAGE AND ADMINISTRATION

Labetalol Hydrochloride Tablets: DOSAGE MUST BE INDIVIDUALIZED. The recommended *initial* dosage is 100 mg *twice* daily whether used alone or added to a diuretic regiment. After 2 or 3 days, using standing blood pressure as an indicator, dosage may be titrated in increments of 100 mg b.i.d. every 2 or 3 days. The usual *maintenance* dosage of Labetalol Hydrochloride is between 200 and 400 mg *twice* daily.

Labetalol Hydrochloride Daily Dose (mg)	200	300	400	600	800	900	1,200	1,600	2,400
Number of patients	522	181	606	608	503	117	411	242	175
Dizziness (%)	2	3	3	3	5	1	9	13	16
Fatigue	2	1	4	4	5	3	7	6	10
Nausea	< 1	0	1	2	4	0	7	11	19
Vomiting	0	0	< 1	< 1	< 1	0	1	2	3
Dyspepsia	1	0	2	2	1	0	2	2	4
Paresthesia	2	0	2	2	1	1	2	5	5
Nasal stuffiness	1	1	2	2	2	2	4	5	6
Ejaculation failure	0	2	1	2	3	0	4	3	5
Impotence	1	1	1	1	1	4	3	4	3
Edema	1	0	1	1	1	0	1	2	2

Since the full antihypertensive effect of Labetalol Hydrochloride is usually seen within the first 1-3 hours of the initial dose or dose increment, the assurance of a lack of an exaggerated hypotensive response can be clinically established in the office setting. The antihypertensive effects of continued dosing can be measured at subsequent visits, approximately 12 hours after a dose, to determine whether further titration is necessary.

Patients with severe hypertension may require from 1,200-2,400 mg per day, with or without thiazide diuretics. Should side effects (principally nausea or dizziness) occur with these doses administered twice daily, the same total daily dose administered three times daily may improve tolerability and facilitate further titration. Titration increments should not exceed 200 mg twice daily.

When a diuretic is added, an additive antihypertensive effect can be expected. In some cases this may necessitate a Labetalol Hydrochloride dosage adjustment. As with most antihypertensive drugs, optimal dosages of Labetalol Hydrochloride Tablets are usually lower in patients also receiving a diuretic.

When transferring patients from other antihypertensive drugs, Labetalol Hydrochloride Tablets should be introduced as recommended and the dosage of the existing therapy progressively decreased.

Labetalol Hydrochloride Injection: Labetalol Hydrochloride Injection is intended for IV use in hospitalized patients. DOSAGE MUST BE INDIVIDUALIZED depending upon the severity of hypertension and the response of the patient during dosing.

Patients should always be kept in a supine position during the period of IV drug administration. A substantial fall in blood pressure on standing should be expected in these patients. The patient's ability to tolerate an upright position should be established before permitting any ambulation, such as using toilet facilities.

Either of two methods of administration of Labetalol Hydrochloride Injection may be used: a) repeated IV injection, or b) slow continuous infusion.

Repeated Intravenous Injection: Initially, Labetalol Hydrochloride Injection should be given in a 20-mg dose (which corresponds to 0.25 mg/kg for an 80-kg patient) by slow IV injection over a 2-minute period.

Immediately before the injection and at 5 and 10 minutes after injection, supine blood pressure should be measured to evaluate response. Additional injections of 40 or 80 mg can be given at 10-minute intervals until a desired supine blood pressure is achieved or a total of 300 mg of Labetalol Hydrochloride has been injected. The maximum effect usually occurs within 5 minutes of each injection.

Slow Continuous Infusion: Labetalol Hydrochloride Injection is prepared for continuous IV infusion by diluting the vial contents with commonly used IV fluids (see below). Examples of two methods of preparing the infusion solution are:

Add 40 mL of Labetalol Hydrochloride Injection to 160 mL of a commonly used IV fluid such that the resultant 200 mL of solution contains 200 mg of Labetalol Hydrochloride, 1 mg/mL. The diluted solution should be administered at a rate of 2 mL per minute to deliver 2 mg per minute.

Alternatively, add 40 mL of Labetalol Hydrochloride Injection to 250 mL of a commonly used IV fluid. The resultant solution will contain 200 mg of Labetalol Hydrochloride, approximately 2 mg/3 mL. The diluted solution should be administered at a rate of 3 mL per minute to deliver approximately 2 mg per minute.

The rate of infusion of the diluted solution may be adjusted according to the blood pressure response, at the discretion of the physician. To facilitate a desired rate of infusion, the diluted solution can be infused using a controlled administration mechanism, e.g., graduated burette or mechanically driven infusion pump.

Since the half-life of Labetalol is 5-8 hours, steady-state blood levels (in the face of a constant rate of infusion) would not be reached during the usual infusion time period. The infusion should be continued until a satisfactory response is obtained and should then be stopped and oral Labetalol Hydrochloride started (see below). The effective IV dose is usually in the range of 50-200 mg. A total dose of up to 300 mg may be required in some patients.

Blood Pressure Monitoring: The blood pressure should be monitored during and after completion of the infusion or IV injection. Rapid or excessive falls in either systolic or diastolic blood pressure during IV treatment should be avoided. In patients with excessive systolic hypertension, the decrease in systolic pressure should be used as an indicator of effectiveness in addition to the response of the diastolic pressure.

Initiation of Dosing with Labetalol Hydrochloride Tablets: Subsequent oral dosing with Labetalol Hydrochloride Tablets should begin when it has been established that the supine diastolic blood pressure has begun to rise. The recommended initial dose is 200 mg, followed in 6-12 hours by an additional dose of 200 or 400 mg, depending on the blood pressure response. Thereafter, *inpatients titration with Labetalol Hydrochloride Tablets* may proceed as follows:

INPATIENT TITRATION INSTRUCTION

Regimen	Daily Dose*
200 mg b.i.d.	400 mg
400 mg b.i.d.	800 mg
800 mg b.i.d.	1,600 mg
1,200 mg b.i.d.	2,400 mg

* *If needed, the total daily dose may be given in three divided doses.*

The dosage of Labetalol Hydrochloride Tablets used in the hospital may be increased at 1-day intervals to achieve the desired blood pressure reduction.

For subsequent outpatient titration or maintenance dosing, see Labetalol Hydrochloride Tablets dosage and administration information above for recommendations.

Compatibility With Commonly Used Intravenous Fluids: Parenteral drug products should be inspected visually for particulate matter and discoloration before administration whenever solution and container permit.

Labetalol Hydrochloride Injection was tested for compatibility with commonly used IV fluids at final concentrations of 1.25-3.75 mg of Labetalol Hydrochloride per milliliter of the mixture. Labetalol Hydrochloride Injection was found to be compatible with and stable (for 24 hours refrigerated or at room temperature) in mixtures with the following solutions: ringer's injection, USP; lactated ringer's injection, USP; 5% dextrose and ringer's injection; 5% lactated ringer's and 5% dextrose injection; 5% dextrose injection, USP; 0.9% sodium chloride injection, USP; 5% dextrose and 0.2% sodium chloride injection, USP; 2.5% dextrose and 0.45% sodium chloride injection, USP; 5% dextrose and 0.9% sodium chloride injection, USP; and 5% dextrose and 0.33% sodium chloride injection, USP.

Labetalol Hydrochloride Injection was NOT compatible with 5% sodium bicarbonate injection, USP.

Labetalol Hydrochloride Tablets should be stored between 2° and 30°C (36° and 86°F). Labetalol Hydrochloride Tablets in the unit dose boxes should be protected from excessive moisture.

Labetalol Hydrochloride Injection: Store between 2° and 30°C (36° and 86°F). Do not freeze. Protect from light.

HOW SUPPLIED
INJECTION: 5 MG/ML

AVERAGE UNIT PRICE (AVAILABLE SIZES)			
BRAND	$1.52		

BRAND/MANUFACTURER	NDC	SIZE	AWP
◆ BRAND			
TRANDATE: Allen & Hanburys	00173-0350-58	20 ml	$30.88
	00173-0350-57	40 ml	$59.82

INJECTION: 20 MG/ML

BRAND/MANUFACTURER	NDC	SIZE	AWP
◆ BRAND			
NORMODYNE: Key	00085-0362-08	4 ml	$13.33

INJECTION: 20 MG

BRAND/MANUFACTURER	NDC	SIZE	AWP
◆ BRAND			
TRANDATE: Allen & Hanburys	00173-0350-00	4 ml	$12.79

INJECTION: 40 MG/ML

BRAND/MANUFACTURER	NDC	SIZE	AWP
◆ BRAND			
NORMODYNE: Key	00085-0362-09	8 ml	$20.00

INJECTION: 40 MG

BRAND/MANUFACTURER	NDC	SIZE	AWP
◆ BRAND			
TRANDATE: Allen & Hanburys	00173-0350-01	8 ml	$19.20

INJECTION: 100 MG

BRAND/MANUFACTURER	NDC	SIZE	AWP
◆ BRAND			
NORMODYNE: Key	00085-0362-07	20 ml	$30.88

INJECTION: 200 MG

BRAND/MANUFACTURER	NDC	SIZE	AWP
◆ BRAND			
NORMODYNE: Key	00085-0362-06	40 ml	$59.82

TABLETS: 100 MG

AVERAGE UNIT PRICE (AVAILABLE SIZES)			
BRAND	$0.42		

BRAND/MANUFACTURER	NDC	SIZE	AWP
◆ BRAND			
➤ NORMODYNE: Key	00085-0244-04	100s	$42.53
➤ TRANDATE: Allen & Hanburys	00173-0346-43	100s	$42.53
➤ NORMODYNE: Key	00085-0244-08	100s ud	$45.16
➤ TRANDATE: Allen & Hanburys	00173-0346-47	100s ud	$45.16
➤ NORMODYNE: Key	00085-0244-05	500s	$201.74
➤ TRANDATE: Allen & Hanburys	00173-0346-44	500s	$201.74
➤ NORMODYNE: Key	00085-0244-07	1000s	$372.04

◆ **RATED THERAPEUTICALLY EQUIVALENT;** ◇ **THERAPEUTIC EQUIVALENCE UNCONFIRMED;** ○ **UNRATED**

TABLETS: 200 MG

AVERAGE UNIT PRICE (AVAILABLE SIZES)

BRAND			$0.59	

BRAND/MANUFACTURER	NDC	SIZE	AWP
◆ BRAND			
➤ NORMODYNE: Key	00085-0752-04	100s	$60.32
➤ TRANDATE: Allen & Hanburys	00173-0347-43	100s	$60.32
➤ NORMODYNE: Key	00085-0752-08	100s ud	$62.95
➤ TRANDATE: Allen & Hanburys	00173-0347-47	100s ud	$62.95
➤ NORMODYNE: Key	00085-0752-05	500s	$286.55
➤ TRANDATE: Allen & Hanburys	00173-0347-44	500s	$286.55
➤ NORMODYNE: Key	00085-0752-07	1000s	$528.23

TABLETS: 300 MG

AVERAGE UNIT PRICE (AVAILABLE SIZES)

BRAND			$0.80	

BRAND/MANUFACTURER	NDC	SIZE	AWP
◆ BRAND			
➤ NORMODYNE: Key	00085-0438-03	100s	$80.23
➤ TRANDATE: Allen & Hanburys	00173-0348-43	100s	$80.23
➤ NORMODYNE: Key	00085-0438-06	100s ud	$82.88
➤ TRANDATE: Allen & Hanburys	00173-0348-47	100s ud	$82.88
➤ NORMODYNE: Key	00085-0438-05	500s	$381.04
➤ TRANDATE: Allen & Hanburys	00173-0348-44	500s	$381.04

Lac-Hydrin SEE AMMONIUM LACTATE

Lacrisert SEE HYDROXYPROPYL CELLULOSE

Lactated Ringer's

DESCRIPTION

This product is a sterile, nonpyrogenic solution of electrolytes without dextrose in water for injection intended for intravenous administration as fluid and nutrient and/or electrolyte replenisher. Lactated Ringer's injection serves as a systemic alkalizer. It contain no bacteriostat, antimicrobial agent or added buffer (except for pH adjustment).

Each 100 ml of Lactated Ringer's injection, USP contains sodium chloride 600 mg, sodium lactate, anhydrous 310 mg, potassium chloride 30 mg and calcium chloride, dihydrate 20 mg. A liter provides 9 calories, sodium (Na^+) 130 mEq, potassium (K^+) 4 mEq, calcium (Ca^{++}) 2.7 mEq, chloride (Cl^-) 109 mEq and lactate [$CH_3CH(OH) COO^-$] 28 mEq. The electrolyte content is isotonic (273 mOsm/liter; calc.) in relation to the extracellular fluid (approx. 280 mOsm/liter). The pH of the solution is 6.7 (approx.). May contain hydrochloric acid or sodium hydroxide for pH adjustment.

Calcium Chloride, USP is chemically designated $CaCl_2 \cdot 2H_2O$, white fragments or granules freely soluble in water.

Potassium Chloride, USP is chemically designated KCl, a white granular powder freely soluble in water.

Sodium Chloride, USP is chemically designated NaCl, a white crystalline compound freely soluble in water.

Sodium Lactate, USP is chemically designated $CH_3CH(OH)COONa$, a 60% aqueous solution miscible in water.

Water for Injection, USP is chemically designated H_2O.

CLINICAL PHARMACOLOGY

When administered intravenously, these solutions provide variable sources of water, electrolytes and carbohydrate calories.

Solutions containing carbohydrate in the form of dextrose restore blood glucose levels and provide calories.

Calcium chloride in water dissociates to provide calcium (Ca^{++}) and chloride (Cl^-) ions. They are normal constituents of the body fluids and are dependent on various physiologic mechanisms for maintenance of balance between intake and output. Approximately 80% of body calcium is excreted in the feces as insoluble salts; urinary excretion accounts for the remaining 20%.

Potassium chloride in water dissociates to provide potassium (K^+) and chloride (Cl^-) ions. Potassium is found in low concentration in plasma and extracellular fluids (3.5 to 5.0 mEq/liter in a healthy adult). It is the chief cation of body cells (160 mEq/liter of intracellular water). Potassium plays an important role in electrolyte balance. Normally about 80 to 90% of the potassium intake is excreted in the urine; the remainder in the stools and to a small extent, in the perspiration. The kidney does not conserve potassium well so that during fasting or in patients on a potassium-free diet, potassium loss from the body continues resulting in potassium depletion.

Sodium chloride in water dissociates to provide sodium (Na^+) and chloride (Cl^-) ions. Sodium (Na^+) is the principal cation of the extracellular fluid and plays a large part in the therapy of fluid and electrolyte disturbances. Chloride (Cl^-) has an integral role in buffering action when oxygen and carbon dioxide exchange occurs in the red blood cells. The distribution and excretion of sodium (Na^+) and chloride (Cl^-) are largely under the control of the kidney which maintains a balance between intake and output.

Sodium lactate provides sodium (Na^+) and lactate ($C_3H_5O_2^-$) ions. The lactate anion is in equilibrium with pyruvate and has an alkalizing effect resulting from simultaneous removal by the liver of lactate and hydrogen ions. In the liver, lactate is metabolized to glycogen which is ultimately converted to carbon dioxide and water by oxidative metabolism. The sodium (Na^+) ion combines with bicarbonate ion produced from carbon dioxide of the body and thus retains bicarbonate to combat metabolic acidosis (bicarbonate deficiency). The normal plasma level of lactate ranges from 0.9 to 1.9 mEq/liter.

Water is an essential constituent of all body tissues and accounts for approximately 70% of total body weight. Average normal adult daily requirement ranges from two to three liters (1.0 to 1.5 liters each for insensible water loss by perspiration and urine production).

Water balance is maintained by various regulatory mechanisms. Water distribution depends primarily on the concentration of electrolytes in the body compartments and sodium (Na^+) plays a major role in maintaining physiologic equilibrium.

INDICATIONS AND USAGE

These solutions are indicated for parenteral replacement of extracellular losses of fluid and electrolytes, plus minimal calories, as required by the clinical condition of the patient.

CONTRAINDICATIONS

Do not administer unless the solution is clear and seal is intact. Discard unused portion.

Solutions containing lactate are *not for use in the treatment of lactic acidosis.*

WARNINGS

Solutions containing calcium ions should not be administered simultaneously through the same administration set as blood because of the likelihood of coagulation.

Solutions which contain potassium should be used with great care, if at all, in patients with hyperkalemia, severe renal failure and in conditions in which potassium retention is present.

Solutions containing sodium ions should be used with great care, if at all, in patients with congestive heart failure, severe renal insufficiency and in clinical states in which there exists edema with sodium retention.

In patients with diminished renal function, administration of solutions containing sodium or potassium ions may result in sodium or potassium retention.

Solutions containing lactate ions should be used with great care in patients with metabolic or respiratory alkalosis. The administration of lactate ions should be done with great care where there is an increased level or an impaired utilization of lactate ions, as in severe hepatic insufficiency.

The intravenous administration of these solutions can cause fluid and/or solute overloading resulting in dilution of serum electrolyte concentrations, overhydration, congested states or pulmonary edema. The risk of dilutional states is inversely proportional to the electrolyte concentrations of administered parenteral solutions.

The risk of solute overload causing congested states with peripheral and pulmonary edema is directly proportional to the electrolyte concentrations of such solutions.

Additives may be incompatible. Consult with pharmacist if available. When introducing additives, use aseptic technique, mix thoroughly and do not store.

PRECAUTIONS

Clinical evaluation and periodic laboratory determinations are necessary to monitor changes in fluid balance, electrolyte concentrations and acid-base balance during prolonged parenteral therapy or whenever the condition of the patient warrants such evaluation.

Solutions containing dextrose should be used with caution in patients with known subclinical or overt diabetes mellitus.

Caution must be exercised in the administration of parenteral fluids, especially those containing sodium ions, to patients receiving corticosteroids or corticotropin.

Potassium containing solutions should be used with caution in the presence of cardiac disease, particularly in digitalized patients or in the presence of renal disease.

Solutions containing lactate ions should be used with caution as excess administration may result in metabolic alkalosis.

Pregnancy Category C. Animal reproduction studies have not been conducted with Ringer's injection, USP, Dextrose and Ringer's injection, Lactated Ringer's injection, USP or Dextrose and Lactated Ringer's injection. It is also not known whether these injections can cause fetal harm when administered to a pregnant woman or can affect reproduction capacity. These injections should be given to a pregnant woman only if clearly needed.

ADVERSE REACTIONS

Reactions which may occur because of the solution or the technique of administration include febrile response, infection at the site of injection, venous thrombosis or phlebitis extending from the site of injection, extravasation and hypervolemia.

➤ SHOWN IN PRODUCT IDENTIFICATION GUIDE

If an adverse reaction does occur, discontinue the infusion, evaluate the patient, institute appropriate therapeutic countermeasures and save the remainder of the fluid for examination if deemed necessary.

OVERDOSAGE

In the event of overhydration or solute overload, re-evaluate the patient and institute appropriate corrective measures. See *"Warnings"* and *"Precautions"*.

DOSAGE AND ADMINISTRATION

The dose is dependent upon the age, weight and clinical condition of the patient.

Parenteral drug products should be inspected visually for particulate matter and discoloration prior to administration, whenever solution and container permit. See *"Contraindications"*.

Protect from freezing and extreme heat.

HOW SUPPLIED
INJECTION:

AVERAGE UNIT PRICE (AVAILABLE SIZES)		GENERIC A-RATED AVERAGE PRICE (GAAP)	
GENERIC	$0.02	1000 ml 12s	$153.64
		500 ml 24s	$267.09

BRAND/MANUFACTURER	NDC	SIZE	AWP
◆ GENERICS			
McGaw	00264-1350-10	500 ml	$10.80
McGaw	00264-1350-00	1000 ml	$12.28
Baxter	00338-0137-04	1000 ml 12s	$148.32
Abbott Hosp	00074-7953-09	1000 ml 12s	$151.19
Baxter	00338-0125-04	1000 ml 12s	$161.42
Abbott Hosp	00074-7953-02	250 ml 24s	$269.33
Baxter	00338-0117-03	500 ml 24s	$264.10
Baxter	00338-0125-03	500 ml 24s	$267.84
Abbott Hosp	00074-7953-03	500 ml 24s	$269.33
Baxter	00338-0117-02	250 ml 36s	$396.15

SOLUTION:

AVERAGE UNIT PRICE (AVAILABLE SIZES)	
GENERIC	$0.02

BRAND/MANUFACTURER	NDC	SIZE	AWP
◆ GENERICS			
Baxter	00338-0137-29	5000 ml 2s	$44.04
Baxter	00338-0137-27	3000 ml 4s	$53.24
Abbott Hosp	00074-7828-08	3000 ml 4s	$69.87
Baxter	00338-0118-44	1000 ml 6s	$307.20
Baxter	00338-0114-04	1000 ml 12s	$205.46

Lactic Acid

DESCRIPTION

Lactic Acid is available as a 10% cream and a 10% and 12% lotion. The cream also contains Vitamin E 3500 u/oz.

Lactic Acid has been reported as an effective naturally occurring humectant in the skin. It has beneficial effects on dry skin and on severe hyperkeratotic conditions. Vitamin E has been used as an aid to control dry or chapped skin. Vitamin E has also found application as an aid in the relief of minor skin disorders such as burns, sunburn, and irritated skin. It has antioxidant properties thus protecting the skin.

INDICATIONS

Lactic Acid is indicated for moisturizing and softening dry, scaly skin (xerosis), ichthyosis vulgaris and itching associated with these conditions.

CONTRAINDICATIONS

Not to be used in patients known to be sensitive to any ingredient in Lactic Acid preparations.

PRECAUTIONS

FOR EXTERNAL USE ONLY. *Patient should be advised to keep this product out of the reach of children.* Avoid contact with eyes, lips and mucous membranes. Irritation may occur when used on the face of fair-skinned patients. A mild stinging, burning or peeling may occur on sensitive, inflamed, or irritated skin areas. If irritation or sensitivity occurs, patient should discontinue use and notify their *Podiatrist, Dermatologist* or *Physician* for appropriate therapy.

Lactic Acid should be given to a pregnant woman only if clearly needed, and caution should be exercised when Lactic Acid is administered to a nursing mother.

DOSAGE AND ADMINISTRATION

Rub thoroughly twice a day to affected areas or as prescribed by your *Podiatrist, Dermatologist* or *Physician.*

Store at controlled room temperature, 15°-30°C (59°-86°F).

HOW SUPPLIED
CREAM:

BRAND/MANUFACTURER	NDC	SIZE	AWP
○ GENERICS			
LACTINOL-E: Pedinol	00884-4990-04	120 gm	$11.00

LIQUID:

BRAND/MANUFACTURER	NDC	SIZE	AWP
○ GENERICS			
	53118-0715-04	120 ml	$8.00
	53118-0715-01	480 ml	$17.50

LOTION:

BRAND/MANUFACTURER	NDC	SIZE	AWP
○ GENERICS			
LACTINOL: Pedinol	00884-5292-08	240 ml	$12.00

Lactulose

DESCRIPTION

Lactulose is a synthetic disaccharide in syrup form for oral or rectal administration. Each 15 mL of Lactulose contains: 10 g Lactulose (and less than 2.2 g galactose, less than 1.2 g lactose, and 1.2 g or less of other sugars). The pH range is 3.0 to 7.0.

Lactulose is a colonic acidifier which promotes laxation and is used for the treatment and prevention of portal-systemic encephalopathy. The chemical name for Lactulose is 4-0-β-D-galactopyranosyl-D-fructofuranose. The molecular weight is 342.30. It is freely soluble in water.

Following is its chemical structure:

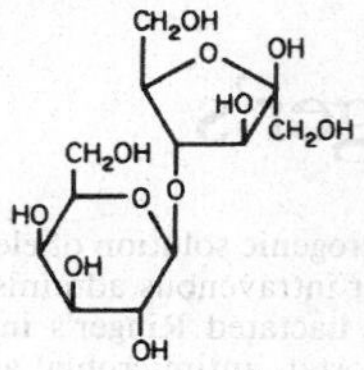

CLINICAL PHARMACOLOGY

Lactulose is poorly absorbed from the gastrointestinal tract and no enzyme capable of hydrolysis of this disaccharide is present in human gastrointestinal tissue. As a result, oral doses of Lactulose reach the colon virtually unchanged. In the colon, Lactulose is broken down primarily to lactic acid, and also to small amounts of formic and acetic acids, by the action of colonic bacteria, which results in an increase in osmotic pressure and slight acidification of the colonic contents. This in turn causes an increase in stool water content and softens the stool.

Lactulose causes a decrease in blood ammonia concentration and reduces the degree of portal-systemic encephalopathy. These actions are considered to be results of the following:

Bacterial degradation of Lactulose in the colon acidifies the colonic contents.

This acidification of colonic contents results in the retention of ammonia in the colon as the ammonium ion. Since the colonic contents are then more acid than the blood, ammonia can be expected to migrate from the blood into the colon to form the ammonium ion.

The acid colonic contents convert NH_3 to the ammonium ion $[NH_4]^-$, trapping it and preventing its absorption.

The laxative action of the metabolites of Lactulose then expels the trapped ammonium ion from the colon.

Since Lactulose does not exert its laxative effect until it reaches the colon, and since transit time through the colon may be slow, 24 to 48 hours may be required to produce the desired bowel movement.

Lactulose given orally to man and experimental animals resulted in only small amounts reaching the blood. Urinary excretion has been determined to be 3% or less and is essentially complete within 24 hours.

INDICATIONS AND USAGE

For the treatment of constipation by oral administration. In patients with a history of chronic constipation, Lactulose syrup therapy increases the number of bowel movements per day and the number of days on which bowel movements occur.

For the prevention and treatment of portal-systemic encephalopathy, including the stages of hepatic pre-coma and coma by oral or rectal administration. Controlled studies have shown that Lactulose syrup therapy reduces the blood ammonia levels by 25-50%; this is generally paralleled by an improvement in the patients' mental state and by an improvement in EEG patterns. The clinical response has been observed in about 75% of patients, which is at least as satisfactory as that resulting from neomycin therapy. An increase in patients' protein tolerance is also frequently observed with Lactulose therapy. In the

---

◆ RATED THERAPEUTICALLY EQUIVALENT; ◇ THERAPEUTIC EQUIVALENCE UNCONFIRMED; ○ UNRATED

treatment of chronic portal-systemic encephalopathy, Lactulose has been given for over 2 years in controlled studies.

CONTRAINDICATIONS

Since Lactulose contains galactose (less than 2.2 g/15 mL), it is contraindicated in patients who require a low galactose diet.

WARNINGS

A theoretical hazard may exist for patients being treated with Lactulose syrup who may be required to undergo electrocautery procedures during proctoscopy or colonoscopy. Accumulation of H_2 gas in significant concentration in the presence of an electrical spark may result in an explosive reaction. Although this complication has not been reported with Lactulose, patients on Lactulose therapy undergoing such procedures should have a thorough bowel cleansing with a non-fermentable solution. Insufflation of CO_2 as an additional safeguard may be pursued but is considered to be a redundant measure.

PRECAUTIONS

GENERAL

Since Lactulose contains galactose (less than 2.2 g/15 mL) and lactose (less than 1.2 g/15 mL), it should be used with caution in diabetics.

In the overall management of portal-systemic encephalopathy, it should be recognized that there is serious underlying liver disease with complications such as electrolyte disturbance (e.g., hypokalemia) for which other specific therapy may be required.

Infants receiving Lactulose may develop hyponatremia and dehydration.

INFORMATION FOR PATIENTS

In the event that an unusual diarrheal condition occurs, contact your physician.

LABORATORY TESTS

Elderly, debilitated patients who receive Lactulose for more than six months should have serum electrolytes (potassium, chloride, carbon dioxide) measured periodically.

DRUG INTERACTIONS

There have been conflicting reports about the concomitant use of neomycin and Lactulose syrup. Theoretically, the elimination of certain colonic bacteria by neomycin and possibly other anti-infective agents may interfere with the desired degradation of Lactulose and thus prevent the acidification of colonic contents. Thus the status of the Lactulose-treated patient should be closely monitored in the event of concomitant oral anti-infective therapy.

Results of preliminary studies in humans and rats suggest that nonabsorble antacids given concurrently with Lactulose may inhibit the desired Lactulose-induced drop in colonic pH. Therefore, a possible lack of desired effect of treatment should be taken into consideration before such drugs are given concomitantly with Lactulose.

Other laxatives should not be used, especially during the initial phase of therapy for portal-systemic encephalopathy, because the loose stools resulting from their use may falsely suggest that adequate Lactulose dosage has been achieved.

CARCINOGENESIS, MUTAGENESIS, IMPAIRMENT OF FERTILITY

There are no known human data on long-term potential for carcinogenicity, mutagenicity, or impairment of fertility. There are no known animal data on long-term potential for mutagenicity.

Administration of Lactulose syrup in the diet of mice for 18 months in concentrations of 3 and 10 percent (V/W) did not produce any evidence of carcinogenicity.

In studies in mice, rats, and rabbits doses of Lactulose syrup up to 6 or 12 mL/kg/day produced no deleterious effects on breeding, conception, or parturition.

PREGNANCY

Teratogenic Effects: Reproduction studies have been performed in mice, rats, and rabbits at doses up to 2 or 3, or 4 or 6 times the usual human oral dose and have revealed no evidence of impaired fertility or harm to the fetus due to Lactulose. There are, however, no adequate and well-controlled studies in pregnant women. Because animal reproduction studies are not always predictive of human response, this drug should be used during pregnancy only if clearly needed.

NURSING MOTHERS

It is not known whether this drug is excreted in human milk. Because many drugs are excreted in human milk, caution should be exercised when Lactulose is administered to a nursing woman.

PEDIATRIC USE

Very little information on the use of Lactulose in young children and adolescents has been recorded. (See *"Dosage and Administration"*.)

Safety and effectiveness in children have not been established.

ADVERSE REACTIONS

Precise frequency data are not available.

Initial dosing may produce gaseous distention with flatulence or belching and abdominal discomfort such as cramping in about 20% of patients. Excessive dosage can lead to diarrhea with potential complications such as loss of fluids, hypokalemia, and hypernatremia.

Nausea and vomiting have been reported.

OVERDOSAGE

SIGNS AND SYMPTOMS

There have been no reports of accidental overdosage. In the event of overdosage, it is expected that diarrhea and abdominal cramps would be the major symptoms. Medication should be terminated.

ORAL LD$_{50}$

The acute oral LD$_{50}$ of the drug is 48.8 mL/kg in mice and greater than 30 mL/kg in rats.

DIALYSIS

Dialysis data are not available for Lactulose. Its molecular similarity to sucrose, however, would suggest that it should be dialyzable.

DOSAGE AND ADMINISTRATION

TREATMENT OF CONSTIPATION

The usual dose is 1 to 2 tablespoonfuls orally (15 to 30 mL, containing 10 g to 20 g of Lactulose) daily. The dose may be increased to 60 mL daily if necessary. Twenty-four to 48 hours may be required to produce a normal bowel movement.

PREVENTION AND TREATMENT OF PORTAL-SYSTEMIC ENCEPHALOPATHY

Oral Adult: The usual adult, oral dosage is 2 to 3 tablespoonfuls (30 to 45 mL, containing 20 g to 30 g of Lactulose) three or four times daily. The dosage may be adjusted every day or two to produce 2 or 3 soft stools daily.

Hourly doses of 30 to 45 mL of Lactulose may be used to induce the rapid laxation indicated in the initial phase of the therapy of portal-systemic encephalopathy. When the laxative effect has been achieved, the dose of Lactulose may then be reduced to the recommended daily dose. Improvement in the patient's condition may occur within 24 hours but may not begin before 48 hours or even later.

Continuous long-term therapy is indicated to lessen the severity and prevent the recurrence of portal-systemic encephalopathy. The dose of Lactulose for this purpose is the same as the recommended daily dose.

Pediatric: Very little information on the use of Lactulose in young children and adolescents has been recorded. As with adults, the subjective goal in proper treatment is to produce 2 or 3 soft stools daily. On the basis of information available, the recommended initial daily oral dose in infants is 2.5 to 10 mL in divided doses. For older children and adolescents, the total daily dose is 40 to 90 mL. If the initial dose causes diarrhea, the dose should be reduced immediately. If diarrhea persists, Lactulose should be discontinued.

Rectal: When the adult patient is in the impending coma or coma stage of portal-systemic encephalopathy and the danger of aspiration exists, or when the necessary endoscopic or intubation procedures physically interfere with the administration of the recommended oral doses, Lactulose may be given as a retention enema via a rectal balloon catheter. Cleansing enemas containing soapsuds or other alkaline agents should not be used.

Three hundred mL of Lactulose should be mixed with 700 mL of water or physiologic saline and retained for 30 to 60 minutes. Lactulose enema may be repeated every 4 to 6 hours. If the enema is inadvertently evacuated too promptly, it may be repeated immediately.

The goal of treatment is reversal of the coma stage in order that the patient may be able to take oral medication. Reversal of coma may take place within 2 hours of the first enema in some patients. Lactulose given orally, in the recommended doses, should be started before Lactulose by enema is stopped entirely.

Note: Some patients have found that Lactulose may be more acceptable when mixed with fruit juice, water, or milk.

STORAGE

Store at room temperature, 59°-86°F (15°-30°C).

Under recommended storage conditions, a normal darkening of color may occur. Such darkening is characteristic of sugar solutions and does not affect therapeutic action. Prolonged exposure to temperatures above 86°F (30°C) or to direct light may cause extreme darkening and turbidity which may be pharmaceutically objectionable. If this condition develops, do not use.

Prolonged exposure to freezing temperatures may cause change to a semisolid, too viscous to pour. Viscosity will return to normal upon warming to room temperature.

HOW SUPPLIED
SOLUTION: 10 GM/15 ML

AVERAGE UNIT PRICE (AVAILABLE SIZES)			
GENERIC	$0.06		
BRAND/MANUFACTURER		NDC	SIZE	AWP
◆ GENERICS				
URL		00677-1334-42	240 ml	$13.70
ENULOSE: URL		00677-1098-33	480 ml	$26.00

SYRUP:

AVERAGE UNIT PRICE (AVAILABLE SIZES)		GENERIC A-RATED AVERAGE PRICE (GAAP)	
BRAND	$0.12	30 ml	$2.09
GENERIC	$0.06	3840 ml	$148.83

BRAND/MANUFACTURER	NDC	SIZE	AWP
◆ BRAND			
CEPHULAC: Marion Merrell Dow	00068-0413-39	30 ml 100s ud	$359.64
CHRONULAC: Marion Merrell Dow	00068-0409-30	30 ml 100s ud	$360.12
◆ GENERICS			
CHOLAC: Alra	51641-0225-61	30 ml	$2.09
CONSTILAC: Alra	51641-0224-61	30 ml	$2.09
CHOLAC: Alra	51641-0225-97	3840 ml	$148.83
CONSTILAC: Alra	51641-0224-97	3840 ml	$148.83
DUPHALAC: Solvay	00032-1602-84	30 ml 10s ud	$26.77

SYRUP: 10 GM/15 ML

AVERAGE UNIT PRICE (AVAILABLE SIZES)		GENERIC A-RATED AVERAGE PRICE (GAAP)	
BRAND	$0.07	240 ml	$13.05
GENERIC	$0.05	960 ml	$36.42
HCFA FUL (240 ml)	$0.04	240 ml	$13.65
HCFA FUL (480 ml)	$0.04	480 ml	$26.39
HCFA FUL (960 ml)	$0.03	960 ml	$48.26
HCFA FUL (1920 ml)	$0.05	1920 ml	$92.13

BRAND/MANUFACTURER	NDC	SIZE	AWP
◆ BRAND			
CHRONULAC: Marion Merrell Dow	00068-0409-08	240 ml	$18.24
CEPHULAC: Marion Merrell Dow	00068-0413-16	480 ml	$36.42
CHRONULAC: Marion Merrell Dow	00068-0409-32	960 ml	$65.16
CEPHULAC: Marion Merrell Dow	00068-0413-64	1920 ml	$130.20
◆ GENERICS			
Major	00904-2117-09	240 ml	$12.60
Geneva	00781-6406-08	240 ml	$12.90
Goldline	00182-6075-44	240 ml	$13.00
Schein	00364-2519-76	240 ml	$13.50
CHOLAC: Alra	51641-0225-68	240 ml	$13.70
CONSTILAC: Alra	51641-0224-68	240 ml	$13.70
Rugby	00536-1418-59	240 ml	$13.73
Moore,H.L.	00839-7199-66	240 ml	$13.84
DUPHALAC: Solvay	00032-1602-08	240 ml	$13.95
Qualitest	00603-1378-56	240 ml	$13.95
CONSTULOSE: Barre	00472-1358-08	240 ml	$14.05
Rugby	00536-1417-85	480 ml	$24.75
Geneva	00781-6405-16	480 ml	$25.65
Schein	00364-2347-16	480 ml	$25.75
Major	00904-2115-16	480 ml	$25.90
Goldline	00182-6072-40	480 ml	$26.00
DUPHALAC: Solvay	00032-1602-78	480 ml	$26.01
Qualitest	00603-1648-58	480 ml	$26.05
ENULOSE: Barre	00472-1360-16	480 ml	$26.11
CHOLAC: Alra	51641-0225-76	480 ml	$26.50
CONSTILAC: Alra	51641-0224-76	480 ml	$26.50
Moore,H.L.	00839-7196-69	480 ml	$30.38
Roxane	00054-3486-63	500 ml	$23.14
CONSTULOSE: Mason Dist	11845-0418-32	960 ml	$26.89
Goldline	00182-6075-58	960 ml	$45.00
Geneva	00781-6406-62	960 ml	$45.79
Schein	00364-2519-32	960 ml	$45.95
Major	00904-2117-69	960 ml	$46.45
Qualitest	00603-1378-59	960 ml	$48.52
CONSTILAC: Alra	51641-0224-82	960 ml	$48.75
Rugby	00536-1418-86	960 ml	$48.75
Moore,L.	00839-7199-62	960 ml	$50.29
DUPHALAC: Solvay	00032-1602-80	960 ml	$50.38
CONSTULOSE: Barre	00472-1358-32	960 ml	$50.45
Roxane	00054-3486-68	1000 ml	$47.00
ENULOSE: Barre	00472-1360-64	1900 ml	$97.77
Major	00904-2115-74	1920 ml	$89.50
Goldline	00182-6072-97	1920 ml	$90.00
CHOLAC: Alra	51641-0225-94	1920 ml	$96.90
Schein	00364-2347-64	1920 ml	$97.75
Roxane	00054-8486-16	30 ml 40s ud	$67.97

SYRUP: 10 GM

BRAND/MANUFACTURER	NDC	SIZE	AWP
◆ GENERICS			
UDL	51079-0636-10	15 ml 50s ud	$73.40

SYRUP: 20 GM

BRAND/MANUFACTURER	NDC	SIZE	AWP
◆ GENERICS			
UDL	51079-0637-10	30 ml 50s ud	$146.80

Lamisil SEE TERBINAFINE HYDROCHLORIDE

Lamprene SEE CLOFAZIMINE

Lanestrin SEE ESTRONE

Lanoxicaps SEE DIGOXIN

Lanoxin SEE DIGOXIN

Lariam SEE MEFLOQUINE HYDROCHLORIDE

Larodopa SEE LEVODOPA

Lasix SEE FUROSEMIDE

Lazer Formalyde SEE FORMALDEHYDE

Lemotussin DM SEE CHLORPHENIRAMINE MALEATE/DEXTROMETHORPHAN HYDROBROMIDE/GUAIFENESIN/PHENYLPROPANOLAMINE HYDROCHLORIDE

Lescol SEE FLUVASTATIN SODIUM

Leucovorin Calcium

DESCRIPTION

Leucovorin Calcium is the calcium salt pentahydrate of N-[4-[[(2-amino-5-formyl-1, 4, 5, 6, 7, 8-hexahydro-4-oxo-6-pteridinyl)-methyl]amino]benzoyl] -L -glutamic acid. Each 5 mg of Leucovorin is equivalent to 5.40 mg of anhydrous Leucovorin Calcium. The formula weight is 511.51.

Leucovorin is a water soluble form of reduced folate in the folate group; it is useful as an antidote to drugs which act as folic acid antagonists. The tablets are intended for oral administration only and contain either 5 mg or 25 mg Leucovorin as the calcium salt. Leucovorin Calcium is available in 50 mg, 100 mg, and 350 mg vials of sterile powder for reconstitution and parenteral administration (intravenous or intramuscular). The dry product contains no preservative. Dilute with Bacteriostatic Water for Injection, USP, which contains benzyl alcohol (see "Warnings" section), or with Sterile Water for Injection, USP. There is 0.004 mEq of Calcium per mg Leucovorin.

Following is its chemical structure:

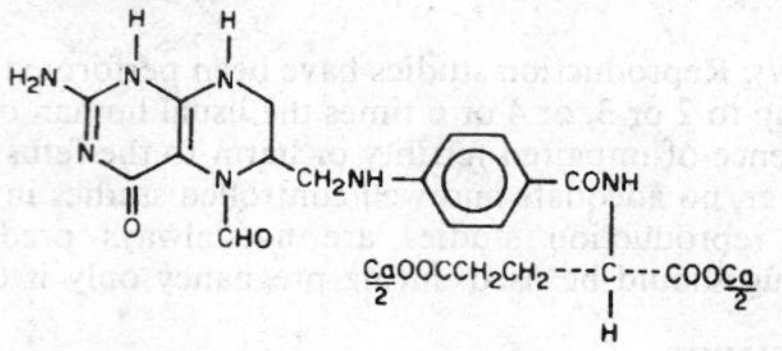

CLINICAL PHARMACOLOGY

Leucovorin Calcium is a racemic mixture of the diastereoisomers of the 5-formyl derivative of tetrahydrofolic acid. The biologically active compound of the mixture is the (-)-L-isomer, known as *Citrovorum factor,* or (-)-folinic acid. Leucovorin Calcium does *not* require reduction by the enzyme dihydrofolate reductase in order to participate in reactions utilizing folates as a source of "one-carbon" moities. l-Leucovrin (l-5-formyltetrahydrofolate) is rapidly metabolized (via 5, 10-methenyltetrahydrofolate then 5,10-methylenetetrahydrofolate) to l-5-methyltetrahydrofolate. l-5-Methyhydrofolate can in turn be metabolized via other pathways back to 5,10-methylenetetrahydrofolate, which is converted to 5-methyltetrahydrofolate by an irreversible, enzyme catalyzed reduction using the cofactors $FADH_2$ and NADPH.

Administration of Leucovorin Calcium can counteract the therapeutic and toxic effects of folic acid antagonists such as methotrexate, which act by inhibiting dihydrofolate reductase. In contrast, Leucovorin Calcium can enhance the

---

◆ RATED THERAPEUTICALLY EQUIVALENT; ◇ THERAPEUTIC EQUIVALENCE UNCONFIRMED; ○ UNRATED

therapeutic and toxic effects of fluoropyrimidines used in cancer therapy, such as 5-fluorouracil. Concurrent administration of Leucovorin Calcium does not appear to alter the plasma pharmacokinetics of 5-fluorouracil. 5-Fluorouracil is metabolized to fluorodeoxyuridylic acid, which binds to and inhibits the enzyme thymidylate synthase (an enzyme important in DNA repair and replication).

Leucovorin Calcium is readily converted to another reduce folate, 5,10-methylenetetrahydrofolate, which acts to stabilize the binding of fluorodeoxyuridylic acid to thymidylate synthase and thereby enhances the inhibition of this enzyme.

After oral administration of Leucovorin Calcium reconstituted with aromatic elixir, the mean peak concentration of serum total reduced folates was 393 ng/mL (range 160 ng/mL to 550 ng/mL). The mean time to peak was 2.3 hours and the terminal half-life was 5.7 hours. The major component was the metabolite 5-methyltetrahydrofolate to which Leucovorin is primarily converted in the intestinal mucosa. The mean peak of 5-methyl-THF was 367 ng/mL at 2.4 hours. The peak level of the parent compound was 51 ng/mL at 1.2 hours. The AUC of total reduced folates after oral administration of the 25 mg dose was 92% of the AUC after intravenous administration.

Following oral administration, Leucovorin Calcium is rapidly absorbed and enters the general body pool of reduced folates. The increase in plasma and serum folate activity (determined microbiologically with *Lactobacillus casei*) seen after oral administration of Leucovorin Calcium is predominantly due to 5-methyltetrahydrofolate.

Twenty normal men were given a single, oral 15 mg dose (7.5 mg/m^2) of Leucovorin Calcium and serum folate concentrations were assayed with *L casei*. Mean values observed (± one standard error) were:

a) Time to peak serum folate concentration: 1.72 ± 0.08 hrs.,
b) Peak serum folate concentration achieved: 268 ± 18 ng/mL,
c) Serum folate half-disappearance time: 3.5 hours.

Oral tablets yielded areas under the serum folate concentration-time curves (AUC's) that were 12% greater than equal amounts of Leucovorin Calcium given intramuscularly and equal to the same amounts given intravenously. At a dose of 25 mg, almost 100% of the *l*-isomer but only 20% of the *d*-isomer is absorbed. Oral absorption of Leucovorin Calcium is saturable at doses above 25 mg. The apparent bioavailability of Leucovorin Calcium was 97% for 25 mg, 75% for 50 mg and 37% for 100 mg.

After intravenous administration of 25 mg Leucovorin Calcium total reduced folate (as measured by *Lactobacillus casei* assay) reached a mean peak of 1259 ng/mL (range 897-1625).

The mean time to peak was 10 minutes. This initial rise in total reduced folate was primarily due to the parent compound 5-formyl THF (measured by S. *faecalis* assay) which rose to 1206 ng/mL at 10 minutes. A sharp drop in parent compound follows and coincides with the appearance of the metabolite (also active) 5-CH$_3$-THF which becomes the predominant circulating form of the drug. The mean peak of 5-CH$_3$-THF was 258 ng/mL occurring at 1.3 hours. The t½ was 6.2 hours for total reduced folates. The area under the concentration versus time curves (AUCs) for *l*-leucovorin, *d*-leucovorin and 5-methyltetrahydrofolate were 28.4 ± 3.5, 956 ± 97 and 129 ± 12 (mg.min/L ± S.E.). When a higher dose of *d,l* - leucovorin (200 mg/m^2) was used, similar results were obtained. The *d* -isomer persisted in plasma at concentrations greatly exceeding those of the *l* -isomer. After intramuscular injection of 25 mg the mean peak total THF was 436 ng/mL (range 240-725) which occurred at a mean time of 52 minutes. Similar to IV administration, the initial sharp rise was due to the parent compound (5-CHO-THF). The mean peak of 5-CHO-THF was 360 ng/mL at 28 minutes and the level of the metabolite 5-CH$_3$-THF increased subsequently over time until at 1.5 hours it represented 50% of the circulating total folate. The mean peak of 5-CH$_3$-THF was 226 ng/mL at 2.8 hours. The t½ of total reduced folate was 6.2 hours. There was no difference of statistical significance between IM and IV administration in the AUC for the total THF, 5-CHO-THF or 5-CH$_3$-THF.

In a randomized clinical study conducted by the Mayo Clinic and the North Central Cancer Treatment Group (Mayo/NCCTG) in patients with advanced metastatic colorectal cancer, three treatment regimens were compared: Leucovorin (LV) 200 mg/m^2 and 5-fluorouracil (5-FU) 370 mg/m^2 versus LV 20 mg/m^2 and 5-FU 425 mg/m^2 versus 5-FU 500 mg/m^2. All drugs were by slow intravenous infusion daily for 5 days repeated every 28 to 35 days. Response rates were 26% (p = 0.04 versus 5-FU alone), 43% (p = 0.001 versus 5-FU alone), and 10% for the high-dose Leucovorin Calcium; low-dose Leucovorin Calcium and 5-FU alone groups, respectively. Respective median survival times were 12.2 months (p = 0.037), 12 months (p = 0.050), and 7.7 months. The low-dose Leukovorin Calcium regimen gave a statistically significant improvement in weight gain of more than 5%, relief of symptoms, and improvement in performance status. The high-dose Leucovorin Calcium regimen gave a statistically significant improvement in performance status and trended toward improvement in weight gain and in relief of symptoms but these were not statistically significant.[1]

In a second Mayo/NCCTG randomized clinical study the 5-FU alone arm was replaced by a regimen of sequentially administered methotrexate (MTX), 5-FU, and Leukovorin Calcium. Response rates with LV 200 mg/m^2 and 5-FU 370 mg/m^2 versus LV 20 mg/m^2 and 5-FU 425 mg/m^2 versus sequential MTX and 5-FU and Leukovorin Calcium were, respectively, 31% (p = <.01), 42% (p = <.01), and 14%. Respective median survival times were 12.7 months (p = <.04), 12.7 months (p = <.01), and 8.4 months. No statistically significant difference in weight gain of more than 5% or in improvement in performance status was seen between the treatment arms.[2]

INDICATIONS AND USAGE

Leucovorin Calcium is indicated to diminish the toxicity and counteract the effects of impaired methotrexate elimination and of inadvertent overdosages of folic acid antagonists. Leukovorin Calcium is also indicated by parenteral administration in the treatment of the megaloblastic anemias due to sprue, nutritional deficiency, pregnancy, and infancy when oral therapy is not feasible. Leukovorin Calcium rescue is indicated after high-dose methotrexate therapy in osteosarcoma. Leucovorin Calcium is also indicated for use in combination with 5-fluorouracil to prolong survival in the palliative treatment of patients with advanced colorectal cancer.

UNLABELED USES

Leucovorin Calcium is used as an adjunct in the treatment of breast carcinoma, including metastatic breast carcinoma, and metastatic colorectal cancer including metastatic adenocarcinoma of the colon and rectum. It is also used, in combination with other antineoplastic agents, in advanced diffuse large-cell lymphoma and stage III and IV carcinoma of the head and neck.

CONTRAINDICATIONS

Leucovorin Calcium is improper therapy for pernicious anemia and other megaloblastic anemias secondary to the lack of vitamin B$_{12}$. A hematologic remission may occur while neurological manifestations continue to progress.

WARNINGS

In the treatment of accidental overdosage of folic acid antagonists, Leucovorin Calcium should be administered as promptly as possible. As the time interval between antifolate administration (e.g., methotrexate [MTX]) and leucovorin rescue increases, Leucovorin Calcium effectiveness in counteracting hematologic toxicity decreases.

Monitoring of the serum MTX concentration is essential in determining the optimal dose and duration of treatment with Leucovorin Calcium which should be such that the resulting levels of tetrahydrofolate are equal to or greater than that of MTX. In determining the dose and duration of Leucovorin Calcium therapy, it should be remembered that there may be a delay of MTX excretion in the presence of a third space fluid accumulation (i.e., ascites, pleural effusion) or if renal insufficiency or inadequate hydration exists. Under such circumstances, high doses of Leucovorin Calcium are recommended. These doses are higher than those recommended for oral use and must be given intravenously. If MTX is administered intrathecally as local therapy and Leucovorin Calcium is administered concurrently, the presence of tetrahydrofolate which diffuses readily into the cerebrospinal fluid may negate the antineoplastic effect of MTX.

Leucovorin Calcium may enhance the toxicity of fluorouracil. Deaths from severe enterocolitis, diarrhea, and dehydration have been reported in elderly patients receiving weekly Leucovorin Calcium and fluorouracil.[3] Concomitant granulocytopenia and fever were present in some but not all of the patients. When these drugs are administered concurrently in the palliative therapy of advanced colorectal cancer, the dosage of 5-fluorouracil must be lower than usually administered. Although the toxicities observed in patients treated with the combination of Leucovorin Calcium plus 5-fluorouracil are qualitatively similar to those observed in patients treated with 5-fluorouracil alone, gastrointestinal toxicities (particularly stomatitis and diarrhea) are observed more commonly and may be more severe and of prolonged duration in patients treated with the combination.

In the first Mayo/NCCTG controlled trial, toxicity, primarily gastrointestinal, resulted in 7% of patients requiring hospitalization when treated with 5-fluorouracil alone or 5-fluorouracil in combination with 200 mg/m^2 of leucovorin and 20% when treated with 5-fluorouracil in combination with 20 mg/m^2 of leucovorin. In the second Mayo/NCCTG trial, hospitalizations related to treatment toxicity also appeared to occur more often in patients treated with the low-dose Leucovorin Calcium/5-fluorouracil combination than in patients treated with the high-dose combination—11% versus 3%. Therapy with Leucovorin Calcium/5-fluorouracil must not be initiated or continued in patients who have symptoms of gastrointestinal toxicity of any severity, until those symptoms have completely resolved. Patients with diarrhea must be monitored with particular care until the diarrhea has resolved, as rapid clinical deterioration leading to death can occur. In an additional study utilizing higher weekly doses of 5-FU and Leucovorin Calcium, elderly and/or debilitated patients were found to be at greater risk for severe gastrointestinal toxicity.[3]

Because of the calcium content of the Leucovorin solution, no more than 160 mg of Leucovorin should be injected intravenously per minute (16 mL of a 10mg/mL, or 8 mL of a 20 mg/mL solution per minute).

Because of the preservative contained in Bacteriostatic Water for Injection, USP (benzyl alcohol preserved), parenteral doses greater than 10 mg/m^2 with this diluent are not recommended. If greater doses are required (see "Dosage and Administration"), the desiccated powder should be reconstituted with Sterile Water for Injection, USP, and used immediately.

PRECAUTIONS

General: Following chemotherapy with folic acid antagonists parenteral administration of Leucovorin Calcium is preferable to oral dosing if there is a possibility that the patient may vomit or not absorb the Leucovorin solution. In the presence of pernicious anemia, a hematologic remission may occur while neurologic manifestations remain progressive. Leucovorin Calcium has no effect on other established toxicities of MTX, such as the nephrotoxicity resulting from drug and/or metabolite precipitation in the kidney. Since Leucovorin enhances the toxicity of fluorouracil, Leucovorin Calcium/5-fluorouracil combination therapy for advanced colorectal cancer should be administered under the supervision of a physician experienced in the use of antimetabolite cancer chemotherapy. Particular care should be taken in the treatment of elderly or debilitated colorectal cancer patients, as these patients may be at increased risk of severe toxicity.

Laboratory Tests: Patients being treated with the Leucovorin Calcium/5-fluorouracil combination should have a CBC with differential and platelets prior to each treatment. During the first two courses a CBC with differential and platelets has to be repeated weekly and thereafter once each cycle at the time of anticipated WBC nadir. Electrolytes and liver function tests should be performed prior to each treatment for the first three cycles, then prior to every other cycle. Dosage modifications of fluorouracil should be instituted as follows, based on the most severe toxicities:

Diarrhea and/or Stomatitis	WBC/mm³ Nadir	Platelets/mm³ Nadir	5-FU Dose
Moderate	1,000-1,900	25-75,000	decrease 20%
Severe	<1,000	<25,000	decrease 30%

If no toxicity occurs, the 5-fluorouracil dose may increase 10%.

Treatment should be deferred until WBC's are 4,000/mm³ and platelets 130,000/mm³. If blood counts do not reach these levels within 2 weeks, treatment should be discontinued. Patients should be followed up with physical examination prior to each treatment course and appropriate radiological examination as needed. Treatment should be discontinued when there is clear evidence of tumor progression.

Drug Interactions: Folic acid in large amounts may counteract the antiepileptic effect of phenobarbital, phenytoin and primidone, and increase the frequency of seizures in susceptible children.

Preliminary animal and human studies have shown that small quantities of systemically administered Leucovorin Calcium enter the CSF primarily as 5-methyltetrahydrofolate and, in humans, remain 1-3 orders of magnitude lower than the usual MTX concentrations following intrathecal administration. However, high doses of Leucovorin Calcium may reduce the efficacy of intrathecally administered MTX.

Leucovorin Calcium may enhance the toxicity of fluorouracil (see "Warnings").

Pregnancy: Teratogenic Effects: Pregnancy Category C. Animal reproduction studies have not been conducted with Leucovorin Calcium. It is also not known whether Leuvorin Calcium can cause fetal harm when administered to a pregnant woman or can affect reproduction capacity. Leucovorin Calcium should be given to a pregnant woman only if clearly needed.

Nursing Mothers: It is not known whether this drug is excreted in human milk. Because many drugs are excreted in human milk, caution should be exercised when Leucovorin Calcium is administered to a nursing mother.

Pediatric Use: See "Drug Interactions".

ADVERSE REACTIONS

Allergic sensitization, including anaphylactoid reactions and urticaria, has been reported following both oral and parenteral administration of Leucovorin Calcium.

No other adverse reactions have been attributed to the use of Leucovorin Calcium *per se*. The following table summarizes significant adverse events occurring in 316 patients treated with the Leucovorin Calcium/5-fluorouracil combinations compared against 70 patients treated with 5-fluorouracil alone for advanced colorectal carcinoma. These data are taken from the Mayo/NCCTG large multicenter prospective trial evaluating the efficacy and safety of the combination regimen. (See related table).

OVERDOSAGE

Excessive amounts of Leucovorin Calcium may nullify the chemotherapeutic effect of frolic acid antagonists.

DOSAGE AND ADMINISTRATION

Leucovorin Calcium tablets are intended for oral administration. Because absorption is saturable, oral administration of doses greater than 25 mg is not recommended.

Leucovorin Rescue After High-Dose Methotrexate Therapy: The recommendations for Leucovorin rescue are based on a methotrexate dose of 12 to 15 grams/m² administered by intravenous infusion over 4 hours (see methotrexate package insert for full Prescribing Information).[4] Leucovorin rescue at a dose of 15 mg (approximately 10 mg/m²) every 6 hours for 10 doses starts 24 hours after the beginning of the methotrexate infusion. In the presence of gastrointestinal toxicity, nausea, or vomiting, Leucovorin should be administered parenterally.

Serum creatinine and methotrexate levels should be determined at least once daily. Leucovorin administration, hydration, and urinary alkalinization (pH of 7.0 or greater) should be continued until the methotrexate level is below 5×10^{-8} M (0.05 micromolar). The Leucovorin dose should be adjusted or Leucovorin rescue extended based on the following guidelines:

GUIDELINES FOR LEUCOVORIN CALCIUM DOSAGE AND ADMINISTRATION

Clinical Situation	Laboratory Findings	Leucovorin Dosage and Duration
Normal Methotrexate Elimination	Serum methotrexate level approximately 10 micromolar at 24 hours after administration, 1 micromolar at 48 hours, and less than 0.3 micromolar at 72 hours.	15 mg PO, IM, or IV q 6 hours for 60 hours (10 doses starting at 24 hours after start of methotrexate infusion).
Delayed Late Methotrexate Elimination	Serum methotrexate level remaining above 0.2 micromolar at 72 hours, and more than 0.05 micromolar at 96 hours after administration.	Continue 15 mg PO, IM, or IV q 6 hours, until methotrexate level is less than 0.05 micromolar.
Delayed Early Methotrexate Elimination and/or Evidence of Acute Renal Injury	Serum methotrexate level of 50 micromolar or more at 24 hours, or 5 micromolar or more at 48 hours after administration, OR; a 100% or greater increase in serum creatinine level at 24 hours after methotrexate administration (eg, an increase from 0.5 mg/dL to a level of 1 mg/dL or more).	150 mg q 3 hours, until methotrexate level is less than 1 micromolar; then 15 mg IV q 3 hours, until methotrexate level is less than 0.05 micromolar.

Patients who experience delayed early methotrexate elimination are likely to develop reversible renal failure. In addition to appropriate Leucovorin therapy, these patients require continuing hydration and urinary alkalinization, and close

PERCENTAGE OF PATIENTS TREATED WITH LEUCOVORIN/FLUOROURACIL FOR ADVANCED COLORECTAL CARCINOMA REPORTING ADVERSE EXPERIENCES OR HOSPITALIZED FOR TOXICITY

	(High LV)/5-FU (N = 155)		(Low LV)/5-FU (N = 161)		5-FU Alone (N = 70)	
	Any (%)	Grade 3+ (%)	Any (%)	Grade 3+ (%)	Any (%)	Grade 3+ (%)
Leukopenia	69	14	83	23	93	48
Thrombocytopenia	8	1	18	1	18	3
Infection	8	1	3	1	7	1
Nausea	74	10	80	9	60	6
Vomiting	46	8	44	9	40	7
Diarrhea	66	18	67	14	43	11
Stomatitis	75	27	84	29	59	16
Constipation	3	0	4	0	1	—
Lethargy/Malaise/ Fatigue	13	3	12	2	6	3
Alopecia	42	5	43	6	37	7
Dermatitis	21	2	25	1	13	—
Anorexia	14	1	22	4	14	—
Hospitalization for Toxicity	5%		15%		7%	

High LV = Leucovorin 200 mg/m², Low LV = Leucovorin 20 mg/m²
Any = percentage of patients reporting toxicity of any severity
Grade 3 + = percentage of patients reporting toxicity of Grade 3 or higher

---

◆ RATED THERAPEUTICALLY EQUIVALENT; ◇ THERAPEUTIC EQUIVALENCE UNCONFIRMED; ○ UNRATED

monitoring of fluid and electrolyte status, until the serum methotrexate level has fallen to below 0.05 micromolar and the renal failure has resolved.

Some patients will have abnormalities in methotrexate elimination or renal function following methotrexate administration, which are significant but less severe than the abnormalities described in the table above. These abnormalities may or may not be associated with significant clinical toxicity. If significant clinical toxicity is observed, leucovorin rescue should be extended for an additional 24 hours (total of 14 doses over 84 hours) in subsequent courses of therapy. The possibility that the patient is taking other medications which interact with methotrexate (eg, medications which may interfere with methotrexate elimination or binding to serum albumin) should always be reconsidered when laboratory abnormalities or clinical toxicities are observed.

Impaired Methotrexate Elimination or Inadvertent Overdosage: Leucovorin rescue should begin as soon as possible after an inadvertent overdosage and within 24 hours of methotrexate administration when there is delayed excretion (see *"Warnings")*. Leucovorin Calcium 15 mg (10 mg/m^2) should be administered I.M., I.V., or P.O. every 6 hours until the serum methotrexate level is less than 10^{-8}M. If there is adequate gastrointestinal function, doses subsequent to the initial dose may be given orally (see labeling of oral product). In the presence of gastrointestinal toxicity, nausea or vomiting, Leucovorin Calcium should be administered parenterally. Concomitant hydration (3L/d) and urinary alkalinization with sodium bicarbonate should be employed. The bicarbonate dose should be adjusted to maintain a urinary pH at 7 or greater.

Serum creatinine and methotrexate levels should be determined at 24 hour intervals. If the 24 hour serum creatinine has increased 50% over baseline or if the 24 hour methotrexate level is greater than $5 + 10^{-6}$M or the 48 hour level is greater than $9 + 10^{-7}$M, the dose of Leucovorin should be increased to 150 mg (100 mg/m^2) I.V. every 3 hours until the methotrexate level is less than 10^{-8}M. Doses greater than 25 mg should be given parenterally (see *"Clinical Pharmacology")*. When such doses are administered, a non-preserved diluent should be used (see *"Warnings")*. Because of the Calcium contents, the rate of injection of Leucovorin Calcium should not exceed 17.5 mL (175 mg leucovorin) per minute.

The recommended dose of Leucovorin Calcium to counteract hematologic toxicity from folic acid antagonists with less affinity for mammalian dihydrofolate reductase than methotrexate (i.e. trimethoprim, pyrimethamine) is substantially less and 5 to 15 mg of Leucovorin per day has been recommended by some investigators.

Patients who experience delayed early methotrexate elimination are likely to develop reversible nonoliguric renal failure. In addition to appropriate leucovorin therapy, these patients require continuing hydration and urinary alkalinization, and close monitoring of fluid and electrolyte status, until the serum methotrexate level has fallen to below 0.05 micromolar and the renal failure has resolved.

Some patients will have abnormalities in methotrexate elimination or renal function following methotrexate administration, which are significant but less severe. These abnormalities may or may not be associated with significant clinical toxicity. If significant clinical toxicity is observed, leucovorin rescue should be extended for an additional 24 hours (total of 14 doses over 84 hours) in subsequent courses of therapy. The possibility that the patient is taking other medications which interact with methotrexate (e.g., medications which may interfere with methotrexate elimination or binding to serum albumin) should always be reconsidered when laboratory abnormalities or clinical toxicities are observed.

Megaloblastic Anemia: No more than or up to 1 mg daily. There is no evidence that doses > 1 mg daily have greater efficacy than those of 1 mg; additionally, loss of folate in urine becomes roughly logarithmic as the amount administered exceeds 1 mg.

Instructions for Reconstitution: Read *"Warnings"* for considerations in choice of diluent. The contents of each vial should be reconstituted with Bacteriostatic Water for Injection, USP (benzyl alcohol preserved) or with Sterile Water for Injection, USP.

Each 50 mg and 100 mg vial of Leucovorin Calcium for Injection when reconstituted with 5 mL and 10 mL, respectively, of sterile diluent yields a leucovorin concentration of 10 mg per mL. Each 350 mg vial of Leucovorin Calcium for Injection when reconstituted with 17 mL of sterile diluent yields a leucovorin concentration of 20 mg leucovorin per mL. Leucovorin Calcium for Injection contains no preservative.

When reconstituted with Bacteriostatic Water for Injection, the resulting solution must be used within 7 days. If reconstituted with Sterile Water for Injection, use immediately and discard any unused portion.

Because of the benzyl alcohol contained in Bacteriostatic Water for Injection, USP, when doses greater than 10 mg/m^2 are administered Leucovorin Calcium should be reconstituted with Sterile Water for Injection, USP, and used immediately (see *"Warnings")*. Because of the calcium content of the leucovorin solution, no more than 160 mg of leucovorin should be injected intravenously per minute (16 mL of a 10 mg/mL, or 8 mL of a 20 mg/mL solution per minute).

Parenteral drug products should be inspected visually for particulate matter and discoloration prior to administration, whenever solution and container permit.

Advanced Colorectal Cancer: Either of the following two regimens is recommended:

1. Leucovorin is administered at 200 mg/m^2 by slow intravenous injection over a minimum of 3 minutes, followed by 5-fluorouracil at 370 mg/m^2 by intravenous injection.

2. Leucovorin is administered at 20 mg/m^2 by intravenous injection followed by 5-fluorouracil at 425 mg/m^2 by intravenous injection.

Treatment is repeated daily for 5 days. This 5-day treatment course may be repeated at 4-week (28 day) intervals, for two courses and then repeated at 1- to 5-week (28- to 35-day) intervals provided that the patient has completely recovered from the toxic effects of the prior treatment course.

In subsequent treatment courses, the dosage of 5-fluorouracil should be adjusted based on patient tolerance of the prior treatment course. The daily dosage of 5-fluorouracil should be reduced by 20% for patients who experienced moderate hematologic or gastrointestinal toxicity in the prior treatment course and by 30% for patients who experienced severe toxicity (see *"Precautions: Laboratory Tests")*. For patients who experienced no toxicity in the prior treatment course, 5-fluorouracil dosage may be increased by 10%. Leucovorin Calcium dosages are not adjusted for toxicity.

Several other doses and schedules of Leucovorin Calcium/5-fluorouracil therapy have also been evaluated in patients with advanced colorectal cancer: some of these alternative regimens may also have efficacy in the treatment of this disease. However, further clinical research will be required to confirm the safety and effectiveness of these alternative Leucovorin Calcium 5-fluorouracil treatment regimens.

Storage: Store tablets at 15° to 25° C (59° to 77° F). Protect from light and moisture. Store dry powder and reconstituted solution at controlled room temperature, 15° to 25° C (59° to 77° F). Protect from light.

REFERENCES

1. Poon MA, et al. Biochemical modulation of fluorouracil: evidence of significant improvement of survival and quality of life in patients with advanced colorectal carcinoma. *J Clin Oncol* 1989; 7:1407-1418. 2. Poon MA, et al. Biochemical modulation of fluorouracil with leucovorin: confirmatory evidence of improved therapeutic efficacy in advanced colorectal cancer. *J Clin Oncol.* 1991; 9, 11:1967-1972. 3. Grem JL, Shoemaker DD, Petrelli NJ, Douglass HO Jr: Severe and fatal toxic effects observed in treatment with high- and low-dose leucovorin plus 5-fluorouracil for colorectal carcinoma. *Cancer Treat Rep* 1987;71:1122. 4. Link MP, Goorin AM, Miser AW, et al. The effect of adjuvant chemotherapy on relapse-free survival patients with osteosarcoma of the extremity. *N Engl J Med.*1986;314:1600-1606.

J CODES
Per 50 mg IM,IV—J0640

HOW SUPPLIED
INJECTION: 50 MG

BRAND/MANUFACTURER	NDC	SIZE	AWP
◆ GENERICS			
Gensia	00703-5130-01	10 ml	$20.56

INJECTION: 100 MG

BRAND/MANUFACTURER	NDC	SIZE	AWP
◆ GENERICS			
Gensia	00703-5140-01	20 ml	$40.63

POWDER FOR INJECTION: 50 MG

AVERAGE UNIT PRICE (AVAILABLE SIZES)		GENERIC A-RATED AVERAGE PRICE (GAAP)	
GENERIC	$29.44	1s	$38.89

BRAND/MANUFACTURER	NDC	SIZE	AWP
◆ GENERICS			
Immunex	00205-5330-92	1s	$21.53
Elkins-Sinn	00641-2369-41	1s	$56.25
Chiron Therapeutics	53905-0051-10	10s	$184.38
Immunex	00205-5330-19	25s	$538.13

POWDER FOR INJECTION: 100 MG

AVERAGE UNIT PRICE (AVAILABLE SIZES)		GENERIC A-RATED AVERAGE PRICE (GAAP)	
GENERIC	$37.47	1s	$38.70

BRAND/MANUFACTURER	NDC	SIZE	AWP
◆ GENERICS			
Burr Wellcome	00081-0638-93	1s	$37.99
Immunex	00205-4646-94	1s	$39.41
Chiron Therapeutics	53905-0052-10	10s	$350.00

TABLETS: 5 MG

AVERAGE UNIT PRICE (AVAILABLE SIZES)		GENERIC A-RATED AVERAGE PRICE (GAAP)	
GENERIC	$3.68	30s	$123.62
HCFA FUL (100s ea)	$2.98	50s	$152.11
		100s	$436.54

BRAND/MANUFACTURER	NDC	SIZE	AWP
◆ GENERICS			
Burr Wellcome	00081-0631-20	20s	$56.48
Roxane	00054-4496-13	30s	$61.48
Barr	00555-0484-01	30s	$70.81
Geneva	00781-1220-31	30s	$149.00
Rugby	00536-4148-07	30s	$151.06
Burr Wellcome	00081-0631-35	50s ud	$141.71

➤ SHOWN IN PRODUCT IDENTIFICATION GUIDE

BRAND/MANUFACTURER	NDC	SIZE	AWP
UDL	51079-0581-06	50s ud	$162.50
Roxane	00054-4496-25	100s	$202.68
Barr	00555-0484-02	100s	$235.20
Burr Wellcome	00081-0631-55	100s	$283.44
Geneva	00781-1220-01	100s	$489.00
Major	00904-2315-60	100s	$493.45
Qualitest	00603-4183-21	100s	$551.87
Goldline	00182-1869-01	100s	$566.30

TABLETS: 5 MG

BRAND/MANUFACTURER	NDC	SIZE	AWP
◇ GENERICS			
Immunex	00005-4536-38	30s	$85.54
Immunex	00005-4536-40	50s ud	$142.56
Immunex	00005-4536-23	100s	$285.00

TABLETS: 10 MG

AVERAGE UNIT PRICE (AVAILABLE SIZES)	
GENERIC	$5.79

BRAND/MANUFACTURER	NDC	SIZE	AWP
◆ GENERICS			
Roxane	00054-4497-05	12s	$69.86
Roxane	00054-4497-10	24s	$138.33

TABLETS: 15 MG

AVERAGE UNIT PRICE (AVAILABLE SIZES)	
GENERIC	$8.44

BRAND/MANUFACTURER	NDC	SIZE	AWP
◆ GENERICS			
Roxane	00054-4498-05	12s	$104.81
Roxane	00054-4498-10	24s	$195.62

TABLETS: 25 MG

AVERAGE UNIT PRICE (AVAILABLE SIZES)		GENERIC A-RATED AVERAGE PRICE (GAAP)	
GENERIC	$22.50	25s	$624.01

BRAND/MANUFACTURER	NDC	SIZE	AWP
◆ GENERICS			
Burr Wellcome	00081-0632-13	10s ud	$200.36
UDL	51079-0582-05	20s ud	$273.75
Roxane	00054-4499-11	25s	$475.07
Burr Wellcome	00081-0632-25	25s	$500.90
Barr	00555-0485-27	25s	$600.00
Geneva	00781-1222-63	25s	$603.00
Rugby	00536-4149-04	25s	$666.79
Qualitest	00603-4184-35	25s	$680.34
Goldline	00182-1870-24	25s	$693.00

Leukeran SEE CHLORAMBUCIL

Leukine SEE SARGRAMOSTIM

Leuprolide Acetate

DESCRIPTION

Leuprolide Acetate is a synthetic nonapeptide analog of naturally occurring gonadotropin-releasing hormone (GnRH or LH-RH). The analog possesses greater potency than the natural hormone. The chemical name is 5-Oxo-L-prolyl-L-histidyl-L- tryptophyl-L-seryl-L- tyrosol-D- leucyl-L-leucyl-L- arginyl-N-ethyl-L-prolinamide acetate (salt).

Leuprolide Acetate solution is a sterile, aqueous solution intended for subcutaneous injection. It is available in a 2.8 mL multiple-dose vial containing 5 mg/mL of Leuprolide Acetate.

Leuprolide Acetate suspension is supplied in a vial containing sterile lyophilized microspheres, which when mixed with diluent, become a suspension, which is intended as an intramuscular injection.

The pediatric suspension is supplied in two strengths, which when combined provide a total dose of 7.5 mg, 11.25 mg, or 15 mg. When one or more vials are combined to provide the proper dosage, this suspension is intended as a single intramuscular injection.

Each vial of Leuprolide Acetate suspension contains:
Leuprolide Acetate ....3.75 mg

Each vial of Leuprolide Acetate pediatric suspension contains:
Leuprolide Acetate ....3.75 or 7.5 mg

Each vial of Leuprolide Acetate Injection contains:
Leuprolide Acetate ....5 mg/ml

Following is its chemical structure:

H—5 - oxoPro - His - Trp - Ser - Tyr - D- Leu - Leu - Arg - Pro—NHEt • CH₃COOH

$$\text{H—5-oxoPro}_1 - \text{His}_2 - \text{Trp}_3 - \text{Ser}_4 - \text{Tyr}_5 - \text{D-Leu}_6 - \text{Leu}_7 - \text{Arg}_8 - \text{Pro}_9\text{—NHEt} \cdot CH_3COOH$$

CLINICAL PHARMACOLOGY

Leuprolide Acetate, an agonist, acts as a potent inhibitor of gonadotropin secretion when given continuously and in therapeutic doses.

Leuprolide Acetate suspension is a long acting GnRH analog. A single injection of Leuprolide Acetate results in an initial stimulation followed by a prolonged suppression of pituitary gonadotropins. Repeated dosing of the suspension at monthly intervals or chronic administration of the solution results in decreased secretion of gonadal steroids; consequently, tissues and functions that depend on gonadal steroids for their maintenance become quiescent. This effect is reversible on discontinuation of drug therapy. Administration of Leuprolide Acetate has resulted in inhibition of the growth of certain hormone dependent tumors (prostatic tumors in Noble and Dunning male rats and DMBA-induced mammary tumors in female rats) as well as atrophy of the reproductive organs.

In humans, subcutaneous administration of single daily doses of Leuprolide Acetate results in an initial increase in circulating levels of luteinizing hormone (LH) and follicle stimulating hormone (FSH), leading to a transient increase in levels of the gonadal steroids (testosterone and dihydrotestosterone in males, and estrone and estradiol in pre-menopausal females). However, continuous daily administration of Leuprolide Acetate results in decreased levels of LH and FSH in all patients. In males, testosterone is reduced to castrate levels. In premenopausal females, estrogens are reduced to postmenopausal levels. These decreases occur within two to four weeks after initiation of treatment, and castrate levels of testosterone in prostatic cancer patients have been demonstrated for periods of up to five years.

Leuprolide Acetate is not active when given orally. In adults, intramuscular injection of the depot formulation provides plasma concentrations of Leuprolide Acetate over a period of one month. The metabolism, distribution and excretion of Leuprolide Acetate in humans have not been determined.

In children with central precocious puberty (CPP) stimulated and basal gonadotropins are reduced to prepubertal levels. Testosterone and estradiol are reduced to prepubertal levels in males and females respectively. Reduction of gonadotropins will allow for normal physical and psychological growth and development. Natural maturation occurs when gonadotropins return to pubertal levels following discontinuation of Leuprolide Acetate.

The following physiologic effects have been noted with the chronic administration of Leuprolide Acetate in the pediatric population.

1. *Skeletal Growth.* A measurable increase in body length can be noted since the epiphyseal plates will not close prematurely.

2. *Organ Growth.* Reproductive organs will return to a prepubertal state.

3. *Menses.* Menses, if present, will cease.

In a study of 22 children with central precocious puberty, doses of Leuprolide Acetate suspension were given every 4 weeks and plasma levels were determined according to weight categories as summarized below:

Patient Weight Range (kg)	Group Weight Average (kg)	Dose (mg)	Trough Plasma Leuprolide Level Mean ± SD (ng/mL)*
20.2-27.0	22.7	7.5	0.77 ± 0.033
28.4-36.8	32.5	11.25	1.25 ± 1.06
39.3-57.5	44.2	15.0	1.59 ± 0.65

* *Group average values determined at Week 4 immediately prior to Leuprolide Acetate injection. Drug levels at 12 and 24 weeks were similar to respective 4 week levels.*

In males receiving a single dose of Leuprolide Acetate suspension 7.5 mg IM, there was an initial burst of Leuprolide Acetate in plasma. Mean plasma Leuprolide levels of about 0.80 ng/mL were maintained which slowly declined over a period of several weeks. In most of the patient volunteers, plasma Leuprolide concentrations were undetected eight weeks after injection. However, three of these men had low, but detectable levels up to 12 weeks.

Absolute bioavailability from a 7.5 mg suspension dose was estimated to be about 90%. Bioavailability by subcutaneous administration is comparable to that by intravenous administration. Leuprolide Acetate has a plasma half-life of approximately three hours.

The metabolism, distribution and excretion of Leuprolide Acetate in humans have not been fully determined.

The pharmacokinetics of the drug in hepatic- and renal-impaired patients have not been determined.

In controlled clinical studies, Leuprolide Acetate suspension 3.75 mg monthly for 6 months was shown to be comparable to danazol, 800 mg/day in relieving the clinical symptoms of endometriosis (pelvic pain, dysmenorrhea, dyspareunia, pelvic tenderness, and induration) and in reducing the size of endometrial implants as evidenced by laparoscopy. The clinical significance of a decrease in endometriotic lesions is not known at this time and in addition, laparoscopic

---

◆ RATED THERAPEUTICALLY EQUIVALENT; ◇ THERAPEUTIC EQUIVALENCE UNCONFIRMED; ○ UNRATED

staging of endometriosis does not necessarily correlate with the severity of symptoms.

Leuprolide Acetate suspension 3.75 mg monthly induced amenorrhea in 74% and 98% of the adult patients after the first and second treatment months respectively. Most of the remaining patients reported episodes of only light bleeding or spotting. In the first, second and third post-treatment months, normal menstrual cycles resumed in 7%, 71% and 95% respectively, of those patients who did not become pregnant.

Figure 1 illustrates the percent of adult patients with symptoms at baseline, final treatment visit and sustained relief at 6 and 12 months following discontinuation of treatment for the various symptoms evaluated during the study. This included all patients at end of treatment and those who elected to participate at the follow-up periods. This might provide a slight bias in the results at follow-up as 75% of the original patients entered the follow-up study, and 36% were evaluated at 6 months and 26% at 12 months respectively.

FIGURE 1
PERCENT OF PATIENTS WITH SYMPTOMS AT BASELINE, FINAL TREATMENT VISIT, AND AFTER 6 AND 12 MONTHS OF FOLLOW-UP

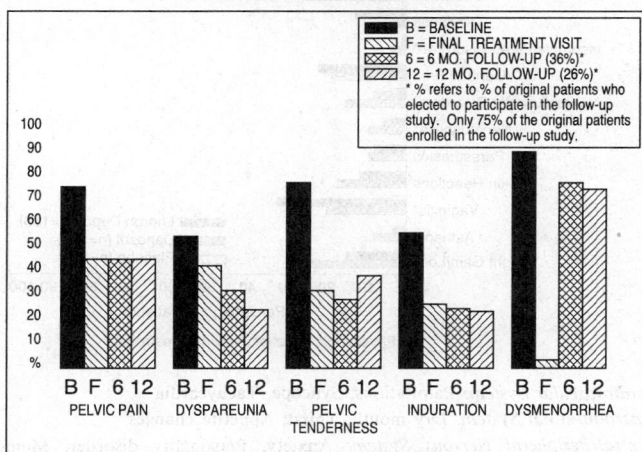

There is no evidence that pregnancy rates are enhanced or adversely affected by the use of Leuprolide Acetate.

INDICATIONS AND USAGE
Leuprolide Acetate solution is indicated in the palliative treatment of advanced prostatic cancer. It offers an alternative treatment of prostatic cancer when orchiectomy or estrogen administration are either not indicated or unacceptable to the patient. In a controlled study comparing Leuprolide Acetate 1 mg/day given subcutaneously to DES (diethyl-stilbestrol), 3 mg/day, the survival rate for the two groups was comparable after two years treatment. The objective response to treatment was also similar for the two groups.

Leuprolide Acetate for depot suspension is indicated for management of endometriosis, including pain relief and reduction of endometriotic lesions in adults. Experience with Leuprolide Acetate for depot suspension for the management of endometriosis has been limited to women 18 years of age and older treated for 6 months.

Leuprolide Acetate suspension is also indicated in the treatment of children with central precocious puberty. Children should be selected using the following criteria:

1. Clinical diagnosis of CPP (idiopathic or neurogenic) with onset of secondary sexual characteristics earlier than 8 years in females and 9 years in males:
2. Clinical diagnosis should be confirmed prior to initiation of therapy:
■ Confirmation of diagnosis by a pubertal response to a GnRH stimulation test. The sensitivity and methodology of this assay must be understood.
■ Bone age advanced one year beyond the chronological age.
3. Baseline evaluation should also include:
■ Height and weight measurements.
■ Sex steroid levels.
■ Adrenal steroid level to exclude congenital adrenal hyperplasia.
■ Beta human chorionic gonadotropin level to rule out a chorionic gonadotropin secreting tumor.
■ Pelvic/adrenal/testicular ultrasound to rule out a steroid secreting tumor.
■ Computerized tomography of the head to rule out intracranial tumor.

UNLABELED USES
Leuprolide is used alone or as an adjunct in the treatment of metastatic breast cancer in premenopausal women and in uterine fibroid tumors (leiomyomata uteri). It is also used for controlled ovarian hyperstimulation during the embryo transfer procedure in *in vitro* fertilization, and is used in the treatment of sexually deviant behavior in male patients with paraphilia.

CONTRAINDICATIONS
1. Hypersensitivity to GnRH. GnRH agonist analogs or any of the excipients in Leuprolide Acetate.
2. Undiagnosed abnormal vaginal bleeding.
3. Leuprolide Acetate is contraindicated in women who are or may become pregnant while receiving the drug. Leuprolide Acetate may cause fetal harm when administered to a pregnant woman. Major dose-related fetal abnormalities were observed in rabbits but not in rats after administration of Leuprolide Acetate throughout gestation. There was increased fetal mortality and decreased fetal weights in rats and rabbits (see "Pregnancy" Section). The effects on fetal mortality are expected consequences of the alterations in hormonal levels brought about by the drug. If this drug is used during pregnancy or if the patient becomes pregnant while taking this drug, she should be apprised of the potential hazard to the fetus.

4. Use in women who are breast feeding (see Nursing Mothers Section).
5. A report of an anaphylactic reaction to synthetic GnRH has been reported in the medical literature.[1]

WARNINGS
Isolated cases of worsening of signs and symptoms during the first weeks of treatment with Leuprolide Acetate solution have been reported. Worsening of symptoms may contribute to paralysis with or without fatal complications.

Safe use of Leuprolide Acetate in pregnancy has not been established clinically. Before starting treatment with Leuprolide Acetate, pregnancy must be excluded.

In adults, when used monthly at the recommended dose, Leuprolide Acetate suspension usually inhibits ovulation and stops menstruation. Contraception is not insured, however, by taking Leuprolide Acetate suspension. Therefore, patients should use nonhormonal methods of contraception. Patients should be advised to see their physician if they believe they may be pregnant. If a patient becomes pregnant during treatment, the drug must be discontinued and the patient must be apprised of the potential risk to the fetus.

During the early phase of therapy, sex steroids temporarily rise above baseline because of the physiologic effect of the drug. Therefore, an increase in clinical signs and symptoms may be observed during the initial days of therapy, but these will dissipate with continued therapy.

In pediatric patients noncompliance with drug regimen or inadequate dosing may result in inadequate control of the pubertal process. The consequences of poor control include the return of pubertal signs such as menses, breast development, and testicular growth. The long-term consequences of inadequate control of gonadal steroid secretion are unknown, but may include a further compromise of adult stature.

PRECAUTIONS
Patients with metastatic vertebral lesions and/or with urinary tract obstruction should be closely observed during the first few weeks of therapy with Leuprolide Acetate solution (see "Adverse Reactions" section).

Patients with known allergies to benzyl alcohol, an ingredient of the drug's vehicle, may present symptoms of hypersensitivity, usually local, in the form of erythema and induration at the injection site.

Information for Adult Patients: An information pamphlet for patients is included with the product. Patients should be aware of the following information:
1. Since menstruation should stop with effective doses of Leuprolide Acetate suspension the patient should notify her physician if regular menstruation persists. Patients missing successive doses of Leuprolide Acetate suspension may experience break-through bleeding.
2. Patients should not use Leuprolide Acetate suspension if they are pregnant, breast feeding, have undiagnosed abnormal vaginal bleeding, or are allergic to any of the ingredients in Leuprolide Acetate suspension.
3. Safe use of the drug in pregnancy has not been established clinically. Therefore, a nonhormonal method of contraception should be used during treatment. Patients should be advised that if they miss successive doses of Leuprolide Acetate suspension, breakthrough bleeding or ovulation may occur with the potential for conception. If a patient becomes pregnant during treatment, she should discontinue treatment and consult her physician.
4. Those adverse events occurring in clinical studies with Leuprolide Acetate suspension are associated with hypoestrogenism; like hot flashes, headaches, emotional lability, decreased libido, acne, myalgia, reduction in breast size, and vaginal dryness. Estrogen levels returned to normal after treatment was discontinued.
5. The induced hypoestrogenic state results in a small loss in bone density over the course of treatment, some of which may not be reversible. During one six-month treatment period, this bone loss should not be important. In patients with major risk factors for decreased bone mineral content such as chronic alcohol and/ or tobacco use, strong family history of osteoporosis, or chronic use of drugs that can reduce bone mass such as anticonvulsants or corticosteroids, Leuprolide Acetate Suspension therapy may pose an additional risk. In these patients the risks and benefits must be weighed carefully before therapy with Leuprolide Acetate suspension is instituted. Repeated courses of treatment with gonadotropin-releasing hormone analogs are not advisable in patients with major risk factors for loss of bone mineral content.
6. Retreatment cannot be recommended since safety data beyond 6 months are not available.

Information for Parents of Pediatric Patients: Prior to starting therapy with Leuprolide Acetate suspension the parent or guardian must be aware of the importance of continuous therapy. Adherence to 4 week drug administration schedules must be accepted if therapy is to be successful.
■ During the first 2 months of therapy, a female may experience menses or spotting. If bleeding continues beyond the second month, notify the physician.
■ Any irritation at the injection site should be reported to the physician immediately.
■ Report any unusual signs or symptoms to the physician.

Laboratory Tests: In adult patients receiving the solution, response to Leuprolide Acetate should be monitored by measuring serum levels of testosterone and acid phosphatase. In the majority of patients, testosterone levels increased above baseline during the first week, declining thereafter to baseline levels or below by the end of the second week of treatment. Castrate levels were reached within two to four weeks and once attained were maintained for as long as drug administration continued. Transient increases in acid phosphatase levels occurred sometimes early in treatment. However, by the fourth week, the elevated levels usually decreased to values at or near baseline.

In pediatric patients, response to Leuprolide Acetate should be monitored 1-2 months after the start of therapy with a GnRH stimulation test and sex steroid levels. Measurement of bone age for advancement should be done every 6-12 months.

Sex steroids may increase or rise above prepubertal levels if the dose is inadequate (see *"Warnings"* section). Once a therapeutic dose has been established, gonadotropin and sex steroid levels will decline to prepubertal levels.

Drug Interactions: No pharmacokinetic-based drug-drug interaction studies have been conducted with Leuprolide Acetate. However, because Leuprolide Acetate is a peptide that is primarily degraded by peptidase and not by cytochrome P-450 enzymes as noted in specific studies, and the drug is only about 46% bound to plasma proteins, drug interactions would not be expected to occur.

Drug/Laboratory Test Interactions: Administration of Leuprolide Acetate depot suspension in therapeutic doses results in suppression of the pituitary gonadal system. Normal function is usually restored within 4 to 12 weeks after treatment is discontinued. Therefore, diagnostic tests of pituitary gonadotropic and gonadal functions conducted during treatment and up to 4 to 8 weeks after discontinuation of Leuprolide Acetate depot suspension therapy may be misleading.

Carcinogenesis, Mutagenesis, Impairment of Fertility: A two-year carcinogenicity study was conducted in rats and mice. In rats, a dose-related increase of benign pituitary hyperplasia and benign pituitary adenomas was noted at 24 months when the drug was administered subcutaneously at high daily doses (0.6 to 4 mg/kg). There was a significant but not dose-related increase of pancreatic islet-cell adenomas in females and of testes interstitial cell adenomas in males (highest incidence in the low dose group). In mice, no Leuprolide Acetate-induced tumors or pituitary abnormalities were observed at a dose as high as 60 mg/kg for two years. Patients have been treated with Leuprolide Acetate for up to three years with doses as high as 10 mg/day and for two years with doses as high as 20 mg/day without demonstrable pituitary abnormalities.

Mutagenicity studies have been performed with Leuprolide Acetate using bacterial and mammalian systems. These studies provided no evidence of a mutagenic potential.

Clinical and pharmacologic studies in adults with Leuprolide Acetate and similar analogs have shown full reversibility of fertility suppression when the drug is discontinued after continuous administration for periods of up to 24 weeks. No clinical studies have been completed with Leuprolide Acetate in children to assess the reversibility of fertility suppression but animal studies (prepubertal and adult rats and monkeys) with Leuprolide Acetate and other GnRH analogs have shown functional recovery. However, following a study with Leuprolide Acetate, immature male rats demonstrated tubular degeneration in the testes even after a recovery period. In spite of the failure to recover histologically, the treated males proved to be as fertile as the controls. Also, no histologic changes were observed in the female rats following the same protocol. In both sexes, the offspring of the treated animals appeared normal. The effect of the treatment of the parents on the reproductive performance of the F1 generation was not tested. The clinical significance of these findings is unknown.

Pregnancy, Teratogenic Effects: Pregnancy Category X. See *"Contraindications"* section. When administered on day 6 of pregnancy at test dosages of 0.00024, 0.0024, and 0.024 mg/kg to rabbits, Leuprolide Acetate produced a dose-related increase in major fetal abnormalities. Similar studies in rats failed to demonstrate an increase in fetal malformations. There was increased fetal mortality and decreased fetal weights with the two higher doses of Leuprolide Acetate in rabbits and with the highest dose (0.024 mg/kg) in rats.

Nursing Mothers: It is not known whether Leuprolide Acetate is excreted in human milk. Because many drugs are excreted in human milk, and because the effects of Leuprolide Acetate on lactation and/or the breastfed child have not been determined, Leuprolide Acetate should not be used by nursing mothers.

Pediatric Use: Safety and effectiveness of adult forms of Leuprolide Acetate in children have not been established.

ADVERSE REACTIONS
LEUPROLIDE ACETATE SUSPENSION
Estradiol levels may increase during the first weeks following the initial injection, but then decline to postmenopausal levels. This transient increase in estradiol can be associated with a temporary worsening of signs and symptoms (see *"Warnings"* section).

As would be expected with a drug that lowers serum estradiol levels, the most frequently reported adverse reactions were those related to hypoestrogenism.

In controlled studies comparing Leuprolide Acetate suspension, 3.75 mg monthly and danazol (800 mg/day), or placebo, adverse reactions most frequently reported and thought to be possibly or probably drug-related are shown in Figure 2.

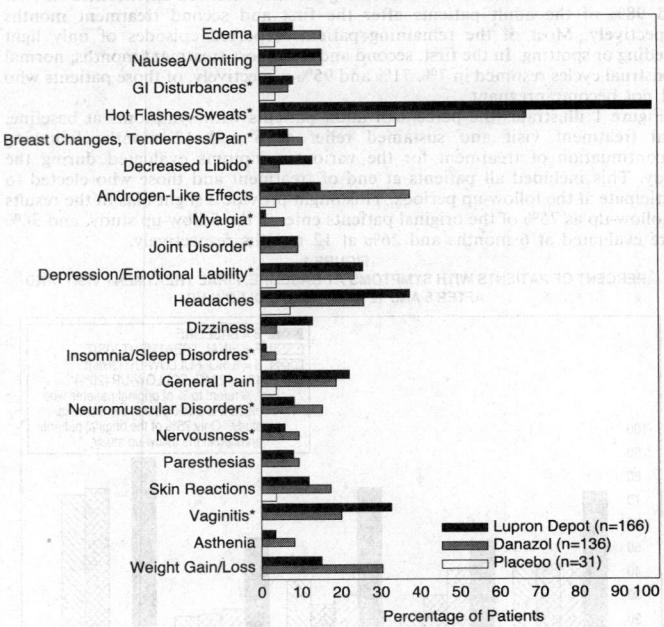

FIGURE 2
ADVERSE EVENTS REPORTED DURING 6 MONTH OF TREATMENT WITH LUPRON DEPOT 3.75 MG

(Legend: ■ Lupron Depot (n=166); ▨ Danazol (n=136); ▢ Placebo (n=31))

Percentage of Patients

* Physiologic effect of decreased estrogen

Cardiovascular System: Palpitations, Syncope, Tachycardia

Gastrointestinal System: Dry mouth, Thirst, Appetite changes

Central/Peripheral Nervous System: Anxiety, Personality disorder, Memory disorder, Delusions

Integumentary System: Ecchymosis, Alopecia, Hair disorder

Urogenital System: Dysuria,* Lactation

Miscellaneous: Ophthalmologic disorders,* Lymphadenopathy

In other clinical trials involving patients with prostate cancer and during postmarketing surveillance, the following adverse reactions were reported to have a possible, probable, or unknown relationship to Leuprolide Acetate solution or suspension as ascribed by the treating physician. Often, it is difficult to assess causality in patients with prostate cancer. Reactions considered not drug related have been excluded.

Cardiovascular System: Congestive heart failure, ECG changes/ischemia, High blood pressure, Murmur, Phlebitis/thrombosis, Angina, Cardiac arrhythmias, Myocardial infarction, Pulmonary emboli, Hypotension, Transient ischemic attack/stroke

Gastrointestinal System: Dysphagia, Gastrointestinal bleeding, Peptic ulcer, Rectal polyps, Hepatic dysfunction

Endocrine System: Decreased testicular size, Gynecomastia, Impotence, Libido increase

Hemic and Lymphatic System: Anemia, Decreased WBC, Hemoptysis

Musculoskeletal System: Bone pain, Ankylosing spondylosis, Pelvic fibrosis

Central/Peripheral Nervous System: Peripheral neuropathy, Syncope/blackouts, Hearing disorder, Spinal fracture/paralysis

Respiratory System: Dyspnea, Sinus congestion, Cough, Pleural rub, Pneumonia, Pulmonary fibrosis Pulmonary infiltrate, Respiratory disorders

Urogenital System: Frequency/urgency, Hematuria, Urinary tract infection, Bladder spasms, Incontinence, Testicular pain, Urinary obstruction, Penile swelling, Prostate Pain

Miscellaneous: Diabetes, Fever, Hypoglycemia, Increased BUN, Increased calcium, Increased creatinine, Inflammation, Hypoproteinemia, Hard nodule in throat, weight gain, increased uric acid.

Changes in Bone Density: After six months of Leuprolide Acetate suspension treatment, vertebral trabecular bone density measured by quantitative computed tomography (QCT) decreased by an average of 13.5% compared to pretreatment levels. A small number of original patients were retested at 6 and 12 months after completion of treatment. At 6 months, 9 patients had an average bone density change from baseline by QCT of –3.2%. At 12 months after completion of treatment, 6 patients had an average bone density change from baseline of –2.4%. These results show that there was partial to complete recovery of bone density in the post-treatment period in a small number of original patients who were retested. Use of Leuprolide Acetate suspension for longer than the recommended six months or in the presence of other known risk factors for decreased bone mineral content may cause additional bone loss.

Changes in Laboratory Values During Treatment:

Plasma enzymes: During clinical trials with Leuprolide Acetate suspension regular laboratory monitoring revealed that SGOT levels were more than twice the upper limit of normal in only one patient. There was no other clinical or laboratory evidence of abnormal liver function.

Lipids: At enrollment, 4% of the Leuprolide Acetate suspension patients and 1% of the danazol patients had total cholesterol values above the normal range. These patients also had cholesterol values above the normal range at the end of treatment.

Of those patients whose pretreatment cholesterol values were in the normal range, 7% of the Leuprolide Acetate suspension patients and 9% of the danazol patients had post-treatment cholesterol values above the normal range.

The mean ($\pm$ SEM) pretreatment values for total cholesterol from all patients were 178.8 (2.9) mg/dL in the Leuprolide Acetate suspension group and 175.3 (3.0) mg/dL in the danazol group. At the end of treatment, the mean values for total cholesterol from all patients were 193.3 mg/dL in the Leuprolide Acetate suspension group and 194.4 mg/dL in the danazol group. These increases from the pretreatment values were statistically significant ($p < 0.03$) in both groups.

Triglycerides were increased above the upper limit of normal in 12% of the patients who received Leuprolide Acetate suspension and in 6% of the patients who received danazol.

At the end of treatment, HDL cholesterol fractions decreased below the lower limit of the normal range in 2% of the Leuprolide Acetate suspension patients compared with 54% of those receiving danazol. LDL cholesterol fractions increased above the upper limit of the normal range in 6% of the patients receiving Leuprolide Acetate suspension compared with 23% of those receiving danazol. There was no increase in the LDL/HDL ratio in patients receiving Leuprolide Acetate suspension, but there was approximately a two-fold increase in the LDL/HDL ratio in patients receiving danazol.

Other Changes: In comparative studies, the following changes were seen in approximately 5% to 8% of patients. Leuprolide Acetate suspension was associated with elevations of LDH and phosphorus, and decreases in WBC counts. Danazol therapy was associated with increases in hematocrit, platelet count, and LDH.

Children: Potential exacerbation of signs and symptoms during the first few weeks of treatment (see *"Precautions"* section) is a concern in patients with rapidly advancing central precocious puberty.

In two studies of children with central precocious puberty, in 2% or more of the patients receiving the drug, the following adverse reactions were reported to have a possible or probable relationship to drug as ascribed by the treating physician. Reactions considered not drug related are excluded.

	Number of Patients N = 395 *(Percent)*
Body as a Whole	
General Pain	7 (2)
Integumentary System	
Acne/Seborrhea	7 (2)
Injection Site Reactions	
Including Abscess	21 (5)
Rash Including	
Erythema Multiforme	8 (2)
Urogenital System	
Vaginitis/Bleeding/Discharge	7 (2)

In those same studies, the following adverse reactions were reported in less than 2% of the patients.

Body as a Whole: Body Odor, Fever, Headache, Infection

Cardiovascular System: Syncope, Vasodilation

Digestive System: Dysphagia, Gingivitis, Nausea/Vomiting

Endocrine System: Accelerated Sexual Maturity

Metabolic and Nutritional Disorders: Peripheral Edema, Weight Gain

Nervous System: Nervousness, Personality Disorder, Somnolence, Emotional Lability

Respiratory System: Epistaxis

Integumentary System: Alopecia, Skin Striae

Urogenital System: Cervix Disorder, Gynecomastia/Breast Disorders, Urinary Incontinence

LEUPROLIDE ACETATE SOLUTION

In the majority of patients testosterone levels increased above baseline during the first week, declining thereafter to baseline levels or below by the end of the second week of treatment. This transient increase was occasionally associated with a temporary worsening of signs and symptoms, usually manifested by an increase in bone pain (see *"Warnings"* section). In a few cases a temporary worsening of existing hematuria and urinary tract obstruction occurred during the first week. Temporary weakness and paresthesia of the lower limbs have been reported in a few cases.

Potential exacerbations of signs and symptoms during the first few weeks of treatment is a concern in patients with vertebral metastases and/or urinary obstruction which, if aggravated, may lead to neurological problems or increase the obstruction.

In a comparative trial of Leuprolide Acetate solution versus DES, in 5% or more of the patients receiving either drug, the following adverse reactions were reported to have a possible or probable relationship to drug as ascribed by the treating physician. Often, causality is difficult to assess in patients with metastatic prostate cancer. Reactions considered not drug related are excluded.

	Leuprolide Acetate (N = 98)	DES (N = 101)
	Number of Reports	
Cardiovascular System		
Congestive heart failure	1	5
ECG changes/ischemia	19	22
High blood pressure	8	5
Murmur	3	8
Peripheral edema	12	30
Phlebitis/thrombosis	2	10
Gastrointestinal System		
Anorexia	6	5
Constipation	7	9
Nausea/vomiting	5	17
Endocrine System		
*Decreased testicular size	7	11
Gynecomastia/breast tenderness or pain	7	63
*Hot flashes	55	12
*Impotence	4	12
Hemic and Lymphatic System		
Anemia	5	5
Musculoskeletal System		
Bone pain	5	2
Myalgia	3	9
Central/Peripheral Nervous System		
Dizziness/lightheadedness	5	7
General pain	13	13
Headache	7	4
Insomnia/sleep disorders	7	5
Respiratory System		
Dyspnea	2	8
Sinus congestion	5	6
Integumentary System		
Dermatitis	5	8
Urogenital System		
Frequency/urgency	6	8
Hematuria	6	4
Urinary tract infection	7	7
Miscellaneous		
Asthenia	10	10

* *Physiologic effect of decreased testosterone.*

In this same study, the following adverse reactions were reported in less than 5% of the patients on Leuprolide Acetate solution.

Cardiovascular System: Angina, Cardiac arrhythmias, Myocardial infarction, Pulmonary emboli

Gastrointestinal System: Diarrhea, Dysphagia, Gastrointestinal bleeding, Gastrointestinal disturbance, Peptic ulcer, Rectal polyps

Endocrine System: Libido decrease, Thyroid enlargement

Musculoskeletal System: Joint pain

Central/Peripheral Nervous System: Anxiety, Blurred vision, Lethargy, Memory disorder, Mood swings, Nervousness, Numbness, Paresthesia, Peripheral neuropathy, Syncope/blackouts, Taste disorders

Respiratory System: Cough, Pleural rub, Pneumonia, Pulmonary fibrosis

Integumentary System: Carcinoma of skin/ear, Dry skin, Ecchymosis, Hair loss, Itching, Local skin reactions, Pigmentation, Skin lesions

Urogenital System: Bladder spasms, Dysuria, Incontinence, Testicular pain, Urinary obstruction

Miscellaneous: Depression, Diabetes, Fatigue, Fever/chills, Hypoglycemia, Increased BUN, Increased calcium, Increased creatinine, Infection/inflammation, Ophthalmologic disorders, Swelling (temporal bone).

OVERDOSAGE

In rats subcutaneous administration of 250 to 500 times the recommended human adult dose, or 125 to 250 times the recommended human pediatric dose, expressed on a per body weight basis, resulted in dyspnea, decreased activity, and local irritation at the injection site. There is no evidence at present that there is a clinical counterpart of this phenomenon. In early clinical trials using daily subcutaneous Leuprolide Acetate in patients with prostate cancer, doses as high as 20 mg/day for up to two years caused no adverse effects differing from those observed with the 1 mg/day dose.

DOSAGE AND ADMINISTRATION

Leuprolide Acetate Suspension: Must Be Administered Under The Supervision of A Physician.

Leuprolide Acetate Solution: The recommended dose is 1 mg (0.2 ml) administered as a single daily subcutaneous injection. As with other drugs administered chronically by subcutaneous injection, the injection site should be varied periodically.

Note: As with all parenteral products, inspect container's solution for discoloration and particulate matter before each use.

Adults: The recommended dose of Leuprolide Acetate suspension is 3.75 mg, incorporated in a depot formulation. The lyophilized microspheres are to be reconstituted and administered monthly as a single intramuscular injection, in accord with the following directions:

1. Using a syringe with a 22 gauge needle, withdraw 1 mL of diluent from the ampule, and inject it into the vial. (Extra diluent is provided; any remaining should be discarded.)
2. Shake well to thoroughly disperse particles to obtain a uniform suspension. The suspension will appear milky.
3. Withdraw the entire contents of the vial into the syringe and inject it at the time of reconstitution.

The recommended duration of administration is six months. Retreatment cannot be recommended since safety data for retreatment are not available. If the symptoms of endometriosis recur after a course of therapy, and further treatment with Leuprolide Acetate is contemplated, it is recommended that bone density be assessed before retreatment begins to ensure that values are within normal limits.

All Patients: Although the suspension has been shown to be stable for 24 hours following reconstitution, since the product does not contain a preservative, the suspension should be discarded if not used immediately. As with other drugs administered by injection, the injection site should be varied periodically.

Children: The dose of Leuprolide Acetate must be individualized for each child. The dose is based on a mg/kg ratio of drug to body weight. Younger children require higher doses on a mg/kg ratio.

After 1-2 months of initiating therapy or changing doses, the child must be monitored with a GnRH stimulation test, sex steroids, and Tanner staging to confirm downregulation. Measurements of bone age for advancement should be monitored every 6-12 months. The dose should be titrated upward until no progression of the condition is noted either clinically and/or by laboratory parameters.

The first dose found to result in adequate downregulation can probably be maintained for the duration of therapy in most children. However, there are insufficient data to guide dosage adjustment as patients move into higher weight categories after beginning therapy at very young ages and low dosages. It is recommended that adequate downregulation be verified in such patients whose weight has increased significantly while on therapy.

As with other drugs administered by injection, the injection site should be varied periodically.

Discontinuation of Leuprolide Acetate should be considered before age 11 for females and age 12 for males.

The recommended starting dose is 0.3 mg/kg/4 weeks (minimum 7.5 mg) administered as a single intramuscular injection. The starting dose will be dictated by the child's weight.

≤ 25 kg	7.5 mg
> 25-37.5 kg	11.25 mg
> 37.5 kg	15 mg

If total downregulation is not achieved, the dose should be titrated upward in increments of 3.75 mg every 4 weeks. This dose will be considered the maintenance dose.

The lyophilized microspheres are to be reconstituted and administered as a single intramuscular injection, in accord with the following directions:

1a. To mix a single vial: Using a syringe with a 22 gauge needle, withdraw 1 mL of diluent from the ampule, and inject it into the vial.
or
1b. To mix two or more vials: Using a syringe with a 22 gauge needle, withdraw approximately 0.5 mL of diluent from the ampule and inject it into each vial. The total volume for administration should be approximately 1 mL.
2. Shake each vial to thoroughly disperse particles to obtain a uniform suspension.
3. Withdraw the entire contents of one vial and then withdraw the contents of the other vial into the same syringe.
4. Inject the medication at the time of reconstitution.

Storage: The vial of Leuprolide Acetate and the ampule of diluent may be stored at room temperature.

No refrigeration necessary for suspension products. Protect from freezing.

Leuprolide Acetate solution should be refrigerated until dispensed. Patient may store unrefrigerated below 86°F. Avoid freezing. Protect from light–store vial in carton until use.

REFERENCE
1. MacLeod TL, et al. Anaphylactic reaction to synthetic luteinizing hormone-releasing hormone. *Fertil Steril* 1987 Sept: 48(3):500-502.

J CODES
Per 1 mg IM,SC—J9218
7.5 mg IM,SC—J9217

HOW SUPPLIED
KIT: 5 MG/ML

BRAND/MANUFACTURER	NDC	SIZE	AWP
○ BRAND			
LUPRON: Tap	00300-3626-28	1s	$256.88
	00300-3626-30	2s	$500.00
	00300-3626-24	6s	$1541.25

KIT: 7.5 MG

BRAND/MANUFACTURER	NDC	SIZE	AWP
○ BRAND			
LUPRON DEPOT-PED: Tap	00300-2106-01	1s	$463.75

KIT: 11.25 MG

BRAND/MANUFACTURER	NDC	SIZE	AWP
○ BRAND			
LUPRON DEPOT-PED: Tap	00300-2270-01	1s	$834.38

KIT: 15 MG

BRAND/MANUFACTURER	NDC	SIZE	AWP
○ BRAND			
LUPRON DEPOT-PED: Tap	00300-2437-01	1s	$927.50

POWDER FOR INJECTION: 3.75 MG

BRAND/MANUFACTURER	NDC	SIZE	AWP
○ BRAND			
LUPRON DEPOT: Tap	00300-3639-01	1s	$370.63
	00300-3639-06	6s	$2223.75

POWDER FOR INJECTION: 7.5 MG

BRAND/MANUFACTURER	NDC	SIZE	AWP
○ BRAND			
LUPRON DEPOT: Tap	00300-3629-01	1s	$463.75
	00300-3629-06	6s	$2782.50

Leustatin *SEE* CLADRIBINE

Levamisole Hydrochloride

DESCRIPTION
Levamisole Hydrochloride is an immunomodulator available in tablets for oral administration containing the equivalent of 50 mg as Levamisole base. Fifty-nine (59) mg of Levamisole HCl is equivalent to 50 mg of Levamisole base.

Levamisole Hydrochloride is (-)-(S)-2,3,5,6-tetrahydro-6-phenylimidazo [2,1-b] thiazole monohydrochloride.

Levamisole Hydrochloride is a white to pale cream colored crystalline powder which is almost odorless and is freely soluble in water. It is quite stable in acid aqueous media but hydrolyzes in alkaline or neutral solutions. It has a molecular weight of 240.75.

Following is its chemical structure:

CLINICAL PHARMACOLOGY
Two clinical trials having essentially the same design have demonstrated an increase in survival and a reduction in recurrence rate in the subset of patients with resected Dukes' C colon cancer treated with a regimen of Levamisole HCl plus fluorouracil[1,2]. After surgery, patients were randomized to no further therapy, Levamisole HCl alone, or Levamisole HCl plus fluorouracil.

In one clinical trial in which 408 Dukes' B and C colorectal cancer patients were studied, 262 Dukes' C patients were evaluated for a minimum follow-up of five years[1]. A subset analysis of these Dukes' C patients showed the estimated reduction in death rate was 27% for Levamisole HCl plus fluorouracil (p = 0.11) and 28% for Levamisole HCl alone (p = 0.11)[3]. The estimated reduction in recurrence rate was 36% for Levamisole HCl plus fluorouracil (p = 0.025) and 28% for Levamisole HCl alone (p = 0.11)[3]. In another clinical trial designed to confirm the above results, 929 Dukes' C colon cancer patients were evaluated for a minimum follow-up of 2 years[2]. The estimated reduction in death rate was 33% for Levamisole HCl plus flurouracil (p = 0.006). The estimated reduction in recurrence rate was 41% for Levamisole HCl plus flurouracil (p < 0.0001). The Levamisole HCl alone group did not show advantage over no treatment on improving recurrence or survival rates. There are presently insufficient data to evaluate the effect of the combination of Levamisole HCl plus fluorouracil in Dukes' B patients. There are also insufficient data to evaluate the effect of Levamisole HCl plus fluorouracil in patients with rectal cancer because only 12

---

patients with rectal cancer were treated with the combination in the first study and none in the second study.

The mechanism of action of Levamisole HCl in combination with fluorouracil is unknown. The effects of Levamisole on the immune system are complex. The drug appears to restore depressed immune function rather than to stimulate response to above-normal levels. Levamisole can stimulate formation of antibodies to various antigens, enhance T-cell responses by stimulating T-cell activation and proliferation, potentiate monocyte and macrophage functions including phagocytosis and chemotaxis, and increase neutrophil mobility, adherence, and chemotaxis. Other drugs have similar short-term effects and the clinical relevance is unclear. p* Besides its immunomodulatory function, Levamisole has other mammalian pharmacologic activities, including inhibition of alkaline phosphatase, and cholinergic activity.

The pharmacokinetics of Levamisole HCl have not been studied in the dosage regimen recommended with fluorouracil nor in patients with hepatic insufficiency. After administration of a single oral dose of 50 mg of a research formulation of Levamisole HCl, it appears that Levamisole is rapidly absorbed from the gastrointestinal tract. Mean peak plasma concentrations of 0.13 mcg/ml are attained within 1.5 to 2 hours.

The plasma elimination half-life of Levamisole is between 3-4 hours. Following a 150-mg radio-labelled dose, Levamisole is extensively metabolized by the liver in humans and the metabolites excreted mainly by the kidneys (70% over 3 days). The elimination half-life of metabolite excretion is 16 hours. Approximately 5% is excreted in the feces. Less than 5% is excreted unchanged in the urine and less than 0.2% in the feces. Approximately 12% is recovered in the urine as the glucuronide of p-hydroxy-levamisole. The clinical significance of these data are unknown since a 150-mg dose may not be proportional to a 50-mg dose.

INDICATIONS AND USAGE
Levamisole HCl is indicated as adjuvant treatment in combination with fluorouracil after surgical resection in patients with Dukes' stage C colon cancer.

UNLABELED USES
Levamisole HCl is also used in the treatment of breast cancer.

CONTRAINDICATIONS
Levamisole HCl is contraindicated in patients with a known hypersensitivity to the drug or its components.

WARNINGS
Levamisole HCl has been associated with agranulocytosis, sometimes fatal. The onset of agranulocytosis is frequently accompanied by a flu-like syndrome (fever, chills, etc.); however, in a small number of patients it is asymptomatic. A flu-like syndrome may also occur in the absence of agranulocytosis. It is essential that appropriate hematological monitoring be done routinely during therapy with Levamisole HCl and fluorouracil. Neutropenia is usually reversible following discontinuation of therapy. Patients should be instructed to report immediately any flu-like symptoms.

Higher than recommended doses of Levamisole HCl may be associated with an increased incidence of agranulocytosis, so the recommended dose should not be exceeded.

The combination of Levamisole HCl and fluorouracil has been associated with frequent neutropenia, anemia and thrombocytopenia.

PRECAUTIONS
Before beginning this combination adjuvant treatment, the physician should become familiar with the labeling for fluorouracil.

Information for Patients: The patient should be informed that if flu-like symptoms or malaise occurs, the physician should be notified immediately.

Drug Interactions: Levamisole HCl has been reported to produce "Antabuse ®"-like side effects when given concomitantly with alcohol. Concomitant administration of phenytoin and Levamisole HCl plus fluorouracil has led to increased plasma levels of phenytoin. The physician is advised to monitor plasma levels of phenytoin and to decrease the dose if necessary.

Because of reports of prolongation of the prothrombin time beyond the therapeutic range in patients taking concurrent Levamisole and warfarin sodium, it is suggested that the prothrombin time be monitored carefully, and the dose of warfarin sodium or other coumarin-like drugs should be adjusted accordingly, in patients taking both drugs.

Laboratory Tests: On the first day of therapy with Levamisole HCl fluorouracil, patients should have a CBC with differential and platelets, electrolytes and liver function tests performed. Thereafter, a CBC with differential and platelets should be performed weekly prior to each treatment with fluorouracil with electrolytes and liver function tests performed every 3 months for a total of one year. Dosage modifications should be instituted as follows: If WBC is 2500-3500/mm³ defer the fluorouracil dose until WBC is > 3500/mm³. If WBC is < 2500/mm³, defer the fluorouracil dose until WBC is > 3500/mm³; then resume the fluorouracil dose reduced by 20%. If WBC remains < 2500/mm³ for over 10 days despite deferring fluorouracil, discontinue administration of Levamisole HCl. Both drugs should be deferred unless enough platelets are present (≥ 100,000/mm³).

Carcinogenesis, Mutagenesis, Impairment of Fertility: Adequate animal carcinogenicity studies have not been conducted with Levamisole. Studies of Levamisole administered in drinking water at 5, 20, and 80 mg/kg/day to mice for up to 18 months or administered to rats in the diet at 5, 20, and 80 mg/kg/day for 24 months showed no evidence of neoplastic effects. These studies were not conducted at the maximum tolerated dose, therefore the animals may not have

been exposed to a reasonable drug challenge. No mutagenic effects were demonstrated in dominant lethal studies in male and female mice, in an Ames test, and in a study to detect chromosomal aberrations in cultured peripheral human lymphocytes.

Adverse effects were not observed on male or female fertility when Levamisole was administered to rats in the diet at doses of 2.5, 10, 40, and 160 mg/kg. In a rat gavage study at doses of 20, 60, and 180 mg/kg, the copulation period was increased, the duration of pregnancy was slightly increased, and fertility, pup viability and weight, lactation index, and number of fetuses were decreased at 60 mg/kg. No negative reproductive effects were present when the offspring were allowed to mate and litter.

Pregnancy: Pregnancy Category C: Teratogenicity studies have been performed in rats and rabbits at oral doses up to 180 mg/kg. Fetal malformations were not observed. In rats, embryotoxicity was present at 160 mg/kg and in rabbits, significant embryotoxicity was observed at 180 mg/kg. There are no adequate and well-controlled studies in pregnant women and Levamisole HCl should not be administered unless the potential benefits outweigh the risks. Women taking the combination of Levamisole HCl and fluorouracil should be advised not to become pregnant.

Nursing Mothers: It is not known whether Levamisole HCl is excreted in human milk; it is excreted in cows' milk. Because of the potential for serious adverse reactions in nursing infants from Levamisole HCl, a decision should be made whether to discontinue nursing or to discontinue the drug, taking into account the importance of the drug to the mother.

Pediatric Use: Safety and effectiveness of Levamisole HCl in children have not been established.

ADVERSE REACTIONS
Almost all patients receiving Levamisole HCl and fluorouracil reported adverse experiences. Tabulated below is the incidence of adverse experiences that occurred in at least 1% of patients enrolled in two clinical trials who were adjuvantly treated with either Levamisole HCl or Levamisole HCl plus fluorouracil following colon surgery. In the larger clinical trial, 66 of 463 patients (14%) discontinued the combination of Levamisole HCl plus fluorouracil because of adverse reactions. Forty-three of these patients (9%) developed isolated or a combination of gastrointestinal toxicities, (e.g., nausea, vomiting, diarrhea, stomatitis and anorexia). Ten patients developed rash and/or pruritus. Five patients discontinued therapy because of flu-like symptoms or fever with chills; ten patients developed central nervous system symptoms such as dizziness, ataxia, depression, confusion, memory loss, weakness, inability to concentrate, and headache; two patients developed reversible neutropenia and sepsis; one patient because of thrombocytopenia; one patient because of hyperbilirubinemia. One patient in the Levamisole HCl plus fluorouracil group developed agranulocytosis and sepsis and died.

In the Levamisole HCl alone arm of the trial, 15 of 310 patients (4.8%) discontinued therapy because of adverse experiences. Six of these (2%) discontinued because of rash, six because of arthralgia/myalgia, and one each for fever and neutropenia, urinary infection, and cough.

Adverse experience	Levamisole HCl N = 440 %	Levamisole HCl plus fluorouracil N = 599 %
Gastrointestinal		
Nausea	22	65
Diarrhea	13	52
Stomatitis	3	39
Vomiting	6	20
Anorexia	2	6
Abdominal pain	2	5
Constipation	2	3
Flatulence	< 1	2
Dyspepsia	< 1	1
Hematological		
Leukopenia		
< 2000/mm³	< 1	1
≥ 2000 to < 4000/mm³	4	19
≥ 4000/mm³	2	33
unscored category	0	< 1
Thrombocytopenia		
< 50,000/mm³	0	0
≥ 50,000 to < 130,000/mm³	1	8
≥ 130,000/mm³	1	10
Anemia	0	6
Granulocytopenia	< 1	2
Epistaxis	0	1
Skin and Appendages		
Dermatitis	8	23
Alopecia	3	22
Pruritus	1	2
Skin		
discoloration	0	2
Urticaria	< 1	0
Body as a Whole		

Adverse experience	Levamisole HCl N = 440 %	Levamisole HCl plus fluorouracil N = 599 %
Fatigue	6	11
Fever	3	5
Rigors	3	5
Chest pain	< 1	1
Edema	1	1
Resistance Mechanisms		
Infection	5	12
Special Senses		
Taste perversion	8	8
Altered sense of smell	1	1
Musculoskeletal System		
Arthralgia	5	4
Myalgia	3	1
Central and Peripheral Nervous System		
Dizziness	3	4
Headache	3	4
Paresthesia	2	1
Ataxia	0	1
Psychiatric		
Somnolence	3	2
Depression	1	2
Nervousness	1	2
Insomnia	1	1
Anxiety	1	1
Forgetfulness	0	1
Vision		
Abnormal tearing	0	4
Blurred vision	1	2
Conjunctivitis	< 1	2
Liver and Biliary System		
Hyperbilirubinemia	< 1	1

In worldwide experience with Levamisole HCl, less frequent adverse experiences included exfoliative dermatitis, periorbital edema, vaginal bleeding, anaphylaxis, confusion, convulsions, hallucinations, impaired concentration, renal failure, elevated serum creatinine, and increased alkaline phosphatase.

Reports of hyperlipidema with marked elevation of triglyceride levels have been observed in patients receiving combination therapy of Levamisole HCl and fluorouracil.

Cases of an encephalopathy-like syndrome associated with demyelination have been reported in patients treated with Levamisole HCl. Worldwide postmarketing experience with the combination therapy of Levamisole HCl and fluorouracil has also included several reports of neurological changes associated with demyelination and several reports of peripheral neuropathy. The onset of symptoms and the clinical presentation in these cases are quite varied. Symptoms may include confusion, speech disturbances, muscle weakness, lethargy, and paresthesia. If an acute neurological syndrome occurs, immediate discontinuation of Levamisole HCl and fluorouracil therapy should be considered.

The following additional adverse experiences have been reported for fluorouracil alone: esophagopharyngitis, pancytopenia, myocardial ischemia, angina, gastrointestinal ulceration and bleeding, anaphylaxis and generalized allergic reactions, acute cerebellar syndrome, nystagmus, dry skin, fissuring, photosensitivity, lacrimal duct stenosis, photophobia, euphoria, thrombophlebitis, and nail changes.

OVERDOSAGE

Fatalities have been reported in a three-year-old child who ingested 15 mg/kg and in an adult who ingested 32 mg/kg. No further clinical information is available. In cases of overdosage, gastric lavage is recommended together with symptomatic and supportive measures.

DOSAGE AND ADMINISTRATION

The adjuvant use of Levamisole HCl and fluorouracil is limited to the following dosage schedule:

Initial Therapy:
Levamisole HCl: 50 mg p.o. q8h for   (starting 7-30 days post-surgery)
   3 days
fluorouracil: 450 mg/m²/day IV for 5   (starting 21-34 days post-surgery)
   days concomitant with a 3-day
   course of Levamisole HCl

Maintenance: Levamisole HCl: 50 mg p.o. q8h for 3 days every 2 weeks.
fluorouracil: 450 mg/m²/day IV once a week beginning 28 days after the initiation of the 5-day course.

Treatment: Levamisole HCl administered orally, should be initiated no earlier than 7 and no later than 30 days post surgery at a dose of 50 mg q8h x 3 days repeated every 14 days for 1 year. Fluorouracil therapy should be initiated no earlier than 21 and no later than 35 days after surgery providing the patient is out of the hospital, ambulatory, maintaining normal oral nutrition, has well-healed wounds, and is fully recovered from any postoperative complications.

If Levamisole HCl has been initiated from 7 to 20 days after surgery, initiation of fluorouracil therapy should be coincident with the second course of Levamisole HCl, i.e., at 21 to 34 days. If Levamisole HCl is initiated from 21 to 30 days after surgery, fluorouracil should be initiated simultaneously with the first course of Levamisole HCl.

Fluorouracil should be administered by rapid IV push at a dosage of 450 mg/m²/day for 5 consecutive days. Dosage calculation is based on actual weight (estimated dry weight if there is evidence of fluid retention). *This course should be discontinued before the full 5 doses are administered if the patient develops any stomatitis or diarrhea* (5 or more loose stools). Twenty-eight days after initiation of this course, weekly fluorouracil should be instituted at a dosage of 450 mg/m²/week and continued for a total treatment time of 1 year. If stomatitis or diarrhea develop during weekly therapy, the next dose of fluorouracil should be deferred until these side effects have subsided. If these side effects are moderate to severe, the fluorouracil dose should be reduced 20% when it is resumed.

Dosage modifications should be instituted as follows: If WBC is 2500-3500/mm³ defer the fluorouracil dose until WBC is > 3500/mm³. If WBC is < 2500/mm³, defer the fluorouracil dose until WBC is > 3500/mm³; then resume the fluorouracil dose reduced by 20%. If WBC remains < 2500/mm³ for over 10 days despite deferring fluorouracil, discontinue administration of Levamisole HCl. Both drugs should be deferred unless platelets are adequate (≥ 100,000/mm³).

Levamisole HCl should not be used at doses exceeding the recommended dose or frequency. Clinical studies suggest a relationship between Levamisole HCl adverse experiences and increasing dose, and since some of these, e.g., agranulocytosis, may be life-threatening, the recommended dosage regimen should not be exceeded (see *"Warnings"*).

Before beginning this combination adjuvant treatment, the physician should become familiar with the labeling for fluorouracil.

Storage: Store at room temperature, 15°-30°C (59°-86°F).
   Protect from moisture.

REFERENCES

1. Laurie JA, Moertel CG, Fleming TR, et al. Surgical adjuvant therapy of large-bowel carcinoma: An evaluation of levamisole and the combination of levamisole and fluorouracil. *J. Clin Oncol.* 1989; 7:1447-1456. 2. Moertel CG, Fleming TR, Macdonald JS, et al. Levamisole and fluorouracil for adjuvant therapy of resected colon carcinoma. *New Engl J Med.* 1990; 322:352-358. 3. Data on file, Janssen Pharmaceutica Inc.

HOW SUPPLIED

TABLETS:

BRAND/MANUFACTURER	NDC	SIZE	AWP
○ **BRAND**			
ERGAMISOL: Janssen	50458-0270-36	36s	$194.40

Levatol SEE PENBUTOLOL SULFATE

Levlen SEE ETHINYL ESTRADIOL WITH LEVONORGESTREL

Levo-Dromoran SEE LEVORPHANOL TARTRATE

Levobunolol Hydrochloride, Ophthalmic

DESCRIPTION

Levobunolol HCl sterile ophthalmic solution is a noncardioselective beta-adrenoceptor blocking agent for ophthalmic use.

Chemical Name: (-)-5-[3-(*tert*-Butylamino)-2-hydroxypropoxy]-3, 4-dihydro-1(2*H*)-naphthalenone hydrochloride.

Contains:

Levobunolol HCl	0.25%
Levobunolol HCl	0.5%

Following is its chemical structure:

CLINICAL PHARMACOLOGY

Levobunolol HCl is a noncardioselective beta-adrenoceptor blocking agent, equipotent at both beta₁ and beta₂ receptors. Levobunolol HCl is greater than 60 times more potent than its dextro isomer in its beta-blocking activity, yet equipotent in its potential for direct myocardial depression. Accordingly, the levo isomer, Levobunolol HCl, is used. Levobunolol HCl does not have significant local anesthetic (membrane-stabilizing) or intrinsic sympathomimetic activity.

Beta-adrenergic receptor blockade reduces cardiac output in both healthy subjects and patients with heart disease. In patients with severe impairment of myocardial function, beta-adrenergic receptor blockade may inhibit the stimulatory effect of the sympathetic nervous system necessary to maintain adequate cardiac function.

Beta-adrenergic receptor blockade in the bronchi and bronchioles results in increased airway resistance from unopposed para-sympathetic activity. Such an effect in patients with asthma or other bronchospastic conditions is potentially dangerous.

Levobunolol HCl has been shown to be an active agent in lowering elevated as well as normal intraocular pressure (IOP) whether or not accompanied by glaucoma. Elevated IOP presents a major risk factor in glaucomatous field loss. The higher the level of IOP, the greater the likelihood of optic nerve damage and visual field loss.

The onset of action with one drop of Levobunolol HCl can be detected within one hour after treatment, with maximum effect seen between 2 and 6 hours.

A significant decrease in IOP can be maintained for up to 24 hours following a single dose.

In two, separate, controlled studies (one three month and one up to 12 months duration) Levobunolol HCl 0.25% b.i.d. controlled the IOP of approximately 64% and 70% of the subjects.

The overall mean decrease from baseline was 5.4 mm Hg and 5.1 mm Hg respectively. In an open-label study, Levobunolol HCl 0.25% q.d. controlled the IOP of 72% of the subjects while achieving an overall mean decrease of 5.9 mm Hg.

In controlled clinical studies of approximately two years duration, intraocular pressure was well-controlled in approximately 80% of subjects treated with Levobunolol HCl 0.5% b.i.d. The mean IOP decrease from baseline was between 6.87 mm Hg and 7.81 mm Hg. No significant effects on pupil size, tear production or corneal sensitivity were observed. Levobunolol HCl at the concentrations tested, when applied topically, decreased heart rate and blood pressure in some patients. The IOP-lowering effect of Levobunolol HCl was well maintained over the course of these studies.

In a three month clinical study, a single daily application of Levobunolol HCl 0.5% controlled the IOP of 72% of subjects achieving an overall mean decrease in IOP of 7.0 mm Hg.

The primary mechanism of the ocular hypotensive action of Levobunolol HCl in reducing IOP is most likely a decrease in aqueous humor production. Levobunolol HCl reduces IOP with little or no effect on pupil size or accommodation in contrast to the miosis which cholinergic agents are known to produce. The blurred vision and night blindness often associated with miotics would not be expected and have not been reported with the use of Levobunolol HCl. This is particularly important in cataract patients with central lens opacities who would experience decreased visual acuity with pupillary constriction.

INDICATIONS AND USAGE
Levobunolol HCl has been shown to be effective in lowering intraocular pressure and may be used in patients with chronic open-angle glaucoma or ocular hypertension.

CONTRAINDICATIONS
Levobunolol HCl is contraindicated in those individuals with bronchial asthma or with a history of bronchial asthma, or severe chronic obstructive pulmonary disease (see "Warnings"); sinus bradycardia; second and third degree atrioventricular block; overt cardiac failure (see "Warnings"); cardiogenic shock; or hypersensitivity to any component of these products.

WARNINGS
As with other topically applied ophthalmic drugs, Levobunolol HCl may be absorbed systemically. The same adverse reactions found with systemic adminstration of beta-adrenergic blocking agents may occur with topical administration. For example, severe respiratory reactions and cardiac reactions, including death due to bronchospasm in patients with asthma, and rarely death in association with cardiac failure, have been reported with topical application of beta-adrenergic blocking agents (see "Contraindications").

Cardiac Failure: Sympathetic stimulation may be essential for support of the circulation in individuals with diminished myocardial contractility, and its inhibition by beta-adrenergic receptor blockade may precipitate more severe failure.

In Patients Without a History of Cardiac Failure: Continued depression of the myocardium with beta-blocking agents over a period of time can, in some cases, lead to cardiac failure. At the first sign or symptom of cardiac failure, Levobunolol HCl should be discontinued.

Obstructive Pulmonary Disease: PATIENTS WITH CHRONIC OBSTRUCTIVE PULMONARY DISEASE (e.g., CHRONIC BRONCHITIS, EMPHYSEMA) OF MILD OR MODERATE SEVERITY, BRONCHOSPASTIC DISEASE OR A HISTORY OF BRONCHOSPASTIC DISEASE (OTHER THAN BRONCHIAL ASTHMA OR A HISTORY OF BRONCHIAL ASTHMA, IN WHICH LEVOBUNOLOL HCL IS CONTRAINDICATED, SEE "CONTRAINDICATIONS"), SHOULD IN GENERAL NOT RECEIVE BETA BLOCKERS, INCLUDING LEVOBUNOLOL HCL. However, if Levobunolol HCL is deemed necessary in such patients, then it should be administered cautiously since it may block

bronchodilation produced by endogenous and exogenous catecholamine stimulation of beta2 receptors.

Major Surgery: The necessity or desirability of withdrawal of beta-adrenergic blocking agents prior to major surgery is controversial.

Beta-adrenergic receptor blockade impairs the ability of the heart to respond to beta-adrenergically mediated reflex stimuli. This may augment the risk of general anesthesia in surgical procedures. Some patients receiving beta-adrenergic receptor blocking agents have been subject to protracted severe hypotension during anesthesia. Difficulty in restarting and maintaining the heartbeat has also been reported. For these reasons, in patients undergoing elective surgery, gradual withdrawal of beta-adrenergic receptor blocking agents may be appropriate.

If necessary during surgery, the effects of beta-adrenergic blocking agents may be reversed by sufficient doses of such agonists as isoproterenol, dopamine, dobutamine or levarterenol (see "Overdosage").

Diabetes Mellitus: Beta-adrenergic blocking agents should be administered with caution in patients subject to spontaneous hypoglycemia or to diabetic patients (especially those with labile diabetes) who are receiving insulin or oral hypoglycemic agents. Beta-adrenergic receptor blocking agents may mask the signs and symptoms of acute hypoglycemia.

Thyrotoxicosis: Beta-adrenergic blocking agents may mask certain clinical signs (e.g., tachycardia) of hyperthyroidism. Patients suspected of developing thyrotoxicosis should be managed carefully to avoid abrupt withdrawal of beta-adrenergic blocking agents, which might precipitate a thyroid storm.

These products contain sodium metabisulfite, a sulfite that may cause allergic-type reactions including anaphylactic symptoms and life-threatening or less severe asthmatic episodes in certain susceptible people. The overall prevalence of sulfite sensitivity in the general population is unknown and probably low. Sulfite sensitivity is seen more frequently in asthmatic than in nonasthmatic people.

PRECAUTIONS
General: Levobunolol HCl should be used with caution in patients with known hypersensitivity to other beta-adrenoceptor blocking agents. Use with caution in patients with known diminished pulmonary function.

Levobunolol HCl should be used with caution in patients who are receiving a beta-adrenergic blocking agent orally, because of the potential for additive effects on systemic beta-blockade or on intraocular pressure. Patients should not typically use two or more topical ophthalmic beta-adrenergic blocking agents simultaneously.

Because of the potential effects of beta-adrenergic blocking agents on blood pressure and pulse rates, these medications must be used cautiously in patients with cerebrovascular insufficiency. Should signs or symptoms develop that suggest reduced cerebral blood flow while using Levobunolol HCl, alternative therapy should be considered.

In patients with angle-closure glaucoma, the immediate objective of treatment is to reopen the angle. This requires, in most cases, constricting the pupil with a miotic. Levobunolol HCl has little or no effect on the pupil. When Levobunolol HCl is used to reduce elevated intraocular pressure in angle-closure glaucoma, it should be followed with a miotic and not alone.

Muscle Weakness: Beta-adrenergic blockade has been reported to potentiate muscle weakness consistent with certain myasthenic symptoms (e.g., diplopia, ptosis and generalized weakness).

DRUG INTERACTIONS
Although Levobunolol HCl used alone has little or no effect on pupil size, mydriasis resulting from concomitant therapy with Levobunolol HCl and epinephrine may occur.

Close observation of the patient is recommended when a beta-blocker is administered to patients receiving catecholamine-depleting drugs such as reserpine, because of possible additive effects and the production of hypotension and/or marked bradycardia, which may produce vertigo, syncope, or postural hypotension.

Patients receiving beta-adrenergic blocking agents along with either oral or intravenous calcium antagonists should be monitored for possible atrioventricular conduction disturbances, left ventricular failure and hypotension. In patients with impaired cardiac function, simultaneous use should be avoided altogether.

The concomitant use of beta-adrenergic blocking agents with digitalis and calcium antagonists may have additive effects on prolonging atrioventricular conduction time.

Phenothiazine-related compounds and beta-adrenergic blocking agents may have additive hypotensive effects due to the inhibition of each other's metabolism.

Risk of Anaphylactic Reaction: While taking beta-blockers, patients with a history of severe anaphylactic reaction to a variety of allergens may be more reactive to repeated challenge, either accidental, diagnostic, or therapeutic. Such patients may be unresponsive to the usual doses of epinephrine used to treat allergic reaction.

Animal Studies: No adverse ocular effects were observed in rabbits administered Levobunolol HCl topically in studies lasting one year in concentrations up to 10 times the human dose concentration.

Carcinogenesis, Mutagenesis, Impairment of Fertility: In a lifetime oral study in mice, there were statistically significant (p ≤ 0.05) increases in the incidence of benign leiomyomas in female mice at 200 mg/kg/day (14,000 times the recommended human dose for glaucoma), but not at 12 or 50 mg/kg/day (850 and 3,500 times the human dose). In a two-year oral study of Levobunolol HCl in rats, there was a statistically significant ($p \leq 0.05$) increase in the incidence of benign hepatomas in male rats administered 12,800 times the recommended human dose for glaucoma. Similar differences were not observed in rats administered oral doses equivalent to 350 times to 2,000 times the recommended human dose for glaucoma.

Levobunolol did not show evidence of mutagenic activity in a battery of microbiological and mammalian *in vitro* and *in vivo* assays. Reproduction and fertility studies in rats showed no adverse effect on male or female fertility at doses up to 1,800 times the recommended human dose for glaucoma.

Pregnancy Category C: Fetotoxicity (as evidenced by a greater number of resorption sites) has been observed in rabbits when doses of Levobunolol HCl equivalent to 200 and 700 times the recommended dose for the treatment of glaucoma were given. No fetotoxic effects have been observed in similar studies with rats at up to 1,800 times the human dose for glaucoma. Teratogenic studies with Levobunolol in rats at doses up to 25 mg/kg/day (1,800 times the recommended human dose for glaucoma) showed no evidence of fetal malformations. There were no adverse effects on postnatal development of offspring. It appears when results from studies using rats and studies with other beta-adrenergic blockers are examined, that the rabbit may be a particularly sensitive species. There are no adequate and well-controlled studies in pregnant women. Levobunolol HCl should be used during pregnancy only if the potential benefit justifies the potential risk to the fetus.

Nursing Mothers: It is not known whether this drug is excreted in human milk. Systemic beta-blockers and topical timolol maleate are known to be excreted in human milk. Caution should be exercised when Levobunolol HCl is administered to a nursing woman.

Pediatric Use: Safety and effectiveness in children have not been established.

ADVERSE REACTIONS

In clinical trials, the use of Levobunolol HCl has been associated with transient ocular burning and stinging in up to 1 in 3 patients, and with blepharoconjunctivitis in up to 1 in 20 patients. Decreases in heart rate and blood pressure have been reported (see *"Contraindications"* and *"Warnings"*).

The following adverse effects have been reported rarely with the use of Levobunolol HCl iridocyclitis, headache, transient ataxia, dizziness, lethargy, urticaria and pruritus.

Decreased corneal sensitivity has been noted in a small number of patients. Although Levobunolol has minimal membrane-stabilizing activity, there remains a possibility of decreased corneal sensitivity after prolonged use. The following additional adverse reactions have been reported either with Levobunolol HCl or ophthalmic use of other beta-adrenergic receptor blocking agents:

Body as a whole: Headache, asthenia, chest pain.

Cardiovascular: Bradycardia, arrhythmia, hypotension, syncope, heart block, cerebral vascular accident, cerebral ischemia, congestive heart failure, palpitation, cardiac arrest.

Digestive: Nausea, diarrhea.

Psychiatric: Depression, increase in signs and symptoms of myasthenia gravis, paresthesia.

Skin: Hypersensitivity, including localized and generalized rash.

Respiratory: Bronchospasm (predominantly in patients with pre-existing bronchospastic disease), respiratory failure, dyspnea, nasal congestion.

Endocrine: Masked symptoms of hypoglycemia in insulin-dependent diabetics (see *"Warnings"*).

Special Senses: Signs and symptoms of keratitis, blepharoptosis, visual disturbances including refractive changes (due to withdrawal of miotic therapy in some cases), diplopia, ptosis.

Other reactions associated with the oral use of non-selective adrenergic receptor blocking agents should be considered potential effects with ophthalmic use of these agents.

OVERDOSAGE

No data are available regarding overdosage in humans. Should accidental ocular overdosage occur, flush eye(s) with water or normal saline. If accidentally ingested, efforts to decrease further absorption may be appropriate (gastric lavage).

The most common signs and symptoms to be expected with overdosage with administration of a systemic beta-adrenergic blocking agent are symptomatic bradycardia, hypotension, bronchospasm, and acute cardiac failure. Should these symptoms occur, discontinue Levobunolol HCl therapy and initiate appropriate supportive therapy. The following supportive measures should be considered:

1. Symptomatic bradycardia: Use atropine sulfate intravenously in a dosage of 0.25 mg to 2 mg to induce vagal blockade. If bradycardia persists, intravenous isoproterenol hydrochloride should be administered cautiously. In refractory cases, the use of a transvenous cardiac pacemaker should be considered.
2. Hypotension: Use sympathomimetic pressor drug therapy, such as dopamine, dobutamine or levarterenol. In refractory cases, the use of glucagon hydrochloride may be useful.
3. Bronchospasm: Use isoproterenol hydrochloride. Additional therapy with aminophylline may be considered.
4. Acute cardiac failure: Conventional therapy with digitalis, diuretics and oxygen should be instituted immediately. In refractory cases, the use of intravenous aminophylline is suggested. This may be followed, if necessary, by glucagon hydrochloride, which may be useful.
5. Heart block (second or third degree): Use isoproterenol hydrochloride or a transvenous cardiac pacemaker.

DOSAGE AND ADMINISTRATION

The recommended starting dose is one to two drops of Levobunolol HCl 0.5% in the affected eye(s) once a day. Typical dosing with Levobunolol HCl 0.25% is one to two drops twice daily. In patients with more severe or uncontrolled glaucoma, Levobunolol HCl 0.5% can be administered b.i.d. As with any new medication, careful monitoring of patients is advised.

Dosages above one drop of Levobunolol HCl 0.5% b.i.d. are not generally more effective. If the patient's IOP is not at a satisfactory level on this regimen, concomitant therapy with dipivefrin and/or epinephrine, and/or pilocarpine and other miotics, and/or systemically administered carbonic anhydrase inhibitors, such as acetazolamide, can be instituted. Patients should not typically use two or more topical ophthalmic beta-adrenergic blocking agents simultaneously.

Protect from light. Store at controlled room temperature 15°-30°C (59°-86°F).

HOW SUPPLIED
DROP: 0.25%

AVERAGE UNIT PRICE (AVAILABLE SIZES)		GENERIC A-RATED AVERAGE PRICE (GAAP)	
GENERIC	$2.39	5 ml	$12.00
		10 ml	$23.85

BRAND/MANUFACTURER	NDC	SIZE	AWP
◆ GENERICS			
Bausch&Lomb Pharm	24208-0545-05	5 ml	$11.00
AKBETA: Akorn	17478-0286-10	5 ml	$11.94
Rugby	00536-2512-65	5 ml	$12.52
Goldline	00182-7003-62	5 ml	$12.52
Bausch&Lomb Pharm	24208-0545-10	10 ml	$22.00
AKBETA: Akorn	17478-0286-11	10 ml	$23.75
Rugby	00536-2512-70	10 ml	$24.83
Goldline	00182-7003-63	10 ml	$24.83

DROP: 0.25%

BRAND/MANUFACTURER	NDC	SIZE	AWP
○ BRAND			
BETAGAN: Allergan Pharm	11980-0469-25	5 ml	$13.91
	11980-0469-20	10 ml	$27.59

DROP: 0.5%

AVERAGE UNIT PRICE (AVAILABLE SIZES)		GENERIC A-RATED AVERAGE PRICE (GAAP)	
GENERIC	$2.91	5 ml	$14.86
		10 ml	$29.04
		15 ml	$42.66

BRAND/MANUFACTURER	NDC	SIZE	AWP
◆ GENERICS			
Schein	00364-3039-53	5 ml	$13.75
Bausch&Lomb Pharm	24208-0505-05	5 ml	$13.75
Major	00904-7887-05	5 ml	$14.95
Rugby	00536-2509-65	5 ml	$14.98
Goldline	00182-7002-62	5 ml	$14.98
AKBETA: Akorn	17478-0287-10	5 ml	$15.00
Qualitest	00603-7168-37	5 ml	$15.35
Aligen	00405-6065-05	5 ml	$16.11
Schein	00364-3039-54	10 ml	$27.50
Bausch&Lomb Pharm	24208-0505-10	10 ml	$27.50
AKBETA: Akorn	17478-0287-11	10 ml	$28.13
Major	00904-7887-10	10 ml	$29.25
Rugby	00536-2509-70	10 ml	$29.28
Goldline	00182-7002-63	10 ml	$29.28
Qualitest	00603-7168-39	10 ml	$29.90
Aligen	00405-6065-10	10 ml	$31.51
AKBETA: Akorn	17478-0287-12	15 ml	$41.25
Schein	00364-3039-72	15 ml	$41.25
Bausch&Lomb Pharm	24208-0505-15	15 ml	$41.25
Major	00904-7887-15	15 ml	$42.65
Rugby	00536-2509-72	15 ml	$42.67
Goldline	00182-7002-64	15 ml	$42.67
Qualitest	00603-7168-41	15 ml	$43.60
Aligen	00405-6065-15	15 ml	$45.92

DROP: 0.5%

BRAND/MANUFACTURER	NDC	SIZE	AWP
○ BRAND			
BETAGAN: Allergan Pharm	11980-0252-02	2 ml	$9.04
	11980-0252-25	5 ml	$16.64
	11980-0252-65	5 ml	$16.64
	11980-0252-20	10 ml	$32.53
	11980-0252-60	10 ml	$32.53
	11980-0252-21	15 ml	$47.41
	11980-0252-61	15 ml	$47.41

◆ RATED THERAPEUTICALLY EQUIVALENT; ◇ THERAPEUTIC EQUIVALENCE UNCONFIRMED; ○ UNRATED

Levocabastine Hydrochloride

DESCRIPTION

Levocabastine Hydrochloride ophthalmic suspension is a selective histamine H_1-receptor antagonist for topical ophthalmic use. Each mL contains 0.54 mg Levocabastine Hydrochloride equivalent to 0.5 mg Levocabastine.

The chemical name for Levocabastine Hydrochloride is (—)-trans-1-[cis-4-Cyano-4-(p-fluorophenyl)cyclohexyl]-3-methyl-4-phenylisonipecotic acid monohydrochloride.

Following is its chemical structure:

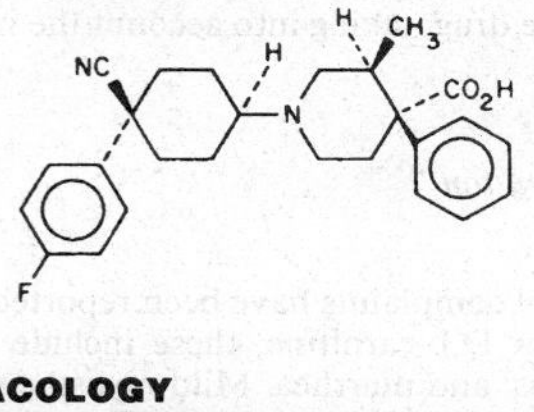

CLINICAL PHARMACOLOGY

Levocabastine is a potent, selective histamine H_1-antagonist.

Antigen challenge studies performed two and four hours after initial drug instillation indicated activity was maintained for at least two hours.

In an environmental study, Levocabastine HCl instilled four times daily was shown to be significantly more effective than its vehicle in reducing ocular itching associated with seasonal allergic conjunctivitis.

After instillation in the eye, Levocabastine is systemically absorbed. However, the amount of systemically absorbed Levocabastine after therapeutic ocular doses is low (mean plasma concentrations in the range of 1—2 ng/mL).

INDICATIONS AND USAGE

Levocabastine HCl ophthalmic suspension is indicated for the temporary relief of the signs and symptoms of seasonal allergic conjunctivitis.

CONTRAINDICATIONS

This product is contraindicated in persons with known or suspected hypersensitivity to any of its components. It should not be used while soft contact lenses are being worn.

WARNINGS

For topical use only. Not for injection.

PRECAUTIONS

Information for Patients: SHAKE WELL BEFORE USING: To prevent contaminating the dropper tip and suspension, care should be taken not to touch the eyelids or surrounding areas with the dropper tip of the bottle. Keep bottle tightly closed when not in use. Do not use if the suspension has discolored. Store at controlled room temperature. Protect from freezing.

Carcinogenesis, Mutagenesis, Impairment of Fertility: Levocabastine was not carcinogenic in male or female rats or in male mice when administered in the diet for up to 24 months. In female mice, Levocabastine doses of 5,000 and 21,500 times the maximum recommended ocular human use level resulted in an increased incidence of pituitary gland adenoma and mammary gland adenocarcinoma possibly produced by increased prolactin levels. The clinical relevance of this finding is unknown with regard to the interspecies differences in prolactin physiology and the very low plasma concentrations of Levocabastine following ocular administration.

Mutagenic potential was not demonstrated for Levocabastine when tested in Ames' Salmonella Reversion test or in *Escherichia coli, Drosophila melanogaster,* a mouse Dominant Lethal Assay or in rat Micronucleus test.

In reproduction studies in rats, Levocabastine showed no effects on fertility at oral doses of 20 mg/kg/day (8,300 times the maximum recommended human ocular dose).

PREGNANCY

Teratogenic Effects: Pregnancy Category C: Levocabastine has been shown to be teratogenic (polydactyly) in rats when given in doses 16,500 times the maximum recommended human ocular dose. Teratogenicity (polydactyly, hydrocephaly, brachygnathia), embryotoxicity, and maternal toxicity were observed in rats at 66,000 times the maximum recommended ocular human dose. There are no adequate and well-controlled studies in pregnant women. Levocabastine should be used during pregnancy only if the potential benefit justifies the potential risk to the fetus.

Nursing Mothers: Based on determinations of Levocabastine in breast milk after ophthalmic administration of the drug to one nursing woman, it was calculated that the daily dose of Levocabastine in the infant was about 0.5 µg.

Pediatric Use: Safety and effectiveness in children below the age of 12 have not been established.

ADVERSE REACTIONS

The most frequent complaint with the use of Levocabastine HCl ophthalmic suspension is that of mild, transient stinging and burning (15%) and headache (5%).

Other adverse experiences which have been reported in approximately 1—3% of patients treated with Levocabastine HCl ophthalmic suspension include visual disturbances, dry mouth, fatigue, pharyngitis, eye pain/dryness, somnolence, red eyes, lacrimation/discharge, cough, nausea, rash/erythema, eyelid edema, and dyspnea.

DOSAGE AND ADMINISTRATION

Shake Well Before Using: The usual dose is one drop instilled in affected eyes four times per day. Treatment may be continued for up to 2 weeks.

Keep tightly closed when not in use.

Do not use if the suspension has discolored.

Stored at controlled room temperature 15° to 30°C (59° to 86°F).

Protect from freezing.

HOW SUPPLIED

DROP: 0.05%

BRAND/MANUFACTURER	NDC	SIZE	AWP
○ BRAND LIVOSTIN: Iolab	00058-2610-05	5 ml	$19.44

Levocarnitine

DESCRIPTION

Chemically, Levocarnitine is (R)-3-carboxy-2-hydroxy-N,N,N-trimethyl-1-propanaminium hydroxide, inner salt. Its impirical formula is $C_7H_{15}NO_3$ and its molecular weight 161.20.

Levocarnitine is a carrier molecule in the transport of long chain fatty acids across the inner mitochondrial membrane. It is available as tablets and solution for oral administration and as a Sterile aqueous solution for injection.

Each tablet contains:	
Levocarnitine	330 mg

Each 10 ml of oral solution contains:	
Levocarnitine	1 gm

Each 5 ml of solution for injection contains:	
Levocarnitine	1 gm

As a bulk drug substance it is a white powder with a melting point of 196-197° C and is readily soluble in water, hot alcohol, and insoluble in acetone. The pH of a solution (1 in 20) is between 6-8; pH of the oral solution is approximately 5, of the solution for injection 6.0-6.5. Its pKa value is 3.8.

Following is its chemical structure:

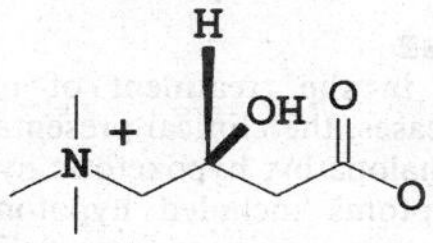

CLINICAL PHARMACOLOGY

Levocarnitine is a naturally occurring substance required in mammalian energy metabolism. It has been shown to facilitate long-chain fatty acid entry into cellular mitochondria, therefore delivering substrate for oxidation and subsequent energy production. Fatty acids are utilized as an energy substrate in all tissues except the brain. In skeletal and cardiac muscle they serve as major fuel. Primary systemic carnitine deficiency is characterized by low plasma, RBC, and/or tissue levels. It has not been possible to determine which symptoms are due to carnitine deficiency and which are due to the underlying organic acidemia, as symptoms of both abnormalities may be expected to improve with carnitine. The literature reports that carnitine can promote the excretion of excess organic or fatty acids in patients with defects in fatty acid metabolism and/or specific organic acidopathies that bioaccumulate acyl CoA esters.[1-6] Secondary Levocarnitine deficiency can be a consequence of inborn errors of metabolism. Levocarnitine may alleviate the metabolic abnormalities of patients with inborn errors that result in accumulation of toxic organic acids. Conditions for which this effect was demonstrated are: glutaric aciduria II, methyl malonic aciduria, propionic acidemia, and medium chain fatty acyl CoA dehydrogenase deficiency.[7,8] Autointoxication occurs in these patients due to the accumulations of acyl CoA components that disrupt intermediary metabolism. The subsequent hydrolysis of the acyl CoA compound to its free acid results in acidosis that can be life threatening. Levocarnitine clears the acyl CoA compound by formation of acyl carnitine which is quickly excreted. Levocarnitine deficiency is defined biochemically as abnormally low plasma levels of free carnitine, less than 20 µM/L at age greater than one week post term and may be associated with low-tissue and/or urine levels. Further, this condition may be associated with a ratio of plasma ester/free Levocarnitine levels greater than 0.4 or abnormally elevated levels of esterified Levocarnitine in the urine. In premature infants and newborns, secondary deficiency is defined as plasma free Levocarnitine levels below age related normal levels.

BIOAVAILABILITY/PHARMACOKINETICS

In a relative bioavailability study in 15 healthy adult male volunteers Levocarnitine tablets were found to be bio-equivalent to Levocarnitine oral solution. Following the administration of 1980 mg b.i.d., the maximum plasma concentration level (C_{max}) was 80 nmol/mL and the time to maximum concentration

➤ SHOWN IN PRODUCT IDENTIFICATION GUIDE

(T_{max}) occurred at 3.3 hours. There were no significant differences for AUC and urinary excretion observed between these two formulations.

In the same bioavailability study of 15 healthy adult males, (Levocarnitine injection administered as a slow 3-minute bolus intravenous injection at a dose of 20 mg/kg showed that free Levocarnitine plasma profiles are best fit by a two-compartment model. Approximately 76% of free Levocarnitine is eliminated in the urine. Using plasma levels uncorrected for endogenous Levocarnitine, the mean distribution half life was 0.585 hours and the mean apparent terminal elimination half life was 17.4 hours following a single intravenous dose.

The absolute bioavailability of L-carnitine from Levocarnitine tablets and oral solution was determined compared to the bioavailability of L-carnitine from Levocarnitine intravenous injection in 15 healthy male volunteers. After correction for circulating endogenous levels of L-carnitine in the plasma, absolute bioavailability was 15.1% ≤ 5.3% for L-carnitine from Levocarnitine tablets and 15.9% ≤ 4.9% from the oral solution.

Total body clearance of L-carnitine (Dose/AUC including endogenous baseline levels) was a mean of 4.00 L/hr. Endogenous baseline levels were not substracted since total body clearance of L-carnitine does not distinguish between exogenous sources of L-carnitine and endogenously synthesized L-carnitine. Volume of distribution of the intravenously administered dose above baseline endogenous levels was calculated to be a mean of 29.0 L ≤ 7.1 L (approximately 0.39 L/kg) which is an underestimate of the true volume of distribution since plasma L-carnitine is known to equilibrate slowly with, for instance, muscle L-carnitine.

L-carnitine was not bound to plasma protein or albumin when tested at any concentration or with any species including the human.[9]

METABOLISM AND EXCRETION

Five normal adult male volunteers, administered a dose of [3H-methyl]-L-carnitine following 15 days of a high carnitine diet and additional carnitine supplement, excreted 58-65% of administered radioactive dose in 5 to 11 days in the urine and feces. Maximum concentration of [³H-methyl]-L-carnitine in serum occurred from 2.0 to 4.5 hr after drug administration. Major metabolites found were trimethylamine N-oxide, primarily in urine (8% to 49% of the administered dose) and [³H]-γ-butyrobetaine, primarily in feces (0.44% to 45% of the administered dose). Urinary excretion of carnitine was 4% to 8% of the dose. Fecal excretion of total carnitine was less than 1% of total carnitine excretion.[10]

After attainment of steady state following 4 days of oral administration of Levocarnitine tablets (1980 mg q12h) or oral solution (2000 mg q12h) to 15 healthy male volunteers, urinary excretion of L-carnitine was a mean of 2107 and 2339 µmoles, respectively, equivalent to 8.6% and 9.4%, respectively, of the orally administered doses (uncorrected for endogenous urinary excretion). After a single intravenous dose (20 mg/kg) prior to multiple oral doses, urinary excretion of L-carnitine was 6974 µmoles equivalent to 75.6% of the intravenously administered dose (uncorrected for endogenous urinary excretion).

INDICATIONS AND USAGE

Levocarnitine is indicated in the treatment of primary systemic carnitine deficiency. In the reported cases, the clinical presentation consisted of recurrent episodes of Reye-like encephalopathy, hypoketotic hypoglycemia, and/or cardiomyopathy. Associated symptoms included hypotonia, muscle weakness and failure to thrive. A diagnosis of primary carnitine deficiency requires that serum, red cell and/or tissue carnitine levels be low and that the patient does not have a primary defect in fatty acid or organic acid oxidation (see "Clinical Pharmacology"). In some patients, particularly those presenting with cardiomyopathy, carnitine supplementation rapidly alleviated signs and symptoms. Treatment should include, in addition to carnitine, supportive and other therapy as indicated by the condition of the patient.

Levocarnitine is also indicated for acute and chronic treatment of patients with an inborn error of metabolism that results in a secondary carnitine deficiency.

UNLABELED USES

Levocarnitine is used alone or as an adjunct in the treatment of Alzheimer's dementia, cardiac hypoxia (angina), and congestive heart failure. It is also used to decrease the incidence of severe forms of myocarditis due to diphtheria and to correct the lipoprotein pattern in uremic patients on hemodialysis. It is prescribed for chronic anemia in patients on long-term maintenance hemodialysis and is used in type IV hyperlipoproteinemia and acute myocardial infarction. It is also prescribed for prophylactic treatment of valproic acid toxicity.

CONTRAINDICATIONS

None known.

WARNINGS

None.

PRECAUTIONS

GENERAL

Levocarnitine oral solution and tablets are for oral/internal use only.

Gastrointestinal reactions may result from too rapid consumption of carnitine. Levocarnitine oral solution may be consumed alone, or dissolved in drinks or other liquid foods to reduce taste fatigue. It should be consumed slowly and doses should be spaced evenly throughout the day to maximize tolerance.

CARCINOGENESIS, MUTAGENESIS, IMPAIRMENT OF FERTILITY

Mutagenicity tests have been performed in *Salmonella typhimurium*, *Saccharomyces cerevisiae*, and *Schizosaccharomyces pombe* that do not indicate that Levocarnitine is mutagenic. Long-term animal studies have not been conducted to evaluate the carcinogenicity of the compound.

PREGNANCY

Pregnancy Category B: Reproductive studies have been performed in rats and rabbits at doses up to 3.8 times the human dose on the basis of surface area and have revealed no evidence of impaired fertility or harm to the fetus due to Levocarnitine. There are, however, no adequate and well controlled studies in pregnant women. Because animal reproduction studies are not always predictive of human response, this drug should be used during pregnancy only if clearly needed.

NURSING MOTHERS

It is not known whether this drug is excreted in human milk. Because many drugs are excreted in human milk, a decision should be made whether to discontinue nursing or to discontinue the drug, taking into account the importance of the drug to the mother.

PEDIATRIC USE

See "Dosage and Administration".

ADVERSE REACTIONS

Various mild gastrointestinal complaints have been reported during the long-term administration of oral L- or D,L-carnitine; these include transient nausea and vomiting, abdominal cramps, and diarrhea. Mild myasthenia has been described only in uremic patients receiving D,L-carnitine. Gastrointestinal adverse reactions with Levocarnitine oral solution dissolved in liquids might be avoided by a slow consumption of the solution or by a greater dilution. Decreasing the dosage often diminishes or eliminates drug-related patient body odor or gastrointestinal symptoms when present. Tolerance should be monitored very closely during the first week of administration, and after any dosage increases.

Transient nausea and vomiting have been observed with intravenous administration. Less frequent adverse reactions are body odor, nausea, and gastritis. An incidence for these reactions is difficult to estimate due to the confounding effects of the underlying pathology.

OVERDOSAGE

There have been no reports of toxicity from Levocarnitine overdosage. The oral LD_{50} of Levocarnitine in mice is 19.2 gm/kg. Large doses of Levocarnitine may cause diarrhea. Overdosage should be treated with supportive care.

DOSAGE AND ADMINISTRATION

LEVOCARNITINE TABLETS

Adults: The recommended oral dosage for adults is 990 mg two or three times a day using the 330 mg tablets, depending on clinical response.

Infants and Children: The recommended oral dosage for infants and children is between 50 and 100 mg/kg/day in divided doses, with a maximum of 3 gm/day. Dosage should begin at 50 mg/kg/day. The exact dosage will depend on clinical response.

Monitoring should include periodic blood chemistries, vital signs, plasma carnitine concentrations and overall clinical condition.

LEVOCARNITINE ORAL SOLUTION

For oral use only. *Not for parenteral use.*

Adults: The recommended dosage of Levocarnitine is 1 to 3 gm/day for a 50 kg subject, which is equivalent to 10 to 30 ml/day of Levocarnitine oral solution. Higher doses should be administered only with caution and only where clinical and biochemical considerations make it seem likely that higher doses will be of benefit. Dosage should start at 1 gm/day, (10 ml/day), and be increased slowly while assessing tolerance and therapeutic response. Monitoring should include periodic blood chemistries, vital signs, plasma carnitine concentrations, and overall clinical condition.

Infants and Children: The recommended dosage of Levocarnitine is 50 to 100 mg/kg/day which is equivalent to 0.5 ml/kg/day Levocarnitine oral solution. Higher doses should be administered only with caution and only where clinical and biochemical considerations make it seem likely that higher doses will be of benefit. Dosage should start at 50 mg/kg/day, and be increased slowly to a maximum of 3 gm/day (30 ml/day) while assessing tolerance and therapeutic responses. Monitoring should include periodic blood chemistries, vital signs, plasma carnitine concentrations, and overall clinical condition.

Levocarnitine oral solution may be consumed alone or dissolved in drink or other liquid food. Doses should be spaced evenly throughout the day (every three or four hours) preferably during or following meals and should be consumed slowly in order to maximize tolerance.

LEVOCARNITINE INJECTION

Levocarnitine injection is administered intravenously. The recommended dose is 50 mg/kg given as a slow 2-3 minute bolus injection or by infusion. Often a loading dose is given in patients with severe metabolic crisis followed by an equivalent dose over the following 24 hours. It should be administered q3h or q4h, and never less than q6h either by infusion or by intravenous injection. All subsequent daily doses are recommended to be in the range of 50 mg/kg or as therapy may require. The highest dose administered has been 300 mg/kg.

It is recommended that a plasma carnitine level be obtained prior to beginning this parenteral therapy. Weekly and monthly monitoring is recommended as well. This monitoring should include blood chemistries, vital signs, plasma carnitine concentrations (the plasma free carnitine level should be between 35 and 60 micromoles/liter) and overall clinical condition.

◆ RATED THERAPEUTICALLY EQUIVALENT; ◇ THERAPEUTIC EQUIVALENCE UNCONFIRMED; ○ UNRATED

Parenteral drug products should be inspected visually for particulate matter and discoloration prior to administration, whenever solution and container permit.

STORAGE
Store solution for injection in carton until their use to protect from light. Discard unused portion of an opened ampoule.

REFERENCES
1. Bohmer T, Ryndling A, Solberg HE: Carnitine levels in human serum in health and disease. *Clin Chim Acta* 57:55-61, 1974. 2. Brooks H, Goldberg L, Holland R et al: Carnitine-induced effects on cardiac and peripheral hemodynamics. *J Clin Pharmacol* 17:561-578, 1977. 3. Christiansen R, Bremer J: Active transport of butyrobetaine and carnitine into isolated liver cells. *Biochem Biophys Acta* 448:562-577, 1977. 4. Lindstedt S, Lindstedt G: Distribution and excretion of carnitine $^{14}CO_2$ in the rat. *Acta Chim Scand* 15: 701-702, 1961. 5. Rebouche CJ, Engel AG: Carnitine metabolism and deficiency syndromes. *Mayo Clin Proc* 58: 533-540, 1983. 6. Rebouche CJ, Paulson DJ: Carnitine metabolism and function in humans. *Ann Rev Nutr* 6: 41-68, 1986. 7. Scriver CR, Beaudet AL, Sly WS, Valle D: *The Metabolic Basis of Inherited Disease*, McGraw-Hill, New York, 1989. 8. Schaub J, Van Hoof F, Vis HL: *Inborn Errors of Metabolism*,Raven Press, New York, 1991. 9. Marzo A, Arrigoni Martelli E, Mancinelli A, Cardace G, Corbelletta C, Bassani E, Solbiati M: Protein binding of L-carnitine family components. *Eur J Drug Met Pharmacokin*, Special Issue III: 364-368, 1992. 10. Rebouche C: Quantitative estimation of absorption and degradation of a carnitine supplement by human adults. *Metabolism*: 1305-1310, 1991.

HOW SUPPLIED
INJECTION: 1 GM/5 ML

BRAND/MANUFACTURER	NDC	SIZE	AWP
◆ BRAND CARNITOR: Sigma-Tau	54482-0146-09	5 ml 5s	$180.00

SOLUTION:

BRAND/MANUFACTURER	NDC	SIZE	AWP
◆ BRAND CARNITOR: Sigma-Tau	54482-0145-08	118 ml 24s	$677.40

TABLETS: 330 MG

BRAND/MANUFACTURER	NDC	SIZE	AWP
○ BRAND CARNITOR: Sigma-Tau	54482-0144-07	90s ud	$71.07

Levodopa

IN ORDER TO REDUCE THE HIGH INCIDENCE OF ADVERSE REACTIONS, IT IS NECESSARY TO INDIVIDUALIZE THE THERAPY AND TO GRADUALLY INCREASE THE DOSAGE TO THE DESIRED THERAPEUTIC LEVEL.

DESCRIPTION
Levodopa is available as tablets or capsules containing 0.1 gm, 0.25 gm or 0.5 gm of drug.
Chemically, Levodopa is (−)-3-(3,4-dihydroxyphenyl)-L-alanine. It is a colorless, crystalline compound, slightly soluble in water and insoluble in alcohol, with a molecular weight of 197.2.

Following is its chemical structure:

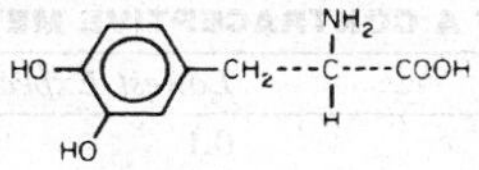

ACTIONS
Evidence indicates that the symptoms of Parkinson's disease are related to depletion of striatal dopamine. Since dopamine apparently does not cross the blood-brain barrier, its administration is ineffective in the treatment of Parkinson's disease. However, Levodopa, the levo-rotatory isomer of dihydroxyphenylalanine (dopa) which is the metabolic precursor of dopamine, does cross the blood-brain barrier. Presumably it is converted into dopamine in the basal ganglia. This is generally thought to be the mechanism whereby oral levodopa acts in relieving the symptoms of Parkinson's disease.
The major urinary metabolites of Levodopa in man appear to be dopamine and homovanillic acid (HVA). In 24-hour urine samples, HVA accounts for 13 to 42 percent of the ingested dose of Levodopa.

INDICATIONS
Levodopa is indicated in the treatment of idiopathic Parkinson's disease (Paralysis Agitans), postencephalitic parkinsonism, symptomatic parkinsonism which may follow injury to the nervous system by carbon monoxide intoxication, and manganese intoxication. It is indicated in those elderly patients believed to develop parkinsonism in association with cerebral arteriosclerosis.

UNLABELED USES
Levodopa is used alone or as an adjunct in the treatment of angina, hypertension, and congestive heart failure. It is also used in the treatment of anorexia nervosa, senile dementia, and severe and persistent tardive dyskinesia in schizophrenic patients who had been maintained on long-term neuroleptic therapy. Levodopa is also prescribed in the treatment of sexual dysfunction in patients with Parkinson's disease, in the treatment of female infertility, and in restless leg syndrome.

CONTRAINDICATIONS
Monoamine oxidase (MAO) inhibitors and Levodopa should not be given concomitantly and these inhibitors must be discontinued two weeks prior to initiating therapy with Levodopa. Levodopa is contraindicated in patients with known hypersensitivity to the drug and in narrow angle glaucoma.
Because Levodopa may activate a malignant melanoma, it should not be used in patients with suspicious, undiagnosed skin lesions or a history of melanoma.

WARNINGS
Levodopa should be administered cautiously to patients with severe cardiovascular or pulmonary disease, bronchial asthma, renal, hepatic or endocrine disease.
Care should be exercised in administering Levodopa to patients with a history of myocardial infarction who have residual atrial, nodal or ventricular arrhythmias. If Levodopa is necessary in this type of patient, it should be used in a facility with a coronary care unit or an intensive care unit.
One must be on the alert for the possibility of upper gastrointestinal hemorrhage in those patients with a past history of active peptic ulcer disease.
All patients should be carefully observed for the development of depression with concomitant suicidal tendencies. Psychotic patients should be treated with caution.
Pyridoxine hydrochloride (vitamin B_6) in oral doses of 10 to 25 mg rapidly reverses the toxic and therapeutic effects of Levodopa. This should be considered before recommending vitamin preparations containing pyridoxine hydrochloride (vitamin B_6).
Usage in Pregnancy: The safety of Levodopa in women who are or who may become pregnant has not been established; hence it should be given only when the potential benefits have been weighed against possible hazards to mother and child. Studies in rodents have shown that Levodopa at dosages in excess of 200 mg/kg/day has an adverse effect on fetal and postnatal growth and viability.
Levodopa should not be used in nursing mothers.
Usage in Children: The safety of Levodopa under the age of 12 has not been established.

PRECAUTIONS
Periodic evaluations of hepatic, hematopoietic, cardiovascular and renal function are recommended during extended therapy in all patients.
Patients with chronic wide angle glaucoma may be treated cautiously with Levodopa provided the intraocular pressure is well controlled and the patient monitored carefully for changes in intraocular pressure during therapy.
Postural hypotensive episodes have been reported as adverse reactions. Therefore, Levodopa should be administered to patients on antihypertensive drug cautiously (for patients receiving pargyline, see note on MAO inhibitors contraindications), and it may be necessary to adjust the dosage of the antihypertensive drugs.

ADVERSE REACTIONS
The most serious adverse reactions associated with the administration of Levodopa having frequent occurrences are: adventitious movements such as choreiform and/or dystonic movements. Other serious adverse reactions with a lower incidence are: cardiac irregularities and/or palpitations, orthostatic hypotensive episodes, bradykinetic episodes (the "on-off" phenomena), mental changes including paranoid ideation and psychotic episodes, depression with or without the development of suicidal tendencies, dementia, and urinary retention.
Rarely, gastrointestinal bleeding, development of duodenal ulcer, hypertension, phlebitis, hemolytic anemia, agranulocytosis, and convulsions have been observed. (The causal relationship between convulsions and Levodopa has not been established.)
Adverse reactions of a less serious nature having a relatively frequent occurrence are the following: anorexia, nausea and vomiting with or without abdominal pain and distress, dry mouth, dysphagia, sialorrhea, ataxia, increased hand tremor, headache, dizziness, numbness, weakness and faintness, bruxism, confusion, insomnia, nightmares, hallucinations and delusions, agitation and anxiety, malaise, fatigue and euphoria. Occurring with a lesser order of frequency are the following: muscle twitching and blepharospasm (which may be taken as an early sign of overdosage; consideration of dosage reduction may be made at this time), trismus, burning sensation of the tongue, bitter taste, diarrhea, constipation, flatulence, flushing, skin rash, increased sweating, bizarre breathing patterns, urinary incontinence, diplopia, blurred vision, dilated pupils, hot flashes, weight gain or loss, dark sweat and/or urine.
Rarely, oculogyric crises, sense of stimulation, hiccups, development of edema, loss of hair, hoarseness, priapism and activation of latent Horner's syndrome have been observed. Elevations of blood urea nitrogen, SGOT, SGPT, LDH, bilirubin, alkaline phosphatase or protein-bound iodine have been reported; and the significance of this is not known. Occasional reductions in WBC, hemoglobin, and hematocrit have been noted.
Leukopenia has occurred and requires cessation, at least temporarily, of Levodopa administration. The Coombs test has occasionally become positive

during extended therapy. Elevations of uric acid have been noted when colorimetric method was used but not when uricase method was used.

OVERDOSAGE

For acute overdosage general supportive measures should be employed, along with immediate gastric lavage. Intravenous fluids should be administered judiciously and an adequate airway maintained.

Electrocardiographic monitoring should be instituted and the patient carefully observed for the possible development of arrhythmias; if required, appropriate antiarrhythmic therapy should be given. Consideration should be given to the possibility of multiple drug ingestion by the patient. To date, no experience has been reported with dialysis; hence its value in Levodopa overdosage is not known. Although pyridoxine hydrochloride (vitamin B_6) has been reported to reverse the antiparkinson effects of Levodopa, its usefulness in the management of acute overdosage has not been established.

DOSAGE AND ADMINISTRATION

The optimal daily dose of Levodopa, *i.e.*, the dose producing maximal improvement with tolerated side effects, must be determined and *carefully titrated for each individual patient*. The usual initial dosage is 0.5 to 1 g daily, divided in two or more doses with food.

The total daily dosage is then increased gradually in increments not more than 0.75 gm every three to seven days as tolerated. The usual optimal therapeutic *dosage should not exceed 8 g.* The exceptional patient may carefully be given more than 8 g as required. In some patients, a significant therapeutic response may not be obtained until six months of treatment.

In the event general anesthesia is required, Levodopa therapy may be continued as long as the patient is able to take fluids and medication by mouth. If therapy is temporarily interrupted, the usual daily dosage may be administered as soon as the patient is able to take oral medication. Whenever therapy has been interrupted for longer periods, dosage should again be adjusted gradually; however, in many cases the patient can be rapidly titrated to his previous therapeutic dosage.

HOW SUPPLIED
TABLETS: 100 MG

BRAND/MANUFACTURER	NDC	SIZE	AWP
◇ **BRAND**			
LARODOPA: Roche Labs	00004-0072-01	100s	$22.14
DOPAR: Roberts Pharm	54092-0060-01	100s	$23.35

TABLETS: 250 MG

BRAND/MANUFACTURER	NDC	SIZE	AWP
◇ **BRAND**			
LARODOPA: Roche Labs	00004-0057-01	100s	$35.36
DOPAR: Roberts Pharm	54092-0061-01	100s	$37.68

TABLETS: 500 MG

BRAND/MANUFACTURER	NDC	SIZE	AWP
◇ **BRAND**			
LARODOPA: Roche Labs	00004-0056-01	100s	$60.75
DOPAR: Roberts Pharm	54092-0062-01	100s	$65.00

Levonorgestrel

Patients should be counseled that this product does not protect against HIV infection (AIDS) and other sexually transmitted diseases.

DESCRIPTION

Levonorgestrel implants are a set of six flexible closed capsules, each containing 36 mg of the progestin Levonorgestrel. The capsules are inserted in a superficial plane beneath the skin of the upper arm.

Evidence indicates that the dose of Levonorgestrel provided by Levonorgestrel implants is initially about 85 mcg/day followed by a decline to about 50 mcg/day by 9 months and to about 35 mcg/day by 18 months with a further decline thereafter to about 30 mcg/day. Levonorgestrel implants is a progestin-only product and does not contain estrogen.

Levonorgestrel, (d(-)-13-beta-ethyl-17-alpha-ethinyl-17-beta-hydroxygon-4-en-3-one), has a molecular weight of 312.46.

Following is its chemical structure:

CLINICAL PHARMACOLOGY

Levonorgestrel is a totally synthetic and biologically active progestin which exhibits no significant estrogenic activity and is highly progestational. The absolute configuration conforms to that of D-natural steroids. Levonorgestrel is not subjected to a "first-pass" effect and is virtually 100% bioavailable. Plasma concentrations average approximately 0.30 ng/mL over 5 years but are highly variable as a function of individual metabolism and body weight.

Diffusion of Levonorgestrel through the wall of each capsule provides a continuous low dose of the progestin. Resulting blood levels are substantially below those generally observed among users of combination oral contraceptives containing the progestins norgestrel or Levonorgestrel. Because of the range of variability in blood levels and variation in individual response, blood levels alone are not predictive of the risk of pregnancy in an individual woman.

At least two mechanisms are active in preventing pregnancy: ovulation inhibition and thickening of the cervical mucus. Other mechanisms may add to these contraceptive effects.

Levonorgestrel concentrations among women show considerable variation depending on individual clearance rates, body weight, and possibly other factors. Levonorgestrel concentrations reach a maximum, or near maximum, within 24 hours after placement with mean values of 1600 ± 1100 pg/mL. They decline rapidly over the first month partially due to a circulating protein, SHBG, that binds Levonorgestrel and which is depressed by the presence of Levonorgestrel. At 3 months, mean levels decline to values of around 400 pg/mL while concentrations normalized to a 60 kg body weight were 327 ± 119 (SD) pg/mL at 12 months with further decline by 1.4 pg/mL/month to reach 258 ± 95 (SD) pg/mL at 60 months.

Concentrations decreased with increasing body weight by a mean of 3.3 pg/mL/kg. After capsule removal, mean concentrations drop to below 100 pg/mL by 96 hours and to below assay sensitivity (50 pg/mL) by 5 to 14 days. Fertility rates return to levels comparable to those seen in the general population of women using no method of contraception. Circulating concentrations can be used to forecast the risk of pregnancy only in a general statistical sense. Mean concentrations associated with pregnancy have been 210 ± 60 (SD) pg/mL. However, in clinical studies, 20 percent of women had one or more values below 200 pg/mL but an average annual gross pregnancy rate of less than 1.0 per 100 women through 5 years.

Although lipoprotein levels were altered in several clinical studies with Levonorgestrel implants, the long-term clinical effects of these changes have not been determined. A decrease in total cholesterol levels has been reported in all lipoprotein studies and reached statistical significance in several. Both increases and decreases in high-density lipoprotein (HDL) levels have been reported in clinical trials. No statistically significant increases have been reported in the ratio of total cholesterol to HDL-cholesterol. Low-density lipoprotein (LDL) levels decreased during Levonorgestrel implant use. Triglyceride levels also decreased from pretreatment values.

INDICATIONS AND USAGE

Levonorgestrel implants are indicated for the prevention of pregnancy and constitute a long-term (up to 5 years) reversible contraceptive system. The capsules should be removed by the end of the 5th year. New capsules may be inserted at that time if continuing contraceptive protection is desired.

In multicenter trials with Levonorgestrel implants, involving 2470 women, the relationship between body weight and efficacy was investigated. Tabulated below is the pregnancy experience as a function of body weight. Because Levonorgestrel implants are a long-term method of contraception, this is reported over five years of use. (See related table).

Typically, pregnancy rates with contraceptive methods are reported for only the first year of use as shown below. The efficacy of these contraceptive methods, except the IUD and sterilization, depends in part on the reliability of use. The efficacy of Levonorgestrel implants does not depend on patient compliance. However, no contraceptive method is 100% effective.

Table 2
LOWEST EXPECTED AND TYPICAL FAILURE RATES (%) DURING THE FIRST YEAR OF USE OF A CONTRACEPTIVE METHOD

Method	Lowest Expected	Typical
Male Sterilization	0.1	0.15
Levonorgestrel implants	0.2	0.2
Female Sterilization	0.2	0.4
DMPA (injectable progestogen)	0.3	0.3
Oral contraceptives		3
Combined	0.1	N/A
Progestin only	0.5	N/A
IUD	< 1	3
Condom without spermicide	2	12
Cervical Cap	6	18
Diaphragm with spermicide cream or jelly	6	18
Vaginal sponge		
nulliparous	6	18
parous	9	28
Spermicides alone (foam. creams, jellies, and vaginal suppositories)	3	21
Periodic abstinence (all methods)	1-9	20
No contraception (planned pregnancy)	85	85
N/A—not available		

◆ RATED THERAPEUTICALLY EQUIVALENT; ◇ THERAPEUTIC EQUIVALENCE UNCONFIRMED; ○ UNRATED

Levonorgestrel implants gross annual discontinuation and continuation rates are summarized in Table 3. (See related table).

CONTRAINDICATIONS
1. Active thrombophlebitis or thromboembolic disorders.
2. Undiagnosed abnormal genital bleeding.
3. Known or suspected pregnancy.
4. Acute liver disease: benign or malignant liver tumors.
5. Known or suspected carcinoma of the breast.

WARNINGS
A. WARNINGS BASED ON EXPERIENCE WITH LEVONORGESTREL IMPLANTS

1. Bleeding Irregularities: Most women can expect some variation in menstrual bleeding patterns. Irregular menstrual bleeding, intermenstrual spotting, prolonged episodes of bleeding and spotting, and amenorrhea occur in some women. Irregular bleeding patterns associated with Levonorgestrel implants could mask symptoms of cervical or endometrial cancer. Overall, these irregularities diminish with continuing use. Since some Levonorgestrel implant users experience periods of amenorrhea, missed menstrual periods cannot serve as the only means of identifying early pregnancy. Pregnancy tests should be performed whenever a pregnancy is suspected. Six (6) weeks or more of amenorrhea after a pattern of regular menses may signal pregnancy. If pregnancy occurs, the capsules must be removed.

Although bleeding irregularities have occurred in clinical trials, proportionately more women had increases rather than decreases in hemoglobin concentrations, a difference that was highly statistically significant. This finding generally indicates that reduced menstrual blood loss is associated with the use of Levonorgestrel implants. In rare instances, blood loss did result in hemoglobin values consistent with anemia.

2. Delayed Follicular Atresia: If follicular development occurs with Levonorgestrel implants, atresia of the follicle is sometimes delayed, and the follicle may continue to grow beyond the size it would attain in a normal cycle. These enlarged follicles cannot be distinguished clinically from ovarian cysts. In the majority of women, enlarged follicles will spontaneously disappear and should not require surgery. Rarely, they may twist or rupture, sometimes causing abdominal pain, and surgical intervention may be required.

3. Ectopic Pregnancies: Ectopic pregnancies have occurred among Levonorgestrel implant users, although clinical studies have shown no increase in the rate of ectopic pregnancies per year among Levonorgestrel implant users as compared with users of no method or of IUDs. The incidence among Levonorgestrel implant users was 1.3 per 1000 woman-years, a rate significantly below the rate that has been estimated for noncontraceptive users in the United States (2.7 to 3.0 per 1000 woman-years). The risk of ectopic pregnancy may increase with the duration of Levonorgestrel implant use and possibly with increased weight of the user. Physicians should be alert to the possibility of an ectopic pregnancy among women using Levonorgestrel implants who become pregnant or complain of lower-abdominal pain. Any patient who presents with lower-abdominal pain must be evaluated to rule out ectopic pregnancy.

4. Foreign-body Carcinogenesis: Rarely, cancers have occurred at the site of foreign-body intrusions or old scars. None has been reported in Levonorgestrel implant clinical trials. In rodents, which are highly susceptible to such cancers, the incidence decreases with decreasing size of the foreign body. Because of the resistance of human beings to these cancers and because of the small size of the capsules, the risk to users of Levonorgestrel implants is judged to be minimal.

5. Thromboembolic Disorders: Patients who develop active thrombophlebitis or thromboembolic disease should have Levonorgestrel capsules removed. Removal should also be considered in women who will be subjected to prolonged immobilization due to surgery or other illnesses.

B. WARNINGS BASED ON EXPERIENCE WITH COMBINATION (PROGESTIN PLUS ESTROGEN) ORAL CONTRACEPTIVES

1. Cigarette Smoking: Cigarette smoking increases the risk of serious cardiovascular side effects from the use of combination oral contraceptives. This risk increases with age and with heavy smoking (15 or more cigarettes per day) and is quite marked in women over 35 years old. While this is believed to be an estrogen-related effects, it is not known whether a similar risk exists with progestin-only methods such as Levonorgestrel implants; however, women who use Levonorgestrel implants should be advised not to smoke.

2. Elevated Blood Pressure: Increased blood pressure has been reported in users of combination oral contraceptives. The prevalence of elevated blood pressure increases with long exposure. Although there were no statistically significant trends among Levonorgestrel implant users in clinical trials, physicians should be aware of the possibility of elevated blood pressure with Levonorgestrel implant.

3. Thromboembolic Disorders and Other Vascular Problems: An increased risk of thromboembolic and thrombotic disease (pulmonary embolism, superficial venous thrombosis, and deep-vein thrombosis) has been found to be associated with the use of combination oral contraceptives. The relative risk has been estimated to be 4- to 11-fold higher for users than for nonusers. While there is evidence of an association between the estrogen content of combination oral contraceptives and thromboembolic risk, the association of the Levonorgestrel implant progestin-only method to this risk is not known.

Cerebrovascular Disorders: Combination oral contraceptives have been shown to increase both the relative and attributable risks of cerebrovascular events (thrombotic and hemorrhagic strokes), although, in general, the risk is greatest among older (> 35 years) hypertensive women who also smoke. Hypertension was found to be a risk factor for both users and nonusers for both types of strokes, while smoking interacted to increase the risk for hemorrhagic strokes. The association of the Levonorgestrel implant progestin-only method to this risk is not known.

Myocardial Infarction: An increased risk of myocardial infarction has been attributed to combination oral-contraceptive use. This is thought to be primarily thrombotic in origin and is related to the estrogen component of combination oral contraceptives. This increased risk occurs primarily in smokers or in women with other underlying risk factors for coronary-artery disease, such as family history of coronary-artery disease, hypertension, hypercholesterolemia, morbid obesity, and diabetes. The current relative risk of heart attack for combination oral-contraceptive users has been estimated as 2 to 6 times the risk for nonusers. The absolute risk is very low for women under 30 years of age.

Studies indicate a significant trend toward higher rates of myocardial infarctions and strokes with increasing doses of progestin in combination oral contraceptives. However, a recent study showed no increased risk of myocardial infarction associated with the past use of Levonorgestrel-containing combination oral contraceptives. The association of the Levonorgestrel implant progestin-only method with the risk of cardiovascular diseases is not known.

4. Carcinoma: Numerous epidemiological studies have been performed to determine the incidence of breast, endometrial, ovarian, and cervical cancer in women using combination oral contraceptives. Recent evidence in the literature suggests that use of combination oral contraceptives is not associated with an increased risk of developing breast cancer in the overall population of users. The Cancer and Steroid Hormone (CASH) study also showed no latent effect on the risk of breast cancer for at least a decade following long-term use. However, some of these same recent studies have shown an increased relative risk of breast cancer in certain subgroups of combination oral-contraceptive users, although no consistent pattern of findings has been identified. This information should be considered when prescribing Levonorgestrel implants.

Some studies suggest that combination oral-contraceptive use has been associated with an increase in the risk of cervical intraepithelial neoplasia in some populations of women. However, there continues to be controversy about the extent to which such findings may be due to differences in sexual behavior and

Table 1
ANNUAL AND FIVE-YEAR CUMULATIVE PREGNANCY RATES PER 100 USERS BY WEIGHT CLASS

Weight class	year 1	year 2	year 3	year 4	year 5	Cumulative
< 50 kg (< 110 lbs)	0.2	0	0	0	0	0.2
50-59 kg (110-130 lbs)	0.2	0.5	0.4	2.0	0.4	3.4
60-69 kg (131-153 lbs)	0.4	0.5	1.6	1.7	0.8	5.0
≥ 70 kg (≥ 154 lbs)	0	1.1	5.1	2.5	0	8.5
All	0.2	0.5	1.2	1.6	0.4	3.9

Table 3
ANNUAL AND FIVE-YEAR CUMULATIVE RATES PER 100 USERS

	year 1	year 2	year 3	year 4	year 5	Cumulative
Pregnancy Bleeding	0.2	0.5	1.2	1.6	0.4	3.9
Irregularities	9.1	7.9	4.9	3.3	2.9	25.1
Medical (excl. bleeding irreg.)	6.0	5.6	4.1	4.0	5.1	22.4
Personal	4.6	7.7	11.7	10.7	11.7	38.7
Continuation	81.0	77.4	79.2	76.7	77.6	29.5

➤ SHOWN IN PRODUCT IDENTIFICATION GUIDE

other factors. In spite of many studies of the relationship between combination oral-contraceptive use and breast and cervical cancers, a cause-and-effect relationship has not been established.

Evidence indicates that combination oral contraceptives may decrease the risk of ovarian and endometrial cancer. Irregular bleeding patterns associated with Levonorgestrel implants could mask symptoms of cervical or endometrial cancer.

5. Hepatic Tumors: Hepatic adenomas have been found to be associated with the use of combination oral contraceptives with an estimated incidence of about 3 occurrences per 100,000 users per year, a risk that increases after 4 or more years of use. Although benign, hepatic adenomas may rupture and cause death through intra-abdominal hemorrhage, the contribution of the progestin component of oral contraceptives to the development of hepatic adenomas is not known.

6. Ocular Lesions: There have been clinical case reports of retinal thrombosis associated with the use of oral contraceptives. Although it is believed that this adverse reaction is related to the estrogen component of oral contraceptives, Levonorgestrel capsules should be removed if there is unexplained partial or complete loss of vision; onset of proptosis or diplopia; papilledema; or retinal vascular lesions. Appropriate diagnostic and therapeutic measures should be undertaken immediately.

7. Use Before or During Early Pregnancy: Extensive epidemiological studies have revealed no increased risk of birth defects in women who have used oral contraceptives prior to pregnancy. Studies also do not suggest a teratogenic effect, particularly insofar as cardiac anomalies and limb-reduction defects are concerned, when taken inadvertently during early pregnancy. There is no evidence suggesting that the risk associated with Levonorgestrel implant use is different.

8. Gallbladder Disease: Earlier studies have reported an increased lifetime relative risk of gallbladder surgery in users of oral contraceptives and estrogens. More recent studies, however, have shown that the relative risk of developing gallbladder disease among oral-contraceptive users may be minimal. The recent findings of minimal risk may be related to the use of oral-contraceptive formulations containing lower hormonal doses of estrogens and progestins. The association of this risk with use of the Levonorgestrel implant progestin-only method is not known.

PRECAUTIONS
Patients should be counseled that this product does not protect against HIV infection (AIDS) and other sexually transmitted diseases.

GENERAL
1. Physical Examination and Follow-Up: A complete medical history and physical examination should be taken prior to the implantation or reimplantation of Levonorgestrel capsules and at least annually during their use. These physical examinations should include special reference to the implant site, blood pressure, breasts, abdomen and pelvic organs, including cervical cytology and relevant laboratory tests. In case of undiagnosed, persistent or recurrent abnormal vaginal bleeding, appropriate diagnostic measures should be conducted to rule out malignancy. Women with a strong family history of breast cancer or who have breast nodules should be monitored with particular care.

2. Carbohydrate Metabolism: An altered glucose tolerance characterized by decreased insulin sensitivity following glucose loading has been found in some users of combination and progestin-only oral contraceptives. The effects of Levonorgestrel implants on carbohydrate metabolism appear to be minimal. In a study in which pretreatment serum-glucose levels were compared with levels after 1 and 2 years of Levonorgestrel implant use, no statistically significant differences in mean serum-glucose levels were evident 2 hours after glucose loading. The clinical significance of these findings is unknown, but diabetic and prediabetic patients should be carefully observed while using Levonorgestrel implants.

Women who are being treated for hyperlipidemias should be followed closely if they elect to use Levonorgestrel implants. Some progestins may elevate LDL levels and may render the control of hyperlipidemias more difficult. (See *"Warnings."*)

3. Liver Function: If jaundice develops in any women while using Levonorgestrel implants. consideration should be given to removing the capsules. Steroid hormones may be poorly metabolized in patients with impaired liver function.

4. Fluid Retention: Steroid contraceptives may cause some degree of fluid retention. They should be prescribed with caution, and only with careful monitoring, in patients with conditions which might be aggravated by fluid retention.

5. Emotional Disorders: Consideration should be given to removing Levonorgestrel capsules in women who become significantly depressed since the symptom may be drug-related. Women with a history of depression should be carefully observed and removal considered if depression recurs to a serious degree.

6. Contact Lenses: Contact-lens wearers who develop visual changes or changes in lens tolerance should be assessed by an ophthalmologist.

7. Idiopathic Intracranial Hypertension: Idiopathic intracranial hypertension (pseudotumor cerebri, benign intracranial hypertension) is a disorder of unknown etiology which is seen most commonly in obese females of reproductive age. There have been reports of idiopathic intracranial hypertension in Levonorgestrel implant users; however, a causal relationship is unclear. A cardinal sign of idiopathic intracranial hypertension is papilledema; early symptoms may include headache (associated with a change in the frequency, pattern, severity, or persistence: of particular importance are those headaches that are unremitting in nature), and visual disturbances. Patients with these symptoms should be

screened for papilledema and, if present, the patient should be referred to a neurologist for further diagnosis and care. Levonorgestrel implants should be removed from patients experiencing this disorder.

8. Insertion and Removal: To be sure that the woman is not pregnant at the time of capsule placement and to assure contraceptive effectiveness during the first cycle of use, it is advisable that insertion be done during the first 7 days of the menstrual cycle or immediately following an abortion. However, Levonorgestrel capsules may be inserted at any time during the cycle provided pregnancy has been excluded and a nonhormonal contraceptive method is used for the remainder of the cycle. Insertion is not recommended before 6 weeks postpartum in breast-feeding women.

Insertion and removal are not difficult procedures but instructions must be followed closely. It is strongly advised that all health-care professionals who insert and remove Levonorgestrel capsules be instructed in the procedures before they attempt them. A proper insertion just under the skin will facilitate removals. Proper Levonorgestrel implant insertion and removal should result in minimal scarring. If the capsules are placed too deeply, they can be harder to remove. If all capsules cannot be removed at the first attempt, removal should be attempted later when the site has healed. Bruising may occur at the implant site during insertion or removal. Other cutaneous reactions that have been reported include ulcerations and sloughing. In some women, hyperpigmentation occurs over the implantation site but is usually reversible following removal. See detailed insertion and removal instructions below.

9. Infections: Infection at the implant, including cellulitis, site has been uncommon. Attention to aseptic technique and proper insertion and removal of Levonorgestrel capsules reduces the possibility of infection. If infection occurs, suitable treatment should be instituted. If infection persists, the capsules should be removed.

10. Expulsion: Expulsion of capsules was uncommon. It occurred more frequently when placement of the capsules was extremely shallow, too close to the incision, or when infection was present. Replacement of an expelled capsule must be accomplished using a new sterile capsule. If infection is present, it should be treated and cured before replacement. Contraceptive efficacy may be inadequate with fewer than 6 capsules.

11. Provisions for Removal: Women should be advised that the capsules will be removed at any time for any reason. The removal should be done on such request or at the end of 5 years of usage by personnel instructed in the removal technique.

Upon removal, Levonorgestrel capsules should be disposed of in accordance with Center for Disease Control Guidelines for the handling of biohazardous waste.

DRUG INTERACTIONS
Reduced efficacy (pregnancy) has been reported for Levonorgestrel implant users taking phenytoin and carbamazepine. Levonorgestrel implant users should be warned of the possibility of decreased efficacy with use of any related drugs.

DRUG/LABORATORY TEST INTERACTIONS
Certain endocrine tests may be affected by Levonorgestrel implant use:
1. Sex-hormone-binding globulin concentrations are decreased.
2. Thyroxine concentrations may be slightly decreased and triiodothyronine uptake increased.

CARCINOGENESIS
See *"Warnings"* section.

PREGNANCY
Pregnancy Category X. See *"Warnings"* section.

NURSING MOTHERS
Steroids are not considered the contraceptives of first choice for lactating women. Levonorgestrel has been identified in the breast milk of lactating women. No significant effects were observed on the growth or health of infants whose mothers used Levonorgestrel implants beginning 6 weeks after parturition in comparative studies with mothers using IUDs or barrier methods. Eighty (80) infants were monitored for three years. No information is available beyond that time. No data are available on use in breastfeeding mothers earlier than 6 weeks after parturition.

INFORMATION FOR THE PATIENT
It is recommended that propective users be fully informed about the risks and benefits associated with use of Levonorgestrel implants, with other forms of contraception, and with no contraception at all. It is also recommended that prospective users be fully informed about the insertion and removal procedures. Health-care providers may wish to obtain informed consent from all patients in light of the techniques involved with insertion and removal.

ADVERSE REACTIONS
The following adverse reactions have been associated with Levonorgestrel implants during the first year of use. They include:

Many bleeding days or prolonged bleeding	27.6%
Spotting	17.1%
Amenorrhea	9.4%
Irregular (onsets of) bleeding	7.6%
Frequent bleeding onsets	7.0%
Scanty bleeding	5.2%

◆ RATED THERAPEUTICALLY EQUIVALENT; ◇ THERAPEUTIC EQUIVALENCE UNCONFIRMED; ○ UNRATED

Pain or itching near implant site (usually transient)	3.7%
Infection at implant site	0.7%
Removal difficulties affecting subject (based on 849 removals)	6.2%

In addition, removal difficulties have been reported with a frequency of 6.2%, which is based on 849 removals occurring through five years of use.

Clinical studies comparing Levonorgestrel implant users with other contraceptive method users suggest that the following adverse reactions occurring during the first year are probably associated with Levonorgestrel implant use:

Headache
Nervousness, Anxiety
Nausea
Dizziness
Adnexal enlargement
Dermatitis, Rash
Acne
Change of appetite
Mastalgia
Weight gain
Hirsutism, hypertrichosis, and scalp-hair loss

In addition, the following adverse reactions have been reported with a frequency of 5% or greater during the first year and possibly may be related to Levonorgestrel implant use:

Breast discharge
Cervicitis
Musculoskeletal pain
Abdominal discomfort
Leukorrhea
Vaginitis

The following adverse reaction has been reported post-marketing with an incidence of less than 1%. This event occurred under circumstances where a causal relationship to Levonorgestrel implants is unknown. This reaction is listed as information for physicians: Emotional lability.

OVERDOSAGE
Overdosage can result if more than six capsules of Levonorgestrel are in situ. All implanted Levonorgestrel capsules should be removed before inserting a new set of Levonorgestrel capsules. Overdosage may cause fluid retention with its associated effects and uterine bleeding irregularities.

DOSAGE AND ADMINISTRATION
Levonorgestrel implants consists of six capsules, each containing 36 mg of the progestin, Levonorgestrel. The total administered (implanted) dose is 216 mg. Implantation of all six capsules should be performed during the first 7 days of the onset of menses by a health-care professional instructed in the Levonorgestrel implant insertion technique. Insertion is subdermal in the midportion of the upper arm about 8 to 10 cm above the elbow crease. Distribution should be in a fanlike pattern, about 15 degrees apart, for a total of 75 degrees. Proper insertion will facilitate later removal. (See section on *"Insertion/Removal"*.)

Store at room temperature away from excess heat and moisture.

Note: Some brands contain chlorofluorocarbons. The indented statement below is required by the Federal government's Clean Air Act for all products containing or manufactured with chlorofluorocarbons (CFCs).

WARNING: Manufactured with dichlorodifluoromethane, a substance which harms public health and environment by destroying ozone in the upper atmosphere.

Dichlorodifluoromethane is a chemical used in the sterilization process and is not contained in the product itself.

INSTRUCTIONS FOR INSERTION AND REMOVAL
Levonorgestrel implants consist of six Levonorgestrel-releasing capsules that are inserted subdermally in the medial aspect of the upper arm.

Levonorgestrel implants provide up to 5 years of effective contraceptive protection.

The basis for successful use and subsequent removal of Levonorgestrel capsules is a correct and carefully performed subdermal insertion of the six capsules. It is recommended that health-care professionals performing insertions or removals of Levonorgestrel capsules avail themselves of instruction and supervision in the proper technique prior to attempting these procedures. During insertion, special attention should be given to the following:
—asepsis.
—correct subdermal placement of the capsules.
—careful technique to minimize tissue trauma.

This will help to avoid infections and excessive scarring at the insertion area and will help keep the capsules from being inserted too deeply in the tissue. If the capsules are placed too deeply, they will be more difficult to remove than correctly placed subdermal capsules.

INSERTION PROCEDURE
Insertion should be performed within seven days from the onset of menses. However, Levonorgestrel capsules may be inserted at any time during the cycle provided pregnancy has been excluded and a nonhormonal contraceptive method is used for the remainder of the cycle. A gynecological examination should be

performed before the insertion of Levonorgestrel capsules, as would be the case before initiating any hormonal contraception. Determine if the subject has any allergies to the antiseptic or anesthetic to be used or contraindications to progestin-only contraception. If none are found, the capsules are inserted using the procedure outlined below.

The insertion is performed under aseptic conditions using a trocar to place the capsules under the skin.

The following equipment is recommended for the insertion:
—an examining table for the patient to lie on.
—sterile surgical drapes, sterile gloves (free of talc), antiseptic solution.
—local anesthetic, needles, and syringe.
—# 11 scalpel, # 10 trocar, forceps.
—skin closure, sterile gauze, and compresses.

Have the patient lie on her back on the examination table with her left arm (if the patient is left-handed, the right arm) flexed at the elbow and externally rotated so that her hand is lying by her head. The capsules will be inserted subdermally through a small 2-mm incision and positioned in a fanlike manner with the fan opening towards the shoulder.

Prep the patient's upper arm with antiseptic solution; cover the arm above and below the insertion area with a sterile cloth. The optimal insertion area is in the inside of the upper arm about 8 to 10 cm above the elbow crease.

After determining the absence of known allergies to the anesthetic agent or related drugs, fill a 5-mL syringe with the local anesthetic. Since blood loss is minimal with this procedure, use of epinephrine-containing anesthetics is not considered necessary. Anesthetize the insertion area by first inserting the needle under the skin and injecting a small amount of anesthetic. Then anesthetize six areas about 4 to 4.5 cm long, to mimic the fanlike position of the implanted capsules.

Use the scalpel to make a small, shallow incision (about 2 mm) just through the dermis of the skin.

The trocar has two marks on it. The first mark is closer to the hub and indicates how far the trocar should be introduced under the skin before the loading of each capsule. The second mark is close to the tip and indicates how much of the trocar should remain under the skin following the insertion of each implant.

Insert the tip of the trocar through the incision beneath the skin at a shallow angle. Once the trocar is inserted, it should be oriented with the bevel up toward the skin to keep the capsules in a superficial plane. It is important to keep the trocar subdermal by tenting the skin with the trocar, as failure to do so may result in deep placement of the capsules and could make removal more difficult.

Advance the trocar gently under the skin to the first mark near the hub of the trocar. The tip of the trocar is now at a distance of about 4 to 4.5 cm from the incision.

Do not force the trocar, and if resistance is felt, try another direction.

When the trocar has been inserted the appropriate distance, remove the obturator and load the first capsule into the trocar using the thumb and forefinger.

Gently advance the capsule with the obturator towards the tip of the trocar until you feel resistance. Never force the obturator.

Hold the obturator steady, and bring the trocar back until it touches the handle of the obturator.

The capsule should have been released under the skin when the mark close to the tip of the trocar is visible in the incision. Release of the capsule can be checked by palpation. It is important to keep the obturator steady and not to push the capsule into the tissue.

Do not remove the trocar from the incision until all capsules have been inserted. The trocar is withdrawn only to the mark close to its tip. Each succeeding capsule is always inserted next to the previous one, to form a fanlike shape. Fix the position of the previous capsule with the forefinger and middle finger of the free hand, and advance the trocar along the tips of the fingers. This will ensure a suitable distance of about 15 degrees between capsules and keep the trocar from puncturing any of the previously inserted capsules.

Leave a distance of about 5 mm between the incision and the tips of the capsules. This will help avoid spontaneous expulsions. The correct position of the capsules can be ensured by feeling them with the fingers after the insertion has been completed.

After the insertion of the sixth capsule, palpate the capsules to make sure that all six have been inserted.

Press the edges of the incision together, and close the incision with a skin closure. Suturing the incision should not be necessary.

Cover the insertion area with a dry compress, and wrap gauze around the arm to ensure hemostasis.

Observe the patient for a few minutes for signs of syncope or bleeding from the incision before she is discharged.

Advise the patient to keep the insertion area dry for 2 to 3 days. The gauze may be removed after 1 day, and the butterfly bandage as soon as the incision has healed, i.e., normally in 3 days.

REMOVAL PROCEDURE
It is recommended that removals be prescheduled so that preparations for carrying out the procedure can be facilitated.

Removal of the capsules should be performed very gently and will take more time than insertion. Capsules are sometimes nicked or cut during removal. The incidence of overall removal difficulties, including damage to capsules, has been 13.2 percent. Less than half of these removal difficulties have caused inconvenience to the patient. If the removal of some of the capsules proves difficult, have the patient return for a second visit. The remaining capsule(s) will be easier to remove after the area is healed. If contraception is still desired, a barrier method should be advised until all capsules are removed.

The position of the patient and the asepsis are the same as for insertion. The following equipment is needed for the removal:
—an examining table for the patient to lie on.
—sterile surgical drapes, sterile gloves (free of talc), antiseptic solution.
—local anesthetic, needles, and syringe.
—# 11 scalpel, forceps (straight and curved mosquito).
—skin closure, sterile gauze, and compresses.

Locate the implanted capsules by palpation, possibly marking their position with a sterile skin marker. Apply a small amount of local anesthetic *under* the capsule ends nearest the original incision site. This will serve to raise the ends of the capsules. Anesthetic injected over the capsules will obscure them and make removal more difficult.

Additional small amounts of the anesthetic can be used for the removal of each of the capsules, if required.

Make a 4-mm incision with the scalpel close to the ends of the capsules. Do not make a large incision.

Push each capsule gently towards the incision with the fingers. When the tip is visible or near to the incision, grasp it with a mosquito forceps.

Use the scalpel very gently to open the tissue sheath that has formed around the capsule.

Remove the capsule from the incision with the second forceps.

After the procedure is completed, the incision is closed and bandaged as with insertion. The upper arm should be kept dry for a few days.

Following removal, a return to the previous level of fertility is usually prompt, and a pregnancy may occur at any time. If the patient wishes to continue using the method, a new set of Levonorgestrel capsules can be inserted through the same incision in the same or opposite direction.

HINTS
Insertion:
—Counselling of the patient on the benefits and side effects of the method prior to insertion will greatly increase patient satisfaction.
—Correct subdermal placement of the capsules will facilitate removal.
—Before insertion, apply the anesthetic just beneath the skin so as to raise the dermis above the underlying tissue.
—Never force the trocar.
—To ensure subdermal placement, the trocar with bevel up should be supported by the index finger and should visibly raise the skin at all times during insertion.
—To avoid damaging the previous implanted capsule, stabilize the capsule with your forefinger and middle finger and advance the trocar alongside the finger tips at an angle of 15 degrees.
—After insertion, make a drawing for the patient's file showing the location of the 6 capsules and describe any variations in placement. This will greatly aid removal.

Removal:
—The removal of the implanted capsules will take a little more time than the insertion.
—Before removal, apply the anesthetic *under* the capsule ends nearest the original incision site.
—If the removal of some of the capsules proves difficult, interrupt the procedure and have the patient return for a second visit. The remaining capsule(s) will be easier to remove after the area is healed.

HOW SUPPLIED
KIT:

BRAND/MANUFACTURER	NDC	SIZE	AWP
○ BRAND			
NORPLANT SYSTEM: Wyeth-Ayerst	00008-2564-01	6s	$456.25

Levophed Bitartrate *SEE* NOREPINEPHRINE BITARTRATE

Levoprome *SEE* METHOTRIMEPRAZINE

Levorphanol Tartrate

DESCRIPTION
Levorphanol Tatrate is a highly potent synthetic analgesic with properties and actions similar to those of morphine. It produces a degree of analgesia at least equal to that of morphine and greater than that of meperidine at far smaller doses than either. It is longer acting than either; from 6 to 8 hours of pain relief can be expected with Levorphanol Tartrate whether given orally or by injection. It is almost as effective orally as it is parenterally. Its safety margin is about equal to that of morphine, but it is less likely to produce nausea, vomiting and constipation.

Following is its chemical structure:

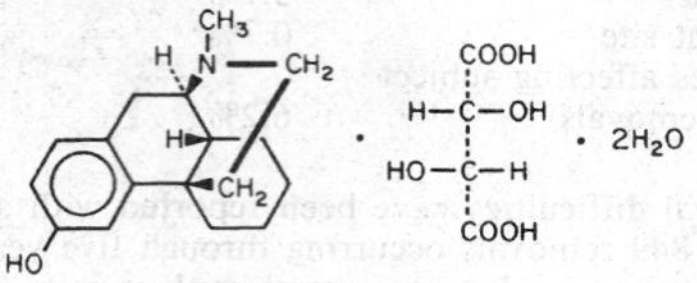

INDICATIONS
Levorphanol Tartrate is recommended whenever a narcotic-analgesic is required. It is recommended for the relief of pain whether moderate or severe. For example, it may be used in alleviating pain due to biliary and renal colic, myocardial infarction, and severe trauma; intractable pain due to cancer and other tumors; and for postoperative pain relief. Used preoperatively, it allays apprehension, provides prolonged analgesia, reduces thiopental requirements and shortens recovery-room time. Levorphanol Tartrate is compatible with a wide range of anesthetic agents. It is a useful supplement to nitrous oxide-oxgen anesthesia. It has been given by slow intravenous injection for special indications.

CONTRAINDICATIONS
As with the use of morphine, Levorphanol Tartrate is contraindicated in acute alcoholism, bronchial asthma, increased intracranial pressure, respiratory depression and anoxia.

WARNING
May be habit forming. Levorphanol Tartrate is a narcotic with an addiction liability similar to that of morphine, and for this reason the same precautions should be taken in administering the drug as with morphine. As with all narcotics, Levorphanol Tartrate should be used in early pregnancy only when expected benefits outweigh risks.

PRECAUTIONS
To counteract narcotic-induced respiratory depression, a narcotic antagonist, such as naloxone hydrochloride, is recommended and should be readily available whenever Levorphanol Tartrate is used by parenteral administration.

ADVERSE REACTIONS
As is true with the use of any narcotic-analgesic, nausea, emesis and dizziness are not uncommon in the ambulatory patient. Respiratory depression, hypotension, urinary retention and various cardiac arrhythmias have been infrequently reported following the use of Levorphanol Tartrate, primarily in surgical patients. Occasional allergic reactions in the form of skin rash or urticaria have been reported. Pruritus or sweating are rarely observed.

ANTIDOTE FOR OVERDOSAGE
In the event of overdosage of Levorphanol Tartrate, an appropriate dose of a narcotic antagonist, such as naloxone HCl, should be administered; consult the prescribing information of the specific narcotic antagonist for details about use.

DOSAGE AND ADMINISTRATION
Good medical practice dictates that the dose of any narcotic-analgesic be appropriate to the degree of pain to be relieved. This is especially important during the postoperative period because (a) residual CNS-depressant effects of anesthetic agents may still be present, and (b) later, gradual lessening of pain may not warrant full narcotizing doses. The average adult dose is 2 mg orally or subcutaneously. The dosage may be increased to 3 mg, if necessary.
Narcotic order required.

J CODES
Up to 2 mg SC,IV—J1960

HOW SUPPLIED
INJECTION (C-II): 2 MG/ML

BRAND/MANUFACTURER	NDC	SIZE	AWP
○ BRAND			
LEVO-DROMORAN: Roche Labs	00004-1911-06	10 ml	$21.05
	00004-1910-06	1 ml 10s	$27.17

TABLETS (C-II): 2 MG

BRAND/MANUFACTURER	NDC	SIZE	AWP
○ BRAND			
LEVO-DROMORAN: Roche Labs	00004-0044-01	100s	$57.51
○ GENERICS			
Roxane	00054-4494-25	100s	$49.71
Roxane	00054-8494-24	100s ud	$66.31

Levothroid *SEE* LEVOTHYROXINE SODIUM

◆ **RATED THERAPEUTICALLY EQUIVALENT;** ◇ **THERAPEUTIC EQUIVALENCE UNCONFIRMED;** ○ **UNRATED**

Levothyroxine Sodium

DESCRIPTION

Levothyroxine Sodium Tablets and injection contain synthetic crystalline L-3,3'5,5'-tetraiodothyronine sodium salt [levothyroxine (T_4) sodium] Synthetic T_4 is similar to that produced in the human thyroid gland. T_4 contains four iodine atoms and is formed by the coupling of two molecules of diiodotyrosine (DIT).

Levothyroxine (T_4) Sodium has an empirical formula of $C_{15}H_{10}I_4NNaO_4xH_2O$, molecular weight of 798.86 (anhydrous).

Following is its chemical structure:

CLINICAL PHARMACOLOGY

The steps in the synthesis of thyroid hormones are controlled by thyrotropin (Thyroid Stimulating Hormone, TSH) secreted by the anterior pituitary. This hormone's secretion is in turn controlled by a feedback mechanism effected by the thyroid hormones themselves and by thyrotropin releasing hormone (TRH), a tripeptide of hypothalamic origin. Endogenous thyroid hormone secretion is suppressed when exogenous thyroid hormones are administered to euthyroid individuals in excess of the normal gland's secretion.

The mechanisms by which thyroid hormones exert their physiologic action are not well understood. These hormones enhance oxygen consumption by most tissues of the body and increase the basal metabolic rate and the metabolism of carbohydrates, lipids, and proteins. Thus they exert a profound influence on every organ system in the body and are of particular importance in the development of the central nervous system.

The normal thyroid gland contains approximately 200 mcg of Levothyroxine (T_4) per gram of gland, and 15 mcg of triiodothyronine (T_3) per gram. The ratio of these two hormones in the circulation does not represent the ratio in the thyroid gland, since about 80 percent of peripheral triiodothyronine comes from monodeiodination of Levothyroxine at the 5 position (outer ring). Perpheral monodeiodination of Levothyroxine at the 5 position (inner ring) results in the formation of reverse triiodothyronine (rT_3), which is calorigenically inactive. These facts would seem to advocate Levothyroxine as the treatment of choice for the hypothyroid patient and to militate against the administration of hormone combinations which, while normalizing thyroxine levels may produce triiodothyronine levels in the thyrotoxic range.

Triiodothyronine (T_3) level is low in the fetus and newborn, in old age, in chronic caloric deprivation, hepatic cirrhosis, renal failure, surgical stress, and chronic illnesses representing what has been called the "low triiodothyronine syndrome."

PHARMACOKINETICS

Animal studies have shown that T_4 is only partially absorbed from the gastrointestinal tract. The degree of absorption is dependent on the vehicle used for its administration and by the character of the intestinal contents, the intestinal flora, including plasma protein, soluble dietary factors, all of which bind thyroid and thereby make it unavailable for diffusion.

Depending on other factors, absorption has varied from 48 to 79 percent of the administered dose. Fasting increases absorption. Malabsorption syndromes, as well as dietary factors, (children's soybean formula, concomitant use of anionic exchange resins such as cholestyramine) cause excessive fecal loss.

More than 99 percent of circulating hormones are bound to serum proteins, including thyroxine-binding globulin (TBG), thyroxine-binding prealbumin (TBPA), and albumin (TBa), whose capacities and affinities vary for the hormones. The higher affinity of Levothyroxine (T_4) for both TBG and TBPA as compared to triiodothyronine (T_3) partially explains the higher serum levels and longer half-life of the former hormone. Both protein-bound hormones exist in equilibrium with minute amounts of free hormone, the latter accounting for the metabolic activity.

Deiodination of Levothyroxine (T_4) occurs at a number of sites, including liver, kidney, and other tissues. The conjugated hormone, in the form of glucuronide or sulfate, is found in the bile and gut where it may complete an enterohepatic circulation. Eighty-five percent of Levothyroxine (T_4) metabolized daily is deiodinated.

INDICATIONS AND USAGE

Levothyroxine Sodium is indicated:

1. As replacement or supplemental therapy in patients with hypothyroidism of any etiology, except transient hypothyroidism during the recovery phase of subacute thyroiditis. This category includes cretinism, myxedema, and ordinary hypothyroidism in patients of any age (children, adults, the elderly), or state (including pregnancy); primary hypothyroidism resulting from functional deficiency, primary atrophy, partial or total absence of thyroid gland, or the effects of surgery, radiation, or drugs, with or without the presence of goiter; and secondary (pituitary), or tertiary (hypothalamic) hypothyroidism. (See "Contraindications" and "Precautions".) Levothyroxine Sodium can be used intravenously whenever a rapid onset of effect is critical and either intravenously or intramuscularly in hypothyroid patients whenever the oral route is precluded for long periods of time.

2. As a pituitary TSH suppressant, in the treatment or prevention of various types of euthyroid goiters, including thyroid nodules, subacute or chronic lymphocytic thyroiditis (Hashimoto's), multinodular goiter, and in the management of thyroid cancer.

3. As a diagnostic agent in suppression tests to aid in the diagnosis of suspected mild hyperthyroidism or thyroid gland autonomy.

UNLABELED USES

Levothyroxine Sodium is used in the treatment of Graves' Disease and by intraamniotic administration, to promote fetal maturation. It is also used in the treatment of amenorrhea secondary to hypothalmic function.

CONTRAINDICATIONS

Thyroid hormone preparations are generally contraindicated in patients with diagnosed but as yet uncorrected adrenal cortical insufficiency, untreated thyrotoxicosis, and apparent hypersensitivity to any of their active or extraneous constituents. There is no well documented evidence from the literature, however, of true allergic or idiosyncratic reactions to thyroid hormone.

WARNINGS

> DRUGS WITH THYROID HORMONE ACTIVITY, ALONE OR TOGETHER WITH OTHER THERAPEUTIC AGENTS, HAVE BEEN USED FOR THE TREATMENT OF OBESITY. IN EUTHYROID PATIENTS, DOSES WITHIN THE RANGE OF DAILY HORMONAL REQUIREMENTS ARE INEFFECTIVE FOR WEIGHT REDUCTION. LARGER DOSES MAY PRODUCE SERIOUS OR EVEN LIFE THREATENING MANIFESTATIONS OF TOXICITY, PARTICULARLY WHEN GIVEN IN ASSOCIATION WITH SYMPATHOMIMETIC AMINES SUCH AS THOSE USED FOR THEIR ANORECTIC EFFECTS.

The use of thyroid hormones in the therapy of obesity, alone or combined with other drugs, is unjustified and has been shown to be ineffective. Neither is their use justified for the treatment of male or female infertility unless this condition is accompanied by hypothyroidism.

PRECAUTIONS

General: Thyroid hormones should be used with great caution in a number of circumstances where the integrity of the cardiovascular system, particularly the coronary arteries, is suspected. These include patients with angina pectoris or the elderly, who have a greater likelihood of occult cardiac disease. In these patients, therapy should be initiated with low doses, ie., 25-50 mcg Levothyroxine (T_4). When, in such patients, a euthyroid state can only be reached at the expense of an aggravation of the cardiovascular disease, thyroid hormone dosage should be reduced.

Thyroid hormone therapy in patients with concomitant diabetes mellitus or insipidus or adrenal cortical insufficiency aggravates the intensity of their symptoms. Appropriate adjustments of the various therapeutic measures directed at these concomitant endocrine diseases are required. The therapy of myxedema coma may require simultaneous administration of glucocorticoids (See "Dosage and Administration").

Hypothyroidism decreases and hyperthyroidism increases the sensitivity to oral anticoagulants. Prothrombin time should be closely monitored in thyroid treated patients on oral anticoagulants and dosage of the latter agents adjusted on the basis of frequent prothrombin time determinations. In infants, excessive doses of thyroid hormone preparations may produce craniosynostosis.

Information for the Patient: Patients on thyroid hormone preparations and parents of children on thyroid therapy should be informed that:

1. Replacement therapy is to be taken essentially for life, with the exception of cases of transient hypothyroidism, usually associated with thyroiditis, and in those patients receiving a therapeutic trial of the drug.

2. They should immediately report during the course of therapy any signs or symptoms of thyroid hormone toxicity, e.g., chest pain, increased pulse rate, palpitations, excessive sweating, heat intolerance, nervousness, or any other unusual event.

3. In case of concomitant diabetes mellitus, the daily dosage of antidiabetic medication may need readjustment as thyroid hormone replacement is achieved. If thyroid medication is stopped, a downward readjustment of the dosage of insulin or oral hypoglycemic agent may be necessary to avoid hypoglycemia. At all times, close monitoring of blood or urinary glucose levels is mandatory in such patients.

4. In case of concomitant oral anticoagulant therapy, the prothrombin time should be measured frequently to determine if the dosage of oral anticoagulants is to be readjusted.

5. Partial loss of hair may be experienced by children in the first few months of thyroid therapy, but this is usually a transient phenomenon and later recovery is usually the rule.

Laboratory Tests: Treatment of patients with thyroid hormones requires the periodic assessment of thyroid status by means of appropriate laboratory tests, by full clinical evaluation, or both. The TSH suppression test can be used to test the effectiveness of any thyroid preparation bearing in mind the relative insensitivity of the infant pituitary to the negative feedback effect of thyroid hormones. Serum T_4 levels can be used to test the effectiveness of Levothyroxine Sodium. When the total serum T_4 is low but TSH is normal, a test specific to assess unbound (free) T_4 levels is warranted. Specific measurements of T_4 and T_3 by competitive protein binding or radioimmunoassay are not influenced by blood levels of organic or inorganic iodine and have essentially replaced older tests of thyroid hormone measurements, i.e., PBI, BEI, and T_4 by column.

Drug Interactions: Oral Anticoagulants: Thyroid hormones appear to increase catabolism of vitamin K-dependent clotting factors. If oral anticoagulants are also being given, compensatory increases in clotting factor synthesis are impaired. Patients stabilized on oral anticoagulants who are found to require thyroid replacement therapy should be watched very closely when thyroid is started. If a patient is truly hypothyroid, it is likely that a reduction in anticoagulant dosage will be required. No special precautions appear to be necessary when oral anticoagulant therapy is begun in a patient already stabilized on maintenance thyroid replacement therapy.

Insulin or Oral Hypoglycemics: Initiating thyroid replacement therapy may cause increases in insulin or oral hypoglycemic requirements. The effects seen are poorly understood and depend upon a variety of factors such as dose and type of thyroid preparations and endocrine status of the patient. Patients receiving insulin or oral hypoglycemics should be closely watched during initiation of thyroid replacement therapy.

Cholestyramine: Cholestyramine binds both T_4 and T_3 in the intestine, thus impairing absorption of these thyroid hormones. *In vitro* studies indicate that the binding is not easily reversed. Therefore, four to five hours should elapse between administration of cholestyramine and thyroid hormones.

Estrogen, Oral Contraceptives: Estrogens tend to increase serum thyroxine-binding globulin (TBG). In a patient with a nonfunctioning thyroid gland who is receiving thyroid replacement therapy, free Levothyroxine may be decreased when estrogens are started thus increasing thyroid requirements. However, if the patient's thyroid gland has sufficient function, the decreased free thyroxine will result in a compensatory increase in thyroxine output by the thyroid. Therefore, patients without a functioning thyroid gland who are on thyroid replacement therapy may need to increase their thyroid dose if estogens or estrogen-containing oral contraceptives are given.

Drug/Laboratory Test Interactions: The following drugs or moieties are known to interfere with some laboratory tests performed in patients on thyroid hormone therapy: Androgens, corticosteroids, estrogens, oral contraceptives containing estrogens, iodine-containing preparations, and the numerous preparations containing salicylates.

1. Changes in TBG concentration should be taken into consideration in the interpretation of T_4 and T_3 values. Pregnancy, estrogens, and estrogen-containing oral contraceptives increase TBG concentrations. TBG may also be increased during infectious hepatitis. Decreases in TBG concentrations are observed in nephrosis, acromegaly, and after androgen or corticosteroid therapy. Familial hyper- or hypo-thyroxine-binding-globulinemias have been described. The incidence of TBG deficiency approximates 1 in 9000. The binding of thyroxine by TBPA is inhibited by salicylates. In such cases, the unbound (free) hormone should be measured. Alternatively, an indirect measure of free thyroxine, such as the Free Thyroxine Index (FTI) may be used.

2. Medicinal or dietary iodine interferes with all *in vivo* tests of radioiodine uptake, producing low uptakes which may not indicate a true decrease in hormone synthesis.

3. The persistence of clinical and laboratory evidence of hypothyroidism in spite of adequate dosage replacement indicates either poor patient compliance, poor absorption, or inactivity of the preparation. Intracellular resistance to thyroid hormone is quite rare, and is suggested by clinical signs and symptoms of hypothyroidism in the presence of high serum T_4 levels.

Carcinogenesis, Mutagenesis, and Impairment of Fertility: A reported association between prolonged thyroid therapy and breast cancer has not been confirmed and patients on thyroid therapy for established indications should not discontinue therapy. No confirmatory long-term studies in animals have been performed to evaluate carcinogenic potential, mutagenicity, or impairment of fertility in either males or females.

Pregnancy: Pregnancy category A. Thyroid hormones do not readily cross the placental barrier. The clinical experience to date does not indicate any adverse effect on fetuses when thyroid hormones are administered to pregnant women. On the basis of current knowledge, thyroid replacement therapy to hypothyroid women should not be discontinued during pregnancy.

Nursing Mothers: Minimal amounts of thyroid hormones are excreted in human milk. Thyroid is not associated with serious adverse reactions and does not have known tumorigenic potential. While caution should be exercised when thyroid is administered to a nursing woman, adequate replacement doses of Levothyroxine are generally needed to maintain normal lactation.

Pediatric Use: Pregnant mothers provide little or no thyroid hormone to the fetus. The incidence of congenital hypothyroidism is relatively high (1 in 4,000) and the hypothyroid fetus would not derive any benefit from the small amounts of hormone crossing the placental barrier. Routine determinations of serum T_4 and/or TSH is strongly advised in neonates in view of the deleterious effects of thyroid deficiency on growth and development.

Treatment should be initiated immediately upon diagnosis, and maintained for life, unless transient hypothyroidism is suspected; in which case, therapy may be interrupted for 2 to 8 weeks after the age of 3 years to reassess the condition. Cessation of therapy is justified in patients who have maintained a normal TSH during those 2 to 8 weeks.

ADVERSE REACTIONS

Adverse reactions other than those indicative of hyperthyroidism because of therapeutic overdosage, either initially or during the maintenance periods, are rare (see *"Overdosage"*).

OVERDOSAGE

Signs and Symptoms: Excessive doses of thyroid result in hypermetabolic state resembling in every respect the condition of endogenous origin. The condition may be self-induced.

Treatment of Overdosage: Dosage should be reduced or therapy temporarily discontinued if signs and symptoms of overdosage appear. Treatment may be reinstated at a low dosage. In normal individuals, normal hypothalamic-pituitary-thyroid axis function is restored in 6 to 8 weeks after thyroid suppression.

Treatment of acute massive thyroid hormone overdosage is aimed at reducing gastrointestinal absorption of the drugs and counteracting central and peripheral effects, mainly those of increased sympathetic activity. Vomiting may be induced initially if further gastrointestinal absorption can reasonably be prevented and barring contraindications such as coma, convulsions, or loss of the gagging reflex. Treatment is symptomatic and supportive. Oxygen may be administered and ventilation maintained. Cardiac glycosides may be indicated if congestive heart failure develops. Measures to control fever, hypoglycemia, or fluid loss should be instituted if needed. Antiadrenergic agents, particularly propranolol, have been used advantageously in the treatment of increased sympathetic activity. Propranolol may be administered intravenously at a dosage of 1 to 3 mg over a 10 minute period or orally, 80 to 160 mg/day, especially when no contraindications exist for its use. Other adjunctive measures may include administration of cholestyramine to interfere with thyroxine absorption, and glucocorticoids to inhibit conversion of T_4 to T_3.

DOSAGE AND ADMINISTRATION

The dosage and rate of administration of Levothyroxine Sodium is determined by the indication and must in every case be individualized according to patient response and laboratory findings.

Hypothyroidism: Levothyroxine Sodium tablets are usually instituted using low doses, with increments which depend on the cardiovascular status of the patient. The usual starting dose is 50 mcg, with increments of 25 mcg every 2 to 3 weeks. A lower starting dosage, 25 mcg/day or less, is recommended in patients with long standing hypothyroidism, particularly if cardiovascular impairment is suspected, in which case extreme caution is recommended. The appearance of angina is an indication for a reduction in dosage. Most patients require not more than 200 mcg/day. Failure to respond to doses of 300 mcg suggests lack of compliance or malabsorption. Adequate therapy usually results in normal TSH and T_4 levels after 2 to 3 weeks of the maintenance dose.

Readjustment of Levothyroxine Sodium tablet dosage should be made within the first four weeks of therapy, after proper clinical and laboratory evaluations.

Levothyroxine Sodium injection by intravenous or intramuscular routes can be substituted for the oral dosage form when ingestion of Levothyroxine Sodium tablet is precluded for long periods of time. The initial parenteral dosage should be approximately one half of the previously established oral dosage of Levothyroxine Sodium tablets. Close observation of the patient, with individual adjustment of the dosage as needed, is recommended.

Myxedema Coma: Myxedema coma is usually precipitated in the hypothyroid patient by intercurrent illness or drugs such as sedatives and anesthetics and should be considered a medical emergency. Therapy should be directed at the correction of electrolyte disturbances and possible infection besides the administration of thyroid hormones. Corticosteroids should be administered routinely. T_4 may be administered via a nasogastric tube but the preferred route of administration is intravenous. Sodium Levothyroxine (T_4) is given at a starting dose of 400 mcg (100 mcg/mL) given rapidly, and is usually well tolerated, even in the elderly. In the presence of concomitant heart disease, the sudden administration of such large doses of L-thyroxine intravenously is clearly not without its cardiovascular risks. Under such circumstances, intravenous therapy should not be undertaken without weighing the alternative risks of the myxedema coma and the cardiovascular disease. Clinical judgement in this situation may dictate smaller intravenous doses of Levothyroxine Sodium injection. The initial dose is followed by daily supplements of 100 to 200 mcg given intravenously. Normal T_4 levels are achieved in 24 hours followed in 3 days by three-fold evaluation of T_3. Continued daily administration of lesser amounts parenterally should be maintained until the patient is fully capable of accepting a daily oral dose. A daily maintenance dose of 50 to 100 mcg parenterally should suffice to maintain the euthyroid state, once established. Oral therapy would be resumed as soon as the clinical situation has been stabilized and the patient is able to take oral medication.

TSH Suppression in Thyroid Cancer, Nodules, and Euthyroid Goiters: Exogenous thyroid hormone may produce regression of metastases from follicular and papillary carcinoma of the thyroid and is used as ancillary therapy of these conditions following surgery or radioactive iodine. Medullary carcinoma of the thyroid is usually unresponsive to this therapy. TSH should be suppressed to low or undetectable levels. Therefore, larger amounts of thyroid hormone than those used for replacement therapy are frequently required. This therapy is also used in treating nontoxic solitary nodules and multinodular goiters, and to prevent thyroid enlargement in chronic (Hashimoto's) thyroiditis.

Thyroid Suppression Therapy: Administration of thyroid hormone in doses higher than those produced physiologically by the gland results in suppression of the production of endogenous hormone. This is the basis for the thyroid suppression

---

◆ RATED THERAPEUTICALLY EQUIVALENT; ◇ THERAPEUTIC EQUIVALENCE UNCONFIRMED; ○ UNRATED

test and is used as an aid in the diagnosis of patients with signs of mild hyperthyroidism in whom base line laboratory tests appear normal, or to demonstrate thyroid gland autonomy in patients with Graves' ophthalmopathy. [131]I uptake is determined before and after the administration of the exogenous hormone. A fifty percent or greater suppression of uptake indicates a normal thyroid-pituitary axis and thus rules out thyroid gland autonomy.

For adults, the average suppressive dose of Levothyroxine (T_4) is 2.6 mcg/kg of body weight per day given for 7 to 10 days. These doses usually yield normal serum T_4 and T_3 levels and lack of response to TSH.

Levothyroxine Sodium should be administered cautiously to patients in whom there is a strong suspicion of thyroid gland autonomy, in view of the fact that the exogenous hormone effects will be additive to the endogenous source.

Pediatric Dosage: Pediatric dosage should follow the recommendations summarized in Table 1. In infants with congenital hypothyroidism, therapy with full doses should be instituted as soon as the diagnosis has been made. Levothyroxine Sodium tablets may be given to infants and children who cannot swallow intact tablets by crushing the proper dose tablet and suspending the *freshly crushed* tablet in a small amount of water or formula. The suspension can be given by spoon or dropper. DO NOT STORE THE SUSPENSION FOR ANY PERIOD OF TIME. The crushed tablet may also be sprinkled over a small amount of food, such as cooked cereal or apple sauce.

Table 1
RECOMMENDED PEDIATRIC DOSAGE FOR CONGENITAL HYPOTHYROIDISM*

| Age | *Levothyroxine Sodium tablets* | |
	Dose per day	*Daily dose per kg of body weight*
0- 6 mos	25- 50 mcg	8-10 mcg
6-12 mos	50- 75 mcg	6- 8 mcg
1- 5 yrs	75-100 mcg	5- 6 mcg
6-12 yrs	100-150 mcg	4- 5 mcg

* *To be adjusted on the basis of clinical response and laboratory tests (see Laboratory Tests).*

STORAGE
Store at controlled room temperature 15°-30°C (59°-86°F).

DIRECTIONS FOR RECONSTITUTION
Reconstitute the lyophilized Levothyroxine Sodium by aseptically adding 5 mL of 0.9% Sodium Chloride Injection, USP or Bacteriostatic Sodium Chloride Injection, USP with Benzyl Alcohol, only. Shake vial to insure complete mixing. *Use immediately* after reconstitution. Do not add to other intravenous fluids. Discard any unused portion.

HOW SUPPLIED
POWDER: 200 MCG

BRAND/MANUFACTURER	NDC	SIZE	AWP
○ GENERICS			
VHA	00702-0880-10	1s	$7.38

POWDER: 500 MCG

BRAND/MANUFACTURER	NDC	SIZE	AWP
○ GENERICS			
VHA	00702-0881-10	1s	$7.38

POWDER FOR INJECTION: 200 MCG

BRAND/MANUFACTURER	NDC	SIZE	AWP
○ BRAND			
SYNTHROID: Boots Pharm	00048-1014-99	1s	$45.24
LEVOTHROID: Forest Pharm	00456-0140-88	1s	$62.56
○ GENERICS			
Gensia	00703-5408-01	1s	$17.19
Schein	00364-2248-54	1s	$17.25
Steris	00402-0835-10	1s	$17.25
UDL	51079-0706-01	1s ud	$12.69

POWDER FOR INJECTION: 500 MCG

BRAND/MANUFACTURER	NDC	SIZE	AWP
○ BRAND			
SYNTHROID: Boots Pharm	00048-1012-99	1s	$49.80
LEVOTHROID: Forest Pharm	00456-0141-88	1s	$89.50
○ GENERICS			
Steris	00402-0732-10	1s	$17.48
Schein	00364-6772-54	1s	$17.48
Fujisawa	00469-2471-30	1s	$42.56
Fujisawa	00469-2481-30	1s	$46.80
UDL	51079-0707-01	1s ud	$12.69

TABLETS:

BRAND/MANUFACTURER	NDC	SIZE	AWP
○ GENERICS			
Ampharco	59015-0833-64	100s	$8.00
Ampharco	59015-0833-65	500s	$33.00

TABLETS: 0.025 MG

BRAND/MANUFACTURER	NDC	SIZE	AWP
○ BRAND			
➤ LEVOTHROID: Forest Pharm	00456-0320-01	100s	$14.50
➤ SYNTHROID: Boots Pharm	00048-1020-03	100s	$16.68
	00048-1020-05	1000s	$141.42
○ GENERICS			
➤ LEVOXYL: Daniels	00689-1117-01	100s	$6.40
Caremark	00339-5923-12	100s	$6.40
Jerome Stevens	50564-0513-01	100s	$10.50
Duramed	51285-0860-02	100s	$11.86
Warner Chilcott	00047-0334-24	100s	$12.30
➤ LEVOXYL: Daniels	00689-1117-05	100s ud	$8.88
Vintage	00254-3911-38	1000s	$19.86
Qualitest	00603-4192-32	1000s	$19.86
Moore,H.L.	00839-7672-16	1000s	$28.07
Moore,H.L.	00839-7823-16	1000s	$28.07
Jerome Stevens	50564-0513-10	1000s	$31.50
Rugby	00536-5503-10	1000s	$38.55
Rugby	00536-5684-10	1000s	$38.55
➤ LEVOXYL: Daniels	00689-1117-10	1000s	$56.17
LEVOTABS: Pecos	59879-0201-10	1000s	$57.00
Duramed	51285-0860-05	1000s	$101.06
Goldline	00182-1529-10	1000s	$101.06

TABLETS: 0.05 MG

BRAND/MANUFACTURER	NDC	SIZE	AWP
○ BRAND			
➤ LEVOTHROID: Forest Pharm	00456-0321-01	100s	$16.28
➤ SYNTHROID: Boots Pharm	00048-1040-03	100s	$18.84
➤ LEVOTHROID: Forest Pharm	00456-0321-63	100s ud	$16.28
➤ SYNTHROID: Boots Pharm	00048-1040-13	100s ud	$20.04
	00048-1040-05	1000s	$158.10
○ GENERICS			
Allscrips	54569-3766-00	30s	$1.36
Southwood	58016-0645-00	100s	$4.64
➤ LEVOXYL: Daniels	00689-1118-01	100s	$7.23
Caremark	00339-5925-12	100s	$7.23
Jerome Stevens	50564-0514-01	100s	$10.70
Duramed	51285-0861-02	100s	$13.38
Warner Chilcott	00047-0336-24	100s	$13.80
➤ LEVOXYL: Daniels	00689-1118-05	100s ud	$9.70
Vintage	00254-3912-38	1000s	$20.15
Qualitest	00603-4193-32	1000s	$20.15
Moore,H.L.	00839-7673-16	1000s	$28.34
Moore,H.L.	00839-7824-16	1000s	$28.34
Jerome Stevens	50564-0514-10	1000s	$36.56
Rugby	00536-5504-10	1000s	$41.40
Rugby	00536-5685-10	1000s	$41.40
LEVOTABS: Pecos	59879-0202-10	1000s	$57.20
➤ LEVOXYL: Daniels	00689-1118-10	1000s	$60.22
Duramed	51285-0861-05	1000s	$113.01
Goldline	00182-1511-10	1000s	$113.01

TABLETS: 0.075 MG

BRAND/MANUFACTURER	NDC	SIZE	AWP
○ BRAND			
➤ LEVOTHROID: Forest Pharm	00456-0322-01	100s	$18.08
➤ SYNTHROID: Boots Pharm	00048-1050-03	100s	$20.88
	00048-1050-13	100s ud	$22.44
	00048-1050-05	1000s	$176.22
○ GENERICS			
Southwood	58016-0185-00	100s	$4.74
➤ LEVOXYL: Daniels	00689-1119-01	100s	$8.00
Caremark	00339-5927-12	100s	$8.00
Jerome Stevens	50564-0515-01	100s	$10.85
Duramed	51285-0862-02	100s	$14.92
Warner Chilcott	00047-0338-24	100s	$15.35
➤ LEVOXYL: Daniels	00689-1119-05	100s ud	$10.50
Vintage	00254-3913-38	1000s	$20.35
Qualitest	00603-4194-32	1000s	$20.35
Moore,H.L.	00839-7674-16	1000s	$28.47
Moore,H.L.	00839-7825-16	1000s	$28.47
Jerome Stevens	50564-0515-10	1000s	$41.15
Rugby	00536-5505-10	1000s	$44.25
Rugby	00536-5686-10	1000s	$44.25
LEVOTABS: Pecos	59879-0203-10	1000s	$57.40
➤ LEVOXYL: Daniels	00689-1119-10	1000s	$67.77
Duramed	51285-0862-05	1000s	$126.00
Goldline	00182-1527-10	1000s	$126.00

➤ SHOWN IN PRODUCT IDENTIFICATION GUIDE

TABLETS: 0.088 MG

BRAND/MANUFACTURER	NDC	SIZE	AWP
○ **BRAND**			
➤ LEVOTHROID: Forest Pharm	00456-0329-01	100s	$18.53
➤ SYNTHROID: Boots Pharm	00048-1060-03	100s	$21.24
○ **GENERICS**			
➤ LEVOXYL: Daniels	00689-1132-01	100s	$8.13
➤ LEVOXYL: Daniels	00689-1132-05	100s ud	$10.60
➤ LEVOXYL: Daniels	00689-1132-10	1000s	$68.75

TABLETS: 0.1 MG

BRAND/MANUFACTURER	NDC	SIZE	AWP
○ **BRAND**			
➤ LEVOTHROID: Forest Pharm	00456-0323-01	100s	$18.56
➤ SYNTHROID: Boots Pharm	00048-1070-03	100s	$21.42
➤ LEVOTHROID: Forest Pharm	00456-0323-63	100s ud	$18.56
➤ SYNTHROID: Boots Pharm	00048-1070-13	100s ud	$23.16
	00048-1070-05	1000s	$181.68
○ **GENERICS**			
Allscrips	54569-0913-01	30s	$1.28
Pharm Corp/America	51655-0091-24	30s	$2.15
Southwood	58016-0931-30	30s	$4.86
Southwood	58016-0931-50	50s	$5.62
Pharm Corp/America	51655-0091-21	100s	$3.05
Allscrips	54569-7078-00	100s	$4.19
Allscrips	54569-0913-00	100s	$4.27
Southwood	58016-0931-00	100s	$6.40
➤ LEVOXYL: Daniels	00689-1110-01	100s	$8.25
Caremark	00339-5579-12	100s	$8.25
Rosemont	00832-0076-00	100s	$10.00
Jerome Stevens	50564-0516-01	100s	$11.05
Warner Chilcott	00047-0341-24	100s	$15.71
Duramed	51285-0863-02	100s	$16.68
R.I.D.	54807-0760-01	100s	$17.25
Auro	55829-0345-10	100s ud	$5.63
Major	00904-2236-61	100s ud	$6.62
U.S. Trading	56126-0468-11	100s ud	$9.75
➤ LEVOXYL: Daniels	00689-1110-05	100s ud	$10.70
Allscrips	54569-0913-02	200s	$7.50
Veratex	17022-5131-06	1000s	$15.95
Vintage	00254-3914-38	1000s	$20.75
Qualitest	00603-4195-32	1000s	$20.75
Goldline	00182-0638-10	1000s	$22.50
Truxton	00463-6299-10	1000s	$25.20
Rosemont	00832-0076-10	1000s	$27.00
Moore,H.L.	00839-7675-16	1000s	$28.74
Moore,H.L.	00839-7826-16	1000s	$28.74
Jerome Stevens	50564-0516-10	1000s	$32.00
Major	00904-2236-80	1000s	$34.25
Aligen	00405-4581-03	1000s	$39.85
➤ L-THYROXIN: Geneva	00781-1905-10	1000s	$41.90
URL	00677-0078-10	1000s	$42.00
➤ Rugby	00536-3952-10	1000s	$42.75
Parmed	00349-2062-10	1000s	$43.30
LEVOTABS: Pecos	59879-0204-10	1000s	$57.60
➤ LEVOXYL: Daniels	00689-1110-10	1000s	$69.75
Duramed	51285-0863-05	1000s	$142.56
Goldline	00182-1116-10	1000s	$142.56
Warner Chilcott	00047-0341-32	1000s	$162.01

TABLETS: 0.112 MG

BRAND/MANUFACTURER	NDC	SIZE	AWP
○ **BRAND**			
➤ LEVOTHROID: Forest Pharm	00456-0330-01	100s	$21.65
➤ SYNTHROID: Boots Pharm	00048-1080-03	100s	$24.84
	00048-1080-05	1000s	$210.78
○ **GENERICS**			
➤ LEVOXYL: Daniels	00689-1130-01	100s	$8.95
➤ LEVOXYL: Daniels	00689-1130-05	100s ud	$11.42
➤ LEVOXYL: Daniels	00689-1130-10	1000s	$73.28

TABLETS: 0.125 MG

BRAND/MANUFACTURER	NDC	SIZE	AWP
○ **BRAND**			
➤ LEVOTHROID: Forest Pharm	00456-0324-01	100s	$21.73
➤ SYNTHROID: Boots Pharm	00048-1130-03	100s	$25.02
➤ LEVOTHROID: Forest Pharm	00456-0324-63	100s ud	$21.73
➤ SYNTHROID: Boots Pharm	00048-1130-13	100s ud	$27.00
	00048-1130-05	1000s	$211.44
○ **GENERICS**			
Allscrips	54569-3767-00	30s	$1.69
Rugby	00536-5506-10	60s	$47.55
Southwood	58016-0644-00	100s	$5.64
➤ LEVOXYL: Daniels	00689-1120-01	100s	$9.60
Caremark	00339-5929-12	100s	$9.60
Jerome Stevens	50564-0519-01	100s	$12.10
Duramed	51285-0864-02	100s	$18.03
Warner Chilcott	00047-0343-24	100s	$18.33
➤ LEVOXYL: Daniels	00689-1120-05	100s ud	$12.08

BRAND/MANUFACTURER	NDC	SIZE	AWP
Moore,H.L.	00839-7676-16	1000s	$32.79
Moore,H.L.	00839-7827-16	1000s	$32.79
L-THYROXIN: Geneva	00781-1088-10	1000s	$43.56
Jerome Stevens	50564-0519-10	1000s	$46.66
LEVOTABS: Pecos	59879-0205-10	1000s	$66.60
➤ LEVOXYL: Daniels	00689-1120-10	1000s	$76.85
Duramed	51285-0864-05	1000s	$153.04
Goldline	00182-1516-10	1000s	$153.04

TABLETS: 0.137 MG

BRAND/MANUFACTURER	NDC	SIZE	AWP
○ **GENERICS**			
LEVOXYL: Daniels	00689-1135-01	100s	$9.73
LEVOXYL: Daniels	00689-1135-05	100s ud	$12.22
LEVOXYL: Daniels	00689-1135-10	1000s	$80.38

TABLETS: 0.15 MG

BRAND/MANUFACTURER	NDC	SIZE	AWP
○ **BRAND**			
➤ LEVOTHROID: Forest Pharm	00456-0325-01	100s	$22.40
➤ SYNTHROID: Boots Pharm	00048-1090-03	100s	$25.80
➤ LEVOTHROID: Forest Pharm	00456-0325-63	100s ud	$22.40
➤ SYNTHROID: Boots Pharm	00048-1090-13	100s ud	$27.66
	00048-1090-05	1000s	$218.16
○ **GENERICS**			
Allscrips	54569-1753-01	30s	$1.53
Pharm Corp/America	51655-0209-21	100s	$3.15
Allscrips	54569-1753-00	100s	$5.09
Southwood	58016-0984-00	100s	$6.75
➤ LEVOXYL: Daniels	00689-1111-01	100s	$9.87
Caremark	00339-5813-12	100s	$9.87
Jerome Stevens	50564-0520-01	100s	$12.25
Rosemont	00832-0082-00	100s	$13.40
Duramed	51285-0865-02	100s	$20.34
Warner Chilcott	00047-0344-24	100s	$22.39
➤ LEVOXYL: Daniels	00689-1111-05	100s ud	$12.35
Vintage	00254-3915-38	1000s	$24.56
Qualitest	00603-4196-32	1000s	$24.56
Goldline	00182-1829-10	1000s	$27.00
Moore,H.L.	00839-7679-16	1000s	$33.87
Moore,H.L.	00839-7828-16	1000s	$33.87
Jerome Stevens	50564-0520-10	1000s	$37.95
Major	00904-2234-80	1000s	$38.95
Parmed	00349-8414-10	1000s	$38.97
➤ L-THYROXIN: Geneva	00781-1908-10	1000s	$45.11
Aligen	00405-4582-03	1000s	$46.57
Rosemont	00832-0082-10	1000s	$48.00
URL	00677-0992-10	1000s	$49.00
➤ Rugby	00536-4380-10	1000s	$51.30
LEVOTABS: Pecos	59879-0206-10	1000s	$67.40
➤ LEVOXYL: Daniels	00689-1111-10	1000s	$83.90
Warner Chilcott	00047-0344-32	1000s	$151.80
Duramed	51285-0865-05	1000s	$173.06
Goldline	00182-1117-10	1000s	$173.06

TABLETS: 0.175 MG

BRAND/MANUFACTURER	NDC	SIZE	AWP
○ **BRAND**			
➤ LEVOTHROID: Forest Pharm	00456-0326-01	100s	$26.63
➤ SYNTHROID: Boots Pharm	00048-1100-03	100s	$30.66
○ **GENERICS**			
➤ LEVOXYL: Daniels	00689-1122-01	100s	$10.90
➤ LEVOXYL: Daniels	00689-1122-05	100s ud	$13.40
➤ LEVOXYL: Daniels	00689-1122-10	1000s	$95.58

TABLETS: 0.2 MG

BRAND/MANUFACTURER	NDC	SIZE	AWP
○ **BRAND**			
➤ LEVOTHROID: Forest Pharm	00456-0327-01	100s	$26.81
➤ SYNTHROID: Boots Pharm	00048-1140-03	100s	$30.84
➤ LEVOTHROID: Forest Pharm	00456-0327-63	100s ud	$26.81
➤ SYNTHROID: Boots Pharm	00048-1140-13	100s ud	$33.30
	00048-1140-05	1000s	$261.24
○ **GENERICS**			
Allscrips	54569-0914-02	30s	$1.68
Southwood	58016-0932-30	30s	$5.60
Pharm Corp/America	51655-0477-01	100s	$3.30
Allscrips	54569-0914-01	100s	$5.59
Southwood	58016-0932-00	100s	$7.57
➤ LEVOXYL: Daniels	00689-1112-01	100s	$11.87
Caremark	00339-5815-12	100s	$11.87
Jerome Stevens	50564-0522-01	100s	$14.70
Rosemont	00832-0077-00	100s	$15.60
Warner Chilcott	00047-0347-24	100s	$22.36
Duramed	51285-0866-02	100s	$24.54
R.I.D.	54807-0761-01	100s	$24.79
Auro	55829-0344-10	100s ud	$7.28
Major	00904-2237-61	100s ud	$7.37
U.S. Trading	56126-0451-11	100s ud	$13.01

◆ RATED THERAPEUTICALLY EQUIVALENT; ◇ THERAPEUTIC EQUIVALENCE UNCONFIRMED; ○ UNRATED

BRAND/MANUFACTURER	NDC	SIZE	AWP
➤ LEVOXYL: Daniels	00689-1112-05	100s ud	$14.33
Veratex	17022-5152-06	1000s	$18.75
Vintage	00254-3916-38	1000s	$27.40
Qualitest	00603-4197-32	1000s	$27.40
Truxton	00463-6300-10	1000s	$30.00
Goldline	00182-0639-10	1000s	$31.50
Moore,H.L.	00839-7677-16	1000s	$34.95
Moore,H.L.	00839-7829-16	1000s	$34.95
Jerome Stevens	50564-0522-10	1000s	$39.20
Major	00904-2237-80	1000s	$41.95
Parmed	00349-8291-10	1000s	$43.86
Rosemont	00832-0077-10	1000s	$49.00
Aligen	00405-4583-03	1000s	$49.50
URL	00677-0079-10	1000s	$50.85
➤ Rugby	00536-4381-10	1000s	$50.85
➤ L-THYROXIN: Geneva	00781-1910-10	1000s	$51.25
Allscrips	54569-0914-00	1000s	$55.93
➤ LEVOTABS: Pecos	59879-0207-10	1000s	$69.20
LEVOXYL: Daniels	00689-1112-10	1000s	$100.45
Warner Chilcott	00047-0347-32	1000s	$183.75
Duramed	51285-0866-05	1000s	$207.31
Goldline	00182-1118-10	1000s	$207.31

TABLETS: 0.3 MG

BRAND/MANUFACTURER	NDC	SIZE	AWP
○ BRAND			
➤ LEVOTHROID: Forest Pharm	00456-0328-01	100s	$36.29
➤ SYNTHROID: Boots Pharm	00048-1170-03	100s	$41.76
➤ LEVOTHROID: Forest Pharm	00456-0328-63	100s ud	$36.29
➤ SYNTHROID: Boots Pharm	00048-1170-05	1000s	$353.04
○ GENERICS			
Allscrips	54569-1644-00	100s	$5.72
Jerome Stevens	50564-0523-01	100s	$15.40
➤ LEVOXYL: Daniels	00689-1121-01	100s	$15.98
Caremark	00339-5817-12	100s	$15.98
Rosemont	00832-0078-00	100s	$17.00
Warner Chilcott	00047-0348-24	100s	$30.33
Duramed	51285-0867-02	100s	$33.56
Auro	55829-0347-10	100s ud	$9.22
➤ LEVOXYL: Daniels	00689-1121-01	100s ud	$18.33
URL	00677-0769-10	1000s	$25.52
Vintage	00254-3917-28	1000s	$29.36
Qualitest	00603-4198-32	1000s	$29.36
Goldline	00182-1498-10	1000s	$36.00
Moore,H.L.	00839-7678-16	1000s	$36.44
Moore,H.L.	00839-7830-16	1000s	$36.44
Jerome Stevens	50564-0523-10	1000s	$40.95
Major	00904-2235-80	1000s	$44.65
Rosemont	00832-0078-10	1000s	$52.00
➤ Rugby	00536-3958-10	1000s	$53.25
Aligen	00405-4584-03	1000s	$53.49
➤ L-THYROXIN: Geneva	00781-1913-10	1000s	$54.50
LEVOTABS: Pecos	59879-0208-10	1000s	$71.80
➤ LEVOXYL: Daniels	00689-1121-10	1000s	$135.70
Duramed	51285-0867-05	1000s	$283.18
Goldline	00182-1119-10	1000s	$283.18

TABLETS: 0.5 MG

BRAND/MANUFACTURER	NDC	SIZE	AWP
○ GENERICS			
L-THYROXIN: Geneva	00781-1074-10	1000s	$32.57

TABLETS: 25 MCG

BRAND/MANUFACTURER	NDC	SIZE	AWP
○ GENERICS			
➤ LEVO-T: Lederle Std Prod	00205-3610-43	100s	$12.74

TABLETS: 50 MCG

BRAND/MANUFACTURER	NDC	SIZE	AWP
○ GENERICS			
ELTROXIN: Roberts Pharm	54092-0105-01	100s	$10.48
➤ LEVO-T: Lederle Std Prod	00205-3611-43	100s	$14.31
➤ LEVO-T: Lederle Std Prod	00205-3611-34	1000s	$120.90

TABLETS: 75 MCG

BRAND/MANUFACTURER	NDC	SIZE	AWP
○ GENERICS			
➤ LEVO-T: Lederle Std Prod	00205-3612-43	100s	$15.90

TABLETS: 100 MCG

BRAND/MANUFACTURER	NDC	SIZE	AWP
○ GENERICS			
ELTROXIN: Roberts Pharm	54092-0108-01	100s	$11.98
➤ LEVO-T: Lederle Std Prod	00205-3613-43	100s	$16.31
ELTROXIN: Roberts Pharm	54092-0108-05	500s	$55.11

BRAND/MANUFACTURER	NDC	SIZE	AWP
➤ LEVO-T: Lederle Std Prod	00205-3613-34	1000s	$138.95

TABLETS: 125 MCG

BRAND/MANUFACTURER	NDC	SIZE	AWP
○ GENERICS			
➤ LEVO-T: Lederle Std Prod	00205-3614-43	100s	$19.10

TABLETS: 137 MCG

BRAND/MANUFACTURER	NDC	SIZE	AWP
○ BRAND			
➤ LEVOTHROID: Forest Pharm	00456-0331-01	100s	$22.08

TABLETS: 150 MCG

BRAND/MANUFACTURER	NDC	SIZE	AWP
○ GENERICS			
ELTROXIN: Roberts Pharm	54092-0112-01	100s	$14.37
➤ LEVO-T: Lederle Std Prod	00205-3615-43	100s	$19.69
➤ LEVO-T: Lederle Std Prod	00205-3615-34	1000s	$166.84

TABLETS: 200 MCG

BRAND/MANUFACTURER	NDC	SIZE	AWP
○ GENERICS			
ELTROXIN: Roberts Pharm	54092-0113-01	100s	$17.25
➤ LEVO-T: Lederle Std Prod	00205-3616-43	100s	$23.58
➤ LEVO-T: Lederle Std Prod	00205-3616-34	1000s	$199.84

TABLETS: 300 MCG

BRAND/MANUFACTURER	NDC	SIZE	AWP
○ GENERICS			
ELTROXIN: Roberts Pharm	54092-0114-01	100s	$23.24
➤ LEVO-T: Lederle Std Prod	00205-3617-43	100s	$31.90

Levsin SEE HYOSCYAMINE SULFATE

Levsin with Phenobarbital
SEE HYOSCYAMINE SULFATE AND PHENOBARBITAL

Levsinex SEE HYOSCYAMINE SULFATE

Librax SEE CHLORDIAZEPOXIDE HYDROCHLORIDE WITH CLIDINIUM BROMIDE

Libritabs SEE CHLORDIAZEPOXIDE

Librium SEE CHLORDIAZEPOXIDE

Lida-Mantle-HC SEE HYDROCORTISONE ACETATE WITH LIDOCAINE

Lidex SEE FLUOCINONIDE

Lidocaine Hydrochloride and Oxytetracycline

DESCRIPTION

Oxytetracycline is a product of the metabolism of *Streptomyces rimosus* and is one of the family of tetracycline antibiotics. Oxytetracycline diffuses readily through the placenta into the fetal circulation, into the pleural fluid and, under some circumstances, into the cerebrospinal fluid. It appears to be concentrated in the hepatic system and excreted in the bile, so that it appears in the feces, as well as in the urine, in a biologically active form.

➤ SHOWN IN PRODUCT IDENTIFICATION GUIDE

COMPOSITION

Lidocaine Hydrochloride/Oxytetracycline Intramuscular Solution is available for *Intramuscular Use Only.*

Each mL contains:

Oxytetracycline ....50 mg or 125 mg
Lidocaine Hydrochloride ....2% w/v

ACTIONS

Lidocaine HCl/Oxytetracycline is primarily bacteriostatic and is thought to exert its antimicrobial effect by the inhibition of protein synthesis. Lidocaine HCl/Oxytetracycline is active against a wide range of gram-negative and gram-positive organisms.

The drugs in the tetracycline class have closely similar antimicrobial spectra, and cross resistance among them is common. Microorganisms may be considered susceptible if the M.I.C. (minimum inhibitory concentration) is not more than 4.0 mcg/ml and intermediate if the M.I.C. is 4.0 to 12.5 mcg/ml.

Susceptibility plate testing: A tetracycline disc may be used to determine microbial susceptibility to drugs in the tetracycline class. If the Kirby-Bauer method of disc susceptibility testing is used, a 30 mcg tetracycline disc should give a zone of at least 19 mm when tested against an oxytetracycline-susceptible bacterial strain.

Tetracyclines are readily absorbed and are bound to plasma proteins in varying degree. They are concentrated by the liver in the bile and excreted in the urine and feces at high concentrations and in a biologically active form.

INDICATIONS

Lidocaine HCl/Oxytetracycline is indicated in infections caused by the following microorganisms:

Rickettsiae (Rocky Mountain spotted fever, typhus fever and the typhus group, Q fever, rickettsialpox and tick fevers).

Mycoplasma pneumoniae (PPLO, Eaton Agent),

Agents of psittacosis and ornithosis,

Agents of lymphogranuloma venereum and granuloma inguinale,

The spirochetal agent of relapsing fever *(Borrelia recurrentis).*

The following gram-negative microorganisms:

Haemophilus ducreyi (chancroid),

Pasteurella pestis, and *Pasteurella tularensis,*

Bartonella bacilliformis,

Bacteroides species,

Vibrio comma and *Vibrio fetus,*

Brucella species (in conjunction with streptomycin).

Because many strains of the following groups of microorganisms have been shown to be resistant to tetracyclines, culture and susceptibility testing are recommended.

Lidocaine HCl/Oxytetracycline is indicated for treatment of infections caused by the following gram-negative microorganisms, when bacteriologic testing indicates appropriate susceptibility to the drug:

Escherichia coli,

Enterobacter aerogenes (formerly *Aerobacter aerogenes*),

Shigella species,

Mima species and *Herellea* species,

Haemophilus influenzae (respiratory infections),

Klebsiella species (respiratory and urinary infections).

Lidocaine HCl/Oxytetracycline is indicated for treatment of infections caused by the following gram-positive microorganisms when bacteriologic testing indicates appropriate susceptibility to the drug:

Streptococcus species:

Up to 44 percent of strains of *Streptococcus pyogenes* and 74 percent of *Streptococcus faecalis* have been found to be resistant to tetracycline drugs. Therefore, tetracyclines should not be used for streptococcal disease unless the organism has been demonstrated to be sensitive.

For upper respiratory infections due to Group A beta-hemolytic streptococci, penicillin is the usual drug of choice, including prophylaxis of rheumatic fever.

Diplococcus pneumoniae,

Staphylococcus aureus, skin and soft tissue infections. Oxytetracycline is not the drug of choice in the treatment of any type of staphylococcal infections.

When penicillin is contraindicated, tetracyclines are alternative drugs in the treatment of infections due to:

Neisseria gonorrhoeae,

Treponema pallidum and *Treponema pertenue* (syphilis and yaws),

Listeria monocytogenes,

Clostridium species,

Bacillus anthracis,

Fusobacterium fusiforme (Vincent's infection),

Actinomyces species.

In acute intestinal amebiasis, the tetracyclines may be a useful adjunct to amebicides.

Tetracyclines are indicated in the treatment of trachoma, although the infectious agent is not always eliminated, as judged by immunofluorescence.

Inclusion conjunctivitis may be treated with oral tetracyclines or with a combination of oral and topical agents.

CONTRAINDICATIONS

This drug is contraindicated in persons who have shown hypersensitivity to any of the tetracyclines.

WARNINGS

THE USE OF TETRACYCLINES DURING TOOTH DEVELOPMENT (LAST HALF OF PREGNANCY, INFANCY, AND CHILDHOOD TO THE AGE OF 8 YEARS) MAY CAUSE PERMANENT DISCOLORATION OF THE TEETH (YELLOW-GRAY-BROWN). This adverse reaction is more common during long-term use of the drugs, but has been observed following repeated short-term courses. Enamel hypoplasia has also been reported. *Tetracyclines, therefore, should not be used in this age group unless other drugs are not likely to be effective or are contraindicated.*

If renal impairment exists, even usual oral or parenteral doses may lead to excessive systemic accumulation of the drug and possible liver toxicity. Under such conditions, lower than usual total doses are indicated and, if therapy is prolonged, serum level determinations of the drug may be advisable. This hazard is of particular importance in the parenteral administration of tetracyclines to pregnant or postpartum patients with pyelonephritis. When used under these circumstances, the blood level should not exceed 15 mcg/ml and liver function tests should be made at frequent intervals. Other potentially hepatotoxic drugs should not be prescribed concomitantly.

(In the presence of renal dysfunction, particularly in pregnancy, intravenous tetracycline therapy in daily doses exceeding 2 grams has been associated with deaths due to liver failure.)

Photosensitivity manifested by an exaggerated sunburn reaction has been observed in some individuals taking tetracyclines. Patients apt to be exposed to direct sunlight or ultraviolet light should be advised that this reaction can occur with tetracycline drugs, and treatment should be discontinued at the first evidence of skin erythema.

The antianabolic action of the tetracyclines may cause an increase in BUN. While this is not a problem in those with normal renal function, in patients with significantly impaired function, higher serum levels of this drug may lead to azotemia, hyperphosphatemia, and acidosis.

The parenteral product may contain sodium formaldehyde sulfoxylate which serves as an antioxidant. Upon oxidation, this compound can form a potential sulfiting agent. Sulfiting agents may cause allergic-type reactions including anaphylactic symptoms and life-threatening or less severe asthmatic episodes in certain susceptible people. The over-all prevalence of sulfite sensitivity in the general population is unknown and probably low. Sulfite sensitivity is seen more frequently in asthmatic than in nonasthmatic people.

Usage in Pregnancy: (See above *"Warning"* about use during tooth development.)

Results of animal studies indicate that tetracyclines cross the placenta, are found in fetal tissues and can have toxic effects on the developing fetus (often related to retardation of skeletal development). Evidence of embryotoxicity has also been noted in animals treated early in pregnancy.

Usage in newborns, infants, and children: (See above *"Warnings"* about use during tooth development.)

All tetracyclines form a stable calcium complex in any bone-forming tissue. A decrease in the fibula growth rate has been observed in prematures given oral tetracycline in doses of 25 mg/kg every 6 hours. This reaction was shown to be reversible when the drug was discontinued.

Tetracyclines are present in the milk of lactating women who are taking a drug in this class.

PRECAUTIONS

As with all intramuscular preparations, Lidocaine HCl/Oxytetracycline for intramuscular use should be injected well within the body of a relatively large muscle.

Adults: The preferred sites are the upper, outer quadrant of the buttock, (i.e., gluteus maximus), and the mid-lateral thigh.

Children: It is recommended that intramuscular injections be given preferably in the mid-lateral muscles of the thigh. In infants and small children the periphery of the upper-outer quadrant of the gluteal region should be used only when necessary, such as in burn patients, in order to minimize the possibility of damage to the sciatic nerve.

The deltoid area should be used only if well developed such as in certain adults and older children, and then only with caution to avoid radial nerve injury. Intramuscular injections should not be made into the lower and mid-thirds of the upper arm. As with all intramuscular injections, aspiration is necessary to help avoid inadvertent injection into a blood vessel.

As with other antibiotic preparations, use of this drug may result in overgrowth of nonsusceptible organisms, including fungi. If superinfection occurs, the antibiotic should be discontinued and appropriate therapy instituted.

In venereal diseases when coexistent syphilis is suspected, a dark field examination should be done before treatment is started and the blood serology repeated monthly for at least 4 months.

Because tetracyclines have been shown to depress plasma prothrombin activity, patients who are on anticoagulant therapy may require downward adjustment of their anticoagulant dosage.

In long term therapy, periodic laboratory evaluation of organ systems, including hematopoietic, renal and hepatic studies should be performed.

All infections due to Group A beta-hemolytic streptococci should be treated for at least 10 days.

Since bacteriostatic drugs may interfere with the bactericidal action of penicillin, it is advisable to avoid giving tetracycline in conjunction with penicillin.

◆ RATED THERAPEUTICALLY EQUIVALENT; ◇ THERAPEUTIC EQUIVALENCE UNCONFIRMED; ○ UNRATED

ADVERSE REACTIONS

Local irritation may be present after intramuscular injection. The injection should be deep, with care taken not to injure the sciatic nerve nor inject intravascularly.

Gastrointestinal: anorexia, nausea, vomiting, diarrhea, glossitis, dysphagia, enterocolitis, and inflammatory lesions (with monilial overgrowth) in the anogenital region. These reactions have been caused by both the oral and parenteral administration of tetracyclines.

Skin: maculopapular and erythematous rashes. Exfoliative dermatitis has been reported but is uncommon. Photosensitivity is discussed above. (See "Warnings").

Renal toxicity: Rise in BUN has been reported and is apparently dose related. (See "Warning").

Hypersensitivity reactions: Urticaria, angioneurotic edema, anaphylaxis, anaphylactoid purpura, pericarditis, and exacerbation of systemic lupus erythematosus.

Bulging fontanels in infants and benign intracranial hypertension in adults have been reported in individuals receiving full therapeutic dosages. These conditions disappeared rapidly when the drug was discontinued.

Blood: Hemolytic anemia, thrombocytopenia, neutropenia, and eosinophilia have been reported.

When given over prolonged periods, tetracyclines have been reported to produce brown-black microscopic discoloration of thyroid glands. No abnormalities of thyroid function studies are known to occur.

DOSAGE AND ADMINISTRATION

INTRAMUSCULAR ADMINISTRATION:

Adults: The usual daily dose is 250 mg administered once every 24 hours or 300 mg given in divided doses at 8-to-12-hour intervals.

For Children above Eight Years of Age: 15-25 mg/kg body weight up to a maximum of 250 mg per single daily injection. Dosage may be divided and given at 8-to-12-hour intervals. Intramuscular therapy should be reserved for situations in which oral therapy is not feasible.

The intramuscular administration of Lidocaine HCl/Oxytetracycline produces lower blood levels than oral administration in the recommended dosages. Patients placed on intramuscular Lidocaine HCl/Oxytetracycline should be changed to the oral dosage form as soon as possible. If rapid, high blood levels are needed. Lidocaine HCl/Oxytetracycline should be administered intravenously.

In Patients with Renal Impairment: (See "Warnings".) Total dosage should be decreased by reduction of recommended individual doses and/or by extending time intervals between doses.

HOW SUPPLIED
INJECTION: 50 MG/ML

BRAND/MANUFACTURER	NDC	SIZE	AWP
○ BRAND			
TERRAMYCIN: Roerig,J.B.	00049-0750-77	10 ml 5s	$47.18

Lidocaine Hydrochloride, Injectable

DESCRIPTION

Lidocaine Hydrochloride is a sterile nonpyrogenic solution of an antiarrhythmic agent administered intravenously by either direct injection or continuous infusion. The specific quantitative composition for each available solution appears in Table 1. (See related table).

Lidocaine Hydrochloride, Injection is composed of an aqueous solution of Lidocaine Hydrochloride. Lidocaine Hydrochloride ($C_{14}H_{22}N_2O \cdot HCl$) is chemically designated acetamide, 2-(diethylamino)-N-(2,6 dimethylphenyl)-, monohydrochloride.

Following is its chemical structure:

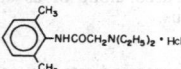

CLINICAL PHARMACOLOGY

MECHANISM OF ACTION AND ELECTROPHYSIOLOGY

Studies of the effects of therapeutic concentrations of Lidocaine Hydrochloride on the electrophysiological properties of mammalian Purkinje fibers have shown that Lidocaine Hydrochloride attenuates phase 4 diastolic depolarization, decreases automaticity, and causes a decrease or no change in excitability and membrane responsiveness. Action potential duration and effective refractory period of Purkinje fibers are decreased, while the ratio of effective refractory period to action potential is increased. Action potential duration and effective refractory period of ventricular muscle are also decreased. Effective refractory period of the AV node may increase, decrease or remain unchanged, and atrial effective refractory period is unchanged. Lidocaine Hydrochloride raises the ventricular fibrillation threshold. No significant interactions between Lidocaine Hydrochloloride and the autonomic nervous system have been described and consequently, Lidocaine Hydrochloride has little or no effect on autonomic tone.

Clinical electrophysiological studies with Lidocaine Hydrochloride have demonstrated no change in sinus node recovery time or sinoatrial conduction time. AV nodal conduction time is unchanged or shortened, and His-Purkinje conduction time is unchanged.

HEMODYNAMICS

At therapeutic doses, Lidocaine Hydrochloride has minimal hemodynamic effects in normal subjects and in patients with heart disease. Lidocaine Hydrochloride has been shown to cause no, or minimal, decrease in ventricular contractility, cardiac output, arterial pressure or heart rate.

PHARMACOKINETICS AND METABOLISM

Lidocaine Hydrochloride is rapidly metabolized by the liver, and less than 10% of a dose is excreted unchanged in the urine. Oxidative N-dealkylation, a major pathway of metabolism, results in the metabolites monoethylglycinexylidide and glycinexylidide. The pharmacological/toxicological activities of these metabolites are similar to, but less than, Lidocaine Hydrochloride. The primary metabolite in urine is a conjugate of 4-hydroxy-2,6-dimethylaniline.

The elimination half-life of Lidocaine Hydrochloride following an intravenous bolus injection is typically 1.5 to 2 hours. There are data that indicate that the half-life may be 3 hours or longer following infusions of greater than 24 hours.

Because of the rapid rate at which Lidocaine Hydrochloride is metabolized, any condition that alters liver function, including changes in liver blood flow, which could result from severe congestive heart failure or shock, may alter Lidocaine Hydrochloride kinetics. The half-life may be two-fold or more greater in patients with liver dysfunction. Renal dysfunction does not affect Lidocaine Hydrochloride kinetics, but may increase the accumulation of metabolites.

Therapeutic effects of Lidocaine Hydrochloride are generally associated with plasma levels of 6 to 25 μmole/L (1.5 to μg free base per mL). The blood to plasma distribution ratio is approximately 0.84. Objective adverse manifestations become increasingly apparent with increasing plasma levels above 6 μg free base per mL.

The plasma protein binding of Lidocaine Hydrochloride is dependent on drug concentration, and the fraction bound decreases with increasing concentration. At concentrations of 1 to 4 μg free base per mL, 60 to 80 percent Lidocaine Hydrochloride is protein bound. In addition to Lidocaine Hydrochloride concentration, the binding is dependent on the plasma concentration of the α-1-acid glycoprotein.

Lidocaine Hydrochloride readily crosses the placental and blood-brain barriers. Dialysis has negligible effects on the kinetics of Lidocaine Hydrochloride.

INDICATIONS AND USAGE

Lidocaine Hydrochloride administered intravenously is specifically indicated in the acute management of ventricular arrhythmias such as those occurring in relation to acute myocardial infarction, or during cardiac manipulation, such as cardiac surgery.

Table 1
COMPOSITION OF AVAILABLE SOLUTIONS

	Dosage Form	Lidocaine Hydrochloride (mg per mL)	Composition* Sodium chloride (mg per mL)
For Direct Intravenous Injection	5 mL (50 mg) prefilled syringe	10	7
	5 mL (100 mg) prefilled syringe	20	6
	5 mL (100 mg) ampule	20	6
For Preparation of Intravenous Infusion Solutions	25 mL (one Gram) single use vial	40	None
	50 mL (Two Grams) single use vial	40	None

* pH of all solutions adjusted to 5.0-7.0 with sodium hydroxide and/or hydrochloric acid. All containers are for single use: solutions do not contain preservatives.

UNLABELED USES

Lidocaine Hydrochloride is used alone or as an adjunct in the treatment of tinnitus and status epilepticus.

CONTRAINDICATIONS

Lidocaine Hydrochloride is contraindicated in patients with a known history of hypersensitivity to local anesthetics of the amide type Lidocaine Hydrochloride should not be used in patients with Stokes-Adams syndrome, Wolff-Parkinson-White syndrome, or with severe degrees of sinoatrial, atrioventricular, or intraventricular block in the absence of an artificial pacemaker.

WARNINGS

IN ORDER TO MANAGE POSSIBLE ADVERSE REACTIONS, RESUSCITATIVE EQUIPMENT, OXYGEN AND OTHER RESUSCITATIVE DRUGS SHOULD BE IMMEDIATELY AVAILABLE WHEN LIDOCAINE HYDROCHLORIDE, INJECTION, USP IS USED.

Systemic toxicity may result in manifestations of central nervous system depression (sedation) or irritability (twitching), which may progress to frank convulsions accompanied by respiratory depression and/or arrest. Early recognition of premonitory signs, assurance of adequate oxygenation and, where necessary, establishment of artificial airway with ventilatory support are essential to management of this problem. Should convulsions persist despite ventilatory therapy with oxygen, *small* increments of anticonvulsant drugs may be used intravenously. Examples of such agents include benzodiazepines (e.g., diazepam), ultrashort-acting barbiturates (e.g., thiopental or thiamylal), or a short-acting barbiturate (e.g., pentobarbital or secobarbital). If the patient is under anesthesia, a short-acting muscle relaxant (e.g., succinylcholine) may be used. Longer-acting drugs should be used only when recurrent convulsions are evidenced.

Should circulatory depression occur, vasopressors may be used.

Constant electrocardiographic monitoring is essential to the proper administration of Lidocaine Hydrochloride. Signs of excessive depression of cardiac electrical activity such as sinus node dysfunction, prolongation of the P-R interval and QRS complex or the appearance or aggravation of arrhythmias, should be followed by flow adjustment and, if necessary, prompt cessation of the intravenous infusion of this agent. Occasionally, acceleration of ventricular rate may occur when Lidocaine Hydrochloride is administered to patients with atrial flutter or fibrillation.

PRECAUTIONS

1. General: Caution should be employed in the use of Lidocaine Hydrochloride in patients with severe liver or kidney disease because accumulation of the drug or metabolites may occur.

Lidocaine Hydrochloride should be used with caution in the treatment of patients with hypovolemia, severe congestive heart failure, shock, and all forms of heart block. In patients with sinus bradycardia or incomplete heart block, the administration of Lidocaine Hydrochloride intravenously for the elimination of ventricular ectopic beats, without prior acceleration in heart rate (e.g., by atropine, isoproterenol or electric pacing), may promote more frequent and serious ventricular arrhythmias or complete heart block (see *"Contraindications"*).

Dosage should be reduced for children and for debilitated and/or elderly patients, commensurate with their age and physical status.

The safety of amide local anesthetic agents in patients with genetic predisposition to malignant hyperthermia has not been fully assessed; therefore, Lidocaine Hydrochloride should be used with caution in such patients.

In hospital environments where drugs known to be triggering agents for malignant hyperthermia (fulminant hypermetabolism) are administered, it is suggested that a standard protocol for management should be available.

It is not known whether Lidocaine Hydrochloride may trigger this reaction; however, large doses resulting in significant plasma concentrations, as may be achieved by intravenous infusion, pose potential risk to these individuals. Recognition of early unexplained signs of tachycardia, tachypnea, labile blood pressure and metabolic acidosis may precede temperature elevation. Successful outcome is dependent on early diagnosis, prompt discontinuance of the triggering agent and institution of treatment including oxygen therapy, supportive measures and dantrolene (for details see dantrolene package insert).

2. Patient Information: The patient should be advised of the possible occurrence of the experiences listed under *"Adverse Reactions"*.

3. Laboratory Tests: None known.

4. Drug Interactions: Lidocaine Hydrochloride should be used with caution in patients with digitalis toxicity accompanied by atrioventricular block. Concomitant use of beta-blocking agents or cimetidine may reduce hepatic blood flow and thereby reduce Lidocaine Hydrochloride clearance.

Lidocaine Hydrochloride and tocainide are pharmacodynamically similar. The concomitant use of these two agents may cause an increased incidence of adverse reactions, including central nervous system adverse reactions such as seizure.

5. Carcinogenesis, Mutagenesis, Impairment of Fertility: Long term studies in animals to evaluate the carcinogenic and mutagenic potential or the effect on fertility of Lidocaine Hydrochloride have not been conducted.

6. Pregnancy: Teratogenic Effects: Pregnancy Category B. Reproduction studies have been performed in rats at doses up to 6.6 times the maximum human doses and have revealed no significant findings. There are, however, no adequate and well-controlled studies in pregnant women. Because animal reproduction studies are not always predictive of human response, this drug should be used during pregnancy only if clearly needed.

7. Labor and Delivery: The effects of Lidocaine Hydrochloride on the mother and the fetus, when used in the management of cardiac arrhythmias during labor and delivery, are not known. Lidocaine Hydrochloride readily crosses the placental barrier.

8. Nursing Mothers: It is not known whether this drug is excreted in human milk. Because many drugs are excreted in human milk, caution should be exercised when Lidocaine Hydrochloride is administered to a nursing woman.

9. Pediatric Use: Safety and effectiveness in children have not been established by controlled clinical studies. (See *"Dosage and Administration"*.)

ADVERSE REACTIONS

Adverse experiences following the administration of Lidocaine Hydrochloride are similar in nature to those observed with other amide local anesthetic agents. Adverse experiences may result from high plasma levels caused by excessive dosage or may result from a hypersensitivity, idiosyncrasy or diminished tolerance on the part of the patient. Serious adverse experiences are generally systemic in nature. The following types are those most commonly reported. The adverse experiences under Central Nervous System and Cardiovascular System are listed, in general, in a progression from mild to severe.

1. Central Nervous System: CNS reactions are excitatory and/or depressant, and may be characterized by light-headedness, nervousness, apprehension, euphoria, confusion, dizziness, drowsiness, tinnitus, blurred or double vision, vomiting, sensations of heat, cold or numbness, twitching, tremors, convulsions, unconsciousness, respiratory depression and arrest. The excitatory reactions may be very brief or may not occur at all, in which case, the first manifestation of toxicity may be drowsiness, merging into unconsciousness and respiratory arrest.

2. Cardiovascular System: Cardiovascular reactions are usually depressant in nature and are characterized by bradycardia, hypotension, and cardiovascular collapse, which may lead to cardiac arrest.

3. Allergic reactions as a result of sensitivity to Lidocaine Hydrochloride are extremely rare and, if they occur, should be managed by conventional means.

DRUG ABUSE AND DEPENDENCE

Although specific studies have not been conducted, Lidocaine Hydrochloride has been used clinically without evidence of abuse of this drug or of psychological or physical dependence as a result of its use.

OVERDOSAGE

Overdosage of Lidocaine Hydrochloride usually results in signs of central nervous system or cardiovascular toxicity. See *"Adverse Reactions"*.

Should convulsions or signs of respiratory depression and arrest develop, the patency of the airway and adequacy of ventilation must be assured immediately. Should convulsions persist despite ventilatory therapy with oxygen, small increments of anticonvulsive agents may be given intravenously. Examples of such agents include a benzodiazepine (e.g., diazepam), an ultrashort-acting barbiturate (e.g., thiopental or thiamylal), or a short-acting barbiturate (e.g., pentobarbital or secobarbital). If the patient is under general anesthesia, a short-acting muscle relaxant (e.g., succinylcholine) may be administered.

Should circulatory depression occur, vasopressors may be used. Should cardiac arrest occur, standard CPR procedures should be instituted. Dialysis is of negligible value in the treatment of acute overdosage from Lidocaine Hydrochloride.

DOSAGE AND ADMINISTRATION

ADULTS

Single Direct Intravenous Injection (bolus): ONLY THE 5 mL, 50 mg OR 100 mg DOSAGE SIZES should be used for direct intravenous injection. The usual dose is 50 to 100 mg of Lidocaine Hydrochloride (0.70 to 1.4 mg/kg; 0.32 to 0.63 mg/lb) administered intravenously under ECG monitoring. This dose may be administered at the rate of approximately 25 to 50 mg/min (0.35 to 0.70 mg/kg/min; 0.16 to 0.32 mg/lb/min). Sufficient time should be allowed to enable a slow circulation to carry the drug to the site of action. If the initial injection of 50 to 100 mg does not produce a desired response, a second dose may be injected after 5 minutes. The syringe should be activated immediately prior to the injection. (See illustrated instructions for use on product package.) NO MORE THAN 200 TO 300 mg OF LIDOCAINE HYDROCHLORIDE SHOULD BE ADMINISTERED DURING A ONE HOUR PERIOD.

Continuous Intravenous Infusion: Following bolus administration, intravenous infusions of Lidocaine Hydrochloride may be initiated at the rate of 1 to 4 mg/min of Lidocaine Hydrochloride (0.014 to 0.057 mg/kg/min; 0.006 to 0.026 mg/lb/min). The rate of intravenous infusions should be reassessed as soon as the patient's basic cardiac rhythm appears to be stable or at the earliest signs of toxicity. It should rarely be necessary to continue intravenous infusions of Lidocaine Hydrochloride for prolonged periods.

Solutions for intravenous infusion may be prepared by the addition of one gram (or two grams) of Lidocaine Hydrochloride to one liter of 5% dextrose in water using aseptic technique. Approximately a 0.1% (or 0.2%) solution will result from this procedure; that is, each milliliter will contain approximately 1 mg (or 2 mg) of Lidocaine Hydrochloride. In those cases in which fluid restriction is medically appropriate, a more concentrated solution may be prepared.

Lidocaine Hydrochloride has been found to be chemically stable for 24 hours after dilution in 5% dextrose in water. However, as with all intravenous admixtures, dilution of the solution should be made just prior to its administration.

◆ RATED THERAPEUTICALLY EQUIVALENT; ◇ THERAPEUTIC EQUIVALENCE UNCONFIRMED; ○ UNRATED

Parenteral drug products should be inspected visually for particulate matter and discoloration prior to administration whenever the solution and container permit. Do not use if solution is discolored or cloudy.

PEDIATRIC
Although controlled clinical studies to establish pediatric dosing schedules have not been conducted, the American Heart Association's *Standards and Guidelines* recommends a bolus dose of 1 mg/kg followed by an infusion rate of 30 μg/kg/min.

Note regarding prolonged infusions: There are data that indicate the half-life may be 3 hours or longer following infusions of greater than 24 hours in duration.

Solutions should be stored at controlled room temperature, 15°-30°C (59°-86°F).

J CODES
50 cc VAR—J2000

HOW SUPPLIED
INJECTION: 1%

BRAND/MANUFACTURER	NDC	SIZE	AWP
○ **BRAND**			
EPIDURAL SINGLE SHOT W/LIDOCAINE: Abbott Hosp	00074-1986-01	2 ml 10s	$379.41

INJECTION: 0.2%

AVERAGE UNIT PRICE (AVAILABLE SIZES)	
GENERIC	$0.04

BRAND/MANUFACTURER	NDC	SIZE	AWP
◆ **GENERICS**			
McGaw	00264-5592-10	500 ml 10s	$173.88
Baxter	00338-0407-03	500 ml 18s	$317.03
Abbott Hosp	00074-7916-24	500 ml 24s	$431.21

INJECTION: 0.4%

AVERAGE UNIT PRICE (AVAILABLE SIZES)	
GENERIC	$0.06

BRAND/MANUFACTURER	NDC	SIZE	AWP
◆ **GENERICS**			
McGaw	00264-9594-20	250 ml	$20.04
McGaw	00264-9594-10	500 ml	$22.44
Abbott Hosp	00074-7931-32	250 ml 12s	$215.60
Baxter	00338-0409-03	500 ml 18s	$409.32
Baxter	00338-0409-02	250 ml 24s	$423.08
Abbott Hosp	00074-7931-24	500 ml 24s	$556.32

INJECTION: 0.5%

AVERAGE UNIT PRICE (AVAILABLE SIZES)		GENERIC A-RATED AVERAGE PRICE (GAAP)	
BRAND	$0.13	50 ml 25s	$77.48
GENERIC	$0.06		

BRAND/MANUFACTURER	NDC	SIZE	AWP
◆ **BRAND**			
XYLOCAINE HCL: Astra	00186-0135-01	50 ml	$3.61
XYLOCAINE-MPF: Astra	00186-0137-01	50 ml	$9.08
◆ **GENERICS**			
Abbott Hosp	00074-4278-01	50 ml 25s	$77.48
Abbott Hosp	00074-4275-01	50 ml 25s	$77.48

INJECTION: 0.8%

AVERAGE UNIT PRICE (AVAILABLE SIZES)	
GENERIC	$0.07

BRAND/MANUFACTURER	NDC	SIZE	AWP
◆ **GENERICS**			
McGaw	00264-9598-20	250 ml	$22.44
McGaw	00264-9598-10	500 ml	$22.96
McGaw	00264-5598-10	500 ml 10s	$229.56
Abbott Hosp	00074-7939-32	250 ml 12s	$278.16
Baxter	00338-0411-03	500 ml 18s	$467.07
Baxter	00338-0411-02	250 ml 24s	$545.76

INJECTION: 1%

AVERAGE UNIT PRICE (AVAILABLE SIZES)		GENERIC A-RATED AVERAGE PRICE (GAAP)	
BRAND	$0.33	50 ml	$3.30
GENERIC	$0.53	20 ml 5s	$42.03
		30 ml 5s	$46.11
		5 ml 10s	$101.20
		5 ml 25s	$113.67
		10 ml 25s	$117.75
		30 ml 25s	$79.02
		50 ml 25s	$38.30

BRAND/MANUFACTURER	NDC	SIZE	AWP
◆ **BRAND**			
XYLOCAINE HCL: Astra	00186-0110-01	20 ml	$2.01
	00186-0145-01	50 ml	$3.31
	00186-0275-12	10 ml 5s	$8.11
XYLOCAINE-MPF: Astra	00186-0278-12	10 ml 5s	$22.45
	00186-0112-01	30 ml 5s	$7.41
	00186-0112-91	30 ml 5s	$39.51
	00186-0255-02	30 ml 5s	$43.30
	00186-0255-92	30 ml 5s	$47.94
	00186-0210-03	2 ml 10s	$14.00
	00186-0276-13	2 ml 10s	$14.05
	00186-0277-13	5 ml 10s	$18.00
	00186-0230-03	5 ml 10s	$18.91
XYLOCAINE HCL: Astra	00186-0615-01	5 ml 10s	$21.13
◆ **GENERICS**			
Fujisawa	00469-1201-15	2 ml	$1.22
Fujisawa	00469-2201-25	10 ml	$0.97
Moore,H.L.	00839-5597-38	50 ml	$1.88
Major	00904-0864-50	50 ml	$2.25
Schein	00364-6549-57	50 ml	$2.25
Steris	00402-0055-50	50 ml	$2.25
URL	00677-0281-24	50 ml	$2.90
Hyrex	00314-0679-50	50 ml	$3.50
Rugby	00536-1450-80	50 ml	$4.88
LIDOJECT-1: Mayrand	00259-0325-50	50 ml	$6.45
Intl Med Sys	00548-1078-00	20 ml 5s	$38.58
Intl Med Sys	00548-1080-00	20 ml 5s	$45.48
Intl Med Sys	00548-1079-00	30 ml 5s	$40.86
Intl Med Sys	00548-1081-00	30 ml 5s	$51.36
Abbott Hosp	00074-4713-01	2 ml 10s	$14.49
Abbott Hosp	00074-4904-01	5 ml 10s	$96.07
Abbott Hosp	00074-4924-01	5 ml 10s	$96.07
Abbott Hosp	00074-8026-01	5 ml 10s	$103.79
Abbott Hosp	00074-4904-23	5 ml 10s	$108.89
Elkins-Sinn	00641-0436-25	5 ml 25s	$16.15
Abbott Hosp	00074-4713-02	5 ml 25s	$49.88
Intl Med Sys	00548-1111-00	5 ml 25s	$114.00
Intl Med Sys	00548-1192-00	5 ml 25s	$116.10
Abbott Hosp	00074-4904-33	5 ml 25s	$272.23
Intl Med Sys	00548-1193-00	10 ml 25s	$106.20
Intl Med Sys	00548-1115-00	10 ml 25s	$129.30
Abbott Hosp	00074-4276-01	20 ml 25s	$54.03
Elkins-Sinn	00641-2380-45	30 ml 25s	$15.00
Abbott Hosp	00074-4279-02	30 ml 25s	$37.41
Abbott Hosp	00074-4270-01	30 ml 25s	$184.66
Elkins-Sinn	00641-2390-45	50 ml 25s	$20.63
Amer Regent	00517-0625-25	50 ml 25s	$27.19
Abbott Hosp	00074-4276-02	50 ml 25s	$67.09

INJECTION: 1.5%

AVERAGE UNIT PRICE (AVAILABLE SIZES)	
BRAND	$1.26
GENERIC	$0.35

BRAND/MANUFACTURER	NDC	SIZE	AWP
◆ **BRAND**			
XYLOCAINE-MPF: Astra	00186-0118-01	20 ml	$10.06
	00186-0244-12	10 ml 5s	$24.69
	00186-0245-02	20 ml 5s	$45.39
	00186-0118-91	20 ml 5s	$49.83
XYLOCAINE HCL: Astra	00186-0212-03	2 ml 10s	$87.36
◆ **GENERICS**			
Abbott Hosp	00074-4056-01	20 ml 5s	$28.68
Abbott Hosp	00074-4776-01	20 ml 25s	$202.77

INJECTION: 2%

AVERAGE UNIT PRICE (AVAILABLE SIZES)		GENERIC A-RATED AVERAGE PRICE (GAAP)	
BRAND	$0.50	50 ml	$3.46
GENERIC	$0.67	5 ml 10s	$100.91
		5 ml 25s	$157.07
		50 ml 25s	$43.33

BRAND/MANUFACTURER	NDC	SIZE	AWP
◆ **BRAND**			
XYLOCAINE HCL: Astra	00186-0120-01	20 ml	$2.16
	00186-0155-01	50 ml	$4.15
	00186-0243-12	10 ml 5s	$9.54

➤ SHOWN IN PRODUCT IDENTIFICATION GUIDE

BRAND/MANUFACTURER	NDC	SIZE	AWP
XYLOCAINE-MPF: Astra	00186-0240-12	10 ml 5s	$26.96
	00186-0240-02	10 ml 5s	$27.71
	00186-0215-03	2 ml 10s	$17.54
	00186-0241-13	2 ml 10s	$19.94
	00186-0242-13	5 ml 10s	$18.81
XYLOCAINE HCL: Astra	00186-0611-01	5 ml 10s	$20.75
XYLOCAINE HCL: Astra	00186-0232-03	5 ml 10s	$43.19
◆ GENERICS			
Fujisawa	00469-1202-25	2 ml	$1.05
Fujisawa	00469-1208-25	5 ml	$1.40
Moore,H.L.	00839-5598-38	50 ml	$2.01
Schein	00364-6551-57	50 ml	$2.25
Steris	00402-0056-50	50 ml	$2.25
Major	00904-0865-50	50 ml	$2.85
Hyrex	00314-0680-50	50 ml	$3.50
Rugby	00536-1460-80	50 ml	$4.88
LIDOJECT-2: Mayrand	00259-0326-50	50 ml	$6.45
Abbott Hosp	00074-8027-01	5 ml 10s	$89.42
Abbott Hosp	00074-4903-01	5 ml 10s	$100.46
Abbott Hosp	00074-4923-01	5 ml 10s	$100.46
Abbott Hosp	00074-4903-23	5 ml 10s	$113.29
Abbott Hosp	00074-4282-01	2 ml 25s	$36.22
Elkins-Sinn	00641-0437-25	5 ml 25s	$16.15
Intl Med Sys	00548-1112-00	5 ml 25s	$114.00
Intl Med Sys	00548-1190-00	5 ml 25s	$120.60
Intl Med Sys	00548-2190-00	5 ml 25s	$251.40
Abbott Hosp	00074-4903-33	5 ml 25s	$283.22
Abbott Hosp	00074-4282-02	10 ml 25s	$60.27
Abbott Hosp	00074-4277-01	20 ml 25s	$54.03
Elkins-Sinn	00641-2400-45	30 ml 25s	$15.94
Elkins-Sinn	00641-2410-45	50 ml 25s	$21.56
Amer Regent	00517-0626-25	50 ml 25s	$30.94
Abbott Hosp	00074-4277-02	50 ml 25s	$77.48

INJECTION: 4%

AVERAGE UNIT PRICE (AVAILABLE SIZES)

BRAND	$0.46		

BRAND/MANUFACTURER	NDC	SIZE	AWP
◆ BRAND			
XYLOCAINE HCL: Astra	00186-0166-01	25 ml	$1.59
	00186-0167-01	25 ml	$2.05
	00186-0169-01	50 ml	$2.03
XYLOCAINE DUO-TRACH KIT: Astra	00186-0235-72	5 ml 5s	$36.40
XYLOCAINE HCL: Astra	00186-0168-01	50 ml 10s	$2.30
XYLOCAINE-MPF: Astra	00186-0235-03	5 ml 10s	$56.59
◆ GENERICS			
Abbott Hosp	00074-4283-01	5 ml 25s	$71.55

INJECTION: 5%

BRAND/MANUFACTURER	NDC	SIZE	AWP
◆ GENERICS			
Abbott Hosp	00074-4712-01	2 ml 25s	$133.00

INJECTION: 5%

BRAND/MANUFACTURER	NDC	SIZE	AWP
○ BRAND			
XYLOCAINE HCL FOR SPINAL: Astra	00186-0225-03	2 ml 10s	$83.46

INJECTION: 10 MG

BRAND/MANUFACTURER	NDC	SIZE	AWP
◆ GENERICS			
Goldline	00182-0565-67	50 ml	$3.00

INJECTION: 10%

BRAND/MANUFACTURER	NDC	SIZE	AWP
◆ GENERICS			
Abbott Hosp	00074-6254-01	10 ml 25s	$207.81

INJECTION: 20 MG

BRAND/MANUFACTURER	NDC	SIZE	AWP
◆ GENERICS			
Goldline	00182-0566-67	50 ml	$3.00

INJECTION: 20%

AVERAGE UNIT PRICE (AVAILABLE SIZES)

GENERIC	$1.32	GENERIC A-RATED AVERAGE PRICE (GAAP)	
		10 ml 25s	$316.66

BRAND/MANUFACTURER	NDC	SIZE	AWP
◆ GENERICS			
Intl Med Sys	00548-6100-00	5 ml 25s	$185.40
Intl Med Sys	00548-6105-00	10 ml 25s	$284.10
Abbott Hosp	00074-6248-01	10 ml 25s	$286.78

BRAND/MANUFACTURER	NDC	SIZE	AWP
Abbott Hosp	00074-6217-02	10 ml 25s	$379.11

Lidocaine Hydrochloride, Local Anesthesia

DESCRIPTION
Lidocaine Hydrochloride is a sterile, non pyrogenic aqueous solution that contains a local anesthetic agent with or without epinephrine and is administered parenterally by injection or topically. See "Indications" for specific uses.

Each ml contains: Lidocaine HCl 5,10,15,20, or 40 mg.
Lidocaine HCl concentration is 0.5%, 1%, 1.5%, 2%, or 4%.
Lidocaine HCl is chemically designated as acetamide 2-(diethylamino)-N-(2,6-dimethylphenyl)-monohydrochloride and has the molecular wt. 270.8. Epinephrine is (-)-3, 4-Dihydroxy-α-[(methylaminomethyl] benzyl alcohol and has the molecular wt. 183.21.

Following is its chemical structure:

CLINICAL PHARMACOLOGY
Mechanism of action: Lidocaine stabilizes the neuronal membrane by inhibiting the ionic fluxes required for the initiation and conduction of impulses, thereby effecting local anesthetic action.

Onset and Duration of Anesthesia: The onset of action is rapid. For retrobulbar injection, 4 ml of 4% Lidocaine HCl, Local Anesthesia, sterile solution provides an average duration of action of 1 to 1 ½ hours. This duration may be extended for ophthalmic surgery by the addition of epinephrine, the usual recommended dilution being 1:50,000 to 1:100,000.

Hemodynamics: Excessive blood levels may cause changes in cardiac output, total peripheral resistance, and mean arterial pressure. With central neural blockade these changes may be attributable to block of autonomic fibers, a direct depressant effect of the local anesthetic agent on various components of the cardiovascular system and/or the beta-adrenergic receptor stimulating action of epinephrine when present. The net effect is normally a modest hypotension when the recommended dosages are not exceeded.

Pharmacokinetics and metabolism: Information derived from diverse formulations, concentrations and usages reveals that Lidocaine is completely absorbed following parenteral administration, its rate of absorption depending, for example, upon various factors such as the site of administration and the presence or absence of a vasoconstrictor agent. Except for intravascular administration, the highest blood levels are obtained following intercostal nerve block and the lowest after subcutaneous administration.

Lidocaine may be absorbed following topical administration to mucous membranes, its rate and extent of absorption depending upon concentration and total dose administered, the specific site of application and duration of exposure. In general, the rate of absorption of local anesthetic agents following topical application occurs most rapidly after intratracheal administration. Lidocaine is also well absorbed from the gastrointestinal tract, but little intact drug appears in the circulation because of biotransformation by the liver.

The plasma binding of Lidocaine is dependent on drug concentration, and the fraction bound decreases with increasing concentration. At concentrations of 1 to 4 µg of free base per ml, 60 to 80 percent of Lidocaine is protein bound. Binding is also dependent on the plasma concentration of the alpha-1-acid glycoprotein.

Lidocaine crosses the blood-brain and placental barriers, presumably by passive diffusion.

Lidocaine is metabolized rapidly by the liver, and metabolites and unchanged drug are excreted by the kidneys. Biotransformation includes oxidative N-dealkylation, ring hydroxylation, cleavage of the amide linkage, and conjugation. N-dealkylation, a major pathway of biotransformation, yields the metabolites monoethylglycinexylidide and glycinexylidide. The pharmacological/toxicological actions of these metabolites are similar to, but less potent than, those of Lidocaine. Approximately 90% of Lidocaine administered is excreted in the form of various metabolites, and less than 10% is excreted unchanged. The primary metabolite in urine is a conjugate of 4-hydroxy-2, 6-dimethylaniline.

Studies have shown that peak blood levels of Lidocaine may occur as early as 5 and as late as 30 minutes after endotracheal administration of a 4% Lidocaine HCl solution.

The elimination half-life of Lidocaine following an intravenous bolus injection is typically 1.5 to 2.0 hours. Because of the rapid rate at which Lidocaine is metabolized, any condition that affects liver function may alter Lidocaine kinetics. The half-life may be prolonged two-fold or more in patients with liver dysfunction. Renal dysfunction does not affect Lidocaine kinetics but may increase the accumulation of metabolites.

Factors such as acidosis and the use of CNS stimulants and depressants affect the CNS levels of Lidocaine required to produce overt systemic effects. Objective adverse manifestations become increasingly apparent with increasing venous

◆ RATED THERAPEUTICALLY EQUIVALENT; ◇ THERAPEUTIC EQUIVALENCE UNCONFIRMED; ○ UNRATED

plasma levels above 6.0 μg free base per ml. In the rhesus monkey arterial blood levels of 18-21 μg/ml have been shown to be threshold for convulsive activity.

INDICATIONS AND USAGE

Lidocaine HCl, Local Anesthesia, is indicated for production of local or regional anesthesia by infiltration techniques such as percutaneous injection and intravenous regional anesthesia by peripheral nerve block techniques such as brachial plexus and intercostal and by central neural techniques such as lumbar and caudal epidural blocks, when the accepted procedures for these techniques as described in standard textbooks are observed.

Lidocaine HCl 4% solution is indicated for the production of topical anesthesia of the mucous membranes of the respiratory tract or the genitourinary tract. It may be injected trans-tracheally to anesthetize the larynx and trachea, and it may be administered by retrobulbar injection to provide anesthesia for ophthalmic surgery.

UNLABELED USES

Lidocaine is used alone or as an adjunct in the treatment of bone pain secondary to bone metastases from cancer, to suppress the cough reflex during cataract surgery, in status epilepticus, and to reduce intracranial hypertension. It is also used in the treatment of pruritus in hemodialysis patients, in diabetic neuropathy, and in tinnitus.

CONTRAINDICATIONS

Lidocaine is contraindicated in patients with a known history of hypersensitivity to local anesthetics of the amide type.

WARNINGS

LIDOCAINE HCL, LOCAL ANESTHESIA, SOLUTION SHOULD BE EMPLOYED ONLY BY CLINICIANS WHO ARE WELL VERSED IN DIAGNOSIS AND MANAGEMENT OF DOSE-RELATED TOXICITY AND OTHER ACUTE EMERGENCIES THAT MIGHT ARISE AND THEN ONLY AFTER ENSURING THE *IMMEDIATE* AVAILABILITY OF OXYGEN. OTHER RESUSCITATIVE DRUGS, CARDIOPULMONARY EQUIPMENT, AND THE PERSONNEL NEEDED FOR PROPER MANAGEMENT OF TOXIC REACTIONS AND RELATED EMERGENCIES (SEE ALSO "ADVERSE REACTIONS" AND "PRECAUTIONS"). DELAY IN PROPER MANAGEMENT OF DOSE-RELATED TOXICITY, UNDERVENTILATION FROM ANY CAUSE AND/OR ALTERED SENSITIVITY MAY LEAD TO THE DEVELOPMENT OF ACIDOSIS, CARDIAC ARREST AND, POSSIBLY, DEATH.

To avoid intravascular injection, aspiration should be performed before the local anesthetic solution is injected. The needle must be repositioned until no return of blood can be elicited by aspiration. Note, however, that the absence of blood in the syringe does not guarantee that intravascular injection has been avoided.

Lidocaine HCl solution should be used with extreme caution if there is sepsis or severely traumatized mucosa in the area of application, since under such conditions there is the potential for rapid systemic absorption.

Local anesthetic solutions containing antimicrobial preservatives (e.g., methylparaben) should not be used for epidural or spinal anesthesia because the safety of these agents has not been established with regard to intrathecal injection, either intentional or accidental.

Some Lidocaine HCl, Local Anesthesia, with epinephrine solutions contain sodium metabisulfite, a sulfite that may cause allergic-type reactions including anaphylactic symptoms and life-threatening or less severe asthmatic episodes in certain susceptible people. The overall prevalence of sulfite sensitivity in the general population is unknown and probably low. Sulfite sensitivity is seen more frequently in asthmatic than in nonasthmatic people.

PRECAUTIONS

General: The safety and effectiveness of Lidocaine depend on proper dosage, correct technique, adequate precautions, and readiness for emergencies. Standard textbooks should be consulted for specific techniques and precautions for various regional anesthetic procedures.

Resuscitative equipment, oxygen, and other resuscitative drugs should be available for immediate use. (See "Warnings" and "Adverse Reactions"). The lowest dosage that results in effective anesthesia should be used to avoid high plasma levels and serious adverse effects. Syringe aspirations should also be performed before and during each supplemental injection when using indwelling catheter techniques. During the administration of epidural anesthesia, it is recommended that a test dose be administered initially and that the patient be monitored for central nervous system toxicity and cardiovascular toxicity, as well as for signs of unintended intrathecal administration, before proceeding. When clinical conditions permit, consideration should be given to employing local anesthetic solutions that contain epinephrine for the test dose because circulatory changes compatible with epinephrine may also serve as a warning sign of unintended intravascular injection. An intravascular injection is still possible even if aspirations for blood are negative. Repeated doses of Lidocaine may cause significant increases in blood levels with each repeated dose because of slow accumulation of the drug or its metabolites. Tolerance to elevated blood levels varies with the status of the patient.

Debilitated, elderly patients, acutely ill patients and children should be given reduced doses commensurate with their age and physical condition. Lidocaine should also be used with caution in patients with severe shock or heart block. Lumbar and caudal epidural anesthesia should be used with extreme caution in persons with the following conditions: existing neurological disease, spinal deformities, septicemia and severe hypertension.

Local anesthetic solutions containing a vasoconstrictor should be used cautiously and in carefully circumscribed quantities in areas of the body supplied by end arteries or having otherwise compromised blood supply. Patients with peripheral vascular disease and those with hypertensive vascular disease may exhibit exaggerated vasoconstrictor response. Ischemic injury or necrosis may result. Preparations containing a vasoconstrictor should be used with caution in patients during or following the administration of potent general anesthetic agents, since cardiac arrhythmias may occur under such conditions.

Careful and constant monitoring of cardiovascular and respiratory (adequacy of ventilation) vital signs and the patient's state of consciousness should be accomplished after each local anesthetic injection. It should be kept in mind at such times that restlessness, anxiety, tinnitus, dizziness, blurred vision, tremors, depression or drowsiness may be early warning signs of central nervous system toxicity.

Since amide-type local anesthetics are metabolized by the liver, HCl, Local Anesthesia, should be used with caution in patients with hepatic disease. Patients with severe hepatic disease, because of their inability to metabolize local anesthetics normally, are at greater risk of developing toxic plasma concentrations. HCl, Local Anesthesia, solution should also be used with caution in patients with impaired cardiovascular function since they may be less able to compensate for functional changes associated with the prolongation of A-V conduction produced by these drugs.

Use in Ophthalmic Surgery: When local anesthetic solutions are employed for retrobulbar block, lack of corneal sensation should not be relied upon to determine whether or not the patient is ready for surgery since corneal sensation usually precedes clinically acceptable external ocular muscle akinesia.

Many drugs used during the conduct of anesthesia are considered potential triggering agents for familial malignant hyperthermia. Since it is not known whether amide-type local anesthetics may trigger this reaction and since the need for supplemental general anesthesia cannot be predicted in advance, it is suggested that a standard protocol for the management of malignant hyperthermia should be available. Early unexplained signs of tachycardia, tachypnea, labile blood pressure and metabolic acidosis may precede temperature elevation. Successful outcome is dependent on early diagnosis, prompt discontinuance of the suspect triggering agent(s) and institution of treatment, including oxygen therapy, indicated supportive measures and dantrolene (consult dantrolene sodium intravenous package insert before using).

Proper tourniquet technique, as described in publications and standard textbooks, is essential in the performance of intravenous regional anesthesia. Solutions containing epinephrine or other vasoconstrictors should not be used for this technique.

Lidocaine should be used with caution in persons with known drug sensitivities. Patients allergic to para-aminobenzoic acid derivatives (procaine, tetracaine, benzocaine, etc.) have not shown cross sensitivity to Lidocaine.

Use in the Head and Neck Area: Small doses of local anesthetics injected into the head and neck area, including retrobulbar, dental and stellate ganglion blocks, may produce adverse reactions similar to systemic toxicity seen with unintentional intravascular injections of larger doses. Confusion, convulsions, respiratory depression and/or respiratory arrest, and cardiovascular stimulation or depression have been reported. These reactions may be due to intra-arterial injection of the local anesthetic with retrograde flow to the cerebral circulation. Patients receiving these blocks should have their circulation and respiration monitored and be constantly observed. Resuscitative equipment and personnel for treating adverse reactions should be immediately available. Dosage recommendations should not be exceeded. (See "Dosage and Administration").

Information for Patients: When appropriate, patients should be informed in advance that they may experience temporary loss of sensation and motor activity, usually in the lower half of the body, following proper administration of epidural anesthesia.

When topical anesthetics are used in the mouth, the patient should be aware that the production of topical anesthesia may impair swallowing and thus enhance the danger of aspiration. For this reason, food should not be ingested for 60 minutes following use of local anesthetic preparations in the mouth or throat area. This is particularly important in children because of their frequency of eating.

Numbness of the tongue or buccal mucosa may enhance the danger of unintentional biting trauma. Food and chewing gum should not be taken while the mouth or throat area is anesthetized.

Clinically Significant Drug Interactions: The administration of local anesthetic solutions containing epinephrine or norepinephrine to patients receiving monoamine oxidase inhibitors or tricyclic antidepressants may produce severe, prolonged hypotension or hypertension.

Phenothiazines and butyrophenones may reduce or reverse the pressor effect of epinephrine.

Concurrent use of these agents should generally be avoided. In situations when concurrent therapy is necessary, careful patient monitoring is essential.

Concurrent administration of vasopressor drugs (for the treatment of hypotension related to obstetric blocks) and ergot-type oxytocic drugs may cause severe, persistent hypertension or cerebrovascular accidents.

Drug Laboratory Test Interactions: The intramuscular injection of Lidocaine may result in an increase in creatine phosphokinase levels. Thus, the use of this enzyme determination without isoenzyme separation, as a diagnostic test for the presence of acute myocardial infarction may be compromised by the intramuscular injection of Lidocaine.

Carcinogenesis, Mutagenesis, Impairment of Fertility: Studies of Lidocaine in animals to evaluate the carcinogenic and mutagenic potential or the effect on fertility have not been conducted.

Pregnancy: Teratogenic Effects. Pregnancy Category B. Reproduction studies have been performed in rats at doses up to 6.6 times the human dose and have revealed no evidence of harm to the fetus caused by Lidocaine. There are, however, no adequate and well-controlled studies in pregnant women. Animal reproduction studies are not always predictive of human response. General consideration should be given to this fact before administering Lidocaine to women of childbearing potential, especially during early pregnancy when maximum organogenesis takes place.

Labor and Delivery: Lidocaine is not contraindicated in labor and delivery. Should Lidocaine HCl solution be used concomitantly with other products containing Lidocaine, the total dose contributed by all formulations must be kept in mind.

Local anesthetics rapidly cross the placenta and when used for epidural, paracervical, pudendal or caudal block anesthesia, can cause varying degrees of maternal, fetal, and neonatal toxicity, (see *"Clinical Pharmacology, Pharmacokinetics"*). The potential for toxicity depends upon the procedure performed, the type and amount of drug used, and the technique of drug administration. Adverse reactions in the parturient, fetus and neonate involve alterations of the central nervous system peripheral vascular tone and cardiac function.

Maternal hypotension has resulted from regional anesthesia. Local anesthetics produce vasodilation by blocking sympathetic nerves. Elevating the patient's legs and positioning her on her left side will help prevent decreases in blood pressure. The fetal heart rate also should be monitored continuously, and electronic fetal monitoring is highly advisable.

Epidural, spinal, paracervical, or pudendal anesthesia may alter the forces of parturition through changes in uterine contractility or maternal expulsive efforts. In one study paracervical block anesthesia was associated with a decrease in the mean duration of first stage labor and facilitation of cervical dilation. However, spinal and epidural anesthesia have also been reported to prolong the second stage of labor by removing the parturient's reflex urge to bear down or by interfering with motor function. The use of obstetrical anesthesia may increase the need for forceps assistance.

The use of some local anesthetic drug products during labor and delivery may be followed by diminished muscle strength and tone for the first day or two of life. The long term significance of these observations is unknown. Fetal bradycardia may occur in 20% to 30% of patients receiving paracervical nerve block anesthesia with the amide-type local anesthetics and may be associated with fetal acidosis. Fetal heart rate should always be monitored during paracervical anesthesia. The physician should weigh the possible advantages against risks when considering paracervical block in prematurity, toxemia of pregnancy, and fetal distress. Careful adherence to recommended dosage is of the utmost importance in obstetrical paracervical block. Failure to achieve adequate analgesia with recommended doses should arouse suspicion of intravascular or fetal intracranial injection. Cases compatible with unintended fetal intracranial injection of local anesthetic solution have been reported following intended paracervical or pudendal block or both. Babies so affected present with unexplained neonatal depression at birth, which correlates with high local anesthetic serum levels, and often manifest seizures within six hours. Prompt use of supportive measures combined with forced urinary excretion of the local anesthetic has been used successfully to manage this complication.

Case reports of maternal convulsions and cardiovascular collapse following use of some local anesthetics for paracervical block in early pregnancy (as anesthesia for elective abortion) suggest that systemic absorption under these circumstances may be rapid. The recommended maximum dose of each drug should not be exceeded. Injection should be made slowly and with frequent aspiration. Allow a 5-minute interval between sides.

Nursing Mothers: It is not known whether this drug is excreted in human milk. Because many drugs are excreted in human milk, caution should be exercised when Lidocaine is administered to a nursing woman.

Pediatric Use: Dosages in children should be reduced, commensurate with age, body weight and physical condition. See *"Dosage and Administration"*.

ADVERSE REACTIONS

Systemic: Adverse experiences following the administration of Lidocaine are similar in nature to those observed with other amide local anesthetic agents. These adverse experiences are, in general, dose-related and may result from high plasma levels caused by excessive dosage, rapid absorption or inadvertent intravascular injection, or may result from a hypersensitivity, idiosyncrasy or diminished tolerance on the part of the patient. Serious adverse experiences are generally systemic in nature. The following types are those most commonly reported:

Central Nervous System: CNS manifestations are excitatory and/or depressant and may be characterized by lightheadedness, nervousness, apprehension, euphoria, confusion, dizziness, drowsiness, tinnitus, blurred or double vision, vomiting, sensations of heat, cold or numbness, twitching, tremors, convulsions, unconsciousness, respiratory depression and arrest. The excitatory manifestations may be very brief or may not occur at all, in which case the first manifestation of toxicity may be drowsiness merging into unconsciousness and respiratory arrest.

Drowsiness following the administration of Lidocaine is usually an early sign of a high blood level of the drug and may occur as a consequence of rapid absorption.

Cardiovascular System: Cardiovascular manifestations are usually depressant and are characterized by bradycardia, hypotension, and cardiovascular collapse, which may lead to cardiac arrest.

Allergic: Allergic reactions are characterized by cutaneous lesions, urticaria, edema or anaphylactoid reactions. Allergic reactions may occur as a result of sensitivity either to local anesthetic agents or to the methylparaben used as a preservative in some brands or formulations. Allergic reactions as a result of sensitivity to Lidocaine are extremely rare and, if they occur, should be managed by conventional means. The detection of sensitivity by skin testing is of doubtful value.

Neurologic: The incidences of adverse reactions associated with the use of local anesthetics may be related to the total dose of local anesthetic administered and are also dependent upon the particular drug used, the route of administration and the physical status of the patient. In a prospective review of 10,440 patients who received Lidocaine for spinal anesthesia, the incidences of adverse reactions were reported to be about 3% each for positional headaches, hypotension and backache; 2% for shivering; and less than 1% each for peripheral nerve symptoms, nausea, respiratory inadequacy and double vision. Many of these observations may be related to local anesthetic techniques, with or without a contribution from the local anesthetic.

In the practice of caudal or lumbar epidural block, occasional unintentional penetration of the subarachnoid space by the catheter may occur. Subsequent adverse effects may depend partially on the amount of drug administered subdurally. These may include spinal block of varying magnitude (including total spinal block), hypotension secondary to spinal block, loss of bladder and bowel control, and loss of perineal sensation and sexual function. Persistent motor, sensory and/or autonomic (sphincter control) deficit of some lower spinal segments with slow recovery (several months) or incomplete recovery have been reported in rare instances when caudal or lumbar epidural block has been attempted.

Backache and headache have also been noted following use of these anesthetic procedures.

OVERDOSAGE

Acute emergencies from local anesthetics are generally related to high plasma levels encountered during therapeutic use of local anesthetics or to unintended subarachnoid injection of local anesthetic solution (see *"Adverse Reactions," "Warnings"* and *"Precautions"*).

Management of Local Anesthetic Emergencies: The first consideration is prevention, best accomplished by careful and constant monitoring of cardiovascular and respiratory vital signs and the patient's state of consciousness after each local anesthetic injection. At the first sign of change, oxygen should be administered.

The first step in the management of convulsions, as well as underventilation or apnea due to unintended subarachnoid injection of drug solution, consists of immediate attention to the maintenance of a patent airway and assisted or controlled ventilation with oxygen and a delivery system capable of permitting immediate positive airway pressure by mask. Immediately after the institution of these ventilatory measures, the adequacy of the circulation should be evaluated, keeping in mind that drugs used to treat convulsions sometimes depress the circulation when administered intravenously. Should convulsions persist despite adequate respiratory support, and if the status of the circulation permits, small increments of an ultra-short acting barbiturate (such as thiopental or thiamylal) or a benzodiazepine (such as diazepam) may be administered intravenously. The clinician should be familiar, prior to the use of local anesthetics, with these anticonvulsant drugs. Supportive treatment of circulatory depression may require administration of intravenous fluids and, when appropriate, a vasopressor as directed by the clinical situation (e.g., ephedrine).

If not treated immediately, both convulsions and cardiovascular depression can result in hypoxia, acidosis, bradycardia, arrhythmias and cardiac arrest. Underventilation or apnea due to unintentional subarachnoid injection of local anesthetic solution may produce these same signs and also lead to cardiac arrest if ventilatory support is not instituted. If cardiac arrest should occur standard cardiopulmonary resuscitative measures should be instituted.

Endotracheal intubation, employing drugs and techniques familiar to the clinician, may be indicated, after initial administration of oxygen by mask, if difficulty is encountered in the maintenance of a patent airway or if prolonged ventilatory support (assisted or controlled) is indicated.

Dialysis is of negligible value in the treatment of acute overdosage with Lidocaine.

The oral LD_{50} of Lidocaine HCl in non-fasted female rats is 459 (346-773) mg/kg (as the salt) and 214 (159-324) mg/kg (as the salt) in fasted female rats.

The intravenous LD_{50} of Lidocaine HCl in female mice is 26 (21-31) mg/kg and subcutaneous LD_{50} is 264 (203-304) mg/kg.

DOSAGE AND ADMINISTRATION

When Lidocaine HCl solution is used concomitantly with other products containing Lidocaine, the total dose contributed by all formulations must be kept in mind.

Table 1 (Recommended Dosages) summarizes the recommended volumes and concentrations of Lidocaine Hydrochloride, Local Anesthesia injection for various types of anesthetic procedures. The dosages suggested in this table are for normal healthy adults and refer to the use of epinephrine-free solutions. When larger volumes are required only solutions containing epinephrine should be used, except in those cases where vasopressor drugs may be contraindicated.

◆ RATED THERAPEUTICALLY EQUIVALENT; ◇ THERAPEUTIC EQUIVALENCE UNCONFIRMED; ○ UNRATED

These recommended doses serve only as a guide to the amount of anesthetic required for most routine procedures. The actual volumes and concentrations to be used depend on a number of factors such as type and extent of surgical procedure, depth of anesthesia and degree of muscular relaxation required, duration of anesthesia required, and the physical condition of the patient, as well as the area to be anesthetized, vascularity of the tissues, individual tolerance, and technique of anesthesia. In all cases the lowest concentration and smallest dose that will produce the desired result should be given. Dosages should be reduced for children and for elderly and debilitated patients and patients with cardiac and/or liver disease.

The onset of anesthesia, the duration of anesthesia and the degree of muscular relaxation are proportional to the volume and concentration (i.e., total dose) of local anesthetic used. Thus, an increase in volume and concentration of Lidocaine Hydrochloride, Local Anesthesia, injection will decrease the onset of anesthesia, prolong the duration of anesthesia, provide a greater degree of muscular relaxation and increase the segmental spread of anesthesia. However, increasing the volume and concentration of Lidocaine Hydrochloride, Local Anesthesia, injection may result in a more profound fall in blood pressure when used in epidural anesthesia. Although the incidence of side effects with Lidocaine is quite low, caution should be exercised when employing large volumes and concentrations, since the incidence of side effects is directly proportional to the total dose of local anesthetic agent injected.

For intravenous regional anesthesia, only the 0.5% injection should be used.

EPIDURAL ANESTHESIA

For epidural anesthesia, only the following dosage forms of Lidocaine Hydrochloride, Local Anesthesia, injection are recommended:

1% without epinephrine . . . . .30 mL ampules
30 ml single dose vials
1% with epinephrine 1:200,000 . . . . .30 mL ampules
30 ml single dose vials
1.5% without epinephrine . . . . .20 mL ampules
20 ml single dose vials
1.5% with epinephrine 1:200,000 . . . . .30 mL ampules
30 ml single dose vials
2% without epinephrine . . . . .10 mL ampules
10 mL single dose vials
2% with epinephrine 1:200,000 . . . . .20 mL ampules
20 ml single dose vials

Although these solutions are intended specifically for epidural anesthesia, they may also be used for infiltration and peripheral nerve block, provided they are employed as single dose units.

In epidural anesthesia, the dosage varies with the number of dermatomes to be anesthetized (generally 2-3 ml of the indicated concentration per dermatome).

Caudal and Lumbar Epidural Block: As a precaution against the adverse experience sometimes observed following unintentional penetration of the subarachnoid space, a test dose such as 2-3 ml of 1.5% Lidocaine should be administered at least 5 minutes prior to injecting the total volume required for a lumbar or caudal epidural block. The test dose should be repeated if the patient is moved in a manner that may have displaced the catheter. Epinephrine, if contained in the test dose (10-15 μg have been suggested), may serve as a warning of unintentional intravascular injection. If injected into a blood vessel, this amount of epinephrine is likely to produce a transient "epinephrine response" within 45 seconds, consisting of an increase in heart rate and systolic blood pressure, circumoral pallor, palpitations and nervousness in the unsedated patient. The sedated patient may exhibit only a pulse rate increase of 20 or more beats per minutes for 15 or more seconds. Patients on beta-blockers may not manifest changes in heart rate, but blood pressure monitoring can detect an evanescent rise in systolic blood pressure. Adequate time should be allowed for onset of anesthesia after administration of each test dose. The rapid injection of a large volume of Lidocaine HCl, Local Anesthesia, injection through the catheter should be avoided, and, when feasible, fractional doses should be administered.

In the event of the known injection of a large volume of local anesthetic solution into the subarachnoid space, after suitable resuscitation and if the catheter is in place, consider attempting the recovery of drug by draining a moderate amount of cerebrospinal fluid (such as 10 mL) through the epidural catheter.

In retrobulbar injection, a portion of the dose is injected retrobulbarly and the rest may be used to block the facial nerve.

In transtracheal injection, the drug should be injected through a large enough needle so that the injection can be made rapidly. By injecting during inspiration some of the drug will be carried into the bronchi and the resulting cough will distribute the rest of the drug over the vocal cords and the epiglottis. Occasionally it may be necessary to spray the pharynx by oropharyngeal spray to achieve complete analgesia. For the combination of the injection and spray, it should rarely be necessary to utilize more than 5 mL (200 mg of lidocaine HCl), i.e., 3 mg/kg or 1.5 mg/lb body weight.

Topical application: For laryngoscopy, bronchoscopy and endotracheal intubation, the pharynx may be sprayed with 1-5 ml (40-200 mg of Lidocaine i.e., 0.6-3 mg/kg or 0.3-1.5 mg/lb body weight.

MAXIMUM RECOMMENDED DOSAGES

Adults: For normal healthy adults, the individual maximum recommended dose of Lidocaine HCl with epinephrine should not exceed 7 mg/kg (3.5 mg/lb) of body weight, and in general it is recommended that the maximum total dose not exceed 500 mg. When used without epinephrine, the maximum individual dose should not exceed 4.5 mg/kg (2 mg per lb) of body weight, and in general it is recommended that the maximum total dose does not exceed 300 mg. For continuous epidural or caudal anesthesia, the maximum recommended dosage should not be administered at intervals of less than 90 minutes. When continuous lumbar or caudal epidural anesthesia is used for non-obstetrical procedures, more drug may be administered if required to produce adequate anesthesia.

The maximum recommended dose per 90 minute period of Lidocaine HCl for paracervical block in obstetrical patients and non-obstetrical patients is 200 mg total. One half of the total dose is usually administered to each side. Inject slowly, five minutes between sides. (See also discussion of paracervical block in "Precautions").

For intravenous regional anesthesia, the dose administered should not exceed 4 mg/kg in adults.

Children: It is difficult to recommend a maximum dose of any drug for children, since this varies as a function of age and weight. For children over 3 years of age but less than ten years who have a normal lean body mass and normal body development the maximum dose is determined by the application of one of the standard pediatric drug formulas (e.g., Clark's rule). For example, in a child of 5 years weighing 50 lbs., the dose of Lidocaine HCl should not exceed 75-100 mg (1.5-2 mg/lb), when calculated according to Clark's rule. In any case, the maximum dose of Lidocaine HCl Solution with epinephrine should not exceed 7 mg/kg (3.2 mg/lb.) of body weight. When used without epinephrine, the amount of Lidocaine HCl Solution administered should be such that the dose of Lidocaine is kept below 300 mg and in any case should not exceed 4.5 mg/kg (2.0 mg/lb) of body weight.

The use of even more dilute solutions (i.e., 0.25-0.5%) and total dosages not to exceed 3 mg/kg (1.4 mg/lb) are recommended for induction of intravenous regional anesthesia in children.

In order to guard against systemic toxicity, the lowest effective concentration and lowest effective dose should be used at all times. In some cases it will be necessary to dilute available concentrations with 0.9% sodium chloride injection in order to obtain the required final concentration.

Note: Parenteral drug products should be inspected visually for particulate matter and discoloration prior to administration whenever the solution and container permit. The injection is not to be used if it is discolored or if it contains a precipitate.

Table 1
RECOMMENDED DOSAGES

| | | Lidocaine HCl injection (without epinephrine) | |
Procedure	Conc (%)	Vol (ml)	Total Dose (mg)
Infiltration			
Percutaneous	0.5 or 1	1-60	5-300
Intravenous regional	0.5	10-60	50-300
Peripheral Nerve Blocks, e.g.,			
Brachial	1.5	15-20	225-300
Dental	2	1-5	20-100
Intercostal	1	3	30
Paravertebral	1	3-5	30-50
Pudendal (each side)	1	10	100
Paracervical			
Obstetrical analgesia (each side)	1	10	100
Sympathetic Nerve Blocks. e.g.,			
Cervical (stellate ganglion)	1	5	50
Lumbar	1	5-10	50-100
Central Neural Blocks			
Epidural†			
Thoracic	1	20-30	200-300
Lumbar			
Analgesia	1	25-30	250-300
Anethesia	1.5	15-20	225-300
	2	10-15	200-300
Caudal			
Obstetrical analgesia	1	20-30	200-300
Surgical anesthesia	1.5	15-20	225-300
Retrobulbar Injection	4	3-5	120-200
Transtracheal Injection	4	2-3	80-120

† Dose determined by number of dermatomes to be anesthetized (2-3 ml/dermatome).

THE ABOVE SUGGESTED CONCENTRATIONS AND VOLUMES SERVE ONLY AS A GUIDE. OTHER VOLUMES AND CONCENTRATIONS MAY BE USED PROVIDED THE TOTAL MAXIMUM RECOMMENDED DOSE IS NOT EXCEEDED.

Sterilization, Storage and Technical Procedures: Disinfecting agents containing heavy metals, which cause release of respective ions (mercury, zinc, copper, etc.) should not be used for skin or mucous membrane disinfection as they have been related to incidents of swelling and edema. When chemical disinfection of multi-dose vials is desired, either isopropyl alcohol (91%) or ethyl alcohol (70%) is recommended. Many commercially available brands of rubbing alcohol, as well as solutions of ethyl alcohol not of U.S.P. grade, contain denaturants which are injurious to rubber and therefore are not to be used.

Storage: All solutions should be stored at controlled room temperature, 15°C-30°C (59°-86°).

HOW SUPPLIED
GEL: 2%

AVERAGE UNIT PRICE (AVAILABLE SIZES)

BRAND	$0.30
GENERIC	$1.09

BRAND/MANUFACTURER	NDC	SIZE	AWP
◆ BRAND			
XYLOCAINE: Astra	00186-0330-01	30 ml	$13.65
ANESTACON: Polymedica	00998-0300-20	240 ml 6s	$134.25
	00998-0300-10	15 ml 12s	$65.25
◆ GENERICS			
Intl Med Sys	00548-3012-00	5 ml 25s	$215.63
Intl Med Sys	00548-3013-00	10 ml 25s	$240.38
Intl Med Sys	00548-3015-00	20 ml 25s	$289.50

GEL: 2%

BRAND/MANUFACTURER	NDC	SIZE	AWP
○ BRAND			
XYLOCAINE: Astra	00186-0330-36	5 ml 10s	$65.63
○ GENERICS			
Copley	38245-0200-11	30 gm	$12.95

INJECTION: 0.5%

AVERAGE UNIT PRICE (AVAILABLE SIZES)

BRAND	$0.13	GENERIC A-RATED AVERAGE PRICE (GAAP)	
GENERIC	$0.06	50 ml 25s	$77.48

BRAND/MANUFACTURER	NDC	SIZE	AWP
◆ BRAND			
XYLOCAINE HCL: Astra	00186-0135-01	50 ml	$3.61
XYLOCAINE-MPF: Astra	00186-0137-01	50 ml	$9.08
◆ GENERICS			
Abbott Hosp	00074-4278-01	50 ml 25s	$77.48
Abbott Hosp	00074-4275-01	50 ml 25s	$77.48

INJECTION: 1%

AVERAGE UNIT PRICE (AVAILABLE SIZES)

BRAND	$0.33	GENERIC A-RATED AVERAGE PRICE (GAAP)	
GENERIC	$0.56	50 ml	$3.39
		20 ml 5s	$52.54
		30 ml 5s	$57.64
		5 ml 10s	$101.20
		5 ml 25s	$125.18
		10 ml 25s	$147.19
		30 ml 25s	$79.02
		50 ml 25s	$38.30

BRAND/MANUFACTURER	NDC	SIZE	AWP
◆ BRAND			
XYLOCAINE HCL: Astra	00186-0110-01	20 ml	$2.01
	00186-0145-01	50 ml	$3.31
	00186-0275-12	10 ml 5s	$8.11
XYLOCAINE-MPF: Astra	00186-0278-12	10 ml 5s	$22.45
	00186-0112-01	30 ml 5s	$7.41
	00186-0112-91	30 ml 5s	$39.51
	00186-0255-02	30 ml 5s	$43.30
	00186-0255-92	30 ml 5s	$47.94
	00186-0210-03	2 ml 10s	$14.00
	00186-0276-13	2 ml 10s	$14.05
	00186-0277-13	5 ml 10s	$18.00
	00186-0230-03	5 ml 10s	$18.91
XYLOCAINE HCL: Astra	00186-0615-01	5 ml 10s	$21.13
◆ GENERICS			
Fujisawa	00469-1201-15	2 ml	$1.22
Fujisawa	00469-2201-25	10 ml	$0.97
Moore,H.L.	00839-5597-38	50 ml	$1.88
Schein	00364-6549-57	50 ml	$2.25
Steris	00402-0055-50	50 ml	$2.25
URL	00677-0281-24	50 ml	$2.90
Goldline	00182-0565-67	50 ml	$3.00
Hyrex	00314-0679-50	50 ml	$3.50
Rugby	00536-1450-80	50 ml	$4.88
LIDOJECT-1: Mayrand	00259-0325-50	50 ml	$6.45
Intl Med Sys	00548-1078-00	20 ml 5s	$48.23
Intl Med Sys	00548-1080-00	20 ml 5s	$56.85
Intl Med Sys	00548-1079-00	30 ml 5s	$51.08
Intl Med Sys	00548-1081-00	30 ml 5s	$64.20
Abbott Hosp	00074-4713-01	2 ml 10s	$14.49
Abbott Hosp	00074-4904-01	5 ml 10s	$96.07
Abbott Hosp	00074-4924-01	5 ml 10s	$96.07
Abbott Hosp	00074-8026-01	5 ml 10s	$103.79

BRAND/MANUFACTURER	NDC	SIZE	AWP
Abbott Hosp	00074-4904-23	5 ml 10s	$108.89
Elkins-Sinn	00641-0436-25	5 ml 25s	$16.15
Abbott Hosp	00074-4713-02	5 ml 25s	$49.88
Intl Med Sys	00548-1111-00	5 ml 25s	$142.50
Intl Med Sys	00548-1192-00	5 ml 25s	$145.13
Abbott Hosp	00074-4904-33	5 ml 25s	$272.23
Intl Med Sys	00548-1193-00	10 ml 25s	$132.75
Intl Med Sys	00548-1115-00	10 ml 25s	$161.63
Abbott Hosp	00074-4276-01	20 ml 25s	$54.03
Elkins-Sinn	00641-2380-45	30 ml 25s	$15.00
Abbott Hosp	00074-4279-02	30 ml 25s	$37.41
Abbott Hosp	00074-4270-01	30 ml 25s	$184.66
Elkins-Sinn	00641-2390-45	50 ml 25s	$20.63
Amer Regent	00517-0625-25	50 ml 25s	$27.19
Abbott Hosp	00074-4276-02	50 ml 25s	$67.09

INJECTION: 1%

BRAND/MANUFACTURER	NDC	SIZE	AWP
○ BRAND			
EPIDURAL SINGLE SHOT W/LIDOCAINE: Abbott Hosp	00074-1986-01	2 ml 10s	$379.41
○ GENERICS			
McGuff	49072-0413-30	30 ml	$1.19
CMC-Cons	00223-7924-30	30 ml	$1.25
McGuff	49072-0415-50	50 ml	$1.39
NERVOCAINE: Keene	00588-5956-95	50 ml	$1.80
Allscrips	54569-2204-00	50 ml	$2.25
TRUXACAINE: Truxton	00463-1077-50	50 ml	$2.35
DILOCAINE: Roberts/Hauck	59441-0564-50	50 ml	$2.50
L-CAINE: Century	00436-0226-79	50 ml	$2.85
Legere	25332-0026-50	50 ml	$2.95
CMC-Cons	00223-7924-50	50 ml	$3.00
ANESTACAINE: Clint	55553-0055-50	50 ml	$3.15
Forest Pharm	00456-0779-83	50 ml	$3.25
Allscrips	54569-3776-00	5 ml 10s	$102.27
Abbott Hosp	00074-4786-01	20 ml 10s	$256.62
Veratex	17022-2176-08	50 ml 10s	$1.25
Allscrips	54569-2356-00	5 ml 25s	$16.15
CMC-Cons	00223-7938-05	5 ml 25s	$35.00
CMC-Cons	00223-7933-30	30 ml 25s	$29.00
Allscrips	54569-2215-00	30 ml 25s	$68.15
CMC-Cons	00223-7924-25	50 ml 25s	$37.50
Allscrips	54569-1415-00	50 ml 25s	$42.89
Allscrips	54569-3198-00	2 ml 100s	$146.40

INJECTION: 1.5%

AVERAGE UNIT PRICE (AVAILABLE SIZES)

BRAND	$1.26
GENERIC	$0.35

BRAND/MANUFACTURER	NDC	SIZE	AWP
◆ BRAND			
XYLOCAINE-MPF: Astra	00186-0118-01	20 ml	$10.06
	00186-0244-12	10 ml 5s	$24.69
	00186-0245-02	20 ml 5s	$45.39
	00186-0118-91	20 ml 5s	$49.83
XYLOCAINE HCL: Astra	00186-0212-03	2 ml 10s	$87.36
◆ GENERICS			
Abbott Hosp	00074-4056-01	20 ml 10s	$28.68
Abbott Hosp	00074-4776-01	20 ml 25s	$202.77

For additional alternatives, turn to the section beginning on page 2859.

Lidocaine with Prilocaine

DESCRIPTION
Lidocaine 2.5% and Prilocaine 2.5% is an emulsion in which the oil phase is a eutectic mixture of Lidocaine and Prilocaine in a ratio of 1:1 by weight. A eutectic mixture has a melting point below room temperature and therefore both local anesthetics exist as a liquid oil rather than as crystals.

Lidocaine is chemically designated as acetamide, 2-(diethylamino)-N(2,6-dimethylphenyl), has an octanol:water partition ratio of 43 at pH 7.4.

Prilocaine is chemically designated as propanamide, N-(2-methyl-phenyl)-2-(propylamino), and has an octanol:water partition ratio of 25 at pH 7.4.

◆ **RATED THERAPEUTICALLY EQUIVALENT;** ◇ **THERAPEUTIC EQUIVALENCE UNCONFIRMED;** ○ **UNRATED**

Each gram of Lidocaine/Prilocaine Cream contains Lidocaine 25 mg, Prilocaine 25 mg. Lidocaine/Prilocaine Cream contains no preservative, however, it passes the USP antimicrobial effectiveness test due to the pH. The specific gravity of Lidocaine/Prilocaine Cream is 1.00.

CLINICAL PHARMACOLOGY

Mechanism of Action: Lidocaine 2.5% and Prilocaine 2.5%, applied to intact skin under occlusive dressing, provides dermal analgesia by the release of Lidocaine and Prilocaine from the cream into the epidermal and dermal layers of the skin and the accumulation of Lidocaine and Prilocaine in the vicinity of dermal pain receptors and nerve endings. Lidocaine and Prilocaine are amide-type local anesthetic agents. Both Lidocaine and Prilocaine stabilize neuronal membranes by inhibiting the ionic fluxes required for the initiation and conduction of impulses, thereby effecting local anesthetic action.

The onset, depth and duration of dermal analgesia provided by Lidocaine/Prilocaine Cream depends primarily on the duration of application. To provide sufficient analgesia for clinical procedures such as intravenous catheter placement and venipuncture, Lidocaine/Prilocaine Cream should be applied under an occlusive dressing for at least 1 hour. To provide dermal analgesia for clinical procedures such as split skin graft harvesting, Lidocaine/Prilocaine Cream should be applied under occlusive dressing for at least 2 hours. Satisfactory dermal analgesia is achieved 1 hour after application, reaches maximum at 2 to 3 hours, and persists for 1 to 2 hours after removal.

Dermal application of Lidocaine/Prilocaine Cream may cause a transient, local blanching followed by a transient, local redness or erythema.

Pharmacokinetics: Lidocaine/Prilocaine Cream is a eutectic mixture of Lidocaine 2.5% and Prilocaine 2.5% formulated as an oil in water emulsion. As a eutectic mixture, both anesthetics are liquid at room temperature (see *"Description"*) and the penetration and subsequent systemic absorption of both Prilocaine and Lidocaine are enhanced over that which would be seen if each component is crystalline form was applied separately as a 2.5% topical cream.

The amount of Lidocaine and Prilocaine systemically absorbed from Lidocaine/Prilocaine Cream is directly related to both the duration of application and to the area over which it is applied. In two pharmacokinetic studies, 60 g of Lidocaine/Prilocaine Cream (1.5 g Lidocaine and 1.5 g Prilocaine) was applied to $400 cm^2$ of intact skin on the lateral thigh and then covered by an occlusive dressing. The subjects were then randomized such that one-half of the subjects had the occlusive dressing and residual cream removed after 3 hours, while the remainder left the dressing in place for 24 hours. The results from these studies are summarized below. (See related table).

When Lidocaine/Prilocaine Cream is used according to the recommended dosing instructions, peak blood levels of Lidocaine are approximately 1/20 the systemic toxic level. Likewise, the maximum Prilocaine level is about 1/36 the toxic level. The application of Lidocaine/Prilocaine Cream to broken or inflamed skin, or to $2,000 cm^2$ or more of skin where more of both anesthetics are absorbed, could result in higher plasma levels that could, in susceptible individuals, produce a systemic pharmacologic response. When each drug is administered intravenously, the steady-state volume of distribution is 1.1 to 2.1 L/kg (mean 1.5, $\pm$ 0.3 SD, n = 13) for Lidocaine and is 0.7 to 4.4 L/kg (mean 2.6, $\pm$ 1.3 SD, n = 13) for Prilocaine. The larger distribution volume for Prilocaine produces the lower plasma concentrations of prilocaine observed when equal amounts of Prilocaine and Lidocaine are administered. At concentrations produced by application of Lidocaine/Prilocaine Cream, Lidocaine is approximately 70% bound to plasma proteins, primarily alpha-1-acid glycoprotein. At much higher plasma concentrations (1 to 4 µg/mL of free base) the plasma protein binding of Lidocaine is concentration dependent. Prilocaine is 55% bound to plasma proteins. Both Lidocaine and Prilocaine cross the placental and blood brain barrier, presumably by passive diffusion.

It is not known if Lidocaine or Prilocaine are metabolized in the skin. Lidocaine is metabolized rapidly by the liver to a number of metabolites including monoethylglycinexylidide (MEGX) and glycinexylidide (GX), both of which have pharmacologic activity similar to, but less potent than that of Lidocaine. The metabolite, 2,6-xylidine, has unknown pharmacologic activity but is carcinogenic in rats (see *"Carcinogenesis"* subsection of *"Precautions"*). Following intravenous administration, MEGX and GX concentrations in serum range from 11 to 36% and from 5 to 11% of Lidocaine concentrations, respectively. Prilocaine is metabolized in both the liver and kidneys by amidases to various metabolites including *ortho*-toluidine and N-n-propylalanine. It is not metabolized by plasma esterases. The *ortho*-toluidine metabolite has been shown to be carcinogenic in several animal models (see *"Carcinogenesis"* subsection of *"Precautions"*). In addition, *ortho*-toluidine can produce methemoglobinemia following systemic doses of prilocaine approximating 8 mg/kg (see *"Adverse Reactions"*). Very young

patients, patients with glucose-6-phosphate deficiencies and patients taking oxidizing drugs such as antimalarials and sulfonamides are more susceptible to methemoglobinemia (see *"Methemoglobinemia"* subsection of *"Precautions"*).

The half-life of Lidocaine elimination from the plasma following IV administration is approximately 65 to 150 minutes (mean 110, $\pm$ 24 SD, n = 13). This half-life may be increased in cardiac or hepatic dysfunction. More than 98% of an absorbed dose of Lidocaine can be recovered in the urine as metabolites or parent drug. The systemic clearance is 10 to 20 mL/min/kg (mean 13, $\pm$ 3 SD, n = 13). The elimination half-life of Prilocaine is approximately 10 to 150 minutes (mean 70, $\pm$ 48 SD, n = 13). The systemic clearance is 18 to 64 mL/min/kg (mean 38, $\pm$ 15 SD, n = 13). Prilocaine's half-life also may be increased in hepatic or renal dysfunction since both of these organs are involved in Prilocaine metabolism.

CLINICAL STUDIES

Lidocaine/Prilocaine Cream application in adults prior to IV cannulation or venipuncture was studied in 200 patients in four clinical studies in Europe. Application for at least 1 hour provided significantly more dermal analgesia than placebo cream or ethyl chloride. Lidocaine/Prilocaine Cream was comparable to subcutaneous Lidocaine, but was less efficacious than intradermal Lidocaine. Most patients found Lidocaine/Prilocaine Cream treatment preferable to Lidocaine infiltration or ethyl chloride spray.

Lidocaine/Prilocaine Cream was compared with 0.5% Lidocaine infiltration prior to skin graft harvesting in one open label study in 80 adult patients in England. Application of Lidocaine/Prilocaine Cream for 2 to 5 hours provided dermal analgesia comparable to Lidocaine infiltration.

Lidocaine/Prilocaine Cream application in children was studied in seven non-US studies (320 patients) and one US study (100 patients). In controlled studies, application of Lidocaine/Prilocaine Cream for at least 1 hour with or without presurgical medication prior to needle insertion provided significantly more pain reduction than placebo. In children under the age of seven years, Lidocaine/Prilocaine Cream was less effective than in older children or adults.

Lidocaine/Prilocaine Cream was compared with placebo in the laser treatment of facial port-wine stains in 72 pediatric patients (ages 5-16). Lidocaine/Prilocaine Cream was effective in providing pain relief during laser treatment.

Local dermal effects associated with Lidocaine/Prilocaine Cream application in these studies on intact skin included paleness, redness and edema and were transient in nature (see *"Adverse Reactions"*).

Individualization of Dose: The dose of Lidocaine/Prilocaine Cream which provides effective analgesia depends on the duration of the application over the treated area.

All pharmacokinetic and clinical studies employed a thick layer of Lidocaine/Prilocaine Cream (1-2 g/10 cm^2). The duration of application prior to venipuncture was 1 hour. The duration of application prior to taking split thickness skin grafts was 2 hours. Although a thinner application may be efficacious, such has not been studied and may result in less complete analgesia or a shorter duration of adequate analgesia.

The systemic absorption of Lidocaine and Prilocaine is a side effect of the desired local effect. The amount of drug absorbed depends on surface area and duration of application. The systemic blood levels depend on the amount absorbed and patient size (weight) and rate of systemic drug elimination. Long duration of application, large treatment area, small patients, or impaired elimination may result in high blood levels. The systemic blood levels are typically a small fraction (1/20 to 1/50) of the blood levels which produce toxicity. Table 2 which follows gives maximum recommended application areas for infants and children.

Table 2

LIDOCAINE/PRILOCAINE CREAM MAXIMUM RECOMMENDED APPLICATION AREA* FOR INFANTS AND CHILDREN BASED ON APPLICATION TO INTACT SKIN

Body Weight (kg)	Maximum Application Area (cm^2)**
up to 10 kg	100
10 to 20 kg	600
above 20 kg	2000

* These are broad guidelines for avoiding systemic toxicity in applying Lidocaine/Prilocaine to patients with normal intact skin and with normal renal and hepatic function.

** For more individualized calculation of how much Lidocaine and Prilocaine may be absorbed, physicians can use the following estimates of

Table 1

ABSORPTION OF LIDOCAINE AND PRILOCAINE FROM EMLA CREAM NORMAL VOLUNTEERS (N = 16)

Lidocaine/Prilocaine (g)	Area (cm^2)	Time on (hrs)	Drug Content (mg)	Absorbed (mg)	Cmax (µg/mL)	Tmax (hr)
60	400	3	Lidocaine 1500	54	0.12	4
			Prilocaine 1500	92	0.07	4
60	400	24*	Lidocaine 1500	243	0.28	10
			Prilocaine 1500	503	0.14	10

* Maximum recommended duration of exposure is 4 hours.

Lidocaine and Prilocaine absorption for children and adults:
The estimated mean (±SD) absorption of Lidocaine is 0.045 (± 0.016) mg/cm²/hr.
The estimated mean (± SD) absorption of Prilocaine is 0.77 (± 0.036) mg/cm²/hr.

An IV antiarrhythmic dose of Lidocaine is 1 mg/kg (70 mg/70 kg) and gives a blood level of about 1 µg/mL. Toxicity would be expected at blood levels above 5 µ/mL. Smaller areas of treatment are recommended in a debilitated patient, a small child or a patient with impaired elimination. Decreasing the duration of application is likely to decrease the analgesia effect.

INDICATION AND USAGE

Lidocaine/Prilocaine Cream (a eutectic mixture of Lidocaine 2.5% and Prilocaine 2.5%) is indicated as a topical anesthetic for use on **normal intact skin** for local analgesia.

Lidocaine/Prilocaine Cream is not recommended for use on mucous membranes because limited studies show much greater absorption of Lidocaine and Prilocaine than through intact skin. Safe dosing recommendations for use on mucous membranes cannot be made because it has not been studied adequately. Lidocaine/Prilocaine Cream is not recommended in any clinical situation in which penetration or migration beyond the tympanic membrane into the middle ear is possible because of the ototoxic effects observed in animal studies (see *"Warnings"*).

CONTRAINDICATIONS

Lidocaine/Prilocaine Cream (Lidocaine 2.5% and Prilocaine 2.5%) is contraindicated in patients with a known history of sensitivity to local anesthetics of the amide type or to any other component of the product.

WARNINGS

Application of Lidocaine/Prilocaine Cream to larger areas or for longer times than those recommended could result in sufficient absorption of Lidocaine and Prilocaine resulting in serious adverse effects (see *"Individualization of Dose"*).

Studies in laboratory animals (guinea pigs) have shown that Lidocaine/Prilocaine Cream has an ototoxic effect when instilled into the middle ear. In these same studies, animals exposed to Lidocaine/Prilocaine Cream in the external auditory canal only, showed no abnormality. Lidocaine/Prilocaine Cream should not be used in any clinical situation in which its penetration or migration beyond the tympanic membrane into the middle ear is possible.

Methemoglobinemia: Lidocaine/Prilocaine Cream should not be used in those rare patients with congenital or idiopathic methemoglobinemia and in infants under the age of twelve months who are receiving treatment with methemoglobin-inducing agents.

Very young patients or patients with glucose-6-phosphate deficiencies are more susceptible to methemoglobinemia. Patients taking drugs associated with drug-induced methemoglobinemia such as sulfonamides, acetaminophen, acetanilid, aniline dyes, benzocaine, chloroquine, dapsone, naphthalene, nitrates and nitrites, nitrofurantoin, nitroglycerin, nitroprusside, pamaquine, para-aminosalicylic acid, phenacetin, phenobarbital, phenytoin, primaquine, quinine, are also at greater risk for developing methemoglobinemia. Methemoglobinemia (28%) developed in a three-month old male infant (5.3 kg) who had 5 grams of Lidocaine/Prilocaine Cream under an occlusive dressing applied to the back of the hands and in the cubital regions for 5 hours. The methemoglobinemia was successfully treated with IV methylene blue. The patient was concomitantly receiving trimethoprim (16 mg/day) and sulfamethoxazole (80 mg/day) for a urinary tract infection.

PRECAUTIONS

General: Repeated doses of Lidocaine/Prilocaine Cream may increase blood levels of Lidocaine and Prilocaine. Lidocaine/Prilocaine Cream should be used with caution in patients who may be more sensitive to the systemic effects of Lidocaine and Prilocaine including acutely ill, debilitated, or elderly patients.

Lidocaine/Prilocaine Cream coming in contact with the eye should be avoided because animal studies have demonstrated severe eye irritation. Also the loss of protective reflexes can permit corneal irritation and potential abrasion. Absorption of Lidocaine/Prilocaine Cream in conjunctival tissues has not been determined. If eye contact occurs, immediately wash out the eye with water or saline and protect the eye until sensation returns.

Patients allergic to para-aminobenzoic acid derivatives (procaine, tetracaine, benzocaine, etc.) have not shown cross sensitivity to Lidocaine and/or Prilocaine, however, Lidocaine/Prilocaine Cream should be used with caution in patients with a history of drug sensitivities, especially if the etiologic agent is uncertain.

Patients with severe hepatic disease, because of their inability to metabolize local anesthetics normally, are at greater risk of developing toxic plasma concentrations of Lidocaine and Prilocaine.

Information for Patients: When Lidocaine/Prilocaine Cream is used, the patient should be aware that the production of dermal analgesia may be accompanied by the block of all sensations in the treated skin. For this reason, the patient should avoid inadvertent trauma to the treated area by scratching, rubbing, or exposure to extreme hot or cold temperatures until complete sensation has returned.

Drug Interactions: Lidocaine/Prilocaine Cream should be used with caution in patients receiving Class I antiarrhythmic drugs (such as tocainide and mexiletine) since the toxic effects are additive and potentially synergistic.

Prilocaine may contribute to the formation of methemoglobin in patients treated with other drugs known to cause this condition (see *"Methemoglobinemia"* subsection of *"Warnings"*).

Carcinogenesis, Mutagenesis, Impairment of Fertility

Carcinogens: Metabolites of both Lidocaine and Prilocaine have been shown to be carcinogenic in laboratory animals. In the animal studies reported below, doses or blood levels are compared to the Single Dermal Administration (SDA) of 60 g of Lidocaine/Prilocaine Cream to 400 cm² for 3 hours to a small person (50 kg). The typical application for one or two treatments for venipuncture sites (2.5 or 5 g) would be 1/24 or 1/12 of that dose in an adult or about the same mg/kg dose in an infant. A two-year oral toxicity study of 2,6-xylidine, a metabolite of lidocaine, has shown that in both male and female rats 2,6-xylidine in daily doses of 900 mg/m² (60 times SDA) resulted in carcinomas and adenomas of the nasal cavity. With daily doses of 300 mg/m² (20 times SDA), the increase in incidence of nasal carcinomas and/or adenomas in each sex of the rat were not statistically greater than the control group. In the low dose (90 mg/m²; 6 times SDA) and control groups, no nasal tumors were observed. A rhabdomyosarcoma, a rare tumor, was observed in the nasal cavity of both male and female rats at the high dose of 900 mg/m². In addition, the compound caused subcutaneous fibromas and/or fibrosarcomas in both male and female rats and neoplastic nodules of the liver in the female rats with a significantly positive trend test; pairwise comparisons using Fisher's Exact Test showed significance only at the high dose of 900 mg/m². The animal study was conducted at oral doses of 15, 50, and 150 mg/kg/day. The dosages have been converted to mg/m² for the SDA calculations above.

Chronic oral toxicity studies of *ortho*-toluidine, a metabolite of Prilocaine, in mice (900 to 14,400 mg/m², 60 to 960 times SDA) and rats (900 to 4,800 mg/m²; 60 to 320 times SDA) have shown that *ortho*-toluidine is a carcinogen in both species. The tumors included hepatocarcinomas/adenomas in female mice, multiple occurrences of hemangiosarcomas/hemangiomas in both sexes of mice, sarcomas of multiple organs, transitional-cell carcinomas/papillomas of urinary bladder in both sexes of rats, subcutaneous fibromas/fibrosarcomas and mesotheliomas in male rats, and mammary gland fibroadenomas/adenomas in female rats. The lowest dose tested (900 mg/m²; 60 times SDA) was carcinogenic in both species. Thus the no-effect dose must be less than 60 times SDA. The animal studies were conducted at 150 to 2,400 mg/kg in mice and at 150 to 800 mg/kg in rats. The dosages have been converted to mg/m² for the SDA calculations above.

Mutagenesis: The mutagenic potential of Lidocaine HCl has been tested in the Ames Salmonella/mammalian microsome test and by analysis of structural chromosome aberrations in human lymphocytes *in vitro*, and by the mouse micronucleus test *in vivo*. There was no indication in these three tests of any mutagenic effects.

The mutagenicity of 2,6-xylidine, a metabolite of Lidocaine, has been studied in different tests with mixed results. The compound was found to be weakly mutagenic in the Ames test only under metabolic activation conditions. In addition, 2,6-xylidine was observed to be mutagenic at the thymidine kinase locus, with or without activation, and induced chromosome aberrations and sister chromatid exchanges at concentrations at which the drug precipitated out of the solution (1.2 mg/mL). No evidence of genotoxicity was found in the *in vivo* assays measuring unscheduled DNA synthesis in rat hepatocytes, chromosome damage in polychromatic erythrocytes or preferential killing of DNA repair-deficient bacteria in liver, lung, kidney, testes and blood extracts from mice. However, covalent binding studies of DNA from liver and ethmoid turbinates in rats indicate that 2,6-xylidine may be genotoxic under certain conditions *in vivo*.

Ortho-toluidine, a metabolite of Prilocaine, (0.5 µg/mL) showed positive results in *Escherichia coli* DNA repair and phage-induction assays. Urine concentrates from rats treated with *ortho*-toluidine (300 mg/kg orally; 300 times SDA) were mutagenic for *Salmonella typhimurium* with metabolic activation. Several other tests on *ortho*-toluidine, including reverse mutations in five different *Salmonella typhimurium* strains with or without metabolic activation and with single strand breaks in DNA of V79 Chinese hamster cells, were negative.

Impairment of Fertility: See *"Use in Pregnancy"*.

Use in Pregnancy: Teratogenic Effects: Pregnancy Category B. Reproduction studies with Lidocaine have been performed in rats and have revealed no evidence of harm to the fetus (30 mg/kg subcutaneously; 22 times SDA). Reproduction studies with Prilocaine have been performed in rats and have revealed no evidence of impaired fertility or harm to the fetus (300 mg/kg intramuscularly; 188 times SDA). There are, however, no adequate and well-controlled studies in pregnant women. Because animal reproduction studies are not always predictive of human response, Lidocaine/Prilocaine Cream should be used during pregnancy only if clearly needed.

Reproduction studies have been performed in rats receiving subcutaneous administration of an aqueous mixture containing Lidocaine HCl and Prilocaine HCl at 1:1 (w/w). At 40 mg/kg each, a dose equivalent to 29 times SDA Lidocaine and 25 times SDA Prilocaine, no teratogenic, embryotoxic or fetotoxic effects were observed.

Labor and Delivery: Neither Lidocaine nor Prilocaine are contraindicated in labor and delivery. Should Lidocaine/Prilocaine Cream be used concomitantly with other products containing Lidocaine and/or Prilocaine, total doses contributed by all formulations must be considered.

Nursing Mothers: Lidocaine and probably Prilocaine, are excreted in human milk. Therefore, caution should be exercised when Lidocaine/Prilocaine Cream is administered to a nursing mother since the milk:plasma ratio of Lidocaine is 0.4 and is not determined for Prilocaine.

◆ RATED THERAPEUTICALLY EQUIVALENT; ◇ THERAPEUTIC EQUIVALENCE UNCONFIRMED; ○ UNRATED

Pediatric Use: Controlled studies of Lidocaine/Prilocaine Cream in children under the age of seven years have shown less overall benefit than in older children or adults. These results illustrate the importance of emotional and psychological support of younger children undergoing medical or surgical procedures.

Lidocaine/Prilocaine Cream should be used with care in patients with conditions or therapy associated with methemoglobinemia (see *"Methemoglobinemia"* subsection of *"Warnings"*).

In children weighing less than 20 kg, the area and duration should be limited (see Table 2 in *"Individualization of Dose"*).

ADVERSE REACTIONS

Localized Reactions: During or immediately after treatment with Lidocaine/Prilocaine Cream, the skin at the site of treatment may develop erythema or edema or may be the locus of abnormal sensation. In clinical studies involving over 1,300 Lidocaine/Prilocaine Cream-treated subjects, one or more such local reactions were noted in 56% of patients, and were generally mild and transient, resolving spontaneously within 1 or 2 hours. There were no serious reactions which were ascribed to Lidocaine/Prilocaine Cream.

In patients treated with Lidocaine/Prilocaine Cream, local effects observed in the trials included: paleness (pallor or blanching) 37%, redness (erythema) 30%, alterations in temperature sensations 7%, edema 6, itching 2% and rash, less than 1%.

Allergic Reactions: Allergic and anaphylactoid reactions associated with Lidocaine or Prilocaine can occur. They are characterized by urticaria, angioedema, bronchospasm, and shock. If they occur they should be managed by conventional means. The detection of sensitivity by skin testing is of doubtful value.

Systemic (Dose Related) Reactions: Systemic adverse reactions following appropriate use of Lidocaine/Prilocaine Cream are unlikely due to the small dose absorbed (see *"Pharmacokinetics"* subsection of *"Clinical Pharmacology"*). Systemic adverse effects of Lidocaine and/or Prilocaine are similar in nature to those observed with other amide local anesthetic agents including CNS excitation and/or depression (light-headedness, nervousness, apprehension, euphoria, confusion, dizziness, drowsiness, tinnitus, blurred or double vision, vomiting, sensations of heat, cold or numbness, twitching, tremors, convulsions, unconsciousness, respiratory depression and arrest). Excitatory CNS reactions may be brief or not occur at all, in which case the first manifestation may be drowsiness merging into unconsciousness. Cardiovascular manifestations may include bradycardia, hypotension and cardiovascular collapse leading to arrest.

OVERDOSAGE

Peak blood levels following a 60 g application to 400 cm^2 for 3 hours are 0.05 to 0.16 μg/mL for Lidocaine and 0.02 to 0.10 μg/mL for Prilocaine. Toxic levels of Lidocaine (> 5 μg/mL) and/or Prilocaine (> 6 μg/mL) cause decreases in cardiac output, total peripheral resistance and mean arterial pressure. These changes may be attributable to direct depressant effects of these local anesthetic agents on the cardiovascular system. In the absence of massive topical overdose or oral ingestion, evaluation should include evaluation of other etiologies for the clinical effects or overdosage from other sources of Lidocaine, Prilocaine or other local anesthetics.

DOSAGE AND ADMINISTRATION

A thick layer of Lidocaine Prilocaine Cream is applied to intact skin and covered with an occlusive dressing:

Minor Dermal Procedures: For minor procedures such as intravenous cannulation and venipuncture, apply 2.5 grams of Lidocaine/Prilocaine Cream (½ the 5 g tube) over 20 to 25 cm^2 of skin surface for at least 1 hour. In controlled clinical trials, two sites were usually prepared in case there was a technical problem with cannulation or venipuncture at the first site.

Major Dermal Procedures: For more painful dermatological procedures involving a larger skin area such as split thickness skin graft harvesting, apply 2 grams of Lidocaine/Prilocaine Cream per 10 cm^2 of skin and allow to remain in contact with the skin for at least 2 hours.

Dermal analgesia can be expected to increase for up to 3 hours under occlusive dressing and persist for 1 to 2 hours after removal of the cream. The amount of Lidocaine and Prilocaine absorbed during the period of application can be estimated from the information in Table 2, ** footnote, in *"Individualization of Dose"*.

A single application of Lidocaine/Prilocaine Cream in a child weighing less than 10 kg should not be applied over an area larger than 100 cm^2. A single application of Lidocaine/Prilocaine Cream in children weighing between 10 kg and 20 kg should not be applied over an area larger than 600 cm^2 (see Table 2 in *"Individualization of Dose"*).

Lidocaine/Prilocaine Cream should not be used in infants under the age of one month or in infants, under the age of twelve months, who are receiving treatment with methemoglobin-inducing agents (see *"Methemoglobinemia"* **subsection of** *"Warnings"*). When Lidocaine/Prilocaine Cream (Lidocaine 2.5% and Prilocaine 2.5%) is used concomitantly with other products containing local anesthetic agents, the amount absorbed from all formulations must be considered (see *"Individualization of Dose"*). The amount absorbed in the case of Lidocaine/Prilocaine Cream is determined by the area over which it is applied and the duration of application under occlusion (see Table 2, ** footnote, in *"Individualization of Dose"*).

Although the incidence of systemic adverse reactions with Lidocaine/Prilocaine Cream is very low, caution should be exercised particularly when applying it over large areas and leaving it on for longer than 2 hours. The incidence of systemic adverse reactions can be expected to be directly proportional to the area and time of exposure (see *"Individualization of Dose"*).

NOT FOR OPHTHALMIC USE. KEEP CONTAINER TIGHTLY CLOSED AT ALL TIMES WHEN NOT IN USE.

Store at controlled room temperature 15°-30°C (59°-86°F).

HOW SUPPLIED
CREAM: 2.5%

BRAND/MANUFACTURER	NDC	SIZE	AWP
○ BRAND			
EMLA: Astra	00186-1516-01	30 gm	$31.89

KIT: 2.5%

BRAND/MANUFACTURER	NDC	SIZE	AWP
○ BRAND			
EMLA: Astra	00186-1515-01	1s	$6.88
	00186-1515-03	1s	$33.13

Lidocaine, Topical

DESCRIPTION

Lidocaine is a local anesthetic agent and is administered topically. See *"Indications"* for specific uses. It is available as an ointment, a solution, a liquid, and a jelly.

Each gm of ointment contains:	
Lidocaine	50 mg

Each ml of solution contains:	
Lidocaine Hydrochloride (HCl)	20 mg

Each ml of liquid contains:	
Lidocaine	50 mg

Each ml of jelly contains:	
Lidocaine HCl	20 mg

Lidocaine is chemically designated as acetamide, 2-(diethylamino)-N-(2,6-dimethylphenyl). Lidocaine HCl is chemically designated as acetamide, 2-(diethylamino)-N-(2,6-dimethylphenyl)-, monohydrochloride.

The molecular formula is $C_{14}H_{22}N_2O$. The molecular weight is 234.34.

The molecular formula of Lidocaine HCl is $C_{14}H_{23}CIN_2O$. The molecular weight is 270.79.

CLINICAL PHARMACOLOGY

MECHANISM OF ACTION
Lidocaine stabilizes the neuronal membrane by inhibiting the ionic fluxes required for the initiation and conduction of impulses, thereby effecting local anesthetic action.

ONSET OF ANESTHESIA
After application of Lidocaine ointment or jelly, local, topical anesthesia appears in 3-5 minutes. It is ineffective when applied to intact skin. Local anesthesia appears within 1-2 minutes after application of Lidocaine liquid and persists for 15-20 minutes in soft tissue.

HEMODYNAMICS
Excessive blood levels may cause changes in cardiac output, total peripheral resistance, and mean arterial pressure. These changes may be attributable to a direct depressant effect of the local anesthetic agent on various components of the cardiovascular system. The net effect is normally a modest hypotension when the recommended dosages are not exceeded.

PHARMACOKINETICS AND METABOLISM
Lidocaine may be absorbed following topical administration to mucous membranes, its rate and extent of absorption depending upon the specific site of application, duration of exposure, concentration, and total dosage. In general, the rate of absorption of local anesthetic agents following topical application occurs most rapidly after intratracheal administration. Lidocaine is also well-absorbed from the gastrointestinal tract, but little intact drug appears in the circulation because of biotransformation in the liver.

Lidocaine is metabolized rapidly by the liver, and metabolites and unchanged drug are excreted by the kidneys. Biotransformation includes oxidative N-dealkylation, ring hydroxylation, cleavage of the amide linkage, and conjugation. N-dealkylation, a major pathway of biotransformation, yields the metabolites monoethylglycinexylidide and glycinexylidide. The pharmacological/toxicological actions of these metabolites are similar to, but less potent than, those of Lidocaine. Approximately 90% of Lidocaine administered is excreted in the form of various metabolites, and less than 10% is excreted unchanged. The primary metabolite in urine is a conjugate of 4-hydroxy-2, 6-dimethylaniline.

The plasma binding of Lidocaine is dependent on drug concentration, and the fraction bound decreases with increasing concentration. At concentrations of 1 to 4 μg of free base per ml, 60 to 80 percent of Lidocaine is protein bound. Binding is also dependent on the plasma concentration of the alpha-1-acid glycoprotein.

Lidocaine crosses the blood-brain and placental barriers, presumably by passive diffusion.

Studies of Lidocaine metabolism following intravenous bolus injections have shown that the elimination half-life of this agent is typically 1.5 to 2.0 hours. Because of the rapid rate at which Lidocaine is metabolized, any condition that affects liver function may alter Lidocaine kinetics. The half-life may be prolonged two-fold or more in patients with liver dysfunction. Renal dysfunction does not affect Lidocaine kinetics but may increase the accumulation of metabolites.

Factors such as acidosis and the use of CNS stimulants and depressants affect the CNS levels of Lidocaine required to produce overt systemic effects. Objective adverse manifestations become increasingly apparent with increasing venous plasma levels above 6.0 μg free base per mL. In the rhesus monkey arterial blood levels 18-21 μg/mL have been shown to be threshold for convulsive activity.

INDICATIONS AND USAGE

Lidocaine ointment and Lidocaine HCl solution are indicated for production of anesthesia of accessible mucous membranes of the oropharynx.

Lidocaine ointment is also useful as an anesthetic lubricant for intubation and for the temporary relief of pain associated with minor burns, including sunburn, abrasions of the skin, and insect bites.

Lidocaine HCl solution is also useful for reducing gagging during the taking of x-ray pictures and dental impressions.

Lidocaine liquid is indicated for the symptomatic relief of painful, irritated or inflamed mucous membranes of the mouth and for anesthesia of these membranes for the performance of minor dental surgical procedures.

Lidocaine HCl jelly is indicated for prevention and control of pain in procedures involving the male and female urethra, for topical treatment of painful urethritis, and as an anesthetic lubricant for endotracheal intubation (oral and nasal).

UNLABELED USES

Lidocaine, topical, is used alone or as an adjunct in the treatment of cough, cluster headache, and as an adjunct in relieving pain due to dyspeptic symptoms.

CONTRAINDICATIONS

Lidocaine and Lidocaine HCl are contraindicated in patients with a known history of hypersensitivity to local anesthetics of the amide type or to other components of the product.

WARNINGS

EXCESSIVE DOSAGE, OR SHORT INTERVALS BETWEEN DOSES, CAN RESULT IN HIGH PLASMA LEVELS AND SERIOUS ADVERSE EFFECTS. PATIENTS SHOULD BE INSTRUCTED TO STRICTLY ADHERE TO THE RECOMMENDED DOSAGE AND ADMINISTRATION GUIDELINES AS SET FORTH HERE.

THE MANAGEMENT OF SERIOUS ADVERSE REACTIONS MAY REQUIRE THE USE OF RESUSCITATIVE EQUIPMENT, OXYGEN, AND OTHER RESUSCITATIVE DRUGS, WHICH SHOULD BE AVAILABLE FOR IMMEDIATE USE WHEN LOCAL ANESTHETIC AGENTS SUCH AS LIDOCAINE ARE ADMINISTERED.

Lidocaine ointment, solution, liquid, and jelly should be used with extreme caution in the presence of sepsis or severely traumatized mucosa in the area of application, since under such conditions there is the potential for rapid systemic absorption.

When Lidocaine jelly is used for endotracheal tube lubrication care should be taken to avoid introducing the product into the lumen of the tube. Do not use the jelly to lubricate the endotracheal stylettes. If allowed into the inner lumen, the jelly may dry on the inner surface leaving a residue which tends to clump with flexion, narrowing the lumen. There have been rare reports in which this residue has caused the lumen to occlude. (See also "Adverse Reactions" and "Dosage and Administration").

PRECAUTIONS

GENERAL

The safety and effectiveness of Lidocaine depend on proper dosage, correct technique, adequate precautions, and readiness for emergencies. (See "Warnings" and "Adverse Reactions"). The lowest dosage that results in effective anesthesia should be used to avoid high plasma levels and serious adverse effects. Repeated doses of Lidocaine may cause significant increases in blood levels with each repeated dose because of slow accumulation of the drug and/or its metabolites. Tolerance to elevated blood levels varies with the status of the patient. Debilitated, elderly patients, acutely ill patients, and children should be given reduced doses commensurate with their age, weight, and physical condition. Lidocaine should also be used with caution in patients with severe shock or heart block.

Lidocaine ointment and liquid, and Lidocaine HCl solution and jelly should be used with caution in patients with known drug sensitivities. Patients allergic to para-aminobenzoic acid derivatives (procaine, tetracaine, benzocaine, etc.) have not shown cross sensitivity to Lidocaine. Many drugs used during the conduct of anesthesia are considered potential triggering agents for familial malignant hyperthermia. Since it is not known whether amide-type local anesthetics may trigger this reaction and since the need for supplemental general anesthesia cannot be predicted in advance, it is suggested that a standard protocol for the management of malignant hyperthermia should be available. Early unexplained signs of tachycardia, tachypnea, labile blood pressure and metabolic acidosis may precede temperature elevation. Successful outcome is dependent on early diagnosis, prompt discontinuance of the suspect triggering agent(s) and institution

of treatment, including oxygen therapy, indicated supportive measures and dantrolene (consult dantrolene sodium intravenous package insert before using).

INFORMATION FOR PATIENTS

When topical anesthetics are used in the mouth or throat, the patient should be aware that the production of topical anesthesia may impair swallowing and thus enhance the danger of aspiration. For this reason, food should not be ingested for 60 minutes following the use of local anesthetic preparations in the mouth or throat area. This is particularly important in children because of their frequency of eating.

Numbness of the tongue or buccal mucosa may enhance the danger of unintentional biting trauma. Food and chewing gum should not be taken while the mouth or throat area is anesthetized.

PATIENTS SHOULD BE INSTRUCTED TO STRICTLY ADHERE TO DOSING INSTRUCTIONS, AND TO KEEP THE SUPPLY OF MEDICATION OUT OF THE REACH OF CHILDREN.

CARCINOGENESIS, MUTAGENESIS, IMPAIRMENT OF FERTILITY

Studies of Lidocaine in animals to evaluate the carcinogenic and mutagenic potential or the effect on fertility have not been conducted.

USE IN PREGNANCY

Teratogenic Effects. Pregnancy Category B. Reproduction studies have been performed in rats at doses up to 6.6 times the human dose and have revealed no evidence of harm to the fetus caused by Lidocaine. There are, however, no adequate and well-controlled studies in pregnant women. Animal reproduction studies are not always predictive of human response. General consideration should be given to this fact before administering Lidocaine to women of childbearing potential, especially during early pregnancy when maximum organogenesis takes place.

LABOR AND DELIVERY

Lidocaine is not contraindicated in labor and delivery. Should Lidocaine ointment or Lidocaine HCl liquid or jelly be used concomitantly with other products containing Lidocaine, the total dose contributed by all formulations must be kept in mind.

NURSING MOTHERS

It is not known whether this drug is excreted in human milk. Because many drugs are excreted in human milk, caution should be exercised when Lidocaine is administered to a nursing woman.

PEDIATRIC USE

Dosages in children should be reduced, commensurate with age, body weight and physical condition. Caution must be taken to avoid overdosage when applying Lidocaine ointment to large areas of injured or abraded skin, since the systemic absorption of Lidocaine may be increased under such conditions. See "Dosage and Administration".

ADVERSE REACTIONS

Adverse experiences following the administration of Lidocaine are similar in nature to those observed with other amide local anesthetic agents. These adverse experiences are, in general, dose-related and may result from high plasma levels caused by excessive dosage or rapid absorption, or may result from a hypersensitivity, idiosyncrasy or diminished tolerance on the part of the patient. Serious adverse experiences are generally systemic in nature. The following types are those most commonly reported:

CENTRAL NERVOUS SYSTEM

CNS manifestations are excitatory and/or depressant and may be characterized by lightheadedness, nervousness, apprehension, euphoria, confusion, dizziness, drowsiness, tinnitus, blurred or double vision, vomiting, sensations of heat, cold or numbness, twitching, tremors, convulsions, unconsciousness, respiratory depression and arrest. The excitatory manifestations may be very brief or may not occur at all, in which case the first manifestation of toxicity may be drowsiness merging into unconsciousness and respiratory arrest.

Drowsiness following the administration of Lidocaine is usually an early sign of a high blood level of the drug and may occur as a consequence of rapid absorption.

CARDIOVASCULAR SYSTEM

Cardiovascular manifestations are usually depressant and are characterized by bradycardia, hypotension, and cardiovascular collapse, which may lead to cardiac arrest.

ALLERGIC

Allergic reactions are characterized by cutaneous lesions, urticaria, edema or anaphylactoid reactions. Allergic reactions may occur as a result of sensitivity either to the local anesthetic agent or to other components in the formulation. Allergic reactions as a result of sensitivity to Lidocaine are extremely rare and, if they occur, should be managed by conventional means. The detection of sensitivity by skin testing is of doubtful value.

There have been rare reports of endotracheal tube occlusion associated with the presence of dried jelly residue in the inner lumen of the tube. (See also "Warnings" and "Dosage and Administration.")

◆ RATED THERAPEUTICALLY EQUIVALENT; ◇ THERAPEUTIC EQUIVALENCE UNCONFIRMED; ○ UNRATED

OVERDOSAGE

Acute emergencies from local anesthetics are generally related to high plasma levels encountered during therapeutic use of local anesthetics. (See *"Adverse Reactions," "Warnings,"* and *"Precautions"*).

MANAGEMENT OF LOCAL ANESTHETIC EMERGENCIES

The first consideration is prevention, best accomplished by careful and constant monitoring of cardiovascular and respiratory vital signs and the patient's state of consciousness after each local anesthetic administration. At the first sign of change, oxygen should be administered.

The first step in the management of convulsions consists of immediate attention to the maintenance of a patent airway and assisted or controlled ventilation with oxygen. In situations where trained personnel are readily available, ventilation should be maintained and oxygen should be delivered by a delivery system capable of permitting immediate positive airway pressure by mask. Immediately after the institution of these ventilatory measures, the adequacy of the circulation should be evaluated, keeping in mind that drugs used to treat convulsions sometimes depress the circulation when administered intravenously. Should convulsions persist despite adequate respiratory support, and if the status of the circulation permits, small increments of an ultra-short acting barbiturate (such as thiopental or thiamylal) or a benzodiazepine (such as diazepam) may be administered intravenously. The clinician should be familiar, prior to use of local anesthetics, with these anticonvulsant drugs. Supportive treatment of circulatory depression may require administration of intravenous fluids and, when appropriate, a vasopressor as directed by the clinical situation (e.g., ephedrine).

If not treated immediately, both convulsions and cardiovascular depression can result in hypoxia, acidosis, bradycardia, arrhythmias and cardiac arrest. If cardiac arrest should occur, standard cardiopulmonary resuscitative measures should be instituted.

Dialysis is of negligible value in the treatment of acute overdosage with Lidocaine.

The oral LD$_{50}$ of Lidocaine HCl in nonfasted female rats is 459 (346-773) mg/kg (as the salt) and 214 (159-324) mg/kg (as the salt) in fasted female rats.

DOSAGE AND ADMINISTRATION

When any Lidocaine formulation is used concomitantly with other products containing Lidocaine, the total dose contributed by all formulations must be kept in mind.

ADULT

A single application should not exceed 5 gm of Lidocaine ointment, containing 250 mg of Lidocaine base (equivalent chemically to approximately 300 mg of Lidocaine HCl). This is roughly equivalent to squeezing a six (6) inch length of ointment from the tube. In a 70 kg adult this dose equals 3.6 mg/kg (1.6 mg/lb) Lidocaine base. No more than one-half tube, approximately 17-20 gm of ointment or 850-1000 mg Lidocaine base, should be administered in any one day.

Although the incidence of adverse effects with Lidocaine ointment is quite low, caution should be exercised, particularly when employing large amounts, since the incidence of adverse effects is directly proportional to the total dose of local anesthetic agent administered.

The maximum recommended single dose of Lidocaine HCl solution for healthy adults should be such that the dose of Lidocaine HCl does not exceed 4.5 mg/kg or 2 mg/lb body weight and does not in any case exceed a total of 300 mg.

For symptomatic treatment of irritated or inflamed mucous membranes of the mouth and pharynx, the usual adult dose is one 15 ml tablespoonful undiluted. For use in the mouth, the solution should be swished around in the mouth and spit out. For use in the pharynx, the undiluted solution should be gargled and may be swallowed. This dose should not be administered at intervals of less than three hours, and not more than eight doses should be given in a 24-hour period.

The dosage should be adjusted commensurate with the patient's age, weight and physical condition (see *"Precautions"*).

The maximum recommended single adult dose of Lidocaine HCl, administered parenterally, is 300 mg (equivalent to 260 mg of Lidocaine). In a 70 kg adult this dose of Lidocaine equals 3.7 mg/kg or 1.7 mg/lb. Thus, a single application of Lidocaine liquid should not exceed a total of 5 ml for all quadrants. In general, however, much smaller volumes are adequate to produce the desired anesthesia. The maximum recommended single adult dose (5 ml) should not be exceeded within any 3-hour interval.

The dosage of Lidocaine HCl jelly varies and depends upon the area to be anesthetized, vascularity of the tissues, individual tolerance, and the technique of anesthesia. The lowest dosage needed to provide effective anesthesia should be administered. Dosages should be reduced for children and for elderly and debilitated patients. Although the incidence of adverse effects with Lidocaine HCl jelly is quite low, caution should be exercised, particularly when employing large amounts, since the incidence of adverse effects is directly proportional to the total dose of local anesthetic agent administered.

For Surface Anesthesia of the Male Adult Urethra: Slowly instill approximately 15 ml (300 mg of Lidocaine HCl) into the urethra or until the patient has a feeling of tension. A penile clamp is then applied for several minutes at the corona. An additional dose of not more than 15 ml (300 mg) can be instilled for adequate anesthesia.

Prior to sounding or cystoscopy, a penile clamp should be applied for 5 to 10 minutes to obtain adequate anesthesia. A total dose of 30 ml (600 mg) is usually required to fill and dilate the male urethra.

Prior to catheterization, smaller volumes of 5-10 ml (100-200 mg) are usually adequate for lubrication.

For Surface Anesthesia of the Female Adult Urethra: Slowly instill 3-5 ml (60-100 mg of Lidocaine HCl) of the jelly into the urethra. If desired, some jelly may be deposited on a cotton swab and introduced into the urethra. In order to obtain adequate anesthesia, several minutes should be allowed prior to performing urological procedures. Care should be taken to prevent contamination of bottle contents (e.g., aspiration of urethral contents into the container when using insertion tip).

Lubrication for Endotracheal Intubation: Apply a moderate amount of jelly to the external surface of the endotracheal tube shortly before use. Care should be taken to avoid introducing the product into the lumen of the tube. Do not use the jelly to lubricate endotracheal stylettes. See *"Warnings"* and *"Adverse Reactions"* concerning rare reports of inner lumen occlusion. It is also recommended that use of endotracheal tubes with dried jelly on the external surface be avoided for lack of lubricating effect.

Maximum Dosage: No more than 600 mg or 30 ml of lidocaine HCl jelly should be given in any 12 hour period.

DOSAGE FOR CHILDREN

Care must be taken to ensure correct dosage in all pediatric patients as there have been cases of overdose due to inappropriate dosing.

It is difficult to recommend a maximum dose of any drug for children since this varies as a function of age and weight. For children from three to ten years who have a normal lean body mass and a normal lean body development, the maximum dose may be determined by the application of one of the standard pediatric drug formulas (e.g., Clark's rule). For example, in a child of five years weighing 50 lbs., the dose of Lidocaine or Lidocaine HCl should not exceed 75-100 mg (¾ to 1 teaspoonful) (1.5 to 2.0 mg/lb) when calculated according to Clark's rule. In any case, the maximum amount of Lidocaine administered should not exceed 4.5 mg/kg (2.0 mg/lb) of body weight.

For infants and in children under 3 years of age, ¼ teaspoon of the solution should be accurately measured and applied to the immediate area with a cotton-tipped applicator. This dose should not be administered at intervals of less than three hours. Not more than four doses should be given in a 12-hour period.

ADMINISTRATION

For medical use, apply Lidocaine ointment topically for adequate control of symptoms. The use of a sterile gauze pad is suggested for application to broken skin tissue. Apply to the tube prior to intubation.

In dentistry, apply to previously dried oral mucosa. Subsequent removal of excess saliva with cotton rolls or saliva ejector minimizes dilution of the ointment, permits maximum penetration, and minimizes the possibility of swallowing the topical ointment.

For use in connection with the insertion of new dentures, apply to all denture surfaces contacting mucosa.

IMPORTANT: Patients should consult a dentist at intervals not exceeding 48 hours throughout the fitting period.

Lidocaine liquid should be applied with a swab, which should be discarded after a single use.

STORAGE

Keep container tightly closed at all times when not in use.

Store at controlled room temperature, 15°-30°C (59°-86°F).

HOW SUPPLIED

LIDOCAINE
OINTMENT: 5%

AVERAGE UNIT PRICE (AVAILABLE SIZES)	
BRAND	$0.48
GENERIC	$0.09

BRAND/MANUFACTURER	NDC	SIZE	AWP
◆ BRAND			
XYLOCAINE: Astra	00186-0315-21	35 gm	$11.63
	00186-0350-01	35 gm	$12.50
	00186-0350-03	3.5 gm 10s	$25.81
◆ GENERICS			
Fougera	00168-0204-37	35 gm	$4.95
Thames	49158-0130-19	50 gm	$2.30

LIDOCAINE HYDROCHLORIDE
GEL: 2%

AVERAGE UNIT PRICE (AVAILABLE SIZES)	
BRAND	$0.30
GENERIC	$0.87

BRAND/MANUFACTURER	NDC	SIZE	AWP
◆ BRAND			
ANESTACON: Polymedica	00998-0300-10	15 ml doz	$65.25
	00998-0300-20	240 ml 6s	$134.25

➤ SHOWN IN PRODUCT IDENTIFICATION GUIDE

BRAND/MANUFACTURER	NDC	SIZE	AWP
◆ GENERICS			
Intl Med Sys	00548-3012-00	5 ml 25s	$172.50
Intl Med Sys	00548-3013-00	10 ml 25s	$192.30
Intl Med Sys	00548-3015-00	20 ml 25s	$231.60

LIQUID: 4%

BRAND/MANUFACTURER	NDC	SIZE	AWP
◆ BRAND			
XYLOCAINE: Astra	00186-0320-01	50 ml	$14.33

OINTMENT: 5%

BRAND/MANUFACTURER	NDC	SIZE	AWP
◆ GENERICS			
Moore,H.L.	00839-5474-81	50 gm	$2.15

SOLUTION: 2%

AVERAGE UNIT PRICE (AVAILABLE SIZES)		GENERIC A-RATED AVERAGE PRICE (GAAP)	
BRAND	$0.12	20 ml	$4.02
GENERIC	$0.07	100 ml	$4.43
HCFA FUL (100 ml)	$0.03		

BRAND/MANUFACTURER	NDC	SIZE	AWP
◆ GENERICS			
Pennex	00832-8464-20	20 ml	$2.44
Pennex	00426-8464-20	20 ml	$5.60
Roxane	00054-3500-49	100 ml	$2.63
Moore,H.L.	00839-6502-40	100 ml	$3.08
Pennex	00832-8464-00	100 ml	$3.30
Schein	00364-7282-61	100 ml	$3.75
Qualitest	00603-1392-64	100 ml	$4.05
Major	00904-0863-04	100 ml	$4.10
Rugby	00536-1331-82	100 ml	$4.12
URL	00677-1015-27	100 ml	$4.60
Barre	00472-0996-33	100 ml	$4.62
Geneva	00781-6190-46	100 ml	$4.65
Pennex	00426-8464-00	100 ml	$5.80
Goldline	00182-1360-70	100 ml	$6.15
LIDOMAR: Marlop	12939-0780-10	100 ml	$6.80
Roxane	00054-8500-16	20 ml 40s ud	$50.50

SOLUTION: 4%

AVERAGE UNIT PRICE (AVAILABLE SIZES)		GENERIC A-RATED AVERAGE PRICE (GAAP)	
GENERIC	$0.72	50 ml	$7.63

BRAND/MANUFACTURER	NDC	SIZE	AWP
◆ GENERICS			
Roxane	00054-3505-47	50 ml	$7.04
Moore,H.L.	00839-7407-99	50 ml	$8.22
Intl Med Sys	00548-6300-00	4 ml 25s	$184.80

SPRAY: 10%

AVERAGE UNIT PRICE (AVAILABLE SIZES)	
BRAND	$0.72

BRAND/MANUFACTURER	NDC	SIZE	AWP
◆ BRAND			
XYLOCAINE HCL 10% ORAL: Astra	00186-0356-01	30 ml	$42.69
	00186-9035-05	30 ml 50s	$26.15

Limbitrol *SEE* AMITRIPTYLINE HYDROCHLORIDE WITH CHLORDIAZEPOXIDE

Lincocin *SEE* LINCOMYCIN HYDROCHLORIDE

Lincomycin Hydrochloride

WARNING

LINCOMYCIN THERAPY HAS BEEN ASSOCIATED WITH SEVERE COLITIS WHICH MAY END FATALLY. THEREFORE, IT SHOULD BE RESERVED FOR SERIOUS INFECTIONS WHERE LESS TOXIC ANTIMICROBIAL AGENTS ARE INAPPROPRIATE, AS DESCRIBED IN THE INDICATIONS SECTION. IT SHOULD NOT BE USED IN PATIENTS WITH NONBACTERIAL INFECTIONS, SUCH AS MOST UPPER RESPIRATORY TRACT INFECTIONS. STUDIES INDICATE A TOXIN(S) PRODUCED BY *CLOSTRIDIA* IS ONE PRIMARY CAUSE OF ANTIBIOTIC ASSOCIATED COLITIS. THE COLITIS IS USUALLY

CHARACTERIZED BY SEVERE, PERSISTENT DIARRHEA AND SEVERE ABDOMINAL CRAMPS AND MAY BE ASSOCIATED WITH THE PASSAGE OF BLOOD AND MUCUS. ENDOSCOPIC EXAMINATION MAY REVEAL PSEUDOMEMBRANOUS COLITIS.

WHEN SIGNIFICANT DIARRHEA OCCURS, THE DRUG SHOULD BE DISCONTINUED OR, IF NECESSARY, CONTINUED ONLY WITH CLOSE OBSERVATION OF THE PATIENT. LARGE BOWEL ENDOSCOPY HAS BEEN RECOMMENDED.

ANTIPERISTALTIC AGENTS SUCH AS OPIATES AND DIPHENOXYLATE WITH ATROPINE (LOMOTIL) MAY PROLONG AND/OR WORSEN THE CONDITION. VANCOMYCIN HAS BEEN FOUND TO BE EFFECTIVE IN THE TREATMENT OF ANTIBIOTIC ASSOCIATED PSEUDO-MEMBRANOUS COLITIS PRODUCED BY *CLOSTRIDIUM DIFFICILE*. THE USUAL ADULT DOSE IS 500 MILLIGRAMS TO 2 GRAMS OF VANCOMYCIN ORALLY PER DAY IN THREE TO FOUR DIVIDED DOSES ADMINISTERED FOR 7 TO 10 DAYS. CHOLESTYRAMINE OR COLESTIPOL RESINS BIND VANCOMYCIN *IN VITRO*. IF BOTH A RESIN AND VANCOMYCIN ARE TO BE ADMINISTERED CONCURRENTLY, IT MAY BE ADVISABLE TO SEPARATE THE TIME OF ADMINISTRATION OF EACH DRUG.

DIARRHEA, COLITIS, AND PSEUDOMEMBRANOUS COLITIS HAVE BEEN OBSERVED TO BEGIN UP TO SEVERAL WEEKS FOLLOWING CESSATION OF THERAPY WITH LINCOMYCIN.

DESCRIPTION

Lincomycin Hydrochloride is the monohydrated salt of Lincomycin, a substance produced by the growth of a member of the *lincolnensis* group of *Streptomyces lincolnensis* (Fam. *Streptomycetaceae*). It is a white, or practically white, crystalline powder and is odorless or has a faint odor. Its solutions are acid and are dextrorotatory. Lincomycin Hydrochloride is freely soluble in water; soluble in dimethylformamide and very slightly soluble in acetone.

Following is its chemical structure:

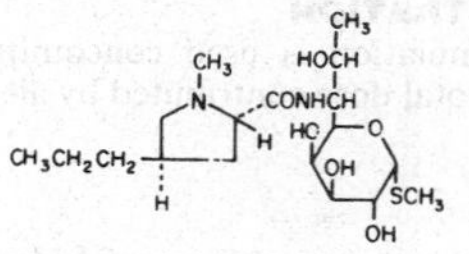

CLINICAL PHARMACOLOGY

Microbiology: Lincomycin has been shown to be effective against most of the common gram-positive pathogens. Depending on the sensitivity of the organism and concentration of the antibiotic, it may be either bactericidal or bacteriostatic. Cross resistance has not been demonstrated with penicillin, chloramphenicol, ampicillin, cephalosporins or the tetracyclines. Despite chemical differences, lincomycin exhibits antibacterial activity similar but not identical to the macrolide antibiotics (eg erythromycin). Some cross resistance (with erythromycin) including a phenomenon known as dissociated cross resistance or macrolide effect has been reported. Microorganisms have not developed resistance to Lincomycin rapidly when tested by *in vitro* or *in vivo* methods. Staphylococci develop resistance to lincomycin in a slow, step-wise manner based on *in vitro*, serial subculture experiments. This pattern of resistance development is unlike that shown for streptomycin.

Studies indicate that Lincomycin does not share antigenicity with penicillin compounds.

Biological Studies: In vitro studies indicate that the spectrum of activity includes *Staphylococcus aureus, Staphylococcus albus, β-hemolytic Streptococcus, Streptococcus viridans, Diplococcus pneumoniae, Clostridium tetani, Clostridium perfringens, Corynebacterium diphtheriae* and *Corynebacterium acnes.*

Note: The drug is not active against most strains of *Streptococcus faecalis*, nor against *Neisseria gonorrhoeae, Neisseria meningitidis, Hemophilus influenzae*, or other gram-negative organisms or yeasts.

Human Pharmacology: Lincomycin is absorbed rapidly after a 500 mg oral dose, reaching peak levels in 2 to 4 hours. Levels are maintained above the MIC (minimum inhibitory concentration) for most gram-positive organisms for 6 to 8 hours. Urinary recovery of drug in a 24-hour period ranges from 1.0 to 31 percent (mean: 4.0) after a single oral dose of 500 mg of Lincomycin. Tissue level studies indicate that bile is an important route of excretion. Significant levels have been demonstrated in the majority of body tissues. Although the drug is not present in significant amounts in the spinal fluid of normal volunteers, it has been demonstrated in the spinal fluid of one patient with pneumococcal meningitis.

Intramuscular administration of a single dose of 600 mg produces a peak serum level at 30 minutes with detectable levels persisting for 24 hours. Urinary excretion after this dose ranges from 1.8 to 24.8 percent (mean: 17.3).

The intravenous infusion over a 2-hour interval of 600 mg of Lincomycin Hydrochloride in 500 mL of 5 percent glucose in distilled water yields therapeutic levels for 14 hours. Urinary excretion ranges from 4.9 to 30.3 percent (mean: 13.8). The biological half-life, after oral, intramuscular or intravenous administration is 5.4 ± 1.0 hours.

Hemodialysis and peritoneal dialysis do not effectively remove Lincomycin from the blood.

◆ RATED THERAPEUTICALLY EQUIVALENT; ◇ THERAPEUTIC EQUIVALENCE UNCONFIRMED; ○ UNRATED

INDICATIONS AND USAGE

Lincomycin Hydrochloride preparations are indicated in the treatment of serious infections due to susceptible strains of streptococci, pneumococci, and staphylococci. Its use should be reserved for penicillin-allergic patients or other patients for whom, in the judgment of the physician, a penicillin is inappropriate. Because of the risk of colitis, as described in the *"Warning"* box, before selecting Lincomycin the physician should consider the nature of the infection and the suitability of less toxic alternatives (eg, erythromycin).

Lincomycin has been demonstrated to be effective in the treatment of staphylococcal infections resistant to other antibiotics and susceptible to lincomycin. Staphylococcal strains resistant to Lincomycin Hydrochloride have been recovered; culture and susceptibility studies should be done in conjunction with therapy with Lincomycin Hydrochloride. In the case of macrolides, partial but not complete cross resistance may occur (see *"Microbiology"*). The drug may be administered concomitantly with other antimicrobial agents when indicated.

CONTRAINDICATIONS

This drug is contraindicated in patients previously found to be hypersensitive to lincomycin or clindamycin. It is not indicated in the treatment of minor bacterial infections or viral infections.

WARNINGS

(See *"Warning"* box). Studies indicate a toxin(s) produced by *Clostridia* is one primary cause of antibiotic associated colitis.[1-5] Mild cases of colitis may respond to drug discontinuance alone. Moderate to severe cases should be managed promptly with fluid, electrolyte and protein supplementation as indicated. Vancomycin has been found to be effective in the treatment of antibiotic associated pseudomembranous colitis produced by *Clostridium difficile*. The usual adult dosage is 500 milligrams to 2 grams of vancomycin orally per day in three to four divided doses administered for 7 to 10 days. Cholestyramine or colestipol resins bind vancomycin *in vitro*. If both a resin and vancomycin are to be administered concurrently, it may be advisable to separate the time of administration of each drug. Systemic corticoids and corticoid retention enemas may help relieve the colitis. Other causes of colitis should also be considered.

A careful inquiry should be made concerning previous sensitivities to drugs and other allergens.

Usage in Pregnancy: Safety for use in pregnancy has not been established.

Usage in Newborn: Until further clinical experience is obtained, Lincomycin Hydrochloride preparations are not indicated in the newborn.

Nursing Mothers: Lincomycin Hydrochloride has been reported to appear in breast milk in ranges of 0.5 to 2.4 mcg/mL.

One form of Lincomycin Hydrochloride Sterile Solution contains benzyl alcohol which has been associated with a fatal gasping syndrome in infants.

PRECAUTIONS

Review of experience to date suggests that a subgroup of older patients with associated severe illness may tolerate diarrhea less well. When Lincomycin Hydrochloride preparations are indicated in these patients, they should be carefully monitored for change in bowel frequency.

Lincomycin Hydrochloride should be prescribed with caution in individuals with a history of gastrointestinal disease, particularly colitis. Lincomycin Hydrochloride like any drug, should be used with caution in patients with a history of asthma or significant allergies. The use of antibiotics occasionally results in overgrowth of nonsusceptible organisms—particularly yeasts. Should superinfections occur, appropriate measures should be taken. When patients with pre-existing monilial infections require therapy with Lincomycin Hydrochloride, concomitant antimonilial treatment should be given.

During prolonged therapy with Lincomycin Hydrochloride, periodic liver and renal function studies and blood counts should be performed.

Since adequate data are not yet available in patients with pre-existing liver disease, its use in such patients is not recommended at this time unless special clinical circumstances so indicate.

Lincomycin has been shown to have neuromuscular blocking properties that may enhance the action of other neuromuscular blocking agents. Therefore, it should be used with caution in patients receiving such agents.

Indicated surgical procedures should be performed in conjunction with antibiotic therapy.

ADVERSE REACTIONS

Gastrointestinal: Glossitis, stomatitis, nausea, vomiting. Persistent diarrhea, enterocolitis and pruritus ani. (See *"Warning"* box).

Hematopoietic: Neutropenia, leukopenia, agranulocytosis and thrombocytopenic purpura have been reported. There have been rare reports of aplastic anemia and pancytopenia in which Lincomycin Hydrochloride preparations could not be ruled out as the causative agent.

Hypersensitivity Reactions: Hypersensitivity reactions such as angioneurotic edema, serum sickness and anaphylaxis have been reported, some of these in patients known to be sensitive to penicillin. Rare instances of erythema multiforme, some resembling Stevens-Johnson syndrome, have been associated with Lincomycin Hydrochloride. If an allergic reaction should occur, the drug should be discontinued and the usual agents (epinephrine, corticosteroids, antihistamines) should be available for emergency treatment.

Skin and Mucous Membranes: Skin rashes, urticaria and vaginitis and rare instances of exfoliative and vesiculobullous dermatitis have been reported.

Liver: Although no direct relationship of Lincomycin Hydrochloride to liver dysfunction has been established, jaundice and abnormal liver function tests (particularly elevations of serum transaminase) have been observed in a few instances.

Renal: Although no direct relationship of lincomycin to renal damage has been established, renal dysfunction as evidenced by azotemia, oliguria, and/or proteinuria has been observed in rare instances.

Cardiovascular: After too rapid intravenous administration, rare instances of cardiopulmonary arrest and hypotension have been reported. (See *"Dosage and Administration"*).

Special Senses: Tinnitus and vertigo have been reported occasionally.

Local Reactions: Patients have demonstrated excellent local tolerance to intramuscularly administered Lincomycin Hydrochloride. Reports of pain following injection have been infrequent. Intravenous administration of Lincomycin Hydrochloride in 250 to 500 mL of 5 percent glucose in distilled water or normal saline produced no local irritation or phlebitis.

DOSAGE AND ADMINISTRATION

If significant diarrhea occurs during therapy, this antibiotic should be discontinued. (See *"Warning"* box).

ORAL

Adults: Serious infections: 500 mg 3 times per day (500 mg approximately every 8 hours). *More severe infections*— 500 mg or more 4 times per day (500 mg or more approximately every 6 hours).

Children over 1 month of age: Serious infections: 30 mg/kg/day (15 mg/lb/day) divided into 3 or 4 equal doses. *More severe infections:* 60 mg/kg/day (30 mg/lb/day) divided into 3 or 4 equal doses.

With β-hemolytic streptococcal infections, treatment should continue for at least 10 days to diminish the likelihood of subsequent rheumatic fever or glomerulonephritis.

Note: For optimal absorption it is recommended that nothing be given by mouth except water for a period of one to two hours before and after oral administration of Lincomycin Hydrochloride preparations.

INTRAMUSCULAR

Adults: Serious infections: 600 mg (2 mL) intramuscularly every 24 hours. *More severe infections:* 600 mg (2 mL) intramuscularly every 12 hours or more often.

Children over 1 month of age: Serious infections: one intramuscular injection of 10 mg/kg (5 mg/lb) every 24 hours. *More severe infections*— one intramuscular injection of 10 mg/kg (5 mg/lb) every 12 hours or more often.

INTRAVENOUS

Adults: The intravenous dose will be determined by the severity of the infection. For serious infections doses of 600 mg of Lincomycin to 1 gram are given every 8-12 hours. For more severe infections these doses may have to be increased. In life-threatening situations daily intravenous doses of as much as 8 grams have been given. Intravenous doses are given on the basis of 1 gram of lincomycin diluted in not less than 100 mL of appropriate solution (see *"Physical Compatibilities"*) and infused over a period of not less than one hour.

Dose	Vol. Diluent	Time
600 mg	100 mL	1 hr
1 gram	100 mL	1 hr
2 grams	200 mL	2 hr
3 grams	300 mL	3 hr
4 grams	400 mL	4 hr

These doses may be repeated as often as required to the limit of the maximum recommended daily dose of 8 grams of Lincomycin.

Children over 1 month of age: 10-20 mg/kg/day (5-10 mg/lb/day) depending on the severity of the infection may be infused in divided doses as described above for adults.

Note: Severe cardiopulmonary reactions have occurred when this drug has been given at greater than the recommended concentration and rate.

Subconjunctival Injection: 0.25 mL (75 mg) injected subconjunctivally will result in ocular fluid levels of antibiotic (lasting for at least 5 hours) with MIC's sufficient for most susceptible pathogens.

Patients with diminished renal function: When therapy with Lincomycin Hydrochloride is required in individuals with severe impairment of renal function, an appropriate dose is 25 to 30% of that recommended for patients with normally functioning kidneys.

Storage: Store at controlled room temperature, 15°-30°C (59°-86°F).

ANIMAL PHARMACOLOGY

In vivo experimental animal studies demonstrated the effectiveness of Lincomycin Hydrochloride preparations in protecting animals infected with *Streptococcus viridans*, β-*hemolytic Streptococcus*, *Staphylococcus aureus*, *Diplococcus pneumoniae* and *Leptospira pomona*. It was ineffective in *Klebsiella*, *Pasteurella*, *Pseudomonas*, *Salmonella* and *Shigella* infections.

➤ SHOWN IN PRODUCT IDENTIFICATION GUIDE

CLINICAL STUDIES

Experience with 345 obstetrical patients receiving this drug revealed no ill effects related to pregnancy.

Physical Compatibilities:

Physically compatible for 24 hours at room temperature unless otherwise indicated.

Infusion Solutions:

Dextrose in Water, 5% and 10%
Dextrose in Saline, 5% and 10%
Ringer's Solution
Sodium Lactate 1/6 Molar
Travert 10% — Electrolyte No. 1
Dextran in Saline 6% w/v

Vitamins in Infusion Solutions:

B-Complex
B-Complex with Ascorbic Acid

Antibiotics in Infusion Solutions:

Penicillin G Sodium (Satisfactory for 4 hours)
Cephalothin
Tetracycline HCl
Cephaloridine
Colistimethate (Satisfactory for 4 hours)
Ampicillin
Methicillin
Chloramphenicol
Polymyxin B Sulfate

Physically Incompatible with:

Novobiocin
Kanamycin

IT SHOULD BE EMPHASIZED THAT THE COMPATIBLE AND INCOMPATIBLE DETERMINATIONS ARE PHYSICAL OBSERVATIONS ONLY, NOT CHEMICAL DETERMINATIONS. ADEQUATE CLINICAL EVALUATION OF THE SAFETY AND EFFICACY OF THESE COMBINATIONS HAS NOT BEEN PERFORMED.

REFERENCES

1. Bailey, WR, Scott, EG, *Diagnostic Microbiology* CV Mosby Company, St. Louis, 1978. 2. Bartlett, JG, et al, "Clindamycin-associated Colitis due to a Toxin-producing Species of *Clostridium* in Hamsters" *J. Inf. Dis.* **136** (5): 701-705, (November) 1977. 3. Larson, HE, Price, AB, "Pseudomembranous Colitis: Presence of Clostridial Toxin," *Lancet,* 1312-1314 (December) 24 and 31, 1977. 4. Lusk, RH, et al, "Clindamycin-Induced Enterocolitis in Hamsters," *J. Inf. Dis.* **137**(4); 464-474 (April) 1978. 5. "Antibiotic-associated Colitis: A Progress Report", *British Med. J.* **1**:669-671 (March 18) 1978.

J CODES

Up to 300 mg IV—J2010

HOW SUPPLIED
CAPSULE: 500 MG

BRAND/MANUFACTURER		NDC	SIZE	AWP
○ **BRAND**				
LINCOCIN: Upjohn		00009-0500-01	24s	$31.76
		00009-0500-02	100s	$126.46

INJECTION: 300 MG/ML

AVERAGE UNIT PRICE (AVAILABLE SIZES)		GENERIC A-RATED AVERAGE PRICE (GAAP)	
BRAND	$2.54	10 ml	$18.94
GENERIC	$1.84		

BRAND/MANUFACTURER	NDC	SIZE	AWP
◆ **BRAND**			
LINCOCIN: Upjohn	00009-0555-01	2 ml	$5.36
	00009-0555-02	10 ml	$24.09
◆ **GENERICS**			
Rugby	00536-3987-70	10 ml	$16.12
Insource	58441-0119-10	10 ml	$19.88
Schein	00364-3002-54	10 ml	$19.88
Genl Inject	52584-0119-10	10 ml	$19.88
LINCOREX: Hyrex	00314-0804-10	10 ml	$12.45
Schein	00364-3002-48	2 ml 25s	$110.63

Lindane

DESCRIPTION

Lindane lotion and shampoo are ectoparasiticides and ovicides. Lindane lotion is effective against *Sarcoptes scabiei* (scabies); Lindane Shampoo is effective against *Pediculosis capitis* (head lice), *Pediculosis pubis* (crab lice) and their ova. Lindane is the highly purified gamma isomer of 1, 2, 3, 4, 5, 6, hexachlorocyclohexane.

The empirical formula is $C_6H_6Cl_6$, and the molecular weight 290.83.

Following is its chemical structure:

CLINICAL PHARMACOLOGY

Lindane exerts its parasiticidal action by being directly absorbed into the parasites and their ova. Feldmann and Mainbach[1] reported approximately 10% absorption of a Lindane acetone solution applied to the forearm and left in place for 24 hours. Dule, et al[2], reported a blood level of 290 ng/ml associated with convulsions following the accidental ingestion of a Lindane containing product. Ginsburg[3] found a mean peak blood level of 28 ng/ml 6 hours after total body application of Lindane lotion to scabietic infants and children. The half-life was determined to be 18 hours. Analysis of blood taken from subjects before and after the use of Lindane shampoo showed a mean peak blood level of only 3 ng/ml which appeared at six hours and disappeared at eight hours after the shampoo was applied.

INDICATIONS AND USAGE

Lindane lotion is indicated for the treatment of patients infested with *Sarcoptes scabiei* (scabies). Lindane shampoo is indicated for the treatment of patients infested with *Pediculus capitis* (head lice), *Pediculus pubis* (crab lice) and their ova.

CONTRAINDICATIONS

Lindane lotion and shampoo are contraindicated for premature neonates because their skin may be more permeable than full term infants and their liver enzymes may not be sufficiently developed. Lindane lotion is also contraindicated for patients with Norwegian (crusted) scabies due to possible increased absorption. The lotion and shampoo are also contraindicated for patients with known seizure disorders and for individuals with a known sensitivity to the product or any of its components.

WARNINGS

LINDANE PENETRATES HUMAN SKIN AND HAS THE POTENTIAL FOR CNS TOXICITY (SEE *"CLINICAL PHARMACOLOGY"* SECTION). LINDANE LOTION AND SHAMPOO SHOULD BE USED ACCORDING TO RECOMMENDED DOSAGE (SEE DIRECTIONS FOR USE) ESPECIALLY ON INFANTS, PREGNANT WOMEN AND NURSING MOTHERS. ANIMAL STUDIES INDICATE THAT POTENTIAL TOXIC EFFECTS OF TOPICALLY APPLIED LINDANE ARE GREATER IN THE YOUNG. SEIZURES, AND, IN RARE INSTANCES, DEATHS HAVE BEEN REPORTED AFTER EXCESS DOSAGE, OVEREXPOSURE, FREQUENT REAPPLICATIONS, AND ACCIDENTIAL AND INTENTIONAL INGESTION OF LINDANE. THESE INSTANCES OF PATIENT MISUSE HAVE BEEN ASSOCIATED WITH LACK OF PATIENT UNDERSTANDING OF DIRECTIONS FOR USE, PRESCRIBING OR DISPENSING EXCESSIVE QUANTITIES, AND IMPROPER REAPPLICATIONS. IN EXCEEDINGLY RARE CASES SEIZURES HAVE BEEN REPORTED WHEN USED ACCORDING TO DIRECTIONS. NO RESIDUAL EFFECTS OF LINDANE TREATMENT HAVE BEEN DEMONSTRATED; THEREFORE, THIS PRODUCT SHOULD NOT BE USED TO WARD OFF A POSSIBLE INFESTATION. If accidental ingestion occurs, prompt gastric lavage is indicated. Because oils may enhance absorption, saline rather than oily cathartics should be used. Central nervous excitation can be controlled by the administration of pentobarbital, phenobarbital or diazepam.

PRECAUTIONS

General: Care should be taken to avoid contact with the eyes. If such contact occurs, eyes should be immediately flushed with water. If irritation or sensitization occurs, the patient should be advised to consult a physician.

Geriatric: Dosage may have to be reduced due to the possibility of increased absorption through elderly skin.

Information for Patients: Patients must be instructed on the proper use of the medication, especially as to amount applied and duration of use.

Laboratory Tests: No laboratory tests are needed for the proper use of this medication.

Drug Interactions: Oils may enhance absorption. Therefore, simultaneous use of Lindane lotion and creams, ointments or oils should be avoided; avoid using oil treatment, or oil based hair dressings or conditioners immediately before and after applying Lindane shampoo.

Carcinogenesis: Although no studies have been conducted with Lindane lotion or shampoo, numerous long-term feeding studies have been conducted in mice and rats to evaluate the carcinogenic potential of the technical grade of hexachlorocyclohexane (BHC) as well as the alpha, beta, gamma (Lindane) and delta isomers. Both oral and topical applications have been evaluated. Nagasaki[4], Gots[6] and Hanada[6] found varying amounts of benign and malignant hepatomas associated with BHC and the alpha, delta and epsilon isomers. None reported a carcinogenic potential for Lindane. Tumors were found only in the animals which had received the alpha isomer. Weisse and Herbst[7] also evaluated the carcinogenic potential of Lindane in mice but could find no evidence of Lindane carcinogenicity. The National Cancer Institute[8] also found no evidence of carcinogenicity.

◆ RATED THERAPEUTICALLY EQUIVALENT; ◇ THERAPEUTIC EQUIVALENCE UNCONFIRMED; ○ UNRATED

Thorpe and Walker compared beta BHC with Lindane, dieldrin. DDT and hexabarbital in mice. Despite the unusually high incidence of tumors in the control group, they concluded that 600 ppm of Lindane was associated with a significant increase in the incidence of hepatoma and thus, considered it a tumorigen.

Orr[10] and Kashyap, et al[11], evaluated the carcinogenic potential in mice of topically applied BHC. In neither study was there any evidence of a tumorigenic or carcinogenic potential associated with topical application of BHC. Mutagenicity tests have been used as predictive information about the carcinogenicity of various chemical compounds. Numerous types of mutagenicity tests have been performed with Lindane. The results of these tests do not indicate that Lindane is mutagenic.

Pregnancy: Teratogenic Effects: Pregnancy Category B: Reproduction, including multigeneration studies have been performed in mice, rats, rabbits, pigs, and dogs at doses up to 10 times the human dose and have revealed no evidence of impaired fertility or harm to the fetus due to orally administered lindane. There are, however, no adequate and well controlled studies in pregnant women. Because animal reproduction studies are not always predictive of human response, the recommended dosage should not be exceeded on pregnant women. They should be treated no more than twice during a pregnancy.

Nursing Mothers: Lindane is secreted in human milk in low concentrations. Studies conducted in the United States as well as in Europe and South America found levels of Lindane in human milk ranging from 0 to 113 pph, as the result of ingestion of foods which had been treated with Lindane. There appeared to be no difference in concentration between country and urban dwellers. Although the levels of Lindane found in blood after topical application with Lindane lotion or shampoo make it unlikely that amounts of Lindane sufficient to cause serious adverse reactions will be excreted in the milk of nursing mothers who have used Lindane lotion or shampoo, if there is any concern, an alternate method of feeding may be used for 4 days.

Pediatric Use: Refer to the *"Contraindications"* and *"Warnings"* sections.

ADVERSE REACTIONS

Lindane has been reported to cause central nervous stimulation ranging from dizziness to convulsions. Cases of convulsions have been reported in connection with Lindane lotion and shampoo therapy. However, these incidents were almost always associated with accidental oral ingestion or misuse of the product, in exceedingly rare cases, seizures have been reported when used according to directions. Eczematous eruptions due to irritation from this product have also been reported. Incidence of these adverse reactions is relatively infrequent, occurring in less than 1 in 100,000 patients.

DRUG ABUSE AND DEPENDENCE

Lindane lotion and shampoo are not subject to abuse, nor is there any dependence on the drug.

OVERDOSAGE

Overdosage or oral ingestion of Lindane lotion or shampoo cause central nervous system excitation and if taken in sufficient quantities, convulsions may occur. If accidental ingestion occurs, prompt gastric lavage should be instituted. However, since oils favor absorption, saline cathartics for intestinal evacuation should be given rather than oil laxatives. If central nervous system manifestations occur, they can be antagonized by the administration of pentobarbital, phenobarbital or diazepam.

DOSAGE AND ADMINISTRATION

Caution: USE ONLY AS DIRECTED. DO NOT EXCEED RECOMMENDED DOSAGE.

No residual effects of Lindane lotion or shampoo treatment have been demonstrated; therefore, this product should not be used to ward off a possible infestation. However, sexual contacts should be treated simultaneously. NOTE: PLEASE READ CAREFULLY.

DIRECTIONS FOR USE
Lindane lotion:
WARNING:
THIS PRODUCT CAN BE POISONOUS IF MISUSED. CHILDREN MUST NOT BE ALLOWED TO APPLY THIS DRUG WITHOUT DIRECT ADULT SUPERVISION. USE LOTION FOR SCABIES ONLY. APPLY ONLY ONCE. USE ONLY ENOUGH TO COVER THE BODY IN A THIN LAYER. 1 OUNCE (HALF OF A 2 OUNCE CONTAINER) SHOULD BE ALL THAT IS NEEDED FOR CHILDREN UNDER 6 YEARS OF AGE; 1 TO 2 OUNCES FOR OLDER CHILDREN AND ADULTS. DO NOT LEAVE ON FOR MORE THAN 12 HOURS. DO NOT INGEST. KEEP AWAY FROM MOUTH AND EYES. COVER INFANTS HANDS AND FEET DURING TREATMENT TO PREVENT SUCKING AND LICKING OF LOTION. DO NOT USE IF OPEN WOUNDS, CUTS OR SORES ARE PRESENT, UNLESS DIRECTED BY YOUR PHYSICIAN.
(LOTION: SHAKE WELL)
1. APPLY THIS PREPARATION TO DRY SKIN IN A THIN LAYER AND RUB IT IN THOROUGHLY.
2. TRIM NAILS AND APPLY UNDER NAILS WITH TOOTHBRUSH (THROW AWAY TOOTHBRUSH AFTER USE).
3. IF A WARM BATH IS TAKEN BEFORE APPLICATION, ALLOW THE SKIN TO DRY AND COOL COMPLETELY BEFORE APPLYING THE MEDICATION.

4. A TOTAL BODY APPLICATION SHOULD BE MADE FROM THE NECK DOWN, INCLUDING SOLES OF FEET, UNLESS OTHERWISE DIRECTED BY YOUR PHYSICIAN.
5. THE LOTION SHOULD BE LEFT ON FOR 8 TO 12 HOURS (USUALLY OVERNIGHT) AND THEN REMOVED BY THOROUGH WASHING (BATH OR SHOWER).
6. AVOID UNNECESSARY CONTACT WITH YOUR SKIN IF YOU ARE APPLYING TO ANOTHER PERSON. IF TREATING MORE THAN ONE PERSON, PERSON APPLYING LOTION (ESPECIALLY PREGNANT OR NURSING WOMEN) SHOULD WEAR RUBBER GLOVES.
7. ALL RECENTLY WORN CLOTHING, UNDERWEAR AND PAJAMAS, AND USED SHEETS, PILLOW CASES, AND TOWELS SHOULD BE WASHED IN VERY HOT WATER OR DRY-CLEANED.
AFTER ONE APPLICATION, ITCHING WILL CONTINUE FOR SEVERAL WEEKS. THIS IS NORMAL AND DOES NOT REQUIRE REAPPLICATION.
IF YOU HAVE ANY QUESTIONS OR CONCERNS ABOUT YOUR CONDITION OR USE OF THE LOTION, CONTACT YOUR PHYSICIAN.

Lindane shampoo:
WARNING:
THIS PRODUCT CAN BE POISONOUS IF MISUSED. CHILDREN MUST NOT BE ALLOWED TO APPLY THIS DRUG WITHOUT DIRECT ADULT SUPERVISION. USE SHAMPOO FOR HEAD AND PUBIC LICE ONLY. DO NOT USE FOR SCABIES. USE ONLY IN AMOUNTS DIRECTED BELOW. IN NO CASE SHOULD MORE THAN 2 OUNCES BE USED BY ONE PERSON IN ONE APPLICATION. DO NOT INGEST. KEEP AWAY FROM MOUTH AND EYES. DO NOT USE IF OPEN WOUNDS, CUTS OR SORES ARE PRESENT ON SCALP OR GROIN, UNLESS DIRECTED BY YOUR PHYSICIAN.
AVOID USING OIL TREATMENTS, OIL BASED HAIR DRESSINGS OR CONDITIONERS IMMEDIATELY BEFORE AND AFTER APPLYING LINDANE SHAMPOO.
(SHAKE WELL)
1. BEFORE APPLYING LINDANE SHAMPOO, USE REGULAR SHAMPOO (WITHOUT CONDITIONERS), RINSE AND COMPLETELY DRY HAIR.
2. USE 1 OUNCE (HALF OF A 2 OUNCE BOTTLE) FOR SHORT HAIR: 1.5 OUNCES (THREE-QUARTERS OF A 2 OUNCE BOTTLE) FOR MEDIUM LENGTH HAIR; AND FULL 2 OUNCE BOTTLE FOR LONG HAIR.
3. APPLY SHAMPOO DIRECTLY TO DRY HAIR WITHOUT ADDING WATER WORK THOROUGHLY INTO THE HAIR AND ALLOW TO REMAIN IN PLACE FOR 4 MINUTES ONLY.
4. AFTER 4 MINUTES, ADD SMALL QUANTITIES OF WATER TO HAIR UNTIL A GOOD LATHER FORMS.
5. IMMEDIATELY RINSE ALL LATHER AWAY. AVOID UNNECESSARY CONTACT OF LATHER WITH OTHER BODY SURFACES.
6. TOWEL BRISKLY AND REMOVE NITS WITH NIT COMB OR TWEEZERS.
7. AVOID UNNECESSARY CONTACT WITH YOUR SKIN IF YOU ARE APPLYING SHAMPOO TO ANOTHER PERSON. IF TREATING MORE THAN ONE PERSON, PERSON APPLYING SHAMPOO (ESPECIALLY PREGNANT AND/OR NURSING WOMEN) SHOULD WEAR RUBBER GLOVES.
RE-TREATMENT IS USUALLY NOT NECESSARY, BUT PRESENCE OF LIVING LICE IN HAIR 7 DAYS AFTER TREATMENT INDICATES THAT RE-TREATMENT MAY BE NECESSARY. DO NOT RE-TREAT WITHOUT THE ADVICE OF A PHYSICIAN.

STORAGE
Store lotion and shampoo at controlled room temperature 15°-30°C (59°-86°F). Dispense in a tight, light-resistant container as defined in the USP, with a child-resistant closure.

REFERENCES
1. Feldmann, R.J. and Maiback, H.I., *Toxicol. Applied, Pharmacol.*, 28:126, 1974. 2. Dale, W.E., Curly, A. and Cueto, C. *Life Sci.* 5:47, 1966. 3. Ginsburg, C.M., et al., *J. Pediatr.* 91:6 998-1000, 1977. 4. Nagasaki, T., Tomii, S., Mepu, T., Murugami, M. and ito. N. *Gann* (Cancer) 63(3):393, 1972. 5. Goto, M., Hatteri, M., Miyugawa, T. and Enomoto, M., *Chemosphere* 6:279, 1972. 6. Hanada, M., Yatani, C., Miyaji, T., *Gann* 64:511, 1973. 7. Weisse, I., and Herbst, M., *Toxicol.* 7:233, 1977. 8. Technical Report Series, NCI-CG-TR-14, *HEW PUBLICATIONS*, No. (NIH) 77-814. 9. Thorpe, E. and Walker, A.I.T., *Food Cosmetic Toxicol.* 11:433, 1978. 10. Orr, J.W., *Nature* 162:189, 1948. 11. Kashyap, S.K. et. al., *J. Environ Sci. Health* 14:305-318, 1979.

HOW SUPPLIED
LIQUID: 1%

AVERAGE UNIT PRICE (AVAILABLE SIZES)		GENERIC A-RATED AVERAGE PRICE (GAAP)	
GENERIC	$0.09	60 ml	$4.75
		480 ml	$45.42

BRAND/MANUFACTURER	NDC	SIZE	AWP
◆ GENERICS			
Rugby	00536-1270-96	60 ml	$3.46
Schein	00364-7327-58	60 ml	$5.15
Geneva	00781-7160-02	60 ml	$5.65

➤ SHOWN IN PRODUCT IDENTIFICATION GUIDE

BRAND/MANUFACTURER	NDC	SIZE	AWP
Rugby	00536-1270-85	480 ml	$17.98
Schein	00364-7327-16	480 ml	$18.90
Geneva	00781-7160-16	480 ml	$28.69
Rugby	00536-1270-90	480 ml	$116.10

LOTION: 1%

AVERAGE UNIT PRICE (AVAILABLE SIZES)		GENERIC A-RATED AVERAGE PRICE (GAAP)	
GENERIC	$0.04	60 ml	$3.52
HCFA FUL (60 ml)	$0.04	480 ml	$17.51
HCFA FUL (480 ml)	$0.03	3840 ml	$100.91

BRAND/MANUFACTURER	NDC	SIZE	AWP
◆ GENERICS			
Barre	00472-0570-02	60 ml	$2.80
Mason Dist	11845-0435-17	60 ml	$2.84
Moore,H.L.	00839-6571-64	60 ml	$2.90
Pennex	00426-8546-60	60 ml	$3.20
Pennex	00832-8546-60	60 ml	$3.20
Qualitest	00603-1404-49	60 ml	$3.31
Rugby	00536-1262-96	60 ml	$3.32
Major	00904-0690-03	60 ml	$3.40
Goldline	00182-1475-43	60 ml	$3.45
Aligen	00405-3175-56	60 ml	$3.50
Schein	00364-7326-58	60 ml	$4.10
Geneva	00781-7150-02	60 ml	$5.55
Qualitest	00603-1404-58	480 ml	$13.45
Pennex	00832-8546-16	480 ml	$14.52
Pennex	00426-8546-16	480 ml	$15.50
Rugby	00536-1262-85	480 ml	$15.60
Goldline	00182-1475-40	480 ml	$15.75
Barre	00472-0570-04	480 ml	$15.90
Moore,H.L.	00839-6571-69	480 ml	$16.05
Major	00904-0690-16	480 ml	$16.10
Mason Dist	11845-0435-13	480 ml	$16.74
Aligen	00405-3175-16	480 ml	$18.20
URL	00677-0808-33	480 ml	$18.95
Schein	00364-7326-16	480 ml	$19.00
Geneva	00781-7150-16	480 ml	$31.15
Major	00904-0690-28	3840 ml	$97.90
Barre	00472-0570-28	3840 ml	$99.90
Rugby	00536-1262-90	3840 ml	$104.94

SHAMPOO: 1%

AVERAGE UNIT PRICE (AVAILABLE SIZES)		GENERIC A-RATED AVERAGE PRICE (GAAP)	
GENERIC	$0.05	60 ml	$3.69
HCFA FUL (60 ml)	$0.04	480 ml	$19.32
HCFA FUL (480 ml)	$0.03	3840 ml	$122.88

BRAND/MANUFACTURER	NDC	SIZE	AWP
◆ GENERICS			
Moore,H.L.	00839-6572-64	60 ml	$3.09
Mason Dist	11845-0436-17	60 ml	$3.16
Qualitest	00603-1406-49	60 ml	$3.47
Barre	00472-0572-02	60 ml	$3.70
Pennex	00426-8547-60	60 ml	$3.80
Pennex	00832-8547-60	60 ml	$3.80
Major	00904-0692-03	60 ml	$4.00
Aligen	00405-3200-56	60 ml	$4.00
Goldline	00182-1476-43	60 ml	$4.20
Qualitest	00603-1406-58	480 ml	$16.78
Pennex	00832-8547-16	480 ml	$16.94
Pennex	00426-8547-16	480 ml	$18.30
Major	00904-0692-16	480 ml	$18.40
Goldline	00182-1476-40	480 ml	$19.50
URL	00677-0809-33	480 ml	$19.68
Mason Dist	11845-0436-13	480 ml	$19.68
Moore,H.L.	00839-6572-69	480 ml	$19.70
Aligen	00405-3200-16	480 ml	$22.10
Barre	00472-0572-16	480 ml	$22.15
Major	00904-0692-28	3840 ml	$115.50
Barre	00472-0572-28	3840 ml	$124.90
Goldline	00182-1476-41	3840 ml	$128.25

Lioresal SEE BACLOFEN

Liothyronine Sodium

DESCRIPTION

Thyroid hormone drugs are natural or synthetic preparations containing tetraiodothyronine (T_4, levothyroxine) sodium or triiodothyronine (T_3, Liothyronine) sodium or both. T_4 and T_3 are produced in the human thyroid gland by the iodination and coupling of the amino acid tyrosine. T_4 contains four iodine atoms and is formed by the coupling of two molecules of diiodotyrosine (DIT). T_3 contains three atoms of iodine and is formed by the coupling of one molecule of DIT with one molecule of monoiodotyrosine (MIT). Both hormones are stored in the thyroid colloid as thyroglobulin and released into the circulation. The major source of T_3 has been shown to be peripheral deiodination of T_4. T_3 is bound less firmly than T_4 in the serum, enters peripheral tissues more readily, and binds to specific nuclear receptor(s) to initiate hormonal, metabolic effects. T_4 is the prohormone which is deiodinated to T_3 for hormone activity.

Thyroid hormone preparations belong to two categories: (1) natural hormonal preparations derived from animal thyroid, and (2) synthetic preparations. Natural preparations include desiccated thyroid and thyroglobulin. Desiccated thyroid is derived from domesticated animals that are used for food by man (either beef or hog thyroid), and thyroglobulin is derived from thyroid glands of the hog. The United States Pharmacopeia (USP) has standardized the total iodine content of natural preparations. Thyroid USP contains not less than (NLT) 0.17 percent and not more than (NMT) 0.23 percent iodine, and thyroglobulin contains not less than (NLT) 0.7 percent of organically bound iodine. Iodine content is only an indirect indicator of true hormonal biologic activity.

Liothyronine Sodium injection and tablets (T_3) contain Liothyronine (L-triiodothyronine or L-T_3), a synthetic form of a natural thyroid hormone, as the sodium salt.

The empirical formula and molecular weight of Liothyronine Sodium are given below.

The empirical formula is $C_{15}H_{11}I_3NNaO_4$ and molecular weight is 672.96. L-Tyrosine, O-(4-hydroxy-3-iodophenyl)-3,5-diiodo-, monosodium salt

In euthyroid patients, 25 mcg of Liothyronine is equivalent to approximately 1 grain of desiccated thyroid or thyroglobulin and 0.1 mg of L-thyroxine.

Each mL of Liothyronine Sodium contains, in sterile non-pyrogenic aqueous solution, Sodium Liothyronine equivalent to 10 mcg of Liothyronine.

Following is its chemical structure:

CLINICAL PHARMACOLOGY

The mechanisms by which thyroid hormones exert their physiologic action are not well understood. Thyroid hormones enhance oxygen consumption by most tissues of the body and increase the basal metabolic rate and the metabolism of carbohydrates, lipids and proteins. In vitro studies indicate that T_3 increases aerobic mitochondrial function, thereby increasing the rates and synthesis and utilization of myocardial high-energy phosphates. This, in turn, stimulates myosin ATPase and reduces tissues lactic acidosis. Thus, thyroid hormones exert a profound influence on virtually every organ system in the body and are of particular importance in the development of the central nervous system.

While the source of levothyroxine (T_4) and some triiodothyronine (T_3) is via secretion from the thyroid gland, it is now well-established that approximately 80% of circulating T_3 arises predominantly by way of the extrathyroidal conversion of T_4. The membrane-bound enzyme responsible for this reaction is iodothyronine 5'-deiodinase. Activity of the enzyme is greatest in the liver and kidney. A second pathway of T_4 to T_3 conversion occurs via a PTU-insensitive 5'-deiodinase located primarily in the pituitary and central nervous system.

The prohormone T_4 must be converted to T_3 in the body before it can exert biological effects. During periods of illness or stress, this conversion is often inhibited and can be diverted to the inactive reverse T_3 (rT_3) moiety. Therefore, correction of the hypothyroid condition in patients with myxedema coma is facilitated by the parenteral administration of triiodothyronine (T_3). T_3 is bound much less firmly to serum binding proteins and therefore penetrates into the cells much more rapidly than T_4. Also, the binding of T_3 to a nuclear thyroid hormone receptor seems to initiate most of the effects of thyroid hormone in tissues. Although most thyroid hormone analogs, both natural and synthetic, will bind to this protein, the affinity of T_3 for this receptor is roughly 10-fold higher than that of T_4. Thus, T_3 is the biologically active thyroid hormone.

PHARMACODYNAMICS

The clinical features of myxedema coma include depression of the cardiovascular, respiratory, gastrointestinal and central nervous systems, impaired diuresis, and hypothermia. Administration of thyroid hormones reverses or attenuates these conditions. Thyroid hormones increase heart rate, ventricular contractility and cardiac output, as well as decrease total systemic vascular resistance. They also increase the rate and depth of respiration, motility of the gastrointestinal tract, rapidity of cerebration, and vasodilatation. Thyroid hormones correct hypothermia by markedly increasing the basal metabolic rate, as well as the number and activity of mitochondria in almost all cells of the body.

PHARMACOKINETICS

Since Liothyronine Sodium (T_3) is not firmly bound to serum protein; it is readily available to body tissues. The onset of activity of Liothyronine Sodium tablets is rapid, occurring within a few hours. Maximum pharmacologic response occurs within two or three days, providing early clinical response. The biological half-life is about 2½ days.

T_3 is almost totally absorbed, 95 percent in four hours. The hormones contained in the natural preparations are absorbed in a manner similar to the synthetic hormones.

Liothyronine Sodium has a rapid cutoff of activity which permits quick dosage adjustment and facilitates control of the effects of overdosage, should they occur.

◆ RATED THERAPEUTICALLY EQUIVALENT; ◇ THERAPEUTIC EQUIVALENCE UNCONFIRMED; ○ UNRATED

The higher affinity of levothyroxine (T_4) as compared to triiodothyronine (T_4) for both thyroid-binding globulin and thyroid-binding prealbumin partially explains the higher serum levels and longer half-life of the former hormone.

Both protein-bound hormones exist in reverse equilibrium with minute amounts of free hormone, the latter accounting for the metabolic activity. T_4 is deiodinated to T_3.

A single dose of Liothyronine Sodium administered intravenously produces a detectable metabolic response in as little as two to four hours and a maximum therapeutic response within two days. However, no pharmacokinetic studies have been performed with intravenous Liothyronine (T_3) in myxedema coma or precoma patients.

INDICATIONS AND USAGE

Liothyronine Sodium injection (T_3) is indicated in the treatment of myxedema coma/precoma.

Liothyronine Sodium injection and tablets can be used in patients allergic to desiccated thyroid or thyroid extract derived from pork or beef.

Thyroid hormone drugs are indicated:

1. As replacement or supplemental therapy in patients with hypothyroidism of any etiology, except transient hypothyroidism during the recovery phase of subacute thyroiditis. This category includes cretinism, myxedema and ordinary hypothyroidism in patients of any age (children, adults, the elderly), or state (including pregnancy); primary hypothyroidism resulting from functional deficiency, primary atrophy, partial or total absence of thyroid gland, or the effects of surgery, radiation, or drugs, with or without the presence of goiter; and secondary (pituitary) or tertiary (hypothalamic) hypothyroidism (see *"Warnings"*).
2. As pituitary thyroid-stimulating hormone (TSH) suppressants, in the treatment or prevention of various types of euthyroid goiters, including thyroid nodules, subacute or chronic lymphocytic thyroiditis (Hashimoto's) and multinodular goiter.
3. As diagnostic agents in suppression tests to differentiate suspected mild hyperthyroidism or thyroid gland autonomy.

UNLABELED USES

Liothyronine is used alone or as an adjunct in the treatment of depression and as thyroid replacement in patients with thyroid cancer.

CONTRAINDICATIONS

Thyroid hormone preparations are generally contraindicated in patients with diagnosed but as yet uncorrected adrenal cortical insufficiency or untreated thyrotoxicosis. Thyroid hormone preparations are also generally contraindicated in patients with hypersensitivity to any of the active or extraneous constituents of these preparations; however, there is no well-documented evidence in the literature of true allergic or idiosyncratic reactions to thyroid hormone.

Concomitant use of Liothyronine Sodium and artificial rewarming of patients is contraindicated. (See *"Precautions"*.)

WARNINGS

DRUGS WITH THYROID HORMONE ACTIVITY, ALONE OR TOGETHER WITH OTHER THERAPEUTIC AGENTS, HAVE BEEN USED FOR THE TREATMENT OF OBESITY. IN EUTHYROID PATIENTS, DOSES WITHIN THE RANGE OF DAILY HORMONAL REQUIREMENTS ARE INEFFECTIVE FOR WEIGHT REDUCTION. LARGER DOSES MAY PRODUCE SERIOUS OR EVEN LIFE-THREATENING MANIFESTATIONS OF TOXICITY, PARTICULARLY WHEN GIVEN IN ASSOCIATION WITH SYMPATHOMIMETIC AMINES SUCH AS THOSE USED FOR THEIR ANORECTIC EFFECTS.

The use of thyroid hormones in the therapy of obesity, alone or combined with other drugs, is unjustified and has been shown to be ineffective. Neither is their use justified for the treatment of male or female infertility unless this condition is accompanied by hypothyroidism.

Thyroid hormones should be used with great caution in a number of circumstances where the integrity of the cardiovascular system, particularly the coronary arteries, is suspected. These include patients with angina pectoris or the elderly, in whom there is a greater likelihood of occult cardiac disease. Therefore, in patients with compromised cardiac function, use thyroid hormones in conjunction with careful cardiac monitoring. In these patients, Liothyronine Sodium therapy should be initiated with low doses, with due consideration for its relatively rapid onset of action. Starting dosage of Liothyronine Sodium tablets is 5 mcg daily, and should be increased by no more than 5 mcg increments at two-week intervals. When, in such patients, a euthyroid state can only be reached at the expense of an aggravation of the cardiovascular disease, thyroid hormone dosage should be reduced.

Morphologic hypogonadism and nephrosis should be ruled out before the drug is administered. If hypopituitarism is present, the adrenal deficiency must be corrected prior to starting the drug. Although the specific dosage of Liothyronine Sodium injection depends upon individual circumstances, in patients with known or suspected cardiovascular disease the extremely rapid onset of action of Liothyronine Sodium injection may warrant initiating therapy at a dose of 10 mcg to 20 mcg. (See *"Dosage and Administration"*.)

Myxedematous patients are very sensitive to thyroid hormones; dosage should be started at a low level and increased gradually as acute changes may precipitate adverse cardiovascular events.

Severe and prolonged hypothyroidism can lead to a decreased level of adrenocortical activity commensurate with the lowered metabolic state. When thyroid-replacement therapy is administered, the metabolism increases at a greater rate than adrenocortical activity. This can precipitate adrenocortical insufficiency. Therefore, in severe and prolonged hypothyroidism, supplemental adrenocortical steroids may be necessary.

In rare instances, the administration of thyroid hormone may precipitate a hyperthyroid state or may aggravate existing hyperthyroidism.

Extreme caution is advised when administering thyroid hormones with digitalis or vasopressors. (See *"Precautions—Drug Interactions"*.)

Fluid therapy should be administered with great care to prevent cardiac decompensation. (See *"Precautions—Adjunctive Therapy"*.)

PRECAUTIONS

GENERAL

Thyroid hormone therapy in patients with concomitant diabetes mellitus (see *"Precautions—Drug Interactions, Insulin or Oral Hypoglycemics"* regarding interaction and dose adjustment with insulin) or insipidus or adrenal cortical insufficiency may aggravate the intensity of their symptoms. Appropriate adjustments of the various therapeutic measures directed at these concomitant endocrine diseases are required.

The therapy of myxedema coma requires simultaneous administration of glucocorticoids. (See *"Precautions—Adjunctive Therapy"*.)

Hypothyroidism decreases and hyperthyroidism increases the sensitivity to oral anticoagulants. Prothrombin time should be closely monitored in thyroid-treated patients on oral anticoagulants and dosage of the latter agents adjusted on the basis of frequent prothrombin time determinations.

In infants, excessive doses of thyroid hormone preparations may produce craniosynostosis.

Oral therapy should be resumed as soon as the clinical situation has been stabilized and the patient is able to take oral medication. If L-thyroxine rather than Liothyronine Sodium is used in initiating oral therapy, the physician should bear in mind that there is a delay of several days in the onset of L-thyroxine activity and that intravenous therapy should be discontinued gradually.

INFORMATION FOR THE PATIENT

Patients on thyroid hormone preparations and parents of children on thyroid therapy should be informed that:

1. Replacement therapy is to be taken essentially for life, with the exception of cases of transient hypothyroidism, usually associated with thyroiditis, and in those patients receiving a therapeutic trial of the drug.
2. They should immediately report during the course of therapy any signs or symptoms of thyroid hormone toxicity, e.g., chest pain, increased pulse rate, palpitations, excessive sweating, heat intolerance, nervousness, or any other unusual event.
3. In case of concomitant diabetes mellitus, the daily dosage of antidiabetic medication may need readjustment as thyroid hormone replacement is achieved. If thyroid medication is stopped, a downward readjustment of the dosage of insulin or oral hypoglycemic agent may be necessary to avoid hypoglycemia. At all times, close monitoring of urinary glucose levels is mandatory in such patients.
4. In case of concomitant oral anticoagulant therapy, the prothrombin time should be measured frequently to determine if the dosage of oral anticoagulants is to be readjusted.
5. Partial loss of hair may be experienced by children in the first few months of thyroid therapy, but this is usually a transient phenomenon and later recovery is usually the rule.

ADJUNCTIVE THERAPY

Many investigators recommend that corticosteroids be administered routinely in the initial emergency treatment of all patients with myxedema coma. Patients with pituitary myxedema should receive adrenocortical hormone replacement therapy at or before the start of Liothyronine Sodium therapy. Similarly, patients with primary myxedema may also require adrenocortical hormone replacement therapy since a rapid return to normal body metabolism from a severely hypothyroid state may result in acute adrenocortical insufficiency and shock.

In considering the need to elevate blood pressure, it should be kept in mind that tissue metabolic requirements are markedly reduced in the hypothyroid patient. Because arrhythmias and circulatory collapse have infrequently occurred following the concomitant administration of thyroid hormones and vasopressor therapies, use caution when administering these therapies concomitantly. (See *"Precautions—Drug Interactions, Vasopressors"*.)

Hyponatremia is frequently present in myxedema coma, but usually resolves without specific therapy as the metabolic status of the patient is improved with thyroid hormone treatment. Fluid therapy should be administered with great care to prevent cardiac decompensation. In addition, some patients with myxedema have inappropriate secretion of ADH and are susceptible to water intoxication.

In some patients, respiratory depression has been a significant factor in the development of persistence of the comatose state. Decreased oxygen saturation and elevated CO_2 levels respond quickly to artificial respiration.

Infection is often present in myxedema coma and should be looked for and treated appropriately.

Concomitant use of Liothyronine Sodium and artificial rewarming of patients is contraindicated. Although patients in myxedema coma are often hypothermic, most investigators believe that artificial rewarming is of little value or may be harmful. The peripheral vasodilation produced by external heat serves to further decrease circulation to vital internal organs and to increase shock if present. It has been reported that the administration of Liothyronine Sodium will restore a

➤ SHOWN IN PRODUCT IDENTIFICATION GUIDE

normal body temperature in 24 to 48 hours if heat loss is prevented by keeping the patient covered with blankets in a warm room.

LABORATORY TESTS

Treatment of patients with thyroid hormone requires the periodic assessment of thyroid status by means of appropriate laboratory tests besides the full clinical evaluation. The TSH suppression test can be used to test the effectiveness of any thyroid preparation, bearing in mind the relative insensitivity of the infant pituitary to the negative feedback effect of thyroid hormones. Serum T_4 levels can be used to test the effectiveness of all thyroid medications except products containing Liothyronine Sodium. When the total serum T_4 is low but TSH is normal, a test specific to assess unbound (free) T_4 levels is warranted. Specific measurements of T_4 and T_3 by competitive protein binding or radioimmunoassay are not influenced by blood levels of organic or inorganic iodine and have essentially replaced older tests of thyroid hormone measurements, i.e., PBI, BEI and T_4 by column.

DRUG INTERACTIONS

Oral Anticoagulants: Thyroid hormones appear to increase catabolism of vitamin K-dependent clotting factors. If oral anticoagulants are also being given, compensatory increases in clotting factor synthesis are impaired. Patients stabilized on oral anticoagulants who are found to require thyroid replacement therapy should be watched very closely when thyroid is started. If a patient is truly hypothyroid, it is likely that a reduction in anticoagulant dosage will be required. No special precautions appear to be necessary when oral anticoagulant therapy is begun in a patient already stabilized on maintenance thyroid replacement therapy.

Insulin or Oral Hypoglycemics: Initiating thyroid replacement therapy may cause increases in insulin or oral hypoglycemic requirements. The effects seen are poorly understood and depend upon a variety of factors such as dose and type of thyroid preparations and endocrine status of the patient.

Patients receiving insulin or oral hypoglycemics should be closely watched during initiation of thyroid replacement therapy.

Cholestyramine: Cholestyramine binds both T_4 and T_3 in the intestine, thus impairing absorption of these thyroid hormones. *In vitro* studies indicate that the binding is not easily removed. Therefore, four to five hours should elapse between administration of cholestyramine and thyroid hormones.

Estrogen, Oral Contraceptives: Estrogens tend to increase serum thyroxine-binding globulin (TBG). In a patient with a nonfunctioning thyroid gland who is receiving thyroid replacement therapy, free levothyroxine may be decreased when estrogens are started thus increasing thyroid requirements. However, if the patient's thyroid gland has sufficient function, the decreased free thyroxine will result in a compensatory increase in thyroxine output by the thyroid. Therefore, patients without a functioning thyroid gland who are on thyroid replacement therapy may need to increase their thyroid dose if estrogens or estrogen-containing oral contraceptives are given.

Tricyclic Antidepressants: Use of thyroid products with imipramine and other tricyclic antidepressants may increase receptor sensitivity and enhance antidepressant activity; transient cardiac arrhythmias have been observed. Thyroid hormone activity may also be enhanced.

Digitalis: Thyroid preparations may potentiate the toxic effects of digitalis. Thyroid hormonal replacement increases metabolic rate, which requires an increase in digitalis dosage.

Ketamine: When administered to patients on a thyroid preparation, this parenteral anesthetic may cause hypertension and tachycardia. Use with caution and be prepared to treat hypertension, if necessary.

Vasopressors: Thyroid hormones increase the adrenergic effect of catecholamines such as epinephrine and norepinephrine. Therefore, use of vasopressors in patients receiving thyroid hormone preparations may increase the risk of precipitating coronary insufficiency, especially in patients with coronary artery disease. Therefore, use caution when administering vasopressors with Liothyronine (T_3).

DRUG/LABORATORY TEST INTERACTIONS

The following drugs or moieties are known to interfere with laboratory tests performed in patients on thyroid hormone therapy: androgens, corticosteroids, estrogens, oral contraceptives containing estrogens, iodine-containing preparations and the numerous preparations containing salicylates.

1. Changes in TBG concentration should be taken into consideration in the interpretation of T_4 and T_3 values. In such cases, the unbound (free) hormone should be measured. Pregnancy, estrogens and estrogen-containing oral contraceptives increase TBG concentrations. TBG may also be increased during infectious hepatitis. Decreases in TBG concentrations are observed in nephrosis, acromegaly and after androgen or corticosteroid therapy. Familial hyper- or hypo-thyroxine-binding globulinemias have been described. The incidence of TBG deficiency approximates 1 in 9000. The binding of thyroxine by thyroxine-binding prealbumin (TBPA) is inhibited by salicylates.

2. Medicinal or dietary iodine interferes with all *in vivo* tests of radioiodine uptake, producing low uptakes which may not be reflective of a true decrease in hormone synthesis.

3. The persistence of clinical and laboratory evidence of hypothyroidism in spite of adequate dosage replacement indicates either poor patient compliance, poor absorption, excessive fecal loss, or inactivity of the preparation. Intracellular resistance to thyroid hormone is quite rare.

CARCINOGENESIS, MUTAGENESIS AND IMPAIRMENT OF FERTILITY

A reportedly apparent association between prolonged thyroid therapy and breast cancer has not been confirmed and patients on thyroid for established indications should not discontinue therapy. No confirmatory long-term studies in animals have been performed to evaluate carcinogenic potential, mutagenicity, or impairment of fertility in either males or females.

PREGNANCY

Pregnancy Category A: Thyroid hormones do not readily cross the placental barrier. The clinical experience to date does not indicate any adverse effect on fetuses when thyroid hormones are administered to pregnant women. On the basis of current knowledge, thyroid replacement therapy to hypothyroid women should not be discontinued during pregnancy.

NURSING MOTHERS

Minimal amounts of thyroid hormones are excreted in human milk. Thyroid hormones are not associated with serious adverse reactions and do not have a known tumorigenic potential. However, caution should be exercised when thyroid hormones are administered to a nursing woman.

PEDIATRIC USE

Pregnant mothers provide little or no thyroid hormone to the fetus. The incidence of congenital hypothyroidism is relatively high (1:4000) and the hypothyroid fetus would not derive any benefits from the small amounts of hormone crossing the placental barrier. Routine determinations of serum T_4 and/or TSH is strongly advised in neonates in view of the deleterious effects of thyroid deficiency on growth and development.

Treatment should be initiated immediately upon diagnosis and maintained for life, unless transient hypothyroidism is suspected, in which case, therapy may be interrupted for two to eight weeks after the age of three years to reassess the condition. Cessation of therapy is justified in patients who have maintained a normal TSH during those two to eight weeks.

ADVERSE REACTIONS

The most frequently reported adverse events were arrhythmia (6% of patients) and tachycardia (3%). Cardiopulmonary arrest, hypotension and myocardial infarction occurred in approximately 2% of patients. The following events occurred in approximately 1% or fewer of patients: angina, congestive heart failure, fever, hypertension, phlebitis and twitching.

Adverse reactions with Liothyronine Sodium tablets other than those indicative of hyperthyroidism because of therapeutic overdosage, either initially or during the maintenance period are rare (see *"Overdosage"*).

In rare instances, allergic skin reactions have been reported with Liothyronine Sodium tablets.

OVERDOSAGE

Signs and Symptoms: Headache, irritability, nervousness, tremor, sweating, increased bowel motility and menstrual irregularities. Angina pectoris, arrhythmia, tachycardia, acute myocardial infarction or congestive heart failure may be induced or aggravated. Shock may also develop if there is untreated pituitary or adrenocortical failure. Massive overdosage may result in symptoms resembling thyroid storm. Chronic excessive dosage will produce the signs and symptoms of hyperthyroidism.

Treatment of Overdosage: Dosage should be reduced or therapy temporarily discontinued if signs and symptoms of overdosage appear. Treatment may be reinstituted at a lower dosage. In normal individuals, normal hypothalamic-pituitary-thyroid axis function is restored in six to eight weeks after cessation of therapy following thyroid suppression.

Treatment of acute massive thyroid hormone overdosage is aimed at reducing gastrointestinal absorption of the drugs and counteracting central and peripheral effects, mainly those of increased sympathetic activity. Vomiting may be induced initially if further gastrointestinal absorption can reasonably be prevented and barring contraindications such as coma, convulsions, or loss of the gagging reflex.

Treatment is symptomatic and supportive. Oxygen may be administered and ventilation maintained. Cardiac glycosides may be indicated if congestive heart failure develops. Antiadrenergic agents, particularly propranolol, have been used advantageously in the treatment of increased sympathetic activity. Propranolol may be administered intravenously at a dosage of 1 to 3 mg over a 10-minute period or orally, 80 to 160 mg/day, especially when no contraindications exist for its use. Measures to control fever, hypoglycemia or fluid loss should be instituted if needed.

DOSAGE AND ADMINISTRATION

LIOTHYRONINE SODIUM INJECTION

Adults: Myxedema coma is usually precipitated in the hypothyroid patient of long standing by intercurrent illness or drugs such as sedatives and anesthetics and should be considered a medical emergency. Therapy should be directed at the correction of electrolyte disturbances, possible infection, or other intercurrent illness in addition to the administration of intravenous Liothyronine (T_3). Simultaneous glucocorticosteroids are required.

Liothyronine Sodium injection (T_3) is for intravenous administration only. It should not be given intramuscularly or subcutaneously.

- Prompt administration of an adequate dose of intravenous Liothyronine (T_3) is important in determining clinical outcome.

◆ RATED THERAPEUTICALLY EQUIVALENT; ◇ THERAPEUTIC EQUIVALENCE UNCONFIRMED; ○ UNRATED

- Initial and subsequent doses of Liothyronine Sodium injection should be based on continuous monitoring of the patient's clinical status and response to therapy.
- Liothyronine Sodium injection doses should normally be administered at least four hours—and not more than 12 hours—apart.
- Administration of at least 65 mcg/day of intravenous Liothyronine (T_3) in the initial days of therapy was associated with lower mortality.
- There is limited clinical experience with intravenous Liothyronine (T_3) at total daily doses exceeding 100 mcg/day.

No controlled clinical studies have been done with Liothyronine Sodium. The following dosing guidelines have been derived from data analysis of myxedema coma/precoma case reports collected since 1963 and from scientific literature since 1956.

An initial intravenous Liothyronine Sodium dose ranging from 25 mcg to 50 mcg is recommended in the emergency treatment of myxedema coma/precoma in adults. In patients with known or suspected cardiovascular disease, an initial dose of 10 mcg to 20 mcg is suggested (see "Warnings"). However, both the initial dose and subsequent doses should be determined on the basis of continuous monitoring of the patient's clinical condition and response to Liothyronine Sodium therapy. Normally at least four hours should be allowed between doses to adequately assess therapeutic response and no more than 12 hours should elapse between doses to avoid fluctuations in hormone levels. Caution should be exercised in adjusting the dose due to the potential of large changes to precipitate adverse cardiovascular events. Review of the myxedema case reports indicates decreased mortality in patients receiving at least 65 mcg/day in the initial days of treatment. However, there is limited clinical experience at total daily doses above 100 mcg. See "Precautions—Drug Interactions" for potential interactions between thyroid hormones and digitalis and vasopressors.

Pediatric Use: There is limited experience with Liothyronine Sodium in children. Safety and effectiveness have not been established. (See "Precautions".)

Switching to Oral Therapy: Oral therapy should be resumed as soon as the clinical situation has been stabilized and the patient is able to take oral medication. When switching a patient to Liothyronine Sodium tablets from Liothyronine Sodium injection discontinue the injection, initiate oral therapy at a low dosage, and increase gradually according to the patient's response.

If L-thyroxine rather than Liothyronine Sodium is used in initiating oral therapy, the physician should bear in mind that there is a delay of several days in the onset of L-thyroxine activity and that intravenous therapy should be discontinued gradually.

LIOTHYRONINE SODIUM TABLETS

The dosage of thyroid hormones is determined by the indication and must in every case be individualized according to patient response and laboratory findings.

Liothyronine Sodium tablets are intended for oral administration; once-a-day dosage is recommended. Although Liothyronine Sodium has a rapid cutoff, its metabolic effects persist for a few days following discontinuance.

Mild Hypothyroidism: Recommended starting dosage is 25 mcg daily. Daily dosage then may be increased by 12.5 or 25 mcg every one or two weeks. Usual maintenance dose is 25-75 mcg daily. Smaller doses may be fully effective in some patients, while dosage of 100 mcg daily may be required in others.

The rapid onset and dissipation of action of Liothyronine Sodium (T_3), as compared with levothyroxine sodium (T_4), has led some clinicians to prefer its use in patients who might be more susceptible to the untoward effects of thyroid medication. However, the wide swings in serum T_3 levels that follow its administration and the possibility of more pronounced cardiovascular side effects tend to counterbalance the stated advantages.

Liothyronine Sodium tablets may be used in preference to levothyroxine (T_4) during radioisotope scanning procedures, since induction of hypothyroidism in those cases is more abrupt and can be of shorter duration. It may also be preferred when impairment of peripheral conversion of T_4 to T_3 is suspected.

Myxedema: Recommended starting dosage is 5 mcg daily. This may be increased by 5 to 10 mcg daily every one or two weeks. When 25 mcg daily is reached, dosage may often be increased by 12.5 or 25 mcg every one or two weeks. Usual maintenance dose is 50 to 100 mcg daily.

Congenital Hypothyroidism: Recommended starting dosage is 5 mcg daily, with a 5 mcg increment every three to four days until the desired response is achieved. Infants a few months old may require only 20 mcg daily for maintenance. At one year, 50 mcg daily may be required. Above three years, full adult dosage may be necessary (see "Precautions, Pediatric Use").

Simple (non-toxic) Goiter: Recommended starting dosage is 5 mcg daily. This dosage may be increased by 5 to 10 mcg daily every one or two weeks. When 25 mcg daily is reached, dosage may be increased every week or two by 12.5 or 25 mcg. Usual maintenance dosage is 75 mcg daily.

In the elderly or in children, therapy should be started with 5 mcg daily and increased only by 5 mcg increments at the recommended intervals.

When switching a patient to Liothyronine Sodium Tablets from thyroid, L-thyroxine or thyroglobulin, discontinue the other medication, initiate Liothyronine Sodium at a low dosage, and increase gradually according to the patient's response. When selecting a starting dosage, bear in mind that this drug has a rapid onset of action, and that residual effects of the other thyroid preparation may persist for the first several weeks of therapy.

Thyroid Suppression Therapy: Administration of thyroid hormone in doses higher than those produced physiologically by the gland results in suppression of the production of endogenous hormone. This is the basis for the thyroid suppression test and is used as an aid in the diagnosis of patients with signs of mild hyperthyroidism in whom baseline laboratory tests appear normal or to demonstrate thyroid gland autonomy in patients with Graves' ophthalmopathy. ^{131}I uptake is determined before and after the administration of the exogenous hormone. A 50 percent or greater suppression of uptake indicates a normal thyroid-pituitary axis and thus rules out thyroid gland autonomy.

Liothyronine Sodium tablets are given in doses of 75-100 mcg/day for seven days, and radioactive iodine uptake is determined before and after administration of the hormone. If thyroid function is under normal control, the radioiodine uptake will drop significantly after treatment. Liothyronine Sodium tablets should be administered cautiously to patients in whom there is a strong suspicion of thyroid gland autonomy, in view of the fact that the exogenous hormone effects will be additive to the endogenous source.

STORAGE
Store between 2° and 8°C.

HOW SUPPLIED
INJECTION: 10 MCG/ML

BRAND/MANUFACTURER	NDC	SIZE	AWP
○ **BRAND** TRIOSTAT: SK Beecham Pharm	00007-5210-06	1 ml 6s	$1373.00

TABLETS: 5 MCG

BRAND/MANUFACTURER	NDC	SIZE	AWP
◆ **BRAND** CYTOMEL: SK Beecham Pharm	00007-3414-20	100s	$13.80

TABLETS: 25 MCG

BRAND/MANUFACTURER	NDC	SIZE	AWP
◆ **BRAND** CYTOMEL: SK Beecham Pharm	00007-3416-20	100s	$16.75

TABLETS: 50 MCG

BRAND/MANUFACTURER	NDC	SIZE	AWP
◆ **BRAND** CYTOMEL: SK Beecham Pharm	00007-3417-20	100s	$25.55

Liotrix

DESCRIPTION
Liotrix Tablets contain Tetraiodothyronine (T_4 levothyroxine) and Triiodothyronine (T_3 liothyronine).

The relative amounts of T_3 to T_4 in each tablet is:

Liotrix-¼	3.1 mcg/12.5 mcg
Liotrix-½	6.25 mcg/25 mcg
Liotrix-1	12.5 mcg/50 mcg
Liotrix-2	25 mcg/100 mcg
Liotrix-3	37.5 mcg/150 mcg

T_3 liothyronine sodium is approximately four times as potent as T_4 thyroxine on a microgram for microgram basis.

CLINICAL PHARMACOLOGY
The steps in the synthesis of the thyroid hormones are controlled by thyrotropin (Thyroid Stimulating Hormone. TSH) secreted by the anterior pituitary. This hormones secretion is in turn controlled by a feedback mechanism effected by the thyroid hormones themselves and by thyrotropin releasing hormone (TRH), a tripeptide of hypothalamic origin. Endogenous thyroid hormone secretion is suppressed when exogenous thyroid hormones are administered to euthyroid individuals in excess of the normal gland's secretion.

The mechanisms by which thyroid hormones exert their physiologic action are not well understood. These hormones enhance oxygen consumption by most tissues of the body, increase the basal metabolic rate, and the metabolism of carbohydrates, lipids, and proteins thus, they exert a profound influence on every organ system in the body and are of particular importance in the development of the central nervous system.

The normal thyroid gland contains approximately 200 mcg of levothyroxine (T_4) per gram of gland, and 15 mcg of triiodothyronine (T_3) per gram. The ratio of these two hormones in the circulation does not represent the ratio in the thyroid gland, since about 80 percent of peripheral triiodothyronine comes from monodeiodination of levothyroxine. Peripheral monodeiodination of levothyroxine at the 5 position (inner ring) also results in the formation of reverse triiodothyronine (T_3), which is calorigenically inactive.

Triiodothyronine (T_3) levels are low in the fetus and newborn in old age, in chronic caloric deprivation, hepatic cirrhosis, renal failure, surgical stress, and chronic illness representing what has been called the low triiodothyronine syndrome.

Pharmacokinetics: Animal studies have shown that T_4 is only partially absorbed from the gastrointestinal tract. The degree of absorption is dependent on the vehicle used for its administration and by the character of the intestinal contents, the intestinal flora including plasma protein soluble dietary factors, all of which bind thyroid and theapy make it unavailable for diffusion. Only 41 percent is absorbed when given in a gelatin capsule as opposed to a 74 percent absorption when given with an albumin carrier.

Depending on other factors, absorption has varied from 48 to 79 percent of the administered dose. Fasting increases absorption. Malabsorption syndromes, as well as dietary factors (children's soybean formula, concomitant use of anionic exchange resins such as cholestyramine) cause excessive fecal loss. T_3 is almost totally absorbed. 95 percent in 4 hours. The hormones contained in the natural preparations are absorbed in a manner similar to the synthetic hormones.

More than 99 percent of circulating hormones are bound to serum proteins, including thyroid-binding globulin (TBg), thyroid-binding prealbumin (TBPA), and albumin (TBa), whose capacities and affinities vary for the hormones. The higher affinity of levothyroxine (T_4) for both TBg and TBPA as compared to triiodothyronine (T_3) partially explains the higher serum levels and longer half-life of the former hormone. Both protein-bound hormones exist in reverse equilibrium with minute amounts of free hormone, the latter accounting for the metabolic activity.

Deiodination of levothyroxine (T_4) occurs at a number of sites, including liver, kidney, and other tissues. The conjugated hormone, in the form of glucuronide or sulfate, is found in the bile and gut where it may complete an enterohepatic circulation. Eighty-five percent of levothyroxine (T_4) metabolized daily is deiodinated.

INDICATIONS AND USAGE

Liotrix Tablets are indicated.

1. As replacement of supplemental therapy in patients with hypothyroidism of any etiology except transient hypothyroidism during the recovery phase of subacute thyroiditis. This category includes cretinism, myxedema, and ordinary hypothyroidism in patients of any age (children, adults the elderly, or state (including pregnancy) primary hypothyroidism resulting from functional deficiency primary atrophy partial or total absence of thyroid gland or the effects of surgery, radiation, or drugs, with or without the presence of goiter, and secondary (pituitary), or tertiary (hypothalamic) hypothyroidism (See *"Warnings"*).

2. As pituitary TSH suppressants in the treatment or prevention of various types of euthyroid goiters, including thyroid nodules, sub-acute or chronic lymphocytic thyroiditis (Hashimoto's), multinodular goiter, and in the management of thyroid cancer.

3. As diagnostic agents in suppression tests to differentiate suspected mild hyperthyroidism of thyroid gland autonomy.

CONTRAINDICATIONS

Thyroid hormone preparations are generally contraindicated in patients with diagnosed but as yet uncorrected adrenal cortical insufficiency, untreated thyrotoxicosis, and apparent hypersensitivity to any of their active or extraneous constituents. There is no well documented evidence from the literature, however, of true allergic or idiosyncratic reactions to thyroid hormone.

WARNINGS

DRUGS WITH THYROID HORMONE ACTIVITY, ALONE OR TOGETHER WITH OTHER THERAPEUTIC AGENTS, HAVE BEEN USED FOR THE TREATMENT OF OBESITY IN EUTHYROID PATIENTS, DOSES WITHIN THE RANGE OF DAILY HORMONAL REQUIREMENTS ARE INEFFECTIVE FOR WEIGHT REDUCTION. LARGER DOSES MAY PRODUCE SERIOUS OR EVEN LIFE-THREATENING MANIFESTATIONS OF TOXICITY, PARTICULARLY WHEN GIVEN IN ASSOCIATION WITH SYMPATHOMIMETIC AMINES SUCH AS THOSE USED FOR THEIR ANORECTIC EFFECTS.

The use of thyroid hormones in the therapy of obesity, alone or combined with other drugs is unjustified and has been shown to be ineffective. Neither is their use justified for the treatment of male or female infertility unless this condition is accompanied by hypothyroidism.

PRECAUTIONS

General: Thyroid hormones should be used with great caution in a number of circumstances where the integrity of the cardiovascular system, particularly the coronary arteries, is suspected. These include patients with angina pectoris or the elderly in whom there is a greater likelihood of occult cardiac disease. In these patients therapy should be initiated with low doses, i.e., one tablet of Liotrix ¼ or Liotrix ½. When, in such patients, a euthyroid state can only be reached at the expense of an aggravation of the cardiovascular disease, thyroid hormone dosage should be reduced.

Thyroid hormone therapy in patients with concomitant diabetes mellitus or diabetes insipidus or adrenal cortical insufficiency aggravates the intensity of their symptoms. Appropriate adjustments of the various therapeutic measures directed at these concomitant endocrine diseases are required. The therapy of myxedema coma requires simultaneous administration of glucocorticoids (See *"Dosage and Administration"*).

Hypothyroidism decreases and hyperthyroidism increases the sensitivity to oral anticoagulants. Prothrombin time should be closely monitored in thyroid treated patients on oral anticoagulants and dosage of the latter agents adjusted on

the basis of frequent prothrombin time determinations. In infants, excessive doses of thyroid hormone preparations may produce craniosynostosis.

Information for the Patient: Patients on thyroid hormone preparations and parents of children on thyroid therapy should be informed that:

1. Replacement therapy is to be taken essentially for life, with the exception of cases of transient hypothyroidism, usually associated with thyroiditis, and in those patients receiving a therapeutic trial of the drug.

2. They should immediately report during the course of therapy any signs or symptoms of thyroid hormone toxicity, e.g. chest pain, increased pulse rate, palpitations, excessive sweating, heat intolerance, nervousness or any other unusual event.

3. In case of concomitant diabetes mellitus, the daily dosage of antidiabetic medication may need readjustment as thyroid hormone replacement is achieved. If thyroid medication is stopped, a downward readjustment of the dosage of insulin or oral hypoglycemic agent may be necessary to avoid hypoglycemia. At all times, close monitoring of urinary glucose levels is mandatory in such patients.

4. In case of concomitant oral anticoagulant therapy, the prothrombin time should be measured frequently to determine if the dosage of oral anticoagulants is to be readjusted.

5. Partial loss of hair may be experienced by children in the first few months of thyroid therapy, but this is usually a transient phenomenon and later recovery is usually the rule.

Laboratory Tests: Treatment of patients with thyroid hormones requires the periodic assessment of thyroid status by means of appropriate laboratory tests besides the full clinical evaluation. The TSH suppression test can be used to test the effectiveness of any thyroid preparation bearing in mind the relative insensitivity of the infant pituitary to the negative feedback effect of thyroid hormones. Serum T_4 levels can be used to test the effectiveness of all thyroid medications except T_3. When the total serum T_4 is low but TSH is normal, a test specific to assess unbound (free) T_4 levels is warranted. Specific measurements of T_4 and T_3 by competitive protein binding or radioimmunoassay are not influenced by blood levels of organic or inorganic iodine.

Drug Interactions: Oral Anticoagulants—Thyroid hormones appear to increase catabolism of vitamin K-dependent clotting factors. If oral anticoagulants are also being given, compensatory increases in clotting factor synthesis are impaired. Patients stabilized on oral anticoagulants who are found to require thyroid replacement therapy should be watched very closely when thyroid is started. If a patient is truly hypothyroid, it is likely that a reduction in anticoagulant dosage will be required. No special precautions appear to be necessary when oral anticoagulant therapy is begun in a patient already stabilized on maintenance thyroid replacement therapy.

Insulin or Oral Hypoglycemics: Initiating thyroid replacement therapy may cause increases in insulin or oral hypoglycemic requirements. The effects seen are poorly understood and depend upon a variety of factors such as dose and type of thyroid preparations and endocrine status of the patient. Patients receiving insulin or oral hypoglycemics should be closely watched during initiation of thyroid replacement therapy.

Cholestyramine or Colestipol: Cholestyramine or colestipol binds both T_4 and T_3 in the intestine thus impairing absorption of these thyroid hormones. *In vitro* studies indicate that the binding is not easily removed. Therefore, four to five hours should elapse between administration of cholestyramine or colestipol and thyroid hormones.

Estrogen, Oral Contraceptives: Estrogens tend to increase serum thyroxine-binding globulin (TBg). In a patient with a nonfunctioning thyroid gland who is receiving thyroid replacement therapy, free levothyroxine may be decreased when estrogens are started, thus increasing thyroid requirements. However, if the patient's thyroid gland has sufficient function, the decreased free thyroxine will result in a compensatory increase in thyroxine output by the thyroid. Therefore, patients without a functioning thyroid gland who are on thyroid replacement therapy may need to increase their thyroid dose if estrogens or estrogen-containing oral contraceptives are given.

Drug/Laboratory Test Interactions: The following drugs or moieties are known to interfere with laboratory tests performed in patients on thyroid hormone therapy: androgens, corticosteroids, estrogens, oral contraceptives containing estrogens, iodine-containing preparations, and the numerous preparations containing salicylates.

1. Changes in TBg concentration should be taken into consideration in the interpretation of T_4 and T_3 values. In such cases the unbound (free) hormone should be measured. Pregnancy, estrogens and estrogen-containing oral contraceptives increase TBg concentrations TBg may also be increased during infectious hepatitis. Decreases in TBg concentrations are observed in nephrosis, acromegaly and after androgen or corticosteroid therapy. Familial hyper- or hypothyroxine-binding-globulinemias have been described. The incidence of TBg deficiency approximates 1 in 9,000. The binding of thyroxine by TBPA is inhibited by salicylates.

2. Medicinal or dietary iodine interferes with all *in vivo* tests of radio-iodine uptake, producing low uptakes which may not be relative of a true decrease in hormone synthesis.

3. The persistence of clinical and laboratory evidence of hypothyroidism in spite of adequate dosage replacement indicates either poor patient compliance, poor absorption, excessive fecal loss or inactivity of the preparation. Intracellular resistance to thyroid hormone is quite rare.

Carcinogenesis, Mutagenesis, and Impairment of Fertility: A reportedly apparent association between prolonged thyroid therapy and breast cancer has not been confirmed and patients on thyroid for established indications should not discontinue therapy. No confirmatory long-term studies in animals have been performed to evaluate carcinogenic potential, mutagenicity, or impairment of fertility in either males or females.

Pregnancy: Category A: Thyroid hormones do not readily cross the placental barrier. The clinical experience to date does not indicate any adverse effect on fetuses when thyroid hormones are administered to pregnant women. On the basis of current knowledge, thyroid replacement therapy to hypothyroid women should not be discontinued during pregnancy.

Nursing Mothers: Minimal amounts of thyroid hormones are excreted in human milk. Thyroid is not associated with serious adverse reactions and does not have a known tumorigenic potential. However, caution should be exercised when thyroid is administered to a nursing woman.

Pediatric Use: Pregnant mothers provide little or no thyroid hormone to the fetus. The incidence of congenital hypothyroidism is relatively high (1,4000) and the hypothyroid fetus would not derive any benefit from the small amounts of hormone crossing the placental barrier. Routine determinations of serum (T_4) and/or TSH is strongly advised in neonates in view of the deleterious effects of thyroid deficiency on growth and development.

Treatment should be initiated immediately upon diagnosis, and maintained for life, unless transient hypothyroidism is suspected, in which case, therapy may be interrupted for 2 to 8 weeks after the age of 3 years to reassess the condition. Cessation of therapy is justified in patients who have maintained a normal TSH during those 2 to 8 weeks.

ADVERSE REACTIONS

Adverse reactions other than those indicative of hyperthyroidism because of therapeutic overdosage, either initially or during the maintenance period, are rare. (See *"Overdosage"*).

OVERDOSAGE

Signs and Symptoms: Excessive doses of thyroid result in a hypermetabolic state resembling in every respect the condition of endogenous origin. The condition may be self-induced.

Treatment of Overdosage: Dosage should be reduced or therapy temporarily discontinued if signs and symptoms of overdosage appear.

Treatment may be reinstituted at a lower dosage in normal individuals, normal hypothalamic-pituitary-thyroid axis function is restored in 6 to 8 weeks after thyroid suppression.

Treatment of acute massive thyroid hormone overdosage is aimed at reducing gastrointestinal absorption of the drugs and counteracting central and peripheral effects, mainly those of increased sympathetic actvity. Vomiting may be induced initially if further gastrointestinal absorption can reasonably be prevented and barring contraindications such as coma, convulsions, or loss of the gagging reflex. Treatment is symptomatic and supportive. Oxygen may be administered and ventilation maintained. Cardiac glycosides may be indicated if congestive heart failure develops. Measures to control fever, hypoglycemia, or fluid loss should be instituted if needed. Antiadrenergic agents, particularly propranolol, have been used advantageously in the treatment of increased sympathetic activity. Propranolol may be administered intravenously at a dosage of 1 to 3 mg over a 10 minute period or orally. 80 to 160 mg/day, initially especially when no contraindications exist for its use.

DOSAGE AND ADMINISTRATION

The dosage of Liotrix USP is determined by the indication and must in every case be individualized according to patient response and laboratory findings.

Thyroid hormones are given orally in acute, emergency conditions, injectable sodium levothyroxine may be given intravenously when oral administration is not feasible or desirable, as in the treatment of myxedema coma, or during total parenteral nutrition. Intramuscular administration is not advisable because of reported poor adsorption.

Hypothyroidism: Therapy is usually instituted using low doses with increments which depend on the cardiovascular status of the patient. The usual starting dose is one tablet of Liotrix ½ with increments of one tablet of Liotrix ¼ every 2 to 3 weeks. A lower starting dosage, one tablet of Liotrix ¼ day, is recommended in patients with long-standing myxedema, particularly if cardiovascular impairment is suspected, in which case extreme caution is recommended. The appearance of angina is an indication for a reduction in dosage. Most patients require one tablet of Liotrix ¼ to one tablet of Liotrix 2 per day. Failure to respond to doses of one tablet of Liotrix 3 suggests lack of compliance or malabsorption. Maintenance dosages of one tablet of Liotrix 1 to one tablet of Liotrix 2 per day usually result in normal serum levothyroxine (T_4) and triiodothyronine (T_3) levels. Adequate therapy usually results in normal TSH and T_4 levels after 2 to 3 weeks of therapy.

Readjustment of thyroid hormone dosage should be made within the first four weeks of therapy, after proper clinical and laboratory evaluations, including serum levels of T_4 bound and free and TSH.

It may be used in preference to levothyroxine (T_4) during radio-isotope scanning procedures since induction of hypothyroidism in those cases is more abrupt and can be of shorter duration. It may also be preferred when impairment of peripheral conversion of T_4 and T_3 is suspected.

Myxedema Coma: Myxedema coma is usually precipitated in the hypothyroid patient of long-standing by intercurrent illness or drugs such as sedatives and anesthetics and should be considered a medical emergency. Therapy should be directed at the correction of electrolyte disturbances and possible infection besides the administration of thyroid hormones. Corticosteroids should be administered routinely. T_4 and T_3 may be administered via a nasogastric tube but the preferred route of administration of both hormones is intravenous. Sodium levothyroxine (T_4) is given at a starting dose of 400 mcg (100 mcg/mL) given rapidly and is usually well tolerated, even in the elderly. This initial dose is followed by daily supplements of 100 to 200 mcg given IV. Normal T_4 levels are achieved in 24 hours followed in 3 days by threefold elevation of T_3. Oral therapy with thyroid hormone would be resumed as soon as the clinical situation has been stabilized and the patient is able to take oral medication.

Thyroid Cancer: Exogenous thyroid hormone may produce regression of metastases from follicular and papillary carcinoma of the thyroid and is used as ancillary therapy of these conditions with radioactive iodine. TSH should be suppressed to low or undetectable levels. Therefore, larger amounts of thyroid hormone than those used for replacement therapy are required. Medullary carcinoma of the thyroid is usually unresponsive to this therapy.

Thyroid Suppression Therapy: Administration of thyroid hormone in doses higher than those produced physiologically by the gland results in suppression of the production of endogenous hormone. This is the basis for the thyroid suppression test and is used as an aid in the diagnosis of patients with signs of mild hyperthyroidism in whom baseline laboratory tests appear normal, or to demonstrate thyroid gland autonomy in patients with Graves ophthalmopathy. 131I uptake is determined before and after the administration of the exogenous hormone. A fifty percent or greater suppression of uptake indicates a normal thyroid-pituitary axis and thus rules out thyroid gland autonomy.

For adults, the usual suppressive dose of levothyroxine (T_4) is 1.56 mg/kg of body weight per day given for 7 to 10 days. These doses usually yield normal serum T_4 and T_3 levels and lack of response to TSH.

Thyroid hormones should be administered cautiously to patients in whom there is strong suspicion of thyroid gland autonomy, in view of the fact that the exogenous hormone effects will be additive to the endogenous source.

Pediatric Dosage: Pediatric dosage should follow the recommendations summarized in Table 1. In infants with congenital hypothyroidism, therapy with full doses should be instituted as soon as the diagnosis has been made.

Table 1

RECOMMENDED PEDIATRIC DOSAGE FOR CONGENITAL HYPOTHYROIDISM

Age	Dose per day in mcg		
	T_3/T_4	to	T_3/T_4
0-6 mos	3.1/12.5	to	6.25/25
6-12 mos	6.25/25	to	9.35/37.5
1-5 yrs	9.35/37.5	to	12.5/50
6-12 yrs	12.5/50	to	18.75/75
Over 12 yrs		over	18.75/75

Tablets should be stored at controlled room temperature. 59°-86°F (15°-30°C) in tight, light-resistant containers.

Note: T_3 liothyronine sodium is approximately four times as potent as T_4 thyroxine on a microgram for microgram basis.

HOW SUPPLIED
TABLETS: 15 MG

BRAND/MANUFACTURER	NDC	SIZE	AWP
○ BRAND ➤ THYROLAR: Forest Pharm	00456-0040-01	100s	$27.05

TABLETS: 30 MG

BRAND/MANUFACTURER	NDC	SIZE	AWP
○ BRAND ➤ THYROLAR: Forest Pharm	00456-0045-01	100s	$30.02

TABLETS: 60 MG

BRAND/MANUFACTURER	NDC	SIZE	AWP
○ BRAND ➤ THYROLAR: Forest Pharm	00456-0050-01	100s	$37.55

TABLETS: 120 MG

BRAND/MANUFACTURER	NDC	SIZE	AWP
○ BRAND ➤ THYROLAR: Forest Pharm	00456-0055-01	100s	$44.12

TABLETS: 180 MG

BRAND/MANUFACTURER	NDC	SIZE	AWP
○ BRAND ➤ THYROLAR: Forest Pharm	00456-0060-01	100s	$53.96

Liquid Pred *SEE* PREDNISONE

➤ SHOWN IN PRODUCT IDENTIFICATION GUIDE

Lisinopril

> **USE IN PREGNANCY**
>
> **WHEN USED IN PREGNANCY DURING THE SECOND AND THIRD TRIMESTERS, ACE INHIBITORS CAN CAUSE INJURY AND EVEN DEATH TO THE DEVELOPING FETUS.** WHEN PREGNANCY IS DETECTED, LISINOPRIL SHOULD BE DISCONTINUED AS SOON AS POSSIBLE. SEE *"WARNINGS. FETAL/NEONATAL MORBIDITY AND MORTALITY."*

DESCRIPTION

Lisinopril, a synthetic peptide derivative, is an oral long-acting angiotensin-converting enzyme inhibitor. Lisinopril is chemically described as (S)-1-[N^2-(1-carboxy-3-phenylpropyl)-L-lysyl]-L-proline dihydrate. Its empirical formula is $C_{21}H_{31}N_3O_5 \cdot 2H_2O$.

Lisinopril is a white to off-white, crystalline powder, with a molecular weight of 441.52. It is soluble in water and sparingly soluble in methanol and practically insoluble in ethanol.

Lisinopril is supplied as 5 mg, 10 mg, 20 mg and 40 mg tablets for oral administration.

Following is its chemical structure:

CLINICAL PHARMACOLOGY

MECHANISM OF ACTION

Lisinopril inhibits angiotensin-converting enzyme (ACE) in human subjects and animals. ACE is a peptidyl dipeptidase that catalyzes the conversion of angiotensin I to the vasoconstrictor substance, angiotensin II. Angiotensin II also stimulates aldosterone secretion by the adrenal cortex. The beneficial effects of Lisinopril in hypertension and heart failure appear to result primarily from suppression of the renin-angiotensin-aldosterone system. Inhibition of ACE results in decreased plasma angiotensin II which leads to decreased vasopressor activity and to decreased aldosterone secretion. The latter decrese may result in a small increase of serum potassium. In hypertensive patients with normal renal function treated with Lisinopril alone for up to 24 weeks, the mean increase in serum potassium was approximately 0.1 mEq/L; however, approximately 15 percent of patients had increases greater than 0.5 mEq/L and approximately six percent had a decrease greater than 0.5 mEq/L. In the same study, patients treated with Lisinopril and hydrochlorothiazide for up to 24 weeks had a mean decrease in serum potassium of 0.1 mEq/L; approximately 4 percent of patients had increases greater than 0.5 mEq/L and approximately 12 percent had a decrease greater than 0.5 mEq/L. (See *"Precautions."*) Removal of angiotensin II negative feedback on renin secretion leads to increased plasma renin activity. ACE is identical to kininase, an enzyme that degrades bradykinin. Whether increased levels of bradykinin, a potent vasodepressor peptide, play a role in the therapeutic effects of Lisinopril remains to be elucidated.

While the mechanism through which Lisinopril lowers blood pressure is believed to be primarily suppression of the renin-angiotensin-aldosterone system, Lisinopril is antihypertensive even in patients with low-renin hypertension. Although Lisinopril was antihypertensive in all races studied, black hypertensive patients (usually a low-renin hypertensive population) had a smaller average response to monotherapy than non-black patients.

Concomitant administration of Lisinopril and hydrochlorothiazide further reduced blood pressure in black and non-black patients and any racial difference in blood pressure response was no longer evident.

PHARMACOKINETICS AND METABOLISM

Following oral administration of Lisinopril, peak serum concentrations of Lisinopril occur within about 7 hours. Declining serum concentrations exhibit a prolonged terminal phase which does not contribute to drug accumulation. This terminal phase probably represents saturable binding to ACE and is not proportional to dose. Lisinopril does not appear to be bound to other serum proteins.

Lisinopril does not undergo metabolism and is excreted unchanged entirely in the urine. Based on urinary recovery, the mean extent of absorption of Lisinopril is approximately 25 percent, with large intersubject variability (6-60 percent) at all doses tested (5-80 mg). Lisinopril absorption is not influenced by the presence of food in the gastrointestinal tract. The absolute bioavailability of Lisinopril is reduced to about 16% in patients with stable NYHA Class II-IV congestive heart failure, and the volume of distribution appears to be slightly smaller than that in normal subjects.

Upon multiple dosing, Lisinopril exhibits an effective half-life of accumulation of 12 hours.

Impaired renal function decreases elimination of Lisinopril, which is excreted principally through the kidneys, but this decrease becomes clinically important only when the glomerular filtration rate is below 30 mL/min. Above this glomerular filtration rate, the elimination half-life is little changed. With greater impairment, however, peak and trough Lisinopril levels increase, time to peak concentration increases and time to attain steady state is prolonged. Older patients, on average, have (approximately doubled) higher blood levels and area under the plasma concentration time curve (AUC) than younger patients. (See *"Dosage and Administration."*) Lisinopril can be removed by hemodialysis.

Studies in rats indicate that Lisinopril crosses the blood-brain barrier poorly. Multiple doses of Lisinopril in rats do not result in accumulation in any tissues. Milk of lactating rats contains radioactivity following administration of ^{14}C Lisinopril. By whole body autoradiography, radioactivity was found in the placenta following administration of labeled drug to pregnant rats, but none was found in the fetuses.

PHARMACODYNAMICS AND CLINICAL EFFECTS

Hypertension: Administration of Lisinopril to patients with hypertension results in a reduction of supine and standing blood pressure to about the same extent with no compensatory tachycardia. Symptomatic postural hypotension is usually not observed although it can occur and should be anticipated in volume and/or salt-depleted patients. (See *"Warnings."*) When given together with thiazide-type diuretics, the blood pressure lowering effects of the two drugs are approximately additive.

In most patients studied, onset of antihypertensive activity was seen at one hour after oral administration of an individual dose of Lisinopril, with peak reduction of blood pressure achieved by six hours. Although an antihypertensive effect was observed 24 hours after dosing with recommended single daily doses, the effect was more consistent and the mean effect was considerably larger in some studies with doses of 20 mg or more than with lower doses. However, at all doses studied, the mean antihypertensive effect was substantially smaller 24 hours after dosing than it was six hours after dosing.

In some patients achievement of optimal blood pressure reduction may require two to four weeks of therapy.

The antihypertensive effects of Lisinopril are maintained during long-term therapy. Abrupt withdrawal of Lisinopril has not been associated with a rapid increase in blood pressure or a significant increase in blood pressure compared to pretreatment levels.

Two dose-response studies utilizing a once daily regimen were conducted in 438 mild to moderate hypertensive patients not on a diuretic. Blood pressure was measured 24 hours after dosing. An antihypertensive effect of Lisinopril was seen with 5 mg in some patients. However, in both studies blood pressure reduction occurred sooner and was greater in patients treated with 10, 20, or 80 mg of Lisinopril. In controlled clinical studies, Lisinopril 20-80 mg has been compared in patients with mild to moderate hypertension to hydrochlorothiazide 12.5-50 mg and with atenolol 50-200 mg; and in patients with moderate to severe hypertension to metoprolol 100-200 mg. It was superior to hydrochlorothiazide in effects on systolic and diastolic blood pressure in a population that was 3/4 Caucasian. Lisinopril was approximately equivalent to atenolol and metoprolol in effects on diastolic blood pressure and had somewhat greater effects on systolic blood pressure.

Lisinopril had similar effectiveness and adverse effects in younger and older (> 65 years) patients. It was less effective in blacks than in Caucasians.

In hemodynamic studies in patients with essential hypertension, blood pressure reduction was accompanied by a reduction in peripheral arterial resistance with little or no change in cardiac output and in heart rate. In a study in nine hypertensive patients, following administration of Lisinopril there was an increase in mean renal blood flow that was not significant. Data from several small studies are inconsistent with respect to the effect of Lisinopril on glomerular filtration rate in hypertensive patients with normal renal function, but suggest that changes, if any, are not larger.

In patients with renovascular hypertension Lisinopril has been shown to be well tolerated and effective in controlling blood pressure (see *"Precautions"*).

Heart Failure: During baseline-controlled clinical trials, in patients receiving digitalis and diuretics, single doses of Lisinopril resulted in decreases in pulmonary capillary wedge pressure, systemic vascular resistance and blood pressure accompanied by an increase in cardiac output and no change in heart rate.

In two placebo controlled, 12-week clinical studies, Lisinopril as adjunctive therapy to digitalis and diuretics improved the following signs and symptoms due to congestive heart failure: edema, rales, paroxysmal nocturnal dyspnea and jugular venous distention. In one of the studies beneficial response was also noted for: orthopnea, presence of third heart sound and the number of patients classified as NYHA Class III and IV. Exercise tolerance was also improved in this one study. The effect of Lisinopril on mortality in patients with heart failure has not been evaluated.

INDICATIONS AND USAGE

HYPERTENSION

Lisinopril is indicated for the treatment of hypertension. It may be used alone as initial therapy or concomitantly with other classes of antihypertensive agents.

HEART FAILURE

Lisinopril is indicated as adjunctive therapy in the management of heart failure in patients who are not responding adequately to diuretics and digitalis.

In using Lisinopril, consideration should be given to the fact that another angiotensin converting enzyme inhibitor, captopril, has caused agranulocytosis, particularly in patients with renal impairment or collagen vascular disease, and that available data are insufficient to show that Lisinopril does not have a similar risk. (See *"Warnings."*)

UNLABELED USES

Lisinopril is used alone or as an adjunct in the treatment of renovascular hypertension.

CONTRAINDICATIONS

Lisinopril is contraindicated in patients who are hypersensitive to this product and in patients with a history of angioedema related to previous treatment with an angiotensin-converting enzyme inhibitor.

WARNINGS

ANGIOEDEMA

Angiodema of the face, extremities, lips, tongue, glottis and/or larynx has been reported in patients treated with angiotensin converting enzyme inhibitors, including Lisinopril This may occur at any time during treatment. In such cases Lisinopril should be promptly discontinued and appropriate therapy and monitoring should be provided until complete and sustained resolution of signs and symptoms has occurred. In instances where swelling has been confined to the face and lips the condition has generally resolved without treatment, although antihistamines have been useful in relieving symptoms. Angioedema associated with laryngeal edema may be fatal. **Where there is involvement of the tongue, glottis or larynx, likely to cause airway obstruction, appropriate therapy, e.g., subcutaneous epinephrine solution 1:1000 (0.3 mL to 0.5 mL) and/or measures necessary to ensure a patent airway, should be provided.** (See *"Adverse Reactions."*)

Patients with a history of angioedema unrelated to ACE inhibitor therapy may be at increased risk of angioedema while receiving an ACE inhibitor (see also *"Contraindications"*).

HYPOTENSION

Excessive hypotension is rare in patients with uncomplicated hypertension treated with Lisinopril alone.

Patients with heart failure given Lisinopril commonly have some reduction in blood pressure with peak blood pressure reduction occurring 6 to 8 hours post dose, but discontinuation of therapy because of continuing symptomatic hypotension usually is not necessary when dosing instructions are followed: caution should be observed when initiating therapy. (See *"Dosage and Administration."*)

Patients at risk of excessive hypotension, sometimes associated with oliguria and/or progressive azotemia, and rarely with acute renal failure and/or death, include those with the following conditions or characteristics: heart failure with systolic blood pressure below 100 mmHg, hyponatremia, high dose diuretic therapy, recent intensive diuresis or increase in diuretic dose, renal dialysis, or severe volume and/or salt depletion of any etiology. It may be advisable to eliminate the diuretic (except in patients with heart failure), reduce the diuretic dose or increase salt intake cautiously before initiating therapy with Lisinopril in patients at risk for excessive hypotension who are able to tolerate such adjustments. (See *"Precautions, Drug Interactions,"* and *"Adverse Reactions."*)

In patients at risk of excessive hypotension, therapy should be started under very close medical supervision and such patients should be followed closely for the first two weeks of treatment and whenever the dose of Lisinopril and/or diuretic is increased. Similar considerations may apply to patients with ischemic heart or cerebrovascular disease, in whom an excessive fall in blood pressure could result in a myocardial infarction or cerebrovascular accident.

If excessive hypotension occurs, the patient should be placed in the supine position and, if necessary, receive an intravenous infusion of normal saline. A transient hypotensive response is not a contraindication to further doses of Lisinopril which usually can be given without difficulty once the blood pressure has stabliized. If symptomatic hypotension develops, a dose reduction or discontinuation of Lisinopril or concomitant diuretic may be necessary.

NEUTROPENIA/AGRANULOCYTOSIS

Another angiotensin-converting enzyme inhibitor, captopril, has been shown to cause agranulocytosis and bone marrow depression, rarely in uncomplicated patients but more frequently in patients with renal impairment especially if they also have a collagen vascular disease. Available data from clinical trials of Lisinopril are insufficient to show that Lisinopril does not cause agranulocytosis at similar rates. Marketing experience has revealed rare cases of neutropenia and bone marrow depression in which a causal relationship to Lisinopril cannot be excluded. Periodic monitoring of white blood cell counts in patients with collagen vascular disease and renal disease should be considered.

FETAL/NEONATAL MORBIDITY AND MORTALITY

ACE inhibitors can cause fetal and neonatal morbidity and death when administered to pregnant women. Several dozen cases have been reported in the world literature. When pregnancy is detected, ACE inhibitors should be discontinued as soon as possible.

The use of ACE inhibitors during the second and third trimesters of pregnancy has been associated with fetal and neonatal injury, including hypotension, neonatal skull hypoplasia, anuria, reversible or irreversible renal failure, and death. Oligohydramnios has also been reported, presumably resulting from decreased fetal renal function; oligohydramnios in this setting has been associated with fetal limb contractures, craniofacial deformation, and hypoplastic lung development. Prematurity, intrauterine growth retardation, and patent ductus arteriosus have also been reported, although it is not clear whether these occurrences were due to the ACE-inhibitor exposure.

These adverse effects do not appear to have resulted from intrauterine ACE-inhibitor exposure that has been limited to the first trimester. Mothers whose embryos and fetuses are exposed to ACE inhibitors only during the first trimester

should be so informed. Nonetheless, when patients become pregnant, physicians should make every effort to discontinue the use of Lisinopril as soon as possible.

Rarely (probably less often than once in every thousand pregnancies), no alternative to ACE inhibitors will be found. In these rare cases, the mothers should be apprised of the potential hazards to their fetuses, and serial ultrasound examinations should be performed to assess the intraamniotic environment.

If oligohydramnios is observed, Lisinopril should be discontinued unless it is considered lifesaving for the mother. Contraction stress testing (CST), a non-stress test (NST), or biophysical profiling (BPP) may be appropriate, depending upon the week of pregnancy. Patients and physicians should be aware, however, that oligohydramnios may not appear until after the fetus has sustained irreversible injury.

Infants with histories of *in utero* exposure to ACE inhibitors should be closely observed for hypotension, oliguria, and hyperkalemia. If oliguria occurs, attention should be directed toward support of blood pressure and renal perfusion. Exchange transfusion or dialysis may be required as means of reversing hypotension and/or substituting for disordered renal function. Lisinopril, which crosses the placenta, has been removed from neonatal circulation by peritoneal dialysis with some clinical benefit, and theoretically may be removed by exchange transfusion, although there is no experience with the latter procedure.

No teratogenic effects of Lisinopril were seen in studies of pregnant rats, mice, and rabbits. On a mg/kg basis, the doses used were up to 625 times (in mice), 188 times (in rats), and 0.6 times (in rabbits) the maximum recommended human dose.

PRECAUTIONS

GENERAL

Impaired Renal Function: As a consequence of inhibiting the renin-angiotensin-aldosterone system, changes in renal function may be anticipated in susceptible individuals. In patients with severe congestive heart failure whose renal function may depend on the activity of the renin-angiotensin-aldosterone system, treatment with angiotensin-converting enzyme inhibitors, including Lisinopril, may be associated with oliguria and/or progressive azotemia and rarely with acute renal failure and/or death.

In hypertensive patients with unilateral or bilateral renal artery stenosis, increases in blood urea nitrogen and serum creatinine may occur. Experience with another angiotensin converting enzyme inhibitor suggests that these increases are usually reversible upon discontinuation of Lisinopril and/or diuretic therapy. In such patients renal function should be monitored during the first few weeks of therapy. Some patients with hypertension or heart failure with no apparent pre-existing renal vascular disease have developed increases in blood urea nitrogen and serum creatinine, usually minor and transient, especially when Lisinopril has been given concomitantly with a diuretic. This is more likely to occur in patients with pre-existing renal impairment. Dosage reduction and/or discontinuation of the diuretic and/or Lisinopril may be required.

Evaluation of patients with hypertension or heart failure should always include assessment of renal function. (See *"Dosage and Administration."*)

Hemodialysis Patients: Anaphylactoid reactions have been reported in patients dialyzed with high-flux membranes (e.g., AN 69*) and treated concomitantly with an ACE inhibitor. In these patients consideration should be given to using a different type of dialysis membrane or a different class of antihypertensive agent.

Hyperkalemia: In clinical trials hyperkalemia (serum potassium greater than 5.7 mEq/L) occurred in approximately 2.2 percent of hypertensive patients and 4.8 percent of patients with heart failure. In most cases these were isolated values which resolved despite continued therapy. Hyperkalemia was a cause of discontinuation of therapy in approximately 0.1 percent of hypertensive patients and 0.6 percent of patients with heart failure. Risk factors for the development of hyperkalemia include renal insufficiency, diabetes mellitus, and the concomitant use of potassium-sparing diuretics, potassium supplements and/or potassium-containing salt substitutes, which should be used cautiously, if at all, with Lisinopril. (See *"Drug Interactions."*)

Cough: Cough has been reported with the use of ACE inhibitors. Characteristically, the cough is nonproductive, persistent and resolves after discontinuation of therapy. ACE inhibitor-induced cough should be considered as part of the differential diagnosis of cough.

Surgery/Anesthesia: In patients undergoing major surgery or during anesthesia with agents that produce hypotension, Lisinopil may block angiotensin II formation secondary to compensatory renin release. If hypotension occurs and is considered to be due to this mechanism, it can be corrected by volume expansion.

INFORMATION FOR PATIENTS

Angioedema: Angioedema, including Laryngeal edema, may occur at any time during treatment with angiotensin converting enzyme inhibitors, including Lisinopril. Patients should be so advised and told to report immediately any signs or symptoms suggesting angioedema (swelling of face, extremities, eyes, lips, tongue, difficulty in swallowing or breathing) and to take no more drug until they have consulted with the prescribing physicians.

Symptomatic Hypotension: Patients should be cautioned to report lightheadedness especially during the first few days of therapy. If actual syncope occurs, the patients should be told to discontinue the drug until they have consulted with the prescribing physician.

---

* Registered trademark of Hospal Ltd.

➤ SHOWN IN PRODUCT IDENTIFICATION GUIDE

All patients should be cautioned that excessive perspiration and dehydration may lead to an excessive fall in blood pressure because of reduction in fluid volume. Other causes of volume depletion such as vomiting or diarrhea may also lead to a fall in blood pressure; patients should be advised to consult with their physician.

Hyperkalemia: Patients should be told tnot use salt substitutes containing potassium without consulting their physician.

Neutropenia: Patients should be told to report promptly any indication of infection (e.g., sore throat, fever) which may be a sign of neutropenia.

Pregnancy: Female patients of childbearing age should be told about the consequences of second- and third-trimester exposure to ACE inhibitors, and they should also be told that these consequences do not appear to have resulted from intrauterine ACE-inhibitor exposure that has been limited to the first trimester. These patients should be asked to report pregnancies to their physicians as soon as possible.

Note: As with many other drugs, certain advice to patients being treated with Lisinopril is warranted. This information is intended to aid in the safe and effective use of this medication. It is not a disclosure of all possible adverse or intended effects.

DRUG INTERACTIONS
Hypotension—Patients on Diuretic Therapy: Patients on diuretics, and especially those in whom diuretic therapy was recently instituted, may occasionally experience an excessive reduction of blood pressure after initiation of therapy with Lisinopril. The possibility of hypotensive effects with Lisinopril can be minimized by either discontinuing the diuretic or increasing the salt intake prior to initiation of treatment with Lisinopril. If it is necessary to continue the diuretic, initiate therapy with Lisinopril at a dose of 5 mg daily, and provide close medical supervision after the initial dose until blood pressure has stabilized. (See *"Warnings"*, and *"Dosage and Administration."*) When a diuretic is added to the therapy of a patient receiving Lisinopril, an additional antihypertensive effect is usually observed. Studies with ACE inhibitors in combination with diuretics indicate that the dose of the ACE inhibitor can be reduced when it is given with a diuretic. (See *"Dosage and Administration."*)

Indomethacin: In a study in 36 patients with mild to moderate hypertension where the antihypertensive effects of Lisinopril alone were compared to Lisinopril given concomitantly with indomethacin, the use of indomethacin was associated with a reduced effect, although the difference between the two regimens was not significant.

Other Agents: Lisinopril has been used concomitantly with nitrates and/or digoxin without evidence of clinically significant adverse interactions. No clinically important pharmacokinetic interactions occurred when Lisinopril was used concomitantly with propranolol or hydrochlorothiazide. The presence of food in the stomach does not alter the bioavailability of Lisinopril.

Agents Increasing Serum Potassium: Lisinopril attenuates potassium loss caused by thiazide-type diuretics. Use of Lisinopril with potassium-sparing diuretics (e.g., spironolactone, triamterene, or amiloride), potassium supplements, or potassium-containing salt substitutes may lead to significant increases in serum potassium. Therefore, if concomitant use of these agents is indicated because of demonstrated hypokalemia, they should be used with caution and with frequent monitoring of serum potassium. Potassium sparing agents should generally not be used in patients with heart failure who are receiving Lisinopril.

Lithium: Lithium toxicity has been reported in patients receiving lithium concomitantly with drugs which cause elimination of sodium, including ACE inhibitors. Lithium toxicity was usually reversible upon discontinuation of lithium and the ACE inhibitor. It is recommended that serum lithium levels be monitored frequently if Lisinopril is administered concomitantly with lithium.

CARCINOGENESIS, MUTAGENESIS, IMPAIRMENT OF FERTILITY
There was no evidence of a tumorigenic effect when Lisinopril was administered for 105 weeks to male and female rats at doses up to 90 mg/kg/day (about 56 times[*] the maximum recommended daily human dose) or when Lisinopril was administered for 92 weeks to (male and female) mice at doses up to 135 mg/kg/day (about 84 times[*] the maximum recommended daily human dose).

Lisinopril was not mutagenic in the Ames microbial mutagen test with or without metabolic activation. It was also negative in a forward mutation assay using Chinese hamster lung cells. Lisinopril did not produce single strand DNA breaks in an *in vitro* alkaline elution rat hepatocyte assay. In addition, Lisinopril did not produce increases in chromosomal aberrations in an *in vitro* test in Chinese hamster ovary cells or in an *in vivo* study in mouse bone marrow.

There were no adverse effects on reproductive performance in male and female rats treated with up to 300 mg/kg/day of Lisinopril.

PREGNANCY
Pregnancy Categories C: (first trimester) *and D:* (second and third trimesters). (See *"Warnings, Fetal/Neonatal Morbidity and Mortality."*)

NURSING MOTHERS
Milk of lactating rats contains radioactivity following administration of ^{14}C Lisinopril. It is not known whether this drug is secreted in human milk. Because

[*] Based on patient weight of 50 kg

many drugs are secreted in human milk, caution should be exercised when Lisinopril is given to a nursing mother.

PEDIATRIC USE
Safety and effectiveness in children have not been established.

ADVERSE REACTIONS
Lisinopril has been found to be generally well tolerated in controlled clinical trials involving 1969 patients. For the most part, adverse experiences were mild and transient.

In clinical trials in patients with hypertension treated with Lisinopril, discontinuation of therapy due to clinical adverse experiences occurred in 5.7 percent of patients. The overall frequency of adverse experiences could not be related to total daily dosage within the recommended therapeutic dosage range.

In patients with heart failure treated with Lisinopril for up to four years, discontinuation of therapy due to clinical adverse experiences occurred in 11.0 percent of patients. In controlled studies in patients with heart failure, therapy was discontinued in 8.1 percent of patients treated with Lisinopril for 12 weeks, compared to 7.7 percent of patients treated with placebo for 12 weeks.

HYPERTENSION
For adverse experiences occurring in greater than one percent of patients with hypertension treated with Lisinopril or Lisinopril plus hydrochlorothiazide in controlled clinical trials, comparative incidence data are listed in the table below: (See related table).

HEART FAILURE
The following table lists those adverse experiences which occurred in greater than one percent of patients with heart failure treated with Lisinopril or placebo for up to 12 weeks in controlled clinical trials. Also listed are those adverse experiences occurring in greater than one percent of patients with heart failure treated with Lisinopril for up to four years. (See related table).

Other clinical adverse experiences occurring in 0.3 to 1.0 percent of patients with hypertension or heart failure treated with Lisinopril in controlled trials and rarer, serious, possibly drug-related events reported in uncontrolled studies or marketing experience are listed below, and within each category, are in order of decreasing severity.

Body as a Whole: Anaphylactoid reactions (see *"Precautions, Hemodialysis Patients"*), chest discomfort, pain, pelvic pain, flank pain, facial edema, peripheral edema, virus infection, chills.

Cardiovascular: Cardiac arrest; myocardial infarction or cerebrovascular accident, possibly secondary to excessive hypotension in high risk patients (see *"Warnings, Hypotension"*); pulmonary embolism and infarction, arrhythmias (including ventricular tachycardia, atrial tachycardia, atrial fibrillation, bradycardia and premature ventricular contractions), transient ischemic attacks, paroxysmal nocturnal dyspnea, decreased blood pressure, peripheral edema, vasculitis.

Digestive: Pancreatitis, hepatitis (hepatocellular or cholestatic jaundice), gastritis, heartburn, gastrointestinal cramps, constipation, flatulence, dry mouth.

Hematologic: Rare cases of bone marrow depression, neutropenia, and thrombocytopenia.

Endocrine: Diabetes mellitus.

Metabolic: Weight loss, dehydration, fluid overload, weight gain.

Musculoskeletal: Arthritis, arthralgia, neck pain, hip pain, low back pain, joint pain, knee pain, shoulder pain, arm pain, lumbago.

Nervous System/Psychiatric: Stroke, ataxia, memory impairment, tremor, peripheral neuropathy (e.g., dysesthesia), spasm, confusion, somnolence, hypersomnia, irritability, and nervousness.

Respiratory System: Malignant lung neoplasms, hemoptysis, pulmonary infiltrates, bronchospasm, asthma, pleural effusion, pneumonia, wheezing, orthopnea, painful respiration, epistaxis, laryngitis, sinusitis, pharyngeal pain, pharyngitis, rhinitis, rhinorrhea.

Skin: Urticaria, alopecia, herpes zoster, photosensitivity, skin lesions, skin infections, erythema, flushing diaphoresis.

Special Senses: Visual loss, diplopia, blurred vision, tinnitus, photophobia.

Urogenital System: Acute renal failure, oliguria, anuria, uremia, progressive azotemia, renal dysfunction (see *"Precautions"* and *"Dosage and Administration"*), pyelonephritis, dysuria, breast pain.

Miscellaneous: A symptom complex has been reported which may include a positive ANA, an elevated erythrocyte sedimentation rate, arthralgia/arthritis, myalgia, fever, vasculitis, leukocytosis, eosinophilia, photosensitivity, rash, and other dermatological manifestations.

Angioedema: Angioedema has been reported in patients receiving Lisinopril (0.1 percent). Angioedema associated with laryngeal edema may be fatal. If angioedema of the face, extremities, lips, tongue, glottis and/or larynx occurs, treatment with Lisinopril should be discontinued and appropriate therapy instituted immediately. (See *"Warnings."*)

Hypotension: In hypertensive patients, hypotension occurred in 1.2 percent and syncope occurred in 0.1 percent of patients. Hypotension or syncope was a cause for discontinuation of therapy in 0.5 percent of hypertensive patients. In patients with heart failure, hypotension occurred in 5.3 percent and syncope occurred in

---

◆ RATED THERAPEUTICALLY EQUIVALENT; ◇ THERAPEUTIC EQUIVALENCE UNCONFIRMED; ○ UNRATED

1.8 percent of patients. These adverse experiences were causes for discontinuation of therapy in 1.8 percent of these patients. (See *"Warnings."*)

Fetal/Neonatal Morbidity and Mortality: see *"Warnings, Fetal/Neonatal Morbidity and Mortality."*

Cough: (See *"Precautions, Cough."*)

CLINICAL LABORATORY TEST FINDINGS

Serum Electrolytes: Hyperkalemia (see *"Precautions"*), hyponatremia.

Creatinine, Blood Urea Nitrogen: Minor increases in blood urea nitrogen and serum creatinine, reversible upon discontinuation of therapy, were observed in about 2.0 percent of patients with essential hypertension treated with Lisinopril alone. Increases were more common in patients receiving concomitant diuretics and in patients with renal artery stenosis. (See *"Precautions."*) Reversible minor increases in blood urea nitrogen and serum creatinine were observed in approximately 11.6 percent of patients with heart failure on concomitant diuretic therapy. Frequently, these abnormalities resolved when the dosage of the diuretic was decreased.

Hemoglobin and Hematocrit: Small decreases in hemoglobin and hematocrit (mean decreases of approximately 0.4 g percent and 1.3 vol percent, respectively) occurred frequently in patients treated with Lisinopril but were rarely of clinical importance in patients without some other cause of anemia. In clinical trials, less than 0.1 percent of patients discontinued therapy due to anemia.

Liver Function Tests: Rarely, elevations of liver enzymes and/or serum bilirubin have occurred.

In hypertensive patients, 2.0 percent discontinued therapy due to laboratory adverse experiences, principally elevations in blood urea nitrogen (0.6 percent), serum creatinine (0.5 percent) and serum potassium (0.4 percent). In the heart failure trials, 3.4 percent of patients discontinued therapy due to laboratory adverse experiences, 1.8 percent due to elevations in blood urea nitrogen and/or creatinine and 0.6 percent due to elevations in serum potassium.

OVERDOSAGE

The oral LD_{50} of Lisinopril is greater than 20 g/kg in mice and rats. The most likely manifestation of overdosage would be hypotension, for which the usual treatment would be intravenous infusion of normal saline solution.

Lisinopril can be removed by hemodialysis.

DOSAGE AND ADMINISTRATION

HYPERTENSION

Initial Therapy: In patients with uncomplicated essential hypertension not on diuretic therapy, the recommended initial dose is 10 mg once a day. Dosage should be adjusted according to blood pressure response. The usual dosage range is 20 to 40 mg per day administered in a single daily dose. The antihypertensive effect may diminish toward the end of the dosing interval regardless of the administered dose, but most commonly with a dose of 10 mg daily. This can be

evaluated by measuring blood pressure just prior to dosing to determine whether satisfactory control is being maintained for 24 hours. If it is not, an increase in dose should be considered. Doses up to 80 mg have been used but do not appear to give a greater effect. If blood pressure is not controlled with Lisinopril alone, a low dose of a diuretic may be added. Hydrochlorothiazide 12.5 mg has been shown to provide an additive effect. After the addition of a diuretic, it may be possible to reduce the dose of Lisinopril.

Diuretic Treated Patients: In hypertensive patients who are currently being treated with a diuretic, symptomatic hypotension may occur occasionally following the initial dose of Lisinopril. The diuretic should be discontinued, if possible, for two to three days before beginning therapy with Lisinopril to reduce the likelihood of hypotension. (See *"Warnings."*) The dosage of Lisinopril should be adjusted according to blood pressure response. If the patient's blood pressure is not controlled with Lisinopril alone, diuretic therapy may be resumed as described above.

If the diuretic cannot be discontinued, an initial dose of 5 mg should be used under medical supervision for at least two hours and until blood pressure has stabilized for at least an additional hour (see *"Warnings"* and *"Precautions, Drug Interactions"*).

Concomitant administration of Lisinopril with potassium supplements, potassium salt substitutes, or potassium-sparing diuretics may lead to increases of serum potassium (see *"Precautions"*).

Dosage Adjustment in Renal Impairment: The usual dose of Lisinopril (10 mg) is recommended for patients with a creatinine clearance > 30 mL/min (serum creatinine of up to approximately 3 mg/dL). For patients with creatinine clearance ≥ 10 mL/min ≤ 30 mL/min (serum creatinine ≥ 3 mg/dL), the first dose is 5 mg once daily. For patients with creatinine clearance < 10 mL/min (usually on hemodialysis) the recommended initial dose is 2.5 mg. The dosage may be titrated upward until blood pressure is controlled or to a maximum of 40 mg daily.

Renal Status	Creatinine-Clearance mL/min	Initial Dose mg/day
Normal Renal Function to Mild Impairment	> 30 mL/min	10 mg
Moderate to Severe Impairment	≥ 10 ≤ mL/min	5 mg
Dialysis Patients*	< 10 mL/min	2.5 mg**

* See *"Precautions, Hemodialysis Patients."*
** Dosage or dosing interval should be adjusted depending on the blood pressure response.

HEART FAILURE

Lisinopril is indicated as adjunctive therapy with diuretics and digitalis. The recommended starting dose is 5 mg once a day.

PERCENT OF PATIENTS IN CONTROLLED STUDIES

	Lisinopril (n = 1349) Incidence (discontinuation)	Lisinopril Hydrochlorothiazide (n = 629) Incidence (discontinuation)	Placebo (n = 207) Incidence (discontinuation)
Body As A Whole			
Fatigue	2.5 (0.3)	4.0 (0.5)	1.0 (0.0)
Asthenia	1.3 (0.5)	2.1 (0.2)	1.0 (0.0)
Chest Pain	1.2 (0.1)	1.3 (0.2)	1.4 (0.0)
Orthostatic Effects	1.2 (0.0)	3.5 (0.2)	1.0 (0.0)
Cardiovascular			
Hypotension	1.2 (0.5)	1.6 (0.5)	0.5 (0.5)
Digestive			
Diarrhea	2.7 (0.2)	2.7 (0.3)	2.4 (0.0)
Nausea	2.0 (0.4)	2.5 (0.2)	2.4 (0.0)
Vomiting	1.1 (0.2)	1.4 (0.1)	0.5 (0.0)
Dyspepsia	0.9 (0.0)	1.9 (0.0)	0.0 (0.0)
Musculoskeletal			
Back Pain	0.6 (0.0)	1.1 (0.1)	1.4 (0.0)
Muscle Cramps	0.5 (0.0)	2.9 (0.8)	0.5 (0.0)
Nervous/Psychiatric			
Headache	5.7 (0.2)	4.5 (0.5)	1.9 (0.0)
Dizziness	5.4 (0.4)	9.2 (1.0)	1.9 (0.0)
Parethesia	0.8 (0.1)	2.1 (0.2)	0.0 (0.0)
Decreased Libido	0.4 (0.1)	1.3 (0.1)	0.0 (0.0)
Vertigo	0.2 (0.1)	1.1 (0.2)	0.0 (0.0)
Respiratory			
Cough	3.5 (0.7)	4.6 (0.8)	1.0 (0.0)
Upper Respiratory Infection	2.1 (0.1)	2.7 (0.1)	0.0 (0.0)
Common Cold	1.1 (0.1)	1.3 (0.0)	0.0 (0.0)
Nasal Congestion	0.4 (0.1)	1.3 (0.1)	0.0 (0.0)
Influenza	0.3 (0.1)	1.1 (0.1)	0.0 (0.0)
Skin			
Rash	1.3 (0.4)	1.6 (0.2)	0.5 (0.5)
Urogenital			
Impotence	1.0 (0.4)	1.6 (0.5)	0.0 (0.0)

➤ SHOWN IN PRODUCT IDENTIFICATION GUIDE

When initiating treatment with Lisinopril in patients with heart failure, the initial dose should be administered under medical observation, especially in those patients with low blood pressure (systolic blood pressure below 100 mmHg). The mean peak blood pressure lowering occurs six to eight hours after dosing. Observation should continue until blood pressure is stable. The concomitant diuretic dose should be reduced, if possible, to help minimize hypovolemia which may contribute to hypotension. (See *"Warnings"* and *"Precautions, Drug Interactions."*) The appearance of hypotension after the initial dose of Lisinopril does not preclude subsequent careful dose titration with the drug, following effective management of the hypotension.

The usual effective dosage range is 5 to 20 mg per day administered as a single daily dose.

Dosage Adjustment in Patients with Heart Failure and Renal Impairment or Hyponatremia: In patients with heart failure who have hyponatremia (serum sodium < 130 mEq/L) or moderate to severe renal impairment (creatinine clearance ≤ 30 mL/min or serum creatinine > 3 mg/dL), therapy with Lisinopril should be initiated at a dose of 2.5 mg once a day under close medical supervision. (See *"Warnings"* and *"Precautions, Drug Interactions."*)

USE IN ELDERLY
In general, blood pressure response and adverse experiences were similar in younger and older patients given similar doses of Lisinopril. Pharmacokinetic studies, however, indicate that maximum blood levels and area under the plasma concentration time curve (AUC) are doubled in older patients so that dosage adjustments should be made with particular caution.

STORAGE
Store at controlled room temperature, 15-30°C (59-86°F), and protect from moisture.

CONTROLLED TRIALS

Dispense in a tight container, if product package is subdivided.

HOW SUPPLIED
TABLETS: 2.5 MG

AVERAGE UNIT PRICE (AVAILABLE SIZES)			
BRAND			$0.50

BRAND/MANUFACTURER	NDC	SIZE	AWP
◆ BRAND			
▶ PRINIVIL: Merck	00006-0015-31	30s	$15.12
	00006-0015-58	100s	$50.39
	00006-0015-28	100s ud	$50.39

TABLETS: 5 MG

AVERAGE UNIT PRICE (AVAILABLE SIZES)			
BRAND			$0.76

BRAND/MANUFACTURER	NDC	SIZE	AWP
◆ BRAND			
▶ ZESTRIL: Stuart	00038-0130-10	100s	$75.46
▶ PRINIVIL: Merck	00006-0019-58	100s	$75.59
▶ ZESTRIL: Stuart	00038-0130-39	100s ud	$75.46
▶ PRINIVIL: Merck	00006-0019-28	100s ud	$75.59
▶ ZESTRIL: Stuart	00038-0130-34	1000s	$745.64
▶ PRINIVIL: Merck	00006-0019-82	1000s	$755.88
	00006-0019-94	1080s	$816.53
	00006-0019-86	5000s	$3936.88
	00006-0019-87	10000s	$7558.80

	Lisinopril (n = 407) Incidence (discontinuation) 12 weeks	Placebo (n = 55) Incidence (discontinuation) 12 weeks	All Trials Lisinopril (n = 620) Incidence (discontinuation) up to 4 years
Body As A Whole			
Chest Pain	3.4 (0.2)	1.3 (0.0)	7.3 (0.3)
Asthenia	3.2 (0.2)	3.2 (0.0)	6.9 (0.3)
Abdominal Pain	2.2 (0.7)	1.9 (0.0)	4.0 (0.5)
Edema	1.0 (0.0)	0.6 (0.0)	2.4 (0.2)
Syncope	1.0 (0.0)	0.6 (0.6)	1.8 (0.0)
Orthostatic Effects	1.0 (0.2)	0.0 (0.0)	1.1 (0.2)
Fever	0.5 (0.0)	0.6 (0.0)	1.1 (0.0)
Malaise	1.0 (0.2)	0.0 (0.0)	1.1 (0.3)
Cardiovascular			
Hypotension	4.4 (1.7)	0.6 (0.6)	5.3 (1.8)
Angina Pectoris	1.5 (0.2)	3.2 (1.3)	3.7 (0.3)
Worsening of Heart Failure	0.0 (0.0)	3.2 (1.9)	2.9 (0.6)
Orthostatic Hypotension	1.0 (0.2)	0.0 (0.0)	1.9 (0.3)
Palpitation	1.0 (0.0)	0.0 (0.0)	1.9 (0.0)
CVA	0.2 (0.0)	0.0 (0.0)	1.6 (0.2)
Myocardial Infarction	0.5 (0.2)	0.6 (0.0)	1.3 (0.5)
Digestive			
Diarrhea	3.7 (0.5)	1.9 (0.0)	6.1 (0.6)
Nausea	2.7 (0.5)	5.2 (0.0)	5.0 (0.5)
Vomiting	1.0 (0.5)	0.6 (0.0)	2.4 (0.3)
Dyspepsia	0.2 (0.2)	0.0 (0.0)	1.8 (0.2)
Anorexia	0.7 (0.2)	1.3 (0.0)	1.5 (0.3)
Increased Salivation	0.0 (0.0)	1.3 (0.0)	0.2 (0.0)
Metabolic			
Gout	0.5 (0.2)	0.0 (0.0)	1.5 (0.2)
Musculoskeletal			
Muscle Cramps	0.5 (0.0)	1.3 (0.0)	2.1 (0.1)
Back Pain	0.5 (0.0)	1.9 (0.0)	1.6 (0.0)
Leg Pain	0.5 (0.0)	0.6 (0.0)	1.3 (0.2)
Myalgia	0.5 (0.0)	1.9 (0.6)	0.6 (0.0)
Nervous/Psychiatric			
Dizziness	11.8 (1.2)	4.5 (1.3)	14.0 (1.8)
Headache	4.4 (0.2)	3.9 (0.0)	4.5 (0.2)
Paresthesia	1.0 (0.0)	0.0 (0.0)	2.6 (0.0)
Insomnia	0.7 (0.0)	0.6 (0.0)	2.3 (0.0)
Depression	0.0 (0.0)	1.3 (0.0)	1.1 (0.0)
Respiratory			
Dyspnea	2.7 (0.2)	4.5 (0.6)	7.6 (0.3)
Cough	1.7 (0.0)	2.6 (0.0)	6.1 (0.2)
Upper Respiratory Infection	1.5 (0.0)	1.3 (0.0)	4.5 (0.0)
Bronchitis	0.5 (0.0)	0.0 (0.0)	1.6 (0.0)
Chest Sound Abnormalities	0.0 (0.0)	1.3 (0.0)	0.3 (0.0)
Pulmonary Edema	0.2 (0.0)	1.3 (0.0)	0.3 (0.0)
Skin			
Rash	1.7 (0.5)	0.6 (0.6)	4.8 (1.0)
Pruritus	1.2 (0.2)	1.9 (0.6)	1.5 (0.2)
Urogenital			
Urinary Tract Infection	0.5 (0.0)	0.0 (0.0)	1.5 (0.0)

TABLETS: 10 MG

AVERAGE UNIT PRICE (AVAILABLE SIZES)

BRAND			$0.78

BRAND/MANUFACTURER	NDC	SIZE	AWP
◆ BRAND			
➤ PRINIVIL: Merck	00006-0106-31	30s	$23.45
➤ ZESTRIL: Stuart	00038-0131-10	100s	$78.01
➤ PRINIVIL: Merck	00006-0106-58	100s	$78.16
➤ ZESTRIL: Stuart	00038-0131-39	100s ud	$78.01
➤ PRINIVIL: Merck	00006-0106-28	100s ud	$78.16
➤ ZESTRIL: Stuart	00038-0131-34	1000s	$770.82
➤ PRINIVIL: Merck	00006-0106-82	1000s	$781.56
	00006-0106-94	1080s	$844.13
	00006-0106-86	5000s	$4070.63
	00006-0106-87	10000s	$7815.60

TABLETS: 20 MG

AVERAGE UNIT PRICE (AVAILABLE SIZES)

BRAND			$0.84

BRAND/MANUFACTURER	NDC	SIZE	AWP
◆ BRAND			
➤ PRINIVIL: Merck	00006-0207-31	30s	$25.08
➤ ZESTRIL: Stuart	00038-0132-10	100s	$83.50
➤ PRINIVIL: Merck	00006-0207-58	100s	$83.64
➤ ZESTRIL: Stuart	00038-0132-39	100s ud	$83.50
➤ PRINIVIL: Merck	00006-0207-28	100s ud	$83.64
➤ ZESTRIL: Stuart	00038-0132-34	1000s	$824.96
➤ PRINIVIL: Merck	00006-0207-82	1000s	$836.40
	00006-0207-94	1080s	$903.44
	00006-0207-86	5000s	$4356.25
	00006-0207-87	10000s	$8364.00

TABLETS: 40 MG

AVERAGE UNIT PRICE (AVAILABLE SIZES)

BRAND			$1.22

BRAND/MANUFACTURER	NDC	SIZE	AWP
◆ BRAND			
➤ ZESTRIL: Stuart	00038-0134-10	100s	$121.96
➤ PRINIVIL: Merck	00006-0237-58	100s	$122.18

Lithium Carbonate

> **WARNING**
> LITHIUM TOXICITY IS CLOSELY RELATED TO SERUM LITHIUM LEVELS, AND CAN OCCUR AT DOSES CLOSE TO THERAPEUTIC LEVELS. FACILITIES FOR PROMPT AND ACCURATE SERUM LITHIUM DETERMINATIONS SHOULD BE AVAILABLE BEFORE INITIATING THERAPY (SEE *"DOSAGE AND ADMINISTRATION"*).

DESCRIPTION

Lithium Carbonate is a white, light alkaline powder with molecular formula Li_2CO_3 and molecular weight 73.89. Lithium is an element of the alkali-metal group with atomic number 3, atomic weight 6.94 and an emission line at 671 nm on the flame photometer. Lithium acts as an antimanic.

Each tablet for oral administration contains:
Lithium Carbonate .... 300 mg

Each capsule for oral administration contains:
Lithium Carbonate .... 150 mg, 300 mg, or 600 mg

Each controlled release tablet for oral administration contains:
Lithium Carbonate .... 450 mg

Lithium Carbonate controlled-release tablets 450 mg are designed to release a portion of the dose initially and the remainder gradually; the release pattern of the controlled release tablets reduces the variability in Lithium blood levels seen with the immediate release dosage forms.

ACTIONS

Preclinical studies have shown that lithium alters sodium transport in nerve and muscle cells and effects a shift toward intraneuronal metabolism of catecholamines, but the specific biochemical mechanism of Lithium action in mania is unknown.

INDICATIONS

Lithium Carbonate is indicated in the treatment of manic episodes of manic-depressive illness. Maintenance therapy prevents or diminishes the intensity of subsequent episodes in those manic-depressive patients with a history of mania.

Typical symptoms of mania include pressure of speech, motor hyperactivity, reduced need for sleep, flight of ideas, grandiosity, elation, poor judgment,

aggressiveness and possibly hostility. When given to a patient experiencing a manic episode Lithium Carbonate may produce a normalization of symptomatology within 1 to 3 weeks.

UNLABELED USES

Lithium Carbonate is used alone or as an adjunct in the treatment of asthma, to reduce aggressiveness in mentally handicapped patients, chronic alcohol withdrawal, and aplastic anemia including Fanconi aplastic anemia. It is also used in anorexia nervosa, bulimia nervosa, cluster headache, cocaine craving, unipolar depressive illness, nonresponsive delusional depression, and to treat seizures in epileptic patients who are poorly controlled on standard anticonvulsant regimens. Lithium Carbonate is also prescribed in Huntington's chorea, in patients with syndrome of inappropriate antidiuretic hormone secretion (SIADH) after brain trauma, as an adjunct in small cell bronchogenic carcinoma, posttraumatic stress disorder, puerperal psychosis, in selected patients with schizophrenia or schizoaffective disorders, and trichotillomania.

WARNINGS

Lithium should generally not be given to patients with significant renal or cardiovascular disease, severe debilitation or dehydration, or sodium depletion, and to patients receiving diuretics, or angiotensin converting enzyme (ACE) inhibitors, since the risk of Lithium toxicity is very high in such patients. If the psychiatric indication is life-threatening, and if such a patient fails to respond to other measures, Lithium treatment may be undertaken with extreme caution, including daily serum Lithium determinations and adjustment to the usually low doses ordinarily tolerated by these individuals. In such instances, hospitalization is a necessity.

Chronic Lithium therapy may be associated with diminution of renal concentrating ability, occasionally presenting as nephrogenic diabetes insipidus, with polyuria and polydipsia. Such patients should be carefully managed to avoid dehydration with resulting Lithium retention and toxicity. This condition is usually reversible when Lithium is discontinued.

Morphologic changes with glomerular and interstitial fibrosis and nephron atrophy have been reported in patients on chronic Lithium therapy. Morphologic changes have also been seen in manic-depressive patients never exposed to Lithium. The relationship between renal functional and morphologic changes and their association with Lithium therapy have not been established. To date, Lithium therapeutic doses have not been reported to cause end-stage renal disease.

When kidney function is assessed, for baseline data prior to starting Lithium therapy or thereafter, routine urinalysis and other tests may be used to evaluate tubular function (e.g., urine specific gravity or osmolality following a period of water deprivation, or 24-hour urine volume) and glomerular function (e.g., serum creatinine or creatinine clearance). During Lithium therapy, progressive or sudden changes in renal function, even within the normal range, indicate the need for reevaluation of treatment.

An encephalopathic syndrome (characterized by weakness, lethargy, fever, tremulousness and confusion, extrapyramidal symptoms, leukocytosis, elevated serum enzymes, BUN and FBS) has occurred in a few patients treated with lithium plus neuroleptic (such as haloperidol) in some instances, the syndrome was followed by irreversible brain damage. Because of a possible causal relationship between these events and the concomitant administration of Lithium and neuroleptics, patients receiving such combined therapy should be monitored closely for early evidence of neurologic toxicity and treatment discontinued promptly if such signs appear. This encephalopathic syndrome may be similar to or the same as neuroleptic malignant syndrome (NMS). The possibility of similar adverse interactions with other antipsychotic medications exists. In addition, concomitant use of Lithium with chlorpromazine and possibly other phenothiazines decreases serum chlorpromazine levels as much as 40%.

Concomitant administration of carbamazepine and Lithium may increase the risk of neurotoxic side effects.

Lithium toxicity is closely related to serum Lithium levels, and can occur at doses close to therapeutic levels (see *"Dosage and Administration"*).

Outpatients and their families should be warned that the patient must discontinue Lithium Carbonate therapy and contact his physician if such clinical signs of Lithium toxicity as diarrhea, vomiting, tremor, mild ataxia, drowsiness or muscular weakness occur.

Lithium Carbonate may impair mental and/or physical abilities. Caution patients about activities requiring alertness (e.g., operating vehicles or machinery).

Lithium may prolong the effects of neuromuscular blocking agents such as decamethonium, pancuronium, and succinylcholine. Therefore, neuromuscular blocking agents should be given with caution to patients receiving Lithium.

Usage in Pregnancy: Pregnancy Category D. Adverse effects on implantation in rats, embryo viability in mice and metabolism *in vitro* of rat testes and human spermatozoa have been attributed to Lithium, as have teratogenicity in submammalian species and cleft palates in mice. Studies in rats, rabbits and monkeys have shown no evidence of lithium-induced teratology.

In humans, Lithium Carbonate may cause fetal harm when administered to a pregnant woman. Data from Lithium birth registries suggest an increase in cardiac and other anomalies, especially Ebstein's anomaly. If this drug is used in women of childbearing potential, or during pregnancy, or if a patient becomes pregnant while taking this drug, the patient should be apprised of the potential hazard to the fetus. If possible, Lithium should be withdrawn for at least the first trimester unless it is determined that this would seriously endanger the mother.

➤ SHOWN IN PRODUCT IDENTIFICATION GUIDE

Usage in Nursing Mothers: Lithium is excreted in human milk. Nursing should not be undertaken during Lithium therapy except in rare and unusual circumstances where, in the view of the physician, the potential benefits to the mother outweigh possible hazards to the child.

Usage in Children: Since information regarding the safety and effectiveness of Lithium Carbonate in children under 12 years of age is not available, its use in such patients is not recommended at this time.

There has been a report of a transient syndrome of acute dystonia and hyperreflexia occurring in a 15 kg child who ingested 300 mg of Lithium Carbonate.

Usage in the Elderly: Elderly patients often require lower Lithium dosages to achieve therapeutic serum levels. They may also exhibit adverse reactions at serum levels ordinarily tolerated by younger patients.

PRECAUTIONS

The ability to tolerate Lithium is greater during the acute manic phase and decreases when manic symptoms subside (see *"Dosage and Administration"*).

Caution should be used when Lithium and diuretics or angiotensin converting enzyme (ACE) inhibitors are used concomitantly because sodium loss may reduce the renal clearance of Lithium and increase serum lithium levels with risk of Lithium toxicity. Patients receiving such combined therapy should have serum Lithium levels monitored closely and the Lithium dosage adjusted if necessary.

The distribution space of Lithium approximates that of total body water. Lithium is primarily excreted in urine with insignificant excretion in feces. Renal excretion of Lithium is proportional to its plasma concentration. The half-life of elimination of Lithium is approximately 24 hours. Lithium decreases sodium reabsorption by the renal tubules which could lead to sodium depletion. Therefore, it is essential for the patient to maintain a normal diet, including salt, and an adequate fluid intake (2500-3500 ml) at least during the initial stabilization period. Decreased tolerance to Lithium has been reported to ensue from protracted sweating or diarrhea and, if such occur, supplemental fluid and salt should be administered under careful medical supervision and Lithium intake reduced or suspended until the condition is resolved. In addition to sweating and diarrhea, concomitant infection with elevated temperatures may also necessitate a temporary reduction or cessation of medication.

Previously existing underlying thyroid disorders do not necessarily constitute a contraindication to Lithium treatment; where hypothyroidism exists, careful monitoring of thyroid function during Lithium stabilization and maintenance allows for correction of changing thyroid parameters, if any; where hypothyroidism occurs during Lithium stabilization and maintenance, supplemental thyroid treatment may be used.

Concomitant extended use of iodide preparations, especially potassium iodide, may produce hypothyroidism. Indomethacin and piroxicam have been reported to increase significantly, steady state plasma Lithium levels. In some cases, Lithium toxicity has resulted from such interactions. There is also some evidence that other nonsteroidal anti-inflammatory agents may have a similar effect. When such combinations are used, increased plasma Lithium level monitoring is recommended. Concurrent use of metronidazole with lithium may provoke lithium toxicity due to reduced renal clearance. Patients receiving such combined therapy should be monitored closely.

Aminophylline, caffeine, dyphylline, oxtriphylline, sodium bicarbonate, or theophylline used concomitantly may decrease the therapeutic effect of Lithium because of its increased urinary excretion.

Concurrent use of calcium channel blocking agents with Lithium may increase the risk of neurotoxicity in the form of ataxia, tremors, nausea, vomiting, diarrhea and/or tinnitus. Caution is recommended.

The following drugs can lower serum Lithium concentrations by increasing urinary Lithium excretion: acetazolamide, urea, xanthine preparations and alkalinizing agents such as sodium bicarbonate.

ADVERSE REACTIONS

The occurrence and severity of adverse reactions are generally directly related to serum Lithium concentrations as well as to individual patient sensitivity to Lithium, and generally occur more frequently and with greater severity at higher concentrations.

Adverse reactions may be encountered at serum Lithium levels below 1.5 mEq/L in patients sensitive to Lithium. Mild to moderate adverse reactions may occur at levels from 1.5 to 2.5 mEq/L, and moderate to severe reactions may be seen at levels of 2.0 mEq/L and above.

Fine hand tremor, polyuria and mild thirst may occur during initial therapy for the acute manic phase, and may persist throughout treatment. Transient and mild nausea and general discomfort may also appear during the first few days of Lithium administration.

These side effects are an inconvenience rather than a disabling condition and usually subside with continued treatment or a temporary reduction or cessation of dosage. If persistent, cessation of Lithium therapy may be required.

Diarrhea, vomiting, drowsiness, muscular weakness and lack of coordination may be early signs of Lithium intoxication, and can occur at Lithium levels below 2.0 mEq/L. At higher levels, ataxia, giddiness, tinnitus, blurred vision and a large output of dilute urine may be seen. Serum Lithium levels above 3.0 mEq/L may produce a complex clinical picture, involving multiple organs and organ systems. Serum Lithium levels should not be permitted to exceed 2.0 mEq/L during the acute treatment phase.

The following reactions have been reported and appear to be related to serum Lithium levels, including levels within the therapeutic range.

Neuromuscular/Central Nervous System: tremor, muscle hyperirritability (fasciculations, twitching, clonic movements of whole limbs), hypertonicity, ataxia, choreo-athetotic movements, hyperactive deep tendon reflex, extrapyramidal symptoms including acute dystonia, cogwheel rigidity, blackout spells, epileptiform seizures, slurred speech, dizziness, vertigo, downbeat nystagmus, incontinence of urine or feces, somnolence, psychomotor retardation, restlessness, confusion, stupor, coma, tongue movements, tics, tinnitus, hallucinations, poor memory, slowed intellectual functioning, startled response, worsening of organic brain syndrome.

Cardiovascular: cardiac arrhythmia, hypotension, peripheral circulatory collapse, bradycardia, sinus node dysfunction with severe bradycardia (which may result in syncope).

Gastrointestinal: anorexia, nausea, vomiting, diarrhea, gastritis, salivary gland swelling, abdominal pain, excessive salivation, flatulence, indigestion;

Genitourinary: glycosuria, decreased creatinine clearance, albuminuria, oliguria, and symptoms of nephrogenic diabetes insipidus including polyuria, thirst and polydipsia.

Dermatologic: drying and thinning of hair, alopecia, anesthesia of skin, acne, chronic folliculitis, xerosis cutis, psoriasis or its exacerbation, generalized pruritus with or without rash, cutaneous ulcers, angioedema.

Autonomic: blurred vision, dry mouth, impotence/sexual dysfunction.

Thyroid Abnormalities: euthyroid goiter and/or hypothyroidism (including myxedema) accompanied by lower T_3 and T_4, I^{131} uptake may be elevated. (See *"Precautions"*.) Paradoxically, rare cases of hyperthyroidism have been reported.

EEG Changes: diffuse slowing, widening of the frequency spectrum, potentiation and disorganization of background rhythm.

EKG Changes: reversible flattening, isoelectricity or inversion of T-waves.

Miscellaneous: fatigue, lethargy, tendency to sleep, transient scotomata, exophthalmos, dehydration, weight loss, leukocytosis, headache, transient hyperglycemia, hypercalcemia, hyperparathyroidism, excessive weight gain, edematous swelling of ankles or wrists, metallic taste, dysgeusia/taste distortion, salty taste, thirst, swollen lips, tightness in chest, swollen and/or painful joints, fever, polyarthralgia, dental caries.

Miscellaneous Reactions Unrelated to Dosage Are: transient, electroencephalographic and electrocardiographic changes, diffuse nontoxic goiter with or without hypothyroidism, generalized pruritus with or without rash, cutaneous ulcers, albuminuria, worsening of organic brain syndromes.

Some reports of nephrogenic diabetes insipidus, hyperparathyroidism and hypothyroidism which persist after lithium discontinuation have been received.

A few reports have been received of the development of painful discoloration of fingers and toes and coldness of the extremities within one day of the starting of treatment with Lithium. The mechanism through which these symptoms (resembling Raynaud's syndrome) developed is not known. Recovery followed discontinuance.

Cases of pseudotumor cerebri (increased intracranial pressure and papilledema) have been reported with Lithium use. If undetected, this condition may result in enlargement of the blind spot, constriction of visual fields and eventual blindness due to optic atrophy.

Lithium should be discontinued, if clinically possible, if this syndrome occurs.

OVERDOSAGE

The toxic levels for lithium are close to the therapeutic levels. It is therefore important that patients and their families be cautioned to watch for early toxic symptoms and to discontinue the drug and inform the physician should they occur. Toxic symptoms are listed in detail under *"Adverse Reactions"*.

TREATMENT
No specific antidote for Lithium poisoning is known. Early symptoms of Lithium toxicity can usually be treated by reduction or cessation of dosage of the drug and resumption of the treatment at a lower dose after 24 to 48 hours. In severe cases of Lithium poisoning, the first and foremost goal of treatment consists of elimination of this ion from the patient. Treatment is especially the same as that used in barbiturate poisoning: 1) gastric lavage, 2) correction of fluid and electrolyte imbalance, and 3) regulation of kidney function. Urea, mannitol and aminophylline all produce significant increases in Lithium excretion. Hemodialysis is an effective and rapid means of removing the ion from the severely toxic patient. Infection prophylaxis, regular chest x-rays and preservation of adequate respiration are essential.

DOSAGE AND ADMINISTRATION
Immediate release capsules and tablets are usually given t.i.d. or q.i.d. Doses of controlled release tablets are usually given b.i.d. (approximately 12-hour intervals). When initiating therapy with immediate release or controlled release Lithium, dosage must be individualized according to serum levels and clinical response.

When switching a patient from immediate release capsules or tablets to the Lithium Carbonate controlled release tablets, give the same total daily dose when possible. Most patients on maintenance therapy are stabilized on 900 mg daily, e.g., 450 mg Lithium Carbonate controlled release b.i.d. When the previous dosage of immediate release Lithium is not a multiple of 450 mg, for example, 1500 mg, initiate Lithium Carbonate controlled release dosage at the multiple of 450 mg nearest to, but *below*, the orginal daily dose, i.e., 1350 mg. When the two doses are unequal, give the larger dose in the evening. In the above example, with a total daily dosage of 1350 mg, generally 450 mg Lithium Carbonate controlled release should be given in the morning and 900 mg Lithium Carbonate controlled release in the evening. If desired, the total daily dosage of 1350 mg can be given in three equal 450 mg Lithium Carbonate controlled release doses. These patients should be monitored at 1-2 week intervals, and dosage adjusted if necessary, until stable and satisfactory serum levels and clinical state are achieved.

When patients require closer titration than that available with Lithium Carbonate controlled release doses in increments of 450 mg, immediate release capsules or tablets should be used.

Acute Mania: Optimal patient response to Lithium Carbonate can usually be established and maintained with 1800 mg per day in divided doses (600 mg per day t.i.d.) Such doses will normally produce the desired serum Lithium level ranging between 1.0 and 1.5 mEq/L.

Dosage must be individualized according to serum levels and clinical response. Regular monitoring of the patient's clinical state and serum Lithium levels is necessary. Serum levels should be determined twice per week during the acute phase, and until the serum level and clinical condition of the patient have been stabilized.

Long-Term Control: The desirable serum Lithium levels are 0.6 to 1.2 mEq/L. Dosage will vary from one individual to another, but usually 900 mg to 1200 mg per day in divided doses (300 mg t.i.d. or q.i.d.) will maintain this level. Serum Lithium levels in uncomplicated cases receiving maintenance therapy during remission should be monitored at least every two months. Patients unusually sensitive to Lithium may exhibit toxic signs at serum levels lowest, 1.0 mEq/l.

N.B.: Blood samples for serum Lithium determinations should be drawn immediately prior to the next dose when Lithium concentrations are relatively stable (i.e., 8-12 hours after the previous dose). Total reliance must not be placed on serum levels alone. Accurate patient evaluation requires both clinical and laboratory analysis.

Elderly patients often respond to reduced dosage, and may exhibit signs of toxicity at serum levels ordinarily tolerated by younger patients.

Storage: Store at controlled room temperature, 15°-30°C (59°-86°F).

HOW SUPPLIED
CAPSULE: 300 MG

AVERAGE UNIT PRICE (AVAILABLE SIZES)		GENERIC A-RATED AVERAGE PRICE (GAAP)	
BRAND	$0.11	100s	$8.00
GENERIC	$0.07	1000s	$64.17
HCFA FUL (100s ea)	$0.04		

BRAND/MANUFACTURER	NDC	SIZE	AWP
◆ BRAND			
➤ LITHONATE: Solvay	00032-7512-01	100s	$7.00
➤ ESKALITH: SK Beecham Pharm	00007-4007-20	100s	$16.10
➤ LITHONATE: Solvay	00032-7512-11	100s ud	$7.94
➤ ESKALITH: SK Beecham Pharm	00007-4007-25	500s	$74.65
➤ LITHONATE: Solvay	00032-7512-10	1000s	$64.78
◆ GENERICS			
Major	00904-2912-89	90s	$5.70
Mason Dist	11845-0236-01	100s	$4.74
Goldline	00182-1781-01	100s	$6.75
Caremark	00339-5773-12	100s	$6.94
Geneva	00781-2100-01	100s	$6.99
Major	00904-2912-60	100s	$7.25
URL	00677-1092-01	100s	$7.38
Qualitest	00603-4220-21	100s	$7.40
Schein	00364-0855-01	100s	$7.43
➤ Roxane	00054-2527-25	100s	$8.13
Intl Labs	00665-4160-06	100s	$8.40
Rugby	00536-3739-01	100s	$8.67
Moore,H.L.	00839-7149-06	100s	$8.71
Geneva	00781-2100-13	100s ud	$7.55
Roxane	00054-8527-25	100s ud	$10.42
Major	00904-2912-61	100s ud	$13.25
Major	00904-2912-18	120s	$7.10
Rugby	00536-3739-05	500s	$42.45
Mason Dist	11845-0236-04	1000s	$36.28
Goldline	00182-1781-10	1000s	$52.50
Major	00904-2912-80	1000s	$60.45
Geneva	00781-2100-10	1000s	$64.75
Qualitest	00603-4220-32	1000s	$67.24
URL	00677-1092-10	1000s	$67.97
Intl Labs	00665-4160-09	1000s	$68.90
➤ Roxane	00054-2527-31	1000s	$69.24
Rugby	00536-3739-10	1000s	$72.20
Moore,H.L.	00839-7149-16	1000s	$82.15

TABLET, EXTENDED RELEASE: 300 MG

BRAND/MANUFACTURER	NDC	SIZE	AWP
○ BRAND			
LITHOBID: Solvay	00032-4492-01	100s	$23.69
	00032-4492-10	1000s	$229.78

TABLET, EXTENDED RELEASE: 450 MG

BRAND/MANUFACTURER	NDC	SIZE	AWP
○ BRAND			
➤ ESKALITH-CR: SK Beecham Pharm	00007-4010-20	100s	$34.10

TABLETS: 300 MG

AVERAGE UNIT PRICE (AVAILABLE SIZES)		GENERIC A-RATED AVERAGE PRICE (GAAP)	
BRAND	$0.07	100s	$8.71
GENERIC	$0.08		

BRAND/MANUFACTURER	NDC	SIZE	AWP
◆ BRAND			
➤ LITHOTABS: Solvay	00032-7516-01	100s	$6.89
	00032-7516-11	100s ud	$8.09
	00032-7516-10	1000s	$63.66
◆ GENERICS			
Caremark	00339-5773-12	100s	$6.89
Roxane	00054-4527-25	100s	$7.99
Roxane	00054-8528-25	100s ud	$11.26
Roxane	00054-4527-31	1000s	$71.29

Lithium Citrate

LITHIUM TOXICITY IS CLOSELY RELATED TO SERIUM LITHIUM LEVELS, AND CAN OCCUR AT DOSES CLOSE TO THERAPEUTIC LEVELS. FACILITIES FOR PROMPT AND ACCURATE SERUM LITHIUM DETERMINATIONS SHOULD BE AVAILABLE BEFORE INITIATING THERAPY.

DESCRIPTION
Lithium Citrate syrup is an oral dosage form of Lithium ion. Lithium Citrate is prepared in solution from Lithium hydroxide and citric acid in a ratio approximating di-lithium citrate:

Each 5 mL of Lithium Citrate syrup, contains 8 mEq or Lithium ion (Li^+), equivalent to the amount of Lithium in 300 mg of Lithium carbonate and alcohol 0.3% v/v. Lithium is an element of the alkali-metal group with atomic number 3, atomic weight 6.94, and an emission line at 671 nm on the flame photometer.

Lithium Citrate is a white, granular or crystalline powder which is soluble in water and slightly soluble in alcohol. Its molecular formula is $C_6H_5li_3O_7 \cdot 4H_2O$. Its chemical name is 1.2.3-Propanetricarboxylic acid, 2-hydroxy-trilithium salt tetrahydrate and its molecular weight is 282.0.

CLINICAL PHARMACOLOGY
Preclinical studies have shown that Lithium alters sodium transport in nerve and muscle cells and effects a shift toward intraneuronal metabolism of catecholamines but the specific biochemical mechanism of Lithium action in mania is unknown.

INDICATIONS AND USAGE
Lithium Citrate is indicated in the treatment of manic episodes of Bipolar Disorder. Bipolar Disorder, Manic (DSM III) is equivalent to Manic Depressive illness, Manic, in the older DSM-II terminology.

Lithium is also indicated as a maintenance treatment for individuals with a diagnosis of Bipolar Disorder. Maintenance therapy reduces the frequency of manic episodes and diminishes the intensity of those episodes which may occur.

Typical symptoms of mania include pressure of speech, motor hyperactivity, reduced need for sleep, flight of ideas, grandiosity, elation, poor judgment, aggressiveness, and possibly hostility. When given to a patient experiencing a manic episode, Lithium may produce a normalization of symptomatology within 1 to 3 weeks.

UNLABELED USES
Lithium Citrate is used alone or as an adjunct in the treatment of aggressive behavior, alcohol withdrawal syndrome, aplastic anemia, and asthma. It is also used in bulimia nervosa, to prevent recurrent unipolar depression, and trichotillomania.

CONTRAINDICATIONS
Lithium should generally not be given to patients with significant renal or cardiovascular disease, severe debilitation or dehydration, or sodium depletion, and to patients receiving diuretics, since the risk of Lithium toxicity is very high in such patients. If the psychiatric indication is life-threatening, and if such a patient fails to respond to other measures, Lithium treatment may be undertaken with extreme caution, including daily serum Lithium determinations and adjustments to the usually low doses ordinarily tolerated by these individuals. In such instances, hospitalization is a necessity.

WARNINGS
Lithium may cause fetal harm when administered to a pregnant woman. There have been reports of Lithium having adverse effects on nidation in rats, embryo viability in mice, and metabolism *in vitro* of rat testis and human spermatozoa have been attributed to Lithium, as have teratogenicity in submammalian species and cleft palates in mice. Studies in rats, rabbits and monkeys have shown no evidence of Lithium-induced teratology. Data from Lithium birth registries suggest an increase in cardiac and other anomalies, especially Ebstein's anomaly. If the patient becomes pregnant while taking Lithium, she should be apprised of the potential risk to the fetus. If possible, Lithium should be withdrawn for at least the first trimester unless it is determined that this would seriously endanger the mother.

➤ SHOWN IN PRODUCT IDENTIFICATION GUIDE

Chronic Lithium therapy may be associated with diminution of renal concentrating ability, occasionally presenting as nephrogenic diabetes insipidus, with polyuria and polyolpsia. Such patients should be carefully managed to avoid dehydration with resulting Lithium retention and toxicity. This condition is usually reversible when Lithium is discontinued.

Morphologic changes with glomerular and interstitial librosis and nephron-atrophy have been reported in patients on chronic Lithium therapy. Morphologic changes have been seen in bipolar patients never exposed to Lithium. The relationship between renal functional and morphologic changes and their association with Lithium therapy has not been established. To date, Lithium in therapeutic doses has not been reported to cause end-stage renal disease.

When kidney function is assessed for baseline data prior to starting Lithium therapy or thereafter, routine urinalysis and other tests may be used to evaluate tubular function (e.g., urine specific gravity or osmolality following a period of water deprivation, or 24-hour urine volume) and glomerular function (e.g., serum creatinine or creatinine clearance). During Lithium therapy, progressive or sudden changes in renal function, even within the normal range, indicate the need for reevaluation of treatment.

Lithium toxicity is closely related to serum Lithium levels, and can occur at doses close to therapeutic levels (see "Dosage and Administration").

PRECAUTIONS

General: The ability to tolerate Lithium is greater during the acute manic phase and decreases when manic symptoms subside (see "Dosage and Administration").

The distribution space of Lithium approximates that of total body water. Lithium is primarily excreted in urine with insignificant excretion in feces. Renal excretion of Lithium is proportional to its plasma concentration. The half-life of elimination of Lithium is approximately 24 hours. Lithium decreases sodium reabsorption by the renal tubules which could lead to sodium depletion. Therefore, it is essential for the patient to maintain a normal diet, including salt, and an adequate fluid intake (2500-3000 mL) at least during the initial stabilization period. Decreased tolerance to Lithium has been reported to ensue from protracted sweating or diarrhea and, if such occur, supplemental fluid and salt should be administered.

In addition to sweating and diarrhea, concomitant infection with elevated temperatures may also necessitate a temporary reduction or cessation of medication.

Previously existing underlying thyroid disorders do not necessarily constitute a contraindication to Lithium treatment; where hypothyroidism exists, careful monitoring of thyroid function during Lithium stabilization and maintenance allows for correction of changing thyroid parameters, if any. Where hypothyroidism occurs during Lithium stabilization and maintenance, supplemental thyroid treatment may be used.

Information for the Patients: Outpatients and their families should be warned that the patient must discontinue Lithium therapy and contact his physician if such clinical signs of Lithium toxicity as diarrhea, vomiting, tremor, mild ataxia, drowsiness or muscular weakness occur.

Lithium may impair mental and/or physical abilities. Caution patients about activities requiring alertness (e.g., operating vehicles or machinery).

Drug Interactions: Combined Use of Haloperidol and Lithium: An encephalopath-ic syndrome (characterized by weakness, lethargy, fever, tremulousness and confusion, extrapyramidal symptoms, leukocytosis, elevated serum enzymes. BUN and FBS) followed by irreversible brain damage has occurred in a few patients treated with Lithium plus halopendol. A causal relationship between these events and the concomitant administration of Lithium and haloperidol has not been established; however, patients receiving such combined therapy should be monitored closely for early evidence of neurologic toxicity and treatment discontinued promptly if such signs appear.

The possibility of similar adverse interactions with other antipsychotic medication exists.

Lithium may prolong the effects of neuromuscular blocking agents. Therefore, neuromuscular blocking agents should be given with caution to patients receiving Lithium.

Indomathacin and piroxicam have been reported to increase significantly steady state plasma Lithium levels. In some cases Lithium toxicity has resulted from such interactions. There is also evidence that other nonsteroidal, anti-inflammatory agents may have a similar effect. When such combinations are used, increased plasma Lithium level monitoring is recommended.

Pregnancy: Teratogenic Effects Pregnancy Category D: See "Warnings" section.

Nursing Mothers: Lithium is excreted in human milk. Nursing should not be undertaken during Lithium therapy except in rare and unusual circumstances where, in the view of the physician, the potential benefits to the mother outweigh possible hazards to the child.

Pediatric Use: Since information regarding the safety and effectiveness of Lithium in children under 12 years of age is not available, its use in such patients is not recommended at this time. There has been a report of a transient syndrome of acute dystonia and hyperreflexia occurring in a 15 kg child who ingested 300 mg of lithium carbonate.

ADVERSE REACTIONS

Lithium Toxicity: The likelihood of toxicity increases with increasing serum Lithium levels. Serum Lithium levels greater than 1.5 mEq/L carry a greater risk than lower levels. However, patients sensitive to Lithium may exhibit toxic signs at serum levels below 1.5 mEq/L.

Diarrhea, vomiting, drowsiness, muscular weakness and lack of coordination may be early signs of Lithium toxicity, and can occur at Lithium levels below 2.0 mEq/L. At higher levels, giddiness, ataxia, blurred vision, tinnitus and a large output of dilute urine may be seen. Serum Lithium levels above 3.0 mEq/L may produce a complex clinical picture involving multiple organs and organ systems. Serum Lithium levels should not be permitted to exceed 2.0 mEq/L during the acute treatment phase.

Fine hand tremor, polyuria and mild thirst may occur during initial therapy for the acute manic phase, and may persist throughout treatment. Transient and mild nausea and general discomfort may also appear during the first few days of Lithium administration.

These side effects are an inconvenience rather than a disabling condition, and usually subside with continued treatment or a temporary reduction or cessation of dosage. If persistent, a cessation of dosage is indicated.

The following adverse reactions have been reported and do not appear to be directly related to serum Lithium levels.

Neuromuscular: tremor, muscle hyperirritability (fasciculations, twitching, clonic movements of whole limbs), ataxia, choreoathetotic movements, hyperactive deep tendon reflexes.

Central Nervous System: blackout spells, epileptiform seizures, slurred speech, dizziness, vertigo, incontinence of urine or feces, somnolence, psychomotor retardation, restlessness, confusion, stupor, coma, acute dystonia, downbeat nystagmus.

Cardiovascular: cardiac arrhythmia, hypotension, peripheral circulatory collapse, sinus node dysfunction with severe bradycardia (which may result in syncope).

Neurological: Cases of pseudotumor cerebral increased intracranial pressure and papilledemal have been reported with Lithium use. If undetected, this condition may result in enlargement of the blind spot, constriction of visual fields and eventual blindness due to optic atrophy. Lithium should be discontinued, if clinically possible, if this syndrome occurs.

Gastrointestinal: anorexia, nausea, vomiting, diarhea.

Genitourinary: albuminuria, pliguria, polyuria, glycosuira.

Dermatologic: drying and thinning of hair, anesthesia of skin, chronic folliculitis, xerosis cults, alopecia and exacerbation of psoriasis.

Autonomic Nervous System: blurred vision, dry mouth.

Miscellaneous: fatigue, lethargy, tendency to sleep, dehydration, weight loss, transient scotomata.

Thyroid Abnormalities: euthyroid goiter and/or hypothyroidism (including myx-odema) accompanied by lower T3 and T4. Iodine 131 uptake may be elevated (See "Precautions"). Paradoxically, rare cases of hyperthyroidism have been reported.

EEG Changes: diffuse slowing, widening of frequency spectrum, potentiation and disorganization of background rhythm.

EKG Changes: reversible flattening, isoelectricity or inversion of T-waves.

Miscellaneous reactions unrelated to dosage are: transient electroencephalographic and electrocardiographic changes, leukocytosis, headache, diffuse nontoxic goiter with or without hypothyroidism, transient hyperglycemia, generalized pruritus with or without rash, cutaneous ulcers, alburimiruria, worsening of organic brain sydromes excessive weight gain, edematous swelling of ankles or wrists, and thirst of polyuria, sometimes resembling diabetes insipidus, and metallic taste.

A single report has been received of the development of painful discoloration of fingers and toes and coldness of the extremities within one day of the starting of treatment of Lithium. The mechanism through which these symptoms (resembling Raynaud's Syndrome) developed, is not known. Recovery followed discontinuance.

OVERDOSAGE

The toxic lovals for Lithium are close to the therapeutic levels. It is therefore important that patients and their families be cautioned to watch for early symptoms and to discontinue the drug and inform the physician should they occur. Toxic symptoms are listed in detail under "Adverse Reactions".

Treatment: No specific antidote for Lithium poisoning is known. Early symptoms of Lithium toxicity can usually be treated by reduction or cessation of dosage of the drug and resumption of the treatment at a lower dose after 24 to 48 hours. In severe cases of Lithium poisoning, the first and foremost goal of treatment consists of elimination of this ion from the patient.

Treatment is essentially the same as that used in barbiturate poisoning: 1) gastric lavage, 2) correction of fluid and electrolyte imbalance and 3) regulation of kidney functioning. Urea, mannitol, and aminophylline all produce significant increases in Lithium excretion. Hemodialysis is an effective and rapid means of removing the ion from the severely toxic patient. Infection prophylaxis, regular chest X-rays, and preservation of adequate respiration are essential.

DOSAGE AND ADMINISTRATION

Acute Menia: Optimal patient response to Lithium Citrate usually can be established and maintained with 600 mg t.i.d. [10 mL (2 teaspoonfuls) (16 mEq of Lithium) t.i.d.]. Such doses will normally produce an effective serum Lithium level ranging between 1.0 and 1.5 mEq/L. Dosage must be individualized according to serum levels and clinical response. Regular monitoring of the patient's clinical state and of serum Lithium levels is necessary. Serum levels should be determined twice per week during the acute phase, and until the serum level and clinical condition of the patient have been stabilized.

Long-Term Control: The desirable serum Lithium levels are 0.6 to 1.2 mEq/L. Dosage will vary from one individual to another, but usually 300 mg t.i.d. or q.i.d. [5 mL (1 teaspoonful) (8 mEq of Lithium) t.i.d. or q.i.d.] will maintain this level. Serum Lithium levels in uncomplicated cases receiving maintenance therapy during remissions should be monitored at least every two months.

Patients abnormally sensitive to Lithium may exhibit toxic signs at serum levels of 1.0 to 1.5 mEq/L. Elderly patients often respond to reduced dosage, and may exhibit signs of toxicity at serum levels ordinarily tolerated by other patients.

N.B.: Blood samples for serum Lithium determination should be drawn immediately prior to the next dose when Lithium concentrations are relatively stable (i.e., 8-12 hours after the previous dose). Total reliance must not be placed on serum levels alone. Accurate patient evaluation requires both clinical and laboratory analysis.

Storage: Store at controlled room temperature, 15°-30°C (59°-85°F).
Dispense in a tight container as defined in the USP.

HOW SUPPLIED
SYRUP:

BRAND/MANUFACTURER	NDC	SIZE	AWP
◆ GENERICS			
Goldline	00182-6148-40	480 ml	$16.20

SYRUP: 8 MEQ

BRAND/MANUFACTURER	NDC	SIZE	AWP
◆ GENERICS			
UDL	51079-0652-10	5 ml 50s ud	$31.50

SYRUP: 16 MEQ

BRAND/MANUFACTURER	NDC	SIZE	AWP
◆ GENERICS			
UDL	51079-0653-10	10 ml 50s ud	$36.20

SYRUP: 300 MG/5 ML

AVERAGE UNIT PRICE (AVAILABLE SIZES)		GENERIC A-RATED AVERAGE PRICE (GAAP)	
GENERIC	$0.05	480 ml	$15.43
HCFA FUL (480 ml)	$0.03		

BRAND/MANUFACTURER	NDC	SIZE	AWP
◆ GENERICS			
Geneva	00781-6100-16	480 ml	$14.25
Pennex	00832-8616-16	480 ml	$14.76
Schein	00364-2140-16	480 ml	$14.80
Major	00904-2914-16	480 ml	$14.95
Qualitest	00603-1410-58	480 ml	$14.98
Pennex	00426-8616-16	480 ml	$15.50
Aligen	00405-3223-16	480 ml	$16.23
Raway	00686-6100-16	480 ml	$17.50
Roxane	00054-3527-63	500 ml	$19.52
Raway	00686-0652-10	5 ml 50s ud	$34.00
Raway	00686-0653-10	10 ml 50s ud	$30.00
Roxane	00054-8529-04	5 ml 100s ud	$71.56

SYRUP: 600 MG/10 ML

BRAND/MANUFACTURER	NDC	SIZE	AWP
◆ GENERICS			
Roxane	00054-8530-04	10 ml 100s ud	$84.09

Lithobid *SEE* LITHIUM CARBONATE

Lithonate *SEE* LITHIUM CARBONATE

Lithostat *SEE* ACETOHYDROXAMIC ACID

Lithotabs *SEE* LITHIUM CARBONATE

Liver Derivative Complex

DESCRIPTION
Liver Derivative Complex Injection is a sterile solution containing 25.5 mg liver derivative complex per mL in water for injection. Liver Derivative Complex Injection is composed of peptides and amino acids. The product contains no protein, is virtually non-allergenic, and does not exhibit anti-anemia activity.

CLINICAL PHARMACOLOGY
The specific action of Liver Derivative Complex is to enhance the resolution of inflammation and edema. In the late 1920s it was demonstrated that liver was of benefit to patients suffering from acne vulgaris. As a consequence, various techniques were employed for isolating the active "factor" from liver. Studies published in the late 1930s and early 1940s showed activity in a specially purified liver fraction. During subsequent years refinements in the isolation of the active material led to the marketing of Liver Derivative Complex.

Initially it was thought that the primary action of Liver Derivative Complex was on the capillaries and precapillary sphincters. However, it is now believed that this effect is a secondary one and that the primary action of Liver Derivative Complex is in response to injury at the cellular level. The capillary changes observed following administration of Liver Derivative Complex appear to be part of a more fundamental anti-inflammatory effect. In the normal animal no consistent pharmacodynamic action has been demonstrated for Liver Derivative Complex. In particular there is no effect on the systemic blood pressure, no action on the autonomic nervous system and no alteration in prothrombin, coagulation or bleeding times. It is concluded that the specific action of the product is only apparent when tissues have been subjected to injury and when inflammation and edema are present.

INDICATIONS AND USAGE
A wide variety of dermatological clinical conditions benefit from Liver Derivative Complex therapy. The common denominator in these varied conditions is the presence of inflammation and edema. Favorable response to administration of Liver Derivative Complex in patients with acne vulgaris, herpes zoster, "poison ivy" dermatitis, pityriasis rosea, seborrheic dermatitis, urticaria and eczema, severe sunburn, and rosacea have been reported.

CONTRAINDICATIONS
Contraindicated in patients with hypersensitivity or intolerance to liver or pork products.

WARNING
Use with caution in patients suspected of being hypersensitive to liver or with other allergic diatheses.

PRECAUTIONS
DRUG INTERACTIONS
No clinically significant drug interactions have been reported.

CARCINOGENESIS, MUTAGENESIS, IMPAIRMENT OF FERTILITY
No long-term animal studies have examined the carcinogenic or mutagenic potential of Liver Derivative Complex. Liver Derivative Complex's effect upon reproductive capacity is similarly unknown.

PREGNANCY—PREGNANCY CATEGORY C
Animal reproduction studies have not been conducted with Liver Derivative Complex. It is also not known whether Liver Derivative Complex can cause fetal harm when administered to a pregnant woman or can affect reproduction capacity. Liver Derivative Complex should be given to a pregnant woman only if clearly needed.

NURSING MOTHERS
It is not known whether this drug is excreted in human milk. Because many drugs are excreted in human milk, caution should be exercised when Liver Derivative Complex is administered to a nursing woman.

ADVERSE REACTIONS
As with all injectable medications, local reactions may occur. Local reactions may include pain, swelling, and erythema.

DRUG ABUSE AND DEPENDENCE
The information on drug abuse and dependence is limited to uncontrolled data derived from marketing experience. Such experience has revealed no evidence of drug abuse and dependence associated with Liver Derivative Complex Injection.

DOSAGE AND ADMINISTRATION
For the management of skin disorders the usual dose of Liver Derivative Complex is 2 mL administered daily or as indicated. The product is given by intramuscular or subcutaneous injection only.

As with all parenteral drug products, Liver Derivative Complex should be inspected visually for particulate matter and discoloration prior to administration, whenever solution and container permit.

Store at controlled room temperature 15°-30°C (59°-86°F).

J CODES
Up to 20 mcg IM—J2050

HOW SUPPLIED
INJECTION:

BRAND/MANUFACTURER	NDC	SIZE	AWP
○ BRAND			
KUTAPRESSIN: Schwarz	00091-1510-21	20 ml	$92.00

➤ SHOWN IN PRODUCT IDENTIFICATION GUIDE

Livostin *SEE* LEVOCABASTINE HYDROCHLORIDE

LMD *SEE* DEXTRAN AND DEXTROSE

Lo/Ovral *SEE* ETHINYL ESTRADIOL AND NORGESTREL

Locoid *SEE* HYDROCORTISONE, TOPICAL

Lodine *SEE* ETODOLAC

Lodoxamide Tromethamine

DESCRIPTION
Ladoxamide Tromethamine is a sterile ophthalmic solution for topical administration to the eyes. Lodoxamide Tromethamine, a mast cell stabilizer, is a white, crystalline, water-soluble powder with a molecular weight of 553.91.

Chemical Name: N,N'-(2-chloro-5-cyano-m-phenylene)dioxamic acid tromethamine salt

   Empirical formula: $C_{19}H_{28}O_{12}N_5Cl$

   Each mL of solution contains: Lodoxamide Tromethamine 1.78 mg (equivalent to 1 mg Lodoxamide)

   Following is its chemical structure:

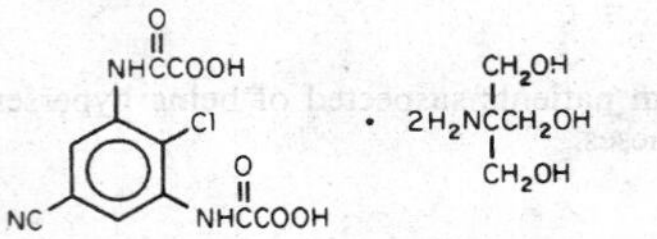

CLINICAL PHARMACOLOGY
Lodoxamide Tromethamine is a mast cell stabilizer that inhibits the *in vivo* Type 1 immediate hypersensitivity reaction. Lodoxamide therapy inhibits the increases in cutaneous vascular permeability that are associated with reagin or IgE and antigen-mediated reactions.

   In vitro studies have demonstrated the ability of Lodoxamide to stabilize rodent mast cells and prevent antigen-stimulated release of histamine. In addition, Lodoxamide prevents the release of other mast cell inflammatory mediators (i.e., SRS-A, slow-reacting substances of anaphylaxis, also known as the peptidoleukotrienes) and inhibits eosinophil chemotaxis. Although Lodoxamide's precise mechanism of action is unknown, the drug has been reported to prevent calcium influx into mast cells upon antigen stimulation.

   Lodoxamide has no intrinsic vasoconstrictor, antihistaminic, cyclooxygenase inhibition, or other anti-inflammatory activity.

   The disposition of ^{14}C-lodoxamide was studied in six healthy adult volunteers receiving a 3 mg (50 μ Ci) oral dose of Lodoxamide. Urinary excretion was the major route of elimination. The elimination half-life of ^{14}C-lodoxamide was 8.5 hours in urine. In a study conducted in twelve healthy adult volunteers, topical administration of Lodoxamide Tromethamine ophthalmic solution, one drop in each eye four times per day for ten days, did not result in any measurable Lodoxamide plasma levels at a detection limit of 2.5 ng/mL.

INDICATIONS AND USAGE
Lodoxamide Tromethamine ophthalmic solution is indicated in the treatment of the ocular disorders referred to by the terms vernal keratoconjunctivitis, vernal conjunctivitis, and vernal keratitis.

CONTRAINDICATIONS
Hypersensitivity to any component of this product.

WARNINGS
Not for injection. Some brands contain benzalkonium chloride; as with all ophthalmic preparations containing benzalkonium chloride, patients should be instructed not to wear soft contact lenses during treatment with Lodoxamide Tromethamine ophthalmic solution.

PRECAUTIONS
General: Patients may experience a transient burning or stinging upon instillation of Lodoxamide Tromethamine ophthalmic solution. Should these symptoms persist, the patient should be advised to contact the prescribing physician.

Carcinogenesis, Mutagenesis, Impairment of Fertility: A long-term study with Lodoxamide Tromethamine in rats (two-year oral administration) showed no neoplastic or tumorigenic effects at doses 100 mg/kg/day (more than 5000 times the proposed human clinical dose). No evidence of mutagenicity or genetic damage was seen in the Ames *Salmonella* Assay, *Chromosomal Aberration in*

CHO Cells Assay, or Mouse Forward Lymphoma Assay. In the BALB/*c*-3T3 Cells Transformation Assay, some increase in the number of transformed foci was seen at high concentrations (greater than 4000 μg/mL). No evidence of impairment of reproductive function was shown in laboratory animal studies.

Pregnancy: Pregnancy Category B: Reproduction studies with Lodoxamide Tromethamine administered orally to rats and rabbits in doses of 100 mg/kg/day (more than 5000 times the proposed human clinical dose) produced no evidence of developmental toxicity. There are, however, no adequate and well-controlled studies in pregnant women. Because animal reproduction studies are not always predictive of human response, Lodoxamide Tromethamine ophthalmic solution should be used during pregnancy only if clearly needed.

Nursing Mothers: It is not known whether Lodoxamide Tromethamine is excreted in human milk. Because many drugs are excreted in human milk, caution should be exercised when Lodoxamide Tromethamine ophthalmic solution is administered to nursing women.

Pediatric Use: Safety and effectiveness in children younger than 2 years of age have not been established.

ADVERSE REACTIONS
During clinical studies of Lodoxamide Tromethamine ophthalmic solution the most frequently reported ocular adverse experiences were transient burning, stinging, or discomfort upon instillation, which occurred in approximately 15% of the subjects. Other ocular events occurring in 1 to 5% of the subjects included ocular itching/pruritus, blurred vision, dry eye, tearing/discharge, hyperemia, crystalline deposits, and foreign body sensation. Events that occurred in less than 1% of the subjects included corneal erosion/ulcer, scales on lid/lash, eye pain, ocular edema/swelling, ocular warming sensation, ocular fatigue, chemosis, corneal abrasion, anterior chamber cells, keratopathy/keratitis, blepharitis, allergy, sticky sensation, and epitheliopathy.

   Nonocular events reported were headache (1.5%) and (at less than 1%) heat sensation, dizziness, somnolence, nausea, stomach discomfort, sneezing, dry nose, and rash.

OVERDOSAGE
There have been no reports of Lodoxamide Tromethamine ophthalmic solution overdose following topical ocular application. Accidental overdose of an oral preparation of 120 to 180 mg of Lodoxamide resulted in a temporary sensation of warmth, profuse sweating, diarrhea, light-headedness, and a feeling of stomach distension; no permanent adverse effects were observed. Side effects reported following systemic oral administration of 0.1 mg to 10.0 mg of Lodoxamide include a feeling of warmth or flushing, headache, dizziness, fatigue, sweating, nausea, loose stools, and urinary frequency/urgency. The physician may consider emesis in the event of accidental ingestion.

DOSAGE AND ADMINISTRATION
The dose for adults and children greater than two years of age is one to two drops in each affected eye four times daily for up to 3 months.
   Store at 15°C-27°C (59°F-80°F).

HOW SUPPLIED
DROP: 0.1%

BRAND/MANUFACTURER	NDC	SIZE	AWP
○ BRAND			
ALOMIDE: Alcon Labs	00065-0345-10	10 ml	$35.00

Lodrane CR *SEE* BROMPHENIRAMINE MALEATE AND PSEUDOEPHEDRINE HYDROCHLORIDE

Loestrin *SEE* ETHINYL ESTRADIOL AND NORETHINDRONE

Lok-Pak-N Kit *SEE* HEPARIN

Lomefloxacin Hydrochloride

DESCRIPTION
Lomefloxacin Hydrochloride is a synthetic broad-spectrum antimicrobial agent for oral administration. Lomefloxacin Hydrochloride, a difluoroquinolone, is the monohydrochloride salt of (±)-1-ethyl-6,8-difluoro-1,4-dihydro-7-(3-methyl -1-piperazinyl)-4-oxo-3-quinolinecarboxylic acid. Its empirical formula is $C_{17}H_{19}F_2N_3O_3$·HCl.

   Lomefloxacin Hydrochloride is a white to pale yellow powder with a molecular weight of 387.8. It is slightly soluble in water and practically insoluble in alcohol. Lomefloxacin Hydrochloride is stable to heat and moisture but is sensitive to light in dilute aqueous solution.

   Lomefloxacin Hydrochloride is available as a film-coated tablet formulation containing 400 mg of Lomefloxacin base.

◆ RATED THERAPEUTICALLY EQUIVALENT; ◇ THERAPEUTIC EQUIVALENCE UNCONFIRMED; ○ UNRATED

Following is its chemical structure:

CLINICAL PHARMACOLOGY

Pharmacokinetics in Healthy Volunteers: In 6 fasting healthy male volunteers, approximately 95% to 98% of a single oral dose of Lomefloxacin was absorbed. Absorption was rapid following single doses of 200 and 400 mg (T_{max} 0.8 to 1.4 hours). Mean plasma concentration increased proportionally between 100 and 400 mg as shown below.

Dose (mg)	Mean Plasma Concentration ($\mu g/mL$)	Area Under Curve (AUC) ($\mu g \cdot h/mL$)
100	0.8	5.6
200	1.4	10.9
400	3.2	26.1

In 6 healthy male volunteers administered 400 mg of Lomefloxacin on an empty stomach qd for 7 days, the following mean pharmacokinetic parameter values were obtained:

C_{max}	2.8 $\mu g/mL$
C_{min}	0.27 $\mu g/mL$
$AUC_{0-24 h}$	25.9 $\mu g \cdot h/mL$
T_{max}	1.5 h
$t_{1/2}$	7.75 h

The elimination half-life in 8 subjects with normal renal function was approximately 8 hours. At 24 hours postdose, subjects with normal renal function receiving single doses of 200 or 400 mg had mean plasma Lomefloxacin concentrations of 0.10 and 0.24 µg/mL, respectively. Steady-state concentrations were achieved within 48 hours of initiating therapy with one-a-day dosing. There was no drug accumulation with single-daily dosing in patients with normal renal function.

Approximately 65% of an orally administered dose was excreted in the urine as unchanged drug in patients with normal renal function. Following a 400-mg dose of Lomefloxacin administered qd for 7 days, the mean urine concentration 4 hours postdose was in excess of 300 µg/mL. The mean urine concentration exceeded 35 µg/mL for at least 24 hours after dosing.

Following a single 400-mg dose, the solubility of Lomefloxacin in urine usually exceeded its peak urinary concentration 2- to 6-fold. In this study, urine pH affected the solubility of Lomefloxacin with solubilities ranging from 7.8 mg/mL at pH 5.2, to 2.4 mg/mL at pH 6.5, and 3.03 mg/mL at pH 8.12.

The urinary excretion of Lomefloxacin was virtually complete within 72 hours after cessation of dosing, with approximately 65% of the dose being recovered as parent drug and 9% as its glucuronide metabolite. The mean renal clearance was 145 mL/min in subjects with normal renal function (GFR = 120 mL/min). This may indicate tubular secretion.

Food Effect: When Lomefloxacin and food were administered concomitantly, the rate of drug absorption was delayed (T_{max} increased to 2 hours [delayed by 41%], C_{max} decreased by 18%), and the extent of absorption (AUC) was decreased by 12%.

Pharmacokinetics in the Geriatric Population: In 16 healthy elderly volunteers (61 to 76 years of age) with normal renal function for their age, the half-life of Lomefloxacin (mean of 8 hours) and its peak plasma concentration (mean of 4.2 µg/mL) following a single 400-mg dose were similar to those in 8 younger subjects dosed with a single 400-mg dose. Thus, drug absorption appears unaffected in the elderly. Plasma clearance was, however, reduced in this elderly population by approximately 25%, and the AUC was increased by approximately 33%. This slower elimination most likely reflects the decreased renal function normally observed in the geriatric population.

Pharmacokinetics in Renally Impaired Patients: In 8 patients with creatinine clearance (Cl_{Cr}) between 10 and 40 mL/min/1.73 m^2, the mean AUC after a single 400-mg dose of Lomefloxacin increased 335% over the AUC demonstrated in patients with a $Cl_{Cr} > 80$ mL/min/1.73 m^2. Also, in these patients, the mean $t_{1/2}$ increased to 21 hours. In 8 patients with $Cl_{Cr} < 10$ mL/min/1.73 m^2, the mean AUC after a single 400-mg dose of Lomefloxacin increased 700% over the AUC demonstrated in patients with a $Cl_{Cr} > 80$ mL/min/1.73 m^2. In these patients with $Cl_{Cr} < 10$ mL/min/1.73 m^2, the mean $t_{1/2}$ increased to 45 hours. The plasma clearance of Lomefloxacin was closely correlated with creatinine clearance, ranging from 31 mL/min/1.73 m^2 when creatinine clearance was zero to 271 mL/min/1.73 m^2 at a normal creatinine clearance of 110 mL/min/1.73 m^2. Peak Lomefloxacin concentrations were not affected by the degree of renal function when single doses of Lomefloxacin were administered. Adjustment of dosage schedules for patients with such decreases in renal function is warranted. (See *"Dosage and Administration."*)

Pharmacokinetics in Patients with Cirrhosis: In 12 patients with histologically confirmed cirrhosis, no significant changes in rate or extent of Lomefloxacin exposure (C_{max}, T_{max}, $t_{1/2}$, or AUC) were observed when they were administered 400 mg of Lomefloxacin as a single dose. No data are available in cirrhotic patients treated with multiple doses of Lomefloxacin. Cirrhosis does not appear to reduce the nonrenal clearance of Lomefloxacin. There does not appear to be a need for a dosage reduction in cirrhotic patients, provided adequate renal function is present.

Metabolism and Pharmacodynamics of Lomefloxacin: Lomefloxacin is minimally metabolized although 5 metabolites have been identified in human urine. The glucuronide metabolite is found in the highest concentration and accounts for approximately 9% of the administered dose. The other 4 metabolites together account for < 0.5% of the dose.

Approximately 10% of an oral dose was recovered as unchanged drug in the feces.

Serum protein binding of Lomefloxacin is approximately 10%.

The following are mean tissue- or fluid-to-plasma ratios of Lomefloxacin following oral administration. Studies have not been conducted to assess the penetration of Lomefloxacin into human cerebrospinal fluid.

Tissue or Body Fluid	Mean Tissue- or Fluid-to-Plasma Ratio
Bronchial mucosa	2.1
Bronchial secretions	0.6
Prostatic tissue	2.0
Sputum	1.3
Urine	140.0

Microbiology: Lomefloxacin is a bactericidal agent with in vitro activity against a wide range of gram-negative and gram-positive organisms. The bactericidal action of Lomefloxacin results from interference with the activity of the bacterial enzyme DNA gyrase, which is needed for the transcription and replication of bacterial DNA. The minimum bactericidal concentration (MBC) generally does not exceed the minimum inhibitory concentration (MIC) by more than a factor of 2, except for staphylococci, which usually have MBCs 2 to 4 times the MIC.

Lomefloxacin has been shown to be active against most strains of the following organisms both in vitro and in clinical infections: (See *"Indications and Usage."*)

GRAM-POSITIVE AEROBES
Staphylococcus saprophyticus

GRAM-NEGATIVE AEROBES
Citrobacter diversus
Enterobacter cloacae
Escherichia coli
Haemophilus influenzae
Klebsiella pneumoniae
Moraxella (Branhamella) catarrhalis
Proteus mirabilis
Pseudomonas aeruginosa. (urinary tract only— See *"Indications and Usage and Warnings"*).

The following in vitro data are available; however, their clinical significance is unknown.

Lomefloxacin exhibits in vitro MICs of 2 µg/mL or less against most strains of the following organisms; however, the safety and effectiveness of Lomefloxacin in treating clinical infections due to these organisms have not been established in adequate and well-controlled trials:

GRAM-POSITIVE AEROBES
Staphylococcus aureus (including methicillin-resistant strains)
Staphylococcus epidermidis (including methicillin-resistant strains)

GRAM-NEGATIVE AEROBES
Aeromonas hydrophila
Citrobacter freundii
Enterobacter aerogenes
Enterobacter agglomerans
Haemophilus parainfluenzae
Hafnia alvei
Klebsiella oxytoca
Klebsiella ozaenae
Morganella morganii
Proteus vulgaris
Providencia alcalifaciens
Providencia rettgeri
Serratia liquefaciens
Serratia marcescens

OTHER ORGANISMS:
Legionella pneumophila

Beta-lactamase production should have no effect on the in vitro activity of Lomefloxacin.

Most group A, B, D, and G streptococci, *Streptococcus pneumoniae*, *Pseudomonas cepacia*, *Ureaplasma urealyticum*, *Mycoplasma hominis*, and anaerobic bacteria are resistant to Lomefloxacin.

Lomefloxacin appears slightly less active in vitro when tested at acidic pH. An increase in inoculum size has little effect on the in vitro activity of Lomefloxacin.

In vitro resistance to Lomefloxacin develops slowly (multiple-step mutation). Rapid one-step development of resistance occurs only rarely ($< 10^{-9}$) in vitro.

Cross-resistance between Lomefloxacin and other quinolone-class antimicrobial agents has been reported; however, cross-resistance between Lomefloxacin and members of other classes of antimicrobial agents, such as aminoglycosides, penicillins, tetracyclines, cephalosporins, or sulfonamides has not yet been reported. Lomefloxacin is active in vitro against some strains of cephalosporin- and aminoglycoside-resistant gram-negative bacteria.

SUSCEPTIBILITY TESTS
Diffusion Techniques: Quantitative methods that require measurement of zone diameters give the most precise estimate of the susceptibility of bacteria to antimicrobial agents. One such standardized procedure[1] that has been recommended for use with disks to test the susceptibility of organisms to Lomefloxacin uses the 10-µg Lomefloxacin disk. Interpretation involves correlation of the diameter obtained in the disk test with the MIC for Lomefloxacin.

Reports from the laboratory giving results of the standard single-disk susceptibility test with a 10-µg Lomefloxacin disk should be interpreted according to the following criteria:

Zone Diameter (mm)	Interpretation
≥ 22	Susceptible (S)
19-21	Intermediate (I)
≤ 18	Resistant (R)

A report of "susceptible" indicates that the pathogen is likely to be inhibited by generally achievable drug concentrations. A report of "intermediate" indicates that the result should be considered equivocal, and, if the organism is not fully susceptible to alternative clinically feasible drugs, the test should be repeated. This category provides a buffer zone that prevents small uncontrolled technical factors from causing major discrepancies in interpretation. A report of "resistant" indicates that achievable drug concentrations are unlikely to be inhibitory, and other therapy should be selected.

Standardized susceptibility test procedures require the use of laboratory control organisms. The 10-µg Lomefloxacin disk should give the following zone diameters:

Organism	Zone Diameter (mm)
S aureus (ATCC 25923)	23-29
E coli (ATCC 25922)	27-33
P aeruginosa (ATCC 27853)	22-28

Dilution Techniques: Use a standardized dilution method (broth, agar, or microdilution) or equivalent with Lomefloxacin powder. The MIC values obtained should be interpreted according to the following criteria:

MIC (µg/mL)	Interpretation
≤ 2	Susceptible (S)
4	Intermediate (I)
≥ 8	Resistant (R)

As with standard diffusion techniques, dilution methods require the use of laboratory control organisms. Standard Lomefloxacin powder should provide the following MIC values:

Organism	MIC (µg/mL)
S aureus (ATCC 29213)	0.25-2.0
E coli (ATCC 25922)	0.03-0.12
P aeruginosa (ATCC 27853)	1.0-4.0

INDICATIONS AND USAGE
TREATMENT
Lomefloxacin Hydrochloride film-coated tablets are indicated for the treatment of adults with mild to moderate infections caused by susceptible strains of the designated microorganisms in the conditions listed below: (See *"Dosage and Administration"* for specific dosing recommendations.)

LOWER RESPIRATORY TRACT
Acute Bacterial Exacerbation of Chronic Bronchitis caused by *Haemophilus influenzae* or *Moraxella (Branhamella) catarrhalis**.

Note: LOMEFLOXACIN IS NOT INDICATED FOR THE EMPIRIC TREATMENT OF ACUTE BACTERIAL EXACERBATION OF CHRONIC BRONCHITIS WHEN IT IS PROBABLE THAT *S PNEUMONIAE* IS A CAUSATIVE PATHOGEN. *S PNEUMONIAE* EXHIBITS IN VITRO RESISTANCE TO LOMEFLOXACIN, AND THE SAFETY AND EFFICACY OF LOMEFLOXACIN IN THE TREATMENT OF PATIENTS WITH ACUTE BACTERIAL EXACERBATION OF CHRONIC BRONCHITIS CAUSED BY *S PNEUMONIAE* HAVE NOT BEEN DEMONSTRATED. IF LOMEFLOXACIN IS TO BE PRESCRIBED FOR GRAM-STAIN-GUIDED EMPIRIC THERAPY OF ACUTE BACTERIAL EXACERBATION OF CHRONIC BRONCHITIS, IT SHOULD BE USED ONLY IF SPUTUM GRAM STAIN DEMONSTRATES AN ADEQUATE QUALITY OF SPECIMEN (> 25 PMNs/LPF) AND THERE IS BOTH A PREDOMINANCE OF GRAM-NEGATIVE ORGANISMS AND NOT A PREDOMINANCE OF GRAM-POSITIVE ORGANISMS.

URINARY TRACT
Uncomplicated Urinary Tract Infections (cystitis) caused by *Escherichia coli, Klebsiella pneumoniae, Proteus mirabilis,* or *Staphylococcus saprophyticus.*

Complicated Urinary Tract Infections caused by *Escherichia coli, Klebsiella pneumoniae, Proteus mirabilis, Pseudomonas aeruginosa, Citrobacter diversus**, or *Enterobacter cloacae**.

Note: In clinical trials with patients experiencing complicated urinary tract infections (UTIs) due to *P aeruginosa,* 12 of 16 patients had the organism eradicated from the urine after therapy with Lomefloxacin. No patients had concomitant bacteremia. Serum levels of Lomefloxacin do not reliably exceed the MIC of *Pseudomonas* isolates. THE SAFETY AND EFFICACY OF LOMEFLOXACIN IN TREATING PATIENTS WITH *PSEUDOMONAS* BACTEREMIA HAVE NOT BEEN ESTABLISHED.

Appropriate culture and susceptibility tests should be performed before antimicrobial treatment in order to isolate and identify organisms causing infection and to determine their susceptibility to Lomefloxacin. In patients with UTIs, therapy with Lomefloxacin film-coated tablets may be initiated before results of these tests are known; once these results become available, appropriate therapy should be continued. In patients with an acute bacterial exacerbation of chronic bronchitis, therapy should not be started empirically with Lomefloxacin when there is a probability the causative pathogen is *S pneumoniae.*

Beta-lactamase production should have no effect on Lomefloxacin activity.

PROPHYLAXIS
Lomefloxacin is indicated preoperatively to reduce the incidence of UTIs in the early postoperative period (3 to 5 days postsurgery) in patients undergoing transurethral surgical procedures. Efficacy in decreasing the incidence of infections other than UTIs in the early postoperative period has not been established. Lomefloxacin, like all drugs for prophylaxis of transurethral surgical procedures, usually should not be used in minor urologic procedures for which prophylaxis is not indicated (eg, simple cystoscopy or retrograde pyelography).

UNLABELED USES
Lomefloxacin is used alone or as an adjunct in the treatment of Neisseria gonorrhea and Chlamydia trachomatis in male urethritis.

CONTRAINDICATIONS
Lomefloxacin is contraindicated in patients with a history of hypersensitivity to Lomefloxacin or to any of the quinolone group of antimicrobial agents.

WARNINGS
MODERATE TO SEVERE PHOTOTOXIC REACTIONS HAVE OCCURRED IN PATIENTS EXPOSED TO DIRECT OR INDIRECT SUNLIGHT OR TO ARTIFICIAL ULTRAVIOLET LIGHT (eg, sunlamps) DURING OR FOLLOWING TREATMENT WITH LOMEFLOXACIN. THESE REACTIONS HAVE ALSO OCCURRED IN PATIENTS EXPOSED TO SHADED OR DIFFUSE LIGHT, INCLUDING EXPOSURE THROUGH GLASS. PATIENTS SHOULD BE ADVISED TO DISCONTINUE LOMEFLOXACIN THERAPY AT THE FIRST SIGNS OR SYMPTOMS OF A PHOTOTOXICITY REACTION SUCH AS A SENSATION OF SKIN BURNING, REDNESS, SWELLING, BLISTERS, RASH, ITCHING, OR DERMATITIS.

These phototoxic reactions have occurred with and without the use of sunscreens or sunblocks. Single doses of Lomefloxacin have been associated with these types of reactions. In a few cases, recovery was prolonged for several weeks. As with some other types of phototoxicity, there is the potential for exacerbation of the reaction on re-exposure to sunlight or artificial ultraviolet light prior to complete recovery from the reaction. In rare cases, reactions have recurred up to several weeks after stopping Lomefloxacin therapy.

EXPOSURE TO DIRECT OR INDIRECT SUNLIGHT (EVEN WHEN USING SUNSCREENS OR SUNBLOCKS) SHOULD BE AVOIDED WHILE TAKING LOMEFLOXACIN AND FOR SEVERAL DAYS FOLLOWING THERAPY. LOMEFLOXACIN THERAPY SHOULD BE DISCONTINUED IMMEDIATELY AT THE FIRST SIGNS OR SYMPTOMS OF PHOTOTOXICITY.

The Safety and Efficacy of Lomefloxacin in Children, Adolescents (Under the Age of 18 Years), Pregnant Women, and Lactating Women have not been Established: (See *"Precautions—Pregnancy; Nursing Mothers; and Pediatric Use."*) The oral administration of multiple doses of Lomefloxacin to juvenile dogs at 0.3 times and to rats at 5.4 times the recommended adult human dose based on mg/m^2 (0.6 and 34 times the recommended adult human dose based on mg/kg, respectively) caused arthropathy and lameness. Histopathologic examination of the weight-bearing joints of these animals revealed permanent lesions of the cartilage. Other quinolones also produce erosions of cartilage of weight-bearing joints and other signs of arthropathy in juvenile animals of various species. (See *"Animal Pharmacology."*)

The safety and efficacy of Lomefloxacin in the treatment of acute bacterial exacerbation of chronic bronchitis due to *S pneumoniae* have not been demonstrated. This product should not be used empirically in the treatment of acute bacterial exacerbation of chronic bronchitis when it is probable that *S pneumoniae* is a causative pathogen.

In clinical trials of complicated UTIs due to *P aeruginosa,* 12 of 16 patients had the organism eradicated from the urine after therapy with Lomefloxacin. No patients had concomitant bacteremia. Serum levels of Lomefloxacin do not reliably exceed the MIC of *Pseudomonas* isolates. THE SAFETY AND EFFICACY OF LOMEFLOXACIN IN TREATING PATIENTS WITH *PSEUDOMONAS* BACTEREMIA HAVE NOT BEEN ESTABLISHED.

* Although treatment of infections due to this organism in this organ system demonstrated a clinically acceptable overall outcome, efficacy was studied in fewer than 10 infections.

◆ RATED THERAPEUTICALLY EQUIVALENT; ◇ THERAPEUTIC EQUIVALENCE UNCONFIRMED; ○ UNRATED

Serious and occasionally fatal hypersensitivity (anaphylactoid or anaphylactic) reactions, some following the first dose, have been reported in patients receiving quinolone therapy. Some reactions were accompanied by cardiovascular collapse, loss of consciousness, tingling, pharyngeal or facial edema, dyspnea, urticaria, or itching. Only a few of these patients had a history of previous hypersensitivity reactions. Serious hypersensitivity reactions have also been reported following treatment with Lomefloxacin. If an allergic reaction to Lomefloxacin occurs, discontinue the drug. Serious acute hypersensitivity reactions may require immediate emergency treatment with epinephrine. Oxygen, intravenous fluids, antihistamines, corticosteroids, pressor amines, and airway management, including intubation, should be administered as indicated.

Convulsions have been reported in patients receiving Lomefloxacin. Whether the convulsions were directly related to Lomefloxacin administration has not yet been established. However, convulsions, increased intracranial pressure, and toxic psychoses have been reported in patients receiving other quinolones. Quinolones may also cause central nervous system (CNS) stimulation, which may lead to tremors, restlessness, lightheadedness, confusion, and hallucinations. If any of these reactions occurs in patients receiving Lomefloxacin, the drug should be discontinued and appropriate measures instituted. No evidence of an effect of Lomefloxacin on the electrical activity of the brain has been demonstrated. Lomefloxacin does not alter cerebral blood flow or cerebral glucose uptake in the CNS based on positron emission tomography. However, until more information becomes available, Lomefloxacin, like all other quinolones, should be used with caution in patients with known or suspected CNS disorders, such as severe cerebral arteriosclerosis, epilepsy, or other factors that predispose to seizures. (See "Adverse Reactions.")

Pseudomembranous colitis has been reported with nearly all antibacterial agents, including quinolones, and may range from mild to life-threatening in severity. Therefore, it is important to consider this diagnosis in patients who present with diarrhea subsequent to the administration of antibacterial agents. Treatment with broad-spectrum antibiotics alters the normal flora of the colon and may permit overgrowth of clostridia. Studies indicate that a toxin produced by *Clostridium difficile* is a primary cause of "antibiotic-associated colitis." After the diagnosis of pseudomembranous colitis has been established, therapeutic measures should be initiated. Mild cases of pseudomembranous colitis usually respond to discontinuation of drug alone. In moderate to severe cases, consideration should be given to management with fluids and electrolytes, protein supplementation, and treatment with an antibacterial drug clinically effective against *C difficile* colitis.

PRECAUTIONS
GENERAL
Alteration of the dosage regimen is recommended for patients with impairment of renal function ($Cl_{Cr} < 40$ mL/min/17.3 m^2). (See "Dosage and Administration.")

INFORMATION FOR PATIENTS
Patients should be advised

■ to avoid to the maximum extent possible direct or indirect sunlight (including exposure through glass and exposure through sunscreens and sunblocks) and artificial ultraviolet light (eg, sunlamps) during treatment with Lomefloxacin and for several days after therapy;
■ to discontinue Lomefloxacin therapy at the first signs or symptoms of phototoxicity reaction such as a sensation of skin burning, redness, swelling, blisters, rash, itching, or dermatitis;
■ that a patient who has experienced a phototoxic reaction should also be advised to avoid re-exposure to sunlight and artificial ultraviolet light until he has completely recovered from the reaction. In rare cases, reactions have recurred up to several weeks after stopping Lomefloxacin therapy.
■ to drink fluids liberally;
■ that Lomefloxacin can be taken without regard to meals;
■ that mineral supplements or vitamins with iron or minerals should not be taken within the 2-hour period before or after taking Lomefloxacin (see "Drug Interactions");
■ that sucralfate or antacids containing magnesium or aluminum should not be taken within 4 hours before or 2 hours after taking Lomefloxacin (see "Drug Interactions");
■ that Lomefloxacin can cause dizziness and light-headedness and, therefore, patients should know how they react to Lomefloxacin before they operate an automobile or machinery or engage in activities requring mental alertness and coordination;
■ that Lomefloxacin may be associated with hypersensitivity reactions, even following the first dose, and to discontinue the drug at the first sign of a skin rash or other allergic reaction.

DRUG INTERACTIONS
Theophylline: In three pharmacokinetic studies including 46 normal, healthy subjects, theophylline clearance and concentration were not significantly altered by the addition of Lomefloxacin. In clinical studies where patients were on chronic theophylline therapy, Lomefloxacin had no measurable effect on the mean distribution of theophylline concentrations or the mean estimates of theophylline clearance. Though individual theophylline levels fluctuated, there were no clinically significant symptoms of drug interaction.

Antacids and Sucralfate: Sucralfate and antacids containing magnesium or aluminum form chelation complexes with Lomefloxacin and interfere with its bioavailability. Sucralfate administered 2 hours before Lomefloxacin resulted in a slower rate of absorption (mean C_{max} decreased by 30% and mean T_{max} increased by 1 hour) and a lesser extent of absorption (mean AUC decreased by

approximately 25%). Magnesium- and aluminum-containing antacids, administered concomitantly with Lomefloxacin, significantly decreased the bioavailability (48%) of Lomefloxacin. Separating the doses of antacid and Lomefloxacin minimizes this decrease in bioavailability; therefore, administration of these agents should precede Lomefloxacin dosing by 4 hours or follow Lomefloxacin dosing by at least 2 hours.

Caffeine: One hundred mg of caffeine (equivalent to 1 to 3 cups of American coffee) was administered to 16 normal, healthy volunteers who had achieved steady-state blood concentrations of Lomefloxacin after being dosed at 400 mg qd. This did not result in any statistically or clinically relevant changes in the pharmacokinetic parameters of either caffeine or Lomefloxacin. No data are available on potential interactions in individuals who consume greater than 100 mg of caffeine per day or in those, such as the geriatric population, who are generally believed to be more susceptible to the development of drug-induced CNS-related adverse effects. Other quinolones have demonstrated moderate to marked interference with the metabolism of caffeine, resulting in a reduced clearance, a prolongation of plasma half-life, and an increase in symptoms that accompany high levels of caffeine.

Cimetidine: Cimetidine has been demonstrated to interfere with the elimination of other quinolones. This interference has resulted in significant increases in half-life and AUC. The interaction between Lomefloxacin and cimetidine has not been studied.

Cyclosporine: Elevated serum levels of cyclosporine have been reported with concomitant use of cyclosporine with other members of the quinolone class. Interaction between Lomefloxacin and cyclosporine has not been studied.

Nonsteroidal Anti-inflammatory Drugs (NSAIDs): Concomitant administration of the NSAID fenbufen with some quinolones has been reported to increase the risk of CNS stimulation and convulsive seizures.

There was an increase in the incidence of seizures in mice treated with fenbufen, when fenbufen was administered to mice that had been concomitantly treated with a dose of Lomefloxacin equivalent to the recommended human dose on a mg/m^2 basis (10 times the recommended human dose on a mg/kg basis). Fenbufen is not presently an approved drug in the United States. (See "Animal Pharmacology".)

Probenecid: Probenecid slows the renal elimination of Lomefloxacin. An increase of 63% in the mean AUC and increases of 50% and 4%, respectively, in the mean T_{max} and mean C_{max} were noted in 1 study of 6 individuals.

Warfarin: Quinolones may enhance the effects of the oral anticoagulant, warfarin, or its derivatives. When these products are administered concomitantly, prothrombin or other suitable coagulation tests should be monitored closely.

CARCINOGENESIS, MUTAGENESIS, IMPAIRMENT OF FERTILITY
Carcinogenesis: Hairless (Skh-1) mice were exposed to UVA light for 3.5 hours five times every 2 weeks for up to 52 weeks while concurrently being administered Lomefloxacin. The Lomefloxacin doses used in this study caused a phototoxic response. In mice treated with both UVA and Lomefloxacin concomitantly, the time to development of skin tumors was 16 weeks. In mice treated concomitantly in this model with both UVA and other quinolones, the times to development of skin tumors ranged from 28 to 52 weeks.

Ninety-two percent (92%) of the mice treated concomitantly with both UVA and Lomefloxacin developed well-differentiated squamous cell carcinomas of the skin. These squamous cell carcinomas were nonmetastatic and were endophytic in character. Two thirds of these squamous cell carcinomas contained large central keratinous inclusion masses and were thought to arise from the vestigial hair follicles in these hairless animals.

In this model, mice treated with Lomefloxacin alone did not develop skin or systemic tumors.

There are no data from similar models using pigmented mice and/or fully haired mice.

The clinical significance of these findings to humans is unknown.

Mutagenesis: One in vitro mutagenicity test (CHO/HGPRT assay) was weakly positive at Lomefloxacin concentrations $\geq$ 226 µg/mL and negative at concentrations < 226 µg/mL. Two other in vitro mutagenicity tests (chromosomal aberrations in Chinese hamster ovary cells, chromosomal aberrations in human lymphocytes) and two in vivo mouse micro-nucleus mutagenicity tests were all negative.

Impairment of Fertility: Lomefloxacin did not affect the fertility of male and female rats at oral doses up to 8 times the recommended human dose based on mg/m^2 (34 times the recommended human dose based on mg/kg).

PREGNANCY: TERATOGENIC EFFECTS. PREGNANCY CATEGORY C
Reproductive function studies have been performed in rats at doses up to 8 times the recommended human dose based on mg/m^2 (34 times the recommended human dose based on mg/kg), and no impaired fertility or harm to the fetus was reported due to Lomefloxacin. Increased incidence of fetal loss in monkeys has been observed at approximately 3 to 6 times the recommended human dose based on mg/m^2 (6 to 12 times the recommended human dose based on mg/kg). No teratogenicity has been observed in rats and monkeys at up to 16 times the recommended human dose exposure. In the rabbit, maternal toxicity and associated fetotoxicity, decreased placental weight, and variations of the coccygeal vertebrae occurred at doses 2 times the recommended human exposure based on mg/m^2. There are, however, no adequate and well-controlled studies in pregnant

women. Lomefloxacin should be used during pregnancy only if the potential benefit justifies the potential risk to the fetus.

NURSING MOTHERS
It is not known whether Lomefloxacin is excreted in human milk. However, it is known that other drugs of this class are excreted in human milk and that Lomefloxacin is excreted in the milk of lactating rats. Because of the potential for serious adverse reactions from Lomefloxacin in nursing infants, a decision should be made whether to discontinue nursing or to discontinue the drug, taking into account the importance of the drug to the mother.

PEDIATRIC USE
The safety and effectiveness of Lomefloxacin in children and adolescents less than 18 years of age have not been established. Lomefloxacin causes arthropathy in juvenile animals of several species. (See *"Warnings and Animal Pharmacology."*)

GERIATRIC USE
Of the total number of patients in clinical trials of Lomefloxacin, 26% were ≥ 65 years of age. No overall differences in effectiveness or safety were observed between these patients and younger patients. (See *"Clinical Pharmacology—Pharmacokinetics in the Geriatric Population."*)

ADVERSE REACTIONS
In clinical trials, most of the adverse events reported were mild to moderate in severity and transient in nature. During these clinical investigations, 2,869 patients received Lomefloxacin Hydrochloride. In 2.6% of the patients, Lomefloxacin was discontinued because of adverse events, primarily involving the gastrointestinal system (0.7%), skin (1.0%), or CNS (0.5%).

ADVERSE CLINICAL EVENTS
The events with the highest incidence (≥ 1%) in patients, regardless of relationship to drug, were nausea (3.7%), headache (3.2%), photosensitivity (2.4%) [see *"Warnings"*], dizziness (2.3%), and diarrhea (1.4%).

Additional clinical events reported in less than 1% of patients treated with Lomefloxacin Hydrochloride, regardless of relationship to drug, are listed below:

Autonomic: dry mouth, flushing, increased sweating.

Body as a Whole: fatigue, back pain, malaise, asthenia, chest pain, chills, allergic reaction, face edema, influenza-like symptoms, decreased heat tolerance.

Cardiovascular: hypotension, hypertension, edema, syncope, tachycardia, bradycardia, arrhythmia, extrasystoles, cyanosis, cardiac failure, angina pectoris, myocardial infarction, pulmonary embolism, cerebrovascular disorder, cardiomyopathy, phlebitis.

Central nervous system: convulsions, coma, hyperkinesia, tremor, vertigo, paresthesias.

Gastrointestinal: abdominal pain, dyspepsia, vomiting, flatulence, constipation, gastrointestinal inflammation, dysphagia, gastrointestinal bleeding, tongue discoloration.

Hearing: earache, tinnitus.

Hematologic: thrombocytopenia, thrombocythemia, purpura, lymphadenopathy, increased fibrinolysis.

Metabolic: thirst, gout, hypoglycemia.

Musculoskeletal: leg cramps, arthralgia, myalgia.

Ophthalmologic: abnormal vision, conjunctivitis, eye pain.

Psychiatric: somnolence, insomnia, nervousness, anorexia, confusion, anxiety, depression, agitation, increased appetite, depersonalization, paroniria.

Reproductive system: Female: vaginitis, leukorrhea, intermenstrual bleeding, perineal pain, vaginal moniliasis. Male; orchitis, epididymitis.

Respiratory: dyspnea, respiratory infection, epistaxis, respiratory disorder, bronchospasm, cough, increased sputum, stridor.

Skin/Allergic: pruritus, rash, urticaria, eczema, skin exfoliation, skin disorder.

Special senses: taste perversion.

Urinary: dysuria, hematuria, strangury, micturition disorder, anuria.

ADVERSE LABORATORY EVENTS
Changes in laboratory parameters, listed as adverse events, without regard to drug relationship include:

Hepatic: elevations of ALT (SGPT) (0.4%), AST (SGOT) (0.3%), bilirubin (0.1%), alkaline phosphatase (0.1%).

Hematologic: monocytosis (0.3%), elevated ESR (0.1%).

Renal: elevated BUN (0.1%), decreased potassium (0.1%).

Additional laboratory changes occurring in ≤ 0.1% in the clinical studies included: elevation of serum gamma glutamyl transferase, decrease in total protein or albumin, prolongation of prothrombin time, anemia, decrease in hemoglobin, leukopenia, eosinophilia, thrombocytopenia, abnormalities of urine specific gravity or serum electrolytes, decrease in blood glucose.

QUINOLONE-CLASS ADVERSE EVENTS
Although not reported in completed clinical studies with Lomefloxacin, a variety of adverse events have been reported with other quinolones.

Clinical adverse events include: anaphylactoid reactions, erythema nodosum, Stevens-Johnson syndrome, exfoliative dermatitis, toxic epidermal necrolysis, hepatic necrosis, possible exacerbation of myasthenia gravis, dysphasia, nystagmus, pseudomembranous colitis, painful oral mucosa, intestinal perforation, hallucinations, manic reaction, ataxia, phobia, hyperpigmentation, diplopia, interstitial nephritis, renal failure, renal calculi, polyuria, urinary retention, acidosis, cardiopulmonary arrest, cerebral thrombosis, laryngeal or pulmonary edema, hiccough, dysgeusia, and photophobia.

Laboratory adverse events include: agranulocytosis, elevation of serum triglycerides, elevation of serum cholesterol, elevation of blood glucose, elevation of serum potassium, albuminuria, candiduria, and crystalluria.

OVERDOSAGE
Information on overdosage in humans is limited. In the event of acute overdosage, the stomach should be emptied by inducing vomiting or by gastric lavage, and the patient should be carefully observed and given supportive treatment. Adequate hydration must be maintained. Hemodialysis or peritoneal dialysis is unlikely to aid in the removal of Lomefloxacin as < 3% is removed by these modalities.

Clinical signs of acute toxicity in rodents progressed from salivation to tremors, decreased activity, dyspnea, and clonic convulsions prior to death. These signs were noted in rats and mice as Lomefloxacin doses were increased.

DOSAGE AND ADMINISTRATION
Lomefloxacin Hydrochloride may be taken without regard to meals. (See *"Clinical Pharmacology."*)

See *"Indications and Usage"* for information on appropriate pathogens and patient populations.

TREATMENT
Patients with Normal Renal Function: The recommended daily dose of Lomefloxacin Hydrochloride is described in the following chart: (See related table).

Elderly Patients: No dosage adjustment is needed for elderly patients with normal renal function (Cl$_{cr}$ ≥ 40 mL/min/1.73 m^2).

Patients with Impaired Renal Function: Lomefloxacin is primarily eliminated by renal excretion. (See *"Clinical Pharmacology."*) Modification of dosage is recommended in patients with renal dysfunction. In patients with a creatinine clearance > 10 mL/min/1.73m^2 but < 40 mL/min/1.73 m^2, the recommended dosage is an initial loading dose of 400 mg followed by daily maintenance doses of 200 mg (1/2 tablet) once daily for the duration of treatment. It is suggested that serial determinations of Lomefloxacin levels be performed to determine any necessary alteration in the appropriate next dosing interval.

If only the serum creatinine is known, the following formula may be used to estimate creatinine clearance.

Men: (weight in kg) × (140 − age)/(72) × serum creatinine (mg/dL)
Women: (0.85) × (calculated value for men)

Dialysis Patients: Hemodialysis removes only a negligible amount of Lomefloxacin (3% in 4 hours). Hemodialysis patients should receive an initial loading dose of 400 mg followed by daily maintenance doses of 200 mg (1/2 tablet) once daily for the duration of treatment.

Patients with Cirrhosis: Cirrhosis does not reduce the non-renal clearance of Lomefloxacin. The need for a dosage reduction in this population should be based on the degree of renal function of the patient and on the plasma concentrations. (See *"Clinical Pharmacology"* and *"Dosage and Administration—Impaired Renal Function."*)

PROPHYLAXIS
A single dose of 400 mg of Lomefloxacin should be administered orally 2 to 6 hours prior to surgery when oral preoperative prophylaxis for transurethral surgical procedures is considered appropriate.

STORAGE
Store at 59° to 86°F (15° to 30°C).

ANIMAL PHARMACOLOGY
Lomefloxacin and other quinolones have been shown to cause arthropathy in juvenile animals. Arthropathy, involving multiple diarthrodial joints, was observed in juvenile dogs administered Lomefloxacin at doses as low as 4.5 mg/kg for 7 to 8 days (0.3 times the recommended human dose based on mg/m^2 or 0.6 times the recommended human dose based on mg/kg). In juvenile rats, no changes were observed in the joints with doses up to 91 mg/kg for 7 days (2 times the recommended human dose based on mg/m^2 or 11 times the recommended human dose based on mg/kg). (See *"Warnings."*)

In a 13-week oral rat study, gamma globulin decreased when Lomefloxacin was administered at less than the recommended human exposure. Beta globulin decreased when Lomefloxacin was administered at 0.6 to 2 times the recommended human dose based on mg/m^2. The A/G ratio increased when Lomefloxacin was administered at 6 to 20 times the human dose. Following a 4-week recovery period, beta globulins in the females and A/G ratios in the females returned to control values. Gamma globulin values in the females and beta and gamma globulins and A/G ratios in the males were still statistically significantly different from control values. No effects on globulins were seen in oral studies in dogs or monkeys in the limited number of specimens collected.

Twenty-seven NSAIDs, administered concomitantly with Lomefloxacin, were tested for seizure induction in mice at approximately 2 times the recommended human dose based on mg/m^2. At a dose of Lomefloxacin equivalent to the

---

◆ RATED THERAPEUTICALLY EQUIVALENT; ◇ THERAPEUTIC EQUIVALENCE UNCONFIRMED; ○ UNRATED

Body System	Infection	Unit Dose	Frequency	Duration	Daily Dose
Lower respiratory tract	Acute bacterial exacerbation of chronic bronchitis	400 mg	qd	10 days	400 mg
Urinary tract	Cystitis	400 mg	qd	10 days	400 mg
	Complicated UTIs	400 mg	qd	14 days	400 mg

recommended human exposure based on mg/m^2 (10 times the human dose based on mg/kg), only fenbufen, when coadministered, produced an increase in seizures.

Crystalluria and ocular toxicity, seen with some related quinolones, were not observed in any Lomefloxacin-treated animals, either in studies designed to look for these effects specifically or in subchronic and chronic toxicity studies in rats, dogs, and monkeys.

Long-term, high-dose systemic use of other quinolones in experimental animals has caused lenticular opacities; however, this finding was not observed with Lomefloxacin.

REFERENCES
1. National Committee for Clinical Laboratory Standards, *Performance Standards for Antimicrobial Disk Susceptibility Tests*—4th ed. Approved Standard NCCLS Document M2-A4, vol 10, No. 7, NCCLS, Villanova, Pa, 1990. 2. National Committee for Clinical Laboratory Standards, *Methods for Dilution Antimicrobial Susceptibility Tests for Bacteria that Grow Aerobically*—2nd ed. Approved Standard NCCLS Document M7-A2, vol 10, No. 8, NCCLS, Villanova, Pa, 1990.

HOW SUPPLIED
TABLETS: 400 MG

BRAND/MANUFACTURER	NDC	SIZE	AWP
○ BRAND			
▶ MAXAQUIN: Searle	00025-1651-20	20s	$117.59
	00025-1651-34	100s ud	$617.36

Lomotil *SEE* ATROPINE SULFATE AND DIPHENOXYLATE HYDROCHLORIDE

Lomustine

> **WARNINGS**
>
> LOMUSTINE SHOULD BE ADMINISTERED UNDER THE SUPERVISION OF A QUALIFIED PHYSICIAN EXPERIENCED IN THE USE OF CANCER CHEMOTHERAPEUTIC AGENTS.
>
> BONE MARROW SUPPRESSION, NOTABLY THROMBOCYTOPENIA AND LEUKOPENIA, WHICH MAY CONTRIBUTE TO BLEEDING AND OVERWHELMING INFECTIONS IN AN ALREADY COMPROMISED PATIENT, IS THE MOST COMMON AND SEVERE OF THE TOXIC EFFECTS OF LOMUSTINE (SEE *"WARNINGS"* AND *"ADVERSE REACTIONS"*).
>
> SINCE THE MAJOR TOXICITY IS DELAYED BONE MARROW SUPPRESSION, BLOOD COUNTS SHOULD BE MONITORED WEEKLY FOR AT LEAST 6 WEEKS AFTER A DOSE (SEE *"ADVERSE REACTIONS"*). AT THE RECOMMENDED DOSAGE, COURSES OF LOMUSTINE SHOULD NOT BE GIVEN MORE FREQUENTLY THAN EVERY 6 WEEKS.
>
> THE BONE MARROW TOXICITY OF LOMUSTINE IS CUMULATIVE AND THEREFORE DOSAGE ADJUSTMENT MUST BE CONSIDERED ON THE BASIS OF NADIR BLOOD COUNTS FROM PRIOR DOSE (SEE *"DOSAGE ADJUSTMENT TABLE"* UNDER *"DOSAGE AND ADMINISTRATION"*).

DESCRIPTION
Lomustine is one of the nitrosoureas used in the treatment of certain neoplastic diseases. It is 1-(2-chloroethyl)-3-cyclohexyl-1-nitrosourea. It is a yellow powder with the empirical formula of $C_9H_{16}ClN_3O_2$ and a molecular weight of 233.71. Lomustine is soluble in 10% ethanol (0.05 mg per mL) and in absolute alcohol (70 mg per mL). Lomustine is relatively insoluble in water (< 0.05 mg per mL).

It is relatively unionized at a physiological pH.

Lomustine is available in 10 mg, 40 mg and 100 mg capsules for oral administration.

Following is its chemical structure:

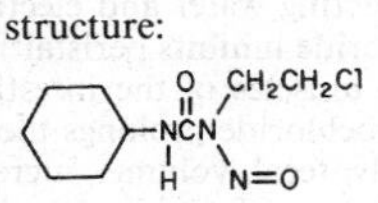

CLINICAL PHARMACOLOGY
Although it is generally agreed that Lomustine alkylates DNA and RNA, it is not cross resistant with other alkylators. As with other nitrosoureas, it may also inhibit several key enzymatic processes by carbamoylation of amino acids in proteins.

Lomustine may be given orally. Following oral administration of radioactive Lomustine at doses ranging from 30 mg/m^2 to 100 mg/m^2, about half of the radioactivity given was excreted in the form of degredation products within 24 hours.

The serum half-life of the metabolites ranges from 16 hours to 2 days. Tissue levels are comparable to plasma levels at 15 minutes after intravenous administration.

Because of the high lipid solubility and the relative lack of ionization at a physiological pH, Lomustine crosses the blood-brain barrier quite effectively. Levels of radioactivity in the CSF are 50% or greater than those measured concurrently in plasma.

INDICATIONS AND USAGE
Lomustine has been shown to be useful as a single agent in addition to other treatment modalities, or in established combination therapy with other approved chemotherapeutic agents in the following:

Brain Tumors: both primary and metastatic, in patients who have already received appropriate surgical and/or radio-therapeutic procedures.

Hodgkin's Disease: secondary therapy in combination with other approved drugs in patients who relapse while being treated with primary therapy, or who fail to respond to primary therapy.

CONTRAINDICATIONS
Lomustine should not be given to individuals who have demonstrated a previous hypersensitivity to it.

WARNINGS
Since the major toxicity is delayed bone marrow suppression, blood counts should be monitored weekly for at least 6 weeks after a dose (see *"Adverse Reactions"*). At the recommended dosage, courses of Lomustine should not be given more frequently than every 6 weeks.

The bone marrow toxicity of Lomustine is cumulative and therefore dosage adjustment must be considered on the basis of nadir blood counts from prior dose (see Dosage Adjustment Table under *"Dosage and Administration"*).

Pulmonary toxicity from Lomustine appears to be dose related (see *"Adverse Reactions"*).

Long term use in nitrosoureas has been reported to be possibly associated with the development of secondary malignancies.

Liver and renal function tests should be monitored periodically (see *"Adverse Reactions"*).

Pregnancy Category D: Lomustine can cause fetal harm when administered to a pregnant woman. Lomustine is embryotoxic and teratogenic in rats and embryotoxic in rabbits at dose levels equivalent to the human dose. There are no adequate and well controlled studies in pregnant women. If this drug is used during pregnancy, or if the patient becomes pregnant while taking (receiving) this drug, the patient should be apprised of the potential hazard to the fetus. Women of childbearing potential should be advised to avoid becoming pregnant.

PRECAUTIONS
General: In all instances where the use of Lomustine is considered for chemotherapy, the physician must evaluate the need and usefulness of the drug against the risks of toxic effects or adverse reactions. Most such adverse reactions are reversible if detected early. When such effects or reactions do occur, the drug should be reduced in dosage or discontinued and appropriate corrective measures should be taken according to the clinical judgment of the physician. Reinstitution of Lomustine therapy should be carried out with caution and with adequate consideration of the further need for the drug and alertness as to possible recurrence of toxicity.

Laboratory Tests: Due to delayed bone marrow suppression, blood counts should be monitored weekly for at least 6 weeks after a dose.

Baseline pulmonary function studies should be conducted along with frequent pulmonary function tests during treatment. Patients with a baseline below 70% of the predicted Forced Vital Capacity (FVC) or Carbon Monoxide Diffusing Capacity (DL$_{CO}$) are particularly at risk.

Since Lomustine may cause liver dysfunction, it is recommended that liver function tests be monitored periodically. Renal function tests should also be monitored periodically.

Carcinogenesis, Mutagenesis, Impairment of Fertility: Lomustine is carcinogenic in rats and mice, producing a marked increase in tumor incidence in doses approximating those employed clinically. Nitrosourea therapy does have carcinogenic potential in humans (see *"Adverse Reactions"*). Lomustine also affects fertility in male rats at doses somewhat higher than the human dose.

Pregnancy: Pregnancy "Category D"— See *"Warnings"* section.

Nursing Mothers: It is not known whether this drug is excreted in human milk. Because many drugs are excreted in human milk and because of the potential for

▶ SHOWN IN PRODUCT IDENTIFICATION GUIDE

serious adverse reactions in nursing infants from Lomustine, a decision should be made whether to discontinue nursing or to discontinue the drug, taking into account the importance of the drug to the mother.

Information for the Patient: Patients receiving Lomustine should be given the following information and instructions by the physicians:

1. Patients should be told that Lomustine is an anticancer drug and belongs to the group of medicines known as alkylating agents.
2. In order to provide the proper dose of Lomustine, patients should be aware that there may be two or more different types and colors of capsules in the container dispensed by the pharmacist.
3. Patients should be told that Lomustine is given as a single oral dose and will not be repeated for at least 6 weeks.
4. Patients should be told that nausea and vomiting usually last less than 24 hours, although loss of appetite may last for several days.
5. If any of the following reactions occur, notify the physician: fever, chills, sore throat, unusual bleeding or bruising, shortness of breath, dry cough, swelling of feet or lower legs, mental confusion or yellowing of eyes and skin.

ADVERSE REACTIONS
Hematologic Toxicity: The most frequent and most serious toxicity of Lomustine is delayed myelosuppression. It usually occurs 4 to 6 weeks after drug administration and is dose related. Thrombocytopenia occurs at about 4 weeks postadministration and persists for 1 to 2 weeks. Leukopenia occurs at 5 to 6 weeks after a dose of Lomustine and persists for 1 to 2 weeks. Approximately 65% of patients receiving 130 mg/m^2 develop white blood counts below 5000 wbc/mm^3. Thirty six percent developed white blood counts below 3000 wbc/mm^3. Thrombocytopenia is generally more severe than leukopenia. However, both may be dose-limiting toxicities.

Lomustine may produce cumulative myelosuppression, manifested by more depressed indices or longer duration of suppression after repeated doses.

The occurrence of acute leukemia and bone marrow dysplasias have been reported in patients following long term nitrosourea therapy.

Anemia also occurs, but is less frequent and less severe than thrombocytopenia or leukopenia.

Pulmonary Toxicity: Pulmonary toxicity characterized by pulmonary infiltrates and/or fibrosis has been reported rarely with Lomustine. Onset of toxicity has occurred after an interval of 6 months or longer from the start of therapy with cumulative doses of Lomustine usually greater than 1100 mg/m^2. There is one report of pulmonary toxicity at a cumulative dose of only 600 mg.

Delayed onset pulmonary fibrosis occurring up to 15 years after treatment has been reported in patients who received related nitrosoureas in childhood and early adolescence combined with cranial radiotherapy for intracranial tumors.

Gastrointestinal Toxicity: Nausea and vomiting may occur 3 to 6 hours after an oral dose and usually lasts less than 24 hours. Prior administration of antiemetics is effective in diminishing and sometimes preventing this side effect. Nausea and vomiting can also be reduced if Lomustine is administered to fasting patients.

Hepatotoxicity: A reversible type of hepatic toxicity, manifested by increased transaminase, alkaline phosphatase and bilirubin levels, has been reported in a small percentage of patients receiving Lomustine.

Nephrotoxicity: Renal abnormalities consisting of progressive azotemia, decrease in kidney size and renal failure have been reported in patients who received large cumulative doses after prolonged therapy with Lomustine. Kidney damage has also been reported occasionally in patients receiving lower total doses.

Other Toxicities: Stomatitis and alopecia have been reported infrequently.

Neurological reactions such as disorientation, lethargy, ataxia, and dysarthria have been noted in some patients receiving Lomustine. However, the relationship to medication in these patients is unclear.

OVERDOSAGE
No proven antidotes have been established for Lomustine overdosage.

DOSAGE AND ADMINISTRATION
The recommended dose of Lomustine in adults and children as a single agent in previously untreated patients is 130 mg/m^2 as a single oral dose every 6 weeks. In individuals with compromised bone marrow function, the dose should be reduced to 100 mg/m^2 every 6 weeks. When Lomustine is used in combination with other myelosuppressive drugs, the doses should be adjusted accordingly.

Doses subsequent to the initial dose should be adjusted according to the hematologic response of the patient to the preceding dose. The following schedule is suggested as a guide to dosage adjustment:

Nadir After Prior Dose		Percentage of Prior Dose to be Given
Leukocytes	Platelets	
> 4000	100,000	100%
3000-3999	75,000-99,999	100%
2000-2999	25,000-74,999	70%
< 2000	(< 25,000) 25,000	50%

A repeat course of Lomustine should not be given until circulating blood elements have returned to acceptable levels (platelets above 100,000/mm^3; leukocytes above 4,000/mm^3) and this is usually in 6 weeks. Adequate number of neutrophils should be present on a peripheral blood smear. Blood counts should be monitored

weekly and repeat courses should not be given before 6 weeks because the hematologic toxicity is delayed and cumulative.

Stability: Lomustine Capsules are stable for the lot life indicated on package labeling when stored at room temperature in well closed containers. Avoid excessive heat (over 40°C).

Procedures for proper handling and disposal of anticancer drugs should be considered. Several guidelines on this subject have been published.[1-7] There is no general agreement that all of the procedures recommended in the guidelines are necessary or appropriate.

REFERENCES
1. Recommendations for the Safe Handling of Parenteral Antineoplastic Drugs. NIH Publication No. 83-2621. For sale by the Superintendent of Documents, U.S. Government Printing Office, Washington, D.C. 20402. 2. AMA Council Report, Guidelines for Handling Parenteral Antineoplastics. *JAMA*. 1985; 253(11):1590-1592. 3. National Study Commission on Cytotoxic Exposure—Recommendations for Handling Cytotoxic Agents. Available from Louis P. Jeffrey, Sc.D., Chairman, National Study Commission on Cytotoxic Exposure, Massachusetts College of Pharmacy and Allied Health Sciences, 179 Longwood Avenue, Boston, Massachusetts 02115. 4. Clinical Oncological Society of Australia: Guidelines and Recommendations for Safe Handling of Antineoplastic Agents. *Med J Australia*. 1983; 1:426-428. 5. Jones, R. B., et. al. Safe Handling of Chemotherapeutic Agents: A report from the Mount Sinai Medical Center, *CA—A Cancer J for Clinicians*. 1983; Sept./Oct., 258-263. 6. American Society of Hospital Pharmacists Technical Assistance Bulletin on Handling Cytotoxic and Hazardous Drugs. *Am J Hosp Pharm*. 1990; 47:1033-1049. 7. OSHA Work-Practice Guidelines for Personnel Dealing with Cytotoxic (Antineoplastic) Drugs. *Am J Hosp Pharm*. 1986; 43:1193-1204.

HOW SUPPLIED
CAPSULE:

BRAND/MANUFACTURER	NDC	SIZE	AWP
○ BRAND CEENU: Bristol-Myer Onc/Hiv	00015-3034-10	6s ud	$78.09

CAPSULE: 10 MG

BRAND/MANUFACTURER	NDC	SIZE	AWP
○ BRAND CEENU: Bristol-Myer Onc/Hiv	00015-3030-20	20s	$84.54

CAPSULE: 40 MG

BRAND/MANUFACTURER	NDC	SIZE	AWP
○ BRAND CEENU: Bristol-Myer Onc/Hiv	00015-3031-20	20s	$254.60

CAPSULE: 100 MG

BRAND/MANUFACTURER	NDC	SIZE	AWP
○ BRAND CEENU: Bristol-Myer Onc/Hiv	00015-3032-20	20s	$483.96

Loniten *SEE* MINOXIDIL, ORAL

Loperamide Hydrochloride

DESCRIPTION
Loperamide Hydrochloride, 4-(p-chlorophenyl)-4-hydroxy-N, N-dimethyl-α,α-diphenyl-1-piperidinebuty-ramide monohydrochloride, is a synthetic antidiarrheal for oral use.

Loperamide Hydrochloride is available in 2 mg capsules.

Following is its chemical structure:

CLINICAL PHARMACOLOGY
In vitro and animal studies show that Loperamide Hydrochloride acts by slowing intestinal motility and by affecting water and electrolyte movement through the bowel. Loperamide Hydrochloride inhibits peristaltic activity by a direct effect on the circular and longitudinal muscles of the intestinal wall.

In man, Loperamide Hydrochloride prolongs the transit time of the intestinal contents. It reduces the daily fecal volume, increases the viscosity and bulk density, and diminishes the loss of fluid and electrolytes. Tolerance to the antidiarrheal effect has not been observed.

Clinical studies have indicated that the apparent elimination half-life of Loperamide in man is 10.8 hours with a range of 9.1-14.4 hours. Plasma levels of unchanged drug remain below 2 nanograms per ml after the intake of a 2 mg capsule of Loperamide Hydrochloride Plasma levels are highest approximately five hours after administration of the capsule and 2.5 hours after the liquid. The peak plasma levels of Loperamide were similar for both formulations. Of the total excreted in urine and feces, most of the administered drug was excreted in feces. In those patients in whom biochemical and hematological parameters were monitored during clinical trials, no trends toward abnormality during Loperamide Hydrochloride therapy were noted. Similarly, urinalyses, EKG and clinical ophthalmological examinations did not show trends toward abnormality.

INDICATIONS AND USAGE

Loperamide Hydrochloride is indicated for the control and symptomatic relief of acute nonspecific diarrhea and of chronic diarrhea associated with inflammatory bowel disease. Loperamide Hydrochloride is also indicated for reducing the volume of discharge from ileostomies.

CONTRAINDICATIONS

Loperamide Hydrochloride is contraindicated in patients with known hypersensitivity to the drug and in those in whom constipation must be avoided.

WARNINGS

Loperamide Hydrochloride should not be used in the case of acute dysentery, which is characterized by blood in stools and high fever.

Fluid and electrolyte depletion often occur in patients who have diarrhea. In such cases, administration of appropriate fluid and electrolytes is very important. The use of Loperamide Hydrochloride does not preclude the need for appropriate fluid and electrolyte therapy.

In some patients with acute ulcerative colitis, and in pseudomembranous colitis associated with broad-spectrum antibiotics, agents which inhibit intestinal motility or delay intestinal transit time have been reported to induce toxic megacolon. Loperamide Hydrochloride therapy should be discontinued promptly if abdominal distention, constipation, or ileus occurs.

Loperamide Hydrochloride should be used with special caution in young children because of the greater variability of response in this age group. Dehydration, particularly in younger children, may further influence the variability of response to Loperamide Hydrochloride.

PRECAUTIONS

General: In acute diarrhea, if clinical improvement is not observed in 48 hours, the administration of Loperamide Hydrochloride should be discontinued.

Patients with hepatic dysfunction should be monitored closely for signs of CNS toxicity because of the apparent large first pass biotransformation.

Information for Patients: Patients should be advised to check with their physician if their diarrhea does not improve after a couple of days or if they note blood in their stools or develop a fever.

Drug Interactions: There was no evidence in clinical trials of drug interactions with concurrent medications.

Carcinogensis, Mutagenesis, Impairment of Fertility: In an 18-month rat study with doses up to 133 times the maximum human dose (on a mg/kg basis), there was no evidence of carcinogenesis. Mutagenicity studies were not conducted. Reproduction studies in rats indicated that high doses (150-200 times the human dose) could cause marked female infertility and reduced male fertility.

PREGNANCY

Teratogenic Effects: Pregnancy Category B: Reproduction studies in rats and rabbits have revealed no evidence of impaired fertility or harm to the fetus at doses up to 30 times the human dose. Higher doses impaired the survival of mothers and nursing young. The studies offered no evidence of teratogenic activity. There are, however, no adequate and well controlled studies in pregnant women. Because animal reproduction studies are not always predictive of human response, this drug should be used during pregnancy only if clearly needed.

Nursing Mothers: It is not known whether this drug is excreted in human milk. Because many drugs are excreted in human milk, caution should be exercised when Loperamide Hydrochloride is administered to a nursing woman.

Pediatric Use: See the *"Warnings"* section for information on the greater variability of response in this age group.

In case of accidental overdosage of Loperamide Hydrochloride by children, see *"Overdosage"* section for suggested treatment.

ADVERSE REACTIONS

The adverse effects reported during clinical investigations of Loperamide Hydrochloride are difficult to distinguish from symptoms associated with the diarrheal syndrome. Adverse experiences recorded during clinical studies with Loperamide Hydrochloride were generally of a minor and self-limiting nature. They were more commonly observed during the treatment of chronic diarrhea.

The following patient complaints have been reported and are listed in decreasing order of frequency with the exception of hypersensitivity reactions which is listed first since it may be the most serious.

■ Hypersensitivity reactions (including skin rash) have been reported with Loperamide Hydrochloride use.
■ Abdominal pain, distention or discomfort
■ Nausea and vomiting
■ Constipation
■ Tiredness
■ Drowsiness or dizziness
■ Dry mouth

In postmarketing experiences, there have been rare reports of paralytic ileus associated with abdominal distention. Most of these reports occurred in the setting of acute dysentery, overdose, and with very young children of less than two years of age.

DRUG ABUSE AND DEPENDENCE

Abuse: A specific clinical study designed to assess the abuse potential of Loperamide at high doses resulted in a finding of extremely low abuse potential.

Dependence: Studies in morphine-dependent monkeys demonstrated that Loperamide Hydrochloride at doses above those recommended for humans prevented signs of morphine withdrawal. However, in humans, the naloxone challenge pupil test, which when positive indicates opiate-like effects, performed after a single high dose, or after more than two years of therapeutic use of Loperamide Hydrochloride was negative. Orally administered Loperamide Hydrochloride is both highly insoluble and penetrates the CNS poorly.

OVERDOSAGE

In case of overdosage, paralytic ileus and CNS depression may occur. Children may be more sensitive to CNS effects than adults. Clinical trials have demonstrated that a slurry of activated charcoal administered promptly after ingestion of Loperamide Hydrochloride can reduce the amount of drug which is absorbed into the systemic circulation by as much as ninefold. If vomiting occurs spontaneously upon ingestion, a slurry of 100 gms of activated charcoal should be administered orally as soon as fluids can be retained.

If vomiting has not occurred, gastric lavage should be performed followed by administration of 100 gms of the activated charcoal slurry through the gastric tube. In the event of overdosage, patients should be monitored for signs of CNS depression for at least 24 hours. Children may be more sensitive to central nervous system effects than adults. If CNS depression is observed, naloxone may be administered. If responsive to naloxone, vital signs must be monitored carefully for recurrence of symptoms of drug overdose for at least 24 hours after the last dose of naloxone.

In view of the prolonged action of Loperamide and the short duration (one to three hours) of naloxone, the patient must be monitored closely and treated repeatedly with naloxone as indicated. Since relatively little drug is excreted in the urine, forced diuresis is not expected to be effective for Loperamide Hydrochloride overdosage.

In clinical trials an adult who took three 20 mg doses within a 24 hour period was nauseated after the second dose and vomited after the third dose. In studies designed to examine the potential for side effects, intentional ingestion of up to 60 mg of Loperamide Hydrochloride in a single dose to healthy subjects resulted in no significant adverse effects.

DOSAGE AND ADMINISTRATION

Patients should receive appropriate fluid and electrolyte replacement as needed.
(1 capsule = 2 mg)

ACUTE DIARRHEA

Adults: The recommended initial dose is 4 mg (two capsules) followed by 2 mg (one capsule) after each unformed stool. Daily dosage should not exceed 16 mg (eight capsules).

Children: Loperamide Hydrochloride use is not recommended for children under 2 years of age. In children 2 to 5 years of age (20 kg or less), the non-prescription liquid formulation should be used: for ages 6 to 12, either Loperamide Hydrochloride capsules or Loperamide Hydrochloride liquid may be used. For children 2 to 12 years of age, the following schedule for capsules or liquid will usually fulfill initial dosage requirements:

Recommended First Day Dosage Schedule

Two to five years:	1 mg t.i.d.
(13 to 20 kg)	(3 mg daily dose)
Six to eight years:	2 mg b.i.d.
(20 to 30 kg)	(4 mg daily dose)
Eight to twelve years:	2 mg t.i.d.
(greater than 30 kg)	(6 mg daily dose)

Recommended Subsequent Daily Dosage

Following the first treatment day, it is recommended that subsequent Loperamide Hydrochloride doses (1 mg/10 kg body weight) be administered only after a loose stool. Total daily dosage should not exceed recommended dosages for the first day.

CHRONIC DIARRHEA

Children: Although Loperamide Hydrochloride has been studied in a limited number of children with chronic diarrhea, the therapeutic dose for the treatment of chronic diarrhea in a pediatric population has not been established.

Adults: The recommended initial dose is 4 mg (two capsules) followed by 2 mg (one capsule) after each unformed stool until diarrhea is controlled, after which the dosage of Loperamide Hydrochloride should be reduced to meet individual requirements. When the optimal daily dosage has been established, this amount may then be administered as a single dose or in divided doses.

The average daily maintenance dosage in clinical trials was 4 to 8 mg (two to four capsules). A dosage of 16 mg (eight capsules) was rarely exceeded. If clinical improvement is not observed after treatment with 16 mg per day for at least 10 days, symptoms are unlikely to be controlled by further administration. Loperamide Hydrochloride administration may be continued if diarrhea cannot be adequately controlled with diet or specific treatment.

➤ SHOWN IN PRODUCT IDENTIFICATION GUIDE

Storage: Store at controlled room temperature, 15°-30°C (59°-86°F)

HOW SUPPLIED
CAPSULE: 2 MG

AVERAGE UNIT PRICE (AVAILABLE SIZES)

		GENERIC A-RATED AVERAGE PRICE (GAAP)	
BRAND	$0.71		
GENERIC	$0.55	100s	$55.32
HCFA FUL (100s ea)	$0.35	500s	$271.97

BRAND/MANUFACTURER	NDC	SIZE	AWP
◆ BRAND			
IMODIUM: Janssen	50458-0400-10	100s	$68.32
	50458-0400-01	100s ud	$76.27
	50458-0400-50	500s	$334.02
◆ GENERICS			
Roxane	00054-2537-25	100s	$37.32
Goldline	00182-1505-01	100s	$52.00
Geneva	00781-2761-01	100s	$54.50
Rugby	00536-3974-01	100s	$54.90
Major	00904-7617-60	100s	$55.10
Novopharm	55953-0020-40	100s	$55.67
URL	00677-1422-01	100s	$55.70
Moore,H.L.	00839-7623-06	100s	$55.74
Schein	00364-2481-01	100s	$55.75
Martec	52555-0519-01	100s	$56.78
Lemmon	00093-0311-01	100s	$57.00
Mylan	00378-2100-01	100s	$57.96
Qualitest	00603-4235-21	100s	$57.96
Aligen	00405-4592-01	100s	$58.60
Du Pont Multi	00056-0200-70	100s	$60.00
Mason Dist	11845-0473-01	100s	$64.97
Roxane	00054-8537-25	100s ud	$39.02
Vangard	00615-0362-13	100s ud	$60.65
UDL	51079-0690-20	100s ud	$61.46
Novopharm	55953-0020-01	100s ud	$62.17
Roxane	00054-2537-29	500s	$176.43
Rugby	00536-3974-05	500s	$266.47
Major	00904-7617-40	500s	$267.10
Novopharm	55953-0020-70	500s	$277.67
Moore,H.L.	00839-7623-12	500s	$277.76
Lemmon	00093-0311-05	500s	$278.50
URL	00677-1422-05	500s	$283.34
Mylan	00378-2100-05	500s	$283.39
Du Pont Multi	00056-0200-85	500s	$290.00
Aligen	00405-4592-02	500s	$292.28
Mason Dist	11845-0473-03	500s	$298.73
Novopharm	55953-0020-80	1000s	$516.17

SOLUTION: 1 MG/5 ML

BRAND/MANUFACTURER	NDC	SIZE	AWP
◆ GENERICS			
Rugby	00536-1610-96	60 ml	$3.30

Lopid *SEE* GEMFIBROZIL

Lopressor *SEE* METOPROLOL

Lopressor HCT *SEE* HYDROCHLOROTHIAZIDE WITH METOPROLOL TARTRATE

Loprox *SEE* CICLOPIROX OLAMINE

Lorabid *SEE* LORACARBEF

Loracarbef

DESCRIPTION

Loracarbef is a synthetic β-lactam antibiotic of the carbacephem class for oral administration. Chemically, carbacephems differ from cephalosporin-class antibiotics in the dihydrothiazine ring where a methylene group has been substituted for a sulfur atom.

The chemical name for Loracarbef is (6R, 7S)-7-[(R)-2-amino-2-phenylacetamino]-3-chloro-8-oxo-1- azabicyclo[4.2.0] oct-2-ene-2-carboxylic acid, monohydrate. It is a white to off-white crystalline compound with a molecular weight of 367.8. The empirical formula is $C_{16}O_4N_3H_{16}Cl.H_2O$.

Loracarbef Pulvules® and Loracarbef for Oral Suspension are intended for oral administration only.

Each pulvule contains Loracarbef equivalent to 200 mg (0.57 mmol) anhydrous loracarbef activity.

After reconstitution, each 5 mL of Loracarbef for Oral Suspension contains Loracarbef equivalent to 100 mg (0.286 mmol) or 200 mg (0.57 mmol) anhydrous Loracarbef activity.

Following is its chemical structure:

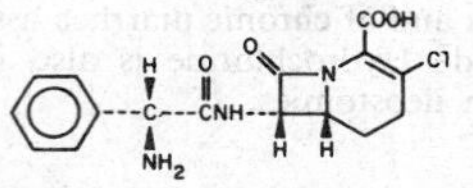

CLINICAL PHARMACOLOGY

Loracarbef, after oral administration, was approximately 90% absorbed from the gastrointestinal tract. When capsules were taken with food, peak plasma concentrations were 50% to 60% of those achieved when the drug was administered to fasting subjects and occurred from 30 to 60 minutes later. Total absorption, as measured by urinary recovery and area under the plasma concentration versus time curve (AUC), was unchanged. The effect of food on the rate and extent of absorption of the suspension formulation has not been studied to date.

The pharmacokinetics of Loracarbef were linear over the recommended dosage range of 200 to 400 mg, with no accumulation of the drug noted when it was given twice daily. Average peak plasma concentrations after administration of 200-mg or 400-mg single doses of Loracarbef as capsules to fasting subjects were approximately 8 and 14 µg/mL, respectively, and were obtained within 1.2 hours after dosing. The average peak plasma concentration in adults following a 400-mg single dose of suspension was 17 µg/mL and was obtained within 0.8 hour after dosing (see *"Table"*).

Dosage (mg)	*Mean Plasma Loracarbef Concentrations (µg/mL)*	
	Peak Cmax	*Time to Peak (Tmax)*
Capsule (single dose)		
200 mg	8	1.2 h
400 mg	14	1.2 h
Suspension (single dose)		
400 mg (adult)	17	0.8 h
7.5 mg/kg (pediatric)	13	0.8 h
15 mg/kg (pediatric)	19	0.8 h

Following administration of 7.5 and 15 mg/kg single doses of oral suspension to children, average peak plasma concentrations were 13 and 19 µg/mL, respectively, and were obtained within 40 to 60 minutes.

This increased rate of absorption (suspension > capsule) should be taken into consideration if the oral suspension is to be substituted for the capsule, and capsules should not be substituted for the oral suspension in the treatment of otitis media (see *"Dosage and Administration"*).

The elimination half-life was an average of 1.0 h in patients with normal renal function. Concomitant administration of probenecid decreased the rate of urinary excretion and increased the half-life to 1.5 hours.

In subjects with moderate impairment of renal function (creatinine clearance 10 to 50 mL/min/1.73 m²), following a single 400-mg dose, the plasma half-life was prolonged to approximately 5.6 hours. In subjects with severe renal impairment (creatinine clearance < 10 mL/min/1.73 m²), the half-life was increased to approximately 32 hours. During hemodialysis the half-life was approximately 4 hours. In patients with severe renal impairment, the C_{max} increased from 15.4 µg/mL to 23 µg/mL (see *"Precautions"* and *"Dosage and Administration"*).

In single-dose studies, plasma half-life and AUC were not significantly altered in healthy elderly subjects with normal renal function.

There is no evidence of metabolism of Loracarbef in humans. Approximately 25% of circulating Loracarbef is bound to plasma proteins.

Middle-ear fluid concentrations of Loracarbef were approximately 48% of the plasma concentration 2 hours after drug administration in children. The peak concentration of Loracarbef in blister fluid was approximately half that obtained in plasma. Adequate data on CSF levels of Loracarbef are not available.

Microbiology: Loracarbef exerts its bactericidal action by binding to essential target proteins of the bacterial cell wall, leading to inhibition of cell-wall synthesis. It is stable in the presence of some bacterial β-lactamases. Loracarbef has been shown to be active against most strains of the following organisms both *in vitro* and in clinical infections (see *"Indications"* and *"Usage"*):

GRAM-POSITIVE AEROBES:
Staphylococcus aureus (including penicillinase-producing strains)

Note: Loracarbef (like most β-lactam antimicrobials) is inactive against methicillin-resistant staphylococci.
Staphylococcus saprophyticus
Streptococcus pneumoniae
Streptococcus pyogenes

◆ RATED THERAPEUTICALLY EQUIVALENT; ◇ THERAPEUTIC EQUIVALENCE UNCONFIRMED; ○ UNRATED

GRAM-NEGATIVE AEROBES:
Escherichia coli
Haemophilus influenzae (including β-lactamase-producing strains)
Moraxella (Branhamella) catarrhalis (including β-lactamase-producing strains)
The following *in vitro* data are available; *however, their clinical significance is unknown.*

Loracarbef exhibits *in vitro* minimum inhibitory concentrations (MIC) of 8 µg/mL or less against most strains of the following organisms; however, the safety and efficacy of Loracarbef in treating clinical infections due to these organisms have not been established in adequate and well-controlled trials.

GRAM-POSITIVE AEROBES:
Staphylococcus epidermidis
Streptococcus agalactiae (group B streptococci)
Streptococcus bovis
Streptococci, groups C, F, and G
viridans group streptococci

GRAM-NEGATIVE AEROBES:
Citrobacter diversus
Haemophilus parainfluenzae
Neisseria gonorrhoeae (including penicillinase-producing strains)
Pasteurella multocida
Proteus mirabilis
Salmonella species
Shigella species
Yersinia enterocolitica

Note: Loracarbef is inactive against most strains of *Acinetobacter, Enterobacter, Morganella morganii, Proteus vulgaris, Providencia, Pseudomonas,* and *Serratia.*

ANAEROBIC ORGANISMS
Clostridium perfringens
Fusobacterium necrophorum
Peptococcus niger
Peptostreptococcus intermedius
Propionibacterium acnes

SUSCEPTIBILITY TESTING
Diffusion Techniques: Quantitative methods that require measurement of zone diameters give the most precise estimate of the susceptibility of bacteria to antimicrobial agents. One such standardized method[1] has been recommended for use with the 30-µg Loracarbef disk. Interpretation involves the correlation of the diameter obtained in the disk test with MIC for Loracarbef.

Reports from the laboratory giving results of the standard single-disk susceptibility test with a 30-µg Loracarbef disk should be interpreted according to the following criteria:

Zone Diameter (mm)	Interpretation
≥ 18	(S) Susceptible
15-17	(MS) Moderately Susceptible
≤ 14	(R) Resistant

A report of "susceptible" implies that the pathogen is likely to be inhibited by generally achievable blood concentrations.

A report of "moderately susceptible" indicates that inhibitory concentrations of the antibiotic may be achieved if high dosage is used or if the infection is confined to tissues and fluids (eg, urine) in which high antibiotic concentrations are attained. A report of "resistant" indicates that achievable concentrations of the antibiotic are unlikely to be inhibitory and other therapy should be selected.

Standardized procedures require the use of laboratory control organisms. The 30-µg Loracarbef disk should give the following zone diameters with the NCCLS approved procedure:

Organism	Zone Diameter (mm)
E. coli ATCC 25922	23-29
S. aureus ATCC 25923	23-31

Dilution Techniques: Use a standardized dilution method[2] (broth, agar, or microdilution) or equivalent with Loracarbef powder. The MIC values obtained should be interpreted according to the following criteria:

MIC (µg/mL)	Interpretation
≤ 8	(S) Susceptible
16	(MS) Moderately Susceptible
≥ 32	(R) Resistant

As with standard diffusion methods, dilution procedures require the use of laboratory control organisms. Standard Loracarbef powder should give the following MIC values with the NCCLS approved procedure:

Organism	MIC Range (µg/mL)
E. coli ATCC 25922	0.5-2
S. aureus ATCC 29213	0.5-2

INDICATIONS AND USAGE
Loracarbef is indicated in the treatment of patients with mild to moderate infections caused by susceptible strains of the designated microorganisms in the conditions listed below. (As recommended dosages, durations of therapy, and applicable patient populations vary among these infections, please (see "Dosage and Administration") for specific recommendations.)

LOWER RESPIRATORY TRACT
Secondary Bacterial Infection of Acute Bronchitis caused by *S. pneumoniae, H. influenzae* (including β-lactamase-producing strains), or *M. catarrhalis* (including β-lactamase-producing strains).

Acute Bacterial Exacerbations of Chronic Bronchitis caused by *S. pneumoniae, H. influenzae* (including β-lactamase-producing strains), or *M. catarrhalis* (including β-lactamase-producing strains).

Pneumonia caused by *S. pneumoniae* or *H. influenzae* (non-β-lactamase-producing strains only). Data are insufficient at this time to establish efficacy in patients with pneumonia caused by β-lactamase-producing strains of *H. influenzae.*

UPPER RESPIRATORY TRACT
Otitis Media† caused by *S. pneumoniae, H. influenzae* (including β-lactamase-producing strains), *M. catarrhalis* (including β-lactamase-producing strains), or *S. pyogenes.*

Acute Maxillary Sinusitis† caused by *S. pneumoniae, H. influenzae* (non β-lactamase-producing strains only), or *M. catarrhalis* (including β-lactamase-producing strains). Data are insufficient at this time to establish efficacy in patients with acute maxillary sinusitis caused by β-lactamase-producing strains of *H. influenzae.*

†Note: In a patient population with significant numbers of β-lactamase-producing organisms, Loracarbef's clinical cure and bacteriological eradication rates were somewhat less than those observed with a product containing a β-lactamase inhibitor. Loracazbef's decreased potential for toxicity compared to products containing β-lactamase inhibitors along with the susceptibility patterns of the common microbes in a given geographic area should be taken into account when considering the use of an antimicrobial (see "Clinical Studies" section).

Pharyngitis and Tonsillitis caused by *S. pyogenes.* (The usual drug of choice in the treatment and prevention of streptococal infections, including the prophylaxis of rheumatic fever, is penicillin administered by the intramuscular route. Loracarbef is generally effective in the eradication of *S. pyogenes* from the nasopharynx; however, data establishing the efficacy of Loracarbef in the subsequent prevention of rheumatic fever are not available at present.)

SKIN AND SKIN STRUCTURE
Uncomplicated Skin and Skin Structure Infections caused by *S. aureus* (including penicillinase-producing strains) or *S. pyogenes.* Abscesses should be surgically drained as clinical indicated.

URINARY TRACT
Uncomplicated Urinary Tract Infections (cystitis) caused by *E. coli* or *S. saprophyticus.**

Note: In considering the use of Loracarbef in the treatment of cystitis, Loracarbef's lower bacterial eradication rates and lower potential for toxicity should be weighted against the increased eradication rates and increased potential for toxicity demonstrated by some other classes of approved agents (see "Clinical Studies" section).

Uncomplicated Pyelonephritis caused by *E. coli*
* Although treatment of infections due to this organism in this organ system demonstrated a clinically acceptable overall outcome, efficacy was studied in fewer than 10 infections.

Culture and sesceptibility testing should be performed when appropriate to determine the causative organism and its susceptibility to Loracarbef. Therapy may be started while awaiting the results of these studies. Once these results become available, antimicrobial therapy should be adjusted accordingly.

CONTRAINDICATION
Loracarbef is contraindicated in patients with known allergy to Loracarbef or cephalosporin-class antibiotics.

WARNINGS
BEFORE THERAPY WITH LORACARBEF IS INSTITUTED, CAREFUL INQUIRY SHOULD BE MADE TO DETERMINE WHETHER THE PATIENT HAS HAD PREVIOUS HYPERSENSITIVITY REACTIONS TO LORACARBEF, CEPHALOSPORINS, PENICILLINS, OR OTHER DRUGS. IF THIS PRODUCT IS TO BE GIVEN TO PENICILLIN-SENSITIVE PATIENTS, CAUTION SHOULD BE EXERCISED BECAUSE CROSS-HYPERSENSITIVITY AMONG β-LACTAM ANTIBIOTICS HAS BEEN CLEARLY DOCUMENTED AND MAY OCCUR IN UP TO 10% OF PATIENTS WITH A HISTORY OF PENCILLIN ALLERGY. IF AN ALLERGIC REACTION TO LORACARBEF OCCURS, DISCONTINUE THE DRUG. SERIOUS ACUTE HYPERSENSITIVITY REACTIONS MAY REQUIRE THE USE OF EPINEPHRINE AND OTHER EMERGENCY MEASURES, INCLUDING OXYGEN, INTRAVENOUS FLUIDS, INTRAVENOUS ANTIHISTAMINES. CORTICOSTEROIDS, PRESSOR AMINES, AND AIRWAY MANAGEMENT, AS CLINICALLY INDICATED.

Pseudomembranous colitis has been reported with nearly all antibacterial agents and may range from mild to life-threatening. Therefore, it is important to consider this diagnosis in patients who present with diarrhea subsequent to the administration of antibacterial agents.

Treatment with broad-spectrum antibiotics alters the normal flora of the colon and may permit overgrowth of clostridia. Studies indicate that a toxin produced by *Clostridium difficile* is a primary cause of "antibiotic-associated colitis."

After the diagnosis of pseudomembranous colitis has been established, therapeutic measures should be initiated. Mild cases of pseudomembranous colitis usually respond to discontinuation of drug alone. In moderate to severe cases, consideration should be given to management with fluids and electrolytes, protein supplementation, and treatment with an antibacterial drug effective against *C. difficile*-associated colitis.

PRECAUTIONS

General: In patients with known or suspected renal impairment (see *"Dosage and Administration"*), careful clinical observation and appropriate laboratory studies should be performed prior to and during therapy. The total daily dose of Loracarbef should be reduced in these patients because high and/or prolonged plasma antibiotic concentrations can occur in such individuals administered the usual doses. Loracarbef, like cephalosporins, should be given with caution to patients receiving concurrent treatment with potent diuretics because these diuretics are suspected of adversely affecting renal function.

As with other broad-spectrum antimicrobials, prolonged use of Loracarbef may result in the overgrowth of nonsusceptible organisms. Careful observation of the patient is essential. If superinfection occurs during therapy, appropriate measures should be taken.

Loracarbef, as with other broad-spectrum antimicrobials, should be prescribed with caution in individuals with a history of colitis.

Information for Patients: Loracarbef should be taken either at least 1 hour prior to eating or at least 2 hours after eating a meal.

Drug Interactions: Probenecid: As with other β-lactam antibiotics, renal excretion of Loracarbef is inhibited by probenecid and resulted in an approximate 80% increase in the AUC for Loracarbef (See *"Clinical Pharmacology"*).

Carcinogenesis, Mutagenesis, Impairment of Fertility: Although lifetime studies in animals have not been performed to evaluate carcinogenic potential, no mutagenic potential was found for Loracarbef in standard tests of genotoxicity, which included bacterial mutation tests and *in vitro* and *in vivo* mammalian systems. In rats, fertility and reproductive performance were not affected by Loracarbef at doses up to 33 times the maximum human exposure in mg/kg (10 times the exposure based on mg/m^2).

Usage in Pregnancy—Pregnancy Category B: Reproduction studies have been performed in mice, rats, and rabbits at doses up to 33 times the maximum human exposure in mg/kg (4, 10, and 4 times the exposure, respectively, based on mg/m^2) and have revealed no evidence of impaired fertility or harm to the fetus due to Loracarbef. There are, however, no adequate and well-controlled studies in pregnant women. Because animal reproduction studies are not always predictive of human response, this drug should be used during pregnancy only if clearly needed.

Labor and Delivery Lozacarbef has not been studied for use during labor and delivery. Treatment should be given only if clearly needed.

Nursing Mothers: It is not known whether this drug is excreted in human milk. Because many drugs are excreted in human milk, caution should be exercised when Loracarbef is administered to a nursing woman.

Pediatric Use: Efficacy and safety in infants less than 6 months of age have not been established.

Geriatric Use: Healthy geriatric volunteers (≥ 65 years old) with normal renal function who received a single 400-mg dose of Loracarbef had no significant differences in AUC or clearance when compared to healthy adult volunteers 20 to 40 years of age. In clinical studies, when geriatric patients received the usual recommended adult doses, clinical efficacy and safety were comparable to results in nongeriatric adult patients. Because significant numbers of elderly patients have decreased renal function, evaluation of renal function in this population is recommended (see *"Dosage and Administration"*).

ADVERSE REACTIONS

The nature of adverse reactions to Loracarbef are similar to those observed with orally administered β-lactam antimicrobials. The majority of adverse reactions observed in clinical trials were of a mild and transient nature: 1.5% of patients discontinued therapy because of drug-related adverse reactions. No one reaction requiring discontinuation accounted for > 0.03% of the total patient population; however, of those reactions resulting in discontinuation, gastrointestinal events (diarrhea and abdominal pain) and skin rashes predominated.

ALL PATIENTS

The following adverse events, irrespective of relationship to drug, have been reported following the use of Loracarbef in clinical trials. Incidence rates (combined for all dosing regimens and dosage forms) were less than 1% for the total patient population, except as otherwise noted:

Gastrointestinal: The most commonly observed adverse reactions were related to the gastrointestinal system. The incidence of gastrointestinal adverse reactions increased in patients treated with higher doses. Individual event rates included diarrhea, 4.1%; nausea, 1.9%; vomiting, 1.4%; abdominal pain, 1.4%; and anorexia.

Hypersensitivity: Hypersensitivity reactions including, skin rashes (1.2%), urticaria, pruritus, and erythema multiforme.

Central Nervous System: Headache (2.9%), somnolence, nervousness, insomnia, and dizziness.

Hemic and Lymphatic Systems: Transient thrombocytopenia, leukopenia, and eosinophilia.

Hepatic: Transient elevations in AST(SGOT), ALT(SGPT), and alkaline phosphatase.

Renal: Transient elevations in BUN and creatinine.

Cardiovascular System: Vasodilatation.

Genitourinary: Vaginitis (1.3%), vaginal moniliasis (1.1%).

PEDIATRIC PATIENTS

The incidences of several adverse events, irrespective of relationship to drug, following treatment with Loracarbef were significantly different in the pediatric population and the adult population as follows:

Event	Pediatric	Adult
Diarrhea	5.8%	3.6%
Headache	0.9%	3.2%
Rhinitis	6.3%	1.6%
Nausea	0.0%	2.5%
Rash	2.9%	0.7%
Vomiting	3.3%	0.5%
Somnolence	2.1%	0.4%
Anorexia	2.3%	0.3%

β-LACTAM ANTIMICROBIAL CLASS LABELING:

Although not observed in patients treated with Loracarbef in clinical trials, the following adverse reactions and altered laboratory test results have been reported in patients treated with β-lactam antibiotics:

Adverse Reactions: Allergic reactions including anaphylaxis, Stevens-Johnson syndrome, serum sickness-like reactions, aplastic anemia, hemolytic anemia, hemorrhage, agranulocytosis, toxic epidermal necrolysis, renal dysfunction, toxic nephropathy, and hepatic dysfunction including cholestasis.

Several β-lactam antibiotics have been implicated in triggering seizures, particularly in patients with renal impairment when the dosage was not reduced. If seizures associated with drug therapy should occur, the drug should be discontinued. Anticonvulsant therapy can be given if clinically indicated.

Altered Laboratory Tests: Increased prothrombin time, positive direct Coombs' test, elevated LDH, pancytopenia, and neutropenia.

OVERDOSAGE

Signs and Symptoms: The toxic symptoms following an overdose of β-lactams may include nausea, vomiting, epigastric distress, and diarrhea.

Loracarbef is eliminated primarily by the kidneys. Forced diuresis, peritoneal dialysis, hemodialysis, or hemoperfusion have not been established as beneficial for an overdose of Loracarbef. Hemodialysis has been shown to be effective in hastening the elimination of Loracarbef from plasma in patients with chronic renal failure.

DOSAGE AND ADMINISTRATION

Loracarbef is administered orally either at least 1 hour prior to eating or at least 2 hours after eating. The recommended dosages, durations of treatment, and applicable patient populations are described in the following chart:

Population/Infection	Dosage (mg)	Duration (days)
ADULTS (13 YEARS AND OLDER)		
Lower Respiratory Tract		
Secondary Bacterial Infection of Acute Bronchitis	200-400 q12h	7
Acute Bacterial Exacerbation of Chronic Bronchitis	400 q12h	7
Pneumonia	400 q12h	14
Upper Respiratory Tract		
Pharyngitis/Tonsillitis	200 q12h	10*
Sinusitis	400 q12h	10
(See *"Clinical Studies"* and *"Indications and Usage"* for further information.)		
Skin and Skin Structure		
Uncomplicated Skin and Skin Structure Infections	200 q12h	7
Urinary Tract		
Uncomplicated cystitis	200 q24h	7
(See *"Clinical Studies"* and *"Indications and Usage"*.)		
Uncomplicated pyelonephritis	400 q12h	14
INFANTS AND CHILDREN (6 MONTHS TO 12 YEARS)		
Upper Respiratory Tract		
Acute Otitis Media**	30 mg/kg/day in divided doses q12h	10

◆ RATED THERAPEUTICALLY EQUIVALENT; ◇ THERAPEUTIC EQUIVALENCE UNCONFIRMED; ○ UNRATED

Population/Infection	Dosage (mg)	Duration (days)
(See "Clinical Studies" and "Indications and Usage" for further information.)		
Pharyngitis/Tonsillitis	15 mg/kg/day in divided doses q12h	10
Skin and Skin Structure Impetigo	15 mg/kg/day in divided doses q12h	7

* *In the treatment of infections due to S. pyogenes, Loracarbef should be administered for at least 10 days.*

** *Otitis media should be treated with the suspension. Clinical studies of otitis media were conducted with the suspension formulation only. The suspension is more rapidly absorbed than the capsules, resulting in higher peak plasma concentrations when administered at the same dose. Therefore, the capsule should not be substituted for the suspension in the treatment of otitis media (see "Clinical Pharmacology").*

PEDIATRIC DOSAGE CHART FOR LORACARBEF
DAILY DOSE 15 mg/kg/day

Weight		100 mg/5 mL Suspension		200 mg/5 mL Suspension	
		Dose given twice daily		Dose given twice daily	
lb	kg	mL	tsp	mL	tsp
15	7	2.6	0.5	—	—
29	13	4.9	1.0	2.5	0.5
44	20	7.5	1.5	3.8	0.75
57	26	9.8	2.0	4.9	1.0

PEDIATRIC DOSAGE CHART
DAILY DOSE 30 mg/kg/day

Weight		100 mg/5 mL Suspension		200 mg/5 mL Suspension	
		Dose given twice daily		Dose given twice daily	
lb	kg	mL	tsp	mL	tsp
15	7	5.2	1.0	2.6	0.5
29	13	9.8	2.0	4.9	1.0
44	20	—	—	7.5	1.5
57	26	—	—	9.8	2.0

Renal Impairment: Loracarbef may be administered to patients with impaired renal function. The usual dose and schedule may be employed in patients with creatinine clearance levels of 50 mL/min or greater. Patients with creatinine clearance between 10 and 49 mL/min may be given half of the recommended dose at the usual dosage interval, or the normal recommended dose at twice the usual dosage interval. Patients with creatinine clearance levels less than 10 mL/min may be treated with the recommended dose given every 3 to 5 days; patients on hemodialysis should receive another dose following dialysis.

When only the serum creatinine is available, the following formula (based on sex, weight, and age of the patient) may be used to convert this value into creatinine clearance (CL_{cr}, mL/min). The equation assumes the patient's renal function is stable.

$$\text{Males} = \frac{(\text{weight in kg}) \times (140 - \text{age})}{(72) \times \text{serum creatinine (mg/100 mL)}}$$

Females = $(0.85) \times$ (above value)

RECONSTITUTION DIRECTIONS FOR ORAL SUSPENSION

Bottle Size	Reconstitution Directions
100 mL	Add 60 mL of water in 2 portions to the dry mixture in the bottle. Shake well after each addition.
50 mL	Add 30 mL of water in 2 portions to the dry mixture in the bottle. Shake well after each addition.

After mixing, the suspension may be kept at room temperature, 59° to 86°F (15° to 30°C), for 14 days without significant loss of potency. Keep tightly closed. Discard unused portion after 14 days.

CLINICAL STUDIES
US ACUTE OTITIS MEDIA STUDY
LORACARBEF (L) VS β-LACTAMASE INHIBITOR-CONTAINING CONTROL DRUG (C)
Efficacy: In a controlled study of acute otitis media performed in the United States where significant rates of β-lactamase-producing organisms were found, Loracarbef was compared to an oral antimicrobial agent that contained a specific β-lactamase inhibitor. In this study, using very strict evaluability criteria and microbiologic and clinical response criteria at the 10-to 16-day posttherapy

follow-up, the following presumptive bacterial eradication/clinical cure outcomes (ie, clinical success) and safety results were obtained:

Pathogen	% of Cases with Pathogens (n = 204)	Success Rate
S. pneumoniae	42.6%	L equivalent to C
H. influenzae	30.4%	L 9% less than C
M. catarrhalis	20.6%	L 19% less than C
S. pyogenes	6.4%	L equivalent to C
Overall	100.0%	L 12% less than C

Safety: The incidences of the following adverse events were clinically and statistically significantly higher in the control arm versus the Loracarbef arm.

Event	Loracarbef	Control
Diarrhea	15%	26%
Rash*	8%	15%

* *The majority of these involved the diaper area in young children.*

EUROPEAN ACUTE OTITIS MEDIA STUDY
LORACARBEF (L) VS AMOXICILLIN (A)
Efficacy: In a controlled clinical study of acute otitis media performed in Europe, Loracarbef was compared to amoxicillin. As expected in a European population, this study population had a lower incidence of β-lactamase-producing organisms than usually seen in US trials. In this study, using very strict evaluability criteria and microbiologic and clinical response criteria at the 10- to 16-day posttherapy follow-up, the following presumptive bacterial eradication/clinical cure outcomes (ie, clinical success) were obtained:

Pathogen	% of Cases With Pathogens (n = 291)	Success Rate
S. pneumoniae	51.5%	L equivalent to A
H. influenzae	29.2%	L 14% greater than A
M. catarrhalis	15.8%	L 31% greater than A
S. pyogenes	3.4%	L equivalent to A
Overall	100.0%	L equivalent to A

EUROPEAN ACUTE MAXILLIARY SINUSITIS STUDY
LORACARBEF (L) VS DOXYCYCLINE (D)
Efficacy: In a controlled clinical study of acute maxillary sinusitis performed in Europe, Loracarbef was compared to doxycycline. In this study, there were 210 sinus-puncture evaluable patients. As expected in a European population, this study population had a lower incidence of β-lactamase-producing organisms than usually seen in US trials. In this study, using very strict evaluability criteria and microbiologic and clinical response criteria at the 1- to 2-week post-therapy follow-up, the following presumptive bacterial eradication/clinical cure outcomes (ie, clinical success) were obtained:

Pathogen	% of Cases With Pathogens (n = 210)	Success Rate
S. pneumoniae	47.6%	L equivalent to D
H. influenzae	41.4%	L equivalent to D
M. catarrhalis	11.0%	L equivalent to D
Overall	100.0%	L equivalent to D

US UNCOMPLICATED CYSTITIS STUDY LORACARBEF (L) VS CEFACLOR (C)
Efficacy: In a controlled clinical study of cystitis performed in the United States, Loracarbef was compared to cefaclor. In this study, using very strict evaluability criteria and microbiologic and clinical response criteria at the 5- to 9-day posttherapy follow-up, the following bacterial eradication rates were obtained:

Pathogen	% of Cases With Pathogens (n = 186)	Eradication Rate
E. coli	77.4%	L 4% greater than C (L = 80%)
Other major Enterobacteriaceae	12.5%	L equivalent to C (L = 61%)
S. saprophyticus	3.8%	L equivalent to C

EUROPEAN UNCOMPLICATED CYSTITIS STUDY
LORACARBEF (L) VS QUINOLONE (Q)
Efficacy: In a second controlled clinical study of cystitis, performed in Europe, Loracarbef was compared to an oral quinolone. In this study, using very strict evaluability criteria and microbiologic and clinical response criteria at the 5- to 9-day posttherapy follow-up, the following bacterial eradication rates were obtained:

Pathogen	% of Cases With Pathogens (n = 189)	Eradication Rate
E. coli	82.0%	L 7% less than Q (L = 81%)

Pathogen	% of Cases With Pathogens (n = 189)	Eradication Rate
Other major Enterobacteriaceae	10.1%	L 32% less than Q (L = 50%)

REFERENCES
1. National Committee for Clinical Laboratory Standards, M2-A4 performance standards for antimicrobial disk susceptibility tests, ed 4, Villanova, PA, April, 1990.   2. National Committee for Clinical Laboratory Standards, M7-A2 methods for dilution antimicrobial susceptibility tests for bacteria that grow aerobically, ed 2, Villanova, PA, April, 1990.

HOW SUPPLIED
CAPSULE: 200 MG

BRAND/MANUFACTURER	NDC	SIZE	AWP
○ BRAND			
▶ LORABID PULVULES: Lilly	00002-3170-30	30s	$94.35

CAPSULE: 400 MG

BRAND/MANUFACTURER	NDC	SIZE	AWP
○ BRAND			
▶ LORABID PULVULES: Lilly	00002-3171-30	30s	$113.40

POWDER FOR RECONSTITUTION: 100 MG/5 ML

BRAND/MANUFACTURER	NDC	SIZE	AWP
○ BRAND			
LORABID: Lilly	00002-5135-87	50 ml	$13.66
	00002-5135-48	100 ml	$24.34

POWDER FOR RECONSTITUTION: 200 MG/5 ML

BRAND/MANUFACTURER	NDC	SIZE	AWP
○ BRAND			
LORABID: Lilly	00002-5136-87	50 ml	$22.80
	00002-5136-48	100 ml	$34.94

Loratadine

DESCRIPTION
Loratadine tablets contain 10 mg micronized Loratadine, an antihistamine, to be administered orally.

Loratadine is a white to off-white powder not soluble in water, but very soluble in acetone, alcohol, and chloroform. It has a molecular weight of 382.89, and empirical formula of $C_{22}H_{23}CIN_2O_2$; its chemical name is ethyl 4-(8-chloro-5,6-dihydro-11H-benzo[5,6]cyclohepta[1,2-b]pyridin-11-ylidene)-1-piperidinecarboxylate.

Following is its chemical structure:

CLINICAL PHARMACOLOGY
Loratadine is a long-acting tricyclic antihistamine with selective peripheral histamine H_1-receptor antagonistic activity.

Human histamine skin wheal studies following single and repeated 10 mg oral doses of Loratadine tablets have shown that the drug exhibits an antihistaminic effect beginning within 1 to 3 hours, reaching a maximum at 8 to 12 hours and lasting in excess of 24 hours. There was no evidence of tolerance to this effect after 28 days of dosing with Loratadine tablets.

Pharmacokinetic studies following single and multiple oral doses of Loratadine in 115 volunteers showed that Loratadine tablets are rapidly absorbed and extensively metabolized to an active metabolite (descarboethoxyloratadine). The specific enzyme systems responsible for metabolism have not been identified. Approximately 80% of the total dose administered can be found equally distributed between urine and feces in the form of metabolic products after 10 days. The mean elimination half-lives found in studies in normal adult subjects (n = 54) were 8.4 hours (range = 3 to 20 hours) for Loratadine tablets and 28 hours (range = 8.8 to 92 hours) for the major active metabolite (descarboethoxyloratadine). In nearly all patients, exposure (AUC) to the metabolite is greater than exposure to parent Loratadine.

In a study involving twelve healthy geriatric subjects (66 to 78 years old), the AUC and peak plasma levels (Cmax) of both Loratadine tablets and descarboethoxyloratadine were significantly higher (approximately 50% increased) than in studies of younger subjects. The mean elimination half-lives for the elderly subjects were 18.2 hours (range = 6.7 to 37 hours) for Loratadine tablets and 17.5 hours (range = 11 to 38 hours) for the active metabolite.

Loratadine tablets, dosed once daily, had reached steady-state by the fifth daily dose. The pharmacokinetics of Loratadine tablets and descarboethoxyloratadine are dose independent over the dose range of 10 to 40 mg and are not significantly altered by the duration of treatment.

In the clinical efficacy studies, Loratidine tablets were administered before meals. In a single-dose study, food increased the AUC of Loratadine tablets by approximately 40% and of descarboethoxyloratadine by approximately 15%. The time to peak plasma concentration (Tmax) of Loratadine tablets and descarboethoxyloratadine was delayed by 1 hour with a meal. Although these differences would not be expected to be clinically important Loratadine tablets should be administered on an empty stomach.

In patients with chronic renal impairment (Creatinine Clearance ≤ 30 mL/min) both the AUC and peak plasma levels (Cmax) increased on average by approximately 73% for Loratadine tablets; and approximately by 120% for descarboethoxyloratadine, compared to individuals with normal renal function. The mean elimination half-lives of Loratadine tablets (7.6 hours) and descarboethoxyloratadine (23.9 hours) were not significantly different from that observed in normal subjects. Hemodialysis does not have an effect on the pharmacokinetics of Loratadine tablets or its active metabolite (descarboethyoxyloratadine) in subjects with chronic renal impairment.

In patients with chronic alcoholic liver disease the AUC and peak plasma levels (Cmax) of Loratadine tablets were double white the pharmacokinetic profile of the active metabolite (descarboethoxyloratadine) was not significantly changed from that in normals. The elimination half-lives for Loratadine tablets and descarboethoxyloratadine were 24 hours and 37 hours, respectively, and increased with increasing severity of liver disease.

There was considerable variability in the pharmacokinetic data in all studies of Loratadine tablets, probably due to the extensive first-pass metabolism. Individual histograms of area under the curve, clearance, and volume of distribution showed a log normal distribution with a 25-fold range in distribution in healthy subjects.

Loratadine tablets are about 97% bound to plasma proteins at the expected concentrations (2.5 to 100 ng/mL) after a therapeutic dose. Loratadine tablets do not affect the plasma protein binding of warfarin and digoxin. The metabolite descarboethoxyloratadine is 73% to 77% bound to plasma proteins (at 0.5 to 100 ng/mL).

Whole body autoradiographic studies in rats and monkeys, radiolabeled tissue distribution studies in mice and rats, and in vivo radioligand studies in mice have shown that neither Loratadine nor its metabolites readily cross the blood-brain barrier. Radioligand binding studies with guinea pig pulmonary and brain H_1-receptors indicate that there was preferential binding to peripheral versus central nervous system H_1-receptors.

Clinical trials of Loratadine tablets involved over 10,700 patients who received either Loratadine tablets or another anithistamine and/or placebo in double-blind randomized controlled studies. In placebo-controlled trials, 10 mg once daily of Loratadine tablets was superior to placebo and similar to clemastine (1 mg BID) or terfenadine (60 mg BID) in effects on nasal and non-nasal symptoms of allergic rhinitis. In these studies, somnolence occurred less frequently with Loratadine tablets than with clemastine and at about the same frequency as terfenadine or placebo. In studies with Loratadine tablets at doses 2 to 4 times higher than the recommended dose of 10 mg, a dose-related increase in the incidence of somnolence was observed. Therefore, some patients, particularly those with hepatic or renal impairment and the elderly, may experience somnolence.

In a study in which Loratadine tablets were administered at 4 times the clinical dose for 90 days, no clinically significant increase in the QTc was seen on ECGs.

INDICATIONS AND USAGE
Loratadine tablets are indicated for the relief of nasal and non-nasal symptoms of seasonal allergic rhinitis.

UNLABELED USES
Loratadine is used alone in the treatment of chronic idiopathic urticaria.

CONTRAINDICATIONS
Loratadine tablets are contraindicated in patients who are hypersensitive to this medication or to any of its ingredients.

PRECAUTIONS
General: Patients with liver impairment should be given a lower initial dose (10 mg every other day) because they have reduced clearance of Loratadine tablets.

Drug Interactions: The coadministration of a single 20 mg dose of Loratadine tablets (double the recommended daily dose) and a 200 mg dose of ketoconazole twice daily to 12 subjects resulted in increased plasma concentrations of Loratadine (180% increase in AUC) and its active metabolite, descarboethoxyloratadine (56% increase in AUC). However, no related changes were noted in the QTc on ECGs taken at 2, 6, and 24 hours after the coadministration of Loratadine and ketoconazole. Also, there were no significant differences in clinical adverse events between Loratadine tablet groups with or without ketoconazole.

Other drugs known to inhibit hepatic metabolism should be coadministered with caution until definitive interaction studies can be completed. The number of subjects who concomitantly received macrolide antibiotics, cimetidine, ranitidine, or theophylline along with Loratadine tablets in controlled clinical trials is too small to rule out possible drug-drug interactions. There does not appear to be an increase in adverse events in subjects who received oral contraceptives and Loratadine tablets compared to placebo.

◆ RATED THERAPEUTICALLY EQUIVALENT; ◇ THERAPEUTIC EQUIVALENCE UNCONFIRMED; ○ UNRATED

Carcinogenesis, Mutagenesis, and Impairment of Fertility: In an 18-month oncogenicity study in mice and a 2-year study in rats, Loratadine was administered in the diet at doses up to 40 mg/kg (mice) and 25 mg/kg (rats). In the carcinogenicity studies, pharmacokinetic assessments were carried out to determine animal exposure to the drug. AUC data demonstrated that the exposure of mice given 40 mg/kg of Loratadine was 3.6 (Loratadine) and 18 (active metabolite) times higher than a human given 10 mg/day. Exposure of rats given 25 mg/kg of Loratadine was 28 (Loratadine) and 67 (active metabolite) times higher than a human given 10 mg/day. Male mice given 40 mg/kg had a significantly higher incidence of hepatocellular tumors (combined adenomas and carcinomas) than concurrent controls. In rats, a significantly higher incidence of hepatocellular tumors (combined adenomas and carcinomas) was observed in males given 10 mg/kg and males and females given 25 mg/kg. The clinical significance of these findings during long-term use of Loratadine tablets is not known.

In mutagenicity studies, there was no evidence of mutagenic potential in reverse (AMES) or forward point mutation (CHO-HGPRT) assays, or in the assay for DNA damage (Rat Primary Hepatocyte Unscheduled DNA Assay) or in two assays for chromosomal aberrations (Human Peripheral Blood Lymphocyte Clastogenesis Assay and the Mouse Bone Marrow Erythrocyte Micronucleus Assay). In the Mouse Lymphoma Assay, a positive finding occurred in the nonactivated but not the activated phase of the study.

Loratadine administration produced hepatic microsomal enzyme induction in the mouse at 40 mg/kg and rat at 25 mg/kg, but not at lower doses.

Decreased fertility in male rats, shown by lower female conception rates, occurred at approximately 64 mg/kg and was reversible with cessation of dosing. Loratadine had no effect on male or female fertility or reproduction in the rat at doses of approximately 24 mg/kg.

Pregnancy Category B: There was no evidence of animal teratogenicity in studies performed in rats and rabbits. There are, however, no adequate and well-controlled studies in pregnant women. Because animal reproduction studies are not always predictive of human response, Loratadine tablets should be used during pregnancy only if clearly needed.

Nursing Mothers: Loratadine and its metabolite, descarboethoxyloratadine, pass easily into breast milk and achieve concentrations that are equivalent to plasma levels with an AUC_{milk}/AUC_{plasma} ratio of 1.17 and 0.85 for the parent and active metabolite, respectively. Following a single oral dose of 40 mg, a small amount of Loratadine and metabolite was excreted into the breast milk (approximately 0.03% of 40 mg over 48 hours). A decision should be made whether to discontinue nursing or to discontinue the drug, taking into account the importance of the drug to the mother. Caution should be exercised when Loratadine tablets are administered to a nursing woman.

Pediatric Use: Safety and effectiveness in children below the age of 12 years have not been established.

ADVERSE REACTIONS

Approximately 90,000 patients received Loratadine tablets 10 mg once daily in controlled and uncontrolled studies. Placebo-controlled clinical trials at the recommended dose of 10 mg once a day varied from 2 weeks' to 6 months' duration. The rate of premature withdrawal from these trials was approximately 2% in both the treated and placebo groups.

REPORTED ADVERSE EVENTS WITH AN INCIDENCE OF MORE THAN 2% IN PLACEBO-CONTROLLED ALLERGIC RHINITIS CLINICAL TRIALS PERCENT OF PATIENTS REPORTING

	Loratadine 10 mg QD n = 1926	Placebo n = 2545	Clemastine 1 mg BID n = 536	Terfenadine 60 mg BID n = 684
Headache	12	11	8	8
Somnolence	8	6	22	9
Fatigue	4	3	10	2
Dry Mouth	3	2	4	3

Adverse event rates did not appear to differ significantly based on age, sex, or race, although the number of nonwhite subjects was relatively small.

In addition to those adverse events reported above, the following adverse events have been reported in 2% or fewer patients.

Autonomic Nervous System: Altered salivation, increased sweating, altered lacrimation, hypoesthesia, impotence, thirst, flushing.

Body as a Whole: Conjunctivitis, blurred vision, earache, eye pain, tinnitus, asthenia, weight gain, back pain, leg cramps, malaise, chest pain, rigors, fever, aggravated allergy, upper respiratory infection, angioneurotic edema.

Cardiovascular System: Hypotension, hypertension, palpitations, syncope, tachycardia.

Central and Peripheral Nervous System: Hyperkinesia, blepharospasm, paresthesia, dizziness, migraine, tremor, vertigo, dysphonia.

Gastrointestinal System: Abdominal distress, nausea, vomiting, flatulence, gastritis, constipation, diarrhea, altered taste, increased appetite, anorexia, dyspepsia, stomatitis, toothache.

Musculoskeletal System: Arthralgia, myalgia.

Psychiatric: Anxiety, depression, agitation, insomnia, paroniria, amnesia, impaired concentration, confusion, decreased libido, nervousness.

Reproductive System: Breast pain, menorrhagia, dysmenorrhea, vaginitis.

Respiratory System: Nasal dryness, epistaxis, pharyngitis, dyspnea, nasal congestion, coughing, rhinitis, hemoptysis, sinusitis, sneezing, bronchospasm, bronchitis, laryngitis.

Skin and Appendages: Dermatitis, dry hair, dry skin, urticaria, rash, pruritus, photosensitivity reaction, purpura.

Urinary System: Urinary discoloration, altered micturition. In addition, the following spontaneous adverse events have been reported rarely during the marketing of Loratadine: peripheral edema; abnormal hepatic function including jaundice, hepatitis, and hepatic necrosis; alopecia; seizures; breast enlargement; erythema multiforme; anaphylaxis.

DRUG ABUSE AND DEPENDENCE

There is no information to indicate that abuse or dependency occurs with Loratadine tablets.

OVERDOSAGE

Somnolence, tachycardia, and headache have been reported with overdoses greater than 10 mg (40 to 180 mg). In the event of overdosage, general symptomatic and supportive measures should be instituted promptly and maintained for as long as necessary.

Treatment of overdosage would reasonably consist of emesis (ipecac syrup), except in patients with impaired consciousness, followed by the administration of activated charcoal to absorb any remaining drug. If vomiting is unsuccessful, or contraindicated, gastric lavage should be performed with normal saline. Saline cathartics may also be of value for rapid dilution of bowel contents. Loratadine is not eliminated by hemodialysis. It is not known if Loratadine is eliminated by peritoneal dialysis.

Oral LD_{50} values for Loratadine were greater than 5000 mg/kg in rats and mice. Doses as high as 10 times the recommended clinical doses showed no effects in rats, mice, and monkeys.

DOSAGE AND ADMINISTRATION

Adults and children 12 years of age and over: One 10 mg tablet daily on an empty stomach.

In patients with liver failure, 10 mg every other day should be the starting dose.

Protect Unit-of-Use packaging and Unit Dose-Hospital Pack from excessive moisture. Store between 2° and 30°C (36° and 86°F).

HOW SUPPLIED
TABLETS: 10 MG

BRAND/MANUFACTURER	NDC	SIZE	AWP
○ BRAND			
▶ CLARITIN: Schering	00085-0458-01	14s	$34.32
	00085-0458-05	30s	$55.30
	00085-0458-03	100s	$184.32
	00085-0458-04	100s ud	$184.32
	00085-0458-06	500s	$921.59

Lorazepam

DESCRIPTION

Lorazepam, a benzodiazepine with anti-anxiety and sedative effects, is available as an intramuscular (IM) or intravenous (IV) injection and as tablets for oral administration.

Each ml for injection contains:
Lorazepam .... 2 or 4mg

Each tablet contains:
Lorazepam .... 0.5, 1, or 2 mg

Lorazepam has the chemical formula: 7-chloro-5-(o-chlorophenyl)-1,3-dihydro-3-hydroxy-2 H-1,4-benzodiazepin-2-one. The molecular weight is 321.2.

Lorazepam is a nearly white powder almost insoluble in water.

Following is its chemical structure:

CLINICAL PHARMACOLOGY

Intravenous or intramuscular administration of the recommended dose of 2 mg to 4 mg of Lorazepam to adult patients is followed by dose-related effects of sedation (sleepiness or drowsiness), relief of preoperative anxiety, and lack of recall of events related to the day of surgery in the majority of patients. The clinical sedation (sleepiness or drowsiness) thus noted is such that the majority of patients are able to respond to simple instructions whether they give the appearance of being awake or asleep. The lack of recall is relative rather than absolute, as determined under conditions of careful patient questioning and testing, using props designed to enhance recall. The majority of patients under these reinforced conditions had difficulty recalling perioperative events or recognizing props from before surgery. The lack of recall and recognition was optimum within 2 hours following intramuscular administration and 15 to 20 minutes after intravenous injection.

The intended effects of the recommended adult dose of Lorazepam injection usually last 6 to 8 hours. In rare instances and where patients received greater than the recommended dose, excessive sleepiness and prolonged lack of recall were noted. As with other benzodiazepines, unsteadiness, enhanced sensitivity to CNS-depressant effects of ethyl alcohol and other drugs were noted in isolated and rare cases for greater than 24 hours.

Studies in healthy adult volunteers reveal that IV Lorazepam in doses up to 3.5 mg/70 kg does not alter sensitivity to the respiratory stimulating effect of carbon dioxide and does not enhance the respiratory depressant effects of doses of meperidine up to 100 mg/70 kg (also determined by carbon dioxide challenge) as long as patients remain sufficiently awake to undergo testing. Upper airway obstruction has been observed in rare instances where the patient received greater than the recommended dose and was excessively sleepy and difficult to arouse. (See "Warnings" and "Adverse Reactions".)

Clinically employed doses of Lorazepam injectable do not greatly affect the circulatory system in the supine position or employing a 70-degree tilt test. Doses of 8 mg to 10 mg of intravenous lorazepam (2 to 2 ½ times the maximum recommended dosage) will produce loss of lid reflexes within 15 minutes.

Studies in six (6) healthy young adults who received Lorazepam injection and no other drugs revealed that visual tracking (the ability to keep a moving line centered) was impaired for a mean of eight (8) hours following administration of 4 mg of IM. Lorazepam and four (4) hours following administration of 2 mg IM with considerable subject variation. Similar findings were noted with pentobarbital, 150 and 75 mg. Although this study showed that both Lorazepam and pentobarbital interfered with eye-hand coordination, the data are insufficient to predict when it would be safe to operate a motor vehicle or engage in a hazardous occupation or sport.

PHARMACOKINETICS

Lorazepam is readily absorbed when given IM. Peak plasma concentrations occur approximately 60 to 90 minutes following administration and appear to be dose-related, e.g., a 2.0 mg dose provides a level of approximately 20 ng/mL and a 4.0 mg dose approximately 40 ng/mL in plasma. The mean half-life of Lorazepam is about 16 hours when given IV or IM. Lorazepam is rapidly conjugated at the 3-hydroxyl group into its major metabolite Lorazepam glucuronide, which is then excreted in the urine. Lorazepam glucuronide has no demonstrable CNS activity in animals. When 5 mg of IV Lorazepam was administered to volunteers once a day for four consecutive days, a steady state of free Lorazepam was achieved by the second day (approximately 52 ng/ml of plasma three hours after the first dose and approximately 62 ng/ml three hours after each subsequent dose, one day apart). At clinically relevant concentrations, Lorazepam is bound 85% to plasma proteins.

Oral Lorazepam studies in healthy volunteers show that in single high oral doses Lorazepam has a tranquilizing action on the central nervous system with no appreciable effect on the respiratory or cardiovascular systems.

Orally administered Lorazepam is readily absorbed with an absolute bioavailability of 90%. Peak concentrations in plasma occur approximately 2 hours following administration. The peak plasma level of Lorazepam from a 2 mg dose is approximately 20 ng/mL.

The mean half-life of unconjugated Lorazepam in human plasma is about 12 hours and for its major metabolite, Lorazepam glucuronide, about 18 hours. At clinically relevant concentrations, Lorazepam is approximately 85% bound to plasma proteins. Lorazepam is rapidly conjugated at its 3-hydroxy group into Lorazepam glucuronide which is then excreted in the urine. Lorazepam glucuronide has no demonstrable CNS activity in animals.

The plasma levels of Lorazepam are proportional to the dose given. There is no evidence of accumulation of Lorazepam on administration up to six months.

Studies comparing young and elderly subjects have shown that the pharmacokinetics of Lorazepam remain unaltered with advancing age.

INDICATIONS AND USAGE

Lorazepam is indicated in adult patients for preanesthetic medication, producing sedation (sleepiness or drowsiness), relief of anxiety, and a decreased ability to recall events related to the day of surgery. It is most useful in those patients who are anxious about their surgical procedure and who would prefer to have diminished recall of the events of the day of surgery (see "Information for Patients").

Lorazepam indicated for the management of anxiety disorders or for the short-term relief of the symptoms of anxiety or anxiety associated with depressive symptoms. Anxiety or tension associated with the stress of everyday life usually does not require treatment with an anxiolytic.

The effectiveness of Lorazepam in long-term use, that is, more than 4 months, has not been assessed by systematic clinical studies. The physician should periodically reassess the usefulness of the drug for the individual patient.

UNLABELED USES

Lorazepam is used alone or as an adjunct in the treatment of acute alcohol withdrawal, and chemotherapy-induced emesis, as well as to control intractable partial complex seizures, and status epilepticus.

CONTRAINDICATIONS

Lorazepam and tablets are contraindicated in patients with a known sensitivity to benzodiazepines or its vehicle and in patients with acute narrow-angle glaucoma.

The use of Lorazepam intra-arterially is contraindicated because, as with other injectable benzodiazepines, inadvertent intra-arterial injection may produce arteriospasm resulting in gangrene which may require amputation (see "Warnings").

WARNINGS

PRIOR TO INTRAVENOUS USE, LORAZEPAM MUST BE DILUTED WITH AN EQUAL AMOUNT OF COMPATIBLE DILUENT (SEE "DOSAGE AND ADMINISTRATION"). INTRAVENOUS INJECTION SHOULD BE MADE SLOWLY AND WITH REPEATED ASPIRATION. CARE SHOULD BE TAKEN TO DETERMINE THAT ANY INJECTION WILL NOT BE INTRA-ARTERIAL AND THAT PERIVASCULAR EXTRAVASATION WILL NOT TAKE PLACE.

PARTIAL AIRWAY OBSTRUCTION MAY OCCUR IN HEAVILY SEDATED PATIENTS. INTRAVENOUS LORAZEPAM, WHEN GIVEN ALONE IN GREATER THAN THE RECOMMENDED DOSE, OR AT THE RECOMMENDED DOSE AND ACCOMPANIED BY OTHER DRUGS USED DURING THE ADMINISTRATION OF ANESTHESIA, MAY PRODUCE HEAVY SEDATION; THEREFORE, EQUIPMENT NECESSARY TO MAINTAIN A PATENT AIRWAY AND TO SUPPORT RESPIRATION/VENTILATION SHOULD BE AVAILABLE.

There is no evidence to support the use of Lorazepam injection in coma, shock, or acute-alcohol intoxication at this time. Since the liver is the most likely site of conjugation of Lorazepam and since excretion of conjugated Lorazepam (glucuronide) is a renal function, this drug is not recommended for use in patients with hepatic and/or renal *failure*. This does not preclude use of the drug in patients with mild-to-moderate hepatic or renal disease. When injectable Lorazepam is selected for use in patients with mild-to-moderate hepatic or renal disease, the lowest effective dose should be considered since drug effect may be prolonged. Experience with other benzodiazepines and with oral and parenteral Lorazepam has demonstrated that tolerance to alcoholic beverages and other central-nervous-system depressants is diminished when used concomitantly.

As is true of similar CNS-acting drugs, patients receiving injectable Lorazepam should not operate machinery or engage in hazardous occupations or drive a motor vehicle for a period of 24 to 48 hours. Impairment of performance may persist for greater intervals because of extremes of age, concomitant use of other drugs, stress of surgery, or the general condition of the patient.

Clinical trials have shown that patients over the age of 50 years may have more profound and prolonged sedation with IV Lorazepam. Ordinarily, an initial dose of 2 mg may be adequate unless a greater degree of lack of recall is desired.

As with all central-nervous-system depressant drugs, care should be exercised in patients given injectable Lorazepam that premature ambulation may result in injury from falling.

There is no added beneficial effect to the addition of scopolamine to injectable Lorazepam, and their combined effect may result in an increased incidence of sedation, hallucination, and irrational behavior.

Lorazepam tablets are not recommended for use in patients with a primary depressive disorder or psychosis.

PREGNANCY

LORAZEPAM MAY CAUSE FETAL DAMAGE WHEN ADMINISTERED TO PREGNANT WOMEN. An increased risk of congenital malformations associated with the use of minor tranquilizers (chlordiazepoxide, diazepam, and meprobamate) during the first trimester of pregnancy has been suggested in several studies. Because the use of these drugs is rarely a matter of urgency, the use of Lorazepam during this period should almost always be avoided. The possibility that a woman of childbearing potential may be pregnant at the time of institution of therapy should be considered. Patients should be advised that if they become pregnant, they should communicate with their physician, about the desirability of discontinuing the drug. In humans, blood levels obtained from umbilical cord blood indicate placental transfer of Lorazepam and Lorazepam glucuronide.

Lorazepam should not be used during pregnancy. There are insufficient data regarding obstetrical safety of parenteral lorazepam, including use in cesarean section. Such use, therefore, is not recommended.

Reproductive studies in animals were performed in mice, rats, and two strains of rabbits. Occasional anomalies (reduction of tarsals, tibia, metatarsals, malrotated limbs, gastroschisis, malformed skull, and microphthalmia) were seen in drug-treated rabbits without relationship to dosage. Although all of these anomalies were not present in the concurrent control group, they have been reported to occur randomly in historical controls. At doses of 40 mg/kg orally or 4 mg/kg intravenously and higher, there was evidence of fetal resorption and increased fetal loss in rabbits which was not seen at lower doses. The clinical significance of these findings is not known.

ENDOSCOPIC PROCEDURES

There are insufficient data to support the use of Lorazepam injection for outpatient endoscopic procedures. Inpatient endoscopic procedures require adequate recovery room observations.

Pharyngeal reflexes are not impaired when Lorazepam injection is used for peroral endoscopic procedures: therefore, adequate topical or regional anesthesia is recommended to minimize reflex activity associated with such procedures.

PRECAUTIONS

GENERAL

The additive central-nervous-system effects of other drugs such as phenothiazines, narcotic analgesics, barbiturates, antidepressants, scopolamine, and monoamine-oxidase inhibitors, should be borne in mind when these other drugs are used

---

◆ RATED THERAPEUTICALLY EQUIVALENT; ◇ THERAPEUTIC EQUIVALENCE UNCONFIRMED; ○ UNRATED

concomitantly with or during the period of recovery from Lorazepam (See *"Clinical Pharmacology"* and *"Warnings"*.)

Extreme care must be used in administering Lorazepam to elderly patients, very ill patients, and to patients with limited pulmonary reserve because of the possibility that underventilation and/or hypoxic cardiac arrest may occur. Resuscitative equipment for ventilatory support should be readily available. (See *"Warnings"* and *"Dosage and Administration"*).

For elderly or debilitated patients, the initial oral daily dosage should not exceed 2 mg in order to avoid oversedation.

When Lorazepam injection is used IV as the premedicant prior to regional or local anesthesia, the possibility of excessive sleepiness or drowsiness may interfere with patient cooperation to determine levels of anesthesia. This is most likely to occur when greater than 0.05 mg/kg is given and when narcotic analgesics are used concomitantly with the recommended dose. (See *"Adverse Reactions"*.)

The patients with depression accompanying anxiety, a possibility for suicide should be borne in mind.

The usual precautions for treating patients with impaired renal or hepatic function should be observed.

In patients where gastrointestinal or cardiovascular disorders coexist with anxiety, it should be noted that Lorazepam has not been shown to be of significant benefit in treating the gastrointestinal or cardiovascular component.

Esophageal dilation occurred in rats treated with Lorazepam for more than one year at 6 mg/kg/day. The no-effect dose was 1.25 mg/kg/day (approximately 6 times the maximum human therapeutic dose of 10 mg per day). The effect was reversible only when the treatment was withdrawn within two months of first observation of the phenomenon. The clinical significance of this is unknown. However, use of Lorazepam for prolonged periods and in geriatric patients requires caution, and there should be frequent monitoring for symptoms of upper G.I. disease.

INFORMATION FOR PATIENTS

As appropriate, the patient should be informed of the pharmacological effects of the drug, such as sedation, relief of anxiety, and lack of recall, and the duration of these effects (about 8 hours), so that they may adequately perceive the risks as well as the benefits to be derived from its use.

Patients who receive Lorazepam as a premedicant should be cautioned that driving an automobile or operating hazardous machinery, or engaging in a hazardous sport, should be delayed for 24 to 48 hours following the injection. Sedatives, tranquilizers, and narcotic analgesics may produce a more prolonged and profound effect when administered along with injectable Lorazepam. This effect may take the form of excessive sleepiness or drowsiness and, on rare occasions, interfere with recall and recognition of events of the day of surgery and the day after.

Getting out of bed unassisted may result in falling and injury if undertaken within 8 hours of receiving Lorazepam injection. Alcoholic beverages should not be consumed for at least 24 to 48 hours after receiving Lorazepam injectable due to the additive effects on central-nervous-system depression seen with benzodiazepines in general. Elderly patients should be told that Lorazapam may make them very sleepy for a period longer than six (6) to eight (8) hours following surgery.

To assure the safe and effective use of Lorazepam), patients should be informed that, since benzodiane pines may produce psychological and physical dependence, it is advisable that they consult with their physician before either increasing the dose or abruptly discontinuing this drug.

LABORATORY TESTS

In clinical trials no laboratory test abnormalities were identified with either single or multiple doses of LORAZEPAM injection. These tests included: CBC, urinarlysis, SCOT, SGPT, bilirubin, alkaline phosphatase, LDH, cholesterol, uric acid, BUN, glucose, calcium, phosphorus, and total proteins.

Some patients on lorazepam have developed leukopenia, and some have had elevations of LDH. As with other benzodiazepines, periodic blood counts and liver-function tests are recommended for patients on long-term therapy.

DRUG INTERACTIONS

Lorazapam, like other benzodiazepines, produces depression of the central nervous system when administered with ethyl alcohol, phenothiszines, barbiturates, MAO inhibitors, and other antidepressants. When scopolamine is used concomitantly with an injectable, Lorazepam, an increased incidence of sedation, hallucinations, and irrational behavior has been observed.

DRUG/LABORATORY TEST INTERACTIONS

No laboratory test abnormalities were identified when Lorazepam was given alone or concomitantly with another drug, such as narcotic analgesic, inhalation anesthetics, scopolamine, atropine, and a variety of tranqquilizing agents.

CARCINOGENESIS, MUTAGENESIS, IMPAIRMENT OF FERTILITY

No evidence of carcinogenic potential emerged in rats and mice during an 15-month study withs oral Lorazepam. No studies regarding mutagenesis have been performed. Pre-implantation study in rats was performed with oral Lorazepam at a 20 mg/kg dose and showed no impairment of fertility.

PREGNANCY

Pregnancy Category D; see *"Warnings"*.

LABOR AND DELIVERY

There are insufficient data to support the use of Lorazepam injection during labor and delivery, including cesarean section; therefore, its use in this situation is not recommended.

NURSING MOTHERS

Lorazepam should not be administered to nursing mothers, because, like other benzodiazepines, the possibility exists that Lorazepam may be excreted in human milk and sedate the infant.

PEDIATRIC USE

There are insufficient data to support efficacy or safety or make dosage recommendations for injectable Lorazepam in patients less than 18 years of age and for Lorazepam tablets in children under 12 years; therefore, such use is not recommended.

ADVERSE REACTIONS

Central Nervous System: The most frequent adverse effects seen with injectable Lorazepam are an extension of the central-nervous-system depressant effects of the drug. The incidence varied from one study to another, depending on the dosage, route of administration, use of other central-nervous-system depressants, and the investigator's opinion concerning the degree and duration of desired sedation. Excessive sleepiness and drowsiness were the main side effects. This interfered with patient cooperation in approximately 6% (25/446) of patients undergoing regional anesthesia in that they were unable to assess levels of anesthesia in regional blocks or with caudal anesthesia. Patients over 50 years of age had a higher incidence of excessive sleepiness or drowsiness when compared with those under 50 (21/106 vs 24/245) when given intravenously (see *"Dosage and Administration"*). On rare occasion (3/1580) the patient was unable to give personal identification in the operating room on arrival, and one patient fell when attempting premature ambulation in the postoperative period.

Symptoms such as restlessness, confusion, depression, crying, sobbing, and delirium occurred in about 1.3% (20/1580). One patient injured himself by picking at his incision during the immediate postoperative period.

Hallucinations were present in about 1% (14/1580) of patients and were visual and self-limiting.

An occasional patient complained of dizziness, diplopia, and/or blurred vision. Depressed hearing was infrequently reported during the peak-effect period.

An occasional patient had a prolonged recovery room stay, either because of excessive sleepiness or because of some form of inappropriate behavior. The latter was seen most commonly when scopolamine was given concomitantly as a premedicant.

Limited information derived from patients who were discharged the day after receiving injectable Lorazepam showed one patient complained of some unsteadiness of gait and a reduced ability to perform complex mental functions. Enhanced sensitivity to alcoholic beverages has been reported more than 24 hours after receiving injectable Lorazepam similar to experience with other benzodiazepine.

Local Effects: Intramuscular injections of Lorazepam has resulted in pain at the injection site, a sensation of burning, or observed redness in the same area in a very variable incidence from one study to another. The overall incidence of pain and burning was about 17% (146/859) at the 24-hour observation time. Reactions at the injection site (redness) occurred in approximately 2% (17/859) in the immediate postinjection period and were present 24 hours later in about 0.8% (7/859).

Intravenous administration of Lorazepam resulted in painful responses in 13/771 patients or approximately 1.6% in the immediate postinjection period, and 24 hours later 4/771 patients or about 0.5% still complained of pain. Redness did not occur immediately following intravenous injection but was noted in 19/771 patients at the 24-hour observation period. This incidence is similar to that observed with an intravenous infusion before Lorazepam is given.

Cardiovascular System: Hypertension (0.1%) and hypotension (0.1%) have occasionally been observed after patients have received injectable Lorazepam.

Respiratory System: Five patients (5/446) who underwent regional anesthesia were observed to have partial airway obstruction. This was believed due to excessive sleepiness at the time of the procedure and resulted in temporary underventilation. Immediate attention to the airway, employing the usual counter-measures will usually suffice to manage this condition (see *"Clinical Pharmacology"*, *"Warnings,"* and *"Precautions"*).

Other Adverse Experiences: Skin rash, nausea, and vomiting have occasionally been noted in patients who have received injectable Lorazepam combined with other drugs during anesthesia and surgery.

Adverse reactions, if they occur, are usually observed at the beginning of therapy and generally disappear on continued medication or upon decreasing the dose. In a sample of about 3,500 anxious patients, the most frequent adverse reaction to Lorazepam is sedation (15.9%), followed by dizziness (6.9%), weakness (4.2%), and unsteadiness (3.4%). Less frequent adverse reactions are disorientation, depression, nausea, change in appetite, headache, sleep disturbance, agitation, dermatological symptoms, eye function disturbance, together with various gastrointestinal symptoms and autonomic manifestations. The incidence of sedation and unsteadiness increased with age.

Small decreases in blood pressure have been noted but are not clinically significant, probably being related to the relief of anxiety produced by Lorazapam.

Transient amnesia or memory impairment has been reported in association with the use of benzodiazepines.

▶ SHOWN IN PRODUCT IDENTIFICATION GUIDE

DRUG ABUSE AND DEPENDENCE

As with other benzodiazepines Lorazepam has a low potential for abuse and may lead to limited dependence. Although there are no clinical data available for injectable Lorazepam in this respect, physicians should be aware that repeated doses over a prolonged period of time may result in limited physical and psychological dependence.

Withdrawal symptoms, similar in character to those noted with barbiturates and alcohol (convulsions, tremor, abdominal and muscle cramps, vomiting, and sweating), have occurred following abrupt discontinuance of Lorazepam. The more severe withdrawal symptoms have usually been limited to those patients who received excessive doses over an extended period of time. Generally milder withdrawal symptoms (e.g., dysphora and insomnia) have been reported following abrupt discontinuance of benzodiazepines taken continuously at therapeutic levels for several months. Consequently, after extended therapy, abrupt discontinuation should generally be avoided and a gradual dosage-tapering schedule followed. Addiction-prone individuals (such as drug addicts or alcoholics) should be under careful surveillance when receiving Lorazepam or other psychotoropic agents because of the predisposition of such patients to habituation and dependence.

OVERDOSAGE

Overdosage of benzodiazepines is usually manifested by varying degrees of central-nervous-system depression, ranging from drowsiness to coma. In mild cases symptoms include drowsiness, mental confusion, and lethargy. In more serious examples, symptoms may include ataxia, hypotonia, hypotension, hypnosis, stages one (1) to three (3) coma, and very rarely death.

Treatment of overdosage is mainly supportive until the drug is eliminated from the body. Vital signs and fluid balance should be carefully monitored. An adequate airway should be maintained and assisted respiration used as needed. With normally functioning kidneys, forced diuresis with intravenous fluids and electrolytes may accelerate elimination of benzodiazepines from the body. In addition, osmotic diuretics, such as mannitol, may be effective as adjunctive measures. In more critical situations, renal dialysis and exchange blood transfusions may be indicated.

In the management of overdosage with any drug, it should be borne in mind that multiple agents may have been taken. Following oral intake, induced vomiting and/or gastric lavage should be undertaken, followed by general supportive care, monitoring of vital signs, and close observation of the patient. Hypotension, though unlikely, usually may be controlled with levarterenol bitartrate injection.

DOSAGE AND ADMINISTRATION

PARENTERAL LORAZEPAM

Intramuscular Injection: For the designated indications as a premedicant, the usual recommended dose of Lorazepam for IM injection is 0.05 mg/kg up to a maximum of 4 mg. As with all premedicant drugs, the dose should be individualized. (See *"Clinical Pharmacology," "Warnings", "Precautions"* and *"Adverse Reactions"*). Doses of other central-nervous-system depressant drugs should be ordinarily reduced (see *"Precautions"*). *For optimum effect, measured as lack of recall, IM Lorazepam should be administered at least 2 hours before the anticipated operative procedure.* Narcotic analgesics should be administered at their usual preoperative time. There are insufficient data to support efficacy to make dosage recommendations for IM Lorazepam in patients less than 18 years of age; therefore, such use is not recommended.

Intravenous Injection: For the primary purpose of sedation and relief of anxiety, the usual recommended initial dose of Lorazepam for IV injection is 2 mg total, or 0.02 mg/lb (0.044 mg/kg), whichever is smaller. This dose will suffice for sedating most adult patients and should not ordinarily be exceeded in patients over 50 years of age. In those patients in whom a greater likelihood of lack of recall for perioperative events would be beneficial, larger doses as high as 0.05 mg/kg up to a total of 4 mg may be administered. (See *"Clinical Pharmacology", "Warnings", "Precautions"*, and *"Adverse Reactions"*). Doses of other injectable central-nervous-system depressant drugs should ordinarily be reduced (see *"Precautions"*). *For optimum effect, measured as lack of recall, IV venous Lorazepam should be administered 15 to 20 minutes before the anticipated operative procedure.*

EQUIPMENT NECESSARY TO MAINTAIN A PATENT AIRWAY SHOULD BE IMMEDIATELY AVAILABLE PRIOR TO IV ADMINISTRATION OF LORAZEPAM (see *"Warnings"*).

There are insufficient data to support efficacy or make dosage recommendations for IV Lorazepam in patients less than 18 years of age; therefore, such use is not recommended.

Administration: When given intramuscularly, Lorazepam injection undiluted, should be injected deep in the muscle mass.

Lorazepam injection can be used with atropine sulfate, narcotic analgesics, other parenterally used analgesics, commonly used anesthetics, and muscle relaxants.

Immediately prior to IV use, Lorazepam injection must be diluted with an equal volume of compatible solution. When properly diluted the drug may be injected directly into a vein or into the tubing of an existing IV infusion. The rate of injection should not exceed 2.0 mg per minute.

Parenteral drug products should be inspected visually for particulate matter and discoloration prior to administration, whenever solution and container permit. Do not use if solution is discolored or contains a precipitate.

Lorazepam is compatible for dilution purposes with the following solutions: sterile water for injection, USP: sodium chloride injection, USP; 5% dextrose injection, USP.

ORAL LORAZEPAM

For optimal results, dose, frequency of administration, and duration of therapy should be individualized according to patient response. To facilitate this, 0.5 mg, 1 mg, and 2 mg tablets are available.

The usual range is 2 to 6 mg/day given in divided doses, the largest dose being taken before bedtime, but the daily dosage may vary from 1 to 10 mg/day.

For anxiety, most patients require an initial dose of 2 to 3 mg/day given b.i.d. or t.i.d.

For insomnia due to anxiety or transient situational stress, a single daily dose of 2 to 4 mg may be given, usually at bedtime.

For elderly or debilitated patients, an initial dosage of 1 to 2 mg/day in divided doses is recommended, to be adjusted as needed and tolerated.

The dosage of Lorazepam should be increased gradually when needed to help avoid adverse effects. When higher dosage is indicated, the evening dose should be increased before the daytime doses.

STORAGE

Injection: Protect from light.
   Store in a refrigerator.
   Use carton to protect contents from light.

Tablets: Store at controlled room temperature.
   Keep bottles tightly closed.
   Dispense in tight container.
   Protect from light.
   Use carton to protect contents from light.

J CODES

2 mg IM,IV—J2060

HOW SUPPLIED

INJECTION (C-IV): 2 MG/ML

AVERAGE UNIT PRICE (AVAILABLE SIZES)

GENERIC	$9.42

BRAND/MANUFACTURER	NDC	SIZE	AWP
◆ GENERICS			
Schein	00364-3048-51	1 ml	$9.78
Schein	00364-3048-54	10 ml	$90.59

INJECTION (C-IV): 2 MG/ML

BRAND/MANUFACTURER	NDC	SIZE	AWP
○ BRAND			
ATIVAN: Wyeth-Ayerst	00008-0581-04	1 ml	$12.01
	00008-0581-01	10 ml	$107.00
	00008-0581-05	0.5 ml 10s	$126.69
	00008-0581-07	0.5 ml 10s	$126.69
	00008-0581-02	1 ml 10s	$126.69
	00008-0581-06	1 ml 10s	$126.69
	00008-0581-52	1 ml 10s	$126.69
	00008-0581-53	1 ml 10s	$126.69

INJECTION (C-IV): 4 MG/ML

AVERAGE UNIT PRICE (AVAILABLE SIZES)

GENERIC	$11.45

BRAND/MANUFACTURER	NDC	SIZE	AWP
◆ GENERICS			
Schein	00364-3049-51	1 ml	$11.49
Schein	00364-3049-54	10 ml	$114.05

INJECTION (C-IV): 4 MG/ML

BRAND/MANUFACTURER	NDC	SIZE	AWP
○ BRAND			
ATIVAN: Wyeth-Ayerst	00008-0570-04	1 ml	$14.69
	00008-0570-01	10 ml	$133.74
	00008-0570-02	1 ml 10s	$126.69
	00008-0570-05	1 ml 10s	$126.69
	00008-0570-50	1 ml 10s	$126.69
	00008-0570-51	1 ml 10s	$126.69

TABLETS: (C-IV): 0.5 MG

AVERAGE UNIT PRICE (AVAILABLE SIZES)		GENERIC A-RATED AVERAGE PRICE (GAAP)	
BRAND	$0.62	100s	$17.38
GENERIC	$0.14	500s	$52.14
HCFA FUL (100s ea)	$0.02	1000s	$72.60

BRAND/MANUFACTURER	NDC	SIZE	AWP
◆ BRAND			
➤ ATIVAN: Wyeth-Ayerst	00008-0081-02	100s	$56.81
	00008-0081-07	100s ud	$66.39
	00008-0081-06	250s	$170.20
	00008-0081-03	500s	$276.13

◆ RATED THERAPEUTICALLY EQUIVALENT; ◇ THERAPEUTIC EQUIVALENCE UNCONFIRMED; ○ UNRATED

BRAND/MANUFACTURER	NDC	SIZE	AWP
◆ GENERICS			
Caraco	57664-0140-08	100s	$3.75
Watson	52544-0332-01	100s	$11.38
Qualitest	00603-4243-21	100s	$12.05
➤ Rugby	00536-3959-01	100s	$12.25
Mutual	53489-0357-01	100s	$12.30
Goldline	00182-1806-01	100s	$12.30
Purepac	00228-2057-10	100s	$12.70
Major	00904-1500-60	100s	$13.10
URL	00677-1056-01	100s	$13.20
➤ Geneva	00781-1403-01	100s	$13.20
Schein	00364-0793-01	100s	$13.22
Aligen	00405-0108-01	100s	$13.36
Moore,H.L.	00839-7902-06	100s	$13.43
Moore,H.L.	00839-7145-06	100s	$13.43
Royce	51875-0240-01	100s	$13.50
Caremark	00339-4017-12	100s	$13.57
Martec	52555-0485-01	100s	$13.75
Warner Chilcott	00047-0431-24	100s	$14.44
Mylan	00378-0321-01	100s	$14.50
Parmed	00349-8461-01	100s	$24.84
Auro	55829-0851-10	100s ud	$25.29
Goldline	00182-1806-89	100s ud	$28.50
Vangard	00615-0450-13	100s ud	$28.66
Vangard	00615-0450-47	100s ud	$28.66
Major	00904-1500-61	100s ud	$28.74
UDL	51079-0417-20	100s ud	$32.61
UDL	51079-0417-21	100s ud	$32.61
➤ Rugby	00536-3959-02	250s	$29.80
Caraco	57664-0140-13	500s	$11.75
Major	00904-1500-40	500s	$31.50
Watson	52544-0332-05	500s	$34.30
Moore,H.L.	00839-7145-12	500s	$48.53
➤ Geneva	00781-1403-05	500s	$49.50
Qualitest	00603-4243-28	500s	$49.81
Goldline	00182-1806-05	500s	$50.00
Mutual	53489-0357-05	500s	$51.60
Mason Dist	11845-0150-03	500s	$51.60
Martec	52555-0485-05	500s	$52.50
Warner Chilcott	00047-0431-30	500s	$52.95
URL	00677-1056-05	500s	$55.93
Purepac	00228-2057-50	500s	$55.98
Aligen	00405-0108-02	500s	$55.99
Mylan	00378-0321-05	500s	$56.25
Schein	00364-0793-05	500s	$56.50
Royce	51875-0240-02	500s	$57.60
Parmed	00349-8461-05	500s	$116.20
Major	00904-1500-80	1000s	$50.40
➤ Rugby	00536-3959-10	1000s	$50.70
Watson	52544-0332-10	1000s	$67.22
Schein	00364-0793-02	1000s	$75.00
Mutual	53489-0357-10	1000s	$77.90
Royce	51875-0240-04	1000s	$79.00
Moore,H.L.	00839-7902-16	1000s	$107.99

TABLETS: (C-IV): 1 MG

AVERAGE UNIT PRICE (AVAILABLE SIZES)		GENERIC A-RATED AVERAGE PRICE (GAAP)	
BRAND	$0.76	100s	$22.43
GENERIC	$0.17	500s	$70.26
HCFA FUL (100s ea)	$0.02	1000s	$102.95

BRAND/MANUFACTURER	NDC	SIZE	AWP
◆ BRAND			
➤ ATIVAN: Wyeth-Ayerst	00008-0064-02	100s	$73.98
	00008-0064-09	100s ud	$80.81
	00008-0064-08	250s	$207.23
	00008-0064-03	500s	$357.98
	00008-0064-05	1000s	$703.48
◆ GENERICS			
Caraco	57664-0141-08	100s	$4.70
Watson	52544-0333-01	100s	$15.15
Qualitest	00603-4244-21	100s	$15.95
➤ Rugby	00536-3960-01	100s	$16.20
Goldline	00182-1807-01	100s	$16.25
Major	00904-1501-60	100s	$16.30
Mutual	53489-0358-01	100s	$16.50
➤ Geneva	00781-1404-01	100s	$16.75
Schein	00364-0794-01	100s	$17.80
Caremark	00339-4019-12	100s	$17.98
Royce	51875-0241-01	100s	$18.25
Martec	52555-0486-01	100s	$18.43
URL	00677-1057-01	100s	$19.22
➤ Purepac	00228-2059-10	100s	$19.26
Moore,H.L.	00839-7903-06	100s	$19.91
Moore,H.L.	00839-7146-06	100s	$19.91
➤ Mylan	00378-0457-01	100s	$19.95
Aligen	00405-0109-01	100s	$19.98
Warner Chilcott	00047-0432-24	100s	$20.13
Parmed	00349-8462-01	100s	$35.96
Auro	55829-0852-10	100s ud	$32.60
Goldline	00182-1807-89	100s ud	$33.00
Vangard	00615-0451-13	100s ud	$34.81
Vangard	00615-0451-47	100s ud	$34.81

BRAND/MANUFACTURER	NDC	SIZE	AWP
UDL	51079-0386-20	100s ud	$35.00
UDL	51079-0386-21	100s ud	$35.00
Major	00904-1501-61	100s ud	$35.76
Caraco	57664-0141-13	500s	$12.60
Watson	52544-0333-05	500s	$42.47
➤ Geneva	00781-1404-05	500s	$43.50
Aligen	00405-0109-02	500s	$53.26
Qualitest	00603-4244-28	500s	$54.35
Moore,H.L.	00839-7146-12	500s	$59.35
Major	00904-1501-40	500s	$63.60
Mutual	53489-0358-05	500s	$75.00
Schein	00364-0794-05	500s	$79.60
➤ Rugby	00536-3960-05	500s	$79.70
Goldline	00182-1807-05	500s	$79.75
Martec	52555-0486-05	500s	$79.85
URL	00677-1057-05	500s	$79.90
Royce	51875-0241-02	500s	$82.00
➤ Purepac	00228-2059-50	500s	$96.30
Warner Chilcott	00047-0432-30	500s	$97.59
➤ Mylan	00378-0457-05	500s	$115.65
Watson	52544-0333-10	1000s	$83.30
➤ Geneva	00781-1404-10	1000s	$83.95
➤ Rugby	00536-3960-10	1000s	$87.40
Goldline	00182-1807-10	1000s	$87.45
Qualitest	00603-4244-32	1000s	$87.78
Major	00904-1501-80	1000s	$89.90
URL	00677-1057-10	1000s	$95.00
Mutual	53489-0358-10	1000s	$95.00
Royce	51875-0241-04	1000s	$97.50
Moore,H.L.	00839-7903-16	1000s	$126.29
Moore,H.L.	00839-7146-16	1000s	$126.29
➤ Mylan	00378-0457-10	1000s	$126.50
Parmed	00349-8462-10	1000s	$151.95

TABLETS: (C-IV): 2 MG

AVERAGE UNIT PRICE (AVAILABLE SIZES)		GENERIC A-RATED AVERAGE PRICE (GAAP)	
BRAND	$1.11	100s	$33.09
GENERIC	$0.26	500s	$102.14
HCFA FUL (100s ea)	$0.03	1000s	$139.98

BRAND/MANUFACTURER	NDC	SIZE	AWP
◆ BRAND			
➤ ATIVAN: Wyeth-Ayerst	00008-0065-02	100s	$107.88
	00008-0065-09	100s ud	$117.68
	00008-0065-08	250s	$301.75
	00008-0065-03	500s	$524.81
	00008-0065-05	1000s	$1024.68
◆ GENERICS			
Caraco	57664-0142-08	100s	$5.25
Watson	52544-0334-01	100s	$22.73
Qualitest	00603-4245-21	100s	$23.40
➤ Rugby	00536-3961-01	100s	$23.50
➤ Geneva	00781-1405-01	100s	$23.50
Mutual	53489-0359-01	100s	$23.55
Goldline	00182-1808-01	100s	$23.55
Major	00904-1502-60	100s	$23.70
Royce	51875-0242-01	100s	$25.15
Martec	52555-0487-01	100s	$25.40
Caremark	00339-4021-12	100s	$25.58
Schein	00364-0795-01	100s	$25.80
URL	00677-1058-01	100s	$26.90
Moore,H.L.	00839-7904-06	100s	$26.93
Moore,H.L.	00839-7147-06	100s	$26.93
Purepac	00228-2063-10	100s	$27.90
➤ Mylan	00378-0777-01	100s	$27.95
Aligen	00405-0110-01	100s	$27.98
Warner Chilcott	00047-0433-24	100s	$28.82
Parmed	00349-8463-01	100s	$49.26
Auro	55829-0853-10	100s ud	$47.86
Goldline	00182-1808-89	100s ud	$52.50
Vangard	00615-0452-13	100s ud	$53.54
Vangard	00615-0452-47	100s ud	$53.54
Major	00904-1502-61	100s ud	$53.70
UDL	51079-0387-20	100s ud	$59.25
UDL	51079-0387-21	100s ud	$59.25
Rugby	00536-3961-02	250s	$57.50
➤ Geneva	00781-1405-05	500s	$65.00
Watson	52544-0334-05	500s	$66.97
Goldline	00182-1808-05	500s	$81.00
Qualitest	00603-4245-28	500s	$82.25
Mutual	53489-0359-05	500s	$85.75
Major	00904-1502-40	500s	$89.20
Royce	51875-0242-02	500s	$90.81
Moore,H.L.	00839-7147-12	500s	$91.19
Martec	52555-0487-05	500s	$91.75
➤ Mylan	00378-0777-05	500s	$96.35
URL	00677-1058-05	500s	$104.20
Schein	00364-0795-05	500s	$104.25
Warner Chilcott	00047-0433-30	500s	$127.85
Aligen	00405-0110-02	500s	$128.90
Purepac	00228-2063-50	500s	$139.50
Parmed	00349-8463-05	500s	$189.31
Watson	52544-0334-10	1000s	$117.60

➤ SHOWN IN PRODUCT IDENTIFICATION GUIDE

BRAND/MANUFACTURER	NDC	SIZE	AWP
➤ Rugby	00536-3961-10	1000s	$118.13
Major	00904-1502-80	1000s	$123.75
Qualitest	00603-4245-32	1000s	$130.40
Mutual	53489-0359-10	1000s	$136.00
Moore,H.L.	00839-7904-16	1000s	$139.04
Royce	51875-0242-04	1000s	$156.00
Purepac	00228-2063-96	1000s	$198.90

TABLETS (C-IV): 0.5 MG

AVERAGE UNIT PRICE (AVAILABLE SIZES)		GENERIC A-RATED AVERAGE PRICE (GAAP)	
BRAND	$0.62	100s	$17.38
GENERIC	$0.14	500s	$52.14
HCFA FUL (100s ea)	$0.02	1000s	$72.60

BRAND/MANUFACTURER	NDC	SIZE	AWP
◆ BRAND			
➤ ATIVAN: Wyeth-Ayerst	00008-0081-02	100s	$56.81
	00008-0081-07	100s ud	$66.39
	00008-0081-06	250s	$170.20
	00008-0081-03	500s	$276.13
◆ GENERICS			
Caraco	57664-0140-08	100s	$3.75
Watson	52544-0332-01	100s	$11.38
Qualitest	00603-4243-21	100s	$12.05
Rugby	00536-3959-01	100s	$12.25
Mutual	53489-0357-01	100s	$12.30
Goldline	00182-1806-01	100s	$12.30
Purepac	00228-2057-10	100s	$12.70
Major	00904-1500-60	100s	$13.10
URL	00677-1056-01	100s	$13.20
Geneva	00781-1403-01	100s	$13.20
Schein	00364-0793-01	100s	$13.22
Aligen	00405-0108-01	100s	$13.36
Moore,H.L.	00839-7902-01	100s	$13.43
Moore,H.L.	00839-7145-06	100s	$13.43
Royce	51875-0240-01	100s	$13.50
Caremark	00339-4017-12	100s	$13.57
Martec	52555-0485-01	100s	$13.75
Warner Chilcott	00047-0431-24	100s	$14.44
Mylan	00378-0321-01	100s	$14.50
Parmed	00349-8461-01	100s	$24.84
Auro	55829-0851-10	100s ud	$25.29
Goldline	00182-1806-89	100s ud	$28.50
Vangard	00615-0450-13	100s ud	$28.66
Vangard	00615-0450-47	100s ud	$28.66
Major	00904-1500-61	100s ud	$28.74
UDL	51079-0417-20	100s ud	$32.61
UDL	51079-0417-21	100s ud	$32.61
Rugby	00536-3959-02	250s	$29.80
Caraco	57664-0140-13	500s	$11.75
Major	00904-1500-40	500s	$31.50
Watson	52544-0332-05	500s	$34.30
Moore,H.L.	00839-7145-12	500s	$48.53
Geneva	00781-1403-05	500s	$49.50
Qualitest	00603-4243-28	500s	$49.81
Goldline	00182-1806-05	500s	$50.00
Mutual	53489-0357-05	500s	$51.60
Mason Dist	11845-0150-03	500s	$51.60
Martec	52555-0485-05	500s	$52.50
Warner Chilcott	00047-0431-30	500s	$52.95
URL	00677-1056-05	500s	$55.93
Purepac	00228-2057-50	500s	$55.98
Aligen	00405-0108-02	500s	$55.99
Mylan	00378-0321-05	500s	$56.25
Schein	00364-0793-05	500s	$56.50
Royce	51875-0240-02	500s	$57.60
Parmed	00349-8461-05	500s	$116.20
Major	00904-1500-80	1000s	$50.40
Rugby	00536-3959-10	1000s	$50.70
Watson	52544-0332-10	1000s	$67.22
Schein	00364-0793-02	1000s	$75.00
Mutual	53489-0357-10	1000s	$77.90
Royce	51875-0240-04	1000s	$79.00
Moore,H.L.	00839-7902-16	1000s	$107.99

TABLETS (C-IV): 1 MG

AVERAGE UNIT PRICE (AVAILABLE SIZES)		GENERIC A-RATED AVERAGE PRICE (GAAP)	
BRAND	$0.76	100s	$22.43
GENERIC	$0.17	500s	$70.26
HCFA FUL (100s ea)	$0.02	1000s	$102.95

BRAND/MANUFACTURER	NDC	SIZE	AWP
◆ BRAND			
➤ ATIVAN: Wyeth-Ayerst	00008-0064-02	100s	$73.98
	00008-0064-09	100s ud	$80.81
	00008-0064-08	250s	$207.23
	00008-0064-05	500s	$357.98
	00008-0064-05	1000s	$703.48

BRAND/MANUFACTURER	NDC	SIZE	AWP
◆ GENERICS			
Caraco	57664-0141-08	100s	$4.70
Watson	52544-0333-01	100s	$15.15
Qualitest	00603-4244-21	100s	$15.95
➤ Rugby	00536-3960-01	100s	$16.20
Goldline	00182-1807-01	100s	$16.25
Major	00904-1501-60	100s	$16.30
Mutual	53489-0358-01	100s	$16.50
➤ Geneva	00781-1404-01	100s	$16.75
Schein	00364-0794-01	100s	$17.80
Caremark	00339-4019-12	100s	$17.98
Royce	51875-0241-01	100s	$18.25
Martec	52555-0486-01	100s	$18.43
URL	00677-1057-01	100s	$19.22
➤ Purepac	00228-2059-10	100s	$19.26
Moore,H.L.	00839-7903-06	100s	$19.91
Moore,H.L.	00839-7146-06	100s	$19.91
➤ Mylan	00378-0457-01	100s	$19.95
Aligen	00405-0109-01	100s	$19.98
Warner Chilcott	00047-0432-24	100s	$20.13
Parmed	00349-8462-01	100s	$35.96
Auro	55829-0852-10	100s ud	$32.60
Goldline	00182-1807-89	100s ud	$33.00
Vangard	00615-0451-13	100s ud	$34.81
Vangard	00615-0451-47	100s ud	$34.81
UDL	51079-0386-20	100s ud	$35.00
UDL	51079-0386-21	100s ud	$35.00
Major	00904-1501-61	100s ud	$35.76
Caraco	57664-0141-13	500s	$12.60
Watson	52544-0333-05	500s	$42.47
➤ Geneva	00781-1404-05	500s	$43.50
Aligen	00405-0109-02	500s	$53.26
Qualitest	00603-4244-28	500s	$54.35
Moore,H.L.	00839-7146-12	500s	$59.35
Major	00904-1501-40	500s	$63.60
Mutual	53489-0358-05	500s	$75.00
Schein	00364-0794-05	500s	$79.60
➤ Rugby	00536-3960-05	500s	$79.70
Goldline	00182-1807-05	500s	$79.75
Martec	52555-0486-05	500s	$79.85
URL	00677-1057-05	500s	$79.90
Royce	51875-0241-02	500s	$82.00
➤ Purepac	00228-2059-50	500s	$96.30
Warner Chilcott	00047-0432-30	500s	$97.59
➤ Mylan	00378-0457-05	500s	$115.65
Watson	52544-0333-10	1000s	$83.30
➤ Geneva	00781-1404-10	1000s	$83.95
➤ Rugby	00536-3960-10	1000s	$87.40
Goldline	00182-1807-10	1000s	$87.45
Qualitest	00603-4244-32	1000s	$87.78
Major	00904-1501-80	1000s	$89.90
URL	00677-1057-10	1000s	$95.00
Mutual	53489-0358-10	1000s	$95.00
Royce	51875-0241-04	1000s	$97.50
Moore,H.L.	00839-7903-16	1000s	$126.29
Moore,H.L.	00839-7146-16	1000s	$126.29
➤ Mylan	00378-0457-10	1000s	$126.50
Parmed	00349-8462-10	1000s	$151.95

TABLETS (C-IV): 2 MG

AVERAGE UNIT PRICE (AVAILABLE SIZES)		GENERIC A-RATED AVERAGE PRICE (GAAP)	
BRAND	$1.11	100s	$33.09
GENERIC	$0.26	500s	$102.14
HCFA FUL (100s ea)	$0.03	1000s	$139.98

BRAND/MANUFACTURER	NDC	SIZE	AWP
◆ BRAND			
➤ ATIVAN: Wyeth-Ayerst	00008-0065-02	100s	$107.88
	00008-0065-09	100s ud	$117.68
	00008-0065-08	250s	$301.75
	00008-0065-03	500s	$524.81
	00008-0065-05	1000s	$1024.68
◆ GENERICS			
Caraco	57664-0142-08	100s	$5.25
Watson	52544-0334-01	100s	$22.73
Qualitest	00603-4245-21	100s	$23.40
Rugby	00536-3961-01	100s	$23.50
Geneva	00781-1405-01	100s	$23.50
Mutual	53489-0359-01	100s	$23.55
Goldline	00182-1808-01	100s	$23.55
Major	00904-1502-60	100s	$23.70
Royce	51875-0242-01	100s	$25.15
Martec	52555-0487-01	100s	$25.40
Caremark	00339-4021-12	100s	$25.58
Schein	00364-0795-01	100s	$25.80
URL	00677-1058-01	100s	$26.90
Moore,H.L.	00839-7904-06	100s	$26.93
Moore,H.L.	00839-7147-06	100s	$26.93
Purepac	00228-2063-10	100s	$27.90
Mylan	00378-0777-01	100s	$27.95
Aligen	00405-0110-01	100s	$27.98

◆ RATED THERAPEUTICALLY EQUIVALENT; ◇ THERAPEUTIC EQUIVALENCE UNCONFIRMED; ○ UNRATED

BRAND/MANUFACTURER	NDC	SIZE	AWP
Warner Chilcott	00047-0433-24	100s	$28.82
Parmed	00349-8463-01	100s	$49.26
Auro	55829-0853-10	100s ud	$47.86
Goldline	00182-1808-89	100s ud	$52.50
Vangard	00615-0452-13	100s ud	$53.54
Vangard	00615-0452-47	100s ud	$53.54
Major	00904-1502-61	100s ud	$53.70
UDL	51079-0387-20	100s ud	$59.25
UDL	51079-0387-21	100s ud	$59.25
Rugby	00536-3961-02	250s	$57.50
Geneva	00781-1405-05	500s	$65.00
Watson	52544-0334-05	500s	$66.97
Goldline	00182-1808-05	500s	$81.00
Qualitest	00603-4245-28	500s	$82.25
Mutual	53489-0359-05	500s	$85.75
Major	00904-1502-40	500s	$89.20
Royce	51875-0242-02	500s	$90.81
Moore,H.L.	00839-7147-12	500s	$91.19
Martec	52555-0487-05	500s	$91.75
Mylan	00378-0777-05	500s	$96.35
URL	00677-1058-05	500s	$104.20
Schein	00364-0795-05	500s	$104.25
Warner Chilcott	00047-0433-30	500s	$127.85
Aligen	00405-0110-02	500s	$128.90
Purepac	00228-2063-50	500s	$139.50
Parmed	00349-8463-05	500s	$189.31
Watson	52544-0334-10	1000s	$117.60
Rugby	00536-3961-10	1000s	$118.13
Major	00904-1502-80	1000s	$123.75
Qualitest	00603-4245-32	1000s	$130.40
Mutual	53489-0359-10	1000s	$136.00
Moore,H.L.	00839-7904-16	1000s	$139.04
Royce	51875-0242-04	1000s	$156.00
Purepac	00228-2063-96	1000s	$198.90

Lorcet SEE ACETAMINOPHEN WITH HYDROCODONE BITARTRATE

Lorelco SEE PROBUCOL

Lortab ASA SEE ACETAMINOPHEN WITH HYDROCODONE BITARTRATE AND ASPIRIN WITH HYDROCODONE BITARTRATE

Lotensin HCT SEE BENAZEPRIL HYDROCHLORIDE AND BENAZEPRIL HYDROCHLORIDE WITH HYDROCHLOROTHIAZIDE

Lotrimin SEE CLOTRIMAZOLE

Lotrisone SEE BETAMETHASONE DIPROPIONATE WITH CLOTRIMAZOLE

Lovastatin

DESCRIPTION

Lovastatin is a cholesterol lowering agent isolated from a strain of *Aspergillus terreus*. After oral ingestion Lovastatin, which is an inactive lactone, is hydrolyzed to the corresponding β-hydroxyacid form. This is a principal metabolite and an inhibitor of 3-hydroxy-3-methylglutaryl-coenzyme A (HMG-CoA) reductase. This enzyme catalyzes the conversion of HMG-CoA to mevalonate, which is an early and rate limiting step in the biosynthesis of cholesterol.

Lovastatin is [1S-[1α(R*),3α,7β,8β(2S*,4S*),8aβ]]-1,2,3,7,8,8a-hexa- hydro-3,7-dimethyl-8-[2-(tetrahydro-4-hydroxy-6-oxo-2H-pyran-2-yl)ethyl]-1-naphthalenyl 2-methylbutanoate. The empirical formula of Lovastatin is $C_{24}H_{36}O_5$ and its molecular weight is 404.55.

Lovastatin is a white, nonhygroscopic crystalline powder that is insoluble in water and sparingly soluble in ethanol, methanol and acetonitrile.

Lovastatin tablets are supplied as 10 mg, 20 mg and 40 mg tablets for oral administration.

Following is its chemical structure:

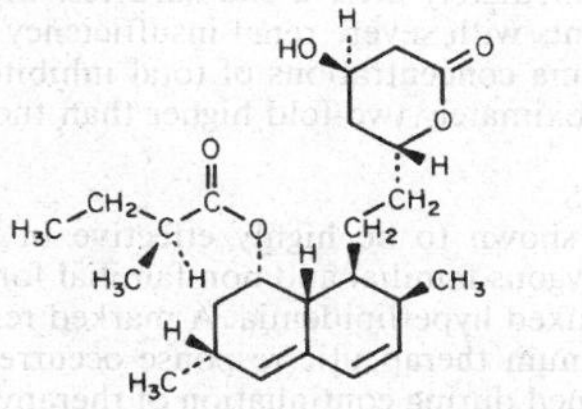

CLINICAL PHARMACOLOGY

The involvement of low-density lipoprotein (LDL) cholesterol in atherogenesis has been well-documented in clinical and pathological studies, as well as in many animal experiments. Epidemiological studies have established that high LDL (low-density lipoprotein) cholesterol and low HDL (high-density lipoprotein) cholesterol are both risk factors for coronary heart disease. The Lipid Research Clinics Coronary Primary Prevention Trial (LRC-CPPT), coordinated by the National Institutes of Health (NIH) studied men aged 35-59 with total cholesterol levels 265 mg/dL (6.8 mmol/L) or greater, LDL cholesterol values 175 mg/dL (4.5 mmol/L) or greater and triglyceride levels not more than 300 mg/dL (3.4 mmol/L). This seven-year, double-blind, placebo-controlled study demonstrated that lowering LDL cholesterol with diet and cholestyramine decreased the combined rate of coronary heart disease death plus non-fatal myocardial infarction.

Lovastatin has been shown to reduce both normal and elevated LDL cholesterol concentrations. The effect of Lovastatin-induced changes in lipoprotein levels, including reduction of serum cholesterol, on cardiovascular morbidity or mortality has not been established.

LDL is formed from VLDL and is catabolized predominantly by the high affinity LDL receptor. The mechanism of the LDL-lowering effect of Lovastatin may involve both reduction of VLDL cholesterol concentration, and induction of the LDL receptor, leading to reduced production and/or increased catabolism of LDL cholesterol. Apolipoprotein B also falls substantially during treatment with Lovastatin. Since each LDL particle contains one molecule of apolipoprotein B, and since little apolipoprotein B is found in other lipoproteins, this strongly suggests that Lovastatin does not merely cause cholesterol to be lost from LDL, but also reduces the concentration of circulating LDL particles. In addition, Lovastatin can produce increases of variable magnitude in HDL cholesterol, and modestly reduces VLDL cholesterol and plasma triglycerides (see Tables 1-4 under "Clinical Studies"). The effects of Lovastatin on Lp(a), fibrinogen, and certain other indpendent biochemical risk markers for coronary heart disease are unknown.

Lovastatin is a specific inhibitor of HMG-CoA reductase, the enzyme which catalyzes the conversion of HMG-CoA to mevalonate. The conversion of HMG-CoA to mevalonate is an early step in the biosynthetic pathway for cholesterol.

PHARMACOKINETICS

Lovastatin is a lactone which is readily hydrolyzed in vivo to the corresponding β-hydroxyacid, a potent inhibitor of HMG-CoA reductase. Inhibition of HMG-CoA reductase is the basis for an assay in pharmacokinetic studies of the β-hydroxyacid metabolites (active inhibitors) and, following base hydrolysis, active plus latent inhibitors (total inhibitors) in plasma following administration of Lovastatin.

Following an oral dose of ^{14}C-labeled Lovastatin in man, 10% of the dose was excreted in urine and 83% in feces. The latter represents absorbed drug equivalents excreted in bile, as well as any unabsorbed drug. Plasma concentrations of total radioactivity (Lovastatin plus ^{14}C-metabolites) peaked at 2 hours and declined rapidly to about 10% of peak by 24 hours postdose. Absorption of Lovastatin, estimated relative to an intravenous reference dose, in each of four animal species tested, averaged about 30% of an oral dose. In animal studies, after oral dosing, Lovastatin had high selectivity for the liver, where it achieved substantially higher concentrations than in non-target tissues. Lovastatin undergoes extensive first-pass extraction in the liver, its primary site of action, with subsequent excretion of drug equivalents in the bile. As a consequence of extensive hepatic extraction of Lovastatin, the availability of drug to the general circulation is low and variable. In a single dose study in four hypercholesterolemic patients, it was estimated that less than 5% of an oral dose of Lovastatin reaches the general circulation as active inhibitors. Following administration of Lovastatin tablets the coefficient of variation, based on between-subject variability, was approximately 40% for the area under the curve (AUC) of total inhibitory activity in the general circulation.

Both Lovastatin and its β-hydroxyacid metabolite are highly bound (> 95%) to human plasma proteins. Animal studies demonstrated that Lovastatin crosses the blood-brain and placental barriers.

The major active metabolites present in human plasma are the β-hydroxyacid of Lovastatin, its 6'-hydroxy derivative, and two additional metabolites. Peak plasma concentrations of both active and total inhibitors were attained within 2 to 4 hours of dose administration. While the recommended therapeutic dose range is 20 to 80 mg/day, linearity of inhibitory activity in the general circulation was established by a single dose study employing Lovastatin tablet dosages from 60 to as high as 120 mg. With a once-a-day dosing regimen, plasma concentrations of total inhibitors over a dosing interval achieved a steady state between the second and third days of therapy and were about 1.5 times those following a single dose. When Lovastatin was given under fasting conditions, plasma concentrations of

➤ SHOWN IN PRODUCT IDENTIFICATION GUIDE

total inhibitors were on average about two-thirds those found when Lovastatin was administered immediately after a standard test meal.

In a study of patients with severe renal insufficiency (creatinine clearance 10-30 mL/min), the plasma concentrations of total inhibitors after a single dose of Lovastatin were approximately two-fold higher than those in healthy volunteers.

CLINICAL STUDIES

Lovastatin has been shown to be highly effective in reducing total and LDL cholesterol in heterozygous familial and non-familial forms of primary hypercholesterolemia and in mixed hyperlipidemia. A marked response was seen within 2 weeks, and the maximum therapeutic response occurred within 4-6 weeks. The response was maintained during continuation of therapy. Single daily doses given in the evening were more effective than the same dose given in the morning, perhaps because cholesterol is synthesized mainly at night.

In multicenter, double-blind studies in patients with familial or non-familial hypercholesterolemia, Lovastatin administered in doses ranging from 20 mg q.p.m. to 40 mg b.i.d., was compared to placebo. Lovastatin consistently and significantly decreased total plasma cholesterol (TOTAL-C), LDL cholesterol (LDL-C), total cholesterol/HDL cholesterol (TOTAL-C/HDL-C) ratio and LDL cholesterol/HDL cholesterol (LDL-C/HDL-C) ratio. In addition, Lovastatin produced increases of variable magnitude in HDL cholesterol (HDL-C), and modestly decreased VLDL cholesterol (VLDL-C) and plasma triglycerides (TRIG.) (see Tables I and IV for dose response results). (See related table).

Lovastatin was compared to cholestyramine in a randomized open parallel study and to probucol in a double-blind, parallel study. Both studies were performed with patients with hypercholesterolemia who were at high risk of myocardial infarction. Summary results of these two comparative studies are presented in Tables 2 & 3. (See related tables).

Lovastatin was studied in controlled trials in hypercholesterolemic patients with well-controlled noninsulin dependent diabetes mellitus with normal renal function. The effect of Lovastatin in lipids and lipoproteins and the safety profile of Lovastatin were similar to that demonstrated in studies in nondiabetics. Lovastatin has no clinically important effect on glycemic control or on the dose requirement of oral hypoglycemic agents.

EXPANDED CLINICAL EVALUATION OF LOVASTATIN (EXCEL) STUDY

Lovastatin was compared to placebo in 8,245 patients with hypercholesterolemia (total cholesterol 240-300 mg/dL [6.2 mmol/L-7.6 mmol/L], LDL cholesterol > 160 mg/dL [4.1 mmol/L]) in the randomized, double-blind, parallel, 48-week EXCEL study. All changes in the lipid measurements (Table 4) in Lovastatin treated patients were dose-related and significantly different from placebo ($p \leq 0.001$). These results were sustained throughout the study. (See related table).

Atherosclerosis: In the Monitored Atherosclerosis Regression Study (MARS), the effect of therapy with Lovastatin on coronary atherosclerosis was assessed by coronary angiography in hyperlipidemic patients. In this randomized double-blind, controlled clinical trial, patients were treated with diet and either Lovastatin 80 mg daily or placebo. Angiograms were evaluated at baseline and at two years by computerized quantitative coronary angiography (QCA). No statistically significant difference between Lovastatin and placebo was seen for the primary endpoint (mean change per patient in percentage diameter stenosis of all lesions), or for most secondary QCA endpoints. Visual assessment by angiographers who formed a consensus opinion of overall angiographic change (Global Change Score) was also a secondary endpoint. By this endpoint, significant slowing of disease was seen, with regression in 23% of patients treated with Lovastatin compared to 11% of placebo patients.

In the Familial Atherosclerosis Treatment Study (FATS), either Lovastatin or niacin in combination with a bile acid sequestrant for 2.5 years in hyperlipidemic subjects significantly reduced the frequency of progression and increased the frequency of regression of coronary atherosclerotic lesions by QCA compared to diet and, in some cases, low-dose resin.

Eye: There was a high prevalence of baseline lenticular opacities in the patient population included in the early clinical trials with Lovastatin. During these trials the appearance of new opacities was noted in both the Lovastatin and placebo groups. There was no clinically significant change in visual acuity in the patients who had new opacities reported nor was any patient, including those with opacities noted at baseline, discontinued from therapy because of a decrease in visual acuity.

A three-year, double-blind, placebo-controlled study in hypercholesterolemic patients to assess the effect of Lovastatin on the human lens demonstrated that there were no clinically or statistically significant differences between the Lovastatin and placebo groups in the incidence, type progression of lenticular opacities.

INDICATIONS AND USAGE

Therapy with lipid-altering agents should be a component of multiple risk factor intervention in those individuals at significantly increased risk for artherosclerotic vascular disease due to hypercholesterolemia. Lovastatin is indicated as an adjunct to diet for the reduction of elevated total and LDL cholesterol levels in patients with primary hypercholesterolemia (Types IIa and IIb[1]), when the response to diet restricted in saturated fat and cholesterol and to other non-pharmacological measures alone has been inadequate.

Table 1
FAMILIAL HYPERCHOLESTEROLEMIA STUDY DOSE RESPONSE OF LOVASTATIN (PERCENT CHANGE FROM BASELINE AFTER 6 WEEKS)

Dosage	N	Total-C (mean)	LDL-C (mean)	HDL-C (mean)	LDL-C/HDL-C (mean)	Total-C/HDL-C (mean)	TRIG (median)
Placebo	21	−1	−2	+1	−1	0	+3
Lovastatin							
20 mg q.p.m.	20	−18	−19	+10	−26	−24	−7
40 mg q.p.m	21	−24	−27	+10	−32	−29	−22
10 mg b.i.d.	19	−22	−25	+6	−28	−25	−11
20 mg b.i.d.	20	−27	−31	+12	−38	−34	−18
40 mg b.i.d.	20	−34	−39	+8	−43	−38	−12

Table 2
LOVASTATIN VS. CHOLESTYRAMINE (PERCENT CHANGE FROM BASELINE AFTER 12 WEEKS)

Treatment	N	Total-C (mean)	LDL-C (mean)	HDL-C (mean)	Total-C/HDL-C (mean)	Total-C/HDL-C (mean)	VLDL-C (median)	TRIG (median)
Lovastatin								
20 mg b.i.d.	85	−27	−32	+9	−36	−31	−34	−21
40 mg b.i.d	88	−34	−42	+8	−44	−37	−31	−27
Cholestyramine								
12 g b.i.d.	88	−17	−23	+8	−27	−21	+2	+11

Table 3
LOVASTATIN VS. PROBUCOL (PERCENT CHANGE FROM BASELINE AFTER 14 WEEKS)

Treatment	N	Total-C (mean)	LDL-C (mean)	HDL-C (mean)	LDL-C/HDL-C (mean)	Total-C/HDL-C (mean)	VLDL-C (median)	TRIG (median)
Lovastatin								
40 mg q.p.m.	47	−25	−32	+9	−38	−31	−37	−18
80 mg q.p.m.	49	−30	−37	+11	−42	−36	−27	−17
40 mg b.i.d.	47	−33	−40	+12	−45	−39	−40	−25
Probucol								
500 mg b.i.d.	97	−10	−8	−23	+26	+23	−13	+1

◆ RATED THERAPEUTICALLY EQUIVALENT; ◇ THERAPEUTIC EQUIVALENCE UNCONFIRMED; ○ UNRATED

Prior to initiating therapy with Lovastatin, secondary causes for hypercholesterolemia (e.g., poorly controlled diabetes mellitus, hypothyroidism, nephrotic syndrome, dysproteinemias, obstructive liver disease, other drug therapy, alcoholism) should be excluded, and a lipid profile performed to measure TOTAL-C, HDL-C, and triglycerides (TG). For patients with TG less than 400 mg/dL (< 4.5 mmol/L), LDL-C can be estimated using the following equation:

$$LDL\text{-}C = Total\ cholesterol - [0.2 \times (triglycerides) + HDL\text{-}C]$$

For TG Levels > 400 mg/dL (> 4.5mmol/L), this equation is less accurate and LDL-C concentrations should be determined by ultracentrifugation. In hypertriglyceridemic patients, LDL-C may be low or normal despite elevated TOTAL-C. In such cases, Lovastatin is not indicated.

The effect of Lovastatin-induced changes in lipoprotein levels, including reduction of serum cholesterol, on cardiovascular morbidity or mortality has not been established.

The National Cholesterol Education Program (NCEP) Treatment Guidelines are summarized below:

Definite Atherosclerotic Disease*	Two or More Other Risk Factors**	LDL-Cholesterol mg/dL (mmol/L)	
		Initiation Level	Goal
No	No	≥ 190 (≥ 4.9)	< 160 (< 4.1)
No	Yes	≥ 160 (≥ 4.1)	< 130 (< 3.4)
Yes	Yes or No	≥ 130 (≥ 3.4)	≤ 100 (≤ 2.6)

* *Coronary heart disease or peripheral vascular disease (including symptomatic carotid artery disease).*

** *Other risk factors for coronary heart disease (CHD) include: age (males: ≥ 45 years; females: ≥ 55 years of premature menopause without estrogen replacement therapy); family history of premature CHD; current cigarette smoking; hypertension; confirmed HDL-C < 35 mg/dL (< 0.91 mmol/ L); and diabetes mellitus. Subtract one risk factor if HDL-C is ≥ 60 mg/dL (≥ 1.6 mmol/L).*

Since the goal of treatment is to lower LDL-C, the NCEP recommends that LDL-C levels be used to initiate and assess treatment response. Only if LDL-C levels are not available, should the TOTAL-C be used to monitor therapy.

Although Lovastatin may be useful to reduce elevated LDL cholesterol levels in patients with combined hypercholesterolemia and hypertriglyceridemia where hypercholesterolemia is the major abnormality (Type IIb hyperlipoproteinemia), it has not been studied in conditions where the major abnormality is elevation of chylomicrons, VLDL or IDL (i.e., hyperlipoproteinemia types I, III, IV, or V).[1]

[1] CLASSIFICATION OF HYPERLIPOPROTEINEMIAS

Type	Lipoproteins elevated	Lipid Elevations	
		major	minor
I (rare)	chylomicrons	TG	→ C
IIa	LDL	C	—
IIb	LDL, VLDL	C	TG
III (rare)	IDL	C/TG	—
IV	VLDL	TG	→ C
V (rare)	chylomicrons, VLDL	TG	→ C

C = cholesterol, TG = triglycerides,
LDL = low-density lipoprotein,
VLDL = very low-density lipoprotein,
IDL = intermediate-density lipoprotein.
† *For adult diabetics, a modification of these guidelines is recommended— see: American Diabetes Association Consensus Statement: Role of cardiovascular risk factors in prevention and treatment of macrovascular disease in diabetes, Diabetes Care 12(8): 573-79, 1989.*

CONTRAINDICATIONS
Hypersensitivity to any component of this medication.

Active liver disease or unexplained persistent elevations of serum transaminases (see "Warnings").

Pregnancy and Lactation: Atherosclerosis is a chronic process and the discontinuation of lipid-lowering drugs during pregnancy should have little impact on the outcome of long-term therapy of primary hypercholesterolemia. Moreover, cholesterol and other products of the cholesterol biosynthesis pathway are essential components for fetal development, including synthesis of steroids and cell membranes. Because of the ability of inhibitors of HMG-CoA reductase such as Lovastatin to decrease the synthesis of cholesterol and possibly other products of the cholesterol biosynthesis pathway, Lovastatin may cause fetal harm when administered to a pregnant woman. Therefore, Lovastatin is contraindicated during pregnancy. **Lovastatin should be administered to women of childbearing age only when such patients are highly unlikely to conceive.** If the patient becomes pregnant while taking this drug, Lovastatin should be discontinued and the patient should be apprised of the potential hazard to the fetus.

WARNINGS
LIVER DYSFUNCTION
Marked persistent increases (to more than 3 times the upper limit of normal) in serum transaminases occurred in 1.9% of adult patients who received Lovastatin for at least one year in early clinical trials (see "Adverse Reactions"). When the drug was interrupted or discontinued in these patients, the transaminase levels usually fell slowly to pretreatment levels. The increases usually appeared 3 to 12 months after the start of therapy with Lovastatin, and were not associated with jaundice or other clinical signs or symptoms. There was no evidence of hypersensitivity. In the EXCEL study (see "Clinical Pharmacology, Clinical Studies"), the incidence of marked persistent increases in serum transaminases over 48 weeks was 0.1% for placebo, 0.1% at 20 mg/day, 0.9% at 40 mg/day, and 1.5% at 80 mg/day in patients on Lovastatin. However, in post-marketing experience with Lovastatin, symptomatic liver disease has been reported rarely at all dosages (see "Adverse Reactions").

It is recommended that liver function tests be performed during therapy with Lovastatin. Serum transaminases, including ALT (SGPT), should be monitored before treatment begins, every 6 weeks during the first 3 months, every 8 weeks during the remainder of the first year, and periodically therafter (e.g., at approximately 6 month intervals). Special attention should be paid to patients who develop elevated serum transaminase levels, and in these patients, measurements should be repeated promptly and then performed more frequently. If the transaminase levels show evidence of progression, particularly if they rise to three times the upper limit of normal and are persistent, the drug should be discontinued. Liver biopsy should be considered if elevations are persistent beyond the discontinuation of the drug.

The drug should be used with caution in patients who consume substantial quantities of alcohol and/or have a past history of liver disease. Active liver disease or unexplained transaminase elevations are contraindications to the use of Lovastatin.

As with other lipid-lowering agents, moderate (less than three times the upper limit of normal) elevations of serum transaminases have been reported following therapy with Lovastatin (see "Adverse Reactions"). These changes appeared soon after initiation of therapy with Lovastatin, were often transient, were not accompanied by any symptoms and interruption of treatment was not required.

SKELETAL MUSCLE
Rhabdomyolysis has been associated with Lovastatin therapy alone, when combined with immunosuppressive therapy including cyclosporine in cardiac transplant patients, and when combined in non-transplant patients with either gemfibrozil or lipid-lowering doses (≥ 1 g/day) of nicotinic acid. Some of the affected patients had pre-existing renal insufficiency, usually as a consequence of long-standing diabetes. Acute renal failure from rhabdomyolysis has been seen more commonly with the Lovastatin-gemfibrozil combination, and has also been reported in transplant patients receiving Lovastatin plus cyclosporine.

Rhabdomyolysis with or without renal impairment has been reported in seriously ill patients receiving erythromycin concomitantly with Lovastatin. Therefore, patients receiving concomitant Lovastatin and erythromycin should be carefully monitored.

Fulminant rhabdomyolysis has been seen as early as three weeks after initiation of combined therapy with gemfibrozil and Lovastatin, but may be seen after several months. For these reasons, it is felt that, in most subjects who have had an unsatisfactory lipid response to either drug alone, the possible benefits of combined therapy with Lovastatin and gemfibrozil do not outweigh the risks of severe myopathy, rhabdomyolysis, and acute renal failure. While it is not known whether this interaction occurs with fibrates other than gemfibrozil, myopathy and rhabdomyolysis have occasionally been associated with the use of other fibrates alone, including clofibrate. Therefore, the combined use of Lovastatin with other fibrates should generally be avoided.

Table 4
**LOVASTATIN VS. PLACEBO
(PERCENT CHANGE FROM BASELINE—AVERAGE VALUES BETWEEN WEEKS 12 AND 48)**

Dosage	N*	Total-C (mean)	LDL-C (mean)	HDL-C (mean)	LDL/C HDL-C (mean)	Total-C/HDL-C (mean)	TRIG. (median)
Placebo	1663	+0.7	+0.4	+2.0	+0.2	+0.6	+4
Lovastatin							
20 mg q.p.m.	1642	−17	−24	+6.6	−27	−21	−10
40 mg q.p.m.	1645	−22	−30	+7.2	−34	−26	−14
20 mg b.i.d.	1646	−24	−34	+8.6	−38	−29	−16
40 mg b.i.d.	1649	−29	−40	+9.5	−44	−34	−19

* *Patients enrolled*

Physicians contemplating combined therapy with Lovastatin and lipid-lowering doses of nicotinic acid or with immunosuppressive drugs should carefully weigh the potential benefits and risks and should carefully monitor patients for any signs and symptoms of muscle pain, tenderness, or weakness, particularly during the initial months of therapy and during any periods of upward dosage titration of either drug. Periodic CPK determinations may be considered in such situations, but there is no assurance that such monitoring will prevent the occurrence of severe myopathy. The monitoring of Lovastatin drug and metabolite levels may be considered in transplant patients who are treated with immunosuppressives and Lovastatin.

Lovastatin therapy should be temporarily withheld or discontinued in any patient with an acute, serious condition suggestive of a myopathy or having a risk factor predisposing to the development of renal failure secondary to rhabdomyolysis, including: severe acute infection, hypotension, major surgery, trauma, severe metabolic, endocrine and electrolyte disorders, and uncontrolled seizures.

Myalgia has been associated with Lovastatin therapy. Transient, mildly elevated creatine phosphokinase levels are commonly seen in Lovastatin-treated patients. However, in early clinical trials, approximately 0.5% of patients developed a myopathy, i.e., myalgia or muscle weakness associated with markedly elevated CPK levels. In the EXCEL study (see *"Clinical Pharmacology, Clinical Studies"*), five (0.1%) patients taking Lovastatin alone (one at 40 mg q.p.m., and four at 40 mg b.i.d.) developed myopathy (muscle symptoms and CPK levels > 10 times the upper limit of normal). Myopathy should be considered in any patient with diffuse myalgias, muscle tenderness or weakness, and/or marked elevation of CPK. Patients should be advised to report promptly unexplained muscle pain, tenderness or weakness, particularly if accompanied by malaise or fever. Lovastatin therapy should be discontinued if markedly elevated CPK levels occur or myopathy is diagnosed or suspected.

Most of the patients who have developed myopathy (including rhabdomyolysis) while taking Lovastatin were receiving concomitant therapy with immunosuppressive drugs, gemfibrozil or lipid-lowering doses of nicotinic acid. In clinical trials, about 30 percent of patients on concomitant immunosuppressive therapy including cyclosporine developed myopathy; the corresponding percentages for gemfibrozil and niacin were approximately 5 percent and 2 percent respectively.

In six patients with cardiac transplants taking immunosuppressive therapy including cyclosporine concomitantly with Lovastatin 20 mg/day, the average plasma level of active metabolites derived from Lovastatin was elevated to approximately four times the expected levels. Because of an apparent relationship between increased plasma levels of active metabolites derived from Lovastatin and myopathy, the daily dosage in patients taking immunosuppressants should not exceed 20 mg/day (see *"Dosage and Administration"*). Even at this dosage, the benefits and risks of using Lovastatin in patients taking immunosuppressants should be carefully considered.

PRECAUTIONS
GENERAL
Before instituting therapy with Lovastatin, an attempt should be made to control hypercholesterolemia with appropriate diet, exercise, weight reduction in obese patients, and to treat other underlying medical problems (see *"Indications and Usage"*).

Lovastatin may elevate creatine phosphokinase and transaminase levels (see *"Warnings"* and *"Adverse Reactions"*). This should be considered in the differential diagnosis of chest pain in a patient on therapy with Lovastatin.

HOMOZYGOUS FAMILIAL HYPERCHOLESTEROLEMIA
Lovastatin is less effective in patients with the rare homozygous familial hypercholesterolemia, possibly because these patients have no functional LDL receptors. Lovastatin appears to be more likely to raise serum transaminases (see *"Adverse Reactions"*) in these homozygous patients.

INFORMATION FOR PATIENTS
Patients should be advised to report promptly unexplained muscle pain, tenderness or weakness, particularly if accompanied by malaise or fever.

DRUG INTERACTIONS
Immunosuppressive Drugs, Gemfibrozil, Niacin (Nicotinic Acid), Erythromycin: See *"Warnings, Skeletal Muscle"*.

Coumarin Anticoagulants: In a small clinical trial in which Lovastatin was administered to warfarin treated patients, no effect on prothrombin time was detected. However, another HMG-CoA reductase inhibitor has been found to produce a less than two seconds increase in prothrombin time in healthy volunteers receiving low doses of warfarin. Also, bleeding and/or increased prothrombin time have been reported in a few patients taking coumarin anticoagulants concomitantly with Lovastatin. It is recommended that in patients taking anticoagulants, prothrombin time be determined before starting Lovastatin and frequently enough during early therapy to insure that no significant alteration of prothrombin time occurs. Once a stable prothrombin time has been documented, prothrombin times can be monitored at the intervals usually recommended for patients on coumarin anticoagulants. If the dose of Lovastatin is changed, the same procedure should be repeated. Lovastatin therapy has not been associated with bleeding or with changes in prothrombin time in patients not taking anticoagulants.

Antipyrine: Because Lovastatin had no effect on the pharmacokinetics of antipyrine or its metabolites, interactions of other drugs metabolized via the same cytochrome isozymes are not expected.

Propranolol: In normal volunteers, there was no clinically significant pharmacokinetic or pharmacodynamic interaction with concomitant administration of single doses of Lovastatin and propranolol.

Digoxin: In patients with hypercholesterolemia, concomitant administration of Lovastatin and digoxin resulted in no effect on digoxin plasma concentrations.

Oral Hypoglycemic Agents: In pharmacokinetic studies of Lovastatin in hypercholesterolemic non-insulin dependent diabetic patients, there was no drug interaction with glipizide or with chlorpropamide (see *"Clinical Pharmacology, Clinical Studies"*).

Other Concomitant Therapy: Although specific interaction studies were not performed, in clinical studies, Lovastatin was used concomitantly with beta blockers, calcium channel blockers, diuretics and nonsteroidal anti-inflammatory drugs (NSAIDs) without evidence of clinically significant adverse interactions.

ENDOCRINE FUNCTION
HMG-CoA reductase inhibitors interfere with cholesterol synthesis and as such might theoretically blunt adrenal and/or gonadal steroid production. Results of clinical trials with drugs in this class have been inconsistent with regard to drug effects on basal and reserve steroid levels. However, clinical studies have shown that Lovastatin does not reduce basal plasma cortisol concentration or impair adrenal reserve, and does not reduce basal plasma testosterone concentration. Another HMG-CoA reductase inhibitor has been shown to reduce the plasma testosterone response to HCG. In the same study, the mean testosterone response to HCG was slightly but not significantly reduced after treatment with Lovastatin 40 mg daily for 16 weeks in 21 men. The effects of HMG-CoA reductase inhibitors on male fertility have not been studied in adequate numbers of male patients. The effects, if any, on the pituitary-gonadal axis in premenopausal women are unknown. Patients treated with Lovastatin who develop clinical evidence of endocrine dysfunction should be evaluated appropriately. Caution should also be exercised if an HMG-CoA reductase inhibitor or other agent used to lower cholesterol levels is administered to patients also receiving other drugs (e.g., ketoconazole, spironolactone, cimetidine) that may decrease the levels or activity of endogenous steroid hormones.

CNS TOXICITY
Lovastatin produced optic nerve degeneration (Wallerian degeneration of retinogeniculate fibers) in clinically normal dogs in a dose-dependent fashion starting at 60 mg/kg/day, a dose that produced mean plasma drug levels about 30 times higher than the mean drug level in humans taking the highest recommended dose (as measured by total enzyme inhibitory activity). Vestibulocochlear Wallerian-like degeneration and retinal ganglion cell chromatolysis were also seen in dogs treated for 14 weeks at 180 mg/kg/day, a dose which resulted in a mean plasma drug level (C_{max}) similar to that seen with the 60 mg/kg/day dose.

CNS vascular lesions, characterized by perivascular hemorrhage and edema, mononuclear cell infiltration of perivascular spaces, perivascular fibrin deposits and necrosis of small vessels, were seen in dogs treated with Lovastatin at a dose of 180 mg/kg/day, a dose which produced plasma drug levels (C_{max}) which were about 30 times higher than the mean values in humans taking 80 mg/day.

Similar optic nerve and CNS vascular lesions have been observed with other drugs of this class.

CARCINOGENESIS, MUTAGENESIS, IMPAIRMENT OF FERTILITY
In a 21-month carcinogenic study in mice, there was a statistically significant increase in the incidence of hepatocellular carcinomas and adenomas in both males and females at 500 mg/kg/day. This dose produced a total plasma drug exposure 3 to 4 times that of humans given the highest recommended dose of Lovastatin (drug exposure was measured as total HMG-CoA reductase inhibitory activity in extracted plasma). Tumor increases were not seen at 20 and 100 mg/kg/day, doses that produced drug exposures of 0.3 to 2 times that of humans at the 80 mg/day dose. A statistically significant increase in pulmonary adenomas was seen in female mice at approximately 4 times the human drug exposure. (Although mice were given 300 times the human dose [HD] on a mg/kg body weight basis, plasma levels of total inhibitory activity were only 4 times higher in mice than in humans given 80 mg of Lovastatin.)

There was an increase in incidence of papilloma in the nonglandular mucosa of the stomach of mice beginning at exposures of 1 to 2 times that of humans. The glandular mucosa was not affected. The human stomach contains only glandular mucosa.

In a 24-month carcinogenicity study in rats, there was a positive dose response relationship for hepatocellular carcinogenicity in males at drug exposures between 2-7 times that of human exposure at 80 mg/day (doses in rats were 5, 30 and 180 mg/kg/day).

A chemically similar drug in this class was administered to mice for 72 weeks at 25, 100, and 400 mg/kg body weight, which resulted in mean serum drug levels approximately 3, 15, and 33 times higher than the mean human serum drug concentration (as total inhibitory activity) after a 40 mg oral dose. Liver carcinomas were significantly increased in high dose females and mid- and high dose males, with a maximum incidence of 90 percent in males. The incidence of adenomas of the liver was significantly increased in mid- and high dose females. Drug treatment also significantly increased the incidence of lung adenomas in mid- and high dose males and females. Adenomas of the Harderian gland (a gland of the eye of rodents) were significantly higher in high dose mice than in controls.

No evidence of mutagenicity was observed in a microbial mutagen test using mutant strains of *Salmonella typhimurium* with or without rat or mouse liver metabolic activation. In addition, no evidence of damage of genetic material was noted in an *in vitro* alkaline elution assay using rat or mouse hepatocytes, a V-79 mammalian cell forward mutation study, an *in vitro* chromosome aberration study in CHO cells, or an *in vivo* chromosomal aberration assay in mouse bone marrow.

Drug-related testicular atrophy, decreased spermatogenesis, spermatocytic degeneration and giant cell formation were seen in dogs starting at 20 mg/kg/day. Similar findings were seen with another drug in this class. No drug-related effects on fertility were found in studies with Lovastatin in rats. However, in studies with a similar drug in this class, there was decreased fertility in male rats treated for 34 weeks at 25 mg/kg body weight, although this effect was not observed in a subsequent fertility study when this same dose was administered for 11 weeks (the entire cycle of spermatogenesis, including epididymal maturation). In rats treated with this same reductase inhibitor at 180 mg/kg/day, seminiferous tubule degeneration (necrosis and loss of spermatogenic epithelium) was observed. No microscopic changes were observed in the testes from rats of either study. The clinical significance of these findings is unclear.

PREGNANCY
Pregnancy Category X: see *"Contraindications"*.

Safety in pregnant women has not been established. Lovastatin has been shown to produce skeletal malformations at plasma levels 40 times the human exposure (for mouse fetus) and 80 times the human exposure (for rat fetus) based on mg/m² surface area (doses were 800 mg/kg/day). No drug-induced changes were seen in either species at multiples of 8 times (rat) or 4 times (mouse) based on surface area. No evidence of malformations was noted in rabbits at exposures up to 3 times the human exposure (dose of 15 mg/kg/day, highest tolerated dose). Rare reports of congenital anomalies have been received following intrauterine exposure to HMG-CoA reductase inhibitors. There has been one report of severe congenital bony deformity, tracheo-esophageal fistula, and anal atresia (VATER association) in a baby born to a woman who took Lovastatin with dextroamphetamine sulfate during the first trimester of pregnancy. Lovastatin should be administered to women of child-bearing potential only when such patients are highly unlikely to conceive and have been informed of the potential hazards. If the woman becomes pregnant while taking Lovastatin, it should be discontinued and the patient advised again as to the potential hazards to the fetus.

NURSING MOTHERS
It is not known whether Lovastatin is excreted in human milk. Because a small amount of another drug in this class is excreted in human breast milk and because of the potential for serious adverse reactions in nursing infants, women taking Lovastatin should not nurse their infants (see *"Contraindications"*).

PEDIATRIC USE
Safety and effectiveness in children and adolescents have not been established. Because children and adolescents are not likely to benefit from cholesterol lowering for at least a decade and because experience with this drug is limited (no studies in subjects below the age of 20 years), treatment of children with Lovastatin is not recommended at this time.

ADVERSE REACTIONS
Lovastatin is generally well tolerated; adverse reactions usually have been mild and transient. Less than 1% of patients were discontinued from controlled clinical studies of up to 14 weeks due to adverse experiences attributable to Lovastatin. About 3% of patients were discontinued from extensions of these studies due to adverse experiences attributable to Lovastatin: about half of these patients were discontinued due to increases in serum transaminases. The median duration of therapy in these extensions was 5.2 years.

In the EXCEL study (see *"Clinical Pharmacology, Clinical Studies"*), 4.6% of the patients treated up to 48 weeks were discontinued due to clinical or laboratory adverse experiences which were rated by the investigator as possibly, probably or definitely related to therapy with Lovastatin. The value for the placebo group was 2.5%.

CLINICAL ADVERSE EXPERIENCES
Adverse experiences reported in patients treated with Lovastatin in controlled clinical studies are shown in the table below: (See related table).

LABORATORY TESTS
Marked persistent increases of serum transaminases have been noted (see *"Warnings"*).

About 11% of patients had elevations of creatine phosphokinase (CPK) levels of at least twice the normal value on one or more occasions. The corresponding values for the control agents were cholestyramine, 9 percent and probucol, 2 percent. This was attributable to the noncardiac fraction of CPK. Large increases in CPK have sometimes been reported (see *"Warnings, Skeletal Muscle"*).

EXPANDED CLINICAL EVALUATION OF LOVASTATIN (EXCEL) STUDY

CLINICAL ADVERSE EXPERIENCES
Lovastatin was compared to placebo in 8.245 patients with hypercholesterolemia (total cholesterol 240-300 mg/dL [6.2-7.8 mmol/L]) in the randomized, double-blind, parallel, 48-week EXCEL study. Clinical adverse experiences reported as possibly, probably or definitely drug-related in ≥ 1% in any treatment group are shown in the table below. For no event was the incidence on drug and placebo statistically different. (See related table).

Other clinical adverse experiences reported as possibly, probably or definitely drug-related in 0.5 to 1.0 percent of patients in any drug-related group are listed below. In all these cases the incidence on drug and placebo was not statistically different.

Body as a Whole: chest pain;

Gastrointestinal: acid regurgitation, dry mouth, vomiting;

Musculoskeletal: leg pain, shoulder pain, arthralgia;

Nervous System/Psychiatric: insomnia, paresthesia;

Skin: alopecia, pruritus;

Special Senses: eye irritation.

CONCOMITANT THERAPY
In controlled clinical studies in which Lovastatin was administered concomitantly with cholestyramine, no adverse reactions peculiar to this concomitant treatment were observed. The adverse reactions that occurred were limited to those reported previously with Lovastatin or cholestyramine. Other lipid-lowering agents were not administered concomitantly with Lovastatin during controlled clinical studies. Preliminary data suggests that the addition of either probucol or gemfibrozil to therapy with Lovastatin is not associated with greater reduction in LDL cholesterol than that achieved with Lovastatin alone. In uncontrolled clinical studies, most of the patients who have developed myopathy were receiving concomitant therapy with immunosuppressive drugs, gemfibrozil or niacin (nicotinic acid) (See *"Warnings, Skeletal Muscle"*).

The following effects have been reported with drugs in this class. Not all the effects listed below have necessarily been associated with Lovastatin therapy.

Skeletal: myopathy, rhabdomyolysis, arthralgias.

Neurological: dysfunction of certain cranial nerves (including alteration of taste, impairment of extra-ocular movement, facial paresis), tremor, vertigo, memory loss, paresthesia, peripheral neuropathy, peripheral nerve palsy, anxiety, insomnia, depression.

Hypersensitivity Reactions: An apparent hypersenstivity syndrome has been reported rarely which has included one or more of the following features: anaphylaxis, angioedema, lupus erythematous-like syndrome, polymyalgia rheumatica, vasculitis, purpura, thrombocytopenia, leukopenia, hemolytic anemia, positive ANA, ESR increase, eosinophilia, arthritis, arthralgia, urticaria, asthenia, photosensitivity, fever, chills, flushing, malaise, dyspnea, toxic epidermal necrolysis, erythema multiforme, including Stevens-Johnson syndrome.

	Lovastatin (N = 613) %	Placebo (N = 82) %	Cholestyramine (N = 88) %	Probucol (N = 97) %
Gastrointestinal				
Constipation	4.9	—	34.1	2.1
Diarrhea	5.5	4.9	8.0	10.3
Dyspepsia	3.9	—	13.6	3.1
Flatus	6.4	2.4	21.6	5.2
Abdominal pain/cramps	5.7	2.4	5.7	5.2
Heartburn	1.6	—	8.0	—
Nausea	4.7	3.7	9.1	6.2
Musculoskeletal				
Muscle cramps	1.1	—	1.1	—
Myalgia	2.4	1.2	—	—
Nervous System/Psychiatric				
Dizziness	2.0	1.2	—	1.0
Headache	9.3	4.9	4.5	8.2
Skin				
Rash/pruritus	5.2	—	4.5	—
Special Senses				
Blurred vision	1.5	—	1.1	3.1
Dysgeusia	0.8	—	1.1	—

	Placebo (N = 1663) %	Lovastatin 20 mg q.p.m. (N = 1642) %	Lovastatin 40 mg q.p.m. (N = 1645) %	Lovastatin 20 mg b.i.d. (N = 1646) %	Lovastatin 40 mg b.i.d. (N = 1649) %
Body As a Whole					
Asthenia	1.4	1.7	1.4	1.5	1.2
Gastrointestinal					
Abdominal pain	1.6	2.0	2.0	2.2	2.5
Constipation	1.9	2.0	3.2	3.2	3.5
Diarrhea	2.3	2.6	2.4	2.2	2.6
Dyspepsia	1.9	1.3	1.3	1.0	1.6
Flatulence	4.2	3.7	4.3	3.9	4.5
Nausea	2.5	1.9	2.5	2.2	2.2
Musculoskeletal					
Muscle cramps	0.5	0.6	0.8	1.1	1.0
Myalgia	1.7	2.6	1.8	2.2	3.0
Nervous System/Psychiatric					
Dizziness	0.7	0.7	1.2	0.5	0.5
Headache	2.7	2.6	2.8	2.1	3.2
Skin					
Rash	0.7	0.8	1.0	1.2	1.3
Special Senses					
Blurred vision	0.8	1.1	0.9	0.9	1.2

Gastrointestinal: pancreatitis, hepatitis, including chronic active hepatitis, cholestatic jaundice, fatty change in liver; and rarely, cirrhosis, fulminant hepatic necrosis, and hepatoma; anorexia, vomiting.

Skin: alopecia, pruritus. A variety of skin changes (e.g., nodules, discoloration, dryness of skin/mucous membranes, changes to hair/nails) has been reported.

Reproductive: gynecomastia, loss of libido, erectile dysfunction.

Eye: progression of cataracts (lens opacities), ophthalmoplegia.

Laboratory, Abnormalities: elevated transaminases, alkaline phosphatase, and bilirubin; thyroid function abnormalities.

OVERDOSAGE
After oral administration of Lovastatin to mice the median lethal dose observed was > 15 g/m^2.

Five healthy human volunteers have received up to 200 mg of Lovastatin as a single dose without clinically significant adverse experiences. A few cases of accidental overdosage have been reported; no patients had any specific symptoms, and all patients recovered without sequelae. The maximum dose taken was 5-6 g.

Until further experience is obtained, no specific treatment of overdosage with Lovastatin can be recommended.

The dialyzability of Lovastatin and its metabolites in man is not known at present.

DOSAGE AND ADMINISTRATION
The patient should be placed on a standard cholesterol-lowering diet before receiving Lovastatin and should continue on this diet during treatment with Lovastatin (see NCEP Treatment Guidelines for details on dietary therapy). Lovastatin should be given with meals.

The recommended starting dose is 20 mg once a day given with the evening meal. The recommended dosing range is 20-80 mg/day in single or divided doses; the maximum recommended dose is 80 mg/day. Adjustments of dosage should be made at intervals of 4 weeks or more. Doses should be individualized according to the patient's response (see *Tables 1 to 4 under "Clinical Pharmacology, Clinical Studies"* for dose response results).

In patients taking immunosuppressive drugs concomitantly with Lovastatin (see *"Warnings, Skeletal Muscle"*), therapy should begin with 10 mg of Lovastatin and should not exceed 20 mg/day.

Cholesterol levels should be monitored periodically and consideration should be given to reducing the dosage of Lovastatin if cholesterol levels fall below the targeted range.

CONCOMITANT THERAPY
Preliminary evidence suggests that the cholesterol-lowering effects of Lovastatin and the bile acid sequestrant, cholestyramine, are additive.

DOSAGE IN PATIENTS WITH RENAL INSUFFICIENCY
In patients with severe renal insufficiency (creatinine clearance < 30 mL/min), dosage increases above 20 mg/day should be carefully considered and, if deemed necessary, implemented cautiously (see *"Clinical Pharmacology"* and *"Warnings, Skeletal Muscle"*).

STORAGE
Store between 5-30°C (41-86°F). Lovastatin Tablets must be protected from light and stored in a well-closed, light-resistant container.

HOW SUPPLIED
TABLETS: 10 MG

BRAND/MANUFACTURER	NDC	SIZE	AWP
○ BRAND			
▶ MEVACOR: Merck	00006-0730-61	60s	$73.69

TABLETS: 20 MG

BRAND/MANUFACTURER	NDC	SIZE	AWP
○ BRAND			
▶ MEVACOR: Merck	00006-0731-61	60s	$119.79
	00006-0731-28	100s ud	$203.23
	00006-0731-37	360s	$718.71
	00006-0731-82	1000s	$1996.58
	00006-0731-94	1080s	$2156.48
	00006-0731-78	1200s	$2396.09
	00006-0731-98	2160s	$4313.41
	00006-0731-87	10000s	$19965.83

TABLETS: 40 MG

BRAND/MANUFACTURER	NDC	SIZE	AWP
○ BRAND			
▶ MEVACOR: Merck	00006-0732-61	60s	$215.61
	00006-0732-82	1000s	$3593.63
	00006-0732-94	1080s	$3881.29
	00006-0732-87	10000s	$35936.33

Lovenox SEE ENOXAPARIN

Loxapine

DESCRIPTION
Loxapine, a dibenzoxazepine compound, represents a new subclass of tricyclic antipsychotic agent, chemically distinct from the thioxanthenes, butyrophenones, and phenothiazines. Chemically, it is 2-chloro-11-(4-methyl-1-piperazinyl)-dibenz[b,f] [1,4]oxazepine. It is present in capsules as the succinate salt, and in the concentrate and parenteral primarily as the hydrochloride salt.

CAPSULES
Each capsule contains Loxapine Succinate equivalent to 5, 10, 25, or 50 mg of Loxapine base.

ORAL CONCENTRATE
Each mL contains Loxapine Hydrochloride equivalent to 25 mg of Loxapine base.

INTRAMUSCULAR (STERILE)
Not for Intravenous Use: Each mL contains Loxapine Hydrochloride equivalent to 50 mg of Loxapine base.

CLINICAL PHARMACOLOGY
Pharmacodynamics: Pharmacologically, Loxapine is a tranquilizer for which the exact mode of action has not been established. However, changes in the level of excitability of subcortical inhibitory areas have been observed in several animal species in association with such manifestations of tranquilization as calming effects and suppression of aggressive behavior.

In normal human volunteers, signs of sedation were seen within 20 to 30 minutes after administration, were most pronounced within 1½ to 3 hours, and lasted through 12 hours. Similar timing of primary pharmacologic effects was seen in animals.

Absorption, Distribution, Metabolism, and Excretion: After administration of Loxapine as an oral solution, systemic bioavailability of the parent drug was only about one third that after an equivalent intramuscular dose (25 mg base) in male volunteers. C$_{max}$ for the parent drug was similar for the IM and oral administrations, whereas T$_{max}$ was significantly longer for the IM administration than the oral administration (approximately 5 v 1 hour). The lower systemic availability of the parent drug after oral administration as compared to the IM administration may be due to first pass metabolism of the oral form. This is supported by the finding that two metabolites found in serum (8-hydroxyloxapine and 8-hydroxy-desmethylloxapine) were formed to a lesser extent after IM administration of Loxapine as compared to oral administration.

The apparent half-life of Loxapine after oral and IM administration is approximately 4 hours (range, 1 to 14 hours) and 12 hours (range, 8 to 23 hours), respectively. The extended half-life for the IM administration as compared to the oral administration may be explained by prolonged absorption of Loxapine from the muscle during the concurrent elimination process.

Loxapine is extensively metabolized, and urinary recovery over 48 hours resulted in recoveries of approximately 30% and 40% of an IM and orally administered Loxapine dose as five metabolites.

INDICATIONS

Loxapine is indicated for the management of the manifestations of psychotic disorders. The antipsychotic efficacy of Loxapine was established in clinical studies which enrolled newly hospitalized and chronically hospitalized acutely ill schizophrenic patients as subjects.

UNLABELED USES
Loxapine is used alone in the treatment of dementia.

CONTRAINDICATIONS

Loxapine is contraindicated in comatose or severe drug-induced depressed states (alcohol, barbiturates, narcotics, etc).

Loxapine is contraindicated in individuals with known hypersensitivity to dibenzoxazepines.

WARNINGS

Tardive Dyskinesia: Tardive dyskinesia, a syndrome consisting of potentially irreversible, involuntary, dyskinetic movements, may develop in patients treated with neuroleptic (antipsychotic) drugs. Although the prevalence of the syndrome appears to be highest among the elderly, especially elderly women, it is impossible to rely upon prevalence estimates to predict, at the inception of neuroleptic treatment, which patients are likely to develop the syndrome. Whether neuroleptic drug products differ in their potential to cause tardive dyskinesia is unknown.

Both the risk of developing the syndrome and the likelihood that it will become irreversible are believed to increase as the duration of treatment and the total cumulative dose of neuroleptic drugs administered to the patient increase. However, the syndrome can develop, although much less commonly, after relatively brief treatment periods at low doses. There is no known treatment for established cases of tardive dyskinesia, although the syndrome may remit, partially or completely, if neuroleptic treatment is withdrawn. Neuroleptic treatment, itself, however, may suppress (or partially suppress) the signs and symptoms of the syndrome, and thereby may possibly mask the underlying disease process. The effect that symptomatic suppression has upon the long-term course of the syndrome is unknown.

Given these considerations, neuroleptics should be prescribed in a manner that is most likely to minimize the occurrence of tardive dyskinesia. Chronic neuroleptic treatment should generally be reserved for patients who suffer from a chronic illness that (1) is known to respond to neuroleptic drugs, and (2) for whom alternative, equally effective, but potentially less harmful treatments are *not* available or appropriate. In patients who do require chronic treatment, the smallest dose and the shortest duration of treatment producing a satisfactory clinical response should be sought. The need for continued treatment should be reassessed periodically.

If signs and symptoms of tardive dyskinesia appear in a patient on neuroleptics, drug discontinuation should be considered. However, some patients may require treatment despite the presence of the syndrome. (see *"Adverse Reactions"* and *"Information for Patients"* sections).

Neuroleptic Malignant Syndrome (NMS): A potentially fatal symptom complex sometimes referred to as Neuroleptic Malignant Syndrome (NMS) has been reported in association with antipsychotic drugs. Clinical manifestations of NMS are hyperpyrexia, muscle rigidity, altered mental status and evidence of autonomic instability (irregular pulse or blood pressure, tachycardia, diaphoresis, and cardiac dysrhythmias).

The diagnostic evaluation of patients with this syndrome is complicated. In arriving at a diagnosis, it is important to identify cases where the clinical presentation includes both serious medical illness (eg, pneumonia, systemic infection, etc) and untreated or inadequately treated extrapyramidal signs and symptoms (EPS). Other important considerations in the differential diagnosis include central anticholinergic toxicity, heat stroke, drug fever and primary central nervous system (CNS) pathology.

The management of NMS should include: (1) immediate discontinuation of antipsychotic drugs and other drugs not essential to concurrent therapy, (2) intensive symptomatic treatment and medical monitoring, and (3) treatment of any concomitant serious medical problems for which specific treatments are available. There is no general agreement about specific pharmacological treatment regimens for uncomplicated NMS.

If a patient requires antipsychotic drug treatment after recovery from NMS, the potential reintroduction of drug therapy should be carefully considered. The patient should be carefully monitored, since recurrences of NMS have been reported.

Loxapine like other tranquilizers, may impair mental and/or physical abilities, especially during the first few days of therapy. Therefore, ambulatory patients should be warned about activities requiring alertness (eg, operating vehicles or machinery) and about concomitant use of alcohol and other CNS depressants.

Loxapine has not been evaluated for the management of behavioral complications in patients with mental retardation, and therefore, it cannot be recommended.

PRECAUTIONS

General: Loxapine should be used with extreme caution in patients with a history of convulsive disorders since it lowers the convulsive threshold. Seizures have been reported in patients receiving Loxapine at antipsychotic dose level, and may occur in epileptic patients even with maintenance of routine anticonvulsant drug therapy.

Loxapine has an antiemetic effect in animals. Since this effect may also occur in man, Loxapine may mask signs of overdosage of toxic drugs and may obscure conditions such as intestinal obstruction and brain tumor.

Loxapine should be used with caution in patients with cardiovascular disease. Increased pulse rates have been reported in the majority of patients receiving antipsychotic doses; transient hypotension has been reported. In the presence of severe hypotension requiring vasopressor therapy, the preferred drugs may be norepinephrine and angiotensin. Usual doses of epinephrine may be ineffective because of inhibition of its vasopressor effect by Loxapine.

The possibility of ocular toxicity from Loxapine cannot be excluded at this time. Therefore, careful observation should be made for pigmentary retinopathy and lenticular pigmentation, since these have been observed in some patients receiving certain other antipsychotic drugs for prolonged periods.

Because of possible anticholinergic action, the drug should be used cautiously in patients with glaucoma or a tendency to urinary retention, particularly with concomitant administration of anticholinergic-type antiparkinson medication.

Experience to date indicates the possibility of a slightly higher incidence of extrapyramidal effects following intramuscular administration than normally anticipated with oral formulations. The increase may be attributable to higher plasma levels following intramuscular injection.

Neuroleptic drugs elevate prolactin levels; the elevation persists during chronic administration. Tissue culture experiments indicate that approximately one third of human breast cancers are prolactin-dependent *in vitro*, a factor of potential importance if the prescription of these drugs is contemplated in a patient with a previously detected breast cancer. Although disturbances such as galactorrhea, amenorrhea, gynecomastia, and impotence have been reported, the clinical significance of elevated serum prolactin levels is unknown for most patients. An increase in mammary neoplasms has been found in rodents after chronic administration of neuroleptic drugs. Neither clinical studies nor epidemiologic studies conducted to date, however, have shown an association between chronic administration of these drugs and mammary tumorigenesis; the available evidence is considered too limited to be conclusive at this time.

Information for Patients: Given the likelihood that some patients exposed chronically to neuroleptics will develop tardive dyskinesia, it is advised that all patients in whom chronic use is contemplated be given, if possible, full information about this risk. The decision to inform patients and/or their guardians must obviously take into account the clinical circumstances and the competency of the patient to understand the information provided.

Usage in Pregnancy: Safe use of Loxapine during pregnancy or lactation has not been established; therefore, its use in pregnancy, in nursing mothers, or in women of childbearing potential requires that the benefits of treatment be weighted against the possible risks to mother and child. No embryotoxicity or teratogenicity was observed in studies in rats, rabbits, or dogs, although, with the exception of one rabbit study, the highest dosage was only two times the maximum recommended human dose and in some studies it was below this dose. Perinatal studies have shown renal papillary abnormalities in offspring of rats treated from midpregnancy with doses of 0.6 and 1.8 mg/kg, doses which approximate the usual human dose, but which are considerably below the maximum recommended human dose.

Nursing Mothers: The extent of the excretion of Loxapine or its metabolites in human milk is not known. However, Loxapine and its metabolites have been shown to be transported into the milk of lactating dogs. Loxapine administration to nursing women should be avoided if clinically possible.

Usage in Children: Studies have not been performed in children; therefore, this drug is not recommended for use in children below the age of 16.

ADVERSE REACTIONS

CNS Effects: Manifestations of adverse effects on the central nervous system, other than extrapyramidal effects, have been seen infrequently. Drowsiness, usually mild, may occur at the beginning of therapy or when dosage is increased. It usually subsides with continued Loxapine therapy. The incidence of sedation has been less than that of certain aliphatic phenothiazines and slightly more than the piperazine phenothiazines. Dizziness, faintness, staggering gait, shuffling gait, muscle twitching, weakness, insomnia, agitation, tension, seizures, akinesia, slurred speech, numbness and confusional states have been reported. Neuroleptic malignant syndrome (NMS) has been reported (see *"Warnings"*).

Extrapyramidal Reactions: Neuromuscular (extrapyramidal) reactions during the administration of Loxapine have been reported frequently, often during the first few days of treatment. In most patients, these reactions involved parkinsonian-like symptoms such as tremor, rigidity, excessive salivation, and masked facies. Akathisia (motor restlessness) also has been reported relatively frequently. These symptoms are usually not severe and can be controlled by reduction of Loxapine dosage or by administration of antiparkinson drugs in usual dosage. Dystonic and dyskinetic reactions have occurred less frequently, but may be more severe. Dystonias include spasms of muscles of the neck and face, tongue protrusion, and oculogyric movement. Dyskinetic reactions have been described in the form of choreoathetoid movements. These reactions sometimes require reduction or temporary withdrawal of Loxapine dosage in addition to appropriate counteractive drugs.

Persistent Tardive Dyskinesia: As with all antipsychotic agents, tardive dyskinesia may appear in some patients on long-term therapy or may appear after drug therapy has been discontinued. The risk appears to be greater in elderly patients on high-dose therapy, especially females. The symptoms are persistent and in some patients appear to be irreversible. The syndrome is characterized by rhythmical involuntary movement of the tongue, face, mouth, or jaw (eg, protrusion of tongue, puffing of cheeks, puckering of mouth, chewing movements). Sometimes these may be accompanied by involuntary movements of extremities.

There is no known effective treatment for tardive dyskinesia; antiparkinson agents usually do not alleviate the symptoms of this syndrome. It is suggested that all antipsychotic agents be discontinued if these symptoms appear. Should it be necessary to reinstitute treatment, or increase the dosage of the agent, or switch to a different antipsychotic agent, the syndrome may be masked. It has been suggested that fine vermicular movements of the tongue may be an early sign of the syndrome, and if the medication is stopped at that time the syndrome may not develop.

Cardiovascular Effects: Tachycardia, hypotension, hypertension, orthostatic hypotension, lightheadedness, and syncope have been reported.

A few cases of ECG changes similar to those seen with phenothiazines have been reported. It is not known whether these were related to Loxapine administration.

Hematologic: Rarely, agranulocytosis, thrombocytopenia, leukopenia.

Skin: Dermatitis, edema (puffiness of face), pruritus, rash, alopecia and seborrhea have been reported with Loxapine.

Anticholinergic Effects: Dry mouth, nasal congestion, constipation, blurred vision, urinary retention and paralytic ileus have occurred.

Gastrointestinal: Nausea and vomiting have been reported in some patients. Hepatocellular injury (ie, SGOT/SGPT elevation) has been reported in association with Loxapine administration and, rarely, jaundice and/or hepatitis questionably related to Loxapine treatment.

Other Adverse Reactions: Weight gain, weight loss, dyspnea, ptosis, hyperpyrexia, flushed facies, headache, paresthesia, and polydipsia have been reported in some patients. Rarely, galactorrhea, amenorrhea, gynecomastia and menstrual irregularity of uncertain etiology have been reported.

OVERDOSAGE

Signs and symptoms of overdosage will depend on the amount ingested and individual patient tolerance. As would be expected from the pharmacologic actions of the drug, the clinical findings may range from mild depression of the CNS and cardiovascular systems to profound hypotension, respiratory depression, and unconsciousness. The possibility of occurrence of extrapyramidal symptoms and/or convulsive seizures should be kept in mind. Renal failure following Loxapine overdosage has also been reported.

The treatment of overdosage is essentially symptomatic and supportive. Early gastric lavage and extended dialysis might be expected to be beneficial. Centrally acting emetics may have little effect because of the antiemetic action of Loxapine. In addition, emesis should be avoided because of the possibility of aspiration of vomitus. Avoid analeptics, such as pentylenetetrazol, which may cause convulsions. Severe hypotension might be expected to respond to the administration of levarterenol or phenylephrine. EPINEPHRINE SHOULD NOT BE USED SINCE ITS USE IN A PATIENT WITH PARTIAL ADRENERGIC BLOCKADE MAY FURTHER LOWER THE BLOOD PRESSURE. Severe extrapyramidal reactions should be treated with anticholinergic antiparkinson agents or diphenhydramine hydrochloride, and anticonvulsant therapy should be initiated as indicated. Additional measures include oxygen and intravenous fluids.

DOSAGE AND ADMINISTRATION

Loxapine is administered, usually in divided doses, two to four times a day. Daily dosage (in terms of base equivalents) should be adjusted to the individual patient's needs as assessed by the severity of symptoms and previous history of response to antipsychotic drugs.

Oral Administration: Initial dosage of 10 mg twice daily is recommended, although in severely disturbed patients initial dosage up to a total of 50 mg daily may be desirable. Dosage should then be increased fairly rapidly over the first 7 to 10 days until there is effective control of psychotic symptoms. The usual therapeutic and maintenance range is 60 to 100 mg daily. However, as with other antipsychotic drugs, some patients respond to lower dosage and others require higher dosage for optimal benefit. Daily dosage higher than 250 mg is not recommended.

One brand of Loxapine Hydrochloride oral solution should be mixed with orange or grapefruit juice shortly before administration.

Maintenance Therapy: For maintenance therapy, dosage should be reduced to the lowest level compatible with symptom control; many patients have been maintained satisfactorily at dosages in the range of 20 to 60 mg daily.

Intramuscular Administration: Loxapine Hydrochloride is utilized for prompt symptomatic control in the acutely agitated patient and in patients whose symptoms render oral medication temporarily impractical. During clinical trial there were only rare reports of significant local tissue reaction. Loxapine Hydrochloride is administered by intramuscular (not intravenous) injection in doses of 12.5 mg at intervals of 4 to 6 hours or longer, both dose and interval depending on patient response. Many patients have responded satisfactorily to twice-daily dosage. As described above for oral administration, attention is directed to the necessity for dosage adjustment on an individual basis over the early days of Loxapine administration.

Once the desired symptomatic control is achieved and the patient is able to take medication orally, Loxapine should be administered in capsule or oral concentrate form. Usually this should occur within 5 days.

Capsules: Store at controlled room temperature, 15°-30° C (59°-86° F).

Oral Solution: Store at controlled room temperature, 15°-30° C (59°-86° F). DO NOT FREEZE.

Injection: Store at controlled room temperature, 15°-30° C (59°-86° F). DO NOT FREEZE.

HOW SUPPLIED

LOXAPINE HYDROCHLORIDE
CONCENTRATE: 25 MG/ML

BRAND/MANUFACTURER	NDC	SIZE	AWP
○ **BRAND**			
LOXITANE C: Lederle Labs	00005-5387-58	120 ml	$234.51

INJECTION: 50 MG/ML

BRAND/MANUFACTURER	NDC	SIZE	AWP
○ **BRAND**			
LOXITANE IM: Lederle Labs	00205-5385-34	10 ml	$96.34

LOXAPINE SUCCINATE
CAPSULE: 5 MG

AVERAGE UNIT PRICE (AVAILABLE SIZES)		GENERIC A-RATED AVERAGE PRICE (GAAP)	
BRAND	$0.86	100s	$53.09
GENERIC	$0.54		
HCFA FUL (100s ea)	$0.43		

BRAND/MANUFACTURER	NDC	SIZE	AWP
◆ **BRAND**			
LOXITANE: Lederle Labs	00005-5359-23	100s	$81.51
	00005-5359-60	100s ud	$89.81
◆ **GENERICS**			
Warner Chilcott	00047-0621-24	100s	$42.86
Schein	00364-2303-01	100s	$43.58
Moore,H.L.	00839-7495-06	100s	$43.86
Major	00904-2310-60	100s	$47.25
Geneva	00781-2710-01	100s	$47.50
Qualitest	00603-4268-21	100s	$49.30
Goldline	00182-1305-01	100s	$52.20
Aligen	00405-5120-01	100s	$67.21
Watson	52544-0369-01	100s	$67.21
Parmed	00349-8839-01	100s	$68.89
Raway	00686-0677-20	100s ud	$44.00
UDL	51079-0677-20	100s ud	$63.27
Watson	52544-0369-10	1000s	$638.50

CAPSULE: 10 MG

AVERAGE UNIT PRICE (AVAILABLE SIZES)		GENERIC A-RATED AVERAGE PRICE (GAAP)	
BRAND	$1.06	100s	$71.94
GENERIC	$0.73		
HCFA FUL (100s ea)	$0.59		

BRAND/MANUFACTURER	NDC	SIZE	AWP
◆ **BRAND**			
LOXITANE: Lederle Labs	00005-5360-23	100s	$105.33
	00005-5360-60	100s ud	$113.68
	00005-5360-34	1000s	$995.34
◆ **GENERICS**			
Warner Chilcott	00047-0632-24	100s	$55.82
Schein	00364-2304-01	100s	$56.18
Geneva	00781-2711-01	100s	$64.75
Qualitest	00603-4269-21	100s	$68.20
Rugby	00536-4834-01	100s	$69.38
Major	00904-2311-60	100s	$69.45
Goldline	00182-1306-01	100s	$69.45
Moore,H.L.	00839-7496-06	100s	$72.62
Aligen	00405-5121-01	100s	$86.85
Watson	52544-0370-01	100s	$86.85
Parmed	00349-8836-01	100s	$88.54
Raway	00686-0678-20	100s ud	$67.00
UDL	51079-0678-20	100s ud	$80.10
Watson	52544-0370-10	1000s	$820.66

◆ RATED THERAPEUTICALLY EQUIVALENT; ◇ THERAPEUTIC EQUIVALENCE UNCONFIRMED; ○ UNRATED

CAPSULE: 25 MG

AVERAGE UNIT PRICE (AVAILABLE SIZES)		GENERIC A-RATED AVERAGE PRICE (GAAP)	
BRAND	$1.59	100s	$111.40
GENERIC	$1.12		
HCFA FUL (100s ea)	$0.85		

BRAND/MANUFACTURER	NDC	SIZE	AWP
◆ BRAND			
LOXITANE: Lederle Labs	00005-5361-23	100s	$159.16
LOXITANE: Lederle Labs	00005-5361-60	100s ud	$167.49
	00005-5361-34	1000s	$1511.45
◆ GENERICS			
Warner Chilcott	00047-0650-24	100s	$87.55
Schein	00364-2305-01	100s	$91.88
Geneva	00781-2712-01	100s	$104.95
URL	00677-1320-01	100s	$107.95
Goldline	00182-1307-01	100s	$108.00
Qualitest	00603-4270-21	100s	$108.05
Rugby	00536-4835-01	100s	$108.68
Major	00904-2312-60	100s	$108.90
Moore,H.L.	00839-7497-06	100s	$114.41
Aligen	00405-5122-01	100s	$131.23
Watson	52544-0371-01	100s	$131.23
Parmed	00349-8837-01	100s	$133.78
Raway	00686-0679-20	100s ud	$105.00
UDL	51079-0679-20	100s ud	$117.99
Watson	52544-0371-10	1000s	$1246.19

CAPSULE: 50 MG

AVERAGE UNIT PRICE (AVAILABLE SIZES)		GENERIC A-RATED AVERAGE PRICE (GAAP)	
BRAND	$2.12	100s	$147.35
GENERIC	$1.49		
HCFA FUL (100s ea)	$1.21		

BRAND/MANUFACTURER	NDC	SIZE	AWP
◆ BRAND			
LOXITANE: Lederle Labs	00005-5362-23	100s	$212.35
	00005-5362-60	100s ud	$220.60
	00005-5362-34	1000s	$2038.25
◆ GENERICS			
Warner Chilcott	00047-0651-24	100s	$114.85
Schein	00364-2306-01	100s	$121.54
Geneva	00781-2713-01	100s	$135.50
Qualitest	00603-4271-21	100s	$138.65
Goldline	00182-1308-01	100s	$139.00
Rugby	00536-4836-01	100s	$139.95
Major	00904-2313-60	100s	$139.95
URL	00677-1321-01	100s	$149.72
Moore,H.L.	00839-7498-06	100s	$164.77
Aligen	00405-5123-01	100s	$175.08
Watson	52544-0372-01	100s	$175.08
Parmed	00349-8838-01	100s	$178.48
Raway	00686-0680-20	100s ud	$135.00
UDL	51079-0680-20	100s ud	$155.38
Watson	52544-0372-10	1000s	$1680.54

Loxitane SEE LOXAPINE

Lozol SEE INDAPAMIDE

Ludiomil SEE MAPROTILINE HYDROCHLORIDE

Lufyllin SEE DYPHYLLINE

Lufyllin GG SEE DYPHYLLINE AND GUAIFENESIN

Luminal Sodium SEE PHENOBARBITAL

Lupron SEE LEUPROLIDE ACETATE

Luride SEE SODIUM FLUORIDE

Lutrepulse SEE GONADORELIN ACETATE

Lymphazurin SEE ISOSULFAN BLUE

Lymphocyte Immune Globulin

> **WARNING**
> ONLY PHYSICIANS EXPERIENCED IN IMMUNOSUPPRESSIVE THERAPY IN THE MANAGEMENT OF RENAL TRANSPLANT OR APLASTIC ANEMIA PATIENTS SHOULD USE LYMPHOCYTE IMMUNE GLOBULIN.
> PATIENTS RECEIVING LYMPHOCYTE IMMUNE GLOBULIN SHOULD BE MANAGED IN FACILITIES EQUIPPED AND STAFFED WITH ADEQUATE LABORATORY AND SUPPORTIVE MEDICAL RESOURCES.

DESCRIPTION

Lymphocyte Immune Globulin Sterile Solution anti-thymocyte globulin [equine], is the purified, concentrated, and sterile gamma globulin, primarily monomeric IgG, from hyperimmune serum of horses immunized with human thymus lymphocytes. Lymphocyte Immune Globulin is a transparent to slightly opalescent aqueous protein solution. It may appear colorless to faintly pink or brown and is nearly odorless. It may develop a slight granular or flaky deposit during storage. (For information about in-line filters, see "Infusion Instructions" in the "Dosage and Administration" section).

Before release for clinical use, each lot of Lymphocyte Immune Globulin is tested to assure its ability to inhibit rosette formation between human peripheral lymphocytes and sheep red blood cells in vitro. In each lot, antibody activity against human red blood cells and platelets is also measured and determined to be within acceptable limits. Only lots that test negative for antihuman serum protein antibody, antiglomerular basement membrane antibody and pyrogens are released.

Each milliliter of Lymphocyte Immune Globulin contains 50 mg of horse gamma globulin.

CLINICAL AND ANIMAL PHARMACOLOGY

Lymphocyte Immune Globulin Sterile Solution is a lymphocyte-selective immunosuppressant as is demonstrated by its ability to reduce the number of circulating, thymus-dependent lymphocytes that form rosettes with sheep erythrocytes. This antilymphocytic effect is believed to reflect an alteration of the function of the T-lymphocytes, which are responsible in part for cell-mediated immunity and are involved in humoral immunity. In addition to its antilymphocytic activity, Lymphocyte Immune Globulin contains low concentrations of antibodies against other formed elements of the blood. In rhesus and cynomolgus monkeys, Lymphocyte Immune Globulin reduces lymphocytes in the thymus-dependent areas of the spleen and lymph nodes. It also decreases the circulating sheep-erythrocyte-rosetting lymphocytes that can be detected, but ordinarily Lymphocyte Immune Globulin does not cause severe lymphopenia.

In general, when Lymphocyte Immune Globulin is given with other immunosuppressive therapy, such as antimetabolites and corticosteroids, the patient's own antibody response to horse gamma globulin is minimal. In a small clinical study, Lymphocyte Immune Globulin administered with other immunosuppressive therapy and measured as horse IgG had a serum half-life of 5.7 ± 3 days.

INDICATIONS AND USAGE

RENAL TRANSPLANTATION

Lymphocyte Immune Globulin Sterile Solution is indicated for the management of allograft rejection in renal transplant patients. When administered with conventional therapy at the time of rejection, it increases the frequency of resolution of the acute rejection episode. The drug has also been administered as an adjunct to other immunosuppressive therapy to delay the onset of the first rejection episode. Data accumulated to date have not consistently demonstrated improvement in functional graft survival associated with therapy to delay the onset of the first rejection episode.

APLASTIC ANEMIA

Lymphocyte Immune Globulin is indicated for the treatment of moderate to severe aplastic anemia in patients who are unsuitable for bone marrow transplantation.

When administered with a regimen of supportive care, Lymphocyte Immune Globulin may induce partial or complete hematologic remission. In a controlled trial, patients receiving Lymphocyte Immune Globulin showed a statistically significant higher improvement rate compared to standard supportive care at 3 months. Improvement was defined in terms of sustained increase in peripheral blood counts and reduced transfusion needs.

Clinical trials conducted at two centers evaluated the one year survival rate for patients with severe and moderate to severe aplastic anemia. Seventy-four of the 83 patients enrolled were evaluable based on response to treatment. The treatment groups studied consisted of: 1) Lymphocyte Immune Globulin and supportive care, 2) Lymphocyte Immune Globulin administered following 3 months of supportive care alone, 3) Lymphocyte Immune Globulin, mismatched marrow infusion, androgens and supportive care, or 4) Lymphocyte Immune Globulin, androgens and supportive care. There were no statistically significant differences between the treatment groups. The one year survival rate for the pooled treatment groups was 69%. These survival results can be compared to a historical survival rate of about 25% for patients receiving standard supportive care alone.

The usefulness of Lymphocyte Immune Globulin has not been demonstrated in patients with aplastic anemia who are suitable candidates for bone marrow transplantation or in patients with aplastic anemia secondary to neoplastic disease, storage disease, myelofibrosis, Fanconi's syndrome or in patients known to have been exposed to myelotoxic agents or radiation.

To date, safety and efficacy have not been established in circumstances other than renal transplantation and aplastic anemia.

SKIN TESTING
Before the first infusion of Lymphocyte Immune Globulin, it is strongly recommended that patients be tested with an intradermal injection of 0.1 mL of a 1:1000 dilution (5 µg horse IgG) of Lymphocyte Immune Globulin in Sodium Chloride Injection, USP and a contralateral Sodium Chloride Injection control. Use only freshly diluted Lymphocyte Immune Globulin for skin testing. The patient and specifically the skin test should be observed every 15 to 20 minutes over the first hour after intradermal injection. A local reaction of 10 mm or greater with a wheal or erythema or both with or without pseudopod formation and itching or a marked local swelling should be considered a positive test.

Note: The predictive value of this test has not been proven clinically. Allergic reactions such as anaphylaxis have occurred in patients whose skin test is negative. In the presence of a locally positive skin test to Lymphocyte Immune Globulin, serious consideration to alternative forms of therapy should be given. The risk to benefit ratio must be carefully weighed. If therapy with Lymphocyte Immune Globulin is deemed appropriate following a locally positive skin test, treatment should be administered in a setting where intensive life support facilities are immediately available and with a physician familiar with the treatment of potentially life threatening allergic reactions in attendance.

A systemic reaction such as a generalized rash, tachycardia, dyspnea, hypotension, or anaphylaxis precludes any additional administration of Lymphocyte Immune Globulin.

See *"Warnings", "Precautions"*, and *"Adverse Reactions"*.

CONTRAINDICATIONS
Do not administer Lymphocyte Immune Globulin Sterile Solution to a patient who has had a severe systemic reaction during prior administration of Lymphocyte Immune Globulin or any other equine gamma globulin preparation.

WARNINGS

> ONLY PHYSICIANS EXPERIENCED IN IMMUNOSUPPRESSIVE THERAPY IN THE MANAGEMENT OF RENAL TRANSPLANT OR APLASTIC ANEMIA PATIENTS SHOULD USE LYMPHOCYTE IMMUNE GLOBULIN.
> PATIENTS RECEIVING LYMPHOCYTE IMMUNE GLOBULIN SHOULD BE MANAGED IN FACILITIES EQUIPPED AND STAFFED WITH ADEQUATE LABORATORY AND SUPPORTIVE MEDICAL RESOURCES.

Precise methods of determining the potency of Lymphocyte Immune Globulin have not been established, thus activity may potentially vary from lot to lot. Discontinue treatment with Lymphocyte Immune Globulin if any of the following occurs:

1. Symptoms of anaphylaxis (see *"Adverse Reactions"*)
2. Severe and unremitting thrombocytopenia in renal transplant patients
3. Severe and unremitting leukopenia in renal transplant patients

In common with products derived from, or purified with human blood components, the possibility of transmission of infectious agents exists.

PRECAUTIONS
Because Lymphocyte Immune Globulin Sterile Solution is an immunosuppressive agent ordinarily given with corticosteroids and antimetabolites, watch patients carefully for signs of leukopenia, thrombocytopenia or concurrent infection. Several studies have suggested an increase in the incidence of cytomegalovirus infection in patients receiving Lymphocyte Immune Globulin. In one study it has been found that it may be possible to reduce this risk by decreasing the dosage of other immunosuppressive agents administered concomitantly with Lymphocyte Immune Globulin. If infection occurs, institute appropriate adjunctive therapy promptly. On the basis of the clinical circumstances, a physician should decide whether or not therapy with Lymphocyte Immune Globulin will continue.

Pregnancy Category C: Lymphocyte Immune Globulin has not been evaluated in either pregnant or lactating women. Animal reproduction studies have not been conducted with Lymphocyte Immune Globulin. It is also not known whether Lymphocyte Immune Globulin can cause fetal harm when administered to a pregnant woman or can affect reproduction capacity. Administration of Lymphocyte Immune Globulin to pregnant women is not recommended and should be considered only under exceptional circumstances.

The safety and effectiveness of Lymphocyte Immune Globulin have been demonstrated only in renal transplant patients who receive concomitant immunosuppressive therapy.

Experience with children has been limited. Lymphocyte Immune Globulin has been administered safely to a small number of pediatric renal allograft recipients

and pediatric aplastic anemia patients at dosage levels comparable to those in adults.

Dilution of Lymphocyte Immune Globulin in Dextrose Injection, USP, is not recommended, as low salt concentrations may result in precipitation. The use of highly acidic infusion solutions is also not recommended because of possible physical instability over time.

DRUG INTERACTIONS
We do not recommend the dilution of Lymphocyte Immune Globulin Sterile Solution in Dextrose Injection, USP, as low salt concentrations may cause precipitation. The use of highly acidic infusion solutions is also not recommended because of possible physical instability over time. When the dose of corticosteroids and other immunosuppressants is being reduced, some previously masked reactions to Lymphocyte Immune Globulin may appear. Under these circumstances, observe patients especially carefully during therapy with Lymphocyte Immune Globulin.

ADVERSE REACTIONS
RENAL TRANSPLANTATION
The primary clinical experience with Lymphocyte Immune Globulin Sterile Solution has been in renal allograft patients who were also receiving concurrent standard immunosuppressive therapy (azathioprine, corticosteroids). In controlled trials, investigators frequently reported the following adverse reactions: fever in 1 patient in 3; chills in 1 patient in 7; leukopenia in 1 patient in 7; thrombocytopenia in 1 patient in 9; and dermatological reactions, such as rash, pruritus, urticaria, wheal, and flare, in 1 patient in 8. The following reactions were reported in more than 1% but less than 5% of the patients: arthralgia, chest or back pain or both, clotted A/V fistula, diarrhea, dyspnea, headache, hypotension, nausea or vomiting or both, night sweats, pain at the infusion site, peripheral thrombophlebitis, and stomatitis.

Reactions reported in less than 1% of the patients in the controlled trials were anaphylaxis, dizziness, weakness or faintness, edema, herpes simplex reactivation, hiccoughs or epigastric pain, hyperglycemia, hypertension, iliac vein obstruction, laryngospasm, localized infection, lymphadenopathy, malaise, myalgia, paresthesia, possible serum sickness, pulmonary edema, renal artery thrombosis, seizures, systemic infection, tachycardia, toxic epidermal necrosis, and wound dehiscence.

APLASTIC ANEMIA
In premarketing clinical trials with Lymphocyte Immune Globulin in the treatment of aplastic anemia, patients were also being concurrently managed with support therapy (transfusions, steroids, antibiotics, antihistamines).

In these trials most patients experienced fever and skin reactions. Other frequently reported adverse reactions were chills, 1 patient in 2; arthralgia, 1 patient in 2; headache, 1 patient in 6; myalgia, 1 patient in 10; nausea, 1 patient in 15; chest pain, 1 patient in 15 and phlebitis, 1 patient in 20.

The following reactions were reported by at least 1 patient, and less than 5% of the total patients: diaphoresis, joint stiffness, periorbital edema, aches, edema, muscle ache, vomiting, agitation/lethargy, listlessness, lightheadedness, seizures, diarrhea, bradycardia, myocarditis, cardiac irregularity, hepatosplenomegaly, possible encephalitis or post viral encephalopathy, hypotension, congestive heart failure, hypertension, burning soles/palms, foot sole pain, lymphadenopathy, post-cervical lymphadenopathy, tender lymph nodes, bilateral pleural effusion, respiratory distress, anaphylactic reaction, and proteinuria.

In other support studies in patients with aplastic anemia and other hematologic abnormalities who have received Lymphocyte Immune Globulin abnormal tests of liver function (SGOT, SGPT, alkaline phosphatase) and renal function (serum creatinine) have been observed. In some trials, clinical and laboratory findings of serum sickness were seen in a majority of patients.

POSTMARKETING EXPERIENCE
During approximately five years of post-approval marketing experience, the frequency of adverse reactions in voluntarily reported cases is as follows: fever 51%; chills 16%; thrombocytopenia 30%; leukopenia 14%; rashes 27%; systemic infection 13%. Events reported in 5 to 10% of reported cases include: abnormal renal function tests, serum sickness-like symptoms, dyspnea/apnea, arthralgia, chest, back or flank pain, diarrhea and nausea and/or vomiting. Events reported with a frequency of less than 5% include: hypertension, Herpes Simplex infection, pain, swelling or redness at infusion site, eosinophilia, headache, myalgias or leg pains, hypotension, anaphylaxis, tachycardia, edema, localized infection, malaise, seizures, GI bleeding or perforation, deep vein thrombosis, sore mouth/throat, hyperglycemia, acute renal failure, abnormal liver function tests, confusion or disorientation, cough, neutropenia or granulocytopenia, anemia, thrombophlebitis, dizziness, epigastric or stomach pain, lymphadenopathy, pulmonary edema or congestive heart failure, abdominal pain, nosebleed, vasculitis, aplasia or pancytopenia, abnormal involuntary movement or tremor, rigidity, sweating, laryngospasm/edema, hemolysis or hemolytic anemia, viral hepatitis, faintness, enlarged or ruptured kidney, paresthesias and renal artery thrombosis.

The recommended management for some of the adverse reactions that could occur with treatment with Lymphocyte Immune Globulin follows:

1. *Anaphylaxis* is uncommon but serious and may occur at any time during therapy with Lymphocyte Immune Globulin. Stop infusion of Lymphocyte Immune Globulin immediately; administer 0.3 mL aqueous epinephrine (1:1000 solution) intramuscularly. Administer steroids, assist respiration, and provide other resuscitative measures. DO NOT resume therapy with Lymphocyte Immune Globulin.

2. *Hemolysis* can usually be detected only in the laboratory. Clinically significant hemolysis has been reported rarely. Appropriate treatment of hemoly-

sis may include transfusion of erythrocytes; if necessary, administer intravenous mannitol, furosemide, sodium bicarbonate, and fluids. Severe and unremitting hemolysis may require discontinuation of therapy with Lymphocyte Immune Globulin.

3. *Thrombocytopenia* is usually transient in renal transplant patients; platelet counts generally return to adequate levels without discontinuing therapy with Lymphocyte Immune Globulin. Platelet transfusions may be necessary in patients with aplastic anemia. (See *"Precautions," "Warnings"* and *"Dosage and Administration".*)

4. *Respiratory distress* may indicate an anaphylactoid reaction. Discontinue infusion of Lymphocyte Immune Globulin. If distress persists, administer an antihistamine or epinephrine or corticosteroids or some combination of the three.

5. *Pain in chest, flank* or *back* may indicate anaphylaxis or hemolysis. Treatment is that indicated above for those conditions.

6. *Hypotension* may indicate anaphylaxis. Stop infusion of Lymphocyte Immune Globulin and stabilize blood pressure with pressors if necessary.

7. *Chills and fever* occur frequently in patients receiving Lymphocyte Immune Globulin. Lymphocyte Immune Globulin may release endogenous leukocyte pyrogens. Prophylactic and/or therapeutic administration of antihistamines, antipyretics or corticosteroids generally controls this reaction.

8. *Chemical phlebitis* can be caused by infusion of Lymphocyte Immune Globulin through peripheral veins. This can often be avoided by administering the infusion solution into a high-flow vein. A subcutaneous arterialized vein produced by a Brescia fistula is also a useful administration site.

9. *Itching and erythema* probably result from the effect of Lymphocyte Immune Globulin on blood elements. Antihistamines generally control the symptoms.

10. *Serum sickness-like symptoms* in aplastic anemia patients have been treated with oral or IV corticosteroids. Resolution of symptoms has generally been prompt and long-term sequelae have not been observed. Prophylactic administration of corticosteroids may decrease the frequency of this reaction.

OVERDOSAGE
Because of its mode of action and because it is a biologic substance, the maximal tolerated dose of Lymphocyte Immune Globulin Sterile Solution would be expected to vary from patient to patient. To date, the largest single daily dose administered to a patient, a renal transplant recipient, was 7000 mg administered at a concentration of approximately 10 mg/mL Sodium Chloride Injection, USP, approximately 7 times the recommended total dose and infusion concentration. In this patient, administration of Lymphocyte Immune Globulin was not associated with any signs of acute intoxication.

The greatest number of doses (10 to 20 mg/kg/dose) that can be administered to a single patient has not yet been determined. Some renal transplant patients have received up to 50 doses in 4 months, and others have received 28-day courses of 21 doses followed by as many as 3 more courses for the treatment of acute rejection. The incidence of toxicologic manifestations did not increase with any of these regimens.

DOSAGE AND ADMINISTRATION
RENAL ALLOGRAFT RECIPIENTS
Adult renal allograft patients have received Lymphocyte Immune Globulin Sterile Solution at the dosage of 10 to 30 mg/kg of body weight daily.

The few children studied received 5 to 25 mg/kg daily. Lymphocyte Immune Globulin has been used to delay the onset of the first rejection episodes[1-4] and at the time of the first rejection episode.[5-9] Most patients who received Lymphocyte Immune Globulin for the treatment of acute rejection had not received it starting at the time of transplantation.

Usually, Lymphocyte Immune Globulin is used concomitantly with azathioprine and corticosteroids, which are commonly used to suppress the immune response. Exercise caution during repeat courses of Lymphocyte Immune Globulin, carefully observe patients for signs of allergic reactions.

Delaying the Onset of Allograft Rejection: Give a fixed dose of 15 mg/kg daily for 14 days, then every other day for 14 days for a total of 21 doses in 28 days. Administer the first dose within 24 hours before or after the transplant.

Treatment of Rejection: The first dose of Lymphocyte Immune Globulin can be delayed until the diagnosis of the first rejection episode. The recommended dose is 10 to 15 mg/kg daily for 14 days. Additional alternative-day therapy up to a total of 21 doses can be given.

APLASTIC ANEMIA
The recommended dosage regimen is 10 to 20 mg/kg daily for 8 to 14 days. Additional alternate-day therapy up to a total of 21 doses can be administered[10-12]. Because thrombocytopenia can be associated with the administration of Lymphocyte Immune Globulin, patients receiving it for the treatment of aplastic anemia may need prophylactic platelet transfusions to maintain platelets at clinically acceptable levels.

PREPARATION OF SOLUTION
Parenteral drug products should be inspected visually for particulate matter and discoloration prior to administration whenever solution and container permit. However, because Lymphocyte Immune Globulin is a gamma globulin product, it can be transparent to slightly opalescent, colorless to faintly pink or brown and may develop a slight granular or flaky deposit during storage. Lymphocyte Immune Globulin (diluted or undiluted) should not be shaken because excessive foaming and/or denaturation of the protein may occur.

Dilute Lymphocyte Immune Globulin for intravenous infusion in an inverted bottle of sterile vehicle so the undiluted Lymphocyte Immune Globulin does not contact the air inside. Add the total daily dose of Lymphocyte Immune Globulin to the sterile vehicle (see *"Compatibility and Stability"*). The concentration should not exceed 4 mg of Lymphocyte Immune Globulin per mL. The diluted solution should be gently rotated or swirled to effect thorough mixing.

ADMINISTRATION
The diluted Lymphocyte Immune Globulin should be allowed to reach room temperature before infusion. Lymphocyte Immune Globulin is appropriate administered into a vascular shunt, arterial venous fistula, or a high-flow central vein through an in-line filter with a pore size of 0.2 to 1.0 micron. The in-line filter should be used with all infusions of Lymphocyte Immune Globulin to prevent the administration of any insoluble material that may develop in the product during storage. The use of high-flow veins will minimize the occurrence of phlebitis and thrombosis. Do not infuse a dose of Lymphocyte Immune Globulin in less than 4 hours. Always keep appropriate resuscitation equipment at the patient's bedside while Lymphocyte Immune Globulin is being administered. Observe the patient continuously for possible allergic reactions throughout the infusions (see *"Adverse Reactions"*).

COMPATIBILITY AND STABILITY
Lymphocyte Immune Globulin, once diluted, has been shown to be physically and chemically stable for up to 24 hours at concentrations of up to 4 mg per mL in the following diluents: 0.9% Sodium Chloride Injection, 5% Dextrose and 0.225% Sodium Chloride Injection, and 5% Dextrose and 0.45% Sodium Chloride Injection.

Adding Lymphocyte Immune Globulin to Dextrose Injection is not recommended, as low salt concentrations can cause precipitation. Highly acidic infusion solutions can also contribute to physical instability over time. It is recommended that diluted Lymphocyte Immune Globulin be stored in a refrigerator if it is prepared prior to the time of infusion. Even if it is stored in a refrigerator, the total time in dilution should not exceed 24 hours (including infusion time).

STORAGE
Store in a refrigerator at 2° to 8° C. DO NOT FREEZE.

ANIMAL TOXICOLOGY
During the development of Lymphocyte Immune Globulin Sterile Solution, aliquots of the various clinical lots were infused intravenously in either *Macaca mulatta or Macaca irus* monkeys. The dosage used was 100 mg/kg on day 0, 200 mg/kg on day 2 and 400 mg/kg on day 4. A 3-week observation period followed. Currently, all marketed lots are similarly tested using a dosage of 50 mg/kg on days 0, 2, 4 and 7 followed by a 3-week observation period.

Many of the changes observed could have been anticipated on the basis of the antilymphocytic activity of Lymphocyte Immune Globulin. They are decreased peripheral blood lymphocytes and increased total leukocyte and neutrophil counts occurring within 24 hours after infusion, decreased thymus size with involution or atrophy or both, and decreased lymphocyte populations in the thymus-dependent areas of the spleen and lymph nodes. The atrophy was particularly common in the animals receiving the higher doses. In animals receiving either dosage regimen, packed cell volume, total erythrocyte counts, and hemoglobin concentrations have decreased and reticulocytes and nucleated erythrocytes have increased enough to be classified as anemia. An occasional animal death believed to have resulted from anemia has occurred. Transient decreases in blood platelet counts have also occurred. Thrombus formation occurred frequently along the routes of infusion, ie, the saphenous and femoral veins. However, the incidence of thrombi has dropped since in-line filters have been used during infusion. In these animals, definitive evidence of DIC (disseminated intravascular coagulation) has not been observed.

REFERENCES
1. Cosimi AB, Wortis HH, Delmonico FL. Russell PS: Randomized clinical trial of antithymocyte globulin in cadaver renal allograft recipients. Importance of T cell monitoring, Surg 80: 155-163 (1976) 2. Wechter WJ, Brodie JA, Morrell RM. Rafi M, Schultz JR: Antithymocyte globulin (ATGAM) in renal allograft recipients. Trans 28(4):294-302 (1979) 3. Kountx SL, Butt KHM, Rao TKS, Zielinski CM, Rafi M, Schultz JR: Antithymocyte globulin (ATG) dosage and graft survival in renal transplantation. Trans Proc 9:1023-1025 (1977) 4. Butt KMH, Zielinski CM, Parsa I, Elberg AJ, Wechter WJ, Kountz SL: Trends in immunosuppression for kidney transplantation. Kidney Int 13(Suppl 8): S95-S98 (1978) 5. Filo RS, Smith EJ, Leapman SB: Reversal of acute renal allograft rejection with adjunctive ATG therapy. Trans Proc 13(1): 482-490 (1981) 6. Nowygrod R, Appel G. Hardy M: Use of ATG for reversal of acute allograft rejection. Trans Proc 13(1): 469-472 (1981). 7. Hardy MA, Nowygrod R, Elberg A, Appel G: Use of ATG in treatment of steroid-resistant rejection. Trans 29:162-164 (1980) 8. Shield CH, Cosimi AB, Tolkoff-Rubin N, Rubin R, Herrin J, Russell PS: Use of antithymocyte globulin for reversal of acute allograft rejection. Trans 28(6): 461-464 (1979) 9. Cosimi AB: The clinical value of antilymphocyte antibodies. Trans Proc 13(1): 462-468 (1981) 10. Cosimi AB, Peters C, Harmon D, Ellman L: Treatment of severe aplastic anemia with a prolonged course of antithymocyte globulin. Trans Proc 14:761-764 (1982) 11. Champlin R, Ho W, Gale R: Antithymocyte globulin treatment in patients with aplastic anemia. NEJM 308(3):113-118 (1983) 12. Doney K, Dahlberg S, Monroe D et al: Therapy of severe aplastic anemia with anti-human thymocyte globulin and androgens: The effect of HLA-haploidentical marrow infusion. Blood 63(2):342-348 (1984) 13. Rubin RH, Cosimi AB, Hirsch MS, Herrin JT: Effects of antithymocyte globulin on cytomegalovirus infection in renal transplant recipients. Trans 31(2):143-145 (1981)

J CODES
50 mg/ml, 5 ml ea IV—J7504

HOW SUPPLIED
INJECTION: 50 MG/ML

BRAND/MANUFACTURER	NDC	SIZE	AWP
○ **BRAND**			
ATGAM: Upjohn	00009-0926-04	5 ml	$262.24

Lypholyte *SEE* DEXTROSE AND ELECTROLYTES *AND* ELECTROLYTES, INJECTABLE

Lypressin

DESCRIPTION
Lypressin nasal solution, USP Nasal Spray contains synthetic lysine-8-vasopressin with an activity of 50 USP Posterior Pituitary (Pressor) Units per mL (0.185 mg/mL).

The molecular formula of lysine-8-vasopressin is $C_{46}H_{65}N_{13}O_{12}S_2$. It is an antidiuretic with vasoconstrictor activity.

Lypressin nasal solution, USP Nasal Spray is provided for intra-nasal administration as a solution containing per 1 mL, 50 USP Posterior Pituitary (Pressor) Units of synthetic lysine-8-vasopressin.

Following is its chemical structure:

$$\text{Cys-Tyr-Phe-Gln-Asn-Cys-Pro-Lys-Gly-NH}_2$$
$$\quad 1 \quad 2 \quad 3 \quad 4 \quad 5 \quad 6 \quad 7 \quad 8 \quad 9$$

CLINICAL PHARMACOLOGY
Lysine-8-vasopressin is a polypeptide and is one of the two known naturally occurring molecular forms of mammalian posterior pituitary antidiuretic hormone. It is identical to the vasopressin produced naturally in swine pituitaries. This synthetic vasopressin differs from that produced in humans in that it contains lysine instead of arginine in its structure. It is present as a protein-free substance in Lypressin nasal solution, USP Nasal Spray. Unlike preparations of posterior pituitary antidiuretic hormone of animal origin, lypressin nasal solution, USP Nasal Spray is completely free of oxytocin and foreign proteins.

The principal pharmacologic action of lysine-8-vasopressin, the active ingredient of Lypressin nasal solution, USP Nasal Spray, is similar to that of arginine-8-vasopressin, the posterior pituitary antidiuretic hormone occurring in man. Lypressin nasal solution, USP Nasal Spray increases the rate of reabsorption of solute free water from the distal renal tubules, without significantly modifying the rate of glomerular filtration, producing a fall in free water clearance and an increase in urinary osmolality. The rates of solute and creatinine excretion noted with therapeutic doses of Lypressin nasal solution, USP Nasal Spray suggest that sodium clearance and glomerular filtration rates are essentially unaltered by this hormone. Lypressin nasal solution, USP Nasal Spray is relatively free of oxytocic activity when used within the recommended therapeutic dose levels.

It possesses little pressor activity, the ratio of pressor to antidiuretic activity being in the range of 1:1000.

The antidiuretic effect produced by Lypressin nasal solution, USP Nasal Spray begins rapidly and usually reaches a peak within 30-120 minutes. Its usual duration of action is 3-8 hours.

INDICATIONS
Lypressin nasal solution, USP Nasal Spray is indicated for the control or prevention of the symptoms and complications of diabetes insipidus due to deficiency of endogenous posterior pituitary antidiuretic hormone in both children and adults. These symptoms and complications include polydipsia, polyuria, and dehydration. It is particularly useful in patients with diabetes insipidus who have become unresponsive to other forms of therapy or who experience various types of local and/or systemic reactions, allergic reactions, or other undesirable effects (e.g., excessive fluid retention) from preparations of posterior pituitary antidiuretic hormone of animal origin.

UNLABELED USES
Lypressin is used alone or as an adjunct in the treatment of idiopathic orthostatic hypotension.

CONTRAINDICATIONS
Hypersensitivity. (See "Precautions".)

WARNINGS
Cardiovascular pressor effects with Lypressin nasal solution, USP Nasal Spray are minimal or absent when it is administered as a nasal spray in therapeutic doses. Nevertheless, it should be used with caution in patients for whom such effects would not be desirable because mild blood pressure elevation has been noted in unanesthetized subjects who received Lypressin intravenously. Large doses intranasally may cause coronary artery constriction and caution should be observed in treating patients with coronary artery disease. There have been reports of acute myocardial infarction in patients taking Lypressin nasal solution, USP Nasal Spray.[1]

PRECAUTIONS
GENERAL
The effectiveness of Lypressin nasal solution, USP Nasal Spray may be lessened in patients with nasal congestion, allergic rhinitis, and upper respiratory infections because these conditions may interfere with absorption of the drug by the nasal mucosa. In this event, larger doses of Lypressin nasal solution, USP Nasal Spray, or adjunctive therapy, may be needed.

Patients with a known sensitivity to antidiuretic hormone should be tested for sensitivity to Lypressin nasal solution, USP Nasal Spray. (See "Contraindications".)

INFORMATION FOR PATIENTS
Lypressin nasal solution, USP Nasal Spray is indicated for the treatment of diabetes insipidus, a disorder in which the lack of a specific hormone, vasopressin, prevents the kidneys from conserving water. As a result, excess urine is produced which can lead to dehydration. The symptoms of this disorder are mainly excessive urination and thirst. Lypressin nasal solution, USP Nasal Spray provides the body with a synthetic form of vasopressin and thus prevents these symptoms.

Patients should be instructed on how to regulate their daily dosage according to their degree of excessive urination and thirst. Once established, daily requirements should remain stable for a long period of time. In case of nasal congestion due to allergic conditions or upper respiratory tract infections which interferes with the absorption of the drug by the nasal mucosa, patients may require larger doses of Lypressin nasal solution, USP Nasal Spray or an alternate form of therapy. Patients should be advised to consult their physician if this circumstance arises.

To assure a uniform delivery of spray with Lypressin nasal solution, USP Nasal Spray, the bottle should be held upright and the patient should be sitting or standing with the head upright.

Lypressin nasal solution, USP Nasal Spray is indicated for use in the treatment of diabetes insipidus *only*. It should not be used in the therapy of other disorders or conditions.

CARCINOGENESIS, MUTAGENESIS, IMPAIRMENT OF FERTILITY
No long-term studies in animals have been performed to evaluate carcinogenic potential. Reproductive studies have not been conducted in animals or humans to test whether Lypressin constitutes a potential problem in relation to mutagenesis or impairment of fertility in either females or males. However, as a posterior pituitary antidiuretic hormone it is unlikely to evoke detrimental reproductive effects. Commercially available since September, 1970, lypressin has not been reported to have been related to any instance of fetal abnormality, infertility or impotence.

PREGNANCY CATEGORY C
Animal reproduction studies have not been conducted with Lypressin nasal solution, USP Nasal Spray. It is not known whether Lypressin nasal solution, USP Nasal Spray can cause fetal harm when administered to a pregnant woman or can affect reproduction capacity. Lypressin nasal solution, USP Nasal Spray should be given to a pregnant woman only if clearly needed.

NURSING MOTHERS
It is not known whether this drug is excreted in human milk. Because many drugs are excreted in human milk, a decision should be made whether to discontinue nursing or to discontinue the drug, taking into account the importance of the drug to the mother.

PEDIATRIC USE
The usual dosage in children is the same as for adults (see "Dosage and Administration"). Safety and efficacy have not been demonstrated in children less than six weeks of age.

ADVERSE REACTIONS
Cardiovascular pressor effects with Lypressin nasal solution, USP Nasal Spray are minimal when it is administered as a nasal spray in therapeutic doses. (See "Warnings".)

With clinical use of Lypressin nasal solution, USP Nasal Spray, adverse reactions, in general, have been infrequent and mild. Such reactions have included rhinorrhea, nasal congestion, irritation and pruritus of the nasal passages, nasal ulceration, headache, conjunctivitis, heartburn secondary to excessive nasal administration with drippage into the pharynx, abdominal and muscle cramps and increased bowel movements. Periorbital edema, with itching, has been reported. Inadvertent inhalation of Lypressin nasal solution, USP Nasal Spray has resulted in substernal tightness, coughing, and transient dyspnea. Tolerance or tachyphylaxis to Lypressin nasal solution, USP Nasal Spray has not been reported to date.

Hypersensitivity manifested by positive skin test has been reported.

DRUG ABUSE AND DEPENDENCE
There have been no reports of drug abuse or dependence with Lypressin nasal solution, USP Nasal Spray.

OVERDOSAGE
The lethal dose of Lypressin nasal solution, USP Nasal Spray has not been established. The I.V. LD_{50} of Lypressin nasal solution, USP in rats is 7266 mg/kg. The oral or intraperitoneal administration of Lypressin nasal solution, USP Nasal Spray to rats in doses up to 20mL (1000 I.U.)/100 gm resulted in no deaths.

◆ RATED THERAPEUTICALLY EQUIVALENT; ◇ THERAPEUTIC EQUIVALENCE UNCONFIRMED; ○ UNRATED

Lypressin nasal solution, USP Nasal Spray is a polypeptide and is therefore subject to inactivation by the proteolytic enzymes of the alimentary tract. Hence, Lypressin nasal solution USP Nasal Spray is NOT ABSORBED from the gastrointestinal tract, and, for this reason, ingestion of this drug is not likely to have toxic effects. The only reasonable route of significant acute overdosage with Lypressin nasal solution, USP Nasal Spray is by excessive use of the nasal spray.

Inadvertent or intentional excessive use of Lypressin nasal solution, USP Nasal Spray may result in significant water retention, and if the overdosage is high enough and associated with a very high fluid intake, the possibility of water intoxication does arise. The symptoms of water intoxication include headache, anorexia, nausea, vomiting, abdominal pain, lethargy, drowsiness, unconsciousness and grand mal-type seizures. The dilution factor associated with marked water retention lowers the electrolyte concentration in the blood.

A patient being treated with Lypressin nasal solution, USP Nasal Spray for diabetes insipidus misunderstood the therapeutic recommendations and used the spray vigorously according to thirst. As a result, marked water retention with related hyponatremia developed. These conditions were relieved by decreasing the frequency of use of the nasal spray.

The treatment of Lypressin nasal solution, USP Nasal Spray overdose should include the following:

1. Discontinue the drug and restrict fluid intake. As the duration of action of Lypressin nasal solution, USP Nasal Spray is from 3-8 hours, these measures alone usually suffice for simple water retention.

2. Correction of electrolyte imbalance as indicated in water intoxication with the I.V. administration of 200-300 mL of 5% saline solution over several hours sufficient to raise the serum sodium to a level at which the symptoms will improve.

3. When there is the possibility of congestive heart failure due to the fluid overload, the simultaneous administration of furosemide with the hypertonic saline usually causes a diuresis sufficient to reduce cardiac overload. Potassium and other electrolyte levels must be monitored with the use of furosemide.

4. If I.V. fluid administration is considered necessary when the serum sodium has been raised to normal, the slow infusion of isotonic saline is advised to maintain normal serum sodium levels.

DOSAGE AND ADMINISTRATION

Patients should be instructed to administer 1 or 2 sprays of Lypressin nasal solution, USP Nasal Spray to one or both nostrils whenever frequency of urination becomes increased or significant thirst develops. (One spray provides approximately 2 USP Posterior Pituitary [Pressor] Units.) The usual dosage for adults and children six weeks and older is 1 or 2 sprays in each nostril four times daily. An additional dose at bedtime is often helpful to eliminate nocturia, if it is not controlled with the regular daily dosage. For patients requiring more than 2 sprays per nostril every 4-6 hours, it is recommended that the time interval between doses be reduced rather than increasing the number of sprays at each dose. (More than 2 or 3 sprays in each nostril usually results in wastage because the unabsorbed excess will drain posteriorly, by way of the nasopharynx, into the digestive tract where it will be inactivated.)

Lypressin nasal solution, USP Nasal Spray permits individualization of dosage necessary to control the symptoms of diabetes insipidus. Patients quickly learn to regulate their dosage in accordance with their degree of polyuria and thirst, and once determined, daily requirements remain fairly stable for months and years. Although most patients require 1 or 2 sprays of Lypressin nasal solution, USP Nasal Spray in each nostril four times daily, dosage has ranged from 1 spray per day at bedtime to 10 sprays in each nostril every 3-4 hours. Requirements of the larger doses may represent greater severity of disease or other phenomena, such as poor nasal absorption. A seeming requirement for larger doses of Lypressin may be due to the presence of mixed hypothalamichypophyseal and nephrogenic diabetes insipidus, the latter condition being unresponsive to administration of antidiuretic hormone.

Lypressin nasal solution, USP Nasal Spray is conveniently administered, from a compact and portable, plastic squeeze bottle, by inserting the nozzle of the bottle into the nostril and squeezing once firmly to deliver each short spray.

Note: To assure that a uniform, well diffused spray is delivered, the bottle of Lypressin nasal solution, USP Nasal Spray should be held upright and the patient should be in a vertical position with head upright.

Store and Dispense: Below 72 °F.

HOW SUPPLIED
SPRAY: 0.185 MG/ML

BRAND/MANUFACTURER	NDC	SIZE	AWP
○ **BRAND**			
DIAPID: Sandoz Pharm	00078-0042-38	8 ml	$41.76

Lysine/Vitamin B Complex/Zinc Sulfate

DESCRIPTION:

Each Tablet contains:

Lysine	200 mg
Vitamin B₁ (Thiamine HCl)	20 mg

Vitamin B₂ (Riboflavin)	6 mg
Vitamin B₅ (Pyridoxine)	4 mg
Vitamin B₁₂ (Cyanocobalamins)	50 mcg
Niacinamide	20 mg
Folic Acid	500 mcg
Vitamin C (Ascorbic Acid)	200 mg
Vitamin E (D L Alpha Tocopheryl Acetate)	40 I.U.
Zinc (Dried Sulfate)	30 mg

Each 15 ml of liquid contains:

L-Lysine	500 mg.
Vitamin B₁ (Thiamine HCl)	4 mg.
Vitamin B₂ (Riboflavin U.S.P.)	4 mg.
Vitamin B₆ (Pyridoxine HCl)	1 mg.
Vitamin B₁₂ (Cyanocobalamin)	8 mcg.
Niacinamide, U.S.P.	50 mg.
Folic Acid	1 mg.
Zinc Sulfate, U.S.P.	30 mg.

INDICATIONS
Appetite stimulant and nutrient supplement of the vitamins found in formula. L-Lysine is an essential amino acid needed in the protein synthesis that takes place in the human body. Folic acid helps in the prevention of concomitant folic acid deficiency in adults, is effective in the treatment of megaloblastic anemias due to a deficiency of folic acid (as may be seen in tropical or nontropical sprue) and in anemias of nutritional origin, pregnancy, infancy or childhood.

Vitamin E: prevents oxidation reactions in the body. It helps red blood cells maintain their shape, slows down platelet clumping and may be an important part of the body's enzyme systems.

Vitamin C: is involved with several functions in the body including utilization of carbohydrates, formation of fats and proteins, maintenance of blood vessels, cell respiration, formation of support tissues, promotion of growth, tissue repair and wound healing, aids in tooth and bone formation, increases iron absorption.

CONTRAINDICATIONS
Folic Acid (pteroylglutamic acid), is contraindicated in patients with untreated and uncomplicated pernicious anemia, and those with anaphylactic sensitivity to Folic Acid.

WARNINGS
Folic Acid alone is improper treatment of pernicious anemia and other megaloblastic anemias where Vitamin B₁₂ is deficient.

PRECAUTIONS
Folic Acid in doses above 0.1 mg daily may obscure pernicious anemia, in that hematologic remission may occur while neurological manifestations remain progressive.

Folic Acid (pteroylglutamic acid) microbiological blood assays are invalidated by the administration of most antibiotics, methotrexate, and pyrimethamine. Folic acid is not effective in reversing the toxic effects of methotrexate. Folinic acid (5-formyl-5,6,6,7,8-tetra hydrofolic acid) must be used in this situation.

ADVERSE REACTIONS
Allergic sensitization has been reported following oral and parenteral administration of Folic Acid.

DOSAGE AND ADMINISTRATION
One or two tablets daily, or as directed by a physician. One tablespoonful two times a day, half (1/2) hour before lunch and dinner or as prescribed by the physician.

HOW SUPPLIED
SYRUP:

BRAND/MANUFACTURER	NDC	SIZE	AWP
○ **GENERICS**			
LYSIPLEX: Kramer Dist	52083-0841-06	180 ml	$8.00

TABLETS:

BRAND/MANUFACTURER	NDC	SIZE	AWP
○ **GENERICS**			
LYSIPLEX: Kramer Dist	52083-0840-30	30s	$8.00

Lysine Hydrochloride/Potassium Bicarbonate/Potassium Chloride

DESCRIPTION
Lysine Hydrochloride/Potassium Bicarbonate/Potassium Chloride is an oral Potassium supplement available as a 20 mEq and 25 mEq effervescent tablet.

Each effervescent tablet contains 20 mEq each of Potassium and Chloride supplied by Potassium Chloride 1.125 g, Potassium Bicarbonate 0.5 g, Lysine Hydrochloride 0.913 g or 25 mEq (1865 mg) Potassium Chloride (supplied by 1.5 g Potassium Chloride, 0.5 g Potassium Bicarbonate and 0.91 g I-lysine monohydrochloride). Dissolution of the tablet in water provides the Potassium and Chloride available for oral ingestion as Potassium Chloride, Potassium Bicarbonate, Potassium citrate and Lysine Hydrochloride.

CLINICAL PHARMACOLOGY

Potassium ion is the principal intracellular cation of most body tissues. Potassium ions participate in many essential physiological processes, such as the maintenance of intracellular tonicity, nerve impulse transmission, enzymatic reactions in intermediary metabolism, cardiac, skeletal and smooth muscle function, and the maintenance of normal renal function.

Potassium depletion may occur whenever the rate of Potassium loss through renal excretion and/or loss from the gastrointestinal tract exceeds the rate of potassium intake. Potassium depletion usually develops slowly as a result of lengthy therapy with oral diuretics, primary or secondary hyperaldosteronism, diabetic kotoacidosis, or inadequate replacement of Potassium in patients on prolonged parenteral nutrition. Depletion is additionally associated with severe diarrhea, accompanied by vomiting. Potassium depletion due to these causes is usually accompanied by a concomitant loss of Chloride and is manifested by hypokalemia and metabolic alkalosis. Potassium depletion may result in fatigue, weakness, nausea, drowsiness, loss of appetite, edema, oliguria, and chronic ileus with distension. Potassium deficiency may be manifested by shallow breathing, lowered blood pressure, disturbances of cardiac rhythm (primarily ectopic beats), prominent U-waves in the electrocardiogram, or other ECG changes, such as lengthened Q-T interval, depressed S-T segment, and depressed or inverted T wave. In advanced cases of Potassium deficiency, flaccid paralysis and/or impaired ability to concentrate urine may be evident.

INDICATIONS

1. For therapeutic use in patients with hypokalemia with or without metabolic alkalosis: in digitalis intoxication and in patients with hypokalemic familial periodic paralysis.

2. For prevention of Potassium depletion when the dietary intake of Potassium is inadequate in the following conditions: patients receiving digitalis and diuretics for congestive heart failure; hepatic cirrhosis with ascites; states of aldosterone excess with normal renal function; Potassium-losing nephropathy, and certain diarrheal states.

3. The use of Potassium salts in patients receiving diuretics for uncomplicated essential hypertension is often unnecessary when such patients have a normal dietary pattern. Serum Potassium should be checked periodically, however, and, if hypokalemia occurs, dietary supplementation with Potassium-containing foods may be adequate to control milder cases. In more severe cases supplementation with Potassium salts may be indicated.

CONTRAINDICATIONS

Severe renal impairment characterized by azotemia or oliguria, untreated Addison's disease, Familial Periodic Paralysis, acute dehydration, heat cramps, or patients receiving aldosterone-inhibiting or Potassium-sparing diuretic agents.

Potassium supplements are contraindicated for patients having hyperkalemia, since a further increase in serum potassium level in these patients can result in cardiac arrest. Hyperkalemia may complicate any of the following conditions: chronic renal failure; systemic acidosis, such as diabetic acidosis; acute dehydration; extensive tissue breakdown, as in severe burns; adrenal insufficiency. Hypokalemia should not be treated by the simultaneous use of Potassium salts and a Potassium-sparing diuretic, such as spironolactone or triamterene, since the concomitant use of these medications can result in severe hyperkalemia.

WARNINGS

The administration of Potassium salts can produce hyperkalemia and cardiac arrest in patients with impaired mechanisms for potassium excretion. Those reactions most commonly occur in patients receiving Potassium intravenously, but may also occur in patients receiving oral Potassium. Potentially fatal hyperkalemia can develop quickly and be asymptomatic. Patients using Potassium salts with chronic renal disease, or any other condition which impairs the excretion of Potassium, require especially carefully monitoring of serum Potassium concentration and appropriate adjustment of dosage.

PRECAUTIONS

In response to a rise in the concentration of body Potassium, renal excretion of the ion is increased. In the presence of normal renal function and hydration, it is difficult to produce Potassium intoxication by oral Potassium salt supplements.

The diagnosis of Potassium depletion is ordinarily made by demonstrating hypokalemia in a patient with a clinical history suggesting a cause for Potassium depletion. When interpreting the serum Potassium concentration, the physician should be aware that acute alkalosis can cause hypokalemia without showing a deficit in total body Potassium. Acute acidosis can increase the serum Potassium level to normal even with a reduced total body Potassium.

Since the extent of Potassium deficiency cannot be accurately determined, it is prudent to proceed cautiously in undertaking Potassium replacement. Periodic evaluations of acid-base balance, the patient's clinical status, serum electrolytes and the EKG should be carried out when replacement therapy is undertaken. This is particularly important in patients with cardiac disease and those patients receiving digitalis.

High serum concentrations of Potassium may cause death through cardiac depression, arrhythmia or cardiac arrest. To minimize gastrointestinal irritation associated with Potassium Chloride preparations, patients should dissolve each Lysine HCl/Potassium Bicarbonate/Potassium Cl tablet in 3 or 4 ounces of cold water or fruit juice. This solution should be ingested slowly with or immediately after meals.

Laboratory Tests: Serum Potassium determinations and ECG should be a part of the frequent clinical evaluation of the patient.

Drug Interactions: Severe hyperkalemia can be produced by the simultaneous administration of Potassium supplements and a Potassium-sparing diuretic. Potassium supplements should be used carefully by patients who are using salt substitutes, because may of these substitutes contain large amounts of Potassium. This simultaneous use could produce hyperkalemia.

Usage in Pregnancy: Pregnancy Category C. Animal reproduction studies have not been conducted with this effervescent Potassium product. It is unknown whether this product can cause fetal harm when given to a pregnant woman or if it can affect reproductive capacity. Pregnant women should be given this product only if it is clearly needed.

Nursing Mothers: Because many drugs are excreted in human milk, there exists the potential for serious adverse reactions in nursing infants from oral Potassium supplements. Therefore, it should be decided whether to discontinue nursing or to discontinue the drug, considering the importance of the drug to the mother.

Pediatric Use: Safety and effectiveness in children have not been established.

ADVERSE REACTIONS

Abdominal discomfort, diarrhea, vomiting, and nausea are the most common adverse reactions to oral Potassium supplements. These adverse reactions occur most frequently when the preparation is not taken with food, is not properly diluted, or not completely dissolved.

Hyperkalemia occurs infrequently in patients with normal renal function who receive oral Potassium supplements.

The symptoms and signs of Potassium intoxication include paresthesias, heaviness, muscle weakness and flaccid paralysis of the extremities. Potassium intoxication can produce listlessness, unexplained anxiety, numbness or tingling in lips, feet, or hands, difficult breathing or shortness of breath, unusual fatigue, mental confusion, a fall in blood pressure, shock, cardiac arrhythmias, heart block and cardiac arrest.

The EKG picture of hyperkalemia is characterized by the early appearance of tall, peaked T waves. The R wave is decreased in amplitude and the S wave deepens; the QRS complex widens progressively. The P wave widens and decreases in amplitude until it disappears. Occasionally, an apparent elevation of the RS-T junction and a cove plane RS-T segment and T wave will be noted in AVL.

OVERDOSAGE

The use of oral Potassium salts by persons with normal renal function rarely results in serious hyperkalemia. However, if excretory mechanisms are impaired or if Potassium is administered too rapidly intravenously, potentially fatal hyperkalemia can result. Hyperkalemia, when detected, must be treated immediately because lethal levels can be reached in a few hours. The earliest clinical signs of hyperkalemia may be only increased serum Potassium concentrations and characteristic ECG changes, such as depression of S-T segment, prolongation of the QT interval, peaking of T-waves and the loss of P-wave. The above mentioned changes in the ECG most frequently occur when the serum Potassium level gets to 7 or 8 mEq per liter. At a level of 9 to 10 mEq per liter, other clinical manifestations may occur, such as muscle paralysis and death due to cardiac arrest.

The focus of the treatment of severe hyperkalemia should be on the reduction of the serum Potassium level by furthering the transfer of Potassium from the extracellular to the intracellular space.

DOSAGE AND ADMINISTRATION

Adults: One Lysine HCl/Potassium Bicarbonate/Potassium Cl effervescent tablet (20 mEq each of Potassium and Chloride) completely dissolved in 3 to 4 ounces of cold water or fruit juice 2 to 4 times daily depending upon the requirements of the patient.

The solution should be ingested slowly over a 5- to 10-minute period with meals or immediately after eating. Deviations from these recommended dosages may be indicated in certain cases of hypokalemia based upon the patient's status. The average total daily dosage must be governed by the patient's response as determined by frequent evaluation of serum electrolytes, EKG and clinical status.

TREATMENT OF HYPERKALEMIA

1. Dextrose solution, 10 or 25% containing 10 units of crystalline insulin per 20 g dextrose, given IV in a dose of 300 to 500 mL in an hour.

2. In the acidolic patient, 150 mEq to 300 mEq of sodium bicarbonate administered intravenously.

3. Adsorption and exchange of Potassium using sodium or ammonium cycle cation exchange resins, orally and as a retention enema. (Caution: Ammonium compounds should not be used in patients with hepatic cirrhosis.)

To make sure that the resin moves rapidly through the gastrointestinal tract, a nonabsorbable polyhydric alcohol such as sorbitol should be administered in sufficient amounts to cause a soft to semiliquid bowel movement to occur every few hours.

4. Hemodialysis and peritoneal dialysis.

5. The use of Potassium-containing foods or medicaments must be eliminated.

In digitalized patients too rapid a lowering of plasma Potassium concentration can cause digitalis toxicity.

◆ RATED THERAPEUTICALLY EQUIVALENT; ◇ THERAPEUTIC EQUIVALENCE UNCONFIRMED; ○ UNRATED

STORAGE
Store and dispense: Below 86°F (30°C).

HOW SUPPLIED
POWDER FOR RECONSTITUTION:

BRAND/MANUFACTURER	NDC	SIZE	AWP
○ GENERICS			
Goldline	00182-1451-17	30s	$6.00

TABLET, EFFERVESCENT:

BRAND/MANUFACTURER	NDC	SIZE	AWP
○ GENERICS			
Goldline	00182-1901-17	30s	$18.70

Lysodren SEE MITOTANE

Macrobid SEE NITROFURANTOIN

Macrodantin SEE NITROFURANTOIN

Mafenide Acetate

DESCRIPTION
Mafenide Acetate Cream is a soft, white, nonstaining, water-miscible, anti-infective cream for topical administration to burn wounds.

Mafenide Acetate Cream spreads easily, and can be washed off readily with water. It has a slight acetic odor. Each gram of Mafenide Acetate Cream contains Mafenide Acetate equivalent to 85 mg of the base.

CLINICAL PHARMACOLOGY
Mafenide Acetate Cream, applied topically, produces a marked reduction in the bacterial population present in the avascular tissues of second- and third-degree burns. Reduction in bacterial growth after application of Mafenide Acetate Cream has also been reported to permit spontaneous healing of deep partial-thickness burns, and thus prevent conversion of burn wounds from partial thickness to full thickness. It should be noted, however, that delayed eschar separation has occurred in some cases.

Absorption and Metabolism: Applied topically, Mafenide Acetate Cream diffuses through devascularized areas, is absorbed, and rapidly converted to a metabolite (ρ-carboxybenzenesulfonamide) which is cleared through the kidneys. Mafenide Acetate is active in the presence of pus and serum, and its activity is not altered by changes in the acidity of the environment.

Antibacterial Activity: Mafenide Acetate exerts bacteriostatic action against many gram-negative and gram-positive organisms, including *Pseudomonas aeruginosa* and certain strains of anaerobes.

INDICATIONS AND USAGE
Mafenide Acetate Cream is a topical agent indicated for adjunctive therapy of patients with second- and third-degree burns.

CONTRAINDICATIONS
Mafenide Acetate is contraindicated in patients who are hypersensitive to it. It is not known whether there is cross sensitivity to other sulfonamides.

WARNINGS
Fatal hemolytic anemia with disseminated intravascular coagulation, presumably related to a glucose-6-phosphate dehydrogenase deficiency, has been reported following therapy with Mafenide Acetate Cream.

Contains sodium metabisulfite, a sulfite that may cause allergic-type reactions including anaphylactic symptoms and life-threatening or less severe asthmatic episodes in certain susceptible people. The overall prevalence of sulfite sensitivity in the general population is unknown and probably low. Sulfite sensitivity is seen more frequently in asthmatic than in nonasthmatic people.

PRECAUTIONS
Mafenide Acetate and its metabolite, ρ-carboxybenzenesulfonamide, inhibit carbonic anhydrase, which may result in metabolic acidosis, usually compensated by hyperventilation. In the presence of impaired renal function, high blood levels of Mafenide Acetate and its metabolite may exaggerate the carbonic anhydrase inhibition. Therefore, close monitoring of acid-base balance is necessary, particularly in patients with extensive second-degree or partial thickness burns and in those with pulmonary or renal dysfunction. Some burn patients treated with Mafenide Acetate Cream have also been reported to manifest an unexplained syndrome of marked hyperventilation with resulting respiratory alkalosis (slightly aklaline blood pH, low arterial pCO_2, and decreased total CO_2); change in arterial pO_2 is variable. The etiology and significance of these findings are unknown.

Mafenide Acetate cream should be used with caution in burn patients with acute renal failure.

Mafenide Acetate Cream should be administered with caution to patients with history of hypersensitivity to Mafenide. It is not known whether there is cross sensitivity to other sulfonamides.

Fungal colonization in and below the eschar may occur concomitantly with reduction of bacterial growth in the burn wound. However, fungal dissemination through the infected burn wound is rare.

Carcinogenesis, Mutagenesis, Impairment of Fertility: No long-term animal studies have been performed to evaluate the drug's potential in these areas.

Pregnancy Category C: Animal reproduction studies have not been conducted with Mafenide Acetate. It is also not known whether Mafenide Acetate can cause fetal harm when administered to a pregnant woman or can affect reproduction capacity. Therefore, the preparation is not recommended for the treatment of women of childbearing potential, unless the burned area covers more than 20% of the total body surface, or the need for the therapeutic benefit of Mafenide Acetate Cream is, in the physician's judgment, greater than the possible risk to the fetus.

Nursing Mothers: It is not known whether Mafenide Acetate is excreted in human milk. Because many drugs are excreted in human milk and because of the potential for serious adverse reaction in nursing infants from Mafenide Acetate, a decision should be made whether to discontinue nursing or to discontinue the drug, taking into account the importance of the drug to the mother.

Pediatric Use: Same as for adults. (See *"Dosage and Administration."*).

ADVERSE REACTIONS
It is frequently difficult to distinguish between an adverse reaction to Mafenide Acetate Cream and the effect of a severe burn. A single case of bone marrow depression and a single case of acute attack of porphyria have been reported following therapy with Mafenide Acetate Cream. Fatal hemolytic anemia with disseminated intravascular coagulation, presumably related to a glucose-6-phosphate dehydrogenase deficiency, has been reported following therapy with Mafenide Acetate Cream.

Dermatologic: The most frequently reported reaction was pain on application or a burning sensation. Rare occurrences are excoriation of new skin, and bleeding of skin.

Allergic: Rash, itching, facial edema, swelling, hives, blisters, erythema, and eosinophilia.

Respiratory: Tachypnea or hyperventilation, decrease in arterial pCO_2.

Metabolic: Acidosis, increase in serum chloride.

Accidental ingestion of Mafenide Acetate Cream has been reported to cause diarrhea.

DOSAGE AND ADMINISTRATION
Prompt institution of appropriate measures for controlling shock and pain is of prime importance. The burn wounds are then cleansed and debrided, and Mafenide Acetate Cream is applied with a sterile gloved hand. Satisfactory results can be achieved with application of the cream once or twice daily, to a thickness of approximately 1/16 inch; thicker application is not recommended. The burned areas should be covered with Mafenide Acetate Cream at all times. Therefore, whenever necessary, the cream should be reapplied to any areas from which it has been removed (e.g., by patient activity). The routine of administration can be accomplished in minimal time, since dressings usually are not required. If individual patient demands make them necessary, however, only a thin layer of dressing should be used.

When feasible, the patient should be bathed daily, to aid in debridement. A whirlpool bath is particularly helpful, but the patient may be bathed in bed or in a shower.

The duration of therapy with Mafenide Acetate Cream depends on each patient's requirements. Treatment is usually continued until healing is progressing well or until the burn site is ready for grafting. *Mafenide Acetate Cream should not be withdrawn from the therapeutic regimen while there is the possibility of infection.* However, if allergic manifestations occur during treatment with Mafenide Acetate Cream, discontinuation of treatment should be considered.

If acidosis occurs and becomes difficult to control, particularly in patients with pulmonary dysfunction, discontinuing therapy with Mafenide Acetate Cream for 24 to 48 hours while continuing fluid therapy may aid in restoring acid-base balance.

Avoid exposure to excessive heat (temperatures above 104°F or 40°C).

HOW SUPPLIED
CREAM:

BRAND/MANUFACTURER	NDC	SIZE	AWP
◇ BRAND			
SULFAMYLON ACETATE: Dow Hickam	00514-0101-50	60 gm	$17.50
	00514-0101-51	120 gm	$32.50
	00514-0101-53	435 gm	$108.50

Magan SEE MAGNESIUM SALICYLATE

➤ SHOWN IN PRODUCT IDENTIFICATION GUIDE

Magnesium Chloride, Injectable

DESCRIPTION

Magnesium Chloride Injection is a sterile solution of Magnesium Chloride Hexahydrate in Water for Injection q.s. Each mL contains Magnesium Chloride Hexahydrate 200 mg; pH adjusted with Hydrochloric Acid and/or Sodium Hydroxide. Total osmolarity equivalent to 2951 mOsm/L. Contains 1.97 mEq of Mg^{++} and Cl^- per mL.

The structural formula is $MgCl_2 \cdot 6H_2O$.

ACTIONS

Magnesium is the second most plentiful cation within cellular fluids. It is an important activator of many enzyme systems, and deficits are accompanied by a variety of functional disturbances.

INDICATIONS

As an electrolyte replenisher in Magnesium deficiencies.

CONTRAINDICATIONS

Magnesium Chloride Injection should not be administered if there is renal impairment, marked myocardial disease or to comatose patients.

WARNING

Do not use if a precipitate is present.

PRECAUTIONS

The usual precautions for parenteral administration should be observed. Administer with caution if flushing and sweating occurs. A preparation of a calcium salt should be readily available for intravenous injection to counteract potential serious signs of Magnesium intoxication. As long as deep tendon reflexes are active it is probable that the patient will not develop respiratory paralysis. Respiration and blood pressure should be carefully observed during and after administration of Magnesium Chloride injection.

Pregnancy: Teratogenic Effects: Pregnancy Category C. Animal reproduction studies have not been conducted with Magnesium Chloride. It is also not known whether Magnesium Chloride can cause fetal harm when administered to a pregnant woman or can affect reproduction capacity. Magnesium Chloride should be given to a pregnant woman only if clearly needed.

ADVERSE REACTIONS

Flushing, sweating, sharply lowered blood pressure, hypothermia, stupor, and ultimately respiratory depression.

DOSAGE AND ADMINISTRATION

For intravenous infusion: 4 grams in 250 mL of 5% Dextrose Injection, at a rate not exceeding 3 mL per minute. Serum Magnesium levels should serve as a guide to continued dosage.

Usual Dosage Range: 1 to 40 grams daily.

Parenteral drug products should be inspected visually for particulate matter and discoloration prior to administration whenever solution and container permit.

Storage: Store at controlled room temperature, 15°-30°C (59°-86°F).

HOW SUPPLIED
INJECTION:

BRAND/MANUFACTURER	NDC	SIZE	AWP
○ GENERICS			
CHLOROMAG: Merit	30727-0304-90	50 ml	$11.85

INJECTION: 20%

BRAND/MANUFACTURER	NDC	SIZE	AWP
○ BRAND			
MAGNESIUM CHLORIDE INJECTION	00517-5034-01	50 ml	$4.38
○ GENERICS			
Amer Regent	00517-5034-01	50 ml	$4.38

INJECTION: 200 MG/ML

BRAND/MANUFACTURER	NDC	SIZE	AWP
○ BRAND			
MAGNESIUM CHLORIDE	00389-0173-50	50 ml	$3.99
	10974-0304-50	50 ml	$4.00
	49072-0473-50	50 ml	$4.19
	00418-5740-44	50 ml	$6.55
○ GENERICS			
Torrance	00389-0173-50	50 ml	$3.99
Pegasus	10974-0304-50	50 ml	$4.00
McGuff	49072-0473-50	50 ml	$4.19

BRAND/MANUFACTURER	NDC	SIZE	AWP
Pasadena	00418-5740-44	50 ml	$6.55

Magnesium Salicylate

DESCRIPTION

Each Magnesium Salicylate tablet for oral administration contains 545 mg of magnesium salicylate equivalent to 500 mg of salicylate. Magnesium Salicylate is a nonsteroidal, anti-inflammatory agent with antipyretic and analgesic properties. Its molecular weight is 298.54.

Magnesium Salicylate is a white odorless, crystalline powder with a sweet taste. It is soluble in water and alcohol.

Following is its chemical structure:

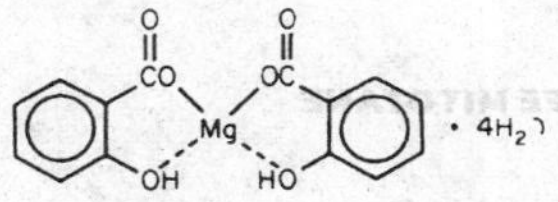

CLINICAL PHARMACOLOGY

Salicylic acid is the active moiety released into the plasma by Magnesium Salicylate. Salicylic acid is enzymatically biotransformed through two pathways to salicyluric acid and salicylphenolic glucuronide and eliminated in the urine.

Oral Salicylates are absorbed rapidly, partly from the stomach but mostly from the upper intestine. Salicylic acid is rapidly distributed throughout all body tissues and most transcellular fluids, mainly by pH-dependent passive processes. It can be detected in synovial, spinal and peritoneal fluid, in saliva and in milk. It readily crosses the placental barrier. From 50% to 90% of salicylic acid is bound to plasma proteins, especially albumin.

Following the ingestion of a single dose of 524 mg of Magnesium Salicylate, a peak concentration of 3.6 mg/dL salicylate acid is reached in 1.5 hours with a m/2 of 2 hours. The major biotransformation paths for the elimination of salicylate acid from the plasma become saturated by low doses of Salicylate acid. As a result, repeated doses of Magnesium Salicylate increase the plasma concentration and markedly prolong the plasma half-life. The plasma concentration of Salicylate acid is increased by conditions that reduce the glomerular filtration rate of tubular secretion such as renal disease or the presence of inhibitors that compete for the transport system such as probenecid.

Therapeutic, plasma concentrations of salicylate acid for an adequate anti-inflammatory effect needed for the treatment of rheumatoid arthritis range between 20-30 mg/dL. Effective analgesia is achieved at lower concentrations. Salicylates relieve pain by both a peripheral and a CNS effect. Salicylates inhibit the synthesis of prostaglandins; the importance of this mechanism in analgesia and anti-inflammation has not been fully elucidated. Salicylates have an antipyretic effect in febrile patients but little in subjects with normal temperatures. This appears to be due to the inhibition of the synthesis of prostaglandins which are powerful pyrogens that affect the hypothalamus. Higher therapeutic concentrations cause reversible tinnitus and high tone hearing loss. Full therapeutic doses of salicylates increase oxygen consumption and CO_2 production. They cause an extracellular and intracellular respiratory, alkalosis which is rapidly compensated. Salicylates irritate the gastric mucosa and frequently lead to blood loss in the stool, this effect is more pronounced with aspirin than Magnesium Salicylate. Salicylates in large doses (over 6 g/day) reduce the plasma prothrombin level. In contrast to aspirin, Magnesium Salicylate does not affect platelets. Salicylic acid increases the urinary excretion of urates at higher doses but may decrease excretion at lower doses.

INDICATIONS AND USAGE

Magnesium Salicylate is indicated for the relief of the signs and symptoms of rheumatoid arthritis, osteoarthritis, bursitis, and other musculoskeletal disorders.

UNLABELED USES

Magnesium Salicylate is used alone or as an adjunct in the treatment of hemophilic arthropathy.

CONTRAINDICATIONS

Magnesium Salicylate is contraindicated in patients with advanced chronic renal insufficiency. It may counteract the effect of uricosuric agents and should not be prescribed for patients on such drugs.

WARNINGS

As with all salicylates, Magnesium Salicylate should be avoided or administered with caution to patients with liver damage, pre-existing hypoprothrombinemia, vitamin K deficiency and before surgery.

PRECAUTIONS

General: Appropriate precautions should be taken in prescribing Magnesium Salicylate for persons known to be sensitive to salicylates and in patients with erosive gastritis or peptic ulcer. If a reaction develops, the drug should be discontinued. Magnesium Salicylate should be used with caution, if at all, concomitantly with anticoagulants. Appropriate precautions should be taken in administering Magnesium Salicylate to patients with any impairment of renal function including discontinuing other drugs containing magnesium and monitoring serum Magnesium levels if dosage levels of Magnesium Salicylate are high.

◆ RATED THERAPEUTICALLY EQUIVALENT; ◇ THERAPEUTIC EQUIVALENCE UNCONFIRMED; ○ UNRATED

Drug Interactions: Even small doses of Magnesium Salicylate should not be given with uricosuric agents such as probenecid that decrease tubular reabsorption because it counteracts their effect. Large doses of Magnesium Salicylate cause hypoprothrombinemia. Lower doses enhance the effects of anticoagulants such as coumadin and must be used with caution in patients receiving anticoagulants that affect the prothrombin time. Caution should also be exercised in patients concurrently treated with a sulfonylurea hypoglycemic agent or methotrexate because of the drug's capability of displacing them from the plasma protein binding sites, resulting in enhanced action of these agents. A similar displacement of barbiturates and diphenylhydantoin may occur; diphenylhydantoin intoxication has been precipitated by the consumption of aspirin. Salicylates inhibit the diuretic action of spironolactone.

Carcinogenesis, Mutagenesis, Impairment of Fertility: There have been no studies in animals or humans to evaluate the carcinogenesis, mutagenesis or impairment of fertility of Magnesium Salicylate. Aspirin causes testicular atrophy and inhibition of spermatogenesis in animals.

Pregnancy: Category C
1. Teratogenic effects: Aspirin has been shown to be teratogenic in animals and to increase the incidence of stillbirths and neonatal deaths in women. There are no adequate or well-controlled studies of Magnesium Salicylate in pregnant women. Magnesium Salicylate should be used during pregnancy only if the potential benefit justifies the potential risk to the fetus.

2. *Nonteratogenic Effects:* Chronic, high dose salicylate therapy of pregnant women increases the length of gestation and the frequency of post maturity and prolongs spontaneous labor. It is recommended Magnesium Salicylate be taken during the last three months of pregnancy only under the close supervision of a physician.

Nursing Mothers: Since salicylates are excreted in human milk, caution should be exercised when Magnesium Salicylate is administered to a nursing woman.

Pediatric Use: Safety end effectiveness of Magnesium Salicylate in children have not been established.

ADVERSE REACTIONS
Magnesium Salicylate in large doses has a hypoprothrombinemic effect and should be given with caution in patients receiving anticoagulant drugs, patients with liver damage, pre-existing hypoprothrombinemia, vitamin K deficiency or before surgery.

Salicylates given in overdose produce stimulation (often manifested as tinnitus) followed by depression of the cental nervous system. The dosage should be lowered at the onset of tinnitus.

Salicylates may cause gastric mucosal irritation and bleeding. However, fecal blood loss in patients taking Magnesium Salicylate is significantly less than in those taking aspirin.

Magnesium Salicylate should not be given to patients with severe renal damage because of the possibility of hypermagnesemia.

In moderate to high doses, Salicylates lower the blood glucose in diabetics. Aspirin-induced hypoglycemia has been described in adults undergoing hemodialysis.

Unlike aspirin, Magnesium Salicylate is not known to affect the platelet adhesiveness involved in the clotting mechanism, and therefore, does not prolong bleeding time. Magnesium Salicylate has not been associated with reactions causing asthmatic attacks in susceptible people.

OVERDOSAGE
Acute overdosage results in Salicylate toxicity. Early signs and symptoms from repeated larger doses as well as a large single dose consist of headache, dizziness, tinnitus (which may be absent in children or the elderly), difficulty in hearing, dimness of vision, mental confusion, lassitude, drowsiness, sweating, thirst, hyperventilation, nausea, vomiting and occasionally diarrhea. More severe salicylate poisoning is manifested by CNS disturbances including EEG abnormalities. Hyperventilation occurs producing initial respiratory alkalosis. This is followed by severe metabolic acidosis with dehydration and loss of potassium. Restlessness, garrulity, incoherent speech, apprehension, vertigo, tremor, diplopia, maniacal delirium, hallucinations, generalized convulsions and coma may occur.

Toxic symptoms may occur at serum levels greater than 20 mg/dL in patients over 60 years of age. Hyperventilation may occur at plasma salicylate levels over 35 mg/dL. Death may result from Salicylate levels between 45-75 mg/dL. As with other Salicylates, 10 to 30 g of the drug may be fatal. Renal or hepatic insufficiency and fever and dehydration in children enhance the acute toxicity of Salicylate overdoses. Treatment of acute poisoning is a medical emergency and should be undertaken in a hospital. Serum salicylate, Na, K, Cl, CO_2 levels, pH, BUN, blood glucose and urine pH and specific gravity should be obtained. Emesis should be induced or gastric lavage performed. Activated charcoal may be administered. Hyperthermia should be controlled with tepid water sponging. Dehydration should be treated and acid-based imbalance corrected. A high concentration of Salicylate acid in the brain may be fatal. Correction of acidosis shifts salicylate from the brain to the plasma. A bicarbonate solution should be infused to maintain an alkaline diuresis. Care should be taken to avoid pulmonary edema. The blood pH, plasma pCO_2 and plasma level should be monitored frequently. Ketosis and hypoglycemia may be corrected by glucose infusions and hypokalemia by potassium chloride added to the intravenous infusate. Avoid respiratory depressants. Shock may be combatted by plasma infusions. Hemorrhagic phenomena may necessitate whole blood transfusions or vitamin K_1. In severe intoxication, exchange transfusion, peritoneal dialysis, hemodialysis or hemoperfusion should be performed to remove plasma salicylate acid. Dialysis should be seriously considered if the patients condition is worsening despite appropriate therapy.

DOSAGE AND ADMINISTRATION
The dosage for Magnesium Salicylate in the treatment of musculoskeletal disorders such as arthritis should be adjusted according to individual patient's needs. The recommended initial regimen is two tablets three times per day. Dosage may be increased, if necessary, to achieve the desired therapeutic effect. In adjusting the dosage, the physician should monitor the dose limiting parameters such as tinnitis and/or serum Salicylate over 30 mg/dL.

Store at controlled room temperature, 15°-30°C (59°-86°F).

HOW SUPPLIED
TABLETS:

BRAND/MANUFACTURER	NDC	SIZE	AWP
GENERICS			
MOBIDIN: Ascher	00225-0310-15	100s	$23.22
MOBIDIN: Ascher	00225-0310-20	500s	$113.16

TABLETS: 545 MG

BRAND/MANUFACTURER	NDC	SIZE	AWP
BRAND			
MAGAN: Savage	00281-4121-17	100s	$50.95

Magnesium Salicylate and Phenyltoloxamine Dihydrogen Citrate

DESCRIPTION
Each tablet for oral administration contains:

Magnesium Salicylate Tetrahydrate .... 600 mg
Phenyltoloxamine Dihydrogen Citrate .... .25 mg

Magnesium Salicylate: Magnesium, bis (2-hydroxybenzoato-0^1, O^2)-, tetrahydrate, with the chemical formula $C_{14}H_{10}MgO_6 4H_2O$, is a white, odorless, crystalline powder with a sweet taste. It is soluble in water and alcohol.

Phenyltoloxamine Dihydrogen Citrate: N,N-Dimethyl-2-[∞phenyltolyloxy ethylamine dihydrogen citrate, with the chemical formula $C_{17}H_{21}NO \cdot C_6H_8O_7$, forms crystals from water or methanol. Its melting point is 138-140°C, and it is soluble in water.

CLINICAL PHARMACOLOGY
MAGNESIUM SALICYLATE
Magnesium Salicylate is a nonsteroidal anti-inflammatory agent with antipyretic and analgesic properties. Salicylic acid is the active moiety released into the plasma by Magnesium Salicylate. Salicylic acid is enzymatically biotransformed through two pathways to salicyluric acid and salicylphenolic glucuronide, and is eliminated in the urine.

Oral Salicylates are absorbed rapidly, party from the stomach, but mostly from the upper intestine. Salicylic acid is rapidly distributed throughout all body tissues and most transcellular fluids, mainly by pH-dependent passive processes. It can be detected in synovial, spinal and peritoneal fluid, in saliva and in milk. It readily crosses the placental barrier. From 50% to 90% of salicylic acid is bound to plasma proteins, especially albumin.

Following the ingestion of a single dose of 524 mg of Magnesium Salicylate, a peak concentration of 3.6 mg/dl salicylic acid is reached in 1.5 hours with a T ½ of 2 hours. The major biotransformation paths for the elimination of salicylic acid from the plasma become saturated by low doses of salicylic acid. As a result, repeated doses increase the plasma concentration and markedly prolong the plasma half-time. The plasma concentration of salicylic acid is increased by conditions that reduce the glomerular filtration rate or tubular secretion such as renal disease or the presence of inhibitors that compete for the transport system such as probenecid.

Therapeutic plasma concentrations of salicylic acid for an adequate anti-inflammatory effect needed for the treatment of rheumatoid arthritis range between 20 - 30 mg/dl. Effective analgesia is achieved at lower concentrations. Salicylates relieve pain by both a peripheral and CNS effect. Salicylates inhibit the synthesis of prostaglandins; the importance of this mechanism in analgesia and anti-inflammation has not been fully elucidated. Salicylates have an antipyretic effect in febrile patients but little in subjects with normal temperatures. This appears to be due to the inhibition of the synthesis of prostaglandins which are powerful pyrogens that affect the hypothalamus. Higher therapeutic concentrations cause reversible tinnitus and high tone hearing loss. Full therapeutic doses of salicylates increase oxygen consumption and CO_2 production. They cause an extracellular and intracellular respiratory alkalosis which is rapidly compensated. Salicylates irritate the gastric mucosa and frequently lead to blood loss in the stool; this effect is more pronounced with aspirin than magnesium salicylate. Salicylate in large doses (over 6 g/day) reduces the plasma prothrombin level. In contrast to aspirin, Magnesium Salicylate does not affect platelets. Salicylic acid

➤ SHOWN IN PRODUCT IDENTIFICATION GUIDE

increases the urinary excretion of urates at higher doses but may decrease excretion at lower doses.

PHENYLTOLOXAMINE

Phenyltoloxamine is an H_1 blocking agent which interfaces with the action of histamine primarily in capillaries surrounding mucous tissue and sensory nerves of nasal and adjacent areas. It has the ability to interfere with certain actions of acetylcholine-inhibiting secretions in the nose, mouth, and pharynx. It commonly causes CNS depression.

INDICATIONS AND USAGE

Magnesium Salicylate/Phenyltoloxamine Dihydrogen Citrate is indicated for the relief of the signs and symptoms of rheumatoid arthritis, osteoarthritis and related diseases and in their daily management.

CONTRAINDICATIONS

Magnesium Salicylate/Phenyltoloxamine Dihydrogen Citrate is contraindicated in patients with advanced chronic renal insufficiency. It may counteract the effect of uricosuric agents and should not be prescribed for patients on such drugs. This drug is contraindicated in patients with hypersensitivity to any of the ingredients.

WARNINGS

As with all salicylates Magnesium Salicylate/Phenyltoloxamine Dihydrogen Citrate should be avoided or administered with caution to patients with liver damage, preexisting hypoprothrombinemia, vitamin K deficiency, and before surgery. Antihistamines may impair mental and physical abilities for the performance of potentially hazardous tasks, such as driving a vehicle or operating machinery, and may impair mental alertness in children. Phenyltoloxamine has an atropine-like action and should be used with caution in patients with increased intraocular pressure, cardiovascular disease, hypertension or in patients with a history of bronchial asthma.

PRECAUTIONS

General: Appropriate precautions should be taken in prescribing Magnesium Salicylate/Phenyltoloxamine Dihydrogen Citrate for persons known to be sensitive to salicylates and in patients with erosive gastritis or peptic ulcer. If a reaction develops, the drug should be discontinued. Magnesium Salicylate/Phenyltoloxamine Dihydrogen Citrate should be used with caution, if at all, concomitantly with anticoagulants. Appropriate precautions should be taken in administering Magnesium Salicylate/Phenyltoloxamine Dihydrogen Citrate to patients with any impairment of renal function including discontinuing other drugs containing magnesium and monitoring serum magnesium levels if dosage levels of Magnesium Salicylate/Phenyltoloxamine Dihydrogen are high.

Drug Interactions: Even small doses of Magnesium Salicylate/Phenyltoloxamine Dihydrogen Citrate should not be given with uricosuric agents such as probenecid that decrease tubular reabsorption because it counteracts their effect. Large doses of Magnesium Salicylate/Phenytoloxamine Dihydrogen Citrate cause hypoprothrombinemia. Lower doses enhance the effects of anticoagulants such as coumadin and must be used with caution in patients receiving anticoagulants that affect the prothrombin time. Caution should also be exercised in patients concurrently treated with a sulfonylurea hypoglycemic agent or methotrexate because of the drug's capability of displacing them from the plasma protein binding sites, resulting in enhanced action of these agents. A similar displacement of barbiturates and diphenylhydantoin may occur; diphenylhydantoin intoxication has been precipitated by the consumption of aspirin. Salicylates inhibit the diuretic action of spironolactone.

Carcinogenesis, Mutogenesis, Impairment of Fertility: There have been no studies in animals or humans to evaluate the carcinogenesis, mutagenesis, or impairment of fertility for Magnesium Salicylate. Aspirin causes testicular atrophy and inhibition of spermatogenesis in animals.

PREGNANCY CATEGORY C

1. Teratogenic Effects: Aspirin has been shown to be teratogenic in animals and to increase the incidence of still births and neonatal deaths in women. There are no adequate or well-controlled studies of Magnesium Salicylate/Phenyltoloxamine Dihydrogen Citrate in pregnant women. Magnesium Salicylate/Phenyltoloxamine Dihydrogen Citrate should be used during pregnancy only if the potential benefit justifies the potential risk to the fetus.

2. Nonteratogenic Effects: Chronic, high dose salicylate therapy of pregnant women increases the length of gestation and the frequency of post maturity, and prolongs spontaneous labor. It is recommended Magnesium Salicylate/Phenyltoloxamine Dihydrogen Citrate be taken during the last three months of pregnancy only under the close supervision of a physician.

Nursing Mothers: Since salicylates are excreted in human milk, caution should be exercised when Magnesium Salicylate/Phenytoloxamine Dihydrogen Citrate is administered to nursing women.

Pediatric Use: Safety and effectiveness of Magnesium Salicylate/Phenyltoloxamine Dihydrogen Citrate in children has not been established.

ADVERSE REACTIONS

Magnesium Salicylate in large doses has a hypoprothrombinemic effect and should be given with caution in patients receiving anticoagulant drugs, patients with liver damage, pre-existing hypoprothrombinemia, vitamin K deficiency or before surgery.

Salicylates given in overdose produce stimulation (often manifested as tinnitus) followed by depression of the central nervous system. The dosage should be lowered at the onset of tinnitus.

Salicylates may cause gastric mucosal irritation and bleeding. However, fecal blood loss in patients taking Magnesium Salicylate/Phenyltoloxamine Dihydrogen Citrate significant less than those taking aspirin.

Magnesium Salicylate/Phenyltoloxamine Dihydrogen Citrate should not be given to patients with severe renal damage because of the possibility of hypermagnesemia.

In moderate to high doses, salicylates lower the blood glucose in diabetics. Aspirin-induced hypoglycemia has been described in adults undergoing hemodialysis.

Unlike aspirin, Magnesium Salicylate is not known to affect the platelet adhesiveness involved in the clotting mechanism; and therefore, does not prolong bleeding time Magnesium Salicylate/Phenyltoloxamine Dihydrogen Citrate has not been associated with reactions causing asthmatic attacks in susceptible people.

Individuals hyperreactive to Phenyltoloxamine Citrate may display ephedrine-like reactions such as tachycardia, palpitations, headache, dizziness or nausea. Patients sensitive to antihistamines may experience mild sedation, drowsiness, restlessness, dizziness, weakness, dry mouth, anorexia, nausea, vomiting, headache, nervousness, blurring of vision, polyuria, heartburn, dysuria and, very rarely, dermatitis.

OVERDOSAGE

Signs and Symptoms: Acute overdosage of Magnesium Salicylate results in salicylate toxicity. Early signs and symptoms from repeated larger doses as well as a large single dose consist of headache, dizziness, tinnitus (which may be absent in children or the elderly), difficulty in hearing, dimness of vision, mental confusion, lassitude, drowsiness, sweating, thirst, hyperventilation, nausea, vomiting and occasionally diarrhea. More severe salicylate poisoning is manifested by CNS disturbances including EEG abnormalities. Hyperventilation occurs producing initial respiratory alkalosis. This is followed by severe metabolic acidosis with dehydration and loss of potassium. Restlessness, garrulity, incoherent speech, apprehension, vertigo, tremor, diplopia, maniacal delirium, hallucinations, generalized convulsions and coma may occur. Toxic symptoms may occur at serum levels greater than 20 mg/dl in patients over 60 years of age. Hyperventilation may occur at serum levels greater than 20 mg/dl in patients over 60 years of age. Hyperventilation may occur at plasma salicylate levels over 35 mg/dl. Death may result from salicylate levels between 45-75 mg/dl. As with other salicylates, 10 to 30 g of the drug may be fatal. Renal or hepatic insufficiency, and fever and dehydration in children enhance the acute toxicity of salicylate overdoses.

Treatment: Treatment of acute poisoning is a medical emergency and should be undertaken in a hospital. Serum Na, K, Cl, CO_2 levels, pH, BUN, blood glucose and urine pH and specific gravity should be obtained. Emesis should be induced or gastric lavage performed. Activated charcoal may be administered. Hyperthermia should be controlled with tepid water sponging. Dehydration should be treated and acid-base imbalance corrected. A high concentration of salicylic acid in the brain may be fatal. Correction of acidosis shifts salicylate from the brain to the plasma. A bicarbonate solution should be infused to maintain an alkaline diuresis. Care should be taken to avoid pulmonary edema. The blood pH, plasma pCO_2 and plasma glucose levels should be monitored frequently. Ketosis and hypoglycemia may be corrected by glucose infusions and hypokalemia by potassium chloride added to the intravenous infusate. Avoid respiratory depressants. Shock may be combatted by plasma infusions. Hemorrhagic phenomena may necessitate whole blood transfusions or vitamin K. In severe intoxication, exchange transfusion, peritoneal dialysis, hemodialysis or hemoperfusion should be performed to remove plasma salicylic acid. Dialysis should be seriously considered if the patient's condition is worsening despite appropriate therapy.

DOSAGE AND ADMINISTRATION

The initial dose is one tablet 3 or 4 times daily. If higher doses are required for optimal effect, the number of tablets may be increased to 6 to 8 tablets daily. As with other therapeutic agents, individual dose titration is advisable and some patients may require higher or lower dosage than the recommended schedules.

Store at controlled room temperature: 15°-30°C (59°-86°F).

Dispense in a tight, light-resistant container as described in the USP/NF, with a child-resistant closure.

HOW SUPPLIED

TABLETS:

BRAND/MANUFACTURER	NDC	SIZE	AWP
○ GENERICS			
MAGSAL TABLETS: U.S. Pharm	52747-0321-60	100s	$34.61

Magnesium Sulfate, Injectable

DESCRIPTION

Magnesium Sulfate Injection or Solution and Dextrose and Magnesium Sulfate Injection are sterile, nonpyrogenic solutions of Magnesium Sulfate heptahydrate (and Dextrose) in water for injection. Magnesium Sulfate Injection for intravenous (IV) or intramuscular (IM) administration is available in 12.5% and 50% concentrations. Magnesium Sulfate solution for IV use is available in 4% and 8% concentrations. Dextrose and Magnesium Sulfate injection for IV use is available in 1% and 2% concentrations.

◆ RATED THERAPEUTICALLY EQUIVALENT; ◇ THERAPEUTIC EQUIVALENCE UNCONFIRMED; ○ UNRATED

Solution characteristics are as follows:

Concentration Magnesium Sulfate (heptahydrate)	Amount of Magnesium	Solution Osmolarity
1%	8.1 mEq/100 mL	333 mOsmol/L (calc.)
2%	16.2 mEq/100 mL	415 mOsmol/L (calc.)
4%	32.4 mEq/100 mL	325 mOsmol/L (calc.)
8%	64.8 mEq/100 mL	649 mOsmol/L (calc.)
12.5%	100 mEq/100 mL	1010 mOsmol/L (calc.)
50%	400 mEq/100 mL	4060 mOsmol/L (calc.)

Each 100 mL of Magnesium Sulfate injection (IV and IM) contains:
Magnesium Sulfate Heptahydrate ....12.5 or 50 g

Each 100 mL of Magnesium Sulfate solution (IV) contains:
Magnesium Sulfate Heptahydrate ....4 or 8 g

Each 100 mL of Dextrose and Magnesium Sulfate contains:
Magnesium Sulfate Heptahydrate ....1 or 2 g
Dextrose, hydrous 5g

Magnesium Sulfate, USP heptahydrate is chemically designated $MgSO_4 \cdot 7H_2O$, colorless crystals or white powder freely soluble in water.

Dextrose (Dextrose Hydrous, USP) is D-glucopyranose monohydrate, a hexose sugar whose empiric formula is $C_6H_{12}O_6 \cdot H_2O$, and whose molecular weight is 198.17.

Water for Injection, USP is chemically designated H_2O.

CLINICAL PHARMACOLOGY

Magnesium (Mg^{++}) is an important cofactor for enzymatic reactions and plays an important role in neurochemical transmission and muscular excitability.

Magnesium prevents or controls convulsions by blocking neuromuscular transmission and decreasing the amount of acetylcholine liberated at the end plate by the motor nerve impulse. Magnesium is said to have a depressant effect on the central nervous system, but it does not adversely affect the mother, fetus or neonate when used as directed in eclampsia or pre-eclampsia. Normal plasma Magnesium levels range from 1.3 to 2.5 or 3.0 mEq/liter.

As plasma Magnesium rises above 4 mEq/liter, the deep tendon reflexes are first decreased and then disappear as the plasma level approaches 10 mEq/liter. At this level respiratory paralysis may occur. Heart block also may occur at this or lower plasma levels of Magnesium.

Magnesium acts peripherally to produce vasodilation. With low doses only flushing and sweating occur, but larger doses cause lowering of blood pressure. The central and peripheral effects of Magnesium poisoning are antagonized to some extent by intravenous administration of calcium.

With intravenous administration the onset of anticonvulsant action is immediate and lasts about 30 minutes. Following intramuscular administration the onset of action occurs in about one hour and persists for three to four hours. Effective anticonvulsant serum levels range from 2.5 to 7.5 mEq/liter. Magnesium is excreted solely by the kidney at a rate proportional to the plasma concentration and glomerular filtration.

As a nutritional adjunct in hyperalimentation, the precise mechanism of action for Magnesium is uncertain. Early symptoms of hypomagnesemia (less than 1.5 mEq/liter) may develop as early as three to four days or within weeks. Predominant deficiency effects are neurological, e.g., muscle irritability, clonic twitching and tremors. Hypocalcemia and hypokalemia often follow low serum levels of Magnesium. While there are large stores of Magnesium present intracellularly and in the bones of adults, these stores often are not mobilized sufficiently to maintain plasma levels. Parenteral Magnesium therapy repairs the plasma deficit and causes deficiency symptoms and signs to cease.

INDICATIONS AND USAGE

Magnesium Sulfate injection and solution and Dextrose and Magnesium Sulfate injection are indicated for use as parenteral anticonvulsants for the prevention and control of seizures (convulsions) in severe toxemia of pregnancy. When used judiciously they effectively prevent and control the convulsions of eclampsia without producing deleterious depression of the central nervous system of the mother or infant. However, other effective drugs are available for this purpose.

Magnesium Sulfate Injection, USP is suitable for replacement therapy in magnesium deficiency, especially in acute hypomagnesemia accompanied by signs of tetany similar to those observed in hypocalcemia. In such cases, the serum Magnesium (Mg^{++}) level is usually below the lower limit of normal (1.5 to 2.5 or 3.0 mEq/liter) and the serum calcium (Ca^{++}) level is normal (4.3 to 5.3 mEq/liter) or elevated.

In total parenteral nutrition, Magnesium Sulfate may be added to the nutrient admixture to correct or prevent hypomagnesemia which can arise during the course of therapy.

Magnesium Sulfate Injection, USP may be used to control hypertension, encephalopathy and convulsions associated with acute nephritis in children. However, other drugs such as barbiturates, reserpine or hydralazine should be tried first.

UNLABELED USES

Magnesium Sulfate is used alone or as an adjunct in the treatment of premature labor, infantile seizures associated with hypomagnesemia, and to control the cardiovascular disturbances associated with severe tetanus. It is also used as an adjunct to soften and dilate the cervix prior to first trimester abortion, to suppress

exercise-induced angina, and bronchial asthma. Magnesium Sulfate is also prescribed in the treatment of cardiac arrhythmias, including torsade de pointes, multifocal atrial tachycardia, ventricular fibrillation, ventricular tachycardia, and supraventricular tachycardia. It is also used to prevent arrhythmias associated with digitoxin toxicity, to reduce mortality and the incidence of arrhythmias after acute myocardial infarction, and to control blood pressure and heart rate during surgery for pheochromocytoma.

CONTRAINDICATIONS

Intravenous Magnesium should not be given to mothers with toxemia of pregnancy during the two hours preceding delivery.

WARNINGS

Intravenous use in eclampsia should be reserved for immediate control of life-threatening convulsions.

Parenteral use in the presence of renal insufficiency may lead to Magnesium intoxication.

PRECAUTIONS

Because Magnesium is removed from the body solely by the kidneys, the drug should be used with caution in patients with renal impairment. Urine output should be maintained at a level of 100 mL every four hours. Monitoring serum Magnesium levels and the patient's clinical status is essential to avoid the consequences of overdosage in toxemia. Clinical indications of a safe dosage regimen include the presence of the patellar reflex (knee jerk) and absence of respiratory depression (approximately 16 breaths or more/minute). Serum Magnesium levels usually sufficient to control convulsions range from 3 to 6 mg/ 100 mL (2.5 to 5 mEq/liter). The strength of the deep tendon reflexes begins to diminish when serum Magnesium levels exceed 4 mEq/liter. Reflexes may be absent at 10 mEq Magnesium/liter, where respiratory paralysis is a potential hazard. An injectable calcium salt should be immediately available to counteract the potential hazards of Magnesium intoxication in eclampsia.

Magnesium Sulfate Solution and Dextrose and Magnesium Sulfate injection should be administered slowly to avoid producing hypermagnesemia.

50% Magnesium Sulfate Injection, USP must be diluted to a concentration of 20% or less prior to I.V. infusion. Rate of administration should be slow and cautions, to avoid producing hypermagnesemia. The 50% solution also should be diluted to 20% or less for intramuscular injection in infants and children.

Pregnancy Category A: Studies in pregnant women have not shown that Magnesium Sulfate injection increases the risk of fetal abnormalities if administered during all trimesters of pregnancy. If this drug is used during pregnancy, the possibility of fetal harm appears remote.

However, because studies cannot rule out the possibility of harm, Magnesium Sulfate injection should be used during pregnancy only if clearly needed.

When administered by continuous intravenous infusion (especially for more than 24 hours preceding delivery) to control convulsions in toxemic mothers, the newborn may show signs of Magnesium toxicity, including neuromuscular or respiratory depression. See *"Overdosage"*.

ADVERSE REACTIONS

The adverse effects of parenterally administered Magnesium usually are the result of Magnesium intoxication. These include flushing, sweating, hypotension, depressed reflexes, flaccid paralysis, hypothermia, circulatory collapse, cardiac and central nervous system depression proceeding to respiratory paralysis. Hypocalcemia with signs of tetany secondary to Magnesium Sulfate therapy for eclampsia has been reported.

OVERDOSAGE

Magnesium intoxication is manifested by a sharp drop in blood pressure and respiratory paralysis. Disappearance of the patellar reflex is a useful clinical sign to detect the onset of Magnesium intoxication. In the event of overdosage artificial ventilation must be provided until a calcium salt can be injected intravenously to antagonize the effects of Magnesium.

In adults intravenous administration of 5 to 10 mEq of 10% calcium gluconate will usually reverse respiratory depression or heart block due to Magnesium intoxication. In extreme cases, peritoneal or hemodialysis may be required.

Hypermagnesemia in the newborn may require resuscitation and assisted ventilation via endotracheal intubation or intermittent positive pressure ventilation as well as intravenous calcium.

DOSAGE AND ADMINISTRATION

Magnesium Sulfate solution and Dextrose and Magnesium Sulfate injection are intended for intravenous use only. For the management of pre-eclampsia or eclampsia, intravenous infusion of dilute solutions of Magnesium (1% to 8%) are often given in combination with intramuscular injections of 50% Magnesium Sulfate Injection, USP. Therefore, in the clinical conditions cited below, both forms of therapy are noted, as appropriate.

Both intravenous and intramuscular administration of Magnesium Sulfate Injection are appropriate. Intramuscular administration of the undiluted 50% solution results in therapeutic plasma levels in 60 minutes, whereas I.V. doses will provide a therapeutic level almost immediately. The rate of I.V. injection should generally not exceed 1.5 mL of a 10% concentration (or its equivalent) per minute, except in severe eclampsia with seizures (see below).

Solutions for intravenous infusion must be diluted to a concentration of 20% or less prior to administration. The diluents commonly used are 5% Dextrose Injection, USP and 0.9% Sodium Chloride Injection, USP. Deep intramuscular injection of the undiluted (50%) solution is appropriate for adults, but the solution should be diluted to a 20% concentration prior to such injection in children.

IN ECLAMPSIA
In severe pre-eclampsia or eclampsia, the total initial dose is 10 to 14 g of Magnesium Sulfate. To initiate therapy, 4 to 5 g of Magnesium Sulfate injection or solution or Dextrose and Magnesium Sulfate injection may be administered intravenously. The rate of I.V. infusion should generally not exceed 150 mg/minute, or 7.5 mL of a 2% concentration (or its equivalent) or 3.75 mL of a 4% concentration (or its equivalent) per minute, except in severe eclampsia with seizures. Simultaneously, 4 to 5 g (32.5 to 40.6 mEq) up to 10g of Magnesium Sulfate may be administered intramuscularly into each buttock using undiluted 50% Magnesium Sulfate Injection, USP. Alternatively, the initial intravenous dose of 4 g may be given by diluting the 50% solution to a 10 or 20% concentration; the diluted fluid (40 mL of a 10% solution or 20 mL of a 20% solution) may then be injected intravenously over a period of three to four minutes. After the initial I.V. dose, some clinicians administer 1-2 g/hour by constant I.V. infusion. Subsequent intramuscular doses of 4 to 5 g of Magnesium Sulfate (8 to 10 mL of the 50% solution) may be injected into alternate buttocks every four hours, depending on the continuing presence of the patellar reflex, adequate respiratory function, and absence of signs of magnesium toxicity. Therapy should continue until paroxysms cease.

A serum magnesium level of 6 mg/100 mL is considered optimal for control of seizures. A total daily (24 hr) dose of 30 to 40 g Magnesium Sulfate should not be exceeded and less should be used if the patient is anuric. In the presence of severe renal insufficiency, frequent serum Magnesium concentrations must be obtained, and the maximum recommended dosage of Magnesium Sulfate is 20 g per 48 hours.

IN MAGNESIUM DEFICIENCY (MAGNESIUM SULFATE INJECTION)
In the treatment of mild Magnesium deficiency, the usual adult dose is 1 g, equivalent to 8.12 mEq of Magnesium (2 mL of the 50% solution) injected intramuscularly every six hours for four doses (equivalent to a total of 32.5 mEq of Magnesium per 24 hours). For severe hypomagnesemia, as much as 2 mEq (0.5 mL of the 50% solution) per kg of body weight may be given intramuscularly within a period of four hours if necessary. Alternatively, 5 g (approximately 40 mEq) can be added to one liter of 5% Dextrose Injection, USP or 0.9% Sodium Chloride Injection, USP for slow intravenous infusion over a three-hour period.

IN HYPERALIMENTATION (MAGNESIUM SULFATE INJECTION)
In total parenteral nutrition, maintenance requirements for Magnesium are not precisely known. The maintenance dose recommended for adults is 5 to 8 mEq Magnesium/liter of TPN solution; typical daily adult intake ranges from 10 to 24 mEq. For infants, the recommended intake ranges from 0.25 to 0.6 mEq/kg/day.

IN NEPHRITIC SEIZURES (MAGNESIUM SULFATE INJECTION)
In children with nephritic seizures, the 50% concentration should be diluted to a 20% solution for intramuscular injection. The dose for children is 20 to 40 mg (0.1 to 0.2 mL of a 20% solution) per kg of body weight administered intramuscularly as needed to control seizures.

Parenteral drug products should be inspected visually for particulate matter and discoloration prior to administration, whenever solution and container permit.

Do not administer unless solution is clear, container undamaged, and vacuum present. Discard unused portion.

Exposure of pharmaceutical products to heat should be minimized. Avoid excessive heat. Protect from freezing. It is recommended that the product be stored at room temperature (25°C); however, brief exposure up to 40°C does not adversely affect the product.

HOW SUPPLIED
INJECTION: 100 MG/ML

BRAND/MANUFACTURER	NDC	SIZE	AWP
○ GENERICS			
Astra	00186-1203-04	20 ml 25s	$30.00
Pasadena	00418-2041-66	20 ml 25s	$87.00
CMC-Cons	00223-8071-20	20 ml 25s	$140.00
Astra	00186-1204-04	50 ml 25s	$92.50

INJECTION: 125 MG/ML

BRAND/MANUFACTURER	NDC	SIZE	AWP
○ GENERICS			
Abbott Hosp	00074-4943-01	8 ml 25s	$69.17

INJECTION: 500 MG/ML

BRAND/MANUFACTURER	NDC	SIZE	AWP
○ GENERICS			
Fujisawa	00469-6400-15	2 ml	$1.18
Fujisawa	00469-6400-30	10 ml	$3.91
Fujisawa	00469-6400-40	20 ml	$7.90
Pegasus	10974-0096-30	30 ml	$2.90
McGuff	49072-0475-50	50 ml	$2.89
CMC-Cons	00223-8072-50	50 ml	$9.75

	NDC	SIZE	AWP
SULFA-MAG: Merit	30727-0383-90	50 ml	$14.85
Fujisawa	00469-4075-60	50 ml	$16.74
Abbott Hosp	00074-4075-02	2 ml 10s	$16.86
Astra	00186-0684-01	5 ml 10s	$30.00
Abbott Hosp	00074-4913-01	5 ml 10s	$120.06
Astra	00186-0685-01	10 ml 10s	$46.88

BRAND/MANUFACTURER	NDC	SIZE	AWP
Abbott Hosp	00074-4914-01	10 ml 10s	$140.13
Gensia	00703-5377-03	50 ml 10s	$55.75
Astra	00186-1209-04	2 ml 25s	$10.50
Amer Regent	00517-2602-25	2 ml 25s	$14.69
Gensia	00703-5372-04	2 ml 25s	$16.25
Solo Pak	39769-0042-01	2 ml 25s	$16.25
UDL	51079-0708-45	2 ml 25s	$23.14
Pasadena	00418-2061-22	2 ml 25s	$23.50
CMC-Cons	00223-8072-02	2 ml 25s	$25.00
Astra	00186-1210-04	10 ml 25s	$13.75
Solo Pak	39769-0042-03	10 ml 25s	$18.44
Amer Regent	00517-2610-25	10 ml 25s	$23.44
Gensia	00703-5374-04	10 ml 25s	$25.63
UDL	51079-0709-45	10 ml 25s	$32.10
CMC-Cons	00223-8072-10	10 ml 25s	$42.50
Abbott Hosp	00074-2168-01	10 ml 25s	$46.31
Intl Med Sys	00548-1034-00	10 ml 25s	$199.88
UDL	51079-0710-45	20 ml 25s	$37.89
Astra	00186-1211-04	20 ml 25s	$42.19
Gensia	00703-5375-04	20 ml 25s	$55.75
Abbott Hosp	00074-2168-02	20 ml 25s	$97.08
UDL	51079-0711-45	50 ml 25s	$54.34
Amer Regent	00517-2650-25	50 ml 25s	$60.94
Abbott Hosp	00074-2168-03	50 ml 25s	$214.64
Pasadena	00418-2081-50	50 ml 25s	$297.00
Raway	00686-2610-25	10 ml 50s	$69.00
Amer Regent	00517-0291-72	2 ml 100s	$68.75
CMC-Cons	00223-8069-02	2 ml 100s	$75.00
Raway	00686-0291-72	2 ml 100s	$110.00

Malathion

DESCRIPTION
Malathion Lotion is a liquid for topical application to the hair and scalp as a lousicide and ovicide. Each mL contains 0.005 g of Malathion Malathion insecticide, has a molecular weight of 330.36 represented by $C_{10}H_{19}O_5PS_2$.

CLINICAL PHARMACOLOGY
Malathion is lousicidal and ovicidal *in vitro*. Louse eggs succumb to 3 seconds of exposure to 0.062% Malathion in acetone and lice to about 0.003% respectively. Resistance to Malathion could not be induced.

Human safety studies included a 21-day cumulative irritancy and others undertaken to determine the potential for contact sensitization, phototoxicity, and photo-contact sensitization and a very low level of irritation.

INDICATIONS AND USAGE
Malathion Lotion is indicated for the treatment of head lice and their ova.

CONTRAINDICATIONS
Malathion Lotion should not be used by individuals with known sensitivity to Malathion Lotion or to any of its components.

WARNINGS
This product is flammable and open flames or hair dryers should be avoided to allow the hair to dry naturally and uncovered.

PRECAUTIONS
If accidentally placed in the eye, flush immediately with water.

Carcinogenesis, Mutagenesis and Fertility: Malathion is neither carcinogenic in male or female F344 rats after 2 years feeding with up to 4000 ppm (0.4%) nor is it tumongenic in Osborn-Mendel rats or B6C3F1 mice after a similar feeding for 80 weeks with 8,000 ppm (0.8%) and 16,000 ppm (1.6%) respectively. Tests for mutagenicity have not been conducted.

Pregnancy Category B: There was no evidence of teratogenicity in studies utilizing single i.p. injections of Malathion at 600 and 900 mg/kg in pregnant rats or oral dosing with up to 300 mg/kg on days 6 through 15 of gestation. A reproduction study in rats failed to show any gross fetal abnormalities attributable to feeding Malathion up to 2,500 ppm in the diet during a three-generation evaluation period. These studies employed at least 50 to 70 times the adult human topical dose.

Because animal reproduction studies are not always predictive of human response, this drug should be used during pregnancy only if clearly needed.

Nursing Mothers: Malathion in an acetone vehicle has been reported to be absorbed through human skin only to the extent of 8% of the applied dose. However, percutaneous absorption from the Malathion Lotion formulation has not been studied and it is not known whether Malathion is excreted in human milk. Caution should be exercised when Malathion Lotion is administered to the nursing mother.

ADVERSE REACTIONS

Irritation of the scalp has been reported.

OVERDOSAGE

Consideration should be given as part of the treatment program to the high concentration of isopropyl alcohol in the vehicle.

Malathion, although a weaker cholinesterase inhibitor and therefore safer than other organophosphates, may be expected to exhibit the same symptoms of cholinesterase depletion after accidental ingestion orally. Vomiting should be induced promptly or the stomach lavaged with 5% sodium bicarbonate solution.

Severe respiratory distress is the major and most serious symptom of organophosphate poisoning requiring artificial respiration and large doses of i.m. or i.v. atropine. The usual starting dose of atropine is 1 to 4 mg with supplementation hourly as needed to counteract the symptoms of cholinesterase depletion.

Repeat analyses of serum and RBC cholinesterase assist in establishing the diagnosis and formulating a long-range prognosis.

DOSAGE AND ADMINISTRATION

1. Sprinkle Malathion Lotion on the hair and rub gently until the scalp is thoroughly moistened.
2. Allow to dry naturally—use no heat and leave uncovered.
3. After 8-12 hours, the hair should be shampooed.
4. Rinse and use a fine-toothed comb to remove dead lice and eggs.
5. If required, repeat with second application of Malathion Lotion in 7 to 9 days.

Further treatment is generally not necessary. Other family members should be evaluated to determine if infested and if so, receive treatment.

HOW SUPPLIED
LOTION:

BRAND/MANUFACTURER	NDC	SIZE	AWP
○ **BRAND**			
OVIDE: Genderm	52761-0637-02	60 ml	$11.91

Mandelamine SEE METHENAMINE MANDELATE

Mandol SEE CEFAMANDOLE NAFATE

Manganese Chloride

DESCRIPTION

Manganese Chloride is a sterile, nonpyrogenic solution intended for use as an additive to intravenous solutions for total parenteral nutrition (TPN). Each mL of solution contains 0.36 mg Manganese Chloride. The solution contains no bacteriostat, antimicrobial agent or added buffer. The pH is 2.0 (1.5 to 2.5); product may contain hydrochloric acid and sodium hydroxide for pH adjustment. The osmolarity is 0.313 mOsmol/mL (calc.).

Manganese Chloride, USP is chemically designated Manganese Chloride, tetrahydrate ($MnCl_2 \cdot 4H_2O$), a deliquescent, crystalline compound soluble in water.

CLINICAL PHARMACOLOGY

Manganese Chloride is an essential nutrient which serves as an activator for enzymes such as polysaccharide polymerase, liver arginase, cholinesterase and pyruvate carboxylase. Providing Manganese during TPN helps prevent development of deficiency symptoms such as nausea and vomiting, weight loss, dermatitis and changes in growth and color of hair.

Under conditions of minimal intake, 20 mcg Manganese/day is retained. Manganese is bound to a specific transport protein, transmanganin, a beta-l-globulin. Manganese is widely distributed but concentrates in the mitochondria rich tissues such as brain, kidney, pancreas, and liver. Assays for Manganese in whole blood result in concentrations ranging from 6 to 12 mcg/Manganese/liter.

Excretion of Manganese occurs mainly through the bile, but in the event of obstruction, ancillary excretion routes include pancreatic juice, or return into the lumen of the duodenum, jejunum, or ileum. Urinary excretion of Manganese is negligible.

INDICATIONS AND USAGE

Manganese Chloride is indicated for use as a supplement to intravenous solutions given for total parenteral nutrition (TPN).

Administration helps to maintain Manganese serum levels and to prevent depletion of endogenous stores and subsequent deficiency symptoms.

CONTRAINDICATIONS

None known.

WARNINGS

Direct intramuscular or intravenous injection of Manganese Chloride is contraindicated as the acidic pH of the solution (2) may cause considerable tissue irritation.

Liver and/or biliary tract dysfunction may require omission or reduction of copper and Manganese doses because these elements are primarily eliminated in the bile.

PRECAUTIONS

GENERAL

Do not use unless solution is clear and seal is intact.

Manganese Chloride should only be used in conjunction with a pharmacy directed admixture program using aseptic technique in a laminar flow environment; it should be used promptly and in a single operation without any repeated penetrations. Solution contains no preservatives; discard unused portion immediately after admixture procedure is completed.

LABORATORY TESTS

Serum Manganese levels can be measured periodically at the discretion of the investigator. Because of the low serum concentration normally present, samples will usually be analyzed by a reference laboratory.

CARCINOGENESIS, MUTAGENESIS, AND IMPAIRMENT OF FERTILITY

Long-term animal studies to evaluate the carcinogenic potential of Manganese Chloride have not been performed, nor have studies been done to assess mutagenesis or impairment of fertility.

NURSING MOTHERS

It is not known whether this drug is excreted in human milk. Because many drugs are excreted in human milk, caution should be exercised when Manganese Chloride additive is administered to a nursing woman.

PEDIATRIC USE

See "Dosage and Administration" section. Safety and effectiveness in children have not been established.

Pregnancy Category C: Animal reproduction studies have not been conducted with Manganese Chloride. It is also not known whether Manganese Chloride can cause fetal harm when administered to a pregnant woman or can affect reproductive capacity. Manganese Chloride should be given to a pregnant woman only if clearly indicated.

ADVERSE REACTIONS

None known.

DRUG ABUSE AND DEPENDENCE

None known.

OVERDOSAGE

Manganese toxicity in TPN patients has not been reported.

DOSAGE AND ADMINISTRATION

Manganese Chloride contains 0.1 mg Manganese/mL and is administered intravenously only after dilution. The additive should be administered in a volume of fluid not less than 100 mL. For the adult receiving TPN, the suggested additive dosage for Manganese is 0.15 to 0.8 mg/day (1.5 to 8 mL/day). For pediatric patients, a dosage of 2 to 10 mcg Manganese/kg/day (0.02 to 0.1 mL/kg/day) is recommended.

Periodic monitoring of Manganese plasma levels is suggested as a guideline for subsequent administration.

Parenteral products should be inspected visually for particulate matter and discoloration prior to administration, whenever solution and container permit. See "Precautions."

Store at controlled room temperature 15° to 30° C (59° to 86° F).

HOW SUPPLIED
INJECTION: 0.1 MG/ML

BRAND/MANUFACTURER	NDC	SIZE	AWP
◆ **GENERICS**			
Abbott Hosp	00074-4091-01	10 ml 25s	$103.61

Mannitol and Sorbitol

DESCRIPTION

Mannitol/Sorbitol Irrigation is a sterile, nonpyrogenic, hypotonic, aqueous solution for urologic nonelectrolyte irrigation during transurethral surgical procedures. Each 100 mL contains Sorbitol 2.70 g and Mannitol 0.54 g in water for injection. The solution is nonelectrolytic and hypotonic (178 mOsmol/liter calc.); pH 5.2 (4.0-7.0).

The solution contains no bacteriostat, antimicrobial agent or added buffer and is intended only for use as a single-dose irrigation. When smaller volumes are required the unused portion should be discarded.

Mannitol/Sorbitol Irrigation is a nonelectrolyte urologic irrigant.

Sorbitol, NF is chemically designated D-glucitol ($C_6H_{14}O_6$), white powder, granules or flakes very soluble in water.

Mannitol, USP is chemically designated D-mannitol ($C_6H_{14}O_6$), white crystalline powder or free-flowing granules, freely soluble in water.

Water for Injection, USP is chemically designated H_2O.

CLINICAL PHARMACOLOGY

Mannitol/Sorbitol are hexitols and are nonelectrolytes. A solution of these constituents in water is therefore nonconductive and suitable for urologic irrigation during electrosurgical procedures. A 3% (approx.) total concentration of Mannitol/Sorbitol contains sufficient solute to minimize the risk of intravascular hemolysis which can occur from absorption of plain water through open prostatic veins during transurethral resection (TUR). Any solution that is absorbed intravascularly during transurethral prostatic or bladder surgery, although variable in amount depending primarily on the extent of surgery, will be excreted by the kidney. When absorbed intravascularly, Sorbitol and Mannitol act as osmotic diuretics.

Intravascular absorption of Sorbitol has been shown to produce elevations of serum lactate after TUR above preoperative values owing to Sorbitol's favored metabolism to lactate from pyruvate. Increased lactate levels were not sufficient to produce evidence of metabolic acidosis. Mannitol is only slightly metabolized and rapidly excreted by the kidney.

INDICATIONS AND USAGE

Mannitol/Sorbitol Irrigation is indicated for use as a urologic irrigating fluid during transurethral prostatic resection and other transurethral surgical procedures.

CONTRAINDICATIONS

NOT FOR INJECTION BY USUAL PARENTERAL ROUTES.

Do not use in patients with anuria.

WARNINGS

FOR UROLOGIC IRRIGATION ONLY.

Solutions for urologic irrigation must be used with caution in patients with severe cardiopulmonary or renal dysfunction.

Irrigating fluids used during transurethral prostatectomy have been demonstrated to enter the systemic circulation in relatively large volumes; thus, Mannitol/Sorbitol irrigant must be regarded as a systemic drug. Absorption of large amounts of fluids containing Mannitol/Sorbitol and the osmotic diuresis it produces may significantly alter cardiopulmonary and renal dynamics.

Hyperglycemia from metabolism of Sorbitol may occur in patients with diabetes mellitus.

Hyperlactatemia from metabolism of sorbitol may potentially produce a significant lactic acidemia in metabolically compromised patients.

The contents of an opened container should be used promptly to minimize the possibility of bacterial growth or pyrogen formation.

Discard the unused portion of irrigation solution since it contains no preservatives. Do not heat over 66° C (150° F).

PRECAUTIONS

Cardiovascular status, especially of the patient with cardiac disease, should be carefully observed before and during transurethral resection of the prostate when using Mannitol/Sorbitol Irrigation, because the quantity of fluid absorbed into the systemic circulation by opened prostatic veins may produce significant expansion of the extracellular fluid and lead to fulminating congestive heart failure.

Shift of sodium-free intracellular fluid into the extracellular compartment following systemic absorption of solution may lower serum sodium concentration and aggravate pre-existing hyponatremia.

Excessive loss of water and electrolytes may lead to serious imbalances. With continuous irrigation, loss of water may occur in excess of electrolytes, producing hypernatremia.

Sustained diuresis that results from transurethral irrigation with Mannitol/Sorbitol Irrigation may obscure and intensify inadequate hydration or hypovolemia.

Aseptic technique is essential for the use of sterile solutions for irrigation. The administration set should be attached promptly. Unused portions should be discarded and a fresh container of appropriate size used for the start-up of each cycle or repeat procedure.

Do not administer unless solution is clear, seal is intact and container is undamaged. Discard unused portion.

ADVERSE REACTIONS

Adverse reactions may result from intravascular absorption of Sorbitol and Mannitol. The literature reports occasional adverse reactions from intravenous Mannitol/Sorbitol infusions. Consequences of absorption of urologic irrigating solutions include fluid and electrolyte disturbances such as acidosis, electrolyte loss, marked diuresis, urinary retention, edema, dryness of mouth, thirst and dehydration; cardiovascular disorders such as hypotension, tachycardia, angina-like pains; pulmonary disorders such as pulmonary congestion; and other general reactions such as blurred vision, convulsions, nausea, vomiting, diarrhea, rhinitis, chills, vertigo, backache and urticaria. Allergic reactions from Mannitol/Sorbitol have also been reported.

Should any adverse reaction occur, discontinue the irrigant, evaluate the patient, institute appropriate therapeutic countermeasures and save the remainder of the fluid for examination if deemed necessary.

OVERDOSAGE

In the event of dehydration, fluid or solute overload, discontinue the irrigation, evaluate the patient and institute corrective measures as indicated. See "Warnings," "Precautions" and "Adverse Reactions".

DOSAGE AND ADMINISTRATION

Mannitol/Sorbitol Irrigation should be administered only by transurethral instillation with appropriate urologic instrumentation. A disposable administration set should be used. The total volume of solution used for irrigation is solely at the discretion of the surgeon.

Height of container(s) above the operating table in excess of 60 cm (approx. 2 ft) has been reported to increase intravascular absorption of the irrigating fluid.

Parenteral drug products should be inspected visually for particulate matter and discoloration prior to administration, whenever container and solution permit. See "Precautions".

Exposure of pharmaceutical products to heat should be minimized. Avoid excessive heat. Protect from freezing. It is recommended that the product be stored at room temperature (25° C); however, brief exposure up to 40° C does not adversely affect the product.

HOW SUPPLIED
SOLUTION:

AVERAGE UNIT PRICE (AVAILABLE SIZES)

GENERIC	$0.02		

BRAND/MANUFACTURER	NDC	SIZE	AWP
◆ GENERICS			
Abbott Hosp	00074-7981-08	3000 ml 4s	$82.94
Abbott Hosp	00074-6144-06	1500 ml 6s	$221.35

Mannitol, Injectable

DESCRIPTION

Mannitol, Injectable, is a sterile, nonpyrogenic solution of Mannitol in water for injection available in concentrations of 5%, 10%, 15% and 20% for administration by intravenous infusion only.

The content and characteristics of the available concentrations are as follows:

Conc. (%)	g/100 mL	mOsmol/liter (calc.)	pH*
5	5	274	6.3 (4.5 to 7.0)
10	10	549	6.3 (4.5 to 7.0)
15	15	823	6.3 (4.5 to 7.0)
20	20	1098	6.3 (4.5 to 7.0)

* *May contain sodium bicarbonate for pH adjustment.*

The solutions contain no bacteriostat, antimicrobial agent or added buffer (except for pH adjustment) and each is intended only as a single-dose injection. When smaller doses are required the unused portion should be discarded.

Mannitol Injection, USP is a parenteral obligatory osmotic diuretic.

The flexible plastic container is fabricated from a specially formulated polyvinylchloride. Water can permeate from inside the container into the overwrap but not in amounts sufficient to affect the solution significantly. Solutions inside the plastic container also can leach out certain of its chemical components in very small amounts before the expiration period is attained. However, the safety of the plastic has been confirmed by tests in animals according to USP biological standards for plastic containers.

Following is its chemical structure:

$$HOCH_2-\overset{\overset{\displaystyle H}{|}}{\underset{\underset{\displaystyle OH}{|}}{C}}-\overset{\overset{\displaystyle H}{|}}{\underset{\underset{\displaystyle OH}{|}}{C}}-\overset{\overset{\displaystyle OH}{|}}{\underset{\underset{\displaystyle H}{|}}{C}}-\overset{\overset{\displaystyle OH}{|}}{\underset{\underset{\displaystyle H}{|}}{C}}-CH_2OH$$

CLINICAL PHARMACOLOGY

When administered intravenously mannitol is confined to the extracellular space, only slightly metabolized and rapidly excreted by the kidney. Approximately 80% of a 100 g dose appears in the urine in 3 hours. The drug is freely filtered by the glomeruli with less than 10% tubular reabsorption; it is not secreted by tubular cells. Mannitol induces diuresis by elevating the osmolarity of the glomerular filtrate and thereby hindering tubular reabsorption of water. Excretion of sodium and chloride is also enhanced.

INDICATIONS AND USAGE

Mannitol is indicated for the following purposes.

THERAPEUTIC USE

1. Promotion of diuresis in the prevention or treatment of the oliguric phase of acute renal failure before irreversible renal failure becomes established.

2. Reduction of intracranial pressure and brain mass.

3. Reduction of high intraocular pressure when the pressure cannot be lowered by other means.

4. Promotion of urinary excretion of toxic materials.

◆ RATED THERAPEUTICALLY EQUIVALENT; ◇ THERAPEUTIC EQUIVALENCE UNCONFIRMED; ○ UNRATED

DIAGNOSTIC USE
Measurement of glomerular filtration rate.

UNLABELED USES
Mannitol is used alone or as an adjunct in the treatment of pregnancy-induced hypertension (preeclampsia), to reduce intracranial pressure associated with Reye's syndrome, and in the induction of abortion.

CONTRAINDICATIONS
1. Well established anuria due to severe renal disease.
2. Severe pulmonary congestion or frank pulmonary edema.
3. Active intracranial bleeding except during craniotomy.
4. Severe dehydration.
5. Progressive renal damage or dysfunction after institution of Mannitol therapy, including increasing oliguria and azotemia.
6. Progressive heart failure or pulmonary congestion after institution of Mannitol therapy.
7. Do not administer to patients with a known hypersensitivity to Mannitol.

WARNINGS
1. In patients with severe impairment of renal function, a test dose should be utilized (see *"Dosage and Administration"*). A second test dose may be tried if there is an inadequate response, but no more than two test doses should be attempted.
2. Excessive loss of water and electrolytes may lead to serious imbalances. Serum sodium and potassium should be carefully monitored during Mannitol administration.
3. If urine output continues to decline during Mannitol infusion, the patient's clinical status should be closely reviewed and Mannitol infusion suspended if necessary. Accumulation of Mannitol may result in overexpansion of the extracellular fluid which may intensify existing or latent congestive heart failure.
4. Excessive loss of water and electrolytes may lead to serious imbalances. With continued administration of Mannitol, loss of water in excess of electrolytes can cause hypernatremia. Electrolyte measurements, including sodium and potassium are therefore of vital importance in monitoring the infusion of Mannitol.
5. Osmotic nephrosis, a reversible vacuolization of the tubules of no known clinical significance, may proceed to severe irreversible nephrosis, so that the renal function must be closely monitored during Mannitol infusion.
6. Mannitol injection may increase cerebral blood flow and the risk of postoperative bleeding in neurosurgical patients.
7. For intravenous use only. Do not administer intramuscularly or subcutaneously. Never add Mannitol in whole blood for transfusion.

PRECAUTIONS
1. The cardiovascular status of the patient should be carefully evaluated before rapidly administering Mannitol since sudden expansion of the extracellular fluid may lead to fulminating congestive heart failure.
2. Shift of sodium-free intracellular fluid into the extracellular compartment following Mannitol infusion may lower serum sodium concentration and aggravate pre-existing hyponatremia.
3. By sustaining diuresis, Mannitol administration may obscure and intensify inadequate hydration or hypovolemia.
4. Electrolyte-free Mannitol solutions should not be given conjointly with blood. If it is essential that blood be given simultaneously, at least 20 mEq of sodium chloride should be added to each liter of Mannitol solution to avoid pseudoagglutination.
5. When exposed to low temperatures, solutions of Mannitol may crystalize. If crystals are observed, the container should be warmed to redissolve, then cooled to body temperature before administering. See *"Note"* under *"Dosage and Administration"*. Do not infuse Mannitol solution if crystals are present.
6. Do not administer unless solution is clear and container is undamaged. Discard unused portion.
Pregnancy Category C. Animal reproduction studies have not been conducted with Mannitol injection. It is also not known whether Mannitol injection can cause fetal harm when given to a pregnant woman or can affect reproduction. Mannitol injection should be given to a pregnant woman only if clearly needed.

ADVERSE REACTIONS
Adverse reactions more commonly reported during or after the infusion of Mannitol include: Pulmonary congestion, fluid and electrolyte imbalance, acidosis, electrolyte loss, dryness of mouth, thirst, marked diuresis, urinary retention, edema, headache, blurred vision, convulsions, nausea, vomiting, rhinitis, arm pain, skin necrosis, thrombophlebitis, chills, dizziness, urticaria, dehydration, hypotension, tachycardia, fever and angina-like chest pains.

Reactions which may occur because of the solution or the technique of administration include febrile response, infection at the site of injection, venous thrombosis or phlebitis extending from the site of injection, extravasation and hypervolemia.

If an adverse reaction does occur, discontinue the infusion, evaluate the patient, institute appropriate therapeutic countermeasures and save the remainder of the fluid for examination if deemed necessary.

OVERDOSAGE
Too rapid infusion of large amounts of Mannitol will cause a shift of intracellular water into the extracellular compartment resulting in cellular dehydration and overexpansion of the intravascular space with hyponatremia, congestive heart failure and pulmonary edema. Repeated doses should not be given to patients with persistent oliguria as this can produce a hyperosmolar state and precipitate

congestive heart failure and pulmonary edema due to volume overload. Dosage must be carefully monitored and adjusted in accordance with the clinical situation to avoid the consequences of overdosage. See *"Contraindications"*, *"Warnings"*, *"Precautions"* and *"Dosage and Administration"*.

DOSAGE AND ADMINISTRATION
Mannitol should be administered only by intravenous infusion. The total dosage, concentration and rate of administration should be governed by the nature and severity of the condition being treated, fluid requirement and urinary output. The usual adult dosage ranges from 50 to 200 g in a 24-hour period, but in most instances an adequate response will be achieved at a dosage of approximately 100 g/24 hours. The rate of administration is usually adjusted to maintain a urine flow of at least 30 to 50 mL/hr. This outline of dosage and administration is only a general guide to therapy.

Test Dose: A test dose of Mannitol should be given prior to instituting Mannitol I.V. therapy for patients with marked oliguria or those believed to have inadequate renal function. Such test dose may be approximately 0.2 g/kg of body weight (about 150 mL of a 10% solution, or 100 mL of 15% solution, or 75 mL of a 20% solution for an adult patient) infused in a period of 3 to 5 minutes to produce a urine flow of at least 30 to 50 mL/hr. If urine flow does not increase, a second test dose may be given; but if there is an inadequate response, the patient should be re-evaluated.

Prevention of Acute Renal Failure (Oliguria): When used during cardiovascular and other types of surgery, 50 to 100 g of Mannitol as a 5%, 10% or 15% solution may be given. The concentration will depend upon the fluid requirements of the patient.

Treatment of Oliguria: The usual dose to promote diuresis in oliguric patients: Adults, 300 to 400 mg/kg of body weight (21 to 28 g for a 70 kg patient) or up to 100 g of solution, given as a single dose (often in conjunction with furosemide); children, 750 mg/kg of body weight. Doses should not be repeated in patients with persistent oliguria.

Reduction of Intracranial Pressure and Brain Mass: In adults or children, a total dose of 1.5 to 2 g/kg (0.75 to 1 g/lb) of body weight is usually infused over a period of 30 to 60 minutes, to reduce brain mass before or after neurosurgery. Careful evaluation must be made of the circulatory and renal reserve prior to and during administration of Mannitol at this relatively high dose and rapid infusion rate. Careful attention must be paid to fluid and electrolyte balance, body weight, and total input and output before and after infusion of Mannitol. Evidence of reduced cerebral spinal fluid pressure must be observed within 15 minutes, after starting infusion.

Reduction of Intraocular Pressure: A dose of 1.5 to 2.0 g/kg may be given over a period as short as 30 minutes in order to obtain a prompt and maximal effect. When used preoperatively, the dose should be given one to one and one half hours before surgery to achieve maximal reduction of intraocular pressure before operation.

Adjunctive Therapy for Intoxications: As an agent to promote urinary excretion of toxic substances: Adults may receive a 5% to 20% solution for as long as indicated if urinary output remains high; children may receive 2 g/kg of body weight of a 5% or 10% solution. The concentration will depend upon the fluid requirement and urinary output of the patient. If benefits are not observed after 200 g of Mannitol are administered, discontinue the Mannitol therapy. Intravenous water and electrolytes must be given to match the loss of these substances in the urine, sweat and expired air.

Measurement of Glomerular Filtration Rate (GFR): 100 mL of a 20% solution (20 g) should be diluted with 180 mL of sodium chloride injection (normal saline) or 200 mL of a 10% solution (20 g) should be diluted with 80 mL of sodium chloride injection (normal saline). The resulting 280 mL of 7.2% solution is infused at a rate of 20 mL per minute. The urine is collected by catheter for a specific period of time and analyzed for Mannitol excreted in mg per minute. A blood sample is drawn at the start and at the end of the time period and the concentration of Mannitol determined in mg/mL of plasma, GFR is the number of mL of plasma that must have been filtered to account for the amount excreted per minute in the urine. Normal clearance rates are approximately 125 mL/minute for men; 116 mL/minute for women.

DRUG INTERACTIONS
Additives may be incompatible. Consult with pharmacist, if available. When introducing additives, use aseptic technique, mix thoroughly and do not store.

Parenteral drug products should be inspected visually for particulate matter and discoloration; whenever container and solution permit. See *"Precautions"*.

PREPARATION FOR ADMINISTRATION
(Use aseptic technique):
1. Close flow control clamp of administration set.
2. Remove cover from outlet port at bottom of container.
3. Insert piercing pin of administration set into port with a twisting motion until the set is firmly seated.

Note: See full directions on administration set carton.
4. Suspend container from hanger.
5. Squeeze and release drip chamber to establish proper fluid level in chamber.
6. Open flow control clamp and clear air from set. Close clamp.
7. Attach set to venipuncture device. If device is not indwelling, prime and make venipuncture.
8. Regulate rate of administration with flow control clamp.

➤ SHOWN IN PRODUCT IDENTIFICATION GUIDE

WARNING: *Do not use flexible container in series connections.*

Note: Crystals may form in Mannitol solutions especially if the solutions are chilled. If crystals are visible redissolve by warming unit to 70°C with agitation. Heat solution by using a dry-heat cabinet with overwrap intact. The use of a water bath is not recommended. Cool to body temperature or less before administering. When infusing concentrated Mannitol the administration set should include a filter.

Exposure of pharmaceutical products to heat should be minimized. Avoid excessive heat. Protect from freezing. It is recommended that the product be stored at room temperature (25°C); however, brief exposure up to 40°C does not adversely affect the product.

J CODES
25% in 50 ml IV—J2150

HOW SUPPLIED
INJECTION: 5%

BRAND/MANUFACTURER	NDC	SIZE	AWP
◆ **BRAND**			
OSMITROL: Baxter	00338-0351-04	1000 ml 12s	$463.03
◆ **GENERICS**			
Abbott Hosp	00074-7712-09	1000 ml 12s	$600.21

INJECTION: 10%

AVERAGE UNIT PRICE (AVAILABLE SIZES)

BRAND	$0.07
GENERIC	$0.07

BRAND/MANUFACTURER	NDC	SIZE	AWP
◆ **BRAND**			
OSMITROL: Baxter	00338-0354-04	1000 ml 12s	$670.48
	00338-0353-03	500 ml 24s	$1011.49
◆ **GENERICS**			
McGaw	00264-1173-00	1000 ml 6s	$414.29
Abbott Hosp	00074-7713-09	1000 ml 12s	$854.15

INJECTION: 15%

BRAND/MANUFACTURER	NDC	SIZE	AWP
◆ **BRAND**			
OSMITROL: Baxter	00338-0355-03	500 ml 24s	$1442.04

INJECTION: 20%

AVERAGE UNIT PRICE (AVAILABLE SIZES)

BRAND	$0.18
GENERIC	$0.16

BRAND/MANUFACTURER	NDC	SIZE	AWP
◆ **BRAND**			
OSMITROL: Baxter	00338-0357-03	500 ml 24s	$1686.82
	00338-0357-02	250 ml 36s	$2028.05
◆ **GENERICS**			
McGaw	00264-1178-10	500 ml	$51.94
McGaw	00264-1178-20	250 ml 12s	$623.23

INJECTION: 25%

AVERAGE UNIT PRICE (AVAILABLE SIZES)

GENERIC	$0.08	50 ml	$2.86
		50 ml 25s	$119.48

BRAND/MANUFACTURER	NDC	SIZE	AWP
◆ **GENERICS**			
Fujisawa	00469-0024-25	50 ml	$2.79
Fujisawa	00469-0014-25	50 ml	$2.93
Astra	00186-1168-04	50 ml 25s	$66.25
Amer Regent	00517-4050-25	50 ml 25s	$85.94
Abbott Hosp	00074-4031-01	50 ml 25s	$121.42
Intl Med Sys	00548-1003-00	50 ml 25s	$204.30

Mantadil *SEE* CHLORCYCLIZINE HYDROCHLORIDE AND HYDROCORTISONE ACETATE

Maolate *SEE* CHLORPHENESIN CARBAMATE

Maprotiline Hydrochloride

DESCRIPTION
Maprotiline Hydrochloride USP, is a tetracyclic antidepressant, available as 25-mg, 50-mg and 75-mg tablets for oral administration. Its chemical name is N-methyl-9,10-ethanoanthracene-9(10H)-propylamine hydrochloride.

Maprotiline Hydrochloride USP is a fine, white to off-white, practically odorless crystalline powder. It is freely soluble in methanol and in chloroform, slightly soluble in water, and practically insoluble in isooctane. Its molecular weight is 313.87.

Following is its chemical structure:

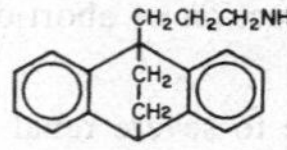

CLINICAL PHARMACOLOGY
The mechanism of action of Maprotiline Hydrochloride is not precisely known. It does not act primarily by stimulation of the central nervous system and is not a monoamine oxidase inhibitor. The postulated mechanism of Maprotiline Hydrochloride is that it acts primarily by potentiation of central adrenergic synapses by blocking reuptake of norepinephrine at nerve endings. This pharmacologic action is thought to be responsible for the drug's antidepressant and anxiolytic effects.

The mean time to peak is 12 hours. The half-life of elimination averages 51 hours.

Steady-state levels measured prior to the morning dose on a one-dosage regimen are summarized as follows:

Regimen	Average Minimum Concentration ng/mL	95% Confidence Limits ng/mL
50 mg x 3 daily	238	181-295

INDICATIONS AND USAGE
Maprotiline Hydrochloride is indicated for the treatment of depressive illness in patients with depressive neurosis (dysthymic disorder) and manic-depressive illness, depressed type (major depressive disorder). Maprotiline Hydrochloride is also effective for the relief of anxiety associated with depression.

UNLABELED USES
Maprotiline Hydrochloride is used alone or as an adjunct in the treatment of bulimia nervosa, enuresis, and micturition difficulties in patients with multiple sclerosis. It is used to inhibit gastric secretion in patients with duodenal ulcer, and is prescribed for chronic pain, and chronic tension headache. It is also used to decrease cocaine craving and to promote abstinence in cocaine abusers.

CONTRAINDICATIONS
Maprotiline Hydrochloride is contraindicated in patients hypersensitive to Maprotiline Hydrochloride and in patients with known or suspected seizure disorders. It should not be given concomitantly with monoamine oxidase (MAO) inhibitors. A minimum of 14 days should be allowed to elapse after discontinuation of MAO inhibitors before treatment with Maprotiline Hydrochloride is initiated. Effects should be monitored with gradual increase in dosage until optimum response is achieved. The drug is not recommended for use during the acute phase of myocardial infarction.

WARNINGS
Seizures have been associated with the use of Maprotiline Hydrochloride. Most of the seizures have occurred in patients without a known history of seizures. However, in some of these cases, other confounding factors were present, including concomitant medications known to lower the seizure threshold, rapid escalation of the dosage of Maprotiline Hydrochloride and dosage that exceeded the recommended therapeutic range. The incidence of direct reports is less than 1/10 of 1%. The risk of seizures may be increased when Maprotiline Hydrochloride is taken concomitantly with phenothiazines, when the dosage of benzodiazepines is rapidly tapered in patients receiving Maprotiline Hydrochloride or when the recommended dosage of Maprotiline Hydrochloride is exceeded. While a cause–and-effect relationship has not been established, the risk of seizures in patients treated with Maprotiline Hydrochloride may be reduced by (1) initiating therapy at a low dosage, (2) maintaining the initial dosage for 2 weeks before raising it gradually in small increments as necessitated by the long half-life of Maprotiline Hydrochloride (average 51 hours), and (3) keeping the dosage at the minimally effective level during maintenance therapy. (See *"Dosage and Administration"*.)

Extreme caution should be used when this drug is given to:
— patients with a history of myocardial infarction;
— patients with a history or presence of cardiovascular disease because of the possibility of conduction defects, arrhythmias, myocardial infarction, strokes and tachycardia.

PRECAUTIONS
General: The possibility of suicide in seriously depressed patients is inherent in their illness and may persist until significant remission occurs. Therefore, patients must be carefully supervised during all phases of treatment with Maprotiline Hydrochloride, and prescriptions should be written for the smallest number of tablets consistent with good patient management.

Hypomanic or manic episodes have been known to occur in some patients taking tricyclic antidepressant drugs, particularly in patients with cyclic disorders. Such occurrences have also been noted, rarely, with Maprotiline Hydrochloride.

Prior to elective surgery, Maprotiline Hydrochloride should be discontinued for as long as clinically feasible, since little is known about the interaction between Maprotiline Hydrochloride and general anesthetics. Maprotiline Hydrochloride should be administered with caution in patients with increased intraocular pressure, history of urinary retention, or history of narrow-angle glaucoma because of the drug's anticholinergic properties.

Information for Patients: Patients should be warned of the association between seizures and the use of Maprotiline Hydrochloride. Moreover, they should be informed that this association is enhanced in patients with a known history of seizures and in those patients who are taking certain other drugs. (See "Warnings".)

Warn patients to exercise caution about potentially hazardous tasks, or operating automobiles or machinery since the drug may impair mental and/or physical abilities.

Maprotiline Hydrochloride may enhance the response to alcohol, barbiturates, and other CNS depressants, requiring appropriate caution of administration.

Laboratory Tests: Maprotiline Hydrochloride should be discontinued if there is evidence of pathological neutrophil depression. Leukocyte and differential counts should be performed in patients who develop fever and sore throat during therapy.

Drug Interactions: Close supervision and careful adjustment of dosage are required when administering Maprotiline Hydrochloride concomitantly with anticholinergic or sympathomimetic drugs because of the possibility of additive atropine-like effects.

Concurrent administration of Maprotiline Hydrochloride with electroshock therapy should be avoided because of the lack of experience in this area.

Caution should be exercised when administering Maprotiline Hydrochloride to hyperthyroid patients or those on thyroid medication because of the possibility of enhanced potential for cardiovascular toxicity of Maprotiline Hydrochloride.

Maprotiline Hydrochloride should be used with caution in patients receiving guanethidine or similar agents since it may block the pharmacologic effects of these drugs.

The risk of seizures may be increased when Maprotiline Hydrochloride is taken concomitantly with phenothiazines or when the dosage of benzodiazepines is rapidly tapered in patients receiving Maprotiline Hydrochloride.

Because of the pharmacologic similarity of Maprotiline Hydrochloride to the tricyclic antidepressants, the plasma concentration of Maprotiline Hydrochloride may be increased when the drug is given concomitantly with hepatic enzyme inhibitors (e.g., cemetidine, fluoxetine) and decreased by concomitant administration with hepatic enzyme enducers (e.g., barbiturates, phenytoin), as has occurred with tricyclic antidepressants. Adjustment of the dosage of Maprotiline Hydrochloride may therefore be necessary in such cases. (See "Information for Patients".)

Carcinogenesis, Mutagenesis, Impairment of Fertility: Carcinogenicity and chronic toxicity studies have been conducted in laboratory rats and dogs. No drug- or dose-related occurrence of carcinogenesis was evident in rats receiving daily oral doses up to 60 mg/kg of Maprotiline Hydrochloride for eighteen months or in dogs receiving daily oral doses up to 30 mg/kg of Maprotiline Hydrochloride for one year. In addition, no evidence of mutagenic activity was found in offspring of female mice mated with males treated with up to 60 times the maximum daily human dose.

Pregnancy Category B: Reproduction studies have been performed in female laboratory rabbits, mice, and rats at doses up to 1.3, 7, and 9 times the maximum daily human dose respectively and have revealed no evidence of impaired fertility or harm to the fetus due to Maprotiline Hydrochloride. There are, however, no adequate and well-controlled studies in pregnant women. Because animal reproduction studies are not always predictive of human response, this drug should be used during pregnancy only if clearly needed.

Labor and Delivery: Although the effect of Maprotiline Hydrochloride on labor and delivery is unknown, caution should be exercised as with any drug with CNS depressant action.

Nursing Mothers: Maprotiline Hydrochloride is excreted in breast milk. At steady state, the concentrations in milk correspond closely to the concentrations in whole blood. Caution should be exercised when Maprotiline Hydrochloride is administered to a nursing woman.

Pediatric Use: Safety and effectiveness in children below the age of 18 have not been established.

ADVERSE REACTIONS

The following adverse reactions have been noted with Maprotiline Hydrochloride and are generally similar to those observed with tricyclic antidepressants.

Cardiovascular: Rare occurrences of hypotension, hypertension, tachycardia, palpitation, arrhythmia, heart block, and syncope have been reported with Maprotiline Hydrochloride.

Psychiatric: Nervousness (6%), anxiety (3%), insomnia (2%), and agitation (2%); rarely, confusional states (especially in the elderly), hallucinations, disorientation, delusions, restlessness, nightmares, hypomania, mania, exacerbation of psychosis, decrease in memory, and feelings of unreality.

Neurological: Drowsiness (16%), dizziness (8%), tremor (3%), and, rarely, numbness, tingling, motor hyperactivity, akathisia, seizures, EEG alterations, tinnitus, extrapyramidal symptoms, ataxia, and dysarthria.

Anticholinergic: Dry mouth (22%), constipation (6%), and blurred vision (4%); rarely, accommodation disturbances, mydriasis, urinary retention, and delayed micturition.

Allergic: Rare instances of skin rash, petechiae, itching, photosensitization, edema, and drug fever.

Gastrointestinal: Nausea (2%) and, rarely, vomiting, epigastric distress, diarrhea, bitter taste, abdominal cramps and dysphagia.

Endocrine: Rare instances of increased or decreased libido, impotence, and elevation or depression of blood sugar levels.

Other: Weakness and fatigue (4%) and headache (4%); rarely, altered liver function, jaundice, weight loss or gain, excessive perspiration, flushing, urinary frequency, increased salivation, nasal congestion and alopecia.

Note: Although there have been only isolated reports of the following adverse reactions with Maprotiline Hydrochloride, its pharmacologic similarity to tricyclic antidepressants requires that each reaction be considered when administering Maprotiline Hydrochloride.

— Bone marrow depression, including agranulocytosis, eosinophilia, purpura, and thrombocytopenia, myocardial infarction, stroke, peripheral neuropathy, sublingual adenitis, black tongue, stomatitis, paralytic ileus, gynecomastia in the male, breast enlargement and galactorrhea in the female, and testicular swelling.

Post-Introduction Reports: Several voluntary reports of interstitial pneumonitis, which were in some cases associated with eosinophilia and increased liver enzymes, have been received since market introduction. However, there is no clear causal relationship.

OVERDOSAGE

Animal Oral LD$_{50}$: The oral LD$_{50}$ of Maprotiline Hydrochloride is 600-750 mg/kg in mice, 760-900 mg/kg in rats, > 1000 mg/kg in rabbits, > 300 mg/kg in cats, and > 30 mg/kg in dogs.

Signs and Symptoms: Data dealing with overdosage in humans are limited with only a few cases on record. Symptoms are drowsiness, tachycardia, ataxia, vomiting, cyanosis, hypotension, shock, restlessness, agitation, hyperpyrexia, muscle rigidity, athetoid movements, mydriasis, cardiac arrhythmias, impaired cardiac condition. In severe cases, loss of consciousness and generalized convulsions may occur. Since congestive heart failure has been seen with overdosages of tricyclic antidepressants, it should be considered with Maprotiline Hydrochloride overdosage.

Treatment: The recommended treatment for overdosage with heterocyclics may change periodically. Therefore, it is recommended that the physician contact a poison control center for current information on treatment. Because CNS involvement, respiratory depression, and cardiac arrhythmia can occur suddenly, hospitalization and close observation may be necessary, even when the amount ingested is thought to be small or the initial degree of intoxication appears slight or moderate. All patients with ECG abnormalities should have continuous cardiac monitoring and be closely observed until well after the cardiac status has returned to normal; relapses may occur after apparent recovery.

In the alert patient, the stomach should be emptied promptly by lavage. In the obtunded patient, the airway should be secured with a cuffed endotracheal tube before beginning lavage (do not induce emesis). Instillation of an activated charcoal slurry may help reduce the absorption of Maprotiline Hydrochloride. The room should be darkened, allowing only minimal external stimulation to reduce the tendency to convulsions. If anticonvulsants are necessary, diazepam and phenytoin may be useful. Adequate respiratory exchange should be maintained, including intubation and artificial respiration, if necessary.

Since it has been reported that physostigmine increases the risk of seizures, its use is not recommended in cases of overdosage with Maprotiline Hydrochloride.

Shock (circulatory collapse) should be treated with supportive measures such as appropriate position, intravenous fluids, and vasopressors if necessary.

Hyperpyrexia should be controlled by whatever means available, including ice packs if necessary.

Digitalis may increase conduction abnormalities and further irritate an already sensitized myocardium. If congestive heart failure necesssitates rapid digitalization, particular care must be exercised.

Dialysis is of little value because of the low plasma concentration of this drug.

DOSAGE AND ADMINISTRATION

A single daily dose is an alternative to divided daily doses. Therapeutic effects are sometimes seen within 3 to 7 days, although as long as 2 to 3 weeks are usually necessary.

Initial Adult Dosage: An initial dosage of 75 mg daily is suggested for outpatients with mild-to-moderate depression. However, in some patients, particularly the elderly, an initial dosage of 25 mg daily may be used. Because of the long half-life of Maprotiline Hydrochloride, the initial dosage should be maintained for two weeks. The dosage may then be increased gradually in 25-mg increments as required and tolerated. In most out-patients a maximum dose of 150 mg daily will result in therapeutic efficacy. It is recommended that this dose not be exceeded except in the most severely depressed patients. In such patients, dosage may be gradually increased to a maximum of 225 mg.

More severely depressed, hospitalized patients should be given an initial daily dose of 100 mg to 150 mg which may be gradually increased as required and tolerated. Most hospitalized patients with moderate-to-severe depression respond to a daily dosage of 150 mg although dosages as high as 225 mg may be required in some cases. Daily dosage of 225 mg should not be exceeded.

Elderly Patients: In general, lower dosages are recommended for patients over 60 years of age. Dosage of 50 mg to 75 mg daily are usually satisfactory as maintenance therapy for elderly patients who do not tolerate higher amounts.

► SHOWN IN PRODUCT IDENTIFICATION GUIDE

Maintenance: Dosage during prolonged maintenance therapy should be kept at the lowest effective level. Dosage may be reduced to levels of 75 mg to 150 mg daily during such periods, with subsequent adjustment depending on therapeutic response.

Storage: Do not store above 86°F (30°C).
   Dispense in tight container (USP).

HOW SUPPLIED
TABLETS: 25 MG

AVERAGE UNIT PRICE (AVAILABLE SIZES)			
BRAND	$0.43	GENERIC A-RATED AVERAGE PRICE (GAAP)	
GENERIC	$0.34		
HCFA FUL (100s ea)	$0.21	100s	$33.48

BRAND/MANUFACTURER	NDC	SIZE	AWP
◆ BRAND			
LUDIOMIL: Ciba Pharm	00083-0110-30	100s	$43.05
◆ GENERICS			
Medirex	57480-0493-06	30s	$13.20
Schein	00364-2294-01	100s	$26.50
Geneva	00781-1631-01	100s	$27.95
Qualitest	00603-4294-21	100s	$30.06
URL	00677-1214-01	100s	$30.65
Rugby	00536-3902-01	100s	$30.69
Major	00904-3323-60	100s	$30.70
Goldline	00182-1882-01	100s	$30.70
Martec	52555-0355-01	100s	$30.95
Watson	52544-0373-01	100s	$35.18
Aligen	00405-4594-01	100s	$35.20
Parmed	00349-8879-01	100s	$35.95
Moore,H.L.	00839-7448-06	100s	$37.19
Mylan	00378-0060-01	100s	$37.50
Major	00904-3323-61	100s ud	$27.56
Raway	00686-0493-20	100s ud	$35.50
UDL	51079-0493-20	100s ud	$42.80
Medirex	57480-0493-01	100s ud	$44.00

TABLETS: 50 MG

AVERAGE UNIT PRICE (AVAILABLE SIZES)			
BRAND	$0.64	100s	$48.42
GENERIC	$0.49	GENERIC A-RATED AVERAGE PRICE (GAAP)	
HCFA FUL (100s ea)	$0.31		

BRAND/MANUFACTURER	NDC	SIZE	AWP
◆ BRAND			
LUDIOMIL: Ciba Pharm	00083-0026-30	100s	$63.70
◆ GENERICS			
Medirex	57480-0494-06	30s	$17.25
Qualitest	00603-4295-21	100s	$39.49
Geneva	00781-1632-01	100s	$40.95
Schein	00364-2295-01	100s	$41.50
Goldline	00182-1883-01	100s	$45.40
URL	00677-1215-01	100s	$47.65
Rugby	00536-3903-01	100s	$47.69
Major	00904-3324-60	100s	$47.70
Martec	52555-0356-01	100s	$48.80
Parmed	00349-8880-01	100s	$49.00
Watson	52544-0374-01	100s	$52.06
Aligen	00405-4595-01	100s	$52.10
Moore,H.L.	00839-7449-06	100s	$52.52
Mylan	00378-0087-01	100s	$55.10
Raway	00686-0494-20	100s ud	$41.50
UDL	51079-0494-20	100s ud	$55.83
Medirex	57480-0494-01	100s ud	$57.50

TABLETS: 75 MG

AVERAGE UNIT PRICE (AVAILABLE SIZES)			
BRAND	$0.88	100s	$63.85
GENERIC	$0.64	GENERIC A-RATED AVERAGE PRICE (GAAP)	
HCFA FUL (100s ea)	$0.44		

BRAND/MANUFACTURER	NDC	SIZE	AWP
◆ BRAND			
LUDIOMIL: Ciba Pharm	00083-0135-30	100s	$87.48
◆ GENERICS			
Qualitest	00603-4296-21	100s	$53.91
Schein	00364-2296-01	100s	$59.50
Goldline	00182-1884-01	100s	$62.25
Major	00904-3325-60	100s	$62.65
Watson	52544-0375-01	100s	$71.50
Aligen	00405-4596-01	100s	$71.62
Mylan	00378-0092-01	100s	$74.85
Major	00904-3322-61	100s ud	$54.48

Marax *SEE* EPHEDRINE SULFATE/HYDROXYZINE
HYDROCHLORIDE/THEOPHYLLINE

Marcaine HCl *SEE* BUPIVACAINE, BUPIVACAINE WITH EPINEPHRINE, AND BUPIVACAINE SPINAL IN DEXTROSE

Marinol *SEE* DRONABINOL

Masoprocol

DESCRIPTION
Masoprocol cream contains Masoprocol 10%, in an emollient cream base. Chemically, Masoprocol is (R*, S*)-4,4'- (2,3-dimethyl-1,4-butanediyl)bis[1,2-benzenediol]. It has a molecular formula of $C_{18}H_{22}O_4$ and has a molecular weight of 302.37. Masoprocol (also known as meso-nordihydroguaiaretic acid) is a white to off-white crystalline powder.

   Following is its chemical structure:

CLINICAL PHARMACOLOGY
The mechanism of action of Masoprocol in the treatment of actinic keratoses is unknown. In tissue culture, Masoprocol has shown antiproliferative activity against keratinocytes. However, the relevance of this activity to its therapeutic effect has not been established.

   A study in 6 male patients with a single topical application of ^{14}C-labeled Masoprocol in the cream formulation demonstrated low absorption (< 1.0%) as measured by ^{14}C content of plasma, urine, and feces over the 96-hour period after application. In a separate study, 6 patients who were treated with unlabeled Actinex cream twice daily for 28 days demonstrated up to 2% absorption after application of ^{14}C-labeled Masoprocol in the cream formulation on day 29, as measured by ^{14}C content of plasma, urine, and feces over the 96-hour period after application.

INDICATIONS AND USAGE
Masoprocol cream is indicated for the topical treatment of actinic (solar) keratoses.

CONTRAINDICATIONS
Masoprocol cream is contraindicated in patients with known hypersensitivity to Masoprocol or other ingredients in this formulation.

WARNINGS
OCCLUSIVE DRESSINGS SHOULD NOT BE USED WITH THIS PRODUCT.
   Masoprocol cream contains sodium metabisulfite, a sulfite that may cause allergic-type reactions including anaphylactic symptoms and life-threatening or less severe asthmatic episodes in certain susceptible people. The overall prevalence of sulfite sensitivity in the general population is unknown and probably low. Sulfite sensitivity is seen more frequently in asthmatic than in nonasthmatic people.

PRECAUTIONS
GENERAL: MASOPROCOL FREQUENTLY INDUCES SENSITIZATION (ALLERGIC CONTACT DERMATITIS). When patients treated with 5% or 10% Masoprocol cream in clinical trials were patch tested with a 1% Masoprocol cream, 9% had reactions indicative of sensitization. In patients rechallenged with 10% Masoprocol cream, dermal reactions were more frequent and more severe. Use of Masoprocol should be discontinued if sensitivity is noted. Masoprocol does not appear to cause photosensitization. However, because solar keratoses are related to exposure to sunlight, the patient should avoid undue sun exposure.

   In applying the product near the eyes, nose, or mouth, patients should be advised to do so with special care. If Masoprocol comes into contact with the eyes (conjunctiva), itching irritation, or transient pain may occur. In case of contact with the eye, wash the eye with water promptly. If Masoprocol is applied with fingers, the hands should be washed immediately after use.

   Masoprocol cream may stain clothing or fabrics.

Information for Patients:
   1. Special care should be taken if Masoprocol cream is to be applied near the eyes, nose, or mouth.
   2. In case of contact with the eye, wash the eye with water promptly.
   3. If Masoprocol cream is applied with fingers, the hands should be washed immediately after use.
   4. Contact physician immediately if a severe reaction occurs, including, for example, oozing or blistering.
   5. While using this product, other skin care products or make-up should not be used without the advice of a physician.

Carcinogenesis, Mutagenesis, Impairment of Fertility: Animal studies have not been performed to evaluate the effect on fertility or the carcinogenic potential of Masoprocol.

   Masoprocol produced mutagenic results in the Ames assay. It was negative with three strains of *Salmonella* and positive with one. In an *in vivo* mouse

---

◆ RATED THERAPEUTICALLY EQUIVALENT; ◇ THERAPEUTIC EQUIVALENCE UNCONFIRMED; ○ UNRATED

estrogenic activity assay conducted using Masoprocol subcutaneously at 2 mg/kg/day for 4 days, treated mice demonstrated no more effects of estrogenic activity than did vehicle controls.

Pregnancy Category B: Teratology studies have been performed in rabbits and rats at doses up to 6 and 16 times the human dose, based on a mg/m^2 basis, respectively. No adverse fetal effects were observed. There are no adequate and well-controlled studies in pregnant women. Because animal reproduction studies are not always predictive of human response, this drug should be used during pregnancy only if clearly needed.

Nursing Mothers: It is not known whether this drug is excreted in human milk. Because many drugs are excreted in human milk, caution should be exercised when Masoprocol cream is administered to a nursing woman.

Pediatric Use: Safety and effectiveness in children have not been established.

ADVERSE REACTIONS
The most frequently occurring adverse reactions considered related or possibly related to Masoprocol cream and their frequency of occurrence are: erythema (46%), flaking (46%), itching (32%), dryness (27%), edema (14%), burning (12%), and soreness (5%). While local skin reactions are frequent, they usually resolve within two weeks of discontinuation. The presence or absence of local skin reactions does not correlate with successful ultimate therapeutic outcome. Reactions reported in 1% to 5% of patients include: bleeding, crusting, eye irritation, oozing, rash, skin irritation, soreness, stinging, tightness, and tingling. Less frequently reported reactions (less than 1%) include: blistering, eczema, excoriation, fissuring, leathery feeling to the skin, skin roughness, and wrinkling. No necrosis, scarring, or ulceration was observed during the initial course of therapy.

OVERDOSAGE
There are no reports of human ingestion overdosage. In animals receiving high oral doses of Masoprocol, the commonly affected systems were the gastrointestinal and hepatic systems. If ingested, evacuate stomach contents, taking care to prevent aspiration.

DOSAGE AND ADMINISTRATION
Wash and dry areas where actinic keratoses are present. Gently massage Masoprocol cream into the area where actinic keratoses are present until it is evenly distributed, avoiding the eyes and mucous membranes of the nose and mouth. Application should be repeated each morning and evening for 28 days.
   OCCLUSIVE DRESSINGS SHOULD NOT BE USED WITH THIS PRODUCT.
   Immediately after applying Masoprocol the patient might experience a transient local burning sensation.
   Masoprocol cream should be stored at controlled room temperature, 15° to 30°C (59° to 86°F).

HOW SUPPLIED
CREAM: 10%

BRAND/MANUFACTURER	NDC	SIZE	AWP
○ **BRAND**			
ACTINEX: Reed & Carnrick	00021-4520-37	30 gm	$48.00

Materna *SEE* VITAMINS, PRENATAL

Matulane *SEE* PROCARBAZINE HYDROCHLORIDE

Maxair *SEE* PIRBUTEROL ACETATE

Maxaquin *SEE* LOMEFLOXACIN HYDROCHLORIDE

Maxidex *SEE* DEXAMETHASONE, OPHTHALMIC

Maxiflor *SEE* DIFLORASONE DIACETATE

Maxitrol *SEE* DEXAMETHASONE/NEOMYCIN SULFATE/POLYMYXIN B SULFATE

Maxzide *SEE* HYDROCHLOROTHIAZIDE AND TRIAMTERENE

Mazanor *SEE* MAZINDOL

Mazindol

DESCRIPTION
Mazindol is an imidazoisoindole anorectic agent. It is chemically designated as 5-(4-chlorophenyl)-2,5-dihydro-3H-imidazo[2,1-a]isoin-dol-5-ol, a tautomeric form of 2-[(2')-(p-chlorobenzoyl) phenyl]-2-imidazoline. Its molecular formula is $C_{16}H_{13}ClN_2O$ and its molecular weight is 284.74.
   Mazindol is available in 1 mg and 2 mg tablets.

   Following is its chemical structure:

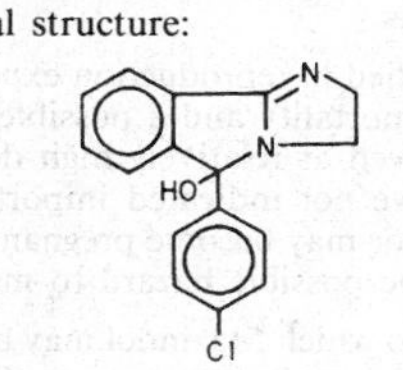

ACTIONS
Mazindol, although an isoindole, has pharmacologic activity similar in many ways to the prototype drugs used in obesity, the amphetamines. Actions include central nervous system stimulation in humans and animals, as well as such amphetamine-like effects in animals as the production of stereotyped behavior. Animal experiments also suggest certain differences from phenethylamine anorectic drugs, e.g., amphetamine, with respect to site and mechanism of action; for example, Mazindol appears to exert its primary effects on the limbic system. The significance of these differences for humans is uncertain. It does not cause brain norepinephrine depletion in animals; on the other hand, it does appear to inhibit storage site uptake of norepinephrine as is suggested by its marked potentiation of the effect of exogenous norepinephrine on blood pressure in dogs (see *"Warnings"*) and on smooth muscle contraction *in vitro*. Tolerance has been demonstrated with all drugs of this class in which this phenomenon has been studied.
   Drugs used in obesity are commonly known as "anorectics" or "anorexigenics." It has not been established, however, that the action of such drugs in treating obesity is exclusively one of appetite suppression. Other central nervous system actions, or metabolic effects may be involved as well. Adult obese subjects instructed in dietary management and treated with anorectic drugs, lose more weight on the average than those treated with placebo and diet, as determined in relatively short-term clinical trials.
   The average magnitude of increased weight loss of drug-treated patients over placebo-treated patients in studies of anorectics in general is ordinarily only a fraction of a pound a week. The rate of weight loss is greatest in the first weeks of therapy for both drug and placebo subjects and tends to decrease in succeeding weeks.
   The amount of weight loss associated with the use of Mazindol as with other anorectic drugs, varies from trial to trial, and the increased weight loss appears to be related in part to variables other than the drugs prescribed, such as the interaction between physician-investigator and the patient, the population treated, and the diet prescribed. The importance of nondrug factors in such weight loss has not been elucidated.
   The natural history of obesity is measured in years, whereas, most studies cited are restricted to a few weeks' duration; thus, the total impact of drug-induced weight loss over that of diet alone must be considered clinically limited.

INDICATIONS AND USAGE
Mazindol is indicated in the management of exogenous obesity as a short-term (a few weeks) adjunct in a regimen of weight reduction based on caloric restriction. The limited usefulness of agents of this class (see *"Actions"*) should be measured against possible risk factors inherent in their use, such as those described below.

UNLABELED USES
Mazindol is used alone or as an adjunct in the treatment of narcolepsy and Duchenne's dystrophy.

CONTRAINDICATIONS
Glaucoma; hypersensitivity or idiosyncrasy to Mazindol.
   Agitated states.
   Patients with a history of drug abuse.
   During or within 14 days following the administration of monoamine oxidase inhibitors (hypertensive crises may result.)

WARNINGS
Tolerance to the effect of many anorectic drugs may develop within a few weeks; if this occurs, the recommended dose should not be exceeded in an attempt to increase the effect; rather, the drug should be discontinued.
   Mazindol is not recommended for severely hypertensive patients or for patients with symptomatic cardiovascular disease including arrhythmias.

➤ SHOWN IN PRODUCT IDENTIFICATION GUIDE

PRECAUTIONS

General: Mazindol may impair the ability of the patient to engage in potentially hazardous activities such as operating machinery or driving a motor vehicle; the patient should therefore be cautioned accordingly.

Drug Interactions: Mazindol may markedly potentiate the pressor effect of exogenous catecholamines. If it should be necessary to give a pressor amine agent (e.g., levarterenol or isoproterenol) to a patient in shock (e.g., from a myocardial infarction) who has recently been taking Mazindol extreme care should be taken in monitoring blood pressure at frequent intervals and initiating pressor therapy with a low initial dose and careful titration.

It should be recognized that reduction in carbohydrate intake may require reduced insulin dosage. However, in diabetic patients treated with insulin and given Mazindol for 12 weeks, no change in insulin requirement was noted.

Mazindol may potentiate blood pressure increases in those patients taking sympathomimetic medications.

Pregnancy: Mazindol was studied in reproduction experiments in rats and rabbits and an increase in neonatal mortality and a possible increased incidence of rib anomalies in rats were observed at relatively high doses.

Although these studies have not indicated important adverse effects, use of Mazindol by women who are or may become pregnant requires that the potential benefit be weighed against the possible hazard to mother and infant.

Nursing Mothers: The extent to which Mazindol may be transferred in breast milk is not known. Therefore, mothers who are nursing should not receive this drug.

Pediatric Use: Safety and effectiveness in children below the age of 12 years have not been established.

ADVERSE REACTIONS

The most common adverse effects of Mazindol are dry mouth, tachycardia, constipation, nervousness and insomnia.

Cardiovascular: Palpitation, tachycardia, edema.

Central Nervous System: Overstimulation, restlessness, dizziness, insomnia, dysphoria, tremor, headache, depression, drowsiness, weakness.

Gastrointestinal: Dryness of the mouth, unpleasant taste, diarrhea, constipation, nausea, vomiting, abdominal discomfort.

Skin: Rash, excessive sweating, clamminess.

Endocrine: Impotence, changes in libido have rarely been observed with Mazindol.

Eye: Treatment of dogs with high doses of Mazindol for long periods resulted in some corneal opacities, reversible on cessation of medication. No such effect has been observed in humans.

Autonomic: Blurred vision, fainting sensation, hot/cold flashes, hyperdipsia, paresthesia.

Genitourinary: Dysuria, pollakiuria.

DRUG ABUSE AND DEPENDENCE

Controlled Studies: Mazindol is controlled by the Drug Enforcement Administration and is classified under Schedule IV.

Abuse or Dependence: In preliminary chronic safety studies in humans, dosages of 2 mg Mazindol t.i.d. were administered for 24 consecutive weeks. Two to three days following abrupt withdrawal of medication the subjects were interviewed and no subject requested or required reinstitution of active medication, and no evidence suggestive of dependence was observed. In widespread clinical use of Mazindol in the United States since 1973, Sandoz Pharmaceuticals has received no reports of development of physical or psychological dependence, drug tolerance, habituation, chronic abuse, or symptoms of withdrawal or abstinence.

OVERDOSAGE

The minimum lethal dose for humans is not known. The oral LD$_{50}$, expressed in mg/kg, is 106 for the mouse, 180-320 for the rat, 98 for the rabbit, and 9-20 for the dog. Fewer than 2 dozen cases of Mazindol overdosage in humans have been reported, and all but 1 of these recovered completely. A 25-year-old female died after ingesting a massive dose of 200 mg of Mazindol and an undetermined amount of ethanol.

The maximum overdosage of Mazindol on record from which the patient recovered is 80 mg. A 20-year-old female ingested 40 Mazindol tablets (2 mg each) and 75-125 mg phenmetrazine in a suicide attempt. The patient was alert during hospitalization and the only clinical finding was frequent premature ventricular contractions. The patient was treated with Lidocaine and recovered completely.

Approximately half of the overdosage cases involved accidental ingestion in children 1-4 years of age. The reported doses ingested ranged from 4-40 mg. All recovered.

In cases in which overdosages have been reported, the symptoms listed below were cited: irritability, agitation, hyperactivity, tachycardia, arrhythmia (premature ventricular contractions occurred in the patient also taking phenmetrazine), tachypnea.

The following symptomatic treatment may include:

Emesis: If the patient is conscious, vomiting should be induced with ipecac syrup (15-30 cc).

Gastric Lavage: Patients should have pharyngeal and laryngeal reflexes. In unconscious patients gastric lavage should not be attempted unless cuffed endotracheal intubation has been performed to prevent aspiration and pulmonary complications.

Sedation: Chlorpromazine (0.5-1 mg/kg, IM) may be given every 30 minutes as needed to control symptoms of central nervous (CNS) overstimulation. A short-acting barbiturate is generally considered the second best choice. Lidocaine may be administered to counteract cardiac arrhythmias.

Forced Acid Diuresis: Sufficient fluids should be given to maintain a urine output of 5-7 L/m^2/day or 2-4 times normal excretion. A 15% solution of mannitol (2.5 mg/kg) given IV every 4-6 hours or whenever the urine specific gravity falls below 1.025 is usually sufficient to produce an acid urine in young people. If necessary, methenamine mandelate or ammonium chloride can be used to acidify the urine. During prolonged forced diuresis, serum electrolytes must be evaluated frequently to avoid hyponatremia or hypokalemia.

Data about treating acute Mazindol overdosage with hemodialysis or peritoneal dialysis are not available. However, Mazindol is soluble only in acid so dialysis with basic or neutral solvents would not remove the drug.

DOSAGE AND ADMINISTRATION

To determine the lowest effective dose, therapy with Mazindol may be initiated at 1 mg once a day and adjusted to the need and response of the patient. Dosage may be increased to a maximum of 3 mg/day given in divided doses with meals.

Store tablets in a tight container, below 77°F (25°C).

HOW SUPPLIED

TABLETS (C-IV): 1 MG

BRAND/MANUFACTURER	NDC	SIZE	AWP
◇ BRAND			
MAZANOR: Wyeth-Ayerst	00008-0071-03	30s	$27.69
SANOREX: Sandoz Pharm	00078-0071-05	100s	$113.40

TABLETS (C-IV): 2 MG

BRAND/MANUFACTURER	NDC	SIZE	AWP
○ BRAND			
SANOREX: Sandoz Pharm	00078-0066-05	100s	$180.00

Measles and Rubella Virus Vaccine Live

DESCRIPTION

Measles and Rubella Virus Vaccine Live is a live virus vaccine for immunization against measles (rubeola) and rubella (German measles). Measles and Rubella Virus Vaccine Live (Measles and Rubella Vaccine) is a sterile lyophilized preparation of (1) Measles Virus Vaccine Live, a more attenuated line of Measles Virus, derived from Enders' attenuated Edmonston strain and grown in cell cultures of chick embryo: and (2) Rubella Virus Vaccine Live, the Wistar RA 27/3 strain of live attenuated Rubella Virus grown in human diploid cell (WI-38) culture. The vaccine viruses are the same as those used in the manufacture of Measles Virus Vaccine Live, and Rubella Virus Vaccine Live. The two viruses are mixed before being lyophilized. The product contains no preservative.

The reconstituted vaccine is for subcutaneous administration. When reconstituted as directed, the dose for injection is 0.5 mL and contains not less than the equivalent of 1,000 TCID$_{50}$ (tissue culture infectious doses) of the U.S. Reference Measles Virus; and 1,000 TCID$_{50}$ of the U.S Reference Rubella Virus. Each dose contains approximately 25 mcg of neomycin. The product contains no preservative. Sorbitol and hydrolized gelatin are added as stabilizers.

CLINICAL PHARMACOLOGY

Clinical studies of 237 double seronegative children, 10 months to 10 years of age, demonstrated that Measles and Rubella Vaccine is highly immunogenic and generally well tolerated. In these studies, a single injection of the vaccine induced Measles hemagglutination-inhibition (HI) antibodies in 95 percent and Rubella HI antibodies in 99 percent of susceptible persons.

The RA 27/3 Rubella strain in Measles and Rubella Vaccine elicits higher immediate post-vaccination HI, complement-fixing and neutralizing antibody levels than other strains of Rubella Vaccine and has been shown to induce a broader profile of circulating antibodies including anti-theta and anti-iota precipitating antibodies. The RA 27/3 Rubella strain immunologically simulates natural infection more closely than other Rubella Vaccine Viruses. The increased levels and broader profile of antibodies produced by RA 27/3 strain Rubella Virus Vaccine appear to correlate with greater resistance to subclinical reinfection with the wild virus, and provide greater confidence for lasting immunity.

Vaccine induced antibody levels following administration of Measles and Rubella Vaccine have been shown to persist up to 11 years without substantial decline. Continued surveillance will be necessary to determine further duration of antibody persistence.

INDICATIONS AND USAGE

Measles and Rubella Vaccine is indicated for simultaneous immunization against Measles and Rubella in persons 15 months of age or older. A second dose of Measles and Rubella Vaccine or monovalent Measles Vaccine is recommended (see *"Revaccination"*).

◆ RATED THERAPEUTICALLY EQUIVALENT; ◇ THERAPEUTIC EQUIVALENCE UNCONFIRMED; ○ UNRATED

Infants who are less than 15 months of age may fail to respond to the measles component of the vaccine due to presence in the circulation of residual measles antibody of maternal origin; the younger the infant, the lower the likelihood of seroconversion. In geographically isolated or other relatively inaccessible populations for whom immunization programs are logistically difficult, and in population groups in which natural measles infection may occur in a significant proportion of infants before 15 months of age, it may be desirable to give the vaccine to infants at an earlier age. Infants vaccinated under these conditions at less than 12 months of age should be revaccinated after reaching 15 months of age. There is some evidence to suggest that infants immunized at less than one year of age may not develop sustained antibody levels when later reimmunized. The advantage of early protection must be weighed against the chance for failure to respond adequately on reimmunization.

Previously unimmunized children of susceptible pregnant women should receive live attenuated Rubella Vaccine, because an immunized child will be less likely to acquire natural rubella and introduce the virus into the household.

Individuals planning travel outside the United States, if not immune, can acquire measles, mumps or rubella and import these diseases to the United States. Therefore, prior to International travel, individuals known to be susceptible to one or more of these diseases can receive either a single antigen vaccine (measles, mumps, or rubella), or a combined antigen vaccine as appropriate. However, Measles Mumps, and Rubella Virus Vaccine Live, is preferred for persons likely to be susceptible to mumps and rubella; and if a single-antigen measles vaccine is not readily available, travelers should receive Measles, Mumps, and Rubella Virus Vaccine Live, regardless of their immune status to mumps or rubella.

NONPREGNANT ADOLESCENT AND ADULT FEMALES

Immunization of susceptible non-pregnant adolescent and adult females of childbearing age with live attenuated Rubella Virus Vaccine is indicated if certain precautions are observed (see below and *"Precautions"*). Vaccinating susceptible postpubertal females confers individual protection against subsequently acquiring rubella infection during pregnancy, which in turn prevents infection of the fetus and consequent congenital rubella injury.

Women of childbearing age should be advised not to become pregnant for three months after vaccination and should be informed of the reason for this precaution.*

It is recommended that rubella susceptibility be determined by serologic testing prior to immunization.** If immune, as evidenced by a specific rubella antibody titer of 1:8 or greater (hemagglutination-inhibition test), vaccination is unnecessary. Congenital malformations do occur in up to seven percent of all live births. Their chance appearance after vaccination could lead to misinterpretation of the cause, particularly if the prior rubella-immune status of vaccines is unknown.

Postpubertal females should be informed of the frequent occurance of generally self-limited arthralgia and/or arthritis beginning 2 to 4 weeks after vaccination (see *"Advertise Reactions).*

POSTPARTUM WOMEN

It has been found convenient in many instances to vaccinate rubella-susceptibel women in the immediate postpartum period. (See *"Nursing Mothers"*.)

Revaccination: Children first vaccinated when younger than 12 months of age should be revaccinated at 15 months age.

The American Academy of Pediatrics (AAP), the Immunization Practices Advisory Committee (ACIP), and some state and local health agencies have recommended guidelines for routine measles revaccination and to help control measles outbreaks.***

Vaccines available for revaccination include monovalent measles vaccine (Measles Virus Vaccine) and polyuvalent vaccines conttaining measles (e.g. Measles, Mumps, and Rubella Virus Vaccine.) If the prevention of sporadic measles outbreaks is the sole objective, revaccination with a monovalent Measles Vaccine should be considered (see appropriate product circular). If concern also exists about immune status regarding mumps or rubella, revaccination with appropriate monovalent or polyvalent vaccines should be considered after consulting the appropriate product circulars. Unnecessary doses of a vaccine are best avoided by ensuring that written documentation of vaccination is preserved and a copy given to each vaccinee's parent or guardian.

---

* *Note:* The Immunization Practices Advisory Committee (ACIP) has recommended "In view of the importance of protecting this age group against rubella, reasonable precautions in a rubella immunization program include asking females if they are pregnant, excluding those who say they are, and explaining the theoretical risks to the others."

** *Note:* The Immunization Practices Advisory Commitee (ACIP) has stated "When practical, and when reliable laboratory services are available, potential vaccinees of childbearing age can have serologic tests to determine susceptibility to rubella.... However, routinely performing serologic tests for all females of childbearing age to determine susceptibility so that vaccine is given only to proven susceptibles is expensive and has been ineffective in some areas. Accordingly, the ACIP believes that rubella vaccination of a woman who is not known to be pregnant and has no history of vaccination is justifiable without serologic testing."

***Note: A primary difference among these recommendations is the timing of revaccination: the ACIP recommends routine revaccination at entry into Kindergarten or first grade, whereas the AAP recommends routine revaccination at entrance to middle school or junior high school. In addition, some public health jurisdictions mandate the age of revaccination. The complete text of applicable guidelines should be consulted.

USE WITH OTHER VACCINES.

Routine administration of DTP (diphteria, tetanus, pertusis) and/or OPV (oral poliovirus vaccine) concomitantly with measles, mumps and rubella vaccines is not recommended because there are insufficient data relating to the simultaneous administration of these antigens. However, the American Academy of Pediatrics had noted that in some circumstances, particualrly when the patient may not return, some practitioners prefer to administer all these antigens on a single day. If done, separate sites and syringes should be used for DTP and Measles and Rubella vaccine.

Measles and Rubella Vaccine should not be given less than one month before or after administration of other virus vaccines.

CONTRAINDICATIONS

Do not give Measles and Rubella vaccine to pregnant females; the possible effects of the vaccine on fetal development are unknown at this time. If vaccination of postpurbertal females is undertaken, pregnancy should be avoided for three months following vaccination. (See *"Precautions, "Pregnancy"*.)

Anaphylactic or anaphylactoid reactions to neomycin (each dose of reconstituted vaccine contains approximately 25 mcg of neomycin).

History of anaphylactic or anaphylactoid reactions to eggs (see *"Hypersensitivity to Eggs,"* below).

Any febrile respiratory illness or other active febrile infection.

Active untreated tuberculosis.

Patients receiving immunosuppressive therapy. This contra-indication does not appy to patients who are receiving corticosteroids as replacement therapy, e.g., for Addison's disease.

Individuals with blood dyscrasias, leukemia, lymphomas of any type, or other malignant neoplasms affecting the bone marrrow or lymphatic systems.

Primary and acquired immunodeficiency states, including patients who are immunosuppressed in association with AIDS or other clinical manifestations of infection with human immunodeficiency viruses; cellular immune deficiencies; and hypogrammaglobulinemic and dysgammaglobulinemic states.

Individuals with a family history of congenital or hereditary immunodeficiency, until the immune competence of the potential vaccine recipient is demonstrated.

HYPERSENSITIVITY TO EGGS

Live measles vaccine is produced in chick embryo cell culture. Persons with a history of anaphylactic, anaphylactoid, or other immediate reactions (e.g., hive, swelling of the mouth and throat, difficulty breathing, hypotension, or shock) subsequent to egg ingestion should not be vaccinated. Evidence indicates that persons are not at increased risk if they have egg allergies that are not anphylactic or anaphylactoid in nature. Such persons may be vaccinated in the usual manner. There is no evidence to indicate that persons with allergies to chicken or feathers are at increased risk of reaction to the vaccine.

PRECAUTIONS

GENERAL

Adequate treatment provisions including epinephrine, should be available for immediate use should an anaphylactic or anaphylactoid reaction occur.

Due caution should be employed in administration of Measles and Rubella Vaccine to persons with a history of cerebral injury, individual or family histories of convulsions, or any other condition in which stress due to fever should be avoided. The physician should be alert to the temperature elevation which may occur following vaccination. (See *"Adverse Reactions"*.) Children and young adults who are known to be infected with human immunodeficiency viruses but without overt clinical manifestations of immunosuppression may be vaccinated; however, the vaccinees should be monitored closely for vaccine-preventable diseases because immunization may be less effective than for uninfected persons.

Vaccination should be deferred for at least 3 months following blood or plasma transfusions, or administration of human immune serum globulin.

Excretion of small amounts of the live attenuated Rubella Virus from the nose or throat has occurred in the majority of susceptible individuals 7-28 days after vaccination. There is no confirmed evidence to indicate that such virus is transmitted to susceptible persons who are in contact with the vaccinated individuals. Consequently, transmission through close personal contact, while accepted as a theoretical possibility, is not regarded as a significant risk. However, transmission of the Rubella Vaccine Virus to infants via breast milk has been documented (see *"Nursing Mothers"*).

There are no reports of transmission of live attenuated Measles Virus from vaccinees to susceptible contacts.

It has been reported that live attenuated Measles and Rubella Virus Vaccines given individually may result in a temporary depression of tuberculin skin sensitivity. Therefore, if a tuberculin test is to be done, it should be administered either before or simultaneously with Measles and Rubella Vaccine.

Children under treatment for tuberculosis have not experienced exacerbation of the disease when immunized with live Measles Virus Vaccine; no studies have been reported to date of the effect of Measles Virus Vaccines on untreated tuberculous children.

As for any vaccine, vaccination with Measles and Rubella Vaccine may not result in seroconversion in 100% of susceptible persons given the vaccine.

PREGNANCY
PREGNANCY CATEGORY C
Animal reproduction studies have not been conducted with Measles and Rubella Vaccine. It is also not known whether Measles and Rubella Vaccine can cause fetal harm when administered to a pregnant woman or can affect reproduction capacity. Therefore, the vaccine should not be administered to pregnant females; furthermore, pregnancy should be avoided for three months following vaccination (see "Contraindications").

In counseling women who are inadvertently vaccinated when pregnant or who become pregnant within 3 months of vaccination, the physician should be aware of the following: (1) In a 10 year survey involving over 700 pregnant women who received Rubella Vaccine within 3 months before or after conception, (of whom 189 received the Wistar RA 27/3 strain), none of the newborns had abnormalities compatible with congenital rubella syndrome: (2) Reports have indicated that contracting of natural measles during pregnancy enhances fetal risk. Increased rates of spontaneous abortion, stillbirth, congenital defects and prematurity have been observed subsequent to natural measles during pregnancy. There are no adequate studies of the attenuated (vaccine) strain of measles virus in pregnancy. However, it would be prudent to assume that the vaccine strain of virus is also capable of inducing adverse fetal effects.

NURSING MOTHERS
It is not known whether measles vaccine virus is secreted in human milk. Recent studies have shown that lactating postpartum women immunized with live attenuated Rubella Vaccine may secrete the virus in breast milk and transmit it to breast-fed infants. In the infants with serological evidence of rubella infection, none exhibited severe disease; however, one exhibited mild clinical illness typical of acquired Rubella. Caution should be exercised when Measles and Rubella Vaccine is administered to a nursing woman.

ADVERSE REACTIONS
Burning and/or stinging of short duration at the injection site have been reported.

The adverse clinical reactions associated with the use of Measles and Rubella Vaccine are those expected to follow administration of the monovalent vaccines given separately. These may include malaise, sore throat, cough, rhinitis, headache, dizziness, fever, rash, nausea, vomiting or diarrhea; mild local reactions such as erythema, induration, tenderness and regional lymphadenopathy; thrombocytopenia and purpura; allergic reactions such as wheal and flare at the injection site or urticaria; polyneuritis, and arthralgia and/or arthritis (usually transient and rarely chronic).

Anaphylaxis and anaphylactoid reactions have been reported.

Vasculitis has been reported rarely.

Moderate fever [101-102.9°F (38.3-39.4°C)] occurs occasionally, and high fever [above 103°F (39.4°C)] occurs less commonly. On rare occasions, children developing fever may exhibit febrile convulsions. Afebrile convulsions or seizures have occurred rarely following vaccination with live attenuated Measles Vaccine. Syncope, particularly at the time of mass vaccination, has been reported. Rash occurs infrequently and is usually minimal, but rarely may be generalized. Erythema multiforme has also been reported rarely. Forms of optic neuritis, including retrobulbar neuritis, papillitis, and retinitis may infrequently follow viral infections, and have been reported to occur 1 to 3 weeks following inoculation with some live virus vaccines.

Clinical experience with live attenuated Measles and Rubella Virus Vaccines given individually indicates that encephalitis and other nervous system reactions have occurred very rarely. These might occur also with Measles and Rubella Vaccine.

Experience from more than 80 million doses of all live Measles Vaccines given in the U.S. through 1975 indicates that significant central nervous system reactions such as encephalitis and encephalopathy, occurring within 30 days after vaccination, have been temporally associated with Measles Vaccine very rarely. In no case has it been shown that reaction were actually caused by vaccine. The Center for Disease Control has pointed out that "a certain number of cases of encephalitis may be expected to occur in a large childhood population in a defined period of time even when no vaccines are administered." However, the data suggest the possibility that some of these cases may have been caused by Measles Vaccines. The risk of such serious neurological disorders following Live Measles Virus Vaccine administration remains far less than that for encephalitis and encephalopathy with natural measles (one per two thousand reported cases).

There have been rare reports of ocular palsies, Guillain-Barré syndrome, or ataxia occurring after immunization with vaccines containing live attenuated Measles Virus. The ocular palsies have occurred approximately 3-24 days following vaccination. No definite causal relationship has been established between these events and vaccination. Isolated reports of polyneuropathy including Guillain-Barré syndrome have also been reported after immunization with rubella-containing vaccines.

There have been reports of subacute sclerosing panencephalitis (SSPE) in children who did not have a history of natural measles but did receive Measles Vaccine. Some of these cases may have resulted from unrecognized measles in the first year of life or possibly from the Measles Vaccination. Based on estimated nationwide Measles Vaccine distribution, the association of SSPE cases to Measles Vaccination is about one case per million vaccine doses distributed. This is far less than the association with natural measles, 6-22 cases of SSPE per million cases of measles. The results of a retrospective case-controlled study conducted by the Center for Disease Control suggest that the overall effect of Measles Vaccine has been to protect against SSPE by preventing measles with its inherent higher risk of SSPE.

Local reactions characterized by marked swelling, redness and vesiculation at the injection site of attenuated Live Measles Virus Vaccines, and systemic reactions including atypical measles, have occurred in persons who received killed measles vaccine previously. Measles and Rubella Vaccine was not given under this condition in clinical trials. Rarely, more severe reactions that require hospitalization, including prolonged high fevers and extensive local reactions, have been reported. Panniculitis has been reported rarely following administration of Measles Vaccine.

Arthralgia and/or arthritis (usually transient and rarely chronic), and polyneuritis are features of natural rubella and vary in frequency and severity with age and sex, being greatest in adult females and least in prepubertal children. This type of involvement as well as myalgia and paresthesia have also been reported following administration of Rubella Virus Vaccine Live.

Chronic arthritis has been associated with natural rubella infection and has been related to persistent virus and/or viral antigen isolated from body tissues. Only rarely have vaccine recipients developed chronic joint symptoms.

Following vaccination in children, reactions in joints are uncommon and generally of brief duration. In women, incidence rates for arthritis and arthralgia are generally higher than those seen in children (children: 0-3%; women: 12-20%), and the reactions tend to be more marked and of longer duration. Symptoms may persist for a matter of months or on rare occasions for years. In adolescent girls, the reactions appear to be intermediate in incidence between those seen in children and in adult women. Even in older women (35-45 years), these reactions are generally well tolerated and rarely interfere with normal activities.

DOSAGE AND ADMINISTRATION
FOR SUBCUTANEOUS ADMINISTRATION
Do not inject intravenously: The dosage of vaccine is the same for all persons. Inject the total volume of the single dose vial (about 0.5 mL) or 0.5 mL of the multiple dose vial of reconstituted vaccine subcutaneously, preferably into the outer aspect of upper arm. *Do not give immune globulin (IG) concurrently with* Measles and Rubella Vaccine. During shipment, to insure that there is no loss of potency, the vaccine must be maintained at a temperature of 10°C (50°F) or less.

Before reconstitution, store Measles and Rubella Vaccine at 2-8°C (36-46°F).

Protect from light.

Caution: A sterile syringe free of preservatives, antiseptics, and detergents should be used for each injection and/or reconstitution of the vaccine because these substances may inactivate the live virus vaccine. A 25 gauge, 5/8" needle is recommended.

To reconstitute, use only the diluent supplied, since it is free of preservatives or other antiviral substances which might inactivate the vaccine.

Single Dose Vial: First withdraw the entire volume of diluent into the siringe to be used for reconstitution. Inject all the diluent in the syringe into the vial of lyophilized vaccine, and agitate to mix thoroughly. Withdraw the entire contents into a syringe and inject the total volume of restored vaccine subcutaneously.

It is important to use a separate sterile syringe and needle for each individual patient to prevent transmission of hepatitis B and other infectious agents from one person to another.

10 Dose Vial (available only to government agencies/institutions): Withdraw the entire contents (7 mL) of the diluent vial into the sterile syringe to be used for reconstitution, and introduce into the 10 dose vial of lyophilized vaccine. Agitate to ensure thorough mixing. The outer labeling suggests "For Jet Injector or Syringe Use". Use with separate sterile syringes is permitted for containers of 10 doses or less. The vaccine and diluent do not contain preservatives; therefore, the user must recognize the potential contamination hazards and exercise special precautions to protect the sterility and potency of the product. The use of aseptic techniques and proper storage prior to and after restoration of the vaccine and subsequent withdrawal of the individual doses is essential. Use 0.5 mL of the reconstituted vaccine for subcutaneous injection.

It is important to use a separate sterile syringe and needle for each individual patient to prevent transmission of hepatitis B and other infectious agents from one person to another.

50 Dose Vial (available only to government agencies/institutions): Withdraw the entire contents (30 mL) of diluent vial into the sterile syringe to be used for reconstitution and introduce into the 50 dose vial of lyophilized vaccine. Agitate to ensure thorough mixing. With full aseptic precautions, attach the vial to the sterilized multidose jet injector apparatus. Use 0.5 mL of the reconstituted vaccine for subcutaneous injection.

Each dose contains not less than the equivalent of 1,000 $TCID_{50}$ of the U.S. Reference Measles Virus and 1,000 $TCID_{50}$ of the U.S. Reference Rubella Virus.

Parenteral drug products should be inspected visually for particulate matter and discoloration prior to administration. Measles and Rubella Vaccine, when reconstituted, is clear yellow.

STORAGE
It is recommended that the vaccine be used as soon as possible after reconstitution. Protect vaccine from light at all times, since such exposure may inactivate the virus. Store reconstituted vaccine in the vaccine vial in a dark place at 2-8°C (36-46°F) and discard if not used within 8 hours.

HOW SUPPLIED
INJECTION:

BRAND/MANUFACTURER	NDC	SIZE	AWP
○ **BRAND**			
M-R-VAX II: Merck	00006-4751-00	1 ml	$20.63
	00006-4677-00	1 ml 10s	$169.88

Measles Virus Vaccine

DESCRIPTION
Measles Virus Vaccine is a live virus vaccine for immunization against measles (rubeola).

Measles Virus Vaccine is a sterile lyophilized preparation of a more attenuated line of measles virus derived from Enders' attenuated Edmonston strain. The further modification of the virus in Measles Virus Vaccine was achieved in the Merck Institute for Therapeutic Research by multiple passage of Edmonston strain virus in cell cultures of chick embryo at low temperature.

The reconstituted vaccine is for subcutaneous administration. When reconstituted as directed, the dose for injection is 0.5 mL and contains not less than the equivalent of 1,000 $TCID_{50}$ (tissue culture infectious doses) of the U.S. Reference Measles Virus. Each dose also contains approximately 25 mcg of neomycin.

CLINICAL PHARMACOLOGY
Measles Virus Vaccine produces a modified measles infection in susceptible persons. Fever and rash may appear. Extensive clinical trials have demonstrated that Measles Virus Vaccine is highly immunogenic and generally well tolerated. A single injection of the vaccine has been shown to induce measles hemagglutination-inhibiting (HI) antibodies in 97 percent or more of susceptible persons. Vaccine-induced antibody levels have been shown to persist for at least 13 years without substantial decline. Continued surveillance will be necessary to determine further duration of antibody persistence.

INDICATIONS AND USAGE
Measles Virus Vaccine is indicated for immunization against measles (rubeola) in persons 15 months of age or older. A second dose of Measles Virus Vaccine is recommended (see "Revaccination"). Infants who are less than 15 months of age may fail to respond to the vaccine due to presence in the circulation of residual measles antibody of maternal origin; the younger the infant, the lower the likelihood of seroconversion. In geographically isolated or other relatively inaccessible populations for whom immunization programs are logistically difficult, and in population groups in which natural measles infection may occur in a significant proportion of infants before 15 months of age, it may be desirable to give the vaccine to infants at an earlier age. Infants vaccinated under these conditiosn at less than 12 months of age should be revaccinated after reaching 15 months of age. There is some evidence to suggest that infants immunized at less than one year of age may not develop sustained antibody levels when later reimmunized. The advantage of early protection must be weighed against the chance for failure to respond adequately on reimmunization.

According to ACIP recommendations, most persons born in 1956 or earlier are likely to have been infected naturally and generally need not be considered susceptible. All children, adolescents, and adults born after 1956 are considered susceptible and should be vaccinated, if there are no contraindications. This includes persons who may be immune to measles but who lack adequate documentation of immunity as evidenced by: (1) physician-diagnosed measles, (2) laboratory evidence of measles immunity, or (3) adequate immunization with live Measles Vaccine on or after the first birthday.

Measles Virus Vaccine given immediately after exposure to natural measles may provide some protection. If, however, the vaccine is given a few days before exposure, substantial protection may be provided.

Individuals planning travel outside the United States, if not immune, can acquire measles, mumps or rubella and import these diseases to the United States. Therefore, prior to international travel, individuals known to be susceptible to one or more of these diseases can receive either a single antigen vaccine (measles, mumps or rubella), or a combined antigen vaccine as appropriate. However, Measles, Mumps, and Rubella Virus Vaccine Live is preferred for persons likely to be susceptible to mumps and rubella; and if single-antigen Measles Vaccine is not readily available, travelers should receive Measles, Mumps, and Rubella Virus Vaccine Live, regardless of their immune status to mumps or rubella.

Revaccination: Children first vaccinated when younger than 12 months of age should be revaccinated at 15 months of age, particularly if vaccine was administered with immune serum globulin or measles immune globulin, a standardized globulin preparation.

The American Academy of Pediatrics (AAP), the Immunization Practices Advisory Committee (ACIP), and some state and local health agencies have recommended guidelines for routine measles revaccination and to help control measles outbreaks.*

---

* *Note:* A primary difference among these recommendations is the timing of revaccination: the ACIP recommends routine revaccination at entry into kindergarten or first grade, whereas the AAP recommends routine revaccination at entrance to middle school or junior high school. In addition, some public health jurisdictions mandate the age for revaccination. The complete text of applicable guidelines should be consulted.

Vaccines available for revaccination include monovalent measles vaccine (Measles Virus Vaccine) and polyvalent vaccines containing measles (e.g., Measles, Mumps, and Rubella Virus Vaccine Live, Measles and Rubella Virus Vaccine Live). If the prevention of sporadic measles outbreaks is the sole objective, revaccination with a monovalent Measles Vaccine should be considered (see appropriate product circular). If concern also exists about immune status regarding mumps or rubella, revaccination with appropriate monovalent or polyvalent vaccines should be considered after consulting the appropriate product circulars. Unnecessary doses of a vaccine are best avoided by ensuring that written documentation of vaccination is preserved and a copy given to each vaccinee's parent or guardian.

Despite the risk of reactions (see "*Adverse Reactions*"), persons born since 1956 who have previously been given inactivated vaccine alone or followed by live vaccine within 3 months should be revaccinated with live vaccine to reduce the risk of the severe atypical form of natural measles that may occur.

USE WITH OTHER VACCINES
Routine administration of DTP (diphtheria, tetanus, pertussis) and/or OPV (oral poliovirus vaccine) concomitantly with measles, mumps and rubella vaccines is not recommended because there are insufficient data relating to the simultaneous administration of these antigens. However, the American Academy of Pediatrics has noted that in some circumstances, particularly when the patient may not return, some practitioners prefer to administer all these antigens on a single day. If done, separate sites and syringes should be used for DTP and Measles Virus Vaccine.

Measles Virus Vaccine should not be given less than one month *before or after* administration of other virus vaccines.

CONTRAINDICATIONS
Do not give Measles Virus Vaccine to pregnant females; the possible effects of the vaccine on fetal development are unknown at this time. If vaccination of postpubertal females is undertaken, pregnancy should be avoided for three months following vaccination (see "*Precautions, Pregnancy*").

Anaphylactic or anaphylactoid reactions to neomycin (each dose of reconstituted vaccine contains approximately 25 mcg of neomycin).

History of anaphylactic or anaphylactoid reactions to eggs (see "*Hypersensitivity to Eggs*" below).

Any febrile respiratory illness or other active febrile infection.

Active untreated tuberculosis.

Patients receiving immunosuppressive therapy. This contraindication does not apply to patients who are receiving corticosteroids as replacement therapy, e.g., for Addison's disease.

Individuals with blood dyscrasias, leukemia, lymphomas of any type, or other malignant neoplasms affecting the bone marrow or lymphatic systems.

Primary and acquired immunodeficiency states, including patients who are immunosuppressed in association with AIDS or other clinical manifestations of infection with human immunodeficiency viruses; cellular immune deficiencies; and hypogammaglobulinemic and dysgammaglobulinemic states.

Individuals with a family history of congenital or hereditary immunodeficiency, until the immune competence of the potential vaccine recipient is demonstrated.

HYPERSENSITIVITY TO EGGS
Live Measles Vaccine is produced in chick embryo cell culture. Persons with a history of anaphylactic, anaphylactoid or other immediate reactions (e.g., hives, swelling of the mouth and throat, difficulty breathing, hypotension and shock) subsequent to egg ingestion should not be vaccinated. Evidence indicates that persons are not at increased risk if they have egg allergies that are not anaphylactic or anaphylactoid in nature. Such persons should be vaccinated in the usual manner. There is no evidence to indicate that persons with allergies to chickens or feathers are at increased risk of reaction to the vaccine.

PRECAUTIONS
GENERAL
Adequate treatment provisions including epinephrine, should be available for immediate use should an anaphylactic or anaphylactoid reaction occur.

Due caution should be employed in administration of Measles Vaccine to persons with a history of cerebral injury, individual or family histories of convulsions, or of any other condition in which stress due to fever should be avoided. The physician should be alert to the temperature elevation which may occur following vaccination. (See "*Adverse Reactions*".)

Children and young adults who are known to be infected with human immunodeficiency viruses but without overt clinical manifestations of immunosuppression may be vaccinated; however, the vaccinees should be monitored closely for vaccine-preventable diseases because immunization may be less effective than for uninfected persons.

Vaccination should be deferred for at least 3 months following blood or plasma transfusions, or administration of human immune serum globulin.

There are no reports of transmission of live attenuated measles virus from vaccinees to susceptible contacts.

It has been reported that attenuated Measles Virus Vaccine, live, may result in a temporary depression of tuberculin skin sensitivity. Therefore, if a tuberculin test is to be done, it should be administered either before or simultaneously with Measles Virus Vaccine.

Children under treatment for tuberculosis have not experienced exacerbation of the disease when immunized with live Measles Virus Vaccine; no studies have been reported to date of the effect of Measles Virus Vaccines on untreated tuberculous children.

As for any vaccine, vaccination with Measles Virus Vaccine may not result in seroconversion in 100% of susceptible persons given the vaccine.

PREGNANCY
PREGNANCY CATEGORY C
Animal reproduction studies have not been conducted with Measles Virus Vaccine. It is also not known whether Measles Virus Vaccine can cause fetal harm when administered to a pregnant woman or can affect reproduction capacity. Therefore, the vaccine should not be administered to pregnant females; furthermore, pregnancy should be avoided for three months following vaccination (see *"Contraindications"*).

Reports have indicated that contracting of natural measles during pregnancy enhances fetal risk. Increased rates of spontaneous abortion, stillbirth, congenital defects and prematurity have been observed subsequent to natural measles during pregnancy. There are no adequate studies of the attenuated (vaccine) strain of measles virus in pregnancy. However, it would be prudent to assume that the vaccine strain of virus is also capable of inducing adverse fetal effects for up to three months following vaccination.

Vaccine administration to postpubertal females entails a potential for inadvertent immunization during pregnancy. Theoretical risks involved should be weighed against the risks that measles poses to the unimmunized adolescent or adult. Advisory committees reviewing this matter have recommended vaccination of postpubertal females who are presumed to be susceptible to measles and not known to be pregnant. If a measles exposure occurs during pregnancy, one should consider the possibility of providing temporary passive immunity through the administration of immune globulin (human).

NURSING MOTHERS
It is not known whether Measles Vaccine Virus is secreted in human milk. Therefore, because many drugs are excreted in human milk, caution should be exercised when Measles Virus Vaccine is administered to a nursing woman.

ADVERSE REACTIONS
Burning and/or stinging of short duration at the injection site have been reported.
Anaphylaxis and anaphylactoid reactions have been reported.

OCCASIONAL
Moderate fever [101-102.9°F (38.3-39.4°C)] may occur during the month after vaccination. Generally, fever, rash, or both appear between the 5th and the 12th days. Cough and rhinitis have also been reported. Rash, when it occurs, is usually minimal, but rarely may be generalized. Erythema multiforme has also been reported rarely.

LESS COMMON
High fever [over 103°F (39.4°C)]. Mild lymphadenopathy has been reported.

RARE
Reactions at injection site. Allergic reactions such as wheal and flare at the injection site or urticaria have been reported.

Diarrhea has been reported after vaccination with measles-containing vaccines.

Children developing fever may, on rare occasions, exhibit febrile convulsions. Afebrile convulsions or seizures have occurred rarely following vaccination with live attenuated Measles Vaccine. Syncope, particularly at the time of mass vaccination, has been reported.

Thrombocytopenia and purpura have occurred rarely.

Vasculitis has been reported rarely.

Forms of optic neuritis, including retrobulbar neuritis, papillitis, and retinitis may infrequently follow viral infections, and have been reported to occur 1 to 3 weeks following inoculation with some live virus vaccines.

Experience from more than 80 million doses of all live Measles Vaccines given in the U.S. through 1975 indicates that significant central nervous system reactions such as encephalitis and encephalopathy, occurring within 30 days after vaccination, have been temporally associated with Measles Vaccine very rarely. In no case has it been shown that reactions were actually caused by vaccine. The Center for Disease Control has pointed out that "a certain number of cases of encephalitis may be expected to occur in a large childhood population in a defined period of time even when no vaccines are administered". However, the data suggest the possibility that some of these cases may have been caused by Measles Vaccines. The risk of such serious neurological disorders following live Measles Virus Vaccine administration remains far less than that for encephalitis and encephalopathy with natural measles (one per two thousand reported cases).

There have been rare reports of ocular palsies, Guillain-Barré syndrome, or ataxia occurring after immunization with vaccines containing live attenuated measles virus. The ocular palsies have occurred approximately 3-24 days following vaccination. No definite causal relationship has been established between either of these events and vaccination. There have been reports of subacute sclerosing panencephalitis (SSPE) in children who did not have a history of natural measles but did receive Measles Vaccine. Some of these cases may have resulted from unrecognized measles in the first year of life or possibly from the measles vaccination. Based on estimated nationwide Measles Vaccine distribution, the association of SSPE cases to measles vaccination is about one case per million vaccine doses distributed. This is far less than the association with natural measles, 6-22 cases of SSPE per million cases of measles. The results of a retrospective case-controlled study conducted by the Center for Disease Control suggest that the overall effect of Measles Vaccine has been to protect against SSPE by preventing measles with its inherent higher risk of SSPE.

Local reactions characterized by marked swelling, redness and vesiculation at the injection site of attenuated live virus Measles Vaccines, and systemic reactions including atypical measles, have occurred in persons who have previously received killed Measles Vaccine. Rarely, more severe reactions that require hospitalization, including prolonged high fevers, panniculitis, and extensive local reactions, have been reported.

DOSAGE AND ADMINISTRATION
FOR SUBCUTANEOUS ADMINISTRATION
Do not inject intravenously: The dosage of vaccine is the same for all persons. Inject the total volume of the single dose vial (about 0.5 mL) or 0.5 mL of the multiple dose vial of reconstituted vaccine subcutaneously, preferably into the outer aspect of upper arm. *Do not give immune globulin (IG) concurrently with* Measles Virus Vaccine. During shipment, to insure that there is no loss of potency, the vaccine must be maintained at a temperature of 10°C (50°F) or less.

Before reconstitution, store Measles Virus Vaccine at 2-8°C (36-46°F). *Protect from light.*

Caution: A sterile syringe free of preservatives, antiseptics, and detergents should be used for each injection and/or reconstitution of the vaccine because these substances may inactivate the live virus vaccine. A 25 gauge, ⅝" needle is recommended.

To reconstitute, use only the diluent supplied, since it is free of preservatives or other antiviral substances which might inactivate the vaccine.

Single Dose Vial: First withdraw the entire volume of diluent into the syringe to be used for reconstitution. Inject all the diluent in the syringe into the vial of lyophilized vaccine, and agitate to mix thoroughly. Withdraw the entire contents into a syringe and inject the total volume of restored vaccine subcutaneously.

It is important to use a separate sterile syringe and needle for each individual patient to prevent transmission of hepatitis B and other infectious agents from one person to another.

10 Dose Vial (available only to government agencies/institutions): Withdraw the entire contents (7 mL) of the diluent vial into the sterile syringe to be used for reconstitution, and introduce into the 10 dose vial of lyophilized vaccine. Agitate to ensure thorough mixing. The outer labeling suggests "For Jet Injector or Syringe Use". Use with separate sterile syringes is permitted for containers of 10 doses or less. The vaccine and diluent do not contain preservatives; therefore, the user must recognize the potential contamination hazards and exercise special precautions to protect the sterility and potency of the product. The use of aseptic techniques and proper storage prior to and after restoration of the vaccine and subsequent withdrawal of the individual doses is essential. Use 0.5 mL of the reconstituted vaccine for subcutaneous injection.

It is important to use a separate sterile syringe and needle for each individual patient to prevent transmission of hepatitis B and other infectious agents from one person to another.

50 Dose Vial (available only to government agencies/institutions): Withdraw the entire contents (30 mL) of diluent vial into the sterile syringe to be used for reconstitution and introduce into the 50 dose vial of lyophilized vaccine. Agitate to ensure thorough mixing. With full aseptic precautions, attach the vial to the sterilized multidose jet injector apparatus. Use 0.5 mL of the reconstituted vaccine for subcutaneous injection.

Each dose of Measles Virus Vaccine contains not less than 1,000 TCID50 (tissue culture infectious doses) of Measles Virus Vaccine expressed in terms of the assigned titer of the U.S. Reference Measles Virus.

Parenteral drug products should be inspected visually for particulate matter and discoloration prior to administration. Measles Virus Vaccine, when reconstituted, is clear yellow.

It is recommended that the vaccine be used as soon as possible after reconstitution. Protect vaccine from light at all times, since such exposure may inactivate the virus. Store reconstituted vaccine in the vaccine vial in a dark place at 2-8°C (36-46°F) and discard if not used within 8 hours.

HOW SUPPLIED
POWDER FOR INJECTION:

BRAND/MANUFACTURER	NDC	SIZE	AWP
○ BRAND			
ATTENUVAX: Merck	00006-4709-00	1s	$12.75
	00006-4589-00	10s	$101.00

Measles/Mumps/Rubella Virus Vaccine Live

DESCRIPTION
Measles/Mumps/Rubella Vaccine Live is a live virus vaccine for immunization against measles (rubeola), mumps and rubella (German measles). Measles/Mumps/Rubella Vaccine Live is a sterile lyophilized preparation of (1) Measles Virus Vaccine Live, a more attenuated line of measles virus, derived from Enders' attenuated Edmonston strain and grown in cell cultures of chick embryo; (2) Mumps Virus Vaccine Live, the Jeryl Lynn (B level) strain of mumps virus grown in cell cultures of chick embryo; and (3) Rubella Virus Vaccine Live, the Wistar RA27/3 strain of live attenuated rubella virus grown in human diploid cell (WI-38) culture. The vaccine viruses are the same as those used in the manufacture of

Measles Virus Vaccine Live, Mumps Virus Vaccine Live, Rubella Virus Vaccine Live. The three viruses are mixed before being lyophilized. The product contains no preservative.

The reconstituted vaccine is for subcutaneous administration. When reconstituted as directed, the dose for injection is 0.5 mL and contains not less than the equivalent of 1,000 $TCID_{50}$ (tissue culture infectious doses) of the U.S. Reference Measles Virus; 20,000 $TCID_{50}$ of the U.S. Reference Mumps Virus; and 1,000 $TCID_{50}$ of the U.S. Reference Rubella Virus. Each dose contains approximately 25 mcg of neomycin. The product contains no preservative.

CLINICAL PHARMACOLOGY

Clinical studies of 279 triple seronegative children, 11 months to 7 years of age, demonstrated that Measles/Mumps/Rubella Vaccine Live is highly immunogenic and generally well tolerated. In these studies, a single injection of the vaccine induced measles hemagglutination-inhibition (HI) antibodies in 95 percent, mumps neutralizing antibodies in 96 percent, and rubella HI antibodies in 99 percent of susceptible persons.

The RA 27/3 rubella strain in Measles/Mumps/Rubella Vaccine Live elicits higher immediate post-vaccination HI, complement-fixing and neutralizing antibody levels than other strains of rubella vaccine and has been shown to induce a broader profile of circulating antibodies including anti-theta and anti-iota precipitating antibodies. The RA 27/3 rubella strain immunologically simulates natural infection more closely than other rubella vaccine viruses. The increased levels and broader profile of antibodies produced by RA 27/3 strain rubella virus vaccine appear to correlate with greater resistance to subclinical reinfection with the wild virus, and provide greater confidence for lasting immunity.

Vaccine induced antibody levels following administration of Measles/Mumps/Rubella Vaccine Live have been shown to persist up to 11 years without substantial decline. Continued surveillance will be necessary to determine further duration of antibody persistence.

INDICATIONS AND USAGE

Measles/Mumps/Rubella Vaccine Live is indicated for simultaneous immunization against measles, mumps, and rubella in persons 15 months of age or older. A second dose of Measles/Mumps/Rubella Vaccine Live or monovalent measles vaccine is recommended (see "Revaccination").

Infants who are less than 15 months of age may fail to respond to the measles component of the vaccine due to presence in the circulation of residual measles antibody of maternal origin, the younger the infant, the lower the likelihood of seroconversion. In geographically isolated or other relatively inaccessible populations for whom immunization programs are logistically difficult, and in population groups in which natural measles infection may occur in a significant proportion of infants before 15 months of age, it may be desirable to give the vaccine to infants at an earlier age. Infants vaccinated under these conditions at less than 12 months of age should be revaccinated after reaching 15 months of age. There is some evidence to suggest that infants immunized at less than one year of age may not develop sustained antibody levels when later reimmunized. The advantage of early protection must be weighed against the chance for failure to respond adequately on reimmunization.

Previously unimmunized children of susceptible pregnant women should receive live attenuated rubella vaccine, because an immunized child will be less likely to acquire natural rubella and introduce the virus into the household.

Individuals planning travel outside the United States, if not immune, can acquire measles, mumps or rubella and import these diseases to the United States. Therefore, prior to international travel, individuals known to be susceptible to one or more of these diseases can receive either a single antigen vaccine (measles, mumps or rubella), or a combined antigen vaccine as appropriate. However, Measles/Mumps/Rubella Vaccine Live is preferred for persons likely to be susceptible to mumps and rubella; and if single-antigen measles vaccine is not readily available, travelers should receive Measles/Mumps/Rubella Vaccine Live regardless of their immune status to mumps or rubella.

NONPREGNANT ADOLESCENT AND ADULT FEMALES

Immunization of susceptible non-pregnant adolescent and adult females of childbearing age with live attenuated Rubella Virus Vaccine is indicated if certain precautions are observed (see below and "Precautions"). Vaccinating susceptible postpubertal females confers individual protection against subsequently acquiring rubella infection during pregnancy, which in turn prevents infection of the fetus and consequent congenital rubella injury.

Women of childbearing age should be advised not to become pregnant for three months after vaccination and should be informed of the reasons for this precaution.*

It is recommended that rubella susceptibility be determined by serologic testing prior to immunization.** If immune, as evidenced by a specific rubella antibody

---

* NOTE: The Immunization Practices Advisory Committee (ACIP) has recommended "In view of the importance of protecting this age group against rubella, reasonable precautions in a rubella immunization program include asking females if they are pregnant, excluding those who say they are, and explaining the theoretical risks to the others."
** NOTE: The Immunization Practices Advisory Committee (ACIP) has stated "When practical, and when reliable laboratory services are available, potential vaccinees of childbearing age can have serologic tests to determine susceptibility to rubella.... However, routinely performing serologic tests for all females of childbearing age to determine susceptibility so that vaccine is given only to proven susceptibles is expensive and has been ineffective in some areas. Accordingly, the ACIP believes that rubella vaccination of a woman who is not known to be pregnant and has no history of vaccination is justifiable without serologic testing."

---

titer of 1:8 or greater (hemagglutination-inhibition test), vaccination is unnecessary. Congenital malformations do occur in up to seven percent of all live births. Their chance appearance after vaccination could lead to misinterprtation of the cause, particularly if the prior rubella-immune status of vaccinees is unknown.

Postpubertal females should be informed of the frequent occurrence of generally self-limited arthralgia and/or arthritis beginning 2 to 4 weeks after vaccination (see "Adverse Reactions").

POSTPARTUM WOMEN
It has been found convenient in many instances to vaccinate rubella-susceptible women in the immediate postpartum period. (See "Nursing Mothers").

Revaccination: Children first vaccinated when younger than 12 months of age should be revaccinated at 15 months of age.

The American Academy of Pediatrics (AAP), the Immunization Practices Advisory Committee (ACIP), and some state and local health agencies have recommended guidelines for routine measles revaccination and to help control measles outbreaks.†

Vaccines available for revaccination include monovalent measles vaccine, Measles Virus Vaccine Live and polyvalent vaccines containing measles [e.g., Measles/Mumps/Rubella Vaccine Live, Measles and Rubella Virus Vaccine Live]. If the prevention of sporadic measles outbreaks is the sole objective, revaccination with a monovalent measles vaccine should be considered (see appropriate product circular). If concern also exists about immune status regarding mumps or rubella, revaccination with appropriate monovalent or polyvalent vaccine should be considered after consulting the appropriate product circulars. Unnecessary doses of a vaccine are best avoided by ensuring that written documentation of vaccination is preserved and a copy given to each vaccinee's parent or guardian.

USE WITH OTHER VACCINES
Routine administration of DTP (diphtheria, tetanus, pertussis) and/or OPV (oral poliovirus vaccine) concomitantly with Measles, Mumps, and Rubella Vaccines is not recommended because there are limited data relating to the simultaneous administration of these antigens. Measles/Mumps/Rubella Vaccine Live should be given one month before or after administration of other vaccines. However, other schedules have been used. For example, the American Academy of Pediatrics has noted that when the patient may not return, some practitioners prefer to administer DTP, OPV, and Measles/Mumps/Rubella Vaccine Live on a single day. If done, separate sites and syringes should be used for DTP and Measles/Mumps/Rubella Vaccine Live. The Immunization Practices Advisory Committee (ACIP) recommends routine simultaneous administration of Measles/Mumps/Rubella Vaccine Live, DTP and OPV or inactivated polio vaccine (IPV) to all children $\geq$ 15 months who are eligible to receive these vaccines on the basis that there are equivalent antibody responses and no clinically significant increases in the frequency of adverse events when DTP, Measles/Mumps/Rubella Vaccine Live and OPV or IPV are administered either simultaneously at different sites or separately.†† Administration of Measles/Mumps/Rubella Vaccine Live at 15 months followed by DTP and OPV (or IPV) at 18 months remains an acceptable alternative, especially for children with caregivers known to be generally compliant with other health-care recommendations.

CONTRAINDICATIONS
Do not give Measles/Mumps/Rubella Vaccine Live to pregnant females; the possible effects of the vaccine on fetal development are unknown at this time. If vaccination of postpubertal females is undertaken, pregnancy should be avoided for three months following vaccination. (See "Precautions, Pregnancy".)

Anaphylactic or anaphylactoid reactions to neomycin (each dose of reconstituted vaccine contains approximately 25 mcg of neomycin).

History of anaphylactic or anaphylactoid reactions to eggs (see "Hypersensitivity to Eggs" below).

Any febrile respiratory illness or other active febrile infection.

Active untreated tuberculosis.

Patients receiving immunosuppressive therapy. This contraindication does not apply to patients who are receiving corticosteroids as replacement therapy, e.g., for Addison's disease.

Individuals with blood dyscrasias, leukemia, lymphomas of any type, or other malignant neoplasms affecting the bone marrow or lymphatic systems.

Primary and acquired immunodeficiency states, including patients who are immunosuppressed in association with AIDS or other clinical manifestations of infection with human immunodeficiency viruses; cellular immune deficiencies; and hypogammaglobulinemic and dysgammaglobulinemic states.

Individuals with a family history of congenital or hereditary immunodeficiency, until the immune competence of the potential vaccine recipient is demonstrated.

---

† NOTE: A primary difference among these recommendations is the timing of revaccination: the ACIP recommends routine revaccination at entry into kindergarten or first grade, whereas the AAP recommends routine revaccination at entrance to middle school or junior high school. In addition, some public health jurisdictions mandate the age for revaccination. The complete text of applicable guidelines should be consulted.
†† The Immunization Practices Advisory Committee (ACIP) recommends administering Measles/Mumps/Rubella Vaccine Live concomitantly with the fourth dose of DTP and the third dose of OPV to children 15 months of age or older providing that 6 months have elapsed since DTP-3; or, if fewer than three DTPs have been received, at least 6 weeks have elapsed since the last dose of DTP and OPV.

HYPERSENSITIVITY TO EGGS

Live Measles Vaccine and live Mumps Vaccine are produced in chick embryo cell culture. Persons with a history of anaphylactic, anaphylactoid, or other immediate reactions (e.g., hives, swelling of the mouth and throat, difficulty breathing, hypotension, or shock) subsequent to egg ingestion should not be vaccinated. Evidence indicates that persons are not at increased risk if they have egg allergies that are not anaphylactic or anaphylactoid in nature. Such persons may be vaccinated in the usual manner. There is no evidence to indicate that persons with allergies to chickens or feathers are at increased risk of reaction to the vaccine.

PRECAUTIONS

GENERAL

Adequate treatment provisions including epinephrine, should be available for immediate use should an anaphylactic or anaphylactoid reaction occur.

Due caution should be employed in administration of Measles/Mumps/Rubella Vaccine Live to persons with a history of cerebral injury, individual or family histories of convulsions, or any other condition in which stress due to fever should be avoided. The physician should be alert to the temperature elevation which may occur following vaccination. (See *"Adverse Reactions"*.)

Children and young adults who are known to be infected with human immunodeficiency viruses but without overt clinical manifestations of immunosuppression may be vaccinated; however, the vaccines should be monitored closely for vaccine-preventable diseases because immunization may be less effective than for uninfected persons.

Vaccination should be deferred for at least 3 months following blood or plasma transfusions, or administration of human immune serum globulin.

Excretion of small amounts of the live attenuated rubella virus from the nose or throat has occurred in the majority of susceptible individuals 7-28 days after vaccination. There is no confirmed evidence to indicate that such virus is transmitted to susceptible persons who are in contact with the vaccinated individuals. Consequently, transmission through close personal contact, while accepted as a theoretical possibility, is not regarded as a significant risk. However, transmission of the rubella vaccine virus to infants via breast milk has been documented (see *"Nursing Mothers"*).

There are no reports of transmission of live attenuated measles or mumps viruses from vaccinees to susceptible contacts. It has been reported that live attenuated Measles, Mumps and Rubella Virus Vaccines given individually may result in a temporary depression of tuberculin skin sensitivity. Therefore, if a tuberculin test is to be done, it should be administered either before or simultaneously with Measles/Mumps/Rubella Vaccine Live.

Children under treatment for tuberculosis have not experienced exacerbation of the disease when immunized with live Measles Virus Vaccine; no studies have been reported to date of the effect of Measles Virus Vaccines on untreated tuberculous children.

As for any vaccine, vaccination with Measles/Mumps/Rubella Vaccine Live may not result in seroconversion in 100% of susceptible persons given the vaccine.

PREGNANCY/PREGNANCY CATEGORY C

Animal reproduction studies have not been conducted with Measles/Mumps/Rubella Vaccine Live. It is also not known whether Measles/Mumps/Rubella Vaccine Live can cause fetal harm when administered to a pregnant woman or can affect reproduction capacity. Therefore, the vaccine should not be administered to pregnant females; furthermore, pregnancy should be avoided for three months following vaccination (see *"Contraindications"*).

In counseling women who are inadvertently vaccinated when pregnant or who become pregnant within 3 months of vaccination, the physician should be aware of the following: (1) In a 10 year survey involving over 700 pregnant women who received Rubella Vaccine within 3 months before or after conception (of whom 189 received the Wistar RA 27/3 strain), none of the newborns had abnormalities compatible with congenital rubella syndrome; (2) Although mumps virus is capable of infecting the placenta and fetus, there is no good evidence that it causes congenital malformations in humans. Mumps Vaccine virus also has been shown to infect the placenta, but the virus has not been isolated from the fetal tissues from susceptible women who were vaccinated and underwent elective abortions; and (3) Reports have indicated that contracting of natural measles during pregnancy enhances fetal risk. Increased rates of spontaneous abortion, stillbirth, congenital defects and prematurity have been observed subsequent to natural measles during pregnancy. There are no adequate studies of the attenuated (vaccine) strain of measles virus in pregnancy. However, it would be prudent to assume that the vaccine strain of virus is also capable of inducing adverse fetal effects.

NURSING MOTHERS

It is not known whether Measles or Mumps Vaccine Virus is secreted in human milk. Recent studies have shown that lactating postpartum women immunized with live attenuated Rubella Vaccine may secrete the virus in breast milk and transmit it to breast-fed infants. In the infants with serological evidence of rubella infection, none exhibited severe disease; however, one exhibited mild clinical illness typical of acquired rubella. Caution should be exercised when Measles/Mumps/Rubella Vaccine Live is administered to a nursing woman.

ADVERSE REACTIONS

Burning and/or stinging of short duration at the injection site have been reported.

The adverse clinical reactions associated with the use of Measles/Mumps/Rubella Vaccine Live are those expected to follow administration of the monovalent vaccines given separately. These may include malaise, sore throat, cough, rhinitis, headache, dizziness, fever, rash, nausea, vomiting or diarrhea; mild local reactions such as erythema, induration, tenderness and regional lymphadenopathy; parotitis, orchitis, nerve deafness, thrombocytopenia and purpura; allergic reactions such as wheal and flare at the injection site or urticaria; polyneuritis; and arthralgia and/or arthritis (usually transient and rarely chronic).

Anaphylaxis and anaphylactoid reactions have been reported.

Vasculitis has been reported rarely.

Otitis media and conjunctivitis have been reported.

Moderate fever [101-102.9°F (38.3-39.4°C)] occurs occasionally, and high fever [above 103°F (39.4°C)] occurs less commonly. On rare occasions, children developing fever may exhibit febrile convulsions. Afebrile convulsions or seizures have occurred rarely following vaccination with live attenuated Measles Vaccine. Syncope, particularly at the time of mass vaccination, has been reported. Rash occurs infrequently and is usually minimal, but rarely may be generalized. Erythema multiforme has also been reported rarely. Forms of optic neuritis, including retrobulbar neuritis, papillitis, and retinitis may infrequently follow viral infections, and have been reported to occur 1 to 3 weeks following inoculation with some live virus vaccines.

Clinical experience with live attenuated Measles, Mumps and Rubella Virus Vaccines given individually indicates that encephalitis and other nervous system reactions have occurred very rarely. These might occur also with Measles/Mumps/Rubella Vaccine Live. Experience from more than 80 million doses of all live Measles Vaccines given in the U.S. through 1975 indicates that significant central nervous system reactions such as encephalitis and encephalopathy, occurring within 30 days after vaccination, have been temporally associated with Measles Vaccine very rarely. In no case has it been shown that reactions were actually caused by vaccine. The Centers for Disease Control and Prevention has pointed out that "a certain number of cases of encephalitis may be expected to occur in a large childhood population in a defined period of time even when no vaccines are administered". However, the data suggest the possibility that some of these cases may have been caused by Measles Vaccines. The risk of such serious neurological disorders following live Measles Virus Vaccine administration remains far less than that for encephalitis and encephalopathy with natural measles (one per two thousand reported cases).

There have been rare reports of ocular palsies, Guillain-Barré syndrome, or ataxia occurring after immunization with vaccines containing live attenuated measles virus. The ocular palsies have occurred approximately 3-24 days following vaccination. No definite causal relationship has been established between these events and vaccination. Isolated reports of polyneuropathy including Guillain-Barré syndrome have also been reported after immunization with Rubella-containing Vaccines.

There have been reports of subacute sclerosing panencephalitis (SSPE) in children who did not have a history of natural measles but did receive Measles Vaccine. Some of these cases may have resulted from unrecognized measles in the first year of life or possibly from the measles vaccination. Based on estimated nationwide Measles Vaccine distribution, the association of SSPE cases to measles vaccination is about one case per million vaccine doses distributed. This is far less than the association with natural measles, 6-22 cases of SSPE per million cases of measles. The results of a retrospective case-controlled study conducted by the Centers for Disease Control and Prevention suggest that the overall effect of measles vaccine has been to protect against SSPE by preventing measles with its inherent higher risk of SSPE.

Local reactions characterized by marked swelling, redness and vesiculation at the injection site of attenuated live Measles Virus Vaccines, and systemic reactions including atypical measles, have occurred in persons who received killed Measles Vaccine previously. Measles/Mumps/Rubella Vaccine Live was not given under this condition in clinical trials. Rarely, more severe reactions that require hospitalization, including prolonged high fevers and extensive local reactions, have been reported. Panniculitis has been reported rarely following administration of Measles Vaccine.

Arthralgia and/or arthritis (usually transient and rarely chronic), and polyneuritis are features of natural rubella and vary in frequency and severity with age and sex, being greatest in adult females and least in prepubertal children. This type of involvement as well as myalgia and paresthesia, have also been reported following administration of Measles/Mumps/Rubella Virus Vaccine Live.

Chronic arthritis has been associated with natural rubella infection and has been related to persistent virus and/or viral antigen isolated from body tissues. Only rarely have vaccine recipients developed chronic joint symptoms.

Following vaccination in children, reactions in joints are uncommon and generally of brief duration. In women, incidence rates for arthritis and arthralgia are generally higher than those seen in children (children: 0-3%; women: 12-20%), and the reactions tend to be more marked and of longer duration. Symptoms may persist for a matter of months or on rare occasions for years. In adolescent girls, the reactions appear to be intermediate in incidence between those seen in children and in adult women. Even in older women (35-45 years), these reactions are generally well tolerated and rarely interfere with normal activities.

DOSAGE AND ADMINISTRATION

FOR SUBCUTANEOUS ADMINISTRATION

DO NOT INJECT INTRAVENOUSLY.

The dosage of vaccine is the same for all persons. Inject the total volume of the single dose vial (about 0.5 mL) or 0.5 mL of the 10 dose vial of reconstituted vaccine subcutaneously, preferably into the outer aspect of upper arm. *Do not give immune globulin (IG) concurrently with* Measles/Mumps/Rubella Vaccine Live.

During shipment, to insure that there is no loss of potency, the vaccine must be maintained at a temperature of 10°C (50°F) or less.

Before reconstitution, store Measles/Mumps/Rubella Vaccine Live at 2-8°C (36-46°F). *Protect from light.*

Caution: A sterile syringe free of preservatives, antiseptics, and detergents should be used for each injection and/or reconstitution of the vaccine because these substances may inactivate the live virus vaccine. A 25 gauge, ⅝″ needle is recommended.

To reconstitute, use only the diluent supplied, since it is free of preservatives or other antiviral substances which might inactivate the vaccine.

Single Dose Vial: First withdraw the entire volume of diluent into the syringe to be used for reconstitution. Inject all the diluent in the syringe into the vial of lyophilized vaccine, and agitate to mix thoroughly. Withdraw the entire contents into a syringe and inject the total volume of restored vaccine subcutaneously.

It is important to use a separate sterile syringe and needle for each individual patient to prevent transmission of hepatitis B and other infectious agents from one person to another.

10 Dose Vial (available only to government agencies/institutions):
Withdraw the entire contents (7 mL) of the diluent vial into the sterile syringe to be used for reconstitution, and introduce into the 10 dose vial of lyophilized vaccine. Agitate to ensure thorough mixing. The outer labeling suggests "For Jet Injector or Syringe Use". Use with separate sterile syringes is permitted for containers of 10 doses or less. The vaccine and diluent do not contain preservatives; therefore, the user must recognize the potential contamination hazards and exercise special precautions to protect the sterility and potency of the product. The use of aseptic techniques and proper storage prior to and after restoration of the vaccine and subsequent withdrawal of the individual doses is essential. Use 0.5 mL of the reconstituted vaccine for subcutaneous injection.

It is important to use a separate sterile syringe and needle for each individual patient to prevent transmission of hepatitis B and other infectious agents from one person to another.

Each dose contains not less than the equivalent of 1,000 $TCID_{50}$ of the U.S. Reference Measles Virus, 20,000 $TCID_{50}$ of the U.S. Reference Mumps Virus and 1,000 $TCID_{50}$ of the U.S. Reference Rubella Virus.

Parenteral drug products should be inspected visually for particulate matter and discoloration prior to administration.

STORAGE
It is recommended that the vaccine be used as soon as possible after reconstitution. Protect vaccine from light at all times, since such exposure may inactivate the virus. Store reconstituted vaccine in the vaccine vial in a dark place at 2-8°C (36-46°F) and discard if not used within 8 hours.

HOW SUPPLIED
INJECTION:

BRAND/MANUFACTURER	NDC	SIZE	AWP
○ **BRAND**			
M-M-R II: Merck	00006-4749-00	1 ml	$31.04
	00006-4681-00	1 ml 10s	$267.91

Mebaral *SEE* MEPHOBARBITAL

Mebendazole

DESCRIPTION
Mebendazole is a (synthetic) broad-spectrum anthelmintic available as chewable tablets, each containing 100 mg of Mebendazole.

Mebendazole is methyl 5-benzoylbenzimidazole-2-carbamate.

Mebendazole is a white to slightly yellow powder with a molecular weight of 295.29. It is less than 0.05% soluble in water, dilute mineral acid solutions, alcohol, ether and chloroform, but is soluble in formic acid.

Following is its chemical structure:

CLINICAL PHARMACOLOGY
Following administration of 100 mg twice daily for three consecutive days, plasma levels of Mebendazole and its primary metabolite, the 2-amine, do not exceed 0.03 µg/ml and 0.09 µg/ml, respectively. All metabolites are devoid of anthelmintic activity. In man, approximately 2% of administered Mebendazole is excreted in urine and the remainder in the feces as unchanged drug or a primary metabolite.

Mode of Action: Mebendazole inhibits the formation of the worms' microtubules and causes the worms' glucose depletion.

INDICATIONS AND USAGE
Mebendazole is indicated for the treatment of *Enterobius vermicularis* (pinworm), *Trichuris trichiura* (whipworm), *Ascaris lumbricoides* (common roundworm), *Ancylostoma duodenale* (common hookworm), *Necator americanus* (American hookworm) in single or mixed infections.

Efficacy varies as a function of such factors as pre-existing diarrhea and gastrointestinal transit time, degree of infection, and helminth strains. Efficacy rates derived from various studies are shown in the table below:

Mebendazole	Pinworm (enterobiasis)	Whipworm (trichuriasis)	Common Roundworm (ascariasis)	Hookworm
Cure rates mean	95%	68%	98%	96%
Egg reduction mean	—	93%	99%	99%

CONTRAINDICATIONS
Mebendazole is contraindicated in persons who have shown hypersensitivity to the drug.

WARNINGS
There is no evidence that Mebendazole even at high doses, is effective for hydatid disease. There have been rare reports of neutropenia and liver function elevations, including hepatitis, when Mebendazole is taken for prolonged periods and at dosages substantially above those recommended.

PRECAUTIONS
Information for Patients: Patients should be informed of the potential risk to the fetus in women taking Mebendazole during pregnancy, especially during the first trimester (see *"Use in Pregnancy"*).

Patients should also be informed that cleanliness is important to prevent reinfection and transmission of the infection.

Drug Interactions: Preliminary evidence suggests that cimetidine inhibits Mebendazole metabolism and may result in an increase in plasma concentrations of Mebendazole.

Carcinogenesis, Mutagenesis: In carcinogenicity tests of Mebendazole in mice and rats, no carcinogenic effects were seen at doses as high as 40 mg/kg given daily over two years. Dominant lethal mutation tests in mice showed no mutagenicity at single doses as high as 640 mg/kg. Neither the spermatocyte test, the F_1 translocation test, nor the Ames test indicated mutagenic properties.

Impairment of Fertility: Doses up to 40 mg/kg in mice, given to males for 60 days and to females for 14 days prior to gestation, had no effect upon fetuses and offspring, though there was slight maternal toxicity.

Use in Pregnancy: Pregnancy Category C. Mebendazole has shown embryotoxic and teratogenic activity in pregnant rats at single oral doses as low as 10 mg/kg. In view of these findings the use of Mebendazole is not recommended in pregnant women. In humans, a post-marketing survey has been done of a limited number of women who inadvertently had consumed Mebendazole during the first trimester of pregnancy. The incidence of spontaneous abortion and malformation did not exceed that in the general population. In 170 deliveries on term, no teratogenic risk of Mebendazole was identified. During pregnancy, especially during the first trimester, Mebendazole should be used only if the potential benefit justifies the potential risk to the fetus.

Nursing Mothers: It is not known whether Mebendazole is excreted in human milk. Because many drugs are excreted in human milk, caution should be exercised when Mebendazole is administered to a nursing woman.

Pediatric Use: The drug has not been extensively studied in children under two years; therefore, in the treatment of children under two years the relative benefit/risk should be considered.

ADVERSE REACTIONS
Transient symptoms of abdominal pain and diarrhea have occurred in cases of massive infection and expulsion of worms. Hypersensitivity reactions such as rash urticaria and angioedema have been observed on rare occasions. Very rare cases of convulsions have been reported.

OVERDOSAGE
In the event of accidental overdosage gastrointestinal complaints lasting up to a few hours may occur. Vomiting and purging should be induced. Activated charcoal may be given.

DOSAGE AND ADMINISTRATION
The same dosage schedule applies to children and adults. The tablet may be chewed, swallowed, or crushed and mixed with food.

➤ SHOWN IN PRODUCT IDENTIFICATION GUIDE

	Pinworm (enterobiasis)	Whipworm (trichuriasis)	Common Roundworm (ascariasis)	Hookworm
Mebendazole Dose	1 tablet, once	1 tablet morning and evening for 3 consecutive days.	1 tablet morning and evening for 3 consecutive days.	1 tablet morning and evening for 3 consecutive days.

If the patient is not cured three weeks after treatment, a second course of treatment is advised. No special procedures, such as fasting or purging, are required.

Store at room temperature 15°-30°C (59°-86°F).

HOW SUPPLIED
CHEW TABLET: 100 MG

BRAND/MANUFACTURER	NDC	SIZE	AWP
○ BRAND			
➤ VERMOX: Janssen	50458-0110-01	12s	$55.50

Mecamylamine Hydrochloride

DESCRIPTION
Mecamylamine Hydrochloride is a potent, oral antihypertensive agent and ganglion blocker, and is a secondary amine. It is N,2,3,3-tetramethylbicyclo[2.2.1] hepatan-2-amine hydrochloride. Its empirical formula is $C_{11}H_{21}N.HCl$.

It is a white, odorless, or practically odorless, crystalline powder, is highly stable, soluble in water and has a molecular weight of 203.75.

Following is its chemical structure:

CLINICAL PHARMACOLOGY
Mecamylamine reduces blood pressure in both normotensive and hypertensive individuals. It has a gradual onset of action (½ to 2 hours) and a long-lasting effect (usually 6 to 12 hours or more). A small oral dosage often produces a smooth and predictable reduction of blood pressure. Although this antihypertensive effect is predominantly orthostatic, the supine blood pressure is also significantly reduced.

Pharmacokinetics and Metabolism: Mecamylamine is almost completely absorbed from the gastrointestinal tract, resulting in consistent lowering of blood pressure in most patients with hypertensive cardiovascular disease. Mecamylamine is excreted slowly in the urine in the unchanged form. The rate of its renal elimination is influenced markedly by urinary pH. Alkalinization of the urine reduces, and acidification promotes, renal excretion of Mecamylamine.

Mecamylamine crosses the blood-brain and placental barriers.

INDICATIONS AND USAGE
For the management of moderately severe to severe essential hypertension and in uncomplicated cases of malignant hypertension.

UNLABELED USES
Mecamylamine is used alone or as an adjunct in the treatment of hyperreflexia in patients with spinal cord injury. It is also used to suppress nicotine craving in patients on smoking cessation programs.

CONTRAINDICATIONS
Mecamylamine Hydrochloride should not be used in mild, moderate, labile hypertension and may prove unsuitable in uncooperative patients. It is contraindicated in coronary insufficiency or recent myocardial infarction.

Mecamylamine Hydrochloride should be given with great discretion, if at all, when renal insufficiency is manifested by a rising or elevated BUN. The drug is contraindicated in uremia. Patients receiving antibiotics and sulfonamides should generally not be treated with ganglion blockers. Other contraindications are glaucoma, organic pyloric stenosis or hypersensitivity to the product.

WARNINGS
Mecamylamine, a secondary amine, readily penetrates into the brain and thus may produce central nervous system effects. Tremor, choreiform movements, mental aberrations, and convulsions may occur rarely. These have occurred most often when large doses of Mecamylamine Hydrochloride were used, especially in patients with cerebral or renal insufficiency.

When ganglion blockers or other potent antihypertensive drugs are discontinued suddenly, hypertensive levels return. In patients with malignant hypertension and others, this may occur abruptly and may cause fatal cerevral vascular accidents or acute congestive heart failure. When Mecamylamine Hydrochloride is withdrawn, this should be done gradually and other antihypertensive therapy usually must be substituted. On the other hand, the effects of Mecamylamine Hydrochloride sometimes may last from hours to days after therapy is discontinued.

PRECAUTIONS
General: The patient's condition should be evaluated carefully, particularly as to renal and cardiovascular function. When renal, cerebral, or coronary blood flow is deficient, any additional impairment, which might result from added hypotension, must be avoided. The use of Mecamylamine Hydrochloride in patients with marked cerebral and coronary arteriosclerosis or after a recent cerebral accident requires caution.

The action of Mecamylamine Hydrochloride may be potentiated by excessive heat, fever, infection, hemorrhage, pregnancy, anesthesia, surgery, vigorous exercise, other antihypertensive drugs, alcohol, and salt depletion as a result of diminished intake or increased excretion due to diarrhea, vomiting, excessive sweating, or diuretics.

During therapy with Mecamylamine Hydrochloride, sodium intake should not be restricted but, if necessary, the dosage of the ganglion blocker must be adjusted.

Since urinary retention may occur in patients on ganglion blockers, caution is required in patients with prostatic hypertrophy, bladder neck obstruction, and urethral stricture. Frequent loose bowel movements with abdominal distention and decreased borborygmi may be the first signs of paralytic ileus. If these are present, Mecamylamine Hydrochloride should be discontinued immediately and remedial steps taken.

Information for Patients: Mecamylamine Hydrochloride may cause dizziness, lightheadedness, or fainting, especially when rising from a lying or sitting position. This effect may be increased by alcoholic beverages, exercise, or during hot weather. Getting up slowly may help alleviate such a reaction.

Drug Interactions: Patients receiving antibiotics and sulfonamides generally should not be treated with ganglion blockers.

The action of Mecamylamine Hydrochloride may be potentiated by anesthesia, other antihypertensive drugs and alcohol.

Carcinogenesis, Mutagenesis, Impairment of Fertility: Long-term studies in animals have not been performed to evaluate the effects upon fertility, mutagenic or carcinogenic potential of Mecamylamine Hydrochloride.

Pregnancy: Pregnancy Category C: Animal reproduction studies have not been conducted with Mecamylamine Hydrochloride. It is not known whether Mecamylamine Hydrochloride can cause fetal harm when given to a pregnant woman or can affect reproductive capacity. Mecamylamine Hydrochloride should be given to a pregnant woman only if clearly needed.

Nursing Mothers: Because of the potential for serious adverse reactions in nursing infants from Mecamylamine Hydrochloride, a decision should be made whether to discontinue nursing or to discontinue the drug, taking into account the importance of the drug to the mother.

ADVERSE REACTIONS
The following adverse reactions have been reported and within each category are listed in order of decreasing severity.

Gastrointestinal: Ileus, constipation (sometimes preceded by small, frequent liquid stools), vomiting, nausea, anorexia, glossitis and dryness of mouth.

Cardiovascular: Orthostatic dizziness and syncope, postural hypotension.

Nervous System/Psychiatric: Convulsions, choreiform movements, mental aberrations, tremor, and paresthesias (see "Warnings").

Respiratory: Interstitial pulmonary edema and fibrosis.

Urogenital: Urinary retention, impotence, decreased libido.

Special Senses: Blurred vision, dilated pupils.

Miscellaneous: Weakness, fatigue, sedation.

OVERDOSAGE
Signs of overdosage include: hypotension (which may progress to peripheral vascular collapse), postural hypotension, nausea, vomiting, diarrhea, constipation, paralytic ileus, urinary retention, dizziness, anxiety, dry mouth, mydriasis, blurred vision, or palpitations. A rise in intraocular pressure may occur.

Pressor amines may be used to counteract excessive hypotension. Since patients being treated with ganglion blockers are more than normally reactive to pressor amines, small doses of the latter are recommended to avoid excessive response. The oral LD_{50} of Mecamylamine in the mouse is 92 mg/kg.

DOSAGE AND ADMINISTRATION
Therapy is usually started with one 2.5 mg tablet of Mecamylamine Hydrochloride twice a day. This initial dosage should be modified by increments of one 2.5 mg tablet at intervals of not less than 2 days until the desired blood pressure response occurs (the criterion being a dosage just under that which causes signs of mild postural hypotension).

The average total daily dosage of Mecamylamine Hydrochloride is 25 mg, usually in three divided doses. However, as little as 2.5 mg daily may be sufficient to control hypertension in some patients. A range of two to four or even more doses may be required in severe cases when smooth control is difficult to obtain.

◆ RATED THERAPEUTICALLY EQUIVALENT; ◇ THERAPEUTIC EQUIVALENCE UNCONFIRMED; ○ UNRATED

In severe or urgent cases, larger increments at smaller intervals may be needed. Partial tolerance may develop in certain patients, requiring an increase in the daily dosage of Mecamylamine Hydrochloride.

Administration of Mecamylamine Hydrochloride after meals may cause a more gradual absorption and smoother control of excessively high blood pressure. The timing of doses in relation to meals should be consistent. Since the blood pressure response to antihypertensive drugs is increased in the early morning, the larger dose should be given at noontime and perhaps in the evening. The morning dose, as a rule, should be relatively small and in some instances may even be omitted.

The *initial regulation of dosage* should be determined by blood pressure readings in the erect position at the time of maximal effect of the drug, as well as by other signs and symptoms of orthostatic hypertension.

The *effective maintenance dosage* should be regulated by blood pressure readings in the erect position and by limitation of dosage to that which causes slight faintness or dizziness in this position. If the patient or a relative can use a sphygmomanometer, instructions may be given to reduce or omit a dose if readings fall below a designated level or if faintness or lightheadedness occurs. *However, no change should be instituted without the knowledge of the physician.* Close supervision and education of the patient, as well as critical adjustment of dosage, are essential to successful therapy.

Other Antihypertensive Agents: When Mecamylamine Hydrochloride is given with other antihypertensive drugs, the dosage of these other agents, as well as that of Mecamylamine Hydrochloride should be reduced to avoid excessive hypotension. However, thiazides should be continued in their usual dosage, while that of Mecamylamine Hydrochloride is decreased by at least 50 percent.

HOW SUPPLIED
TABLETS: 2.5 MG

BRAND/MANUFACTURER	NDC	SIZE	AWP
○ BRAND			
INVERSINE: Merck	00006-0052-68	100s	$12.61

Mechlorethamine Hydrochloride

DESCRIPTION
Mechlorethamine Hydrochloride, an antineoplastic nitrogen mustard also known as HN2 Hydrochloride, is a nitrogen analog of sulfur mustard. It is a white, crystalline, hygroscopic powder that is very soluble in water and also soluble in alcohol.

Mechlorethamine Hydrochloride is designated chemically as 2-chloro-N-(2-chloroethyl)-N-methylethanamine hydrochloride. The molecular weight is 192.52 and the melting point is 108-111°C. The empirical formula is $C_5H_{11}Cl_2N\cdot HCl$.

Trituration of Mechlorethamine Hydrochloride is a sterile, white crystalline powder for injection by the intravenous or intracavitary routes after dissolution. Each vial of Mechlorethamine Hydrochloride contains 10 mg of Mechlorethamine Hydrochloride triturated with sodium chloride q.s. 100 mg. When dissolved with 10 mL Sterile Water for Injection or 0.9% Sodium Chloride Injection, the resulting solution has a pH of 3-5 at a concentration of 1 mg Mechlorethamine Hydrochloride per mL.

Following is its chemical structure:

$$CH_3N(CH_2CH_2Cl)_2 \cdot HCl$$

CLINICAL PHARMACOLOGY
Mechlorethamine, a biologic alkylating agent, has a cytotoxic action which inhibits rapidly proliferating cells.

Pharmacokinetics and Metabolism: In water or body fluids, Mechlorethamine undergoes rapid chemical transformation and combines with water or reactive compounds of cells, so that the drug is no longer present in active form a few minutes after administration.

INDICATIONS AND USAGE
Before using Mechlorethamine Hydrochloride see *"Contraindications," "Warnings," "Precautions," "Adverse Reactions,"* and *"Dosage and Administration."*

Special Handling: Mechlorethamine Hydrochloride, administered intravenously, is indicated for the palliative treatment of Hodgkin's disease (Stages III and IV), lymphosarcoma, chronic myelocytic or chronic lymphocytic leukemia, polycythemia vera, mycosis fungoides, and bronchogenic carcinoma.

Mechlorethamine Hydrochloride, administered intrapleurally, intraperitoneally, or intrapericardially, is indicated for the palliative treatment of metastatic carcinoma resulting in effusion.

UNLABELED USES
Mechlorethamine Hydrochloride is used alone or as an adjunct in the treatment of nonHodgkin's lymphoma.

CONTRAINDICATIONS
The use of Mechlorethamine Hydrochloride is contraindicated in the presence of known infectious diseases and in patients who have had previous anaphylactic reactions to Mechlorethamine Hydrochloride.

WARNINGS

> EXTRAVASATION OF THE DRUG INTO SUBCUTANEOUS TISSUES RESULTS IN A PAINFUL INFLAMMATION. THE AREA USUALLY BECOMES INDURATED AND SLOUGHING MAY OCCUR. IF LEAKAGE OF DRUG IS OBVIOUS, PROMPT INFILTRATION OF THE AREA WITH STERILE ISOTONIC SODIUM THIOSULFATE (1/6 MOLAR) AND APPLICATION OF AN ICE COMPRESS FOR 6 TO 12 HOURS MAY MINIMIZE THE LOCAL REACTION. FOR A 1/6 MOLAR SOLUTION OF SODIUM THIOSULFATE, USE 4.14 G OF SODIUM THIOSULFATE PER 100 ML OF STERILE WATER FOR INJECTION OR 2.64 G OF ANHYDROUS SODIUM THIOSULFATE PER 100 ML OR DILUTE 4 ML OF SODIUM THIOSULFATE INJECTION (10%) WITH 6 ML OF STERILE WATER FOR INJECTION.

Before using Mechlorethamine Hydrochloride, an accurate histologic diagnosis of the disease, a knowledge of its natural course, and an adequate clinical history are important. The hematologic status of the patient must first be determined. It is essential to understand the hazards and therapeutic effects to be expected. Careful clinical judgment must be exercised in selecting patients. If the indication for its use is not clear, the drug should not be used.

As nitrogen mustard therapy may contribute to extensive and rapid development of amyloidosis; it should be used only if foci of acute and chronic suppurative inflammation are absent.

USAGE IN PREGNANCY
Mechlorethamine Hydrochloride can cause fetal harm when administered to a pregnant woman. Mechlorethamine Hydrochloride has been shown to produce fetal malformations in the rat and ferret when given as single subcutaneous injections of 1 mg/kg (2-3 times the maximum recommended human dose). There are no adequate and well controlled studies in pregnant women. If this drug is used during pregnancy, or if the patient becomes pregnant while taking this drug, the patient should be apprised of the potential hazard to the fetus. Women of childbearing potential should be advised to avoid becoming pregnant.

PRECAUTIONS
GENERAL
This drug is highly toxic and both powder and solution must be handled and administered with care. Since Mechlorethamine Hydrochloride is a powerful vesicant, it is intended primarily for intravenous use, and in most instances is given by this route. Inhalation of dust or vapors and contact with skin or mucous membranes, especially those of the eyes, must be avoided. Rubber gloves should be worn when handling Mechlorethamine Hydrochloride (See *"Dosage and Administration"* and *"How Supplied, Special Handling"*).

Because of the toxicity of Mechlorethamine Hydrochloride, and the unpleasant side effects following its use, the potential risk and discomfort from the use of this drug in patients with inoperable neoplasms or in the terminal stage of the disease must be balanced against the limited gain obtainable. These gains will vary with the nature and the status of the disease under treatment. The routine use of Mechlorethamine Hydrochloride in all cases of widely disseminated neoplasms is to be discouraged.

The use of Mechlorethamine Hydrochloride in patients with leukopenia, thrombocytopenia, and anemia, due to invasion of the bone marrow by tumor carries a greater risk. In such patients a good response to treatment with disappearance of the tumor from the bone marrow may be associated with improvement of bone marrow function. However, in the absence of a good response or in patients who have been previously treated with chemotherapeutic agents, hematopoiesis may be further compromised, and leukopenia, thrombocytopenia and anemia may become more severe and lead to the demise of the patient.

Tumors of bone and nervous tissue have responded poorly to therapy. Results are unpredictable in disseminated and malignant tumors of different types.

Precautions must be observed with the use of Mechlorethamine Hydrochloride and x-ray therapy or other chemotherapy in alternating courses. Hematopoietic function is characteristically depressed by either form of therapy, and neither Mechlorethamine Hydrochloride following x-ray therapy nor x-ray therapy subsequent to the drug should be given until bone marrow function has recovered. In particular, irradiation of such areas as sternum, ribs, and vertebrae shortly after a course of nitrogen mustard may lead to hematologic complications.

Mechlorethamine Hydrochloride has been reported to have immunosuppressive activity. Therefore, it should be borne in mind that use of the drug may predispose the patient to bacterial, viral or fungal infection.

Hyperuricemia may develop during therapy with Mechlorethamine Hydrochloride. The problem of urate precipitation should be anticipated, particularly in the treatment of the lymphomas, and adequate methods for control of hyperuricemia should be instituted and careful attention directed toward adequate fluid intake before treatment.

Since drug toxicity, especially sensitivity to bone marrow failure, seems to be more common in chronic lymphatic leukemia than in other conditions, the drug should be given in this condition with great caution, if at all.

► SHOWN IN PRODUCT IDENTIFICATION GUIDE

Extreme caution must be used in exceeding the average recommended dose. (See "Overdosage".)

LABORATORY TESTS

Many abnormalities of renal, hepatic, and bone marrow function have been reported in patients with neoplastic disease and receiving Mechlorethamine. It is advisable to check renal, hepatic, and bone marrow functions frequently.

CARCINOGENSIS, MUTAGENESIS, IMPAIRMENT OF FERTILITY

Therapy with alkylating agents such as Mechlorethamine Hydrochloride may be associated with an increased incidence of a second malignant tumor, especially when such therapy is combined with other antineoplastic agents or radiation therapy.

Young-adult female RF mice were injected intravenously with four doses of 2.4 mg/kg of Mechlorethamine (0.1% solution) at 2-week intervals with observations for up to 2 years. An increased incidence of thymic lymphomas and pulmonary adenomas was observed. Painting Mechlorethamine on the skin of mice for periods up to 33 weeks resulted in squamous cell tumors in 9 of 33 mice.

Mechlorethamine induced mutations in the Ames test, in *E. coli*, and *Neurospora crassa*. Mechlorethamine caused chromosome aberrations in a variety of plant and mammalian cells. Dominant lethal mutations were produced in ICR/ Ha Swiss mice.

Mechlorethamine impaired fertility in the rat at a daily dose of 500 mg/kg intravenously for two weeks.

PREGNANCY

Pregnancy Category D. See *"Warnings"*.

NURSING MOTHERS

It is not known whether this drug is excreted in human milk. Because many drugs are excreted in human milk and because of the potential for serious adverse reactions in nursing infants from Mechlorethamine Hydrochloride, a decision should be made whether to discontinue nursing or to discontinue the drug, taking into account the importance of the drug to the mother.

PEDIATRIC USE

Safety and effectiveness in children have not been established by well-controlled studies. Use of Mechlorethamine Hydrochloride in children has been quite limited. Mechlorethamine Hydrochloride has been used in Hodgkin's disease, stages III and IV, in combination with other oncolytic agents (MOPP schedule). The MOPP chemotherapy combination includes Mechlorethamine, vincristine, procarbazine, and prednisone or prednisolone.

ADVERSE REACTIONS

Clinical use of Mechlorethamine Hydrochloride usually is accompanied by toxic manifestations.

LOCAL TOXICITY

Thrombosis and thrombophlebitis may result from direct contact of the drug with the intima of the injected vein. Avoid high concentration and prolonged contact with the drug, especially in cases of elevated pressure in the antebrachial vein (e.g., in mediastinal tumor compression from severe vena cava syndrome).

SYSTEMIC TOXICITY

General: Hypersensitivity reactions, including anaphylaxis, have been reported. Nausea, vomiting and depression of formed elements in the circulating blood are dose-limiting side effects and usually occur with the use of full doses of Mechlorethamine Hydrochloride. Jaundice, alopecia, vertigo, tinnitus and diminished hearing may occur infrequently. Rarely, hemolytic anemia associated with such diseases as the lymphomas and chronic lymphocytic leukemia may be precipitated by treatment with alkylating agents including Mechlorethamine Hydrochloride. Also, various chromosomal abnormalities have been reported in association with nitrogen mustard therapy.

Mechlorethamine Hydrochloride is given preferably at night in case sedation for side effects is required. Nausea and vomiting usually occur 1 to 3 hours after use of the drug. Emesis may disappear in the first 8 hours, but nausea may persist for 24 hours. Nausea and vomiting may be so severe as to precipitate vascular accidents in patients with a hemorrhagic tendency. Premedication with antiemetics, in addition to sedatives, may help control severe nausea and vomiting. Anorexia, weakness and diarrhea may also occur.

Hematologic: The usual course of Mechlorethamine Hydrochloride (total dose of 0.4 mg/kg either given as a single intravenous dose or divided into two or four daily doses of 0.2 or 0.1 mg/kg respectively) generally produces a lymphocytopenia within 24 hours after the first injection; significant granulocytopenia occurs within 6 to 8 days and lasts for 10 days to 3 weeks. Agranulocytosis appears to be relatively infrequent and recovery from leukopenia in most cases is complete within two weeks of the maximum reduction. Thrombocytopenia is variable but the time course of the appearance and recovery from reduced platelet counts generally parallels the sequence of granulocyte levels. In some cases severe thrombocytopenia may lead to bleeding from the gums and gastrointestinal tract, petechiae, and small subcutaneous hemorrhages; these symptoms appear to be transient and in most cases disappear with return to a normal platelet count. However, a severe and even uncontrollable depression of the hematopoietic system occasionally may follow the usual dose of Mechlorethamine Hydrochloride, particularly in patients with widespread disease and debility and in patients previously treated with other antineoplastic agents or x-ray. Persistent pancytopenia has been reported. In rare instances, hemorrhagic complications may be due to hyperheparinemia. Erythrocyte and hemoglobin levels may decline during the first 2 weeks after therapy but rarely significantly. Depression of the hematopoietic system may be found up to 50 days or more after starting therapy.

Integumentary: Occasionally, a maculopapular skin eruption occurs, but this may be idiosyncratic and does not necessarily recur with subsequent courses of the drug. Erythema multiforme has been observed. Herpes zoster, a common complicating infection in patients with lymphomas, may first appear after therapy is instituted and on occasion may be precipitated by treatment. Further treatment should be discontinued during the acute phase of this illness to avoid progression to generalized herpes zoster.

Reproductive: Since the gonads are susceptible to Mechlorethamine Hydrochloride, treatment may be followed by delayed catamenia, oligomenorrhea, or temporary or permanent amenorrhea. Impaired spermatogenesis, azoospermia, and total germinal aplasia have been reported in male patients treated with alkylating agents, especially in combination with other drugs. In some instances spermatogenesis may return in patients in remission, but this may occur only several years after intensive chemotherapy has been discontinued. Patients should be warned of the potential risk to their reproductive capacity.

OVERDOSAGE

With total doses exceeding 0.4 mg/kg of body weight for a single course, severe leukopenia, anemia, thrombocytopenia and a hemorrhagic diathesis with subsequent delayed bleeding may develop. Death may follow. The only treatment in instances of excessive dosage appears to be repeated blood product transfusions, antibiotic treatment of complicating infections and general supportive measures.

The intravenous LD_{50} of Mechlorethamine Hydrochloride is 2 mg/kg and 1.6 mg/kg in the mouse and rat, respectively.

DOSAGE AND ADMINISTRATION

INTRAVENOUS ADMINISTRATION

The dosage of Mechlorethamine Hydrochloride varies with the clinical situation, the therapeutic response and the magnitude of hematologic depression. A total dose of 0.4 mg/kg of body weight for each course usually is given either as a single dose or in divided doses of 0.1 to 0.2 mg/kg per day. Dosage should be based on ideal dry body weight. The presence of edema or ascites must be considered so that dosage will be based on actual weight unaugmented by these conditions.

The margin of safety in therapy with Mechlorethamine Hydrochloride is narrow and considerable care must be exercised in the matter of dosage. Repeated examinations of blood are *mandatory* as a guide to subsequent therapy. (See *"Overdosage".*)

Within a few minutes after intravenous injection, Mechlorethamine Hydrochloride undergoes chemical transformation, combines with reactive compounds, and is no longer present in its active form in the blood stream. Subsequent courses should not be given until the patient has recovered hematologically from the previous course; this is best determined by repeated studies of the peripheral blood elements awaiting their return to normal levels. It is often possible to give repeated courses of Mechlorethamine Hydrochloride as early as three weeks after treatment.

PREPARATION OF SOLUTION FOR INTRAVENOUS ADMINISTRATION

This drug is highly toxic and both powder and solution must be handled and administered with care. Since Mechlorethamine Hydrochloride is a powerful vesicant, it is intended primarily for intravenous use, and in most instances is given by this route. Inhalation of dust or vapors and contact with skin or mucous membranes, especially those of the eyes, must be avoided. Rubber gloves should be worn when handling Mechlorethamine Hydrochloride. Should accidental eye contact occur, copious irrigation with water, normal saline or a balanced salt ophthalmic irrigating solution should be instituted immediately, followed by prompt ophthalmologic consultation. Should accidental skin contact occur, the affected part must be irrigated immediately with copious amounts of water, for at least 15 minutes followed by 2 percent sodium thiosulfate solution. (See also *"Box Warning"* and *"Special Handling".*)

Each vial of Mechlorethamine Hydrochloride contains 10 mg of Mechlorethamine Hydrochloride triturated with sodium chloride q.s. 100 mg. In neutral or alkaline aqueous solution it undergoes rapid chemical transformation and is highly unstable. Although solutions prepared according to instructions are acidic and do not decompose as rapidly, they should be prepared immediately before each injection since they will decompose on standing. When reconstituted, Mechlorethamine Hydrochloride is a clear colorless solution. *Do not use if the solution is discolored or if droplets of water are visible within the vial prior to reconstitution.*

Using a sterile 10 mL syringe, inject 10 mL of Sterile Water for Injection or 10 mL Sodium Chloride Injection into a vial of Mechlorethamine Hydrochloride. With the needle (syringe attached) still in the rubber stopper, shake the vial several times to dissolve the drug completely. The resultant solution contains 1 mg of Mechlorethamine Hydrochloride per mL.

Parenteral drug products should be inspected visually for particulate matter and discoloration prior to administration whenever solution and container permit.

SPECIAL HANDLING

Due to the drug's toxic and mutagenic properties, appropriate precautions including the use of appropriate safety equipment are recommended for the preparation of Mechlorethamine Hydrochloride for parenteral administration.

The National Institutes of Health presently recommends that the preparation of injectable anti-neoplastic drugs should be performed in a Class II laminar flow biological safety cabinet and that personnel preparing drugs of this class should wear surgical gloves and a closed front surgical-type gown with knit cuffs. Several other guidelines for proper handling and disposal of anticancer drugs have been published and should be considered. There is no general agreement that all of the procedures recommended in the guidelines are necessary or appropriate.

Accidental contact: Should accidental eye contact occur, copious irrigation with water, normal saline or a balanced salt ophthalmic irrigating solution should be instituted immediately, followed by prompt ophthalmologic consultation. Should accidental skin contact occur, the affected part must be irrigated immediately with copious amounts of water, for at least 15 minutes, followed by 2 percent sodium thiosulfate solution. (See also box *"Warning"*).

TECHNIQUE FOR INTRAVENOUS ADMINISTRATION
Withdraw into the syringe the calculated volume of solution required for a single injection. *Dispose of any remaining solution after neutralization* (see below). Although the drug may be injected directly into any suitable vein, it is injected preferably into the rubber or plastic tubing of a flowing intravenous infusion set. This reduces the possibility of severe local reactions due to extravasation or high concentration of the drug. Injecting the drug into the tubing rather than adding it to the entire volume of the infusion fluid minimizes a chemical reaction between the drug and the solution. The rate of injection apparently is not critical provided it is completed within a few minutes.

INTRACAVITARY ADMINISTRATION
Nitrogen mustard has been used by intracavitary administration with varying success in certain malignant conditions for the control of pleural, peritoneal, and pericardial effusions caused by malignant cells.

The technic and the dose used by any of these routes varies. Therefore, if Mechlorethamine Hydrochloride is given by the intracavitary route, the published articles concerning such use should be consulted. *Because of the inherent risks involved, the physician should be experienced in the appropriate injection technics, and be thoroughly aware of the indications, dosages, hazards, and precautions as set forth in the published literature. When using Mechlorethamine Hydrochloride by the intracavitary route, the general precautions concerning this agent should be borne in mind.*

As a general guide, reference is made especially to the technics of Weisberger et al. Intracavitary use is indicated in the presence of pleural, peritoneal, or pericardial effusion due to metastatic tumors. Local therapy with nitrogen mustard is used only when malignant cells are demonstrated in the effusion. Intracavitary injection is not recommended when the accumulated fluid is chylous in nature, since results are likely to be poor.

Paracentesis is first performed with most of the fluid being removed from the pleural or peritoneal cavity. The intracavitary use of Mechlorethamine Hydrochloride may exert at least some of its effect through production of a chemical poudrage. Therefore, the removal of excess fluid allows the drug to more easily contact the peritoneal and pleural linings. For intrapleural or intrapericardial injection nitrogen mustard is introduced directly through the thoracentesis needle. For intraperitoneal injection it is given through a rubber catheter inserted into the trocar used for paracentesis or through a No. 18 gauge needle inserted at another site. This drug should be injected slowly, with frequent aspiration to ensure that a free flow of fluid is present. If fluid cannot be aspirated, pain and necrosis due to injection of solution outside the cavity may occur. Free flow of fluid also is necessary to prevent injection into a loculated pocket and to ensure adequate dissemination of nitrogen mustard.

The usual dose of nitrogen mustard for intracavitary injection is 0.4 mg/kg of body weight, though 0.2 mg/kg (or 10 to 20 mg) has been used by the intrapericardial route. The solution is prepared, as previously described for intravenous injection, by adding 10 mL of Sterile Water for Injection or 10 mL of Sodium Chloride Injection to the vial containing 10 mg of Mechlorethamine Hydrochloride. (Amounts of diluent of 50 to 100 mL of normal saline have also been used.) The position of the patient should be changed every 5 to 10 minutes for an hour after injection to obtain more uniform distribution of the drug throughout the serous cavity. The remaining fluid may be removed from the pleural or peritoneal cavity by paracentesis 24 to 36 hours later. The patient should be followed carefully by clinical and x-ray examination to detect reaccumulation of fluid.

Pain occurs rarely with intrapleural use; it is common with intraperitoneal injection and is often associated with nausea, vomiting, and diarrhea of 2 to 3 days duration. Transient cardiac irregularities may occur with intrapericardial injection. Death, possibly accelerated by nitrogen mustard, has been reported following the use of this agent by the intracavitary route. Although absorption of Mechlorethamine Hydrochloride when given by the intracavitary route is probably not complete because of its rapid deactivation by body fluids, the systemic effect is unpredictable. The acute side effects such as nausea and vomiting are usually mild. Bone marrow depression is generally milder than when the drug is given intravenously. Care should be taken to avoid use by the intracavitary route when other agents which may suppress bone marrow function are being used systemically.

NEUTRALIZATION OF EQUIPMENT AND UNUSED SOLUTION
To clean rubber gloves, tubing, glassware, etc., after giving Mechlorethamine Hydrochloride, soak them in an aqueous solution containing equal volumes of sodium thiosulfate (5%) and sodium bicarbonate (5%) for 45 minutes. Excess reagents and reaction products are washed away easily with water. Any unused injection solution should be neutralized by mixing with an equal volume of sodium thiosulfate/sodium bicarbonate solution. Allow the mixture to stand for 45 minutes. Vials that have contained Mechlorethamine Hydrochloride should be treated in the same way with thiosulfate/bicarbonate solution before disposal.

J CODES
10 mg IV—J9230

HOW SUPPLIED
POWDER FOR INJECTION: 10 MG

BRAND/MANUFACTURER	NDC	SIZE	AWP
○ BRAND			
MUSTARGEN: Merck	00006-7753-31	4s	$40.41

Meclan *SEE* MECLOCYCLINE SULFOSALICYLATE

Meclizine Hydrochloride

DESCRIPTION
Chemically, Meclizine Hydrochloride (*p*-chloro-α-phenylbenzyl)-4-(*m*-methylbenzyl)piperazine dihydrochloride monohydrate.

Following is its chemical structure:

ACTIONS
Meclizine Hydrochloride is an antihistamine which shows marked protective activity against nebulized histamine and lethal doses of intravenously injected histamine in guinea pigs. It has a marked effect in blocking the vasodepressor response to histamine, but only a slight blocking action against acetylcholine. Its activity is relatively weak in inhibiting the spasmogenic action of histamine on isolated guinea pig ileum.

INDICATIONS
BASED ON A REVIEW OF THIS DRUG BY THE NATIONAL ACADEMY OF SCIENCES-NATIONAL RESEARCH COUNCIL AND/OR OTHER INFORMATION, FDA HAS CLASSIFIED THE INDICATIONS AS FOLLOWS:

EFFECTIVE: MANAGEMENT OF NAUSEA AND VOMITING, AND DIZZINESS ASSOCIATED WITH MOTION SICKNESS.

POSSIBLY EFFECTIVE: MANAGEMENT OF VERTIGO ASSOCIATED WITH DISEASES AFFECTING THE VESTIBULAR SYSTEM.

FINAL CLASSIFICATION OF THE LESS THAN EFFECTIVE INDICATIONS REQUIRES FURTHER INVESTIGATION.

CONTRAINDICATIONS
Meclizine Hydrochloride is contraindicated in individuals who have shown a previous hypersensitivity to it.

WARNINGS
Since drowsiness may, on occasion, occur with use of this drug, patients should be warned of this possibility and cautioned against driving a car or operating dangerous machinery.

Patients should avoid alcoholic beverages while taking the drug. Due to its potential anticholinergic action, this drug should be used with caution in patients with asthma, glaucoma, or enlargement of the prostate gland.

USAGE IN CHILDREN
Clinical studies establishing safety and effectiveness in children have not been done; therefore, usage is not recommended in children under 12 years of age.

USAGE IN PREGNANCY
Pregnancy Category B: Reproduction studies in rats have shown cleft palates at 25-50 times the human dose. Epidemiological studies in pregnant women, however, do not indicate that meclizine increases the risk of abnormalities when administered during pregnancy. Despite the animal findings, it would appear that the possibility of fetal harm is remote. Nevertheless, meclizine, or any other medication, should be used during pregnancy only if clearly necessary.

ADVERSE REACTIONS
Drowsiness, dry mouth and, on rare occasions, blurred vision have been reported.

DOSAGE AND ADMINISTRATION
VERTIGO
For the control of vertigo associated with diseases affecting the vestibular system, the recommended dose is 25 to 100 mg daily, in divided dosage, depending upon clinical response.

MOTION SICKNESS

The initial dose of 25 to 50 mg of Meclizine Hydrochloride should be taken one hour prior to embarkation for protection against motion sickness. Thereafter, the dose may be repeated every 24 hours for the duration of the journey.

HOW SUPPLIED
CHEW TABLET: 25 MG

AVERAGE UNIT PRICE (AVAILABLE SIZES)		GENERIC A-RATED AVERAGE PRICE (GAAP)	
GENERIC	$0.03	100s	$3.29
HCFA FUL (100s ea)	$0.03	1000s	$24.96

BRAND/MANUFACTURER	NDC	SIZE	AWP
◆ GENERICS			
Richlyn	00115-3875-01	100s	$2.77
➤ Sidmak	50111-0355-01	100s	$3.50
Goldline	00182-0571-01	100s	$3.60
Goldline	00182-0571-10	1000s	$19.15
Richlyn	00115-3875-03	1000s	$21.30
Sidmak	50111-0355-03	1000s	$23.40
URL	00677-0416-10	1000s	$36.00

TABLETS: 12.5 MG

AVERAGE UNIT PRICE (AVAILABLE SIZES)		GENERIC A-RATED AVERAGE PRICE (GAAP)	
BRAND	$0.33	100s	$5.33
GENERIC	$0.05	1000s	$24.97
HCFA FUL (100s ea)	$0.02		

BRAND/MANUFACTURER	NDC	SIZE	AWP
◆ BRAND			
➤ ANTIVERT: Roerig	00662-2100-66	100s	$34.28
	00662-2100-82	1000s	$325.20
◆ GENERICS			
Medirex	57480-0346-06	30s	$5.54
Richlyn	00115-3870-01	100s	$1.76
Camall	00147-0137-10	100s	$2.64
Major	00904-2384-60	100s	$3.10
Schein	00364-0411-01	100s	$3.56
Par	49884-0034-01	100s	$3.70
Goldline	00182-0871-01	100s	$3.85
Martec	52555-0509-01	100s	$4.38
Qualitest	00603-4319-21	100s	$4.40
Moore,H.L.	00839-6009-06	100s	$4.46
URL	00677-0418-01	100s	$4.52
Purepac	00228-2575-10	100s	$4.57
➤ Rugby	00536-3986-01	100s	$4.65
Geneva	00781-1542-01	100s	$4.95
Parmed	00349-2084-01	100s	$5.00
Aligen	00405-4601-01	100s	$5.00
Raway	00686-0089-20	100s ud	$5.50
Major	00904-2384-61	100s ud	$5.84
Goldline	00182-0871-89	100s ud	$6.75
Vangard	00615-1553-13	100s ud	$6.91
Auro	55829-0354-10	100s ud	$7.78
Medirex	57480-0346-01	100s ud	$8.25
UDL	51079-0089-20	100s ud	$15.75
Major	00904-2384-40	500s	$6.80
Camall	00147-0137-20	1000s	$11.41
Richlyn	00115-3870-03	1000s	$13.50
Major	00904-2384-80	1000s	$18.95
Schein	00364-0411-02	1000s	$19.00
URL	00677-0418-10	1000s	$20.53
Purepac	00228-2575-96	1000s	$20.58
Geneva	00781-1542-10	1000s	$25.95
Goldline	00182-0871-10	1000s	$25.95
Parmed	00349-2084-10	1000s	$28.15
Qualitest	00603-4319-32	1000s	$29.80
➤ Rugby	00536-3986-10	1000s	$29.85
Par	49884-0034-10	1000s	$32.19
Aligen	00405-4601-03	1000s	$32.19
Martec	52555-0509-10	1000s	$32.80
Moore,H.L.	00839-6009-16	1000s	$33.75

TABLETS: 25 MG

AVERAGE UNIT PRICE (AVAILABLE SIZES)		GENERIC A-RATED AVERAGE PRICE (GAAP)	
BRAND	$0.53	100s	$6.88
GENERIC	$0.06	1000s	$34.82
HCFA FUL (100s ea)	$0.02		

BRAND/MANUFACTURER	NDC	SIZE	AWP
◆ BRAND			
➤ ANTIVERT/25: Roerig	00662-2110-66	100s	$54.20
	00662-2110-82	1000s	$514.48
◆ GENERICS			
Allscrips	54569-0349-09	15s	$0.81
Medirex	57480-0347-06	30s	$8.67
Camall	00147-0101-01	100s	$3.05
Major	00904-2350-60	100s	$4.10
Schein	00364-0412-01	100s	$4.18
Par	49884-0035-01	100s	$4.70

BRAND/MANUFACTURER	NDC	SIZE	AWP
Goldline	00182-0872-01	100s	$4.90
Martec	52555-0510-01	100s	$5.35
URL	00677-0419-01	100s	$5.69
Moore,H.L.	00839-6010-06	100s	$5.74
Parmed	00349-2087-01	100s	$5.75
➤ Rugby	00536-3988-01	100s	$5.85
Qualitest	00603-4320-21	100s	$5.88
➤ Geneva	00781-1544-01	100s	$5.90
Aligen	00405-4602-01	100s	$6.54
Purepac	00228-2576-10	100s	$7.94
Major	00904-2350-61	100s ud	$6.39
Vangard	00615-1554-13	100s ud	$7.81
➤ Goldline	00182-0872-89	100s ud	$7.85
Medirex	57480-0347-01	100s ud	$9.25
Auro	55829-0355-10	100s ud	$9.64
Raway	00686-0090-20	100s ud	$10.50
UDL	51079-0090-20	100s ud	$17.50
Camall	00147-0101-20	1000s	$16.11
Schein	00364-0412-02	1000s	$25.15
Major	00904-2350-80	1000s	$27.90
Parmed	00349-2087-10	1000s	$29.20
➤ Rugby	00536-3988-10	1000s	$31.49
➤ Goldline	00182-0872-10	1000s	$32.25
URL	00677-0419-10	1000s	$37.48
Qualitest	00603-4320-32	1000s	$37.48
➤ Geneva	00781-1544-10	1000s	$37.50
Martec	52555-0510-10	1000s	$39.60
Par	49884-0035-10	1000s	$40.89
Aligen	00405-4602-03	1000s	$40.89
Moore,H.L.	00839-6010-16	1000s	$42.93
Purepac	00228-2576-96	1000s	$48.57

TABLETS: 30 MG

BRAND/MANUFACTURER	NDC	SIZE	AWP
◆ GENERICS			
MEDIVERT: Med-Tek	52349-0220-10	100s	$24.65

TABLETS: 50 MG

BRAND/MANUFACTURER	NDC	SIZE	AWP
◆ BRAND			
➤ ANTIVERT: Roerig	00662-2140-66	100s	$102.99

Meclocycline Sulfosalicylate

DESCRIPTION

Meclocycline Sulfosalicylate Cream 1% is a homogeneous smooth yellow cream, each gram of which contains Meclocycline Sulfosalicylate equivalent to 10 mg. of Meclocycline activity in an aqueous cream vehicle consisting of glyceryl stearate, propylene glycol stearate, caprylic/capric triglyceride, paraffin, trihydroxystearin, polysorbate 40, sorbitol solution, propyl gallate, sorbic acid, sodium formaldehyde sulfoxylate, perfume, and water. The vehicle is pharmaceutically compatible with both oil- and water-based systems.

Chemically Meclocycline Sulfosalicylate is $[4\underline{S}\text{-}(4\alpha,4a\alpha,5\alpha, 5a\alpha,12a\alpha)]$-7-chloro-4-(dimethyl-amino)-1,4,4a,5,5a,6,11, -12a-,octahydro-3,5,10,12,12a- pentahydroxy-6-methylene-1,-11-dioxo -2- naphthacenecarboxamide 5-sulfosalicylate.

Following is its chemical structure:

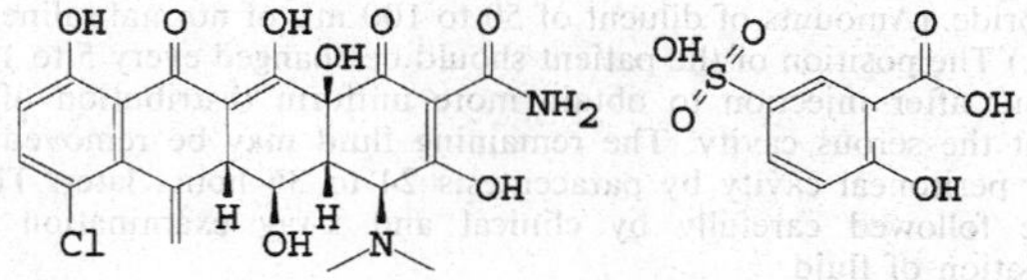

ACTIONS (CLINICAL PHARMACOLOGY)

The mode of action of Meclocycline Sulfosalicylate Cream in the treatment of acne is not fully understood. However, it appears that Meclocycline possesses a localized effect, since it is not absorbed through the skin in sufficient quantities to be detected systemically. In subtotal body inunction studies, up to 40 times the average treatment dose was applied to 20 human subjects daily for 28 days. No measurable amounts of Meclocycline appeared in the blood (0.1 microgram/ml. level of detectability) or urine (0.02 microgram/ml level of detectability).

INDICATION

Meclocycline Sulfosalicylate Cream is indicated for topical application in the treatment of acne vulgaris.

CONTRAINDICATIONS

Meclocycline Sulfosalicylate is contraindicated in persons who have shown hypersensitivity to any of its ingredients or to any of the other tetracyclines.

◆ RATED THERAPEUTICALLY EQUIVALENT; ◇ THERAPEUTIC EQUIVALENCE UNCONFIRMED; ○ UNRATED

WARNINGS

Although no absorption has been demonstrated by 28-day inunction studies in humans, the possibility exists that significant percutaneous absorption may result from prolonged use. Therefore, caution is advised in administering Meclocycline Sulfosalicylate to persons with hepatic or renal dysfunction.

Contains sodium formaldehyde sulfoxylate, a sulfite-producing agent that may cause allergic-type reactions including anaphylactic symptoms and life-threatening or less severe asthmatic episodes in certain susceptible people. The overall prevalence of sulfite sensitivity in the general population is unknown and probably low. Sulfite sensitivity is seen more frequently in asthmatic than in nonasthmatic people.

PRECAUTIONS

This drug is for external use only and should be kept out of the eyes, nose, and mouth. It should be used with caution by patients who are sensitive to formaldehyde.

Pregnancy: Pregnancy Category B. Reproduction studies have been performed in rats and rabbits at oral doses up to 1000 times the human dose (assuming the human dose to be one gram of cream per day) and have revealed no evidence of impaired fertility or harm to the fetus due to Meclocycline Sulfosalicylate. There was, however, a slight delay in ossification in rabbits when Meclocycline was applied topically. There are no adequate and well-controlled studies in pregnant women. Because animal reproduction studies are not always predictive of human response, this drug should be used during pregnancy only if clearly needed.

Nursing Mothers: It is not known whether this drug is excreted in human milk. Because many drugs are excreted in human milk, caution should be exercised when Meclocycline Sulfosalicylate is administered to a nursing woman.

ADVERSE REACTIONS

Meclocycline Sulfosalicylate is well tolerated by the skin. In the clinical trials there was one report of acute contact dermatitis. There were isolated reports of skin irritation. Temporary follicular staining may occur with excessive application. Patch testing has demonstrated no photosensitivity or contact allergy potential.

DOSAGE AND ADMINISTRATION

It is recommended that Meclocycline Sulfosalicylate be applied to the affected area twice daily, morning and evening. Less frequent application may be used depending on patient response. Excessive use of Meclocycline Sulfosalicylate Cream may cause staining of some fabrics.

HOW SUPPLIED
CREAM: 1%

BRAND/MANUFACTURER	NDC	SIZE	AWP
○ BRAND			
MECLAN: Ortho Pharm	00062-0675-80	20 gm	$20.40
	00062-0675-01	45 gm	$35.16

Meclofenamate Sodium

DESCRIPTION

Meclofenamate Sodium is N-(2, 6-dichloro-m-tolyl) anthranilic acid, sodium salt, monohydrate. It is an anti-inflammatory drug for oral administration. Meclofenamate Sodium capsules contain 50 mg or 100 mg meclofenamic acid as the sodium salt.

It is a white powder with melting point 287° to 291°C, molecular weight 336.15, and water solubility greater than 250 mg/mL.

Following is its chemical structure:

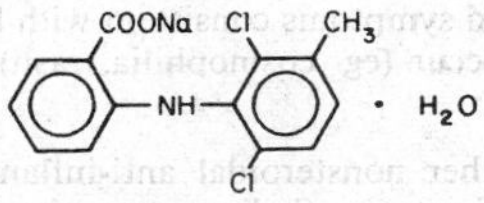

CLINICAL PHARMACOLOGY
PHARMACODYNAMICS

Meclofenamate Sodium is a nonsteroidal agent which has demonstrated anti-inflammatory, analgesic, and antipyretic activity in laboratory animals. The mode of action, like that of other nonsteroidal anti-inflammatory agents, is not known. Therapeutic action does not result from pituitary-adrenal stimulation. In animal studies, Meclofenamate Sodium was found to inhibit prostaglandin synthesis and to compete for binding at the prostaglandin receptor site. In vitro, Meclofenamate Sodium was found to be an inhibitor of human leukocyte-5-lipoxygenase activity. These properties may be responsible for the anti-inflammatory action of Meclofenamate Sodium. There is no evidence that Meclofenamate Sodium alters the course of the underlying disease.

In several human isotope studies, Meclofenamate Sodium at a dosage of 300 mg/day, produced a fecal blood loss of 1 to 2 ml per day and 2 to 3 ml per day at 400 mg/day. Aspirin, at a dosage of 3.6 g/day, caused a fecal blood loss of 6 ml per day.

In a multiple-dose, one-week study in normal human volunteers, Meclofenamate Sodium had little or no effect on collagen-induced platelet aggregation, platelet count, or bleeding time. In comparison, aspirin suppressed collagen-induced platelet aggregation and increased bleeding time. The concomitant administration of antacids (aluminum and magnesium hydroxides) does not interfere with absorption of Meclofenamate Sodium.

PHARMACOKINETICS

Meclofenamate Sodium is rapidly absorbed in man following single and multiple oral doses with peak plasma concentrations occurring in 0.5 to 2 hours. Based on a comparison to a suspension of meclofenamic acid, Meclofenamate Sodium is completely bioavailable. The plasma concentrations of meclofenamic acid decline monoexponentially following oral administration. In a study in 10 healthy subjects following a single oral dose the apparent elimination half-life ranged from 0.8 to 5.3 hours. After the administration of Meclofenamate Sodium for 14 days every 8 hours, the apparent elimination half-life ranged from 0.8 to 2.1 hours with no evidence of accumulation of meclofenamic acid in plasma (see Table). (See related table).

Meclofenamic acid is extensively metabolized to an active metabolite (Metabolite I; 3-hydroxymethyl metabolite of meclofenamic acid) and at least six other less well characterized minor metabolites.

Only this Metabolite I has been shown *in vitro* to inhibit cyclooxygenase activity with approximately one fifth the activity of Meclofenamate Sodium Metabolite I (3-hydroxymethyl metabolite of meclofenamic acid) with a mean half-life of approximately 15 hours did accumulate following multiple dosing. After the administration of 100 mg Meclofenamate Sodium for 14 days every 8 hours, Metabolite I reached a peak plasma concentration of only 1 µg/mL. By contrast, the peak concentration was 4.8 µg/mL for the parent compound on both days 1 and 14. Therefore, the accumulation of Metabolite I is probably not clinically significant.

Approximately 70% of the administered dose is excreted by the kidneys with 8-35% excreted as predominantly conjugated species of meclofenamic acid and Metabolite I (see Table). Other metabolites, whose excretion rates are unknown, account for the remaining 35-62% of the dose excreted in the urine. The remainder of the administered dose (approximately 30%) is eliminated in the feces (apparently through biliary excretion). There is insufficient experience to know if Meclofenamate Sodium or its metabolites accumulate in patients with compromised renal or hepatic function. Therefore, Meclofenamate Sodium should be used with caution in these patients. (See *"Precautions."*) Trace amounts of Meclofenamate Sodium are excreted in human breast milk.

Meclofenamic acid is greater than 99% bound to plasma proteins over a wide drug concentration range.

Unlike most NSAIDs, which when administered with food have a decrease in rate but not in extent of absorption, meclofenamic acid is decreased in both. Following the administration of Meclofenamate Sodium capsules one half-hour after a meal, the average extent of bioavailability decreased by 26%, the average age peak concentration (Cmax) decreased 4 fold and the time to Cmax was delayed by 3 hours.

CLINICAL STUDIES

Controlled clinical trials comparing Meclofenamate with aspirin demonstrated comparable efficacy in rheumatoid arthritis. The Meclofenamate-treated patients had fewer reactions involving the special senses, specifically tinnitus, but more gastrointestinal reactions, specifically diarrhea.

The incidence of patients who discontinued therapy due to adverse reactions was similar for both the Meclofenamate and aspirin-treated groups.

The improvement with Meclofenamate reported by patients and the reduction of the disease activity as evaluated by both physicians and patients with rheumatoid arthritis are associated with a significant reduction in number of tender joints, severity of tenderness, and duration of morning stiffness.

The improvement reported by patients and as evaluated by physicians in patients treated with Meclofenamate for osteoarthritis is associated with a significant reduction in night pain, pain on walking, degree of starting pain, and pain on passive motion. The function of knee joints also improved significantly.

Meclofenamate has been used in combination with gold salts or corticosteroids in patients with rheumatoid arthritis. Studies have demonstrated that Meclofenamate contributes to the improvement of patients' conditions while maintained on gold salts or corticosteroids. Data are inadequate to demonstrate that Meclofenamate in combination with salicylates produces greater improvement than that achieved with Meclofenamate alone.

In controlled clinical trials of patients with mild to moderate pain, Meclofenamate 50 mg provided significant pain relief. In these studies of episiotomy and dental pain, Meclofenamate 100 mg demonstrated additional benefit in some patients. The onset of analgesic effect was generally within one hour and the duration of action was 4 to 6 hours.

In controlled clinical trials of patients with dysmenorrhea, Meclofenamate 100 mg t.i.d. provided significant reduction in the symptoms associated with dysmenorrhea.

In randomized double-blind crossover trials of Meclofenamate 100 mg t.i.d. versus placebo in women with heavy menstrual blood loss (MBL), Meclofenamate treatment was usually associated with a reduction in menstrual flow.

The graph below is a scatter plot of menstrual flow from the average of two menstrual periods on Meclofenamate treatments (x-axis) versus two menstrual periods on placebo (y-axis) for 55 women. Of note, although the amount of reduction in MBL was variable, some degree of reduction occurred in 90% of women in this study.

Scattergram of Menstrual Flow
Average of Two Periods on Each Treatment
of 55 Women from Three Clinical Trials

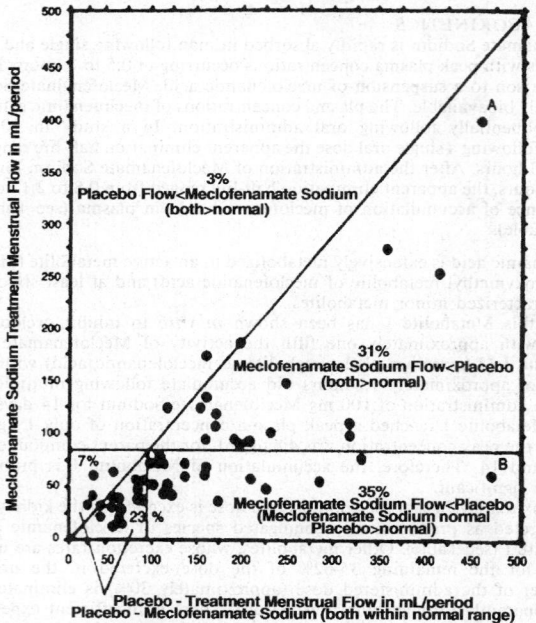

Placebo - Treatment Menstrual Flow in mL/period
Placebo - Meclofenamate Sodium (both within normal range)

The points on the graph represent the mean MBL for each subject when treated for two periods with placebo and two periods with Meclofenamate Sodium. To ease in interpretation, the following examples may be helpful. Point A represents a woman who had MBL of 459 mL while on placebo, and 405 mL on Meclofenamate Sodium. Point B represents a woman who had MBL of 472 mL while on placebo, and 64 mL when treated with Meclofenamate Sodium.

In association with this reduction in menstrual blood loss, the duration of menses was decreased by 1 day, tampon/pad usage was decreased by an average of 2 per day on the two days of heaviest flow, and symptoms of dysmenorrhea were significantly reduced.

INDICATIONS AND USAGE
Meclofenamate Sodium is indicated for the relief of mild to moderate pain. Meclofenamate Sodium is also indicated for the treatment of primary dysmenorrhea and for the treatment of idiopathic heavy menstrual blood loss. (See "Clinical Pharmacology" and "Precautions" sections.)

Meclofenamate Sodium is also indicated for relief of the signs and symptoms of acute and chronic rheumatoid arthritis and osteoarthritis. As with all nonsteroidal anti-inflammatory drugs, selection of Meclofenamate Sodium requires a careful assessment of the benefit/risk ratio. (See "Warnings," "Precautions" and "Adverse Reactions" sections.)

Meclofenamate Sodium is not recommended in children because adequate studies to demonstrate safety and efficacy have not been carried out.

UNLABELED USES
Meclofenamate Sodium is used alone or as an adjunct in the treatment of ankylosing spondylitis, hypermenorrhea, and episiotomy pain. It is also used in acute gout and eosinophilic cystitis.

CONTRAINDICATIONS
Meclofenamate should not be used in patients who have previously exhibited hypersensitivity to it.

Because the potential exists for cross-sensitivity to aspirin or other nonsteroidal anti-inflammatory drugs, Meclofenamate Sodium should not be given to patients in whom these drugs induce symptoms of bronchospasm, allergic rhinitis, or urticaria.

WARNINGS
Risk of GI Ulceration, Bleeding and Perforation with NSAID Therapy: Serious gastrointestinal toxicity, such as bleeding, ulceration, and perforation, can occur at any time, with or without warning symptoms, in patients treated chronically with NSAID therapy. Although minor upper gastrointestinal problems, such as dyspepsia, are common, usually developing early in therapy, physicians should remain alert for ulceration and bleeding in patients treated chronically with NSAIDs even in the absence of previous GI tract symptoms. In patients observed in clinical trials of several months to two years' duration, symptomatic upper GI ulcers, gross bleeding or perforation appear to occur in approximately 1% of patients treated for 3-6 months, and in about 2-4% of patients treated for one year. Physicians should inform patients about the signs and/or symptoms of serious GI toxicity and what steps to take if they occur.

Studies to date have not identified any subset of patients not at risk of developing peptic ulceration and bleeding. Except for a prior history of serious GI

events and other risks factors known to be associated with peptic ulcer disease, such as alcoholism, smoking, etc, no risk factors (e.g., age, sex) have been associated with increased risk. Elderly or debilitated patients seem to tolerate ulceration or bleeding less well than other individuals, and most spontaneous reports of fatal GI events are in this population. Studies to date are inconclusive concerning the relative risk of various NSAIDs in causing such reactions. High doses of any NSAID probably carry a greater risk of these reactions, although controlled clinical trials showing this do not exist in most cases. In considering the use of relatively large doses (within the recommended dosage range), sufficient benefit should be anticipated to offset the potential increased risk of GI toxicity.

PRECAUTIONS
General: Patients receiving nonsteroidal anti-inflammatory agents, such as Meclofenamate Sodium should be evaluated periodically to insure that the drug is still necessary and well tolerated. (See other "Precautions," "Warnings," and "Adverse Reactions.")

Diarrhea, gastrointestinal irritation and abdominal pain may be associated with Meclofenamate Sodium therapy. Dosage reduction or temporarily stopping the drug have generally controlled these symptoms. (See "Adverse Reactions" and "Dosage and Administration" sections.)

Decreases in hemoglobin and/or hematocrit levels have occurred in approximately 1 of 6 patients, but rarely required discontinuation of Meclofenamate Sodium therapy. The clinical data revealed no evidence of increased chronic blood loss, bone-marrow suppression, or hemolysis to account for the decreases in hemoglobin or hematocrit levels. Patients who are receiving long-term Meclofenamate Sodium therapy should have hemoglobin and hematocrit values determined if anemia is suspected on clinical grounds.

If a patient develops visual symptoms (see "Adverse Reactions") during Meclofenamate Sodium therapy, the drug should be discontinued and the patient should have a complete ophthalmologic examination.

When Meclofenamate Sodium is used in combination with steroid therapy, any reduction in steroid dosage should be gradual to avoid the possible complications of sudden steroid withdrawal.

Elderly: Adverse effects are seen more commonly in the elderly; therefore, a lower starting dose and careful follow-up are advised.

Evaluation of Patients with Heavy Menstrual Blood Loss: Prior to prescribing Meclofenamate Sodium for heavy blood flow and primary dysmenorrhea, a thorough risk/benefit assessment should be made that takes into account the results described in the "Clinical Pharmacology" section. It is recommended that Meclofenamate Sodium treatment not be prescribed for heavy menstrual flow without establishing its idiopathic nature. Spotting or bleeding between cycles should be evaluated fully and not treated with Meclofenamate Sodium. Worsening of menstrual blood loss or excessive blood loss failing to respond to Meclofenamate Sodium should also be evaluated by an appropriate work-up and not treated with Meclofenamate Sodium.

Hepatic Reactions: As with other nonsteroidal anti-inflammatory drugs, borderline evaluations of one or more liver tests may occur in some patients. These abnormalities may progress, may remain essentially unchanged, or may be transient with continued therapy. The SGPT (ALT) test is probably the most sensitive indicator of liver dysfunction. Meaningful (3 times the upper limit of normal) elevations of SGPT or SGOT (AST) occurred in controlled clinical trials in less than 1% of patients. A patient with symptoms and/or signs suggesting liver dysfunction, or in whom an abnormal liver test has occurred, should be evaluated for evidence of the development of more severe hepatic reaction while on therapy with Meclofenamate Sodium. Severe hepatic reactions, including jaundice and cases of fatal hepatitis, have been reported with other nonsteroidal anti-inflammatory drugs. Although such reactions are rare, if abnormal liver tests persist or worsen, if clinical signs and symptoms consistent with liver disease develop, or if systemic manifestations occur (eg. eosinophilia, rash), Meclofenamate Sodium should be discontinued.

Renal Effects: As with other nonsteroidal anti-inflammatory drugs, long-term administration of Meclofenamate Sodium to animals has resulted in renal papillary necrosis and other abnormal renal pathology. In humans, there have been reports of acute interstitial nephritis with hematuria, proteinuria, and occasionally nephrotic syndrome.

A second form of renal toxicity has been seen in patients with prerenal conditions leading to a reduction in renal blood flow or blood volume, where the renal prostaglandins have a supportive role in the maintenance of renal perfusion. In these patients administration of an NSAID may cause a dose-dependent reduction in prostaglandin formation and may precipitate overt renal decompensation. Patients at greatest risk of this reaction are those with impaired renal function, heart failure, liver dysfunction, those taking diuretics, and the elderly. Discontinuation of NSAID therapy is typically followed by recovery to the pretreatment state. Since Meclofenamate Sodium metabolites are eliminated primarily by the kidneys, patients with significantly impaired renal function should be closely monitored; a lower daily dosage should be employed to avoid excessive drug accumulation.

Information for Patients: Patients should be advised that nausea, vomiting, diarrhea, and abdominal pain have been associated with the use of Meclofenamate Sodium. The patient should be made aware of a possible drug connection and accordingly should consider discontinuing the drug and contacting his or her physician if any of these conditions are severe.

Women who are taking Meclofenamate Sodium for heavy menstrual flow should be advised to consult their doctor if they have spotting or bleeding between cycles or worsening of their menstrual blood flow. These symptoms may be signs of the development of a more serious condition that is not appropriately treated with Meclofenamate Sodium.

Meclofenamate Sodium may be taken with meals or milk to control gastrointestinal complaints. Concomitant administration of an antacid (specifically, aluminum and magnesium hydroxides) does not interfere with the absorption of the drug.

Meclofenamate Sodium like other drugs of its class, is not free of side effects. The side effects of these drugs can cause discomfort and, rarely, there are more serious side effects, such as gastrointestinal bleeding, which may result in hospitalization and even fatal outcomes.

NSAIDs (nonsteroidal anti-inflammatory drugs) are often essential agents in the management of arthritis and have a major role in the treatment of pain, but they also may be commonly employed for conditions which are less serious. Physicians may wish to discuss with their patients the potential risks (see "Warnings," "Precautions," and "Adverse Reactions" sections) and likely benefits of NSAID treatment, particularly when the drugs are used for less serious conditions where treatment without NSAIDs may represent an acceptable alternative to both the patient and physician.

Laboratory Tests: Patients receiving long-term Meclofenamate Sodium therapy should have hemoglobin and hematocrit values determined if signs or symptoms of anemia occur.

Low white blood cell counts were rarely observed in clinical trials. These low counts were transient and usually returned to normal while the patient continued on Meclofenamate Sodium therapy. Persistent leukopenia, granulocytopenia, or thrombocytopenia warrant further clinical evaluation and may require discontinuation of the drug.

When abnormal blood chemistry values are obtained, follow-up studies are indicated.

Elevations of serum transaminase levels and of alkaline phosphatase levels occurred in approximately 4% of patients. An occasional patient had elevations of serum creatinine or BUN levels.

Because serious GI tract ulceration and bleeding can occur without warning symptoms, physicians should follow chronically treated patients for the signs and symptoms of ulceration and bleeding and should inform them of the importance of this follow-up (see "Risk of GI Ulcerations, Bleeding and Perforation with NSAID Therapy").

DRUG INTERACTIONS

1. Warfarin: Meclofenamate Sodium enhances the effect of warfarin. Therefore, when Meclofenamate Sodium is given to a patient receiving warfarin, the dosage of warfarin should be reduced to prevent excessive prolongation of the prothrombin time.

2. Aspirin: Concurrent administration of aspirin may lower Meclofenamate Sodium plasma levels, possibly by competing for protein-binding sites. The urinary excretion of Meclofenamate Sodium is unaffected by aspirin, indicating no change in Meclofenamate Sodium absorption. Meclofenamate Sodium does not affect serum salicylate levels. Greater fecal blood loss results from concomitant administration of both drugs than from either drug alone.

3. Propoxyphene: The concurrent administration of propoxyphene hydrochloride does not affect the bioavailability of Meclofenamate Sodium.

4. Antacids: Concomitant administration of aluminum and magnesium hydroxides does not interfere with absorption of Meclofenamate Sodium.

Carcinogenesis: An 18-month study in rats revealed no evidence of carcinogenicity.

Usage in Pregnancy: Meclofenamate Sodium like aspirin and other non-steroidal anti-inflammatory drugs, causes fetotoxicity, minor skeletal malformations, eg, supernumerary ribs, and delayed ossification in rodent reproduction trials, but no major teratogenicity. Similarly, it prolongs gestation and interferes with parturition and with normal development of young before weaning. Meclofenamate Sodium is not recommended for use during pregnancy, particularly in the 1st and 3rd trimesters, based on these animal findings. There are, however, no adequate and well-controlled studies in pregnant women.

Usage in Nursing Mothers: Trace amounts of meclofenamic acid are excreted in human milk. Because of the possible adverse effects of prostaglandin-inhibiting drugs on neonates, Meclofenamate Sodium is not recommended for nursing women.

Pediatric Use: Safety and effectiveness in children below the age of 14 have not been established.

ADVERSE REACTIONS
INCIDENCE GREATER THAN 1%
The following adverse reactions were observed in clinical trials and included observations from more than 2,700 patients, 594 of whom were treated for one year and 248 for at least two years.

Gastrointestinal: The most frequently reported adverse reactions associated with Meclofenamate Sodium involve the gastrointestinal system. In controlled studies of up to six months duration, these disturbances occurred in the following decreasing order of frequency with the approximate incidences in parentheses: diarrhea (10-33%), nausea with or without vomiting (11%), other gastrointestinal disorders (10%), and abdominal pain.* In long-term uncontrolled studies of up to four years duration, one third of the patients had at least one episode of diarrhea some time during Meclofenamate Sodium therapy. In approximately 4% of the patients in controlled studies, diarrhea was severe enough to require discontinuation of Meclofenamate Sodium. The occurrence of diarrhea is dose related, generally subsides with dose reduction, and clears with termination of therapy. The incidence of diarrhea in patients with osteoarthritis is generally lower than that reported in patients with rheumatoid arthritis.

Other reactions less frequently reported were pyrosis,* flatulence,* anorexia, constipation, stomatitis, and peptic ulcer. The majority of the patients with peptic ulcer had either a history of ulcer disease or were receiving concomitant anti-inflammatory drugs, including corticosteroids, which are known to produce peptic ulceration.

Cardiovascular: edema

Dermatologic: rash,* urticaria, pruritus

Central Nervous System: headache,* dizziness*

Special Senses: tinnitus

INCIDENCE LESS THAN 1%
Probably Causally Related: The following adverse reactions were reported less frequently than 1% during controlled clinical trials and through voluntary reports since marketing. The probability of a causal relationship exists between the drug and these adverse reactions.

Gastrointestinal: bleeding and/or perforation with or without obvious ulcer formation, colitis, cholestatic jaundice

Renal: renal failure.

Hematologic: neutropenia, thrombocytopenic purpura, leukopenia, agranulocytosis, hemolytic anemia, eosinophilia, decrease in hemoglobin and/or hematocrit

Dermatologic: erythema multiforme, Stevens-Johnson syndrome, exfoliative dermatitis

* Incidence between 3% and 9%. Those reactions occurring in 1% to 3% of patients are not marked with an asterisk.

Table
SUMMARY OF MECLOFENAMATE SODIUM PHARMACOKINETIC PARAMETERS

	Mean (Range) Parameter Values (n = 10)	
	Meclofenamic Acid	Metabolite I[a]
	100-mg[c]	
Cmax µg/mL[1]	4.8 (1.8-7.2)	1.0 (0.5-1.5)
tmax hr[2]	0.9 (0.5-1.5)	2.4 (0.5-4.0)
Cmin µg/mL[3]	0.2 (0.5-1.5)	0.4 (0.2-1.1)
Cl/F mL/min[4]	206.0 (126-342)	-
Vd/F liters[5]	23.3 (9.1-43.2)	-
t$_{1/2}$ hr[6]	1.3 (0.8-2.1)	15.3[b]
% of Dose in Urine Unconjugated	0.0 -	0.5 (0-1.2)
Total	2.7 (0-4.5)	21.6 (7.5-32.6)

[a] 3-Hydroxymethyl metabolite of meclofenamic acid with 20% activity of Meclomen in vitro
[b] Estimated from mean data
[c] Administered every 8 hours for 14 days
[1] Peak plasma concentration
[2] Time to peak plasma concentration
[3] Trough plasma concentration
[4] Oral clearance
[5] Oral distribution volume
[6] Elimination half-life

Hepatic: alteration of liver function tests

Allergic: lupus and serum sickness-like symptoms

INCIDENCE LESS THAN 1%

Causal Relationship Unknown: Other reactions have been reported but under conditions where a causal relationship could not be established. However, in these rarely reported events, that possibility cannot be excluded. Therefore, these observations are listed to alert physicians.

Cardiovascular: palpitations

Central Nervous System: malaise, fatigue, paresthesia, insomnia, depression

Special Senses: blurred vision, taste disturbances, decreased visual acuity, temporary loss of vision, reversible loss of color vision, retinal changes including macular fibrosis, macular and perimacular edema, conjunctivitis, iritis

Renal: nocturia

Gastrointestinal: paralytic ileus

Dermatologic: erythema nodosum, hair loss

OVERDOSAGE

The following is based on the little information available concerning overdosage with Meclofenamate Sodium and related compounds. After a massive overdose, CNS stimulation may be manifested by irrational behavior, marked agitation and generalized seizures. Following this phase, renal toxicity (falling urine output, rising creatinine, abnormal urinary cellular elements) may be noted with possible oliguria or anuria and azotemia. A 24-year-old male was anuric for approximately 1 week after ingesting an overdose of 6-7 grams of Meclofenamate Sodium. Spontaneous diuresis and recovery subsequently occurred.

Management consists of emptying the stomach by emesis or lavage and instilling an ample dose of activated charcoal into the stomach. There is some evidence that charcoal will actively absorb Meclofenamate Sodium but dialysis or hemoperfusion may be less effective because of plasma protein binding. The seizures should be controlled by an appropriate anticonvulsant regimen. Attention should be directed throughout, by careful monitoring, to the preservation of vital functions and fluid-electrolyte balance. Dialysis may be required to correct serious azotemia or electrolyte imbalance.

DOSAGE AND ADMINISTRATION

Usual Dosage: For mild to moderate pain, the recommended dose is 50 mg every 4 to 6 hours. Doses of 100 mg may be needed in some patients for optimal pain relief. (See *"Clinical Pharmacology"* section.) However, the daily dose should not exceed 400 mg. (See *"Adverse Reactions"* section.)

For excessive menstrual blood loss and primary dysmenorrhea, the recommended dose of Meclofenamate Sodium is 100 mg three times a day, for up to six days, starting at the onset of menstrual flow.

For rheumatoid arthritis and osteoarthritis, including acute exacerbations of chronic disease, the dosage is 200 to 400 mg per day, administered in three or four equal doses.

Therapy should be initiated at the lower dosage, then increased as necessary to improve clinical response. The dosage should be individually adjusted for each patient depending on the severity of the symptoms and the clinical response. The daily dosage should not exceed 400 mg per day. The smallest dosage of Meclofenamate Sodium that yields clinical control should be employed.

Although improvement may be seen in some patients in a few days, two to three weeks of treatment may be required to obtain the optimum therapeutic benefit.

After a satisfactory response has been achieved, the dosage should be adjusted as required. A lower dosage may suffice for long-term administration.

If gastrointestinal complaints occur, see *"Warnings"* and *"Precautions."* Meclofenamate Sodium may be administered with meals or with milk. (See *"Clinical Pharmacology"* for a description of food effects.) If intolerance occurs, the dosage may need to be reduced. Therapy should be terminated if any severe adverse reactions occur.

Storage: Store at room temperature below 30°C (86°F). Protect from moisture and light.

HOW SUPPLIED

CAPSULE: 50 MG

AVERAGE UNIT PRICE (AVAILABLE SIZES)			
BRAND	$0.74	*GENERIC A-RATED AVERAGE PRICE (GAAP)*	
GENERIC	$0.34	100s	$35.07
HCFA FUL (100s ea)	$0.16	500s	$151.20

BRAND/MANUFACTURER	*NDC*	*SIZE*	*AWP*
◆ **BRAND**			
MECLOMEN: Parke-Davis	00071-0268-24	100s	$74.12
◆ **GENERICS**			
Goldline	00182-1270-01	100s	$28.50
Aligen	00405-4612-01	100s	$29.69
Schein	00364-2155-01	100s	$33.50
Qualitest	00603-4344-21	100s	$34.08
Major	00904-1413-60	100s	$35.50
Mylan	00378-2150-01	100s	$36.25
Geneva	00781-2702-01	100s	$36.25
Moore,H.L.	00839-7274-06	100s	$39.69
Parmed	00349-8637-01	100s	$51.00

BRAND/MANUFACTURER	*NDC*	*SIZE*	*AWP*
U.S. Trading	56126-0414-11	100s ud	$22.50
Raway	00686-0496-20	100s ud	$31.00
UDL	51079-0496-20	100s ud	$42.88
Major	00904-1413-40	500s	$98.40
Qualitest	00603-4344-28	500s	$148.60
Mylan	00378-2150-05	500s	$174.75
Moore,H.L.	00839-7274-12	500s	$183.06

CAPSULE: 100 MG

AVERAGE UNIT PRICE (AVAILABLE SIZES)		*GENERIC A-RATED AVERAGE PRICE (GAAP)*	
BRAND	$1.03	100s	$49.15
GENERIC	$0.48	500s	$227.66
HCFA FUL (100s ea)	$0.24		

BRAND/MANUFACTURER	*NDC*	*SIZE*	*AWP*
◆ **BRAND**			
MECLOMEN: Parke-Davis	00071-0269-24	100s	$102.62
◆ **GENERICS**			
Goldline	00182-1271-01	100s	$39.00
Qualitest	00603-4345-21	100s	$45.40
Schein	00364-2156-01	100s	$45.80
Major	00904-1414-60	100s	$45.90
Mylan	00378-3000-01	100s	$48.25
Geneva	00781-2703-01	100s	$48.29
Purepac	00228-2256-10	100s	$48.48
Aligen	00405-4613-01	100s	$48.92
Moore,H.L.	00839-7275-06	100s	$52.31
Parmed	00349-8638-01	100s	$75.30
Raway	00686-0497-20	100s ud	$39.00
UDL	51079-0497-20	100s ud	$53.18
Major	00904-1414-40	500s	$132.40
Qualitest	00603-4345-28	500s	$219.47
Mylan	00378-3000-05	500s	$235.20
Moore,H.L.	00839-7275-12	500s	$261.35
Parmed	00349-8638-05	500s	$289.90

TABLETS: 100 MG

BRAND/MANUFACTURER	*NDC*	*SIZE*	*AWP*
◆ **GENERICS**			
Schein	00364-2156-05	500s	$157.50

Meclomen *SEE* MECLOFENAMATE SODIUM

Medent *SEE* GUAIFENESIN AND PSEUDOEPHEDRINE HYDROCHLORIDE

Medihaler-Iso *SEE* ISOPROTERENOL

Medrol *SEE* METHYLPREDNISOLONE

Medroxyprogesterone Acetate, Contraceptive

Patients should be counseled that this product does not protect against HIV infection (AIDS) and other sexually transmitted diseases.

DESCRIPTION

Medroxyprogesterone Acetate Contraceptive Injection contains a derivative of progesterone, as its active ingredient. Medroxyprogesterone Acetate is active by the parenteral and oral routes of administration. It is a white to off-white, odorless crystalline powder that is stable in air and that melts between 200° C and 210° C. It is freely soluble in chloroform, soluble in acetone and dioxane, sparingly soluble in alcohol and methanol, slightly soluble in ether, and insoluble in water.

The chemical name for Medroxyprogesterone Acetate is pregn-4-ene-3.20-dione, 17-(acetyloxy)-6-methyl-,(6α)-. Medroxyprogesterone Acetate Contraceptive Injection for intramuscular injection is available in 150 mg/mL vials each containing 1 mL Medroxyprogesterone Acetate sterile aqueous suspension.

Each mL contains:	
Medroxyprogesterone Acetate	150 mg
Polyethylene glycol 3350	28.9 mg
Polysorbate 80	2.41 mg
Sodium chloride	8.68 mg
Methylparaben	1.37 mg
Propylparaben	0.150 mg
Water for injection	q.s.

When necessary, pH is adjusted with sodium hydroxide and/or hydrochloric acid.

Following is its chemical structure:

CLINICAL PHARMACOLOGY

Medroxyprogesterone Acetate Contraceptive Injection, when administered at the recommended dose to women every 3 months, inhibits the secretion of gonadotropins which, in turn, prevents follicular maturation and ovulation and results in endometrial thinning. These actions produce its contraceptive effect.

Following a single 150 mg IM dose of Medroxyprogesterone Acetate Contraceptive Injection, Medroxyprogesterone Acetate concentrations, measured by an extracted radioimmunoassay procedure, increase for approximately three weeks to reach peak plasma concentrations of 1 to 7 ng/mL. The levels then decrease exponentially until they become undetectable (< 100 pg/mL) between 120 to 200 days following injection. Using an unextracted radioimmunoassay procedure for the assay of Medroxyprogesterone Acetate in serum, the apparent half-life for Medroxyprogesterone Acetate following IM administration of Medroxyprogesterone Acetate Contraceptive Injection is approximately 50 days.

Women with lower body weights conceive sooner than women with higher body weights after discontinuing Medroxyprogesterone Acetate.

The effect of hepatic and/or renal disease on the pharmacokinetics of Medroxyprogesterone Acetate Contraceptive Injection is unknown.

INDICATIONS AND USAGE

Medroxyprogesterone Acetate Contraceptive Injection is indicated only for the prevention of pregnancy. It is a long-term injectable contraceptive in women when administered at 3-month intervals. Dosage does not need to be adjusted for body weight. In five Medroxyprogesterone Acetate clinical studies the 12 month failure rate for the group of women treated with Medroxyprogesterone Acetate was zero (no pregnancies reported) to 0.7 by Life-Table method. Pregnancy rates with contraceptive measures are typically reported for only the first year of use as shown in Table 1. Except for intrauterine devices (IUD), implants, sterilization, and Medroxyprogesterone Acetate, the efficacy of these contraceptive measures depends in part on the reliability of use. The effectiveness of Medroxyprogesterone Acetate is dependent on the patient returning every 3 months for re-injection.

Table 1
LOWEST EXPECTED AND TYPICAL FAILURE RATES* EXPRESSED AS PERCENT OF WOMEN EXPERIENCING AN ACCIDENTAL PREGNANCY IN THE FIRST YEAR OF CONTINUOUS USE

Method	Lowest Expected	Typical
Injectable progestogen		
Medroxyprogesterone Acetate	0.3	0.3
Implants		
Norplant (6 capsules)	0.2†	0.2†
Female sterilization	0.2	0.4
Male sterilization	0.1	0.15
Pill		3
Combined	0.1	
Progestogen only	0.5	
IUD		
Progestasert		3
Copper T 380A	0.8	1
Condom	2	12
Diaphragm	6	18
Cap	6	18
Spermicides	3	21
Sponge		
Parous women	9	28
Nulliparous women	6	18
Periodic abstinence	1-9	20
Withdrawal	4	18
No Method	85	85

Source: Trussell et al[1]*
Lowest expected - when used exactly as directed.
Typical - includes those not following directions exactly.

CONTRAINDICATIONS

1. Known or suspected pregnancy or as a diagnostic test for pregnancy.
2. Undiagnosed vaginal bleeding.
3. Known or suspected malignancy of breast.
4. Active thrombophlebitis, or current or past history of thromboembolic disorders, or cerebral vascular disease.
5. Liver dysfunction or disease.

6. Known sensitivity to Medroxyprogesterone Acetate or any of its other ingredients.

WARNINGS

1. Bleeding Irregularities: Most women using Medroxyprogesterone Acetate Contraceptive Injection experience disruption of menstrual bleeding patterns. Altered menstrual bleeding patterns include irregular or unpredictable bleeding or spotting, or rarely, heavy or continuous bleeding. If abnormal bleeding persists or is severe, appropriate investigation should be instituted to rule out the possibility of organic pathology, and appropriate treatment should be instituted when necessary.

As women continue using Medroxyprogesterone Acetate, fewer experience intermenstrual bleeding and more experience amenorrhea. By month 12 amenorrhea was reported by 55% of women, and by month 24 amenorrhea was reported by 68% of women using Medroxyprogesterone Acetate.[2]

2. Bone Mineral Density Changes: Use of Medroxyprogesterone Acetate may be considered among the risk factors for development of osteoporosis. The rate of bone loss is greatest in the early years of use and then subsequently approaches the normal rate of age related fall.

3. Cancer Risks: Long-term case-controlled surveillance of Medroxyprogesterone Acetate Contraceptive Injection users found slight or no increased overall risk of breast cancer[4] and no overall increased risk of ovarian,[5] liver,[6] or cervical[7] cancer and a prolonged, protective effect of reducing the risk of endometrial[8] cancer in the population of users.

An increased relative risk (RR) of 2.19 (95% C.I. 1.23-3.89)[4] of breast cancer has been associated with use of Medroxyprogesterone Acetate in women whose first exposure to drug was within the previous 4 years and who were under 35 years of age [C.I. = Confidence Interval]. However, the overall relative risk for ever-users of Medroxyprogesterone Acetate was only 1.2 (95% C.I. 0.96-1.52).

(Note: A relative risk of 1.0 indicates neither an increased nor a decreased risk of cancer associated with the use of the drug, relative to no use of the drug. In the case of subpopulation with a relative risk of 2.19, the 95% C.I. is fairly wide and does not include the value of 1.0, thus inferring an increased risk of breast cancer in the defined sub-group relative to non-users. The value of 2.19 means that women whose first exposure to drug was within the previous 4 years and who are under 35 years of age have a 2.19-fold [95% C.I. 1.23-3.89-fold] increased risk of breast cancer relative to non-users. The National Cancer Institute[9] reports an average annual incidence rate for breast cancer for U.S. women, all races, ages 30-34 years of 26.7/100,000. A relative risk of 2.19 thus increases the possible risk from 26.7 to 58.5 cases per 100,000 women. The attributable risk, thus, is 3.18 per 10,000 women per year.)

A statistically insignificant increase in relative risk estimates of invasive squamous cell cervical cancer has been associated with the use of Medroxyprogesterone Acetate in women who were first exposed before the age of 35 years (RR 1.22 to 1.28 and 95% C.I. 0.93-1.70). The overall, non-significant relative rate of invasive squamous cell cervical cancer in women who never used Medroxyprogesterone Acetate was estimated to be 1.11 (95% C.I. 0.96-1.29). No trends in risk with duration of use or times since initial or most recent exposure were observed.

4. Thromboembolic Disorders: The physician should be alert to the earliest manifestations of thrombotic disorders (thrombophlebitis, pulmonary embolism, cerebrovascular disorders, and retinal thrombosis). Should any of these occur or be suspected, the drug should not be readministered.

5. Ocular Disorders: Medication should not be readministered pending examination if there is a sudden partial or complete loss of vision or if there is a sudden onset of proptosis, diplopia, or migraine. If examination reveals papilledema or retinal vascular lesions, medication should not be readministered.

6. Accidental Pregnancies: Infants from accidental pregnancy that occur 1-2 months after injection of Medroxyprogesterone Acetate Contraceptive Injection may be at an increased risk of low birth weight, which in turn is associated with an increased risk of neonatal death. The attributable risk is low because such pregnancies are uncommon.[10,11]

A significant increase in incidence of polysyndactyly and chromosomal anomalies were observed among infants of Medroxyprogesterone Acetate users, the former being most pronounced in women under 30 years of age. The unrelated nature of these defects, the lack of confirmation from other studies, the distant preconceptual exposure to Medroxyprogesterone Acetate, and the chance effects due to multiple statistical comparisons, make a causal association unlikely.[12]

Children exposed to Medroxyprogesterone Acetate in utero and followed to adolescence, showed no evidence of any adverse effects on their health including their physical, intellectual, sexual or social development.

Several reports suggest an association between intrauterine exposure to progestational drugs in the first trimester of pregnancy and genital abnormalities in male and female fetuses. The risk of hypospadias (5 to 8 per 1000 male births in the general population) may be approximately doubled with exposure to these drugs. There are insufficient data to quantify the risk to exposed female fetuses, but because some of these drugs include mild virilization of the external genitalia of the female fetus and because of the increased association of hypospadias in the male fetus, it is prudent to avoid the use of these drugs during the first trimester of pregnancy.

To ensure that Medroxyprogesterone Acetate is not administered inadvertently to a pregnant woman, it is important that the first injection be given only during the first 5 days after the onset of a normal menstrual period; within five days postpartum if not breast feeding; and if breast feeding, at the sixth week postpartum (see *"Dosage and Administration"*).

7. Ectopic Pregnancy: Health-care providers should be alert to be the possibility of an ectopic pregnancy among women using Medroxyprogesterone Acetate Contraceptive Injection who become pregnant or complain of severe abdominal pain.

8. Lactation: Detectable amounts of drug have been identified in the milk of mothers receiving Medroxyprogesterone Acetate. In nursing mothers treated with Medroxyprogesterone Acetate Contraceptive Injection, milk composition, quality, and amount are not adversely affected. Infants exposed to Medroxyprogesterone Acetate via breast milk have been studied for developmental and behavioral effects through puberty. No adverse effects have been noted.

PRECAUTIONS
GENERAL
1. Physical Examination: The pretreatment and annual history and physical examination should include special reference to breast and pelvic organs, as well as a Papanicolaou smear.

2. Fluid Retention: Because progestation drugs may cause some degree of fluid retention, conditions that might be influenced by this condition, such as epilepsy, migraine, asthma, and cardiac or renal dysfunction, require careful observation.

3. Weight Changes: There is a tendency for women to gain weight while on Medroxyprogesterone Acetate therapy. From an initial average body weight of 136 lbs, women who completed 1 year of therapy with Medroxyprogesterone Acetate gained an average of 5.4 lbs. Women who completed 2 years of therapy gained an average of 8.1 lbs.

Women who completed 4 years gained an average of 13.8 lbs. Women who completed 6 years gained an average of 16.5 lbs. Two percent of women withdrew from a large-scale clinical trial because of excessive weight gain.

4. Return of Fertility: Medroxyprogesterone Acetate Contraceptive Injection has a prolonged contraceptive effect. In a large U.S. study of women who discontinued use of Medroxyprogesterone Acetate to become pregnant, data are available for 61% of them. Based on Life-Table analysis of these data, it is expected that 68% of women who do become pregnant may conceive within 12 months, 83% may conceive within 15 months, and 93% may conceive within 18 months from the last injection. The median time to conception for those who do conceive is 10 months following the last injection with a range of 4 to 31 months, and is unrelated to the duration of use. No data are available for 39% of the patients who discontinue Medroxyprogesterone Acetate to become pregnant and who were lost to follow-up or changed their mind.

5. CNS Disorders and Convulsions: Patients who have a history of psychic depression should be carefully observed and the drug not be readministered if the depression recurs.

There have been a few reported cases of convulsions in patients who were treated with Medroxyprogesterone Acetate Contraceptive Injection. Association with drug use or pre-existing conditions is not clear.

6. Carbohydrate Metabolism: A decrease in glucose tolerance has been observed in some patients on Medroxyprogesterone Acetate treatment. The mechanism of this decrease is obscure. For this reason, diabetic patients should be carefully observed while receiving such therapy.

7. Liver Function: If jaundice develops, consideration should be given to not readministering the drug.

DRUG INTERACTIONS
Aminoglutethimide administered concomitantly with the Medroxyprogesterone Acetate Contraceptive Injection may significantly depress the serum concentrations of Medroxyprogesterone Acetate.[13] Medroxyprogesterone Acetate users should be warned of the possibility of decreased efficacy with the use of this or any related drugs.

Laboratory Test Interactions: The pathologist should be advised of progestin therapy when relevant specimens are submitted.

The following laboratory tests may be affected by progestins including Medroxyprogesterone Acetate Contraceptive Injection:

a) Plasma and urinary steroid levels are decreased (e.g., progesterone, estradiol, pregnanediol, testosterone, cortisol).

b) Gonadotropin levels are decreased.

c) Sex-hormone binding globulin concentrations are decreased.

d) Protein bound iodine and butanol extractable protein bound iodine may increase. T_3 uptake values may decrease.

e) Coagulation test values for prothrombin (Factor II), and Factors VII, VIII, IX, and X may increase.

f) Sulfobromophthalein and other liver function test values may be increased.

g) The effects of Medroxyprogesterone Acetate on lipid metabolism are inconsistent. Both increases and decreases in total cholesterol, triglycerides, low-density lipoprotein (LDL) cholesterol, and high-density lipoprotein (HDL) cholesterol have been observed in studies.

Carcinogenesis: See "Warnings" section 3.

Pregnancy: Pregnancy Category X. See "Warnings" section 6.

Nursing Mothers: See "Warnings" section 8.

Information for the Patient: Patient labeling is included with each single dose vial of Medroxyprogesterone Acetate Contraceptive Injection to help describe its characteristics to the patient. It is recommended that prospective users be given this labeling and be informed about the risks and benefits associated with the use of Medroxyprogesterone Acetate, as compared with other forms of contraception or with no contraception at all. It is recommended that physicians or other health

care providers responsible for those patients advise them at the beginning of treatment that their menstrual cycle may be disrupted and that irregular and unpredictable bleeding or spotting results, and that this usually decreases to the point of amenorrhea as treatment with Medroxyprogesterone Acetate continues, without other therapy being required.

ADVERSE REACTIONS
In the largest clinical trial with Medroxyprogesterone Acetate Contraceptive Injection, over 3900 women, who were treated for up to 7 years, reported the following adverse reactions, which may or may not be related to the use of Medroxyprogesterone Acetate. The following adverse reactions were reported by more than 5% of subjects:

Menstrual irregularities (bleeding and/or amenorrhea)
Weight changes
Headache
Nervousness
Abdominal pain or discomfort
Dizziness
Asthenia (weakness or fatigue)

Adverse reactions reported by 1% to 5% of subjects using Medroxyprogesterone Acetate were:

Decreased libido or anorgasmia
Backache
Leg cramps
Depression
Nausea
Insomnia
Leukorrhea
Acne
Vaginitis
Pelvic pain
Breast pain
No hair growth or alopecia
Bloating
Rash
Edema
Hot flashes
Arthralgia

Events reported by fewer than 1% of subjects included: galactorrhea, melasma, chloasma, convulsions, changes in appetite, gastrointestinal disturbances, jaundice, genitourinary infections, vaginal cysts, dyspareunia, paresthesia, chest pain, pulmonary embolus, allergic reactions, anemia, drowsiness, syncope, dyspnea and asthma, tachycardia, fever, excessive sweating and body odor, dry skin, chills, increased libido, excessive thirst, hoarseness, pain at injection site, blood dyscrasia, rectal bleeding, changes in breast size, breast lumps or nipple bleeding, axillary swelling, breast cancer, prevention of lactation, sensation of pregnancy, lack of return to fertility, paralysis, facial palsy, scleroderma, osteoporosis, uterine hyperplasia, cervical cancer, varicose veins, dysmenorrhea, hirsutism, accidental pregnancy, thrombophlebitis, deep vein thrombosis.

In addition, voluntary reports have been received of anaphylaxis and anaphylactoid reaction with use of Medroxyprogesterone Acetate.

DOSAGE AND ADMINISTRATION
The Medroxyprogesterone Acetate Contraceptive Injection one mL vial should be vigorously shaken just before use to ensure that the dose being administered represents a uniform suspension.

The recommended dose is 150 mg of Medroxyprogesterone Acetate Contraceptive Injection every 3 months administered by deep, intramuscular injection in the gluteal or deltoid muscle. To increase assurance that the patient is not pregnant at the time of the first administration, it is recommended that this injection be given only during the first 5 days after the onset of a normal menstrual period; within 5 days postpartum if not breast-feeding; or, if breast-feeding, at 6 weeks postpartum. If the period between injection is greater than 14 weeks, the physician should determine that the patient is not pregnant before administering the drug.

REFERENCES
1. Trussell J. Hatcher RA, Cates W Jr. Stewart FH, Kost K: A guide to interpreting contraceptive efficacy studies, Obstet Gynecol 76:558-567, 1990. 2. Trussell J, Kost K: Contraceptive failure in the United States: A critical review of the literature. Stud Fam Plan 18:237-283, 1987. 3. Schwallie PC, Assenzo JR: Contraceptive use-efficacy study utilizing medroxyprogesterone acetate administered as an intramuscular injection once every 90 days. Fertil Steril 24:331-339, 1973. 4. WHO Collaborative Study of Neoplasia and Steroid Contraceptives: Breast cancer and depot-medroxyprogesterone acetate: A multi-national study. Lancet 338 833-838, 1991. 5. WHO Collaborative Study of Neoplasia and Steroid Contraceptives: Depot-medroxyprogesterone acetate (DMPA) and risk of epithelial ovarian cancer. Int J Cancer 49:191-95, 1991. 6. WHO Collaborative Study of Neoplasia and Steroid Contraceptives: Depot-medroxyprogesterone acetate (DMPA) and risk of liver cancer. Int J Cancer 49:182-85, 1991. 7. WHO Collaborative Study of Neoplasia and Steroid Contraceptives: Depot-medroxyprogesterone acetate (DMPA) and risk of invasive squamous cell cervical cancer. Contraception, 45:299-312, 1992. 8. WHO Collaborative Study of Neoplasia and Steroid Contraceptives: Depot-medroxyprogesterone acetate (DMPA) and risk of endometrial cancer, Int J Cancer 49:186-190, 1991. 9. Surveillance, Epidemiology, and End Results: Incidence and Mortality Data, 1973-77, National Cancer Institute Monograph 57, June 1981, (NIH publication No. 81-2330). 10. Gray, RH, Pardthaisong T: In Utero Exposure to Steroid Contraceptives and Survival During Infancy. Am J Epidemiol 134:795-803, 1991. 11. Pardthaisong T, Gray RH: In Utero Exposure to Steroid Contraceptives and

Outcome of Pregnancy, Am J Epidemiol *134*:795-803, 1991. 12. Pardthaisong T, Gray RH, McDaniel EB, Chandacham A: Steroid Contraceptive Use and Pregnancy Outcome, Teratology *38*:51-58, 1988. 13. Van Deijk WA, Biljham GH, Mellink WAM, and Meulenberg PMM: Influence of Aminoglutethimide on Plasma Levels of Medroxyprogesterone Acetate: Its Correlation With Serum Cortisol. Cancer Treatment Reports *69*:1, 85-90, January 1985.

HOW SUPPLIED
INJECTION: 150 MG/ML

BRAND/MANUFACTURER	NDC	SIZE	AWP
○ **BRAND**			
DEPO-PROVERA CONTRACEPTIVE: Upjohn	00009-0746-30	1 ml	$36.87
	00009-0746-31	1 ml	$36.88

INJECTION: 400 MG/ML

BRAND/MANUFACTURER	NDC	SIZE	AWP
○ **BRAND**			
DEPO-PROVERA: Upjohn	00009-0626-01	2.5 ml	$82.69
	00009-0626-02	10 ml	$313.95

Medroxyprogesterone Acetate, Injectable

WARNING

THE USE OF STERILE AQUEOUS SUSPENSION OF MEDROXY- PROGESTERONE ACETATE DURING THE FIRST FOUR MONTHS OF PREGNANCY IS NOT RECOMMENDED.

PROGESTATIONAL AGENTS HAVE BEEN USED BEGINNING WITH THE FIRST TRIMESTER OF PREGNANCY IN AN ATTEMPT TO PREVENT HABITUAL ABORTION. THERE IS NO ADEQUATE EVIDENCE THAT SUCH USE IS EFFECTIVE WHEN SUCH DRUGS ARE GIVEN DURING THE FIRST FOUR MONTHS OF PREGNANCY. FURTHERMORE, IN THE VAST MAJORITY OF WOMEN, THE CAUSE OF ABORTION IS A DEFECTIVE OVUM, WHICH PROGESTATIONAL AGENTS COULD NOT BE EXPECTED TO INFLUENCE. IN ADDITION, THE USE OF PROGESTATIONAL AGENTS, WITH THEIR UTERINE-RELAXANT PROPERTIES, IN PATIENTS WITH FERTILIZED DEFECTIVE OVA MAY CAUSE A DELAY IN SPONTANEOUS ABORTION. THEREFORE, THE USE OF SUCH DRUGS DURING THE FIRST FOUR MONTHS OF PREGNANCY IS NOT RECOMMENDED.

SEVERAL REPORTS SUGGEST AN ASSOCIATION BETWEEN INTRAUTERINE EXPOSURE TO PROGESTATIONAL DRUGS IN THE FIRST TRIMESTER OF PREGNANCY AND GENITAL ABNORMALITIES IN MALE AND FEMALE FETUSES. THE RISK OF HYPOSPADIAS, 5 TO 8 PER 1,000 MALE BIRTHS IN THE GENERAL POPULATION, MAY BE APPROXIMATELY DOUBLED WITH EXPOSURE TO THESE DRUGS. THERE ARE INSUFFICIENT DATA TO QUANTIFY THE RISK TO EXPOSED FEMALE FETUSES, BUT INSOFAR AS SOME OF THESE DRUGS INDUCE MILD VIRILIZATION OF THE EXTERNAL GENITALIA OF THE FEMALE FETUS, AND BECAUSE OF THE INCREASED ASSOCIATION OF HYPOSPADIAS IN THE MALE FETUS, IT IS PRUDENT TO AVOID THE USE OF THESE DRUGS DURING THE FIRST TRIMESTER OF PREGNANCY.

IF THE PATIENT IS EXPOSED TO STERILE AQUEOUS SUSPENSION OF MEDROXYPROGESTERONE ACETATE DURING THE FIRST FOUR MONTHS OF PREGNANCY OR IF SHE BECOMES PREGNANT WHILE TAKING THIS DRUG, SHE SHOULD BE APPRISED OF THE POTENTIAL RISKS TO THE FETUS.

DESCRIPTION

Sterile Aqueous Suspension of Medroxyprogesterone Acetate a derivative of progesterone and is active by the parenteral and oral routes of administration. It is a white to off-white, odorless crystalline powder, stable in air, melting between 200 and 210°C. It is freely soluble in chloroform, soluble in acetone and dioxane, sparingly soluble in alcohol and methanol, slightly soluble in ether and insoluble in water.

The chemical name for Medroxyprogesterone Acetate is Pregn-4-ene-3,20-dione, 17-(acetyloxy)-6-methyl-, (6α)-.

Medroxyprogesterone Acetate for intramuscular injection is available in 2 strengths, 100 mg/mL and 400 mg/mL.

Each mL of the 100 mg/mL suspension contains:
Medroxyprogesterone Acetate ....100 mg

Each mL of the 400 mg/mL suspension contains:
Medroxyprogesterone Acetate ....400 mg

Following is its chemical structure:

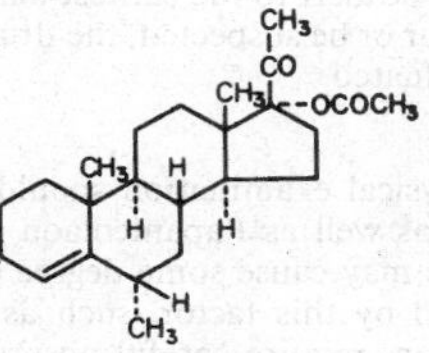

ACTIONS

Medroxyprogesterone Acetate administered parenterally in the recommended doses to women with adequate endogenous estrogen transforms proliferative endometrium into secretory endometrium.

Medroxyprogesterone Acetate inhibits (in the usual dose range) the secretion of pituitary gonadotropin which, in turn, prevents follicular maturation and ovulation.

Because of its prolonged action and the resulting difficulty in predicting the time of withdrawal bleeding following injection, Medroxyprogesterone Acetate is not recommended in secondary amenorrhea or dysfunctional uterine bleeding. In these conditions oral therapy is recommended.

INDICATIONS AND USAGE

Adjunctive therapy and palliative treatment of inoperable, recurrent, and metastatic endometrial or renal carcinoma.

UNLABELED USES

Medroxyprogesterone Acetate is used alone or as an adjunct in the treatment of breast cancer, catamenial seizures, hirsutism, menorrhagia, and pelvic congestion. It is also used to increase ventilatory capacity in patients with Pickwickian syndrome, precocious puberty, premenstrual syndrome, prostate cancer, schizophrenia, and hypersexuality, including deviant sexual behavior.

CONTRAINDICATIONS

1. Thrombophlebitis, thromboembolic disorders, cerebral apoplexy or patients with a past history of these conditions.
2. Carcinoma of the breast.
3. Undiagnosed vaginal bleeding.
4. Missed abortion.
5. As a diagnostic test for pregnancy.
6. Known sensitivity to Medroxyprogesterone Acetate Sterile Aqueous Suspension.

WARNINGS

1. The physician should be alert to the earliest manifestations of thrombotic disorders (thrombophlebitis, cerebrovascular disorders, pulmonary embolism, and retinal thrombosis). Should any of these occur or be suspected, the drug should be discontinued immediately.

2. Long term toxicology studies in the monkey, dog and rat disclose:

1) Beagle dogs receiving 75 mg/kg and 3 mg/kg every 90 days developed mammary nodules, as did some of the control animals. The nodules appearing in the control animals were intermittent in nature, whereas the nodules in the drug treated animals were larger, more numerous, persistent, and there were two high dose animals that developed breast malignancies.

2) Two of the monkeys receiving 150 mg/kg every 90 days developed undifferentiated carcinoma of the uterus. No uterine malignancies were found in monkeys receiving 30 mg/kg, 3 mg/kg, or placebo every 90 days. Transient mammary nodules were found during the study in the control, 3 mg/kg and 30 mg/kg groups, but not in the 150 mg/kg group. At sacrifice, the only nodules extant were in three of the monkeys in the 30 mg/kg group. Upon histopathologic examination these nodules have been determined to be hyperplastic.

3) No uterine or breast abnormalities were revealed in the rat.

The relevance of any of these findings with respect to humans has not been established.

3. The use of Medroxyprogesterone Acetate Sterile Aqueous Suspension for contraception is investigational since there are unresolved questions relating to its safety for this indication. Therefore, this is not an approved indication.

4. Discontinue medication pending examination if there is sudden partial or complete loss of vision, or if there is a sudden onset of proptosis, diplopia or migraine. If examination reveals papilledema or retinal vascular lesions, medication should be withdrawn.

5. Usage in pregnancy (See *"Warning"* box).

6. Retrospective studies of morbidity and mortality in Great Britain and studies of morbidity in the United States have shown a statistically significant association between thrombophlebitis, pulmonary embolism, and cerebral thrombosis and embolism and the use of oral contraceptives.[1-4] The estimate of the relative risk of thromboembolism in the study by Vessey and Doll[3] was about sevenfold, while Sartwell and associates[4] in the United States found a relative risk of 4.4, meaning that the users are several times as likely to undergo thromboembolic disease without evident cause as non-users. The American study also indicated that the risk did not persist after discontinuation of administration, and that it was not enhanced by long continued administration. The American study was not designed to evaluate a difference between products.

➤ SHOWN IN PRODUCT IDENTIFICATION GUIDE

7. Following repeated injections, amenorrhea and infertility may persist for periods up to 18 months and occasionally longer.

8. The physician should be alert to the earliest manifestations of impaired liver function. Should these occur or be suspected, the drug should be discontinued and the patient's status re-evaluated.

PRECAUTIONS

1. The pretreatment physical examination should include special reference to breast and pelvic organs, as well as Papanicolaou smear.

2. Because progestogens may cause some degree of fluid retention, conditions which might be influenced by this factor, such as epilepsy, migraine, asthma, cardiac or renal dysfunction, require careful observation.

3. In cases of breakthrough bleeding, as in all cases of irregular bleeding per vaginum, nonfunctional causes should be borne in mind. In cases of undiagnosed vaginal bleeding, adequate diagnostic measures are indicated.

4. Patients who have a history of psychic depression should be carefully observed and the drug discontinued if the depression recurs to a serious degree.

5. Any possible influence of prolonged progestin therapy on pituitary, ovarian, adrenal, hepatic or uterine functions awaits further study.

6. A decrease in glucose tolerance has been observed in a small percentage of patients on estrogen-progestin combination drugs. The mechanism of this decrease is obscure. For this reason, diabetic patients should be carefully observed while receiving progestin therapy.

7. The age of the patient constitutes no absolute limiting factor although treatment with progestins may mask the onset of the climacteric.

8. The pathologist should be advised of progestin therapy when relevant specimens are submitted.

9. Because of the occasional occurrence of thrombotic disorders, (thrombophlebitis, pulmonary embolism, retinal thrombosis, and cerebrovascular disorders) in patients taking estrogen-progestin combinations and since the mechanism is obscure, the physician should be alert to the earliest manifestation of these disorders.

10. Aminoglutethimide administered concomitantly with Medroxyprogesterone Acetate may significantly depress the bioavailability of Medroxyprogesterone Acetate.

INFORMATION FOR THE PATIENT
The manufacturer's patient insert should be given to all premenopausal women, except those in whom childbearing is impossible.

ADVERSE REACTIONS
(See *"Warning"* box for possible adverse effects on the fetus).

In a few instances there have been undesirable sequelae at the site of injection, such as residual lump, change in color of skin or sterile abscess.

The following adverse reactions have been associated with the use of Medroxyprogesterone Acetate Sterile Aqueous Suspension.

Breast: In a few instances, breast tenderness or galactorrhea have occurred.

Psychic: An occasional patient has experienced nervousness, insomnia, somnolence, fatigue or dizziness.

Thromboembolic Phenomena: Thromboembolic phenomena including thrombophlebitis and pulmonary embolism have been reported.

Skin and Mucous Membranes: Sensitivity reactions ranging from pruritus, urticaria, angioneurotic edema to generalized rash and anaphylaxis and/or anaphylactoid reactions have occasionally been reported. Acne, alopecia, or hirsutism have been reported in a few cases.

Gastrointestinal: Rarely, nausea has been reported. Jaundice, including neonatal jaundice, has been noted in a few instances.

Miscellaneous: Rare cases of headache and hyperpyrexia have been reported.

The following adverse reactions have been observed in women taking progestins including Medroxyprogesterone Acetate:
breakthrough bleeding
spotting
change in menstrual flow
amenorrhea
edema
change in weight (increase or decrease)
changes in cervical erosion and cervical secretions
cholestatic jaundice
rash (allergic) with and without pruritus
melasma or chloasma
mental depression

A statistically significant association has been demonstrated between use of estrogen-progestin combination drugs and the following serious adverse reactions: thrombophlebitis; pulmonary embolism and cerebral thrombosis and embolism. For this reason patients on progestin therapy should be carefully observed.

Although available evidence is suggestive of an association, such a relationship has been neither confirmed nor refuted for the following serious adverse reactions; neuro-ocular lesions, eg, retinal thrombosis and optic neuritis.

The following adverse reactions have been observed in patients receiving estrogen-progestin combination drugs:
rise in blood pressure in susceptible individuals
premenstrual-like syndrome
changes in libido
changes in appetite
cystitis-like syndrome
headache
nervousness
dizziness
fatigue
backache
hirsutism
loss of scalp hair
erythema multiforme
erythema nodosum
hemorrhagic eruption
itching

In view of these observations, patients on progestin therapy should be carefully observed.

The following laboratory results may be altered by the use of estrogen-progestin combination drugs:
Increased sulfobromophthalein retention and other hepatic function tests.
Coagulation tests: increase in prothrombin factors VII, VIII, IX and X.
Metyrapone test.
Pregnanediol determination.
Thyroid function; increase in PBI, and butanol extractable protein bound iodine and decrease in T^3 uptake values.

DOSAGE AND ADMINISTRATION
The suspension is intended for intramuscular administration only.

Endometrial or renal carcinoma: doses of 400 mg to 1000 mg of Medroxyprogesterone Acetate Sterile Aqueous Suspension per week are recommended initially. If improvement is noted within a few weeks or months and the disease appears stabilized, it may be possible to maintain improvement with as little as 400 mg per month. Medroxyprogesterone Acetate is not recommended as primary therapy, but as adjunctive and palliative treatment in advanced inoperable cases including those with recurrent or metastatic disease.

REFERENCES
1. Royal College of General Practitioners: Oral contraception and thromboembolic disease. J Coll Gen Pract 13:267-279, 1967. 2. Inman WHW, Vessey MP: Investigation of deaths from pulmonary, coronary, and cerebral thrombosis and embolism in women of child-bearing age. Br Med J 2:193-199, 1968. 3. Vessey MP, Doll R: Investigation of relation between use of oral contraceptives and thromboembolic disease. A further report. Br Med J 2:651-657, 1969. 4. Sartwell PE, Masi AT, Arthes FG. et al: Thromboembolism and oral contraceptives: An epidemiological case-control study. Am J Epidemiol 90:365-380, 1969.

J CODES
150 mg IM—J1055
100 mg IM—J1050

HOW SUPPLIED
INJECTION: 150 MG/ML

BRAND/MANUFACTURER	NDC	SIZE	AWP
○ BRAND			
DEPO-PROVERA CONTRACEPTIVE: Upjohn	00009-0746-30	1 ml	$36.87
	00009-0746-31	1 ml	$36.88

INJECTION: 400 MG/ML

BRAND/MANUFACTURER	NDC	SIZE	AWP
○ BRAND			
DEPO-PROVERA: Upjohn	00009-0626-01	2.5 ml	$82.69
	00009-0626-02	10 ml	$313.95

Medroxyprogesterone Acetate, Oral

WARNING
THE USE OF MEDROXYPROGESTERONE ACETATE DURING THE FIRST FOUR MONTHS OF PREGNANCY IS NOT RECOMMENDED.

PROGESTATIONAL AGENTS HAVE BEEN USED BEGINNING WITH THE FIRST TRIMESTER OF PREGNANCY IN AN ATTEMPT TO PREVENT HABITUAL ABORTION. THERE IS NO ADEQUATE EVIDENCE THAT SUCH USE IS EFFECTIVE WHEN SUCH DRUGS ARE GIVEN DURING THE FIRST FOUR MONTHS OF PREGNANCY. FURTHERMORE, IN THE VAST MAJORITY OF WOMEN, THE CAUSE OF ABORTION IS A DEFECTIVE OVUM, WHICH PROGESTATIONAL AGENTS COULD NOT BE EXPECTED TO INFLUENCE. IN ADDITION, THE USE OF PROGESTATIONAL AGENTS WITH THEIR UTERINE-RELAXANT PROPERTIES, IN PATIENTS WITH FERTILIZED DEFECTIVE OVA MAY CAUSE A DELAY IN SPONTANEOUS

ABORTION. THEREFORE, THE USE OF SUCH DRUGS DURING THE FIRST FOUR MONTHS OF PREGNANCY IS NOT RECOMMENDED.

SEVERAL REPORTS SUGGEST AN ASSOCIATION BETWEEN INTRA-UTERINE EXPOSURE TO PROGESTATIONAL DRUGS IN THE FIRST TRIMESTER OF PREGNANCY AND GENITAL ABNORMALITIES IN MALE AND FEMALE FETUSES. THE RISK OF HYPOSPADIAS, 5 TO 8 PER 1,000 MALE BIRTHS IN THE GENERAL POPULATION, MAY BE APPROXIMATELY DOUBLED WITH EXPOSURE TO THESE DRUGS. THERE ARE INSUFFICIENT DATA TO QUANTIFY THE RISK TO EXPOSED FEMALE FETUSES, BUT INSOFAR AS SOME OF THESE DRUGS INDUCE MILD VIRILIZATION OF THE EXTERNAL GENITALIA OF THE FEMALE FETUS, AND BECAUSE OF THE INCREASED ASSOCIATION OF HYPOSPADIAS IN THE MALE FETUS, IT IS PRUDENT TO AVOID THE USE OF THESE DRUGS DURING THE FIRST TRIMESTER OF PREGNANCY.

IF THE PATIENT IS EXPOSED TO MEDROXYPROGESTERONE ACETATE DURING THE FIRST FOUR MONTHS OF PREGNANCY OR IF SHE BECOMES PREGNANT WHILE TAKING THIS DRUG, SHE SHOULD BE APPRISED OF THE POTENTIAL RISKS TO THE FETUS.

DESCRIPTION
Medroxyprogesterone Acetate, is a derivative of progesterone. It is a white to off-white, odorless crystalline powder, stable in air, melting between 200 and 210° C. It is freely soluble in chloroform, soluble in acetone and in dioxane, sparingly soluble in alcohol and in methanol, slightly soluble in ether, and insoluble in water.

The chemical name for Medroxyprogesterone Acetate is Pregn-4-ene-3,20-dione, 17-(acetyloxy)-6-methyl-, (6α)-.

Each tablet for oral administration contains 2.5 mg, 5 mg or 10 mg of Medroxyprogesterone Acetate.

Following is its chemical structure:

ACTIONS
Medroxyprogesterone Acetate, administered orally or parenterally in the recommended doses to women with adequate endogenous estrogen, transforms proliferative into secretory endometrium. Androgenic and anabolic effects have been noted, but the drug is apparently devoid of significant estrogenic activity. While parenterally administered Medroxyprogesterone Acetate inhibits gonadotropin production, which in turn prevents follicular maturation and ovulation, available data indicate that this does not occur when the usually recommended oral dosage is given as single daily doses.

INDICATIONS AND USAGE
Secondary amenorrhea; abnormal uterine bleeding due to hormonal imbalance in the absence of organic pathology, such as fibroids or uterine cancer.

UNLABELED USES
Medroxyprogesterone Acetate is used alone or as an adjunct in the treatment of breast cancer, catamenial seizures, hirsutism, menorrhagia, and pelvic congestion. It is also used to increase ventilatory capacity in patients with Pickwickian syndrome, precocious puberty, premenstrual syndrome, prostate cancer, schizophrenia, and hypersexuality, including deviant sexual behavior. Oral Medroxyprogesterone is also used to relieve menopausal symptoms and endometriosis.

CONTRAINDICATIONS
1. Thrombophlebitis, thromboembolic disorders, cerebral apoplexy or patients with a past history of these conditions.
2. Liver dysfunction or disease.
3. Known or suspected malignancy of breast or genital organs.
4. Undiagnosed vaginal bleeding.
5. Missed abortion.
6. As a diagnostic test for pregnancy.
7. Known sensitivity to Medroxyprogesterone Acetate Tablets.

WARNINGS
1. The physician should be alert to the earliest manifestations of thrombotic disorders (thrombophlebitis, cerebrovascular disorders, pulmonary embolism, and retinal thrombosis). Should any of these occur or be suspected, the drug should be discontinued immediately.
2. Beagle dogs treated with Medroxyprogesterone Acetate developed mammary nodules some of which were malignant. Although nodules occasionally appeared in control animals, they were intermittent in nature, whereas the nodules in the drug-treated animals were larger, more numerous, persistent, and there were some breast malignancies with metastases. Their significance with respect to humans has not been established.

3. Discontinue medication pending examination if there is sudden partial or complete loss of vision, or if there is a sudden onset of proptosis, diplopia or migraine. If examination reveals papilledema or retinal vascular lesions, medication should be withdrawn.
4. Detectable amounts of progestin have been identified in the milk of mothers receiving the drug. The effect of this on the nursing infant has not been determined.
5. Usage in pregnancy is not recommended (See "Warning" box).
6. Retrospective studies of morbidity and mortality in Great Britain and studies of morbidity in the United States have shown a statistically significant association between thrombophlebitis, pulmonary embolism, and cerebral thrombosis and embolism and the use of oral contraceptives.[1-4] The estimate of the relative risk of thromboembolism in the study by Vessey and Doll[3] was about sevenfold, while Sartwell and associates[4] in the United States found a relative risk of 4.4, meaning that the users are several times as likely to undergo thromboembolic disease without evident cause as nonusers. The American study also indicated that the risk did not persist after discontinuation of administration, and that it was not enhanced by long continued administration. The American study was not designed to evaluate a difference between products.

PRECAUTIONS
1. The pretreatment physical examination should include special reference to breast and pelvic organs, as well as Papanicolaou smear.
2. Because progestogens may cause some degree of fluid retention, conditions which might be influenced by this factor, such as epilepsy, migraine, asthma, cardiac or renal dysfunction, require careful observation.
3. In cases of breakthrough bleeding, as in all cases of irregular bleeding per vaginum, nonfunctional causes should be borne in mind. In cases of undiagnosed vaginal bleeding, adequate diagnostic measures are indicated.
4. Patients who have a history of psychic depression should be carefully observed and the drug discontinued if the depression recurs to a serious degree.
5. Any possible influence of prolonged progestin therapy on pituitary, ovarian, adrenal, hepatic or uterine functions awaits further study.
6. A decrease in glucose tolerance has been observed in a small percentage of patients on estrogen-progestin combination drugs. The mechanism of this decrease is obscure. For this reason, diabetic patients should be carefully observed while receiving progestin therapy.
7. The age of the patient constitutes no absolute limiting factor although treatment with progestins may mask the onset of the climacteric.
8. The pathologist should be advised of progestin therapy when relevant specimens are submitted.
9. Because of the occasional occurrence of thrombotic disorders, (thrombophlebitis, pulmonary embolism, retinal thrombosis, and cerebrovascular disorders) in patients taking estrogen-progestin combinations and since the mechanism is obscure, the physician should be alert to the earliest manifestation of these disorders.
10. Studies of the addition of a progestin product to an estrogen replacement regimen for seven or more days of a cycle of estrogen administration have reported a lowered incidence of endometrial hyperplasia. Morphological and biochemical studies of endometrium suggest that 10-13 days of a progestin are needed to provide maximal maturation of the endometrium and to eliminate any hyperplastic changes. Whether this will provide protection from endometrial carcinoma has not been clearly established. There are possible additional risks which may be associated with the inclusion of progestin in estrogen replacement regimen. The potential risks include adverse effects on carbohydrate and lipid metabolism. The dosage used may be important in minimizing these adverse effects.
11. Aminoglutethimide administered concomitantly with Medroxyprogesterone Acetate may significantly depress the bioavailability of Medroxyprogesterone Acetate.

CARCINOGENESIS, MUTAGENESIS, IMPAIRMENT OF FERTILITY
Long-term intramuscular administration of Medroxyprogesterone Acetate has been shown to produce mammary tumors in beagle dogs (see "Warnings"). There was no evidence of a carcinogenic effect associated with the oral administration of Medroxyprogesterone Acetate to rats and mice. Medroxyprogesterone Acetate was not mutagenic in a battery of in vitro or in vivo genetic toxicity assays.

Medroxyprogesterone Acetate at high doses is an antifertility drug and high dose would be expected to impair fertility until the cessation of treatment.

INFORMATION FOR THE PATIENT
See manufacturer's patient information.

ADVERSE REACTIONS
Pregnancy: See "Warning" box for possible adverse effects on the fetus).

Breast: Breast tenderness or galactorrhea has been reported rarely.

Skin: Sensitivity reactions consisting of urticaria, pruritus, edema and generalized rash have occurred in an occasional patient. Acne, alopecia and hirsutism have been reported in a few cases.

Thromboembolic Phenomena: Thromboembolic phenomena including thrombophlebitis and pulmonary embolism have been reported.

The following adverse reactions have been observed in women taking progestins including Medroxyprogesterone Acetate Tablets:
breakthrough bleeding
spotting
change in menstrual flow

amenorrhea
edema
change in weight (increase or decrease)
changes in cervical erosin and cervical secretions
cholestatic jaundice
anaphylactoid reactions and anaphylaxis
rash (allergic) with and without pruritus
mental depression
pyrexia
insomnia
nausea
somnolence

A statistically significant association has been demonstrated between use of estrogen-progestin combination drugs and the following serious adverse reactions: thrombophlebitis; pulmonary embolism and cerebral thrombosis and embolism. For this reason patients on progestin therapy should be carefully observed.

Although available evidence is suggestive of an association. such a relationship has been neither confirmed nor refuted for the following serious adverse reactions:

neuro-ocular lesions, eg, retinal thrombosis and optic neuritis.

The following adverse reactions have been observed in patients receiving estrogen progestin combination drugs:
rise in blood pressure in susceptible individuals
premenstrual-like syndrome
changes in libido
changes in appetite
cystitis-like syndrome
headache
nervousness
fatigue
backache
hirsutism
loss of scalp hair
erythema multiforme
erythema nodosum
hemorrhagic eruption
itching
dizziness

In view of these observations, patients on progestin therapy should be carefully observed.

The following laboratory results may be altered by the use of estrogen-progestin combination drugs:
Increased sulfobromophthalein retention and other hepatic function tests.
Coagulation tests: increase in prothrombin factors VII, VIII, IX and X.
Metyrapone test
Pregnanediol determination.
Thyroid function: increase in PBI and butanol extractable protein bound iodine and decrease in T^3 uptake values.

DOSAGE AND ADMINISTRATION

Secondary Amenorrhea: Medroxyprogesterone Acetate Tablets may be given in dosages of 5 to 10 mg daily for from 5 to 10 days. A dose for inducing an optimum secretory transformation of an endometrium that has been adequately primed with either endogenous or exogenous estrogen is 10 mg of Medroxyprogesterone Acetate daily for 10 days. In case of secondary amenorrhea, therapy may be started at any time. Progestin withdrawal bleeding usually occurs within three to seven days after discontinuing Medroxyprogesterone Acetate therapy.

Abnormal Uterine Bleeding Due to Hormonal Imbalance in the Absence of Organic Pathology: Beginning on the calculated 16th or 21st day of the menstrual cycle, 5 to 10 mg of Medroxyprogesterone Acetate may be given daily for from 5 to 10 days. To produce an optimum secretory transformation of an endometrium that has been adequately primed with either endogenous or exogenous estrogen, 10 mg of Medroxyprogesterone Acetate daily for 10 days beginning on the 16th day of the cycle is suggested. Progestin withdrawal bleeding usually occurs within three to seven days after discontinuing therapy with Medroxyprogesterone Acetate. Patients with a past history of recurrent episodes of abnormal uterine bleeding may benefit from planned menstrual cycling with Medroxyprogesterone Acetate.

Storage: Store at controlled room temperature, 15°-30°C (59°-86°F).

REFERENCES
1. Royal College of General Practitioners: Oral contraception and thromboembolic disease. J Coll Gen Pract **13**:267-279, 1967. 2. Inman WHW, Vessey MP: Investigation of deaths from pulmonary, coronary, and cerebral thrombosis and embolism in women of child-bearing age. Br Med J **2**:193-199, 1968. 3. Vessey MP, Doll R: Investigation of relation between use of oral contraceptives and thromboembolic disease. A further report. Br Med J **2**:651-657, 1969. 4. Sartwell PE, Masi AT, Arthes FG, et al: Thromboembolism and oral contraceptives: An epidemiological case-control study. Am J Epidemiol **90**:365-380, 1969.

HOW SUPPLIED
TABLETS: 2.5 MG

AVERAGE UNIT PRICE (AVAILABLE SIZES)		GENERIC A-RATED AVERAGE PRICE (GAAP)	
BRAND	$0.33	100s	$29.59
GENERIC	$0.30		

BRAND/MANUFACTURER	NDC	SIZE	AWP
◆ BRAND			
➤ PROVERA: Upjohn	00009-0064-06	30s	$10.21
	00009-0064-04	100s	$33.90
	00009-0064-12	20000s	$6272.24
◆ GENERICS			
Allscrips	54569-3806-00	10s	$2.98
Allscrips	54569-8570-00	60s	$17.90
Allscrips	54569-8570-01	90s	$26.85
➤ CYCRIN: Esi Pharma	59911-5898-01	100s	$29.34
Allscrips	54569-3806-01	100s	$29.83

TABLETS: 5 MG

AVERAGE UNIT PRICE (AVAILABLE SIZES)			
BRAND	$0.50		
GENERIC	$0.45		

BRAND/MANUFACTURER	NDC	SIZE	AWP
◆ BRAND			
➤ PROVERA: Upjohn	00009-0286-32	30s	$15.58
	00009-0286-03	100s	$51.15
	00009-0286-42	20000s	$9463.03
◆ GENERICS			
Allscrips	54569-3807-00	10s	$4.50
Allscrips	54569-8571-00	90s	$40.51
➤ CYCRIN: Esi Pharma	59911-5897-01	100s	$44.32

TABLETS: 10 MG

AVERAGE UNIT PRICE (AVAILABLE SIZES)		GENERIC A-RATED AVERAGE PRICE (GAAP)	
BRAND	$0.61	100s	$35.18
GENERIC	$0.30		

BRAND/MANUFACTURER	NDC	SIZE	AWP
◆ BRAND			
➤ PROVERA: Upjohn	00009-0050-09	30s	$20.01
	00009-0050-02	100s	$63.38
	00009-0050-11	500s	$301.19
	00009-0050-27	20000s	$10842.63
◆ GENERICS			
Allscrips	54569-8572-00	30s	$7.97
➤ CYCRIN: Esi Pharma	59911-5896-01	100s	$53.80
U.S. Trading	56126-0480-11	100s ud	$16.56
Mason Dist	11845-0341-02	250s	$53.00

TABLETS: 10 MG

BRAND/MANUFACTURER	NDC	SIZE	AWP
◇ BRAND			
AMEN: Carrnick	00086-0049-05	50s	$16.90
CURRETAB: Solvay	00032-1007-42	50s	$25.79
AMEN: Carrnick	00086-0049-10	100s	$28.10
	00086-0049-90	1000s	$214.70
◇ GENERICS			
Major	00904-2690-51	50s	$7.50
Moore,H.L.	00839-6610-04	50s	$10.11
Warner Chilcott	00047-0874-19	50s	$11.81
Intl Labs	00665-4001-42	50s	$11.90
Geneva	00781-1680-50	50s	$12.40
Goldline	00182-1196-19	50s	$12.40
Qualitest	00603-4368-19	50s	$12.41
URL	00677-0803-02	50s	$13.10
Rugby	00536-3995-06	50s	$13.12
Martec	52555-0463-00	50s	$13.20
Schein	00364-0521-50	50s	$13.73
Parmed	00349-2309-50	50s	$13.95
Rosemont	00832-0087-26	50s	$14.00
Aligen	00405-4618-50	50s	$14.82
Moore,H.L.	00839-6610-06	100s	$13.08
URL	00677-0803-01	100s	$24.00
Rosemont	00832-0087-00	100s	$25.65
Intl Labs	00665-4001-06	100s	$26.90
Parmed	00349-2309-01	100s	$26.95
R.I.D.	54807-0550-01	100s	$59.04
Auro	55829-0356-10	100s ud	$22.01
Moore,H.L.	00839-6610-09	250s	$29.15
Major	00904-2690-70	250s	$33.75
Goldline	00182-1196-02	250s	$37.50
Martec	52555-0463-02	250s	$42.75
Rugby	00536-3995-02	250s	$52.43
Qualitest	00603-4368-24	250s	$54.40
Rosemont	00832-0087-25	250s	$55.00
URL	00677-0803-03	250s	$58.75
Schein	00364-0521-04	250s	$58.80

◆ RATED THERAPEUTICALLY EQUIVALENT; ◇ THERAPEUTIC EQUIVALENCE UNCONFIRMED; ○ UNRATED

BRAND/MANUFACTURER	NDC	SIZE	AWP
Geneva	00781-1680-25	250s	$58.90
Warner Chilcott	00047-0874-29	250s	$59.05
Intl Labs	00665-4001-07	250s	$59.75
Parmed	00349-2309-25	250s	$60.05
Major	00904-2690-40	500s	$53.80
Parmed	00349-2309-05	500s	$83.46

Medrysone

DESCRIPTION
Medrysone sterile ophthalmic suspension is a topical anti-inflammatory agent for ophthalmic use.

Chemical Name: 11β-Hydroxy-6α-methylpregn-4-ene-3,20-dione.

Following is its chemical structure:

CLINICAL PHARMACOLOGY
Medrysone is a synthetic corticosteroid with topical anti-inflammatory and anti-allergic activity. Corticosteroids inhibit the inflammatory response to inciting agents of mechanical, chemical or immunological nature of edema, fibrin deposition, capillary dilation and leukocyte migration, capillary proliferation, deposition of collagen and scar formation. Medrysone has less anti-inflammatory potency than 0.1% dexamethasone. Data from 2 uncontrolled studies[1-2] indicate that in patients with increased intraocular pressure and in those susceptible to a rise in intraocular pressure, there is less effect on pressure with Medrysone than with dexamethasone or betamethasone.

INDICATIONS AND USAGE
Medrysone is indicated for the treatment of allergic conjunctivitis, vernal conjunctivitis, episcleritis, and epinephrine sensitivity.

UNLABELED USES
Medrysone is used alone or as an adjunct in the anti-inflammatory therapy of superficial pingueculitis.

CONTRAINDICATIONS
Medrysone is contraindicated in the following conditions:

Acute superficial herpes simplex
Viral diseases of the conjunctiva and cornea
Ocular tuberculosis
Fungal diseases of the eye
Hypersensitivity to any of the components of the drug

WARNINGS
Acute purulent untreated infections of the eye may be masked, enhanced or activated by the presence of corticosteroid medication.

Corneal or scleral perforation occasionally has been reported with prolonged use of topical corticosteroids. In high dosages they have been associated with corneal thinning.

Prolonged use of topical corticosteroids may increase intraocular pressure, with resultant glaucoma, damage to the optic nerve, and defects in visual acuity and fields of vision. However, data from 2 uncontrolled studies[1-2] indicate that in patients with increased intraocular pressure and in those susceptible to a rise in intraocular pressure upon application of topical corticosteroids, there is less effect on pressure with Medrysone than with dexamethasone or betamethasone.

Prolonged use of topical corticosteroids may rarely be associated with development of posterior subcapsular cataracts.

Systemic absorption and systemic side effects may result with the use of topical corticosteroids.

Medrysone sterile ophthalmic suspension is not recommended for use in iritis and uveitis as its therapeutic effectiveness has not been demonstrated in these conditions.

Corticosteroid medication in the presence of stromal herpes simplex requires great caution; frequent slit-lamp microscopy is suggested.

Prolonged use may aid in the establishment of secondary ocular infections from fungi and viruses liberated from ocular tissue.

PRECAUTIONS
General: With prolonged use of Medrysone, the intraocular pressure and the lens should be examined periodically. In persistent corneal ulceration where a corticosteroid has been used, or is in use, fungal infection should be suspected.

Carcinogenesis, Mutagenesis, Impairment of Fertility: No studies have been conducted in animals or in humans to evaluate the potential of these effects.

Pregnancy Category C: Medrysone has been shown to be embryocidal in rabbits when given in doses 10 and 30 times the human dose. Medrysone was ocularly applied to both eyes of pregnant rabbits 2 drops 4 times per day on day 6 through 18 of gestation. A significant increase in early resorptions was observed in the treated rabbits. There are no adequate or well-controlled studies in pregnant women. Medrysone should be used during pregnancy only if the potential benefit justifies the potential risk to the fetus.

Pediatric Use: Safety and effectiveness in children have not been established.

ADVERSE REACTIONS
Adverse reactions include occasional transient stinging and burning upon instillation. Increased intraocular pressure, which may be associated with optic nerve damage and defects in the visual fields, and posterior subcapsular cataract formation have been reported rarely with the use of Medrysone.

OVERDOSAGE
Overdosage will not ordinarily cause acute problems. If accidentally ingested, drink fluids to dilute.

DOSAGE AND ADMINISTRATION
Shake well before using. Instill one drop in the conjunctival sac up to every four hours.

Protect from freezing.

REFERENCES
1. Becker B, Kolker AE. Intraocular pressure response to topical corticosteroids. In: Leopold IH, ed. Ocular therapy, complications and management. St. Louis: C.V. Mosby, 1967. 2. Spaeth G. Hydroxymethylprogesterone. Arch Ophthalmol 1966; 75:783-787.

HOW SUPPLIED
DROP:

BRAND/MANUFACTURER	NDC	SIZE	AWP
○ **BRAND**			
HMS: Allergan Optical	11980-0074-05	5 ml	$13.05
	11980-0074-10	10 ml	$20.04

Mefenamic Acid

DESCRIPTION
Mefenamic Acid is N-(2,3-xylyl)-anthranilic acid. It is an analgesic agent for oral administration. Mefenamic Acid is available in capsules containing 250 mg.

It is a white powder with a melting point of 230-231°C, molecular weight 241.28, and water solubility of 0.004% at pH 7.1.

Following is its chemical structure:

CLINICAL PHARMACOLOGY
Mefenamic Acid is a nonsteroidal agent with demonstrated antiinflammatory, analgesic, and antipyretic activity in laboratory animals.[1,2] The mode of action is not known. In animal studies, Mefenamic Acid was found to inhibit prostaglandin synthesis and to compete for binding at the prostaglandin receptor site.[3] Pharmacologic studies show Mefenamic Acid did not relieve morphine abstinence signs in abstinent, morphine-habituated monkeys.[1]

Following a single 1-gram oral dose, peak plasma levels of 10 μg/ml occurred in 2 to 4 hours with a half-life of 2 hours. Following multiple doses, plasma levels are proportional to dose with no evidence of drug accumulation. One gram of Mefenamic Acid given four times daily produces peak blood levels of 20 μg/ml by the second day of administration.[4]

Following a single dose, sixty-seven percent of the total dose is excreted in the urine as unchanged drug or as one of two metabolites. Twenty to twenty-five percent of the dose is excreted in the feces during the first three days.[4]

In controlled, double-blind, clinical trials, Mefenamic Acid was evaluated for the treatment of primary spasmodic dysmenorrhea. The parameters used in determining efficacy included pain assessment by both patient and investigator; the need for concurrent analgesic medication; and evaluation of change in frequency and severity of symptoms characteristic of spasmodic dysmenorrhea. Patients received either Mefenamic Acid, 500 mg (2 capsules) as an initial dose and 250 mg every 6 hours, or placebo at onset of bleeding or of pain, whichever began first. After three menstrual cycles, patients were crossed over to the alternate treatment for an additional three cycles. Mefenamic Acid was significantly superior to placebo in all parameters, and both treatments (drug and placebo) were equally tolerated.

INDICATIONS AND USAGE
Mefenamic Acid is indicated for the relief of moderate pain[5] when therapy will not exceed one week. Mefenamic Acid is also indicated for the treatment of primary dysmenorrhea.[5,6]

Studies in children under 14 years of age have been inadequate to evaluate the safety and effectiveness of Mefenamic Acid.

➤ SHOWN IN PRODUCT IDENTIFICATION GUIDE

UNLABELED USES
Mefenamic Acid is used alone in the treatment of fever, osteoarthritis, rheumatoid arthritis, menorrhagia, and premenstrual syndrome.

CONTRAINDICATIONS
Mefenamic Acid should not be used in patients who have previously exhibited hypersensitivity to it.

Because the potential exists for cross-sensitivity to aspirin or other nonsteroidal antiinflammatory drugs, Mefenamic Acid should not be given to patients in whom these drugs induce symptoms of bronchospasm, allergic rhinitis, or urticaria.

Mefenamic Acid is contraindicated in patients with active ulceration or chronic inflammation of either the upper or lower gastrointestinal tract.

Mefenamic Acid should be avoided in patients with preexisting renal disease.

WARNINGS
If diarrhea occurs, the dosage should be reduced or temporarily suspended (see "*Adverse Reactions*" and "*Dosage and Administration*"). Certain patients who develop diarrhea may be unable to tolerate the drug because of recurrence of the symptoms on subsequent exposure.

Risk of GI Ulceration, Bleeding and Perforation with NSAID Therapy: Serious gastrointestinal toxicity such as bleeding, ulceration, and perforation, can occur at any time, with or without warning symptoms, in patients treated chronically with NSAID therapy. Although minor upper gastrointestinal problems, such as dyspepsia, are common, usually developing early in therapy, physicians should remain alert for ulceration and bleeding in patients treated chronically with NSAIDs even in the absence of previous GI tract symptoms. In patients observed in clinical trials of several months to two years duration, symptomatic upper GI ulcers, gross bleeding or perforation appear to occur in approximately 1% of patients treated for 3-6 months, and in about 2-4% of patients treated for one year. Physicians should inform patients about the signs and/or symptoms of serious GI toxicity and what steps to take if they occur.

Studies to date have not identified any subset of patients not at risk of developing peptic ulceration and bleeding. Except for a prior history of serious GI events and other risk factors known to be associated with peptic ulcer disease, such as alcoholism, smoking, etc., no risk factors (eg, age, sex) have been associated with increased risk. Elderly or debilitated patients seem to tolerate ulceration or bleeding less well than other individuals and most spontaneous reports of fatal GI events are in this population. Studies to date are inconclusive concerning the relative risk of various NSAIDs in causing such reactions. High doses of any NSAID probably carry a greater risk of these reactions, although controlled clinical trials showing this do not exist in most cases. In considering the use of relatively large doses (within the recommended dosage range), sufficient benefit should be anticipated to offset the potential increased risk of GI toxicity.

PRECAUTIONS
If rash occurs, administration of the drug should be stopped. A false-positive reaction for urinary bile, using the diazo tablet test, may result after Mefenamic Acid administration. If biliuria is suspected, other diagnostic procedures, such as the Harrison spot test, should be performed.

Renal Effects: As with other nonsteroidal antiinflammatory drugs, long-term administration of Mefenamic Acid to animals has resulted in renal papillary necrosis and other abnormal renal pathology. In humans, there have been reports of acute interstitial nephritis with hematuria, proteinuria and occasionally nephrotic syndrome.

A second form of renal toxicity has been seen in patients with prerenal conditions leading to a reduction in renal blood flow or blood volume, where the renal prostaglandins have a supportive role in the maintenance of renal perfusion. In these patients administration of an NSAID may cause a dose-dependent reduction in prostaglandin formation and may precipitate overt renal decompensation. Patients at greatest risk of this reaction are those with impaired renal function, heart failure, liver dysfunction, those taking diuretics, and the elderly Discontinuation of NAID therapy is typically followed by recovery to the pretreatment state. Since Mefenamic Acid is eliminated primarily by the kidneys, the drug should not be administered to patients with significantly impaired renal functions.

As with other nonsteroidal antiinflammatory drugs, borderline elevations of one or more liver tests may occur in some patients. These abnormalities may progress, may remain essentially unchanged, or may be transient with continued therapy. The SGPT (ALT) test is probably the most sensitive indicator of liver dysfunction. Meaningful (3 times the upper limit of normal) elevations of SGPT or SGOT (AST) occurred in controlled clinical trials in less than 1% of patients. A patient with symptoms and/or signs suggesting liver dysfunction, or in whom an abnormal liver test has occurred, should be evaluated for evidence of the development of more severe hepatic reaction while on therapy with Mefenamic Acid. Severe hepatic reactions, including jaundice and cases of fatal hepatitis, have been reported with other nonsteroidal antiinflammatory drugs. Although such reactions are rare, if abnormal liver tests persist or worsen, if clinical signs and symptoms consistent with liver disease develop, or if systemic manifestations occur (eg eosinophilia, rash, etc.), Mefenamic Acid should be discontinued.

Information for Patients: Patients should be advised that if rash, diarrhea or other digestive problems arise, they should stop the drug and consult their physician.

Patients in whom aspirin or other nonsteroidal antiinflammatory drugs induce symptoms of bronchospasm, allergic rhinitis, or urticaria should be made aware that the potential exists for cross-sensitivity to Mefenamic Acid.

The long-term effects, if any, of intermittent Mefenamic Acid therapy for dysmenorrhea are not known. Women on such therapy should consult their physician if they should decide to become pregnant.

Mefenamic Acid like other drugs of its class, is not free of side effects. The side effects of these drugs can cause discomfort and, rarely, there are more serious side effects, such as gastrointestinal bleeding, which may result in hospitalization and even fatal outcomes.

NSAIDs (nonsteroidal antiinflammatory drugs) are often essential agents in the management of arthritis and have a major role in the treatment of pain, but they also may be commonly employed for conditions which are less serious. Physicians may wish to discuss with their patients the potential risks (see "*Warnings*", "*Precautions*", and "*Adverse Reactions*" sections) and likely benefits of NSAID treatment, particularly when the drugs are used for less serious conditions where treatment without NSAIDs may represent an acceptable alternative to both the patient and physician.

Laboratory Tests: Because serious GI tract ulceration and bleeding can occur without warning symptoms, physicians should follow chronically treated patients for the signs and symptoms of ulceration and bleeding and should inform them of the importance of this follow-up (see "*Warnings, Risk of GI Ulcerations, Bleeding and Perforation with NSAID Therapy*").

Drug Interactions: Mefenamic Acid may prolong prothrombin time.[5] Therefore, when the drug is administered to patients receiving oral anticoagulant drugs, frequent monitoring of prothrombin time is necessary.

Use in Pregnancy: Pregnancy Category C. Reproduction studies have been performed in rats, rabbits and dogs. Rats given up to 10 times the human dose showed decreased fertility, delay in parturition, and a decreased rate of survival to weaning. Rabbits at 2.5 times the human dose showed an increase in the number of resorptions. There were no fetal anomalies observed in these studies nor in dogs at up to 10 times the human dose.[5]

There are no adequate and well-controlled studies in pregnant women. Because animal reproduction studies are not always predictive of human response, this drug should be used only if clearly needed.

The use of Mefenamic Acid in late pregnancy is not recommended because of the effects on the fetal cardiovascular system of drugs of this class.

Nursing Mothers: Trace amounts of Mefenamic Acid may be present in breast milk and transmitted to the nursing infant[7]; thus Mefenamic Acid should not be taken by the nursing mother because of the effects on the infant cardiovascular system of drugs of this class.

Use in Children: Safety and effectiveness in children below the age of 14 have not been established.

ADVERSE REACTIONS
Gastrointestinal: The most frequently reported adverse reactions associated with the use of Mefenamic Acid involve the gastrointestinal tract. In controlled studies for up to eight months, the following disturbances were reported in decreasing order of frequency: diarrhea (approximately 5% of patients), nausea with or without vomiting, other gastrointestinal symptoms, and abdominal pain.

In certain patients, the diarrhea was of sufficient severity to require discontinuation of medication. The occurrence of the diarrhea is usually dose related, generally subsides on reduction of dosage, and rapidly disappears on termination of therapy.

Other gastrointestinal reactions less frequently reported were anorexia, pyrosis, flatulence, and constipation.

Gastrointestinal ulceration with and without hemorrhage has been reported.

Hematopoietic: Cases of autoimmune hemolytic anemia have been associated with the continuous administration of Mefenamic Acid for 12 months or longer. In such cases the Coombs test results are positive with evidence of both accelerated RBC production and RBC destruction. The process is reversible upon termination of Mefenamic Acid administration.

Decreases in hematocrit have been noted in 2-5% of patients and primarily in those who have received prolonged therapy. Leukopenia, eosinophilia, thrombocytopenic purpura, agranulocytosis, pancytopenia, and bone marrow hypoplasia have also been reported on occasion.

Nervous System: Drowsiness, dizziness, nervousness, headache, blurred vision, and insomnia have occurred.

Integumentary: Urticaria, rash, and facial edema have been reported.

Renal: As with other nonsteroidal antiinflammatory agents, renal failure, including papillary necrosis, has been reported. In elderly patients renal failure has occurred after taking Mefenamic Acid for 2-6 weeks. The renal damage may not be completely reversible. Hematuria and dysuria have also been reported with Mefenamic Acid.

Other: Eye irritation, ear pain, perspiration, mild hepatic toxicity, and increased need for insulin in a diabetic have been reported. There have been rare reports of palpitation, dyspnea, and reversible loss of color vision.

OVERDOSAGE
Although doses up to 6000 mg/day have been given, no specific information is available on the management of acute massive overdosage.

Should accidental overdosage occur, the stomach should be emptied by inducing emesis or by careful gastric lavage followed by the administration of activated charcoal.[8] Laboratory studies indicate that Mefenamic Acid should be adsorbed from the gastrointestinal tract by activated charcoal.[4] Vital functions should be monitored and supported. Because Mefenamic Acid and its metabolities are firmly bound to plasma proteins, hemodialysis and peritoneal dialysis may be of little value.[4]

DOSAGE AND ADMINISTRATION

Administration is by the oral route, preferably with food. The recommended regimen in acute pain for adults and children over 14 years of age is 500 mg as an initial dose followed by 250 mg every six hours as needed, usually not to exceed one week.[5]

For the treatment of primary dysmenorrhea, the recommended dosage is 500 mg as an initial dose followed by 250 mg every 6 hours, starting with the onset of bleeding and associated symptoms. Clinical studies indicate that effective treatment can be initiated with the start of menses and should not be necessary for more than 2 to 3 days.[6]

REFERENCES

1. Winder CV, et al: Antiinflammatory, antipyretic and antinociceptive properties of N-(2,3-xylyl) anthranilic acid (mefenamic acid). *J Pharmacol Exp Ther* 138: 405-413, 1962. 2. Wax J, et al: Comparative activities, tolerances and safety of nonsteroidal antiinflammatory agents in rats. *J Pharmacol Exp Ther* 192: 172-178, 1975. 3. Ferreira SH, Vane JR: Aspirin and prostaglandins, in *The Prostaglandins*, Ramwell PW Ed. Plenum Press, NY, vol. 2, 1974, pp 1-47. 4. Glazko AJ: Experimental observations of flufenamic, mefenamic, and meclofenamic acids. Part III. Metabolic disposition, in *Fenamates in Medicine*. A Symposium, London 1966; *Annals of Physical Medicine*, supplement, pp 23-36. 1967. 5. Data on file, Medical Affairs Dept. Parke-Davis.

HOW SUPPLIED
CAPSULE: 250 MG

BRAND/MANUFACTURER	NDC	SIZE	AWP
○ **BRAND**			
PONSTEL: Parke-Davis	00071-0540-24	100s	$91.51

Mefloquine Hydrochloride

DESCRIPTION

Mefloquine Hydrochloride is an antimalarial agent available as 250-mg tablets of mefloquine hydrochloride (equivalent to 228.0 mg of the free base) for oral administration.

Mefloquine Hydrochloride is a 4-quinolinemethanol derivative with the specific chemical name of (R*, S*)-(±)-α-2-piperidinyl-2,8-bis (trifluoromethyl)-4-quinolinemethanol hydrochloride. It is a 2-aryl substituted chemical structural analog of quinine. The drug is a white to almost white crystalline compound, slightly soluble in water.

Mefloquine Hydrochloride has a calculated molecular weight of 414.78.

Following is its chemical structure:

CLINICAL PHARMACOLOGY

Mefloquine is an antimalarial agent which acts as a blood schizonticide. Its exact mechanism of action is not known. Pharmacokinetic studies of Mefloquine in healthy male subjects showed that a significant lagtime occurred after drug administration, and the terminal elimination half-life varied widely (13 to 24 days) with a mean of about 3 weeks. Mefloquine is a mixture of enantiomeric molecules whose rates of release, absorption, transport, action, degradation and elimination may differ. A valid pharmacokinetic model may not exist in such a case.

Additional studies in European subjects showed slightly greater concentrations of drug for longer periods of time. The absorption half-life was 0.36 to 2 hours, and the terminal elimination half-life was 15 to 33 days. The primary metabolite was identified and its concentrations were found to surpass the concentrations of Mefloquine.

Multiple-dose kinetic studies confirmed the long elimination half-lives previously observed. The mean metabolite to Mefloquine ratio measured at steady-state was found to range between 2.3 and 8.6.

The total clearance of the drug, which is essentially all hepatic, is approximately 30 mL/min. The volume of distribution, approximately 20L/kg, indicates extensive distribution. The drug is highly bound (98%) to plasma proteins and concentrated in blood erythrocytes, the target cells in malaria, at a relatively constant erythrocyte-to-plasma concentration ratio of about 2.

The pharmacokinetics of Mefloquine in patients with compromised renal function and compromised hepatic function have not been studied.

In vitro and *in vivo* studies showed no hemolysis associated with glucose-6-phosphate dehydrogenase deficiency. (See *"Animal Toxicology"* for additional information.)

Microbiology: Strains of *Plasmodium falciparum* resistant to Mefloquine have been reported.

INDICATIONS AND USAGE

Treatment of Acute Malaria Infections: Mefloquine Hydrochloride is indicated for the treatment of mild to moderate acute malaria caused by Mefloquine-susceptible strains of *P. fulciparum* (both chloroquine-susceptible and resistant strains) or by *Plasmodium vivax*. There are insufficient clinical data to document the effect of Mefloquine in malaria caused by *P. oval* or *P. malariae*.

Note: Patients with acute *P. vivax* malaria, treated with Mefloquine Hydrochloride are at high risk of relapse because Mefloquine Hydrochloride does not eliminate exoerythrocytic (hepatic phase) parasites. To avoid relapse, after initial treatment of the acute infection with Mefloquine Hydrochloride patients should subsequently be treated with an 8-aminoquinoline (e.g., primaquine).

Prevention of Malaria: Mefloquine Hydrochloride is indicated for the prophylaxis of *P. falciparum* and *P. vivax* malaria infections, including prophylaxis of chloroquine-resistant strains of *P. falciparum*.

CONTRAINDICATIONS

Use of this drug is contraindicated in patients with a known hypersensitivity to Mefloquine or related compounds (e.g., quinine).

WARNINGS

If case of life-threatening, serious or overwhelming malaria infections due to *P. falciparum*, patients should be treated with an intravenous antimalarial drug. Following completion of intravenous treatment, Mefloquine Hydrochloride may be given orally to complete the course of therapy.

Concomitant administration of Mefloquine Hydrochloride and quinine, quinidine or drugs producing beta-adrenergic blockade may produce electrocardiographic abnormalities or cardiac arrest. Concomitant administration of Mefloquine Hydrochloride and quinine or chloroquine may increase the risk of convulsions. (See *"Precautions:* Drug Interactions".)

PRECAUTIONS

General: Caution should be exercised with regard to driving, piloting airplanes and operating machines, as dizziness, a disturbed sense of balance, neurological or psychiatric reactions have been reported during and following the use of Mefloquine Hydrochloride. These effects may occur after therapy is discontinued due to the long half-life of the drug. During prophylactic use, if signs of unexplained anxiety, depression, restlessness or confusion are noticed, these may be considered prodromal to a more serious event. In these cases, the drug must be discontinued. Mefloquine Hydrochloride should be used with caution in patients with psychiatric disturbances because Mefloquine use has been associated with emotional disturbances (see *"Adverse Reactions"* section).

This drug has not been administered for longer than 1 year. If the drug is to be administered for a prolonged period, periodic evaluations including liver function tests should be performed. Although retinal abnormalities seen in humans with long-term chloroquine use have not been observed with Mefloquine use, long-term feeding of Mefloquine to rats resulted in dose-related ocular lesions (retinal degeneration, retinal edema and lenticular opacity at 12.5 mg/kg/day and higher). (See *"Animal Toxicology"*.) Therefore, periodic ophthalmic examinations are recommended.

Parenteral studies in animals show that Mefloquine, a myocardial depressant, possesses 20% of the antifibrillatory action of quinidine and produces 50% of the increase in the PR interval reported with quinine. The effect of Mefloquine on the compromised cardiovascular system has not been evaluated. However, transitory and clinically silent ECG alterations have been reported during the use of Mefloquine. Alterations included sinus bradycardia, sinus arrhythmia, first degree AV-block, prolongation of the QTc interval and abnormal T waves (see also cardiovascular effects under *"Precautions: Drug Interactions"* and *"Adverse Reactions"*). The benefits of Mefloquine Hydrochloride therapy should be weighed against the possibility of adverse effects in patients with cardiac disease.

Laboratory Tests: Periodic evaluation of hepatic function should be performed during prolonged prophylaxis.

Drug Interactions: Drug-drug interactions with Mefloquine Hydrochloride have not been explored in detail. There is one report of cardiopulmonary arrest, with full recovery, in a patient who was taking a beta blocker (propranolol), (see also *"Warnings"* and *"Precautions: General"*). The effects of Mefloquine on the compromised cardiovascular system have not been evaluated. The benefits of Mefloquine Hydrochloride therapy should be weighted against the possibility of adverse effects in patients with cardiac disease.

Mefloquine Hydrochloride should not be used concurrently with quinine or quinidine. If these drugs are to be used in the initial treatment of severe malaria, Mefloquine Hydrochloride administration should be delayed at least 12 hours after the last dose.

Patients taking Mefloquine Hydrochloride while taking valproic acid had loss of seizure control and lower than expected valproic acid blood levels. Therefore, patients concurrently taking antiseizure medication and Mefloquine Hydrochloride should have the blood level of their antiseizure medication monitored and the dosage adjusted appropriately.

In clinical trials the concomitant administration of sulfadoxine and pyrimethamine did not alter the adverse reaction profile.

Carcinogenesis, Mutagenesis, Impairment of Fertility:

➤ SHOWN IN PRODUCT IDENTIFICATION GUIDE

Carcinogenesis: The carcinogenic potential of Mefloquine was studied in rats and mice in 2-year feeding studies at doses up to 30 mg/kg/day. No treatment-related increases in tumor of any type were noted.

Mutagenesis: The mutagenic potential of Mefloquine was studied in a variety of assay systems including: Ames test, a host-mediated assay in mice, fluctuation tests and a mouse micronucleus assay. Several of these assays were performed with and without prior metabolic activation. In no instance was evidence obtained for the mutagenicity of Mefloquine.

Impairment of Fertility: Fertility studies in rats at doses of 5, 20 and 50 mg/kg/day of Mefloquine have demonstrated adverse effects on fertility in the male at the high dose of 50 mg/kg/day, and in the female at doses of 20 and 50 mg/kg/day. Histopathological lesions were noted in the epididymides from male rats at doses of 20 and 50 mg/kg/day. Administration of 250 mg/week of Mefloquine (base) in adult males for 22 weeks failed to reveal any deleterious effects on human spermatozoa.

Pregnancy: Teratogenic Effects. Pregnancy Category C. Mefloquine has been demonstrated to be teratogenic in rats and mice at a dose of 100 mg/kg/day. In rabbits, a high dose of 160 mg/kg/day was embryotoxic and teratogenic, and a dose of 80 mg/kg/day was teratogenic but not embryotoxic. There are no adequate and well-controlled studies in pregnant women. Mefloquine should be used during pregnancy only if the potential benefit justifies the potential risk to the fetus. Women of childbearing potential who are traveling to areas where malaria is endemic should be warned against becoming pregnant.

Nursing Mothers: Mefloquine is excreted in human milk. Based on a study in a few subjects, low concentrations (3% to 4%) of Mefloquine were excreted in human milk following a dose equivalent to 250 mg of the free base. Because of the potential for serious adverse reactions in nursing infants from Mefloquine, a decision should be made whether to discontinue the drug, taking into account the importance of the drug to the mother.

Pediatric Use: Safety and effectiveness in children have not been established. Two studies of Mefloquine in children living in endemic areas for *P. falciparum* were conducted. All children in these studies had at least a low level of parasitemia and 18% to 40% had significant parasitemia with or without mild malaria symptoms. When given 20 to 30 mg/kg of Mefloquine as a single dose, all children with fever became afebrile, and 92% of those with significant parasitemia had a satisfactory response to treatment. While incomplete followup was obtained in these studies, nausea and vomiting occurred in approximately 10% and 20%, respectively, and dizziness was seen in approximately 40% of children.

ADVERSE REACTIONS

Clinical: At the doses used for treatment of acute malaria infections, the symptoms possibly attributable to drug administration cannot be distinguished from those symptoms usually attributable to the disease itself.

Among subjects who received Mefloquine for prophylaxis of malaria, the most frequently observed adverse experience was vomiting (3%). Dizziness, syncope, extrasystoles and other complaints affecting less than 1% were also reported.

Among subjects who received Mefloquine for treatment, the most frequently observed adverse experiences included: dizziness, myalgia, nausea, fever, headache, vomiting, chills, diarrhea, skin rash, abdominal pain, fatigue, loss of appetite and tinnitus. Those side effects occurring in less than 1% included bradycardia, hair loss, emotional problems, pruritus, asthenia, transient emotional disturbances and telogen effluvium (loss of resting hair). Seizures have also been reported.

Two serious adverse reactions were cardiopulmonary arrest in one patient shortly after ingesting a single prophylactic dose of Mefloquine while concomitantly using propranolol (see *"Warnings"* and *"Precautions"*) and encephalopathy of unknown etiology during prophylactic Mefloquine administration. The relationship of encephalopathy to drug administration could not be clearly established.

Postmarketing: Postmarketing surveillance indicates that the same adverse experiences are reported during prophylaxis, as well as acute treatment.

The following additional adverse reactions have been reported during postmarketing surveillance; vertigo, visual disturbances, central nervous system disturbances (e.g., psychotic manifestations, hallucinations, confusion, anxiety and depression) and Stevens-Johnson syndrome and erythema multiforma.

Laboratory: The most frequently observed laboratory alterations which could be possibly attributable to drug administration were decreased hematocrit, transient elevation of transaminases, leukopenia and thrombocytopenia. These alterations were observed in patients with acute malaria who received treatment doses of the drug and were attributed to the disease itself.

During prophylactic administration of Mefloquine to indigenous populations in malaria-endemic areas, the following occasional alterations in laboratory values were observed: transient elevation of transaminases, leukocytosis or thrombocytopenia.

OVERDOSAGE

The following procedure is recommended in case of overdosage: Induce vomiting or perform gastric lavage, as appropriate. Monitor cardiac function and neurologic and psychiatric status for at least 24 hours. Provide symptomatic and intensive supportive treatment as required, particularly for cardiovascular disturbances. Treat vomiting or diarrhea with standard fluid therapy.

DOSAGE AND ADMINISTRATION

(See *"Indications and Usage"* section):

(a) Treatment of mild to moderate malaria in adults caused by *P. vivax* or Mefloquine-susceptible strains of *P. falciparum*—5 tablets (1250 mg) Mefloquine Hydrochloride to be given as a single oral dose. The drug should not be taken on an empty stomach and should be administered with at least 8 oz (240 mL) of water.

If a full treatment course has been administered without clinical cure, alternative treatment should be given. Similarly, if previous prophylaxis with Mefloquine has failed, Mefloquine Hydrochloride should not be used for curative treatment.

Note: Patients with acute *P. vivax* malaria, treated with Mefloquine Hydrochloride are at high risk of relapse because Mefloquine Hydrochloride does not eliminate exoerythrocytic (hepatic phase) parasites. To avoid relapse after initial treatment of the acute infection with Mefloquine Hydrochloride patients should subsequently be treated with an 8-aminoquinoline (e.g., primaquine).

(b) Malaria prophylaxis—one 250 mg Mefloquine Hydrochloride tablet once weekly.

Prophylactic drug administration should begin 1 week before departure to an endemic area. Subsequent weekly doses should always be taken on the same day of the week. To reduce the risk of malaria after leaving an endemic area, prophylaxis should be continued for 4 additional weeks. Tablets should not be taken on an empty stomach and should be administered with at least 8 oz (240 mL) of water.

Tablets should be stored at 15°–30°C (59°–86°F).

ANIMAL TOXICOLOGY

Ocular lesions were observed in rats fed Mefloquine daily for 2 years. All surviving rats given 30 mg/kg/day had ocular lesions in both eyes characterized by retinal degeneration, opacity of the lens and retinal edema. Similar but less severe lesions were observed in 80% of female and 22% of male rats fed 12.5 mg/kg/day for 2 years. At doses of 5 mg/kg/day, only corneal lesions were observed. They occurred in 9% of rats studied.

HOW SUPPLIED
TABLETS: 250 MG

BRAND/MANUFACTURER	NDC	SIZE	AWP
○ BRAND LARIAM: Roche Labs	00004-0172-02	25s	$154.24

Mefoxin *SEE* CEFOXITIN SODIUM

Megace *SEE* MEGESTROL ACETATE

Megestrol Acetate

WARNING

THE USE OF MEGESTROL ACETATE ORAL SUSPENSION IS CONTRAINDICATED IN PREGNANCY; THE USE OF MEGESTROL ACETATE TABLETS DURING THE FIRST 4 MONTHS OF PREGNANCY IS NOT RECOMMENDED.

PROGESTATIONAL AGENTS HAVE BEEN USED BEGINNING WITH THE FIRST TRIMESTER OF PREGNANCY IN AN ATTEMPT TO PREVENT HABITUAL ABORTION. THERE IS NO EVIDENCE THAT SUCH USE IS EFFECTIVE WHEN SUCH DRUGS ARE GIVEN DURING THE FIRST 4 MONTHS OF PREGNANCY OR THAT THE USE OF A HIGH DOSE PROGESTATIONAL AGENT SUCH AS MEGESTROL ACETATE ORAL SUSPENSION DURING ANY PHASE OF PREGNANCY IS EFFECTIVE FOR THIS PURPOSE. FURTHERMORE, IN THE VAST MAJORITY OF WOMEN, THE CAUSE OF ABORTION IS A DEFECTIVE OVUM, WHICH PROGESTATIONAL AGENTS COULD NOT BE EXPECTED TO INFLUENCE. IN ADDITION, THE USE OF PROGESTATIONAL AGENTS, WITH THEIR UTERINE-RELAXANT PROPERTIES, IN PATIENTS WITH FERTILIZED DEFECTIVE OVA MAY CAUSE A DELAY IN SPONTANEOUS ABORTION.

SEVERAL REPORTS SUGGEST AN ASSOCIATION BETWEEN INTRAUTERINE EXPOSURE TO PROGESTATIONAL DRUGS IN THE FIRST TRIMESTER OF PREGNANCY AND GENITAL ABNORMALITIES IN MALE AND FEMALE FETUSES. THE RISK OF HYPOSPADIAS, 5 TO 8 PER 1,000 MALE BIRTHS IN THE GENERAL POPULATION, MAY BE APPROXIMATELY DOUBLED WITH EXPOSURE TO THESE DRUGS.

THERE ARE INSUFFICIENT DATA TO QUANTIFY THE RISK TO EXPOSED FEMALE FETUSES, BUT INSOFAR AS SOME OF THESE DRUGS INDUCE MILD VIRILIZATION OF THE EXTERNAL GENITALIA OF THE FEMALE FETUS, AND BECAUSE OF THE INCREASED ASSOCIATION OF HYPOSPADIAS IN THE MALE FETUS, IT IS PRUDENT TO AVOID THE USE OF THESE DRUGS DURING THE FIRST TRIMESTER OF PREGNANCY AND

THE USE OF MEGESTROL ACETATE ORAL SUSPENSION DURING PREGNANCY.

IF THE PATIENT IS EXPOSED TO MEGESTROL ACETATE ORAL SUSPENSION DURING PREGNANCY, OR MEGESTROL ACETATE TABLETS DURING THE FIRST 4 MONTHS OF PREGNANCY, OR IF SHE BECOMES PREGNANT WHILE TAKING THIS DRUG, SHE SHOULD BE APPRISED OF THE POTENTIAL RISKS TO THE FETUS.

DESCRIPTION

Megestrol Acetate is a synthetic derivative of the naturally occurring steroid hormone, progesterone. It is an antineoplastic, progestational drug available as an oral suspension and tablets.

Each ml of oral suspension contains:
Megestrol Acetate ....40 mg

Each tablet contains:
Megestrol Acetate ....20 or 40 mg

Megestrol Acetate is a white, crystalline solid chemically designated as 17 α-(acetyloxy)-6-methylpregna-4,6-diene-3,20-dione. Solubility at 37°C in water is 2 µg per mL, solubility in plasma is 24 µg per mL. Its molecular weight is 384.51. The empirical formula is $C_{24}H_{32}O_4$.

Following is its chemical structure:

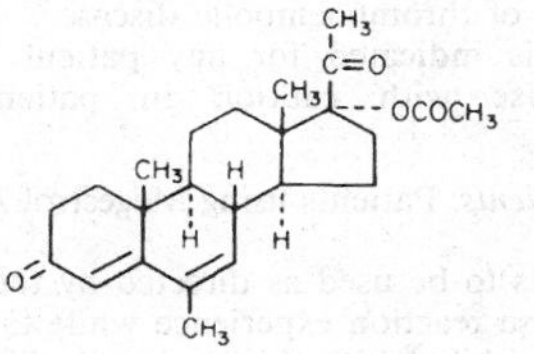

CLINICAL PHARMACOLOGY

Several investigators have reported on the appetite enhancing property of Megestrol Acetate and its possible use in cachexia. The precise mechanism by which Megestrol Acetate produces effects in anorexia and cachexia is unknown at the present time.

While the precise mechanism by which Megestrol Acetate produces its antineoplastic effects against endometrial carcinoma is unknown at the present time, inhibition of pituitary gonadotropin production and resultant decrease in estrogen secretions may be factors. There is evidence to suggest a local effect as a result of the marked changes brought about by the direct instillation of progestational agents into the endometrial cavity. The antineoplastic action of Megestrol Acetate on carcinoma of the breast is effected by modifying the action of other steroid hormones and by exerting a direct cytotoxic effect on tumor cells.[1] In metastatic cancer, hormone receptors may be present in some tissues but not others. The receptor mechanism is a cyclic process whereby estrogen produced by the ovaries enters the target cell, forms a complex with cytoplasmic receptor and is transported into the cell nucleus. There it induces gene transcription and leads to the alteration of normal cell functions. Pharmacologic doses of Megestrol Acetate not only decrease the number of hormone-dependent human breast cancer cells but also is capable of modifying and abolishing the stimulatory effects of estrogen on these cells. It has been suggested[2] that progestins may inhibit in one of two ways: by interfering with either the stability, availability, or turnover of the estrogen receptor complex in its interaction with genes or in conjunction with the progestin receptor complex, by interacting directly with the genome to turn off specific estrogen-responsive genes.

There are several analytical methods used to estimate Megestrol Acetate plasma concentrations, including gas chromatography-mass fragmentography (GC-MF), high pressure liquid chromatography (HPLC) and radioimmunoassay (RIA). The GC-MF and HPLC methods are specific for Megestrol Acetate and yield equivalent concentrations. The RIA method reacts to Megestrol Acetate metabolites and is, therefore, non-specific and indicates higher concentrations than the GC-MF and HPLC methods. Plasma concentrations are dependent, not only on the method used, but also on intestinal and hepatic inactivation of the drug, which may be affected by factors such as intestinal tract motility, intestinal bacteria, antibiotics administered, body weight, diet and liver function.[3,4]

The major route of drug elimination in humans is urine. When radiolabeled Megestrol Acetate was administered to humans in doses of 4 to 90 mg, the urinary excretion within 10 days ranged from 56.5% to 78.4% (mean 66.4%) and fecal excretion ranged from 7.7% to 30.3% (mean 19.8%). The total recovered radioactivity varied between 83.1% and 94.7% (mean 86.2%). Megestrol Acetate metabolites which were identified in urine constituted 5% to 8% of the dose administered and were considered negligible.[5] Respiratory excretion as labeled carbon dioxide and fat storage may have accounted for at least part of the radioactivity not found in urine and feces.

Plasma steady state pharmacokinetics of Megestrol Acetate were evaluated in 10 adult, cachectic male patients with acquired immunodeficiency syndrome (AIDS) and an involuntary weight loss greater than 10% of baseline. Patients received single oral doses of 800 mg/day of Megestrol Acetate oral suspension for 21 days. Plasma concentration data obtained on day 21 were evaluated for up to 48 hours past the last dose.

Mean (± 1SD) peak plasma concentration (C_{max}) of Megestrol Acetate was 753 (± 539) ng/ml. Mean area under the concentration time-curve (AUC) was 10476 (± 7788) ng × hr/ml. Median TMAX value was five hours. Seven of 10 patients gained weight in three weeks.

Additionally, 24 adult, asymptomatic HIV seropositive male subjects were dosed once daily with 750 mg of Megestrol Acetate oral suspension. The treatment was administered for 14 days. Mean C_{max} and AUC values 490 (± 238) ng/ml and 6779 (± 3048) hr × ng/ml respectively. The median TMAX value was three hours. The mean C_{min} value was 202 (± 101) ng/ml. The mean % FL value was 107 (± 40).

In normal male volunteers (N-23) who received 160 mg of Megestrol Acetate given as a 40 mg qid regimen, the oral absorption of Megestrol Acetate appeared to be variable. Plasma levels were assayed by a high pressure liquid chromatographic (HPLC) procedure. Peak drug levels for the first 40 mg dose ranged from 10 to 56 ng/ml (mean 27.6 ng/ml) and the times to peak concentrations ranged from 1.0 to 3.0 hours (mean 2.2 hours). Plasma elimination half-life ranged from 13.0 to 104.9 hours (mean 34.2 hours). The steady state plasma concentrations for a 40 mg qid regimen have not been established.

The relative bioavailability of Megestrol Acetate tablets, 40 mg tablets and Megestrol Acetate oral suspension has not been evaluated. The effect of food on the bioavailability of Megestrol Acetate oral suspension has not been evaluated.

DESCRIPTION OF CLINICAL STUDIES

The clinical efficacy of Megestrol Acetate oral suspension was assessed in two clinical trials. One was a multicenter, randomized, double-blind, placebo-controlled study comparing Megestrol Acetate at doses of 100 mg, 400 mg, and 800 mg per day versus placebo in AIDS patients with anorexia/cachexia and significant weight loss. Of the 270 patients entered on study, 195 met all inclusion/exclusion criteria, had at least two additional post baseline weight measurements over a 12 week period or had one post baseline weight measurement but dropped out for therapeutic failure. The percent of patients gaining five or more lb. at maximum weight gain in 12 study weeks was statistically significantly greater for the 800 mg (64%) and 400 mg (57%) Megestrol Acetate-treated groups than for the placebo group (24%). Mean weight increased from baseline to last evaluation in 12 study weeks in the 800 mg Megestrol Acetate-treated group by 7.8 lbs., the 400 mg Megestrol Acetate group by 4.2 lbs., the 100 mg Megestrol Acetate group by 1.9 lbs. and decreased in the placebo group by 1.6 lbs. Mean weight changes at 4, 8 and 12 weeks for patients evaluable for efficacy in the two clinical trials are shown graphically. Changes in body composition during the 12 study weeks as measured by bioelectrical impedance analysis showed increases in non-water body weight in the Megestrol Acetate-treated groups (see "Clinical Studies" table). In addition, edema developed or worsened in only 3 patients.

Greater percentages of Megestrol Acetate-treated patients in the 800 mg group (89%), the 400 mg group (68%) and the 100 mg group (72%), than in the placebo group (50%), showed an improvement in appetite at last evaluation during the 12 study weeks. A statistically significant difference was observed between the 800 mg Megestrol Acetate-treated group and the placebo group in the change in caloric intake from baseline to time of maximum weight change. Patients were asked to assess weight change, appetite, appearance, and overall perception of well-being in 9 question survey. At maximum weight change only the 800 mg Megestrol Acetate-treated group gave responses that were statistically significantly more favorable to all questions when compared to the placebo-treated group. A dose response was noted in the survey with positive responses correlating with higher dose for all questions.

The second trial was a multicenter, randomized, double-blind, placebo-controlled study comparing Megestrol Acetate 800 mg/day versus placebo in AIDS patients with anorexia/cachexia and significant weight loss. Of the 100 patients entered on study, 65 met all inclusion/exclusion criteria, had at least two additional post baseline weight measurements over a 12 week period or had one post baseline weight measurement but dropped out for therapeutic failure. Patients in the 800 mg Megestrol Acetate-treated group had a statistically significantly larger increase in mean maximum weight change than patients in the placebo group. From baseline to study week 12, mean weight increased by 11.2 lbs. in the Megestrol Acetate-treated group and decreased 21 lbs. in the placebo group.

Changes in body composition as measured by bioelectrical impedance analysis showed increases in non-water weight in the Megestrol Acetate-treated group (see "Clinical Studies" table). No edema was reported in the Megestrol Acetate-treated group. A greater percentage of Megestrol Acetate-treated patients (67%) than placebo-treated patients (38%) showed an improvement in appetite at last evaluation during the 12 study weeks; this difference was statistically significant. There were no statistically significant differences between treatment groups in mean caloric change or in daily caloric intake at time to maximum weight change. In the same 9 question survey referenced in the first trial, patients' assessments of weight change, appetite, appearance, and overall perception of well-being showed increases in mean scores in Megestrol Acetate-treated patients as compared to the placebo group.

In both trials, patients tolerated the drug well and no statistically significant differences were seen between the treatment groups with regard to laboratory abnormalities, new opportunistic infections, lymphocyte counts, T_4 counts, T_8 counts, or skin reactivity tests (see "Adverse Reactions").

CLINICAL STUDIES (SEE RELATED TABLE).

Presented below are the results of mean weight changes for patients evaluable for efficacy in trials 1 and 2.

➤ SHOWN IN PRODUCT IDENTIFICATION GUIDE

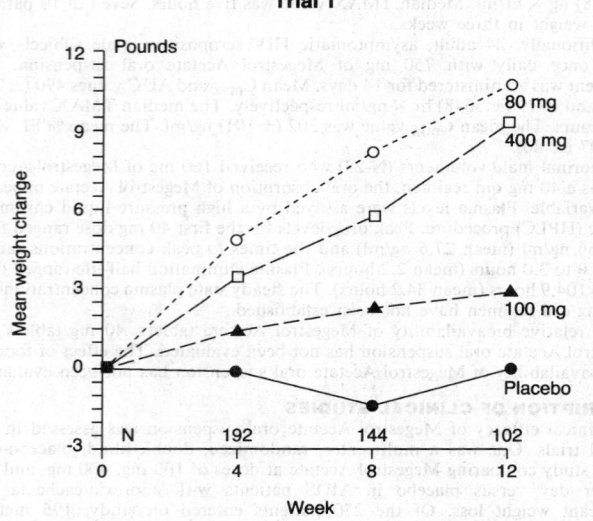

Trial 1

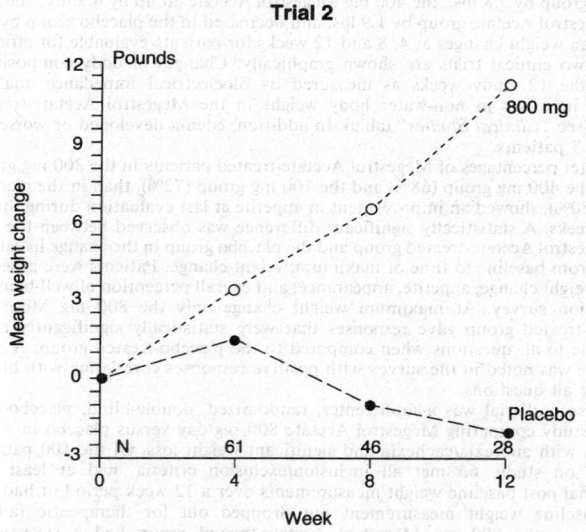

Trial 2

INDICATIONS AND USAGE

Megestrol Acetate oral suspension is indicated for the treatment of anorexia, cachexia, or an unexplained, significant weight loss in patients with a diagnosis of acquired immunodeficiency syndrome (AIDS).

Megestrol Acetate tablets are indicated for the palliative treatment of advanced carcinoma of the breast or endometrium (ie, recurrent, inoperable, or metastatic disease). Megestrol Acetate should not be used in lieu of currently accepted procedures such as surgery, radiation, or chemotherapy.

UNLABELED USES

Megestrol Acetate is used alone or as an adjunct to reduce levels of gonadotropins and the secretion of testosterone in benign prostatic hypertrophy. It is used in the treatment of ovarian carcinoma, and to relieve symptoms of endometriosis. It is also prescribed for patients with symptomatic stage D prostatic cancer, and is used as a contraceptive.

CONTRAINDICATIONS

As a diagnostic test for pregnancy.
Known or suspected pregnancy.

WARNINGS

Megestrol Acetate may cause fetal harm when administered to a pregnant woman. Fertility and reproduction studies with high doses of Megestrol Acetate have shown a reversible feminizing effect on some male rat fetuses.[6] For other animal data on fetal effects, see the "Impairment of Fertility" section under "Precautions". There are no adequate and well-controlled studies in pregnant women. If this drug is used during pregnancy, or if the patient becomes pregnant while taking (receiving) this drug, the patient should be apprised of the potential hazard to the fetus. Women of childbearing potential should be advised to avoid becoming pregnant.

Megestrol Acetate oral suspension is not intended for prophylactic use to avoid weight loss.

The use of Megestrol Acetate tablets in other types of neoplastic disease is not recommended. See also "Carcinogenesis, Mutagenesis, and Impairment of Fertility" section under "Precautions".

PRECAUTIONS

General: Therapy with Megestrol Acetate oral suspension for weight loss should only be instituted after treatable causes of weight loss are sought and addressed. These treatable causes include possible malignancies, systemic infections, gastrointestinal disorders affecting absorption, endocrine disease and renal or psychiatric diseases.

Although the glucocorticoid effects of Megestrol Acetate oral suspension in HIV-infected individuals have not been evaluated, laboratory evidence of adrenal suppression has been observed which is clinically insignificant.

Effects on HIV viral replication have not been determined. Use with caution in patients with a history of thromboembolic disease.

Close surveillance is indicated for any patient treated for recurrent or metastatic cancer. Use with caution in patients with a history of thrombophlebitis.

Information for the Patients: Patients using Megestrol Acetate should receive the following instructions.
1. This medication is to be used as directed by the physician.
2. Report any adverse reaction experience while taking this medication.
3. Use contraception while taking this medication if you are a woman capable of becoming pregnant.
4. Notify your physician if you become pregnant while taking this medication.

Drug Interactions: Possible interactions of Megestrol Acetate with concomitant medications have not been investigated.

Animal Toxicology: Long-term treatment with Megestrol Acetate may increase the risk of respiratory infections. A trend toward increased frequency of respiratory infections, decreased lymphocyte counts and increased neutrophil counts was observed in a two-year chronic toxicity/carcinogenicity study of Megestrol Acetate conducted in rats.

Laboratory Tests: Breast malignancies in which estrogen and/or progesterone receptors are positive are more likely to respond to Megestrol Acetate.[7,8,9]

Carinogenesis, Mutagenesis, and Impairment of Fertility:

Carcinogenesis: Data on carcinogenesis were obtained from studies conducted in dogs, monkeys and rats treated with Megestrol Acetate at doses 53.2, 26.6 and 1.3 times *lower* than the proposed dose (13.3 mg/kg/day) for humans. No males were used in the dog and monkey studies. In female beagles, Megestrol Acetate (0.01, 0.1 or 0.25 mg/kg/day) administered for up to 7 years induced both benign and malignant tumors of the breast.[10] In female monkeys, no tumors were found following 10 years of treatment with 0.01, 0.1, or 0.5 mg/kg/day Megestrol Acetate. Pituitary tumors were observed in female rats treated with 3.9 or 10 mg/kg/day of Megestrol Acetate for 2 years. The relationship of these tumors in rats and dogs to humans is unknown but should be considered in assessing the risk-to-benefit ratio when prescribing Megestrol Acetate and in surveillance of patients on therapy.[10,11] Also see "Warnings" section.

Mutagenesis: No mutagenesis data are currently available.

Impairment of Fertility: Perinatal/postnatal (segment III) toxicity studies were performed in rats at doses (0.05—12.5 mg/kg) *less* than that indicated for humans (13.3 mg/kg); in these low dose studies, the reproductive capability of male offspring of Megestrol Acetate-treated females was impaired. Similar results were obtained in dogs. Pregnant rats treated with Megestrol Acetate showed a reduction in fetal weight and number of live births. No toxicity data are currently available on male reproduction (spermatogenesis).

Pregnancy:

Oral Suspension: Pregnancy Category X. (See "Warnings" and "Impairment of Fertility" section.) No adequate animal teratology information is available at clinically relevant doses.

Tablets: Pregnancy Category D. See "Warnings" section.

Nursing Mothers: Because of the potential for adverse effects on the newborn, nursing should be discontinued if Megestrol Acetate is required.

Use in HIV-Infected Women: Although Megestrol Acetate has been used extensively in women for the treatment of endometrial and breast cancers, its use in HIV-infected women has been limited.

All 10 women in the clinical trials reported breakthrough bleeding.

Pediatric Use: Safety and effectiveness in children have not been established.

◆ **RATED THERAPEUTICALLY EQUIVALENT;** ◇ **THERAPEUTIC EQUIVALENCE UNCONFIRMED;** ○ **UNRATED**

ADVERSE REACTIONS

Clinical Adverse Events: Adverse events which occurred in at least 5% of patients in any arm of the two clinical efficacy trials and the open trial are listed below by treatment group. All patients listed had at least one post baseline visit during the 12 study weeks. These adverse events should be considered by the physician when prescribing Megestrol Acetate oral suspension. (See related table).

Adverse events which occurred in 1% to 3% of all patients enrolled in the two clinical efficacy trials with at least one follow-up visit during the first 12 weeks of the study are listed below by body system. Adverse events occurring less than 1% are not included. There were no significant differences between incidence of these events in patients treated with Megestrol Acetate and patients treated with placebo.

Body as a Whole: abdominal pain, chest pain, infection, moniliasis and sarcoma

Cardiovascular System: cardiomyopathy, palpitation, thromboembolic phenomena including thrombophlebitis and pulmonary embolism.

Digestive System: constipation, dry mouth, hepatomegaly, increased salivation and oral moniliasis

Hemic and Lymphatic System: leukopenia

Metabolic and Nutritional: LDH increased, edema and peripheral edema

Nervous System: parethesia, confusion, convulsion, depression, neuropathy, hypesthesia and thinking abnormal

Respiratory System: dyspnea, cough, pharyngitis and lung disorder

Skin and Appendages: alopecia, herpes, pruritus, vesiculobulous rash, sweating and skin disorder

Special Senses: amblyopia

Urogenital System: albuminuria, urinary incontinence, urinary tract infection, breakthrough bleeding and gynecomastia

Other: carpal tunnel syndrome, tumor flare (with or without hypercalcemia)

OVERDOSAGE

No serious unexpected side effects have resulted from studies involving Megestrol Acetate oral suspension administered in dosages as high as 1200 mg/day or Megestrol Acetate tablets in doses as high as 1600 mg/day. Oral administration of large, single doses of Megestrol Acetate (5 g/kg) did not produce toxic effects in mice.[6] Megestrol Acetate has not been tested for dialyzability; however, due to its low solubility it is postulated that dialysis would not be an effective means of treating overdose.

DOSAGE AND ADMINISTRATION

ORAL SUSPENSION

The recommended adult initial dosage of Megestrol Acetate oral suspension is 800 mg/day (20 ml/day). Shake container well before using.

In clinical trials evaluating different dose schedules, daily doses of 400 and 800 mg/day were found to be clinically effective.

TABLETS

Breast Cancer: 160 mg/day (40 mg qid)

Endometrial Carcinoma: 40 to 320 mg/day in divided doses. At least 2 months of continuous treatment is considered an adequate period for determining the efficacy of Megestrol Acetate.

STORAGE

Store Megestrol Acetate oral suspension at or below 25°C and dispense in a tight container. Protect from heat.

Store Megestrol Acetate tablets at room temperature; protect from temperatures above 40°C (104°F).

SPECIAL HANDLING

Health Hazard Data: There is no threshold limit value established by OSHA, NIOSH, or ACGIH.

Exposure or "overdose" at levels approaching recommended dosage levels could result in side effects described above ("Warnings", "Adverse Reactions"). Women at risk of pregnancy should avoid such exposure.

MEGESTROL ACETATE ORAL SUSPENSION CLINICAL EFFICACY TRIALS

	Trial 1 Study Accrual Dates 11/88 to 12/90				Trial 2 Study Accrual Dates 5/89 to 4/91	
Megestrol Acetate, mg/day	0	100	400	800	0	800
Entered Patients	38	82	75	75	48	52
Evaluable Patients	28	61	53	53	29	36
Mean Change in Weight (lb.)						
Baseline to 12 Weeks	0.0	2.9	9.3	10.7	−2.1	11.2
% Patients ≥ 5 lbs Gain						
at Last Evaluation in 12 weeks	21	44	57	64	28	47
Mean Changes in Body Composition*:						
Fat Body Mass (lb.)	0.0	2.2	2.9	5.5	1.5	5.7
Lean Body Mass (lb.)	−1.7	−0.3	1.5	2.5	−1.6	−0.6
Water (liters)	−1.3	−0.3	0.0	0.0	−0.1	−0.1
% Patients With Improved Appetite						
At Time of Max. Wt. Change	50	72	72	93	48	69
At Last Evaluation in 12 Wk	50	72	68	89	38	67
Mean Change in Daily Caloric Intake:						
Baseline to Time of Maximum						
Weight Change	−107	326	308	646	30	464

* *Based on bioelectrical impedance analysis determination at last evaluation in 12 weeks*

ADVERSE EVENTS % OF PATIENTS REPORTING

Megestrol Acetate mg/day No. of Patients	Trial 1 (N = 236)				Trial 2 (N = 87)			Open Label Trial
	Placebo 0 N = 34	100 N = 68	400 N = 69	800 N = 65	Placebo 0 N = 38	800 N = 49		1200 N = 176
Diarrhea	15	13	8	15	8	6		10
Impotence	3	4	6	4	0	4		7
Rash	9	4	4	12	3	2		6
Flatulence	9	0	1	9	3	10		6
Hypertension	0	0	0	8	0	0		4
Asthenia	0	3	3	6	8	4		5
Insomnia	0	3	4	6	0	0		1
Nausea	9	4	0	5	3	4		5
Anemia	6	3	3	5	0	0		0
Fever	6	1	1	5	3	2		1
Libido								
Decreased	3	4	1	5	0	2		1
Dyspepsia	0	0	1	3	5	4		2
Hyperglycemia	3	0	0	3	0	0		3
Headache	6	10	1	3	3	0		3
Pain	6	0	0	2	5	6		4
Vomiting	6	3	0	2	3	6		4
Pneumonia	6	2	0	2	3	0		2
Urinary Freq.	0	0	1	2	5	2		1

➤ SHOWN IN PRODUCT IDENTIFICATION GUIDE

REFERENCES

1. Allegra JC, Kiefer SM. Mechanisms of Action of Progestational Agents. *Semin Oncol.* 1985; 12(Suppl 1):3. 2. DeSombre ER, Kuivanen PC. Progestin Modulation of Estrogen-Dependent Marker Protein Synthesis in the Endometrium, *Semin Oncol.* 1985; 12(Suppl 1):6. 3. Alexieva-Figusch J, Blankenstein MA. Hop WCJ, et al. Treatment of Metastatic Breast Cancer Patients with Different Dosages of Megestrol Acetate: Dose Relations, Metabolic and Endocrine Effects. *Eur J Cancer Clin Oncol.* 1984; 20:33-40. 4. Gaver RC, Movahhed HS, Farmen RH, Pittman KA. Liquid Chromatographic Procedure for the Quantitative Analysis of Megestrol Acetate in Human Plasma. *J Pharm Sci.* 1985;74:664. 5. Cooper JM, Kellie AE. The Metabolism of Megestrol Acetate (17-alpha-acetoxy-6-methylprega-4,6-diene-3,20-dione) in Women. *Steroids.* 1968;11:133. 6. David A, Edwards K, Fellowes KP, Plummer JM. Anti-Ovulatory and Other Biological Properties of Megestrol Acetate. *J Reprod Fertil.* 1963;5:331. 7. McGuire WL, Clark GM. The Prognostic Role of Progesterone Receptors in Human Breast Cancer. *Semin Oncol.* 1983;10(Suppl 4):2. 8. Horwitz KB. The Central Role of Progesterone Receptors and Progestational Agents in the Management and Treatment of Breast Cancer. *Semin Oncol.* 1988;15(Suppl 1):14. 9. Bonomi P, Johnson P, Anderson K, Wolter J, Bunting N, Strauss A, Roseman D, Shorey W, Econonou S. Primary Hormonal Therapy of Advanced Breast Cancer with Megestrol Acetate: Predictive Value of Estrogen Receptor and Progesterone Receptor Levels. *Semin Oncol.* 1985;12(1 Suppl 1):48-54. 10. Nelson LW, Weikel JH Jr., Reno FE. Mammary Nodules in Dogs during Four Years' Treatment with Megestrol Acetate or Chlormadione Acetate. *J Natl Cancer Inst.* 1973;51:1303. 11. Owen LN, Briggs MH. Contraceptive Steroid Toxicology in the Beagle Dog and its Relevance to Human Carcinogenicity. *Curr Med Res Opin.* 1976;4:309.

HOW SUPPLIED
SUSPENSION: 40 MG/ML

BRAND/MANUFACTURER	NDC	SIZE	AWP
○ BRAND			
MEGACE: Bristol-Myer Onc/Hiv	00015-0508-42	240 ml	$103.80

TABLETS: 20 MG

AVERAGE UNIT PRICE (AVAILABLE SIZES)		GENERIC A-RATED AVERAGE PRICE (GAAP)	
BRAND	$0.70	100s	$60.16
GENERIC	$0.60		
HCFA FUL (100s ea)	$0.37		

BRAND/MANUFACTURER	NDC	SIZE	AWP
◆ BRAND			
MEGACE: Bristol-Myer Onc/Hiv	00015-0595-01	100s	$69.96
◆ GENERICS			
Major	00904-3570-60	100s	$52.50
Goldline	00182-1863-01	100s	$52.50
Rugby	00536-4821-01	100s	$54.38
Qualitest	00603-4391-21	100s	$56.60
Schein	00364-2235-01	100s	$59.00
Martec	52555-0375-01	100s	$59.90
Moore,H.L.	00839-7405-06	100s	$61.16
Par	49884-0289-01	100s	$62.36
Parmed	00349-8766-01	100s	$66.66
Aligen	00405-4623-01	100s	$66.66
Goldline	00182-1863-89	100s ud	$64.50
UDL	51079-0434-20	100s ud	$65.65

TABLETS: 40 MG

AVERAGE UNIT PRICE (AVAILABLE SIZES)		GENERIC A-RATED AVERAGE PRICE (GAAP)	
BRAND	$1.22	100s	$95.71
GENERIC	$0.93	250s	$221.69
HCFA FUL (100s ea)	$0.67	500s	$444.56

BRAND/MANUFACTURER	NDC	SIZE	AWP
◆ BRAND			
MEGACE: Bristol-Myer Onc/Hiv	00015-0596-41	100s	$124.79
	00015-0596-46	250s	$305.74
	00015-0596-45	500s	$599.00
◆ GENERICS			
Goldline	00182-1864-01	100s	$87.00
Major	00904-3571-60	100s	$87.40
Rugby	00536-4822-01	100s	$89.55
Qualitest	00603-4392-21	100s	$89.55
URL	00677-1206-01	100s	$92.43
Aligen	00405-4624-01	100s	$95.99
Mason Dist	11845-0287-01	100s	$95.99
Schein	00364-2234-01	100s	$96.00
Lemmon	00093-0674-01	100s	$99.00
Parmed	00349-8767-01	100s	$99.00
Par	49884-0290-01	100s	$101.75
Martec	52555-0376-01	100s	$102.88
Moore,H.L.	00839-7406-06	100s	$106.37
Major	00904-3571-61	100s ud	$76.52
Goldline	00182-1864-89	100s ud	$105.00
UDL	51079-0435-20	100s ud	$106.95
Major	00904-3571-70	250s	$192.75
Aligen	00405-4624-04	250s	$207.75
Parmed	00349-8767-25	250s	$215.00
Rugby	00536-4822-02	250s	$220.28
Mason Dist	11845-0287-02	250s	$239.98
Par	49884-0290-04	250s	$254.38
Major	00904-3571-40	500s	$371.25
Qualitest	00603-4392-28	500s	$423.81

◆ RATED THERAPEUTICALLY EQUIVALENT; ◇ THERAPEUTIC EQUIVALENCE UNCONFIRMED; ○ UNRATED

BRAND/MANUFACTURER	NDC	SIZE	AWP
Mason Dist	11845-0287-03	500s	$447.30
Par	49884-0290-05	500s	$474.14
Moore,H.L.	00839-7406-12	500s	$506.32

Melanex *SEE* HYDROQUINONE

Melfiat *SEE* PHENDIMETRAZINE TARTRATE

Mellaril *SEE* THIORIDAZINE HYDROCHLORIDE

Melphalan

> WARNING: MELPHALAN SHOULD BE ADMINISTERED UNDER THE SUPERVISION OF A QUALIFIED PHYSICIAN EXPERIENCED IN THE USE OF CANCER CHEMOTHERAPEUTIC AGENTS. SEVERE BONE MARROW SUPPRESSION WITH RESULTING INFECTION OR BLEEDING MAY OCCUR. CONTROLLED TRIALS COMPARING INTRAVENOUS TO ORAL MELPHALAN HAVE SHOWN MORE MYELOSUPPRESSION WITH THE INTRAVENOUS FORMULATION. HYPERSENSITIVITY REACTIONS, INCLUDING ANAPHYLAXIS, HAVE OCCURRED IN APPROXIMATELY 2% OF PATIENTS WHO RECEIVED THE INTRAVENOUS FORMULATION. MELPHALAN IS LEUKEMOGENIC IN HUMANS. MELPHALAN PRODUCES CHROMOSOMAL ABERRATIONS *IN VITRO* AND *IN VIVO* AND, THEREFORE, SHOULD BE CONSIDERED POTENTIALLY MUTAGENIC IN HUMANS.

DESCRIPTION

Melphalan, also known as L-phenylalanine mustard, phenylalanine mustard, L-PAM, or L-sarcolysin, is a phenylalanine derivative of nitrogen mustard. Melphalan is a bifunctional alkylating agent which is active against selected human neoplastic diseases. It is known chemically as 4-[bis(2-chloroethyl)amino]-*L*-phenylalanine. The molecular formula is $C_{13}H_{18}Cl_2N_2O_2$ and the molecular weight is 305.20.

Melphalan is the active L-isomer of the compound and was first synthesized in 1953 by Bergel and Stock; the D-isomer, known as medphalan, is less active against certain animal tumors, and the dose needed to produce effects on chromosomes is larger than that required with the L-isomer. The racemic (DL-) form is known as merphalan or sarcolysin.

Melphalan is practically insoluble in water and has a pKa_1 of ~ 2.5.

Melphalan for Injection is supplied as a sterile, non-pyrogenic, freeze-dried powder. Each single-use vial contains Melphalan Hydrochloride, equivalent to 50 mg Melphalan and 20 mg povidone. Melphalan for Injection is reconstituted using the sterile diluent provided. Melphalan for Injection is administered intravenously.

Melphalan is available in tablet form for oral administration. Each scored tablet contains 2 mg Melphalan.

Following is its chemical structure:

$$(ClCH_2CH_2)_2N \text{—} \bigcirc \text{—} CH_2 \text{---} \overset{\overset{NH_2}{|}}{\underset{\underset{H}{|}}{C}} \text{---} COOH$$

CLINICAL PHARMACOLOGY

Melphalan is an alkylating agent of the bischloroethylamine type. As a result, its cytotoxicity appears to be related to the extent of its interstrand cross-linking with DNA, probably by binding at the N^7 position of guanine. Like other bifunctional alkylating agents, it is active against both resting and rapidly dividing tumor cells.

Pharmacokinetics: The pharmacokinetics of Melphalan after intravenous and oral administration has been extensively studied in adult patients. Following injection, drug plasma concentrations declined rapidly in a biexponential manner with distribution phase and terminal elimination phase half-lives of approximately 10 and 75 minutes, respectively. Estimates of average total body clearance varied among studies, but typical values of approximately 7 to 9 mL/min/kg (250 to 325 mL/min/m²) were observed. One study has reported that on repeat dosing of 0.5 mg/kg every 6 weeks, the clearance of Melphalan decreased from 8.1 mL/min/kg after the first course, to 5.5 mL/min/kg after the third course, but did not decrease appreciably after the third course. Mean (± SD) peak Melphalan plasma concentrations in myeloma patients given Melphalan intravenously at doses of 10 or 20 mg/m² were 1.2 ± 0.4 and 2.8 ± 1.9 ng/mL, respectively.

Plasma Melphalan levels are highly variable after oral dosing, both with respect to the time of the first appearance of Melphalan in plasma (range 0 to 336 minutes) and to the peak plasma concentration (range 0.166 to 3.741 μg/mL) achieved. These results may be due to incomplete intestinal absorption, a variable "first pass" hepatic metabolism, or to rapid hydrolysis. Five patients were studied after both oral and intravenous dosing with 0.6 mg/kg as a single bolus dose by each route. The areas under the plasma concentration-time curves after oral administration averaged 61 ± 26% (± standard deviation; range 25% to 89%) of those following intravenous administration. In 18 patients given a single oral dose of 0.6 mg/kg of Melphalan, the terminal plasma half-disappearance time of parent drug was 89.5 ± 50 minutes. The 24-hour urinary excretion of parent drug in these patients was 10 ± 4.5%, suggesting that renal clearance is not a major route of elimination of parent drug.

One study using universally labeled ^{14}C-melphalan found substantially less radioactivity in the urine of patients given the drug by mouth (30% of administered dose in nine days) than in the urine of those given it intravenously (35% to 65% in seven days). Following either oral or intravenous administration, the pattern of label recovery was similar, with the majority being recovered in the first 24 hours. Following oral administration, peak radioactivity occurred in plasma at two hours and then disappeared with a half-life of approximately 160 hours. In one patient where parent drug (rather than just radiolabel) was determined, the Melphalan half-disappearance time was 67 minutes.

The steady-state volume of distribution of Melphalan is 0.5 L/kg. Penetration into cerebrospinal fluid (CSF) is low. The extent of Melphalan binding to plasma proteins ranges from 60% to 90%. Serum albumin is the major binding protein, while α_1-acid glycoprotein appears to account for about 20% of the plasma protein binding. Approximately 30% of the drug is (covalently) irreversibly bound to plasma proteins. Interactions with immunoglobulins have been found to be negligible.

Melphalan is eliminated from plasma primarily by chemical hydrolysis to monohydroxy- and dihydroxymelphalan. Aside from these hydrolysis products, no other Melphalan metabolites have been observed in humans. Although the contribution of renal elimination to Melphalan clearance appears to be low, one study noted an increase in the occurrence of severe leukopenia in patients with elevated BUN after 10 weeks of therapy and one pharmacokinetic study showed a significant positive correlation between the elimination rate constant for Melphalan and renal function and a significant negative correlation between renal function and the area under the plasma Melphalan concentration/time curve.

Clincial Trial: A randomized trial compared prednisone plus intravenous Melphalan to prednisone plus oral Melphalan in the treatment of myeloma. As discussed below, overall response rates at week 22 were comparable; however, because of changes in trial design, conclusions as to the relative activity of the two formulations after week 22 are impossible to make.

Both arms received oral prednisone starting at 0.8 mg/kg/day with doses tapered over 6 weeks. Melphalan doses in each arm were:

Arm 1 Oral Melphalan 0.15 mg/kg/day × 7 followed by 0.05 mg/kg/day when WBC began to rise.

Arm 2 Intravenous Melphalan 16 mg/m^2 q 2 weeks × 4 (over 6 weeks) followed by the same dose every 4 weeks.

Doses of Melphalan were adjusted according to the following criteria:

WBC/mm^3	Platelets	% of full dose
≥ 4000	≥ 100,000	100
≥ 3000	≥ 75,000	75
≥ 2000	≥ 50,000	50
< 2000	< 50,000	0

107 patients were randomized to the oral Melphalan arm and 203 patients to the intravenous Melphalan arm. More patients had a poor-risk classification (58% vs 44%) and high tumor load (51% vs 34%) on the oral compared to the I.V. arm (P < 0.04). Response rates at week 22 are shown in the following table:

Initial arm	Evaluable patients	Responders n (%)	P
Oral Melphalan	100	44 (44%)	P > 0.2
I.V. Melphalan	195	74 (38%)	

Because of changes in protocol design after week 22, other efficacy parameters such as response duration and survival cannot be compared.

Severe myelotoxicity (WBC ≤ 1000 and/or platelets ≥ 25,000) was more common in the intravenous Melphalan arm (28%) than in the oral Melphalan arm (11%).

An association was noted between poor renal function and myelosuppression; consequently, an amendment to the protocol required a 50% reduction in I.V. Melphalan dose if the BUN was ≥ 30 mg/dL. The rate of severe leukopenia in the I.V. arm in the patients with BUN over 30 mg/dL decreased from 50% (8/16) before protocol amendment to 11% (3/28) (P = .01) after the amendment.

Before the dosing amendment, there was a 10% (8/77) incidence of drug-related death in the I.V. arm. After the dosing amendment, this incidence was 3% (3/108). This compares to an overall 1% (1/100) incidence of drug-related death in the oral arm.

INDICATIONS AND USAGE

Melphalan for Injection is indicated for the palliative treatment of patients with multiple myeloma for whom oral therapy is not appropriate.

Melphalan Tablets are indicated for the palliative treatment of multiple myeloma and for the palliation of nonresectable epithelial carcinoma of the ovary.

UNLABELED USES

Melphalan is used alone or as an adjunct in the treatment of amyloidosis, breast carcinoma, and chronic myelogenous leukemia.

CONTRAINDICATIONS

Melphalan should not be used in patients whose disease has demonstrated prior resistance to this agent. Patients who have demonstrated hypersensitivity to Melphalan should not be given the drug.

WARNINGS

Melphalan should be administered in carefully adjusted dosage by or under the supervision of experienced physicians who are familiar with the drug's actions and the possible complications of its use.

As with other nitrogen mustard drugs, excessive dosage will produce marked bone marrow suppression. Bone marrow suppression is the most significant toxicity associated with Melphalan for Injection or oral Melphalan in most patients. Therefore, the following tests should be performed at the start of therapy and prior to each subsequent dose or course of Melphalan: platelet count, hemoglobin, white blood cell count, and differential. Thrombocytopenia and/or leukopenia are indications to withhold further therapy until the blood counts have sufficiently recovered. Frequent blood counts are essential to determine optimal dosage and to avoid toxicity. (See *"Precautions: Laboratory Tests"*). Dose adjustment on the basis of blood counts at the nadir and day of treatment should be considered.

Hypersensitivity reactions including anaphylaxis have occurred in approximately 2% of patients who received the intravenous formulation and rarely after oral administration (see *"Adverse Reactions"*). These reactions usually occur after multiple courses of treatment and have recurred in patients who experienced a hypersensitivity reaction to intravenous Melphalan. Treatment is symptomatic. The intravenous infusion should be terminated immediately, followed by the administration of volume expanders, pressor agents, corticosteroids, or antihistamines at the discretion of the physician. If a hypersensitivity reaction occurs, intravenous or oral Melphalan should not be readministered.

Carcinogenesis: Secondary malignancies, including acute nonlymphocytic leukemia, myeloproliferative syndrome, and carcinoma, have been reported in patients with cancer treated with alkylating agents (including Melphalan). Some patients also received other chemotherapeutic agents or radiation therapy. Precise quantitation of the risk of acute leukemia, myeloproliferative syndrome, or carcinoma is not possible. Published reports of leukemia in patients who have received Melphalan (and other alkylating agents) suggest that the risk of leukemogenesis increases with chronicity of treatment and with cumulative dose. In one study, the 10-year cumulative risk of developing acute leukemia or myeloproliferative syndrome after oral Melphalan therapy was 19.5% for cumulative doses ranging from 730 mg to 9652 mg. In this same study, as well as in an additional study, the 10-year cumulative risk of developing acute leukemia or myeloproliferative syndrome after oral Melphalan therapy was less than 2% for cumulative doses under 600 mg. This does not mean that there is a cumulative dose below which there is not risk of the induction of secondary malignancy. The potential benefits from Melphalan therapy must be weighed on an individual basis against the possible risk of the induction of a second malignancy.

Adequate and well-controlled carcinogenicity studies have not been conducted in animals. However, i.p. administration of Melphalan in rats (5.4 to 10.8 mg/m^2) and in mice (2.25 to 4.5 mg/m^2) 3 times per week for 6 months followed by 12 months post-dose observation produced peritoneal sarcoma and lung tumors, respectively.

Mutagenesis: Melphalan has been shown to cause chromatid or chromosome damage in humans. Intramuscular administration of Melphalan at 6 and 60 mg/m^2 produced structural aberrations to the chromatid and chromosomes in bone marrow cells of Wistar rats.

Impairment of Fertility: Melphalan causes suppression of ovarian function in premenopausal women, resulting in amenorrhea in a significant number of patients. Reversible and irreversible testicular suppression have also been reported.

Pregnancy: Pregnancy Category D. Melphalan may cause fetal harm when administered to a pregnant woman. While adequate animal studies have not been conducted with intravenous Melphalan, oral (6 to 18 mg/m^2/day for 10 days) and i.p. (18 Mg/m^2 kg single dose) administration in rats was embryolethal and teratogenic. Malformations resulting from Melphalan included alterations of the brain (underdevelopment, deformation, meningocele, and encephalocele) and eye (anophthalmia and microphthalmos), reduction of the mandible and tail, as well as hepatocele (exomphaly). There are no adequate and well-controlled studies in pregnant women. If this drug is used during pregnancy, or if the patient becomes pregnant while taking this drug, the patient should be apprised of the potential hazard to the fetus.

Women of childbearing potential should be advised to avoid becoming pregnant.

PRECAUTIONS

General: In all instances where the use of Melphalan is considered for chemotherapy, the physician must evaluate the need and usefulness of the drug against the risk of adverse events. Melphalan should be used with extreme caution in patients whose bone marrow reserve may have been compromised by prior irradiation or chemotherapy or whose marrow function is recovering from previous cytotoxic therapy. If the leukocyte count falls below 3,000 cells/μL, or the platelet count below 100,000 cells/µL, Melphalan should be discontinued until the peripheral blood cell counts have recovered.

Dose reduction should be considered in patients with renal insufficiency receiving I.V. Melphalan. In one trial, increased bone marrow suppression was observed in patients with BUN levels $\geq$ 30 mg/dL. A 50% reduction in the I.V. Melphalan dose decreased the incidence of severe bone marrow suppression in the latter portion of this study.

A recommendation as to whether or not dosage reduction of oral Melphalan should be made routinely in patients with renal insufficiency cannot be made because:

(a) There is considerable inherent patient-to-patient variability in the systemic availability of Melphalan in patients with normal renal function.

(b) Only a small amount of the administered dose appears as parent drug in the urine of patients with normal renal function.

Patients with azotemia should be closely observed, however, in order to make dosage reductions, if required, at the earliest possible time.

Information for Patients: Patients should be informed that the major acute toxicities of Melphalan are related to bone marrow suppression, hypersensitivity reactions, gastrointestinal toxicity and pulmonary toxicity. The major long-term toxicities are related to infertility and secondary malignancies. Patients should never be allowed to take the drug without close medical supervision and should be advised to consult their physicians if they experience skin rash, signs or symptoms of vasculitis, bleeding, fever, persistent cough, nausea, vomiting, amenorrhea, weight loss, or unusual lumps/masses. Women of childbearing potential should be advised to avoid becoming pregnant.

Laboratory Tests: Periodic complete blood counts with differentials should be performed during the course of treatment with Melphalan. At least one determination should be obtained prior to each dose or treatment course. Patients should be observed closely for consequences of bone marrow suppression, which include severe infections, bleeding, and symptomatic anemia (see *"Warnings"*).

Drug Interactions: The development of severe renal failure has been reported in patients treated with a single dose of intravenous Melphalan followed by standard oral doses of cyclosporine. Cisplatin may affect Melphalan kinetics by inducing renal dysfunction and subsequently altering Melphalan clearance. Intravenous Melphalan may also reduce the threshold for carmustine lung toxicity. When nalidixic acid and intravenous Melphalan are given simultaneously, the incidence of severe hemorrhagic necrotic enterocolitis has been reported to increase in pediatric patients.

There are no known drug/drug interactions with oral Melphalan.

Carcinogenesis, Mutagenesis, Impairment of Fertility: See *"Warnings"* section.

Pregnancy: Teratogenic Effects: Pregnancy Category D: See *"Warnings"* section.

Nursing Mothers: It is not known whether this drug is excreted in human milk. Melphalan should not be given to nursing mothers.

Pediatric Use: The safety and effectiveness in children have not been established.

Geriatric Use: Clinical experience with Melphalan has not identified differences in responses between the elderly and younger patients. In general, dose selection for an elderly patient should be cautious, reflecting the greater frequency of decreased hepatic, renal, or cardiac function, and of concomitant disease or other drug therapy.

ADVERSE REACTIONS
(See *"Overdosage"*):

The following information on adverse reactions is based on data from both oral and intravenous administration of Melphalan as a single agent, using several different dose schedules for treatment of a wide variety of malignancies.

Hematologic: The most common side effect is bone marrow suppression. White blood cell count and platelet count nadirs usually occur 2 to 3 weeks after treatment, with intravenous Melphalan with recovery in 4 to 5 weeks after treatment. Irreversible bone marrow failure has been reported. Although bone marrow suppression frequently occurs, it is usually reversible if Melphalan is withdrawn early enough.

Gastrointestinal: Gastrointestinal disturbances such as nausea and vomiting, diarrhea, and oral ulceration occur infrequently. Hepatic toxicity, including veno-occlusive disease, has been reported.

Hypersensitivity: Acute hypersensitivity reactions including anaphylaxis were reported in 2.4% of 425 patients receiving Melphalan for Injection for myeloma (see *"Warnings"*). These reactions were characterized by urticaria, pruritus, edema, and in some patients, tachycardia, bronchospasm, dyspnea, and hypotension. These patients appeared to respond to antihistamine and corticosteroid therapy. If a hypersensitivity reaction occurs, intravenous or oral Melphalan should not be readministered since hypersensitivity reactions have also been reported with oral Melphalan.

Miscellaneous: Other reported adverse reactions include skin hypersensitivity, skin ulceration at injection site, skin necrosis rarely requiring skin grafting, vasculitis, alopecia, hemolytic anemia, pulmonary fibrosis, and interstitial pneumonitis. Allergic reactions, including rare anaphylaxis, have occurred after multiple courses of treatment.

OVERDOSAGE
Overdoses of intravenous Melphalan resulting in death have been reported. Overdoses, including doses up to 290 mg/m^2, have produced the following symptoms: severe nausea and vomiting, decreased consciousness, convulsions,

muscular paralysis, and cholinomimetic effects. Severe mucositis, stomatitis, colitis, diarrhea, and hemorrhage of the gastrointestinal tract occur at high doses (> 100 mg/m^2). Elevations in liver enzymes and veno-occlusive disease occur infrequently. Significant hyponatremia caused by an associated inappropriate secretion of ADH syndrome has been observed. Nephrotoxicity and adult respiratory distress syndrome have been reported rarely. The principal toxic effect is bone marrow suppression.

Overdoses of oral Melphalan, including doses up to 50 mg/day for 16 days, have been reported. Immediate effects are likely to be vomiting, ulceration of the mouth, diarrhea and hemorrhage of the gastrointestinal tract. The principal toxic effect is bone marrow suppression.

Hematologic parameters should be closely followed for three to six weeks. An uncontrolled study suggests that administration of autologous bone marrow or hematopoietic growth factors (i.e., sargramostim, filgrastim) may shorten the period of pancytopenia. General supportive measures together with appropriate blood transfusions and antibiotics should be instituted as deemed necessary by the physician. This drug is not removed from plasma to any significant degree by hemodialysis or hemoperfusion. A pediatric patient survived a 254 mg/m^2 intravenous overdose treated with standard supportive care.

DOSAGE AND ADMINISTRATION
MELPHALAN FOR INJECTION
The usual intravenous dose is 16 mg/m^2. Dosage reduction of up to 50% should be considered in patients with renal insufficiency (BUN $\geq$ 30 mg/dL) (see *"Precautions: General"*). The drug is administered as a single infusion over 15 to 20 minutes. Melphalan is administered at 2-week intervals for 4 doses, then, after adequate recovery from toxicity, at 4-week intervals. Available evidence suggests about one-third to one-half of the patients with multiple myeloma show a favorable response to the drug.

Dose adjustment on the basis of blood cell counts at the nadir and day of treatment should be considered.

Administration Precautions: As with other toxic compounds, caution should be exercised in handling and preparing the solution of Melphalan. Skin reactions associated with accidental exposure may occur. The use of gloves is recommended. If the solution of Melphalan contacts the skin or mucosa, immediately wash the skin or mucosa thoroughly with soap and water.

Procedures for proper handling and disposal of anticancer drugs should be considered. Several guidelines on this subject have been published.[1-7] There is no general agreement that all of the procedures recommended in the guidelines are necessary or appropriate.

Parenteral drug products should be visually inspected for particulate matter and discoloration prior to administration whenever solution and container permit. If either occurs, do not use this product.

PREPARATION FOR ADMINISTRATION/STABILITY
1. Melphalan for Injection must be reconstituted by rapidly injecting 10 mL of the supplied diluent directly into the vial of lyophilized powder using a sterile needle (20 gauge or larger needle diameter) and syringe. Immediately shake vial vigorously until a clear solution is obtained. This provides a 5 mg/mL solution of Melphalan. Rapid addition of the diluent followed by immediate vigorous shaking is important for proper dissolution.

2. *Immediately* dilute the dose to be administered in 0.9% sodium chloride injection, U.S.P., to a concentration not greater than 0.45 mg/mL.

3. Administer the diluted product over a minimum of 15 minutes.

4. Complete administration within 60 minutes of reconstitution.

The time between reconstitution/dilution and administration of Melphalan should be kept to a minimum because reconstituted and diluted solutions of Melphalan are unstable. Over as short a time as 30 minutes, a citrate derivative of Melphalan has been detected in reconstituted material from the reaction of Melphalan with Sterile Diluent for Melphalan. Upon further dilution with saline, nearly 1% label strength of Melphalan hydrolyzes every 10 minutes. A precipitate forms if the reconstituted solution is stored at 5°C. DO NOT REFRIGERATE THE RECONSTITUTED PRODUCT.

Store at controlled room temperature 15° to 30°C (59° to 86°F) and protect from light.

MELPHALAN TABLETS
Multiple Myeloma: The usual oral dose is 6 mg (3 tablets) daily. The entire daily dose may be given at one time. The dose is adjusted, as required, on the basis of blood counts done at approximately weekly intervals. After two to three weeks of treatment the drug should be discontinued for up to four weeks during which time the blood count should be followed carefully. When the white blood cell and platelet counts are rising, a maintenance dose of 2 mg daily may be instituted. Because of the patient-to-patient variation in Melphalan plasma levels following oral administration of the drug, several investigators have recommended that the dosage of Melphalan Hydrochloride be cautiously escalated until some myelosuppression is observed in order to assure that potentially therapeutic levels of the drug have been reached.

Other dosage regimens have been used by various investigators. Osserman and Takatsuki have used an initial course of 10 mg/day for seven to ten days.[2,3] They report that maximal suppression of the leukocyte and platelet counts occurs within three to five weeks and recovery within four to eight weeks. Continuous maintenance therapy with 2 mg/day is instituted when the white blood cell count is greater than 4,000 cells/µL and the platelet count is greater than 100,000 cells/µL. Dosage is adjusted to between 1 and 3 mg/day depending upon the hematological response. It is desirable to try to maintain a significant degree of bone marrow depression so as to keep the leukocyte count in the range of 3,000 to 3,500 cells/μL.

Hoogstraten *et al* have started treatment with 0.15 mg/kg/day for seven days.[4] This is followed by a rest period of at least 14 days, but it may be as long as five to six weeks. Maintenance therapy is started when the white blood cell and platelet counts are rising. The maintenance dose is 0.05 mg/kg per day or less and is adjusted according to the blood count.

Available evidence suggests that about one third to one half of the patients with multiple myeloma show a favorable response to oral administration of the drug.

One study by Alexanian *et al* has shown that the use of Melphalan in combination with prednisone significantly improves the percentage of patients with multiple myeloma who achieve palliation.[5] One regimen has been to administer courses of Melphalan at 0.25 mg/kg/day for four consecutive days (or, 0.20 mg/kg/day for five consecutive days) for a total dose of 1 mg/kg per course. These four- to five-day courses are then repeated every four to six weeks if the granulocyte count and the platelet count have returned to normal levels.

It is to be emphasized that response may be very gradual over many months; it is important that repeated courses or continuous therapy be given since improvement may continue slowly over many months, and the maximum benefit may be missed if treatment is abandoned too soon.

In patients with moderate to severe renal impairment, currently available pharmacokinetic data does not justify an absolute recommendation on dosage reduction to those patients, but it may be prudent to use a reduced dose initially.

Epithelial Ovarian Cancer: One commonly employed regimen for the treatment of ovarian carcinoma has been to administer Melphalan at a dose of 0.2 mg/kg daily for five days as a single course. Courses are repeated every four to five weeks depending upon hematologic tolerance.[6,7]

Store at 15° to 25°C (59° to 77°F) in a dry place, protect from light, and dispense in glass.

REFERENCES
1. Recommendations for the safe handling of parenteral antineoplastic drugs. Washington, DC: Division of Safety, National Institutes of Health; 1983. US Dept of Health and Human Services, Public Health Service publication NIH 83-2621. 2. AMA Council on Scientific Affairs. Guidelines for handling parenteral antineoplastics. *JAMA.* 1985; 253:1590-1591. 3. National Study Commission on Cytotoxic Exposure. Recommendations for handling cytotoxic agents. 1987. Available from Louis P. Jeffrey, ScD, Director of Pharmacy Services, Rhode Island Hospital, 593 Eddy Street, Providence, RI 02902. 4. Clinical Oncological Society of Australia. Guidelines and recommendations for safe handling of antineoplastic agents. *Med J Australia.* 1983;1:426-428. 5. Jones RB, Frank R, Mass T. Safe handling of chemotherapeutic agents: a report from the Mount Sinai Medical Center. *CA-A Cancer J for Clin.* 1983;33:258-263. 6. American Society of Hospital Pharmacists. ASHP technical assistance bulletin on handling cytotoxic and hazardous drugs. *Am J Hosp Pharm.* 1990;47:1033-1049. 7. Yodaiken RE, Bennett D. OSHA work-practice guidelines for personnel dealing with cytotoxic (antineoplastic) drugs. *Am J Hosp Pharm.* 1986;43:1193-1204. 8. Pallante SL, Fenselau C, Mennel RG, et al. Quantitation by gas chromatography-chemical ionization-mass spectrometry of phenylalanine mustard in plasma of patients. *Cancer Res.* 1980;40:2268-2272. 9. Osserman EF. Therapy of plasma cell myeloma with melphalan (1-phenylalanine mustard). *Proc Am Assoc Cancer Res.* 1963;4:50. Abstract. 10. Osserman EF, Takatsuki K. Plasma cell myeloma: gamma globulin synthesis and structure. A review of biochemical and clinical data, with the description of a newly-recognized and related syndrome, "H-gamma-2-chain" (Franklin's) disease. *Medicine* (Balt). 1963;42:357-384. 11. Hoogstraten B, Sheehe PR, Cuttner J, et al. Melphalan in multiple myeloma. *Blood.* 1967;30:74-83. 12. Alexanian R, Haut A, Khan AU, et al. Treatment for multiple myeloma; combination chemotherapy with different melphalan dose regimens. *JAMA.* 1969;208:1680-1685. 13. Smith JP, Rutledge FN: Chemotherapy in advanced ovarian cancer. *Natl Cancer Inst Monog.* 1975; 42:141-143. 14. Young RC, Chabner BA, Hubbard SP, et al. Advanced ovarian adenocarcinoma: a prospective clinical trial of melphalan (L-PAM) versus combination chemotherapy. *N Engl J Med.* 1978;299:1261-1266.

HOW SUPPLIED
POWDER FOR INJECTION: 50 MG

BRAND/MANUFACTURER	NDC	SIZE	AWP
○ BRAND			
ALKERAN I.V.: Burr Wellcome	00081-0130-93	1s	$260.50

TABLETS: 2 MG

BRAND/MANUFACTURER	NDC	SIZE	AWP
○ BRAND			
ALKERAN: Burr Wellcome	00081-0045-35	50s	$74.35

Melquin-3 *SEE* HYDROQUINONE

Menest *SEE* ESTROGENS, ESTERIFIED

Meningococcal Polysaccharide Vaccine

DESCRIPTION
Meningococcal Polysaccharide Vaccine, Groups A, C, Y and W-135 Combined, is a freeze-dried preparation of the group-specific polysaccharide antigens from *Neisseria meningitidis*, Group A, Group C, Group Y and Group W-135 for subcutaneous use. The diluent is sterile pyrogen-free distilled water to which thimerosal (mercury derivative) 1:10,000 is added as a preservative. After reconstitution with diluent as indicated on the label, each 0.5 ml dose contains 50 mcg of "isolated product" from each of Groups A, C, Y and W-135 in isotonic sodium chloride solution preserved with thimerosal (mercury derivative). Each dose of vaccine also contains 2.5 mg to 5 mg of lactose added as a stabilizer.[1] The vaccine when reconstituted is a clear colorless liquid.

THIS VACCINE CONFORMS TO W.H.O. REQUIREMENTS.

CLINICAL PHARMACOLOGY
N. meningitidis causes both endemic and epidemic disease, principally meningitis and Meningococcemia. It is the second most common cause of bacterial meningitis in the United States (approximately 20% of all cases), affecting an estimated 3,000-4,000 people each year. The case-fatality rate is approximately 10% for meningococcal meningitis and 20% for meningococcemia, despite therapy with antimicrobial agents,such as penicillin, to which all strains remain highly sensitive.[2]

Within the United States, serogroup B, for which a vaccine is not yet available, accounts for 50%-55% of all cases; serogroup C, for 20%-25%; and serogroup W-135, for 15%. Serogroups Y (10%) and A (1%-2%) account for nearly all remaining cases. Serogroup W-135 has emerged as a major cause of disease only since 1975. While serogroup A causes only a small proportion of endemic disease in the United States, it is the most common cause of epidemics elsewhere.[2] A study performed using 4 lots of Meningococcal Polysaccharide Vaccine, Groups A, C, Y and W-135 Combined in 150 adults showed at least a 4-fold increase in bactericidal antibodies to all groups in greater than 90 percent of the subjects.[3,4]

A study was conducted in 73 children 2 to 12 years of age. Post-immunization sera were not obtained on four children. Therefore, the seroconversion rates were based on 69 paired samples. Seroconversion rates as measured by bactericial antibody were: Group A—72 percent, Group C—58 percent, Group Y—90 percent and Group W-135—82 percent. Seroconversion rates as measured by a 2-fold rise in antibody titers based on Solid Phase Radioimmunoassay were: Group A—99 percent, Group C—99 percent, Group Y—97 percent and Group W-135—89 percent.[5]

As with any vaccine, vaccination with Meningococcal Polysaccharide Vaccine, Groups A, C, Y and W-135 Combined may not protect 100% of susceptible individuals.

Vaccine Efficacy: Numerous studies have demonstrated the immunogenicity and clinical efficacy of the A and C vaccines. The serogroup A Polysaccharide induces antibody in some children as young as 3 months of age, although a response comparable to that seen in adults is not achieved until 4 or 5 years of age; the serogroup C component does not induce a good antibody response before age 18-24 months. The serogroup A vaccine has been shown to have a clinical efficacy of 85%-95% and to be of use in controlling epidemics.[6] A similar level of clinical efficacy has been demonstrated for the serogroup C vaccine, both in American military recruits and in an epidemic. The group Y and W-135 Polysaccharides have been shown to be safe and immunogenic in adults and in children over 2 years of age; clinical protection has not been demonstrated directly, but is assumed, based on the production of bactericidal antibody, which for group C has been correlated with clinical protection. The antibody responses to each of the four Polysaccharides in the quadrivalent vaccine are serogroup-specific and independent.[2]

Duration of Efficacy. Antibodies against the group A and C Polysaccharides decline markedly over the first 3 years following a single dose of vaccine. This antibody decline is more rapid in infants and young children than in adults. Similarly, while vaccine-induced clinical protection probably persists in school-children and adults for at least 3 years, a recent study in Africa has demonstrated a marked decline in the efficacy of the group A vaccine in young children over time. In this study, efficacy declined from greater than 90% to less than 10% over 3 years in those under 4 years of age at the time of vaccination; in older children, efficacy was still 67%, 3 years after vaccination.[2,7]

INDICATIONS AND USAGE
Meningococcal Polysaccharide Vaccine, Groups A, C, Y and W-135 Combined, is indicated for the following individuals:

1. Persons 2 years of age and above in epidemic or endemic areas as might be determined in a population delineated by neighborhood, school, dormitory, or other reasonable boundary. The prevalent serogroup in such a situation should match a serogroup in the vaccine.
2. Individuals at particular high-risk to include persons with terminal component complement deficiencies and those with anatomic or functional asplenia.
3. Travelers to countries recognized as having hyperendemic or epidemic disease such as the part of Sub-Saharan Africa known as the "meningitis belt", which extends from Mauritania in the west to Ethiopia in the east.

Vaccinations also should be considered for household or institutional contacts of persons with Meningococcal disease as an adjunct to appropriate antibiotic chemoprophylaxis as well as medical and laboratory personnel at risk of exposure to Meningococcal disease.

This vaccine will not stimulate protection against infections caused by organisms other than Groups A, C, Y and W-135 Meningococci.

► SHOWN IN PRODUCT IDENTIFICATION GUIDE

CONTRAINDICATIONS
Immunization should be deferred during the course of any acute illness. Pregnant women should not be immunized since effects of vaccine on the fetus are unknown.

IT IS A CONTRAINDICATION TO ADMINISTER MENINGOCOCCAL POLYSACCHARIDE VACCINE A/C/Y/W-135 TO INDIVIDUALS KNOWN TO BE SENSITIVE TO THIMEROSAL OR AN OTHER COMPONENT OF THE VACCINE.

WARNING
If the vaccine is used in persons receiving immunosuppressive therapy, the expected immune response may not be obtained.

PRECAUTIONS
GENERAL
Epinephrine Injection (1:1000) must be immediately available to combat unexpected anaphylactic or other allergic reactions.

Prior to an injection of any vaccine, all known precautions should be taken to prevent side reactions. This includes a review of the patient's history with respect to possible sensitivity to the vaccine or similar vaccines.

As with any vaccine, vaccination with Meningococcal Polysaccharide Vaccine, Groups A, C, Y and W-135 Combined may not protect 100% of susceptible individuals. Protective antibody levels may be achieved within 10-14 days after vaccination.[2]

Special care should be taken to avoid injecting the vaccine intradermally, intramuscularly, or intravenously since clinical studies have not been done to establish safety and efficacy of the vaccine using these routes of administration.

A separate, sterile syringe and needle or a sterile disposable unit should be used for each individual patient to prevent transmission of hepatitis and other infectious agents from one person to another.

During use it is possible that the nozzle of the Jet Injector Apparatus may become contaminated with blood or serum. In one instance, such contamination has been reported to be associated with transmission of hepatitis b disease. Therefore, if blood or serum contamination occurs, the nozzle should be dissambled, cleansed and sterilized before continued use to prevent the possibility of transmission of hepatitis or other infectious agents from one person to another.[8]

PREGNANCY[9]
REPRODUCTIVE STUDIES—PREGNANCY CATEGORY C
Animal reproduction studies have not been conducted with Meningococcal Polysaccharide Vaccine, Groups A, C, Y and W-135. It is also not known whether Meningococcal Polysaccharide Vaccine, Groups A, C, Y and W-135 can cause fetal harm when administered to a pregnant woman or can affect reproduction capacity.

EXPERIENCE IN HUMANS
There is no data on the safety of Meningococcal Polysaccharide Vaccine when administered to a pregnant woman. Therefore, Meningococcal Polysaccharide Vaccine should not be administered to a pregnant woman, particularly in the first trimester.

PEDIATRIC USE
THERE ARE NO DATA ON SAFETY AND EFFICACY OF MENINGOCOC-CAL POLYSACCHARIDE VACCINE WHEN ADMININSTERED TO CHILDREN UNDER 2 YEARS OF AGE.

ADVERSE REACTIONS
Adverse reactions to Meningococcal Vaccine are mild and infrequent, consisting of localized erythema lasting 1-2 days. Up to 2% of young children develop fever transiently after vaccination.[2]

As with the administration of any vaccine, one should expect possible hypersensitivity reactions.

DOSAGE AND ADMINISTRATION
Parenteral drug products should be inspected visually for extraneous particulate matter and/or discoloration prior to administration whenever solution and container permit. If these conditions exist, vaccine should not be administered. Reconstitute the vaccine using only the diluent supplied for this purpose. Draw the volume of diluent shown on the diluent label into a suitable size syringe and inject into the vial containing the vaccine. Shake vial until the vaccine is dissolved. Administer the vaccine subcutaneously.

The immunizing dose is a single injection of 0.5 ml given subcutaneously.

PRIMARY IMMUNIZATION
For both adults and children, vaccine is administered subcutaneously as a single 0.5 ml dose. The vaccine can be given at the same time as other immunizations, if needed. Protective antibody levels may be achieved within 10-14 days after vaccination.[2]

REVACCINATION
Revaccination may be indicated for individuals at high risk of infection, particularly children who were first immunized under 4 years of age; such children should be considered for revaccination after 2 or 3 years if they remain at high risk. The need for revaccination in older children and adults remains unknown.[2]

STORAGE
Store freeze-dried vaccine and reconstituted vaccine, when not in use, between 2°-8°C (35°-46°F). Discard remainder of multidose vials of vaccine within 5 days after reconstitution. The single dose vial should be used within 24 hours of reconstitution.

SPECIAL INSTRUCTIONS FOR 50 DOSE VIAL OF MENINGOCOCCAL POLY-SACCHARIDE VACCINE, A, C, Y AND W-135 COMBINED, FOR JET INJECTOR USE.

DOSAGE AND ADMINISTRATION
PARENTERAL DRUG PRODUCTS SHOULD BE INSPECTED VISUALLY FOR EXTRANEOUS PARTICULAR MATTER AND/OR DISCOLORATION PRIOR TO ADMINISTRATION WHENEVER SOLUTION AND CONTAINER PERMIT. IF THESE CONDITIONS EXIST, VACCINE SHOULD NOT BE ADMINISTERED.

USING A SUITABLE SIZE SYRINGE AND NEEDLE AND ASEPTIC PRE-CAUTIONS, TRANSFER THE VOLUME OF DILUENT SHOWN ON THE DILUENT LABEL INTO THE VIAL CONTAINING THE VACCINE. SHAKE VIAL UNTIL THE VACCINE IS DISSOLVED.

ADMINISTER ONLY WITH AUTOMATIC HYPODERMIC JET APPARA-TUS. 50 DOSE VIAL NOT TO BE UTILIZED IN NEEDLE AND SYRINGE METHOD OF IMMUNIZATION. IF ABSOLUTELY NECESSARY, SYRINGES AND NEEDLES MAY BE USED WITH SUCH CONTAINERS WITH CAUTION. HOWEVER, DUE TO CORING OF THE STOPPER DO NOT INSERT NEEDLE INTO VIAL MORE THAN 20 TIMES. DISCARD PARTIALLY USED VIAL OF VACCINE. IMMUNIZATION CONSISTS OF A SINGLE INJECTION OF 0.5 ML GIVEN SUBCUTANEOUSLY. SPECIAL CARE SHOULD BE TAKEN TO AVOID INJECTING THE VACCINE INTRADERMALLY, INTRAMUSCULARLY, OR INTRAVENOUSLY BY USING THE DELTOID AREA, SINCE CLINICAL STUD-IES HAVE NOT BEEN DONE TO ESTABLISH THE SAFETY AND EFFICACY OF THE VACCINE USING THESE ROUTES OF ADMINISTRATION.

ANY PARTIALLY USED RECONSTITUTED VACCINE WHICH HAS BEEN ADMINISTERED WITH A JET INJECTOR APPARATUS SHOULD NOT BE REUSED AND SHOULD BE DISCARDED.

CAUTION
DURING USE IT IS POSSIBLE THAT THE NOZZLE OF JET INJECTOR APPARATUS MAY BECOME CONTAMINATED WITH BLOOD OR SERUM. IN ONE INSTANCE, SUCH CONTAMINATION HAS BEEN REPORTED TO BE ASSOCIATED WITH TRANSMISSION OF HEPATITIS B DISEASE. THERE-FORE, IF BLOOD OR SERUM CONTAMINATION OCCURS, THE NOZZLE SHOULD BE DISASSEMBLED, CLEANSED AND STERILIZED BEFORE CON-TINUED USE TO PREVENT THE POSSIBILITY OF TRANSMISSION OF HEPATITIS OR OTHER INFECTIOUS AGENTS FROM ONE PERSON TO ANOTHER.[8]

REFERENCES
1. Tiesjema, R.H., et al: Enhanced stability of Meningococcal Polysaccharide Vaccines by using lactose as a menstruum for lyophilization. *Bull WHO* 55: 43-48, 1977 2. Recommendation of the Immunization Practices Advisory Committee (ACIP). Meningococcal Vaccines. *MMWR* 34: 255-259, 1985 3. Hankins, W.A., et al: Clinical and serological evaluation of a Meningococcal Polysaccharide vaccine groups A, C, Y and W-135. *Proc Soc Exper Biol Med* 169: 54-57, 1982 4. Lepow, M.L., et al: Reactogenicity and immunogenicity of a quadrivalent combined Meningococcal Polysaccharide Vaccine in children. *J Infect Dis* 154: 1033-1036, 1986 5. Unpublished data available from Connaught Laboratories, Inc., compiled 1982 6. Peltola, H., et al: Clinical efficacy of Meningococcus Group A capsular Polysaccharide Vaccine in children three months to five years of age. *N Engl J Med* 297: 686-691, 1977 7. Reingold, A. L., et al: Age-specific differences in duration of clinical protection after vaccination with Meningococcal Polysaccharide A Vaccine. *Lancet*. No. 8447: 114-118, 1985 8. CDC. Hepatitis B associated with jet gun injection—California. *MMWR* 35: 373-376, 1986 9. Code of Federal Regulations. 21CFR201.57 (f) (6) (c), 1989

HOW SUPPLIED
POWDER FOR INJECTION:

BRAND/MANUFACTURER	NDC	SIZE	AWP
○ BRAND			
MENOMUNE A/C/Y/W-135: Connaught	49281-0489-01	1s	$48.50
	49281-0489-91	1s	$260.50

Menomune A/C/Y/W-135 *SEE*
MENINGOCOCCAL POLYSACCHARIDE VACCINE

Menotropins
DESCRIPTION
Menotropins are a purified preparation of gonadotropins extracted from the urine of postmenopausal women. Each ampule of Menotropins contains 75 IU or 150

IU of follicle-stimulating hormone (FSH) activity and 75 IU or 150 IU of luteinizing hormone (LH) activity, respectively, plus 10 mg lactose in a sterile, lyophilized form. Menotropins are administered by intramuscular injection.

Menotropins are biologically standard for FSH and LH (ICSH) gonadotropin activities in terms of the Second International Reference Preparation for Human Menopausal Gonadotropins established in September, 1964 by the Expert Committee on Biological Standards of the World Health Organization.

Both FSH and LH are glycoproteins that are acidic and water soluble.

Therapeutic class: Infertility.

CLINICAL PHARMACOLOGY
WOMEN
Menotropins administered for seven to twelve days produce ovarian follicular growth in women who do not have primary ovarian failure. Treatment with Menotropins in most instances results only in follicular growth and maturation. In order to effect ovulation, human chorionic gonadotropin (hCG) must be given following the administration of Menotropins when clinical assessment of the patient indicates that sufficient follicular maturation has occurred.

MEN
Menotropins administered concomitantly with human chorionic gonadotropin (hCG) for at least three months induce spermatogenesis in men with primary or secondary pituitary hypofunction who have achieved adequate masculinization with prior hCG therapy.

INDICATIONS AND USAGE
WOMEN
Menotropins and hCG given in a sequential manner are indicated for the induction of ovulation and pregnancy in the anovulatory infertile patient, in whom the cause of anovulation is functional and is not due to primary ovarian failure.

Menotropins and hCG may also be used to stimulate the development of multiple follicles in ovulatory patients participating in an in vitro fertilization program.

MEN
Menotropins with concomitant hCG are indicated for the stimulation of spermatogenesis in men who have primary or secondary hypogonadotropic hypogonadism.

Menotropins with concomitant hCG have proven effective in inducing spermatogenesis in men with primary hypogonadotropic hypogonadism due to a congenital factor or prepubertal hypophysectomy and in men with secondary hypogonadotropic hypogonadism due to hypophysectomy, craniopharyngioma, cerebral aneurysm or chromophobe adenoma.

SELECTION OF PATIENTS
WOMEN
1. Before treatment with Menotropins is instituted, a thorough gynecologic and endocrinologic evaluation must be performed. Except for those patients enrolled in an in vitro fertilization program, this should include a hysterosalpingogram (to rule out uterine and tubal pathology) and documentation of anovulation by means of basal body temperature, serial vaginal smears, examination of cervical mucus, determination of serum (or urinary) progesterone, urinary pregnanediol and endometrial biopsy. Patients with tubal pathology should receive Menotropins only if enrolled in an in vitro fertilization program.
2. Primary ovarian failure should be excluded by the determination of gonadotropin levels.
3. Careful examination should be made to rule out the presence of an early pregnancy.
4. Patients in late reproductive life have a greater predilection to endometrial carcinoma as well as a higher incidence of anovulatory disorders. Cervical dilation and curettage should always be done for diagnosis before starting Menotropin therapy in such patients who demonstrate abnormal uterine bleeding or other signs of endometrial abnormalities.
5. Evaluation of the husband's fertility potential should be included in the workup.

MEN
Patient selection should be made based on a documented lack of pituitary function. Prior to hormonal therapy, these patients will have low testosterone levels and low or absent gonadotropin levels. Patients with primary hypogonadotropic hypogonadism will have a subnormal development of masculinization, and those with secondary hypogonadotropic hypogonadism will have decreased masculinization.

CONTRAINDICATIONS
WOMEN
Menotropins are contraindicated in women who have:

1. A high FSH level indicating primary ovarian failure.
2. Uncontrolled thyroid and adrenal dysfunction.
3. An organic intracranial lesion such as a pituitary tumor.
4. The presence of any cause of infertility other than anovulation, unless they are candidates for in vitro fertilization.
5. Abnormal bleeding of undetermined origin.
6. Ovarian cysts or enlargement not due to polycystic ovary syndrome.
7. Prior hypersensitivity to Menotropins.

8. Menotropins are contraindicated in women who are pregnant and may cause fetal harm when administered to a pregnant woman. There are limited human data on the effects of Menotropins when administered during pregnancy.

MEN
Menotropins are contraindicated in men who have:

1. Normal gonadotropin levels indicating normal pituitary function.
2. Elevated gonadotropin levels indicating primary testicular failure.
3. Infertility disorders other than hypogonadotropic hypogonadism.

WARNINGS
Menotropins are a drug that should only be used by physicians who are thoroughly familiar with infertility problems. It is a potent gonadotropic substance capable of causing mild to severe adverse reactions in women. Gonadotropin therapy requires a certain time commitment by physicians and supportive health professionals, and its use requires the availability of appropriate monitoring facilities (see *"Precautions—Laboratory Tests"*). In female patients it must be used with a great deal of care.

Overstimulation of the Ovary During Menotropin Therapy: Ovarian Enlargement: Mild to moderate uncomplicated ovarian enlargement which may be accompanied by abdominal distension and/or abdominal pain occurs in approximately 20% of those treated with Menotropins and hCG, and generally regresses without treatment within two or three weeks.

In order to minimize the hazard associated with the occasional abnormal ovarian enlargement which may occur with Menotropin hCG therapy, the lowest dose consistent with expectation of good results should be used. Careful monitoring of ovarian response can further minimize the risk of overstimulation.

If the ovaries are abnormally enlarged on the last day of Menotropin therapy, hCG should not be administered in this course of therapy; this will reduce the chances of development of the Ovarian Hyperstimulation Syndrome.

The Ovarian Hyperstimulation Syndrome (OHSS): OHSS is a medical event distinct from uncomplicated ovarian enlargement. OHSS may progress rapidly to become a serious medical event. It is characterized by an apparent dramatic increase in vascular permeability which can result in a rapid accumulation of fluid in the peritoneal cavity, thorax, and potentially, the pericardium. The early warning signs of development of OHSS are severe pelvic pain, nausea, vomiting, and weight gain. The following symptomatology has been seen with cases of OHSS: abdominal pain, abdominal distension, gastrointestinal symptoms including nausea, vomiting and diarrhea, severe ovarian enlargement, weight gain, dyspnea, and oliguria. Clinical evaluation may reveal hypovolemia, hemoconcentration, electrolyte imbalances, ascites, hemoperitoneum, pleural effusions, hydrothorax, acute pulmonary distress, and thromboembolic events (see *"Pulmonary and Vascular Complications"* below). Transient liver function test abnormalities suggestive of hepatic dysfunction, which may be accompanied by morphologic changes on liver biopsy, have been reported in association with the Ovarian Hyperstimulation Syndrome (OHSS).

OHSS occurs in approximately 0.4% of patients when the recommended dose is administered and in 1.3% of patients when higher than recommended doses are administered. Cases of OHSS are more common, more severe and more protracted if pregnancy occurs. OHSS develops rapidly; therefore patients should be followed for at least two weeks after hCG administration. Most often, OHSS occurs after treatment has been discontinued and reaches its maximum at about seven to ten days following treatment. Usually, OHSS resolves spontaneously with the onset of menses. If there is evidence that OHSS may be developing prior to hCG administration (see *"Precautions—Laboratory Tests"*), the hCG should be withheld.

If OHSS occurs, treatment should be stopped and the patient hospitalized. Treatment is primarily symptomatic, consisting of bed rest, fluid and electrolyte management, and analgesics if needed. The phenomenon of hemoconcentration associated with fluid loss into the peritoneal cavity, pleural cavity, and the pericardial cavity has been seen to occur and should be thoroughly assessed in the following manner: 1) fluid intake and output, 2) weight, 3) hematocrit, 4) serum and urinary electrolytes, 5) urine specific gravity, 6) BUN and creatinine, and 7) abdominal girth. These determinations are to be performed daily or more often if the need arises.

With OHSS there is an increased risk of injury to the ovary. The ascitic, pleural, and pericardial fluid should not be removed unless absolutely necessary to relieve symptoms such as pulmonary distress or cardiac tamponade. Pelvic examination may cause rupture of an ovarian cyst, which may result in hemoperitoneum, and should therefore be avoided. If this does occur, and if bleeding becomes such that surgery is required, the surgical treatment should be designed to control bleeding and to retain as much ovarian tissue as possible. Intercourse should be prohibited in those patients in whom significant ovarian enlargement occurs after ovulation because of the danger of hemoperitoneum resulting from ruptured ovarian cysts.

The management of OHSS may be divided into three phases: the acute, the chronic, and the resolution phases. Because the use of diuretics can accentuate the diminished intravascular volume, diuretics should be avoided except in the late phase of resolution as described below.

Acute Phase: Management during the acute phase should be designed to prevent hemoconcentration due to loss of intravascular volume to the third space and to minimize the risk of thromboembolic phenomena and kidney damage. Treatment is designed to normalize electrolytes while maintaining an acceptable but somewhat reduced intravascular volume. Full correction of the intravascular volume deficit may lead to an unacceptable increase in the amount of third space fluid accumulation. Management includes administration of limited intravenous fluids, electrolytes, and human serum albumin. Monitoring for the development of hyperkalemia is recommended.

Chronic Phase: After stabilizing the patinet during the acute phase, excessive fluid accumulation in the third space should be limited by instituting severe potassium, sodium, and fluid restriction.

Resolution Phase: A fall in hematocrit and an increasing urinary output without an increased intake are observed due to the return of third space fluid to the intravascular compartment. Peripheral and/or pulmonary edema may result if the kidneys are unable to excrete third space fluid as rapidly as it is mobilized. Diuretics may be indicated during the resolution phase if necessary to combat pulmonary edema.

Pulmonary and Vascular Complications: Serious pulmonary conditions (e.g., atelectasis, acute respiratory distress syndrome) have been reported. In addition, thromboembolic events both in association with, and separate from, the Ovarian Hyperstimulation Syndrome have been reported following Menotropin therapy. Intravascular thrombosis and embolism, which may originate in venous or arterial vessels, can result in reduced blood flow to critical organs or the extremities. Sequelae of such events have included venous thrombophlebitis, pulmonary embolism, pulmonary infarction, cerebral vascular occlusion (stroke), and arterial occlusion resulting in loss of limb. In rare cases, pulmonary complications and/or thromboembolic events have resulted in death.

Multiple Births: Data from a clinical trial revealed the following results regarding multiple births: Of the pregnancies following therapy with Menotropins and hCG, 80% resulted in single births, 15% in twins, and 5% of the total pregnancies resulted in three or more concepti. The patient and her husband should be advised of the frequency and potential hazards of multiple gestation before starting treatment.

Hypersensitivity/Anaphylactic Reactions: Hypersensitivity/anaphylactic reactions associated with Menotropins administration have been reported in some patients. These reactions presented as generalized urticaria, facial edema, angioneurotic edema, and/or dyspnea suggestive of laryngeal edema. The relationship of these symptoms to uncharacterized urinary proteins is uncertain.

PRECAUTIONS

General: Careful attention should be given to diagnosis in the selection of candidate for Menotropin therapy (see *"Indications and Usage—Selection of Patients"*).

Information for Patients: Prior to therapy with Mentropins, patients should be informed of the duration of treatment and the monitoring of their condition that will be required. Possible adverse reactions (see *"Adverse Reactions"* section) and the risk of multiple births should be also discussed.

Laboratory Tests: Women: Treatment for Induction of Ovulation.

In most instances, treatment with Menotropins results only in follicular growth and maturation. In order to effect ovulation, hCG must be given following the administration of Menotropins when clinical assessment of the patient indicates that sufficient follicular maturation has occurred. This may be directly estimated by measuring serum (or urinary) estrogen levels and sonographic visualization of the ovaries. The combination of both estradiol levels and ultrasonography are useful for monitoring the growth and development of follicles, timing hCG administration, as well as minimizing the risk of the Ovarian Hyperstimulation Syndrome and multiple gestation.

Other clinical parameters which may have potential use for monitoring menotropins therapy include:

a) Changes in the vaginal cytology;
b) Appearance and volume of the cervical mucus;
c) Spinnbarkeit; and
d) Ferning of the cervical mucus.

The above clinical indices provide an indirect estimate of the estrogenic effect upon the target organs, and therefore should be used adjunctively with more direct estimates of follicular development, i.e., serum estradiol and ultrasonography.

The clinical confirmation of ovulation, with the exception of pregnancy, is obtained by direct and indirect indices of progesterone production. The indices most generally used are as follows:

a) A rise in basal body temperature;
b) Increase in serum progesterone; and
c) Menstruation following the shift in basal body temperature.

When used in conjunction with indices of progesterone production, sonographic visualization of the ovaries will assist in determining if ovulation has occurred. Sonographic evidence of ovulation may include the following:

a) Fluid in the cul-de-sac;
b) Ovarian stigmata; and
c) Collapsed follicle.

Because of the subjectivity of the various tests for the determination of follicular maturation and ovulation, it cannot be overemphasized that the physician should choose tests with which he/she is thoroughly familiar.

Drug Interactions: No clinically significant drug/drug or drug/food adverse interactions have been reported during Menotropin therapy.

Carcinogenesis and Mutagenesis: Long-term toxicity studies in animals have not been performed to evaluate the carcinogenic potential of Menotropins.

Pregnancy: Pregnancy Category X. See *"Contraindications"* section.

Nursing Mothers: It is not known whether this drug is excreted in human milk. Because many drugs are excreted in human milk, caution should be exercised if Menotropins are administered to a nursing woman.

ADVERSE REACTIONS

WOMEN
The following adverse reactions, reported during Menotropin therapy, are listed in decreasing order of potential severity:

1. Pulmonary and vascular complications (see *"Warnings"*)
2. Ovarian Hyperstimulation Syndrome (see *"Warnings"*)
3. Hemoperitoneum
4. Adnexal torsion (as a complication of ovarian enlargement)
5. Mild to moderate ovarian enlargement
6. Ovarian cysts
7. Abdominal pain
8. Sensitivity to Menotropins (Febrile reactions suggestive of allergic response have been reported following the administration of Menotropins. Reports of flu-like symptoms including fever, chills, musculoskeletal aches, joint pains, nausea, headaches and malaise have also been reported).
9. Gastrointestinal symptoms (nausea, vomiting, diarrhea, abdominal cramps, bloating)
10. Pain, rash, swelling and/or irritation at the site of injection
11. Body rashes
12. Dizziness, tachycardia, dyspnea, tachypnea

The following medical events have been reported subsequent to pregnancies resulting from Menotropin therapy:

1. Ectopic pregnancy
2. Congenital abnormalities: From a study of 287 completed pregnancies following Menotropin-hCG therapy five incidents of birth defects were reported (1.7%). One infant had multiple congenital anomalies consisting of imperforate anus, aplasia of the sigmoid colon, third degree hypospadias, cecovesicle fistula, bifid scrotum, meningocele, bilateral internal tibial torsion, and right metatarsus adductus. Another infant was born with an imperforate anus and possible congenital heart lesions; another had a supernumerary digit; another was born with hypospadias and exstrophy of the bladder; and the fifth child had Down's syndrome. None of the investigators felt that these defects were drug-related. Subsequently one report of an infant death due to hydrocephalus and cardiac anomalies has been received.

MEN
1. Gynecomastia may occur occasionally during Menotropin-hCG therapy. This is a known effect of hCG treatment.
2. Erythrocytosis (hct 50%, hgb 17.8 g%) was recorded in one patient.

DRUG ABUSE AND DEPENDENCE

There have been no reports of abuse or dependence with Menotropins.

OVERDOSAGE

Aside from possible ovarian hyperstimulation (see *"Warnings"*), little is known concerning the consequences of acute overdosage with Menotropins.

DOSAGE AND ADMINISTRATION

WOMEN
1. Dosage: The dose of Menotropins to produce maturation of the follicle must be individualized for each patient. It is recommended that the initial dose to any patient should be 75 IU of FSH/LH per day, *Administered Intramuscularly,* for seven to twelve days followed by hCG, 5,000 U to 10,000 U, one day after the last dose of Menotropins. Administration of Menotropins should not exceed 12 days in a single course of therapy. The patient should be treated until indices of estrogenic activity, as indicated under *"Precautions"* above, are equivalent to or greater than those of the normal individual. If serum or urinary estradiol determinations or ultrasonographic visualizations are available, they may be useful as a guide to therapy. If the ovaries are abnormally enlarged on the last day of Menotropin therapy, hCG should not be administered in this course of therapy; this will reduce the chances of development of the Ovarian Hyperstimulation Syndrome. If there is evidence of ovulation but no pregnancy, repeat this dosage regime for at least two more courses before increasing the dose of Menotropins to 150 IU of FSH/LH per day for seven to twelve days. As before, this dose should be followed by 5,000 U to 10,000 U of hCG one day after the last dose of Menotropins. A Menotropin dose of 150 IU of FSH/LH per day has proven to be the most effective dose especially for in vitro fertilization. If evidence of ovulation is present, but pregnancy does not ensue, repeat the same dose for two more courses. Doses larger than this are not routinely recommended.

During treatment with both Menotropins and hCG and during a two-week post-treatment period, patients should be examined at least every other day for signs of excessive ovarian stimulation. It is recommended that Menotropin administration be stopped if the ovaries become abnormally enlarged or abdominal pain occurs. Most of the Ovarian Hyperstimulation Syndrome occurs after treatment has been discontinued and reaches its maximum at about seven to ten days post-ovulation. Patients should be followed for at least two weeks after hCG administration.

The couple should be encouraged to have intercourse daily, beginning on the day prior to the administration of hCG until ovulation becomes apparent from the indices employed for the determination of progestational activity. Care should be taken to insure insemination. In the light of the foregoing indices and parameters mentioned, it should become obvious that, unless a physician is

	% Pts. Ovul.	% Pts. Preg.	% Abort.	% Multi Preg.	% Twins	% 3 or More Concepti	% Hyperstim. Syndr.
Primary Amenorrhea	62	22	14	25	26	0	0
Secondary Amenorrhea	61	28	24	28	18	10	1.9
Secondary Amen. with Galactorrhea	77	42	21	41	31	10	1.2
Polycystic Ovaries	76	26	39	17	17	0	1.1
Anovulatory Cycles	77	24	15	14	9	5	2.0
Miscellaneous	83	20	36	2	2	0	0.1

willing to devote considerable time to these patients and be familiar with and conduct the necessary laboratory studies, he/she should not use Menotropins.

2. Administration: Dissolve the contents of one ampule of Menotropins in one to two ml of sterile saline and *Administer Intramuscularly* immediately. Any unused reconstituted material should be discarded. Parenteral drug products should be inspected visually for particulate matter and discoloration prior to administration, whenever solution and container permit.

MEN

1. Dosage: Prior to concomitant therapy with Mentropins and hCG, pretreatment with hCG alone (5,000 U three times a week) is required. Treatment should continue for a period sufficient to achieve serum testosterone levels within the normal range and masculinization as judged by the appearance of secondary sex characteristics. Such pretreatment may require four to six months, then the recommended dose of Menotropins is 75 IU FSH/LH *Administered Intramuscularly* , three times a week and the recommended dose of hCG is 2,000 U twice a week. Therapy should be carried on for a minimum of four more months to insure detecting spermatozoa in the ejaculate, as it takes 74 ± 4 days in the human male for germ cells to reach the spermatozoa stage.

If the patient has not responded with evidence of increased spermatogenesis at the end of four months of therapy, treatment may continue with 75 IU FSH/LH three times a week, or the dose can be increased to 150 IU FSH/LH three times a week, with the hCG dose unchanged.

2. Administration: Dissolve the contents of one ampule of Menotropins in one to two ml of sterile saline and *Administer Intramuscularly* immediately. Any unused reconstituted material should be discarded. Parenteral drug products should be inspected visually for particulate matter and discoloration prior to administration, whenever solution and container permit.

Lyophilized powder may be stored refrigerated or at room temperature (3°-25°C/37°-77°F). Protect from light. Use immediately after reconstitution. Discard unused material.

CLINICAL STUDIES

WOMEN

The results of the clinical experience and effectiveness of the administration of Menotropins to 1,286 patients in 3,002 courses of therapy are summarized below. The values include patients who were treated with other than the recommended dosage regime. The values for the presently recommended dosage regime are essentially the same.

	%
Patients ovulating	75
Patients pregnant	25
Patients aborting	25*
Multiple pregnancies	20†
Twins	15†
Three or more concepti	5†
Fetal abnormalities	1.7†
Hyperstimulation syndrome	1.3

*   *Based on total pregnancies*
†   *Based on total deliveries*

Results by diagnosis group are summarized below (these values include patients who were treated with other than the present recommended dosage regime): (See related table).

MEN

Clinical results of the treatment of men with primary or secondary hypogonadotropic hypogonadism are as follows:

In the Serono Cooperative study, with an adequate treatment period of 3 to 8 months, 60 of 70 men with primary hypogonadotropic hypogonadism and 8 of 11 men with secondary hypogonadotropic hypogonadism responded with mean increases in their sperm counts from less than 5 to 24 million spermatozoa per milliliter of ejaculate. Forty-one wives of 54 men with primary hypogonadotropic hypogonadism desiring offspring and 7 wives of men with secondary hypogonadotropic hypogonadism conceived. Patients treated with Menotropins and hCG for less than 3 months or with Menotropins alone did not respond to therapy.

A world-wide data search revealed that of 160 recorded pregnancies as the result of use of Menotropins-hCG in men, there were 7 spontaneous abortions, one ectopic pregnancy and 3 congenital anomalies at birth (esophageal atresia in a female infant which was later corrected by surgery, unilateral cryptorchidism, inguinal hernia).

HOW SUPPLIED
POWDER FOR INJECTION: 75 IU

BRAND/MANUFACTURER	NDC	SIZE	AWP
○ **BRAND** PERGONAL: Serono	44087-0571-07	1s	$64.94
	44087-5075-03	10s	$606.87

POWDER FOR INJECTION: 150 IU

BRAND/MANUFACTURER	NDC	SIZE	AWP
○ **BRAND** PERGONAL: Serono	44087-5150-01	1s	$124.67

Mepenzolate Bromide

DESCRIPTION

Mepenzolate Bromide chemically is 3-[(hydroxydiphenylacetyl) oxy]-1,1-dimethylpiperidinium bromide.

Mepenzolate Bromide occurs as a white or light cream-colored powder, which is freely soluble in methanol, slightly soluble in water and chloroform, and practically insoluble in ether.

Each yellow tablet contains 25 mg Mepenzolate Bromide USP.

Following is its chemical structure:

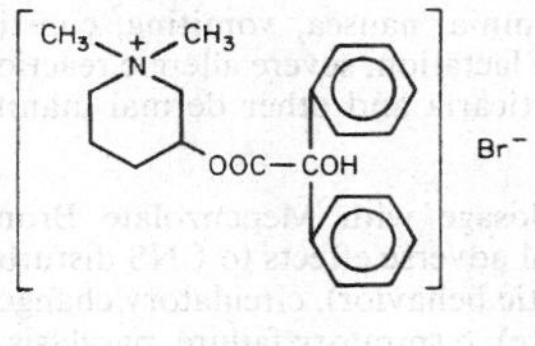

CLINICAL PHARMACOLOGY

Mepenzolate Bromide diminishes gastric acid and pepsin secretion. Mepenzolate Bromide also suppresses spontaneous contractions of the colon. Pharmacologically, it is a post-ganglionic parasympathetic inhibitor.

Radiotracer studies in which Mepenzolate Bromide -^{14}C was used in animals and humans indicate that absorption following oral administration, as with other quaternary ammonium compounds, is low. Between 3 and 22% of an orally administered dose is excreted in the urine over a 5-day period, with the majority of the radioactivity appearing on Day 1. The remainder appears in the next 5 days in the feces and presumably has not been absorbed.

INDICATION

Mepenzolate Bromide is indicated for use as adjunctive therapy in the treatment of peptic ulcer. Mepenzolate Bromide has not been shown to be effective in contributing to the healing of peptic ulcer, decreasing the rate of recurrence or preventing complications.

CONTRAINDICATIONS

Glaucoma obstructive uropathy (for example, bladder neck obstruction due to prostatic hypertrophy), obstructive disease of the gastrointestinal tract (for example, pyloroduodenal stenosis, achalasia), paralytic ileus, intestinal atony of the elderly or debilitated patient, unstable cardiovascular status in acute hemorrhage, severe ulcerative colitis, toxic megacolon complicating ulcerative colitis, myasthenia gravis, allergic or idiosyncratic reactions to Mepenzolate Bromide or related compounds.

WARNINGS

In the presence of high environmental temperature, heat prostration (fever and heat stroke due to decreased sweating) can occur with use of Mepenzolate Bromide.

Mepenzolate Bromide may produce drowsiness or blurred vision. The patient should be cautioned regarding activities requiring mental alertness such as operating a motor vehicle or other machinery or performing hazardous work while taking this drug.

With overdosage, a curare-like action may occur, i.e., neuromuscular blockage leading to muscular weakness and possible paralysis.

It should be noted that the use of anticholinergic drugs in the treatment of gastric ulcer may produce a delay in gastric emptying time and may complicate such therapy (antral stasis).

PREGNANCY
Reproduction studies in rats and rabbits have shown no evidence of impaired fertility or harm to the animal fetus. Information on possible adverse effects in the pregnant female is limited to uncontrolled data derived from marketing experience. Such experience has revealed no reports of the effect of Mepenzolate Bromide on human pregnancies. No controlled studies to establish the safety of the drug in pregnancy have been performed.

PEDIATRIC USE
Since there is no adequate experience in children who have received this drug, safety and efficacy in children have not been established. Newborn animal studies have been undertaken that show that younger animals are more sensitive to the toxic effects of Mepenzolate Bromide than are older animals.

PRECAUTIONS
Use Mepenzolate Bromide with caution in the elderly and in all patients with:

Autonomic neuropathy, hepatic or renal disease.
Ulcerative colitis. Large doses may suppress intestinal motility to the point of producing a paralytic ileus and for this reason precipitate or aggravate "toxic megacolon," a serious complication of the disease.
Hyperthyroidism, coronary heart disease, congestive heart failure, "cardiac tachyarrhythmias," tachycardia, hypertension, and prostatic hypertrophy.
Hiatal hernia associated with reflux esophagitis, since anticholinergic drugs may aggravate this condition.
This product contains FD&C Yellow No. 5 (tartrazine), which may cause allergic-type reactions (including bronchial asthma) in certain susceptible individuals. Although the overall incidence of FD&C Yellow No. 5 (tartrazine) sensitivity in the general population is low, it is frequently seen in patients who also have aspirin hypersensitivity.

NURSING MOTHERS
It is not known whether this drug is secreted in human milk. As a general rule, nursing should not be undertaken while a patient is on a drug since many drugs are excreted in human milk.

ADVERSE REACTIONS
Xerostomia, decreased sweating, urinary hesistancy and retention, blurred vision, tachycardia, palpitations, dilatation of the pupil, cycloplegia, increased ocular tension, loss of taste, headaches, nervousness, mental confusion, drowsiness, weakness, dizziness, insomnia, nausea, vomiting, constipation, bloated feeling, impotence, suppression of lactation, severe allergic reaction or drug idiosyncrasies including anaphylaxis, urticaria and other dermal manifestations.

OVERDOSAGE
The symptoms of overdosage with Mepenzolate Bromide progress from an intensification of the usual adverse effects to CNS disturbances (from restlessness and excitement to psychotic behavior), circulatory changes (flushing, fall in blood pressure, circulatory failure), respiratory failure, paralysis, and coma. Measures to be taken are (1) immediate lavage of the stomach and (2) injection of physostigmine 0.5 to 2 mg intravenously, repeated as necessary up to a total of 5 mg. Fever may be treated symptomatically (alcohol sponging, ice packs). Excitement of a degree that demands attention may be managed with sodium thiopental 2% solution given slowly intravenously or chloral hydrate (100-200 ml of a 2% solution) by rectal infusion. In the event of progression of the curare-like effect to paralysis of the respiratory muscles, artificial respiration should be instituted and maintained until effective respiratory action returns.

DOSAGE AND ADMINISTRATION
Usual Adult Dose: 1 or 2 tablets three times a day preferably with meals and 1 or 2 tablets at bedtime. Begin with the lower dosage when possible and adjust subsequently according to the patient's response.

Since there is no adequate experience in children who have received this drug, safety and efficacy in children have not been established.

DRUG INTERACTIONS
Concomitant administration of anticholinergic drugs and any other drugs which would increase the anticholinergic effects of Mepenzolate Bromide is to be avoided.

HOW SUPPLIED
TABLETS:

BRAND/MANUFACTURER	NDC	SIZE	AWP
○ **BRAND**			
CANTIL: Marion Merrell Dow	00068-0037-01	100s	$77.40

Mepergan *SEE* MEPERIDINE HYDROCHLORIDE WITH PROMETHAZINE HYDROCHLORIDE

Meperidine Hydrochloride

DESCRIPTION
Meperidine Hydrochloride is ethyl 1-methyl-4-phenylisonipecotate hydrochloride, a white crystalline substance with a melting point of 186°C to 189°C. It is readily soluble in water and has a neutral reaction and a slightly bitter taste. The solution is not decomposed by a short period of boiling.

The syrup contains 50 mg of Meperidine Hydrochloride per 5 mL teaspoon (25 drops contain 13 mg of Meperidine Hydrochloride). The tablets contain 50 mg or 100 mg of the analgesic.

The pH of Meperidine Hydrochloride solution is adjusted between 3.5 and 6 with sodium hydroxide or hydrochloric acid.

Meperidine Hydrochloride, 5 percent solution has a specific gravity of 1.0086 at 20°C and 10 percent solution, a specific gravity of 1.0165 at 20°C.

Following is its chemical structure:

CLINICAL PHARMACOLOGY
Meperidine Hydrochloride is a narcotic analgesic with multiple actions qualitatively similar to those of morphine; the most prominent of these involve the central nervous system and organs composed of smooth muscle. The principal actions of therapeutic value are analgesia and sedation.

There is some evidence which suggests that Meperidine may produce less smooth muscle spasm, constipation, and depression of the cough reflex than equianalgesic doses of morphine. Meperidine, in 60 mg to 80 mg parenteral doses, is approximately equivalent in analgesic effect to 10 mg of morphine. The onset of action is slightly more rapid than with morphine, and the duration of action is slightly shorter. Meperidine is significantly less effective by the oral than by the parenteral route, but the exact ratio of oral to parenteral effectiveness is unknown.

INDICATIONS AND USAGE
For the relief of moderate to severe pain (parenteral and oral forms)
   For preoperative medication (parenteral form only)
   For support of anesthesia (parenteral form only)
   For obstetrical analgesia (parenteral form only)

UNLABELED USES
Meperidine is used alone or as an adjunct in the treatment of migraine headaches during pregnancy, and chills and fever induced by amphotericin-B. It is also used to control postanesthetic shivering.

CONTRAINDICATIONS
Hypersensitivity to Meperidine.

Meperidine is contraindicated in patients who are receiving monoamine oxidase (MAO) inhibitors or those who have recently received such agents. Therapeutic doses of Meperidine have occasionally precipitated unpredictable, severe, and occasionally fatal reactions in patients who have received such agents within 14 days. The mechanism of these reactions is unclear, but may be related to a preexisting hyperphenylalaninemia. Some have been characterized by coma, severe respiratory depression, cyanosis, and hypotension, and have resembled the syndrome of acute narcotic overdose. In other reactions the predominant manifestations have been hyperexcitability, convulsions, tachycardia, hyperpyrexia, and hypertension. Although it is not known that other narcotics are free of the risk of such reactions, virtually all of the reported reactions have occurred with Meperidine. If a narcotic is needed in such patients, a sensitivity test should be performed in which repeated, small, incremental doses of morphine are administered over the course of several hours while the patient's condition and vital signs are under careful observation. (Intravenous hydrocortisone or prednisolone have been used to treat severe reactions, with the addition of intravenous chlorpromazine in those cases exhibiting hypertension and hyperpyrexia. The usefulness and safety of narcotic antagonists in the treatment of these reactions is unknown.) Solutions of Meperidine Hydrochloride and barbiturates are chemically incompatible.

WARNINGS
Drug Dependence: Meperidine can produce drug dependence of the morphine type and therefore has the potential for being abused. Psychic dependence, physical dependence, and tolerance may develop upon repeated administration of Meperidine, and it should be prescribed and administered with the same degree of caution appropriate to the use of morphine. Like other narcotics, Meperidine is subject to the provisions of the Federal narcotic laws.

Interaction with Other Central Nervous System Depressants: MEPERIDINE SHOULD BE USED WITH GREAT CAUTION AND IN REDUCED DOSAGE IN PATIENTS WHO ARE CONCURRENTLY RECEIVING OTHER NARCOTIC ANALGESICS, GENERAL ANETHETICS, PHENOTHIAZINES, OTHER TRANQUILIZERS (SEE *"Dosage and Administration"*), SEDATIVE-HYPNOTICS (INCLUDING BARBITURATES), TRICYCLIC ANTIDEPRESSANTS, AND OTHER CNS DEPRESSANTS (INCLUDING

ALCOHOL), RESPIRATORY DEPRESSION, HYPOTENSION, AND PROFOUND SEDATION OR COMA MAY RESULT.

Head Injury and Increased Intracranial Pressure: The respiratory depressant effects of Meperidine and its capacity to elevate cerebrospinal fluid pressure may be markedly exaggerated in the presence of head injury, other intracranial lesions, or a preexisting increase in intracranial pressure. Furthermore, narcotics produce adverse reactions which may obscure the clinical course of patients with head injuries. In such patients, Meperidine must be used with extreme caution and only if its use is deemed essential.

Intravenous Use: If necessary, Meperidine may be given intravenously, but the injection should be given very slowly, preferably in the form of a diluted solution. Rapid intravenous injection of narcotic analgesics, including Meperidine, increases the incidence of adverse reactions; severe respiratory depression, apnea, hypotension, peripheral circulatory collapse, and cardiac arrest have occurred. Meperidine should not be administered intravenously unless a narcotic antagonist and the facilities for assisted or controlled respiration are immediately available. When Meperidine is given parenterally, especially intravenously, the patient should be lying down.

Asthma and Other Respiratory Conditions: Meperidine should be used with extreme caution in patients having an acute asthmatic attack, patients with chronic obstructive pulmonary disease or cor pulmonale, patients having a substantially decreased respiratory reserve, and patients with preexisting respiratory depression, hypoxia, or hypercapnia. In such patients, even usual therapeutic doses of narcotics may decrease respiratory drive while simultaneously increasing airway resistance to the point of apnea.

Hypotensive Effect: The administration of Meperidine may result in severe hypotension in the postoperative patient or any individual whose ability to maintain blood pressure has been compromised by a depleted blood volume or the administration of drugs such as the phenothiazines or certain anesthetics.

Usage in Ambulatory Patients: Meperidine may impair the mental and/or physical abilities required for the performance of potentially hazardous tasks such as driving a car or operating machinery. The patient should be cautioned accordingly.

Meperidine, like other narcotics, may produce orthostatic hypotension in ambulatory patients.

Usage in Pregnancy and Lactation: Meperidine should not be used in pregnant women prior to the labor period, unless in the judgment of the physician the potential benefits outweigh the possible hazards, because safe use in pregnancy prior to labor has not been established relative to possible adverse effects on fetal development.

When used as an obstetrical analgesic, Meperidine crosses the placental barrier and can produce depression of respiration and psychophysiologic functions in the newborn. Resuscitation may be required (see section on *"Overdosage"*). Meperidine appears in the milk of nursing mothers receiving the drug.

PRECAUTIONS

As with all intramuscular preparations Meperidine Hydrochloride intramuscular injection should be injected well within the body of a large muscle.

Supraventricular Tachycardias: Meperidine should be used with caution in patients with atrial flutter and other supraventricular tachycardias because of a possible vagolytic action which may produce a significant increase in the ventricular response rate.

Convulsions: Meperidine may aggravate preexisting convulsions in patients with convulsive disorders. If dosage is escalated substantially above recommended levels because of tolerance development, convulsions may occur in individuals without a history of convulsive disorders.

Acute Abdominal Conditions: The administration of Meperidine or other narcotics may obscure the diagnosis or clinical course in patients with acute abdominal conditions.

Special Risk Patients: Meperidine should be given with caution and the initial dose should be reduced in certain patients such as the elderly or debilitated, and those with severe impairment of hepatic or renal function, hypothyroidism, Addison's disease, and prostatic hypertrophy or urethral stricture.

ADVERSE REACTIONS

The major hazards of Meperidine, as with other narcotic analgesics, are respiratory depression and, to a lesser degree, circulatory depression; respiratory arrest, shock, and cardiac arrest have occurred.

The most frequently observed adverse reactions include lightheadedness, dizziness, sedation, nausea, vomiting, and sweating. These effects seem to be more prominent in ambulatory patients and in those who are not experiencing severe pain. In such individuals, lower doses are advisable. Some adverse reactions in ambulatory patients may be alleviated if the patient lies down.

Other adverse reactions include:

Nervous System: Euphoria, dysphoria, weakness, headache, agitation, tremor, uncoordinated muscle movements, severe convulsions, transient hallucinations and disorientation, visual disturbances. Inadvertent injection about a nerve trunk may result in sensory-motor paralysis which is usually, though not always, transitory.

Gastrointestinal: Dry mouth, constipation, biliary tract spasm.

Cardiovascular: Flushing of the face, tachycardia, bradycardia, palpitation, hypotension (see *"Warnings"*), syncope, phlebitis following intravenous injection.

Genitourinary: Urinary retention.

Allergic: Pruritus, urticaria, other skin rashes, wheal and flare over the vein with intravenous injection.

Other: Pain at injection site; local tissue irritation and induration following subcutaneous injection, particularly when repeated; antidiuretic effect.

OVERDOSAGE

Symptoms: Serious overdosage with Meperidine is characterized by respiratory depression (a decrease in respiratory rate and/or tidal volume, Cheyne-Stokes respiration, cyanosis), extreme somnolence progressing to stupor or coma, skeletal muscle flaccidity, cold and clammy skin, and sometimes bradycardia and hypotension. In severe overdosage, particularly by the intravenous route, apnea, circulatory collapse, cardiac arrest, and death may occur.

Treatment: Primary attention should be given to the reestablishment of adequate respiratory exchange through provision of a patent airway and institution of assisted or controlled ventilation. The narcotic antagonist, naloxone hydrochloride, is a specific antidote against respiratory depression which may result from overdosage or unusual sensitivity to narcotics, including Meperidine. Therefore, an appropriate dose of this antagonists should be administered, preferably by the intravenous route, simultaneously with efforts at respiratory resuscitation.

An antagonist should not be administered in the absence of clinically significant respiratory or cardiovascular depression.

Oxygen, intravenous fluids, vasopressors, and other supportive measures should be employed as indicated.

In cases of overdosage with Meperidine Hydrochloride tablets, the stomach should be evacuated by emesis or gastric lavage.

Note: In an individual physically dependent on narcotics, the administration of the usual dose of a narcotic antagonist will precipitate an acute withdrawal syndrome. The severity of this syndrome will depend on the degree of physical dependence and the dose of antagonist administered. The use of narcotic antagonists in such individuals should be avoided if possible. If a narcotic antagonist must be used to treat serious respiratory depression in the physically dependent patient the antagonist should be administered with extreme care and only one-fifth to one-tenth the usual initial dose administered.

DOSAGE AND ADMINISTRATION

FOR RELIEF OF PAIN

Dosage should be adjusted according to the severity of the pain and the response of the patient. While subcutaneous administration is suitable for occasional use, intramuscular administration is preferred when repeated doses are required. If intravenous administration is required, dosage should be decreased and the injection made very slowly, preferably utilizing a diluted solution. Meperidine is less effective orally than on parenteral administration. The dose of Meperidine Hydrochloride should be proportionately reduced (usually by 25 to 50 percent) when administered concomitantly with phenothiazines and many other tranquilizers since they potentiate the action of Meperidine Hydrochloride.

Adults: The usual dosage is 50 mg to 150 mg intramuscularly, subcutaneously, or orally, every 3 or 4 hours as necessary.

Children: The usual dosage is 0.5 mg/lb to 0.8 mg/lb intramuscularly, subcutaneously, or orally up to the adult dose, every 3 or 4 hours as necessary.

Each dose of the syrup should be taken in one-half glass of water, since if taken undiluted, it may exert a slight topical anesthetic effect on mucous membranes.

FOR PREOPERATIVE MEDICATION

Adults: The usual dosage is 50 mg to 100 mg intramuscularly or subcutaneously, 30 to 90 minutes before the beginning of anesthesia.

Children: The usual dosage is 0.5 mg/lb to 1 mg/lb intramuscularly or subcutaneously up to the adult dose, 30 to 90 minutes before the beginning of anesthesia.

FOR SUPPORT OF ANESTHESIA

Repeated slow intravenous injections of fractional doses (e.g., 10 mg/mL) or continuous intravenous infusion of a more dilute solution (e.g., 1 mg/mL) should be used. The dose should be titrated to the needs of the patient and will depend on the premedication and type of anesthesia being employed, the characteristics of the particular patient, and the nature and duration of the operative procedure.

FOR OBSTETRICAL ANALGESIA

The usual dosage is 50 mg to 100 mg intramuscularly or subcutaneously when pain becomes regular, and may be repeated at 1- to 3-hour intervals.

J CODES

IM,IV,SC—J2175

HOW SUPPLIED
INJECTION (C-II): 10 MG/ML

BRAND/MANUFACTURER	NDC	SIZE	AWP
◆ GENERICS			
Schein	00364-3022-56	30 ml	$13.80

INJECTION (C-II): 25 MG/ML

BRAND/MANUFACTURER	NDC	SIZE	AWP
◆ GENERICS			
Wyeth-Ayerst	00008-0601-50	1 ml 10s	$9.11

➤ SHOWN IN PRODUCT IDENTIFICATION GUIDE

INJECTION (C-II): 25 MG

AVERAGE UNIT PRICE (AVAILABLE SIZES)		GENERIC A-RATED AVERAGE PRICE (GAAP)	
BRAND	$0.51	1 ml 25s	$9.65
GENERIC	$0.44		

BRAND/MANUFACTURER	NDC	SIZE	AWP
◆ BRAND			
DEMEROL HCL: Sanofi Winthrop	00024-0324-02	1 ml 10s	$5.36
	00024-0371-04	1 ml 25s	$12.46
	00024-0361-04	1 ml 25s ud	$12.46
◆ GENERICS			
Wyeth-Ayerst	00008-0601-02	1 ml 10s	$5.36
Elkins-Sinn	00641-1120-35	1 ml 25s	$8.86
Elkins-Sinn	00641-0130-25	1 ml 25s	$10.44

INJECTION (C-II): 50 MG/ML

AVERAGE UNIT PRICE (AVAILABLE SIZES)		GENERIC A-RATED AVERAGE PRICE (GAAP)	
BRAND	$0.65	30 ml	$10.60
GENERIC	$0.48		

BRAND/MANUFACTURER	NDC	SIZE	AWP
◆ BRAND			
DEMEROL HCL: Sanofi Winthrop	00024-0329-01	30 ml	$19.59
◆ GENERICS			
Schein	00364-3026-56	30 ml	$10.56
Steris	00402-0947-30	30 ml	$10.56
Wyeth-Ayerst	00008-0258-01	30 ml	$10.69
Astra	00186-1284-01	30 ml 5s	$55.98
Wyeth-Ayerst	00008-0602-50	1 ml 10s	$9.63

INJECTION (C-II): 50 MG

AVERAGE UNIT PRICE (AVAILABLE SIZES)		GENERIC A-RATED AVERAGE PRICE (GAAP)	
BRAND	$0.53	1 ml 25s	$10.46
GENERIC	$0.50		

BRAND/MANUFACTURER	NDC	SIZE	AWP
◆ BRAND			
DEMEROL HCL: Sanofi Winthrop	00024-0325-02	1 ml 10s	$5.87
	00024-0372-04	1 ml 25s	$12.65
	00024-0362-04	1 ml 25s ud	$12.65
◆ GENERICS			
Goldline	00182-9130-66	30 ml	$17.40
Wyeth-Ayerst	00008-0602-02	1 ml 10s	$5.88
Elkins-Sinn	00641-1130-35	1 ml 25s	$9.41
Elkins-Sinn	00641-0140-25	1 ml 25s	$11.50

INJECTION (C-II): 75 MG/ML

BRAND/MANUFACTURER	NDC	SIZE	AWP
◆ GENERICS			
Wyeth-Ayerst	00008-0605-50	1 ml 10s	$10.10

INJECTION (C-II): 75 MG

AVERAGE UNIT PRICE (AVAILABLE SIZES)		GENERIC A-RATED AVERAGE PRICE (GAAP)	
BRAND	$0.44	1 ml 25s	$10.91
GENERIC	$0.51		

BRAND/MANUFACTURER	NDC	SIZE	AWP
◆ BRAND			
DEMEROL HCL: Sanofi Winthrop	00024-0326-02	1 ml 10s	$6.34
	00024-0373-04	1.5 ml 25s	$12.89
	00024-0363-04	1.5 ml 25s ud	$12.89
◆ GENERICS			
Wyeth-Ayerst	00008-0605-02	1 ml 10s	$6.35
Elkins-Sinn	00641-1140-35	1 ml 25s	$9.56
Elkins-Sinn	00641-0150-25	1 ml 25s	$12.25
Elkins-Sinn	00641-0150-26	1 ml 100s	$51.19

INJECTION (C-II): 100 MG/ML

AVERAGE UNIT PRICE (AVAILABLE SIZES)		GENERIC A-RATED AVERAGE PRICE (GAAP)	
BRAND	$1.28	20 ml	$14.06
GENERIC	$0.72		

BRAND/MANUFACTURER	NDC	SIZE	AWP
◆ BRAND			
DEMEROL HCL: Sanofi Winthrop	00024-0331-01	20 ml	$25.68
◆ GENERICS			
Schein	00364-3027-55	20 ml	$13.97
Steris	00402-0948-20	20 ml	$13.97
Wyeth-Ayerst	00008-0259-01	20 ml	$14.23
Astra	00186-1283-01	20 ml 5s	$45.15
Wyeth-Ayerst	00008-0613-50	1 ml 10s	$10.60

INJECTION (C-II): 100 MG

AVERAGE UNIT PRICE (AVAILABLE SIZES)		GENERIC A-RATED AVERAGE PRICE (GAAP)	
BRAND	$0.45	1 ml 25s	$11.66
GENERIC	$0.69		

BRAND/MANUFACTURER	NDC	SIZE	AWP
◆ BRAND			
DEMEROL HCL: Sanofi Winthrop	00024-0328-02	1 ml 10s	$6.84
	00024-0375-04	1 ml 25s	$13.16
	00024-0365-04	1 ml 25s ud	$13.16
	00024-0374-04	2 ml 25s	$13.16
	00024-0364-04	2 ml 25s ud	$13.16
◆ GENERICS			
Goldline	00182-9131-65	20 ml	$22.50
Wyeth-Ayerst	00008-0613-02	1 ml 10s	$6.85
Elkins-Sinn	00641-1150-35	1 ml 25s	$10.19
Elkins-Sinn	00641-0160-25	1 ml 25s	$13.13

SYRUP (C-II): 50 MG/5 ML

BRAND/MANUFACTURER	NDC	SIZE	AWP
◆ BRAND			
DEMEROL HCL: Sanofi Winthrop	00024-0332-06	480 ml	$77.60
◆ GENERICS			
Roxane	00054-3545-63	500 ml	$31.87

TABLETS (C-II): 50 MG

AVERAGE UNIT PRICE (AVAILABLE SIZES)		GENERIC A-RATED AVERAGE PRICE (GAAP)	
BRAND	$0.61	100s	$26.13
GENERIC	$0.27		

BRAND/MANUFACTURER	NDC	SIZE	AWP
▶ BRAND			
DEMEROL HCL: Sanofi Winthrop	00024-0335-02	25s ud	$12.98
	00024-0335-04	100s	$69.12
	00024-0335-06	500s	$316.46
◆ GENERICS			
Goldline	00182-9140-01	100s	$25.50
Major	00904-1977-60	100s	$25.95
Parmed	00349-8965-01	100s	$26.95
Wyeth-Ayerst	00008-0308-03	250s	$70.64

TABLETS (C-II): 100 MG

AVERAGE UNIT PRICE (AVAILABLE SIZES)		GENERIC A-RATED AVERAGE PRICE (GAAP)	
BRAND	$1.18	100s	$42.30
GENERIC	$0.42		

BRAND/MANUFACTURER	NDC	SIZE	AWP
▶ BRAND			
DEMEROL HCL: Sanofi Winthrop	00024-0337-02	25s ud	$24.55
	00024-0337-04	100s	$131.47
	00024-0337-06	500s	$620.45
◆ GENERICS			
Major	00904-1978-60	100s	$38.70
Goldline	00182-9141-01	100s	$45.90

Meperidine Hydrochloride with Promethazine Hydrochloride

DESCRIPTION
This product is available in concentration providing 25 mg each of Meperidine Hydrochloride and Promethazine Hydrochloride per mL.

ACTIONS
Meperidine Hydrochloride is a narcotic analgesic with multiple actions qualitatively similar to those of morphine. Promethazine HCl is a phenothiazine derivative that has several different pharmacologic properties including antihistaminic, sedative, and antiemetic actions.

INDICATIONS
As a preanesthetic medication when analgesia and sedation are indicated. As an adjunct to local and general anesthesia.

CONTRAINDICATIONS
Hypersensitivity to Meperidine or Promethazine.

Under no circumstances should Meperidine Hydrochloride/Promethazine Hydrochloride be given by intraarterial injection, due to the likelihood of severe arteriospasm and the possibility of resultant gangrene (see "Warnings").

Meperidine Hydrochloride/Promethazine Hydrochloride should not be given by the subcutaneous route; evidence of chemical irritation has been noted, and necrotic lesions have resulted on rare occasions following subcutaneous injection. The preferred parenteral route of administration is by deep, intramuscular injection.

◆ RATED THERAPEUTICALLY EQUIVALENT; ◇ THERAPEUTIC EQUIVALENCE UNCONFIRMED; ○ UNRATED

Meperidine is contraindicated in patients who are receiving monoamine-oxidase inhibitors (MAOI) or those who have received such agents within 14 days.

Therapeutic doses of Meperidine have inconsistently precipitated unpredictable, severe, and occasionally fatal reactions in patients who have received such agents within 14 days. The mechanism of these reactions is unclear. Some have been characterized by coma, severe respiratory depression, cyanosis, and hypotension and have resembled the syndrome of acute narcotic overdose. In other reactions the predominant manifestations have been hyperexcitability, convulsions, tachycardia, hyperpyrexia, and hypertension. Although it is not known that other narcotics are free of the risk of such reactions, virtually all of the reported reactions have occurred with Meperidine. If a narcotic is needed in such patients, a sensitivity test should be performed in which repeated, small, incremental doses of morphine are administered over the course of several hours while the patient's condition and vital signs are under careful observation.

(Intravenous hydrocortisone or prednisolone have been used to treat severe reactions, with the addition of intravenous chlorpromazine in those cases exhibiting hypertension and hyperpyrexia. The usefulness and safety of narcotic antagonists in the treatment of these reactions is unknown.)

WARNINGS

Meperidine Hydrochloride/Promethazine Hydrochloride Injection contains sodium metabisulfite, a sulfite that may cause allergic-type reactions, including anaphylactic symptoms and life-threatening or less severe asthmatic episodes, in certain susceptible people. The overall prevalence of sulfite sensitivity in the general population is unknown and probably low. Sulfite sensitivity is seen more frequently in asthmatic than in nonasthmatic people.

TOLERANCE AND ADDICTION LIABILITY
Warning—may be habit forming.

Drug Dependence: Meperidine can produce drug dependence of the morphine type and therefore has the potential for being abused. Psychic dependence, physical dependence, and tolerance may develop upon repeated administration of Meperidine, and it should be prescribed and administered with the same degree of caution appropriate to the use of morphine. Like other narcotics, Meperidine is subject to the provisions of the Federal narcotic laws.

Interactions with other Central Nervous System Depressants: Meperidine should be used with great caution and in reduced dosage in patients who are concurrently receiving other narcotic analgesics, general anesthetics, phenothiazines, other tranquilizers, sedative-hypnotics, tricyclic antidepressants, and other CNS depressants (including alcohol). Respiratory depression, hypotension, and profound sedation or coma may result.

The sedative action of Promethazine Hydrochloride is additive to the sedative effects of central nervous system depressants; therefore, agents such as alcohol, barbiturates, and narcotic analgesics should either be eliminated or given in reduced dosage in the presence of Promethazine Hydrochloride. When given concomitantly with Promethazine Hydrochloride, the dose of barbiturates should be reduced by at least one-half and the dose of analgesic depressants, such as morphine or Meperidine, should be reduced by one-quarter to one-half.

Head Injury and Increased Intracranial Pressure: The respiratory-depressant effects of Meperidine and its capacity to elevate cerebrospinal-fluid pressure may be markedly exaggerated in the presence of head injury, other intracranial lesions, or a preexisting increase in intracranial pressure. Furthermore, narcotics produce adverse reactions which may obscure the clinical course of patients with head injuries. In such patients, Meperidine must be used with extreme caution and only if its use is deemed essential.

Inadvertent Intra-arterial Injection: Due to the close proximity of arteries and veins in the areas most commonly used for intravenous injection, extreme care should be exercised to avoid perivascular extravasation or inadvertent intra-arterial injection of Meperidine Hydrochloride/Promethazine Hydrochloride. Reports compatible with inadvertent intra-arterial injection suggest that pain, severe chemical irritation, severe spasm of distal vessels, and resultant gangrene requiring amputation is likely under such circumstances. Intravenous injection was intended in all the cases reported, but perivascular extravasation or arterial placement of the needle is now suspect. There is no proven successful management of this condition after it occurs, although sympathetic block and heparinization are commonly employed during the acute management because of the results of animal experiments with other known arteriolar irritants. Aspiration of dark blood does not preclude intra-arterial needle placement, because blood is discolored upon contact with Promethazine. Use of syringes with rigid plungers or of small bore needles might obscure typical arterial backflow if this is relied upon alone.

Intravenous Use: If necessary, Meperidine may be given intravenously, but the injection should be given very slowly, preferably in the form of a diluted solution. Rapid intravenous injection of narcotic analgesics, including Meperidine, increases the incidence of adverse reactions: severe respiratory depression, apnea, hypotension, peripheral circulatory collapse, and cardiac arrest have occurred. Meperidine should not be administered intravenously unless a narcotic antagonist and the facilities for assisted or controlled respiration are immediately available. When Meperidine is given parenterally, especially intravenously, the patient should be lying down.

When used intravenously, Meperidine Hydrochloride/Promethazine Hydrochloride should be given at a rate not to exceed 1 mL (25 mg of each component) per minute. When administering any irritant drug intravenously, it is usually preferable to inject it through the tubing of an intravenous infusion set that is known to be functioning satisfactorily. In the event that a patient complains of pain during intended intravenous injection of Meperidine Hydrochloride/Promethazine Hydrochloride, the injection should immediately be stopped to provide for evaluation of possible arterial placement or perivascular extravasation.

Asthma and Other Respiratory Conditions: Meperidine should be used with extreme caution in patients having an acute asthmatic attack, patients with chronic obstructive pulmonary disease or cor pulmonale, patients having a substantially decreased respiratory reserve, and patients with preexisting respiratory depression, hypoxia, or hypercapnia. In such patients, even usual therapeutic doses of narcotics may decrease respiratory drive while simultaneously increasing airway resistance to the point of apnea.

Hypotensive Effect: The administration of Meperidine may result in severe hypotension in an individual whose ability to maintain his blood pressure has already been compromised by a depleted blood volume or concurrent administration of drugs such as the phenothiazines or certain anesthetics.

Usage in Ambulatory Patients: Meperidine may impair the mental and/or physical abilities required for the performance of potentially hazardous tasks, such as driving a car or operating machinery. The patient should be cautioned accordingly.

Meperidine, like other narcotics, may produce orthostatic hypotension in ambulatory patients.

Usage in Pregnancy and Lactation: Meperidine should not be used in pregnant women prior to the labor period, unless in the judgment of the physician the potential benefits outweigh the possible hazards, because safe use in pregnancy prior to labor has not been established relative to possible adverse effects on fetal development.

When used as an obstetrical analgesic, Meperidine crosses the placental barrier and can produce respiratory depression in the newborn: resuscitation may be required (see *"Overdosage"*).

Meperidine appears in the milk of nursing mothers receiving the drug.

PRECAUTIONS

Supraventricular Tachycardias: Meperidine should be used with caution in patients with atrial flutter and other supraventricular tachycardias because of a possible vagolytic action which may produce a significant increase in the ventricular response rate.

Convulsions: Meperidine may aggravate preexisting convulsions in patients with convulsive disorders. If dosage is escalated substantially above recommended levels because of tolerance development, convulsions may occur in individuals without a history of convulsive disorders.

Acute Abdominal Conditions: The administration of Meperidine or other narcotics may obscure the diagnosis or clinical course in patients with acute abdominal conditions.

Special-Risk Patients: Meperidine should be given with caution, and the initial dose should be reduced in certain patients, such as the elderly or debilitated, and those with severe impairment of hepatic or renal function, hypothyroidism, Addison's disease, and prostatic hypertrophy or urethral stricture.

Antiemetics may mask the symptoms of an unrecognized disease and thereby interfere with diagnosis.

Patients in pain who have received inadequate or no analgesia have been noted to develop "athetoidlike" movements of the upper extremities following the parenteral administration of Promethazine. These symptoms usually disappear upon adequate control of the pain.

Ambulatory patients should be cautioned against driving automobiles or operating dangerous machinery until it is known that they do not become drowsy or dizzy from Promethazine Hydrochloride therapy.

ADVERSE REACTIONS

The major hazards of Meperidine, as with other narcotic analgesics, are respiratory depression and, to a lesser degree, circulatory depression: respiratory arrest, shock, and cardiac arrest have occurred.

The most frequently observed adverse reactions include light-headedness, dizziness, sedation, nausea, vomiting, and sweating. These effects seem to be more prominent in ambulatory patients and in those who are not experiencing severe pain. In such individuals, lower doses are advisable. Some adverse reactions in ambulatory patients may be alleviated if the patient lies down.

Other adverse reactions include:

Central Nervous System: Euphoria, dysphoria, weakness, headache, agitation, tremor, uncoordinated muscle movements, transient hallucinations and disorientation, visual disturbances and, rarely, extrapyramidal reactions.

Gastrointestinal: Dry mouth, constipation, biliary-tract spasm.

Cardiovascular: Flushing of the face, tachycardia, bradycardia, palpitation, faintness, syncope.

Cardiovascular effects from Promethazine have been rare. Minor increases in blood pressure and occasional mild hypotension have been reported. Venous thrombosis at the injection site has been reported. Intra-arterial injection of Meperidine Hydrochloride/Promethazine Hydrochloride may result in gangrene of the affected extremity (see *"Warnings"*).

Genitourinary: Urinary retention.

Allergic: Pruritus, urticaria, other skin rashes, wheal and flare over the vein with IV injection.

Photosensitivity, although extremely rare, has been reported. Occurrence of photosensitivity may be a contraindication to further treatment with Promethazine or related drugs.

Other: Pain at injection site; local tissue irritation, induration, and possible tissue necrosis, particularly when injection is repeated at same site; antidiuretic effect.

Patients may occasionally complain of autonomic reactions, such as dryness of the mouth, blurring of vision and, rarely, dizziness following the use of Promethazine.

Very rare cases have been reported where patients receiving Promethazine have developed leukopenia. In one instance agranulocytosis has been reported. In nearly every instance reported, other toxic agents known to have caused these conditions have been associated with the administration of Promethazine.

OVERDOSAGE

Symptoms: Serious overdose with Meperidine is characterized by respiratory depression (a decrease in respiratory rate and/or tidal volume. Cheyne-Stokes respiration, cyanosis), extreme somnolence progressing to stupor or coma, skeletal muscle flaccidity, cold and clammy skin, and sometimes bradycardia and hypotension. In severe overdosage, particularly by the intravenous route, apnea, circulatory collapse, cardiac arrest, and death may occur.

Treatment: Primary attention should be given to the reestablishment of adequate respiratory exchange through provision of a patent airway and institution of assisted or controlled ventilation. The narcotic antagonist, naloxone hydrochloride, is a specific antidote against respiratory depression which may result from overdosage or unusual sensitivity to narcotics, including Meperidine. The usual initial adult dose of naloxone is 0.4 to 2.0 mg, administered intravenously. If the desired degree of counteraction and improvement in respiratory functions is not obtained, this dosage can be repeated at two- to three-minute intervals while resuscitation efforts continue. If 10 mg of naloxone have been administered without an improvement in the clinical situation, the diagnosis of Meperidine Hydrochloride/Promethazine Hydrochloride overdose should be questioned.

An antagonist should not be administered in absence of clinically significant respiratory or cardiovascular depression. Oxygen, intravenous fluids, vasopressors, and other supportive measures should be employed as indicated.

Note: In an individual physically dependent on narcotics, the administration of the usual dose of a narcotic antagonist will precipitate an acute withdrawal syndrome. The severity of this syndrome will depend on the degree of physical dependence and the dose of antagonist administered. The use of narcotic antagonists in such individuals should be avoided if possible. If a narcotic antagonist must be used to treat serious respiratory depression in the physically dependent patient, the antagonist should be administered with extreme care and only one-tenth to one-fifth the usual initial dose administered.

Attempted suicides with Promethazine have resulted in deep sedation, coma, rarely convulsions and cardiorespiratory symptoms compatible with the depth of sedation present. Extrapyramidal reactions may be treated with anticholinergic antiparkinson agents, diphenhydramine, or barbiturates.

If severe hypotension occurs, levarterenol or phenylephrine may be indicated. Epinephrine is probably best avoided, since it has been suggested that Promethazine overdosage could produce a partial alpha-adrenergic blockade.

A paradoxical reaction, characterized by hyperexcitability and nightmares, has been reported in children receiving large single doses of Promethazine.

DOSAGE AND ADMINISTRATION

Parenteral drug products should be inspected visually for particulate matter and discoloration prior to administration, whenever solution and container permit.

WARNING—BARBITURATES ARE NOT CHEMICALLY COMPATIBLE IN SOLUTION WITH MEPERIDINE HYDROCHLORIDE/PROMETHAZINE HYDROCHLORIDE AND SHOULD NOT BE MIXED IN THE SAME SYRINGE.

The TUBEX® Sterile Cartridge-Needle Unit is designed for single-dose use. VIALS should be used when required doses are fractions of a milliliter, as indicated below.

Meperidine Hydrochloride/Promethazine Hydrochloride is usually administered intramuscularly. However, in certain specific situations, the intravenous route may be employed. INADVERTENT INTRA-ARTERIAL INJECTION CAN RESULT IN GANGRENE OF THE AFFECTED EXTREMITY (SEE *"WARNINGS"*). SUBCUTANEOUS ADMINISTRATION IS CONTRAINDICATED, AS IT MAY RESULT IN TISSUE NECROSIS (SEE *"CONTRAINDICATIONS"*). INJECTION INTO OR NEAR PERIPHERAL NERVES MAY RESULT IN PERMANENT NEUROLOGICAL DEFICIT.

When used intravenously, the rate should not be greater than 1 mL of Meperidine Hydrochloride/Promethazine Hydrochloride (25 mg of each component) per minute; it is preferable to inject through the tubing of an intravenous infusion set that is known to be functioning satisfactorily.

Adult Dose: 1 to 2 mL (25 to 50 mg of each component) per single injection, which can be repeated every 3 to 4 hours.

Children 12 Years of Age and Under: 0.5 mg of each component per pound of body weight. The dosage may be repeated every 3 to 4 hours as necessary. For preanesthetic medication the usual adult dose is 2 mL (50 mg of each component) intramuscularly with or without appropriate atropinelike drug. Atropine sulfate, 0.3 to 0.4 mg, or scopolamine hydrobromide, 0.25 to 0.4 mg, in sterile solution may be mixed in the same syringe with Meperidine Hydrochloride/Promethazine Hydrochloride. Repeat doses of 50 mg or less of both Promethazine and Meperidine may be administered by either route at 3 to 4 hour intervals, as

necessary. As an adjunct to local or general anesthesia, the usual dose is 2 mL (50 mg each of Meperidine and Promethazine).

Do not use if solution is discolored or contains a precipitate.
Protect from light.
Use carton to protect contents from light.
Store at room temperature, approximately 25° C (77° F).

J CODES
Up to 50 mg IM,IV—J2180

HOW SUPPLIED
CAPSULE (C-II):

BRAND/MANUFACTURER	NDC	SIZE	AWP
○ **BRAND**			
MEPERGAN FORTIS: Wyeth-Ayerst	00008-0261-02	100s	$50.61

CAPSULE (C-II): 50 MG-25 MG

BRAND/MANUFACTURER	NDC	SIZE	AWP
○ **GENERICS**			
MEPROZINE: Vintage	00254-4206-28	100s	$36.50
Qualitest	00603-4424-21	100s	$36.50

INJECTION (C-II): 25 MG/ML

BRAND/MANUFACTURER	NDC	SIZE	AWP
○ **BRAND**			
MEPERGAN: Wyeth-Ayerst	00008-0234-01	10 ml	$13.75
	00008-0235-01	2 ml 10s	$36.20

Mephentermine Sulfate

DESCRIPTION
Mephentermine Sulfate is a synthetic sympathomimetic drug which is intended for intramuscular or intravenous administration. In addition to the stated quantity of the active ingredient (15 or 30 mg/mL), each mL of the sterile injection solution is buffered to a pH of 5 (pH range of 4 to 6.5).

Mephentermine Sulfate occurs as white, usually odorless crystals.
It is soluble in water and slightly soluble in alcohol.
The chemical name of Mephentermine Sulfate is N,α,α-trimethyl-benzeneethanamine sulfate (2:1).

Following is its chemical structure:

$$\left[\begin{array}{c} \text{CH}_3 \\ | \\ \text{CH}_2-\text{C}-\text{NH} \\ | \quad | \\ \text{CH}_3 \ \text{CH}_3 \end{array} \right]_2 \cdot \text{H}_2\text{SO}_4$$

CLINICAL PHARMACOLOGY
Mephentermine Sulfate is a sympathomimetic amine that acts indirectly by releasing norepinephrine. Cardiac contraction is enhanced, and cardiac output and systolic and diastolic pressures are usually increased. The pressor response also involves peripheral vasoconstriction. The change in heart rate is variable, depending on the degree of vagal tone; large doses can depress the heart. In some cases the net vascular effect may be vasodilation, which appears not to involve beta-adrenergic receptors.

Coronary blood flow is increased, forearm blood flow is reduced, and venous tone is increased. Marked mucosal vasoconstriction can be produced by local application of the drug. CNS effects may occur with large doses of Mephentermine. The main effect of therapeutic doses of Mephentermine is cardiac stimulation.

Mephentermine is metabolized in the liver by N-demethylation to normephentermine (or phentermine) with subsequent p-hydroxylation to p-hydroxynormephentermine (or p-hydroxyphentermine).

The excretion rate of the drug and its metabolites is more rapid in an acidic urine and is only slightly influenced by urine output.

The half-life in humans is reported to be between 17 and 18 hours.

A pressor response occurs almost immediately and persists for 15 to 30 minutes following intravenous injection of therapeutic doses of Mephentermine Sulfate. Pressor activity occurs within 5 to 15 minutes following intramuscular administration and persists for 1 to 4 hours.

INDICATIONS AND USAGE
Mephentermine Sulfate Injection is indicated in the treatment of hypotension secondary to ganglionic blockade and that occurring with spinal anesthesia.

CONTRAINDICATIONS
Mephentermine Sulfate should not be used in patients with a past history of sensitivity to the drug.

Mephentermine Sulfate, like epinephrine and ephedrine, is contraindicated in the treatment of hypotension induced by chlorpromazine, since sympathomimetic amines act to potentiate, rather than to correct, hypotension secondary to the adrenolytic effects of chlorpromazine.

Mephentermine Sulfate should not be administered in combination with a monoamine oxidase inhibitor.

◆ RATED THERAPEUTICALLY EQUIVALENT; ◇ THERAPEUTIC EQUIVALENCE UNCONFIRMED; ○ UNRATED

WARNINGS

Persistent hypotension during or after surgery usually indicates hypovolemia and should be treated by replacement of blood volume, rather than with a sympathomimetic such as Mephentermine Sulfate.

Cyclopropane and halothane are known to sensitize the heart to the arrhythmic action of catecholamines. Serious ventricular arrhythmias may occur in patients under general anesthesia with these agents if sympathomimetic drugs such as Mephentermine are given to control hypotension.

PRECAUTIONS

GENERAL
Patients with hyperthyroidism may show an increased responsiveness to vasopressor agents.

Mephentermine Sulfate must be used with caution in patients with known cardiovascular diseases and in chronically ill patients, since the drug's action on the cardiovascular system may be profound.

If Mephentermine Sulfate is to be given to known hypertensives, careful monitoring of the blood pressure is advisable.

DRUG INTERACTIONS
Administration of Mephentermine Sulfate to patients who are receiving cyclopropane or halogenated hydrocarbon general anesthetics which increase cardiac irritability may result in serious ventricular arrhythmias. The possibility that digitalis or mercurial diuretics can also sensitize the myocardium to the effects of sympathomimetic drugs should be considered.

Phenothiazines, including chlorpromazine, may antagonize the pressor effects of Mephentermine.

Monoamine oxidase inhibitors may potentiate the pressor effects of Mephentermine by inhibiting the metabolism of catecholamines.

Drugs such as reserpine and guanethidine, which reduce the quantity of norepinephrine in sympathetic nerve endings, may significantly reduce the pressor response to mephentermine.

CARCINOGENESIS, MUTAGENESIS, IMPAIRMENT OF FERTILITY
Long-term animal studies have not been performed to evaluate the carcinogenic potential of Mephentermine Sulfate, nor are there relevant data with regard to mutagenicity or impairment of fertility.

PREGNANCY
It is not known whether Mephentermine Sulfate crosses the placental barrier.

Teratogenic Effects: Pregnancy Category C. Animal reproduction studies have not been conducted with Mephentermine Sulfate. It is also not known whether Mephentermine Sulfate can cause fetal harm when administered to a pregnant woman or can affect reproduction capacity. Mephentermine Sulfate should be given to a pregnant woman only if clearly needed.

Nonteratogenic Effects: Mephentermine Sulfate may increase uterine contractions especially during the third trimester of pregnancy.

LABOR AND DELIVERY
Animal studies indicated that Mephentermine Sulfate, used during labor, caused a decrease in uterine blood flow. Fetal hypoxia from decreased uterine blood flow secondary to uterine vasoconstriction may occur. Transient fetal hypertension (mean arterial blood pressure more than 20% of control) has also been reported with Mephentermine Sulfate in animal experiments.

NURSING MOTHERS
It is not known whether Mephentermine Sulfate is excreted in human milk. Because many drugs are excreted in human milk, caution should be exercised when Mephentermine Sulfate is administered to a nursing woman.

PEDIATRIC USE
Safety and effectiveness of Mephentermine Sulfate in children have not been established.

ADVERSE REACTIONS
Adverse reactions to Mephentermine Sulfate may be especially likely to occur in patients with cardiovascular diseases, hypertension, hyperthyroidism, or other chronic illnesses.

Following the administration of recommended doses of Mephentermine Sulfate, CNS stimulating effects may result in nervousness and anxiety.

Mephentermine Sulfate may produce arrhythmias, including transient extrasystoles, AV block, and hypertension.

OVERDOSAGE
Effects of overdosage are an extension of the pharmacological activity of Mephentermine. In therapy with Mephentermine Sulfate, cardiac contractility, cardiac output, systolic and diastolic blood pressure are usually raised. The increase in heart rate is variable, depending on vagal tone. Large doses may depress the heart. Doses in the range of 3 mg/kg of body weight may alter myocardial conduction by decreasing conduction time and shortening the refractory period. Tachycardia may also be present. Central nervous system effects may occur with large doses: hyperexcitability, prolonged wakefulness, weeping, incoherence, convulsions, flushing, tremor, and hallucinations.

TREATMENT
Therapy of overdosage is symptomatic and supportive. Side effects, in general, disappear rapidly on withdrawal of the drug. Sedation may help to control CNS hyperexcitability. Blood pressure should be followed closely, and cardiac excitability should be monitored by EKG.

Convulsions or cardiac arrhythmias should be treated promptly if they occur. Since arrhythmias produced by Mephentermine Sulfate may be due to excessive beta-adrenergic stimulation, a beta-blocking agent such as propranolol may be considered.

DOSAGE AND ADMINISTRATION
Parenteral drug products should be inspected visually for particulate matter and discoloration prior to administration, whenever solution and container permit.

Mephentermine Sulfate can be administered intramuscularly without fear of irritation or abnormal tissue reaction. Pressor response is evident 5 to 15 minutes after intramuscular injection and has a duration of 1 to 2 hours. Injection of an injectable parenteral solution of Mephentermine Sulfate, containing 30 mg/mL, or a continuous infusion of a solution of Mephentermine Sulfate, in 5% dextrose in water, with a concentration of approximately 1 mg/mL, directly into the vein, is the preferred route for treatment of shock. Intravenous administration of undiluted Mephentermine Sulfate does not produce vascular irritation, and should extravasation occur, no untoward tissue reaction will develop. Dosage of Mephentermine Sulfate used in the treatment of shock and hypotension is based on experimental observations that 0.5 mg/kg produces a positive inotropic action, the pharmacologic action of Mephentermine Sulfate responsible for the pressor effect.

Treatment of hypotension occurring following spinal anesthesia is accomplished by the administration of 30 to 45 mg Mephentermine Sulfate intravenously in a single injection. Doses of 30 mg may be repeated as necessary to maintain the desired level of blood pressure. An immediate response and maintenance of blood pressure can be accomplished by the continuous intravenous infusion of a 0.1% solution of Mephentermine Sulfate in 5% dextrose in water (1 mg Mephentermine Sulfate/mL solution). The rate of flow and duration of this intravenous therapy should be regulated according to the response of the patient.

Treatment of hypotension secondary to spinal anesthesia in the obstetrical patient undergoing Caesarean section, who is known to react more positively to drugs, is accomplished by the administration of an initial dose of 15 mg of Mephentermine Sulfate intravenously. This dose may be repeated if the response is not adequate.

Prevention of hypotension attendant to spinal anesthesia can be accomplished by the administration of 30 to 45 mg Mephentermine Sulfate intramuscularly 10 to 20 minutes prior to anesthesia, operation, or termination of the operative procedure.

PREPARATION OF INTRAVENOUS SOLUTION
The 0.1% solution of Mephentermine Sulfate recommended for continuous intravenous administration can be conveniently prepared in the approximate concentration (0.115%) by adding two 10 mL vials of Mephentermine Sulfate, 30 mg/mL, to 500 mL of 5% dextrose in water.

STORAGE
Store at room temperature, approximately 25° C (77° F).

Do not use if solution is discolored or contains a precipitate.

J CODES
Up to 30 mg IM,IV—J3450

HOW SUPPLIED
INJECTION: 15 MG/ML

BRAND/MANUFACTURER	NDC	SIZE	AWP
○ BRAND			
WYAMINE SULFATE INJECTION: Wyeth-Ayerst	00008-0159-02	10 ml	$10.83
	00008-0159-03	2 ml 25s	$64.65

INJECTION: 30 MG/ML

BRAND/MANUFACTURER	NDC	SIZE	AWP
○ BRAND			
WYAMINE SULFATE INJECTION: Wyeth-Ayerst	00008-0224-02	10 ml	$17.18

Mephenytoin

DESCRIPTION
Mephenytoin is 3-methyl 5,5-phenyl-ethyl-hydantoin. It may be considered to be the hydantoin homolog of the barbiturate mephobarbital.

Active Ingredient: mephenytoin, USP

Following is its chemical structure:

ACTIONS
Mephenytoin exhibits pharmacologic effects similar to both diphenylhydantoin and the barbiturates in antagonizing experimental seizures in laboratory animals. Mephenytoin produces behavioral and electroencephalographic effects in man which are similar to those produced by barbiturates.

INDICATIONS

For the control of grand mal, focal, Jacksonian, and psychomotor seizures in those patients who have been refractory to less toxic anticonvulsants.

CONTRAINDICATIONS

Hypersensitivity to hydantoin products.

WARNINGS

Mephenytoin should be used only after safer anticonvulsants have been given an adequate trial and have failed.

As with all anticonvulsants, dose reduction must be gradual so as to minimize the risk of precipitating seizures.

Patients should be cautioned about possible additive effects of alcohol and other CNS depressants. Acute alcohol intoxication may increase the anticonvulsant effect due to decreased metabolic breakdown. Chronic alcohol abuse may result in decreased anticonvulsant effect due to enzyme induction.

USAGE IN PREGNANCY

The effects of Mephenytoin in human pregnancy and nursing infants are unknown.

Recent reports suggest an association between the use of anticonvulsant drugs by women with epilepsy and an elevated incidence of birth defects in children born to these women. Data are more extensive with respect to diphenylhydantoin and phenobarbital, but these are also the most commonly prescribed anticonvulsants; less systematic or anecdotal reports suggest a possible similar association with the use of all known anticonvulsant drugs.

The reports suggesting an elevated incidence of birth defects in children of drug-treated epileptic women cannot be regarded as adequate to prove a definite cause and effect relationship. There are intrinsic methodologic problems in obtaining adequate data on drug teratogenicity in humans; the possibility also exists that other factors, e.g., genetic factors or the epileptic condition itself, may be more important than drug therapy in leading to birth defects. The great majority of mothers on anticonvulsant medication deliver normal infants. It is important to note that anticonvulsant drugs should not be discontinued in patients in whom the drug is administered to prevent major seizures because of the strong possibility of precipitating status epilepticus with attendant hypoxia and threat to life. In individual cases where the severity and frequency of the seizure disorder are such that the removal of medication does not pose a serious threat to the patient, discontinuation of the drug may be considered prior to and during pregnancy, although it cannot be said with any confidence that even minor seizures do not pose some hazards to the developing embryo or fetus.

The prescribing physician will wish to weigh these considerations in treating or counseling epileptic women of childbearing potential.

PRECAUTIONS

The patient taking Mephenytoin must be kept under close medical supervision at all times since serious adverse reactions may emerge.

Because the primary site of degradation is the liver, it is recommended that screening tests of liver function precede introduction of the drug.

Some patients may show side reactions as the result of individual sensitivity. These reactions can be broken down into three types respectively according to severity: 1) blood dyscrasias; 2) skin and mucous membrane manifestations; and 3) central effects. The blood, skin and mucous membrane manifestations are the more important since they can be more serious in nature. Since Mephenytoin has been reported to produce blood dyscrasia in certain instances, the patient must be instructed that in the event any unusual symptoms develop (e.g., sore throat, fever, mucous membrane bleeding, glandular swelling, cutaneous reaction), he must discontinue the drug and report for examination immediately. It is recommended that blood examinations be made (total white cell count and differential count) during the initial phase of administration. Such tests are best made: a) before starting medication; b) after 2 weeks on a low dosage; c) again after 2 weeks when full dosage is reached; d) thereafter, monthly for a year; e) from then on, every 3 months. If the neutrophils drop to between 2500 and 1600/cu.mm., counts are made every 2 weeks. Stop medication if the count drops to 1600.

ADVERSE REACTIONS

A number of side effects and toxic reactions have been reported with Mephenytoin as well as with other hydantoin compounds. Many of these appear to be dose related while others seem to be a manifestation of a hypersensitivity reaction to these drugs.

BLOOD DYSCRASIAS

Leukopenia, neutropenia, agranulocytosis, thrombocytopenia and pancytopenia have occurred. Eosinophilia, monocytosis, and leukocytosis have been described. Simple anemia, hemolytic anemia, megaloblastic anemia and aplastic anemia have occurred but are uncommon.

SKIN AND MUCOUS MEMBRANCE MANIFESTATIONS

Maculopapular, morbilliform, scarlatiniform, urticarial, purpuric (associated with thrombocytopenia) and non-specific skin rashes have been reported. Exfoliative dermatitis, erythema multiforme (Stevens-Johnson Syndrome), toxic epidermal necrolysis and fatal dermatitides have been described on rare occasions. Skin pigmentation and rashes associated with a lupus erythematosus syndrome have also been reported.

CENTRAL EFFECTS

Drowsiness is dose-related and may be reduced by a reduction in dose. Ataxia, diplopia, nystagmus, dysarthria, fatigue, irritability, choreiform movements, depression and tremor have been encountered.

Nervousness, nausea, vomiting, sleeplessness and dizziness may occur during the initial stages of therapy. Generally, these symptoms are transient, often disappearing with continued treatment.

Mental confusion and psychotic disturbances and increased seizures have been reported, but a definite causal relationship with the drug is uncertain.

MISCELLANEOUS

Hepatitis, jaundice and nephrosis have been reported but a definite cause and effect relationship between the drug and these effects has not been established.

Alopecia, weight gain, edema, photophobia, conjunctivitis and gum hyperplasia have been encountered.

Polyarthropathy, pulmonary fibrosis, lupus erythematosus syndrome and lymphadenopathy which simulates Hodgkin's Disease have also been observed.

DOSAGE AND ADMINISTRATION

Dosage of antiepileptic therapy should be adjusted to the needs of the individual patient. Maintenance dosage is that smallest amount of antiepileptic necessary to suppress seizures completely or reduce their frequency. Optimum dosage is attained by starting with ½ or 1 tablet of Mephenytoin per day during the first week and thereafter increasing the daily dose by ½ or 1 tablet at weekly intervals. No dose should be increased until it has been taken for at least 1 week.

The average dose of Mephenytoin for adults ranges from 2-6 tablets (0.2-0.6 gm) daily. In some instances it may be necessary to administer as much as 8 tablets or more daily in order to obtain full seizure control. Children usually require from 1-4 tablets (0.1-0.4 gm) according to nature of seizures and age.

When the physician wishes to replace the anticonvulsant now being employed with Mephenytoin, he should give ½-1 tablet of Mephenytoin daily during the first week and gradually increase the daily dose at weekly intervals while gradually reducing that of the drug being discontinued. The transition can be made smoothly over a period of 3-6 weeks. If seizures are not completely controlled with the dose so attained, the daily dose should then be increased by a one-tablet increment at weekly intervals to the point of maximum effect. If the patient had also been receiving phenobarbital, it is well to continue it until the transition is completed, at which time gradual withdrawal of the phenobarbital may be tried.

Store and dispense below 86°F (30°C); tight container.

HOW SUPPLIED
TABLETS: 100 MG

BRAND/MANUFACTURER	NDC	SIZE	AWP
◆ **BRAND**			
MESANTOIN: Sandoz Pharm	00078-0052-05	100s	$25.50

Mephobarbital

DESCRIPTION

Mephobarbital, 5-Ethyl-1-methyl-5-phenylbarbituric acid, is a barbiturate with sedative, hypnotic, and anticonvulsant properties. It occurs as a white, nearly odorless, tasteless powder and is slightly soluble in water and in alcohol.

Following is its chemical structure:

CLINICAL PHARMACOLOGY

Barbiturates are capable of producing all levels of CNS mood alteration from excitation to mild sedation, to hypnosis, and deep coma. Overdosage can produce death. In high enough therapeutic doses, barbiturates induce anesthesia.

Barbiturates depress the sensory cortex, decrease motor activity, alter cerebellar function, and produce drowsiness, sedation, and hypnosis.

Barbiturates are respiratory depressants. The degree of respiratory depression is dependent upon dose. With hypnotic doses, respiratory depression produced by barbiturates is similar to that which occurs during physiologic sleep with slight decrease in blood pressure and heart rate.

Studies in laboratory animals have shown that barbiturates cause reduction in the tone and contractility of the uterus, ureters, and urinary bladder. However, concentrations of the drugs required to produce this effect in humans are not reached with sedative-hypnotic doses.

Barbiturates do not impair normal hepatic function, but have been shown to induce liver microsomal enzymes, thus increasing and/or altering the metabolism of barbiturates and other drugs. (See "Precautions—Drug Interactions"). Mephobarbital exerts a strong sedative and anticonvulsant action but has a relatively mild hypnotic effect. It reduces the incidence of epileptic seizures in grand mal and petit mal. Mephobarbital usually causes little or no drowsiness or lassitude. Hence, when it is used as a sedative or anticonvulsant, patients usually become more calm, more cheerful, and better adjusted to their surroundings without clouding of mental faculties. Mephobarbital is reported to produce less sedation than does phenobarbital.

Barbiturates are weak acids that are absorbed and rapidly distributed to all tissues and fluids with high concentrations in the brain, liver, and kidneys. Lipid solubility of the barbiturates is the dominant factor in their distribution within the body. Barbiturates are bound to plasma and tissue proteins to a varying degree with the degree of binding increasing directly as a function of lipid solubility.

Approximately 50% of an oral dose of Mephobarbital is absorbed from the gastrointestinal tract. Therapeutic plasma concentrations for Mephobarbital have not been established nor has the half-life been determined. Following oral administration, the onset of action of the drug is 30 to 60 minutes and the duration of action is 10 to 16 hours. The primary route of Mephobarbital metabolism is N-demethylation by the microsomal enzymes of the liver to form phenobarbital. Phenobarbital may be excreted in the urine unchanged or further metabolized to *p*-hydroxyphenobarbital and excreted in the urine as glucuronide or sulfate conjugates. About 75% of a single oral dose of Mephobarbital is converted to phenobarbital in 24 hours.

Therefore, chronic administration of Mephobarbital may lead to an accumulation of phenobarbital (not Mephobarbital) in plasma. It has not been determined whether Mephobarbital or phenobarbital is the active agent during long-time Mephobarbital therapy.

INDICATIONS AND USAGE
Mephobarbital is indicated for use as a sedative for the relief of anxiety, tension, and apprehension, and as an anticonvulsant for the treatment of grand mal and petit mal epilepsy.

CONTRAINDICATIONS
Hypersensitivity to any barbiturate. Manifest or latent porphyria.

WARNINGS
HABIT FORMING
Barbiturates may be habit forming. Tolerance, psychological, and physical dependence may occur with continued use. (See *"Drug Abuse and Dependence"* and "Clinical Pharmacology"). Patients who have psychological dependence on barbiturates may increase the dosage or decrease the dosage interval without consulting a physician and may subsequently develop a physical dependence on barbiturates. To minimize the possibility of overdosage or the development of dependence, the prescribing and dispensing of sedative-hypnotic barbiturates should be limited to the amount required for the interval until the next appointment. Abrupt cessation after prolonged use in the dependent person may result in withdrawal symptoms, including delirium, convulsions, and possibly death. Barbiturates should be withdrawn gradually from any patient known to be taking excessive dosage over long periods of time. (See *"Drug Abuse and Dependence."*)

ACUTE OR CHRONIC PAIN
Caution should be exercised when barbiturates are administered to patients with acute or chronic pain, because paradoxical excitement could be induced or important symptoms could be masked. However, the use of barbiturates as sedatives in the postoperative surgical period and as adjuncts to cancer chemotherapy is well established.

USE IN PREGNANCY
Barbiturates can cause fetal damage when administered to a pregnant woman. Retrospective, case-controlled studies have suggested a connection between the maternal consumption of barbiturates and a higher than expected incidence of fetal abnormalities. Following oral or parenteral administration, barbiturates readily cross the placental barrier and are distributed throughout fetal tissues with highest concentrations found in the placenta, fetal liver, and brain. Fetal blood levels approach maternal blood levels following parenteral administration.

Withdrawal symptoms occur in infants born to mothers who receive barbiturates throughout the last trimester of pregnancy. (See *"Drug Abuse and Dependence"*). If this drug is used during pregnancy, or if the patient becomes pregnant while taking this drug, the patient should be apprised of the potential hazard to the fetus.

SYNERGISTIC EFFECTS
The concomitant use of alcohol or other CNS depressants may produce additive CNS depressant effects.

PRECAUTIONS
GENERAL
Barbiturates may be habit forming. Tolerance and psychological and physical dependence may occur with continuing use. (See *"Drug Abuse and Dependence"*). Barbiturates should be administered with caution, if at all, to patients who are mentally depressed, have suicidal tendencies, or a history of drug abuse.

Elderly or debilitated patients may react to barbiturates with marked excitement, depression, and confusion. In some persons, barbiturates repeatedly produce excitement rather than depression.

In patients with hepatic damage, barbiturates should be administered with caution and initially in reduced doses. Barbiturates should not be administered to patients showing the premonitory signs of hepatic coma.

Status epilepticus may result from the abrupt discontinuation of Mephobarbital even when administered in small daily doses in the treatment of epilepsy.

Caution and careful adjustment of dosage are required when Mephobarbital is used in patients with impaired renal, cardiac, or respiratory function and in patients with myasthenia gravis and myxedema. The least quantity feasible should be prescribed or dispensed at any one time in order to minimize the possibility of acute or chronic overdosage.

Vitamin D Deficiency: Mephobarbital may increase vitamin D requirements, possibly by increasing vitamin D metabolism via enzyme induction. Rarely, rickets and osteomalacia have been reported following prolonged use of barbiturates.

Vitamin K: Bleeding in the early neonatal period due to coagulation defects may follow exposure to anticonvulsant drugs *in utero*; therefore, vitamin K should be given to the mother before delivery or to the child at birth.

INFORMATION FOR THE PATIENT
Practitioners should give the following information and instructions to patients receiving barbiturates.

1. The use of barbiturates carries with it an associated risk of psychological and/or physical dependence. The patient should be warned against increasing the dose of the drug without consulting a physician.

2. Barbiturates may impair mental and/or physical abilities required for the performance of potentially hazardous tasks (e.g., driving, operating machinery, etc).

3. Alcohol should not be consumed while taking barbiturates. Concurrent use of the barbiturates with other CNS depressants (e.g. alcohol, narcotics, tranquilizers, and antihistamines) may result in additional CNS depressant effects.

LABORATORY TESTS
Prolonged therapy with barbiturates should be accompanied by periodic laboratory evaluation of organ systems, including hematopoietic, renal, and hepatic systems. (See *"Precautions: General"* and *"Adverse Reactions."*)

DRUG INTERACTIONS
Most reports of clinically significant drug interactions occurring with the barbiturates have involved phenobarbital. However, the application of these data to other barbiturates appears valid and warrants serial blood level determinations of the relevant drugs when there are multiple therapies.

1. Anticoagulants: Phenobarbital lowers the plasma levels of dicumarol (name previously used: bishydroxycoumarin) and causes a decrease in anticoagulant activity as measured by the prothrombin time. Barbiturates can induce hepatic microsomal enzymes resulting in increased metabolism and decreased anticoagulant response of oral anticoagulants (e.g. warfarin, acenocoumarol, dicumarol, and phenprocoumon). Patients stabilized on anticoagulant therapy may require dosage adjustments if barbiturates are added to or withdrawn from their dosage regimen.

2. Corticosteroids: Barbiturates appear to enhance the metabolism of exogenous corticosteroids probably through the induction of hepatic microsomal enzymes. Patients stabilized on corticosteroid therapy may require dosage adjustments if barbiturates are added to or withdrawn from their dosage regimen.

3. Griseofulvin: Phenobarbital appears to interfere with the absorption of orally administered griseofulvin, thus decreasing its blood level. The effect of the resultant decreased blood levels of griseofulvin on therapeutic response has not been established. However, it would be preferable to avoid concomitant administration of these drugs.

4. Doxycycline: Phenobarbital has been shown to shorten the half-life of doxycycline for as long as 2 weeks after barbiturate therapy is discontinued.

This mechanism is probably through the induction of hepatic microsomal enzymes that metabolize the antibiotic. If phenobarbital and doxycycline are administered concurrently, the clinical response to doxycycline should be monitored closely.

5. Phenytoin, Sodium Valproate, Valproic Acid: The effect of barbiturates on the metabolism of phenytoin appears to be variable. Some investigators report an accelerating effect, while others report no effect. Because the effect of barbiturates on the metabolism of phenytoin is not predictable, phenytoin and barbiturate blood levels should be monitored more frequently if these drugs are given concurrently. Sodium valproate and valproic acid appear to decrease barbiturate metabolism; therefore, barbiturate blood levels should be monitored and appropriate dosage adjustments made as indicated.

6. Central Nervous System Depressants: The concomitant use of other central nervous system depressants, including other sedatives or hypnotics, antihistamines, tranquilizers, or alcohol, may produce additive depressant effects.

7. Monoamine Oxidase Inhibitors (MAOI): MAOI prolong the effects of barbiturates probably because metabolism of the barbiturate is inhibited.

8. Estradiol, Estone, Progesterone, and other Steroidal Hormones: Pretreatment with or concurrent administration of phenobarbital may decrease the effect of estradiol by increasing its metabolism. There have been reports of patients treated with antiepileptic drugs (e.g. phenobarbital) who become pregnant while taking oral contraceptives. An alternate contraceptive method might be suggested to women taking phenobarbital.

CARCINOGENESIS
Animal Data: Phenobarbital sodium is carcinogenic in mice and rats after lifetime administration. In mice, it produced benign and malignant liver cell tumors. In rats, benign liver cell tumors were observed very late in life. Phenobarbital is the major metabolite of Mephobarbital.

Human Data: In a 29-year epidemiological study of 9,136 patients who were treated on an anticonvulsant protocol which included phenobarbital, results indicated a higher than normal incidence of hepatic carcinoma. Previously, some of these patients were treated with thorotrast, a drug which is known to produce hepatic carcinomas. Thus, this study did not provide sufficient evidence that phenobarbital sodium is carcinogenic in humans. Phenobarbital is the major metabolite of Mephobarbital.

A retrospective study of 84 children with brain tumors matched to 73 normal controls and 78 cancer controls (malignant disease other than brain tumors) suggested an association between exposure to barbiturates prenatally and an increased incidence of brain tumors.

PREGNANCY

Teratogenic Effects: Pregnancy Category D— See *"Warnings—Use in Pregnancy."*

Nonteratogenic Effects: Reports of infants suffering from long-term barbiturate exposure *in utero* included the acute withdrawal syndrome of seizures and hyperirritability from birth to a delayed onset of up to 14 days. (See *"Drug Abuse and Dependence"*).

LABOR AND DELIVERY

Hypnotic doses of these barbiturates do not appear to significantly impair uterine activity during labor. Full anesthetic doses of barbiturates decrease the force and frequency of uterine contractions. Administration of sedative-hypnotic barbiturates to the mother during labor may result in respiratory depression in the newborn. Premature infants are particularly susceptible to the depressant effects of barbiturates. If barbiturates are used during labor and delivery, resuscitation equipment should be available.

Data are currently not available to evaluate the effect of these barbiturates when forceps delivery or other intervention is necessary. Also, data are not available to determine the effect of these barbiturates on the later growth, development, and functional maturation of the child.

NURSING MOTHERS

Caution should be exercised when a barbiturate is administered to a nursing woman since small amounts of barbiturates are excreted in the milk.

ADVERSE REACTIONS

The following adverse reactions and their incidence were compiled from surveillance of thousands of hospitalized patients. Because such patients may be less aware of certain of the milder adverse effects of barbiturates, the incidence of these reactions may be somewhat higher in fully ambulatory patients.

More than 1 in 100 Patients: The most common adverse reaction estimated to occur at a rate of 1 to 3 patients per 100 is:

Nervous System: Somnolence.

Less than 1 in 100 Patients: Adverse reactions estimated to occur at a rate of less than 1 in 100 patients listed below, grouped by organ system, and by decreasing order of occurrence are:

Nervous System: Agitation, confusion, hyperkinesia, ataxia, CNS depression, nightmares, nervousness, psychiatric disturbance, hallucinations, insomnia, anxiety, dizziness, thinking abnormality.

Respiratory System: Hypoventilation, apnea.

Cardiovascular System: Bradycardia, hypotension, syncope.

Digestive System: Nausea, vomiting, constipation.

Other Reported Reactions: Headache, hypersensitivity reactions (angioedema, skin rashes, exfoliative dermatitis), fever, liver damage, megaloblastic anemia following chronic phenobarbital use.

DRUG ABUSE AND DEPENDENCE

Mephobarbital is a controlled substance in Narcotic Schedule IV. Barbiturates may be habit forming. Tolerance, psychological dependence, and physical dependence may occur especially following prolonged use of high doses of barbiturates. As tolerance to barbiturates develops, the amount needed to maintain the same level of intoxication increases; tolerance to a fatal dosage, however, does not increase more than two-fold. As this occurs, the margin between an intoxicating dosage and fatal dosage becomes smaller.

Symptoms of acute intoxication with barbiturates include unsteady gait, slurred speech, and sustained nystagmus. Mental signs of chronic intoxication include confusion, poor judgment, irritability, insomnia, and somatic complaints. Symptoms of barbiturate dependence are similar to those of chronic alcoholism. If an individual appears to be intoxicated with alcohol to a degree that is radically disproportionate to the amount of alcohol in his or her blood the use of barbiturates should be suspected. The lethal dose of a barbiturate is far less if alcohol is also ingested.

The symptoms of barbiturate withdrawal can be severe and may cause death. Minor withdrawal symptoms may appear 8 to 12 hours after the last dose of a barbiturate. These symptoms usually appear in the following order: anxiety, muscle twitching, tremor of hands and fingers, progressive weakness, dizziness, distortion in visual perception, nausea, vomiting, insomnia, and orthostatic hypotension. Major withdrawal symptoms (convulsions and delirium) may occur within 16 hours and last up to 5 days after abrupt cessation of these drugs. Intensity of withdrawal symptoms gradually declines over a period of approximately 15 days. Individuals susceptible to a barbiturate abuse and dependence include alcoholics and opiate abusers, as well as other sedative-hypnotic and amphetamine abusers.

Drug dependence to barbiturates arises from repeated administration of a barbiturate or agent with barbiturate-like effect on a continuous basis, generally in amounts exceeding therapeutic dose levels. The characteristics of drug dependence to barbiturates include: (a) a strong desire or need to continue taking the drug; (b) a tendency to increase the dose; (c) a psychic dependence on the effects of the drug related to subjective and individual appreciation of those effects; and (d) a physical dependence on the effects of the drug requiring its presence for maintenance of homeostasis and resulting in a definite, characteristic, and self-limited abstinence syndrome when the drug is withdrawn.

Treatment of barbiturate dependence consists of cautious and gradual withdrawal of the drug. Barbiturate-dependent patients can be withdrawn by using a number of different withdrawal regimens. In all cases withdrawal takes an extended period of time. One method involves substituting a 30 mg dose of phenobarbital for each 100 mg to 200 mg dose of barbiturate that the patient has been taking. The total daily amount of phenobarbital is then administered in 3 to 4 divided doses, not to exceed 600 mg daily. Should signs of withdrawal occur on the first day of treatment, a loading dose of 100 mg to 200 mg of phenobarbital may be administered IM in addition to the oral dose. After stabilization on phenobarbital, the total daily dose is decreased by 30 mg a day as long as withdrawal is proceeding smoothly. A modification of this regimen involves initiating treatment at the patient's regular dosage level and decreasing the daily dosage by 10% if tolerated by the patient.

Infants physically dependent on barbiturates may be given phenobarbital 3 mg/kg/day to 10 mg/kg/day. After withdrawal symptoms (hyperactivity, disturbed sleep, tremors, hyperreflexia) are relieved, the dosage of phenobarbital should be gradually decreased and completely withdrawn over a 2-week period.

OVERDOSAGE

The toxic dose of barbiturates varies considerably. In general, an oral dose of 1 g of most barbiturates produces serious poisoning in an adult. Death commonly occurs after 2 g to 10 g of ingested barbiturate. Barbiturate intoxication may be confused with alcoholism, bromide intoxication, and with various neurological disorders.

Acute overdosage with barbiturates is manifested by CNS and respiratory depression which may progress to Cheyne-Stokes respiration, areflexia, constriction of the pupils to a slight degree (though in severe poisoning they may show paralytic dilation), oliguria, tachycardia, hypotension, lowered body temperature, and coma. Typical shock syndrome (apnea, circulatory collapse, respiratory arrest, and death) may occur.

In extreme overdose, all electrical activity in the brain may cease, in which case a "flat" EEG normally equated with clinical death cannot be accepted. This effect is fully reversible unless hypoxic damage occurs. Consideration should be given to the possibility of barbiturate intoxication even in situations that appear to involve trauma.

Complications such as pneumonia, pulmonary edema, cardiac arrhythmias, congestive heart failure, and renal failure may occur. Uremia may increase CNS sensitivity to barbiturates if renal function is impaired. Differential diagnosis should include hypoglycemia, head trauma, cerebrovascular accidents, convulsive states, and diabetic coma.

Treatment of overdosage is mainly supportive and consists of the following:
1. Maintenance of an adequate airway, with assisted respiration and oxygen administration as necessary.
2. Monitoring of vital signs and fluid balance.
3. If the patient is conscious and has not lost the gag reflex, emesis may be induced with ipecac. Care should be taken to prevent pulmonary aspiration of vomitus. After completion of vomiting, 30 g activated charcoal in a glass of water may be administered.
4. If emesis is contraindicated, gastric lavage may be performed with a cuffed endotracheal tube in place with the patient in the face down position. Activated charcoal may be left in the emptied stomach and a saline cathartic administered.
5. Fluid therapy and other standard treatment for shock, if needed.
6. If renal function is normal, forced diuresis may aid in the elimination of the barbiturate. Alkalinization of the urine increases renal excretion of some barbiturates, including mephobarbital (which is metabolized to phenobarbital).
7. Although not recommended as a routine procedure, hemodialysis may be used in severe barbiturate intoxications or if the patient is anuric or in shock.
8. Patient should be rolled from side to side every 30 minutes.
9. Antibiotics should be given if pneumonia is suspected.
10. Appropriate nursing care to prevent hypostatic pneumonia, decubiti aspiration, and other complications of patients with altered states of consciousness.

DOSAGE AND ADMINISTRATION

Epilepsy: Average dose for adults: 400 mg to 600 mg (6 grains to 9 grains) daily; children under 5 years: 16 mg to 32 mg (¼ grain to ½ grain) three or four times daily; children over 5 years: 32 mg to 64 mg (½ grain to 1 grain) three or four times daily. Mephobarbital is best taken at bedtime if seizures generally occur at night, and during the day if attacks are diurnal. Treatment should be started with a small dose which is gradually increased over four or five days until the optimum dosage is determined. If the patient has been taking some other antiepileptic drug, it should be tapered off as the doses of Mephobarbital are increased, to guard against the temporary marked attacks that may occur when any treatment for epilepsy is changed abruptly. Similarly, when the dose is to be lowered to a maintenance level or to be discontinued, the amount should be reduced gradually over four or five days.

◆ RATED THERAPEUTICALLY EQUIVALENT; ◇ THERAPEUTIC EQUIVALENCE UNCONFIRMED; ○ UNRATED

Special Patient Population: Dosage should be reduced in the elderly or debilitated because these patients may be more sensitive to barbiturates. Dosage should be reduced for patients with impaired renal function or hepatic disease.

Combination with Other Drugs: Mephobarbital may be used in combination with phenobarbital, either in the form of alternating courses or concurrently. When the two drugs are used at the same time, the dose should be about one-half the amount of each used alone. The average daily dose for an adult is from 50 mg to 100 mg (¾ grain to 1 ½ grains) of phenobarbital and from 200 mg to 300 mg (3 grains to 4 ½ grains) of Mephobarbital tablets.

Mephobarbital may also be used with phenytoin sodium; in some cases, combined therapy appears to give better results than either agent used alone, since phenytoin sodium is particularly effective for the psychomotor types of seizure but relatively ineffective for petit mal. When the drugs are employed concurrently, a reduced dose of phenytoin sodium is advisable, but the full dose of Mephobarbital may be given. Satisfactory results have been obtained with an average daily dose of 230 mg (3 ½ grains) of phenytoin sodium plus about 600 mg (9 grains) of Mephobarbital.

Sedation: Adults: 32 mg to 100 mg (½ grain to 1 ½ grains) —optimum dose, 50 mg (¾ grain)—three to four times daily. Children: 16 mg to 32 mg (¼ grain to ½ grain) three to four times daily.

HOW SUPPLIED
TABLETS (C-IV): 32 MG

BRAND/MANUFACTURER	NDC	SIZE	AWP
○ BRAND			
MEBARAL: Sanofi Winthrop	00024-1231-05	250s	$40.36

TABLETS (C-IV): 50 MG

BRAND/MANUFACTURER	NDC	SIZE	AWP
○ BRAND			
MEBARAL: Sanofi Winthrop	00024-1232-05	250s	$57.78

TABLETS (C-IV): 100 MG

BRAND/MANUFACTURER	NDC	SIZE	AWP
○ BRAND			
MEBARAL: Sanofi Winthrop	00024-1233-05	250s	$77.45

Mephyton SEE PHYTONADIONE

Mepivacaine Hydrochloride

THESE SOLUTIONS ARE NOT INTENDED FOR SPINAL ANESTHESIA OR DENTAL USE.

DESCRIPTION
Mepivacaine Hydrochloride is 2-Piperidinecarboxamide, N-(2,6-dimethylphenyl)-1-methyl-, monohydrochloride.

It is a white crystalline odorless powder, soluble in water, but very resistant to both acid and alkaline hydrolysis.

Mepivacaine HCl is a local anesthetic available as sterile isotonic solutions in concentrations of 1%, 1.5%, and 2% for injection via local infiltration, peripheral nerve block, and caudal and lumbar epidural blocks.

Mepivacaine HCl is related chemically and pharmacologically to the amide-type local anesthetics. It contains an amide linkage between the aromatic nucleus and the amino group. (See related table).

Following is its chemical structure:

CLINICAL PHARMACOLOGY
Local anesthetics block the generation and the conduction of nerve impulses, presumably by increasing the threshold for electrical excitation in the nerve, by slowing the propagation of the nerve impulse, and by reducing the rate of rise of the action potential. In general, the progression of anesthesia is related to the diameter, myelination, and conduction velocity of affected nerve fibers. Clinically, the order of loss of nerve function is as follows: pain, temperature, touch, proprioception, and skeletal muscle tone.

Systemic absorption of local anesthetics produces effects on the cardiovascular and central nervous systems. At blood concentrations achieved with normal therapeutic doses, changes in cardiac conduction, excitability, refractoriness, contractility, and peripheral vascular resistance are minimal. However, toxic blood concentrations depress cardiac conduction and excitability, which may lead to atrioventricular block and ultimately to cardiac arrest. In addition, myocardial contractility is depressed and peripheral vasodilation occurs, leading to decreased cardiac output and arterial blood pressure.

Following systemic absorption, local anesthetics can produce central nervous system stimulation, depression, or both. Apparent central stimulation is manifested as restlessness, tremors, and shivering, progressing to convulsions, followed by depression and coma progressing ultimately to respiratory arrest. However, the local anesthetics have a primary depressant effect on the medulla and on higher centers. The depressed stage may occur without a prior excited stage.

PHARMACOKINETICS
The rate of systemic absorption of local anesthetics is dependent upon the total dose and concentration of drug administered, the route of administration, the vascularity of the administration site, and the presence or absence of epinephrine in the anesthetic solution. A dilute concentration of epinephrine (1:200,000 or 5 µg/mL) usually reduces the rate of absorption and plasma concentration of Mepivacaine HCl, however it has been reported that vasoconstrictors do not significantly prolong anesthesia with Mepivacaine HCl.

Onset of anesthesia with Mepivacaine HCl is rapid, the time of onset for sensory block ranging from about 3 to 20 minutes depending upon such factors as the anesthetic technique, the type of block, the concentration of the solution, and the individual patient. The degree of motor blockade produced is dependent on the concentration of the solution. A 0.5% solution will be effective in small superficial nerve blocks while the 1% concentration will block sensory and sympathetic conduction without loss of motor function. The 1.5% solution will provide extensive and often complete motor block and the 2% concentration of Mepivacaine HCl will produce complete sensory and motor block of any nerve group.

The duration of anesthesia also varies depending upon the technique and type of block, the concentration, and the individual. Mepivacaine HCl will normally provide anesthesia which is adequate for 2 to 2 ½ hours of surgery.

Local anesthetics are bound to plasma proteins in varying degrees. Generally, the lower the plasma concentration of drug, the higher the percentage of drug bound to plasma. Local anesthetics appear to cross the placenta by passive diffusion. The rate and degree of diffusion is governed by the degree of plasma protein binding, the degree of ionization, and the degree of lipid solubility. Fetal/maternal ratios of local anesthetics appear to be inversely related to the degree of plasma protein binding, because only the free, unbound drug is available for placental transfer. Mepivacaine HCl is approximately 75% bound to plasma proteins. The extent of placental transfer is also determined by the degree of ionization and lipid solubility of the drug. Lipid soluble, nonionized drugs readily enter the fetal blood from the maternal circulation.

Depending upon the route of administration, local anesthetics are distributed to some extent to all body tissues, with high concentrations found in highly perfused organs such as the liver, lungs, heart, and brain.

Various pharmacokinetic parameters of the local anesthetics can be significantly altered by the presence of hepatic or renal disease, addition of epinephrine, factors affecting urinary pH, renal blood flow, the route of drug administration, and the age of the patient. The half-life of Mepivacaine HCl in adults is 1.9 to 3.2 hours and in neonates 8.7 to 9 hours.

Mepivacaine HCl, because of its amide structure, is not detoxified by the circulating plasma esterases. It is rapidly metabolized, with only a small percentage of the anesthetic (5 percent to 10 percent) being excreted unchanged in the urine. The liver is the principal site of metabolism, with over 50% of the administered dose being excreted into the bile as metabolites. Most of the metabolized Mepivacaine HCl is probably resorbed in the intestine and then excreted into the urine since only a small percentage is found in the feces. The principal route of excretion is via the kidney. Most of the anesthetic and its metabolites are eliminated within 30 hours. It has been shown that hydroxylation and N-demethylation, which are detoxification reactions, play important roles in the metabolism of the anesthetic. Three metabolites of Mepivacaine HCl have

COMPOSITION OF AVAILABLE SOLUTIONS(*)

	1% Single-Dose 30 mL Vial mg/mL	1% Multiple-Dose 50 mL Vial mg/mL	1.5% Single-Dose 30 mL Vial mg/mL	2% Single-Dose 20 mL Vial mg/mL	2% Multiple-Dose 50 mL Vial mg/mL
Mepivacaine Hydrochloride	10	10	15	20	20
Sodium chloride	6.6	7	5.6	4.6	5
Potassium chloride	0.3		0.3	0.3	
Calcium chloride	0.33		0.33	0.33	
Methylparaben		1			1

* In Water for Injection
The pH of the solutions is adjusted between 4.5 and 6.8 with sodium hydroxide or hydrochloric acid.

been identified from human adults: two phenols, which are excreted almost exclusively as their glucuronide conjugates, and the N-demethylated compound (2′,6′-pipecoloxylidide).

Mepivacaine HCl does not ordinarily produce irritation or tissue damage, and does not cause methemoglobinemia when administered in recommended doses and concentrations.

INDICATIONS AND USAGE
Mepivacaine HCl is indicated for production of local or regional analgesia and anesthesia by local infiltration, peripheral nerve block techniques, and central neural techniques including epidural and caudal blocks.

The routes of administration and indicated concentrations for Mepivacaine HCl are:

local infiltration	0.5% (via dilution) or 1%
peripheral nerve blocks	1% and 2%
epidural block	1%, 1.5%, 2%
caudal block	1%, 1.5%, 2%

See *"Dosage and Administration"* for additional information. Standard textbooks should be consulted to determine the accepted procedures and techniques for the administration of Mepivacaine HCl.

CONTRAINDICATIONS
Mepivacaine HCl is contraindicated in patients with a known hypersensitivity to it or to any local anesthetic agent of the amide-type or to other components of solutions of Mepivacaine HCl.

WARNINGS
LOCAL ANESTHETICS SHOULD ONLY BE EMPLOYED BY CLINICIANS WHO ARE WELL VERSED IN DIAGNOSIS AND MANAGEMENT OF DOSE-RELATED TOXICITY AND OTHER ACUTE EMERGENCIES WHICH MIGHT ARISE FROM THE BLOCK TO BE EMPLOYED, AND THEN ONLY AFTER INSURING THE *IMMEDIATE* AVAILABILITY OF OXYGEN, OTHER RESUSCITATIVE DRUGS, CARDIOPULMONARY RESUSCITATIVE EQUIPMENT, AND THE PERSONNEL RESOURCES NEEDED FOR PROPER MANAGEMENT OF TOXIC REACTIONS AND RELATED EMERGENCIES. (*SEE ALSO "ADVERSE REACTIONS* AND *PRECAUTIONS"*.) DELAY IN PROPER MANAGEMENT OF DOSE-RELATED TOXICITY, UNDERVENTILATION FROM ANY CAUSE, AND/OR ALTERED SENSITIVITY MAY LEAD TO THE DEVELOPMENT OF ACIDOSIS, CARDIAC ARREST AND, POSSIBLY, DEATH.

Local anesthetic solutions containing antimicrobial preservatives (ie, those supplied in multiple-dose vials) should not be used for epidural or caudal anesthesia because safety has *not* been established with regard to intrathecal injection, either intentionally or inadvertently, of such preservatives. It is essential that aspiration for blood or cerebrospinal fluid (where applicable) be done prior to injecting any local anesthetic, both the original dose and all subsequent doses, to avoid intravascular or subarachnoid injection. However, a negative aspiration does not ensure against an intravascular or subarachnoid injection.

Reactions resulting in fatality have occurred on rare occasions with the use of local anesthetics.

Mepivacaine HCl with epinephrine or other vasopressors should not be used concomitantly with ergot-type oxytocic drugs, because a severe persistent hypertension may occur. Likewise, solutions of Mepivacaine HCl containing a vasoconstrictor, such as epinephrine, should be used with extreme caution in patients receiving monoamine oxidase inhibitors (MAOI) or antidepressants of the triptyline or imipramine types, because severe prolonged hypertension may result. Local anesthetic procedures should be used with caution when there is inflammation and/or sepsis in the region of the proposed injection.

Mixing or the prior or intercurrent use of any local anesthetic with Mepivacaine HCl cannot be recommended because of insufficient data on the clinical use of such mixtures.

PRECAUTIONS
GENERAL
The safety and effectiveness of local anesthetics depend on proper dosage, correct technique, adequate precautions, and readiness for emergencies. Resuscitative equipment, oxygen, and other resuscitative drugs should be available for immediate use. (See *"Warnings"* and *"Adverse Reactions"*.) During major regional nerve blocks, the patient should have IV fluids running via an indwelling catheter to assure a functioning intravenous pathway. The lowest dosage of local anesthetic that results in effective anesthesia should be used to avoid high plasma levels and serious adverse effects. Injections should be made slowly, with frequent aspirations before and during the injection to avoid intravascular injection. Current opinion favors fractional administration with constant attention to the patient, rather than rapid bolus injection. Syringe aspirations should also be performed before and during each supplemental injection in continuous (intermittent) catheter techniques. An intravascular injection is still possible even if aspirations for blood are negative. During the administration of epidural anesthesia, it is recommended that a test dose be administered initially and the effects monitored before the full dose is given. When using a "continuous" catheter technique, test doses should be given prior to both the original and all reinforcing doses, because plastic tubing in the epidural space can migrate into a blood vessel or through the dura. When clinical conditions permit, an effective test dose should contain epinephrine (10 µg to 15 µg have been suggested) to serve as a warning of unintended intravascular injection. If injected into a blood vessel, this amount of epinephrine is likely to produce an "epinephrine response" within 45 seconds, consisting of an increase of pulse and blood pressure, circumoral

pallor, palpitations, and nervousness in the unsedated patient. The sedated patient may exhibit only a pulse rate increase of 20 or more beats per minute for 15 or more seconds. Therefore, following the test dose, the heart rate should be monitored for a heart rate increase. The test dose should also contain 45 mg to 50 mg of Mepivacaine HCl to detect an unintended intrathecal administration. This will be evidenced within a few minutes by signs of spinal block (eg, decreased sensation of the buttocks, paresis of the legs, or, in the sedated patient, absent knee jerk).

Injection of repeated doses of local anesthetics may cause significant increases in plasma levels with each repeated dose due to slow accumulation of the drug or its metabolites or to slow metabolic degradation. Tolerance to elevated blood levels varies with the status of the patient. Debilitated, elderly patients, and acutely ill patients should be given reduced doses commensurate with their age and physical status. Local anesthetics should also be used with caution in patients with severe disturbances of cardiac rhythm, shock, heart block, or hypotension.

Careful and constant monitoring of cardiovascular and respiratory (adequacy of ventilation) vital signs, and the patient's state of consciousness should be performed after each local anesthetic injection. It should be kept in mind at such times that restlessness, anxiety, incoherent speech, lightheadedness, numbness and tingling of the mouth and lips, metallic taste, tinnitus, dizziness, blurred vision, tremors, twitching, depression, or drowsiness may be early warning signs of central nervous system toxicity.

Local anesthetic solutions containing a vasoconstrictor should be used cautiously and in carefully restricted quantities in areas of the body supplied by end arteries or having otherwise compromised blood supply such as digits, nose, external ear, penis. Patients with hypertensive vascular disease may exhibit exaggerated vasoconstrictor response. Ischemic injury or necrosis may result.

Mepivacaine HCl should be used with caution in patients with known allergies and sensitivities.

Because amide-type local anesthetics such as Mepivacaine HCl are metabolized by the liver and excreted by the kidneys, these drugs, especially repeat doses, should be used cautiously in patients with hepatic and renal disease. Patients with severe hepatic disease, because of their inability to metabolize local anesthetics normally, are at a greater risk of developing toxic plasma concentrations. Local anesthetics should also be used with caution in patients with impaired cardiovascular function because there may be less able to compensate for functional changes associated with the prolongation of AV conduction produced by these drugs.

Serious dose-related cardiac arrhythmias may occur if preparations containing a vasoconstrictor such as epinephrine are employed in patients during or following the administration of potent inhalation anesthetics. In deciding whether to use these products concurrently in the same patient, the combined action of both agents upon the myocardium, the concentration and volume of vasoconstrictor used, and the time since injection, when applicable, should be taken into account.

Many drugs used during the conduct of anesthesia are considered potential triggering agents for familial malignant hyperthermia. Because it is not known whether amide-type local anesthetics may trigger this reaction and because the need for supplemental general anesthesia cannot be predicted in advance, it is suggested that a standard protocol for management should be available. Early unexplained signs of tachycardia, tachypnea, labile blood pressure, and metabolic acidosis may precede temperature elevation. Successful outcome is dependent on early diagnosis, prompt discontinuance of the suspect triggering agent(s), and institution of treatment, including oxygen therapy, indicated supportive measures, and dantrolene. (Consult dantrolene sodium intravenous package insert before using.)

USE IN HEAD AND NECK AREA
Small doses of local anesthetics injected into the head and neck area may produce adverse reactions similar to systemic toxicity seen with unintentional intravascular injections of larger doses. The injection procedures require the utmost care.

Confusion, convulsions, respiratory depression, and/or respiratory arrest, and cardiovascular stimulation or depression have been reported. These reactions may be due to intraarterial injection of the local anesthetic with retrograde flow to the cerebral circulation. Patients receiving these blocks should have their circulation and respiration monitored and be constantly observed. Resuscitative equipment and personnel for treating adverse reactions should be immediately available. Dosage recommendations should not be exceeded.

INFORMATION FOR PATIENTS
When appropriate, patients should be informed in advance that they may experience temporary loss of sensation and motor activity, usually in the lower half of the body, following proper administration of caudal or epidural anesthesia. Also, when appropriate, the physician should discuss other information including adverse reactions listed in the package insert on Mepivacaine HCl.

CLINICALLY SIGNIFICANT DRUG INTERACTIONS
The administration of local anesthetic solutions containing epinephrine or norepinephrine to patients receiving monoamine oxidase inhibitors or tricyclic antidepressants may produce severe, prolonged hypertension. Concurrent use of these agents should generally be avoided. In situations when concurrent therapy is necessary, careful patient monitoring is essential.

Concurrent administration of vasopressor drugs and of ergot-type oxytocic drugs may cause severe, persistent hypertension or cerebrovascular accidents.

Phenothiazines and butyrophenones may reduce or reverse the pressor effect of epinephrine.

CARCINOGENESIS, MUTAGENESIS, AND IMPAIRMENT OF FERTILITY

Long-term studies in animals of most local anesthetics including Mepivacaine HCl to evaluate the carcinogenic potential have not been conducted. Mutagenic potential or the effect on fertility has not been determined. There is no evidence from human data that Mepivacaine HCl may be carcinogenic or mutagenic or that it impairs fertility.

PREGNANCY CATEGORY C

Animal reproduction studies have not been conducted with Mepivacaine HCl. There are no adequate and well-controlled studies in pregnant women of the effect of Mepivacaine HCl on the developing fetus. Mepivacaine HCl should be used during pregnancy only if the potential benefit justifies the potential risk to the fetus. This does not preclude the use of Mepivacaine HCl at term for obstetrical anesthesia or analgesia. (See *"Labor and Delivery"*.)

Mepivacaine HCl has been used for obstetrical analgesia by the epidural, caudal, and paracervical routes without evidence of adverse effects on the fetus when no more than the maximum safe dosages are used and strict adherence to technique is followed.

LABOR AND DELIVERY

Local anesthetics rapidly cross the placenta, and when used for epidural, paracervical, caudal, or pudendal block anesthesia, can cause varying degrees of maternal, fetal, and neonatal toxicity. (See *"Pharmacokinetics, Clinical Pharmacology"*.) The incidence and degree of toxicity depend upon the procedure performed, the type and amount of drug used, and the technique of drug administration. Adverse reactions in the parturient, fetus, and neonate involve alternations of the central nervous system, peripheral vascular tone and cardiac function.

Maternal hypotension has resulted from regional anesthesia. Local anesthetics produce vasodilation by blocking sympathetic nerves. Elevating the patient's legs and positioning her on her left side will help prevent decreases in blood pressure. The fetal heart rate also should be monitored continuously and electronic fetal monitoring is highly advisable.

Epidural, paracervical, caudal, or pudendal anesthesia may alter the forces of parturition through changes in uterine contractility or maternal expulsive efforts. In one study, paracervical block anesthesia was associated with a decrease in the mean duration of first stage labor and facilitation of cervical dilation. Epidural anesthesia has been reported to prolong the second stage of labor by removing the parturient's reflex urge to bear down or by interfering with motor function. The use of obstetrical anesthesia may increase the need for forceps assistance.

The use of some local anesthetic drug products during labor and delivery may be followed by diminished muscle strength and tone for the first day or two of life. The long-term significance of these observations is unknown.

Fetal bradycardia may occur in 20 to 30 percent of patients receiving paracervical block anesthesia with the amide-type local anesthetics and may be associated with fetal acidosis. Fetal heart rate should always be monitored during paracervical anesthesia. Added risk appears to be present in prematurity, postmaturity, toxemia of pregnancy, and fetal distress. The physician should weigh the possible advantages against dangers when considering paracervical block in these conditions. Careful adherence to recommended dosage is of the utmost importance in obstetrical paracervical block. Failure to achieve adequate analgesia with recommended doses should arouse suspicion of intravascular or fetal intracranial injection.

Cases compatible with unintended fetal intracranial injection of local anesthetic solution have been reported following intended paracervical or pudendal block or both. Babies so affected present with unexplained neonatal depression at birth which correlates with high local anesthetic serum levels and usually manifest seizures within six hours. Prompt use of supportive measures combined with forced urinary excretion of the local anesthetic has been used successfully to manage this complication.

Case reports of maternal convulsions and cardiovascular collapse following use of some local anesthetics for paracervical block in early pregnancy (as anesthesia for elective abortion) suggest that systemic absorption under these circumstances may be rapid. The recommended maximum dose of the local anesthetic should not be exceeded. Injection should be made slowly and with frequent aspiration. Allow a five-minute interval between sides.

It is extremely important to avoid aortocaval compression by the gravid uterus during administration of regional block to parturients. To do this, the patient must be maintained in the left lateral decubitus position or a blanket roll or sandbag may be placed beneath the right hip and the gravid uterus displaced to the left.

NURSING MOTHERS

It is not known whether local anesthetic drugs are excreted in human milk. Because many drugs are excreted in human milk, caution should be exercised when local anesthetics are administered to a nursing woman.

PEDIATRIC USE

Guidelines for the administration of Mepivacaine HCl to children are presented in *"Dosage and Administration"*.

ADVERSE REACTIONS

Reactions to Mepivacaine HCl are characteristic of those associated with other amide-type local anesthetics. A major cause of adverse reactions to this group of drugs is excessive plasma levels, which may be due to overdosage, inadvertent intravascular injection, or slow metabolic degradation.

SYSTEMIC

The most commonly encountered acute adverse experiences which demand immediate countermeasures are related to the central nervous system and the cardiovascular system. These adverse experiences are generally dose related and due to high plasma levels which may result from overdosage, rapid absorption from the injection site, diminished tolerance, or from unintentional intravascular injection of the local anesthetic solution. In addition to systemic dose-related toxicity, unintentional subarachnoid injection of drug during the intended performance of caudal or lumbar epidural block or nerve blocks near the vertebral column (especially in the head and neck region) may result in underventilation or apnea ("Total or High Spinal"). Also, hypotension due to loss of sympathetic tone and respiratory paralysis or under-ventilation due to cephalad extension of the motor level of anesthesia may occur. This may lead to secondary cardiac arrest if untreated. Factors influencing plasma protein binding, such as acidosis, systemic diseases which alter protein production, or competition of other drugs for protein binding sites, may diminish individual tolerance.

CENTRAL NERVOUS SYSTEM REACTIONS

These are characterized by excitation and/or depression. Restlessness, anxiety, dizziness, tinnitus, blurred vision, or tremors may occur, possibly proceeding to convulsions. However, excitement may be transient or absent, with depression being the first manifestation of an adverse reaction. This may quickly be followed by drowsiness merging into unconsciousness and respiratory arrest. Other central nervous system effects may be nausea, vomiting, chills, and constriction of the pupils.

The incidence of convulsions associated with the use of local anesthetics varies with the procedure used and the total dose administered. In a survey of studies of epidural anesthesia, overt toxicity progressing to convulsions occurred in approximately 0.1% of local anesthetic administrations.

CARDIOVASCULAR REACTIONS

High doses or, inadvertent intravascular injection, may lead to high plasma levels and related depression of the myocardium, decreased cardiac output, heart block, hypotension (or sometimes hypertension), bradycardia, ventricular arrhythmias, and possibly cardiac arrest. (See *"Warnings" "Precautions"* and *"Overdosage"* sections).

ALLERGIC

Allergic-type reactions are rare and may occur as a result of sensitivity to the local anesthetic or to other formulation ingredients, such as the antimicrobial preservative methylparaben, contained in multiple-dose vials. These reactions are characterized by signs such as urticaria, pruritus, erythema, angioneurotic edema (including laryngeal edema), tachycardia, sneezing, nausea, vomiting, dizziness, syncope, excessive sweating, elevated temperature, and possibly, anaphylactoid-like symptomatology (including severe hypotension). Cross sensitivity among members of the amide-type local anesthetic group has been reported. The usefulness of screening for sensitivity has not been definitely established.

NEUROLOGIC

The incidences of adverse neurologic reactions associated with the use of local anesthetics may be related to the total dose of local anesthetic administered and are also dependent upon the particular drug used, the route of administration, and the physical status of the patient. Many of these effects may be related to local anesthetic techniques, with or without a contribution from the drug.

In the practice of caudal or lumbar epidural block, occasional unintentional penetration of the subarachnoid space by the catheter or needle may occur. Subsequent adverse effects may depend partially on the amount of drug administered intrathecally and the physiological and physical effects of a dural puncture. A high spinal is characterized by paralysis of the legs, loss of consciousness, respiratory paralysis, and bradycardia.

Neurologic effects following epidural or caudal anesthesia may include spinal block of varying magnitude (including high or total spinal block); hypotension secondary to spinal block; urinary retention; fecal and urinary incontinence; loss of perineal sensation and sexual function; persistent anesthesia, paresthesia, weakness, paralysis of the lower extremities, and loss of sphincter control all of which may have slow, incomplete, or no recovery; headache; backache; septic meningitis; meningismus; slowing of labor; increased incidence of forceps delivery; cranial nerve palsies due to traction on nerves from loss of cerebrospinal fluid.

Neurologic effects following other procedures or routes of administration may include persistent anesthesia, paresthesia, weakness, paralysis, all of which may have slow, incomplete, or no recovery.

OVERDOSAGE

Acute emergencies from local anesthetics are generally related to high plasma levels encountered during therapeutic use of local anesthetics or to unintended subarachnoid injection of local anesthetic solution. (See *"Adverse Reactions"*, *"Warnings"*, and *"Precautions"*).

MANAGEMENT OF LOCAL ANESTHETIC EMERGENCIES

The first consideration is prevention, best accomplished by careful and constant monitoring of cardiovascular and respiratory vital signs and the patient's state of consciousness after each local anesthetic injection. At the first sign of change, oxygen should be administered.

The first step in the management of systemic toxic reactions, as well as underventilation or apnea due to unintentional subarachnoid injection of drug solution, consists of *immediate* attention to the establishment and maintenance of a patent airway and effective assisted or

RECOMMENDED CONCENTRATIONS AND DOSES OF MEPIVACAINE HCL

Procedure	Concentration	Total Dose mL	Total Dose mg	Comments
Cervical, brachial, intercostal, pudendal nerve block	1%	5-40	50-400	Pudendal block: one half of total dose injected each side.
	2%	5-20	100-400	
Transvaginal block (paracervical plus pudendal)	1%	up to 30 (both sides)	up to 300 (both sides)	One half of total dose injected each side. See "Precautions".
Paracervical block	1%	up to 20 (both sides)	up to 200 (both sides)	One half of total dose injected each side. This is maximum recommended dose per 90-minute period in obstetrical and nonobstetrical patients. Inject slowly, 5 minutes between sides. See "Precautions".
Caudal and Epidural block	1%	15-30	150-300	Use only single-dose vials which do not contain a preservative.
	1.5%	10-25	150-375	
	2%	10-20	200-400	
Infiltration	1%	up to 40	up to 400	An equivalent amount of a 0.5% solution (prepared by diluting the 1% solution with Sodium Chloride Injection, USP) may be used for large areas.
Therapeutic block (pain management)	1%	1-5	10-50	
	2%	1-5	20-100	

Unused portions of solutions not containing preservatives should be discarded.

controlled ventilation with 100% oxygen with a delivery system capable of permitting immediate positive airway pressure by mask.

This may prevent convulsions if they have not already occurred.

If necessary, use drugs to control the convulsions. A 50 mg to 100 mg bolus IV injection of succinylcholine will paralyze the patient without depressing the central nervous or cardiovascular systems and facilitate ventilation. A bolus IV dose of 5 mg to 10 mg of diazepam or 50 mg to 100 mg of thiopental will permit ventilation and counteract central nervous system stimulation, but these drugs also depress central nervous system, respiratory, and cardiac function, add to postictal depression and may result in apnea. Intravenous barbiturates, anticonvulsant agents, or muscle relaxants should only be administered by those familiar with their use. Immediately after the institution of these ventilatory measures, the adequacy of the circulation should be evaluated. Supportive treatment of circulatory depression may require administration of intravenous fluids, and when appropriate, a vasopressor dictated by the clinical situation (such as ephedrine or epinephrine to enhance myocardial contractile force).

Endotracheal intubation, employing drugs and techniques familiar to the clinician may be indicated after initial administration of oxygen by mask, if difficulty is encountered in the maintenance of a patent airway or if prolonged ventilatory support (assisted or controlled) is indicated.

Recent clinical data from patients experiencing local anesthetic induced convulsions demonstrated rapid development of hypoxia, hypercarbia, and acidosis within a minute of the onset of convulsions. These observations suggest that oxygen consumption and carbon dioxide production are greatly increased during local anesthetic convulsions and emphasize the importance of immediate and effective ventilation with oxygen which may avoid cardiac arrest.

If not treated immediately, convulsions with simultaneous hypoxia, hypercarbia, and acidosis, plus myocardial depression from the direct effects of the local anesthetic may result in cardiac arrhythmias, bradycardia, asystole, ventricular fibrillation, or cardiac arrest. Respiratory abnormalities, including apnea, may occur. Underventilation or apnea due to unintentional subarachnoid injection of local anesthetic solution may produce these same signs and also lead to cardiac arrest if ventilatory support is not instituted. If cardiac arrest should occur, standard cardiopulmonary resuscitative measures should be instituted and maintained for a prolonged period if necessary. Recovery has been reported after prolonged resuscitative efforts.

The supine position is dangerous in pregnant women at term because of aortocaval compression by the gravid uterus. Therefore during treatment of systemic toxicity, maternal hypotension, or fetal bradycardia following regional block, the parturient should be maintained in the left lateral decubitus position if possible, or manual displacement of the uterus off the great vessels be accomplished.

The mean seizure dosage of Mepivacaine HCl in rhesus monkeys was found to be 18.8 mg/kg with mean arterial plasma concentration of 24.4 µg/mL. The intravenous and subcutaneous LD_{50} in mice is 23 mg/kg to 35 mg/kg and 280 mg/kg respectively.

DOSAGE AND ADMINISTRATION

The dose of any local anesthetic administered varies with the anesthetic procedure, the area to be anesthetized, the vascularity of the tissues, the number of neuronal segments to be blocked, the depth of anesthesia and degree of muscle relaxation required, the duration of anesthesia desired, individual tolerance and the physical condition of the patient. The smallest dose and concentration required to produce the desired result should be administered. Dosages of Mepivacaine HCl should be reduced for elderly and debilitated patients and patients with cardiac and/or liver disease. The rapid injection of a large volume of local anesthetic solution should be avoided and fractional doses should be used when feasible.

For specific techniques and procedures, refer to standard textbooks.

The recommended single *adult* dose (or the total of a series of doses given in one procedure) of Mepivacaine HCl, for unsedated, healthy, normal-sized individuals should not usually exceed 400 mg. The recommended dosage is based on requirements for the average adult and should be reduced for elderly or debilitated patients.

While maximum doses of 7 mg/kg (550 mg) have been administered without adverse effect, these are not recommended, except in exceptional circumstances and under no circumstances should the administration be repeated at intervals of less than 1 1/2 hours. The total dose for any 24-hour period should not exceed 1000 mg because of a slow accumulation of the anesthetic or its derivatives or slower than normal metabolic degradation or detoxification with repeat administration (see "Clinical Pharmacology" and "Precautions").

Children tolerate the local anesthetic as well as adults. However, the pediatric dose should be *carefully measured* as a percentage of the total adult dose *based on weight*, and should not exceed 5 mg/kg to 6 mg/kg (2.5 mg/lb to 3 mg/lb) in children, especially those weighing less than 30 lb. In children *under 3 years of age or weighing less than 30 lb* concentrations less than 2% (eg, 0.5% to 1.5%) should be employed. **Unused portions of solutions not containing preservatives, ie, those supplied in single-dose vials, should be discarded following initial use.**

This product should be inspected visually for particulate matter and discoloration prior to administration whenever solution and container permit. Solutions which are discolored or which contain particulate matter should not be administered.

THESE SOLUTIONS ARE NOT INTENDED FOR SPINAL ANESTHESIA OR DENTAL USE.

Store at controlled room temperature between 15°C to 30°C (59°F to 86°F); brief exposure up to 40°C (104°F) does not adversely affect the product. (See related table).

J CODES
VAR—J0670

HOW SUPPLIED
INJECTION: 1%

AVERAGE UNIT PRICE (AVAILABLE SIZES)

BRAND	$0.16	*GENERIC A-RATED AVERAGE PRICE (GAAP)*		
GENERIC	$0.22	50 ml		$8.18

BRAND/MANUFACTURER	NDC	SIZE	AWP
◆ **BRAND**			
CARBOCAINE HCL: Sanofi Winthrop	00024-0231-01	30 ml	$9.98
	00024-0232-01	50 ml	$14.29
POLOCAINE-MPF: Astra	00186-0412-01	30 ml 50s	$6.50
POLOCAINE: Astra	00186-0410-01	50 ml 50s	$9.21
◆ **GENERICS**			
Schein	00364-6770-57	50 ml	$6.00
Rugby	00536-5281-80	50 ml	$10.35
Intl Med Sys	00548-1102-00	30 ml 5s	$51.00

◆ RATED THERAPEUTICALLY EQUIVALENT; ◇ THERAPEUTIC EQUIVALENCE UNCONFIRMED; ○ UNRATED

INJECTION: 1.5%

AVERAGE UNIT PRICE (AVAILABLE SIZES)			
BRAND	$0.23		

BRAND/MANUFACTURER	NDC	SIZE	AWP
◆ BRAND			
CARBOCAINE HCL: Sanofi Winthrop	00024-0234-01	30 ml	$13.59
POLOCAINE: Astra	00186-0418-01	30 ml 50s	$8.81

INJECTION: 2%

AVERAGE UNIT PRICE (AVAILABLE SIZES)		GENERIC A-RATED AVERAGE PRICE (GAAP)	
BRAND	$0.22	50 ml	$5.82
GENERIC	$0.12		

BRAND/MANUFACTURER	NDC	SIZE	AWP
◆ BRAND			
CARBOCAINE HCL: Sanofi Winthrop	00024-0236-01	20 ml	$11.19
	00024-0237-01	50 ml	$16.72
POLOCAINE: Astra	00186-0422-01	20 ml 50s	$7.23
	00186-0420-01	50 ml 50s	$10.64
	00186-0460-14	1.8 ml 100s	$35.00
◆ GENERICS			
Moore,H.L.	00839-6798-38	50 ml	$4.74
Schein	00364-6771-57	50 ml	$6.90

INJECTION: 3%

BRAND/MANUFACTURER	NDC	SIZE	AWP
◆ BRAND			
POLOCAINE: Astra	00186-0440-14	1.8 ml 100s	$35.00

INJECTION: 10 MG/ML

BRAND/MANUFACTURER	NDC	SIZE	AWP
◆ GENERICS			
Steris	00402-0756-50	50 ml	$6.00

INJECTION: 10 MG

BRAND/MANUFACTURER	NDC	SIZE	AWP
◆ GENERICS			
Goldline	00182-3053-67	50 ml	$6.60

INJECTION: 20 MG/ML

BRAND/MANUFACTURER	NDC	SIZE	AWP
◆ GENERICS			
Steris	00402-0757-50	50 ml	$6.90

Meprobamate

DESCRIPTION
Meprobamate is a white powder with a characteristic odor and a bitter taste. It is slightly soluble in water, freely soluble in acetone and alcohol, and sparingly soluble in ether. Meprobamate is available as 200 mg, 400 mg and 600 mg tablets.

Following is its chemical structure:

$$NH_2COOCH_2 \underset{CH_2CH_2CH_3}{\overset{CH_3}{C}} CH_2OOCNH_2$$

ACTIONS
Meprobamate is a carbamate derivative which has been shown in animal studies to have effects at multiple sites in the central nervous system, including the thalamus and limbic system.

INDICATIONS
Meprobamate is indicated for the management of anxiety disorders or for the short-term relief of the symptoms of anxiety. Anxiety or tension associated with the stress of everyday life usually do not require treatment with an anxiolytic.

The effectiveness of Meprobamate in long-term use, that is, more than 4 months, has not been assessed by systematic clinical studies. The physician should periodically reassess the usefulness of the drug for the individual patient.

UNLABELED USES
Meprobamate is used alone or as an adjunct in the treatment of muscle contraction headache (migraine headache) and premenstrual tension.

CONTRAINDICATIONS
Acute intermittent porphyria as well as allergic or idiosyncratic reactions to Meprobamate or related compounds such as carisoprodol, mebutamate, tybamate or carbromal.

WARNINGS
DRUG DEPENDENCE
Physical dependence, psychological dependence, and abuse have occurred. When chronic intoxication from prolonged use occurs, it usually involves ingestion of greater than recommended doses and is manifested by ataxia, slurred speech, and vertigo. Therefore, careful supervision of dose and amounts prescribed is advised, as well as avoidance of prolonged administration, especially for alcoholics and other patients with a known propensity for taking excessive quantities of drugs.

Sudden withdrawal of the drug after prolonged and excessive use may precipitate recurrence of pre-existing symptoms, such as anxiety, anorexia, or insomnia, or withdrawal reactions, such as vomiting, ataxia, tremors, muscle twiching, confusional states, hallucinosis, and, rarely, convulsive seizures. Such seizures are more likely to occur in persons with central nervous system damage or pre-existent or latent convulsive disorders. Onset of withdrawal symptoms occurs usually within 12 to 48 hours after discontinuation of Meprobamate; symptoms usually cease within the next 12 to 48 hours.

When excessive dosage has continued for weeks or months, dosage should be reduced gradually over a period of one or two weeks rather than abruptly stopped. Alternatively, a short-acting barbiturate may be substituted, then gradually withdrawn.

POTENTIALLY HAZARDOUS TASKS
Patients should be warned that this drug may impair the mental and/or physical abilities required for the performance of potentially hazardous tasks such as driving a motor vehicle or operating machinery.

ADDITIVE EFFECTS
Since the effects of Meprobamate and alcohol or Meprobamate and other CNS depressants or psychotropic drugs may be additive, appropriate caution should be exercised with patients who take more than one of these agents simultaneously.

USAGE IN PREGNANCY AND LACTATION
An increased risk of congenital malformations associated with the use of minor tranquilizers (Meprobamate, chlordiazepoxide, and diazepam) during the first trimester of pregnancy has been suggested in several studies. Because use of these drugs is rarely a matter of urgency, their use during this period should almost always be avoided. The possibility that a woman of childbearing potential may be pregnant at the time of institution of therapy should be considered. Patients should be advised that if they become pregnant during therapy or intend to become pregnant they should communicate with their physician about the desirability of discontinuing the drug.

Meprobamate passes the placental barrier. It is present both in umbilical cord blood at or near maternal plasma levels and in breast milk of lactating mothers at concentrations two to four times that of maternal plasma. When use of Meprobamate is contemplated in breast-feeding patients, the drug's higher concentration in breast milk as compared to maternal plasma levels should be considered.

USAGE IN CHILDREN
Meprobamate 200 mg and 400 mg tablets should not be administered to children under age six, since there is a lack of documented evidence for safety and effectiveness in this age group. Meprobamate 600mg tablets are not intended for use in children.

PRECAUTIONS
The lowest effective dose should be administered, particularly to elderly and/or debilitated patients, in order to preclude oversedation.

The possibility of suicide attempts should be considered and the least amount of drug feasible should be dispensed at any one time.

Meprobamate is metabolized in the liver and excreted by the kidney; to avoid its excess accumulation, caution should be exercised in administration to patients with compromised liver or kidney function.

Meprobamate occasionally may precipitate seizures in epileptic patients.

ADVERSE REACTIONS
CENTRAL NERVOUS SYSTEM
Drowsiness, ataxia, dizziness, slurred speech, headache, vertigo, weakness, paresthesias, impairment of visual accomodation, euphoria, overstimulation, paradoxical excitement, fast EEG activity.

GASTROINTESTINAL
Nausea, vomiting, diarrhea.

CARDIOVASCULAR
Palpitations, tachycardia, various forms of arrhythmia, transient ECG changes, syncope; also, hypotensive crises (including one fatal case).

ALLERGIC OR IDIOSYNCRATIC
Allergic or idiosyncratic reactions are usually seen within the period of the first to fourth dose in patients having had no previous contact with the drug. Milder reactions are characterized by an itchy, urticarial, or erythematous maculopapular rash which may be generalized or confined to the groin. Other reactions have included leukopenia, acute non-thrombocytopenic purpura, petechiae, ecchymoses, eosinophilia, peripheral edema, adenopathy, fever, fixed drug eruption with cross reaction to carisoprodol, and cross sensitivity between Meprobamate/mebutamate and Meprobamate/carbromal.

➤ SHOWN IN PRODUCT IDENTIFICATION GUIDE

More severe hypersensitivity reactions, rarely reported, include hyperpyrexia, chills, angioneurotic edema, bronchospasm, oliguria, and anuria. Also, anaphylaxis, erythema multiforme, exfoliative dermatitis, stomatitis, proctitis, Stevens-Johnson syndrome, and bullous dermatitis, including one fatal case of the latter following administration of Meprobamate in combination with prednisolone.

In case of allergic or idiosyncratic reactions to Meprobamate, discontinue the drug and initiate appropriate symptomatic therapy, which may include epinephrine, antihistamines, and in severe cases corticosteroids. In evaluating possible allergic reactions, also consider allergy to excipients.

HEMATOLOGIC
(See also "Allergic or Idiosyncratic".) Agranulocytosis and aplastic anemia have been reported. These cases rarely were fatal. Rare cases of thrombocytopenic purpura have been reported.

OTHER
Exacerbation of porphyric symptoms.

DOSAGE AND ADMINISTRATION
Meprobamate 200 mg and 400 mg tablets:
The usual adult daily dosage is 1200 mg to 1600 mg, in three or four divided doses; a daily dosage above 2400 mg is not recommended. The usual daily dosage for children ages six to twelve is 200 mg to 600 mg, in two or three divided doses.
Not recommended for children under age 6 (see "Usage in Children").
Meprobamate 600 mg tablets:

Adults: One tablet twice a day. Doses of Meprobamate above 2400 mg daily are not recommended.
Not recommended for use in children (see "Usage in Children").

Storage: Store at controlled room temperature 15°-30°C (59°-86°F). Dispense in a tight container.

OVERDOSAGE
Suicidal attempts with Meprobamate have resulted in drowsiness, lethargy, stupor, ataxia, coma, shock, vasomotor and respiratory collapse. Some suicidal attempts have been fatal. The following data on Meprobamate tablets have been reported in the literature and from other sources. These data are not expected to correlate with each case (considering factors such as individual susceptibility and length of time from ingestion to treatment), but represent the usual ranges reported.

Acute simple overdose: Meprobamate alone): Death has been reported with ingestion of as little as 12 mg Meprobamate and survival with as much as 40 gm.

Blood Levels:
0.5-2.0 mg% represents the usual blood level range of Meprobamate after therapeutic doses. The level may occasionally be as high as 3.0 mg%.
3-10 mg% usually corresponds to finds of mild to moderate symptoms of overdosage, such as stupor or light coma.
10-20 mg% usually corresponds to deeper coma, requiring more intensive treatment. Some fatalities occur.
At levels greater than 20%, more fatalities than survivals can be expected.

Acute combined overdose: (Meprobamate with alcohol or other CNS depressants or psychotropic drugs): Since effects can be additive, a history of ingestion of a low dose of Meprobamate plus any of these compounds (or of a relative low blood or tissue level) cannot be used as a prognostic indicator. In cases where excessive doses have been taken, sleep ensues rapidly and blood pressure, pulse, and respiratory rates are reduced to basal levels. Any drug remaining in the stomach should be removed and symptomatic therapy given. Should respiration or blood pressure become compromised, respiratory assistance, central nervous system stimulants, and pressor agents should be administered cautiously as indicated. Meprobamate is metabolized in the liver and excreted by the kidney. Diuresis, osmotic (mannitol) diuresis, peritoneal dialysis, and hemodialysis have been used successfully. Careful monitoring of urinary output is necessary and caution should be taken to avoid overhydration. Relapse and death, after initial recovery, have been attributed to incomplete gastric emptying and delayed absorption. Meprobamate can be measured in biological fluids by two methods: colorimetric (Hoffman, A.J. and Ludwig, B.J.: J Amer Pharm Assn 48: 740, 1959) and gas chromatographic (Douglas, J.F. et al.: Anal Chem 39: 956, 1967).

HOW SUPPLIED
CAPSULE, EXTENDED RELEASE (C-IV): 200 MG

BRAND/MANUFACTURER	NDC	SIZE	AWP
○ BRAND			
MEPROSPAN-200: Wallace	00037-1401-01	100s	$179.44

CAPSULE, EXTENDED RELEASE (C-IV): 400 MG

BRAND/MANUFACTURER	NDC	SIZE	AWP
○ BRAND			
MEPROSPAN-400: Wallace	00037-1301-01	100s	$283.55

TABLETS (C-IV): 200 MG

AVERAGE UNIT PRICE (AVAILABLE SIZES)		GENERIC A-RATED AVERAGE PRICE (GAAP)	
BRAND	$0.63	100s	$4.29
GENERIC	$0.04	1000s	$29.89
HCFA FUL (100s ea)	$0.04		

BRAND/MANUFACTURER	NDC	SIZE	AWP
◆ BRAND			
EQUANIL: Wyeth-Ayerst	00008-0002-03	100s	$21.33
MILTOWN: Wallace	00037-1101-01	100s	$103.60
◆ GENERICS			
MB-TAB: Alra	51641-0327-01	100s	$3.10
Richlyn	00115-3888-01	100s	$3.37
Rugby	00536-4005-01	100s	$3.98
Schein	00364-0160-01	100s	$4.02
Eon	00185-0716-01	100s	$4.10
Major	00904-0044-60	100s	$4.25
URL	00677-0232-01	100s	$4.66
Moore,H.L.	00839-5070-06	100s	$4.71
Qualitest	00603-4439-21	100s	$5.35
Aligen	00405-0115-01	100s	$5.38
MB-TAB: Alra	51641-0327-10	1000s	$15.75
Schein	00364-0160-02	1000s	$25.82
Richlyn	00115-3888-03	1000s	$25.95
URL	00677-0232-10	1000s	$30.64
Rugby	00536-4005-10	1000s	$30.69
Eon	00185-0716-10	1000s	$32.50
Aligen	00405-0115-03	1000s	$38.04
Major	00904-0044-80	1000s	$39.75

TABLETS (C-IV): 400 MG

AVERAGE UNIT PRICE (AVAILABLE SIZES)		GENERIC A-RATED AVERAGE PRICE (GAAP)	
BRAND	$0.85	100s	$7.40
GENERIC	$0.06	1000s	$50.60
HCFA FUL (100s ea)	$0.05		

BRAND/MANUFACTURER	NDC	SIZE	AWP
◆ BRAND			
EQUANIL: Wyeth-Ayerst	00008-0001-05	100s	$26.70
MILTOWN: Wallace	00037-1001-01	100s	$127.03
EQUANIL: Wyeth-Ayerst	00008-0001-07	500s	$131.19
MILTOWN: Wallace	00037-1001-03	500s	$623.71
	00037-1001-02	1000s	$1223.35
◆ GENERICS			
MB-TAB: Alra	51641-0325-01	100s	$4.50
Richlyn	00115-3890-01	100s	$5.23
Eon	00185-0717-01	100s	$5.25
➤ Schein	00364-0161-01	100s	$6.06
Geneva	00781-1410-01	100s	$6.25
Major	00904-0045-60	100s	$7.00
Rugby	00536-4006-01	100s	$7.43
URL	00677-0233-01	100s	$8.80
Goldline	00182-0294-01	100s	$8.85
Moore,H.L.	00839-5004-06	100s	$9.25
Qualitest	00603-4440-21	100s	$9.36
Aligen	00405-0116-01	100s	$9.40
Major	00904-0045-61	100s ud	$7.98
Vangard	00615-0447-13	100s ud	$8.29
MB-TAB: Alra	51641-0325-10	1000s	$28.50
Geneva	00781-1410-10	1000s	$37.50
➤ Schein	00364-0161-02	1000s	$38.35
Richlyn	00115-3890-03	1000s	$40.20
Eon	00185-0717-10	1000s	$44.80
Major	00904-0045-80	1000s	$47.95
Aligen	00405-0116-03	1000s	$57.34
Parmed	00349-8830-10	1000s	$57.50
Rugby	00536-4006-10	1000s	$59.25
URL	00677-0233-10	1000s	$59.75
Qualitest	00603-4440-32	1000s	$59.80
Goldline	00182-0294-10	1000s	$60.75
Moore,H.L.	00839-5004-16	1000s	$66.14

TABLETS (C-IV): 600 MG

BRAND/MANUFACTURER	NDC	SIZE	AWP
◆ BRAND			
MILTOWN 600: Wallace	00037-1601-01	100s	$197.90

Mepron SEE ATOVAQUONE

Meprospan SEE MEPROBAMATE

Mercaptopurine

Caution: Mercaptopurine is a potent drug. It should not be used unless a diagnosis of acute lymphatic leukemia has been adequately established and the responsible physician is knowledgeable in assessing response to chemotherapy.

◆ RATED THERAPEUTICALLY EQUIVALENT; ◇ THERAPEUTIC EQUIVALENCE UNCONFIRMED; ○ UNRATED

DESCRIPTION

Mercaptopurine is one of a large series of purine analogues which interfere with nucleic acid biosynthesis and has been found active against human leukemias.

Mercaptopurine, known chemically as 1,7-dihydro-6H-purine-6-thione monohydrate, is an analogue of the purine bases adenine and hypoxanthine.

Mercaptopurine is available in tablet form for oral administration. Each scored tablet contains 50 mg Mercaptopurine.

Following is its chemical structure:

CLINICAL PHARMACOLOGY

Clinical studies have shown that the absorption of an oral dose of Mercaptopurine in man is incomplete and variable, averaging approximately 50% of the administered dose.[2] The factors influencing absorption are unknown. Intravenous administration of an investigational preparation of Mercaptopurine revealed a plasma half-disappearance time of 21 minutes in children and 47 minutes in adults. The volume of distribution usually exceeded that of the total body water.[2]

Following the oral administration of ^{35}S-6-Mercaptopurine in one subject, a total of 46% of the dose could be accounted for in the urine (as parent drug and metabolites) in the first 24 hours. Metabolites of Mercaptopurine were found in urine within the first 2 hours after administration. Radioactivity (in the form of sulfate) could be found in the urine for weeks afterwards.[3]

There is negligible entry of Mercaptopurine into cerebrospinal fluid.

Plasma protein binding averages 19% over the concentration range 10 to 50 mcg per mL (a concentration only achieved by intravenous administration of Mercaptopurine at doses exceeding 5 to 10 mg/kg).[2]

Monitoring of plasma levels of Mercaptopurine during therapy is of questionable value.[3] There is technical difficulty in determining plasma concentrations which are seldom greater than 1 to 2 mcg per mL after a therapeutic oral dose. More significantly, Mercaptopurine enters rapidly into the anabolic and catabolic pathways for purines, and the active intracellular metabolites have appreciably longer half-lives than the parent drug. The biochemical effects of a single dose of Mercaptopurine are evident long after the parent drug has disappeared from plasma. Because of this rapid metabolism of Mercaptopurine to active intracellular derivatives, hemodialysis would not be expected to appreciably reduce toxicity of the drug. There is no known pharmacologic antagonist to the biochemical actions of Mercaptopurine in vivo.

Mercaptopurine competes with hypoxanthine and guanine for the enzyme hypoxanthine-guanine phosphoribosyltransferase (HGPRTase) and is itself converted to thioinosinic acid (TIMP). This intracellular nucleotide inhibits several reactions involving inosinic acid (IMP), including the conversion of IMP to xanthylic acid (XMP) and the conversion of IMP to adenylic acid (AMP) via adenylosuccinate (SAMP). In addition, 6-methylthioinosinate (MTIMP) is formed by the methylation of TIMP. Both TIMP and MTIMP have been reported to inhibit glutamine-5-phosphoribosylpyrophosphate amidotransferase, the first enzyme unique to the de novo pathway for purine ribonucleotide synthesis.[3]

Experiments indicate that radiolabeled Mercaptopurine may be recovered from the DNA in the form of deoxythioguanosine.[4] Some Mercaptopurine is converted to nucleotide derivatives of 6-thioguanine (6-TG) by the sequential actions of inosinate (IMP) dehydrogenase and xanthylate (XMP) aminase, converting TIMP to thioguanylic acid (TGMP).

Animal tumors that are resistant to Mercaptopurine often have lost the ability to convert Mercaptopurine to TIMP. However, it is clear that resistance to Mercaptopurine may be acquired by other means as well, particularly in human leukemias.

It is not known exactly which of any one or more of the biochemical effects of Mercaptopurine and its metabolites are directly or predominantly responsible for cell death.[5]

The catabolism of Mercaptopurine and its metabolites is complex. In man, after oral administration of ^{35}S-6-Mercaptopurine, urine contains intact Mercaptopurine, thiouric acid (formed by direct oxidation by xanthine oxidase, probably via 6-mercapto-8-hydroxypurine), and a number of 6-methylated thiopurines. The methylthiopurines yield appreciable amounts of inorganic sulfate.[3] The importance of the metabolism by xanthine oxidase relates to the fact that Zyloprim® (allopurinol) inhibits this enzyme and retards the catabolism of Mercaptopurine and its active metabolites. A significant reduction in Mercaptopurine dosage is mandatory if a potent xanthine oxidase inhibitor and Mercaptopurine are used simultaneously in a patient (see "Precautions").

INDICATIONS AND USAGE

Mercaptopurine is indicated for remission induction and maintenance therapy of acute lymphatic leukemia. The response to this agent depends upon the particular subclassification of acute lymphatic leukemia and the age of the patient (child or adult).

Acute Lymphatic (Lymphocytic, Lymphoblastic) Leukemia: Given as a single agent for remission induction, Mercaptopurine induces complete remission in approximately 25% of children and 10% of adults. However, reliance upon Mercaptopurine alone is not justified for initial remission induction of acute lymphatic leukemia since combination chemotherapy with vincristine, prednisone, and L-asparaginase results in more frequent complete remission induction than with Mercaptopurine alone or in combination. The duration of complete remission induced in acute lymphatic leukemia is so brief without the use of maintenance therapy that some form of drug therapy is considered essential. Mercaptopurine, as a single agent, is capable of significantly prolonging complete remission duration; however, combination therapy has produced remission duration longer than that achieved with Mercaptopurine alone.

Acute Myelogenous (and Acute Myelomonocytic) Leukemia: As a single agent, Mercaptopurine will induce complete remission in approximately 10% of children and adults with acute myelogenous leukemia or its subclassifications. These results are inferior to those achieved with combination chemotherapy employing optimum treatment schedules.

Central Nervous System Leukemia: Mercaptopurine is not effective for prophylaxis or treatment of central nervous system leukemia.

Other Neoplasms: Mercaptopurine is not effective in chronic lymphatic leukemia, the lymphomas (including Hodgkin's Disease), or solid tumors.

UNLABELED USES

Mercaptopurine is used alone or as an adjunct in the treatment of Crohn's Disease.

CONTRAINDICATIONS

Mercaptopurine should not be used unless a diagnosis of acute lymphatic leukemia has been adequately established and the responsible physician is knowledgeable in assessing response to chemotherapy.

Mercaptopurine should not be used in patients whose disease has demonstrated prior resistance to this drug. In animals and man, there is usually complete cross-resistance between Mercaptopurine and thioguanine.

WARNINGS

SINCE DRUGS USED IN CANCER CHEMOTHERAPY ARE POTENTIALLY HAZARDOUS, IT IS RECOMMENDED THAT ONLY PHYSICIANS EXPERIENCED WITH THE RISKS OF MERCAPTOPURINE AND KNOWLEDGEABLE IN THE NATURAL HISTORY OF ACUTE LEUKEMIAS ADMINISTER THIS DRUG.

Bone Marrow Toxicity: The most consistent, dose-related toxicity is bone marrow suppression. This may be manifest by anemia, leukopenia, thrombocytopenia, or any combination of these. Any of these findings may also reflect progression of the underlying disease. Since Mercaptopurine may have a delayed effect, it is important to withdraw the medication temporarily at the first sign of an abnormally large fall in any of the formed elements of the blood.

Hepatotoxicity: Mercaptopurine is hepatotoxic in animals and man. A small number of deaths have been reported which may have been attributed to hepatic necrosis due to administration of Mercaptopurine. Hepatic injury can occur with any dosage, but seems to occur with more frequency when doses of 2.5 mg/kg/day are exceeded. The histologic pattern of Mercaptopurine hepatotoxicity includes features of both intrahepatic cholestasis and parenchymal cell necrosis, either of which may predominate. It is not clear how much of the hepatic damage is due to direct toxicity from the drug and how much may be due to a hypersensitivity reaction. In some patients jaundice has cleared following withdrawal of Mercaptopurine and reappeared with its reintroduction.[6]

Published reports have cited widely varying incidences of overt hepatotoxicity. In a large series of patients with various neoplastic diseases, Mercaptopurine was administered orally in doses ranging from 2.5 mg/kg to 5.0 mg/kg without any evidence of hepatotoxicity. It was noted by the authors that no definite clinical evidence of liver damage could be ascribed to the drug, although an occasional case of serum hepatitis did occur in patients receiving 6-MP who previously had transfusions.[6] In reports of smaller cohorts of adult and pediatric leukemic patients, the incidence of hepatotoxicity ranged from 0 to 6%.[7,8,9] In an isolated report by Einhorn and Davidsohn, jaundice was observed more frequently (40%), especially when doses exceeded 2.5 mg/kg.[10] Usually, clinically detectable jaundice appears early in the course of treatment (one to two months). However, jaundice has been reported as early as one week and as late as eight years after the start of treatment with Mercaptopurine.[11] Monitoring of serum transaminase levels, alkaline phosphatase, and bilirubin levels may allow early detection of hepatotoxicity. It is advisable to monitor these liver function tests at weekly intervals when first beginning therapy and at monthly intervals thereafter. Liver function tests may be advisable more frequently in patients who are receiving Mercaptopurine with other hepatotoxic drugs or with known pre-existing liver disease.

The concomitant administration of Mercaptopurine with other hepatotoxic agents requires especially careful clinical and biochemical monitoring of hepatic function. Combination therapy involving Mercaptopurine with other drugs not felt to be hepatotoxic should nevertheless be approached with caution. The combination of Mercaptopurine with doxorubicin (Adriamycin) was reported to be hepatotoxic in 19 of 20 patients undergoing remission-induction therapy for leukemia resistant to previous therapy.[12]

The hepatotoxicity has been associated in some cases with anorexia, diarrhea, jaundice, and ascites. Hepatic encephalopathy has occurred.

The onset of clinical jaundice, hepatomegaly, or anorexia with tenderness in the right hypochondrium are immediate indications for withholding Mercaptopurine until the exact etiology can be identified. Likewise, any evidence of deterioration in liver function studies, toxic hepatitis, or biliary stasis should prompt discontinuation of the drug and a search for an etiology of the hepatotoxicity.

Immunosuppression: Mercaptopurine recipients may manifest decreased cellular hypersensitivities and impaired allograft rejection. Induction of immunity to infectious agents or vaccines will be subnormal in these patients; the degree of immunosuppression will depend on antigen dose and temporal relationship to drug. This immunosuppressive effect should be carefully considered with regard to intercurrent infections and risk of subsequent neoplasia.

Pregnancy: "Pregnancy Category D." Mercaptopurine can cause fetal harm when administered to a pregnant woman. Women receiving Mercaptopurine in the first trimester of pregnancy have an increased incidence of abortion; the risk of malformation in offspring surviving first trimester exposure is not accurately known.[13] In a series of twenty-eight women receiving Mercaptopurine after the first trimester of pregnancy, three mothers died undelivered, one delivered a stillborn child, and one aborted; there were no cases of macroscopically abnormal fetuses.[14] Since such experience cannot exclude the possibility of fetal damage, Mercaptopurine should be used during pregnancy only if the benefit clearly justifies the possible risk to the fetus, and particular caution should be given to the use of Mercaptopurine in the first trimester of pregnancy.

There are no adequate and well controlled studies in pregnant women. If this drug is used during pregnancy or if the patient becomes pregnant while taking the drug, the patient should be apprised of the potential hazard to the fetus. Women of childbearing potential should be advised to avoid becoming pregnant.

PRECAUTIONS

General: The safe and effective use of Mercaptopurine demands a thorough knowledge of the natural history of the condition being treated. After selection of an initial dosage schedule, therapy will frequently need to be modified depending upon the patient's response and manifestations of toxicity.

The most frequent, serious, toxic effect of Mercaptopurine is myelosuppression resulting in leukopenia, thrombocytopenia, and anemia. These toxic effects are often unavoidable during the induction phase of adult acute leukemia if remission induction is to be successful. Whether or not these manifestations demand modification or cessation of dosage depends both upon the response of the underlying disease and a careful consideration of supportive facilities (granulocyte and platelet transfusions) which may be available. Life-threatening infections and bleeding have been observed as a consequence of Mercaptopurine-induced granulocytopenia and thrombocytopenia. Severe hematologic toxicity may require supportive therapy with platelet transfusions for bleeding, and antibiotics and granulocyte transfusions if sepsis is documented.

If it is not the intent of deliberately induce bone marrow hypoplasia, it is important to discontinue the drug temporarily at the first evidence of an abnormally large fall in white blood cell count, platelet count, or hemoglobin concentration. In many patients with severe depression of the formed elements of the blood due to Mercaptopurine, the bone marrow appears hypoplastic on aspiration or biopsy, whereas in other cases it may appear normocellular. The qualitative changes in the erythroid elements toward the megaloblastic series, characteristically seen with the folic acid antagonists and some other antimetabolites, are not seen with this drug. It is probably advisable to start with smaller dosages in patients with impaired renal function, since the latter might result in slower elimination of the drug and metabolites and a greater cumulative effect.

Information for Patients: Patients should be informed that the major toxicities of Mercaptopurine are related to myelosuppression, hepatotoxicity and gastrointestinal toxicity. Patients should never be allowed to take the drug without medical supervision and should be advised to consult their physician if they experience fever, sore throat, jaundice, nausea, vomiting, signs of local infection, bleeding from any site, or symptoms suggestive of anemia. Women of childbearing potential should be advised to avoid becoming pregnant.

Laboratory Tests: It is recommended that evaluation of the hemoglobin or hematocrit, total white blood cell count and differential count, and quantitative platelet count be obtained weekly while the patient is on Mercaptopurine therapy. In cases where the cause of fluctuations in the formed elements in the peripheral blood is obscure, bone marrow examination may be useful for the evaluation of marrow status. The decision to increase, decrease, continue, or discontinue a given dosage of Mercaptopurine must be based not only on the absolute hematologic values, but also upon the rapidity with which changes are occurring. In many instances, particularly during the induction phase of acute leukemia, complete blood counts will need to be done more frequently than once weekly in order to evaluate the effect of the therapy.

Drug Interactions:

Interaction with allopurinol: When allopurinol and Mercaptopurine are administered concomitantly, it is imperative that the dose of Mercaptopurine be reduced to one-third to one-quarter of the usual dose. Failure to observe this dosage reduction will result in a delayed catabolism of Mercaptopurine and the strong likelihood of inducing severe toxicity.

There is usually complete cross-resistance between Mercaptopurine and thioguanine.

The dosage of Mercaptopurine may need to be reduced when this agent is combined with other drugs whose primary or secondary toxicity is myelosuppression. Enhanced marrow suppression has been noted in some patients also receiving trimethoprim-sulfamethoxazole.[15,16]

Carcinogenesis, Mutagenesis, Impairment of Fertility: Mercaptopurine causes chromosomal aberrations in animals and man and induces dominant-lethal mutations in male mice. In mice, surviving female offspring of mothers who received chronic low doses of Mercaptopurine during pregnancy were found sterile or if they became pregnant had smaller litters and more dead fetuses as compared to control animals.[17] Carcinogenic potential exists in man, but the extent of the risk is unknown.

The effect of Mercaptopurine on human fertility is unknown for either males or females.

Pregnancy: Teratogenic Effects: Pregnancy Category D. See *"Warnings"* section.

Nursing Mothers: It is not known whether this drug is excreted in human milk. Because many drugs are excreted in human milk, and because of the potential for serious adverse reactions in nursing infants from Mercaptopurine, a decision should be made whether to discontinue nursing or to discontinue the drug, taking into account the importance of the drug to the mother.

ADVERSE REACTIONS

The principal and potentially serious toxic effects of Mercaptopurine are bone marrow toxicity and hepatotoxicity (see *"Warnings"*).

Hematologic: The most frequent adverse reaction to Mercaptopurine is myelosuppression. The induction of complete remission of acute lymphatic leukemia frequently is associated with marrow hypoplasia. Maintenance of remission generally involves multiple drug regimens whose component agents cause myelosuppression. Anemia, leukopenia, and thrombocytopenia are frequently observed. Dosages and schedules are adjusted to prevent life-threatening cytopenias.

Renal: Hyperuricemia may occur in patients receiving Mercaptopurine as a consequence of rapid cell lysis accompanying the antineoplastic effect. Adverse effects can be minimized by increased hydration, urine alkalinization, and the prohylactic administration of a xanthine oxidase inhibitor such as allopurinol. The dosage of Mercaptopurine should be reduced to one-third to one-quarter of the usual dose if allopurinol is given concurrently.

Gastrointestinal: Intestinal ulceration has been reported.[18] Nausea, vomiting and anorexia are uncommon during initial administration. Mild diarrhea and sprue-like symptoms have been noted occasionally, but it is difficult at present to attribute these to the medication. Oral lesions are rarely seen, and when they occur they resemble thrush rather than antifolic ulcerations.

An increased risk of pancreatitis may be associated with the investigational use of Mercaptopurine in inflammatory bowel disease.[19,20,21]

Miscellaneous: While dermatologic reactions can occur as a consequence of disease, the administration of Mercaptopurine has been associated with skin rashes and hyperpigmentation.[22] Drug fever has been very rarely reported with Mercaptopurine. Before attributing fever to Mercaptopurine, every attempt should be made to exclude more common causes of pyrexia, such as sepsis, in patients with acute leukemia.

OVERDOSAGE

Signs and symptoms of overdosage may be immediate such as anorexia, nausea, vomiting and diarrhea; or delayed such as myelosuppression, liver dysfunction and gastroenteritis. Dialysis cannot be expected to clear Mercaptopurine. Hemodialysis is thought to be of marginal use due to the rapid intracellular incorporation of Mercaptopurine into active metabolites with long persistence. The oral LD_{50} of Mercaptopurine was determined to be 480 mg/kg in the mouse and 425 mg/kg in the rat.[23]

There is no known pharmacologic antagonist of Mercaptopurine. The drug should be discontinued immediately if unintended toxicity occurs during treatment. If a patient is seen immediately following an acidental overdosage of the drug, it may be useful to induce emesis.

DOSAGE AND ADMINISTRATION

Induction Therapy: Mercaptopurine is administered orally. The dosage which will be tolerated and be effective varies from patient to patient, and therefore careful titration is necessary to obtain the optimum therapeutic effect without incurring excessive, unintended toxicity. The usual initial dosage for children and adults is 2.5 mg/kg of body weight per day (100 to 200 mg in the average adult and 50 mg in an average 5-year-old child). Children with acute leukemia have tolerated this dose without difficulty in most cases; it may be continued daily for several weeks or more in some patients. If, after four weeks at this dosage, there is no clinical improvement and no definite evidence of leukocyte or platelet depression, the dosage may be increased up to 5 mg/kg daily. A dosage of 2.5 mg/kg per day may result in a rapid fall in leukocyte count within 1 to 2 weeks in some adults with acute lymphatic leukemia and high total leukocyte counts.

The total daily dosage may be given at one time. It is calculated to the nearest multiple of 25 mg. The dosage of Mercaptopurine should be reduced to one-third to one-quarter of the usual dose if allopurinol is given concurrently. Because the drug may have a delayed action, it should be discontinued at the first sign of an abnormally large or rapid fall in the leukocyte or platelet count. If subsequently the leukocyte count or platelet count remains constant for two or three days, or rises, treatment may be resumed.

Maintenance Therapy: Once a complete hematologic remission is obtained, maintenance therapy is considered essential. Maintenance doses will vary from patient to patient. A usual daily maintenance dose of Mercaptopurine is 1.5 to 2.5 mg/kg/day as a single dose. It is to be emphasized that in children with acute lymphatic leukemia in remission, superior results have been obtained when Mercaptopurine has been combined with other agents (most frequently with methotrexate) for remission maintenance. Mercaptopurine should rarely be relied

---

◆ RATED THERAPEUTICALLY EQUIVALENT; ◇ THERAPEUTIC EQUIVALENCE UNCONFIRMED; ○ UNRATED

upon as a single agent for the maintenance of remissions induced in acute leukemia.

Procedures for proper handling and disposal of anti-cancer drugs should be considered. Several guidelines on this subject have been published.[24-30]

There is no general agreement that all of the procedures recommended in the guidelines are necessary or appropriate.

Store at 15° to 25°C (59° to 77°F) in a dry place.

REFERENCES

1. Hitchings GH, Elion GB. The chemistry and biochemistry of purine analogs. *Ann NY Acad Sci.* 1954; 60:195-199. 2. Loo TL, Luce JK, Sullivan MP, Frei E III. Clinical pharmacologic observations on 6-mercaptopurine and 6-methylthiopurine ribonucleoside. *Clin Pharmacol Ther.* 1968; 9:180-194. 3. Elion GB. Biochemistry and pharmacology of purine analogs. *Fed Proc.* 1967; 26:898-904. 4. Scannell JP, Hitchings GH. Thioguanine in deoxyribonucleic acid from tumors of 6-mercaptopurine-treated mice. *Proc Soc Exp Biol Med.* 1966; 122:627-629. 5. Paterson ARP, Tidd DM. 6-thiopurines. In Sartorelli AC, Johns DG eds. *Antineoplastic and Immunosuppressive Agents*, Part II. Berlin, Springer-Verlag; 1975; 384-403. 6. Burchenal JH, Ellison RR, Murphy ML, et al. Clinical studies on 6-mercaptopurine. *Ann NY Acad Sc.* 1954; 60:359-368. 7. Farber S. Summary of experience with 6-mercaptopurine. *Ann NY Acad Sc.* 1954; 60:412-414. 8. Fountain JR. Clinical observations of the treatment of leukemia and allied disorders with 6-mercaptopurine. *Ann NY Acad Sc.* 1954; 60:439-446. 9. Hyman GA, Gellhorn A, Wolff JA. The therapeutic effect of mercaptopurine in a variety of human neoplastic diseases. *Ann NY Acad Sc.* 1954; 60:430-435. 10. Einhorn M, Davidsohn I. Hepatotoxicity of mercaptopurine *JAMA.* 1964: 188:802-806. 11. Schein PS, Winokur SH. Immunosuppressive and cytotoxic chemotherapy: long-term, complications. *Ann Intern Med.* 1975; 82:84-95. 12. Stern MH, Minow RA, Casey JH, Luna MA. Hepatoxicity in patients treated with adriamycin and 6-mercaptopurine for refractory leukemia. *Am J Clin Pathol.* 1975; 63:758-759. Abstract. 13. Blatt J, Mulvihill JJ, Ziegler JL, Young RC, Poplack DG. Pregnancy outcome following cancer chemotherapy. *Am J Med.* 1980; 69:828-832. 14. Nicholson HO. Cytotoxic drugs in pregnancy: review of reported cases. *J Obstet Gynaecol Br Commonw.* 1968; 75:307-312. 15. Woods WG, Daigle AE, Hutchinson RJ, Robison LL. Myelosuppression associated with co-trimoxazole as a prophylactic antibiotic in the maintenance phase of childhood acute lymphocytic leukemia. *J Pediatr.* 1984; 105:639-644. 16. Rees CA, Lennard L, Lilleyman JS, Maddocks JL. Disturbance of 6-mercaptopurine metabolism by cotrimoxazole in childhood lymphoblastic leukemia. *Cancer Chemother Pharmacol.* 1984; 12:87-89. 17. Reimers TJ, Sluss PM. 6-mercaptopurine treatment of pregnant mice: effects on second and third generations. *Science.* 1978; 201:65-67. 18. Clark PA, Hsia YE, Huntsman RG. Toxic complications of treatment with 6-mercaptopurine. *Br Med J [Clin Res].* 1960; 1:393-395. 19. Present DH, Meltzer SJ, Wolke A, Korelitz BI. Short and long term toxicity to 6-mercaptopurine in the management of inflammatory bowel disease. *Gastroenterology.* 1985; 88:1545. Abstract. 20. Bank L, Wright JP. 6-mercaptopurine-related pancreatitis in 2 patients with inflammatory bowel disease. *Dig Dis Sci.* 1984; 29:357-359. 21. Singleton JW, Law DH, Kelley ML Jr, Mekhjian HS, Sturdevant RAL. National Cooperative Crohn's disease study: adverse reactions to study drugs. *Gastroenterology.* 1979; 77:870-882. 22. Dreizen S, Bodey GP, Rodriguez V, McCredie KB. Cutaneous complications of cancer chemotherapy. *Postgrad Med.* 1975; 58(Nov):150-158. 23. Unpublished data on file with Burroughs Wellcome Co. 24. Recommendations for the safe handling of parenteral antineoplastic drugs. Washington, DC: Division of Safety: National Institutes of Health; 1983. US Dept of Health and Human Services. Public Health Service publication NIH 83-2621. 25. AMA Council Report on Scientific Affairs. Guidelines for handling parenteral antineoplastics, *JAMA.* 1985; 253:1590-1591. 26. National Study Commission on Cytotoxic Exposure. Recommendations for handling cytotoxic agents. 1984. Available from Louis P. Jeffrey, ScD, Director of Pharmacy Services, Rhode Island Hospital, 593 Eddy Street, Providence, RI 02902. 27. Clinical Oncological Society of Australia. Guidelines and recommendations for safe handling of antineoplastic agents. *Med J Australia.* 1983; 1:426-428. 28. Jones RB, Frank R, Mass T. Safe handling of chemotherapeutic agents: A report from the Mount Sinai Medical Center. *CA—A Cancer J for Clinicians.* 1983; 33:258-263. 29. American Society of Hospital Pharmacists. ASHP technical assistance bulletin on handling cytotoxic and hazardous drugs in hospitals. *Am J Hosp Pharm.* 1990; 47:1033-1049. 30. Yodaiken RE, Bennett D. OSHA work-practice guidelines for personnel dealing with cytotoxic (antineoplastic) drugs. *Am J Hosp Pharm.* 1986; 43:1193-1204.

HOW SUPPLIED
TABLETS: 50 MG

BRAND/MANUFACTURER	NDC	SIZE	AWP
○ **BRAND**			
PURINETHOL: Burr Wellcome	00081-0807-25	25s	$53.60
	00081-0807-65	250s	$510.64

Meruvax II *SEE* RUBELLA VIRUS VACCINE

Mesalamine

DESCRIPTION
The active ingredient Mesalamine is also known as 5-aminosalicylic acid (5-ASA). Chemically, Mesalamine is 5-amino-2-hydroxybenzoic acid, and is classified as an anti-inflammatory drug.

The empirical formula is $C_7H_7NO_3$, representing a molecular weight of 153.14.

Enema: Each rectal suspension enema unit contains 4 grams of Mesalamine.

Suppository: Each suppository contains 500 mg of Mesalamine in a base of Hard Fat, NF.

Controlled release capsule: each capsule contains 250 mg of Mesalamine.

Delayed release tablet: each tablet contains 400 mg of Mesalamine.

Following is its chemical structure:

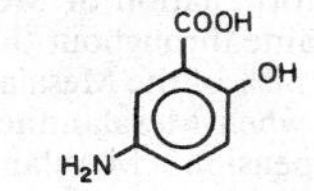

CLINICAL PHARMACOLOGY
Sulfasalazine is split by bacterial action in the colon into sulfapyridine (SP) and Mesalamine (5-ASA). It is thought that the Mesalamine component is therapeutically active in ulcerative colitis [A.K. Azad Khan et al, *Lancet* 2:892-895 (1977)]. The usual oral dose of sulfasalazine for active ulcerative colitis in adults is two to four grams per day in divided doses. Four grams of sulfasalazine provide 1.6 g of free Mesalamine to the colon. Each Mesalamine enema delivers up to 4 g of Mesalamine to the left side of the colon. Each Mesalamine suppository delivers 500 mg of Mesalamine to the rectum.

The mechanism of action of Mesalamine (and sulfasalazine) is unknown, but appears to be topical rather than systemic. Mucosal production of arachidonic acid (AA) metabolites, both through the cyclooxygenase pathways, i.e., prostanoids, and through the lipoxygenase pathways, i.e., leukotrienes (LTs) and hydroxyeicosatetraenoic acids (HETEs) is increased in patients with chronic inflammatory bowel disease, and it is possible that Mesalamine diminishes inflammation by blocking cyclooxygenase and inhibiting prostaglandin (PG) production in the colon.

PRECLINICAL TOXICOLOGY
Preclinical studies have shown the kidney to be the major target organ for Mesalamine toxicity. Adverse renal function changes were observed in rats after a single 600 mg/kg oral dose, but not after a 200 mg/kg dose. Gross kidney lesions, including papillary necrosis, were observed after a single oral > 900 mg/kg dose, and after i.v. doses of > 214 mg/kg. Mice responded similarly. In a 13-week oral (gavage) dose study in rats, the high dose of 640 mg/kg/day Mesalamine caused deaths, probably due to renal failure, and dose-related renal lesions (papillary necrosis and/or multifocal tubular injury) were seen in most rats given the high dose (males and females) as well as in males receiving lower doses 160 mg/kg/day. Renal lesions were not observed in the 160 mg/kg/day female rats. Minimal tubular epithelial damage was seen in the 40 mg/kg/day males and was reversible. In a six-month oral study in dogs, the no-observable dose level of Mesalamine was 40 mg/kg/day and doses of 80 mg/kg/day and higher caused renal pathology similar to that described for the rat. In a combined 52-week toxicity and 127-week carcinogenicity study in rats, degeneration in kidneys was observed at doses of 100 mg/kg/day and above admixed with diet for 52 weeks, and at 127 weeks increased incidence of kidney degeneration and hyalinization of basement membranes and Bowman's capsules was seen at 100 mg/kg/day and above. In the 12 month eye toxicity study in dogs, Keratocon junctivitis Sicca (KCS) occurred at oral doses of 40 mg/kg/day and above. The oral preclinical studies were done with a highly bioavailable suspension where absorption throughout the gastrointestinal tract occurred. The human dose of 4 grams represents approximately 80 mg/kg but when Mesalamine is given rectally as a suspension, absorption is poor and limited to the distal colon (see *"Pharmacokinetics"*). Overt renal toxicity has not been observed (see *"Adverse Reactions"* and *"Precautions"*), but the potential must be considered.

PHARMACOKINETICS
Enema and Suppository: Mesalamine administered rectally as Mesalamine suspension enema is poorly absorbed from the colon and is excreted principally in the feces through subsequent bowel movements. The extent of absorption is dependent upon the retention time of the drug product, and there is considerable individual variation. At steady state, approximately 10 to 30% of the daily 4-gram dose can be recovered in cumulative 24-hour urine collections. Other than the kidney, the organ distribution and other bioavailability characteristics of absorbed Mesalamine in man are not known. It is known that the compound undergoes acetylation but whether this process takes place at colonic or systemic sites has not been elucidated. Whatever the metabolic site, most of the absorbed Mesalamine is excreted in the urine as the N-acetyl-5-ASA metabolite. The poor colonic absorption of rectally administered Mesalamine is substantiated by the low serum concentration of 5-ASA and N-acetyl-5-ASA seen in ulcerative colitis patients after dosage with Mesalamine. Under clinical conditions patients demonstrated plasma levels 10 to 12 hours post Mesalamine administration of 2 µg/mL, about two-thirds of which was the N-acetyl metabolite. While the elimination half-life of Mesalamine is short (0.5 to 1.5 h), the acetylated metabolite exhibits a half-life of 5 to 10 hours [U. Klotz. *Clin. Pharmacokin,* 10:285-302 (1985)]. In addition, steady state plasma levels demonstrated a lack of accumulation of either free or metabolized drug during repeated daily administrations. Following single doses of Mesalamine 500 mg suppository in normal volunteers, 24-hr urines contained (only) N-acetylmesalamine equivalent to 15 to 38% (avg. 24%) of the administered dose. This is commensurate with the finding of 3 to 36% (avg. 10%) in urine in a study of Mesalamine 4 g enema in normals. In that study, 40 to 107% (avg 75%) of the administered dose was recovered in feces. At steady state in ulcerative colitis patients (n = 38) being treated with Mesalamine enema, 24-hr urines contained 0 to 41% (avg. 8%) of the 4 g daily dose and plasma levels 10 to 12 hr post administration ranged from 0 to 2.1 mcg/mL (avg. 0.37 mcg/mL) of Mesalamine equivalent (84% as N-acetyl metabolite). Multiple dose pharmacokinetic studies have not been conducted with Mesalamine suppository nor have plasma levels been reported from single dose studies.

➤ SHOWN IN PRODUCT IDENTIFICATION GUIDE

Controlled Release Capsule: Mesalamine controlled release capsule is an ethylcellulose-coated, controlled-release formulation of Mesalamine designed to release therapeutic quantities of Mesalamine throughout the gastrointestinal tract. Based on urinary excretion data, 20% to 30% of the Mesalamine in the controlled release capsule is absorbed. In contrast, when Mesalamine is administered orally as an unformulated 1-g aqueous suspension, Mesalamine is approximately 80% absorbed.

Plasma Mesalamine concentration peaked at approximately 1 µg/mL 3 hours following a 1-g Mesalamine dose and declined in a biphasic manner. The literature describes a mean terminal half-life of 42 minutes for Mesalamine following intravenous administration. Because of the continuous release and absorption of Mesalamine from Mesalamine throughout the gastrointestinal tract, the true elimination half-life cannot be determined after oral administration. N-acetylmesalamine, the major metabolite of Mesalamine, peaked at approximately 3 hours at 1.8 µg/mL, and its concentration followed a biphasic decline. Pharmacological activities of N-acetylmesalamine are unknown, and other metabolites have not been identified.

Oral Mesalamine pharmacokinetics were nonlinear when Mesalamine capsules were dosed from 250 mg to 1 g four times daily, with steady-state Mesalamine plasma concentrations increasing about nine times, from 0.14 µg/mL to 1.21 µg/mL, suggesting saturable first-pass metabolism. N-acetylmesalamine pharmacokinetics were linear.

Elimination: About 130 mg free Mesalamine was recovered in the feces following a single 1-g Mesalamine dose, which was comparable to the 140 mg of Mesalamine recovered from the molar equivalent sulfasalazine tablet dose of 2.5 g. Elimination of free Mesalamine and salicylates in feces increased proportionately with Mesalamine dose. N-acetylmesalamine was the primary compound excreted in the urine (19% to 30%) following Mesalamine dosing.

Delayed Release Tablets: Mesalamine tablets are coated with an acrylic-based resin that delays release of Mesalamine until it reaches the terminal ileum and beyond. This has been demonstrated in human studies conducted with radiological and serum markers. Approximately 28% of the Mesalamine in Mesalamine tablets is absorbed after oral ingestion, leaving the remainder available for topical action and excretion in the feces. Absorption of Mesalamine is similar in fasted and fed subjects. The absorbed Mesalamine is rapidly acetylated in the gut mucosal wall and by the liver. It is excreted mainly by the kidney as N-acetyl-5-aminosalicylic acid.

Mesalamine from orally administered Mesalamine tablets appears to be more extensively absorbed than the Mesalamine released from sulfasalazine. Maximum plasma levels of Mesalamine and N-acetyl-5-aminosalicylic acid following multiple Mesalamine doses are about 1.5 to 2 times higher than those following an equivalent dose of Mesalamine in the form of sulfasalazine. Combined Mesalamine and N-acetyl-5-aminosalicylic acid AUC's and urine drug dose recoveries following multiple doses of Mesalamine tablets are about 1.3 to 1.5 times higher than those following an equivalent dose of Mesalamine in the form of sulfasalazine.

The t_{max} for Mesalamine and its metabolite, N-acetyl-5-aminosalicyclic acid, is usually delayed, reflecting the delayed release, and ranges from 4 to 12 hours. The half-lives of elimination ($t_{1/2elm}$) for Mesalamine and N-acetyl-5-aminosalicylic acid are usually about 12 hours, but are variable, ranging from 2 to 15 hours. There is a large inter subject variability in the plasma concentrations of Mesalamine and N-acetyl-5-aminosalicyclic acid and in their elimination half-lives following administration of Mesalamine tablets.

EFFICACY

Mesalamine Suspension Enema: In a placebo-controlled, international, multicenter trial of 153 patients with active distal ulcerative colitis, proctosigmoiditis or proctitis, Mesalamine suspension enema reduced the overall disease activity index (DAI) and individual components as follows: (See related table).

Differences between Mesalamine Suspension Enema and placebo were also statistically different in subgroups of patients on concurrent sulfasalazine and in those having an upper disease boundary between 5 and 20 or 20 and 40 cm. Significant differences between Mesalamine Suspension Enema and placebo were not achieved in those subgroups of patients on concurrent prednisone or with an upper disease boundary between 40 and 50 cm.

Mesalamine Suppositories: Two double-blind placebo-controlled, multicenter studies were conducted in North America in patients with active ulcerative proctitis. The primary measures of efficacy were the same in both trials. The main difference between the two studies was the dosage regimen: 500 mg three times daily (1.5 g/d) in Study 1 and 500 mg twice daily (1.0 g/d) in Study 2. A total of 173 patients were studied (Study 1, n = 79; Study 2, n = 94) Patients were evaluated clinically and sigmoidoscopically after three and six weeks of suppository treatment.

Compared to placebo, Mesalamine suppository treatment was statistically (P < .01) superior in both trials with respect to stool frequency, rectal bleeding, mucosal appearance, disease severity and overall disease activity after both three and six weeks of treatment. Daily diary records indicated significant improvement in rectal bleeding in the first week of therapy while tenesmus and diarrhea improved significantly within two weeks. Investigators rated patients much improved in 84% and 79% with Mesalamine in Studies 1 and 2, respectively compared to 41% and 26% with placebo (P < .001, P < .001).

Normalization of rectal mucosa was achieved by 62% and 60% of Mesalamine-treated patients in Studies 1 and 2 compared to 25% and 10% of placebo-treated patients (P < .001, P < .001). The effectiveness of Mesalamine suppositories was statistically significant irrespective of sex, extent of proctitis, duration, of current episode or duration of disease. Overall the efficacy demonstrated with the twice daily regimen (Study 2) was comparable to that observed with three times daily dosing (Study 1).

Controlled Release Capsule: In two randomized, double-blind, placebo-controlled, dose-response trials (UC-1 and UC-2) of 625 patients with active mild to moderate ulcerative colitis, Mesalamine at an oral dose of 4 g/day given 1 g four times daily, produced consistent improvement in prospectively identified primary efficacy parameters, PGA, Tx F, and SI as shown in the table below.

The 4-g dose of Mesalamine also gave consistent improvement in secondary efficacy parameters, namely the frequency of trips to the toilet, stool consistency, rectal bleeding, abdominal/rectal pain, and urgency. The 4-g dose of Mesalamine induced remission as assessed by endoscopic and symptomatic endpoints.

In some patients, the 2-g dose of Mesalamine was observed to improve efficacy parameters measured. However, the 2-g dose gave inconsistent results in primary efficacy parameters across the two adequate and well-controlled trials. (See related table).

Delayed Release Tablet: Two placebo-controlled studies have demonstrated the efficacy of Mesalamine tablets in patients with mildly to moderately active ulcerative colitis. In one randomized, double-blind, multicenter trial of 158 patients, Mesalamine doses of 1.6 g/day and 2.4 g/day were compared to placebo. At the dose of 2.4 g/day, Mesalamine tablets reduced the disease activity, with 21 of 43 (49%. Mesalamine patients showing improvement in sigmoidoscopic appearance of the bowel compared to 12 of 44 (27%) placebo patients (p = 0.048). In addition, significantly more patients in the Mesalamine 2.4 g/day group showed improvement in rectal bleeding and stool frequency. The 1.6 g/day dose did not produce consistent evidence of effectiveness.

In a second randomized, double-blind, placebo-controlled clinical trial of 6 weeks duration in 87 ulcerative colitis patients, Mesalamine tablets, at a dose of 4.8 g/day, gave sigmoidoscopic improvement in 28 of 38 (74%) patients compared to 10 of 38 (26%) placebo patients (p < 0.001). Also, more patients in the Mesalamine 4.8 g/day group showed improvement in overall symptoms.

The effect of Mesalamine on sulfasalazine-induced impairment of male fertility was examined in an open-label study. Nine patients (age < 40 years) with chronic ulcerative colitis in clinical remission on sulfasalazine 2-3 g/day were crossed over to an equivalent Mesalamine dose (0.8-1.2 g/day) for 3 months. Improvement in sperm count (p < 0.02) and morphology (p < 0.02) occurred in all caes. Improvement in sperm motility (p < 0.001) occurred in 8 of the 9 patients.

INDICATIONS AND USAGE

Mesalamine suspension enema is indicated for the treatment of active mild to moderate distal ulcerative colitis, proctosigmoiditis or proctitis.

Mesalamine suppositories are indicated for the treatment of active ulcerative proctitis.

Mesalamine controlled release capsules is indicated for the induction of remission and for the treatment of patients with mildly to moderately active ulcerative colitis.

Mesalamine tablets are indicated for the treatment of mildly to moderately active ulcerative colitis.

CONTRAINDICATIONS

Mesalamine suspension enema is contraindicated for patients known to have hypersensitivity to the drug or any component of this medication, or salicylates.

Mesalamine suppositories are contraindicated for patients known to have hypersensitivity to mesalamine (5-aminosalicylic acid) or to the suppository vehicle (Hard Fat, NF).

WARNINGS

Mesalamine suspension enema contains potassium metabisulfite, a sulfite that may cause allergic-type reactions including anaphylactic symptoms and life-threatening or less severe asthmatic episodes in certain susceptible people. The overall prevalence of sulfite sensitivity in the general population is unknown but probably low. Sulfite sensitivity is seen more frequently in asthmatic or in atopic nonasthmatic persons.

Epinephrine is the preferred treatment for serious allergic or emergency situations even though epinephrine injection contains sodium or potassium metabisulfite with the above mentioned potential liabilities. The alternatives to using epinephrine in a life-threatening situation may not be satisfactory. The presence of a sulfite(s) in epinephrine injection should not deter the administration of the drug for treatment of serious allergic or other emergency situations.

PRECAUTIONS

Mesalamine has been implicated in the production of an acute intolerance syndrome characterized by cramping, acute abdominal pain and bloody diarrhea, sometimes fever, headache and a rash; in such cases prompt withdrawal is required. The patient's history of sulfasalazine intolerance, if any, should be re-evaluated. If a rechallenge is performed later in order to validate the hypersensitivity it should be carried out under close supervision and only if clearly needed, giving consideration to reduced dosage. In the literature one patient previously sensitive to sulfasalazine was rechallenged with 400 mg oral Mesalamine, within eight hours she experienced headache, fever, intensive abdominal colic, profuse diarrhea and was readmitted as an emergency. She responded poorly to steroid therapy and two weeks later a pancolectomy was required.

Caution should be exercised if Mesalamine controlled release capsules are administered to patients with impaired renal function. Single reports of nephrotic syndrome and interstitial nephritis associated with Mesalamine therapy have been described in the foreign literature. There have been rare reports of interstitial nephritis in patients receiving Mesalamine controlled release capsules. In animal studies, a 13-week oral toxicity study in mice and 13-week and 52-week oral toxicity studies in rats and cynomolgus monkeys have shown the kidney to be the major target organ of Mesalamine toxicity. Oral daily doses of 2400 mg/kg in mice and 1150 mg/kg in rats produced renal lesions including granular and hyaline casts, tubular degeneration, tubular dilation, renal infarct, papillary necrosis, tubular necrosis, and interstitial nephritis. In cynomolgus monkeys, oral daily doses of 250 mg/kg or higher produced nephrosis, papillary edema, and interstitial fibrosis. Patients with preexisting renal disease, increased BUN or serum creatinine, or proteinuria should be carefully monitored.

Although renal abnormalities were not noted in the clinical trials with Mesalamine suspension enema, the possibility of increased absorption of Mesalamine and concomitant renal tubular damage as noted in the preclinical studies must be kept in mind. Patients on Mesalamine especially those on concurrent oral products which liberate Mesalamine and those with preexisting renal disease, should be carefully monitored with urinalysis, BUN and creatinine studies.

Therefore, caution should be exercised when using Mesalamine or other compounds converted to Mesalamine or its metabolites in patients with known renal dysfunction or history of renal disease. It is recommended that all patients have an evaluation of renal function prior to initiation of Mesalamine tablets and periodically while on Mesalamine therapy.

In a clinical trial most patients who were hypersensitive to sulfasalazine were able to take Mesalamine rectally without evidence of any allergic reaction. Nevertheless, caution should be exercised when Mesalamine is initially used in patients known to be allergic to sulfasalazine. These patients should be instructed to discontinue therapy if signs of rash or fever become apparent.

While using Mesalamine some patients have developed pancolitis. However, extension of upper disease boundary and/or flare-ups occurred less often in the Mesalamine treated group than in the placebo-treated group.

Rare instances of pericarditis have been reported with Mesalamine containing products including sulfasalazine. Cases of pericarditis have also been reported as manifestations of inflammatory bowel disease. In the cases reported with Mesalamine Rectal Suspension Enema there have been positive rechallenges with Mesalamine or Mesalamine containing products. In one of these cases, however, a second rechallenge with sulfasalazine was negative throughout a 2 month follow-up. Chest pain or dypsnea in patients treated with Mesalamine should be investigated with this information in mind. Discontinuation of Mesalamine may be warranted in some cases, but rechallenge with Mesalamine can be performed under careful clinical observation should the continued therapeutic need for Mesalamine be present.

CARCINOGENESIS, MUTAGENESIS, IMPAIRMENT OF FERTILITY
Mesalamine caused no increase in the incidence of neoplastic lesions over controls in a two-year study of Wistar rats fed up to 300 mg/kg/day of Mesalamine admixed with diet. Mesalamine is not mutagenic to Salmonella typhimurium tester strains TA98, TA100, TA1535, TA1537, TA1538. There were no reverse mutations in an assay using E. coli strain WP2UVRA. There were no effects in an in vivo mouse micro nucleus assay at 600 mg/kg and in an in vivo sister chromatid exchange at I.P. doses up to 610 mg/kg. No effects on fertility were observed in rats receiving oral doses up to 320 mg/kg/day. The oligospermia and infertility in men associated with sulfasalazine have not been reported with Mesalamine.

EFFECT OF TREATMENT ON SEVERITY OF DISEASE DATA FROM U.S.-CANADA TRIAL COMBINED RESULTS OF EIGHT CENTERS

			Activity Indices, mean			
		n	Baseline	Day 22	End-Point	Change Baseline To End-Point†
Overall DAI	Mesalamine Suspension Enema	76	7.42	4.05**	3.37***	-55.07%***
	Placebo	77	7.40	6.03	5.83	-21.58%
Stool Frequency	Mesalamine Suspension Enema		1.58	1.11*	1.01**	-0.57*
	Placebo		1.92	1.47	1.50	-0.41
Rectal Bleeding	Mesalamine Suspension Enema		1.82	0.59***	0.51***	-1.30***
	Placebo		1.73	1.21	1.11	-0.61
Mucosal Inflammation	Mesalamine Suspension Enema		2.17	1.22**	0.96***	-1.21**
	Placebo		2.18	1.74	1.61	-0.56
Physician's Assessment of Disease Severity	Mesalamine Suspension Enema		1.86	1.13***	0.88***	-0.97***
	Placebo		1.87	1.62	1.55	-0.30

Each parameter has a 4-point scale with a numerical rating: 0 = normal, 1 = mild, 2 = moderate, 3 = severe. The four parameters are added together to produce a maximum overall DAI of 12.
† Percent change for overall DAI only (calculated by taking the average of the change for each individual patient).
* Significant Mesalamine Suspension Enema/placebo difference. p < 0.05
** Significant Mesalamine Suspension Enema/placebo difference. p < 0.01
*** Significant/ placebo difference, p < 0.001

	Clinical Trial UC.1			Clinical Trial UC.2		
	Mesalamine Controlled Release Capsules			Mesalamine Controlled Release Capsules		
Parameter Evaluated	PL (n = 90)	4 g/day (n = 95)	2 g/day PL (n = 97)	(n = 83)	4 g/day (n = 85)	2 g/day (n = 83)
PGA	36%	59%*	57%*	31%	55%*	41%
Tx F	22%	9%*	18%	31*	9%*	17%*
SI	-2.5	-5.0*	-4.3*	-1.6	-3.8*	-2.6
Remission†	12%	26%*	24%*	12%	27%*	12%

* p < 0.05 vs placebo.
PGA: Physician Global Assessment: proportion of patients with complete or marked improvement.
Tx F: Treatment Failure: proportion of patients developing severe or fulminant UC requiring steroid therapy or hospitalization or worsening of the disease at 7 days of therapy, or lack of significant improvement by 14 days of therapy.
SI: Sigmoidoscopic Index: an objective measure of disease activity rated by a standard (15-point) scale that includes mucosal vascular pattern, erythema, friability, granularity/ulcerations, and mucopus: improvement over baseline.
† Defined as complete resolution of symptoms plus improvement of endoscopic endpoints. To be considered in remission, patients had a "1" score for one of the endoscopic components (mucosal vascular pattern, erythema, granularity, or friability) and "0" for the others.

► SHOWN IN PRODUCT IDENTIFICATION GUIDE

PREGNANCY (CATEGORY B)

Teratologic studies have been performed in rats and rabbits at oral doses of up to ten and sixteen times respectively, the maximum recommended human rectal suppository dose, and have revealed no evidence of harm to the embryo or the fetus. There are, however, no adequate and well controlled studies in pregnant women for either sulfasalazine or Mesalamine. Because animal reproduction studies are not always predictive of human response Mesalamine should be used during pregnancy only if clearly needed.

NURSING MOTHERS

Minute quantities of Mesalamine were distributed to breast milk and amniotic fluid of pregnant women following sulfasalazine therapy. When treated with sulfasalazine at a dose equivalent to 1.25 g/day of Mesalamine, 0.02 µg/mL to 0.08 µg/mL and trace amounts of Mesalamine were measured in amniotic fluid and breast milk, respectively. N-acetylmesalamine, in quantities of 0.07 µg/mL to 0.77 µg/mL and 1.13 µg/mL to 3.44 µg/mL, was identified in the same fluids, respectively.

Caution should be exercised when Mesalamine is administered to a nursing woman.

PEDIATRIC USE

Safety and effectiveness in children have not been established.

ADVERSE REACTIONS

CLINICAL ADVERSE EXPERIENCE

Enema: Mesalamine suspension enema is usually well tolerated. Most adverse effects have been mild and transient.

ADVERSE REACTIONS OCCURRING IN MORE THAN 0.1% OF MESALAMINE SUSPENSION ENEMA TREATED PATIENTS (COMPARISON TO PLACEBO)

Symptom	Mesalamine (n = 815) n	%	Placebo (n = 128) n	%
Abdominal Pain/ Cramps/Discomfort	66	8.10	10	7.81
Headache	53	6.50	16	12.50
Gas/Flatulence	50	6.13	5	3.91
Nausea	47	5.77	12	9.38
Flu	43	5.28	1	0.78
Tired/Weak/Malaise/ Fatigue	28	3.44	8	6.25
Fever	26	3.19	0	0.00
Rash/Spots	23	2.82	4	3.12
Cold/Sore Throat	19	2.33	9	7.03
Diarrhea	17	2.09	5	3.91
Leg/Joint Pain	17	2.09	1	0.78
Dizziness	15	1.84	3	2.34
Bloating	12	1.47	2	1.56
Back Pain	11	1.35	1	0.78
Pain on Insertion of Enema Tip	11	1.35	1	0.78
Hemorrhoids	11	1.35	0	0.00
Itching	10	1.23	1	0.78
Rectal Pain	10	1.23	0	0.00
Constipation	8	0.98	4	3.12
Hair Loss	7	0.86	0	0.00
Peripheral Edema	5	0.61	11	8.59
UTI/Urinary Burning	5	0.61	4	3.12
Rectal Pain/Soreness/Burning	5	0.61	3	2.34
Asthenia	1	0.12	4	3.12
Insomnia	1	0.12	3	2.34

HAIR LOSS

Mild hair loss characterized by "more hair in the comb" but no withdrawal from clinical trials has been observed in seven of 815 Mesalamine patients but none of the placebo-treated patients. In the literature there are at least six additional patients with mild hair loss who received either Mesalamine or sulfasalazine. Retreatment is not always associated with repeated hair loss.

SUPPOSITORY: ADVERSE REACTIONS OCCURRING IN MORE THAN 1% OF MESALAMINE SUPPOSITORY-TREATED PATIENTS (COMPARISON TO PLACEBO)

Symptom	Mesalamine (n = 168) n	%	Placebo (n = 84) n	%
Headache	11	6.5	10	11.9
Flatulence	6	3.6	6	7.1
Abdominal Pain	5	3.0	7	8.3
Diarrhea	5	3.0	5	6.0
Dizziness	5	3.0	2	2.4
Rectal Pain	3	1.8	0	0.0
Upper Resp. Infection	3	1.8	2	2.4
Acne	2	1.2	0	0.0

Symptom	Mesalamine (n = 168) n	%	Placebo (n = 84) n	%
Asthenia	2	1.2	4	4.8
Colitis	2	1.2	0	0.0
Fever	2	1.2	0	0.0
Generalized Edema	2	1.2	1	1.2
Nausea	2	1.2	6	7.1
Rash	2	1.2	0	0.0

In addition, the following adverse events have been associated with Mesalamine: nephrotoxicity, pancreatitis, fibrosing alveolitis and elevated liver enzymes. Cases of pancreatitis and fibrosing alveolitis have been reported as manifestations of inflammatory bowel disease as well.

Controlled Release Capsules: In combined domestic and foreign clinical trials, more than 2100 patients with ulcerative colitis or Crohn's disease received Mesalamine therapy. Generally Mesalamine therapy was well tolerated. The most common events (ie, greater than or equal to 1%) were diarrhea (3.4%), headache (2.0%), nausea (1.8%), abdominal pain (1.7%), dyspepsia (1.6%), vomiting (1.5%), and rash (1.0%).

In two domestic placebo-controlled trials involving over 600 ulcerative colitis patients, adverse events were fewer in Mesalamine treated patients than in the placebo group Mesalamine 14% vs placedo 18%) and were not dose-related. Events occurring at 1% or more are shown in the table below. Of these, only nausea and vomiting were more frequent in the Mesalamine group. Withdrawal from therapy due to adverse events was more common on placebo than Mesalamine (7% vs 4%).

ADVERSE EVENTS OCCURRING IN MORE THAN 1% OF EITHER PLACEBO OR MESALAMINE CONTROLLED RELEASE CAPSULES PATIENTS IN DOMESTIC PLACEBO-CONTROLLED ULCERATIVE COLITIS TRIALS. (MESALAMINE CONTROLLED RELEASE CAPSULES COMPARISON TO PLACEBO)

Event	Capsules n = 451	Placebo n = 173
Diarrhea	16 (3.5%)	13 (7.5%)
Headache	10 (2.2%)	6 (3.5%)
Nausea	14 (3.1%)	—
Abdominal Pain	5 (1.1%)	7 (4.0%)
Melena (Bloody Diarrhea)	4 (0.9%)	6 (3.5%)
Rash	6 (1.3%)	2 (1.2%)
Anorexia	5 (1.1%)	2 (1.2%)
Fever	4 (0.9%)	2 (1.2%)
Rectal Urgency	1 (0.2%)	4 (2.3%)
Nausea and Vomiting	5 (1.1%)	—
Worsening of Ulcerative Colitis	2 (0.4%)	2 (1.2%)
Acne	1 (0.2%)	2 (1.2%)

Clinical laboratory measurements showed no significant abnormal trends for any test, including measurement of hematologic, liver, and kidney function.

The following adverse events, presented by body system, were reported infrequently (ie, less than 1%) during domestic ulcerative colitis and Crohn's disease trials. In many cases, the relationship to Mesalamine has not been established.

Gastrointestinal: abdominal distention, anorexia, constipation, duodenal ulcer, dysphagia, eructation, esophageal ulcer, fecal incontinence, GGTP increase, GI bleeding, increased alkaline phosphatase, LDH increase, mouth ulcer, oral moniliases, pancreatitis, rectal bleeding, SGOT increase, SGPT increase, stool abnormalities (color or texture change), thirst.

Dermatological: acne, alopecia, dry skin, eczema, erythema nodosum, nail disorder, photosensitivity, pruritus, sweating, urticaria.

Nervous System: depression, dizziness, insomnia, somnolence, paresthesia.

Cardiovascular: palpitations, pericarditis, vasodilation.

Other: albuminuria, amenorrhea, amylase increase, arthralgia, asthenia, breast pain, conjunctivitis, ecchymosis, edema, fever, hematuria, hypomenorrhea, Kawasaki-like syndrome, leg cramps, lichen planus, lipase increase, malaise, menorrhagia, metrorrhagia, myalgia, pulmonary infiltrates, thrombocythemia, thrombocytopenia, urinary frequency.

One week after completion of an 8-week ulcerative colitis study, a 72-year-old male, with no previous history of pulmonary problems, developed dyspnea. The patient was subsequently diagnosed with interstitial pulmonary fibrosis without eosinophilia by one physician and bronchiolitis obliterans with organizing pneumonitis by a second physician. A causal relationship between this event and Mesalamine therapy has not been established.

Published case reports have described infrequent instances of pericarditis, fatal myocarditis, chest pain and T-wave abnormalities, hypersensitivity pneumonitis, pancreatitis, nephrotic syndrome, interstitial nephritis, or hepatitis while receiving Mesalamine therapy.

Delayed Release Tablets: Mesalamine tablets have been evaluated in about 1830 inflammatory bowel disease patients (most patients with ulcerative colitis)

◆ RATED THERAPEUTICALLY EQUIVALENT; ◇ THERAPEUTIC EQUIVALENCE UNCONFIRMED; ○ UNRATED

in controlled and open-label studies. Adverse events seen in clinical trials with Mesalamine tablets have generally been mild and reversible. In two short-term (6 weeks) placebo-controlled clinical studies involving 245 patients, 155 of whom were randomized to Mesalamine tablets, five (3.2%) of the Mesalamine patients discontinued Mesalamine therapy because of adverse events as compared to two (2.2%) of the placebo patients. Adverse reactions leading to withdrawal from Mesalamine tablets included (each in one patient): diarrhea and colitis flare; dizziness, nausea, joint pain, and headache; rash, lethargy and constipation; dry mouth, malaise, lower back discomfort, mild disorientation, mild indigestion and cramping; headache, nausea, malaise, aching, vomiting, muscle cramps, a stuffy head, plugged ears, and fever.

Adverse events occurring at a frequency of 2% or greater in the two short-term, double-blind, placebo-controlled trials mentioned above are listed in the table below. Overall, the incidence of adverse events seen with Mesalamine tablets was similar to placebo.

FREQUENCY (%) OF COMMON ADVERSE EVENTS REPORTED IN ULCERATIVE COLITIS PATIENTS TREATED WITH MESALAMINE TABLETS OR PLACEBO IN DOUBLE-BLIND CONTROLLED STUDIES

	Percent of Patients with Adverse Events	
Event	Placebo (n = 87)	Mesalamine tablets (n = 152)
Headache	36	35
Abdominal pain	14	18
Eructation	15	16
Pain	8	14
Nausea	15	13
Pharyngitis	9	11
Dizziness	8	8
Asthenia	15	7
Diarrhea	9	7
Back pain	5	7
Fever	8	6
Rash	3	6
Dyspepsia	1	6
Rhinitis	5	5
Arthralgia	3	5
Vomiting	2	5
Constipation	1	5
Hypertonia	3	5
Flatulence	7	3
Flu syndrome	2	3
Chills	2	3
Colitis exacerbation	0	3
Chest pain	2	3
Peripheral edema	2	3
Myalgia	1	3
Pruritus	0	3
Sweating	1	3
Dysmenorrhea	3	3

Of these adverse events, only rash showed a consistently higher frequency with increasing Mesalamine dose in these studies. In uncontrolled data, fever, flu syndrome, and headache also seemed dose-related.

In addition, the following adverse reactions were seen in 1-2% of the patients in the controlled studies: malaise, arthritis, increased cough, acne, and conjunctivitis.

Over 1800 patients have been treated with Mesalamine tablets in clinical studies. In addition to the adverse events listed above, the following adverse events also have been reported in controlled clinical studies, open-label studies, or foreign marketing experience. The relationship of the reported events to Mesalamine administration is unclear in many cases. Some complaints, including anorexia, joint pains, pyoderma gangrenosum, oral ulcers, and anemia could be part of the clinical presentation of inflammatory bowel disease.

Body as a Whole: Weakness, neck pain, abdominal enlargement, facial edema, edema.

Cardiovascular: Pericarditis (rare), myocarditis (rare), vasodilation, migraine.

Digestive: Anorexia, hepatitis (rare), pancreatitis, gastroenteritis, gastritis, increased appetite, cholecystitis, dry mouth, oral ulcers, perforated peptic ulcer (rare), bloody diarrhea, tenesmus.

Hematologic: Agranulocytosis (rare), thrombocytopenia, eosinophilia, leukopenia, anemia, lymphadenopathy.

Musculoskeletal: Gout.

Nervous: Anxiety, insomnia, depression, somnolence, emotional lability, hyperesthesia, vertigo, nervousness, confusion, paresthesia, tremor, peripheral neuropathy (rare), transverse myelitis (rare), Guillain-Barre syndrome (rare).

Respiratory/Pulmonary: Sinusitis, interstitial pneumonitis, asthma exacerbation.

Skin: Alopecia, psoriasis (rare), pyoderma gangrenosum (rare), dry skin, erythema nodosum, urticaria.

Special Senses: Ear pain, eye pain, taste perversion, blurred vision, tinnitus.

Urogenital: Interstitial nephritis (see also "Renal" subsection in "Precautions") minimal change nephropathy (see also "Renal" subsection in "Precaution"), dysuria, urinary urgency, hematuria, epididymitis, menorrhagia.

Laboratory Abnormalities: Elevated AST (SGPT) or ALT (SGOT), elevated alkaline phosphatase, elevated serum creatinine and BUN.

Hepatitis has been reported to occur rarely with Mesalamine tablets. More commonly, asymptomatic elevations of liver enzymes have occurred which usually resolve during continued use or with discontinuation of the drug.

OVERDOSAGE

Single oral doses of Mesalamine up to 5 g/kg in pigs or a single intravenous dose of Mesalamine at 920 mg/kg in rats were not lethal.

There is no clinical experience with Mesalamine overdosage. Mesalamine is an aminosalicylate, and symptoms of salicylate toxicity may be possible, such as: tinnitus, vertigo, headache, confusion, drowsiness, sweating, hyperventilation, vomiting, and diarrhea. Severe intoxication with salicylates can lead to disruption of electrolyte balance and blood pH, hyperthermia, and dehydration.

Treatment of Overdosage: Since Mesalamine is an aminosalicylate, conventional therapy for salicylate toxicity may be beneficial in the event of acute overdosage. This includes prevention of further gastrointestinal tract absorption by emesis and, if necessary, by gastric lavage. Fluid and electrolyte imbalance should be corrected by the administration of appropriate intravenous therapy. Adequate renal function should be maintained.

One case of overdosage has been reported. A 3-year-old male ingested 2 grams of Mesalamine tablets. He was treated with ipecac and activated charcoal. No adverse events occurred. Oral doses of mesalamine in mice and rats of 5000 mg/kg and 4595 mg/kg, respectively, cause significant lethality.

DOSAGE AND ADMINISTRATION

Mesalamine Suspension Enema: The usual dosage of Mesalamine suspension enema in 60 mL units is one rectal instillation (4 grams) once a day, preferably at bedtime, and retained for approximately eight hours. While the effect of Mesalamine may be seen within three to twenty-one days, the usual course of therapy would be from three to six weeks depending on symptoms and sigmoidoscopic findings. Studies available to date have not assessed if Mesalamine suspension enema will modify relapse rates after the 6-week short-term treatment.

Patients should be instructed to shake the bottle well to make sure the suspension is homogeneous. The patient should remove the protective sheath from the applicator tip. Holding the bottle at the neck will not cause any of the medication to be discharged. The position most often used is obtained by lying on the left side (to facilitate migration into the sigmoid colon); with the lower leg extended and the upper right leg flexed forward for balance. An alternative is the knee-chest position. The applicator tip should be gently inserted in the rectum pointing toward the umbilicus. A steady squeezing of the bottle will discharge most of the preparation. The preparation should be taken at bedtime with the objective of retaining it all night. Patient instructions are included with every seven units.

Mesalamine Suppositories: The usual dosage of Mesalamine suppositories 500 mg is one rectal suppository 2 times daily. The suppository should be retained for one to three hours or longer, if possible, to achieve the maximum benefit. While the effect of Mesalamine suppositories may be seen within three to twenty-one days, the usual course of therapy would be from three to six weeks depending on symptoms and sigmoidoscopic findings. Studies available to date have not assessed if Mesalamine suppositories will modify relapse rates after the six-week short-term treatment.

Patient Instructions:
1. Detach one suppository from strip of suppositories.
2. Hold suppository upright and carefully remove the foil wrapper.
3. Avoid excessive handling of suppository, which is designed to melt at body temperature.
4. Insert suppository completely into rectum with gentle pressure, pointed end first.

Controlled Release Capsules: The recommended dosage for the induction of remission and the symptomatic treatment of mildly to moderately active ulcerative colitis is 1 g (4 Mesalamine capsules) four times a day for a total daily dose of 4 g. Treatment duration in controlled trials was up to 8 weeks.

Delayed Release Tablets: The usual dosage in adults is two 400-mg tablets to be taken three times a day for a total daily dose of 2.4 grams for a duration of 6 weeks.

STORAGE

Mesalamine Suspension Enema: Store at controlled room temperature 15° to 30°C (59° to 86°F). Once the foil-wrapped unit of seven bottles is opened, all enemas should be used promptly as directed by your physician. **Contents of enemas removed from the foil pouch may darken with time. Slight darkening will not affect potency, however enemas with dark brown contents should be discarded.**

Note: Mesalamine suspension enema may cause staining of garments, fabrics, painted surfaces, marble, granite, vinyl or other direct contact surfaces.

Controlled Release Capsules and Delayed Release Tablets: Store at controlled room temperature 59°-86°F (15°-30°C).

➤ SHOWN IN PRODUCT IDENTIFICATION GUIDE

HOW SUPPLIED
CAPSULE, EXTENDED RELEASE: 250 MG

BRAND/MANUFACTURER	NDC	SIZE	AWP
○ BRAND			
PENTASA: Marion Merrell Dow	00088-2010-80	80s	$26.94
	00088-2010-46	240s	$80.82
	00088-2010-90	5000s	$1590.00

LIQUID: 4 GM

BRAND/MANUFACTURER	NDC	SIZE	AWP
○ BRAND			
ROWASA: Solvay	00032-1924-82	60 ml 7s	$61.12

SUPPOSITORY: 500 MG

BRAND/MANUFACTURER	NDC	SIZE	AWP
○ BRAND			
ROWASA: Solvay	00032-1928-46	12s	$33.28
	00032-1928-24	24s	$63.21

TABLET, EXTENDED RELEASE: 400 MG

BRAND/MANUFACTURER	NDC	SIZE	AWP
○ BRAND			
ASACOL: P&G Pharm	00149-0752-02	100s	$57.13

Mesantoin SEE MEPHENYTOIN

Mesna

DESCRIPTION
Mesna Injection is a detoxifying agent to inhibit the hemorrhagic cystitis induced by ifosfamide. Mesna is a synthetic sulfhydryl compound designated as sodium 2-mercaptoethanesulfonate with a molecular formula of $C_2H_5NaO_3S_2$ and a molecular weight of 164.18.

Mesna Injection is a sterile preservative-free aqueous solution of clear and colorless appearance in clear glass ampules for intravenous administration. The Injection contains 100 mg/mL Mesna, 0.25 mg/mL edetate disodium and sodium hydroxide for pH adjustment. The solution has a pH range of 6.5-8.5.

CLINICAL PHARMACOLOGY
Mesna was developed as a prophylactic agent to prevent the hemorrhagic cystitis induced by ifosfamide.

Analogous to the physiological cysteine-cystine system, following intravenous administration, Mesna is rapidly oxidized to its only metabolite, Mesna disulfide (dimesna). Mesna disulfide remains in the intravascular compartment and is rapidly eliminated by the kidneys.

In the kidney, the Mesna disulfide is reduced to the free thiol compound Mesna, which reacts chemically with the urotoxic ifosfamide metabolites (acrolein and 4-hydroxy-ifosfamide) resulting in their detoxification. The first step in the detoxification process is the binding of Mesna to 4-hydroxy-ifosfamide forming a nonurotoxic 4-sulfoethylthioifosfamide. Mesna also binds to the double bonds of acrolein and other urotoxic metabolites.

After administration of an 800 mg dose the half-lives of Mesna and diMesna in the blood are 0.36 hours and 1.17 hours, respectively. Approximately 32% and 33% of the administered dose was eliminated in the urine in 24 hours as Mesna and diMesna, respectively. The majority of the dose recovered was eliminated within 4 hours. Mesna has a volume of distribution of 0.652 L/kg and a plasma clearance of 1.23 L/kg/hour.

Ifosfamide has been shown to have dose-dependent pharmacokinetics in humans. At doses of 2-4 g, its terminal elimination half-life is about 7 hours. As a result, in order to maintain adequate levels of Mesna in the urinary bladder during the course of elimination of the urotoxic ifosfamide metabolites, repeated doses of Mesna are required.

Based on the pharmacokinetic profiles of Mesna and ifosfamide as discussed above, Mesna was given as bolus doses prior to ifosfamide and at 4 and 8 hours after ifosfamide administration. The hemorrhagic cystitis produced by ifosfamide is dose dependent. At a dose of 1.2 g/m^2 ifosfamide administered daily for 5 days, 16% to 26% of the patients who received conventional uroprophylaxis (high fluid intake, alkalinization of the urine and the administration of diuretics) developed hematuria (> 50 rbc/hpf or macrohematuria). In contrast none of the patients who received Mesna together with this dose of ifosfamide developed hematuria. Higher doses of ifosfamide from 2 to 4 g/m^2 administered for 3 to 5 days, produced hematuria in 31% to 100% of the patients. When Mesna was administered together with these doses of ifosfamide the incidence of hematuria was less than 7%.

INDICATIONS AND USAGE
Mesna has been shown to be effective as a prophylactic agent in reducing the incidence of ifosfamide-induced hemorrhagic cystitis.

CONTRAINDICATIONS
Mesna is contraindicated in patients known to be hypersensitive to Mesna or other thiol compounds.

WARNINGS
Mesna has been developed as an agent to prevent ifosfamide-induced hemorrhagic cystitis. It will not prevent or alleviate any of the other adverse reactions or toxicities associated with ifosfamide therapy.

Mesna does not prevent hemorrhagic cystitis in all patients. Up to 6% of patients treated with Mesna have developed hematuria (> 50 rbc/hpf or WHO grade 2 and above). As a result, a morning specimen of urine should be examined for the presence of hematuria (red blood cells) each day prior to ifosfamide therapy. If hematuria develops when Mesna is given with ifosfamide according to the recommended dosage schedule, depending on the severity of the hematuria, dosage reductions or discontinuation of ifosfamide therapy may be initiated.

In order to obtain adequate protection, Mesna must be administered with each dose of ifosfamide as outlined in the Dosage and Administration section. Mesna is not effective in preventing hematuria due to other pathological conditions such as thrombocytopenia.

PRECAUTIONS
LABORATORY TESTS
A false positive test for urinary ketones may arise in patients treated with Mesna. In this test, a red-violet color develops which, with the addition of glacial acetic acid, will return to violet.

DRUG INTERACTIONS
In vitro and in vivo animal tumor models have shown that Mesna does not have any effect on the antitumor efficacy of concomitantly administered cytotoxic agents.

CARCINOGENESIS, MUTAGENESIS AND IMPAIRMENT OF FERTILITY
No long term animal studies have been performed to evaluate the carcinogenic potential of Mesna. The Ames Salmonella typhimurium test, mouse micronucleus assay and frequency of sister chromatid exchange and chromosomal aberrations in PHA-stimulated lymphocytes in vitro assays revealed no mutagenic activity.

PREGNANCY
Pregnancy Category B: Reproduction studies in rats and rabbits with oral doses up to 1000 mg/kg have revealed no harm to the fetus due to Mesna. It is not known whether Mesna can cause fetal harm when administered to a pregnant woman or can affect reproductive capacity. Mesna should be given to a pregnant woman only if the benefits clearly outweigh any possible risks.

Teratology studies in rats and rabbits have shown no effects.

NURSING MOTHERS
It is not known whether Mesna or diMesna is excreted in human milk. Because many drugs are excreted in human milk and because of the potential for adverse reactions in nursing infants, a decision should be made whether to discontinue nursing or discontinue the drug, taking into account the importance of the drug to the mother.

ADVERSE REACTIONS
Because Mesna is used in combination with ifosfamide and other chemotherapeutic agents with documented toxicities, it is difficult to distinguish the adverse reactions which may be due to Mesna from those caused by the concomitantly administered cytostatic agents. As a result, the adverse reaction profile of Mesna was determined in three Phase I studies (16 subjects) utilizing intravenous and oral administration and two controlled studies in which ifosfamide and Mesna were compared to ifosfamide and standard prophylaxis.

In Phase I studies in which IV bolus doses of 0.8 to 1.6 g/m^2 Mesna were administered as single or three repeated doses to a total of 10 patients, a bad taste in the mouth (100%) and soft stools (70%) were reported. At intravenous and oral bolus doses of 2.4 g/m^2 which are approximately 10 times the recommended clinical doses (0.24 g/m^2) headache (50%), fatigue (33%), nausea (33%), diarrhea (83%), limb pain (50%), hypotension (17%), and allergy (17%) have also been reported in the 6 patients who participated in this study. In controlled clinical studies, adverse reactions which can be reasonably associated with Mesna were vomiting, diarrhea and nausea.

OVERDOSAGE
There is no known antidote for Mesna.

DOSAGE AND ADMINISTRATION
For the prophylaxis of ifosfamide-induced hemorrhagic cystitis, Mesna may be given on a fractionated dosing schedule of bolus intravenous injections as outlined below.

Mesna is given as intravenous bolus injections in a dosage equal to 20% of the ifosfamide dosage (w/w) at the time of ifosfamide administration and 4 and 8 hours after each dose of ifosfamide. The total daily dose of Mesna is 60% of the ifosfamide dose.

◆ RATED THERAPEUTICALLY EQUIVALENT; ◇ THERAPEUTIC EQUIVALENCE UNCONFIRMED; ○ UNRATED

The recommended dosing schedule is outlined below:

	0 Hours	4 Hours	8 Hours
Ifosfamide	1.2 g/m^2	-	-
Mesna	240 mg/m^2	240 mg/m^2	240 mg/m^2

In order to maintain adequate protection, this dosing schedule should be repeated on each day that ifosfamide is administered. When the dosage of ifosfamide is adjusted (either increased or decreased), the dose of Mesna should be modified accordingly. When exposed to oxygen Mesna is oxidized to the disulfide, diMesna. As a result, any unused drug remaining in the ampules after dosing should be discarded and new ampules used for each administration.

PREPARATION OF INTRAVENOUS SOLUTIONS/STABILITY

For IV administration the drug can be diluted by adding the contents of a Mesna ampule to any of the following fluids obtaining final concentrations of 20 mg Mesna/mL fluid:

5% Dextrose Injection, USP
5% Dextrose and Sodium Chloride Injection, USP
0.9% Sodium Chloride Injection, USP
Lactated Ringer's Injection, USP
For example:
One ampule of Mesna Injection 200 mg/2 mL may be added to 8 mL, or one ampule of Mesna Injection 400 mg/4 mL may be added to 16 mL of any of the solutions listed above to create a final concentration of 20 mg Mesna mL fluid.

Diluted solutions are chemically and physically stable for 24 hours at 25°C (77°F).

It is recommended that solutions of Mesna be refrigerated and used within 6 hours.

Mesna is not compatible with cisplatin.

Parenteral drug products should be inspected visually for particulate matter and discoloration prior to administration.

Store at room temperature.

HOW SUPPLIED
KIT:

BRAND/MANUFACTURER	NDC	SIZE	AWP
BRAND			
IFEX/MESNEX: Bristol-Myer Onc/Hiv	00015-3558-41	1s	$741.13
	00015-3559-41	1s	$889.38
	00015-3557-41	1s	$1790.86

Mesoridazine Besylate

DESCRIPTION
Mesoridazine Besylate, the besylate salt of a metabolite of thioridazine, is a phenothiazine tranquilizer that is effective in the treatment of schizophrenia, organic brain disorders, alcoholism and psychoneuroses.

Mesoridazine Besylate is 10-[2(1-methyl-2-piperidyl) ethyl]-2- (methyl-sulfinyl)-phenothiazine [as the Besylate].

Mesoridazine Besylate is available in 10 mg, 25 mg, 50 mg, and 100 mg tablets; in a 25 mg per mL oral concentrate; and in 1 mL ampuls providing 25 mg for intramuscular injection.

Following is its chemical structure:

ACTIONS
Based upon animal studies, Mesoridazine Besylate as with other phenothiazines, acts indirectly on reticular formation, whereby neuronal activity into reticular formation is reduced without affecting its intrinsic ability to activate the cerebral cortex. In addition, the phenothiazines exhibit at least part of their activities through depression of hypothalamic centers. Neurochemically, the phenothiazines are thought to exert their effects by a central adrenergic blocking action.

INDICATIONS
In clinical studies Mesoridazine Besylate has been found useful in the following disease states:

Schizophrenia: Mesoridazine Besylate is effective in the treatment of schizophrenia. It substantially reduces the severity of emotional withdrawal, conceptual disorganization, anxiety, tension, hallucinatory behavior, suspiciousness and blunted affect in schizophrenic patients. As with other phenothiazines, patients refractory to previous medication may respond to Mesoridazine Besylate.

Behavioral Problems in Mental Deficiency and Chronic Brain Syndrome: The effect of Mesoridazine Besylate was found to be excellent or good in the management of hyperactivity and uncooperativeness associated with mental deficiency and chronic brain syndrome.

Alcoholism—Acute and Chronic: Mesoridazine Besylate ameliorates anxiety, tension, depression, nausea and vomiting in both acute and chronic alcoholics without producing hepatic dysfunction or hindering the functional recovery of the impaired liver.

Psychoneurotic Manifestations: Mesoridazine Besylate reduces the symptoms of anxiety and tension, prevalent symptoms often associated with neurotic components of many disorders, and benefits personality disorders in general.

CONTRAINDICATIONS
As with other phenothiazines, Mesoridazine Besylate is contraindicated in severe central nervous system depression or comatose states from any cause. Mesoridazine Besylate is contraindicated in individuals who have previously shown hypersensitivity to the drug.

WARNINGS
Tardive Dyskinesia: Tardive dyskinesia, a syndrome consisting of potentially irreversible, involuntary, dyskinetic movements may develop in patients treated with neuroleptic (antipsychotic) drugs. Although the prevalence of the syndrome appears to be highest among the elderly, especially elderly women, it is impossible to rely upon prevalence estimates to predict, at the inception of neuroleptic treatment, which patients are likely to develop the syndrome. Whether neuroleptic drug products differ in their potential to cause tardive dyskinesia is unknown.

Both the risk of developing the syndrome and the likelihood that it will become irreversible are believed to increase as the duration of treatment and the total cumulative dose of neuroleptic drugs administered to the patient increase. However, the syndrome can develop, although much less commonly, after relatively brief treatment periods at low doses. There is no known treatment for established cases of tardive dyskinesia, although the syndrome may remit, partially or completely, if neuroleptic treatment is withdrawn. Neuroleptic treatment, itself, however, may suppress (or partially suppress) the signs and symptoms of the syndrome and thereby may possibly mask the underlying disease process. The effect that symptomatic suppression has upon the longterm course of the syndrome is unknown.

Given these considerations, neuroleptics should be prescribed in a manner that is most likely to minimize the occurrence of tardive dyskinesia. Chronic neuroleptic treatment should generally be reserved for patients who suffer from a chronic illness 1) that is known to respond to neuroleptic drugs, and 2) for which alternative, equally effective but potentially less harmful treatments are *not* available or appropriate. In patients who do require chronic treatment, the smallest dose and the shortest duration of treatment producing a satisfactory clinical response should be sought. The need for continued treatment should be reassessed periodically.

If signs and symptoms of tardive dyskinesia appear in a patient on neuroleptics, drug discontinuation should be considered. However, some patients may require treatment despite the presence of the syndrome.

(For further information about the description of tardive dyskinesia and its clinical detection, please refer to the sections on *"Information for Patients"* and *"Adverse Reactions."*)

Neuroleptic Malignant Syndrome (NMS): A potentially fatal symptom complex sometimes referred to as Neuroleptic Malignant Syndrome (NMS) has been reported in association with antipsychotic drugs. Clinical manifestations of NMS are hyperpyrexia, muscle rigidity, altered mental status and evidence of autonomic instability (irregular pulse or blood pressure, tachycardia, diaphoresis, and cardiac dysrhythmias).

The diagnostic evaluation of patients with this syndrome is complicated. In arriving at a diagnosis, it is important to identify cases where the clinical presentation includes both serious medical illness (e.g., pneumonia, systemic infection, etc.) and untreated or inadequately treated extrapyramidal signs and symptoms (EPS). Other important considerations in the differential diagnosis include central anticholinergic toxicity, heat stroke, drug fever and primary central nervous system (CNS) pathology.

The management of NMS should include 1) immediate discontinuation of antipsychotic drugs and other drugs not essential to concurrent therapy, 2) intensive symptomatic treatment and medical monitoring, and, 3) treatment of any concomitant serious medical problems for which specific treatments are available. There is no general agreement about specific pharmacological treatment regimens for uncomplicated NMS. If a patient requires antipsychotic drug treatment after recovery from NMS, the potential reintroduction of drug therapy should be carefully considered. The patient should be carefully monitored, since recurrences of NMS have been reported.

Where patients are participating in activities requiring complete mental alertness (e.g., driving), it is advisable to administer the phenothiazines cautiously and to increase the dosage gradually.

Usage in Pregnancy: The safety of this drug in pregnancy has not been established; hence, it should be given only when the anticipated benefits to be derived from treatment exceed the possible risks to mother and fetus.

Usage in Children: The use of Mesoridazine Besylate in children under 12 years of age is not recommended, because safe conditions for its use have not been established.

Attention should be paid to the fact that phenothiazines are capable of potentiating central nervous system depressants (e.g., anesthetics, opiates, alcohol, etc.) as well as atropine and phosphorus insecticides.

➤ SHOWN IN PRODUCT IDENTIFICATION GUIDE

PRECAUTIONS

While ocular changes have not to date been related to Mesoridazine Besylate, one should be aware that such changes have been seen with other drugs of this class. Because of possible hypotensive effects, reserve parenteral administration for bedfast patients or for acute ambulatory cases, and keep patient lying down for at least one-half hour after injection.

Leukopenia and/or agranulocytosis have been attributed to phenothiazine therapy. A single case of transient granulocytopenia has been associated with Mesoridazine Besylate. Since convulsive seizures have been reported, patients receiving anticonvulsant medication should be maintained on that regimen while receiving Mesoridazine Besylate.

Neuroleptic drugs elevate prolactin levels; the elevation persists during chronic administration. Tissue culture experiments indicate that approximately one-third of human breast cancers are prolactin dependent *in vitro*, a factor of potential importance if the prescription of these drugs is contemplated in a patient with a previously detected breast cancer. Although disturbances such as galactorrhea, amenorrhea, gynecomastia, and impotence have been reported, the clinical significance of elevated serum prolactin levels is unknown for most patients. An increase in mammary neoplasms has been found in rodents after chronic administration of neuroleptic drugs. Neither clinical studies nor epidemiologic studies conducted to date, however, have shown an association between chronic administration of these drugs and mammary tumorigenesis; the available evidence is considered too limited to be conclusive at this time.

Information for Patients: Given the likelihood that some patients exposed chronically to neuroleptics will develop tardive dyskinesia, it is advised that all patients in whom chronic use is contemplated be given, if possible, full information about this risk.

ADVERSE REACTIONS

Drowsiness and hypotension were the most prevalent side effects encountered. Side effects tended to reach their maximum level of severity early with the exception of a few (rigidity and motoric effects) which occurred later in therapy.

With the exceptions of tremor and rigidity, adverse reactions were generally found among those patients who received relatively high doses early in treatment. Clinical data showed no tendency for the investigators to terminate treatment because of side effects.

Mesoridazine Besylate has demonstrated a remarkably low incidence of adverse reactions when compared with other phenothiazine compounds.

Central Nervous System: Drowsiness, Parkinson's syndrome, dizziness, weakness, tremor, restlessness, ataxia, dystonia, rigidity, slurring, akathisia, and motoric reactions (opisthotonos) have been reported.

Autonomic Nervous System: Dry mouth, nausea and vomiting, fainting, stuffy nose, photophobia, constipation and blurred vision have occurred in some instances.

Genitourinary System: Inhibition of ejaculation, impotence, enuresis, and incontinence have been reported.

Skin: Itching, rash, hypertrophic papillae of the tongue and angioneurotic edema have been reported.

Cardiovascular System: Hypotension and tachycardia have been reported. EKG changes have occurred in some instances (see *"Phenothiazine Derivatives: Cardiovascular Effects"*).

Phenothiazine Derivatives: It should be noted that efficacy, indications and untoward effects have varied with the different phenothiazines. The physician should be aware that the following have occurred with one or more phenothiazines and should be considered whenever one of these drugs is used:

Autonomic Reactions: Miosis, obstipation, anorexia, paralytic ileus.

Cutaneous Reactions: Erythema, exfoliative dermatitis, contact dermatitis.

Blood Dyscrasias: Agranulocytosis, leukopenia, eosinophilia, thrombocytopenia, anemia, aplastic anemia, pancytopenia.

Allergic Reactions: Fever, laryngeal edema, angioneurotic edema, asthma.

Hepatotoxicity: Jaundice, biliary stasis.

Cardiovascular Effects: Changes in the terminal portion of the electrocardiogram, including prolongation of the Q-T interval, lowering and inversion of the T wave and appearance of a wave tentatively identified as a bifid T or a U wave have been observed in some patients receiving the phenothiazine tranquilizers, including Mesoridazine Besylate. To date, these appear to be due to altered repolarization and not related to myocardial damage. They appear to be reversible. While there is no evidence at present that these changes are in any way precursors of any significant disturbance of cardiac rhythm, it should be noted that sudden and unexpected deaths apparently due to cardiac arrest have occurred in patients previously showing characteristic electrocardiographic changes while taking the drug. The use of periodic electrocardiograms has been proposed but would appear to be of questionable value as a predictive device.

Hypotension, rarely resulting in cardiac arrest, has been noted.

Extrapyramidal Symptoms: Akathisia, agitation, motor restlessness, dystonic reactions, trismus, torticollis, opisthotonos, oculogyric crises, tremor, muscular rigidity, akinesia.

Tardive Dyskinesia: Chronic use of neuroleptics may be associated with the development of tardive dyskinesia. The salient features of this syndrome are described in the *"Warnings"* section and below.

The syndrome is characterized by involuntary choreoathetoid movements which variously involve the tongue, face, mouth, lips, or jaw (e.g., protrusion of the tongue, puffing of cheeks, puckering of the mouth, chewing movements), trunk and extremities. The severity of the syndrome and the degree of impairment produced vary widely.

The syndrome may become clinically recognizable either during treatment, upon dosage reduction, or upon withdrawal of treatment. Movements may decrease in intensity and may disappear altogether if further treatment with neuroleptics is withheld. It is generally believed that reversibility is more likely after short- rather than long-term neuroleptic exposure. Consequently, early detection of tardive dyskinesia is important. To increase the likelihood of detecting the syndrome at the earliest possible time, the dosage of neuroleptic drug should be reduced periodically (if clinically possible) and the patient observed for signs of the disorder. This maneuver is critical, for neuroleptic drugs may mask the signs of the syndrome.

Endocrine Disturbances: Menstrual irregularities, altered libido, gynecomastia, lactation, weight gain, edema. False positive pregnancy tests have been reported.

Urinary Disturbances: Retention, incontinence.

Others: Hyperpyrexia. Behavioral effects suggestive of a paradoxical reaction have been reported. These include excitement, bizarre dreams, aggravation of psychoses and toxic confusional states. More recently, a peculiar skin-eye syndrome has been recognized as a side effect following long-term treatment with phenothiazines. This reaction is marked by progressive pigmentation of areas of the skin or conjunctiva and/or accompanied by discoloration of the exposed sclera and cornea. Opacities of the anterior lens and cornea described as irregular or stellate in shape have also been reported. Systemic lupus erythematosus-like syndrome.

OVERDOSAGE

SYMPTOMS OF ACUTE OVERDOSAGE

—Drowsiness, confusion, disorientation, agitation, coma, death.
—Dryness of mouth, edema of glottis, laryngeal spasms, nasal congestion, blurred vision, vomiting.
—Hyperpyrexia, dilated pupils, muscle rigidity, hyperactive reflexes, areflexia.
—Stupor, and CNS depression or stimulation with convulsions followed by respiratory depression.
—Cardiac abnormalities, including QRS changes, tachycardia, hypotension, bilateral bundle branch block, ventricular fibrillation, shock, cardiac arrest and congestive heart failure. (See case description below.)

TREATMENT OF ACUTE OVERDOSAGE

No specific antidote is known. The drug is not dialyzable. Treatment should include:

—*General supportive:* measures with *emesis* and *gastric lavage.*

—*Respiratory assistance:* is apparently the most effective measure when indicated.

—*The administration of barbiturates:* for control of convulsions alleviates an increase in the cardiac work load, but should be undertaken with caution to avoid potentiation of respiratory depression.

—*Intramuscular paraldehyde* or *diazepam* provides anticonvulsant activity with less respiratory depression than do the barbiturates; diazepam seems to be preferred.

—*The use of digitalis and/or physostignine* may be considered in case of serious cardiovascular abnormalities or cardiac failure.

—Due to several cases of severe cardiotoxicity following Serentil® (mesoridazine besylate USP) overdose, *continuous ECG monitoring* of these patients is recommended. Two cases are described below:

Marrs-Simon et al (Cardiotoxic manifestations of Mesoridazine overdose. *Ann Emerg Med.* 1988;17:1074-1078) describes the management of a 20-year-old female who experienced severe cardiotoxicity following an overdose of Mesoridazine. The paper also describes similar cases from the published literature.

The serum Mesoridazine level in a 115-lb patient following ingestion of 4.5 g to 6.0 g of Serentil was 2.5 mcg/mL. She was comatose, hypotensive, convulsing, and had ECG changes. Twenty-four hours later, after hemoperfusion with activated charcoal, the Mesoridazine blood levels fell to 1.3 mcg/mL and the patient was normotensive and responsive.

DOSAGE AND ADMINISTRATION

The dosage of Mesoridazine Besylate, as in most medications, should be adjusted to the needs of the individual. The lowest effective dosage should always be used. When maximum response is achieved, dosage may be reduced gradually to a maintenance level.

Schizophrenia: For most patients, regardless of severity, a starting dose of 50 mg t.i.d. is recommended. The usual optimum total daily dose range is 100-400 mg per day.

Behavioral Problems in Mental Deficiency and Chronic Brain Syndrome: For most patients a starting dose of 25 mg t.i.d. is recommended. The usual optimum total daily dose range is 75-300 mg per day.

Alcoholism: For most patients the usual starting dose is 25 mg b.i.d. The usual optimum total daily dose range is 50-200 mg per day.

Psychoneurotic Manifestations: For most patients the usual starting dose is 10 mg t.i.d. The usual optimum total daily dose range is 30-150 mg per day.

◆ RATED THERAPEUTICALLY EQUIVALENT; ◇ THERAPEUTIC EQUIVALENCE UNCONFIRMED; ○ UNRATED

Injectable Form: In those situations in which an intramuscular form of medication is indicated, Mesoridazine Besylate injectable is available. For most patients a starting dose of 25 mg is recommended. The dose may be repeated in 30 to 60 minutes, if necessary. The usual optimum total daily dose range is 25-200 mg per day.

STORAGE
Tablets: Below 86°F (30°C).

Injection: Below 86°F (30° C); protect from light.

Oral Solution: Below 77°F (25°C). Protect from light. Dispense in amber glass bottles only.

The concentrate may be diluted with distilled water, acidified tap water, orange juice or grape juice.

Each dose should be diluted just prior to administration. Preparation and storage of bulk dilutions is not recommended.

PHARMACOLOGY
Pharmacological studies in laboratory animals have established that Mesoridazine Besylate has a spectrum of pharmacodynamic actions typical of a major tranquilizer. In common with other tranquilizers it inhibits spontaneous motor activity in mice, prolongs thiopental and hexobarbital sleeping time in mice and produces spindles and block of arousal reaction in the EEG of rabbits. It is effective in blocking spinal reflexes in the cat and antagonizes damphetamine excitation and toxicity in grouped mice. It shows a moderate adrenergic blocking activity *in vitro* and *in vivo* and antagonizes 5-hydroxytryptamine *in vivo*. Intravenously administered, it lowers the blood pressure of anesthetized dogs. It has a weak antiacetylcholine effect *in vitro*. The most outstanding activity of Mesoridazine Besylate is seen in tests developed to investigate antiemotive activity of drugs. Such tests are those in which the rat reacts to acute or chronic stress by increased defecation (emotogenic defecation) or tests in which "emotional mydriasis" is elicited in the mouse by an electric shock. In both of these tests Mesoridazine Besylate is effective in reducing emotive reactions. Its ED_{50} in inhibiting emotogenic defecation in the rat is 0.053 mg/kg (subcutaneous administration) Mesoridazine Besylate has a potent antiemetic action. The intravenous ED_{50} against apomorphine-induced emesis in the dog is 0.64 mg/kg Mesoridazine Besylate, in common with other phenothiazines, demonstrates antiarrhythmic activity in anesthetized dogs.

Metabolic studies in the dog and rabbit with tritium labeled Mesoridazine Besylate demonstrate that the compound is well absorbed from the gastrointestinal tract. The biological half-life of Mesoridazine Besylate in these studies appears to be somewhere between 24 and 48 hours. Although significant urinary excretion was observed following the administration of Mesoridazine Besylate, these studies also suggest that biliary excretion is an important excretion route for Mesoridazine Besylate and/or its metabolites.

TOXICITY STUDIES ACUTE LD$_{50}$ (mg/kg):

Route	Mouse	Rat	Rabbit	Dog
Oral	560 ± 62.5	644 ± 48	MLD = 800	MLD = 800
I.M.	—	509M 584F	405	—
I.V.	26 ± 0.08	—	—	—

Chronic toxicity studies were conducted in rats and dogs. Rats were administered Mesoridazine Besylate orally seven days per week for a period of 17 months in doses up to 160 mg/kg per day. Dogs were administered Mesoridazine Besylate orally seven days per week for a period of 13 months. The daily dosage of the drug was increased during the period of this test such that the "top-dose" group received a daily dose of 120 mg/kg of Mesoridazine Besylate for the last month of the study.

Untoward effects that occurred upon chronic administration of high dose levels included:

Rats: Reduction of food intake, slowed weight gain, morphological changes in pituitary-supported endocrine organs, and melanin-like pigment deposition in renal tissues.

Dogs: Emesis, muscle tremors, decreased food intake and death associated with aspiration of oral-gastric contents into the respiratory system.

Increased intrauterine resorptions were seen with Mesoridazine Besylate in rats at 70 mg/kg and in rabbits at 125 mg/kg but not at 60 and 100 mg/kg, respectively. No drug-related teratology was suggested by these reproductive studies.

Local irritation from the intramuscular injection of Mesoridazine Besylate was of the same order of magnitude as with other phenothiazines.

HOW SUPPLIED
CONCENTRATE: 25 MG/ML

BRAND/MANUFACTURER	NDC	SIZE	AWP
○ **BRAND** SERENTIL: Boehr Ingelheim	00597-0025-04	120 ml	$44.98

INJECTION: 25 MG

BRAND/MANUFACTURER	NDC	SIZE	AWP
○ **BRAND** SERENTIL: Boehr Ingelheim	00597-0027-02	1 ml 20s	$82.82

TABLETS: 10 MG

BRAND/MANUFACTURER	NDC	SIZE	AWP
○ **BRAND** SERENTIL: Boehr Ingelheim	00597-0020-01	100s	$51.32

TABLETS: 25 MG

BRAND/MANUFACTURER	NDC	SIZE	AWP
○ **BRAND** SERENTIL: Boehr Ingelheim	00597-0021-01	100s	$68.69

TABLETS: 50 MG

BRAND/MANUFACTURER	NDC	SIZE	AWP
○ **BRAND** SERENTIL: Boehr Ingelheim	00597-0022-01	100s	$77.56

TABLETS: 100 MG

BRAND/MANUFACTURER	NDC	SIZE	AWP
○ **BRAND** SERENTIL: Boehr Ingelheim	00597-0023-01	100s	$94.80

Mestinon *SEE* PYRIDOSTIGMINE BROMIDE

Mestranol and Norethindrone

DESCRIPTION
Patients should be counseled that this product does not protect against HIV infection (AIDS) and other sexually transmitted diseases.

Tablets provide a continuous oral contraceptive regimen consisting of 21 white tablets containing norethindrone 1 mg and mestranol 0.05 mg.

Norethindrone is a potent progestational agent with the chemical name 17-Hydroxy-19-Nor-17α-pregn-4-en-20-yn-3-one. Ethinyl estradiol is an estrogen with the chemical name 19-nor-17α-pregna-1, 3, 5(10)-trien-20-yne-3, 17-diol. Mestranol is an estrogen with the chemical name 3-Methoxy-19-nor-17α-pregna-1, 3, 5(10) -trien-20-yn-17-ol.

CLINICAL PHARMACOLOGY
Combination oral contraceptives act by suppression of gonadotrophins. Although the primary mechanism of this action is inhibition of ovulation, other alterations include changes in the cervical mucus (which increase the difficulty of sperm entry into the uterus) and the endometrium (which may reduce the likelihood of implantation).

INDICATIONS AND USAGE
Oral contraceptives are indicated for the prevention of pregnancy in women who elect to use these products as a method of contraception.

Oral contraceptives are highly effective. Table 1 lists the typical accidental pregnancy rates for users of combination oral contraceptives and other methods of contraception.[1] The efficacy of these contraceptive methods, except sterilization, depends upon the reliability with which they are used. Correct and consistent use of methods can result in lower failure rates.

Table 1
LOWEST EXPECTED AND TYPICAL FAILURE RATES DURING THE FIRST YEAR OF CONTINUOUS USE OF A METHOD

Method	% of Women Experiencing an Accidental Pregnancy in the First Year of Continuous Use	
	Lowest Expected[a]	Typical[b]
(No contraception)	(85)	(85)
Oral contraceptives		3
combined	0.1	N/A[c]
progestogen only	0.5	N/A[c]
Diaphragm with spermicidal cream or jelly	6	18
Spermicides alone (foam, creams, jellies and vaginal suppositories)	3	21
Vaginal sponge		
Nulliparous	6	18
Multiparous	>9	>28
IUD (medicated)	2	3[d]
Condom without spermicides	2	12
Periodic abstinence (all methods)	1-9	20
Injectable progestogen[e]	0.4	0.4
Implants	0.04	0.04

► **SHOWN IN PRODUCT IDENTIFICATION GUIDE**

Method	Lowest Expected[a]	Typical[b]
Female sterilization	0.2	0.4
Male sterilization	0.1	0.15

Adapted from J. Trussell, Table I[1]

[a] *The authors' best guess of the percentage of women expected to experience an accidental pregnancy among couples who initiate a method (not necessarily for the first time) and who use it consistently and correctly during the first year if they do not stop for any other reason.*

[b] *This term represents "typical" couples who initiate use of a method (not necessarily for the first time), who experience an accidental pregnancy during the first year if they do not stop use for any other reason. The authors derive these data largely from the National Surveys of Family Growth (NSFG), 1976 and 1982.*

[c] *N/A—Data not available from the NSFG, 1976 and 1982.*

[d] *Combined typical rate for both medicated and nonmedicated IUD. The rate for medicated IUD alone is not available.*

[e] *All forms.*

CONTRAINDICATIONS

Oral contraceptives should not be used in women who have the following conditions:

- Thrombophlebitis or thromboembolic disorders
- A past history of deep vein thrombophlebitis or thromboembolic disorders
- Cerebral vascular or coronary artery disease
- Known or suspected carcinoma of the breast
- Carcinoma of the endometrium, and known or suspected estrogen-dependent neoplasia
- Undiagnosed abnormal genital bleeding
- Cholestatic jaundice of pregnancy or jaundice with prior pill use
- Hepatic adenomas, carcinomas or benign liver tumors
- Known or suspected pregnancy

WARNINGS

CIGARETTE SMOKING INCREASES THE RISK OF SERIOUS CARDIOVASCULAR SIDE EFFECTS FROM ORAL CONTRACEPTIVE USE. THIS RISK INCREASES WITH AGE AND WITH HEAVY SMOKING (15 OR MORE CIGARETTES PER DAY) AND IS QUITE MARKED IN WOMEN OVER 35 YEARS OF AGE. WOMEN WHO USE ORAL CONTRACEPTIVES ARE STRONGLY ADVISED NOT TO SMOKE.

The use of oral contraceptives is associated with increased risks of several serious conditions including myocardial infarction, thromboembolism, stroke, hepatic neoplasia and gallbladder disease, although the risk of serious morbidity and mortality increases significantly in the presence of other underlying risk factors such as hypertension, hyperlipidemias, hypercholesterolemia, obesity and diabetes.[2-5]

Practitioners prescribing oral contraceptives should be familiar with the following information relating to these risks. The information contained in this package insert is principally based on studies carried out in patients who used oral contraceptives with formulations containing 0.05 mg or higher of estrogen.[6-11] The effects of long-term use with lower dose formulations of both estrogens and progestogens remain to be determined.

Throughout this labeling, epidemiological studies reported are of two types: retrospective or case control studies and prospective or cohort studies. Case control studies provide a measure of the relative risk of a disease. Relative risk, the *ratio* of the incidence of a disease among oral contraceptive users to that among non-users, cannot be assessed directly from case control studies, but the odds ratio obtained is a measure of relative risk. The relative risk does not provide information on the actual clinical occurrence of a disease. Cohort studies provide not only a measure of the relative risk but a measure of attributable risk, which is the *difference* in the incidence of disease between oral contraceptive users and non-users. The attributable risk does provide information about the actual occurrence of a disease in the population.[12-13]

1. THROMBOEMBOLIC DISORDERS AND OTHER VASCULAR PROBLEMS

a. Myocardial Infarction: An increased risk of myocardial infarction has been attributed to oral contraceptive use. This risk is primarily in smokers or women with other underlying risk factors for coronary artery disease such as hypertension, hypercholesterolemia, morbid obesity and diabetes.[2-5,13] The relative risk of heart attack for current oral contraceptive users has been estimated to be 2 to 6.[2,14-19] The risk is very low under the age of 30. However, there is the possibility of a risk of cardiovascular disease even in very young women who take oral contraceptives.

Smoking in combination with oral contraceptive use has been shown to contribute substantially to the incidence of myocardial infarctions in women 35 or older, with smoking accounting for the majority of excess cases.[20]

Mortality rates associated with circulatory disease have been shown to increase substantially in smokers over the age of 35 and non-smokers over the age of 40 among women who use oral contraceptives (see Table 2).[16]

Table 2

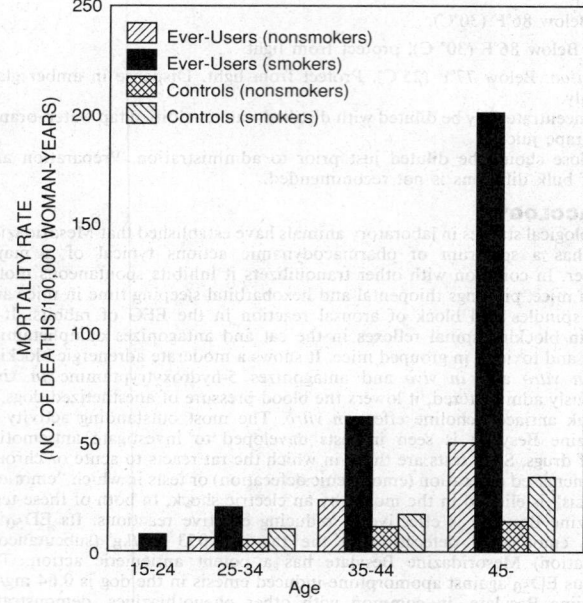

CIRCULATORY DISEASE MORTALITY RATES PER 100,000 WOMAN-YEARS BY AGE, SMOKING STATUS AND ORAL CONTRACEPTIVE USE

Oral contraceptives may compound the effects of well-known risk factors for coronary artery disease, such as hypertension, diabetes, hyperlipidemias, hypercholesterolemia, age and obesity.[3,13,21] In particular, some progestogens are known to decrease HDL cholesterol and impair oral glucose tolerance, while estrogens may create a state of hyperinsulinism.[21-25] Oral contraceptives have been shown to increase blood pressure among users (see *"Warnings"*, section 9). Similar effects on risk factors have been associated with an increased risk of heart disease. Oral contraceptives must be used with caution in women with cardiovascular disease risk factors.

b. Thromboembolism: An increased risk of thromboembolic and thrombotic disease associated with the use of oral contraceptives is well established. Case control studies have found the relative risk of users compared to non-users to be 3 for the first episode of superficial venous thrombosis, 4 to 11 for deep vein thrombosis or pulmonary embolism, and 1.5 to 6 for women with predisposing conditions for venous thromboembolic disease.[12,13,26-31] One cohort study has shown the relative risk to be somewhat lower, about 3 for new cases (subjects with no past history of venous thrombosis or varicose veins) and about 4.5 for new cases requiring hospitalization.[32] The risk of thromboembolic disease due to oral contraceptives is not related to length of use and disappears after pill use is stopped.[12]

A 2- to 6-fold increase in relative risk of post-operative thromboembolic complications has been reported with the use of oral contraceptives.[18] If feasible, oral contraceptives should be discontinued at least 4 weeks prior to and for 2 weeks after elective surgery and during and following prolonged immobilization. Since the immediate postpartum period also is associated with an increased risk of thromboembolism, oral contraceptives should be started no earlier than 4 to 6 weeks after delivery in women who elect not to breast feed.[33]

c. Cerebrovascular diseases: An increase in both the relative and attributable risks of cerebrovascular events (thrombotic and hemorrhagic strokes) has been shown in users of oral contraceptives. In general, the risk is greatest among older (> 35 years), hypertensive women who also smoke. Hypertension was found to be a risk factor for both users and non-users for both types of strokes while smoking interacted to increase the risk for hemorrhagic strokes.[34]

In a large study, the relative risk of thrombotic strokes has been shown to range from 3 for normotensive users to 14 for users with severe hypertension.[35] The relative risk of hemorrhagic stroke is reported to be 1.2 for non-smokers who used oral contraceptives, 2.6 for smokers who did not use oral contraceptives, 7.6 for smokers who used oral contraceptives, 1.8 for normotensive users and 25.7 for users with severe hypertension.[35] The attributable risk also is greater in women 35 or older and among smokers.[13]

d. Dose-related risk of vascular disease from oral contraceptives: A positive association has been observed between the amount of estrogen and progestogen in oral contraceptives and the risk of vascular disease.[36-38] A decline in serum high density lipoproteins (HDL) has been reported with some progestational agents.[22-24] A decline in serum high density lipoproteins has been associated with an increased incidence of ischemic heart disease.[39] Because estrogens increase HDL cholesterol, the net effect of an oral contraceptive depends on a balance achieved between doses of estrogen and progestogen and the nature and absolute amount of progestogens used in the contraceptives. The amount of both hormones should be considered in the choice of an oral contraceptive.[37] Minimizing exposure to estrogen and progestogen is in keeping with good principles of therapeutics. For any particular estrogen/progestogen combination, the dosage regimen prescribed should be one which contains the least amount of estrogen and progestogen that is compatible with a low failure rate and the needs of the individual patient. New acceptors of oral contraceptive agents should be started on preparations containing the lowest estrogen content that produces satisfactory results for the individual.

e. Persistence of risk of vascular disease: There are three studies which have shown persistence of risk of vascular disease for ever-users of oral contraceptives.[17,34,40] In a study in the United States, the risk of developing myocardial infarction after discontinuing oral contraceptives persists for at least 9 years for women 40-49 years who had used oral contraceptives for 5 or more years, but this increased risk was not demonstrated in other age groups.[17] In another study in Great Britain, the risk of developing cerebrovascular disease persisted for at least 6 years after discontinuation of oral contraceptives, although excess risk was very small.[40] Subarachnoid hemorrhage also has a significantly increased relative risk after termination of use of oral contraceptives.[34] However, these studies were performed with oral contraceptive formulations containing 0.05 mg or higher of estrogen.

2. ESTIMATES OF MORTALITY FROM CONTRACEPTIVE USE
One study gathered data from a variety of sources which have estimated the mortality rates associated with different methods of contraception at different ages (see Table III).[41] These estimates include the combined risk of death associated with contraceptive methods plus the risk attributable to pregnancy in the event of method failure. Each method of contraception has its specific benefits and risks. The study concluded that with the exception of oral contraceptive users 35 and older who smoke and 40 and older who do not smoke, mortality associated with all methods of birth control is low and below that associated with childbirth. The observation of a possible increase in risk of mortality with age for oral contraceptive users is based on data gathered in the 1970's—but not reported in the U.S. until 1983.[16,41] However, current clinical practice involves the use of lower estrogen dose formulations combined with careful restriction of oral contraceptive use to women who do not have the various risk factors listed in this labeling.

Because of these changes in practice and, also, because of some limited new data which suggest that the risk of cardiovascular disease with the use of oral contraceptives may now be less than previously observed[78,79] the Fertility and Maternal Health Drugs Advisory Committee was asked to review the topic in 1989. The Committee concluded that although cardiovascular disease risks may be increased with oral contraceptive use after age 40 in healthy non-smoking women (even with the newer low-dose formulations), there are greater potential health risks associated with pregnancy in older women and with the alternative surgical and medical procedures which may be necessary if such women do not have access to effective and acceptable means of contraception.

Therefore, the Committee recommended that the benefits of oral contraceptive use by healthy non-smoking women over 40 may outweigh the possible risks. Of course, older women, as all women who take oral contraceptives, should take the lowest possible dose formulation that is effective.[80]

Table 3
ESTIMATED ANNUAL NUMBER OF BIRTH-RELATED OR METHOD-RELATED DEATHS ASSOCIATED WITH CONTROL OF FERTILITY PER 100,000 NONSTERILE WOMEN, BY FERTILITY CONTROL METHOD ACCORDING TO AGE

Method of control and outcome	15-19	30-24	25-29	30-34	35-69	40-44
No fertility control methods*	7.0	7.4	9.1	14.8	25.7	28.2
Oral contraceptives non-smoker**	0.3	0.5	0.9	1.9	13.8	31.6
Oral contraceptives smoker **	2.2	3.4	6.6	13.5	51.1	117.2
IUD**	0.8	0.8	1.0	1.0	1.4	1.4
Condom*	1.1	1.6	0.7	0.2	0.3	0.4
Diaphragm/ Spermicide*	1.9	1.2	1.2	1.3	2.2	2.8
Periodic abstinence*	2.5	1.6	1.6	1.7	2.9	3.6

* *Deaths are birth related*
** *Deaths are method related*

Estimates adapted from H.W. Ory, Table 3[41]

3. CARCINOMA OF THE BREAST AND REPRODUCTIVE ORGANS
Numerous epidemiological studies have been performed on the incidence of breast, endometrial, ovarian and cervical cancer in women using oral contraceptives. The evidence in the literature suggests that use of oral contraceptives is not associated with an increase in the risk of developing breast cancer, regardless of the age and parity of first use or with most of the marketed brands and doses.[42,43]

The Cancer and Steroid Hormone study also showed no latent effect on the risk of breast cancer for at least a decade following long-term use.[43] A few studies have shown a slightly increased relative risk of developing breast cancer,[44-47] although the methodology of these studies, which included differences in examination of users and non-users and differences in age at start of use, has been questioned.[47-49] Some studies have reported an increased relative risk of developing breast cancer, particularly at a younger age. This increased relative risk appears to be related to duration of use.[81,82]

Some studies suggest that oral contraceptive use has been associated with an increase in the risk of cervical intraepithelial neoplasia in some populations of women.[50-53] However, there continues to be controversy about the extent to which such findings may be due to differences in sexual behavior and other factors.

In spite of many studies of the relationship between oral contraceptive use and breast or cervical cancers, a cause and effect relationship has not been established.

4. HEPATIC NEOPLASIA
Benign hepatic adenomas are associated with oral contraceptive use although the incidence of benign tumors is rare in the United States. Indirect calculations have estimated the attributable risk to be in the range of 3.3 cases per 100,000 for users, a risk that increases after 4 or more years of use.[54] Rupture of rare, benign, hepatic adenomas may cause death through intra-abdominal hemorrhage.[55-56]

Studies in the United States and Britain have shown an increased risk of developing hepatocellular carcinoma in long-term (> 8 years) oral contraceptive users.[57-59] However, these cancers are extremely rare in the United States and the attributable risk (the excess incidence) of liver cancers in oral contraceptive users is less than 1 per 1,000,000 users.

5. OCULAR LESIONS
There have been clinical case reports of retinal thrombosis associated with the use of oral contraceptives. Oral contraceptives should be discontinued if there is unexplained partial or complete loss of vision; onset of proptosis or diplopia; papilledema; or retinal vascular lesions. Appropriate diagnostic and therapeutic measures should be undertaken immediately.

6. ORAL CONTRACEPTIVE USE BEFORE OR DURING EARLY PREGNANCY
Extensive epidemiological studies have revealed no increased risk of birth defects in women who have used oral contraceptives prior to pregnancy.[60-62] More recent studies do not suggest a teratogenic effect, particularly insofar as cardiac anomalies and limb reduction defects are concerned, when taken inadvertently during early pregnancy.[60,61,63,64]

The administration of oral contraceptives to induce withdrawal bleeding should not be used as a test for pregnancy. Oral contraceptives should not be used during pregnancy to treat threatened or habitual abortion.

It is recommended that for any patient who has missed 2 consecutive periods, pregnancy should be ruled out before continuing oral contraceptive use. If the patient has not adhered to the prescribed schedule, the possibility of pregnancy should be considered at the time of the first missed period. Oral contraceptive use should be discontinued if pregnancy is confirmed.

7. GALLBLADDER DISEASE
Earlier studies have reported an increased lifetime relative risk of gallbladder surgery in users of oral contraceptives and estrogens.[65-66] More recent studies, however, have shown that the relative risk of developing gallbladder disease among oral contraceptive users may be minimal.[67] The recent findings of minimal risk may be related to the use of oral contraceptive formulations containing lower hormonal doses of estrogens and progestogens.[68]

8. CARBOHYDRATE AND LIPID METABOLIC EFFECTS
Oral contraceptives have been shown to impair glucose tolerance.[69] Oral contraceptives containing greater than 0.075 mg of estrogen cause glucose intolerance with impaired insulin secretion, while lower doses of estrogen may produce less glucose intolerance.[70] Progestogens increase insulin secretion and create insulin, resistance, this effect varying with different progestational agents.[25,71] However, in the non-diabetic woman, oral contraceptives appear to have no effect on fasting blood glucose.[69] Because of these demonstrated effects, prediabetic and diabetic women should be carefully observed while taking oral contraceptives.

Some women may develop persistent hypertriglyceridemia while on the pill.[72] As discussed earlier (see *"Warnings"* sections *"1a,"* and *"1d."*), changes in serum triglycerides and lipoprotein levels have been reported in oral contraceptive users.[23]

9. ELEVATED BLOOD PRESSURE
An increase in blood pressure has been reported in women taking oral contraceptives. The incidence of risk also was reported to increase with continued use and among older women.[66] Data from the Royal College of General Practitioners and subsequent randomized trials have shown that the incidence of hypertension increases with increasing concentrations of progestogens.

Women with a history of hypertension or hypertension-related diseases, or renal disease should be encouraged to use another method of contraception. If women elect to use oral contraceptives, they should be monitored closely and if significant elevation of blood pressure occurs oral contraceptives should be discontinued. For most women, elevated blood pressure will return to normal after stopping oral contraceptives and there is no difference in the occurrence of hypertension among ever-and never-users.[73-75]

10. HEADACHE
The onset of exacerbation of migraine or development of headache with a new pattern which is recurrent, persistent or severe requires discontinuation of oral contraceptives and evaluation of the cause.

11. BLEEDING IRREGULARITIES
Breakthrough bleeding and spotting are sometimes encountered in patients on oral contraceptives, especially during the first 3 months of use. Non-hormonal causes should be considered and adequate diagnostic measures taken to rule out malignancy or pregnancy in the event of breakthrough bleeding, as in the case of any abnormal vaginal bleeding. If pathology has been excluded, time or a change to another formulation may solve the problem. In the event of amenorrhea, pregnancy should be ruled out.

Some women may encounter post-pill amenorrhea or oligomenorrhea, especially when such a condition was pre-existent.

PRECAUTIONS
GENERAL
Patients should be counseled that this product does not protect against HIV (AIDS) and other sexually transmitted diseases:

1. PHYSICAL EXAMINATION AND FOLLOW UP
It is good medical practice for all women to have annual history and physical examinations, including women using oral contraceptives. The physical examination, however, may be deferred until after initiation of oral contraceptives if requested by the woman and judged appropriate by the clinician. The physical examination should include special reference to blood pressure, breasts, abdomen and pelvic organs, including cervical cytology and relevant laboratory tests. In case of undiagnosed, persistent or recurrent abnormal vaginal bleeding, appropriate measures should be conducted to rule out malignancy. Women with a strong family history of breast cancer or who have breast nodules should be monitored with particular care.

2. LIPID DISORDERS
Women who are being treated for hyperlipidemias should be followed closely if they elect to use oral contraceptives. Some progestogens may elevate LDL levels and may render the control of hyperlipidemias more difficult.

3. LIVER FUNCTION
If jaundice develops in any woman receiving oral contraceptives the medication should be discontinued. Steroid hormones may be poorly metabolized in patients with impaired liver function.

4. FLUID RETENTION
Oral contraceptives may cause some degree of fluid retention. They should be prescribed with caution, and only with careful monitoring, in patients with conditions which might be aggravated by fluid retention.

5. EMOTIONAL DISORDERS
Women with a history of depression should be carefully observed and the drug discontinued if depression recurs to a serious degree.

6. CONTACT LENSES
Contact lens wearers who develop visual changes or changes in lens tolerance should be assessed by an ophthalmologist.

7. DRUG INTERACTIONS
Reduced efficacy and increased incidence of breakthrough bleeding and menstrual irregularities have been associated with concomitant use of rifampin. A similar association though less marked, has been suggested with barbiturates, phenylbutazone, phenytoin sodium, and possibly with griseofulvin, ampicillin and tetracyclines.[76]

8. INTERACTIONS WITH LABORATORY TESTS
Certain endocrine and liver function tests and blood components may be affected by oral contraceptives:

a. Increased prothrombin and factors VII, VIII, IX, and X; decreased antithrombin 3; increased norepinephrine-induced platelet aggregability.

b. Increased thyroid binding globulin (TBG) leading to increased circulating total thyroid hormone, as measured by protein-bound iodine (PBI), T4 by column or by radioimmunoassay. Free T3 resin uptake is decreased, reflecting the elevated TBG. Free T4 concentration is unaltered.

c. Other binding proteins may be elevated in serum.

d. Sex steroid binding globulins are increased and result in elevated levels of total circulating sex steroids and corticoids; however, free or biologically active levels remain unchanged.

e. Triglycerides may be increased.

f. Glucose tolerance may be decreased.

g. Serum folate levels may be depressed by oral contraceptive therapy. This may be of clinical significance if a woman becomes pregnant shortly after discontinuing oral contraceptives.

9. CARCINOGENESIS
(See *"Warnings"* section.)

10. PREGNANCY
Pregnancy Category X. See *"Contraindications"* and *"Warnings"* sections.

11. NURSING MOTHERS
Small amounts of oral contraceptive steroids have been identified in the milk of nursing mothers and a few adverse effects on the child have been reported, including jaundice and breast enlargement. In addition, oral contraceptives given in the postpartum period may interfere with lactation by decreasing the quantity and quality of breast milk. If possible, the nursing mother should be advised not to use oral contraceptives but to use other forms of contraception until she has completely weaned her child.

INFORMATION FOR THE PATIENT
See patient labeling supplied with this product.

ADVERSE REACTIONS
An increased risk of the following serious adverse reactions has been associated with the use of oral contraceptives (see *"Warnings"* section).

- Thrombophlebitis
- Arterial thromboembolism
- Pulmonary embolism
- Myocardial infarction
- Cerebral hemorrhage
- Cerebral thrombosis
- Hypertension
- Gallbladder disease
- Hepatic adenomas, carcinomas or benign liver tumors

There is evidence of an association between the following conditions and the use of oral contraceptives, although additional confirmatory studies are needed:
- Mesenteric thrombosis
- Retinal thrombosis

The following adverse reactions have been reported in patients receiving oral contraceptives and are believed to be drug-related:
- Nausea
- Vomiting
- Gastrointestinal symptoms (such as abdominal cramps and bloating)
- Breakthrough bleeding
- Spotting
- Change in menstrual flow
- Amenorrhea
- Temporary infertility after discontinuation of treatment
- Edema
- Melasma which may persist
- Breast changes: tenderness, enlargement, secretion
- Change in weight (increase or decrease)
- Change in cervical erosion and secretion
- Diminution in lactation when given immediately postpartum
- Cholestatic jaundice
- Migraine
- Rash (allergic)
- Mental depression
- Reduced tolerance to carbohydrates
- Vaginal candidiasis
- Change in corneal curvature (steepening)
- Intolerance to contact lenses

The following adverse reactions have been reported in users of oral contraceptives and the association has been neither confirmed nor refuted:
- Pre-menstrual syndrome
- Cataracts
- Changes in appetite
- Cystitis-like syndrome
- Headache
- Nervousness
- Dizziness
- Hirsutism
- Loss of scalp hair
- Erythema multiforme
- Erythema nodosum
- Hemorrhagic eruption
- Vaginitis
- Porphyria
- Impaired renal function
- Hemolytic uremic syndrome
- Budd-Chiari syndrome
- Acne
- Changes in libido
- Colitis

OVERDOSAGE
Serious ill effects have not been reported following acute ingestion of large doses of oral contraceptives by young children. Overdosage may cause nausea, and withdrawal bleeding may occur in females.

NON-CONTRACEPTIVE HEALTH BENEFITS
The following noncontraceptive health benefits related to the use of oral contraceptives are supported by epidemiological studies which largely utilized

---

◆ RATED THERAPEUTICALLY EQUIVALENT; ◇ THERAPEUTIC EQUIVALENCE UNCONFIRMED; ○ UNRATED

oral contraceptive formulations containing estrogen doses exceeding 0.035 mg of ethinyl estradiol or 0.05 mg of mestranol.[6-11]

Effects on menses:

- Increased menstrual cycle regularity
- Decreased blood loss and decreased incidence of iron deficiency anemia
- Decreased incidence of dysmenorrhea

Effects related to inhibition of ovulation:

- Decreased incidence of functional ovarian cysts
- Decreased incidence of ectopic pregnancies

Effects from long-term use:

- Decreased incidence of fibroadenomas and fibrocystic disease of the breast
- Decreased incidence of acute pelvic inflammatory disease
- Decreased incidence of endometrial cancer
- Decreased incidence of ovarian cancer

DOSAGE AND ADMINISTRATION

To achieve maximum contraceptive effectiveness, oral contraceptives must be taken exactly as described and at intervals not exceeding 24 hours.

21-Day Schedule: For a SUNDAY START when menstrual flow begins on or before Sunday, the first tablet (white or yellow-green or blue) is taken on that day. For a Day 5 start, count the first day of menstrual flow as Day 1 and the first tablet (white or yellow-green or blue) is then taken on Day 5. With either a SUNDAY START or DAY 5 START, 1 tablet is taken each day at the same time for 21 days. No tablets are taken for 7 days, then, whether bleeding has stopped or not, a new course is started of 1 tablet a day for 21 days. This institutes a 3 weeks on, 1 week off dosage regimen.

28-Day Schedule: For a SUNDAY START when menstrual flow begins on or before Sunday, the first tablet (white or yellow-green or blue) is taken on that day. For a Day 5 start, count the first day of menstrual flow as Day 1 and the first tablet (white or yellow-green or blue) is then taken on Day 5. With either a SUNDAY START or DAY 5 START, 1 tablet (white or yellow-green or blue) is taken each day at the same time for 21 days. Then the orange tablets are taken for 7 days, whether bleeding has stopped or not. After all 28 tablets have been taken, whether bleeding has stopped or not, the same dosage schedule is repeated beginning on the following day.

INSTRUCTIONS TO PATIENTS

- To achieve maximum contraceptive effectiveness, the oral contraceptive pill must be taken exactly as directed and at intervals not exceeding 24 hours.
- Important: Women should be instructed to use an additional method of protection until after the first 7 days of administration *in the initial cycle.*
- Due to the normally increased risk of thromboembolism occurring postpartum, women should be instructed not to initiate treatment with oral contraceptives earlier than 4 weeks after a full-term delivery. If pregnancy is terminated in the first 12 weeks, the patient should be instructed to start oral contraceptives immediately or within 7 days. If pregnancy is terminated after 12 weeks, the patient should be instructed to start oral contraceptives after 2 weeks.[33,77]
- If spotting or breakthrough bleeding should occur, the patient should continue the medication according to the schedule. Should spotting or breakthrough bleeding persist, the patient should notify her physician.
- If the patient misses 1 pill, she should be instructed to take it as soon as she remembers and then take the next pill at the regular time. The patient should be advised that missing a pill can cause spotting or light bleeding and that she may be a little sick to her stomach on the days she takes the missed pill with her regularly scheduled pill. If the patient has missed more than one pill, she should not take the missed pills and they should be discarded. She should be advised to take the next pill at the next regular time and continue to take them as scheduled. Furthermore, she should use an additional method of contraception in addition to taking her pills for the remainder of the cycle.
- Use of oral contraceptives in the event of a missed menstrual period:

1. If the patient has not adhered to the prescribed dosage regimen, the possibility of pregnancy should be considered after the first missed period and oral contraceptives should be withheld until pregnancy has been ruled out.

2. If the patient has adhered to the prescribed regimen and misses 2 consecutive periods, pregnancy should be ruled out before continuing the contraceptive regimen.

REFERENCES

1. Trussell, J., et al: *Stud Fam Plann* 21(1):51-54, 1990 2. Mann, J., et al.: *Br Med J* 2(5956):241-245, 1975. 3. Knopp, R.H.: *J Reprod Med* 31(9):913-921, 1986. 4. Mann, J.I., et al.: *Br Med J* 2:445-447, 1976. 5. Ory, H: *JAMA* 237:2619-2622, 1977. 6. The Cancer and Steroid Hormone Study of the Centers for Disease Control: *JAMA* 249(2):1596-1599, 1983. 7. The Cancer and Steroid Hormone Study of the Centers for Disease Control: *JAMA* 257(6):796-800, 1987. 8. Ory, H.W.: *JAMA* 228(1):68-69, 1974. 9. Ory, H.W., et al.: *N Engl J Med* 294:419-422, 1976. 10. Ory, H.W.: *Fam Plann Perspect* 14:182-184, 1982. 11. Ory, H.W., et al.: *Making Choices,* New York, The Alan Guttmacher Institute, 1983. 12. Stadel, B.: *N Engl J Med* 305(11):612-618, 1981. 13. Stadel, B.: *N Engl J Med* 305(12):672-677, 1981. 14. Adam, S., et al.: *Br J Obstet Gynaecol* 88:838-845, 1975. 15. Mann, J., et al.: *Br Med J* 2(5965):245-248, 1975. 16. Royal College of General Practitioners' Oral Contraceptive Study: *Lanzet* 1:541-546, 1981. 17. Slone, D., et al.: *N Engl J Med* 305(8):420-424, 1981. 18. Vessey, M.P.: *Br J Fam Plann* 6 (supplement):1-12, 1980. 19. Russell-Briefel, R., et al.: *Prev Med* 15:352-362, 1986. 20. Goldbaum, G., et al.: *JAMA* 258(10):1339-1342, 1987. 21. LaRosa, J.C.: *J Reprod Med* 31(9):906-912, 1986. 22. Krauss, R.M., et al.: *Am J Obstet Gynecol* 145:446-452, 1983. 23. Wahl, P., et al.: *N Engl J Med* 308(15):862-867, 1983. 24. Wynn, V., et al.: *Am J Obstet Gynecol* 142(6):766-771,1982. 25. Wynn V., et al.: *J Reprod Med* 31(9):892-897, 1986. 26. Inman, W.H., et al.: *Br Med J* 2I5599):193-199, 1968. 27. Maguire, M.G., et al.: *Am J Epidemiol* 110(2):188-195, 1979. 28. Petitti, D., et al.: *JAMA* 242(11):1150-1154, 1979. 29. Vessey, M.P., et al.: *Br Med J* 2(5599):199-205, 1968. 30. Vessey, M.P., et al.: *Br Med J* 2(5658):651-657, 1969. 31. Porter, J.B., et al.: *Obstet Gynecol* 59(3):299-302, 1982. 32. Vessey, M.P., et al.: *J Biosoc Sci* 8:373-427, 1976. 33.Mishell, D.R., et al.: *Reproductive Endocrinology,* Philadelphia, F.A. Davis Co., 1979. 34. Petitti, D.B., et al.: *Lancet* 2:234-236, 1978. 35. Collaborative Group for the Study of Stroke in Young Women: *JAMA* 231(7):718-722, 1975. 36.Inman, W.H., et al.: *Br Med J* 2:203-209, 1970. 37. Meade, T.W., et al.: *Br Med J* 280 (6224): 1157-1161, 1980. 38Kay, C.R.: *Am J Obstet Gynecol* 142(6):762-765, 1982. 39. Gordon, T., et al.: *Am J Med* 62:707-714, 1977. 40. Royal College of General Practitioners' Oral Contraception Study: *J Coll Gen Proct* 33:75-82, 1983. 41. Ory, H.W.: *Fam Plann Perspect* 15(2):57-63, 1983. 42. Paul, C., et al.: *Br Med J* 293:723-725, 1986. **43.** 43. The Cancer and Steroid Hormone Study of the Centers for Disease Control: *N Engl J Med* 315(7):405-411. 1986. 44. Pike, M.C., et al.: *Lancet* 2:926-929, 1983. 45. Miller, D.R., et al.: *Lancet* 2:748-749, 68:863-868, 1986. 46. Olsson, H., et al.: *Lancet* 2:748-749, 1985. 47. McPherson, K., et al.: *Br J Cancer* 56:653-660, 1987. 48. Huggins, G.R., et al.: *Fetil Steril* 47(5):733-761, 1987. 49. McPherson. K., et al.: *Br Med J* 293:709-710. 1986. 50.Ory, H., et al.: *Am J Obstet Gynecol* 124(6):573-577, 1976. 51. Vessey, M.P., et al.: *Lancet,* 2:930, 1983. 52. Brinton, L.A., et al.: *Int J Cancer* 38:339-344, 1986. 53. WHO Collaborative Study of Neoplasia and Steroid Contraceptives: *Br Med J* 290:961-965, 1985. 54. Rooks, J.B., et al.: *JAMA* 242(7):644-648, 1977. 55. Bein, N.N., et al.: *Br J Surg* 64:433-435, 1977. 56. Klatskin, G.: *Gastroenterology* 73:386-394, 1977. 57. Henderson, B.E., et al.: *Br J Cancer* 48:437-440, 1983. 58. Neuberger, J., et al.: *Br Med J* 292:1355-1357, 1986. 59.Forman, D., et al.: *Br Med J* 292:1357-1361, 1986. 60.Harlap, S., et al.: *Obstet Gynecol* 55(4):447-452, 1980. 61. Savolainen, E., et al.: *Am J Obstet Gynecol* 140(5):521-524, 1981. 62. Janerich, D.T., et al.: *Am J Epidermiol* 112(1):73-79, 1980. 63. Ferencz, C., et al.: *Teratology* 21:225-239, 1980. 64. Rothman, J., et al.: *Am J Epidermiol* 109(4):433-439, 1979. 65. Boston Collaborative Drug Surveillance Program: *Lancet* 1:1399-1404. 1973. 66. Royal College of General Practitioners: *Oral contraceptives and health* New York, Pittman, 1974. 67. Rome Group for the Epidermiology and Prevention of Cholelithiasis: *Am J Epidermiol* 119(5):796-805, 1984. 68. Strom, B.L., et al.: *Clin Pharmacol Ther* 39(3):335-341, 1986. 69. Perlman, J.A., et al.: *J Chronic Dis* 38(10):857-864, 1985. 70. Wynn, V., et al.: *Lancet* 1:1045-1049, 1979. 71. Wynn, V.: *Progesterone and Progestin,* New York, Raven Press, 1983. 72. Wynn, V.: *Lancet* 2:720-723, 1966. 73. Fisch, I.R., et al.: *JAMA Lancet* 2*:720-723, 19866. 74. Laragh, J.H.: *Am J Obstet Gynecol* 126(1):141-147, 1976. 75. Ramcharan, S., et al.: *Pharmacology of Steroid Contraceptive Drugs,* New York, Raven Press, 1977. 76. Stockley, L: *Pharm J* 216:140-143, 1976. 77. Dickey, R.P.:*Managing Contraceptive Pill Patients,* Oklahoma, Creative Informatics Inc., 1984. 78. Porter J.B., Hunter J., Jick H., et al: *Obstet Gynecol* 1985:66:1-4. 79. Porter J.B., Hershel J., Walker A.M.: *Obstet gynecol* 1987;70:29-32. 80. Fertility and Maternal Health Drugs Advisory Committee, F.D.A., October, 1989. 81. Schlesselman J., Stadel B.V., Murray V., Lai S.: *Breast cancer in relation to early use of oral contraceptives.* JAMA 1988;259:1828-1833. 82. Hennekens C.H., Speizer F.E., Lipnick R.J., Rosner B. Bain C., Belanger C., Stampfer M.J., Willett W., Peto R.: *A case-control study of ora contraceptive use and breast cancer.* JNCl 1984:72:39-42.

HOW SUPPLIED

TABLETS: 1 MG-0.05 MG

HCFA FUL (21s ea) — $0.49

BRAND/MANUFACTURER	NDC	SIZE	AWP
◆ **BRAND**			
▶ NORINYL 1/50: Syntex/F.P.	42987-0101-61	672s	$533.93

TABLETS: 50 MCG-1 MG

AVERAGE UNIT PRICE (AVAILABLE SIZES)		GENERIC A-RATED AVERAGE PRICE (GAAP)	
BRAND	$0.92	168s	$73.67
GENERIC	$0.51		
HCFA FUL (63s ea)	$0.49		

BRAND/MANUFACTURER	NDC	SIZE	AWP
◆ **BRAND**			
▶ ORTHO-NOVUM 1/50: Ortho Pharm	00062-1331-15	126s	$132.36
▶ NORINYL 1/50: Syntex/F.P.	42987-0100-23	126s	$133.45
ORTHO-NOVUM 1/50: Ortho Pharm	00062-1332-15	168s	$133.08
▶ NORINYL 1/50: Syntex/F.P.	42987-0101-24	168s	$133.45
◆ **GENERICS**			
GENORA 1/50: Rugby	00536-4059-44	63s	$36.30
NELOVA 1/50 M: Warner Chilcott	00047-0942-11	126s	$74.30
GENORA 1/50: Rugby	00536-4056-48	168s	$72.60
NELOVA 1/50 M: Warner Chilcott	00047-0947-35	168s	$74.74

Metahydrin SEE TRICHLORMETHIAZIDE

Metaprel SEE METAPROTERENOL SULFATE

Metaproterenol Sulfate

DESCRIPTION

Metaproterenol Sulfate Inhalation Aerosol is administered by oral inhalation. The Inhalation Aerosol containing 150 mg of Metaproterenol Sulfate as micronized powder is sufficient medication for 200 inhalations. Each metered dose delivers through the mouthpiece 0.65 mg of Metaproterenol Sulfate (each mL contains 15 mg).

▶ SHOWN IN PRODUCT IDENTIFICATION GUIDE

Metaproterenol Sulfate Inhalation Solution is administered by oral inhalation with the aid of a hand-bulb nebulizer or an intermittent positive pressure breathing apparatus (IPPB). It contains Metaproterenol Sulfate 5% in a pH-adjusted aqueous solution containing benzalkonium chloride and edetate disodium as preservatives.

Metaproterenol Sulfate Inhalation Solution unit-dose vial is administered by oral inhalation with the aid of an intermittent positive pressure breathing apparatus (IPPB). It contains Metaproterenol Sulfate 0.4% or 0.6%.

Metaproterenol Sulfate Syrup is administered orally. Each teaspoonful (5 mL) of syrup contains Metaproterenol Sulfate 10 mg.

Metaproterenol Sulfate Tablets are administered orally. Each tablet contains Metaproterenol Sulfate 10 mg or 20 mg.

Chemically, Metaproterenol Sulfate is 1-(3,5 dihydroxyphenyl)-2-isopropylaminoethanol sulfate, a white crystalline, racemic mixture of two optically active isomers. It differs from isoproterenol hydrochloride by having two hydroxyl groups attached at the meta positions on the benzene ring rather than one at the meta and one at the para position. Its molecular formula is $(C_{11}H_{17}NO_3)_2 \cdot H_2SO_4$ and molecular weight is 520.59.

Following is its chemical structure:

$$\text{HO} - \bigcirc - \text{CHCH}_2\text{NHCH} \begin{matrix} CH_3 \\ CH_3 \end{matrix} \cdot H_2SO_4$$

CLINICAL PHARMACOLOGY

Metaproterenol Sulfate is a potent beta-adrenergic stimulator. *In vitro* studies and *in vivo* pharamacologic studies have demonstrated that Metaproterenol Sulfate has a preferential effect on beta-2 adrenergic receptors compared with isoproterenol. While it is recognized that beta-2 adrenergic receptors are the predominant receptors in bronchial smooth muscle, recent data indicate that there is a population of beta-2 receptors in the human heart existing in a concentration between 10%-50%. The precise function of these, however, is not yet established. Metaproterenol Sulfate Inhalation Aerosol and Inhalation Solution have a rapid onset of action.

The pharmacologic effects of beta adrenergic agonist drugs, including Metaproterenol Sulfate, are at least in part attributable to stimulation through beta adrenergic receptors of intracellular adenyl cyclase, the enzyme which catalyzes the conversion of adenosine triphosphate (ATP) to cyclic-3', 5'-adenosine monophosphate (c-AMP). Increased c-AMP levels are associated with relaxation of bronchial smooth muscle and inhibition of release of mediators of immediate hypersensitivity from cells, especially from mast cells.

Pharmacokinetics: Absorption, biotransformation and excretion studies in humans following administration by inhalation have shown that approximately 3 percent of the actuated dose is absorbed intact through the lungs. The major metabolite, metaproterenol-3-O-sulfate, is produced in the gastrointestinal tract. Metaproterenol Sulfate is not metabolized by catechol-O-methyltransferase nor have glucuronide conjugates been isolated to date.

Following oral administration in humans, an average of 40% of the drug is absorbed; it is not metabolized by catechol-O-methyltransferase or sulfatase enzymes in the gut, but is excreted primarily as glucuronic acid conjugates.

When administered orally or by inhalation, Metaproterenol Sulfate decreases reversible bronchospasm. Pulmonary function tests performed concomitantly usually show improvement following aerosol Metaproterenol Sulfate administration, e.g., an increase in the one-second forced expiratory volume (FEV_1), an increase in maximum expiratory flow rate, an increase in peak expiratory flow rate, an increase in forced vital capacity, and/or a decrease in airway resistance. The resultant decrease in airway obstruction may relieve the dyspnea associated with bronchospasm.

Controlled single- and multiple-dose studies have been performed with pulmonary function monitoring. The duration of effect of a single dose of Metaproterenol Sulfate Tablets 20 mg or Metaproterenol Sulfate Syrup (that is, the period of time during which there is a 15% or greater increase in FEV_1) was up to 4 hours. Four controlled multiple-dose 60-day studies, comparing the effectiveness of Metaproterenol Sulfate Tablets with ephedrine tablets, have been performed. Because of difficulties in study design, only one study was available which could be analyzed in depth. This study showed a loss of efficacy with time for both Metaproterenol Sulfate and ephedrine. Therefore, the physician should take this phenomenon into account in evaluating the individual patient's overall management. Further studies are in progress to adequately explain these results.

Controlled single- and multiple-dose studies have been performed with pulmonary function monitoring. The duration of effect of a single dose of two to three inhalations of Metaproterenol Sulfate Inhalation Aerosol (that is, the period of time during which there is a 20% or greater increase in FEV_1) has varied from 1 to 5 hours.

In repetitive-dosing studies (up to q.i.d.) the duration of effect for a similar dose of Metaproterenol Sulfate Inhalation Aerosol has ranged from about 1 to 2.5 hours. Present studies are inadequate to explain the divergence in duration of the FEV_1 effect between single- and repetitive-dosing studies, respectively. Following controlled single dose studies with Metaproterenol Sulfate Inhalation Solution by an intermittent positive pressure breathing apparatus (IPPB) and by hand-bulb nebulizers, significant improvement (15% or greater increase in FEV_1) occurred within 5 to 30 minutes and persisted for periods varying from 2 to 6 hours.

In these studies, the longer duration of effect occurred in the studies in which the drug was administered by IPPB, i.e., 6 hours, versus 2 to 3 hours when administered by hand-bulb nebulizer. In these studies, the doses used were 0.3 ml by IPPB and 10 inhalations by hand-bulb nebulizer.

In controlled repetitive-dosing studies with Metaproterenol Sulfate Inhalation Solution by IPPB and by hand-bulb nebulizer the onset of effect occurred within 5 to 30 minutes and duration ranged from 4 to 6 hours. In these studies, the doses used were 0.3 ml b.i.d. or t.i.d. when given by IPPB, and 10 inhalations q.i.d. (no more often than q4h) when given by hand-bulb nebulizer. As in the single dose studies, effectiveness was measured as a sustained increase in FEV_1 of 15% or greater. In these repetitive-dosing studies there was no apparent difference in duration between the two methods of delivery. Clinical studies were conducted in which the effectiveness of Metaproterenol Sulfate Inhalation Solution was evaluated by comparison with that of isoproterenol hydrochloride over periods of two to three months. Both drugs continued to produce significant improvement in pulmonary function throughout this period of treatment.

In two well-controlled studies in children 6 to 12 years of age with acute exacerbation of asthma, 70% of patients receiving Metaproterenol Sulfate Inhalation Solution (0.1 mL to 0.2 mL) showed improvement in pulmonary function as demonstrated by a 15% increase in FEV_1 above baseline.

Recent studies in laboratory animals (minipigs, rodents and dogs) recorded the occurrence of cardiac arrhythmias and sudden death (with histologic evidence of myocardial necrosis) when beta agonists and methylxanthines were administered concurrently. The significance of these findings when applied to humans is currently unknown.

INDICATIONS AND USAGE

Metaproterenol Sulfate is indicated as a bronchodilator for bronchial asthma and for reversible bronchospasm which may occur in association with bronchitis and emphysema. Metaproterenol Sulfate Inhalation Solution 5% is additionally indicated for the treatment of acute asthmatic attacks in children age 6 years and older.

Following controlled single dose studies by an intermittent positive pressure breathing apparatus (IPPB) and by hand bulb nebulizers, significant improvement (15% or greater increase in FEV_1) occurred within 5 to 30 minutes and persisted for periods varying from 2 to 6 hours.

In these studies, the longer duration of effect occurred in the studies in which the drug was administered by IPPB, i.e., 6 hours versus 2 to 3 hours when administered by hand bulb nebulizer. In these studies the doses used were 0.3 mL by IPPB and 10 inhalations by hand bulb nebulizer.

In controlled repetitive dosing studies by IPPB and by hand bulb nebulizer the onset of effect occurred within 5 to 30 minutes and duration ranged from 4 to 6 hours. In these studies the doses used were 0.3 mL b.i.d. or t.i.d. when given by IPPB, and 10 inhalations q.i.d. (no more often than q4h) when given by hand bulb nebulizer. As in the single-dose studies, effectiveness was measured as a sustained increase in FEV_1 of 15% or greater. In these repetitive dosing studies there was no apparent difference in duration between the two methods of delivery.

During recent clinical tolerance studies Metaproterenol Sulfate was administered q.i.d. (by nebulizer) for periods of 60 and 90 days. On specified days before, during, and after these open label trials, patients were referred to a laboratory where the effects of single doses of Metaproterenol Sulfate and isoproterenol on pulmonary function were recorded (in a double blind cross-over controlled setting). Both drugs continued to exert significant improvement in function throughout this period of treatment.

Clinical studies were conducted in which the effectiveness of Metaproterenol Sulfate Inhalation Solution was evaluated by comparison with that of isoproterenol hydrochloride over periods of 2-3 months. Both drugs continued to produce significant improvement in pulmonary function throughout this period of treatment.

CONTRAINDICATIONS

Use in patients with cardiac arrhythmias associated with tachycardia is contraindicated.

Although rare, immediate, hypersensitivity reactions can occur. Therefore, Metaproterenol Sulfate is contraindicated in patients with a history of hypersensitivity to any of its components.

WARNINGS

Excessive use of adrenergic aerosols is potentially dangerous. Fatalities have been reported following excessive use of Metaproterenol Sulfate as with other sympathomimetic inhalation preparations, and the exact cause is unknown. Cardiac arrest was noted in several cases.

Metaproterenol Sulfate, like other beta adrenergic agonists, can produce a significant cardiovascular effect in some patients, as measured by pulse rate, blood pressure, symptoms and/or ECG changes. As with other beta adrenergic aerosols, Metaproterenol Sulfate can produce paradoxical bronchospasm (which can be life threatening). If it occurs, the preparation should be discontinued immediately and alternative therapy instituted.

Metaproterenol Sulfate should not be used more often than prescribed. Patients should be advised to contact their physician in the event that they do not respond to their usual dose of a sympathomimetic amine aerosol.

PRECAUTIONS

General: Extreme care must be exercised with respect to the administration of additional sympathomimetic agents. Since Metaproterenol Sulfate is a sympathomimetic amine it should be used with caution in patients with cardiovascular disorders, including ischemic heart disease, hypertension or cardiac arrhythmias, in patients with hyperthyroidism or diabetes mellitus, and in patients who are unusually responsive to sympathomimetic amines or who have convulsive disorders. Significant changes in systolic and diastolic blood pressure could be expected to occur in some patients after use of any beta adrenergic bronchodilator.

Physicians should recognize that a single dose of nebulized Metaproterenol Sulfate in the treatment of acute asthma may alleviate symptoms and improve pulmonary function temporarily but fail to completely abort an attack.

Information for Patients: Extreme care must be exercised with respect to the administration of additional sympathomimetic agents. A sufficient interval of time should elapse prior to administration of another sympathomimetic agent. Metaproterenol Sulfate Inhalation Solution 5% effects may last up to 6 hours or longer. It should not be used more often than recommended and the patient should not increase the number of inhalations or frequency of use without first consulting the physician. If symptoms of asthma get worse, adverse reactions occur, or the patient does not respond to the usual dose, the patient should be instructed to contact the physician immediately.

Metaproterenol Sulfate Tablets and Metaproterenol Sulfate Syrup should not be used more often than prescribed. If symptoms persist, patients should consult a physician promptly.

A single dose of nebulized Metaproterenol Sulfate in the treatment of an acute attack of asthma may not completely abort an attack.

Drug Interactions: Other beta adrenergic aerosol bronchodilators should not be used concomitantly with Metaproterenol Sulfate because they may have additive effects. Beta adrenergic agonists should be administered with caution to patients being treated with monoamine oxidase inhibitors or tricyclic antidepressants, since the action of beta adrenergic agonists on the vascular system may be potentiated.

Carcinogenesis, Mutagenesis, Impairment of Fertility: In an 18-month study in mice, Metaproterenol Sulfate produced a significant increase in benign hepatic adenomas in males and in benign ovarian tumors in females at doses corresponding to 31 and 62 (320 and 640 for Metaproterenol Sulfate Inhalation Aerosol) times the maximum recommended dose (based on a 50 kg individual). In a 2-year study in rats, a nonsignificant incidence of benign leiomyomata of the mesovarium was noted at 62 (640 for Metaproterenol Sulfate Inhalation Aerosol) times the maximum recommended dose. The relevance of these findings to man is not known. Mutagenic studies with Metaproterenol Sulfate have not been conducted. Reproduction studies in rats revealed no evidence of impaired fertility.

PREGNANCY/TERATOGENIC EFFECTS
Pregnancy Category C: Metaproterenol Sulfate has been shown to be teratogenic and embryotoxic in rabbits when given orally in doses 620 times the human inhalation dose and 100 mg/kg or 62 times the human oral dose. These effects included skeletal abnormalities, hydrocephalus and skull bone separation.

Embryotoxicity has also been shown in mice when given orally at doses of 50 mg/kg or 31 times the maximum recommended human oral dose. Results of other oral reproduction studies in rats (40 mg/kg) and rabbits (50 mg/kg) have not revealed any teratogenic, embryotoxic or fetotoxic effects. There are no adequate and well-controlled studies in pregnant women. Metaproterenol Sulfate should be used during pregnancy only if the potential benefit justifies the potential risk to the fetus.

Nursing Mothers: It is not known whether Metaproterenol Sulfate is excreted in human milk; therefore Metaproterenol Sulfate should be used during nursing only if the potential benefit justifies the possible risk to the newborn.

Pediatric Use: See "Dosage and Administration."

ADVERSE REACTIONS
Adverse reactions are similar to those noted with other sympathomimetic agents. Adverse reactions such as tachycardia, hypertension, palpitations, nervousness, tremor, nausea and vomiting have been reported.

The most frequent adverse reaction to Metaproterenol Sulfate administered by metered-dose inhaler among 251 patients in 90-day controlled clinical trials was nervousness. This was reported in 6.8% of patients. Less frequent adverse experiences, occurring in 1-4% of patients were headache, dizziness, palpitations, gastrointestinal distress, tremor, throat irritation, nausea, vomiting, cough and asthma exacerbation. Tachycardia occurred in less than 1% of patients.

Adverse experiences associated with Metaproterenol Sulfate Inhalation Solution 5% in at least 2% of 120 patients participating in multiple-dose clinical trial of 60- and 90-day duration included nervousness (14.1%; n = 17), cough (3.3%; n = 4) headache (3.3%; n = 4), tachycardia (2.5%; n = 3) and tremor (2.5%; n = 3).

Metaproterenol Sulfate Inhalation Solution 5% may be associated with a somewhat higher incidence of adverse reactions in children. In controlled clinical trials conducted in 160 patients the incidence of adverse reactions observed at the recommended doses was as follows: tachycardia, 16.6%; tremor, 33%; nausea, 14%; vomiting, 7.7%. The corresponding incidence in placebo-treated patients was: tachycardia, 7.6%; tremor, 20%; nausea, 7.7%; vomiting, 2.5%.

In two well-controlled studies in children 6 to 12 years of age with acute exacerbation of asthma, Metaproterenol Sulfate Inhalation Solution 5% was not efficacious in approximately 30% of patients, where efficacy was defined as a 15% increase in FEV_1 above baseline at two or more time points during the 1-hour testing period. In 8% of patients there was a decrease in FEV_1 of 10% or more from baseline at two or more time points during the testing period. Insufficient information exists to assess the relationship of drug administration to the decline in pulmonary function observed in these patients, but paradoxical bronchospasm is one possibility.

Adverse events associated with Metaproterenol Sulfate Tablets with an incidence rate of 2% or more in 496 patients participating in 26 controlled clinical trials included nervousness (20.2%; n = 100), tachycardia (17.1%; n = 85), tremor (16.9%; n = 84), headache (7.0%; n = 35), palpitations (3.8%; n = 19), nausea (3.6% n = 18), gastrointestinal distress (3.0%; n = 15), dizziness (2.4%; n = 12) and asthma exacerbation (2.0%; n = 10). Adverse events with an incidence rate of less than 2% in 3 to 9 patients are: insomnia (n = 9), fatigue (n = 7), diarrhea (n = 6), bad taste (n = 4), vomiting (n = 4), drowsiness (n = 3). Adverse events with an incidence rate of less than 2% in one patient are: chest pain, edema, sensory disturbances, weakness, diaphoresis, hives, pain, spasms, blurred vision, laryngeal changes, chattiness, chills, clonus noted on flexing foot, flu symptoms, and facial and finger puffiness.

The incidence of adverse events occurring in at least 1% of the 1,120 patients treated with Metaproterenol Sulfate Syrup in 44 clinical trials are tachycardia (6.1%; n = 68), nervousness (4.8%; n = 54), tremor (1.6%; n = 18), nausea (1.3%; n = 15) and headache (1.1%; n = 12).

It is important to recognize that adverse reactions from beta agonist bronchodilator solutions for nebulization may occur with the use of a new container of a product in patients who have previously tolerated that same product without adverse effect. There have been reports that indicate that such patients may subsequently tolerate replacement containers of the same product without adverse effect.

OVERDOSAGE
The expected symptoms with overdosage are those of excessive beta-adrenergic stimulation and/or any of the symptoms listed under adverse reactions, e.g. angina, hypertension or hypotension, arrhythmias, nervousness, headache, tremor, dry mouth, palpitation, nausea, dizziness, fatigue, malaise and insomnia.

Treatment consists of discontinuation of Metaproterenol Sulfate together with appropriate symptomatic therapy.

DOSAGE AND ADMINISTRATION
If Metaproterenol Sulfate is administered before or after other sympathomimetic bronchodilators, caution should be exercised with respect to possible potentiation of adrenergic effects.

Inhalation Aerosol: The usual single dose is two to three inhalations. With repetitive dosing, inhalation should usually not be repeated more often than about every three to four hours. Total dosage per day should not exceed 12 inhalations. Metaproterenol Sulfate Inhalation Aerosol is not recommended for use in children under 12 years of age.

Inhalation Solution: Usually, treatment need not be repeated more often than every four hours to relieve acute attacks of bronchospasm.

As with all medications, the physician should begin therapy with the lowest effective dose and then titrate the dosage according to the individual patient's requirements.

Inhalation Solution 5%: Metaproterenol Sulfate Inhalation Solution is administered by oral inhalation with the aid of a hand-bulb nebulizer or an intermittent positive pressure breathing apparatus (IPPB).

Metaproterenol Sulfate Inhalation Solution may be administered three to four times a day for the treatment of reversible airways disease in adults. A single dose of nebulized Metaproterenol Sulfate in the treatment of an acute attack of asthma may not completely abort an attack. (See related table).

Inhalation Solution 0.4% and 0.6% Unit-dose Vials; Metaproterenol Sulfate Inhalation Solution Unit-dose Vial is administered by oral inhalation using an IPPB device. The usual adult dose is one vial per nebulization treatment. Each vial of Metaproterenol Sulfate Inhalation Solution 0.4% is equivalent to 0.2 mL Metaproterenol Sulfate Inhalation Solution 5% diluted to 2.5 mL with normal saline; each vial of Metaprotenol Sulfate Inhalation Solution 0.6% is equivalent to 0.3 mL Metaproterenol Sulfate Inhalation Solution 5% diluted to 2.5 mL with normal saline.

Usually, treatment need not be repeated more often than every 4 hours to relieve acute attacks of bronchospasm. As part of a total treatment program in chronic bronchospastic pulmonary diseases, Metaproterenol Sulfate Inhalation Solution Unit-dose Vials may be administered three to four times a day.

As with all medications, the physician should begin therapy with the lowest effective dose and then titrate the dosage according to the individual patient's requirements.

Metaproterenol Sulfate Inhalation Solution Unit-dose Vial is not recommended for use in children under 12 years of age.

As part of a total treatment program in chronic bronchospastic pulmonary diseases, Metaproterenol Sulfate Inhalation Solution may be administered three to four times a day.

Metaproterenol Sulfate Inhalation Solution Unit-dose Vial is not recomended for use in children under 12 years of age.

Syrup: Children: Aged six to nine years or weight under 60 lbs—one teaspoonful three or four times a day. Children over nine years or weight over 60 lbs—two teaspoonfuls three or four times a day. Clinical trial experience in children under the age of 6 is limited. Of 40 children treated with Metaproterenol Sulfate Syrup for at least 1 month, daily doses of approximatel 1.3 to 2.6 mg/kg were well tolerated. *Adults:* two teaspoonfuls three or four times a day. It is recommended that the physician titrate the dosage according to each individual patient's response to therapy.

Tablets: Adults: The usual dose is 20 mg three or four times a day. *Children:* Aged six to nine years or weight under 60 lbs—10 mg three or four times a day. Over nine years or weight over 60 lbs—20 mg three or four times a day. Metaproterenol Sulfate tablets are not recommended for use in children under six years at this time. It is recommended that the physician titrate the dosage according to each individual patient's response to therapy.

INSTRUCTIONS FOR USE OF INHALATION AEROSOL
1. Insert metal canister into clear end of mouthpiece.
2. Remove protective cap, invert canister and *shake well before each use*.
3. Enclose mouthpiece with the lips. The base of the canister should be held vertically.
4. Exhale deeply, then inhale slowly through the mouth and at the same time firmly press once on the upended canister base; continue to inhale deeply. Hold your breath for a few seconds and then remove the mouthpiece from the mouth and exhale slowly.
5. One inhalation is often enough to obtain relief. The inhalation can be repeated once or twice, if necessary, or as your physician directs. Wait at least 2 minutes before repeating the inhalation. In most cases, the dose should not be repeated more often than every 3-4 hours. No more than 12 inhalations should be taken in 1 day.
6. Replace protective cap after use.

WARNING: Do not exceed the dose prescribed by your physician. If difficulty in breathing persists, contact your physician immediately.

Note: When full, the container holds enough medication for at least 200 inhalations. Check regularly, by shaking the cylinder or container, to determine whether it contains any medication. When it first seems empty, there are still about 10 doses left. Refill containers for the plastic mouthpiece are available when prescribed by your physician.

Keep the mouthpiece clean. Wash with hot water. If soap is used, rinse thoroughly with plain water.

Never open the container holding the medication. Opening it is dangerous and renders the contents useless.

Caution: Contents under pressure. Do not puncture or incinerate container. Do not expose to heat or store at temperatures above 120°F. Keep out of reach of small children.

WARNING: Inhalation Aerosol
Contains trichloromonofluoromethane (CFC-11), dichlorodifluoromethane (CFC-12) and dichlorotetrafluoroethane (CFC-114), substances which harm public health and the environment by destroying ozone in the upper atmosphere. Store between 59°F (15°C) and 77°F (25°C). Avoid excessive humidity.

Inhalation Solution: Store between 59°F (15°C) and 77°F (25°C).

Inhalation Solution Unit-dose Vial: Protect from light. Do not use the solution if it is pinkish or darker than slightly yellow or contains a precipitate. Store vials in pouch until ready for use.

Syrup: Store between 59°F (15°C) and 86°F (30°C). Protect from light.

Tablets: Storage for bottles: Store between 59°F (15°C) and 86°F (30°C). Protect from light.

Blister samples: Store between 59°F (15°C) and 77°F (25°C). Protect from light.*

J CODES
5.0%, per ml INH—J7675
0.6%, per 2.5 ml INH—J7672
0.4%, per 2.5 ml INH—J7670

HOW SUPPLIED
AEROSOL LIQUID: 0.65 MG/INH

BRAND/MANUFACTURER	NDC	SIZE	AWP
○ BRAND			
ALUPENT: Boehr Ingelheim	00597-0070-18	10 ml	$17.92

AEROSOL LIQUID W/ADAPTER: 0.65 MG/INH

BRAND/MANUFACTURER	NDC	SIZE	AWP
○ BRAND			
ALUPENT: Boehr Ingelheim	00597-0070-17	10 ml	$20.02

SOLUTION: 0.4%

AVERAGE UNIT PRICE (AVAILABLE SIZES)		GENERIC A-RATED AVERAGE PRICE (GAAP)	
BRAND	$0.67	2.5 ml 25s	$23.96
GENERIC	$0.36		

BRAND/MANUFACTURER	NDC	SIZE	AWP
◆ BRAND			
ALUPENT: Boehr Ingelheim	00597-0078-62	2.5 ml 25s ud	$41.76

DOSAGE AND ADMINISTRATION

Population	Method of Administration	Usual Single Dose	Range	Dilution
Adult 12 years and older	Hand-bulb nebulizer	10 inhalations	5-15 inhalations	No dilution
	IPPB or nebulizer	0.3 mL	0.2-0.3 mL	Diluted in approx. 2.5 mL saline solution or other diluent
Pediatric 6-12 years	Nebulizer	0.1 mL	0.1-0.2 mL	Diluted in saline solution to a total volume of 3 mL

BRAND/MANUFACTURER	NDC	SIZE	AWP
◆ GENERICS			
Par	49884-0360-48	2.5 ml 25s	$29.95
Dey	49502-0678-03	2.5 ml 25s	$30.75
Roxane	00054-8613-11	2.5 ml 25s ud	$11.18
Astra	00186-4131-01	2.5 ml 100s ud	$68.69

SOLUTION: 0.6%

AVERAGE UNIT PRICE (AVAILABLE SIZES)		GENERIC A-RATED AVERAGE PRICE (GAAP)	
BRAND	$0.67	2.5 ml 25s	$23.96
GENERIC	$0.36		

BRAND/MANUFACTURER	NDC	SIZE	AWP
◆ BRAND			
ALUPENT: Boehr Ingelheim	00597-0069-62	2.5 ml 25s ud	$41.76
◆ GENERICS			
Par	49884-0361-48	2.5 ml 25s	$29.95
Dey	49502-0676-03	2.5 ml 25s	$30.75
Roxane	00054-8614-11	2.5 ml 25s	$11.18
Astra	00186-4130-01	2.5 ml 100s ud	$68.69

SOLUTION: 5%

AVERAGE UNIT PRICE (AVAILABLE SIZES)	
BRAND	$1.18

BRAND/MANUFACTURER	NDC	SIZE	AWP
◆ BRAND			
METAPREL: Sandoz Pharm	00078-0210-26	10 ml	$7.56
ALUPENT: Boehr Ingelheim	00597-0071-75	10 ml	$14.58
	00597-0071-30	30 ml	$40.15

SOLUTION: 6%

BRAND/MANUFACTURER	NDC	SIZE	AWP
◆ GENERICS			
Moore,H.L.	00839-7639-07	2.5 ml 25s	$31.44

SYRUP: 10 MG/5 ML

AVERAGE UNIT PRICE (AVAILABLE SIZES)		GENERIC A-RATED AVERAGE PRICE (GAAP)	
BRAND	$0.05	480 ml	$16.05
GENERIC	$0.03		
HCFA FUL (480 ml)	$0.02		

BRAND/MANUFACTURER	NDC	SIZE	AWP
◆ BRAND			
METAPREL: Sandoz Pharm	00078-0211-33	480 ml	$13.08
ALUPENT: Boehr Ingelheim	00597-0073-16	480 ml	$33.37
◆ GENERICS			
Raway	00686-6117-38	480 ml	$8.50
Pennex	00426-8650-16	480 ml	$13.00
Pennex	00832-8650-16	480 ml	$13.00
Moore,H.L.	00839-7442-69	480 ml	$13.49
Aligen	00405-3255-16	480 ml	$13.50
Mason Dist	11845-0412-13	480 ml	$14.50
Silarx	54838-0507-80	480 ml	$15.54
Schein	00364-2417-16	480 ml	$15.80
Rugby	00536-1462-85	480 ml	$16.04
Qualitest	00603-1422-58	480 ml	$16.45
Major	00904-2880-16	480 ml	$17.25
Goldline	00182-6080-40	480 ml	$17.25
Copley	38245-0138-07	480 ml	$17.90
URL	00677-1445-33	480 ml	$18.89
Geneva	00781-6404-16	480 ml	$20.43
Biocraft	00332-6117-38	480 ml	$23.70

TABLETS: 10 MG

AVERAGE UNIT PRICE (AVAILABLE SIZES)		GENERIC A-RATED AVERAGE PRICE (GAAP)	
BRAND	$0.23	100s	$14.54
GENERIC	$0.15		
HCFA FUL (100s ea)	$0.07		

BRAND/MANUFACTURER	NDC	SIZE	AWP
◆ BRAND			
METAPREL: Sandoz Pharm	00078-0212-05	100s	$12.36
▶ ALUPENT: Boehr Ingelheim	00597-0074-01	100s	$34.20

◆ RATED THERAPEUTICALLY EQUIVALENT; ◇ THERAPEUTIC EQUIVALENCE UNCONFIRMED; ○ UNRATED

BRAND/MANUFACTURER	NDC	SIZE	AWP
◆ GENERICS			
Raway	00686-2230-09	100s	$6.75
Qualitest	00603-4464-21	100s	$12.51
Moore,H.L.	00839-7485-06	100s	$13.43
Biocraft	00332-2230-09	100s	$14.00
Mason Dist	11845-0144-01	100s	$15.60
URL	00677-1253-01	100s	$15.62
Rugby	00536-4437-01	100s	$15.67
Par	49884-0258-01	100s	$15.70
Major	00904-2878-60	100s	$15.70
Schein	00364-2283-01	100s	$15.75
Goldline	00182-1283-01	100s	$15.75
Aligen	00405-4629-01	100s	$16.42
Major	00904-2878-61	100s ud	$16.13

TABLETS: 20 MG

AVERAGE UNIT PRICE (AVAILABLE SIZES)		GENERIC A-RATED AVERAGE PRICE (GAAP)	
BRAND	$0.33	100s	$19.76
GENERIC	$0.20		
HCFA FUL (100s ea)	$0.11		

BRAND/MANUFACTURER	NDC	SIZE	AWP
◆ BRAND			
METAPREL: Sandoz Pharm	00078-0213-05	100s	$16.50
ALUPENT: Boehr Ingelheim	00597-0072-01	100s	$48.59
◆ GENERICS			
Raway	00686-2232-09	100s	$9.75
Biocraft	00332-2232-09	100s	$17.75
Moore,H.L.	00839-7486-06	100s	$18.23
Rugby	00536-4438-01	100s	$19.35
Major	00904-2879-60	100s	$19.60
Qualitest	00603-4465-21	100s	$19.90
URL	00677-1254-01	100s	$20.90
Goldline	00182-1284-01	100s	$21.00
Par	49884-0259-01	100s	$23.19
Schein	00364-2284-01	100s	$23.25
Aligen	00405-4630-01	100s	$23.25
Major	00904-2879-61	100s ud	$20.94

Metaraminol Bitartrate

DESCRIPTION
Metaraminol Bitartrate is a potent sympathomimetic amine that increases both systolic and diastolic blood pressure.

Metaraminol Bitartrate is [R-(R*,S*)]-α-(1-aminoethyl)-3-hydroxybenzenem-ethanol [R-(R*,K*)]-2,3-dihydroxybutanedioate (1:1) (salt), which is levorotatory. Its empirical formula is $C_9H_{13}NO_2 \cdot C_4H_6O_6$.

Metaraminol Bitartrate is a white, crystalline powder with a molecular weight of 317.29, is freely soluble in water, slightly soluble in alcohol, and practically insoluble in chloroform and in ether.

Injection Metaraminol Bitartrate is a sterile solution.

Each mL contains:

Metaraminol Bitartrate equivalent to Metaraminol ....10 mg

Following is its chemical structure:

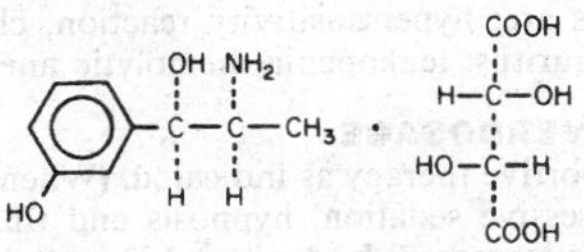

CLINICAL PHARMACOLOGY
The pressor effect of Metaraminol Bitartrate begins in 1 to 2 minutes after intravenous infusion, in about 10 minutes after intramuscular injection, and in 5 to 20 minutes after subcutaneous injection. The effect lasts from about 20 minutes to one hour. Metaraminol Bitartrate has a positive inotropic effect on the heart and a peripheral vasoconstrictor action.

Renal, coronary, and cerebral blood flow are a function of perfusion pressure and regional resistance. In patients with insufficient or failing vasoconstriction, there is additional advantage to the peripheral action of Metaraminol Bitartrate, but in most patients with shock, vasoconstriction is adequate and any further increase is unnecessary. Blood flow to vital organs may decrease with Metaraminol Bitartrate if regional resistance increases excessively.

The pressor effect of Mataraminol Bitartrate is decreased but not reversed by alpha-adrenergic blocking agents. Primary or secondary fall in blood pressure and tachyphylactic response to repeated use are uncommon.

INDICATIONS AND USAGE
Mataraminol Bitartrate is indicated for prevention and treatment of the acute hypotensive state occurring with spinal anesthesia. It is also indicated as adjunctive treatment of hypotension due to hemorrhage, reactions to medications, surgical complications, and shock associated with brain damage due to trauma or tumor.

UNLABELED USES
Metaraminol Bitartrate is used alone or as an adjunct in the treatment of priapism.

CONTRAINDICATIONS
Use of Metaraminol Bitartrate with cyclopropane or halothane anesthesia should be avoided, unless clinical circumstances demand such use.

Hypersensitivity to any component of this product, including sulfites (see "Warnings").

WARNINGS
Use of sympathomimetic amines with monoamine oxidase inhibitors or tricyclic antidepressants may result in potentiation of the pressor effect. (See "Precautions, Drug Interactions.")

Metaraminol Bitartrate contains sodium bisulfite, a sulfite that may cause allergic-type reactions including anaphylactic symptoms and life-threatening or less severe asthmatic episodes in certain susceptible people. The overall prevalence of sulfite sensitivity in the general population is unknown and probably low. Sulfite sensitivity is seen more frequently in asthmatic than in nonasthmatic people.

PRECAUTIONS
GENERAL
Caution should be used to avoid excessive blood pressure response. Rapidly induced hypertensive responses have been reported to cause acute pulmonary edema, arrhythmias, cerebral hemorrhage, or cardiac arrest.

Patients with cirrhosis should be treated with caution, with adequate restoration of electrolytes if diuresis ensues. Fatal ventricular arrhythmia was reported in one patient with Laennec's cirrhosis while receiving Metaraminol Bitartrate. In several instances, ventricular extrasystoles that appeared during infusion of this vasopressor subsided promptly when the rate of infusion was reduced.

With the prolonged action of Metaraminol Bitartrate, a cumulative effect is possible. If there is an excessive vasopressor response there may be a prolonged elevation of blood pressure even after discontinuation of therapy.

When vasopressor amines are used for long periods, the resulting vasoconstriction may prevent adequate expansion of circulating volume and may cause perpetuation of shock. There is evidence that plasma volume may be reduced in all types of shock, and that the measurement of central venous pressure is useful in assessing the adequacy of the circulating blood volume. Therefore, blood or plasma volume expanders should be used when the principal reason for hypotension or shock is decreased circulating volume.

Because of its vasoconstrictor effect Metaraminol Bitartrate should be given with caution in heart or thyroid disease, hypertension, or diabetes. Sympathomimetic amines may provoke a relapse in patients with a history of malaria.

DRUG INTERACTIONS
Metaraminol Bitartrate should be used with caution in digitalized patients, since the combination of digitals and sympathomimetic amines may cause ectopic arrhythmias.

Monoamine oxidase inhibitors or tricyclic antidepressants may potentiate the action of sympathomimetic amines. Therefore, when irritating pressor therapy in patients receiving these drugs, the initial dose should be small and given with caution. (See "Warnings.")

CARCINOGENESIS, MUTAGENESIS, IMPAIRMENT OF FERTILITY
Studies in animals have not been performed to evaluate the mutagenic or carcinogenic potential of Metaraminol Bitartrate or its potential to affect fertility.

PREGNANCY
Pregnancy Category C: Animal reproduction studies have not been conducted with Metaraminol Bitartrate. It is not known whether Metaraminol Bitartrate can cause fetal harm when given to a pregnant woman or can affect reproduction capacity. Metaraminol Bitartrate should be given to a pregnant woman only if clearly needed.

NURSING MOTHERS
It is not known whether this drug is secreted in human milk. Because many drugs are secreted in human milk, caution should be exercised when Metaraminol Bitartrate is given to a nursing woman.

PEDIATRIC USE
Safety and effectiveness in children have not been established.

ADVERSE REACTIONS
Sympathomimetic amines, including Metaraminol Bitartrate, may cause sinus or ventricular tachycardia, or other arrhythmias, especially in patients with myocardial infarction. (See "Precautions.")

In patients with a history of malaria, these compounds may provoke a relapse.

Abscess formation, tissue necrosis, or sloughing rarely may follow the use of Metaraminol Bitartrate. In choosing the site of injection, it is important to avoid those areas recognized as *not* suitable for use of any pressor agent and to discontinue the infusion immediately if infiltration or thrombosis occurs. Although the physician may be forced by the urgent nature of the patient's condition to choose injection sites that are not recognized as suitable, he should, when possible, use the preferred areas of injection. The larger veins of the antecubital fossa or the thigh are preferred to veins in the dorsum of the hand or ankle veins, particularly in patients with peripheral vascular disease, diabetes mellitus. Buerger's disease, or conditions with coexistent hypercoagulability.

OVERDOSAGE

Overdosage may result in severe hypertension accompanied by headache, constricting sensation in the chest, nausea, vomiting, euphoria, diaphoresis, pulmonary edema, tachycardia, bradycardia, sinus arrhythmia, atrial or ventricualr arrhythmias, cerebral hemorrhage, myocardial infarction, cardiac arrest or convulsions.

Should an excessive elevation of blood pressure occur, it may be immediately relieved by a sympatholytic agent, e.g. phentolamine. An appropriate antiarrhythmic agent may also be required.

The oral LD_{50} in the rat and mouse is 240 mg/kg and 99 mg/kg, respectively.

DOSAGE AND ADMINISTRATION

Metaraminol Bitartrate may be given intramuscularly, subcutaneously, or intravenously, the route depending on the nature and severity of the indication.

Parenteral drug products should be inspected visually for particulate matter and discoloration prior to use, whenever solution and container permit.

Allow at least 10 minutes to elapse before increasing the dose because the maximum effect is not immediately apparent. When the vasopressor is discontinued, observe the patient carefully as the effect of the drug tapers off, so that therapy can be reinitiated promptly if the blood pressure falls too rapidly. The response to vasopressors may be poor in patients with coexistent shock and acidosis. When indicated, established methods of shock management should be used, such as blood or fluid replacement.

Intramuscular or Subcutaneous Injection: (for prevention of hypotension, see *"Indications"*): The recommended dose is 2 to 10 mg (0.2 to 1 mL). As with other agents given subcutaneously, only the preferred sites of injection, as set forth in standard texts, should be used.

Intravenous Infusion: (for adjunctive treatment of hypotension, see *"Indications"*): The recommended dose is 15 to 100 mg (1.5 to 10 mL) in 500 mL of Sodium Chloride Injection or 5% Dextrose Injection, adjusting the rate of infusion to maintain the blood pressure at the desired level. Higher concentrations of Metaraminol Bitartrate, 150 to 500 mg per 500 mL of infusion fluid, have been used.

If the patient needs more saline or dextrose solution at a rate of flow that would provide an excessive dose of the vasopressor, the recommended volume of infusion fluid (500 mL) should be increased accordingly. Metaraminol Bitartrate may also be added to *less* than 500 mL of infusion fluid if a smaller volume is desired.

COMPATIBILITY INFORMATION

In addition to Sodium Chloride Injection and Dextrose Injection 5%, the following infusion solutions were found physically and chemically compatible with Injection Metaraminol Bitartrate when 5 mL of Injection Metaraminol Bitartrate, 10 mg/mL Metaraminol equivalent), was added to 500 mL of infusion solution: Ringer's Injection, Lactated Ringer's Injection, Dextran 6% in Saline[†], Normosol®-R pH 7.4[†], and Normosol®-M in D5-W[†].

When Injection Metaraminol Bitartrate is mixed with an infusion solution, sterile precautions should be observed. Since infusion solutions generally do not contain preservatives, mixtures should be used within 24 hours.

Direct Intravenous Injection: In severe shock, when time is of great importance, this agent should be given by direct intravenous injection. The suggested dose is 0.5 to 5 mg (0.05 to 0.5 mL), followed by an infusion of 15 to 100 mg (1.5 to 10 mL) in 500 mL of infusion fluid as described previously. Vials may be sterilized by autoclaving or by immersion in a sterilizing solution.

STORAGE

Protect from light. Store container in carton until contents have been used.

Avoid storage at temperatures below −20°C (−4°F) and above 40°C (104°F).

J CODES

Up to 10 mg IV,IM,SC—J0380

HOW SUPPLIED

INJECTION: 1%

BRAND/MANUFACTURER	NDC	SIZE	AWP
◆ BRAND			
ARAMINE: Merck	00006-3222-10	10 ml	$11.48

Metastron *SEE* STRONTIUM-89 CHLORIDE

Metatensin *SEE* RESERPINE AND TRICHLORMETHIAZIDE

† Product of Abbott Laboratories

Metaxalone

DESCRIPTION

Each tablet contains: Metaxalone, 400 mg. The chemical name of Metaxalone is 5-[(3,4-dimethylphenoxy)methyl]-2 oxazolidinone.

Following is its chemical structure:

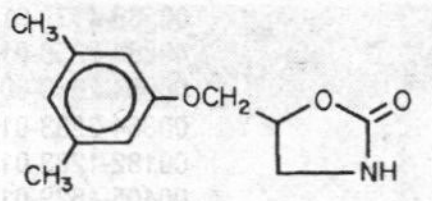

ACTIONS

The mechanism of action of Metaxalone in humans has not been established, but may be due to general central nervous system depression. It has no direct action on the contractile mechanism of striated muscle, the motor end plate or the nerve fiber.

INDICATIONS

Metaxalone is indicated as an adjunct to rest, physical therapy, and other measures for the relief of discomforts associated with acute, painful musculoskeletal conditions. The mode of action of this drug has not been clearly identified, but may be related to its sedative properties. Metaxalone does not directly relax tense skeletal muscles in man.

CONTRAINDICATIONS

Metaxalone is contraindicated in individuals who have shown hypersensitivity to the drug. Metaxalone should not be administered to patients with a known tendency to drug-induced, hemolytic, or other anemias. It is contraindicated in patients with significantly impaired renal or hepatic function.

PRECAUTIONS

Elevation in cephalin flocculation tests without concurrent changes in other liver function parameters have been noted. Hence, it is recommended that Metaxalone be administered with great care to patients with pre-existing liver damage and that serial liver function studies be performed as required.

False-positive Benedict's tests, due to an unknown reducing substance, have been noted. A glucose-specific test will differentiate findings.

Pregnancy: Reproduction studies have been performed in rats and have revealed no evidence of impaired fertility or harm to the fetus due to Metaxalone. Reactions reports from marketing experience have not revealed evidence of fetal injury, but such experience cannot exclude the possibility of infrequent or subtle damage to the human fetus. Safe use of Metaxalone has not been established with regard to possible adverse effects upon fetal development. Therefore, Metaxalone tablets should not be used in women who are or may become pregnant and particularly during early pregnancy unless in the judgment of the physician the potential benefits outweigh the possible hazards.

Nursing Mothers: It is not known whether this drug is secreted in human milk. As a general rule, nursing should not be undertaken while a patient is on a drug since many drugs are excreted in human milk.

Pediatric Use: Safety and effectiveness in children 12 years of age and below have not been established.

ADVERSE REACTIONS

The most frequent reactions to Metaxalone include nausea, vomiting, gastrointestinal upset, drowsiness, dizziness, headache, and nervousness or "irritability." Other adverse reactions are: hypersensitivity reaction, characterized by a light rash with or without pruritus; leukopenia; hemolytic anemia; jaundice.

MANAGEMENT OF OVERDOSAGE

Gastric lavage and supportive therapy as indicated. (When determining the LD_{50} in rats and mice, progressive sedation, hypnosis and finally respiratory failure were noted as the dosage increased. In dogs, no LD_{50} could be determined as the higher doses produced an emetic action in 15 to 30 minutes.) No documented case of major toxicity has been reported.

DOSAGE

The recommended dose for adults and children over 12 years of age is two tablets (800 mg) three to four times a day.

Store at controlled room temperature, between 15°C and 30°C (59°F and 86°F).

HOW SUPPLIED

TABLETS: 400 MG

BRAND/MANUFACTURER	NDC	SIZE	AWP
◇ BRAND			
SKELAXIN: Carnrick	00086-0062-10	100s	$33.75
	00086-0062-50	500s	$138.80

Methacholine Chloride

METHACHOLINE CHLORIDE IS A BRONCHOCONSTRICTOR AGENT FOR DIAGNOSTIC PURPOSES ONLY AND SHOULD NOT BE USED AS A

◆ RATED THERAPEUTICALLY EQUIVALENT; ◇ THERAPEUTIC EQUIVALENCE UNCONFIRMED; ○ UNRATED

THERAPEUTIC AGENT. METHACHOLINE CHLORIDE INHALATION CHALLENGE SHOULD BE PERFORMED ONLY UNDER THE SUPERVISION OF A PHYSICIAN TRAINED IN AND THOROUGHLY FAMILIAR WITH ALL ASPECTS OF THE TECHNIQUE OF METHACHOLINE CHALLENGE, ALL CONTRAINDICATIONS, WARNINGS AND PRECAUTIONS, AND THE MANAGEMENT OF RESPIRATORY DISTRESS.

EMERGENCY EQUIPMENT AND MEDICATION SHOULD BE IMMEDIATELY AVAILABLE TO TREAT ACUTE RESPIRATORY DISTRESS.

METHACHOLINE CHLORIDE SHOULD BE ADMINISTERED ONLY BY INHALATION. SEVERE BRONCHOCONSTRICTION AND REDUCTION IN RESPIRATORY FUNCTION CAN RESULT FROM THE ADMINISTRATION OF METHACHOLINE CHLORIDE. PATIENTS WITH SEVERE HYPER-REACTIVITY OF THE AIRWAYS CAN EXPERIENCE BRONCHOCONSTRICTION AT A DOSAGE AS LOW AS 0.025 MG/ML (0.125 CUMULATIVE UNITS). IF SEVERE BRONCHOCONSTRICTION OCCURS, IT SHOULD BE REVERSED IMMEDIATELY BY THE ADMINISTRATION OF A RAPID-ACTING INHALED BRONCHODILATOR AGENT (BETA AGONIST). BECAUSE OF THE POTENTIAL FOR SEVERE BRONCHOCONSTRICTION, METHACHOLINE CHLORIDE CHALLENGE SHOULD NOT BE PERFORMED IN ANY PATIENT WITH CLINICALLY APPARENT ASTHMA, WHEEZING, OR VERY LOW BASELINE PULMONARY FUNCTION TESTS (E.G., FEV$_1$ LESS THAN 1 TO 1.5 LITER OR LESS THAN 70% OF THE PREDICTED VALUES). PLEASE CONSULT STANDARD NOMOGRAMS FOR PREDICTED VALUES.[1]

DESCRIPTION

Methacholine Chloride is a parasympathomimetic (cholinergic) bronchoconstrictor agent to be administered in solution only, by inhalation, for diagnostic purposes. Each 5-mL vial contains 100 mg of Methacholine Cl powder which is to be reconstituted with 0.9% sodium chloride injection containing 0.4% phenol (pH 7.0). See *"Dosage and Administration"* for dilution procedures, concentrations and schedule of administration.

Chemically, Methacholine Cl (the active ingredient) is 1-propanaminium, 2-(acetyloxy)-*N,N,N,*-trimethyl,-chloride. It is a white to practically white deliquescent compound, soluble in water. Methacholine Cl has an empirical formula of $C_8H_{18}ClNO_2$ and a calculated molecular weight of 195.69.

Following is its chemical structure:

$$[CH_3COOCHCH_2N^+(CH_3)_3] \ Cl^-$$
$$\quad\quad\quad | \quad\quad\quad\quad\quad$$
$$\quad\quad\quad CH_3 \quad\quad\quad\quad\quad$$

CLINICAL PHARMACOLOGY

Methacholine Cl is the β-methyl homolog of acetylcholine and differs from the latter primarily in its greater duration and selectivity of action. Bronchial smooth muscle contains significant parasympathetic (cholinergic) innervation. Bronchoconstriction occurs when the vagus nerve is stimulated and acetylcholine is released from the nerve endings. Muscle constriction is essentially confined to the local site of release because acetylcholine is rapidly inactivated by acetylcholinesterase.

Compared with acetylcholine, Methacholine Cl is more slowly hydrolyzed by acetylcholinesterase and is almost totally resistant to inactivation by nonspecific cholinesterase or pseudocholinesterase.

When a sodium chloride solution containing Methacholine Cl is inhaled, subjects with asthma are markedly more sensitive to Methacholine-induced bronchoconstriction than are healthy subjects. This difference in response is the pharmacologic basis for the Methacholine Cl inhalation diagnostic challenge. However, it should be recognized that Methacholine challenge may occasionally be positive after influenza, upper respiratory infections or immunizations, in very young or very old patients, or in patients with chronic lung disease (cystic fibrosis, sarcoidosis, tuberculosis, chronic obstructive pulmonary disease). The challenge may also be positive in patients with allergic rhinitis without asthma, in smokers, in patients after exposure to air pollutants, or in patients who have had or will in the future develop asthma.

There are no metabolic and pharmacokinetic data available on Methacholine Cl.

INDICATIONS AND USAGE

Methacholine Cl is indicated for the diagnosis of bronchial airway hyperreactivity in subjects who do not have clinically apparent asthma.

CONTRAINDICATIONS

Methacholine Cl is contraindicated in patients with known hypersensitivity to this drug or to other parasympathomimetic agents.

Repeated administration of Methacholine Cl by inhalation other than on the day that a patient undergoes challenge with increasing doses is contraindicated.

Inhalation challenge should not be performed in patients receiving any beta-adrenergic blocking agent because in such patients responses to Methacholine Cl can be exaggerated or prolonged, and may not respond as readily to accepted modalities of treatment (see *"Warnings"*).

PRECAUTIONS

General: Administration of Methacholine Cl to patients with epilepsy, cardiovascular disease accompanied by bradycardia, vagotonia, peptic ulcer disease, thyroid disease, urinary tract obstruction or other condition that could be adversely affected by a cholinergic agent should be undertaken only if the physician feels benefit to the individual outweighs the potential risks.

Information for Patients: To assure the safe and effective use of Methacholine Cl inhalation challenge, the following instructions and information should be given to patients:

1. Patients should be instructed regarding symptoms that may occur as a result of the test and how such symptoms can be managed.
2. A female patient should inform her physician if she is pregnant, or the date of her last onset of menses, or the date and result of her last pregnancy test. (See *"Precautions: Pregnancy."*)

Carcinogenesis, Mutagenesis, Impairment of Fertility: There have been no studies with Methacholine Cl that would permit an evaluation of its carcinogenic or mutagenic potential or of its effect on fertility.

Pregnancy: Teratogenic Effects: Pregnancy Category C. Animal reproduction studies have not been conducted with Methacholine Cl. It is not known whether Methacholine Cl can cause fetal harm when administered to a pregnant patient or affect reproductive capacity. Methacholine Cl should be given to a pregnant woman only if clearly needed.

IN FEMALES OF CHILDBEARING POTENTIAL, METHACHOLINE CL INHALATION CHALLENGE SHOULD BE PERFORMED EITHER WITHIN TEN DAYS FOLLOWING THE ONSET OF MENSES OR WITHIN 2 WEEKS OF A NEGATIVE PREGNANCY TEST.

Nursing Mothers: Methacholine Cl inhalation challenge should not be administered to a nursing mother since it is not known whether Methacholine Cl when inhaled is excreted in breast milk.

Pediatric Use: The safety and efficacy of Methacholine Cl inhalation challenge have not been established in children below the age of 5 years.

ADVERSE REACTIONS

Adverse reactions associated with 153 inhaled Methacholine Cl challenges include one occurrence each of headache, throat irritation, lightheadedness and itching.

Methacholine Cl is to be administered only by inhalation. When administered orally or by injection, Methacholine Cl is reported to be associated with nausea and vomiting, substernal pain or pressure, hypotension, fainting and transient complete heart block. (See *"Overdosage."*)

OVERDOSAGE

Methacholine Cl is to be administered only by inhalation. When administered orally or by injection, overdosage with Methacholine Cl can result in a syncopal reaction, with cardiac arrest and loss of consciousness. Serious toxic reactions should be treated with 0.5 mg to 1 mg of atropine sulfate, administered IM or IV.

The acute (24-hour) oral LD$_{50}$ of Methacholine Cl and related compounds is 1100 mg/kg in the mouse and 750 mg/kg in the rat.

Cynomolgus monkeys were exposed to a 2% (20 mg/mL) aerosol of Methacholine Cl in acute (10-minute) and subchronic (7-day) inhalation toxicity studies. In the former study, animals exposed to the aerosol for up to 10 minutes demonstrated an increase in respiratory rate and decrease in tidal volume after 30 seconds. These changes peaked at 2-minutes and were followed by a rise in pulmonary resistance and a decrease in compliance. Pulmonary function returned to normal 20 to 25 minutes after exposure ended. In the 7-day study, monkeys were given daily inhalations equivalent to the maximum and roughly five times the maximum standard human dose. Although the typical pulmonary response/recovery sequence was observed, distinct changes in airway resistance were noted at the end of the study. These changes were not rapidly reversed in the maximum equivalent standard-dose group, which was observed for 9 weeks.

DOSAGE AND ADMINISTRATION

Before Methacholine Cl inhalation challenge is begun, baseline pulmonary function tests must be performed. A subject to be challenged must have an FEV$_1$ of at least 70% of the predicted value.

The target level for a positive challenge is a 20% reduction in the FEV$_1$ compared with the baseline value after inhalation of the control sodium chloride solution. This target value should be calculated and recorded before Methacholine Cl challenge is started.

Dilutions: (Note: Do not inhale powder. Do not handle this material if you have asthma or hay fever.) All dilutions should be made with 0.9% sodium chloride injection containing 0.4% phenol (pH 7.0). After adding the sodium chloride solution, shake each vial to obtain a clear solution.

DILUTION SEQUENCE-MULTIPLE PATIENT TESTING (2-5 PATIENTS) (REQUIRES 2 VIALS OF METHACHOLINE CL)

Vials		Concentrations
A$_1$ & A$_2$	Add 4 mL of 0.9% sodium chloride injection containing 0.4% phenol (pH 7.0) to each of two 5 mL vials containing 110 mg of Methacholine Cl. These will be designated vials A$_1$ and A$_2$.	25 mg/mL

Serial Concentration	Number of Breaths	Cumulative Units per Concentration	Total Cumulative Units
0.025 mg/mL	5	0.125	0.125
0.25 mg/mL	5	1.25	1.375
2.5 mg/mL	5	12.5	13.88
10.0 mg/mL	5	50.0	63.88
25.0 mg/mL	5	125.0	188.88

Vials		Concentrations
B	Remove 3 mL from vial A₁, transfer to another vial and add 4.5 mL of 0.9% sodium chloride injection containing 0.4% phenol (pH 7.0). This is vial B.	10 mg/mL
C	Remove 1 mL from vial A₂, transfer to another vial and add 9 mL of 0.9% sodium chloride injection containing 0.4% phenol (pH 7.0). This is vial C.	2.5 mg/mL
D	Remove 1 mL from vial C, transfer to another vial and add 9 mL of 0.9% sodium chloride injection containing 0.4% phenol (pH 7.0). This is vial D.	0.25 mg/mL
E	Remove 1 mL from vial D, transfer to another vial and add 9 mL of 0.9% sodium chloride injection containing 0.4% phenol (pH 7.0) This is vial E. Vial E must be prepared on the day of challenge.	0.025 mg/mL

DILUTION SEQUENCE—SINGLE PATIENT TESTING

Vials		Concentrations
A	Add 4 mL of 0.9% sodium chloride injection containing 0.4% phenol (pH 7.0) to the 5 mL vial containing 100 mg of Methacholine Cl. This is vial A.	25 mg/mL
B	Remove 1 mL from vial A, transfer to another vial and add 1.5 mL of 0.9% sodium chloride injection containing 0.4% phenol (pH 7.0). This is vial B.	10 mg/mL
C	Remove 1 mL from vial A, transfer to another vial and add 9 mL of 0.9% sodium chloride injection containing 0.4% phenol (pH 7.0). This is vial C.	2.5 mg/mL
D	Remove 1 mL from vial C, transfer to another vial and add 9 mL of 0.9% sodium chloride injection containing 0.4% phenol (pH 7.0). This is vial D.	0.25 mg/mL
E	Remove 1 mL from vial D, transfer to another vial and and add 9 mL of 0.9% sodium chloride injection containing 0.4% phenol (pH 7.0). This is vial E. Vial E must be prepared on the day of challenge.	0.025 mg/mL

Dilutions A through D should be stored at 36° to 46°F in a refrigerator and can be stored for up to 2 weeks. (The unreconstituted powder should be stored at 59° to 86°F.) After this time, discard the vials and prepare new dilutions. Freezing does not affect the stability of dilutions A through D. Vial E must be prepared on the day of challenge. A bacterial-retentive filter (porosity 0.22μ) should be used when transferring a solution from each vial to a nebulizer.

Procedure: A standardized procedure for inhalation has been developed.

The challenge is performed by giving a subject ascending serial concentrations of Methacholine Cl. At each concentration, five breaths are administered by a nebulizer that permits intermittent delivery time of 0.6 seconds by either a Y-tube or a breath-actuated timing device (dosimeter).

At each of five inhalations of a serial concentration, the subject begins at functional residual capacity (FRC) and slowly and completely inhales the dose delivered. Within 5 minutes, FEV_1 values are determined. The procedure ends either when there is a 20% or greater reduction in the FEV_1 compared with the baseline sodium chloride solution value (i.e., a positive response) or if 188.88 total cumulative units has been administered (see table below) and the FEV_1 has been reduced by 14% or less (ie, a negative response). If there is a reduction of 15% to 19% in the FEV_1 compared with baseline, either the challenge may be repeated at that concentration or a higher concentration may be given as long as the dosage administered does not result in total cumulative units exceeding 188.88.

The following is a suggested schedule for the administration of Methacholine Cl challenge. Cumulative units are calculated by multiplying the number of breaths by the concentration administered.

Total cumulative units is the sum of cumulative units for each concentration administered. (See related table).

An inhaled beta-agonist may be administered after Methacholine Cl challenge to expedite the return of the FEV_1 to baseline and to relieve the discomfort of the subject. Most patients revert to normal pulmonary function within 5 minutes following bronchodilators or within 30 to 45 minutes without any bronchodilator.

Storage
Store the powder at 59° to 86°F. Refrigerate the reconstituted solutions at 36° to 46°F.

REFERENCE
1. Morris JF, Koski WA, Johnson LC. Spirometric standards for healthy nonsmoking adults. *Am Rev Resp Dis.* Jan 1971; 103:57-67.

HOW SUPPLIED
POWDER FOR RECONSTITUTION: 100 MG

BRAND/MANUFACTURER	NDC	SIZE	AWP
○ **BRAND**			
PROVOCHOLINE: Roche Labs	00004-6102-01	5 gm	$51.27

Methadone Hydrochloride

> **CONDITIONS FOR DISTRIBUTION AND USE OF METHADONE PRODUCTS: CODE OF FEDERAL REGULATIONS, TITLE 21, SEC. 291.505**
>
> METHADONE PRODUCTS, WHEN USED FOR THE TREATMENT OF NARCOTIC ADDICTION IN DETOXIFICATION OR MAINTENANCE PROGRAMS, SHALL BE DISPENSED ONLY BY APPROVED HOSPITAL PHARMACIES, APPROVED COMMUNITY PHARMACIES, AND MAINTENANCE PROGRAMS APPROVED BY THE FOOD AND DRUG ADMINISTRATION AND THE DESIGNATED STATE AUTHORITY.
>
> APPROVED MAINTENANCE PROGRAMS SHALL DISPENSE AND USE METHADONE IN ORAL FORM ONLY AND ACCORDING TO THE TREATMENT REQUIREMENTS STIPULATED IN THE FEDERAL METHADONE REGULATIONS (21 CFR 291.505).
>
> FAILURE TO ABIDE BY THE REQUIREMENTS IN THESE REGULATIONS MAY RESULT IN CRIMINAL PROSECUTION, SEIZURE OF THE DRUG SUPPLY, REVOCATION OF THE PROGRAM APPROVAL, AND INJUNCTION PRECLUDING OPERATION OF THE PROGRAM.
>
> A METHADONE PRODUCT, WHEN USED AS AN ANALGESIC, MAY BE DISPENSED IN ANY LICENSED PHARMACY.

DESCRIPTION
Methadone Hydrochloride (3-heptanone, 6-(dimethylamino)-4,4-diphenyl-,hydrochloride), is a white, crystalline material that is water soluble. The dispersable tablets of some brands have been formulated with insoluble excipients to deter use of this drug by injection. Its molecular weight is 345.91.

Injection: Each mL contains Methadone 10 mg (0.029 mmol).

Tablets: Each tablet contains 5 mg (0.015 mmol) or 10 mg (0.029 mmol Methadone Hydrochloride.

Oral Solution: Each 5 mL solution contains Methadone Hydrochloride 5 mg or 10 mg.

Dispersible Tablets: Each tablet contains 40 mg (0.116 mmol) Methadone Hydrochloride.

ACTIONS
Methadone HCl is a synthetic narcotic analgesic with multiple actions quantatively similar to those of morphine, the most prominent of which involve the central nervous system and organs composed of smooth muscle. The principal actions of therapeutic value are analgesia and sedation and detoxification or temporary maintenance in narcotic addiction. The Methadone abstinence syn-

drome, although qualitatively similar to that of morphine, differs in that the onset is slower, the course is more prolonged, and the symptoms are less severe.

A parenteral dose of 8 to 10 mg of Methadone HCl is approximately equivalent in analgesic effect to 10 mg of morphine. With single-dose administration, the onset and duration of analgesic action of the 2 drugs are similar.

When administered orally, Methadone is approximately one-half as potent as when given parenterally. Oral administration results in a delay of the onset, a lowering of the peak, and an increase in the duration of analgesic effect.

Following is its chemical structure:

INDICATIONS
(See boxed *"Note"*.)
For relief of severe pain (except dispersable tablets).
For detoxification treatment of narcotic addiction.
For temporary maintenance treatment of narcotic addiction.

NOTE

IF METHADONE IS ADMINISTERED FOR TREATMENT OF HEROIN DEPENDENCE FOR MORE THAN 3 WEEKS, THE PROCEDURE PASSES FROM TREATMENT OF THE ACUTE WITHDRAWAL SYNDROME (DETOXIFICATION) TO MAINTENANCE THERAPY. MAINTENANCE TREATMENT IS PERMITTED TO BE UNDERTAKEN ONLY BY APPROVED METHADONE PROGRAMS. THIS DOES NOT PRECLUDE THE MAINTENANCE TREATMENT OF AN ADDICT WHO IS HOSPITALIZED FOR MEDICAL CONDITIONS OTHER THAN ADDICTION AND WHO REQUIRES TEMPORARY MAINTENANCE DURING THE CRITICAL PERIOD OF HIS/HER STAY OR WHOSE ENROLLMENT HAS BEEN VERIFIED IN A PROGRAM APPROVED FOR MAINTENANCE TREATMENT WITH METHADONE.

UNLABELED USES
Methadone is used alone or as an adjunct in the treatment of restless leg syndrome.

CONTRAINDICATION
Hypersensitivity to Methadone.

WARNINGS
Methadone tablets and dispersible tablets are for oral administration only and *must not* be used for injection. The dispersible tablets contain insoluble excipients and therefore *must not* be injected. It is recommended that Methadone HCl tablets and dispersible tablets, if dispensed, be packaged in child-resistant containers and kept out of the reach of children to prevent accidental ingestion.

Methadone HCl a narcotic, is a Schedule II controlled substance under the Federal Controlled Substances Act. Appropriate security measures should be taken to safeguard stocks of Methadone against diversion.

Drug Dependence: METHADONE CAN PRODUCE DRUG DEPENDENCE OF THE MORPHINE TYPE AND, THEREFORE, HAS THE POTENTIAL FOR BEING ABUSED. PSYCHIC DEPENDENCE, PHYSICAL DEPENDENCE, AND TOLERANCE MAY DEVELOP ON REPEATED ADMINISTRATION OF METHADONE AND IT SHOULD BE PRESCRIBED AND ADMINISTERED WITH THE SAME DEGREE OF CAUTION APPROPRIATE TO THE USE OF MORPHINE.

Interaction With Other Central Nervous System Depressants: Methadone should be used with caution and in reduced dosage in patients who are concurrently receiving other narcotic analgesics, general anesthetics, phenothiazines, other tranquilizers, sedative-hypnotics, tricyclic anti-depressants, and other CNS depressants (including alcohol). Respiratory depression, hypotension, and profound sedation or coma may result.

Anxiety: Since Methadone, as used by tolerant subjects at a constant maintenance dosage, is not a tranquilizer, patients who are maintained on this drug will react to life problems and stresses with the same symptoms of anxiety as do other individuals. The physician should not confuse such symptoms with those of narcotic abstinence and should not attempt to treat anxiety by increasing the dosage of Methadone. The action of Methadone in maintenance treatment is limited to the control of narcotic symptoms and is ineffective for relief of general anxiety.

Head Injury and Increased Intracranial Pressure: The respiratory depressant effects of Methadone and its capacity to elevate cerebrospinal-fluid pressure may be markedly exaggerated in the presence of increased intracranial pressure. Furthermore, narcotics produce side effects that may obscure the clinical course of patients with head injuries. In such patients, Methadone must be used with caution and only if it is deemed essential.

Asthma and Other Respiratory Conditions: Methadone HCl should be used with caution in patients having an acute asthmatic attack, in those with chronic obstructive pulmonary disease or cor pulmonale, and in individuals with a substantially decreased respiratory reserve, preexisting respiratory depression,

hypoxia, or hypercapnia. In such patients, even usual therapeutic doses of narcotics may decrease respiratory drive while simultaneously increasing airway resistance to the point of apnea.

Hypotensive Effect: The administration of Methadone may result in severe hypotension in an individual whose ability to maintain normal blood pressure has already been compromised by a depleted blood volume or concurrent administration of such drugs as the phenothiazines or certain anesthetics.

Use in Ambulatory Patients: Methadone may impair the mental and/or physical abilities required for the performance of potentially hazardous tasks, such as driving a car or operating machinery. The patient should be cautioned accordingly.

Methadone like other narcotics, may produce orthostatic hypotension in ambulatory patients.

Use in Pregnancy: Safe use in pregnancy has not been established in relation to possible adverse effects on fetal development. Therefore, Methadone should not be used in pregnant women unless, in the judgment of the physician, the potential benefits outweigh the possible hazards.

Methadone is not recommended for obstetric analgesia because its long duration of action increases the probability of respiratory depression in the newborn.

Use in Children: Methadone is not recommended for use as an analgesic in children, since documented clinical experience has been insufficient to establish a suitable dosage regimen for the pediatric age group.

PRECAUTIONS
DRUG INTERACTIONS
Pentazocine: Patients who are addicted to heroin or who are on the Methadone maintenance program may experience withdrawal symptoms when given an opioid agonist-antagonist, such as pentazocine.

Rifampin: The concurrent administration of rifampin may possibly reduce the blood concentration of Methadone to a degree sufficient to produce withdrawal symptoms. The mechanism by which rifampin may decrease blood concentrations of Methadone is not fully understood, although enhanced microsomal drug-metabolized enzymes may influence drug disposition.

Monoamine Oxidase (MAO) Inhibitors: Therapeutic doses of meperidine have precipitated severe reactions in patients concurrently receiving monoamine oxidase inhibitors or those who have received such agents within 14 days. Similar reactions thus far have not been reported with Methadone; but if the use of Methadone is necessary in such patients, a sensitivity test should be performed in which repeated small incremental doses are administered over the course of several hours while the patient's condition and vital signs are under careful observation.

Desipramine: Blood levels of desipramine have increased with concurrent methadone therapy.

Special-Risk Patients: Methadone HCl should be given with caution and the initial dose should be reduced in certain patients, such as the elderly or debilitated and those with severe impairment of hepatic or renal function, hypothyroidism, Addison's disease, prostatic hypertrophy, or urethral stricture.

Acute Abdominal Conditions: The administration of Methadone or other narcotics may obscure the diagnosis or clinical course in patients with acute abdominal conditions.

ADVERSE REACTIONS
Heroin Withdrawal: During the induction phase of Methadone maintenance treatment, patients are being withdrawn from heroin and may therefore show typical withdrawal symptoms, which should be differentiated from Methadone-induced side effects. They may exhibit some or all of the following symptoms associated with acute withdrawal from heroin or other opiates: lacrimation, rhinorrhea, sneezing, yawning, excessive perspiration, goose-flesh, fever, chilliness alternating with flushing, restlessness, irritability, "sleepy yen," weakness, anxiety, depression, dilated pupils, tremors, tachycardia, abdominal cramps, body aches, involuntary twitching and kicking movements, anorexia, nausea, vomiting, diarrhea, intestinal spasms, and weight loss.

Initial Administration: Initially, the dosage of Methadone should be carefully titrated to the individual. Induction too rapid for the patient's sensitivity is more likely to produce the following effects.

THE MAJOR HAZARDS OF METHADONE HCl AS OF OTHER NARCOTIC ANALGESICS, ARE RESPIRATORY DEPRESSION AND, TO A LESSER DEGREE, CIRCULATORY DEPRESSION. RESPIRATORY ARREST, SHOCK, AND CARDIAC ARREST HAVE OCCURRED.

The most frequently observed adverse reactions include lightheadedness, dizziness, sedation, nausea, vomiting, and sweating. These effects seem to be more prominent in ambulatory patients and in those who are not suffering severe pain. In such individuals, lower doses are advisable. Some adverse reactions may be alleviated if the ambulatory patient lies down.

Other adverse reactions include the following:

Central Nervous System: Euphoria, dysphoria, weakness, headache, insomnia, agitation, disorientation, and visual disturbances.

Gastrointestinal: Dry mouth, anorexia, constipation, and biliary tract spasm.

Cardiovascular: Flushing of the face, bradycardia, palpitation, faintness, and syncope.

Genitourinary: Urinary retention or hesitancy, antidiuretic effect, and reduced libido and/or potency.

Allergic: Pruritus, urticaria, other skin rashes, edema, and rarely, hemorrhagic urticaria.

Hematologic: Reversible thrombocytopenia has been described in a narcotics addict with chronic hepatitis.

In addition, pain at injection site; local tissue irritation and induration following subcutaneous injection, particularly when repeated.

Maintenance on a Stabilized Dose: During prolonged administration of Methadone, as in a Methadone maintenance treatment program, there is a gradual, yet progressive, disappearance of side effects over a period of several weeks. However, constipation and sweating often persist.

OVERDOSAGE

Signs and Symptoms: Methadone HCl is an opioid and produces effects similar to those of morphine. Symptoms of overdose begin within seconds after intravenous administration and within minutes of nasal, oral, or rectal administration. Prominent symptoms are miosis, respiratory depression (a decrease in respiratory rate and/or tidal volume, Cheyne-Stokes respiration, cyanosis), somnolence coma, cool clammy skin, skeletal muscle flaccidity that may progress to hypotension, apnea, bradycardia, and death. Noncardiac pulmonary edema may occur and monitoring of heart filling pressures may be helpful.

Treatment: To obtain up-to-date information about the treatment of overdose, a good resource is your certified Regional Poison Control Center. Telephone numbers of certified poison control centers are listed in the *Physicians' Desk Reference (PDR).* In managing overdosage, consider the possibility of multiple drug overdoses, interaction among drugs, and unusual drug kinetics in your patient.

Initial management of opioid overdose should include establishment of a secure airway and support of ventilation and perfusion. Naloxone may be given to antagonize opioid effects, but the airway must be secured as vomiting may ensue. **The duration of Methadone effect is much longer (36 to 48 hours) than the duration of naloxone effect (1 to 3 hours) and repeated doses (or continuous intravenous infusion) of naloxone may be required.** The patient must, therefore, be monitored continuously for recurrence of respiratory depression and treated repeatedly with the narcotic antagonist as needed. If the diagnosis is correct and respiratory depression is due only to overdosage of Methadone, the use of other respiratory stimulants is not indicated.

An antagonist should not be administered in the absence of clinically significant respiratory or cardiovascular depression. Intravenously administered narcotic antagonists (naloxone and nalorphine) are the drugs of choice to reverse signs of intoxication. These agents should be given repeatedly until the patient's status remains satisfactory. The hazard that the narcotic agent will further depress respiration is less likely with the use of naloxone.

Oxygen, intravenous fluids, vasopressors, and other supportive measures should be employed as indicated.

If the patient has chronically abused opioids, administration of naloxone may precipitate a withdrawal syndrome that may include yawning, tearing, restlessness, sweating, dilated pupils, piloerection, vomiting, diarrhea, and abdominal cramps. If these symptoms develop, they should abate quickly as the effects of naloxone dissipate.

If Methadone has been taken by mouth, protect the patient's airway and support ventilation and perfusion. Meticulously monitor and maintain, within acceptable limits, the patient's vital signs, blood gases, serum electrolytes, etc. Absorption of drugs from the gastrointestinal tract may be decreased by giving activated charcoal, which, in many cases, is more effective than emesis or lavage; consider charcoal instead of or in addition to gastric emptying. Repeated doses of charcoal over time may hasten elimination of some drugs that have been absorbed. Safeguard the patient's airway when employing gastric emptying or charcoal.

Forced diuresis, peritoneal dialysis, hemodialysis, or charcoal hemoperfusion have not been established as beneficial for an overdose of Methadone.

> NOTE: IN AN INDIVIDUAL PHYSICALLY DEPENDENT ON NARCOTICS, THE ADMINISTRATION OF THE USUAL DOSE OF A NARCOTIC ANTAGONIST WILL PRECIPITATE AN ACUTE WITHDRAWAL SYNDROME. THE SEVERITY OF THIS SYNDROME WILL DEPEND ON THE DEGREE OF PHYSICAL DEPENDENCE AND THE DOSE OF THE ANTAGONIST ADMINISTERED. THE USE OF A NARCOTIC ANTAGONIST IN SUCH A PERSON SHOULD BE AVOIDED IF POSSIBLE. IF IT MUST BE USED TO TREAT SERIOUS RESPIRATORY DEPRESSION IN THE PHYSICALLY DEPENDENT PATIENT, THE ANTAGONIST SHOULD BE ADMINISTERED WITH EXTREME CARE AND BY TITRATION WITH SMALLER THAN USUAL DOSES OF THE ANTAGONIST.

DOSAGE AND ADMINISTRATION

For Relief of Pain: Dosage should be adjusted according to the severity of the pain and the response of the patient. Occasionally, it may be necessary to exceed the usual dosage recommended in cases of exceptionally severe pain or in those patients who have become tolerant to the analgesic effect of narcotics.

Although subcutaneous administration is suitable for occasional use, intramuscular injection is preferred when repeated doses are required.

The usual adult dosage is 2.5 to 10 mg intramuscularly or subcutaneously or orally, every 3 or 4 hours as necessary.

For Detoxification Treatment: THE DRUG SHALL BE ADMINISTERED DAILY UNDER CLOSE SUPERVISION AS FOLLOWS:

A detoxification treatment course shall not exceed 21 days and may not be repeated earlier than 4 weeks after completion of the preceding course.

The oral form of administration is preferred. However, if the patient is unable to ingest oral medication, parenteral administration may be substituted.

In detoxification, the patient may receive Methadone when there are significant symptoms of withdrawal. The dosage schedules indicated below are recommended but could be varied in accordance with clinical judgment. Initially, a single dose of 15 to 20 mg of Methadone will often be sufficient to suppress withdrawal symptoms. Additional Methadone may be provided if withdrawal symptoms are not suppressed or if symptoms reappear. When patients are physically dependent on high doses, it may be necessary to exceed these levels. Forty mg/day in single or divided doses will usually constitute an adequate stabilizing dosage level. Stabilization can be continued for 2 to 3 days, and then the amount of Methadone normally will be gradually decreased. The rate at which Methadone is decreased will be determined separately for each patient. The dose of Methadone can be decreased on a daily basis or at 2-day intervals, but the amount of intake shall always be sufficient to keep withdrawal symptoms at a tolerable level. In hospitalized patients, a daily reduction of 20% of the total daily dose may be tolerated and may cause little discomfort. In ambulatory patients, a somewhat slower schedule may be needed. If Methadone is administered for more than 3 weeks, the procedure is considered to have progressed from detoxification or treatment of the acute withdrawal syndrome to maintenance treatment, even though the goal and intent may be eventual total withdrawal.

For Maintenance Treatment: In maintenance treatment, the initial dosage of Methadone should control the abstinence symptoms that follow withdrawal of narcotic drugs but should not be so great as to cause sedation, respiratory depression, or other effects of acute intoxication. It is important that the initial dosage be adjusted on an individual basis to the narcotic tolerance of the new patient. If such a patient has been a heavy user of heroin up to the day of admission, he/she may be given 20 mg 4 to 8 hours later or 40 mg in a single or dose. If the patient enters treatment with little or no narcotic tolerance (e.g., if he/she has recently been released from jail or other confinement), the initial dosage may be one half these quantities. When there is any doubt, the smaller dose should be used initially. The patient should then be kept under observation, and, if symptoms of abstinence are distressing, additional 10-mg doses may be administered as needed. Subsequently, the dosage should be adjusted individually, as tolerated and required, up to a level of 120 mg daily. The patient will initially ingest the drug under observation daily, or at least 6 days a week, for the first 3 months. After demonstrating satisfactory adherence to the program regulations for at least 3 months, the patient may be permitted to reduce to 3 times weekly the occasions when he/she must ingest the drug under observation. The patient shall receive no more than a 2-day take-home supply. With continuing adherence to the program's requirements for at least 2 years, he/she may then be permitted twice-weekly visits to the program for drug ingestion under observation, with a 3-day take-home supply. A daily dose of 120 mg or more shall be justified in the medical record. Prior approval from state authority and the Food and Drug Administration is required for any dose above 120 mg administered at the clinic and for any dose above 100 mg to be taken at home. A regular review of dosage level should be made by the responsible physician, with careful consideration given to reduction of dosage as indicated on an individual basis. A new dosage level is only a test level until stability is achieved.

Special Considerations for a Pregnant Patient: Caution shall be taken in the maintenance treatment of pregnant patients. Dosage levels shall be kept as low as possible if continued Methadone treatment is deemed necessary. It is the responsibility of the program sponsor to assure that each female patient be fully informed concerning the possible risks to a pregnant woman or her unborn child from the use of Methadone.

Special Limitations: Treatment of Patients under Age 18:

1. The safety and effectiveness of Methadone for use in the treatment of adolescents have not been proved by adequate clinical study. Special procedures are therefore necessary to assure that patients under age 16 will not be admitted to a program and that patients between 16 and 18 years of age will be admitted to maintenance treatment only under limited conditions.

2. No patients between 16 and 18 years of age may be admitted to a maintenance treatment program unless a parent, legal guardian, or responsible adult designated by the state authority completes and signs Form FD 2635, "Consent for Methadone Treatment."

Methadone treatment of new patients between the ages of 16 and 18 years will be permitted with a documented history of 2 or more unsuccessful attempts at detoxification and a documented history of dependence on heroin or other morphine-like drugs beginning 2 years or more prior to application for treatment. No patient under age 16 may be continued or started on Methadone treatment, but these patients may be detoxified and retained in the program in a drug-free state for follow-up and aftercare.

3. Patients under age 18 who are not placed on maintenance treatment may be detoxified.

Storage: Store at controlled room temperature, 59° to 86°F (15° to 30°C).

J CODES
Up to 10 mg IM,SC—J1230

◆ RATED THERAPEUTICALLY EQUIVALENT; ◇ THERAPEUTIC EQUIVALENCE UNCONFIRMED; ○ UNRATED

HOW SUPPLIED
CONCENTRATE: 10 MG/ML

AVERAGE UNIT PRICE (AVAILABLE SIZES)

GENERIC	$0.33		

BRAND/MANUFACTURER	NDC	SIZE	AWP
◆ GENERICS			
Roxane	00054-3553-44	30 ml	$17.46
Roxane	00054-3553-67	946 ml	$70.00

CONCENTRATE (C-II):

BRAND/MANUFACTURER	NDC	SIZE	AWP
◆ GENERICS			
METHADOSE: Mallinckrodt-II	00406-0527-05	960 ml	$74.00

CONCENTRATE (C-II): 10 MG/ML

AVERAGE UNIT PRICE (AVAILABLE SIZES)

GENERIC	$0.33		

BRAND/MANUFACTURER	NDC	SIZE	AWP
◆ GENERICS			
Roxane	00054-3553-44	30 ml	$17.46
Roxane	00054-3553-67	946 ml	$70.00

INJECTION (C-II): 10 MG/ML

BRAND/MANUFACTURER	NDC	SIZE	AWP
○ BRAND			
DOLOPHINE HCL: Lilly	00002-1682-01	20 ml	$12.56
	00002-1682-25	20 ml 25s	$278.00

TABLETS (C-II) 5 MG

AVERAGE UNIT PRICE (AVAILABLE SIZES)		GENERIC A-RATED AVERAGE PRICE (GAAP)	
BRAND	$0.09	100s	$14.12
GENERIC	$0.14		

BRAND/MANUFACTURER	NDC	SIZE	AWP
◆ BRAND			
DOLOPHINE HCL: Lilly	00002-1064-02	100s	$8.68
◆ GENERICS			
METHADOSE: Mallinckrodt-II	00406-6974-34	100s	$5.75
Roxane	00054-4570-25	100s	$7.44
Roxane	00054-8553-24	100s ud	$29.17

TABLETS (C-II) 10 MG

AVERAGE UNIT PRICE (AVAILABLE SIZES)		GENERIC A-RATED AVERAGE PRICE (GAAP)	
BRAND	$0.14	100s	$18.33
GENERIC	$0.18		

BRAND/MANUFACTURER	NDC	SIZE	AWP
◆ BRAND			
DOLOPHINE HCL: Lilly	00002-1072-02	100s	$14.10
◆ GENERICS			
METHADOSE: Mallinckrodt-II	00406-3454-34	100s	$9.42
Roxane	00054-4571-25	100s	$12.35
Roxane	00054-8554-24	100s ud	$33.21

TABLETS (C-II) 40 MG

AVERAGE UNIT PRICE (AVAILABLE SIZES)		GENERIC A-RATED AVERAGE PRICE (GAAP)	
GENERIC	$0.29	100s	$28.75

BRAND/MANUFACTURER	NDC	SIZE	AWP
◆ GENERICS			
METHADOSE: Mallinckrodt-II	00406-0540-34	100s	$25.95
Lilly	00002-2153-02	100s	$31.55

Methamphetamine Hydrochloride

METHAMPHETAMINE HAS A HIGH POTENTIAL FOR ABUSE. IT SHOULD THUS BE TRIED ONLY IN WEIGHT REDUCTION PROGRAMS FOR PATIENTS IN WHOM ALTERNATIVE THERAPY HAS BEEN INEFFECTIVE. ADMINISTRATION OF METHAMPHETAMINE FOR PROLONGED PERIODS OF TIME IN OBESITY MAY LEAD TO DRUG DEPENDENCE AND MUST BE AVOIDED. PARTICULAR ATTENTION SHOULD BE PAID TO THE POSSIBILITY OF SUBJECTS OBTAINING METHAMPHETAMINE FOR NON-THERAPEUTIC USE OF DISTRIBUTION TO OTHERS, AND THE DRUG SHOULD BE PRESCRIBED OR DISPENSED SPARINGLY.

DESCRIPTION
Methamphetamine Hydrochloride, chemically known as (S)-N, α-dimethylben-zeneethanamine hydrochloride, is a member of the amphetamine group of sympathomimetic amines.

Methamphetamine Hydrochloride sustained-release tablets are available containing 5 mg, 10 mg or 15 mg of methamphetamine hydrochloride for oral administration. The sustained-release tablet is an inert, porous, plastic matrix, which is impregnated with Methamphetamine Hydrochloride. The drug is leached slowly from the sustained-release tablet as it passes through the gastrointestinal tract. The expended matrix is not absorbed and is excreted in the stool.

Following is its chemical structure:

$$CH_2CHNHCH_3 \cdot HCl$$
$$CH_3$$

CLINICAL PHARMACOLOGY
Methamphetamine HCl is a sympathomimetic amine with CNS stimulant activity. Peripheral actions include elevation of systolic and diastolic blood pressures and weak bronchodilator and respiratory stimulant action. Drugs of this class used in obesity are commonly known as "anorectics" or "anorexigenics". It has not been established, however, that the action of such drugs in treating obesity is primarily one of appetite suppression. Other central nervous system actions, or metabolic effects, may be involved, for example.

Adult obese subjects instructed in dietary management and treated with "anorectic" drugs, lose more weight on the average than those treated with placebo and diet, as determined in relatively short-term clinical trials.

The magnitude of increased weight loss of drug-treated patients over placebo-treated patients is only a fraction of a pound a week. The rate of weight loss is greatest in the first weeks of therapy for both drug and placebo subjects and tends to decrease in succeeding weeks. The origins of the increased weight loss due to the various possible drug effects are not established. The amount of weight loss associated with the use of an "anorectic" drug varies from trial to trial, and the increased weight loss appears to be related in part to variables other than the drug prescribed, such as the physician-investigator, the population treated, and the diet prescribed. Studies do not permit conclusions as to the relative importance of the drug and non-drug factors on weight loss. The natural history of obesity is measured in years, whereas the studies cited are restricted to a few weeks duration; thus, the total impact of drug-induced weight loss over that of diet alone must be considered clinically limited.

The mechanism of action involved in producing the beneficial behavioral changes seen in hyperkinetic children receiving Methamphetamine is unknown.

In humans, Methamphetamine HCl is rapidly absorbed from the gastrointestinal tract. The primary site of metabolism is in the liver by aromatic hydroxyl-ation, N-dealkylation and deamination. At least seven metabolites have been identified in the urine. The biological half-life has been reported in the range of 4 to 5 hours. Excretion occurs primarily in the urine and is dependent on urine pH. Alkaline urine will significantly increase the drug half-life. Approximately 62% of an oral dose is eliminated in the urine within the first 24 hours with about one-third as intact drug and the remainder as metabolites.

INDICATIONS AND USAGE
Attention Deficit Disorder with Hyperactivity: Methamphetamine HCl is indicated as an integral part of a total treatment program which typically includes other remedial measures (psychological, educational, social) for a stabilizing effect in children over 6 years of age with a behavioral syndrome characterized by the following group of developmentally inappropriate symptoms: moderate to severe distractibility, short attention span, hyperactivity, emotional lability, and impulsivity. The diagnosis of this syndrome should not be made with finality when these symptoms are only of comparatively recent origin. Nonlocalizing (soft) neurological signs, learning disability, and abnormal EEG may or may not be present, and a diagnosis of central nervous system dysfunction may or may not be warranted.

Exogenous Obesity: As a short-term (i.e., a few weeks) adjunct in a regimen of weight reduction based on caloric restriction, for patients in whom obesity is refractory to alternative therapy, e.g., repeated diets, group programs, and other drugs. The limited usefulness of Methamphetamine HCl (see "Clinical Pharmacology" section) should be weighed against possible risks inherent in use of the drug, such as those described below.

CONTRAINDICATIONS
Methamphetamine HCl is contraindicated during or within 14 days following the administration of monoamine oxidase inhibitors; hypertensive crises may result. It is also contraindicated in patients with glaucoma, advanced arteriosclerosis, symptomatic cardiovascular disease, moderate to severe hypertension, hyperthyroidism or known hypersensitivity or idiosyncrasy to sympathomimetic amines. Methamphetamine HCl should not be given to patients who are in an agitated state or who have a history of drug abuse.

WARNINGS
Tolerance to the anorectic effect usually develops within a few weeks. When this occurs, the recommended dose should not be exceeded in an attempt to increase the effect; rather, the drug should be discontinued (see "Drug Abuse and Dependence" section).

➤ SHOWN IN PRODUCT IDENTIFICATION GUIDE

Decrements in the predicted growth (i.e., weight gain and/or height) rate have been reported with the long-term use of stimulants in children. Therefore, patients requiring long-term therapy should be carefully monitored.

Usage in Nursing Mothers: Amphetamines are excreted in human milk. Mothers taking amphetamines should be advised to refrain from nursing.

PRECAUTIONS

General: Methamphetamine HCl should be used with caution in patients with even mild hypertension.

Methamphetamine HCl should not be used to combat fatigue or to replace rest in normal persons.

Prescribing and dispensing of Methamphetamine HCl should be limited to the smallest amount that is feasible at one time in order to minimize the possibility of overdosage.

The 15 mg dosage strength of Methamphetamine HCl contains FD&C Yellow No. 5 (tartrazine) which may cause allergic-type reactions (including bronchial asthma) in certain susceptible individuals. Although the overall incidence of FD&C Yellow No. 5 (tartrazine) sensitivity in the general population is low, it is frequently seen in patients who also have aspirin hypersensitivity.

Information for Patients: The patient should be informed that Methamphetamine HCl may impair the ability to engage in potentially hazardous activities, such as, operating machinery or driving a motor vehicle.

The patient should be cautioned not to increase dosage, except on advice of the physician.

Drug Interactions: Insulin requirements in diabetes mellitus may be altered in association with the use of Methamphetamine HCl and concomitant dietary regimen.

Methamphetamine HCl may decrease the hypotensive effect of *guanethidine.*
Methamphetamine HCl should not be used concurrently with *monoamine oxidase inhibitors* (see "Contraindications" section).

Concurrent administration of *tricyclic antidepressants* and indirect-acting sympathomimetic amines such as amphetamines, should be closely supervised and dosage carefully adjusted.

Phenothiazines are reported in the literature to antagonize the CNS stimulant action of the amphetamines.

Drug/Laboratory Test Interactions: Literature reports suggest that amphetamines may be associated with significant elevation of plasma corticosteroids. This should be considered if determination of plasma corticosteroid levels is desired in a person receiving amphetamines.

Carcinogensis, Mutagenesis, Impairment of Fertility: Data are not available on long-term potential for carcinogenicity, mutagenicity, or impairment of fertility.

Pregnancy: Teratogenic effects: Pregnancy Category C. Methamphetamine HCl has been shown to have teratogenic and embryocidal effects in mammals given high multiples of the human dose. There are no adequate and well-controlled studies in pregnant women. Methamphetamine HCl should not be used during pregnancy unless the potential benefit justifies the potential risk to the fetus.

Nonteratogenic effects: Infants born to mothers dependent on amphetamines have an increased risk of premature delivery and low birth weight. Also, these infants may experience symptoms of withdrawal as demonstrated by dysphoria, including agitation and significant lassitude.

Nursing Mothers: See "Warnings" section.

Pediatric Use: Safety and effectiveness for use as an anorectic agent in children below the age of 12 years have not been established.

Long-term effects of Methamphetamine in children have not been established (see "Warnings" section).

Drug treatment is not indicated in all cases of the behavioral syndrome characterized by moderate to severe distractibility, short attention span, hyperactivity, emotional lability and impulsivity. It should be considered only in light of the complete history and evaluation of the child. The decision to prescribe Methamphetamine HCl should depend on the physician's assessment of the chronicity and severity of the child's symptoms and their appropriateness for his/her age. Prescription should not depend solely on the presence of one or more of the behavioral characteristics.

When these symptoms are associated with acute stress reactions, treatment with Methamphetamine HCl is usually not indicated.

Clinical experience suggests that in psychotic children, administration of Methamphetamine HCl may exacerbate symptoms of behavior disturbance and thought disorder.

Amphetamines have been reported to exacerbate motor and phonic tics and Tourette's syndrome. Therefore, clinical evaluation for tics and Tourette's syndrome in children and their families should precede use of stimulant medications.

ADVERSE REACTIONS

The following are adverse reactions in decreasing order of severity within each category that have been reported:

Cardiovascular: Elevation of blood pressure, tachycardia and palpitation.

Central Nervous System: Psychotic episodes have been rarely reported at recommended doses. Dizziness, dysphoria, overstimulation, euphoria, insomnia, tremor, restlessness and headache. Exacerbation of motor and phonic tics and Tourette's syndrome.

Gastrointestinal: Diarrhea, constipation, dryness of mouth, unpleasant taste and other gastrointestinal disturbances.

Hypersensitivity: Urticaria.

Endocrine: Impotence and changes in libido.

Miscellaneous: Suppression of growth has been reported with the long-term use of stimulants in children (see "Warnings" section).

DRUG ABUSE AND DEPENDENCE

Controlled Substance: Methamphetamine HCl is subject to control under DEA schedule II.

Abuse: Methamphetamine HCl has been extensively abused. Tolerance, extreme psychological dependence, and severe social disability have occurred. There are reports of patients who have increased the dosage to many times that recommended. Abrupt cessation following prolonged high dosage administration results in extreme fatigue and mental depression; changes are also noted on the sleep EEG. Manifestations of chronic intoxication with Methamphetamine HCl include severe dermatoses, marked insomnia, irritability, hyperactivity, and personality changes. The most severe manifestation of chronic intoxication is psychosis, often clinically indistinguishable from schizophrenia.

OVERDOSAGE

Manifestations of acute overdosage with Methamphetamine HCl include restlessness, tremor, hyperreflexia, rapid respiration, confusion, assaultiveness, hallucinations, panic states, hyperpyrexia, and rhabdomyolysis. Fatigue and depression usually follow the central stimulation. Cardiovascular effects include arrhythmias, hypertension or hypotension, and circulatory collapse. Gastrointestinal symptoms include nausea, vomiting, diarrhea, and abdominal cramps. Fatal poisoning usually terminates in convuslions and coma.

Management of acute Methamphetamine HCl intoxication is largely symptomatic and includes gastric evacuation and sedation with a barbiturate. Experience with hemodialysis or peritoneal dialysis is inadequate to permit recommendations in this regard.

Acidification of urine increases Methamphetamine HCl excretion. Intravenous phentolamine (Regitine®) has been suggested for possible acute, severe hypertension, if this complicates Methamphetamine HCl overdosage. Usually a gradual drop in blood pressure will result when sufficient sedation has been achieved. Chlorpromazine has been reported to be useful in decreasing CNS stimulation and sympathomimetic effects.

Since the extended release tablet releases Methamphetamine gradually, therapy should be directed at reversing the effects of the ingested drug and at supporting the patient until symptoms subside. Saline cathartics are useful for hastening the evacuation of the tablets that have not already released medication.

DOSAGE AND ADMINISTRATION

Methamphetamine HCl tablets are given orally. Methamphetamine HCl should be administered at the lowest effective dosage, and dosage should be indivdually adjusted. Late evening medication should be avoided because of the resulting insomnia.

ATTENTION DEFICIT DISORDER WITH HYPERACTIVITY

For treatment of children 6 years or older with a behavioral syndrome characterized by moderate to severe distractibility, short attention span, hyperactivity, emotional lability and impulsivity: an initial dose of 5 mg Methamphetamine HCl once or twice a day is recommended. Daily dosage may be raised in increments of 5 mg at weekly intervals until optimum clinical response is achieved. The usual effective dose is 20 to 25 mg daily. The total daily dose may be given once daily using the extended release dosage tablet. The extended release dosage form should not be utilized for initiation of dosage nor until the titrated daily dosage is equal to or greater than the dosage provided in a extended release tablet.

Where possible, drug administration should be interrupted occasionally to determine if there is a recurrence of behavioral symptoms sufficient to require continued therapy.

For obesity: one extended release tablet, 10 or 15 mg, once a day in the morning. Treatment should not exceed a few weeks in duration. Methamphetamine HCl is not recommended for use as an anorectic agent in children under 12 years of age.

Recommended Storage: Store below 86°F (30°C).

HOW SUPPLIED
TABLETS (C-II): 5 MG

BRAND/MANUFACTURER	NDC	SIZE	AWP
◆ **BRAND**			
DESOXYN: Abbott Pharm	00074-3377-04	100s	$64.20

Methenamine Mandelate

DESCRIPTION

Methenamine Mandelate, a urinary anti-bacterial agent, is the chemical combination of mandelic acid with Methenamine. Methenamine Mandelate is available for oral use as film-coated tablets and suspension.

Active Ingredient: Methenamine Mandelate: 500 mg or 0.5gm.
Methenamine Mandelate: 1000 mg or 1.0 gm.

◆ RATED THERAPEUTICALLY EQUIVALENT; ◇ THERAPEUTIC EQUIVALENCE UNCONFIRMED; ○ UNRATED

Following is its chemical structure:

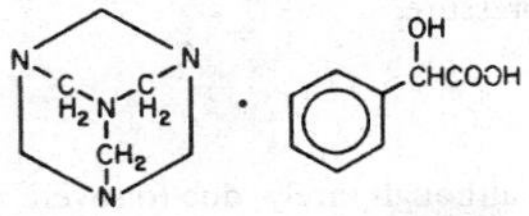

CLINICAL PHARMACOLOGY
Methenamine Mandelate is readily absorbed but remains essentially inactive until it is excreted by the kidney and concentrated in the urine. An acid urine is essential for antibacterial action, with maximum efficacy occurring at pH5.5 or less. In an acid urine, mandelic acid exerts its antibacterial action and also contributes to the acidification of the urine. Mandelic acid is excreted by both glomerular filtration and tubular excretion. The methanamine component, in an acid urine, is hydrolyzed to ammonia and to the bactericidal agent formaldehyde. There is equally effective antibacterial activity against both gram-positive and gram-negative organisms, since the antibacterial action of mandelic acid and formaldehyde is non-specific. There are reports that Methenanine Mandelate is ineffective in some infections with *Proteus vulgaris* and urea-splitting strains of *Pseudomonas aeruginosa* and *A aerogenes*. Since urea-splitting strains may raise the pH of the urine, particular attention to supplementary acidification is required. However, results in any single case will depend to a large extent on the underlying pathology and the overall management.

INDICATIONS AND USAGE
Methenamine Mandelate is indicated for the suppression or elimination of bacteriuria associated with pyelonephritis, cystitiss, and other chronic urinary tract infections; also for infected residual urine sometimes accompanying neurologic diseases. When used as recommended, Methhenamine Mandelate is particularly suitable for long-term therapy because of its safety and because resistance to the nonspecific bactericidal action of formaldehyde does not develop. Pathogens resistant to other antibacterial agents may respond to Methenamine Mandelate because of the nonspecific effect of formaldehyde formed in an acid urine.

Prophylactic Use Rationale: Urine is a good culture medium for many urinary pathogens. Inoculation by a few organisms (relapse or reinfection) may lead to bacteriuria in susceptible individuals. Thus, the rationale of management in recurring urinary tract infection (bacteriuria) is to change the urine from a growth-supporting to a growth-inhibiting medium. There is a growing body of evidence that long-term administration of Methenamine Mandelate can prevent the recurrence of bacteriuria in patients with chronic pyelonephritis.

Therapeutic Use Rationale: Methenamine Mandelate helps to sterilize the urine, and in some situations in which underlying pathologic conditions prevent sterilization by any means, it can help to suppress the bacteriuria Methenamine Mandelate should not be used alone for acute infections with parenchymal involvement causing systemic symptoms such as chills and fever. A thorough diagnostic investigation as a part of the overall management of the urinary tract infection should accompany the use of Methanamine Mandelate.

CONTRAINDICATIONS
Contraindicated in renal insufficiency.
Methenamine Mandelate should not be used in patients who have previously exhibited hypersentivity to it.

PRECAUTIONS
General: Dysuria may occur (usually at higher than recommended dosage). This can be controlled by reducing the dosage and the acidification. When urine acidification is contraindicated or unattainable (as with some urea-splitting bacteria), the drug is not recommended.
To avoid inducing lipid pneumonia, administer Methenamine Mandelate Suspension with care to elderly, debilitated, or otherwise susceptible patients.

Drug Interactions: Formaldehyde and sulfamethizole form an insoluble precipitate in acid urine; therefore, Methenamine Mandelate should not be administered concurrently with sulfamethizole.

Drug/Laboratory Test Interactions: Formaldehyde interferes with fluorometric procedures for determination of urinary catecholamines and vanillylmandeic acid (VMA), causing erroneously high results. Formaldehyde also causes falsely decreased urine estriol levels by reacting with estriol when acid hydrolysis techniques are used; estriol determinations which use enzymatic hydrolysis are unaffected by formaldehyde. Formaldehyde causes falsely elevated 17-hydroxy-corticosteroid levels when the Porter-Siber method is used and falsely decreased 5-hydroxyindoleacetic acid (5HIAA) levels by inhibiting color development when nitrosonaphthol methods are used.

Pregnancy Category C: Animal reproduction studies have not been conducted with Methenamine Mandelate. It is also not known whether Methenamine Mandelate can cause fetal harm when administered to a pregnant women or can affect reproduction capacity. Methenamine Mandelate should be given to a pregnant women only if clearly needed.

Since introduction, published reports on the use of Methenamine Mandelate in pregnant women have not shown an increased risk of fetal abnormalities from use during pregnancy.

ADVERSE REACTIONS
An occasional patient may experience gastrointestinal disturbance or a generalized skin rash. Microscopic and rarely gross hematuria have been described.

DOSAGE AND ADMINISTRATION
Suspension: Shake well before using.
The average adult dosage is 4 grams daily given as 1 gram after each meal and at bedtime. Children 6 to 12 should receive half the adult dose, and children under 6 years of age should receive 250 mg per 30 lb. body weight, four times daily. (See chart.) Since an acid urine is essential for antibacterial activity, with maximum efficacy occurring at pH 5.5 or below, restriction of alkalinizing foods and medication is thus desirable. If testing of urine pH reveals the need, supplemental acidification should be given.

DOSAGES

Dosage	Adults	Children
Tablets		
1 gram	1 tablet qid	—
0.5 gram	2 tablets qid	(Ages 6-12) 1 tablet qid
Suspension Forte		
500 mg/5 mL teasp.	2 teaspoonfuls (10 mL) qid	(Ages 6-12) 1 teaspoonful (5 mL) qid

Store between 15°-30°C (59°-86°F).

HOW SUPPLIED
ENTERIC COATED TABLETS: 0.5 GM

BRAND/MANUFACTURER	NDC	SIZE	AWP
○ BRAND			
MANDELAMINE HAFGRAMS: Parke-Davis	00071-0166-24	100s	$31.35
○ GENERICS			
Richlyn	00115-3976-01	100s	$5.05
Amide	52152-0111-02	100s	$13.75
Rugby	00536-4022-01	100s	$15.68
Jerome Stevens	50564-0540-01	100s	$16.75
Major	00904-2267-70	250s	$33.80
Truxton	00463-6120-10	1000s	$30.00
Richlyn	00115-3976-03	1000s	$38.85
Amide	52152-0111-05	1000s	$127.95
Rugby	00536-4022-10	1000s	$139.26
Jerome Stevens	50564-0540-10	1000s	$140.00

ENTERIC COATED TABLETS: 1 GM

BRAND/MANUFACTURER	NDC	SIZE	AWP
○ BRAND			
MANDELAMINE 1 GM.: Parke-Davis	00071-0167-24	100s	$50.13
○ GENERICS			
Richlyn	00115-3977-01	100s	$9.36
Amide	52152-0112-02	100s	$21.40
Jerome Stevens	50564-0541-01	100s	$26.10
Rugby	00536-4024-01	100s	$26.12
Goldline	00182-0187-01	100s	$27.00
URL	00677-0775-01	100s	$27.50
Truxton	00463-6121-10	1000s	$45.00
Richlyn	00115-3977-03	1000s	$72.00
Jerome Stevens	50564-0541-10	1000s	$195.00
Amide	52152-0112-05	1000s	$206.25
Rugby	00536-4024-10	1000s	$248.16

SUSPENSION: 0.5 GM/5 ML

BRAND/MANUFACTURER	NDC	SIZE	AWP
○ GENERICS			
Goldline	00182-0764-40	480 ml	$39.00
Schein	00364-7194-16	480 ml	$44.89
Barre	00472-0783-16	480 ml	$48.50
Mikart	46672-0621-16	480 ml	$55.05

➤ SHOWN IN PRODUCT IDENTIFICATION GUIDE

TABLET: 0.5 GM

BRAND/MANUFACTURER	NDC	SIZE	AWP
○ GENERICS			
Aligen	00405-4637-01	100s	$14.47

TABLET: 1 GM

BRAND/MANUFACTURER	NDC	SIZE	AWP
○ GENERICS			
Aligen	00405-4638-01	100s	$22.53

Methazolamide

DESCRIPTION

Methazolamide, a sulfonamide derivative, is a white crystalline powder, weakly acidic, slightly soluble in water, alcohol and acetone. The chemical name for Methazolamide is: N-[5-(aminosulfonyl)-3-methyl-1,3,4-thiadiazol-2 (3H)-yli-dene]-acetamide.

Methazolamide is available for oral administration as 25 mg and 50 mg tablets.

Following is its chemical structure:

$$CH_3CON \quad SO_2NH_2$$
$$CH_3-N \quad N$$

CLINICAL PHARMACOLOGY

Methazolamide is a potent inhibitor of carbonic anhydrase. Methazolamide is well absorbed from the gastrointestinal tract. Peak plasma concentrations are observed 1 to 2 hours after dosing. In a multiple-dose, pharmacokinetic study, administration of Methazolamide 25 mg bid, 50 mg bid, and 100 mg bid demonstrated a linear relationship between plasma Methazolamide levels and Methazolamide dose. Peak plasma concentrations (C_{max}) for the 25 mg, 50 mg, and 100 mg bid regimens were 2.5 mcg/mL, 5.1 mcg/mL, and 10.7 mcg/mL, respectively. The area under the plasma concentration-time curves (AUC) was 1130 mcg.min/mL, 2571 mcg.min/mL, and 5418 mcg.min/mL for the 25 mg, 50 mg, and 100 mg dosage regimens, respectively. Methazolamide is distributed throughout the body including the plasma, cerebrospinal fluid, aqueous humor of the eye, red blood cells, bile and extracellular fluid. The mean apparent volume of distribution (V_{area}/F) ranges from 17 L to 23 L. Approximately 55% is bound to plasma proteins. The steady-state Methazolamide red blood cell: plasma ratio varies with dose and was found to be 27:1, 16:1, and 10:1 following the administration of Methazolamide 25 mg bid, 50 mg bid, and 100 mg bid, respectively.

The mean steady-state plasma elimination half-life for Methazolamide is approximately 14 hours. At steady state approximately 25% of the dose is recovered unchanged in the urine over the dosing interval. Renal clearance accounts for 20% to 25% of the total clearance of drug. After repeated bid-tid dosing, Methazolamide accumulates to steady-state concentrations in 7 days.

Methazolamide's inhibitory action on carbonic anhydrase decreases the secretion of aqueous humor and results in a decrease in intraocular pressure. The onset of the decrease in intraocular pressure generally occurs within 2 to 4 hours, has a peak effect in 6 to 8 hours, and a total duration of 10 to 18 hours.

Methazolamide is a sulfonamide derivative; however, it does not have any clinically significant antimicrobial properties. Although Methazolamide achieves a high concentration in the cerebrospinal fluid, it is not considered an effective anticonvulsant.

Methazolamide has a weak and transient diuretic effect; therefore use results in an increase in urinary volume, with excretion of sodium, potassium, and chloride. The drug should not be used as a diuretic. Inhibition of renal bicarbonate reabsorption produces an alkaline urine. Plasma bicarbonate decreases, and a relative, transient metabolic acidosis may occur due to a disequilibrium in carbon dioxide transport in the red cell. Urinary citrate excretion is decreased by approximately 40% after doses of 100 mg every 8 hours. Uric acid output has been shown to decrease 36% in the first 24-hour period.

INDICATIONS AND USAGE

Methazolamide is indicated in the treatment of ocular conditions where lowering intraocular pressure is likely to be of therapeutic benefit, such as chronic open-angle glaucoma, secondary glaucoma, and preoperatively in acute angle-closure glaucoma where lowering the intraocular pressure is desired before surgery.

CONTRAINDICATIONS

Methazolamide therapy is contraindicated in situations in which sodium and/or potassium serum levels are depressed, in cases of marked kidney or liver disease or dysfunction, in adrenal gland failure, and in hyperchloremic acidosis. In patients with cirrhosis, use may precipitate the development of hepatic encephalopathy.

Long-term administration of Methazolamide is contraindicated in patients with angle-closure glaucoma, since organic closure of the angle may occur in spite of lowered intraocular pressure.

WARNINGS

Fatalities have occurred, although rarely, due to severe reactions to sulfonamides including Stevens-Johnson syndrome, toxic epidermal necrolysis, fulminant hepatic necrosis, agranulocytosis, aplastic anemia, and other blood dyscrasias. Hypersensitivity reactions may recur when a sulfonamide is readministered, irrespective of the route of administration. If hypersensitivity or other serious reactions occur, the use of this drug should be discontinued.

Caution is advised for patients receiving high-dose aspirin and Methazolamide concomitantly, as anorexia, tachypnea, lethargy, coma, and death have been reported with concomitant use of high-dose aspirin and carbonic anhydrase inhibitors.

PRECAUTIONS

General: Potassium excretion is increased initially upon administration of Methazolamide and in patients with cirrhosis or hepatic insufficiency could precipitate a hepatic coma. In patients with pulmonary obstruction or emphysema, where alveolar ventilation may be impaired, Methazolamide should be used with caution because it may precipitate or aggravate acidosis.

Information for Patients: Adverse reactions common to all sulfonamide derivatives may occur: anaphylaxis, fever, rash (including erythema multiforme, Stevens-Johnson syndrome, toxic epidermal necrolysis), crystalluria, renal calculus, bone marrow depression, thrombocytopenic purpura, hemolytic anemia, leukopenia, pancytopenia, and agranulocytosis. Precaution is advised for early detection of such reactions, and the drug should be discontinued and appropriate therapy instituted.

Caution is advised for patients receiving high-dose aspirin and Methazolamide concomitantly.

Laboratory Tests: To monitor for hematologic reactions common to all sulfonamides, it is recommended that a baseline CBC and platelet count be obtained on patients prior to initiating Methazolamide therapy and at regular intervals during therapy. If significant changes occur, early discontinuance and institution of appropriate therapy are important. Periodic monitoring of serum electrolytes is also recommended.

Drug Interactions: Methazolamide should be used with caution in patients on steroid therapy because of the potential for developing hypokalemia.

Caution is advised for patients receiving high-dose aspirin and Methazolamide concomitantly, as anorexia, tachypnea, lethargy, coma, and death have been reported with concomitant use of high-dose aspirin and carbonic anhydrase inhibitors (see "Warnings").

Carcinogenesis, Mutagenesis, Impairment of Fertility: Long-term studies in animals to evaluate the carcinogenic potential of Methazolamide and its effect on fertility have not been conducted. Methazolamide was not mutagenic in the Ames bacterial test.

Pregnancy: Teratogenic effects: Pregnancy Category C. Methazolamide has been shown to be teratogenic (skeletal anomalies) in rats when given in doses approximately 40 times the human dose. There are no adequate and well-controlled studies in pregnant women. Methazolamide should be used during pregnancy only if the potential benefit justifies the potential risk to the fetus.

Nursing Mothers: It is not known whether this drug is excreted in human milk. Because many drugs are excreted in human milk and because of the potential for serious adverse reactions in nursing infants from Methazolamide, a decision should be made whether to discontinue nursing or to discontinue the drug, taking into account the importance of the drug to the mother.

Pediatric Use: The safety and effectiveness of Methazolamide in children have not been established.

ADVERSE REACTIONS

Adverse reactions, occurring most often early in therapy, include paresthesias, particularly a "tingling" feeling in the extremities; hearing dysfunction or tinnitus; fatigue; malaise; loss of appetite; taste alteration; gastrointestinal disturbances such as nausea, vomiting, and diarrhea; polyuria; and occasional instances of drowsiness and confusion.

Metabolic acidosis and electrolyte imbalance may occur. Transient myopia has been reported. This condition invariably subsides upon diminution or discontinuance of the medication.

Other occasional adverse reactions include urticaria, melena, hematuria, glycosuria, hepatic insufficiency, flaccid paralysis, photosensitivity, convulsions, and, rarely, crystalluria and renal calculi. Also see "Precautions".

Information for Patients for possible reactions common to sulfonamide derivatives. Fatalities have occurred, although rarely, due to severe reactions to sulfonamides including Stevens-Johnson syndrome, toxic epidermal necrolysis, fulminant hepatic necrosis, agranulocytosis, aplastic anemia, and other blood dyscrasis (see "Warnings").

◆ RATED THERAPEUTICALLY EQUIVALENT; ◇ THERAPEUTIC EQUIVALENCE UNCONFIRMED; ○ UNRATED

OVERDOSAGE

No data are available regarding Methazolamide overdosage in humans as no cases of acute poisoning with this drug have been reported. Animal data suggest that even a high dose of Methazolamide is nontoxic. No specific antidote is known. Treatment should be symptomatic and supportive.

Electrolyte imbalance, development of an acidotic state, and central nervous system effects might be expected to occur. Serum electrolyte levels (particularly potassium) and blood pH levels should be monitored.

Supportive measures may be required to restore electrolyte and pH balance.

DOSAGE AND ADMINISTRATION

The effective therapeutic dose administered varies from 50 mg to 100 mg two to three times daily. The drug may be used concomitantly with miotic and osmotic agents.

Store at controlled room temperature 15° to 30°C (59° to 86°F).

HOW SUPPLIED
TABLETS: 25 MG

AVERAGE UNIT PRICE (AVAILABLE SIZES)		GENERIC A-RATED AVERAGE PRICE (GAAP)		
BRAND	$0.53	100s		$45.66
GENERIC	$0.46			

BRAND/MANUFACTURER	NDC	SIZE	AWP
◆ BRAND			
➤ NEPTAZANE: Storz/Lederle	57706-0756-23	100s	$53.13
◆ GENERICS			
GLAUCTABS: Akorn	17478-0525-01	100s	$38.13
Effcon	55806-0021-03	100s	$43.40
Goldline	00182-1075-01	100s	$45.00
Rugby	00536-5615-01	100s	$45.02
Major	00904-7781-60	100s	$45.70
Qualitest	00603-4470-21	100s	$47.43
Geneva	00781-1072-01	100s	$47.76
Copley	38245-0411-10	100s	$48.00
Aligen	00405-4631-01	100s	$50.53

TABLETS: 50 MG

AVERAGE UNIT PRICE (AVAILABLE SIZES)		GENERIC A-RATED AVERAGE PRICE (GAAP)		
BRAND	$0.79	100s		$68.62
GENERIC	$0.69			

BRAND/MANUFACTURER	NDC	SIZE	AWP
◆ BRAND			
➤ NEPTAZANE: Storz/Lederle	57706-0757-23	100s	$79.30
◆ GENERICS			
GLAUCTABS: Akorn	17478-0550-01	100s	$57.50
Effcon	55806-0020-03	100s	$66.58
Rugby	00536-5616-01	100s	$67.21
Goldline	00182-1076-01	100s	$67.50
Qualitest	00603-4471-21	100s	$67.60
Major	00904-7782-60	100s	$68.20
Geneva	00781-1071-01	100s	$71.29
Copley	38245-0424-10	100s	$72.00
Moore,H.L.	00839-7835-06	100s	$72.48
Aligen	00405-4632-01	100s	$75.79

Methdilazine Hydrochloride

DESCRIPTION

Methdilazine Hydrochloride is an antihistamine antipruritic with the following chemical structure: 10[(1-methyl-3-pyrrolidinyl) methyl] phenothiazine.

Methdilazine and its Hydrochloride salt occur as light tan, crystalline powders with respectively poor and free solubility in water.

Methdilazine or Methdilazine HCl is a phenothiazine derivative available as:

Tablets: Each tablet contains 8 mg Methdilazine HCl.

Syrup: Each 5 ml (one teaspoonful) contains 4 mg Methdilazine HCl.

Chewable Tablets: Each tablet contains Methdilazine equivalent to 4 mg Methdilazine HCl.

Following is its chemical structure:

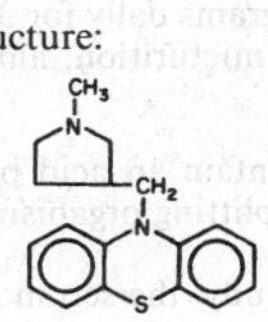

CLINICAL PHARMACOLOGY

No information is currently available which assess the disposition of Methdilazine.

INDICATIONS AND USAGE

Methdilazine and Methdilazine HCl are indicated for the treatment of pruritic symptoms in urticaria, symptomatic relief in the management of nasal allergies (hayfever, allergic rhinitis, etc.), relief of pruritic symptoms in a variety of allergic and non-allergic conditions including: atopic dermatitis, neurodermatitis, contact dermatitis, pityriasis rosea, poison ivy dermatitis, eczamatous dermatitis, pruritus ani and vulvae, and drug rash.

CONTRAINDICATIONS

Methdilazine is contraindicated in patients who are comatose, those who have received large amounts of CNS depressants, patients with bone marrow depression, jaundice or those who have demonstrated an idiosyncrasy or hypersensitivity to Methdilazine or other phenothiazines.

This drug is contraindicated in newborn or premature infants and nursing mothers as well as in children who are acutely ill and dehydrated, since there may be an increased susceptibility to dystonias.

WARNINGS

Phenothiazines with antihistaminic and anticholinergic effects, including Methdilazine and Methdilazine HCl, should be used with extreme caution in patients with: asthmatic attack, narrow-angle glaucoma, prostatic hypertrophy, stenosing peptic ulcer, pyloroduodenal obstruction, bladder neck obstruction, as well as in patients receiving monoamine oxidase inhibitors. Phenothiazine should not be used with alcohol ingestion.

Methdilazine HCl syrup contains sodium bisulfite, a sulfite that may cause allergic-type reactions including anaphylactic symptoms and life-threatening or less severe asthmatic episodes in certain susceptible people. The overall prevalence of sulfite sensitivity in the general population is unknown and probably low. Sulfite sensitivity is seen more frequently in asthmatic than in nonasthmatic people.

Usage in Pregnancy: There are reports of jaundice and prolonged extrapyramidal symptoms in infants whose mothers received phenothiazines during pregnancy.

Hyperreflexia has been reported in the newborn when a phenothiazine was used during pregnancy.

Use in Children: Methdilazine should be used with caution, as administration in the young child may result in excitation. Overdosage may produce hallucinations, convulsions, and sudden death.

Use in the Elderly (60 Years or Older): The elderly are more prone to develop the following side effects from phenothiazines; hypertension, syncope, toxic confusional states, excessive sedation, extrapyramidal signs (especially parkinsonism), akathisia and persistent dyskinesia.

PRECAUTIONS

General: Phenothiazines may block and even reverse some of the actions of epinephrine. Methdilazine should be used cautiously in persons with acute or chronic respiratory impairment, particularly children, as it may supress the cough reflex.

The drug should be used cautiously in persons with cardiovascular disease, impairment of liver function or those with a history of ulcer disease.

Information for Patients: Patients should be cautioned that Methdilazine or Methdilazine HCl may impair the mental and/or physical ability required for the performance of potentially hazardous tasks, such as driving a vehicle or operating machinery. Similarly, it may impair mental alertness in children. The concomitant use of alcohol or other central nervous system depressants may have an additive effect.

DRUG INTERACTIONS

■ CNS Depressants/Narcotics — Phenothiazines may increase, prolong or intensify the sedative action of nervous system depressants such as anesthetics, barbiturates or alcohol. The dose of a narcotic or barbiturate may be reduced to 1/4 or 1/2 the usual amount when Methdilazine is administered concomitantly. Excessive amounts of Methdilazine, relative to a narcotic, may lead to restlessness and motor hyperactivity in the patient with pain.

■ Epinephrine — Phenothiazines may block and even reverse some of the actions of epinephrine.

■ MAO Inhibitors — Combined use of MAO inhibitors and phenothiazines may result in hypotension and extrapyramidal reactions.

■ Thiazide Diuretics — The anticholinergic effects of phenothiazines may be prolonged and intensified by the concomitant use of thiazide diuretics.

■ Oral Contraceptives, Progesterone, Reserpine, Nylidrin Hydrochloride — These drugs potentiate the effects of phenothiazines.

DRUG/LABORATORY TEST INTERACTIONS

The following changes in laboratory determinations have been reported in patients taking phenothiazines:

■ increased serum cholesterol, blood glucose, spinal fluid protein, and urinary urobilinogen levels

■ decreased protein bound iodine (PBI)

■ false positives in urine bilirubin tests

■ interference with urinary ketone determinations, pregnancy tests and steroid determinations.

Carcinogenesis/Mutagenesis/Impairment of Fertility: Mutagenicity and long-term carcinogenicity studies in animals have not been performed. Mutagenicity has been evaluated using the Ames Salmonella/Microsome Plate test. Methdilazine HCl tablets and syrup were found to be nonmutagenic.

Pregnancy Category B: Reproduction studies have been performed in rats at doses up to 70 times the usual human dose and have revealed no evidence of impaired fertility or harm to the fetus due to Methdilazine. There are, however, no

➤ SHOWN IN PRODUCT IDENTIFICATION GUIDE

adequate and well controlled studies in pregnant women. Because animal reproduction studies are not always predictive of human response, this drug should be used during pregnancy only if clearly needed.

Nonteratogenic Effects: There are reports of jaundice and prolonged extrapyramidal symptoms in infants whose mothers received phenothiazines during pregnancy.

Nursing Mothers: It is not known whether this drug is excreted in human milk. Because many drugs are excreted in human milk, caution should be exercised when Methdilazine is administered to a nursing woman. (See *"Contraindications"*).

Pediatric Usage: Safety and effectiveness in children below the age of 3 years have not been established. (See *"Contraindications" "Warnings"* and *"Dosage and Administration."*)

ADVERSE REACTIONS

This drug may produce adverse reactions common to both phenothiazines and antihistamines.

Note: Not all of the following adverse reactions have been reported with this specific drug; however, pharmacological similarities among the phenothiazine derivatives require that each be considered when Methdilazine is administered. There have been occasional reports of sudden death in patients receiving phenothiazine derivatives chronically.

CNS: Drowsiness is the most prominent CNS effect of the drug. Extrapyramidal reactions occur, particularly with high doses. Other reported reactions include dizziness, lassitude, tinnitus, incoordination, fatigue, blurred vision, euphoria diplopia, nervousness, insomnia, tremors and grand mal seizures, excitation, catatonic-like states, neuritis and hysteria.

Cardiovasular: Postural hypotension is the most common cardiovascular effect of the phenothiazines. Reflex tachycardia may be seen. Bradycardia, faintness, dizziness and cardiac arrest have been reported. ECG changes, including blunting of T waves and prolongation of the Q-T interval may be seen.

Gastrointestinal: Anorexia, nausea, vomiting, epigastric distress, constipation and dry mouth may occur. Diarrhea has also been reported as well as increased appetite and weight gain.

Genitourinary: Urinary frequency, dysuria and urinary retention have been reported.

Respiratory: Thickening of bronchial secretions, tightness of the chest, wheezing and nasal stuffiness may occur.

Allergic Reactions: These include urticaria, dermatitis, asthma, laryngeal edema, angioneurotic edema, photosensitivity, lupus erythematosus-like syndrome and anaphylactoid reactions.

Other Reported Reactions: Leukopenia, agranulocytosis, thrombocytopenic purpura and jaundice of the obstructive type have been reported. The jaundice is usually reversible, but chronic jaundice has been reported.

Long-term Therapy Considerations: After prolonged administration at high dosage, pigmentation of the skin has occurred, chiefly in the exposed areas. Ocular changes consist of the appearance of lenticular and corneal opacities, epithelial keratopathies and pigmentary retinopathy. Vision may be impaired.

Endocrine: Early menses, induced lactation, gynecomastia, decreased libido and inhibition of ejaculation have been reported.

OVERDOSAGE

Signs and symptoms of overdosage range from mild depression of the central nervous system and cardiovascular system, to profound hypotension, respiratory depression and unconsciousness. Stimulation may be evident, especially in children and geriatric patients. Atropine-like signs and symptoms — dry mouth, fixed dilated pupils, flushing, etc. — as well as gastrointestinal symptoms may occur. The treatment of overdosage is essentially symptomatic and supportive. Early gastric lavage may be beneficial. Centrally acting emetics are of little use.

Avoid analeptics, which may cause convulsions. Severe hypotension usually responds to the administration of levarterenol or phenylephrine. **EPINEPHRINE SHOULD NOT BE USED**, since its use in the patient with partial adrenorgic blockade may further lower the blood pressure. Additional measures include oxygen and intravenous fluids. Limited experience with dialysis indicates that it is not helpful. The oral LD_{50} of Methdilazine HCl is approximately 225 mg/kg in mice, 448 mg/kg in rats and 269 mg/kg in guinea pigs.

DOSAGE AND ADMINISTRATION

METHDILAZINE HCL TABLETS
Adults: 1 tablet (8 mg) 2 to 4 times daily.
Children over 3 years: 1/2 tablet (4 mg) 2 to 4 times daily.

METHDILAZINE HCL SYRUP
Adults: 2 teaspoons (8 mg) 2 to 4 times daily.
Children over 3 years: 1 teaspoon (4 mg) 2 to 4 times daily.

METHDILAZINE CHEWABLE TABLETS
Adults: 2 tablets (7.2 mg) 2 to 4 times daily.
Children over 3 years: 1 tablet (3.6 mg) 2 to 4 times daily. This product form should be chewed and swallowed promptly.

STORAGE
Dispense in tight, light-resistant container. Store at room temperature away from strong light.

HOW SUPPLIED
CHEW TABLET: 3.6 MG

BRAND/MANUFACTURER	NDC	SIZE	AWP
○ BRAND TACARYL: Westwood-Squibb	00072-7300-01	100s	$44.92

SYRUP: 4 MG/5 ML

BRAND/MANUFACTURER	NDC	SIZE	AWP
○ BRAND TACARYL: Westwood-Squibb	00072-7500-01	480 ml	$53.59

TABLETS: 8 MG

BRAND/MANUFACTURER	NDC	SIZE	AWP
○ BRAND TACARYL: Westwood-Squibb	00072-7400-01	100s	$57.24

Methenamine Hippurate

DESCRIPTION

Each contains 1 g Methenamine Hippurate which is the Hippuric Acid Salt of Methenamine (hexamethylenetetramine). Certain brands of Methenenamine Hippurate also contain inactive ingredients: FD&C Yellow No. 5 (tartrazine, see *"Precautions"*).

Following is its chemical structure:

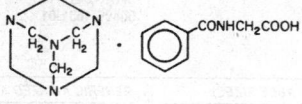

ACTIONS

Microbiology: Methenamine Hippurate has antibacterial activity because the Methanamine component is hydrolyzed to formaldehyde in acid urine. Hippuric acid, the other component, has some antibacterial activity and also acts to keep the urine acid. The drug is generally active against *E. coli*, enterococci and staphylococci. *Enterobacter aerogenes* is generally resistant. The urine must be kept sufficiently acid for urea-splitting organisms such as *Proteus* and *Pseudomonas* to be inhibited.

Human Pharmacology: Within ½ hour after ingestion of a single 1-gram dose of Methenamine Hippurate, antibacterial activity is demonstrable in the urine. Urine has continuous antibacterial activity when Methenamine Hippurate is administered at the recommended dosage schedule of 1 gram twice daily. Over 90% of Methenamine moiety is excreted in the urine within 24 hours after administration of a single 1-gram dose. Similarly, the Hippurate moiety is rapidly absorbed and excreted, and it reaches the urine by both tubular secretion and glomerular filtration. This action may be important in older patients or in those with some degree of renal impairment.

INDICATIONS

Methenamine Hippurate is indicated for prophylactic or suppressive treatment of frequently recurring urinary tract infections when long-term therapy is considered necessary. This drug should only be used after eradication of the infection by other appropriate antimicrobial agents.

CONTRAINDICATIONS

Methenamine Hippurate is contraindicated in patients with renal insufficiency, severe hepatic insufficiency, or severe dehydration. Methenamine preparations should not be given to patients taking sulfonamides because some sulfonamides may form an insoluble precipitate with formaldehyde in the urine.

WARNING

Large doses of Methenamine (8 grams daily for 3 to 4 weeks) have caused bladder irritation, painful and frequent micturition, albuminuria, and gross hematuria.

PRECAUTIONS

1. Care should be taken to maintain an acid pH of the urine, especially when treating infections due to urea-splitting organisms such as *Proteus* and strains of *Pseudomonas*.

2. In a few instances in one study, the serum transaminase levels were slightly elevated during treatment but returned to normal while the patients were still taking Methenamine Hippurate. Because of this report, it is recommended that liver function studies be performed periodically on patients taking the drug, especially those with liver dysfunction.

3. *Use in Pregnancy:* In early pregnancy the safe use of Methenamine Hippurate is not established. In the last trimester, safety is suggested, but not definitely proved. No adverse effects on the fetus were seen in studies in pregnant rats and rabbits. Methenamine Hippurate taken during pregnancy can interfere with laboratory

tests of urine estriol (resulting in unmeasurably low values) when acid hydrolysis is used in the laboratory procedure. This interference is due to the presence in the urine of Methenamine and/or formaldehyde. Enzymatic hydrolysis, in place of acid hydrolysis, will circumvent this problem.

4. This product contains FD&C Yellow No. 5 (tartrazine), which may cause allergic-type reactions (including bronchial asthma) in certain susceptible individuals. Although the overall incidence of FD&C Yellow No. 5 (tartrazine) sensitivity in the general population is low, it is frequently seen in patients who also have aspirin hypersensitivity.

ADVERSE REACTIONS
Minor adverse reactions have been reported in less than 3.5% of patients treated. These reactions have included nausea, upset stomach, dysuria, and rash.

DOSAGE AND ADMINISTRATION
1 tablet (1.0 g) twice daily (morning and night) for adults and children over 12 years of age.

½ to 1 tablet (0.5 to 1.0 g) twice daily (morning and night) for children 6 to 12 years of age.

Since the antibacterial activity of Methenamine Hippurate is greater in acid urine, restriction of alkalinizing foods and medications is desirable. If necessary, as indicated by urinary pH and clinical response, supplemental acidification of the urine should be instituted. The efficacy of therapy should be monitored by repeated urine cultures.

HOW SUPPLIED
TABLETS: 1 GM

AVERAGE UNIT PRICE (AVAILABLE SIZES)

BRAND			$1.03

BRAND/MANUFACTURER	NDC	SIZE	AWP
◆ BRAND			
UREX: 3M Pharm	00089-0371-10	100s	$102.60
HIPREX: Marion Merrell Dow	00068-0277-61	100s	$103.62

Methenamine Mandelate and Sodium Acid Phosphate

DESCRIPTION
Each tablet contains:

Methenamine Mandelate .... 350 mg
Sodium Acid Phosphate, monohydrate .... 200 mg
No. 2 Methenamine Mandelate .... 500 mg
Sodium Acid Phosphate, monohydrate .... 500 mg

CLINICAL PHARMACOLOGY
Methenamine Mandelate is rapidly absorbed and excreted in the urine. Formaldehyde is released by acid hydrolysis from methenamine with bactericidal levels rapidly reached at pH 5.0-5.5. Proportionally less formaldehyde is released as urinary pH approaches 6.0 and insufficient quantities are released above this level for therapeutic response. In acid urine, mandelic acid exerts its antibacterial action and also contributes to the acidification of the urine. Mandelic acid is excreted by both glomerular filtration and tubular excretion. In acid urine, there is equally effective antibacterial activity against both gram-positive and gram-negative organisms, since the antibacterial action of mandelic acid and formaldehyde is nonspecific. With Proteus vulgaris and urea splitting strains of Pseudomonas and Aerobacter, results may be discouraging and particular attention is required in monitoring urinary pH and overall management.

INDICATIONS AND USAGE
For the suppression or elimination of bacteriuria associated with chronic and recurrent infections of the urinary tract, including pyelitis, pyelonephritis, cystitis, and infected residual urine accompanying neurogenic bladder. When used as recommended, Methenamine Mandelate/Sodium Acid Phosphate and Methenamine Mandelate/Sodium Acid Phosphate No. 2 are particularly suitable for long-term therapy because of their relative safety and because resistance to the nonspecific bactericidal action of formaldehyde does not develop. Pathogens resistant to other antibacterial agents may respond because of the nonspecific effect of formaldehyde formed in an acid urine.

Prophylactic Use Rationale: Urine is a good culture medium for many urinary pathogens. Inoculation by a few organisms (relapse or reinfection) may lead to bacteriuria in susceptible individuals. Thus, the rationale of management in recurring urinary tract infection (bacteriuria) is to change the urine from a growth-supporting to a growth-inhibiting medium. There is a growing body of evidence that long-term administration of methenamine can prevent recurrence of bacteriuria in patients with chronic pyelonephritis.

Therapeutic Use Rationale: Helps to sterilize the urine and, in some situations in which underlying pathologic conditions prevent sterilization by any means, they can help to suppress bacteriuria. As part of the overall management of the urinary tract infection, a thorough diagnostic evaluation should accompany the use of these products.

CONTRAINDICATIONS
Methenamine Mandelate/Sodium Acid Phosphate and Methenamine Mandelate/Sodium Acid Phosphate No. 2 are contraindicated in patients with renal insufficiency, severe hepatic disease, severe dehydration, hyperphosphatemia, and in patients who have exhibited hypersensitivity to any components of these products.

PRECAUTIONS
General: These products should not be used as the sole therapeutic agent in acute parenchymal infections causing systemic symptoms such as chills and fever.

Methenamine Mandelate/Sodium Acid Phosphate and Methenamine Mandelate/Sodium Acid Phosphate No. 2 contain approximately 33 mg and 83 mg of sodium per tablet, respectively, and should be used with caution in patients on a sodium-restricted diet.

Sodium Phosphates should be used with caution in the following conditions: cardiac failure; peripheral or pulmonary edema; hypernatremia; hypertension; toxemia of pregnancy; hypoparathyroidism; and acute pancreatitis. High serum phosphate levels increase the incidence of extraskeletal calcification.

Large doses of Methenamine (8 grams daily for 3 to 4 weeks) have caused bladder irritation, painful and frequent micturation, albuminuria and gross hematuria. Dysuria may occur, although usually at higher than recommended doses, and can be controlled by reducing the dosage. These products contain a urinary acidifier and can cause metabolic acidosis. Care should be taken to maintain an acid urinary pH (below 5.5), especially when treating infections due to urea-splitting organisms such as Proteus and strains of Pseudomonas. Drugs and/or foods which produce an alkaline urine should be restricted. Frequent urine pH tests are essential. If acidification of the urine is contraindicated or unattainable, use of these products should be discontinued.

Information for Patients: To assure an acidic pH, patients should be instructed to restrict or avoid most fruits, milk and milk products, and antacids containing sodium carbonate or bicarbonate.

Laboratory Tests: As with all urinary tract infections, the efficacy of therapy should be monitored by repeated urine cultures. During long-term therapy, careful monitoring of renal function, serum phosphorous and Sodium may be required at periodic intervals.

Drug Interactions: Formaldehyde and sulfonamides form an insoluble precipitate in acid urine and increase the risk of crystalliuria; therefore, these products should not be used concurrently. Thiazide diuretics, carbonic anhydrase inhibitors, antacids, or urinary alkalinizing agents should not be used concurrently since they may cause the urine to become alkaline and reduce the effectiveness of Methenamine by inhibiting its conversion to formaldehyde. Concurrent use of antihypertensives, especially diazoxide, guanethidine, hydralazine, methyldopa, or rauwolfia alkaloids; or corticosteroids, especially mineralocorticoids or corticotropin, with sodium phosphates may result in hypernatremia. Concurrent use of salicylates may lead to increased serum salicylate levels since excretion of salicylates is reduced in acidified urine. Serum salicylate levels should be closely monitored to avoid toxicity.

Laboratory Test Interactions: Formaldehyde interferes with fluorometric procedures for determination of urinary catecholamines and vanilmandelic acid (VMA) causing erroneously high results. Formaldehyde also causes falsely decreased urine estriol levels by reacting with estriol when acid hydrolysis techniques are used; estriol determinations which use enzymatic hydrolysis are unaffected by formaldehyde. Formaldehyde causes falsely elevated 17-hydroxycorticosteroid levels when the Porter-Silber method is used and falsely decreased 5-hydroxyindoleacetic acid (5HIAA) levels by inhibiting color development when nitrosonaphthol methods are used.

Carcinogenesis, Mutagenesis, Impairment of Fertility: Long-term animal studies to evaluate the carcinogenic, mutagenic, or impairment of fertility potential of these products have not been performed.

Pregnancy: Pregnancy Category C. Animal reproduction studies have not been conducted with these products. It is also not known whether these products can cause fetal harm when administered to a pregnant woman or can affect reproduction capacity. Since Methenamine is known to cross the placental barrier, these products should be given to a pregnant woman only if clearly needed.

Nursing Mothers: Methenamine is excreted in breast milk. Caution should be exercised when these products are administered to a nursing woman.

ADVERSE REACTIONS
Gastrointestinal disturbances (nausea, stomach upset), generalized skin rash, dysuria, painful or difficult urination may occur occasionally with the use of Methenamine preparations. Microscopic and rarely, gross hematuria have also been reported.

Gastrointestinal upsets (diarrhea, nausea, stomach pain, and vomiting) may occur with the use of Sodium Phosphates. Also, bone or joint pain (possible phosphate induced osteomalacia) could occur. The following adverse effects may be observed (primarily from Sodium or potassium): headaches; dizziness; mental confusion; seizures; weakness or heaviness of legs; unusual tiredness or weakness; muscle cramps; numbness, tingling, pain or weakness of hands or feet; numbness or tingling around lips; fast or irregular heartbeat; shortness of breath or troubled breathing; swelling of feet or lower legs; unusual weight gain; low urine output; unusual thirst.

DIRECTIONS

Methenamine Mandelate/Sodium Acid Phosphates: Initially, 3 tablets 4 times daily. For maintenance, 1 or 2 tablets 4 times daily. Methenamine Mandelate/Sodium Acid Phosphates No. 2 Initially, 2 tablets 4 times daily. For maintenance, 2 to 4 tablets daily, in divided doses. Give these products with a full glass of water.

HOW SUPPLIED
TABLETS:

BRAND/MANUFACTURER	NDC	SIZE	AWP
○ **BRAND**			
URO-PHOSPHATE: Poythress	00095-0031-01	100s	$16.25
URISEDAMINE: Polymedica	00998-2210-10	100s	$53.75
○ **GENERICS**			
URL	00677-1393-01	100s	$8.95
Eon	00185-0230-01	100s	$8.95
Alphagen	59743-0016-01	100s	$9.05
Qualitest	00603-6311-21	100s	$9.78
Qualitest	00603-6311-32	1000s	$65.11
Eon	00185-0230-10	1000s	$84.95
Alphagen	59743-0016-10	1000s	$86.40

Methergine *SEE* METHYLERGONOVINE MALEATE

Methicillin Sodium

DESCRIPTION

Methicillin Sodium is a semisynthetic antibiotic substance derived from 6-amino-penicillanic acid. It is the Sodium salt in a sterile parenteral dosage form for intramuscular or intravenous use.

4-Thia-1-azabicyclo[3.2.0]heptane-2-carboxylic acid. 6-[(2,6-dimethoxyben-zoyl)amino]-3,3-dimethyl-7-oxo-monosodium salt, monohydrate, [2S-(2α, 5α, 6β)]-.

Following is its chemical structure:

CLINICAL PHARMACOLOGY

Microbiology: Penicillinase-resistant penicillins exert a bactericidal action against penicillin-susceptible microorganisms during the state of active multiplication. All penicillins inhibit the biosynthesis of the bacterial cell wall.

The drugs in this class are highly resistant to inactivation by staphylococcal penicillinase and are active against penicillinase producing and nonpenicillinase producing strains of *Staphylococcus aureus.*

The penicillinase-resistant penicillins are active *in vitro* against a variety of other bacteria.

Susceptibility Plate Testing: Quantitative methods of susceptibility testing that require measurement of zone diameters or minimal inhibitory concentrations (MICs) give the most precise estimates of antibiotic susceptibility. One such procedure has been recommended for use with discs to test susceptibility to this class of drugs. Interpretations correlate diameters on the disc test with MIC values. A penicillinase-resistant class disc may be used to determine microbial susceptibility to cloxacillin, dicloxacillin, methicillin, nafcillin, and oxacillin. With this procedure, employing a 5 microgram methicillin sodium disc, a report from the laboratory of "susceptible" (zone of at least 14 mm) indicates that the infecting organism is likely to respond to therapy. A report of "resistant" (zone of less than 10 mm) indicates that the infecting organism is not likely to respond to therapy. A report of "intermediate susceptibility" (zone of 10 to 13 mm) suggests that the organism might be susceptible if high doses of the antibiotic are used, or if the infection is confined to tissues and fluids (eg, urine), in which high antibiotic levels are attained.

In general, all staphylococci should be tested against the penicillin G disc and against the Methicillin disc. Routine methods of antibiotic susceptibility testing may fail to detect strains of organisms resistant to the penicillinase-resistant penicillins. For this reason, the use of large inocula and 48-hour incubation periods may be necessary to obtain accurate susceptibility studies with these antibiotics. Bacterial strains which are resistant to one of the penicillinase-resistant penicillins should be considered resistant to all of the drugs in the class.

Pharmacokinetics: Methicillin Sodium is not acid-resistant and must be administered by intramuscular or intravenous injection. A 1-gram intramuscular dose gives a peak blood level of approximately 12 μg/mL which drops off to about 1 μg/mL within a 4-hour period. Methicillin is rapidly excreted unchanged in the urine in individuals with normal kidney function. Impairment in kidney function results in elevated blood levels which may require adjustment of dosage and treatment intervals. Protein binding of Methicillin is approximately 40%. The drug penetrates body tissues well, and diffuses readily into pleural, pericardial, and synovial fluids. As with all penicillins, absorption into spinal fluids is poor

under normal conditions. However, higher concentrations may be attained in the presence of meningeal inflammation.

INDICATIONS AND USAGE

The penicillinase-resistant penicillins are indicated in the treatment of infections caused by penicillinase-producing staphylococci which have demonstrated susceptibility to the drugs. Culture and susceptibility tests should be performed initially to determine the causative organism and their sensitivity to the drug (see "*Clinical Pharmacology—Susceptibility Plate Testing*").

The penicillinase-resistant penicillins may be used to initiate therapy in suspected cases of resistant staphylococcal infections prior to the availability of laboratory test results. The penicillinase-resistant penicillins should not be used in infections caused by organisms susceptible to penicillin G. If the susceptibility tests indicate that the infection is due to an organism other than a resistant staphylococcus, therapy should not be continued with a penicillinase-resistant penicillin.

CONTRAINDICATIONS

A history of a hypersensitivity (anaphylactic) reaction to any penicillin is a contraindication.

WARNINGS

Serious and occasionally fatal hypersensitivity (anaphylactic shock with collapse) reactions have occurred in patients receiving penicillin. The incidence of anaphylactic shock in all penicillin-treated patients is between 0.015 and 0.04 percent. Anaphylactic shock resulting in death has occurred in approximately 0.002 percent of the patients treated. Although anaphylaxis is more frequent following parenteral administration, it has occurred in patients receiving oral penicillins.

When penicillin therapy is indicated, it should be initiated only after a comprehensive patient drug and allergy history has been obtained. If an allergic reaction occurs, the drug should be discontinued and the patient should receive supportive treatment, eg, artificial maintenance of ventilation, pressor amines, antihistamines, and corticosteroids. Individuals with a history of penicillin hypersensitivity may also experience allergic reactions when treated with a cephalosporin.

PRECAUTIONS

General: Penicillinase-resistant penicillins should generally not be administered to patients with a history of sensitivity to any penicillin.

Penicillin should be used with caution in individuals with histories of significant allergies and/or asthma. Whenever allergic reactions occur, penicillin should be withdrawn unless, in the opinion of the physician, the condition being treated is life-threatening and amenable only to penicillin therapy.

The oral route of administration should not be relied upon in patients with severe illness, or with nausea, vomiting, gastric dilation, cardiospasm, or intestinal hypermotility. Occasionally patients will not absorb therapeutic amounts of orally administered penicillin.

The use of antibiotics may result in overgrowth of nonsusceptible organisms. If new infections due to bacteria or fungi occur, the drug should be discontinued and appropriate measures taken.

Laboratory Tests: Bacteriologic studies to determine the causative organisms and their susceptibility to the penicillinase-resistant penicillins should be performed (see "*Clinical Pharmacology-Microbiology*"). In the treatment of suspected staphylococcal infections, therapy should be changed to another active agent if culture tests fail to demonstrate the presence of staphylococci.

Periodic assessment of organ system function including renal, hepatic, and hematopoietic should be made during prolonged therapy with the penicillinase-resistant penicillins.

Blood cultures, white blood cell, and differential cell counts should be obtained prior to initiation of therapy and at least weekly during therapy with penicillinase-resistant penicillins.

Periodic urinalysis, blood urea nitrogen, and creatinine determinations should be performed during therapy with the penicillinase-resistant penicillins and dosage alterations should be considered if these values become elevated. If any impairment of renal function is suspected or known to exist, a reduction in the total dosage should be considered and blood levels monitored to avoid possible neurotoxic reactions (see "*Dosage and Administration*").

SGOT and SGPT values should be obtained periodically during therapy to monitor for possible liver function abnormalities.

Drug Interactions: Tetracycline, a bacteriostatic antibiotic, may antagonize the bactericidal effect of penicillin and concurrent use of these drugs should be avoided.

Carcinogenesis, Mutagenesis, Impairment of Fertility: No long-term animal studies have been conducted with these drugs.

Studies on reproduction (nafcillin) in rats and rabbits reveal no fetal or maternal abnormalities before conception and continuously through weaning (one generation).

Pregnancy Category B: Reproduction studies performed in the mouse, rat, and rabbit have revealed no evidence of impaired fertility or harm to the fetus due to the penicillinase-resistant penicillins. Human experience with the penicillins during pregnancy has not shown any positive evidence of adverse effects on the fetus. There are, however, no adequate or well-controlled studies in pregnant women showing conclusively that harmful effects of these drugs on the fetus can be excluded. Because animal reproduction studies are not always predictive of human response, this drug should be used during pregnancy only if clearly needed.

Nursing Mothers: Penicillins are excreted in breast milk. Caution should be exercised when penicillins are administered to a nursing woman.

Pediatric Use: Because of incompletely developed renal function in newborns, penicillinase-resistant penicillins (especially Methicillin) may not be completely excreted, with abnormally high blood levels resulting. Frequent blood levels are advisable in this group with dosage adjustments when necessary. All newborns treated with penicillins should be monitored closely for clinical and laboratory evidence of toxic or adverse effects (see *"Dosage and Administration"*).

ADVERSE REACTIONS
Body as a Whole: The reported incidence of allergic reactions to penicillins ranges from 0.7 to 10 percent (see *"Warnings"*). Sensitization is usually the result of treatment but some individuals have had immediate reactions to penicillin when first treated. In such cases, it is thought that the patients may have had prior exposure to the drug via trace amounts present in milk and vaccines.

Two types of allergic reactions to penicillin are noted clinically, immediate and delayed.

Immediate reactions usually occur within 20 minutes of administration and range in severity from urticaria and pruritus to angioneurotic edema, laryngospasm, bronchospasm, hypotension, vascular collapse, and death. Such immediate anaphylactic reactions are very rare (see *"Warnings"*) and usually occur after parenteral therapy but have occurred in patients receiving oral therapy. Another type of immediate reaction, an accelerated reaction, may occur between 20 minutes and 48 hours after administration and may include urticaria, pruritus, and fever. Although laryngeal edema, laryngospasm, and hypotension occasionally occur, fatality is uncommon.

Delayed allergic reactions to penicillin therapy usually occur after 48 hours and sometimes as late as 2 to 4 weeks after initiation of therapy. Manifestations of this type of reaction include serum sickness like symptoms (ie, fever, malaise, urticaria, myalgia, arthralgia, abdominal pain) and various skin rashes. Nausea, vomiting diarrhea, stomatitis, black or hairy tongue, and other symptoms of gastrointestinal irritation may occur, especially during oral penicillin therapy.

Nervous System Reactions: Neurotoxic reactions similar to those observed with penicillin G may occur with large intravenous doses of the penicillinase-resistant penicillins especially in patients with renal insufficiency.

Urogenital Reactions: Renal tubular damage and interstitial nephritis have been associated with the administration of methicillin sodium and infrequently with the administration of nafcillin and oxacillin. Manifestations of this reaction may include rash, fever, eosinophilla, hematuria, proteinuria, and renal insufficiency. Methicillin-induced nephropathy does not appear to be dose-related and is generally reversible upon prompt discontinuation of therapy.

Metabolic Reactions: Agranulocytosis, neutropenia, and bone marrow depression have been associated with the use of Methicillin Sodium, nafcillin, oxacillin, and cloxacillin. Hepatotoxicity, characterized by fever, nausea, and vomiting associated with abnormal liver function tests, mainly elevated SGOT levels, has been associated with the use of oxacillin and cloxacillin.

DOSAGE AND ADMINISTRATION
The penicillinase-resistant penicillins are available for oral administration and for intramuscular and intravenous injection. The sodium salts of Methicillin, oxacillin, and nafcillin may be administered parenterally and the sodium salts of cloxacillin, dicloxacillin, oxacillin, and nafcillin are available for oral use.

Bacteriologic studies to determine the causative organisms and their sensitivity to the penicillinase-resistant penicillins should always be performed. Duration of therapy varies with the type and severity of infection as well as the overall condition of the patient, therefore, it should be determined by the clinical and bacteriological response of the patient. In severe staphylococcal infections, therapy with penicillinase-resistant penicillins should be continued for at least 14 days. Therapy should be continued for at least 48 hours after the patient has become afebrile, asymptomatic, and cultures are negative. The treatment of endocarditis and osteomyelitis may require a longer term of therapy.

Concurrent administration of the penicillinase-resistant penicillins and probenecid increases and prolongs serum penicillin levels. Probenecid decreases the apparent volume of distribution and slows the rate of excretion by competitively inhibiting renal tubular secretion of penicillin. Penicillin-probenecid therapy is generally limited to those infections where very high serum levels of penicillin are necessary.

Oral preparations of the penicillinase-resistant penicillins should not be used as initial therapy in serious, life-threatening infections (see *"Precautions-General"*). Oral therapy with the penicillinase-resistant penicillins may be used to follow-up the previous use of a parenteral agent as soon as the clinical condition warrants. For intramuscular gluteal injections, care should be taken to avoid sciatic nerve injury. With intravenous administration, particularly in elderly patients, care should be taken because of the possibility of thrombophlebitis. When using this product for direct IV administration inject at the rate of 10 mL per minute.

RECOMMENDED DOSAGES FOR METHICILLIN SODIUM

Drug	Adults	Infants and Children <40 kg (88 lbs)
Methicillin Sodium	1 gram IM every 4 or 6 hours IV every 6 hours	25 mg/kg IM every 6 hours IV not recommended

DIRECTIONS FOR USE (SEE RELATED TABLE).

IMPORTANT: This chemical stability information in no way indicates that it would be acceptable practice to use this product well after the preparation time. Good professional practice suggests that a product should be used as soon after preparation as feasible.

Stability: Studies of Methicillin Sodium concentrations of 2 mg/mL, 10 mg/mL and 20 mg/mL in various intravenous solutions listed below indicate the drug will lose less than 10% activity at room temperature (70°F) during an 8-hour period.

IV Solution:
Dextrose 5% and NaCl 0.9% Injection
10% D-Fructose in Water
10% D-Fructose in Normal Saline
Lactated Potassic Saline Injection
5% Plasma Hydrolysate in Water
* 10% Invert Sugar in Normal Saline
10% Invert Sugar Plus 0.3% Potassium Chloride in Water
Travert 10% Electrolyte #1
Travert 10% Electrolyte #2
Travert 10% Electrolyte #3

Only those solutions listed above should be used for the intravenous infusion of Methicillin Sodium. The concentration of the antibiotic should fall within the range specified. The drug concentration and the rate and volume of the infusion should be adjusted so that the total dose of Methicillin is administered before the drug loses its stability in the solution in use.

If another agent is used in conjunction with Methicillin therapy, it should not be physically mixed with Methicillin but should be administered separately.

Parenteral drug products should be inspected visually for particulate matter and discoloration prior to administration, whenever solution and container permit.

*At a concentration of 2 mg/mL Methicillin Sodium stable for only 4 hours in this solution. Concentrations between 10 mg/mL and 30 mg/mL are stable for 8 hours.

J CODES
Up to 1 g IM,IV—J2970

HOW SUPPLIED
POWDER FOR INJECTION: 1 GM

BRAND/MANUFACTURER	NDC	SIZE	AWP
○ BRAND			
STAPHCILLIN: Apothecon	00015-7961-20	1s	$5.53

STABILITY PERIODS FOR METHICILLIN SODIUM

Concentration mg/mL	Sterile H₂O for Injection	Sodium Chloride Injection 0.9%	M/6 Molar Sodium Lactate Injection	Dextrose Injection 5%	5% Dextrose in 0.45% NaCl	10% Invert Sugar	Lactated Ringers Injection
Room Temperature (25°C)							
10-200	24 Hrs	24 Hrs					
2-20			8 Hrs	8 Hrs		8 Hrs	8 Hrs
10-30					24 Hrs		
Refrigeration (4°C)							
10-200	7 Days	7 Days		7 Days	7 Days	7 Days	7 Days
10-30			7 Days				
Frozen (-15°C)							
19-500	30 Days						
20-100		30 Days	30 Days	30 Days	30 Days	30 Days	30 Days

► SHOWN IN PRODUCT IDENTIFICATION GUIDE

POWDER FOR INJECTION: 4 GM

BRAND/MANUFACTURER	NDC	SIZE	AWP
○ **BRAND**			
STAPHCILLIN: Apothecon	00015-7964-20	1s	$20.15

POWDER FOR INJECTION: 10 GM

BRAND/MANUFACTURER	NDC	SIZE	AWP
○ **BRAND**			
STAPHCILLIN: Apothecon	00015-7102-28	1s	$53.33

Methimazole

DESCRIPTION

Methimazole (1-methylimidazole-2-thiol) is a white, crystalline substance that is freely soluble in water. It differs chemically from the drugs of the thiouracil series primarily because it has a 5- instead of a 6-membered ring.

Each tablet contains 5 or 10 mg (43.8 or 87.6 µmol) Methimazole, an orally administered antithyroid drug.

The molecular weight is 114.16, and the empirical formula is $C_4H_6N_2S$.

Following is its chemical structure:

CLINICAL PHARMACOLOGY

Methimazole inhibits the synthesis of thyroid hormones and thus is effective in the treatment of hyperthyroidism. The drug does not inactivate existing thyroxine and triiodothyronine that are stored in the thyroid or circulating in the blood nor does it interfere with the effectiveness of thyroid hormones given by mouth or by injection.

The actions and use of Methimazole are similar to those of propylthiouracil. On a weight basis, the drug is at least 10 times as potent as Propylthiouracil, but Methimazole may be less consistent in action.

Methimazole is readily absorbed from the gastrointestinal tract. It is metabolized rapidly and requires frequent administration. Methimazole is excreted in the urine.

In laboratory animals, various regimens that continuously suppress thyroid function and thereby increase TSH secretion result in thyroid tissue hypertrophy. Under such conditions, the appearance of thyroid and pituitary neoplasms has also been reported. Regimens that have been studied in this regard include antithyroid agents, such as Methimazole, as well as dietary iodine deficiency, subtotal thyroidectomy, implantation of autonomous thyrotropic hormone-secreting pituitary tumors, and administration of chemical goitrogens.

INDICATIONS AND USAGE

Methimazole is indicated in the medical treatment of hyperthyroidism. Long-term therapy may lead to remission of the disease. Methimazole may be used to ameliorate hyperthyroidism in preparation for subtotal thyroidectomy or radioactive iodine therapy. Methimazole is also used when thyroidectomy is contraindicated or not advisable.

CONTRAINDICATIONS

Methimazole is contraindicated in the presence of hypersensitivity to the drug and in nursing mothers because the drug is excreted in milk.

WARNINGS

Agranulocytosis is potentially a serious side effect. Patients should be instructed to report to their physicians any symptoms of agranulocytosis, such as fever or sore throat. Leukopenia, thrombocytopenia, and aplastic anemia (pancytopenia) may also occur. The drug should be discontinued in the presence of agranulocytosis, aplastic anemia (pancytopenia), hepatitis, or exfoliative dermatitis. The patient's bone marrow function should be monitored.

Due to the similar hepatic toxicity profiles of Methimazole and Propylthiouracil, attention is drawn to the severe hepatic reactions which have occurred with both drugs. There have been rare reports of fulminant hepatitis, hepatic necrosis, encephalopathy, and death. Symptoms suggestive of hepatic dysfunction (anorexia, pruritus, right upper quadrant pain, etc) should prompt evaluation of liver function. Drug treatment should be discontinued promptly in the event of clinically significant evidence of liver abnormality including hepatic transaminase values exceeding 3 times the upper limit of normal.

Methimazole can cause fetal harm when administered to a pregnant woman. Methimazole readily crosses the placental membranes and can induce goiter and even cretinism in the developing fetus. In addition, rare instances of aplasia cutis, as manifested by scalp defects, have occurred in infants born to mothers who received Methimazole during pregnancy. If Methimazole is used during pregnancy or if the patient becomes pregnant while taking this drug, the patient should be warned of the potential hazard to the fetus.

Since scalp defects have not been reported in offspring of patients treated with Propylthiouracil, that agent may be preferable to Methimazole in pregnant women requiring treatment with antithyroid drugs.

Postpartum patients receiving Methimazole should not nurse their babies.

PRECAUTIONS

General: Patients who receive Methimazole should be under close surveillance and should be cautioned to report immediately any evidence of illness, particularly sore throat, skin eruptions, fever, headache, or general malaise. In such cases, white-blood-cell and differential counts should be made to determine whether agranulocytosis has developed. Particular care should be exercised with patients who are receiving additional drugs known to cause agranulocytosis.

Laboratory Tests: Because Methimazole may cause hypoprothrombinemia and bleeding, prothrombin time should be monitored during therapy with the drug, especially before surgical procedures (see "General" under "Precautions").

Periodic monitoring of thyroid function is warranted, and the finding of an elevated TSH warrants a decrease in the dosage of Methimazole.

Drug Interactions: The activity of anticoagulants may be potentiated by anti-vitamin-K activity attributed to Methimazole.

Carcinogenesis, Mutagenesis, Impairment of Fertility: Rats treated for 2 years with Methimazole demonstrated thyroid hyperplasia and thyroid adenoma and carcinoma formation. Such findings are seen with continuous suppression of thyroid function by sufficient doses of a variety of antithyroid agents. Pituitary adenomas have also been observed (see "Clinical Pharmacology").

Pregnancy Category D: see "Warnings". Methimazole used judiciously is an effective drug in hyperthyroidism complicated by pregnancy. In many pregnant women, the thyroid dysfunction diminishes as the pregnancy proceeds; consequently, a reduction in dosage may be possible. In some instances, use of Methimazole can be discontinued 2 or 3 weeks before delivery.

Nursing Mothers: The drug appears in human breast milk and its use is contraindicated in nursing mothers (see "Warnings").

Usage in Children: See "Dosage and Administration."

ADVERSE REACTIONS

Major adverse reactions (which occur with much less frequency than the minor adverse reactions) include inhibition of myelopoiesis (agranulocytosis, granulocytopenia, and thrombocytopenia), aplastic anemia, drug fever, a lupuslike syndrome, insulin autoimmune syndrome (which can result in hypoglycemic coma), hepatitis (jaundice may persist for several weeks after discontinuation of the drug), periarteritis, and hypoprothrombinemia. Nephritis occurs very rarely. Minor adverse reactions include skin rash, urticaria, nausea, vomiting, epigastric distress, arthralgia, paresthesia, loss of taste, abnormal loss of hair, myalgia, headache, pruritus, drowsiness, neuritis, edema, vertigo, skin pigmentation, jaundice, sialadenopathy, and lymphadenopathy.

It should be noted that about 10% of patients with untreated hyperthyroidism have leukopenia (white-blood-cell count of less than 4,000/mm³), often with relative granulopenia.

OVERDOSAGE

Signs and Symptoms: Symptoms may include nausea, vomiting, epigastric distress, headache, fever, joint pain, pruritus, and edema. Aplastic anemia (pancytopenia) or agranulocytosis may be manifested in hours to days. Less frequent events are hepatitis, nephrotic syndrome, exfoliative dermatitis, neuropathies, and CNS stimulation or depression. Although not well studied Methimazole-induced agranulocytosis is generally associated with doses of 40 mg or more in patients older than 40 years of age.

No information is available on the median lethal dose of the drug or the concentration of Methimazole in biologic fluids associated with toxicity and/or death.

Treatment: To obtain up-to-date information about the treatment of overdose, a good resource is your certified Regional Poison Control Center. Telephone numbers of certified poison control centers are listed in the *Physicians' Desk Reference (PDR)*. In managing overdosage, consider the possibility of multiple drug overdoses, interaction among drugs, and unusual drug kinetics in your patient.

Protect the patient's airway and support ventilation and perfusion. Meticulously monitor and maintain, within acceptable limits, the patient's vital signs, blood gases, serum electrolytes, etc. The patient's bone marrow function should be monitored. Absorption of drugs from the gastrointestinal tract may be decreased by giving activated charcoal, which, in many cases, is more effective than emesis or lavage; consider charcoal instead of or in addition to gastric emptying. Repeated doses of charcoal over time may hasten elimination of some drugs that have been absorbed. Safeguard the patient's airway when employing gastric emptying or charcoal.

Forced diuresis, peritoneal dialysis, hemodialysis, or charcoal hemoperfusion have not been established as beneficial for an overdose of methimazole.

DOSAGE AND ADMINISTRATION

Methimazole is administered orally. It is usually given in 3 equal doses at approximately 8-hour intervals.

Adult: The initial daily dosage is 15 mg for mild hyperthyroidism, 30 to 40 mg for moderately severe hyperthyroidism, and 60 mg for severe hyperthyroidism, divided into 3 doses at 8-hour intervals. The maintenance dosage is 5 to 15 mg daily.

Pediatric: Initially, the daily dosage is 0.4 mg/kg of body weight divided into 3 doses and given at 8-hour intervals. The maintenance dosage is approximately 1/2 of the initial dose.

◆ RATED THERAPEUTICALLY EQUIVALENT; ◇ THERAPEUTIC EQUIVALENCE UNCONFIRMED; ○ UNRATED

HOW SUPPLIED
TABLETS: 5 MG

BRAND/MANUFACTURER	NDC	SIZE	AWP
○ **BRAND** TAPAZOLE: Lilly	00002-1094-02	100s	$13.35

TABLETS: 10 MG

BRAND/MANUFACTURER	NDC	SIZE	AWP
○ **BRAND** TAPAZOLE: Lilly	00002-1095-02	100s	$21.30

Methocarbamol

Methocarbamol is available in tablet and injectable form.

Each tablet contains:

Methocarbamol	500 mg
Methocarbamol-750	750 mg

Each mL of the injectable solution contains:

Methocarbamol	100 mg

AFTER MIXING WITH I.V. INFUSION FLUIDS, **DO NOT REFRIGERATE.**

Methocarbamol is a central nervous system depressant used as an adjunct in the treatment of painful musculoskeletal conditions.

Following is its chemical structure:

$$ \text{OCH}_2\text{CHCH}_2\text{OOCNH}_2 $$

(with OH and OCH$_3$ substituents on the benzene ring)

ACTIONS
The mechanism of action of Methocarbamol in humans has not been established, but may be due to general central nervous system depression. It has no direct action on the contractile mechanism of striated muscle, the motor end plate or the nerve fiber.

INDICATIONS
Methocarbamol is indicated as an adjunct to rest, physical therapy, and other measures for the relief of discomforts associated with acute, painful musculoskeletal conditions. The mode of action of this drug has not been clearly identified, but may be related to its sedative properties. Methocarbamol does not directly relax tense skeletal muscles in man.

CONTRAINDICATIONS
Methocarbamol is contraindicated in patients hypersensitive to any of the ingredients.

Methocarbamol injectable should not be administered to patients with known or suspected renal pathology. This caution is necessary because of the presence of polyethylene glycol 300 in the vehicle.

A much larger amount of polyethylene glycol 300 than is present in recommended doses of Methocarbamol injectable is known to have increased pre-existing acidosis and urea retention in patients with renal impairment. Although the amount present in this preparation is well within the limits of safety, caution dictates this contraindication.

Methocarbamol injectable is contraindicated in patients hypersensitive to any of the ingredients.

WARNINGS
Since Methocarbamol may possess a general central nervous system depressant effect, patients receiving Methocarbamol tablets or injection should be cautioned about combined effects with alcohol and other CNS depressants.

Safe use of Methocarbamol has not been established with regard to possible adverse effects upon fetal development. Therefore, Methocarbamol should not be used in women who are or may become pregnant and particularly during early pregnancy unless in the judgment of the physician the potential benefits outweigh the possible hazards.

PRECAUTIONS
Safety and effectiveness in children below the age of 12 years have not been established.

It is not known whether this drug is secreted in human milk. As a general rule, nursing should not be undertaken while a patient is on a drug since many drugs are excreted in human milk.

As with other agents administered either intravenously or intramuscularly, careful supervision of dose and rate of injection should be observed. Rate of injection should not exceed 3 mL per minute—i.e., one 10 mL via in approximately three minutes. Since Methocarbamol injectable is hypertonic, vascular extravasation must be avoided. A recumbent position will reduce the likelihood of side reactions.

Blood aspirated into the syringe does not mix with the hypertonic solution. This phenomenon occurs with many other intravenous preparations. The blood may be safely injected with the Methocarbamol, or the injection may be stopped when the plunger reaches the blood, whichever the physician prefers.

The total dosage should not exceed 30 mL (three vials) a day for more than three consecutive days except in the treatment of tetanus.

Caution should be observed in using the injectable form in suspected or known epileptic patients.

Safety and effectiveness in children below the age of 12 years have not been established except in tetanus. See special directions for use in tetanus.

Methocarbamol may cause a color interference in certain screening tests for 5-hydroxyindoleacetic acid (5-HIAA) and vanillylmandelic acid (VMA).

ADVERSE REACTIONS
Light-headedness, dizziness, drowsiness, nausea, allergic manifestations such as urticaria, pruritus, rash, conjunctivitis with nasal congestion, blurred vision, headache, fever.

DOSAGE AND ADMINISTRATION
METHOCARBAMOL TABLETS
Methocarbamol: 500 mg—Adults: initial dosage, 3 tablets q.i.d.; maintenance dosage, 2 tablets q.i.d.

Methocarbamol-750: 750 mg—Adults: initial dosage, 2 tablets q.i.d.; maintenance dosage, 1 tablet q.4h. or 2 tablets t.i.d.

Six grams a day are recommended for the first 48 to 72 hours of treatment. (For severe conditions 8 grams a day may be administered.) Thereafter, the dosage can usually be reduced to approximately 4 grams a day.

METHOCARBAMOL INJECTABLE
For Intravenous and Intramuscular Use Only: Total adult dosage should not exceed 30 mL (3 vials) a day for more than 3 consecutive days except in the treatment of tetanus. A like course may be repeated after a lapse of 48 hours if the condition persists. Dosage and frequency of injection should be based on the severity of the condition being treated and therapeutic response noted.

For the relief of symptoms of moderate degree, 10 mL (one vial) may be adequate. Ordinarily this injection need not be repeated, as the administration of the oral form will usually sustain the relief initiated by the injection. For the severest cases or in postoperative conditions in which oral administration is not feasible, 20 to 30 mL (two to three vials) may be required.

Directions for Intravenous Use: Methocarbamol injectable may be administered undiluted directly into the vein at a **maximum rate of three mL per minute.** It may also be added to an intravenous drip of sodium chloride injection (sterile isotonic sodium chloride solution for parenteral use) or five per cent dextrose injection (sterile 5 per cent dextrose solution); one vial given as a single dose should not be diluted to more than 250 mL for I.V. infusion. Care should be exercised to avoid vascular extravasation of this hypertonic solution which may result in thrombophlebitis. It is preferable that the patient be in a recumbent position during and for at least 10 to 15 minutes following the injection.

Directions for Intramuscular Use: When the intramuscular route is indicated, not more than five mL (one-half vial) should be injected into each gluteal region. The injections may be repeated at eight hour intervals, if necessary. When satisfactory relief of symptoms is achieved, it can usually be maintained with tablets.

NOT RECOMMENDED FOR SUBCUTANEOUS ADMINISTRATION
Special Directions for Use in Tetanus: There is clinical evidence which suggests that methocarbamol may have a beneficial effect in the control of the neuromuscular manifestations of tetanus. It does not, however, replace the usual procedure of debridement, tetanus antitoxin, penicillin, tracheotomy, attention to fluid balance, and supportive care. Methocarbamol injectable should be added to the regimen as soon as possible.

For adults: Inject one or two vials directly into the tubing of a previously inserted indwelling needle. An additional 10 mL or 20 mL may be added to the infusion bottle so that a total of up to 30 mL (three vials) is given as the initial dose (note Precautions). This procedure should be repeated every six hours until conditions allow for the insertion of a nasogastric tube. Crushed Methocarbamol tablets suspended in water or saline may then be given through this tube. Total daily oral doses up to 24 grams may be required as judged by patient response.

For children: A minimum initial dose of 15 mg/kg is recommended. This dosage may be repeated every six hours as indicated. The maintenance dosage may be given by injection into the tubing or by I.V. infusion with an appropriate quantity of fluid. See directions for I.V. use.

STORAGE
Store at controlled room temperature, between 15°C and 30°C (59°F and 86°F).
Dispense in tight container.

HOW SUPPLIED
INJECTION: 100 MG/ML

AVERAGE UNIT PRICE (AVAILABLE SIZES)		GENERIC A-RATED AVERAGE PRICE (GAAP)	
BRAND	$0.45	10 ml	$4.32
GENERIC	$0.43		

BRAND/MANUFACTURER	NDC	SIZE	AWP
◆ **BRAND** ROBAXIN: Robins Pharm	00031-7409-87	10 ml 5s	$23.63
	00031-7409-94	10 ml 25s	$106.84

► SHOWN IN PRODUCT IDENTIFICATION GUIDE

BRAND/MANUFACTURER	NDC	SIZE	AWP
◆ GENERICS			
Schein	00364-6726-54	10 ml	$2.93
Steris	00402-0131-10	10 ml	$2.93
Moore,H.L.	00839-6359-30	10 ml	$3.63
Rugby	00536-5331-70	10 ml	$7.80

TABLETS: 500 MG

AVERAGE UNIT PRICE (AVAILABLE SIZES)		GENERIC A-RATED AVERAGE PRICE (GAAP)	
BRAND	$0.44	100s	$10.51
GENERIC	$0.09	500s	$37.48
HCFA FUL (100s ea)	$0.07		

BRAND/MANUFACTURER	NDC	SIZE	AWP
◆ BRAND			
➤ ROBAXIN: Robins Pharm	00031-7429-63	100s	$43.50
	00031-7429-64	100s ud	$46.00
	00031-7429-70	500s	$205.28
◆ GENERICS			
Lederle Std Prod	00005-3562-23	100s	$6.39
West-Ward	00143-1290-01	100s	$7.10
Pioneer	60104-6036-02	100s	$7.15
Rugby	00536-4026-01	100s	$8.25
Qualitest	00603-4487-21	100s	$8.48
URL	00677-0430-01	100s	$8.95
Major	00904-2364-60	100s	$8.95
Schein	00364-0346-01	100s	$8.95
Geneva	00781-1760-01	100s	$8.97
Goldline	00182-0572-01	100s	$9.00
Aligen	00405-4635-01	100s	$9.57
Richlyn	00115-3900-01	100s	$9.63
Moore,H.L.	00839-5132-06	100s	$10.46
Parmed	00349-8041-01	100s	$12.14
Raway	00686-0091-20	100s ud	$9.95
UDL	51079-0091-20	100s ud	$10.64
Auro	55829-0360-10	100s ud	$11.83
Goldline	00182-0572-89	100s ud	$12.00
Major	00904-2364-61	100s ud	$13.77
West-Ward	00143-1290-25	100s ud	$14.50
Schein	00364-0346-90	100s ud	$16.50
Geneva	00781-1760-13	100s ud	$18.00
Pioneer	60104-6036-06	500s	$29.92
Lederle Std Prod	00005-3562-31	500s	$31.58
West-Ward	00143-1290-05	500s	$31.60
Aligen	00405-4635-02	500s	$33.85
Rugby	00536-4026-05	500s	$34.42
Qualitest	00603-4487-28	500s	$35.50
Major	00904-2364-40	500s	$36.20
Schein	00364-0346-05	500s	$37.45
Geneva	00781-1760-05	500s	$37.49
URL	00677-0430-05	500s	$38.95
Goldline	00182-0572-05	500s	$39.00
Richlyn	00115-3900-02	500s	$40.84
Parmed	00349-8041-05	500s	$48.26
Moore,H.L.	00839-5132-12	500s	$49.61
Rugby	00536-4026-10	1000s	$67.75

TABLETS: 750 MG

AVERAGE UNIT PRICE (AVAILABLE SIZES)		GENERIC A-RATED AVERAGE PRICE (GAAP)	
BRAND	$0.62	100s	$13.52
GENERIC	$0.12	500s	$50.29
HCFA FUL (100s ea)	$0.09		

BRAND/MANUFACTURER	NDC	SIZE	AWP
◆ BRAND			
➤ ROBAXIN-750: Robins Pharm	00031-7449-63	100s	$62.19
	00031-7449-64	100s ud	$64.46
	00031-7449-70	500s	$292.86
◆ GENERICS			
Lederle Std Prod	00005-3563-23	100s	$8.24
West-Ward	00143-1292-01	100s	$9.50
Major	00904-2365-60	100s	$10.25
Qualitest	00603-4488-21	100s	$10.40
Geneva	00781-1750-01	100s	$10.42
URL	00677-0431-01	100s	$10.45
➤ Schein	00364-0347-01	100s	$10.45
Pioneer	60104-6038-02	100s	$10.45
Goldline	00182-0573-01	100s	$10.45
Aligen	00405-4636-01	100s	$10.78
Rugby	00536-4027-01	100s	$11.39
Richlyn	00115-3902-01	100s	$14.16
Moore,H.L.	00839-5101-06	100s	$18.56
Raway	00686-0092-20	100s ud	$11.95
West-Ward	00143-1292-25	100s ud	$16.25
Goldline	00182-0573-89	100s ud	$16.50
Auro	55829-0361-10	100s ud	$16.53
UDL	51079-0092-20	100s ud	$16.75
➤ Schein	00364-0347-90	100s ud	$21.75
Geneva	00781-1750-13	100s ud	$25.20
West-Ward	00143-1292-05	500s	$40.25

BRAND/MANUFACTURER	NDC	SIZE	AWP
Lederle Std Prod	00005-3563-31	500s	$40.74
➤ Schein	00364-0347-05	500s	$43.20
Goldline	00182-0573-05	500s	$45.90
Pioneer	60104-6038-06	500s	$45.98
Geneva	00781-1750-05	500s	$47.19
Rugby	00536-4027-05	500s	$47.25
Major	00904-2365-40	500s	$47.30
URL	00677-0431-05	500s	$47.35
Qualitest	00603-4488-28	500s	$47.40
Aligen	00405-4636-02	500s	$50.30
Richlyn	00115-3902-02	500s	$59.90
Moore,H.L.	00839-5101-12	500s	$90.98
Rugby	00536-4027-10	1000s	$95.55

Methohexital Sodium

> **WARNING**
>
> THIS DRUG SHOULD BE ADMINISTERED BY PERSONS QUALIFIED IN THE USE OF INTRAVENOUS ANESTHETICS. CARDIAC LIFE SUPPORT EQUIPMENT MUST BE IMMEDIATELY AVAILABLE DURING USE OF METHOHEXITAL.

DESCRIPTION

Methohexital Sodium for Injection, USP is 2,4,6 (1H,3H,5H)-Pyrimidinetrione, 1-methyl-5-(1-methyl-2-pentynyl)-5- (2-propenyl)-, (±)-, monosodium salt. Methohexital Sodium for Injection is a freeze-dried, sterile, nonpyrogenic mixture of Methohexital Sodium and anhydrous sodium carbonate added as a buffer, which is prepared from an aqueous solution of Methohexital, sodium hydroxide, and sodium carbonate. It contains not less than 90% and not more than 110% of the labeled amount of $C_{14}H_{17}NaO_3$. This mixture is ordinarily intended to be reconstituted so as to contain 1% Methohexital Sodium in Sterile Water for Injection for direct intravenous injection or 0.2% Methohexital Sodium in 5% dextrose injection (or 0.9% sodium chloride injection) for administration by continuous intravenous drip. The pH of the 1% solution is between 10 and 11: the pH of the 0.2% solution in 5% dextrose is between 9.5 and 10.5.

Methohexital Sodium is a rapid, ultrashort-acting barbiturate anesthetic. It occurs as a white, crystalline powder that is freely soluble in water.

Following is its chemical structure:

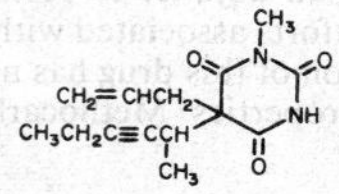

CLINICAL PHARMACOLOGY

Compared with Thiamylal and Thiopental, Methohexital is at least twice as potent on a weight basis, and its duration of action is only about half as long. Although the metabolic fate of Methohexital in the body is not clear, the drug does not appear to concentrate in fat depots to the extent that other barbiturate anesthetics do. Thus, cumulative effects are fewer and recovery is more rapid with Methohexital than with thiobarbiturates. In experimental animals, the drug cannot be detected in the blood 24 hours after administration.

Methohexital differs chemically from the established barbiturate anesthetics in that it contains no sulfur. Little analgesia is conferred by barbiturates; their use in the presence of pain may result in excitation.

Intravenous administration of Methohexital results in rapid uptake by the brain (within 30 seconds) and rapid induction of sleep. With single doses, the rate of redistribution determines duration of pharmacologic effect. Metabolism occurs in the liver through demethylation and oxidation. Side-chain oxidation is the most important biotransformation involved in termination of biologic activity. Excretion occurs via the kidneys through glomerular filtration.

INDICATIONS AND USAGE

Methohexital Sodium can be used as follows:

1. For intravenous induction of anesthesia prior to the use of other general anesthetic agents.
2. For intravenous induction of anesthesia and as an adjunct to subpotent inhalational anesthetic agents (such as nitrous oxide in oxygen) for short surgical procedures Methohexital Sodium may be given by infusion or intermittent injection.
3. For use along with other parenteral agents, usually narcotic analgesics, to supplement subpotent inhalational anesthetic agents (such as nitrous oxide in oxygen) for longer surgical procedures.
4. As intravenous anesthesia for short surgical, diagnostic, or therapeutic procedures associated with minimal painful stimuli (see *"Precautions"*).
5. As an agent for inducing a hypnotic state.

UNLABELED USES

Methohexital Sodium is used alone or as adjunct in the diagnosis of epilepsy (seizure disorders) and the activation of electroencephalograms.

◆ RATED THERAPEUTICALLY EQUIVALENT; ◇ THERAPEUTIC EQUIVALENCE UNCONFIRMED; ○ UNRATED

CONTRAINDICATIONS

Methohexital Sodium is contraindicated in patients in whom general anesthesia is contraindicated, in those with latent or manifest porphyria, or in patients with a known hypersensitivity to barbiturates.

WARNINGS

See boxed *"Warning"*.

AS WITH ALL POTENT ANESTHETIC AGENTS AND ADJUNCTS, THIS DRUG SHOULD BE ADMINISTERED ONLY BY THOSE TRAINED IN THE ADMINISTRATION OF GENERAL ANESTHESIA, THE MAINTENANCE OF A PATENT AIRWAY AND VENTILATION, AND THE MANAGEMENT OF CARDIOVASCULAR DEPRESSION ENCOUNTERED DURING ANESTHESIA AND SURGERY.

Because the liver is involved in demethylation and oxidation of Methohexital and because barbiturates may enhance preexisting circulatory depression, severe hepatic dysfunction, severe cardiovascular instabilty, or a shock-like condition may be reason for selecting another induction agent.

Psychomotor seizures may be elicited in susceptible individuals.[1]

Prolonged administration may result in cumulative effects, including extended somnolence, protracted unconsciousness, and respiratory and cardiovascular depression. Respiratory depression in the presence of an impaired airway may lead to hypoxia, cardiac arrest, and death.

The CNS-depressant effect of Methohexital Sodium may be additive with that of other CNS depressants, including ethyl alcohol and propylene glycol.

DANGER OF INTRA-ARTERIAL INJECTION

Unintended intra-arterial injection of barbiturate solutions may be followed by the production of platelet aggregates and thrombosis, starting in arterioles distal to the site of injection. The resulting necrosis may lead to gangrene, which may require amputation. The first sign in conscious patients may be a complaint of fiery burning that roughly follows the distribution path of the injected artery; if noted, the injection should be stopped immediately and the situation reevaluated. *Transient* blanching *may* or may not be noted very early; blotchy cyanosis and dark discoloration may then be the first sign in anesthetized patients. There is no established treatment other than prevention. The following should be considered prior to injection.

1. The extent of injury is related to concentration. Concentrations of 1% Methohexital will usually suffice; higher concentrations should ordinarily be avoided.
2. Check the infusion to ensure that the catheter is in the lumen of a vein before injection. Injection through a running intravenous infusion may enhance the possibility of detecting arterial placement; however, it should be remembered that the characteristic bright-red color of arterial blood is often altered by contact with drugs. The possibility of aberrant arteries should always be considered.

Postinjury arterial injection of vasodilators and/or arterial infusion of parenteral fluids are generally regarded to be of no value in altering outcome. Animal experiments and published individual case reports concerned with a variety of arteriolar irritants, including barbiturates, suggest that 1 or more of the following *may* be of benefit in reducing the area of necrosis:

1. Arterial injection of heparin at the site of injury, followed by systemic anticoagulation.
2. Sympathetic blockade (or brachial plexus blockade in the arm).
3. Intra-arterial glucocorticoid injection at the site of injury, followed by systemic steroids.
4. A recent case report (nonbarbiturate injury) suggests that intra-arterial urokinase may promote fibrinolysis, even if administered late in treatment.

If extravasation is noted during injection of Methohexital, the injection should be discontinued until the situation is remedied. Local irritation may result from extravasation; subcutaneous swelling may also serve as a sign of arterial or periarterial placement of the catheter.

PRECAUTIONS

General: Maintenance of a patent airway and adequacy of ventilation must be ensured during induction and maintenance of anesthesia with Methohexital Sodium solution. Laryngospasm is common during induction with all barbiturates and may be due to a combination of secretions and accentuated reflexes following induction or may result from painful stimuli during light anesthesia. Transient apnea may be noted during induction, which may impair pulmonary ventilation; the duration of apnea may be longer than that produced by other barbiturate anesthetics. Cardiorespiratory arrest may occur. Intravenous administration of Methohexital Sodium is often associated with hiccups, coughing, and/or muscle twitching, which may also impair pulmonary ventilation.

Following induction, temporary hypotension and tachycardia may occur.

Recovery from Methohexital anesthesia is rapid and smooth. The incidence of postoperative nausea and vomiting is low if the drug is administered to fasting patients. Postanesthetic shivering has occurred in a few instances.

The usual precautions taken with any barbiturate anesthetic should be observed with Methohexital Sodium. The drug should be used with caution in patients with asthma, obstructive pulmonary disease, severe hypertension or hypotension, myocardial disease, congestive heart failure, severe anemia, or extreme obesity.

Methohexital Sodium should be used with extreme caution in patients in status asthmaticus.

Caution should be exercised in debilitated patients or in those with impaired function of respiratory, circulatory, renal, hepatic, or endocrine systems.

Information for Patients: When appropriate, patients should be instructed as to the hazards of drowsiness that may follow use of Methohexital Sodium. Outpatients should be released in the company of another individual, and no skilled activities, such as operating machinery or driving a motor vehicle, should be engaged in for 8 to 12 hours.

Laboratory Tests: BSP and liver function studies may be influenced by administration of a single dose of barbiturates.

Drug Interactions: Barbiturates may influence the absorption and elimination of other concomitantly used drugs, such as Diphenylhydantoin, halothane, anticoagulants, corticosteroids, ethyl alcohol,[2] and propylene glycol-containing solutions.

Carcinogenesis, Mutagenesis, Impairment of Fertility: Studies in animals to evaluate the carcinogenic and mutagenic potential of Methohexital Sodium have not been conducted. Reproduction studies in animals have revealed no evidence of impaired fertility.[3]

Usage in Pregnancy—Pregnancy Category B: Reproduction studies have been performed in rabbits and rats at doses up to 4 and 7 times the human dose respectively and have revealed no evidence of harm to the fetus due to Methohexital Sodium.[3] There are, however, no adequate and well-controlled studies in pregnant women. Because animal reproduction studies are not always predictive of human response, this drug should be used during pregnancy only if clearly needed.

Labor and Delivery: Methohexital Sodium has been used in cesarean section delivery but, because of its solubility and lack of protein binding, it readily and rapidly traverses the placenta.

Nursing Mothers: Caution should be exercised when Methohexital Sodium is administered to a nursing woman.

Usage in Children: Safety and effectiveness in children have not been established.

ADVERSE REACTIONS

Side effects associated with Methohexital Sodium are extensions of pharmacologic effects and include:

Cardiovascular: Circulatory depression, thrombophlebitis, hypotension, peripheral vascular collapse, and convulsions in association with cardiorespiratory arrest.

Respiratory: Respiratory depression (including apnea), cardiorespiratory arrest, laryngospasm, bronchospasm, hiccups, and dyspnea.

Neurologic: Skeletal muscle hyperactivity (twitching), injury to nerves adjacent to injection site, and seizures.

Psychiatric: Emergence delirium, restlessness, and anxiety may occur, especially in the presence of postoperative pain.

Gastrointestinal: Nausea, emesis, and abdominal pain.

Allergic: Erythema, pruritus, urticaria, and cases of anaphylaxis have been reported.

Other: Other adverse reactions include pain at injection site, salivation, headache, and rhinitis.

DRUG ABUSE AND DEPENDENCE

Controlled Substance—Methohexital Sodium is a Schedule IV drug.

Methohexital Sodium may be habit-forming.

OVERDOSAGE

Signs and Symptoms: The onset of toxicity following an overdose of intravenously administered Methohexital will be within seconds of the infusion. If Methohexital is administered rectally or is ingested, the onset of toxicity may be delayed. The manifestations of an ultrashort-acting barbiturate in overdose include central nervous system depression, respiratory depression, hypotension, loss of peripheral vascular resistance, and muscular hyperactivity ranging from twitching to convulsive-like movements. Other findings may include convulsions and allergic reactions. Following massive exposure to any barbiturate, pulmonary edema, circulatory collapse with loss of peripheral vascular tone, and cardiac arrest may occur.

Treatment: To obtain up-to-date information about the treatment of overdose, a good resource is your certified Regional Poison Control Center. Telephone numbers of certified poison control centers are listed in the *Physicians' Desk Reference (PDR)*. In managing overdosage, consider the possibility of multiple drug overdoses, interaction among drugs, and unusual drug kinetics in your patient.

Establish an airway and ensure oxygenation and ventilation. Resuscitative measures should be initiated promptly. For hypotension, intravenous fluids should be administered and the patient's legs raised. If desirable increase in blood pressure is not obtained, vasopressor and/or inotropic drugs may be used as dictated by the clinical situation.

For convulsions diazepam intravenously and phenytoin may be required. If seizures are refractory to diazepam and phenytoin, general anesthesia and paralysis with a neuromuscular blocking agent may be necessary.

Protect the patient's airway and support ventilation and perfusion. Meticulously monitor and maintain, within acceptable limits, the patient's vital signs, blood gases, serum electrolytes, etc. Absorption of drugs from the gastrointestinal tract may be decreased by giving activated charcoal, which, in many cases, is more

PREPARATION OF SOLUTIONS OF METHOHEXITAL SODIUM

Preparation of Solution—Follow Diluting Instructions Exactly. Diluents—Do Not Use Diluents Containing Bacteriostats. Sterile Water for Injection is the preferred diluent. Five percent Dextrose Injection or 0.9% Sodium Chloride Injection may be used. (Methohexital Sodium is not compatible with Lactated Ringer's Injection.)

Vial	Amount of Diluent to Be Added to the Vial	For 1% Solution Dilute to
(2.5 g)	15 mL	250 mL
(5 g)	30 mL	500 mL

When the first dilution is made the solution in the vial will be yellow. When further diluted to make a 1% solution, it must be clear and colorless or should not be used. Solutions of Methohexital should be freshly prepared and used promptly. Reconstituted solutions of Methohexital are chemically stable at room temperature for 24 hours.

COMPATIBILITY OF METHOHEXITAL SODIUM WITH SOLUTIONS HAVING A LOW pH

Active Ingredient	Potency per mL	Volume Used	Immediate	Physical Change		
				15 min	30 min	1 h
Methohexital Sodium	10 mg	10 mL			CONTROL	
Atropine sulfate	1/150 gr	1 mL	None	Haze		
Atropine sulfate	1/100 gr	1 mL	None	Ppt	Ppt	
Succinylcholine chloride	0.5 mg	4 mL	None	None	Haze	
Succinylcholine chloride	1 mg	4 mL	None	None	Haze	
Metocurine iodide	0.5 mg	4 mL	None	None	Ppt	
Metocurine iodide	1 mg	4 mL	None	None	Ppt	
Scopolamine hydrobromide	1/120 gr	1 mL	None	None	None	Haze
Tubocurarine chloride	3 mg	4 mL	None	Haze		

effective than emesis or lavage; consider charcoal instead of or in addition to gastric emptying. Repeated doses of charcoal over time may hasten elimination of some drugs that have been absorbed. Safeguard the patient's airway when employing gastric emptying or charcoal.

DOSAGE AND ADMINISTRATION
Preanesthetic medication is generally advisable. Methohexital Sodium may be used with any of the recognized preanesthetic medications, but the phenothiazines are less satisfactory than the combination of an opiate and a belladonna derivative.

Facilities for assisting respiration and administering oxygen are necessary adjuncts for intravenous anesthesia. Since cardiorespiratory arrest may occur, patients should be observed carefully during and after use of Methohexital Sodium. Resuscitative equipment (i.e., intubation and cardioversion equipment, oxygen, suction, and a secure intravenous line) and personnel qualified in its use must be immediately available. (See related table).

For continuous drip anesthesia, prepare a 0.2% solution by adding 500 mg of Methohexital to 250 mL of diluent. For this dilution, either 5% glucose solution or isotonic (0.9%) sodium chloride solution is recommended instead of distilled water in order to avoid extreme hypotonicity.

ADMINISTRATION
Methohexital is administered intravenously in a concentration of no higher than 1%. Higher concentrations markedly increase the incidence of muscular movements and irregularities in respiration and blood pressure. Dosage is highly individualized; the drug should be administered only by those completely familiar with its quantitative differences from other barbiturate anesthetics.

Methohexital may be dissolved in Sterile Water for Injection, 5% Dextrose Injection, or Sodium Chloride Injection. For induction of anesthesia, a 1% solution is administered at a rate of about 1 mL/5 seconds. Gaseous anesthetics and/or skeletal muscle relaxants may be administered concomitantly. The dose required for induction may range from 50 to 120 mg or more but averages about 70 mg. The induction dose usually provides anesthesia for 5 to 7 minutes.

The usual dosage in adults ranges from 1 to 1.5 mg/kg. Data on dosage requirements in children are not available.

Maintenance of anesthesia may be accomplished by intermittent injections of the 1% solution or, more easily, by continuous intravenous drip of a 0.2% solution. Intermittent injections of about 20 to 40 mg (2 to 4 mL of a 1% solution) may be given as required, usually every 4 to 7 minutes. For continuous drip, the average rate of administration is about 3 mL of a 0.2% solution/minute (1 drop/second). The rate of flow must be individualized for each patient. For longer surgical procedures, gradual reduction in the rate of administration is recommended (see discussion of prolonged administration in *"Warnings"*). Other parenteral agents, usually narcotic analgesics, are ordinarily employed along with Methohexital Sodium during longer procedures.

Parenteral drug products should be inspected visually for particulate matter and discoloration prior to administration, whenever solution and container permit.

COMPATIBILITY INFORMATION
Solutions of Methohexital Sodium should not be mixed in the same syringe or administered simultaneously during intravenous infusion through the same needle with acid solutions, such as Atropine sulfate, Metocurine Iodide Injection, USP and succinylcholine chloride. Alteration of pH may cause free barbituric acid

to be precipitated. Solubility of the soluble sodium salts of barbiturates, including Methohexital Sodium, is maintained only at a relatively high (basic) pH.

Because of numerous requests for anesthesiologists for information regarding the chemical compatibility of these mixtures, the following chart contains information obtained from compatibility studies in which a 1% solution of Methohexital Sodium was mixed with therapeutic amounts of agents whose solutions have a low (acid) pH. (See related table).

STORAGE
The vials may be stored at room temperature, 77°F (25°C or below). The expiration period for the vials is 2 years.

REFERENCES
1. Rockoff MA, Goudsouzian NG: Seizures induced by methohexital. *Anesthesiology* 1981; 54:333.   2. Hansten PD: *Drug Interactions*, ed 4. Philadelphia, Lea & Febiger, 1979, p 224.   3. Gibson WR, et al: Reproduction and teratology studies in rats and rabbits using sodium methohexital, Lilly Toxicology Laboratories, Eli Lilly and Company, Greenfield, Indiana 46140, unpublished manuscript, August 1970.

HOW SUPPLIED
POWDER FOR INJECTION (C-IV): 2.5 MG

BRAND/MANUFACTURER	NDC	SIZE	AWP
○ BRAND BREVITAL SODIUM: Lilly	00002-1448-25	25s	$517.04

POWDER FOR INJECTION (C-IV): 500 MG

BRAND/MANUFACTURER	NDC	SIZE	AWP
○ BRAND BREVITAL SODIUM: Lilly	00002-1446-01	1s	$7.61
	00002-1465-01	1s	$11.49
	00002-1446-25	25s	$181.10

POWDER FOR INJECTION (C-IV): 5 GM

BRAND/MANUFACTURER	NDC	SIZE	AWP
○ BRAND BREVITAL SODIUM: Lilly	00002-1445-01	1s	$44.25

Methotrexate

WARNINGS
METHOTREXATE SHOULD BE USED ONLY BY PHYSICIANS WHOSE KNOWLEDGE AND EXPERIENCE INCLUDES THE USE OF ANTIMETABOLITE THERAPY.

THE USE OF METHOTREXATE HIGH-DOSE REGIMENS RECOMMENDED FOR OSTEOSARCOMA REQUIRES METICULOUS CARE (SEE *"DOSAGE AND ADMINISTRATION"*). HIGH-DOSAGE REGIMENS FOR OTHER NEOPLASTIC DISEASES ARE INVESTIGATIONAL AND A THERAPEUTIC ADVANTAGE HAS NOT BEEN ESTABLISHED.

◆ RATED THERAPEUTICALLY EQUIVALENT; ◇ THERAPEUTIC EQUIVALENCE UNCONFIRMED; ○ UNRATED

BECAUSE OF THE POSSIBILITY OF SERIOUS TOXIC REACTIONS, THE PATIENT SHOULD BE INFORMED BY THE PHYSICIAN OF THE RISKS INVOLVED AND SHOULD BE UNDER A PHYSICIAN'S CONSTANT SUPERVISION.

DEATHS HAVE BEEN REPORTED WITH THE USE OF METHOTREXATE IN THE TREATMENT OF MALIGNANCY, PSORIASIS, AND RHEUMATOID ARTHRITIS.

IN THE TREATMENT OF PSORIASIS OR RHEUMATOID ARTHRITIS, METHOTREXATE USE SHOULD BE RESTRICTED TO PATIENTS WITH SEVERE, RECALCITRANT, DISABLING DISEASE, WHICH IS NOT ADEQUATELY RESPONSIVE TO OTHER FORMS OF THERAPY, AND ONLY WHEN THE DIAGNOSIS HAS BEEN ESTABLISHED AND AFTER APPROPRIATE CONSULTATION.

1. METHOTREXATE HAS BEEN REPORTED TO CAUSE FETAL DEATH AND/OR CONGENITAL ANOMALIES. THEREFORE, IT IS NOT RECOMMENDED FOR WOMEN OF CHILDBEARING POTENTIAL UNLESS THERE IS CLEAR MEDICAL EVIDENCE THAT THE BENEFITS CAN BE EXPECTED TO OUTWEIGH THE CONSIDERED RISKS. PREGNANT PATIENTS WITH PSORIASIS OR RHEUMATOID ARTHRITIS SHOULD NOT RECEIVE METHOTREXATE (SEE *"CONTRAINDICATIONS"*.)

2. PERIODIC MONITORING FOR TOXICITY, INCLUDING CBC WITH DIFFERENTIAL AND PLATELET COUNTS, AND LIVER AND RENAL FUNCTION TESTS IS A MANDATORY PART OF METHOTREXATE THERAPY. PERIODIC LIVER BIOPSIES MAY BE INDICATED IN SOME SITUATIONS. PATIENTS AT INCREASED RISK FOR IMPAIRED METHOTREXATE ELIMINATION (EG, RENAL DYSFUNCTION, PLEURAL EFFUSIONS, OR ASCITES) SHOULD BE MONITORED MORE FREQUENTLY. (SEE *"PRECAUTIONS"*.)

3. METHOTREXATE CAUSES HEPATOTOXICITY, FIBROSIS, AND CIRRHOSIS, BUT GENERALLY ONLY AFTER PROLONGED USE. ACUTELY, LIVER ENZYME ELEVATIONS ARE FREQUENTLY SEEN; THESE ARE USUALLY TRANSIENT AND ASYMPTOMATIC, AND ALSO DO NOT APPEAR PREDICTIVE OF SUBSEQUENT HEPATIC DISEASE. LIVER BIOPSY AFTER SUSTAINED USE OFTEN SHOWS HISTOLOGIC CHANGES, AND FIBROSIS AND CIRRHOSIS HAVE BEEN REPORTED; THESE LATTER LESIONS OFTEN ARE NOT PRECEDED BY SYMPTOMS OR ABNORMAL LIVER FUNCTION TESTS. (SEE *"PRECAUTIONS"*).

4. METHOTREXATE-INDUCED LUNG DISEASE IS A POTENTIALLY DANGEROUS LESION, WHICH MAY OCCUR ACUTELY AT ANY TIME DURING THERAPY AND WHICH HAS BEEN REPORTED AT DOSES AS LOW AS 7.5 MG/WEEK. IT IS NOT ALWAYS FULLY REVERSIBLE. PULMONARY SYMPTOMS (ESPECIALLY A DRY, NONPRODUCTIVE COUGH) MAY REQUIRE INTERRUPTION OF TREATMENT AND CAREFUL INVESTIGATION.

5. METHOTREXATE MAY PRODUCE MARKED BONE MARROW DEPRESSION, WITH RESULTANT ANEMIA, LEUKOPENIA, AND/OR THROMBOCYTOPENIA.

6. DIARRHEA AND ULCERATIVE STOMATITIS REQUIRE INTERRUPTION OF THERAPY; OTHERWISE, HEMORRHAGIC ENTERITIS AND DEATH FROM INTESTINAL PERFORATION MAY OCCUR.

7. METHOTREXATE THERAPY IN PATIENTS WITH IMPAIRED RENAL FUNCTION SHOULD BE UNDERTAKEN WITH EXTREME CAUTION, AND AT REDUCED DOSAGES, BECAUSE RENAL DYSFUNCTION WILL PROLONG METHOTREXATE ELIMINATION.

8. UNEXPECTEDLY SEVERE (SOMETIMES FATAL) MARROW SUPPRESSION AND GASTROINTESTINAL TOXICITY HAVE BEEN REPORTED WITH CONCOMITANT ADMINISTRATION OF METHOTREXATE (USUALLY IN HIGH DOSAGE) ALONG WITH SOME NONSTEROIDAL ANTI-INFLAMMATORY DRUGS (NSAIDS). (SEE *"PRECAUTIONS, DRUG INTERACTIONS"*.)

METHOTREXATE FORMULATIONS AND DILUENTS CONTAINING PRESERVATIVES MUST NOT BE USED FOR INTRATHECAL OR HIGH-DOSE METHOTREXATE THERAPY.

DESCRIPTION

Methotrexate is an antimetabolite used in the treatment of certain neoplastic diseases, severe psoriasis, and adult rheumatoid arthritis.

Chemically Methotrexate is N-[4-[[(2,4-diamino-6-pteridinyl)-methyl] methylamino]benzoyl]-L-glutamic acid. The molecular formula is $C_{26}H_{22}N_2O_5$ and the molecular weight 454.44.

It is available as tablets and injection. The liquid for injection may or may not contain a preservative. Each tablet contains Methotrexate Sodium equivalent to 2.5 mg Methotrexate. The liquid for injection contains Methotrexate Sodium equivalent to 20, 50, 100, 200, 250, or 1,000 mg Methotrexate.

Following is its chemical structure:

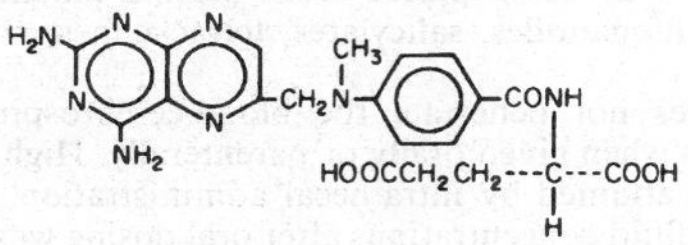

CLINICAL PHARMACOLOGY

Methotrexate inhibits dihydrofolic acid reductase. Dihydrofolates must be reduced to tetrahydrofolates by this enzyme before they can be utilized as carriers of one-carbon groups in the synthesis of purine nucleotides and thymidylate. Therefore, Methotrexate interferes with DNA synthesis, repair, and cellular replication. Actively proliferating tissues such as malignant cells, bone marrow, fetal cells, buccal and intestinal mucosa, and cells of the urinary bladder are in general more sensitive to this effect of Methotrexate. When cellular proliferation in malignant tissues is greater than in most normal tissues, Methotrexate may impair malignant growth without irreversible damage to normal tissues.

The mechanism of action in rheumatoid arthritis is unknown; it may affect immune function. Two reports describe *in vitro* Methotrexate inhibition of DNA precursor uptake by stimulated mononuclear cells, and another describes, in animal polyarthritis, partial correction by Methotrexate of spleen cell hyporesponsiveness and suppressed IL 2 production. Other laboratories, however, have been unable to demonstrate similar effects. Clarification of Methotrexate's effect on immune activity and its relation to rheumatoid immunopathogenesis await further studies.

In patients with rheumatoid arthritis, effects of Methotrexate on articular swelling and tenderness can be seen as early as 3 to 6 weeks. Although Methotrexate clearly ameliorates symptoms of inflammation (pain, swelling, stiffness), there is no evidence that it induces remission of rheumatoid arthritis nor has a beneficial effect been demonstrated on bone erosions and other radiologic changes which result in impaired joint use, functional disability, and deformity.

Most studies of Methotrexate in patients with rheumatoid arthritis are relatively short term (3 to 6 months). Limited data from long-term studies indicate that an initial clinical improvement is maintained for at least 2 years with continued therapy.

In psoriasis, the rate of production of epithelial cells in the skin is greatly increased over normal skin. This differential in proliferation rates is the basis for the use of Methotrexate to control the psoriatic process.

Methotrexate in high doses, followed by leucovorin rescue, is used as a part of the treatment of patients with nonmetastatic osteosarcoma. The original rationale for high-dose Methotrexate therapy was based on the concept of selective rescue of normal tissues by leucovorin. More recent evidence suggests that high-dose Methotrexate may also overcome Methotrexate resistance caused by impaired active transport, decreased affinity of dihydrofolic acid reductase for Methotrexate, increased levels of dihydrofolic acid reductase resulting from gene amplification, or decreased polyglutamation of Methotrexate. The actual mechanism of action is unknown.

Two Pediatric Oncology Group studies (one randomized and one nonrandomized) demonstrated a significant improvement in relapse-free survival in patients with nonmetastatic osteosarcoma, when high-dose Methotrexate with leucovorin rescue was used in combination with other chemotherapeutic agents following surgical resection of the primary tumor. These studies were not designed to demonstrate the specific contribution of high-dose Methotrexate/leucovorin rescue therapy to the efficacy of the combination. However, a contribution can be inferred from the reports of objective responses to this therapy in patients with metastatic osteosarcoma, and from reports of extensive tumor necrosis following preoperative administration of this therapy to patients with nonmetastatic osteosarcoma.

PHARMACOKINETICS

Absorption: In adults, oral absorption appears to be dose dependent. Peak serum levels are reached within 1 to 2 hours. At doses of 30 mg/m² or less, Methotrexate is generally well absorbed with a mean bioavailability of about 60%. The absorption of doses greater than 80 mg/m² is significantly less, possibly due to a saturation effect.

In leukemic children, oral absorption has been reported to vary widely (23% to 95%). A twenty-fold difference between highest and lowest peak levels (C_{max}: 0.11 to 2.3 micromolar after a 20 mg/m² dose) has been reported. Significant interindividual variability has also been noted in time to peak concentration (T_{max}: 0.67 to 4h after a 15 mg/m² dose) and fraction of dose absorbed. Food has been shown to delay absorption and reduce peak concentration.

Methotrexate is generally completely absorbed from parenteral routes of injection. After intramuscular injection, peak serum concentrations occur in 30 to 60 minutes.

Distribution: After intravenous administration, the initial volume of distribution is approximately 0.18 L/kg (18% of body weight) and steady-state volume of distribution is approximately 0.4 to 0.8 L/kg (40% to 80% of body weight). Methotrexate competes with reduced folates for active transport across cell membranes by means of a single carrier-mediated active transport process. At serum concentrations greater than 100 micromolar, passive diffusion becomes a major pathway by which effective intracellular concentrations can be achieved.

Methotrexate in serum is approximately 50% protein bound. Laboratory studies demonstrate that it may be displaced from plasma albumin by various compounds including sulfonamides, salicylates, tetracyclines, chloramphenicol, and phenytoin.

Methotrexate does not penetrate the blood-cerebrospinal fluid barrier in therapeutic amounts when given orally or parenterally. High CSF concentrations of the drug may be attained by intrathecal administration.

In dogs, synovial fluid concentrations after oral dosing were higher in inflamed than uninflamed joints. Although salicylates did not interfere with this penetration, prior prednisone treatment reduced penetration into inflamed joints to the level of normal joints.

Metabolism: After absorption, Methotrexate undergoes hepatic and intracellular metabolism to polyglutamated forms which can be converted back to Methotrexate by hydrolase enzymes. These polyglutamates act as inhibitors of dihydrofolate reductase and thymidylate synthetase. Small amounts of Methotrexate polyglutamates may remain in tissues for extended periods. The retention and prolonged drug action of these active metabolites vary among different cells, tissues, and tumors. A small amount of metabolism to 7-hydroxymethotrexate may occur at doses commonly prescribed. Accumulation of this metabolite may become significant at the high doses used in osteogenic sarcoma. The aqueous solubility of 7-hydroxymethotrexate is three- to fivefold lower than the parent compound. Methotrexate is partially metabolized by intestinal flora after oral administration.

Half-Life: The terminal half-life reported for Methotrexate is approximately 3 to 10 hours for patients receiving treatment for psoriasis, or rheumatoid arthritis or low-dose antineoplastic therapy (less than 30 mg/m^2). For patients receiving high doses of Methotrexate the terminal half-life is 8 to 15 hours.

Excretion: Renal excretion is the primary route of elimination and is dependent upon dosage and route of administration. With IV administration, 80% to 90% of the administered dose is excreted unchanged in the urine within 24 hours. There is limited biliary excretion amounting to 10% or less of the administered dose. Enterohepatic recirculation of Methotrexate has been proposed.

Renal excretion occurs by glomerular filtration and active tubular secretion. Nonlinear elimination due to saturation of renal tubular reabsorption has been observed in psoriatic patients at doses between 7.5 and 30 mg. Impaired renal function, as well as concurrent use of drugs such as weak organic acids that also undergo tubular secretion, can markedly increase Methotrexate serum levels. Excellent correlation has been reported between Methotrexate clearance and endogenous creatinine clearance.

Methotrexate clearance rates vary widely and are generally decreased at higher doses. Delayed drug clearance has been identified as one of the major factors responsible for Methotrexate toxicity. It has been postulated that the toxicity of Methotrexate for normal tissues is more dependent upon the duration of exposure to the drug rather than the peak level achieved. When a patient has delayed drug elimination due to compromised renal function, a third-space effusion, or other causes, Methotrexate serum concentrations may remain elevated for prolonged periods.

The potential for toxicity from high-dose regimens or delayed excretion is reduced by the administration of leucovorin calcium during the final phase of Methotrexate plasma elimination. Pharmacokinetic monitoring of Methotrexate serum concentrations may help identify those patients at high risk for Methotrexate toxicity and aid in proper adjustment of leucovorin dosing. Guidelines for monitoring serum Methotrexate levels, and for adjustment of leucovorin dosing to reduce the risk of Methotrexate toxicity, are provided below in *"Dosage and Administration".*

Methotrexate has been detected in human breast milk. The highest breast milk to plasma concentration ratio reached was 0.08:1.

INDICATIONS AND USAGE

Neoplastic Diseases: Methotrexate is indicated in the treatment of gestational choriocarcinoma, choriadenoma destruens, and hydatidiform mole.

In acute lymphocytic leukemia, Methotrexate is indicated in the prophylaxis of meningeal leukemia and is used in maintenance therapy in combination with other chemotherapeutic agents. Methotrexate is also indicated in the treatment of meningeal leukemia.

Methotrexate is used alone or in combination with other anticancer agents in the treatment of breast cancer, epidermoid cancers of the head and neck, advanced mycosis fungoides, and lung cancer, particularly squamous cell and small cell types. Methotrexate is also used in combination with other chemotherapeutic agents in the treatment of advanced stage non-Hodgkin's lymphomas.

Methotrexate in high doses followed by leucovorin rescue in combination with other chemotherapeutic agents is effective in prolonging relapse-free survival in patients with nonmetastatic osteosarcoma who have undergone surgical resection or amputation for the primary tumor.

Psoriasis: Methotrexate is indicated in the symptomatic control of severe, recalcitrant, disabling psoriasis that is not adequately responsive to other forms of therapy, *but only when the diagnosis has been established, as by biopsy and/or after dermatologic consultation.* It is important to ensure that a psoriasis "flare" is not due to an undiagnosed concomitant disease affecting immune responses.

Rheumatoid Arthritis: Methotrexate is indicated in the management of selected adults with severe, active, classical, or definite rheumatoid arthritis (ARA criteria) who have had an insufficient therapeutic response to, or are intolerant of, an adequate trial of first-line therapy including full dose NSAIDs and usually a trial of at least one or more disease-modifying antirheumatic drugs.

Aspirin, nonsteroidal anti-inflammatory agents, and/or low-dose steroids may be continued, although the possibility of increased toxicity with concomitant use of NSAIDs including salicylates has not been fully explored (see *"Precautions, Drug Interactions").* Steroids may be reduced gradually in patients who respond to Methotrexate. Combined use of Methotrexate with gold, penicillamine, hydroxychloroquine, sulfasalazine, or cytotoxic agents, has not been studied and may increase the incidence of adverse effects. Rest and physiotherapy as indicated should be continued.

UNLABELED USES
Methotrexate is used alone or as an adjunct in the treatment of steroid-dependent asthma, juvenile rheumatoid arthritis, osteogenic sarcoma, and advanced transitional cell carcinoma. It is also used in the treatment of unruptured ectopic pregnancy, Felty's syndrome, and in the prevention of graft-versus-host disease. Methotrexate is also prescribed in the treatment of refractory inflammatory bowel disease including Crohn's disease and chronic ulcerative colitis; childhood acute lymphocytic leukemia, Hodgkin's lymphoma, and as a topical treatment of mycosis fungoides. In addition, Methotrexate is also used in severe disabling pityriasis rubra pilaris, psoriatic arthritis, Reiter's syndrome, and Sézary syndrome.

CONTRAINDICATIONS

Methotrexate can cause fetal death or teratogenic effects when administered to a pregnant woman. Methotrexate is contraindicated in pregnant patients with psoriasis or rheumatoid arthritis and should be used in the treatment of neoplastic diseases only when the potential benefit outweighs the risk to the fetus. Women of childbearing potential should not be started on Methotrexate until pregnancy is excluded and should be fully counseled on the serious risk to the fetus (see *"Precautions")* should they become pregnant while undergoing treatment. Pregnancy should be avoided if either partner is receiving Methotrexate during and for a minimum of 3 months after therapy for male patients, and during and for at least one ovulatory cycle after therapy for female patients. (See boxed *"Warnings".)*

Because of the potential for serious adverse reactions from Metho- trexate in breast fed infants, it is contraindicated in nursing mothers.

Patients with psoriasis or rheumatoid arthritis with alcoholism, alcoholic liver disease, or other chronic liver disease should not receive Methotrexate.

Patients with psoriasis or rheumatoid arthritis who have overt or laboratory evidence of immunodeficiency syndromes should not receive Methotrexate.

Patients with psoriasis or rheumatoid arthritis who have preexisting blood dyscrasias, such as bone marrow hypoplasia, leukopenia, thrombocytopenia, or significant anemia, should not receive Methotrexate.

Patients with a known hypersensitivity to Methotrexate should not receive the drug.

WARNING
See boxed *"Warnings".*

PRECAUTIONS
General: Methotrexate has the potential for serious adverse reactions (see boxed *"Warnings").* Toxic effects may be related in frequency and severity to dose or frequency of administration but have been seen at all doses. Because they can occur at any time during therapy, it is necessary to follow patients on Methotrexate closely. Most adverse reactions are reversible if detected early. When such reactions do occur, the drug should be reduced in dosage or discontinued and appropriate corrective measures should be taken. If necessary, this could include the use of leucovorin calcium (see *"Overdosage").* If Methotrexate therapy is reinstituted, it should be carried out with caution, with adequate consideration of further need for the drug, and with increased alertness as to possible recurrence of toxicity.

The clinical pharmacology of Methotrexate has not been well studied in older individuals. Due to diminished hepatic and renal function as well as decreased folate stores in this population, relatively low doses should be considered, and these patients should be closely monitored for early signs of toxicity.

Information for Patients: Patients should be informed of the early signs and symptoms of toxicity, of the need to see their physician promptly if they occur, and the need for close follow-up, including periodic laboratory tests to monitor toxicity.

Both the physician and pharmacist should emphasize to the patient that the recommended dose is taken weekly in rheumatoid arthritis and psoriasis, and that mistaken daily use of the recommended dose has led to fatal toxicity. Prescriptions should not be written or refilled on a PRN basis.

Patients should be informed of the potential benefit and risk in the use of Methotrexate. The risk of effects on reproduction should be discussed with both male and female patients taking Methotrexate.

Laboratory Tests: Patients undergoing Methotrexate therapy should be closely monitored so that toxic effects are detected promptly. Baseline assessment should include a complete blood count with differential and platelet counts, hepatic enzymes, renal function tests, and a chest X-ray. During therapy of rheumatoid arthritis and psoriasis, monitoring of these parameters is recommended: hematology at least monthly, and liver and renal function every 1 to 3 months. More frequent monitoring is usually indicated during antineoplastic therapy. *During initial or changing doses,* or during periods of increased risk of elevated Methotrexate blood levels (eg, dehydration), more frequent monitoring may also be indicated.

A relationship between abnormal liver function tests and fibrosis or cirrhosis of the liver has not been established. Transient liver function test abnormalities are

---

◆ RATED THERAPEUTICALLY EQUIVALENT; ◇ THERAPEUTIC EQUIVALENCE UNCONFIRMED; ○ UNRATED

observed frequently after Methotrexate administration and are usually not cause for modification of Methotrexate therapy. Persistent liver function test abnormalities just prior to dosing and/or depression of serum albumin may be indicators of serious liver toxicity and require evaluation.

Pulmonary function tests may be useful if Methotrexate-induced lung disease is suspected, especially if baseline measurements are available.

Drug Interactions: Nonsteroidal anti-inflammatory drugs should not be administered prior to or concomitantly with the high doses of Methotrexate used in the treatment of osteosarcoma. Concomitant administration of some NSAIDs with high-dose Methotrexate therapy has been reported to elevate and prolong serum Methotrexate levels, resulting in deaths from severe hematologic and gastrointestinal toxicity.

Caution should be used when NSAIDs and salicylates are administered concomitantly with lower doses of Methotrexate. These drugs have been reported to reduce the tubular secretion of Methotrexate in an animal model and may enhance its toxicity.

Despite the potential interactions, studies of Methotrexate in patients with rheumatoid arthritis have usually included concurrent use of constant dosage regimens of NSAIDs, without apparent problems. It should be appreciated however, that the doses used in rheumatoid arthritis (7.5 to 15 mg/week) are somewhat lower than those used in psoriasis and that larger doses could lead to unexpected toxicity. Methotrexate is partially bound to serum albumin, and toxicity may be increased because of displacement by certain drugs, such as salicylates, phenylbutazone, phenytoin, and sulfonamides. Renal tubular transport is also diminished by probenecid; use of Methotrexate with this drug should be carefully monitored.

In the treatment of patients with osteosarcoma, caution must be exercised if high-dose Methotrexate is administered in combination with a potentially nephrotoxic chemotherapeutic agent (eg, cisplatin).

Oral antibiotics such as tetracycline, chloramphenicol, and nonabsorbable broad-spectrum antibiotics, may decrease intestinal absorption of Methotrexate or interfere with the enterohepatic circulation by inhibiting bowel flora and suppressing metabolism of the drug by bacteria.

Vitamin preparations containing folic acid or its derivatives may decrease responses to systemically administered Methotrexate. Preliminary animal and human studies have shown that small quantities of intravenously administered leucovorin enter the CSF primarily as 5-methyltetrahydrofolate and, in humans, remain 1 to 3 orders of magnitude lower than the usual Methotrexate concentrations following intrathecal administration. However, high doses of leucovorin may reduce the efficacy of intrathecally administered Methotrexate.

Folate deficiency states may increase Methotrexate toxicity. Trimethoprim/sulfamethoxazole has been reported rarely to increase bone marrow suppression in patients receiving Methotrexate probably by an additive antifolate effect.

Carcinogenesis, Mutagenesis, and Impairment of Fertility: No controlled human data exist regarding the risk of neoplasia with Methotrexate. Methotrexate has been evaluated in a number of animal studies for carcinogenic potential with inconclusive results. Although there is evidence that Methotrexate causes chromosomal damage to animal somatic cells and human bone marrow cells, the clinical significance remains uncertain. Assessment of the carcinogenic potential of Methotrexate is complicated by conflicting evidence of an increased risk of certain tumors in rheumatoid arthritis. Benefit should be weighed against this potential risk before using Methotrexate alone or in combination with other drugs, especially in children or young adults. Methotrexate causes embryotoxicity, abortion, and fetal defects in humans. It has also been reported to cause impairment of fertility, oligospermia, and menstrual dysfunction in humans, during and for a short period after cessation of therapy.

Pregnancy: Psoriasis and rheumatoid arthritis: Methotrexate is in Pregnancy Category X. See *"Contraindications"*.

Nursing Mothers: See *"Contraindications"*.

Pediatric Use: Safety and effectiveness in children have not been established, other than in cancer chemotherapy.

ORGAN SYSTEM TOXICITY
Gastrointestinal: If vomiting, diarrhea, or stomatitis occur, which may result in dehydration, Methotrexate should be discontinued until recovery occurs; Methotrexate should be used with extreme caution in the presence of peptic ulcer disease or ulcerative colitis.

Hematologic: Methotrexate can suppress hematopoiesis and cause anemia, leukopenia, and/or thrombocytopenia. In patients with malignancy and preexisting hematopoietic impairment, the drug should be used with caution, if at all. In controlled clinical trials in rheumatoid arthritis (n = 128), leukopenia (WBC < 3000/mm^3) was seen in two patients, thrombocytopenia (platelets < 100,000/mm^3) in six patients, and pancytopenia in two patients.

In psoriasis and rheumatoid arthritis Methotrexate should be stopped immediately if there is a significant drop in blood counts. In the treatment of neoplastic diseases, Methotrexate should be continued only if the potential benefit warrants the risk of severe myelosuppression. Patients with profound granulocytopenia and fever should be evaluated immediately and usually require parenteral broad-spectrum antibiotic therapy.

Hepatic: Methotrexate has the potential for acute (elevated transaminases) and chronic (fibrosis and cirrhosis) hepatotoxicity. Chronic toxicity is potentially fatal; it generally has occurred after prolonged use (generally 2 years or more) and after a total dose of at least 1.5 grams. In studies in psoriatic patients,

hepatotoxicity appeared to be a function of total cumulative dose and appeared to be enhanced by alcoholism, obesity, diabetes, and advanced age. An accurate incidence rate has not been determined; the rate of progression and reversibility of lesions is not known. Special caution is indicated in the presence of preexisting liver damage or impaired hepatic function.

Liver function tests, including serum albumin, should be performed periodically prior to dosing but are often normal in the face of developing fibrosis or cirrhosis. These lesions may be detectable only by biopsy.

In psoriasis, the usual recommendation is to obtain a liver biopsy at a total cumulative dose of 1.5 grams. Moderate fibrosis or any cirrhosis normally leads to discontinuation of the drug: mild fibrosis normally suggests a repeat biopsy in 6 months. Milder histologic findings, such as fatty change and low grade portal inflammation, are relatively common pretherapy. Although these mild changes are usually not a reason to avoid or discontinue Methotrexate therapy, the drug should be used with caution.

Clinical experience with liver disease in rheumatoid arthritis is limited, but the same risk factors would be anticipated. Liver function tests are also usually not reliable predictors of histological changes in this population.

When to perform a liver biopsy in rheumatoid arthritis patients has not been established, either in terms of cumulative Methotrexate dose or duration of therapy. There is a combined reported experience in 217 rheumatoid arthritis patients with liver biopsies both before and during treatment (after a cumulative dose of at least 1500 mg) and in 714 patients with a biopsy only during treatment. There are 64 (7%) cases of fibrosis and 1 (0.1%) case of cirrhosis. Of the 64 cases of fibrosis, 60 were deemed mild. The reticulin stain is more sensitive for early fibrosis and its use may increase these figures. It is unknown whether even longer use will increase these risks.

Infection or Immunologic States: Methotrexate should be used with extreme caution in the presence of active infection, and is usually contraindicated in patients with overt or laboratory evidence of immunodeficiency syndromes. Immunization may be ineffective when given during Methotrexate therapy. Immunization with live virus vaccines is generally not recommended. There have been reports of disseminated vaccinia infections after smallpox immunization in patients receiving Methotrexate therapy. Hypogammaglobulinemia has been reported rarely.

Neurologic: There have been reports of leukoencephalopathy following intravenous administration of Methotrexate to patients who have had craniospinal irradiation. Chronic leukoencephalopathy has also been reported in patients with osteosarcoma who received repeated doses of high-dose Methotrexate with leucovorin rescue even without cranial irradiation. Discontinuation of Methotrexate does not always result in complete recovery.

A transient acute neurologic syndrome has been observed in patients treated with high-dosage regimens. Manifestations of this neurologic disorder may include behavioral abnormalities, focal sensorimotor signs, and abnormal reflexes. The exact cause is unknown.

After the intrathecal use of Methotrexate the central nervous system toxicity which may occur can be classified as follows: chemical arachnoiditis manifested by such symptoms as headache, back pain, nuchal rigidity, and fever; paresis, usually transient, manifested by paraplegia associated with involvement with one or more spinal nerve roots; leukoencephalopathy manifested by confusion, irritability, somnolence, ataxia, dementia, and occasionally major convulsions.

Pulmonary: Pulmonary symptoms (especially a dry, nonproductive cough) or a nonspecific pneumonitis occurring during Methotrexate therapy may be indicative of a potentially dangerous lesion and require interruption of treatment and careful investigation. Although clinically variable, the typical patient with Methotrexate-induced lung disease presents with fever, cough, dyspnea, hypoxemia, and an infiltrate on chest x-ray; infection needs to be excluded. This lesion can occur at all dosages.

Renal: High doses of Methotrexate used in the treatment of osteosarcoma may cause renal damage leading to acute renal failure. Nephrotoxicity is due primarily to the precipitation of Methotrexate and 7-hydroxymethotrexate in the renal tubules. Close attention to renal function including adequate hydration, urine alkalinization and measurement of serum Methotrexate and creatinine levels are essential for safe administration.

Other Precautions: Methotrexate should be used with extreme caution in the presence of debility.

Methotrexate exits slowly from third-space compartments (eg, pleural effusions or ascites). This results in a prolonged terminal plasma half-life and unexpected toxicity. In patients with significant third-space accumulations, it is advisable to evacuate the fluid before treatment and to monitor plasma Methotrexate levels.

Lesions of psoriasis may be aggravated by concomitant exposure to ultraviolet radiation. Radiation dermatitis and sunburn may be "recalled" by the use of Methotrexate.

ADVERSE REACTIONS
In general, the incidence and severity of acute side effects are related to dose and frequency of administration. The most serious reactions are discussed above under "organ system toxicity" in the "Precautions" section. That section should also be consulted when looking for information about adverse reactions with Methotrexate.

The most frequently reported adverse reactions include ulcerative stomatitis, leukopenia, nausea, and abdominal distress. Other frequently reported adverse effects are malaise, undue fatigue, chills and fever, dizziness, and decreased resistance to infection.

Other adverse reactions that have been reported with Methotrexate are listed below by organ system. In the oncology setting, concomitant treatment and the underlying disease make specific attribution of a reaction of Methotrexate difficult.

Alimentary System: Gingivitis, pharyngitis, stomatitis, anorexia, nausea, vomiting, diarrhea, hematemesis, melena, gastrointestinal ulceration and bleeding, enteritis.

Central Nervous System: Headaches, drowsiness, blurred vision. Aphasia, hemiparesis, paresis, and convulsions have also occurred following administration of Methotrexate. **Following low doses, occasional patients have reported transient subtle cognitive dysfunction, mood alteration, or unusual cranial sensations.**

Pulmonary System: Interstitial pneumonitis deaths have been reported, and chronic interstitial obstructive pulmonary disease has occasionally occurred.

Skin: Erythematous rashes, pruritus, urticaria, photosensitivity, pigmentary changes, alopecia, ecchymosis, telangiectasia, acne, furunculosis.

Urogenital System: Severe nephropathy or renal failure, azotemia, cystitis, hematuria; defective oogenesis or spermatogenesis, transient oligospermia, menstrual dysfunction and vaginal discharge; infertility, abortion, fetal defects.

Other rarer reactions related to or attributed to the use of Methotrexate such as opportunistic infection, arthralgia/myalgia, loss of libido/impotence, diabetes, osteoporosis, and sudden death. A few cases of anaphylactoid reactions have been reported.

Adverse Reactions in Double-Blind Rheumatoid Arthritis Studies: The approximate incidences of Methotrexate attributed (ie, placebo rate subtracted) adverse reactions in 12- to 18-week double-blind studies of patients (n = 128) with rheumatoid arthritis treated with low-dose oral (7.5 to 15 mg/week) pulse Methotrexate are listed below. Virtually all of these patients were on concomitant nonsteroidal anti-inflammatory drugs and some were also taking low dosages of corticosteroids.

Incidence greater than 10%: Elevated liver function tests 15%, nausea/vomiting 10%.

Incidence 3% to 10%: Stomatitis, thrombocytopenia (platelet count less than 100,000/mm^3).

Incidence 1% to 3%: Rash/pruritus/dermatitis, diarrhea, alopecia, leukopenia (WBC < 3000/mm^3), pancytopenia, dizziness.

No pulmonary toxicity was seen in these two trials. Thus, the incidence is probably less than 2.5% (95% C.L.). Hepatic histology was not examined in these short-term studies (see *"Precautions"*).

Other less common reactions included decreased hematocrit, headache, upper respiratory infection, anorexia, arthralgias, chest pain, coughing, dysuria, eye discomfort, epistaxis, fever, infection, sweating, tinnitus, and vaginal discharge.

Adverse Reactions in Psoriasis: There are no recent placebo-controlled trials in patients with psoriasis. There are two literature reports (Roenigk, 1969 and Nyfors, 1978) describing large series (n = 204, 248) of psoriasis patients treated with Methotrexate. Dosages ranged up to 25 mg per week, and treatment was administered for up to 4 years. With the exception of alopecia, photosensitivity, and "burning of skin lesions" (each 3% to 10%), the adverse reaction rates in these reports were very similar to those in the rheumatoid arthritis studies.

OVERDOSAGE

Leucovorin is indicated to diminish the toxicity and counteract the effect of inadvertently administered overdosages of Methotrexate. Leucovorin administration should begin as promptly as possible. As the time interval between Methotrexate administration and leucovorin initiation increases, the effectiveness of leucovorin in counteracting toxicity decreases. Monitoring of the serum Methotrexate concentration is essential in determining the optimal dose and duration of treatment with leucovorin.

In cases of massive overdosage, hydration and urinary alkalinization may be necessary to prevent the precipitation of Methotrexate and/or its metabolites in the renal tubules. Neither hemodialysis nor peritoneal dialysis has been shown to improve Methotrexate elimination.

DOSAGE AND ADMINISTRATION

NEOPLASTIC DISEASES

Oral administration in tablet form is often preferred when low doses are being administered since absorption is rapid and effective serum levels are obtained. Methotrexate sodium injection and for injection may be given by the intramuscular, intravenous, intra-arterial, or intrathecal route. However, the preserved formulation contains Benzyl Alcohol and must not be used for intrathecal or high-dose therapy. Parenteral drug products should be inspected visually for particulate matter and discoloration prior to administration, whenever solution and container permit.

Choriocarcinoma and Similar Trophoblastic Disease: Methotrexate is administered orally or intramuscularly in doses of 15 to 30 mg daily for a 5-day course. Such courses are usually repeated for three to five times as required, with rest periods of 1 or more weeks interposed between courses, until any manifesting toxic symptoms subside. The effectiveness of therapy is ordinarily evaluated by 24-hour quantitative analysis of urinary chorionic gonadotropin (hCG), which should return to normal or less than 50 IU/24h usually after the third or fourth course and usually be followed by a complete resolution of measurable lesions in 4 to 6 weeks. One to two courses of Methotrexate after normalization of hCG is usually recommended. Before each course of the drug careful clinical assessment

is essential. Cyclic combination therapy of Methotrexate with other antitumor drugs has been reported as being useful.

Since hydatidiform mole may precede choriocarcinoma, prophylactic chemotherapy with Methotrexate has been recommended.

Chorioadenoma destruens is considered to be an invasive form of hydatidiform mole. Methotrexate is administered in these disease states in doses similar to those recommended for choriocarcinoma.

Leukemia: Acute lymphoblastic leukemia in children and young adolescents is the most responsive to present-day chemotherapy. In young adults and older patients, clinical remission is more difficult to obtain and early relapse is more common.

Methotrexate alone or in combination with steroids was used initially for induction of remission in acute lymphoblastic leukemias. More recently corticosteroid therapy, in combination with other antileukemic drugs or in cyclic combinations with Methotrexate included, has appeared to produce rapid and effective remissions. When used for induction, Methotrexate in doses of 3.3 mg/m^2 in combination with 60 mg/m^2 of prednisone, given daily, produced remissions in 50% of patients treated, usually within a period of 4 to 6 weeks. Methotrexate in combination with other agents appears to be the drug of choice for securing maintenance of drug-induced remissions. When remission is achieved and supportive care has produced general clinical improvement, maintenance therapy is initiated, as follows: Methotrexate is administered two times weekly either by mouth or intramuscularly in total weekly doses of 30 mg/m^2. It has also been given in doses of 2.5 mg/kg intravenously every 14 days. If and when relapse does occur, reinduction of remission can again usually be obtained by repeating the initial induction regimen.

A variety of combination chemotherapy regimens have been used for both induction and maintenance therapy in acute lymphoblastic leukemia. The physician should be familiar with the new advances in antileukemic therapy.

Meningeal Leukemia: In the treatment or prophylaxis of meningeal leukemia, Methotrexate must be administered intrathecally. Preservative-free Methotrexate is diluted to a concentration of 1 mg/ml in an appropriate sterile, preservative-free medium such as 0.9% Sodium Chloride Injection, USP.

The cerebrospinal fluid volume is dependent on age and not on body surface area. The CSF is at 40% of the adult volume at birth and reaches the adult volume in several years.

Intrathecal Methotrexate administration at a dose of 12 mg/m^2 (maximum 15 mg) has been reported to result in low CSF Methotrexate concentrations and reduced efficacy in children and high concentrations and neurotoxicity in adults. The following dosage regimen is based on age instead of body surface area:

Age (years)	Dose (mg)
< 1	6
1	8
2	10
3 or older	12

In one study in patients under the age of 40, this dosage regimen appeared to result in more consistent CSF Methotrexate concentrations and less neurotoxicity. Another study in children with acute lymphocytic leukemia compared this regimen to a dose of 12 mg/m^2 (maximum 15 mg). A significant reduction in the rate of CNS relapse was observed in the group whose dose was based on age.

Because the CSF volume and turnover may decrease with age, a dose reduction may be indicated in elderly patients. For the treatment of meningeal leukemia, intrathecal Methotrexate may be given at intervals of 2 to 5 days. However, administration at intervals of less than 1 week may result in increased subacute toxicity. Methotrexate is administered until the cell count of the cerebrospinal fluid returns to normal. At this point one additional dose is advisable. For prophylaxis against meningeal leukemia, the dosage is the same as for treatment except for the intervals of administration. On this subject, it is advisable for the physician to consult the medical literature.

Untoward side effects may occur with any given intrathecal injection and are commonly neurological in character. Large doses may cause convulsions. Methotrexate given by the intrathecal route appears significantly in the systemic circulation and may cause systemic Methotrexate toxicity. Therefore, systemic antileukemic therapy with the drug should be appropriately adjusted, reduced, or discontinued. Focal leukemic involvement of the CNS may not respond to intrathecal chemotherapy and is best treated with radiotherapy.

Lymphomas: In Burkitt's tumor, Stages I to II, Methotrexate has produced prolonged remissions in some cases. Recommended dosage is 10 to 25 mg/day orally for 4 to 8 days. In Stage III, Methotrexate is commonly given concomitantly with other antitumor agents. Treatment in all stages usually consists of several courses of the drug interposed with 7- to 10-day rest periods. Lymphosarcomas in Stage III may respond to combined drug therapy with Methotrexate given in doses of 0.625 to 2.5 mg/kg daily.

Mycosis Fungoides: Therapy with Methotrexate appears to produce clinical remissions in one half of the cases treated. Dosage is usually 2.5 to 10 mg daily by mouth for weeks or months. Dose levels of drug and adjustment of dose regimen by reduction or cessation of drug are guided by patient response and hematologic monitoring. Methotrexate has also been given intramuscularly in doses of 50 mg once weekly or 25 mg two times weekly.

Osteosarcoma: An effective adjuvant chemotherapy regimen requires the administration of several cytotoxic chemotherapeutic agents. In addition to high-dose Methotrexate with leucovorin rescue, these agents may include doxorubicin,

---

◆ RATED THERAPEUTICALLY EQUIVALENT; ◇ THERAPEUTIC EQUIVALENCE UNCONFIRMED; ○ UNRATED

cisplatin, and the combination of bleomycin, cyclophosphamide and dactinomycin (BCD) in the doses and schedule shown in the table below. The starting dose for high-dose Methotrexate treatment is 12 grams/m². If this dose is not sufficient to produce a peak serum Methotrexate concentration of 1,000 micromolar (10^{-3} mol/L) at the end of the Methotrexate infusion, the dose may be escalated to 15 grams/m² in subsequent treatments. If the patient is vomiting or is unable to tolerate oral medication, leucovorin is given IV or IM at the same dose and schedule. (See related table).

When these higher doses of Methotrexate are to be administered, the following safety guidelines should be closely observed.

GUIDELINES FOR METHOTREXATE THERAPY WITH LEUCOVORIN RESCUE

1. Administration of Methotrexate should be delayed until recovery if:
- the WBC count is < 1500/microliter
- the neutrophil count is < 200/microliter
- the platelet count is < 75,000/microliter
- the serum bilirubin level is > 1.2 mg/dL
- the SGPT level is > 450 U
- mucositis is present, until there is evidence of healing
- persistent pleural effusion is present; this should be drained dry prior to infusion.

2. Adequate renal function must be documented.

a. Serum creatinine must be normal, and creatinine clearance must be greater than 60 mL/min, before initiation of therapy.

b. Serum creatinine must be measured prior to each subsequent course of therapy. If serum creatinine has increased by 50% or more compared to a prior value, the creatinine clearance must be measured and documented to be greater than 60 mL/min (even if the serum creatinine is still within the normal range).

3. Patients must be well hydrated, and must be treated with sodium bicarbonate for urinary alkalinization.

a. Administer 1,000 ml/m² of intravenous fluid over 6 hours prior to initiation of the Methotrexate infusion. Continue hydration at 125 ml/m²/hr (3 liters/m²/day) during the Methotrexate infusion, and for 2 days after the infusion has been completed.

b. Alkalinize urine to maintain pH above 7.0 during Methotrexate infusion and leucovorin calcium therapy. This can be accomplished by the administration of sodium bicarbonate orally or by incorporation into a separate intravenous solution.

4. Repeat serum creatinine and serum Methotrexate 24 hours after starting Methotrexate and at least once daily until the Methotrexate level is below 5 × 10^{-8} mol/L (0.05 micromolar).

5. The table below provides guidelines for leucovorin calcium dosage based upon serum Methotrexate levels. (See table below.‡)

‡ LEUCOVORIN RESCUE SCHEDULES FOLLOWING TREATMENT WITH HIGHER DOSES OF METHOTREXATE

Clinical Situation	Laboratory Findings	Leucovorin Dosage and Duration
Normal Methotrexate Elimination	Serum Methotrexate level approximately 10 micromolar at 24 hours after administration, 1 micromolar at 48 hours, and less than 0.2 micromolar at 72 hours.	15 mg PO, IM, or IV q6h for 60 hours (10 doses starting at 24 hours after start of Methotrexate infusion).
Delayed Late Methotrexate Elimination	Serum Methotrexate level remaining above 0.2 micromolar at 72 hours, and more than 0.05 micromolar at 96 hours after administration.	Continue 15 mg PO, IM, or IV q6h, until Methotrexate level is less than 0.05 micromolar.
Delayed Early Methotrexate Elimination and/or	Serum Methotrexate level of 50 micromolar or more at 24 hours, or	150 mg IV q3h, until Methotrexate level is less than 1 micromolar;

Clinical Situation	Laboratory Findings	Leucovorin Dosage and Duration
Evidence of Acute Renal Injury	5 micromolar or more at 48 hours after administration, OR; a 100% or greater increase in serum creatinine level at 24 hours after Methotrexate administration (eg, an increase from 0.5 mg/dL to a level of 1.0 mg/dL or more).	then 15 mg IV q3h, until Methotrexate level is less than 0.05 micromolar.

Patients who experience delayed early Methotrexate elimination are likely to develop nonreversible oliguric renal failure. In addition to appropriate leucovorin therapy, these patients require continuing hydration and urinary alkalinization, and close monitoring of fluid and electrolyte status, until the serum Methotrexate level has fallen to below 0.05 micromolar and the renal failure has resolved.

6. Some patients will have abnormalities in Methotrexate elimination, or abnormalities in renal function following Methotrexate administration, which are significant but less severe than the abnormalities described in the table below. These abnormalities may or may not be associated with significant clinical toxicity. If significant clinical toxicity is observed, leucovorin rescue should be extended for an additional 24 hours (total 14 doses over 84 hours) in subsequent courses of therapy. The possibility that the patient is taking other medications which interact with Methotrexate (e.g., medications which may interfere with Methotrexate binding to serum albumin, or elimination) should always be reconsidered when laboratory abnormalities or clinical toxicities are observed.

PSORIASIS AND RHEUMATOID ARTHRITIS

The patient should be fully informed of the risks involved and should be under constant supervision of the physician. (See "Information for Patients" and "Precautions".) Assessment of hematologic, hepatic, renal, and pulmonary function should be made by history, physical examination, and laboratory tests before beginning, periodically during, and before reinstituting Methotrexate therapy (see "Precautions"). Appropriate steps should be taken to avoid conception during Methotrexate therapy. (See "Precautions" and "Contraindications".)

Weekly therapy may be instituted with the Methotrexate doses over a range of 5 mg to 15 mg administered as a single weekly dose. All schedules should be continually tailored to the individual patient. An initial test dose may be given prior to the regular dosing schedule to detect any extreme sensitivity to adverse effects (see "Adverse Reactions"). Maximal myelosuppression usually occurs in 7 to 10 days.

Psoriasis: Recommended Starting Dose Schedules

1. Weekly single oral, IM, or IV dose schedule: 10 to 25 mg per week until adequate response is achieved.

2. Divided oral dose schedule: 2.5 mg at 12-hour intervals for three doses.

Dosages in each schedule may be gradually adjusted to achieve optimal clinical response; 30 mg/week should not ordinarily be exceeded.

Once optimal clinical response has been achieved, each dosage schedule should be reduced to the lowest possible amount of drug and to the longest possible rest period. The use of Methotrexate may permit the return to conventional topical therapy, which should be encouraged.

Rheumatoid Arthritis: Recommended Starting Dosage Schedules

1. Single oral doses of 7.5 mg once weekly.

2. Divided oral dosages of 2.5 mg at 12-hour intervals for three doses given as a course once weekly.

Dosages in each schedule may be adjusted gradually to achieve an optimal response, but not ordinarily to exceed a total weekly dose of 20 mg. Limited experience shows a significant increase in the incidence and severity of serious toxic reactions, especially bone marrow suppression, at doses greater than 20 mg/wk.

Once response has been achieved, each schedule should be reduced, if possible, to the lowest possible effective dose.

Drug*	Dose*	Treatment Week After Surgery
Methotrexate	12 g/m² IV as 4 hour infusion (starting dose)	4, 5, 6, 7, 11, 12, 15, 16, 29, 30, 44, 45
Leucovorin	15 mg orally every 6 hours for 10 doses starting at 24 hours after start of Methotrexate infusion	
Doxorubicin† as a single drug	30 mg/m²/day IV × 3 days	8, 17
Doxorubicin†	50 mg/m² IV	20, 23, 33, 36
Cisplatin†	100 mg/m² IV	20, 23, 33, 36
Bleomycin†	15 units/m² IV × 2 days	2, 13, 26, 39, 42
Cyclophosphamide†	600 mg/m² IV × 2 days	2, 13, 26, 39, 42
Dactinomycin†	0.6 mg/m² IV × 2 days	2, 13, 26, 39, 42

* Link MP, Goorin AM, Miser AW, et al: The effect of adjuvant chemotherapy on relapse-free survival in patients with osteosarcoma of the extremity. N Engl J Med 1986; 314(no. 25):1600–1606.
† See each respective package insert for full prescribing information. Dosage modification may be necessary because of drug-induced toxicity.

Therapeutic response usually begins within 3 to 6 weeks and the patient may continue to improve for another 12 weeks or more.

The optimal duration of therapy is unknown. Limited data available from long-term studies indicate that the initial clinical improvement is maintained for at least 2 years with continued therapy. When Methotrexate is discontinued, the arthritis usually worsens within 3 to 6 weeks.

HANDLING AND DISPOSAL
Procedures for proper handling and disposal of anticancer drugs should be considered. Several guidelines on this subject have been pub- lished.[1-6] There is no general agreement that all of the procedures recommended in the guidelines are necessary or appropriate.

RECONSTITUTION OF LOW SODIUM CRYODESICCATED POWDERS
Reconstitute immediately prior to use.

Methotrexate Sodium for Injection should be reconstituted with an appropriate sterile, preservative-free medium such as 5% dextrose solution, USP, or sodium chloride injection USP. Reconstitute the 20 mg and 50 mg vials to a concentration no greater than 25 mg/ml. *The 1 gm vial should be reconstituted with 19.4 ml to a concentration of 50 mg/mL.* When high doses of Methotrexate are administered by IV infusion, the total dose is diluted in 5% dextrose solution. For intrathecal injection, reconstitute to a concentration of 1 mg/ml with an appropriate sterile, preservative-free medium such as sodium chloride injection, USP.

DILUTION INSTRUCTIONS FOR LIQUID METHOTREXATE SODIUM INJECTION PRODUCTS
Methotrexate Sodium Injection, Preservative Protected: If desired, the solution may be further diluted with a compatible medium such as sodium chloride injection. Storage for 24 hours at a temperature of 21° to 25° C results in a product which is within 90% of label potency.

Methotrexate Sodium Injection, Isotonic, Preservative Free, for Single Use Only: If desired, the solution may be further diluted immediately prior to use with an appropriate sterile, preservative-free medium such as 5% dextrose solution. USP or sodium chloride injection, USP.

STORAGE
Parenteral: Storage between 15° C (59° F) and 25° C (77° F) is recommended.

Oral: Store at controlled room temperature 15°-30° C (59°-86° F). Protect from light.

REFERENCES
1. Recommendations for the Safe Handling of Parenteral Antineoplastic Drugs. NIH Publication No. 83-2621. For sale by the Superintendent of Documents, U.S. Government Printing Office, Washington, D.C. 20402. 2. AMA Council Report. Guidelines for Handling Parenteral Antineoplastics. *JAMA*, March 15, 1985. 3. National Study Commission on Cytotoxic Exposure-Recommendations for Handling Cytotoxic Agents. Available from Louis P. Jeffrey, ScD, Director of Pharmacy Services, Rhode Island Hospital, 593 Eddy Street, Providence, Rhode Island 02902. 4. Clinical Oncological Society of Australia: Guidelines and recommendations for safe handling of antineoplastic agents. *Med J Australia* 1983;1;426-428. 5. Jones RB, et al. Safe handling of chemotherapeutic agents: A report from the Mount Sinai Medical Center, *CA:A Cancer Journal for Clinicians* Sept/Oct, 1983: 258-263. 6. American Society of Hospital Pharmacists. Technical assistance bulletin on handling cytotoxic drugs in hospitals. *Am J Hosp Pharm* 1985;42:131-137.

J CODES
50 mg IV,IM,IT,IA—J9260
5 mg IV,IM,IT,IA—J9250

HOW SUPPLIED
INJECTION: 25 MG/ML

AVERAGE UNIT PRICE (AVAILABLE SIZES)		GENERIC A-RATED AVERAGE PRICE (GAAP)	
BRAND	$7.39	2 ml	$4.75
GENERIC	$2.28	10 ml	$20.48

BRAND/MANUFACTURER	NDC	SIZE	AWP
◆ **BRAND**			
FOLEX PFS: Pharmacia	00013-2266-91	2 ml	$15.20
	00013-2276-91	4 ml	$30.18
	00013-2286-91	8 ml	$59.10
	00013-2296-91	10 ml	$70.19
◆ **GENERICS**			
Immunex	00205-4556-26	2 ml	$4.75
Immunex	00205-5325-26	2 ml	$4.75
Immunex	00205-5326-18	4 ml	$8.50
Immunex	00205-5327-30	8 ml	$16.73
Immunex	00205-5338-34	10 ml	$20.48
Immunex	00205-5337-34	10 ml	$20.48
Chiron Therapeutics	53905-0031-10	2 ml 10s	$68.75
Chiron Therapeutics	53905-0032-10	4 ml 10s	$87.50
Chiron Therapeutics	53905-0033-10	8 ml 10s	$175.00
Chiron Therapeutics	53905-0034-10	10 ml 10s	$268.75
Immunex	00205-5337-98	10 ml 25s	$364.79

POWDER FOR INJECTION: 20 MG

BRAND/MANUFACTURER	NDC	SIZE	AWP
◆ **GENERICS**			
Immunex	00205-4654-90	1s	$2.78

POWDER FOR INJECTION: 50 MG

BRAND/MANUFACTURER	NDC	SIZE	AWP
◆ **GENERICS**			
Immunex	00205-9337-92	1s	$4.75

TABLET: 2.5 MG

AVERAGE UNIT PRICE (AVAILABLE SIZES)		GENERIC A-RATED AVERAGE PRICE (GAAP)	
GENERIC	$3.06	8s	$24.41
HCFA FUL (100s)	$2.99	12s	$36.41
		16s	$49.65
		20s	$61.29
		24s	$73.87
		36s	$114.01
		100s	$299.88

BRAND/MANUFACTURER	NDC	SIZE	AWP
◆ **GENERICS**			
Roxane	00054-8550-03	8s	$23.00
RHEUMATREX DOSE PACK: Lederle Labs	00005-4507-04	8s	$26.43
Barr	00555-0572-45	8s ud	$23.79
Roxane	00054-8550-05	12s	$35.00
RHEUMATREX DOSE PACK: Lederle Labs	00005-4507-05	12s	$39.59
UDL	51079-0670-86	12s ud	$35.43
Barr	00555-0572-46	12s ud	$35.63
Roxane	00054-8550-06	16s	$49.00
RHEUMATREX DOSE PACK: Lederle Labs	00005-4507-07	16s	$52.81
UDL	51079-0670-87	16s ud	$47.26
Barr	00555-0572-47	16s ud	$49.53
Roxane	00054-8550-07	20s	$61.00
RHEUMATREX DOSE PACK: Lederle Labs	00005-4507-09	20s	$66.04
UDL	51079-0670-05	20s ud	$58.85
UDL	51079-0670-88	20s ud	$59.11
Barr	00555-0572-48	20s ud	$61.44
Roxane	00054-8550-10	24s	$72.00
RHEUMATREX DOSE PACK: Lederle Labs	00005-4507-91	24s	$79.24
UDL	51079-0670-89	24s ud	$70.92
Barr	00555-0572-49	24s ud	$73.32
Barr	00555-0572-35	36s	$91.56
Aligen	00405-4643-36	36s	$91.56
Geneva	00781-1076-36	36s	$103.11
Major	00904-1749-73	36s	$106.45
Roxane	00054-4550-15	36s	$133.88
Rugby	00536-3998-36	36s	$157.50
Barr	00555-0572-02	100s	$269.45
Aligen	00405-4643-01	100s	$269.45
Qualitest	00603-4499-21	100s	$269.45
Schein	00364-2499-01	100s	$285.00
Geneva	00781-1076-01	100s	$285.00
Major	00904-1749-60	100s	$299.95
Rugby	00536-3998-01	100s	$299.99
Roxane	00054-4550-25	100s	$305.16
Mylan	00378-0014-01	100s	$314.34
Goldline	00182-1539-01	100s	$314.34
Lederle Labs	00005-4507-23	100s	$381.21
Roxane	00054-8550-25	100s ud	$305.16

Methotrimeprazine

Caution: Following administration of this drug, orthostatic hypotension, fainting, or dizziness may occur. Ambulation should be avoided or carefully supervised for at least 6 hours following the initial dose. Tolerance to this effect usually develops with continued administration.

DESCRIPTION
Methotrimeprazine is 10*H*-phenothiazine-10-propanamine, 2-methoxy-*N,N*,β-tri-methyl-, (-)-. It was formerly called levomepromazine. The empirical formula is $C_{19}H_{24}N_2OS$.

It is available as a clear transparent solution of the hydrochloride salt containing 20 mg of Methotrimeprazine per mL.

Following is its chemical structure:

ACTIONS

Methotrimeprazine, a phenothiazine derivative, is a potent central nervous system depressant with sites of action postulated in the thalamus, hypothalamus, reticular and limbic systems, producing suppression of sensory impulses, reduction of motor activity, sedation and tranquilization. It raises the pain threshold and produces amnesia. Methotrimeprazine also has antihistamine, anticholinergic, and antiadrenalin effects. It is actively metabolized into sulfoxides and glucuronic conjugates and largely excreted into the urine as such. Small amounts of unchanged drug are excreted in the feces and in the urine (1%). Low concentrations of drug occur in the blood serum in man. Elimination into the urine usually continues for several days after intramuscular administration of the drug is discontinued.

Methotrimeprazine produces an analgesic effect in both animals and man comparable to morphine and meperidine. A sedative effect is produced as well. Its use thus far has not been reported to result in signs of addiction, dependence or withdrawal symptoms even with large doses or with prolonged administration. Maximum analgesic effect usually occurs within 20 to 40 minutes after intramuscular injection and is maintained for about 4 hours.

Respiratory depression in the patient or in the newborn during or following preanesthetic or obstetrical use occurs infrequently with Methotrimeprazine. The drug does not appear to affect the cough reflex.

INDICATIONS

Methotrimeprazine is indicated for the relief of pain of moderate to marked degree of severity in nonambulatory patients.

It is indicated for obstetrical analgesia and sedation where respiratory depression is to be avoided.

Methotrimeprazine is indicated as a preanesthetic medication for producing sedation, somnolence, and relief of apprehension and anxiety.

CONTRAINDICATIONS

Methotrimeprazine should not be used:

1. Concurrently with antihypertensive drugs including monoamine oxidase inhibitors.
2. In patients with a history of phenothiazine hypersensitivity.
3. In the presence of overdosage of CNS depressants or comatose states.
4. In the presence of severe myocardial, renal or hepatic disease.
5. In the presence of clinically significant hypotension.
6. In patients under 12 years of age, since safe and effective use has not been established in children under this age.

WARNINGS

Methotrimeprazine should be used with caution in women of child-bearing potential and during early pregnancy since its safety for the developing embryo has not been clearly established. A possible antifertility effect has been suggested in that successive generations of animals dosed with this drug have shown a diminution of litter size over the controls. There is no evidence of adverse developmental effect when administered during late pregnancy and labor.

Methotrimeprazine, as with other phenothiazine derivatives, has been found to depress spermatogenesis in experimental animals in doses greatly exceeding the recommended human dose.

Methotrimeprazine exerts additive effects with central nervous system depressant drugs including narcotics, barbiturates, general anesthetics, and certain drugs such as acetylsalicylic acid, meprobamate, and reserpine. Consequently, the dosage of Methotrimeprazine and of each such drug should be reduced and critically adjusted when used concomitantly or when sequence of use results in overlapping of drug effects.

Some brands contain sodium metabisulfite, a sulfite that may cause allergic-type reactions including anaphylactic symptoms and life-threatening or less severe asthmatic episodes in certain susceptible people. The overall prevalence of sulfite sensitivity in the general population is unknown and probably low. Sulfite sensitivity is seen more frequently in asthmatic than in nonasthmatic people.

PRECAUTIONS

Methotrimeprazine should be used with caution when given concomitantly with atropine, scopolamine, and succinylcholine in that tachycardia and fall in blood pressure may occur, and undesirable central nervous system effects such as stimulation, delirium, and extrapyramidal symptoms may be aggravated.

Elderly and debilitated patients with heart disease are more sensitive to phenothiazine effects. Therefore, a low initial dose is recommended with adjustment of subsequent doses according to response and tolerance of the patient. The pulse, blood pressure, and general circulatory status should be checked frequently until dosage requirements and response are stabilized.

Continued administration for more than 30 days has usually been unnecessary, and is advised only when narcotic drugs are contraindicated or in terminal illnesses. When long-term use is anticipated, periodic blood counts and liver function studies are recommended.

Patients should remain in bed or be closely supervised for about 6 hours after each of the first several injections, and not be ambulatory because of the possibility of orthostatic hypotension. Once tolerance to this effect is obtained, tolerance will usually be maintained unless more than several days elapse between subsequent doses. Therapy with vasopressor drugs has been required very rarely. Phenylephrine and methoxamine are suitable vasopressor agents; however, epinephrine should not be used, since a paradoxical decrease in blood pressure may result. Levarterenol should be reserved for hypotension not reversed by other vasopressors.

ADVERSE REACTIONS

The most important side effects have been those associated with orthostatic hypotension. These effects, which include fainting or syncope, and weakness, usually can be avoided by keeping the patient in a supine position for about 6 hours (occasionally as much as 12 hours) after injection. A drop in blood pressure (usually within the physiological range) often occurs, beginning generally within 10 to 20 minutes following intramuscular injection, and may last 4 to 6 hours (occasionally up to 12 hours). This effect usually diminishes or disappears with continued or intermittent administration. Occasionally, fall in blood pressure may be profound and require immediate restorative measures.

Adverse reactions sometimes encountered include disorientation, dizziness, excessive sedation, weakness, slurring of speech; abdominal discomfort, nausea, and vomiting, dry mouth, nasal congestion, difficulties in urination; chills; rarely uterine inertia.

Pain at the site of injection is frequently observed following administration of this drug. Local inflammation and swelling have occurred.

Agranulocytosis and jaundice have been reported following long-term, high-dosage use of this drug. Other adverse effects reported following the use of the phenothiazine family of drugs usually during their administration as psychotherapeutic agents have included: blood dyscrasias (agranulocytosis, pancytopenia, leukopenia, eosinophilia, thrombocytopenia); hepatotoxicity (jaundice, biliary stasis); extrapyramidal symptoms (dyskinesia, tilting stance, dystonia, parkinsonism, opisthotonos, hyperreflexia, especially in patients with previous brain damage); grand mal convulsions; potentiation of CNS depressants (opiates, barbiturates, antihistamines, alcohol, analgesics), atropine, phosphorous insecticides, heat; cerebral edema and altered cerebral spinal fluid proteins; reactivation of psychotic processes, catatonia; autonomic reactions (dryness of mouth, constipation), cardiac arrest, tachycardia; hyperpyrexia; endocrine disturbances (menstrual and lactation irregularities); dermatological disorders (photosensitivity, itching, erythema, urticaria, pigmentation, rash, exfoliative dermatitis) ocular changes (lenticular and corneal deposits and pigmentary retinopathy); hypersensitivity reactions (angioneurotic, laryngeal, and peripheral edema, anaphylactoid reactions, and asthma). There is considerable individual variation in type and frequency to these effects and although some are dose-related, many involve individual patient sensitivity. Most of these effects have occurred only on long-term, high-dosage administration and have not necessarily been reported with the recommended analgesic doses of Methotrimeprazine.

ADMINISTRATION AND DOSAGE

Adult Administration: Methotrimeprazine should be administered by deep intramuscular injection into a large muscle mass. As with other intramuscularly administered drugs, proper injection technique is important to prevent inadvertent injection into a blood vessel, into, or in the region of, a peripheral nerve trunk, and to avoid leakage along the needle tract. When multiple injections are used, rotation of the injection sites is advisable. Methotrimeprazine should not be administered subcutaneously as local irritation may occur. Until more experience is obtained, intravenous administration is not recommended.

Methotrimeprazine may be given intramuscularly in the same syringe with either atropine sulfate or scopolamine hydrobromide. It should NOT be mixed in the same syringe with other drugs.

The usual adult dose for analgesia is 10 to 20 mg (0.5 to 1.0 mL) administered deeply into a large muscle every 4 to 6 hours as required for pain relief. The dose per injection has varied from 5 to 40 mg (0.25 to 2.0 mL) at intervals of from 1 to 24 hours. A flexible dosage schedule and low initial dose of 10 mg are advisable until individual patient response and tolerance have been determined.

In elderly patients who are more sensitive to phenothiazine effects, an initial dose of 5 to 10 mg (0.25 to 0.5 mL) is suggested. If the patient tolerates the drug, and requires greater pain relief, subsequent doses may be slowly increased.

Analgesia for Acute or Intractable Pain: Initial dose of 10 to 20 mg, with adjustment of subsequent doses, at intervals of 4 to 6 hours as required for relief of pain.

Obstetrical Analgesia: During labor, an initial dose of 15 to 20 mg is usually satisfactory. Methotrimeprazine may be repeated in similar or adjusted amounts at intervals as needed for analgesia and sedation.

Preanesthetic Medication: The preoperative dose has varied from 2 to 20 mg administered 45 minutes to 3 hours before surgery. A dose of 10 mg is often satisfactory, and 15 to 20 mg, may be used when more sedation is desired. Atropine sulfate or scopolamine hydrobromide may be used concurrently but in lower than usual dosage (see also under "Precautions").

Postoperative Analgesia: In the immediate postoperative period, initial dosage of 2.5 to 7.5 mg is suggested, since residual effects of anesthetic agents and other medications may be additive to the actions of Methotrimeprazine. Subsequent doses should be adjusted and administered at intervals of 4 to 6 hours as needed for pain relief. Ambulation must be avoided or carefully supervised (see also under *"Caution," "Adverse Reactions", and "Precautions"*).

Storage: Store at controlled room temperature, 15°-30°C (59°-86°F).

J CODES
Up to 20 mg IM—J1970

HOW SUPPLIED
INJECTION: 20 MG/ML

BRAND/MANUFACTURER	NDC	SIZE	AWP
○ **BRAND**			
LEVOPROME: Immunex	00205-4534-34	10 ml	$226.89

Methoxamine Hydrochloride

DESCRIPTION
Methoxamine Hydrochloride Injection is a sterile solution for intravenous or intramuscular injection, made isotonic with sodium chloride. Each 1 ml ampul contains 20 mg Methoxamine HCl.

Methoxamine HCl is a sympathomimetic amine. It has the empirical formula $C_{11}H_{17}NO_3 \cdot HCl$ and a molecular weight of 247.72. The drug is very soluble in water, soluble in ethanol, but practically insoluble in ether, benzene or chloroform. It is known chemically as α-(1-aminoethyl)-2,5-dimethoxybenzenemethanol hydrochloride.

Following is its chemical structure:

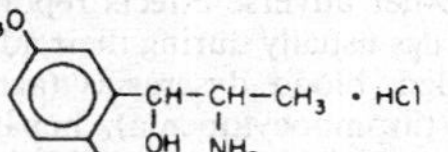

CLINICAL PHARMACOLOGY
Methoxamine HCl is an alpha-receptor stimulant which produces a prompt and prolonged rise in blood pressure following parenteral administration. It is especially useful for maintaining blood pressure during operations under spinal anesthesia[1,2,3] and may also be used safely during general anesthesia. Methoxamine HCl does not increase the irritability of the cyclopropane-sensitized heart, making it useful during cyclopropane anesthesia.[4,5] Tachyphylaxis has not been a clinical problem.[1]

The major pharmacological effect of Methoxamine HCl is a potent, prolonged pressor action following parenteral administration. Methoxamine HCl differs from most other sympathomimetic amines both in animals[4,6,7] and in man[1,8] by having a predominantly peripheral action and lacking inotropic and chronotropic effects. Methoxamine HCl has less arrhythmogenic potential than other sympathomimetic amines and rarely causes ventricular tachycardia, fibrillation, or increased sinoatrial rate.[4] On occasion, a decrease in rate occurs as blood pressure increases,[1,9,10] apparently caused by a carotid sinus reflex. This bradycardia can be abolished by atropine.[9] The pressor action appears to be due to peripheral vasoconstriction rather than a centrally mediated effect. Evidence for direct action on blood vessels is provided in part by the observation of intense constriction along the course of a vein into which Methoxamine HCl has been injected.[1] Methoxamine HCl also increases venous pressure.[8]

Following intravenous administration of Methoxamine HCl in dogs[11] and humans,[9,12] the peak pressor effect occurs within 0.5 to 2 minutes. In a group of human surgical patients,[13] the duration of the pressor effect following a single intravenous dose of 2 to 4 mg of Methoxamine HCl was 10 to 15 minutes. No clinical pharmacology studies are available concerning the onset and duration of action after administration of recommended intramuscular doses (10 to 15 mg). With administration of 10 to 40 mg Methoxamine HCl intramuscularly to patients, however, the peak effect occurs within 15 to 20 minutes, and the duration of action is approximately one and a half hours.[14]

Data from pharmacokinetic studies of Methoxamine HCl following either intravenous or intramuscular administration are not available.

INDICATIONS AND USAGE
Methoxamine HCl is intended for supporting, restoring or maintaining blood pressure during anesthesia (including cyclopropane anesthesia). It can be used to terminate some episodes of supraventricular tachycardia.

CONTRAINDICATIONS
Methoxamine HCl is contraindicated in patients with severe hypertension, or in patients who are hypersensitive to Methoxamine.

WARNINGS
The use of Methoxamine HCl in patients receiving monoamine oxidase inhibitors, tricyclic antidepressants or oxytocic agents such as vasopressin or certain ergot alkaloids may result in potentiation of the pressor effect (see *"Drug Interactions"* under *"Precautions"*).

Contains potassium metabisulfite, a sulfite that may cause allergic-type reactions including anaphylactic symptoms and life-threatening or less severe asthmatic episodes in certain susceptible people. The overall prevalence of sulfite sensitivity in the general population is unknown and probably low. Sulfite sensitivity is seen more frequently in asthmatic than in nonasthmatic people.

PRECAUTIONS
General: Methoxamine HCl, like other vasopressor agents, should be used with caution in patients with hyperthyroidism, bradycardia, partial heart block, myocardial disease, or severe arteriosclerosis. Caution should be exercised to avoid overdosage, preventing undesirable high blood pressure and/or bradycardia. Note: Bradycardia may be abolished with atropine (see *"Overdosage"*). Also, caution should be taken when Methoxamine HCl is used closely following the parenteral injection of ergot alkaloids to avoid an excessive rise in blood pressure.

Drug Interactions: The pressor effect of Methoxamine HCl may be markedly potentiated when Methoxamine HCl is used in conjunction with monoamine oxidase inhibitors, tricyclic antidepressants, vasopressin or ergot alkaloids such as ergotamine, ergonovine or methylergonovine. Therefore, when initiating pressor therapy in patients receiving these drugs the initial dose should be small and given with caution (see *"Warnings"*).

Drug/Laboratory Test Interactions: Methoxamine HCl may increase plasma cortisol and ACTH levels. Caution should be used when interpreting plasma cortisol and ACTH levels in a patient concurrently receiving Methoxamine HCl.[15,16]

Carcinogenesis, Mutagenesis, Impairment of Fertility: No long-term animal studies have been performed to evaluate the potential of Methoxamine HCl in these areas.

Pregnancy: Teratogenic Effects: Pregnancy Category C: Methoxamine HCl has been shown to decrease uterine blood flow, decrease fetal heart rate and adversely affect the fetal acid-base status in pregnant ewes and monkeys at doses comparable to those used in humans. There are no adequate and well-controlled studies in pregnant women. There has been one report of a fetal death; the mother received Methoxamine HCl concomitantly with several other drugs. A direct causal relationship to Methoxamine HCl was not established. Methoxamine HCl should be used during pregnancy only if the potential benefit justifies the potential risk to the fetus.

Methoxamine HCl (2.5 mg I.V., 1 to 3 times over a 45 min. period) given to 7 pregnant ewes showed a significant deterioration in fetal acid-base status as evidenced by hypoxia, hypercarbia and metabolic acidosis.[17] An inverse relationship between pressor response to Methoxamine HCl and uteroplacental blood flow has been shown in 16 pregnant ewes studied at doses ranging from 0.025 mg/kg to 0.2 mg/kg.[18] Uterine blood flow was decreased at all doses, but no significant change in fetal blood gas or acid-base status was demonstrated. Methoxamine HCl administration to 4 fetuses (50 mcg/kg/min for 60 min) and to 4 ewes (25 mcg/kg/min for 30 min) was associated with a decrease in fetal heart rate and uterine blood flow.[19] Nine monkeys studied at an average Methoxamine HCl dose of 1.3 mg/kg administered over 57 min showed a decrease in uterine blood flow and a possible association with fetal asphyxia.[20]

Labor and Delivery: If vasopressor drugs are used to correct hypotension or added to the local anesthetic solution during labor and delivery, some oxytocic drugs (vasopressin, ergotamine, ergonovine, methylergonovine) may cause severe persistent hypertension (see *"Warnings"* and *"Drug Interactions"* under *"Precautions"*).

"Note": In pregnant animals, Methoxamine HCl has been shown to decrease uterine blood flow, possibly resulting in fetal asphyxia. Uterine hypertonus and fetal bradycardia may also be produced. (See *"Adverse Reactions"* and *"Pregnancy"* under *"Precautions"*).

Nursing Mothers: It is not known whether this drug is excreted in human milk. Because many drugs are excreted in human milk, caution should be exercised when Methoxamine HCl is administered to a nursing woman.

Pediatric Use: Safety and effectiveness in children have not been established.

ADVERSE REACTIONS
The following adverse reactions have been observed, but there are insufficient data to support an estimate of their frequency:

Cardiovascular: Excessive blood pressure elevations particularly with high dosage, ventricular ectopic beats.

Gastrointestinal: Nausea, vomiting (often projectile)

Central Nervous System: Headache (often severe), anxiety

Integumentary: Sweating, pilomotor response

Genitourinary: Uterine hypertonus, fetal bradycardia (see *"Labor and Delivery"* under *"Precautions"*), urinary urgency

OVERDOSAGE
Overdosage of Methoxamine HCl may be manifested as an undesirable elevation in blood pressure and/or bradycardia. Should a clinically significant elevation of blood pressure occur that requires treatment, it may be immediately reversed with an alpha-adrenergic blocking agent (e.g., phentolamine). Bradycardia may be abolished by atropine.

DOSAGE AND ADMINISTRATION
Blood volume depletion should always be corrected before any vasopressor is administered. The usual intravenous dose of Methoxamine HCl for emergencies is 3 to 5 mg, injected slowly. Intravenous injection may be supplemented by intramuscular injections to provide a more prolonged effect. The usual intramuscular dose is 10 to 15 mg given shortly before or at the time of administering spinal anesthesia to prevent a fall in blood pressure. The tendency for the blood pressure to fall is greater with higher levels of spinal anesthesia, hence the dosage

---

◆ RATED THERAPEUTICALLY EQUIVALENT; ◇ THERAPEUTIC EQUIVALENCE UNCONFIRMED; ○ UNRATED

may be adjusted accordingly; 10 mg may be adequate at lower spinal levels while 15 to 20 mg may be required at high levels of spinal anesthesia. Repeated doses may be given if necessary, but time should be allowed for the previous dose to act (about 15 minutes, see *"Clinical Pharmacology"*). For cases of only moderate hypotension, 5 to 10 mg intramuscularly may be adequate.

For purposes of correcting a fall in blood pressure, an intramuscular injection of 10 to 15 mg of Methoxamine HCl may be given depending upon the degree of fall. In cases where the systolic pressure falls to 60 mmHg or less, or whenever an emergency exists, an intravenous injection of 3 to 5 mg Methoxamine HCl is indicated. This intravenous dose may be accompanied by 10 to 15 mg intramuscularly to provide more prolonged effect. For termination of episodes of supraventricular tachycardia not responsive to other modes of therapy, the usual dose of Methoxamine HCl is 10 mg intravenously, administered by slow push (i.e., 3 to 5 min).

Parenteral drug products should be inspected visually for particulate matter and discoloration prior to administration whenever solution and container permit.

Store at 15° to 30°C (59° to 86°F) and protect from light.

REFERENCES

1. King BD, Dripps RD: The use of methoxamine for maintenance of the circulation during spinal anesthesia. *Surg Gynecol Obstet* 1950;90:659-665. 2. Kistler EM, Ruben JE: Methoxamine in 1 percent procaine as a prophylactic vasopressor in spinal anesthesia. *Arch Surg* 1951;62:64-69. 3. Poe MF: Use of methoxamine hydrochloride as a pressor agent during spinal analgesia. *Anesthesiology* 1952; 13:89-93. 4. Lahti RE, Brill IC, McCawley EL: The effect of methoxamine hydrochloride (Vasoxyl) on cardiac rhythm. *J Pharmacol Exp Ther* 1955;115:268-274. 5. Stutzman JW, Pettinga FL, Fruggiero EJ: Cardiac effects of methoxamine (β-[2,5-dimethoxy-phenyl]-β-hydroxyiso-propylamine HCl) and desoxyephedrine during cyclopropane anesthesia. *J Pharmacol Exp Ther* 1949; 97:385-387. 6. West JW, Faulk AT, Guzman SV: Comparative study of effects of levarterenol and methoxamine in shock associated with acute myocardial ischemia in dogs. *Circ Res* 1962;10:712-721. 7. Goldberg LI, Cotten M, Darby TD, Howell EV: Comparative heart contractile force effects of equipressor doses of several sympathomimetic amines. *J Pharmacol Exp Ther* 1953;108:177-185. 8. Aviado DM, Wnuck AL: Mechanisms for cardiac slowing by methoxamine. *J Pharmacol Exp Ther* 1957; 119:99-106. 9. Nathanson MH, Miller H: Clinical observations on a new epinephrin-like compound, methoxamine. *Am J Med Sci* 1952;223:270-279. 10. Stanfield CA, Yu PN: Hemodynamic effects of methoxamine in mitral valve disease. *Circ Res* 1960;8:859-864. 11. Imai S, Shigei T, Hashimoto K: Cardiac actions of methoxamine with special reference to its antagonist action to epinephrine. *Circ Res* 1961;9:552-560. 12. *The Extra Pharmacopoeia, Martindale* 28th Ed., Reynolds, JEF, ed., Pharmaceutical Press (London), pp. 19. 13. Goldberg LI, Bloodwell RD, Braunwald E, *et al.* The direct effects of norepinephrine, epinephrine, and methoxamine on myocardial contractile force in man. *Circ* 1960;22:1125-1132. 14. Data on File, Burroughs Wellcome Co. 15. Laurian L, Oberman Z, Hoerer E, *et al.*: Low cortisol and growth hormone secretion in response to methoxamine administration in obese subjects. *Isr J Med Sci* 1977;13:477-481. 16. Nakai Y, Imura H, Yoshimi T, Matsukura S: Adrenergic control mechanism for ACTH secretion in man. *Acta Endocrinol* 1973;74:263-270. 17. Shnider SM, DeLorimier AA, Asling JH, Morishima HO: Vasopressors in obstetrics. II. Fetal hazards of methoxamine administration during obstetric spinal anesthesia. *J Obstet Gynecol* 1970;106:680-686. 18. Ralston DH, Shnider SM, DeLorimier AA: Effects of equipotent ephedrine, metaraminol, mephentermine and methoxamine on uterine blood flow in the pregnant ewe. *Anesthesiology* 1974;40:354-370. 19. Oakes GK, Ehrenkranz RA, Walker AM, *et al.*: Effect of α-adrenergic agonist and antagonist infusion on the umbilical and uterine circulations of pregnant sheep. *Biol Neonate* 1980;38:229-237. 20. Eng M, Berges PU, Ueland K, *et al.*: The effects of methoxamine and ephedrine in normotensive pregnant primates. *Anesthesiology* 1971;35:354-360.

J CODES
Up to 20 mg IM,IV—J3390

HOW SUPPLIED
INJECTION: 20 MG/ML

BRAND/MANUFACTURER	NDC	SIZE	AWP
○ **BRAND**			
VASOXYL: Burr Wellcome	00081-0957-10	1 ml 10s	$213.41

Methoxsalen

Caution: METHOXSALEN IS A POTENT DRUG. READ ENTIRE MONO-GRAPH PRIOR TO PRESCRIBING OR DISPENSING THIS MEDICATION.

METHOXSALEN WITH UV RADIATION SHOULD BE USED ONLY BY PHYSICIANS WHO HAVE SPECIAL COMPETENCE IN THE DIAGNOSIS AND TREATMENT OF PSORIASIS AND WHO HAVE SPECIAL TRAINING AND EXPERIENCE IN PHOTOCHEMOTHERAPY. THE USE OF PSORALEN AND ULTRAVIOLET RADIATION THERAPY SHOULD BE UNDER CONSTANT SUPERVISION OF SUCH A PHYSICIAN. FOR THE TREATMENT OF PATIENTS WITH PSORIASIS, PHOTOCHEMOTHERAPY SHOULD BE RESTRICTED TO PATIENTS WITH SEVERE, RECALCITRANT, DISABLING PSORIASIS WHICH IS NOT ADEQUATELY RESPONSIVE TO OTHER FORMS OF THERAPY, AND ONLY WHEN THE DIAGNOSIS HAS BEEN SUPPORTED BY BIOPSY. BECAUSE OF THE POSSIBILITIES OF OCULAR DAMAGE, AGING OF THE SKIN, AND SKIN CANCER (INCLUDING MELANOMA), THE PATIENT SHOULD BE FULLY INFORMED BY THE PHYSICIAN OF THE RISKS INHERENT IN THIS THERAPY.

WARNING: METHOXSALEN LOTION IS A POTENT DRUG CAPABLE OF PRODUCING SEVERE BURNS IF IMPROPERLY USED. IT SHOULD BE APPLIED ONLY BY A PHYSICIAN UNDER CONTROLLED CONDITIONS FOR LIGHT EXPOSURE AND SUBSEQUENT LIGHT SHIELDING.
THIS PREPARATION SHOULD NEVER BE DISPENSED TO A PATIENT.

CAUTION: METHOXSALEN CAPSULES SHOULD NOT BE USED INTERCHANGEABLY WITH METHOXSALEN LOTION. THIS NEW DOSAGE FORM OF METHOXSALEN EXHIBITS SIGNIFICANTLY GREATER BIOAVAILABILITY AND EARLIER PHOTOSENSITIZATION ONSET TIME THAN PREVIOUS METHOXSALEN DOSAGE FORMS.

PATIENTS SHOULD BE TREATED IN ACCORDANCE WITH THE DOSIMETRY SPECIFICALLY RECOMMENDED FOR THIS PRODUCT. THE MINIMUM PHOTOTOXIC DOSE (MPD) AND PHOTOTOXIC PEAK TIME AFTER DRUG ADMINISTRATION PRIOR TO ONSET OF PHOTOCHEMOTHERAPY WITH THIS DOSAGE FORM SHOULD BE DETERMINED.

DESCRIPTION
Methoxsalen is a naturally occurring photoactive substance found in the seeds of the *Ammi majus* (Umbelliferae) plant. It belongs to a group of compounds known as psoralens, or furocoumarins. The chemical name of Methoxsalen is 9-methoxy-7H-furo [3,2-g] [1]benzopyran-7-one.

Each capsule contains:
Methoxsalen ....10 mg

Each ml of lotion contains:
Methoxsalen ....10 mg

Following is its chemical structure:

CLINICAL PHARMACOLOGY
The combination treatment regimen of psoralen (P) and ultraviolet radiation of 320—400 nm wavelength commonly referred to as UVA is known by the acronym, PUVA. Skin reactivity to UVA (320—400 nm) radiation is markedly enhanced by the ingestion of Methoxsalen. In a well controlled bioavailability study, Methoxsalen capsules reached peak drug levels in the blood of test subjects between 0.5 and 4 hours (Mean = 1.8 hours) as compared to between 1.5 and 6 hours (Mean = 3.0 hours) for regular Methoxsalen when administered with 8 ounces of milk. Peak drug levels were 2 to 3 fold greater when the overall extent of drug absorption was approximately two fold greater for Methoxsalen capsules as compared to regular Methoxsalen capsules. Detectable Methoxsalen levels were observed up to 12 hours post dose.

The drug half-life is approximately 2 hours. Photosensitivity studies demonstrate a shorter time of peak photosensitivity of 1.5 to 2.1 hours vs. 3.9 to 4.25 hours for Methoxsalen capsules. In addition, the mean minimal erythema dose (MED), J/cm^2, for the Methoxsalen capsules is substantially less than that required for regular Methoxsalen capsules (Levins et al., 1984 and private communication[1]).

Methoxsalen is reversibly bound to serum albumin and is also preferentially taken up by epidermal cells (Artuc et al., 1979[2]). At a dose which is six times larger than that used in humans, it induces mixed function oxidases in the liver of mice (Mandula et al., 1978[3]). In both mice and man, Methoxsalen is rapidly metabolized. Approximately 95% of the drug is excreted as a series of metabolites in the urine within 24 hours (Pathak et al., 1977[4]). The exact mechanism of action of Methoxsalen with the epidermal melanocytes and keratinocytes is not known. The best known biochemical reaction of Methoxsalen is with DNA. Methoxsalen, upon photoactivation, conjugates and forms covalent bonds with DNA which leads to the formation of both monofunctional (addition to a single strand of DNA) and bifunctional (cross-linking of psoralen to both strands of DNA) adducts (Dall' Acqua et al., 1971[5]; Cole, 1970[6]; Musajo et al., 1974[7]; Dall' Acqua et al., 1979[8]). Reactions with proteins have also been described (Yoshikawa, et al., 1979[9]).

Methoxsalen acts as a photosensitizer. Administration or topical application of the drug and subsequent exposure to UVA, whether artificial or sunlight, can lead to cell injury. Orally administered Methoxsalen reaches the skin via the blood and UVA penetrates well into the skin. If sufficient cell injury occurs in the skin, an inflammatory reaction occurs. The most obvious manifestation of this reaction is delayed erythema, which may not begin for several hours and peaks at 48—72 hours or longer. It is crucial to realize that the length of time the skin remains sensitized or when the maximum erythema will occur is quite variable from person to person. The inflammation is followed, over several days to weeks, by repair which is manifested by increased melanization of the epidermis and thickening of the stratum corneum. The mechanisms of therapy are not known, but it has been suggested melanocytes in the hair follicles are stimulated to move up the follicle and to repopulate the epidermis. (Ortonne, et al, 1979[10]). In the treatment of psoriasis, the mechanism is most often assumed to be DNA photodamage and resulting decrease in cell proliferation but other vascular, leukocyte, or cell regulatory mechanisms may also be playing some role. Psoriasis is a hyper-proliferative disorder and other agents known to be therapeutic for psoriasis are known to inhibit DNA systhesis.

INDICATIONS AND USAGE

CAPSULES

Photochemotherapy (Methoxsalen with long wave UVA radiation) is indicated for the symptomatic control of severe, recalcitrant, disabling psoriasis not adequately responsive to other forms of therapy and when the diagnosis has been supported by biopsy. Methoxsalen is intended to be administered only in conjunction with a schedule of controlled doses of long wave ultraviolet radiation.

LOTION

As a topical repigmenting agent in vitiligo in conjunction with controlled doses of ultraviolet A (320-400 nm) or sunlight.

CONTRAINDICATIONS

A. Patients exhibiting idiosyncratic reactions to psoralen compounds or having a history of sensitivity reactions to them.

B. Patients possessing a specific history of light sensitive disease states should not initiate Methoxsalen therapy except under special circumstances. Diseases associated with photosensitivity include lupus erythematosus, porphyria cutanea tarda, erythropoietic protoporphyria, variegate porphyria, xeroderma pigmentosum, and albinism.

C. Patients with melanoma or with a history of melanoma.

D. Patients with invasive squamous cell carcinomas.

E. Patients with aphakia, because of the significantly increased risk of retinal damage due to the absence of lenses.

F. Children under 12 since clinical studies to determine the efficacy and safety of treatment in this age group have not been done.

WARNINGS

A. SKIN BURNING

Serious burns from either UVA or sunlight (even through window glass) can result if the recommended dosage of the drug and/or exposure schedules are exceeded and/or protective covering or sunscreens are not used. The blistering of the skin sometimes encountered after UVA exposure generally heals without complication or scarring. Suitable covering of the area of application or a topical sunblock should follow the therapeutic UVA exposure.

B. CARCINOGENICITY

1. Animal Studies: Topical or intraperitoneal Methoxsalen has been reported to be a potent photocarcinogen in albino mice and hairless mice (Hakim et al., 1960[11]). However, Methoxsalen given by the oral route to Swiss albino mice suggests this agent exerts a protective effect against ultraviolet carcinogenesis; mice given 8-methoxypsoralen in their diet showed 38% ear tumors 180 days after the start of ultraviolet therapy compared to 62% for controls (O'Neal et al., 1957[12]).

2. Human Studies: A 5.7 year prospective study of 1380 psoriasis patients treated with oral Methoxsalen and ultraviolet A photochemotherapy (PUVA) demonstrated that the risk of cutaneous squamous-cell carcinoma developing at least 22 months following the first PUVA exposure was approximately 12.8 times higher in the high dose patients than in the low dose patients (Stern et al., 1979[13], Stern et al., 1980[14], and Stern et al., 1984[15]). The substantial dose-dependent increase was observed in patients with neither a prior history of skin cancer nor significant exposure to cutaneous carcinogens. Reduction in PUVA dosage significantly reduces the risk. No substantial dose related increase was noted for basal cell carcinoma according to Stern et al., 1984[15]. Increases appear greatest in patients who have pre-PUVA exposure to 1) prolonged tar and UVB treatment, 2) ionizing radiation, or 3) arsenic.

Roenigk et al., 1980[16], studied 690 patients for up to 4 years and found no increase in the risk of non-melanoma skin cancer, although patients in this cohort had significantly less exposure to PUVA than in the Stern et al. study. After 5 years, two of 1380 patients in the Stern et al. PUVA study have developed malignant melanoma. In addition, more than 1/5 of the patients in this cohort have developed macular pigmented lesions on the buttocks. While there is no evidence that an increased risk of melanoma exists in PUVA treated patients, these observations indicate the need for continued evaluation of melanoma risk of PUVA treated patients.

In a study in Indian patients treated for 4 years for vitiligo, 12 patients developed keratoses, but not cancer, in the depigmented, vitiliginous areas (Mosher, 1980[17]).

Clinically, the keratoses were keratotic papules, actinic keratosis-like macules, nonscaling dome-shaped papules, and lichenoid porokeratotic-like papules. Clinical investigators have not reported skin cancers as a complication of topical treatment for vitiligo. However, it is recommended that caution be exercised when the patient is fair-skinned or has a history of prior coal tar UVA treatment, or has had ionizing radiation or taken arsenical compounds.

C. CATARACTOGENICITY

1. Animal Studies: Exposure to large doses of UVA causes cataracts in animals, and this effect is enhanced by the administration of Methoxsalen (Cloud et al, 1960[18]; Cloud et al, 1961[19]; Freeman et al, 1969[20]).

2. Human Studies: It has been found that the concentration of Methoxsalen in the lens is proportional to the serum level. If the lens is exposed to UVA during the time Methoxsalen is present in the lens, photochemical action may lead to irreversible binding of Methoxsalen to proteins and the DNA components of the lens (Lerman et al, 1980[20]). However, if the lens is shielded from UVA, the Methoxsalen will diffuse out of the lens in a 24 hour period (Lerman et al.,

1980[21]). Patients should be told emphatically to wear UVA-absorbing, wrap-around sunglasses for the twenty-four (24) hour period following ingestion of Methoxsalen, whether exposed to direct or indirect sunlight in the open or through a window glass.

Among patients using proper eye protection, there is no evidence for a significantly increased risk of cataracts in association with PUVA therapy (Stern et al., 1979[13]). Thirty-five of 1380 patients have developed cataracts in the five years since their first PUVA treatment. This incidence is comparable to that expected in a population of this size and age distribution. No relationship between PUVA dose and cataract risk in this group has been noted.

D. ACTINIC DEGENERATION

Exposure to sunlight and/or ultraviolet radiation may result in "premature aging" of the skin.

E. BASAL CELL CARCINOMAS

Patients exhibiting multiple basal cell carcinomas or having a history of basal cell carcinomas should be diligently observed and treated.

F. RADIATION THERAPY

Patients having a history of previous x-ray therapy or grenz ray therapy should be diligently observed for signs of carcinoma.

G. ARSENIC THERAPY

Patients having a history of previous arsenic therapy should be diligently observed for signs of carcinoma.

H. HEPATIC DISEASES

Patients with hepatic insufficiency should be treated with caution since hepatic biotransformation is necessary for drug urinary excretion.

I. CARDIAC DISEASES

Patients with cardiac diseases or others who may be unable to tolerate prolonged standing or exposure to heat stress should not be treated in a vertical UVA chamber.

J. TOTAL DOSAGE

The total cumulative dose of UVA that can be given over long periods of time with safety has not as yet been established.

K. CONCOMITANT THERAPY

Special care should be exercised in treating patients who are receiving concomitant therapy (either topically or systemically) with known photosensitizing agents such as anthralin, coal tar or coal tar derivatives, griseofulvin, phenothiazines, nalidixic acid, halogenated salicylanilides (bacteriostatic soaps), sulfonamides, tetracyclines, thiazides and certain organic staining dyes such as methylene blue, toluidine blue, rose bengal, and methyl orange.

PRECAUTIONS

A. GENERAL — APPLICABLE TO PSORIASIS TREATMENT

1. Before Methoxsalen Ingestion: Patients must not sunbathe during the 24 hours prior to Methoxsalen ingestion and UV exposure. The presence of a sunburn may prevent an accurate evaluation of the patient's response to photochemotherapy.

2. After Methoxsalen Ingestion:

a. UVA-absorbing wrap-around sunglasses should be worn during daylight for 24 hours after Methoxsalen ingestion. The protective eyewear must be designed to prevent entry of stray radiation to the eyes, including that which may enter from the sides of the eyewear. The protective eyewear is used to prevent the irreversible binding of Methoxsalen to the proteins and DNA components of the lens. Cataracts form when enough of the binding occurs. Visual discrimination should be permitted by the eyewear for patient well-being and comfort.

b. Patients must avoid sun exposure, even through window glass or cloud cover, for at least 8 hours after Methoxsalen ingestion. If sun exposure cannot be avoided, the patient should wear protective devices such as a hat and gloves, and/ or apply sunscreens which contain ingredients that filter out UVA radiation (e.g., sunscreens containing benzophenone and/or PABA esters which exhibit a sun protective factor equal to or greater than 15). These chemical sunscreens should be applied to all areas that might be exposed to the sun (including lips). Sunscreens should not be applied to areas affected by psoriasis until after the patient has been treated in the UVA chamber.

3. During PUVA Therapy:

a. Total UVA-absorbing/blocking goggles mechanically designed to give maximal ocular protection must be worn. Failure to do so may increase the risk of cataract formation. A reliable radiometer can be used to verify elimination of UVA transmission through the goggles.

b. Abdominal skin, breasts, genitalia, and other sensitive areas should be protected for approximately 1/3 of the initial exposure time until tanning occurs.

c. Unless affected by disease, male genitalia should be shielded.

4. After Combined Methoxsalen/UVA Therapy:

a. UVA-absorbing wrap-around sunglasses should be worn during daylight for 24 hours after combined Methoxsalen/UVA therapy.

b. Patients must not sunbathe for 48 hours after therapy. Erythema and/or burning due to photochemotherapy and sunburn due to sun exposure are additive.

B. VITILIGO TREATMENT

Methoxsalen lotion should be applied only in small, well-defined lesions and preferably on lesions which can be protected by clothing or a sunscreen from subsequent exposure to radiant UVA. If this product is used to treat vitiligo of

---

face or hands, be very emphatic when instructing patient to keep the treated areas protected from light by use of protective clothing or sunscreening agents. The area of application may be highly photosensitive for several days and may result in severe burn injury if exposed to additional UVA or sunlight.

C. LABORATORY TESTS
1. Patients should have an ophthalmologic examination prior to start of therapy with Methoxsalen capsules, and thence yearly.
2. Patients should have routine laboratory tests prior to the start of therapy and at regular periods thereafter if patients are on extended treatments.

D. DRUG INTERACTIONS
See *"Warnings"* section.

E. CARCINOGENESIS
See *"Warnings"* section.

F. PREGNANCY
Pregnancy Category C.: Animal reproduction studies have not been conducted with oral or topical Methoxsalen. It is also not known whether Methoxsalen can cause fetal harm when administered to or used topically on a pregnant woman or can affect reproduction capacity. It is not known to what degree, if any, topical Methoxsalen is absorbed systemically. Methoxsalen should be used in a woman with reproductive capacity or a pregnant woman only if clearly needed.

G. NURSING MOTHERS
It is not known whether this drug is excreted in human milk or whether topical Methoxsalen is absorbed or excreted in milk. Because many drugs are excreted in human milk, either Methoxsalen ingestion or nursing should be discontinued. Caution is advised when topical Methoxsalen is used in a nursing mother.

H. PEDIATRIC USE
Safety of oral Methoxsalen in children has not been established. Potential hazards of long-term therapy include the possibilities of carcinogenicity and cataractogenicity as described in the *"Warnings"* section as well as the probability of actinic degeneration which is also described in the *"Warnings"* section. Safety and effectiveness of topical Methoxsalen in children below the age of 12 years have not been established.

ADVERSE REACTIONS
A. METHOXSALEN CAPSULES
The most commonly reported side effect of Methoxsalen alone is nausea, which occurs with approximately 10% of all patients. This effect may be minimized or avoided by instructing the patient to take Methoxsalen with milk or food, or to divide the dose into two portions, taken approximately one-half hour apart. Other effects include nervousness, insomnia, and psychological depression.

B. COMBINED METHOXSALEN CAPSULES/UVA THERAPY
1. Pruritus: This adverse reaction occurs with approximately 10% of all patients. In most cases, pruritus can be alleviated with frequent application of bland emollients or other topical agents; severe pruritus may require systemic treatment. If pruritus is unresponsive to these measures, shield pruritic areas from further UVA exposure until the condition resolves. If intractable pruritus is generalized, UVA treatment should be discontinued until the pruritus disappears.

2. Erythema: Mild, transient erythema at 24-48 hours after PUVA therapy is an expected reaction and indicates that a therapeutic interaction between Methoxsalen and UVA occurred. Any area showing moderate erythema (greater than Grade 2 — See Table 1 for grades of erythema) should be shielded during subsequent UVA exposures until the erythema has resolved. Erythema greater than Grade 2 which appears within 24 hours after UVA treatment may signal a potentially severe burn. Erythema may become progressively worse over the next 24 hours, since the peak erythemal reaction characteristically occurs 48 hours or later after Methoxsalen ingestion. The patient should be protected from further UVA exposures and sunlight, and should be monitored closely.

3. Important Differences between PUVA Erythema and Sunburn: PUVA-induced inflammation differs from sunburn or UVB phototherapy in several ways. The percent transmission of UVB varies between 0% to 34% through skin whereas UVA varies between 1% to 80% transmission; thus, UVA is transmitted to a larger percent through the skin. (Diffey, 1982[22]).
The DNA lesions induced by PUVA are very different from UV-induced thymine dimers and may lead to a DNA crosslink. This DNA lesion may be more problematic to the cell because crosslinks are more lethal and psoralen-DNA photoproducts may be "new" or unfamiliar substrates for DNA repair enzymes. DNA synthesis is also suppressed longer after PUVA. The time course of delayed erythema is different with PUVA and may not involve the usual mediators seen in sunburn. PUVA-induced redness may be just beginning at 24 hours, when UVB erythema has already passed its peak. The erythema dose-response curve is also steeper for PUVA. Compared to equally erythemogenic doses of UVB, the histologic alterations induced by PUVA show more dermal vessel damage and longer duration of epidermal and dermal abnormalities.

4. Other Adverse Reactions: Those reported include edema, dizziness, headache, malaise, depression, hypopigmentation, vesiculation and bullae formation, non-specific rash, herpes simplex, miliaria, urticaria, folliculitis, gastrointestinal disturbances, cutaneous tenderness, leg cramps, hypotension, and extension of psoriasis.

C. METHOXSALEN LOTION
Systemic adverse reactions have not been reported. The most common adverse reaction is severe burns of the treated area from overexposure to UVA, including sunlight. *Treatment must be individualized.* Minor blistering of the skin is not a contraindication to further treatment and generally heals without incident. Treatment would be the standard for burn therapy. Since 1953, many studies have demonstrated the safety and effectiveness of topical Methoxsalen and UVA for the treatment of vitiligo when used as directed. (Lerner, A.B., et al, 1953[23]) (Fitzpatrick, T.B. et al, 1966[24]) (Fulton, James F. et al, 1969[25])

OVERDOSAGE
In the event of Methoxsalen overdosage, induce emesis and keep the patient in a darkened room for at least 24 hours. Emesis is most beneficial within the first 2 to 3 hours after ingestion of Methoxsalen, since maximum blood levels are reached by this time.
This does not apply to topical usage. In the unlikely event that the lotion is ingested, standard procedures for poisoning should be followed.

DRUG DOSAGE AND ADMINISTRATION
METHOXSALEN CAPSULES

> THE CAPSULES REPRESENT A NEW DOSE FORM OF METHOXSALEN. THIS NEW DOSAGE FORM OF METHOXSALEN EXHIBITS SIGNIFICANTLY GREATER BIOAVAILABILITY AND EARLIER PHOTOSENSITIZATION ONSET TIME THAN PREVIOUS METHOXSALEN DOSAGE FORMS. EACH PATIENT SHOULD BE EVALUATED BY DETERMINING THE MINIMUM PHOTOTOXIC DOSE (MPD) AND PHOTOTOXIC PEAK TIME AFTER DRUG ADMINISTRATION PRIOR TO ONSET OF PHOTOCHEMOTHERAPY WITH THIS DOSAGE FORM. HUMAN BIOAVAILABILITY STUDIES HAVE INDICATED THE FOLLOWING DRUG DOSAGE AND ADMINISTRATION DIRECTIONS ARE TO BE USED AS A GUIDELINE ONLY.

PSORIASIS THERAPY
1. Drug Dosage: Initial Therapy: The Methoxsalen capsules should be taken 1½ to 2 hours before UVA exposure with some low fat food or milk according to the following table:

Patient's Weight (kg)	Dose (lbs)	(mg)
< 30	< 65	10
30-50	65-100	20
51-65	101-145	30
66-80	146-175	40
81-90	176-200	50
91-115	201-250	60
> 115	> 250	70

2. Initial Exposure: The initial UVA exposure energy level and corresponding time of exposure is determined by the patient's skin characteristics for sunburning and tanning as follows:

Skin Type	History	Recommended Joules/cm²
I	Always burn, never tan (patients with erythodermic psoriasis are to be classed as Type 1 for determination of UVA dosage.)	0.5 J/cm²
II	always burn, but sometimes tan	1.0 J/cm²
III	Sometimes burn, but always tan	1.5 J/cm²
IV	Never burn, always tan	2.0 J/cm²

Skin Type	Physician Examination	Joules/cm²
V*	Moderately pigmented	2.5 J/cm²
VI*	Blacks	3.0 J/cm²

(* *Patients with natural pigmentation of these types should be classified into a lower skin type category if the sunburning history so indicates.*)

If the MPD is done, start at ½ MPD.
Additional drug dosage directions are as follows:

a. Weight Change: In the event that the weight of a patient changes during treatment such that he/she falls into an adjacent weight range/dose category, no change in the dose of Methoxsalen is usually required. If, in the physician's opinion, however, a weight change is sufficiently great to modify the drug dose, then an adjustment in the time of exposure to UVA should be made.

b. Dose/Week: The number of doses per week of Methoxsalen capsules will be determined by the patient's schedule of UVA exposures. In no case should treatments be given more often than once every other day because the full extent of phototoxic reactions may not be evident until 48 hours after each exposure.

c. *Dosage Increase:* Dosage may be increased by 10 mg after the fifteenth treatment under the conditions outlined under PUVA treatment protocol, clearing phase, miscellaneous situations.

UVA RADIATION SOURCE SPECIFICATIONS & INFORMATION
A. Irradiance Uniformity: The following specifications should be met with the window of the detector held in a vertical plane:

1. Vertical variation: For readings taken at any point along the vertical center axis of the chamber (to within 15 cm from the top and bottom), the lowest reading should not be less than 70 percent of the highest reading.

2. Horizontal variation: Throughout any specific horizontal plane, the lowest reading must be at least 80 percent of the highest reading, excluding the peripheral 3 cm of the patient treatment space.

B. Patient Safety Features: The following safety features should be present: (1) Protection from electrical hazard: All units should be grounded and conform to applicable electrical codes. The patient or operator should not be able to touch any live electrical parts. There should be ground fault protection. (2) Protective shielding of lamps: The patient should not be able to come in contact with the bare lamps. In the event of lamp breakage, the patient should not be exposed to broken lamp components, (3) Hand rails and hand holds: Appropriate supports should be available to the patient. (4) Patient viewing window: A window which blocks UV should be provided for viewing the patient during treatment. (5) Door and latches: Patients should be able to open the door from the inside with only slight pressure to the door. (6) Non-skid floor: The floor should be of a non-skid nature. (7) Thermoregulation: Sufficient air flow should be provided for patient safety and comfort, limiting temperature within the UVA radiator cabinet to approximately less than 100°F. (8) Timer: The irradiator should be equipped with an automatic timer which terminates the exposure at the conclusion of a pre-set time interval. (9) Patient alarm device: An alarm device within the UVA irradiator chamber should be accessible to the patient for emergency activation. (10) Danger label: The unit should have a label prominently displayed which reads as follows:

DANGER—Ultraviolet Radiation—Follow your physicians instructions— Failure to use protective eyewear may result in eye injury.

C. UVA Exposure Dosimetry Measurements: The maximum radiant exposure or irradiance (within ± 15 percent) of UVA (320-400 nm) delivered to the patient should be determined by using an appropriate radiometer calibrated to be read in Joules/cm² or mW/cm². In the absence of a standard measuring technique approved by the National Bureau of Standards, the system should use a detector corrected to a cosine spatial response. The use and recalibration frequency of such a radiometer for a specific UVA irradiator chamber should be specified by the manufacturer because the UVA dose (exposure) is determined by the design of the irradiator, the number of lamps, and the age of the lamps. If irradiance is measured, the radiometer reading in mW/cm² is used to calculate the exposure time in minutes to deliver the required UVA in Joules/cm² to a patient in the UVA irradiator cabinet. The equation is:

$$\text{Exposure Time (minutes)} = \frac{\text{Desired UVA Dose (J/cm}^2)}{0.06 \times \text{Irradiance (mW/cm}^2)}$$

Overexposure due to human error should be minimized by using an accurate automatic timing device, which is set by the operator and controlled by energizing and deenergizing the UVA irradiator lamp. The timing device calibration interval should be specified by the manufacturer. Safety systems should be included to minimize the possibility of delivering a UVA exposure which exceeds the prescribed dose, in the event the timer or radiometer should malfunction.

D. UVA Spectral Output Distribution: The spectral distributions of the lamps should meet the following specifications:

Wavelength band (nanometers)	Output[1]
< 310	< 1
310 to 320	1 to 3
320 to 330	4 to 8
330 to 340	11 to 17
340 to 350	18 to 25
350 to 360	19 to 28
360 to 370	15 to 23
370 to 380	8 to 12
380 to 390	3 to 7
390 to 400	1 to 3

[1] *As a percentage of total irradiance between 320 and 400 nanometers.*

PUVA TREATMENT PROTOCOL INTRODUCTION
Methoxsalen capsules reach their maximum bioavailability in 1½ to 2 hours after ingestion.

On average, the serum level achieved with Methoxsalen is twice that obtained with regular Methoxsalen and reach their peak concentration in less than ½ the time of the regular capsules.

As a result the mean MED J/cm² for the Methoxsalen capsules is substantially less than that required for regular Methoxsalen capsules[1] (Levins et al., 1984 and private communications.[1])

Photosensitivity studies demonstrate a shorter time of peak photosensitivity of 1.5 to 2.1 hours vs. 3.9 to 4.25 hours for regular Methoxsalen capsules.

A. INITIAL EXPOSURE
The initial UVA exposures should be conducted according to the guidelines presented previously under *"Drug Dosage and Administration — Initial Therapy and Exposure"*.

B. CLEARING PHASE
Specific recommendations for patient treatment are as follows:

1. Skin Types I, II, & III: Patients with skin types I, II, and III may be treated 2 or 3 times per week. UVA exposure may be held constant or increased by up to 1.0 Joule/cm² at each treatment, according to the patient's response. If erythema occurs, however, do not increase exposure time until erythema resolves. The severity and extent of the patient's erythema may be used to determine whether the next exposure should be shortened, omitted, or maintained at the previous dosage. See *"Adverse Reactions"* section for additional information.

2. Skin Types IV, V, & VI: Patients with skin types IV, V, and VI may be treated 2 or 3 times per week. UVA exposure may be held constant or increased by up to 1.5 Joules/cm² at each treatment unless erhthema occurs. If erythema occurs, follow instructions outlined above in the procedures for patients with skin types, I, II, and III.

3. Erythrodermic Psoriasis: Patients with erythrodermic psoriasis should be treated with special attention because pre-existing erythema may obscure observations of possible treatment-related phototoxic erythema. These patients may be treated 2 or 3 times per week, as a Type I patient.

4. Miscellaneous Situations:
a. If there is no response after a total of 10 treatments, the exposure of UVA energy may be increased by an additional 0.5-1.0 Joules/cm² above the prior incremental increases for each treatment. (Example: a patient whose exposure dose is being increased by 1.0 Joule/cm² may now have all subsequent doses increased by 1.5-2.0 Joules/cm².)

b. If there is no response, or only minimal response, after 15 treatments, the dosage of Methoxsalen may be increased by 10 mg (a one-time increase in dosage). This increased dosage may be continued for the remainder of the course of treatment but should not be exceeded.

c. If a patient misses a treatment, the UVA exposure time of the next treatment should not be increased. If more than one treatment is missed, reduced the exposure by 0.5 Joule/cm² for each treatment missed.

d. If the lower extremities are not responding as well as the rest of the body and do not show erythema, cover all other body areas and give 25 percent of the present exposure dose as an additional exposure to the lower extremities. This additional exposure to the lower extremities should be terminated if erythema develops on these areas.

e. Non-responsive psoriasis: If a patient's generalized psoriasis is not responding, or if the condition appears to be worsening during treatment, the possibility of a generalized phototoxic reaction should be considered. This may be confirmed by the improvement of the condition following temporary discontinuance of this therapy for two weeks. If no improvement occurs during the interruption of treatment, this patient may be considered a treatment failure.

C. ALTERNATIVE EXPOSURE SCHEDULE
As an alternative to increasing the UVA exposure at each treatment, the following schedule may be followed; this schedule may reduce the total number of Joules/cm² received by the patient over the entire course of therapy.

1. Incremental increases in UVA exposure for all patients may range from 0.5 to 1.5 Joules/cm², according to the patient's response to therapy.

2. Once Grade 2 clearing (see Table 2) has been reached and the patient is progressing adequately, UVA dosage is held constant. The dosage is maintained until Grade 4 clearing is reached.

3. If the rate of clearing significantly decreases, exposure dosage may be increased at each treatment (0.1-1.5 Joules/cm²) until Grade 3 clearing and a satisfactory progress rate is attained. The UVA exposure will be held constant again until Grade 4 clearing is attained. These increases may be used also if the rate of clearing significantly decreases between Grade 3 and Grade 4 response. However, the possibility of a phototoxic reaction should be considered; see Non-responsive Psoriasis, above.

4. In summary, this schedule raises slightly the increments (Joules/cm²) of UVA dosage, but limits these increases to those periods when the patient is not responding adequately. Otherwise, the UVA exposure is held at the lowest effective dose.

D. MAINTENANCE PHASE
The goal of maintenance treatment is to keep the patient symptom-free as possible with the least amount of UVA exposure.

1. Schedule of Exposures: When patients have achieved 95 percent clearing, or Grade 4 response (Table 2), they may be placed on the following maintenance schedules (M₁—M₄), in sequence. It is recommended that each maintenance schedule be adhered to for at least 2 treatments (unless erythema or psoriatic flare occurs, in which case see (2a) and (2b) below).

MAINTENANCE SCHEDULES
M$_1$—once/week
M$_2$—once/2 weeks
M$_3$—once/3 weeks
M$_4$—p.r.n. (i.e. for flares)

2. *Length of Exposure:* The UVA exposure for the first maintenance treatment of any schedule (except M₄ as noted below) is the same as that as the patient's last treatment under the previous schedule. For skin types I-IV, however, it is recommended that the maximum UVA dosage during maintenance treatments not exceed the following:

Skin Types	$Joules/cm^2/treatment$
I	12
II	14
III	18
IV	22

If the patient develops erythema or new lesions of psoriasis, proceed as follows:

a. Erythema: During maintenance therapy, the patient's tan and threshold dose for erythema may gradually decrease. If maintenance of treatments produce significant erythema, the exposure to UVA should be decreased by 25 percent until further treatments no longer produce erythema.

b. Psoriasis: If the patient develops new areas of psoriasis during maintenance therapy (but still is classified as having a Grade 4 response), the exposure to UVA may be increased by 0.5-1.5 $Joules/cm^2$ at each treatment; this is appropriate for all types of patients. These increases are continued until the psoriasis is brought under control and the patient is again clear. The exposure being administered when this clearing is reached should be used for further maintenance treatment.

3. Flares During Maintenance: If the patient flares during maintenance treatment (i.e., develops psoriasis on more than 5 percent of the originally involved areas of the body) his maintenance treatment schedule may be changed to the preceding maintenance or clearing schedule. The patient may be kept on his schedule until again 95 percent clear. If the original maintenance treatment schedule is unable to control the psoriasis, the schedule may be changed to a more frequent regimen. If a flare occurs less than 6 weeks after the last treatment, 25 percent of the maximum exposure received during the clearing phase, with the clearing schedule received during the clearing phase, may be used and then proceed with the clearing schedule previously followed for this patient. (At 95 percent clearing, follow regular maintenance until the optimum maintenance schedule is determined for the patient.) If more than 6 weeks have elapsed since the last treatment was given, treat patients as if they were beginning therapy insofar as exposure dosages are concerned, since their threshold for erythema may have decreased.

Table 1
GRADES OF ERYTHEMA

Grades	Erythema
0	No erythema
1	Minimally perceptible erythema—faint pink
2	Marked erythema but with no edema
3	Fiery erythema with edema
4	Fiery erythema with edema and blistering

Table 2
RESPONSE TO THERAPY

Grade	Criteria	Percent Improvement (compared to original extent of disease)
1	Psoriasis worse	0
0	No change	0
1	Minimal improvement—slightly less scale and/or erythema	5–20
2	Definite improvement—partial flattening of all plaques—less scaling and less erythema	20–50
3	Considerable improvement—nearly complete flattening of all plaques but borders of plaques still palpable	50–95
4	Clearing; complete flattening of plaques including borders; plaques may be outlined by pigmentation	95

METHOXSALEN LOTION
The Methoxsalen lotion is applied to a well-defined area of vitiligo by the physician and the area is then exposed to a suitable source of UVA. Initial exposure time should be conservative and not exceed that which is predicted to be one-half the minimal erythema dose. Treatment intervals should be regulated by the erythema response; generally once a week is recommended or less often depending on the results. The hands and fingers of the person applying the medication should be protected by gloves or finger cots to avoid photo-sensitization and possible burns.

Pigmentation may begin after a few weeks but significant repigmentation may require up to 6 to 9 months of treatment. Periodic re-treatment may be necessary to retain all of the new pigment. Idiopathic vitiligo is reversible but not equally reversible in every patient. Treatment must be individualized. Repigmentation will vary in completeness, time of onset, and duration. Repigmentation occurs more rapidly in fleshy areas such as face, abdomen, and buttocks and less rapidly over less fleshy areas such as the dorsum of the hands or feet.

Methoxsalen lotion should be stored at controlled room temperature (15-30°C; 59-86°F).

REFERENCES
1. Levins, P.C., Gauge, R.W., Momtaz-T.K., Parrish, J.A., and Fitzpatrick, T.B.: A New Liquid Formulation of 8-Methoxypsoralen: Bioactivity and Effect of Diet: JID, *82*, No. 2, pp. 185-187 (1984) and private communication. 2. Artuc, M., Stuettgen, G. Schalla, W., Schaefer, H., and Gazith, J.: Reversible binding of 5- and 8-methoxypsoralen to human serum proteins (albumin) and to epidermis in vitro: Brit. J. Dermat. *101*, pp. 669-677 (1979). 3. Mandula, B.B., Pathak, M.A. Nakayama, T., and Davidson, S.J.: Induction of mixed-function oxidases in mouse liver by psoralens, Ibid. *99*, pp. 687-692 (1978). 4. Pathak, M.A., Fitzpatrick, T.B., Parrish, J.A.: PSORIASIS, Proceedings of the Second International Symposium. Edited by E.M. Farber, A.J. Cox, Yorke Medical Books, pp. 262-265 (1977). 5. Dall'Acqua, F., Marciani, S., Ciavatta, L., Rodighiero, G.: Formation of interstrand cross-linkings in the photoreactions between furocoumarins and DNA; Z Naturforsch (B), *26*, pp. 561-569 (1971). 6. Cole, R.S.: Light-induced cross-linkings of DNA in the presence of a furocoumarin (psoralen), Biochem. Biophys. Acta, *217*, pp. 30-39 (1970). 7. Musajo, L, Rodighiero, G., Caporale, G., Dall'Acqua, F, Marciani, S., Bordin, F., Baccichetti, F., Bevilacqua, R.: Photoreactions between Skin-Photosentizing Furocoumarins and Nucleic Acids, *Sunlight and Man*; Normal and Abnormal Photobiologic Responses. Edited by M.A. Pathak, LC, Harber, M. Seiji et al. University of Tokyo Press, pp. 369-387 (1974). 8. Dall'Acqua, F., Vedaldi, D., Bordin, F., and Rodighiero, G.: New studies in the interaction between 8-methoxypsoralen and DNA in vitro: JID, *73*, pp. 191-197 (1979). 9. Yoshikawa, K., Mori, N., Sakakibara, S., Mizuno, N. Song. P.: Photo Conjugation of 8-methoxypsoralen with Proteins: Photochem. & Photobiol. *29*, pp. 1127-1133 (1979). 10. Ortonne, J.P.: MacDonald, D.M.: Micoud, A.: Thivolet, J.: PUVA-induced repigmentation of vitiligo: a histochemical (split-DOPA) and ultra-structural study: *Brit, J. Dermat., 101,* , pp. 1-12 (1979). 11. Hakim, R.D., Griffin, A.C.: Knox, J.M.: Erythema and tumor formation in methoxsalen treated mice exposed to fluorescent light; Arch. Dermatol. *82*, pp. 572-577 (1960). 12. O'Neal, M.A., Griffin, A.C.: The Effect of Oxypsoralen upon Ultraviolet Carcinogenesis in Albino Mice, Cancer Res., *17*, pp. 911-916 (1957). 13. Stern, R.S., Unpublished personal communication. 14. Stern, R.S., Parrish, J.A., Zierler, S.: Skin Carcinoma in Patients with Psoriasis Treated with Topical Tar and Artificial Ultraviolet Radiation. Lancet, *1*, pp. 732-735 (1980). 15. Stern, R.S., Laird, N., Melski, J. Parrish, J.A., Fitzpatrick, T.B., Bleich, H.L.: Cutaneous Squamous-Cell Carcinoma in Patients Treated with PUVA: NEJM, *310*, No. 18, pp. 1156-1161 (1984). 16. Roenigk, Jr., H.H., and 12 Cooperating Investigators: Skin Cancer in the PUVA-48 Cooperative Study of Psoriasis. Program for Forty-First Annual Meeting for The Society of Investigative Dermatology, Inc., Sheraton Washington Hotel, Washington, D.C., May 12, 13, and 14, 1980. Abstracts JID, *74*, No. 4, p. 250 (April, 1980). 17. Mosher, D.B., Pathak, M.A., Harris, T.J., Fitzpatrick, T.B.: Development of Cutaneous Lesions in Vitiligo During Long-Term PUVA Therapy. Program for Forty-First Annual Meeting for the Society for Investigative Dermatology, Inc., Sheraton Washington Hotel, Washington, D.C., May 12, 13, and 14, 1980. Abstracts JID, *74*, No. 4, p 259 (April, 1980). 18. Cloud, TM. Hakim, R., Griffin, A.C.: Photosensitization of the eye with methoxsalen. I. Acute effects: Arch. Ophthalmol, *64*, pp. 346-352 (1960). 19. Cloud, T.M. Hakim, R., Griffin, A.C.: Photosensitization of the eye with methoxsalen. II. Chronic effects, Ibid. *66*, pp. 689-694 (1961). 20. Freeman, R.G., Troll, D.: Photosensitization of the eye by 8-methoxypsoralen, JID, *53*, p. 449-453 (1969). 21. Lerman, S., Megaw, J., Willis, I.: Potential ocular complications from PUVA therapy and their prevention; JID, *74*, pp. 197-199 (1980). 22. Diffey, B.L., Medical Physics Handbook 11, Ultraviolet Radiation in Medicine, Adam Hilger, Ltd., Bristol, p. 86 (1982). 23. Lerner, A.B.; Denton, C.R.: Fitzpatrick, T.B.: Clinical and experimental studies with 8-methoxypsoralen in vitiligo; J. Invest, Derm., 20, pp. 299-314 (April, 1953). 24. Fitzpatrick, T.B.; Arndt, K.A.: El Mofty, A.M.: Hydroquinone and psoralens in the therapy of hypermelanosis and vitiligo: Arch Derm., 93, pp. 589-599 (May, 1966). 25. Fulton, James F.; Leyden, James; Papa, Christopher: Treatment of vitiligo with topical methoxsalen and blacklite; Arch, Derm., 101, pp. 224-229 (1969).
Rev. Jan., 1990.

HOW SUPPLIED
CAPSULE: 10 MG

BRAND/MANUFACTURER	NDC	SIZE	AWP
BRAND			
8-MOP: ICN	00187-0651-42	50s	$169.00
OXSORALEN-ULTRA: ICN	00187-0650-42	50s	$202.80

LOTION:

BRAND/MANUFACTURER	NDC	SIZE	AWP
BRAND			
OXSORALEN: ICN	00187-0402-31	30 ml	$81.90

Methoxyflurane

DESCRIPTION
Methoxyflurane, a volatile liquid, is intended only for vaporization at suitable concentrations for administration by inhalation with appropriate anesthesia equipment or devices.

Methoxyflurane is an inhalation anesthetic/analgesic which belongs to the fluorinated hydrocarbon group of volatile anesthetics. It is chemically designated 2,2-dichloro-1, 1-difluoroethyl methyl ether.

Methoxyflurane has a mildly pungent odor.
Some of the physical constants are:

Molecular weight 164.97
Boiling point at 760 mm Hg .... 104.6°C
Partition coefficients at 37°C
  Water/gas 4.5

Blood/gas (mean range) ....10.20 to 14.06
Oil/gas 825
Vapor Pressure 17.7°C ....20 mm Hg
Flash points
  in air ....62.8°C
  in oxygen (closed system) ....32.8°C
  in nitrous oxide 50% with 50% oxygen ....28.2°C
Lower limits of flammability of vapor concentration
  in air 7.0%
  in oxygen 5.4%
  in N₂O 50% 4.6%

Methoxyflurane is stable and does not decompose in contact with soda lime. An antioxidant, butylated hydroxytoluene 0.01% w/w is added to insure stability on standing. This slowly oxidizes to a yellow pigment that progressively turns to brown, and which may accumulate on the vaporizer wick. The colored matter may be removed by rinsing the wick with diethyl ether. The wick must be dried after cleaning to avoid introducing diethyl ether into the system.

Polyvinyl chloride plastics are extracted by Methoxyflurane, therefore, contact should be avoided. Methoxyflurane does not extract polyethylene plastics, polypropylene plastics, fluorinated hydrocarbon plastics or nylon. It is very soluble in rubber and soda lime. Disposable conductive plastic circuits should be discarded after a single use to avoid cross contamination and because Methoxyflurane may reduce conductivity of such materials below safe limits for subsequent administration of a flammable anesthetic.

The vapor concentration of Methoxyflurane is limited by its vapor pressure at room temperature to a maximum of about 3.5% at 23°C. In practice, this concentration is not easily reached due to the cooling effect of vaporization. Methoxyflurane is not flammable except at vapor concentrations well above those recommended for its use. Recommended concentrations are nonflammable and nonexplosive in air, oxygen and nitrous oxide mixtures at ordinary room temperature.

CLINICAL PHARMACOLOGY

Methoxyflurane provides anesthesia and/or analgesia.

After surgical anesthesia with Methoxyflurane, analgesia and drowsiness may persist after consciousness has returned. This may obviate or reduce the need for narcotics in the immediate postoperative period.

When used alone in safe concentration, Methoxyflurane, will not produce appreciable skeletal muscle relaxation. A muscle relaxing agent, e.g., succinylcholine chloride or tubocurarine chloride should be used as an adjunct.

Bronchiolar constriction or laryngeal spasm is not ordinarily provoked by Methoxyflurane.

During Methoxyflurane anesthesia, the cardiac rhythm is usually regular. The myocardium is only minimally sensitized by Methoxyflurane to epinephrine. Some decrease in blood pressure often accompanies light planes of anesthesia. This may be accompanied by bradycardia. The hypotension noted is accompanied by reduced cardiac contractile force and reduced cardiac output.

When used for obstetrical delivery, light planes of Methoxyflurane anesthesia have little effect on uterine contractions. There are no known contraindications to the concomitant use of Methoxyflurane and oxytocic agents.

Biotransformation of Methoxyflurane occurs in man. Approximately 20% of Methoxyflurane uptake is recovered in the exhaled air, while urinary excretion of organic fluorine, fluoride and oxalic acid accounts for about 30% of the Methoxyflurane uptake.

Studies have shown that higher peak blood fluoride levels are obtained earlier in obese patients than in nonobese.

INDICATIONS AND USAGE

1. Methoxyflurane is indicated usually in combination with oxygen and nitrous oxide to provide anesthesia for surgical procedures in which total duration of Methoxyflurane administration is anticipated to be 4 hours or less, and in which Methoxyflurane is not to be used in concentrations that will provide skeletal muscle relaxation; see "Warnings" regarding time and dose relationships.

2. Methoxyflurane, may be used alone with hand held inhalers or in combination with oxygen and nitrous oxide for analgesia in obstetrics and in minor surgical procedures.

CONTRAINDICATIONS

See "Warnings."

WARNINGS

SEQUENTIAL ANESTHESIA WITH METHOXYFLURANE AND HALOTHANE, OR HALOTHANE AND METHOXYFLURANE, IN EITHER ORDER, HAS BEEN FOLLOWED BY JAUNDICE IN A FEW RARE CASES. WHEN A PREVIOUS EXPOSURE TO METHOXYFLURANE, OR HALOTHANE HAS BEEN FOLLOWED BY UNEXPLAINED HEPATIC DYSFUNCTION AND/OR JAUNDICE, CONSIDERATION SHOULD BE GIVEN TO THE USE OF OTHER AGENTS.

THE NEPHROTOXICITY ASSOCIATED WITH METHOXYFLURANE ADMINISTRATION APPEARS TO BE RELATED TO THE TOTAL DOSE (TIME AND CONCENTRATION). SEE PARAGRAPH 5. THE MANIFESTATIONS RANGE IN SEVERITY FROM REVERSIBLE ALTERATIONS IN LABORATORY FINDINGS TO POLYURIC OR OLIGURIC RENAL FAILURE, SOMETIMES FATAL.

POLYURIC RENAL FAILURE IS CHARACTERIZED BY THE DEVELOPMENT, EARLY IN THE POSTOPERATIVE PERIOD, OF THE FOLLOWING:

WEIGHT LOSS
URINE: LOW SPECIFIC GRAVITY, LARGE VOLUME EQUAL TO OR IN EXCESS OF FLUID INTAKE, DECREASED OSMOLALITY.
SERUM/BLOOD: ELEVATION OF SODIUM, CHLORIDE, URIC ACID, BUN, CREATININE.

THIS SYNDROME IS BELIEVED TO BE RELATED TO RELEASE OF THE FLUORIDE ION, A METABOLIC PRODUCT OF PENTHRANE AND TO BE RELATED TO THE TOTAL DOSAGE ADMINISTERED. THEREFORE, THE LOWEST EFFECTIVE DOSAGE SHOULD BE ADMINISTERED, ESPECIALLY IN AGED OR OBESE PATIENTS AND IN SURGICAL PROCEDURES OF LONG DURATION, BEARING IN MIND THAT THE TOTAL DOSE DELIVERED TO THE PATIENT IS A FACTOR OF DURATION OF ADMINISTRATION AND CONCENTRATION OF VAPOR.

OXALATE CRYSTALS AND/OR ACUTE TUBULAR NECROSIS HAVE BEEN NOTED AT AUTOPSY.

The guiding principles in minimizing the possibility of renal injury are:

1. AVOID USING METHOXYFLURANE AS THE SOLE OR PRINCIPAL AGENT TO ACHIEVE MUSCULAR RELAXATION.

2. PATIENTS WITH PRE-EXISTING RENAL DISEASE, IMPAIRMENT OF RENAL FUNCTION, TOXEMIA OF PREGNANCY, AND PATIENTS UNDERGOING VASCULAR SURGERY AT OR NEAR THE RENAL VESSELS SHOULD NOT RECEIVE METHOXYFLURANE UNLESS IN THE JUDGMENT OF THE PHYSICIAN THE BENEFITS OUTWEIGH THE INCREASED RISK OF NEPHROTOXIC EFFECT.

3. URINARY OUTPUT SHOULD BE MONITORED IN ALL PATIENTS IF EXCESSIVE URINE OUTPUT OCCURS, APPROPRIATE LABORATORY STUDIES SHOULD BE DONE TO ASSESS RENAL FUNCTION. IN HIGH RISK PATIENTS (SEE 2, ABOVE) SERIAL TESTS OF RENAL FUNCTION AND MEASUREMENTS OF FLUID AND ELECTROLYTE BALANCE ARE IMPERATIVE. ALL FLUID AND ELECTROLYTE LOSSES SHOULD BE PROMPTLY REPLACED.

4. THE CONCURRENT USE OF TETRACYCLINE AND METHOXYFLURANE HAS BEEN REPORTED TO RESULT IN FATAL RENAL TOXICITY. THE POSSIBILITY EXISTS THAT METHOXYFLURANE MAY ENHANCE THE ADVERSE RENAL EFFECTS OF OTHER DRUGS INCLUDING CERTAIN ANTIBIOTICS OF KNOWN NEPHROTOXIC POTENTIAL SUCH AS GENTAMICIN, KANAMYCIN, COLISTIN, POLYMYXIN B, CEPHALORIDINE AND AMPHOTERICIN B. THIS SHOULD BE CAREFULLY CONSIDERED WHEN PRESCRIBING SUCH DRUGS DURING THE PREOPERATIVE, OPERATIVE AND POSTOPERATIVE PERIODS.

5. BECAUSE OF THE DOSE-RELATED NEPHROTOXICITY POTENTIAL OF METHOXYFLURANE IT IS SUGGESTED THAT THE TOTAL DURATION OF LIGHT ANESTHETIC DEPTH WITH METHOXYFLURANE NOT EXCEED APPROXIMATELY 4 HOURS AT A SINGLE ADMINISTRATION.

PRECAUTIONS

Diabetic patients may have an increased likelihood of developing nephropathy if they have impaired renal function or polyuria, are obese, or are not optimally controlled.

Caution should be exercised in using Methoxyflurane in patients under treatment with enzyme inducing drugs (e.g., barbiturates) as such agents may enhance the metabolism of Methoxyflurane resulting in increased fluoride levels.

Ventilation should be assessed carefully and, if depressed, should be augmented to insure adequate oxygenation and carbon dioxide removal. Parenteral anesthetic adjuncts (e.g., barbiturates, narcotics and neuromuscular blocking agents) may also cause depression of respiration requiring assisted or controlled ventilation. A sufficient reduction in respiratory minute volume occurs during deep anesthesia to produce a significant respiratory acidosis if ventilation is not adequately assisted. Methoxyflurane causes a slight metabolic acidosis.

Methoxyflurane augments the effect of nondepolarizing muscle relaxants so that their usual dosage should be reduced by approximately one-half.

Epinephrine or levarterenol (norepinephrine) should be employed cautiously during Methoxyflurane anesthesia.

When Methoxyflurane is used under the conditions of dosage and administration shown below, in surgery or obstetrics, inorganic fluoride levels may infrequently reach those at which changes in renal laboratory values have been seen.

General anesthesia, including general anesthesia with Methoxyflurane has been associated in susceptible individuals with the acute onset of fulminant hypermetabolism of skeletal muscle known as *malignant hyperthermic crisis*. This syndrome is characterized by the acute onset of skeletal muscle overactivity and resulting high oxygen demand which usually exceeds supply. *Tachycardia* and *Tachypnea* are the most important early signs; these may be associated with increased utilization of anesthesia circuit carbon dioxide absorber, arrhythmias, cyanosis, skin mottling, profuse sweating, unstable blood pressure, rapidly rising body temperature (usually appearing sometime after the first signs, when noted) and other indications of markedly increased oxygen demand. Laboratory tests usually confirm the excessive oxygen demand and resulting metabolic acidosis (blood gases); hyperkalemia and myoglobinemia are also frequently noted. Hypoglobinuria and renal failure may develop later. When these signs suggests a diagnosis of malignant hyperthermic crisis, it is important to terminate the anesthetic, cancel the surgery when possible, confirm the diagnosis and initiate management of the condition.

◆ RATED THERAPEUTICALLY EQUIVALENT; ◇ THERAPEUTIC EQUIVALENCE UNCONFIRMED; ○ UNRATED

Dantrolene sodium intravenous is indicated, along with supportive measures, in the management of malignant hyperthermic crisis. These necessary supportive measures must be individualized, but will usually involve discontinuance of the suspect triggering agents, attendance to increased oxygen requirements and carbon dioxide production, management of metabolic acidosis, assurance of adequate urinary output, management of electrolyte imbalance and institution of measures to control rising temperature, when indicated. Consult literature references and the prescribing information for dantrolene sodium intravenous for additional information about the management of malignant hyperthermic crisis.

INFORMATION FOR PATIENTS
When appropriate, as in some cases where discharge is anticipated soon after Methoxyflurane anesthesia, patients should be cautioned not to drive an automobile, operate hazardous machinery or engage in hazardous sports for 24 hours or more (depending upon total dosage of Methoxyflurane, condition of the patient and consideration given to other drugs administered) after anesthesia.

CARCINOGENESIS, MUTAGENESIS, IMPAIRMENT OF FERTILITY
A 15 month transplacental inhalation study of Methoxyflurane at a subanesthetic concentration of 0.13% in the mouse revealed no evidence of anesthetic-related carcinogenesis. This concentration is equivalent to 36 hours of 0.2% Methoxyflurane.

Mutagenesis testing of Methoxyflurane was negative. Tests included: Ames bacterial assay, mouse sperm morphology assay and sister chromatid exchange in Chinese hamster ovary cells.

Studies of the effect on fertility have not been reported.

Pregnancy Category C: Methoxyflurane has been shown to cause fetal growth retardation in the rat at levels equivalent to 67 hours exposure of 0.2% Methoxyflurane. There are no adequate and well-controlled studies in pregnant women. Methoxyflurane should be used during pregnancy only if the potential benefit justifies the potential risk to the fetus.

Nursing Mothers: Caution should be exercised when Methoxyflurane is administered to a nursing mother.

Labor and Delivery: In obstetrics attention should be given to the directions for *Dosage and Administration* shown below. Fluoride levels in cord blood are usually less than, but may equal those of the mother at delivery. The effect of inorganic fluoride on the infant is not known. However, clinical experience has demonstrated that cases of high output renal failure in either mother or child must be considered unlikely.

Pediatric Use: Safety and effectiveness of Methoxyflurane in children have not been established.

ADVERSE REACTIONS
Renal Dysfunction: See "Warnings."

Hepatic dysfunction, jaundice, and fatal hepatic necrosis have occurred following Methoxyflurane anesthesia. Also as with other anesthetics, transient alterations in liver function tests may follow Methoxyflurane administration. Hepatic complications rarely have involved reported cross reactions between Methoxyflurane and Halothane.

Some patients exhibit pallor during recovery from Methoxyflurane anesthesia.

Other adverse reactions which have been reported include cardiac arrest, malignant hyperpyrexia, prolonged postoperative somnolence, respiratory depression laryngospasm, bronchospasm, nausea, vomiting postoperative headache, hypotension and emergence delirium.

OVERDOSAGE
Patients should be closely observed for signs of excessive dosage during administration of Methoxyflurane. Methoxyflurane overdosage is characterized by decrease in tidal and minute volume; decrease in blood pressure, pallor, cyanosis and muscle relaxation. If the above signs are observed, turn off vaporizer and increase ventilation. If anesthesia exceeds light levels, vapor concentration should be reduced promptly. Prolonged administration (beyond four hours) and/or excessive vapor concentration beyond the equivalent of four hours of 0.25% delivered Methoxyflurane may cause nephrotoxic effects attributable to metabolic release of free fluoride ion. See "Warnings," "Precautions" and "Dosage and Administration."

In the event of postoperative excessive urine output, fluid and electrolyte losses should be promptly replaced.

DOSAGE AND ADMINISTRATION
THE LOWEST EFFECTIVE DOSAGE OF METHOXYFLURANE SHOULD BE USED IN ORDER TO MINIMIZE THE POSSIBILITY OF NEPHROPATHY AND TO ALLOW FOR OPTIMAL RECOVERY TIME. IN CASES OF UNUSUALLY HIGH MAINTENANCE REQUIREMENTS, THE USE OF ANESTHETIC ADJUNCTS OR ANOTHER AGENT MAY BE INDICATED. THE ABSENCE OF HYPOTENSION CANNOT BE RELIED UPON AS EVIDENCE THAT DOSAGE HAS NOT BEEN EXCESSIVE DURING MAINTENANCE.

ANALGESIA
For analgesia, intermittent inhalation of vapor concentrations in the range of 0.3 to 0.8% are recommended. Methoxyflurane may be self administered by hand-held inhalers (e.g., Analgizer, Cyprane) if the patient is kept under close observation.

For intermittent administration from the hand-held inhaler, dosage for each patient is limited to not more than a single 15 ml charge of liquid Methoxyflurane. Such analgesia in labor should not be instituted before relief becomes necessary.

Use of the hand-held inhaler does not preclude transfer of the patient to a conventional anesthesia machine for inhalation anesthesia, but concentrations should be kept at the lowest effective dosage. Total time for anesthesia combined with analgesia should be as short as possible, bearing in mind the recommended duration for continuous anesthesia (four hours).

ANESTHESIA
A light level of anesthesia should be used. The use of deeper levels to achieve muscle relaxation should be avoided.

Apparatus: Methoxyflurane should be vaporized by calibrated, temperature compensated, out of circle vaporizers (e.g., Pentec II, Pentomatic) or other methods which provide accurate delivered vapor concentration. Anesthetic uptake by rubber tubing, bags and soda lime which may prolong induction and recovery time can be reduced by the use of nonabsorptive plastic circuit material (not polyvinyl chloride) and fresh moist Baralyme. The fresh gas inlet should be located downstream of the CO_2 absorber in order to avoid excessive anesthetic absorption, and the rebreathing bag and pop-off valve should be located on the expiratory side.

Premedication: The usual preanesthetic medications may be administered prior to Methoxyflurane, anesthesia, see "Precautions."

Induction: Use of a parenteral induction agent (such as an ultrashort acting barbiturate) is recommended unless contraindicated in an individual patient.

Carrier Gases: For general surgery, Methoxyflurane should usually be administered with a carrier gas flow consisting of oxygen and at least 50% nitrous oxide in order to minimize the total Methoxyflurane dose unless nitrous oxide is contraindicated.

Muscle Relaxation: Methoxyflurane should not be administered at levels required to achieve muscle relaxation. Adequate relaxation should be obtained from adjunctive use of a muscle relaxant, e.g., succinylcholine chloride or tubocurarine chloride. The usual dosage of nondepolarizing muscle relaxants should be reduced by approximately one-half.

Vapor Concentrations: Initially Methoxyflurane concentrations may be increased as tolerated to a maximum of approximately 2.0%. This concentration should only be continued for about two to five minutes, or until patient signs of light anesthesia are evident. The concentration of Methoxyflurane should then be reduced by frequent decrements to the lowest possible levels consistent with the maintenance of adequate anesthesia. For example, in a 70 kg patient, the following sequential reduction in the delivered vapor concentration of Methoxyflurane may be appropriate:

Elapsed Minutes	0 to 5	5 to 20	20 to 60	60 to 120	120 to 240
Vapor Conc.*	2.0%	0.6%	0.4%	0.2%	0.1%

* *Concentrations are approximate and subject to adjustment according to patient signs of anesthesia. Based on 5 liters per minute gas flow and ventilation rate throughout procedure, 50/50 N_2O and oxygen.*

Concentration may be increased or decreased according to the requirements of the individual patient. Four hours of 0.25% delivered Methoxyflurane should not be exceeded in normal adult patients unless in the opinion of the clinician, the anticipated benefits outweigh the increase risk of dose related nephrotoxicity. The product of these two factors (four hours of 0.25% delivered Methoxyflurane) may be used to estimate other combinations of time and dose: Thus two hours of 0.5%, for example, should not ordinarily be exceeded. In sufficiently long cases, Methoxyflurane should be discontinued 30 to 40 minutes before the end of surgery. Rapid flushing will not remove Methoxyflurane absorbed by rubber circuit components.

Patient signs and levels: The Methoxyflurane level of conscious analgesia is suited for pain relief, as in labor and uncomplicated vaginal deliveries. The level of unconscious analgesia is suitable for many minor surgical procedures. The level of light anesthesia is recommended for general surgical use. Deep anesthesia with Methoxyflurane is not recommended.

Appropriate patient signs of Methoxyflurane anesthesia should be observed closely as a guide to proper depth. A blood pressure decrease of about 22 mm Hg may be seen during induction. A greater decrease may occur in hypertensive patients. Blood pressure usually recovers as a level of light anesthesia is reached. The absence of hypotension cannot be relied upon as evidence that dosage has not been excessive during maintenance.

Storage: Preserve in tight, light-resistant containers and avoid exposure to excessive heat.

Protect from light. Protect from freezing and extreme heat.

HOW SUPPLIED
SOLUTION:

BRAND/MANUFACTURER	NDC	SIZE	AWP
○ **BRAND**			
PENTHRANE: Abbott Hosp	00074-6864-03	125 ml 4s	$2049.72
	00074-6864-08	15 ml 20s	$1643.74

➤ SHOWN IN PRODUCT IDENTIFICATION GUIDE

Methscopolamine Bromide

DESCRIPTION

Methscopolamine Bromide, an anticholinergic, occurs as white crystals, or as a white odorless crystalline powder. Methscopolamine Bromide melts at about 225° with decomposition. The drug is freely soluble in water, slightly soluble in alcohol, and insoluble in acetone and in chloroform.

The chemical name for Methscopolamine Bromide is 3-Oxa-9-azoniatricyclo [$3.3.1.0^{2,4}$]nonane, 7-(3-hydroxy-1-oxo-2-phenylpropoxy)-9, 9-dimethyl-, bromide, [7(S)-(1α, 2β, 4β 5α, 7β)]-and the molecular weight is 389.30.

Each Methscopolamine Bromide tablet for oral administration contains 2.5 mg of Methscopolamine Bromide.

Following is its chemical structure:

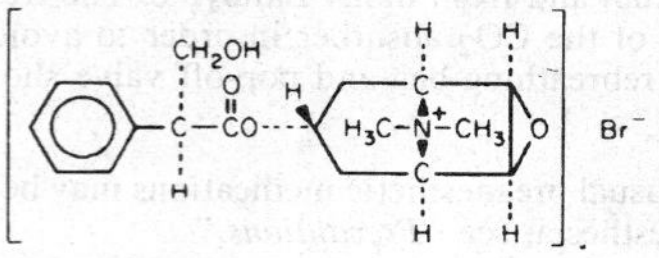

CLINICAL PHARMACOLOGY

Methscopolamine Bromide is an anticholergic agent which possesses most of the pharmacologic actions of that drug class. These include reduction in volume and total acid content of gastric secretion, inhibition of gastrointestinal motility, inhibition of salivary excretion, dilation of the pupil and inhibition of accommodation with resulting blurring of vision. Large doses may result in tachycardia.

PHARMACOKINETICS

Methscopolamine Bromide is a quaternary ammonium derivative of scopolamine. As a class, these agents are poorly and unreliably absorbed.[1,2] Total absorption of quaternary ammonium derivatives of the alkaloids is 10-25%. Rate of absorption is not available. Quaternary ammonium salts have limited absorption from intact skin, and conjunctival penetration is poor.[1] Little is known of the fate and excretion of most of these agents.[1] Following oral administration, drug effects appear in about one hour and persist for 4 to 6 hours.[2] Methscopolamine Bromide has limited ability to cross the blood-brain-barrier.[3,4,5] The drug is excreted primarily in the urine and bile, or as unabsorbed drug in feces.[2] There is no data on the presence of Methscopolamine in breast milk; traces of atropine have been found after administration of atropine.[1]

INDICATIONS AND USAGE

Adjunctive therapy for the treatment of peptic ulcer.

METHSCOPOLAMINE BROMIDE HAS NOT BEEN SHOWN TO BE EFFECTIVE IN CONTRIBUTING TO THE HEALING OF PEPTIC ULCER, DECREASING THE RATE OF RECURRENCE OR PREVENTING COMPLICATIONS.

CONTRAINDICATIONS

Glaucoma; obstructive uropathy (eg, bladder neck obstruction due to prostatic hypertrophy); obstructive disease of the gastrointestinal tract (eg, pyloroduodenal stenosis); paralytic ileus; intestinal atony of the elderly or debilitated patient; unstable cardiovascular status in acute hemorrhage; severe ulcerative colitis; toxic megacolon complicating ulcerative colitis; myasthenia gravis.

Methscopolamine Bromide is contraindicated in patients who are hypersensitive to it or related drugs.

WARNINGS

In the presence of high environmental temperature, heat prostration (fever and heat stroke due to decreased sweating) can occur with drug use.

Diarrhea may be an early symptom of incomplete intestinal obstruction, especially in patients with ileostomy or colostomy. In this instance treatment with this drug would be inappropriate and possibly harmful.

Methscopolamine Bromide may produce drowsiness or blurred vision. The patient should be cautioned regarding activities requiring mental alertness such as operating a motor vehicle or other machinery or performing hazardous work while taking this drug.

With overdosage, a curare-like action may occur, ie, neuromuscular blockade leading to muscular weakness and possible paralysis.

PRECAUTIONS

1. GENERAL PRECAUTIONS

Use Methscopolamine Bromide Tablets with caution in the elderly and in all patients with: autonomic neuropathy; hepatic or renal disease; or ulcerative colitis—large doses may suppress intestinal motility to the point of producing a paralytic ileus and for this reason precipitate or aggravate "toxic megacolon", a serious complication of the disease.

The drug should also be used with caution in patients having hyperthyroidism, coronary heart disease, congestive heart failure, tachyrhythmia, tachycardia, hypertension, or prostatic hypertrophy.

2. INFORMATION FOR PATIENT

See statement under "Warnings".

3. LABORATORY TESTS

Progress of the peptic ulcer under treatment should be followed by upper gastrointestinal contrast radiology or endoscopy to insure healing. Stool tests for occult blood and blood hemoglobin or hematocrit values should be followed to rule out bleeding from the ulcer.

4. CARCINOGENESIS, MUTAGENESIS, IMPAIRMENT OF FERTILITY

No long-term studies in animals have been performed to evaluate carcinogenic potential.

5. PREGNANCY

Teratogenic Effects: Pregnancy Category C. Animal reproduction studies have not been conducted with Methscopolamine Bromide. It is also not known whether Methscopolamine Bromide can cause fetal harm when administered to a pregnant woman or can affect reproduction capacity. Methscopolamine Bromide should be given to a pregnant woman only if clearly needed.

6. NURSING MOTHERS

It is not known whether this drug is excreted in human milk. Because many drugs are excreted in human milk, caution should be exercised when Methscopolamine Bromide is administered to a nursing woman.

Anticholinergic drugs may suppress lactation.

7. PEDIATRIC USE

Safety and efficacy in children have not been established.

8. DRUG INTERACTIONS

Additive anticholinergic effects may result from concomitant use with antipsychotics, tricyclic antidepressants, and other drugs with anticholinergic effects. Concomitant administration with antacids may interfere with the absorption of Methscopolamine Bromide.

ADVERSE REACTIONS

The following adverse reactions have been observed, but there are not enough data to support an estimate of frequency.

Cardiovascular: Tachycardia, palpitation.

Allergic: Severe allergic reaction or drug idiosyncrasies including anaphylaxis.

CNS: Headaches, nervousness, mental confusion, drowsiness, dizziness.

Special Senses: Blurred vision, dilatation of the pupil, cycloplegia, increased ocular tension, loss of taste.

Renal: Urinary hesitancy and retention.

Gastrointestinal: Nausea, vomiting, constipation, bloated feeling.

Dermatologic: Decreased sweating, urticaria and other dermal manifestations.

Miscellaneous: Xerostomia, weakness, insomnia, impotence, suppression of lactation.

DRUG ABUSE AND DEPENDENCE

Not applicable.

OVERDOSAGE

The symptoms of overdosage with Methscopolamine Bromide Tablets progress from intensification of the usual side effects to CNS disturbances (from restlessness and excitement to psychotic behavior), circulatory changes (flushing, fall in blood pressure, circulatory failure), respiratory failure, paralysis, and coma.

Measures to be taken are (1) induction of emesis and (2) injection of physostigmine 0.5 to 2 mg intravenously, and repeated as necessary up to a total of 5 mg. Fever may be treated symptomatically (alcohol sponging, ice packs). Excitement of a degree which demands attention may be managed with sodium thiopental 2% solution given slowly intravenously or chloral hydrate (100-200 mL of a 2% solution) by rectal infusion. In the event of progression of the curare-like effect to paralysis of the respiratory muscles, artificial respiration should be instituted and maintained until effective respiratory action returns.

The oral LD_{50} in rats is 1,352 to 2,617 mg/kg.

No data is available on the dialyzability of Methscopolamine.

DOSAGE AND ADMINISTRATION

The average dosage of Methscopolamine Bromide Tablets is 2.5 mg one-half hour before meals and 2.5 to 5 mg at bedtime. A starting dose of 12.5 mg daily will be clinically effective in most patients without the production of appreciable side effects.

Patients whose dosage has been reduced to eliminate or modify side effects often continue to show adequate response both subjectively in relief of symptoms and objectively as measured by antisecretory effects.

If the patient is having severe symptoms which demand prompt relief, the drug may be started on a daily dosage of 20 mg, administered in doses of 5 mg one-half hour before meals and at bedtime. If very unpleasant side effects develop promptly, the daily dosage should be reduced. If neither symptomatic relief nor side effects appear, the daily dosage may be increased. Some patients have tolerated 30 mg daily with no unpleasant reactions.

The ultimate aim of therapy is to arrive at a dosage which provides maximal clinical effectiveness with a minimum of unpleasant side effects. Many patients report no side effects on a dosage which gives complete relief of symptoms. On the other hand, some patients have reported severe side effects without appreciable symptomatic relief. Such patients must be considered unsuited for this therapy. Usually they have been or will prove to be similarly intolerant to other

---

◆ RATED THERAPEUTICALLY EQUIVALENT; ◇ THERAPEUTIC EQUIVALENCE UNCONFIRMED; ○ UNRATED

anticholinergic drugs. If Methscopolamine Bromide is to be used in a patient who gives a history of such intolerance, it should be started at a low dosage.

Store at controlled room temperature 15°—30° C (59°—86° F).

REFERENCES

1. *The Pharmacological Basis of Therapeutics*, Gilman and Goodman, MacMillan Publ. Co., New York, 6th Ed., 1980. 2. *American Hospital Formulary Service*, American Society of Hospital Pharmacists, Bethesda, Maryland. 3. Domino, E.F., Corasen, G.: Central and Peripheral Effects of Muscarinic Cholinergic Blocking Agents in Man. *Anesthesiology* 28:568-574 (1967). 4. Mogensen, L. and Orinius, E.: Arrhythmic Complications after Parasympathetic Treatment of Bradyarrhythmias in a Coronary Care Unit, *Acta Med. Scand.* 190:495-498 (1971). 5. Neeld, J.B., Jr., et al: Cardiac Rate and Rhythm Changes with Atropine and Methscopolamine, *Clin. Pharmacol. Ther.* 17(3):290-295 (March) 1975.

HOW SUPPLIED

TABLETS: 2.5 MG

BRAND/MANUFACTURER	NDC	SIZE	AWP
◆ BRAND PAMINE: Kenwood	00482-0061-01	100s	$26.29

Methsuximide

DESCRIPTION

Methsuximide is an anticonvulsant succinimide, chemically designated as N,2-Dimethyl-2-phenylsuccinimide.

Each Methsuximide capsule contains 150 mg or 300 mg Methsuximide, USP.

Following is its chemical structure:

ACTION

Methsuximide suppresses the paroxysmal three-cycle-per-second spike and wave activity associated with lapses of consciousness which is common in absence (petit mal) seizures. The frequency of epileptiform attacks is reduced, apparently by depression of the motor cortex and elevation of the threshold of the central nervous system to convulsive stimuli.

INDICATION

Methsuximide is indicated for the control of absence (petit mal) seizures that are refractory to other drugs.

CONTRAINDICATION

Methsuximide should not be used in patients with a history of hypersensitivity to succinimides.

WARNINGS

Blood dyscrasias, including some with fatal outcome, have been reported to be associated with the use of succinimides; therefore, periodic blood counts should be performed. Should signs and/or symptoms of infection (eg sore throat, fever) develop, blood counts should be considered at that point.

It has been reported that succinimides have produced morphological and functional changes in animal liver. For this reason, Methsuximide should be administered with extreme caution to patients with known liver or renal disease. Periodic urinalysis and liver function studies are advised for all patients receiving the drug.

Cases of systemic lupus erythematosus have been reported with the use of succinimides. The physician should be alert to this possibility.

USAGE IN PREGNANCY

The effects of Methsuximide in human pregnancy and nursing infants are unknown.

Recent reports suggest an association between the use of anticonvulsant drugs by women with epilepsy and an elevated incidence of birth defects in children born to these women. Data are more extensive with respect to phenytoin and phenobarbital, but these are also the most commonly prescribed anticonvulsants; less systematic or anecdotal reports suggest a possible similar association with the use of all known anticonvulsant drugs.

The reports suggesting an elevated incidence of birth defects in children of drug-treated epileptic women cannot be regarded as adequate to prove a definite cause-and-effect relationship. There are intrinsic methodologic problems in obtaining adequate data on drug teratogenicity in humans; the possibility also exists that other factors, eg, genetic factors or the epileptic condition itself, may be more important than drug therapy in leading to birth defects. The great majority of mothers on anticonvulsant medication deliver normal infants. It is important to note that anticonvulsant drugs should not be discontinued in patients in whom the drug is administered to prevent major seizures because of the strong possibility of precipitating status epilepticus with attendant hypoxia and threat to life. In individual cases where the severity and frequency of the seizure disorder are such that the removal of medication does not pose a serious threat to the patient, discontinuation of the drug may be considered prior to and during pregnancy, although it cannot be said with any confidence that even minor seizures do not pose some hazard to the developing embryo or fetus.

The prescribing physician will wish to weigh these considerations in treating or counseling epileptic women of childbearing potential.

Hazardous Activities: Methsuximide may impair the mental and/or physical abilities required for the performance of potentially hazardous tasks, such as driving a motor vehicle or other such activity requiring alertness; therefore, the patient should be cautioned accordingly.

PRECAUTIONS

GENERAL

It is recommended that the physician withdraw the drug slowly on the appearance of unusual depression, aggressiveness, or other behavioral alterations.

As with other anticonvulsants, it is important to proceed slowly when increasing or decreasing dosage, as well as when adding or eliminating other medication. Abrupt withdrawal of anticonvulsant medication may precipitate absence (petit mal) status.

Methsuximide, when used alone in mixed types of epilepsy, may increase the frequency of grand mal seizures in some patients.

INFORMATION FOR PATIENTS

Methsuximide may impair the mental and/or physical abilities required for the performance of potentially hazardous tasks, such as driving a motor vehicle or other such activity requiring alertness, therefore, the patient should be cautioned accordingly.

Patients taking Methsuximide should be advised of the importance of adhering strictly to the prescribed dosage regimen.

Patients should be instructed to promptly contact their physician if they develop signs and/or symptoms suggesting an infection (eg sore throat, fever).

ADVICE TO THE PHARMACIST AND PATIENT

Since Methsuximide has a relatively low melting temperature (124°F), storage conditions which may promote high temperatures (closed cars, delivery vans, or storage near steam pipes) should be avoided. Do not dispense or use capsules that are not full or in which contents have melted. Effectiveness may be reduced. Protect from excessive heat (104°F).

DRUG INTERACTIONS

Since Methsuximide may interact with concurrently administered antiepileptic drugs, periodic serum level determinations of these drugs may be necessary (eg Methsuximide may increase the plasma concentrations of phenytoin and phenobarbital).

PREGNANCY

See *"Warnings."*

ADVERSE REACTIONS

Gastrointestinal System: Gastrointestinal symptoms occur frequently and have included nausea or vomiting, anorexia, diarrhea, weight loss, epigastric and abdominal pain, and constipation.

Hemopoietic System: Hemopoietic complications associated with the administration of Methsuximide have included eosinophilia, leukopenia, monocytosis, and pancytopenia.

Nervous System: Neurologic and sensory reactions reported during therapy with Methsuximide have included drowsiness, ataxia or dizziness, irritability and nervousness, headache, blurred vision, photophobia, hiccups, and insomnia. Drowsiness, ataxia, and dizziness have been the most frequent side effects noted. Psychologic abnormalities have included confusion, instability, mental slowness, depression, hypochondriacal behavior, and aggressiveness. There have been rare reports of psychosis, suicidal behavior, and auditory hallucinations.

Integumentary System: Dermatologic manifestations which have occurred with the administration of Methsuximide have included urticaria, Stevens-Johnson syndrome, and pruritic erythematous rashes.

Cardiovascular: Hyperemia.

Genitourinary system: Proteinuria, microscopic hematuria.

Body as a Whole: Periorbital edema.

OVERDOSAGE

Acute overdoses may produce nausea, vomiting, and CNS depression including coma with respiratory depression. Methsuximide poisoning may follow a biphasic course. Following an initial comatose state, patients have awakened and then relapsed into a coma within 24 hours. It is believed that an active metabolite of Methsuximide, N-desmethylMethsuximide, is responsible for this biphasic profile. It is important to follow plasma levels of N-desmethylmethsuximide in Methsuximide poisonings. Levels greater than 40 µg/mL have caused toxicity and coma has been seen at levels of 150 µg/mL.

TREATMENT

Treatment should include emesis (unless the patient is or could rapidly become obtunded, comatose, or convulsing) or gastric lavage, activated charcoal, cathartics and general supportive measures. Charcoal hemoperfusion may be useful in removing the N-desmethyl metabolite of Methsuximide. Forced diuresis and exchange transfusions are ineffective.

➤ SHOWN IN PRODUCT IDENTIFICATION GUIDE

DOSAGE AND ADMINISTRATION

Optimum dosage of Methsuximide must be determined by trial. A suggested dosage schedule is 300 mg per day for the first week. If required, dosage may be increased thereafter at weekly intervals by 300 mg per day for the three weeks following to a daily dosage of 1.2 g. Because therapeutic effect and tolerance vary among patients, therapy with Methsuximide must be individualized according to the response of each patient. Optimal dosage is that amount of Methsuximide which is barely sufficient to control seizures so that side effects may be kept to a minimum. The smaller capsule (150 mg) facilitates administration to small children.

Methsuximide may be administered in combination with other anticonvulsants when other forms of epilepsy coexist with absence (petit mal).

Store at controlled room temperature 15°-30°C (59°-86°F). Protect from light and moisture.

HOW SUPPLIED
CAPSULE: 300 MG

BRAND/MANUFACTURER	NDC	SIZE	AWP
○ BRAND			
CELONTIN: Parke-Davis	00071-0525-24	100s	$70.40

Methyclothiazide

DESCRIPTION

Methyclothiazide is a member of the benzothiadiazine (thiazide) class of drugs. It is an analogue of hydrochlorothiazide and occurs as a white to practically white crystalline powder which is basically odorless. Methyclothiazide is very slightly soluble in water and chloroform, and slightly soluble in alcohol. Chemically, Methyclothiazide is represented as 6-chloro-3-(chloromethyl)-3, 4-dihydro-2-methyl-2H-1,2,4-benzothiadiazine-7-sulfonamide 1,1-dioxide.

Clinically, Methyclothiazide is an oral diuretic-antihypertensive agent.

Following is its chemical structure:

CLINICAL PHARMACOLOGY

The diuretic and saluretic effects of Methyclothiazide result from a drug-induced inhibition of the renal tubular reabsorption of electrolytes. The excretion of sodium and chloride is greatly enhanced. Potassium excretion is also enhanced to a variable degree, as it is with the other thiazides. Although urinary excretion of bicarbonate is increased slightly, there is usually no significant change in urinary pH. Methyclothiazide has a per mg natriuretic activity approximately 100 times that of the prototype thiazide, chlorothiazide. At maximal therapeutic dosages, all thiazides are approximately equal in their diuretic/natriuretic effects.

There is significant natriuresis and diuresis within two hours after administration of a single dose of Methyclothiazide. These effects reach a peak in about six hours and persist for 24 hours following oral administration of a single dose. Like other benzothiadiazines, Methyclothiazide also has antihypertensive properties, and may be used for this purpose either alone or to enhance the antihypertensive action of other drugs. The mechanism by which the benzothiadiazines, including Methyclothiazide, produce a reduction of elevated blood pressure is not known. However, sodium depletion appears to be involved.

Methyclothiazide is rapidly absorbed and slowly eliminated by the kidneys as intact drug but primarily as an inactive metabolite. Additional information on the pharmacokinetics is not known at this time.

INDICATIONS AND USAGE

Methyclothiazide is indicated in the management of hypertension either as the sole therapeutic agent or to enhance the effect of other antihypertensive drugs in the more severe forms of hypertension.

Methyclothiazide tablets are indicated as adjunctive therapy in edema associated with congestive heart failure, hepatic cirrhosis, and corticosteroid and estrogen therapy.

Methyclothiazide tablets have also been found useful in edema due to various forms of renal dysfunction such as the nephrotic syndrome, acute glomerulonephritis, and chronic renal failure.

Usage in Pregnancy: The routine use of diuretics in an otherwise healthy pregnant woman is inappropriate and exposes mother and fetus to unnecessary hazard. Diuretics do not prevent development of toxemia of pregnancy, and there is no satisfactory evidence that they are useful in the treatment of developed toxemia.

Edema during pregnancy may arise from pathological causes or from the physiological and mechanical consequences of pregnancy. Thiazides are indicated in pregnancy when edema is due to pathological causes, just as they are in the absence of pregnancy (see *"Precautions—Pregnancy"*). Dependent edema in pregnancy, resulting from restriction of venous return by the expanded uterus, is properly treated through elevation of the lower extremities and use of support hose; use of diuretics to lower intravascular volume in this case is illogical and unnecessary. There is hypervolemia during normal pregnancy that is harmful to neither the fetus nor the mother (in the absence of cardiovascular disease), but

that is associated with edema, including generalized edema, in the majority of pregnant women. If this edema produces discomfort, increased recumbency will often provide relief. In rare instances, this edema may cause extreme discomfort that is not relieved by rest. In these cases, a short course of diuretics may provide relief and may be appropriate.

CONTRAINDICATIONS

Methyclothiazide is contraindicated in patients with anuria and in patients with a history of hypersensitivity to this compound or other sulfonamide-derived drugs.

WARNINGS

Methyclothiazide shares with other thiazides the propensity to deplete potassium reserves to an unpredictable degree. There have been isolated reports that certain non-edematous individuals developed severe fluid and electrolyte derangements after only brief exposure to normal doses of thiazide and non-thiazide diuretics.

Thiazides should be used with caution in patients with renal disease or significant impairment of renal function, since azotemia may be precipitated and cumulative drug effects may occur.

Thiazides should be used with caution in patients with impaired hepatic function or progressive liver disease, since minor alterations of fluid and electrolyte balance may precipitate hepatic coma.

Sensitivity reactions may occur in patients with a history of allergy or bronchial asthma.

The possibility of exacerbation or activation of systemic lupus erythematosus has been reported.

Hyperuricemia may occur or frank gout may be precipitated in certain patients receiving thiazide therapy.

PRECAUTIONS

Laboratory Tests: Initial and periodic determinations of serum electrolytes should be performed at appropriate intervals for the purpose of detecting possible electrolyte imbalances such as hyponatremia, hypochloremic alkalosis, and hypokalemia. Serum and urine electrolyte determinations are particularly important when a patient is vomiting excessively or receiving parenteral fluids.

General: All patients should be observed for clinical signs of electrolyte imbalances such as dryness of mouth, thirst, weakness, lethargy, drowsiness, restlessness, muscle pains or cramps, muscular fatigue, hypotension, oliguria, tachycardia, and gastrointestinal disturbances such as nausea and vomiting.

Hypokalemia may develop, especially with brisk diuresis, when severe cirrhosis is present, during concomitant use of corticosteroids or ACTH, or after prolonged therapy.

Interference with adequate oral electrolyte intake will also contribute to hypokalemia. Hypokalemia may be avoided or treated by use of potassium supplements or foods with a high potassium content.

Any chloride deficit is generally mild and usually does not require specific treatment except under extraordinary circumstances (as in liver disease or renal disease). Dilutional hyponatremia may occur in edematous patients in hot weather; appropriate therapy is water restriction rather than administration of salt, except in rare instances when the hyponatremia is life threatening. In actual salt depletion, appropriate replacement is the therapy of choice.

Latent diabetes mellitus may become manifest during thiazide administration.

The antihypertensive effects of the drug may be enhanced in the postsympathectomy patient.

If progressive renal impairment becomes evident as indicated by a rising nonprotein nitrogen or blood urea nitrogen, a careful reappraisal of therapy is necessary with consideration given to withholding or discontinuing diuretic therapy. Thiazides may decrease urinary calcium excretion. Thiazides may cause intermittent and slight elevation of serum calcium in the absence of known disorders of calcium metabolism. Marked hypercalcemia may be evidence of hidden hyperparathyroidism. Thiazides should be discontinued before carrying out tests for parathyroid function.

Thiazides may cause increased concentrations of total serum cholesterol, total triglycerides, and low-density lipoproteins in some patients. Use thiazides with caution in patients with moderate or high cholesterol concentrations and in patients with elevated triglyceride levels.

Information for Patients: Patients should inform their doctor if they have: 1) had an allergic reaction to Methyclothiazide or other diuretics 2) asthma 3) kidney disease 4) liver disease 5) gout 6) systemic lupus erythematosus, or 7) been taking other drugs such as cortisone, digitalis, lithium carbonate, or drugs for diabetes.

The physician should inform patients of possible side effects and caution the patient to report any of the following symptoms of electrolyte imbalance; dryness of mouth, thirst, weakness, tiredness, drowsiness, restlessness, muscle pains or cramps, nausea, vomiting or increased heart rate.

The physician should advise the patient to take this medication every day as directed. Physicians should also caution patients that drinking alcohol can increase the chance of dizziness.

Drug Interactions: Hypokalemia can sensitize or exaggerate the response of the heart to the toxic effects of *digitalis* (e.g., increased ventricular irritability).

Hypokalemia may develop during concomitant use of *steroids* or ACTH.

Insulin requirements in diabetic patients may be increased, decreased, or unchanged.

Thiazides may decrease arterial responsiveness to *norepinephrine*. This diminution is not sufficient to preclude effectiveness of the pressor agent for therapeutic use.

Thiazide drugs may increase the responsiveness to *tubocurarine*.

◆ RATED THERAPEUTICALLY EQUIVALENT; ◇ THERAPEUTIC EQUIVALENCE UNCONFIRMED; ○ UNRATED

Lithium renal clearance is reduced by thiazides, increasing the risk of lithium toxicity.

Thiazides may add to or potentiate the action of *other antihypertensive* drugs. Potentiation occurs with ganglionic or peripheral adrenergic blocking drugs.

Drug/Laboratory Test Interactions: Thiazides may decrease serum PBI levels without signs of thyroid disturbance.

Thiazides should be discontinued before carrying out tests for parathyroid function.

Carcinogenesis, Mutagenesis, Impairment of Fertility: No data are available concerning the potential for carcinogenicity or mutagenicity in animals or humans. Methyclothiazide did not impair fertility in rats receiving up to 4 mg/kg/day (at least 20 times the maximum recommended human dose of 10 mg, assuming patient weight equal to or greater than 50 kg).

Pregnancy—Teratogenic Effects: Pregnancy Category B. Reproduction studies performed in rats and rabbits at doses up to 4 mg/kg/day have revealed no evidence of harm to the fetus due to Methyclothiazide. There are, however, no adequate and well-controlled studies in pregnant women. Because animal reproduction studies are not always predictive of human response, this drug should be used during pregnancy only if clearly needed.

Nonteratogenic Effects: Thiazides cross the placental barrier and appear in cord blood. The use of thiazides in pregnant women requires that the anticipated benefit be weighed against possible hazards to the fetus. These hazards include fetal or neonatal jaundice, thrombocytopenia and possible other adverse reactions that have occurred in the adult.

Nursing Mothers: Thiazides are excreted in breast milk. Because of the potential for serious adverse reactions in nursing infants, a decision should be made whether to discontinue nursing or to discontinue the drug taking into account the importance of the drug to the mother.

Pediatric Use: Safety and effectiveness in children have not been established.

ADVERSE REACTIONS

Adverse reactions are usually reversible upon reduction of dosage or discontinuation of Methyclothiazide tablets. Whenever adverse reactions are moderate or severe, it may be necessary to discontinue the drug.

The following adverse reactions have been observed, but there has not been enough systematic collection of data to support an estimate of their frequency. Consequently the reactions are categorized by organ system and are listed in decreasing order of severity and not frequency.

Body as a Whole: Headache, cramping, weakness.

Cardiovascular System: Orthostatic hypotension (may be potentiated by alcohol, barbiturates, or narcotics).

Digestive System: Pancreatitis, jaundice (intrahepatic cholestatic), sialadenitis, vomiting, diarrhea, nausea, gastric irritation, constipation, anorexia.

Hemic and Lymphatic System: Aplastic anemia, hemolytic anemia, agranulocytosis, leukopenia, thrombocytopenia.

Hypersensitivity Reactions: Anaphylactic reactions, necrotizing angiitis (vasculitis, cutaneous vasculitis), Stevens-Johnson syndrome, respiratory distress including pneumonitis and pulmonary edema, fever, purpura, urticaria, rash, photosensitivity.

Metabolic and Nutritional Disorders: Hyperglycemia, hyperuricemia, electrolyte imbalance (see "Precautions" section), hypercalcemia.

Nervous System: Vertigo, dizziness, paresthesias, muscle spasm, restlessness.

Special Senses: Transient blurred vision, xanthopsia.

Urogenital System: Glycosuria.

OVERDOSAGE

Symptoms of overdosage include electrolyte imbalance and signs of potassium deficiency such as confusion, dizziness, muscular weakness, and gastrointestinal disturbances. General supportive measures including replacement of fluids and electrolytes may be indicated in treatment of overdosage.

DOSAGE AND ADMINISTRATION

Methyclothiazide is administered orally. Therapy should be individualized according to patient response. This therapy should be titrated to gain maximal therapeutic response as well as the minimal dose possible to maintain that therapeutic response.

For edematous conditions: The usual adult dose ranges from 2.5 to 10 mg once daily. Maximum effective single dose is 10 mg; larger single doses do not accomplish greater diuresis, and are not recommended.

For the treatment of hypertension: The usual adult dose ranges from 2.5 to 5 mg once daily.

If control of blood pressure is not satisfactory after 8 to 12 weeks of therapy with 5 mg once daily, another antihypertensive drug should be added. Increasing the dosage of Methyclothiazide will usually not result in further lowering of blood pressure.

Methyclothiazide may be either employed alone for mild to moderate hypertension or concurrently with other antihypertensive drugs in the management of more severe forms of hypertension. Combined therapy may provide adequate control of hypertension with lower dosage of the component drugs and fewer or less severe side effects. An enhanced response frequently follows its

concurrent administration with deserpidine so that dosage of both drugs may be reduced.

When other antihypertensive agents are to be added to the regimen, this should be accomplished gradually. Ganglionic blocking agents should be given at only half the usual dose since their effect is potentiated by pretreatment with Methyclothiazide tablets.

Dispense in a USP tight container.

Store below 86°F (30°C).

HOW SUPPLIED
TABLETS: 2.5 MG

AVERAGE UNIT PRICE (AVAILABLE SIZES)		GENERIC A-RATED AVERAGE PRICE (GAAP)	
BRAND	$0.40	100s	$7.95
GENERIC	$0.08		
HCFA FUL (100s ea)	$0.08		

BRAND/MANUFACTURER	NDC	SIZE	AWP
◆ BRAND			
ENDURON: Abbott Pharm	00074-6827-01	100s	$39.89
◆ GENERICS			
Major	00904-2692-60	100s	$6.60
Moore,H.L.	00839-6580-06	100s	$8.09
Zenith	00172-2986-60	100s	$8.25
Geneva	00781-1803-01	100s	$8.85
Zenith	00172-2986-80	1000s	$78.38

TABLETS: 5 MG

AVERAGE UNIT PRICE (AVAILABLE SIZES)		GENERIC A-RATED AVERAGE PRICE (GAAP)	
BRAND	$0.77	100s	$10.14
GENERIC	$0.09	1000s	$68.40
HCFA FUL (100s ea)	$0.06		

BRAND/MANUFACTURER	NDC	SIZE	AWP
◆ BRAND			
ENDURON: Abbott Pharm	00074-6812-01	100s	$52.78
AQUATENSEN: Wallace	00037-0153-92	100s	$105.25
ENDURON: Abbott Pharm	00074-6812-10	100s ud	$57.43
AQUATENSEN: Wallace	00037-0153-96	500s	$494.81
ENDURON: Abbott Pharm	00074-6812-02	1000s	$511.90
AQUATENSEN: Wallace	00037-0153-99	4500s	$4264.54
◆ GENERICS			
Goldline	00182-1491-01	100s	$7.45
Major	00904-2693-60	100s	$7.95
Rugby	00536-4025-01	100s	$8.67
Geneva	00781-1810-01	100s	$9.25
Mylan	00378-0160-01	100s	$9.50
Moore,H.L.	00839-6581-06	100s	$9.50
Moore,H.L.	00839-7938-06	100s	$9.98
Major	00904-2693-61	100s ud	$18.85
Major	00904-2693-80	1000s	$56.55
Rugby	00536-4025-10	1000s	$68.69
Parmed	00349-8264-10	1000s	$79.95

Methyclothiazide with Reserpine

> WARNING: THIS FIXED COMBINATION DRUG IS NOT INDICATED FOR INITIAL THERAPY OF HYPERTENSION. HYPERTENSION REQUIRES THERAPY TITRATED TO THE INDIVIDUAL PATIENT. IF THE FIXED COMBINATION REPRESENTS THE DOSAGE SO DETERMINED, ITS USE MAY BE MORE CONVENIENT IN PATIENT MANAGEMENT. THE TREATMENT OF HYPERTENSION IS NOT STATIC, BUT MUST BE RE-EVALUATED AS CONDITIONS IN EACH PATIENT WARRANT.

DESCRIPTION

Methyclothiazide/Reserpine is a combination of two active antihypertensive agents: Methyclothiazide, an analogue of hydrochlorothiazide; and Reserpine, an alkaloid of *Rauwolfia serpentina*. Methyclothiazide/Reserpine is available as tablets for oral administration. Each round, white, pink-mottled, monogrammed tablet contains 2.5 mg Methyclothiazide and 0.1 mg Reserpine.

Methyclothiazide is 6-chloro-3-(chloromethyl)-3,4-dihydro-2-methyl-2H-1,2,4-benzothiadiazine-7-sulfonamide, 1,1-dioxide. It is insoluble in water, chloroform, or benzene, sparingly soluble in methanol and alcohol, slightly soluble in ether, and very soluble in acetone and pyridine. The molecular formula is $C_9H_{11}Cl_2N_3O_4S_2$, with a molecular weight of 360.23.

Reserpine is 11, 17-dimethoxy-18-[(3,4, 5-trimethoxybenzoyl)oxy]-yohimban-16-carboxylic acid methyl ester. It is insoluble in water, slightly soluble in alcohol, methanol, acetone and ether, and freely soluble in chloroform, methylene chloride, and glacial acetic acid, and soluble in benzene and ethyl acetate. The molecular formula is $C_{33}H_{40}N_2O_9$ with a molecular weight of 608.69.

CLINICAL PHARMACOLOGY

Methyclothiazide: The diuretic and saluretic effects of Methyclothiazide result from a drug-induced inhibition of the renal tubular reabsorption of electrolytes. The excretion of sodium and chloride is greatly enhanced. Potassium excretion is also enhanced to a variable degree, as it is with the other thiazides. Although urinary excretion of bicarbonate is increased slightly, there is usually no significant change in urinary pH. Methyclothiazide has a per mg natriuretic activity approximately 100 times that of the prototype thiazide, chlorothiazide. At maximal therapeutic dosages, all thiazides are approximately equal in their diuretic/natriuretic effects.

There is significant natriuresis and diuresis within 2 hours after administration of a single dose of Methyclothiazide. These effects reach a peak in about 6 hours and persist for 24 hours following oral administration of a single dose.

Like other benzothiadiazines, Methyclothiazide also has antihypertensive properties, and may be used for this purpose either alone or to enhance the antihypertensive action of other drugs. The mechanism by which the benzothiadiazines, including Methyclothiazide, produce a reduction of elevated blood pressure is not known. However, sodium depletion appears to be involved.

Reserpine: Reserpine has antihypertensive, bradycardic, and tranquilizing properties. It lowers arterial blood pressure by depletion of catecholamines. Reserpine is beneficial in relieving anxiety, tension, and headache in the hypertensive patient. It acts at the hypothalamic level of the central nervous system to promote relaxation without hypnosis or analgesia. The sleep pattern shown by the electroencephalogram following barbiturates does not occur with this drug. In laboratory animals spontaneous activity and response to external stimuli are decreased, but confusion or difficulty of movement is not evident.

The bradycardic action of Reserpine promotes relaxation and may eliminate sinus bradycardia. It is most pronounced in subjects with sinus tachycardia and usually is not prominent in persons with a normal pulse rate.

Miosis, relaxation of the nictitating membrane, ptosis, hypothermia, and increased gastrointestinal activity are noted in animals given Reserpine, sometimes in subclinical doses. None of these effects, except increased gastrointestinal activity, have been found to be clinically significant in man with therapeutic doses.

PHARMACOKINETICS AND METABOLISM
Methyclothiazide: Methyclothiazide is rapidly absorbed and slowly eliminated by the kidneys as intact drug but primarily as an inactive metabolite. Additional information on the pharmacokinetics is not known at this time.

Reserpine: Oral Reserpine is rapidly absorbed from the gastrointestinal tract. Methylreserpate and trimethoxybenzoic acid are the primary metabolites which result from the hydrolytic cleavage of Reserpine. Maximal blood levels are achieved approximately 2 hours after the oral dosage of ^{3}H-reserpine to six normal volunteers; within 96 hours approximately 8 percent was excreted in urine and 62 percent in feces.

INDICATIONS AND USAGE
Hypertension (See box *"Warning"*).

CONTRAINDICATIONS
Methyclothiazide: Methyclothiazide is contraindicated in patients with anuria and in patients with a history of hypersensitivity to this or other sulfonamide-derived drugs.

Reserpine: Known hypersensitivity; mental depression or a history of mental depression, especially with suicidal tendencies; active peptic ulcer; ulcerative colitis; and patients receiving electroconvulsive therapy.

WARNINGS
Methyclothiazide: Methyclothiazide shares with other thiazides the propensity to deplete potassium reserves to an unpredictable degree.

There have been isolated reports that certain nonedematous individuals developed severe fluid and electrolyte derangements after only brief exposure to normal doses of thiazide and nonthiazide diuretics.

Thiazides should be used with caution in patients with renal disease or significant impairment of renal function, since azotemia may be precipitated and cumulative drug effects may occur.

Thiazides should be used with caution in patients with impaired hepatic function or progressive liver disease, since minor alterations of fluid and electrolyte balance may precipitate hepatic coma.

Sensitivity reactions may occur in patients with a history of allergy or bronchial asthma.

The possibility of exacerbation or activation of systemic lupus erythematosus has been reported.

Hyperuricemia may occur or frank gout may be precipitated in certain patients receiving thiazide therapy.

Reserpine: Reserpine may cause mental depression. Recognition of depression may be difficult because this condition may often be disguised by somatic complaints (Masked Depression). The drug should be discontinued at first signs of depression such as despondency, early morning insomnia, loss of appetite, impotence, or self-deprecation. Drug induced depression may persist for several months after drug withdrawal and may be severe enough to result in suicide.

MAO inhibitors should be avoided or used with extreme caution.

Electroshock therapy should not be given to patients under treatment with Reserpine since severe and even fatal reactions to such therapy have been reported in patients receiving Reserpine. Reserpine should be discontinued for two weeks before electroshock therapy is given.

PRECAUTIONS
GENERAL
Methyclothiazide: All patients should be observed for other clinical signs of electrolyte imbalances such as dryness of mouth, thirst, weakness, lethargy, drowsiness, restlessness, muscle pains or cramps, muscular fatigue, hypotension, oliguria, tachycardia, and gastrointestinal disturbances such as nausea and vomiting.

Hypokalemia may develop, especially with brisk diuresis, when severe cirrhosis is present, during concomitant use of corticosteroids or ACTH, or after prolonged therapy.

Interference with adequate oral electrolyte intake will also contribute to hypokalemia. Hypokalemia may be avoided or treated with the intake of potassium supplements or foods containing a high potassium content.

Any chloride deficit is generally mild and usually does not require specific treatment except under extraordinary circumstance (as in liver disease or renal disease). Dilutional hyponatremia may occur in edematous patients in hot weather. Appropriate therapy is water restriction rather than administration of salt, except in rare instances when the hyponatremia is life threatening. In actual salt depletion, appropriate replacement is the therapy of choice.

Latent diabetes mellitus may become manifest during thiazide administration.

The antihypertensive effects of the drug may be enhanced in the postsympathectomy patient.

If progressive renal impairment becomes evident as indicated by a rising nonprotein nitrogen or blood urea nitrogen, a careful reappraisal of therapy is necessary with consideration given to withholding or discontinuing diuretic therapy.

Thiazides have been shown to increase the urinary excretion of magnesium which may result in hypomagnesemia.

Thiazides may decrease urinary calcium excretion and may cause intermittent and slight elevation of serum calcium in the absence of known disorders of calcium metabolism. Marked hypercalcemia may be evidence of hidden hyperparathyroidism. Thiazides should be discontinued before carrying out tests for parathyroid function.

Thiazides may cause increased concentration of total serum cholesterol, total triglycerides, and low-density lipoproteins in some patients. Use thiazides with caution in patients with moderate or high cholesterol concentrations and in patients with elevated triglyceride levels.

Reserpine: Since Reserpine may increase gastric secretion and motility, it should be used cautiously in patients with a history of peptic ulcer, ulcerative colitis, or other gastrointestinal disorder. This compound may precipitate biliary colic in patients with gallstones, or bronchial asthma in susceptible persons.

Reserpine may cause hypotension including orthostatic hypotension.

Anxiety or depression, as well as psychosis, may develop during Reserpine therapy. If depression is present when therapy is begun, it may be aggravated. Mental depression is unusual with Reserpine doses of 0.25 mg daily or less. In any case, Methyclothiazide/Reserpine should be discontinued at the first sign of depression. Extreme caution should be used in treating patients with a history of mental depression, and the possibility of suicide should be kept in mind.

Caution should be exercised when treating hypertensive patients with renal insufficiency since they adjust poorly to lowered blood pressure levels.

INFORMATION FOR PATIENTS
Methyclothiazide: Caution patients that thiazides cause the body to lose mineral salts such as sodium, chloride, and especially potassium, and advise them to report any of the following without delay: excessive thirst, tiredness, drowsiness, muscle pains or cramps, nausea, vomiting, increased heart rate or pulse.

Reserpine: Advise patients to report promptly the onset of any of the following symptoms, especially if they have a history of mental depression: despondency, difficulty sleeping, loss of appetite, impotence, or feelings of worthlessness.

LABORATORY TESTS
Initial and periodic determination of serum electrolytes should be performed at appropriate intervals for the purpose of detecting possible electrolyte imbalances such as hyponatremia, hypochloremic alkalosis, and hypokalemia. Serum and urine electrolyte determinations are particularly important when a patient is vomiting excessively or receiving parenteral fluids.

DRUG INTERACTIONS
Methyclothiazide: Hypokalemia can sensitize or exaggerate the response of the heart to the toxic effects of *digitalis* (e.g., increased ventricular irritability).

Hypokalemia may develop during concomitant use of *steroids* or *ACTH*.

Insulin requirements in diabetic patients may be increased, decreased, or unchanged.

Thiazides may decrease arterial responsiveness to *norepinephrine*. This diminution is not sufficient to preclude effectiveness of the pressor agent for therapeutic use.

Nonsteroidal Anti-Inflammatory Drugs: In some patients the administration of a nonsteroidal anti-inflammatory agent can reduce the diuretic, natriuretic, and anti-hypertensive effects of loop, potassium-sparing, and thiazide diuretics. Therefore, when Methyclothiazide/Reserpine tablets and nonsteroidal anti-inflammatory agents are used concomitantly, the patient should be observed closely to determine if the desired effect of the diuretic is obtained.

Thiazide drugs may increase the responsiveness to *tubocurarine*.

Lithium renal clearance is reduced by thiazides, increasing the risk of lithium toxicity.

◆ RATED THERAPEUTICALLY EQUIVALENT; ◇ THERAPEUTIC EQUIVALENCE UNCONFIRMED; ○ UNRATED

Thiazides may add to or potentiate the action of *other antihypertensive drugs*. Potentiation occurs with ganglionic or peripheral adrenergic blocking agents.

Reserpine: Use Reserpine cautiously with digitalis and quinidine since cardiac arrhythmias have occurred with the concurrent use of rauwolfia preparations. Concomitant use of Reserpine with other antihypertensive agents necessitates careful titration of dosage with each agent. In hypertensive patients with coronary artery disease, it is important to avoid a precipitous drop in blood pressure.

Preoperative withdrawal of Reserpine does not assure that circulatory instability will not occur. It is important that the anesthesiologist be aware of the patient's drug intake and consider this in the overall management, since hypotension has occurred in patients receiving rauwolfia preparations. Anticholinergic and/or adrenergic drugs (e.g., metaraminol, norepinephrine) have been employed to treat adverse vagocirculatory effects. Concurrent use of Reserpine and direct or indirect acting sympathomimetics should be closely monitored. The action of direct acting amines (epinephrine, isoproterenol, phenylephrine, metaraminol) may be prolonged when given to patients taking Reserpine. The action of indirect acting amines (ephedrine, tyramine, amphetamines) is inhibited.

Concurrent use of tricyclic antidepressants may decrease the antihypertensive effect of Reserpine (see *"Contraindications"*).

Barbiturates enhance the central nervous system depressant effect of Reserpine.

DRUG/LABORATORY TEST INTERACTIONS
Thiazides may decrease serum PBI levels without signs of thyroid disturbance.

Thiazides decrease calcium excretion and, on rare occasions, serum calcium has been elevated to hypercalcemic levels. The serum calcium levels have returned to normal when the medication was stopped. Thiazides should be discontinued before carrying out tests for parathyroid function.

CARCINOGENESIS, MUTAGENESIS, AND IMPAIRMENT OF FERTILITY
No long-term studies have been done with Methyclothiazide/Reserpine and information is not available to evaluate its potential for these effects.

Reserpine: Reserpine at a concentration of 1 to 5000 mcg/plate had no mutagenic activity against four strains of S. typhimurium *in vitro* in the Ames microbial mutagen test with or without metabolic activation. Reserpine did not induce malignant transformation of mouse fibroblasts *in vitro* at concentrations of 0.3 to 10 mcg/mL.

A few chromosomal aberrations were induced by Reserpine *in vitro* in cultured mouse mammary carcinoma cells but were considered negative in this study. The drug did not produce chromosomal aberrations in human peripheral leucocyte cultures although an increase in mitotic figures occurred. One study reported chromosomal aberrations and dominant lethal mutations in mice at doses up to 10 mg/kg of Reserpine in the form of a pharmaceutical preparation. Another study did not show dominant lethal mutations in mice at IP doses of 0.92 and 4.6 mg/kg of Reserpine.

Reserpine did not impair fertility in rats at an oral dose of 0.025 mg/kg. Rodent studies have shown that Reserpine is an animal tumorigen, causing an increased incidence of mammary fibroadenomas in female mice, malignant tumors of seminal vesicles in male mice, and malignant adrenal medullary tumors in male rats. These findings arose in 2 year studies in which the drug was administered in the feed at concentrations of 5 and 10 ppm — about 100 to 300 times the usual human dose. The breast neoplasmas are thought to be related to Reserpine's prolactin-elevating effect. Several other prolactin-elevating drugs have also been associated with an increased incidence of mammary neoplasia in rodents.

The extent to which these findings indicate a risk to humans is uncertain. Tissue culture experiments show that about one-third of human breast tumors are prolactin-dependent *in vitro*, a factor of considerable importance if the use of the drug is contemplated in a patient with previously detected breast cancer. The possibility of an increased risk of breast cancer in Reserpine users has been studied extensively; however, no firm conclusion has emerged. Although a few epidemiologic studies have suggested a slightly increased risk (less than twofold in all studies except one) in women who have used Reserpine, other studies of generally similar design have not confirmed this. Epidemiologic studies conducted using other drugs (neuroleptic agents) that, like Reserpine, increase prolactin levels and therefore would be considered rodent mammary carcinogens, have not shown an association between chronic administration of the drug and human mammary tumorigenesis. While long-term clinical observation has not suggested such an association, the available evidence is considered too limited to be conclusive at this time. An association of Reserpine intake with pheochromocytoma or tumors of the seminal vesicles has not been explored.

PREGNANCY: TERATOGENIC EFFECTS
Pregnancy Category C. Animal reproduction studies have not been conducted with Methyclothiazide/Reserpine. It is also not known whether Methyclothiazide/Reserpine can cause fetal harm when administered to a pregnant woman or can affect reproduction capacity. Methyclothiazide/Reserpine should be given to a pregnant woman only if clearly needed.

Reserpine: Reproduction studies in rats have shown that Reserpine is teratogenic at doses of 1-2 mg/kg (125-250 times the maximum recommended human dose) IM or IP given early in pregnancy. A variety of abnormalities was produced including anophthalmia, absence of the axial skeleton, hydronephrosis, etc. Pregnancy in rabbits was interrupted when doses as low as 0.04 mg/kg (10 times the maximum recommended human dose) were given early or late in pregnancy.

PREGNANCY: NON-TERATOGENIC EFFECTS
The use of Methyclothiazide/Reserpine in pregnant women requires that the anticipated benefits be weighed against possible hazards to the fetus. These hazards include: fetal or neonatal jaundice, thrombocytopenia, increased respiratory secretions, nasal congestion, cyanosis, anorexia, and possibly other adverse reactions that have occurred in the adult.

Methyclothiazide: Thiazides cross the placental barrier and appear in cord blood.

Reserpine: Reserpine has been demonstrated to cross the placental barrier in guinea pigs with depression of adrenal catecholamine stores in the newborn. There is some evidence that side effects such as nasal congestion, lethargy, depressed Moro reflex, and bradycardia may appear in infants born of Reserpine-treated mothers.

NURSING MOTHERS
Thiazides and Reserpine appear in breast milk. Because of the potential for serious adverse reactions in nursing infants from Methyclothiazide/Reserpine, a decision should be made whether to discontinue the drug, taking into account the importance of the drug to the mother.

Pediatric Use: Safety and effectiveness in children have not been established.

ADVERSE REACTIONS
The following adverse reactions have been observed, but there is not enough systematic collection of data to support an estimate of their frequency. They are listed by organ systems in decreasing order of severity for each ingredient.

METHYCLOTHIAZIDE
Body as a Whole: Headache, cramping, weakness.

Cardiovascular System: Orthostatic hypotension (may be potentiated by alcohol, barbiturates, or narcotics).

Digestive System: Pancreatitis, jaundice (intrahepatic cholestatic), sialadenitis, vomiting, diarrhea, nausea, gastric irritation, constipation, anorexia.

Hemic and Lymphatic System: Aplastic anemia, hemolytic anemia, agranulocytosis, leukopenia, thrombocytopenia.

Hypersensitivity Reactions: Anaphylactic reactions, necrotizing angiitis (vasculitis, cutaneous vasculitis), Stevens Johnson syndrome, respiratory distress (including pneumonitis and pulmonary edema), fever, purpura, urticaria, rash, photosensitivity.

Metabolic and Nutritional Disorders: Hyperglycemia, hyperuricemia, electrolyte imbalance (see *"Precautions"*), hypercalcemia.

Nervous System: Vertigo, dizziness, paresthesias, muscle spasm, restlessness.

Special Senses: Transient blurred vision, xanthopsia.

Urogential System: Glycosuria.

RESERPINE
Cardiovascular: Angina pectoris, arrythmia, premature ventricular contractions, other direct cardiac effects (e.g., fluid retention, congestive heart failure), bradycardia.

Digestive: Vomiting, diarrhea, nausea, hypersecretion and increased motility, anorexia, dryness of mouth, increased salivation.

Hematologic: Thrombocytopenic purpura, excessive bleeding following prostatic surgery.

Hypersensitivity: Pruritus, rush, flushing of skin.

Metabolic: Weight gain.

Musculoskeletal: Muscular aches.

Nervous System/Psychiatric: Mental depression, dull sensorium, syncope, paradoxical anxiety, excessive sedation, nightmares, headache, dizziness, nervousness, parkinsonism (usually reversible with decreased dosage or discontinuance of therapy).

Respiratory: Dyspnea, epistaxis, nasal congestion, enhanced susceptibility to colds.

Special Senses: Optic atrophy, uveitis, deafness, glaucoma, conjunctival injection, blurred vision.

Urogenital: Dysuria, impotence, decreased libido, nonpuerperal lactation, gynecomastia, breast engorgement.

OVERDOSAGE
METHYCLOTHIAZIDE
Signs and Symptoms: Diuresis is to be expected. Lethargy of varying degree may appear and may progress to coma within a few hours, even in the absence of significant changes in serum electrolytes or dehydration and with minimal depression of respiration and cardiovascular function. The mechanism of CNS depression with thiazide overdosage is not known. GI irritation, hypermotility, and signs of potassium deficiency such as confusion, dizziness, and muscular weakness may occur. A temporary rise in BUN and changes in serum electrolytes could occur, especially in patients with compromised renal function.

Treatment: Evacuate stomach contents using appropriate caution and procedures to guard against aspiration and to protect the airway, especially in the stuporous or comatose patient. Monitor serum electrolyte levels, blood gases, and renal function. Institute general supportive measures as required individually to maintain hydration, electrolyte balance, respiration, and cardiovascular-renal function.

GI side effects are usually of short duration but may require symptomatic treatment.

RESERPINE

Signs and Symptoms: CNS depression manifested by impairment of consciousness may occur and may range from drowsiness to coma. Pupillary constriction, peripheral vasodilation with flushing of the skin, and conjunctival injection are to be expected. Hypotension, hypothermia, central nervous system depression, and bradycardia may develop in cases of severe overdosage. Diarrhea may also occur.

Treatment: General supportive measures and symptomatic treatment is indicated. Since Reserpine is long-acting, observe patients for at least 72 hours and treat accordingly.

Evacuate stomach contents using appropriate caution and procedures to guard against aspiration and to protect the airway, especially in the stuporous or comatose patient.

Hypotension, especially if excessive, may require the use of a vasopressor. In such cases, use a vasopressor having a direct action on vascular smooth muscle (e.g., phenylephrine, metaraminol).

DOSAGE AND ADMINISTRATION
As determined by individual titration (see box *"Warning"*).

Usual Adult Dosage: 1 to 2 tablets once daily in a single dose.

Up to 4 tablets may be given in single or divided doses, if indicated.

Since antihypertensive effects of Reserpine are not immediately apparent, maximal reduction in blood pressure from a given dosage may not occur for 2 weeks. For maintenance, reduce dosage to lowest effective level; as little as 1 tablet daily may suffice.

When necessary, other antihypertensive agents may be added gradually in reduced dosages. Watch effects carefully.

Storage: Store at controlled room temperature, 15°-30°C (59°-86°F).

Dispense in tight, light-resistant container.

HOW SUPPLIED
TABLETS:

BRAND/MANUFACTURER	NDC	SIZE	AWP
○ **BRAND**			
DIUTENSEN-R: Wallace	00037-0274-92	100s	$224.33
	00037-0274-96	500s	$1055.21
	00037-0274-99	5000s	$9793.82

Methyldopa

DESCRIPTION
Methyldopa is an antihypertensive drug. Methyldopate Hydrochloride is an antihypertensive agent for intravenous use.

Methyldopa, the *L*-isomer of alpha-methyldopa is levo-3-(3,4-dihydroxyphenyl)-2-methylalanine. Its empirical formula is $C_{10}H_{13}NO_4$, with a molecular weight of 211.22.

Methyldopa HCl [levo-3-(3,4-dihydroxyphenyl)-2-methylalanine, ethyl ester hydrochloride] is the ethyl ester of Methyldopa, supplied as the hydrochloride salt with a molecular weight of 275.73. Methyldopate HCl is more soluble and stable in solution than Methyldopa and is the preferred form for intravenous use.

The empirical formula for Methyldopate HCl is $C_{12}H_{17}NO_4 \cdot HCl$.

Methyldopa is a white to yellowish white, odorless fine power, and is soluble in water.

Methyldopa is supplied as tablets, for oral use, and oral suspension.

Each tablet contains:
Methyldopa ....125, 250, or 500 mg

Each 5 ml of oral suspension contains:
Methyldopa ....250 mg

Each 5 ml of intravenous solution contains:
Methyldopate HCl ....250 mg

Following is its chemical structure:

CLINICAL PHARMACOLOGY
Methyldopa is an aromatic-amino-acid decarboxylase inhibitor in animals and in man. Although the mechanism of action has yet to be conclusively demonstrated, the antihypertensive effect of Methyldopa probably is due to its metabolism to alpha-methylnorepinephrine, which then lowers arterial pressure by stimulation of central inhibitory alpha-adrenergic receptors, false neurotransmission, and/or reduction of plasma renin activity. Methyldopa has been shown to cause a net

reduction in the tissue concentration of serotonin, dopamine, norepinephrine, and epinephrine.

Only Methyldopa, the *L*-isomer of alpha Methyldopa, has the ability to inhibit dopa decarboxylase and to deplete animal tissues of norepinephrine. In man the antihypertensive activity appears to be due solely to the *L*-isomer. About twice the dose of the racemate (*DL*-alpha-methyldopa) is required for equal antihypertensive effect.

Methyldopa has no direct effect on cardiac function and usually does not reduce glomerular filtration rate, renal blood flow, or filtration fraction. Cardiac output usually is maintained without cardiac acceleration. In some patients the heart rate is slowed.

Normal or elevated plasma renin activity may decrease in the course of Methyldopa therapy.

Methyldopa reduces both supine and standing blood pressure. It usually produces highly effective lowering of the supine pressure with infrequent symptomatic postural hypotension. Exercise hypotension and diurnal blood pressure variations rarely occur.

PHARMACOKINETICS AND METABOLISM
The maximum decrease in blood pressure occurs four to six hours after oral dosage. Once an effective dosage level is attained, a smooth blood pressure response occurs in most patients in 12 to 24 hours. After withdrawal, blood pressure usually returns to pretreatment levels within 24-48 hours. Following intravenous administration of Methyldopate HCl a decrease in blood pressure may occur in four to six hours and last 10 to 16 hours.

Methyldopa is extensively metabolized. The known urinary metabolites are; α-methyldopa mono-0-sulfate; 3-0-methyl-α-methyldopa; 3,4-dihydroxyphenylacetone; α-methyldopamine; 3-0-methyl-α-methyldopamine and their conjugates. Approximately 70% of the drug which is absorbed is excreted in the urine as Methyldopa and its mono-0-sulfate conjugate. The renal clearance is about 130 mL/min in normal subjects and is diminished in renal insufficiency. The plasma half-life of Methyldopa is 105 minutes. After oral doses, excretion is essentially complete in 36 hours.

Methyldopate HCl is the ethyl ester of Methyldopa HCl and possesses the same pharmacologic attributes.

Approximately 49 percent of the dose of Methyldopate HCl is excreted in the urine as Methyldopa and its mono-0-sulfate. The renal clearance of Methyldopa following Methyldopate HCl is about 156 mL/min in normal subjects and is diminished in renal insufficiency. Following Methyldopate HCl injection the plasma half-life of Methyldopa is 90-127 mins. Approximately 17 percent of a dose of Methyldopate HCl given to normal subjects appears in plasma as free Methyldopa.

Methyldopa crosses the placental barrier, appears in cord blood and appears in breast milk.

INDICATION AND USAGE
Hypertension.

Methyldopate HCl is used in hypertension, when parenteral medication is indicated. The treatment of hypertensive crises may be initiated with Methyldopate HCl injection.

UNLABELED USES
Methyldopa is used alone or as an adjunct in the treatment of congestive heart failure, hyperhidrosis, Raynaud's disease, menopausal hot flushes, and in tardive dyskinesia secondary to chronic psychotropic medication.

CONTRAINDICATIONS
Active hepatic disease, such as acute hepatitis and active cirrhosis.

If previous Methyldopa therapy has been associated with liver disorders (see *"Warnings"*).

Hypersensitivity to any component of these products including sulfites contained in some formulations.

WARNINGS
It is important to recognize that a positive Coombs test, hemolytic anemia, and liver disorders may occur with Methyldopa therapy. The rare occurrences of hemolytic anemia or liver disorders could lead to potentially fatal complications unless properly recognized and managed. Read this section carefully to understand these reactions.

With prolonged Methyldopa therapy, 10 to 20 percent of patients develop a positive direct Coombs test which usually occurs between 6 and 12 months of Methyldopa therapy. Lowest incidence is at daily dosage of 1 g or less. This on rare occasions may be associated with hemolytic anemia, which could lead to potentially fatal complications. One cannot predict which patients with a positive direct Coombs test may develop hemolytic anemia.

Prior existence or development of a positive direct Coombs test is not in itself a contraindication to use of Methyldopa. If a positive Coombs test develops during Methyldopa therapy, the physician should determine whether hemolytic anemia exists and whether the positive Coombs test may be a problem. For example, in addition to a positive direct Coombs test there is less often a positive indirect Coombs test which may interfere with cross matching of blood.

Before treatment is started, it is desirable to do a blood count (hematocrit, hemoglobin, or red cell count) for a baseline or to establish whether there is anemia. Periodic blood counts should be done during therapy to detect hemolytic anemia. It may be useful to do a direct Coombs test before therapy and at 6 and 12 months after the start of therapy.

If Coombs-positive hemolytic anemia occurs, the cause may be Methyldopa and the drug should be discontinued. Usually the anemia remits promptly. If not, corticosteroids may be given and other causes of anemia should be considered. If

---

◆ RATED THERAPEUTICALLY EQUIVALENT; ◇ THERAPEUTIC EQUIVALENCE UNCONFIRMED; ○ UNRATED

the hemolytic anemia is related to Methyldopa, the drug should not be reinstituted.

When Methyldopa causes Coombs positivity alone or with hemolytic anemia, the red cell is usually coated with gamma globulin of the IgG (gamma G) class only. The positive Coombs test may not revert to normal until weeks to months after Methyldopa is stopped.

Should the need for transfusion arise in a patient receiving Methyldopa, both a direct and an indirect Coombs test should be performed. In the absence of hemolytic anemia, usually only the direct Coombs test will be positive. A positive direct Coombs test alone will not interfere with typing or cross matching. If the indirect Coombs test is also positive, problems may arise in the major cross match and the assistance of a hematologist or transfusion expert will be needed. Occasionally, fever has occurred within the first 3 weeks of Methyldopa therapy, associated in some cases with eosinophilia or abnormalities in one or more liver function tests, such as serum alkaline phosphatase, serum transaminases (SGOT, SGPT), bilirubin, and prothrombin time. Jaundice, with or without fever, may occur with onset usually within the first 2 to 3 months of therapy. In some patients the findings are consistent with those of cholestasis. In others the findings are consistent with hepatitis and hepatocellular injury.

Rarely, fatal hepatic necrosis has been reported after use of Methyldopa. These hepatic changes may represent hypersensitivity reactions. Periodic determinations of hepatic function should be done particularly during the first 6 to 12 weeks of therapy or whenever an unexplained fever occurs. If fever, abnormalities in liver function tests, or jaundice appear, stop therapy with Methyldopa. If caused by Methyldopa, the temperature and abnormalities in liver function characteristically have reverted to normal when the drug was discontinued. Methyldopa should not be reinstituted in such patients.

Rarely, a reversible reduction of the white blood cell count with a primary effect on the granulocytes has been seen. The granulocyte count returned promptly to normal on discontinuance of the drug. Rare cases of granulocytopenia have been reported. In each instance, upon stopping the drug, the white cell count returned to normal. Reversible thrombocytopenia has occurred rarely.

Some formulations contain sodium bisulfite, a sulfite that may cause allergic-type reactions including anaphylactic symptoms and life-threatening or less severe asthmatic episodes in certain susceptible people. The overall prevalence of sulfite sensitivity in the general population is unknown and probably low. Sulfite sensitivity is seen more frequently in asthmatic than in nonasthmatic people.

PRECAUTIONS

GENERAL

Methyldopa should be used with caution in patients with a history of previous liver disease or dysfunction (see "Warnings").

Some patients taking Methyldopa experience clinical edema or weight gain which may be controlled by use of a diuretic. Methyldopa should not be continued if edema progresses or signs of heart failure appear.

A paradoxical pressor response has been reported with intravenous administration of Methyldopate HCl.

Hypertension has recurred occasionally after dialysis in patients given Methyldopa because the drug is removed by this procedure.

Rarely involuntary choreoathetotic movements have been observed during therapy with Methyldopa in patients with severe bilateral cerebrovascular disease. Should these movements occur, stop therapy.

LABORATORY TESTS

Blood count, Coombs test, and liver function tests are recommended before initiating therapy and at periodic intervals (see "Warnings").

DRUG INTERACTIONS

When Methyldopa is used with other antihypertensive drugs, potentiation of antihypertensive effect may occur. Patients should be followed carefully to detect side reactions or unusual manifestations of drug idiosyncrasy.

Patients may require reduced doses of anesthetics when on Methyldopa. If hypotension does occur during anesthesia, it usually can be controlled by vasopressors. The adrenergic receptors remain sensitive during treatment with Methyldopa.

When Methyldopa and lithium are given concomitantly the patient should be carefully monitored for symptoms of lithium toxicity. Read the circular for lithium preparations.

DRUG/LABORATORY TEST INTERACTIONS

Methyldopa may interfere with measurement of urinary uric acid by the phosphotungstate method, serum creatinine by the alkaline picrate method, and SGOT by colorimetric methods. Interference with spectrophotometric methods for SGOT analysis has not been reported.

Since Methyldopa causes fluorescence in urine samples at the same wave lengths as catecholamines, falsely high levels of urinary catecholamines may be reported. This will interfere with the diagnosis of pheochromocytoma. It is important to recognize this phenomenon before a patient with a possible pheochromocytoma is subjected to surgery. Methyldopa does not interfere with measurement of VMA (vanillylmandelic acid), a test for pheochromocytoma, by those methods which convert VMA to vanillin. Methyldopa is not recommended for the treatment of patients with pheochromocytoma. Rarely, when urine is exposed to air after voiding, it may darken because of breakdown of Methyldopa or its metabolites.

CARCINOGENESIS, MUTAGENESIS, IMPAIRMENT OF FERTILITY

No evidence of a tumorigenic effect was seen when Methyldopa was given for two years to mice at doses up to 1800 mg/kg/day or to rats at doses up to 240 mg/kg/day (30 and 4 times the maximum recommended human dose in mice and rats, respectively, when compared on the basis of body weight; 2.5 and 0.6 times the maximum recommended human dose in mice and rats, respectively, when compared on the basis of body surface area; calculations assume a patient weight of 50 kg).

Methyldopa was not mutagenic in the Ames Test and did not increase chromosomal aberration or sister chromatid exchanges in Chinese hamster ovary cells. These *in vitro* studies were carried out both with and without exogenous metabolic activation.

Fertility was unaffected when Methyldopa was given to male and female rats at 100 mg/kg/day (1.7 times the maximum daily human dose when compared on the basis of body weight; 0.2 times the maximum daily human dose when compared on the basis of body surface area). Methyldopa decreased sperm count, sperm motility, the number of late spermatids and the male fertility index when given to male rats at 200 and 400 mg/kg/day (3.3 and 6.7 times the maximum daily human dose when compared on the basis of body weight; 0.5 and 1 times the maximum daily human dose when compared on the basis of body surface area.)

Long-term studies in animals have not been performed to evaluate the carcinogenic potential of Methyldopate HCl; nor have evaluations of this ester's mutagenic potential or potential to affect fertility been carried out.

PREGNANCY

Methyldopa: Pregnancy Category B. Reproduction studies performed with Methyldopa at oral doses up to 1000 mg/kg in mice, 200 mg/kg in rabbits and 100 mg/kg in rats revealed no evidence of harm to the fetus. These doses are 16.6 times, 3.3 times and 1.7 times, respectively, the maximum daily human dose when compared on the basis of body weight: 1.4 times, 1.1 times and 0.2 times, respectively, when compared on the basis of body surface area; calculations assume a patient weight of 50 kg. There are, however, no adequate and well-controlled studies in pregnant women in the first trimester of pregnancy. Because animal reproduction studies are not always predictive of human response, Methyldopa should be used during pregnancy only if clearly needed.

Published reports of the use of Methyldopa during all trimesters indicate that if this drug is used during pregnancy the possibility of fetal harm appears remote. In five studies, three of which were controlled, involving 332 pregnant hypertensive women, treatment with Methyldopa was associated with an improved fetal outcome. The majority of these women were in the third trimester when Methyldopa therapy was begun.

In one study, women who had begun Methyldopa treatment between weeks 16 and 20 of pregnancy gave birth to infants whose average head circumference was reduced by a small amount (34.2 ± 1.7 cm vs. 34.6 ± 1.3 cm [mean ± 1 S.D.]). Long-term follow up of 195 (97.5%) of the children born to Methyldopa-treated pregnant women (including those who began treatment between weeks 16 and 20) failed to uncover any significant adverse effect on the children. At four years of age, the developmental delay commonly seen in children born to hypertensive mothers was less evident in those whose mothers were treated with Methyldopa during pregnancy than those whose mothers were untreated. The children of the treated group scored consistently higher than the children of the untreated group on five major indices of intellectual and motor development. At age seven and one-half developmental scores and intelligence indices showed no significant differences in children of treated or untreated hypertensive women.

Methyldopate HCl: Pregnancy Category C.: Animal reproduction studies have not been conducted with Methyldopate HCl. It is also not known whether Methyldopate HCl can affect reproduction capacity or can cause fetal harm when given to a pregnant woman. Methyldopate HCl should be given to a pregnant woman only if clearly needed.

NURSING MOTHERS

Methyldopa appears in breast milk. Therefore, caution should be exercised when Methyldopa is given to a nursing woman.

ADVERSE REACTIONS

Sedation, usually transient, may occur during the initial period of therapy or whenever the dose is increased. Headache, asthenia, or weakness may be noted as early and transient symptoms. However, significant adverse effects due to Methyldopa have been infrequent and this agent usually is well tolerated.

The following adverse reactions have been reported and, within each category, are listed in order of decreasing severity.

Cardiovascular: Aggravation of angina pectoris, congestive heart failure, prolonged carotid sinus hypersensitivity, paradoxical pressor response with intravenous use, orthostatic hypotension (decrease daily dosage), edema or weight gain, bradycardia.

Digestive: Pancreatitis, colitis, vomiting, diarrhea, sialadenitis, sore or "black" tongue, nausea, constipation, distension, flatus, dryness of mouth.

Endocrine: Hyperprolactinemia.

Hematologic: Bone marrow depression, leukopenia, granulocytopenia, thrombocytopenia, hemolytic anemia; positive tests for antinuclear antibody, LE cells, and rheumatoid factor, positive Coombs test.

Hepatic: Liver disorders including hepatitis, jaundice, abnormal liver function tests (see "Warnings").

Hypersensitivity: Myocarditis, pericarditis, vasculitis, lupus-like syndrome, drug-related fever.

Nervous System/Psychiatric: Parkinsonism, Bell's palsy, decreased mental acuity, involuntary choreoathetotic movements, symptoms of cerebrovascular insufficiency, psychic disturbances including nightmares and reversible mild psychoses or depression, headache, sedation, asthenia or weakness, dizziness, lightheadedness, paresthesias.

Metabolic: Rise in BUN.

Musculoskeletal: Arthralgia, with or without joint swelling; myalgia.

Respiratory: Nasal stuffiness.

Skin: Toxic epidermal necrolysis, rash.

Urogenital: Amenorrhea, breast enlargement, gynecomastia, lactation, impotence, decreased libido.

OVERDOSAGE

Acute overdosage may produce acute hypotension with other responses attributable to brain and gastrointestinal malfunction (excessive sedation, weakness, bradycardia, dizziness, lightheadedness, constipation, distention, flatus, diarrhea, nausea, vomiting).

In the event of overdosage, symptomatic and supportive measures should be employed. When ingestion is recent, gastric lavage or emesis may reduce absorption. When ingestion has been earlier, infusions may be helpful to promote urinary excretion. Otherwise, management includes special attention to cardiac rate and output, blood volume, electrolyte balance, paralytic ileus, urinary function and cerebral activity.

Sympathomimetic drugs (e.g., levarterenol, epinephrine, metaraminol bitartrate) may be indicated. Methyldopa is dialyzable.

The oral LD$_{50}$ of Methyldopa is greater than 1.5 g/kg in both the mouse and the rat. The acute intravenous LD$_{50}$ of Methyldopate HCl in the mouse is 321 mg/kg.

DOSAGE AND ADMINISTRATION

ORAL METHYLDOPA

ADULTS

Initiation of Therapy: The usual starting dosage of Methyldopa is 250 mg two or three times a day in the first 48 hours. The daily dosage then may be increased or decreased, preferably at intervals of not less than two days, until an adequate response is achieved. To minimize the sedation, start dosage increases in the evening. By adjustment of dosage, morning hypotension may be prevented without sacrificing control of afternoon blood pressure.

When Methyldopa is given to patients on other antihypertensives, the dose of these agents may need to be adjusted to effect a smooth transition. When Methyldopa is given with antihypertensives other than thiazides, the initial dosage of Methyldopa should be limited to 500 mg daily in divided doses; when Methyldopa is added to a thiazide, the dosage of thiazide need not be changed.

Maintenance Therapy: The usual dosage of Methyldopa is 500 mg to 2 g in two to four doses. Although occasional patients have responded to higher doses, the maximum recommended daily dosage is 3 g. Once an effective dosage range is attained, a smooth blood pressure response occurs in most patients in 12 to 24 hours. Since Methyldopa has a relatively short duration of action, withdrawal is followed by return of hypertension usually within 48 hours. This is not complicated by an overshoot of blood pressure.

Occasionally tolerance may occur, usually between the second and third month of therapy. Adding a diuretic or increasing the dosage of Methyldopa frequently will restore effective control of blood pressure. A thiazide may be added at any time during Methyldopa therapy and is recommended if therapy has not been started with a thiazide or if effective control of blood pressure cannot be maintained on 2 g of Methyldopa daily.

Methyldopa is largely excreted by the kidney and patients with impaired renal function may respond to smaller doses. Syncope in older patients may be related to an increased sensitivity and advanced arteriosclerotic vascular disease. This may be avoided by lower doses.

CHILDREN

Initial dosage is based on 10 mg/kg of body weight daily in two to four doses. The daily dosage then is increased or decreased until an adequate response is achieved. The maximum dosage is 65 mg/kg or 3 g daily, whichever is less.

INTRAVENOUS METHYLDOPATE HCL

Methyldopate HCl, when given intravenously in effective doses, causes a decline in blood pressure that may begin in four to six hours and last 10 to 16 hours after injection.

Add the desired dose of Methyldopate HCl to 100 mL of 5 percent dextrose injection. Alternatively the desired dose may be given in 5% dextrose in water in a concentration of 100 mg/10 mL. Give this intravenous infusion slowly over a period of 30 to 60 minutes.

The vial containing Methyldopate HCl should be inspected visually for particulate matter and discoloration before use whenever solution and container permit.

ADULTS

The usual adult dosage intravenously is 250 to 500 mg at six hour intervals as required. The maximum recommended intravenous dose is 1 g every six hours.

When control has been obtained, oral therapy with Methyldopa HCl may be substituted for intravenous therapy, starting with the same dosage schedule used for the parenteral route.

CHILDREN

The recommended daily dosage is 20 to 40 mg/kg of body weight in divided doses every six hours. The maximum dosage is 65 mg/kg or 3 g daily, whichever is less. When the blood pressure is under control, continue with oral therapy using Methyldopa tablets in the same dosage as for the parenteral route.

STORAGE

Store Methyldopa oral suspension below 26°C (78°F) in a tight, light-resistant container. Protect from freezing.

Store Methyldopate HCl injection below 30°C (86°F). Protect from freezing.

HOW SUPPLIED

METHYLDOPA

SUSPENSION: 250 MG/5 ML

BRAND/MANUFACTURER	NDC	SIZE	AWP
○ BRAND			
ALDOMET: Merck	00006-3382-74	473 ml	$58.61

TABLETS: 125 MG

AVERAGE UNIT PRICE (AVAILABLE SIZES)		GENERIC A-RATED AVERAGE PRICE (GAAP)	
BRAND	$0.26	100s	$12.56
GENERIC	$0.13		
HCFA FUL (100s ea)	$0.06		

BRAND/MANUFACTURER	NDC	SIZE	AWP
◆ BRAND			
► ALDOMET: Merck	00006-0135-68	100s	$26.04
◆ GENERICS			
Qualitest	00603-4535-21	100s	$10.41
Major	00904-2399-60	100s	$11.75
Aligen	00405-4651-01	100s	$12.33
Sidmak	50111-0475-01	100s	$12.65
Rugby	00536-5680-01	100s	$13.75
Geneva	00781-1317-01	100s	$13.95
Moore,H.L.	00839-7217-06	100s	$14.84
U.S. Trading	56126-0374-11	100s ud	$6.75
Major	00904-2399-61	100s ud	$16.65

TABLETS: 250 MG

AVERAGE UNIT PRICE (AVAILABLE SIZES)		GENERIC A-RATED AVERAGE PRICE (GAAP)	
BRAND	$0.34	100s	$18.15
GENERIC	$0.16	1000s	$136.13
HCFA FUL (100s ea)	$0.07		

BRAND/MANUFACTURER	NDC	SIZE	AWP
◆ BRAND			
► ALDOMET: Merck	00006-0401-68	100s	$33.14
	00006-0401-28	100s ud	$35.73
	00006-0401-82	1000s	$321.68
	00006-0401-78	1200s	$397.80
◆ GENERICS			
Medirex	57480-0349-06	30s	$8.12
Vangard	00615-2530-06	60s	$7.70
Major	00904-2410-60	100s	$13.25
Novopharm	55953-0164-40	100s	$13.37
Novopharm	55953-0471-40	100s	$13.37
Schein	00364-0707-01	100s	$13.75
Rugby	00536-4553-01	100s	$13.88
Rugby	00536-5681-01	100s	$13.88
Major	00904-2400-60	100s	$13.90
Goldline	00182-1732-01	100s	$13.90
Goldline	00182-1785-01	100s	$13.90
Qualitest	00603-4536-21	100s	$13.90
Moore,H.L.	00839-7692-06	100s	$13.95
Moore,H.L.	00839-7778-06	100s	$13.95
Warner Chilcott	00047-0323-24	100s	$14.96
Sidmak	50111-0476-01	100s	$15.40
Zenith	00172-2931-60	100s	$15.65
Moore,H.L.	00839-7119-06	100s	$18.97
Aligen	00405-4652-01	100s	$21.22
URL	00677-0973-01	100s	$21.95
Geneva	00781-1320-01	100s	$22.00
Mylan	00378-0611-01	100s	$22.50
Vangard	00615-2530-01	100s	$22.96
Lederle Std Prod	00005-3850-43	100s	$29.50
U.S. Trading	56126-0343-11	100s ud	$7.86
Raway	00686-0200-20	100s ud	$13.25
Major	00904-2410-61	100s ud	$16.89
Schein	00364-0707-90	100s ud	$19.25
Geneva	00781-1320-13	100s ud	$19.70
Goldline	00182-1732-89	100s ud	$21.20
Vangard	00615-2530-13	100s ud	$24.04
Major	00904-2400-61	100s ud	$24.12
Auro	55829-0371-10	100s ud	$26.03

◆ RATED THERAPEUTICALLY EQUIVALENT; ◇ THERAPEUTIC EQUIVALENCE UNCONFIRMED; ○ UNRATED

BRAND/MANUFACTURER	NDC	SIZE	AWP
UDL	51079-0200-20	100s ud	$27.90
Medirex	57480-0349-01	100s ud	$28.75
Vangard	00615-2530-12	120s	$14.36
Lederle Std Prod	00005-3850-31	500s	$81.03
Major	00904-2410-80	1000s	$99.10
Novopharm	55953-0164-80	1000s	$102.50
Novopharm	55953-0471-80	1000s	$102.50
Mason Dist	11845-0142-04	1000s	$103.75
Rugby	00536-4553-10	1000s	$108.68
Rugby	00536-5681-10	1000s	$108.68
Major	00904-2400-80	1000s	$111.10
Goldline	00182-1732-10	1000s	$119.95
Goldline	00182-1785-10	1000s	$119.95
Moore,H.L.	00839-7778-16	1000s	$121.43
Warner Chilcott	00047-0323-32	1000s	$122.48
Schein	00364-0707-02	1000s	$135.00
Qualitest	00603-4536-32	1000s	$136.11
Zenith	00172-2931-80	1000s	$137.15
Sidmak	50111-0476-03	1000s	$143.00
Aligen	00405-4652-03	1000s	$168.90
URL	00677-0973-10	1000s	$169.72
Geneva	00781-1320-10	1000s	$169.77
Parmed	00349-8950-10	1000s	$176.06
Moore,H.L.	00839-7119-16	1000s	$179.54
Moore,H.L.	00839-7692-16	1000s	$179.54
Mylan	00378-0611-10	1000s	$179.95

TABLETS: 500 MG

AVERAGE UNIT PRICE (AVAILABLE SIZES)		GENERIC A-RATED AVERAGE PRICE (GAAP)	
BRAND	$0.61	100s	$31.96
GENERIC	$0.30	500s	$136.02
HCFA FUL (100s ea)	$0.13		

BRAND/MANUFACTURER	NDC	SIZE	AWP
◆ BRAND			
➤ ALDOMET: Merck	00006-0516-68	100s	$60.54
	00006-0516-28	100s ud	$62.24
	00006-0516-74	500s	$298.45
	00006-0516-78	1200s	$726.58
◆ GENERICS			
Medirex	57480-0350-06	30s	$13.78
Vangard	00615-2531-06	60s	$17.30
Vangard	00615-2531-90	90s	$19.89
Major	00904-2411-60	100s	$24.20
Sidmak	50111-0477-01	100s	$25.08
Novopharm	55953-0165-40	100s	$25.48
Novopharm	55953-0498-40	100s	$25.48
Rugby	00536-4554-01	100s	$25.90
Rugby	00536-5682-01	100s	$25.90
Goldline	00182-1733-01	100s	$25.90
Goldline	00182-1786-01	100s	$25.90
Moore,H.L.	00839-7693-06	100s	$25.95
Moore,H.L.	00839-7779-06	100s	$25.95
Major	00904-2401-60	100s	$26.20
Warner Chilcott	00047-0324-24	100s	$26.35
Schein	00364-0708-01	100s	$28.07
Zenith	00172-2932-60	100s	$29.70
Qualitest	00603-4537-21	100s	$31.40
URL	00677-0974-01	100s	$35.86
Moore,H.L.	00839-7120-06	100s	$35.91
Geneva	00781-1322-01	100s	$36.80
Mylan	00378-0421-01	100s	$36.95
Vangard	00615-2531-01	100s	$37.33
Aligen	00405-4653-01	100s	$44.30
Lederle Std Prod	00005-3851-43	100s	$47.99
U.S. Trading	56126-0344-11	100s ud	$18.68
Raway	00686-0201-20	100s ud	$24.00
Major	00904-2411-61	100s ud	$29.90
Schein	00364-0708-90	100s ud	$32.25
Geneva	00781-1322-13	100s ud	$32.64
Goldline	00182-1733-89	100s ud	$34.25
Vangard	00615-2531-13	100s ud	$39.04
Major	00904-2401-61	100s ud	$39.30
Auro	55829-0372-10	100s ud	$40.20
UDL	51079-0201-20	100s ud	$45.19
Medirex	57480-0350-01	100s ud	$46.50
Major	00904-2411-40	500s	$99.10
Novopharm	55953-0165-70	500s	$102.50
Novopharm	55953-0498-70	500s	$102.50
Mason Dist	11845-0143-03	500s	$103.75
Rugby	00536-4554-05	500s	$108.68
Rugby	00536-5682-05	500s	$108.68
Major	00904-2401-40	500s	$111.10
Goldline	00182-1733-05	500s	$119.95
Goldline	00182-1786-05	500s	$119.95
Moore,H.L.	00839-7779-12	500s	$121.43
Warner Chilcott	00047-0324-30	500s	$121.51
Schein	00364-0708-05	500s	$136.87
Zenith	00172-2932-70	500s	$137.15
Sidmak	50111-0477-02	500s	$137.50
Qualitest	00603-4537-28	500s	$137.88

BRAND/MANUFACTURER	NDC	SIZE	AWP
Lederle Std Prod	00005-3851-31	500s	$153.03
URL	00677-0974-05	500s	$169.78
Moore,H.L.	00839-7120-12	500s	$169.83
Moore,H.L.	00839-7693-12	500s	$169.83
Parmed	00349-8951-05	500s	$170.50
Geneva	00781-1322-05	500s	$171.10
Mylan	00378-0421-05	500s	$171.50
Aligen	00405-4653-02	500s	$184.28

METHYLDOPATE HYDROCHLORIDE
INJECTION: 50 MG/ML

AVERAGE UNIT PRICE (AVAILABLE SIZES)		GENERIC A-RATED AVERAGE PRICE (GAAP)	
GENERIC	$1.36	5 ml 25s	$210.19
		10 ml 25s	$417.55

BRAND/MANUFACTURER	NDC	SIZE	AWP
◆ GENERICS			
Amer Regent	00517-8905-01	5 ml	$6.24
Du Pont Multi	00590-5529-63	5 ml 20s	$87.50
Du Pont Multi	00590-5529-71	10 ml 20s	$140.00
Abbott Hosp	00074-3030-01	5 ml 25s	$209.30
Abbott Hosp	00074-3405-02	5 ml 25s	$211.08
Abbott Hosp	00074-3030-02	10 ml 25s	$417.41
Abbott Hosp	00074-3406-02	10 ml 25s	$417.70

INJECTION: 250 MG/5 ML

AVERAGE UNIT PRICE (AVAILABLE SIZES)	
BRAND	$2.43
GENERIC	$1.61

BRAND/MANUFACTURER	NDC	SIZE	AWP
◆ BRAND			
ALDOMET: Merck	00006-3293-05	5 ml	$12.13
◆ GENERICS			
Elkins-Sinn	00641-2501-41	5 ml	$8.06
Elkins-Sinn	00641-2502-41	10 ml	$16.13

Methylene Blue

DESCRIPTION
Methylene Blue Injection, USP is a sterile solution of Phenothiazin-5-ium, 3, 7-bis (dimethylamino)-, chloride, trihydrate. Each mL contains 10 mg of Methylene Blue, USP in Water for Injection q.s. pH adjusted with Sodium Hydroxide and/or Hydrochloric Acid.

The molecular formula is $C_{16}H_{18}ClN_3S•3H_2O$ and molecular weight is 373.90.

CLINICAL PHARMACOLOGY
Methylene Blue is Phenothiazin-5-ium, 3, 7-bis (dimethylamino)-, chloride, trihydrate. It will produce two opposite actions on hemoglobin. Low concentrations will convert methemoglobin to hemoglobin. High concentrations convert the ferrous iron of reduced hemoglobin to ferric iron which results in the formation of methemoglobin.

INDICATIONS AND USAGE
Drug-induced methemoglobinemia.

UNLABELED USES
Methylene Blue is used alone or as an adjunct in the treatment of genital herpes infections, pruritus ani, and in the surgical exploration of patients with hyperparathyroidism.

CONTRAINDICATION
Intraspinal injection is contraindicated.

WARNINGS
Methylene Blue should not be given by subcutaneous or intrathecal injection.

PRECAUTIONS
Methylene Blue must be injected intravenously very slowly over a period of several minutes to prevent local high concentration of the compound from producing additional methemoglobin. Do not exceed recommended dosage.

ADVERSE REACTIONS
Large intravenous doses of Methylene Blue produce nausea, abdominal and precordial pain, dizziness, headache, profuse sweating, mental confusion and the formation of methemoglobin.

Use in Pregnancy: Safety for use in pregnancy has not been established. Use of Methylene Blue in women of childbearing potential requires that anticipated benefits be weighed against possible hazards.

DOSAGE AND ADMINISTRATION
0.1 to 0.2 mL per kg body weight (0.045 to 0.09 mL per pound body weight). Inject Methylene Blue intravenously very slowly over a period of several minutes.

➤ SHOWN IN PRODUCT IDENTIFICATION GUIDE

Parenteral drug products should be inspected visually for particulate matter and discoloration, whenever solution and container permit.

HOW SUPPLIED
INJECTION: 1%

BRAND/MANUFACTURER	NDC	SIZE	AWP
○ GENERICS			
Amer Regent	00517-0310-10	10 ml	$10.18
Hope	60267-0400-44	1 ml 10s	$44.95
Amer Regent	00517-0301-10	1 ml 10s	$78.13
Hope	60267-0500-55	10 ml 10s	$62.40
Pasadena	00418-6521-36	1 ml 25s	$68.75
Amer Regent	00517-0372-71	1 ml 25s	$175.00
Raway	00686-0732-71	1 ml 25s	$239.00
CMC-Cons	00223-8173-25	1 ml 25s	$245.00
Pasadena	00418-6521-46	10 ml 25s	$207.50
Amer Regent	00517-0373-70	10 ml 25s	$293.75
CMC-Cons	00223-8175-10	10 ml 25s	$325.00
Raway	00686-0373-70	10 ml 25s	$335.00

Methylergonovine Maleate

DESCRIPTION
Methylergonovine Maleate is a semi-synthetic ergot alkaloid used for the prevention and control of postpartum hemorrhage.

Methylergonovine Maleate is available in sterile ampuls of 1 mL, containing 0.2 mg Methylergonovine Maleate for intramuscular or intravenous injection and in tablets for oral ingestion containing 0.2 mg Methylergonovine Maleate.

Tablets: Methylergonovine Maleate USP, 0.2 mg

Ampuls: 1 mL, clear, colorless solution, Methylergonovine Maleate USP, 0.2 mg

Chemically, Methylergonovine Maleate is designated as ergoline-8-carboxamide, 9,10-didehydro-N-[(1-(hydroxymethyl) propyl)-6-methyl-, [8β(S)]-, (Z)-2-butenedioate (1:1) (salt).

Its molecular formula is $C_{20}H_{25}N_3O_2 \cdot C_4H_4O_4$ and molecular weight is 455.51.

Following is its chemical structure:

CLINICAL PHARMACOLOGY
Methylergonovine Maleate acts directly on the smooth muscle of the uterus and increases the tone, rate, and amplitude of rhythmic contractions. Thus, it induces a rapid and sustained tetanic uterotonic effect which shortens the third stage of labor and reduces blood loss. The onset of action after IV administration is immediate; after i.m. administration, 2-5 minutes, and after oral administration, 5-10 minutes.

Pharmacokinetic studies have utilized radioimmunoassay techniques. After IV injection of 0.2 mg, Methylergonovine Maleate is rapidly distributed from plasma to peripheral tissues within an alpha-phase half-life of 2-3 minutes or less. The beta-phase elimination half-life is 20-30 minutes or more, but clinical effects continue for about 3 hours.[1,2]

Intramuscular injection of 0.2 mg afforded peak plasma concentrations of over 3 ng/mL at t_{max} of 0.5 hours. After 2 hours, total plasma clearance was 120-240 mL/minute.

After oral administration, bioavailability was reported as 60% with no cumulation after repeated doses. During delivery, with parenteral injection, bioavailability increased to 78%.

Excretion is rapid and appears to be partially renal and partially hepatic. Whether the drug is able to penetrate the blood/brain barrier has not been determined.

INDICATIONS AND USAGE
For routine management after delivery of the placenta; postpartum atony and hemorrhage; subinvolution. Under full obstetric supervision, it may be given in the second stage of labor following delivery of the anterior shoulder.

CONTRAINDICATIONS
Hypertension; toxemia; pregnancy; and hypersensitivity.

WARNINGS
This drug should not be administered i.v. routinely because of the possibility of inducing sudden hypertensive and cerebrovascular accidents. If i.v. administration is considered essential as a lifesaving measure, Methylergonovine Maleate should be given slowly over a period of no less than 60 seconds with careful monitoring of blood pressure.

PRECAUTION
GENERAL
Caution should be exercised in the presence of sepsis, obliterative vascular disease, hepatic or renal involvement. Also use with caution during the second stage of labor. The necessity for manual removal of a retained placenta should occur only rarely with proper technique and adequate allowance of time for its spontaneous separation.

DRUG INTERACTIONS
Caution should be exercised when Methylergonovine Maleate is used concurrently with other vasoconstrictors or ergot alkaloids.

CARCINOGENESIS, MUTAGENESIS, IMPAIRMENT OF FERTILITY
No long-term studies have been performed in animals to evaluate carcinogenic potential. The effect of the drug on fertility has not been determined.

PREGNANCY
Category C. Animal reproductive studies have not been conducted with Methylergonovine Maleate. It is also not known whether Methylergonovine Maleate can cause fetal harm or can affect reproductive capacity. Use of Methylergonovine Maleate is contraindicated during pregnancy. (See "Indications and Usage".)

LABOR AND DELIVERY
The uterotonic effect of Methylergonovine Maleate is utilized after delivery to assist involution and decrease hemorrhage, shortening the third stage of labor.

NURSING MOTHERS
Methylergonovine Maleate may be administered orally for a maximum of 1 week postpartum to control uterine bleeding. Recommended dosage is 1 tablet (0.2 mg) 3 or 4 times daily. At this dosage level a small quantity of drug appears in mothers' milk.

Adverse effects have not been described, but caution should be exercised when Methylergonovine Maleate is administered to a nursing woman.

ADVERSE REACTIONS
The most common adverse reaction is hypertension associated in several cases with seizure and/or headache. Hypotension has also been reported. Nausea and vomiting have occurred occasionally. Rarely observed reactions have included, in order of severity: transient chest pains, dyspnea, hematuria, thrombophlebitis, water intoxication, hallucinations, leg cramps, dizziness, tinnitus, nasal congestion, diarrhea, diaphoresis, palpitation, and foul taste.[3]

There have been rare isolated reports of anaphylaxis, without a proven causal relationship to the drug product.

DRUG ABUSE AND DEPENDENCE
Methylergonovine Maleate has not been associated with drug abuse or dependence of either a physical or psychological nature.

OVERDOSE
Symptoms of acute overdose may include: nausea, vomiting, abdominal pain, numbness, tingling of the extremities, rise in blood pressure, in severe cases followed by hypotension, respiratory depression, hypothermia, convulsions, and coma. Because reports of overdosage with Methylergonovine Maleate are infrequent, the lethal dose in humans has not been established. The oral LD_{50} (in mg/kg) for the mouse is 187, the rat 93, and the rabbit 4.5.[4] Several cases of accidental Methylergonovine Maleate injection in newborn infants have been reported, and in such cases 0.2 mg represents an overdose of great magnitude. However, recovery occurred in all but one case following a period of respiratory depression, hypothermia, hypertonicity with jerking movements and, in one case, a single convulsion.

Also, several children 1-3 years of age have accidentally ingested up to 10 tablets (2 mg) with no apparent ill effects. A postpartum patient took 4 tablets at one time in error and reported paresthesias and clamminess as her only symptoms. Treatment of acute overdosage is symptomatic and includes the usual procedures of:
1. removal of offending drug by inducing emesis, gastric lavage, catharsis, and supportive diuresis.
2. maintenance of adequate pulmonary ventilation, especially if convulsions or coma develop.
3. correction of hypotension with pressor drugs as needed.
4. control of convulsions with standard anticonvulsant agents.
5. control of peripheral vasospasm with warmth to the extremities if needed.[5]

DOSAGE AND ADMINISTRATION
Parenteral drug products should be inspected visually for particulate matter and discoloration prior to administration.

INTRAMUSCULARLY
1 mL, 0.2 mg, after delivery of the anterior shoulder, after delivery of the placenta, or during the puerperium. May be repeated as required, at intervals of 2-4 hours.

INTRAVENOUSLY
Dosage same as intramuscular. (See "Warnings".)

ORALLY
One tablet, 0.2 mg, 3 or 4 times daily in the puerperium for a maximum of 1 week.

◆ RATED THERAPEUTICALLY EQUIVALENT; ◇ THERAPEUTIC EQUIVALENCE UNCONFIRMED; ○ UNRATED

STORE AND DISPENSE

Tablets: Below 77°F (25°C); tight, light-resistant container.

Ampuls: Below 77°F (25°C); protect from light—administer only if solution is clear and colorless.

REFERENCES

1. Mantyla, R. and Kants, J.: Clinical Pharmacokinetics of Methylergometrine (Methylergonovine). Int. J. Clin. Pharmacol. Ther. Toxicol. 19(9): 386-391, 1981 2. Iwamura, S. and Kambegawa, A.: Determination of Methylergometrine and Dihydroergotoxine in Biological Fluids. J. Pharm. Dyn. 4: 275-281, 1981 3. Information on Adverse Reactions supplied by Medical Services Dept., Sandoz Pharmaceuticals, E. Hanover, N.J., based on computerized clinical reports. 4. Berde, B. and Schild, H.O.: *Ergot Alkaloids and Related Compounds*, Springer-Verlag, New York, 1978, p. 810 5. Treatment of Acute Overdosage. Sandoz Dorsey Rx Products. Sandoz Inc., Medical Services Department.

J CODES

Up to 2.0 mg IM,IV—J2210

HOW SUPPLIED
INJECTION: 0.2 MG

AVERAGE UNIT PRICE (AVAILABLE SIZES)			
BRAND	$2.55		

BRAND/MANUFACTURER	NDC	SIZE	AWP
◆ BRAND			
METHERGINE: Sandoz Pharm	00078-0053-03	1 ml 20s	$51.96
	00078-0053-04	1 ml 50s	$125.04

TABLETS: 0.2 MG

AVERAGE UNIT PRICE (AVAILABLE SIZES)			
BRAND	$0.47		

BRAND/MANUFACTURER	NDC	SIZE	AWP
◆ BRAND			
METHERGINE: Sandoz Pharm	00078-0054-05	100s	$47.04
	00078-0054-06	100s ud	$49.32
	00078-0054-09	1000s	$458.94

Methylphenidate Hydrochloride

DESCRIPTION

Methylphenidate Hydrochloride is a mild central nervous system (CNS) stimulant available in immediate-release and sustained-release tablets for oral administration. Methylphenidate Hydrochloride is methyl ∝-phenyl-2-piperidineacetate Hydrochloride.

Methylphenidate Hydrochloride USP is a white, odorless, fine crystalline powder. Its solutions are acid to litmus. It is freely soluble in water and in methanol, soluble in alcohol, and slightly soluble in chloroform and in acetone. Its molecular weight is 269.77.

Following is its chemical structure:

CLINICAL PHARMACOLOGY

Methylphenidate HCl is a mild central nervous system stimulant. The mode of action in man is not completely understood, but Methylphenidate HCl presumably activates the brain stem arousal system and cortex to produce its stimulant effect.

There is neither specific evidence which clearly establishes the mechanism whereby Methylphenidate HCl produces its mental and behavioral effects in children, nor conclusive evidence regarding how these effects relate to the condition of the central nervous system.

Methylphenidate HCl in sustained release tablets is more slowly but as extensively absorbed as in the regular tablets. Relative bioavailability of the sustained release tablet compared to the Methylphenidate HCl tablet, measured by the urinary excretion of Methylphenidate HCl major metabolite (∝-phenyl-2-piperidine acetic acid) was 105% (49-168%) in children and 101% (85-152%) in adults. The time to peak rate in children was 4.7 hours (1.3-8.2 hours) for the sustained release tablets and 1.9 hours (0.3-4.4 hours) for the tablets. An average of 67% of sustained release tablet dose was excreted in children as compared to 86% in adults.

INDICATIONS
ATTENTION DEFICIT DISORDERS, NARCOLEPSY

Attention Deficit Disorders (previously known as Minimal Brain Dysfunction in Children). Other terms being used to describe the behavioral syndrome below include: Hyperkinetic Child Syndrome, Minimal Brain Damage, Minimal Cerebral Dysfunction, Minor Cerebral Dysfunction.

Methylphenidate HCl is indicated as an integral part of a total treatment program which typically includes other remedial measures (psychological, educational, social) for a stabilizing effect in children with a behavioral syndrome characterized by the following group of developmentally inappropriate symptoms: moderate-to-severe distractibility, short attention span, hyperactivity, emotional lability, and impulsivity. The diagnosis of this syndrome should not be made with finality when these symptoms are only of comparatively recent origin. Nonlocalizing (soft) neurological signs, learning disability, and abnormal EEG may or may not be present, and a diagnosis of central nervous system dysfunction may or may not be warranted.

SPECIAL DIAGNOSTIC CONSIDERATIONS

Specific etiology of this syndrome is unknown, and there is no single diagnostic test. Adequate diagnosis requires the use not only of medical but of special psychological, educational, and social resources.

Characteristics commonly reported include: chronic history of short attention span, distractibility, emotional lability, impulsivity, and moderate-to-severe hyperactivity; minor neurological signs and abnormal EEG. Learning may or may not be impaired. The diagnosis must be based upon a complete history and evaluation of the child and not solely on the presence of one or more of these characteristics.

Drug treatment is not indicated for all children with this syndrome. Stimulants are not intended for use in the child who exhibits symptoms secondary to environmental factors and/or primary psychiatric disorders, including psychosis. Appropriate educational placement is essential and psychosocial intervention is generally necessary. When remedial measures alone are insufficient, the decision to prescribe stimulant medication will depend upon the physician's assessment of the chronicity and severity of the child's symptoms.

CONTRAINDICATIONS

Marked anxiety, tension, and agitation are contraindications to Methylphenidate HCl, since the drug may aggravate these symptoms. Methylphenidate HCl is contraindicated also in patients known to be hypersensitive to the drug, in patients with glaucoma, and in patients with motor tics or with a family history or diagnosis of Tourette's syndrome.

WARNINGS

Methylphenidate HCl should not be used in children under six years, since safety and efficacy in this age group have not been established.

Sufficient data on safety and efficacy of long-term use of Methylphenidate HCl in children are not yet available. Although a causal relationship has not been established, suppression of growth (*ie*, weight gain, and/or height) has been reported with the long-term use of stimulants in children. Therefore, patients requiring long-term therapy should be carefully monitored. Methylphenidate HCl should not be used for severe depression of either exogenous or endogenous origin. Clinical experience suggests that in psychotic children, administration of Methylphenidate HCl may exacerbate symptoms of behavior disturbance and thought disorder.

Methylphenidate HCl should not be used for the prevention or treatment of normal fatigue states.

There is some clinical evidence that Methylphenidate HCl may lower the convulsive threshold in patients with prior history of seizures, with prior EEG abnormalities in absence of seizures, and, very rarely, in absence of history of seizures and no prior EEG evidence of seizures. Safe concomitant use of anticonvulsants and Methylphemdate HCl has not been established. In the presence of seizures, the drug should be discontinued.

Use cautiously in patients with hypertension. Blood pressure should be monitored at appropriate intervals in all patients taking Methylphenidate HCl, especially those with hypertension.

Symptoms of visual disturbances have been encountered in rare cases. Difficulties with accommodation and blurring of vision have been reported.

DRUG INTERACTIONS

Methylphenidate HCl may decrease the hypotensive effect of guanethidine. Use cautiously with pressor agents and MAO inhibitors. Human pharmacologic studies have shown that Methylphenidate HCl may inhibit the metabolism of coumarin anticoagulants, anticonvulsants (phenobarbital, diphenylhydantoin, primidone), phenylbutazone, and tricyclic drugs (imipramine, clomipramine, desipramine). Downward dosage adjustments of these drugs may be required when given concomitantly with Methylphenidate HCl.

USAGE IN PREGNANCY

Adequate animal reproduction studies to establish safe use of Methylphenidate HCl during pregnancy have not been conducted. Therefore, until more information is available, Methylphenidate HCl should not be prescribed for women of childbearing age unless, in the opinion of the physician, the potential benefits outweigh the possible risks.

DRUG DEPENDENCE

METHYLPHENIDATE HCL SHOULD BE GIVEN CAUTIOUSLY TO EMOTIONALLY UNSTABLE PATIENTS, SUCH AS THOSE WITH A HISTORY OF DRUG DEPENDENCE OR ALCOHOLISM, BECAUSE SUCH PATIENTS MAY INCREASE DOSAGE ON THEIR OWN INITIATIVE.

CHRONICALLY ABUSIVE USE CAN LEAD TO MARKED TOLERANCE AND PSYCHIC DEPENDENCE WITH VARYING DEGREES OF ABNORMAL BEHAVIOR. FRANK PSYCHOTIC EPISODES CAN OCCUR, ESPECIALLY WITH PARENTERAL ABUSE. CAREFUL SUPERVISION IS REQUIRED DURING DRUG WITHDRAWAL, SINCE SEVERE DEPRESSION AS WELL AS THE

► SHOWN IN PRODUCT IDENTIFICATION GUIDE

EFFECTS OF CHRONIC OVERACTIVITY CAN BE UNMASKED. LONG-TERM FOLLOW-UP MAY BE REQUIRED BECAUSE OF THE PATIENT'S BASIC PERSONALITY DISTURBANCES.

PRECAUTIONS

Patients with an element of agitation may react adversely; discontinue therapy if necessary.

Periodic CBC, differential, and platelet counts are advised during prolonged therapy.

Drug treatment is not indicated in all cases of this behavioral syndrome and should be considered only in light of the complete history and evaluation of the child. The decision to prescribe Methylphenidate HCl should depend on the physician's assessment of the chronicity and severity of the child's symptoms and their appropriateness for his/her age. Prescription should not depend solely on the presence of one or more of the behavioral characteristics.

When these symptoms are associated with acute stress reactions, treatment with Methylphenidate HCl is usually not indicated.

Long-term effects of Methylphenidate HCl in children have not been well established.

ADVERSE REACTIONS

Nervousness and insomnia are the most common adverse reactions but are usually controlled by reducing dosage and omitting the drug in the afternoon or evening. Other reactions include hypersensitivity (including skin rash, urticaria, fever, arthralgia, exfoliative dermatitis, erythema multiforme with histopathological findings of necrotizing vasculitis, and thrombocytopenic purpura); anorexia; nausea; dizziness; palpitations; headache; dyskinesia; drowsiness; blood pressure and pulse changes, both up and down; tachycardia; angina; cardiac arrhythmia; abdominal pain; weight loss during prolonged therapy. There have been rare reports of Tourette's syndrome. Toxic psychosis has been reported. Although a definite causal relationship has not been established, the following have been reported in patients taking this drug; isolated cases of cerebral arteritis and/or occlusion; leukopenia and/or anemia; transient depressed mood, a few instances of scalp hair loss.

In children, loss of appetite, abdominal pain, weight loss during prolonged therapy, insomnia, and tachycardia may occur more frequently; however, any of the other adverse reactions listed above may also occur.

DOSAGE AND ADMINISTRATION

Dosage should be individualized according to the needs and responses of the patient.

ADULTS

Tablets: Administer in divided doses 2 or 3 times daily, preferably 30 to 45 minutes before meals. Average dosage is 20 to 30 mg daily. Some patients may require 40 to 60 mg daily. In others, 10 to 15 mg daily will be adequate. Patients who are unable to sleep if medication is taken late in the day should take the last dose before 6 p.m.

Sustained Release Tablets: Methylphenidate HCl sustained release tablets have a duration of action of approximately 8 hours. Therefore, Methylphenidate HCl sustained release tablets may be used in place of Methylphenidate HCl tablets when the 8-hour dosage of Methylphenidate HCl Sustained release corresponds to the titrated 8-hour dosage of Methylphenidate HCl. Methylphenidate HCl sustained release tablets must be swallowed whole and never crushed or chewed.

CHILDREN (6 YEARS AND OVER)

Methylphenidate HCl should be initiated in small doses, with gradual weekly increments. Daily dosage above 60 mg is not recommended.

If improvement is not observed after appropriate dosage adjustment over a one-month period, the drug should be discontinued.

Tablets: Start with 5 mg twice daily (before breakfast and lunch) with gradual increments of 5 to 10 mg weekly.

Sustained Release Tablets: Sustained release tablets have a duration of action of approximately 8 hours. Therefore, Methylphenidate HCl sustained release tablets may be used in place of Methylphenidate HCl tablets when the 8-hour dosage of Methylphenidate HCl sustained release corresponds to the titrated 8-hour dosage of Methylphenidate HCl. Methylphenidate HCl sustained release tablets must be swallowed whole and never crushed or chewed.

If paradoxical aggravation of symptoms or other adverse effects occur, reduce dosage, or, if necessary, discontinue the drug.

Methylphenidate HCl should be periodically discontinued to assess the child's condition. Improvement may be sustained when the drug is either temporarily or permanently discontinued.

Drug treatment should not and need not be indefinite and usually may be discontinued after puberty.

OVERDOSAGE

Signs and symptoms of acute overdosage, resulting principally from overstimulation of the central nervous system and from excessive sympathomimetic effects, may include the following: vomiting, agitation, tremors, hyperreflexia, muscle twitching, convulsions (may be followed by coma), euphoria, confusion, hallucinations, delirium, sweating, flushing, headache, hyperpyrexia, tachycardia, palpitations, cardiac arrhythmias, hypertension, mydriasis, and dryness of mucous membranes.

Treatment consists of appropriate supportive measures. The patient must be protected against self-injury and against external stimuli that would aggravate overstimulation already present. If signs and symptoms are not too severe and the patient is conscious, gastric contents may be evacuated by induction of emesis or gastric lavage. In the presence of severe intoxication, use a carefully titrated dosage of a *short-acting* barbiturate *before* performing gastric lavage.

Intensive care must be provided to maintain adequate circulation and respiratory exchange; external cooling procedures may be required for hyperpyrexia.

Efficacy of peritoneal dialysis or extracorporeal hemodialysis for Methylphenidate HCl overdosage has not been established.

Dispense in tight, light-resistant container (USP): Do not store above 86°F (30°C). Protect from moisture.

HOW SUPPLIED
TABLET, EXTENDED RELEASE (C-II): 20 MG

AVERAGE UNIT PRICE (AVAILABLE SIZES)		GENERIC A-RATED AVERAGE PRICE (GAAP)	
BRAND	$0.94	100s	$83.44
GENERIC	$0.83		
HCFA FUL (100s ea)	$0.90		

BRAND/MANUFACTURER	NDC	SIZE	AWP
◆ **BRAND**			
➤ RITALIN-SR: Ciba Pharm	00083-0016-30	100s	$93.72
◆ **GENERICS**			
➤ MD Pharm	43567-0562-07	100s	$71.41
Aligen	00405-0128-01	100s	$78.92
Goldline	00182-9147-01	100s	$83.50
Rugby	00536-4039-01	100s	$84.35
Major	00904-2773-60	100s	$84.55
Purepac	00228-2089-10	100s	$84.58
Qualitest	00603-4572-21	100s	$84.65
Parmed	00349-8834-01	100s	$89.00
Schein	00364-2329-01	100s	$89.99

TABLETS (C-II): 5 MG

AVERAGE UNIT PRICE (AVAILABLE SIZES)		GENERIC A-RATED AVERAGE PRICE (GAAP)	
BRAND	$0.30	100s	$27.08
GENERIC	$0.27	1000s	$260.09
HCFA FUL (100s ea)	$0.27		

BRAND/MANUFACTURER	NDC	SIZE	AWP
◆ **BRAND**			
➤ RITALIN: Ciba Pharm	00083-0007-30	100s	$29.83
◆ **GENERICS**			
➤ MD Pharm	43567-0531-07	100s	$22.73
Aligen	00405-0125-01	100s	$25.12
Goldline	00182-1173-01	100s	$26.50
Purepac	00228-2091-10	100s	$27.01
Major	00904-2768-60	100s	$27.90
Qualitest	00603-4569-21	100s	$28.25
Rugby	00536-4029-01	100s	$28.27
Parmed	00349-8365-01	100s	$28.35
Schein	00364-0561-01	100s	$29.61
➤ MD Pharm	43567-0531-12	1000s	$211.10
Aligen	00405-0125-03	1000s	$233.33
Major	00904-2768-80	1000s	$259.00
Rugby	00536-4029-10	1000s	$268.86
Qualitest	00603-4569-32	1000s	$270.30
Parmed	00349-8365-10	1000s	$275.00
Goldline	00182-1173-10	1000s	$277.50
Schein	00364-0561-02	1000s	$285.60

TABLETS (C-II): 10 MG

AVERAGE UNIT PRICE (AVAILABLE SIZES)		GENERIC A-RATED AVERAGE PRICE (GAAP)	
BRAND	$0.43	100s	$37.90
GENERIC	$0.37	1000s	$360.19
HCFA FUL (100s ea)	$0.38		

BRAND/MANUFACTURER	NDC	SIZE	AWP
◆ **BRAND**			
➤ RITALIN: Ciba Pharm	00083-0003-30	100s	$42.57
◆ **GENERICS**			
➤ MD Pharm	43567-0530-07	100s	$32.50
Aligen	00405-0126-01	100s	$35.85
Goldline	00182-1066-01	100s	$37.00
Purepac	00228-2092-10	100s	$37.49
Major	00904-2769-60	100s	$38.55
Rugby	00536-4035-01	100s	$39.49
Qualitest	00603-4570-21	100s	$39.50
Schein	00364-0479-01	100s	$40.32
Parmed	00349-8366-01	100s	$40.40
➤ MD Pharm	43567-0530-12	1000s	$290.70
Aligen	00405-0126-03	1000s	$321.31
Major	00904-2769-80	1000s	$352.20
Rugby	00536-4035-10	1000s	$375.15
Qualitest	00603-4570-32	1000s	$380.12
Goldline	00182-1066-10	1000s	$381.00

◆ RATED THERAPEUTICALLY EQUIVALENT; ◇ THERAPEUTIC EQUIVALENCE UNCONFIRMED; ○ UNRATED

BRAND/MANUFACTURER	NDC	SIZE	AWP
Parmed	00349-8366-10	1000s	$390.00
Schein	00364-0479-02	1000s	$391.00

TABLETS (C-II): 20 MG

AVERAGE UNIT PRICE (AVAILABLE SIZES)		GENERIC A-RATED AVERAGE PRICE (GAAP)	
BRAND	$0.61	100s	$54.63
GENERIC	$0.54	1000s	$519.24
HCFA FUL (100s ea)	$0.55		

BRAND/MANUFACTURER	NDC	SIZE	AWP
◆ BRAND			
➤ RITALIN: Ciba Pharm	00083-0034-30	100s	$61.24
◆ GENERICS			
➤ MD Pharm	43567-0532-07	100s	$46.66
Major	00904-2770-60	100s	$52.15
Purepac	00228-2093-10	100s	$54.26
Aligen	00405-0127-01	100s	$54.95
Rugby	00536-4030-01	100s	$55.72
Qualitest	00603-4571-21	100s	$56.80
Parmed	00349-8367-01	100s	$57.00
Goldline	00182-1174-01	100s	$57.00
Schein	00364-0562-01	100s	$57.12
Major	00904-2770-80	1000s	$428.40
➤ MD Pharm	43567-0532-12	1000s	$434.50
Parmed	00349-8367-10	1000s	$550.00
Goldline	00182-1174-10	1000s	$562.50
Qualitest	00603-4571-32	1000s	$565.01
Schein	00364-0562-02	1000s	$575.00

Methylprednisolone

DESCRIPTION

Methylprednisolone Tablets contain Methylprednisolone which is a glucocorticoid. Glucocorticoids are adrenocortical steroids, both naturally occurring and synthetic, which are readily absorbed from the gastrointestinal tract. Methylprednisolone occurs as a white to practically white, odorless, crystalline powder. It is sparingly soluble in alcohol, in dioxane, and in methanol, slightly soluble in acetone, and in chloroform, and very slightly soluble in ether. It is practically insoluble in water.

The chemical name for Methylprednisolone is pregna-1, 4-diene-3, 20-dione,11, 17, 21-trihydroxy-6-methyl-,(6α, 11β)-and the molecular weight is 374.48.

Methylprednisolone Sterile Aqueous Suspension contains Methylprednisolone Acetate which is the 6-methyl derivative of prednisolone. Methylprednisolone Acetate is a white or practically white, odorless, crystalline powder which melts at about 215° with some decomposition. It is soluble in dioxane, sparingly soluble in acetone, in alcohol, in chloroform, and in methanol, and slightly soluble in ether. It is practically insoluble in water.

The chemical name for Methylprednisolone Acetate is pregna-1,4-diene-3,20-dione, 21-(acetyloxy)-11,17-dihy-droxy-6-methyl-,(6α, 11β)- and the molecular weight is 416.51.

Methylprednisolone Acetate Sterile Aqueous Suspension is an anti-inflammatory glucocorticoid for intramuscular, intrasynovial, soft tissue or intralesional injection, not for intravenous use. It is available in three strengths: 20 mg/mL; 40 mg/mL; 80 mg/mL and as single-dose vials in two strengths: 40 mg/mL; 80 mg/mL.

Methylprednisolone Sodium Succinate Sterile Powder for Injection contains Methylprednisolone Sodium Succinate as the active ingredient. Methylprednisolone Sodium Succinate, USP, occurs as a white, or nearly white, odorless hygroscopic, amorphous solid. It is very soluble in water and in alcohol: it is insoluble in chloroform and is very slightly soluble in acetone.

The chemical name for Methylprednisolone Sodium Succinate is pregna-1,4-diene-3,20-dione,21-(3-carboxy-1-oxopropoxy)-11,17-dihy-   droxy-6-methyl-,monosodium salt, (6α, 11β), and the molecular weight is 496.53.

Methylprednisolone Sodium Succinate is so extremely soluble in water that it may be administered in a small volume of diluent and is especially well suited for intravenous use in situations in which high blood levels of Methylprednisolone are required rapidly.

Methylprednisolone Sodium Succinate for Injection is available in several strengths and packages for intravenous or intramuscular administration.

Each Tablet for oral administration contains: Methylprednisolone 2 mg, 4 mg, 8 mg, 16 mg, 24 mg, or 32 mg

Each mL of Aqueous Suspension contains: Methylprednisolone Acetate 20 mg, 40 mg, or 80 mg. When necessary, pH was adjusted with sodium hydroxide and/or hydrochloric acid. The pH of the finished product remains within the USP specified range; i.e., 3.5 to 7.0.

Sterile powder for injection, mixed:

Each mL contains: Methylprednisolone Sodium Succinate equivalent to 40 mg Methylprednisolone

Each 2 mL contains: Methylprednisolone Sodium Succinate equivalent to 125 mg Methylprednisolone

Each 8 mL contains: Methylprednisolone Sodium Succinate equivalent to 500 mg or 1 gm Methylprednisolone

Each 16 mL contains: Methylprednisolone Sodium Succinate equivalent to 1 gm Methylprednisolone

Each 30.6 mL contains: Methylprednisolone Sodium Succinate equivalent to 2 gm Methylprednisolone

When necessary, the pH of each formula was adjusted with sodium hydroxide so that the pH of the reconstituted solution is within the USP specified range of 7 to 8 and the tonicities are, for the 40 mg per mL solution, 0.50 osmolar; for the 125 mg per 2 mL, 500 mg per 8 mL and 1 gram per 16 mL solutions, 0.40 osmolar; for the 2 gram per 30.6 mL solutions, 0.42 osmolar. (Isotonic saline = 0.28 osmolar).

Important —Use only the accompanying diluent or Bacteriostatic Water For Injection with Benzyl Alcohol when reconstituting Methylprednisolone Sodium Succinate.

"Use within 48 hours after mixing"

Following is its chemical structure:

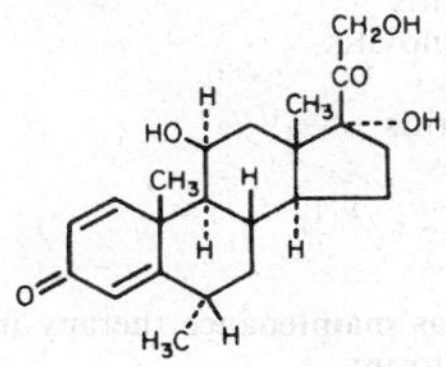

ACTIONS

Naturally occurring glucocorticoids (hydrocortisone and cortisone), which also have salt-retaining properties, are used as replacement therapy in adrenocortical deficiency states. Their synthetic analogs are primarily used for their potent anti-inflammatory effects in disorders of many organ systems.

Glucocorticoids cause profound and varied metabolic effects. In addition, they modify the body's immune responses to diverse stimuli.

As of November, 1990, the formulation for Methylprednisolone Acetate Sterile Aqueous Suspension was revised. In a bioavailability study with thirty subjects, the new formulation was found to be more bioavailable than the previous formulation. An increase in the extent of Methylprednisolone absorption was observed for the new formulation as indicated by significantly increased values for area under the serum Methylprednisolone concentration curve and maximum serum Methylprednisolone concentration (see table below). No difference in elimination half-life ($t_{1/2}$, calculated from the mean terminal elimination rate) was observed between the two formulations. No medically meaningful differences between the two formulations were seen in relation to vital signs, safety laboratory analyses, formulation effects, local tolerance, or side effects. This increase in absorption is not considered clinically significant.

	Previous Formulation	Current Formulation
AUC 0-240 hrs	1053 (47.3)*	1286 (39.2)
(ng × hr/mL)	[133-2297]**	[208-2225]
C_{max} (ng/mL)	8.98 (65.9)	11.8 (44.1)
	[0-28.5]	[3.37-23.4]
$T_{1/2}$ (hr)	139	139
	[46-990]	[58-866]

* *Coefficient of variation (%)*
** *Range of values*

Methylprednisolone is a potent anti-inflammatory steroid. It has a greater anti-inflammatory potency than prednisone and even less tendency than prednisolone to induce sodium and water retention.

Methylprednisolone Sodium Succinate has the same metabolic and anti-inflammatory actions as Methylprednisolone. When given parenterally and in equimolar quantities, the two compounds are equivalent in biologic activity. The relative potency of Methylprednisolone Sodium Succinate and hydrocortisone sodium succinate, as indicated by depression of eosinophil count, following intravenous administration, is at least four to one. This is in good agreement with the relative oral potency of Methylprednisolone and hydrocortisone.

INDICATIONS

Methylprednisolone Tablets are indicated in the following conditions.

When oral therapy is not feasible and the strength, dosage form, and route of administration of the drug reasonably lend the preparation to the treatment of the condition, the intramuscular use of Methylprednisolone Acetate Sterile Aqueous Suspensions or the intravenous or intramuscular use of Methylprednisolone Sodium Succinate Sterile Powder is indicated.

1. ENDOCRINE DISORDERS

Primary or secondary adrenocortical insufficiency (hydrocortisone or cortisone is the first choice; synthetic analogs may be used in conjunction with mineralocorticoids where applicable; in infancy mineralocorticoid supplementation is of particular importance).

  Congenital adrenal hyperplasia
  Nonsuppurative thyroiditis
  Hypercalcemia associated with cancer

Methylprednisolone Acetate Suspension and Methylprednisolone Sodium Succinate Powder are also indicated in: Acute adrenocortical insufficiency (hydrocortisone or cortisone is the drug of choice; mineralocorticoid supplementation may be necessary, particularly when synthetic analogs are used)

Preoperatively and in the event of serious trauma or illness, in patients with known adrenal insufficiency or when adrenocortical reserve is doubtful.

Methylprednisolone Sodium Succinate Powder is also indicated in: Shock unresponsive to conventional therapy if adrenocortical insufficiency exists or is suspected.

2. RHEUMATIC DISORDERS
As adjunctive therapy for short-term administration (to tide the patient over an acute episode or exacerbation) in:
Psoriatic arthritis
Rheumatoid arthritis, including juvenile rheumatoid arthritis (selected cases may require low-dose maintenance therapy)
Ankylosing spondylitis
Acute and subacute bursitis
Acute nonspecific tenosynovitis
Acute gouty arthritis
Post-traumatic osteoarthritis
Synovitis of osteoarthritis
Epicondylitis

3. COLLAGEN DISEASES
During an exacerbation or as maintenance therapy in selected cases of:
Systemic lupus erythematosus
Acute rheumatic carditis
Systemic dermatomyositis (polymyositis)

4. DERMATOLOGIC DISEASES
Pemphigus
Bullous dermatitis herpetiformis
Severe erythema multiforme (Stevens-Johnson syndrome)
Exfoliative dermatitis
Mycosis fungoides
Severe psoriasis
Severe seborrheic dermatitis

5. ALLERGIC STATES
Control of severe or incapacitating allergic conditions intractable to adequate trials of conventional treatment:
Seasonal or perennial allergic rhinitis
Serum sickness
Bronchial asthma
Drug hypersensitivity reactions
Contact dermatitis
Atopic dermatitis

Methylprednisolone Acetate Suspension and Methylprednisolone Sodium Succinate Powder are also indicated in:
Urticarial transfusion reactions
Acute noninfectious laryngeal edema (epinephrine is the drug of first choice)

6. OPHTHALMIC DISEASES
Severe acute and chronic allergic and inflammatory processes involving the eye and its adnexa such as:
Allergic corneal marginal ulcers
Herpes zoster ophthalmicus
Anterior segment inflammation
Diffuse posterior uveitis and choroiditis
Sympathetic ophthalmia
Allergic conjunctivitis
Keratitis
Chorioretinitis
Optic neuritis
Iritis and iridocyclitis

7. RESPIRATORY DISEASES
Symptomatic sarcoidosis
Loeffler's syndrome not manageable by other means
Berylliosis
Fulminating or disseminated pulmonary tuberculosis when used concurrently with appropriate antituberculous chemotherapy
Aspiration pneumonitis

8. HEMATOLOGIC DISORDERS
Idiopathic thrombocytopenic purpura in adults (IV only; IM administration is contraindicated)
Secondary thrombocytopenia in adults
Acquired (autoimmune) hemolytic anemia
Erythroblastopenia (RBC anemia)
Congenital (erythroid) hypoplastic anemia

9. NEOPLASTIC DISEASES
For palliative management of:
Leukemias and lymphomas in adults
Acute leukemia of childhood

10. EDEMATOUS STATES
To induce a diuresis or remission of proteinuria in the nephrotic syndrome, without uremia, of the idiopathic type or that due to lupus erythematosus.

11. GASTROINTESTINAL DISEASES
To tide the patient over a critical period of the disease in:
Ulcerative colitis (Systemic for Methylprednisolone Acetate and Methylprednisolone Sodium Succinate)
Regional enteritis (Systemic for Methylprednisolone Acetate and Methylprednisolone Sodium Succinate)

12. NERVOUS SYSTEM
Acute exacerbations of multiple sclerosis

13. MISCELLANEOUS
Tuberculous meningitis with subarachnoid block or impending block when used concurrently with appropriate antituberculous chemotherapy.
Trichinosis with neurologic or myocardial involvement

For intrasynovial or soft tissue administration (see *"Warnings"*). Methylprednisolone Acetate Sterile Aqueous Suspension is indicated as adjunctive therapy for short-term administration (to tide the patient over an acute episode or exacerbation) in:
Synovitis of osteoarthritis
Rheumatoid arthritis
Acute and subacute bursitis
Acute gouty arthritis
Epicondylitis
Acute nonspecific tenosynovitis
Posttraumatic osteoarthritis
For Intralesional Administration, Methylprednisolone Acetate Sterile Aqueous Suspension is indicated for intralesional use in the following conditions:
Keloids
Localized hypertrophic infiltrated, inflammatory lesions of:
lichen planus, psoriatic plaques, granuloma annulare, and lichen simplex chronicus (neurodermatitis)
Discoid lupus erythematosus
Necrobiosis lipoidica diabeticorum
Alopecia areata
Methylprednisolone Acetate Sterile Aqueous Suspension also may be useful in cystic tumors of an aponeurosis or tendon (ganglia).

UNLABELED USES
Methylprednisolone is used alone or as an adjunct in the treatment of male infertility, chemotherapy-induced emesis, and acute crescentic glomerulonephritis. It is also used in AIDS patients with *pneumocystis carinii* pneumonia and is prescribed in the treatment of adult respiratory distress syndrome, polymyalgia rheumatica, and congenital pure red cell aplasia (Diamond-Blackfan syndrome). It is also used to control symptoms of De Quervain's tenosynovitis.

CONTRAINDICATIONS
Systemic fungal infections and known hypersensitivity to components.

Methylprednisolone Acetate Sterile Aqueous Suspension is contraindicated for intrathecal administration. Reports of severe medical events have been associated with this route of administration. Methylprednisolone Acetate (except the single dose vial) and some forms of Methylprednisolone Sodium Succinate are contraindicated for use in premature infants because the formulation contains benzyl alcohol. Benzyl alcohol has been reported to be associated with a fatal "gasping syndrome" in premature infants.

WARNINGS
Methylprednisolone Acetate Sterile Aqueous Suspension and some forms of Methylprednisolone Sodium Succinate Sterile Powder may contain benzyl alcohol which is potentially toxic when administered locally to neural tissue.

Multidose use of Methylprednisolone Acetate Sterile Aqueous Suspension from a single vial requires special care to avoid contamination. The single dose vial is not suitable for multi-dose use. Following administration of the desired dose, any remaining suspension should be discarded.

Although essentially sterile, any multidose use of vials may lead to contamination unless strict aseptic technique is observed. Particular care, such as use of disposable sterile syringes and needles is necessary.

While crystals of adrenal steroids in the dermis suppress inflammatory reactions, their presence may cause disintegration of the cellular elements and physiochemical changes in the ground substance of the connective tissue. The resultant infrequently occurring dermal and/or subdermal changes may form depressions in the skin at the injection site. The degree to which this reaction occurs will vary with the amount of adrenal steroid injected. Regeneration is usually complete within a few months or after all crystals of the adrenal steroid have been absorbed.

In order to minimize the incidence of dermal and subdermal atrophy, care must be exercised not to exceed recommended doses in injections. Multiple small injections into the area of the lesion should be made whenever possible. The technique of intrasynovial and intramuscular injection should include precautions against injection or leakage into the dermis. Injection into the deltoid muscle should be avoided because of a high incidence of subcutaneous atrophy.

It is critical that, during administration of Methylprednisolone Acetate, appropriate technique be used and care taken to assure proper placement of drug.

◆ RATED THERAPEUTICALLY EQUIVALENT; ◇ THERAPEUTIC EQUIVALENCE UNCONFIRMED; ○ UNRATED

In patients on corticosteroid therapy subjected to unusual stress, increased dosage of rapidly acting corticosteroids before, during, and after the stressful situation is indicated.

Corticosteroids may mask some signs of infection and new infections may appear during their use. There may be decreased resistance and inability to localize infection when corticosteroids are used. Do not use Methylprednisolone Acetate Suspension intra-articularly, intrabursally or for intratendinous administration for local effect in the presence of acute infection.

A study has failed to establish the efficacy of Methylprednisolone Sodium Succinate in the treatment of sepsis syndrome and septic shock. The study also suggests that treatment of these conditions with Methylprednisolone Sodium Succinate may increase the risk of mortality in certain patients (ie, patients with elevated serum creatinine levels or patients who develop secondary infections after Methylprednisolone Sodium Succinate).

Prolonged use of corticosteroids may produce posterior subcapsular cataracts, glaucoma with possible damage to the optic nerves, and may enhance the establishment of secondary ocular infections due to fungi or viruses.

Usage in pregnancy: Since adequate human reproduction studies have not been done with corticosteroids, the use of these drugs in pregnancy, nursing mothers or women of childbearing potential requires that the possible benefits of the drug be weighed against the potential hazards to the mother and embryo or fetus. Infants born of mothers who have received substantial doses of corticosteroids during pregnancy should be carefully observed for signs of hypoadrenalism.

Average and large doses of hydrocortisone or cortisone can cause elevation of blood pressure, salt and water retention, and increased excretion of potassium. These effects are less likely to occur with the synthetic derivatives except when used in large doses. Dietary salt restriction and potassium supplementation may be necessary. All corticosteroids increase calcium excretion.

While on corticosteroid therapy patients should not be vaccinated against smallpox. Other immunization procedures should not be undertaken in patients who are on corticosteroids, especially on high dose, because of possible hazards of neurological complications and a lack of antibody response.

The use of Methylprednisolone products in active tuberculosis should be restricted to those cases of fulminating or disseminated tuberculosis in which the corticosteroid is used for the management of the disease in conjunction with an appropriate antituberculous regimen.

If corticosteroids are indicated in patients with latent tuberculosis or tuberculin reactivity, close observation is necessary as reactivation of the disease may occur. During prolonged corticosteroid therapy, these patients should receive chemoprophylaxis.

Because rare instances of anaphylactic (eg. bronchospasm) reactions have occurred in patients receiving parenteral corticosteroid therapy, appropriate precautionary measures should be taken prior to administration, especially when the patient has a history of allergy to any drug.

There are reports of cardiac arrhythmias and/or circulatory collapse and/or cardiac arrest following the rapid administration of large IV doses of Methylprednisolone Sodium Succinate (greater than 0.5 gram administered over a period of less than 10 minutes). Bradycardia has been reported during or after the administration of large doses of Methylprednisolone Sodium Succinate, and may be unrelated to the speed or duration of infusion.

Persons who are on drugs which suppress the immune system are more susceptible to infections than healthy individuals. Chicken pox and measles, for example, can have a more serious or even fatal course in non-immune children or adults on corticosteroids. In such children or adults who have not had these diseases particular care should be taken to avoid exposure. How the dose, route and duration of corticosteroid administration affects the risk of developing a disseminated infection is not known. The contribution of the underlying disease and/or prior corticosteroid treatment to the risk is also not known. If exposed to chicken pox, prophylaxis with varicella zoster immune globulin (VZIG) may be indicated. If exposed to measles, prophylaxis with pooled intramuscular immunoglobulin (IG) may be indicated. (See the respective package inserts for complete VZIG and IG prescribing information.) If chicken pox develops, treatment with antiviral agents may be considered.

PRECAUTIONS

Drug-induced secondary adrenocortical insufficiency may be minimized by gradual reduction of dosage. This type of relative insufficiency may persist for months after discontinuation of therapy: therefore, in any situation of stress occurring during that period, hormone therapy should be reinstituted. Since mineralocorticoid secretion may be impaired, salt and/or a mineralocorticoid should be administered concurrently.

When multidose vials are used, special care to prevent contamination of the contents is essential. There is some evidence that benzalkonium chloride is not an adequate antiseptic for sterilizing Methylprednisolone Acetate Sterile Aqueous Suspension multidose vials. A povidone-iodine solution or similar product is recommended to cleanse the vial top prior to aspiration of contents. (See "Warnings").

There is an enhanced effect of corticosteroids on patients with hypothyroidism and in those with cirrhosis.

Corticosteroids should be used cautiously in patients with ocular herpes simplex because of possible corneal perforation.

The lowest possible dose of corticosteroid should be used to control the condition under treatment, and when reduction in dosage is possible, the reduction should be gradual.

Psychic derangements may appear when corticosteroids are used, ranging from euphoria, insomnia, mood swings, personality changes and severe depression, to frank psychotic manifestations. Also, existing emotional instability or psychotic tendencies may be aggravated by corticosteroids.

Steroids should be used with caution in nonspecific ulcerative colitis, if there is a probability of impending perforation, abscess or other pyogenic infection. Caution must also be used in diverticulitis; fresh intestinal anastomoses; active or latent peptic ulcer; renal insufficiency; hypertension; osteoporosis; and myasthenia gravis when steroids are used as direct or adjunctive therapy.

Growth and development of infants and children on prolonged corticosteroid therapy should be carefully observed. Although controlled clinical trials have shown corticosteroids to be effective in speeding the resolution of acute exacerbations of multiple sclerosis, they do not show that corticosteroids affect the ultimate outcome or natural history of the disease. The studies do show that relatively high doses of corticosteroids are necessary to demonstrate a significant effect. (See "Dosage and Administration".)

Since complications of treatment with glucocorticoids are dependent on the size of the dose and the duration of treatment, a risk/benefit decision must be made in each individual case as to dose and duration of treatment and as to whether daily or intermittent therapy should be used.

Some strengths of some tablet brands may contain FD&C Yellow No. 5 (tartrazine) which may cause allergic-type reactions (including bronchial asthma) in certain susceptible individuals. Although the overall incidence of FD&C Yellow No. 5 (tartrazine) sensitivity in the general population is low, it is frequently seen in patients who also have aspirin hypersensitivity.

The following additional precautions apply for parenteral corticosteroids. Intrasynovial injection of a corticosteroid may produce systemic as well as local effects.

Appropriate examination of any joint fluid present is necessary to exclude a septic process.

A marked increase in pain accompanied by local swelling, further restriction of joint motion, fever, and malaise are suggestive of septic arthritis. If this complication occurs and the diagnosis of sepsis is confirmed, appropriate antimicrobial therapy should be instituted.

Local injection of a steroid into a previously infected joint is to be avoided.

Corticosteroids should not be injected into unstable joints. The slower rate of absorption by intramuscular administration should be recognized.

Information for the Patient: Persons who are on immunosuppressant doses of corticosteroids should be warned to avoid exposure to chicken pox or measles. Patients should also be advised that if they are exposed, medical advice should be sought without delay.

DRUG INTERACTIONS

The pharmacokinetic interactions listed below are potentially clinically important. Mutual inhibition of metabolism occurs with concurrent use of cyclosporine and Methylprednisolone; therefore, it is possible that adverse events associated with the individual use of either drug may be more apt to occur. Convulsions have been reported with concurrent use of Methylprednisolone and cyclosporine. Since concurrent use of these agents results in a mutual inhibition of metabolism, it is possible that adverse events associated with the individual use of either drug may be more apt to occur. Drugs that induce hepatic enzymes such as phenobarbital, phenytoin and rifampin may increase the clearance of Methylprednisolone and may require increases in Methylprednisolone dose to achieve the desired response. Drugs such as troleandomycin and ketoconazole may inhibit the metabolism of Methylprednisolone and thus decrease its clearance. Therefore, the dose of Methylprednisolone should be titrated to avoid steroid toxicity.

Methylprednisolone may increase the clearance of chronic high dose aspirin. This could lead to decreased salicylate serum levels or increase the risk of salicylate toxicity when Methylprednisolone is withdrawn. Aspirin should be used cautiously in conjunction with corticosteroids in patients suffering from hypoprothrombinemia.

The effect of Methylprednisolone on oral anticoagulants is variable. There are reports of enhanced as well as diminished effects of anticoagulant when given concurrently with corticosteroids. Therefore, coagulation indices should be monitored to maintain the desired anticoagulant effect.

ADVERSE REACTIONS
FLUID AND ELECTROLYTE DISTURBANCES
Sodium retention
Fluid retention
Congestive heart failure in susceptible patients
Potassium loss
Hypokalemic alkalosis
Hypertension

MUSCULOSKELETAL
Muscle weakness
Steroid myopathy
Loss of muscle mass
Osteoporosis
Severe arthralgia (Methylprednisolone Sodium Succinate)
Vertebral compression fractures
Aseptic necrosis of femoral and humeral heads
Pathologic fracture of long bones

GASTROINTESTINAL
Peptic ulcer with possible perforation and hemorrhage
Pancreatitis
Abdominal distention

Ulcerative esophagitis

Increases in alanine transaminase (ALT, SGPT) aspartate transaminase (AST, SGOT) and alkaline phosphatase have been observed following corticosteroid treatment. These changes are usually small, not associated with any clinical syndrome and are reversible upon discontinuation.

DERMATOLOGIC
Impaired wound healing
Thin fragile skin
Petechiae and ecchymoses
Facial erythema
Increased sweating
May suppress reactions to skin tests

NEUROLOGICAL
Increased intracranial pressure with papilledema (pseudotumor cerebri) usually after treatment
Convulsions
Vertigo
Headache

ENDOCRINE
Development of Cushingoid state
Suppression of growth in children
Secondary adrenocortical and pituitary unresponsiveness, particularly in times of stress, as in trauma, surgery or illness
Menstrual irregularities
Decreased carbohydrate tolerance
Manifestations of latent diabetes mellitus
Increased requirements for insulin or oral hypoglycemic agents in diabetics

OPHTHALMIC
Posterior subcapsular cataracts
Increased intraocular pressure
Glaucoma
Exophthalmos

METABOLIC
Negative nitrogen balance due to protein catabolism

The following additional reactions have been reported following oral as well as parenteral therapy: Urticaria and other allergic, anaphylactic or hypersensitivity reactions.

The following *additional* adverse reactions are related to parenteral corticosteroid therapy:
Hyperpigmentation or hypopigmentation
Subcutaneous and cutaneous atrophy
Sterile abscess
Injection site infections following non-sterile administration (see "*Warnings*")
Postinjection flare, following intra-articular use
Charcot-like arthropathy
Nausea and vomiting
Cardiac arrhythmias; hypotension or hypertension

ADVERSE REACTIONS REPORTED WITH THE FOLLOWING ROUTES OF ADMINISTRATION FOR METHYLPREDNISOLONE ACETATE SUSPENSION.

INTRATHECAL/EPIDURAL
Arachnoiditis
Meningitis
Paraparesis/paraplegia
Sensory disturbances
Bowel/bladder dysfunction
Headache
Seizures

INTRANASAL
Temporary/permanent visual impairment including blindness
Allergic reactions
Rhinitis

OPHTHALMIC
Temporary/permanent visual impairment including blindness
Increased intraocular pressure
Ocular and periocular inflammation including allergic reactions
Infection
Residue or slough at injection site

MISCELLANEOUS INJECTION SITES
(Scalp, tonsilar fauces, sphenopalatine ganglion-blindness

DOSAGE AND ADMINISTRATION
Methylprednisolone Tablets: The initial dosage of Methylprednisolone Tablets may vary from 4 to 48 mg per day depending on the specific disease entity being treated. In situations of less severity lower doses will generally suffice while in selected patients higher initial doses may be required. The initial dosage should be maintained or adjusted until a satisfactory response is noted. If after a reasonable

period of time there is a lack of satisfactory clinical response, Methylprednisolone should be discontinued and the patient transferred to other appropriate therapy. **IT SHOULD BE EMPHASIZED THAT DOSAGE REQUIREMENTS ARE VARIABLE AND MUST BE INDIVIDUALIZED ON THE BASIS OF THE DISEASE UNDER TREATMENT AND THE RESPONSE OF THE PATIENT.** After a favorable response is noted, the proper maintenance dosage should be determined by decreasing the initial drug dosage in small decrements at appropriate time intervals until the lowest dosage which will maintain an adequate clinical response is reached. It should be kept in mind that constant monitoring is needed in regard to drug dosage. Included in the situations which may make dosage adjustments necessary are changes in clinical status secondary to remissions or exacerbations in the disease process, the patient's individual drug responsiveness, and the effect of patient exposure to stressful situations not directly related to the disease entity under treatment: in this latter situation it may be necessary to increase the dosage of Methylprednisolone for a period of time consistent with the patient's condition. If after long-term therapy the drug is to be stopped, it is recommended that it be withdrawn gradually rather than abruptly.

Multiple Sclerosis: In treatment of acute exacerbations of multiple sclerosis daily doses of 200 mg of prednisolone for a week followed by 80 mg every other day for 1 month have been shown to be effective (4 mg of Methylprednisolone is equivalent to 5 mg of prednisolone).

ALTERNATE DAY THERAPY
Alternate day therapy is a corticosteroid dosing regimen in which twice the usual daily dose of corticoid is administered every other morning. The purpose of this mode of therapy is to provide the patient requiring long-term pharmacologic dose treatment with the beneficial effects of corticoids while minimizing certain undesirable effects, including pituitary-adrenal suppression, the Cushingoid state, corticoid withdrawal symptoms, and growth suppression in children.

The rationale for this treatment schedule is based on two major premises: (a) the anti-inflammatory or therapeutic effect of corticoids persists longer than their physical presence and metabolic effects and (b) administration of the corticosteroid every other morning allows for re-establishment of more nearly normal hypothalamic-pituitary-adrenal (HPA) activity on the off-steroid day.

A brief review of the HPA physiology may be helpful in understanding this rationale. Acting primarily through the hypothalamus a fall in free cortisol stimulates the pituitary gland to produce increasing amounts of corticotropin (ACTH) while a rise in free cortisol inhibits ACTH secretion. Normally the HPA system is characterized by diurnal (circadian) rhythm. Serum levels of ACTH rise from a low point about 10 pm to a peak level about 6 am. Increasing levels of ACTH stimulate adrenal cortical activity resulting in a rise in plasma cortisol with maximal levels occurring between 2 am and 8 am. This rise in cortisol dampens ACTH production and in turn adrenal cortical activity. There is a gradual fall in plasma corticoids during the day with lowest levels occurring about midnight.

The diurnal rhythm of the HPA axis is lost in Cushing's disease, a syndrome of adrenal cortical hyperfunction characterized by obesity with centripetal fat distribution, thinning of the skin with easy bruisability, muscle wasting with weakness, hypertension, latent diabetes, osteoporosis, electrolyte imbalance, etc. The same clinical findings of hyperadrenocorticism may be noted during long-term pharmacologic dose corticoid therapy administered in conventional daily divided doses. It would appear, then, that a disturbance in the diurnal cycle with maintenance of elevated corticoid values during the night may play a significant role in the development of undesirable corticoid effects. Escape from these constantly elevated plasma levels for even short periods of time may be instrumental in protecting against undesirable pharmacologic effects.

During conventional pharmacologic dose corticosteroid therapy, ACTH production is inhibited with subsequent suppression of cortisol production by the adrenal cortex. Recovery time for normal HPA activity is variable depending upon the dose and duration of treatment. During this time the patient is vulnerable to any stressful situation. Although it has been shown that there is considerably less adrenal suppression following a single morning dose of prednisolone (10 mg) as opposed to a quarter of that dose administered every 6 hours, there is evidence that some suppressive effect on adrenal activity may be carried over into the following day when pharmacologic doses are used. Further, it has been shown that a single dose of certain corticosteroids will produce adrenal cortical suppression for two or more days. Other corticoids, including Methylprednisolone, hydrocortisone, prednisone, and prednisolone, are considered to be short acting (producing adrenal cortical suppression for 1 1/4 to 1 1/2 days following a single dose) and thus are recommended for alternate day therapy.

The following should be kept in mind when considering alternate day therapy:

1) Basic principles and indications for corticosteroid therapy should apply. The benefits of Alternate Day Therapy (ADT) should not encourage the indiscriminate use of steroids.

2) ADT is a therapeutic technique primarily designed for patients in whom long-term pharmacologic corticoid therapy is anticipated.

3) In less severe disease processes in which corticoid therapy is indicated, it may be possible to initiate treatment with ADT. More severe disease states usually will require daily divided high dose therapy for initial control of the disease process. The initial suppressive dose level should be continued until satisfactory clinical response is obtained, usually four to ten days in the case of many allergic and collagen diseases. It is important to keep the period of initial suppressive dose as brief as possible particularly when subsequent use of alternate day therapy is intended.

Once control has been established, two courses are available: (a) change to ADT and then gradually reduce the amount of corticoid given every other day *or* (b) following control of the disease process reduce the daily dose of corticoid to the lowest effective level as rapidly as possible and then change over to an alternate day schedule. Theoretically, course (a) may be preferable.

4) Because of the advantages of ADT, it may be desirable to try patients on this form of therapy who have been on daily corticoids for long periods of time (eg. patients with rheumatoid arthritis). Since these patients may already have a suppressed HPA axis, establishing them on ADT may be difficult and not always successful. However, it is recommended that regular attempts be made to change them over. It may be helpful to triple or even quadruple the daily maintenance dose and administer this every other day rather than just doubling the daily dose if difficulty is encountered. Once the patient is again controlled, an attempt should be made to reduce this dose to a minimum.

5) As indicated above, certain corticosteroids, because of their prolonged suppressive effect on adrenal activity, are not recommended for alternate day therapy (eg. dexamethasome and betamethasone).

6) The maximal activity of the adrenal cortex is between 2 am and 8 am, and it is minimal between 4 pm and midnight. Exogenous corticosteroids suppress adrenocortical activity the least, when given at the time of maximal activity (am).

7) In using ADT it is important, as in all therapeutic situations, to individualize and tailor the therapy to each patient. Complete control of symptoms will not be possible in all patients. An explanation of the benefits of ADT will help the patient to understand and tolerate the possible flare-up in symptoms which may occur in the latter part of the off-steroid day. Other symptomatic therapy may be added or increased at this time if needed.

8) In the event of an acute flare-up of the disease process, it may be necessary to return to a full suppressive daily divided corticoid dose for control. Once control is again established alternate day therapy may be reinstituted.

9) Although many of the undesirable features of corticosteroid therapy can be minimized by ADT, as in any therapeutic situation, the physician must carefully weigh the benefit-risk ratio for each patient in whom corticoid therapy is being considered.

Methylprednisolone Acetate Sterile Aqueous Suspension: Because of possible physical incompatibilities, Methylprednisolone Acetate Sterile Aqueous Suspension should not be diluted or mixed with other solutions.

A. ADMINISTRATION FOR LOCAL EFFECT
Therapy with Methylprednisolone Acetate does not obviate the need for the conventional measures usually employed. Although this method of treatment will ameliorate symptoms, it is in no sense a cure and the hormone has no effect on the cause of the inflammation.

1. Rheumatoid and Osteoarthritis. The dose for intra-articular administration depends upon the size of the joint and varies with the severity of the condition in the individual patient. In chronic cases, injections may be repeated at intervals ranging from one to five or more weeks depending upon the degree of relief obtained from the initial injection. The doses in the following table are given as a general guide:

Size of Joint	Examples	Range of Dosage
Large	Knees Ankles Shoulders	20 to 80 mg
Medium	Elbows Wrists	10 to 40 mg
Small	Metacarpophalangeal Interphalangeal Sternoclavicular Acromioclavicular	4 to 10 mg

Procedure: It is recommended that the anatomy of the joint involved be reviewed before attempting intra-articular injection. In order to obtain the full anti-inflammatory effect it is important that the injection be made into the synovial space. Employing the same sterile technique as for a lumbar puncture, a sterile 20 to 24 gauge needle (on a dry syringe) is quickly inserted into the synovial cavity. Procaine infiltration is elective. The aspiration of only a few drops of joint fluid proves the joint space has been entered by the needle. *The injection site for each joint is determined by that location where the synovial cavity is most superficial and most free of large vessels and nerves.* With the needle in place, the aspirating syringe is removed and replaced by a second syringe containing the desired amount of Methylprednisolone Acetate Sterile Aqueous Suspension. The plunger is then pulled outward slightly to aspirate synovial fluid and to make sure the needle is still in the synovial space. After injection, the joint is moved gently a few times to aid mixing of the synovial fluid and the suspension. The site is covered with a small sterile dressing.

Suitable sites for intra-articular injection are the knee, ankle, wrist, elbow, shoulder, phalangeal, and hip joints. Since difficulty is not infrequently encountered in entering the hip joint, precautions should be taken to avoid any large blood vessels in the area. Joints not suitable for injection are those that are anatomically inaccessible such as the spinal joints and those like the sacroiliac joints that are devoid of synovial space. Treatment failures are most frequently the result of failure to enter the joint space. Little or no benefit follows injection into surrounding tissue. If failures occur when injections into the synovial spaces are certain, as determined by aspiration of fluid, repeated injections are usually futile. Local therapy does not alter the underlying disease process, and whenever possible comprehensive therapy including physiotherapy and orthopedic correction should be employed.

Following intra-articular steroid therapy, care should be taken to avoid overuse of joints in which symptomatic benefit has been obtained. Negligence in this matter may permit an increase in joint deterioration that will more than offset the beneficial effects of the steroid.

Unstable joints should not be injected. Repeated intra-articular injection may in some cases result in instability of the joint. X-ray follow-up is suggested in selected cases to detect deterioration.

If a local anesthetic is used prior to injection of Methylprednisolone Acetate the anesthetic package insert should be read carefully and all the precautions observed.

2. Bursitis. The area around the injection site is prepared in a sterile way and a wheal at the site made with 1 percent procaine hydrochloride solution. A 20 to 24 gauge needle attached to a dry syringe is inserted into the bursa and the fluid aspirated. The needle is left in place and the aspirating syringe changed for a small syringe containing the desired dose. After injection, the needle is withdrawn and a small dressing applied.

3. Miscellaneous: Ganglion, Tendinitis, Epicondylitis. In the treatment of conditions such as tendinitis or tenosynovitis, care should be taken, following application of a suitable antiseptic to the overlying skin, to inject the suspension into the tendon sheath rather than into the substance of the tendon. The tendon may be readily palpated when placed on a stretch. When treating conditions such as epicondylitis, the area of greatest tenderness should be outlined carefully and the suspension infiltrated into the area. For ganglia of the tendon sheaths, the suspension is injected directly into the cyst. In many cases, a single injection causes a marked decrease in the size of the cystic tumor and may effect disappearance. The usual sterile precautions should be observed, of course, with each injection.

The dose in the treatment of the various conditions of the tendinous or bursal structures listed above varies with the condition being treated and ranges from 4 to 30 mg. In recurrent or chronic conditions, repeated injections may be necessary.

4. Injections for Local Effect in Dermatologic Conditions. Following cleansing with an appropriate antiseptic such as 70% alcohol, 20 to 60 mg of the suspension is injected into the lesion. It may be necessary to distribute doses ranging from 20 to 40 mg by repeated local injections in the case of large lesions. Care should be taken to avoid injection of sufficient material to cause blanching since this may be followed by a small slough. One to four injections are usually employed, the intervals between injections varying with the type of lesion being treated and the duration of improvement produced by the initial injection.

When multidose vials are used, special care to prevent contamination of the contents is essential (See "*Warnings*".)

B. ADMINISTRATION FOR SYSTEMIC EFFECT
The intramuscular dosage will vary with the condition being treated. When employed as a temporary substitute for oral therapy, a single injection during each 24-hour period of a dose of the suspension equal to the total daily oral dose of Methylprednisolone Tablets is usually sufficient. When a prolonged effect is desired, the weekly dose may be calculated by multiplying the daily oral dose by 7 and given as a single intramuscular injection.

Dosage must be individualized according to the severity of the disease and response of the patient. For infants and children, the recommended dosage will have to be reduced, but dosage should be governed by the severity of the condition rather than by strict adherence to the ratio indicated by age or body weight.

Hormone therapy is an adjunct to, and not a replacement for, conventional therapy. Dosage must be decreased or discontinued gradually when the drug has been administered for more than a few days. The severity, prognosis and expected duration of the disease and the reaction of the patient to medication are primary factors in determining dosage. If a period of spontaneous remission occurs in a chronic condition, treatment should be discontinued. Routine laboratory studies, such as urinalysis, two-hour postprandial blood sugar, determination of blood pressure and body weight, and a chest X-ray should be made at regular intervals during prolonged therapy. Upper GI x-rays are desirable in patients with an ulcer history or significant dyspepsia.

In patients with the *adrenogenital syndrome*, a single intramuscular injection of 40 mg every two weeks may be adequate. For maintenance of patients with *rheumatoid arthritis*, the weekly intramuscular dose will vary from 40 to 120 mg. The usual dosage for patients with *dermatologic lesions* benefited by systemic corticoid therapy is 40 to 120 mg of Methylprednisolone Acetate administered intramuscularly at weekly intervals for one to four weeks. In acute severe dermatitis due to poison ivy, relief may result within 8 to 12 hours following intramuscular administration of a single dose of 80 to 120 mg. In chronic contact dermatitis repeated injections at 5 to 10 day intervals may be necessary. In seborrheic dermatitis, a weekly dose of 80 mg may be adequate to control the condition.

Following intramuscular administration of 80 to 120 mg to asthmatic patients, relief may result within 6 to 48 hours and persist for several days to two weeks. Similarly in patients with allergic rhinitis (hay fever) an intramuscular dose of 80 to 120 mg may be followed by relief of coryzal symptoms within six hours persisting for several days to three weeks.

If signs of stress are associated with the condition being treated, the dosage of the suspension should be increased. If a rapid hormonal effect of maximum intensity is required, the intravenous administration of highly soluble Methylprednisolone Sodium Succinate is indicated.

► SHOWN IN PRODUCT IDENTIFICATION GUIDE

Methylprednisolone Sodium Succinate Sterile Powder: When high dose therapy is desired, the recommended dose of Methylprednisolone Sodium Succinate is 30 mg/kg administered intravenously over at least 30 minutes. This dose may be repeated every 4 to 6 hours for 48 hours.

In general, high dose corticosteroid therapy should be continued only until the patient's condition has stabilized; usually not beyond 48 to 72 hours.

Although adverse effects associated with high dose short-term corticoid therapy are uncommon, peptic ulceration may occur. Prophylactic antacid therapy may be indicated.

In other indications initial dosage will vary from 10 to 40 mg of Methylprednisolone depending on the clinical problem being treated. The larger doses may be required for short-term management of severe, acute conditions. The initial dose usually should be given intravenously over a period of one to several minutes. Subsequent doses may be given intravenously or intramuscularly at intervals dictated by the patient's response and clinical condition. Corticoid therapy is an adjunct to, and not replacement for conventional therapy.

Dosage may be reduced for infants and children but should be governed more by the severity of the condition and response of the patient than by age or size. It should not be less than 0.5 mg per kg every 24 hours.

Dosage must be decreased or discontinued gradually when the drug has been administered for more than a few days. If a period of spontaneous remission occurs in a chronic condition, treatment should be discontinued. Routine laboratory studies, such as urinalysis, two-hour postprandial blood sugar, determination of blood pressure and body weight, and a chest x-ray should be made at regular intervals during prolonged therapy. Upper GI x-rays are desirable in patients with an ulcer history or significant dyspepsia.

Methylprednisolone Sodium Succinate may be administered by intravenous or intramuscular injection or by intravenous infusion, the preferred method for initial emergency use being intravenous injection. To administer by intravenous (or intramuscular) injection, prepare solution as directed. The desired dose may be administered intravenously over a period of several minutes. Subsequent doses may be withdrawn and administered similarly. If desired, the medication may be administered in diluted solutions by adding Water for Injection or other suitable diluent.

To prepare solutions for intravenous infusion, first prepare the solution for injection as directed. This solution may then be added to indicated amounts of 5% dextrose in water, isotonic saline solution or 5% dextrose in isotonic saline solution.

Multiple Sclerosis: In treatment of acute exacerbations of multiple sclerosis, daily doses of 200 mg of prednisolone for a week followed by 80 mg every other day for 1 month have been shown to be effective (4 mg of Methylprednisolone is equivalent to 5 mg of prednisolone).

STORAGE

Methylprednisolone Tablets and Suspension: Store at controlled room temperature, 15° to 30°C (59° to 86°F.)

Methylprednisolone Acetate Injection: Store at controlled room temperature, 15° - 30°C (59-86°F).

Methylprednisolone Sodium Succinate Injection: Store unreconstituted product at controlled room temperature, 15° to 30°C (59°-86°F).

Store solution at controlled room temperature, 15°-30°C (59°-86°F).

Use solution within 48 hours after mixing.

J CODES
4 mg ORAL K0166
Up to 125 mg IM,IV—J2930
Up to 40 mg IM,IV—J2920
80 mg IM—J1040
40 mg IM—J1030
20 mg IM—J1020

HOW SUPPLIED

METHYLPREDNISOLONE
TABLETS: 2 MG

BRAND/MANUFACTURER	NDC	SIZE	AWP
◆ BRAND			
➤ MEDROL: Upjohn	00009-0049-02	100s	$29.50

TABLETS: 4 MG

AVERAGE UNIT PRICE (AVAILABLE SIZES)		GENERIC A-RATED AVERAGE PRICE (GAAP)	
BRAND	$0.55	21s	$11.50
GENERIC	$0.55	100s	$54.30

BRAND/MANUFACTURER	NDC	SIZE	AWP
◆ BRAND			
➤ MEDROL: Upjohn	00009-0056-04	21s	$11.31
	00009-0056-02	100s	$55.80
	00009-0056-05	100s ud	$56.11
	00009-0056-03	500s	$275.99
◆ GENERICS			
Geneva	00781-1402-07	21s	$9.98
Mason Dist	11845-0120-19	21s	$10.45
Major	00904-2175-19	21s	$10.55
Qualitest	00603-4593-15	21s	$10.65
URL	00677-0565-13	21s	$10.89
Rugby	00536-4036-44	21s	$10.90
Moore,H.L.	00839-6224-58	21s	$10.94
➤ Duramed	51285-0301-21	21s	$11.00
Parmed	00349-8279-21	21s	$11.30
Goldline	00182-1050-03	21s	$14.00
Aligen	00405-4666-21	21s	$15.87
Rugby	00536-4036-01	100s	$45.50
Geneva	00781-1402-01	100s	$48.14
URL	00677-0565-01	100s	$48.35
Qualitest	00603-4593-21	100s	$48.40
Major	00904-2175-60	100s	$50.25
Moore,H.L.	00839-6224-06	100s	$53.31
➤ Duramed	51285-0301-02	100s	$54.00
Parmed	00349-8279-01	100s	$59.95
Goldline	00182-1050-01	100s	$62.00
Aligen	00405-4666-01	100s	$97.51
U.S. Trading	56126-0326-11	100s ud	$29.87

TABLETS: 4 MG

BRAND/MANUFACTURER	NDC	SIZE	AWP
◇ GENERICS			
Schein	00364-0467-21	21s	$10.19
Schein	00364-0467-01	100s	$50.26

TABLETS: 8 MG

BRAND/MANUFACTURER	NDC	SIZE	AWP
◆ BRAND			
➤ MEDROL: Upjohn	00009-0022-01	25s	$19.58

TABLETS: 16 MG

AVERAGE UNIT PRICE (AVAILABLE SIZES)	
BRAND	$1.21

BRAND/MANUFACTURER	NDC	SIZE	AWP
◆ BRAND			
➤ MEDROL: Upjohn	00009-0073-02	14s	$16.98
	00009-0073-01	50s	$60.51

TABLETS: 24 MG

BRAND/MANUFACTURER	NDC	SIZE	AWP
◆ BRAND			
➤ MEDROL: Upjohn	00009-0155-01	25s	$35.68

TABLETS: 32 MG

BRAND/MANUFACTURER	NDC	SIZE	AWP
◆ BRAND			
➤ MEDROL: Upjohn	00009-0176-01	25s	$43.43

METHYLPREDNISOLONE ACETATE
INJECTION: 20 MG/ML

BRAND/MANUFACTURER	NDC	SIZE	AWP
◇ BRAND			
DEPO-MEDROL: Upjohn	00009-0274-01	5 ml	$10.30
◇ GENERICS			
Schein	00364-6748-54	10 ml	$5.25
Steris	00402-0195-10	10 ml	$5.25
Rugby	00536-5370-70	10 ml	$10.26

INJECTION: 40 MG/ML

BRAND/MANUFACTURER	NDC	SIZE	AWP
◇ BRAND			
DEPO-MEDROL: Upjohn	00009-3073-01	1 ml	$5.18
	00009-3073-02	1 ml	$5.18
	00009-0280-02	5 ml	$18.80
	00009-0280-32	5 ml	$18.80
	00009-0280-03	10 ml	$34.21
	00009-0280-33	10 ml	$34.21
◇ GENERICS			
Schein	00364-6705-53	5 ml	$5.48
Steris	00402-0196-05	5 ml	$5.48
Insource	58441-1122-05	5 ml	$7.32
Genl Inject	52584-0196-05	5 ml	$7.32
Major	00904-0898-05	5 ml	$7.45
Moore,H.L.	00839-6200-25	5 ml	$8.22
Moore,H.L.	00839-7946-25	5 ml	$8.22
URL	00677-0492-20	5 ml	$8.42
Geneva	00781-3055-75	5 ml	$8.47
DEPOPRED: Hyrex	00314-0840-75	5 ml	$9.90
Rugby	00536-5340-65	5 ml	$10.26
Goldline	00182-1067-62	5 ml	$12.00

◆ RATED THERAPEUTICALLY EQUIVALENT; ◇ THERAPEUTIC EQUIVALENCE UNCONFIRMED; ○ UNRATED

BRAND/MANUFACTURER	NDC	SIZE	AWP
Schein	00364-6705-54	10 ml	$8.37
Steris	00402-0196-10	10 ml	$8.37
DEPOPRED: Hyrex	00314-0842-70	10 ml	$15.66
Rugby	00536-5340-70	10 ml	$15.66
DEPOJECT-40: Mayrand	00259-0387-10	10 ml	$26.60

INJECTION: 80 MG/ML

BRAND/MANUFACTURER	NDC	SIZE	AWP
◇ **BRAND**			
DEPO-MEDROL: Upjohn	00009-3475-01	1 ml	$8.56
	00009-3475-02	1 ml	$8.56
	00009-0306-02	5 ml	$34.21
	00009-0306-10	5 ml	$34.21
◇ **GENERICS**			
Schein	00364-6713-53	5 ml	$8.37
Steris	00402-0197-05	5 ml	$8.37
Moore,H.L.	00839-6201-25	5 ml	$12.41
Moore,H.L.	00839-7947-25	5 ml	$12.41
Insource	58441-1123-05	5 ml	$12.57
Genl Inject	52584-0197-05	5 ml	$12.57
URL	00677-0631-20	5 ml	$15.50
DEPOPRED: Hyrex	00314-0841-75	5 ml	$15.60
Rugby	00536-5351-65	5 ml	$15.66
Major	00904-0897-05	5 ml	$15.70
Goldline	00182-1068-62	5 ml	$17.40
DEPOJECT-80: Mayrand	00259-0388-05	5 ml	$26.60

INJECTION: 80 MG/5 ML

BRAND/MANUFACTURER	NDC	SIZE	AWP
◆ **GENERICS**			
Geneva	00781-3065-75	5 ml	$15.41

METHYLPREDNISOLONE SODIUM SUCCINATE

POWDER FOR INJECTION: 25 MG

AVERAGE UNIT PRICE (AVAILABLE SIZES)

BRAND	$6.04		

BRAND/MANUFACTURER	NDC	SIZE	AWP
◆ **BRAND**			
SOLU-MEDROL: Upjohn	00009-0190-09	1s	$5.31
	00009-0190-10	1s	$5.31
A-METHAPRED: Abbott Hosp	00074-5685-02	10s	$74.93

POWDER FOR INJECTION: 40 MG

AVERAGE UNIT PRICE (AVAILABLE SIZES)

BRAND	$2.28		

BRAND/MANUFACTURER	NDC	SIZE	AWP
◆ **BRAND**			
SOLU-MEDROL: Upjohn	00009-0113-12	1s	$2.00
	00009-0113-13	1s	$2.00
A-METHAPRED: Abbott Hosp	00074-5684-01	10s	$28.26

POWDER FOR INJECTION: 500 MG

AVERAGE UNIT PRICE (AVAILABLE SIZES)

BRAND	$23.20		

BRAND/MANUFACTURER	NDC	SIZE	AWP
◆ **BRAND**			
SOLU-MEDROL: Upjohn	00009-0758-01	1s	$17.88
	00009-0765-02	1s	$20.06
	00009-0887-01	1s	$20.06
A-METHAPRED: Abbott Hosp	00074-5601-44	1s	$28.80
	00074-5630-04	25s	$729.72

POWDER FOR INJECTION: 1000 MG

AVERAGE UNIT PRICE (AVAILABLE SIZES)

BRAND	$49.21		

BRAND/MANUFACTURER	NDC	SIZE	AWP
◆ **BRAND**			
A-METHAPRED: Abbott Hosp	00074-5603-44	1s	$48.74
	00074-5631-08	25s	$1242.13

POWDER FOR INJECTION: 1 GM

AVERAGE UNIT PRICE (AVAILABLE SIZES)

BRAND	$31.10		

BRAND/MANUFACTURER	NDC	SIZE	AWP
◆ **BRAND**			
SOLU-MEDROL: Upjohn	00009-0698-01	1s	$30.00
	00009-3389-01	1s	$32.19

POWDER FOR INJECTION: 2 GM

AVERAGE UNIT PRICE (AVAILABLE SIZES)

BRAND	$54.69		

BRAND/MANUFACTURER	NDC	SIZE	AWP
◆ **BRAND**			
SOLU-MEDROL: Upjohn	00009-0796-01	1s	$54.69
	00009-0988-01	1s	$54.69

Methylprednisolone Acetate and Neomycin Sulfate

DESCRIPTION

Methylprednisolone is a markedly effective anti-inflammatory corticosteroid. Clinical studies indicate that topically applied Methylprednisolone is highly active. Methylprednisolone/Neomycin Topical contains Methylprednisolone Acetate in a concentration of 0.25% and the broad-spectrum antibiotic, Neomycin Sulfate, equivalent to 3.5 mg Neomycin. Each gram of this preparation contains methylparaben 0.4% and butylparaben 0.3%.

CLINICAL PHARMACOLOGY

Topical steroids are primarily effective because of their anti-inflammatory, antipruritic and vasoconstrictive actions.

Methylprednisolone, one of the most potent corticosteroids, exerts a profound anti-inflammatory action at the tissue level. Studies of anti-inflammatory activity, using the granuloma pouch assay, have shown it to be more potent, on a weight basis, than prednisolone. Similarly a high order of activity has been observed following local application of Methylprednisolone. Because of this high order of activity, it is effective topically in the available low concentrations. Prompt control of excessive tissue reaction to allergens, irritants, and trauma may be anticipated following the use of these topical preparations.

Mothylprednisolone applied locally has been found to be rapidly effective in acute uncomplicated allergic dermatitis. In many instances objective signs of improvement, subsidence of erythema and edema, as well as symptomatic relief occur within a few hours of the first application. With symptomatic relief, further damage to the skin, with subsequent possible injection, is prevented. Following discontinuance of applications no "rebound" activation of lesions has been observed.

Neomycin is an antibacterial substance derived from cultures of the soil organism *Streptomyces fradiae*. It exhibits a wider spectrum of antibacterial activity than does bacitracin, streptomycin, or penicillin and is active against a variety of gram-positive and gram-negative organisms including *staphylococci*, *Escherichia coli*, and *Hemophilus influenzae*. It is not active against fungi. Neomycin rarely causes resistant strains of microorganisms to develop; in addition, it is unusually nontoxic for human epithelial cells in tissue culture and is nonirritating topically in therapeutic concentrations.

INDICATIONS AND USAGE

For the treatment of corticosteroid-responsive dermatoses with secondary infection. It has not been demonstrated that this steroid-antibiotic combination provides greater benefit than the steroid component alone after seven days of treatment. (See *"Warnings"* section.)

CONTRAINDICATIONS

Local application is contraindicated in tuberculosis of the skin, herpes simplex, vaccinia, varicella, and in other cutaneous infections for which an effective antibiotic or chemotherapeutic agent is not available for simultaneous application.

Methylprednisolone/Neomycin Topical should not be used in individuals with a history of hypersensitivity to any of its components.

WARNINGS

Because of the potential hazard of nephrotoxicity and ototoxicity, prolonged use or use of large amounts of this product should be avoided in the treatment of skin injections following extensive burns, trophic ulceration and other conditions where absorption of Neomycin is possible.

Because of the concern of nephrotoxicity and ototoxicity associated with Neomycin, this combination product should not be used over a wide area or for extended periods of time.

PRECAUTIONS

This preparation is usually well tolerated. However, Neomycin may occasionally induce sensitivity reactions. If signs of irritation or sensitivity should develop, application should be discontinued.

If extensive areas are treated or if the occlusive technique is used, the possibility exists of increased absorption of the corticoid and suitable precautions should be taken.

The safety of the use of topical steroid preparations during pregnancy has not been fully established. Therefore, they should not be used unnecessarily during pregnancy, on extended areas, in large amounts, or for prolonged periods of time.

This product should not be put in the eyes or, if the ear drum is perforated, in the external ear canal.

► SHOWN IN PRODUCT IDENTIFICATION GUIDE

Note: The prolonged use of antibiotic-containing preparations may result in overgrowth of nonsusceptible organisms, particularly fungi. If new infections appear during treatment, appropriate therapy should be instituted.

ADVERSE REACTIONS
When steroid preparations are used for long periods in intertriginous areas or under occlusive dressing, localized atrophy and striae may occur.

Other local adverse reactions associated with topically applied corticoids either with or without occlusive dressings include: burning sensations, itching, irritation, dryness, folliculitis, secondary infection, atrophy of the skin, acneiform eruption and hypopigmentation.

Ototoxicity and nephrotoxicity have been reported following absorption of topically applied Neomycin.

According to current medical literature there has been an increase in the prevalence of Neomycin hypersensitivity.

DOSAGE AND ADMINISTRATION
After careful cleansing of the affected skin to minimize the possibility of introducing infection, a small amount is applied and rubbed gently into the involved areas. Application should be made initially one to three times daily. Once control is achieved—usually within a few hours—the frequency of application should be reduced to the minimum necessary to avoid relapses.

HOW SUPPLIED
OINTMENT: 0.25%

BRAND/MANUFACTURER	NDC	SIZE	AWP
○ **BRAND**			
NEO-MEDROL ACETATE: Upjohn	00009-0888-02	30 gm	$17.08

Methyltestosterone

DESCRIPTION
Methyltestosterone is a synthetic androgen. Androgens are steroids that develop and maintain primary and secondary male sex characteristics.

Methyltestosterone is available for oral administration as tablets or capsules.

Each tablet contains:
Methyltestosterone ....10 or 25 mg

Each capsule contains:
Methyltestosterone ....10 mg

Androgens are derivatives of cyclopentanoperhydrophenanthrene. Endogenous androgens are C-19 steroids with a side chain at C-17, and with two angular methyl groups. Testosterone is the primary endogenous androgen. In their active form, all drugs in the class have a 17-beta-hydroxy group. 17-alpha alkylation (Methyltestosterone) increases the pharmacologic activity per unit weight compared to testosterone when given orally.

Methyltestosterone is the 17α-methyl derivative of testosterone, the true testicular hormone. Chemically, methyltestosterone is 17β-hydroxy-17-methyl-landrost-4-en-3-one, with the empirical formula $C_{20}H_{30}O_2$, and a molecular weight of 302.5.

Methyltestosterone is a white or creamy white, odorless, and slightly hygroscopic powder or crystals. It is practically insoluble in water, and is soluble in alcohol, and other organic solvents.

Following is its chemical structure:

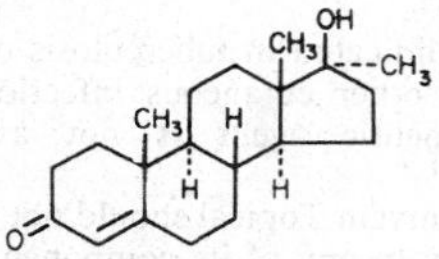

CLINICAL PHARMACOLOGY
Endogenous androgens are responsible for the normal growth and development of the male sex organs and for maintenance of secondary sex characteristics. These effects include the growth and maturation of prostate, seminal vesicles, penis and scrotum; the development of male hair distribution, such as beard, pubic, chest, and axillary hair; laryngeal enlargement, vocal cord thickening; alterations in body musculature and fat distribution. Drugs in this class also cause retention of nitrogen, sodium, potassium, phosphorus, and decreased urinary excretion of calcium. Androgens have been reported to increase protein anabolism and decrease protein catabolism. Nitrogen balance is improved only when there is sufficient intake of calories and protein. Androgens are responsible for the growth spurt of adolescence and for the eventual termination of linear growth which is brought about by fusion of the epiphyseal growth centers. In children, exogenous androgens accelerate linear growth rates, but may cause a disproportionate advancement in bone maturation. Use over long periods may result in fusion of the epiphyseal growth centers and termination of growth process. Androgens have been reported to stimulate the production of red blood cells by enhancing the production of erythropoietic stimulating factor.

During exogenous administration of androgens, endogenous testosterone release is inhibited through feedback inhibition of pituitary luteinizing hormone (LH). With large doses of exogenous androgens, spermatogenesis may also be suppressed through feedback inhibition of pituitary follicle stimulating hormone (FSH).

There is a lack of substantial evidence that androgens are effective in fractures, surgery, convalescence, and functional uterine bleeding.

Pharmacokinetics: Testosterone given orally is metabolized by the gut and 44% is cleared by the liver in the first pass. Oral doses as high as 400 mg per day are needed to achieve clinically effective blood levels for full replacement therapy. The synthetic androgen Methyltestosterone is less extensively metabolized by the liver and has a longer half-life. It is more suitable than testosterone for oral administration.

Testosterone in plasma is 98% bound to a specific testosterone-estradiol binding globulin, and about 1 to 2% is free. Generally, the amount of this sex-hormone binding globulin in the plasma will determine the distribution of testosterone between free and bound forms, and the free testosterone concentration will determine its half-life.

About 90% of a dose of testosterone is excreted in the urine as glucuronic and sulfuric acid conjugates of testosterone and its metabolites; about 6% of a dose is excreted in the feces, mostly in the unconjugated form. Inactivation of testosterone occurs primarily in the liver. Testosterone is metabolized to various 17-keto steroids through two different pathways. As reported in the literature, the half-life of testosterone varies considerably, ranging from 10 to 100 minutes.

In many tissues the activity of testosterone appears to depend on reduction to dihydrotestosterone, which binds to cytosol receptor proteins. The steroid-receptor complex is transported to the nucleus where it initiates transcription events and cellular changes related to androgen action.

INDICATIONS AND USAGE
IN THE MALE
Methyltestosterone tablets are indicated for replacement therapy in conditions associated with a deficiency or absence of endogenous testosterone:

Primary Hypogonadism (congenital or acquired): Testicular failure due to cryptorchidism, bilateral torsion, orchitis, vanishing testis syndrome or orchidectomy.

Hypogonadotropic Hypogonadism (congenital or acquired): Idiopathic gonadotropin or LHRH deficiency, or pituitary-hypothalamic injury from tumors, trauma or radiation.

If the above conditions occur prior to puberty, androgen replacement therapy will be needed during the adolescent years for development of secondary sexual characteristics. Prolonged androgen treatment will be required to maintain sexual characteristics in these and other males who develop testosterone deficiency after puberty.

Androgens may be used to stimulate puberty in carefully selected males with clearly delayed puberty. These patients usually have a familial pattern of delayed puberty that is not secondary to a pathological disorder: puberty is expected to occur spontaneously at a relatively late date. Brief treatment with conservative doses may occasionally be justified in these patients if they do not respond to psychological support. The potential adverse effect on bone maturation should be discussed with the patient and parents prior to androgen administration. An x-ray of the hand and wrist to determine bone age should be obtained every 6 months to assess the effect of treatment on the epiphyseal centers. (See *"Warnings".*)

IN THE FEMALE
Methyltestosterone tablets may be used secondarily in women with advancing inoperable metastatic (skeletal) breast cancer who are 1 to 5 years postmenopausal. Primary goals of therapy in these women include ablation of the ovaries. Other methods of counteracting estrogen activity are adrenalectomy, hypophysectomy, and/or anti-estrogen therapy. This treatment has also been used in premenopausal women with breast cancer who have benefited from oophorectomy and are considered to have a hormone-responsive tumor. Judgment concerning androgen therapy should be made by an oncologist with expertise in this field.

UNLABLED USES
Methyltestosterone is used alone or as an adjunct in the treatment of hereditary angioedema.

CONTRAINDICATIONS
Methyltestosterone tablets are contraindicated for use in men with carcinomas of the breast or with known or suspected carcinomas of the prostate, and in women who are or may become pregnant.

When administered to pregnant women, androgens cause virilization of the external genitalia of the female fetus. This virilization includes clitoromegaly, abnormal vaginal development, and fusion of genital folds to form a scrotal-like structure. The degree of masculinization is related to the amount of drug given and the age of the fetus, and is most likely to occur in the female fetus when the drugs are given in the first trimester. If the patient becomes pregnant while taking these drugs, she should be apprised of the potential hazard to the fetus.

WARNINGS
In patients with breast cancer, androgen therapy may cause hypercalcemia by stimulating osteolysis. In this case, the drug should be discontinued.

Prolonged use of high doses of androgens has been associated with the development of peliosis hepatis and hepatic neoplasms including hepatocellular carcinoma. (See *"Precautions: Carcinogenesis, Mutagenesis, Impairment of Fertility".*) Peliosis hepatis can be a life-threatening or fatal complication.

Cholestatic hepatitis and jaundice occur with 17-alpha-alkylandrogens (such as Methyltestosterone) at a relatively low dose. If cholestatic hepatitis with jaundice appears or if liver function tests become abnormal, the androgen should be discontinued and the etiology should be determined. Drug-induced jaundice is reversible when the medication is discontinued.

Geriatric patients treated with androgens may be at an increased risk for the development of prostatic hypertrophy and prostatic carcinoma.

Edema with or without congestive heart failure may be a serious complication in patients with pre-existing cardiac, renal or hepatic disease. In addition to discontinuation of the drug, diuretic therapy may be required.

Gynecomastia frequently develops and occasionally persists in patients being treated for hypogonadism.

Androgen therapy should be used cautiously in healthy males with delayed puberty. The effect on bone maturation should be monitored by assessing bone age of the wrist and hand every 6 months. In children, androgen treatment may accelerate bone maturation without producing compensatory gain in linear growth. This adverse effect may result in compromised adult stature. The younger the child the greater the risk of compromising final mature height.

This drug has not been shown to be safe and effective for the enhancement of athletic performance. Because of the potential risk of serious adverse health effects, this drug should not be used for such purpose.

PRECAUTIONS
GENERAL
Women should be observed for signs of virilization (deepening of the voice, hirsutism, acne, clitoromegaly and menstrual irregularities). Discontinuation of drug therapy at the time of evidence of mild virilism is necessary to prevent irreversible virilization. Such virilization is usual following androgen use at high doses. A decision may be made by the patient and the physician that some virilization will be tolerated during treatment for breast carcinoma.

Priapism or excessive sexual stimulation may develop. Males, especially the elderly, may become overstimulated. In treating males for symptoms of climacteric, avoid stimulation to the point of increasing the nervous, mental, and physical activities beyond the patient's cardiovascular capacity. Oligospermia and reduced ejaculatory volume may occur after prolonged administration of excessive dosage.

INFORMATION FOR PATIENTS
The physician should instruct patients to report any of the following side effects of androgens:

Adult or Adolescent Males: Too frequent or persistent erections of the penis.

Women: Hoarseness, acne, changes in menstrual periods, or more hair on the face.

All Patients: Any nausea, vomiting, changes in skin color or ankle swelling.

Any male adolescent patient receiving androgens for delayed puberty should have bone development checked every 6 months.

LABORATORY TESTS:
Women with disseminated breast carcinoma should have frequent determination of urine and serum calcium levels during the course of androgen therapy. (See *"Warnings".*)

Because of the hepatotoxicity associated with the use of 17-alpha-alkylated androgens, liver function tests should be obtained periodically.

Periodic (every 6 months) x-ray examinations of bone age should be made during treatment of pre-pubertal males to determine the rate of bone maturation and the effects of androgen therapy on the epiphyseal centers.

Hemoglobin and hematocrit should be checked periodically for polycythemia in patients who are receiving high doses of androgens.

DRUG INTERACTIONS
Anticoagulants: C-17 substituted derivatives of testosterone, such as methandrostenolone, have been reported to decrease the anticoagulant requirements of patients receiving oral anticoagulants. Patients receiving oral anticoagulant therapy require close monitoring, especially when androgens are started or stopped.

Oxyphenbutazone: Concurrent administration of oxyphenbutazone and androgens may result in elevated serum levels of oxyphenbutazone.

Insulin: In diabetic patients the metabolic effects of androgens may decrease blood glucose and insulin requirements.

DRUG/LABORATORY TEST INTERFERENCES
Androgens may decrease levels of thyroxine-binding globulin, resulting in decreased total T_4 serum levels and increased resin uptake of T_3 and T_4. Free thyroid hormone levels remain unchanged, however, and there is no clinical evidence of thyroid dysfunction.

CARCINOGENESIS, MUTAGENESIS, IMPAIRMENT OF FERTILITY
Animal Data: Testosterone has been tested by subcutaneous injection and implantation in mice and rats. The implant induced cervical-uterine tumors in mice, which metastasized in some cases. There is suggestive evidence that injection of testosterone into some strains of female mice increases their susceptibility to hepatoma. Testosterone is also known to increase the number of tumors and decrease the degree of differentiation of chemically induced carcinomas of the liver in rats.

Human Data: There are rare reports of hepatocellular carcinoma in patients receiving long-term therapy with androgens in high doses. Withdrawal of the drugs did not lead to regression of the tumors in all cases.

Geriatric patients treated with androgens may be at an increased risk for the development of prostatic hypertrophy and prostatic carcinoma.

Information of mutagenesis is unknown.

PREGNANCY
Teratogenic Effects—Pregnancy Category X: See *"Contraindications".*

Nursing Mothers: It is not known whether androgens are excreted in human milk. Because many drugs are excreted in human milk and because of the potential for serious adverse reactions in nursing infants from androgens, a decision should be made whether to discontinue nursing or to discontinue the drug, taking into account the importance of the drug to the mother.

Pediatric Use: Androgen therapy should be used very cautiously in children and only by specialists who are aware of the adverse effects on bone maturation. Skeletal maturation must be monitored every six months by an x-ray of the hand and wrist. (See *"Indications and Usage"* and *"Warnings".*)

ADVERSE REACTIONS
ENDOCRINE AND UROGENITAL
Female: The most common side effects of androgen therapy are amenorrhea and other menstrual irregularities, inhibition of gonadotropin secretion, and virilization, including deepening of the voice and clitoral enlargement. The latter usually is not reversible after androgens are discontinued. When administered to a pregnant woman, androgens cause virilization of external genitalia of the female fetus.

Male: Gynecomastia, and excessive frequency and duration of penile erections. Oligospermia may occur at high dosages. (See *"Clinical Pharmacology".*)

Skin and Appendages: Hirsutism, male pattern of baldness, and acne.

Fluid and Electrolyte Disturbances: Retention of sodium, chloride, water, potassium, calcium, and inorganic phosphates.

Gastrointestinal: Nausea, cholestatic jaundice, alterations in liver function tests, rarely hepatocellular neoplasms and peliosis hepatis. (See *"Warnings".*)

Hematologic: Suppression of clotting factors, II, V, VII, and X, bleeding in patients on concomitant anticoagulant therapy, and polycythemia.

Nervous System: Increased or decreased libido, headache, anxiety, depression, and generalized paresthesia.

Metabolic: Increased serum cholesterol.

Miscellaneous: Rarely anaphylactoid reactions.

DRUG ABUSE AND DEPENDENCE
Controlled Substance Class: Methyltestosterone tablets are classified as controlled substances under the Anabolic Steroids Control Act of 1990 and have been assigned to Schedule III.

OVERDOSAGE
Overdose of medication may be reflected in the occurrence of the signs and symptoms associated with testosterone-anabolic drugs. Nausea and appearance of the early manifestations of edema should be looked for. However, there has been no report of acute overdosage with androgens.

DOSAGE AND ADMINISTRATION
Methyltestosterone tablets and capsules are administered orally. Dosage must be strictly individualized. The suggested dosage for androgens varies depending on the age, sex, and diagnosis of the individual patient. Adjustments and duration of dosage will depend upon the patient's response and the appearance of adverse reactions.

Males: In the androgen-deficient male the following guideline for replacement therapy indicates the usual initial dosages.

	Route	Dose	Frequency
Methyltestosterone tablets	Oral	10-50 mg	Daily

Various dosage regimens have been used to induce pubertal changes in hypogonadal males; some experts have advocated lower dosages initially, gradually increasing the dose as puberty progresses, with or without a decrease to maintenance levels. Other experts emphasize that higher dosages are needed to induce pubertal changes and lower dosages can be used for maintenance after puberty. The chronological and skeletal ages must be taken into consideration, both in determining the initial dose and in adjusting the dose.

Dosages used in delayed puberty generally are in the lower ranges of those given above, and are for limited duration, for example, 4 to 6 months.

Females: Women with metastatic breast carcinoma must be followed closely because androgen therapy occasionally appears to accelerate the disease. Thus, many experts prefer to use the shorter acting androgen preparations rather than those with prolonged activity for treating breast carcinoma particularly during the early stages of androgen therapy.

Guideline dosages and adrogens for use in the palliative treatment of women with metastatic breast cancer:

	Route	Dose	Frequency
Methyltestosterone tablets breast cancer	Oral	50-200 mg	Daily

HOW SUPPLIED
CAPSULE (C-III): 10 MG

BRAND/MANUFACTURER	NDC	SIZE	AWP
◇ **GENERICS**			
TESTRED: ICN	00187-0901-01	100s	$124.86

CAPSULE, EXTENDED RELEASE (C-III): 10 MG

BRAND/MANUFACTURER	NDC	SIZE	AWP
◇ **BRAND**			
VIRILON: Star	00076-0301-03	100s	$43.20
	00076-0301-04	1000s	$402.24

TABLETS (C-III): 10 MG

BRAND/MANUFACTURER	NDC	SIZE	AWP
◇ **BRAND**			
ANDROID-10: ICN	00187-0311-06	100s	$124.86
ORETON METHYL: ICN	00187-0311-01	100s	$124.86
◇ **GENERICS**			
Major	00904-0807-60	100s	$5.50
Major	00904-0808-60	100s	$5.95
Richlyn	00115-3982-01	100s	$6.38
Richlyn	00115-3984-01	100s	$6.38
Goldline	00182-0185-01	100s	$24.75
Goldline	00182-0582-01	100s	$24.75
Richlyn	00115-3982-03	1000s	$49.05
Richlyn	00115-3984-03	1000s	$49.05

TABLETS (C-III): 25 MG

BRAND/MANUFACTURER	NDC	SIZE	AWP
◇ **BRAND**			
ANDROID-25: ICN	00187-0499-06	100s	$312.12
◇ **GENERICS**			
Major	00904-0809-60	100s	$10.30
Richlyn	00115-3986-01	100s	$14.53
Goldline	00182-0583-01	100s	$48.75
Major	00904-0809-80	1000s	$55.45
Richlyn	00115-3986-03	1000s	$111.75

Methysergide Maleate

> **WARNING**
> RETROPERITONEAL FIBROSIS, PLEUROPULMONARY FIBROSIS AND FIBROTIC THICKENING OF CARDIAC VALVES MAY OCCUR IN PATIENTS RECEIVING LONG-TERM METHYSERGIDE MALEATE THERAPY. THEREFORE, THIS PREPARATION MUST BE RESERVED FOR PROPHYLAXIS IN PATIENTS WHOSE VASCULAR HEADACHES ARE FREQUENT AND/OR SEVERE AND UNCONTROLLABLE AND WHO ARE UNDER CLOSE MEDICAL SUPERVISION. (SEE ALSO *"WARNINGS"* SECTION)

DESCRIPTION
(Methysergide Maleate) is a partially synthetic compound structurally related to lysergic acid butanolamide, well-known as methylergonovine in obstetrical practice as an oxytocic agent.

Chemically, Methysergide Maleate is designated as ergoline-8-carboxamide, 9,10-didehydro-N-[1-(hydroxymethyl)propyl]-1,6-dimethyl-, (8β)-, (Z)-2-butenedioate (1:1) (salt). Its molecular formula is $C_{21}H_{27}N_3O_2 \cdot C_4H_4O_4$ and its molecular weight is 469.54.

Methylation in the number 1 position of the ring structure enormously enhances the antagonism to serotonin which is present to a much lesser degree in the partially methylated compound (methylergonovine maleate) as well as profoundly altering other pharmacologic properties.

Active Ingredient: Methysergide Maleate, USP.

Following is its chemical structure:

ACTIONS
(Methysergide Maleate) has been shown, *in vitro* and *in vivo*, to inhibit or block the effects of serotonin, a substance which may be involved in the mechanisms of vascular headaches. Serotonin has been variously described as a central neurohumoral agent or chemical mediator, as a "headache substance" acting directly or indirectly to lower pain threshold (others in this category include tyramine; polypeptides, such as bradykinin: histamine; and acetylcholine), as an intrinsic 'motor hormone' of the gastrointestinal tract, and as a 'hormone' involved in connective tissue reparative processes. Suggestions have been made by investigators as to the mechanism whereby methysergide produces its clinical effects, but this has not been finally established.

INDICATIONS
For the prevention or reduction of intensity and frequency of vascular headaches in the following kinds of patients:
1. Patients suffering from one or more severe vascular headaches per week.
2. Patients suffering from vascular headaches that are uncontrollable or so severe that preventive therapy is indicated regardless of the frequency of the attack.

UNLABELED USES
Methysergide Maleate is used alone or as an adjunct in the treatment of histaminic cephalalgia (cluster headache).

CONTRAINDICATIONS
Pregnancy, peripheral vascular disease, severe arteriosclerosis, severe hypertension, coronary artery disease, phlebitis or cellulitis of the lower limbs, pulmonary disease, collagen diseases or fibrotic processes, impaired liver or renal function, valvular heart disease, debilitated states and serious infections.

WARNINGS
With long-term, uninterrupted administration, retroperitoneal fibrosis or related conditions—pleuropulmonary fibrosis and cardiovascular disorders with murmurs or vascular bruits have been reported. Patients must be warned to report immediately the following symptoms: cold, numb, and painful hands and feet; leg cramps on walking: any type of girdle, flank, or chest pain, or any associated symptomatology. Should any of these symptoms develop, methysergide should be discontinued. Continuous administration should not exceed 6 months. There must be a drug-free interval of 3-4 weeks after each 6-month course of treatment. The dosage should be reduced gradually during the last 2-3 weeks of each treatment course to avoid "headache rebound."

The drug is not recommended for use in children.

PRECAUTIONS
All patients receiving Methysergide Maleate should remain under constant supervision of the physician and be examined regularly for the development of fibrotic or vascular complications. (See *"Adverse Reactions"*.)

The manifestations of retroperitoneal fibrosis, pleuropulmonary fibrosis, and vascular shutdown have shown a high incidence of regression once Methysergide Maleate is withdrawn. These facts should be borne in mind to avoid unnecessary surgical intervention. Cardiac murmurs, which may indicate endocardial fibrosis, have shown varying degrees of regression, with complete disappearance in some and persistence in others.

Methysergide Maleate has been specifically designed for the prophylaxis of vascular headache and has no place in the management of the acute attack.

ADVERSE REACTIONS
Within the recommended dose levels, the following side effects have been reported:

1) FIBROTIC COMPLICATIONS
Fibrotic changes have been observed in the retropritoneal, pleuropulmonary, cardiac, and other tissues, either singly or, very rarely, in combination.

Retroperitoneal Fibrosis: This nonspecific fibrotic process is usually confined to the retroperitoneal connective tissue above the pelvic brim and may present clinically with one or more symptoms such as general malaise, fatigue, weight loss, backache, low grade fever (elevated sedimentation rate), urinary obstruction (girdle or flank pain, dysuria, polyuria, oliguria, elevated BUN), vascular insufficiency of the lower limbs (leg pain, Leriche syndrome, edema of legs, thrombophlebitis). The single most useful diagnostic procedure in suspected cases of retroperitoneal fibrosis is intravenous pyelography. Typical deviation and obstruction of one or both ureters may be observed.

Pleuropulmonary Complications: A similar nonspecific fibrotic process, limited to the pleural and immediately subjacent pulmonary tissues, usually presents clinically with dyspnea, tightness and pain in the chest, pleural friction rubs, and pleural effusion. These findings may be confirmed by chest x-ray.

Cardiac Complications: Nonrheumatic fibrotic thickenings of the aortic root and of the aortic and mitral valves usually present clinically with cardiac murmurs and dyspnea.

Other Fibrotic Complications: Several cases of fibrotic plaques, simulating Peyronie's Disease, have been described.

2) CARDIOVASCULAR COMPLICATIONS
Encroachment of retroperitoneal fibrosis on the aorta, inferior vena cava and their common iliac branches may result in vascular insufficiency of the lower limbs, the presenting features of which are mentioned under *"Retroperitoneal Fibrosis"*.

Intrinsic vasoconstriction of large and small arteries, involving one or more vessels or merely a segment of a vessel, may occur at any stage of therapy. Depending on the vessel involved, this complication may present with chest pain, abdominal pain, or cold, numb, painful extremities with or without paresthesias and diminished or absent pulses. Progression to ischemic tissue damage has rarely been reported. Prompt withdrawal of the drug at the first signs of impaired circulation is recommended (see "Warnings") to obviate such effects.

Postural hypotension and tachycardia have also been observed.

3) GASTROINTESTINAL SYMPTOMS

Nausea, vomiting, diarrhea, heartburn, abdominal pain. These effects tend to appear early and can frequently be obviated by gradual introduction of the medication and by administration of the drug with meals. Constipation and elevation of gastric hydrochloride have also been reported.

4) CNS SYMPTOMS

Insomnia, drowsiness, mild euphoria, dizziness, ataxia, light-headedness, hyperesthesia, unworldly feelings (described variously as "dissociation", "hallucinatory experiences", etc.). Some of these symptoms may be associated with vascular headaches per se, and may, therefore, be unrelated to the drug.

5) DERMATOLOGICAL MANIFESTATIONS

Facial flush, telangiectasia, and nonspecific rashes have rarely been reported. Increased hair loss may occur, but in many instances the tendency has abated despite continued therapy.

6) EDEMA

Peripheral edema, and, more rarely, localized brawny edema may occur.

Dependent edema has responded to lowered doses, salt restriction, or diuretics.

7) WEIGHT GAIN

Weight gain may be a reason to caution patients regarding their caloric intake.

8) HEMATOLOGICAL MANIFESTATIONS

Neutropenia, eosinophilia.

9) MISCELLANEOUS

Weakness, arthralgia, myalgia.

DOSAGE AND ADMINISTRATION

Usual adult dose 4-8 mg daily. Tablets to be given with meals.

Note: There must be a medication-free interval of 3-4 weeks after every 6 month course of treatment. (See "Warnings".) No pediatric dosage has been established.

If after a 3-week trial period, efficacy has not been demonstrated, longer administration of Methysergide Maleate is unlikely to be of benefit.

HOW SUPPLIED
TABLETS: 2 MG

BRAND/MANUFACTURER	NDC	SIZE	AWP
○ BRAND			
SANSERT: Sandoz Pharm	00078-0058-05	100s	$155.04

Meticorten SEE PREDNISONE

Metimyd SEE PREDNISOLONE AND SULFACETAMIDE
SODIUM

Metipranolol

DESCRIPTION

Metipranolol Sterile Ophthalmic Solution contains Metipranolol, a nonselective beta-adrenergic receptor blocking agent. Metipranolol is a white, odorless, crystalline powder. The molecular weight is 309.40.

The empiric chemical formula of Metipranolol is $C_{17}H_{27}NO_4$.

The chemical name of Metipranolol is ($\pm$)-1-(4-Hydroxyl-2, 3, 5-trimethylphenoxyl)-3-(iso-propylamino)-2-propanol-4-acetate.

Following is its chemical structure:

CLINICAL PHARMACOLOGY

Metipranolol blocks beta$_1$ and beta$_2$ (nonselective adrenergic receptors. It does not have significant intrinsic sympathomimetic activity, and has only weak local anesthetic (membrane-stabilizing) and myocardial depressant activity.

Orally administered beta-adrenergic blocking agents reduce cardiac output in both healthy subjects and patients with heart disease. In patients with severe impairment of myocardial function, beta-adrenergic receptor antagonists may inhibit the sympathetic stimulatory effect necessary to maintain adequate cardiac output.

Beta-adrenergic receptor blockade in the bronchi and bronchioles may result in significantly increased airway resistance from unopposed para-sympathetic activity. Such an effect is potentially dangerous in patients with asthma or other bronchospastic conditions (see "Contraindications" and "Warnings").

Metipranolol Ophthalmic Solution, when applied topically in the eye, has the action of reducing elevated as well as normal intraocular pressure (IOP), whether or not accompanied by glaucoma. Elevated intraocular pressure is a major risk factor in the pathogenesis of glaucomatous visual field loss. The higher the level of intraocular pressure, the greater the likelihood of glaucomatous visual field loss and optic nerve damage.

The primary mechanism of the ocular hypotensive action of Metipranolol is most likely due to a reduction in aqueous humor production. A slight increase in outflow may be an additional mechanism. Metipranolol Ophthalmic Solution reduces IOP with little or no effect on pupil size or accommodation.

ANIMAL PHARMACOLOGY

In rabbits administered Metipranolol one eye at 2 to 4 fold increased concentrations, multi-focal interstitial nephritis was observed in male animals, and lymphohysticocytic and heterophilic interstitial pneumonia was observed in female animals. The clinical relevance of these findings is unknown.

INDICATIONS AND USAGE

Metipranolol Ophthalmic Solution is indicated in the treatment of ocular conditions where lowering intraocular pressure is likely to be of therapeutic benefit; including patients with ocular hypertension, and patients with chronic open-angle glaucoma.

In controlled studies of patients with intraocular pressure greater than 24 mmHg at base line, Metipranolol Ophthalmic Solution reduced the average intraocular pressure approximately 20-26%.

The onset of action of Metipranolol Ophthalmic Solution, as measured by a reduction in intraocular pressure, occurs within 30 minutes after a single administration. The maximum effect occurs at about 2 hours. A reduction in intraocular pressure can be demonstrated 24 hours after a single dose. Clinical studies in patients with glaucoma treated for up to two years indicate that an intraocular pressure lowering effect is maintained.

In clinical trials, Metipranolol Ophthalmic Solution was safely used during concommitant therapy with pilocarpine, epinephrine or acetazolamide.

UNLABELED USES

Metipranolol is used as an adjunct to lower intraocular pressure in cataract surgery. The oral form of Metipranolol is used alone or as an adjunct in the treatment of mild-to-moderate hypertension.

CONTRAINDICATIONS

Hypersensitivity to any component of this product.

Metipranolol Ophthalmic Solution is contraindicated in patients with bronchial asthma or a history of bronchial asthma, or severe chronic obstructive pulmonary disease; symptomatic sinus bradycardia; greater than a first degree atrioventricular block; cardiogenic shock; or overt cardiac failure.

WARNINGS

As with other topically applied ophthalmic drugs, this drug may be absorbed systemically. Thus, the same adverse reactions found with systemic administration of beta-adrenergic blocking agents may occur with topical administration. For example, severe respiratory reactions and cardiac reactions, including death due to bronchospasm in patients with asthma, and rarely, death in association with cardiac failure, have been reported following topical application of beta-adrenergic blocking agents (see "Contraindications").

Since Metipranolol Ophthalmic Solution had a minor effect on heart rate and blood pressure in clinical studies, caution should be observed in treating patients with a history of cardiac failure. Treatment with Metipranolol Ophthalmic Solution should be discontinued at the first evidence of cardiac failure.

Metipranolol Ophthalmic Solution, or other beta-blockers, should not, in general, be administered to patients with chronic obstructive pulmonary disease (e.g., chronic bronchitis, emphysema) of mild or moderate severity (see "Contraindications"). However, if the drug is necessary in such patients, then it should be administered with caution since it may block bronchodilation produced by endrogenous and exogenous catecholamine stimulation of beta$_2$ receptors.

PRECAUTIONS

General: Because of potential effects of beta-adrenergic receptor blocking agents relative to blood pressure and pulse, these agents should be used with caution in patients with cerebrovascular insufficiency. If signs or symptoms suggesting reduced cerebral blood flow develop following initiation of therapy with Metipranolol Ophthalmic Solution, alternative therapy should be considered.

Some authorities recommend gradual withdrawal of beta-adrenergic receptor blocking agents in patients undergoing elective surgery. If necessary during surgery, the effects of beta-adrenergic receptor blocking agents may be reversed by sufficient doses of such agonists as isoproterenol, dopamine, dobutamine or levarterenol.

While Metipranolol Ophthalmic Solution has demonstrated a low potential for systemic effect, it should be used with caution in patients with diabetes (especially labile diabetes) because of possible masking of signs and symptoms of acute hypoglycemia.

Beta-adrenergic receptor blocking agents may mask certain signs and symptoms of hyperthyroidism, and their abrupt withdrawal might precipitate a thyroid storm.

Beta-adrenergic blockade has been reported to potentiate muscle weakness consistent with certain myasthenic symptoms (e.g., diplopia, ptosis, and generalized weakness).

Risk of anaphylactic reaction: While taking beta-blockers, patients with a history of severe anaphylactic reaction to a variety of allergens may be more reactive to repeated challenge, either accidental, diagnostic, or therapeutic. Such patients may be unresponsive to the usual doses of epinephrine used to treat allergic reaction.

Drug Interactions: Metipranolol Ophthalmic Solution should be used with caution in patients who are receiving a beta-adrenergic blocking agent orally, because of the potential for additive effects on systemic beta-blockade.

Close observation of the patient is recommended when a beta-blocker is administered to patients receiving catecholamine-depleting drugs such as reserpine, because of possible additive effects and the production of hypotension and/or bradycardia.

Caution should be used in the coadministration of beta-adrenergic receptor blocking agents, such as Metipranolol and oral or intravenous calcium channel antagonists, because of possible precipitation of left ventricular failure, and hypotension. In patients with impaired cardiac function, who are receiving calcium channel antagonists, coadministration should be avoided.

The concomitant use of beta-adrenergic receptor blocking agents with digitalis and calcium channel antagonists may have additive effects, prolonging arterioventricular conduction time.

Caution should be used in patients using concomitant adrenergic psychotropic drugs.

Ocular: In patients with angle-closure glaucoma, the immediate treatment objective is to re-open the angle by constriction of the pupil with a miotic agent. Metipranolol Ophthalmic Solution has little or no effect on the pupil, therefore, when it is used to reduce intraocular pressure in angle-closure glaucoma, it should be used only with concomitant administration of a miotic agent.

Carcinogenesis, Mutagenesis, Impairment of Fertility: Lifetime studies with Metipranolol have been conducted in mice at oral doses of 5, 50 and 100 mg/kg/day and in rats at oral doses of up to 70 mg/kg/day. Metipranolol demonstrated no carcinogenic effect. In the mouse study, female animals receiving the low, but not the intermediate or high dose had an increased number of pulmonary adenomas. The significance of this observation is unknown. In a variety of *in vitro* and *in vivo* bacterial and mammalian cell assays, Metipranolol was non-mutagenic.

Reproduction and fertility studies of Metipranolol in rats and mice showed no adverse effect on male fertility at oral doses of up to 50 mg/kg/day, and female fertility at oral doses of up to 25 mg/kg/day.

Pregnancy: Pregnancy Category C: No drug related effects were reported for the segment II teratology study in fetal rats after administration, during organogenesis, to dams of up to 50 mg/kg/day. Metipranolol Ophthalmic Solution has been shown to increase fetal resorption, fetal death, and delayed development when administered orally to rabbits at 50 mg/kg during organogenesis.

There are no adequate and well-controlled studies in pregnant women. Metipranolol Ophthalmic Solution should be used during pregnancy only if the potential benefit justifies the potential risk to the fetus.

Nursing Mothers: It is not known whether Metipranolol Ophthalmic Solution is excreted in human milk. Because many drugs are excreted in human milk, caution should be exercised when Metipranolol Ophthalmic Solution is administered to nursing women.

Pediatric Use: Safety and effectiveness in children have not been established.

ADVERSE REACTIONS

In clinical trials the use of Metipranolol Ophthalmic Solution has been associated with transient local discomfort.

Other ocular adverse reactions, such as conjunctivitis, eyelid dermatitis, blepharitis, blurred vision, tearing, browache, abnormal vision, photophobia, and edema have been reported in small numbers of patients, either in U.S. clinical trials or from post-marketing experience in Europe.

Other systemic adverse reactions, such as allergic reaction, headache, asthenia, hypertension, myocardial infarct, atrial fibrillation, angina, papitation, bradycardia, nausea, rhinitis, dyspnea, epistaxis, bronchitis, coughing, dizziness, anxiety, depression, somnolence, nervousness, arthritis, myalgia, and rash have also been reported, in small numbers of patients.

OVERDOSAGE

No information is available on overdosage of Metipranolol Ophthalmic Solution in humans. The symptoms which might be expected with an overdose of a systemically administered beta-adrenergic receptor blocking agent are bradycardia, hypotension and acute cardiac failure.

DOSAGE AND ADMINISTRATION

The recommended dose is one drop of Metipranolol Ophthalmic Solution in the affected eye(s) twice a day.

If the patient's IOP is not at a satisfactory level on this regimen, use of more frequent administration or a larger dose of Metipranolol Ophthalmic Solution is not known to be of benefit. Concomitant therapy to lower intraocular pressure can be instituted.

Store at controlled room temperature, 15°-30°C (59°-86°F).

HOW SUPPLIED
DROP: 0.3%

BRAND/MANUFACTURER	NDC	SIZE	AWP
○ **BRAND**			
OPTIPRANOLOL HCL: Bausch&Lomb Pharm	24208-0275-07	5 ml	$10.75
	24208-0275-09	10 ml	$17.31

Metoclopramide Hydrochloride

DESCRIPTION

For oral administration, Metoclopramide Hydrochloride is available as tablets containing 5 mg or 10 mg of Metoclopramide as the monohydrochloride monohydrate and as syrup containing 5 mg of Metoclopramide as the monohydrochloride monohydrate per 5 mL.

Each 1 mL of Metoclopramide injectable contains Metoclopramide 5 mg as the monohydrochloride monohydrate.

Metoclopramide Hydrochloride is a white crystalline, odorless substance, freely soluble in water. Chemically, it is 4-amino-5-chloro-N-[2-(diethylamino)ethyl]-2-methoxy benzamide monohydrochloride monohydrate. Molecular weight is 354.3.

Following is its chemical structure:

$$Cl \text{—} C_6H_2(NH_2)(OCH_3) \text{—} CONHCH_2CH_2N(C_2H_5)_2$$

CLINICAL PHARMACOLOGY

Metoclopramide stimulates motility of the upper gastrointestinal tract without stimulating gastric, biliary, or pancreatic secretions. Its mode of action is unclear. It seems to sensitize tissues to the action of acetylcholine. The effect of Metoclopramide on motility is not dependent on intact vagal innervation, but it can be abolished by anticholinergic drugs. Metoclopramide increases the tone and amplitude of gastric (especially antral) contractions, relaxes the pyloric sphincter and the duodenal bulb, and increases peristalsis of the duodenum and jejunum resulting in accelerated gastric emptying and intestinal transit. It increases the resting tone of the lower esophageal sphincter. It has little, if any effect on the motility of the colon or gallbladder.

In patients with gastroesophageal reflux and low LESP (lower esophageal sphincter pressure), single oral doses of Metoclopramide produce dose-related increases in LESP. Effects begin at about 5 mg and increase through 20 mg (the largest dose tested). The increase in LESP from a 5 mg dose lasts about 45 minutes and that of 20 mg lasts between 2 and 3 hours. Increased rate of stomach emptying has been observed with single oral doses of 10 mg.

The antiemetic properties of metoclopramide appear to be a result of its antagonism of central and peripheral dopamine receptors. Dopamine produces nausea and vomiting by stimulation of the medullary chemoreceptor trigger zone (CTZ), and Metoclopramide blocks stimulation of the CTZ by agents like 1-dopa or apomorphine which are known to increase dopamine levels or to possess dopamine-like effects. Metoclopramide also abolishes the slowing of gastric emptying caused by apomorphine.

Like the phenothiazines and related drugs, which are also dopamine antagonists, Metoclopramide produces sedation and may produce extrapyramidal reactions, although these are comparatively rare (see *"Warnings"*). Metoclopramide inhibits the central and peripheral effects of apomorphine, induces release of prolactin and causes a transient increase in circulating aldosterone levels, which may be associated with transient fluid retention.

The onset of pharmacological action of Metoclopramide is 1 to 3 minutes following an intravenous dose, 10 to 15 minutes following intramuscular administration, and 30 to 60 minutes following an oral dose; pharmacological effects persist for 1 to 2 hours.

Pharmacokinetics: Metoclopramide is rapidly and well absorbed. Relative to an intravenous dose of 20 mg, the absolute oral bioavailability of metoclopramide is 80% ± 15.5% as demonstrated in a crossover study of 18 subjects. Peak plasma concentrations occur at about 1-2 hr after a single oral dose. Similar time to peak is observed after individual doses at steady state.

In a single dose study of 12 subjects the area under the drug concentration-time curve increases linearly with doses from 20 to 100 mg. Peak concentrations increase linearly with dose; time to peak concentrations remains the same; whole body clearance is unchanged; and the elimination rate remains the same. The average elimination half-life in individuals with normal renal function is 5-6 hr. Linear kinetic processes adequately describe the absorption and elimination of Metoclopramide.

Approximately 85% of the radioactivity of an orally administered dose appears in the urine within 72 hr. Of the 85% eliminated in the urine, about half is present as free or conjugated Metoclopramide.

The drug is not extensively bound to plasma proteins (about 30%). The whole body volume of distribution is high (about 3.5 L/kg) which suggests extensive distribution of drug to the tissues.

Renal impairment affects the clearance of Metoclopramide. In a study with patients with varying degrees of renal impairment, a reduction in creatinine clearance was correlated with a reduction in plasma clearance, renal clearance, nonrenal clearance, and increase in elimination half-life. The kinetics of Metoclopramide in the presence of renal impairment remained linear however.

◆ RATED THERAPEUTICALLY EQUIVALENT; ◇ THERAPEUTIC EQUIVALENCE UNCONFIRMED; ○ UNRATED

The reduction in clearance as a result of renal impairment suggests that adjustment downward of maintenance dosage should be done to avoid drug cumulation.

INDICATIONS AND USAGE

Symptomatic Gastroesophageal Reflux: Metoclopramide tablets and Syrup are indicated as short-term (4 to 12 weeks) therapy for adults with symptomatic, documented gastroesophageal reflux who fail to respond to conventional therapy.

The principal effect of Metoclopramide is on symptoms of postprandial and daytime heartburn with less observed effect on nocturnal symptoms. If symptoms are confined to particular situations, such as following the evening meal, use of Metoclopramide as single doses prior to the provocative situation should be considered, rather than using the drug throughout the day. Healing of esophageal ulcers and erosions has been endoscopically demonstrated at the end of a 12-week trial using doses of 15 mg q.i.d. As there is no documented correlation between symptoms and healing of esophageal lesions, patients with documented lesions should be monitored endoscopically.

Diabetic Gastroparesis (diabetic gastric stasis): Metoclopramide Hydrochloride, USP is indicated for the relief of symptoms associated with acute and recurrent diabetic gastric stasis. The usual manifestations of delayed gastric emptying (e.g., nausea, vomiting, heartburn, persistent fullness after meals and anorexia) appear to respond to Metoclopramide within different time intervals. Significant relief of nausea occurs early and continues to improve over a three-week period. Relief of vomiting and anorexia may precede the relief of abdominal fullness by one week or more.

The Prevention of Nausea and Vomiting Associated with Emetogenic Cancer Chemotherapy: Metoclopramide injectable is indicated for the prophylaxis of vomiting associated with emetogenic cancer chemotherapy.

The Prevention of Postoperative Nausea and Vomiting: Metoclopramide injectable is indicated for the prophylaxis of postoperative nausea and vomiting in those circumstances where nasogastric suction is undesirable.

Small Bowel Intubation: Metoclopramide injectable may be used to facilitate small bowel intubation in adults and children in whom the tube does not pass the pylorus with conventional maneuvers.

Radiological Examination: Metoclopramide injectable may be used to stimulate gastric emptying and intestinal transit of barium in cases where delayed emptying interferes with radiological examination of the stomach and/or small intestine.

UNLABELED USES

Metoclopramide HCl is used alone or as an adjunct in the treatment of postoperative or drug-induced adynamic ileus and amenorrhea associated with normoprolactinemia and normal or low plasma concentrations of gonadotropins. It is used as an adjunct in the treatment of pain from arthritis, hip surgery, and prostaglandin induced abortion. It is also used with acetaminophen as an adjunct in the treatment of osteoarthritis and rheumatoid arthritis. Metoclopramide is prescribed to improve gastrointestinal symptoms in patients with anorexia nervosa, to lower mean gastric volume and decrease the risk of aspiration pneumonitis, and to reduce bezoar formation in patients with diabetic gastroparesis or a complication of vagotomy. It is also used in nondiabetic gastroparesis, lactation insufficiency, migraine headache, orthostatic hypotension, gastric and duodenal ulcer, tardive dyskinesia, hiccups, and vomiting occurring during pregnancy.

CONTRAINDICATIONS

Metoclopramide should not be used whenever stimulation of gastrointestinal motility might be dangerous, e.g., in the presence of gastrointestinal hemorrhage, mechanical obstruction, or perforation.

Metoclopramide is contraindicated in patients with pheochromocytoma because the drug may cause a hypertensive crisis, probably due to release of catecholamines from the tumor. Such hypertensive crises may be controlled by phentolamine.

Metoclopramide is contraindicated in patients with known sensitivity or intolerance to the drug.

Metoclopramide should not be used in epileptics or patients receiving other drugs which are likely to cause extrapyramidal reactions, since the frequency and severity of seizures or extrapyramidal reactions may be increased.

WARNINGS

Mental depression has occurred in patients with and without prior history of depression. Symptoms have ranged from mild to severe and have included suicidal ideation and suicide. Metoclopramide should be given to patients with a prior history of depression only if the expected benefits outweigh the potential risks.

Extrapyramidal symptoms, manifested primarily as acute dystonic reactions, occur in approximately 1 in 500 patients treated with the usual adult dosages of 30-40 mg/day of Metoclopramide. These usually are seen during the first 24-48 hours of treatment with Metoclopramide, occur more frequently in children and young adults, and are even more frequent at the higher doses used in prophylaxis of vomiting due to cancer chemotherapy. These symptoms may include involuntary movements of limbs and facial grimacing, torticollis, oculogyric crisis, rhythmic protrusion of tongue, bulbar type of speech, trismus, or dystonic reactions resembling tetanus. Rarely, dystonic reactions may present as stridor and dyspnea, possibly due to laryngospasm. If these symptoms should occur, inject 50 mg (diphenhydramine hydrochloride) intramuscularly, and they usually will subside. Benztropine Mesylate, 1 to 2 mg intramuscularly, may also be used to reverse these reactions.

Parkinsonian-like symptoms have occurred, more commonly within the first 6 months after beginning treatment with Metoclopramide, but occasionally after longer periods. These symptoms generally subside within 2-3 months following discontinuance of Metoclopramide. Patients with preexisting Parkinson's disease should be given Metoclopramide cautiously, if at all, since such patients may experience exacerbation of parkinsonian symptoms when taking Metoclopramide.

Tardive Dyskinesia: Tardive dyskinesia, a syndrome consisting of potentially irreversible, involuntary, dyskinetic movements may develop in patients treated with Metoclopramide. Although the prevalence of the syndrome appears to be highest among the elderly, especially elderly women, it is impossible to predict which patients are likely to develop the syndrome. Both the risk of developing the syndrome and the likelihood that it will become irreversible are believed to increase with the duration of treatment and the total cumulative dose.

Less commonly, the syndrome can develop after relatively brief treatment periods at low doses; in these cases, symptoms appear more likely to be reversible.

There is no known treatment for established cases of tardive dyskinesia although the syndrome may remit, partially or completely, within several weeks-to-months after Metoclopramide is withdrawn. Metoclopramide itself, however, may suppress (or partially suppress) the signs of tardive dyskinesia, thereby masking the underlying disease process. The effect of this symptomatic suppression upon the long-term course of the syndrome is unknown. Therefore, the use of Metoclopramide for the symptomatic control of tardive dyskenesia is not recommended.

PRECAUTIONS

General: In one study in hypertensive patients, intravenously administered metoclopramide was shown to release catecholamines; hence, caution should be exercised when Metoclopramide is used in patients with hypertension.

Intravenous injections of undiluted Metoclopramide should be made slowly allowing 1 to 2 minutes for 10 mg since a transient but intense feeling of anxiety and restlessness, followed by drowsiness, may occur with rapid administration.

Intravenous administration of Metoclopramide injectable diluted in a parenteral solution should be made slowly over a period of not less than 15 minutes.

Giving a promotility drug such as Metoclopramide theoretically could put increased pressure on suture lines following a gut anastomosis or closure. Although adverse events related to this possibility have not been reported to date, the possibility should be considered and weighed when deciding whether to use Metoclopramide or nasogastric suction in the prevention of postoperative nausea and vomiting.

Information for Patients: Metoclopramide may impair the mental and/or physical abilities required for the performance of hazardous tasks such as operating machinery or driving a motor vehicle. The ambulatory patient should be cautioned accordingly.

Drug Interactions: The effects of Metoclopramide on gastrointestinal motility are antagonized by anticholinergic drugs and narcotic analgesics. Additive sedative effects can occur when Metoclopramide is given with alcohol, sedatives, hypnotics, narcotics or tranquilizers.

The finding that Metoclopramide releases catecholamines in patients with essential hypertension suggests that it should be used cautiously, if at all, in patients receiving monoamine oxidase inhibitors.

Absorption of drugs from the stomach may be diminished (e.g., digoxin) by Metoclopramide, whereas absorption of drugs from the small bowel may be accelerated (e.g., acetaminophen, tetracycline, levodopa, ethanol).

Gastroparesis (gastric stasis) may be responsible for poor diabetic control in some patients. Exogenously administered insulin may begin to act before food has left the stomach and lead to hypoglycemia. Because the action of Metoclopramide will influence the delivery of food to the intestines and thus the rate of absorption, insulin dosage or timing of dosage may require adjustment.

Carcinogenesis, Mutagenesis, Impairment of Fertility: A 77-week study was conducted in rats with oral doses up to about 40 times the maximum recommended human daily dose. Metoclopramide elevates prolactin levels and the elevation persists during chronic administration. Tissue culture experiments indicate that approximately one-third of human breast cancers are prolactin-dependent *in vitro*, a factor of potential importance if the prescription of Metoclopramide is contemplated in a patient with previously detected breast cancer. Although disturbances such as galactorrhea, amenorrhea, gynecomastia, and impotence have been reported with prolactin-elevating drugs, the clinical significance of elevated serum prolactin levels is unknown for most patients. An increase in mammary neoplasms has been found in rodents after chronic administration of prolactin-stimulating neuroleptic drugs and Metoclopramide. Neither clinical studies nor epidemiologic studies conducted to date, however, have shown an association between chronic administration of these drugs and mammary tumorigenesis; the available evidence is too limited to be conclusive at this time.

An Ames mutagenicity test performed on Metoclopramide was negative.

Pregnancy Category B: Reproduction studies performed in rats, mice, and rabbits by the i.v., i.m., s.c. and oral routes at maximum levels ranging from 12 to 250 times the human dose have demonstrated no impairment of fertility or significant harm to the fetus due to Metoclopramide. There are, however, no adequate and well-controlled studies in pregnant women. Because animal reproduction studies are not always predictive of human response, this drug should be used during pregnancy only if clearly needed.

Nursing Mothers: Metoclopramide is excreted in human milk. Caution should be exercised when Metoclopramide is administered to a nursing mother.

ADVERSE REACTIONS

In general, the incidence of adverse reactions correlates with the dose and duration of Metoclopramide administration. The following reactions have been reported, although in most instances, data do not permit an estimate of frequency.

CNS Effects: Restlessness, drowsiness, fatigue and lassitude occur in approximately 10% of patients receiving the most commonly prescribed dosage of 10 mg q.i.d. (see *"Precautions"*). Insomnia, headache, confusion, dizziness or mental depression with suicidal ideation (see *"Warnings"*) occur less frequently. In cancer chemotherapy patients being treated with 1-2 mg/kg per dose, incidence of drowsiness is about 70%. There are isolated reports of convulsive seizures without clearcut relationship to metoclopramide. Rarely, hallucinations have been reported.

Extrapyramidal Reactions (EPS): Acute dystonic reactions, the most common type of EPS associated with Metoclopramide, occur in approximately 0.2% of patients (1 in 500) treated with 30 to 40 mg of Metoclopramide per day. In cancer chemotherapy patients receiving 1-2 mg/kg per dose, the incidence is 2% in patients over the ages of 30-35, and 25% or higher in children and young adults who have not had prophylactic administration of diphenhydramine. Symptoms include involuntary movements of limbs, facial grimacing, torticollis, oculogyric crisis, rhythmic protrusion of tongue, bulbar type of speech, trismus, opisthotonus (tetanus-like reactions) and rarely, stridor and dyspnea, possibly due to laryngospasm; ordinarily these symptoms are readily reversed by diphenhydramine (see *"Warnings"*).

Parkinsonian-like symptoms may include bradykinesia, tremor, cogwheel rigidity, mask-like facies (see *"Warnings"*). Tardive dyskinesia most frequently is characterized by involuntary movements of the tongue, face, mouth or jaw, and sometimes by involuntary movements of the trunk and/or extremities; movements may be choreoathetotic in appearance (see *"Warnings"*).

Motor restlessness (akathisia) may consist of feelings of anxiety, agitation, jitteriness, and insomnia, as well as inability to sit still, pacing, foot-tapping. These symptoms may disappear spontaneously or respond to a reduction in dosage.

Endocrine Disturbances: Galactorrhea, amenorrhea, gynecomastia, impotence secondary to hyperprolactinemia (see *"Precautions"*). Fluid retention secondary to transient elevation of aldosterone (see *"Clinical Pharmacology"*).

Cardiovascular: Hypotension, hypertension supraventricular tachycardia, and bradycardia (see *"Contraindications", Precautions"*).

Gastrointestinal: Nausea and bowel disturbances, primarily diarrhea.

Hepatic: Rarely, cases of hepatotoxicity, characterized by such findings as jaundice and altered liver function tests, when Metoclopramide was administered with other drugs with known hepatotoxic potential.

Renal: Urinary frequency and incontinence.

Hematologic: A few cases of neutropenia, leukopenia, or agranulocytosis, generally without clearcut relationship to Metoclopramide. Methemoglobinemia, especially with overdosage in neonates (see *"Overdosage"*).

Allergic Reactions: A few cases of rash, urticaria, or bronchospasm, especially in patients with a history of asthma. Rarely, angioneurotic edema, including glossal or laryngeal edema.

Miscellaneous: Visual disturbances, Porphyria, Rare occurrences of neuroleptic malignant syndrome (NMS) have been reported. This potentially fatal syndrome is comprised of the symptom complex of hyperthermia, altered consciousness, muscular rigidity and autonomic dysfunction.

Transient flushing of the face and upper body, without alterations in vital signs, following high doses intravenously.

OVERDOSAGE

Symptoms of overdosage may include drowsiness, disorientation and extrapyramidal reactions. Anticholinergic or antiparkinson drugs or antihistamines with anticholinergic properties may be helpful in controlling the extrapyramidal reactions. Symptoms are self-limiting and usually disappear within 24 hours.

Hemodialysis removes relatively little Metoclopramide, probably because of the small amount of the drug in blood relative to tissues. Similarly, continuous ambulatory peritoneal dialysis does not remove significant amounts of drug. It is unlikely that dosage would need to be adjusted to compensate for losses through dialysis. Dialysis is not likely to be an effective method of drug removal in overdose situations.

Methemoglobinemia has occurred in premature and full-term neonates who were given overdoses of Metoclopramide (1-4 mg/kg/day orally, intramuscularly or intravenously for 1-3 or more days). Methemoglobinemia has not been reported in neonates treated with 0.5 mg/kg/day in divided doses. Methemoglobinemia can be reversed by the intravenous administration of methylene blue.

DOSAGE AND ADMINISTRATION

For the Relief of Symptomatic Gastroesophageal Reflux: Administer from 10 mg to 15 mg Metoclopramide Hydrochloride, USP orally up to q.i.d. 30 minutes before each meal and at bedtime, depending upon symptoms being treated and clinical response (see *"Clinical Pharmacology"* and *"Indications"*). If symptoms occur only intermittently or at specific times of the day, use of Metoclopramide in single doses up to 20 mg prior to the provoking situation may be preferred rather than continuous treatment. Occasionally, patients (such as elderly patients) who

are more sensitive to the therapeutic or adverse effects of Metoclopramide will require only 5 mg per dose.

Experience with esophageal erosions and ulcerations is limited, but healing has thus far been documented in one controlled trial using q.i.d. therapy at 15 mg/dose, and this regimen should be used when lesions are present, so long as it is tolerated (see *"Adverse Reactions"*). Because of the poor correlation between symptoms and endoscopic appearance of the esophagus, therapy directed at esophageal lesions is best guided by endoscopic evaluation.

Therapy longer than 12 weeks has not been evaluated and cannot be recommended.

For the Relief of Symptoms Associated with Diabetic Gastroparesis (diabetic gastric stasis): Administer 10 mg of Metoclopramide 30 minutes before each meal and at bedtime for two to eight weeks, depending upon response and the likelihood of continued well-being upon drug discontinuation.

The initial route of administration should be determined by the severity of the presenting symptoms. If only the earliest manifestations of diabetic gastric stasis are present, oral administration of Metoclopramide may be initiated. However, if severe symptoms are present, therapy should begin with Metoclopramide injectable (I.M. or I.V.). Doses of 10 mg may be administered slowly by the intravenous route over a 1- to 2-minute period.

Administration of Metoclopramide injectable up to 10 days may be required before symptoms subside, at which time oral administration may be instituted. Since diabetic gastric stasis is frequently recurrent, Metoclopramide therapy should be reinstituted at the earliest manifestation.

For the Prevention of Nausea and Vomiting Associated with Emetogenic Cancer Chemotherapy: For doses in excess of 10 mg Metoclopramide injectable should be diluted in 50 mL of a parenteral solution.

The preferred parenteral solution is Sodium Chloride Injection (normal saline), which when combined with Metoclopramide injectable, can be stored frozen for up to 4 weeks. Metoclopramide injectable is degraded when admixed and frozen with Dextrose-5% in Water. Metoclopramide injectable diluted in Sodium Chloride Injection, Dextrose-5% in Water, Dextrose-5% in 0.45% Sodium Chloride, Ringer's Injection or Lactated Ringer's Injection may be stored up to 48 hours (without freezing) after preparation if protected from light. All dilutions may be stored unprotected from light under normal light conditions up to 24 hours after preparation.

Intravenous infusions should be made slowly over a period of not less than 15 minutes, 30 minutes before beginning cancer chemotherapy and repeated every 2 hours for two doses, then every 3 hours for three doses.

The initial two doses should be 2 mg/kg if highly emetogenic drugs such as cisplatin or dacarbazine are used alone or in combination. For less emetogenic regimens, 1 mg/kg per dose may be adequate.

If extrapyramidal symptoms should occur, inject 50 mg diphenhydramine hydrochloride, intramuscularly, and EPS usually will subside.

For the Prevention of Postoperative Nausea and Vomiting: Metoclopramide injectable should be given intramuscularly near the end of surgery. The usual adult dose is 10 mg; however, doses of 20 mg may be used.

To Facilitate Small Bowel Intubation: If the tube has not passed the pylorus with conventional maneuvers in 10 minutes, a single dose (undiluted) may be administered slowly by the intravenous route over a 1- to 2-minute period.

The recommended single dose is: Adults—10 mg Metoclopramide base. Children (6-14 years of age)—2.5 to 5 mg Metoclopramide base; (under 6 years of age)—0.1 mg/kg Metoclopramide base.

To Aid in Radiological Examinations: In patients where delayed gastric emptying interferes with radiological examination of the stomach and/or small intestine, a single dose may be administered slowly by the intravenous route over a 1- to 2-minute period.

For dosage, see intubation, above.

Use in Patients with Renal or Hepatic Impairment: Since Metoclopramide is excreted principally through the kidneys, in those patients whose creatinine clearance is below 40 ml/min, therapy should be initiated at approximately one-half the recommended dosage. Depending upon clinical efficacy and safety considerations, the dosage may be increased or decreased as appropriate.

See *"Overdosage"* section for information regarding dialysis. Metoclopramide undergoes minimal hepatic metabolism, except for simple conjugation. Its safe use has been described in patients with advanced liver disease whose renal function was normal.

Note: Parenteral drug products should be inspected visually for particulate matter and discoloration prior to administration, whenever solution and container permit.

Admixture Compatibilities: Metoclopramide injectable is compatible for mixing and injection with the following dosage forms to the extent indicated below:

Physically and Chemically Compatible up to 48 hours: Cimetidine Hydrochloride (SK&F), Mannitol, USP (Abbott), Potassium Acetate, USP (Invenex), Potassium Chloride, USP (ESI), Potassium Phosphate, USP (Invenex).

Physically Compatible up to 48 hours: Ascorbic Acid, USP (Abbott), Benztropine Mesylate, USP (MS&D). Cytarabine, USP (Upjohn), Dexamethasone Sodium Phosphate, USP (ESI, MS&D), Diphenhydramine Hydrochloride, USP (Parke-Davis), Doxorubicin Hydrochloride, USP (Adria), Heparin Sodium, USP (ESI), Hydrocortisone Sodium Phosphate (MS&D), Lidocaine Hydrochloride, USP (ESI), Magnesium Sulfate, USP (ESI), Multi-Vitamin Infusion (must be refrigerated-USV), Vitamin B Complex with Ascorbic Acid (Roche).

◆ RATED THERAPEUTICALLY EQUIVALENT; ◇ THERAPEUTIC EQUIVALENCE UNCONFIRMED; ○ UNRATED

Physically Compatible up to 24 hours (Do not use if precipitation occurs): Aminophylline, USP (ESI), Clindamycin Phosphate, USP (Upjohn), Cyclophosphamide, USP (Mead-Johnson), Insulin, USP (Lilly), Methylprednisolone Sodium Succinate, USP (ESI).

Conditionally Compatible (Use within one hour after mixing or may be infused directly into the same running IV line): Ampicillin sodium, USP (Bristol), Calcium Gluconate, USP (ESI), Cisplatin (Bristol), Erythromycin Lactobionate, USP (Abbott), Methotrexate Sodium, USP (Lederle), Penicillin G Potassium, USP (Squibb), Tetracycline Hydrochloride, USP (Lederle).

Incompatible (Do Not Mix): Cephalothin Sodium, USP (Lilly), Chloramphenicol Sodium, USP (Parke-Davis), Sodium Bicarbonate, USP (Abbott).

Storage: Store vials and ampuls in carton until used. Do not store open single dose vials or ampuls for later use, as they contain no preservative.

Dilutions may be stored unprotected from light under normal light conditions up to 24 hours after preparation.

Tablets, syrup and injectable should be stored at controlled room temperature between 15°C and 30°C (59°F and 86°F).

J CODES
Up to 10 mg IV—J2765

HOW SUPPLIED

INJECTION: 5 MG/ML

AVERAGE UNIT PRICE (AVAILABLE SIZES)		GENERIC A-RATED AVERAGE PRICE (GAAP)	
BRAND	$0.97	2 ml 25s	$52.19
GENERIC	$0.85	10 ml 25s	$191.10

BRAND/MANUFACTURER	NDC	SIZE	AWP
◆ BRAND			
REGLAN: Robins Pharm	00031-6709-90	2 ml 5s	$11.09
	00031-6709-95	2 ml 25s	$52.55
	00031-6709-78	10 ml 25s	$227.09
	00031-6709-24	30 ml 25s	$613.03
◆ GENERICS			
OCTAMIDE PFS: Pharmacia	00013-6126-70	30 ml 6s	$147.00
Du Pont Multi	00590-5709-77	20 ml 10s	$118.13
Du Pont Multi	00590-5709-85	30 ml 10s	$175.00
Du Pont Multi	00590-5709-57	2 ml 25s	$41.56
Gensia	00703-4502-04	2 ml 25s	$51.88
OCTAMIDE PFS: Pharmacia	00013-6106-95	2 ml 25s	$56.56
Solo Pak	39769-0066-02	2 ml 25s	$58.75
Du Pont Multi	00590-5709-73	10 ml 25s	$164.06
OCTAMIDE PFS: Pharmacia	00013-6116-95	10 ml 25s	$218.13
OCTAMIDE PFS: Pharmacia	00013-6126-95	30 ml 25s	$588.44

INJECTION: 10 MG

AVERAGE UNIT PRICE (AVAILABLE SIZES)		GENERIC A-RATED AVERAGE PRICE (GAAP)	
GENERIC	$1.70	2 ml 25s	$84.76

BRAND/MANUFACTURER	NDC	SIZE	AWP
◆ GENERICS			
Abbott Hosp	00074-3413-01	2 ml 25s	$79.27
Abbott Hosp	00074-3414-01	2 ml 25s	$90.25

SOLUTION: 5 MG/5 ML

AVERAGE UNIT PRICE (AVAILABLE SIZES)	
GENERIC	$0.03

BRAND/MANUFACTURER	NDC	SIZE	AWP
◆ GENERICS			
Silarx	54838-0508-40	120 ml	$4.10
Silarx	54838-0508-80	480 ml	$11.98
Roxane	00054-3563-63	500 ml	$21.24
Silarx	54838-0508-00	3840 ml	$88.20

SOLUTION: 5 MG

BRAND/MANUFACTURER	NDC	SIZE	AWP
◆ GENERICS			
UDL	51079-0429-10	5 ml 50s ud	$25.30

SOLUTION: 10 MG/10 ML

BRAND/MANUFACTURER	NDC	SIZE	AWP
◆ GENERICS			
Roxane	00054-8563-04	10 ml 100s	$61.89

SOLUTION: 10 MG

BRAND/MANUFACTURER	NDC	SIZE	AWP
◆ GENERICS			
UDL	51079-0590-10	10 ml 50s ud	$28.12

SYRUP: 5 MG/5 ML

AVERAGE UNIT PRICE (AVAILABLE SIZES)		GENERIC A-RATED AVERAGE PRICE (GAAP)	
BRAND	$0.09	480 ml	$16.99
GENERIC	$0.04		

BRAND/MANUFACTURER	NDC	SIZE	AWP
◆ BRAND			
REGLAN: Robins Pharm	00031-6706-25	480 ml	$43.36
◆ GENERICS			
Moore,H.L.	00839-7359-69	480 ml	$11.87
Barre	00472-0454-16	480 ml	$11.97
Raway	00686-6105-38	480 ml	$14.00
Schein	00364-2195-16	480 ml	$14.75
Rugby	00536-1463-85	480 ml	$14.88
Biocraft	00332-6105-38	480 ml	$16.00
Qualitest	00603-1435-58	480 ml	$16.70
Pennex	00426-8622-16	480 ml	$17.00
Pennex	00832-8622-16	480 ml	$17.00
Major	00904-1073-16	480 ml	$17.35
URL	00677-1256-33	480 ml	$17.75
Goldline	00182-6082-40	480 ml	$17.95
Geneva	00781-6301-16	480 ml	$18.26
Pharm Assoc	00121-0576-16	480 ml	$19.27
Aligen	00405-3260-16	480 ml	$22.35
Warner Chilcott	00047-2996-23	480 ml	$24.72
Major	00904-1073-28	3840 ml	$118.00
Pharm Assoc	00121-0576-10	10 ml 100s ud	$56.15

SYRUP: 5 MG

BRAND/MANUFACTURER	NDC	SIZE	AWP
◆ GENERICS			
Goldline	00182-6150-40	480 ml	$17.95

TABLETS: 5 MG

AVERAGE UNIT PRICE (AVAILABLE SIZES)		GENERIC A-RATED AVERAGE PRICE (GAAP)	
BRAND	$0.39	100s	$31.24
GENERIC	$0.30	500s	$122.17
HCFA FUL (100s ea)	$0.21		

BRAND/MANUFACTURER	NDC	SIZE	AWP
◆ BRAND			
▶ REGLAN: Robins Pharm	00031-6705-63	100s	$37.15
	00031-6705-64	100s ud	$40.64
◆ GENERICS			
Allscrips	54569-3851-00	12s	$3.26
Medirex	57480-0475-06	30s	$15.75
▶ Invamed	52189-0227-24	100s	$19.80
Parmed	00349-8841-01	100s	$24.50
Schein	00364-2549-01	100s	$24.75
Qualitest	00603-4616-21	100s	$24.80
Biocraft	00332-2204-09	100s	$25.50
Caremark	00339-5232-12	100s	$26.96
Goldline	00182-1898-01	100s	$27.00
Duramed	51285-0834-02	100s	$27.16
Martec	52555-0523-01	100s	$27.25
Major	00904-1069-60	100s	$29.90
URL	00677-1323-01	100s	$31.00
Aligen	00405-4671-01	100s	$31.02
Moore,H.L.	00839-7530-06	100s	$31.04
Rugby	00536-4038-01	100s	$33.20
UDL	51079-0629-20	100s ud	$36.17
Vangard	00615-3546-13	100s ud	$38.85
Goldline	00182-1898-89	100s ud	$40.50
Medirex	57480-0475-01	100s ud	$42.00
Major	00904-1069-61	100s ud	$52.12
Invamed	52189-0227-29	500s	$99.00
Qualitest	00603-4616-29	500s	$103.93
Biocraft	00332-2204-13	500s	$124.00
Rugby	00536-4038-05	500s	$125.25
Parmed	00349-8841-05	500s	$125.80
Goldline	00182-1898-05	500s	$130.00
Duramed	51285-0834-04	500s	$134.55
Major	00904-1069-40	500s	$134.80

▶ SHOWN IN PRODUCT IDENTIFICATION GUIDE

TABLETS: 10 MG

AVERAGE UNIT PRICE (AVAILABLE SIZES)		GENERIC A-RATED AVERAGE PRICE (GAAP)	
BRAND	$0.59	100s	$17.05
GENERIC	$0.15	500s	$64.75
HCFA FUL (100s ea)	$0.02	1000s	$127.60

BRAND/MANUFACTURER	NDC	SIZE	AWP
◆ **BRAND**			
➤ REGLAN: Robins Pharm	00031-6701-63	100s	$58.05
	00031-6701-64	100s ud	$63.80
	00031-6701-70	500s	$272.93
◆ **GENERICS**			
Allscrips	54569-0434-08	12s	$1.72
Medirex	57480-0348-06	30s	$8.29
Goldline	00182-1789-01	100s	$2.85
Raway	00686-2203-09	100s	$3.55
Watson	52544-0312-01	100s	$6.75
Schein	00364-0769-01	100s	$9.25
Geneva	00781-1301-01	100s	$9.45
Invamed	52189-0207-24	100s	$9.45
Qualitest	00603-4617-21	100s	$9.60
Duramed	51285-0805-02	100s	$9.75
Warner Chilcott	00047-0878-24	100s	$9.88
Martec	52555-0120-01	100s	$9.98
Caremark	00339-5233-12	100s	$14.35
➤ Purepac	00228-2269-10	100s	$15.61
Moore,H.L.	00839-7127-06	100s	$17.21
URL	00677-1039-01	100s	$17.30
Rugby	00536-4042-01	100s	$17.31
Major	00904-1070-60	100s	$17.35
Aligen	00405-4672-01	100s	$19.82
Biocraft	00332-2203-09	100s	$21.66
Sidmak	50111-0430-01	100s	$22.00
Lederle Std Prod	00005-4542-23	100s	$25.48
Parmed	00349-8442-01	100s	$27.84
Raway	00686-0283-20	100s ud	$9.00
Major	00904-1070-61	100s ud	$12.85
Goldline	00182-1789-89	100s ud	$23.50
Auro	55829-0378-10	100s ud	$25.87
Vangard	00615-2536-13	100s ud	$27.31
Geneva	00781-1301-13	100s ud	$28.50
UDL	51079-0283-20	100s ud	$28.54
Schein	00364-0769-90	100s ud	$29.60
Medirex	57480-0348-01	100s ud	$29.75
Goldline	00182-1789-05	500s	$10.50
Watson	52544-0312-05	500s	$27.95
Major	00904-1070-40	500s	$39.00
Qualitest	00603-4617-28	500s	$40.86
Schein	00364-0769-05	500s	$41.40
Martec	52555-0120-05	500s	$42.85
Geneva	00781-1301-05	500s	$44.80
Warner Chilcott	00047-0878-30	500s	$45.27
Duramed	51285-0805-04	500s	$47.50
Rugby	00536-4042-05	500s	$77.38
URL	00677-1039-05	500s	$78.00
➤ Purepac	00228-2269-50	500s	$78.05
Parmed	00349-8442-05	500s	$86.11
Aligen	00405-4672-02	500s	$89.19
Invamed	52189-0207-29	500s	$91.50
Biocraft	00332-2203-13	500s	$101.84
Sidmak	50111-0430-02	500s	$102.50
Lederle Std Prod	00005-4542-31	500s	$120.85
Watson	52544-0312-10	1000s	$54.00
Moore,H.L.	00839-7127-16	1000s	$88.43
Duramed	51285-0805-05	1000s	$94.25
Qualitest	00603-4617-32	1000s	$124.12
Rugby	00536-4042-10	1000s	$130.75
Major	00904-1070-80	1000s	$131.60
Parmed	00349-8442-10	1000s	$132.75
Biocraft	00332-2203-15	1000s	$195.53
Sidmak	50111-0430-03	1000s	$197.00
Parmed	00349-8442-52	2500s	$181.74

Metocurine Iodide

THIS DRUG SHOULD BE ADMINISTERED ONLY BY ADEQUATELY TRAINED INDIVIDUALS WHO ARE FAMILIAR WITH ITS ACTIONS, CHARACTERISTICS, AND HAZARDS.

DESCRIPTION

Metocurine Iodide is a nondepolarizing muscle relaxant and is presented as a sterile isotonic solution for intravenous injection. It is (+)-*O, O'*-Dimethylchondrocurarine diiodide.

The empirical formula is $C_{40}H_{48}I_2N_2O_6$, and the molecular weight is 906.64.

Following is its chemical structure:

CLINICAL PHARMACOLOGY

Metocurine Iodide is a methyl analogue of tubocurarine which produces nondepolarizing (competitive) neuromuscular blockade at the myoneural junction. Recent animal studies suggest that Metocurine Iodide does not produce the autonomic ganglionic blockade seen with other nondepolarizing muscle relaxants. Recent clinical findings suggest that Metocurine Iodide reaches the neuromuscular junction more rapidly than does tubocurarine. After intravenous injection, there is rapid onset (1 to 4 minutes) of muscle relaxation with maximum twitch inhibition (96%) in 1.5 to 10 minutes. The maximum effect lasts 35 to 60 minutes. The time for recovery to 50% of control twitch response is in excess of 3 hours.

Following bolus injection of 0.05 mg/kg, the mean terminal half-life of Metocurine Iodide was 3.6 hours (217 minutes). Approximately 50% of the dose was excreted as unchanged drug in the urine over 48 hours, and 2% was excreted unchanged in the bile. Approximately 35% is protein bound, mainly to the beta and gamma globulins.

The use of repeated doses may be accompanied by a cumulative effect. The duration of action and degree of muscle relaxation may be altered by dehydration, body temperature changes, hypocalcemia, excess magnesium, or acid-base imbalance. Concurrently administered general anesthetics, certain antibiotics, and neuromuscular disease may potentiate the neuromuscular blocking action of Metocurine Iodide. Histamine release with Metocurine Iodide occurs less frequently than with *d*-tubocurarine and is related to dosage and rapidity of administration. Effects on the cardiovascular system (eg, changes in pulse rate, hypotension) are less than those reported with equipotent doses of *d*-tubocurarine and gallamine.

Because the main excretory pathway for Metocurine Iodide is through the kidneys, severe renal disease or conditions associated with poor renal perfusion (shock states) may result in prolonged neuromuscular blockade.

Following intravenous injection in the mother, placental transfer of Metocurine Iodide occurs rapidly, and, after 6 minutes, the fetal plasma concentration is approximately one-tenth the maternal level.

INDICATIONS AND USAGE

Metocurine Iodide is indicated as an adjunct to anesthesia to induce skeletal-muscle relaxation. It may be employed to reduce the intensity of muscle contractions in pharmacologically or electrically induced convulsions. It may also be employed to facilitate the management of patients undergoing mechanical ventilation.

CONTRAINDICATIONS

Metocurine Iodide is contraindicated in those persons with known hypersensitivity to the drug or to its Iodide content.

WARNINGS

METOCURINE IODIDE SHOULD BE ADMINISTERED IN CAREFULLY ADJUSTED DOSES BY OR UNDER THE SUPERVISION OF EXPERIENCED CLINICIANS WHO ARE FAMILIAR WITH THE COMPLICATIONS WHICH MAY OCCUR WITH THE USE OF THIS DRUG. Metocurine Iodide should not be administered unless facilities for intubation, artificial ventilation, oxygen therapy, and reversal agents are immediately available. The clinician must be prepared to assist or control respiration.

Metocurine Iodide should be used with extreme caution in patients with myasthenia gravis. In such patients, a peripheral nerve stimulator may be valuable in assessing the effects of administration.

PRECAUTIONS

General: Metocurine Iodide should be used with caution in patients with poor renal perfusion or severe renal disease (see *"Clinical Pharmacology"*).

Rapid administration of large doses of Metocurine Iodide may produce changes in blood pressure or heart rate or signs of histamine release.

Metocurine Iodide has no effect on consciousness, pain threshold, or cerebration; therefore, it should be used with adequate anesthesia.

Drug Interactions: Synergistic or antagonistic effects may result when depolarizing and nondepolarizing muscle relaxants are administered simultaneously or sequentially.

Parenteral administration of high doses of certain antibiotics may intensify or resemble the neuroblocking action of muscle relaxants. These include neomycin, streptomycin, bacitracin, kanamycin, gentamicin, dihydrostreptomycin, polymyxin B, colistin, sodium colistimethate, and tetracyclines. If muscle relaxants and antibiotics must be administered simultaneously, the patient should be observed closely for any unexpected prolongation of respiratory depression. Certain general anesthetics have a synergistic action with neuromuscular blocking agents. Diethyl ether, halothane, and isoflurane potentiate the neuromuscular blocking action of other nondepolarizing agents and may be presumed to do so with Metocurine Iodide.

◆ RATED THERAPEUTICALLY EQUIVALENT; ◇ THERAPEUTIC EQUIVALENCE UNCONFIRMED; ○ UNRATED

Administration of quinidine shortly after recovery may produce recurrent paralysis.

The effect of diazepam on neuromuscular blockade by Metocurine Iodide is not clear. Until more information is available, patients should be carefully monitored for unexpected drug response and prolongation of action.

The use of magnesium sulfate in preeclamptic patients potentiates the effects of both depolarizing and nondepolarizing muscle relaxants.

Usage in Pregnancy—Pregnancy Category C: Intrauterine growth retardation and limb deformities resembling club-foot were produced by *d*-tubocurarine chloride and succinylcholine chloride when administered to the rat fetus between the 16th and 19th days of gestation or when injected in chick embryos from the 5th to the 15th day of incubation. When *d*-tubocurarine was injected intramuscularly into the interscapular region of the fetuses on the 16th to the 19th day of gestation, the incidence of growth retardation and limb deformity ranged from 21 to 23% and 7 to 8% respectively. There are no adequate and well-controlled studies of Metocurine Iodide in pregnant women. Metocurine Iodide should be used during pregnancy only if the potential benefit justifies the risk to the fetus.

Labor and Delivery: It is not known whether the use of muscle relaxants during labor or delivery has immediate or delayed adverse effects on the fetus, prolongs the duration of labor, or increases the likelihood that forceps delivery, obstetric intervention, or resuscitation of the newborn will be necessary.

Nursing Mothers: It is not known whether Metocurine Iodide is excreted in human milk. Because many drugs are excreted in human milk, caution should be exercised when Metocurine Iodide is administered to a nursing woman.

Usage in Children: A clinical study has shown that Metocurine Iodide is twice as potent as *d*-tubocurarine in children, but the rate of recovery is the same. There may be a slight increase in heart rate, but no change occurs in blood pressure or ECG. Doses calculated on the basis of body weight or body surface area may be applicable when the advantages of nondepolarizing neuromuscular blockade are desired.

ADVERSE REACTIONS

The most frequently noted adverse reaction is prolongation of the drug's pharmacologic action. Neuromuscular effects may range from skeletal-muscle weakness to a profound relaxation that produces respiratory insufficiency or apnea. Possible adverse reactions include allergic or hypersensitivity reactions to the drug or its iodide content and histamine release when large doses are administered rapidly. Signs of histamine release include erythema, edema, flushing, tachycardia, arterial hypotension, bronchospasm, and circulatory collapse.

Prolonged apnea and respiratory depression have occurred following the use of muscle relaxants. Many physiologic factors, drug interactions, and individual sensitivities may contribute to the development of respiratory paralysis (see "Clinical Pharmacology" and "Precautions").

OVERDOSAGE

To obtain up-to-date information about the treatment of overdose, a good resource is your certified Regional Poison Control Center. Telephone numbers of certified poison control centers are listed in the *Physicians' Desk Reference (PDR).* In managing overdosage, consider the possibility of multiple drug overdoses, interaction among drugs, and unusual drug kinetics in your patient.

An overdose of Metocurine Iodide may result in prolonged apnea, cardiovascular collapse, and sudden release of histamine.

Massive doses of Metocurine are not reversible by the antagonists edrophonium or neostigmine and atropine.

Overdosage may be avoided by the careful monitoring of response by means of a peripheral nerve stimulator.

The primary treatment for residual neuromuscular blockade with respiratory paralysis or inadequate ventilation is maintenance of the patient's airway and manual or mechanical ventilation.

Accompanying derangements of blood pressure, electrolyte imbalance, or circulating blood volume should be determined and corrected by appropriate fluid and electrolyte therapy.

Residual neuromuscular blockade following surgery may be reversed by the use of anticholinesterase inhibitors such as neostigmine or pyridostigmine bromide and atropine. Prescribing information should be consulted for the appropriate drug selection based on dosage and desired duration of action.

DOSAGE AND ADMINISTRATION

Metocurine Iodide should be administered intravenously as a sustained injection over a period of 30 to 60 seconds. *Intramuscular Administration of Metocurine Iodide is not Recommended.* Care must be taken to avoid overdosage. The use of a peripheral nerve stimulator to monitor response will minimize the risk of overdosage. The type of anesthetic used and nature of the surgical procedure will influence the amount of Metocurine Iodide required. Doses of 0.2 to 0.4 mg/kg have been found satisfactory for endotracheal intubation. Relaxation following the initial dose may be expected to be effective for periods of 25 to 90 minutes, with an average of approximately 60 minutes. Supplemental administration may be made as indicated to provide needed surgical relaxation. Supplemental doses average 0.5 to 1 mg. The use of strong anesthetics that potentiate the effect of neuromuscular blocking drugs such as halothane, diethyl ether, isoflurane, or enflurane reduces the requirement for Metocurine Iodide. Incremental doses should be reduced by approximately one-third to one-half.

Recommended Doses for Use During Electroshock Therapy: Doses required for satisfactory relaxation range from 1.75 to 5.5 mg. When the patient is treated for

the 1st time, the drug is administered slowly by the intravenous route as a sustained injection until a head-drop response ensues. After dosage has been established, subsequent injections are completed in 15 to 50 seconds. The average dose ranges from 2 to 3 mg.

Drug Incompatibilities: Metocurine Iodide is unstable in alkaline solutions. When it is combined with barbiturate solutions, precipitation may occur. Solutions of barbiturates, meperidine, and morphine sulfate should not be administered from the same syringe.

Parenteral drug products should be inspected visually for particulate matter and discoloration prior to administration, whenever solution and container permit.

Store at controlled room temperature, 59° to 86°F (15° to 30°C).

J CODES

Up to 2 mg IV—J2240

HOW SUPPLIED
INJECTION: 2 MG/ML

BRAND/MANUFACTURER	NDC	SIZE	AWP
BRAND			
METUBINE IODIDE: Dista	00777-1421-01	20 ml	$24.18

Metolazone

DO NOT INTERCHANGE FORMULATIONS OF METOLAZONE THAT HAVE A SLOW AND INCOMPLETE BIOAVAILABILITY WITH MORE RAPIDLY AVAILABLE AND COMPLETELY BIOAVAILABLE METOLAZONE FORMULATIONS. THEY ARE NOT THERAPEUTICALLY EQUIVALENT.

DESCRIPTION

Metolazone tablets for oral administration contain ½ mg (rapid availability) or 2½, 5 or 10 mg (slow availability) of Metolazone, USP, a diuretic/saluretic/antihypertensive drug of the quinazoline class.

Metolazone has the molecular formula $C_{16}H_{16}ClN_3O_3S$, the chemical name 7-chloro-1,2,3,4-tetrahydro-2-methyl-3-(2-methylphenyl)-4-oxo-6- quinazolinesulfonamide and a molecular weight of 365.83.

Metolazone is only sparingly soluble in water, but more soluble in plasma, blood, alkali and organic solvents.

Following is its chemical structure:

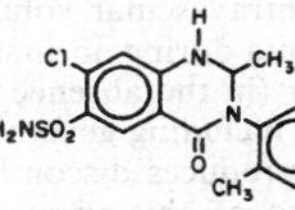

CLINICAL PHARMACOLOGY

Metolazone is a quinazoline diuretic, with properties generally similar to the thiazide diuretics. The actions of Metolazone result from interference with the renal tubular mechanism of electrolyte reabsorption.

Metolazone acts primarily to inhibit sodium reabsorption at the cortical diluting site and to a lesser extent in the proximal convoluted tubule. Sodium and chloride ions are excreted in approximately equivalent amounts. The increased delivery of sodium to the distal-tubular exchange site results in increased potassium excretion. Metolazone does not inhibit carbonic anhydrase. A proximal action of Metolazone has been shown in humans by increased excretion of phosphate and magnesium ions and by a markedly increased fractional excretion of sodium in patients with severely compromised glomerular filtration. This action has been demonstrated in animals by micropuncture studies.

The antihypertensive mechanism of action of Metolazone is not fully understood but is presumed to be related to its saluretic and diuretic properties.

When Metolazone slow availability Tablets are given, diuresis and saluresis usually begin within one hour and may persist for 24 hours or more. For most patients, the duration of effect can be varied by adjusting the daily dose. High doses may prolong the effect. A single daily dose is recommended. When a desired therapeutic effect has been obtained, it may be possible to reduce dosage to a lower maintenance level.

In two double-blind, controlled clinical trials of Metolazone rapid availability tablets, the maximum effect on mean blood pressure was achieved within 2 weeks of treatment and showed some evidence of an increased response at 1mg compared to ½ mg. There was no indication of an increased response with 2 mg. After six weeks of treatment, the mean fall in serum potassium was 0.42 mEq/L at ½ mg, 0.66 mEq/l at 1 mg and 0.7 mEq/L at 2 mg. Serum uric acid increased by 1.1 to 1.4 mg/dL at increasing doses. There were small falls in serum sodium and chloride and a 1.3-2.1 mg/dL increase in BUN at increasing doses.

The diuretic potency of Metolazone slow availability at maximum therapeutic dosage is approximately equal to thiazide diuretics. However, unlike thiazides, Metolazone slow availability may produce diuresis in patients with glomerular filtration rates below 20 mL/min.

Metolazone slow availability and furosemide administered concurrently have produced marked diuresis in some patients where edema or ascites was refractory to treatment with maximum recommended doses of these or other diuretics administered alone. The mechanism of this interaction is unknown (see *"Drug Interactions"* and *"Warnings"*).

With slow availability formulations, maximum blood levels of Metolazone are found approximately eight hours after dosing; absorption continues for an additional 12 hours. A small fraction of Metolazone is metabolized. Most of the drug is excreted in the unconverted form in the urine.

The rate and extent of absorption of Metolazone from rapid availability tablets were equivalent to those from an oral solution of Metolazone. Peak blood levels are obtained within 2 to 4 hours of oral administration with an elimination half-life of approximately 14 hours. Metolazone rapid availability tablets have been shown to produce blood levels that are dose proportional between ½-2 mg. Steady state blood levels are usually reached in 4-5 days.

INDICATIONS AND USAGE

Metolazone slow availability is indicated for the treatment of salt and water retention including:

-edema accompanying congestive heart failure;

-edema accompanying renal diseases, including the nephrotic syndrome and states of diminished renal function. Metolazone slow availability is also indicated for the treatment of hypertension, alone or in combination with other antihypertensive drugs of a different class. Metolazone rapid availability tablets are intended for the treatment of new patients with mild to moderate hypertension, alone or in combination with other antihypertensive drugs of a different class.

Metolazone rapid availability tablets have not been evaluated for the treatment of congestive heart failure or fluid retention due to renal or hepatic disease and the correct dosage for these conditions and other edema states has not been established.

Since a safe and effective diuretic dose has not been established, Metolazone rapid availability tablets should not be used when diuresis is desired. A dose titration is necessary if Metolazone rapid availability tablets are to be substituted for Metolazone slow availability tablets in the treatment of hypertension.

USAGE IN PREGNANCY

The routine use of diuretics in an otherwise healthy woman is inappropriate and exposes mother and fetus to unnecessary hazard. Diuretics do not prevent development of toxemia of pregnancy, and there is no evidence that they are useful in the treatment of developed toxemia.

Edema during pregnancy may arise from pathologic causes or from the physiologic and mechanical consequences of pregnancy. Metolazone slow availability is indicated in pregnancy when edema is due to pathologic causes, just as it is in the absence of pregnancy (see *"Precautions"*). Metolazone rapid availability is not indicated for the treatment of edema in pregnancy. Dependent edema in pregnancy resulting from restriction of venous return by the expanded uterus is properly treated through elevation of the lower extremities and use of support hose; use of diuretics to lower intravascular volume in this case is illogical and unnecessary. There is hypervolemia during normal pregnancy which is harmful to neither the fetus nor the mother (in the absence of cardiovascular disease), but which is associated with edema, including generalized edema, in the majority of pregnant women. If this edema produces discomfort, increased recumbency will often provide relief. In rare instances, this edema may cause extreme discomfort which is not relieved by rest. In these cases, a short course of diuretics may be appropriate.

UNLABELED USES

Metolazone is used alone or as an adjunct in the treatment of calcium nephralithiases, premanagement of menstrual syndrome and the adjunct treatment of renal failure.

CONTRAINDICATIONS

Anuria, hepatic coma or pre-coma, known allergy or hypersensitivity to Metolazone.

WARNINGS

RAPID ONSET HYPONATREMIA

Rarely, the rapid onset of severe hyponatremia and/or hypokalemia has been reported following initial doses of thiazide and nonthiazide diuretics. When symptoms consistent with severe electrolyte imbalance appear rapidly, drug should be discontinued and supportive measures should be initiated immediately. Parenteral electrolytes may be required. Appropriateness of therapy with this class of drugs should be carefully re-evaluated.

HYPOKALEMIA

Hypokalemia may occur with consequent weakness, cramps, and cardiac dysrhythmias. Serum potassium should be determined at regular intervals, and dose reduction, potassium supplementation or addition of a potassium-sparing diuretic instituted whenever indicated. Hypokalemia is a particular hazard in patients who are digitalized or who have or have had a ventricular arrhythmia: dangerous or fatal arrhythmias may be precipitated. Hypokalemia is dose related.

In controlled clinical trials, 1.5% of patients taking ½ mg and 3.1% of patients taking 1 mg of daily developed clinical hypokalemia (defined as hypokalemia accompanied by signs or symptoms); 21% of the patients taking ½ mg and 30% of the patients taking 1 mg of Metolazone rapid availability daily developed hypokalemia (defined as a serum potassium concentration below 3.5 mEq/L); in another controlled clinical trial in which the patients started therapy with a serum potassium level greater than 4.0 mEq/L, 8% of patients taking ½ mg of Metolazone rapid availability daily developed hypokalemia (defined as a serum potassium concentration below 3.5 mEq/L).

CONCOMITANT THERAPY

Lithium: In general, diuretics should not be given concomitantly with lithium because they reduce its renal clearance and add a high risk of lithium toxicity. Read prescribing information for lithium preparations before use of such concomitant therapy.

Furosemide: Unusually large or prolonged losses of fluids and electrolytes may result when Metolazone is administered concomitantly to patients receiving furosemide (see *"Precautions, Drug Interactions"*).

Other Antihypertensive Drugs: When Metolazone is used with other antihypertensive drugs, particular care must be taken to avoid excessive reduction of blood pressure, especially during initial therapy.

CROSS-ALLERGY

Cross-allergy, while not reported to date, theoretically may occur when Metolazone is given to patients known to be allergic to sulfonamide-derived drugs, thiazides, or quinethazone.

SENSITIVITY REACTIONS

Sensitivity reactions may occur with or without a history of allergy or bronchial asthma.

PRECAUTIONS

DO NOT INTERCHANGE FORMULATIONS OF METOLAZONE THAT HAVE A SLOW AND INCOMPLETE BIOAVAILABILITY WITH MORE RAPIDLY AVAILABLE AND COMPLETELY BIOAVAILABLE METOLAZONE FORMULATIONS. THEY ARE NOT THERAPEUTICALLY EQUIVALENT.

A. GENERAL

Fluid and Electrolytes: All patients receiving therapy with Metolazone Tablets should have serum electrolyte measurements done at appropriate intervals and be observed for clinical signs of fluid and/or electrolyte imbalance: namely, hyponatremia, hypochloremic alkalosis, and hypokalemia. In patients with severe edema accompanying cardiac failure or renal disease, a low-salt syndrome may be produced, especially with hot weather and a low-salt diet. Serum and urine electrolyte determinations are particularly important when the patient has protracted vomiting, severe diarrhea, or is receiving parenteral fluids. Warning signs of imbalance are: dryness of mouth, thirst, weakness, lethargy, drowsiness, restlessness, muscle pains or cramps, muscle fatigue, hypotension, oliguria, tachycardia, and gastrointestinal disturbances such as nausea and vomiting. Hyponatremia may occur at any time during long term therapy and, on rare occasions, may be life threatening.

The risk of hypokalemia is increased when larger doses are used, when diuresis is rapid, when severe liver disease is present, when corticosteroids are given concomitantly, when oral intake is inadequate or when excess potassium is being lost extrarenally, such as with vomiting or diarrhea.

Thiazide-like diuretics have been shown to increase the urinary excretion of magnesium: this may result in hypomagnesemia.

Glucose Tolerance: Metolazone may raise blood glucose concentrations possibly causing hyperglycemia and glycosuria in patients with diabetes or latent diabetes.

Hyperuricemia: Metolazone regularly causes an increase in serum uric acid and can occasionally precipitate gouty attacks even in patients without a prior history of them.

Azotemia: Azotemia, presumably pre-renal azotemia may be precipitated during the administration of Metolazone. If azotemia and oliguria worsen during treatment of patients with severe renal disease, Metolazone should be discontinued.

Renal Impairment: Use caution when administering Metolazone tablets to patients with severely impaired renal function. As most of the drug is excreted by the renal route, accumulation may occur.

Orthostatic Hypotension: Orthostatic hypotension may occur; this may be potentiated by alcohol, barbiturates, narcotics, or concurrent therapy with other antihypertensive drugs. In controlled clinical trials, 1.4% of patients treated with Metolazone rapid availability tablets (½ mg) had orthostatic hypotension; this effect was not reported in the placebo group.

Hypercalcemia: Hypercalcemia may infrequently occur with Metolazone, especially in patients taking high doses of vitamin D or with high bone turnover states, and may signify hidden hyperparathyroidism. Metolazone should be discontinued before tests for parathyroid function are performed.

Systemic Lupus Erythematosus: Thiazide diuretics have exacerbated or activated systemic lupus erythematosus and this possibility should be considered with Metolazone tablets.

B. INFORMATION FOR PATIENTS

Patients should be informed of possible adverse effects, advised to take the medication as directed and promptly report any possible adverse reactions to the treating physician.

C. DRUG INTERACTIONS

Diuretics: Furosemide and probably other loop diuretics given concomitantly with Metolazone can cause unusually large or prolonged losses of fluid and electrolytes (see *"Warnings"*).

◆ RATED THERAPEUTICALLY EQUIVALENT; ◇ THERAPEUTIC EQUIVALENCE UNCONFIRMED; ○ UNRATED

Other Antihypertensives: When Metolazone Tablets are used with other antihypertensive drugs, care must be taken, especially during initial therapy. Dosage adjustments of other antihypertensives may be necessary.

Alcohol, Barbiturates, and Narcotics: The hypotensive effects of these drugs may be potentiated by the volume contraction that may be associated with Metolazone therapy.

Digitalis Glycosides: Diuretic-induced hypokalemia can increase the sensitivity of the myocardium to digitialis. Serious arrhythmias can result.

Corticosteroids or ACTH: May increase the risk of hypokalemia and increase salt and water retention.

Lithium: Serum lithium levels may increase (see "Warnings").

Curariform Drugs: Diuretic-induced hypokalemia may enhance neuromuscular blocking effects of curariform drugs (such as tubocurarine) - the most serious effect would be respiratory depression which could proceed to apnea. Accordingly, it may be advisable to discontinue Metolazone Tablets three days before elective surgery.

Salicylates and Other Non-Steroidal Anti-Inflammatory Drugs: May decrease the antihypertensive effects of Metolazone Tablets.

Sympathomimetics: Metolazone may decrease arterial responsiveness to norepinephrine, but this diminution is not sufficient to preclude effectiveness of the pressor agent for therapeutic use.

Insulin and Oral Antidiabetic Agents: See "Glucose Tolerance" under "Precautions, General".

Methenamine: Efficacy may be decreased due to urinary alkalizing effect of Metolazone.

Anticoagulants: Thiazide-like diuretics may affect the hypoprothrombinemic response to anticoagulants; dosage adjustments may be necessary.

D. DRUG/LABORATORY TEST INTERACTIONS
None reported.

E. CARCINOGENESIS, MUTAGENESIS, IMPAIRMENT OF FERTILITY
Mice and rats administered Metolazone 5 days/week for up to 18 and 24 months, respectively, at daily doses of 2, 10 and 50 mg/kg, exhibited no evidence of a tumorigenic effect of the drug. The small number of animals examined histologically and poor survival in the mice limit the conclusions that can be reached from these studies.

Metolazone was not mutagenic *in vitro* in the Ames Test using Salmonella typhimurium strains TA-97, TA-98, TA-100, TA-102 and TA-1535.

Reproductive performance has been evaluated in mice and rats. There is no evidence that Metolazone possesses the potential for altering reproductive capacity in mice. In a rat study, in which males were treated orally with Metolazone at doses of 2, 10 and 50 mg/kg for 127 days prior to mating with untreated females, an increased number of resorption sites was observed in dams mated with males from the 50 mg/kg group. In addition, the birth weight of offspring was decreased and the pregnancy rate was reduced in dams mated with males from the 10 and 50 mg/kg groups.

F. PREGNANCY
Teratogenic Effects—Pregnancy Category B: Reproduction studies performed in mice, rabbits and rats treated during the appropriate period of gestation at doses up to 50 mg/kg/day have revealed no evidence of harm to the fetus due to Metolazone. There are, however, no adequate and well-controlled studies in pregnant women. Because animal reproduction studies are not always predictive of human response, Metolazone tablets should be used during pregnancy only if clearly needed. Metolazone crosses the placental barrier and appears in cord blood.

Nonteratogenic Effects: The use of Metolazone tablets in pregnant women requires that the anticipated benefit be weighed against possible hazards to the fetus. These hazards include fetal or neonatal jaundice, thrombocytopenia, and possibly other adverse reactions which have occurred in the adult. It is not known what effect the use of the drug during pregnancy has on the later growth, development and functional maturation of the child. No such effects have been reported with Metolazone.

G. LABOR AND DELIVERY
Based on clinical studies in which women received Metolazone in late pregnancy until the time of delivery, there is no evidence that the drug has any adverse effects on the normal course of labor or delivery.

H. NURSING MOTHERS
Metolazone appears in breast milk. Because of the potential for serious adverse reactions in nursing infants from Metolazone, a decision should be made whether to discontinue nursing or to discontinue the drug, taking into account the importance of the drug to the mother.

I. PEDIATRIC USE
Safety and effectiveness in children have not been established and such use is not recommended.

ADVERSE REACTIONS
Metolazone is usually well tolerated, and most reported adverse reactions have been mild and transient. Many Metolazone slow availability related adverse reactions represent extensions of its expected pharmacologic activity and can be attributed to either its antihypertensive action or its renal/metabolic actions. The following adverse reactions have been reported. Several are single or comparably rare occurrences. Adverse reactions are listed in decreasing order of severity within body systems.

Cardiovascular: Chest pain/discomfort, orthostatic hypotension, excessive volume depletion, hemoconcentration, venous thrombosis, palpitations.

Central and Peripheral Nervous System: Syncope, neuropathy, vertigo, paresthesias, psychotic depression, impotence, dizziness/light-headedness, drowsiness, fatigue, weakness, restlessness (sometimes resulting in insomnia), headache.

Dermatologic/Hypersensitivity: Necrotizing angiitis (cutaneous vasculitis), purpura, dermatitis (photosensitivity), urticaria and skin rashes.

Gastrointestinal: Hepatitis, intrahepatic cholestatic jaundice, pancreatitis, vomiting, nausea, epigastric distress, diarrhea, constipation, anorexia, abdominal bloating.

Hematologic: Aplastic/hypoplastic anemia, agranulocytosis, leukopenia.

Metabolic: Hypokalemia, hyponatremia, hyperuricemia, hypochloremia, hypochloremic alkalosis, hyperglycemia, glycosuria, increase in serum urea nitrogen (BUN) or creatinine, hypophosphatemia, hypomagnesemia, hypercalcemia.

Musculoskeletal: Joint pain, acute gouty attacks, muscle cramps or spasm.

Other: Transient blurred vision, chills.

Adverse experience information is available from more than 14 years of accumulated marketing experience with other formulations of Metolazone for which reliable quantitative information is lacking and from controlled clinical trials with Metolazone rapid availability from which incidences can be calculated. In controlled clinical trails with Metolazone rapid availability, adverse experiences resulted in discontinuation of therapy in 6.7-6.8% of patients given ½ to 1 mg of Metolazone rapid availability.

Adverse experiences occurring in controlled clinical trials with Metolazone rapid availability with an incidence of > 2%, whether or not considered drug-related, are summarized in the following table.

INCIDENCE OF ADVERSE EXPERIENCES VOLUNTEERED OR ELICITED (BY PATIENT IN PERCENT)*

	Metolazone Rapid Availability $n = 226$[†]
Dizziness (light-headedness)	10.2
Headaches	9.3
Muscle Cramps	5.8
Fatigue (malaise, lethargy, lassitude)	4.4
Joint Pain, swelling	3.1
Chest Pain (precordial discomfor)	2.7

*   *Percent of patients reporting an adverse experience one or more times.*
†   *All doses combined (½, 1 and 2 mg).*

Some of the adverse effects reported in association with Metolazone rapid availability also occur frequently in untreated hypertensive patients, such as headache and dizziness, which occured in 14.8 and 7.4% of patients in a smaller parallel placebo group. The following adverse effects were reported in less than 2% of the Metolazone rapid availability treated patients.

Cardiovascular: Cold extremities, edema, orthostatic hypotension, palpitations.

Central and Peripheral Nervous System: Anxiety, depression, dry mouth, impotence, nervousness, neuropathy, weakness, "weird" feeling.

Dermatological: Pruritus, rash, skin dryness.

Eyes, Ears, Nose, Throat: Cough, epistaxis, eye itching, sinus congestion, sore throat, tinnitus.

Gastrointestinal: Abdominal discomfort (pain, bloating, bitter taste, constipation, diarrhea, nausea, vomiting.

Genitourinary: Nocturia.

Musculoskeletal: Back pain.

Other Adverse Experiences: Adverse experiences reported with other marketed Metolazone formulations and most thiazide diuretics, for which quantitative data are not available, are listed in decreasing order of severity within body systems. Several are single or rare occurrences.

Cardiovascular: excessive volume depletion, hemoconcentration, venous thrombosis.

Central and Peripheral Nervous System: syncope, paresthesias, drowsiness, restlessness (sometimes resulting in insomnia).

Dermatologic/Hypersensitivity: necrotizing angiitis (cutaneous vasculitis), purpura, dermatitis, photosensitivity, urticaria.

Gastrointestinal: hepatitis, intrahepatic cholestitic jaundice, pancreatitis, anorexia.

Hematologic: aplastic (hypoplastic) anemia, agranulocytosis, leukopenia.

Metabolic: hypokalemia (see "Warning, Hypokalemia"), hyponatremia, hyperuricenia, hypochloremia, hypochloremic alkalosis, hyperglycemia, glycosuria, increase in serum urea nitrogen (BUN) or creatinine, hypophophatemia, hypomagnesemia, hypercalcemia.

Musculoskeletal: acute gouty attacks.

Other: transient blurred vision, chills.

In addition, adverse reactions reported with similar antihypertensive-diuretics, but which have not been reported to date for Metolazone include: bitter taste, dry mouth, sialadenitis, xanthopsia, respiratory distress (including pneumonitis), thrombocytopenia and anaphylactic reactions. These reactions should be considered as possible occurrences with clinical usage of Metolazone.

Whenever adverse reactions are moderate or severe, Metolazone dosage should be reduced or therapy withdrawn.

OVERDOSAGE

Intentional overdosage has been reported rarely with Metolazone and similar diuretic drugs.

Signs and Symptoms: Orthostatic hypotension, dizziness, drowsiness, syncope, electrolyte abnormalities, hemoconcentration and hemodynamic changes due to plasma volume depletion may occur. In some instances depressed respiration may be observed. At high doses, lethargy of varying degree may progress to coma within a few hours. The mechanism of CNS depression with thiazide overdosage is unknown. Also, GI irritation and hypermotility may occur. Temporary elevation of BUN has been reported, especially in patients with impairment of renal function. Serum electrolyte changes and cardiovascular and renal function should be closely monitored.

Treatment: There is no specific antidote available but immediate evacuation of the stomach contents is advised. Dialysis is not likely to be effective. Care should be taken when evacuating the gastric contents to prevent aspiration, especially in the stuporous or comatose patient. Supportive measures should be initiated as required to maintain hydration, electrolyte balance, respiration and cardiovascular and renal function.

DOSAGE AND ADMINISTRATION

Effective dosage of Metolazone should be individualized according to indication and patient response. A single daily dose is recommended. Therapy with Metolazone should be titrated to gain an initial therapeutic response and to determine the minimal dose possible to maintain the desired therapeutic response.

METOLAZONE SLOW AVAILABILITY

Usual Single Daily Dosage Schedules: Suitable initial dosages will usually fall in the ranges given. Edema of cardiac failure: Metolazone slow availability 5 to 20 mg once daily. Edema of renal disease. Metolazone slow availability 5 to 20 mg once daily. Mild to moderate essential hypertension: Metolazone slow availability 2½ to 5 mg once daily.

Treatment of Edematous States: The time interval required for the initial dosage to produce an effect may vary. Diuresis and saluresis usually begin within one hour and persist for 24 hours or longer. When a desired therapeutic effect has been obtained, it may be advisable to reduce the dose if possible. The daily dose depends on the severity of the patient's condition, sodium intake and responsiveness. A decision to change the daily dose should be based on the results of thorough clinical and laboratory evaluations. If antihypertensive drugs or diuretics are given concurrently with Metolazone slow availability, more careful dosage adjustment may be necessary. For patients who tend to experience paroxysmal nocturnal dyspnea, it may be advisable to employ a larger dose to ensure prolongation of diuresis and saluresis for a full 24-hour period.

Treatment of Hypertension: The time interval required for the initial dosage regimen to show effect may vary from three or four days to three to six weeks in the treatment of elevated blood pressure. Doses should be adjusted at appropriate intervals to achieve maximum therapeutic effect.

METOLAZONE RAPID AVAILABILITY

For initial treatment of mild to moderate hypertension, the recommended dose is one Metolazone rapid availability tablet (½ mg) once daily, usually in the morning. If patients are inadequately controlled with one ½ mg tablet, the dose can be increased to two Metolazone rapid availability Tablets (1 mg) once a day. An increase in hypokalemia may occur. Doses larger than 1 mg do not give increased effectiveness. The same dose titration is necessary if Metolazone rapid availability tablets are to be substituted for other dosage forms of Metolazone in the treatment of hypertension. If blood pressure is not adequately controlled with two Metolazone rapid availability tablets alone, the dose should not be increased; rather, another antihypertensive agent with a different mechanism of action should be added to therapy with Metolazone rapid availability tablets.

STORAGE

Store at room temperature. Dispense in a tight, light-resistant container.

HOW SUPPLIED
TABLETS: 2.5 MG

AVERAGE UNIT PRICE (AVAILABLE SIZES)			
BRAND			$0.45

BRAND/MANUFACTURER	NDC	SIZE	AWP
◆ BRAND			
➤ ZAROXOLYN: Fisons Presc	00585-0975-71	100s	$42.86
	00585-0975-72	100s ud	$50.95
	00585-0975-90	1000s	$397.10

TABLETS: 5 MG

AVERAGE UNIT PRICE (AVAILABLE SIZES)			
BRAND			$0.50

BRAND/MANUFACTURER	NDC	SIZE	AWP
◆ BRAND			
➤ ZAROXOLYN: Fisons Presc	00585-0850-71	100s	$48.73
	00585-0850-72	100s ud	$56.72
	00585-0850-90	1000s	$452.62

TABLETS: 10 MG

AVERAGE UNIT PRICE (AVAILABLE SIZES)			
BRAND			$0.59

BRAND/MANUFACTURER	NDC	SIZE	AWP
◆ BRAND			
➤ ZAROXOLYN: Fisons Presc	00585-0835-71	100s	$58.32
	00585-0835-72	100s ud	$65.80
	00585-0835-90	1000s	$541.60

Metoprolol

DESCRIPTION

Metoprolol Tartrate is a selective beta$_1$-adrenoreceptor blocking agent, available as 50- and 100-mg tablets for oral administration and in 5-ml ampuls for intravenous administration. Each ampul contains a sterile solution of Metoprolol 5 mg, and sodium chloride USP, 45 mg. Metoprolol is 1-(isopropylamino)-3-[p-(2-methoxyethyl) phenoxy]-2-propanol (2:1) *dextro*-tartrate salt.

Metoprolol Tartrate is a white, practically odorless, crystalline powder with a molecular weight of 684.82. It is very soluble in water; freely soluble in methylene chloride, in chloroform, and in alcohol; slightly soluble in acetone; and insoluble in either.

Metoprolol Succinate, is a beta$_1$-selective (cardioselective) adrenoceptor blocking agent, for oral administration, available as extended release tablets. Metoprolol Succinate has been formulated to provide a controlled and predictable release of metoprolol for once daily administration. The tablets comprise a multiple unit system containing Metoprolol Succinate in a multitude of controlled release pellets. Each pellet acts as a separate drug delivery unit and is designed to deliver metoprolol continuously over the dosage interval. The tablets contain 47.5 mg, 95 mg and 190 mg of Metoprolol Succinate equivalent to 50, 100 and 200 mg of Metoprolol Tartrate, USP, respectively. Its chemical name is (±)1-(isopropyl-amino)-3-[p-(2-methoxyethyl)phenoxy]-2-propa nol succinate (2:1) (salt).

CLINICAL PHARMACOLOGY

Metoprolol Tartrate (Metoprolol) is a beta-adrenergic receptor blocking agent. *In vitro* and *in vivo* animal studies have shown that it has a preferential effect on beta$_1$ adrenoreceptors, chiefly located in cardiac muscle. This preferential effect is not absolute, however, and at higher doses, Metoprolol also inhibits beta$_2$ adrenoreceptors, chiefly located in the bronchial and vascular musculature.

Clinical pharmacology studies have confirmed the beta-blocking activity of Metoprolol in man, as shown by (1) reduction in heart rate and cardiac output at rest and upon exercise, (2) reduction of systolic blood pressure upon exercise, (3) inhibition of isoproterenol-induced tachycardia, and (4) reduction of reflex orthostatic tachycardia.

Relative beta$_1$ selectivity has been confirmed by the following: (1) In normal subjects, Metoprolol is unable to reverse the beta$_2$-mediated vasodilating effects of epinephrine. This contrasts with the effect of nonselective (beta$_1$ plus beta$_2$) beta blockers, which completely reverse the vasodilating effects of epinephrine. (2) In asthmatic patients, Metoprolol reduces FEV$_1$ and FVC significantly less than a nonselective beta blocker, propranolol, at equivalent beta$_1$-receptor blocking doses.

Metoprolol has no intrinsic sympathomimetic activity, and membrane-stabilizing activity is detectable only at doses much greater than required for beta blockade. Metoprolol crosses the blood-brain barrier and has been reported in the CSF in a concentration 78% of the simultaneous plasma concentration. Animal and human experiments indicate that Metoprolol slows the sinus rate and decreases AV nodal conduction.

In controlled clinical studies, Metoprolol has been shown to be an effective antihypertensive agent when used alone or as concomitant therapy with thiazide-type diuretics, at dosages of 100-450 mg daily. In controlled, comparative, clinical studies, Metoprolol has been shown to be as effective an antihypertensive agent as propranolol, methyldopa, and thiazide-type diuretics, and to be equally effective in supine and standing positions.

The mechanism of the antihypertensive effects of beta-blocking agents has not been elucidated. However, several possible mechanisms have been proposed: (1) competitive antagonism of catecholamines at peripheral (especially cardiac) adrenergic neuron sites, leading to decreased cardiac output; (2) a central effect leading to reduced sympathetic outflow to the periphery; and (3) suppression of renin activity.

In controlled clinical studies, an immediate release dosage form of Metoprolol has been shown to be an effective antihypertensive agent when used alone or as concomitant therapy with thiazide-type diuretics at dosages of 100-450 mg daily. Metoprolol Succinate in dosages of 100 to 400 mg once daily, has been shown to possess comparable β_1-blockade as conventional Metoprolol tablets administered two to four times daily. In addition, Metoprolol Succinate administered at a dose of 50 mg once daily has been shown to lower blood pressure 24-hours post-dosing in placebo controlled studies. In controlled, comparative, clinical studies, immediate release Metoprolol appeared comparable as an antihypertensive agent to propranolol, methyldopa, and thiazide-type diuretics, and affected both supine and standing blood pressure. Because of variable plasma levels attained with a given dose and lack of a consistent relationship of antihypertensive activity to drug plasma concentration, selection of proper dosage requires individual titration.

By blocking catecholamine-induced increases in heart rate, in velocity and extent of myocardial contraction, and in blood pressure, Metoprolol reduces the oxygen requirements of the heart at any given level of effort, thus making it useful in the long-term management of angina pectoris. However, in patients with heart failure, beta-adrenergic blockade may increase oxygen requirements by increasing left ventricular fiber length and end-diastolic pressure.

Although beta-adrenergic receptor blockade is useful in the treatment of angina and hypertension, there are situations in which sympathetic stimulation is vital. In patients with severely damaged hearts, adequate ventricular function may depend on sympathetic drive. In the presence of AV block, beta blockade may prevent the necessary facilitating effect of sympathetic activity on conduction. Beta$_2$-adrenergic blockade results in passive bronchial constriction by interfering with endogenous adrenergic bronchodilator activity in patients subject to bronchospasm and may also interfere with exogenous bronchodilators in such patients.

In controlled clinical trials, Metoprolol, administered two or four times daily, has been shown to be an effective antianginal agent, reducing the number of angina attacks and increasing exercise tolerance. The dosage used in these studies ranged from 100 to 400 mg daily. Metoprolol Succinate in dosages of 100 to 400 mg once daily, has been shown to possess comparable β_1-blockade as conventional metoprolol tablets administered two to four times daily. A controlled, comparative, clinical trial showed that Metoprolol was indistinguishable from propranolol in the treatment of angina pectoris.

In a large (1,395 patients randomized), double-blind, placebo-controlled clinical study, Metoprolol was shown to reduce 3-month mortality by 36% in patients with suspected or definite myocardial infarction.

Patients were randomized and treated as soon as possible after their arrival in the hospital, once their clinical condition had stabilized and their hemodynamic status had been carefully evaluated. Subjects were ineligible if they had hypotension, bradycardia, peripheral signs of shock, and/or more than minimal basal rales as signs of congestive heart failure. Initial treatment consisted of intravenous followed by oral administration of Metoprolol or placebo, given in a coronary care or comparable unit. Oral maintenance therapy with Metoprolol or placebo was then continued for 3 months. After this double-blind period, all patients were given Metoprolol and followed up to 1 year.

The median delay from the onset of symptoms to the initiation of therapy was 8 hours in both the Metoprolol and placebo treatment groups. Among patients treated with Metoprolol, there were comparable reductions in 3-month mortality for those treated early ($\leq$ 8 hours) and those in whom treatment was started later. Significant reductions in the incidence of ventricular fibrillation and in chest pain following initial intravenous therapy were also observed with Metoprolol and were independent of the interval between onset of symptoms and initiation of therapy.

The precise mechanism of action of Metoprolol in patients with suspected or definite myocardial infarction is not known.

In this study, patients treated with Metoprolol received the drug both very early (intravenously) and during a subsequent 3-month period, while placebo patients received no beta-blocker treatment for this period. The study thus was able to show a benefit from the overall Metoprolol regimen but cannot separate the benefit of very early intravenous treatment from the benefit of later beta-blocker therapy. Nonetheless, because the overall regimen showed a clear beneficial effect on survival without evidence of an early adverse effect on survival, one acceptable dosage regimen is the precise regimen used in the trial. Because the specific benefit of very early treatment remains to be defined however, it is also reasonable to administer the drug orally to patients at a later time as is recommended for certain other beta blockers.

In five controlled studies in normal healthy subjects, the same daily doses of Metoprolol Succinate and immediate release Metoprolol were compared in terms of the extent and duration of beta$_1$-blockade produced. Both formulations were given in a dose range equivalent to 100-400 mg of immediate release Metoprolol per day. In these studies, Metoprolol Succinate was administered once a day and immediate release Metoprolol was administered once to four times a day. A sixth controlled study compared the beta$_1$-blocking effects of a 50 mg daily dose of the two formulations. In each study, beta$_1$-blockade was expressed as the percent change from baseline, in exercise heart rate following standardized submaximal exercise tolerance tests at steady state. Metoprolol Succinate administered once a day, and immediate release Metoprolol administered once to four times a day, provided comparable total beta$_1$-blockade over 24 hours (area under the beta$_1$-blockade versus time curve) in the dose range 100-400 mg. At a dosage of 50 mg once daily, Metoprolol Succinate produced significantly higher total beta$_1$-blockade over 24 hours than immediate release Metoprolol. For Metoprolol Succinate, the percent reduction in exercise heart rate was relatively stable throughout the entire dosage interval and the level of beta$_1$-blockade increased with increasing doses from 50 to 300 mg daily. The effects at peak/trough (i.e. at 24 hours post dosing) were; 14/9, 16/10, 24/14, 27/22 and 27/20% reduction in exercise heart rate for doses of 50, 100, 200, 300 and 400 mg Metoprolol Succinate once a day, respectively. In contrast to Metoprolol Succinate immediate release Metoprolol given at a dose of 50-100 mg once a day, produced a significantly larger peak effect on exercise tachycardia, but the effect was not evident at 24 hours. To match the peak to trough ratio obtained with Metoprolol Succinate over the dosing range of 200 to 400 mg, a t.i.d. to q.i.d. divided dosing regimen was required for immediate release Metoprolol.

The relationship between plasma Metoprolol levels and reduction in exercise heart rate is independent of the pharmaceutical formulation. Using the E_{max} model, the maximal beta$_1$-blocking effect has been estimated to produce a 28.3% reduction in exercise heart rate. Beta$_1$-blocking effects in the range of 30-80% of the maximal effect (corresponding to approximately 8-23% reduction in exercise heart rate) are expected to occur at Metoprolol plasma concentrations ranging from 30-540 nmol/L. The concentration-effect curve begins reaching a plateau between 200-300 nmol/L, and higher plasma levels produce little additional beta$_1$-blocking effect. The relative beta$_1$-selectivity of Metoprolol diminishes and blockade of beta$_2$-adrenoceptors increases at higher plasma concentrations.

PHARMACOKINETICS

In man, absorption of Metoprolol is rapid and complete. Plasma levels following oral administration, however, approximate 50% of levels following intravenous administration, indicating about 50% first-pass metabolism.

Plasma levels achieved are highly variable after oral administration. Only a small fraction of the drug (about 12%) is bound to human serum albumin. Elimination is mainly by biotransformation in the liver, and the plasma half-life ranges from approximately 3 to 7 hours. Less than 5% of an oral dose of Metoprolol is recovered unchanged in the urine; the rest is excreted by the kidneys as metabolites that appear to have no clinical significance. The systemic availability and half-life of Metoprolol in patients with renal failure do not differ to a clinically significant degree from those in normal subjects. Consequently, no reduction in dosage is usually needed in patients with chronic renal failure.

In comparison to conventional Metoprolol, the plasma Metoprolol levels following administration of Metoprolol Succinate are characterized by lower peaks, longer time to peak and significantly lower peak to trough variation. The peak plasma levels following once daily administration of Metoprolol Succinate average one-fourth to one-half the peak plasma levels obtained following a corresponding dose of conventional Metoprolol, administered once daily or in divided doses. At steady state the average bioavailability of Metoprolol following administration of Metoprolol Succinate across the dosage range of 50 to 400 mg once daily, was 77% relative to the corresponding single or divided doses of conventional metoprolol. Nevertheless, over the 24 hour dosing interval, β_1-blockade is comparable and dose-related (see *"Clinical Pharmacology"*). The bioavailability of Metoprolol shows a dose-related, although not directly proportional increase with dose and is not significantly affected by food following Metoprolol Succinate administration.

Significant beta-blocking effect (as measured by reduction of exercise heart rate) occurs within 1 hour after oral administration, and its duration is dose-related. For example, a 50% reduction of the maximum registered effect after single oral doses of 20, 50, and 100 mg occurred at 3.3, 5.0, and 6.4 hours, respectively, in normal subjects. After repeated oral dosages of 100 mg twice daily, a significant reduction in exercise systolic blood pressure was evident at 12 hours.

Following intravenous administration of Metoprolol, the urinary recovery of unchanged drug is approximately 10%. When the drug was infused over a 10-minute period, in normal volunteers, maximum beta blockade was achieved at approximately 20 minutes. Doses of 5 mg and 15 mg yielded a maximal reduction in exercise-induced heart rate of approximately 10% and 15%, respectively. The effect on exercise heart rate decreased linearly with time at the same rate for both doses, and disappeared at approximately 5 hours and 8 hours for the 5-mg and 15-mg doses, respectively.

Equivalent maximal beta-blocking effect is achieved with oral and intravenous doses in the ratio of approximately 2.5:1.

There is a linear relationship between the log of plasma levels and reduction of exercise heart rate. However, antihypertensive activity does not appear to be related to plasma levels. Because of variable plasma levels attained with a given dose and lack of a consistent relationship of antihypertensive activity to dose, selection of proper dosage requires individual titration.

In several studies of patients with acute myocardial infarction, intravenous followed by oral administration of Metoprolol caused a reduction in heart rate, systolic blood pressure, and cardiac output. Stroke volume, diastolic blood pressure, and pulmonary artery end diastolic pressure remained unchanged.

In patients with angina pectoris, plasma concentration measured at 1 hour is linearly related to the oral dose within the range of 50 to 400 mg. Exercise heart rate and systolic blood pressure are reduced in relation to the logarithm of the oral dose of metoprolol. The increase in exercise capacity and the reduction in left ventricular ischemia are also significantly related to the logarithm of the oral dose.

INDICATIONS AND USAGE

HYPERTENSION

Metoprolol tablets are indicated for the treatment of hypertension. They may be used alone or in combination with other antihypertensive agents.

ANGINA PECTORIS

Metoprolol is indicated in the long-term treatment of angina pectoris.

MYOCARDIAL INFARCTION

Metoprolol ampuls and tablets are indicated in the treatment of hemodynamically stable patients with definite or suspected acute myocardial infarction to reduce cardiovascular mortality. Treatment with intravenous Metoprolol can be initiated as soon as the patient's clinical condition allows (see *"Dosage and Administration," "Contraindications,"* and *"Warnings"*). Alternatively, treatment can begin within 3 to 10 days of the acute event (see *"Dosage and Administration"*).

UNLABELED USES
Metoprolol is used alone or as an adjunct in the treatment of unstable angina pectoris and supraventricular and ventricular arrhythmias. Metoprolol is also used for the prophylaxis of migraine headache.

CONTRAINDICATIONS
HYPERTENSION AND ANGINA
Metoprolol is contraindicated in sinus bradycardia, heart block greater than first degree, cardiogenic shock, and overt cardiac failure (see *"Warnings"*).

MYOCARDIAL INFARCTION
Metoprolol is contraindicated in patients with a heart rate < 45 beats/min; second- and third-degree heart block; significant first-degree heart block (P-R interval ≥ 0.24 sec); systolic blood pressure < 100 mmHg; or moderate-to-severe cardiac failure (see *"Warnings"*).

WARNINGS
HYPERTENSION AND ANGINA
Cardiac Failure: Sympathetic stimulation is a vital component supporting circulatory function in congestive heart failure, and beta blockade carries the potential hazard of further depressing myocardial contractility and precipitating more severe failure. In hypertensive and angina patients who have congestive heart failure controlled by digitalis and diuretics, Metoprolol should be administered cautiously. Both digitalis and Metoprolol slow AV conduction.

In Patients Without a History of Cardiac Failure: Continued depression of the myocardium with beta-blocking agents over a period of time can, in some cases, lead to cardiac failure. At the first sign or symptom of impending cardiac failure, patients should be fully digitalized and/or given a diuretic. The response should be observed closely. If cardiac failure continues, despite adequate digitalization and diuretic therapy, Metoprolol should be withdrawn.

> *ISCHEMIC HEART DISEASE:* FOLLOWING ABRUPT CESSATION OF THERA-PY WITH CERTAIN BETA-BLOCKING AGENTS, EXACERBATIONS OF ANGI-NA PECTORIS AND, IN SOME CASES, MYOCARDIAL INFARCTION HAVE OCCURRED. WHEN DISCONTINUING CHRONICALLY ADMINISTERED ME-TOPROLOL, PARTICULARLY IN PATIENTS WITH ISCHEMIC HEART DIS-EASE, THE DOSAGE SHOULD BE GRADUALLY REDUCED OVER A PERIOD OF 1-2 WEEKS AND THE PATIENT SHOULD BE CAREFULLY MONITORED. IF ANGINA MARKEDLY WORSENS OR ACUTE CORONARY INSUFFICIEN-CY DEVELOPS METOPROLOL ADMINISTRATION SHOULD BE REINSTAT-ED PROMPTLY, AT LEAST TEMPORARILY, AND OTHER MEASURES APPROPRIATE FOR THE MANAGEMENT OF UNSTABLE ANGINA SHOULD BE TAKEN. PATIENTS SHOULD BE WARNED AGAINST INTERRUPTION OR DISCONTINUATION OF THERAPY WITHOUT THE PHYSICIAN'S ADVICE. BECAUSE CORONARY ARTERY DISEASE IS COMMON AND MAY BE UN-RECOGNIZED, IT MAY BE PRUDENT NOT TO DISCONTINUE METOPRO-LOL THERAPY ABRUPTLY EVEN IN PATIENTS TREATED ONLY FOR HYPERTENSION.

Bronchospastic Diseases: **PATIENTS WITH BRONCHOSPASTIC DISEASE SHOULD, IN GEN-ERAL, NOT RECEIVE BETA-BLOCKERS. Because of its relative beta$_1$ selectivity, however, Metoprolol may be used with caution in patients with bronchospastic disease who do not respond to, or cannot tolerate, other antihypertensive treatment. Since beta$_1$ selectivity is not absolute, a beta$_2$-stimulating agent should be administered concomitantly, and the lowest possible dose of Metoprolol should be used. In these circumstances it would be prudent initially to administer Metoprolol in small doses three times daily, instead of larger doses two times daily, to avoid the higher plasma levels associated with the longer dosing interval.** (See *"Dosage and Administration."*)

Major Surgery: The necessity or desirability of withdrawing beta-blocking therapy prior to major surgery is controversial; the impaired ability of the heart to respond to reflex adrenergic stimuli may augment the risks of general anesthesia and surgical procedures.

Metoprolol like other beta blockers, is a competitive inhibitor of beta-receptor agonists, and its effects can be reversed by administration of such agents, e.g., dobutamine or isoproterenol. However, such patients may be subject to protract-ed severe hypotension. Difficulty in restarting and maintaining the heart beat has also been reported with beta blockers.

Diabetes and Hypoglycemia: Metoprolol should be used with caution in diabetic patients if a beta-blocking agent is required. Beta blockers may mask tachycardia occurring with hypoglycemia, but other manifestations such as dizziness and sweating may not be significantly affected.

Thyrotoxicosis: Beta-adrenergic blockade may mask certain clinical signs (e.g., tachycardia) of hyperthyroidism. Patients suspected of developing thyrotoxicosis should be managed carefully to avoid abrupt withdrawal of beta blockade, which might precipitate a thyroid storm.

MYOCARDIAL INFARCTION
Cardiac Failure: Sympathetic stimulation is a vital component supporting circulatory function, and beta blockade carries the potential hazard of depressing myocardial contractility and precipitating or exacerbating minimal cardiac failure.

During treatment with Metoprolol the hemodynamic status of the patient should be carefully monitored. If heart failure occurs or persists despite appropriate treatment, Metoprolol should be discontinued.

Bradycardia: Metoprolol produces a decrease in sinus heart rate in most patients; this decrease is greatest among patients with low initial heart rates and least among patients with low initial heart rates. Acute myocardial infarction (particu-larly inferior infarction) may in itself produce significant lowering of the sinus rate. If the sinus rate decreases to < 40 beats/min, particularly if associated with evidence of lowered cardiac output, atropine (0.25-0.5 mg) should be adminis-tered intravenously. If treatment with atropine is not successful, Metoprolol should be discontinued, and cautious administration of isoproterenol or installa-tion of a cardiac pacemaker should be considered.

AV Block: Metoprolol slows AV conduction and may produce significant first- (P-R interval ≥ 0.26 sec), second-, or third-degree heart block. Acute myocardial infarction also produces heart block.

If heart block occurs Metoprolol should be discontinued and atropine (0.25-0.5 mg) should be administered intravenously. If treatment with atropine is not successful, cautious administration of isoproterenol or installation of a cardiac pacemaker should be considered.

Hypotension: If hypotension (systolic blood pressure ≤ 90 mmHg) occurs Metoprolol should be discontinued, and the hemodynamic status of the patient and the extent of myocardial damage carefully assessed. Invasive monitoring of central venous, pulmonary capillary wedge, and arterial pressures may be required. Appropriate therapy with fluids, positive inotropic agents, balloon counterpulsation, or other treatment modalities should be instituted. If hypoten-sion is associated with sinus bradycardia or AV block, treatment should be directed at reversing these (see above).

Bronchospastic Diseases: **PATIENTS WITH BRONCHOSPASTIC DISEASES SHOULD, IN GENERAL, NOT RECEIVE BETA BLOCKERS. Because of its relative beta$_1$ selectivity, Metoprolol may be used with extreme caution in patients with bronchospastic disease. Because it is unknown to what extent beta$_2$-stimulating agents may exacerbate myocardial ischemia and the extent of infarction, these agents should *not* be used prophylactically. If bronchospasm not related to congestive heart failure occurs Metoprolol should be discontinued. A theophylline deriva-tive or a beta$_2$ agonist may be administered cautiously, depending on the clinical condition of the patient. Both theophylline derivatives and beta$_2$ agonists may produce serious cardiac arrhythmias.**

PRECAUTIONS
GENERAL
Metoprolol should be used with caution in patients with impaired paired hepatic function.

INFORMATION FOR PATIENTS
Patients should be advised to take Metoprolol regularly and continuously, as directed, with or immediately following meals. If a dose should be missed, the patients should take only the next scheduled dose (without doubling it). Patients should not discontinue Metoprolol without consulting the physician.

Patients should be advised (1) to avoid operating automobiles and machinery or engaging in other tasks requiring alertness until the patient's response to therapy with Metoprolol has been determined; (2) to contact the physician if any difficulty in breathing occurs; (3) to inform the physician or dentist before any type of surgery that he or she is taking Metoprolol.

LABORATORY TESTS
Clinical laboratory findings may include elevated levels of serum transaminase, alkaline phosphatase, and lactate dehydrogenase.

DRUG INTERACTIONS
Catecholamine-depleting drugs (e.g., reserpine) may have an additive effect when given with beta-blocking agents. Patients treated with Metoprolol plus a catecholamine depletor should therefore be closely observed for evidence of hypotension or marked bradycardia, which may produce vertigo, syncope, or postural hypotension.

Risk of Anaphylactic Reaction: While taking beta-blockers, patients with a history of severe anaphylactic reaction to a variety of allergens may be more reactive to repeated challenge, either accidental, diagnostic, or therapeutic. Such patients may be unresponsive to the usual doses of epinephrine used to treat allergic reactions.

CARCINOGENESIS, MUTAGENESIS, IMPAIRMENT OF FERTILITY
Long-term studies in animals have been conducted to evaluate carcinogenic potential. In 2-year studies in rats at three oral dosage levels of up to 800 mg/kg per day, there was no increase in the development of spontaneously occurring benign or malignant neoplasms of any type. The only histologic changes that appeared to be drug related were an increased incidence of generally mild focal accumulation of foamy macrophages in pulmonary alveoli and a slight increase in biliary hyperplasia. In a 21-month study in Swiss albino mice at three oral dosage levels of up to 750 mg/kg per day, benign lung tumors (small adenomas) occurred more frequently in female mice receiving the highest dose than in untreated control animals. There was no increase in malignant or total (benign plus

malignant) lung tumors, nor in the overall incidence of tumors or malignant tumors. This 21-month study was repeated in CD-1 mice, and no statistically or biologically significant differences were observed between treated and control mice of either sex for any type or tumor.

All mutagenicity tests performed (a dominant lethal study in mice, chromosome studies in somatic cells, a Salmonella/ mammalian-microsome mutagenicity test, and a nucleus anomaly test in somatic interphase nuclei) were negative. No evidence of impaired fertility due to Metoprolol was observed in a study performed in rats at doses up to 55.5 times the maximum daily human dose of 450 mg.

PREGNANCY CATEGORY C
Metoprolol has been shown to increase postimplantation loss and decrease neonatal survival in rats at doses up to 55.5 times the maximum daily human dose of 450 mg. Distribution studies in mice confirm exposure of the fetus when Metoprolol is administered to the pregnant animal. These studies have revealed no evidence of impaired fertility or teratogenicity. There are no adequate and well-controlled studies in pregnant women. Because animal reproduction studies are not always predictive of human response, this drug should be used during pregnancy only if clearly needed.

NURSING MOTHERS
Metoprolol is excreted in breast milk in very small quantity. An infant consuming 1 liter of breast milk daily would receive a dose of less than 1 mg of the drug. Caution should be exercised when Metoprolol is administered to a nursing woman.

PEDIATRIC USE
Safety and effectiveness in children have not been established.

ADVERSE REACTIONS
HYPERTENSION AND ANGINA
Most adverse effects have been mild and transient.

Central Nervous System: Tiredness and dizziness have occurred in about 10 of 100 patients. Depression has been reported in about 5 of 100 patients. Mental confusion and short-term memory loss have been reported. Headache, nightmares, and insomnia have also been reported.

Cardiovascular: Shortness of breath and bradycardia have occurred in approximately 3 of 100 patients. Cold extremities; arterial insufficiency, usually of the Raynaud type; palpitations; congestive heart failure; peripheral edema; and hypotension have been reported in about 1 of 100 patients. (See *"Contraindications, Warnings, and Precautions."*)

Respiratory: Wheezing (bronchospasm) and dyspnea have been reported in about 1 of 100 patients (see *"Warnings"*).

Gastrointestinal: Diarrhea has occurred in about 5 of 100 patients. Nausea, dry mouth, gastric pain, constipation, flatulence, and heartburn have been reported in about 1 of 100 patients.

Hypersensitive Reactions: Pruritus or rash have occurred in about 5 of 100 patients. Worsening of psoriasis has also been reported.

Miscellaneous: Peyronie's disease has been reported in fewer than 1 of 100,000 patients. Musculoskeletal pain, blurred vision, and tinnitus have also been reported.

There have been rare reports of reversible alopecia, agranulocytosis, and dry eyes. Discontinuation of the drug should be considered if any such reaction is not otherwise explicable. The oculomucocutaneous syndrome associated with the beta blocker practolol has not been reported with Metoprolol.

MYOCARDIAL INFARCTION
Central Nervous System: Tiredness has been reported in about 1 of 100 patients. Vertigo, sleep disturbances, hallucinations, headache, dizziness, visual disturbances, confusion, and reduced libido have also been reported, but a drug relationship is not clear.

Cardiovascular: In the randomized comparison of Metoprolol and placebo described in the *"Clinical Pharmacology"* section, the following adverse reactions were reported:

	Metoprolol	Placebo
Hypotension (systolic BP < 90 mmHg)	27.4%	23.2%
Bradycardia (heart rate < 40 beats/min)	15.9%	6.7%
Second- or third-degree heart block	4.7%	4.7%
First-degree heart block (P-R ≥ 0.26 sec)	5.3%	1.9%
Heart failure	27.5%	29.6%

Respiratory: Dyspnea of pulmonary origin has been reported in fewer than 1 of 100 patients.

Gastrointestinal: Nausea and abdominal pain have been reported in fewer than 1 of 100 patients.

Dermatologic: Rash and worsened psoriasis have been reported, but a drug relationship is not clear.

Miscellaneous: Unstable diabetes and claudication have been reported, but a drug relationship is not clear.

POTENTIAL ADVERSE REACTIONS
A variety of adverse reactions not listed above have been reported with other beta-adrenergic blocking agents and should be considered potential adverse reactions to Lopressor.

Central Nervous System: Reversible mental depression progressing to catatonia; an acute reversible syndrome characterized by disorienta- tion for time and place, short-term memory loss, emotional lability, slightly clouded sensorium, and decreased performance on neuropsychometrics.

Cardiovascular: Intensification of AV block (see *"Contraindications"*).

Hematologic: Agranulocytosis, nonthrombocytopenic purpura, thrombocytopenic purpura.

Hypersensitivie Reactions: Fever combined with aching and sore throat, laryngospasm, and respiratory distress.

OVERDOSAGE
ACUTE TOXICITY
Several cases of overdosage have been reported, some leading to death.
Oral LD$_{50}$'s (mg/kg): mice, 1158-2460; rats, 3090-4670.

SIGNS AND SYMPTOMS
Potential signs and symptoms associated with overdosage with Metoprolol are bradycardia, hypotension, bronchospasm, and cardiac failure.

TREATMENT
There is no specific antidote.

In general, patients with acute or recent myocardial infarction may be more hemodynamically unstable than other patients and should be treated accordingly (see *"Warnings, Myocarial Infarction"*).

On the basis of the pharmacologic actions of Metoprolol, the following general measures should be employed:

Elimination of the Drug: Gastric lavage should be performed.

Bradycardia: Atropine should be administered. If there is no response to vagal blockade, isoproterenol should be administered cautiously.

Hypotension: A vasopressor should be administered, e.g., levarterenol or dopamine.

Bronchospasm: A beta$_2$-stimulating agent and/or a theophylline derivative should be administered.

Cardiac Failure: A digitalis glycoside and diuretic should be administered. In shock resulting from inadequate cardiac contractility, administration of dobutamine, isoproterenol, or glucagon may be considered.

DOSAGE AND ADMINISTRATION
HYPERTENSION
The dosage of Metoprolol should be individualized. Lopressor should be taken with or immediately following meals.

The usual initial dosage is 100 mg daily in single or divided doses, whether used alone or added to a diuretic. The dosage may be increased at weekly (or longer) intervals until optimum blood pressure reduction is achieved. In general, the maximum effect of any given dosage level will be apparent after 1 week of therapy. The effective dosage range is 100 to 450 mg per day. Dosages above 450 mg per day have not been studied. While once-daily dosing is effective and can maintain a reduction in blood pressure throughout the day, lower doses (especially 100 mg) may not maintain a full effect at the end of the 24-hour period, and larger or more frequent daily doses may be required. This can be evaluated by measuring blood pressure near the end of the dosing interval to determine whether satisfactory control is being maintained throughout the day. Beta$_1$ selectivity diminishes as the dose of Metoprolol is increased.

ANGINA PECTORIS
The dosage of Metoprolol should be individualized. Metoprolol should be taken with or immediately following meals.

The usual initial dosage is 100 mg daily, given in two divided doses. The dosage may be gradually increased at weekly intervals until optimum clinical response has been obtained or there is pronounced slowing of the heart rate. The effective dosage range is 100 to 400 mg per day. Dosages above 400 mg per day have not been studied. If treatment is to be discontinued, the dosage should be reduced gradually over a period of 1-2 weeks (see *"Warnings"*).

MYOCARDIAL INFARCTION
Early Treatment: During the early phase of definite or suspected acute myocardial infarction, treatment with Metoprolol can be initiated as soon as possible after the patient's arrival in the hospital. Such treatment should be initiated in a coronary care or similar unit immediately after the patient's hemodynamic condition has stabilized.

Treatment in this early phase should begin with the intravenous administration of three bolus injections of 5 mg of Metoprolol each; the injections should be given at approximately 2-minute intervals. During the intravenous administration of Metoprolol, blood pressure, heart rate, and electrocardiogram should be carefully monitored.

In patients who tolerate the full intravenous dose (15 mg), Metoprolol tablets, 50 mg every 6 hours, should be initiated 15 minutes after the last intravenous dose and continued for 48 hours. Thereafter, patients should receive a maintenance dosage of 100 mg twice daily (see *"Late Treatment"* below).

Patients who appear not to tolerate the full intravenous dose should be started on Metoprolol tablets either 25 mg or 50 mg every 6 hours (depending on the degree of intolerance) 15 minutes after the last intravenous dose or as soon as their clinical condition allows. In patients with severe intolerance, treatment with Metoprolol should be discontinued (see *"Warnings"*).

Late Treatment: Patients with contraindications to treatment during the early phase of suspected or definite myocardial infarction, patients who appear not to tolerate the full early treatment, and patients in whom the physician wishes to delay therapy for any other reason should be started on Metoprolol tablets, 100 mg twice daily, as soon as their clinical condition allows. Therapy should be continued for at least 3 months. Although the efficacy of Metoprolol beyond 3 months has not been conclusively established, data from studies with other beta blockers suggest that treatment should be continued for 1-3 years.

Metoprolol Succinate is an extended release tablet intended for once-a-day administration. When switching from immediate release Metoprolol tablet to Metoprolol Succinate, the same total daily dose of Toprol XL should be used.

As with immediate release Metoprolol, dosages of Metoprolol Succinate should be individualized and titration may be needed in some patients.

Metoprolol Succinate tablets are scored and can be divided; however, the whole or half tablet should be swallowed whole and not chewed or crushed.

HYPERTENSION

The usual initial dosage is 50 to 100 mg daily in a single dose, whether used alone or added to a diuretic. The dosage may be increased at weekly (or longer) intervals until optimum blood pressure reduction is achieved. In general, the maximum effect of any given dosage level will be apparent after 1 week of therapy. Dosages above 400 mg per day have not been studied.

ANGINA PECTORIS

The dosage of Metoprolol Succinate should be individualized. The usual initial dosage is 100 mg daily, given in a single dose. The dosage may be gradually increased at weekly intervals until optimum clinical response has been obtained or there is a pronounced slowing of the heart rate. Dosages above 400 mg per day have not been studied. If treatment is to be discontinued, the dosage should be reduced gradually over a period of 1-2 weeks (see *"Warnings"*).

Note: **Parenteral drug products should be inspected visually for particulate matter and discoloration prior to administration, whenever solution and container permit.**

STORAGE

Store between 59°-86°F (15°-30°C). Protect from moisture. Dispense in tight, light-resistant container (USP).

HOW SUPPLIED

METOPROLOL SUCCINATE
TABLET, EXTENDED RELEASE: 50 MG

BRAND/MANUFACTURER	NDC	SIZE	AWP
○ **BRAND**			
➤ TOPROL XL: Astra	00186-1090-05	100s	$42.59

TABLET, EXTENDED RELEASE: 100 MG

BRAND/MANUFACTURER	NDC	SIZE	AWP
○ **BRAND**			
➤ TOPROL XL: Astra	00186-1092-05	100s	$64.01

TABLET, EXTENDED RELEASE: 200 MG

BRAND/MANUFACTURER	NDC	SIZE	AWP
○ **BRAND**			
➤ TOPROL XL: Astra	00186-1094-05	100s	$128.02

METOPROLOL TARTRATE
INJECTION: 1 MG/ML

BRAND/MANUFACTURER	NDC	SIZE	AWP
◆ **GENERICS**			
Schein	00364-3036-25	5 ml 3s	$14.67

INJECTION: 5 MG/5 ML

BRAND/MANUFACTURER	NDC	SIZE	AWP
◆ **BRAND**			
LOPRESSOR: Geigy	00028-4201-33	5 ml 12s	$63.36

TABLETS: 50 MG

AVERAGE UNIT PRICE (AVAILABLE SIZES)		GENERIC A-RATED AVERAGE PRICE (GAAP)	
BRAND	$0.51	100s	$45.05
GENERIC	$0.44	500s	$216.70
HCFA FUL (100s each)	$0.20	1000s	$435.54

BRAND/MANUFACTURER	NDC	SIZE	AWP
◆ **BRAND**			
➤ LOPRESSOR: Geigy	00028-0051-01	100s	$49.57
	00028-0051-61	100s ud	$53.85
	00028-0051-10	1000s	$490.56
	00028-0051-65	1200s	$596.99
◆ **GENERICS**			
Allscrips	54569-3787-00	30s	$13.43
Allscrips	54569-8574-00	90s	$40.67
Novopharm	55953-0727-40	100s	$41.75
Apothecon	59772-3692-02	100s	$41.78
Goldline	00182-1966-01	100s	$43.00
Goldline	00182-1987-01	100s	$43.00
Schein	00364-2560-01	100s	$43.05
Major	00904-7772-60	100s	$43.50
Qualitest	00603-4627-21	100s	$44.51
Purepac	00228-2554-10	100s	$45.35
Rugby	00536-5604-01	100s	$45.94
Aligen	00405-5673-01	100s	$47.23
Martec	52555-0499-01	100s	$47.50
Major	00904-7772-61	100s ud	$49.39
UDL	51079-0801-20	100s ud	$49.70
Novopharm	55953-0727-70	500s	$206.65
Purepac	00228-2554-50	500s	$226.75
Novopharm	55953-0727-80	1000s	$413.50
Apothecon	59772-3692-05	1000s	$413.51
Goldline	00182-1966-10	1000s	$425.90
Goldline	00182-1987-10	1000s	$425.90
Schein	00364-2560-02	1000s	$425.96
Major	00904-7772-80	1000s	$430.70
Rugby	00536-5604-10	1000s	$441.50
Purepac	00228-2554-96	1000s	$445.99
Qualitest	00603-4627-32	1000s	$448.11
Aligen	00405-5673-03	1000s	$458.32
Martec	52555-0499-10	1000s	$461.50

TABLETS: 100 MG

AVERAGE UNIT PRICE (AVAILABLE SIZES)		GENERIC A-RATED AVERAGE PRICE (GAAP)	
BRAND	$0.74	100s	$67.46
GENERIC	$0.66	500s	$322.95
HCFA FUL (100s each)	$0.31	1000s	$653.54

BRAND/MANUFACTURER	NDC	SIZE	AWP
◆ **GENERICS**			
Allscrips	54569-3788-00	30s	$20.09
Novopharm	55953-0734-40	100s	$62.75
Apothecon	59772-3693-02	100s	$62.78
Goldline	00182-1967-01	100s	$64.60
Goldline	00182-1988-01	100s	$64.60
Schein	00364-2561-01	100s	$64.68
Major	00904-7773-60	100s	$65.40
Purepac	00228-2555-10	100s	$67.41
Qualitest	00603-4628-21	100s	$67.86
Rugby	00536-5605-01	100s	$69.04
Aligen	00405-4674-01	100s	$70.82
Martec	52555-0500-01	100s	$71.20
Major	00904-7773-61	100s ud	$71.68
UDL	51079-0802-20	100s ud	$74.20
Novopharm	55953-0734-70	500s	$310.60
Purepac	00228-2555-50	500s	$335.30
Novopharm	55953-0734-80	1000s	$621.40
Apothecon	59772-3693-05	1000s	$621.41
Goldline	00182-1967-10	1000s	$640.00
Goldline	00182-1988-10	1000s	$640.00
Schein	00364-2561-02	1000s	$640.11
Major	00904-7773-80	1000s	$647.25
Rugby	00536-5605-10	1000s	$663.48
Purepac	00228-2555-96	1000s	$665.54
Qualitest	00603-4628-32	1000s	$668.40
Aligen	00405-4674-03	1000s	$688.35
Martec	52555-0500-10	1000s	$693.00

TABLETS: 100 MG

BRAND/MANUFACTURER	NDC	SIZE	AWP
○ **BRAND**			
➤ LOPRESSOR: Geigy	00028-0071-01	100s	$74.49
	00028-0071-61	100s ud	$78.16
	00028-0071-73	720s	$537.14
	00028-0071-10	1000s	$737.20
	00028-0071-65	1200s	$895.79

Metrizamide

DESCRIPTION

Metrizamide, 2-[3-Acetamido-2,4,6-triodo-5-(N-methylacetamido)ben-zamido]-2-deoxy-D-glucopyranose, is a compound derived from metrizoic acid and glucosamine. It is a nonionic water-soluble contrast medium with a molecular weight of 789 (iodine content: 48.25%).

The viscosity in centipoise of the "use" concentration ranges from 2.9 at 170 mgI/mL to 12.7 at 300 mgI/mL at room temperature (20°C) and from 1.8 to 6.2 at body temperature (37°C), respectively. Osmolality in mosm/kg at 37°C ranges from 300 at 170 mgI/mL concentration to 484 at 300 mgI/mL. CSF is approximately 301. Specific gravity ranges from 1.184 at 170 mgI/mL to 1.329 at

◆ RATED THERAPEUTICALLY EQUIVALENT; ◇ THERAPEUTIC EQUIVALENCE UNCONFIRMED; ○ UNRATED

300 mgI/mL. (CSF normal range is 1.005 to 1.009.) The pH of the solution reconstituted from the diluent is approximately 7.4.

In the following text, intrathecal use is discussed in full, followed by a complete discussion of intravascular use.

Metrizamide solution and powder is sensitive to heat or light and, therefore, should be protected from exposure.

Following is its chemical structure:

CLINICAL PHARMACOLOGY

INTRATHECAL

Metrizamide is absorbed from cerebrospinal fluid into the bloodstream in adults. Approximately 60 percent of the administered dose is excreted unchanged through the kidneys within 48 hours.

The initial concentration and volume of the medium, in conjunction with appropriate patient manipulation, will determine the extent of the diagnostic contrast that can be achieved. This can be monitored by fluoroscopy.

Following subarachnoid injection conventional radiography will continue to provide good diagnostic contrast for at least 30 minutes. At about 1 hour diagnostic degree of contrast will not usually be available. However, sufficient contrast for CT myelography will be available for several hours. CT myelography, following conventional myelography, should be deferred for at least 4 hours to reduce the degree of contrast.

In a multi-centered study, Metrizamide was used in 502 pediatric patients for a variety of procedures. The results and effects of the medium were similar to that in adults.

Following subarachnoid placement, irrespective of the position in which the patient is later maintained, slow upward diffusion of Metrizamide takes place through the CSF. After introduction into the lumbar subarachnoid space, without special positioning of the patient, computerized tomography (CT) shows CSF contrast enhancement in the thoracic region in about 1 hour, in the cervical region in about 2 hours, and in the basal cisterns in 3 to 4 hours.

When low doses (4 mL to 6 mL of 170 mgI/mL to 190 mgI/mL) of Metrizamide are introduced into the lumbar CSF and moved cephalad under gravity control and examined by CT scanning, they will provide immediate CSF contrast in the basal cisterns. Depending on the specific technique used, the lateral, third, and fourth ventricles may also be visualized. The contrast in this area will markedly diminish at 6 hours and disappear by 24 hours. CSF enhancement will be evident at the cortical sulci and interhemispheric fissures at 6 hours.

Between 12 and 24 hours the surfaces of the cerebrum and cerebellum, in contact with the subarachnoid spaces, will develop a "blush" effect on the scan which will normally disappear in 36 to 48 hours. The rate, time, extent of diffusion, and the disappearance or stasis of Metrizamide as demonstrated with CT scanning, can be used to detect or infer the presence of CNS or CSF circulation abnormalities.

INDICATIONS AND USAGE

INTRATHECAL

Metrizamide is indicated in adults and pediatric patients for lumbar, thoracic, cervical, and total columnar myelography and for use in computerized tomography of the intracranial subarachnoid spaces following spinal subarachnoid injection.

In pediatric patients Metrizamide is also indicated for cisternography and ventriculography by direct injection using standard radiologic techniques.

CONTRAINDICATIONS

INTRATHECAL

Metrizamide should not be administered to patients with a known hypersensitivity to Metrizamide.

Intrathecal administration of corticosteroids with Metrizamide is contraindicated.

Immediate repeat myelography, in the event of technical failure, is contraindicated because of overdosage considerations. (See interval recommendation under "Dosage and Administration".)

Lumbar puncture should not be performed in the presence of significant local or systemic infection where bacteremia is likely.

WARNINGS

INTRATHECAL

If grossly bloody CSF is encountered, the possible benefits of a myelographic procedure should be considered in terms of the risk to the patient.

Fatal reactions have been associated with the administration of water-soluble contrast media. Therefore, it is of utmost importance that a course of action be carefully planned in advance for the immediate treatment of serious reactions, and that adequate and appropriate facilities and personnel be readily available in case of a severe reaction.

Caution is advised in patients with a history of epilepsy, severe cardiovascular disease, chronic alcoholism or multiple sclerosis.

Elderly patients may present a greater risk following myelography. The need for the procedure in these patients should be evaluated carefully. Special attention must be paid to dose and concentration of the medium, hydration, and technique used.

Patients who are receiving anticonvulsants should be maintained on this therapy. Should a seizure occur, intravenous diazepam or phenobarbital sodium is recommended. In patients with a history of seizure activity who are not on anticonvulsant therapy, premedication with barbiturates or phenytoin should be considered.

Prophylactic anticonvulsant treatment with barbiturates should be considered in patients with evidence of inadvertent intracranial entry of a large or concentrated bolus of the contrast medium since there is an increased risk of seizures in such cases.

Drugs which lower the seizure threshold, especially phenothiazine derivatives, including those used for their antihistamine properties should not be used with Metrizamide. Others include MAO inhibitors, tricylic antidepressants, CNS stimulants, psychoactive drugs described as analeptics, major tranquilizers, or antipsychotic drugs. Such medication should be discontinued at least 48 hours before myelography, should not be used for the control of nausea and vomiting, and should not be resumed for at least 24 hours postprocedure.

Care is required in patient management to prevent inadvertent intracranial entry of a large dose or concentrated bolus of the medium. Also, effort should be directed to avoid rapid dispersion of the medium causing inadvertent rise to intracranial levels (eg, by active patient movement). Direct intracisternal or ventricular administration for standard radiography (not CT) is not recommended.

In most reported cases of *major motor seizures* one or more of the following factors were present. Therefore *avoid*:

- Deviations from recommended procedure or in myelographic management.
- Use in patients with a history of epilepsy.
- Inadvertent overdosage.
- Intracranial entry of a bolus or premature diffusion of a high concentration of the medium.
- Medication with neuroleptic drugs or phenothiazine antinauseants.
- Failure to maintain elevation of the head during the procedure, on the stretcher, or in bed.
- Excessive and particularly active patient movement or straining.

At concentrations of 200 mgI/mL or less, these seizures have been noted only very rarely.

Treatment with intravenous diazepam or administration of phenobarbital sodium has provided rapid control of seizures. (See "Patient Management".)

PRECAUTIONS

INTRATHECAL

Before a contrast medium is injected, the patient should be questioned for a history of allergy. Although a history of allergy, including asthma, may imply a greater than usual risk, it does not arbitrarily contraindicate the use of the medium. No conclusive relationship between severe reactions and antigen-antibody reactions or other manifestations of allergy has been established.

In patients with severe renal insufficiency or failure, the drug is excreted by the liver into the bile at a much slower rate. Patients with hepatorenal insufficiency should not be examined unless the possibility of benefit clearly outweighs the additional risk.

For "Repeat Procedure" see "Dosage and Administration".

If nondisposable equipment is used, scrupulous care should be taken to prevent residual contamination with traces of cleansing agents.

Pregnancy Category B: Reproduction studies have been performed in rats and rabbits up to 70 times the human dose and have revealed no evidence of impaired fertility or harm to the fetus due to Metrizamide. There are, however, no adequate and well controlled studies in pregnant women. Because animal reproduction studies are not always predictive of human response, this drug should be used during pregnancy only if clearly needed.

Nursing Mothers: Caution should be exercised when Metrizamide is administered to a nursing woman. Metrizamide is excreted in milk to the extent of 1 mg of the injected myelographic dose over 2 days.

ADVERSE REACTIONS

INTRATHECAL

The most frequently occurring adverse reactions are headache, nausea, and vomiting. These reactions occur 3 to 8 hours postinjection, almost all occurring within 24 hours. They are usually mild to moderate in degree lasting for a few hours and usually disappearing within 24 hours. Rarely, headaches may be severe or persist for days. The reported incidence of headaches varies from 20 to over 60 percent and they are often accompanied by nausea and vomiting. Headaches tend to be more frequent and persistent in patients not optimally hydrated. (See "Patient Management.")

Backache, neck stiffness, numbness and paresthesias, leg or sciatic-type pain occurred less frequently, often in the form of a transient exacerbation of preexisting symptomatology. Temperature elevations constitute the fourth most common reaction in individuals under 18 years of age. Dizziness has also been reported.

The incidence and nature of adverse reactions in pediatric patients is similar to adult patients except for the occurrence of a higher incidence of fever (19%) and occasional incidence of croup, breast feeding problems, and crying spells. Of the 42 percent of pediatric patients who received general anesthesia, the incidence of nausea and vomiting was generally higher.

Cardiovascular: Chest pain, tachycardia, bradycardia and other arrhythmias, hypertension or hypotension, cardiac arrest, vasculitis, hemorrhage, collapse, and shock have also been reported.

Transient alterations in *vital signs* may occur. Their significance must be assessed on an individual basis.

Other rarely occurring adverse reactions include the following:

Major Motor Seizures: Focal or generalized grand mal seizures have occurred with an incidence reported between 0.1 and 0.3 percent. They have usually occurred 4 to 12 hours following injection, and have consisted of one or two episodes 1 or more hours apart, which have responded promptly to the intravenous injection of diazepam. For prolonged prophylaxis barbiturates have been recommended.

Early onset of seizures (less than 2 hours) is indicative of early substantial intracranial entry.

Transitory EEG changes are frequent and usually take the form of slow wave activity, although sharp activity and paroxysmal activity have been reported up to 24 hours after the procedure. The incidence of EEG changes may be as high as 30 percent.

An *aseptic meningitis* syndrome has been reported rarely (less than 0.1%). It was usually preceded by pronounced headaches, nausea and vomiting. Onset usually occurred about 12 to 18 hours postprocedure. Prominent features were meningismus, fever, sometimes with oculomotor signs and mental confusion. Lumbar puncture revealed a high white cell count, high protein content often with a low glucose level and with absence of organisms. The condition usually started to clear spontaneously about 10 hours after onset, with complete recovery over 2 to 3 days.

Allergy or Idiosyncrasy: Chills, fever, profuse diaphoresis, pruritus, urticaria, nasal congestion, dyspnea, and a case of Guillian-Barre syndrome.

CNS Irritation: Mild and transitory perceptual aberrations such as hallucinations, depersonalization, amnesia, hostility, amblyopia, photophobia, psychosis, insomnia, anxiety, depression, hyperesthesia, visual, auditory or speech disturbances, confusion and disorientation. In addition, malaise, weakness, EEG changes, meningismus, hyperreflexia or areflexia, hypertonia or flaccidity, hemiplegia, paralysis, quadriplegia, restlessness, tremor, echoacousia, echolalia, asterixis or dysphasia have occurred.

Profound mental disturbances have also rarely been reported. They have usually consisted of various forms and degrees of aphasia, mental confusion or disorientation. The onset is usually at 8 to 10 hours and lasts for about 24 hours, without aftereffects. However, occasionally they have been manifest as apprehension, agitation, or progressive withdrawal in several instances to the point of somnolence, stupor and coma. In a few cases these have been accompanied by transitory hearing loss or other auditory symptoms and visual disturbances (believed subjective or delusional), including unilateral or bilateral loss of vision which may last for hours. In one case persistent cortical loss of vision has been reported in association with convulsions. Ventricular block has been reported in two cases; amnesia of varying degrees may be present for the reaction event.

Rarely, persistent though transitory weakness in the leg or ocular muscles has been reported.

Neuropathies: Neuropathies have been rare and almost always transitory. They include sensory and/or motor or nerve root disturbances, myelitis, persistent leg muscle pain or weakness, or 6th nerve palsy, or cauda equina syndrome. Muscle cramps, fasciculation or myoclonia, spinal convulsion, or spasticity are unusual and have responded promptly to a small intravenous dose of diazepam.

Respiratory: Apnea and pulmonary edema have been reported.

Body-General: Asthenia, cellulitis, hyponatremia, hemolytic anemia, generalized angioedema with marked dsypnea and stridor, and deaths have been reported.

Urogential: Renal failure, polyuria, hematuria, and urinary retention have been reported.

OVERDOSAGE
INTRATHECAL
There is clinical evidence that reactions, particularly seizures and mental aberrations, following the administration of myelographic doses in excess of those recommended tend to be dose related. Even use of a recommended dose can produce effects tantamount to overdosage, if incorrect management of the patient during or immediately following the procedure permits inadvertent early intracranial entry of a large portion of the medium.

Treatment: See "Adverse Reactions—Major motor seizures."
The subarachnoid LD_{50} in mice is greater than 1,500 mgI/kg.

DOSAGE AND ADMINISTRATION
INTRATHECAL
See also "Patient management."
The dosage and concentration of Metrizamide will depend on the degree and extent of contrast required in the area(s) under examinination and on the equipment and technique employed. Concentrations which are approximately isotonic (170 mgI/mL to 190 mgI/mL) are recommended for examination in the lumbar region. For movement of the medium to distant target areas, higher concentrations are recommended to compensate for dilution of Metrizamide with CSF.

A total dose of 3000 mg iodine or a concentration of 300 mgI/mL should not be exceeded. As in all diagnostic procedures, the least amount to produce adequate visualization should be used. Most procedures do not require either maximum dose or concentration. The incidence of serious adverse reactions is considerably less with concentrations of 200 mgI/mL or less. The dose and concentration used in the spinal area influence ultimate intracranial concentrations.

Anesthesia is not necessary. Premedication sedatives or tranquilizers are usually not needed (see "Precautions"). Patients should be well hydrated. Epileptic patients should be maintained on their anticonvulsant medication.

As with any lumbar puncture, sterile technique must be employed. The lumbar puncture is usually made between L3 and L4, but if pathology is suspected at this level the interspace immediately above or below may be selected. A lateral cervical puncture may also be used.

Rate of Injection: To avoid excessive mixing with CSF and consequent loss of contrast as well as premature dispersion upward, injection must be made slowly over 1 to 2 minutes.

The lumbar puncture needle is removed immediately following injection since it is not necessary to remove Metrizamide after injection into subarachnoid spaces.

Repeat Procedure: An interval of at least 48 hours should be allowed before repeat examination; however, whenever possible 5 to 7 days is recommended.

The recommended usual and maximum doses of Metrizamide are summarized in the following tables:

ADULT DOSAGE TABLE—IODINE CONTENT

Procedure	Conc. of Solution (mgI/mL)	Usual Recommended Dose* (mL)	Max. Dose Total (mgI)
Lumbar myelogram	170-190	10-15	2850
Thoracic myelogram	220	12	2640
Cervical myelogram (lumbar injection)	250-300	10	3000
Cervical myelogram (lateral cervical injection)	220	10	2200
Total columnar myelography	250-280	10	2800
CT cisternography (lumbar injection)	170-190	4-6	1140

* Refer to "Dilution Table for Intrathecal Use" for preparation of solution

PEDIATRIC DOSAGE TABLE—IODINE CONTENT

Conventional Radiography

Procedure	Age	Conc. of Solution (mgI/mL)	Usual Recommended Dose* (mL)
Lumbar, thoracic myelography (lumbar injection)	Less than 2 months	170-190	2-3
	2 months to 2 years	170-190	2-4
	3 to 7 years	170-190	4-8
	8 to 12 years	170-190	7-9
	13 to 18 years	170-190	8-10
Cervical myelography (lumbar injection)	Less than 2 months	170-210	2-3
	2 months to 2 years	170-200	2-4
	3 to 7 years	170-210	4-8
	8 to 12 years	170-230	7-9
	13 to 18 years	170-230	8-10
Cervical myelography (lateral cervical injection)	8 to 18 years	200-220	3-5
Cisternography (direct injection)	Less than 2 months	170-220	2-3
	8 to 18 years	170-220	2-5
Cisternography (lumbar injection)	2 months to 2 years	170-220	2-3
	3 to 7 years	170-190	3-5
	8 to 12 years	170-190	5-6

Conventional Radiography			
Procedure	Age	Conc. of Solution (mgI/mL)	Usual Recommended Dose* (mL)
Ventriculography (direct injection)	Less than 2 months	170-220	2-3
	2 months to 2 years	170-220	2-3
	3 to 12 years	170-220	2-4
	13 to 18 years	190-220	2-5
Ventriculography (lumbar injection)	2 months to 2 years	170-220	2-3
CT Radiography			
CT cistermography (lumbar injection)	3 to 7 years	170-190	3-5
	8 to 12 years	180-190	3-5
	13 to 18 years	170-190	3-5
CT ventriculography (direct injection)	Less than 2 months	170-220	2
	2 months to 2 years	170-220	2
	3 to 7 years	170-220	3
CT ventriculography (lumbar injection)	3 to 7 years	170-220	3

* Refer to "Dilution Table for Intrathecal Use" for preparation of solution

The above pediatric doses, intended as guidelines, are based on age range rather than weight because brain or CSF capacity is independent of weight. Variations will depend on such factors as height, nature of pathology, condition of the patient, technique used, etc. (eg, whether for CSF contrast for CT scan or for standard radiography, or whether movement of the medium is to be directed to an area distal to the site of injection). Direct intracranial placement will require particular care in planning to maintain total dose and concentration as low as practical to avoid convulsive response. Whenever possible (eg, for CT scan) the use of the isotonic concentration (170 mgI/mL) is preferable. In children, loss of contrast due to mixing on movement of the medium is less apt to occur because of their shorter spinal cord. Therefore, the use of relatively lower dosages may be feasible.

The medium disperses in about 60 minutes following direct ventricular placement.

Young children may require general anesthesia for technical reasons.

Convulsions occurred in a few patients, only one attributed to the medium, at these dosage schedules.

Prophylactic barbiturates are suggested for inadvertent overdosage. Parenteral diazepam or barbiturates is suggested for treatment of seizures and barbiturates and/or phenytoin for continued suppression.

PREPARATION OF THE SOLUTION—INTRATHECAL

1. Select the correct iodine concentration recommended for the procedure in the "Dosage Tables."
2. The volume of diluent required to obtain that iodine concentration can be obtained from the "Dilution Table."
3. Using a sterile technique with a small guage transfer needle (approximately 22 guage to help prevent coring), withdraw the required amount of diluent.
4. Insert this volume of diluent into the lyophil vial also using the fine needle. Contents under vacuum. Use only if vacuum is present as evidenced by diluent being drawn into vial when stopper is punctured. Leave syringe and needle in place.
5. Gently swirl the vial (without shaking) until its contents are dissolved (approximately 3 to 10 minutes) to insure complete dissolution of the lyophil. The resulting solution should be clear and colorless to slightly yellow. Do not use if undissolved particulate matter or bubbles are present.
6. Withdraw the volume of Metrizamide recommended for the procedure in the "Dosage Tables."
7. Detach syringe and attach to myelographic injection unit. Use immediately after reconstitution. Discard any unused portion. (See "Individual Indications and Usage—Intravascular" section "Preparation of the Solution-Intravascular Use #7.")

DILUTION FOR INTRATHECAL USE

Conc. of Solution (mgI/mL)	Volume of Diluent to be Added	
	3.75 g vial (mL)*	6.75 g vial (mL)**
170	8.9	16.1
180	8.3	15.0
190	7.8	14.0
200	7.3	13.2
210	6.9	12.4
220	6.5	11.7
230	6.1	11.1

Conc. of Solution (mgI/mL)	Volume of Diluent to be Added	
	3.75 g vial (mL)*	6.75 g vial (mL)**
240	5.8	10.5
250	5.5	10.0
260	5.2	9.4
270	5.0	9.0
280	4.7	8.5
290	4.5	8.1
300	4.3	7.8

* The volume of the final solution will equal the volume of the diluent + 1.7 mL
** The volume of the final solution will equal the volume of the diluent + 3.1 mL

The volume of the final solution will exceed the amount required to achieve the recommended dosage. For volume for injection refer to "Dosage Tables."

PATIENT MANAGEMENT—INTRATHECAL
Suggestions for usual patient management

PREPROCEDURE
■ Discontinue neuroleptic drugs (including phenothiazines, eg, chlorpromazine, prochlorperazine, and promethazine) 48 hours beforehand.
■ Maintain normal diet up to 2 hours before.
■ Ensure hydration—fluids up to procedure.

DURING PROCEDURE
■ Use minimum dose and concentration required for satisfactory contrast. (See "Dosage And Administration".)
■ In all positioning techniques keep the patient's head elevated above highest level of spine.
■ Do not lower head of table more than 15° during thoraco-cervical procedures.
■ In patients with excessive lordosis consider lateral position for injection and movement of the medium cephalad.
■ Avoid intracranial entry of a bolus.
■ Avoid early and high cephalad dispersion of the medium.
■ Inject slowly over 1 to 2 minutes to avoid excessive mixing.
■ Abrupt or active patient movement causes excessive mixing with CSF. Instruct patient to remain passive. Move patient slowly and only as necessary.
■ To maintain as a bolus, move medium to distal area very slowly under fluoroscopic control.
■ At completion of direct cervical or lumbo-cervical procedures, raise head of table steeply (45 °) for about 2 minutes to restore medium to lower levels.

POSTPROCEDURE
■ Raise head of stretcher to at least 15° before moving patient onto it.
■ Movement onto stretcher, and off the stretcher bed, should be done slowly with patient completely passive, maintaining head up position.
■ Before moving patient onto bed, raise head of bed 15° to 30°.
■ Advise patient to remain still in bed, in head up position, especially in first few hours.
■ Maintain close observation for at least 12 hours after myelogram.
■ After 8 hours, patient may be lowered to a horizontal position for further 16 hours.
■ Obtain visitors' cooperation in keeping the patient quiet and in head up position, especially in first few hours.
■ Encourage oral fluids and diet as tolerated.
■ If nausea or vomiting occurs, do not use phenothiazine antinauseants. Persistent nausea and vomiting will result in dehydration. Therefore, prompt consideration of replacement by intravenous fluids is recommended.

ALTERNATIVE POSTPROCEDURE METHOD
Recent evidence suggests that maintaining the patient postmyelography in an upright position (via wheelchair or ambulation) may help minimize adverse effects. The upright position may help to delay upward dispersion of the medium and to maximize the spinal arachnoid absorption.

CLINICAL PHARMACOLOGY
INTRAVASCULAR
Intravascular injection of a radiopaque diagnostic agent opacifies those vessels in the path of flow of the contrast medium permitting radiographic visualization of the internal structures of the human body until significant hemodilution occurs. The pharmacokinetics of the intravenously administered radiopaque contrast media are usually best described by a two compartment model with a rapid alpha phase for drug distribution and a slow beta phase for drug elimination. In patients with renal functional impairment, the elimination half-life for the beta phase may be prolonged for up to several days.

Following intravenous injection, Metrizamide is distributed and excreted in a manner similar to the diatriazoates, ie, following initial high serum levels, the level falls rapidly as the medium becomes distributed throughout the extravascular compartment. Thereafter, it is excreted unchanged principally by glomerular filtration. It is not metabolized. About 94% of the medium is excreted in this manner in 24 hours and a further 5% by hepatobiliary excretion via the bowel.

➤ SHOWN IN PRODUCT IDENTIFICATION GUIDE

INDICATIONS AND USAGE
INTRAVASCULAR
Metrizamide is indicated for intravenous digital arteriography for head and neck, adult peripheral arteriography, and pediatric angiocardiography.

CONTRAINDICATIONS
INTRAVASCULAR
Known hypersensitivity to Metrizamide.

WARNINGS
INTRAVASCULAR
Nonionic iodinated contrast media inhibit blood coagulation, *in vitro*, less than ionic contrast media. Clotting has been reported when blood remains in contact with syringes containing nonionic contrast media.

Serious, rarely fatal, thromboembolic events causing myocardial infarction and stroke have been reported during angiographic procedures with both ionic and nonionic contrast media. Therefore, meticulous intravascular administration technique is necessary, particularly during angiographic procedures, to minimize thromboembolic events. Numerous factors, including length of procedure, catheter and syringe material, underlying disease state, and concomitant medications may contribute to the development of thromboembolic events. For these reasons, meticulous angiographic techniques are recommended including close attention to guidewire and catheter manipulation, use of manifold systems and/or three-way stopcocks, frequent catheter flushing with heparinized saline solutions and minimizing the length of the procedure. The use of plastic syringes in place of glass syringes has been reported to decrease but not eliminate the likelihood of *in vitro* clotting.

In patients with myelomatosis, the effects of nonionic media on renal function is unknown. If a decision to use Metrizamide is made, the patient should be well hydrated beforehand, a minimal diagnostic dose used, and renal function and extent of urinary precipitation of the myeloma protein checked for a few days afterwards.

Contrast media may promote sickling in individuals who are homozygous for sickle cell disease when the material is injected intravenously or intra-arterially.

Administration of radiopaque materials to patients known or suspected of having pheochromocytoma should be performed with extreme caution. If, in the opinion of the physician, the possible benefits of such procedures outweigh the considered risks, the procedures may be performed; however, the amount of radiopaque medium injected should be kept to an absolute minimum. The blood pressure should be assessed throughout the procedure and measures for treatment of a hypertensive crisis should be available.

Recent reports of thyroid storm occurring following the intravascular use of iodinated radiopaque diagnostic agents in patients with hyperthyroidism or with an autonomously functioning thyroid nodule suggest that this additional risk be evaluated in such patients before use of these drugs.

Arteriography should be performed with caution in patients with severely impaired renal function and patients with combined renal and hepatic disease.

PRECAUTIONS
INTRAVASCULAR
Diagnostic procedures which involve the use of radiopaque diagnostic agents should be carried out under the direction of personnel with the prerequisite training and with a thorough knowledge of the particular procedure to be performed. Appropriate facilities should be available for coping with any complication of the procedure, as well as for emergency treatment of severe reactions to the contrast agent itself. After parenteral administration of a radiopaque agent, competent personnel and emergency facilities should be available for at least 30 to 60 minutes since severe delayed reactions have occurred (see *"Adverse Reactions"*).

Since allergic response can occur with the nonionic media, similar preparations to those recommended for ionic media should be planned to handle severe or potentially fatal complications. These measures are to ensure the ready availability of appropriate resuscitative drugs, equipment, and personnel.

A history of allergy to the intravascular use of Metrizamide, or other contrast agents, may indicate a greater likelihood of allergic response. However, such history is not a contraindication but calls for caution in use.

The possibility of an idiosyncratic reaction in susceptible patients should always be considered (see *"Adverse Reactions"*). The susceptible population includes patients with a history of a previous reaction to a contrast media, patients with a known sensitivity to iodine per se, and patients with a known clinical hypersensitivity: bronchial asthma, hay fever and food allergies.

The occurrence of severe idiosyncratic reactions has prompted the use of several pretesting methods. However, pretesting cannot be relied upon to predict severe reactions and may itself be hazardous for the patient. It is suggested that a thorough medical history with emphasis on alergy and hypersensitivity, prior to the injection of any contrast media, may be more accurate than pretesting in predicting potential adverse reactions.

A positive history of allergies or hypersensitivity does not arbitrarily contraindicate the use of a contrast agent, where a diagnostic procedure is thought essential, but caution should be exercised (see *"Adverse Reactions"*). Premedication with antihistamines or corticosteroids to avoid or minimize possible allergic reactions in such patients should be considered. Recent reports indicate that such pretreatment does not prevent serious life-threatening reactions, but may reduce both their incidence and severity.

Azotemia is not a contraindication. Care should be taken regarding dosage and hydration status and the patient's renal status should be monitored for days afterwards.

Acute renal failure has been reported in diabetic patients with diabetic nephropathy and in susceptible nondiabetic patients (often elderly with preexisting renal disease) following intravascular use of contrast media. Therefore, careful consideration of the potential risks should be given before performing this radiographic procedure in these patients.

Preparatory dehydration is dangerous and may contribute to acute renal failure in infants, young children, elderly, patients with preexisting renal insufficiency, and patients with advanced vascular disease. Dehydration in these patients seems to be enhanced by the osmotic diuretic action of contrast agents. It is believed that overnight fluid restriction prior to angiography does not provide better visualization in normal patients. Therefore, preparatory dehydration is unnecessary, and is usually contraindicated, in association with the angiographic use of Metrizamide.

Angiography should be avoided whenever possible in patients with homocystinuria, because of the risk of inducing thrombosis and embolism.

Drug/Laboratory Test Interactions: It is expected that the results of thyroid function tests, which depend on iodine estimations, will not reflect true function for about 16 days. Tests which directly determine thyroxine levels should not be affected.

Pregnancy Category B: See *"Precautions, Intrathecal."*

Nursing Mothers: Caution should be exercised when Metrizamide is administered to a nursing woman. Metrizamide is excreted in milk to the extent of 1 mg of the injected myelographic dose over 2 days.

The nature of the adverse effects which occur following intravascular administration of Metrizamide is similar to that following corresponding ionic media although their incidence and severity may be less.

The following is based on general vascular experience with both ionic and nonionic media.

ADVERSE REACTIONS
INTRAVASCULAR
Reactions which have been observed are similar in nature to those following the use of ionic media.

Cardiovascular: Various arrhythmias, bradycardia being the most frequent, as well as peripheral vasodilation with brief hypotension have occurred.

Hemodynamic: A feeling of heat, usually mild but which may be moderate in degree, may be evident particularly following selective arterial procedures. Frank pain is very unusual.

Renal: Mild diuresis and transitory mild increase in urine osmolarity.

Allergic: Dermal urticaria or erythemata have occurred. Therefore, other allergic manifestations such as rigors, broncho or laryngospastic attacks with serious cardiopulmonary complications resulting in fatality must be considered a possibility.

Respiratory: Pulmonary or laryngeal edema, dyspnea.

Nervous System: Restlessness, tremors.

Technical Factors: Hematoma, ecchymosis, extravasation of the medium particularly on mechanical high pressure injection, venous rupture or hemorrhage from arterial injection sites (observe areas for at least 24 hours).

INDIVIDUAL INDICATIONS AND USAGE
INTRAVASCULAR
INTRAVENOUS DIGITAL ARTERIOGRAPHY FOR
THE HEAD AND NECK
Metrizamide solution can be injected intravenously as a rapid bolus to provide arterial visualization using digital subtraction radiography. Preprocedural medications are not considered necessary. Metrizamide will provide diagnostic arterial radiographs in about 90% of patients. In almost all cases in which poor arterial visualization occurs (10%), it can be attributed to patient movement. Metrizamide is very well tolerated in the vascular system. There is very little subjective or objective evidence of patient discomfort (general sensation of heat) following the injection as compared with ionic media. Very few of the reactions are moderate to severe in degree. In about 87% of patients discomfort is either absent or is mild. Some patients exhibit mild nausea which does not appear to be dose related.

PRECAUTIONS
Since the dose is usually administered mechanically under high pressure, rupture of smaller peripheral veins has occurred. It has been suggested that this can be avoided by using an intravenous catheter threaded proximally beyond larger tributaries or in the case of the antecubital vein, into the superior vena cava. Sometimes the femoral vein is used.

DOSAGE AND ADMINISTRATION
The maximum total dose administered to the patient should not exceed 87.5 g of iodine. See *"Description"* section for iodine content.

Metrizamide is administered intravenously as a bolus injection in a concentration of 370 mgI/mL.

The usual individual volume is about 40 mL (range 30 mL to 60 mL).

Frequently three injections may be required, up to a total volume of about 120 mL (range 40 mL to 165 mL).

The patient is urged not to move during, or immediately after, the injection. In the case of carotid-cerebral arteriography, the patient is also asked not to swallow during this period. Metrizamide is usually administered via 16-18 gauge catheter by mechanical injection at a rate of about 12 mL/sec.

A dextrose solution may be layered over the contrast medium in the injector with the purpose of pushing the remnant of the bolus forward into the main circulation, and to flush out the vein.

ADULT PERIPHERAL ARTERIOGRAPHY

Metrizamide solution in a concentration of 370 mgI/mL is recommended for arteriography of the lower limbs. The injection is usually through a catheter introduced into the femoral artery with the tip placed as to achieve lower aortic or aorto-iliac runoff or visualization of individual femoral artery or its distribution throughout the lower limb. When necessary, the catheter tip may be advanced to the level of the renal artery. Pressure injection is usually employed. Visualization is similar to that achieved with ionic media of similar dose and concentration. Sedative premedication may be employed with Metrizamide; however, anesthesia is usually not considered necessary.

ADVERSE REACTIONS

Very brief (seconds to minutes) nausea immediately following the injection or mild urticaria starting within minutes and of a few hours duration, has been reported in about 3% of patients; these reactions have not interfered with the procedure. Patient discomfort during and immediately following the injection is substantially less than the discomfort which follows injection of ionic media of similar volume and concentrations. Severe discomfort is very unusual.

DOSAGE AND ADMINISTRATION

The maximum total dose administered to the patient should not exceed 87.5 g of iodine. See *"Description"* section for iodine content.

The volume required will depend on the size, flow rate and disease status of the injected artery, and on the size and condition of the patient as well as the imaging technique used. The usual individual volume is about 50 mL (range 25 mL to 65 mL). Two injections are usually required, sometimes three, and rarely up to five.

PEDIATRIC ANGIOCARDIOGRAPHY

Metrizamide at a maximum concentration of 370 mgI/mL may be used for angiocardiography in infants and young children.

DOSAGE AND ADMINISTRATION

The recommended single dose of Metrizamide in 370 mgI/mL concentration is about 1.5 mL/kg (range 1 mL/kg to 2 mL/kg). In addition, small test volumes of about 2 mL may be used for catheter placement.

The usual total dose of Metrizamide per procedure, which includes diagnostic and test doses, is about 4 mL/kg (range 1.5 mL/kg to 6 mL/kg). Analgesics and/or sedative tranquilizers may be required in these young patients.

PREPARATION OF THE SOLUTION — INTRAVASCULAR USE

1. Determine the concentration required for the vascular procedure.
2. The volume of diluent required to obtain that iodine concentration can be obtained from the *"Dilution Table."*
3. Using a sterile technique with a small gauge transfer needle (approximately 22 gauge to help prevent coring), withdraw the required amount of diluent.
4. Insert this volume of diluent into the lyophil vial also using the fine needle. Contents under vacuum. Use only if vacuum is present as evidenced by diluent being drawn into vial when stopper is punctured. Leave syringe and needle in place.
5. Gently swirl the vial (without shaking) until its contents are dissolved (approximately 3 to 22 minutes) to insure complete dissolution of the lyophil. The resulting solution should be clear and colorless to slightly yellow. Do not use if undissolved particulate matter or bubbles are present.
6. Withdraw the volume of Metrizamide required.
7 Do not prefill plastic syringes with Metrizamide for prolonged periods (ie, for several hours or longer) before use. Use immediately after reconstitution. Discard any unused portion.

DILUTION TABLE FOR INTRAVASCULAR USE

Conc. of Solution (mgI/mL)	Volume of Diluent to be Added 6.75 g vial (mL)
300	7.8
310	7.4
320	7.1
330	6.8
340	6.5
350	6.2
360	6.0
370	5.7

The volume of the final solution will equal the volume of the diluent + 3.1 mL

The volume of the final solution will exceed the amount required to achieve the recommended dosage. For volume for injection refer to individual *"Dosage and Administration"* sections.

STORAGE

Protect vials of Metrizamide from light or excessive heat, 40°C (104° F).

POWDER FOR INJECTION: 13.5%

BRAND/MANUFACTURER	NDC	SIZE	AWP
○ **BRAND**			
AMIPAQUE: Sanofi Winthrop	00024-0046-01	1s	$127.62

POWDER FOR INJECTION: 18.75%

BRAND/MANUFACTURER	NDC	SIZE	AWP
○ **BRAND**			
AMIPAQUE: Sanofi Winthrop	00024-0044-01	1s	$76.56

Metrodin SEE UROFOLLITROPIN

MetroGel SEE METRONIDAZOLE, TOPICAL AND
METRONIDAZOLE, VAGINAL

Metronidazole, Systemic

> **WARNING**
>
> METRONIDAZOLE HAS BEEN SHOWN TO BE CARCINOGENIC IN MICE AND RATS (SEE *"PRECAUTIONS"*). UNNECESSARY USE OF THE DRUG SHOULD BE AVOIDED. ITS USE SHOULD BE RESERVED FOR THE CONDITIONS DESCRIBED IN THE *"INDICATIONS AND USAGE"* SECTION BELOW.

DESCRIPTION

Metronidazole and Metronidazole Hydrochloride (HCl) are synthetic antiprotozoal and antibacterial agent, 1-(β-hydroxyethyl)-2-methyl-nitroimidazole and 1-(β-hydroxyethyl)-2-methyl-5-nitroimidazole hydrochloride.

Each Metronidazole tablet contains:

Metronidazole	250 mg
Metronidazole	500 mg

Each Vial of Metronidazole I.V. contains:
Metronidazole HCl hyophilized ....500 mg Metronidazole equivalent

Each ready-to-use container of Metronidazole I.V. contains:
Metronidazole ....500 mg /100 mL

Following is its chemical structure:

$$O_2N \underset{\displaystyle \text{N}}{\overset{\displaystyle CH_2CH_2OH}{\bigwedge}} CH_3$$

CLINICAL PHARMACOLOGY

Metronidazole is a synthetic antibacterial compound. Disposition of Metronidazole in the body is similar for both oral and intravenous dosage forms, with an average elimination half-life in healthy humans of eight hours.

The major route of elimination of Metronidazole and its metabolites is via the urine (60-80% of the dose), with fecal excretion accounting for 6-15% of the dose. The metabolites that appear in the urine result primarily from side-chain oxidation [1-(β-hydroxyethyl)-2-hydroxymethyl-5-nitroimidazole and 2-methyl-5-nitroimidazole-1-yl-acetic acid] and glucuronide conjugation, with unchanged Metronidazole accounting for approximately 20% of the total. Renal clearance of Metronidazole is approximately 10 ml/min/1.73 m^2.

Metronidazole is the major component appearing in the plasma, with lesser quantities of the 2-hydroxymethyl metabolite also being present. Less than 20% of the circulating Metronidazole is bound to plasma proteins. Both the parent compound and the metabolite possess *in vitro* bactericidal activity against most strains of anaerobic bacteria and *in vitro* trichomanacidal activity.

Metronidazole appears in cerebrospinal fluid, saliva, and breast milk in concentrations similar to those found in plasma. Bactericidal concentrations of Metronidazole have also been detected in pus from hepatic abscesses.

Following oral administration, Metronidazole is well absorbed, with peak plasma concentrations occurring between one and two hours after administration. Plasma concentrations of Metronidazole are proportional to the administered dose. Oral administration of 250 mg, 500 mg, or 2,000 mg produced peak plasma concentrations of 6 mcg/ml, 12 mcg/ml, and 40 mcg/ml, respectively. Studies reveal no significant bioavailability differences between males and females; however, because of weight differences, the resulting plasma levels in males are generally lower.

Plasma concentrations of Metronidazole are proportional to the administered dose. An eight-hour intravenous infusion of 100-4,000 mg of Metronidazole in normal subjects showed a linear relationship between dose and peak plasma concentration.

In patients treated with Metronidazole I.V., using a dosage regimen of 15 mg/kg loading dose followed six hours later by 7.5 mg/kg every six hours, peak steady-state plasma concentrations of Metronidazole averaged 25 meg/ml with trough (minimum) concentrations averaging 18 mcg/ml.

Decreased renal function does not alter the single-dose pharmacokinetics of Metronidazole. However, plasma clearance of Metronidazole is decreased in patients with decreased liver function.

In one study newborn infants appeared to demonstrate diminished capacity to eliminate Metronidazole. The elimination half-life, measured during the first three days of life, was inversely related to gestational age. In infants whose gestational ages were between 28 and 40 weeks, the corresponding elimination half-lives ranged from 109 to 22.5 hours.

Microbiology: Trichomonas cagindis, Entamoeba histolytica. Oral Metronidazole possesses direct trichomonacidal and amebacidal activity against *T. vaginalis* and *E. histolytica.* The *in vitro* minimal inhibitory concentration (MIC) for most strains of these organisms is 1 mcg/ml or less.

Metronidazole is active *in vitro* against most obligate anaerobes, but does not appear to possess any clinically relevant activity against facultative anaerobes or obligate aerobes. Against susceptible organisms, Metronidazole is generally bactericidal at concentrations equal to or slightly higher than the minimal inhibitory concentrations. Metronidazole has been shown to have *in vitro* and clinical activity against the following organisms:

Anaerobic gram-negative bacilli, including: *Bacteroides* species, including the *Bacteroides fragilis* group (*B. fragilis, B. distasonis, B. ovatus, B. thetaiotaomicron, B. vulgatus) Fusobacterium* species.

Anaerobic gram-positive bacilli, including: *Clostridium* species and susceptible strains of *Eubacterium.*

Anaerobic gram-positive cocci, including: *Peptococcus* species. *Peptostreptococcus* species

Susceptibility Tests: Bacteriologic studies should be performed to determine the causative organisms and their susceptibility to Metronidazole; however, the rapid, routine susceptibility testing of individual isolates of anaerobic bacteria is not always practical, and therapy may be started while awaiting these results.

Quantitative methods give the most accurate estimates of susceptibility to antibacterial drugs. A standardized agar dilution method and a broth microdilution method are recommended.[1]

Control strains are recommended for standardized susceptibility testing. Each time the test is performed, one or more of the following strains should be included: *Clostridium perfringens* ATCC 13124, *Bacteroides fragilis* ATCC 25285, and *Bacteroides thetaiotaomicron* ATCC 29741. The mode Metronidazole MICs for those three strains are reported to be 0.25, 0.25, and 0.5 mcg/ml, respectively.

A clinical laboratory test is considered under acceptable control if the results of the control strains are within one doubling dilution of the mode MICs reported for Metronidazole.

A bacterial isolate may be considered susceptible if the MIC value for Metronidazole is not more than 16 mcg/ml. An organism is considered resistant if the MIC is greater than 16 mcg/ml. A report of "resistant" from the laboratory indicates that the infecting organism is not likely to respond to therapy.

INDICATIONS AND USAGE

Symptomatic Trichomoniasis: Metronidazole is indicated for the treatment of symptomatic trichomoniasis in females and males when the presence of the trichomonad has been confirmed by appropriate laboratory procedures (wet smears and/or cultures).

Asymptomatic Trichomoniasis: Oral Metronidazole is indicated in the treatment of asymptomatic females when the organism is associated with endocervicitis, cervicitis, or cervical erosion. Since there is evidence that presence of the trichomonad can interfere with accurate assessment of abnormal cytological smears, additional smears should be performed after eradication of the parasite.

Treatment of Asymptomatic Consorts: T. vaginalis infection is a veneral disease. Therefore, asymptomatic sexual partners of treated patients should be treated simultaneously if the organism has been found to be present, in order to prevent reinfection of the partner. The decision as to whether to treat an asymptomatic male partner who has a negative culture or one for whom no culture has been attempted is an individual one. In making this decision, it should be noted that there is evidence that a woman may become reinfected if her consort is not treated. Also, since there can be considerable difficulty in isolating the organism from the asymptomatic male carrier, negative smears and cultures cannot be relied upon in this regard. In any event, the consort should be treated with Oral Metronidazole in cases of reinfection.

Amebiasis: Oral Metronidazole is indicated in the treatment of acute intestinal amebiasis (amebic dysentery) and amebic liver abscess.

In amebic liver abscess, oral Metronidazole therapy does not obviate the need for aspiration or drainage of pus.

TREATMENT OF ANAEROBIC INFECTIONS

Metronidazole is indicated in the treatment of serious infections caused by susceptible anaerobic bacteria. Indicated surgical procedures should be performed in conjunction with Metronidazole therapy. In a mixed aerobic and anaerobic infection, antibiotics appropriate for the treatment of the aerobic infection should be used in addition to Metronidazole.

In the treatment of most serious anaerobic infections, Metronidazole HCl I.V. or Metronidazole I.V. is usually administered initially. This may be followed by oral therapy with Metronidazole at the discretion of the physician.

Metronidazole Systemic I.V. is effective in *Bacteroides fragilis* infections resistant to clindamycin, chloramphenicol, and penicillin.

Intra-Abdominal Infections: including peritonitis, intra-abdominal abscess, and liver abscess, caused by *Bacteroides* species including the *B. fragilis* group (*B. fragilis, B. distasonis, B. ovatus, B. thetaiotaomicron, B. vulgatus). Clostridium* species, *Eubacterium* species, *Peptococcus* species, and *Peptostreptococcus* species.

Skin and Skin Structure Infections caused by *Bacteroides* species including the *B. fragilis* group, *Clostridium* species, *Peptococcus* species, *Peptostreptococcus* species, and *Fusobacterium* species.

Gynecologic Infections including endometritis, endomyometritis, tubo-ovarian abscess, and postsurgical vaginal cuff infection, caused by *Bacteroides* species including the *B. fragilis* group, *Clostridium* species, *Peptococcus* species, and *Peptostreptococcus* species.

Bacterial Septioemia caused by *Bacteroides* species including the *B. fragilis* group, and *Clostridium* species.

Bone and Joint Infections as adjunctive therapy, caused by *Bacteroides* species including the *B. fragilis* group.

Central Nervous System (CNS) Infections including meningitis and brain abscess, caused by *Bacteroides* species including the *B. fragilis* group.

Lower Respiratory Tract Infections including pneumonia, empyema, and lung abscess, caused by *Bacteroides* species including the *B. fragilis* group.

Endocarditis caused by *Bacteroides* species including the *B. fragilis* group.

PROPHYLAXIS
The prophylactic administration of Metronidazole Systemic I.V. preoperatively, intraoperatively, and postoperatively may reduce the incidence of postoperative infection in patients undergoing elective colorectal surgery which is classified as contaminated or potentially contaminated.

Prophylactic use of Metronidazole Systemic I.V. should be discontinued within 12 hours after surgery. If there are signs of infection, specimens for cultures should be obtained for the identification of the causative organism(s) so that appropriate therapy may be given (see *"Dosage and Administration"*).

UNLABELED USES
Metronidazole is used alone or as an adjunct in the treatment of Crohn's disease, renal cell carcinoma in combination with mitomycin-C, infectious diarrhea and giardiasis.

CONTRAINDICATIONS

Metronidazole Systemic is contraindicated in patients with a prior history of hypersensitivity to Metronidazole or other nitroimidazole derivatives.

In patients with trichomoniasis, Oral Metronidazole is contraindicated during the first trimester of pregnancy. (See *"Warnings"*.)

WARNINGS

Convulsive Seizures and Peripheral Neuropathy: Convulsive seizures and peripheral neuropathy, the latter characterized mainly by numbness or paresthesia of an extremity, have been reported in patients treated with Metronidazole. The appearance of abnormal neurologic signs demands the prompt evaluation of the benefit/risk ratio of the continuation of therapy or the prompt discontinuation of Oral Metronidazole therapy. Metronidazole should be administered with caution to patients with central nervous system diseases.

PRECAUTIONS

General: Patients with severe hepatic disease metabolize Metronidazole slowly, with resultant accumulation of Metronidazole and its metabolites in the plasma. Accordingly, for such patients, doses below those usually recommended should be administered cautiously.

Administration of solutions containing sodium ions may result in sodium retention. Care should be taken when administering Metronidazole Systemic I.V., ready to use, to patients receiving corticosteroids or to patients predisposed to edema.

Known or previously unrecognized candidiasis may present more prominent symptoms during therapy with Metronidazole and requires treatment with a candicidal agent.

Laboratory Tests: Metronidazole is a nitroimidazole, and should be used with care in patients with evidence of or history of blood dyscrasia. A mild leukopenia has been observed during its administration; however, no persistent hematologic abnormalities attributable to Metronidazole have been observed in clinical studies. Total and differential leukocyte counts are recommended before and after therapy for trichomoniasis and amebiasis, especially if a second course of therapy is necessary, and before and after therapy for anaerobic infection.

Drug Interactions: Metronidazole has been reported to potentiate the anticoagulant effect of warfarin and other oral coumarin anticoagulants, resulting in a prolongation of prothrombin time. This possible drug interaction should be considered when Metronidazole is prescribed for patients on this type of anticoagulant therapy.

The simultaneous administration of drugs that induce microsomal liver enzymes, such as phenytein or phenobarbital, may accelerate the elimination of Metronidazole, resulting in reduced plasma levels; impaired clearance of phenytoin has also been reported.

The simultaneous administration of drugs that decrease microsomal liver enzyme activity, such as cimetidine, may prolong the half-life and decrease plasma clearance of Metronidazole.

In patients stabilized on relatively high doses of lithium, short-term oral Metronidazole therapy has been associated with elevation of serum lithium and, in a few cases, signs of lithium toxicity. Serum lithium and serum creatinine levels should be obtained several days after beginning Metronidazole to detect any increase that may precede clinical symptoms of lithium intoxication.

Alcoholic beverages should not be consumed during Metronidazole therapy and for at least one day afterward because abdominal cramps, nausea, vomiting, headaches, and flushing may occur.

Psychotic reactions have been reported in alcoholic patients who are using Metronidazole and disulfiram concurrently. Metronidazole should not be given to patients who have taken disulfiram within the last two weeks.

Drug/Laboratory Test Interactions: Metronidazole may interfere with certain types of determinations of serum chemistry values, such as aspartate aminotransferase (AST, SGOT), alanine aminotransferase (ALT, SGPT), lactate dehydrogenase (LDH), triglycerides, and hexokinase glucose. Values of zero may be observed. All of the assays in which interference has been reported involve enzymatic coupling of the assay to oxidation-reduction of nicotine adenine dinucleotide (NAD+ $\rightleftharpoons$ NADH). Interference is due to the similarity in absorbance peaks of NADH (340 nm) and Metronidazole (322 nm) at pH 7.

Carcinogenesis, Mutagenesis, Impairment of Fertility: Tumorigenicity in Rodents—Metronidazole has shown evidence of carcinogenic activity in studies involving chronic, oral administration in mice and rats. Prominent among the effects in the mouse was the promotion of pulmonary tumorigenesis. This has been observed in all six reported studies in that species, including one study in which the animals were dosed on an intermittent schedule (administration during every fourth week only). At very high dose levels (approx. 500 mg/kg/day) there was a statistically significant increase in the incidence of malignant liver tumors in males. Also, the published results of one of the mouse studies indicate an increase in the incidence of malignant lymphomas as well as pulmonary neoplasms associated with lifetime feeding of the drug. All these effects are statistically significant.

Several long-term, oral-dosing studies in the rat have been completed. There were statistically significant increases in the incidence of various neoplasms, particularly in mammary and hepatic tumors, among female rats administered Metronidazole over those noted in the concurrent female control groups.

Two lifetime tumorigenicity studies in hamsters have been performed and reported to be negative. Also, Metronidazole has shown mutagenic activity in a number of *in vitro* assay systems, but studies in mammals (*in vivo*) failed to demonstrate a potential for genetic damage.

Pregnancy: Teratogenic Effects—Pregnancy Category B. Metronidazole crosses the placental barrier and enters the fetal circulation rapidly. Reproduction studies have been performed in rats at doses up to five times the human dose and have revealed no evidence of impaired fertility or harm to the fetus due to Metronidazole. Metronidazole administered intraperitoneally to pregnant mice at approximately the human dose caused fetotoxicity; administered orally to pregnant mice, no fetotoxicity was observed. There are, however, no adequate and well-controlled studies in pregnant women. Because animal reproduction studies are not always predictive of human response, and because Metronidazole is a carcinogen in rodents, these drugs should be used during pregnancy only if clearly needed (see *"Contraindications"*).

Use of oral Metronidazole for trichomoniasis in the second and third trimesters should be restricted to those in whom local palliative treatment has been inadequate to control symptoms.

Nursing Mothers: Because of the potential for tumorigenicity shown for Metronidazole in mouse and rat studies, a decision should be made whether to discontinue nursing or to discontinue the drug, taking into account the importance of the drug to the mother. Metronidazole is secreted in breast milk in concentrations similar to those found in plasma.

Pediatric Use: Safety and effectiveness in children have not been established, except for the treatment of amebiasis.

ADVERSE REACTIONS

Two serious adverse reactions reported in patients treated with Metronidazole have been convulsive seizures and peripheral neuropathy, the latter characterized mainly by numbness or paresthesia of an extremity. Since persistent peripheral neuropathy has been reported in some patients receiving prolonged oral administration of Metronidazole, patients should be specifically warned about these reactions and should be told to stop the drug and report immediately to their physicians if any neurologic symptoms occur. If neurologic symptoms occur, a prompt evaluation should be made of the benefit/risk ratio of the continuation of therapy.

The following reactions have also been reported during treatment with Metronidazole HCl I.V. and Metronidazole.

Gastrointestinal: Nausea, vomiting, abdominal discomfort, diarrhea, and an unpleasant metallic taste.

Hematopoietic: Reversible neutropenia (leukopenia).

Dermatologic: Erythematous rash and pruritus.

Central Nervous System: Headache, dizziness, syncope, ataxia, and confusion.

Local Reactions: Thrombophlebitis after intravenous infusion. This reaction can be minimized or avoided by avoiding prolonged use of indwelling intravenous catheters.

Other: Fever. Instances of a darkened urine have also been reported, and this manifestation has been the subject of a special investigation. Although the pigment which is probably responsible for this phenomenon has not been positively identified, it is almost certainly a metabolite of Metronidazole and seems to have no clinical significance.

The following adverse reactions have been reported during treatment with oral Metronidazole:

Gastrointestinal: Nausea, sometimes accompanied by headache, anorexia, and occasionally vomiting; diarrhea, epigastric distress, abdominal cramping, and constipation.

Mouth: A sharp, unpleasant metallic taste is not unusual. Furry tongue, glossitis, and stomatitis have occurred; these may be associated with a sudden overgrowth of *Candida* which may occur during effective therapy.

Hematopoietic: Reversible neutropenia (leukopenia); rarely, reversible thrombocytopenia.

Cardiovascular: Flattening of the T-wave may be seen in electrocardiographic tracings.

Central Nervous System: Convulsive seizures, peripheral neuropathy, dizziness, vertigo, incoordination, ataxia, confusion, irritability, depression, weakness, and insomnia.

Hypersensitivity: Urticaria, erythematous rash, flushing, nasal congestion, dryness of mouth (or vagina or vulva), and fever.

Renal: Dysuria, cystitis, polyuria, incontinence, and a sense of pelvic pressure. Instances of darkened urine have been reported by approximately one patient in 100,000. Although the pigment which is probably responsible for this phenomenon has not been positively identified, it is almost certainly a metabolite of Metronidazole and seems to have no clinical significance.

Other: Proliferation of *Candida* in the vagina, dyspareunia, decrease of libido, proctitis, and fleeting joint pains sometimes resembling "serum sickness." If patients receiving Metronidazole drink alcoholic beverages, they may experience abdominal distress, nausea, vomiting, flushing, or headache. A modification of the taste of alcoholic beverages has also been reported. Rare cases of pancreatitis, which abated on withdrawal of the drug, have been reported.

Crohn's disease patients are known to have an increased incidence of gastrointestinal and certain extraintestinal cancers. There have been some reports in the medical literature of breast and colon cancer in Crohn's disease patients who have been treated with Metronidazole at high doses for extended periods of time. A cause and effect relationship has not been established. Crohn's disease is not an approved indication for Metronidazole.

OVERDOSAGE

Use of dosages of Metronidazole Systemic I.V. higher than those recommended has been reported. These include the use of 27 mg/kg three times a day for 20 days, and the use of 75 mg/kg as a single loading dose followed by 7.5 mg/kg maintenance doses. No adverse reactions were reported in either of the two cases.

Single oral doses of Metronidazole, up to 15 g, have been reported in suicide attempts and accidental overdoses. Symptoms reported include nausea, vomiting, and ataxia.

Oral Metronidazole has been studied as a radiation sensitizer in the treatment of malignant tumors. Neurotoxic effects, including seizures and peripheral neuropathy, have been reported after 5 to 7 days of doses of 6 to 10.4 g every other day.

Treatment: There is no specific antidote for overdose; therefore, management of the patient should consist of symptomatic and supportive therapy.

DOSAGE AND ADMINISTRATION

In elderly patients the pharmacokinetics of Metronidazole may be altered and therefore monitoring of serum levels may be necessary to adjust the Metronidazole dosage accordingly.

ORAL METRONIDAZOLE
Trichomoniasis
In the Female:

One-day Treatment: two grams of oral Metronidazole given either as a single dose or in two divided doses of one gram each given in the same day.

Seven-day Course of Treatment: 250 mg three times daily for seven consecutive days. There is some indication from controlled comparative studies that cure rates as determined by vaginal smears, signs and symptoms, may be higher after a seven-day course of treatment than after a one-day treatment regimen.

The dosage regimen should be individualized. Singledose treatment can assure compliance, especially if administered under supervision, in those patients who cannot be relied on to continue the seven-day regimen. A seven-day course of treatment may minimize reinfection of the female long enough to treat sexual contacts. Further, some patients may tolerate one course of therapy better than the other.

Pregnant patients should not be treated during the first trimester with either regimen. If treated during the second or third trimester, the one-day course of therapy should not be used, as it results in higher serum levels which reach the fetal circulation. (See *"Contraindications"* and *"Precautions"*.)

When repeat courses of the drug are required, it is recommended that an interval of four to six weeks elapse between courses and that the presence of the trichomonad be reconfirmed by appropriate laboratory measures. Total and differential leukocyte counts should be made before and after re-treatment.

In the Male: Treatment should be individualized as for the female.

Amebiasis:

Adults:

For acute intestinal amebiasis (acute amebic dysentery): 750 mg orally three times daily for 5 to 10 days.

For amebic liver abscess: 500 mg or 750 mg orally three times daily for 5 to 10 days.

Children: 35 to 50 mg/kg/24 hours, divided into three doses, orally for 10 days.

Treatment of Anaerobic Infections: In the treatment of most serious anaerobic infections, Metronidazole HCl I.V. or Metronidazole I.V. is usually administered initially.

The recommended dosage schedule for *adults* is:

Loading dose: 15 mg/kg infused over one hour (approximately 1 g for a 70-kg adult).

Maintenance Dose: 7.5 mg/kg infused over one hour every six hours (approximately 500 mg for a 70-kg adult). The first maintenance dose should be instituted six hours following the initiation of the loading dose.

Parenteral therapy may be changed to oral Metronidazole when conditions warrant, based upon the severity of the disease and the response of the patient to Metronidazole Systemic I.V. treatment. The usual adult oral dosage is 7.5 mg/kg every six hours (approx. 500 mg for a 70-kg adult).

A maximum of 4 g should not be exceeded during a 24-hour period.

Patients with severe hepatic disease metabolize Metronidazole slowly, with resultant accumulation of Metronidazole and its metabolites in the plasma. Accordingly, for such patients, doses below those usually recommended should be administered cautiously. Close monitoring of plasma Metronidazole levels[2] and toxicity is recommended.

In patients receiving Metronidazole Systemic I.V. in whom gastric secretions are continuously removed by nasogastric aspiration, sufficient Metronidazole may be removed in the aspirate to cause a reduction in serum levels.

The dose of Metronidazole should not be specifically reduced in anuric patients since accumulated metabolites may be rapidly removed by dialysis.

The usual duration of therapy is 7 to 10 days; however, infections of the bone and joint, lower respiratory tract, and endocardium may require longer treatment.

Prophylaxis: For surgical prophylactic use, to prevent postoperative infection in contaminated or potentially contaminated colorectal surgery, the recommended dosage schedule of Metronidazole HCl I.V. and Metronidazole I.V. for adults is:

a. 15 mg/kg infused over 30 to 60 minutes and completed approximately one hour before surgery; followed by

b. 7.5 mg/kg infused over 30 to 60 minutes at 6 and 12 hours after the initial dose.

It is important that (1) administration of the initial preoperative dose be completed approximately one hour before surgery so that adequate drug levels are present in the serum and tissues at the time of initial incision, and (2) Metronidazole Systemic I.V. be administered, if necessary, at 6-hour intervals to maintain effective drug levels. Prophylactic use of Metronidazole Systemic I.V. should be limited to the day of surgery only, following the above guidelines.

Caution: **Metronidazole HCl I.V or Metronidazole I.V. is to be administered by slow intravenous drip infusion only, either as a continuous or intermittent infusion. I.V. admixtures containing Metronidazole and other drugs should be avoided. Additives should not be introduced into the Metronidazole I.V. solution. If used with a primary intravenous fluid system, the primary solution should be discontinued during Metronidazole infusion. DO NOT USE EQUIPMENT CONTAINING ALUMINUM (EG, NEEDLES, CANNULAE) THAT WOULD COME IN CONTACT WITH THE DRUG SOLUTION.**

METRONIDAZOLE HCL I.V.

Metronidazole HCl I.V.: *cannot* **be given by direct intravenous injection (I.V. bolus) because of the low pH (0.5 to 2.0) of the reconstituted product. Metronidazole HCl I.V. MUST BE FURTHER DILUTED AND NEUTRALIZED FOR I.V. INFUSION.**

Metronidazole HCl I.V.: is prepared for use in two steps:

NOTE: ORDER OF MIXING IS IMPORTANT

A. Reconstitution

B. Dilution in intravenous solution followed by pH neutralization with sodium bicarbonate injection into the dilution.

Reconstitution: To prepare the solution, add 4.4 ml of one of the following diluents and mix thoroughly: Sterile Water for Injection, USP, Bacteriostatic Water for Injection, USP; 0.9% Sodium Chloride Injection, USP; or Bacteriostatic 0.9% Sodium Chloride Injection, USP. The resultant approximate withdrawal volume is 5.0 ml with an approximate concentration of 100 mg/ml.

The pH of the reconstituted product will be in the range of 0.5 to 2.0. Reconstituted Metronidazole HCl I.V. is clear, and pale yellow to yellow-green in color.

Dilution in Intravenous Solutions: Properly reconstituted Metronidazole HCl I.V. may be added to a glass or plastic I.V. container not to exceed a concentration of 8 mg/ml. Any of the following intravenous solutions may be used: 0.9% Sodium Chloride Injection, USP; 5% Dextrose Injection, USP; or Lactated Ringer's Injection, USP.

NEUTRALIZATION IS REQUIRED PRIOR TO ADMINISTRATION.

The final product should be mixed thoroughly and used within 24 hours.

Neutralization For Intravenous Infusion: Neutralize the intravenous solution containing Metronidazole HCl I.V. with approximately 5 mEq of sodium bicarbonate injection for each 500 mg of Metronidazole HCl I.V. used. Mix thoroughly. The pH of the neutralized intravenous solution will be approximately 6.0 to 7.0. Carbon dioxide gas will be generated with neutralization. It may be necessary to relieve gas pressures within the container.

Note: When the contents of one vial (500 mg) are diluted and neutralized to 100 ml, the resultant concentration is 5 mg/ml. Do not exceed an 8 mg/ml concentration of Metronidazole HCl I.V. in the neutralized intravenous solution, since neutralization will decrease the aqueous solubility and precipitation may occur. DO NOT REFRIGERATE NEUTRALIZED SOLUTIONS: otherwise, precipitation may occur.

Storage and Stability: Reconstituted vials of Metronidazole HCl I.V. are chemically stable for 96 hours when stored below 86°F (30°C) in room light.

Use diluted and neutralized intravenous solutions containing Metronidazole HCl I.V. within 24 hours of mixing.

METRONIDAZOLE I.V.

Metronidazole I.V. is a ready-to-use isotonic solution. **NO DILUTION OR BUFFERING IS REQUIRED.** Do not refrigerate. Each container of Metronidazole I.V. contains 14 mEq of sodium.

DIRECTIONS FOR USE OF PLASTIC CONTAINER

Caution: **Do not use plastic containers in series connections. Such use could result in air embolism due to residual air (approximately 15 ml) being drawn from the primary container before administration of the fluid from the secondary container is complete.**

To open. Tear overwrap down side at slit and remove solution container. Some opacity of the plastic due to moisture absorption during the sterilization process may be observed. This is normal and does not affect the solution quality or safety. The opacity will diminish gradually. Check for minute leaks by squeezing inner bag firmly. If leaks are found discard solution as sterility may be impaired.

Preparation for administration:

1. Suspend container from eyelet support.
2. Remove plastic protector from outlet port at bottom of container.
3. Attach administration set. Refer to complete directions accompanying set.

Parenteral drug products should be inspected visually for particulate matter and discoloration prior to administration, whenever solution and container permit. Do not use if cloudy or precipitated or if the seal is not intact.

Use sterile equipment. It is recommended that the intravenous administration apparatus be replaced at least once every 24 hours.

STORAGE

Store oral Metronidazole below 86°F (30°C) and protect from light.

Metronidazole HCl I.V., prior to reconstitution, should be stored below 86°F (30°C) and protected from light.

Metronidazole I.V. should be stored at controlled room temperature, 59° to 86° F (15° to 30°C), and protected from light during storage.

REFERENCE

1. Proposed standard: PSM-11—Proposed Reference Dilution Procedure for Antimicrobic Susceptibility Testing of Anaerobic Bacteria, National Committee for Clinical Laboratory Standards; and Sutter, et al.: Collaborative Evaluation of a Proposed Reference Dilution Method of Susceptibility Testing of Anaerobic Bacteria, Antimicrob. Agents Chemother. 16: 495-502 (Oct.) 1979; and Tally, et al.: *In Vitro* Activity of Thienamycin, Antimicrob. Agents Chemother. 14: 436-438 (Sept.) 1978. 2. Ralph, E.D., and Kirby, W.M.M.: Bioassay of Metronidazole With Either Anaerobic or Aerobic Incubation, J. Infect. Dis. 132: 587-591 (Nov.) 1975; or Gulaid, et al.: Determination of Metronidazole and Its Major Metabolites in Biological Fluids by High Pressure Liquid Chromatography, Br. J. Clin. Pharmacol. 6: 430-432, 1978.

HOW SUPPLIED
INJECTION: 5 MG/ML

BRAND/MANUFACTURER		NDC	SIZE	AWP
◆ **GENERICS**				
METRO I.V.: McGaw		00264-5535-32	100 ml 24s	$645.12

INJECTION: 500 MG/100 ML

AVERAGE UNIT PRICE (AVAILABLE SIZES)		GENERIC A-RATED AVERAGE PRICE (GAAP)	
BRAND	$0.08	100 ml	$8.33
GENERIC	$0.11		

BRAND/MANUFACTURER	NDC	SIZE	AWP
◆ **BRAND**			
FLAGYL I.V. RTU: SCS Pharm	00905-1847-24	100 ml 24s	$196.33
◆ **GENERICS**			
Elkins-Sinn	00641-2337-41	100 ml	$7.81
Elkins-Sinn	00641-2337-61	100 ml	$8.85
Baxter	00338-1055-48	100 ml 24s	$368.16

◆ **RATED THERAPEUTICALLY EQUIVALENT;** ◇ **THERAPEUTIC EQUIVALENCE UNCONFIRMED;** ○ **UNRATED**

INJECTION: 500 MG

BRAND/MANUFACTURER		NDC	SIZE	AWP
◆ GENERICS				
Abbott Hosp		00074-7811-37	100 ml 80s	$2225.85

POWDER FOR INJECTION: 500 MG

BRAND/MANUFACTURER		NDC	SIZE	AWP
◆ BRAND				
FLAGYL I.V.: SCS Pharm		00905-1804-10	10s	$161.38

TABLETS: 250 MG

AVERAGE UNIT PRICE (AVAILABLE SIZES)		GENERIC A-RATED AVERAGE PRICE (GAAP)	
BRAND	$1.23	100s	$28.70
GENERIC	$0.20	250s	$28.81
HCFA FUL (100s ea)	$0.04	500s	$49.67
		1000s	$112.68

BRAND/MANUFACTURER	NDC	SIZE	AWP
◆ BRAND			
➤ FLAGYL: Searle	00025-1831-50	50s	$65.36
	00025-1831-31	100s	$125.74
	00025-1831-34	100s ud	$131.03
	00025-1831-41	250s	$296.73
	00025-1831-55	2500s	$2655.80
◆ GENERICS			
Allscrips	54569-0965-07	56s	$11.02
Qualitest	00603-4640-21	100s	$7.11
Schein	00364-0595-01	100s	$7.25
Rugby	00536-4032-01	100s	$8.20
Mason Dist	11845-0241-01	100s	$8.24
Martec	52555-0095-01	100s	$8.50
Major	00904-1453-60	100s	$8.75
Moore,H.L.	00839-6415-06	100s	$10.38
Geneva	00781-1742-01	100s	$12.95
Goldline	00182-1330-01	100s	$12.95
Parmed	00349-2363-01	100s	$13.75
Zenith	00172-2971-60	100s	$13.90
Eon	00185-0551-01	100s	$15.00
Lemmon	00093-0851-01	100s	$18.50
Sidmak	50111-0333-01	100s	$18.50
Par	49884-0095-01	100s	$19.10
URL	00677-0690-01	100s	$20.00
Mutual	53489-0135-01	100s	$20.00
Purepac	00228-2258-10	100s	$20.39
Aligen	00405-4677-01	100s	$21.82
➤ PROTOSTAT: Ortho Pharm	00062-1570-01	100s	$108.54
U.S. Trading	56126-0095-11	100s ud	$5.52
Raway	00686-0122-20	100s ud	$10.25
Major	00904-1453-61	100s ud	$18.80
Goldline	00182-1330-89	100s ud	$53.65
Vangard	00615-1576-13	100s ud	$54.22
UDL	51079-0122-20	100s ud	$55.45
Auro	55829-0364-10	100s ud	$70.06
Geneva	00781-1742-13	100s ud	$72.00
Medirex	57480-0432-01	100s ud	$72.00
Schein	00364-0595-90	100s ud	$75.30
Qualitest	00603-4640-24	250s	$16.15
Rugby	00536-4032-02	250s	$16.95
Major	00904-1453-70	250s	$16.95
Schein	00364-0595-04	250s	$17.25
Martec	52555-0095-02	250s	$17.40
Goldline	00182-1330-02	250s	$25.20
Moore,H.L.	00839-6415-09	250s	$25.23
Parmed	00349-2363-25	250s	$30.91
URL	00677-0690-03	250s	$31.95
Geneva	00781-1742-25	250s	$31.95
Zenith	00172-2971-65	250s	$32.10
Lemmon	00093-0851-52	250s	$34.75
Par	49884-0095-04	250s	$35.00
Eon	00185-0551-52	250s	$35.50
Mutual	53489-0135-03	250s	$35.50
Sidmak	50111-0333-06	250s	$43.41
Aligen	00405-4677-04	250s	$43.50
Major	00904-1453-40	500s	$25.65
Goldline	00182-1330-05	500s	$32.95
Qualitest	00603-4640-28	500s	$34.90
Martec	52555-0095-05	500s	$35.45
Mason Dist	11845-0241-03	500s	$41.51
Rugby	00536-4032-05	500s	$43.70
Sidmak	50111-0333-02	500s	$53.00
Parmed	00349-2363-05	500s	$53.91
Zenith	00172-2971-70	500s	$55.10
Geneva	00781-1742-05	500s	$62.90
Lemmon	00093-0851-05	500s	$67.75
Par	49884-0095-05	500s	$67.90
Eon	00185-0551-05	500s	$71.00
Zenith	00172-2971-80	1000s	$105.35
Par	49884-0095-10	1000s	$120.00

TABLETS: 500 MG

AVERAGE UNIT PRICE (AVAILABLE SIZES)		GENERIC A-RATED AVERAGE PRICE (GAAP)	
BRAND	$2.27	50s	$26.02
GENERIC	$0.47	100s	$50.99
HCFA FUL (100s ea)	$0.08	500s	$138.74

BRAND/MANUFACTURER	NDC	SIZE	AWP
◆ BRAND			
➤ FLAGYL: Searle	00025-1821-50	50s	$116.81
	00025-1821-31	100s	$229.05
	00025-1821-34	100s ud	$235.14
	00025-1821-51	500s	$1056.17
◆ GENERICS			
Vangard	00615-1577-16	4s	$2.79
Vangard	00615-1577-11	14s	$3.29
Parmed	00349-2383-50	50s	$8.95
Moore,H.L.	00839-6620-04	50s	$10.73
➤ Schein	00364-0687-50	50s	$12.85
Zenith	00172-3007-48	50s	$13.25
Lemmon	00093-0852-53	50s	$18.50
Par	49884-0114-03	50s	$18.75
➤ PROTOSTAT: Ortho Pharm	00062-1571-01	50s	$99.12
Mason Dist	11845-0238-01	100s	$13.98
Martec	52555-0114-01	100s	$16.20
Goldline	00182-1517-01	100s	$24.60
Zenith	00172-3007-60	100s	$25.45
Moore,H.L.	00839-6620-06	100s	$26.18
Qualitest	00603-4641-21	100s	$29.86
Major	00904-2694-60	100s	$29.95
Geneva	00781-1747-01	100s	$29.95
Rugby	00536-4033-01	100s	$30.38
Parmed	00349-2383-01	100s	$30.91
URL	00677-0816-01	100s	$31.50
Mutual	53489-0136-01	100s	$31.50
Sidmak	50111-0334-01	100s	$31.75
Aligen	00405-4678-01	100s	$31.82
Par	49884-0114-01	100s	$33.15
Eon	00185-0555-01	100s	$34.75
Raway	00686-0126-20	100s ud	$18.00
Major	00904-2694-61	100s ud	$39.96
UDL	51079-0126-20	100s ud	$82.94
Vangard	00615-1577-13	100s ud	$85.02
Auro	55829-0365-10	100s ud	$98.03
Goldline	00182-1517-89	100s ud	$104.95
Geneva	00781-1747-13	100s ud	$128.70
Medirex	57480-0433-01	100s ud	$130.00
➤ Schein	00364-0687-90	100s ud	$135.15
Rugby	00536-4033-32	200s	$67.43
Par	49884-0114-04	250s	$80.38
Parmed	00349-2383-05	500s	$93.04
Qualitest	00603-4641-28	500s	$130.11
Sidmak	50111-0334-02	500s	$132.00
Par	49884-0114-05	500s	$160.78
Lemmon	00093-0852-05	500s	$177.75

Metronidazole, Topical

DESCRIPTION

Metronidazole, Topical gel contains Metronidazole, USP, at a concentration of 7.5 mg per gram (0.75%) in a gel. Metronidazole is classified therapeutically as an antiprotozoal and antibacterial agent. Chemically, Metronidazole is named 2-methyl-5-nitro-1*H*-Imidazole-1 -ethanol.

Following is its chemical structure:

CLINICAL PHARMACOLOGY

Bioavailability studies on the topical administration of 1 gram of Metronidazole, Topical to the face (7.5 mg of Metronidazole) of 10 rosacea patients showed a maximum serum concentration of 66 nanograms per milliliter in one patient. This concentration is approximately 100 times less than concentrations afforded by a single 250 mg oral tablet. The serum Metronidazole concentrations were below the detectable limits of the assay at the majority of time points in all patients. Three of the patients had no detectable serum concentrations of Metronidazole at any time point. The mean dose of gel applied during clinical studies was 600 mg which represents 4.5 mg of Metronidazole per application. Therefore, under normal usage levels, the formulation affords minimal serum concentrations of Metronidazole.

The mechanisms by which Metronidazole, Topical acts in reducing inflammatory lesions of rosacea are unknown, but may include an antibacterial and/or an anti-inflammatory effect.

INDICATIONS AND USAGE

Metronidazole, Topical is indicated for topical application in the treatment of inflammatory papules, pustules, and erythema of rosacea.

➤ SHOWN IN PRODUCT IDENTIFICATION GUIDE

CONTRAINDICATIONS

Metronidazole, Topical is contraindicated in individuals with a history of hypersensitivity to Metronidazole, parabens, or other ingredients of the formulations.

PRECAUTIONS

Because of the minimal absorption of Metronidazole and consequently its insignificant plasma concentration after topical administration, the adverse experiences reported with the oral form of the drug have not been reported with Metronidazole, Topical.

GENERAL

Metronidazole, Topical has been reported to cause tearing of the eyes. Therefore, contact with the eyes should be avoided. If a reaction suggesting local irritation occurs, patients should be directed to use the medication less frequently, discontinue use temporarily, or discontinue use until further instructions. Metronidazole is a nitroimidazole and should be used with care in patients with evidence of, or history of, blood dyscrasia.

INFORMATION FOR THE PATIENT

This medication is to be used as directed by the physician. It is for external use only. Avoid contact with the eyes.

DRUG INTERACTIONS

Drug interactions are less likely with topical administration but should be kept in mind when Metronidazole, Topical is prescribed for patients who are receiving anticoagulant treatment. Oral Metronidazole has been reported to potentiate the anticoagulant effect of coumarin and warfarin resulting in a prolongation of prothrombin time.

CARCINOGENESIS

Tumorigenicity in Rats: Metronidazole has shown evidence of carcinogenic activity in a number of studies involving chronic, oral administration in mice and rats but not in studies involving hamsters. These studies have not been conducted with 0.75% Metronidazole gel, which would result in significantly lower systemic blood levels than oral formulations.

MUTAGENICITY STUDIES

Although Metronidazole has shown mutagenic activity in a number of *in vitro* bacterial assay systems, studies in mammals (*in vivo*) have failed to demonstrate a potential for genetic damage.

PREGNANCY

Pregnancy Category B

There has been no experience to date with the use of Metronidazole, Topical in pregnant patients. Metronidazole crosses the placental barrier and enters the fetal circulation rapidly. No fetotoxicity was observed after oral Metronidazole in rats or mice. However, because animal reproduction studies are not always predictive of human response and since oral Metronidazole has been shown to be a carcinogen in some rodents, this drug should be used during pregnancy only if clearly needed.

NURSING MOTHERS

After oral administration, Metronidazole is secreted in breast milk in concentrations similar to those found in the plasma. Even though Metronidazole, Topical blood levels are significantly lower than those achieved after oral Metronidazole, a decision should be made whether to discontinue nursing or to discontinue the drug, taking into account the importance of the drug to the mother.

PEDIATRIC USE

Safety and effectiveness in children have not been established.

ADVERSE REACTIONS

Adverse conditions reported include watery (tearing) eyes if the gel is applied too closely to this area, transient redness, and mild dryness, burning, and skin irritation. None of the side effects exceeded an incidence of 2% of patients.

OVERDOSAGE

There is no human experience with overdosage of Metronidazole, Topical. The acute oral toxicity of the Metronidazole, Topical formulation was determined to be greater than 5 g/kg (the highest dose given) in albino rats.

DOSAGE AND ADMINISTRATION

Apply and rub in a thin film of Metronidazole, Topical twice daily, morning and evening, to entire affected areas after washing. Significant therapeutic results should be noticed within three weeks. Clinical studies have demonstrated continuing improvement through nine weeks of therapy.

Areas to be treated should be cleansed before application of Metronidazole, Topical. Patients may use cosmetics after application of Metronidazole, Topical.

Store at controlled room temperatures: 59° to 86°F; 15° to 30°C.

HOW SUPPLIED
GEL: 0.75%

BRAND/MANUFACTURER	NDC	SIZE	AWP
○ **BRAND**			
METROGEL: Galderma	00299-3835-28	30 gm	$23.00
	00299-3835-45	45 gm	$31.06
METROGEL-VAGINAL: Curatek	55326-0200-25	70 gm	$24.00

Metronidazole, Vaginal

DESCRIPTION

Metronidazole, Vaginal, is the intravaginal dosage form of the synthetic antibacterial agent, Metronidazole, USP at a concentration of 0.75%. Metronidazole is a member of the imidazole class of antibacterial agents and is classified therapeutically as an anti-protozoal and anti-bacterial agent. Chemically, Metronidazole is 2-methyl-5-nitroimidazole-1-ethanol. It has a chemical formula of $C_6H_9N_3O_3$, and a molecular weight of 171.16.

Metronidazole, Vaginal, is a gelled, purified water solution, containing Metronidazole at a concentration of 7.5 mg/g (0.75%). The gel is formulated at pH 4.0. The gel also contains carbomer 934P, edetate disodium, methyl paraben, propyl paraben, propylene glycol, and sodium hydroxide. Each applicator full of 5 grams of vaginal gel contains approximately 37.5 mg of Metronidazole.

Following is its chemical structure:

CLINICAL PHARMACOLOGY

NORMAL SUBJECTS

Following a single, intravaginal 5-gram dose of Metronidazole Vaginal gel (equivalent to 37.5 mg of Metronidazole) to 12 normal subjects, a mean maximum serum Metronidazole concentration of 237 ng/mL was reported (range: 152 to 368 ng/mL). This is approximately 2% of the mean maximum serum Metronidazole concentration reported in the same subjects administered a single, oral 500-mg dose of Metronidazole (mean C_{max}=12,785 ng/mL, range: 10,013 to 17,400 ng/mL). These peak concentrations were obtained in 6 to 12 hours after dosing with Metronidazole, Vaginal, gel and 1 to 3 hours after dosing with oral Metronidazole.

The extent of exposure [area under the curve (A.U.C.)] of metronidazole, when administered as a single intravaginal 5-gram dose of Metronidazole Vaginal, gel (equivalent to 37.5 mg of Metronidazole), was approximately 4% of the A.U.C. of a single oral 500 mg Metronidazole dose (4977 ng-hr/mL and approximately 125,000 ng-hr/mL, respectively). Dose adjusted comparisons of A.U.C.'s demonstrated that, on a mg to mg comparison basis, the absorption of Metronidazole, when administered vaginally, was approximately half that of an equivalent oral dosage.

PATIENTS WITH BACTERIAL VAGINOSIS:

Following single and multiple 5-gram doses of Metronidazole, Vaginal, gel to 4 patients with bacterial vaginosis, a mean maximum serum Metronidazole concentration of 214 ng/mL on day 1 and 294 ng/mL (range: 228 to 349 ng/mL) on day five were reported. Steady state Metronidazole serum concentrations following oral dosages of 400 to 500 mg B.I.D. have been reported to range from 6,000 to 20,000 ng/mL.

MICROBIOLOGY

The intracellular targets of action of Metronidazole on anaerobes are largely unknown. The 5-nitro group of Metronidazole is reduced by metabolically active anaerobes, and studies have demonstrated that the reduced form of the drug interacts with bacterial DNA. However, it is not clear whether interaction with DNA alone is an important component in the bactericidal action of Metronidazole on anaerobic organisms.

Culture and sensitivity testing of bacteria are not routinely performed to establish the diagnosis of bacterial vaginosis. (See *"Indications and Usage"*.)

Standard methodology for the susceptibility testing of the potential bacterial vaginosis pathogens. *Gardnerella vaginalis, Mobiluncus* spp., and *Mycoplasma hominis*, has not been defined. Nonetheless, metronidazole is an antimicrobial agent active *in vitro* against most strains of the following organisms that have been reported to be associated with bacterial vaginosis:

Bacteroides spp.
Gardnerella vaginalis
Mobiluncus spp.
Peptostreptococcus spp.

INDICATIONS AND USAGE

Metronidazole, Vaginal, is indicated in the treatment of bacterial vaginosis (formerly referred to as *Haemophilus* vaginitis, *Gardnerella* vaginitis, nonspecific vaginitis, *Corynebacterium* vaginitis, or anerobic vaginosis).

Note: For purposes of this indication, a clinical diagnosis of bacterial vaginosis is usually defined by the presence of a homogeneous vaginal discharge that (a) has a pH of greater than 4.5 (b) emits a "fishy" amine odor when mixed with a 10% KOH solution, and (c) contains clue cells on microscopic examination. Gram's stain results consistent with a diagnosis of bacterial vaginosis include (a) markedly reduced or absent *Lactobacillus* morphology, (b) predominance of *Gardnerella* morphotype, and (c) absent or few white blood cells. Other pathogens commonly associated with vulvovaginitis, e.g., *Trichomonas vaginalis, Chlamydia trachomatis, N. gonorrhoeae, Candida albicans,* and *Herpes simplex* virus should be ruled out.

◆ RATED THERAPEUTICALLY EQUIVALENT; ◇ THERAPEUTIC EQUIVALENCE UNCONFIRMED; ○ UNRATED

CONTRAINDICATIONS

Metronidazole, Vaginal, is contraindicated in patients with a prior history of hypersensitivity to metronidazole, parabens, other ingredients of the formulation, or other nitroimidazole derivatives.

WARNINGS

CONVULSIVE SEIZURES AND PERIPHERAL NEUROPATHY

Convulsive seizures and peripheral neuropathy, the latter characterized mainly by numbness or paresthesia of an extremity, have been reported in patients treated with oral Metronidazole. The appearance of abnormal neurologic signs demands the prompt discontinuation of Metronidazole, Vaginal, gel therapy. Metronidazole, Vaginal, gel should be administered with caution to patients with central nervous system diseases.

PSYCHOTIC REACTIONS

Psychotic reactions have been reported in alcoholic patients who were using oral Metronidazole and disulfiram concurrently. Metronidazole, Vaginal, gel should not be administered to patients who have taken disulfiram within the last two weeks.

PRECAUTIONS

Metronidazole, Vaginal, affords minimal peak serum levels and systemic exposure (A.U.C.'s) of Metronidazole compared to 500 mg oral metronidazole dosing. Although these lower levels of exposure are less likely to produce the common reactions seen with oral Metronidazole, the possibility of these and other reactions cannot be excluded presently. Data from well-controlled trials directly comparing Metronidazole administered orally to Metronidazole administered vaginally are not available.

GENERAL

Patients with severe hepatic disease metabolize Metronidazole slowly. This results in the accumulation of Metronidazole and its metabolites in the plasma. Accordingly, for such patients, Metronidazole, Vaginal, gel should be administered cautiously.

Known or previously unrecognized vaginal candidiasis may present more prominent symptoms during therapy with Metronidazole Vaginal gel. Approximately 6% of patients treated with Metronidazole, Vaginal developed symptomatic *candida* vaginitis during or immediately after therapy. Disulfiram-like reaction to alcohol has been reported with oral Metronidazole, thus the possibility of such a reaction occurring while on Metronidazole, Vaginal, gel therapy cannot be excluded.

Metronidazole, Vaginal, contains ingredients that may cause burning and irritation of the eye. In the event of accidental contact with the eye, rinse the eye with copious amounts of cool tap water.

INFORMATION FOR THE PATIENT

The patient should be informed not to drink alcohol while being treated with Metronidazole, Vaginal, gel. While blood levels are significantly lower with Metronidazole, Vaginal, than with usual doses of oral Metronidazole, a possible interaction with alcohol cannot be excluded.

The patient should also be instructed not to engage in vaginal intercourse during treatment with this product.

DRUG INTERACTIONS

Oral Metronidazole has been reported to potentiate the anticoagulant effect of warfarin and other coumarin anticoagulants, resulting in a prolongation of prothrombin time. This possible drug interaction should be considered when Metronidazole, Vaginal, gel is prescribed for patients on this type of anticoagulant therapy.

DRUG/LABORATORY TEST INTERACTIONS

Metronidazole may interfere with certain types of determinations of serum chemistry values, such as aspartate aminotransferase (AST, SGOT), alanine aminotransferase (ALT, SGPT), lactate dehydrogenase (LDH), triglycerides, and glucose hexokinase. Values of zero may be observed. All of the assays in which interference has been reported involve enzymatic coupling of the assay to oxidation-reduction of nicotinamide-adenine dinucleotide (NAD+NADH). Interference is due to the similarity in absorbance peaks of NADH (340 nm) and Metronidazole (322 nm) at pH 7.

CARCINOGENESIS, MUTAGENECIS, IMPAIRMENT OF FERTILITY

Metronidazole has shown evidence of carcinogenic activity in a number of studies involving chronic oral administration in mice and rats. Prominent among the effects in the mouse was the promotion of pulmonary tumorigenesis. This has been observed in all six reported studies in that species, including one study in which the animals were dosed on an intermittent schedule (administration during every fourth week only). At very high dose levels (approx. 500 mg/kg/day), there was a statistically significant increase in the incidence of malignant liver tumors in males. Also, the published results of one of the mouse studies indicate an increase in the incidence of malignant lymphomas as well as pulmonary neoplasms associated with lifetime feeding of the drug. All these effects are statistically significant. Several long-term oral dosing studies in the rat have been completed. There were statistically signficant increases in the incidence of various neoplasms, particularly in mammary and hepatic tumors, among female rats administered Metronidazole over those noted in the concurrent female control groups.

Two lifetime tumorigenicity studies in hamsters have been performed and reported to be negative. These studies have not been conducted with 0.75%

Metronidazole Vaginal gel, which would result in significantly lower systemic blood levels than those obtained with oral formulations.

Although Metronidazole has shown mutagenic activity in a number of *in vitro* assay systems, studies in mammals (*in vivo*) have failed to demonstrate a potential for genetic damage.

Fertility studies have been performed in mice up to six times the recommended human vaginal dose (based on mg/m^2) and have revealed no evidence of impaired fertility.

PREGNANCY: TERATOGENIC EFFECTS

Pregnancy Category B: There has been no experience to date with the use of Metronidazole, Vaginal, in pregnant patients. Metronidazole crosses the placental barrier and enters the fetal circulation rapidly. No fetotoxicity or teratogenicity was observed when Metronidazole was administered orally to pregnant mice at six times the recommended human vaginal dose (based on mg/m^2); however, in a single small study where the drug was administered intraperitoneally, some intrauterine deaths were observed. The relationship of these findings to the drug is unknown.

There are, however, no adequate and well-controlled studies in pregnant women. Because animal reproduction studies are not always predictive of human response, and because Metronidazole is a carcinogen in rodents, this drug should be used during pregnancy only if clearly needed.

NURSING MOTHERS

Specific studies of Metronidazole levels in human milk following intravaginally administered metronidazole have not been performed. However, Metronidazole is secreted in human milk in concentrations similar to those found in plasma following oral administration of metronidazole.

Because of the potential for tumorigenicity shown for Metronidazole in mouse and rat studies, a decision should be made whether to discontinue nursing or to discontinue the drug, taking into account the importance of the drug to the mother.

PEDIATRIC USE

Safety and effectiveness in children have not been established.

ADVERSE REACTIONS

CLINICAL TRIALS

There were no deaths or serious adverse events in clinical trials involving 295 patients; however, approximately 1% of non-pregnant patients treated with Metronidazole, Vaginal, discontinued therapy early due to drug-related adverse events. One patient discontinued therapy due to abdominal pain after 2 days of therapy and one patient discontinued therapy due to a severe headache after 5 doses. Similar headaches of uncertain cause had been reported in the past by this patient.

Medical events judged to be related, probably related, or possibly related to administration of Metronidazole, Vaginal, were reported for 50/295 (17%) non-pregnant patients. Unless percentages are otherwise stipulated, the incidence of individual adverse reactions listed below was less than 1%:

Genital tract:
Symptomatic *Candida* cervicitis/vaginitis (6.1%),
Vaginal, perineal, or vulvar itching (1.4%),
Urinary frequency, vaginal or vulvar burning or irritation, vaginal discharge (not *candida*), and vulvar swelling.

Gastrointestinal:
Cramps/pain (abdominal/uterine) (3.4%),
Nausea (2.0%),
Metallic or bad taste (1.7%),
Constipation, decreased appetite, and diarrhea.

Central Nervous System:
Dizziness, headache, and lightheadedness.

Dermatologic:
Rash.

Laboratory:
Incresed/decreased white blood cell counts (1.7%).

OTHER METRONIDAZOLE FORMULATIONS

Other effects that have been reported in association with the use of *topical (dermal)* formulations of Metronidazole include skin irritation, transient skin erythema, and mild skin dryness and burning. None of these adverse events exceeded an incidence of 2% of patients.

Metronidazole, Vaginal affords minimal peak serum levels and systemic exposure (AUC's) of Metronidazole compared to 500 mg oral Metronidazole dosing. Although these lower levels of exposure are less likely to produce the common reactions seen with oral metronidazole, the possibility of these and other reactions cannot be excluded presently. Data from well-controlled trials directly comparing metronidazole administered orally to Metronidazole administered vaginally are not available.

The following adverse reactions and altered laboratory tests have been reported with the *oral or parenteral* use of Metronidazole:

Cardiovascular: Flattening of the T-wave may be seen in electrocardiographic tracings.

Central Nervous System: (See *"Warnings."*) Headache, dizziness, syncope, ataxia, confusion, convulsive seizures, peripheral neuropathy, vertigo, incoordination, irritability, depression, weakness, insomnia.

► SHOWN IN PRODUCT IDENTIFICATION GUIDE

Gastrointestinal: Abdominal discomfort; nausea; vomiting; diarrhea; an unpleasant metallic taste; anorexia; epigastric distress; abdominal cramping; constipation; "furry" tongue glossitis and stomatitis; pancreatitis; modification of taste of alcoholic beverages.

Genitourinary: Overgrowth of *Candida* in the vagina, dyspareunia, decreased libido, proctitis.

Hematopoietic: Reversible neutropenia, reversible thrombocytopenia.

Hypersensitivity Reactions: Urticaria; erythematous rash; flushing; nasal congestion; dryness of the mouth, vagina, or vulva; fever; pruritus; fleeting joint pains.

Renal: Dysuria, cystitis, polyuria, incontinence, a sense of pelvic pressure, darkened urine.

OVERDOSAGE

There is no human experience with overdosage of Metronidazole Vaginal gel. Vaginally applied Metronidazole, 0.75% could be absorbed in sufficient amounts to produce systemic effect. (See *"Warnings."*)

DOSAGE AND ADMINISTRATION

The recommended dose is one applicator full of Metronidazole, Vaginal (approximately 5 grams containing approximately 37.5 mg of Metronidazole) intravaginally twice daily for 5 days. The medication should be applied once in the morning and once in the evening.

Store at controlled room temperature, 15° to 30°C (59° to 86°F). Protect from freezing.

HOW SUPPLIED
GEL: 0.75%

BRAND/MANUFACTURER	NDC	SIZE	AWP
○ **BRAND**			
METROGEL: Galderma	00299-3835-28	30 gm	$23.00
	00299-3835-45	45 gm	$31.06
METROGEL-VAGINAL: Curatek	55326-0200-25	70 gm	$24.00

Metubine Iodide *SEE* METOCURINE IODIDE

Metyrosine

DESCRIPTION

Metyrosine is (-)-α-methyl-L-tyrosine or (α-MPT).

Metyrosine is a white, crystalline compound of molecular weight 195. It is very slightly soluble in water, acetone, and methanol, and insoluble in chloroform and benzene. It is soluble in acidic aqueous solutions. It is also soluble in alkaline aqueous solutions, but is subject to oxidative degradation under these conditions.

Metyrosine is supplied as capsules, for oral administration. Each capsule contains 250 mg Metyrosine.

Following is its chemical structure:

$$HO-\text{C}_6\text{H}_4-CH_2-\underset{\underset{NH_2}{|}}{\overset{\overset{CH_3}{|}}{C}}-COOH$$

CLINICAL PHARMACOLOGY

Metyrosine inhibits tyrosine hydroxylase, which catalyzes the first transformation in catecholamine biosynthesis, i.e., the conversion of tyrosine to dihydroxyphenylalanine (DOPA). Because the first step is also the rate-limiting step, blockade of tyrosine hydroxylase activity results in decreased endogenous levels of catecholamines, usually measured as decreased urinary excretion of catecholamines and their metabolites.

In patients with pheochromocytoma, who produce excessive amounts of norepinephrine and epinephrine, administration of one to four grams of Metyrosine per day has reduced catecholamine biosynthesis from about 35 to 80 percent as measured by the total excretion of catecholamines and their metabolites (metanephrine and vanillylmandelic acid). The maximum biochemical effect usually occurs within two to three days, and the urinary concentration of catecholamines and their metabolites usually returns to pretreatment levels within three to four days after Metyrosine is discontinued. In some patients the total excretion of catecholamines and catecholamine metabolites may be lowered to normal or near normal levels (less than 10 mg/24 hours). In most patients the duration of treatment has been two to eight weeks, but several patients have received Metyrosine for periods of one to 10 years.

Most patients with pheochromocytoma treated with Metyrosine experience decreased frequency and severity of hypertensive attacks with their associated headache, nausea, sweating, and tachycardia. In patients who respond, blood pressure decreases progressively during the first two days of therapy with Metyrosine after withdrawal, blood pressure usually increases gradually to pretreatment values within two to three days.

Metyrosine is well absorbed from the gastrointestinal tract. From 53 to 88 percent (mean 69 percent) was recovered in the urine as unchanged drug following maintenance oral doses of 600 to 4000 mg/24 hours in patients with pheochromocytoma or essential hypertension. Less than 1% of the dose was recovered as catechol metabolites. These metabolites are probably not present in sufficient amounts to contribute to the biochemical effects of Metyrosine. The quantities excreted, however, are sufficient to interfere with accurate determination of urinary catecholamines determined by routine techniques.

Plasma half-life of Metyrosine determined over an 8-hour period after single oral doses was 3.4-3.7 hours in three patients.

For further information, refer to: Sjoersdma, A.: Engelman, K.: Waldman, T. A.: Cooperman, L. H.: Hammond, W. G.: *Pheochromocytoma: Current concepts of diagnosis and treatment.* Ann. Intern. Med. 65:1302-1326, Dec. 1966.

INDICATIONS AND USAGE

Metyrosine is indicated in the treatment of patients with pheochromocytoma for:

1. Preoperative preparation of patients for surgery
2. Management of patients when surgery is contraindicated
3. Chronic treatment of patients with malignant pheochromocytoma.

Metyrosine is not recommended for the control of essential hypertension.

CONTRAINDICATIONS

Metyrosine is contraindicated in persons known to be hypersensitive to this compound.

WARNINGS

Maintain Fluid Volume During and After Surgery: When Metyrosine is used preoperatively, alone or especially in combination with alpha-adrenergic blocking drugs, adequate intravascular volume must be maintained intraoperatively (especially after tumor removal) and postoperatively to avoid hypotension and decreased perfusion of vital organs resulting from vasodilatation and expanded volume capacity. Following tumor removal, large volumes of plasma may be needed to maintain blood pressure and central venous pressure within the normal range.

In addition, life-threatening arrhythmias may occur during anesthesia and surgery, and may require treatment with a beta blocker or lidocaine. During surgery, patients should have continuous monitoring of blood pressure and electrocardiogram.

Intraoperative Effects: While the preoperative use of Metyrosine in patients with pheochromocytoma is thought to decrease intraoperative problems with blood pressure control, Metyrosine does not eliminate the danger of hypertensive crises or arrhythmias during manipulation of the tumor, and the alpha-adrenergic blocking drug, phentolamine, may be needed.

Interaction with Alcohol: Metyrosine may add to the sedative effects of alcohol and other CNS depressants, e.g., hypnotics, sedatives, and tranquilizers. (See *"Precautions, Information for Patients"* and *"Drug Interactions".*)

PRECAUTIONS

General: **Metyrosine Crystalluria:** Crystalluria and urolithiasis have been found in dogs treated with Metyrosine at doses similar to those used in humans, and crystalluria has also been observed in a few patients. To minimize the risk of crystalluria, patients should be urged to maintain water intake sufficient to achieve a daily urine volume of 2000 mL or more, particularly when doses greater than 2 g per day are given. Routine examination of the urine should be carried out. Metyrosine will crystallize as needles or rods. If Metyrosine crystalluria occurs, fluid intake should be increased further. If crystalluria persists, the dosage should be reduced or the drug discontinued.

Relatively Little Data Regarding Long-term Use: The total human experience with the drug is quite limited and few patients have been studied long-term. Chronic animal studies have not been carried out. Therefore, suitable laboratory tests should be carried out periodically in patients requiring prolonged use of Metyrosine and caution should be observed in patients with impaired hepatic or renal function.

Information for Patients: When receiving Metyrosine patients should be warned about engaging in activities requiring mental alertness and motor coordination, such as driving a motor vehicle or operating machinery. Metyrosine may have additive sedative effects with alcohol and other CNS depressants, e.g., hypnotics, sedatives, and tranquilizers.

Patients should be advised to maintain a liberal fluid intake. (See *"Precautions, General".*)

Drug Interactions: Caution should be observed in administering Metyrosine to patients receiving phenothiazines or haloperidol because the extrapyramidal effects of these drugs can be expected to be potentiated by inhibition of catecholamine synthesis.

Concurrent use of Metyrosine with alcohol or other CNS depressants can increase their sedative effects. (See *"Warnings"* and *"Precautions, Information for Patients".*)

Laboratory Test Interference: Spurious increases in urinary catecholamines may be observed in patients receiving Metyrosine due to the presence of metabolites of the drug.

Carcinogenesis, Mutagenesis, Impairment of Fertility: Long-term carcinogenic studies in animals and studies on mutagenesis and impairment of fertility have not been performed with Metyrosine.

Pregnancy: Pregnancy Category C: Animal reproduction studies have not been conducted with Metyrosine. It is also not known whether Metyrosine can cause fetal harm when administered to a pregnant woman or can affect reproduction capacity. Metyrosine should be given to a pregnant woman only if clearly needed.

Nursing Mothers: It is not known whether Metyrosine is excreted in human milk. Because many drugs are excreted in human milk, caution should be exercised when Metyrosine is administered to a nursing woman.

Pediatric Use: Safety and effectiveness in children under 12 years of age have not been established.

ADVERSE REACTIONS
CENTRAL NERVOUS SYSTEM
Sedation: The most common adverse reaction to Metyrosine is moderate to severe sedation, which has been observed in almost all patients. It occurs at both low and high dosages. Sedative effects begin within the first 24 hours of therapy, are maximal after two to three days, and tend to wane during the next few days. Sedation usually is not obvious after one week unless the dosage is increased, but at dosages greater than 2000 mg/day some degree of sedation or fatigue may persist.

In most patients who experience sedation, temporary changes in sleep pattern occur following withdrawal of the drug. Changes consist of insomnia that may last for two or three days and feelings of increased alertness and ambition. Even patients who do not experience sedation while on Metyrosine may report symptoms of psychic stimulation when the drug is discontinued.

Extrapyramidal Signs: Extrapyramidal signs such as drooling, speech difficulty, and tremor have been reported in approximately 10 percent of patients. These occasionally have been accompanied by trismus and frank parkinsonism.

Anxiety and Psychic Disturbances: Anxiety and psychic disturbances such as depression, hallucinations, disorientation, and confusion may occur. These effects seem to be dose-dependent and may disappear with reduction of dosage.

DIARRHEA
Diarrhea occurs in about 10 percent of patients and may be severe. Antidiarrheal agents may be required if continuation of Metyrosine is necessary.

MISCELLANEOUS
Infrequently, slight swelling of the breast, galactorrhea, nasal stuffiness, decreased salivation, dry mouth, headache, nausea, vomiting, abdominal pain and impotence or failure of ejaculation may occur. Crystalluria (see *"Precautions"*) and transient dysuria and hematuria have been observed in a few patients. Hematologic disorders (including eosinophilia, anemia, thrombocytopenia, and thrombocytosis), increased SGOT levels, peripheral edema, and hypersensitivity reactions such as urticaria and pharyngeal edema have been reported rarely.

OVERDOSAGE
Signs of Metyrosine overdosage include those central nervous system effects observed in some patients even at low dosages.

At doses exceeding 2000 mg/day, some degree of sedation or feeling of fatigue may persist. Doses of 2000-4000 mg/day can result in anxiety or agitated depression, neuromuscular effects (including fine tremor of the hands, gross tremor of the trunk, tightening of the jaw with trismus), diarrhea, and decreased salivation with dry mouth.

Reduction of drug dose or cessation of treatment results in the disappearance of these symptoms.

The acute toxicity of Metyrosine was 442 mg/kg and 752 mg/kg in the female mouse and rat respectively.

DOSAGE AND ADMINISTRATION
The recommended initial dosage of Metyrosine for adults and children 12 years of age and older is 250 mg orally four times daily. This may be increased by 250 mg to 500 mg every day to a maximum of 4.0 g/day in divided doses. When used for preoperative preparation, the optimally effective dosage of Metyrosine should be given for at least five to seven days. Optimally effective dosages of Metyrosine usually are between 2.0 and 3.0 g/day, and the dose should be titrated by monitoring clinical symptoms and catecholamine excretion. In patients who are hypertensive, dosage should be titrated to achieve normalization of blood pressure and control of clinical symptoms. In patients who are usually normotensive, dosage should be titrated to the amount that will reduce urinary metanephrines and/or vanillylmandelic acid by 50 percent or more.

If patients are not adequately controlled by the use of Metyrosine, an alpha-adrenergic blocking agent (phenoxybenzamine) should be added.

Use of Metyrosine in children under 12 years of age has been limited and a dosage schedule for this age group cannot be given.

HOW SUPPLIED
CAPSULE: 250 MG

BRAND/MANUFACTURER	NDC	SIZE	AWP
○ **BRAND**			
DEMSER: Merck	00006-0690-68	100s	$137.94

Mevacor *SEE* LOVASTATIN

Mexiletine Hydrochloride

DESCRIPTION
Mexiletine Hydrochloride is an orally active antiarrhythmic agent available as 150 mg, 200 mg and 250 mg capsules. 100 mg of Mexiletine Hydrochloride is equivalent to 83.31 mg of Mexiletine base. It is a white to off-white crystalline powder with a slightly bitter taste, freely soluble in water and in alcohol. Mexiletine Hydrochloride has a pKa of 9.2.

Chemically, Mexiletine Hydrochloride is 1-methyl-2-(2,6-xylyloxy)-ethylamine hydrochloride. Its molecular formula is $C_{11}H_{17}NO \cdot HCl$ and molecular weight is 215.73.

Following is its chemical structure:

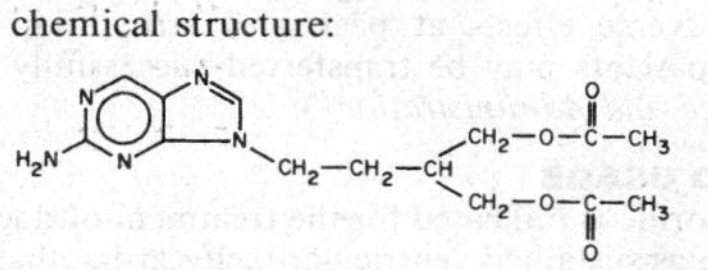

CLINICAL PHARMACOLOGY
Mechanism of Action: Mexiletine Hydrochoride is a local anesthetic, antiarrhythmic agent, structurally similar to lidocaine, but orally active. In animal studies, Mexiletine Hydrochloride has been shown to be effective in the suppression of induced ventricular arrhythmias, including those induced by glycoside toxicity and coronary artery ligation. Mexiletine Hydrochloride, like lidocaine, inhibits the inward sodium current, thus reducing the rate of rise of the action potential, Phase 0. Mexiletine Hydrochloride decreased the effective refractory period (ERP) in Purkinje fibers. The decrease in ERP was of lesser magnitude than the decrease in action potential duration (APD), with a resulting increase in the ERP/APD ratio.

Electrophysiology in Man: Mexiletine Hydrochloride is a Class IB antiarrhythmic compound with electrophysiologic properties in man similar to those of lidocaine, but dissimilar from quinidine, procainamide, and disopyramide.

In patients with normal conduction systems, Mexiletine Hydrochloride has a minimal effect on cardiac impulse generation and propagation. In clinical trials, no development of second-degree or third-degree AV block was observed. Mexiletine Hydrochloride did not prolong ventricular depolarization (QRS duration) or repolarization (QT intervals) as measured by electrocardiography. Theoretically, therefore, Mexiletine Hydrochloride may be useful in the treatment of ventricular arrhythmias associated with a prolonged QT interval.

In patients with pre-existing conduction defects, depression of the sinus rate, prolongation of sinus node recovery time, decreased conduction velocity and increased effective refractory period of the intraventricular conduction system have occasionally been observed.

The antiarrhythmic effect of Mexiletine Hydrochloride has been established in controlled comparative trials against placebo, quinidine, procainamide and disopyramide. Mexiletine Hydrochloride, at doses of 200-400 mg q8h, produced a significant reduction of ventricular premature beats, paired beats, and episodes of non-sustained ventricular tachycardia compared to placebo and was similar in effectiveness to the active agents. Among all patients entered into the studies, about 30% in each treatment group had a 70% or greater reduction in PVC count and about 40% failed to complete the three-month studies because of adverse effects. Follow-up of patients from the controlled trials has demonstrated continued effectiveness of Mexiletine Hydrochloride in long-term use.

Hemodynamics: Hemodynamic studies in a limited number of patients, with normal or abnormal myocardial function, following oral administration of Mexiletine Hydrochloride, have shown small, not statistically significant, decreases in cardiac output and increases in systemic vascular resistance, but no significant negative inotropic effect. Blood pressure and pulse rate remain essentially unchanged. Mild depression of myocardial function, similar to that produced by lidocaine, has occasionally been observed following intravenous Mexiletine Hydrochloride therapy in patients with cardiac disease.

Pharmacokinetics: Mexiletine Hydrochloride is well absorbed (~ 90%) from the gastrointestinal tract. Unlike lidocaine, its first-pass metabolism is low. Peak blood levels are reached in two to three hours. In normal subjects, the plasma elimination half-life of Mexiletine Hydrochloride is approximately 10-12 hours. It is 50-60% bound to plasma protein, with a volume of distribution of 5-7 liters/kg. Mexiletine Hydrochloride is metabolized in the liver. Approximately 10% is excreted unchanged by the kidney. While urinary pH does not normally have much influence on elimination, marked changes in urinary pH influence the rate of excretion: acidification accelerates excretion, while alkalinization retards it.

Several metabolites of Mexiletine have shown minimal antiarrhythmic activity in animal models. The most active is the minor metabolite N-methylmexiletine, which is less than 20% as potent as Mexiletine. The urinary excretion of N-methylmexiletine in man is less than 0.5%. Thus the therapeutic activity of Mexiletine Hydrochloride is due to the parent compound.

Hepatic impairment prolongs the elimination half-life of Mexiletine Hydrochloride. In eight patients with moderate to severe liver disease, the mean half-life was approximately 25 hours.

Consistent with the limited renal elimination of Mexiletine Hydrochloride, little change in the half-life has been detected in patients with reduced renal function. In eight patients with creatinine clearance less than 10 ml/min, the mean plasma elimination half-life was 15.7 hours; in seven patients with creatinine clearance between 11-40 ml/min, the mean half-life was 13.4 hours.

The absorption rate of Mexiletine Hydrochloride is reduced in clinical situations such as acute myocardial infarction in which gastric emptying time is increased. Narcotics, atropine and magnesium-aluminum hydroxide have also been reported to slow the absorption of Mexiletine Hydrochloride. Metoclopramide has been reported to accelerate absorption.

Mexiletine plasma levels of at least 0.5 mcg/ml are generally required for therapeutic response. An increase in the frequency of central nervous system adverse effects has been observed when plasma levels exceed 2.0 mcg/ml. Thus the therapeutic range is approximately 0.5 to 2.0 mcg/ml. Plasma levels within the therapeutic range can be attained with either three times daily or twice daily dosing but peak to trough differences are greater with the latter regimen, creating the possibility of adverse effects at peak and arrhythmic escape at trough. Nevertheless, some patients may be transferred successfully to the twice daily regimen (see *"Dosage and Administration"*).

INDICATIONS AND USAGE

Mexiletine Hydrochloride is indicated for the treatment of documented ventricular arrhythmias, such as sustained ventricular tachycardia, that, in the judgement of the physician, are life-threatening. Because of the proarrhythmic effects of Mexiletine Hydrochloride, its use with lesser arrhythmias is generally not recommended. Treatment of patients with asymptomatic ventricular premature contractions should be avoided.

Initiation of Mexiletine Hydrochloride treatment, as with other antiarrhythmic agents used to treat life-threatening arrhythmias, should be carried out in the hospital.

Antiarrhythmic drugs have not been shown to enhance survival in patients with ventricular arrhythmias.

UNLABELED USES

Mexiletine Hydrochloride is used alone or as an adjunct in the treatment of supraventricular tachycardia, diabetic neuropathy, and arrhythmias complicating acute myocardial infarction. It is also used as an adjunct in Wolf-Parkinson-White syndrome.

CONTRAINDICATIONS

Mexiletine Hydrochloride is contraindicated in the presence of cardiogenic shock or pre-existing second- or third-degree AV block (if no pacemaker is present).

WARNINGS

Mortality: In the National Heart, Lung and Blood Institute's Cardiac Arrhythmia Suppression Trial (CAST), a long-term, multicentered, randomized, double-blind study in patients with asymptomatic non-life-threatening ventricular arrhythmias who had had myocardial infarctions more than six days but less than two years previously, an excessive mortality or non-fatal cardiac arrest rate was seen in patients treated with encainide or flecainide (56/730) compared with that seen in patients assigned to matched placebo-treated groups (22/725). The average duration of treatment with encainide or flecainide in this study was ten months.

The applicability of these results to other populations (e.g., those without recent myocardial infarction) or to other antiarrhythmic drugs is uncertain, but at present it is prudent to consider any antiarrhythmic agent to have a significant risk in patients with structural heart disease.

Acute Liver Injury: In postmarketing experience abnormal liver function tests have been reported, some in the first few weeks of therapy with Mexiletine Hydrochloride. Most of these have been observed in the setting of congestive heart failure or ischemia and their relationship to Mexiletine Hydrochloride has not been established.

PRECAUTIONS

General: If a ventricular pacemaker is operative, patients with second or third degree heart block may be treated with Mexiletine Hydrochloride if continuously monitored. A limited number of patients (45 of 475 in controlled clinical trials) with pre-existing first degree AV block were treated with Mexiletine Hydrochloride; none of these patients developed second or third degree AV block. Caution should be exercised when it is used in such patients or in patients with pre-existing sinus node dysfunction or intraventricular conduction abnormalities.

Like other antiarrhythmics Mexiletine Hydrochloride can cause worsening of arrhythmias. This has been uncommon in patients with less serious arrhythmias (frequent premature beats or non-sustained ventricular tachycardia: (see *"Adverse Reactions"*), but is of greater concern in patients with life-threatening arrhythmias such as sustained ventricular tachycardia. In patients with such arrhythmias subjected to programmed electrical stimulation or to exercise provocation, 10-15% of patients had exacerbation of the arrhythmia, a rate not greater than that of other agents.

Mexiletine Hydrochloride should be used with caution in patients with hypotension and severe congestive heart failure because of the potential for aggravating these conditions.

Since Mexiletine Hydrochloride is metabolized in the liver, and hepatic impairment has been reported to prolong the elimination half-life of Mexiletine Hydrochloride, patients with liver disease should be followed carefully while receiving Mexiletine Hydrochloride. The same caution should be observed in patients with hepatic dysfunction secondary to congestive heart failure.

Concurrent drug therapy or dietary regimens which may markedly alter urinary pH should be avoided during Mexiletine Hydrochloride therapy. The minor fluctuations in urinary pH associated with normal diet do not affect the excretion of Mexiletine Hydrochloride.

SGOT Elevation and Liver Injury: In three-month controlled trials, elevations of SGOT greater than three times the upper limit of normal occurred in about 1% of

both Mexiletine-treated and control patients. Approximately 2% of patients in the Mexiletine compassionate use program had elevations of SGOT greater than or equal to three times the upper limit of normal. These elevations frequently occurred in association with identifiable clinical events and therapeutic measures such as congestive heart failure, acute myocardial infarction, blood transfusions and other medications. These elevations were often asymptomatic and transient, usually not associated with elevated bilirubin levels and usually did not require discontinuation of therapy. Marked elevations of SGOT (> 1000 U/L) were seen before death in four patients with end-stage cardiac disease (severe congestive heart failure, cardiogenic shock).

Rare instances of severe liver injury, including hepatic necrosis, have been reported in association with Mexiletine Hydrochloride treatment. It is recommended that patients in whom an abnormal liver test has occurred, or who have signs or symptoms suggesting liver dysfunction, be carefully evaluated. If persistent or worsening elevation of hepatic enzymes is detected, consideration should be given to discontinuing therapy.

Blood Dyscrasias: Among 10,867 patients treated with Mexiletine in the compassionate use program, marked leukopenia (neutrophils less than 1000/mm^3) or agranulocytosis were seen in 0.06%, and milder depressions of leukocytes were seen in 0.08%, and thrombocytopenia was observed in 0.16%. Many of these patients were seriously ill and receiving concomitant medications with known hematologic adverse effects. Rechallenge with Mexiletine in several cases was negative. Marked leukopenia or agranulocytosis did not occur in any patient receiving Mexiletine Hydrochloride alone; five of the six cases of agranulocytosis were associated with procainamide (sustained release preparations in four) and one with vinblastine. If significant hematologic changes are observed, the patient should be carefully evaluated, and, if warranted, Mexiletine Hydrochloride should be discontinued. Blood counts usually return to normal within one month of discontinuation. (See *"Adverse Reactions"*.)

Convulsions (seizures) did not occur in Mexiletine Hydrochloride controlled clinical trials. In the compassionate use program, convulsions were reported in about 2 of 1000 patients. Twenty-eight percent of these patients discontinued therapy. Convulsions were reported in patients with and without a prior history of seizures. Mexiletine should be used with caution in patients with known seizure disorder.

Drug Interactions: In a large compassionate use program Mexiletine Hydrochloride has been used concurrently with commonly employed antianginal, antihypertensive, and anticoagulant drugs without observed interactions. A variety of antiarrhythmics such as quinidine or propranolol were also added, sometimes with improved control of ventricular ectopy. When phenytoin or other hepatic enzyme inducers such as rifampin and phenobarbital have been taken concurrently with Mexiletine Hydrochloride, lowered Mexiletine Hydrochloride plasma levels have been reported. Monitoring of Mexiletine Hydrochloride plasma levels is recommended during such concurrent use to avoid ineffective therapy.

In a formal study, benzodiazepines were shown not to affect Mexiletine Hydrochloride plasma concentrations. ECG intervals (PR, QRS and QT) were not affected by concurrent Mexiletine Hydrochloride and digoxin, diuretics, or propranolol.

Concurrent administration of cimetidine and Mexiletine Hydrochloride has been reported to increase, decrease, or leave unchanged Mexiletine Hydrochloride plasma levels; therefore patients should be followed carefully during concurrent therapy.

Mexiletine Hydrochloride does not alter serum digoxin levels, but magnesium-aluminum hydroxide, when used to treat gastrointestinal symptoms due to Mexiletine Hydrochloride has been reported to lower serum digoxin levels.

Concurrent use of Mexiletine Hydrochloride and theophylline may lead to increased plasma theophylline levels. One controlled study in eight normal subjects showed a 72% mean increase (range 35-136%) in plasma theophylline levels. This increase was observed at the first test point which was the second day after starting Mexiletine Hydrochloride. Theophylline plasma levels returned to pre-Mexiletine Hydrochloride values within 48 hours after discontinuing Mexiletine Hydrochloride. If Mexiletine Hydrochloride and theophylline are to be used concurrently, theophylline blood levels should be monitored, particularly when the Mexiletine Hydrochloride dose is changed. An appropriate adjustment in theophylline dose should be considered.

Additionally, in one controlled study in five normal subjects and seven patients, the clearance of caffeine was decreased 50% following the administration of Mexiletine Hydrochloride.

Carcinogenesis, Mutagenesis and Impairment of Fertility: Studies of carcinogenesis in rats (24 months) and mice (18 months) did not demonstrate any tumorigenic potential. Mexiletine Hydrochloride was found to be non-mutagenic in the Ames test. Mexiletine Hydrochloride did not impair fertility in the rat.

Pregnancy/Teratogenic Effects: Pregnancy Category C: Reproduction studies performed with Mexiletine Hydrochloride in rats, mice and rabbits at doses up to four times the maximum human oral dose (24 mg/kg in a 50 kg patient) revealed no evidence of teratogenicity or impaired fertility but did show an increase in fetal resorption. There are no adequate and well-controlled studies in pregnant women; this drug should be used in pregnancy only if the potential benefit justifies the potential risk to the fetus.

Nursing Mothers: Mexiletine Hydrochloride appears in human milk in concentrations similar to those observed in plasma. Therefore, if the use of Mexiletine Hydrochloride is deemed essential, an alternative method of infant feeding should be considered.

Pediatric Use: Safety and effectiveness in children have not been established.

ADVERSE REACTIONS

Mexiletine Hydrochloride commonly produces reversible gastrointestinal and nervous system adverse reactions but is otherwise well tolerated. Mexiletine Hydrochloride has been evaluated in 483 patients in one-month and three-month controlled studies and in over 10,000 patients in a large compassionate use program. Dosages in the controlled studies ranged from 600-1200 mg/day; some patients (8%) in the compassionate use program were treated with higher daily doses (1600-3200 mg/day). In the three-month controlled trials comparing Mexiletine Hydrochloride to quinidine, procainamide and disopyramide, the most frequent adverse reactions were upper gastrointestinal distress (41%), lightheadedness (10.5%), tremor (12.6%) and coordination difficulties (10.2%). Similar frequency and incidence were observed in the one-month placebo-controlled trial. Although these reactions were generally not serious, and were dose-related and reversible with a reduction in dosage, by taking the drug with food or antacid or by therapy discontinuation, they led to therapy discontinuation in 40% of patients in the controlled trials. A tabulation of the adverse events reported in the one-month placebo-controlled trial follows:

COMPARATIVE INCIDENCE (%) OF ADVERSE EVENTS AMONG PATIENTS TREATED WITH MEXILETINE AND PLACEBO IN THE 4-WEEK, DOUBLE-BLIND CROSSOVER TRIAL

	Mexiletine N = 53	Placebo N = 49
Cardiovascular		
Palpitations	7.5	10.2
Chest Pain	7.5	4.1
Increased Ventricular Arrhythmias/PVCs	1.9	—
Digestive		
Nausea/Vomiting/ Heartburn	39.6	6.1
Central Nervous System		
Dizziness/Light-headedness	26.4	14.3
Tremor	13.2	—
Nervousness	11.3	6.1
Coordination Difficulties	9.4	—
Changes in Sleep Habits	7.5	16.3
Paresthesias/Numbness	3.8	2.0
Weakness	1.9	4.1
Fatigue	1.9	2.0
Tinnitus	1.9	4.1
Confusion/Clouded Sensorium	1.9	2.0
Other		
Headache	7.5	6.1
Blurred Vision/ Visual/Disturbances	7.5	2.0
Dyspnea/Respiratory	5.7	10.2
Rash	3.8	2.0
Non-specific Edema	3.8	—

A tabulation of adverse reactions occurring in one percent or more of patients in the three-month controlled studies follows: (See related table).

Less than 1%: Syncope, edema, hot flashes, hypertension, short-term memory loss, loss of consciousness, other psychological changes, diaphoresis, urinary hestancy/retention, malaise, impotence/decreased libido, pharyngitis, congestive heart failure.

An additional group of over 10,000 patients has been treated in a program allowing administration of Mexiletine Hydrochloride under compassionate use circumstances. These patients were seriously ill with the large majority on multiple drug therapy. Twenty-four percent of the patients continued in the program for one year or longer. Adverse reactions leading to therapy discontinuation occurred in 15 percent of patients (usually upper gastrointestinal system or nervous system effects). In general, the more common adverse reactions were similar to those in the controlled trials. Less common adverse events possibly related to Mexiletine Hydrochloride use include:

Cardiovascular System: Syncope and hypotension, each about 6 in 1000; bradycardia, about 4 in 1000; angina/angina-like pain, about 3 in 1000; edema, atrioventricular block/conduction disturbances and hot flashes, each about 2 in 1000; atrial arrhythmias, hypertension and cardiogenic shock, each about 1 in 1000.

Central Nervous System: Short-term memory loss, about 9 in 1000 patients; hallucinations and other psychological changes, each about 3 in 1000; psychosis and convulsions/seizures, each about 2 in 1000; loss of consciousness, about 6 in 10,000.

Digestive: Dysphagia, about 2 in 1000; peptic ulcer, about 8 in 10,000; upper gastrointestinal bleeding, about 7 in 10,000; esophageal ulceration, about 1 in 10,000. Rare cases of severe hepatitis/acute hepatic necrosis.

Skin: Rare cases of exfoliative dermatitis and Stevens-Johnson Syndrome with Mexiletine Hydrochloride treatment have been reported.

Laboratory: Abnormal liver function tests, about 5 in 1000 patients; positive ANA and thrombocytopenia, each about 2 in 1000; leukopenia (including neutropenia and agranulocytosis), about 1 in 1000; myelofibrosis, about 2 in 10,000 patients.

Other: Diaphoresis, about 6 in 1000; altered taste, about 5 in 1000; salivary changes, hair loss and impotence/decreased libido, each about 4 in 1000; malaise, about 3 in 1000; urinary hesitancy/retention, each about 2 in 1000; hiccups, dry skin, laryngeal and pharyngeal changes and changes in oral mucous membranes, each about 1 in 1000; SLE syndrome, about 4 in 10,000.

Hematology: Blood dyscrasias were not seen in the controlled trials but did occur among the 10,867 patients treated with Mexiletine in the compassionate use program (see "Precautions").

Myelofibrosis was reported in two patients in the compassionate use program: one was receiving long-term thiotepa therapy and the other had pretreatment myeloid abnormalities.

In postmarketing experience, there have been isolated, spontaneous reports of pulmonary changes including pulmonary fibrosis during Mexiletine Hydrochloride therapy with or without other drugs or diseases that are known to produce pulmonary toxicity. A causal relationship to Mexiletine Hydrochloride therapy has not been established. In addition, there have been isolated reports of exacerbation of congestive heart failure in patients with preexisting compromised ventricular function.

OVERDOSAGE

Nine cases of Mexiletine Hydrochloride overdosage have been reported; two were fatal. In one fatality, 4400 mg of the drug was ingested. In the other death, the dose ingested was unknown. There has been a report of non-fatal ingestion of 8000 mg. Symptoms associated with overdosage include nausea, hypotension, sinus bradycardia, paresthesia, seizures, intermittent left bundle branch block and temporary asystole.

There is no specific antidote for Mexiletine Hydrochloride. Acidification of the urine, which will accelerate the excretion of Mexiletine, may be useful. Treatment of overdosage should be supportive, and may include the administration of atropine if hypotension or bradycardia occurs.

DOSAGE AND ADMINISTRATION

The dosage of Mexiletine Hydrochloride must be individualized on the basis of response and tolerance, both of which are dose-related. Administration with food or antacid is recommended. Initiate Mexiletine Hydrochloride therapy with 200 mg every eight hours when rapid control of arrhythmia is not essential A minimum of two to three days between dose adjustments is recommended. Dose may be adjusted in 50 or 100 mg increments up or down.

As with any antiarrhythmic drug, clinical and electrocardiographic evaluation (including Holter monitoring if necessary for evaluation) are needed to determine whether the desired antiarrhythmic effect has been obtained and to guide titration and dose adjustment.

Satisfactory control can be achieved in most patients by 200 to 300 mg given every eight hours with food or antacid. If satisfactory response has not been achieved at 300 mg q8h, and the patient tolerates Mexiletine Hydrochloride well, a dose of 400 mg q8h may be tried. As the severity of CNS side effects increase with total daily dose, the dose should not exceed 1200 mg/day.

In general, patients with renal failure will require the usual doses of Mexiletine Hydrochloride. Patients with severe liver disease, however, may require lower doses and must be monitored closely. Similarly, marked right-sided congestive heart failure can reduce hepatic metabolism and reduce the needed dose. Plasma level may also be affected by certain concomitant drugs (see "Precautions: Drug Interactions").

Loading Dose: When rapid control of ventricular arrhythmia is essential, an initial loading dose of 400 mg of Mexiletine Hydrochloride may be administered, followed by a 200 mg dose in eight hours. Onset of therapeutic effect is usually observed within 30 minutes to two hours.

Q12H Dosage Schedule: Some patients responding to Mexiletine Hydrochloride may be transferred to a 12-hour dosage schedule to improve convenience and compliance. If adequate suppression is achieved on a Mexiletine Hydrochloride dose of 300 mg or less every eight hours, the same total daily dose may be given in divided doses every 12 hours while carefully monitoring the degree of suppression of ventricular ectopy. This dose may be adjusted up to a maximum of 450 mg every 12 hours to achieve the desired response.

Transferring to Mexiletine Hydrochloride: The following dosage schedule based on theoretical considerations rather than experimental data, is suggested for transferring patients from other Class I oral antiarrhythmic agents to Mexiletine Hydrochloride: Mexiletine Hydrochloride treatment may be initiated with a 200 mg dose, and titrated to response as described above, 6-12 hours after the last dose of quinidine sulfate, 3-6 hours after the last dose of procainamide, 6-12 hours after the last dose of disopyramide or 8-12 hours after the last dose of tocainide.

In patients in whom withdrawal of the previous antiarrhythmic agent is likely to produce life-threatening arrhythmias, hospitalization of the patient is recommended.

When transferring from lidocaine to Mexiletine Hydrochloride, the lidocaine infusion should be stopped when the first oral dose of Mexiletine Hydrochloride is administered. The infusion line should be left open until suppression of the arrhythmia appears to be satisfactorily maintained. Consideration should be given to the similarity of the adverse effects of lidocaine and Mexiletine Hydrochloride and the possibility that they may be additive.

Storage: Store below 86°F (30°C).

COMPARATIVE INCIDENCE (%) OF ADVERSE EVENTS AMONG PATIENTS TREATED WITH MEXILETINE OR CONTROL DRUGS IN THE 12-WEEK DOUBLE-BLIND TRIALS

	Mexiletine N = 430	Quinidine N = 262	Procainamide N = 78	Disopyramide N = 69
Cardiovascular				
Palpitations	4.3	4.6	1.3	5.8
Chest Pain	2.6	3.4	1.3	2.9
Angina/Angina-like Pain	1.7	1.9	2.6	2.9
Increased Ventricular Arrhythmias/PVCs	1.0	2.7	2.6	
Digestive				
Nausea/Vomiting/Heartburn	39.3	21.4	33.3	14.5
Diarrhea	5.2	33.2	2.6	8.7
Constipation	4.0	—	6.4	11.6
Changes in Appetite	2.6	1.9		
Abdominal Pain/Cramps/Discomfort	1.2	1.5	—	1.4
Central Nervous System				
Dizziness/Light-headedness	18.9	14.1	14.1	2.9
Tremor	13.2	2.3	3.8	1.4
Coordination Difficulties	9.7	1.1	1.3	—
Changes in Sleep Habits	7.1	2.7	11.5	8.7
Weakness	5.0	5.3	7.7	2.9
Nervousness	5.0	1.9	6.4	5.8
Fatigue	3.8	5.7	5.1	1.4
Speech Difficulties Confusion/Clouded Sensorium	2.6	—	3.8	—
Paresthesias/Numbness	2.4	2.3	2.6	—
Tinnitus	2.4	1.5	—	—
Depression	2.4	1.1	1.3	1.4
Other				
Blurred Vision/Visual Disturbances	5.7	3.1	5.1	7.2
Headache	5.7	6.9	7.7	4.3
Rash	4.2	3.8	10.3	1.4
Dyspnea/Respiratory	3.3	3.1	5.1	2.9
Dry Mouth	2.8	1.9	5.1	14.5
Arthralgia	1.7	2.3	5.1	1.4
Fever	1.2	3.1	2.6	—

HOW SUPPLIED
CAPSULE: 150 MG

BRAND/MANUFACTURER	NDC	SIZE	AWP
○ BRAND			
MEXITIL: Boehr Ingelheim	00597-0066-01	100s	$73.73
	00597-0066-61	100s ud	$77.41

CAPSULE: 200 MG

BRAND/MANUFACTURER	NDC	SIZE	AWP
○ BRAND			
MEXITIL: Boehr Ingelheim	00597-0067-01	100s	$87.94
	00597-0067-61	100s ud	$92.30

CAPSULE: 250 MG

BRAND/MANUFACTURER	NDC	SIZE	AWP
○ BRAND			
MEXITIL: Boehr Ingelheim	00597-0068-01	100s	$102.11
	00597-0068-61	100s ud	$107.18

Mexitil *SEE* MEXILETINE HYDROCHLORIDE

Mezlin *SEE* MEZLOCILLIN SODIUM

Mezlocillin Sodium

DESCRIPTION
Mezlocillin Sodium is a semisynthetic broad spectrum penicillin antibiotic for parenteral administration. It is the monohydrate sodium salt of 6-{D-2[3-(methyl-sulfonyl) -2- OXO-imidazolidine -1-carboxamido]-2-phenyl acetamido} penicillanic acid.

Empirical Formula: $C_{21}H_{24}N_5O_8S_2Na \cdot H_2O$

Mezlocillin Sodium has a molecular weight of 579.6 and contains 42.6 mg (1.85 mEq) of sodium per one gram of Mezlocillin activity. The dosage form is supplied as a sterile white to pale yellow crystalline powder, which is freely soluble in water. When reconstituted, solutions of Mezlocillin Sodium are clear and range from colorless to pale yellow with a pH of 4.5 to 8.0.

Following is its chemical structure:

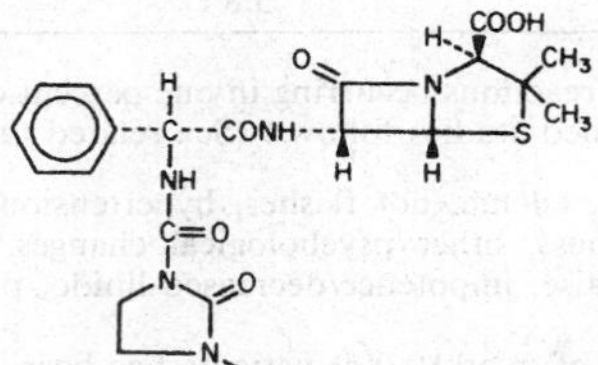

CLINICAL PHARMACOLOGY
Intravenous Administration: In healthy adult volunteers, mean serum levels of Mezlocillin 5 minutes after a 5-minute intravenous injection of 1 g, 2 g, or 5 g are 100, 253, or 411 mcg/mL, respectively. Serum levels, as noted below, lack dose proportionality. (See related table).

Fifteen minutes after a 4 g intravenous injection (2-5 min.), the concentration in serum is 254 mcg/mL; 1 hour and 4 hours later levels are 93 mcg/mL and 9.1 mcg/mL, respectively. (See related table).
After an intravenous infusion (15 min.) of 3 g, mean levels 15 minutes after dosing are 269 mcg/mL (170-280).

A 30-minute intravenous infusion of 3 g produces mean peak concentrations of 263 mcg/mL; 1 hour and 4 hours later the concentrations are 57 mcg/mL and 4.4 mcg/mL, respectively: (See related table).

Following intravenous infusion (2 hr.) of a 3 g dose of Mezlocillin every 4 hours for 7 days, mean peak serum concentrations are higher than 100 mcg/mL, and levels above 50 mcg/mL are maintained throughout dosing.

Intramuscular Administration: Mezlocillin Sodium is rapidly absorbed after intramuscular injection. In healthy volunteers, the mean peak serum concentration occurs approximately 45 minutes after a single dose of 1 g and is about 15 mcg/mL. The oral administration of 1 g probenecid before injection produces an increase in Mezlocillin serum levels of about 50%. After repetitive intramuscular doses of 1 g Mezlocillin every 6 hours, peak levels in the serum generally range

◆ RATED THERAPEUTICALLY EQUIVALENT; ◇ THERAPEUTIC EQUIVALENCE UNCONFIRMED; ○ UNRATED

between 35 and 45 mcg/mL. The relationship between the pharmacokinetics of intramuscular and intravenous dosing has not yet been clearly established.

General. As with other penicillins, Mezlocillin is excreted primarily by glomerular filtration and tubular secretion. The rate of elimination is dose dependent and related to the degree of renal functional impairment. In patients with normal renal function, approximately 55% of the administered dose is recovered from the urine within the first 6 hours after dosing. Two hours after an intravenous injection of 2 g, concentrations of active drug in urine generally exceed 4000 mcg/mL. By 4-6 hours after injection, concentrations usually decline to a range of about 50 to 200 mcg/mL. The serum elimination half-life of Mezlocillin after intravenous dosing is approximately 55 minutes.

In patients with reduced renal function, the half-life is only slightly prolonged. Dosage adjustments are usually not necessary except in patients with severe renal impairment. (See *"Dosage and Administration"*.) As with other penicillins, Mezlocillin is metabolized only slightly; less than 10% of the drug excreted in the urine is in the form of the penicilloate or penilloate. The drug is readily removed from the serum by hemodialysis and, to a lesser extent, by peritoneal dialysis. Up to 26% of a dose of Mezlocillin is recovered from the bile of patients with normal liver function. Following intravenous doses of 2 g to 5 g, concentrations of active drug in bile generally range from 500 to 2500 mcg/mL. The biliary excretion of Mezlocillin is reduced in patients with common bile duct obstruction.

Mezlocillin is not appreciably absorbed when given orally. Following parenteral administration, the apparent volume of distribution is approximately equal to the extracellular fluid volume. The drug is present in active form in the serum, urine, bile, peritoneal fluid, pleural fluid, bronchial and wound secretions, bone and other tissues. As with other penicillins, penetration into the cerebrospinal fluid (CSF) is generally poor, however higher CSF concentrations are obtained in the presence of meningeal inflammation.

Protein binding studies indicate that the degree of Mezlocillin binding is low (16-42%) and depends upon testing methods and concentrations of drug studied.

MICROBIOLOGY

Mezlocillin is a bactericidal antibiotic which acts by interfering with synthesis of cell wall components. It is active against a variety of gram-negative and gram-positive bacteria, including aerobic and anaerobic strains. Mezlocillin is usually active *in vitro* against most strains of the following organisms:

GRAM-NEGATIVE BACTERIA

Escherichia coli
Proteus mirabilis
Proteus vulgaris
Morganella morganii (formerly *P. morganii*)
Providencia rettgeri (formerly *Proteus rettgeri*)
Providencia stuartii
Citrobacter species*
Klebsiella species (including *K. pneumoniae*)
Enterobacter species
*Shigella species**
Pseudomonas aeruginosa(and other species)
Haemophilus influenzae
Haemophilus parainfluenzae
Neisseria species
Many strains of *Serratia, Salmonella**, and *Acinetobacter** are also susceptible.

GRAM-POSITIVE BACTERIA

Staphylococcus aureus (non-penicillinase producing strains)
Beta-hemolytic *streptococci* (Groups A and B)
Streptococcus pneumoniae (formerly *Diplococcus pneumoniae*)
Streptococcus faecalis (enterococcus)

ANAEROBIC ORGANISMS

Peptococcus species
Peptostreptococcus species
Clostridium species
Fusobacterium species*
Veillonella species*
Eubacterium species*
Bacteroides species (including *B. fragilis* group)
Noteworthy is Mezlocillin's broadened spectrum of *in vitro* activity against important pathogenic aerobic gram-negative bacteria, including strains of *Pseudomonas, Klebsiella, Enterobacter, Serratia, Proteus, Escherichia* and *Haemophilus*, as well as *Bacteroides* and other anaerobes; and its excellent inhibitory effect against gram-positive organisms including *Streptococcus faecalis* (enterococcus). It is inactive against penicillinase-producing strains of *Staphylococcus aureus*.

In vitro studies have shown that Mezlocillin combined with an aminoglycoside (e.g., gentamicin, tobramycin, amikacin, sisomicin) acts synergistically against strains of *Streptococcus faecalis* and *Pseudomonas aeruginosa*. In some instances, this combination also acts synergistically *in vitro* against other gram-negative bacteria such as *Serratia, Klebsiella* and *Acinetobacter* species.

Mezlocillin is slightly more active when tested at alkaline pH and, as with other penicillins, has reduced activity when tested *in vitro* with increasing inoculum. The minimum bactericidal concentration (MBC) generally exceeds the minimum inhibitory concentration (MIC) by a factor of 2 or 3. Resistance to Mezlocillin *in vitro* develops slowly (multiple step mutation). Some strains of *Pseudomonas aeruginosa* have developed resistance fairly rapidly. Mezlocillin is not stable in the presence of penicillinase and strains of *Staphylococcus aureus* resistant to penicillin are also resistant to Mezlocillin.

SUSCEPTIBILITY TESTS

Quantitative methods that require measurement of zone diameters give good estimates of bacterial susceptibility. One such procedure* has been recommended for use with discs to test susceptibility to antimicrobials. When the causative organism is tested by the Kirby-Bauer method of disc susceptibility, a 75 mcg Mezlocillin disc should give a zone of 18 mm or greater to indicate susceptibility. Zone sizes of 14 mm or less indicate resistance. Zone sizes of 15 to 17 mm indicate intermediate susceptibility. Susceptible strains of *Haemophilus* and *Neisseria* species give zones of ≥ 29 mm, resistant strains ≤ 28 mm. With this procedure, a report from the laboratory of "Susceptible" indicates that the infecting organism is likely to respond to therapy. A report of "Resistant" indicates that the infecting organism is not likely to respond to therapy; other therapy should be selected. A report of "Intermediate Susceptibility" suggests that the organism may be susceptible if the infection is confined to tissues and fluids (e.g., urine), in which high antibiotic levels are attained. The Mezlocillin disc should be used for testing susceptibility to Mezlocillin. In certain conditions, it may be desirable to do additional susceptibility testing by broth or agar dilution techniques. Dilution methods, preferably the agar plate dilution procedure, are most accurate for susceptibility testing of obligate anaerobes. *Enterobacteriaceae, Pseudomonas* species and *Acinetobacter* species are considered susceptible if the MIC of Mezlocillin is no greater than 64 mcg/mL and are considered resistant if the MIC is greater than 128 mcg/mL. *Haemophilus* species and *Neisseria* species are considered susceptible if the MIC of Mezlocillin is less than or equal to 1 mcg/mL. Mezlocillin standard is available for broth or agar dilution studies.

* Bauer, A.W., Kirby, W.M., Sherris, J.C., and Turck, M.: Antibiotic Testing by a Standardized Single Disc Method, Am. J. Clin. Pathol., 45:493, 1966; Standardized Disc Susceptibility Test, *FEDERAL REGISTER*, 39:19182-19184, 1974.

---

* Mezlocillin has been shown to be active *in vitro* against these organisms, however clinical efficacy has not yet been established.

MEZLOCILLIN SERUM LEVELS IN ADULTS (MCG/ML) 5 MIN. IV INJECTION

Dose	0	5 min.	10 min.	20 min.	30 min.	1 hr.	2 hr.	3 hr.	4 hr.	6 hr.	8 hr.
1 g	149 (132-185)	100 (64-143)	66 (47-87)	50 (31-87)	40 (22-83)	18 (8-31)	5.3 (3.3-7.7)	2.5 (1.7-3.7)	1.7 (0.7-2.8)	0.5 (0-1.2)	0.1 (0-0.2)
2 g	314 (207-362)	253 (161-364)	161 (113-214)	117 (76-174)	82 (55-112)	56 (23-88)	20 (7.5-32)	11 (3.8-16)	4.4 (1.6-8.7)	1.5 (0.5-2.6)	0.6 (0.1-1.4)
5 g	547 (268-854)	411 (199-597)	357 (246-456)	250 (203-353)	226 (190-333)	131 (104-193)	76 (59-104)	31 (20-40)	13 (6.4-17)	4.6 (2.1-9.4)	1.9 (1.1-3.6)

MEZLOCILLIN SERUM LEVELS IN ADULTS (MCG/ML) 2-5 MIN. IV INJECTION

DOSE	0	15 min.	30 min.	45 min.	1 hr.	2 hr.	3 hr.	4 hr.	6 hr.
4 g	—	254 (155-400)	163 (99-260)	122 (78-215)	93 (67-133)	47 (22-96)	20 (8-45)	9.1 (6-13)	8.4 (5-17)

MEZLOCILLIN SERUM LEVELS IN ADULTS (MCG/ML) 30 MIN. IV INFUSION

DOSE	0	5 min.	15 min.	30 min.	45 min.	1 hr.	2 hr.	3 hr.	4 hr.	6 hr.	8 hr.
3 g	263 (87-489)	170 (63-371)	141 (75-301)	109 (56-288)	79 (41-135)	57 (28-100)	26 (14-55)	12 (5.8-26)	4.4 (2.2-6.5)	1.6 (1.0-3.4)	< 1

➤ SHOWN IN PRODUCT IDENTIFICATION GUIDE

INDICATIONS AND USAGE

Mezlocillin Sodium is indicated for the treatment of serious infections caused by susceptible strains of the designated microorganisms in the conditions listed below:

Lower Respiratory Tract Infections including pneumonia and lung abscess caused by *Haemophilus influenzae, Klebsiella* species including *K. pneumoniae, Proteus mirabilis, Pseudomonas* species including *P. aeruginosa, E. coli,* and *Bacteroides* species including *B. fragilis.*

Intra-Abdominal Infections including acute cholecystitis, cholangitis, peritonitis, hepatic abscess and intraabdominal abscess caused by susceptible *E. coli, Proteus mirabilis, Klebsiella* species, *Pseudomonas* species, *S. faecalis* (enterococcus), *Bacteroides* species, *Peptococcus* species, and *Peptostreptococcus* species.

Urinary Tract Infections caused by susceptible *E. coli, Proteus mirabilis,* the indole positive *Proteus* species, *Morganella morganii; Klebsiella* species, *Enterobacter* species, *Serratia* species, *Pseudomonas* species, *S. faecalis* (enterococcus).
Uncomplicated gonorrhea due to susceptible *Neisseria gonorrhoeae.*

Gynecological Infections including endometritis, pelvic cellulitis, and pelvic inflammatory disease associated with susceptible *Neisseria gonorrhoeae, Peptococcus* species, *Peptostreptococcus* species, *Bacteroides* species, *E. coli, Proteus mirabilis, Klebsiella* species, and *Enterobacter* species.

Skin And Skin Structure Infections caused by susceptible *S. faecalis* (enterococcus), *E. coli, Proteus mirabilis,* the indole positive *Proteus* species, *Proteus vulgaris,* and *Providencia rettgeri; Klebsiella* species, *Enterobacter* species, *Pseudomonas* species, *Peptococcus* species, and *Bacteroides* species.

Septicimia: including bacteremia caused by susceptible *E. coli, Klebsiella* species, *Enterobacter* species, *Pseudomonas* species, *Bacteroides* species, and *Peptococcus* species.

Mezlocillin has also been shown to be effective for the treatment of infections caused by *Streptococcus* species including Group A Beta-hemolytic *Streptococcus* and *Streptococcus pneumoniae* (formerly *Diplococcus pneumoniae*) however, infections caused by these organisms are ordinarily treated with more narrow spectrum penicillins.

Appropriate culture and susceptibility tests should be performed before treatment in order to isolate and identify organisms causing infection and to determine their susceptibility to Mezlocillin. Therapy with Mezlocillin Sodium may be initiated before results of these tests are known; once results become available, appropriate therapy should be continued.

Mezlocillin's broad spectrum of activity makes it particularly useful for treating mixed infections caused by susceptible strains of both gram-negative and gram-positive aerobic or anaerobic bacteria. It is not effective, however, against infections caused by penicillinase-producing *Staphylococcus aureus.*

In certain severe infections, when the causative organisms are unknown, Mezlocillin Sodium may be administered in conjunction with an aminoglycoside or a cephalosporin antibiotic as initial therapy. As soon as results of culture and susceptibility tests become available, antimicrobial therapy should be adjusted if indicated. Culture and sensitivity testing, performed periodically during therapy, will provide information on the therapeutic effect of the antimicrobial and will monitor for the possible emergence of bacterial resistance.

Mezlocillin Sodium has been used effectively in combination with an aminoglycoside antibiotic for the treatment of life-threatening infections caused by *Pseudomonas aeruginosa.* For the treatment of febrile episodes in immunosuppressed patients with granulocytopenia, Mezlocillin Sodium should be combined with an aminoglycoside or a cephalosporin antibiotic.

Prevention: The administration of Mezlocillin Sodium perioperatively (preoperatively, intraoperatively, and postoperatively) may reduce the incidence of infections in patients undergoing surgical procedures (e.g. vaginal hysterectomy and colorectal surgery) that may be classified as contaminated or potentially contaminated. Effective perioperative use for surgery depends on the time of administration. To achieve effective tissue levels, Mezlocillin Sodium should be given ½ hour to 1 ½ hours before surgery.

In patients undergoing Caesarean section, intraoperative (after clamping the umbilical cord) and postoperative use of Mezlocillin Sodium may reduce the incidence of certain postoperative infections. (see *"Dosage and Administration"* section).

For patients undergoing colorectal surgery, preoperative bowel preparation by mechanical cleansing as well as with a non-absorbable antibiotic (e.g. neomycin) is recommended.

If there are signs of infection, specimens for culture should be obtained for identification of the causative organism so that appropriate therapy may be instituted.

CONTRAINDICATIONS

Mezlocillin Sodium is contraindicated in patients with a history of hypersensitivity reactions to any of the penicillins.

WARNINGS

Serious and occasionally fatal hypersensitivity (anaphylactic) reactions have occurred in patients receiving a penicillin. These reactions are more apt to occur in individuals with a history of sensitivity to multiple allergens. There have been reports of individuals with a history of penicillin hypersensitivity reactions who have experienced severe hypersensitivity reactions when treated with cephalosporin. Before therapy with Mezlocillin is instituted, careful inquiry should be made to determine whether the patient has had previous hypersensitivity reactions to

penicillins, cephalosporins or other drugs. Antibiotics should be used with caution in any patient who has demonstrated some form of allergy, particularly to drugs.

If an allergic reaction occurs during therapy with Mezlocillin, the drug should be discontinued. SERIOUS ANAPHYLACTOID REACTIONS REQUIRE IMMEDIATE EMERGENCY TREATMENT. EPINEPHRINE, OXYGEN, INTRAVENOUS STEROIDS, AND AIRWAY MANAGEMENT, INCLUDING INTUBATION, SHOULD BE PROVIDED AS INDICATED.

PRECAUTIONS

GENERAL

Although Mezlocillin Sodium shares with other penicillins the low potential for toxicity, as with any potent drug, periodic assessment of organ system functions, including renal, hepatic and hematopoietic, is advisable during prolonged therapy. Mezlocillin Sodium has been reported rarely to cause acute interstitial nephritis.

Bleeding manifestations have occurred in some patients receiving beta-lactam antibiotics. These reactions have been associated with abnormalities of coagulation tests, such as clotting time, platelet aggregation and prothrombin time and are more likely to occur in patients with renal impairment. Although Mezlocillin Sodium has rarely been associated with clinical bleeding, the possibility of this occurring should be kept in mind, particularly in patients with severe renal impairment receiving maximum doses of the drug.

Mezlocillin Sodium has only rarely been reported to cause hypokalemia; however, the possibility of this occurring should also be kept in mind, particularly when treating patients with fluid and electrolyte imbalance. Periodic monitoring of serum potassium may be advisable in patients receiving prolonged therapy.

Mezlocillin Sodium as a monosodium salt containing only 42.6 mg (1.85 mEq) of sodium per gram of Mezlocillin. This should be considered when treating patients requiring restricted salt intake.

As with any penicillin, an allergic reaction, including anaphylaxis, may occur during Mezlocillin Sodium administration, particularly in a hypersensitive individual.

As with other antibiotics, prolonged use of Mezlocillin Sodium may result in overgrowth of non-susceptible organisms. If this occurs, appropriate measures should be taken.

Mezlocillin Sodium along with other ureidopenicillins, has been reported in one study to prolong neuromuscular blockage of vecuronium. Caution is indicated when Mezlocillin is used perioperatively.

Antimicrobials used in high doses for short periods to treat gonorrhea may mask or delay the symptoms of incubating syphilis. Therefore, prior to treatment, patients with gonorrhea should also be evaluated for syphilis. Specimens for dark field examination should be obtained from any suspected primary lesion and serologic tests should be performed. Patients treated with Mezlocillin Sodium should undergo follow-up serologic tests three months after therapy.

INTERACTIONS WITH DRUGS AND LABORATORY TESTS

As with other penicillins, the mixing of Mezlocillin with an aminoglycoside in solutions for parenteral administration can result in substantial inactivation of the aminoglycoside. Probenecid interferes with the renal tubular secretion of Mezlocillin, thereby increasing serum concentrations and prolonging serum half-life of the antibiotic.

High urine concentrations of Mezlocillin may produce false positive protein reactions (pseudoproteinuria) with the following methods: sulfosalicylic acid and boiling test, acetic acid test, biuret reaction, and nitric acid test. The bromphenol blue (Multi-stix® reagent strip test has been reported to be reliable.

PREGNANCY CATEGORY B

Reproduction studies have been performed in rats and mice at doses up to 2 times the human dose, and have revealed no evidence of impaired fertility or harm to the fetus, due to Mezlocillin Sodium. There are however no adequate and well-controlled studies in pregnant women. Because animal reproductive studies are not always predictive of human response, this drug should be used during pregnancy only if clearly needed. Mezlocillin crosses the placenta and is found in low concentrations in cord blood and amniotic fluid.

NURSING MOTHERS

Mezlocillin is detected in low concentrations in the milk of nursing mothers, therefore caution should be exercised when Mezlocillin Sodium is administered to a nursing woman.

ADVERSE REACTIONS

As with other penicillins, the following adverse reactions may occur:

Hypersensitivity Reactions: skin rash, pruritus, urticaria, drug fever, acute interstitial nephritis and anaphylactic reactions.

Gastrointestinal Disturbances: abnormal taste sensation, nausea, vomiting and diarrhea. If diarrhea persists, pseudomembranous colitis should be considered.

Hemic and Lymphatic Systems: thrombocytopenia, leukopenia, neutropenia, eosinophilia, reduction of hemoglobin or hematocrit, and positive Coombs' test.

Abnormalities of Hepatic and Renal Function Tests: elevation of serum aspartate aminotransferase (SGOT), serum alanine aminotransferase (SGPT), serum alkaline phosphatase, serum bilirubin. Elevation of serum creatinine and/or BUN. Reduction in serum potassium.

Central Nervous System: convulsive seizures or neuromuscular hyperirritability.

Local Reactions: thrombophlebitis with intravenous administration, pain with intramuscular injection.

◆ RATED THERAPEUTICALLY EQUIVALENT; ◇ THERAPEUTIC EQUIVALENCE UNCONFIRMED; ○ UNRATED

OVERDOSAGE

As with other penicillins Mezlocillin Sodium in overdosage has the potential to cause neuromuscular hyperirritability or convulsive seizures. Hemodialysis, if necessary, will aid in the removal of drug from the blood.

DOSAGE AND ADMINISTRATION

Mezlocillin Sodium may be administered intravenously or intramuscularly. For serious infections, the intravenous route of administration should be used. Intramuscular doses should not exceed 2 g per injection.

The 20 g pharmacy bulk package is intended for the preparation of solutions for intravenous use. When intramuscular administration is required, the Mezlocillin Sodium vial should be used.

The recommended adult dosage for serious infections is 200-300 mg/kg per day given in 4 to 6 divided doses. The usual dose is 3 g given every 4 hours (18g/day) or 4 g given every 6 hours (16g/day). For life-threatening infections, up to 350 mg/kg per day may be administered, but the total daily dosage should ordinarily not exceed 24 g. (See related table).

For patients with life-threatening infections, 4 g may be administered every 4 hours (24 g/day).

Dosage for any individual patient must take into consideration the site and severity of infection, the susceptibility of the organisms causing infection, and the status of the patient's host defense mechanism.

The duration of therapy depends upon the severity of infection. Generally, Mezlocillin Sodium should be discontinued for at least 2 days after the signs and symptoms of infection have disappeared. The usual duration is 7 to 10 days; however, in difficult and complicated infections, more prolonged therapy may be required. Antibiotic therapy for Group A Beta-hemolytic streptococcal infections should be maintained for at least 10 days to reduce the risk of rheumatic fever or glomerulonephritis.

In certain deep-seated infections, involving abscess formation, appropriate surgical drainage should be performed in conjunction with antimicrobial therapy.

For acute, uncomplicated gonococcal urethritis, the usual dose is 1-2 g given once intravenously or by intramuscular injection. Probenecid 1 g may be given orally at the time of dosing or up to ½-hour before. (For full prescribing information, refer to probenecid package insert.)

PREVENTION

To prevent postoperative infection in contaminated or potentially contaminated surgery, the following doses are recommended:

4 g IV given ½ hour to 1½ hours prior to the start of surgery.
4 g IV given 6 hours and 12 hours later.
Caesarean Section Patients.

The first dose of 4 g is given intravenously as soon as the umbilical cord is clamped. The second and third doses of 4 g should be given intravenously 4 and 8 hours, respectively, after the first dose.

PATIENTS WITH IMPAIRED RENAL FUNCTION

The rate of elimination of Mezlocillin is dose dependent and related to the degree of renal function impairment. After an intravenous dose of 3 g, the serum half-life is approximately 1 hour in patients with creatinine clearances above 60 mL/min., 1.3 hr. in those with clearances of 30-59 mL/min., 1.6 hr. in those with clearances of 10-29 mL/min, and approximately 3.6 hr. in patients with clearances of less than 10 mL/min. Dosage adjustments of Mezlocillin Sodium are not required in patients with mild impairment of renal function. For patients with a creatinine clearance of ≤ 30 mL/min. (serum creatinine of approximately 3.0 mg% or greater), the following dosage guide may be used: (See related table).

For life-threatening infections, 3 g may be given every 6 hours to patients with creatinine clearances between 10-30 mL/min. and 2 g every 6 hours to those with clearances less than 10 mL/min.

For patients with serious systemic infection undergoing hemodialysis for renal failure, 3-4 g may be administered after each dialysis and then every 12 hours. Patients undergoing peritoneal dialysis may receive 3 g every 12 hours.

For patients with renal failure and hepatic insufficiency, measurement of serum levels of Mezlocillin will provide additional guidance for adjusting dosage.

DIRECTIONS FOR PROPER USE OF 20 GRAM PHARMACY BULK PACKAGE

A pharmacy bulk package is a container of a sterile preparation for parenteral use that contains many single doses. The contents are intended for use in a pharmacy admixture program and are restricted to the preparation of admixtures for intravenous infusion, or the filling of empty sterile syringes for intravenous injection for patients with individualized dosing requirements.

The Closure Shall be Penetrated Only One Time After Reconstitution with a suitable sterile transfer set or dispensing device which allows measured dispensing of the contents. The pharmacy bulk package is to be used only in a suitable work area such as a laminar flow hood or an equivalent clean air compounding area.

Reconstitute by vigorous shaking with 186 mL of Sterile Water for Injection, 5% Dextrose Injection or 0.9% Sodium Chloride Injection resulting in a solution containing approximately 100 mg/mL which should be stored at controlled room temperature or under refrigeration. Within 8 hours of reconstitution, the desired dosages should be withdrawn and may be further diluted with an appropriate intravenous solution (see "Compatibility and Stability" section).

INTRAVENOUS ADMINISTRATION

Mezlocillin Sodium may be administered intravenously by intermittent infusion or by direct intravenous injection.

Infusion: Each gram of Mezlocillin should be reconstituted by vigorous shaking with at least 9-10 mL of Sterile Water for Injection, 5% Dextrose Injection or 0.9% Sodium Chloride Injection. The dissolved drug should be further diluted to desired volume (50-100 mL) with an appropriate intravenous solution. (See "Compatibility and Stability" section.) The solution of reconstituted drug may then be administered over a period of 30 minutes by direct infusion, or through a Y-type intravenous infusion set which may already be in place. If this method or the "piggyback" method of administration is used, it is advisable to discontinue temporarily the administration of any other solutions during the infusion of Mezlocillin Sodium.

Injection: The reconstituted solution of Mezlocillin Sodium may also be injected directly into a vein or into intravenous tubing; when administered this way, the injection should be given slowly over a period of 3-5 minutes. To minimize venous irritation, the concentration of drug should not exceed 10%.

When Mezlocillin Sodium is given in combination with another antimicrobial, such as an aminoglycoside, each drug should be given separately in accordance with the recommended dosage and routes of administration for each drug.

INTRAMUSCULAR ADMINISTRATION

Each gram of Mezlocillin may be reconstituted by vigorous shaking with 3-4 mL of sterile water for injection or with 3-4 mL of 0.5 or 1.0% lidocaine hydrochloride solution (without epinephrine). (For full prescribing information, refer to lidocaine package insert.) Intramuscular doses of Mezlocillin Sodium should not exceed 2 g per injection.

As with all intramuscular preparations, Mezlocillin Sodium should be injected well within the body of a relatively large muscle, such as the upper outer quadrant of the buttock (i.e., gluteus maximus); aspiration will help avoid unintentional

MEZLOCILLIN SODIUM DOSAGE GUIDE (ADULTS)

Condition	Daily Dosage Range	Usual Daily Dosage	Frequency and Route of Administration
Urinary tract infection (uncomplicated)	100-125 mg/kg	6-8 g	1.5-2 g every 6 hours IV or IM
Urinary tract infection (complicated)	150-200 mg/kg	12 g	3 g every 6 hours IV
Lower respiratory tract infection			
Intra-abdominal infection Gynecological infection Skin & skin structure infection Septicemia	225-300 mg/kg	16-18 g	4 g every 6 hours or 3 g every 4 hours IV

MEZLOCILLIN SODIUM DOSAGE GUIDE FOR PATIENTS WITH IMPAIRED RENAL FUNCTION

Creatinine Clearance mL/min.	Urinary Tract Infection (Uncomplicated)	Urinary Tract Infection (Complicated)	Serious Systemic Infection
> 30		Usual Recommended Dosage	
10-30	1.5 g every 8 hours	1.5 g every 6 hours	3 g every 8 hours
< 10	1.5 g every 8 hours	1.5 g every 8 hours	2 g every 8 hours

► SHOWN IN PRODUCT IDENTIFICATION GUIDE

MEZLOCILLIN SODIUM DOSAGE GUIDE (NEWBORNS)

BODY WEIGHT (grams)	AGE	
	≤ 7 DAYS	> 7 DAYS
≤ 2000	75 mg/kg every 12 hours (150 mg/kg/day)	75 mg/kg every 8 hours (225 mg/kg/day)
> 2000	75 mg/kg every 12 hours (150 mg/kg/day)	75 mg/kg every 6 hours (300 mg/kg/day)

	STABILITY	
Intravenous Solution	Controlled Room Temperature	Refrigeration
Sterile Water for Injection, USP	48 hours	7 days
0.9% Sodium Chloride Injection, USP	48 hours	7 days
5% Dextrose Injection, USP	48 hours	7 days
5% Dextrose in 0.225% Sodium Chloride Injection, USP	72 hours	7 days
Lactated Ringer's Injection, USP	24 hours	7 days
5% Dextrose in Electrolyte # 75 Injection	72 hours	7 days
5% Dextrose in 0.45% Sodium Chloride Injection, USP*	48 hours	48 hours
Ringer's Injection	24 hours	24 hours
10% Dextrose Injection	24 hours	24 hours
5% Fructose Injection	24 hours	24 hours

If precipitation should occur under refrigeration, the product should be warmed to 37°C for 20 minutes in a water bath and shaken well.
*This solution is stable from 10 mg/mL to 50 mg/mL under refrigeration.

injection into a blood vessel. Slow injection (12-15 sec.) will minimize the discomfort associated with intramuscular administration.

INFANTS AND CHILDREN
Only limited data are available on the safety and effectiveness of Mezlocillin Sodium in the treatment of infants and children with documented serious infection. In the event a child has an infection for which Mezlocillin Sodium may be judged particularly appropriate, the following dosage guide may be used: (See related table).

For infants beyond one month of age and children up to the age of 12 years, *50 mg/kg may be administered every 4 hours (300 mg/kg/day).*

The drug may be infused intravenously over 30-minutes or be given by intramuscular injection.

COMPATIBILITY AND STABILITY
Mezlocillin Sodium at concentrations of 10 mg/mL and 100 mg/mL is stable (loss of potency less than 10%) in the following intravenous solutions for the time periods stated (includes time retained in pharmacy bulk package after reconstitution): (See related table).

Mezlocillin Sodium at concentrations up to 250 mg/mL is stable for 24 hours at room temperature in the following diluents:
sterile water for injection, USP
0.9% sodium chloride injection, USP
0.5% and 1.0% lidocaine hydrochloride solution (without epinephrine)
Mezlocillin Sodium is stable for up to 28 days when frozen at —12°C at concentrations up to 100 mg/mL in the following diluents: Sterile Water for Injection, USP
0.9% sodium chloride injection, USP or 5% dextrose injection, USP.

STORAGE
Unreconstituted Mezlocillin Sodium should be stored at temperatures not exceeding 86°F (30°C). The powder as well as the reconstituted solution of drug may darken slightly, depending upon storage conditions, but potency is not affected.

HOW SUPPLIED
POWDER FOR INJECTION: 1 GM

BRAND/MANUFACTURER	NDC	SIZE	AWP
○ BRAND			
MEZLIN: Miles Pharm	00026-8211-30	10s	$42.77

POWDER FOR INJECTION: 2 GM

BRAND/MANUFACTURER	NDC	SIZE	AWP
○ BRAND			
MEZLIN: Miles Pharm	00026-8212-30	10s	$82.93
	00026-8212-36	10s	$89.15

POWDER FOR INJECTION: 3 GM

BRAND/MANUFACTURER	NDC	SIZE	AWP
○ BRAND			
MEZLIN: Miles Pharm	00026-8213-35	10s	$122.47
	00026-8213-19	10s	$125.06
	00026-8213-36	10s	$128.30

POWDER FOR INJECTION: 4 GM

BRAND/MANUFACTURER	NDC	SIZE	AWP
○ BRAND			
MEZLIN: Miles Pharm	00026-8214-35	10s	$155.51
	00026-8214-19	10s	$158.11
	00026-8214-36	10s	$163.28

POWDER FOR INJECTION: 20 GM

BRAND/MANUFACTURER	NDC	SIZE	AWP
○ BRAND			
MEZLIN: Miles Pharm	00026-8220-31	6s	$443.20

Miacalcin *SEE* CALCITONIN

Miconazole Nitrate

DESCRIPTION
Miconazole Nitrate Cream contains Miconazole Nitrate 2%, formulated into a water-miscible base.

Miconazole Nitrate Vaginal Suppositories are white to off-white suppositories, each containing the antifungal agent, Miconazole Nitrate 200 mg.

The Chemical Name of Miconazole Nitrate is 1-[2,4-dichloro-β-[-(2,4-dichloro-benzyl)oxy] phenethyl] imidazole mononitrate.

Following is its chemical structure:

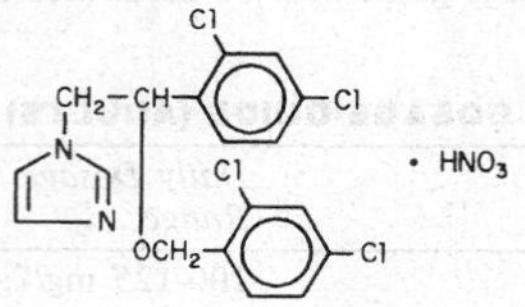

ACTIONS
Miconazole Nitrate is a synthetic antifungal agent which inhibits the growth of the common dermatophytes, *Trichophyton rubrum, Trichophyton mentagrophytes,* and *Epidermophyton floccosum,* the yeast-like fungus, *Candida albicans,* and the organism responsible for tinea versicolor (*Malassezia furfur*).

CLINICAL PHARMACOLOGY
The pharmacologic mode of action is unknown. Following intravaginal administration of Miconazole Nitrate, small amounts are absorbed. Administration of a single dose of Miconazole Nitrate suppositories (100mg) to healthy subjects resulted in a total recovery from the urine and feces of 0.85% (±0.43%) of the administered dose.

Animal studies indicate that the drug crossed the placenta and doses above those used in humans result in embryo- and fetotoxicity (80 mg/kg, orally), although this has not been reported in human subjects (see "Precautions").

In multi-center clinical trials in 440 women with vulvovaginal candidiasis, the efficacy of treatment with the Miconazole Nitrate Vaginal Suppository for 3 days was compared with treatment for 7 days with Miconazole Nitrate Vaginal Cream.

◆ RATED THERAPEUTICALLY EQUIVALENT; ◇ THERAPEUTIC EQUIVALENCE UNCONFIRMED; ○ UNRATED

The clinical cure rates (free of microbiological evidence and clinical signs and symptoms of candidiasis at 8-10 days and 30-35 days posttherapy) were numerically lower, although not statistically different, with the 3-Day Suppository when compared with the 7-Day Cream.

INDICATIONS

Miconazole Nitrate Cream is indicated for topical application in the treatment of tinea pedis (athlete's foot), tinea cruris, and tinea corporis caused by *Trichophyton rubrum*, *Trichophyton mentagrophytes*, and *Epidermophyton floccosum*, in the treatment of cutaneous candidiasis (moniliasis), and in the treatment of tinea versicolor.

Miconazole Nitrate Vaginal Suppositories are indicated for the local treatment of vulvovaginal candidiasis (moniliasis). Effectiveness in pregnancy and in diabetic patients has not been established. As Miconazole Nitrate Vaginal Suppositories are effective only for candidal vulvovaginitis, the diagnosis should be confirmed by KOH smear and/or cultures. Other pathogens commonly associated with vulvovaginitis (*Trichomonas* and *Haemophilus vaginalis [Gardnerella]*) should be ruled out by appropriate laboratory methods.

CONTRAINDICATIONS

Miconazole Nitrate Cream has no known contraindications. Miconazole Nitrate Vaginal Suppositories are contraindicated in patients known to be hypersensitive to this drug.

PRECAUTIONS

If a reaction suggesting sensitivity or chemical irritation should occur, use of the medication should be discontinued. The cream is for external use only. Avoid introduction of Miconazole Nitrate Cream into the eyes.

The base contained in the suppository formulation may interact with certain latex products, such as that used in vaginal contraceptive diaphragms. Concurrent use is not recommended. Miconazole Nitrate 7-Day Vaginal Cream may be considered for use under these conditions.

Laboratory Tests: If there is a lack of response to Miconazole Nitrate Vaginal Suppositories, appropriate microbiological studies (standard KOH smear and/or cultures) should be repeated to confirm the diagnosis and rule out other pathogens.

Carcinogenesis, Mutagenesis, Impairment of Fertility: Long-term animal studies to determine carcinogenic potential have not been performed.

Fertility (Reproduction): Oral administration of Miconazole Nitrate in rats has been reported to produce prolonged gestation. However, this effect was not observed in oral rabbit studies. In addition, signs of fetal and embryo toxicity were reported in rat and rabbit studies, and dystocia was reported in rat studies after oral doses at and above 80 mg per kg. Intravaginal administration did not produce these effects in rats.

Pregnancy: Since imidazoles are absorbed in small amounts from the human vagina, they should not be used in the first trimester of pregnancy unless the physician considers it essential to the welfare of the patient.

Clinical studies, during which Miconazole Nitrate Vaginal Cream and Suppositories were used for up to 14 days, were reported to include 514 pregnant patients. Follow-up reports available in 471 of these patients reveal no adverse effects or complications attributable to Miconazole Nitrate therapy in infants born to these women.

Nursing Mothers: It is not known whether Miconazole Nitrate is excreted in human milk. Because many drugs are excreted in human milk, caution should be exercised when Miconazole Nitrate is administered to a nursing woman.

ADVERSE REACTIONS

There have been isolated reports of irritation, burning, maceration, and allergic contact dermatitis associated with application of Miconazole Nitrate Cream.

During clinical studies with the Miconazole Nitrate Vaginal Suppository 301 patients were treated. The incidence of vulvovaginal burning, itching or irritation was 2%. Complaints of cramping (2%) and headaches (1.3%) were also reported. Other complaints (hives, skin rash) occurred with less than a 0.5% incidence. The therapy-related dropout rate was 0.3%.

OVERDOSAGE

Overdose of Miconazole Nitrate in humans has not been reported to date. In mice, rats, guinea pigs and dogs, the oral LD 50 values were found to be 578.1, > 640, 275.9 and > 160 mg/kg, respectively.

DOSAGE AND ADMINISTRATION

Sufficient Miconazole Nitrate Cream should be applied to cover affected areas twice daily (morning and evening) in patients with tinea pedis, tinea cruris, tinea corporis, and cutaneous candidiasis, and once daily in patients with tinea versicolor. If Miconazole Nitrate Cream is used in intertriginous areas, it should be applied sparingly and smoothed in well to avoid maceration effects.

Early relief of symptoms (2 to 3 days) is experienced by the majority of patients and clinical improvement may be seen fairly soon after treatment is begun; however, *Candida* infections and tinea cruris and corporis should be treated for two weeks and tinea pedis for one month in order to reduce the possibility of recurrence. If a patient shows no clinical improvement after a month of treatment, the diagnosis should be redetermined. Patients with tinea versicolor usually exhibit clinical and mycological clearing after two weeks of treatment.

Miconazole Nitrate Vaginal Suppositories: One suppository (Miconazole Nitrate, 200 mg) is inserted intravaginally once daily at bedtime for three consecutive days. Before prescribing another course of therapy, the diagnosis should be reconfirmed by smears and/or cultures to rule out other pathogens.

HOW SUPPLIED

AEROSOL LIQUID: 2%

BRAND/MANUFACTURER	NDC	SIZE	AWP
BRAND			
ONY-CLEAR NAIL: Pedinol	00884-4893-45	45 ml	$14.75

CREAM:

BRAND/MANUFACTURER	NDC	SIZE	AWP
BRAND			
FUNGOID: Pedinol	00884-2493-60	60 gm	$16.00

CREAM: 2%

BRAND/MANUFACTURER	NDC	SIZE	AWP
BRAND			
MONISTAT-DERM: Ortho Pharm	00062-5434-02	15 gm	$11.88
	00062-5434-01	30 gm	$20.04
	00062-5434-03	85 gm	$38.82

SUPPOSITORY: 200 MG

BRAND/MANUFACTURER	NDC	SIZE	AWP
BRAND			
MONISTAT 3: Ortho Pharm	00062-5437-01	3s	$23.22

TAMPON:

BRAND/MANUFACTURER	NDC	SIZE	AWP
BRAND			
MONISTAT 5: Ortho Advanced	00062-5436-01	5s	$15.96

TINCTURE LIQUID:

BRAND/MANUFACTURER	NDC	SIZE	AWP
BRAND			
FUNGOID: Pedinol	00884-0293-01	30 ml	$8.50

Miconazole, Injectable

DESCRIPTION

Miconazole, 1-[2-(2,4-dichlorophenyl)-2-[(2,4-dichlorophenyl) methoxyl] ethyl]-1H-imidazole, is a synthetic antifungal agent supplied as a sterile solution for intravenous infusion. Each mL of this solution contains 10 mg of Miconazole with 0.115 mL PEG 40 castor oil, 1.0 mg lactic acid USP, 0.5 mg methylparaben USP, 0.05 mg propylparaben USP in water for injection. Miconazole IV is a clear, colorless to slightly yellow solution having a pH of 3.7 to 5.7.

Following is its chemical structure:

CLINICAL PHARMACOLOGY

Miconazole IV is rapidly metabolized in the liver and about 14% to 22% of the administered dose is excreted in the urine, mainly as inactive metabolites. The pharmacokinetic profile fits a three compartment open model with the following biologic half life: 0.4, 2.1, and 24.1 hours for each phase respectively. The pharmacokinetic profile of Miconazole IV is unaltered in patients with renal insufficiency, including those patients on hemodialysis. The *in vitro* antifungal activity of Miconazole IV is very broad. Clinical efficacy has been demonstrated in patients with the following species of fungi: *Coccidioides immitis*, *Candida albicans*, *Cryptococcus neoformans*, *Pseudoallescheria boydii (Petriellidium boydii; Allescheria boydii)*, and *Paracoccidioides brasiliensis*.

Recommended doses of Miconazole IV produce serum concentrations of drug which exceed the in vitro minimum inhibitory concentration (MIC) values listed below.

MEDIAN MINIMAL INHIBITORY CONCENTRATIONS OF MICONAZOLE IN MCG/ML

Clinical Isolates	Median	Range
Coccidioides immitis	0.4	0.1-1.6
Candida albicans	0.2	0.1-0.8
Cryptococcus neoformans	0.8	0.4-1.3
Paracoccidioides brasiliensis	0.24	0.16-0.31
Pseudoallescheria boydii (Petriellidium boydii)	1.0	0.16-10

➤ SHOWN IN PRODUCT IDENTIFICATION GUIDE

Doses above 9 mg/kg of Miconazole IV produce peak blood levels above 1 mcg/ml in most cases. The drug penetrates into joints.

INDICATIONS AND USAGE

Miconazole IV is indicated for the treatment of the following severe systemic fungal infections, based on data derived from open clinical trials: coccidioidomycosis (N = 52[*]), candidiasis (N = 151), cryptococcosis (N = 13), pseudoallescheriosis (petriellidiosis; allescheriosis) (N = 12), paracoccidioidomycosis (N = 12), and for the treatment of chronic mucocutaneous candidiasis (N = 16).

[*] Represents treatment courses, as some patients were treated more than once.

However, in the treatment of fungal meningitis and *Candida* urinary bladder infections an intravenous infusion alone is inadequate. It must be supplemented with intrathecal administration or bladder irrigation. Appropriate diagnostic procedures should be performed and MIC's should be measured to determine if the organism is susceptible to Miconazole.

Miconazole IV should only be used to treat severe systemic fungal diseases.

CONTRAINDICATIONS

Miconazole IV is contraindicated in those patients who have shown hypersensitivity to it, or to its components.

WARNINGS

There have been several reports of cardiorespiratory arrest and/or anaphylaxis in patients receiving Miconazole IV Excessively rapid administration of the drug may have been responsible in some cases. Rapid injection of undiluted Miconazole IV may produce transient tachycardia or dysrhythmia. (See *"Dosage and Administration".*)

Miconazole IV should only be used to treat severe systemic fungal diseases.

PRECAUTIONS

General: Before a treatment course of Miconazole IV is started, the physician should ascertain insofar as possible that the patient is not hypersensitive to the drug product. Miconazole IV should be given by intravenous infusion. The treatment should be started under stringent conditions of hospitalization but subsequently may be administered to suitable patients under ambulatory conditions with close clinical monitoring. It is recommended that an initial dose of 200 mg be administered with the physician in attendance. It is also recommended that clinical laboratory monitoring including hemoglobin, hematocrit, electrolytes and lipids be performed.

It should be borne in mind that systemic fungal mycoses may be complications of chronic underlying conditions which in themselves may require appropriate measures.

Since *Pseudoallescheria boydii* is difficult to distinguish histologically from species of *Aspergillus*, it is strongly recommended that cultures be planted.

Drug Interactions: Drugs containing cremophor type vehicles are known to cause electrophoretic abnormalities of the lipoprotein; for example, the values and/or patterns may be altered. These effects are reversible upon discontinuation of treatment but are usually not an indication that treatment should be discontinued.

Interaction with oral and IV anticoagulant drugs, resulting in an enhancement of the anticoagulant effect, may occur. However, this has only been reported with oral (coumadin) administration. In cases of simultaneous treatment with Miconazole IV and anticoagulant drugs, the anticoagulant effect should be carefully titrated since reductions of the anticoagulant doses may be indicated.

Interactions between oral miconazole and oral hypoglycemic agents leading to severe hypoglycemia have been reported. Since concomitant administration of rifampin and ketoconazole (an imidazole) reduces the blood levels of the latter, the concurrent administration of Miconazole IV (an imidazole) and rifampin should be avoided.

Ketoconazole (an imidazole) increases the blood level of cyclosporine; therefore, there is the possibility of a similar drug interaction involving cyclosporine and Miconazole IV (an imidazole). Blood levels of cyclosporine should be monitored if the two drugs must be given concurrently.

Concomitant administration of Miconazole with CNS-active drugs such as carbamazepine or phenytoin may alter the metabolism of one or both of the drugs. Therefore, consideration should be given to the advisability of monitoring plasma levels of these drugs. It is not known whether Miconazole may affect the metabolism of other CNS-active drugs.

Pregnancy Category C: Reproduction studies using Miconazole IV were performed in rats and rabbits. At intravenous doses of 40 mg/kg in the rat and 20 mg/kg in the rabbit, no evidence of impaired fertilty or harm to the fetus appeared. There are no adequate and well-controlled studies using Miconazole IV in pregnant women. Miconazole IV should be given to a pregnant woman only if clearly needed.

Pediatric Use: The safety of Miconazole IV in children under one year has not been extensively studied. However, reports in the literature describe the treatment of 21 neonates for periods ranging from 1 to 56 days at doses ranging from 3 to 50 mg/kg per day in 3 or 4 divided doses. No unanticipated adverse events occurred in children who received these doses. The majority of use was a daily dose in the 15 to 30 mg/kg range. Seven of the eleven evaluable children recovered or improved.

ADVERSE REACTIONS

Adverse reactions which have been observed with Miconazole IV therapy include phlebitis, pruritus, rash, nausea, vomiting, febrile reactions, drowsiness, diarrhea, anorexia and flushes. In the U.S. studies, 29% of 209 patients studied had phlebitis, 21% pruritus, 18% nausea, 10% fever and chills, 9% rash, and 7%

emesis. Transient decreases in hematocrit and serum sodium values have been observed following infusion of Miconazole IV.

In rare cases, anaphylaxis has occured.

Thrombocytopenia has also been reported. No serious renal or hepatic toxicity has been reported. If pruritus and skin rashes are severe, discontinuation of treatment may be necessary. Nausea and vomiting can be lessened with antihistaminic or antiemetic drugs given prior to Miconazole i.v. infusion, or by reducing the dose, slowing the rate of infusion, or avoiding administration with foods.

Aggregation of erythrocytes or rouleau formation on blood smears has been reported. Hyperlipemia has occurred in patients and is reported to be due to the vehicle. Cremophor EL (PEG 40 castor oil).

DOSAGE AND ADMINISTRATION

DOSAGE

Adults: Doses may vary from 200 to 1200 mg per infusion depending on severity of infection and sensitivity of the organism. The following daily doses, which may be divided over 3 infusions, are recommended:

Organism	Dosage Range[*]	Duration of Successful Therapy (weeks)
Candidiasis	600 to 1800 mg per day	1 to > 20
Cryptococosis	1200 to 2400 mg per day	3 to > 12
Coccidioidomycosis	1800 to 3600 mg per day	3 to > 20
Pseudoallescheriosis (Petriellidiosis; Allescheriosis)	600 to 3000 mg per day	5 to > 20
Paracoccidioidomycosis	200 to 1200 mg per day	2 to > 16

[*] *May be divided over 3 infusions*

Repeated courses may be necessitated by relapse or reinfection.

Children:

Children under one year: Total daily doses of 15 to 30 mg/kg have been used (See Pediatric Use).

Children 1 to 12 years: Total daily doses of 20 to 40 mg/kg have generally been adequate.

However, a dose of 15 mg/kg body weight per infusion should not be exceeded.

ADMINISTRATION

For daily doses of up to 2400 mg, Miconazole IV should be diluted in at least 200 ml of diluent per ampoule and should be administered at a rate of approximately 2 hours per ampoule. For daily doses higher than 2400 mg adjust the rate of infusion and the diluent in terms of patient tolerability (see *"Warnings"*).

It is recommended that 0.9% Sodium Chloride Injection be used as the diluent to minimize the possibility of transient hyponatremia following an infusion of Miconazole IV. Alternatively, if clinically indicated, 5% Dextrose Injection may be used.

Generally, treatment should be continued until all clinical and laboratory tests no longer indicate that active fungal infection is present. Inadequate periods of treatment may yield poor response and lead to early recurrence of clinical symptoms. The dosing intervals and sites and the duration of treatment vary from patient to patient and depend on the causative organism.

OTHER MODES OF ADMINISTRATION

Intrathecal: Administration of the undiluted injectable solution of Miconazole IV by the various intrathecal routes (20 mg per dose) is indicated as an adjunct to intravenous treatment in fungal meningitis. Succeeding intrathecal injections may be alternated between lumbar, cervical, and cisternal punctures every 3 to 7 days.

Bladder instillation: 200 mg of Miconazole in a diluted solution is indicated in the treatment of *Candida* of the urinary bladder.

Store at Controlled room temperature (15° to 30°C/59° to 86°F).

HOW SUPPLIED
INJECTION: 10 MG/ML

BRAND/MANUFACTURER	NDC	SIZE	AWP
○ BRAND			
MONISTAT I.V.: Janssen	50458-0200-20	20 ml	$38.47

Micrainin *SEE* ASPIRIN WITH MEPROBAMATE

MICRhoGAM *SEE* GLOBULIN, IMMUNE RHO$_O$(D) *AND* RH$_O$(D) IMMUNE GLOBULIN

◆ RATED THERAPEUTICALLY EQUIVALENT; ◇ THERAPEUTIC EQUIVALENCE UNCONFIRMED; ○ UNRATED

Micro-K *SEE* **POTASSIUM CHLORIDE, ORAL**

Micronase *SEE* **GLYBURIDE**

Micronor *SEE* **NORETHINDRONE**

Micrurus Fulvius

DESCRIPTION
COMPOSITION
Micrurus Fulvius antivenin, is a refined, concentrated, and lyophilized preparation of serum globulins obtained by fractionating blood from healthy horses that have been immunized with eastern coral snake (Micrurus fulvius fulvius) venom.

Micrurus Fulvius antivenin is standardized for potency in mice in terms of its LD_{50} neutralizing capacity per milliliter as determined by intravenous injection of a graded series of Antivenin—M.f. fulvius venom mixtures. Based on this assay system, the reconstituted contents of each vial (10 ml) will neutralize approximately 250 mouse LD_{50} or approximately 2 mg of M.f. fulvius venom.

The results of cross-neutralization tests indicate that Micrurus fulvius antivenin will neutralize the venom of M. fulvius tenere (Texas coral snake) but will *not* neutralize the venom of Micruroides euryxanthus (Arizona or Sonoran coral snake).

INDICATIONS AND USAGE
CORAL SNAKES AND BITES
Two genera of coral snakes are found in the United States—Micrurus (including the eastern and Texas varieties) and Micruroides (the Sonoran or Arizona variety), found only in southeastern Arizona and southwestern New Mexico.

There are two subspecies of Micrurus Fulvius native to the United States: 1) M.f. fulvius, found in the area from eastern North Carolina through the tip of Florida and in the Gulf coastal plain to the Mississippi River; 2) M.f. tenere, the Texas coral snake, found west of the Mississippi River in Louisiana, Arkansas, and Texas. These subspecies can be differentiated by experts but are very similar in appearance. The adult coral snake (M. fulvius) may vary between 20 to 44 inches in length, has a black snout, and yellow, black, and red bands encircling the body. The red and black rings are wider than the *interposed* yellow rings. However, melanistic (all black), albino (all white), and partially pigmented forms may be rarely seen. In contrast to the pit vipers (rattlesnakes, copper-heads, cottonmouths), coral snakes have round pupils and lack facial pits. They are secretive and rarely bite unless disturbed or *handled*. The fanges are short, erect, and fixed to the maxilla. Venom flows through the fang from a duct at its base. Pit vipers usually strike and then rapidly withdraw the head after insertion of the fangs. However, coral snakes, with their less efficient biting mechanism, may strike, hold on, and "chew", presumably so a sufficient amount of venom can be introduced to immobilize the prey. This "chewing" action may result in more than one "bite", and the victim *may* recall the colorful snake "hanging on" for a "minute" or so. Permitted to bite under laboratory conditions, M.f.fulvius have yielded 1 to 28 mg of venom. [1,2] Fix and Minton,[2] after measuring the venom yields of 14 M.f.fulvius and the length of the individual snakes, found a positive linear relationship; six snakes measuring between 29 and 44 inches in length yielded 14 to 28 mg of dried venom, whereas eight measuring 21 to 28 inches in length yielded 2 to 10 mg. The adult human LD_{100} of M.f.fulvius venom has been estimated to be 4 to 5 mg of dried venom. Coral snake venom is chiefly paralytic (neurotoxic) in action, and usually only minimal-to-moderate tissue reaction and pain occur at the site of bite. Most coral snakebites are inflicted upon the upper extremities, especially the hands and fingers. The limited size of the biting apparatus makes it difficult for the coral snake to penetrate clothing or to successfully grasp any part of the body except the hands and feet. Hence, in areas where coral snakes are found, adherence to the simple practices of *never* picking up colorful snakes, *never* putting the hands where they cannot be seen (reaching behind rocks, logs, flowers, etc.), and always wearing leather shoes would substantially reduce the chances of a bite.

There are few published reports describing envenomation caused by coral snakebites.[1, 3-7] It has been estimated that only 20 ± 5 coral snakebites occur in the United States each year.[3] Although those persons who exhibit one or more fang punctures seem most likely to develop envenomation, there is NO way to predict which victim may be envenomated by a coral snakebite. Even a reliable observation that the biting snake did or did not "hang on" should *not* be used to predict the likelihood or possible severity of envenomation. Coral snakebites, like bites by crotalids, are not always followed by envenomation. However, in contradistinction to crotalid bites, in which moderate-to-severe envenomation usually can be predicted by rapid onset of the local effects (e.g., pain, discoloration, edema), severe and even fatal envenomation from a coral snakebite can be present without any significant local tissue reaction.

Systemic signs and symptoms of envenomation usually begin from one to seven hours after the bite but may be delayed for as long as 18 hours. If envenomation occurs, the symptoms and signs may progress rapidly and precipitously. Paralysis has been observed within 2-½ hours post bite and appears to be of a bulbar type, involving cranial motor nerves. Death from respiratory paralysis has occurred within four hours of the accident.

Systemic: signs and symptoms of envenomation may include euphoria, lethargy, weakness, nausea, vomiting, excessive salivation, ptosis of the eyelids, dyspnea, abnormal reflexes, convulsions, and motor weakness or paralysis, including complete respiratory paralysis. *Local* signs and symptoms may include scratch marks or fang puncture wounds, no-to-moderate edema, erythema, pain at the bite site, and paresthesia in the bitten extremity.

Treatment of Coral Snakebite: If practical, immobilize victim immediately and completely. Carry the victim to the nearest hospital as soon as possible. If complete immobilization is not practical, splint the bitten extremity to limit spread of venom. If the biting snake was killed, bring it to the hospital also.

ANY victim of a bite by a coral snake with ANY evidence of a break in the skin caused by the snake's teeth or fangs should be *hospitalized* for observation and/or treatment. Cleanse the bite area with germicidal soap and water to remove any venom remaining on the skin. If fang puncture wounds are present, application of a tourniquet and incision and suction over the fang punctures has been recommended,[1,3] even though there is no evidence to indicate that incision and suction are or are not of value in removing coral snake venom. In addition to maintaining close observation of the patient for 24 hours, which should include checking the respiratory rate every 30 minutes, make sure the following will be available and ready for immediate use should need arise:
—a supply of Micrurus Fulvius
—an oxygen supply
—a mechanical respirator
—facilities and equipment for a tracheostomy
—the services of an anesthesiologist

Appropriate horse-serum sensitivity tests should be done so that, in case administration of Antivenin is subsequently required, a decision on how to proceed will have been made. Parrish and Khan[3] have recommended intravenous administration of coral snake antivenin to patients with one or more fang puncture wounds as soon as possible and before onset of symptoms and signs of envenomation.

If symptoms or signs of envenomation occur in a patient under observation or are already present at the time the patient is first seen, give Micrurus Fulvius promptly by the intravenous route. With vigorous treatment and careful observation, patients with complete respiratory paralysis have recovered, indicating that the respiratory paralysis is reversible.[4,5] Hemoglobinuria has been observed in experimental animals envenomated by coral snakes. Hence, continuous bladder drainage is recommended with careful attention to urinary output and blood electrolyte balance.

Appropriate tetanus prophylaxis is indicated as for any other potentially contaminated puncture wound.

PRECAUTIONS
GENERAL PRECAUTIONS
Morphine or other narcotics that depress respiration are contraindicated. Sedatives should be used with extreme caution.

The physician should be familiar with the package brochure and the pertinent published medical literature concerning envenomation resulting from coral snakebites, as well as the currently acceptable concepts of nonspecific treatment for venomous snakebites.

PRECAUTIONS TO BE TAKEN IN ADMINISTRATION OF HORSE SERUM
Before administration of any product prepared from horse serum, appropriate measures must be taken in an effort to detect the presence of dangerous sensitivity: (1) A careful review of the patient's history, including any report of (a) asthma, hay fever, urticaria, or other allergic manifestations; (b) allergic reactions upon exposure to horses; and (c) prior injections of horse serum. (2) A suitable test for detection of sensitivity. A skin test should be performed in every patient prior to administration, regardless of clinical history.

Skin Test: Inject intracutaneously 0.02 to 0.03 ml of a 1:10 dilution of Normal Horse Serum or antivenin. A control test on the opposite extremity, using sodium chloride injection, USP, facilitates interpretation. Use of larger amounts for the skin-test dose increases the likelihood of false-positive reactions, and in the exquisitely sensitive patient, increases the risk of a systemic reaction from the skin-test dose. A 1:100 or greater dilution should be used for preliminary skin testing if the history suggests sensitivity. A positive reaction to a skin test occurs within five to thirty minutes and is manifested by a wheal with or without pseudopodia and surrounding erythema. In general, the shorter the interval between injection and the beginning of the skin reaction, the greater the sensitivity.

If the history is negative for allergy and the result of a skin test is negative, proceed with administration of Antivenin as outlined above. If the history is positive and a skin test is strongly positive, administration may be dangerous, especially if the positive sensitivity test is accompanied by systemic allergic manifestations. In such instances, the risk of administering Antivenin must be weighed against the risk of withholding it, keeping in mind that severe envenomation can be fatal. (See last paragraph of this section.)

A negative allergic history and absence of reaction to a properly applied skin test do not rule out the possibility of an immediate reaction. Also, a negative skin test has no bearing on whether or not delayed serum reactions (serum sickness) will occur after administration of the full dose.

If the history is negative, and the skin test is mildly or questionably positive, administer as follows to reduce the risk of a severe immediate systemic reaction: (a) Prepare, in separate sterile vials or syringes, 1:100 and 1:10 dilutions of Antivenin. (b) Allow at least 15 minutes between injections and proceed with the next dose if no reaction follows the previous dose. (c) Inject subcutaneously, using a tuberculin-type syringe, 0.1, 0.2, and 0.5 ml of the 1:100 dilution at 15-minute intervals; repeat with the 1:10 dilution, and finally undiluted Antivenin. (d) If a systemic reaction occurs after any injection, place a tourniquet proximal to the site of injections and administer an appropriate dose of epinephrine, 1:1000, proximal to the tourniquet or into another extremity. Wait at least 30 minutes before injecting another dose. The amount of the next dose should be the same as the last that did not evoke a reaction. (e) If no reaction occurs after 0.5 ml of undiluted antivenin has been administered, switch to the intramuscular route and continue doubling the dose at 15-minute intervals until the entire dose has been injected intramuscularly or proceed to the intravenous route as described above under "Dosage and Administration".

ADVERSE REACTIONS

SYSTEMIC REACTIONS

A. The immediate reaction (shock, anaphylaxis) usually occurs within 30 minutes. Symptoms and signs may develop before the needle is withdrawn and may include apprehension, flushing, itching, urticaria; edema of the face, tongue, and throat; cough, dyspnea, cyanosis, vomiting, and collapse.

B. Serum sickness usually occurs 5 to 24 days after administration. The incubation period may be less than 5 days, especially in those who have received horse-serum-containing preparations in the past. The usual symptoms and signs are malaise, fever, urticaria, lymphadenopathy, edema, arthralgia, nausea, and vomiting. Occasionally, neurological manifestations develop, such as meningismus or peripheral neuritis. Peripheral neuritis usually involves the shoulders and arms. Pain and muscle weakness are frequently present, and permanent atrophy may develop.

DOSAGE AND ADMINISTRATION

TECHNIC FOR RECONSTITUTION OF ANTIVENIN

Pry off the small metal disc in the cap over the diaphragms of the vials of Antivenin and diluent. Swab the exposed surface of the rubber diaphragms of both vials with an appropriate germicide. With a sterile 10 ml syringe and needle, withdraw the diluent (Water for Injection, USP, containing phenylmercuric nitrate 1:100,000) from the vial of diluent and inject it into the vial of Antivenin. Gentle agitation will hasten complete dissolution of the lyophilized Antivenin.

IMPORTANT

1. Before administration, read sections on "Precautions to be Taken in Administration of Horse Serum" and "Systemic Reactions". Since the possibility of a severe immediate reaction (anaphylaxis) always exists whenever horse serum is administered, appropriate therapeutic agents, such as tourniquet, oxygen supply, epinephrine 1:1000, and another injectable pressor amine (NOT corticosteroids), must be ready for immediate use.

2. Constant attendance and observation for untoward response is *mandatory* whenever horse serum is administered intravenously so that, should such occur, injection may be discontinued and appropriate treatment instituted immediately.

Start an intravenous drip of 250 to 500 ml of Sodium Chloride Injection, USP. If the results of appropriate tests have indicated the patient is not dangerously hypersensitive to horse serum, and depending on the nature and severity of the signs and symptoms of envenomation, administer the contents of 3 to 5 vials (30 to 50 ml) *intravenously* by slow injection directly into the intravenous tubing or by adding to the reservoir bottle of the intravenous drip. (If added to reservoir bottle, mix by gentle swirling—*Do Not Shake*.) In either case, the first 1 or 2 ml should be injected over a 3- to 5-minute period with careful observation of the patient for evidence of allergic reaction. If no signs or symptoms of anaphylaxis appear, continue the injection or intravenous infusion. The rate of delivery is regulated by the severity of signs and symptoms of envenomation and tolerance of Antivenin. However, until the equivalent of 30 to 50 ml of undiluted Antivenin has been given, administer at the maximum safe rate for intravenous fluids, based on body weight and general condition of the patient. For instance, if given by intravenous drip to a previously healthy adult, allow 250 or 500 ml to run in within 30 minutes; in small children, allow the first 100 ml to run in rapidly but then decrease to a rate not to exceed 4 ml per minute. Response to treatment may be rapid and dramatic. Observe the patient carefully and administer additional Antivenin intravenously as required.

According to the data reported by Fix and Minton[2] and cited above concerning venom yields obtained under artificial but probably physiological biting conditions, some envenomated patients may require administration of the contents of 10 or more vials to neutralize the venom dose injected by the biting snake if the entire venom load were delivered by the bite(s).

BIBLIOGRAPHY

1. Mc Collough, N. and Gennaro, J.: Coral snakebites in the United States, J. Florida Med. Assn. 49:968, 1963. 2. Fix, J. and Minton, S.: Venom extraction and yields from the North American Coral Snake, Micrurus fulvius. Toxicon 14:143, 1976. 3. Parrish, H. and Kahn, M.: Bites by coral snakes: Report of 11 representative cases. Am. J. Med. Sci. 253:561, 1967. 4. Mosely, T.: Coral snakebite: Recovery following symptoms of respiratory paralysis. Ann. Surg. 163:943, 1966. 5. Ramsey, G. and Klickstein, G.: Coral snakebite. Report of a case and suggested therapy. JAMA 182:949, 1962. 6. Neill, W.: Some misconceptions regarding the eastern coral snake, Micrurus fulvius. Herpetologica 13:111, 1957. 7. Russell, F.: Bites by the Sonoran coral snake, Micruroides euryxanthus. Toxicon 5:39, 1967.

HOW SUPPLIED

KIT:

BRAND/MANUFACTURER	NDC	SIZE	AWP
○ **BRAND**			
ANTIVENIN: Wyeth-Ayerst	00008-0407-03	1s	$275.29

Midamor *SEE* AMILORIDE HYDROCHLORIDE

Midazolam Hydrochloride

INTRAVENOUS MIDAZOLAM HYDROCHLORIDE HAS BEEN ASSOCIATED WITH RESPIRATORY DEPRESSION AND RESPIRATORY ARREST, ESPECIALLY WHEN USED FOR CONSCIOUS SEDATION. IN SOME CASES, WHERE THIS WAS NOT RECOGNIZED PROMPTLY AND TREATED EFFECTIVELY, DEATH OR HYPOXIC ENCEPHALOPATHY HAS RESULTED. INTRAVENOUS MIDAZOLAM HYDROCHLORIDE SHOULD BE USED ONLY IN HOSPITAL OR AMBULATORY CARE SETTINGS, INCLUDING PHYSICIANS' OFFICES, THAT PROVIDE FOR CONTINUOUS MONITORING OF RESPIRATORY AND CARDIAC FUNCTION. IMMEDIATE AVAILABILITY OF RESUSCITATIVE DRUGS AND EQUIPMENT AND PERSONNEL TRAINED IN THEIR USE SHOULD BE ASSURED. (SEE "WARNINGS".)

THE INITIAL INTRAVENOUS DOSE FOR CONSCIOUS SEDATION MAY BE AS LITTLE AS 1 MG, BUT SHOULD NOT EXCEED 2.5 MG IN A NORMAL HEALTHY ADULT. LOWER DOSES ARE NECESSARY FOR OLDER (OVER 60 YEARS) OR DEBILITATED PATIENTS AND IN PATIENTS RECEIVING CONCOMITANT NARCOTICS OR OTHER CNS DEPRESSANTS. THE INITIAL DOSE AND ALL SUBSEQUENT DOSES SHOULD NEVER BE GIVEN AS A BOLUS; ADMINISTER OVER AT LEAST 2 MINUTES AND ALLOW AN ADDITIONAL 2 OR MORE MINUTES TO FULLY EVALUATE THE SEDATIVE EFFECT. THE USE OF THE 1 MG/ML FORMULATION OR DILUTION OF THE 1 MG/ML OR 5 MG/ML FORMULATION IS RECOMMENDED TO FACILITATE SLOWER INJECTION. SEE "DOSAGE AND ADMINISTRATION" FOR COMPLETE DOSING INFORMATION.

DESCRIPTION

Midazolam Hydrochloride is a water-soluble benzodiazepine available as a sterile, nonpyrogenic parenteral dosage form for intravenous or intramuscular injection. Each mL contains Midazolam Hydrochloride equivalent to 1 mg or 5 mg Midazolam.

Midazolam is a white to light yellow crystalline compound, insoluble in water. The Hydrochloride salt of Midazolam, which is formed *in situ*, is soluble in aqueous solutions. Chemically, Midazolam HCl is 8-chloro-6-(2-fluorophenyl)-1-methyl-4H-imidazo[1,5-a] [1,4] benzodiazepine hydrochloride. Midazolam Hydrochloride has the empirical formula $C_{18}H_{13}ClFN_3 \cdot HCl$ and a calculated molecular weight of 362.25.

Following is its chemical structure:

CLINICAL PHARMACOLOGY

Midazolam Hydrochloride is a short-acting benzodiazepine central nervous system depressant.

The effects of Midazolam Hydrochloride on the CNS are dependent on the dose administered, the route of administration, and the presence or absence of other premedications. Onset time of sedative effects after IM administration was 15 minutes, with peak sedation occurring 30 to 60 minutes following injection.

In one study, when tested the following day, 73% of the patients who received Midazolam Hydrochloride intramuscularly had no recall of memory cards shown 30 minutes following drug administration; 40% had no recall of the memory cards shown 60 minutes following drug administration.

Sedation after IV injection was achieved within 3 to 5 minutes; the time of onset is affected by total dose administered and the concurrent administration of narcotic premedication. Seventy-one percent of the patients in the endoscopy studies had no recall of introduction of the endoscope; 82% of the patients had no recall of withdrawal of the endoscope.

When Midazolam Hydrochloride is given intravenously as an anesthetic induction agent, induction of anesthesia occurs in approximately 1.5 minutes when narcotic premedication has been administered and in 2 to 2.5 minutes without narcotic premedication or with sedative premedication. Some impairment in a test of memory was noted in 90% of the patients studied.

◆ RATED THERAPEUTICALLY EQUIVALENT; ◇ THERAPEUTIC EQUIVALENCE UNCONFIRMED; ○ UNRATED

Midazolam Hydrochloride used as directed, does not delay awakening from general anesthesia. Gross tests of recovery after awakening (orientation, ability to stand and walk, suitability for discharge from the recovery room, return to baseline Trieger competency) usually indicate recovery within 2 hours but recovery may take up to 6 hours in some cases. When compared with patients who received thiopental, patients who received Midazolam generally recovered at a slightly slower rate.

In patients without intracranial lesions, induction with Midazolam Hydrochloride is associated with a moderate decrease in cerebrospinal fluid pressure (lumbar puncture measurements), similar to that seen following use of thiopental. Preliminary data in intracranial surgical patients with normal intracranial pressure but decreased compliance (subarachnoid screw measurements) show comparable elevations of intracranial pressure with Midazolam Hydrochloride and with thiopental during intubation.

Usual intramuscular premedicating doses of Midazolam Hydrochloride do not depress the ventilatory response to carbon dioxide stimulation to a clinically significant extent. Induction doses of Midazolam Hydrochloride depress the ventilatory response to carbon dioxide stimulation for 15 minutes or more beyond the duration of ventilatory depression following administration of thiopental. Impairment of ventilatory response to carbon dioxide is more marked in patients with chronic obstructive pulmonary disease (COPD). Sedation with intravenous Midazolam Hydrochloride does not adversely affect the mechanics of respiration (resistance, static recoil, most lung volume measurements); total lung capacity and peak expiratory flow decrease significantly but static compliance and maximum expiratory flow at 50% of awake total lung capacity (Vmax) increase.

In cardiac hemodynamic studies, induction with Midazolam Hydrochloride was associated with a slight to moderate decrease in mean arterial pressure, cardiac output, stroke volume and systemic vascular resistance. Slow heart rates (less than 65/minute), particularly in patients taking propranolol for angina, tended to rise slightly; faster heart rates (eg, 85/minute) tended to slow slightly.

The following preliminary pharmacokinetic data for Midazolam have been reported. In normal subjects and healthy patients intravenous Midazolam exhibited an elimination half-life of 1.2 to 12.3 hours, a large volume of distribution (0.95 to 6.6 L/kg) and a plasma clearance of 0.15 to 0.77 L/hr/kg. Clinical effects of Midazolam Hydrochloride do not directly correlate with the blood concentrations of Midazolam.

Following intravenous administration, less than 0.03% of the dose is excreted in the urine as intact Midazolam. Midazolam is rapidly metabolized to 1-hydroxymethyl Midazolam, which is conjugated, with subsequent excretion in the urine. Approximately 45% to 57% of the dose is excreted in the urine as the conjugate of 1-hydroxymethyl Midazolam, the major metabolite of Midazolam. The half-life of elimination of 1-hydroxymethyl Midazolam is similar to the parent compound. The concentration of Midazolam is 10-to 30-fold greater than that of 1-hydroxymethyl Midazolam after single IV administration.

In a small group of patients ($n = 11$) with congestive heart failure, there appeared to be a 2- to 3-fold increase in the elimination half-life and volume of distribution of Midazolam; however, the total body clearance of Midazolam appeared to remain unchanged at a single 5-mg intravenous dose. There was no apparent change in the pharmacokinetic profile following the intravenous administration of 5 mg of Midazolam to a small group of patients ($n = 12$) with hepatic dysfunction. There was a 1.5- to 2-fold increase in elimination half-life, total body clearance and volume of distribution in a small group of patients ($n = 15$) with chronic renal failure.

In a small group ($n = 12$) of surgical patients, aged 49 to 60 years old, given 0.2 mg/kg Midazolam intravenously, there appeared to be a small increase in the volume of distribution and elimination half-life with little change in total body clearance compared to an equal number of younger surgical patients (aged 18 to 30).

The mean absolute bioavailability of Midazolam following intramuscular administration is greater than 90%. The mean time of maximum Midazolam plasma concentrations following intramuscular dosing occurs within 45 minutes postadministration. Peak concentrations of Midazolam as well as 1-hydroxymethyl Midazolam after intramuscular administration are about one-half of those achieved after equivalent intravenous doses. The pharmacokinetic profile of elimination after intramuscularly administered Midazolam is comparable to that observed following intravenous administration of the drug. Dose-linearity relationships have not been adequately defined.

Midazolam is approximately 97% plasma protein-bound in normal subjects and patients with renal failure. In animals, Midazolam has been shown to cross the blood-brain barrier. In animals and in humans, Midazolam has been shown to cross the placenta and enter into fetal circulation. Midazolam is excreted in human milk. (See *"Precautions: Nursing Mothers"*.)

INDICATIONS

Injectable Midazolam Hydrochloride is indicated—

- intramuscularly for preoperative sedation (induction of sleepiness or drowsiness and relief of apprehension) and to impair memory of perioperative events;
- intravenously as an agent for conscious sedation prior to short diagnostic or endoscopic procedures, such as bronchoscopy, gastroscopy, cystoscopy, coronary angiography and cardiac catheterization, either alone or with a narcotic;
- intravenously for induction of general anesthesia, before administration of other anesthetic agents. With the use of narcotic premedication, induction of anesthesia can be attained within a relatively narrow dose range and in a short period of time. Intravenous Midazolam Hydrochloride can also be used as a component of intravenous supplementation of nitrous oxide and oxygen (balanced anesthesia) *for short surgical procedures*; longer procedures have not been studied.

When used intravenously, Midazolam Hydrochloride is associated with a high incidence of partial or complete impairment of recall for the next several hours. (See *"Clinical Pharmacology"*.)

CONTRAINDICATIONS

Injectable Midazolam Hydrochloride is contraindicated in patients with a known hypersensitivity to the drug. Benzodiazepines are contraindicated in patients with acute narrow angle glaucoma. Benzodiazepines may be used in patients with open-angle glaucoma only if they are receiving appropriate therapy. Measurements of intraocular pressure in patients without eye disease show a moderate lowering following induction with Midazolam Hydrochloride; patients with glaucoma have not been studied.

Midazolam Hydrochloride is not intended for intrathecal or epidural administration due to the presence of the preservative benzyl alcohol in dosage form.

WARNINGS

Midazolam Hydrochloride must never be used without individualization of dosage. Prior to the intravenous administration of Midazolam Hydrochloride in any dose, the immediate availability of oxygen, resuscitative equipment and skilled personnel for the maintenance of a patent airway and support of ventilation should be ensured. Patients should be continuously monitored for early signs of underventilation or apnea, which can lead to hypoxia/cardiac arrest unless effective countermeasures are taken immediately. Vital signs should continue to be monitored during the recovery period. Because intravenous Midazolam Hydrochloride depresses respiration (see *"Clinical Pharmacology"*) and because opioid agonists and other sedatives can add to this depression, Midazolam Hydrochloride should be administered as an induction agent only by a person trained in general anesthesia and should be used for conscious sedation only in the presence of personnel skilled in early detection of under-ventilation, maintaining a patent airway and supporting ventilation. **When used for conscious sedation, Midazolam Hydrochloride should not be administered by rapid or single bolus intravenous administration.**

Serious cardiorespiratory adverse events have occurred. These have included respiratory depression, apnea, respiratory arrest and/or cardiac arrest, sometimes resulting in death. There have also been rare reports of hypotensive episodes requiring treatment during or after diagnostic or surgical manipulations in patients who have received Midazolam Hydrochloride. Hypotension occurred more frequently in the conscious sedation studies in patients premedicated with a narcotic.

Reactions such as agitation, involuntary movements (including tonic/clonic movements and muscle tremor), hyperactivity and combativeness have been reported. These reactions may be due to inadequate or excessive dosing or improper administration of Midazolam Hydrochloride; however, consideration should be given to the possibility of cerebral hypoxia or true paradoxical reactions. Should such reactions occur, the response to each dose of Midazolam Hydrochloride and all other drugs, including local anesthetics, should be evaluated before proceeding.

Concomitant use of barbiturates, alcohol or other central nervous system depressants may increase the risk of under-ventilation or apnea and may contribute to profound and/or prolonged drug effect. Narcotic premedication also depresses the ventilatory response to carbon dioxide stimulation.

Higher risk surgical patients, elderly patients and debilitated patients require lower dosages, whether premedicated or not. Patients with chronic obstructive pulmonary disease are unusually sensitive to the respiratory depressant effect of Midazolam Hydrochloride. Patients with chronic renal failure and patients with congestive heart failure eliminate Midazolam more slowly. (See *"Clinical Pharmacology"*.) Because elderly patients frequently have inefficient function of one or more organ systems, and because dosage requirements have been shown to decrease with age, reduced initial dosage of Midazolam Hydrochloride is recommended and the possibility of profound and/or prolonged effect should be considered.

Injectable Midazolam Hydrochloride should not be administered to patients in shock or coma, or in acute alcohol intoxication with depression of vital signs. Particular care should be exercised in the use of intravenous Midazolam Hydrochloride in patients with uncompensated acute illnesses, such as severe fluid or electrolyte disturbances.

The hazards of intra-arterial injection of Midazolam Hydrochloride solutions in humans are unknown; therefore, precautions against unintended intra-arterial injection should be taken. Extravasation should also be avoided.

The safety and efficacy of Midazolam Hydrochloride following non-intravenous and non-intramuscular routes of administration have not been established. Midazolam Hydrochloride should only be administered intramuscularly or intravenously.

The decision as to when patients who have received injectable Midazolam Hydrochloride, particularly on an outpatient basis, may again engage in activities requiring complete mental alertness, operate hazardous machinery or drive a motor vehicle must be individualized. Gross tests of recovery from the effects of Midazolam Hydrochloride (see *"Clinical Pharmacology"*) cannot be relied upon alone to predict reaction time under stress. This drug is never used alone during anesthesia and the contribution of other perioperative drugs and events can vary. It is recommended that no patient operate hazardous machinery or a motor vehicle until the effects of the drug, such as drowsiness, have subsided or until the day after anesthesia and surgery, whichever is longer.

Usage in Pregnancy: **An increased risk of congenital malformations associated with the use of benzodiazepine drugs (diazepam and chlordiazepoxide) has been suggested in several studies. If this drug is used during pregnancy, the patient should be apprised of the potential hazard to the fetus.**

PRECAUTIONS

General: Intravenous doses of Midazolam Hydrochloride should be decreased for elderly and for debilitated patients. (See *"Warnings"* and *"Dosage and Administration"*.) These patients will also probably take longer to recover completely after Midazolam Hydrochloride administration for the induction of anesthesia.

Midazolam Hydrochloride does not protect against the increase in intracranial pressure or against the heart rate rise and/or blood pressure rise associated with endotracheal intubation under light general anesthesia.

Information for Patients: To assure safe and effective use of benzodiazepines, the following information and instructions should be communicated to the patient when appropriate:

1. Inform your physician about any alcohol consumption and medicine you are now taking, including drugs you buy without a prescription. Alcohol has an increased effect when consumed with benzodiazepines; therefore, caution should be exercised regarding simultaneous ingestion of alcohol during benzodiazepine treatment.

2. Inform your physician if you are pregnant or are planning to become pregnant.

3. Inform your physician if you are nursing.

Drug Interactions: The sedative effect of intravenous Midazolam Hydrochloride is accentuated by premedication, particularly narcotics (eg, morphine, meperidine and fentanyl) and also secobarbital and Innovar (fentanyl and droperidol). Consequently, the dosage of Midazolam Hydrochloride should be adjusted according to the type and amount of premedication administered. (See *"Dosage and Administration".*)

A moderate reduction in induction dosage requirements of thiopental (about 15%) has been noted following use of intramuscular Midazolam Hydrochloride for premedication.

The intravenous administration of Midazolam Hydrochloride decreases the minimum alveolar concentration (MAC) of halothane required for general anesthesia. This decrease correlates with the dose of Midazolam Hydrochloride administered.

Although the possibility of minor interactive effects has not been fully studied, Midazolam Hydrochloride and pancuronium have been used together in patients without noting clinically significant changes in dosage, onset or duration. Midazolam Hydrochloride does not protect against the characteristic circulatory changes noted after administration of succinylcholine or pancuronium and does not protect against the increased intracranial pressure noted following administration of succinylcholine. Midazolam Hydrochloride does not cause a clinically significant change in dosage, onset or duration of a single intubating dose of succinylcholine.

No significant adverse interactions with commonly used premedications or drugs used during anesthesia and surgery (including atropine, scopolamine, glycopyrrolate, diazepam, hydroxyzine, d-tubocurarine, succinylcholine and non-depolarizing muscle relaxants) or topical local anesthetics (including lidocaine, dyclonine HCl and Cetacaine) have been observed.

The clearance of Midazolam and certain other benzodiazepines may be delayed with the concomitant administration of cimetidine (but not ranitidine). The clinical significance of this interaction is unclear.

Drug/Laboratory Test Interactions: Midazolam has not been shown to interfere with results obtained in clinical laboratory tests.

Carcinogenesis, Mutagenesis, Impairment of Fertility: Carcinogenesis: Midazolam maleate was administered with diet in mice and rats for 2 years at dosages of 1, 9 and 80 mg/kg/day. In female mice in the highest dose group there was a marked increase in the incidence of hepatic tumors. In high dose male rats there was a small but statistically significant increase in benign thyroid follicular cell tumors. Dosages of 9 mg/kg/day of Midazolam maleate (25 times a human dose of 0.35 mg/kg) do not increase the incidence of tumors. The pathogenesis of induction of these tumors is not known. These tumors were found after chronic administration, whereas human use will ordinarily be of single or several doses.

Mutagenesis: Midazolam did not have mutagenic activity in *Salmonella typhimurium* (5 bacterial strains), Chinese hamster lung cells (V79), human lymphocytes, or in the micronucleus test in mice.

Impairment of Fertility: A reproduction study in male and female rats did not show any impairment of fertility at dosages up to ten times the human IV dose of 0.35 mg/kg.

Pregnancy: Teratogenic Effects: Pregnancy Category D. See *"Warnings"* section.

Segment II teratology studies, performed with Midazolam maleate injectable in rabbits and rats at 5 and 10 times the human dose of 0.35 mg/kg, did not show evidence of teratogenicity.

Nonteratogenic Effects: Studies in rats showed no adverse effects on reproductive parameters during gestation and lactation. Dosages tested were approximately 10 times the human dose of 0.35 mg/kg.

Labor and Delivery: In humans, measurable levels of Midazolam were found in maternal venous serum, umbilical venous and arterial serum and amniotic fluid, indicating placental transfer of the drug. Following intramuscular administration of 0.05 mg/kg of Midazolam, both the venous and the umbilical arterial serum concentrations were lower than maternal concentrations.

The use of injectable Midazolam Hydrochloride in obstetrics has not been evaluated in clinical studies. Because Midazolam is transferred transplacentally and because other benzodiazepines given in the last weeks of pregnancy have resulted in neonatal CNS depression, Midazolam Hydrochloride is not recommended for obstetrical use.

Nursing Mothers: Midazolam is excreted in human milk. Midazolam Hydrochloride is not recommended for use in nursing mothers.

Pediatric Use: Safety and effectiveness of Midazolam Hydrochloride in children below the age of 18 years have not been established.

ADVERSE REACTIONS

See *"Warnings"* concerning serious cardiorespiratory events and possible paradoxical reactions. Fluctuations in vital signs were the most frequently seen findings following parenteral administration of Midazolam Hydrochloride and included decreased tidal volume and/or respiratory rate decrease (23.3% of patients following IV and 10.8% of patients following IM administration) and apnea (15.4% of patients following IV administration), as well as variations in blood pressure and pulse rate.

The following additional adverse reactions were reported after intramuscular administration:

headache (1.3%)

Local effects at IM injection site
pain (3.7%)
induration (0.5%)
redness (0.5%)
muscle stiffness (0.3%)

Administration of IM Midazolam Hydrochloride to elderly and/or higher risk surgical patients has been associated with rare reports of death under circumstances compatible with cardiorespiratory depression. In most of these cases, the patients also received other central nervous system depressants capable of depressing respiration, especially narcotics (see *"Dosage and Administration"*).

The following additional adverse reactions were reported subsequent to intravenous administration:

hiccoughs (3.9%)
nausea (2.8%)
vomiting (2.6%)
coughing (1.3%)
"oversedation" (1.6%)
headache (1.5%)
drowsiness (1.2%)

Local effects at the IV site
tenderness (5.6%)
pain during injection (5.0%)
redness (2.6%)
induration (1.7%)
phlebitis (0.4%)

Other adverse experiences, observed mainly following IV injection and occurring at an incidence of less than 1.0%, are as follows:

Respiratory: Laryngospasm, bronchospasm, dyspnea, hyperventilation, wheezing, shallow respirations, airway obstruction, tachypnea.

Cardiovascular: Bigeminy, premature ventricular contractions, vasovagal episode, bradycardia, tachycardia, nodal rhythm.

Gastrointestinal: Acid taste, excessive salivation, retching.

CNS/Neuromuscular: Retrograde amnesia, euphoria, hallucination, confusion, argumentativeness, nervousness, anxiety, grogginess, restlessness, emergence delirium or agitation, prolonged emergence from anesthesia, dreaming during emergence, sleep disturbance, insomnia, nightmares, athetoid movements, seizure-like activity, ataxia, dizziness, dysphoria, slurred speech, dysphonia, paresthesia.

Special Sense: Blurred vision, diplopia, nystagmus, pin-point pupils, cyclic movements of eyelids, visual disturbance, difficulty focusing eyes, ears blocked, loss of balance, light-headedness.

Integumentary: Hive-like elevation at injection site, swelling or feeling of burning, warmth or coldness at injection site.

Hypersensitivity: Allergic reactions including anaphylactoid reactions, hives, rash, pruritus.

Miscellaneous: Yawning, lethargy, chills, weakness, toothache, faint feeling, hematoma.

DRUG ABUSE AND DEPENDENCE
Midazolam is subject to Schedule IV control under the Controlled Substances Act of 1970.

Midazolam was actively self-administered in primate models used to assess the positive reinforcing effects of psychoactive drugs.

Midazolam produced physical dependence of a mild to moderate intensity in cynomolgus monkeys after 5 to 10 weeks of administration. Available data concerning the drug abuse and dependence potential of Midazolam suggest that its abuse potential is at least equivalent to that of diazepam.

OVERDOSAGE
While there is insufficient human data on overdosage with Midazolam Hydrochloride, the manifestations of Midazolam Hydrochloride overdosage are expected to be similar to those observed with other benzodiazepines and include sedation, somnolence, confusion, impaired coordination, diminished reflexes, coma and untoward effects on vital signs. No evidence of specific organ toxicity from Midazolam Hydrochloride overdosage would be expected.

◆ RATED THERAPEUTICALLY EQUIVALENT; ◇ THERAPEUTIC EQUIVALENCE UNCONFIRMED; ○ UNRATED

Treatment of Overdosage: Treatment of injectable Midazolam Hydrochloride overdosage is the same as that followed for overdosage with other benzodiazepines. Respiration, pulse rate and blood pressure should be monitored and general supportive measures should be employed. Attention should be given to the maintenance of a patent airway and support of ventilation. An intravenous infusion should be started. Should hypotension develop, treatment may include intravenous fluid therapy, repositioning, judicious use of vasopressors appropriate to the clinical situation, if indicated, and other appropriate countermeasures. There is no information as to whether peritoneal dialysis, forced diuresis or hemodialysis are of any value in the treatment of Midazolam overdosage.

Flumazenil, a specific benzodiazepine-receptor antagonist, is indicated for the complete or partial reversal of the sedative effects of benzodiazepines and may be used in situations when an overdose with a benzodiazepine is known or suspected. Prior to the administration of flumazenil, necessary measures should be instituted to secure airway, ventilation, and intravenous access. Flumazenil is intended as an adjunct to, not as a substitute for, proper management of benzodiazepine overdose. Patients treated with flumazenil should be monitored for resedation, respiratory depression and other residual benzodiazepine effects for an appropriate period after treatment. **The prescriber should be aware of a risk of seizure in association with flumazenil treatment, particularly in long-term benzodiazepine users and in cyclic antidepressant overdose.** The complete flumazenil package insert, including *"Contraindications"*, *"Warnings"*, and *"Precautions"*, should be consulted prior to use.

DOSAGE AND ADMINISTRATION

Midazolam Hydrochloride is a potent sedative agent which requires slow administration and individualization of dosage. Clinical experience has shown Midazolam Hydrochloride to be 3 to 4 times as potent per mg as diazepam. BECAUSE SERIOUS AND LIFE-THREATENING CARDIORESPIRATORY ADVERSE EVENTS HAVE BEEN REPORTED, PROVISION FOR MONITORING, DETECTION AND CORRECTION OF THESE REACTIONS MUST BE MADE FOR EVERY PATIENT TO WHOM MIDAZOLAM HYDROCHLORIDE INJECTION IS ADMINISTERED, REGARDLESS OF AGE OR HEALTH STATUS. Excess doses or rapid or single bolus intravenous administration may result in respiratory depression and/or arrest. (See *"Warnings"*.)

Reactions such as agitation, involuntary movements, hyperactivity and combativeness have been reported. Should such reactions occur, caution should be exercised before continuing administration of Midazolam Hydrochloride. (See *"Warnings"*.)

Midazolam Hydrochloride should only be administered IM or IV (See *"Warnings"*.)

Care should be taken to avoid intra-arterial injection or extravasation. (See *"Warnings"*.)

Midazolam Hydrochloride Injection may be mixed in the same syringe with the following frequently used premedications: morphine sulfate, meperidine, atropine sulfate or scopolamine. Midazolam Hydrochloride at a concentration of 0.6 mg/mL, is compatible with 5% dextrose in water and 0.9% sodium chloride for up to 24 hours and with lactated Ringer's solution for up to 4 hours. Both the 1 mg/mL and 5 mg/mL formulations of Midazolam Hydrochloride may be diluted with 0.9% sodium chloride or 5% dextrose in water.

Intramuscularly	*Usual Adult Dose*
For preoperative sedation (induction of sleepiness or drowsiness and relief of apprehension) and to impair memory of perioperative events.	The recommended premedication dose of Midazolam Hydrochloride for good risk (ASA Physical Status I & II) adult patients below the age of 60 years is 0.07 to 0.08 mg/kg IM (approximately 5 mg IM) administered approximately 1 hour before surgery.
For intramuscular use, Midazolam Hydrochloride should be injected deep in a large muscle mass.	The dose must be individualized and reduced when IM Midazolam Hydrochloride is administered to patients with chronic obstructive pulmonary disease, other higher risk surgical patients, patients 60 or more years of age, and patients who have received concomitant narcotics or other CNS depressants (see *"Adverse Reactions"*). In a study of patients 60 years or older, who did not receive concomitant administration of narcotics, 2 to 3 mg (0.02 to 0.05 mg/kg) of Midazolam Hydrochloride produced adequate sedation during the preoperative period. The dose of 1 mg IM Midazolam Hydrochloride may suffice for some older patients if the anticipated intensity and duration of sedation is less critical. As with any potential respiratory depressant, these patients require observation for signs of cardiorespiratory depression after receiving IM Midazolam Hydrochloride.
	Onset is within 15 minutes, peaking at 30 to 60 minutes. It can be administered concomitantly with atropine sulfate or scopolamine hydrochloride and reduced doses of narcotics.

Intravenously

Conscious Sedation (See *"Indications"*):

Intramuscularly	*Usual Adult Dose*
Narcotic premedication results in less variability in patient response and a reduction in dosage of Midazolam Hydrochloride. For peroral procedures, the use of an appropriate topical anesthetic is recommended. For bronchoscopic procedures, the use of narcotic premedication is recommended.	**When used for conscious sedation, dosage must be individualized and titrated. Midazolam Hydrochloride should not be administered by rapid or single bolus intravenous administration. Individual response will vary with age, physical status and concomitant medications, but may also vary independent of these factors. (See *"Warnings concerning cardiac/respiratory arrest"*.)**
Midazolam Hydrochloride 1 mg/mL formulation is recommended for conscious sedation, to facilitate slower injection. Both the 1 mg/mL and the 5 mg/mL formulations may be diluted with 0.9% sodium chloride or 5% dextrose in water.	

1. Healthy Adults Below the Age of 60:
Titrate slowly to the desired effect, eg. the initiation of slurred speech. Some patients may respond to as little as 1 mg. No more than 2.5 mg should be given over a period of at least 2 minutes. Wait an additional 2 or more minutes to fully evaluate the sedative effect. If further titration is necessary, continue to titrate, using small increments, to the appropriate level of sedation. Wait an additional 2 or more minutes after each increment to fully evaluate the sedative effect. A total dose-greater than 5 mg is not usually necessary to reach the desired endpoint. If narcotic premedication or other CNS depressants are used, patients will require approximately 30% less Midazolam Hydrochloride than unpremedicated patients.

2. Patients Age 60 or Older, and Debilitated or Chronically Ill Patients:
Because the danger of under-ventilation or apnea is greater in elderly patients and those with chronic disease states or decreased pulmonary reserve, and because the peak effect may take longer in these patients, increments should be smaller and the rate of injection slower. Titrate *slowly* to the desired effect, eg, the initiation of slurred speech. Some patients may respond to as little as 1 mg. No more than 1.5 mg should be given over a period of no less than 2 minutes. Wait an additional 2 or more minutes to fully evaluate the sedative effect. If additional titration is necessary, it should be given at a rate of no more than 1 mg over a period of 2 minutes, waiting an additional 2 or more minutes each time to fully evaluate the sedative effect. Total doses greater than 3.5 mg are not usually necessary.
If concomitant CNS depressant premedications are used in these patients, they will require at least 50% less Midazolan Hydrochloride than healthy young unpremedicated patients.

3. Maintenance Dose:
Additional doses to maintain the desired level of sedation may be given in increments of 25% of the dose used to first reach the sedative endpoint, but again only by slow titration, especially in the elderly and chronically ill or debilitated patient. These additional doses should be given *only* after a thorough clinical evaluation clearly indicates the need for additional sedation.

Induction of Anesthesia: For induction of general anesthesia, before administration of other anesthetic agents.	Individual response to the drug is variable, particularly when a narcotic premedication is not used. The dosage should be titrated to the desired effect according to the patient's age and clinical status. When Midazolan Hydrochloride is used before other intravenous agents for induction of anesthesia, the initial dose of each agent may be significantly reduced, at times to as low as 25% of the usual initial dose of the individual agents.

Unpremedicated Patients:
In the absence of premedication, an average adult under the age of 55 years will usually require an initial dose of 0.3 to 0.35 mg/kg for induction, administered over 20 to 30 seconds and allowing 2 minutes for effect. If needed to complete

Intramuscularly	Usual Adult Dose
	induction, increments of approximately 25% of the patients initial dose may be used; induction may instead be completed with volatile liquid inhalational anesthetics. In resistant cases, up to 0.6 mg/kg total dose may be used for induction, but such larger doses may be prolong recovery. Unpremedicated patients over the age of 55 years usually require less Midazolam Hydrochloride induction; an initial dose of 0.3 mg/kg is recommended. Unpremedicated patients with severe systemic disease or other debilitation usually require less Midazolam Hydrochloride for induction. An initial dose of 0.2 to 0.25 mg/kg will usually suffice; in some cases, as little as 0.15 mg/kg may suffice.
	Premedicated Patients:
	When the patient has received sedative or narcotic premedication, particularly narcotic premedication, the range of recommended doses is 0.15 to 0.35 mg/kg.
	In average adults below the age of 55 years, a dose of 0.25 mg/kg, administered over 20 to 30 seconds and allowing 2 minutes for effect, will usually suffice.
	The initial dose of 0.2 mg/kg is recommended for good risk (ASA I & II) sugical patients over the age 55 years.
	In some patients with severe systemic disease or debilitation, as little as 0.15 mg/kg may suffice. Narcotic premedication frequently used during clinical trials included fentanyl (1.5 to 2 µg/kg IV, administered 5 minutes before induction), morphine (dosage individualized, up to 0.15 mg/kg IM), meperidine (dosage individualized, up to 1 mg/kg IM) and Innovar (0.02 mL/kg IM). Sedative premedications were hydroxyzine pamoate (100 mg orally) and sodium secobarbital (200 mg orally). Except for intravenous fentanyl, administered 5 minutes before induction, all other premedications should be administered approximately 1 hour prior to the time anticipated for Midazolam Hydrochloride induction.
Injectable Midazolam Hydrochloride can also be used during maintenance of anesthesia, *for short surgical procedures,* as a component of balanced anesthesia. Effective narcotic premedication is especially recommended in such cases. Long surgical procedures have not been studied.	Incremental injections of approximately 25% of the induction dose should be given in response to signs of lightening of anesthesia and repeated as necessary.

Note: Parenteral drug products should be inspected visually for particulate matter and discoloration prior to administration, whenever solution and container permit.

Store at 59° to 86°F (15° to 30°C).

HOW SUPPLIED
INJECTION (C-IV): 1 MG/ML

BRAND/MANUFACTURER	NDC	SIZE	AWP
○ **BRAND**			
VERSED: Roche Labs	00004-1998-06	2 ml 10s	$41.20
	00004-1999-01	5 ml 10s	$90.57
	00004-2000-06	10 ml 10s	$161.97

INJECTION (C-IV): 5 MG/ML

BRAND/MANUFACTURER	NDC	SIZE	AWP
○ **BRAND**			
VERSED: Roche Labs	00004-1974-01	1 ml 10s	$90.57
	00004-1973-01	2 ml 10s	$161.97
	00004-1947-01	2 ml 10s	$203.49
	00004-1975-01	5 ml 10s	$382.48
	00004-1946-01	10 ml 10s	$726.71

Midrin *SEE ACETAMINOPHEN/DICHLORALPHENAZONE/ ISOMETHEPTENE MUCATE*

Migergot *SEE ERGOTAMINE TARTRATE WITH CAFFEINE*

Milontin *SEE PHENSUXIMIDE*

Milrinone Lactate

DESCRIPTION
Milrinone Lactate is a member of a new class of bipyridine inotropic/vasodilator agents with phosphodiesterase inhibitor activity, distinct from digitalis glycosides or catecholamines.

Milirinone Lactate is designated as 1,6-dihydro-2-methyl-6-oxo-[3,4'-bipyridine]-5-carbonitrile lactate.

Milrinone is an off-white to tan crystalline compound with a molecular weight of 211.2 and an empirical formula of $C_{12}H_9N_3O$. It is slightly soluble in methanol, and very slightly soluble in chloroform and in water. As the lactate salt, it is stable and colorless to pale yellow in solution. Milrinone Lactate is available as a sterile solution of the Lactate salt of Milrinone. Each mL contains Milrinone Lactate equivalent to 1 mg Milrinone.

Following is its chemical structure:

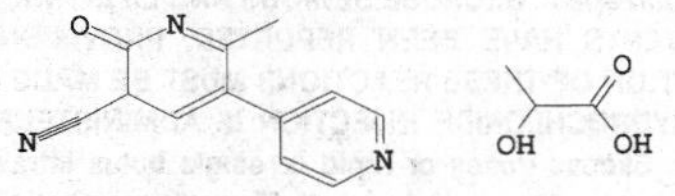

CLINICAL PHARMACOLOGY
Milrinone Lactate is a positive inotrope and vasodilator, with little chronotropic activity different in structure and mode of action from either the digitalis glycosides or catecholamines. Milrinone Lactate at relevant inotropic and vasorelaxant concentrations, is a selective inhibitor of peak III cAMP phosphodiesterase isozyme in cardiac and vascular muscle. This inhibitory action is consistent with cAMP mediated increases in intracellular ionized calcium and contractile force in cardiac muscle, as well as with cAMP dependent contractile protein phosphorylation and relaxation in vascular muscle. Additional experimental evidence also indicates that Milrinone Lactate is not a beta-adrenergic agonist nor does it inhibit sodium-potassium adenosine triphosphatase activity as do the digitalis glycosides.

Clinical studies in patients with congestive heart failure have shown that Milrinone Lactate produces dose-related and plasma drug concentration-related increases in the maximum rate of increase of left ventricular pressure. Studies in normal subjects have shown that Milrinone Lactate produces increases in the slope of the left ventricular pressure-dimension relationship, indicating a direct inotropic effect of the drug. Milrinone Lactate also produces dose-related and plasma concentration-related increases in forearm blood flow in patients with congestive heart failure, indicating a direct arterial vasodilator activity of the drug.

Both the inotropic and vasodilatory effects have been observed over the therapeutic range of plasma Milrinone concentrations of 100 ng/mL to 300 ng/mL.

In addition to increasing myocardial contractility, Milrinone Lactate improves diastolic function as evidenced by improvements in left ventricular diastolic relaxation.

PHARMACOKINETICS
Following intravenous injections of 12.5 µg/kg to 125 µg/kg to congestive heart failure patients, Milrinone Lactate had a volume of distribution of 0.38 liters/kg, a mean terminal elimination half-life of 2.3 hours, and a clearance of 0.13 liters/kg/hr. Following intravenous infusions of 0.20 µg/kg/min to 0.70 µg/kg/min to congestive heart failure patients, the drug had a volume of distribution of about 0.45 liters/kg, a mean terminal elimination half-life of 2.4 hours, and a clearance of 0.14 liters/kg/hr. These pharmacokinetic parameters were not dose-dependent, and the area under the plasma concentration versus time curve following injections was significantly dose-dependent.

Milrinone Lactate has been shown (by equilibrium dialysis) to be approximately 70% bound to human plasma protein.

The primary route of excretion of Milrinone Lactate in man is via the urine. The major urinary excretion of orally administered Milrinone Lactate in man are Milrinone (83%) and its 0-glucuronide metabolite (12%). Elimination in normal subjects via the urine is rapid, with approximately 60% recovered within the first two hours following dosing and approximately 90% recovered within the first eight hours following dosing. The mean renal clearance of Milrinone Lactate is approximately 0.3 liters/min, indicative of active secretion.

PHARMACODYNAMICS
In patients with depressed myocardial function, Milrinone Lactate injection, produced a prompt increase in cardiac output and decreases in pulmonary capillary wedge pressure and vascular resistance, without a significant increase in heart rate or myocardial oxygen consumption. These hemodynamic improve-

ments were dose and plasma Milrinone concentration related. Hemodynamic improvement during intravenous therapy with Milrinone Lactate was accompanied by clinical symptomatic improvement, as measured by changes in New York Heart Association classification. The great majority of patients experience improvements in hemodynamic function within 5 to 15 minutes of the initiation of therapy.

In studies in congestive heart failure patients, Milirnone Lactate when administered as a loading injection followed by a maintenance infusion produced significant mean initial increases in cardiac index of 25 percent, 38 percent, and 42 percent at dose regimens of 37.5 µg/kg/0.375 µg/kg/min, 50 µg/kg/0.50 µg/kg/min, and 75 µg/kg/0.75 µg/kg/min, respectively. Over the same range of loading injections and maintenance infusions, pulmonary capillary wedge pressure significantly decreased by 20 percent, 23 percent, and 36 percent, respectively, while systemic vascular resistance significantly decreased by 17 percent, 21 percent, and 37 percent. The heart rate was generally unchanged (increases of 3, 3 and 10 percent, respectively). Mean arterial pressure fell by up to 5 percent at the two lower dose regimens, but by 17 percent at the highest dose. Patients evaluated for 48 hours maintained improvements in hemodynamic function, with no evidence of diminished response (tachyphylaxis). A smaller number of patients have received infusions of Milrinone Lactate for periods up to 72 hours without evidence of tachyphylaxis.

The duration of therapy should depend upon patient responsiveness. Patients have been maintained on infusions of Milrinone Lactate for up to 5 days.

Milrinone Lactate has a favorable inotropic effect in fully digitalized patients without causing signs of glycoside toxicity. Theoretically, in cases of atrial flutter/fibrillation, it is possible that Milrinone Lactate may increase ventricular response rate because of its slight enhancement of AV node conduction. In these cases, digitalis should be considered prior to the institution of therapy with Milrinone Lactate.

Improvement in left ventricular function in patients with ischemic heart disease has been observed. The improvement has occurred without inducing symptoms or electrocardiographic signs of myocardial ischemia.

The steady-state plasma Milrinone Lactate concentrations after approximately 6 to 12 hours of unchanging maintenance infusion of 0.50 µg/kg/min are approximately 200 ng/mL. Near maximum favorable effects of Milrinone Lactate on cardiac output and pulmonary capillary wedge pressure are seen at plasma Milrinone concentrations in the 150 ng/mL to 250 ng/mL range.

INDICATIONS AND USAGE
Milrinone Lactate is indicated for the short-term intravenous therapy of congestive heart failure. The majority of experience with intravenous Milrinone Lactate has been in patients receiving digoxin and diuretics.

In some patients injections of Milrinone Lactate and oral Milrinone Lactate have been shown to increase ventricular ectopy, including nonsustained ventricular tachycardia. Patients receiving Milrinone Lactate should be closely monitored during infusion.

CONTRAINDICATIONS
Milrinone Lactate is contraindicated in patients who are hypersensitive to it.

PRECAUTIONS
GENERAL
Milrinone Lactate should not be used in patients with severe obstructive aortic or pulmonic valvular disease in lieu of surgical relief of the obstruction. Like other inotropic agents, it may aggravate outflow tract obstruction in hypertrophic subaortic stenosis.

Supraventricular and ventricular arrhythmias have been observed in the high-risk population treated. In some patients, injections of Milrinone Lactate and oral Milrinone Lactate have been shown to increase ventricular ectopy, including nonsustained ventricular tachycardia. The potential for arrhythmia, present in congestive heart failure itself, may be increased by many drugs or combinations of drugs. Patients receiving Milrinone Lactate should be closely monitored during infusion.

Milrinone Lactate produces a slight shortening of AV node conduction time, indicating a potential for an increased ventricular response rate in patients with atrial flutter/fibrillation which is not controlled with digitalis therapy.

During therapy with Milrinone Lactate, blood pressure and heart rate should be monitored and the rate of infusion slowed or stopped in patients showing excessive decreases in blood pressure.

If prior vigorous diuretic therapy is suspected to have caused significant decreases in cardiac filling pressure Milrinone Lactate should be cautiously administered with monitoring of blood pressure, heart rate, and clinical symptomatology.

USE IN ACUTE MYOCARDIAL INFARCTION
No clinical studies have been conducted in patients in the acute phase of post myocardial infarction. Until further clinical experience with this class of drugs is gained, Milrinone Lactate is not recommended in these patients.

LABORATORY TESTS
Fluid and Electroyltes: Fluid and electrolyte changes and renal function should be carefully monitored during therapy with Milrinone Lactate. Improvement in cardiac output with resultant diuresis may necessitate a reduction in the dose of diuretic. Potassium loss due to excessive diuresis may predispose digitalized patients to arrhythmias. Therefore, hypokalemia should be corrected by potassium supplementation in advance of or during use of Milrinone Lactate.

DRUG INTERACTIONS
No untoward clinical manifestations have been observed in limited experience where patients in whom Milrinone Lactate was used concurrently with the following drugs: digitalis glycosides; lidocaine, quinidine; hydralazine, prazosin; isosorbide dinitrate, nitroglycerin; chlorthalidone, furosemide, hydrochlorothiazide, spironolactone; captopril; heparin, warfarin, diazepam, insulin; and potassium supplements.

CHEMICAL INTERACTIONS
There is an immediate chemical interaction which is evidenced by the formation of a precipitate when furosemide is injected into an intravenous line of an infusion of Milrinone Lactate. Therefore, furosemide should not be administered in intravenous lines containing Milrinone Lactate injection.

CARCINOGENESIS, MUTAGENESIS, IMPAIRMENT OF FERTILITY
Twenty-four months of oral administration of Milrinone Lactate to mice at doses up to 40 mg/kg/day (about 50 times the human oral therapeutic dose in a 50 kg patient) was unassociated with evidence of carcinogenic potential. Neither was there evidence of carcinogenic potential when Milrinone Lactate was orally administered to rats at doses up to 5 mg/kg/day (about 6 times the human oral therapeutic dose) for twenty-four months or at 25 mg/kg/day (about 30 times the human oral therapeutic dose) for up to 18 months in males and 20 months in females. Whereas the Chinese Hamster Ovary Chromosome Aberration Assay was positive in the presence of a metabolic activation system, results from the Ames Test, the Mouse Lymphoma Assay, the Micronucleus Test, and the in vivo Rat Bone Marrow Metaphase Analysis indicated an absence of mutagenic potential. In reproductive performance studies in rats, Milrinone Lactate had no effect on male or female fertility at oral doses up to 32 mg/kg/day.

ANIMAL TOXICITY
Oral and intravenous administration of toxic dosages of Milrinone Lactate to rats and dogs resulted in myocardial degeneration/fibrosis and endocardial hemorrhage, principally affecting the left ventricular papillary muscles. Coronary vascular lesions characterized by periarterial edema and inflammation have been observed in dogs only. The myocardial/endocardial changes are similar to those produced by beta-adrenergic receptor agonists such as isoproterenol, while the vascular changes are similar to those produced by minoxidil and hydralazine. Doses within the recommended clinical dose range (up to 1.13 mg/kg/day) for congestive heart failure patients have not produced significant adverse effects in animals.

PREGNANCY CATEGORY C
Oral administration of Milrinone Lactate to pregnant rats and rabbits during organogenesis produced no evidence of teratogenicity at dose levels up to 40 mg/kg/day and 12 mg/kg/day, respectively. Milrinone Lactate did not appear to be teratogenic when administered intravenously to pregnant rats at doses up to 3 mg/kg/day (about 2.5 times the maximum recommended clinical intravenous dose) or pregnant rabbits at doses up to 12 mg/kg/day, although an increased resorption rate was apparent at both 8 mg/kg/day and 12 mg/kg/day (intravenous) in the latter species. There are no adequate and well-controlled studies in pregnant women. Milrinone Lactate should be used during pregnancy only if the potential benefit justifies the potential risk to the fetus.

NURSING MOTHERS
Caution should be exercised when Milrinone Lactate is administered to nursing women, since it is not known whether it is excreted in human milk.

PEDIATRIC USE
Safety and effectiveness in children have not been established.

USE IN ELDERLY PATIENTS
There are no special dosage recommendations for the elderly patient. Ninety percent of all patients administered Milrinone Lactate in clinical studies were within the age range of 45 to 70 years, with a mean age of 61 years. Patients in all age groups demonstrated clinically and statistically significant responses. No age-related effects on the incidence of adverse reactions have been observed. Controlled pharmacokinetic studies have not disclosed any age-related effects on the distribution and elimination of Milrinone Lactate injection.

ADVERSE REACTIONS
Cardiovascular Effects: In patients receiving Milrinone Lactate in Phase II and III clinical trials, ventricular arrhythmias were reported in 12.1%: Ventricular ectopic activity, 8.5%; nonsustained ventricular tachycardia, 2.8%; sustained ventricular tachycardia, 1% and, ventricular fibrillation, 0.2% (2 patients experienced more than one type of arrhythmia). Holter recordings demonstrated that in some patients injection of Milrinone Lactate increased ventricular ectopy, including nonsustained ventricular tachycardia. Life-threatening arrhythmias were infrequent and when present have been associated with certain underlying factors such as preexisting arrhythmias, metabolic abnormalities (e.g., hypokalemia), abnormal digoxin levels and catheter insertion. Milrinone Lactate was not shown to be arrhythmogenic in an electrophysiology study. Supraventricular arrhythmias were reported in 3.8% of the patients receiving Milrinone Lactate. The incidence of both supraventricular and ventricular arrhythmias has not been related to the dose or plasma Milrinone concentration.

Other cardiovascular adverse reactions include hypotension, 2.9% and angina/chest pain, 1.2%.

CNS EFFECTS

Headaches, usually mild to moderate in severity, have been reported in 2.9% of patients receiving Milrinone Lactate.

OTHER EFFECTS

Other adverse reactions reported, but not definitely related to the administration of Milrinone Lactate include hypokalemia, 0.6%; tremor, 0.4%; and thrombocytopenia, 0.4%.

OVERDOSAGE

Doses of Milrinone Lactate may produce hypotension because of its vasodilator effect. If this occurs, administration of Milrinone Lactate should be reduced or temporarily discontinued until the patient's condition stabilizes. No specific antidote is known, but general measures for circulatory support should be taken.

DOSAGE AND ADMINISTRATION

Milrinone Lactate should be administered with a loading dose followed by a continuous infusion (maintenance dose) according to the following guidelines:

LOADING DOSE

50 µg/kg: Administer Slowly Over 10 Minutes

MAINTENANCE DOSE

	Infusion Rate	Total Daily Dose/ (24 Hours)	
Minimum	0.375 µg/kg/min	0.59 mg/kg	Administer as
Standard	0.50 µg/kg/min	0.77 mg/kg	a continuous
Maximum	0.75 µg/kg/min	1.13 mg/kg	intravenous
			infusion.

The infusion rate should be adjusted according to hemodynamic and clinical response. Patients should be closely monitored. In controlled clinical studies, most patients showed an improvement in hemodynamic status as evidenced by increases in cardiac output and reductions in pulmonary capillary wedge pressure.

Note: See *"Dosage Adjustment in Renally Impaired Patients."* Dosage may be titrated to the maximum hemodynamic effect and should not exceed 1.13 mg/kg/day. Duration of therapy should depend upon patient responsiveness. Intravenous infusions of Milrinone Lactate injection should be administered as described in the following chart.

MILRINONE LACTATE RATES OF INFUSION FOR CONCENTRATIONS OF 100 µg/mL, 150 µg/mL, AND 200 µg/mL
INFUSION DELIVERY RATE

Milrinone Lactate (µg/kg/min)	100 µg/mL* (mL/kg/hr)	150 µg/mL** (mL/kg/hr)	200 µg/mL/+ (mL/kg/hr)
0.375	0.22	0.15	0.11
0.400	0.24	0.16	0.12
0.500	0.30	0.20	0.15
0.600	0.36	0.24	0.18
0.700	0.42	0.28	0.21
0.750	0.45	0.30	0.22

In order to calculate flow rate (milliliters per hour), multiply infusion delivery rate times patient weight (in kilograms).
* *Prepare by adding 180 mL diluent per 20 mg vial (20 mL) Milrinone Lactate.*
** *Prepare by adding 113 mL diluent per 20 mg vial (20 mL) Milrinone Lactate.*
+ *Prepare by adding 80 mL diluent per 20 mg vial (20 mL) Milrinone Lactate.*

Note: Diluents which may be used to prepare dilutions of Milrinone Lactate for intravenous infusion are 0.45% Sodium Chloride Injection, USP, 0.9% Sodium Chloride Injection, USP, or 5% Dextrose Injection, USP.

Intravenous drug products should be inspected visually and should not be used if particulate matter or discoloration is present.

DOSAGE ADJUSTMENT IN RENALLY IMPAIRED PATIENTS

Data obtained from patients with severe renal impairment (creatinine clearance = 0 to 30 mL/min) but without congestive heart failure have demonstrated that the presence of renal impairment significantly increases the terminal elimination half-life of Milrinone Lactate injection. Reductions in infusion rate may be necessary in patients with renal impairment. For patients with clinical evidence of renal impairment, the recommended infusion rate can be obtained from the following table:

Creatinine Clearance (mL/min/1.73 m²)	Infusion Rate (µg/kg/min)
5	0.20
10	0.23
20	0.28
30	0.33
40	0.38
50	0.43

Store at controlled room temperature 15°C to 30°C (59°F to 86°F). Avoid freezing.

HOW SUPPLIED
INJECTION: 5 MG

BRAND/MANUFACTURER	NDC	SIZE	AWP
○ **BRAND**			
PRIMACOR I.V.: Sanofi Winthrop	00024-1200-06	5 ml 10s	$305.88
	00024-1200-10	10 ml 40s	$578.12
	00024-1200-20	20 ml 40s	$1092.00

Miltown SEE MEPROBAMATE

Mini-Gamulin Rh SEE GLOBULIN, IMMUNE RHO₀(D)

Mini-Gamulin Rh SEE RHO(D) IMMUNE GLOBULIN

Minipress SEE PRAZOSIN HYDROCHLORIDE

Minitran SEE NITROGLYCERIN

Minizide SEE

Minocin SEE MINOCYCLINE HYDROCHLORIDE

Minocycline Hydrochloride

DESCRIPTION

Minocycline Hydrochloride a semisynthetic derivative of tetracycline, is [4S-(4α,4aα,5aα,12aα)]-4, 7-bis(dimethylamino)-1,4,4a,5,5a,6,11,12a-octahydro-3,10,12,12a-tetrahydroxy-1,11-dioxo-2-naphthacenecarboxamide monohydrochloride.

Minocycline HCl pellet-filled capsules for oral administration contain pellets of Minocycline HCl equivalent to 50 mg or 100 mg of Minocycline.

Each vial dried by cryodesiccation, contains sterile Minocycline HCl equivalent to 100 mg Minocycline. When reconstituted with 5 mL of Sterile Water for Injection, the pH ranges from 2.0 to 2.8.

Minocycline HCl oral suspension contains Minocycline HCl equivalent to 50 mg of Minocycline per 5 mL (10 mg/mL).

Following is its chemical structure:

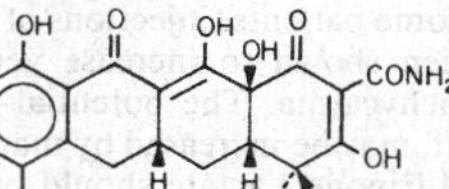

CLINICAL PHARMACOLOGY

Minocycline HCl pellet-filled capsules are rapidly absorbed from the gastrointestinal tract following oral administration. Following a single dose of two 100 mg pellet-filled capsules of Minocycline HCl administered to 18 normal fasting adult volunteers, maximum serum concentrations were attained in 1 to 4 hours (average 2.1 hours) and ranged from 2.1 to 5.1 mcg/mL (average 3.5 mcg/mL). The serum half-life in the normal volunteers ranged from 11.1 to 22.1 hours (average 15.5 hours).

Following a single dose of two 100 mg Minocycline HCl capsules administered to 10 normal adult volunteers, serum levels ranged from 0.74 to 4.45 mcg/mL in 1 hour (average 2.24), after 12 hours, they ranged from 0.34 to 2.36 mcg/mL (average 1.25).

When Minocycline HCl pellet-filled capsules were given concomitantly with a meal which included dairy products, the extent of absorption of Minocycline HCl pellet-filled capsules was not noticeably influenced. The peak plasma concentrations were slightly decreased (11.2%) and delayed by 1 hour when administered with food, compared to dosing under fasting conditions.

Following a single dose of 200 mg administered intravenously to 10 healthy male volunteers, serum levels ranged from 2.52 to 6.63 mcg/mL (average 4.18), after 12 hours they ranged from 0.82 to 2.64 mcg/mL (average 1.38). In a group of five healthy male volunteers, serum levels of 1.4 to 1.8 mcg/mL were maintained at 12 and 24 hours with doses of 100 mg every 12 hours for 3 days. When given

200 mg once daily for 3 days, the serum levels had fallen to approximately 1 mcg/mL at 24 hours. The serum half-life following IV doses of 100 mg every 12 hours or 200 mg once daily did not differ significantly and ranged from 15 to 23 hours.

Intravenously administered Minocycline appears similar to oral doses in excretion. The urinary and fecal recovery of oral Minocycline when administered to 12 normal volunteers is one-half to one-third that of other tetracyclines.

In previous studies, the Minocycline serum half-life ranged from 11 to 17 hours in 12 essentially normal volunteers following a single 200 mg oral dose, from 11 to 16 hours in 7 patients with hepatic dysfunction, and from 18 to 69 hours in 5 patients with renal dysfunction. The urinary and fecal recovery of Minocycline when administered to 12 normal volunteers is one-half to one-third that of other tetracyclines.

Microbiology: The tetracyclines are primarily bacteriostatic and are thought to exert their antimicrobial effect by the inhibition of protein synthesis. The tetracyclines, including Minocycline, have similar antimicrobial spectra of activity against a wide range of gram-positive and gram-negative organisms. Cross-resistance of these organisms to tetracyclines is common.

While *in vitro* studies have demonstrated the susceptibility of most strains of the following microorganisms, clinical efficacy for infections other than those included in the *"Indications and Usage"* section has not been documented.

GRAM-NEGATIVE BACTERIA
Bartonella bacilliformis
Brucella species
Campylobacter fetus
Francisella tularensis
Haemophilus ducreyi
Haemophilus influenzae
Listeria monocytogenes
Neisseria gonorrhoeae
Vibrio cholerae
Yersinia pestis

Because many strains of the following groups of gram-negative microorganisms have been shown to be resistant to tetracyclines, culture and susceptibility tests are especially recommended:

Acinetobacter species
Bacteroides species
Enterobacter aerogenes
Escherichia coli
Klebsiella species
Shigella species

GRAM-POSITIVE BACTERIA
Because many strains of the following groups of gram-positive microorganisms have been shown to be resistant to tetracyclines, culture and susceptibility testing are especially recommended. Up to 44 percent of *Streptococcus pyogenes* strains have been found to be resistant to tetracycline drugs. Therefore, tetracyclines should not be used for streptococcal disease unless the organism has been demonstrated to be susceptible.

Alpha-hemolytic streptococci (viridans group)
Streptococcus pneumoniae
Streptococcus pyogenes

OTHER MICROORGANISMS
Actinomyces species
Bacillus anthracis
Balantidium coli
Borrelia recurrentis
Chlamydia psittaci
Chlamydia trachomatis
Clostridium species
Entamoeba species
Fusobacterium fusiforme
Propionibacterium acnes
Treponema pallidum
Treponema pertenue
Ureaplasma urealyticum

Susceptibility Tests: Diffusion Techniques: The use of antibiotic disk susceptibility test methods which measure zone diameter gives an accurate estimation of susceptibility of microorganisms to Minocycline HCl *pellet-filled capsules.* One such standard procedure[1] has been recommended for use with disks for testing antimicrobials. Either the 30 mcg tetracycline-class disk or the 30 mcg Minocycline disk should be used for the determination of the susceptibility of microorganisms to Minocycline.

With this type of procedure a report of "susceptible" from the laboratory indicates that the infecting organism is likely to respond to therapy. A report of "intermediate susceptibility" suggests that the organism would be susceptible if a high dosage is used or if the infection is confined to tissues and fluids (eg, urine) in which high antibiotic levels are attained. A report of 'resistant' indicates that the infecting organism is not likely to respond to therapy. With either the tetracycline-class disk or the Minocycline disk, zone sizes of 19 mm or greater indicate susceptibility, zone sizes of 14 mm or less indicate resistance, and zone sizes of 15 to 18 mm indicate intermediate susceptibility.

If the Kirby-Bauer method of susceptibility testing (using a 30 mcg tetracycline disc) gives a zone of 18 mm or greater, the bacterial strain is considered to be susceptible to any tetracycline. Minocycline shows moderate *in vitro* activity against certain strains of staphylococci which have been found resistant to other tetracyclines. For such strains, Minocycline susceptibility powder may be used for additional susceptibility testing.

If the Kirby-Bauer method of susceptibility testing (using a 30 mcg tetracycline disc) gives a zone of 18mm or greater, the bacterial strain is considered to be susceptible to any tetracycline. Minocycline shows moderate *in vitro* activity against certain strains of staphylococci which have been found resistant to other tetracyclines. For such strains, Minocycline susceptibility powder may be used for additional susceptibility testing.

Standardized procedures require the use of laboratory control organisms. The 30 mcg tetracycline disk should give zone diameters between 19 and 28 mm for *Straphylococcus aureus* ATCC 25923 and between 18 and 25 mm for *Escherichia coli* ATCC 25922. The 30 mcg Minocycline disk should give zone diameters between 25 and 30 mm for *S aureus* ATCC 25923 and between 19 and 25 mm for *E coli* ATCC 25922.

Dilution Techniques: When using the NCCLS agar dilution or broth dilution (including microdilution) method[2] or equivalent, a bacterial isolate may be considered susceptible if the MIC (minimal inhibitory concentration) of Minocycline is 4 mcg/mL or less. Organisms are considered resistant if the MIC is 16 mcg/mL or greater. Organisms with an MIC value of less than 16 mcg/mL but greater than 4 mcg/mL are expected to be susceptible if a high dosage is used or if the infection is confined to tissues and fluids (eg, urine) in which high antibiotic levels are attained.

Tube dilution testing: Microorganisms may be considered susceptible (likely to respond to Minocycline therapy) if the minimum inhibitory concentration (MIC) is not more than 4 mcg/mL. Microorganisms may be considered intermediate (harboring partial resistance) if the MIC is 4 to 12.5 mcg/mL and resistant (not likely to respond to Minocycline therapy) if the MIC is greater than 12.5 mcg/mL.

As with standard diffusion methods, dilution procedures require the use of laboratory control organisms. Standard tetracycline or Minocycline powder should give MIC values of 0.25 mcg/mL to 1.0 mcg/mL for *S aureus* ATCC 25923, and 1.0 mcg/mL to 4.0 mcg/mL for *E coli* ATCC 25922.

INDICATIONS AND USAGE
Minocycline HCl *pellet-filled capsules* are indicated in the treatment of the following infections due to susceptible strains of the designated microorganisms:

Rocky Mountain spotted fever, typhus fever and the typhus group, Q fever, rickettsialpox and tick fevers caused by Rickettsiae
Respiratory tract infections caused by *Mycoplasma pneumoniae*
Lymphogranuloma venereum caused by *Chlamydia trachomatis*
Psittacosis (Ornithosis) due to *Chlamydia psittaci*
Trachoma caused by *Chlamydia trachomatis*, although the infectious agent is not always eliminated, as judged by immunofluorescence.
Inclusion conjunctivitis caused by *Chlamydia trachomatis*; may be treated with oral tetracyclines or with a combination of oral and topical agents
Nongonococcal urethritis or uncomplicated urethral, endocervical, or rectal infections in adults caused by *Ureaplasma urealyticum* or *Chlamydia trachomatis*
Minocycline HCl is indicated for the treatment of uncomplicated gonococcal urethritis in men due to *Neisseria gonorrhoeae*
Relapsing fever due to *Borrelia recurrentis*
Chancroid caused by *Haemophilus ducreyi*
Plague due to *Yersinia pestis*
Tularemia due to *Francisella tularensis*
Cholera caused by *Vibrio cholerae*
Campylobacter fetus infections caused by *Campylobacter fetus*
Brucellosis due to *Brucella* species (in conjunction with streptomycin)
Bartonellosis due to *Bartonella bacilliformis*
Granuloma inguinale caused by *Calymmatobacterium granulomatis*

Minocycline is indicated for treatment of infections caused by the following gram-negative microorganisms, when bacteriologic testing indicates appropriate susceptibility to the drug:

Escherichia coli
Enterobacter aerogenes
Shigella species
Acinetobacter calcoaceticus
Respiratory tract infections caused by *Haemophilus influenzae*
Respiratory tract and urinary tract infections caused by *Klebsiell Influenzae*

Minocycline HCl *pellet-filled capsules* are indicated for the treatment of infections caused by the following gram-positive microorganisms when bacteriologic testing indicates appropriate susceptibility to the drug:

Streptococcus species:
Up to 44% of strains of *Streptococcus pyogenes* and 74% of *Streptococcus faecalis* have been found to be resistant to drugs. Therefore, tetracyclines should not be used for streptococcal disease unless the organism has been demonstrated to be sensitive.
For upper respiratory infections due to Group A betahemolytic streptococci, penicillin is the usual drug of choice, including prophylaxis of rheumatic fever.
Upper respiratory tract infections caused by *Streptococcus pneumoniae*
Skin and skin structure infections caused by *Staptococcus aureus*. (Note: Minocycline is not the drug of choice in the treatment of any type of staphylococcal infection.)
Uncomplicated urethritis in men due to *Neisseria gonorrhoeae* and for the treatment of other gonococcal infections when penicillin is contraindicated.

When penicillin is contraindicated, Minocycline is an alternative drug in the treatment of the following infections:

Infections in women caused by *Neisseria gonorrhoeae*
Syphilis caused by *Treponema pallidum*
Yaws caused by *Treponema pertenue*
Listeriosis due to *Listeria monocytogenes*
Anthrax due to *Bacillus anthracis*
Vincent's infection caused by *Fusobacterium fusiforme*
Actinomycosis caused by *Actinomyces israelii*
Infections caused by *Clostridium* species

In *acute intestinal amebiasis*, Minocycline may be a useful adjunct to amebicides.
In severe *acne*, Minocycline may be useful adjunctive therapy.

Oral Minocycline is indicated in the treatment of asymptomatic carriers of *Neisseria meningitidis* to eliminate meningococci from the nasopharynx. In order to preserve the usefulness of Minocycline in the treatment of asymptomatic meningococcal carrier, diagnostic laboratory procedures, including serotyping and susceptibility testing, should be performed to establish the carrier state and the correct treatment. It is recommended that the prophylactic use of Minocycline be reserved for situations in which the risk of Meningococcal meningitis is high.

Oral Minocycline is not indicated for the treatment of meningococcal infection.

Although no controlled clinical efficacy studies have been conducted, limited clinical data show that oral Minocycline hydrochloride has been used successfully in the treatment of infections caused by *Mycobacterium marinum*.

UNLABELED USES
Minocycline HCL is used alone or as an adjunct in the treatment of anaerobic infections, cystic fibrosis, gingivitis, and plasmodium falciparum infections (malaria). Minocycline HCL is also used in the treatment of leprosy.

CONTRAINDICATIONS
This drug is contraindicated in persons who have shown hypersensitivity to any of the tetracyclines.

WARNINGS
MINOCYCLINE HCL PELLET-FILLED CAPSULES, LIKE OTHER TETRA-CYCLINE-CLASS ANTIBIOTICS, CAN CAUSE FETAL HARM WHEN ADMINISTERED TO A PREGNANT WOMAN IF ANY TETRACYCLINE IS USED DURING PREGNANCY OR IF THE PATIENT BECOMES PREGNANT WHILE TAKING THESE DRUGS, THE PATIENT SHOULD BE APRISED OF THE POTENTIAL HAZARD TO THE FETUS. THE USE OF DRUGS OF THE TETRACYCLINE CLASS DURING TOOTH DEVELOPMENT (LAST HALF OF PREGNANCY, INFANCY, AND CHILDHOOD TO THE AGE OF 8 YEARS) MAY CAUSE PERMANENT DISCOLORATION OF THE TEETH (YELLOW-GRAY-BROWN).

This adverse reaction is more common during long-term use of the drug but has been observed following repeated short-term courses. Enamel hypoplasia has also been reported. TETRACYCLINE DRUGS, THEREFORE, SHOULD NOT BE USED DURING TOOTH DEVELOPMENT UNLESS OTHER DRUGS ARE NOT LIKELY TO BE EFFECTIVE OR ARE CONTRAINDICATED.

All tetracyclines form a stable calcium complex in any bone-forming tissue. A decrease in fibula growth rate has been observed in young animals (rats and rabbits) and prematures given oral tetracycline in doses of 25 mg/kg every 6 hours. This reaction was shown to be reversible when the drug was discontinued.

Results of animal studies indicate that tetracyclines cross the placenta, are found in fetal tissues, and can have toxic effects on the developing fetus (often related to retardation of skeletal development). Evidence of embryotoxicity has been noted in animals treated early in pregnancy.

In the presence of renal dysfunction, particularly in pregnancy, intravenous tetracycline therapy in daily doses exceeding 2 g has been associated with deaths through liver failure.

When the need for intensive treatment outweighs its potential dangers (mostly during pregnancy or in individuals with known or suspected renal or liver impairment), it is advisable to perform renal and liver function tests before and during therapy. Also, tetracycline serum concentrations should be followed.

The anti-anabolic action of the tetracyclines may cause an increase in BUN. While this is not a problem in those with normal renal function, in patients with significantly impaired function, higher serum levels of tetracycline may lead to azotemia, hyperphosphatemia, and acidosis. If renal impairment exists, even usual oral or parenteral doses may lead to excessive systemic accumulations of the drug and possible liver toxicity. Under such conditions, lower than usual total doses are indicated, and if therapy is prolonged, serum level determinations of the drug may be advisable. This hazard is of particular importance in the parenteral administration of tetracyclines to pregnant or postpartum patients with pyelonephritis. When used under these circumstances, the blood level should not exceed 15 mcg/mL and liver function tests should be made at frequent intervals. Other potentially hepatotoxic drugs should not be prescribed concomitantly.

Photosensitivity manifested by an exaggerated sunburn reaction has been observed in some individuals taking tetracyclines. Patients apt to be exposed to direct sunlight or ultraviolet light should be advised that this reaction can occur with tetracycline drugs, and treatment should be discontinued at the first evidence of skin erythema. This has been reported rarely with Minocycline.

Central nervous system side effects including light-headedness, dizziness, or vertigo have been reported with Minocycline therapy. Patients who experience these symptoms should be cautioned about driving vehicles or using hazardous machinery while on Minocycline therapy. These symptoms may disappear during therapy and usually disappear rapidly when the drug is discontinued.

Some brands of oral suspension contain sodium sulfite a sulfite that may cause allergic-type reactions including anaphylactic symptoms and life-threatening or less severe asthmatic episodes in certain susceptible people. The overall prevalence of sulfite sensitivity in the general population is unknown and probably low. Sulfite sensitivity is seen more frequently in asthmatic than in nonasthmatic people.

PRECAUTIONS
General: As with other antibiotic preparations, use of this drug may result in overgrowth of nonsusceptible organisms, including fungi. If superinfection occurs, the antibiotic should be discontinued and appropriate therapy instituted. Pseudotumor cerebri (benign intracranial hypertension) in adults has been associated with the use of tetracyclines. The usual clinical manifestations are headache and blurred vision. Bulging fontanels have been associated with the use of tetracyclines in infants. While both of these conditions and related symptoms usually resolve after discontinuation of the tetracycline, the possibility for permanent sequelae exists.

Incision and drainage or other surgical procedures should be performed in conjunction with antibiotic therapy when indicated.

All infections due to Group A beta-hemolytic streptococci should be treated for at least 10 days.

Information for Patients: Photosensitivity manifested by an exaggerated sunburn reaction has been observed in some individuals taking tetracyclines. Patients apt to be exposed to direct sunlight or ultraviolet light should be advised that this reaction can occur with tetracycline drugs, and treatment should be discontinued at the first evidence of skin erythema. This reaction has been reported rarely with use of minocycline.

Patients who experience central nervous system symptoms (see *"Warnings"*) should be cautioned about driving vehicles or using hazardous machinery while on minocycline therapy.

Concurrent use of tetracycline may render oral contraceptives less effective (see *"Drug Interactions"*).

Laboratory Tests: In veneral disease when coexistent syphilis is suspected, a darkfield examination should be done before treatment is started and the blood serology repeated monthly for at least 4 months.

In long-term therapy, periodic laboratory evaluations of organ systems, including hematopoietic, renal, and hepatic studies should be performed.

Drug Interactions: Because tetracyclines have been shown to depress plasma prothrombin activity, patients who are on anticoagulant therapy may require downward adjustment of their anticoagulant dosage.

Since bacteriostatic drugs may interfere with the bactericidal action of penicillin, it is advisable to avoid giving tetracycline-class drugs in conjunction with penicillin.

Absorption of tetracyclines is impaired by antacids containing aluminum, calcium, or magnesium, and iron-containing preparations.

The concurrent use of tetracycline and methoxyflurane has been reported to result in fatal renal toxicity.

Concurrent use of tetracyclines may render oral contraceptives less effective.

Drug/Laboratory Test Interactions: False elevations of urinary catecholamine levels may occur due to interference with the fluorescence test.

Carcinogenesis, Mutagenesis, Impairment of Fertility: Dietary administration of Minocycline in long-term tumorigenicity studies in rats resulted in evidence of thyroid tumor production. Minocycline has also been found to produce thyroid hyperplasia in rats and dogs. In addition, there has been evidence of oncogenic activity in rats in studies with a related antibiotic, oxytetracycline (ie, adrenal and pituitary tumors). Likewise, although mutagenicity studies of minocycline have not been conducted, positive results in *in vitro* mammalian cell assays (ie, mouse lymphoma and Chinese hamster lung cells) have been reported for related antibiotics (tetracycline hydrochloride and oxytetracycline). Segment I (fertility and general reproduction) studies have provided evidence that Minocycline impairs fertility in male rats.

Teratogenic Effects: Pregnancy: Pregnancy Category D: (see *"Warnings"*).

Results of animal studies indicate that tetracyclines cross the placenta, are found in fetal tissues, and can have toxic effects on the developing fetus (often related to retardation of skeletal development). Evidence of embryotoxicity has also been noted in animals treated early in pregnancy.

The safety of Minocycline HCl for use during pregnancy has not been established.

Labor and Delivery: The effect of tetracyclines on labor and delivery is unknown.

Nursing Mothers: Tetracyclines are excreted in human milk. Because of the potential for serious adverse reactions in nursing infants from the tetracyclines, a decision should be made whether to discontinue nursing or discontinue the drug, taking into account the importance of the drug to the mother (see *"Warnings"*).

Pediatric Use: See *"Warnings"*.

ADVERSE REACTIONS
Due to oral Minocycline's virtually complete absorption, side effects to the lower bowel, particularly diarrhea, have been infrequent. The following adverse reactions have been observed in patients receiving tetracyclines.

Gastrointestinal: Anorexia, nausea, vomiting, diarrhea, glossitis, dysphagia, enterocolitis, pancreatitis, and inflammatory lesions (with monilial overgrowth) in the anogenital region, increases in liver enzymes, and rarely hepatitis have been reported. These reactions have been caused by both the oral and parenteral administration of tetracyclines. Rare instances of esophagitis and esophageal ulcerations have been reported in patients taking the tetracycline-class antibiotics in capsule and tablet form. Most of these patients took the medication immediately before going to bed (see *"Dosage and Administration"*).

Skin: Maculopapular and erythematous rashes. Exfoliative dermatitis has been reported but is uncommon. Fixed drug eruptions, including balanitis, have been rarely reported. Erythema multiforme and rarely Stevens-Johnson syndrome have been reported. Photosensitivity is discussed above (see *"Warnings"*). Pigmentation of the skin and mucous membranes has been reported.

Renal Toxicity: Elevations in BUN have been reported and are apparently dose related (see *"Warnings"*).

Hypersensitivity reactions: Urticaria, angioneurotic edema, polyarthralgia, anaphylaxis, anaphylactoid purpura, pericarditis, exacerabation of systemic lupus erythematosus and rarely pulmonary infiltrates with eosinophilia have been reported.

Blood: Hemolytic anemia, thrombocytopenia, neutropenia, and eosinophilia have been reported.

Central Nervous System: Bulging fontanels in infants and benign intracranial hypertension (pseudotumor cerebri) in adults (see *"Precautions—General"*) have been reported. Headache has also been reported.

Other: When given over prolonged periods, tetracyclines have been reported to produce brown-black microscopic discoloration of the thyroid glands. No abnormalities of thyroid function are known to occur in man.

Decreased hearing has been rarely reported in patients on Minocycline HCl.

Tooth discoloration in children less than 8 years of age (see *"Warnings"*) and also, rarely, in adults has been reported.

OVERDOSAGE
In case of overdosage, discontinue medication, treat symptomatically, and institute supportive measures.

DOSAGE AND ADMINISTRATION
CAPSULES
THE USUAL DOSAGE AND FREQUENCY OF ADMINISTRATION OF MINOCYCLINE DIFFERS FROM THAT OF THE OTHER TETRACYCLINES. EXCEEDING THE RECOMMENDED DOSAGE MAY RESULT IN AN INCREASED INCIDENCE OF SIDE EFFECTS.

Minocycline HCl pellet-filled capsules may be taken with or without food (see *"Clinical Pharmacology"*).

Adults: The usual dosage of Minocycline HCl pellet-filled capsules is 200 mg initially followed by 100 mg every 12 hours. Alternatively, if more frequent doses are preferred, two or four 50 mg pellet-filled capsules may be given initially followed by one 50 mg capsule four times daily.

For children above 8 years of age: The usual dosage of Minocycline HCl is 4 mg/kg initially followed by 2 mg/kg every 12 hours.

Uncomplicated gonococcal infections other than urethritis and anorectal infections in men: 200 mg initially, followed by 100 mg every 12 hours for a minimum of 4 days, with post-therapy cultures within 2 to 3 days.

In the treatment of uncomplicated gonococcal urethritis in men, 100 mg every 12 hours for 5 days is recommended.

For the treatment of syphilis, the usual dosage of Minocycline HCl *pellet-filled capsules* should be administered over a period of 10 to 15 days. Close follow-up, including laboratory tests, is recommended.

In the treatment of meningococcal carrier state, the recommended dosage is 100 mg every 12 hours for 5 days.

Mycobacterium marinum infections: Although optimal doses have not been established, 100 mg every 12 hours for 6 to 8 weeks have been used successfully in a limited number of cases.

Uncomplicated nongonococcal urethral infection in adults caused by *Chlamydia trachomatis* or *Ureaplasma urealyticum*: 100 mg orally, every 12 hours for at least 7 days.

Ingestion of adequate amounts of fluids along with capsule and tablet forms of drugs in the tetracycline-class is recommended to reduce the risk of esophageal irritation and ulceration.

In patients with renal impairment (see *"Warnings"*), the total dosage should be decreased by either reducing the recommended individual doses and/or by extending the time intervals between doses.

INTRAVENOUS
Note: Rapid administration is to be avoided. Parenteral therapy is indicated only when oral therapy is not adequate or tolerated. Oral therapy should be instituted as soon as possible. If intravenous therapy is given over prolonged periods of time, thrombophlebitis may result.

Adults: Usual adult dose: 200 mg followed by 100 mg every 12 hours and should not exceed 400 mg in 24 hours. The cryodesiccated powder should be reconstituted with 5 mL Sterile Water for Injection USP and immediately further diluted to 500 mL to 1,000 mL with Sodium Chloride Injection USP, Dextrose Injection USP, Dextrose and Sodium Chloride Injection USP, Ringer's Injection USP, or Lactated Ringer's Injection USP, but not other solutions containing calcium because a precipitate may form.

Final dilutions (500 mL to 1,000 mL) should be administered immediately but product and diluents are compatible at room temperature for 24 hours without a

significant loss of potency. Any unused portions must be discarded after that period.

For children above 8 years of age: Usual pediatric dose: 4 mg/kg followed by 2 mg/kg every 12 hours.

In patients with renal impairment: (See *"Warnings"*.) Total dosage should be decreased by reduction of recommended individual doses and/or extending time intervals between doses.

Parenteral drug products should be inspected visually for particulate matter and discoloration prior to administration, whenever solution and container permit.

ORAL SUSPENSION
Therapy should be continued for at least 24 to 48 hours after symptoms and fever have subsided.

Concomitant Therapy: Antacids containing aluminum, calcium, or magnesium impair absorption and should not be given to patients taking oral tetracycline.

Studies to date have indicated that the absorption of Minocycline HCl is not notably influenced by foods and dairy products.

In patients with Renal Impairment: (See *"Warnings"*.) Total dosage should be decreased by reduction of recommended individual doses and/or extending time intervals between doses.

In the treatment of streptococcal infections, a therapeutic dosage of tetracycline should be administered for at least 10 days.

Adults: The usual dosage of Minocycline HCl is 200 mg initially followed by 100 mg every 12 hours.

For Children above 8 Years of Age: The usual dosage of Minocycline HCl is 4 mg/kg initially followed by 2 mg/kg every 12 hours.

For treatment of syphilis, the usual dosage of Minocycline HCl should be administered over a period of 10 to 15 days. Close follow-up, including laboratory tests, is recommended.

Gonorrhea patients sensitive to penicillin may be treated with Minocycline HCl administered as 200 mg initially, followed by 100 mg every 12 hours for a minimum of 4 days, with post-therapy cultures within 2 to 3 days.

In the treatment of meningococcal carrier state, recommended dosage is 100 mg every 12 hours for 5 days.

Mycobacterium marinum infections: Although optimal doses have not been established, 100 mg twice a day for 6 to 8 weeks have been used successfully in a limited number of cases.

Uncomplicated urethral, endocervical, or rectal infection in adults caused by *Chlamydia trachomatis* or *Ureaplasma urealyticum*: 100 mg, by mouth, 2 times a day for at least 7 days.[1]

In the treatment of uncomplicated gonococcal urethritis in men, 100 mg twice a day orally for 5 days is recommended.

STORAGE
Store at controlled room temperature, 15°-30°C (59°-86°F). Protect from light, moisture and excessive heat. Do not freeze oral suspension.

ANIMAL PHARMACOLOGY AND TOXICOLOGY
Minocycline HCl has been found to produce high blood concentrations following oral dosage to various animal species and to be extensively distributed to all tissues examined in ^{14}C-labeled drug studies in dogs.

Minocycline HCl has been observed to cause a dark discoloration of the thyroid in experimental animals (rats, minipigs, dogs, and monkeys). In the rat, chronic treatment with Minocycline HCl has resulted in goiter accompanied by elevated radioactive iodine uptake, and evidence of thyroid tumor production. Minocycline HCl has also been found to produce thyroid hyperplasia in rats and dogs.

REFERENCES
1. National Committee for Clinical Laboratory Standards, Approved Standard: *Performance Standards for Antimicrobial Disk Susceptibility Tests*, 3rd Edition, Vol. 4(16):M2-A3, Villanova, PA, December 1984. 2. National Committee for Clinical Laboratory Standards, Approved Standard: *Methods for Dilution Antimicrobial Susceptibility Tests for Bacteria that Grow Aerobically*, 2nd Edition, Vol. 5(22):M7-A, Villanova, PA, December 1985.

HOW SUPPLIED
CAPSULE: 50 MG

AVERAGE UNIT PRICE (AVAILABLE SIZES)		GENERIC A-RATED AVERAGE PRICE (GAAP)	
BRAND	$1.04	100s	$118.29
GENERIC	$1.17		
HCFA FUL (100s ea)	$0.67		

BRAND/MANUFACTURER	NDC	SIZE	AWP
◆ BRAND			
DYNACIN: Medicis	99207-0497-10	100s	$103.58
◆ GENERICS			
Moore,H.L.	00839-7649-06	100s	$105.18
Rugby	00536-1382-01	100s	$115.18
Schein	00364-2497-01	100s	$118.00
Goldline	00182-1102-01	100s	$118.00
Geneva	00781-2333-01	100s	$118.40
Qualitest	00603-4678-21	100s	$119.86
URL	00677-1435-01	100s	$119.95
Aligen	00405-4680-01	100s	$120.00
Goldline	00182-1430-01	100s	$120.00

BRAND/MANUFACTURER	NDC	SIZE	AWP
Biocraft	00332-3165-09	100s	$120.00
Warner Chilcott	00047-0615-24	100s	$120.00
Major	00904-2413-60	100s	$120.55
Major	00904-7682-60	100s	$120.55
Major	00904-2413-61	100s ud	$120.36
Warner Chilcott	00047-0615-32	1000s	$1051.80

CAPSULE: 50 MG

BRAND/MANUFACTURER	NDC	SIZE	AWP
○ BRAND			
DYNACIN: Medicis	99207-0497-05	500s	$492.02

CAPSULE: 100 MG

AVERAGE UNIT PRICE (AVAILABLE SIZES)		GENERIC A-RATED AVERAGE PRICE (GAAP)	
BRAND	$1.81	50s	$96.85
GENERIC	$1.93		

BRAND/MANUFACTURER	NDC	SIZE	AWP
◆ BRAND			
DYNACIN: Medicis	99207-0498-50	50s	$90.64
◆ GENERICS			
Moore, H.L.	00839-7650-04	50s	$87.60
➤ Warner Chilcott	00047-0616-19	50s	$96.36
Schein	00364-2498-50	50s	$97.00
Goldline	00182-1103-19	50s	$97.00
Major	00904-2414-51	50s	$97.45
Major	00904-7683-51	50s	$97.45
Geneva	00781-2341-50	50s	$97.80
Goldline	00182-1431-19	50s	$98.00
Biocraft	00332-3167-07	50s	$98.00
Qualitest	00603-4679-19	50s	$98.00
URL	00677-1436-02	50s	$98.10
Rugby	00536-1392-06	50s	$98.12
Aligen	00405-4681-50	50s	$98.20
Major	00904-2414-61	100s ud	$196.25
➤ Warner Chilcott	00047-0616-32	1000s	$1754.40

CAPSULE: 100 MG

BRAND/MANUFACTURER	NDC	SIZE	AWP
○ BRAND			
DYNACIN: Medicis	99207-0498-05	500s	$861.05

CAPSULE, COATED PELLETS: 50 MG

AVERAGE UNIT PRICE (AVAILABLE SIZES)	
BRAND	$1.55

BRAND/MANUFACTURER	NDC	SIZE	AWP
◆ BRAND			
➤ MINOCIN: Lederle Labs	00005-5343-23	100s	$155.58
	00005-5343-27	250s	$387.99

CAPSULE, COATED PELLETS: 100 MG

AVERAGE UNIT PRICE (AVAILABLE SIZES)	
BRAND	$2.59

BRAND/MANUFACTURER	NDC	SIZE	AWP
◆ BRAND			
MINOCIN: Lederle Labs	00005-5344-18	50s	$129.59
	00005-5344-27	250s	$646.30

POWDER FOR INJECTION: 100 MG

BRAND/MANUFACTURER	NDC	SIZE	AWP
◆ BRAND			
MINOCIN: Lederle Labs	00205-5305-94	1s	$31.23

SUSPENSION: 50 MG/5 ML

BRAND/MANUFACTURER	NDC	SIZE	AWP
○ BRAND			
MINOCIN: Lederle Labs	00005-5313-56	60 ml	$29.04

Minoxidil, Oral

WARNINGS

MINOXIDIL TABLETS CONTAIN THE POWERFUL ANTIHYPERTENSIVE AGENT, MINOXIDIL, WHICH MAY PRODUCE SERIOUS ADVERSE EFFECTS. IT CAN CAUSE PERICARDIAL EFFUSION, OCCASIONALLY PROGRESSING TO TAMPONADE, AND ANGINA PECTORIS MAY BE EXACERBATED. MINOXIDIL SHOULD BE RESERVED FOR HYPERTENSIVE PATIENTS WHO DO NOT RESPOND ADEQUATELY TO MAXIMUM THERAPEUTIC DOSES OF A DIURETIC AND TWO OTHER ANTIHYPERTENSIVE AGENTS.

IN EXPERIMENTAL ANIMALS, MINOXIDIL CAUSED SEVERAL KINDS OF MYOCARDIAL LESIONS AS WELL AS OTHER ADVERSE CARDIAC EFFECTS (SEE "CARDIAC LESIONS IN ANIMALS").

MINOXIDIL MUST BE ADMINISTERED UNDER CLOSE SUPERVISION, USUALLY CONCOMITANTLY WITH THERAPEUTIC DOSES OF A BETA-ADRENERGIC BLOCKING AGENT TO PREVENT TACHYCARDIA AND INCREASED MYOCARDIAL WORKLOAD. IT MUST ALSO USUALLY BE GIVEN WITH A DIURETIC, FREQUENTLY ONE ACTING IN THE ASCENDING LIMB OF THE LOOP OF HENLE, TO PREVENT SERIOUS FLUID ACCUMULATION. PATIENTS WITH MALIGNANT HYPERTENSION AND THOSE ALREADY RECEIVING GUANETHIDINE (SEE "WARNINGS") SHOULD BE HOSPITALIZED WHEN MINOXIDIL IS FIRST ADMINISTERED SO THAT THEY CAN BE MONITORED TO AVOID TOO RAPID, OR LARGE ORTHOSTATIC, DECREASES IN BLOOD PRESSURE.

DESCRIPTION

Minoxidil Tablets contain Minoxidil, an antihypertensive peripheral vasodilator. Minoxidil occurs as a white or off-white, odorless, crystalline solid that is soluble in water to the extent of approximately 2 mg/ml; is readily soluble in propylene glycol or ethanol; and is almost insoluble in acetone, chloroform or ethyl acetate. The chemical name for Minoxidil is 2,4-pyrimidinediamine, 6-(1-piperidinyl)-, 3-oxide (mw = 209.25).

Minoxidil Tablets for oral administration contain either 2.5 mg or 10 mg of Minoxidil.

Following is its chemical structure:

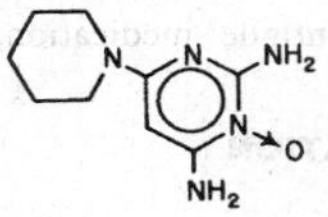

CLINICAL PHARMACOLOGY

1. GENERAL PHARMACOLOGIC PROPERTIES

Minoxidil is an orally effective direct acting peripheral vasodilator that reduces elevated systolic and diastolic blood pressure by decreasing peripheral vascular resistance. Microcirculatory blood flow in animals is enhanced or maintained in all systemic vascular beds. In man, forearm and renal vascular resistance decline; forearm blood flow increases while renal blood flow and glomerular filtration rate are preserved.

Because it causes peripheral vasodilation, Minoxidil elicits a number of predictable reactions. Reduction of peripheral arteriolar resistance and the associated fall in blood pressure trigger sympathetic, vagal inhibitory, and renal homeostatic mechanisms, including an increase in renin secretion, that lead to increased cardiac rate and output and salt and water retention. These adverse effects can usually be minimized by concomitant administration of a diuretic and a beta-adrenergic blocking agent or other sympathetic nervous system suppressant.

Minoxidil does not interfere with vasomotor reflexes and therefore does not produce orthostatic hypotension. The drug does not enter the central nervous system in experimental animals in significant amounts, and it does not affect CNS function in man.

2. EFFECTS ON BLOOD PRESSURE AND TARGET ORGANS

The extent and time-course of blood pressure reduction by Minoxidil do not correspond closely to its concentration in plasma. After an effective single oral dose, blood pressure usually starts to decline within one-half hour, reaches a minimum between 2 and 3 hours and recovers at an arithmetically linear rate of about 30%/day. The total duration of effect is approximately 75 hours. When Minoxidil is administered chronically, once or twice a day, the time required to achieve maximum effect on blood pressure with a given daily dose is inversely related to the size of the dose. Thus, maximum effect is achieved on 10 mg/day within 7 days, on 20 mg/day within 5 days, and on 40 mg/day within 3 days.

The blood pressure response to Minoxidil is linearly related to the logarithm of the dose administered. The slope of this log-linear dose-response relationship is proportional to the extent of hypertension and approaches zero at a supine diastolic blood pressure of approximately 85 mmHg.

When used in severely hypertensive patients resistant to other therapy, frequently with an accompanying diuretic and beta blocker, Minoxidil Tablets usually decreased the blood pressure and reversed encephalopathy and retinopathy.

3. ABSORPTION AND METABOLISM

Minoxidil is at least 90% absorbed from the GI tract in experimental animals and man. Plasma levels of the parent drug reach maximum within the first hour and decline rapidly thereafter. The average plasma half-life in man is 4.2 hours. Approximately 90% of the administered drug is metabolized, predominantly by conjugation with glucuronic acid at the N-oxide position in the pyrimidine ring, but also by conversion to more polar products. Known metabolites exert much less pharmacologic effect than Minoxidil itself; all are excreted principally in the urine. Minoxidil does not bind to plasma proteins, and its renal clearance corresponds to the glomerular filtration rate. In the absence of functional renal tissue, Minoxidil and its metabolites can be removed by hemodialysis.

4. CARDIAC LESIONS IN ANIMALS
Minoxidil produced two types of cardiac lesions in non-primate species:

(a) Dog atrial lesion— Daily oral doses of 0.5 mg/kg for several days to 1 month or longer produced a grossly visible hemorrhagic lesion of the right atrium of the dog. This lesion has not been seen in other species. Microscopic examination showed replacement of myocardial cells by proliferating fibroblasts and angioblasts; phagocytosis; and hemosiderin accumulation in macrophages.

(b) Papillary muscle lesion— Short term treatment (about 3 days) in several species (dog, rat, minipig) produced necrosis of the papillary muscles and, in some cases subendocardial areas of the left ventricle, lesions similar to those produced by other peripheral dilators and by beta-adrenergic receptor agonists such as isoproterenol and epinephrine. These are thought to result from myocardial ischemia resulting from reflex sympathetic or vagal withdrawal-induced tachycardia in combination with hypotension. These lesions were reduced in incidence and severity by beta-adrenergic receptor blockade.

(c) Epicarditis A less fully studied lesion is focal epicarditis, seen in dogs after 2 days of oral Minoxidil. More recently, chronic proliferative epicarditis was observed in dogs treated topically twice a day for 90 days. In a one-year oral dog study, serosanguinous pericardial fluid was seen.

In addition to these lesions, longer term studies in rats, dogs, and monkeys showed cardiac hypertrophy and (in rats) cardiac dilation. In monkeys, hydrochlorothiazide partly reversed the increased heart weight, suggesting it may be related to fluid overload. In a one-year dog study, serosanguinous pericardial fluid was seen.

Autopsies of 79 patients who died from various causes and who had received Minoxidil did not reveal right atrial or other hemorrhagic pathology of the kind seen in dogs. Instances of necrotic areas in the papillary muscles were seen, but these occurred in the presence of known pre-existing ischemic heart disease and did not appear different from, or more common than, lesions seen in patients never exposed to Minoxidil. Studies to date cannot rule out the possibility that Minoxidil can be associated with cardiac damage in humans.

INDICATIONS AND USAGE
Because of the potential for serious adverse effects, Minoxidil Tablets are indicated only in the treatment of hypertension that is symptomatic or associated with target organ damage and is not manageable with maximum therapeutic doses of a diuretic plus two other antihypertensive drugs. At the present time use in milder degrees of hypertension is not recommended because the benefit-risk relationship in such patients has not been defined.

Minoxidil reduced supine diastolic blood pressure by 20 mm Hg or to 90 mm Hg or less in approximately 75% of patients, most of whom had hypertension that could not be controlled by other drugs.

CONTRAINDICATIONS
Tablets are contraindicated in pheochromocytoma, because Minoxidil may stimulate secretion of catecholamines from the tumor through its antihypertensive action.

WARNINGS
1. *Salt and Water Retention: Congestive Heart Failure:* concomitant use of an adequate diuretic is required—Minoxidil Tablets must usually be administered concomitantly with a diuretic adequate to prevent fluid retention and possible congestive heart failure; a high ceiling (loop) diuretic is *almost always* required. Body weight should be monitored closely. If Minoxidil is used without a diuretic, retention of several hundred milli-equivalents of salt and corresponding volumes of water can occur within a few days, leading to increased plasma and interstitial fluid volume and local or generalized edema. Diuretic treatment alone, or in combination with restricted salt intake, will usually minimize fluid retention, although reversible edema did develop in approximately 10% of nondialysis patients so treated. Ascites has also been reported. Diuretic effectiveness was limited mostly by disease-related impaired renal function. The condition of patients with preexisting congestive heart failure occasionally deteriorated in association with fluid retention although because of the fall in blood pressure (reduction of afterload), more than twice as many improved than worsened. Rarely, refractory fluid retention may require discontinuation of Minoxidil. Provided that the patient is under close medical supervision, it may be possible to resolve refractory salt retention by discontinuing Minoxidil for 1 or 2 days and then resuming treatment in conjunction with vigorous diuretic therapy.

2. *Concomitant Treatment to Prevent Tachycardia is Usually Required:* Minoxidil increases the heart rate. Angina may worsen or appear for the first time during treatment with Minoxidil, probably because of the increased oxygen demands associated with increased heart rate and cardiac output. The increase in rate and the occurrence of angina generally can be prevented by the concomitant administration of a beta-adrenergic blocking drug or other sympathetic nervous system suppressant. The ability of beta-adrenergic blocking agents to minimize papillary muscle lesions in animals is further reason to utilize such an agent concomitantly. Round-the-clock effectiveness of the sympathetic suppressant should be ensured.

3. *Pericarditis, Pericardial Effusion and Tamponade:* There have been reports of pericarditis occurring in association with the use of Minoxidil. The relationship of this association to renal status is uncertain. Pericardial effusion, occasionally with tamponade, has been observed in about 3% of treated patients not on dialysis, especially those with inadequate or compromised renal function. Although in many cases, the pericardial effusion was associated with a connective tissue disease, the uremic syndrome, congestive heart failure, or marked fluid retention, there have been instances in which these potential causes of effusion were not present. Patients should be observed closely for any suggestion of a pericardial disorder, and echocardiographic studies should be carried out if suspicion arises. More vigorous diuretic therapy, dialysis, pericardiocentesis, or surgery may be required. If the effusion persists, withdrawal of Minoxidil should be considered in light of other means of controlling the hypertension and the patient's clinical status.

4. *Interaction with Guanethidine:* Although Minoxidil does not itself cause orthostatic hypotension, its administration to patients already receiving guanethidine can result in profound orthostatic effects. If at all possible, guanethidine should be discontinued well before Minoxidil is begun. Where this is not possible, Minoxidil therapy should be started in the hospital and the patient should remain institutionalized until severe orthostatic effects are no longer present or the patient has learned to avoid activities that provoke them.

5. *Hazard of Rapid Control of Blood Pressure:* In patients with very severe blood pressure elevation, too rapid control of blood pressure, especially with intravenous agents, can precipitate syncope, cerebrovascular accidents, myocardial infarction and ischemia of special sense organs with resulting decrease or loss of vision or hearing. Patients with compromised circulation or cryoglobulinemia may also suffer ischemic episodes of the affected organs. Although such events have not been unequivocally associated with Minoxidil use, total experience is limited at present.

Any patient with malignant hypertension should have initial treatment with Minoxidil carried out in a hospital setting, both to assure that blood pressure is falling and to assure that it is not falling more rapidly than intended.

PRECAUTIONS
1. GENERAL PRECAUTIONS:
(a) *Monitor fluid and electrolyte balance and body weight* (see "Warnings: Salt and Water Retention").

(b) *Observe for signs and symptoms of pericardial effusion* (see "Warnings: Pericardial Effusion and Tamponade").

(c) *Use after myocardial infarction:* Minoxidil Tablets have not been used in patients who have had a myocardial infarction within the preceding month. It is possible that a reduction of arterial pressure with Minoxidil might further limit blood flow to the myocardium, although this might be compensated by decreased oxygen demand because of lower blood pressure.

(d) *Hypersensitivity*: Possible hypersensitivity to Minoxidil manifested as a skin rash, has been seen in less than 1% of patients: whether the drug should be discontinued when this occurs depends on treatment alternatives.

(e) *Renal failure or dialysis patients:* May require smaller doses of Minoxidil and should have close medical supervision to prevent exacerbation of renal failure or precipitation of cardiac failure.

2. INFORMATION FOR PATIENT
The patient should be made fully aware of the importance of continuing all of his antihypertensive medications and of the nature of symptoms that would suggest fluid overload. A patient brochure has been prepared and is included with each package of Minoxidil. The text of this brochure is reprinted at the end of the insert.

3. LABORATORY TESTS
Those laboratory tests which are abnormal at the time of initiation of Minoxidil therapy, such as urinalysis, renal function tests, EKG, chest x-ray, echocardiogram, etc., should be repeated at intervals to ascertain whether improvement or deterioration is occurring under Minoxidil therapy. Initially, such tests should be performed frequently, e.g., 1-3 month intervals; later as stabilization occurs, at intervals of 6-12 months.

4. DRUG INTERACTIONS
See "Interaction with Guanethidine" under "Warnings".

5. CARCINOGENESIS, MUTAGENESIS AND IMPAIRMENT OF FERTILITY
Twenty-two month carcinogenicity studies in rats at doses 15 times the human dose did not provide evidence of tumorigenicity. The drug was not mutagenic in the Salmonella (Ames) test.

Rats receiving up to five times the human dose of Minoxidil had a reduction in conception rate, possibly related to drug treatment. There was no evidence of increased fetal resorptions in rats but they did occur in rabbits.

6. PREGNANCY-TERATOGENIC EFFECTS
Pregnancy Category C. Minoxidil has been shown to reduce the conception rate in rats and to show evidence of increased fetal absorption in rabbits when administered at five times the human dose. There was no evidence of teratogenic effects in rats and rabbits. There are no adequate and well controlled studies in pregnant women. Minoxidil should be used during pregnancy only if the potential benefit justifies the potential risk to the fetus.

7. LABOR AND DELIVERY
The effects on labor and delivery are unknown.

8. NURSING MOTHERS

Minoxidil has been reported to be secreted in human milk. As a general rule, nursing should not be undertaken while a patient is on Minoxidil.

9. PEDIATRIC USE

Use in children has been limited to date, particularly in infants. The recommendations under *"Dosage and Administration"* can be considered only a rough guide at present and careful titration is essential.

10. UNAPPROVED USE

Use of Minoxidil Tablets, in any formulation, to promote hair growth is not an approved indication. While clinical trials with Minoxidil Topical Solution 2% demonstrated that formulation and dosage were safe and effective, the effects of extemporaneous formulations and dosages have not been shown to be safe or effective. Because systemic absorption of topically applied drug may occur and is dependent on vehicle and/or method of use, extemporaneous topical formulations made from Minoxidil should be considered to share in the full range of *"Contraindications"*, *"Warnings"*, *"Precautions"*, and *"Adverse Reactions"* listed in this insert.

In addition, skin intolerance to drug and/or vehicle may occur.

ADVERSE REACTIONS

1. Salt and Water Retention:" (see *"Warnings: Concomitant Use of Adequate Diuretic is Required"*): Temporary edema developed in 7% of patients who were not edematous at the start of therapy.

2. Pericarditis, Pericardial Effusion and Tamponade: (see *"Warnings"*).

3. Dermatologic: Hypertrichosis—Elongation, thickening, and enhanced pigmentation of fine body hair are seen in about 80% of patients taking Minoxidil Tablets. This develops within 3 to 6 weeks after starting therapy. It is usually first noticed on the temples, between the eyebrows, between the hairline and the eyebrows, or in the side-burn area of the upper lateral cheek, later extending to the back, arms, legs, and scalp. Upon discontinuation of Minoxidil, new hair growth stops, but 1 to 6 months may be required for restoration to pretreatment appearance. No endocrine abnormalities have been found to explain the abnormal hair growth: thus, it is hypertrichosis without virilism. Hair growth is especially disturbing to children and women and such patients should be thoroughly informed about this effect before therapy with Minoxidil is begun.

Allergic—Rashes have been reported, including rare reports of bullous eruptions, and Stevens-Johnson Syndrome.

4. Hematologic: Thrombocytopenia and leukopenia (WBC < 3000/mm³) have rarely been reported.

5. Gastrointestinal: Nausea and/or vomiting has been reported. In clinical trials the incidence of nausea and vomiting associated with the underlying disease has shown a decrease from pretrial levels.

6. Miscellaneous: Breast tenderness—This developed in less than 1% of patients.

7. Altered Laboratory Findings: (a) ECG changes—changes in direction and magnitude of the ECG T-waves occur in approximately 60% of patients treated with Minoxidil. In rare instances a large negative amplitude of the T-wave may encroach upon the S-T segment, but the S-T segment is not independently altered. These changes usually disappear with continuance of treatment and revert to the pretreatment state if Minoxidil is discontinued. No symptoms have been associated with these changes, nor have there been alterations in blood cell counts or in plasma enzyme concentrations that would suggest myocardial damage. Long-term treatment of patients manifesting such changes has provided no evidence of deteriorating cardiac function. At present the changes appear to be nonspecific and without identifiable clinical significance. (b) Effects of hemodilution—hematocrit, hemoglobin and erythrocyte count usually fall about 7% initially and then recover to pretreatment levels. (c) Other—Alkaline phosphatase increased varyingly without other evidence of liver or bone abnormality. Serum creatinine increased an average of 6% and BUN slightly more, but later declined to pretreatment levels.

OVERDOSAGE

There have been only a few instances of deliberate or accidental overdosage with Minoxidil Tablets. One patient recovered after taking 50 mg of Minoxidil together with 500 mg of a barbiturate. When exaggerated hypotension is encountered, it is most likely to occur in association with residual sympathetic nervous system blockade from previous therapy (guanethidine-like effects or alpha-adrenergic blockage), which prevents the usual compensatory maintenance of blood pressure. Intravenous administration of normal saline will help to maintain blood pressure and facilitate urine formation in these patients. Sympathomimetic drugs such as norepinephrine or epinephrine should be avoided because of their excessive cardiac stimulating action. Phenylephrine, angiotensin II, vasopressin, and dopamine all reverse hypotension due to Minoxidil, but should only be used if underperfusion of a vital organ is evident. Radioimmunoassay can be performed to determine the concentration of Minoxidil in the blood. At the maximum adult dosage of 100 mg/day, peak blood levels of 1641 ng/ml and 2441 ng/ml were observed in two patients, respectively. Due to patient-to-patient variation in blood levels, it is difficult to establish an overdosage warning level. In general, a substantial increase above 2000 ng/ml should be regarded as overdosage, unless the physician is aware that the patient has taken no more than the maximum dose.

Oral LD₅₀ in rats has ranged from 1321-3492 mg/kg; in mice, 2456-2648 mg/kg.

DOSAGE AND ADMINISTRATION

Patients over 12 Years of Age: The recommended initial dosage of Minoxidil Tablets is 5 mg given as a single daily dose. Daily dosage can be increased to 10, 20 and then to 40 mg in single or divided doses if required for optimum blood pressure control. The effective dosage range is usually 10 to 40 mg per day. The maximum recommended dosage is 100 mg per day.

Patients under 12 Years of Age: The initial dosage is 0.2 mg/kg Minoxidil as a single daily dose. The dosage may be increased in 50 to 100% increments until optimum blood pressure control is achieved. The effective dosage range is usually 0.25 to 1.0 mg/kg/day. The maximum recommended dosage is 50 mg daily, (see *"9. Pediatric Use"* under *"Precautions"*).

Dose Frequency: The magnitude of within-day fluctuation of arterial pressure during therapy with Minoxidil is directly proportional to the extent of pressure reduction. If supine diastolic pressure has been reduced less than 30 mmHg, the drug need be administered only once a day; if supine diastolic pressure has been reduced more than 30 mmHg, the daily dosage should be divided into two equal parts.

Frequency of Dosage Adjustment: Dosage must be titrated carefully according to individual response. Intervals between dosage adjustments normally should be at least 3 days since the full response to a given dose is not obtained for at least that amount of time. *Where a more rapid management of hypertension is required, dose adjustments can be made every 6 hours if the patient is carefully monitored.*

Concomitant therapy: Diuretic and beta blocker or other sympathetic nervous system suppressant.

Diuretics: Minoxidil must be used in conjunction with a diuretic in patients relying on renal function for maintaining salt and water balance. Diuretics have been used at the following dosages when starting therapy with Minoxidil: hydrochlorothiazide (50 mg, b.i.d.) or other thiazides at equieffective dosage; chlorthalidone (50 to 100 mg, once daily): furosemide (40 mg, b.i.d.). If excessive salt and water retention results in a weight gain of more than 5 pounds, diuretic therapy should be changed to furosemide; if the patient is already taking furosemide, dosage should be increased in accordance with the patient's requirements.

Beta Blockers or Other Sympathetic Nervous System Suppressants: When therapy with Minoxidil is begun, the dosage of a beta-adrenergic receptor blocking drug should be the equivalent of 80 to 160 mg of propranolol per day in divided doses.

If beta blockers are contraindicated, Methyldopa (250 to 750 mg, b.i.d.) may be used instead. Methyldopa must be given for at least 24 hours before starting therapy with Minoxidil because of the delay in the onset of Methyldopa's action. Limited clinical experience indicates that clonidine may also be used to prevent tachycardia induced by Minoxidil; the usual dosage is 0.1 to 0.2 mg twice daily.

Sympathetic nervous system suppressants may not completely prevent an increase in heart rate due to Minoxidil but usually do prevent tachycardia. Typically, patients receiving a beta blocker prior to initiation of therapy with Minoxidil have a bradycardia and can be expected to have an increase in heart rate toward normal when Minoxidil is added. When treatment with Minoxidil and beta blocker or other sympathetic nervous system suppressant are begun simultaneously, their opposing cardiac effects usually nullify each other, leading to little change in heart rate.

Store at controlled room temperature 15°-30°C (59°-86°F).

PATIENT INFORMATION

Minoxidil Tablets contain Minoxidil, a medicine for the treatment of high blood pressure in the patient who has not been controlled or is experiencing unacceptable side effects with other medications. It must usually be taken with other medicines.

Be absolutely sure to take all of your medicines for high blood pressure according to your doctor's instructions. Do not stop taking Minoxidil unless your doctor tells you to. Do not give any of your medicine to other people.

It is important that you look for the warning signals of certain undesired effects of Minoxidil. Call your doctor if they occur. Your doctor will need to see you regularly while you are taking Minoxidil. Be sure to keep all your appointments or to arrange for new ones if you must miss one.

Do not hesitate to call your doctor if any discomforts or problems occur.

The information here is intended to help you take Minoxidil properly. It does not tell you all there is to know about Minoxidil. There is a more technical leaflet that you may request from the pharmacist: you may need your doctor's help in understanding parts of that leaflet.

WHAT IS MINOXIDIL?

Minoxidil Tablets contain Minoxidil, which is a drug for lowering the blood pressure. It works by relaxing and enlarging certain small blood vessels so that blood flows through them more easily.

WHY LOWER BLOOD PRESSURE?

Your doctor has prescribed Minoxidil to lower your blood pressure and protect vital parts of your body. Uncontrolled blood pressure can cause stroke, heart failure, blindness, kidney failure, and heart attacks.

Most people with high blood pressure need to take medicines to treat it for their whole lives.

WHO SHOULD TAKE MINOXIDIL?

There are many people with high blood pressure, but most of them do not need Minoxidil. Minoxidil is used ONLY when your doctor decides that:
  1. your high blood pressure is severe;

2. your high blood pressure is causing symptoms or damage to vital organs; and
3. other medicines did not work well enough or had very disturbing side effects.
Minoxidil should be taken only when a doctor prescribes it. Never give any of your Minoxidil Tablets, or any other high blood pressure medicine, to a friend or relative.

Pregnancy: In some cases doctors may prescribe Minoxidil for women who are pregnant or who are planning to have children. However, its safe use in pregnancy has not been established. Laboratory animals had a reduced ability to become pregnant and a reduced survival of offspring while taking Minoxidil. If you are pregnant or are planning to become pregnant, be sure to tell your doctor.

HOW TO TAKE MINOXIDIL
Usually, your doctor will prescribe two other medicines along with Minoxidil. These will help lower blood pressure and will help prevent undesired effects of Minoxidil.

Often, when a medicine like Minoxidil lowers blood pressure, your body tries to return the blood pressure to the original, higher level. It does this by holding on to water and salt (so there will be more fluid to pump) and by making your heart beat faster. To prevent this, your doctor will usually prescribe a water tablet to remove the extra salt and water from your body (a diuretic: dye-u-RET-tic) and another medicine to slow your heart beat.

You must follow your doctor's instructions exactly, taking all the prescribed medicines, in the right amounts, each day.

These medicines will help keep your blood pressure down. The water tablet and heart beat medicine will help prevent the undesired effects of Minoxidil.

Minoxidil Tablets come in two strengths (2 1/2 milligrams and 10 milligrams) that are marked on each tablet. Pay close attention to the tablet markings to be sure you are taking the correct strength. Your doctor may prescribe half a tablet: the tablets are scored (partly cut on one side) so that you can easily break them.

When you first start taking Minoxidil your doctor may need to see you often in order to adjust your dosage. Take all your medicine according to the schedule prescribed by your doctor. **Do not skip any doses. If you should forget a dose of Minoxidil wait until it is time for your next dose, then continue with your regular schedule. Remember: do not stop taking Minoxidil or any of your other high blood pressure medicines, without checking with your doctor.** Make sure that any doctor treating or examining you knows that you are taking high blood pressure medicines, including Minoxidil.

WARNING SIGNALS
Even if you take all your medicines correctly, Minoxidil Tablets may cause undesired effects. Some of these are serious and you should be on the lookout for them. **If any of the following warning signals occur, you must call your doctor immediately:**

1. Increase in Heart Rate: You should measure your heart rate by counting your pulse rate **while you are resting.** If you have an increase of 20 beats or more a minute over your normal pulse contact your doctor immediately. If you do not know how to take your pulse rate, ask your doctor. Also ask your doctor how often to check your pulse.

2. Rapid Weight Gain of More than 5 Pounds: You should weigh yourself daily. If you quickly gain five or more pounds, or if there is any swelling or puffiness in the face, hands, ankles, or stomach area, this could be a sign that you are retaining body fluids. Your doctor may have to change your drugs or change the dose of your drugs. You may also need to reduce the amount of salt you eat. A smaller weight gain (2 to 3 pounds) often occurs when treatment is started. You may lose this extra weight with continued treatment.

3. Increased Difficulty in Breathing: especially when lying down. This too may be due to an increase of body fluids. It can also happen because your high blood pressure is getting worse. In either case, you might require treatment with other medicines.

4. New or Worsening of Pain in the Chest, Arm, or Shoulder or Signs of Severe Indigestion: These could be signs of serious heart problems.

5. Dizziness, Light-headedness or Fainting: These can be signs of high blood pressure or they may be side effects from one of the medicines. Your doctor may need to change or adjust the dosage of the medicines you are taking.

OTHER UNDESIRED EFFECTS
Minoxidil Tablets can cause other undesired effects such as nausea and/or vomiting that are annoying but not dangerous. Do not stop taking the drug because of these other undesired effects without talking to your doctor.

Hair Growth: About 8 out of every 10 patients who have taken Minoxidil noticed that fine **body hair grew darker or longer** on certain parts of the body. This happened about three to six weeks after beginning treatment. The hair may first be noticed on the forehead and temples, between the eyebrows, or on the upper part of the cheeks. Later, hair may grow on the back, arms, legs, or scalp. Although hair growth may not be noticeable to some patients, it often is bothersome in women and children. **Unwanted hair can be controlled with a hair remover or by shaving.** The extra hair is not permanent, it disappears within 1 to 6 months of stopping Minoxidil. Nevertheless, **you should not stop taking Minoxidil without first talking to your doctor.**

A few patients have developed a rash or breast tenderness while taking Minoxidil Tablets, but this is unusual.

HOW SUPPLIED
TABLETS: 2.5 MG

AVERAGE UNIT PRICE (AVAILABLE SIZES)		GENERIC A-RATED AVERAGE PRICE (GAAP)	
BRAND	$0.40	100s	$29.24
GENERIC	$0.29		
HCFA FUL (100s ea)	$0.15		

BRAND/MANUFACTURER	NDC	SIZE	AWP
◆ BRAND			
LONITEN: Upjohn	00009-0121-01	100s	$39.80
◆ GENERICS			
Parmed	00349-4038-01	100s	$15.44
Qualitest	00603-4687-21	100s	$22.01
Rugby	00536-4045-01	100s	$22.88
URL	00677-1444-01	100s	$23.20
Schein	00364-2172-01	100s	$23.25
Martec	52555-0444-01	100s	$25.32
Goldline	00182-1602-01	100s	$25.50
Major	00904-1279-60	100s	$26.80
Par	49884-0256-01	100s	$45.00
Aligen	00405-4683-01	100s	$45.00
Moore,H.L.	00839-7353-06	100s	$47.25
Schein	00364-2172-05	500s	$102.25

TABLETS: 10 MG

AVERAGE UNIT PRICE (AVAILABLE SIZES)		GENERIC A-RATED AVERAGE PRICE (GAAP)	
BRAND	$0.87	100s	$48.81
GENERIC	$0.47	500s	$204.20
HCFA FUL (100s ea)	$0.19		

BRAND/MANUFACTURER	NDC	SIZE	AWP
◆ BRAND			
LONITEN: Upjohn	00009-0137-01	100s	$87.45
	00009-0137-02	500s	$433.39
◆ GENERICS			
Goldline	00182-1280-01	100s	$39.45
Qualitest	00603-4688-21	100s	$40.00
Major	00904-1280-60	100s	$44.50
URL	00677-1162-01	100s	$45.95
Schein	00364-2173-01	100s	$46.00
Rugby	00536-4043-01	100s	$47.25
Par	49884-0257-01	100s	$54.00
Parmed	00349-8949-01	100s	$54.00
Aligen	00405-4684-01	100s	$54.00
Martec	52555-0445-01	100s	$55.10
Moore,H.L.	00839-7342-06	100s	$56.70
Major	00904-1280-40	500s	$182.80
Schein	00364-2173-05	500s	$192.00
Parmed	00349-8949-05	500s	$199.00
Par	49884-0257-05	500s	$243.00

Minoxidil, Topical

DESCRIPTION
Minoxidil Topical Solution is a hair growth stimulant. Minoxidil, Topical contains the active ingredient Minoxidil. Minoxidil appears as a white or off-white, odorless crystalline solid that is soluble in water to the extent of approximately 2 mg/mL, is readily soluble in propylene glycol or ethanol, and is almost insoluble in acetone, chloroform or ethyl acetate.

The chemical name for Minoxidil is 2,4-pyrimidinediamine, 6-(l-piperidinyl)-, 3-oxide (MW = 209.25).

Topical Solution is available at a concentration of 2% (20 mg Minoxidil per milliliter).

Following is its chemical structure:

CLINICAL PHARMACOLOGY
PHARMACOLOGIC PROPERTIES AND PHARMACOKINETICS
Minoxidil Topical Solution stimulates hair growth in individuals with androgenetic alopecia, expressed in males as baldness of the vertex of the scalp and in females as diffuse hair loss or thinning of the frontoparietal areas. The mechanism by which Minoxidil stimulates hair growth is not known but like Minoxidil some other arterial dilating drugs also stimulate hair growth when given systematically.

Because of its serious side effects oral Minoxidil is indicated only for the treatment of hypertension that is symptomatic or associated with target organ damage and is not manageable with maximum therapeutic doses of a diuretic plus two other antihypertensive drugs. It is a direct acting peripheral arterial dilator that reduces blood pressure by decreasing peripheral vascular resistance. Reduction of peripheral arteriolar resistance and the resulting fall in blood pressure trigger sympathetic, vagal inhibitory, and renal homeostatic mechanisms, including increased renin secretion, that lead to increased heart rate and cardiac output and salt and water retention.

The major side effects of oral Minoxidil, aside from unwelcome generalized hair growth, result from fluid retention, often profound, and tachycardia, and require that Minoxidil be administered in most cases with a beta blocker or other agent to reduce heart rate and a diuretic, almost always a high ceiling (loop) diuretic. Fluid retention can lead to marked weight gain, local or generalized edema, heart failure, and pleural or pericardial effusion, including cardiac tamponade. Pericarditis has been reported, usually in patients with renal failure or collagen vascular disease, but in some cases these causes of pericarditis do not seem to have been present. The tachycardia and increased cardiac output caused by Minoxidil can lead to exacerbation of existing angina or the onset of angina in persons with compromised coronary circulation. It is these serious side effects that have restricted use of oral Minoxidil to patients with severe hypertension not controllable with other agents.

In placebo controlled trials involving over 3500 male patients given topical Minoxidil for 4 months (longer treatment was given after the placebo group was discontinued), and in over 300 female patients given topical Minoxidil for eight months, the typical systemic effects of oral Minoxidil (weight gain, edema, tachycardia, fall in blood pressure, and their more serious consequences) were not seen more frequently in patients given topical Minoxidil than in those given topical placebo (see "Adverse Reactions"). The mean changes from baseline in weight, heart rate, and blood pressure in the treated and placebo groups were similar, and the number of patients experiencing significant changes, such as a blood pressure decrease of 15 mmHg or more diastolic or 30 mmHg or more systolic, a heart rate increase of 15 beats/minute or more, or weight gain of at least 5 pounds, was also similar. In an effort to explore the potential for systemic effects of topical Minoxidil, three concentrations of topical Minoxidil (1, 2 and 5%) applied twice daily were compared to low oral doses (2.5 and 5 mg given once daily), and placebo in hypertensive patients (normotensive patients have little or no blood pressure response to Minoxidil at dose of 10 mg per day) in a double-blind controlled trial. The 5 mg oral dose had readily detectable effects, a fall in diastolic pressure of about 5 mmHg and an increase in heart rate of 7 beats/minute. No other group had a clear effect, although there was some evidence of a weak and inconsistent effect in the 2.5 mg oral, and possibly the 5% topical, treatments.

The failure to detect evidence of systemic effects during treatment with topical Minoxidil reflects the poor absorption of topical Minoxidil, which averages about 1.4% (range 0.3 to 4.5%) from normal intact scalp, and was about 2% in the hypertensive patients, whose scalps were shaved.

In a comparison of topical and oral absorption, peak serum levels of unchanged Minoxidil after 1 mL b.i.d. of 2% Minoxidil solution (the maximum recommended dose) averaged 5.8% (range 1.4% to 12.7%) of the level observed after 2.5 mg b.i.d. oral doses (5 mg is the recommended starting dose of oral Minoxidil). Similarly, in the hypertension study, where patients had shaved scalps, mean Minoxidil concentrations after 1 mL b.i.d. of 2% topical Minoxidil (1.7 ng/mL) were 1/20 the concentrations seen after daily oral doses of 2.5 mg (32.8 ng/mL) or 5 mg (59.2 ng/mL). Blood levels obtained in the large controlled hair growth trials averaged less than 2 ng/mL for the 2% solution. There were, however, occasional values that were higher; about 1% of the patients on 2% Minoxidil had serum levels of 5 ng/mL or greater and a few approached 30 ng/mL. It is possible, therefore, that if more than the recommended dose were applied to inflamed skin in an individual with relatively high absorption, blood levels with systemic effects might rarely be obtained. Physicians and patients need to be aware of the possibility.

Serum Minoxidil levels resulting from administration of Minoxidil, Topical are governed by the drug's percutaneous absorption rate. Following cessation of topical dosing of Minoxidil, Topical approximately 95% of systemically absorbed Minoxidil is eliminated within four days. The metabolic biotransformation of Minoxidil absorbed following administration of Minoxidil, Topical has not been fully determined.

Minoxidil absorbed following oral administration is metabolized predominantly by conjugation with glucuronic acid at the N-oxide position in the pyrimidine ring but also by conversion to more polar products. Known metabolites exert much less pharmacologic effect than the parent compound. Minoxidil and its metabolites are excreted principally in the urine. Minoxidil does not bind to plasma proteins and its renal clearance corresponds to the glomerular filtration rate. Minoxidil does not enter the central nervous system (CNS) of experimental animals in significant amounts and it does not affect CNS function in man.

CARDIAC LESIONS IN ANIMALS

Minoxidil produces several cardiac lesions in animals. Some are characteristic of agents that cause tachycardia and diastolic hypotension (beta-agonists like isoproterenol, arterial dilators like hydralazine) while others are produced by a narrower range of agents with arterial dilating properties. The significance of these lesions for humans is not clear, as they have not been recognized in patients treated with oral Minoxidil at systemically active doses, despite formal review of over 150 autopsies of treated patients.

(a) Papillary muscle/subendocardial necrosis

The most characteristic lesion of Minoxidil, seen in rat, dog, and minipig (but not monkeys), is focal necrosis of the papillary muscle and subendocardial areas of the left ventricle. These lesions appear rapidly, within a few days of treatment with doses of 0.5 to 10 mg/kg/day in the dog and minipig, and are not progressive, although they leave residual scars. They are similar to lesions produced by other peripheral arterial dilators, by theobromine, and by beta-adrenergic receptor agonists such as isoproterenol, epinephrine, and albuterol. The lesions are thought

to reflect ischemia provoked by increased oxygen demand (tachycardia, increased cardiac output) and relative decrease in coronary flow (decreased diastolic pressure and decreased time in diastole) caused by the vasodilatory effects of these agents coupled with reflex or directly induced tachycardia.

(b) Hemorrhagic lesions

After acute oral Minoxidil treatment (0.5 to 10 mg/kg/day) in dogs and minipigs, hemorrhagic lesions are seen in many parts of the heart, mainly in the epicardium, endocardium, and walls of small coronary arteries and arterioles. In minipigs the lesions occur primarily in the left atrium while in dogs they are most prominent in the right atrium, frequently appearing as grossly visible hemorrhagic lesions. With exposure of 1-20 mg/kg/day in the dog for 30 days or longer, there is replacement of myocardial cells by proliferating fibroblasts and angioblasts, hemorrhage and hemosiderin accumulation. These lesions can be produced by topical Minoxidil administration that gives systemic absorption of 0.5 to 1 mg/kg/day. Other peripheral dilators, including an experimental agent, nicorandil, and theobromine, have produced similar lesions.

(c) Epicarditis

A less fully studied lesion is focal epicarditis, seen in dogs after 2 days of oral Minoxidil. More recently, chronic proliferative epicarditis was observed in dogs treated topically twice a day for 90 days. In a one year oral dog study, serosanguinous percardial fluid was seen.

(d) Hypertrophy and Dilation

Oral and topical studies in rats, dogs, monkeys (oral only), and rabbits (dermal only) show cardiac hypertrophy and dilation. This is presumed to represent the consequences of prolonged fluid overload; there is preliminary evidence in monkeys that diuretics partly reverse these effects.

Autopsies of over 150 patients who died of various causes after receiving oral Minoxidil for hypertension have not revealed the characteristics hemorrhagic (especially atrial) lesions seen in dogs and minipigs. While areas of papillary muscle and subendocardial necrosis were occasionally seen, they occurred in the presence of known pre-existing coronary artery disease and were also seen in patients never exposed to Minoxidil in another series using similar, but not identical, autopsy methods.

CLINICAL TRIAL EXPERIENCE
MALES

In clinical trials in *males*, three main parameters of efficacy were used: hair counts in a one inch diameter circle on the vertex of the scalp; investigator evaluation of terminal hair regrowth; and patient evaluation of hair regrowth. At the end of four-month placebo-controlled portions of 12-month clinical studies (i.e., baseline to Month 4), Minoxidil Topical Solution (20 mg Minoxidil per mL) demonstrated the following efficacy:

A. Hair Counts: Minoxidil, Topical was significantly more effective than placebo in producing hair regrowth as assessed by hair counts. Patients using Minoxidil, Topical had a mean increase from baseline of 72 non-vellus hairs in the one inch diameter circle compared with a mean increase of 39 non-vellus hairs in patients using the placebo (P < 0.0005).

B. Investigator Evaluation: Based on the investigators' evaluation, there was no statistically significant difference in terminal hair regrowth between treatment groups. Eight percent (8%) of the patients using Minoxidil, Topical demonstrated moderate to dense terminal hair regrowth compared with 4% using the placebo. During the initial four months of treatment, however, very little regrowth of terminal hair can be expected. Although most patients did not demonstrate cosmetically significant regrowth of hair, 26% of the patients showed minimal terminal hair regrowth using Minoxidil, Topical compared with 16% of those using placebo as assessed by the investigator.

C. Patient Evaluation: Based on the patients' self-evaluation, 26% using Minoxidil, Topical demonstrated moderate to dense hair regrowth compared with 11% using the placebo (P < 0.0005).

Patients who continued on Minoxidil, Topical during the remaining eight months of the 12-month clinical studies (i.e., the non-placebo-controlled portion of the studies) continued to sustain a regrowth response as evaluated by hair counts, investigator evaluation, and patient evaluation.

At the end of the eight month non-placebo-controlled portion of the 12-month clinical studies (i.e., Months 4 to 12), the following results were obtained.

A. Hair Count: Patients using Minoxidil, Topical had a mean increase of 112 non-vellus hairs in the same one inch diameter circle as compared to Month 4 (P < 0.0005).

B. Investigator Evaluation: Based on the investigators' evaluation, 39% of the patients achieved moderate to dense terminal hair by Month 12.

C. Patient Evaluation: Based on the patients' assessment, 48% felt they had achieved moderate to dense hair regrowth at Month 12.

Trends in the data suggest that those patients who are older, who have been balding for a longer period of time, or who have a larger area of baldness, may do less well.

CLINICAL TRIAL EXPERIENCE
FEMALES

In clinical trials in *females* (age range 18-45 years, 90% who were Caucasian) with Ludwig grade I and II diffuse frontoparietal hair thinning, the main parameters of efficacy were: non-vellus hair counts in a designated 1.0 cm^2 site on the frontoparietal areas of the scalp; investigator evaluation of hair regrowth; and patient evaluation of hair regrowth. Data demonstrate that 44% to 63%

(investigators' evaluation from the international and US multicenter trials, respectively) of women with androgenetic alopecia will have discernible growth of non-vellus hair when treated with Minoxidil, Topical for 32 weeks versus 29% to 39% for vehicle control treated women.

Two 8-month placebo-controlled studies in females (US multicenter trial and an international multicenter trial) produced the following results:

A. Hair Counts: Minoxidil, Topical was significantly more effective than placebo in producing hair regrowth as assessed by hair counts in both studies. Patients using Minoxidil, Topical had a mean increase from baseline of 22.7 and 33.2 non-vellus hairs, respectively, in the same $1.0 cm^2$ site compared with a mean increase of 11.0 and 19.1 non-vellus hairs, respectively, in patients using placebo (p = 0.0004 and p = 0.0001, respectively).

B. Investigator Evaluation: Based on the investigators' evaluation 63% (13% moderate and 50% minimal) and 44% (12% moderate and 32% minimal), respectively, of the patients using Minoxidil, Topical in the two studies achieved hair regrowth at Week 32, compared with 39% (6% moderate and 33% minimal) and 29% (5% moderate and 24% minimal), respectively, of those using placebo (p < 0.0005 and p = 0.008, respectively).

C. Patient Evaluation: Based on the patients' self evaluation, 59% (19% moderate and 40% minimal) and 55% (1% dense, 24% moderate and 30% minimal), respectively, of the patients using Minoxidil, Topical reported hair regrowth at Week 32, compared with 40% (7% moderate and 33% minimal) and 41% (12% moderate and 29% minimal), respectively, of those using placebo (p = 0.002 and p = 0.013, respectively).

Hair growth was defined as follows:

Investigator Evaluation of Growth: No visible new hair growth
  Minimal growth: Definite growth but no substantial covering of thinning areas.
  Moderate growth: New growth partially covering thinning areas, less dense than non-thinning areas (readily discernible)
  Dense Growth: Full covering of thinning areas: density of hair similar to non-thinning areas

Patient Evaluation of Growth: No visible hair growth
  Minimal hair growth: Barely discernible
  Moderate new hair growth: Readily discernible
  Dense new hair growth

INDICATIONS AND USAGE

Minoxidil Topical Solution is indicated for the treatment of androgenetic alopecia, expressed in males as baldness of the vertex of the scalp and in females as diffuse hair loss or thinning of the frontoparietal areas. At least four months of twice daily applications of Minoxidil, Topical are generally required before evidence of hair growth can be expected.

CONTRAINDICATIONS

Minoxidil Topical Solution is contraindicated in those patients with a history of hypersensitivity to any of the components of the preparation.

WARNINGS

1. Need for normal scalp

The majority of clinical studies included only healthy patients with normal scalps and no cardiovascular disease. Before starting a patient on Minoxidil, Topical the physician should ascertain that the patient has a healthy, normal scalp. Local abrasion or dermatitis may increase absorption and hence increase the risk of side effects.

2. Potential adverse effects

Although extensive use of topical Minoxidil has not revealed evidence that enough Minoxidil is absorbed to have systemic effects, greater absorption because of misuse or individual variability or unusual sensitivity could lead, at least theoretically, to a systemic effect, and physicians and patients need to be aware of this.

Experience with oral Minoxidil has shown the following major cardiovascular effects (the package insert for Minoxidil, Topical tablets should be reviewed for details):
—salt and water retention, generalized and local edema
—pericardial effusion, pericarditis, tamponade
—tachycardia
—increased frequency of angina or new onset of angina

If systemic effects were to occur, patients with underlying heart disease, including coronary artery disease and congestive heart failure, would be at particular risk. Minoxidil could also have additive effects with other therapy in patients being treated for hypertension.

Patients being considered for Minoxidil Topical Solution should have a history and physical examination. Patients should be advised of the potential risk and a decision should be made by the patient and physician that the benefits outweigh the risks. Patients with a history of underlying heart disease should be aware that adverse effects in them might be especially serious. Patients should be alerted to the possibility of tachycardia and fluid retention and should watch for, and be monitored for, increased heart rate and weight gain or other systemic effects.

PRECAUTIONS

GENERAL PRECAUTIONS

Patients treated with Minoxidil Topical Solution should be monitored one month after starting Minoxidil, Topical and at least every six months thereafter. If systemic effects should occur, discontinue use of Minoxidil, Topical.

Minoxidil, Topical contains an alcohol base which will cause burning and irritation of the eye. In the event of accidental contact with sensitive surfaces (eye, abraded skin, and mucous membranes), the area should be bathed with large amounts of cool tap water.

Inhalation of the spray mist should be avoided.

Minoxidil, Topical should not be used in conjunction with other topical agents including topical corticosteroids, retinoids, and petrolatum or agents that are known to enhance cutaneous drug absorption.

Minoxidil is for topical use only. Each milliliter contains 20 mg minoxidil. Accidental ingestion of the solution could lead to possible adverse systemic effects (see *"Overdosage"*).

As is the case with other topically applied drugs, decreased integrity of the epidermal barrier caused by inflammation or disease processes in the skin (e.g., excoriations of the scalp, scalp psoriasis, or severe sunburn) may increase percutaneous absorption of Minoxidil.

INFORMATION FOR THE PATIENT

A patient information leaflet has been prepared and is included with each package of Minoxidil, Topical.

DRUG INTERACTIONS

There are currently no known drug interactions associated with the use of Minoxidil Topical Solution. Although it has not been clinically demonstrated, there exists the theoretical possibility of absorbed Minoxidil potentiating orthostatic hypotension in patients concurrently taking guanethidine.

CARCINOGENESIS, MUTAGENESIS, AND IMPAIRMENT OF FERTILITY

No evidence of carcinogenicity was detected in rats and rabbits when Minoxidil Topical Solution was applied to the skin for up to one year. Dietary administration of Minoxidil to mice for up to 24 months was associated with an increased incidence of malignant lymphomas in females and an increased incidence of hepatic nodules in males. The lymphoma incidence was unrelated to dose levels and at all doses was within the range seen in control groups from other studies employing mice from the same colony. The incidence of hepatic nodules was dose dependent, with a significant increase observed at 63 but not at 25 or 10 mg/kg/day. There was no effect of drug on the incidence of malignant tumors of the liver. As with the lymphomas, the incidence of hepatic nodules was within the historical control range for the subject mouse colony. No evidence of carcinogenic potential was obtained from a dietary administration study of Minoxidil in rats. However, the rat study involved only ⅓ the number of animals and half the maximum dosage level evaluated in the mouse experiment, and shorter durations of administration (up to 15 months in males and up to 22 months in females). Minoxidil was not mutagenic in the salmonella (Ames) test, the DNA damage/alkaline elution assay or the rat micronucleus test.

In a study in which male and female rats received one or five times the maximum recommended human oral antihypertensive dose of Minoxidil (multiples based on a 50 kg patient) there was a dose-dependent reduction in conception rate.

PREGNANCY

Pregnancy Category C. Adequate and well-controlled studies have not been conducted in pregnant women treated with Minoxidil Topical Solution nor in pregnant women treated with oral Minoxidil for hypertension. Oral administration of Minoxidil has been associated with evidence of increased fetal resorption in rabbits, but not rats, when administered at five times the oral antihypertensive human dose. There was no evidence of teratogenic effects of ORALLY administered Minoxidil in rats or rabbits. Subcutaneous administration of Minoxidil to pregnant rats at 80 mg/kg/day (approximately 2000 times the maximal systemic human exposure from daily topical administration) was maternally toxic but not teratogenic. Higher subcutaneous doses produced evidence of developmental toxicity. Minoxidil, Topical should not be administered to pregnant women.

LABOR AND DELIVERY

The effects on labor and delivery are unknown.

NURSING MOTHERS

There has been one report of Minoxidil excretion in the breast milk of a woman treated with 5 mg oral minoxidil twice daily for hypertension. Because of the potential for adverse effects in nursing infants from Minoxidil absorption, Minoxidil, Topical should not be administered to a nursing woman.

PEDIATRIC USE

Safety and effectiveness in patients under 18 years of age have not been established.

POST-MENOPAUSAL USE

Efficacy in postmenopausal women has not been studied.

ADVERSE REACTIONS

Minoxidil Topical Solution has been used by 3,857 patients (347 females) enrolled in placebo-controlled trials. The rate of adverse events, grouped by body system, is shown in the following table. Except dermatologic events, which were more common in the Minoxidil group, no individual reaction or body system grouping seemed to be increased in the Minoxidil-treated group. (See related table).

Patients have been followed for up to 5 years and there has been no change in incidence or severity of reported reactions. Additional events reported in

MEDICAL EVENT PERCENT OCCURRENCE BY BODY SYSTEM IN THE PLACEBO-CONTROL CLINICAL TRIALS INVOLVING MINOXIDIL TOPICAL SOLUTION—ALL PATIENTS ENROLLED

Body System	Minoxidil Solution n = 3857 (4-8 months)		Placebo n = 2717 (4-8 months)	
	# Pats.	% Occ.	# Pats.	% Occ.
Dermatological (irritant dermatitis, allergic contact dermatitis)	284	7.36	1.47	5.41
Respiratory (bronchitis, upper respiratory infection, sinusitis)	276	7.16	233	8.58
Gastrointestinal (diarrhea, nausea, vomitting)	167	4.33	178	6.55
Neurology (headache, dizziness, faintness, light-headedness)	132	3.42	94	3.46
Musculoskeletal (fractures, back pain, tendinitis, aches and pains)	100	2.59	60	2.21
Cardiovascular (edema, chest pain, blood pressure increases/ decreases, palpitations, pulse rate increases/ decreases)	59	1.53	42	1.55
Allergy (nonspecific allergic reactions, hives, allergic rhinitis, facial swelling, and sensitivity)	49	1.27	26	0.96
Metabolic-Nutritiona (edema, weight gain)	48	1.24	35	1.29
Special Senses (conjunctivitis, ear infections, vertigo)	45	1.17	33	1.21
Genital Tract (prostatitis, epididymitis, pregnancy, vaginitis, vulvitis, vaginal discharge and itching)	35	0.91	22	0.81
Urinary tract (urinary tract infections, renal calculi, urethitis)	36	0.93	31	1.14
Endocrine (menstrual changes, breast symptoms)	18	0.47	14	0.52
Psychiatric (anxiety, depression, fatigue)	14	0.36	26	0.96
Hematology (lymphadenopathy, thrombocytopenia, anemia)	12	0.31	15	0.55

postmarketing clinical experience include: eczema, hypertrichosis, local erythema, pruritus, dry skin/scalp flaking, sexual dysfunction, visual disturbances including decreased visual acuity, exacerbation of hair loss, alopecia.

OVERDOSAGE

Increased systemic absorption of Minoxidil may potentially occur if more frequent or larger doses of Minoxidil, Topical (than directed) are used or if Minoxidil, Topical is applied to large surface areas of the body or areas other than the scalp. There are no known cases of Minoxidil overdosage resulting from topical administration of Minoxidil, Topical.

In a 14-day controlled clinical trial, 1 mL of 3% Minoxidil Topical Solution was applied eight times daily (six times the recommended dose) to the scalp of 11 normal male volunteers and to the chest of 11 other volunteers. No significant systemic effects were observed in these subjects when compared with a similar number of placebo-treated subjects. All subjects in the study were monitored for vital sign, electrocardiographic, and echocardiographic changes.

In a reported case of accidental ingestion, a 3-year-old male swallowed 1 to 2 mL of a 3% concentration of topical Minoxidil solution. After vomiting he was treated in an emergency room. The child was found to be alert and active with no obvious signs of distress. His temperature was 37°C, pulse 152 bpm, respiration 32, and systolic blood pressure 110 by palpation. Cardiovascular, chest, lungs, abdomen, head, skin, and neurological examinations were normal. Blood levels taken indicated a total Minoxidil level (glucuronide and unchanged) of 320.6 ng/ mL. The child was discharged without sequelae.

Because of the high concentration of Minoxidil in Minoxidil Topical Solution, accidental ingestion has the potential of producing systemic effects related to the pharmacologic action of the drug (5 mL of Minoxidil Topical Solution contains 100 mg Minoxidil, the maximum adult dose for oral Minoxidil administration when used to treat hypertension). Signs and symptoms of Minoxidil overdosage would most likely be cardiovascular effects associated with fluid retention and tachycardia. Fluid retention can be managed with appropriate diuretic therapy. Clinically significant tachycardia can be controlled by administration of a beta-adrenergic blocking agent. If encountered, hypotension should be treated by intravenous administration of normal saline. Sympathomimetic drugs, such as norepinephrine and epinephrine, should be avoided because of their excessive cardiac stimulating activity.

Oral LD$_{50}$ in rats has ranged from 1321 to 3492 mg/kg; in mice 2457 to 2648 mg/kg. Minoxidil and its metabolites are hemodialyzable.

DOSAGE AND ADMINISTRATION

Hair and scalp should be dry prior to topical application of Minoxidil Topical Solution. A dose of 1 mL Minoxidil Topical Solution should be applied to the total affected areas of the scalp twice daily. The total daily dosage should not exceed 2 mL. If finger tips are used to facilitate drug application, hands should be washed afterwards. Twice daily application for four months or longer may be

required before evidence of hair regrowth is observed. Onset and degree of hair regrowth may be variable among patients. If hair regrowth is realized, twice daily applications of Minoxidil, Topical appear necessary for additional or continued hair regrowth. Some anecdotal patient reports indicate that regrown hair and the balding process return to their untreated state three to four months following cessation of the drug.

Store at controlled room temperature 15° to 30°C (59°-86°F).

HOW SUPPLIED
SOLUTION: 2%

BRAND/MANUFACTURER	NDC	SIZE	AWP
○ BRAND ROGAINE: Upjohn	00009-3367-05	60 ml	$57.74
	00009-3367-19	180 ml	$152.99

Mintezol *SEE* THIABENDAZOLE

Miochol *SEE* ACETYLCHOLINE CHLORIDE

Miostat *SEE* CARBACHOL

Miradon *SEE* ANISINDIONE

Misoprostol

CONTRAINDICATIONS AND WARNINGS

MISOPROSTOL IS CONTRAINDICATED, BECAUSE OF ITS ABORTIFACIENT PROPERTY, IN WOMEN WHO ARE PREGNANT. (SEE "PRECAUTIONS.") PATIENTS MUST BE ADVISED OF THE ABORTIFACIENT PROPERTY AND WARNED NOT TO GIVE THE DRUG TO OTHERS. MISOPROSTOL SHOULD NOT BE USED IN WOMEN OF CHILDBEARING POTENTIAL UNLESS THE PATIENT REQUIRES NONSTEROIDAL ANTI-INFLAMMATORY DRUG

◆ RATED THERAPEUTICALLY EQUIVALENT; ◇ THERAPEUTIC EQUIVALENCE UNCONFIRMED; ○ UNRATED

(NSAID) THERAPY AND IS AT HIGH RISK OF COMPLICATIONS FROM GASTRIC ULCERS ASSOCIATED WITH USE OF THE NSAID, OR IS AT HIGH RISK OF DEVELOPING GASTRIC ULCERATION. IN SUCH PATIENTS, MISOPROSTOL MAY BE PRESCRIBED IF THE PATIENT

■ IS CAPABLE OF COMPLYING WITH EFFECTIVE CONTRACEPTIVE MEASURES.

■ HAS RECEIVED BOTH ORAL AND WRITTEN WARNINGS OF THE HAZARDS OF MISOPROSTOL, THE RISK OF POSSIBLE CONTRACEPTION FAILURE, AND THE DANGER TO OTHER WOMEN OF CHILDBEARING POTENTIAL SHOULD THE DRUG BE TAKEN BY MISTAKE.

■ HAS HAD A NEGATIVE *SERUM* PREGNANCY TEST WITHIN TWO WEEKS PRIOR TO BEGINNING THERAPY.

■ WILL BEGIN MISOPROSTOL ONLY ON THE SECOND OR THIRD DAY OF THE NEXT NORMAL MENSTRUAL PERIOD.

DESCRIPTION

Misoprostol oral tablets contain either 100 mcg or 200 mcg of Misoprostol, a synthetic prostaglandin E_1 analog.

Misoprostol contains approximately equal amounts of the two diastereomers.

Its molecular formula is $C_{22}H_{38}O_5$ and molecular weight is 382.5. The chemical name of Misoprostol is (±)methyl 11α, 16-dihydroxy-16-methyl-9-oxoprost-13E-en-1-oate

Misoprostol is a water-soluble, viscous liquid hydroxypropyl methylcellulose, microcrystalline cellulose, and sodium starch glycolate.

Following is its chemical structure:

CLINICAL PHARMACOLOGY

Pharmacokinetics: Misoprostol is extensively absorbed, and undergoes rapid de-esterification to its free acid, which is responsible for its clinical activity and, unlike the parent compound, is detectable in plasma. The alpha side chain undergoes beta oxidation and the beta side chain undergoes omega oxidation followed by reduction of the ketone to give prostaglandin F analogs.

In normal volunteers, Misoprostol is rapidly absorbed after oral administration with a T_{max} of Misoprostol acid of 12 ± 3 minutes and a terminal half-life of 20-40 minutes.

There is high variability of plasma levels of Misoprostol acid between and within studies but mean values after single doses show a linear relationship with dose over the range of 200-400 mcg. No accumulation of Misoprostol acid was noted in multiple dose studies; plasma steady state was achieved within two days.

Maximum plasma concentrations of Misoprostol acid are diminished when the dose is taken with food and total availability of Misoprostol acid is reduced by use of concomitant antacid. Clinical trials were conducted with concomitant antacid, however, so this effect does not appear to be clinically important.

Mean ± SD	C_{max}(pg/ml)	AUC (0-4) (pg·hr/ml)	T_{max}(min)
Fasting	811 ± 317	417 ± 135	14 ± 8
With Antacid	689 ± 315	349 ± 108*	20 ± 14
With High Fat Breakfast	303 ± 176*	373 ± 111	64 ± 79*

* *Comparisons with fasting results statistically significant, $p < 0.05$.*

After oral administration of radiolabeled Misoprostol, about 80% of detected radioactivity appears in urine. Pharmacokinetic studies in patients with varying degrees of renal impairment showed an approximate doubling of $T_{1/2}$, C_{max}, and AUC compared to normals, but no clear correlation between the degree of impairment and AUC. In subjects over 64 years of age, the AUC for Misoprostol acid is increased. No routine dosage adjustment is recommended in older patients or patients with renal impairment, but dosage may need to be reduced if the usual dose is not tolerated.

Misoprostol does not affect the hepatic mixed function oxidase (cytochrome P-450) enzyme systems in animals.

Drug interaction studies between Misoprostol and several nonsteroidal anti-inflammatory drugs showed no effect on the kinetics of ibuprofen or diclofenac, and a 20% decrease in aspirin AUC, not thought to be clinically significant.

Pharmacokinetic studies also showed a lack of drug interaction with antipyrine and propranolol when these drugs were given with Misoprostol. Misoprostol given for one week had no effect on the steady state pharmacokinetics of diazepam when the two drugs were administered two hours apart.

The serum protein binding of Misoprostol acid is less than 90% and is concentration-independent in the therapeutic range.

Pharmacodynamics: Misoprostol has both antisecretory (inhibiting gastric acid secretion) and (in animals) mucosal protective properties. NSAIDs inhibit prostaglandin synthesis, and a deficiency of prostaglandins within the gastric mucosa may lead to diminishing bicarbonate and mucus secretion and may contribute to the mucosal damage caused by these agents. Misoprostol can increase bicarbonate and mucus production, but in man this has been shown at doses 200 mcg and above that are also antisecretory. It is therefore not possible to tell whether the ability of Misoprostol to prevent gastric ulcer is the result of its antisecretory effect, its mucosal protective effect, or both.

In vitro studies on canine parietal cells using tritiated Misoprostol acid as the ligand have led to the identification and characterization of specific prostaglandin receptors. Receptor binding is saturable, reversible, and stereospecific. The sites have a high affinity for Misoprostol, for its acid metabolite, and for other E type prostaglandins, but not for F or I prostaglandins and other unrelated compounds, such as histamine or cimetidine. Receptor-site affinity for Misoprostol correlates well with an indirect index of antisecretory activity. It is likely that these specific receptors allow Misoprostol taken with food to be effective topically, despite the lower serum concentrations attained.

Misoprostol produces a moderate decrease in pepsin concentration during basal conditions, but not during histamine stimulation. It has no significant effect on fasting or postprandial gastrin nor on intrinsic factor output.

Effects on Gastric Acid Secretion: Misoprostol, over the range of 50-200 mcg, inhibits basal and nocturnal gastric acid secretion, and acid secretion in response to a variety of stimuli, including meals, histamine, pentagastrin, and coffee. Activity is apparent 30 minutes after oral administration and persists for at least 3 hours. In general, the effects of 50 mcg were modest and shorter lived, and only the 200-mcg dose had substantial effects on nocturnal secretion or on histamine and meal-stimulated secretion.

Uterine Effects: Misoprostol has been shown to produce uterine contractions that may endanger pregnancy. (See "Contraindications" and "Warnings"). In studies in women undergoing elective termination of pregnancy during the first trimester, Misoprostol caused partial or complete expulsion of the uterine contents in 11% of the subjects and increased uterine bleeding in 41%.

Other Pharmacologic Effects: Misoprostol does not produce clinically significant effects on serum levels of prolactin, gonadotropins, thyroid-stimulating hormone, growth hormone, thyroxine, cortisol, gastrointestinal hormones (somatostatin, gastrin, vasoactive intestinal polypeptide, and motilin), creatinine, or uric acid. Gastric emptying, immunologic competence, platelet aggregation, pulmonary function, or the cardiovascular system are not modified by recommended doses of Misoprostol.

Clinical Studies: In a series of small short-term (about one week) placebo-controlled studies in healthy human volunteers, doses of Misoprostol were evaluated for their ability to prevent NSAID-induced mucosal injury. Studies of 200 mcg q.i.d. of Misoprostol with tolmetin and naproxen, and of 100 and 200 mcg q.i.d. with ibuprofen, all showed reduction of the rate of significant endoscopic injury from about 70-75% on placebo to 10-30% on Misoprostol. Doses of 25-200 mcg q.i.d. reduced aspirin-induced mucosal injury and bleeding.

Preventing Gastric Ulcers Caused by Nonsteroidal Anti-Inflammatory Drugs (NSAIDs): Two 12-week, randomized, double-blind trials in osteoarthritic patients who had gastrointestinal symptoms but no ulcer on endoscopy while taking an NSAID compared the ability of 200 mcg of Misoprostol, 100 mcg of Misoprostol, and placebo to prevent gastric ulcer (GU) formation. Patients were approximately equally divided between ibuprofen, piroxicam, and naproxen, and continued this treatment throughout the 12 weeks. The 200-mcg dose caused a marked, statistically significant reduction in gastric ulcers in both studies. The lower dose was somewhat less effective, with a significant result in only one of the studies. (See related table).

In these trials there were no significant differences between Misoprostol and placebo in relief of day or night abdominal pain. No effect of Misoprostol in preventing duodenal ulcers was demonstrated, but relatively few duodenal lesions were seen. In another clinical trial, 239 patients receiving aspirin 650-1300 mg q.i.d. for rheumatoid arthritis who had endoscopic evidence of duodenal and/or gastric inflammation were randomized to Misoprostol 200 mcg q.i.d. or placebo for eight weeks while continuing to receive aspirin. The study evaluated the possible interference of Misoprostol on the efficacy of aspirin in these patients with rheumatoid arthritis by analyzing joint tenderness, joint swelling, physician's clinical assessment, patient's assessment, change in ARA classification, change in handgrip strength, change in duration of morning stiffness, patient's assessment of pain at rest, movement, interference with daily activity, and ESR. Misoprostol did not interfere with the efficacy of aspirin in these patients with rheumatoid arthritis.

INDICATIONS AND USAGE

Misoprostol is indicated for the prevention of NSAID (nonsteroidal anti-inflammatory drugs, including aspirin)-induced gastric ulcers in patients at high risk of complications from gastric ulcer, eg, the elderly and patients with concomitant debilitating disease, as well as patients at high risk of developing gastric ulceration, such as patients with a history of ulcer. Misoprostol has not been shown to prevent duodenal ulcers in patients taking NSAIDs. Misoprostol should be taken for the duration of NSAID therapy. Misoprostol has been shown to prevent gastric ulcers in controlled studies of three months' duration. It had no effect, compared to placebo, on gastrointestinal pain or discomfort associated with NSAID use.

UNLABELED USES

Misoprostol is used alone or as an adjunct in the treatment of gastric ulcer and duodenal ulcer. It is also used to promote cervical ripening for vaginal delivery and to terminate pregnancy as an abortifacient.

CONTRAINDICATIONS

See boxed *"Contraindications"* and *"Warnings."* Misoprostol should not be taken by anyone with a history of allergy to prostaglandins.

WARNINGS

See boxed *"Contraindications"* and *"Warnings."*

PRECAUTIONS

Information for Patients: Misoprostol is contraindicated in women who are pregnant, and should not be used in women of childbearing potential unless the patient requires nonsteroidal anti-inflammatory drug (NSAID) therapy and is at high risk of complications from gastric ulcers associated with the use of the NSAID, or is at high risk of developing gastric ulceration. Women of childbearing potential should be told that they must not be pregnant when Misoprostol therapy is initiated, and that they must use an effective contraception method while taking Misoprostol.

See boxed *"Contraindications"* and *"Warnings."*

Patients should be advised of the following:

Misoprostol is intended for administration along with nonsteroidal anti-inflammatory drugs (NSAIDs), including aspirin, to decrease the chance of developing an NSAID-induced gastric ulcer.

Misoprostol should be taken only according to the directions given by a physician.

If the patient has questions about or problems with Misoprostol the physician should be contacted promptly.

THE PATIENT SHOULD NOT GIVE MISOPROSTOL TO ANYONE ELSE. Misoprostol has been prescribed for the patient's specific condition, may not be the correct treatment for another person, and may be dangerous to the other person if she were to become pregnant.

The Misoprostol package the patient receives from the pharmacist will include a leaflet containing patient information. The patient should read the leaflet before taking Misoprostol and each time the prescription is renewed because the leaflet may have been revised.

Keep Misoprostol out of reach of children.

Special Note for Women: **Misoprostol must not be used by pregnant women. Misoprostol may cause miscarriage. Miscarriages caused by Misoprostol may be incomplete, which could lead to potentially dangerous bleeding, hospitalization, surgery, infertility, or maternal or fetal death.**

Misoprostol is available only as a unit-of-use package that includes a leaflet containing patient information. See *"Patient Information"* at the end of this labeling.

Drug Interactions: See *"Clinical Pharmacology."* Misoprostol has not been shown to interfere with the beneficial effects of aspirin on signs and symptoms of rheumatoid arthritis. Misoprostol does not exert clinically significant effects on the absorption, blood levels, and antiplatelet effects of therapeutic doses of aspirin. Misoprostol has no clinically significant effect on the kinetics of diclofenac or ibuprofen.

Animal Toxicology: A reversible increase in the number of normal surface gastric epithelial cells occurred in the dog, rat, and mouse. No such increase has been observed in humans administered Misoprostol for up to one year.

An apparent response of the female mouse to Misoprostol in long-term studies at 100 to 1000 times the human dose was hyperostosis, mainly of the medulla of sternebrae. Hyperostosis did not occur in long-term studies in the dog and rat and has not been seen in humans treated with Misoprostol.

Carcinogenesis, Mutagenesis, Impairment of Fertility: There was no evidence of an effect of Misoprostol on tumor occurrence or incidence in rats receiving daily doses up to 150 times the human dose for 24 months. Similarly, there was no effect of Misoprostol on tumor occurrence or incidence in mice receiving daily doses up to 1000 times the human dose for 21 months. The mutagenic potential of Misoprostol was tested in several *in vitro* assays, all of which were negative.

Misoprostol, when administered to breeding male and female rats at doses 6.25 times to 625 times the maximum recommended human therapeutic dose, produced dose-related pre- and postimplantation losses and a significant decrease in the number of live pups born at the highest dose. These findings suggest the possibility of a general adverse effect on fertility in males and females.

Pregnancy: Pregnancy Category X: See boxed *"Contraindications"* and *"Warnings."*

Nonteratogenic Effects: Misoprostol may endanger pregnancy (may cause miscarriage) and thereby cause harm to the fetus when administered to a pregnant woman. Misoprostol produces uterine contractions, uterine bleeding, and expulsion of the products of conception. Miscarriages caused by Misoprostol may be incomplete. In studies in women undergoing elective termination of pregnancy during the first trimester, Misoprostol caused partial or complete expulsion of the products of conception in 11% of the subjects and increased uterine bleeding in 41%. If a woman is or becomes pregnant while taking this drug, the drug should be discontinued and the patient apprised of the potential hazard to the fetus.

Teratogenic effects: Misoprostol is not fetotoxic or teratogenic in rats and rabbits at doses 625 and 63 times the human dose, respectively.

Nursing Mothers: See *"Contraindications."* It is unlikely that Misoprostol is excreted in human milk since it is rapidly metabolized throughout the body. However, it is not known if the active metabolite (Misoprostol acid) is excreted in human milk. Therefore, Misoprostol should not be administered to nursing mothers because the potential excretion of Misoprostol acid could cause significant diarrhea in nursing infants.

Pediatric use: Safety and effectiveness in children below the age of 18 years have not been established.

ADVERSE REACTIONS

The following have been reported as adverse events in subjects receiving Misoprostol:

Gastrointestinal: In subjects receiving Misoprostol 400 or 800 mcg daily in clinical trials, the most frequent gastrointestinal adverse events were diarrhea and abdominal pain. The incidence of diarrhea at 800 mcg in controlled trials in patients on NSAIDs ranged from 14-40% and in all studies (over 5,000 patients) averaged 13%. Abdominal pain occurred in 13-20% of patients in NSAID trials and about 7% in all studies, but there was no consistent difference from placebo.

Diarrhea was dose related and usually developed early in the course of therapy (after 13 days), usually was self-limiting (often resolving after 8 days), but sometimes required discontinuation of Misoprostol (2% of the patients). Rare instances of profound diarrhea leading to severe dehydration have been reported. Patients with an underlying condition such as inflammatory bowel disease, or those in whom dehydration, were it to occur, would be dangerous, should be monitored carefully if Misoprostol is prescribed. The incidence of diarrhea can be minimized by administering after meals and at bedtime, and by avoiding coadministration of Misoprostol with magnesium-containing antacids.

Gynecological: Women who received Misoprostol during clinical trials reported the following gynecological disorders: spotting (0.7%), cramps (0.6%), hypermenorrhea (0.5%), menstrual disorder (0.3%) and dysmenorrhea (0.1%). Postmenopausal vaginal bleeding may be related to Misoprostol administration. If it

PREVENTION OF GASTRIC ULCERS INDUCED BY IBUPROFEN, PIROXICAM, OR NAPROXEN
[No. of Patients with Ulcer(s)(%)]

Therapy	Therapy Duration		
	4 weeks	8 weeks	12 weeks
Study No. 1			
Misoprostol 200 mcg q.i.d. (n = 74)	1 (1.4)	0	1 (1.14)*
Misoprostol 100 mcg q.i.d. (n = 77)	3 (3.9)	1 (1.3)	1 (1.3)	5 (6.5)*
Placebo (n = 76)	11 (14.5)	4 (5.3)	4 (5.3)	19 (25.0)
Study No. 2			
Misoprostol 200 mcg q.i.d. (n = 65)	1 (1.5)	1 (1.5)	0	2 (3.1)*
Misoprostol 100 mcg q.i.d. (n = 66)	2 (3.0)	2 (3.0)	1 (1.5)	5 (7.6)
Placebo (n = 62)	6 (9.7)	2 (3.2)	3 (4.8)	11 (17.7)
Studies No. 1 & No. 2**			
Misoprostol 200 mcg q.i.d. (n = 139)	2 (1.4)	1 (0.7)	0	3 (2.2)*
Misoprostol 100 mcg q.i.d. (n = 143)	5 (3.5)	3 (2.1)	2 (1.4)	10 (7.0)*
Placebo (n = 138)	17 (12.3)	6 (4.3)	7 (5.1)	30 (21.7)

* *Statistically significantly different from placebo at the 5% level.*
** *Combined data from Study No. 1 and Study No. 2.*

occurs, diagnostic workup should be undertaken to rule out gynecological pathology.

Elderly: There were no significant differences in the safety profile of Misoprostol in approximately 500 ulcer patients who were 65 years of age or older compared with younger patients.

Additional adverse events which were reported are categorized as follows:

Incidence Greater than 1%: In clinical trials, the following adverse reactions were reported by more than 1% of the subjects receiving Misoprostol and may be causally related to the drug: nausea (3.2%), flatulence (2.9%), headache (2.4%), dyspepsia (2.0%), vomiting (1.3%), and constipation (1.1%). However, there were no significant differences between the incidences of these events for Misoprostol and placebo.

Causal Relationship Unknown: The following adverse events were infrequently reported. Causal relationships between Misoprostol and these events have not been established but cannot be excluded:

Body as a Whole: aches/pains, asthenia, fatigue, fever, rigors, weight changes.

Skin: rash, dermatitis, alopecia, pallor, breast pain.

Special Senses: abnormal taste, abnormal vision, conjunctivitis, deafness, tinnitus, earache.

Respiratory: upper respiratory tract infection, bronchitis, bronchospasm, dyspnea, pneumonia, epistaxis.

Cardiovascular: chest pain, edema, diaphoresis, hypotension, hypertension, arrhythmia, phlebitis, increased cardiac enzymes, syncope.

Gastrointestinal: GI bleeding, GI inflammation/infection, rectal disorder, abnormal hepatobiliary function, gingivitis, reflux, dysphagia, amylase increase.

Hypersensitivity: Anaphylaxis.

Metabolic: glycosuria, gout, increased nitrogen, increased alkaline phosphatase.

Genitourinary: polyuria, dysuria, hematuria, urinary tract infection.

Nervous System/Psychiatric: anxiety, change in appetite, depression, drowsiness, dizziness, thirst, impotence, loss of libido, sweating increase, neuropathy, neurosis, confusion.

Musculoskeletal: arthralgia, myalgia, muscle cramps, stiffness, back pain.

Blood/Coagulation: anemia, abnormal differential, thrombocytopenia, purpura, ESR increased.

OVERDOSAGE

The toxic dose of Misoprostol in humans has not been determined. Cumulative total daily doses of 1600 mcg have been tolerated, with only symptoms of gastrointestinal discomfort being reported. In animals, the acute toxic effects are diarrhea, gastrointestinal lesions, focal cardiac necrosis, hepatic necrosis, renal tubular necrosis, testicular atrophy, respiratory difficulties, and depression of the central nervous system. Clinical signs that may indicate an overdose are sedation, tremor, convulsions, dyspnea, abdominal pain, diarrhea, fever, palpitations, hypotension, or bradycardia. Symptoms should be treated with supportive therapy.

It is not known if Misoprostol acid is dialyzable. However, because Misoprostol is metabolized like a fatty acid, it is unlikely that dialysis would be appropriate treatment for overdosage.

DOSAGE AND ADMINISTRATION

The recommended adult oral dose of Misoprostol for the prevention of NSAID-induced gastric ulcers is 200 mcg four times daily with food. If this dose cannot be tolerated, a dose of 100 mcg can be used. (See *"Clinical Pharmacology; Clinical Studies."*) Misoprostol should be taken for the duration of NSAID therapy as prescribed by the physician. Misoprostol should be taken with a meal, and the last dose of the day should be at bedtime.

Renal Impairment: Adjustment of the dosing schedule in renally impaired patients is not routinely needed, but dosage can be reduced if the 200-mcg dose is not tolerated. (See *"Clinical Pharmacology."*)

Store below 86°F (30°C) in a dry area.

PATIENT INFORMATION

Read this leaflet before taking Misoprostol and each time your prescription is renewed, because the leaflet may be changed.

Misoprostol is being prescribed by your doctor to decrease the chance of getting stomach ulcers related to the arthritis/pain medication that you take.

Misoprostol can cause miscarriage, often associated with potentially dangerous bleeding. This may result in hospitalization, surgery, infertility, or death. **Do not take it if you are pregnant and do not become pregnant while taking this medicine.**

If you become pregnant during Misoprostol therapy, stop taking Misoprostol and contact your physician immediately. Remember that even if you are on a means of birth control it is still possible to become pregnant. Should this occur, stop taking Misoprostol and contact your physician immediately.

Misoprostol may cause diarrhea, abdominal cramping, and/or nausea in some people. In most cases these problems develop during the first few weeks of therapy and stop after about a week. You can minimize possible diarrhea by making sure you take Misoprostol with food.

Because these side effects are usually mild to moderate and usually go away in a matter of days, most patients can continue to take Misoprostol. If you have prolonged difficulty (more than 8 days), or if you have severe diarrhea, cramping and/or nausea, call your doctor.

Take Misoprostol only according to the directions given by your physician. Do not give Misoprostol to anyone else. It has been prescribed for your specific condition, may not be the correct treatment for another person, and would be dangerous if the other person were pregnant.

This information sheet does not cover all possible side effects of Misoprostol. This patient information leaflet does not address the side effects of your arthritis/pain medication. See your doctor if you have questions.

Keep out of reach of children.

HOW SUPPLIED
TABLETS: 100 MCG

BRAND/MANUFACTURER	NDC	SIZE	AWP
○ BRAND			
▶ CYTOTEC: Searle	0025-1451-60	60s	$28.04
	0025-1451-34	100s ud	$49.02
	0025-1451-20	120s	$56.04

TABLETS: 200 MCG

BRAND/MANUFACTURER	NDC	SIZE	AWP
○ BRAND			
▶ CYTOTEC: Searle	0025-1461-60	60s	$40.80
	0025-1461-31	100s	$68.01
	0025-1461-34	100s ud	$71.41

Mithracin *SEE* PLICAMYCIN

Mitomycin

WARNING

MITOMYCIN SHOULD BE ADMINISTERED UNDER THE SUPERVISION OF A QUALIFIED PHYSICIAN EXPERIENCED IN THE USE OF CANCER CHEMOTHERAPEUTIC AGENTS. APPROPRIATE MANAGEMENT OF THERAPY AND COMPLICATIONS IS POSSIBLE ONLY WHEN ADEQUATE DIAGNOSTIC AND TREATMENT FACILITIES ARE READILY AVAILABLE.

BONE MARROW SUPPRESSION, NOTABLY THROMBOCYTOPENIA AND LEUKOPENIA, WHICH MAY CONTRIBUTE TO OVERWHELMING INFECTIONS IN AN ALREADY COMPROMISED PATIENT, IS THE MOST COMMON AND SEVERE OF THE TOXIC EFFECTS OF MITOMYCIN (SEE *"WARNINGS"* AND *"ADVERSE REACTIONS"* SECTIONS).

HEMOLYTIC UREMIC SYNDROME (HUS), A SERIOUS COMPLICATION OF CHEMOTHERAPY, CONSISTING PRIMARILY OF MICROANGIOPATHIC HEMOLYTIC ANEMIA, THROMBOCYTOPENIA, AND IRREVERSIBLE RENAL FAILURE, HAS BEEN REPORTED IN PATIENTS RECEIVING SYSTEMIC MITOMYCIN. THE SYNDROME MAY OCCUR AT ANY TIME DURING SYSTEMIC THERAPY WITH MITOMYCIN AS A SINGLE AGENT OR IN COMBINATION WITH OTHER CYTOTOXIC DRUGS, HOWEVER, MOST CASES OCCUR AT DOSES ≥ 60 MG OF MITOMYCIN. BLOOD PRODUCT TRANSFUSION MAY EXACERBATE THE SYMPTOMS ASSOCIATED WITH THIS SYNDROME.

THE INCIDENCE OF THE SYNDROME HAS NOT BEEN DEFINED.

DESCRIPTION

Mitomycin is an antibiotic isolated from the broth of *Streptomyces caespitosus* which has been shown to have antitumor activity. The compound is heat stable, has a high melting point, and is freely soluble in organic solvents.

Following is its chemical structure:

ACTION

Mitomycin selectively inhibits the synthesis of deoxyribonucleic acid (DNA). The guanine and cytosine content correlates with the degree of Mitomycin-induced cross-linking. At high concentrations of the drug, cellular RNA and protein synthesis are also suppressed.

In humans, Mitomycin is rapidly cleared from the serum after intravenous administration. Time required to reduce the serum concentration by 50% after a 30 mg. bolus injection is 17 minutes. After injection of 30 mg., 20 mg., or 10 mg. I.V., the maximal serum concentrations were 2.4 µg./mL, 1.7 µg./mL, and 0.52 µg./mL, respectively. Clearance is effected primarily by metabolism in the liver, but metabolism occurs in other tissues as well. The rate of clearance is inversely proportional to the maximal serum concentration because, it is thought, of saturation of the degradative pathways.

Approximately 10% of a dose of Mitomycin is excreted unchanged in the urine. Since metabolic pathways are saturated at relatively low doses, the percent of a dose excreted in urine increases with increasing dose. In children, excretion of intravenously administered Mitomycin is similar.

ANIMAL TOXICOLOGY

Mitomycin has been found to be carcinogenic in rats and mice. At doses approximating the recommended clinical dose in man, it produces a greater than 100% increase in tumor incidence in male Sprague-Dawley rats, and a greater than 50% increase in tumor incidence in female Swiss mice.

INDICATIONS

Mitomycin is not recommended as single-agent, primary therapy. It has been shown to be useful in the therapy of disseminated adenocarcinoma of the stomach or pancreas in proven combinations with other approved chemotherapeutic agents and as palliative treatment when other modalities have failed. Mitomycin is not recommended to replace appropriate surgery and/or radiotherapy.

UNLABELED USES
Mitomycin is used alone or as an adjunct in the treatment of bladder, breast, cervical, and esophageal carcinoma.

CONTRAINDICATIONS

Mitomycin is contraindicated in patients who have demonstrated a hypersensitive or idiosyncratic reaction to it in the past.

Mitomycin is contraindicated in patients with thrombocytopenia, coagulation disorder, or an increase in bleeding tendency due to other causes.

WARNINGS

Patients being treated with Mitomycin must be observed carefully and frequently during and after therapy.

The use of Mitomycin results in a high incidence of bone marrow suppression, particularly thrombocytopenia and leukopenia. Therefore, the following studies should be obtained repeatedly during therapy and for at least 8 weeks following therapy: platelet count, white blood cell count, differential, and hemoglobin. The occurrence of a platelet count below 100,000/mm^3 or a WBC below 4,000/mm^3 or a progressive decline in either is an indication to withhold further therapy until blood counts have recovered above these levels.

Patients should be advised of the potential toxicity of this drug, particularly bone marrow suppression. Deaths have been reported due to septicemia as a result of leukopenia due to the drug.

Patients receiving Mitomycin should be observed for evidence of renal toxicity. Mitomycin should not be given to patients with a serum creatinine greater than 1.7 mg %.

Usage in Pregnancy: Safe use of Mitomycin in pregnant women has not been established. Teratological changes have been noted in animal studies. The effect of Mitomycin on fertility is unknown.

PRECAUTIONS

Acute shortness of breath and severe bronchospasm have been reported following the administration of vinca alkaloids in patients who had previously or simultaneously received Mitomycin. The onset of this acute respiratory distress occurred within minutes to hours after the vinca alkaloid injection. The total number of doses for each drug has varied considerably. Bronchodilators, steroids and/or oxygen have produced symptomatic relief.

A few cases of adult respiratory distress syndrome have been reported in patients receiving Mitomycin in combination with other chemotherapy and maintained at F1O$_2$ concentrations greater than 50% perioperatively. Therefore, caution should be exercised using only enough oxygen to provide adequate arterial saturation since oxygen itself is toxic to the lungs. Careful attention should be paid to fluid balance and overhydration should be avoided.

ADVERSE REACTIONS

Bone Marrow Toxicity: This was the most common and most serious toxicity, occurring in 605 of 937 patients (64.4%). Thrombocytopenia and/or leukopenia may occur anytime within 8 weeks after onset of therapy with an average time of 4 weeks. Recovery after cessation of therapy was within 10 weeks. About 25% of the leukopenic or thrombocytopenic episodes did not recover. Mitomycin produces cumulative myelosuppression.

Integument and Mucous Membrane Toxicity: This has occurred in approximately 4% of patients treated with Mitomycin. Cellulitis at the injection site has been reported and is occasionally severe. Stomatitis and alopecia also occur frequently. Rashes are rarely reported. The most important dermatological problem with this drug, however, is the necrosis and consequent sloughing of tissue which results if the drug is extravasated during injection. Extravasation may occur with or without an accompanying stinging or burning sensation and even if there is adequate blood return when the injection needle is aspirated. There have been reports of delayed erythema and/or ulceration occurring either at or distant from the injection site, weeks to months after Mitomycin, even when no obvious evidence of extravasation was observed during administration. Skin grafting has been required in some of the cases.

Renal Toxicity: 2% of 1,281 patients demonstrated a statistically significant rise in creatinine. There appeared to be no correlation between total dose administered or duration of therapy and the degree of renal impairment.

Pulmonary Toxicity: This has occurred infrequently but can be severe and may be life threatening. Dyspnea with a non-productive cough and radiographic evidence of pulmonary infiltrates may be indicative of Mitomycin-induced pulmonary

toxicity. If other etiologies are eliminated, Mitomycin therapy should be discontinued. Steroids have been employed as treatment of this toxicity, but the therapeutic value has not been determined. A few cases of adult respiratory distress syndrome have been reported in patients receiving Mitomycin in combination with other chemotherapy and maintained at F1O$_2$ concentrations greater than 50% perioperatively.

Hemolytic Uremic Syndrome (HUS): This serious complication of chemotherapy, consisting primarily of microangiopathic hemolytic anemia (hematocrit ≤ 25%), thrombocytopenia (≤ 100,000/mm^3), and irreversible renal failure (serum creatinine ≥ 1.6 mg/dL) has been reported in patients receiving systemic Mitomycin. Microangiopathic hemolysis with fragmented red blood cells on peripheral blood smears has occurred in 98% of patients with the syndrome. Other less frequent complications of the syndrome may include pulmonary edema (65%), neurologic abnormalities (16%), and hypertension. Exacerbation of the symptoms associated with HUS has been reported in some patients receiving blood product transfusions. A high mortality rate (52%) has been associated with this syndrome.

The syndrome may occur at any time during systemic therapy with Mitomycin as a single agent or in combination with other cytotoxic drugs. Less frequently, HUS has also been reported in patients receiving combinations of cytotoxic drugs not including Mitomycin. Of 83 patients studied, 72 developed the syndrome at total doses exceeding 60 mg of Mitomycin. Consequently, patients receiving ≥ 60 mg of Mitomycin should be monitored closely for unexplained anemia with fragmented cells on peripheral blood smear, thrombocytopenia, and decreased renal function.

The incidence of the syndrome has not been defined.
Therapy for the syndrome is investigational.

Cardiac Toxicity: Congestive heart failure, often treated effectively with diuretics and cardiac glycosides, has rarely been reported. Almost all patients who experienced this side effect had received prior doxorubicin therapy.

Acute Side Effects Due to Mitomycin were fever, anorexia, nausea, and vomiting. They occurred in about 14% of 1,281 patients.

Other Undesirable Side Effects that have been reported during Mitomycin therapy have been headache, blurring of vision, confusion, drowsiness, syncope, fatigue, edema, thrombophlebitis, hematemesis, diarrhea, and pain. These did not appear to be dose related and were not unequivocally drug related. They may have been due to the primary or metastatic disease processes.

DOSAGE AND ADMINISTRATION

Mitomycin should be given intravenously only, using care to avoid extravasation of the compound. If extravasation occurs, cellulitis, ulceration, and slough may result.

Each vial contains either Mitomycin 5 mg and mannitol 10 mg, Mitomycin 20 mg and mannitol 40 mg, or Mitomycin 40 mg and mannitol 80 mg. To administer, add Sterile Water for Injection, 10 mL, 40 mL or 80 mL, respectively. Shake to dissolve. If product does not dissolve immediately, allow to stand at room temperature until solution is obtained.

After full hematological recovery (see guide to *"Dosage Adjustment"*) from any previous chemotherapy, the following dosage schedule may be used at 6- to 8-week intervals:

20 mg/m^2 intravenously as a single dose via a functioning intravenous catheter.

Because of cumulative myelosuppression, patients should be fully reevaluated after each course of Mitomycin, and the dose reduced if the patient has experienced any toxicities. Doses greater than 20 mg/m^2 have not been shown to be more effective, and are more toxic than lower doses.

The following schedule is suggested as a guide to dosage adjustment:

NADIR AFTER PRIOR DOSE

Leukocytes/ mm^3	Platelets/ mm^3	Percentage of Prior Dose To be Given
> 4000	> 100,000	100%
3000-3999	75,000-99,999	100%
2000-2999	25,000-74,999	70%
< 2000	< 25,000	50%

No repeat dosage should be given until leukocyte count has returned to 4000/mm^3 and platelet count to 100,000/mm^3. When Mitomycin is used in combination with other myelo-suppressive agents, the doses should be adjusted accordingly. If the disease continues to progress after two courses of Mitomycin, the drug should be stopped since chances of response are minimal.

STABILITY

1. Unreconstituted Mitomycin stored at room temperature is stable for the lot life indicated on the package. Avoid excessive heat (over 40°C).

2. Reconstituted with Sterile Water for Injection to a concentration of 0.5 mg. per mL, Mitomycin is stable for 14 days refrigerated or 7 days at room temperature.

3. Diluted in various IV fluids at room temperature, to a concentration of 20 to 40 micrograms per mL:

IV Fluid	Stability
5% Dextrose Injection	3 hours
0.9% Sodium Chloride Injection	12 hours
Sodium Lactate Injection	24 hours

◆ RATED THERAPEUTICALLY EQUIVALENT; ◇ THERAPEUTIC EQUIVALENCE UNCONFIRMED; ○ UNRATED

4. *The combination* of Mitomycin (5 mg. to 15 mg.) and heparin (1,000 units to 10,000 units) in 30 mL of 0.9% Sodium Chloride Injection is stable for 48 hours at room temperature.

Procedures for proper handling and disposal of anticancer drugs should be considered. Several guidelines on this subject have been published.[1-7] There is no general agreement that all of the procedures recommended in the guidelines are necessary or appropriate.

REFERENCES
1. Recommendations for the Safe Handling of Parenteral Antineoplastic Drugs. NIH Publication No. 83-2621. For sale by the Superintendent of Documents, U.S. Government Printing Office, Washington, D.C. 20402. 2. AMA Council Report. Guidelines for Handling Parenteral Antineoplastics, *JAMA.* 1985; 253(11):1590-1592. 3. National Study Commission on Cytotoxic Exposure—Recommendations for Handling Cytotoxic Agents. Available from Louis P. Jeffrey, Sc.D., Chairman, National Study Commission on Cytotoxic Exposure, Massachusetts College of Pharmacy and Allied Health Sciences, 179 Longwood Avenue, Boston, Massachusetts 02115. 4. Clinical Oncological Society of Australia: Guidelines and Recommendations for Safe Handling of Antineoplastic Agents. *Med J Australia.* 1983; 1:426-428. 5. Jones, R. B., et al. Safe Handling of Chemotherapeutic Agents: A Report from the Mount Sinai Medical Center, *CA—A Cancer J for Clinicians.* 1983; Sept./Oct., 258-263. 6. American Society of Hospital Pharmacists Technical Assistance Bulletin on Handling Cytotoxic and Hazardous Drugs. *Am J Hosp Pharm.* 1990; 47:1033-1049. 7. OSHA Work-Practice Guidelines for Personnel Dealing with Cytotoxic (antineoplastic) Drugs. *Am J Hosp Pharm.* 1986; 43:1193-1204.

J CODES
40 mg IV—J9291
20 mg IV—J9290
5 mg IV—J9280

HOW SUPPLIED
POWDER FOR INJECTION: 5 MG

BRAND/MANUFACTURER	NDC	SIZE	AWP
◆ BRAND MUTAMYCIN: Bristol-Myer Onc/Hiv	00015-3001-20	1s	$128.95

POWDER FOR INJECTION: 20 MG

BRAND/MANUFACTURER	NDC	SIZE	AWP
◆ BRAND MUTAMYCIN: Bristol-Myer Onc/Hiv	00015-3002-20	1s	$435.49

POWDER FOR INJECTION: 40 MG

BRAND/MANUFACTURER	NDC	SIZE	AWP
◆ BRAND MUTAMYCIN: Bristol-Myer Onc/Hiv	00015-3059-20	1s	$879.89

Mitotane

WARNINGS
MITOTANE SHOULD BE ADMINISTERED UNDER THE SUPERVISION OF A QUALIFIED PHYSICIAN EXPERIENCED IN THE USES OF CANCER CHEMOTHERAPEUTIC AGENTS. MITOTANE SHOULD BE TEMPORARILY DISCONTINUED IMMEDIATELY FOLLOWING SHOCK OR SEVERE TRAUMA SINCE ADRENAL SUPPRESSION IS ITS PRIME ACTION. EXOGENOUS STEROIDS SHOULD BE ADMINISTERED IN SUCH CIRCUMSTANCES, SINCE THE DEPRESSED ADRENAL MAY NOT IMMEDIATELY START TO SECRETE STEROIDS.

DESCRIPTION
Mitotane is an oral chemotherapeutic agent. It is best known by its trivial name, o,p'-DDD, and is chemically, 1,1-dichloro-2-(o-chlorophenyl)-2-(p-chlorophenyl) ethane. Mitotane is a white granular solid composed of clear colorless crystals. It is tasteless and has a slight pleasant aromatic odor. It is soluble in ethanol, isoctane and carbon tetrachloride. It has a molecular weight of 320.05.

Following is its chemical structure:

CLINICAL PHARMACOLOGY
Mitotane can best be described as an adrenal cytotoxic agent, although it can cause adrenal inhibition, apparently without cellular destruction. Its biochemical mechanism of action is unknown. Data are available to suggest that the drug modifies the peripheral metabolism of steroids as well as directly suppressing the adrenal cortex. The administration of Mitotane alters the extra-adrenal metabolism of cortisol in man, leading to a reduction in measurable 17-hydroxy corticosteroids, even though plasma levels of corticosteroids do not fall. The drug apparently causes increased formation of 6-β-betahydroxyl cortisol.

Data in adrenal carcinoma patients indicate that about 40% of oral Mitotane is absorbed and approximately 10% of administered dose is recovered in the urine as a water-soluble metabolite. A variable amount of metabolite (1 to 17%) is excreted in the bile and the balance is apparently stored in the tissues.

Following discontinuation of Mitotane, the plasma terminal half life has ranged from 18 to 159 days. In most patients blood levels become undetectable after 6 to 9 weeks. Autopsy data have provided evidence that Mitotane is found in most tissues of the body; however, fat tissues are the primary site of storage. Mitotane is converted to a water-soluble metabolite.

No unchanged Mitotane has been found in urine or bile.

INDICATIONS AND USAGE
Mitotane is indicated in the treatment of inoperable adrenal cortical carcinoma of both functional and nonfunctional types.

UNLABELED USES
Mitotane is used, with and without concomitant pituitary irradiation, in the treatment of Cushing's syndrome.

CONTRAINDICATIONS
Mitotane should not be given to individuals who have demonstrated a previous hypersensitivity to it.

WARNINGS
Mitotane should be temporarily discontinued immediately following shock or severe trauma, since adrenal suppression is its prime action. Exogenous steroids should be administered in such circumstances, since the depressed adrenal may not immediately start to secrete steroids.

Mitotane should be administered with care to patients with liver disease other than metastatic lesions from the adrenal cortex, since the metabolism of Mitotane may be interfered with and the drug may accumulate.

All possible tumor tissues should be surgically removed from large metastatic masses before Mitotane administration is instituted. This is necessary to minimize the possibility of infarction and hemorrhage in the tumor due to a rapid cytotoxic effect of the drug.

Long-term continuous administration of high doses of Mitotane may lead to brain damage and impairment of function. Behavioral and neurological assessments should be made at regular intervals when continuous Mitotane treatment exceeds 2 years.

A substantial percentage of the patients treated show signs of adrenal insufficiency. It therefore appears necessary to watch for and institute steroid replacement in those patients. However, some investigators have recommended that steroid replacement therapy be administered concomitantly with Mitotane. It has been shown that the metabolism of exogenous steroids is modified and consequently somewhat higher doses than normal replacement therapy may be required.

PRECAUTIONS
General: Adrenal insufficiency may develop in patients treated with Mitotane, and adrenal steroid replacement should be considered for these patients.

Since sedation, lethargy, vertigo, and other CNS side effects can occur, ambulatory patients should be cautioned about driving, operating machinery, and other hazardous pursuits requiring mental and physical alertness.

Drug Interactions: Mitotane has been reported to accelerate the metabolism of warfarin by the mechanism of hepatic microsomal enzyme induction, leading to an increase in dosage requirements for warfarin. Therefore, physicians should closely monitor patients for a change in anticoagulant dosage requirements when administering Mitotane to patients on coumarin-type anticoagulants. In addition, Mitotane should be given with caution to patients receiving other drugs susceptible to the influence of hepatic enzyme induction.

Carcinogenesis, Mutagenesis, Impairment of Fertility: The carcinogenic and mutagenic potentials of Mitotane are unknown. However, the mechanism of action of this compound suggests that it probably has less carcinogenic potential than other cytotoxic chemotherapeutic drugs.

Pregnancy: Pregnancy "Category C." Animal reproduction studies have not been conducted with Mitotane. It is also not known whether Mitotane can cause fetal harm when administered to a pregnant woman or can affect reproduction capacity. Mitotane should be given to a pregnant woman only if clearly needed.

Nursing Mothers: It is not known whether this drug is excreted in human milk. Because many drugs are excreted in human milk and because of the potential for adverse reactions in nursing infants from Mitotane, a decision should be made whether to discontinue nursing or to discontinue the drug, taking into account the importance of the drug to the mother.

ADVERSE REACTIONS
A very high percentage of patients treated with Mitotane has shown at least one type of side effect. The main types of adverse reactions consist of the following:
1. Gastrointestinal disturbances, which consist of anorexia, nausea or vomiting, and in some cases diarrhea, occur in about 80% of the patients.
2. Central nervous system side effects occur in 40% of the patients. These consist primarily of depression as manifested by lethargy and somnolence (25%), and dizziness or vertigo (15%).
3. Skin toxicity has been observed in about 15% of the cases. These skin changes consist primarily of transient skin rashes which do not seem to be dose

related. In some instances, this side effect subsided while the patients were maintained on the drug without a change of dose.

Infrequently occurring side effects involve the eye (visual blurring, diplopia, lens opacity, toxic retinopathy); the genitourinary system (hematuria, hemorrhagic cystitis, and albuminuria); cardiovascular system (hypertension, orthostatic hypotension, and flushing); and some miscellaneous effects including generalized aching, hyperpyrexia, and lowered protein bound iodine (PBI).

OVERDOSAGE

No proven antidotes have been established for Mitotane overdosage.

DOSAGE AND ADMINISTRATION

The recommended treatment schedule is to start the patient at 2 to 6 g of Mitotane per day in divided doses, either three or four times a day. Doses are usually increased incrementally to 9 to 10 g per day. If severe side effects appear, the dose should be reduced until the maximum tolerated dose is achieved. If the patient can tolerate higher doses and improved clinical response appears possible, the dose should be increased until adverse reactions interfere. Experience has shown that the maximum tolerated dose (MTD) will vary from 2 to 16 g per day, but has usually been 9 to 10 g per day. The highest doses used in the studies to date were 18 to 19 g per day.

Treatment should be instituted in the hospital until a stable dosage regimen is achieved.

Treatment should be continued as long as clinical benefits are observed. Maintenance of clinical status or slowing of growth of metastatic lesions can be considered clinical benefits if they can clearly be shown to have occurred.

If no clinical benefits are observed after 3 months at the maximum tolerated dose, the case would generally be considered a clinical failure. However, 10% of the patients who showed a measurable response required more than 3 months at the MTD. Early diagnosis and prompt institution of treatment improve the probability of a positive clinical response. Clinical effectiveness can be shown by reduction in tumor mass; reduction in pain, weakness or anorexia; and reduction of symptoms and signs due to excessive steroid production.

A number of patients have been treated intermittently with treatment being restarted when severe symptoms have reappeared. Patients often do not respond after the third or fourth such course. Experience accumulated to date suggests that continuous treatment with the maximum possible dosage of Mitotane is the best approach.

Procedures for proper handling and disposal of anticancer drugs should be considered. Several guidelines on this subject have been published.[1-7] There is no general agreement that all of the procedures recommended in the guidelines are necessary or appropriate.

Tablets may be stored at room temperature.

REFERENCES

1. Recommendations for the Safe Handling of Parenteral Antineoplastic Drugs. NIH Publication No. 83-2621. For sale by the Superintendent of Documents, U.S. Government Printing Office, Washington, D.C. 20402. 2. AMA Council Report. Guidelines for Handling Parenteral Antineoplastics. *JAMA*. 1985; 253(11):1590-1592. 3. National Study Commission on Cytotoxic Exposure—Recommendations for Handling Cytotoxic Agents. Available from Louis P. Jeffrey, Sc.D., Chairman, National Study Commission on Cytotoxic Exposure, Massachusetts College of Pharmacy and Allied Health Sciences, 179 Longwood Avenue, Boston, Massachusetts 02115. 4. Clinical Oncological Society of Australia: Guidelines and Recommendations for Safe Handling of Antineoplastic Agents, *Med J Australia*. 1983; 1:426-428. 5. Jones, R. B., et. al. Safe Handling of Chemotherapeutic Agents: A Report from the Mount Sinai Medical Center, *CA—A Cancer J for Clinicians*. 1983; Sept./Oct., 258-263. 6. American Society of Hospital Pharmacists Technical Assistance Bulletin on Handling Cytotoxic and Hazardous Drugs. *Am J Hosp Pharm*. 1990; 47:1033-1049. 7. OSHA Work-Practice Guidelines for Personnel Dealing with Cytotoxic (Antineoplastic) Drugs. *Am J Hosp Pharm*. 1986; 43:1193-1204.

HOW SUPPLIED
TABLETS: 500 MG

BRAND/MANUFACTURER	NDC	SIZE	AWP
○ **BRAND**			
LYSODREN: Bristol-Myer Onc/Hiv	00015-3080-60	100s	$204.68

Mitoxantrone Hydrochloride

DESCRIPTION

Mitoxantrone Hydrochloride is a synthetic antineoplastic anthracenedione for intravenous use. Its molecular formula is $C_{22}H_{28}N_4O_6.2HCl$ and its molecular weight is 517.41. It is supplied as a concentrate which *must be diluted prior to injection*. The concentrate is a sterile, nonpyrogenic, dark blue aqueous solution containing Mitoxantrone Hydrochloride equivalent to 2 mg/mL Mitoxantrone free base. The solution has a pH of 3.0 to 4.5 and contains 0.14 mEq of sodium per mL. The product does not contain preservatives. Its chemical name is: 1,4-Dihydroxy-5,8-bis [[2-[(2-hydroxyethyl) amino] ethyl]] amino]-9, 10-anthracenedione dihydrochloride.

Following is its chemical structure:

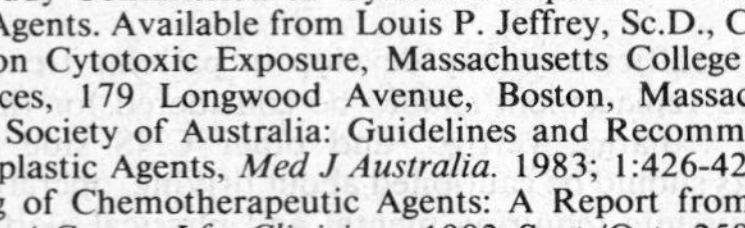

CLINICAL PHARMACOLOGY

Although its mechanism of action is not fully elucidated, Mitoxantrone Hydrochloride is a DNA-reactive agent. It has a cytocidal effect on both proliferating and nonproliferating cultured human cells, suggesting lack of cell cycle phase specificity. Pharmacokinetic studies have not been performed in humans receiving multiple daily doses. Pharmacokinetic studies in adult patients following a single intravenous administration of Mitoxantrone Hydrochloride have demonstrated multi-exponential plasma clearance. Distribution to tissues is rapid and extensive. Distribution to the brain, spinal cord, eye, and spinal fluid in the monkey is low. The apparent steady-state volume of distribution exceeds 1000L/m2. Elimination of drug is slow with an apparent mean terminal plasma half-life of 5.8 days (range 2.3 to 13.0). The half-life in tissues may be longer. Multiple intravenous doses in dogs daily for 5 days resulted in significant accumulation in plasma and tissue. The extent of accumulation was fourfold. Mitoxantrone Hydrochloride is 78% bound to plasma proteins in the observed concentration range of 26 to 455 ng/mL. This binding is independent of concentration and was not affected by the presence of diphenylhydantoin, doxorubicin, methotrexate, prednisone, prednisolone, heparin, or acetylsalicylic acid.

Mitoxantrone Hydrochloride is excreted via the renal and hepatobiliary systems. Renal excretion is limited: only 6% to 11% of the dose is recovered in the urine within 5 days after drug administration. Of the material recovered in the urine, 65% is unchanged drug; the remaining 35% is comprised primarily of two inactive metabolites and their glucuronide conjugates. The metabolites are mono- and dicarboxylic acid derivatives. Hepatobiliary elimination of drug appears to be of greater significance with as much as 25% of the dose recovered in the feces within 5 days of intravenous dosing. No significant difference in the pharmacokinetics of Mitoxantrone Hydrochoride was observed in seven patients with moderately impaired liver function (serum bilirubin 1.3 to 3.4 mg/dL) as compared with 16 patients without hepatic dysfunction. Results of pharmacokinetic studies on four patients with severe hepatic dysfunction (bilirubin greater than 3.4 mg/dL) suggest that these patients have a lower total body clearance and a larger Area Under Curve than other patients at a comparable Mitoxantrone Hydrochloride dose.

In two large randomized multicenter trials, remission induction therapy for ANLL with Mitoxantrone Hydrochloride 12 mg/m2 daily for 3 days as a 10-minute intravenous infusion and cytosine arabinoside 100 mg/m2 for 7 days given as a continuous 24-hour infusion was compared with daunorubicin 45 mg/m2 daily by intravenous infusion for 3 days plus the same dose and schedule of cytosine arabinoside used with Mitoxantrone Hydrochloride. Patients who had an incomplete antileukemic response received a second induction course in which Mitoxantrone Hydrochloride or daunorubicin was given for 2 days and cytosine arabinoside for 5 days using the same daily dosage schedule. Response rates and median survival information for both the US and international multicenter trials are given in the following table:

Trial	% Complete Response (CR)		Median Time to CR (days)		Median Survival (days)	
	MIT	DAUN	MIT	DAUN	MIT	DAUN
US	63 (62/98)	53 (54/102)	35	42	312	237
Foreign	50 (56/112)	51 (62/123)	36	42	192	230

MIT = Mitoxantrone Hydrochloride + Cytosine Arabinoside
DAUN = Daunorubicin + Cytosine Arabinoside

In these studies, two consolidation courses were administered to complete responders on each arm. Consolidation therapy consisted of the same drug and daily dosage used for remission induction but only 5 days of cytosine arabinoside and 2 days of Mitoxantrone Hydrochloride or daunorubicin were given. The first consolidation course was administered 6 weeks after the start of the final induction course if the patient achieved a complete remission. The second consolidation course was generally administered 4 weeks later. Full hematologic recovery was necessary for patients to receive consolidation therapy. For the US trial, median granulocyte nadirs for patients receiving Mitoxantrone Hydrochloride + cytosine arabinoside for consolidation course 1 and 2 were 10/mm3 for both courses, and for those patients receiving daunorubicin + cytosine arabinoside were 170/mm3 and 260/mm3, respectively. Median platelet nadirs for patients who received Mitoxantrone Hydrochloride + cytosine arabinoside for consolidation courses 1 and 2 were 17,000/mm3 and 14,000/mm3, respectively, and were 33,000/mm3 and 22,000/ mm3 in courses 1 and 2 for those patients who received daunorubicin + cytosine arabinoside. The benefit of consolidation therapy in ANLL patients who achieve a complete remission remains controversial. However, in the only well-controlled prospective, randomized multicenter trials with Mitoxantrone Hydrochloride in ANLL, consolidation therapy was given to all patients who achieved a complete remission. During consolidation in the US study, two myelosuppression-related deaths occurred on the Mitoxantrone Hydrochloride arm and one on the daunorubicin arm. However, in the foreign study there were eight deaths on the Mitoxantrone Hydrochloride arm during consolidation which were related to the myelosuppression and none on the daunorubicin arm where less myelosuppression occurred.

INDICATIONS AND USAGE

Mitoxantrone Hydrochloride in combination with other approved drugs(s) is indicated in the initial therapy of acute nonlymphocytic leukemia (ANLL) in

---

adults. This category includes myelogenous, promyelocytic, monocytic, and erythroid acute leukemias.

UNLABELED USES
Mitoxantrone Hydrochloride is used alone or as an adjunct in the treatment of non-Hodgkin's lymphoma, acute lymphoblastic leukemia, Hodgkin's disease, and nasopharyngeal carcinoma.

CONTRAINDICATIONS
Mitoxantrone Hydrochloride is contraindicated in patients who have demonstrated prior hypersensitivity to it.

WARNINGS
WHEN MITOXANTRONE HYDROCHLORIDE IS USED IN DOSES INDICATED FOR THE TREATMENT OF LEUKEMIA, SEVERE MYELOSUPPRESSION WILL OCCUR. THEREFORE, IT IS RECOMMENDED THAT MITOXANTRONE HYDROCHLORIDE BE ADMINISTERED ONLY BY PHYSICANS EXPERIENCED IN THE CHEMOTHERAPY OF THIS DISEASE. LABORATORY AND SUPPORTIVE SERVICES MUST BE AVAILABLE FOR HEMATOLOGIC AND CHEMISTRY MONITORING AND ADJUNCTIVE THERAPIES, INCLUDING ANTIBIOTICS. BLOOD AND BLOOD PRODUCTS MUST BE AVAILABLE TO SUPPORT PATIENTS DURING THE EXPECTED PERIOD OF MEDULLARY HYPOPLASIA AND SEVERE MYELOSUPPRESSION. PARTICULAR CARE SHOULD BE GIVEN TO ASSURING FULL HEMATOLOGIC RECOVERY BEFORE UNDERTAKING CONSOLIDATION THERAPY (IF THIS TREATMENT IS USED) AND PATIENTS SHOULD BE MONITORED CLOSELY DURING THIS PHASE.

Patients with preexisting myelosuppression as the result of prior drug therapy should not receive Mitoxantrone Hydrochloride unless it is felt that the possible benefit from such treatment warrants the risk of further medullary suppression. Because of the possible danger of cardiac effects in patients previously treated with daunorubicin or doxorubicin, the benefit-to-risk ratio of Mitoxantrone Hydrochloride therapy in such patients should be determined before starting therapy.

The safety of Mitroxantrone Hydrochloride in patients with hepatic insufficiency is not established. (See "Clinical Pharmacology".)

Cardiac Effects: General: Functional cardiac changes including congestive heart failure and decrease in left ventricular ejection fraction (LVEF) occur with Mitoxantrone Hydrochloride. Cardiac toxicity may be more common in patients with prior treatment with anthracyclines, prior mediastinal radiotherapy, or with preexisting cardiovascular disease. Such patients should have regular cardiac monitoring of LVEF from the initiation of therapy. In investigational trials of intermittent single dose in other tumor types, patients who received up to the cumulative dose of 140 mg/m^2 had a cumulative 2.6% probability of clinical congestive heart failure. The overall cumulative probability rate of moderate or serious decreases in LVEF at this dose was 13% in comparative trials.

Leukemia: Acute CHF may occasionally occur in patients treated with Mitoxantrone Hydrochloride for ANLL. In first-line comparative trials of Mitoxantrone Hydrochloride + cytosine arabinoside v daunorubicin + cytosine arabinoside in adult patients with previously untreated ANLL, therapy was associated with congestive heart failure in 6.5% of patients on each arm. A causal relationship between drug therapy and cardiac effects is difficult to establish in this setting since myocardial function is frequently depressed by the anemia, fever and infection, and hemorrhage, which often accompany the underlying disease.

Pregnancy Category D: Mitoxantrone Hydrochloride may cause fetal harm when administered to a pregnant woman. In treated rats, low fetal birth weight and retarded development of the fetal kidney were seen in greater frequency. In rabbits an increased incidence of premature delivery was observed. Mitoxantrone Hydrochloride was not teratogenic in rabbits. There are no adequate and well-controlled studies in pregnant women. If this drug is used during pregnancy, or if the patient becomes pregnant while taking this drug, the patient should be apprised of the potential hazard to the fetus. Women of childbearing potential should be advised to avoid becoming pregnant. Safety for use by routes other than intravenous administration has not been established.

PRECAUTIONS
General: Therapy with Mitoxantrone Hydrochloride should be accompanied by close and frequent monitoring of hematologic and chemical laboratory parameters, as well as frequent patient observation.

Hyperuricemia may occur as a result of rapid lysis of tumor cells by Mitoxantrone Hydrochloride. Serum uric acid levels should be monitored and hypouricemic therapy instituted prior to the initiation of antileukemic therapy.

Systemic infections should be treated concomitantly with or just prior to commencing therapy with Mitoxantrone Hydrochloride.

Information for Patients: Mitoxantrone Hydrochloride may impart a blue-green color to the urine for 24 hours after administration, and patients should be advised to expect this during therapy. Bluish discoloration of the sclera may also occur. Patients should be advised of the signs and symptoms of myelosuppression.

Laboratory Tests: Serial complete blood counts and liver function tests are necessary for appropriate dose adjustments. (See "Dosage and Administration".)

Carcinogenesis, Mutagenesis: Mitoxantrone Hydrochloride can result in chromosomal aberrations in animals and it is mutagenic in bacterial systems. Mitoxantrone Hydrochloride caused DNA damage and sister chromatid exchanges *in vitro*.

Pregnancy Category D: (See "Warnings".)

Nursing Mothers: It is not known whether Mitoxantrone Hydrochloride is excreted in human milk. Because of the potential for serious adverse reactions in infants from Mitoxantrone Hydrochloride, breast feeding should be discontinued before starting treatment.

Pediatric Use: Safety and effectiveness in children have not been established.

ADVERSE REACTIONS
Mitoxantrone Hydrochloride has been studied in approximately 600 patients with acute nonlymphocytic leukemia. The table below represents the adverse reaction experience in the large US comparative study of Mitoxantrone Hydrochloride + cytosine arabinoside v daunorubicin + cytosine arabinoside. Experience in the large foreign study was similar. A much wider experience in a variety of other tumor types revealed no additional important reactions other than cardiomyopathy (see "Warnings"). It should be appreciated that the listed adverse reaction categories include overlapping clinical symptoms related to the same condition, e.g. dyspnea, cough, and pneumonia. In addition, the listed adverse reactions cannot all necessarily be attributed to chemotherapy as it is often impossible to distinguish effects of the drug and effects of the underlying disease. It is clear, however, that the combination of Mitoxantrone Hydrochloride + cytosine arabinoside was responsible for nausea and vomiting, alopecia, mucositis/stomatitis, and myelosuppression.

The following table summarizes adverse reactions occurring in patients treated with Mitoxantrone Hydrochloride + cytosine arabinoside in comparison with those who received daunorubicin + cytosine arabinoside for therapy of ANLL in a large, multicenter, randomized prospective US trial. Adverse reactions are presented as major categories and selected examples of clinically significant subcategories. (See related table.)

Allergic Reaction: Hypotension, urticaria, dyspnea, and rashes have been reported occasionally.

Cutaneous: Phlebitis has been reported infrequently at the site of infusion. There have been rare reports of tissue necrosis following extravasation.

Hematologic: Myelosuppression is rapid in onset and is consistent with the requirement to produce significant marrow hypoplasia in order to achieve a response. The incidences of infection and bleeding seen in the US trial are consistent with those reported for other standard induction regimens.

Gastrointestinal: Nausea and vomiting occurred acutely in most patients, but were generally mild to moderate and could be controlled through the use of antiemetics. Stematitis/mucositis occurs within 1 week of therapy.

Cardiovascular: Congestive heart failure, tachycardia, EKG changes including arrhythmias, chest pain, and asymptomatic decreases in left ventricular ejection fraction have occurred (see "Warnings".)

OVERDOSAGE
There is no known specific antidote for Mitoxantrone Hydrochloride. Accidental overdoses have been reported. Four patients receiving 140 to 180 mg/m^2 as a single bolus injection died as a result of severe leukopenia with infection. Hematologic support and antimicrobial therapy may be required during prolonged periods of medullary hypoplasia.

Although patients with severe renal failure have not been studied, Mitoxantrone Hydrochloride is extensively tissue bound and it is unlikely that the therapeutic effect or toxicity would be mitigated by peritoneal or hemodialysis.

DOSAGE AND ADMINISTRATION
(See "Warnings".)
MITOXANTRONE HYDROCHLORIDE SOLUTION MUST BE DILUTED PRIOR TO USE.

Combination Initial Therapy for ANLL in Adults: For induction, the recommended dosage is 12 mg/m^2 of Mitoxantrone Hydrochloride daily on days 1 to 3 given as an intravenous infusion, and 100 mg/m^2 cytosine arabinoside for 7 days given as a continuous 24-hour infusion on days 1 to 7.

Most complete remissions will occur following the initial course of induction therapy. In the event of an incomplete antileukemic response, a second induction course may be given. Mitoxantrone Hydrochloride should be given for 2 days and cytosine arabinoside for 5 days using the same daily dosage levels.

If severe or life-threatening nonhematologic toxicity is observed during the first induction course, the second induction course should be withheld until toxicity clears.

Consolidation therapy which was used in two large, randomized, multicenter trials consisted of Mitoxantrone Hydrochloride 12 mg/m^2 given by intravenous infusion daily for days 1 and 2 and cytosine arabinoside 100 mg/m^2 for 5 days given as a continuous 24-hour infusion on days 1 to 5. The first course was given approximately 6 weeks after the final induction course; the second was generally administered 4 weeks after the first. Severe myelosuppression occurred. (See "Clinical Pharmacology".)

The dose of Mitoxantrone Hydrochloride should be diluted to at least 50 mL with either 0.9% Sodium Chloride Injection (USP) or 5% Dextrose Injection (USP). This solution should be introduced slowly into the tubing as a freely running intravenous infusion of 0.9% Sodium Chloride Injection (USP) or 5% Dextrose Injection (USP) over a period of not less than 3 minutes. Unused infusion solutions should be discarded immediately in an appropriate fashion. In the case of multidose use, the remaining portion of the undiluted Mitoxantrone Hydrochloride concentrate should be stored not longer than 7 days between 15°C (59°F) and 25°C (77°F) or 14 days under refrigeration. If extravasation occurs, the administration should be stopped immediately and restarted in another vein. The

	All Induction (percentage of pts entering induction)		All Consolidation (percentage of pts entering consolidation)	
	Mit N = 102	Daun N = 102	Mit N = 55	Daun N = 49
Cardiovascular	26	28	11	24
CHF	5	6	0	0
Arrhythmias	3	3	4	4
Bleeding	37	41	20	6
GI	16	12	2	2
Petechiae/Ecchymoses	7	9	11	2
Gastrointestinal	88	85	58	51
Nausea/Vomiting	72	67	31	31
Diarrhea	47	47	18	8
Abdominal Pain	15	9	9	4
Mucositis/Stomatitis	29	33	18	2
Hepatic	10	11	14	2
Jaundice	3	8	7	0
Infections	66	73	60	43
UTI	7	2	7	0
Pneumonia	9	7	9	2
Sepsis	34	36	31	18
Fungal Infections	15	13	9	6
Renal Failure	8	6	0	2
Fever	78	71	24	18
Alopecia	37	40	22	16
Pulmonary	43	43	24	14
Cough	13	9	9	2
Dyspnea	18	20	6	0
CNS	30	30	34	35
Seizures	4	4	2	8
Headache	10	9	13	4
Eye	7	6	2	0
Conjunctivitis	5	1	0	0

nonvesicant properties of Mitoxantrone Hydrochloride minimize the possibility of severe local reactions following extravasation. However, care should be taken to avoid extravasation at the infusion site and to avoid contact of Mitoxantrone Hydrochloride with the skin, mucous membranes, or eyes.

Skin accidentally exposed to Mitoxantrone Hydrochloride should be rinsed copiously with warm water and if the eyes are involved, standard irrigation techniques should be used immediately. The use of goggles, gloves, and protective gowns is recommended during preparation and administration of the drug. Spills on equipment and environmental surfaces may be cleaned using an aqueous solution of calcium hypochlorite (5.5 parts calcium hypochlorite in 13 parts by weight of water for each 1 part of Mitoxantrone Hydrochloride. Absorb the solution with gauze or towels and dispose of these in a safe manner. Appropriate safety equipment such as goggles and gloves should be worn while working with calcium hypochlorite.

Mitoxantrone Hydrochloride should not be mixed in the same infusion as heparin since a precipitate may form. Because specific compatibility data are not available, it is recommended that Mitoxantrone Hydrochloride not be mixed in the same infusion with other drugs.

STORAGE AND HANDLING
Procedures for proper handling and disposal of anticancer drugs should be considered. Several guidelines on this subject have been published.[1-6] There is no general agreement that all of the procedures recommended in the guidelines are necessary or appropriate.

Mitoxantrone Hydrochloride should be stored between 15°C (59°F) and 25°C (77°F). DO NOT FREEZE.

After the penetration of the stopper, the remaining portion of Mitoxantrone Hydrochloride may be stored no longer than 7 days between 15°C (59°F) and 25°C (77°F) or 14 days under refrigeration. CONTAINS NO PRESERVATIVE.

Mitoxantrone Hydrochloride may be further diluted into Dextrose 5% in Water, Normal Saline, or Dextrose 5% with Normal Saline and used immediately. DO NOT FREEZE.

Parenteral drug products should be inspected visually for particulate matter and discoloration prior to administration whenever solution and container permit.

REFERENCES
1. Recommendations for the Safe Handling of Parenteral Antineoplastic Drugs. NIH Publication No. 83-2621. For sale by the Superintendent of Documents, U.S. Government Printing Office, Washington, DC 20402. 2. AMA Council Report. Guidelines for Handling Parenteral Antineoplastics. JAMA. March 15, 1985. 3. National Study Commission on Cytotoxic Exposure—Recommendations for Handling Cytotoxic Agents. Available from Louis P. Jeffrey, Sc. D., Director of Pharmacy Services, Rhode Island Hospital, 593 Eddy Street, Providence, RI 02902. 4. Clinical Oncological Society of Australia: Guidelines and recommendations for safe handling of antineoplastic agents. *Med J Australia.*1983; 1:426-428. 5. Jones RB, et al. Safe handling of chemotherapeutic agents: A report from the Mount Sinai Medical Center. *Ca—A Cancer Journal for Clinicians.* Sept/Oct. 1983; 258-263. 6. American Society of Hospital Pharmacists: Technical assistance bulletin on handling cytotoxic drugs in hospitals. *Am J Hosp Pharm.*1985; 42:131-137.

J CODES
20 mg IV—J9293

HOW SUPPLIED
INJECTION: 2 MG/ML

BRAND/MANUFACTURER	NDC	SIZE	AWP
○ BRAND			
NOVANTRONE: Immunex	00205-9393-34	10 ml	$616.18
	00205-9393-72	12.5 ml	$770.20
	00205-9393-36	15 ml	$924.26

Mivacron SEE MIVACURIUM CHLORIDE

Mivacurium Chloride

This drug should be administered only by adequately trained individuals familiar with its actions, characteristics, and hazards.

DESCRIPTION
Mivacurium Chloride is a short-acting, non-depolarizing skeletal muscle relaxant for intravenous administration. Mivacurium Chloride is $[R[R*,R*-(E)]]$-2, 2'-[(1,8-dioxo-4-octene-1,8-diyl)bis(oxy-3,1-propanediyl)]b is[1,2, 3,4-tetrahydro-6,7-dimethoxy-2-methyl-1-[(3,4,5-trimethoxyphenyl) methyl]isoquinolinium]dichloride. The molecular formula is $C_{58}H_{80}Cl_2N_2O_{14}$ and the molecular weight is 1100.18.

The partition coefficient of the compound is 0.015 in a 1-octanol/distilled water system at 25°C.

Mivacurium Chloride is a mixture of three stereoisomers: $(1R, 1'R, 2S, 2'S)$, the *trans-trans* diester; $(1R, 1'R, 2R, 2'S)$, the *cis-trans* diester; and $(1R, 1'R, 2R, 2'R)$, the *cis-cis* diester. The *trans-trans* and *cis-trans* stereoisomers comprise 92% to 96% of Mivacurium Chloride and their neuromuscular blocking potencies are not significantly different from each other or from Mivacurium Chloride. The *cis-cis* diester has been estimated from studies in cats to have one-tenth the neuromuscular blocking potency of the other two stereoisomers. Mivacurium Chloride Injection is a sterile, non-pyrogenic solution (pH 3.5 to 5.0) containing Mivacurium Chloride equivalent to 2 mg/mL Mivacurium in Water for Injection. Hydrochloric acid may have been added to adjust pH. Mivacurium Premixed Infusion is a sterile, non-pyrogenic solution (pH 3.5 to 5.0; 260 mOsmol/L-measured) containing Mivacurium Chloride equivalent to 0.5 mg/mL

Mivacurium in 5% Dextrose Injection USP. Hydrochloric acid may have been added to adjust pH.

Following is its chemical structure:

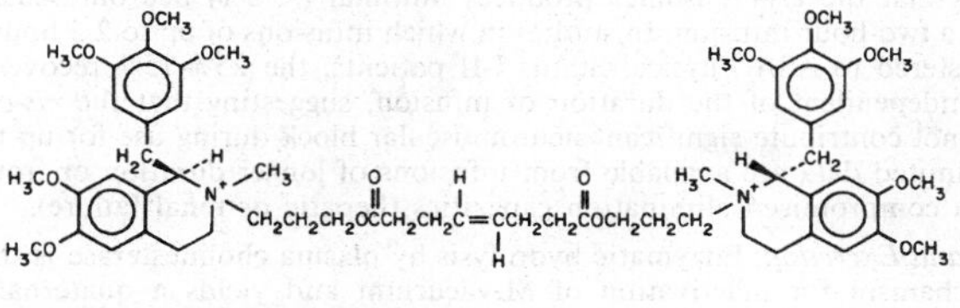

CLINICAL PHARMACOLOGY

Mivacurium Chloride (a mixture of three stereoisomers) binds competitively to cholinergic receptors on the motor end-plate to antagonize the action of acetylcholine, resulting in a block of neuromuscular transmission. This action is antagonized by acetylcholinesterase inhibitors, such as neostigmine.

Pharmacodynamics: The time to maximum neuromuscular block is similar for recommended doses of Mivacurium Chloride and intermediate-acting agents (e.g., atracurium), but longer than for the ultra-short-acting agent, succinylcholine. The clinically effective duration of action of the stereoisomers in Mivacurium Chloride (a mixture of three stereoisomers) is one-third to one-half that of intermediate-acting agents and 2 to 2.5 times that of succinylcholine.

The average ED_{95} (dose required to produce 95% suppression of the adductor pollicis muscle twitch response to ulnar nerve stimulation) of Mivacurium Chloride is 0.07 mg/kg (range: 0.06 to 0.09) in adults receiving opioid/nitrous oxide/oxygen an esthesia. The pharmacodynamics of doses of Mivacurium Chloride $\geq ED_{95}$ administered over 5 to 15 seconds during opioid/nitrous oxide/oxygen anesthesia are summarized in Table 1. The mean time for spontaneous recovery of the twitch response from 25% to 75% of control amplitude is about 6 minutes (range: 3 to 9, n = 32) following an initial dose of 0.15 mg/kg Mivacurium Chloride and 7 to 8 minutes (range: 4 to 24, n = 85) following initial doses of 0.20 or 0.25 mg/kg Mivacurium Chloride.

Volatile anesthetics may decrease the dosing requirement for Mivacurium Chloride and prolong the duration of action; the magnitude of these effects may be increased as the concentration of the volatile agent is increased. Isoflurane and enflurane (administered with nitrous oxide/oxygen to achieve 1.25 MAC [Minimum Alveolar Concentration]) may decrease the effective dose of Mivacurium Chloride by as much as 25%, and may prolong the clinically effective duration of action and decrease the average infusion requirement by as much as 35% to 40%. At equivalent MAC values, halothane has little or no effect on the ED_{50} of Mivacurium Chloride, but may prolong the duration of action and decrease the average infusion requirement by as much as 20% (see *"Individualization of Dosage"* subsection of *"Clinical Pharmacology"* and *"Drug Interaction"* subsection of *"Precautions"*). (See related table.)

Administration of Mivacurium Chloride over 30 to 60 seconds does not alter the time to maximum neuromuscular block or the duration of action. The duration of action of the stereoisomers in Mivacurium Chloride may be prolonged in patients with reduced plasma cholinesterase (pseudocholinesterase) activity (see *"Reduced Plasma Cholinesterase Activity"* subsection of *"Precautions"* and *"Individualization of Dosages"* subsection of *"Clinical Pharmacology"*).

Interpatient variability in duration of action occurs with Mivacurium Chloride as with other neuromuscular blocking agents. However, analysis of data from 224 patients in clinical studies receiving various doses of Mivacurium Chloride during opioid/nitrous oxide/oxygen anesthesia with a variety of premedicants and varying lengths of surgery indicated that approximately 90% of the patients had clinically effective durations of block within 8 minutes of the median duration predicted from the dose-response data shown in Table 1. Variations in plasma cholinesterase activity, including values within the normal range and values as low as 20% below the lower limit of the normal range, were not associated with clinically significant effects on duration. The variability in duration, however, was greater in patients with plasma cholinesterase activity at or slightly below the lower limit of the normal range.

When administered during the induction of adequate anesthesia using thiopental or propofol, nitrous oxide/oxygen, and co-induction agents such as fentanyl and/or midazolam, doses of 0.15 mg/kg ($2 \times ED_{95}$) Mivacurium Chloride administered over 5 to 15 seconds or 0.20 mg/kg Mivacurium Chloride administered over 30 seconds produced generally good-to-excellent tracheal intubation conditions in 2.5 to 3 and 2 to 2.5 minutes, respectively. A dose of 0.25 mg/kg Mivacurium Chloride administered as a divided dose (0.15 mg/kg followed 30 sec later by 0.10 mg/kg) produced generally good-to-excellent intubation conditions in 1.5 to 2 minutes after initiating the dosing regimen.

Repeated administration of maintenance doses or continuous infusion of Mivacurium Chloride for up to 2.5 hours is not associated with development of tachyphylaxis or cumulative neuromuscular blocking effects in ASA Physical Status I-II patients. Limited data are available from patients receiving infusions for longer than 2.5 hours. Spontaneous recovery of neuromuscular function after infusion is independent of the duration of infusion and comparable to recovery reported for single doses (Table 1).

The neuromuscular block produced by the stereoisomers in Mivacurium Chloride is readily antagonized by anticholinesterase agents. As seen with other nondepolarizing neuromuscular blocking agents, the more profound the neuromuscular block at the time of reversal, the longer the time and the greater the dose of anticholinesterase agent required for recovery of neuromuscular function.

In children (2 to 12 years) Mivacurium Chloride has a higher ED_{95} (0.10 mg/kg), faster onset, and shorter duration of action than in adults. The mean time for spontaneous recovery of the twitch response from 25% to 75% of control amplitude is about 5 minutes (n = 4) following an initial dose of 0.20 mg/kg Mivacurium Chloride. Recovery following reversal is faster in children than in adults (Table 1).

Hemodynamics: Administration of Mivacurium Chloride in doses up to and including 0.15 mg/kg ($2 \times ED_{95}$) over 5 to 15 seconds to ASA Physical Status I-II patients during opioid/nitrous oxide/oxygen anesthesia is associated with minimal changes in mean arterial blood pressure (MAP) or heart rate (HR) (Table 2).

Table 2

CARDIOVASCULAR DOSE RESPONSE DURING OPIOID/NITROUS OXIDE/OXYGEN ANESTHESIA

Initial Mivacurium Chloride Dose* (mg/kg)		% of Patients With $\geq 30\%$ Change			
		MAP		HR	
		Dec	Inc	Dec	Inc
Adults 0.07 to					
0.10	[n = 49]	0%	2%	0%	0%
0.15	[n = 53]	4%	4%	4%	2%
0.20†	[n = 53]	30%	0%	0%	8%
0.25†	[n = 44]	39%	2%	0%	14%

Table 1

PHARMACODYNAMIC DOSE RESPONSE DURING OPIOID/NITROUS OXIDE/OXYGEN ANESTHESIA

Initial Mivacurium Chloride Dose* (mg/kg)		Time to Maximum Block† (min)	Time to Spontaneous Recovery*			
			5% Recovery (min)	25% Recovery‡ (min)	95% Recovery§ (min)	T_4/T_1 Ratio $\geq 75\%$§ (min)
Adults						
0.07 to 0.10	[n = 47]	4.9 (2.0-7.6)	11 (7-19)	13 (8-24)	21 (10-36)	21 (10-36)
0.15	[n = 50]	3.3 (1.5-8.8)	13 (6-31)	16 (9-38)	26 (16-41)	26 (15-45)
0.20″	[n = 50]	2.5 (1.2-6.0)	16 (10-29)	20 (10-36)	31 (15-51)	34 (19-56)
0.25″	[n = 48]	2.3 (1.0-4.8)	19 (11-29)	23 (14-38)	34 (22-64)	43 (26-75)
Children 2 to 12 Years						
0.11 to 0.12	[n = 17]	2.8 (1.2-4.6)	5 (3-9)	7 (4-10)	—	—
0.20	[n = 18]	1.9 (1.3-3.3)	7 (3-12)	10 (6-15)	19 (14-26)	16 (12-23)
0.25	[n = 9]	1.6 (1.0-2.2)	7 (4-9)	9 (5-12)	—	—

* *Doses administered over 5 to 15 seconds.*
† *Values shown are medians of means from individual studies (range of individual patient values).*
‡ *Clinically effective duration of neuromuscular block.*
§ *Data available for as few as 40% of adults in specific dose groups and for 22% of children in the 0.20 mg/kg dose group due to administration of reversal agents or additional doses of Mivacurium Chloride prior to 95% recovery or T_4/T_1 ratio recovery to $\leq 75\%$.*
″ *Rapid administration not recommended due to possibility of decreased blood pressure. Administrator 0.20 mg/kg over 30 sec; administer 0.25 mg/kg as divided dose (0.15 mg/kg followed 30 sec later by 0.10 mg/kg). See "Dosage and Administration".*

	% of Patients With ≥ 30% Change			
Initial Mivacurium Chloride Dose* (mg/kg)	MAP		HR	
	Dec	Inc	Dec	Inc
Children 2 to 12 years				
0.11 to 0.12 [n = 17]	0%	6%	0%	0%
0.20 [n = 17]	0%	0%	0%	0%
0.25 [n = 8]	13%	0%	0%	0%

* *Doses administered over 5 to 15 seconds.*

† *Rapid administration not recommended due to possibility of decreased blood pressure. Administer 0.20 mg/kg over 30 sec; administer 0.25 mg/kg as divided dose (0.15 mg/kg followed 30 sec later by 0.10 mg/kg). See "Dosage and Administration".*

Higher doses of ≥ 0.20 mg/kg (≥ $3 \times ED_{95}$) may be associated with transient decreases in MAP and increases in HR in some patients. These decreases in MAP are usually maximal within 1 to 3 minutes following the dose, typically resolve without treatment in an additional 1 to 3 minutes, and are usually associated with increases in plasma histamine concentration. Decreases in MAP can be minimized by administering Mivacurium Chloride over 30 to 60 seconds (see *"Individualization of Dosages"* subsection of *"Clinical Pharmacology"* and *"General"* subsection of *"Precautions"*).

Analysis of 426 patients in clinical studies receiving initial doses of Mivacurium Chloride up to and including 0.30 mg/kg during opioid/nitrous oxide/oxygen anethesia showed that high initial doses and a rapid rate of injection contributed to a greater probability of experiencing a decrease of ≥ 30% in MAP after Mivacurium Chloride administration. Obese patients also had a greater probability of experiencing a decrease of ≥ 30% in MAP when dosed on the basis of actual body weight, thereby receiving a larger dose than if dosed on the basis of ideal body weight (see *"Individualization of Dosages"* subsection of *"Clinical Pharmacology"* and the *"General"* subsection of *"Precautions"*).

Children experience minimal changes in MAP or HR after administration of Mivacurium Chloride doses up to and including 0.20 mg/kg over 5 to 15 seconds, but higher doses (≥ 0.25 mg/kg) may be associated with transient decreases in MAP (Table 2).

Following a dose of 0.15 mg/kg Mivacurium Chloride administered over 60 seconds, adult patients with significant cardiovascular disease undergoing coronary artery bypass grafting or valve replacement procedures showed no clinically important changes in MAP or HR. Transient decreases in MAP were observed in some patients after doses of 0.20 to 0.25 mg/kg Mivacurium Chloride administered over 60 seconds. The number of patients in whom these decreases in MAP required treatment was small.

Pharmacokinetics: Table 3 describes the results from a study of 9 ASA Physical Status I-II adult patients (31 to 48 years) receiving an infusion of Mivacurium Chloride at 5 µg/kg/min for 60 minutes followed by 10 µg/kg/min for 60 minutes. Mivacurium Chloride is a mixture of isomers which do not interconvert in vivo. The Mivacurium pharmacokinetic parameters presented in Table 3 were determined using a stereospecific assay. The two more potent isomers, *cis-trans* (36% of the mixture) and *trans-trans* (57% of the mixture), have very high clearances that exceed cardiac output, reflecting the extensive metabolism by plasma cholinesterase. The volume of distribution is relatively small, reflecting limited tissue distribution secondary to the polarity and large molecular weight of Mivacurium. The combination of high metabolic clearance and low distribution volume results in the short elimination half-life of approximately 2 minutes for the two active isomers. The short elimination half-lives and high metabolic clearances of the active isomers are consistent with the short duration of action of Mivacurium Chloride. The steady-state concentrations of the *cis-trans* and *trans-trans* isomers doubled after the infusion rate was increased from 5 to 10 µg/kg/min, indicating that their pharmacokinetics are dose-proportional.

Table 3

STEREOISOMER PHARMACOKINETIC PARAMETERS* OF MIVACURIUM CHLORIDE IN ASA PHYSICAL STATUS I-II ADULT PATIENTS [n = 9] DURING OPIOID/NITROUS OXIDE/OXYGEN ANESTHESIA

Parameter	trans-trans isomer	cis-trans isomer
Elimination Half-life ($t_{1/2}$, min)	2.3 (1.4-3.6)	2.1 (0.8-4.8)
Volume of Distribution (L/kg)	0.15 (0.06-0.24)	0.27 (0.08-0.56)
Plasma Clearance (mL/min/kg)	53 (32-105)	99 (52-230)

* *Values shown are mean (range).*

† *Ages 31 to 48 years.*

The *cis-cis* isomer (6% of the mixture) has approximately one-tenth the neuromuscular blocking potency of the *trans-trans* and *cis-trans* isomers in cats. In the nine patients shown in Table 3, the volume of distribution of the *cis-cis* isomer averaged 0.31 L/kg (range: 0.18 to 0.46), the clearance averaged 4.2 mL/min/kg

(range: 2.4 to 5.4), and the half-life averaged 55 minutes (range: 32 to 102). The neuromuscular blocking potency of the *cis-cis* isomer in humans has not been established; however, modeling of clinical pharmacokinetic-pharmacodynamic data suggests that the *cis-cis* isomer produces minimal (< 5%) neuromuscular block during a two-hour infusion. In studies in which infusions of up to 2.5 hours were administered to ASA Physical Status I-II patients, the 25%-75% recovery times were independent of the duration of infusion, suggesting that the *cis-cis* isomer does not contribute significant neuromuscular block during use for up to 2.5 hours. Limited data are available from infusions of longer duration or from patients with compromised elimination capacities (hepatic or renal failure).

Metabolism and Excretion: Enzymatic hydrolysis by plasma cholinesterase is the primary mechanism for inactivation of Mivacurium and yields a quaternary alcohol and a quaternary monoester metabolite. Renal and biliary excretion of unchanged Mivacurium are minor elimination pathways: urine and bile are important elimination pathways for the two metabolites. Tests in which these two metabolites were administered to cats and dogs suggest that each metabolite is unlikely to produce clinically significant neuromuscular, autonomic or cardiovascular effects following administration of Mivacurium Chloride.

Special Populations: The pharmacokinetics of Mivacurium isomers has not been studied in the elderly or in patients with renal or hepatic disease using a stereospecific assay. The non-stereospecific, total Mivacurium assay used in pharmacokinetic-pharmacodynamic studies in these populations provided preliminary evidence that reduced clearance of one or more isomers is responsible for the longer duration of action of Mivacurium Chloride seen in patients with end-stage kidney or liver disease. The data did not provide a pharmacokinetic explanation for the 15% to 20% longer duration of block seen in the elderly. Tables 4 and 5 summarize the pharmacodynamic results in these special populations as compared with young adults (ages 18 to 49 years). No data are available from patients with kidney or liver disease not requiring transplantation. (See related table).

Renal: The clinically effective duration of action of 0.15 mg/kg Mivacurium Chloride was about 1.5 times longer in patients with end-stage kidney disease than in healthy patients, presumably due to reduced clearance of one or more isomers.

Hepatic: The clinically effective duration of action of 0.15 mg/kg Mivacurium Chloride was three times longer in patients with end-stage liver disease than in healthy patients and is likely related to the markedly decreased plasma cholinesterase activity (30% of healthy patient values) which could decrease the clearance of one or more isomers (see *"Reduced Plasma Cholinesterase Activity"* subsection of *"Precautions"*). (See related table).

Individualization of Dosages: DOSES OF MIVACURIUM CHLORIDE SHOULD BE INDIVIDUALIZED AND A PERIPHERAL NERVE STIMULATOR SHOULD BE USED TO MEASURE NEUROMUSCULAR FUNCTION DURING MIVACURIUM CHLORIDE ADMINISTRATION IN ORDER TO MONITOR DRUG EFFECT. DETERMINE THE NEED FOR ADDITIONAL DOSES, AND CONFIRM RECOVERY FROM NEUROMUSCULAR BLOCK.

Based on the known actions of Mivacurium Chloride (a mixture of three stereoisomers) and other neuromuscular blocking agents, the following factors should be considered when administering Mivacurium Chloride.

Renal or Hepatic Impairment: A dose of 0.15 mg/kg Mivacurium Chloride is recommended for facilitation of tracheal intubation in patients with renal or hepatic impairment. However, the clinically effective duration of block produced by this dose is about 1.5 times longer in patients with end-stage kidney disease and about 3 times longer in patients with end-stage liver disease than in patients with normal renal and hepatic function. Infusion rates should be decreased by as much as 50% in these patients depending on the degree of renal or hepatic impairment (see *"Renal and Hepatic Disease"* subsection of *"Precautions"*).

Reduced Plasma Cholinesterase Activity: The possibility of prolonged neuromuscular block following administration of Mivacurium Chloride must be considered in patients with reduced plasma cholinesterase (pseudocholinesterase) activity. Mivacurium Chloride should be used with great caution, if at all, in patients known or suspected of being homozygous for the atypical plasma cholinesterase gene (see *"Warnings"*). Doses of 0.03 mg/kg produced complete neuromuscular block for 26 to 128 minutes in three such patients: thus initial doses greater than 0.03 mg/kg are not recommended in homozygous patients. Infusion of Mivacurium Chloride are not recommended in homozygous patients.

Mivacurium Chloride has been used safely in patients heterozygous for the atypical plasma cholinesterase gene and in genotypically normal patients with reduced plasma cholinesterase activity. After an initial dose of 0.15 mg/kg Mivacurium Chloride the clinically effective duration of block in heterozygous patients may be approximately 10 minutes longer than in patients with normal genotype and normal plasma cholinesterase activity. Lower Mivacurium Chloride infusion rates are recommended in these patients (see *"Reduced Plasma Cholinesterase Activity"* subsection of *"Precautions"*).

Drugs or Conditions Causing Potentiation of or Resistance to Neuromuscular Block: As with other neuromuscular blocking agents Mivacurium Chloride may have profound neuromuscular blocking effects in cachectic or debilitated patients, patients with neuromuscular diseases, and patients with carcinomatosis. In these or other patients in whom potentiation of neuromuscular block or difficulty with reversal may be anticipated, the initial dose should be decreased. A test dose of not more than 0.015 to 0.020 mg/kg, which represents the lower end of the dose-response curve for Mivacurium Chloride is recommended in such patients (see *"General"* subsection of *"Precautions"*).

The neuromuscular blocking action of the stereoisomers in Mivacurium Chloride is potentiated by isoflurane or enflurane anesthesia. Recommended initial Mivacurium Chloride doses (see "Dosage and Administration") may be used for intubation prior to the administration of these agents. If Mivacurium Chloride is first administered after establishment of stable-state isoflurane or enflurane anesthesia (administered with nitrous oxide/oxygen to achieve 1.25 MAC), the initial Mivacurium Chloride dose should be reduced by as much as 25%, and the infusion rate reduced by as much as 35% to 40%. A greater potentiation of the neuromuscular blocking action of the stereoisomers in Mivacurium Chloride may be expected with higher concentrations of enflurane or isoflurane. The use of halothane requires no adjustment of the initial dose of Mivacurium Chloride but may prolong the duration of action and decrease the average infusion rate by as much as 20% (see "Drug Interactions" subsection of "Precautions").

When Mivacurium Chloride is administered to patients receiving certain antibiotics, magnesium salts, lithium, local anesthetics, procainamide and quinidine, longer durations of neuromuscular block may be expected and infusion requirements may be lower (see "Drug Interactions" subsection of "Precautions").

When Mivacurium Chloride is administered to patients chronically receiving phenytoin or carbamazepine, slightly shorter durations of neuromuscular block may be anticipated and infusion rate requirements may be higher (see "Drug Interactions" subsection of "Precautions").

Severe acid-base and/or electrolyte abnormalities may potentiate or cause resistance to the neuromuscular blocking action of the stereoisomers in Mivacurium Chloride. No data are available in such patients and no dosing recommendations can be made (see "General" subsection of "Precautions").

Burns: While patients with burns are known to develop resistance to nondepolarizing neuromuscular blocking agents, they may also have reduced plasma cholinesterase activity. Consequently, in these patients, a test dose of not more than 0.015 to 0.020 mg/kg Mivacurium Chloride is recommended, followed by additional appropriate dosing guided by the use of a neuromuscular block monitor (see "General" subsection of "Precautions").

Cardiovascular Disease: In patients with clinically significant cardiovascular disease, the initial dose of Mivacurium Chloride should be 0.15 mg/kg or less, administered over 60 seconds (see "Hemodynamics" subsection of "Clinical Pharmacology" and General subsection of "Precautions").

Obesity: Obese patients (patients weighing ≥ 30% more than their ideal body weight) dosed on the basis of actual body weight, thereby receiving a larger dose than if dosed on the basis of ideal body weight, had a greater probability of experiencing a decrease of ≥ 30% in MAP (see "Hemodynamics" subsection of "Clinical Pharmacology" and "General" subsection of "Precautions"). Therefore, in obese patients, the initial dose should be determined using the patient's ideal body weight (IBW), according to the following formulae:

Men: IBW in kg = [106 + (6 × inches in height above 5 feet)]/2.2
Women: IBW in kg = [100 + (5 × inches in height above 5 feet)]/2.2

Allergy and Sensitivity: In patients with any history suggestive of a greater sensitivity to the release of histamine or related mediators (e.g., asthma), the initial dose of Mivacurium Chloride should be 0.15 mg/kg or less, administered over 60 seconds (see General subsection of "Precautions").

INDICATIONS AND USAGE

Mivacurium Chloride is a short-acting neuromuscular blocking agent indicated for inpatients and outpatients, as an adjunct to general anesthesia, to facilitate tracheal intubation and to provide skeletal muscle relaxation during surgery or mechanical ventilation.

CONTRAINDICATIONS

Mivacurium Chloride is contraindicated in patients known to have an allergic hypersensitivity to Mivacurium Chloride or other benzylisoquinolinium agents, as manifested by reactions such as urticaria or severe respiratory distress or hypotension. Use of Mivacurium Chloride from multi-dose vials is contraindicated in patients with a known allergy to benzyl alcohol.

WARNINGS

MIVACURIUM CHLORIDE SHOULD BE ADMINISTERED IN CAREFULLY ADJUSTED DOSAGE BY OR UNDER THE SUPERVISION OF EXPERIENCED CLINICIANS WHO ARE FAMILIAR WITH THE DRUG'S ACTIONS AND THE POSSIBLE COMPLICATIONS OF ITS USE. THE DRUG SHOULD NOT BE ADMINISTERED UNLESS PERSONNEL AND FACILITIES FOR RESUSCITATION AND LIFE SUPPORT (TRACHEAL INTUBATION, ARTIFICIAL VENTILATION, OXYGEN THERAPY), AND AN ANTAGONIST OF MIVACURIUM CHLORIDE ARE IMMEDIATELY AVAILABLE. IT IS RECOMMENDED THAT A PERIPHERAL NERVE STIMULATOR BE USED TO MEASURE NEUROMUSCULAR FUNCTION DURING THE ADMINISTRATION OF MIVACURIUM CHLORIDE IN ORDER TO MONITOR DRUG EFFECT, DETERMINE THE NEED FOR ADDITIONAL DRUG, AND CONFIRM RECOVERY FROM NEUROMUSCULAR BLOCK.

MIVACURIUM CHLORIDE HAS NO KNOWN EFFECT ON CONSCIOUSNESS, PAIN THRESHOLD, OR CEREBRATION. TO AVOID DISTRESS TO THE PATIENT, NEUROMUSCULAR BLOCK SHOULD NOT BE INDUCED BEFORE UNCONSCIOUSNESS.

MIVACURIUM CHLORIDE IS METABOLIZED BY PLASMA CHOLINESTERASE AND SHOULD BE USED WITH GREAT CAUTION, IF AT ALL, IN PATIENTS KNOWN TO BE OR SUSPECTED OF BEING HOMOZYGOUS FOR THE ATYPICAL PLASMA CHOLINESTERASE GENE.

Mivacurium Chloride Injection and Mivacurium Chloride Premixed Infusion are acidic (pH 3.5 to 5.0) and may not be compatible with alkaline solutions having a pH greater than 8.5 (e.g., barbiturate solutions).

Multiple dose vials of Mivacurium Chloride contain benzyl alcohol. In newborn infants, benzyl alcohol has been associated with an increased incidence of neurological and other complications which are sometimes fatal. Single use vials and Mivacurium Chloride Premixed Infusion do not contain benzyl alcohol.

Table 4

PHARMACODYNAMIC PARAMETERS* OF MIVACURIUM CHLORIDE IN ASA PHYSICAL STATUS I-II YOUNG ADULT PATIENTS AND ELDERLY PATIENTS DURING ISOFLURANE/NITROUS OXIDE/OXYGEN ANESTHESIA

Parameter	Young Adult Patients (18-49 years)		Elderly Patients (68-77 years)
Initial Dose†	0.10 mg/kg [n = 9]	0.25 mg/kg‡ [n = 9]	0.10 mg/kg [n = 8]
Maximum Block (%)	98 (83-100)	100 (100-100)	99 (95-100)
Time to Maximum Block (min)	3.2 (2.0-6.0)	1.7 (1.3-2.5)	4.8 (3.0-7.0)
Clinically Effective Duration of Block§ (min)	17 (9-29)	27 (18-34)	20 (14-28)

* Values shown are mean (range).
† Doses administered over 5 to 15 seconds.
‡ Rapid administration not recommended due to possibility of decreased blood pressure. Administer 0.25 mg/kg as divided dose (0.15 mg/kg followed 30 sec later by 0.10 mg/kg). (See "Dosage and Administration").
§ Time from injection to 25% recovery of the control twitch height.

Table 5

PHARMACODYNAMIC PARAMETERS* OF MIVACURIUM CHLORIDE IN ASA PHYSICAL STATUS I-II PATIENTS AND IN PATIENTS UNDERGOING KIDNEY OR LIVER TRANSPLANTATION DURING ISOFLURANE/NITROUS OXIDE/OXYGEN ANESTHESIA

Parameter	Young Adult Patients	Kidney Transplant Patients	Liver Transplant Patients‡
Initial Dose	0.15 mg/kg [n = 8]	0.15 mg/kg [n = 9]	0.15 mg/kg [n = 8]
Maximum Block (%)	99.8 (98-100)	100 (100-100)	100 (100-100)
Time to Maximum Block (min)	1.9 (0.8-3.5)	2.6 (1.0-4.5)	2.1 (1.0-4.0)
Clinically Effective Duration of Block† (min)	19 (12-30)	30 (19-58)	57 (29-80)

* Values shown are mean (range).
† Time from injection to 25% recovery of the control twitch height.
§ Liver transplant patients received isoflurane without nitrous oxide.

PRECAUTIONS

General: Although Mivacurium Chloride (a mixture of three stereoisomers) is not a potent histamine releaser, the possibility of substantial histamine release must be considered. Release of histamine is related to the dose and speed of injection.

Caution should be exercised in administering Mivacurium Chloride to patients with clinically significant cardiovascular disease and patients with any history suggesting a greater sensitivity to the release of histamine or related mediators (e.g., asthma). In such patients, the initial dose of Mivacurium Chloride should be 0.15 mg/kg or less, administered over 60 seconds; assurance of adequate hydration and careful monitoring of hemodynamic status are important (see *"Hemodynamics"* and *"Individualization of Dosages"* subsection of *"Clinical Pharmacology"*).

Obese patients may be more likely to experience clinically significant transient decreases in MAP than non-obese patients when the dose of Mivacurium Chloride is based on actual rather than ideal body weight. Therefore, in obese patients, the initial dose should be determined using the patient's ideal body weight (see *"Hemodynamics"* and *"Individualization of Dosages"* subsection of *"Clinical Pharmacology"*).

Recommended doses of Mivacurium Chloride have no clinically significant effects on heart rate; therefore, Mivacurium Chloride will not counteract the bradycardia produced by many anesthetic agents or by vagal stimulation.

Neuromuscular blocking agents may have a profound effect in patients with neuromuscular diseases (e.g., myasthenia gravis and the myasthenic syndrome). In these and other conditions in which prolonged neuromuscular block is a possibility (e.g., carcinomatosis), the use of a peripheral nerve stimulator and a dose of not more than 0.015 to 0.020 mg/kg Mivacurium Chloride is recommended to assess the level of neuromuscular block and to monitor dosage requirements (see *"Individualization of Dosages"* subsection of *"Clinical Pharmacology"*).

Mivacurium Chloride has not been studied in patients with burns. Resistance to nondepolarizing neuromuscular blocking agents may develop in patients with burns, depending upon the time elapsed since the injury and the size of the burn. Patients with burns may have reduced plasma cholinesterase activity which may offset this resistance (see *"Individualization of Dosages"* subsection of *"Clinical Pharmacology"*).

Acid-base and/or serum electrolyte abnormalities may potentiate or antagonize the action of neuromuscular blocking agents. The action of neuromuscular blocking agents may be enhanced by magnesium salts administered for the management of toxemia of pregnancy (see *"Individualization of Dosages"* subsection of *"Clinical Pharmacology"*).

No data are available to support the use of Mivacurium Chloride by intramuscular injection.

Renal and Hepatic Disease: The possibility of prolonged neuromuscular block must be considered when Mivacurium Chloride is used in patients with renal or hepatic disease (see *"Pharmacokinetics"* subsection of *"Clinical Pharmacology"*). Most patients with chronic hepatic disease such as hepatitis, liver abscess, and cirrhosis of the liver exhibit a marked reduction in plasma cholinesterase activity. Patients with acute or chronic renal disease may also show a reduction in plasma cholinesterase activity (see *"Individualization of Dosages"* subsection of *"Clinical Pharmacology"*).

Reduced Plasma Cholinesterase Activity: The possibility of prolonged neuromuscular block following administration of Mivacurium Chloride must be considered in patients with reduced plasma cholinesterase (pseudocholinesterase) activity.

Plasma cholinesterase activity may be diminished in the presence of genetic abnormalities of plasma cholinesterase (e.g., patients heterozygous or homozygous for the atypical plasma cholinesterase gene), pregnancy, liver or kidney disease, malignant tumors, infections, burns, anemia, decompensated heart disease, peptic ulcer, or myxedema. Plasma cholinesterase activity may also be diminished by chronic administration of oral contraceptives, glucocorticoids, or certain monoamine oxidase inhibitors and by irreversible inhibitors of plasma cholinesterase (e.g., organophosphate insecticides, echothiophate, and certain antineoplastic drugs).

Mivacurium Chloride has been used safely in patients heterozygous for the atypical plasma cholinesterase gene. At doses of 0.10 to 0.20 mg/kg Mivacurium Chloride, the clinically effective duration of action was 8 to 11 minutes longer in patients heterozygous for the atypical gene than in genotypically normal patients. As with succinylcholine, patients homozygous for the atypical plasma cholinesterase gene (1 in 2500 patients) are extremely sensitive to the neuromuscular blocking effect of Mivacurium Chloride. In three such adult patients, a small dose of 0.03 mg/kg (approximately the ED_{10-20} in genotypically normal patients) produced complete neuromuscular block for 26 to 128 minutes. Once spontaneous recovery had begun, neuromuscular block in these patients was antagonized with conventional doses of neostigmine. One adult patient, who was homozygous for the atypical plasma cholinesterase gene, received a dose of 0.18 mg/kg Mivacurium Chloride and exhibited complete neuromuscular block for about 4 hours. Response to post-tetanic stimulation was present after 4 hours, all four responses to train-of-four stimulation were present after 6 hours, and the patient was extubated after 8 hours. Reversal was not attempted in this patient.

Malignant Hyperthermia (MH): In a study of MH-susceptible pigs, Mivacurium Chloride did not trigger MH. Mivacurium Chloride has not been studied in MH-susceptible patients. Because MH can develop in the absence of established triggering agents, the clinician should be prepared to recognize and treat MH in any patient undergoing general anethesia.

Long-Term Use in the Intensive Care Unit (ICU): No data are available on the long-term use of Mivacurium Chloride in patients undergoing mechanical ventilation in the ICU.

Drug Interactions: Although Mivacurium Chloride (a mixture of three stereoisomers) has been administered safely following succinylcholine-facilitated tracheal intubation, the interaction between the stereoisomers in Mivacurium Chloride and succinylcholine has not been systematically studied. Prior administration of succinylcholine can potentiate the neuromuscular blocking effects of nondepolarizing agents. Evidence of spontaneous recovery from succinylcholine should be observed before the administration of Mivacurium Chloride. The use of Mivacurium Chloride before succinylcholine to attenuate some of the side effects of succinylcholine has not been studied.

There are no clinical data on the use of Mivacurium Chloride with other nondepolarizing neuromuscular blocking agents.

Isoflurane and enflurane (administered with nitrous oxide/oxygen to achieve 1.25 MAC) decrease the ED_{50} of Mivacurium Chloride by as much as 25% (see *"Pharmacodynamics and Individualization of Dosages"* subsections of *"Clinical Pharmacology"*). These agents may also prolong the clinically effective duration of action and decrease the average infusion requirement of Mivacurium Chloride by as much as 35% to 40%. A greater potentiation of the neuromuscular blocking effects of the stereoisomers in Mivacurium Chloride may be expected with higher concentrations of enflurane or isoflurane. Halothane has little or no effect on the ED_{50}, but may prolong the duration of action and decrease the average infusion requirement by as much as 20%.

Other drugs which may enhance the neuromuscular blocking action of nondepolarizing agents such as the stereoisomers in Mivacurium Chloride include certain antibiotics (e.g., aminoglycosides, tetracyclines, bacitracin, polymyxins, lincomycin, clindamycin, colistin, and sodium colistimethate), magnesium salts, lithium, local anesthetics, procainamide, and quinidine. The neuromuscular blocking effect of Mivacurium Chloride may be enhanced by drugs that reduce plasma cholinesterase activity (e.g., chronically administered oral contraceptives, glucocorticoids, or certain monoamine oxidase inhibitors) or by drugs that irreversibly inhibit plasma cholinesterase (see *"Reduced Plasma Cholinesterase Activity"* subsection of *"Precautions"*).

Resistance to the neuromuscular blocking action of non-depolarizing neuromuscular blocking agents has been demonstrated in patients chronically administered phenytoin or carbamazepine. While the effects of chronic phenytoin or carbamazepine therapy on the action of the stereoisomers in Mivacurium Chloride are unknown, slightly shorter durations of neuromuscular block may be anticipated; and infusion rate requirements may be higher.

Carcinogenesis, Mutagenesis, Impairment of Fertility: Carcinogenesis and fertility studies have not been performed. Mivacurium Chloride was evaluated in a battery of four short-term mutagenicity tests. It was non-mutagenic in the Ames Salmonella assay, the mouse lymphoma assay, the human lymphocyte assay, and the in vivo rat bone marrow cytogenic assay.

Pregnancy: Teratogenic Effects: Pregnancy Category C. Teratology testing in nonventilated pregnant rats and mice treated subcutaneously with maximum subparalyzing doses of Mivacurium Chloride revealed no maternal or fetal toxicity or teratogenic effects. There are no adequate and well-controlled studies of Mivacurium Chloride in pregnant women. Because animal studies are not always predictive of human response, and the doses used were subparalyzing, Mivacurium Chloride should be used during pregnancy only if the potential benefit justifies the potential risk to the fetus.

Labor and Delivery: The use of Mivacurium Chloride during labor, vaginal delivery, or cesarean section has not been studied in humans and it is not known whether Mivacurium Chloride administered to the mother has effects on the fetus. Doses of 0.08 and 0.20 mg/kg Mivacurium Chloride given to female beagles undergoing cesarean section resulted in negligible levels of the stereoisomers in Mivacurium Chloride in umbilical vessel blood of neonates and no deleterious effects on the puppies.

Nursing Mothers: It is not known whether any of the stereoisomers of Mivacurium are excreted in human milk. Because many drugs are excreted in human milk, caution should be exercised following administration of Mivacurium Chloride to a nursing woman.

Pediatric Use: Mivacurium Chloride has not been studied in children below the age of 2 years (see *"Clinical Pharmacology"* and *"Dosage and Administration"* for clinical experience and recommendations for use in children 2 to 12 years of age).

Geriatric Use: Mivacurium Chloride was safely administered during clinical trials to 64 elderly ($\geq$ 65 years) patients, including 31 patients with significant cardiovascular disease (see *"General"* subsection of *"Precautions"*). The duration of neuromuscular block may be slightly longer in elderly patients than in young adult patients (see *"Clinical Pharmacology"*).

ADVERSE REACTIONS

Observed in Clinical Trials: Mivacurium Chloride (a mixture of three stereoisomers) was well tolerated during extensive clinical trials in inpatients and outpatients. Prolonged neuromuscular block, which is an important adverse experience associated with neuromuscular blocking agents as a class, was reported as an adverse experience in 3 of 2074 patients administered Mivacurium Chloride. The most commonly reported adverse experience following the administration of Mivacurium Chloride was transient, dose-dependent cutaneous flushing about the face, neck, and/or chest. Flushing was most frequently noted after the initial dose of Mivacurium Chloride and was reported in about 25% of adult patients who received 0.15 mg/kg Mivacurium Chloride over 5 to 15 seconds. When present, flushing typically began within 1 to 2 minutes after the dose of Mivacurium Chloride and lasted for 3 to 5 minutes. Of 105 patients who experienced flushing after 0.15 mg/kg Mivacurium Chloride two patients also experienced mild hypotension that was not treated, and one patient experienced moderate wheezing that was successfully treated.

Overall, hypotension was infrequently reported as an adverse experience in the clinical trials of Mivacurium Chloride. One of 332 (0.3%) healthy adults who received 0.15 mg/kg Mivacurium Chloride over 5 to 15 seconds and none of 37 cardiac surgery patients who received 0.15 mg/kg Mivacurium Chloride over 60 seconds was treated for a decrease in blood pressure in association with the administration of Mivacurium Chloride. One to two percent of healthy adults given ≥ 0.20 mg/kg Mivacurium Chloride over 5 to 15 seconds, 2% to 3% of healthy adults given 0.20 mg/kg over 30 seconds, none of 100 healthy adults given 0.25 mg/kg as a divided dose (0.15 mg/kg followed in 30 sec by 0.10 mg/kg), and 2% to 4% of cardiac surgery patients given ≥ 0.20 mg/kg over 60 seconds were treated for a decrease in blood pressure. None of the 63 children who received the recommended dose of 0.20 mg/kg Mivacurium Chloride was treated for a decrease in blood pressure in association with the administration of Mivacurium Chloride.

The following adverse experiences were reported in patients administered Mivacurium Chloride (all events judged by investigators during the clinical trials to have a possible causal relationship):

INCIDENCE GREATER THAN 1%—
Cardiovascular: Flushing (16%)

INCIDENCE LESS THAN 1%—
Cardiovascular: Hypotension, Tachycardia, Bradycardia,

Cardiac: Arrhythmia, Phlebitis

Respiratory: Bronchospasm, Wheezing, Hypoxemia

Dermatological: Rash, Urticaria, Erythema, Injection Site Reaction

Nonspecific: Prolonged Drug Effect

Neurologic: Dizziness

Musculoskeletal: Muscle Spasms

Observed in Clinical Practice: Based on initial clinical practice experience in patients who received Mivacurium Chloride, spontaneously reported adverse events are uncommon. Some of these events occurred at recommended doses and required treatment. There are insufficient data to establish a causal relationship or to support an estimate of their incidence. Adverse events reported during clinical practice include:

General: Allergic Reactions which, in rare instances, were severe

Musculoskeletal: Diminished Drug Effect, Prolonged Drug Effect

Cardiovascular: Hypotension (rarely severe), Flushing

Respiratory: Bronchospasm

Integumentary: Rash

OVERDOSAGE
Overdosage with neuromuscular blocking agents may result in neuromuscular block beyond the time needed for surgery and anesthesia. The primary treatment is maintenance of a patent airway and controlled ventilation until recovery of normal neuromuscular function is assured. Once evidence of recovery from neuromuscular block is observed, further recovery may be facilitated by administration of an anticholinesterase agent (e.g., neostigmine, edrophonium) in conjunction with an appropriate anticholinergic agent (see *"Antagonism of Neuromuscular Block"*). Overdosage may increase the risk of hemodynamic side effects, especially decreases in blood pressure. If needed, cardiovascular support may be provided by proper positioning of the patient, fluid administration, and/or vasopressor agent administration.

ANTAGONISM OF NEUROMUSCULAR BLOCK:
ANTAGONISTS (SUCH AS NEOSTIGMINE) SHOULD NOT BE ADMINISTERED WHEN COMPLETE NEUROMUSCULAR BLOCK IS EVIDENT OR SUSPECTED. THE USE OF A PERIPHERAL NERVE STIMULATOR TO EVALUATE RECOVERY AND ANTAGONISM OF NEUROMUSCULAR BLOCK IS RECOMMENDED.

Administration of 0.030 to 0.064 mg/kg neostigmine or 0.5 mg/kg edrophonium at approximately 10% recovery from neuromuscular block (range: 1 to 15) produced 95% recovery of the muscle twitch response and a T_4/T_1 ratio ≥ 75% in about 10 minutes. The times from 25% recovery of the muscle twitch response to T_4/T_1 ratio ≥ 75% following these doses of antagonists averaged about 7 to 9 minutes. In comparison, average times for spontaneous recovery from 25% to T_4/T_1 ≥ 75% were 12 to 13 minutes.

Patients administered antagonists should be evaluated for adequate clinical evidence of antagonism, e.g., 5-second head lift and grip strength. Ventilation must be supported until no longer required.

Antagonism may be delayed in the presence of debilitation, carcinomatosis, and the concomitant use of certain broad spectrum antibiotics, or anesthetic agents and other drugs which enhance neuromuscular block or separately cause respiratory depression (see *"Drug Interactions"* subsection of *"Precautions"*). Under such circumstances the management is the same as that of prolonged neuromuscular block (see *"Overdosage"*).

DOSAGE AND ADMINISTRATION
MIVACURIUM CHLORIDE SHOULD ONLY BE ADMINISTERED INTRAVENOUSLY.

The dosage information provided below is intended as a guide only. Doses of Mivacurium Chloride should be individualized (see *"Individualization of Dos-*

ages" subsection of *"Clinical Pharmacology"*). Factors that may warrant dosage adjustment include but may not be limited to: the presence of significant kidney, liver, or cardiovascular disease, obesity (patients weighing ≥ 30% more than ideal body weight for height), asthma, reduction in plasma cholinesterase activity, and the presence of inhalational anesthetic agents. When using Mivacurium Chloride or other neuromuscular blocking agents to facilitate tracheal intubation, it is important to recognize that the most important factors affecting intubation are the depth of general anesthesia and the level of neuromuscular block. Satisfactory intubating conditions can usually be achieved before complete neuromuscular block is attained if there is adequate anesthesia.

The use of a peripheral nerve stimulator will permit the most advantageous use of Mivacurium Chloride, minimize the possibility of overdosage or underdosage, and assist in the evaluation of recovery. When using a stimulator to monitor onset of neuromuscular block, clinical studies have shown that all four twitches of the train-of-four response may be present, with little or no fade, at the times recommended for intubation. Therefore, as with other neuromuscular blocking agents, it is important to use other criteria, such as clinical evaluation of the status of relaxation of jaw muscles and vocal cords, in conjunction with peripheral muscle twitch monitoring, to guide the appropriate time of intubation.

The onset of conditions suitable for tracheal intubation occurs earlier after a conventional intubating dose of succinylcholine than after recommended doses of Mivacurium Chloride.

ADULTS
Initial Doses: Doses of 0.15 mg/kg administered over 5 to 15 seconds, 0.20 mg/kg administered over 30 seconds, or 0.25 mg/kg administered in divided doses (0.15 mg/kg followed in 30 sec by 0.10 mg/kg) are recommended for facilitation of tracheal intubation for most patients (see Table 6). (See related table).

The purpose of slowed or divided dosing of Mivacurium Chloride at doses above 0.15 mg/kg is to minimize the transient decreases in blood pressure observed in some patients given these doses over 5 to 15 seconds (see *"Clinical Pharmacology"*, *"Precautions"*, and *"Adverse Reactions"*). The quality of intubation conditions does not significantly differ for the times and doses of Mivacurium Chloride recommended in Table 6, but the onset of suitable intubation conditions may be reached earlier with higher doses. The choice of a particular dose and regimen should be based on individual circumstances and patient requirements (see *"Individualization of Dosages"* subsection of *"Clinical Pharmacology"*).

In patients with clinically significant cardiovascular disease and in patients with any history suggesting a greater sensitivity to the release of histamine or other mediators (e.g., asthma), the dose of Mivacurium Chloride should be 0.15 mg/kg or less, administered over 60 seconds (see *"Precautions"*). No data are available on the use of doses of Mivacurium Chloride above 0.15 mg/kg in patients with clinically significant kidney or liver disease.

Clinically effective neuromuscular block may be expected to last for 15 to 20 minutes (range: 9 to 38) and spontaneous recovery may be expected to be 95% complete in 25 to 30 minutes (range: 16 to 41) following 0.15 mg/kg Mivacurium Chloride administered to patients receiving opioid/nitrous oxide/oxygen anesthesia. The expected duration of clinically effective block and time to 95% spontaneous recovery following 0.20 mg/kg Mivacurium Chloride are approximately 20 and 30 minutes, respectively, and following 0.25 mg/kg Mivacurium Chloride are approximately 25 and 35 minutes. Initiation of maintenance dosing during opioid nitrous oxide/oxygen anesthesia is generally required approximately 15, 20 and 25 minutes following initial doses of 0.15, 0.20, and 0.25 mg/kg Mivacurium Chloride, respectively (see Table 1). Maintenance doses of 0.10 mg/kg each provide approximately 15 minutes of additional clinically effective block. For shorter or longer durations of action, smaller or larger maintenance doses may be administered.

The neuromuscular blocking action of Mivacurium Chloride is potentiated by isoflurane or enflurane anesthesia. Recommended initial doses of Mivacurium Chloride may be used to facilitate tracheal intubation prior to the administration of these agents; however, if Mivacurium Chloride is first administered after establishment of stable-state isoflurane or enflurane anesthesia (administered with nitrous oxide/oxygen to achieve 1.25 MAC), the initial Mivacurium Chloride dose may be reduced by as much as 25%. Greater reductions in the Mivacurium Chloride dose may be required with higher concentrations of enflurane or isoflurane. With halothane, which has only a minimal potentiating effect on Mivacurium Chloride, a smaller dosage reduction may be considered.

Continuous Infusion: Continuous infusion of Mivacurium Chloride may be used to maintain neuromuscular block. Upon early evidence of spontaneous recovery from an initial dose, an initial infusion rate of 9 to 10 µg/kg/min is recommended. If continuous infusion is initiated simultaneously with the administration of an initial dose, a lower initial infusion rate should be used (e.g., 4 µg/kg/min). In either case, the initial infusion rate should be adjusted according to the response to peripheral nerve stimulation and to clinical criteria. On average, an infusion rate of 6 to 7 µg/kg/min (range: 1 to 15) may be expected to maintain neuromuscular block within the range of 89% to 99% for extended periods in adults receiving opioid/nitrous oxide/oxygen anesthesia. Reduction of the infusion rate by up to 35% to 40% should be considered when Mivacurium Chloride is administered during stable-state conditions of isoflurane or enflurane anesthesia (administered with nitrous oxide/oxygen to achieve 1.25 MAC). Greater reductions in the Mivacurium Chloride infusion rate may be required with greater concentrations of enflurane or isoflurane. With halothane, smaller reductions in infusion rate may be required.

CHILDREN

Initial Doses: Dosage requirements for Mivacurium Chloride on a mg/kg basis are higher in children than adults. Onset and recovery of neuromuscular block occur more rapidly in children than adults (see "Clinical Pharmacology").

The recommended dose of Mivacurium Chloride for facilitating tracheal intubation in children 2 to 12 years of age is 0.20 mg/kg administered over 5 to 15 seconds. When administered during stable opioid nitrous oxide/oxygen anesthesia, 0.20 mg/kg of Mivacurium Chloride produces maximum neuromuscular block in an average of 1.9 minutes (range: 1.3 to 3.3) and clinically effective block for 10 minutes (range: 6 to 15). Maintenance doses are generally required more frequently in children than in adults. Administration of Mivacurium Chloride doses above the recommended range (> 0.20 mg/kg) is associated with transient decreases in MAP in some children (see "Hemodynamics" subsection of "Clinical Pharmacology").

Mivacurium Chloride has not been studied in children below the age of 2 years.

Continuous Infusion: Children require higher Mivacurium Chloride infusion rates than adults. During opioid/nitrous oxide/oxygen anesthesia the infusion rate required to maintain 89% to 99% neuromuscular block averages 14 µg/kg/min (range: 5 to 31). The principles for infusion of Mivacurium Chloride in adults are also applicable to children (see above).

INFUSION RATE TABLES

For adults and children the amount of infusion solution required per hour depends upon the clinical requirements of the patient, the concentration of Mivacurium Chloride in the infusion solution, and the patient's weight. The contribution of the infusion solution to the fluid requirements of the patient must be considered. Tables 7 and 8 provide guidelines for delivery in mL/hr (equivalent to microdrops/min when 60 microdrops = 1 mL) of Mivacurium Chloride Premixed Infusion (0.5 mg/mL) and of Mivacurium Chloride Injection (2 mg/mL). (See related table).

MIVACURIUM CHLORIDE PREMIXED INFUSION IN FLEXIBLE PLASTIC CONTAINERS

The flexible plastic container is fabricated from a specially formulated, nonplasticized, thermoplastic co-polyester (CR3). Water can permeate from inside the container into the overwrap but not in amounts sufficient to affect the solution significantly. Solutions inside the plastic container also can leach out certain of the chemical components in very small amounts before the expiration period is attained. However, the safety of the plastic has been confirmed by tests in animals according to USP biological standards for plastic containers.

INSTRUCTIONS FOR USE

1. Tear outer wrap at notch and remove solution container. Check for minute leaks by squeezing container firmly. If leaks are found, discard solution as sterility may be impaired.
2. Close flow control clamp of administration set.
3. Remove cover from outlet port at bottom of container.
4. Insert piercing pin of administration set into port with a twisting motion until the pin is firmly seated. *Note:* See full directions on administration set carton.
5. Suspend container from hanger.
6. Squeeze and release drip chamber to establish proper fluid level in chamber during infusion.
7. Open flow control clamp to expel air from set. Close clamp.
8. Attach set to intravenous tubing.
9. Regulate rate of administration with flow control clamp.

Additives should not be introduced into this solution. Do not administer unless solution is clear and container is undamaged. Mivacurium Chloride Premixed Infusion is intended for single patient use only. The unused portion of the solution should be discarded.

Warning: Do not use flexible plastic container in series connections.
Mivacurium Chloride Injection Compatibility and Admixtures:

Y-site Administration: Mivacurium Chloride Injection may not be compatible with alkaline solutions having a pH greater than 8.5 (e.g., barbiturate solutions).

Studies have shown that Mivacurium Chloride Injection is compatible with:

- 5% Dextrose Injection USP
- 0.9% Sodium Chloride Injection USP
- 5% Dextrose and 0.9% Sodium Chloride Injection USP
- Lactated Ringer's Injection USP
- 5% Dextrose in Lactated Ringer's Injection
- Sufentanil citrate Injection, diluted as directed
- Alfentanil hydrochloride injection, diluted as directed
- Fentanyl citrate injection, diluted as directed
- Midazolam hydrochloride injection, diluted as directed
- Droperidol Injection, diluted as directed

Compatibility studies with other parenteral products have not been conducted.

Dilution Stability: Mivacurium Chloride Injection diluted to 0.5 mg Mivacurium per mL in 5% Dextrose Injection USP, 5% Dextrose and 0.9% Sodium Chloride Injection USP, 0.9% Sodium Chloride Injection USP, Lactated Ringer's Injection USP, or 5% Dextrose in Lactated Ringer's Injection is physically and chemically stable when stored in PVC (polyvinyl chloride) bags at 5° to 25°C (41° to 77°F) for up to 24 hours. Aseptic techniques should be used to prepare the diluted product. Admixtures of Mivacurium Chloride should be prepared for single patient use only and used within 24 hours of preparation. The unused portion of diluted Mivacurium Chloride should be discarded after each case.

Note: Parenteral drug products should be inspected visually for particulate matter and discoloration prior to administration whenever solution and container permit. Solutions which are not clear and colorless should not be used.

Table 6
RECOMMENDED INITIAL DOSING REGIMENS FOR ADULTS

Dosing Paradigm[a]	Anesthetic Induction Technique Studied	Time to Generally Good-to-Excellent Intubating Conditions
0.15 mg/kg, IV (over 5 to 15 sec)	Thiopental/opioid/ N2O/ O2 or propofol/opioid	2.5 to 3 min after completion of dose
0.20 mg/kg, IV (over 30 sec)	Thiopental/opioid/ N2O/ O2 or propofol/opioid	2 to 2.5 min after completion of dose
0.25 mg/kg, IV (0.15 mg/kg followed in 30 sec by 0.10 mg/kg)	Propofol/opioid	1.5 to 2 min after completion of 0.15 mg/kg dose

[a] *Dosing instituted after induction of adequate general anesthesia.*

Table 7
INFUSION RATES FOR MAINTENANCE OF NEUROMUSCULAR BLOCK DURING OPIOID/NITROUS OXIDE/OXYGEN ANESTHESIA USING MIVACURIUM CHLORIDE PREMIXED INFUSION (0.5 MG/ML)

Patient Weight (kg)	Drug Delivery Rate (µg/kg/min)									
	4	5	6	7	8	10	14	16	18	20
	Infusion Delivery Rate (mL/hr)									
10	5	6	7	8	10	12	17	19	22	24
15	7	9	11	13	14	18	25	29	32	36
20	10	12	15	17	19	24	34	38	43	48
25	12	15	18	21	24	30	42	48	54	60
35	17	21	26	29	34	42	59	67	76	84
50	24	30	36	42	48	60	84	96	108	120
60	29	36	43	50	58	72	101	115	130	144
70	34	42	50	59	67	84	118	134	151	168
80	39	48	58	67	77	96	134	154	173	192
90	44	54	65	76	86	108	151	173	194	216
100	48	60	72	84	96	120	168	192	216	240

◆ RATED THERAPEUTICALLY EQUIVALENT; ◇ THERAPEUTIC EQUIVALENCE UNCONFIRMED; ○ UNRATED

Table 8
INFUSION RATES FOR MAINTENANCE OF NEUROMUSCULAR BLOCK DURING OPIOID/NITROUS OXIDE/OXYGEN ANESTHESIA USING MIVACURIUM CHLORIDE INJECTION (2 MG/ML)

Patient Weight (kg)	Drug Delivery Rate (µg/kg/min)									
	4	5	6	7	8	10	14	16	18	20
	Infusion Delivery Rate (mL/hr)									
10	1.2	1.5	1.8	2.1	2.4	3.0	4.2	4.8	5.4	6.0
15	1.8	2.3	2.7	3.2	3.6	4.5	6.3	7.2	8.1	9.0
20	2.4	3.0	3.6	4.2	4.8	6.0	8.4	9.6	10.8	12.0
25	3.0	3.8	4.5	5.3	6.0	7.5	10.5	12.0	13.5	15.0
35	4.2	5.3	6.3	7.4	8.4	10.5	14.7	16.8	18.9	21.0
50	6.0	7.5	9.0	10.5	12.0	15.0	21.0	24.0	27.0	30.0
60	7.2	9.0	10.8	12.6	14.4	18.0	25.2	28.8	32.4	36.0
70	8.4	10.5	12.6	14.7	16.8	21.0	29.4	33.6	37.8	42.0
80	9.6	12.0	14.4	16.8	19.2	24.0	33.6	38.4	43.2	48.0
90	10.8	13.5	16.2	18.9	21.6	27.0	37.8	43.2	48.6	54.0
100	12.0	15.0	18.0	21.0	24.0	30.0	42.0	48.0	54.0	60.0

STORAGE

Store Mivacurium Chloride Injection at room temperature of 15° to 25°C (59° to 77°F). Avoid exposure to direct ultraviolet light. DO NOT FREEZE.

Recommended storage for Mivacurium Chloride Premixed Infusion is room temperature (15° to 25°C/59° to 77°F). Avoid excessive heat. Avoid exposure to direct ultraviolet light. Protect from freezing.

HOW SUPPLIED
INJECTION: 0.5 MG/ML

BRAND/MANUFACTURER	NDC	SIZE	AWP
○ **BRAND**			
MIVACRON: Burr Wellcome	00081-0709-01	50 ml 24s	$360.00
	00081-0709-02	100 ml 24s	$633.60

INJECTION: 2 MG/ML

BRAND/MANUFACTURER	NDC	SIZE	AWP
○ **BRAND**			
MIVACRON: Burr Wellcome	00081-0705-02	50 ml	$50.40
	00081-0705-44	5 ml 10s	$96.00
	00081-0705-95	10 ml 10s	$150.00
	00081-0705-01	20 ml 10s	$252.00

M-M-R II *SEE* MEASLES/MUMPS/RUBELLA VIRUS VACCINE LIVE

Moban *SEE* MOLINDONE HYDROCHLORIDE

Moctanin *SEE* MONOCTANOIN

Modicon *SEE* ETHINYL ESTRADIOL AND NORETHINDRONE

Moduretic 5-50 *SEE* AMILORIDE HYDROCHLORIDE WITH HYDROCHLOROTHIAZIDE

Molindone Hydrochloride

DESCRIPTION

Molindone Hydrochloride is a dihydroindolone compound which is not structurally related to the phenothiazines, the butyrophenones or the thioxanthenes.

Molindone Hydrochloride is 3-ethyl-6, 7-dihydro-2-methyl-5-(morpholinomethyl) indol-4 (5H)-one Hydrochloride. It is a white to off-white crystalline powder, freely soluble in water and alcohol and has a molecular weight of 312.67.

Molindone Hydrochloride in available in 5 mg, 10 mg, 25 mg, 50 mg, and 100 mg tablets for oral administration. It is also available in concentrate form.

Following is its chemical structure:

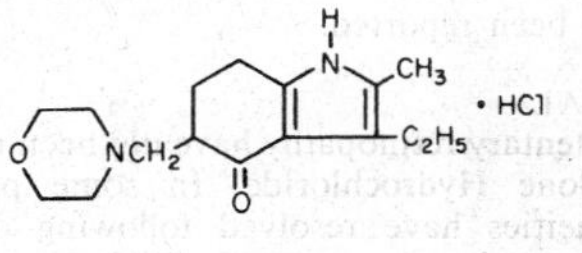

ACTIONS

Molidone Hydrochloride has a pharmacological profile in laboratory animals which predominantly resembles that of major tranquilizers causing reduction of spontaneous locomotion and aggressiveness, suppression of a conditioned response and antagonism of the bizarre stereotyped behavior and hyperactivity induced by amphetamines. In addition, Molidone Hydrochloride antagonizes the depression caused by the tranquilizing agent tetrabenazine.

In human clinical studies tranquilization is achieved in the absence of muscle relaxing or incoordinating effects. Based on EEG studies, Molidone Hydrochloride exerts its effect on the ascending reticular activating system.

Human metabolic studies show Molidone Hydrochloride to be rapidly absorbed and metabolized when given orally. Unmetabolized drug reached a peak blood level at 1.5 hours. Pharmacological effect from a single oral dose persists for 24-36 hours. There are 36 recognized metabolites with less than 2-3% unmetabolized Molidone Hydrochloride being excreted in urine and feces.

INDICATIONS

Molindone Hydrochloride is indicated for the management of the manifestations of psychotic disorders. The antipsychotic efficacy of Molindone Hydrochloride was established in clinical studies which enrolled newly hospitalized and chronically hospitalized, acutely ill, schizophrenic patients as subjects.

UNLABELED USES
Molindone is used alone or as an adjunct in the treatment of anxiety associated with premenstrual tension.

CONTRAINDICATIONS

Molindone Hydrochloride is contraindicated in severe central nervous system depression (alcohol, barbiturates, narcotics, etc.) or comatose states, and in patients with known hypersensitivity to the drug.

WARNINGS

TARDIVE DYSKINESIA
Tardive dyskinesia, a syndrome consisting of potentially irreversible, involuntary, dyskinetic movements may develop in patients treated with neuroleptic (antipsychotic) drugs. Although the prevalence of the syndrome appears to be highest among the elderly, especially elderly women, it is impossible to rely upon prevalence estimates to predict, at the inception of neuroleptic treatment, which patients are likely to develop the syndrome. Whether neuroleptic drug products differ in their potential to cause tardive dyskinesia is unknown.

Both the risk of developing the syndrome and the likelihood that it will become irreversible are believed to increase as the duration of treatment and the total cumulative dose of neuroleptic drugs administered to the patient increase. However, the syndrome can develop, although much less commonly, after relatively brief treatment periods at low doses. There is no known treatment for established cases of tardive dyskinesia, although the syndrome may remit, partially or completely, if neuroleptic treatment is withdrawn. Neuroleptic treatment, itself, however, may suppress (or partially suppress) the signs and symptoms of the syndrome and thereby may possibly mask the underlying disease process. The effect that symptomatic suppression has upon the long-term course of the syndrome is unknown.

Given these considerations, neuroleptics should be prescribed in a manner that is most likely to minimize the occurrence of tardive dyskinesia. Chronic neuroleptic treatment should generally be reserved for patients who suffer from a chronic illness that, 1) is known to respond to neuroleptic drugs, and 2) for whom alternative, equally effective, but potentially less harmful treatments are *not* available or appropriate. In patients who do require chronic treatment, the smallest dose and the shortest duration of treatment producing a satisfactory clinical response should be sought. The need for continued treatment should be reassessed periodically.

If signs and symptoms of tardive dyskinesia appear in a patient on neuroleptics, drug discontinuation should be considered. However, some patients may require treatment despite the presence of the syndrome.

(For further information about the description of tardive dyskinesia and its clinical detection, please refer to the section on *"Adverse Reactions"*).

NEUROLEPTIC MALIGNANT SYNDROME (NMS)

A potentially fatal symptom complex sometimes referred to as Neuroleptic Malignant Syndrome (NMS) has been reported in association with antipsychotic drugs. Clinical manifestations of NMS are hyperpyrexia, muscle rigidity, altered mental status and evidence of autonomic instability (irregular pulse or blood pressure, tachycardia, diaphoresis, and cardiac dysrhythmias).

The diagnostic evaluation of patients with this syndrome is complicated. In arriving at a diagnosis, it is important to identify cases where the clinical presentation includes both serious medical illness (e.g., pneumonia, systemic infection, etc.) and untreated or inadequately treated extrapyramidal signs and symptoms (EPS). Other important considerations in the differential diagnosis include central anticholinergic toxicity, heat stroke, drug fever and primary central nervous system (CNS) pathology.

The management of NMS should include: 1) immediate discontinuation of antipsychotic drugs and other drugs not essential to concurrent therapy, 2) intensive symptomatic treatment and medical monitoring, and 3) treatment of any concomitant serious medical problems for which specific treatments are available. There is no general agreement about specific pharmacological treatment regimens for uncomplicated NMS.

If a patient requires antipsychotic drug treatment after recovery from NMS, the potential reintroduction of drug therapy should be carefully considered. The patient should be carefully monitored, since recurrences of NMS have been reported.

Usage in Pregnancy: Studies in pregnant patients have not been carried out. Reproduction studies have been performed in the following animals:

Pregnant Rats Oral Dose:
no adverse effect   20 mg/kg/day-10 days
no adverse effect   40 mg/kg/day-10 days

Pregnant Mice Oral Dose:
slight increase resorptions   20 mg/kg/day-10 days
slight increase resorptions   40 mg/kg/day-10 days

Pregnant Rabbits Oral Dose:
no adverse effect   5 mg/kg/day-12 days
no adverse effect   10 mg/kg/day-12 days
no adverse effect   20 mg/kg/day-12 days

Animal reproductive studies have not demonstrated a teratogenic potential. The anticipated benefits must be weighed against the unknown risks to the fetus if used in pregnant patients.

Nursing Mothers: Data are not available on the content of Molindone Hydrochloride in the milk of nursing mothers.

Usage in Children: Use of Molindone Hydrochloride in children below the age of twelve years is not recommended because safe and effective conditions for its usage have not been established.

Molindone Hydrochloride has not been shown effective in the management of behavioral complications in patients with mental retardation.

Sulfite Sensitivity: Molindone Hydrochloride Concentrate contains sodium metabisulfite, a sulfite that may cause allergic-type reactions including anaphylactic symptoms and life-threatening or less severe asthmatic episodes in certain susceptible people. The overall prevalence of sulfite sensitivity in the general population is unknown and probably low. Sulfite sensitivity is seen more frequently in asthmatic than in nonasthmatic people.

PRECAUTIONS

Some patients receiving Molindone Hydrochloride may note drowsiness initially and they should be advised against activities requiring mental alertness until their response to the drug has been established.

Increased activity has been noted in patients receiving Molindone Hydrochloride. Caution should be exercised where increased activity may be harmful.

Molindone Hydrochloride does not lower the seizure threshold in experimental animals to the degree noted with more sedating antipsychotic drugs. However, in humans convulsive seizures have been reported in a few instances.

The physician should be aware that certain brands of Molindone Hydrochloride contain calcium sulfate as an excipient and that calcium ions may interfere with the absorption of preparations containing phenytoin sodium and tetracyclines.

Molindone Hydrochloride has an antiemetic effect in animals. A similar effect may occur in humans and may obscure signs of intestinal obstruction or brain tumor.

Neuroleptic drugs elevate prolactin levels; the elevation persists during chronic administration. Tissue culture experiments indicate that approximately one-third of human breast cancers are prolactin dependent *in vitro*, a factor of potential importance if the prescription of these drugs is contemplated in a patient with a previously detected breast cancer. Although disturbances such as galactorrhea, amenorrhea, gynecomastia, and impotence have been reported, the clinical significance of elevated serum prolactin levels is unknown for most patients. An increase in mammary neoplasms has been found in rodents after chronic administration of neuroleptic drugs. Neither clinical studies nor epidemiologic studies conducted to date, however, have shown an association between chronic administration of these drugs and mammary tumorigenesis; the available evidence is considered too limited to be conclusive at this time.

ADVERSE REACTIONS

CNS EFFECTS

The most frequently occurring effect is initial drowsiness that generally subsides with continued usage of the drug or lowering of the dose.

Noted less frequently were depression, hyperactivity and euphoria.

NEUROLOGICAL EXTRAPYRAMIDAL REACTIONS

Extrapyramidal reactions noted below may occur in susceptible individuals and are usually reversible with appropriate management.

AKATHISIA

Motor restlessness may occur early.

PARKINSON SYNDROME

Akinesia, characterized by rigidity, immobility and reduction of voluntary movements and tremor, have been observed. Occurrence is less frequent than akathisia.

DYSTONIC SYNDROME

Prolonged abnormal contractions of muscle groups occur infrequently. These symptoms may be managed by the addition of a synthetic antiparkinson agent (other than L-dopa), small doses of sedative drugs, and/or reduction in dosage.

TARDIVE DYSKINESIA

Neuroleptic drugs are known to cause a syndrome of dyskinetic movements commonly referred to as tardive dyskinesia. The movements may appear during treatment or upon withdrawal of treatment and may be either reversible or irreversible (i.e., persistent) upon cessation of further neuroleptic administration.

The syndrome is known to have a variable latency for development and the duration of the latency cannot be determined reliably. It is thus wise to assume that any neuroleptic agent has the capacity to induce the syndrome and act accordingly until sufficient data has been collected to settle the issue definitively for a specific drug product. In the case of neuroleptics known to produce the irreversible syndrome, the following has been observed:

Tardive dyskinesia has appeared in some patients on long-term therapy and has also appeared after drug therapy has been discontinued. The risk appears to be greater in elderly patients on high-dose therapy, especially females. The symptoms are persistent and in some patients appear to be irreversible. The syndrome is characterized by rhythmical involuntary movements of the tongue, face, mouth or jaw (e.g., protrusion of tongue, puffing of cheeks, puckering of mouth, chewing movements). There may be involuntary movements of extremities.

There is no known treatment of tardive dyskinesia; antiparkinsonism agents usually do not alleviate the symptoms of this syndrome. It is suggested that all antipsychotic agents be discontinued if these symptoms appear. Should it be necessary to reinstitute treatment, or increase the dosage of the agent, or switch to a different antipsychotic agent, the syndrome may be masked. It has been reported that fine vermicular movements of the tongue may be an early sign of the syndrome and if the mechanism is stopped at that time the syndrome may not develop (see *"Warnings"*).

AUTONOMIC NERVOUS SYSTEM

Occasionally blurring of vision, tachycardia, nausea, dry mouth and salivation have been reported. Urinary retention and constipation may occur particularly if anticholinergic drugs are used to treat extrapyramidal symptoms. One patient being treated with Molindone Hydrochloride experienced priapism which required surgical intervention, apparently resulting in residual impairment of erectile function.

LABORATORY TESTS

There have been rare reports of leucopenia and leucocytosis. If such reactions occur, treatment with Molindone Hydrochloride may continue if clinical symptoms are absent. Alterations of blood glucose, B.U.N., and red blood cells have not been considered clinically significant.

METABOLIC AND ENDOCRINE EFFECTS

Alteration of thyroid function has not been significant. Amenorrhea has been reported infrequently. Resumption of menses in previously amenorrheic women has been reported. Initially heavy menses may occur. Galactorrhea and gynecomastia have been reported infrequently. Increase in libido has been noted in some patients. Impotence has not been reported. Although both weight gain and weight loss have been in the direction of normal or ideal weight, excessive weight gain has not occurred with Molindone Hydrochloride.

HEPATIC EFFECTS

There have been rare reports of clinically significant alternations in liver function in association with Molindone Hydrochloride use.

CARDIOVASCULAR

Rare, transient, non-specific T wave changes have been reported on E.K.G. Association with a clinical syndrome has not been established. Rarely has significant hypotension been reported.

OPHTHALMOLOGICAL

Lens opacities and pigmentary retinopathy have not been reported where patients have received Molindone Hydrochloride. In some patients, phenothiazine induced lenticular opacities have resolved following discontinuation of the phenothiazine while continuing therapy with Molindone Hydrochloride.

◆ RATED THERAPEUTICALLY EQUIVALENT; ◇ THERAPEUTIC EQUIVALENCE UNCONFIRMED; ○ UNRATED

SKIN

Early, non-specific skin rash, probably of allergic origin, has occasionally been reported. Skin pigmentation has not been seen with Molindone Hydrochloride usage alone.

Molindone Hydrochloride has certain pharmacological similarities to other antipsychotic agents. Because adverse reactions are often extensions of the pharmacological activity of drug, all of the known pharmacological effects associated with other antipsychotic drugs should be kept in mind when Molindone Hydrochloride is used. Upon abrupt withdrawal after prolonged high dosage an abstinence syndrome has not been noted.

DRUG INTERACTIONS

Potentiation of drugs administered concurrently with Molindone Hydrochloride has not been reported. Additionally, animal studies have not shown increased toxicity when Molindone Hydrochloride is given concurrently with representative members of three classes of drugs (i.e., barbiturates, chloral hydrate and antiparkinson drugs).

MANAGEMENT OF OVERDOSAGE

Symptomatic, supportive therapy should be the rule. Gastric lavage is indicated for the reduction of absorption of Molindone Hydrochloride which is freely soluble in water.

Since the adsorption of Molindone Hydrochloride in activated charcoal has not been determined, the use of this antidote must be considered of theoretical value.

Emesis in a comatose patient is contraindicated. Additionally, while the emetic effect of apomorphine is blocked by Molindone Hydrochloride in animals, this blocking effect has not been determined in humans.

A significant increase in the rate of removal of unmetabolized Molindone Hydrochloride from the body by forced diuresis, peritoneal or renal dialysis would not be expected. (Only 2% of a single ingested dose of Molindone Hydrochloride is excreted unmetabolized in the urine). However, poor response of the patient may justify use of these procedures.

While the use of laxatives or enemas might be based on general principles, the amount of unmetabolized Molindone Hydrochloride in feces is less than 1%. Extrapyramidal symptoms have responded to the use of diphenhydramine, Amantadine HCl and the synthetic anticholinergic antiparkinson agents, (i.e., Artane, Cogentin, Akineton).

DOSAGE AND ADMINISTRATION

Initial and maintenance doses of Molindone Hydrochloride should be individualized.

INITIAL DOSAGE SCHEDULE
The usual starting dosage is 50-75 mg/day.
—Increase to 100 mg/day in 3 or 4 days.
—Based on severity of symptomatology, dosage may be titrated up or down depending on individual patient response.
—An increase to 225 mg/day may be required in patients with severe symptomatology.
Elderly and debilitated patients should be started on lower dosage.

MAINTENANCE DOSAGE SCHEDULE
1. Mid: 5 mg—15 mg three or four times a day.
2. Moderate: 10 mg—25 mg three or four times a day.
3. Severe: 225 mg/day may be required.

Store concentrate at controlled room temperature (59°-86°F, 15°-30° C). Protect from light.

HOW SUPPLIED
CONCENTRATE: 20 MG/ML

BRAND/MANUFACTURER	NDC	SIZE	AWP
○ BRAND MOBAN: Gate	57844-0920-12	120 ml	$110.09

TABLETS: 5 MG

BRAND/MANUFACTURER	NDC	SIZE	AWP
○ BRAND MOBAN: Gate	57844-0914-01	100s	$51.88

TABLETS: 10 MG

BRAND/MANUFACTURER	NDC	SIZE	AWP
○ BRAND MOBAN: Gate	57844-0915-01	100s	$74.53

TABLETS: 25 MG

BRAND/MANUFACTURER	NDC	SIZE	AWP
○ BRAND MOBAN: Gate	57844-0916-01	100s	$111.17

TABLETS: 50 MG

BRAND/MANUFACTURER	NDC	SIZE	AWP
○ BRAND MOBAN: Gate	57844-0917-01	100s	$148.46

TABLETS: 100 MG

BRAND/MANUFACTURER	NDC	SIZE	AWP
○ BRAND MOBAN: Gate	57844-0918-01	100s	$198.33

Molypen SEE AMMONIUM MOLYBDATE

Mometasone Furoate

DESCRIPTION
Mometasone Furoate products contain Mometasone Furoate for dermatologic use. Mometasone Furoate is a synthetic corticosteroid with anti-inflammatory activity.

Chemically, Mometasone Furoate is 9α,21-Dichloro-11β,17-dihydroxy-16α-methylpregna-1,4-diene- 3,20-dione 17-(2-furoate), with the empirical formula $C_{27}H_{30}Cl_2O_6$ and a molecular weight of 521.4.

Mometasone Furoate is a white to off-white powder practically insoluble in water, slightly soluble in octanol, and moderately soluble in ethyl alcohol. Each gram of Mometasone Furoate Cream 0.1% contains: 1 mg Mometasone Furoate in a cream base of hexylene glycol, phosphoric acid, propylene glycol stearate, stearyl alcohol and ceteareth-20, titanium dioxide, aluminum starch octenylsuccinate, white wax, white petrolatum and purified water. Each gram of Mometasone Furoate Ointment 0.1% contains: 1 mg Mometasone Furoate in an ointment base of hexylene glycol, propylene glycol stearate, white wax, white petrolatum and purified water. May also contain phosphoric acid. Each gram of Mometasone Furoate Lotion 0.1% contains: 1 mg of Mometasone Furoate in a lotion base of isopropyl alcohol (40%), propylene glycol, hydroxypropylcellulose, sodium phosphate and water. May also contain phosphoric acid and sodium hydroxide used to adjust the pH to approximately 4.5.

Following is its chemical structure:

CLINICAL PHARMACOLOGY
The corticosteroids are a class of compounds comprising steroid hormones secreted by the adrenal cortex and their synthetic analogs. In pharmacologic doses corticosteroids are used primarily for their anti-inflammatory and/or immunosuppressive effects. Topical corticosteroids, such as Mometasone Furoate, are effective in the treatment of corticosteroid-responsive dermatoses primarily because of their anti-inflammatory, anti-pruritic, and vasoconstrictive actions. However, while the physiologic, pharmacologic, and clinical effects of the corticosteroids are well known, the exact mechanisms of their actions in each disease are uncertain. Mometasone Furoate has been shown to have topical (dermatologic) and systemic pharmacologic and metabolic effects characteristic of this class of drugs.

Pharmacokinetics: The extent of percutaneous absorption of topical corticosteroids is determined by many factors including the vehicle, the integrity of the epidermal barrier, and the use of occlusive dressings. (See *"Dosage and Administration"*.) Topical corticosteroids can be absorbed from normal intact skin.

The percutaneous absorption of ^{3}H-Mometasone Furoate was evaluated in rabbits following topical application of both cream (0.1%) and ointment (0.1%) formulations. Approximately 5% of the topically applied dose was systemically absorbed following topical application of the cream and 6% following application of the ointment formulation. Based upon these results, it was concluded that Mometasone Furoate is absorbed to a similar extent following application of either the cream or ointment formulations. Percutaneous absorption studies of ^{3}H-Mometasone Furoate ointment in rats and dogs have shown that approximately 2.5% of a topically applied dose was absorbed by rats and 2% by dogs.

The percutaneous absorption of ^{3}H-Mometasone Furoate was also studied in man following topical application of an ointment (0.1%) formulation. Results showed that only about 0.7% of the steroid was systemically absorbed following 8 hours of contact without occlusion. Minimal absorption would be anticipated with the cream and lotion formulations.

Inflammation and/or other disease processes in the skin increase percutaneous absorption. Occlusive dressings substantially increase the percutaneous absorption of topical corticosteroids. (See *"Dosage and Administration"*.)

In studies of the effects of Mometasone Furoate on the hypothalamic-pituitary-adrenal (HPA) axis (one with the cream and one with the ointment), 15 grams was applied twice daily for seven days to six patients with psoriasis or atopic dermatitis. The cream or ointment was applied without occlusion to at least 30% of the body surface. The results suggest that the drug caused a slight lowering of adrenal corticosteroid secretion, although in no case did plasma cortisol levels go below the lower limit of the normal range.

➤ SHOWN IN PRODUCT IDENTIFICATION GUIDE

Mometasone Furoate lotion was applied at 15 mL twice daily (30 mL per day) to diseased skin (patients with scalp and body psoriasis) of four patients for seven days, to study its effects on the hypothalamic-pituitary-adrenal (HPA) axis. Plasma cortisol levels for each of the four patients remained well within the normal range and changed little from baseline.

Once absorbed through the skin, topical corticosteroids are handled through pharmacokinetic pathways similar to systemically administered corticosteroids. Corticosteroids are bound to plasma proteins in varying degrees. Corticosteroids are metabolized primarily in the liver and are then excreted by the kidneys. Some of the topical corticosteroids and their metabolites are also excreted into the bile.

INDICATIONS AND USAGE
Mometasone Furoate products are indicated for the relief of the inflammatory and pruritic manifestations of corticosteroid-responsive dermatoses.

CONTRAINDICATIONS
Mometasone Furoate products are contraindicated in patients who are hypersensitive to Mometasone Furoate, to other corticosteroids, or to any ingredient in these preparations.

PRECAUTIONS
General: Systemic absorption of potent topical corticosteroids has produced reversible hypothalamic-pituitary-adrenal (HPA) axis suppression, manifestations of Cushing's syndrome, hyperglycemia, and glucosuria in some patients. Conditions which augment systemic absorption include application of steroids in optimized vehicles, application of more potent steroids, use over large surface areas, prolonged use, use in areas where the epidermal barrier is disrupted, and the use of occlusive dressings. (See *"Dosage and Administration"*.)

Patients receiving a large dose of a potent topical steroid applied to a large surface area or under an occlusive dressing should be evaluated periodically for evidence of HPA axis suppression by using the urinary free cortisol and ACTH stimulation tests. If HPA axis suppression is noted, an attempt should be made to withdraw the drug, to reduce the frequency of application, or to substitute a less potent steroid.

Recovery of HPA axis function is generally prompt and complete upon discontinuation of the drug. Infrequently, signs and symptoms of steroid withdrawal may occur, requiring supplemental systemic corticosteroids.

Children may absorb proportionally larger amounts of topical corticosteroids and thus be more susceptible to systemic toxicity. (See *"Precautions—Pediatric Use."*) If irritation develops, topical corticosteroids should be discontinued and appropriate therapy instituted.

In the presence of dermatological infections, use of an appropriate antifungal or antibacterial agent should be instituted. If a favorable response does not occur promptly, the corticosteroid should be discontinued until the infection has been adequately controlled.

Information for Patients: Patients using topical corticosteroids should receive the following information and instructions. This information is intended to aid in the safe and effective use of this medication. It is not a disclosure of all possible adverse or intended effects.

1. This medication is to be used as directed by the physician. It is for external use only. Avoid contact with the eyes.

2. Patients should be advised not to use this medication for any disorder other than that for which it was prescribed.

3. The treated skin area should not be bandaged or otherwise covered or wrapped so as to be occlusive unless directed by the physician. (See *"Dosage and Administration"*.)

4. Patients should report any signs of local adverse reactions.

5. Parents of pediatric patients should be advised not to use tight-fitting diapers or plastic pants on a child being treated in the diaper area, as these garments may constitute occlusive dressing. (See *"Dosage and Administration"*.)

Laboratory Tests: The following tests may be helpful in evaluating HPA axis suppression:
Urinary free cortisol test
ACTH stimulation test

Carcinogenesis, Mutagenesis, and Impairment of Fertility: Long-term animal studies have not been performed to evaluate the carcinogenic potential or the effect on fertility of topical corticosteroids.

Genetic toxicity studies with Mometasone Furoate, which included the Ames test, mouse lymphoma assay, and a micronucleus test, did not reveal any mutagenic potential.

Pregnancy Category C: Corticosteroids are generally teratogenic in laboratory animals when administered systemically at relatively low dosage levels. Corticosteroids have been shown to be teratogenic after dermal application in laboratory animals. There are no adequate and well-controlled studies of teratogenic effects from topically applied corticosteroids in pregnant women. Therefore, topical corticosteroids should be used during pregnancy only if the potential benefit justifies the potential risk to the fetus. Drugs of this class should not be used extensively on pregnant patients, in large amounts, or for prolonged periods.

Nursing Mothers: It is not known whether topical administration of corticosteroids could result in sufficient systemic absorption to produce detectable quantities in breast milk. Systemically administered corticosteroids are secreted into breast milk in quantities not likely to have a deleterious effect on the infant. Nevertheless, a decision should be made whether to discontinue nursing or to discontinue the drug taking into account the importance of the drug to the mother.

Pediatric Use: Pediatric patients may demonstrate greater susceptibility to topical corticosteroid-induced HPA axis suppression and Cushing's syndrome than mature patients because of a larger skin surface area to body weight ratio.

Hypothalamic-pituitary-adrenal (HPA) axis suppression, Cushing's syndrome, and intracranial hypertension have been reported in children receiving topical corticosteroids. Manifestations of adrenal suppression in children include linear growth retardation, delayed weight gain, low plasma cortisol levels, and absence of response to ACTH stimulation. Manifestations of intracranial hypertension include bulging fontanelles, headaches, and bilateral papilledema.

Administration of topical corticosteroids to children should be limited to the least amount compatible with an effective therapeutic regimen. Chronic corticosteroid therapy may interfere with the growth and development of children.

ADVERSE REACTIONS
The following local adverse reactions were reported with Mometasone Furoate **Cream** during clinical studies with 319 patients: burning, 1; pruritus, 1; and signs of skin atrophy, 3.

The following local adverse reactions were reported with Mometasone Furoate **Ointment** during clinical studies with 812 patients: burning, 13; pruritus, 8; skin atrophy, 8; tingling/stinging, 7; and furunculosis, 3.

The following local adverse reactions were reported with Mometasone Furoate **Lotion** during clinical studies with 209 patients: acneiform reaction, 2; burning, 4; and itching, 1. In an irritation/sensitization study with 156 normal subjects, folliculitis was reported in 4.

The following local adverse reactions have been reported infrequently when other topical dermatologic corticosteroids have been used as recommended. These reactions are listed in an approximate decreasing order of occurrence; burning, itching, irritation, dryness, folliculitis, hypertrichosis, acneiform eruptions, hypopigmentation, perioral dermatitis, allergic contact dermatitis, maceration of the skin, secondary infection, skin atrophy, striae, miliaria.

OVERDOSAGE
Topically applied corticosteroids can be absorbed in sufficient amounts to produce systemic effects. (See *"Precautions"*.)

DOSAGE AND ADMINISTRATION
Apply a thin film of Mometasone Furoate **Cream** or **Ointment** to the affected skin areas once daily. Do not use occlusive dressings. Apply a few drops of Mometasone Furoate **Lotion** to the affected areas once daily and massage lightly until it disappears. For the most effective and economical use, hold the nozzle of the bottle very close to the affected areas and gently squeeze.

Store Mometasone Furoate between 2° and 30°C (36° and 86°F).

HOW SUPPLIED
CREAM: 0.1%

BRAND/MANUFACTURER	NDC	SIZE	AWP
○ **BRAND**			
ELOCON: Schering	00085-0567-01	15 gm	$14.05
	00085-0567-02	45 gm	$25.74

LOTION: 0.1%

BRAND/MANUFACTURER	NDC	SIZE	AWP
○ **BRAND**			
ELOCON: Schering	00085-0854-01	30 ml	$15.23
	00085-0854-02	60 ml	$29.06

OINTMENT: 0.1%

BRAND/MANUFACTURER	NDC	SIZE	AWP
○ **BRAND**			
ELOCON: Schering	00085-0370-01	15 gm	$14.05
	00085-0370-02	45 gm	$25.74

Monistat *SEE* MICONAZOLE NITRATE *AND* MICONAZOLE, INJECTABLE

Mono-Gesic *SEE* SALSALATE

Mono-Vacc Test (O.T.) *SEE* TUBERCULIN

Monobenzone

DESCRIPTION
Each gram of Monobenzone Cream contains 200 mg of Monobenzone, USP, in a water-washable base.

◆ RATED THERAPEUTICALLY EQUIVALENT; ◇ THERAPEUTIC EQUIVALENCE UNCONFIRMED; ○ UNRATED

Following is its chemical structure:

CLINICAL PHARMACOLOGY

The mechanism of action of Monobenzone is not fully understood. Denton et al.[1] suggested that Monobenzone may be converted to hydroquinone, which they found to inhibit the enzymatic oxidation of tyrosine to DOPA.

Iijima and Watanabe[2] suggested a direct action on tyrosinase.

Another suggestion by Denton and his group was that Monobenzone acts as an anti-oxidant to prevent SH-group oxidation so that more SH groups are available to inhibit tyrosinase. The primary role of inflammation in the depigmentation process was studied by Becker and Spencer[3] who suggested that increased cell permeability allows Monobenzone to enter the melanocyte to form an antigenic substance which attached to the melanin granule enters the dermis where antibodies are produced, remote positive patch-testing may result.

INDICATIONS AND USAGE

Monobenzone Cream is indicated for final depigmentation in extensive vitiligo.

Monobenzone Cream is not recommended for freckling, hyperpigmentation due to photosensitization following use of certain perfumes (berlock dermatitis), melasma (chloasma) of pregnancy, and hyperpigmentation following inflammation of the skin. Monobenzone Cream is of no value in the treatment of cafe-au-lait spots, pigmented nevi, malignant melanoma, or pigment resulting from pigments other than melanin, including bile, silver, and artificial pigments.

CONTRAINDICATIONS

Prior history of sensitivity or allergic reaction to this product or any of its ingredients. The safety of topical Monobenzone use during pregnancy or in children (12 years and under) has not been established.

WARNINGS

A. Monobenzone Cream is a potent depigmenting agent, not a mild cosmetic bleach. Do not use except for final depigmentation in extensive vitiligo.
B. Keep this and all medication out of the reach of children. In case of accidental ingestion, call a physician or a poison control center immediately.

PRECAUTIONS

See "Warnings".

A. Pregnancy Category C. Animal reproduction studies have not been conducted with topical Monobenzone. It is also not known whether Monobenzone can cause fetal harm when used topically on a pregnant woman or affect reproductive capacity. It is not known to what degree, if any, topical Monobenzone is absorbed systemically. Topical Monobenzone should be used in pregnant women only when clearly indicated.
B. Nursing mothers. It is not known whether topical Monobenzone is absorbed or excreted in human milk. Caution is advised when topical Monobenzone is used by a nursing mother.
C. Pediatric usage. Safety and effectiveness in children below the age of 12 years have not been established.

ADVERSE REACTIONS

Occasional irritation, a burning sensation, or dermatitis may occur in which case medication should be discontinued and the physician notified immediately.

DOSAGE AND ADMINISTRATION

Menobenzone should be applied to the pigmented area and rubbed in well two or three times daily or as directed by physician. There is no recommended dosage for children under 12 years of age except under the advice and supervision of a physician.

NOTE
Depigmentation is usually observed after one to four months of therapy. If satisfactory results have not been obtained within four months, treatment should be discontinued.

Monobenzone Cream should be stored at controlled room temperature (15-30°C) (59-86°F).

REFERENCES
1. Denton, C.R.; A.B. Lerner; and T.B. Fitzpatrick; "Inhibition of Melanin Formation by Chemical Agents", *The Journal of Investigative Dermatology*, Vol. 18, No. 2, February, 1952.   2. Iijima, Susumu and Kazu Watanabe: "Studies or DOPA Reaction: II, Effect of Chemicals on the Reaction", *The Journal of Investigative Dermatology*, Vol. 28, No. 1, January, 1957.   3. Becker, S.W. and Malcolm C. Spencer: "Evaluation of Monobenzone", *The Journal of American Medical Association*, Vol. 180, No. 4, April 28, 1962.

HOW SUPPLIED
CREAM: 20%

BRAND/MANUFACTURER	NDC	SIZE	AWP
○ BRAND BENOQUIN: ICN	00187-0380-34	37.5 gm	$41.34

Monocid *SEE* **CEFONICID SODIUM**

Monoctanoin

DESCRIPTION
Monoctanoin is a semi-synthetic esterified glycerol. The mixed mono-di-glyceride has the following approximate composition:

Glyceryl-l-mono-octanoate	80-85%
Glyceryl-l-mono-decanoate	10-15%
Glyceryl-2-di-octanoate	10-15%
Free Glycerol	max.2.5%

Monoctanoin is a clear, viscous, sterile liquid intended for perfusion into the bile ducts. By virtue of its ability to dissolve cholesterol, it is effective for dissolving cholesterol (radiolucent) gallstones.

CLINICAL PHARMACOLOGY
Monoctanoin has been shown, *in vitro,* to have 2.5 times greater dissolution capacity for cholesterol (about 120 mg cholesterol/mL of Monoctanoin) than does sodium cholate.

Monoctanoin is readily hydrolyzed by pancreatic and other digestive lipases. The liberated fatty acids are excreted or absorbed and metabolized in a normal fashion. Monoctanoin is irritating to the gastrointestinal and biliary tracts in animals and man. Such irritation was found to be reversible and disappeared 2 to 7 days after therapy was completed.

These effects are closely related to biliary tract pressure and rate of perfusion; both should be closely monitored.

Administration to dogs via a Heidenhain pouch resulted in a disruption of the ionic mucosal barrier, similar to that seen with bile acid reflux.

The rat model was used to evaluate the potential toxic effects of gallstone solvents. Direct intrahepatic injection of low doses of Monoctanoin into the left lobe of rat livers produced fibrotic areas with hyalinized, necrotic centers. Large doses of Monoctanoin directly injected into rat livers caused hemorrhagic pneumonitis resulting in high mortality. This study emphasized the need for a manometer to be placed in the delivery pathway to limit biliary pressure and prevent reflux into the substance of the liver.

In man, a study incorporating endoscopic examination and mucosal biopsies from the gastric antrum, duodenum and bile ducts showed diffuse erythema in the antral and duodenal mucosa plus mucosal erosions of duodenum. There was no significant histologic alteration in gastric mucosa, but duodenum showed significant inflammatory cell infiltration and ulceration in 3 of 5 patients. In one patient, multiple duodenal ulcerations adjacent to the infusion catheter were observed.

Mucosal abnormalities were not seen one month after discontinuation of therapy in all patients in the study.

INDICATIONS AND USAGE
Monoctanoin is indicated as a solubilizing agent for cholesterol (radiolucent) gallstones retained in the bile ducts following cholecystectomy, when other means of removing cholesterol (radiolucent) stones retained in the bile ducts have failed or cannot be undertaken.

When reduced in size the stones may pass spontaneously or may become susceptible to physical extraction. Complete dissolution is much more likely when there is a single stone (almost 50%) than when there are multiple stones (about 20%). For unclear reasons, complete dissolution is lower in diabetic patients (about 10%).

In the clinical study that was used to support the U.S. New Drug Application 326 patients completed the study. In 1/3 of the patients, the stone or stones completely disappeared plus another 1/3 became smaller or softer so that they were able to be easily removed by either the basket technique or some other means of removal that had been unsuccessful earlier. The patient population used in this study had either already been treated by other methods of stone removal that had failed and were thus already traumatized, or were considered too ill for other methods to be attempted.

Significantly higher success rates may be expected in other patient populations due to:

1. Smaller stone size than original study.
2. Healthier patients with less traumatized biliary tracts.
3. Updated Set-Up and Administration instructions for physicians to follow.
4. Better solvent placement due to greater experience.
5. The institution of closer follow-up examination to determine if friability has increased, or softening of the stone has occurred.

However, the influence of these factors, alone or in combination, on efficacy and safety, has not been convincingly established.

CONTRAINDICATIONS
Monoctanoin should not be used in patients with significant biliary tract infection or with a history of recent duodenal ulcer or jejunitis, or in patients with impaired hepatic function and patients with porto-systemic shunting, such that there is a saturation of the hepatic uptake and metabolism of material absorbed from the gut lumen. Monoctanoin should not be used in patients with acute pancreatitis.

WARNING
MONOCTANOIN IS INTENDED FOR BILIARY TRACT PERFUSION ONLY AND IS *NOT* FOR PARENTERAL USE. It is not intended for perfusion into the gallbladder. Monoctanoin must NOT be administered IV or IM.

Monoctanoin is irritating to the gastrointestinal and biliary tracts of animals and humans. These effects are closely related to biliary tract pressure and rate of perfusion. Such irritation was found to be reversible and disappeared 2 to 7 days after therapy was completed.

Biliary pressure during perfusion must be kept below 20 cm through the use of a manometer in the delivery pathway. Cut off the stem of the manometer at 20 cm, which should preclude elevated intraductal pressures which could lead to adverse reactions such as pulmonary edema.

Biliary pressure over 30 cm of H_2O during Monoctanoin perfusion in dogs caused reflux which resulted in acute respiratory failure and a high mortality rate. Pressure in excess of 20 cm must be avoided.

When Monoctanoin is perfused through a T-tube or a nasobiliary catheter after papillotomy, extravasation into the peritoneal cavity must be avoided or peritonitis may occur. Ascending cholangitis has been reported with Monoctanoin therapy, possibly related to obstruction in the common bile duct.

If fever, chills, leukocytosis, severe right upper quadrant abdominal pain or increasing jaundice occur, discontinue treatment.

PRECAUTIONS

Liver function tests should be monitored in all patients. Monoctanoin therapy should be undertaken with caution in patients with obstructive jaundice due to stones. The use of the second catheter for drainage should prevent any problems due to back pressure. (See *"Dosage and Administration".*)

CARCINOGENESIS, MUTATAGENESIS, IMPAIRMENT OF FERTILITY
No data available.

Pregnancy: Teratogenic Effects: Pregnancy Category C. Animal reproduction studies have not been conducted with Monoctanoin. It is not known whether Monoctanoin can cause fetal harm when administered to a pregnant woman or can affect reproduction capacity.

Monoctanoin should be given to a pregnant woman only if clearly needed.

Nursing Mothers: It is not known whether this drug is excreted in human milk. Because many drugs are excreted in human milk, caution should be exercised when Monoctanoin is administered to a nursing woman.

Pediatric Use: Safety and effectiveness in children have not been established.

ADVERSE REACTION

Aside from improper placement of catheter, the adverse reactions of Monoctanoin are related to the perfusion rate and biliary pressure. Most symptoms can be alleviated by temporarily stopping perfusion and restarting at a lower rate. Abdominal pain, nausea, vomiting and diarrhea were the most common side effects reported by patients receiving Monoctanoin therapy.

The incidence of adverse reactions listed in the following tables are based on observations of 326 patients treated with Monoctanoin in the multicenter clinical study. In that study the rate of perfusion varied from 5 - 15 mL/hr, and the biliary pressure was not monitored or reported.

The reactions are arranged in order of decreasing frequency.

ADVERSE REACTIONS OCCURRING IN MORE THAN 1% OF MONOCTANOIN TREATED PATIENTS.

N = 326

Reactions Gastrointestinal	No. of reactions	Frequency (%)
Pain	139	43
Nausea	104	32
Emesis	65	20
Diarrhea	63	19
Discomfort	24	7.3
Fever	19	6.3
Anorexia	10	3.0
Loose stool	5	1.5
Indigestion	4	1.2

Most of the adverse reactions were mild gastrointestinal symptoms. Some were tolerated, some abated with reduced perfusion rate and some by discontinuing perfusion during meals.

ADVERSE REACTIONS OCCURRING IN LESS THAN 1% OF MONOCTANOIN TREATED PATIENTS

Adverse reactions which occurred in 0.3% to 0.9% of treated patients included burning epigastrium, increased drainage from fistula, increased serum amylase, "bile shock", persistent leucopenia, hypokalemia, pruritus, fatigue/lethargy, intolerance, chills, depression, diaphoresis, headache and allergic reaction.

The following table identifies those reactions which were considered severe enough to discontinue therapy.

REASONS FOR PATIENT DISCONTINUATION

Number of Patients Enrolled = 326
Number of Patients Discontinued = 39

Reason	Number of Patients
Severe and/or immediate gastrointestinal side effects	25
Patient refused further treatment	4
No reason given	2
Stone impacted, obstructive jaundice	2
Bile shock, diaphoresis	1

Number of Patients Enrolled = 326
Number of Patients Discontinued = 39

Reason	Number of Patients
Allergic reaction	1
Pressure > 15 cm	1
Liver function enzymes elevated	1
Patient had cerebrovascular accident	1
Patients with sepsis, CHF and renal failure died after 24-hour perfusion[1]	1

[1] *Patient had these symptoms prior to entering the trial.*

One patient with lupus erythematosus developed upper right quadrant abdominal pain, dyspnea and hypotension with hyperventilation. The symptoms abated when the drug was discontinued.

Also reported in the literature are the following instances of death having occurred among patients treated with Monoctanoin. Causal to effect relationship has not been established.

—One patient admitted to the hospital with severe unremitting cholangitis.
—One patient with pre-existing biliary peritonitis secondary to gallbladder perforation.
—One patient with pulmonary embolism.
—One obese female patient with pre-existing jaundice and pancreatitis.
—One patient with symptoms of sepsis, CHF and renal failure.[2]

Ductal perfusion of Monoctanoin has been associated with non-cardiogenic pulmonary edema, but the exact incidence is not known. Patients treated with Monoctanoin should be observed carefully for early signs or symptoms of pulmonary edema, the occurrence of which should prompt consideration of discontinuation of the perfusion.

One elderly patient developed adult respiratory distress syndrome (ARDS) but improved when Monoctanoin was discontinued. A cause and effect relationship has not been established.

DOSAGE AND ADMINISTRATION

In order to determine if Monoctanoin will be of value in treating gallstones of a particular patient, the following tests are recommended:

1. Chemical analysis of gallstones (removed from the gallbladder or common bile duct, saved and kept dry without preservatives) to determine the percentage of cholesterol contained in the stones.

a. Monoctanoin has been found to be approximately 70% effective if the cholesterol content is between 20% and 40%. Higher cholesterol content may increase effectiveness.

2. Incubation of gallstones removed from the gallbladder or common bile duct which were saved and kept dry without a preservative are then immersed in 30 mL of ether for 6 hours with stirring. This can be done while the patient's sutures are healing in order to save time.

a. Monoctanoin has been found to be approximately 70% effective if incubation shows dissolution, reduction in size, softening or increased crushability in 2 hours.

A suitable method is described in an article entitled: "Pigment vs. Cholesterol Cholelithiasis: Comparison of Stone and Bile Composition" in *A J Dig Dis*, 19, 585, July, 1974.

3. A cholangiogram is performed.

a. Monoctanoin has been found to be 70% effective if stones are partially radiolucent. Higher radiolucency may increase effectiveness.

If all of the above are negative, Monoctanoin treatment should not be instituted or should be discontinued.

ROUTES OF ADMINISTRATION
Monoctanoin is perfused into the biliary tract utilizing one of the following routes of administration:

1. directly through a catheter inserted through the T-Tube, or a catheter inserted through the mature sinus tract.

2. through a nasobiliary tube placed endoscopically.

The tip of the catheter must be placed as close to the stone(s) as possible to insure stone contact and bathing.

SET-UP FOR ADMINISTRATION
The 'Gravity Feed' method is utilized if a proper positive pressure infusion pump is not available.

If the proper pump is available, insert it between the vented IV set and the manometer. Remove the controller.

The bottom of the IV set primer must be at least 3" above the top of the manometer tube.

Pressure in the biliary tract is limited by using an open manometer cut off at 20 cm in the delivery pathway between the vented IV set and the delivery catheter or the T-Tube.

For the manometer to measure the pressure accurately, care must be taken to position the stopcock of the manometer at the mid-axillary line of the reclining patient. For patients who are sitting or standing, the stopcock should be at the same horizontal level as the stone or the delivery top of the catheter delivering Monoctanoin within the duct. Attach an overflow cup (paper or plastic) to the IV pole to catch any overflow if it occurs.

---

[2] Patient had these symptoms prior to entering the trial.

If the manometer overflows repeatedly, it indicates the possibility of an obstruction. The use of a second catheter for drainage usually relieves this excessive pressure so that treatment can be continued. The use of a second catheter to provide drainage has also been found to be effective in relieving pain from distension of the biliary tree or reflux into the pancreatic duct if the sphincter of Oddi is blocked by the impacted stone. For a description of methods see Crummy and Mack, AJR, March, 1981, 136: 622 - 623 and Baskin et al AJR, 148: 185 - 188.

Monoctanoin is effective only when in direct contact with the stone(s). For example, a pigtail catheter with multiple distal sideholes can be used for perfusion and placed such that the stone(s) lie in the curve of the pigtail, adjacent to the sideholes to ensure maximum drug-stone contact.

Add 13 mL of Sterile Water for Injection to each 120 mL vial (a 10% dilution) to reduce the viscosity and enhance the bathing of the stone(s).

The addition of Sterile Water for Injection reduces the viscosity by almost 50%. Monoctanoin should be at 37° C (98.6° F) as it enters the body.

Monoctanoin is continuously perfused on a 24 hour basis at a rate of 3 to 5 mL/hour.

Continuous perfusion of Monoctanoin usually requires 2 to 10 days for elimination or size reduction of stones. If, after 10 days, cholangiography shows neither elimination nor reduction in size or density of stones, endoscopy should be performed to determine advisability of additional perfusion based on friability, softness or reduction of the density of the stone.

If nausea, diarrhea or pain occur, temporarily interrupting the perfusion will usually resolve these symptoms. If the symptoms persist, the perfusion may have to be resumed at a lower rate. Also, alleviation of the above symptoms can be obtained by temporarily stopping the perfusion during mealtime.

STORAGE
Store at controlled room temperature, 15° to 30°C (59° to 86°F).

When stored at temperatures below 15°C (59°F) Monoctanoin may form a semi-solid; this semi-solid can be reliquified by heating to 21° to 27°C (70° to 80°F). Before use, warm Monoctanoin to 37° C (98.6°F) and maintain at this temperature during administration. (See *"Dosage and Administration".*)

HOW SUPPLIED
SOLUTION:

BRAND/MANUFACTURER	NDC	SIZE	AWP
BRAND MOCTANIN: Ethitek	54686-0399-18	120 ml	$120.00

Monodox *SEE* DOXYCYCLINE

Monoket *SEE* ISOSORBIDE MONONITRATE

Mononine *SEE* FACTOR IX (HUMAN)

Monopril *SEE* FOSINOPRIL SODIUM

8-MOP *SEE* METHOXSALEN

Moricizine Hydrochloride

DESCRIPTION
Moricizine Hydrochloride is an orally active antiarrhythmic drug available for administration in tablets containing 200 mg, 250 mg and 300 mg of Moricizine Hydrochloride. The chemical name of Moricizine Hydrochloride is 10-(3-morpholinopropionyl) phenothiazine-2-carbamic acid ethyl ester hydrochloride.

Moricizine Hydrochloride is a white to tan crystalline powder, freely soluble in water and has a pKa of 6.4 (weak acid).

Following is its chemical structure:

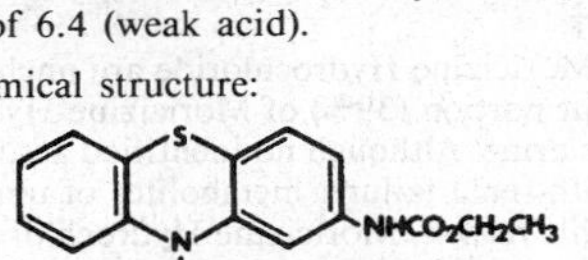

CLINICAL PHARMACOLOGY
MECHANISM OF ACTION
Moricizine Hydrochloride is a Class I antiarrhythmic agent with potent local anesthetic activity and myocardial membrane stabilizing effects. Moricizine Hydrochloride reduces the fast inward current carried by sodium ions.

In isolated dog Purkinje fibers, Moricizine Hydrochloride shortens Phase II and III repolarization, resulting in a decreased action potential duration and effective refractory period. A dose-related decrease in the maximum rate of Phase 0 depolarization (V_{max}) occurs without effect on maximum diastolic potential or action potential amplitude. The sinus node and atrial tissue of the dog are not affected.

ELECTROPHYSIOLOGY
Electrophysiology studies in patients with ventricular tachycardia have shown that Moricizine Hydrochloride at daily doses of 750 mg and 900 mg, prolongs atrioventricular conduction. Both AV nodal conduction time (AH interval) and His-Purkinje conduction time (HV interval) are prolonged by 10-13% and 21-26%, respectively. The PR interval is prolonged by 16-20% and the QRS by 7-18%. Prolongations of 2-5% in the corrected QT interval result from widening of the QRS interval, but there is shortening of the JT interval, indicating an absence of significant effect on ventricular repolarization. Intra-atrial conduction or atrial effective refractory periods are not consistently affected. In patients without sinus node dysfunction, Moricizine Hydrochloride has minimal effects on sinus cycle length and sinus node recovery time. These effects may be significant in patients with sinus node dysfunction (see *"Precautions: Electrocardiographic Changes/ Conduction Abnormalities"*).

HEMODYNAMICS
In patients with impaired left ventricular function, Moricizine Hydrochloride has minimal effects on measurements of cardiac performance such as cardiac index, stroke volume index, pulmonary capillary wedge pressure, systemic or pulmonary vascular resistance or ejection fraction, either at rest or during exercise. Moricizine Hydrochloride is associated with a small, but consistent increase in resting blood pressure and heart rate. Exercise tolerance in patients with ventricular arrhythmias is unaffected. In patients with a history of congestive heart failure or angina pectoris, exercise duration and rate-pressure product at maximal exercise are unchanged during Moricizine Hydrochloride administration. Nonetheless, in some cases worsened heart failure in patients with severe underlying heart disease has been attributed to Moricizine Hydrochloride.

OTHER PHARMACOLOGIC EFFECTS
Although Moricizine Hydrochloride is chemically related to the neuroleptic phenothiazines, it has no demonstrated central or peripheral dopaminergic activity in animals. Moreover, in patients on chronic Moricizine Hydrochloride, serum prolactin levels did not increase.

PHARMACOKINETICS/PHARMACODYNAMICS
The antiarrhythmic and electrophysiologic effects of Moricizine Hydrochloride are not related in time course or intensity to plasma moricizine concentrations or to the concentrations of any identified metabolite, all of which have short (2-3 hours) half-lives. Following single doses of Moricizine Hydrochloride, there is a prompt prolongation of the PR interval, which becomes normal within 2 hours, consistent with the rapid fall of plasma moricizine. JT interval shortening, however, peaks at about 6 hours and persists for at least 10 hours. Although an effect on VPD rates is seen within 2 hours after dosing, the full effect is seen after 10-14 hours and persists in full, when therapy is terminated, for more than 10 hours, after which the effect decays slowly, and is still substantial at 24 hours. This suggests either an unidentified, active, long half-life metabolite or a structural or functional "deep compartment" with slow entry from, and release to, the plasma. The following description of parent compound pharmacokinetics is therefore of uncertain relevance to clinical actions.

Following oral administration, Moricizine Hydrochloride undergoes significant first-past metabolism resulting in an absolute bioavailability of approximately 38%. Peak plasma concentrations of Moricizine Hydrochloride are usually reached within 0.5-2 hours. Administration 30 minutes after a meal delays the rate of absorption, resulting in lower peak plasma concentrations, but the extent of absorption is not altered. Moricizine Hydrochloride plasma levels are proportional to dose over the recommended therapeutic dose range.

The apparent volume of distribution after oral administration is very large ($\geq$ 300L) and is not significantly related to body weight. Moricizine Hydrochloride is approximately 95% bound to human plasma proteins. This binding interaction is independent of Moricizine Hydrochloride plasma concentration.

Moricizine Hydrochloride undergoes extensive biotransformation. Less than 1% of orally administered Moricizine Hydrochloride is excreted unchanged in the urine. There are at least 26 metabolites, but no single metabolite has been found to represent as much as 1% of the administered dose, and as stated above, antiarrhythmic response has relatively slow onset and offset. Two metabolites are pharmacologically active in at least one animal model: moricizine sulfoxide and phenothiazine-2-carbamic acid ethyl ester sulfoxide. Each of these metabolites represents a small percentage of the administered dose (< 0.6%), is present in lower concentrations in the plasma than the parent drug, and has a plasma elimination half-life of approximately three hours.

Moricizine Hydrochloride has been shown to induce its own metabolism. Average Moricizine Hydrochloride plasma concentrations in patients decrease with multiple dosing. This decrease in plasma levels of parent drug does not appear to affect clinical outcome for patients receiving chronic Moricizine Hydrochloride therapy.

➤ SHOWN IN PRODUCT IDENTIFICATION GUIDE

The plasma half-life of Moricizine Hydrochloride is 1.5-3.5 hours (most values about 2 hours) following single or multiple oral doses in patients with ventricular ectopy. Approximately 56% of the administered dose is excreted in the feces and 39% is excreted in the urine. Some Moricizine Hydrochloride is also recycled through enterohepatic circulation.

CLINICAL ACTIONS

Moricizine Hydrochloride at daily doses of 600-900 mg procedures a dose-related in the occurrence of frequent ventricular premature depolarizations (VPDs) and reduces the incidence of nonsustained and sustained ventricular tachycardia (VT). In controlled clinical trials, Moricizine Hydrochloride has been shown to have antiarrhythmic activity that is generally similar to that of disopyramide, propranolol, and quinidine at the doses studied. In controlled and compassionate use programmed electrical stimulation studies (PES), Moricizine Hydrochloride prevented the induction of sustained ventricular tachycardia in approximately 25% of patients. In a post-marketing randomized comparative PES study, Moricizine Hydrochloride had a response rate of approximately 12% (7/59). Activity of Moricizine Hydrochloride is maintained during long-term use.

Moricizine Hydrochloride is effective in treating ventricular arrhythmias in patients with and without organic heart disease. Moricizine Hydrochloride may be effective in patients in whom other antiarrhythmic agents are ineffective, not tolerated, and/or contraindicated.

Arrhythmia exacerbation or "rebound" is not noted following discontinuation of Moricizine Hydrochloride therapy.

INDICATIONS AND USAGE

Moricizine Hydrochloride is indicated for the treatment of documented ventricular arrhythmias, such as sustained ventricular tachycardia, that in the judgement of the physician are life-threatening. Because of the proarrhythmic effects of Moricizine Hydrochloride its use with lesser arrhythmias is generally not recommended. Treatment of patients with asymptomatic ventricular premature contractions should be avoided.

Initiation of Moricizine Hydrochloride treatment, as with other antiarrhythmic agents used to treat life-threatening arrhythmias, should be carried out in the hospital.

Antiarrhythmic drugs have not been shown to enhance survival in patients with ventricular arrhythmias.

UNLABELED USES

Moricizine Hydrochloride is used alone or as an adjunct in the treatment of superventricular arrhythmias.

CONTRAINDICATIONS

Moricizine Hydrochloride is contraindicated in patients with pre-existing second- or third-degree AV block and in patients with right bundle branch block when associated with left hemi-block (bifasicular block) unless a pacemaker is present. Moricizine Hydrochloride also contraindicated in the presence of cardiogenic shock or known hypersensitivity to the drug.

WARNINGS

MORTALITY

Moricizine Hydrochloride was one of three antiarrhythmic drugs included in the National Heart Lung and Blood Institute's Cardiac Arrhythmia Suppression Trial (CAST I), a long-term multicenter, randomized, double-blind study in patients with asymptomatic non-life-threatening ventricular arrhythmias who had a myocardial infarction more than 6 days, but less than 2 years previously. An excessive mortality or nonfatal cardiac arrest rate was seen in patients treated with both of the Class IC agents included in the trial, which led to discontinuation of those 2 arms of the trial. The average duration of treatment with these agents was 10 months. The Moricizine Hydrochloride and placebo arms of the trial were continued in the NHLBI sponsored CAST II. In this randomized, double-blind trial, patients with asymptomatic, non-life-threatening arrhythmias who had had a myocardial infarction within 4 to 90 days and left ventricular ejection fraction ≤ 0.40 prior to enrollment were evaluated. The average duration of treatment with Moricizine Hydrochloride in this study was 18 months. The study was discontinued because there was no possibility of demonstrating a benefit toward improved survival with Moricizine Hydrochloride and because of an evolving adverse trend after long-term treatment.

The applicability of the CAST results to other populations (e.g., those without recent myocardial infarction) is uncertain. Considering the known proarrhythmic properties of Moricizine Hydrochloride and the lack of evidence of improved survival for any antiarrhythmic drug in patients without life-threatening arrhythmias, the use of Moricizine Hydrochloride as well as other antiarrhythmic agents, should be reserved for patients with life-threatening ventricular arrhythmias.

PROARRHYTHMIA

Like other antiarrhythmic drugs, Moricizine Hydrochloride can provoke new rhythm disturbances or make existing arrhythmias worse. These proarrhythmic effects can range from an increase in the frequency of VPDs to the development of new or more severe ventricular tachycardia, e.g., tachycardia that is more sustained or more resistant to conversion to sinus rhythm, with potentially fatal consequences. It is often not possible to distinguish a proarrhythmic effect from the patient's underlying rhythm disorder, so that the occurrence rates given below must be considered approximations. Note also that drug-induced arrhythmias can generally be identified only when they occur early after starting the drug and when the rhythm can be identified, usually because the patient is being monitored. It is clear from the NIH sponsored CAST (Cardiac Arrhythmia Suppression Trial) that some antiarrhythmic drugs can cause increased sudden death mortality, presumably due to new arrhythmias or asystole that do not appear early after treatment but that represent a sustained increased risk.

Domestic premarketing trials included 1072 patients given Moricizine Hydrochloride 397 had baseline lethal arrhythmias (sustained VT or VF and nonsustained VT with hemodynamic symptoms) and 576 had potentially lethal arrhythmias (increased VPDs or NSVT in patients with known structural heart disease, active ischemia, congestive heart failure or an LVEF < 40% and/or CI < 2.0 1/min/m^2). In this population there were 40 (3.7%) identified proarrhythmic events, 26 (2.5%) of which were serious, either fatal (6), new hemodynamically significant sustained VT or VF (4), new sustained VT that was not hemodynamically significant (11) or sustained VT that became syncopal/presyncopal when it had not been before (5). Proarrhythmic effects described as incessant ventricular tachycardia were observed in the post-marketing PES study and in post-marketing adverse event reports.

In general, serious proarrhythmic effects in the domestic premarketing trials were equally common in patients with more and less severe arrhythmias, 2.5% in the patients with baseline lethal arrhythmias vs. 2.8% in patients with potentially lethal arrhythmias, although the patients with serious effects were more likely to have a history of sustained VT (38% vs. 23%). In the post-marketing comparative PES study, patients treated with Moricizine Hydrochloride (250-300 mg TID) had a proarrhythmia rate of 14% (8/59).

Five of the six fatal proarrhythmic events were in patients with baseline lethal arrhythmias; four had prior cardiac arrests. Rates and severity of proarrhythmic events were similar in patients given 600-900 mg of Moricizine Hydrochloride per day and those given higher doses. Patients with proarrhythmic events were more likely than the overall population to have coronary artery disease (85% vs. 67%), history of acute myocardial infarction (75% vs. 53%), congestive heart failure (60% vs. 43%), and cardiomegaly (55% vs. 33%). All of the six proarrhythmic deaths were in patients with coronary artery disease; 5/6 each had documented acute myocardial infarction, congestive heart failure, and cardiomegaly.

ELECTROLYTE DISTURBANCES

Hypokalemia, hyperkalemia, or hypomagnesemia may alter the effects of Class I antiarrhythmic drugs. Electrolyte imbalances should be corrected before administration of Moricizine Hydrochloride.

SICK SINUS SYNDROME

Moricizine Hydrochloride should be used only with extreme caution in patients with sick sinus syndrome, as it may cause sinus bradycardia, sinus pause, or sinus arrest.

PRECAUTIONS

GENERAL
ELECTROCARDIOGRAPHIC CHANGES/CONDUCTION
ABNORMALITIES

Moricizine Hydrochloride slows AV nodal and intraventricular conduction, producing dose-related increases in the PR and QRS intervals. In clinical trials, the average increase in the PR interval was 12% and the QRS interval was 14%. Although the QTC interval is increased, this is wholly because of QRS prolongation; the JT interval is shortened, indicating the absence of significant slowing of ventricular repolarization. The degree of lengthening of PR and QRS intervals does not predict efficacy.

In controlled clinical trials and in open studies, the overall incidence of delayed ventricular conduction, including new bundle branch block pattern, was approximately 9.4%. In patients without baseline conduction abnormalities, the frequency of second-degree AV block was 0.2% and third-degree AV block did not occur. In patients with baseline conduction abnormalities, the frequencies of second-degree AV block and third-degree AV block were 0.9% and 1.4% respectively.

Moricizine Hydrochloride therapy was discontinued in 1.6% of patients due to electrocardiographic changes (0.6% due to sinus pause or asystole, 0.2% to AV block, 0.2% to junctional rhythm, 0.4% to intraventricular conduction delay, and 0.2% to wide QRS and/or PR interval).

In patients with pre-existing conduction abnormalities, Moricizine Hydrochloride therapy should be initiated cautiously. If second- or third-degree AV block occurs, Moricizine Hydrochloride therapy should be discontinued unless a ventricular pacemaker is in place. When changing the dose of Moricizine Hydrochloride or adding concomitant medications which may also affect cardiac conduction, patients should be monitored electrocardiographically.

HEPATIC IMPAIRMENT

Patients with significant liver dysfunction have reduced plasma clearance and an increased half-life of Moricizine Hydrochloride. Although the precise relationship of Moricizine Hydrochloride levels to effect is not clear, patients with hepatic disease should be treated with lower doses and closely monitored for excessive pharmacological effects, including effects on ECG intervals, before dosage adjustment. Patients with severe liver disease should be administered Moricizine Hydrochloride with particular care, if at all. (See "Dosage and Administration.")

RENAL IMPAIRMENT

Plasma levels of intact Moricizine Hydrochloride are unchanged in hemodialysis patients, but a significant portion (39%) of Moricizine Hydrochloride is metabolized and excreted in the urine. Although no identified active metabolite is known to increase in people with renal failure, metabolites of unrecognized importance could be affected. For this reason, Moricizine Hydrochloride should be administered cautiously in patients with impaired renal function. Patients with significant renal dysfunction should be started on lower doses and monitored for excessive pharmacologic effects, including ECG intervals, before dosage adjustment. (See "Dosage and Administration.")

CONGESTIVE HEART FAILURE

Most patients with congestive heart failure have tolerated the recommended Moricizine Hydrochloride daily doses without unusual toxicity or change in effect. Pharmacokinetic differences between Moricizine Hydrochloride patients with and without congestive heart failure were not apparent (See Hepatic Impairment above). In some cases, worsened heart failure has been attributed to Moricizine Hydrochloride. Patients with pre-existing heart failure should be monitored carefully when Moricizine Hydrochloride is initiated.

EFFECTS ON PACEMAKER THRESHOLD

The effect of Moricizine Hydrochloride on the sensing and pacing thresholds of artificial pacemakers has not been sufficiently studied. In such patients, pacing parameters must be monitored, if Moricizine Hydrochloride is used.

DRUG INTERACTIONS

No significant changes in serum digoxin levels or pharmacokinetics have been observed in patients or healthy subjects receiving concomitant Moricizine Hydrochloride therapy. Concomitant use was associated with additive prolongation of the PR interval, but not with a significant increase in the rate of second- or third-degree AV block.

Concomitant administration of cimetidine resulted in a decrease in Moricizine Hydrochloride clearance of 49% and a 1.4 fold increase in plasma levels in healthy subjects. During clinical trials, no significant changes in the efficacy or tolerance of Moricizine Hydrochloride have been observed in patients receiving concomitant cimetidine therapy. Patients on cimetidine should have Moricizine Hydrochloride therapy initiated at relatively low doses: not more than 600 mg/day. Patients should be monitored when concomitant cimetidine therapy is instituted or discontinued or when the Moricizine Hydrochloride dose is changed. Concomitant administration of beta blocker therapy did not reveal significant changes in overall electrocardiographic intervals in patients. In one controlled study, Moricizine Hydrochloride and propranolol administered concomitantly produced a small additive increase in the PR interval.

Theophylline clearance and plasma half-life were significantly affected by multiple dose Moricizine Hydrochloride administration when both conventional and sustained release theophylline were given to healthy subjects (clearance increased 44-66% and plasma half-life decreased 19-33%). Plasma theophylline levels should be monitored when concomitant Moricizine Hydrochloride is initiated or discontinued.

Because of possible additive pharmacologic effects, caution is indicated when Moricizine Hydrochloride is used with any drug that affects cardiac electrophysiology. Uncontrolled experience in patients indicates no serious adverse interaction during the concomitant use of Moricizine Hydrochloride and diuretics, vasodilators, antihypertensive drugs, calcium channel blockers, beta-blockers, angiotensin-converting enzyme inhibitors, or warfarin. Plasma warfarin levels, warfarin pharmacokinetics, and prothrombin times were unaffected during multiple dose Moricizine Hydrochloride administration to young, healthy, male subjects in a controlled study. However, there are isolated reports of the need to either increase or decrease warfarin doses after initiation of Moricizine Hydrochloride. Some patients who were taking warfarin with a stable prothrombin time experienced excessive prolongation of the prothrombin time following the initiation of Moricizine Hydrochloride. In some cases, liver enzymes also were elevated. Bleeding or bruising may occur. When Moricizine Hydrochloride is started or stopped in a patient stabilized on warfarin, more frequent prothrombin time monitoring is advisable.

Results from *in vitro* studies do not suggest alterations in Moricizine Hydrochloride plasma protein binding in the presence of other highly plasma protein bound drugs.

CARCINOGENESIS, MUTAGENESIS, IMPAIRMENT OF FERTILITY

In a 24-month mouse study in which Moricizine Hydrochloride was administered in the feed at concentrations calculated to provide doses ranging up to 320 mg/kg/day, ovarian tubular adenomas and granulosa cell tumors were limited in occurrence to Moricizine Hydrochloride treated animals. Although the findings were of borderline statistical significance, or not statistically significant, historical control data indicate that both of these tumors are uncommon in the strain of mouse studied. In a 24-month study in which Moricizine Hydrochloride was administered by gavage to rats at doses of 25, 50 and 100 mg/kg/day, Zymbal's Gland Carcinoma was observed in one mid-dose and two high dose males. This tumor appears to be uncommon in the strain of rat studied. Rats of both sexes showed a dose-related increase in hepatocellular cholangioma (also described as bile ductile cystadenoma or cystic hyperplasia) along with fatty metamorphosis, possibly due to disruption of hepatic choline utilization for phospholipid biosynthesis. The rat is known to be uniquely sensitive to alteration in choline metabolism.

Moricizine Hydrochloride was not mutagenic when assayed for genotoxicity in *in vitro* bacterial (Ames test) and mammalian (Chinese hamster ovary/hypoxanthine-guanine phosphoribosyl transferase and sister chromatid exchange) cell systems or in *in vivo* mammalian systems (rat bone cytogenicity and mouse micronucleus).

A general reproduction and fertility study was conducted in rats at dose levels up to 6.7 times the maximum recommended human dose of 900 mg/day (based upon 50 kg human body weight) and revealed no evidence of impaired male or female fertility.

PREGNANCY—TERATOGENIC EFFECTS

Pregnancy Category B: Teratology studies have been performed with Moricizine Hydrochloride in rats and in rabbits at doses up to 6.7 and 4.7 times the maximum recommended human daily dose, respectively, and have revealed no evidence of harm to the fetus. There are, however, no adequate and well-controlled studies in pregnant women. Because animal reproduction studies are not always predictive of human response, Moricizine Hydrochloride should be used during pregnancy only if clearly needed.

PREGNANCY—NONTERATOGENIC EFFECTS

In a study in which rats were dosed with Moricizine Hydrochloride prior to mating, during mating and throughout gestation and lactation, dose levels 3.4 and 6.7 times the maximum recommended human daily dose produced a dose-related decrease in pup and maternal weight gain, possibly related to a larger litter size. In a study in which dosing was begun on Day 15 of gestation, Moricizine Hydrochloride at a level 6.7 times the maximum recommended human daily dose, produced a retardation in maternal weight gain but no effect on pup growth.

NURSING MOTHERS

Moricizine Hydrochloride is secreted in the milk of laboratory animals and has been reported to be present in human milk. Because of the potential for serious adverse reactions in nursing infants from Moricizine Hydrochloride a decision should be made whether to discontinue the drug, taking into account the importance of the drug to the mother.

PEDIATRIC USE

The safety and effectiveness of Moricizine Hydrochloride in children less than 18 years of age have not been established.

ADVERSE REACTIONS

The most serious adverse reaction reported for Moricizine Hydrochloride is proarrhythmia (see *"Warnings"*). This occurred in 3.7% of 1072 patients with ventricular arrhythmias who received a wide range of doses under a variety of circumstances.

In addition to discontinuations because of proarrhythmias, in controlled clinical trials and in open studies, adverse reactions led to discontinuation of Moricizine Hydrochloride in 7% of 1105 patients with ventricular and supraventricular arrhythmias, including 3.2% due to nausea, 1.6% due to ECG abnormalities (principally conduction defects, sinus pause, junctional rhythm, or AV block), 1% due to congestive heart failure, and 0.3-0.4% due to dizziness, anxiety, drug fever, urinary retention, blurred vision, gastrointestinal upset, rash, and laboratory abnormalities.

The most frequently occurring adverse reactions in the 1072 patients (including all adverse experiences whether or not considered Moricizine Hydrochloride related by the investigator) were dizziness (15.1%), nausea (9.6%), headache (8.0%), fatigue (5.9%), palpitations (5.8%), and dyspnea (5.7%). Dizziness appears to be related to the size of each dose. In a comparison of 900 mg/day given at 450 mg b.i.d. or 300 mg t.i.d., more than 20% of patients experienced dizziness on the b.i.d. regimen vs. 12% on the t.i.d. regimen.

Adverse reactions reported by less than 5%, but in 2% or greater of the patients, were sustained ventricular tachycardia, hypesthesias, abdominal pain, dyspepsia, vomiting, sweating, cardiac chest pain, asthenia, nervousness, paresthesias, congestive heart failure, musculoskeletal pain, diarrhea, dry mouth, cardiac death, sleep disorders, and blurred vision.

Adverse reactions infrequently reported (in less than 2% of the patients) were:

Cardiovascular: hypotension, hypertension, syncope, supraventricular arrhythmias (including atrial fibrillation/flutter), cardiac arrest, bradycardia, pulmonary embolism, myocardial infarction, vasodilation, cerebrovascular events, thrombophlebitis;

Nervous System: tremor, anxiety, depression, euphoria, confusion, somnolence, agitation, seizure, coma, abnormal gait, hallucinations, nystagmus, diplopia, speech disorder, akathisia, loss of memory, ataxia, abnormal coordination, dyskinesia, vertigo tinnitus;

Genitourinary: urinary retention or frequency, dysuria, urinary incontinence, kidney pain, impotence, decreased libido;

Respiratory: hyperventilation, apnea, asthma, pharyngitis, cough, sinusitus;

Gastrointestinal: anorexia, bitter taste, dysphagia, flatulence, ileus;

Other: drug fever, hypothermia, temperature intolerance, eye pain, rash, pruritus, dry skin, urticaria, swelling of the lips and tongue, periorbital edema.

During Moricizine Hydrochloride therapy, two patients developed thrombocytopenia that may have been drug-related. Clinically significant elevations in liver function tests (bilirubin, serum transaminases) and jaundice consistent with hepatitis were rarely reported. Although a cause and effect relationship has not been established, caution is advised in patients who develop unexplained signs of hepatic dysfunction, and consideration should be given to discontinuing therapy.

Three patients developed rechallenge-confirmed drug fever, with one patient experiencing an elevation above 103°F (to 105°F. with rigors). Fevers occurred at about 2 weeks in 2 cases, and after 21 weeks in the third. Fevers resolved within 48 hours of discontinuation of moricizine.

Adverse reactions were generally similar in patients over 65 (n = 375) and under 65 (n = 697), although discontinuation of therapy for reasons other than proarrhythmia was more common in older patients (13.9% vs. 7.7%). Overall mortality was greater in older patients (9.3% vs. 3.9%), but those were not deaths attributed to treatment and the older patients had more serious underlying heart disease.

The following table compares the most common (occurrence in more than 2% of the patients) non-cardiac adverse reactions (i.e., drug-related or of unknown relationship) in controlled clinical trials during the first one to two weeks of

INCIDENCE (%) OF THE MOST COMMON ADVERSE REACTIONS (THERAPY DURATION = 1-14 DAYS)

Adverse Reactions	> 2% Moricizine No.	%	> 2% Placebo No.	%	> 2% Quinidine No.	%	> 5% Disopyramide No.	%	> 5% Propranolol No.	%
Total No. of Patients	1072		618		110		31		24	
Dizziness	121	11.3	33	5.3	8	7.3	—		2	8.3
Nausea	74	6.9	18	2.9	7	6.4	3	9.7	—	
Headache	62	5.8	27	4.4	—		—		4	16.7
Pain	41	3.8	31	5.0	6	5.5	2	6.5	—	
Dyspnea	41	3.8	22	3.6	—		—		—	
Hypesthesia	40	3.7	—		3	2.7	—		—	
Fatigue	33	3.1	16	2.6	6	5.5	2	6.5	3	12.5
Vomiting	22	2.1	—		—		—		—	
Dry Mouth	—		—		—		11	35.5	—	
Nervousness	—		—		—		3	9.7	—	
Blurred vision	—		—		3	2.7	2	6.5	3	12.5
Diarrhea	—		—		25	22.7	—		—	
Constipation	—		—		—		2	6.5	—	
Somnolence	—		—		—		—		2	8.3
Urinary Retention	—		—		—		4	12.9	—	

therapy with Moricizine Hydrochloride quinidine, placebo, disopyramide, or propranolol in patients with ventricular arrhythmias. (See related table).

OVERDOSAGE
Deaths have occurred after accidental or intentional overdosages of 2,250 and 10,000 mg of Moricizine Hydrochloride respectively.

SIGNS, SYMPTOMS AND LABORATORY FINDINGS ASSOCIATED WITH AN OVERDOSAGE OF DRUG
Overdosage with Moricizine Hydrochloride may produce emesis, lethargy, coma, syncope, hypotension, conduction disturbances, exacerbation of congestive heart failure, myocardial infarction, sinus arrest, arrhythmias (including junctional bradycardia, ventricular tachycardia, ventricular fibrillation and asystole), and respiratory failure.

LETHAL DOSE IN ANIMALS
Oral doses of Moricizine Hydrochloride of about 200 mg/kg in dogs, 250 mg/kg in monkeys, 420 mg/kg in mice and 905 mg/kg in rats were lethal to about one-half of the animals exposed. Death was usually preceded by tremors, convulsions and respiratory depression.

RECOMMENDED GENERAL TREATMENT PROCEDURES
A specific antidote for Moricizine Hydrochloride has not been identified. In the event of overdosage, treatments should be supportive. Patients should be hospitalized and monitored for cardiac, respiratory and CNS changes. Advanced life support systems, including an intracardiac pacing catheter, should be provided where necessary. Acute overdosage should be treated with appropriate gastric evacuation, and with special care to avoid aspiration. Accidental introduction of Moricizine Hydrochloride into the lungs of monkeys resulted in rapid arrhythmic death.

DOSAGE AND ADMINISTRATION
The dosage of Moricizine Hydrochloride must be individualized on the basis of antiarrhythmic response and tolerance. Clinical, cardiac rhythm monitoring, electrocardiogram intervals, exercise testing, and/or programmed electrical stimulation testing may be used to guide antiarrhythmic response and dosage adjustment. In general, the patients will be at high risk and should be hospitalized for the initiation of therapy (see "Indications and Usage").

The usual adult dosage is between 600 and 900 mg per day, given every 8 hours in three equally divided doses. Within this range, the dosage can be adjusted as tolerated, in increments of 150 mg/day at 3-day intervals, until the desired effect is obtained. Patients with life-threatening arrhythmias who exhibit a beneficial response as judged by objective criteria (Holter monitoring, programmed electrical stimulation, exercise testing, etc.) can be maintained on chronic Moricizine Hydrochloride therapy. As the antiarrhythmic effect of Moricizine Hydrochloride persists for more than 12 hours, some patients whose arrhythmias are well-controlled on a Q8H regimen may be given the same total daily dose in a Q12H regimen to increase convenience and help assure compliance. When higher doses are used, patients may experience more dizziness and nausea on the Q12 hour regimen.

PATIENTS WITH HEPATIC IMPAIRMENT
Patients with hepatic disease should be started at 600 mg/day or lower and monitored closely, including measurement of ECG intervals, before dosage adjustment.

PATIENTS WITH RENAL IMPAIRMENT
Patients with significant renal dysfunction should be started at 600mg/day or lower and monitored closely, including measurement of ECG intervals, before dosage adjustment.

TRANSFER TO MORICIZINE HYDROCHLORIDE
Recommendations for transferring patients from another antiarrhythmic to Moricizine Hydrochloride can be given based on theoretical considerations. Previous antiarrhythmic therapy should be withdrawn for 1-2 plasma half-lives before starting Moricizine Hydrochloride at the recommended dosages. In patients in whom withdrawal of a previous antiarrhythmic is likely to produce life-threatening arrhythmias, hospitalization is recommended.

Transferred From	Start Moricizine Hydrochloride
Quinidine, Disopyramide	6-12 hours after last dose
Procainamide	3-6 hours after last dose
Encainide, Propafenone, Tocainide or Mexiletine	8-12 hours after last dose
Flecainide	12-24 hours after last dose

Store at controlled room temperature (59°-86°F, 15°-30°C) in a tightly-closed, light resistant container. Keep in carton until dispensed. Protect from light.

HOW SUPPLIED
TABLETS: 200 MG

BRAND/MANUFACTURER	NDC	SIZE	AWP
○ BRAND			
ETHMOZINE: Roberts Pharm	54092-0046-01	100s	$83.87
	54092-0046-52	100s ud	$83.87

TABLETS: 250 MG

BRAND/MANUFACTURER	NDC	SIZE	AWP
○ BRAND			
ETHMOZINE: Roberts Pharm	54092-0047-01	100s	$101.55
	54092-0047-52	100s ud	$101.55

TABLETS: 300 MG

BRAND/MANUFACTURER	NDC	SIZE	AWP
○ BRAND			
ETHMOZINE: Roberts Pharm	54092-0048-01	100s	$117.30
	54092-0048-52	100s ud	$117.30

Morphine Sulfate

WARNING: May be habit forming

> FOR THE SUSTAINED RELEASE DOSAGE FORM: PATIENT SHOULD BE INSTRUCTED TO SWALLOW THE TABLET AS A WHOLE; THE TABLET SHOULD NOT BE BROKEN IN HALF, NOR SHOULD IT BE CRUSHED OR CHEWED.
> THE SUSTAINED RELEASE OF MORPHINE FROM MORPHINE SULFATE SUSTAINED RELEASE SHOULD BE TAKEN INTO CONSIDERATION IN EVENT OF ADVERSE REACTIONS OR OVERDOSAGE.

DESCRIPTION
Morphine is the most important alkaloid of opium and is a phenanthrene derivative. It is available as the sulfate.

◆ RATED THERAPEUTICALLY EQUIVALENT; ◇ THERAPEUTIC EQUIVALENCE UNCONFIRMED; ○ UNRATED

Chemically, Morphine Sulfate is 7,8-didehydro-4,5α-epoxy-17- methylmorphinan-3,6 α-diol sulfate (2:1) (salt) pentahydrate. The empirical formula is $(C_{17}H_{19}NO_3)_2 \cdot H_2SO_4 \cdot 5H_2O$ and the molecular weight is 758.83.

Each tablet or capsule contains:
Morphine Sulfate ....15 or 30 mg

Each Sustained or Controlled Release Tablet contains:
Morphine Sulfate ....15, 30, 60, or 100 mg

Morphine Sulfate Injection, High Potency, is intended for use in continuous microinfusion devices for intraspinal administration in the management of pain.

Each 20 mL ampul of Morphine Sulfate Injection, High Potency, 200 contains:
Morphine Sulfate, USP ....200 mg or 10 mg/mL

Each 20 mL ampul of Morphine Sulfate Injection, High Potency, 500 contains:
Morphine Sulfate, USP ....500 mg or 25 mg/mL

Each 20 mL ampul of Morphine Sulfate Injection, High Potency, is intended for **single use only.** *Discard any unused portion.* DO NOT HEAT-STERILIZE.

Each 5 mL of Morphine Sulfate Oral Solution contains:
Morphine Sulfate ....10 or 20 mg

Each 1 mL of Morphine Sulfate Oral Solution Concentrate contains:
Morphine Sulfate ....20 mg

Each mL of Morphine Sulfate Immediate Release Concentrated Oral Solution contains:
Morphine Sulfate ....20 mg

Each 1.5 mL of Morphine Sulfate Immediate Release Concentrated Oral Solution contains:
Morphine Sulfate ....30 mg

Each 5 mL of Morphine Sulfate Immediate Release Concentrated Oral Solution contains:
Morphine Sulfate ....100 mg

Each 2.5 mL of Morphine Sulfate Immediate Release Oral Solution contains:
Morphine Sulfate ....10 mg

Each 5 mL of Morphine Sulfate Immediate Release Oral Solution contains:
Morphine Sulfate ....20 mg

Morphine Sulfate occurs as white, feathery, silky crystals, cubical masses of crystals, or white crystalline powder; it is soluble in water and slightly soluble in alcohol. Morphine has a pKa of 7.9, with an octanol/water partition coefficient of 1.42 at pH 7.4. At this pH, the tertiary amino group is mostly ionized, making the molecule water-soluble. Morphine is significantly more water-soluble than any other opioid in clinical use.

Following is its chemical structure:

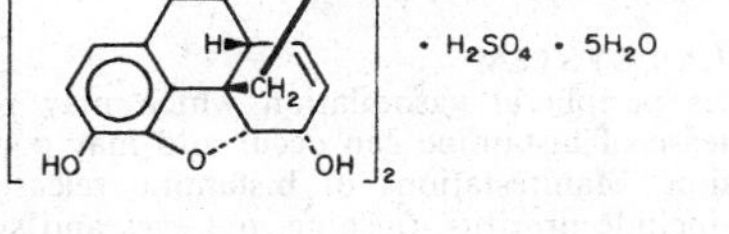

CLINICAL PHARMACOLOGY
METABOLISM AND PHARMACOKINETICS
Morphine exerts its primary effects on the central nervous system and organs containing smooth muscle. Pharmacologic effects include analgesia, drowsiness or somnolence, alteration in mood (euphoria or dysphoria), reduction in body temperature (at low doses), dose-related depression of respiration, diminished gastrointestinal motility, interference with adrenocortical response to stress (at high doses), reduction in peripheral resistance with little or no effect on cardiac index, miosis, and physical dependence.

Morphine, as other opioids, acts as an agonist interacting with stereo-specific and saturable binding sites/receptors in the brain, spinal cord and other tissues. These sites have been classified as μ receptors and are widely distributed throughout the central nervous system being present in highest concentration in the limbic system (frontal and temporal cortex, amygdala and hippocampus), thalamus, striatum, hypothalamus, midbrain and laminae I, II, IV and V of the dorsal horn in the spinal cord. It has been postulated that exogenously administered morphine exerts its analgesic effect, in part, by altering the central release of neurotransmitter from afferent nerves sensitive to noxious stimuli. Peripheral threshold or responsiveness to noxious stimuli is unaffected leaving monosynaptic reflexes such as the patellar or the Achilles tendon reflex intact.

Following oral administration of a given dose of Morphine, the amount ultimately absorbed is essentially the same whether the source is Morphine Sulfate controlled release or a conventional formulation. Morphine is released from Morphine Sulfate controlled release somewhat more slowly than from conventional oral preparations. Because of pre-systemic elimination (i.e., metabolism in the gut wall and liver) only about 40% of the administered dose reaches the central compartment.

Once absorbed, Morphine is distributed to skeletal muscle, kidneys, liver, intestinal tract, lungs, spleen and brain. Morphine also crosses the placental membranes and has been found in breast milk.

Although a small fraction (less than 5%) of Morphine is demethylated, for all practical purposes, virtually all Morphine is converted to glucuronide metabolites; among these, morphine-3-glucuronide is present in the highest plasma concentration following oral administration.

The glucuronide system has a very high capacity and is not easily saturated even in disease. Therefore, rate of delivery of Morphine to the gut and liver should not influence the total and, probably, the relative quantities of the various metabolites formed. Moreover, even if rate affected the relative amounts of each metabolite formed, it should be unimportant clinically because Morphine's metabolites are ordinarily inactive.

The following pharmacokinetic parameters show considerable inter-subject variation but are representative of average values reported in the literature. The volume of distribution (Vd) for Morphine is 4 liters per kilogram, and its terminal elimination half-life is normally 2 to 4 hours.

Following the administration of conventional oral Morphine products, approximately fifty percent of the Morphine that will reach the central compartment intact reaches it within 30 minutes. Following the administration of an equal amount of Morphine Sulfate Controlled or Sustained Release to normal volunteers, however, this extent of absorption occurs, on average, after 1.5 hours.

The possible effect of food upon the systemic bioavailability of Morphine Sulfate Controlled or Sustained Release has not been evaluated.

Variation in the physical/mechanical properties of a formulation of an oral Morphine drug product can affect both its absolute bioavailability and its absorption rate constant (k_a). The formulation employed in Morphine Sulfate Controlled or Sustained Release has not been shown to affect Morphine's oral bioavailability, but does decrease its apparent k_a. Other basic pharmacokinetic parameters (e.g., volume of distribution [Vd], elimination rate constant [k_e], clearance [Cl]), are unchanged as they are fundamental properties of Morphine in the organism. However, in chronic use, the possibility that shifts in metabolite to parent drug ratios may occur cannot be excluded.

When immediate-release, controlled-release, or sustained-release oral Morphine is given on a fixed dosing regimen, steady state is achieved in about a day.

For a given dose and dosing interval, the AUC and average blood concentration of Morphine at steady state (Css) will be independent of the specific type of oral formulation administered so long as the formulations have the same absolute bioavailability. The absorption rate of a formulation will, however, affect the maximum (Cmax) and minimum (Cmin) blood levels and the times of their occurrence.

While there is no predictable relationship between Morphine blood levels and analgesic response, effective analgesia will not occur below some minimum blood level in a given patient. The minimum effective blood level for analgesia will, of course, vary among patients, especially among patients who have been previously treated with potent mu agonist opioids. Similarly, there is no predictable relationship between blood Morphine concentration and untoward clinical responses; again, however, higher concentrations are more likely to be toxic than lower ones.

For any fixed dose and dosing interval Morphine Sulfate Controlled or Sustained Release will have at steady state, a lower Cmax and a higher Cmin than conventional Morphine. This is a potential advantage: a reduced fluctuation in Morphine concentration during the dosing interval should keep Morphine blood levels more centered within the theoretical "therapeutic window." (Fluctuation for a dosing interval is defined as [Cmax-Cmin]/[Css-average].) On the other hand, the degree of fluctuation in serum Morphine concentration might conceivably affect other phenomena. For example, reduced fluctuations in blood Morphine concentrations might influence the rate of tolerance induction.

The elimination of Morphine occurs primarily as renal excretion of 3-morphine glucuronide. A small amount of the glucuronide conjugate is excreted in the bile, and there is some minor enterohepatic recycling; about 10% of the glucuronide conjugate is excreted in the feces. The elimination half-life of Morphine is reported to vary between 2 and 4 hours. Thus, steady-state is probably achieved on most regimens within a day. Because Morphine is primarily metabolized to inactive metabolites, the effects of renal disease on Morphine's elimination are not likely to be pronounced. However, as with any drug, caution should be taken to guard against unanticipated accumulation if renal and/or hepatic function is seriously impaired.

Autonomic reflexes are not affected by epidural or intrathecal Morphine.

Central nervous system effects of intravenously administered Morphine Sulfate are influenced by ability to cross the blood-brain barrier. When Morphine is introduced outside of the CNS (e.g., *intravenously*), plasma concentrations of Morphine remain higher than the corresponding CSF Morphine levels. Conversely, when Morphine is injected into the *intrathecal space*, it diffuses out into the systemic circulation slowly, accounting for the long duration of action of Morphine administered by this route.

The delay in the onset of analgesia following epidural or intrathecal injection may be attributed to its relatively poor liquid solubility (i.e., an oil/water partition coefficient of 1.42), and its slow access to the receptor sites. The hydrophilic character of Morphine may also explain its retention in the CNS and its low release into the systemic circulation, resulting in a prolonged effect.

Nausea and vomiting may be prominent and are thought to be the result of central stimulation of the chemoreceptor trigger zone. Histamine release is common; allergic manifestations of urticaria and, rarely, anaphylaxis may occur. Bronchoconstriction may occur either as an idiosyncratic reaction or from large dosages.

Morphine has a total plasma clearance which ranges from 0.9 to 1.2 L/kg/h (liters/kilogram/hour) in postoperative patients, but shows considerable interindividual variation. The major pathway of clearance is hepatic glucuronidation to morphine-3-glucuronide, which is pharmacologically inactive. Free Morphine is rapidly redistributed in parenchymatous tissues. For intravenously administered Morphine, 90% is excreted in the urine within 24 hours and traces are detectable in urine up to 48 hours. About 7-10% of administered Morphine eventually appears in the feces as conjugated Morphine. Terminal half-life is commonly reported to vary from 1.5 to 4.5 hours, although the longer half-lives were obtained when Morphine levels were monitored over protracted periods with very sensitive radioimmunoassay methods. The accepted elimination half-life in normal subjects is 1.5 to 2 hours.

Peak serum levels following epidural or intrathecal administration of Morphine Sulfate Injection are reached within 30 minutes in most subjects and decline to very low levels during the next 2 to 4 hours. The onset of action occurs in 15 to 60 minutes following epidural administration or intrathecal administration: analgesia may last up to 24 hours. Due to this extended duration of action, sustained pain relief can be provided with lower daily doses (by these two routes) than are usually required with intravenous or intramuscular Morphine administration.

"Selective" blockade of pain sensation is possible by neuraxial application of Morphine. In addition, duration of analgesia may be much longer by this route compared to systemic administration. However, CNS effects, associated with systemic administration, are still seen. These include respiratory depression, sedation, nausea and vomiting, pruritis and urinary retention. In particular, both early and late respiratory depression (up to 24 hours post dosing) have been reported following neuraxial administration. Circulation of the spinal fluid may also result in high concentrations of Morphine reaching the brain stem directly.

The incidence of unwanted CNS effects, including delayed respiratory depression, associated with neuraxial application of Morphine, is related to the circulatory dynamics of the epidural venous plexus and the spinal fluid. The lipid solubility and degree of ionization of Morphine plays an important part in both the onset and duration of analgesia and the CNS effects. Morphine has a pH_a 7.9, with an octanol/water partition coefficient of 1.42 at pH 7.4. At this pH, the tertiary amino group in each of the opioids is mostly ionized, making the molecule water soluble. Morphine, with additional hydroxyl groups on the molecule, is significantly more water soluble than any other opioid in clinical use.

Morphine, injected into the *epidural space*, is rapidly absorbed into the general circulation. Absorption is so rapid that the plasma concentration-time profiles closely resembled those obtained after intravenous or intramuscular administration. Peak plasma concentrations averaging 33-40 ng/mL (range 5-62 ng/mL) are achieved within 10 to 15 minutes after administration of 3 mg of Morphine. Plasma concentrations decline in a multiexponential fashion. The terminal half-life is reported to range from 39 to 249 minutes (mean of 90 ± 34.3 min) and, though somewhat shorter, is similar in magnitude as values reported after intravenous and intramuscular administration (1.5-4.5 h). CSF concentrations of Morphine, after epidural doses of 2 to 6 mg in post-operative patients, have been reported to be 50 to 250 times higher than corresponding plasma concentrations. The CSF levels of Morphine exceed those in plasma after only 15 minutes and are detectable for as long as 20 hours after the injection of 2 mg of epidural Morphine. Approximately 4% of the dose injected epidurally reaches the CSF. This corresponds to the relative minimum effective epidural and intrathecal doses of 5 mg and 0.25 mg, respectively. The disposition of Morphine in the CSF follows a biphasic pattern, with an early half-life of 1.5 h and a late phase half-life of about 6 h. Morphine crosses the dura slowly, with an absorption half-life across the dura averaging 22 minutes. Maximum CSF concentrations are seen 60-90 minutes after injection. Minimum effective CSF concentrations for postoperative analgesia average 150 ng/mL (range < 1-380 ng/mL).

The *intrathecal route* of administration circumvents meningeal diffusion barriers and, therefore, lower doses of Morphine produce comparable analgesia to that induced by the epidural route. After intrathecal bolus injection of Morphine, there is a rapid initial distribution phase lasting 15-30 minutes and a half-life in the CSF of 42-136 min (mean 90 ± 16 min). Derived from limited data, it appears that the disposition of Morphine in the CSF, from 15 minutes postintrathecal administration to the end of a six-hour observation period, represents a combination of the distribution and elimination phases. Morphine concentrations in the CSF averaged 332 ± 137 ng/mL at 6 hours, following a bolus dose of 0.3 mg of morphine. The apparent volume of distribution of Morphine in the intrathecal space is about 22 ± 8 mL.

Time-to-peak plasma concentrations, however, is similar (5-10 min) after either epidural or intrathecal bolus administration of Morphine. Maximum plasma Morphine concentrations after 0.3 mg intrathecal Morphine have been reported from < 1 to 7.8 ng/mL. The minimum analgesic Morphine plasma concentration during Patient-Controlled Analgesia (PCA) has been reported as 20-40 ng/mL, suggesting that any analgesic contribution from systemic redistribution would be minimal after the first 30-60 minutes with epidural administration and virtually absent with intrathecal administration of Morphine.

The pharmacokinetic parameters following oral administration of Morphine Sulfate sustained release, presented in the table below, show considerable intersubject variation, but are representative of average values reported in the literature. (See related table).

PHARMACODYNAMICS
The effects described below are common to all Morphine containing products.

CENTRAL NERVOUS SYSTEM
The principal actions of therapeutic value of Morphine are analgesia and sedation (i.e., sleepiness and anxiolysis).

The precise mechanism of the analgesic action is unknown. However, specific CNS opiate receptors and endogenous compounds with Morphine-like activity have been identified in at least three anatomical areas of the central nervous system—the periaqueductal-periventricular gray matter, the ventromedial medulla, and the spinal cord—and are likely to play a role in the expression of analgesic effects. Morphine appears to increase the patient's tolerance for pain, and to decrease the discomfort, although the presence of pain itself may still be recognized.

Morphine produces respiratory depression by direct action on brain stem respiratory centers. The mechanism of respiratory depression involves a reduction in the responsiveness of the brain stem respiratory centers to increases in carbon dioxide tension, and to electrical stimulation.

Morphine depresses the cough reflex by direct effect on the cough center in the medulla. Antitussive effects may occur with doses lower than those usually required for analgesia. Morphine causes miosis, even in total darkness. Pinpoint pupils are a sign of narcotic overdose but are not pathognomonic (e.g., pontine lesions of hemorrhagic or ischemic origins may produce similar findings). Marked mydriasis rather than miosis may be seen with worsening hypoxia.

While there is considerable variability in the relationship between Morphine blood concentration and analgesic response, effective analgesia probably will not occur below some minimum blood level in a given patient. The minimum effective blood level for analgesia will vary among patients, especially among patients who have been previously treated with potent μ-agonist opioids. Similarly, there is a considerable variability in the relationship between Morphine plasma concentration and untoward clinical responses, but higher concentrations are more likely to be toxic.

In contrast to immediate-release Morphine, after dosing with Morphine Sulfate, Sustained Release, the Morphine blood levels show reduced fluctuation between peak and trough plasma levels: that means that they are more centered within the theoretical "therapeutic window". On the other hand, the reduced fluctuation in Morphine plasma concentration might conceivably affect other phenomena, as for example, the rate of tolerance induction.

Morphine Sulfate, sustained release is an analgesic intended for patients who require chronic Morphine analgesia and who will have, in consequence, markedly different degrees of pharmacodynamic tolerance for opioid drugs. Morphine and similar opioids induce tolerance to their effects, so that a shortening of the duration of satisfactory analgesia may be the first sign of an increase in tolerance.

Once patients are started on Morphine, the dose required for satisfactory analgesia will rise, with the rate of development of tolerance varying, depending on the patient's prior narcotic use, level of pain, degree of anxiety, use of other CNS-active drugs, circulatory status, total daily dose, and the dosing interval.

GASTROINTESTINAL TRACT AND OTHER SMOOTH MUSCLE
Gastric, biliary and pancreatic secretions are decreased by morphine. Morphine causes a reduction in motility associated with an increase in tone in the antrum of the stomach and duodenum. Digestion of food in the small intestine is delayed and propulsive contractions are decreased. Propulative peristaltic waves in the colon are decreased, while tone is increased to the point of spasm. The end result is constipation. Morphine can cause a marked increase in biliary tract pressure as a result of spasm of sphincter of Oddi.

CARDIOVASCULAR SYSTEM
Morphine produces peripheral vasodilation which may result in orthostatic hypothension. Release of histamine can occur and may contribute to narcotic-induced hypotension. Manifestations of histamine release and/or peripheral vasodilation may include pruritus, flushing, red eyes and sweating.

INDICATIONS AND USAGE
Morphine is indicated for the relief of severe acute and severe chronic pain. Morphine Sulfate Controlled or Sustained Release is intended for use in patients who require repeated dosing with potent opioid analgesics over periods of more than a few days.

Morphine Sulfate injection is a systemic narcotic analgesic for administration by the intravenous, epidural or intrathecal routes. It is used for the management of pain not responsive to non-narcotic analgesics. Morphine Sulfate, administered epidurally or intrathecally, provides pain relief for extended periods without attendant loss of motor, sensory or sympathetic function.

Morphine Sulfate solution that is indicated only for intrathecal or epidural infusion in the treatment of intractable chronic pain was developed for use in continuous microinfusion devices and may require dilution before use as dictated by the characteristics of the device and the dosage requirements of the individual patient.

MORPHINE SULFATE SOLUTION FOR INTRATHECAL OR EPIDURAL INFUSION IS NOT RECOMMENDED FOR SINGLE-DOSE INTRAVENOUS, INTRAMUSCULAR OR SUBCUTANEOUS ADMINISTRATION DUE TO THE VERY LARGE AMOUNT OF MORPHINE IN THE AMPUL AND THE ASSOCIATED RISK OF OVERDOSAGE.

CONTRAINDICATIONS
Morphine Sulfate is contraindicated in patients with known hypersensitivity to the drug, in patients with respiratory insufficiency or depression in the absence of

resuscitative equipment, and in patients with acute or severe bronchial asthma. It is also contraindicated in patients with severe CNS depression; heart failure secondary to chronic lung disease; cardiac arrhythmias; increased intracranial or cerebrospinal pressure; head injuries; brain tumor; acute alcoholism; delirium tremens; convulsive disorders; after biliary tract surgery; suspected surgical abdomen; surgical anastomosis; concomitantly with MAO inhibitors or within 14 days of such treatment.

Morphine Sulfate is contraindicated in any patient who has or is suspected of having a paralytic ileus.

Morphine Sulfate Injection is contraindicated in those medical conditions which would preclude the administration of opioids by the intravenous route—allergy to Morphine or other opiates, acute bronchial asthma, upper airway obstruction. Administration of Morphine by the epidural or intrathecal route is contraindicated in the presence of infection at the injection site, anticoagulant therapy, bleeding diathesis, parenterally administered corticosteroids within a two week period or other concomitant drug therapy or medical condition which would contraindicate the technique of epidural or intrathecal analgesia.

WARNINGS
(See also "Clinical Pharmacology".)

IMPAIRED RESPIRATION
Respiratory depression is the chief hazard of all Morphine preparations. Respiratory depression occurs most frequently in the elderly and debilitated patients, as well as in those suffering from conditions accompanied by hypoxia or hypercapnia when even moderate therapeutic doses may dangerously decrease pulmonary ventilation.

Morphine should be used with extreme caution in patients with chronic obstructive pulmonary disease or cor pulmonale, and in patients having a substantially decreased respiratory reserve (e.g., emphysema, severe obesity, kyphoscoliosis, or paralysis of the phrenic nerve) hypoxia; hypercapnia; or preexisting respiratory depression. In such patients, even usual therapeutic doses of Morphine may decrease respiratory drive while simultaneously increasing airway resistance to the point of apnea.

Morphine Sulfate should not be given in cases of chronic asthma, upper airway obstruction, or in any other chronic pulmonary disorder without due consideration of the known risk of acute respiratory failure following Morphine administration in such patients.

HEAD INJURY AND INCREASED INTRACRANIAL PRESSURE
The respiratory depressant effects of Morphine with carbon dioxide retention and secondary elevation of cerebrospinal fluid pressure may be markedly exaggerated in the presence of head injury, other intracranial lesions, or preexisting increase in intracranial or intraocular pressure. Morphine produces effects which may obscure neurologic signs of further increases in pressure in patients with head injuries; pupillary changes (miosis) from Morphine may obscure the existence, extent and course of intracranial pathology. High doses of neuraxial Morphine may produce myoclonic events (see "Adverse Reactions"). Clinicians should maintain a high index of suspicion for adverse drug reactions when evaluating altered mental status or movement abnormalities in patients receiving this modality of treatment.

HYPOTENSIVE EFFECT
Morphine Sulfate, like all opioid analgesics, may cause severe hypotension in an individual whose ability to maintain his blood pressure has already been compromised by a depleted blood volume, impaired myocardial function, or a concurrent administration of drugs such as phenothiazines or general anesthetics. (See also "Precautions: Drug Interactions".) Morphine Sulfate may produce orthostatic hypotension in ambulatory patients.

Morphine Sulfate, like all opioid analgesics, should be administered with caution to patients in circulatory shock, since vasodilation produced by the drug may further reduce cardiac output and blood pressure.

HEPATIC OR RENAL DISEASE
The clearance of Morphine may be reduced in patients with hepatic dysfunction, while the clearance of its metabolites may be decreased in renal dysfunction. This will be manifested by both, a prolonged elimination half-life and the accumulation of levels of either Morphine or its metabolites in excess of those produced in normals, with the potential for an increase of adverse effects.

These changes in Morphine pharmacodynamics, in patients with hepatic and renal dysfunctions, should be considered when adjusting the dose and dosage intervals of Morphine Sulfate Sustained Release.

Care should also be exercised in administering Morphine Sulfate epidurally to patients with these conditions, since high blood Morphine levels, due to reduced clearance, may take several days to develop.

BILIARY SURGERY OR DISORDERS OF THE BILIARY TRACT
As significant Morphine is released into the systemic circulation from neuraxial administration, the ensuing smooth muscle hypertonicity may result in biliary colic.

DISORDERS OF THE URINARY SYSTEM
Initiation of neuraxial opiate analgesia is frequently associated with disturbances of micturition, especially in males with prostatic enlargement. Early recognition of difficulty in urination and prompt intervention in cases of urinary retention is indicated.

INTERACTIONS WITH OTHER CNS DEPRESSANTS
Morphine Sulfate, like all opioid analgesics, should be used with great caution and in reduced dosage in patients who are concurrently receiving other central nervous system depressants including sedatives or hypnotics, general anesthetics, phenothiazines, other tranquilizers and alcohol because respiratory depression, hypotension and profound sedation or coma may result.

INTERACTIONS WITH MIXED AGONIST/ANTAGONIST OPIOID ANALGESICS
From a theoretical perspective, agonist/antagonist analgesics (i.e., pentazocine, nalbuphine, butorphanol and buprenorphine) should NOT be administered to a patient who has received or is receiving a course of therapy with a pure opioid agonist analgesic. In these patients, mixed agonist/antagonist analgesics may reduce the analgesic effect or may precipitate withdrawal symptoms.

DRUG DEPENDENCE
Morphine Sulfate is a Schedule II narcotic under the United States Controlled Substance Act (21 U.S.C. 801-886).

Morphine can produce drug dependence and has a potential for being abused. Tolerance as well as psychological and physical dependence may develop upon repeated administration irrespective of the route of administration (oral, intravenous, intramuscular, intrathecal, epidural). Individuals with a prior history of opioid or other substance abuse or dependence, being more apt to respond to eurphorogenic and reinforcing properties of Morphine, would be considered to be at greater risk. Physical dependence, however, is not of paramount importance in the management of terminally ill patients or any patients in severe pain. Abrupt cessation or a sudden reduction in dose after prolonged use may result in withdrawal symptoms. After prolonged exposure to opioid analgesics, if withdrawal is necessary, it must be undertaken gradually. (See "Drug Abuse and Dependence".)

Infants born to mothers physically dependent on opioid analgesics may also be physically dependent and exhibit respiratory depression and withdrawal symptoms. (See "Drug Abuse and Dependence".)

Morphine Sulfate Injection administration should be limited to use by those familiar with the management of respiratory depression, and in the case of epidural or intrathecal administration, familiar with the techniques and patient management problems associated with epidural or intrathecal drug administration. Because epidural administration has been associated with lessened potential for immediate or late adverse effects than intrathecal administration, the epidural

APPROXIMATE[1] AVERAGE PHARMACOKINETIC PARAMETERS FOLLOWING ORAL DOSING OF MORPHINE SULFATE SUSTAINED RELEASE

Pharmacokinetic Parameter (scientific notation) (unit)		Dose of Morphine Sulfate Sustained Release		
		30 mg	60 mg	100 mg
Bioavailability (oral compared to injectable)		approximately 40%		
Time-to-peak plasma concentration $[T_{max}]$(h)	mean (range)	3.8 (1-7)	3.8 (2-7)	3.6 (1.5-12)
Peak plasma concentration $[C_{max}]$ (ng/mL) [single dose]	mean (range)	9.9 (5.0-18.6)	16.1 (10.0-25.3)	27.4 (14.1-46.1)
Volume of distribution (calculated from mean clearance and terminal half-life) $[Vd(\beta)]$ (L/kg)	mean	4 L/kg		

Dose metabolized = approximately 90%
Morphine metabolites (%) = morphine-3-glucuronide (55-75%), morphine-6-glucuronide (1-5%)

[1] Derived from pharmacokinetic studies in 24 normal volunteers

➤ SHOWN IN PRODUCT IDENTIFICATION GUIDE

route should be used whenever possible. Rapid intravenous administration may result in chest wall rigidity.

FACILITIES WHERE MORPHINE SULFATE INJECTION OR INFUSION IS ADMINISTERED MUST BE EQUIPPED WITH RESUSCITATIVE EQUIPMENT, OXYGEN, NALOXONE INJECTION, AND OTHER RESUSCITATIVE DRUGS. WHEN THE EPIDURAL OR INTRATHECAL ROUTE OF ADMINISTRATION IS EMPLOYED, PATIENTS MUST BE OBSERVED IN A FULLY EQUIPPED AND STAFFED ENVIRONMENT FOR AT LEAST 24 HOURS. AFTER THE INITIAL (SINGLE) TEST DOSE AND, AS APPROPRIATE, FOR THE FIRST SEVERAL DAYS AFTER CATHETER IMPLANTATION.

SEVERE RESPIRATORY DEPRESSION UP TO 24 HOURS FOLLOWING EPIDURAL OR INTRATHECAL ADMINISTRATION HAS BEEN REPORTED.

MORPHINE SULFATE SOLUTION FOR INTRATHECAL OR EPIDURAL INFUSION WAS DEVELOPED FOR USE (AFTER APPROPRIATE DILUTION, IF NECESSARY) IN CONTINUOUS MICROINFUSION DEVICES FOR INTRATHECAL OR EPIDURAL INFUSION OF NARCOTICS TO CONTROL SEVERE CANCER PAIN, CHRONIC NEURAXIAL OPIOID ANALGESIA IS APPROPRIATE ONLY WHEN LESS INVASIVE MEANS OF CONTROLLING PAIN HAVE FAILED AND SHOULD ONLY BE UNDERTAKEN BY THOSE WHO ARE EXPERIENCED IN APPLYING THE TREATMENT IN A SETTING WHERE ITS COMPLICATIONS CAN BE ADEQUATELY MANAGED.

RESERVOIR FILLING MUST BE PERFORMED BY FULLY TRAINED AND QUALIFIED PERSONNEL FOLLOWING THE DIRECTIONS PROVIDED BY THE DEVICE MANUFACTURER. CARE SHOULD BE TAKEN IN SELECTING THE PROPER REFILL FREQUENCY TO PREVENT DEPLETION OF THE RESERVOIR, WHICH WOULD RESULT IN EXACERBATION OF SEVERE PAIN AND/OR REFLUX OF CSF INTO SOME DEVICES. STRICT ASEPTIC TECHNIQUE IN FILLING IS REQUIRED TO AVOID BACTERIAL CONTAMINATION AND SERIOUS INFECTION. EXTREME CARE MUST BE TAKEN TO ENSURE THAT THE NEEDLE IS PROPERTY IN THE FILLING PORT OF THE DEVICE BEFORE ATTEMPTING TO REFILL THE RESERVOIR. INJECTING THE SOLUTION INTO THE TISSUE AROUND THE DEVICE OR (IN THE CASE OF DEVICES THAT HAVE MORE THAN ONE PORT) ATTEMPTING TO INJECT THE REFILL DOSE INTO THE DIRECT INJECTION PORT WILL RESULT IN A LARGE, CLINICALLY SIGNIFICANT, OVERDOSAGE TO THE PATIENT.

A PERIOD OF OBSERVATION APPROPRIATE TO THE CLINICAL SITUATION SHOULD FOLLOW EACH REFILL OR MANIPULATION OF THE DRUG RESERVOIR. BEFORE DISCHARGE. THE PATIENT AND ATTENDANT(S) SHOULD RECEIVE INSTRUCTION IN THE PROPER HOME CARE OF THE DEVICE AND INSERTION SITE AND IN THE RECOGNITION AND PRACTICAL TREATMENT OF AN OVERDOSE OF NEURAXIAL MORPHINE.

TOLERANCE AND MYOCLONIC ACTIVITY
PATIENTS SOMETIMES MANIFEST UNUSUAL ACCELERATION OF NEURAXIAL MORPHINE REQUIREMENTS, WHICH MAY CAUSE CONCERN REGARDING SYSTEMIC ABSORPTION AND THE HAZARDS OF LARGE DOSES; THESE PATIENTS MAY BENEFIT FROM HOSPITALIZATION AND DETOXIFICATION. TWO CASES OF MYOCLONIC-LIKE SPASM OF THE LOWER EXTREMITIES HAVE BEEN REPORTED IN PATIENTS RECEIVING MORE THAN 20 MG/DAY OF INTRATHECAL MORPHINE AFTER DETOXIFICATION. IT MIGHT POSSIBLE TO RESUME TREATMENT AT LOWER DOSES, AND SOME PATIENTS HAVE BEEN SUCCESSFULLY CHANGED FROM CONTINUOUS EPIDURAL MORPHINE TO CONTINUOUS INTRATHECAL MORPHINE. REPEAT DETOXIFICATION MAY BE INDICATED AT A LATER DATE. THE UPPER DAILY DOSAGE LIMIT FOR EACH PATIENT DURING CONTINUING TREATMENT MUST BE INDIVIDUALIZED.

PRECAUTIONS
(See also "Clinical Pharmacology.")

GENERAL
Morphine Sulfate Oral Solutions, Tablets and Capsules are intended for use in patients who require a potent opioid analgesic for relief of moderate to severe pain.

Morphine Sulfate Controlled Release is intended for use in patients who require more than several days continuous treatment with a potent opioid analgesic. The controlled-release nature of the formulation allows it to be administered on a more convenient schedule than conventional immediate-release oral Morphine products. (See "Clinical Pharmacology: Metabolism and Pharmacokinetics".) However, Morphine Sulfate Controlled Release does not release Morphine continuously over the course of a dosing interval. The administration of single doses of Morphine Sulfate Controlled Release on a q12 hour dosing schedule will result in higher peak and lower trough plasma levels than those that occur when an identical daily dose of Morphine is administered using conventional oral formulations on a q4h regimen. The clinical significance of greater fluctuations in Morphine plasma level has not been systematically evaluated. (See "Dosage and Administration".)

As with any potent opioid, it is critical to adjust the dosing regimen for each patient individually, taking into account the patient's prior analgesic treatment experience. Although it is clearly impossible to enumerate every consideration that is important to the selection of the initial dose and dosing interval of Morphine Sulfate controlled release, attention should be given to 1) the daily dose, potency, and characteristics of the opioid the patient has been taking previously (e.g., whether it is a pure agonist or mixed agonist/antagonist), 2) the reliability of the relative potency estimate used to calculate the dose of Morphine needed [N.B. potency estimates may vary with the route of administration], 3) the

degree of opioid tolerance, if any, and 4) the general condition and medical status of the patient.

Selection of patients for treatment with Morphine Sulfate should be governed by the same principles that apply to the use of Morphine or other potent opioid analgesics. Specifically, the increased risks associated with its use in the following population should be considered: the elderly or debilitated and those with severe impairment of hepatic, pulmonary or renal function: myxedema or hypothyroidism; adrenocortical insufficiency (e.g., Addison's Disease); CNS depression or coma; toxic psychosis; prostatic hypertrophy or urethral stricture; acute alcoholism; delirium tremens; kyphoscoliosis, or inability to swallow.

The administration of Morphine, like all opioid analgesics, may obscure the diagnosis or clinical course in patients with acute abdominal conditions. Morphine may aggravate preexisting convulsions in patients with convulsive disorders.

Morphine should be used with caution in patients about to undergo surgery of the biliary tract since it may cause spasm of the sphincter of Oddi. Similarly, Morphine should be used with caution in patients with acute pancreatitis secondary to biliary tract disease.

It is recommended that administration of Morphine Sulfate by the epidural or intrathecal routes be limited to the lumbar area. Intrathecal use has been associated with a higher incidence of respiratory depression than epidural use. Smooth muscle hypertonicity may result in biliary colic, difficulty in urination and possible urinary retention requiring catheterization. Consideration should be given to risks inherent in urethral catheterization, e.g., sepsis, when epidural or intrathecal administration is considered, especially in the perioperative period.

Elimination half-life may be prolonged in patients with reduced metabolic rates and with hepatic or renal dysfunction. Hence, care should be exercised in administering Morphine in these conditions, particularly with repeated dosing.

Control of pain by neuraxial opiate delivery, using a continuous microinfusion device, is always accompanied by considerable risk to the patients and requires a high level of skill to be successfully accomplished. The task of treating these patients must be undertaken by experienced clinical teams, well-versed in patient selection, evolving technology and emerging standards of care. For reasons of safety, it is recommended that administration of Morphine Sulfate Solution 200 and 500 (10 and 25 mg/mL, respectively) by the intrathecal route be limited to the lumbar area.

INFORMATION FOR PATIENTS
If clinically advisable, patients receiving Morphine Sulfate should be given the following instructions by the physician:

1. Morphine may produce psychological and/or physical dependence. For this reason, the dose of the drug should not be adjusted without consulting a physician.
2. Morphine may impair mental and/or physical ability required for the performance of potentially hazardous tasks (e.g., driving, operating machinery).
3. Morphine should not be taken with alcohol or other CNS depressants (sleep aids, tranquilizers) because addictive effects including CNS depression may occur. A physician should be consulted if other prescription medications are currently being used or are prescribed for future use.
4. For women of childbearing potential who become or are planning to become pregnant, a physician should be consulted regarding analgesics and other drug use.

DRUG INTERACTIONS
(See "Warnings".)

Generally, effects of Morphine may be potentiated by alkalizing agents and antagonized by acidifying agents. Analgesic effect of Morphine is potentiated by chlorpromazine and methocarbamol.

Morphine may increase anticoagulant activity of coumarin and other anticoagulants.

The concomitant use of other central nervous system depressants including sedatives or hypnotics, barbiturates, general anesthetics, phenothiazines, tranquilizers, MAO inhibitors, butyrophenones, tricyclic antidepressants, chloral hydrate, glutethimide, beta-blockers, furazolidone, and alcohol may produce additive depressant effects. Respiratory depression, hypotension and profound sedation or coma may occur. When such combined therapy is contemplated, the dose of one or both agents should be reduced. Opioid analgesics, including Morphine Sulfate may enhance the neuromuscular blocking action of skeletal muscle relaxants and produce an increased degree of respiratory depression. Premedication or intra-anesthetic use of neuroleptics with Morphine may increase the risk of respiratory depression.

CARCINOGENICITY/MUTAGENICITY/IMPAIRMENT OF FERTILITY
Studies of Morphine Sulfate in animals to evaluate the drug's carcinogenic and mutagenic potential or the effect on fertility have not been conducted.

PREGNANCY
Teratogenic Effects—Category C: Adequate animal studies on reproduction have not been performed to determine whether Morphine affects fertility in males or females. Morphine Sulfate is not teratogenic in rats at 35 mg/kg/day (thirty-five times the usual human dose) but does result in increased pup mortality and growth retardation at doses that narcotize the animal (> 10 mg/kg/day, ten times the usual human dose). There are no well-controlled studies in women, but marketing experience does not include any evidence of adverse effects on the fetus following routine (short-term) clinical use of Morphine Sulfate products. Although there is no clearly defined risk, such experience can not exclude the possibility of infrequent or subtle damage to the human fetus.

Morphine Sulfate should be used in pregnant women only when clearly needed. (See also *"Precautions: Labor and Delivery"* and *"Drug Abuse and Dependence"*.)

Nonteratogenic Effects: Infants born from mothers who have been taking Morphine chronically may exhibit withdrawal symptoms.

LABOR AND DELIVERY
Morphine Sulfate is not recommended for use in women during and immediately prior to labor. Occasionally, opioid analgesics may prolong labor through actions which temporarily reduce the strength, duration and frequency of uterine contractions. However, this effect is not consistent and may be offset by an increased rate of cervical dilatation which tends to shorten labor.

Neonates whose mothers received opioid analgesics during labor should be observed closely for signs of respiratory depression. A specific narcotic antagonist, naloxone, should be available for reversal of narcotic-induced respiratory depression in the neonate.

Intravenous Morphine readily passes into the fetal circulation and may result in respiratory depression in the neonate. Naloxone and resuscitative equipment should be available for reversal of narcotic-induced respiratory depression in the neonate. In addition, intravenous Morphine may reduce the strength, duration and frequency of uterine contraction resulting in prolonged labor.

Epidurally and intrathecally administered morphine readily passes into the fetal circulation and may result in respiratory depression of the neonate. Controlled clinical studies have shown that *epidural* administration has little or no effect on the relief of labor pain.

However, studies have suggested that in most cases 0.2 to 1 mg of Morphine *intrathecally* provides adequate pain relief with little effect on the duration of first stage labor. The second stage labor, though, may be prolonged if the parturient is not encouraged to bear down. A continuous intravenous infusion of naloxone, 0.6 mg/hr, for 24 hours after intrathecal injection may be employed to reduce the incidence of potential side effects.

Morphine Sulfate Injection, Preservative Free 200 and 500 (10 and 25 mg/mL, respectively) are too highly concentrated for routine use in obstetric neuraxial analgesia.

NURSING MOTHERS
Low levels of *Morphine* have been detected in the breast milk. Withdrawal symptoms can occur in breast-feeding infants when maternal administration of Morphine Sulfate is stopped. Ordinarily, nursing should not be undertaken while a patient is receiving Morphine Sulfate since Morphine may be excreted in the milk.

PEDIATRIC USE
Morphine Sulfate has not been evaluated systematically in children.

The pharmacodynamic effects of Morphine Sulfate in the aged are more variable than in the younger population. Patients will vary widely in the effective initial dose, rate of development of tolerance and the frequency and magnitude of associated adverse effects as the dose is increased. Initial doses should be based on careful clinical observation following "test doses", after making due allowances for the effects of the patient's age and infirmity on their ability to clear the drug, particularly in patients receiving epidural Morphine.

ADVERSE REACTIONS
The adverse reactions caused by Morphine are essentially those observed with other opioid analgesics. They include the following major hazards: respiratory depression, apnea, and to a lesser degree, circulatory depression; respiratory arrest, shock and cardiac arrest.

Note: THE SUSTAINED RELEASE OF MORPHINE FROM MORPHINE SULFATE SUSTAINED RELEASE SHOULD BE TAKEN INTO CONSIDERATION IN THE EVENT OF OCCURRING ADVERSE EFFECTS.

In general, side effects are amenable to reversal by narcotic antagonists. **NALOXONE HYDROCHLORIDE INJECTION AND RESUSCITATIVE EQUIPMENT SHOULD BE IMMEDIATELY AVAILABLE FOR ADMINISTRATION IN CASE OF LIFE THREATENING OR INTOLERABLE SIDE EFFECTS AND WHENEVER MORPHINE SULFATE SOLUTION THERAPY IS BEING INITIATED, THE RESERVOIR IS BEING REFILLED OR ANY MANIPULATION OF THE RESERVOIR SYSTEM IS TAKING PLACE.**

MOST FREQUENTLY OBSERVED
Constipation, light-headedness, dizziness, sedation, nausea, vomiting, sweating, dysphoria and euphoria.

Some of these effects seem to be more prominent in ambulatory patients and in those not experiencing severe pain. Some adverse reactions in ambulatory patients may be alleviated if the patient lies down.

LESS FREQUENTLY OBSERVED REACTIONS
Central Nervous System: Weakness, headache, agitation, tremor, uncoordinated muscle movements, seizure, paresthesia, alterations of mood (nervousness, apprehension, depression, floating feelings), dreams, muscle rigidity, transient hallucinations and disorientation, visual disturbances, insomnia and increased intracranial pressure.

Gastrointestinal: Dry mouth, constipation, biliary tract spasm, laryngospasm, anorexia, diarrhea, cramps and taste alterations.

Cardiovascular: Flushing of the face, chills, tachycardia, bradycardia, palpitation, faintness, syncope, hypotension and hypertension.

Genitourinary: Urine retention or hesitance, oliguria, reduced libido and/or potency.

Dermatologic: Pruritus, urticaria, other skin rashes, edema and diaphoresis.

Other: Antidiuretic effect, paresthesia, muscle tremor, blurred vision, depression of cough reflex, interference with thermal regulation, nystagmus, diplopia and miosis.

The most serious side effect is respiratory depression. Because of delay in maximum CNS effect with intravenously administered drug (30 min), rapid administration may result in overdosing. Bolus administration by the epidural or intrathecal route may result in early respiratory depression due to direct venous redistribution of Morphine to the respiratory centers in the brain. Late (up to 24 hours) onset of acute respiratory depression has been reported with administration by the epidural or intrathecal route and is believed to be the result of rostral spread. Reports of respiratory depression following intrathecal administration have been more frequent, but the dosage used in most of these cases has been considerably higher than that recommended. This depression may be severe and could require intervention (see *"Warning"* and *"Overdosage"* sections). Even without clinical evidence of ventilatory inadequacy, a diminished CO_2 ventilation response may be noted for up to 22 hours following epidural or intrathecal administration.

While low doses of intravenously administered Morphine have little effect on cardiovascular stability, high doses are excitatory, resulting from sympathetic hyperactivity and increase in circulating catecholamines. Excitation of the central nervous system resulting in convulsions may accompany high doses of Morphine given intravenously. Dysphoric reactions may occur and toxic psychoses have been reported. Epidural or intrathecal administration is accompanied by a high incidence of pruritus which is dose related but not confined to site of administration. Nausea and vomiting are frequently seen in patients following Morphine administration. Urinary retention which may persist for 10-20 hours following single epidural or intrathecal administration has been reported in approximately 90% of males. Incidence is somewhat lower in females. Patients may require catheterization (see *"Precautions"*). Pruritus, nausea/vomiting and urinary retention frequently can be alleviated by the intravenous administration of low doses of naloxone (0.2 mg).

Tolerance and dependence to chronically administered Morphine, by whatever route, is known to occur (see *"Drug Abuse and Dependence"* section).

> IMPROPER OR ERRONEOUS SUBSTITUTION OF MORPHINE SULFATE SOLUTION IN 200 OR 500 (10 OR 25 MG/ML, RESPECTIVELY) FOR REGULAR MORPHINE SULFATE SOLUTION (0.5 OR 1 MG/ML) IS LIKELY TO RESULT IN SERIOUS OVERDOSAGE, LEADING TO SEIZURES, RESPIRATORY DEPRESSION AND, POSSIBLY, FATAL OUTCOME.

The most serious adverse experiences encountered during continuous intrathecal or epidural infusion of Morphine Sulfate Solution are respiratory depression and myoclonus.

1. Single-dose neuraxial administration may result in acute or delayed respiratory depression for periods at least as long as 24 hours. **Severe respiratory depression, potentially life-threatening, can result from technical errors during refill, e.g., injection of Morphine Sulfate Solution outside the filling port, unintentional injection into the direct bypass-dosing port featured on some devices or local infiltration.**

2. *Tolerance and Myoclonus:* See *"Warnings"* for discussion of these and related hazards.

While low doses of intravenously administered Morphine have little effect on cardiovascular stability, high doses are excitatory, resulting from *sympathetic hyperactivity* and increase in circulatory catecholamines. Excitation of the central nervous system, resulting in *convulsions*, may accompany high doses of Morphine given intravenously.

Dysphoric reactions may occur after any size dose and *toxic psychoses* have been reported.

Pruritus: Single-dose epidural or intrathecal administration is accompanied by a high incidence of *pruritus* that is dose-related but not confined to the site of administration. Pruritus, following continuous infusion of epidural or intrathecal Morphine, is occasionally reported in the literature; these reactions are poorly understood as to their cause.

Urinary Retention: Urinary retention, which may persist 10 to 20 hours following single epidural or intrathecal administration, is a frequent side effect and must be anticipated primarily in male patients, with a somewhat lower incidence in females. Also frequently reported in the literature is the occurrence of urinary retention during the first several days of hospitalization for the initiation of continuous intrathecal or epidural Morphine therapy. Patients who develop urinary retention have responded to cholinomimetic treatment and/or judicious use of catheters (see *"Precautions"*).

Constipation: Constipation is frequently encountered during continuous infusion of Morphine; this can usually be managed by conventional therapy.

Headache: Lumbar puncture-type headache is encountered in a significant minority of cases for several days following intrathecal catheter implantation; this, generally, responds to bed rest and/or other conventional therapy.

Peripheral Edema: There are several reports of peripheral edema, including unexplained genital swelling in male patients, following infusion-device implant surgery.

TREATMENT OF THE MOST FREQUENT ADVERSE REACTIONS:
Constipation: Ample intake of water or other liquids should be encouraged. Concomitant administration of a stool softener and a peristaltic stimulant with the narcotic analgesic can be an effective preventive measure for those patients in need of therapeutics. If elimination does not occur for two days, an enema should be administered to prevent impaction.

In the event diarrhea occurs, seepage around a fecal impaction is a possible cause to consider before antidiarrheal measures are employed.

Nausea and Vomiting: Phenothiazines and antihistamines can be effective treatments for nausea of the medullary and vestibular sources respectively. However, these drugs may potentiate the side effects of the narcotic or the antinauseant.

Drowsiness (Sedation): Once pain control is achieved, undesirable sedation can be minimized by titrating the dosage to a level that just maintains a tolerable pain or pain free state.

DRUG ABUSE AND DEPENDENCE

Morphine Sulfate is a Schedule II substance under the Drug Enforcement Administration classification. Opioid analgesics may cause psychological and physical dependence (see *"Warnings"*). Cerebral and spinal receptors may develop tolerance/dependence independently, as a function of local dosage. Physical dependence results in withdrawal symptoms in patients who abruptly discontinue the drug or may be precipitated through the administration of drugs with narcotic antagonist activity, e.g., naloxone or mixed agonist/antagonist analgesics (pentazocine, etc.; see also *"Overdosage"*). Care must be taken to avert withdrawal in those patients who have been maintained on parenteral/oral narcotics when epidural or intrathecal administration is considered. Physical dependence usually does not occur to a clinically significant degree until after several weeks of continued narcotic usage. Tolerance, in which increasingly large doses are required in order to produce the same degree of analgesia, is initially manifested by a shortened duration of analgesic effect, and, subsequently, by decreases in the intensity of analgesia. Tolerance and psychological and physical dependence to Morphine may develop irrespective of the route of administration (intravenous, intramuscular, intrathecal, epidural or oral). Individuals with a prior history of opioid or other substance abuse or dependence, being more apt to respond to the euphorogenic and reinforcing properties of morphine, would be considered to be a greater risk.

In chronic pain patients, and in narcotic-tolerant cancer patients, the administration of Morphine Sulfate should be guided by the degree of tolerance manifested. Physical dependence, per se, is not ordinarily a concern when one is dealing with opioid-tolerant patients whose pain and suffering is associated with an irreversible illness.

If Morphine Sulfate is abruptly discontinued, a moderate to severe abstinence syndrome may occur. The opioid agonist abstinence syndrome is characterized by some or all of the following: restlessness, lacrimation, rhinorrhea, yawning, perspiration, gooseflesh, restless sleep or "yen" and mydriasis during the first 24 hours. These symptoms often increase in severity and over the next 72 hours may be accompanied by increasing irritability, anxiety, weakness, twitching and spasms of muscles: kicking movements; severe backache, abdominal and leg pains; abdominal and muscle cramps; hot and cold flashes, insomnia; nausea, anorexia, vomiting, intestinal spasm, diarrhea; coryza and repetitive sneezing; increase in body temperature, blood pressure, respiratory rate and heart rate. Because of excessive loss of fluids through sweating, vomiting and diarrhea, there is usually marked weight loss, dehydration, ketosis, and disturbances in acid-base balance. Cardiovascular collapse can occur. Without treatment most observable symptoms disappear in 5-14 days; however, there appears to be a phase of secondary or chronic abstinence which may last for 2-6 months characterized by insomnia, irritability, and muscular aches.

If treatment of physical dependence of patients on Morphine Sulfate is necessary, the patient may be detoxified by gradual reduction of the dosage. Gastrointestinal disturbances or dehydration should be treated accordingly.

Treatment of the abstinence syndrome is primarily symptomatic and supportive, including maintenance of proper fluid and electrolyte balance. If withdrawal has inadvertently been precipitated in a patient who requires narcotics for pain management, the withdrawal syndrome can be terminated rapidly by the administration of an appropriate dose of a pure agonist opioid, such as Morphine. The degree of physical dependence of a patient on Morphine Sulfate can be intentionally reduced by a gradual reduction of dosage and symptomatic treatment of withdrawal symptomatology.

The chance of drug dependence is substantially reduced when the patient is placed on scheduled narcotic programs instead of a "pain to relief-of-pain" cycle typical of a PRN regimen.

OVERDOSAGE

Note: THE SUSTAINED RELEASE OF MORPHINE FROM MORPHINE SULFATE SUSTAINED RELEASE SHOULD BE TAKEN INTO CONSIDERATION IN THE EVENT OF AN OVERDOSAGE.

Acute overdosage with Morphine is manifested by respiratory depression (a decrease in respiratory rate and/or tidal volume, Cheyne-Stokes respiration, cyanosis), with or without concomitant CNS depression, somnolence progressing to stupor or coma, skeletal muscle flaccidity, cold and clammy skin, constricted pupils, and, sometimes, bradycardia and hypotension.

In the treatment of overdosage, since respiratory arrest may result either through direct depression of the respiratory center or as the result of hypoxia, primary attention should be given to the re-establishment of a patent airway and institution of assisted or controlled ventilation. The pure opioid antagonist, naloxone, is a specific antidote against respiratory depression which results from opioid overdose. Naloxone (usually 0.4 to 2.0 mg) should be administered intravenously, simultaneously with respiratory resuscitation; however, because its duration of action is relatively short, the patient must be carefully monitored until spontaneous respiration is reliably re-established. If the response to naloxone is suboptimal or not sustained, additional naloxone may be re-administered, as needed, or given by continuous infusion to maintain alertness and respiratory function; however, there is no information available about the cumulative dose of naloxone that may be safely administered. If no response is observed after 10 mg of naloxone has been administered, the diagnosis of narcotic-induced, or partial narcotic-induced, toxicity should be questioned. Intramuscular or subcutaneous administration may be used if the intravenous route is not a available.

As the duration of effect of naloxone is considerably shorter than that of epidural or intrathecal Morphine, repeated administration may be necessary. Patients should be closely observed for evidence of renarcotization.

Naloxone should not be administered in the absence of clinically significant respiratory or circulatory depression secondary to Morphine overdose. Naloxone should be administered cautiously to persons who are known, or suspected to be physically dependent on Morphine Sulfate. In such cases, an abrupt or complete reversal of narcotic effects may precipitate an acute abstinence syndrome.

Note: In an individual physically dependent on opioids, administration of the usual dose of the antagonist will precipitate an acute withdrawal syndrome. The severity of the withdrawal syndrome produced will depend on the degree of physical dependence and the dose of the antagonist administered. Use of a narcotic antagonist in such a person should be avoided. If necessary to treat serious respiratory depression in the physically dependent patient, the antagonist should be administered with extreme care and by titration with smaller than usual doses of the antagonist.

Respiratory depression may be delayed in onset up to 24 hours following epidural or intrathecal administration. In painful conditions, reversal of narcotic effect may result in acute onset of pain and release of catecholamines. Careful administration of naloxone may permit reversal of side effects without affecting analgesia. Parenteral administration of narcotics in patients receiving epidural or intrathecal Morphine may result in overdosage.

Supportive measures (including oxygen, vasopressors) should be employed in the management of circulatory shock and pulmonary edema accompanying overdose as indicated. Cardiac arrest or arrhythmias may require cardiac massage or defibrillation.

When indicated, gut decontamination should be performed via emesis and/or activated charcoal (60 to 100 g in adults, 1 to 2 g/kg in children) with cathartic. With Morphine Sulfate sustained release, absorption may be expected to continue for many hours, particularly following an overdose, combined with decreased peristaltic activity of the gastrointestinal tract.

DOSAGE AND ADMINISTRATION

(See also *"Clinical Pharmacology," "Warnings"* and *"Precautions"* sections.)

Dosage of Morphine is a patient-dependent variable, which must be individualized according to patient metabolism, age and disease state and also response to Morphine. Each patient should be maintained at the lowest dosage level that will produce acceptable analgesia. As the patient's well-being improves after successful relief of moderate to severe pain, periodic reduction of dosage and/or extension of dosing interval should be attempted to minimize exposure to Morphine.

Note: Medication may supress respiration in the elderly, the very ill, and those patients with respiratory problems, therefore lower doses may be required.

IMMEDIATE RELEASE ORAL TABLETS, CAPSULES, SOLUTION, AND CONCENTRATED SOLUTION
Usual Adult Oral Dose: 5 to 30 mg every four (4) hours or as directed by physician. For control of pain in terminal illness, it is recommended that the appropriate dose of Morphine Sulfate, Immediate Release Oral Solutions, Morphine Sulfate, Immediate Release Oral Tablets or Morphine Sulfate, Immediate Release Oral Capsules be given on a regularly scheduled basis every four hours at the minimum dose to achieve acceptable analgesia. If converting a patient from another narcotic to Morphine Sulfate on the basis of standard equivalence tables, a 1 to 3 ratio of parenteral to oral Morphine equivalence is suggested. This ratio is conservative and may underestimate the amount of Morphine required. If this is the case, the dose of Morphine Sulfate, Immediate Release Oral Solutions. Morphine Sulfate, Immediate Release Oral Tablets or Morphine Sulfate, Immediate Release Oral Capsules should be gradually increased to achieve acceptable analgesia and tolerable side effects.

SPRINKLING CONTENTS OF CAPSULE ON FOOD OR LIQUIDS
Morphine Sulfate, Immediate Release Oral Capsules may be carefully opened and the entire beaded contents added to a small amount of cool, soft food, such as applesauce or pudding, or a liquid, such as water or orange juice. The bead-food mixture should be swallowed immediately and not stored for future use.

MORPHINE SULFATE CONTROLLED OR SUSTAINED RELEASE TABLETS
MORPHINE SULFATE CONTROLLED OR SUSTAINED RELEASE TABLETS ARE TO BE TAKEN WHOLE, AND ARE NOT TO BE BROKEN, CHEWED OR CRUSHED. TAKING BROKEN, CHEWED OR CRUSHED MORPHINE SULFATE CONTROLLED OR SUSTAINED RELEASE TABLETS COULD LEAD TO THE RAPID RELEASE AND ABSORPTION OF A POTENTIALLY TOXIC DOSE OF MORPHINE.

Morphine Sulfate controlled or sustained release is intended for use in patients who require more than several days continuous treatment with a potent opioid analgesic. The controlled- or sustained-release nature of the formulation allows it to be administered on a more convenient schedule than conventional immediate-release oral Morphine products. (See *"Clinical Pharmacology, Metabolism and Pharmacokinetics".*) However, Morphine Sulfate Controlled or Sustained Release does not release Morphine continuously over the course of the dosing interval. The administration of single doses of Morphine Sulfate Controlled or Sustained Release on a q12h dosing schedule will result in higher peak and lower trough plasma levels than those that occur when an identical daily dose of Morphine is administered using conventional oral formulations on a q4h regimen. The clinical significance of greater fluctuations in Morphine plasma level has not been systematically evaluated. If pain is not controlled for a full 12 hours, then the dosing interval should be shortened, but to no less than 8 hours.

As with any potent opioid drug product, it is critical to adjust the dosing regimen for each patient individually, taking into account the patient's prior analgesic treatment experience. Although it is clearly impossible to enumerate every consideration that is important to the selection of initial dose and dosing interval of Morphine Sulfate, controlled or sustained release, attention should be given to 1) the daily dose, potency and precise characteristics of the opioid the patient has been taking previously (e.g., whether it is a pure agonist or mixed agonist/antagonist), 2) the reliability ability of the relative potency estimate used to calculate the dose of Morphine needed [N.B. potency estimates may vary with the route of administration], 3) the fact that roughly only 40% of the Morphine Sulfate in Morphine Sulfate controlled or sustained release becomes available after pre-systemic metabolization in the intestinal wall and liver, 4) the degree of opioid tolerance, if any, and 5) the general condition and medical status of the patient.

The following dosing recommendations, therefore, can only be considered suggested approaches to what is actually a series of clinical decisions in the management of the pain of an individual patient.

CONVERSION FROM CONVENTIONAL ORAL MORPHINE TO MORPHINE SULFATE CONTROLLED OR SUSTAINED RELEASE
A patient's daily Morphine requirement is established using immediate-release oral Morphine (dosing every 4 to 6 hours). The patient is then converted to Morphine Sulfate Controlled or Sustained Release in either of two ways: 1) by administering one-half of the patient's 24-hour requirement as Morphine Sulfate Controlled or Sustained Release on an every 12-hour schedule; or, 2) by administering one-third of the patient's daily requirement as Morphine Sulfate Controlled or Sustained Release on an every eight hour schedule. With either method, dose and dosing interval is then adjusted as needed (see discussion below.) The 15 mg tablet should be used for initial conversion for patients whose total daily requirement is expected to be less than 60 mg. The 30 mg tablet strength is recommended for patients with a daily Morphine requirement of 60 to 120 mg. When the total daily dose is expected to be greater than 120 mg, the appropriate combination of tablet strengths should be employed.

CONVERSION FROM PARENTERAL MORPHINE OR OTHER OPIOIDS (PARENTERAL OR ORAL) TO MORPHINE SULFATE CONTROLLED OR SUSTAINED RELEASE
Morphine Sulfate Controlled or Sustained Release can be administered as the initial oral Morphine drug product; in this case, however, particular care must be exercised in the conversion process. Because of uncertainty about, and intersubject variation in, relative estimates of opioid potency and cross tolerance, initial dosing regimens should be conservative; that is, an underestimation of the 24 hour oral Morphine requirement is preferred to an overestimate. To this end, initial individual doses of Morphine Sulfate Controlled or Sustained Release should be estimated conservatively. In patients whose daily Morphine requirements are expected to be less than or equal to 120 mg per day, the 30 mg tablet strength is recommended for the initial titration period. Once a stable dose regimen is reached, the patient can be converted to the 60 mg or 100 mg tablet strength, or appropriate combination of tablet strengths, if desired.

Estimates of the relative potency of opioids are only approximate and are influenced by route of administration, individual patient differences, and possibly, by an individual's medical condition. Consequently, it is difficult to recommend any fixed rule for converting a patient to Morphine Sulfate Controlled or Sustained Release directly. The following general points should be considered, however.

1. Parenteral to Oral Morphine Ratio: Estimates of the oral to parenteral potency of Morphine vary. Some authorities suggest that a dose of oral Morphine only three times the daily parenteral Morphine requirement may be sufficient in chronic use settings.

2. Other Parenteral or Oral Opioids to Oral Morphine: Because there is lack of systemic evidence bearing on these types of analgesic substitutions, specific recommendations are not possible. Physicians are advised to refer to published relative potency data, keeping in mind that such ratios are only approximate. In general, it is safer to underestimate the daily dose of Morphine Sulfate Controlled or Sustained Release required and rely upon ad hoc supplementation to deal with inadequate analgesia. (See discussion which follows.)

USE OF MORPHINE SULFATE CONTROLLED OR SUSTAINED RELEASE AS THE FIRST OPIOID ANALGESIC
There has been no systematic evaluation of Morphine Sulfate Controlled or Sustained Release as an initial opioid analgesic in the management of pain.

Because it may be more difficult to titrate a patient using a controlled- or sustained-release morphine, it is ordinarily advisable to begin treatment using an immediate-release formulation.

CONSIDERATIONS IN THE ADJUSTMENT OF DOSING REGIMENS
Whatever the approach, if signs of excessive opioid effects are observed early in a dosing interval, the next dose should be reduced. If this adjustment leads to inadequate analgesia, that is, "breakthrough" pain occurs late in the dosing interval, the dosing interval may be shortened. Alternatively, a supplemental dose of a short-acting analgesic may be given. As experience is gained, adjustments can be made to obtain an appropriate balance between pain relief, opioid side effects, and the convenience of the dosing schedule.

In adjusting dosing requirements, it is recommended that the dosing interval never be extended beyond 12 hours because the administration of very large single doses may lead to acute overdose. (N.B. Morphine Sulfate Controlled or Sustained Release does not release Morphine continuously over the dosing interval.)

For patients with low daily Morphine requirements, the 15 mg tablet should be used.

CONVERSION FROM MORPHINE SULFATE CONTROLLED OR SUSTAINED RELEASE TO PARENTERAL OPIOIDS
When converting a patient from Morphine Sulfate Controlled or Sustained Release to parenteral opioids, it is best to assume that the parenteral to oral potency relationship is high. *Note that this is the converse of the strategy used when the direction of conversion is from the parenteral to oral formulations. In both cases, however, the aim is to estimate the new dose conservatively.* For example, to estimate the required 24-hour dose of Morphine for IM use, one could employ a conversion of 1 mg of Morphine IM for every 6 mg of Morphine as Morphine Sulfate Controlled or Sustained Release. Of course, the IM 24-hour dose would have to be divided by six and administered on a q4h regimen. This approach is recommended because it is least likely to cause overdose.

Note: MORPHINE SULFATE CONTROLLED OR SUSTAINED RELEASE TABLET MUST BE SWALLOWED WHOLE. DO NOT BREAK THE TABLET IN HALF. DO NOT CRUSH OR CHEW.

MORPHINE SULFATE INJECTION
Morphine Sulfate Injection is intended for intravenous, epidural or intrathecal administration.

INTRAVENOUS ADMINISTRATION
Dosage: The initial dose of Morphine should be 2 mg to 10 mg/70 kg of body weight. Patients under the age of 18; no information available.

EPIDURAL ADMINISTRATION
MORPHINE SULFATE INJECTION SHOULD BE ADMINISTERED EPIDURALLY ONLY BY PHYSICIANS EXPERIENCED IN THE TECHNIQUES OF EPIDURAL ADMINISTRATION AND WHO ARE THOROUGHLY FAMILIAR WITH THE LABELING. IT SHOULD BE ADMINISTERED ONLY IN SETTINGS WHERE ADEQUATE PATIENT MONITORING IS POSSIBLE. RESUSCITATIVE EQUIPMENT AND A SPECIFIC ANTAGONIST (NALOXONE HYDROCHLORIDE INJECTION) SHOULD BE IMMEDIATELY AVAILABLE FOR THE MANAGEMENT OF RESPIRATORY DEPRESSION AS WELL AS COMPLICATIONS WHICH MIGHT RESULT FROM INADVERTENT INTRATHECAL OR INTRAVASCULAR INJECTION. (NOTE: INTRATHECAL DOSAGE IS USUALLY 1/10 THAT OF EPIDURAL DOSAGE). PATIENT MONITORING SHOULD BE CONTINUED FOR AT LEAST 24 HOURS AFTER EACH DOSE, SINCE DELAYED RESPIRATORY DEPRESSION MAY OCCUR.

Proper placement of a needle or catheter in the epidural space should be verified before Morphine Sulfate Injection is injected. Acceptable techniques for verifying proper placement include: a) aspiration to check for absence of blood or cerebrospinal fluid, or b) administration of 5 mL (3 mL in obstetric patients) of 1.5% UNPRESERVED Lidocaine and Epinephrine (1:200,000) Injection and then observe the patient for lack of tachycardia (this indicates that vascular injection has *not* been made) and lack of sudden onset of segmental anesthesia (this indicates that intrathecal injection has *not* been made).

Epidural Adult Dosage: Initial injection of 5 mg in the lumbar region may provide satisfactory pain relief for up to 24 hours. If adequate pain relief is not achieved within one hour, careful administration of incremental doses of 1 to 2 mg at intervals sufficient to assess effectiveness may be given. No more than 10 mg/24 hr should be administered.

Thoracic administration has been shown to dramatically increase the incidence of early and late respiratory depression even at doses of 1 to 2 mg.

For continuous infusion an initial dose of 2 to 4 mg/24 hours is recommended. Further doses of 1 to 2 mg may be given if pain relief is not achieved initially.

Aged or debilitated patients—Administer with extreme caution (see *"Precautions"* section). Doses of less than 5 mg may provide satisfactory pain relief for up to 24 hours.

Epidural Pediatric Use: No information on use in pediatric patients is available.

INTRATHECAL ADMINISTRATION

NOTE: INTRATHECAL DOSAGE IS USUALLY 1/10 THAT OF EPIDURAL DOSAGE

MORPHINE SULFATE INJECTION SHOULD BE ADMINISTERED INTRATHECALLY ONLY BY PHYSICIANS EXPERIENCED IN THE TECHNIQUES OF INTRATHECAL ADMINISTRATION AND WHO ARE THOROUGHLY FAMILIAR WITH THE LABELING. IT SHOULD BE ADMINISTERED ONLY IN SETTINGS WHERE ADEQUATE PATIENT MONITORING IS POSSIBLE RESUSCITATIVE EQUIPMENT AND A SPECIFIC ANTAGONIST (NALOXONE HYDROCHLORIDE INJECTION) SHOULD BE IMMEDIATELY AVAILABLE FOR THE MANAGEMENT OF RESPIRATORY DEPRESSION AS WELL AS COMPLICATIONS WHICH MIGHT RESULT FROM INADVERTENT INTRAVASCULAR INJECTION. **PATIENT MONITORING SHOULD BE CONTINUED FOR AT LEAST 24 HOURS AFTER EACH DOSE, SINCE DELAYED RESPIRATORY DEPRESSION MAY OCCUR. RESPIRATORY DEPRESSION (BOTH EARLY AND LATE ONSET) HAS OCCURRED MORE FREQUENTLY FOLLOWING INTRATHECAL ADMINISTRATION.**

Intrathecal Adult Dosage: A single injection of 0.2 to 1 mg may provide satisfactory pain relief for up to 24 hours. **(CAUTION: THIS IS ONLY 0.4 TO 2 ML OF THE 0.5 MG/ML POTENCY OR 0.2 TO 1 ML OF THE 1 MG/ML POTENCY OF MORPHINE SULFATE INJECTION. DO NOT INJECT INTRATHECALLY MORE THAN 2 ML OF THE 0.5 MG/ML POTENCY OR 1 ML OF THE 1 MG/ML POTENCY. USE IN THE LUMBAR AREA ONLY IS RECOMMENDED.** Repeated intrathecal injections of Morphine Sulfate Injection are not recommended. A constant intravenous infusion of naloxone hydrochloride, 0.6 mg/hr, for 24 hours after intrathecal injection may be used to reduce the incidence of potential side effects.

Aged or debilitated patients — Administer with extreme caution (see *"Precautions"* section). A lower dosage is usually satisfactory.

Repeat Dosage: If pain recurs, alternative routes of administration should be considered, since experience with repeated doses of Morphine by the intrathecal route is limited.

Intrathecal Pediatric Use: No information on use in pediatric patients is available.

Parenteral drug products should be inspected for particulate matter and discoloration prior to administration, whenever solution and container permit.

Do not use if color is darker than pale yellow, if it is discolored in any way or if it contains a precipitate.

MORPHINE SULFATE SOLUTION FOR MICROINFUSION

MORPHINE SULFATE SOLUTION FOR MICROINFUSION 200 AND 500 (10 AND 25 MG/ML RESPECTIVELY) SHOULD NOT BE USED FOR SINGLE-DOSE NEURAXIAL INJECTION BECAUSE LOWER DOSES CAN BE MORE RELIABLY ADMINISTERED WITH THE STANDARD PREPARATION OF MORPHINE SULFATE SOLUTION FOR MICROINFUSION (0.5 AND 1 MG/ML).

CANDIDATES FOR NEURAXIAL ADMINISTRATION OF MORPHINE SULFATE SOLUTION FOR MICROINFUSION IN A CONTINUOUS MICROINFUSION DEVICE SHOULD BE HOSPITALIZED TO PROVIDE FOR ADEQUATE PATIENT MONITORING DURING ASSESSMENT OF RESPONSE TO SINGLE DOSES OF INTRATHECAL OR EPIDURAL MORPHINE. HOSPITALIZATION SHOULD BE MAINTAINED FOR SEVERAL DAYS AFTER SURGERY INVOLVING THE INFUSION DEVICE FOR ADDITIONAL MONITORING AND ADJUSTMENT OF DAILY DOSAGE. THE FACILITY MUST BE EQUIPPED WITH RESUSCITATIVE EQUIPMENT, OXYGEN, NALOXONE INJECTION AND OTHER RESUSCITATIVE DRUGS. BECAUSE OF THE RISK OF DELAYED RESPIRATORY DEPRESSION, PATIENTS SHOULD BE OBSERVED IN A FULLY EQUIPPED AND STAFFED ENVIRONMENT FOR AT LEAST 24 HOURS AFTER EACH TEST DOSE AND, AS INDICATED, FOR THE FIRST SEVERAL DAYS AFTER SURGERY.

Familiarization with the continuous microinfusion device is essential. The desired amount of Morphine should be withdrawn from the ampul through a microfilter. *To minimize risk from glass or other particles, the product must be filtered through a 5 μ (or smaller) microfilter before injecting into the microinfusion device.* If dilution is required, 0.9% Sodium Chloride Injection is recommended.

Intrathecal Dosage: The starting dose must be individualized, based upon in-hospital evaluation of the response to serial single-dose intrathecal bolus injections of regular Morphine Sulfate injection 0.5 mg/mL or 1 mg/mL, with close observation of the analgesic efficacy and adverse effects *prior* to surgery involving the continuous microinfusion device.

The recommended initial lumbar intrathecal dose range in patients with no tolerance to opioids is 0.2 to 1 mg/day. The published range of doses for individuals who have some degree of opioid tolerance varies from 1 to 10 mg/day. The upper daily dosage limit for each patient must be individualized.

Limited experience with continuous intrathecal infusion of Morphine has shown that the daily doses have to be increased over time. Although the rate of increase, over time, in the dose required to sustain analgesia is highly variable, an estimate of the expected rate of increase is shown in the following Figure.

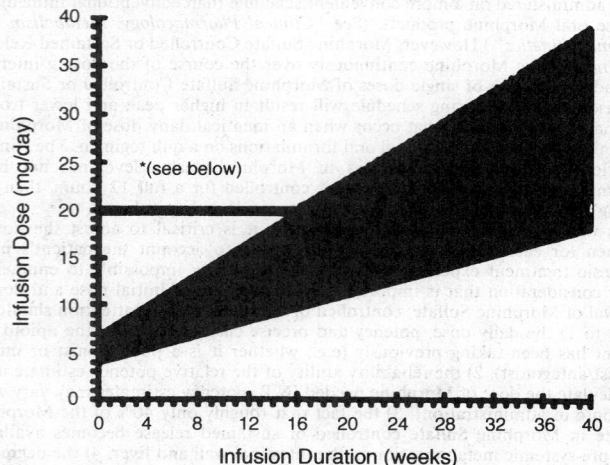

Figure:
DOSE TREND IN CONTINUOUS INFUSIONS OF INTRATHECAL MORPHINE (MEAN AND 95% CONFIDENCE INTERVALS)

*20 mg/day is the lowest dose for which regional myoclonus has been reported. The rate of occurrence cannot be estimated.

Doses above 20 mg/day should be employed with caution since they may be associated with a higher likelihood of serious side effects (see *"Warnings"*) concerning potential neurological hazards and *"Adverse Reactions"*.

Epidural Dosage: The starting dose must be individualized, based upon in-hospital evaluation of the response to serial single dose epidural bolus injections of regular Morphine Sulfate Solution for Microinfusion 0.5 mg/mL or 1 mg/mL, with dose observation for analgesic efficacy and adverse effects *prior* to surgery involving the continuous microinfusion device.

The recommended initial epidural dose in patients who are not tolerant to opioids ranges from 3.5 to 7.5 mg/day. The usual starting dose for continuous epidural infusion, based upon limited data in patients who have some degree of opioid tolerance, is 4.5 to 10 mg/day. The dose requirements may increase significantly during treatment, frequently to 20-30 mg/day. The upper daily limit for each patient must be individualized.

SAFETY AND HANDLING INFORMATION

> MORPHINE SULFATE SOLUTION FOR MICROINFUSION IS SUPPLIED IN SEALED AMPULS. ACCIDENTAL DERMAL EXPOSURE SHOULD BE TREATED BY THE REMOVAL OF ANY CONTAMINATED CLOTHING AND RINSING THE AFFECTED AREA WITH WATER.
>
> EACH AMPUL OF MORPHINE SULFATE SOLUTION FOR MICROINFUSION CONTAINS A LARGE AMOUNT OF POTENT NARCOTIC WHICH HAS BEEN ASSOCIATED WITH ABUSE AND DEPENDENCE AMONG HEALTH CARE PROVIDERS. **DUE TO THE LIMITED INDICATIONS FOR THIS PRODUCT, THE RISK OF OVERDOSAGE AND THE RISK OF ITS DIVERSION AND ABUSE, IT IS RECOMMENDED THAT SPECIAL MEASURES BE TAKEN TO CONTROL THIS PRODUCT WITHIN THE HOSPITAL OR CLINIC.** *MORPHINE SULFATE SOLUTION FOR MICROINFUSION SHOULD BE SUBJECT TO RIGID ACCOUNTING, RIGOROUS CONTROL OF WASTAGE AND RESTRICTIVE ACCESS.*
>
> **THIS PARENTERAL DRUG PRODUCT MUST BE INSPECTED FOR PARTICULATE MATTER BEFORE OPENING THE AMBER AMPUL AND AGAIN FOR COLOR AFTER REMOVING CONTENTS FROM THE AMPUL. DO NOT USE IF THE SOLUTION IN THE UNOPENED AMPUL CONTAINS A PRECIPITATE WHICH DOES NOT DISAPPEAR UPON SHAKING. AFTER REMOVAL, DO NOT USE UNLESS THE SOLUTION IS COLORLESS OR PALE YELLOW.**

Morphine Dosage Reduction: During the first two to three days of effective pain relief, the patient may sleep for many hours. This can be misinterpreted as the effect of excessive analgesic dosing rather than the first sign of relief in a pain exhausted patient. The dose, therefore, should be maintained for at least three days before reduction, if respiratory activity and other vital signs are adequate.

Following successful relief of severe pain, periodic attempts to reduce the narcotic dose should be made. Smaller doses or complete discontinuation of the narcotic analgesic may become feasible due to a physiologic change or the improved mental state of the patient.

STORAGE

Store tablets, capsules, and oral solutions at controlled room temperature 15°-30°C (59°-86°F).

Dispense in tight, light-resistant container.

Morphine Sulfate Injection and Solution for Microinfusion contain no preservative. **DISCARD ANY UNUSED PORTION. DO NOT AUTOCLAVE.**

Morphine Sulfate Controlled or Sustained Release is supplied as tablets that pose little risk of direct exposure to health care personnel and should be handled and disposed of in accordance with hospital policy. Patients and their families should be instructed to dispose of Morphine Sulfate Controlled or Sustained Release tablets, that are no longer needed, down the toilet.

J CODES
Per 10 mg SC,IM,IV—J2275
Up to 10 mg IM,IV,SC—J2270

HOW SUPPLIED
CAPSULE (C-II): 15 MG

BRAND/MANUFACTURER	NDC	SIZE	AWP
○ BRAND			
MSIR: Purdue Frederick	00034-1025-15	50s	$13.51

CAPSULE (C-II): 30 MG

BRAND/MANUFACTURER	NDC	SIZE	AWP
○ BRAND			
MSIR: Purdue Frederick	00034-1026-30	50s	$25.21

CONCENTRATE (C-II): 20 MG/ML

BRAND/MANUFACTURER	NDC	SIZE	AWP
○ BRAND			
MSIR: Purdue Frederick	00034-0523-01	30 ml	$15.83
	00034-0523-02	120 ml	$59.50

INJECTION (C-II):

AVERAGE UNIT PRICE (AVAILABLE SIZES)	
GENERIC	$0.89

BRAND/MANUFACTURER	NDC	SIZE	AWP
◆ GENERICS			
Goldline	00182-9139-65	20 ml	$16.50
ASTRAMORPH PF: Astra	00186-1150-02	10 ml 5s	$47.75

INJECTION (C-II): 0.5 MG/ML

AVERAGE UNIT PRICE (AVAILABLE SIZES)		GENERIC A-RATED AVERAGE PRICE (GAAP)	
GENERIC	$1.97	2 ml 10s	$80.19
		10 ml 10s	$116.59
		10 ml 25s	$313.50

BRAND/MANUFACTURER	NDC	SIZE	AWP
◆ GENERICS			
Schein	00364-3015-54	10 ml	$9.29
Schein	00364-3015-28	2 ml 10s	$76.78
ASTRAMORPH PF: Astra	00186-1159-03	2 ml 10s	$83.60
DURAMORPH PF: Elkins-Sinn	00641-1112-33	10 ml 10s	$86.04
Abbott Hosp	00074-2028-02	10 ml 10s	$147.13
Abbott Hosp	00074-4057-02	10 ml 10s	$298.66
Abbott Hosp	00074-3814-12	10 ml 25s	$328.34

INJECTION (C-II): 1 MG/ML

AVERAGE UNIT PRICE (AVAILABLE SIZES)		GENERIC A-RATED AVERAGE PRICE (GAAP)	
GENERIC	$1.31	10 ml 5s	$52.78
		2 ml 10s	$87.56
		10 ml 10s	$140.98
		10 ml 25s	$334.13

BRAND/MANUFACTURER	NDC	SIZE	AWP
◆ GENERICS			
Schein	00364-3016-54	10 ml	$9.80
Schein	00364-2469-58	60 ml	$11.55
Abbott Hosp	00074-6062-11	100 ml	$14.77
Abbott Hosp	00074-6062-02	250 ml	$19.74
Abbott Hosp	00074-6062-03	500 ml	$26.54
ASTRAMORPH PF: Astra	00186-1151-02	10 ml 5s	$51.00
ASTRAMORPH PF: Astra	00186-1153-12	10 ml 5s	$54.56
Schein	00364-3016-28	2 ml 10s	$82.98
ASTRAMORPH PF: Astra	00186-1160-03	2 ml 10s	$92.13
DURAMORPH PF: Elkins-Sinn	00641-1114-33	10 ml 10s	$92.19
Abbott Hosp	00074-2029-02	10 ml 10s	$189.76
Abbott Hosp	00074-6023-04	30 ml 10s	$164.35
Abbott Hosp	00074-4058-02	10 ml 25s	$318.25
Abbott Hosp	00074-3815-02	10 ml 25s	$350.02

INJECTION (C-II): 5 MG/10 ML

BRAND/MANUFACTURER	NDC	SIZE	AWP
◆ GENERICS			
ASTRAMORPH PF: Astra	00186-1152-12	10 ml 5s	$51.19

INJECTION (C-II): 10 MG/ML

BRAND/MANUFACTURER	NDC	SIZE	AWP
◆ BRAND			
INFUMORPH: Wyeth-Ayerst	00641-1131-31	20 ml	$156.00
◆ GENERICS			
Abbott Hosp	00074-3817-02	10 ml 25s	$408.80

INJECTION (C-II): 15 MG/ML

BRAND/MANUFACTURER	NDC	SIZE	AWP
◆ GENERICS			
Abbott Hosp	00074-3819-02	20 ml 25s	$531.41

INJECTION (C-II): 25 MG/ML

BRAND/MANUFACTURER	NDC	SIZE	AWP
◆ BRAND			
INFUMORPH: Wyeth-Ayerst	00641-1132-31	20 ml	$281.00

SOLUTION (C-II): 10 MG/5 ML

BRAND/MANUFACTURER	NDC	SIZE	AWP
○ BRAND			
MSIR: Purdue Frederick	00034-0521-02	120 ml	$8.33
	00034-0521-01	5 ml 10s ud	$4.75

SOLUTION (C-II): 20 MG/5 ML

BRAND/MANUFACTURER	NDC	SIZE	AWP
○ BRAND			
MSIR: Purdue Frederick	00034-0522-02	120 ml	$11.42

TABLET, EXTENDED RELEASE (C-II): 15 MG

BRAND/MANUFACTURER	NDC	SIZE	AWP
○ BRAND			
MS CONTIN: Purdue Frederick	00034-0514-25	25s ud	$19.81
	00034-0514-10	100s	$72.87
	00034-0514-90	500s	$346.18

TABLET, EXTENDED RELEASE (C-II): 30 MG

BRAND/MANUFACTURER	NDC	SIZE	AWP
◇ BRAND			
MS CONTIN: Purdue Frederick	00034-0515-25	25s	$39.57
ORAMORPH SR: Roxane	00054-4805-19	50s	$59.85
MS CONTIN: Purdue Frederick	00034-0515-50	50s	$72.87
ORAMORPH SR: Roxane	00054-4805-25	100s	$113.75
MS CONTIN: Purdue Frederick	00034-0515-10	100s	$138.49
ORAMORPH SR: Roxane	00054-4805-27	250s	$275.80
MS CONTIN: Purdue Frederick	00034-0515-45	250s	$335.76
	00034-0515-90	500s	$636.96

TABLET, EXTENDED RELEASE (C-II): 60 MG

BRAND/MANUFACTURER	NDC	SIZE	AWP
◇ BRAND			
MS CONTIN: Purdue Frederick	00034-0516-25	25s ud	$79.11
ORAMORPH SR: Roxane	00054-4792-25	100s	$221.90
MS CONTIN: Purdue Frederick	00034-0516-10	100s	$270.23
	00034-0516-90	500s	$1243.01

TABLET, EXTENDED RELEASE (C-II): 100 MG

BRAND/MANUFACTURER	NDC	SIZE	AWP
◇ BRAND			
MS CONTIN: Purdue Frederick	00034-0517-25	25s	$123.23
ORAMORPH SR: Roxane	00054-4793-25	100s	$359.80
MS CONTIN: Purdue Frederick	00034-0517-10	100s	$409.70
	00034-0517-90	500s	$1669.14

TABLET, EXTENDED RELEASE (C-II): 200 MG

BRAND/MANUFACTURER	NDC	SIZE	AWP
○ BRAND			
MS CONTIN: Purdue Frederick	00034-0513-25	25s ud	$230.43
	00034-0513-10	100s	$750.30

TABLETS (C-II): 15 MG

BRAND/MANUFACTURER	NDC	SIZE	AWP
○ BRAND			
MSIR: Purdue Frederick	00034-0518-15	50s	$7.89

TABLETS (C-II): 30 MG

BRAND/MANUFACTURER	NDC	SIZE	AWP
◇ BRAND			
ORAMORPH SR: Roxane	00054-8805-24	100s ud	$131.95

➤ SHOWN IN PRODUCT IDENTIFICATION GUIDE

TABLETS (C-II): 30 MG

BRAND/MANUFACTURER	NDC	SIZE	AWP
○ **BRAND**			
MSIR: Purdue Frederick	00034-0519-30	50s	$13.33

TABLETS (C-II): 60 MG

BRAND/MANUFACTURER	NDC	SIZE	AWP
◇ **BRAND**			
ORAMORPH SR: Roxane	00054-8792-11	25s ud	$65.10

TABLETS (C-II): 100 MG

BRAND/MANUFACTURER	NDC	SIZE	AWP
◇ **BRAND**			
ORAMORPH SR: Roxane	00054-8793-11	25s ud	$108.15

Morrhuate Sodium

DESCRIPTION

Morrhuate Sodium Injection, USP is a mixture of the sodium salts of the saturated and unsaturated fatty acids of cod liver oil. Morrhuate Sodium Injection, USP is prepared by the saponification of selected cod liver oils, it is overlaid with filtered Nitrogen to prevent discoloration that occurs on exposure to oxygen. Morrhuate Sodium occurs as a pale-yellowish, granular powder with a slight fishy odor and is soluble in water and in alcohol.

NOTE: Solid matter may develop a hazy appearance on standing and the injection should not be used if the solid matter does not dissolve completely on warming. The pH of the injection is adjusted to approximately 9.5.

CLINICAL PHARMACOLOGY

Morrhuate Sodium, when injected into the vein, causes inflammation of the intima and formation of a thrombus. This blood clot occludes the injected vein and fibrous tissue develops, resulting in the obliteration of the vein.

INDICATIONS AND USAGE

Morrhuate Sodium is used for the obliteration of primary varicosed veins that consist of simple dilation with competent valves.

Sclerotherapy should not be used in patients with significant valvular or deep vein incompetence. (See *"Precautions".*)

Although Morrhuate Sodium has been used as a sclerosing agent for the treatment of internal hemorrhoids, there is no substantial evidence that the drug is useful for this purpose. Most patients with symptomatic primary varicosed veins should be treated initially with compression stockings. If this treatment is inadequate, surgery may be required. Sclerosing agents may be useful as a supplement to venous ligation to obliterate residual varicosed veins or in patients who have conditions which increase the risk of surgery. However, many clinicians consider sclerotherapy if not effective may decrease the potential success of later surgery, should this be required.

CONTRAINDICATIONS

Morrhuate Sodium is contraindicated in patients who have shown a previous hypersensitivity reaction to the drug or to the fatty acids of cod liver oil. Continued administration of the drug is contraindicated when an unusual local reaction at the injection site or a systemic reaction occurs.

Thrombosis induced by Morrhuate Sodium may extend into the deep venous system in patients with significant valvular incompetence, therefore, valvular competency, deep vein patency, and deep vein competency should be determined by angiogrphy and/or by tests such as the Trendelenberg and Perthes before injection of sclerosing agents. The drug is contraindicated for obliterations of superficial veins in patients with persistent occlusion of the deep veins. Morrhuate Sodium is also contraindicated in patients with acute superficial thrombophlebitis; underlying arterial disease; varicosities caused by abdominal and pelvic tumors, uncontrolled diabetes mellitus, thyrotoxicosis, tuberculosis, neoplasms, asthma, sepsis, blood dyscrasias, acute respiratory or skin disease; and in bedridden patients. Treatment with Morrhuate Sodium should be delayed in patients with acute local or systemic infections (including infected ulcers). Extensive therapy with the drug is inadvisable in patients who are severely debilitated or senile.

PRECAUTIONS

Burning or cramping sensations indicate local reactions. Urticaria may result. Sloughing and necrosis of tissue may occur with extravasation of the drug. Technique development is essential for optimal success in sclerotherapy, therefore the drug should be administered only by a physician familiar with proper injection technique. Drowsiness and headache may occur rarely. Pulmonary embolism has been reported.

Rarely, patients may have, or may develop hypersensitivity to Morrhuate Sodium, characterized by dizziness, weakness, vascular collapse, asthma, respiratory depression, gastrointestinal disturbances (i.e., nausea, vomiting), and urticaria. Anaphylactic reactions may occur within a few minutes after injection of the drug and are most likely to occur when therapy is reinstituted after an interval of several weeks. Morrhuate Sodium should only be administered when adequate facilities, drugs (i.e., epinephrine, antihistamines, corticosteroids), and personnel are available for the treatment of anaphylactic reactions.

PREGNANCY

Safety in use of Morrhuate Sodium during pregnancy has not been established.

DOSAGE

Morrhuate Sodium is administered only by *Intravenous* Injection. Care must be taken to avoid extravasation. (See *"Precautions".*) Specialized references should be consulted for specific procedures and techniques of administration. When small veins are injected, or the injection solution is cold, or if solid matter has separated in the solution, the ampul or vial should be warmed by immersing in hot water. The solution should become clear on warming; only a clear solution should be used. Because the solution froths easily, a large bore needle should be used to fill the syringe, however, a small bore needle should be used for the injection.

To determine possible sensitivity to the drug, some clinicians recommend injection of 0.25-1 mL of 5% Morrhuate Sodium injection into a varicosity 24 hours before administration of a large dose.

Dosage of Morrhuate Sodium depends on the size and degree of varicosity. The usual adult dose for obliteration of small or medium veins is 50-100mg (1-2mL of the 5% injection). For large veins, 150-250 (3-5mL of the injection) is used. The drug may be given as multiple injections at one time or in single doses. Therapy may be repeated at 5-7 day intervals, according to the patient's response. Following injection of Morrhuate Sodium, the vein promptly becomes hard and swollen for 2-4 inches, depending on the size and response of the vein. After 24 hours, the vein is hard and slightly tender to the touch (with little or no periphlebitis). The skin around the injection becomes light-bronze; this color usually disappears shortly. An aching sensation and feeling of stiffness usually occur and last approximately 48 hours.

STORAGE

Store below 40° C (104° F) preferably in a refrigerator, or between 15-30° C (59-86° F).

HOW SUPPLIED
INJECTION: 5%

BRAND/MANUFACTURER	NDC	SIZE	AWP
○ **GENERICS**			
Palisades	53159-0003-01	30 ml	$30.18
CMC-Cons	00223-8541-30	30 ml	$49.50
Pasadena	00418-5411-30	30 ml 25s	$28.93

INJECTION: 50 MG/ML

BRAND/MANUFACTURER	NDC	SIZE	AWP
○ **GENERICS**			
Amer Regent	00517-3065-01	30 ml	$31.19

Motofen SEE ATROPINE SULFATE AND DIFENOXIN HYDROCHLORIDE

Motrin SEE IBUPROFEN

MRV SEE RESPIRATORY VACCINE, MIXED

M-R-Vax II SEE MEASLES AND RUBELLA VIRUS VACCINE LIVE

MS Contin SEE MORPHINE SULFATE

MSIR SEE MORPHINE SULFATE

MSTA Mumps Skin Test Antigen SEE MUMPS SKIN TEST ANTIGEN

Mucomyst SEE ACETYLCYSTEINE

Mudrane GG-2 SEE AMINOPHYLLINE/EPHEDRINE HYDROCHLORIDE/GUAIFENESIN/PHENOBARBITAL

◆ RATED THERAPEUTICALLY EQUIVALENT; ◇ THERAPEUTIC EQUIVALENCE UNCONFIRMED; ○ UNRATED

Multitest CMI *SEE* SKIN TEST ANTIGENS, MULTIPLE

Mulvidren-F *SEE* SODIUM FLUORIDE AND VITAMINS, MULTI

Mumps Skin Test Antigen

DESCRIPTION
NOT FOR IMMUNIZATION, DIAGNOSIS, OR TREATMENT
NOT FOR DIAGNOSIS OF IMMUNITY TO MUMPS

Mumps Skin Test Antigen, is a sterile suspension of killed mumps virus for intradermal use. It is prepared from the extraembryonic fluid of the virus-infected chicken embryo and is concentrated and purified by differential centrifugation. The virus is killed with formaldehyde solution, 1:1000, and is then diluted with isotonic sodium chloride solution. The resultant product contains approximately 0.012 molar glycine and less than 1:8,000 formaldehyde solution. Thimerosal (mercury derivative) 1:10,000 is added as a preservative. Each ml of the skin test antigen contains 40 complement-fixing units. This product after shaking is slightly opalescent in color.

CLINICAL PHARMACOLOGY
Information is available concerning the pharmacologic mode of action of skin test antigens.[1] Skin testing is a widely employed and readily available method of clinically assessing the cellular immune response. A positive skin-test reaction indicates previous antigen exposure, T-cell competence, an intact inflammatory response, and is an assessment of the cellular integrity of the immune response.[2]

Skin testing with Mumps Skin Test Antigen detects delayed-hypersensitivity.[2] Since most of the population (except for the very young) have had contact or infection with mumps virus,[3] they usually demonstrate a delayed-hypersensitivity reaction to Mumps Skin Test Antigen if an adequate cellular immune system exists.[4]

A single masked placebo-controlled study involving 90 cancer subjects was performed using Mumps Skin Test Antigen, Tetanus Toxoid Fluid, Mixed Respiratory Vaccine, Dermatophyton O, staphage lysate and PPD (Tubersol®). The injection sites were read at 48 and 72 hours. The number of positive reactors to Mumps Skin Test Antigen was greater than the number of positive subjects receiving the other antigens. None of the patients experienced any sloughing, necrosis, abscess formation, or painful lymphadenopathy as a result of the Mumps Skin Test Antigen skin test. This study demonstrated that Mumps Skin Test Antigen evoked a positive delayed-hypersensitivity (DH) reaction in immuno-competent individuals. The frequency of reactions in subjects with an impaired immune system was reduced. The sensitivity of Mumps Skin Test Antigen has been demonstrated by the fact that: 1) in all instances when any of the other test antigens were positive, Mumps Skin Test Antigen was also positive; and 2) several subjects showed a DH reaction to Mumps Skin Test Antigen but did not show a DH reaction to the other antigens.[2]

INDICATIONS AND USAGE
Mumps Skin Test Antigen, is indicated when detection of a delayed-hypersensitivity (DH) reaction is desired.

Mumps Skin Test Antigen has not been tested in persons immunized with live mumps vaccine; therefore, its safety and efficacy in this population group has not been established.

CONTRAINDICATIONS
MUMPS VIRUS FOR THE PREPARATION OF MUMPS SKIN TEST ANTIGEN IS PROPAGATED IN EGGS. THEREFORE, THIS PRODUCT SHOULD NOT BE ADMINISTERED TO ANYONE WITH A HISTORY OF HYPERSENSITIVITY (ALLERGY), ESPECIALLY ANAPHYLACTIC REACTIONS TO EGGS OR EGG PRODUCTS. IT IS ALSO A CONTRAINDICATION TO ADMINISTER MUMPS SKIN TEST ANTIGEN TO INDIVIDUALS KNOWN TO BE SENSITIVE TO THIMEROSAL. IN ANY CASE, EPINEPHRINE INJECTION (1:1000) MUST BE IMMEDIATELY AVAILABLE TO COMBAT UNEXPECTED ANAPHYLACTIC OR OTHER ALLERGIC REACTIONS.

WARNINGS
Neurologic complications, such as encephalopathies or peripheral-nervous systems disorders, or anaphylactic reactions have followed the administration of almost all biologics, although these have not been reported after the injection of Mumps Skin Test Antigen.

PRECAUTIONS
GENERAL
Epinephrine Injection (1:1000) must be immediately available to combat unexpected anaphylactic or other allergic reactions.

A separate, sterile syring and needle or a sterile disposable unit should be used for each individual patient to prevent transmission of hepatitis or other infectious agents from one person to another.

The antigen must be given intradermally. If it is injected subcutaneously, no reaction or an unreliable reaction may occur.

PREGNANCY
Reproductive Studies - Pregnancy Category C: Animal reproduction studies have not been conducted with Mumps Skin Test Antigen. It is not known whether Mumps Skin Test Antigen can cause fetal harm when administered to a pregnant woman or can affect reproduction capacity. Mumps Skin Test Antigen should be given to a pregnant woman only if clearly needed. There are no carefully done studies available on the effect of the drug on later growth, development, and functional maturation of the child.

USAGE IN NURSING MOTHERS
It is not known whether this drug is excreted in human milk. Because many drugs are excreted in human milk, caution should be exercised when Mumps Skin Test Antigen is administered to a nursing woman.

PEDIATRIC USE
Safety and effectiveness in children have not been established.

USAGE IN YOUNG ADULTS
Safety and effectiveness have not been established in young adults who have been immunized with live mumps vaccine.

ADVERSE REACTIONS
Local reactions may include tenderness, pruritis, vesiculation and rash. Sloughing, necrosis, abscess formation, or regional lymphadenopathy may be associated with unusually large DH reactions. Adverse reactions may include nausea, anorexia, headache, unsteadiness, drowsiness, sweating, sensation of warmth and lymphadenopathy. None of these reactions were noted in the clinical study.[2]

Epinephrine Injection (1:1000) must be immediately available to combat unexpected anaphylactic and other allergic reactions.

DOSAGE AND ADMINSTRATION
Parenteral drug products should be inspected visually for extraneous particulate matter and/or discoloration prior to administration.

SHAKE VIAL WELL before withdrawing each dose.

A separate, sterile syringe and needle or a sterile disposable unit should be used for each individual patient to prevent transmission of hepatitis or other infectious agents from one person to another.

An injection of 0.1 ml of the antigen is made on the inner surface of the forearm. Before injection, the skin over the site to be injected should be cleansed with a suitable germicide. Care should be taken to inject the test antigen intradermally.

Interpretation of Reactions: The reaction should be examined in 48 to 72 hours. A mean diameter (i.e., the longest width plus the longest length, divided by 2) of induration of 5 mm or more indicates a positive DH reaction to the antigen. A negative reaction, if the test dose has been given corrected, usually indicates either anergy or nonsensitivity. Pseudopositive reactions may develop in persons highly sensitive to egg protein.

Storage: Store between 2°-8°C (35°-46°F). DO NOT FREEZE.

REFERENCES
1. Holborow, E.J., et al: Immunology in Medicine. Second Edition, pp 19 and 121. Grune & Stratton, 1983. 2. Unpublished data available from Connaught Laboratories, Inc., compiled 1983. 3. Petersdorf, R.G.: Mumps. in Harrison's Principles of Internal Medicine, Ed. 7 (edited by M.M. Wintrobe, G.W. Thorn, R.D. Adams, E.Braunwald, K.J. Isselbacher, and R.G. Petersdorf) p 985. New York: McGraw-Hill Book Company, 1974. 4. Dempster, G.: Mumps in Textbook of Virology, Ed. 5 (edited by A.J. Rhodes and C.E. Van Rooyen) p 461 Baltimore: The Williams & Wilkins Co., 1968.

HOW SUPPLIED
INJECTION:

BRAND/MANUFACTURER	NDC	SIZE	AWP
○ BRAND			
MSTA MUMPS SKIN TEST ANTIGEN: Connaught	49281-0240-10	1 ml	$42.88

Mumps Virus Vaccine Live

DESCRIPTION
Mumps Virus Vaccine Live is a live virus vaccine for immunization against mumps.

Mumps Virus Vaccine Live is a sterile lyophilized preparation of the Jeryl Lynn (B level) strain of Mumps Virus. The virus was adapted to and propagated in cell cultures of chick embryo free of avian leukosis virus and other adventitious agents.

The reconstituted vaccine is for subcutaneous administration. When reconstituted as directed, the dose for injection is 0.5 ml and contains not less than the equivalent of 20,000 $TCID_{50}$ (tissue culture infectious doses) of the U.S. Reference Mumps Virus. Each dose contains approximately 25 mcg of neomycin. The product contains no preservative. Sorbitol and hydrolized gelatin are added as stabilizers.

CLINICAL PHARMACOLOGY
Mumps Virus Vaccine Live produces a modified, non-communicable mumps infection in susceptible persons. Extensive clinical trials have demonstrated that Mumps Virus Vaccine Live is highly immunogenic and well tolerated. A single injection of the vaccine has been shown to induce mumps neutralizing antibodies in approximately 97 percent of susceptible children and approximately 93 percent

of susceptible adults. The pattern of antibody response closely resembles that observed for natural mumps. Although the antibody level is significantly lower than that following natural infection, it is protective and long lasting. Vaccine-induced antibody levels have been shown to persist for at least 15 years with a rate of decline comparable to that seen in natural infection. If the present pattern continues, it will provide a basis for the expectation that immunity following vaccination will be permanent. However, continued surveillance will be required to demonstrate this point.

INDICATIONS AND USAGE

Mumps Virus Vaccine Live is indicated for immunization against mumps in persons 12 months of age or older. Most adults are likely to have been infected naturally and generally may be considered immune, even if they did not have clinically recognizable disease. A booster is not needed. It is not recommended for infants younger than 12 months because they may retain maternal mumps neutralizing antibodies which may interfere with the immune response.

Evidence indicates that the vaccine will not offer protection when given after exposure to natural mumps. Passively acquired antibody can interfere with the response to live, attenuated-virus vaccines. Therefore, administration of Mumps Virus Vaccine should be deferred until approximately three months after passive immunization.

Individuals planning travel outside the United States, if not immune, can acquire measles, mumps or rubella and import these diseases to the United States. Therefore, prior to International travel, individuals known to be susceptible to one or more of these diseases can receive either a single antigen vaccine (measles, mumps or rubella), or a combined antigen vaccine as appropriate. However Measles, Mumps, and Rubella Virus Vaccine Live is preferred for persons likely to be susceptible to mumps and rubella; and if single-antigen measles vaccine is not readily available travelers should receive Measles, Mumps, and Rubella Virus Vaccine Live regardless of their immune status to mumps or rubella.

Revaccination: Children vaccinated when younger than 12 months of age should be revaccinated. Based on available evidence, there is no reason to routinely revaccinate persons who were vaccinated originally when 12 months of age or older. However, persons should be revaccinated if there is evidence to suggest that initial immunization was ineffective.

USE WITH OTHER VACCINES

Routine administration of DTP (diphtheria, tetanus, pertussis) and/or OPV (oral poliovirus vaccine) concomitantly with measles, mumps and rubella vaccines is not recommended because there are insufficient data relating to the simultaneous administration of these antigens. However, the American Academy of Pediatrics has noted that in some circumstances, particularly when the patient may not return, some practitioners prefer to administer all these antigens on a single day. If done, separate sites and syringes should be used for DTP and Mumps Virus Vaccine Live.

Mumps Virus Vaccine Live should not be given less than one month before or after administration of other virus vaccines.

CONTRAINDICATIONS

Do not give Mumps Virus Vaccine Live to pregnant females; the possible effects of the vaccine on fetal development are unknown at this time. If vaccination of postpubertal females is undertaken, pregnancy should be avoided for three months following vaccination (see "*Precautions, Pregnancy*").

Anaphylactic or anaphylactoid reactions to neomycin (each dose of reconstituted vaccine contains approximately 25 mcg of neomycin).

History of anaphylactic or anaphylactoid reactions to eggs (see "*Hypersensitivity To Eggs*" below).

Any febrile respiratory illness or other active febrile infection.

Active untreated tuberculosis.

Patients receiving immunosuppressive therapy. This contraindication does not apply to patients who are receiving corticosteroids as replacement therapy, e.g., for Addison's disease.

Individuals with blood dyscrasias, leukemia, lymphomas of any type, or other malignant neoplasms affecting the bone marrow or lymphatic systems.

Primary and acquired immunodeficiency states, including patients who are immunosuppressed in association with AIDS or other clinical manifestations of infection with human immunodeficiency viruses; cellular immune deficiencies; and hypogammaglobulinemic and dysgammaglobulinemic states.

Individuals with a family history of congenital or hereditary immunodeficiency, until the immune competence of the potential vaccine recipient is demonstrated.

HYPERSENSITIVITY TO EGGS

Live mumps vaccine is produced in chick embryo cell culture. Persons with a history of anaphylactic, anaphylactoid, or other immediate reactions (e.g., hives, swelling of the mouth and throat, difficulty breathing, hypotension, or shock) subsequent to egg ingestion should be vaccinated only with extreme caution. Evidence indicates that persons are not at increased risk if they have egg allergies that are not anaphylactic or anaphylactoid in nature. Such persons may be vaccinated in the usual manner. There is no evidence to indicate that persons with allergies to chickens or feathers are at increased risk of reaction to the vaccine.

PRECAUTIONS
GENERAL
Adequate treatment provisions including epinephrine, should be available for immediate use should an anaphylactic or anaphylactoid reaction occur.

Children and young adults who are known to be infected with human immunodeficiency viruses but without overt clinical manifestations of immuno-suppression may be vaccinated; however, the vaccinees should be monitored closely for vaccine-preventable diseases because immunization may be less effective than for uninfected persons.

Vaccnation should be deferred for at least 3 months following blood or plasma transfusions, or administration of human immune serum globulin.

There are no reports of transmission of live Mumps Virus from vaccinees to susceptible contacts.

It has been reported that Mumps Virus Vaccine Live, may result in a temporary depression of tuberculin skin sensitivity. Therefore, if a tuberculin test is to be done, it should be administered either before or simultaneously with Mumps Virus Vaccine Live.

As with any vaccine, vaccination with Mumps Virus Vaccine Live may not result in seroconversion in 100% of susceptible persons given the vaccine.

PREGNANCY

Pregnancy Category C: Animal reproduction studies have not been conducted with Mumps Virus Vaccine Live. It is also not known whether Mumps Virus Vaccine Live can cause fetal harm when administered to a pregnant woman or can affect reproduction capacity. Therefore, Mumps Virus Vaccine should not be given to persons known to be pregnant; furthermore, pregnancy should be avoided for three months following vaccination. Although Mumps Virus is capable of infecting the placental and fetus, there is no good evidence that it causes congenital malformations in humans. Mumps Vaccine Virus also has been shown to infect the placenta, but the virus has not been isolated from the fetal tissues from susceptible women who were vaccinated and underwent elective abortions.

NURSING MOTHERS

It is not known whether Mumps Vaccine Virus is secreted in human milk. Therefore, because many drugs are excreted in human milk, caution should be exercised when Mumps Virus Vaccine Live is administered to a nursing woman.

ADVERSE REACTIONS

Burning and/or stinging of short duration at the injection site have been reported.

Anaphylaxis and anaphylactoid reactions have been reported.

Mild fever occurs occasionally. Fever above 103°F (39.4°C) is uncommon.

Mild lymphadenopathy has been reported.

Cough and rhinitis have been reported after vaccination with other mumps-containing vaccines.

Diarrhea has been reported after vaccination with mumps-containing vaccines.

Vasculitis has been reported rarely after vaccination with other mumps-containing vaccines.

Parotitis has been reported to occur in very low incidence, and orchitis rarely, in persons who were vaccinated. In most instances investigated, prior exposure to natural mumps was established. In other instances, whether or not this was due to vaccine or to prior natural mumps exposure or to other causes has not been established.

Reports of purpura and allergic reactions such as wheal and flare at the injection site or urticaria have been extremely rare. Erythema multiforme has also been reported rarely.

Forms of optic neuritis, including retrobulbar neuritis and papillitis may infrequently follow viral infections, and have been reported to occur 1 to 3 weeks following inoculation with some live virus vaccines.

Syncope, particularly at the time of mass vaccination, has been reported.

Very rarely encephalitis, febrile seizures, nerve deafness and other nervous system reactions have occurred in vaccinees. A cause-effect relationship has not been established.

DOSAGE AND ADMINISTRATION

FOR SUBCUTANEOUS ADMINISTRATION
Do not inject intravenously

The dosage of vaccine is the same for all persons. Inject the total volume (about 0.5 mL) of reconstituted vaccine subcutaneously, preferably into the outer aspect of upper arm. *Do not give immune serum globulin (ISG) concurrently with* Mumps Virus Vaccine Live.

Before reconstitution, store Mumps Virus Vaccine Live at 2-8°C(36-46°F). *Protect from light.*

CAUTION: A sterile syringe free of preservatives, antiseptics, and detergents should be used for each injection and/or reconstitution of the vaccine because these substances may inactivate the live virus vaccine. A 25 gauge, 5/8" needle is recommended. To reconstitute, use only the diluent supplied, since it is free of preservatives or other antiviral substances which might inactivate the vaccine.

Single Dose Vial: First withdraw the entire volume of diluent into the syringe to be used for reconstitution. Inject all the diluent in the syringe into the vial of lyophilized vaccine, and agitate to mix thoroughly. Withdraw the entire contents into a syringe and inject the total volume of restored vaccine subcutaneously.

It is important to use a separate sterile syringe and needle for each individual patient to prevent transmission of hepatitis B and other infectious agents from one person to another.

10 Dose Vial (available only to government agencies/institutions): Withdrawal the entire contents (7 mL) of the diluent vial into the sterile syringe to be used for reconstitution, and introduce into the 10 dose vial of lyophilized vaccine. Agitate to ensure thorough mixing. The outer labeling suggests "For Jet Injector or Syringe Use." Use with separate sterile syringes is permitted for containers of 10 doses or less. The vaccine and diluent do not contain preservatives; therefore, the user must recognize the potential contamination hazards and exercise special precautions to protect the sterility and potency of the product. The use of aseptic techniques and proper storage prior to and after restoration of the vaccine and subsequent withdrawal of the individual doses is essential. Use 0.5 mL of the reconstituted vaccine for subcutaneous injection.

It is important to use a separate sterile syringe and needle for each individual patient to prevent transmission of hepatitis B and other infectious agents from one person to another.

50 Dose Vial (available only to government agencies/institutions): Withdraw the entire contents (30 mL) of the diluent vial into the sterile syringe to be used for reconstitution and introduce into the 50 dose vial of lyophilized vaccine. Agitate to ensure thorough mixing. With full aseptic precautions, attach the vial to the sterilized multidose jet injector apparatus. Use 0.5 mL of the reconstituted vaccine for subcutaneous injection.

Each dose of Mumps Virus Vaccine Live contains not less than the equivalent of 20,000 $TCID_{50}$ of the U.S. Reference Mumps Virus. Parenteral drug products should be inspected visually for particulate matter and discoloration prior to administration. Mumps Virus Vaccine Live when reconstituted is clear yellow.

STORAGE
It is recommended that the vaccine be used as soon as possible after reconstitution. Protect vaccine from light at all times, since such exposure may inactivate the virus. Store reconstituted vaccine in the vaccine vial in a dark place at 2-8°C (36-46°F) and discard if not used within 8 hours.

HOW SUPPLIED
INJECTION:

BRAND/MANUFACTURER	NDC	SIZE	AWP
○ BRAND			
MUMPSVAX: Merck	00006-4753-00	1 ml	$14.76
	00006-4584-00	1 ml 10s	$132.00

Mumpsvax *SEE* MUMPS VIRUS VACCINE LIVE

Mupirocin

DESCRIPTION
Each gram of Mupirocin Ointment 2% contains 20 mg Mupirocin in a bland water miscible ointment base (polyethylene glycol ointment, N.F.) consisting of polyethylene glycol 400 and polyethylene glycol 3350. Mupirocin is a naturally occurring antibiotic. The chemical name is (E)-(2S, 3R, 4R, 5S)-5-[(2S, 3S, 4S, 5S)-2, 3-Epoxy-5-hydroxy-4-methyl-hexyl] tetrahydro -3,4- dihydroxy-β-methyl -2H-pyran-2-crotonic acid, ester with 9-hydroxynonanoic acid.

Following is its chemical structure:

CLINICAL PHARMACOLOGY
Mupirocin is produced by fermentation of the organism *Pseudomonas fluorescens.* Mupirocin inhibits bacterial protein synthesis by reversibly and specifically binding to bacterial isoleucyl transfer-RNA synthetase. Due to this mode of action, Mupirocin shows no cross resistance with chloramphenicol, erythromycin, fusidic acid, gentamicin, lincomycin, methicillin, neomycin, novobiocin, penicillin, streptomycin, and tetracycline.

Application of ^{14}C-labeled Mupirocin ointment to the lower arm of normal male subjects followed by occlusion for 24 hours showed no measurable systemic absorption (<1.1 nanogram Mupirocin per milliliter of whole blood). Measurable radioactivity was present in the stratum corneum of these subjects 72 hours after application.

Microbiology: The following bacteria are susceptible to the action of Mupirocin *in vitro:* the aerobic isolates of *Staphylococcus aureus* (including methicillin-resistant and β-lactamase producing strains), *Staphylococcus epidermidis, Staphylococcus saprophyticus,* and *Streptococcus pyogenes.*

Only the organisms listed in the *"Indications and Usage"* section have been shown to be clinically susceptible to Mupirocin.

INDICATIONS AND USAGE
Mupirocin Ointment is indicated for the topical treatment of impetigo due to: *Staphylococcus aureus,* beta hemolytic *Streptococcus**, and *Streptococcus pyogenes.*

CONTRAINDICATIONS
This drug is contraindicated in individuals with a history of sensitivity reactions to any of its components.

* Efficacy for this organism in this organ system was studied in fewer than ten infections.

WARNINGS
Mupirocin Ointment is not for ophthalmic use.

PRECAUTIONS
If a reaction suggesting sensitivity or chemical irritation should occur with the use of Mupirocin Ointment, treatment should be discontinued and appropriate alternative therapy for the infection instituted.

As with other antibacterial products prolonged use may result in overgrowth of nonsusceptible organisms, including fungi.

Mupirocin is not formulated for use on mucosal surfaces. Intranasal use has been associated with isolated reports of stinging and drying.

Polyethylene glycol can be absorbed from open wounds and damaged skin and is excreted by the kidneys. In common with other polyethylene glycol-based ointments, Mupirocin should not be used in conditions where absorption of large quantities of polyethylene glycol is possible, especially if there is evidence of moderate or severe renal impairment.

Pregnancy Category B: Reproduction studies have been performed in rats and rabbits at systemic doses, i.e., orally, subcutaneously, and intramuscularly, up to 100 times the human topical dose and have revealed no evidence of impaired fertility or harm to the fetus due to Mupirocin. There are, however, no adequate and well-controlled studies in pregnant women. Because animal studies are not always predictive of human response, this drug should be used during pregnancy only if clearly needed.

Nursing Mothers: It is not known whether Mupirocin is present in breast milk. Nursing should be temporarily discontinued while using Mupirocin.

ADVERSE REACTIONS
The following local adverse reactions have been reported in connection with the use of Mupirocin Ointment: burning, stinging, or pain in 1.5% of patients; itching in 1% of patients; rash, nausea, erythema, dry skin, tenderness, swelling, contact dermatitis, and increased exudate in less than 1% of patients.

DOSAGE AND ADMINISTRATION
A small amount of Mupirocin Ointment should be applied to the affected area three times daily. The area treated may be covered with a gauze dressing if desired. Patients not showing a clinical response within 3 to 5 days should be re-evaluated.

Store between 15° and 30°C (59° and 86°F).

HOW SUPPLIED
OINTMENT: 2%

BRAND/MANUFACTURER	NDC	SIZE	AWP
○ BRAND			
BACTROBAN: SK Beecham Pharm	00029-1525-22	15 gm	$14.50
	00029-1525-25	30 gm	$27.30

Muromonab-CD3

> **WARNING**
> ONLY PHYSICIANS EXPERIENCED IN IMMUNOSUPPRESSIVE THERAPY AND MANAGEMENT OF SOLID ORGAN TRANSPLANT PATIENTS SHOULD USE MUROMONAB-CD3.
> ANAPHYLACTIC OR ANAPHYLACTOID REACTIONS MAY OCCUR FOLLOWING ADMINISTRATION OF ANY DOSE OR COURSE OF MUROMONAB-CD3. SERIOUS AND OCCASIONALLY LIFE-THREATENING SYSTEMIC, CARDIOVASCULAR, AND CENTRAL NERVOUS SYSTEM REACTIONS HAVE BEEN REPORTED FOLLOWING ADMINISTRATION OF MUROMONAB-CD3. THESE HAVE INCLUDED: PULMONARY EDEMA, ESPECIALLY IN PATIENTS WITH VOLUME OVERLOAD; SHOCK; CARDIOVASCULAR COLLAPSE; CARDIAC OR RESPIRATORY ARREST; SEIZURES; AND COMA. HENCE, A PATIENT BEING TREATED WITH MUROMONAB-CD3 MUST BE MANAGED IN A FACILITY EQUIPPED AND STAFFED FOR CARDIO-PULMONARY RESUSCITATION. (SEE *"WARNINGS: CYTOKINE RELEASE SYNDROME, NEURO-PSYCHIATRIC EVENTS, ANAPHYLACTIC REACTIONS"*.)

DESCRIPTION
Muromonab-CD3 Sterile Solution is a murine monoclonal antibody to the CD3 antigen of human T cells which functions as an immunosuppressant. It is for intravenous use only. The antibody is a biochemically purified IgG_{2a} immunoglobulin with a heavy chain of approximately 50,000 daltons and a light chain of approximately 25,000 daltons. It is directed to a glycoprotein with a molecular weight of 20,000 in the human T cell surface which is essential for T cell functions. Because it is a monoclonal antibody preparation, Muromonab-CD3 Sterile Solution is a homogeneous, reproducible antibody product with consistent, measurable reactivity to human T cells.

Each 5 mL ampule of Muromonab-CD3 Sterile Solution contains 5 mg (1 mg/mL) of Muromonab-CD3 in a clear colorless solution which may contain a few fine translucent protein particles. Each ampule contains a buffered solution (pH 7.0 ± 0.5) of monobasic sodium phosphate (2.25 mg), dibasic sodium phosphate

(9.0 mg), sodium chloride (43 mg), and polysorbate 80 (1.0 mg) in water for injection.

The proper name, Muromonab-CD3, is derived from the descriptive term murine monoclonal antibody. The CD3 designation identifies the specificity of the antibody as the Cell Differentiation (CD) cluster 3 defined by the First International Workshop on Human Leukocyte Differentiation Antigens.

CLINICAL PHARMACOLOGY

Muromonab-CD3 reverses graft rejection, most probably by blocking the function of all T cells which play a major role in acute allograft rejection. Muromonab-CD3 reacts with and blocks the function of a 20,000 dalton molecule (CD3) in the membrane of human T cells that has been associated *in vitro* with the antigen recognition structure of T cells and is essential for signal transduction. In *in vitro* cytolytic assays, Muromonab-CD3 blocks both the generation and function of effector cells. Binding of Muromonab-CD3 to T lymphocytes results in early activation of T cells, which leads to cytokine release, followed by blocking T cell functions. After termination of Muromonab-CD3 therapy, T cell function usually returns to normal within one week.

In vivo, Muromonab-CD3 reacts with most peripheral blood T cells and T cells in body tissues, but has not been found to react with other hematopoietic elements or other tissues of the body.

A rapid and concomitant decrease in the number of circulating CD2 positive, CD3 positive, CD4 positive, and CD8 positive T cells has been observed within minutes after the administration of Muromonab-CD3. This decrease in the number of CD3 positive T cells results from the specific interaction between Muromonab-CD3 and the CD3 antigen on the surface of all T lymphocytes. T cell activation results in the release of numerous cytokines/lymphokines, which are felt to be responsible for many of the acute clinical manifestations seen following Muromonab-CD3 administration (see *"Warnings: Cytokine Release Syndrome, Neuro-Psychiatric Events"*).

While CD3 positive cells are not detectable between days two and seven, increasing numbers of circulating CD4 and CD8 positive cells have been observed. The presence of these CD4 and CD8 positive cells has not been shown to affect reversal of rejection. After termination of Muromonab-CD3 therapy, CD3 positive cells reappear rapidly and reach pretreatment levels within a week. In some patients however, increasing numbers of CD3 positive cells have been observed prior to termination of Muromonab-CD3 therapy. This reappearance of CD3 positive cells has been attributed to the development of neutralizing antibodies to Muromonab-CD3, which in turn block its ability to bind to the CD3 antigen on T lymphocytes (see *"Precautions: Sensitization"*). In the initial clinical trials using low doses of prednisone and azathioprine during Muromonab-CD3 therapy for renal allograft rejection, antibodies to Muromonab-CD3 were observed with an incidence of 21% (n = 43) for IgM, 86% (n = 43) for IgG and 29% (n = 35) for IgE. The mean time of appearance of IgG antibodies was 20±2 (mean ±SD) days. Early IgG antibodies appeared towards the end of the second week of treatment in 3% (n = 86) of the patients.

Subsequent clinical experience has shown that the dose, duration, and type of immunosuppressive medications used in combination with Muromonab-CD3 may affect both the incidence and magnitude of the host antibody response. Furthermore, immunosuppressive agents used concomitantly with Muromonab-CD3 (i.e., steroids, azathioprine, prednisone, or cyclosporine) have altered the time course of anti-mouse antibody development and the specificity of the antibodies formed (i.e., idiotypic, isotypic, allotypic).

Serum levels of Muromonab-CD3 are measurable using an enzyme-linked immunosorbent assay (ELISA). During the initial clinical trials in renal allograft rejection, in patients treated with 5 mg per day for 14 days, mean serum trough levels of the drug rose over the first three days and then averaged 900 ng/mL on days 3 to 14. Subsequent clinical experience has demonstrated that circulating serum levels greater than 800 ng/mL of Muromonab-CD3 blocks the function of cytotoxic T cells *in vitro* and *in vivo* (see *"Precautions: Laboratory Tests"*).

Following administration of Muromonab-CD3 *in vivo*, leukocytes have been observed in cerebrospinal and peritoneal fluids. The mechanism for this effect is not completely understood, but probably is related to cytokines altering membrane permeability, rather than an active inflammatory process (see *"Warnings: Cytokine Release Syndrome, Neuro-Psychiatric Events"*).

INDICATIONS AND USAGE

Muromonab-CD3 is indicated for the treatment of acute allograft rejection in renal transplant patients.

Muromonab-CD3 is also indicated for the treatment of steroid-resistant acute allograft rejection in cardiac and hepatic transplant patients.

ACUTE RENAL REJECTION

In a controlled randomized clinical trial, Muromonab-CD3 was significantly more effective than conventional high-dose steroid therapy in reversing acute renal allograft rejection. In this trial, 122 evaluable patients undergoing acute rejection of cadaveric renal transplants were treated either with Muromonab-CD3 daily for a mean of 14 days, with concomitant lowering of the dosage of azathioprine and maintenance steroids (62 patients), or with conventional high dose steroids (60 patients) Muromonab-CD3 reversed 94% of the rejections compared to a 75% reversal rate obtained with conventional high-dose steroid treatment (p = 0.006). The one year Kaplan-Meier (actuarial) estimates of graft survival rates for these patients who had acute rejection were 62% and 45% for Muromonab-CD3 and steroid-treated patients, respectively (p = 0.04). At two years the rates were 56% and 42%, respectively (p = 0.06).

One- and two-year patient survivals were not significantly different between the two groups, being 85% and 75% for Muromonab-CD3 treated patients and 90% and 85% for steroid-treated patients.

In additional open clinical trials, the observed rate of reversal of acute renal allograft rejection was 92% (n = 126) for Muromonab-CD3 therapy Muromonab-CD3 was also effective in reversing acute renal allograft rejections in 65% (n = 225) of cases where steroids and lymphocyte immune globulin preparations were contraindicated or were not successful (rescue).

ACUTE CARDIAC OR HEPATIC ALLOGRAFT REJECTION

Muromonab-CD3 has also been shown to be effective in reversing acute cardiac and hepatic allograft rejection in patients who are unresponsive to high-doses of steroids. Controlled randomized trials have not been conducted to evaluate the effectiveness of Muromonab-CD3 compared to conventional therapy as first line treatment for acute cardiac and hepatic allograft rejection.

The rate of reversal in acute cardiac allograft rejection was 90% (n = 61) and was 83% for hepatic allograft rejection (n = 124) in patients unresponsive to treatment with steroids. The dosage of other immunosuppressive agents used in conjunction with Muromonab-CD3 should be reduced to the lowest level compatible with an effective immunosuppressive response (see *"Warnings"* and *"Adverse Reactions: Infections, Neoplasia; Dosage and Administration"*).

UNLABELED USES

Muromonab-CD3 is used alone or as an adjunct in the treatment of allogeneic bone marrow transplantation prophylaxis and reversal of pancreas transplantation rejection.

CONTRAINDICATIONS

Muromonab-CD3 should not be given to patients who:

- are hypersensitive to this or any other product of murine origin;
- have anti-mouse antibody titers ≥ 1:1000;
- are in (uncompensated) heart failure or in fluid overload, as evidenced by chest X-ray or a greater than 3 percent weight gain within the week prior to planned Muromonab-CD3 administration;
- have a history of seizures, or are predisposed to seizures;
- are determined and/or suspected to be pregnant, or who are breast-feeding (see *"Precautions: Pregnancy, Nursing Mothers"*).

WARNINGS

See *"Boxed Warning"*.

CYTOKINE RELEASE SYNDROME

Temporarily associated with the administration of the first few doses of Muromonab-CD3 (particularly, the first two to three doses), most patients have developed an acute clinical syndrome [i.e., Cytokine Release Syndrome (CRS)] that has been attributed to the release of cytokines by activated lymphocytes or monocytes. This clinical syndrome has ranged from a more frequently reported mild, self-limited, "flu-like" illness to a less frequently reported severe, life-threatening, shock-like reaction, which may include serious cardiovascular and central nervous system manifestations. The syndrome typically begins approximately 30 to 60 minutes after administration of a dose of Muromonab-CD3 but may occur later) and may persist for several hours. The frequency and severity of this symptom complex is usually greatest with the first dose. With each successive dose of Muromonab-CD3, both the frequency and severity of the Cytokine Release Syndrome tends to diminish. Increasing the amount of a dose or resuming treatment after a hiatus may result in a reappearance of the CRS.

Common Clinical Manifestations of the Cytokine Release Syndrome may include: high (often spiking, up to 107°F) fever, chills/rigors, headache, tremor, nausea/ vomiting, diarrhea, abdominal pain, malaise, muscle/joint aches and pains, and generalized weakness. Less frequently reported adverse experiences include; minor dermatologic reactions (e.g., rash, pruritus, etc.) and a spectrum of often serious, occasionally fatal, cardiorespiratory and neuro-psychiatric adverse experiences (see *"Warnings,"* *"Precautions,"* and *"Adverse Reactions: Neuro-Psychiatric Events"*).

Cardiorespiratory Findings may include: dyspnea, shortness of breath, bronchospasm/wheezing, tachypnea, respiratory arrest/failure/distress, cardiovascular collapse, cardiac arrest, angina/myocardial infarction, chest pain/tightness, tachycardia, hypertension, hemodynamic instability, hypotension including profound shock, heart failure, pulmonary edema (cardiogenic and non-cardiogenic), adult respiratory distress syndrome, hypoxemia, apnea, and arrhythmias (see *"Boxed Warning;"* *"Precautions;"* and *"Adverse Reactions"*).

In the initial renal rejection studies, the most serious post-dose reaction-potentially fatal, severe *pulmonary edema*—occurred in 4.7% of the initial 107 patients. Fluid overload was present before treatment in all of these cases. However, it occurred in 0.0% of the subsequent 311 patients treated with first-dose volume/weight restrictions. In subsequent trials and in post-marketing experience, severe pulmonary edema has occurred in patients who appeared to be euvolemic. The pathogenesis of pulmonary edema may involve all or some of the following: volume overload; increased pulmonary vascular permeability; and/or reduced left ventricular compliance/contractility.

During the first 1 to 3 days of Muromonab-CD3 therapy, some patients have experienced an acute and transient decline in the glomerular filtration rate (GFR) and diminished urine output with a resulting *increase in the level of serum creatinine.* Massive release of cytokines appears to lead to reversible renal functional impairment and/or delayed renal allograft function. Similarly, transient elevations in hepatic transaminases have been reported following administration of the first few doses of Muromonab-CD3.

Patients at Risk for more serious complications of the Cytokine Release Syndrome may include those with the following conditions: unstable angina; recent myocardial infarction or symptomatic ischemic heart disease; heart failure of any etiology; pulmonary edema of any etiology; any form of chronic obstructive pulmonary disease; intravascular volume overload or depletion of any etiology (e.g., excessive dialysis, recent intensive diuresis, blood loss, etc.); cerebrovascular disease; patients with advanced symptomatic vascular disease or neuropathy; a history of seizures; and septic shock. Efforts should be made to correct or stabilize background conditions prior to the initiation of therapy.

Prior to administration of Muromonab-CD3, the patient's volume (fluid) status should be assessed carefully. It is imperative, especially prior to the first few doses, that there be no clinical evidence of volume overload or uncompensated heart failure, including a clear chest X-ray and weight restriction of $\leq$ 3% above the patient's minimum weight during the week prior to injection.

Manifestations of the Cytokine Release Syndrome may be prevented or minimized: by pretreatment with 8 mg/kg of methylprednisolone (i.e., high-dose steroids), given 1 to 4 hours prior to administration of the first dose of Muromonab-CD3, and by closely following recommendations for dosage and treatment duration. (see *"Dosage and Administration"*).

The administration of Muromonab-CD3 should be performed in a facility that is equipped and staffed for cardiopulmonary resuscitation and where a patient can be closely monitored for an appropriate period based on the patient's status.

If any of the more serious presentations of the Cytokine Release Syndrome occur, intensive treatment including oxygen, intravenous fluids, corticosteroids, pressor amines, antihistamines, intubation, etc., may be required.

ANAPHYLACTIC REACTIONS

Serious and occasionally fatal, immediate (usually within 10 minutes) hypersensitivity (anaphylactic) reactions have been reported in patients treated with Muromonab-CD3. **Manifestations of anaphylaxis may appear similar to manifestations of the Cytokine Release Syndrome (described above). It may be impossible to determine the mechanism responsible for any systemic reaction(s).** Reactions attributed to hypersensitivity have been reported less frequently than those attributed to cytokine release. Acute hypersensitivity reactions may be characterized by: cardiovascular collapse, cardiorespiratory arrest, loss of consciousness, hypotension/shock, tachycardia, tingling, angioedema (including laryngeal, pharyngeal, or facial edema), airway obstruction, bronchospasm, dyspnea, urticaria, and pruritus.

Serious allergic events, including anaphylactic or anaphylactoid reactions, have been reported in patients re-exposed to Muromonab-CD3 subsequent to their initial course of therapy. Pretreatment with antihistamines and/or steroids may not reliably prevent anaphylaxis in this setting. Possible allergic hazards of retreatment should be weighed against expected therapeutic benefits and alternatives. If retreatment with Muromonab-CD3 is employed, epinephrine and other emergency life-support equipment should be available, and the patient should be monitored closely.

If hypersensitivity is suspected, discontinue the drug immediately, do not resume therapy or re-expose the patient to Muromonab-CD3. Serious acute hypersensitivity reactions may require emergency treatment with 0.3 mL to 0.5 mL aqueous epinephrine (1:1000 dilution) subcutaneously and other resuscitative measures including oxygen, intravenous fluids, antihistamines, corticosteroids, pressor amines, and airway management, as clinically indicated (see *"Precautions: Cytokine Release Syndrome vs. Anaphylactic Reactions", "Adverse Reactions: Hypersensitivity Reactions"*).

NEURO-PSYCHIATRIC EVENTS

Seizures, encephalopathy, cerebral edema, aseptic meningitis, and headache have been reported, even following the first dose, during therapy with Muromonab-CD3, resulting in part from T cell activation and subsequent systemic release of cytokines.

Seizures: some accompanied by loss of consciousness or cardiorespiratory arrest, or death, have occurred independently or in conjunction with any of the neurologic syndromes described below. Patients predisposed to seizures may include those with the following conditions: acute tubular necrosis/uremia, fever, infection, a precipitous fall in serum calcium, fluid overload, hypertension, hypoglycemia, history of seizures, and electrolyte imbalances or those who are taking a medication concomitantly that may, by itself, cause seizures. Between 1987 and 1992, 75 post-marketing reports described seizures, averaging about 12 per year, and including 23 fatalities. More than two-thirds of these reports (53) were of domestic spontaneous origin, and their age and sex distributions were broad. Post-licensure reports generally do not provide sufficient basis for estimation of actual risks (incidence rates for specific adverse events), due to the typically substantial but unknown extent of under-ascertainment of incident events. Nonetheless, the number and regularity of seizure reports with Muromonab-CD3 indicate that this hazard appears not to be rare. Convulsions should be anticipated clinically with appropriate patient monitoring.

Manifestations of encephalopathy may include: impaired cognition, confusion, obtundation, altered mental status, auditory/visual hallucinations, psychosis (delirium, paranoia), mood changes (e.g., mania, agitation, combativeness, etc.), diffuse hypotonus, hyperreflexia, myoclonus, tremor, asterixis, involuntary movements, major motor seizures, lethargy/stupor/coma, and diffuse weakness. Approximately one-third of patients with a diagnosis of encephalopathy may have had coexisting aseptic meningitis syndrome.

Cerebral edema (and other signs of increased vascular permeability e.g., otitis media, nasal and ear stuffiness, etc.): has been seen in patients treated with Muromonab-CD3 and may accompany some of the other neurologic manifestations.

Signs and symptoms of the *aseptic meningitis syndrome* described in association with the use of Muromonab-CD3 have included: fever, headache, meningismus (stiff neck), and photophobia. In a post-marketing survey involving 214 renal transplant patients, the incidence of this syndrome was 6%. Fever (89%), headache (44%), neck stiffness (14%), and photophobia (10%) were the most commonly reported symptoms: a combination of these four symptoms occurred in 5% of patients. Diagnosis is confirmed by cerebrospinal fluid (CSF) analysis demonstrating leukocytosis with pleocytosis, elevated protein and normal or decreased glucose, with negative viral, bacterial and fungal cultures. In any immunosuppressed transplant patient with clinical findings suggesting meningitis, the possibility of infection should be evaluated. Approximately one-third of the patients with a diagnosis of aseptic meningitis had coexisting signs and symptoms of encephalopathy. Most patients with the aseptic meningitis syndrome had a benign course and recovered without any permanent sequelae during therapy or subsequent to its completion or discontinuation.

Headache: is frequently seen after any of the first few doses and may occur in any of the aforementioned neurologic syndromes or by itself.

The following additional neurologic events have each been reported occasionally in post-licensure reports: irreversible blindness, impaired vision, quadri or paraparesis/plegia, cerebrovascular accident (hemiparesis/plegia), aphasia, transient ischemic attack, subarachnoid hemorrhage, palsy of the VI cranial nerve, and hearing loss.

Signs or symptoms of encephalopathy, meningitis, seizures, and cerebral edema, with or without headache, have typically been reversible. Headache, aseptic meningitis, seizures, and less severe forms of encephalopathy resolved in most patients despite continued treatment. However, some events have been irreversible.

Other neurologic events observed in patients treated with Muromonab-CD3 include: post-therapy encephalopathy with or without coexisting metabolic disturbances, post-therapy meningitis, CNS lymphoproliferative disorders and infections. Since these patients usually had both serious and multiple coexisting medical conditions and were also receiving multiple concomitant medications the association of these events with Muromonab-CD3 treatment is unclear.

Patients who may be at greater risk for CNS adverse experiences include those: with known or suspected CNS disorders (e.g., history of seizure disorder, etc.); with cerebrovascular disease (small or large vessel); with conditions having associated neurologic problems (e.g., head trauma, uremia, etc.); with underlying vascular diseases; or who are receiving a medication concomitantly that may, by itself, affect the central nervous system (see *"Warnings", "Precautions"* and *"Adverse Reactions: Cytokine Release Syndrome"; "Precautions: Drug Interactions"*).

CONSEQUENCES OF IMMUNOSUPPRESSION

Serious and sometimes fatal infections and neoplasias have been reported in association with all immunosuppressive therapies, including those regimens containing Muromonab-CD3.

Infections: Muromonab-CD3 is usually added to immunosuppressive therapeutic regimens, thereby augmenting the degree of immunosuppression. This increase in the total burden of immunosuppression may alter the spectrum of infections observed and increase the risk, the severity, and the potential gravity (morbidity) of infectious complications. During the first month post-transplant, patients are at greatest risk for the following infections: (1) those present prior to transplant, perhaps exacerbated by post-transplant immunosuppression; (2) infection conveyed by the donor organ; and (3) the usual post-operative urinary tract, intravenous line-related, wound, or pulmonary infections due to bacterial pathogens.

Approximately one to six months post-transplant, patients are at risk for viral infections [e.g., Cytomegalovirus (CMV), Epstein-Barr Virus (EBV), Herpes simplex virus (HSV), etc.] which produce serious systemic disease and which also increase the overall state of immunosuppression. Clinically significant infections (e.g., pneumonia, sepsis, etc.) may occur with any microorganisms including: *Pneumocystis carinii, Listeria monocytogenes, Aspergillus* species, *Candida species, Nocardia asteroids, Legionella*, mycobacteria, gram-negative rods, and gram-positive cocci (staphylococci and streptococci), etc. Opportunistic infections, related to decreased T cell function, are associated with all immunosuppressive modalities employed to treat transplant rejection. Multiple or intensive courses of any anti-T cell antibody preparation, including Muromonab-CD3, which produce profound impairment of cell-mediated immunity, further increase the risk of (opportunistic) infection, especially with the Herpes viruses (HSV, CMV, EBV) and fungi.

Reactivation (1 to 4 months post-transplant) of EBV and CMV has been reported. Infectious syndromes due to CMV have included: fever of unknown origin, pneumonia, viremia, hepatitis, liver/renal dysfunction, gastritis or gastrointestinal ulcerations, pancreatitis, chorioretinitiş, leukopenia, and thrombocytopenia. When administration of an antilymphocyte antibody, including Muromonab-CD3, is followed by an immunosuppressive regimen including cyclosporine, there is an increased risk of reactivating CMV and impaired ability to limit its proliferation, resulting in symptomatic and disseminated disease. EBV infection, either primary or reactivated, may play an important role in the development of post-transplant lymphoproliferative disorders (see *"Warnings"* and *"Adverse Reactions: Neoplasia"*).

Anti-infective prophylaxis may reduce the morbidity associated with certain potential pathogens and should be considered for high-risk patients. Judicious use of immunosuppressive drugs, including type, dosage, and duration, may limit the risk and seriousness of some opportunistic infections. It is also possible to reduce the risk of serious CMV infection by avoiding transplantation of a CMV-seropositive (donor) organ into a seronegative patient.

Neoplasia: As a result of depressed cell-mediated immunity, organ transplant patients have an increased risk of developing malignancies. This risk is evidenced almost exclusively by the occurrence of lymphoproliferative disorders (LPD), lymphomas, and skin cancers. In immunosuppressed patients, T cell cytotoxicity is impaired allowing for transformation and proliferation of EBV-infected B lymphocytes. Transformed B lymphocytes are thought to initiate the oncogenic process that ultimately culminates in the development of most post-transplant lymphoproliferative disorders (see *"Adverse Reactions: Neoplasia"*).

Following the initiation of Muromonab-CD3 therapy, patients should be continuously monitored for evidence of LPD, through physical examination and histological evaluation of any suspect lymphoid tissue. Vigilant surveillance is advised, since early detection with subsequent reduction of total immunosuppression may result in regression of some of these lymphoproliferative disorders. Since the potential for the development of LPD is related to the duration and extent (intensity) of total immunosuppression, physicians are advised; to adhere to the recommended dosage and duration of Muromonab-CD-3 therapy; to limit the number of courses of Muromonab-CD3 and other anti-T lymphocyte antibody preparations administered within a short period of time; and, if appropriate, to reduce the dosage(s) of immunosuppressive drugs used concomitantly to the lowest level compatible with an effective therapeutic response (see *"Dosage and Administration"*).

The long-term risk of neoplastic events in patients being treated with Muromonab-CD3 has not been determined.

PRECAUTIONS
GENERAL
PRIOR TO TREATMENT WITH MUROMONAB-CD3
Fluid Status: The patient's volume (fluid) status should be assessed carefully. It is imperative, especially prior to the first few doses, that there be no clinical evidence of volume overload or uncompensated heart failure, including a clear chest X-ray and weight restriction of $\leq$ 3% above the patient's minimum weight during the week prior to injection. *Fever:* If the temperature of the patient exceeds 37.8°C (100°F), it should be lowered by antipyretics before administration of each dose of Muromonab-CD3. The possibility of infection should be evaluated.

Blood Tests: Periodic assessment of organ system functions (renal, hepatic, and hematopoietic) should be performed.

During therapy with Muromonab-CD3: Periodic monitoring to ensure plasma Muromonab-CD3 levels (> 800 ng/mL) or T cell clearance (CD3 positive T cells < 25 cells/mm^2) is recommended.

Severe Cytokine Release Syndrome Versus Anaphylactic Reactions: **It may be very difficult, even impossible, to distinguish between an acute hypersensitivity reaction (e.g., anaphylaxis, angioedema, etc.) and the Cytokine Release Syndrome. Potentially serious signs and symptoms having an** *immediate* **onset (usually within 10 minutes) following administration of Muromonab-CD3 are more likely due to acute hypersensitivity; discontinue the drug immediately. If hypersensitivity is suspected, do not resume therapy or re-expose the patient to Muromonab-CD3.** Clinical manifestations beginning approximately 30 to 60 minutes (or later) following administration of Muromonab-CD3, are more likely cytokine-mediated (see *"Warnings: Cytokine Release Syndrome, Anaphylactic Reactions"*).

Neuro-Psychiatric Events: Since some seizures (and other serious central nervous system events) following Muromonab-CD3 administration have been life-threatening, anti-seizure precautions (e.g., an airway ready for use, if needed) should be taken (see *"Warnings"* and *"Adverse Reactions: Neuro-Psychiatric Events"*).

Infection/Viral-Induced Lymphoproliferative Disorders: Patients must be observed carefully for any signs and symptoms suggesting infection or viral-induced lymphoproliferative disorders (LPD). Anti-infective prophylaxis should be considered for patients at high risk. If infection or viral-induced LPD occur, culture or biopsy as soon as possible, institute promptly appropriate anti-infective therapy, and (if possible) reduce/discontinue immunosuppressive therapy.

When using combinations of immunosuppressive agents, the dose of each agent, including Muromonab-CD3 should be reduced to the lowest level compatible with an effective therapeutic response so as to reduce the potential for and severity of infections and malignant transformations (see: *"Warnings: Infections, Neoplasia"*).

Low Protein-Binding Filter: Use a low protein-binding 0.2 or 0.22 micrometer (μm) filter to prepare the injections (see *"Administration Instructions"*).

Sensitization: Muromonab-CD3 is a mouse (immunoglobulin) protein that can induce human antimouse antibody production (i.e., sensitization) in patients following exposure (see *"Clinical Pharmacology"*). Monitoring for human antibody titers after Muromonab-CD3 therapy is strongly recommended (see *"Contraindications"*).

Reduced T cell clearance or impaired ability to maintain adequate Muromonab-CD3 levels provides a basis for adjusting Muromonab-CD3 dosage or for discontinuing therapy (see *"Warnings: Anaphylactic Reactions;" Precautions: Laboratory Tests"; "Adverse Reactions: Hypersensitivity Reactions"*).

Intravascular Thrombosis: As with other immunosuppressive therapies, arterial or venous thromboses of allografts and other vascular beds (e.g., heart, lungs, brain, bowel, etc.) have been reported in patients treated with Muromonab-CD3. The decision to use Muromonab-CD3 in patients with a history of thrombotic events or underlying vascular disease should take these findings into consideration. Concomitant use of prophylactic anti-thrombotic interventions (e.g., mini-dose heparin etc.) should be considered (see *"Adverse Reactions"*).

INFORMATION FOR PATIENTS
Patients should be advised:

■ of the signs and symptoms associated with the Cytokine Release Syndrome, including the potentially serious nature of this symptom complex (e.g., systemic, cardiovascular, neuro-psychiatric events).
■ to seek medical attention at the first sign of skin rash, urticaria, rapid heartbeat, difficulty in swallowing and breathing, or any swelling that may suggest angioedema, or other allergic reaction.
■ to know how they might react to Muromonab-CD3 before operating an automobile or machinery, or engaging in activities requiring mental alertness and coordination.
■ of the potential benefits and other risks attendant to the use of Muromonab-CD3 (see *"Boxed Warning"; "Warnings"; "Precautions"; "Adverse Reactions"*).

Drug Interactions: The following medications are frequently used with Muromonab-CD3 and the information provided below may be helpful in evaluating any adverse events reported in Muromonab-CD3 treated patients.

With *indomethacin*: Encephalopathy and other CNS effects have been reported in patients treated with indomethacin alone and in conjunction with Muromonab-CD3. The mechanism of these effects is unknown.

With *corticosteroids*: Psychosis and infections have been seen in patients treated with corticosteroids alone and in conjunction with Muromonab-CD3.

With *azathioprine*: Infections or malignancies have been reported with azathioprine alone and in conjunction with Muromonab-CD3.

With *cyclosporine*: Seizures, encephalopathy, infections, malignancies, and thrombotic events have been reported in patients receiving cyclosporine alone and in conjunction with Muromonab-CD3.

LABORATORY TESTS
As with many potent drugs, periodic assessment of organ system functions should be performed during treatment with Muromonab-CD3.

The following tests should be monitored prior to and during Muromonab-CD3 therapy.

■ Renal: BUN, serum creatinine, etc.:
■ Hepatic: transaminases, alkaline phosphatase bilirubin:
■ Hematopoietic: WBCs and differential, platelet count, etc.:
■ Chest X-ray within 24 hours *before* initiating Muromonab-CD3 treatment. *Recommendation: chest X-ray should be free of any evidence of heart failure or fluid overload.*

One of the following immunologic tests should be monitored *during* Muromonab-CD3 therapy:

■ Plasma Muromonab-CD3 levels (as determined by an ELISA); *target Muromonab-CD3 levels should be $\geq$ 800 ng/mL*; or
■ Quantitative T lymphocyte surface phenotyping (CD3, CD4, CD8); target CD3 positive T cells < 25 cells/mm^3.

Testing for human-mouse antibody titers is strongly recommended: *a titer $\geq$ 1:1000 is a contraindication for use* (see *"Contraindications;" "Precautions; Sensitization"*).

CARCINOGENESIS
Long-term studies have not been performed in laboratory animals to evaluate the carcinogenic potential of Muromonab-CD3 (see *"Warnings"* and *"Adverse Reactions: Neoplasia"*).

PREGNANCY CATEGORY C
Animal reproductive studies have not been conducted with Muromonab-CD3. It is also not known whether Muromonab-CD3 can cause fetal harm when administered to a pregnant woman or can affect reproduction capacity. However, Muromonab-CD3 is an IgG antibody and may cross the human placenta. The effect on the fetus of the release of cytokines and/or immunosuppression after treatment with Muromonab-CD3 is not known. If this drug is used during pregnancy, or the patient becomes pregnant while taking this drug, the patient should be apprised of the potential hazard to the fetus (see *"Contraindications", "Warnings", and "Adverse Reactions"*).

NURSING MOTHERS
It is not known whether Muromonab-CD3 is excreted in human milk. Because many drugs are excreted in human milk and because of the potential for serious adverse reactions/oncogenesis shown for Muromonab-CD3 in human studies, a decision should be made to discontinue nursing or to discontinue the drug, taking into account the importance of the drug to the mother (see *"Contraindications"*).

PEDIATRIC USE
Safety and effectiveness in children have not been established. No adequately controlled clinical studies have been conducted in children. Published literature[4,10] has reported the use of Muromonab-CD3 in infants/children, beginning with a dose of $\leq$ 5 mg. Based on immunologic monitoring, the dosage has been adjusted accordingly (see *"Precautions: Laboratory Tests"*). Pediatric recipients

are reported to be significantly immunosuppressed for a prolonged period of time and therefore, require close monitoring post-therapy for opportunistic infections, particularly varicella (VZV), which poses an infectious complication unique to this population. Gastrointestinal fluid loss secondary to diarrhea and/or vomiting resulting from the Cytokine Release Syndrome may be significant when treating small children and may require parenteral hydration. It is unknown whether there may be significant long-term sequelae (e.g., neurodevelopmental language difficulties in infants under 1 year of age) related to the occurrence of seizures, high fever, CNS infections, aseptic meningitis, etc., following Murumonab-CD3 treatment. In cases where administration of Muromonab-CD3 would be deemed medically appropriate, more vigilant and frequent monitoring is required for children than in adults (see *"Boxed Warning"; "Warnings"; "Precautions"; "Adverse Reactions"*).

ADVERSE REACTIONS
CYTOKINE RELEASE SYNDROME
In controlled clinical trials for treatment of acute renal allograft rejection, patients treated with Muromonab-CD3 plus concomitant low-dose immunosuppressive therapy (primarily azathioprine and corticosteroids) were observed to have an increased incidence of adverse experiences during the first two days of treatment, as compared with the group receiving azathioprine and high-dose steroid therapy. During this period the majority of patients experienced pyrexia (90%), of which 19% were 40.0°C (104°F) or above and chills (59%). In addition, other adverse experiences occurring in 8% or more of the patients during the first two days of Muromonab-CD3 therapy included: dyspnea (21%), nausea (19%), vomiting (19%), chest pain (14%), diarrhea (14%), tremor (13%), wheezing (13%), headache (11%), tachycardia (10%), rigor (8%), and hypertension (8%). A similar spectrum of clinical manifestations has been observed in open clinical studies and in post-marketing experience involving patients treated with Muromonab-CD3 for rejection following renal, cardiac, and hepatic transplantation.

Additional serious and occasionally fatal cardiorespiratory manifestations have been reported following any of the first few doses (see *"Warnings: Cytokine Release Syndrome"; "Adverse Reactions: Cardiovascular Respiratory"*).

In the acute renal allograft rejection trials, potentially fatal pulmonary edema had been reported following the first two doses in less than 2% of the patients treated with Muromonab-CD3. Pulmonary edema was usually associated with fluid overload. However, post-marketing experience revealed that pulmonary edema has occurred in patients who appeared to be euvolemic, presumably as a consequence of cytokine-mediated increased vascular permeability ("leaky capillaries") and/or reduced myocardial contractility/compliance (i.e., left ventricular dysfunction). (See *"Warnings Cytokine Release Syndrome"; "Dosage and Administration"*.)

INFECTIONS
In the controlled randomized renal rejection trial conducted during the pre-cyclosporine era, the most common infections during the first 45 days of Muromonab-CD3 therapy were due to Herpes simplex (27%) and cytomegalovirus (19%). Other severe and life-threatening infections were *Staphylococcus epidermidis* (4.8%), *Pneumocystis carinii* (3.1%), *Legionella* (1.6%), *Cryptococcus* (1.6%), *Serratia* (1.6%) and gram-negative bacteria (1.6%). The incidence of infections was similar in patients treated with Muromonab-CD3 and in patients treated with high-dose steroids.

In a clinical trial of acute hepatic rejection refractory to conventional treatment, the most common infections reported in patients treated with Muromonab-CD3 during the first 45 days of the study were cytomegalovirus (15.7% of patients, of which 43% of infections were severe), fungal infections (14.9% of patients, of which 30% were severe), and Herpes simplex (7.5% of patients, of which 10% were severe). Other severe and life-threatening infections were gram-positive infections (9.0% of patients), gram-negative infections (7.5% of patients), viral infections (1.5% of patients), and *Legionella* (0.7% of patients). In another hepatic rejection trial the incidence of fungal infections was 34% and infections with the Herpes simplex virus was 31%.

In a clinical trial of acute cardiac rejection refractory to conventional treatment, the most common infections reported in the Muromonab-CD3 group during the first 45 days of the study were Herpes simplex (5% of patients, of which 20% were severe), fungal infections (4% of patients, of which 75% were severe), and cytomegalovirus (3% of patients, of which 33% were severe). No other severe or life-threatening infections were reported during this period.

Clinically significant infections (e.g., pneumonia, sepsis, etc.) due to the following pathogens have been reported:

Bacterial: Clostridium species (including perfringens), Corynebacterium, *Enterococcus, Enterobacter aerogenes, Escherichia coli, Klebsiella* species, *Lactobacillus, Legionella, Listeria monocytogenes, Mycobacteria* species, *Nocardia asteroides, Proteus* species, *Providencia* species, *Pseudomonas aeruginosa, Serratia* species, *Staphylococcus* species, *Streptococcus* species, *Yersinia enterocolitica,* and other gram-negative bacteria.

Fungal:* Aspergillus, Candida, Cryptococcal, Dermatophytes.*

Protozoa: Pneumocystis carinii, Toxoplasma gondii.

Viral: Cytomegalovirus* (CMV), Epstein-Barr virus* (EBV), Herpes simplex virus* (HSV), Hepatitis viruses, Varicella zoster virus (VZV).

As a consequence of being a potent immunosuppressive, the incidence and severity of infections with designated(*) pathogens, especially the Herpes family of viruses, may be increased (see *"Warnings: Infections"*).

NEOPLASIA
In patients treated with Muromonab-CD3, post-transplant lymphoproliferative disorders (LPD) reported have ranged from lymphadenopathy or benign polyclonal B cell hyperplasias to malignant and often fatal monoclonal B cell lymphomas. In post-marketing experience, approximately one-third of the lymphoproliferations reported were benign, and two-thirds were malignant. Classification of these lymphomas has induced: B cell, large cell, polyclonal, non-Hodgkin's, lymphocytic, T cell, Burkitt's; the majority have not been classified histologically. When malignant lymphomas have been reported, they have appeared to develop soon after transplantation, the majority within the first four months post-treatment. Many of these have been rapidly progressive, widely disseminated at time of diagnosis, and fatal. Carcinomas of the skin have included: basal cell, squamous cell, Kaposi's sarcoma, malanoma, and keratocanthoma. Other neoplasms infrequently reported include: multiple myeloma, leukemia, carcinoma of the breast, adenocarcinoma, cholangiocarcinoma, and recurrences of pre-existing hepatoma and renal cell carcinoma (see *"Warnings: Neoplasia"*).

HYPERSENSITIVITY REACTIONS
Reported adverse reactions resulting from the formation of antibodies to Muromonab-CD3 have included antigen-antibody (immune complex) mediated syndromes and IgE-mediated reactions. Reported hypersensivity reactions have ranged from a mild, self-limited rash or pruritus to severe, life-threatening anaphylactic reactions/shock or angioedema (including: swelling of lips, eyelids, laryngeal spasm and airway obstruction with hypoxia). (See *"Warnings: Anaphylactic Reactions"*.)

Other hypersensitivity reactions have included: ineffectiveness of treatment, serum sickness, arthritis, allergic interstitial nephritis, immune complex deposition resulting in glomerulonephritis, vasculitis, and temporal arteritis, and eosinophilia.

Clinical adverse events occurring in clinical trials and post-marketing experience are listed below by body system:

Body as a Whole: fever (including, spiking temperatures as high as 107°F), chills/rigors, flu-like syndrome, fatigue/malaise, generalized weakness, anorexia.

Cardiovascular: cardiac arrest, hypotension/shock, heart failure, cardiovascular collapse, angina/myocardial infarction, tachycardia, bradycardia, hemodynamic instability, hypertension, left ventricular dysfunction, arrhythmias, chest pain/tightness.

Respiratory: respiratory arrest, adult respiratory distress syndrome (ARDS), respiratory failure, pulmonary edema (cardiogenic or noncardiogenic), apnea, dyspnea, bronchospasm, wheezing, shortness of breath, hypoxemia, tachypnea/hyperventilation, abnormal chest sounds, and pneumonia/pneumonitis (bacterial, viral, P. *carinii*, etc.).

Dermatologic: rash, urticaria, pruritus, erythema, flushing, diaphoresis.

Gastrointestinal: diarrhea, nausea/vomiting, abdominal pain, bowel infarction.

Hematopoietic: pancytopenia, aplastic anemia, neutropenia, leukopenia, thrombocytopenia, lymphopenia, leukocytosis, lymphadenopathy; arterial and venous thrombosis of allografts and other vascular beds (e.g., heart, lung, brain, bowel, etc.); disturbances of coagulation.

Hepatobiliary: increases in transaminases (SGOT, SGPT, etc.); hepato/splenomegaly or hepatitis, usually secondary to viral infection or lymphoma.

Neuro-Psychiatric: seizures, lethargy/stupor/coma, encephalopathy, psychotic reactions (delirium), encephalitis, meningitis, cerebral edema, headache, dizziness, tremor, aphasia, quadri- or paraparesis/plegia, obtundation, confusion, altered mental status (e.g., paranoia, etc.), impaired cognition, disorientation, auditory and visual hallucinations, agitation/combativeness, mood changes (e.g., mania, etc.), hypotonus, hyperreflexia, myoclonus, asterixis, involuntary movements, CNS infections, CNS malignancies, cerebrovascular accident/hemiparesis/plegia, transient ischemic attack, subarachnoid hemorrhage.

Musculoskeletal: arthralgia, arthritis, myalgia, stiffness/aches/pains.

Special Senses: blindness, blurred vision, diplopia, hearing loss, otitis media, tinnitus, vertigo, VI cranial nerve palsy, photophobia, conjunctivitis, nasal and ear stuffiness.

Renal: anuria/oliguria; delayed graft function; transient and reversible increases in BUN and serum creatinine; abnormal urinary cytology including exfoliation of damaged lymphocytes, collecting duct cells and cellular casts.

OVERDOSAGE
The maximum amount of Muromonab-CD3 that can be safely administered in single or multiple doses has not been determined.

DOSAGE AND ADMINISTRATION
The recommended dose of Muromonab-CD3 for the treatment of acute renal, steroid-resistant cardiac, or steroid-resistant hepatic allograft rejection is 5 mg per day in a single *(bolus)* intravenous injection for 10 to 14 days. For acute renal rejection, treatment should begin upon diagnosis. For steroid-resistant cardiac or hepatic allograft rejection, treatment should begin when the treating physician deems a rejection has not been reversed by an adequate course of corticosteroid therapy (see *"Clinical Pharmacology"; "Precautions: Sensitization, Laboratory Tests"*). For the first few doses, patients should be monitored in a facility equipped and staffed for cardiopulmonary resuscitation with frequent determinations of vital signs. With subsequent doses, the patient should be monitored following Muromonab-CD3 therapy in a facility equipped and staffed for CPR for an appropriate period of time based on the patient's clinical status. Since the Cytokine Release Syndrome may also occur following a treatment hiatus and resumption of therapy, as with the first few doses, exercise vigilant care.

Prior to the administration of any dose of Murumonab-CD3 the patient's temperature should be lowered to < 37.8°C (100°F).

Prior to administration of Muromonab-CD3, the patient's volume status should be assessed carefully. It is imperative, especially prior to the first few doses, that there be no clinical evidence of volume overload or uncompensated heart failure, including a clear chest X-ray and weight restriction of ≤ 3% above the patient's minimum weight during the week prior to injection (see *"Warnings"* and *"Adverse Reactions: Cytokine Release Syndrome"*). Intravenous methylprednisolone sodium succinate 8.0 mg/kg given 1 to 4 hours prior to administering the first dose of Muromonab-CD3 is strongly recommended to decrease the incidence and severity of reactions to the first dose, which have been attributed to the Muromonab-CD3 mediated Cytokine Release Syndrome. Acetaminophen and antihistamines given concomitantly with Muromonab-CD3 may also help to reduce some early reactions (see *"Warnings"* and *"Adverse Reactions: Cytokine Release Syndrome"*).

When using concomitant immunosuppressive drugs, the dose of each should be reduced to the lowest level compatible with an effective therapeutic response in order to reduce the potential for malignant transformations and the incidence and/or severity of infections. Maintenance immunosuppression should be resumed approximately three days prior to the cessation of Muromonab-CD3 therapy (see *"Warnings"* and *"Adverse Reactions: Infection, Neoplasia"*).

ADMINISTRATION INSTRUCTIONS
1. Prior to administration, parenteral drug products should be inspected visually for particulate matter and discoloration. Because Muromonab-CD3 is a protein solution, it may develop a few fine translucent particles which have been shown not to affect its potency.

2. No bacteriostatic agent is present in this product: adherence to aseptic technique is advised. Once the ampule is opened, use immediately and discard the unused portion.

3. Prepare Muromonab-CD3 for injection by drawing solution into a syringe through a low protein-binding 0.2 or 0.22 micrometer (μm) filter. Discard filter and attach a new needle for intravenous bolus injection.

4. Since no data is available on compatibility of Muromonab-CD3 with other intravenous substances or additives, other medications/substances should not be added or infused simultaneously through the same intravenous line. If the same intravenous line is used for sequential infusion of several different drugs, the line should be flushed with saline before and after infusion of Muromonab-CD3.

5. Administer Muromonab-CD3 as an intravenous bolus in less than one minute. Do not administer by intravenous infusion or in conjunction with other drug solutions.

STORAGE
Store in a refrigerator at 2° to 8°C (36° to 46°F). DO NOT FREEZE OR SHAKE.

HOW SUPPLIED
INJECTION: 1 MG/ML

BRAND/MANUFACTURER	NDC	SIZE	AWP
○ BRAND			
ORTHOCLONE OKT 3: Ortho Biotech	00062-7102-01	5 ml	$535.00

Mustargen SEE MECHLORETHAMINE HYDROCHLORIDE

Mutamycin SEE MITOMYCIN

M.V.I. SEE VITAMINS, MULTI, INJECTABLE

Myambutol SEE ETHAMBUTOL HYDROCHLORIDE

Mycelex SEE CLOTRIMAZOLE

Mycifradin SEE NEOMYCIN SULFATE

Mycobutin SEE RIFABUTIN

Mycolog-II SEE NYSTATIN AND TRIAMCINOLONE ACETONIDE

Mycostatin SEE NYSTATIN, ORAL AND NYSTATIN, TOPICAL

Mydriacyl SEE TROPICAMIDE

Myelo-Kit SEE IOHEXOL

Myleran SEE BUSULFAN

Myochrysine SEE GOLD SODIUM THIOMALATE

Mysoline SEE PRIMIDONE

Mytelase Chloride SEE AMBENONIUM CHLORIDE

Nabumetone

DESCRIPTION
Nabumetone is a naphthylalkanone designated chemically as 4-(6-methoxy-2-naphthalenyl)-2-butanone.

Nabumetone is a white to off-white crystalline substance with a molecular weight of 228.3. It is nonacidic and practically insoluble in water, but soluble in alcohol and most organic solvents. It has an n-octanol: phosphate buffer partition coefficient of 2400 at pH 7.4.

Tablets for Oral Administration: Each oval-shaped, film-coated tablet contains 500 mg or 750 mg of Nabumetone.

Following is its chemical structure:

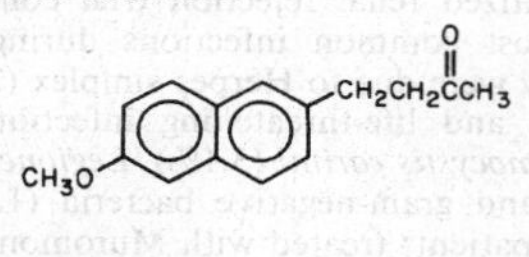

CLINICAL PHARMACOLOGY
Nabumetone is a nonsteroidal anti-inflammatory drug (NSAID) that exhibits anti-inflammatory, analgesic and antipyretic properties in pharmacologic studies. As with other nonsteroidal anti-inflammatory agents, its mode of action is not known. However, the ability to inhibit prostaglandin synthesis may be involved in the anti-inflammatory effect.

The parent compound is a prodrug, which undergoes hepatic biotransformation to the active component, 6-methoxy-2-naphthylacetic acid (6MNA), that is a potent inhibitor of prostaglandin synthesis.

It is acidic and has an n-octanol: phosphate buffer partition coefficient of 0.5 at pH 7.4.

PHARMACOKINETICS
After oral administration, approximately 80% of a radio-labelled dose of Nabumetone is found in the urine, indicating that Nabumetone is well absorbed from the gastrointestinal tract. Nabumetone itself is not detected in the plasma because, after absorption, it undergoes rapid biotransformation to the principal active metabolite, 6-methoxy-2-naphthylacetic acid (6MNA). Approximately 35% of a 1000 mg oral dose of Nabumetone is converted to 6MNA and 50% is converted into unidentified metabolites which are subsequently excreted in the urine. Following oral administration of Nabumetone, 6MNA exhibits pharmacokinetic characteristics that generally follow a one-compartment model with first order input and first order elimination.

6MNA is more than 99% bound to plasma proteins. The free fraction is dependent on total concentration of 6MNA and is proportional to dose over the range of 1000 mg to 2000 mg. It is 0.2% to 0.3% at concentrations typically achieved following administration of Nabumetone 1000 mg and is approximately 0.6% to 0.8% of the total concentrations at steady state following daily administration of 2000 mg.

Steady-state plasma concentrations of 6MNA are slightly lower than predicted from single-dose data. This may result from the higher fraction of unbound 6MNA which undergoes greater hepatic clearance.

Coadministration of food increases the rate of absorption and subsequent appearance of 6MNA in the plasma but does not affect the extent of conversion of Nabumetone into 6MNA. Peak plasma concentrations of 6MNA are increased by approximately one-third.

Coadministration with an aluminum-containing antacid had no significant effect on the bioavailability of 6MNA. (See related table).

The stimulated curves in the graph below illustrate the range of active metabolite plasma concentrations that would be expected from 95% of patients following 1000 mg to 2000 mg doses to steady state. The cross-hatched area represents the expected overlap in plasma concentrations due to intersubject variation following oral administration of 100 mg to 2000 mg of Nabumetone.

6MNA undergoes biotransformation in the liver, producing inactive metabolites that are eliminated as both free metabolites and conjugates. None of the known metabolites of 6MNA has been detected in plasma. Preliminary in vivo and in vitro studies suggest that unlike other NSAIDs, there is no evidence of enterohepatic recirculation of the active metabolite. Approximately 75% of a radiolabelled dose was recovered in urine in 48 hours. Approximately 80% was recovered in 168 hours. A further 9% appeared in the feces. In the first 48 hours, metabolites consisted of:

—Nabumetone, unchanged	not detectable
—6-methoxy-2-naphthylacetic acid (6MNA), unchanged	< 1%
—6MNA, conjugated	11%
—6-hydroxy-2-naphthylacetic acid (6HNA), unchanged	5%
—6HNA, conjugated	7%
—4-(6-methoxy-2-naphthyl)-butan-2-ol, conjugated	9%
—O-desmethyl-nabumetone, conjugated	7%
—unidentified minor metabolites	34%
Total % Dose:	73%

Following oral administration of dosages of 1000 mg to 2000 mg to steady state, the mean plasma clearance of 6MNA is 20 to 30 mL/min. and the elimination half-life is approximately 24 hours.

Elderly Patients: Steady-state plasma concentrations in elderly patients were generally higher than in young healthy subjects. (See *"Table 1"* for summary of pharmacokinetic parameters).

Renal Insufficiency: In studies of patients with renal insufficiency, the mean terminal half-life of 6MNA was increased in patients with severe renal dysfunction (creatine clearance <30 mL/min./1.73 m^2). In patients undergoing hemodialysis, steady-state plasma concentrations of the active metabolite were similar to those observed in healthy subjects. Due to extensive protein-binding, 6MNA is not dialyzable.

Hepatic Impairment: Data in patients with severe hepatic impairment are limited. Biotransformation of Nabumetone to 6MNA and the further metabolism of 6MNA to inactive metabolites is dependent on hepatic function and could be reduced in patients with severe hepatic impairment (history of or biopsy-proven cirrhosis).

SPECIAL STUDIES

Gastrointestinal: Nabumetone was compared to Aspirin in inducing gastrointestinal blood loss. Food intake was not monitored. Studies utilizing ^{51}Cr-tagged red blood cells in healthy males showed no difference in fecal blood loss after 3 or 4 weeks' administration of Nabumetone 1000 mg or 2000 mg daily when compared to either placebo-treated or nontreated subjects. In contrast, Aspirin 3600 mg daily produced an increase in fecal blood loss when compared to the Nabumetone treated, placebo-treated or nontreated subjects. The clinical relevance of the data is unknown.

The following endoscopy trials entered patients who had been previously treated with NSAIDs. These patients had varying baseline scores and different courses of treatment. The trials were not designed to correlate symptoms and endoscopy scores. The clinical relevance of these endoscopy trials, i.e., either G.I. symptoms or serious G.I. events, is not known.

Ten endoscopy studies were conducted in 488 patients who had baseline and post-treatment endoscopy. In 5 clinical trials that compared a total of 194 patients on Nabumetone 1000 mg daily or Naproxen 250 mg or 500 mg twice daily for 3 to 12 weeks, Nabumetone treatment resulted in fewer patients with endoscopically detected lesions (> 3 mm). In 2 trials a total of 101 patients on Nabumetone 1000 mg or 2000 mg daily or piroxicam 10 mg to 20 mg for 7 to 10 days, there were fewer Nabumetone patients with endoscopically detected lesions. In 3 trials of a total of 47 patients on Nabumetone 1000 mg daily or Indomethacin 100 mg to 150 mg daily for 3 or 4 weeks, the endoscopy scores were higher with

Indomethacin. Another 12-week trial in a total of 171 patients compared the results of treatment with Nabumetone 1000 mg/day to Ibuprofen 2400 mg/day and Ibuprofen 2400 mg/day plus Misoprostol 800 mcg/day. The results showed that patients treated with Nabumetone had a lower number of endoscopically detected lesions (> 5 mm) than patients treated with Ibuprofen alone but comparable to the combination of Ibuprofen plus Misoprostol. The results did not correlate with abdominal pain.

Other: In 1-week repeat-dose studies in healthy volunteers, Nabumetone 1000 mg daily had little effect on collagen-induced platelet aggregation and no effect on bleeding time. In comparison Naproxen 500 mg daily suppressed collagen-induced platelet aggregation and significantly increased bleeding time.

CLINICAL TRIALS

Osteoarthritis: The use of Nabumetone in relieving the signs and symptoms of osteoarthritis was assessed in double-blind controlled trials in which 1,047 patients were treated for 6 weeks to 6 months. In these trials, Nabumetone in a dose of 1000 mg/day administered at night was comparable to Naproxen 500 mg/day and to Aspirin 3600 mg/day.

Rheumatoid Arthritis: The use of Nabumetone in relieving the signs and symptoms of rheumatoid arthritis was assessed in double-blind, randomized, controlled trials in which 770 patients were treated for 3 weeks to 6 months. Nabumetone, in a dose of 1000 mg/day administered at night, was comparable to Naproxen 500 mg/day and to Aspirin 3600 mg/day.

In controlled clinical trials of rheumatoid arthritis patients, Nabumetone has been used in combination with Gold, d-Penicillamine and corticosteroids.

INDIVIDUALIZATION OF DOSING

There is considerable interpatient variation in response to Nabumetone. Therapy is usually initiated at a Nabumetone dose of 1000 mg daily, then adjusted, if needed, based on clinical response.

In clinical trials with osteoarthritis and rheumatoid arthritis patients, most patients responded to Nabumetone in doses of 1000 mg/day administered nightly; total daily dosages up to 2000 mg were used. In open-labelled studies, 1,490 patients were permitted dosage increases and were followed for approximately 1 year (mode). Twenty percent of patients (n = 294) were withdrawn for lack of effectiveness during the first year of these open-labelled studies. The following table provides patient-exposure to doses used in the U.S. clinical trials:

Table 2

CLINICAL DOUBLE-BLIND AND OPEN-LABELLED TRIALS OF NABUMETONE IN OSTEOARTHRITIS AND RHEUMATOID ARTHRITIS

Nabumetone Dose	Number of Patients		Mean/Mode Duration of Treatment (years)	
	OA	RA	OA	RA
500 mg	17	6	0.4/-	0.2/-
1000 mg	917	701	1.2/1	1.4/1
1500 mg	645	224	2.3/1	1.7/1
2000 mg	15	100	0.6/1	1.3/1

As with other NSAIDs, the lowest dose should be sought for each patient. Patients weighing under 50 kg may be less likely to require dosages beyond 1000 mg. Therefore, after observing the response to initial therapy, the dose should be adjusted to meet individual patients' requirements.

INDICATIONS AND USAGE

Nabumetone is indicated for acute and chronic treatment of signs and symptoms of osteoarthritis and rheumatoid arthritis.

UNLABELED USES

Nabumetone is used alone or as an adjunct in the treatment of skin and soft tissue injuries.

CONTRAINDICATIONS

Nabumetone is contraindicated in patients who have previously exhibited hypersensitivity to it.

Nabumetone is contraindicated in patients in whom Nabumetone Aspirin or other NSAIDs induce asthma, urticaria or other allergic-type reactions. Fatal asthmatic reactions have been reported in such patients receiving NSAIDs.

Table 1

MEAN PHARMACOKINETIC PARAMETERS OF NABUMETONE ACTIVE METABOLITE (6MNA) AT STEADY STATE FOLLOWING ORAL ADMINISTRATION OF 1000 MG OR 2000 MG DOSES OF NABUMETONE

Abbreviation (units)	Young Adults Mean ± SD 1000 mg n = 31	Young Adults Mean ± SD 2000 mg n = 12	Elderly Mean ± SD 1000 mg n = 27
t_{max} (hours)	3.0 (1.0 to 12.0)	2.5 (1.0 to 8.0)	4.0 (1.0 to 10.0)
$t\frac{1}{2}$ (hours)	22.5 ± 3.7	26.2 ± 3.7	29.8 ± 8.1
CL_{SS}/F (mL/min.)	26.1 ± 17.3	21.0 ± 4.0	18.6 ± 13.4
Vd_{SS}/F (L)	55.4 ± 26.4	53.4 ± 11.3	50.2 ± 25.3

WARNINGS

Risk of G.I. Ulceration, Bleeding and Perforation with NSAID Therapy: Serious gastrointestinal toxicity such as bleeding, ulceration and perforation can occur at any time, with or without warning symptoms, in patients treated chronically with NSAID therapy. Although minor upper gastrointestinal problems, such as dyspepsia, are common, usually developing early in therapy, physicians should remain alert for ulceration and bleeding in patients treated chronically with NSAIDs even in the absence of previous G.I. tract symptoms. In controlled clinical trials involving 1,677 patients treated with Nabumetone (1,140 followed for 1 year and 927 for 2 years), the cumulative incidence of peptic ulcers was 0.3% (95% CI; 0%, 0.6%) at 3 to 6 months, 0.5% (95% CI; 0.1%, 0.9%) at 1 year and 0.8% (95% CI; 0.3%, 1.3%) at 2 years. Physicians should inform patients about the signs and symptoms of serious G.I. toxicity and what steps to take if they occur. In patients with active peptic ulcer, physicians must weigh the benefits of Nabumetone therapy against possible hazards, institute an appropriate ulcer treatment regimen and monitor the patients' progress carefully.

Studies to date have not identified any subset of patients not at risk of developing peptic ulceration and bleeding. Except for a prior history of serious G.I. events and other risk factors known to be associated with peptic ulcer disease, such as alcoholism, smoking, etc., no risk factors (e.g., age, sex) have been associated with increased risk. Elderly or debilitated patients seem to tolerate ulceration or bleeding less well than other individuals and most spontaneous reports of fatal G.I. events are in this population.

High doses of an NSAID probably carry a greater risk of these reactions, although controlled clinical trials showing this do not exist in most cases. In considering the use of relatively large doses (within the recommended dosage range), sufficient benefit should be anticipated to offset the potential increased risk of G.I. toxicity.

PRECAUTIONS

GENERAL

Renal Effects: As a class, NSAIDs have been associated with renal papillary necrosis and other abnormal renal pathology during long-term administration to animals.

A second form of renal toxicity often associated with NSAIDs is seen in patients with conditions leading to a reduction in renal blood flow or blood volume, where renal prostaglandins have a supportive role in the maintenance of renal perfusion. In these patients, administration of an NSAID results in a dose-dependent decrease in prostaglandin synthesis and, secondarily, in a reduction of renal blood flow, which may precipitate overt renal decompensation. Patients at greatest risk of this reaction are those with impaired renal function, heart failure, liver dysfunction, those taking diuretics, and the elderly. Discontinuation of NSAID therapy is typically followed by recovery to the pretreatment state.

Because Nabumetone undergoes extensive hepatic metabolism, no adjustment of Nabumetone dosage is generally necessary in patients with renal insufficiency. However, as with all NSAIDs, patients with impaired renal function should be monitored more closely than patients with normal renal function (see *"Clinical Pharmacology: Special Studies"*). The oxidized and conjugated metabolites of 6MNA are eliminated primarily by the kidneys. The extent to which these largely inactive metabolites may accumulate in patients with renal failure has not been studied. As with other drugs whose metabolites are excreted by the kidneys, the possibility that adverse reactions (not listed in *"Adverse Reactions"*) may be attributable to these metabolites should be considered.

Hepatic Function: As with other NSAIDs, borderline elevations of one or more liver function tests may occur in up to 15% of patients. These abnormalities may progress, may remain essentially unchanged, or may return to normal with continued therapy. The ALT (SGPT) test is probably the most sensitive indicator of liver dysfunction. Meaningful (3 times the upper limit of normal) elevations of ALT (SGPT) or AST (SGOT) have occurred in controlled clinical trials of Nabumetone in less than 1% of patients. A patient with symptoms and/or signs suggesting liver dysfunction, or in whom an abnormal liver test has occurred, should be evaluated for evidence of the development of a more severe hepatic reaction while on Nabumetone therapy. Severe hepatic reactions, including jaundice and fatal hepatitis, have been reported with other NSAIDs. Although such reactions are rare, if abnormal liver tests persist or worsen, if clinical signs and symptoms consistent with liver disease develop, or if systemic manifestations occur (e.g., eosinophilia, rash, etc.), Nabumetone should be discontinued. Because Nabumetone's biotransformation to 6MNA is dependent upon hepatic function, the biotransformation could be decreased in patients with severe hepatic dysfunction. Therefore, Nabumetone should be used with caution in patients with severe hepatic impairment (see *"Pharmacokinetics: Hepatic Impairment"*).

Fluid Retention and Edema: Fluid retention and edema have been observed in some patients taking Nabumetone. Therefore, as with other NSAIDs, Nabumetone should be used cautiously in patients with a history of congestive heart failure, hypertension or other conditions predisposing to fluid retention.

Photosensitivity: Based on U.V. light photosensitivity testing, Nabumetone may be associated with more reactions to sun exposure than might be expected based on skin tanning types.

INFORMATION FOR PATIENTS

Nabumetone, like other drugs of its class, is not free of side effects. The side effects of these drugs can cause discomfort and, rarely, there are more serious side effects, such as gastrointestinal bleeding, which may result in hospitalization and even fatal outcome.

NSAIDs are often essential agents in the management of arthritis, but they also may be commonly employed for conditions which are less serious. Physicians may wish to discuss with their patients the potential risk (see *"Warnings, Precautions"* and *"Adverse Reactions"*) and likely benefits of NSAID treatment, particularly when the drugs are used for less serious conditions where treatment without NSAIDs may represent an acceptable alternative to both the patient and the physician.

LABORATORY TESTS

Because severe G.I. tract ulceration and bleeding can occur without warning symptoms, physicians should follow chronically treated patients for signs and symptoms of ulceration and bleeding, and should inform them of the importance of this follow-up (see *"Warnings: Risk of G.I. Ulceration, Bleeding and Perforation with NSAID Therapy"*).

DRUG INTERACTIONS

In vitro studies have shown that, because of its affinity for protein, 6MNA may displace other protein-bound drugs from their binding site. Caution should be exercised when administering Nabumetone with warfarin since interactions have been seen with other NSAIDs.

Concomitant administration of an aluminum-containing antacid had no significant effect on the bioavailability of 6MNA. When administered with food or milk, there is more rapid absorption; however, the total amount of 6MNA in the plasma is unchanged (see *"Pharmacokinetics"*).

CARCINOGENESIS, MUTAGENESIS

In two-year studies conducted in mice and rats, Nabumetone had no statistically significant tumorigenic effect. Nabumetone did not show mutagenic potential in the Ames test and mouse micronucleus test *in vivo*. However, Nabumetone- and 6MNA-treated lymphocytes in culture showed chromosomal aberrations at 80 mcg/mL and higher concentrations (equal to the average human exposure to Nabumetone at the maximum recommended dose).

IMPAIRMENT OF FERTILITY

Nabumetone did not impair fertility of male or female rats treated orally at doses of 320 mg/kg/day (1888 mg/m^2) before mating.

PREGNANCY

Teratogenic Effects. Pregnancy Category C. Nabumetone did not cause any teratogenic effect in rats given up to 400 mg/kg (2360 mg/m^2) and in rabbits up to 300 mg/kg (3540 mg/m^2) orally. However, increased post-implantation loss was observed in rats at 100 mg/kg (590 mg/m^2) orally and at higher doses (equal to the average human exposure to 6MNA at the maximum recommended human dose). There are no adequate, well-controlled studies in pregnant women. This drug should be used during pregnancy only if clearly needed.

Because of the known effect of prostaglandin-synthesis-inhibiting drugs on the human fetal cardiovascular system (closure of ductus arteriosus), use of Nabumetone during the third trimester of pregnancy is not recommended.

LABOR AND DELIVERY

The effects of Nabumetone on labor and delivery in women are not known. As with other drugs known to inhibit prostaglandin synthesis, an increased incidence of dystocia and delayed parturition occurred in rats treated throughout pregnancy.

NURSING MOTHERS

Nabumetone is not recommended for use in nursing mothers because of the possible adverse effects of prostaglandin-synthesis-inhibiting drugs on neonates. It is not known whether Nabumetone or its metabolites are excreted in human milk; however, 6MNA is excreted in the milk of lactating rats.

PEDIATRIC USE

Nabumetone is not recommended for use in children because the safety and efficacy in children have not been established.

GERIATRIC USE

Of the 1,677 patients in U.S. clinical studies who were treated with Nabumetone 411 patients (24%) were 65 years of age or older: 22 patients (1%) were 75 years of age or older. No overall differences in efficacy or safety were observed between these older patients and younger ones. Similar results were observed in a 1-year, non-U.S. postmarketing surveillance study of 10,800 Nabumetone patients, of whom 4,577 patients (42%) were 65 years of age or older.

ADVERSE REACTIONS

Adverse reaction information was derived from blinded-controlled and open-labelled clinical trials and from worldwide marketing experience. In the description below, rates of the more common events (greater than 1%) and many of the less common events (less than 1%) represent results of U.S. clinical studies.

Of the 1,677 patients who received Nabumetone during U.S. clinical trials, 1,524 were treated for at least 1 month, 1,327 for at least 3 months, 929 for at least a year and 750 for at least 2 years. Over 300 patients have been treated for 5 years or longer.

The most frequently reported adverse reactions were related to the gastrointestinal tract. They were diarrhea, dyspepsia and abdominal pain.

◆ RATED THERAPEUTICALLY EQUIVALENT; ◇ THERAPEUTIC EQUIVALENCE UNCONFIRMED; ○ UNRATED

INCIDENCE ≥ 1% — PROBABLY CAUSALLY RELATED

Gastrointestinal: Diarrhea (14%), dyspepsia (13%), abdominal pain (12%), constipation*, flatulence*, nausea*, positive stool guaiac*, dry mouth, gastritis, stomatitis, vomiting.

Central Nervous System: Dizziness*, headache*, fatigue, increased sweating, insomnia, nervousness, somnolence.

Dermatologic: Pruritus*, rash*.

Special Senses: Tinnitus*.

Miscellaneous: Edema*.

INCIDENCE < 1% — PROBABLY CAUSALLY RELATED†

Gastrointestinal: Anorexia, cholestatic jaundice, duodenal ulcer, dysphagia, gastric ulcer, gastroenteritis, gastrointestinal bleeding, increased appetite, liver function abnormalities, melena.

Central Nervous System: Asthenia, agitation, anxiety, confusion, depression, malaise, paresthesia, tremor, vertigo.

Dermatologic: Bullous eruptions, photosensitivity, urticaria, pseudoporphyria cutanea tarda, *toxic epidermal necrolysis*.

Cardiovascular: Vasculitis.

Metabolic: Weight gain.

Respiratory: Dyspnea, *eosinophilic pneumonia, hypersensitivity pneumonitis*.

Genitourinary: Albuminuria, azotemia, *hyperuricemia, interstitial nephritis, nephrotic syndrome, vaginal bleeding*.

Special Senses: Abnormal vision.

Hypersensitivity: *Anaphylactoid reaction, anaphylaxis*, angioneurotic edema.

INCIDENCE < 1% — CAUSAL RELATIONSHIP UNKNOWN†

Gastrointestinal: Bilirubinuria, duodenitis, eructation, gallstones, gingivitis, glossitis, pancreatitis, rectal bleeding.

Central Nervous System: Nightmares.

Dermatologic : Acne, alopecia, erythema multiforme, Stevens-Johnson Syndrome.

Cardiovascular: Angina, arrhythmia, hypertension, myocardial infarction, palpitations, syncope, thrombophlebitis.

Respiratory: Asthma, cough.

Genitourinary: Dysuria, hematuria, impotence, renal stones.

Special Senses: Taste disorder.

Body as a Whole: Fever, chills.

Hematologic/Lymphatic: Anemia, leukopenia, granulocytopenia, thrombocytopenia.

Metabolic/Nutritional: Hyperglycemia, hypokalemia, weight loss.

OVERDOSAGE

Since only 1 case of Nabumetone overdose has been reported, the experience is limited. If acute overdose occurs, it is recommended that the stomach be emptied by vomiting or lavage and general supportive measures be instituted, as necessary. In addition, the use of activated charcoal, up to 60 grams, may effectively reduce Nabumetone absorption. Coadministration of Nabumetone with charcoal to man has resulted in an 80% decrease in maximum plasma concentrations of the active metabolite.

The 1 overdose occurred in a 17-year-old female patient who had a history of abdominal pain and was hospitalized for increased abdominal pain following ingestion of 30 Nabumetone tablets (15 grams total). Stools were negative for occult blood and there was no fall in serum hemoglobin concentration.

The patient had no other symptoms. She was given an H_2-receptor antagonist and discharged from the hospital without sequelae.

DOSAGE AND ADMINISTRATION

OSTEOARTHRITIS AND RHEUMATOID ARTHRITIS

The recommended starting dose is 1000 mg taken as a single dose with or without food. Some patients may obtain more symptomatic relief from 1500 mg to 2000 mg per day. Nabumetone can be given in either a single or twice-daily dose. Dosages over 2000 mg per day have not been studied. The lowest effective dose should be used for chronic treatment.

Store at controlled room temperature (59° to 86°F) in well-closed container; dispense in light-resistant container.

HOW SUPPLIED
TABLETS: 500 MG

BRAND/MANUFACTURER	NDC	SIZE	AWP
○ BRAND			
➤ RELAFEN: SK Beecham Pharm	00029-4851-20	100s	$97.80
	00029-4851-21	100s	$97.80

---

* Incidence of reported reaction between 3% and 9%. Reactions occurring in 1% to 3% of the patients are unmarked.
† Adverse reactions reported only in worldwide postmarketing experience or in the literature, not seen in clinical trials, are considered rarer and are italicized.

TABLETS: 750 MG

BRAND/MANUFACTURER	NDC	SIZE	AWP
○ BRAND			
➤ RELAFEN: SK Beecham Pharm	00029-4852-20	100s	$123.15

Nadolol

DESCRIPTION

Nadolol is a synthetic nonselective beta-adrenergic receptor blocking agent designated chemically as 1-(*tert*-butylamino)-3-[(5,6,7,8-tetrahydro-*cis*-6,7-dihydroxy-1-naphthyl)oxy]-2-propanol.

Its molecular formula is $C_{17}H_{22}NO_4$ and its molecular weight is 309.40. The CAS number of Nadolol is 42200-33-9.

Nadolol is a white crystalline powder. It is freely soluble in ethanol, soluble in hydrochloric acid, slightly soluble in water and in chloroform, and very slightly soluble in sodium hydroxide.

Nadolol is available for oral administration as 20 mg, 40 mg, 80 mg, 120 mg, and 160 mg tablets.

Following is its chemical structure:

$$OCH_2CHCH_2NHC(CH_3)_3$$

CLINICAL PHARMACOLOGY

Nadolol is a nonselective beta-adrenergic receptor blocking agent. Clinical pharmacology studies have demonstrated beta-blocking activity by showing (1) reduction in heart rate and cardiac output at rest and on exercise, (2) reduction of systolic and diastolic blood pressure at rest and on exercise, (3) inhibition of isoproterenol-induced tachycardia, and (4) reduction of relfex orthostatic tachycardia.

Nadolol specifically competes with beta-adrenergic receptor agonists for available beta receptor sites; it inhibits both the $beta_1$ receptors located chiefly in cardiac muscle and the $beta_2$ receptors located chiefly in the bronchial and vascular musculature, inhibiting the chronotropic, inotropic, and vasodilator responses to beta-adrenergic stimulation proportionally. Nadolol has no intrinsic sympathomimetic activity and, unlike some other beta-adrenergic blocking agents Nadolol has little direct myocardial depressant activity and does not have an anesthetic-like membrance-stabilizing action. Animal and human studies show that Nadolol slows the sinus rate and depresses AV conduction. In dogs, only minimal amounts of Nadolol were detected in the brain relative to amounts in blood and other organs and tissues. Nadolol has low lipophilicity as determined by octanol/water partition coefficient, a characteristic of certain beta-blocking agents that has been correlated with the limited extent to which these agents cross the blood-brain barrier, their low concentration in the brain, and low incidence of CNS-related side effects.

In controlled clinical studies, Nadolol at doses of 40 to 320 mg/day has been shown to decrease both standing and supine blood pressure, the effect persisting for approximately 24 hours after dosing.

The mechanism of the antihypertensive effects of beta-adrenergic receptor blocking agents has not been established; however, factors that may be involved include (1) competitive antagonism of catecholamines at peripheral (non-CNS) adrenergic neuron sites (especially cardiac) leading to decreased cardiac output, (2) a central effect leading to reduced tonic-sympathetic nerve outflow to the periphery, and (3) suppression of renin secretion by blockade of the beta-adrenergic receptors responsible for renin release from the kidneys.

While cardiac output and arterial pressure are reduced by Nadolol therapy, renal hemodynamics are stable, with preservation of renal blood flow and glomerular filtration rate. By blocking catecholamine-induced increases in heart rate, velocity and extent of myocardial contraction, and blood pressure, Nadolol generally reduces the oxygen requirements of the heart at any given level of effort, making it useful for many patients in the long-term management of angina pectoris. On the other hand, Nadolol can increase oxygen requirements by increasing left ventricular fiber length and end diastolic pressure, particularly in patients with heart failure.

Although beta-adrenergic receptor blockade is useful in treatment of angina and hypertension, there are also situations in which sympathetic stimulation is vital. For example, in patients with severely damaged hearts, adequate ventricular function may depend on sympathetic drive. Beta-adrenergic blockade may worsen AV block by preventing the necessary facilitating effects of sympathetic acivity on conduction. $Beta_2$-adrenergic blockade results in passive bronchial constriction by interfering with endogenous adrenergic bronchodilator activity in patients subject to bronchospasm and may also interfere with exogenous bronchodilators in such patients.

Absorption of Nadolol after oral dosing is variable, averaging about 30%. Peak serum concentrations of Nadolol usually occur in 3 to 4 hours after oral administration and the presence of food in the gastrointestinal tract does not affect the rate or extent of Nadolol absorption. Approximately 30% of the Nadolol present in serum is reversibly bound to plasma protein.

Unlike many other beta-adrenergic blocking agents Nadolol is not metabolized by the liver and is excreted unchanged, principally by the kidneys.

➤ SHOWN IN PRODUCT IDENTIFICATION GUIDE

The half-life of therapeutic doses of Nadolol is about 20 to 24 hours, permitting once-daily dosage. Because Nadolol is excreted predominantly in the urine, its half-life increases in renal failure (see *"Precautions"* and *"Dosage and Administration"*). Steady-state serum concentrations of Nadolol are attained in 6 to 9 days with once-daily dosage in persons with normal renal function. Because of variable absorption and different individual responsiveness, the proper dosage must be determined by titration.

Exacerbation of angina and, in some cases, myocardial infarction and ventricular dysrhythmias have been reported after abrupt discontinuation of therapy with beta-adrenergic blocking agents in patients with coronary artery disease. Abrupt withdrawal of these agents in patients without coronary artery disease has resulted in transient symptoms, including tremulousness, sweating, palpitaion, headache, and malaise. Several mechanisms have been proposed to explain these phenomena, among them increased sensitivity to catecholamines because of increased numbers of beta receptors.

INDICATIONS AND USAGE

Angina Pectoris: Nadolol is indicated for the long-term management of patients with angina pectoris.

Hypertension: Nadolol is indicated in the management of hypertension; it may be used alone or in combination with other antihypertensive agents, especially thiazide-type diuretics.

UNLABELED USES

Nadolol is used alone or as an adjunct in the treatment of arrhythmias, including sustained supraventricular tachycardia. It is also used for the treatment of initial bleeding in cirrhosis, and for prophylaxis of migraine headache. It is also used in the acute phase of myocardial infarction.

CONTRAINDICATIONS

Nadolol is contraindicated in bronchial asthma, sinus bradycardia and greater than first degree conduction block, cardiogenic shock, and overt cardiac failure (see *"Warnings"*).

WARNINGS

Cardiac Failure: Sympathetic stimulation may be a vital component supporting circulatory function in patients with congestive heart failure, and its inhibition by beta-blockade may precipitate more severe failure. Although beta-blockers should be avoided in overt congestive heart failure, if necessary, they can be used with caution in patients with a history of failure who are well compensated, usually with digitalis and diuretics. Beta-adrenergic blocking agents do not abolish the inotropic action of digitalis on heart muscle.

In Patients Without A History Of Heart Failure, continued use of beta-blockers can, in some cases, lead to cardiac failure. Therefore, at the first sign or symptom of heart failure, the patient should be digitalized and/or treated with diuretics, and the response observed closely, or Nadolol should be discontinued (gradually, if possible).

EXACERBATION OF ISCHEMIC HEART DISEASE FOLLOWING ABRUPT WITHDRAWAL:

HYPERSENSITIVITY TO CATECHOLAMINES HAS BEEN OBSERVED IN PATIENTS WITHDRAWN FROM BETA-BLOCKER THERAPY; EXACERBATION OF ANGINA AND, IN SOME CASES, MYOCARDIAL INFARCTION HAVE OCCURRED AFTER *ABRUPT* DISCONTINUATION OF SUCH THERAPY. WHEN DISCONTINUING CHRONICALLY ADMINISTERED NADOLOL, PARTICULARLY IN PATIENTS WITH ISCHEMIC HEART DISEASE, THE DOSAGE SHOULD BE GRADUALLY REDUCED OVER A PERIOD OF 1 TO 2 WEEKS AND THE PATIENT SHOULD BE CAREFULLY MONITORED. IF ANGINA MARKEDLY WORSENS OR ACUTE CORONARY INSUFFICIENCY DEVELOPS, NADOLOL ADMINISTRATION SHOULD BE REINSTITUTED PROMPTLY, AT LEAST TEMPORARILY, AND OTHER MEASURES APPROPRIATE FOR THE MANAGEMENT OF UNSTABLE ANGINA SHOULD BE TAKEN. PATIENTS SHOULD BE WARNED AGAINST INTERRUPTION OR DISCONTINUATION OF THERAPY WITHOUT THE PHYSICIAN'S ADVICE. BECAUSE CORONARY ARTERY DISEASE IS COMMON AND MAY BE UNRECOGNIZED, IT MAY BE PRUDENT NOT TO DISCONTINUE NADOLOL THERAPY ABRUPTLY EVEN IN PATIENTS TREATED ONLY FOR HYPERTENSION.

Nonallergic Bronchospasm (eg, Chronic Bronchitis, Emphysema): PATIENTS WITH BRONCHOSPASTIC DISEASES SHOULD IN GENERAL NOT RECEIVE BETA-BLOCKERS. Nadolol should be administered with caution since it may block bronchodilation produced by endogenous or exogenous catecholamine stimulation of beta$_2$ receptors.

Major Surgery: Because beta-blockade impairs the ability of the heart to respond to reflex stimuli and may increase the risks of general anesthesia and surgical procedures, resulting in protracted hypotension or low cardiac output, it has generally been suggested that such therapy should be withdrawn several days prior to surgery. Recognition of the increased sensitivity to catecholamines of patients recently withdrawn from beta-blocker therapy, however, has made this recommendation controversial. If possible, beta-blockers should be withdrawn well before surgery takes place. In the event of emergency surgery, the anesthesiologist should be informed that the patient is on beta-blocker therapy. The effects of Nadolol can be reversed by administration of beta-receptor agonists such as isoproterenol, dopamine, dobutamine, or levarterenol. Difficulty in restarting and maintaining the heart beat has also been reported with beta-adrenergic receptor blocking agents.

Diabetes and Hypoglycemia: Beta-adrenergic blockade may prevent the appearance of premonitory signs and symptoms (eg, tachycardia and blood pressure changes) of acute hypoglycemia. This is especially important with labile diabetics. Beta-blockade also reduces the release of insulin in response to hyperglycemia; therefore, it may be necessary to adjust the dose of antidiabetic drugs.

Thyrotoxicosis: Beta-adrenergic blockade may mask certain clinical signs (eg, tachycardia) of hyperthyroidism. Patients suspected of developing thyrotoxicosis should be managed carefully to avoid abrupt withdrawal of beta-adrenergic blockade which might precipitate a thyroid storm.

PRECAUTIONS

IMPAIRED RENAL FUNCTION
Nadolol should be used with caution in patients with impaired renal function (see *"Dosage and Administration"*).

INFORMATION FOR PATIENTS
Patients, especially those with evidence of coronary artery insufficiency, should be warned against interruption or discontinuation of Nadolol therapy without the physician's advice. Although cardiac failure rarely occurs in properly selected patients, patients being treated with beta-adrenergic blocking agents should be advised to consult the physician at the first sign or symptom of impending failure. The patient should also be advised of a proper course in the event of an inadvertently missed dose.

DRUG INTERACTIONS
When administered concurrently, the following drugs may interact with beta-adrenergic receptor blocking agents:

Anesthetics, General: exaggeration of the hypotension induced by general anesthetics (see *"Warnings, Major Surgery"*).

Antidiabetic Drugs (oral agents and insulin): hypoglycemia or hyperglycemia; adjust dosage of antidiabetic drug accordingly (see *"Warnings, Diabetes and Hypoglycemia"*).

Catecholamine-depleting Drugs (eg, reserpine): additive effect; monitor closely for evidence of hypotension and/or excessive bradycardia (eg, vertigo, syncope, postural hypotension).

Response to Treatment for Anaphylactic Reaction: While taking beta-blockers, patients with a history of severe anaphylactic reaction to a variety of allergens may be more reactive to repeated challenge, either accidental, diagnostic, or therapeutic. Such patients may be unresponsive to the usual doses of epinephrine used to treat allergic reaction.

CARCINOGENESIS, MUTAGENESIS, IMPAIRMENT OF FERTILITY
In chronic oral toxicologic studies (1 to 2 years) in mice, rats, and dogs, Nadolol did not produce any significant toxic effects. In 2-year oral carcinogenic studies in rats and mice, Nadolol did not produce any neoplastic, preneoplastic, or nonneoplastic pathologic lesions. In fertility and general reproductive perforance studies in rats, Nadolol caused no adverse effects.

PREGNANCY CATEGORY C
In animal reproduction studies with Nadolol, evidence of embryo- and fetotoxicity was found in rabbits, but not in rats or hamsters, at doses 5 to 10 times greater (on a mg/kg basis) than the maximum indicated human dose. No teratogenic potential was observed in any of these species.

There are no adequate and well-controlled studies in pregnant women. Nadolol should be used during pregnancy only if the potential benefit justifies the potential risk to the fetus. Neonates whose mothers are receiving Nadolol at parturition have exhibited bradycardia, hypoglycemia, and associated symptoms.

NURSING MOTHERS
Nadolol is excreted in human milk. Because of the potential for adverse effects in nursing infants, a decision should be made whether to discontinue nursing or to discontinue therapy taking into account the importance of Nadolol to the mother.

PEDIATRIC USE
Safety and effectiveness in children have not been established.

ADVERSE REACTIONS
Most adverse effects have been mild and transient and have rarely required withdrawal of therapy.

Cardiovascular: Bradycardia with heart rates of less than 60 beats per minute occurs commonly, and heart rates below 40 beats per minute and/or symptomatic bradycardia were seen in about 2 of 100 patients. Symptoms of peripheral vascular insufficiency, usually of the Raynaud type, have occurred in approximately 2 of 100 patients. Cardiac failure, hypotension, and rhythm/conduction disturbances have each occurred in about 1 of 100 patients. Single instances of first degree and third degree heart block have been reported: intensification of AV block is a known effect of beta-blockers (see also *"Contraindications"*, *"Warnings"* and *"Precautions"*).

Central Nervous System: Dizziness or fatigue has been reported in approximately 2 of 100 patients; paresthesias, sedation, and change in behavior have each been reported in approximately 6 of 1000 patients.

◆ RATED THERAPEUTICALLY EQUIVALENT; ◇ THERAPEUTIC EQUIVALENCE UNCONFIRMED; ○ UNRATED

Respiratory: Bronchospasm has been reported in approximately 1 of 1000 patients (see *"Contraindications"* and *"Warnings"*).

Gastrointestinal: Nausea, diarrhea, abdominal discomfort, constipation, vomiting, indigestion, anorexia, bloating, and flatulence have been reported in 1 to 5 of 1000 patients.

Miscellaneous: Each of the following has been reported in 1 to 5 of 1000 patients: rash; pruritus; headache; dry mouth, eyes, or skin; impotence or decreased libido; facial swelling; weight gain; slurred speech; cough; nasal stuffiness; sweating; tinnitus; blurred vision. Reversible alopecia has been reported infrequently.

The following adverse reactions have been reported in patients taking Nadolol and/or other beta-adrenergic blocking agents, but no causal relationship to Nadolol has been established.

Central Nervous System: Reversible mental depression progressing to catatonia; visual disturbances; hallucinations; an acute reversible syndrome characterized by disorientation for time and place, short-term memory loss, emotional lability with slightly clouded sensorium, and decreased performance on neuropsychometrics.

Gastrointestinal: Mesenteric arterial thrombosis; ischemic colitis; elevated liver enzymes.

Hematologic: Agranulocytosis; thrombocytopenic or nonthrombocytopenic purpura.

Allergic: Fever combined with aching and sore throat; laryngospasm; respiratory distress.

Miscellaneous: Pemphigoid rash; hypertensive reaction in patients with pheochromocytoma; sleep disturbances; Peyronie's disease.

The oculomucocutaneous syndrome associated with the beta-blocker practolol has not been reported with Nadolol.

OVERDOSAGE
Nadolol can be removed from the general circulation by hemodialysis.

In addition to gastric lavage, the following measures should be employed, as appropriate. In determining the duration of corrective therapy, note must be taken of the long duration of the effect of Nadolol.

Excessive Bradycardia: Administer atropine (0.25 to 1.0 mg). If there is no response to vagal blockade, administer isoproterenol cautiously.

Cardiac Failure: Administer a digitalis glycoside and diuretic. It has been reported that glucagon may also be useful in this situation.

Hypotension: Administer vasopressors, eg, epinephrine or levarterenol. (There is evidence that epinephrine may be the drug of choice.)

Bronchospasm: Administer a beta₂-stimulating agent and/or a theophylline derivative.

DOSAGE AND ADMINISTRATION
DOSAGE MUST BE INDIVIDUALIZED. NADOLOL MAY BE ADMINISTERED WITHOUT REGARD TO MEALS.

Angina Pectoris: The usual initial dose is 40 mg Nadolol once daily. Dosage may be gradually increased in 40 to 80 mg increments at 3- to 7-day intervals until optimum clinical response is obtained or there is pronounced slowing of the heart rate. The usual maintenance dose is 40 or 80 mg administered once daily. Doses up to 160 or 240 mg administered once daily may be needed.

The usefulness and safety in angina pectoris of dosage exceeding 240 mg per day have not been established. If treatment is to be discontinued, reduce the dosage gradually over a period of 1 to 2 weeks (see *"Warnings"*).

Hypertension: The usual initial dose is 40 mg Nadolol once daily, whether it is used alone or in addition to diuretic therapy. Dosage may be gradually increased in 40 to 80 mg increments until optimum blood pressure reduction is achieved. The usual maintenance dose is 40 or 80 mg administered once daily. Doses up to 240 or 320 mg administered once daily may be needed.

Dosage Adjustment in Renal Failure: Absorbed Nadolol is excreted principally by the kidneys and, although nonrenal elimination does occur, dosage adjustments are necessary in patients with renal impairment. The following dose intervals are recommended:

Creatinine Clearance (mL/min/1.73m²)	Dosage Interval (hours)
> 50	24
31-50	24-36
10-30	24-48
< 10	40-60

Storage: Store at room temperature; avoid excessive heat. Protect from light. Keep bottle tightly closed.

HOW SUPPLIED
TABLET: 20 MG

AVERAGE UNIT PRICE (AVAILABLE SIZES)		GENERIC A-RATED AVERAGE PRICE (GAAP)		
GENERIC	$0.76	100s		$76.13
BRAND/MANUFACTURER		NDC	SIZE	AWP
◆ BRAND				
➤ CORGARD: B/M Squibb U.S. Phar		00003-0232-50	100s	$85.40
		00003-0232-51	100s ud	$92.21
◆ GENERICS				
Allscrips		54569-3789-00	30s	$22.80
Apothecon		59772-2461-01	100s	$69.50
Moore,H.L.		00839-7869-06	100s	$72.40
Major		00904-7816-60	100s	$73.60
Qualitest		00603-4740-21	100s	$74.42
Apothecon		59772-2461-02	100s	$75.05
Mylan		00378-0028-01	100s	$76.00
UDL		51079-0812-20	100s ud	$84.23

TABLET: 40 MG

AVERAGE UNIT PRICE (AVAILABLE SIZES)		GENERIC A-RATED AVERAGE PRICE (GAAP)		
GENERIC	$0.88	100s		$86.80
BRAND/MANUFACTURER		NDC	SIZE	AWP
◆ BRAND				
➤ CORGARD: B/M Squibb U.S. Phar		00003-0207-50	100s	$100.11
		00003-0207-53	100s ud	$108.06
		00003-0207-76	1000s	$980.74
◆ GENERICS				
Allscrips		54569-3790-00	30s	$26.73
Allscrips		54569-8591-00	90s	$80.18
Apothecon		59772-2462-01	100s	$81.48
Qualitest		00603-4741-21	100s	$84.67
Moore,H.L.		00839-7870-06	100s	$84.88
Major		00904-7817-60	100s	$86.25
Mylan		00378-1171-01	100s	$89.09
Apothecon		59772-2462-02	100s ud	$87.95
UDL		51079-0813-20	100s ud	$89.10
Apothecon		59772-2462-03	1000s	$798.24
Mylan		00378-1171-10	1000s	$881.75

TABLET: 80 MG

AVERAGE UNIT PRICE (AVAILABLE SIZES)		GENERIC A-RATED AVERAGE PRICE (GAAP)		
GENERIC	$1.18	100s		$118.32
		1000s		$1167.40
BRAND/MANUFACTURER		NDC	SIZE	AWP
◆ BRAND				
➤ CORGARD: B/M Squibb U.S. Phar		00003-0241-50	100s	$137.26
		00003-0241-55	100s ud	$145.02
		00003-0241-76	1000s	$1344.56
◆ GENERICS				
Allscrips		54569-3791-00	30s	$36.65
Apothecon		59772-2463-01	100s	$111.72
Qualitest		00603-4742-21	100s	$116.09
Copley		38245-0724-10	100s	$116.20
Moore,H.L.		00839-7871-06	100s	$116.38
Major		00904-7818-60	100s	$118.30
Mylan		00378-1132-01	100s	$122.16
Apothecon		59772-2463-02	100s ud	$118.03
UDL		51079-0814-20	100s ud	$120.80
Apothecon		59772-2463-03	1000s	$1094.35
Copley		38245-0724-20	1000s	$1138.15
Mylan		00378-1132-10	1000s	$1196.65

TABLET: 120 MG

AVERAGE UNIT PRICE (AVAILABLE SIZES)				
GENERIC	$1.50			
BRAND/MANUFACTURER		NDC	SIZE	AWP
◆ BRAND				
➤ CORGARD: B/M Squibb U.S. Phar		00003-0208-50	100s	$178.91
		00003-0208-76	1000s	$1749.76
◆ GENERICS				
Apothecon		59772-2464-01	100s	$145.61
Copley		38245-0727-10	100s	$151.45
Apothecon		59772-2464-03	1000s	$1424.16
Copley		38245-0727-20	1000s	$1481.15

For additional alternatives, turn to the section beginning on page 2859.

Nafarelin Acetate

DESCRIPTION
Nafarelin Acetate Nasal Solution is intended for administration as a spray to the nasal mucosa. Nafarelin Acetate is a decapeptide with the chemical name: 5-oxo-*L*-prolyl-*L*-histidyl-*L*-tryptophyl-*L*-seryl-*L*-tyrosyl-3-(2-naphthyl)-*D*-alanyl-*L*-leucyl-*L*-arginyl-*L*-prolyl-glycinamide acetate. Nafarelin Acetate is a

➤ SHOWN IN PRODUCT IDENTIFICATION GUIDE

synthetic analog of the naturally occurring gonadotropin-releasing hormone (GnRH).

The Nasal Solution contains Nafarelin Acetate (2 mg/mL, content expressed as Nafarelin base).

After priming the pump unit for Nafarelin Acetate, each actuation of the unit delivers approximately 100 µL of the spray containing approximately 200 µg Nafarelin base. The contents of one spray bottle are intended to deliver at least 60 sprays.

Following is its chemical structure:

H-5-oxo-L-Pro-L-His-L-Trp-L-Ser-L-Tyr—N---C--C—

L-Leu-L-Arg-L-Pro-Gly—NH_2 · x CH_3COOH · y H_2O

CLINICAL PHARMACOLOGY

Nafarelin Acetate is a potent agonistic analog of gonadotropin-releasing hormone (GnRH). At the onset of administration, Nafarelin stimulates the release of the pituitary gonadotropins, LH and FSH, resulting in a temporary increase of steroidogenesis. Repeated dosing abolishes the stimulatory effect on the pituitary gland. Twice daily administration leads to decreased secretion of gonadal steroids by about 4 weeks; consequently, tissues and functions that depend on gonadal steroids for their maintenance become quiescent. Nafarelin Acetate is rapidly absorbed into the systemic circulation after intranasal administration. Maximum serum concentrations (measured by RIA) were achieved between 10 and 45 minutes. Following a single dose of 400 µg base, the observed peak concentration was 2.2 ng/mL, whereas following a single dose of 600 µg base, the observed peak concentration was 6.6 ng/mL. The average serum half-life of Nafarelin following intranasal administration of a 400 µg dose was approximately 2.5 hours. It is not known and cannot be predicted what the pharmacokinetics of Nafarelin will be in children given a dose above 600 µg.

In adult women, maximum serum concentrations (measured by RIA) were achieved between 10 and 40 minutes. Following a single dose of 200 µg base, the observed average peak concentration was 0.6 ng/mL (range 0.2 to 1.4 ng/mL), whereas following a single dose of 400 µg base, the observed average peak concentration was 1.8 ng/mL (range 0.5 to 5.3 ng/mL). Bioavailability from a 400 µg dose averaged 2.8% (range 1.2 to 5.6%). The average serum half-life of Nafarelin following intranasal administration was approximately 3 hours. About 80% of Nafarelin Acetate was bound to plasma proteins at 4°C. Twice daily intranasal administration of 200 or 400 µg of Nafarelin Acetate in 18 healthy women for 22 days did not lead to significant accumulation of the drug. Based on the mean Cmin levels on Days 15 and 22, there appears to be dose proportionality across the two dose levels. After subcutaneous administration of ^{14}C-Nafarelin Acetate to men, 44-55% of the dose was recovered in urine and 18.5-44.2% was recovered in feces. Approximately 3% of the administered dose appeared as unchanged Nafarelin in urine. The ^{14}C serum half-life of the metabolites was about 85.5 hours. Six metabolites of Nafarelin have been identified of which the major metabolite is Tyr-D(2)-Nal-Leu-Arg-Pro-Gly-NH_2(5-10). The activity of the metabolites, the metabolism of Nafarelin by nasal mucosa, and the pharmacokinetics of the drug in hepatically- and renally-impaired patients have not been determined.

There appeared to be no significant effect of rhinitis, i.e. nasal congestion, on the systemic bioavailability of Nafarelin Acetate; however, if the use of a nasal decongestant for rhinitis is necessary during treatment with Nafarelin Acetate, the decongestant should not be used until at least 2 hours following dosing of Nafarelin Acetate.

When used regularly in girls and boys with **central precocious puberty (CPP)** at the recommended dose, Nafarelin Acetate suppresses LH and sex steroid hormone levels to prepubertal levels, affects a corresponding arrest of secondary sexual development, and slows linear growth and skeletal maturation. In some cases, initial estrogen withdrawal bleeding may occur, generally within 6 weeks after initiation of therapy. Thereafter, menstruation should cease.

In clinical studies the peak response of LH to GnRH stimulation was reduced from a pubertal response to a prepubertal response (< 15 mIU/mL) within one month of treatment.

Linear growth velocity, which is commonly pubertal in children with CPP, is reduced in most children within the first year of treatment to values of 5 to 6 cm/year or less. Children with CPP are frequently taller than their chronological age peers; height for chronological age approaches normal in most children during the second or third year of treatment with Nafarelin Acetate. Skeletal maturation rate (bone age velocity—change in bone age divided by change in chronological age) is usually abnormal (greater than 1) in children with CPP; in most children, bone age velocity approaches normal (1) during the first year of treatment. This results in a narrowing of the gap between bone age and chronological age, usually by the second or third year of treatment. The mean predicted adult height increases.

In clinical trials, breast development was arrested or regressed in 82% of girls, and genital development was arrested or regressed in 100% of boys. Because pubic hair growth is largely controlled by adrenal androgens, which are unaffected by Nafarelin, pubic hair development was arrested or regressed only in 54% of girls and boys.

Reversal of the suppressive effects of Nafarelin Acetate has been demonstrated to occur in all children with CPP for whom one-year post-treatment follow-up is available (n = 69). This demonstration consisted of the appearance or return of menses, the return of pubertal gonadotropin and gonadal sex steroid levels, and/or the advancement of secondary sexual development. Semen analysis was normal in the two ejaculated specimens obtained thus far from boys who have been taken off therapy to resume puberty. Fertility has not been documented by pregnancies and the effect of long term use of the drug on fertility is not known.

In controlled clinical studies in adult women, Nafarelin Acetate at doses of 400 and 800 µg/day for 6 months was shown to be comparable to danazol, 800 mg/day, in relieving the clinical symptoms of endometriosis (pelvic pain, dysmenorrhea, and dyspareunia) and in reducing the size of endometrial implants as determined by laparoscopy. The clinical significance of a decrease in endometriotic lesions is not known at this time and in addition, laparoscopic staging of endometriosis does not necessarily correlate with severity of symptoms.

Nafarelin Acetate 400 µg daily induced amenorrhea in approximately 65%, 80%, and 90% of the patients after 60, 90, and 120 days, respectively. In the first, second, and third post-treatment months, normal menstrual cycles resumed in 4%, 82%, and 100%, respectively, of those patients who did not become pregnant.

At the end of treatment, 60% of patients who received Nafarelin Acetate, 400 µg/day, were symptom free, 32% had mild symptoms, 7% had moderate symptoms and 1% had severe symptoms. Of the 60% of patients who had complete relief of symptoms at the end of treatment, 17% had moderate symptoms 6 months after treatment was discontinued, 33% had mild symptoms, 50% remained symptom free, and no patient had severe symptoms.

During the first two months use of Nafarelin Acetate, some women experience vaginal bleeding of variable duration and intensity. In all likelihood, this bleeding represents estrogen withdrawal bleeding, and is expected to stop spontaneously. If vaginal bleeding continues, the possibility of lack of compliance with the dosing regimen should be considered. If the patient is complying carefully with the regimen, an increase in dose to 400 µg twice a day should be considered.

There is no evidence that pregnancy rates are enhanced or adversely affected by the use of Nafarelin Acetate.

INDICATIONS AND USAGE
INDICATIONS AND USAGE FOR CENTRAL PRECOCIOUS PUBERTY
Nafarelin Acetate is indicated for treatment of central precocious puberty (CPP) (gonadotropin-dependent precocious puberty) in children of both sexes.

The diagnosis of central precocious puberty (CPP) is suspected when premature development of secondary sexual characteristics occurs at or before the age of 8 years in girls and 9 years in boys, and is accompanied by significant advancement of bone age and/or a poor adult height prediction. The diagnosis should be confirmed by pubertal gonadal sex steroid levels and a pubertal LH response to stimulation by native GnRH. Pelvic ultrasound assessment in girls usually reveals enlarged uterus and ovaries, the latter often with multiple cystic formations. Magnetic resonance imaging or CT-scanning of the brain is recommended to detect hypothalamic or pituitary tumors, or anatomical changes associated with increased intracranial pressure. Other causes of sexual precocity, such as congenital adrenal hyperplasia, testotoxicosis, testicular tumors and/or other autonomous feminizing or masculinizing disorders must be excluded by proper clinical hormonal and diagnostic imaging examinations.

INDICATIONS AND USAGE FOR ENDOMETRIOSIS
Nafarelin Acetate is indicated for management of endometriosis, including pain relief and reduction of endometriotic lesions. Experience with Nafarelin Acetate for the management of endometriosis has been limited to women 18 years of age and older treated for 6 months.

UNLABELED USES
Nafarelin Acetate is used alone or as an adjunct in the treatment of hirsutism and uterine leiomyomata. It is also used to provide symptomatic relief of benign prostatic hyperplasia and for suppression of spermatogenesis (male contraception).

CONTRAINDICATIONS
1. Hypersensitivity to GnRH, GnRH agonist analogs or any of the excipients in Nafarelin Acetate.
2. Undiagnosed abnormal vaginal bleeding;
3. Use in pregnancy or in women who may become pregnant while receiving the drug. Nafarelin Acetate may cause fetal harm when administered to a pregnant woman. Major fetal abnormalities were observed in rats, but not in mice or rabbits after administration of Nafarelin Acetate during the period of organogenesis. There was a dose-related increase in fetal mortality and a decrease in fetal weight in rats (see *"Pregnancy"* section). The effects on rat fetal mortality are expected consequences of the alterations in hormonal levels brought about by the drug. If this drug is used during pregnancy or if the patient becomes pregnant while taking this drug, she should be apprised of the potential hazard to the fetus:
4. Use in women who are breast feeding (see *"Nursing Mothers"* section).

WARNINGS
CENTRAL PRECOCIOUS PUBERTY
The diagnosis of central precocious puberty (CPP) must be established before treatment is initiated. Regular monitoring of CPP patients is needed to assess both patient response as well as compliance. This is particularly important during the first 6 to 8 weeks of treatment to assure that suppression of pituitary-gonadal function is rapid. Testing may include LH response to GnRH stimulation and circulating gonadal sex steroid levels. Assessment of growth velocity and bone age velocity should begin within 3 to 6 months of treatment initiation.

Some patients may not show suppression of the pituitary-gonadal axis by clinical and/or biochemical parameters. This may be due to lack of compliance with the recommended treatment regimen and may be rectified by recommending that the dosing be done by caregivers. If compliance problems are excluded, the possibility of gonadotropin independent sexual precocity should be reconsidered and appropriate examinations should be conducted. If compliance problems are excluded and if gonadotropin independent sexual precocity is not present, the dose of Nafarelin Acetate may be increased to 1800 µg/day administered as 600 µg tid.

ENDOMETRIOSIS

Safe use of Nafarelin Acetate in pregnancy has not been established clinically. Before starting treatment with Nafarelin Acetate, pregnancy must be excluded.

When used regularly at the recommended dose, Nafarelin Acetate usually inhibits ovulation and stops menstruation. Contraception is not insured, however, by taking Nafarelin Acetate, particularly if patients miss successive doses. Therefore, patients should use nonhormonal methods of contraception. Patients should be advised to see their physician if they believe they may be pregnant. If a patient becomes pregnant during treatment, the drug must be discontinued and the patient must be apprised of the potential risk to the fetus.

PRECAUTIONS
GENERAL
As with other drugs that stimulate the release of gonadotrophins or that induce ovulation in adult women with endometriosis, ovarian cysts have been reported to occur in the first two months of therapy with Nafarelin Acetate. Many, but not all, of these events occurred in women with polycystic ovarian disease. These cystic enlargements may resolve spontaneously, generally by about four to six weeks of therapy, but in some cases may require discontinuation of drug and/or surgical intervention. The relevance, if any, of such events in children is unknown.

INFORMATION FOR PATIENTS, PATIENTS' PARENTS OR GUARDIANS
An information pamphlet for patients is included with the product. Patients and their caregivers should be aware of the following information:

CENTRAL PRECOCIOUS PUBERTY
1. Reversibility of the suppressive effects of Nafarelin has been demonstrated by the appearance or return of menses, by the return of pubertal gonadotropin and gonadal sex steroid levels, and/or by advancement of secondary sexual development. Semen analysis was normal in the two ejaculated specimens obtained thus far from boys who have been taken off therapy to resume puberty. Fertility has not been documented by pregnancies and the effect of long term use of the drug on fertility is not known.
2. Patients and their caregivers should be adequately counselled to assure full compliance; irregular or incomplete daily doses may result in stimulation of the pituitary-gonadal axis.
3. During the first month of treatment with Nafarelin Acetate, some signs of puberty, e.g., vaginal bleeding or breast enlargement, may occur. This is the expected initial effect of the drug. Such changes should resolve soon after the first month. If such resolution does not occur within the first two months of treatment, this may be due to lack of compliance or the presence of gonadotropin independent sexual precocity. If both possibilities are definitively excluded, the dose of Nafarelin Acetate may be increased to 1800 µg/day administered as 600 µg tid.
4. Patients with intercurrent rhinitis should consult their physician for the use of a topical nasal decongestant. If the use of a topical nasal decongestant is required during treatment with Nafarelin Acetate, the decongestant should not be used until at least 2 hours following dosing with Nafarelin Acetate.

Sneezing during or immediately after dosing with Nafarelin Acetate should be avoided, if possible, since this may impair drug absorption.

ENDOMETRIOSIS
1. Since menstruation should stop with effective doses of Nafarelin Acetate, the patient should notify her physician if regular menstruation persists. The cause of vaginal spotting, bleeding or menstruation could be noncompliance with the treatment regimen, or it could be that a higher dose of the drug is required to achieve amenorrhea. The patient should be questioned regarding her compliance. If she is careful and compliant, and menstruation persists to the second month, consideration should be given to doubling the dose of Nafarelin Acetate. If the patient has missed several doses, she should be counseled on the importance of taking Nafarelin Acetate regularly as prescribed.
2. Patients should not use Nafarelin Acetate if they are pregnant, breast feeding, have undiagnosed abnormal vaginal bleeding, or are allergic to any of the ingredients in Nafarelin Acetate.
3. Safe use of the drug in pregnancy has not been established clinically. Therefore, a nonhormonal method of contraception should be used during treatment. Patients should be advised that if they miss successive doses of Nafarelin Acetate, breakthrough bleeding or ovulation may occur with the potential for conception. If a patient becomes pregnant during treatment, she should discontinue treatment and consult her physician.
4. Those adverse events occurring most frequently in clinical studies with Nafarelin Acetate are associated with hypoestrogenism; the most frequently reported are hot flashes, headaches, emotional lability, decreased libido, vaginal dryness, acne, myalgia, and reduction in breast size. Estrogen levels returned to normal after treatment was discontinued. Nasal irritation occurred in about 10% of all patients who used intranasal Nafarelin.

5. The induced hypoestrogenic state results in a small loss in bone density over the course of treatment, some of which may not be reversible. During one six-month treatment period, this bone loss should not be important. In patients with major risk factors for decreased bone mineral content such as chronic alcohol and/or tobacco use, strong family history of osteoporosis, or chronic use of drugs that can reduce bone mass such as anticonvulsants or corticosteroids, therapy with Nafarelin Acetate may pose an additional risk. In these patients the risks and benefits must be weighed carefully before therapy with Nafarelin Acetate is instituted. Repeated courses of treatment with gonadotropin-releasing hormone analogs are not advisable in patients with major risk factors for loss of bone mineral content.
6. Patients with intercurrent rhinitis should consult their physician for the use of a topical nasal decongestant. If the use of a topical nasal decongestant is required during treatment with Nafarelin Acetate, the decongestant should not be used until at least 2 hours following dosing with Nafarelin Acetate.

Sneezing during or immediately after dosing with Nafarelin Acetate should be avoided if possible, since this may impair drug absorption.

7. Retreatment cannot be recommended since safety data beyond 6 months are not available.

DRUG INTERACTIONS
No pharmacokinetic-based drug-drug interaction studies have been conducted with Nafarelin Acetate. However, because Nafarelin Acetate is a peptide that is primarily degraded by peptidase and not by cytochrome P-450 enzymes, and the drug is only about 80% bound to plasma proteins at 4°C, drug interactions would not be expected to occur.

DRUG/LABORATORY TEST INTERACTIONS
Administration of Nafarelin Acetate in therapeutic doses results in suppression of the pituitary-gonadal system. Normal function is usually restored within 4 to 8 weeks after treatment is discontinued. Therefore, diagnostic tests of pituitary gonadotropic and gonadal functions conducted during treatment and up to 4 to 8 weeks after discontinuation of therapy with Nafarelin Acetate may be misleading.

CARCINOGENESIS, MUTAGENESIS, IMPAIRMENT OF FERTILITY
Carcinogenicity studies of Nafarelin were conducted in rats (24 months) at doses up to 100 µg/kg/day and mice (18 months) at doses up to 500 µg/kg/day using intramuscular doses (up to 110 times and 560 times the maximum recommended human intranasal dose, respectively). These multiples of the human dose are based on the relative bioavailability of the drug by the two routes of administration. As seen with other GnRH agonists, Nafarelin Acetate given to laboratory rodents at high doses for prolonged periods induced proliferative responses (hyperplasia and/or neoplasia) of endocrine organs. At 24 months, there was an increase in the incidence of pituitary tumors (adenoma/carcinoma) in high-dose female rats and a dose-related increase in male rats. There was an increase in pancreatic islet cell adenomas in both sexes, and in benign testicular and ovarian tumors in the treated groups. There was a dose-related increase in benign adrenal medullary tumors in treated female rats. In mice, there was a dose-related increase in Harderian gland tumors in males and an increase in pituitary adenomas in high-dose females. No metastases of these tumors were observed. It is known that tumorigenicity in rodents is particularly sensitive to hormonal stimulation.

Mutagenicity studies have been performed with Nafarelin Acetate using bacterial, yeast, and mammalian systems. These studies provided no evidence of mutagenic potential. Reproduction studies in male and female rats have shown full reversibility of fertility suppression when drug treatment was discontinued after continuous administration for up to 6 months. The effect of treatment of prepubertal rats on the subsequent reproductive performance of mature animals has not been investigated.

PREGNANCY, TERATOGENIC EFFECTS
Pregnancy Category X. See " Contraindications". Intramuscular Nafarelin Acetate was administered to rats during the period of organogenesis at 0.4, 1.6, and 6.4 µg/kg/day (about 0.5, 2, and 7 times the maximum recommended human intranasal dose based on the relative bioavailability by the two routes of administration). An increase in major fetal abnormalities was observed in 4/80 fetuses at the highest dose. A similar, repeat study at the same doses in rats and studies in mice and rabbits at doses up to 600 µg/kg/day and 0.18 µg/kg/day, respectively, failed to demonstrate an increase in fetal abnormalities after administration during the period of organogenesis. In rats and rabbits, there was a dose-related increase in fetal mortality and a decrease in fetal weight with the highest dose.

NURSING MOTHERS
It is not known whether Nafarelin Acetate is excreted in human milk. Because many drugs are excreted in human milk, and because the effects of Nafarelin Acetate on lactation and/or the breastfed child have not been determined, Nafarelin Acetate should not be used by nursing mothers.

PEDIATRIC USE
Safety and effectiveness of Nafarelin Acetate for endometriosis in patients younger than 18 years have not been established.

ADVERSE REACTIONS
CENTRAL PRECOCIOUS PUBERTY
In clinical trials of 155 pediatric patients, 2.6% reported symptoms suggestive of drug sensitivity, such as shortness of breath, chest pain, urticaria, rash and pruritus.

In these 155 patients treated for an average of 41 months and as long as 80 months (6.7 years), adverse events most frequently reported (> 3% of patients) consisted largely of episodes occurring during the first 6 weeks of treatment as a result of the transient stimulatory action of Nafarelin upon the pituitary-gonadal axis:

acne (10%)
transient breast enlargement (8%)
vaginal bleeding (8%)
emotional lability (6%)
transient increase in pubic hair (5%)
body odor (4%)
seborrhea (3%)

Hot flashes, common in adult women treated for endometriosis, occurred in only 3% of treated children and were transient. Other adverse events thought to be drug-related, and occurring in > 3% of patients were rhinitis (5%) and white or brownish vaginal discharge (3%). Approximately 3% of patients withdrew from clinical trials due to adverse events. In one male patient with concomitant congenital adrenal hyperplasia, and who had discontinued treatment 8 months previously to resume puberty, adrenal rest tumors were found in the left testis. Relationship to Nafarlin Acetate is unlikely.

Regular examinations of the pituitary gland by magnetic resonance imaging (MRI) or computer assisted tomography (CT) of children during long-term Nafarelin therapy as well as during the posttreatment period has occasionally revealed changes in the shape and size of the pituitary gland. These changes include asymmetry and enlargement of the pituitary gland, and a pituitary microadenoma has been suspected in a few children. The relationship of these findings to Nafarelin Acetate is not known.

ENDOMETRIOSIS

As would be expected with a drug which lowers serum estradiol levels, the most frequently reported adverse reactions were those related to hypoestrogenism.

In controlled studies comparing Nafarelin Acetate (400 µg/day) and danazol (600 or 800 mg/day), adverse reactions most frequently reported and thought to be drug-related are shown in the figure below.

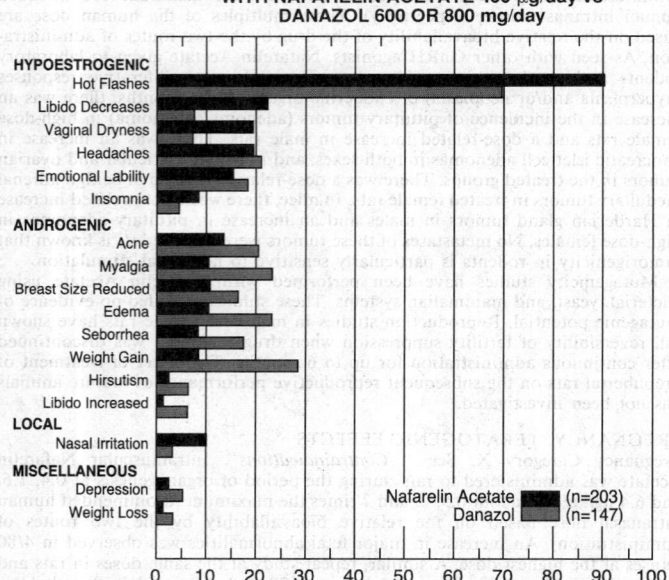

ADVERSE EVENTS DURING 6 MONTH TREATMENT WITH NAFARELIN ACETATE 400 µg/day vs DANAZOL 600 OR 800 mg/day

In addition, less than 1% of patients experienced paresthesia, palpitations, chloasma, maculopapular rash, eye, pain, urticaria, asthenia, lactation, breast engorgement, and arthralgia. In formal clinical trials, immediate hypersensitivity thought to be possibly or probably related to Nafarelin occurred in 3 (0.2%) of 1509 healthy subjects or patients.

CHANGES IN BONE DENSITY

After six months of treatment with Nafarelin Acetate, vertebral trabecular bone density and total vertebral bone mass, measured by quantitative computed tomography (QCT), decreased by an average of 8.7% and 4.3%, respectively, compared to pretreatment levels. There was partial recovery of bone density in the post-treatment period; the average trabecular bone density and total bone mass were 4.9% and 3.3% less than the pretreatment levels, respectively. Total vertebral bone mass, measured by dual photon absorptiometry (DPA), decreased by a mean of 5.9% at the end of treatment. Mean total vertebral mass, re-examined by DPA six months after completion of treatment, was 1.4% below pretreatment levels. There was little, if any, decrease in the mineral content in compact bone of the distal radius and second metacarpal. Use of Nafarelin Acetate for longer than the recommended six months or in the presence of other

known risk factors for decreased bone mineral content may cause additional bone loss.

CHANGES IN LABORATORY VALUES DURING TREATMENT

Plasma Enzymes: During clinical trials with Nafarelin Acetate, regular laboratory monitoring revealed that SGOT and SGPT levels were more than twice the upper limit of normal in only one patient each. There was no other clinical or laboratory evidence of abnormal liver function and levels returned to normal in both patients after treatment was stopped.

Lipids: At enrollment, 9% of the patients in the group taking Nafarelin Acetate 400 µg/day and 2% of the patients in the danazol group had total cholesterol values above 250 mg/dL. These patients also had cholesterol values above 250 mg/dL at the end of treatment.

Of those patients whose pretreatment cholesterol values were below 250 mg/dL, 6% in the group treated with Nafarelin Acetate and 18% in the danazol group, had post-treatment values above 250 mg/dL.

The mean (±SEM) pretreatment values for total cholesterol from all patients were 191.8 (4.3) mg/dL in the group treated with Nafarelin Acetate and 193.1 (4.6) mg/dL in the danazol group. At the end of treatment, the mean values for total cholesterol from all patients were 204.5 (4.8) mg/dL in the group treated with Nafarelin Acetate and 207.7 (5.1) mg/dL in the danazol group. These increases from the pretreatment values were statistically significant (p < 0.05) in both groups.

Triglycerides were increased above the upper limit of 150 mg/dL in 12% of the patients who received Nafarelin Acetate and in 7% of the patients who received danazol.

At the end of treatment, no patients receiving Nafarelin Acetate had abnormally low HDL cholesterol fractions (less than 30 mg/dL) compared with 43% receiving danazol. None of the patients receiving Nafarelin Acetate had abnormally high LDL cholesterol fractions (greater than 190 mg/dL) compared with 15% of those receiving danazol. There was no increase in the LDL/HDL ratio in patients receiving Nafarelin Acetate, but there was approximately a 2-fold increase in the LDL/HDL ratio in patients receiving danazol.

Other Changes: In comparative studies, the following changes were seen in approximately 10% to 15% of patients. Treatment with Nafarelin Acetate was associated with elevations of plasma phosphorus and eosinophil counts, and decreases in serum calcium and WBC counts. Danazol therapy was associated with an increase of hematocrit and WBC.

OVERDOSAGE

In experimental animals, a single subcutaneous administration of up to 60 times the recommended human dose (on a µg/kg basis, not adjusted for bioavailability) had no adverse effects. At present, there is no clinical evidence of adverse effects following overdosage of GnRH analogs.

Based on studies in monkeys, Nafarelin Acetate is not absorbed after oral administration.

DOSAGE AND ADMINISTRATION

For the treatment of central precocious puberty (CPP), the recommended daily dose of Nafarelin Acetate is 1600 µg. The dose can be increased to 1800 µg daily if adequate suppression cannot be achieved at 1600 µg/day.

The 1600 µg dose is achieved by two sprays (400 µg) into each nostril in the morning (4 sprays) and two sprays into each nostril in the evening (4 sprays), a total of 8 sprays per day. The 1800 µg dose is achieved by 3 sprays (600 µg) into alternating nostrils three times a day, a total of 9 sprays per day. The patient's head should be tilted back slightly, and 30 seconds should elapse between sprays.

If the prescribed therapy has been well tolerated by the patient, treatment of CPP with Nafarelin Acetate should continue until resumption of puberty is desired.

There appeared to be no significant effect of rhinitis, i.e. nasal congestion, on the systemic bioavailability of Nafarelin Acetate; however, if the use of a nasal decongestant for rhinitis is necessary during treatment with Nafarelin Acetate, the decongestant should not be used until at least 2 hours following dosing with Nafarelin Acetate.

Sneezing during or immediately after dosing with Nafarelin Acetate should be avoided, if possible, since this may impair drug absorption.

At 1600 µg/day, a bottle of Nafarelin Acetate provides about a 7-day supply (about 56 sprays). If the daily dose is increased, increase the supply to the patient to ensure uninterrupted treatment for the duration of therapy.

For the management of endometriosis, the recommended daily dose of Nafarelin Acetate is 400 µg. This is achieved by one spray (200 µg) into one nostril in the morning and one spray into the other nostril in the evening. Treatment should be started between days 2 and 4 of the menstrual cycle.

In an occasional patient, the 400 µg daily dose may not produce amenorrhea. For these patients with persistent regular menstruation after 2 months of treatment, the dose of Nafarelin Acetate may be increased to 800 µg daily. The 800 µg dose is administered as one spray into each nostril in the morning (a total of two sprays) and again in the evening. The recommended duration of administration is six months. Retreatment cannot be recommended since safety data for retreatment are not available. If the symptoms of endometriosis recur after a course of therapy, and further treatment with Nafarelin Acetate is contemplated, it is recommended that bone density be assessed before retreatment begins to ensure that values are within normal limits.

At 400 µg/day, a bottle of Nafarelin Acetate provides a 30-day (about 60 sprays) supply. If the daily dose is increased, increase the supply to the patient to ensure uninterrupted treatment for the recommended duration of therapy.

Store upright at room temperature. Avoid heat above 30°C (86°F). Protect from light. Protect from freezing.

HOW SUPPLIED

SOLUTION: 2 MG/ML

BRAND/MANUFACTURER	NDC	SIZE	AWP
○ **BRAND**			
SYNAREL: Syntex	00033-2260-40	10 ml	$323.32

Nafcillin Sodium

DESCRIPTION

Nafcillin Sodium is a semisynthetic penicillin. Although primarily designed as an antistaphylococcal penicillin, in limited clinical trials it has been shown to be effective in the treatment of infections caused by pneumococci and Group A beta-hemolytic streptococci. Because of this wide gram-positive spectrum, this product is particularly suitable for initial therapy in severe or potentially severe infections before definitive culture results are known and in which staphylococci are suspected.

This product is readily soluble and can be conveniently administered in both oral and parenteral dosage forms. It is resistant to inactivation by staphylococcal penicillinase. Following intramuscular administration in humans, it rapidly appears in the plasma, penetrates body tissues in high concentration, and diffuses well into pleural, pericardial, and synovial fluids.

Nafcillin Sodium capsules contain Nafcillin Sodium as the monohydrate equivalent to 250 mg Nafcillin.

Nafcillin Sodium tablets contain Nafcillin Sodium as the monohydrate equivalent to 500 mg Nafcillin.

Nafcillin Sodium as the monohydrate is available for parenteral administration in vials of 1 gram or 2 grams Nafcillin. When reconstituted as directed, each vial contains, respectively, 4 mL, or 8 mL of solution. Each mL contains Nafcillin Sodium equivalent to 250 mg Nafcillin buffered with 10 mg Sodium citrate.

Note: Nafcillin Sodium contains 2.9 milliequivalents of Sodium per gram of Nafcillin as the Sodium salt.

Following is its chemical structure:

CLINICAL PHARMACOLOGY

MICROBIOLOGY

Nafcillin Sodium is a bactericidal penicillin which has shown activity *in vitro* against both penicillin-G-sensitive and penicillin-G-resistant strains of *Staphylococcus aureus* as well as against pneumococcus, beta-hemolytic streptococcus, and alpha streptococcus (viridans).

In experimental mouse infections induced with pneumococci, beta-hemolytic streptococci, and both penicillin-G-susceptible and penicillin-G-resistant strains of *Staph. aureus*, Nafcillin Sodium was compared with methicillin and oxacillin. Regardless of the route of drug administration (intramuscular or oral), Nafcillin Sodium was consistently and significantly more effective than the other two penicillins.

The fate of a penicillin-G-resistant strain of *Staph. aureus* was determined in the kidneys of mice treated with penicillin G, methicillin, and Nafcillin Sodium. Animals injected with the Nafcillin Sodium showed negative cultures after the fourteenth day, whereas positive kidney cultures were obtained during the entire 28-day period from mice treated with penicillin G and methicillin.

PHARMACOLOGY

Nafcillin Sodium is relatively nontoxic for animals. The acute LD50 of this product by oral administration in rats and mice was greater than 5 g/kg; by intramuscular administration in rats, 2800 mg/kg; by intraperitoneal administration in rats, 1240 mg/kg; and by intravenous administration in mice, 1140 mg/kg. The intraperitoneal LD50 in dogs is 600 mg/kg. Animal studies indicated that local tissue responses following intramuscular administration of 25% solutions were minimal and resembled those of penicillin G rather than methicillin.

Animal studies indicate that antibacterial amounts are concentrated in the bile, kidney, lung, heart, spleen, and liver. Eighty-four percent of an intravenously administered dose can be recovered by biliary cannulation and 13 percent by renal excretion in 24 hours. High and prolonged tissue levels can be demonstrated by both biological activity assays and C^{14} distribution patterns.

At comparable dosage, intramuscular absorption of this product is nearly equivalent to that of intramuscular methicillin, and oral absorption to that of oral oxacillin. Blood concentrations may be tripled by the concurrent use of probenecid. Clinical studies with Nafcillin Sodium monohydrate in infants under three days of age and prematures have revealed higher blood levels and slower rates of urinary excretion than in older children and adults.

Studies of the effect of this product on reproduction in rats and rabbits have been completed and reveal no fetal or maternal abnormalities. These studies include the observation of the effects of administration of the drug before conception and continuously through weaning (one generation).

DISC SUSCEPTIBILITY TESTS

Quantitative methods that require measurement of zone diameters give the most precise estimates of antibiotic susceptibility. One such procedure[*] has been recommended for use with discs for testing susceptibility to penicillinase-resistant penicillin-class antibiotics. Interpretations correlate diameters on the disc test with MIC values for penicillinase-resistant penicillins. With this procedure, a report from the laboratory of "susceptible" indicates that the infecting organism is likely to respond to therapy. A report of "resistant" indicates that the infecting organism is not likely to respond to therapy. A report of "intermediate susceptibility" suggests that the organism would be susceptible if high dosage is used, or if the infection is confined to tissues and fluids (e.g., urine) in which high antibiotic levels are attained.

INDICATIONS

Although the principal indication for Nafcillin Sodium is in the treatment of infections due to penicillinase-producing staphylococci, it may be used to initiate therapy in such patients in whom a staphylococcal infection is suspected (see *"Important Note"*).

Bacteriologic studies to determine the causative organisms and their sensitivity to Nafcillin Sodium should be performed.

In serious, life-threatening infections, oral preparations of the penicillinase-resistance penicillins should not be relied on for initial therapy.

IMPORTANT NOTE

When it is judged necessary that treatment be initiated before definitive culture and sensitivity results are known, the choice of Nafcillin Sodium should take into consideration the fact that it has been shown to be effective only in the treatment of infections caused by pneumococci, Group A beta-hemolytic streptococci, and penicillin-G-resistant and penicillin-G-sensitive staphylococci. If the bacteriology report later indicates the infection is due to an organism other than a penicillin-G-resistant staphylococcus sensitive to Nafcillin Sodium, the physician is advised to continue therapy with a drug other than Nafcillin Sodium or any other penicillinase-resistant, semisynthetic penicillin.

Recent studies have reported that the percentage of staphylococcal isolates resistant to penicillin G outside the hospital is increasing, approximating the high percentage of resistant staphylococcal isolates found in the hospital. For this reason, it is recommended that a penicillinase-resistant penicillin be used as initial therapy for any suspected staphylococcal infection until culture and sensitivity results are known.

Methicillin is a compound that acts through a mechanism similar to that of Nafcillin Sodium against penicillin-G-resistant staphylococci. Strains of staphylococci resistant to methicillin have existed in nature, and it is known that the number of these strains reported has been increasing. Such strains of staphylococci have been capable of producing serious disease, in some instances resulting in fatality. Because of this there is concern that widespread use of the penicillinase-resistant penicillins may result in the appearance of an increasing number of staphylococcal strains which are resistant to these penicillins.

Methicillin-resistant strains are almost always resistant to all other penicillinase-resistant penicillins (cross-resistance with cephalosporin derivatives also occurs frequently). Resistance to any penicillinase-resistant penicillin should be interpreted as evidence of clinical resistance to all, in spite of the fact that minor variations in *in vitro* sensitivity may be encountered when more than one penicillinase-resistant penicillin is tested against the same strain of staphylococcus.

CONTRAINDICATIONS

A history of allergic reaction to any of the penicillins is a contraindication.

WARNINGS

Serious and occasionally fatal hypersensitivity (anaphylactoid) reactions have been reported in patients on penicillin therapy. Although anaphylaxis is more frequent following parenteral therapy, it has occurred in patients on oral penicillins. These reactions are more apt to occur in individuals with a history of sensitivity to multiple allergens.

There have been reports of individuals with a history of penicillin hypersensitivity reactions who have experienced severe hypersensitivity reactions when treated with a cephalosporin. Before therapy with a penicillin, careful inquiry should be made concerning previous hypersensitivity reactions to penicillins, cephalosporins, and other allergens. If an allergic reaction occurs, appropriate therapy should be instituted, and discontinuation of Nafcillin therapy considered. The usual agents (antihistamines, pressor amines, corticosteroids) should be readily available.

Nafcillin Sodium injection should be used with caution when administered by the intravenous route because of the possibility of thrombophlebitis. To help minimize the risk of thrombophlebitis, it is important to administer Nafcillin Sodium through the tubing of an intravenous infusion set that is known to be functioning satisfactorily and to administer it in recommended concentrations (see *"Dosage and Administration"*). Caution should also be exercised to avoid

---

[*] Bauer, A.W., Kirby, W.M.M., Sherris, J.C., and Turck, M.: Antibiotic Testing by a Standardized Single-Discs Method, *Am. J. Clin. Pathol.*, 45:493, 1966; Standardized Disc Susceptibility Test, *FEDERAL REGISTER* 37:20527-29, 1972.

➤ SHOWN IN PRODUCT IDENTIFICATION GUIDE

extravasation, since under such circumstances chemical irritation of perivascular tissues may be severe. Reports of injuries following extravasation have included ulceration, tissue necrosis, sloughing, and gangrene which, in some cases, required surgical debridement and skin grafting. In the event that a patient complains of pain during intravenous infusion of Nafcillin Sodium, the infusion should immediately be stopped to provide for evaluation of possible thrombophlebitis or perivascular extravasation.

PRECAUTIONS

As with any potent drug, periodic assessment of organ-system function, including renal, hepatic, and hematopoietic, should be made during prolonged therapy.

The possibility of bacterial and fungal overgrowth should be kept in mind during long-term therapy. If overgrowth of resistant organisms occurs, appropriate measures should be taken.

The oral route of administration should not be relied upon in patients with severe illness, or with nausea, vomiting, gastric dilatation, cardiospasm, or intestinal hypermotility. Safety for use in pregnancy has not been established.

ADVERSE REACTIONS

Reactions to Nafcillin Sodium have been infrequent and mild in nature. As with other penicillins, the possibility of an anaphylactic reaction or serum-sickness like reactions should be considered. A careful history should be taken. Patients with histories of hay fever, asthma, urticaria, or previous sensitivity to penicillin are more likely to react adversely.

Transient leukopenia, neutropenia with evidence of granulocytopenia or thrombocytopenia are infrequent and usually associated with prolonged therapy with high doses of penicillin. These alterations have been noted to return to normal after cessation of therapy.

The few reactions associated with the intramuscular use of Nafcillin Sodium have been skin rash, pruritus, and possible drug fever. As with other penicillins, reactions from oral use of the drug have included nausea, vomiting, diarrhea, urticaria, and pruritus.

DOSAGE AND ADMINISTRATION

Parenteral drug products should be inspected visually for particulate matter and discoloration prior to administration, whenever solution and container permit.

It is recommended that parenteral therapy be used initially in severe infections. The patient should be placed on oral therapy with this product as soon as the clinical condition warrants. Very severe infections may require very high doses.

INTRAVENOUS ROUTE

500 mg every 4 hours; double the dose if necessary in very severe infections.

The required amount of drug should be diluted in 15 to 30 mL of Sterile Water for Injection, USP, or Sodium Chloride Injection, USP, and injected over a 5- to 10-minute period. This may be accomplished through the tubing of an intravenous infusion if desirable.

To add Nafcillin Sodium to an intravenous solution, reconstitute the vials as directed under *"How Supplied"—"For Parenteral Administration."* Add the reconstituted vial contents immediately to the intravenous solution or within 8 hours following reconstitution if the vials are kept at room temperature (25° C) or within 48 hours following reconstitution if the vials are kept at refrigeration (2°-8° C).

Stability studies on Nafcillin Sodium at concentrations of 2 mg/mL to 40 mg/mL in the following intravenous solutions indicate the drug will lose less than 10% activity at room temperature (70° F) or, if kept under refrigeration, during the time period stipulated:

Stability of	Room Temperature	Refrigerated
Sterile Water for Injection	24 hours	96 hours
Isotonic Sodium Chloride	24 hours	96 hours
5% dextrose in water	24 hours	96 hours
5% dextrose in 0.4% solution chloride solution	24 hours	96 hours
Ringer's solution	24 hours	96 hours
M/6 Sodium lactate solution	24 hours	96 hours

Discard any unused portions of intravenous solutions after 24 hours if kept at room temperature or after 96 hours if kept under refrigeration.

Only those solutions listed above should be used for the intravenous infusion of Nafcillin Sodium. The concentration of the antibiotic should fall within the range of 2 to 40 mg/mL. The drug concentrate and the rate and volume of the infusion should be adjusted so that the total dose of Nafcillin is administered before the drug loses its stability in the solution in use.

There is no clinical experience available on the use of this agent in neonates or infants for this route of administration. This route of administration should be used for relatively short-term therapy (24 to 48 hours) because of the occasional occurrence of thrombophlebitis, particularly in elderly patients.

This route of administration requires care be taken not to allow perivascular extravasation (see *"Warnings"*).

PIGGYBACK UNITS (FOR INTRAVENOUS DRIP USE)

As diluents, use the following solutions, Sterile Water for Injection, Isotonic Sodium Chloride, 5% dextrose in water, 5% dextrose in 0.4% Sodium chloride solution, Ringer's solution, or M/6 Sodium lactate solution.

1-GRAM BOTTLE

Add a minimum of 49 mL diluent and shake well. If lower concentrations are desired, the solution could be further diluted with up to a total of 99 mL of diluent.

Amount of Diluent	Concentration of Solution
49 mL	20 mg/mL
99 mL	10 mg/mL

2-Gram Bottle

Add a minimum of 49 mL diluent and shake well. If lower concentrations are desired, the solution could be further diluted with up to a total of 99 mL of diluent.

Amount of Diluent	Concentration of Solution
49 mL	40 mg/mL
99 mL	20 mg/mL

The resulting solutions may then be administered alone or with the intravenous solutions listed above. Discard unused solution after 24 hours at room temperature (70°F) or 96 hours if kept under refrigeration. Administer piggyback through an IV tubing very slowly (at least 30 to 60 minutes) to avoid vein irritation.

At times it may be desired to use the contents of the piggyback bottles for addition to large-volume IV fluids. In this case the entire vial contents should be dissolved in not less than 25 mL of Sterile Water for Injection. Use the resulting concentration within 24 hours when kept at room temperature or within 96 hours when kept under refrigeration.

TEN-GRAM BOTTLE

Add 94 mL Sterile Water for Injection, USP, or Sodium Chloride Injection, USP, and shake well. For ease of reconstitution, the amount of diluent should be added in two portions; the first portion should not exceed 25 mL. Shake gently after each addition and before using. The final concentration will be approximately 100 mg/mL. After reconstitution, use within 8 hours if kept at room temperature or within 48 hours if kept under refrigeration.

The closure shall be penetrated only one time after reconstitution with a suitable sterile transfer device or dispensing set which allows measured dispensing of the contents. The Pharmacy Bulk Package is to be used only in a suitable work area, such as a laminar flow hood (or an equivalent clean-air compounding area).

IV INFUSION

The recommended dosage should be withdrawn from the stock solution and further diluted with water or saline to a maximum concentration of 40 mg/mL or less. The solution thus diluted will remain stable for 24 hours at room temperature or 96 hours under refrigeration. Any unused portion of the above-mentioned solutions must be discarded after the time periods specified above.

Caution: Administer slowly by intravenous route over a period of at least 30 to 60 minutes to avoid vein irritation.

INTRAMUSCULAR ROUTE

500 mg every 6 hours in adults; decrease the interval to 4 hours if necessary in severe infections. In infants and children, a dose of 25 mg/kg (about 12 mg/lb) twice daily is usually adequate.

For neonates, 10 mg/kg is recommended twice daily.

ORAL ROUTE

In adults a dose of 250 to 500 mg every 4 to 6 hours is sufficient for mild-to-moderate infections. In severe infections 1 gram every 4 to 6 hours may be necessary.

In children, streptococcal pharyngitis cases have responded to a dosage of 250 mg t.i.d. Beta-hemolytic streptococcal infections should be treated for at least ten days to prevent development of acute rheumatic fever or glomerulonephritis.

Children and infants with scarlet fever and pneumonia should receive 25 mg/kg/day in four divided doses. For staphylococcal infections, 50 mg/kg/day in four divided doses is recommended. For neonates, 10 mg/kg three to four times daily is recommended. If inadequate, resort to parenteral Nafcillin Sodium.

Capsules and Tablets: Store at room temperature, approx. 25° C (77° F).
Keep tightly closed.
Dispense in tight container.

Parenteral Solution: Store at room temperature, approximately 25°C (77°F), before reconstitution.
Shake vial well after adding diluent and before using.
Use solution within 8 hours if kept at room temperature or 48 hours if kept under refrigeration.

HOW SUPPLIED
CAPSULE: 250 MG

BRAND/MANUFACTURER	NDC	SIZE	AWP
○ **BRAND**			
UNIPEN: Wyeth-Ayerst	00008-0057-03	100s	$98.65

◆ RATED THERAPEUTICALLY EQUIVALENT; ◇ THERAPEUTIC EQUIVALENCE UNCONFIRMED; ○ UNRATED

POWDER FOR INJECTION: 500 MG

AVERAGE UNIT PRICE (AVAILABLE SIZES)		GENERIC A-RATED AVERAGE PRICE (GAAP)	
BRAND	$3.26	1s	$2.10
GENERIC	$2.10		

BRAND/MANUFACTURER	NDC	SIZE	AWP
◆ BRAND			
UNIPEN: Wyeth-Ayerst	00008-0751-01	1s	$3.26
◆ GENERICS			
NALLPEN: Abbott Hosp	00029-6370-25	1s	$1.75
Apothecon	00015-7224-20	1s	$2.45

POWDER FOR INJECTION: 1 GM

AVERAGE UNIT PRICE (AVAILABLE SIZES)		GENERIC A-RATED AVERAGE PRICE (GAAP)	
BRAND	$6.42	1s	$4.28
GENERIC	$5.68	10s	$98.85

BRAND/MANUFACTURER	NDC	SIZE	AWP
◆ BRAND			
UNIPEN: Wyeth-Ayerst	00008-0751-02	1s	$6.10
	00008-0751-15	1s	$6.55
	00008-0751-24	10s	$64.70
	00008-0751-16	10s	$65.46
◆ GENERICS			
NALLPEN: Abbott Hosp	00029-6372-22	1s	$2.75
NALLPEN: Abbott Hosp	00029-6372-40	1s	$3.05
NALLPEN: Abbott Hosp	00029-6372-21	1s	$3.35
Apothecon	00015-7225-20	1s	$4.63
Apothecon	00015-7225-18	1s	$5.45
Apothecon	00015-7195-28	1s	$6.43
VHA	00015-7225-22	10s	$82.70
VHA	00015-7225-21	10s	$115.00

POWDER FOR INJECTION: 2 GM

AVERAGE UNIT PRICE (AVAILABLE SIZES)		GENERIC A-RATED AVERAGE PRICE (GAAP)	
BRAND	$12.08	1s	$8.05
GENERIC	$10.45	10s	$176.30

BRAND/MANUFACTURER	NDC	SIZE	AWP
◆ BRAND			
UNIPEN: Wyeth-Ayerst	00008-0751-03	1s	$11.83
	00008-0751-13	1s	$12.28
	00008-0751-10	10s	$118.20
	00008-0751-28	10s	$121.95
	00008-0751-14	10s	$122.79
◆ GENERICS			
NALLPEN: Abbott Hosp	00029-6374-27	1s	$5.30
NALLPEN: Abbott Hosp	00029-6374-40	1s	$5.60
NALLPEN: Abbott Hosp	00029-6374-21	1s	$5.80
Apothecon	00015-7226-20	1s	$8.98
Apothecon	00015-7226-18	1s	$9.18
Apothecon	00015-7196-28	1s	$13.46
VHA	00015-7226-22	10s	$160.20
VHA	00015-7226-21	10s	$192.40

POWDER FOR INJECTION: 10 GM

AVERAGE UNIT PRICE (AVAILABLE SIZES)		GENERIC A-RATED AVERAGE PRICE (GAAP)	
BRAND	$52.66	1s	$36.30
GENERIC	$36.30		

BRAND/MANUFACTURER	NDC	SIZE	AWP
◆ BRAND			
UNIPEN: Wyeth-Ayerst	00008-0751-30	10s	$526.63
◆ GENERICS			
NALLPEN: Abbott Hosp	00029-6376-21	1s	$21.85
Apothecon	00015-7101-28	1s	$50.74

Naftifine Hydrochloride

DESCRIPTION

Naftifine Hydrochloride is a synthetic, broad-spectrum, antifungal agent. Naftifine HCl 1% Gel and Cream are for topical use only.

Chemical Name: (E)-N-Cinnamyl-N-methyl-1-naphthalene-methylamine hydrochloride. Naftifine Hydrochloride has an empirical formula of $C_{21}H_{21}N \cdot HCl$ and a molecular weight of 323.86.

Active Ingredient: Naftifine Hydrochloride 1%

Following is its chemical structure:

CLINICAL PHARMACOLOGY

Naftifine Hydrochloride is a synthetic allylamine derivative. The following *in vitro* data are available but their clinical significance is unknown. Naftifine HCl has been shown to exhibit fungicidal activity *in vitro* against a broad spectrum of organisms including *Trichophyton rubrum, Trichophyton mentagrophytes, Trichophyton tonsurans, Epidermophyton floccosum,* and *Microsporum canis, Microsporum audouini,* and *Microsporum gypseum*; and fungistatic activity against *Candida* species including *Candida albicans* . Naftifine HCl Gel and Cream have only been shown to be clinically effective against the disease entities listed in the *"Indications and Usage"* section.

Although the exact mechanism of action against fungi is not known, Naftifine HCl appears to interfere with sterol biosynthesis by inhibiting the enzyme squalene 2,3-epoxidase. This inhibition of enzyme activity results in decreased amounts of sterols, especially ergosterol, and a corresponding accumulation of squalene in the cells.

Pharmacokinetics: In vitro and *in vivo* bioavailability studies have demonstrated that Naftifine penetrates the stratum corneum in sufficient concentration to inhibit the growth of dermatophytes.

Following single topical application of ^{3}H-labeled Naftifine gel 1% to the skin of healthy subjects, up to 4.2% of the applied dose was absorbed. Following a single topical application of 1% Naftifine Cream to the skin of healthy subjects, systemic absorption of Naftifine was approximately 6% of the applied dose. Naftifine and/or its metabolites are excreted via the urine and feces with a half-life of approximately two to three days.

INDICATION AND USUAGE

Naftifine HCl Gel is indicated for the topical treatment of tinea pedis, tinea cruris and tinea corporis caused by the organisms *Trichophyton rubrum, Trichophyton mentagrophytes. Trichophyton tonsurans[*]* and *Epidermophyton floccosum.[*]*

Naftifine HCl Cream is indicated for the topical application in the treatment of tinea pedis, tinea cruris and tinea corporis caused by the organisms *Tricophyton rubrum, Tricophyton mentagrophytes,* and *Epidermophyton floccosum.*

CONTRAINDICATIONS

Naftifine HCl Gel and Cream are contraindicated in individuals who have shown hypersensitivity to any of its components.

WARNINGS

Naftifine HCl Gel and Cream are for topical use only and not for ophthalmic use.

PRECAUTIONS

General: Naftifine HCl Gel and Cream are for external use only. If irritation or sensitivity develops with the use of Naftifine HCl Gel and Cream, treatment should be discontinued and appropriate therapy instituted. Diagnosis of the disease should be confirmed either by direct microscopic examination of a mounting of infected tissue in a solution of potassium hydroxide or by culture on an appropriate medium.

Information for Patients: The patient should be told to:

1. Avoid the use of occlusive dressings or wrappings unless otherwise directed by the physician.
2. Keep Naftifine HCl Gel and Cream away from the eyes, nose, mouth and other mucous membranes.

Carcinogenesis, Mutagenesis, Impairment of Fertility: Long-term animal studies to evaluate the carcinogenic potential of Naftifine HCl Gel and Cream have not been performed. *In vitro* and animal studies have not demonstrated any mutagenic effect or effect on fertility.

Pregnancy: Teratogenic Effects: Pregnancy Category B: Reproduction studies have been performed in rats and rabbits (via oral administration) at doses 150 times or more than the topical human dose and have revealed no significant evidence of impaired fertility or harm to the fetus due to Naftifine. There are, however, no adequate and well-controlled studies in pregnant women. Because animal reproduction studies are not always predictive of human response, this drug should be used during pregnancy only if clearly needed.

Nursing Mothers: It is not known whether this drug is excreted in human milk. Because many drugs are excreted in human milk, caution should be exercised when Naftifine HCl Gel or Cream is administered to a nursing woman.

Pediatric Use: Safety and effectiveness in children have not been established.

ADVERSE REACTIONS

During clinical trials with Naftifine HCl Gel, the incidence of adverse reactions was as follows: burning/stinging (5.0%), itching (1.0%), erythema (0.5%), rash (0.5%), skin tenderness (0.5%).

During clinical trials with Naftifine HCl Cream, the incidence of adverse reactions was as follows: burning/stinging (6%), dryness (3%), erythema (2%), itching (2%), local irritation (2%).

DOSAGE AND ADMINISTRATION

A sufficient quantity of Naftifine HCl should be gently massaged into the affected and surrounding skin areas twice a day, in the morning and evening, for the gel, once a day for the cream. The hands should be washed after application.

---

[*] Efficacy for this organism in this organ system was studied in fewer than 10 infections.

► SHOWN IN PRODUCT IDENTIFICATION GUIDE

If no clinical improvement is seen after four weeks of treatment with Naftifine HCl, the patient should be reevaluated.

Store the gel at room temperature, the cream below 30°C (86°F).

HOW SUPPLIED
CREAM: 1%

BRAND/MANUFACTURER	NDC	SIZE	AWP
○ **BRAND**			
NAFTIN: Allergan Herbert	00023-4126-15	15 gm	$13.09
	00023-4126-30	30 gm	$21.83
	00023-4126-60	60 gm	$33.35

GEL: 1%

BRAND/MANUFACTURER	NDC	SIZE	AWP
○ **BRAND**			
NAFTIN: Allergan Herbert	00023-4770-20	20 gm	$18.25
	00023-4770-40	40 gm	$28.98
	00023-4770-60	60 gm	$33.96

Naftin SEE NAFTIFINE HYDROCHLORIDE

Nalbuphine Hydrochloride

DESCRIPTION
Nalbuphine Hydrochloride a synthetic narcotic agonist-antagonist analgesic of the phenanthrene series. It is chemically related to both the widely used narcotic antagonist, naloxone, and the potent narcotic analgesic, oxymorphone.

Nalbuphine Hydrochloride is (-)-17-(cyclobutylmethyl)-4,5 α-epoxymorphinan-3,6α, 14-triol hydrochloride. Nalbuphine Hydrochloride is available in two concentrations, 10 mg and 20 mg of nalbuphine hydrochloride per mL.

Nalbuphine Hydrochloride is also available in a sulfite and paraben-free formulation in two concentrations, 10 mg and 20 mg of nalbuphine hydrochloride per mL.

Following is its chemical structure:

ACTIONS
Nalbuphine Hydrochloride is a potent analgesic. Its analgesic potency is essentially equivalent to that of morphine on a milligram basis. Its onset of action occurs within 2 to 3 minutes after intravenous administration, and in less than 15 minutes following subcutaneous or intramuscular injection. The plasma half-life of Nalbuphine is 5 hours and in clinical studies the duration of analgesic activity has been reported to range from 3 to 6 hours.

The narcotic antagonist activity of Nalbuphine Hydrochloride is one-fourth as potent as nalorphine and 10 times that of pentazocine.

INDICATIONS
Nalbuphine Hydrochloride is indicated for the relief of moderate to severe pain. Nalbuphine Hydrochloride can also be used as a supplement to balanced anesthesia, for preoperative and postoperative analgesia, and for obstetrical analgesia during labor and delivery.

CONTRAINDICATIONS
Nalbuphine Hydrochloride should not be administered to patients who are hypersensitive to it.

WARNINGS
Nalbuphine Hydrochloride should be administered as a supplement to general anesthesia only by persons specifically trained in the use of intravenous anesthetics and management of the respiratory effects of potent opioids.

Naloxone, resuscitative and intubation equipment and oxygen should be readily available.

Drug Dependence. Nalbuphine Hydrochloride has been shown to have a low abuse potential. When compared with drugs which are not mixed agonist-antagonists, it has been reported that nalbuphine's potential for abuse would be less than that of codeine and propoxyphene. Psychological and physical dependence and tolerance may follow the abuse or misuse of nalbuphine. Therefore, caution should be observed in prescribing it for emotionally unstable patients, or for individuals with a history of narcotic abuse. Such patients should be closely supervised when long-term therapy is contemplated.

Care should be taken to avoid increases in dosage or frequency of administration which in susceptible individuals might result in physical dependence.

Abrupt discontinuation of Nalbuphine Hydrochloride following prolonged use has been followed by symptoms of narcotic withdrawal, i.e., abdominal cramps, nausea and vomiting, rhinorrhea, lacrimation, restlessness, anxiety, elevated temperature and piloerection.

Use in Ambulatory Patients: Nalbuphine Hydrochloride may impair the mental or physical abilities required for the performance of potentially dangerous tasks such as driving a car or operating machinery. Therefore, Nalbuphine Hydrochloride should be administered with caution to ambulatory patients who should be warned to avoid such hazards.

Use in Emergency Procedures: Maintain patient under observation until recovered from Nalbuphine Hydrochloride effects that would affect driving or other potentially dangerous tasks.

Use in Children: Clinical experience to support administration to patients under 18 years is not available at present.

Use in Pregnancy (other than labor): Safe use Nalbuphine Hydrochloride in pregnancy has not been established. Although animal reproductive studies have not revealed teratogenic or embryotoxic effects, Nalbuphine should only be administered to pregnant women when, in the judgement of the physician, the potential benefits outweigh the possible hazards.

Use During Labor and Delivery: Nalbuphine Hydrochloride can produce respiratory depression in the neonate. It should be used with caution in women delivering premature infants.

Head Injury and Increased Intracranial Pressure: The possible respiratory depressant effects and the potential of potent analgesics to elevate cerebrospinal fluid pressure (resulting from vasodilation following CO_2 retention) may be markedly exaggerated in the presence of head injury, intracranial lesions or a preexisting increase in intracranial pressure. Furthermore, potent analgesics can produce effects which may obscure the clinical course of patients with head injuries. Therefore Nalbuphine Hydrochloride should be used in these circumstances only when essential, and then should be administered with extreme caution.

Interaction With Other Central Nervous System Depressants: Although Nalbuphine Hydrochloride possesses narcotic antagonist activity, there is evidence that in nondependent patients it will not antagonize a narcotic analgesic administered just before, concurrently, or just after an injection of Nalbuphine Hydrochloride. Therefore, patients receiving a narcotic analgesic, general anesthetics, phenothiazines, or other tranquilizers, sedatives, hypnotics, or other CNS depressants (including alcohol) concomitantly with Nalbuphine Hydrochloride may exhibit an additive effect. When such combined therapy is contemplated, the dose of one or both agents should be reduced.

Sulfites Sensitivity: Nalbuphine Hydrochloride contains sodium metabisulfite, a sulfite that may cause allergic-type reactions including anaphylactic symptoms and life-threatening or less severe asthmatic episodes in certain susceptible people. The overall prevalence of sulfite sensitivity in the general population is unknown and probably low. Sulfite sensitivity is seen more frequently in asthmatic than in nonasthmatic people.

PRECAUTIONS
Impaired Respiration: At the usual adult dose of 10 mg/70 kg. Nalbuphine Hydrochloride causes some respiratory depression approximately equal to that produced by equal doses of morphine. However, in contrast to morphine, respiratory depression is not appreciably increased with higher doses of Nalbuphine Hydrochloride. Respiratory depression induced by Nalbuphine Hydrochloride can be reversed by naloxone hydrochloride when indicated. Nalbuphine Hydrochloride should be administered with caution at low doses to patients with impaired respiration (e.g., from other medication, uremia, bronchial asthma, severe infection, cyanosis or respiratory obstructions).

Impaired Renal or Hepatic Function: Because Nalbuphine Hydrochloride is metabolized in the liver and excreted by the kidneys, patients with renal or liver dysfunction may over-react to customary doses. Therefore, in these individuals Nalbuphine Hydrochloride should be used with caution and administered in reduced amounts.

Myocardial Infarction: As with all potent analgesics, Nalbuphine Hydrochloride should be used with caution in patients with myocardial infarction who have nausea or vomiting.

Biliary Tract Surgery: As with all narcotic analgesics, Nalbuphine Hydrochloride should be used with caution in patients about to undergo surgery of the biliary tract since it may cause spasm of the sphincter of Oddi.

Cardiovascular System: During evaluation of Nalbuphine Hydrochloride in anesthesia, a higher incidence of bradycardia has been reported in patients who did not receive atropine pre-operatively or in the pre-operative period.

ADVERSE REACTIONS
The most frequent adverse reaction in 1066 patients treated with Nalbuphine Hydrochloride is sedation 381(36%).

Less frequent reactions are: sweaty/clammy 99(9%), nausea/vomiting 68(6%), dizziness/ vertigo 58(5%), dry mouth 44(4%), and headache 27(3%).

Other adverse reactions which may occur (reported incidence of 1% or less) are:

CNS Effects: Nervousness, depression, restlessness, crying, euphoria, floating, hostility, unusual dreams, confusion, faintness, hallucinations, dysphoria, feeling of heaviness, numbness, tingling, unreality. The incidence of psychotomimetic effects, such as unreality, depersonalization, delusions, dysphoria and hallucinations has been shown to be less than that which occurs with pentazocine.

◆ RATED THERAPEUTICALLY EQUIVALENT; ◇ THERAPEUTIC EQUIVALENCE UNCONFIRMED; ○ UNRATED

Cardiovascular: Hypertension, hypotension, bradycardia, tachycardia, pulmonary edema.

Gastrointestinal: Cramps, dyspepsia, bitter taste.

Respiration: Depression, dyspnea, asthma.

Dermatological: Itching, burning, urticaria.

Miscellaneous: Speech difficulty, urinary urgency, blurred vision, flushing and warmth.

DOSAGE AND ADMINISTRATION

The usual recommended adult dose is 10 mg for a 70 kg individual, administered subcutaneously, intramuscularly or intravenously; this dose may be repeated every 3 to 6 hours as necessary. Dosage should be adjusted according to the severity of the pain, physical status of the patient and other medications which the patient may be receiving. (See *"Interaction with Other Central Nervous System Depressants"* under *"Warnings"*). In nontolerant individuals, the recommended single maximum dose is 20 mg, with a maximum total daily dose of 160 mg.

The use of Nalbuphine Hydrochloride as a supplement to balanced anesthesia requires larger doses than those recommended for analgesia. Induction doses of Nalbuphine Hydrochloride range from 0.3 mg/kg to 3.0 mg/kg intravenously to be administered over a 10 to 15 minute period with maintenance doses of 0.25 to 0.50 mg/kg in single intravenous administrations as required. The use of Nalbuphine Hydrochloride may be followed by respiratory depression which can be reversed with the narcotic antagonist naloxone hydrochloride.

Patients Dependent on Narcotics. Patients who have been taking narcotics chronically may experience withdrawal symptoms upon the administration of Nalbuphine Hydrochloride. If unduly troublesome, narcotic withdrawal symptoms can be controlled by the slow intravenous administration of small increments of morphine, until relief occurs. If the previous analgesic was morphine, meperidine, codeine, or other narcotic with similar duration of activity, one-fourth of the anticipated dose of Nalbuphine Hydrochloride can be administered initially and the patient observed for signs of withdrawal, i.e., abdominal cramps, nausea and vomiting, lacrimation, rhinorrhea, anxiety, restlessness, elevation of temperature or piloerection. If untoward symptoms do not occur, progressively larger doses may be tried at appropriate intervals until the desired level of analgesia is obtained with Nalbuphine Hydrochloride.

Management of Overdosage: The immediate intravenous administration of naloxone hydrochloride is a specific antidote. Oxygen, intravenous fluids, vasopressors and other supportive measures should be used as indicated. The administration of single doses of 72 mg of Nalbuphine Hydrochloride subcutaneously to eight normal subjects has been reported to have resulted primarily in symptoms of sleepiness and mild dysphoria.

Store at controlled room temperature (59°-86°F, 15°-30°C).

HOW SUPPLIED
INJECTION: 10 MG/ML

AVERAGE UNIT PRICE (AVAILABLE SIZES)

BRAND	$1.64
GENERIC	$2.50

BRAND/MANUFACTURER	NDC	SIZE	AWP
◆ **BRAND**			
NUBAIN: Du Pont Multi	00590-0386-01	10 ml	$21.60
	00590-0395-10	1 ml 10s	$11.16
◆ **GENERICS**			
Astra	00186-1262-12	10 ml 5s	$49.23
Abbott Hosp	00074-1463-01	1 ml 10s	$39.43
Abbott Hosp	00074-1464-01	10 ml 25s	$643.92

INJECTION: 20 MG/ML

AVERAGE UNIT PRICE (AVAILABLE SIZES)

BRAND	$2.97
GENERIC	$3.32

BRAND/MANUFACTURER	NDC	SIZE	AWP
◆ **BRAND**			
NUBAIN: Du Pont Multi	00590-0399-01	10 ml	$33.54
	00590-0398-10	1 ml 10s	$12.36
	00590-0396-15	1 ml 10s	$43.25
◆ **GENERICS**			
Astra	00186-1266-12	10 ml 5s	$56.25
Abbott Hosp	00074-1465-01	1 ml 10s	$48.45
Abbott Hosp	00074-1467-01	10 ml 25s	$996.31

Naldecon *SEE* CHLORPHENIRAMINE MALEATE/
PHENYLEPHRINE HYDROCHLORIDE/PHENYLPROPANOLAMINE
HYDROCHLORIDE/PHENYLTOLOXAMINE CITRATE

Naldecon-CX Adult *SEE* CODEINE PHOSPHATE/
GUAIFENESIN/PHENYLPROPANOLAMINE HYDROCHLORIDE

Nalex A *SEE* CHLORPHENIRAMINE MALEATE/
PHENYLEPHRINE HYDROCHLORIDE/PHENYLTOLOXAMINE CITRATE

Nalex DH *SEE* HYDROCODONE BITARTRATE WITH
PHENYLEPHRINE HYDROCHLORIDE

Nalex JR *SEE* GUAIFENESIN AND PSEUDOEPHEDRINE
HYDROCHLORIDE

Nalfon *SEE* FENOPROFEN CALCIUM

Nalidixic Acid

DESCRIPTION

Nalidixic Acid, an oral antibacterial agent, is 1-Ethyl-1,4-dihydro-7-methyl-4-oxo-1, 8-naphthyridine-3-carboxylic acid. It is a pale yellow, crystalline substance and a very weak organic acid.

Following is its chemical structure:

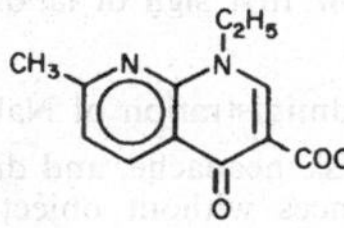

CLINICAL PHARMACOLOGY

Nalidixic Acid has marked antibacterial activity against gram-negative bacteria including *Proteus mirabilis, P. morganii, P. vulgaris,* and *P. rettgeri; Echerichia coli;* Enterobacter (Aerobacter), and Klebsiella. Pseudomonas strains are generally resistant to the drug. Nalidixic Acid is bactericidal and is effective over the entire urinary pH range. Conventional chromosomal resistance to Nalidixic Acid taken in full dosage has been reported to emerge in approximately 2 to 14 percent of patients during treatment; however, bacterial resistance to Nalidixic Acid has not been shown to be transferable via R factor.

INDICATIONS AND USAGE

Nalidixic Acid is indicated for the treatment of urinary tract infections caused by susceptible gram-negative microorganisms, including the majority of Proteus strains, Klebsiella, Enterobacter (Aerobacter), and *E. coli.* Disc susceptibility testing with the 30 µg disc should be performed prior to administration of the drug, and during treatment if clinical response warrants.

CONTRAINDICATIONS

Nalidixic Acid is contraindicated in patients with known hypersensitivity to Nalidixic Acid and in patients with a history of convulsive disorders.

WARNINGS

CNS effects including brief convulsions, increased intracranial pressure, and toxic psychosis have been reported rarely. These have occurred in infants and children or in geriatric patients, usually from overdosage or in patients with predisposing factors, and have been completely and rapidly reversible pon discontinuation of the drug. If these reactions occur, Nalidixic Acid should be discontinued and appropriate therapeutic measures instituted; only if rapid disappearance of CNS symptoms does not occur within 48 hours should diagnostic procedures involving risk to the patient be undertaken. (See *"Adverse Reactions"* and *"Overdosage"*.)

PRECAUTIONS

Blood counts and renal and liver function tests should be performed periodically if treatment is continued for more than two weeks. Nalidixic Acid should be used with caution in patients with liver disease, epilepsy, or severe cerebral arteriosclerosis. While caution should be used in patients with severe renal failure, therapeutic concentrations of Nalidixic Acid in the urine, without increased toxicity due to drug accumulation in the blood, have been observed in patients on full dosage with creatinine clearances as low as 2 mL/minute to 8 mL/minute.

Patients should be cautioned to avoid undue exposure to direct sunlight while receiving Nalidixic Acid. Therapy should be discontinued if photosensitivity occurs.

If bacterial resistance to Nalidixic Acid emerges during treatment, it usually does so within 48 hours, permitting rapid change to another antimicrobial. Therefore, if the clinical response is unsatisfactory or if relapse occurs, cultures and sensitivity tests should be repeated. Underdosage with Nalidixic Acid during initial treatment (with less than 4 g per day for adults) may predispose to emergence of bacterial resistance. (See *"Dosage and Administration".*)

Drug Interactions: Nitrofurantoin interferes with the therapeutic action of Nalidixic Acid.

➤ SHOWN IN PRODUCT IDENTIFICATION GUIDE

Cross resistance between Nalidixic Acid and other antimicrobials has been observed only with oxolinic acid.

Nalidixic Acid may enhance the effects of oral anticoagulants, warfarin or bishydroxycoumarin, by displacing significant amounts from serum albumin binding sites.

When Benedict's or Fehling's solutions or Clinitest® Reagent Tablets are used to test the urine of patients taking Nalidixic Acid, a false-positive reaction for glucose may be obtained, due to the liberation of glucuronic acid from the metabolites excreted. However, a colorimetric test for glucose based on an enzyme reaction (eg, with Clinistix® Reagent Strips or Tes-Tape®) does not give a false-positive reaction to the liberated glucuronic acid.

Incorrect values may be obtained for urinary 17-keto and ketogenic steroids in patients receiving Nalidixic Acid because of an interaction between the drug and the *m*-dinitrobenzene used in the usual assay method. In such cases, the Porter-Silber test for 17-hydroxycorticoids may be used.

Usage in Prepubertal Children: Recent toxicological studies have shown that Nalidixic Acid and related drugs can produce erosions of the cartilage in weight-bearing joints and other signs of arthropathy in immature animals of most species tested. No such joint lesions have been reported in man to date. Nevertheless, until the significance of this finding is clarified, care should be exercised when prescribing this product for prepubertal children.

Usage in Pregnancy: Safe use of Nalidixic Acid during the first trimester of pregnancy has not been established. However, the drug has been used during the last two trimesters without producing apparent ill effects in mother or child.

Caution should be used in administering Nalidixic Acid in the days prior to delivery because of the theoretical risk that exposure to maternal Nalidixic Acid in utero may lead to significant blood levels of Nalidixic Acid in the neonate immediately after birth. Patients using Nalidixic Acid during pregnancy should be advised to discontinue use at the first sign of labor.

ADVERSE REACTIONS
Reactions reported after oral administration of Nalidixic Acid include:

CNS effects: drowsiness, weakness, headache, and dizziness and vertigo. Reversible subjective visual disturbances without objective findings have occurred infrequently (generally with each dose during the first few days of treatment). These reactions include overbrightness of lights, change in color perception, difficulty in focusing, decrease in visual acuity, and double vision. They usually disappeared promptly when dosage was reduced or therapy was discontinued. Toxic psychosis or brief convulsions have been reported rarely, usually following excessive doses. In general, the convulsions have occurred in patients with predisposing factors such as epilepsy or cerebral arteriosclerosis. In infants and children receiving therapeutic doses of Nalidixic Acid, increased intracranial pressure with bulging anterior fontanel, papilledema, and headache has occasionally been observed. A few cases of 6th cranial nerve palsy have been reported. Although the mechanisms of these reactions are unknown, the signs and symptoms usually disappeared rapidly with no sequelae when treatment was discontinued.

Gastrointestinal: abdominal pain, nausea, vomiting, and diarrhea.

Allergic: rash, pruritus, urticaria, angioedema, eosinophilia, arthralgia with joint stiffness and swelling, and rarely, anaphylactoid reaction. Photosensitivity reactions consisting of erythema and bullae on exposed skin surfaces usually resolve completely in 2 weeks to 2 months after Nalidixic Acid is discontinued; however, bullae may continue to appear with successive exposures to sunlight or with mild skin trauma for up to 3 months after discontinuation of drug. (See *"Precautions"*.)

Other: rarely, cholestasis, paresthesia, metabolic acidosis, thrombocytopenia, leukopenia, or hemolytic anemia, sometimes associated with glucose-6-phosphate dehydrogenase deficiency.

DOSAGE AND ADMINISTRATION
Adults: The recommended dosage for initial therapy in adults is 1 g administered four times daily for one or two weeks (total daily dose, 4 g). For prolonged therapy, the total daily dose may be reduced to 2 g after the initial treatment period. Underdosage during initial treatment may predispose to emergence of bacterial resistance.

Children: Until further experience is gained, Nalidixic Acid should not be administered to infants younger than three months. Dosage in children 12 years of age and under should be calculated on the basis of body weight. The recommended total daily dosage for initial therapy is 25 mg/lb/day (55 mg/kg/day), administered in four equally divided doses. For prolonged therapy, the total daily dose may be reduced to 15 mg/lb/day (33 mg/kg/day). Nalidixic Acid Suspension or Nalidixic Acid Caplets of 250 mg may be used. One 250 mg tablet is equivalent to one teaspoon (5 mL) of the Suspension.

OVERDOSAGE
Manifestations: Toxic psychosis, convulsions, increased intracranial pressure, or metabolic acidosis may occur in patients taking more than the recommended dosage. Vomiting, nausea, and lethargy may also occur following overdosage.

Treatment: Reactions are short-lived (two to three hours) because the drug is rapidly excreted. If overdosage is noted early, gastric lavage is indicated. If absorption has occurred, increased fluid administration is advisable and supportive measures such as oxygen and means of artificial respiration should be available. Although anticonvulsant therapy has not been used in the few instances of overdosage reported, it may be indicated in a severe case.

PHARMACOLOGY
Following oral administration Nalidixic Acid, is rapidly absorbed from the gastrointestinal tract, partially metabolized in the liver, and rapidly excreted through the kidneys. Unchanged Nalidixic Acid appears in the urine along with an active metabolite, hydroxynalidixic acid, which has antibacterial activity similar to that of Nalidixic Acid. Other metabolites include glucuronic acid conjugates of Nalidixic Acid and hydroxynalidixic acid, and the dicarboxylic acid derivative. The hydroxy metabolite represents 30 percent of the biologically active drug in the blood and 85 percent in the urine. Peak serum levels of active drug average approximately 20 µg to 40 µg per mL (90 percent protein bound), one to two hours after administration of a 1 g dose to a fasting normal individual, with a half-life of about 90 minutes. Peak urine levels of active drug average approximately 150 µg to 200 µg per mL, three to four hours after administration, with a half-life of about six hours. Approximately four percent of Nalidixic Acid is excreted in the feces. Traces of Nalidixic Acid were found in blood and urine of an infant whose mother had received the drug during the last trimester of pregnancy.

ANIMAL PHARMACOLOGY
Nalidixic Acid and related drugs have been shown to cause anthropathy in juvenile animals of most species tested. (See *"Precautions"*.)

Hydroxynalidixic acid, the principal metabolite of Nalidixic Acid, did not produce any oculotoxic effects at any dosage level in seven species of animals including three primate species. However, oral administration of this metabolite in high doses has been shown to have oculotoxic potential, namely in dogs and cats where it produced retinal degeneration upon prolonged administration leading, in some cases, to blindness.

In experiments with Nalidixic Acid itself, little if any such activity could be elicited in either dogs or cats. Sensitivity to CNS side effects in these species limited the doses of Nalidixic Acid that could be used; this factor, together with a low conversion rate to the hydroxy metabolite in these species, may explain the absence of these effects.

HOW SUPPLIED
SUSPENSION: 250 MG/5 ML

BRAND/MANUFACTURER	NDC	SIZE	AWP
◆ **BRAND**			
NEGGRAM: Sanofi Winthrop	00024-1318-06	480 ml	$106.81

TABLETS: 250 MG

BRAND/MANUFACTURER	NDC	SIZE	AWP
◆ **BRAND**			
NEGGRAM: Sanofi Winthrop	00024-1321-03	56s	$41.53

TABLETS: 500 MG

AVERAGE UNIT PRICE (AVAILABLE SIZES)		GENERIC A-RATED AVERAGE PRICE (GAAP)	
BRAND	$1.21	100s	$66.88
GENERIC	$0.69		
HCFA FUL (100s ea)	$0.65		

BRAND/MANUFACTURER	NDC	SIZE	AWP
◆ **BRAND**			
NEGGRAM: Sanofi Winthrop	00024-1322-03	56s	$68.59
	00024-1322-06	500s	$598.75
◆ **GENERICS**			
Schein	00364-2324-50	50s	$38.50
Aligen	00405-4691-01	100s	$43.45
Schein	00364-2324-01	100s	$75.50
Moore,H.L.	00839-7528-06	100s	$81.68

TABLETS: 1 GM
HCFA FUL (100s ea) $0.92

BRAND/MANUFACTURER	NDC	SIZE	AWP
◆ **BRAND**			
NEGGRAM: Sanofi Winthrop	00024-1323-04	100s	$184.85
◆ **GENERICS**			
Schein	00364-2325-01	100s	$102.50

Naloxone Hydrochloride

DESCRIPTION
Naloxone Hydrochloride injection, USP a narcotic antagonist, is a synthetic congener of oxymorphone. In structure it differs from oxymorphone in that the methyl group on the nitrogen atom is replaced by an allyl group. Naloxone Hydrochloride occurs as a white to slightly off-white powder, and is soluble in water, in dilute acids, and in strong alkali; slightly soluble in alcohol; practically insoluble in either and in chloroform.

Naloxone Hydrochloride injection is available as a sterile solution for intravenous, intramuscular and subcutaneous administration in three concentrations, 0.02 mg, 0.4 mg and 1.0 mg of Naloxone Hydrochloride per mL. One mL of the 0.02 mg and 0.4 mg strengths contains 8.6 mg of sodium chloride. One mL of the 1.0 mg strength contains 8.35 mg of sodium chloride. One mL of the 0.4 mg and 1.0 mg strengths also contains 2.0 mg of methylparaben and propylparaben as perservatives in a ratio of 9 to 1. pH is adjusted to 3.5 ± 0.5 with hydrochloric acid.

Naloxone Hydrochloride injection is also available in a paraben-free formulation in three concentrations: 0.02 mg and 0.4 mg and 1.0 mg of Naloxone Hydrochloride per mL. One mL of each strength contains 9.0 mg of sodium chloride. pH is adjusted to 3.5 ± 0.5 with hydrochloric acid.

Following is its chemical structure:

CLINICAL PHARMACOLOGY

Naloxone Hydrochloride injection, USP prevents or reverses the effects of opioids including respiratory depression, sedation and hypotension. Also, it can reverse the psychotomimetic and dysphoric effects of agonist-antagonists such as pentazocine.

Naloxone Hydrochloride injection, USP is an essentially pure narcotic antagonist, i.e., it does not possess the "agonistic" or morphine-like properties characteristic of other narcotic antagonists; Naloxone Hydrochloride does not produces respiratory depression, psychotomimetic effects of pupillary constriction. In the absence of narcotics or agonistic effects of other narcotic antagonists it exhibits essentially no pharmacologic activity.

Naloxone Hydrochloride has not been shown to produce tolerance nor to cause physical or psychological dependence.

In the presence of physical dependence on narcotics Naloxone Hydrochloride will produce withdrawal symptoms.

Mechanisms of Action: While the mechanism of action of Naloxone Hydrochloride is not fully understood, the preponderance of evidence suggests that Naloxone Hydrochloride antagonizes the opioid effects by competing for the same receptor sites.

When Naloxone Hydrochloride is administered intravenously the onset of action is generally apparent within two minutes; the onset of action is only slightly less rapid when it is administered subcutaneously or intramuscularly. The duration of action is dependent upon the dose and route of administration of Naloxone Hydrochloride. Intramuscular administration produces a more prolonged effect than intravenous administration. The requirement for repeat doses of Naloxone Hydrochloride, however, will also be dependent upon the amount, type and route of administration of the narcotic being antagonized.

Following parenteral administration Naloxone Hydrochloride is rapidly distributed in the body. It is metabolized in the liver, primarily by glucuronide conjugation and excreted in urine. In one study the serum half-life in adults ranged from 30 to 81 minutes (mean 64 ± 12 minutes). In a neonatal study the mean plasma half-life was observed to be 3.1 ± 0.5 hours.

INDICATIONS AND USAGE

Naloxone Hydrochloride is indicated for the complete or partial reversal of narcotic depression, including respiratory depression, induced by opioids including natural and synthetic narcotics, propoxyphene, methadone and certain narcotic-antagonist analgesics; nalbuphine, pentazocine and butorphanol. Naloxone Hydrochloride is also indicated for the diagnosis of suspected acute opioid overdosage.

CONTRAINDICATIONS

Naloxone Hydrochloride is contraindicated in patients known to be hypersensitive to it.

WARNINGS

Naloxone Hydrochloride should be administered cautiously to persons including newborns of mothers who are known or suspected to be physically dependent on opioids. In such cases an abrupt and complete reversal of narcotic effects may precipitate an acute abstinence syndrome.

The patient who has satisfactorily responded to Naloxone Hydrochloride should be kept under continued surveillance and repeated doses of Naloxone Hydrochloride should be administered, as necessary, since the duration of action of some narcotics may exceed that of Naloxone Hydrochloride.

Naloxone Hydrochloride is not effective against respiratory depression due to nonopioid drugs. Reversal of buprenorphine-induced respiratory depression may be incomplete. If an incomplete response occurs, respirations should be mechanically assisted.

PRECAUTIONS

In addition to Naloxone Hydrochloride other resuscitative measures such as maintenance of a free airway, artificial ventilation, cardiac massage, and vasopressor agents should be available and employed when necessary to counteract acute narcotic poisoning.

Several instances of hypotension, hypertension, ventricular tachycardia and fibrillation, and pulmonary edema have been reported. These have occurred in postoperative patients most of whom had pre-existing cardiovascular disorders or received other drugs which may have similar adverse cardiovascular effects. Although a direct cause and effection relationship has not been established,

Naloxone Hydrochloride should be used with caution in patients with pre-existing cardiac disease or patients who have received potentially cardiotoxic drugs.

Carcinogenesis, Mutagenesis, Impairment of Fertility: Carcinogenicity and mutagenicity studies have not been performed with Naloxone Hydrochloride. Reproductive studies in mice and rats demonstrated no impairment of fertility.

Use in Pregnancy: Pregnancy Catagory B: Reproduction studies performed in mice and rats at doses up to 1,000 times the human dose, revealed no evidence of impaired fertility or harm to the fetus due to Naloxone Hydrochloride. There are, however, no adequate and well controlled studies in pregnant women. Because animal reproduction studies are not always predictive of human response, Naloxone Hydrochloride should be used during pregnancy only if clearly needed.

Nursing Mothers: It is not known whether Naloxone Hydrochloride is excreted in human milk. Because many drugs are excreted in human milk, caution should be exercised when Naloxone Hydrochloride is administered to a nursing woman.

ADVERSE REACTIONS

Abrupt reversal of narcotic depression may result in nausea, vomiting, sweating, tachycardia, increased blood pressure, tremulousness, seizures and cardiac arrest. In postoperative patients, larger than necessary dosage of Naloxone Hydrochloride may result in significant reversal of analgesia, and in excitement. Hypotension, hypertension, ventricular tachycardia and fibrillation, and pulmonary edema have been associated with the use of Naloxone Hydrochloride postoperatively (see *"Precautions"* and *"Usage in Adults-Postoperative Narcotic Depression"*).

OVERDOSAGE

There is no clinical experience with Naloxone Hydrochloride overdosage in humans.

In the mouse and rat the intravenous LD_{50} is 150 ± 5 mg/kg and 109 ± 4 mg/kg respectively. In acute subcutaneous toxicity studies in newborn rats the LD_{50} (95% CL) is 260 (228-296) mg/kg. Subcutaneous injection of 100 mg/kg/day in rats for 3 weeks produced only transient salivation and partial ptosis following injection; no toxic effects were seen at 10 mg/kg/day for 3 weeks.

DOSAGE AND ADMINISTRATION

Naloxone Hydrochloride injection, USP may be administered intravenously, intramuscularly, or subcutaneously. The most rapid onset of action is achieved by intravenous administration and it is recommended in emergency situations.

Since the duration of action of some narcotics may exceed that of Naloxone Hydrochloride the patient should be kept under continued surveillance and repeated doses of Naloxone Hydrochloride should be administered, as necessary.

Intravenous Infusion: Naloxone Hydrochloride may be diluted for intravenous infusion in normal saline or 5% dextrose solutions. The addition of 2 mg of Naloxone Hydrochloride in 500 mL of either solution provides a concentration of 0.004 mg/mL. Mixtures should be used within 24 hours. After 24 hours, the remaining unused solution must be discarded. The rate of administration should be titrated in accordance with the patient's response. Parenteral drug products should be inspected visually for particular matter and discoloration prior to administration whenever solution and container permit. Naloxone Hydrochloride should not be mixed with preparations containing bisulfite, metabisulfite, long-chain or high molecular weight anions, or any solution having an alkaline pH. No drug or chemical agent should be added to Naloxone Hydrochloride unless its effect on the chemical and physical stability of the solution has first been established.

USAGE IN ADULTS

Narcotic Overdose—Known or Suspected: An initial dose of 0.4 mg to 2 mg of Naloxone Hydrochloride may be administered intravenously. If the desired degree of counteraction and improvement in respiratory functions is not obtained, it may be repeated at 2 to 3 minute intervals. If no response is observed after 10 mg of Naloxone Hydrochloride have been administered, the diagnosis of narcotic induced or partial narcotic induced toxicity should be questioned. Intramuscular or subcutaneous administration may be necessary if the intravenous route is not available.

Postoperative Narcotic Depression: For the partial reversal of narcotic depression following the use of narcotics during surgery, smaller doses of Naloxone Hydrochloride are usually sufficient. The dose of Naloxone Hydrochloride should be titrated according to the patient's response. For the initial reversal of respiratory depression, Naloxone Hydrochloride should be injected in increments of 0.1 to 0.2 mg intravenously at two to three minute intervals to the desired degree of reversal i.e. adequate ventilation and alertness without significant pain or discomfort. Larger than necessary dosage of Naloxone Hydrochloride may result in significant reversal of analgesia and increase in blood pressure. Similarly, too rapid reversal may induce nausea, vomiting, sweating or circulatory stress.

Repeat doses of Naloxone Hydrochloride may be required within one to two hour intervals depending upon the amount, type (i.e., short or long acting) and time interval since last administration of narcotic. Supplemental intramuscular doses have been shown to produce a longer lasting effect.

USAGE IN CHILDREN

Narcotic Overdose—Known or Suspected: The usual initial dose in children is 0.01 mg/kg body weight given I.V. If this dose does not result in the desired degree of clinical improvement, a subsequent dose of 0.1 mg/kg body weight may be administered. If an I.V. route of administration is not available, Naloxone

Hydrochloride may be administered I.M. or S.C. in divided doses. If necessary, Naloxone Hydrochloride can be diluted with sterile water for injection.

Postoperative Narcotic Depression: Follow the recommendations and cautions under *"Adult Postoperative Depression".* For the initial reversal of respiratory depression Naloxone Hydrochloride should be injected in increments of 0.005 mg to 0.01 mg intravenously at two to three minute intervals to the desired degree of reversal.

USAGE IN NEONATES

Narcotic-induced Depression: The usual initial dose is 0.01 mg/kg body weight administered I.V., I.M., or S.C. This dose may be repeated in accordance with adult administration guidelines for postoperative narcotic depression.

Store at controlled room temperature (59°-86°F, 15°-30°C).

HOW SUPPLIED
INJECTION: 0.02 MG/ML

AVERAGE UNIT PRICE (AVAILABLE SIZES)		GENERIC A-RATED AVERAGE PRICE (GAAP)		
GENERIC	$3.14	2 ml 10s		$62.76

BRAND/MANUFACTURER		NDC	SIZE	AWP
◆ GENERICS				
Astra		00186-1252-13	2 ml 10s	$16.88
NARCAN: Du Pont Multi		00590-0359-10	2 ml 10s	$56.63
Abbott Hosp		00074-1211-01	2 ml 10s	$84.43
Abbott Hosp		00074-1216-01	2 ml 10s	$93.10

INJECTION: 0.4 MG/ML

AVERAGE UNIT PRICE (AVAILABLE SIZES)		GENERIC A-RATED AVERAGE PRICE (GAAP)		
GENERIC	$6.16	10 ml		$47.88
		1 ml 10s		$58.31
		1 ml 25s		$259.22

BRAND/MANUFACTURER		NDC	SIZE	AWP
◆ GENERICS				
Elkins-Sinn		00641-2521-41	10 ml	$45.00
NARCAN: Du Pont Multi		00590-0365-05	10 ml	$50.75
Astra		00186-1254-12	10 ml 5s	$27.50
Astra		00186-1250-13	1 ml 10s	$11.88
NARCAN: Du Pont Multi		00590-0358-10	1 ml 10s	$31.12
Solo Pak		39769-0129-01	1 ml 10s	$50.00
Elkins-Sinn		00641-1451-33	1 ml 10s	$52.50
Elkins-Sinn		00641-0447-23	1 ml 10s	$59.75
NARCAN: Du Pont Multi		00590-0365-15	1 ml 10s	$75.25
Abbott Hosp		00074-1212-01	1 ml 10s	$88.47
Abbott Hosp		00074-1215-01	1 ml 10s	$97.49
Intl Med Sys		00548-1466-00	1 ml 25s	$208.50
Abbott Hosp		00074-1213-01	1 ml 25s	$309.94
Intl Med Sys		00548-1467-00	2 ml 25s	$417.00
Abbott Hosp		00074-1219-01	10 ml 25s	$1637.86

INJECTION: 1 MG/ML

AVERAGE UNIT PRICE (AVAILABLE SIZES)		GENERIC A-RATED AVERAGE PRICE (GAAP)		
GENERIC	$7.12	1 ml 10s		$73.27
		2 ml 10s		$189.17

BRAND/MANUFACTURER		NDC	SIZE	AWP
◆ GENERICS				
NARCAN: Du Pont Multi		00590-0368-05	10 ml	$75.81
Astra		00186-1253-13	5 ml 5s	$64.13
Astra		00186-1255-12	10 ml 5s	$153.00
Astra		00186-1251-13	1 ml 10s	$34.13
NARCAN: Du Pont Multi		00590-0368-15	1 ml 10s	$112.40
NARCAN: Du Pont Pharma		00590-0377-10	2 ml 10s	$170.88
NARCAN: Du Pont Multi		00590-0368-13	2 ml 10s	$207.45
Intl Med Sys		00548-1469-00	2 ml 25s	$508.50

Naloxone Hydrochloride and Pentazocine Hydrochloride

> NALOXONE HCL/PENTAZOCINE HCL IS INTENDED FOR ORAL USE ONLY. SEVERE, POTENTIALLY LETHAL, REACTIONS MAY RESULT FROM MISUSE OF NALOXONE HCL/PENTAZOCINE HCL BY INJECTION EITHER ALONE OR IN COMBINATION WITH OTHER SUBSTANCES. (SEE *"DRUG ABUSE AND DEPENDENCE"* SECTION.)

DESCRIPTION

Each tablet contains Pentazocine Hydrochloride, USP, equivalent to 50 mg base and is a member of the benzazocine series (also known as the benzomorphan series). Each tablet also contains Naloxone Hydrochloride, USP, equivalent to 0.5 mg base.

Naloxone HCl/Pentazocine HCl is an analgesic for oral administration.

Chemically, Pentazocine Hydrochloride is 1,2,3,4,5,6-Hexahydro -6,11-di-methyl -3-(3-methyl-2-butenyl)-2, 6-methano-3-benzazocin-8-ol hydrochloride, a white, crystalline substance soluble in acidic aqueous solutions.

Chemically, Naloxone Hydrochloride is Morphinan-6-one, 4, 5-epoxy-3, 14-dihydroxy-17-(2-propenyl)-, hydrochloride, (5α)-. It is a slightly off-white power, and is soluble in water and dilute acids.

CLINICAL PHARMACOLOGY

Pentazocine is a potent analgesic which when administered orally in a 50 mg dose appears equivalent in analgesic effect to 60 mg (1 grain) of codeine. Onset of significant analgesia usually occurs between 15 and 30 minutes after oral administration, and duration of action is usually three hours or longer. Onset and duration of action and the degree of pain relief are related both to dose and the severity of pretreatment pain. Pentazocine weakly antagonizes the analgesic effects of morphine and meperidine; in addition, it produces incomplete reversal of cardiovascular, respiratory, and behavioral depression induced by morphine and meperidine. Pentazocine has about 1/50 the antagonistic activity of nalorphine. It also has sedative activity.

Pentazocine is well absorbed from the gastrointestinal tract. Concentrations in plasma coincide closely with the onset, duration, and intensity of analgesia; peak values occur 1 to 3 hours after oral administration. The half-life in plasma is 2 to 3 hours.

Pentazocine is metabolized in the liver and excreted primarily in the urine. Pentazocine passes into the fetal circulation. Naloxone when administered orally at 0.5 mg has no pharmacologic activity. Naloxone Hydrochloride administered parenterally at the same dose is an effective antagonist to Pentazocine and a pure antagonist to narcotic analgesics.

Naloxone HCl/Pentazocine HCl is a potent analgesic when administered orally. However, the presence of Naloxone in Naloxone HCl/Pentazocine HCl will prevent the effect of Pentazocine if the product is misused by injection.

Studies in animals indicate that the presence of Naloxone does not affect Pentazocine analgesia when the combination is given orally. If the combination is given by injection the action of Pentazocine is neutralized.

INDICATIONS AND USAGE

> NALOXONE HCL/PENTAZOCINE HCL IS INTENDED FOR ORAL USE ONLY. SEVERE, POTENTIALLY LETHAL, REACTIONS MAY RESULT FROM MISUSE OF NALOXONE HCL/PENTAZOCINE HCL BY INJECTION EITHER ALONE OR IN COMBINATION WITH OTHER SUBSTANCES. (SEE *"DRUG ABUSE AND DEPENDENCE"* SECTION.)

Naloxone HCl/Pentazocine HCl is indicated for the relief of moderate to severe pain.

Naloxone HCl/Pentazocine HCl is indicated for oral use only.

CONTRAINDICATIONS

Naloxone HCl/Pentazocine HCl should not be administered to patients who are hypersensitive to either Pentazocine or Naloxone.

WARNINGS

> NALOXONE HCL/PENTAZOCINE HCL IS INTENDED FOR ORAL USE ONLY. SEVERE, POTENTIALLY LETHAL, REACTIONS MAY RESULT FROM MISUSE OF NALOXONE HCL/PENTAZOCINE HCL BY INJECTION EITHER ALONE OR IN COMBINATION WITH OTHER SUBSTANCES. (SEE *"DRUG ABUSE AND DEPENDENCE"* SECTION.)

Drug Dependence: Pentazocine can cause a physical and psychological dependence. (See *"Drug Abuse And Dependence".*)

Head Injury and Increased Intracranial Pressure: As in the case of other potent analgesics, the potential of Pentazocine for elevating cerebrospinal fluid pressure may be attributed to CO_2 retention due to the respiratory depressant effects of the drug. These effects may be markedly exaggerated in the presence of head injury, other intracranial lesions, or a preexisting increase in intracranial pressure. Furthermore, Pentazocine can produce effects which may obscure the clinical course of patients with head injuries. In such patients, Pentazocine must be used with extreme caution and only if its use in deemed essential.

Usage with Alcohol: Due to the potential for increased CNS depressant effects, alcohol should be used with caution in patients who are currently receiving Pentazocine.

Patients Receiving Narcotics: Pentazocine is a mild narcotic antagonist. Some patients previously given narcotics, including methadone for the daily treatment of narcotic dependence, have experienced withdrawal symptoms after receiving Pentazocine.

Certain Respiratory Conditions: Although respiratory depression has rarely been reported after oral administration of Pentazocine, the drug should be administered with caution to patients with respiratory depression from any cause, severely limited respiratory reserve, severe bronchial asthma, and other obstructive respiratory conditions, or cyanosis.

Acute CNS Manifestations: Patients receiving therapeutic doses of Pentazocine have experienced hallucinations (usually visual), disorientation, and confusion which have cleared spontaneously within a period of hours. The mechanism of this reaction is not known. Such patients should be very closely observed and vital signs checked. If the drug is reinstituted, it should be done with caution since these acute CNS manifestations may recur.

PRECAUTIONS

CNS Effect: Caution should be used when Pentazocine is administered to patients prone to seizures; seizures have occurred in a few such patients in association with the use of pentazocine though no cause and effect relationship has been established.

Impaired Renal or Hepatic Function: Decreased metabolism of Pentazocine by the liver in extensive liver disease may predispose to accentuation of side effects. Although laboratory tests have not indicated that Pentazocine causes or increases renal or hepatic impairment, the drug should be administered with caution to patients with such impairment.

In prescribing Pentazocine for long-term use, the physician should take precautions to avoid increases in dose by the patient.

Biliary Surgery: Narcotic drug products are generally considered to elevate biliary tract pressure for varying periods following their administration. Some evidence suggests that Pentazocine may differ from other marketed narcotics in this respect (ie, it causes little or no elevation in biliary tract pressures). The clinical significance of these findings, however, is not yet known.

Information for Patients: Since sedation, dizziness, and occasional euphoria have been noted, ambulatory patients should be warned not to operate machinery, drive cars, or unnecessarily expose themselves to hazards. Pentazocine may cause physical and psychological dependence when taken alone and may have additive CNS depressant properties when taken in combination with alcohol or other CNS depressants.

Myocardial Infarction: As with all drugs, Pentazocine should be used with caution in patients with myocardial infarction who have nausea or vomiting.

Drug Interactions. Usage with Alcohol: See "Warnings".

Carcinogenesis, Mutagenesis, Impairment of Fertility: No long-term studies in animals to test for carcinogenesis have been performed with the components of Naloxone HCl/Pentazocine HCl, brand of Pentazocine and Naloxone Hydrochloride tablets.

Pregnancy Category C: Animal reproduction studies have not been conducted with Naloxone HCl/Pentazocine HCl. It is also not known whether Naloxone HCl/Pentazocine HCl can cause fetal harm when administered to pregnant women or can affect reproduction capacity. Naloxone HCl/Pentazocine HCl should be given to pregnant women only if clearly needed. However, animal reproduction studies with Pentazocine have not demonstrated teratogenic or embryotoxic effects.

Labor and Delivery: Patients receiving Pentazocine during labor have experienced no adverse effects other than those that occur with commonly used analgesics. Naloxone HCl/Pentazocine HCl should be used with caution in women delivering premature infants. The effect of Naloxone HCl/Pentazocine HCl on the mother and fetus, the duration of labor or delivery, the possibility that forceps delivery or other intervention or resuscitation of the newborn may be necessary, or the effect of Naloxone HCl/Pentazocine HCl on the later growth, development, and functional maturation of the child are unknown at the present time.

Nursing Mothers: It is not known whether this drug is excreted in human milk. Because many drugs are excreted in human milk, caution should be exercised when Naloxone HCl/Pentazocine HCl is administered to a nursing woman.

Pediatric Use: Safety and effectiveness in children below the age of 12 years have not been established.

ADVERSE REACTIONS

Cardiovascular: Hypotension, tachycardia, syncope.

Respiratory: Rarely, respiratory depression.

Acute CNS Manifestations: Patients receiving therapeutic doses of Pentazocine have experienced hallucinations (usually visual), disorientation, and confusion which have cleared spontaneously within a period of hours. The mechanism of this reaction is not known. Such patients should be closely observed and vital signs checked. If the drug is reinstituted it should be done with caution since these acute CNS manifestations may recur.

Other CNS Effects: Dizziness, light headedness, hallucinations, sedation, euphoria, headache, confusion, disorientation; infrequently weakness, disturbed dreams, insomnia, syncope, visual blurring and focusing difficulty, depression; and rarely tremor, irritability, excitement, tinnitus.

Autonomic: Sweating; infrequently flushing; and rarely chills.

Gastrointestinal: Nausea, vomiting, constipation, diarrhea, anorexia, rarely abdominal distress.

Allergic: Edema of the face; dermatitis, including pruritus; flushed skin, including plethora; infrequently rash, and rarely urticaria.

Ophthalmic: Visual blurring and focusing difficulty.

Hematologic: Depression of white blood cells (especially granulocytes), which is usually reversible, moderate transient eosinophilia.

Other: Headache, chills, insomnia, weakness, urinary retention, paresthesia.

DRUG ABUSE AND DEPENDENCE

Controlled Substance: Naloxone HCl/Pentazocine HCl is a Schedule IV controlled substance.

There have been some reports of dependence and of withdrawal symptoms with orally administered Pentazocine. Patients with a history of drug dependence should be under close supervision while receiving Pentazocine orally. There have been rare reports of possible abstinence syndromes in newborns after prolonged use of Pentazocine during pregnancy.

There have been instances of psychological and physical dependence on parenteral Pentazocine in patients with a history of drug abuse and rarely, in patients without such a history. Abrupt discontinuance following the extended use of parenteral Pentazocine has resulted it, withdrawal symptoms.

In prescribing Pentazocine for chronic use, the physician should take precautions to avoid increases in dose by the patient.

The amount of Naloxone present in Naloxone HCl/Pentazocine HCl (0.5 mg per tablet) has no action when taken orally and will not interfere with the pharmacologic action of Pentazocine. However, this amount of Naloxone given by injection has profound antagonistic action to narcotic analgesics.

Severe, even lethal, consequences may result from misuse of tablets by injection either alone or in combination with other substances, such as pulmonary emboli, vascular occlusion, ulceration and abscesses, and withdrawal symptoms in narcotic dependent individuals.

Naloxone HCl/Pentazocine HCl contains an opioid antagonist, Naloxone (0.5 mg). Naloxone is inactive when administered orally at this dose, and its inclusion in Naloxone HCl/Pentazocine HCl is intended to curb a form of misuse of oral Pentazocine. Parenterally Naloxone is an active narcotic antagonist. Thus, Naloxone HCl/Pentazocine HCl has a lower potential for parenteral misuse than the previous oral Pentazocine formulation. However, it is still subject to patient misuse and abuse by the oral route.

OVERDOSAGE

Manifestations: Clinical experience of overdosage with this oral medication has been insufficient to define the signs of this condition.

Treatment: Oxygen, intravenous fluids, vasopressors, and other supportive measures should be employed as indicated. Assisted or controlled ventilation should also be considered. For respiratory depression due to overdosage or unusual sensitivity to Pentazocine, parenteral Naloxone is a specific and effective antagonist.

DOSAGE AND ADMINISTRATION

> NALOXONE HCL/PENTAZOCINE HCL IS INTENDED FOR ORAL USE ONLY. SEVERE, POTENTIALLY LETHAL, REACTIONS MAY RESULT FROM MISUSE OF NALOXONE HCL/PENTAZOCINE HCL BY INJECTION EITHER ALONE OR IN COMBINATION WITH OTHER SUBSTANCES. (SEE *"DRUG ABUSE AND DEPENDENCE"* SECTION.)

Adults: The usual initial adult dose is 1 tablet every three or four hours. This may be increased to 2 tablets when needed. Total daily dosage should not exceed 12 tablets.

When anti-inflammatory or antipyretic effects are desired in addition to analgesia, aspirin can be administered concomitantly with this product.

Children Under 12 Years of Age: Since clinical experience in children under 12 years of age is limited, administration of this product in this age group is not recommended.

Duration of Therapy: Patients with chronic pain who receive Naloxone HCl/Pentazocine HCl orally for prolonged periods have only rarely been reported to experience withdrawal symptoms when administration was abruptly discontinued (see "Warnings"). Tolerance to the analgesic effect of Pentazocine has also been reported only rarely. However, there is no long–term experience with the oral administration of Naloxone HCl/Pentazocine HCl.

HOW SUPPLIED
TABLETS (C-IV): 0.5 MG-50 MG

BRAND/MANUFACTURER	NDC	SIZE	AWP
○ BRAND			
▶ TALWIN NX: Sanofi Winthrop	00024-1951-04	100s	$79.88
	00024-1951-24	250s ud	$219.15

Naltrexone Hydrochloride

DESCRIPTION

Naltrexone Hydrochloride, an opioid antagonist, is a synthetic congener of oxymorphone, and is technically, therefore, a thebaine derivative. However, it has no opioid agonist properties. Naltrexone differs in structure from oxymorphone in that the methyl group on the nitrogen atom is replaced by a cyclopropylmethyl group. Naltrexone Hydrochloride is also related to the potent opioid antagonist, naloxone, or nallylnoroxymorphone.

Naltrexone Hydrochloride is a white, crystalline compound. The hydrochloride salt is soluble in water to the extent of about 100 mg/cc. Each tablet contains 50 mg of Naltrexone Hydrochloride.

Following is its chemical structure:

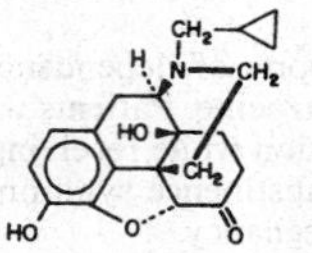

CLINICAL PHARMACOLOGY

Pharmacodynamic Actions: Naltrexone Hydrochloride is a pure opioid antagonist. It markedly attenuates or completely blocks, reversibly, the subjective effects of intravenously administered opioids. [In this context, the term opioid is used to describe 1) classic morphine-like agonists and 2) analgesics possessing agonist and antagonist activity (e.g., butorphanol, nalbuphine and pentazocine).]

When co-administered with morphine, on a chronic basis, Naltrexone Hydrochloride blocks the physical dependence to morphine and presumably other opioids.

Naltrexone Hydrochloride has few, if any, intrinsic actions besides its opioid blocking properties. However, it does produce some pupillary constriction, by an unknown mechanism.

The administration of Naltrexone Hydrochloride is not associated with the development of tolerance or dependence.

In subjects physically dependent on opioids, Naltrexone Hydrochloride will precipitate withdrawal symptomatology.

Clinical studies indicate that 50 mg of Naltrexone Hydrochloride will block the pharmacologic effects of 25 mg of intravenously administered heroin for periods as long as 24 hours. Other data suggest that doubling the dose of Naltrexone Hydrochloride provides blockade for 48 hours, and tripling the dose of Naltrexone Hydrochloride provides blockade for about 72 hours.

While the mechanism of action is not fully understood, the preponderance of evidence suggests that Naltrexone Hydrochloride blocks the effects of opioids by competitive binding (i.e., analogous to competitive inhibition of enzymes) at opioid receptors. This makes the blockade produced potentially surmountable.

Bioavailability/Pharmacokinetics: Following oral administration, Naltrexone Hydrochloride is subject to extensive "first pass" hepatic metabolism (its major route of elimination) with approximately 95% of the absorbed drug being converted to several metabolites. The major metabolite, 6-β-naltrexol, like Naltrexone Hydrochloride, is believed to be a pure antagonist and may contribute to the pharmacological blockade of opioid receptors. A minor metabolite is 2-hydroxy-3-methoxy-6-β-naltrexol. Naltrexone Hydrochloride and its metabolites are also conjugated to form additional metabolic products. Naltrexone Hydrochloride and its metabolites are excreted primarily by the kidney, with fecal excretion being a minor elimination pathway. The urinary excretion of unchanged Naltrexone Hydrochloride accounts for less than 1% of an oral dose; urinary excretion of unchanged and conjugated 6-β-naltrexol accounts for approximately 38% of an oral dose. The pharmacokinetic profile of Naltrexone Hydrochloride suggests that Naltrexone Hydrochloride and its metabolites undergo enterohepatic recycling.

Following the administration of 50 mg Naltrexone Hydrochloride tablets to 24 healthy adult male volunteers, the C_{max} for Naltrexone Hydrochloride and its major metabolite, 6-β-naltrexol were 8.6 ng/ml and 99.3 ng/ml, respectively. The maximum concentration (C_{max}), area under the curve (AUC), and amount excreted in the urine for both Naltrexone Hydrochloride and 6-β-naltrexol increased proportionally as the amount of Naltrexone Hydrochloride administered increased from 50 mg to 200 mg. The time to maximum concentration (T_{max}) is one hour for both Naltrexone Hydrochloride and 6-β-naltrexol. The mean elimination half-life (T-1/2) values for Naltrexone Hydrochloride and 6-β-naltrexol are 3.9 hours and 12.9 hours, respectively. The mean elimination half-life (T-1/2) and time to maximum concentration (T_{max}) for Naltrexone Hydrochloride and 6-β-naltrexol are independent of dose. Naltrexone Hydrochloride does not accumulate during chronic dosing. As predicted by its longer half-life, plasma levels of 6-β-naltrexol increase by 40% during chronic Naltrexone Hydrochloride dosing.

The total body clearance of Naltrexone Hydrochloride is 1.5 L/min which approximates liver blood flow, and suggests Naltrexone Hydrochloride is a highly extracted compound. A renal clearance of 127 ml/min for Naltrexone Hydrochloride suggests it is solely cleared by glomerular filtration. A renal clearance of 283 ml/min for 6-β-naltrexol suggests an additional renal tubular secretory mechanism. The volume of distribution for Naltrexone Hydrochloride following intravenous administration is estimated to be 1350 liters. *In vitro* tests with human plasma show Naltrexone Hydrochloride to be 21% bound to plasma protein over the therapeutic dose range.

In a relative bioavailability study in 24 healthy adult male volunteers Naltrexone Hydrochloride tablets were found to be bioequivalent to Naltrexone Hydrochloride syrup: no differences were observed for C_{max}, AUC, and urinary excretion. As expected, the time to maximum concentration (T_{max}) occurred slightly earlier for the syrup (0.6 hours) than for the tablet (1.0 hr).

INDICATIONS AND USAGE

Naltrexone Hydrochloride is indicated to provide blockade of the pharmacologic effects of exogenously administered opioids as an adjunct to the maintenance of the opioid free-state in detoxified formerly opioid-dependent individuals.

There are no data that demonstrate an unequivocally beneficial effect of Naltrexone Hydrochloride on rates of recidivism among detoxified, formerly opioid-dependent individuals.

UNLABELED USES

Naltrexone is used alone or as an adjunct in the treatment of alcohol dependence, amenorrhea, and bulimia nervosa. It is also used in the treatment of erectile dysfunction, premenstrual syndrome, and autism associated with inattentiveness and self-injurious behavior. It is also prescribed in the treatment of Tourette's syndrome.

CONTRAINDICATIONS

Naltrexone Hydrochloride is contraindicated in:

1) Patients receiving opioid analgesics.
2) Opioid dependent patients.
3) Patients in acute opioid withdrawal (see *"Warnings"*).
4) Any individual who has failed to pass the Naloxone challenge (see *"Dosage and Administration"* section).
5) Any individual who has a positive urine screen for opioids.
6) Any individual with a history of sensitivity to Naltrexone Hydrochloride. It is not known if there is any cross-sensitivity with naloxone or other phenanthrene containing opioids.
7) Any individual with acute hepatitis or liver failure.

WARNINGS

HEPATOTOXICITY

NALTREXONE HYDROCHLORIDE HAS THE CAPACITY TO CAUSE DOSE RELATED HEPATOCELLULAR INJURY.

PRIOR TO MAKING A DECISION TO INITIATE TREATMENT WITH NALTREXONE HYDROCHLORIDE, THE PHYSICIAN SHOULD ESTABLISH WHETHER THE PATIENT HAS SUBCLINICAL LIVER INJURY OR DISEASE. (SEE *"PRECAUTIONS," LABORATORY TESTS*). NALTREXONE HYDROCHLORIDE IS CONTRAINDICATED IN ACUTE HEPATITIS OR LIVER FAILURE, BUT ITS USE EVEN IN PATIENTS WITH EVIDENCE OF LESS SEVERE LIVER DISEASE OR A HISTORY OF RECENT LIVER DISEASE MUST BE CAREFULLY CONSIDERED IN LIGHT OF ITS HEPATOTOXIC POTENTIAL.

THE EVIDENCE THAT IDENTIFIED NALTREXONE HYDROCHLORIDE AS A HEPATOTOXIN WAS *NOT* OBTAINED IN STUDIES INVOLVING ITS USE AT THE DOSES RECOMMENDED FOR OPIATE BLOCKADE, WHERE THE CHANGES IN SERUM LEVELS OF LIVER ENZYMES SEEN WERE SIMILAR TO THOSE PRESENT AT BASELINE IN THE STUDY POPULATION. HOWEVER, THE MARGIN OF SEPARATION BETWEEN THE APPARENTLY SAFE AND THE HEPATOTOXIC DOSES APPEARS TO BE ONLY FIVE-FOLD OR LESS.

Evidence of Naltrexone Hydrochloride's hepatotoxic potential is derived primarily from a placebo controlled study in which Naltrexone Hydrochloride was administered to obese subjects at a dose approximately five-fold that recommended for the blockade of opiate receptors (300 mg per day). In the study, 5 of 26 Naltrexone Hydrochloride recipients developed elevations of serum transaminases (i.e., peak SGPT values ranging from a low of 121 to a high of 532; or 3 to 19 times their baseline values) after three to eight weeks of treatment. Although the patients involved were generally clinically asymptomatic and the transaminase levels of all patients on whom follow-up was obtained returned to (or toward) baseline values in a matter of weeks, the lack of any transaminase elevations of similar magnitude in any of the 24 placebo patients in the same study is persuasive evidence that Naltrexone Hydrochloride is a direct (i.e., not an idiosyncratic) hepatotoxin. This conclusion is also supported by evidence from other placebo controlled studies in which exposure to Naltrexone Hydrochloride at doses from one to two-fold the amount recommended for opiate blockade consistently produced more numerous and more significant elevations of serum transaminases than did placebo, and reports of transaminase elevations in 3 of 9 patients with Alzheimer's Disease who received Naltrexone Hydrochloride (up to 300 mg/day) for 5 to 8 weeks in an open clinical trial.

Unintended Precipitation of Abstinence: To prevent occurrence of an acute absence syndrome, or exacerbation of a pre-existing sub-clinical abstinence syndrome, patients should remain opioid-free for a minimum of 7-10 days before starting Naltrexone Hydrochloride. Since the absence of an opioid drug in the urine is often not sufficient proof that a patient is opioid-free, a Naloxone, challenge should be employed to exclude the possibility of precipitating a withdrawal reaction following administration of Naltrexone Hydrochloride. The Naloxone challenge test is described in the *"Dosage and Administration"* section.

While Naltrexone Hydrochloride is a potent antagonist with a prolonged pharmacologic effect (24 to 72 hours), the blockade produced by Naltrexone Hydrochloride is surmountable. This is useful in patients who may require analgesia, but poses a potential risk to individuals who attempt, on their own, to overcome the blockade by administering large amounts of exogenous opioids. Indeed, any attempt by a patient to overcome the antagonism by taking opioids is very dangerous and may lead to a fatal overdose. Injury may arise because the plasma concentration of exogenous opioids attained immediately following their acute administration may be sufficient to overcome the competitive receptor blockade. As a consequence, the patient may be in immediate danger of suffering life endangering opioid intoxication (e.g., respiratory arrest, circulatory collapse). Also, lesser amounts of exogenous opioids may prove dangerous if they are taken in a manner (i.e., relatively long after the last dose of Naltrexone) and in an amount so that they persist in the body longer than effective concentrations of

---

Naltrexone and its metabolites. *Patients should be told of the serious consequences of surmounting the opiate blockade.* See *"Information for Patients"* section.

PRECAUTIONS
GENERAL
Actions Suggested When Reversal of Naltrexone Hydrochloride Blockade is Required: In an emergency situation requiring analgesia which can only be achieved with opioids, the amount of opioid required may be greater than usual, and the resulting respiratory depression may be deeper and more prolonged. No methods to reverse overdose have been established by controlled clinical trials; therefore in such circumstances, a rapidly acting analgesic which minimizes respiratory depression is preferred. The amount of analgesic administered should be titrated to the needs of the patient.

Additionally, non-receptor mediated actions may occur (e.g., facial swelling, itching, generalized erythema presumably due to histamine release).

Irrespective of the drug chosen to reverse Naltrexone Hydrochloride blockade, the patient should be monitored closely by appropriately trained personnel in a hospital setting.

Actions Suggested When Withdrawal is Accidentally Precipitated With Naltrexone Hydrochloride: Severe opioid withdrawal syndromes precipitated by the accidental ingestion of Naltrexone Hydrochloride have been reported in opioid-dependent individuals. Symptoms of withdrawal have usually appeared within five minutes of ingestion of Naltrexone Hydrochloride and have lasted for up to 48 hours. Mental status changes including confusion, somnolence and visual hallucinations have occurred. Significant fluid losses from vomiting and diarrhea have required intravenous fluid administration. In all cases patients were closely monitored and therapy tailored to meet individual requirements.

Interference With the Action of Narcotic Containing Drug Product: Patients taking Naltrexone Hydrochloride may not benefit from opioid containing medicines, such as cough and cold preparations, antidiarrheal preparations, and opioid analgesics. Where a non-opioid containing alternative is available, it should be used.

INFORMATION FOR PATIENTS
It is suggested that the prescribing physician relate the following information to patients being treated with Naltrexone Hydrochloride:

You have been prescribed Naltrexone Hydrochloride as part of the comprehensive treatment for your drug dependence. You should carry identification to alert medical personnel to the fact that you are taking Naltrexone Hydrochloride. A Naltrexone Hydrochloride medication card may be obtained from your physician and can be used for this purpose. Carrying the identification card should help to ensure that you can obtain adequate treatment in an emergency. If you require medical treatment, be sure to tell the treating physician that you are receiving Naltrexone Hydrochloride therapy.

You should take Naltrexone Hydrochloride as directed by your physician. If you attempt to self-administer heroin or any other opiate drug, in small doses, you will not perceive any effect. *Most important, however, if you attempt to self-administer large doses of heroin or any other narcotic, you may die or sustain serious injury, including coma.*

LABORATORY TESTS
Tests designed to detect hepatic injury should be obtained prior to initiation of Naltrexone Hydrochloride therapy and periodically thereafter (see *"Warnings"* section on *"Hepatotoxicity"*).

Periodic testing of all patients after initiation of treatment is critical if the occurrence of Naltrexone Hydrochloride induced liver damage is to be detected at the earliest possible time. Evaluations, using appropriate batteries of tests to detect liver injury are recommended on a monthly basis during the first six months of use; thereafter, clinical judgment about the frequency of monitoring must be relied upon.

Laboratory tests which may be used for the separation and detection of morphine, methadone or quinine in the urine and with which Naltrexone Hydrochloride does not interfere include thin-layer, gas-liquid, and high pressure liquid chromatographic methods.

CARCINOGENESIS, MUTAGENESIS AND IMPAIRMENT OF FERTILITY
Carcinogenesis: In a two-year carcinogenicity study in rats, there were small increases in the numbers of mesotheliomas in males, and tumors of vascular origin in both sexes. The number of tumors were within the range seen in historical control groups, except for the vascular tumors in females, where the 4% incidence exceeded the historical maximum of 2%.

Mutagenesis: A total of twenty-two distinct tests were performed using bacterial, mamalian, and tissue culture systems. All tests were negative except for weakly positive findings in the Drosophila recessive lethal assay and non-specific DNA repair tests with *E. coli*. The significance of these findings is undetermined.

Impairment of Fertility: Naltrexone Hydrochloride (100 mg/kg, approximately 140 times the human therapeutic dose) caused a significant increase in pseudopregnancy in the rat. A decrease in the pregnancy rate of mated female rats also occurred. The relevance of these observations to human fertility is not known.

PREGNANCY: CATEGORY C
Naltrexone Hydrochloride has been shown to have an embryocidal effect in the rat and rabbit when given in doses approximately 140 times the human therapeutic dose. This effect was demonstrated in rats dosed with Naltrexone Hydrochloride (100 mg/kg) prior to and throughout gestation, and rabbits treated with 60 mg/kg of Naltrexone Hydrochloride during the period of organogenesis. There are no adequate and well-controlled studies in pregnant women. Naltrexone Hydrochloride should be used in pregnancy only when the potential benefit justifies the potential risk to the fetus.

Labor and Delivery: Whether or not Naltrexone Hydrochloride affects the duration of labor and delivery is unknown.

NURSING MOTHERS
Whether or not Naltrexone Hydrochloride is excreted in human milk is unknown. Because many drugs are excreted in human milk, caution should be exercised when Naltrexone Hydrochloride is administered to a nursing mother.

PEDIATRIC USE
The safe use of Naltrexone Hydrochloride in subjects younger than 18 years old has not been established.

ADVERSE REACTIONS
While extensive clinical studies evaluating the use of Naltrexone Hydrochloride in detoxified, formerly opioid dependent individuals failed to identify any single, serious untoward risk of Naltrexone Hydrochloride use, placebo controlled studies employing up to five-fold higher doses of Naltrexone Hydrochloride (up to 300 mg per day) than that recommended for use in opiate receptor blockade have shown that Naltrexone Hydrochloride causes hepatocellular injury in a substantial proportion of patients exposed at this higher dose (see *"Warnings"* and *"Precautions: Laboratory Tests"*).

Aside from this finding, however, available evidence does not incriminate Naltrexone Hydrochloride used at any dose, as a cause of any other serious untoward event for the patient who is "opioid free." It is critical to recognize that Naltrexone Hydrochloride can precipitate or exacerbate abstinence signs and symptoms in any individual who is not completely free of exogenous opioids.

Naltrexone Hydrochloride used at the doses recommended to produce opiate receptor blockade does *not* appear to be the cause of any of the numerous adverse events and abnormal laboratory findings, *including liver function abnormalities*, that were observed in the course of the clinical trials that enrolled individuals with a history of both alcohol and substance abuse. In the one placebo controlled trial intended to assess the effects of opiate receptor blockade on drug abuse recidivism, observed untoward events and laboratory abnormalities occurred with nearly equal frequency among placebo and Naltrexone Hydrochloride recipients. In all open studies, the untoward events observed (e.g., lymphocytosis, transaminase elevations, GI disturbances) were findings that would be anticipated in any similar population *not* treated with Naltrexone. Supporting this judgment, many of the abnormalities detected during the course of the clinical trials were present at baseline, and in some instances, baseline abnormalities, including transaminase elevations, improved or returned to normal during the course of treatment with Naltrexone.

In summary, among opioid free individuals, Naltrexone Hydrochloride administration at the recommended dose has not been associated with a predictable profile of serious adverse or untoward events. However, as mentioned above, among individuals using opioids, Naltrexone Hydrochloride may cause serious reactions (see *"Contraindications"*, *"Warnings"*, *"Dosage and Administration"*).

Events other than hepatocellular injury reported during clinical testing:

The following adverse reactions have been reported both at baseline and during the Naltrexone Hydrochloride medication period at an incidence rate of more than 10%:

Difficulty sleeping, anxiety, nervousness, abdominal pain/cramps, nausea and/or vomiting, low energy, joint and muscle pain, and headache.

The incidence was less than 10% for:

Loss of appetite, diarrhea, constipation, increased thirst, increased energy, feeling down, irritability, dizziness, skin rash, delayed ejaculation, decreased potency, and chills.

The following events occurred in less than 1% of subjects:

Respiratory: nasal congestion, itching, rhinorrhea, sneezing, sore throat, excess mucus or phlegm, sinus trouble, heavy breathing, hoarseness, cough, shortness of breath.

Cardiovascular: nose bleeds, phlebitis, edema, increased blood pressure, non-specific ECG changes, palpitations, tachycardia.

Gastrointestinal: excessive gas, hemorrhoids, diarrhea, ulcer.

Musculoskeletal: painful shoulders, legs or knees; tremors, twitching.

Genitourinary: increased frequency of, or discomfort during, urination; increased or decreased sexual interest.

Dermatologic: oily skin, pruritus, acne, athlete's foot, cold sores, alopecia.

Psychiatric: depression, paranoia, fatigue, restlessness, confusion, disorientation, hallucinations, nightmares, bad dreams.

Special senses: eyes-blurred, burning, light sensitive, swollen, aching, strained; ears-"clogged", aching, tinnitus.

General: increased appetite, weight loss, weight gain, yawning, somnolence, fever, dry mouth, head "pounding", inguinal pain, swollen glands, "side" pains, cold feet, "hot spells." Lethargy and somnolence have been reported following dosing of Naltrexone Hydrochloride and thioridazine.

Laboratory tests: With the exception of liver test abnormalities in investigator studies (see *"Warnings,"* *"Precautions,"* etc), results of laboratory tests, like adverse reaction reports, have not shown consistent patterns of abnormalities that can be attributed to treatment with Naltrexone Hydrochloride.

In the trials evaluating Naltrexone Hydrochloride for the blockade of opiate receptors, abnormal liver function tests and lymphocytosis were the two most common categories of abnormalities reported. As noted earlier, these abnormalities are common among populations of parenteral opioid users and alcoholics. As is the case with the untoward events described above, a large proportion of patients had abnormal laboratory tests at baseline, further supporting the conclusion that the abnormalities observed are not attributable to Naltrexone Hydrochloride.

Idiopathic thrombocytopenic purpura was reported in one patient who may have been sensitized to Naltrexone Hydrochloride in a previous course of treatment with Naltrexone Hydrochloride. The condition cleared without sequelae after discontinuation of Naltrexone Hydrochloride and corticosteroid treatment.

DRUG ABUSE AND DEPENDENCE

Naltrexone Hydrochloride is a pure opioid antagonist. It does not lead to physical or psychological dependence. Tolerance to the opioid antagonist effect is not known to occur.

OVERDOSAGE

There is no clinical experience with Naltrexone Hydrochloride overdosage in humans. In one study, subjects who received 800 mg daily Naltrexone Hydrochloride for up to one week showed no evidence of toxicity. In the mouse, rat, and guinea pig, the oral LD_{50}S were $1,100 \pm 96$ mg/kg; $1,450 \pm 265$ mg/kg; and $1,490 \pm 102$ mg/kg, respectively.

In acute toxicity studies in the mouse, rat, and dog, cause of death was due to clonictonic convulsions and/or respiratory failure.

TREATMENT OF OVERDOSAGE

Consideration should be given to contacting a poison control center for the most up-to-date information.

In view of the lack of actual experience in the treatment of Naltrexone Hydrochloride overdose, patients should be treated symptomatically in a closely supervised environment.

DOSAGE AND ADMINISTRATION

Induction of Naltrexone Hydrochloride Therapy: DO NOT ATTEMPT TREATMENT UNTIL NALOXONE CHALLENGE IS NEGATIVE (see below). Initiate treatment with Naltrexone Hydrochloride using the following guidelines.

1. Treatment should not be attempted until the patient has remained opioid-free for 7–10 days. Self-reporting of abstinence from opioids should be verified by analysis of the patient's urine for absence of opioids. The patient should not be manifesting withdrawal signs or reporting withdrawal symptoms.
2. A Naloxone challenge test (see below) should be administered to the patient. If signs of opioid withdrawal are still observed following Naloxone challenge, treatment with Naltrexone Hydrochloride should not be attempted. The naloxone challenge can be repeated in 24 hours.
3. Treatment should be initiated carefully, slowly increasing the dose of Naltrexone Hydrochloride administered. This can be accomplished by administration of 25 mg of Naltrexone Hydrochloride initially. The patient should be observed for 1 hour. If no withdrawal signs occur, the patient may be given the rest of the daily dose.

Naloxone Challenge Test: The naloxone challenge test should *not* be performed in a patient showing clinical signs or symptoms of opioid withdrawal, or in a patient whose urine contains opioids.

The naloxone challenge test may be administered by either the intravenous or subcutaneous routes.

Intravenous challenge: Following appropriate screening of the patient, 0.8 mg of naloxone should be drawn into a sterile syringe. If the intravenous route of administration is selected, 0.2 mg of naloxone should be injected, and while the needle is still in the patient's vein, the patient should be observed for 30 seconds for evidence of withdrawal signs or symptoms. If there is no evidence of withdrawal, the remaining 0.6 mg of naloxone should be injected, and the patient observed for an additional period of 20 minutes for signs and symptoms of withdrawal.

Subcutaneous challenge: If the subcutaneous route is selected, 0.8 mg should be administered subcutaneously, and the patient observed for signs and symptoms of withdrawal for 45 minutes.

Conditions and technique for observation of patient: During the appropriate period of observation, the patient's vital signs should be monitored and the patient should be monitored for signs of withdrawal. It is also important to question the patient carefully. The signs and symptoms of opioid withdrawal include, but are not limited to, the following:

Withdrawal Signs: Stuffiness or running nose, tearing, yawning, sweating, tremor, vomiting or piloerection.

Withdrawal Symptoms: feeling of temperature change, joint or bone and muscle pain, abdominal cramps, skin crawling, etc.

Interpretation of the Challenge: Warning: the elicitation of the enumerated signs or symptoms indicates a potential risk for the subject, and Naltrexone Hydrochloride should not be administered. If no signs or symptoms of withdrawal are observed, elicited, or reported, Naltrexone Hydrochloride MAY BE ADMINISTERED. If there is any doubt in the observer's mind that the patient is not in an opioid-free

state, or is in continuing withdrawal, naloxone should be readministered as follows:

Confirmatory rechallenge (if necessary): 1.6 mg of naloxone should be injected intravenously and the patient again observed for signs and symptoms of withdrawal. If none are present, Naltrexone Hydrochloride may be administered. *If signs and symptoms of withdrawal are present, administration of Naltrexone Hydrochloride should be delayed until repeated naloxone challenge indicates the patient is no longer at risk.*

Maintenance Treatment: Once the patient has been started on Naltrexone Hydrochloride 50 mg every 24 hours will produce adequate clinical blockade of the actions of parenterally administered opioids (i.e., this dose will block the effects of a 25 mg intravenous heroin challenge). A flexible approach to a dosing regimen may be employed. Thus, patients may receive 50 mg of Naltrexone Hydrochloride every weekday with a 100 mg dose on Saturday or patients may receive 100 mg every other day, or 150 mg every third day. While the degree of opioid blockade may be somewhat reduced by using higher doses at longer dosing intervals, improved patient compliance may result from dosing every 48–72 hours.

Several of the clinical studies reported in the literature have employed the following dosing regimen: 100 mg on Monday, 100 mg on Wednesday, and 150 mg on Friday. This dosing schedule appeared to be acceptable to many Naltrexone Hydrochloride patients successfully maintaining their opioid free state.

Storage: Protect from excessive light.

HOW SUPPLIED
TABLETS: 50 MG

BRAND/MANUFACTURER	NDC	SIZE	AWP
○ BRAND			
TREXAN: Du Pont Pharma	00056-0080-50	50s	$227.58

Nandrolone

DESCRIPTION

Nandrolone injection is available as a sterile solution of Nandrolone Decanoate, a long-acting anabolic agent, or Nandrolone Phenpropionate, a short-acting anabolic agent, for intramuscular injection. *Each ml contains*: Nandrolone Decanoate 50, 100, or 200 mg or Nandrolone Phenpropionate 25 or 50 mg. Chemically, Nandrolone Decanoate is 17β-hydroxyestr-4-en-3-one 17-decanoate; Nandrolone Phenpropionate is Estr-4-en-3-one, 17(1-oxo-3-phenylpropoxy)-, (17β)-.

Following is its chemical structure:

CLINICAL PHARMACOLOGY

Anabolic steroids are synthetic derivatives of testosterone. Certain clinical effects and adverse reactions demonstrate the androgenic properties of this class of drugs. No dissociation of androgenic and anabolic potency has been demonstrated clinically for any anabolic steroid although there is some suggestion from animal studies that such dissociation may be possible.

The actions of anabolic steroids are therefore similar to those of male sex hormones with the possibility of causing serious disturbances of growth and sexual development if given to young children. Anabolic steroids suppress the gonadotropic functions of the pituitary and may exert a direct effect upon the testes.

During exogenous administration of anabolic androgens, endogenous testosterone release is inhibited through inhibition of pituitary luteinizing hormone (LH). At large doses, spermatogenesis may be suppressed through feedback inhibition of pituitary follicle-stimulating hormone (FSH).

Anabolic steroids increase low-density lipoproteins and decrease high-density lipoproteins. These changes revert to normal on discontinuation of treatment.

INDICATIONS AND USAGE

Nandrolone Decanoate injection is indicated for the management of the anemia of renal insufficiency and has been shown to increase hemoglobin and red cell mass. Surgically induced anephric patients have been reported to be less responsive.

Nandrolone Phenpropionate injection is indicated for the control of metastatic breast cancer in women.

UNLABELED USES

Nondrolone Decanoate is used alone or as an adjunct in the treatment of anemia secondary to bone marrow failure, breast cancer in postmenopausal women, non-small cell lung cancer, and postmenopausal osteoporosis.

CONTRAINDICATIONS

1. Known or suspected carcinoma of the prostate or the male breast.

2. Carcinoma of the breast in females with hypercalcemia (androgenic anabolic steroids may stimulate osteolytic bone resorption).

3. Pregnancy, because of possible masculinization of the female fetus. Androgenic anabolic steroids are known to cause embryotoxicity, fetotoxicity, and masculinization of female animal offspring. Nandrolone injection is contraindicated in women who are or may become pregnant. If this drug is used during pregnancy, or if the patient becomes pregnant while taking this drug, she should be apprised of the potential hazard to the fetus.

4. Nephrosis or the nephrotic phase of nephritis.

WARNINGS

PELIOSIS HEPATIS, A CONDITION IN WHICH LIVER AND SOMETIMES SPLENIC TISSUE IS REPLACED WITH BLOOD-FILLED CYSTS, HAS BEEN REPORTED IN PATIENTS RECEIVING ANDROGENIC ANABOLIC STEROID THERAPY, PARTICULARLY IN THOSE ON PROLONGED TREATMENT WITH 17-ALPHA-ALKYLATED STEROIDS. THESE CYSTS ARE SOMETIMES PRESENT WITH MINIMAL HEPATIC DYSFUNCTION, BUT AT OTHER TIMES THEY HAVE BEEN ASSOCIATED WITH LIVER FAILURE. THEY ARE OFTEN NOT RECOGNIZED UNTIL LIFE-THREATENING LIVER FAILURE OR INTRA-ABDOMINAL HEMORRHAGE DEVELOPS. WITHDRAWAL OF DRUG USUALLY RESULTS IN COMPLETE DISAPPEARANCE OF LESIONS.

LIVER CELL TUMORS ARE ALSO REPORTED. MOST OFTEN THESE TUMORS ARE BENIGN AND ANDROGEN-DEPENDENT, BUT FETAL MALIGNANT TUMORS HAVE BEEN REPORTED. WITHDRAWAL OF DRUG OFTEN RESULTS IN REGRESSION OR CESSATION OF PROGRESSION OF THE TUMOR. HOWEVER, HEPATIC TUMORS ASSOCIATED WITH ANDROGENS OR ANABOLIC STEROIDS ARE MUCH MORE VASCULAR THAN OTHER HEPATIC TUMORS AND MAY BE SILENT UNTIL LIFE-THREATENING INTRA-ABDOMINAL HEMORRHAGE DEVELOPS.

BLOOD LIPID CHANGES THAT ARE KNOWN TO BE ASSOCIATED WITH INCREASED RISK OF ATHEROSCLEROSIS ARE SEEN IN PATIENTS TREATED WITH ANDROGENS AND ANABOLIC STEROIDS. THESE CHANGES INCLUDE DECREASED HIGH-DENSITY LIPOPROTEIN AND SOMETIMES INCREASED LOW-DENSITY LIPOPROTEIN. THE CHANGES MAY BE VERY MARKED AND COULD HAVE SERIOUS IMPACT ON THE RISK OF ATHEROSCLEROSIS AND CORONARY ARTERY DISEASE.

Cholestatic hepatitis and jaundice occur with 17-alpha-alkylated androgens at a relatively low dose. If cholestatic hepatitis with jaundice appears or if liver function tests become abnormal, Nandrolone injection should be discontinued, and the etiology should be determined. Drug-induced jaundice is reversible when the medication is discontinued.

In patients with breast cancer, anabolic steroid therapy may cause hypercalcemia by stimulating osteolysis. Nandrolone therapy should be discontinued if hypercalcemia occurs.

Edema with or without congestive heart failure may be a serious complication in patients with pre-existing cardiac, renal, or hepatic disease. Concomitant administration of adrenal cortical steroid or ACTH may add to the edema.

In children, androgen therapy may accelerate bone maturation without producing compensatory gain in linear growth. This adverse effect results in compromised adult stature. The younger the child, the greater the risk of compromising final mature height. The effect on bone maturation should be monitored by assessing bone age of the wrist and hand every six months.

Geriatric patients treated with androgenic anabolic steroids may be at an increased risk for the development of prostatic hypertrophy and prostatic carcinoma.

THERE IS NO PERSUASIVE EVIDENCE THAT ATHLETIC PERFORMANCE IS IMPROVED BY USING ANABOLIC STEROIDS.

PRECAUTIONS

GENERAL

Women should be observed for signs of virilization (deepening of the voice, hirsutism, acne, clitoromegaly). Such virilization is usual following anabolic steroid use in high doses. Discontinuation of drug therapy at time of evidence of mild virilism is necessary to prevent irreversible virilization. Some virilizing changes (facial hair growth, clitoromegaly, deepening of the voice) in women are irreversible even after prompt discontinuation of therapy and are not prevented by concomitant use of estrogens. Menstrual irregularities may also occur.

Anabolic steroids may cause suppression of clotting factors II, V, VII, and X, and an increase in prothrombin time.

Insulin or oral hypoglycemic dosage may need adjustment in diabetic patients who receive anabolic steroids.

INFORMATION FOR PATIENTS

The physician should instruct patients to report any of the following side effects of androgens:

Adult or Adolescent Males: Too frequent or persistent erections of the penis, appearance of or aggravation of acne.

Females: Hoarseness, acne, changes in menstrual periods, or more facial hair.

All patients: Nausea, vomiting, changes in skin color, or ankle swelling.

LABORATORY TESTS

Women with disseminated breast carcinoma should have frequent determination of urine and serum calcium levels during the course of therapy (see *"Warnings"*).

Because of the hepatotoxicity associated with the use of 17-alpha-alkylated androgens, liver function tests should be obtained periodically.

Periodic (every six months) x-ray examinations of bone age should be made during treatment of prepubertal males and females to determine the rate of bone maturation and the effects of androgen therapy on the epiphyseal centers.

Serum lipids and high-density lipoprotein cholesterol determinations should be done periodically as anabolic androgenic steroids have been reported to increase low-density lipoproteins and decrease high-density lipoproteins. Serum cholesterol levels may increase during therapy. Therefore, caution is required when administering these agents to patients with a history of myocardial infarction or coronary artery disease. Serial determinations of serum cholesterol should be made and therapy adjusted accordingly.

Hemoglobin and hematocrit should be checked periodically for polycythemia in patients who are receiving high doses of anabolic steroids.

DRUG INTERACTIONS

Anticoagulants: Anabolic steroids, in particular 17-alpha-alkylated steroids, may increase sensitivity to oral anticoagulants. Dosage of the anticoagulant may have to be decreased in order to maintain prothrombin time at the desired therapeutic level. Patients receiving oral anticoagulant therapy require close monitoring, especially when anabolic steroids are started or stopped.

Oral Hypoglycemic Agents: Nandrolone Decanoate injection, may inhibit the metabolism of oral hypoglycemic agents.

DRUG/LABORATORY TEST INTERACTIONS

Anabolic steroids may decrease levels of thyroxine-binding globulin, resulting in decreased total T_4 serum levels and increased resin uptake of T_3 and T_4. Free thyroid hormone levels remain unchanged.

Anabolic steroids, in particular 17-alpha-alkylated steroids, may cause an increase in prothrombin time.

CARCINOGENESIS, MUTAGENESIS, IMPAIRMENT OF FERTILITY

Animal Data: Testosterone has been tested by subcutaneous injection and implantation in mice and rats. The implant induced cervical-uterine tumors in mice, which metastasized in some cases. There is suggestive evidence that injection of testosterone into some strains of female mice increases their susceptibility to hepatoma. Testosterone is also known to increase the number of tumors and decrease the degree of differentiation of chemically-induced carcinomas of the liver in rats.

Human Data: There are rare reports of hepatocellular carcinoma in patients receiving long-term therapy with androgens in high doses. Withdrawal of the drugs did not lead to regression of the tumors in all cases.

Geriatric patients treated with androgens may be at an increased risk of developing prostatic hypertrophy and prostatic carcinoma although conclusive evidence to support this concept is lacking.

This compound has not been tested for mutagenic potential. However, as noted above, carcinogenic effects have been attributed to treatment with androgenic hormones. The potential carcinogenic effects likely occur through a hormonal mechanism rather than by a direct chemical interaction mechanism.

Impairment of fertility was not tested directly in animal species. However, oligospermia in males and amenorrhea in females have been seen with several other drugs in this class. Therefore, impairment of fertility is a possible outcome of treatment with Nandrolone injection.

PREGNANCY

Teratogenic Effects: Pregnancy Category X. See *"Contraindications"*.

NURSING MOTHERS

It is not known whether anabolic steroids are excreted in human milk. Many drugs are excreted in human milk and because of the potential for serious adverse reactions in nursing infants from anabolic steroids, a decision should be made whether to discontinue nursing or to discontinue the drug, taking into account the importance of the drug to the mother.

PEDIATRIC USE

Anabolic agents may accelerate epiphyseal maturation more rapidly than linear growth in children, and the effect may continue for six months after the drug has been stopped. Therefore, therapy should be monitored by x-ray studies at six-month intervals in order to avoid the risk of compromising adult height. Anabolic androgenic steroid therapy should be used very cautiously in children and only by specialists who are aware of the effects on bone maturation.

The safety and efficacy of Nandrolone Phenpropionate in children with metastatic breast cancer (rarely found) has not been established. (See *"Warnings"* section.)

ADVERSE REACTIONS

Hepatic: Cholestatic jaundice with, rarely, hepatic necrosis and death. Hepatocellular neoplasms and peliosis hepatitis have been reported in association with long-term use of androgenic anabolic steroids, particularly those that are 17-alpha-alkylated (see *"Warnings"*). Reversible changes in liver function tests also occur including increased bromsulphalein (BSP) retention, and increases in serum bilirubin, glutamic oxaloacetic transaminase (SGOT), and alkaline phosphatase.

Genitourinary System:

In men:
Prepubertal: Phallic enlargement and increased frequency of erections.

Postpubertal: Inhibition of testicular function, testicular atrophy and oligospermia, impotence, chronic priapism, epididymitis and bladder irritability.

In women: Clitoral enlargement, menstrual irregularities.

In both sexes: Increased or decreased libido.

CNS: Habituation, excitation, insomnia, depression.

Gastrointestinal: Nausea, vomiting, diarrhea.

Hematologic: Bleeding in patients on concomitant anticoagulant therapy (see *"Precautions, Drug Interactions"*).

Breast: Gynecomastia.

Larynx: Deepening of the voice in women.

Hair: Hirsutism and male pattern baldness in women.

Skin: Acne (especially in women and prepubertal boys).

Skeletal: Premature closure of epiphyses in children (see *"Precautions, Pediatric Use"*).

Fluid and Electrolytes: Edema, retention of serum electrolytes (sodium chloride, potassium phosphate, calcium).

Metabolic/Endocrine: Decreased glucose tolerance (see *"Precations, Drug Interactions"*), increased serum levels of low-density lipoproteins and decreased levels of high-density lipoproteins (see *"Precautions, Laboratory Tests"*), increased creatine and creatinine excretion, increased serum levels of creatine phosphokinase (CPK). Some virilizing changes in women are irreversible even after prompt discontinuance of therapy and are not prevented by concomitant use of estrogens (see *"Precautions"* section).

DRUG ABUSE AND DEPENDENCE
Controlled Substance Class: Nandrolone is classified as a controlled substance under the Anabolic Steroids Control Act of 1990 and has been assigned to Schedule III.

OVERDOSAGE
There have been no reports of acute overdosage with the anabolics.

DOSAGE AND ADMINISTRATION
Nandrolone injection is intended only for deep intramuscular injection preferably into the gluteal muscle. Dosage should be based on therapeutic response and consideration of the benefit/risk ratio. Duration of therapy will depend on the response of the condition and the appearance of adverse reactions. If possible, therapy should be intermittent.

Nandrolone Decanoate should be regarded as adjunctive therapy and adequate quantities of nutrients should be consumed in order to obtain maximal therapeutic effects. When it is used in the treatment of refractory anemias, for example, adequate iron intake is required for a maximal response.

ANEMIA OF RENAL DISEASE
A dose of 50-100 mg per week Nandrolone Decanoate is recommended for women and 100-200 mg per week for men. Drug therapy should be discontinued if no hematologic improvement is seen within the first six months. When used in the treatment of renal insufficiency, adequate iron intake is required for maximal response. For children from 2 to 13 years of age, the average dose is 25-50 mg every 3 to 4 weeks.

METASTATIC BREAST CANCER
The recommended dosage of Nandrolone Phenpropionate injection in metastatic breast cancer is 50-100 mg/week based on therapeutic response, and consideration of the benefit-to-risk ratio.

Parenteral drug products should be inspected visually for particulate matter and discoloration prior to administration, whenever solution and container permit.

STORAGE
Store at 15°-30°C (59°-86°F). Protect from bright light.

J CODES
Up to 200 mg IM—J2322
Up to 100 mg IM—J2321
Up to 50 mg IM—J2320
Up to 50 mg IM—J0340

HOW SUPPLIED
NANDROLONE DECANOATE
INJECTION (C-III): 50 MG/ML

AVERAGE UNIT PRICE (AVAILABLE SIZES)		GENERIC A-RATED AVERAGE PRICE (GAAP)	
BRAND	$5.89	2 ml	$8.65
GENERIC	$3.86		

BRAND/MANUFACTURER	NDC	SIZE	AWP
◆ BRAND			
DECA-DURABOLIN: Organon	00052-0696-02	2 ml	$11.77

BRAND/MANUFACTURER	NDC	SIZE	AWP
◆ GENERICS			
Steris	00402-0407-02	2 ml	$4.95
HYBOLIN DECANOATE: Hyrex	00314-3520-02	2 ml	$9.90
Goldline	00182-1142-61	2 ml	$11.10
Schein	00364-6716-47	2 ml 10s	$49.50

INJECTION (C-III): 100 MG/ML

AVERAGE UNIT PRICE (AVAILABLE SIZES)		GENERIC A-RATED AVERAGE PRICE (GAAP)	
BRAND	$9.77	2 ml	$11.22
GENERIC	$5.16		

BRAND/MANUFACTURER	NDC	SIZE	AWP
◆ BRAND			
DECA-DURABOLIN: Organon	00052-0697-02	2 ml	$20.14
	00052-0697-71	1 ml 25s	$236.84
◆ GENERICS			
Steris	00402-0432-02	2 ml	$4.95
Major	00904-1196-98	2 ml	$7.50
URL	00677-0798-19	2 ml	$11.98
Goldline	00182-1143-61	2 ml	$12.00
HYBOLIN DECANOATE: Hyrex	00314-3525-02	2 ml	$12.90
Rugby	00536-5411-67	2 ml	$18.00
Schein	00364-6717-47	2 ml 10s	$49.50

INJECTION (C-III): 200 MG/ML

AVERAGE UNIT PRICE (AVAILABLE SIZES)	
BRAND	$16.88
GENERIC	$4.33

BRAND/MANUFACTURER	NDC	SIZE	AWP
◆ BRAND			
DECA-DURABOLIN: Organon	00052-0698-01	1 ml	$19.30
	00052-0698-25	1 ml 25s	$382.58
	00052-0698-71	1 ml 25s	$400.75
◆ GENERICS			
Steris	00402-0710-01	1 ml	$4.33
Schein	00364-2186-46	1 ml 25s	$108.38

NANDROLONE PHENPROPIONATE
INJECTION (C-III): 25 MG/ML

BRAND/MANUFACTURER	NDC	SIZE	AWP
◆ BRAND			
DURABOLIN: Organon	00052-0691-05	5 ml	$16.26
◆ GENERICS			
Major	00904-1207-05	5 ml	$5.00

INJECTION (C-III): 50 MG/ML

AVERAGE UNIT PRICE (AVAILABLE SIZES)		GENERIC A-RATED AVERAGE PRICE (GAAP)	
BRAND	$7.08	2 ml	$6.70
GENERIC	$2.67		

BRAND/MANUFACTURER	NDC	SIZE	AWP
◆ BRAND			
DURABOLIN-50: Organon	00052-0695-02	2 ml	$14.15
◆ GENERICS			
Major	00904-1206-98	2 ml	$4.90
HYBOLIN-IMPROVED: Hyrex	00314-3501-02	2 ml	$8.50
Major	00904-1206-05	5 ml	$6.55

Naphazoline Hydrochloride

DESCRIPTION
Naphazoline Hydrochloride, an ocular vasoconstrictor, is an imidazoline derivative sympathomimetic amine.

The chemical name is 2-(1-naphthylmethyl)-2-imidazoline monohydrochloride. The empirical formula is $C_{14}H_{14}N_2 \cdot HCl$.

Naphazoline Hydrochloride ophthalmic solution is a sterile solution containing 1 mg/mL Naphazoline Hydrochloride in an isotonic solution.

Following is its chemical structure:

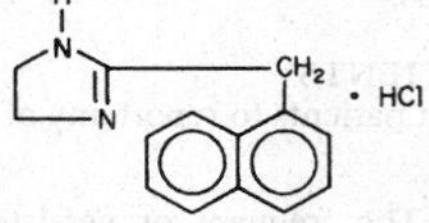

CLINICAL PHARMACOLOGY
Naphazoline constricts the vascular system of the conjunctiva. It is presumed that this effect is due to direct stimulation action of the drug upon the alpha adrenergic

---

◆ RATED THERAPEUTICALLY EQUIVALENT; ◇ THERAPEUTIC EQUIVALENCE UNCONFIRMED; ○ UNRATED

receptors in the arterioles of the conjunctiva resulting in decreased conjunctival congestion. Naphazoline belongs to the imidazoline class of sympathomimetics.

INDICATIONS AND USAGE:
Naphazoline HCl is indicated for use as a topical ocular vasoconstrictor.

CONTRAINDICATIONS:
Contraindicated in the presence of an anatomically narrow angle or in narrow angle glaucoma or in persons who have shown hypersensitivity to any component of this preparation.

WARNINGS
Patients under therapy with MAO inhibitors may experience a severe hypertensive crisis if given a sympathomimetic drug. Use in children, especially infants, may result in CNS depression leading to coma and marked reduction in body temperature.

PRECAUTIONS
General: Use with caution in the presence of hypertension, cardiovascular abnormalities, hyperglycemia (diabetes), hyperthyroidism, ocular infection or injury and when other medications are being used.

Patient Information: Patients should be advised to discontinue the drug and consult a physician if relief is not obtained within 48 hours of therapy, if irritation, blurring, or redness persists or increases, or if symptoms of systemic absorption occur, i.e., dizziness, headache, nausea, decrease in body temperature, or drowsiness.

To prevent contaminating the dropper tip and solution, do not touch the eyelids or the surrounding area with the dropper tip of the bottle. If solution changes color or becomes cloudy, do not use.

Drug Interactions: Concurrent use of maprotiline or tricyclic antidepressants and Naphazoline may potentiate the pressor effect of Naphazoline. Patients under therapy with MAO inhibitors may experience a severe hypertensive crisis if given a sympathomimetic drug. (See *"Warnings"*.)

Pregnancy Category C: Animal reproduction studies have not been conducted with Naphazoline. It is also not known whether Naphazoline can cause fetal harm when administered to a pregnant woman or can affect reproduction capacity. Naphazoline should be given to a pregnant woman only if clearly needed.

Nursing Mothers: It is not known whether Naphazoline is excreted in human milk. Because many drugs are excreted in human milk, caution should be exercised when Naphazoline is administered to a nursing woman.

Pediatric Use: Safety and effectiveness in children have not been established. See *"Warnings"* and *"Contraindications"*.

ADVERSE REACTIONS
Ocular: Mydriasis, increased redness, irritation, discomfort, blurring, punctate keratitis, lacrimation, increased intraocular pressure.

Systemic: Dizziness, headache, nausea, sweating, nervousness, drowsiness, weakness, hypertension, cardiac irregularities, and hyperglycemia.

DOSAGE AND ADMINISTRATION
Instill one or two drops in the conjunctival sac(s) every three to four hours as needed.
Store at controlled room temperature, 15°-30°C (59°-86°F).

HOW SUPPLIED
DROP: 0.1%

AVERAGE UNIT PRICE (AVAILABLE SIZES)		GENERIC A-RATED AVERAGE PRICE (GAAP)	
BRAND	$0.90	15 ml	$5.58
GENERIC	$0.37		

BRAND/MANUFACTURER	NDC	SIZE	AWP
◆ **BRAND**			
ALBALON: Allergan Pharm	11980-0154-15	15 ml	$13.16
VASOCON: Iolab	00058-2884-15	15 ml	$13.32
NAPHCON FORTE: Alcon Ophthalmic	00998-0079-15	15 ml	$14.00
◆ **GENERICS**			
Logen	00820-0112-25	15 ml	$2.25
NAFAZAIR: Genetco	00302-3114-15	15 ml	$4.65
AK-CON: Akorn	17478-0216-12	15 ml	$4.88
Aligen	00405-6081-15	15 ml	$5.19
Schein	00364-7421-72	15 ml	$5.35
Qualitest	00603-7178-41	15 ml	$5.49
Bausch&Lomb Pharm	24208-0725-06	15 ml	$5.65
Parmed	00349-8641-85	15 ml	$5.99
Moore,H.L.	00839-6692-31	15 ml	$6.06
Goldline	00182-7032-64	15 ml	$6.30
Rugby	00536-1702-72	15 ml	$6.36
Major	00904-1906-35	15 ml	$6.40
MURO'S OPCON: Bausch&Lomb Pharm	00303-9910-15	15 ml	$8.00

Naphazoline Hydrochloride and Pheniramine Maleate

DESCRIPTION
Naphazoline Hydrochloride/Pheniramine Maleate is a combination of an antihistamine and a decongestant prepared as a sterile topical ophthalmic solution.
Established name: Naphazoline Hydrochloride
Chemical name: 1*H*-Imidazole, 4,5-dihydro- 2-(1-naphthalenylmethyl)-, monohydrochloride.
Established name: Pheniramine Maleate
Chemical name: *N,N*-Dimethyl-y-phenyl-2-pyridine-propanamine, (Z)-Butenedioic acid.

CLINICAL PHARMACOLOGY
Naphazoline Hydrochloride/Pheniramine Maleate combines the effects of the antihistamine, Pheniramine Maleate, and the decongestant, Naphazoline.

INDICATIONS AND USAGE

BASED ON A REVIEW OF A RELATED COMBINATION OF DRUGS BY THE NATIONAL ACADEMY OF SCIENCES—NATIONAL RESEARCH COUNCIL AND/OR OTHER INFORMATION. FDA HAS CLASSIFIED THE INDICATIONS AS FOLLOWS: "POSSIBLY" EFFECTIVE: FOR RELIEF OF OCULAR IRRITATION AND/OR CONGESTION OR FOR THE TREATMENT OF ALLERGIC OR INFLAMMATORY OCULAR CONDITIONS. FINAL CLASSIFICATION OF THE LESS-THAN-EFFECTIVE INDICATION REQUIRES FURTHER INVESTIGATION.

CONTRAINDICATIONS
Hypersensitivity to one or more of the components of this preparation.
Do not use in the presence of narrow angle glaucoma or in patients predisposed to narrow angle glaucoma.

WARNINGS
Patients under MAO inhibitors may experience a severe hypertensive crisis if given a sympathomimetic drug such as Naphazoline Hydrochloride. Use in infants and children may result in CNS depression leading to coma and marked reduction in body temperature.

PRECAUTIONS
GENERAL
For topical eye use only—not for injection. This preparation should be used with caution in patients with severe cardiovascular disease including cardiac arrhythmias, patients with poorly controlled hypertension, patients with diabetes, especially those with a tendency toward diabetic ketoacidosis.

Information For Patients: To prevent contaminating the dropper tip and solution, care should be taken not to touch the eyelids or surrounding area with the dropper tip of the bottle.

Carcinogenesis, Mutagenesis, Impairment of Fertility: There have been no long-term studies done using Naphazoline Hydrochloride and/or Pheniramine Maleate in animals to evaluate carcinogenic potential.

Pregnancy: Pregnancy Category C. Animal reproduction studies have not been conducted with Naphazoline Hydrochloride and/or Pheniramine Maleate. It is also not known whether Naphazolien Hydrochloride and/or Pheniramine Maleate can cause fetal harm when administered to a pregnant woman or can affect reproduction capacity. Naphazoline Hydrochloride/Pheniramine Ophthalmic Solution should be given to a pregnant woman only if clearly needed.

Nursing Mothers: It is not known whether these drugs are excreted in human milk. Because many drugs are excreted in human milk, caution should be exercised when Naphazoline Hydrochloride/Pheniramine Ophthalmic Solution is administered to a nursing woman.

ADVERSE REACTIONS
The following adverse reactions may occur. Pupillary dilation, increase in intraocular pressure, systemic effects due to absorption (i.e., hypertension, cardiac irregularities, hyperglycemia). Drowsiness may be experienced by some patients.

DOSAGE AND ADMINISTRATION
One or two drops instilled in each eye every 3 to 4 hours or less frequently, as required to relieve symptoms.
Store at 2°-27°C (36°-80°F). Keep bottle tightly closed when not in use. Protect from light and excessive heat.

HOW SUPPLIED
DROP: 0.025%-0.3%

AVERAGE UNIT PRICE (AVAILABLE SIZES)		GENERIC A-RATED AVERAGE PRICE (GAAP)	
GENERIC	$0.41	15 ml	$6.11

BRAND/MANUFACTURER	NDC	SIZE	AWP
◆ **GENERICS**			
ALLERSOL: Ocusoft	54799-0860-15	15 ml	$5.30
Parmed	00349-8642-85	15 ml	$5.99
ALLERSOL-A: Ocusoft	54799-0863-15	15 ml	$7.05

➤ SHOWN IN PRODUCT IDENTIFICATION GUIDE

DROP: 0.025%-0.3%

BRAND/MANUFACTURER	NDC	SIZE	AWP
○ **BRAND**			
NAPHCON-A: Alcon Ophthalmic	00998-0080-15	15 ml	$14.00

Naphcon *SEE* NAPHAZOLINE HYDROCHLORIDE *AND* NAPHAZOLINE HYDROCHLORIDE AND PHENIRAMINE MALEATE

Naprosyn *SEE* NAPROXEN

Naproxen

DESCRIPTION

Naproxen tablets for oral administration each contain 250 mg, 375 mg or 500 mg of naproxen. Naproxen suspension for oral administration contains 125 mg/5 mL of Naproxen. Naproxen is a member of the arylacetic acid group of nonsteroidal anti-inflammatory drugs.

The chemical name for Naproxen is 2-naphthaleneacetic acid, 6-methoxy-α-methyl-,(+).

Naproxen is an odorless, white to off-white crystalline substance. It is lipid soluble, practically insoluble in water at low pH and freely soluble in water at high pH.

Naproxen Sodium tablets for oral administration each contain 275 mg of Naproxen Sodium, which is equivalent to 250 mg Naproxen with 25 mg (about 1 mEq) Sodium. Naproxen Sodium tablets for oral administration each contain 550 mg of Naproxen Sodium, which is equivalent to 500 mg Naproxen with 50 mg (about 2 mEq) Sodium. Naproxen Sodium is a member of the arylacetic acid group of nonsteroidal anti-inflammatory drugs.

The chemical name of Naproxen Sodium is 2-naphthaleneacetic acid, 6-methoxy-α-methyl-, sodium salt, (—)-.

Naproxen Sodium is a white to creamy white, crystalline solid, freely soluble in water.

Naproxen suspension for oral administration contains 125 mg/5 mL of Naproxen.

Following is its chemical structure:

CLINICAL PHARMACOLOGY

Naproxen is a nonsteroidal anti-inflammatory drug with analgesic and antipyretic properties. Naproxen Sodium, the sodium salt of Naproxen, has been developed as an analgesic because it is more rapidly absorbed. The Naproxen anion inhibits prostaglandin synthesis but beyond this its mode of action is unknown.

Naproxen is rapidly and completely absorbed from the gastrointestinal tract. After administration of Naproxen, peak plasma levels of Naproxen anion are attained in 2 to 4 hours (1 to 2 hours for Naproxen Sodium), with steady-state conditions normally achieved after 4-5 doses. The mean biological half-life of the anion in humans is approximately 13 hours, and at therapeutic levels it is greater than 99% albumin bound. At doses of Naproxen greater than 500 mg/day there is a lack of dose proportionality due to an increase in clearance caused by saturation of proteins at higher doses. Approximately 95% of the dose is excreted in the urine, primarily as Naproxen, 6-0-desmethyl Naproxen or their conjugates. The rate of excretion has been found to coincide closely with the rate of drug disappearance from the plasma. The drug does not induce metabolizing enzymes.

In children of 5 to 16 years of age with arthritis, plasma Naproxen levels following a 5 mg/kg single dose of suspension were found to be similar to those found in normal adults following a 500 mg dose. The terminal half-life appears to be similar in children and adults. Pharmacokinetic studies of Naproxen were not performed in children of less than 5 years of age.

The drug was studied in patients with rheumatoid arthritis, osteoarthritis, juvenile arthritis, ankylosing spondylitis, tendinitis and bursitis, and acute gout. It is not a corticosteroid. Improvement in patients treated for rheumatoid arthritis has been demonstrated by a reduction in joint swelling, a reduction in pain, a reduction in duration of morning stiffness, a reduction in disease activity as assessed by both the investigator and patient, and by increased mobility as demonstrated by a reduction in walking time.

In patients with osteoarthritis, the therapeutic action of the drug has been shown by a reduction in joint pain or tenderness, an increase in range of motion in knee joints, increased mobility as demonstrated by a reduction in walking time, and improvement in capacity to perform activities of daily living impaired by the disease.

In clinical studies in patients with rheumatoid arthritis, osteoarthritis, and juvenile arthritis, the drug has been shown to be comparable to aspirin and indomethacin in controlling the aforementioned measures of disease activity, but the frequency and severity of the milder gastrointestinal adverse effects (nausea, dyspepsia, heartburn) and nervous system adverse effects (tinnitus, dizziness, light-headedness) were less than in both the aspirin- and indomethacin-treated patients. It is not known whether the drug causes less peptic ulceration than aspirin.

In patients with ankylosing spondylitis, the drug has been shown to decrease night pain, morning stiffness and pain at rest. In double-blind studies the drug was shown to be as effective as aspirin, but with fewer side effects.

In patients with acute gout, a favorable response to the drug was shown by significant clearing of inflammatory changes (e.g., decrease in swelling, heat) within 24-48 hours, as well as by relief of pain and tenderness.

The drug may be used safely in combination with gold salts and/or corticosteroids; however, in controlled clinical trials, when added to the regimen of patients receiving corticosteroids it did not appear to cause greater improvement over that seen with corticosteroids alone. Whether the drug could be used in conjunction with partially effective doses of corticosteroid for a "steroid-sparing" effect has not been adequately studied. When added to the regimen of patients receiving gold salts the drug did result in greater improvement. Its use in combination with salicylates is not recommended because data are inadequate to demonstrate that the drug produces greater improvement over that achieved with aspirin alone. Further, there is some evidence that aspirin increases the rate of excretion of the drug.

Generally, improvement due to the drug has not been found to be dependent on age, sex, severity or duration of disease.

In clinical trials in patients with osteoarthritis and rheumatoid arthritis comparing treatments of 750 mg per day (825 mg for Naproxen Sodium) with 1,500 mg per day (1,650 mg for Naproxen Sodium), there were trends toward increased efficacy with the higher dose and a more clearcut increase in adverse reactions, particularly gastrointestinal reactions severe enough to cause the patient to leave the trial, which approximately doubled.

The drug was studied in patients with mild to moderate pain, and pain relief was obtained within 1 hour. It is not a narcotic and is not a CNS-acting drug. Controlled double-blind studies have demonstrated the analgesic properties of the drug in, for example, postoperative, postpartum, orthopedic and uterine contraction pain and dysmenorrhea. In dysmenorrheic patients, the drug reduces the level of prostaglandins in the uterus, which correlates with a reduction in the frequency and severity of uterine contractions. Analgesic action has been shown by such measures as a reduction of pain intensity scores, increase in pain relief scores, decrease in numbers of patients requiring additional analgesic medication, and delay in time for required remedication. The analgesic effect has been found to last for up to 7 hours.

In ^{51}Cr blood loss and gastroscopy studies with normal volunteers, daily administration of 1,000 mg of Naproxen or 1,100 mg of Naproxen Sodium the drug has been demonstrated to cause statistically significantly less gastric bleeding and erosion than 3,250 mg of aspirin.

INDICATIONS AND USAGE

Naproxen is indicated for the treatment of rheumatoid arthritis, osteoarthritis, juvenile arthritis, ankylosing spondylitis, tendinitis and bursitis, and acute gout. It is also indicated in the relief of mild to moderate pain and for the treatment of primary dysmenorrhea.

UNLABELED USES

Naproxen is used alone or as an adjunct in the treatment and prevention of migraine.

CONTRAINDICATIONS

The drug is contraindicated in patients who have had allergic reactions to Naproxen or Naproxen Sodium. It is also contraindicated in patients in whom aspirin or other nonsteroidal anti-inflammatory/analgesic drugs induce the syndrome of asthma, rhinitis, and nasal polyps. Both types of reactions have the potential of being fatal. Anaphylactoid reactions to Naproxen Sodium or Naproxen, whether of the true allergic type or the pharmacologic idiosyneratic (e.g., aspirin syndrome) type, usually but not always occur in patients with a known history of such reactions. Therefore, careful questioning of patients for such things as asthma, nasal polyps, urticaria, and hypotension associated with nonsteroidal anti-inflammatory drugs before starting therapy is important. In addition, if such symptoms occur during therapy, treatment should be discontinued.

WARNINGS

Risk of GI Ulceration, Bleeding and Perforation with NSAID Therapy: Serious gastrointestinal toxicity such as bleeding, ulceration, and perforation, can occur at any time, with or without warning symptoms, in patients treated chronically with NSAID therapy. Although minor upper gastrointestinal problems, such as dyspepsia, are common, usually developing early in therapy, physicians should remain alert for ulceration and bleeding in patients treated chronically with NSAIDs even in the absence of previous GI tract symptoms. In patients observed in clinical trials of several months to two years duration, symptomatic upper GI ulcers, gross bleeding or perforation appear to occur in approximately 1% of patients treated for 3-6 months, and in about 2-4% of patients treated for one year. Physicians should inform patients about the signs and/or symptoms of serious GI toxicity and what steps to take if they occur.

Studies to date have not identified any subset of patients not at risk of developing peptic ulceration and bleeding. Except for a prior history of serious GI events and other risk factors known to be associated with peptic ulcer disease, such as alcoholism, smoking, etc., no risk factors (e.g., age, sex) have been associated with increased risk. Elderly or debilitated patients seem to tolerate ulceration or bleeding less well than other individuals and most spontaneous

---

reports of fatal GI events are in this population. Studies to date are inconclusive concerning the relative risk of various NSAIDs in causing such reactions. High doses of any NSAID probably carry a greater risk of these reactions, although controlled clinical trials showing this do not exist in most cases. In considering the use of relatively large doses (within the recommended dosage range), sufficient benefit should be anticipated to offset the potential increased risk of GI toxicity.

PRECAUTIONS
GENERAL
SHOULD NOT BE USED CONCOMITANTLY WITH THE RELATED DRUG NAPROXEN SODIUM SINCE THEY BOTH CIRCULATE IN PLASMA AS THE NAPROXEN ANION.

Renal Effects: As with other nonsteroidal anti-inflammatory drugs, long-term administration of Naproxen to animals has resulted in renal papillary necrosis and other abnormal renal pathology. In humans, there have been reports of acute interstitial nephritis with hematuria, proteinuria, and occasionally nephrotic syndrome.

A second form of renal toxicity has been seen in patients with prerenal conditions leading to a reduction in renal blood flow or blood volume, where the renal prostaglandins have a supportive role in the maintenance of renal perfusion. In these patients, administration of a nonsteroidal anti-inflammatory drug may cause a dose-dependent reduction in prostaglandin formation and may precipitate overt renal decompensation. Patients at greatest risk of this reaction are those with impaired renal function, heart failure, liver dysfunction, those taking diuretics, and the elderly. Discontinuation of nonsteroidal anti-inflammatory therapy is typically followed by recovery to the pretreatment state.

Naproxen and its metabolites are eliminated primarily by the kidneys, therefore the drug should be used with great caution in patients with significantly impaired renal function and the monitoring of serum creatinine and/or creatinine clearance is advised in these patients. Caution should be used if the drug is given to patients with creatinine clearance of less than 20 mL/minute because accumulation of Naproxen metabolites has been seen in such patients.

Chronic alcoholic liver disease and probably other forms of cirrhosis reduce the total plasma concentration of Naproxen, but the plasma concentration of unbound Naproxen is increased. Caution is advised when high doses are required and some adjustment of dosage may be required in these patients. It is prudent to use the lowest effective dose.

Studies indicate that although total plasma concentration of Naproxen is unchanged, the unbound plasma fraction of Naproxen is increased in the elderly. Caution is advised when high doses are required and some adjustment of dosage may be required in elderly patients. As with other drugs used in the elderly, it is prudent to use the lowest effective dose.

As with other nonsteroidal anti-inflammatory drugs, borderline elevations of one or more liver tests may occur in up to 15% of patients. These abnormalities may progress, may remain essentially unchanged, or may be transient with continued therapy. The SGPT (ALT) test is probably the most sensitive indicator of liver dysfunction. Meaningful (3 times the upper limit of normal) elevations of SGPT or SGOT (AST) occurred in controlled clinical trials in less than 1% of patients. A patient with symptoms and/or signs suggesting liver dysfunction, or in whom an abnormal liver test has occurred, should be evaluated for evidence of the development of more severe hepatic reaction while on therapy with this drug. Severe hepatic reactions, including jaundice and cases of fetal hepatitis, have been reported with this drug as with other nonsteroidal anti-inflammatory drugs. Although such reactions are rare, if abnormal liver tests persist or worsen, if clinical signs and symptoms consistent with liver disease develop, or if systemic manifestations occur (e.g. eosinophilia, rash, etc.), this drug should be discontinued.

If steroid dosage is reduced or eliminated during therapy, the steroid dosage should be reduced slowly and the patients must be observed closely for any evidence of adverse effects, including adrenal insufficiency and exacerbation of symptoms of arthritis.

Patients with initial hemoglobin values of 10 grams or less who are to receive long-term therapy should have hemoglobin values determined periodically.

Peripheral edema has been observed in some patients. Since each Naproxen Sodium tablet contains approximately 25 mg or 50 mg (about 1 or 2 mEq) of Sodium, and Naproxen Suspension contains 8 mg/mL of sodium, this should be considered in patients whose overall intake of sodium must be markedly restricted. For these reasons, the drug should be used with caution in patients with fluid retention, hypertension or heart failure.

The antipyretic and anti-inflammatory activities of the drug may reduce fever and inflammation, thus diminishing its utility as diagnostic signs in detecting complications of presumed non-infectious, non-inflammatory painful conditions.

Because of adverse eye findings in animal studies with drugs of this class, it is recommended that ophthalmic studies be carried out if any change or disturbance in vision occurs.

INFORMATION FOR PATIENTS
Naproxen, like other drugs of its class, is not free of side effects. The side effects of these drugs can cause discomfort and, rarely, there are more serious side effects, such as gastrointestinal bleeding, which may result in hospitalization and even fatal outcomes.

NSAIDs (Nonsteroidal Anti-Inflammatory Drugs) are often essential agents in the management of arthritis and have a major role in the treatment of pain, but they also may be commonly employed for conditions which are less serious. Physicians may wish to discuss with their patients the potential risks (see *"Warnings"*, *"Precautions"*, and *"Adverse Reactions"* sections) and likely benefits of NSAID treatment, particularly when the drugs are used for less serious conditions where treatment without NSAIDs may represent an acceptable alternative to both the patients and physician.

Caution should be exercised by patients whose activities require alertness if they experience drowsiness, dizziness, vertigo or depression during therapy with the drug.

LABORATORY TESTS
Because serious GI tract ulceration and bleeding can occur without warning symptoms, physicians should follow chronically treated patients for the signs and symptoms of ulceration and bleeding and should inform them of the importance of this follow-up (see *"Risk of GI Ulcerations, Bleeding and Perforation with NSAID Therapy"*).

DRUG INTERACTIONS
In vitro studies have shown that Naproxen anion, because of its affinity for protein, may displace from their binding sites other drugs which are also albumin-bound. Theoretically, the Naproxen anion itself could likewise be displaced. Short-term controlled studies failed to show that taking the drug significantly affects prothrombin times when administered to individuals on coumarin-type anticoagulants. Caution is advised nonetheless, since interactions have been seen with other nonsteroidal agents of this class. Similarly, patients receiving the drug and a hydantoin, sulfonamide or sulfonylurea should be observed for signs of toxicity to these drugs. The natriuretic effect of furosemide has been reported to be inhibited by some drugs of this class. Inhibition of renal lithium clearance leading to increases in plasma lithium concentrations has also been reported.

This and other nonsteroidal anti-inflammatory drugs can reduce the antihypertensive effect of propranolol and other beta-blockers.

Probenecid given concurrently increases Naproxen anion plasma levels and extends its plasma half-life significantly.

Caution should be used if this drug is administered concomitantly with methotrexate. Naproxen and other nonsteroidal anti-inflammatory drugs have been reported to reduce the tubular secretion of methotrexate in an animal model, possibly enhancing the toxicity of that drug.

DRUG/LABORATORY TEST INTERACTIONS
The drug may decrease platelet aggregation and prolong bleeding time. This effect should be kept in mind when bleeding times are determined.

The administration of the drug may result in increased urinary values for 17-ketogenic steroids because of an interaction between the drug and/or its metabolites with m-dinitrobenzene used in this assay. Although 17-hydroxy-corticosteroid measurements (Porter-Silber test) do not appear to be artifactually altered, it is suggested that therapy with the drug be temporarily discontinued 72 hours before adrenal function tests are performed.

The drug may interfere with some urinary assays of 5-hydroxy indoleacetic acid (5HIAA).

CARCINOGENESIS
A two-year study was performed in rats to evaluate the carcinogenic potential of the drug. No evidence of carcinogenicity was found.

PREGNANCY
Teratogenic Effects: Pregnancy Category B: Reproduction studies have been performed in rats, rabbits and mice at doses up to six times the human dose and have revealed no evidence of impaired fertility or harm to the fetus due to the drug. There are, however, no adequate and well-controlled studies in pregnant women. Because animal reproduction studies are not always predictive of human response, the drug should not be used during pregnancy unless clearly needed. Because of the known effect of drugs of this class on the human fetal cardiovascular system (closure of ductus arteriosus), use during late pregnancy should be avoided.

Non-teratogenic Effects: As with other drugs known to inhibit prostaglandin synthesis, an increased incidence of dystocia and delayed parturition occurred in rats.

NURSING MOTHERS
The Naproxen anion has been found in the milk of lactating women at a concentration of approximately 1% of that found in the plasma. Because of the possible adverse effects of prostaglandin-inhibiting drugs on neonates, use in nursing mothers should be avoided.

PEDIATRIC USE
Safety and effectiveness in children below the age of 2 years have not been established. Pediatric dosing recommendations for juvenile arthritis are based on well-controlled studies (see *"Dosage and Administration"*). There are no adequate effectiveness or dose-response data for other pediatric conditions, but the experience in juvenile arthritis and other use experience have established that single doses of 2.5-5 mg/kg (as Naproxen Suspension; see *"Dosage and Administration"*), with total daily dose not exceeding 15 mg/kg/day, are safe in children over 2 years of age.

ADVERSE REACTIONS
The following adverse reactions are divided into 3 parts based on frequency and likelihood of causal relationship to Naproxen.

INCIDENCE GREATER THAN 1%
Probable Causal Relationship: Adverse reactions reported in controlled clinical trials in 960 patients treated for rheumatoid arthritis or osteoarthritis are listed below. In general, these reactions were reported 2 to 10 times more frequently

than they were in studies in the 962 patients treated for mild to moderate pain or for dysmenorrhea.

A clinical study found gastrointestinal reactions to be more frequent and more severe in rheumatoid arthritis patients taking 1,500 mg Naproxen or 1,650 mg Naproxen Sodium daily compared to those taking 750 mg Naproxen or 825 mg Naproxen Sodium daily (see *"Clinical Pharmacology"*).

In controlled clinical trials with about 80 children and in well-monitored open studies with about 400 children with juvenile arthritis, the incidences of rash and prolonged bleeding times were increased, the incidences of gastrointestinal and central nervous system reactions were about the same, and the incidences of other reactions were lower in children than in adults.

Gastrointestinal: The most frequent complaints reported related to the gastrointestinal tract. They were: constipation*, heartburn*, abdominal pain*, nausea*, dyspepsia, diarrhea, stomatitis.

Central Nervous System: Headache*, dizziness*, drowsiness*, lightheadedness, vertigo.

Dermatologic: Itching (pruritus)*, skin eruptions*, ecchymoses*, sweating, purpura.

Special Senses: Tinnitus*, hearing disturbances, visual disturbances.

Cardiovascular: Edema*, dyspnea*, palpitations.

General: Thirst.

INCIDENCE LESS THAN 1%
Probable Causal Relationship: The following adverse reactions were reported less frequently than 1% during controlled clinical trials and through voluntary reports since marketing. The probability of a causal relationship exists between the drug and these adverse reactions.

Gastrointestinal: Abnormal liver function tests, colitis, gastrointestinal bleeding and/or perforation, hematemesis, jaundice, melena, peptic ulceration with bleeding and/or perforation, vomiting.

Renal: Glomerular nephritis, hematuria, hyperkalemia, interstitial nephritis, nephrotic syndrome, renal disease, renal failure, renal papillary necrosis.

Hematologic: Agranulocytosis, eosinophilia, granulocytopenia, leukopenia, thrombocytopenia.

Central Nervous System: Depression, dream abnormalities, inability to concentrate, insomnia, malaise, myalgia and muscle weakness.

Dermatologic: Alopecia, photosensitive dermatitis, skin rashes.

Special Senses: Hearing impairment.

Cardiovascular: Congestive heart failure.

Respiratory: Eosinophilic pneumonitis.

General: Anaphylactoid reactions, menstrual disorders, pyrexia (chills and fever).

CAUSAL RELATIONSHIP UNKNOWN
Other reactions have been reported in circumstances in which a causal relationship could not be established. However, in these rarely reported events, the possibility cannot be excluded. Therefore, these observations are being listed to serve as alerting information to the physicians:

Hematologic: Aplastic anemia, hemolytic anemia.

Central Nervous System: Aseptic meningitis, cognitive dysfunction.

Dermatologic: Epidermal necrolysis, erythema multiforme, photosensitivity reactions resembling porphyria cutanea tarda and epidermolysis bullosa, Stevens-Johnson syndrome, urticaria.

Gastrointestinal: Non-peptic gastrointestinal ulceration, ulcerative stomatitis.

Cardiovascular: Vasculitis.

General: Angioneurotic edema, hyperglycemia, hypoglycemia.

OVERDOSAGE
Significant overdosage may be characterized by drowsiness, heartburn, indigestion, nausea or vomiting. Because Naproxen Sodium may be rapidly absorbed, high and early blood levels should be anticipated. A few patients have experienced seizures, but it is not clear whether or not these were drug related. It is not known what dose of the drug would be life threatening. The oral LD$_{50}$ of the drug is 543 mg/kg in rats, 1,234 mg/kg in mice, 4,110 mg/kg in hamsters and greater than 1,000 mg/kg in dogs.

Should a patient ingest a large number of tablets or a large volume of suspension, accidentally or purposefully, the stomach may be emptied and usual supportive measures employed. In animals 0.5 g/kg of activated charcoal was effective in reducing plasma levels of Naproxen. Hemodialysis does not decrease the plasma concentration of Naproxen because of the high degree of its protein binding.

DOSAGE AND ADMINISTRATION
NAPROXEN
A measuring cup marked in ½ teaspoon and 2.5 milliliter increments is provided with the suspension. This cup or a teaspoon may be used to measure the appropriate dose.

* Incidence of reported reactions between 3% and 9%. Those reactions occurring in less than 3% of the patients are unmarked.

FOR RHEUMATOID ARTHRITIS, OSTEOARTHRITIS, AND ANKYLOSING SPONDYLITIS
The recommended dose of Naproxen in adults is 250 mg (10 mL or 2 tsp of suspension), 375 mg (15 mL or 3 tsp), or 500 mg (20 mL or 4 tsp) twice daily (morning and evening). During long-term administration, the dose may be adjusted up or down depending on the clinical response of the patient. A lower daily dose may suffice for long-term administration. The morning and evening doses do not have to be equal in size and the administration of the drug more frequently than twice daily is not necessary. In patients who tolerate lower doses well, the dose may be increased to 1,500 mg per day for limited periods when a higher level of anti-inflammatory/analgesic activity is required. When treating such patients with the 1,500 mg/day dose, the physician should observe sufficient increased clinical benefits to offset the potential increased risk (see *"Clinical Pharmacology"*).

Symptomatic improvement in arthritis usually begins within 2 weeks. However, if improvement is not seen within this period, a trial for an additional 2 weeks should be considered.

FOR JUVENILE ARTHRITIS
The recommended total daily dose of Naproxen is approximately 10 mg/kg given in 2 divided doses. One half of the 250 mg tablet may be used to approximate this dose. The following table may be used as a guide for the suspension:

Child's Weight	Dose
13 kg (29 lb)	2.5 mL (½ tsp) b.i.d.
25 kg (55 lb)	5 mL (1 tsp) b.i.d.
38 kg (84 lb)	7.5 mL (1½ tsp) b.i.d.

FOR ACUTE GOUT
The recommended starting dose of Naproxen is 750 mg (30 mL or 6 tsp), followed by 250 mg (10 mL or 2 tsp) every 8 hours until the attack has subsided.

FOR MILD TO MODERATE PAIN, PRIMARY DYSMENORRHEA AND ACUTE TENDINITIS AND BURSITIS
The recommended starting dose of Naproxen is 500 mg (20 mL or 4 tsp), followed by 250 mg (10 mL or 2 tsp) every 6 to 8 hours as required. The total daily dose should not exceed 1,250 mg (50 mL or 10 tsp).

NAPROXEN SODIUM
FOR MILD TO MODERATE PAIN, PRIMARY DYSMENORRHEA AND ACUTE TENDINITIS AND BURSITIS
The recommended starting dose is 550 mg, followed by 275 mg every 6 to 8 hours, as required. The total daily dose should not exceed 1,375 mg.

FOR RHEUMATOID ARTHRITIS, OSTEOARTHRITIS, AND ANKYLOSING SPONDYLITIS
The recommended dose in adults is 275 mg or 550 mg twice daily (morning and evening). During long-term administration, the dose may be adjusted up or down depending on the clinical response of the patient. A lower daily dose may suffice for long-term administration. The morning and evening doses do not have to be equal in size and the administration of the drug more frequently than twice daily is not necessary.

In patients who tolerate lower doses well, the dose may be increased to 1,650 mg per day for limited periods when a higher level of anti-inflammatory/analgesic activity is required. When treating such patients with the 1,650 mg/day dose, the physician should observe sufficient increased clinical benefits to offset the potential increased risk (see *"Clinical Pharmacology"*).

Symptomatic improvement in arthritis usually begins within two weeks. However, if improvement is not seen within this period, a trial for an additional two weeks should be considered.

FOR ACUTE GOUT
The recommended starting dose is 825 mg, followed by 275 mg every eight hours until the attack has subsided.

FOR JUVENILE ARTHRITIS
The recommended total daily dose is approximately 10 mg/kg given in two divided doses. The 275 mg Naproxen Sodium tablet is not well suited to this dosage so use of the related drug Naproxen as the 250 mg scored tablet or the 125 mg/5 mL suspension is recommended for this indication.

STORAGE
Store tablets at room temperature in well-closed containers; dispense in light-resistant containers.

Store suspension at room temperature; avoid excessive heat, above 40°C (104°F). Dispense in light-resistant container.

HOW SUPPLIED
NAPROXEN
SUSPENSION: 25 MG/ML

AVERAGE UNIT PRICE (AVAILABLE SIZES)			
GENERIC	$0.11		
BRAND/MANUFACTURER	NDC	SIZE	AWP
◆ GENERICS			
Roxane	00054-3630-63	500 ml	$34.75
Roxane	00054-8632-11	15 ml 25s ud	$50.00
Roxane	00054-8633-11	20 ml 25s ud	$66.65

◆ RATED THERAPEUTICALLY EQUIVALENT; ◇ THERAPEUTIC EQUIVALENCE UNCONFIRMED; ○ UNRATED

SUSPENSION: 25 MG/ML

BRAND/MANUFACTURER	NDC	SIZE	AWP
○ **BRAND** NAPROSYN: Syntex/PR	18393-0278-20	480 ml	$39.30

TABLETS: 250 MG

AVERAGE UNIT PRICE (AVAILABLE SIZES)		GENERIC A-RATED AVERAGE PRICE (GAAP)	
BRAND	$0.78	100s	$66.44
GENERIC	$0.67	500s	$329.32
HCFA FUL (100s ea)	$0.19	1000s	$630.65

BRAND/MANUFACTURER	NDC	SIZE	AWP
◆ **BRAND**			
➤ NAPROSYN: Syntex/PR	18393-0272-42	100s	$77.44
	18393-0272-53	100s ud	$80.39
	18393-0272-62	500s	$377.34
◆ **GENERICS**			
Allscrips	54569-3758-00	20s	$13.67
Allscrips	54569-3758-02	28s	$19.14
Allscrips	54569-3758-01	60s	$41.00
URL	00677-1515-01	75s	$75.00
Roxane	00054-4641-25	100s	$66.10
Major	00904-7745-60	100s	$67.05
Lemmon	00093-0147-01	100s	$67.05
Qualitest	00603-4730-21	100s	$67.05
West Point	59591-0253-68	100s	$67.05
Mylan	00378-0377-01	100s	$67.08
Rugby	00536-5612-01	100s	$67.08
Schein	00364-2562-01	100s	$67.08
Goldline	00182-1971-01	100s	$67.08
Hamilton	60322-0282-42	100s	$67.08
Novopharm	55953-0517-40	100s	$67.10
Copley	38245-0146-10	100s	$69.00
➤ Lederle Std Prod	00005-3300-43	100s	$69.13
Geneva	00781-1163-01	100s	$69.62
Martec	52555-0488-01	100s	$71.75
Vangard	00615-3562-13	100s ud	$34.84
Roxane	00054-8641-25	100s ud	$68.75
Geneva	00781-1163-13	100s ud	$69.64
UDL	51079-0793-20	100s ud	$72.80
Roxane	00054-4641-29	500s	$325.90
URL	00677-1515-05	500s	$326.85
Major	00904-7745-40	500s	$326.85
Lemmon	00093-0147-05	500s	$326.85
Mylan	00378-0377-05	500s	$326.86
Schein	00364-2562-05	500s	$326.86
Goldline	00182-1971-05	500s	$326.86
Hamilton	60322-0282-62	500s	$326.86
Novopharm	55953-0517-70	500s	$326.90
Copley	38245-0146-50	500s	$335.00
➤ Lederle Std Prod	00005-3300-31	500s	$336.83
Geneva	00781-1163-05	500s	$339.23
Lemmon	00093-0147-10	1000s	$630.50
Hamilton	60322-0282-66	1000s	$630.54
Novopharm	55953-0517-80	1000s	$630.60
Geneva	00781-1163-10	1000s	$630.97

TABLETS: 375 MG

AVERAGE UNIT PRICE (AVAILABLE SIZES)		GENERIC A-RATED AVERAGE PRICE (GAAP)	
BRAND	$1.00	100s	$84.88
GENERIC	$0.85	500s	$422.29
HCFA FUL (100s ea)	$0.24	1000s	$803.28

BRAND/MANUFACTURER	NDC	SIZE	AWP
◆ **BRAND**			
➤ NAPROSYN: Syntex/PR	18393-0273-42	100s	$99.54
	18393-0273-53	100s ud	$102.32
	18393-0273-62	500s	$482.82
◆ **GENERICS**			
Allscrips	54569-3759-00	10s	$8.69
Allscrips	54569-3759-03	14s	$12.17
Allscrips	54569-3759-05	15s	$13.04
Allscrips	54569-3759-04	20s	$17.38
Allscrips	54569-3759-01	21s	$18.25
Allscrips	54569-3759-02	30s	$26.08
Allscrips	54569-3759-07	40s	$34.87
Allscrips	54569-3759-06	45s	$39.11
Roxane	00054-4642-25	100s	$85.40
Major	00904-7746-60	100s	$86.20
Lemmon	00093-0148-01	100s	$86.20
Qualitest	00603-4731-21	100s	$86.20
West Point	59591-0254-68	100s	$86.20
Mylan	00378-0555-01	100s	$86.23
Rugby	00536-5613-01	100s	$86.23
Schein	00364-2563-01	100s	$86.23
Goldline	00182-1972-01	100s	$86.23
Hamilton	60322-0283-42	100s	$86.23

BRAND/MANUFACTURER	NDC	SIZE	AWP
Novopharm	55953-0518-40	100s	$86.25
URL	00677-1516-01	100s	$87.90
➤ Lederle Std Prod	00005-3301-43	100s	$88.81
Copley	38245-0443-10	100s	$89.00
Geneva	00781-1164-01	100s	$89.49
Martec	52555-0489-01	100s	$92.56
Vangard	00615-1504-13	100s ud	$32.60
Roxane	00054-8642-25	100s ud	$88.00
Geneva	00781-1164-13	100s ud	$88.63
UDL	51079-0794-20	100s ud	$93.05
Roxane	00054-4642-29	500s	$417.20
Qualitest	00603-4731-28	500s	$418.15
Major	00904-7746-40	500s	$418.20
Lemmon	00093-0148-05	500s	$418.20
Mylan	00378-0555-05	500s	$418.23
Rugby	00536-5613-05	500s	$418.23
Schein	00364-2563-05	500s	$418.23
Goldline	00182-1972-05	500s	$418.23
Hamilton	60322-0283-62	500s	$418.23
Novopharm	55953-0518-70	500s	$418.25
URL	00677-1516-05	500s	$425.00
Copley	38245-0443-50	500s	$425.00
➤ Lederle Std Prod	00005-3301-31	500s	$431.10
Geneva	00781-1164-05	500s	$434.06
Martec	52555-0489-05	500s	$438.00
Lemmon	00093-0148-10	1000s	$801.90
Hamilton	60322-0283-66	1000s	$801.91
Novopharm	55953-0518-80	1000s	$801.95
Geneva	00781-1164-10	1000s	$807.35

TABLETS: 500 MG

AVERAGE UNIT PRICE (AVAILABLE SIZES)		GENERIC A-RATED AVERAGE PRICE (GAAP)	
GENERIC	$1.02	100s	$103.40
HCFA FUL (100s ea)	$0.29	500s	$492.91
		1000s	$980.95

BRAND/MANUFACTURER	NDC	SIZE	AWP
◆ **GENERICS**			
Allscrips	54569-3760-03	10s	$10.61
Allscrips	54569-3760-04	14s	$14.85
Allscrips	54569-3760-00	15s	$15.92
Allscrips	54569-3760-01	20s	$21.22
Allscrips	54569-3760-02	30s	$31.83
Allscrips	54569-3760-05	40s	$42.44
Roxane	00054-4643-25	100s	$104.30
Rugby	00536-5614-01	100s	$105.30
Major	00904-7747-60	100s	$105.30
Lemmon	00093-0149-01	100s	$105.30
Qualitest	00603-4732-21	100s	$105.30
West Point	59591-0255-68	100s	$105.30
Mylan	00378-0451-01	100s	$105.31
Schein	00364-2564-01	100s	$105.31
Goldline	00182-1973-01	100s	$105.31
➤ Hamilton	60322-0287-42	100s	$105.31
Novopharm	55953-0520-40	100s	$105.35
Copley	38245-0150-10	100s	$108.00
➤ Lederle Std Prod	00005-3302-43	100s	$108.45
Geneva	00781-1165-01	100s	$109.29
Martec	52555-0490-01	100s	$112.35
Vangard	00615-3563-13	100s ud	$37.55
Geneva	00781-1165-13	100s ud	$108.47
Roxane	00054-8643-25	100s ud	$109.00
UDL	51079-0795-20	100s ud	$114.15
Allscrips	54569-8582-00	180s	$190.98
URL	00677-1517-01	500s	$107.51
Roxane	00054-4643-29	500s	$509.60
Qualitest	00603-4732-28	500s	$510.48
Major	00904-7747-40	500s	$510.55
Lemmon	00093-0149-05	500s	$510.55
Mylan	00378-0451-05	500s	$510.57
Rugby	00536-5614-05	500s	$510.57
Schein	00364-2564-05	500s	$510.57
Goldline	00182-1973-05	500s	$510.57
➤ Hamilton	60322-0287-62	500s	$510.57
Novopharm	55953-0520-70	500s	$510.60
URL	00677-1517-05	500s	$520.00
Copley	38245-0150-50	500s	$525.00
Aligen	00405-4695-02	500s	$525.10
➤ Lederle Std Prod	00005-3302-31	500s	$526.19
Geneva	00781-1165-05	500s	$529.90
Martec	52555-0490-05	500s	$541.00
Lemmon	00093-0149-10	1000s	$979.35
➤ Hamilton	60322-0287-66	1000s	$979.39
Novopharm	55953-0520-80	1000s	$979.45
Geneva	00781-1165-10	1000s	$985.61

TABLETS: 500 MG

BRAND/MANUFACTURER	NDC	SIZE	AWP
○ **BRAND**			
➤ NAPROSYN: Syntex/PR	18393-0277-42	100s	$121.57
	18393-0277-53	100s ud	$125.22
	18393-0277-62	500s	$589.43

NAPROXEN SODIUM
TABLETS: 275 MG

AVERAGE UNIT PRICE (AVAILABLE SIZES)		GENERIC A-RATED AVERAGE PRICE (GAAP)	
BRAND	$0.77	100s	$66.60
GENERIC	$0.66	500s	$321.50
		1000s	$621.76

BRAND/MANUFACTURER	NDC	SIZE	AWP
◆ **BRAND**			
➤ ANAPROX: Syntex/PR	18393-0274-42	100s	$77.18
	18393-0274-53	100s ud	$80.38
	18393-0274-62	500s	$372.54
◆ **GENERICS**			
Allscrips	54569-3761-00	20s	$13.37
Allscrips	54569-3761-01	21s	$14.04
Allscrips	54569-3761-02	30s	$20.06
Roxane	00054-4638-25	100s	$60.00
Major	00904-7802-60	100s	$66.85
Lemmon	00093-0536-01	100s	$66.85
Schein	00364-2553-01	100s	$66.86
Goldline	00182-1974-01	100s	$66.86
Hamilton	63322-0284-42	100s	$66.86
URL	00677-1513-01	100s	$66.90
Qualitest	00603-4733-21	100s	$66.90
Novopharm	55953-0531-40	100s	$66.90
West Point	59591-0256-68	100s	$66.90
Geneva	00781-1187-01	100s	$69.38
Mylan	00378-0537-01	100s	$69.45
Roxane	00054-8638-25	100s ud	$60.00
Novopharm	55953-0531-01	100s ud	$68.65
Geneva	00781-1187-13	100s ud	$69.62
Roxane	00054-4638-29	500s	$300.00
URL	00677-1513-05	500s	$322.00
Major	00904-7802-40	500s	$322.70
Lemmon	00093-0536-05	500s	$322.70
Schein	00364-2553-05	500s	$322.70
Goldline	00182-1974-05	500s	$322.70
Hamilton	63322-0284-62	500s	$322.70
Novopharm	55953-0531-70	500s	$322.75
Mylan	00378-0537-05	500s	$335.25
Novopharm	55953-0531-80	1000s	$613.25
Lemmon	00093-0536-10	1000s	$626.00
Geneva	00781-1187-10	1000s	$626.04

TABLETS: 550 MG

AVERAGE UNIT PRICE (AVAILABLE SIZES)		GENERIC A-RATED AVERAGE PRICE (GAAP)	
BRAND	$1.21	100s	$103.46
GENERIC	$1.02	500s	$500.20
		1000s	$968.29

BRAND/MANUFACTURER	NDC	SIZE	AWP
◆ **BRAND**			
➤ ANAPROX-DS: Syntex/PR	18393-0276-42	100s	$120.17
	18393-0276-53	100s ud	$125.20
	18393-0276-62	500s	$580.18
◆ **GENERICS**			
Allscrips	54569-3762-00	10s	$10.41
Allscrips	54569-3762-01	12s	$12.49
Allscrips	54569-3762-07	14s	$14.57
Allscrips	54569-3762-02	16s	$16.65
Allscrips	54569-3762-03	20s	$20.82
Allscrips	54569-3762-04	21s	$21.86
Allscrips	54569-3762-05	30s	$31.23
Allscrips	54569-3762-06	60s	$62.45
Roxane	00054-4639-25	100s	$90.00
Qualitest	00603-4734-21	100s	$103.65
Major	00904-7803-60	100s	$104.05
Lemmon	00093-0537-01	100s	$104.05
Schein	00364-2554-01	100s	$104.09
Goldline	00182-1975-01	100s	$104.09
Hamilton	63322-0286-42	100s	$104.09
West Point	59591-0258-68	100s	$104.10
Novopharm	55953-0533-40	100s	$104.15
URL	00677-1514-01	100s	$104.20
Geneva	00781-1188-01	100s	$108.03
Mylan	00378-0733-01	100s	$108.10
Roxane	00054-8639-25	100s ud	$100.00
Novopharm	55953-0533-01	100s ud	$105.90
Roxane	00054-4639-29	500s	$450.00
Qualitest	00603-4734-28	500s	$494.37
Major	00904-7803-40	500s	$502.55
Lemmon	00093-0537-05	500s	$502.55
Schein	00364-2554-05	500s	$502.56
Goldline	00182-1975-05	500s	$502.56
Hamilton	63322-0286-62	500s	$502.56
Novopharm	55953-0533-70	500s	$502.65
URL	00677-1514-05	500s	$520.00
Mylan	00378-0733-05	500s	$522.15
Novopharm	55953-0533-80	1000s	$955.00
Lemmon	00093-0537-10	1000s	$974.90
Geneva	00781-1188-10	1000s	$974.97

Naqua *SEE* TRICHLORMETHIAZIDE

Nardil *SEE* PHENELZINE SULFATE

Nasalcrom *SEE* CROMOLYN SODIUM

Nasalide *SEE* FLUNISOLIDE

Natacyn *SEE* NATAMYCIN

Natalins Rx *SEE* VITAMINS, PRENATAL

Natamycin

DESCRIPTION
Natamycin 5% Ophthalmic Suspension is a sterile, antifungal drug for topical ophthalmic administration.

Each mL of the suspension contains Natamycin 5% (50mg).

Following is its chemical structure:

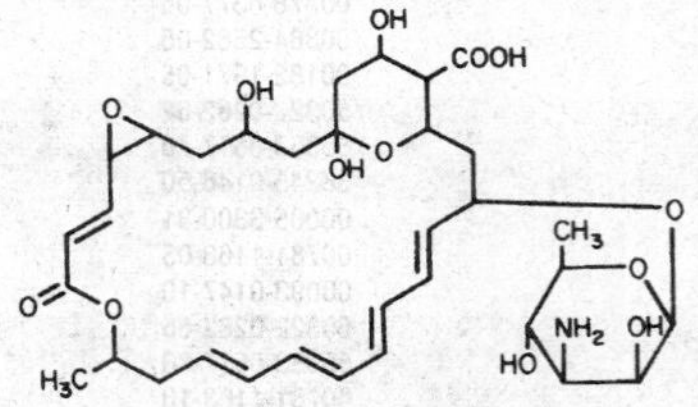

CLINICAL PHARMACOLOGY
Natamycin is a tetraene polyene antibiotic derived from *Streptomyces natalensis*. It possesses *in vitro* activity against a variety of yeast and filamentous fungi, including *Candida, Aspergillus, Cephalosporium, Fusarium and Penicillium*.

The mechanism of action appears to be through binding of the molecule to the sterol moiety of the fungal cell membrane. The polyenesterol complex alters the permeability of the membrane to produce depletion of essential cellular constituents. Although the activity against fungi is dose-related, Natamycin is predominantly fungicidal.* Natamycin is not effective *in vitro* against gram-positive or gram-negative bacteria. Topical administration appears to produce effective concentrations of Natamycin within the corneal stroma, but not in intraocular fluid. Systemic absorption should not be expected following topical administration of Natamycin 5% Ophthalmic Suspension. As with other polyene antibiotics, absorption from the gastrointestinal tract is very poor. Studies in rabbits receiving topical Natamycin revealed no measurable compound in the aqueous humor or sera, but the sensitivity of the measurement was no greater than 2 mg/mL.

INDICATIONS AND USAGE
Natamycin 5% Ophthalmic Suspension is indicated for the treatment of fungal blepharitis, conjunctivitis, and keratitis caused by susceptible organisms including *Fusarium solani* keratitis. As in other forms of suppurative keratitis, initial and sustained therapy of fungal keratitis should be determined by the clinical diagnosis, laboratory diagnosis by smear and culture of corneal scrapings and drug response.

Whenever possible, the *in vitro* activity of Natamycin against the responsible fungus should be determined. The effectiveness of Natamycin as a single agent in fungal endophthalmitis has not been established.

CONTRAINDICATION
Natamycin 5% Ophthalmic Suspension is contraindicated in individuals with a history of hypersensitivity to any of its components.

◆ RATED THERAPEUTICALLY EQUIVALENT; ◇ THERAPEUTIC EQUIVALENCE UNCONFIRMED; ○ UNRATED

PRECAUTIONS
GENERAL
For topical eye use only—*Not For Injection*. Failure of improvement of keratitis following 7-10 days of administration of the drug suggests that the infection may be caused by a microorganism not susceptible to Natamycin.

Continuation of therapy should be based on clinical re-evaluation and additional laboratory studies.

Adherence of the suspension to areas of epithelial ulceration or retention of the suspension in the fornices occurs regularly. There has only been a limited number of cases in which Natamycin has been used; therefore, it is possible that adverse reactions of which we have no knowledge at present may occur. For this reason, patients on this drug should be monitored at least twice weekly. Should suspicion of drug toxicity occur, the drug should be discontinued.

INFORMATION FOR PATIENTS
Do not touch dropper tip to any surface, as this may contaminate the suspension.

Carcinogenesis, Mutagenesis, Impairment of Fertility: There have been no long term studies done using Natamycin in animals to evaluate carcinogenesis, mutagenesis, or impairment of fertility.

Pregnancy: Pregnancy Category C. Animal reproduction studies have not been conducted with Natamycin. It is also not known whether Natamycin can cause fetal harm when administered to a pregnant woman or can affect reproduction capacity. Natamycin 5% Ophthalmic Suspension should be given to a pregnant woman only if clearly needed.

Nursing Mothers: It is not known whether these drugs are excreted in human milk. Because many drugs are excreted in human milk, caution should be exercised when Natamycin is administered to a nursing woman.

Pediatric Use: Safety and effectiveness in children have not been established.

ADVERSE REACTIONS
One case of conjunctival chemosis and hyperemia, thought to be allergic in nature, has been reported.

DOSAGE AND ADMINISTRATION
Shake Well Before Using. The preferred initial dosage in fungal keratitis is one drop of Natamycin 5% Ophthamic Suspension instilled in the conjunctival sac at hourly or two-hourly intervals. The frequency of application can usually be reduced to one drop 6 to 8 times daily after the first 3 to 4 days. Therapy should generally be continued for 14 to 21 days or until there is resolution of active fungal keratitis. In many cases, it may be helpful to reduce the dosage gradually at 4 to 7 day intervals to assure that the replicating organism has been eliminated. Less frequent initial dosage (4 to 6 daily applications) may be sufficient in fungal blepharitis and conjunctivitis.

May be stored in refrigerator [(36°-46° F) (2°-8°C)] or at room temperature [(46°-75° F) (8°-24°C)]. *Do not freeze.* Avoid exposure to light and excessive heat.

REFERENCES
* Laupen, J.O.; McLellan, W.L.; El Nakeeb, M.A.: "Antibiotics and Fungal Physiology," Antimicrobial Agents and Chemotherapy, 1965:1006, 1965. 1. Barckhausen, B.: Die Behandlung der Probleminfektionen das vorderen Augenabschnittes in der Praxis. Landarzt 46:842, 1970. 2. Cuendet, J.F.; Nour, A.: Traitement local en ophthalmologie par un nouvel antibiotique fungicide, la "pimaricin". Ophthalmologica 145:297, 1963. 3. Forster, R.K.; Rebell, G.: "The Diagnosis and Management of Keratomycoses" Arch. Ophth. 93:1134, 1975. 4. Francois, J.; de Vos, El: Traitement des mycoses oculaires par la pimaricine. Bull. Soc. Belge Ophthal. 131:382, 1962. 5. Jones, D.B.; Sexton, R.; Rebell, G.: "Mycotic keratitis in South Florida: A Review of Thirty-nine Cases." Transactions ophthal. Soc. U.K. 89:781, 1969. 6. Jones, D.B.; Forster, R.K.; Rebell, G.: *"Fusarium solani* keratitis treated with Natamycin (pimaricin), 18 consecutive cases." Arch. Ophth. 88:147, 1972. 7. L'Editeur: Traitement des mycoses oculaires. Presse med. 77:147, 1969. 8. Vozza, R.; Bagolini, B.: Su di un caso di grave ulcerazione bilaterale delle palpebre de Candida albicans. Bol. Oculist. 43:433, 1964.

HOW SUPPLIED
DROP: 5%

BRAND/MANUFACTURER	NDC	SIZE	AWP
○ BRAND NATACYN: Alcon Labs	00065-0645-15	15 ml	$93.75

Naturetin *SEE* BENDROFLUMETHIAZIDE

Navane *SEE* THIOTHIXENE

Navogan Ped *SEE* TRIMETHOBENZAMIDE
HYDROCHLORIDE

Nebcin *SEE* TOBRAMYCIN SULFATE, INJECTABLE

Nebupent *SEE* PENTAMIDINE ISETHIONATE

Nedocromil Sodium

DESCRIPTION
Nedocromil Sodium is an inhaled anti-inflammatory agent for the preventive management of asthma. Nedocromil Sodium is a pyranoquinoline with the chemical name 4H-Pyrano[3,2-g]quinoline-2,8-dicarboxylic acid, 9-ethyl-6,9-di-hydro-4, 6-dioxo-10-propyl-, disodium salt, and it has a molecular weight of 415.3. The empirical formula is $C_{19}H_{15}NNa_2O_7$. Nedocromil Sodium, a yellow powder, is soluble in water.

Chemical Class: Pyranoquinoline

Nedocromil Sodium inhalation aerosol is a pressurized metered-dose aerosol suspension for oral inhalation.

Each actuation delivers from the mouthpiece 1.75 mg Nedocromil Sodium. Each 16.2 g canister provides at least 112 metered inhalations.

Following is its chemical structure:

CLINICAL PHARMACOLOGY
Cellular and Animal Studies: Nedocromil Sodium has been shown to inhibit the *in vitro* activation of, and mediator release from, a variety of inflammatory cell types associated with asthma, including eosinphils, neutrophils, macrophages, mast cells, monocytes, and platelets. *In vitro* studies on cells obtained by bronchoalveolar lavage from antigensensitized macaque monkeys show that Nedocromil Sodium inhibits the release of mediators including histamine, leukotriene C_4 and prostaglandin D_2. Similar studies with human bronchoalveolar cells showed inhibition of histamine release from mast cells and beta-glucuronidase release from macrophages.

Nedocromil Sodium has been tested in experimental models of asthma using allergic animals and shown to inhibit the development of early and late bronchoconstriction responses to inhaled antigen. The development of airway hyper-responsiveness to nonspecific bronchoconstrictors was also inhibited. Nedocromil Sodium reduced antigen-induced increases in airway microvasculature leakage when administered intravenously in a model system.

Clinical Studies: Nedocromil Sodium has been shown to inhibit acutely the bronchoconstrictor response to several kinds of challenge. Pretreatment with single doses of Nedocromil Sodium inhibited the bronchoconstriction caused by sulfur dioxide, inhaled neurokinin A, various antigens, exercise, cold air, fog, and adenosine monophosphate.

Nedocromil Sodium has no intrinsic bronchodilator, antihistamine, or glucocorticoid activity.

Nedocromil Sodium, when delivered by inhalation at the recommended dose, has no known therapeutic systemic activity.

Pharmacokinetics and Bioavailability: Systemic bioavailability of Nedocromil Sodium administered as an inhaled aerosol is low. In a single dose study involving 20 healthy subjects who were administered a 3.5 mg dose of Nedocromil Sodium (2 actuations of 1.75 mg each), the mean AUC was 5.0 ng × hr/mL and the mean Cmax was 1.6 ng/mL attained about 28 minutes after dosing. The mean half life was 3.3 hours. Urinary excretion over 12 hours averaged 3.4% of the administered dose, of which approximately 75% was excreted in the first six hours of dosing.

In a multiple dose study, six healthy volunteers (3 males and 3 females) received a 3.5 mg single dose followed by 3.5 mg four times a day for seven consecutive days. Accumulation of the drug was not observed. Following single and multiple dose inhalations, urinary excretion of Nedocromil accounted for 5.6% and 12% of the drug administered, respectively. After intravenous administration, urinary excretion of Nedocromil was approximately 70%. The absolute bioavailability of Nedocromil was thus 8% (5.6/70) for single and 17% (12/70) for multiple inhaled doses.

Similarly, in a multiple dose study of 12 asthmatic patients, each given a 3.5 mg single dose followed by 3.5 mg four times a day for one month, both single dose and multiple dose inhalation gave a mean high plasma concentration of 2.8 ng/mL between 5 and 90 minutes, mean AUC of 5.6 ng × hr/mL, and a mean terminal half life of 1.5 hours. The mean 24-hour urinary excretion after either single or multiple dose administration represented approximately 5% of the administered dose.

Studies involving very high oral doses of Nedocromil (600 mg single dose, and subsequently 200 mg three times a day for seven days), showed an absolute bioavailability of less than 2%. In a radiolabeled (^{14}C) Nedocromil study involving two healthy males, urinary excretion accounted for 64% of the dose, fecal excretion for 36%.

Protein binding—Nedocromil is approximately 89% protein bound to human plasma over a concentration range of 0.5 to 50 μg/mL. This binding is reversible.

Metabolism—Nedocromil is not metabolized after IV administration and is excreted unchanged.

CLINICAL STUDIES

The worldwide clinical trial experience with Nedocromil Sodium comprises 5352 patients. Studies have been conducted both at twice daily and at four times daily dosage regimens. Evidence from these studies indicates that the four times daily regimen has been more effective than the twice daily regimen. A lower dose (two or three times daily) can be considered in patients under good control on the four times daily regimen (see *"Dosage and Administration"*).

1. Nedocromil Sodium vs. Placebo: The effectiveness of Nedocromil Sodium given four times daily was examined in a 14 week double-blind, placebo-controlled, parallel group trial in five centers in 120 patients (60/treatment). To be eligible for entry, the asthmatic patients had to be controlled using only sustained-release theophylline (SRT) and beta-agonists. Two weeks after the test therapies were begun the SRT was discontinued and four weeks after that oral beta-agonists were stopped. Beta-agonist metered dose inhalers could still be used after 6 weeks. Efficacy was assessed by symptom scores recorded on diary cards completed on a daily basis by the patients. Each morning the patient recorded nightime asthma on a 0-2 scale, (0 = slept well, no asthma; 1 = woke once because of asthma: 2 = woke more than once because of asthma). Before bedtime the patients recorded daytime asthma and cough on a 0-5 scale (0 = no symptoms of asthma/cough today: 5 = asthma/cough symptoms were noticed most of the day and caused a lot of trouble). At the end of the treatment phase, patients and clinicians were asked for their opinions on the effectiveness of the treatment based on a five point scale (1 = very effective; 5 = made condition worse). The results of these evaluations are shown in Table 1: Nedocromil Sodium was significantly superior to placebo for all measurements.

Table 1

Variable	Time Period	Nedocromil Sodium Mean	Placebo Mean
Daytime Asthma[1]	Weeks 7-14	1.26	2.08
Nightime Asthma[2]	Weeks 7-14	0.67	0.96
Cough[1]	Weeks 7-14	0.68	1.49
Patient's Opinion[2]	Week 14	2.27	3.55
Clinician's Opinion[2]	Week 14	2.13	3.48
FEV_1[2] (liters)	Week 2	2.69	2.18
FEV_1[2] (liters)	Week 6	2.65	2.15
FEV_1[2] (liters)	Week 10	2.55	2.15
FEV_1[2] (liters)	Week 14	2.59	2.10

1. Nedocromil Sodium significantly better than Placebo, $p < 0.05$
2. Nedocromil Sodium significantly better than Placebo, $p < 0.01$

The FEV_1 percentage change relative to baseline is shown in Figure 1; these also favored Nedocromil Sodium over placebo throughout the study, with an effect seen first at the two week measurement.

FIGURE 1

Nedocromil Sodium vs. Placebo
Percentage Chenge from Baseline FEV_1

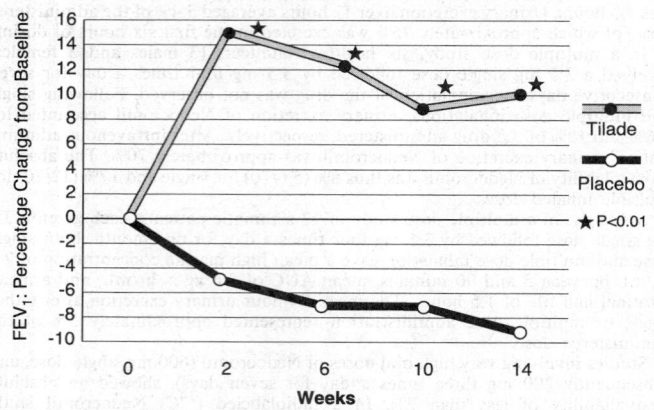

Note: SRT discontinued after 2 weeks
Oral b2 discontinued after 6 weeks

This study shows that Nedocromil Sodium improves symptom control and pulmonary function when it is added to a prn inhaled beta-adrenergic bronchodilator regimen and that a beneficial effect could be detected within two weeks.

2. Nedocromil Sodium vs. Cromolyn Sodium vs. Placebo: The effectiveness of Nedocromil Sodium was compared to cromolyn sodium and placebo in an eight week, double-blind, parallel group, 12 center trial during which medication was given four times daily. Three hundred and six patients were randomized to treatment (103 Nedocromil Sodium 104/cromolyn sodium: 99/placebo). All patients were SRT dependent and this drug was stopped prior to starting the test treatment. Efficacy was assessed on the basis of diary card symptom scores and FEV_1. The diary scores were the same as used in the 14 week study except that nighttime symptoms were recorded on a 0-3 scale. The primary efficacy variable was a summary symptom score derived by averaging the scores for daytime asthma, nighttime asthma and cough. The results of the study are shown in Table 2.

Table 2

Variable	Time Period	Nedocromil Sodium Mean	Placebo Mean	Cromolyn Sodium Mean
Summary Score[1]	Weeks 3-8	1.30	1.76	1.13
Daytime Asthma[1]	Weeks 3-8	1.59	2.05	1.41
Nighttime Asthma[2]	Weeks 3-8	0.91	1.23	0.77
Cough[3]	Weeks 3-8	1.11	1.58	0.93
FEV_1[2]	Weeks 3-8	2.46	2.23	2.56
Patient's Opinion[1]	Week 8	2.54	3.39	2.22
Clinician's Opinion[1]	Week 8	2.60	3.43	2.39

1. Nedocromil Sodium significantly better than Placebo, $p < 0.001$
2. Nedocromil Sodium significantly better than Placebo, $p < 0.01$, cromolyn sodium significantly better than Nedocromil Sodium, $p < 0.05$
3. Nedocromil Sodium significantly better than Placebo, $p < 0.05$

This study corroborates the findings of the 14 week study, showing that Nedocromil Sodium is effective in the management of symptoms and pulmonary function in primarily atopic mild to moderate asthmatics. Both active treatments were statistically significantly better than placebo for the primary efficacy variable (summary symptom score): Nedocromil Sodium and cromolyn sodium were not significantly different for this parameter. A statistically significant difference favoring cromolyn sodium was, however, seen for nighttime asthma and FEV_1.

In laboratory studies, pretreatment with Nedocromil Sodium before an anticipated challenge can prevent the bronchoconstriction associated with sulfur dioxide, cold air, fog, exercise, allergen challenge, adenosine monophospate, and neurokinin A. Controlled studies have not been carried out to assess the clinical significance of these findings.

In allergic asthmatics who are well controlled on cromolyn sodium, there is no evidence that the substitution of Nedocromil Sodium for cromolyn sodium would confer additional benefit to the patient. Efficacy with one agent is not known to be predictive of efficacy with the other.

The presently available data on the relative efficacy of Nedocromil Sodium and cromolyn sodium are inconclusive.

INDICATIONS AND USAGE

Nedocromil Sodium Inhaler is indicated for maintenance therapy in the management of patients with mild to moderate bronchial asthma. Nedocromil Sodium is not indicated for the reversal of acute bronchospasm.

UNLABELED USES

Nedocromil Sodium is used alone or as an adjunct in the treatment of seasonal allergic rhinitis, allergic conjunctivitis, and vernal conjunctivitis.

CONTRAINDICATIONS

Nedocromil Sodium Inhaler is contraindicated in those patients who have shown hypersensitivity to Medocromil Sodium or other ingredients in this preparation.

WARNINGS

Nedocromil Sodium Inhaler is not a bronchodilator and, therefore, should not be used for the reversal of acute bronchospasm, particularly status asthmaticus Nedocromil Sodium should ordinarily be continued during acute exacerbations, unless the patient becomes intolerant to the use of inhaled dosage forms.

PRECAUTIONS

General: Inhaled medications can cause coughing and bronchospasm in some patients. If this should occur with Nedocromil Sodium, its use should be discontinued and alternative therapy instituted as appropriate.

If systemic or inhaled steroid therapy is at all reduced, patients must be monitored carefully. Nedocromil Sodium has not been shown to be able to substitute for the total dose of steroids.

Information for Patients: Nedocromil Sodium must be taken regularly to achieve benefit, even during symptom-free periods. Because the therapeutic effect depends upon topical application to the lungs, it is essential that patients be properly instructed in the correct method of use (see *"Patient Instruction"* leaflet).

◆ RATED THERAPEUTICALLY EQUIVALENT; ◇ THERAPEUTIC EQUIVALENCE UNCONFIRMED; ○ UNRATED

	Adverse Events (AE)			
	% Experiencing AE		% Withdrawing	
	Nedocromil Sodium (n = 2042)	Placebo (n = 1875)	Nedocromil Sodium	Placebo
Special Senses				
Unpleasant Taste*	12.6%	3.6%	2.1%	0.4%
Respiratory System Disorders				
Coughing	7.0	7.2	1.4	1.4
Pharyngitis	5.7	5.0	0.6	0.5
Rhinitis*	4.6	3.0	0.1	0.1
Upper Respiratory Tract Infection*	3.9	2.4	0.1	0.1
Sputum Increased	1.7	1.4	0.1	0.2
Bronchitis	1.2	1.3	0.1	0.1
Dyspnea	2.8	3.8	0.9	1.3
Bronchospasm**	5.4	8.2	1.5	2.3
Gastro-Intestinal Tract				
Nausea*	4.0	2.1	1.3	0.7
Vomiting*	1.7	0.9	0.2	0.4
Dyspepsia*	1.3	0.6	0.1	0.1
Mouth Dry	1.0	0.9	0.1	0.2
Diarrhea	0.9	0.6	0.1	0.0
Abdominal Pain*	1.2	0.5	0.2	0.1
Central and Peripheral Nervous System				
Dizziness	0.9	1.2	0.1	0.2
Dysphonia	1.0	0.6	0.1	0.1
Body as a Whole				
Headache	6.0	4.7	0.5	0.3
Chest Pain	4.0	3.9	0.9	0.6
Fatigue	1.1	0.7	0.2	0.1
Resistance Mechanism Disorders				
Infection Viral	2.4	3.4	0.1	0.1

Table includes data from double-bind group comparative studies at four times per day dosing.
* Statistically significant (p ≤ 0.05) higher frequency of events on Nedocromil Sodium
** Statistically significant (p ≤ 0.05) higher frequency of events on Placebo.

An illustrated leaflet for the patient is included in each Nedocromil Sodium Inhaler pack.

Drug Interactions: Nedocromil Sodium has been co-administered with other anti-asthma therapies including inhaled and oral bronchodilators and inhaled corticosteroids. There are no known adverse drug interactions.

Carcinogenesis, Mutagenesis, Impairment of Fertility: A two-year inhalation chronic/carcinogenicity study of Nedocromil Sodium in Wistar rats showed no carcinogenic potential. The maximum achievable daily dose of 24 mg/kg corresponded to 86 times the maximum human daily aerosol dose of 0.28 mg/kg (based on eight actuations of 1.75 mg to a 50 kg person). Assuming 5% systemic absorption in man, and comparing calculated exposure to measured exposure in rats, systemic exposure in rats in this study was about 40 times human exposure. A 21-month oral dietary carcinogenicity study of Nedocromil Sodium performed in B6C3F1 mice with daily doses up to 180 mg/kg showed no carcinogenic potential. Systemic exposure in the mouse, calculated as above for the rats, was about six times that in humans, or about 20 times that in humans based on free drug concentrations in plasma. The exposure of the GI tract in top dose animals corresponded to 643 times the human daily dose since, in man, most of an inhaled dose is subsequently swallowed.

Nedocromil Sodium showed no mutagenic potential in the Ames Salmonella/microsome plate assay, mitotic gene conversion in *S. cevisiae*, mouse lymphoma forward mutation and mouse micronucleus assays.

Reproduction and fertility studies in mice and rats showed no effects on male or female fertility at subcutaneous doses of 100 mg/kg/day.

Pregnancy: Pregnancy Category B. Reproduction studies performed in mice, rats and rabbits using subcutaneous doses of 100 mg/kg/day, revealed no evidence of impaired fertility or harm to the fetus due to Nedocromil Sodium. There are, however, no adequate and well-controlled studies in pregnant women. Because animal reproduction studies are not always predictive of human response, this drug should be used during pregnancy only if clearly needed.

Nursing Mothers: It is not known whether this drug is excreted in human milk. Because many drugs are excreted in human milk, caution should be exercised when Nedocromil Sodium is administered to a nursing woman.

Pediatric Use: Safety and effectiveness in children below the age of 12 years have not been established.

ADVERSE REACTIONS

Nedocromil Sodium is generally well tolerated. Adverse event information was derived from 5352 patients receiving Nedocromil Sodium in controlled and open-label clinical trials of 2-52 weeks in duration. A total of 3538 patients received two inhalations four times a day. An additional 1814 patients received two inhalations twice daily or some other dose regimen. Seventy-three percent of patients were exposed to study drug for eight weeks or longer.

Of the 3538 patients who received two inhalations of Nedocromil Sodium four times a day, 2042 were in placebo-controlled trials and of these 7% withdrew from the trials due to adverse events, compared to 6% of the 1875 patients who received placebo.

The reasons for withdrawal were generally similar in the Nedocromil Sodium and placebo-treated groups, except that patients withdrew due to bad taste statistically more frequently on Nedocromil Sodium than on placebo. Headache reported as severe or very severe was experienced by 1.2 percent of Nedocromil Sodium patients and 0.9 percent of placebo patients, some with nausea and ill feeling.

The events reported with a frequency of 1% or greater across all placebo-controlled studies are displayed below for all patients who received Nedocromil Sodium or placebo at two inhalations four times daily. (See related table.)

Other adverse events present at less than the 1% level of occurrence, but that might be related to Nedocromil Sodium administration, include rash, arthritis, tremor and a sensation of warmth.

Elevations of SGPT were noted in 3.3% of patients on Nedocromil Sodium vs. 1.7% on placebo. The average elevation over placebo was 10 I.U. with only two patients increasing by more than 100 I.U. and none becoming ill. The clinical significance of these elevations is unclear.

One case of pneumonitis with eosinophilia and one case of anaphylaxis have been reported in foreign post-marketing experience in which the relationship to drug is undetermined.

OVERDOSAGE

There is no experience to date with overdose of Nedocromil Sodium in humans. Animal studies by several routes of administration (inhalation, oral, intravenous, subcutaneous) have demonstrated little potential for significant toxicity in humans from inhalation of high doses of Nedocromil Sodium. Head shaking/tremor and salivation were observed in beagle dogs following daily inhalation doses of 5 mg/kg and transient hypotension was detected following daily subcutaneous doses of 8 mg/kg. In addition, clonic convulsions were observed in dogs following daily inhalation doses of 20 mg/kg plus subcutaneous doses of 20 mg/kg giving peak plasma levels of 7.6 µg/mL, some three orders of magnitude greater than peak plasma levels (2.5 ng/mL) of the human daily dose. Specific tests designed to evaluate CNS activity demonstrated no effects due to Nedocromil Sodium, and Nedocromil Sodium does not pass the blood brain barrier. Therefore, overdosage is unlikely to result in clinical manifestations requiring more than observation and discontinuation of the drug where appropriate.

DOSAGE AND ADMINISTRATION

The recommended dosage for symptomatic adults and children (12 years of age and over) is two inhalations four times a day at regular intervals to provide 14 mg of Nedocromil Sodium per day. Maintenance therapy should be initiated at the same dose. In patients under good control on four times daily dosing (i.e., patients whose only medication need is occasional [not more than twice a week] inhaled or oral beta-agonists, and who have no serious exacerbations with respiratory infections) a lower dose can be tried. If use of lower doses is attempted, Nedocromil Sodium should be first reduced to a three times daily regimen (10.5

mg of Nedocromil Sodium per day) then, after several weeks on continued good control, to twice a day (7 mg of Nedocromil Sodium per day).

Nedocromil Sodium Inhaler should be added to the patient's existing treatment regimen (e.g., bronchodilators). When a clinical response to Nedocromil Sodium Inhaler is evident and if the asthma is under good control, an attempt may be made to decrease concomitant medication usage gradually.

Proper inhalational technique is essential (see *"Patient Instruction"* leaflet).

Patients should be advised that the optimal effect of Nedocromil Sodium therapy depends upon its administration at regular intervals, even during symptom-free periods.

Store between 2°-30°C (36°-86°F). Do not freeze. Contents under pressure. Do not puncture, incinerate, place near sources of heat or use with other mouthpieces. Keep out of the reach of children.

Note: the indented statement below is required by the Federal government's Clean Air Act for all products containing or manufactured with chlorofluorocarbons (CFC's).

Warning: Contains CFC-12 and CFC-114, substances which harm public health an environment by destroying ozone in the upper atmosphere.

A notice similar to the above *"Warning"* has been placed in the "Patient Instructions for Use" portion of this package circular pursuant to EPA regulations.

HOW SUPPLIED
AEROSOL SOLID W/ADAPTER: 1.75 MG/INH

BRAND/MANUFACTURER	NDC	SIZE	AWP
○ BRAND TILADE: Fisons Presc	00585-0685-02	16.2 gm	$26.15

NegGram *SEE* NALIDIXIC ACID

Nembutal *SEE* PENTOBARBITAL SODIUM

Neo-Cortef *SEE* HYDROCORTISONE ACETATE WITH NEOMYCIN SULFATE

Neo-Medrol Acetate *SEE* METHYLPREDNISOLONE ACETATE AND NEOMYCIN SULFATE

Neo-Synephrine *SEE* PHENYLEPHRINE HYDROCHLORIDE

NeoDecadron *SEE* DEXAMETHASONE SODIUM PHOSPHATE AND NEOMYCIN SULFATE, TOPICAL *AND* DEXAMETHASONE SODIUM PHOSPHATE WITH NEOMYCIN SULFATE, OPHTHALMIC

Neomycin Sulfate

WARNINGS
SYSTEMIC ABSORPTION OF NEOMYCIN OCCURS FOLLOWING ORAL ADMINISTRATION AND TOXIC REACTIONS MAY OCCUR. PATIENTS TREATED WITH NEOMYCIN SHOULD BE UNDER CLOSE CLINICAL OBSERVATION BECAUSE OF THE POTENTIAL TOXICITY ASSOCIATED WITH ITS USE. NEUROTOXICITY (INCLUDING OTOTOXICITY) AND NEPHROTOXICITY FOLLOWING PARENTERAL AEROSOL, AND ORAL ADMINISTRATION: INTRA-OPERATIVE, WOUND, AND BOWEL IRRIGATION; INJECTION INTO PLEURAL AND SYNOVIAL SPACES; IMPLANTATION OF IMPREGNATED GRAFTS; AND CUTANEOUS APPLICATION OF NEOMYCIN HAVE BEEN REPORTED, EVEN WHEN USED IN RECOMMENDED DOSES. THE POTENTIAL FOR NEPHROTOXICITY, PERMANENT BILATERAL AUDITORY OTOTOXICITY AND SOMETIMES VESTIBULAR TOXICITY IS PRESENT OR INCREASED IN PATIENTS WITH NORMAL RENAL FUNCTION WHEN TREATED WITH HIGHER DOSES OF NEOMYCIN AND/OR FOR LONGER PERIODS THAN RECOMMENDED. SERIAL, VESTIBULAR, AND AUDIOMETRIC TESTS, AS WELL AS TESTS OF RENAL FUNCTION, SHOULD BE PERFORMED (ESPECIALLY IN HIGH RISK PATIENTS). THE RISK OF NEPHROTOXICITY AND OTOTOXICITY IS

GREATER IN PATIENTS WITH IMPAIRED RENAL FUNCTION. HOWEVER, RENAL IMPAIRMENT IS NOT A PREREQUISITE FOR OTOTOXICITY. ABSORPTION IS UNPREDICTABLE AND OTOTOXICITY IS NOT ALWAYS STRICTLY DOSE RELATED. THE LIKELIHOOD OF THE OCCURRENCE OF TOXICITY DEPENDS UPON THE AMOUNT ABSORBED, THE CUMULATIVE LEVELS IN THE INNER EAR, AND THE DURATION OF TREATMENT. OTOTOXICITY IS OFTEN DELAYED IN ONSET AND PATIENTS DEVELOPING COCHLEAR DAMAGE WILL NOT HAVE SYMPTOMS DURING THERAPY TO WARN THEM OF DEVELOPING EIGHTH NERVE DESTRUCTION AND TOTAL OR PARTIAL DEAFNESS MAY OCCUR LONG AFTER NEOMYCIN HAS BEEN DISCONTINUED.

NEUROMUSCULAR BLOCKAGE AND RESPIRATORY PARALYSIS HAVE BEEN REPORTED FOLLOWING THE ORAL USE OF NEOMYCIN. THE POSSIBILITY OF THE OCCURRENCE OF NEUROMUSCULAR BLOCKAGE AND RESPIRATORY PARALYSIS SHOULD BE CONSIDERED IF NEOMYCIN IS ADMINISTERED, ESPECIALLY TO PATIENTS RECEIVING ANESTHETICS, NEUROMUSCULAR BLOCKING AGENTS SUCH AS TUBOCURARINE, SUCCINYLCHOLINE, DECAMETHONIUM, OR IN PATIENTS RECEIVING MASSIVE TRANSFUSIONS OF CITRATE ANTICOAGULATED BLOOD. IF BLOCKAGE OCCURS, CALCIUM SALTS MAY REVERSE THESE PHENOMENA BUT MECHANICAL RESPIRATORY ASSISTANCE MAY BE NECESSARY.

FATAL AND IRREVERSIBLE TOXIC REACTIONS MAY FOLLOW THE LOCAL INTRA-OPERATIVE USE OF NEOMYCIN (E.G. INTRAPERITONEAL, ORTHOPEDIC, INTRANEURAL, INTRAPLEURAL IRRIGATIONS AND INSTALLATIONS), AND THE APPLICATION OF NEOMYCIN-CONTAINING PRODUCTS TO FULL THICKNESS BURNS AND WHERE THE AREA OF A BURN EXCEEDS 5% OF THE BODY SURFACE. THESE ROUTES OF ADMINISTRATION SHOULD BE AVOIDED BECAUSE THEY MAY BE EQUIVALENT TO PARENTERAL ADMINISTRATION AND TOXIC BLOOD LEVELS CAN EQUAL THOSE FOLLOWING INTRAMUSCULAR INJECTION. FATALITIES HAVE BEEN REPORTED FOLLOWING A SINGLE INTRAPERITONEAL INSTILLATION OF A SOLUTION CONTAINING NEOMYCIN AND BACITRACIN, AND FOLLOWING ENTERAL USE. SIGNIFICANT TOXICITY WILL OCCUR IF THE NEOMYCIN CONTENT OF THE LUMEN OF THE GUT IS ALLOWED TO SPILL INTO THE PERITONEAL CAVITY AS DURING SURGICAL PROCEDURES ON THE GASTRO-INTESTINAL TRACT.

CONCURRENT AND/OR SEQUENTIAL SYSTEMIC, (INCLUDING INTRA-OPERATIVE), ORAL, CUTANEOUS, OR TOPICAL USE OF OTHER AMINOGLYCOSIDES (GENTAMICIN, TOBRAMYCIN, AMIKACIN, NETILMICIN, KANAMYCIN, STREPTOMYCIN, INCLUDING PAROMOMYCIN) AND OTHER POTENTIALLY NEUROTOXIC AND/OR NEPHROTOXIC DRUGS SUCH AS BACITRACIN, CISPLATIN, VANCOMYCIN, AMPHOTERICIN B, POLYMYXIN B, COLISTIN, AND VIOMYCIN SHOULD BE AVOIDED BECAUSE THEIR TOXICITIES MAY BE ADDITIVE.

OTHER FACTORS WHICH INCREASE THE RISK OF TOXICITY ARE ADVANCED AGE AND DEHYDRATION.

THE CONCURRENT USE OF NEOMYCIN WITH POTENT DIURETICS SUCH AS ETHACRYNIC ACID OR FUROSEMIDE SHOULD BE AVOIDED SINCE CERTAIN DIURETICS BY THEMSELVES MAY CAUSE OTOTOXICITY. IN ADDITION, WHEN ADMINISTERED INTRAVENOUSLY, DIURETICS MAY ENHANCE NEOMYCIN TOXICITY BY ALTERING THE ANTIBIOTIC CONCENTRATION IN SERUM AND TISSUE.

DESCRIPTION
Neomycin Sulfate oral solution for oral administration contains Neomycin which is an antibiotic obtained from the metabolic products of the actinomycete *Streptomyces fradiae.* Each 5 ml of Neomycin Sulfate oral solution contains 125 mg of Neomycin Sulfate.

The empirical formula of Neomycin Sulfate is $C_{23}H_{46}N_6O_{13} \cdot 2\frac{1}{2}H_2SO_4$.

Following is its chemical structure:

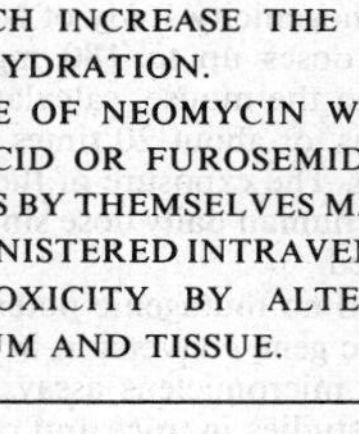

CLINICAL PHARMACOLOGY
Neomycin Sulfate is poorly absorbed from the normal gastrointestinal tract. Absorption can be unpredictable and subject to considerable variability. The small absorbed fraction is rapidly distributed in the tissues and is excreted by the

kidney in keeping with the degree of kidney function. The unabsorbed portion of the drug (approximately 97%) is eliminated unchanged in the feces.

Growth of most intestinal bacteria is rapidly suppressed following oral administration of Neomycin Sulfate, with the suppression persisting for 48-72 hours. Nonpathogenic yeasts and occasionally resistant strains of *Enterobacter aerogenes* (formerly *Aerobacter aerogenes*) replace the intestinal bacteria.

As with other aminoglycosides, the amount of systemically absorbed Neomycin transferred to the tissues increases cumulatively with each repeated dose administered until a steady state is achieved. The kidney functions as the primary excretory path as well as the tissue binding site with the highest concentration found in the renal cortex. With repeated dosings, significant accumulation occurs in the renal cortex and cochlear tissues. Release of tissue bound Neomycin occurs slowly over a period of several weeks after dosing has been discontinued.

Protein binding studies have shown that the degree of aminoglycoside protein binding is low and, depending upon the methods used for testing, this may be between 0% and 30%.

MICROBIOLOGY
In vitro tests have demonstrated that Neomycin is bactericidal and acts by inhibiting the synthesis of protein in susceptible bacterial cells. It is effective primarily against gram-negative bacilli but does have some activity against gram-positive organisms. Neomycin is active *in vitro* against *Escherichia coli* and the *Klebsiella-Enterobacter* group. Neomycin is not active against anaerobic bowel flora.

If susceptibility testing is needed, using a 30 mcg disc, organisms producing zones of 16 mm or greater are considered susceptible. Resistant organisms produce zones of 13 mm or less. Zones greater than 13 mm and less than 16 mm indicate intermediate susceptibility.

INDICATIONS AND USAGE
SUPPRESSION OF INTESTINAL BACTERIA
Oral Neomycin Sulfate is indicated as adjunctive therapy as part of a regimen for the suppression of the normal bacterial flora of the bowel, eg, preoperative preparation of the bowel. It is given concomitantly with erythromycin enteric coated base (see *"Dosage and Administration"* section).

HEPATIC COMA (PORTAL-SYSTEMIC ENCEPHALOPATHY)
Neomycin Sulfate has been shown to be effective adjunctive therapy in hepatic coma by reduction of the ammonia forming bacteria in the intestinal tract. The subsequent reduction in blood ammonia has resulted in neurologic improvement.

In the past, Neomycin had been administered through lower enteral routes, i.e. through the distal portion of the colon to prepare the colon in staged colonic resection, and through the rectum as an enema to treat acute hepatic coma. Evidence to establish effectiveness of Neomycin by these routes is lacking, and considerable toxicity has been documented.

UNLABELED USES
Neomycin Sulfate is used alone or as an adjunct in the treatment of infectious diarrhea and hypercholesterolemia, as well as in the prophylaxis of traveler's diarrhea.

CONTRAINDICATIONS
Neomycin Sulfate oral preparations are contraindicated in the presence of intestinal obstruction and in individuals with a history of hypersensitivity to the drug.

Patients with a history of hypersensitivity or serious toxic reaction to other aminoglycosides may have a cross-sensitivity to Neomycin.

WARNINGS
(See boxed *"Warnings"*.)

Absorbed Neomycin accumulates in the inner ear where it is retained in perilymph, and where it destroys outer and inner hair cells, supporting cells in the organ of Corti, and the distal ends of the fibers of the cochlear nerve. It is eliminated slowly from the inner ear and cochleotoxicity is often delayed in onset. Patients who subsequently develop cochlear damage usually have no symptoms during therapy to warn them of eighth nerve destruction. Progressive cochlear destruction continues for several months after symptoms appear and total or partial deafness may occur long after Neomycin has been discontinued. Serial audiometric tests, as well as tests of renal function, should be performed (especially in high risk patients). The absence of symptoms and a report of a normal audiogram at the end of therapy does not mean that Neomycin-induced hearing loss will not develop at a later time or that hearing loss has not already developed at frequencies above 8,000 KHz, higher than the conventional audiometer is capable of detecting.

Neomycin-induced nephrotoxicity is usually manifested as proximal tubular necrosis and is not dependent upon the presence of renal dysfunction. Aminoglycoside-induced nephrotoxicity is usually reversible after short-term treatment when the drug has been discontinued.

Neuromuscular blockade and respiratory paralysis have been reported following the use of Neomycin. Blockade and paralysis may occur immediately or may be delayed in onset. These possibilities should be considered when Neomycin is administered, especially to patients receiving anesthetics, neuromuscular blocking agents such as tubocurarine, succinylcholine, decamethonium, or in patients receiving massive transfusions of citrate-anticoagulated blood. If blockade occurs resuscitative equipment should be immediately available. Calcium salts may reverse these phenomena but mechanical respiratory assistance may be necessary.

Additional manifestations of neurotoxicity may include numbness, skin tingling, muscle twitching, and convulsions.

Systemic absorption may occur following cutaneous application to denuded skin and caution should be exercised when using any formulation containing Neomycin Sulfate for the treatment of lacerations, ulcers, biopsy or skin donor sites, and other skin conditions where the lesion may be deep and/or extensive in order to avoid toxicity due to systemic absorption.

The use of Neomycin Sulfate formulations in the external auditory canal may cause cochleotoxicity when the tympanic membrane has been perforated.

Aminoglycosides can cause fetal harm when administered to a pregnant woman. Aminoglycoside antibiotics cross the placenta and there have been several reports of total irreversible bilateral congenital deafness in children whose mothers received streptomycin during pregnancy. Although serious side effects to fetus or newborn have not been reported in the treatment of pregnant women with other aminoglycosides, the potential for harm exists when Neomycin is given. Animal reproduction studies of Neomycin have not been conducted. If Neomycin is used during pregnancy, or if the patient becomes pregnant while taking this drug, the patient should be apprised of the potential hazard to the fetus.

PRECAUTIONS
GENERAL
As with other antibiotics, use of oral Neomycin may result in overgrowth of nonsusceptible organisms, particularly fungi. If this occurs, appropriate therapy should be instituted.

Neomycin is quickly and almost totally absorbed from body surfaces (except the urinary bladder) after local irrigation and when applied topically in association with surgical procedures. Delayed-onset, irreversible deafness, renal failure, and death due to neuromuscular blockade (regardless of the status of renal function) have been reported following irrigation of both small and large surgical fields with minute quantities of Neomycin.

Cross-allergenicity among aminoglycosides has been demonstrated.

Aminoglycosides should be used with caution in patients with muscular disorders such as myasthenia gravis or parkinsonism since these drugs may aggravate muscle weakness because of their potential curare-like effect on the neuromuscular junction.

Small amounts of orally administered Neomycin are absorbed through intact intestinal mucosa and the drug may be absorbed from ulcerated or denuded areas.

If Neomycin has been used for the preoperative preparation of the gut, spillage into the peritoneal cavity during the operative procedure may be extremely hazardous.

There have been many reports in the literature of nephrotoxicity and/or ototoxicity with the oral use of Neomycin. If renal insufficiency develops during oral therapy, consideration should be given to reducing the drug dosage or discontinuing therapy.

An oral Neomycin dose of 12 g per day produces a malabsorption syndrome for a variety of substances including fat, nitrogen, cholesterol, carotene, glucose, xylose, lactose, sodium, calcium, cyanocobalamin and iron.

Orally administered Neomycin increases fecal bile acid excretion and reduces intestinal lactase activity.

INFORMATION FOR THE PATIENT
Before administering the drug, patients or members of their families should be informed of possible toxic effects on the eighth nerve. The possibility of acute toxicity increases in premature infants and neonates.

LABORATORY TESTS
Patients with renal insufficiency may develop toxic Neomycin blood levels unless doses are properly regulated. If renal insufficiency develops during treatment, the dosage should be reduced or the antibiotic discontinued. To avoid nephrotoxicity and eighth nerve damage associated with high doses, accumulation, and prolonged treatment, the following should be performed prior to and periodically during therapy: urinalysis for increased excretion of protein, decreased specific gravity, casts and cells; renal function tests such as serum creatinine, BUN or creatinine clearance; tests of the vestibulocochlearis nerve (eighth cranial nerve) function.

Serial, vestibular and audiometric tests should be performed (especially in high risk patients) and should be repeated periodically. Since elderly patients may have reduced renal function which may not be evident in the results of routine screening tests such as BUN or serum creatinine, a creatinine clearance determination may be more useful.

DRUG INTERACTIONS
Caution should be taken in concurrent or serial use of other neurotoxic and/or nephrotoxic drugs because of possible enhancement of the nephrotoxicity and/or ototoxicity of Neomycin (see boxed *"Warnings"*).

Caution should also be taken in concurrent or serial use of other aminoglycosides and polymyxins because they may enhance Neomycin's nephrotoxicity and/or ototoxicity and potentiate Neomycin Sulfate's neuromuscular blocking effects.

Neomycin, polymyxin B, and bacitracin are nephrotoxic and, when combined, these nephrotoxicities are additive. These drug-induced nephrotoxicities are usually proximal tubular necrosis or tubular degeneration. Bacitracin also depresses the glomerular filtration rate. The renal damage induced by each antibiotic after short-term treatment is usually reversible when the drug has been discontinued; however, the safety of the additive (or synergistic) effects on the kidney of the three antibiotics in combination apparently has not been studied.

Both Neomycin and polymyxin B may induce neuromuscular blockade and respiratory paralysis. In cats the blocks produced by these two antibiotics in combination are additive, not only in terms of potency and duration but also in terms of the characteristics of the block.

Oral Neomycin inhibits the gastrointestinal absorption of penicillin V, oral vitamin B-12, methotrexate and 5-fluorouracil. The gastrointestinal absorption of digoxin also appears to be inhibited. Therefore, digoxin serum levels should be monitored.

Oral Neomycin Sulfate may enhance the effect of coumarin in anticoagulants by decreasing vitamin K availability.

CARCINOGENESIS, MUTAGENESIS, IMPAIRMENT OF FERTILITY
No long-term animal studies have been performed with Neomycin Sulfate to evaluate carcinogenic or mutagenic potential or impairment of fertility.

PREGNANCY CATEGORY D
(See "Warnings" section.)

NURSING MOTHERS
It is not known whether Neomycin is excreted in human milk but it has been shown to be excreted in cow milk following a single intramuscular injection. Other aminoglycosides have been shown to be excreted in human milk. Because of the potential for serious adverse reactions from the aminoglycosides in nursing infants, a decision should be made whether to discontinue nursing or to discontinue the drug, taking into account the importance of the drug to the mother.

PEDIATRIC USE
The safety and efficacy of oral Neomycin Sulfate in patients less than eighteen years of age have not been established. If treatment of a patient less than eighteen years of age is necessary, Neomycin should be used with caution and the period of treatment should not exceed three weeks because of absorption from the gastrointestinal tract.

ADVERSE REACTIONS
The most common adverse reactions to oral Neomycin Sulfate are nausea, vomiting, and diarrhea. The "Malabsorption Syndrome" characterized by increased fecal fat, decreased serum carotene and fall in xylose absorption has been reported with prolonged therapy. Nephrotoxicity, ototoxicity, and neuromuscular blockage have been reported (see boxed "Warnings" and "Precautions" sections).

OVERDOSAGE
Because of low absorption, it is unlikely that acute overdosage would occur with oral Neomycin Sulfate. However, prolonged administration could result in sufficient systemic drug levels to produce neurotoxicity, ototoxicity, and/or nephrotoxicity.

Hemodialysis will remove Neomycin Sulfate from the blood.

DOSAGE AND ADMINISTRATION
To minimize the risk of toxicity use the lowest possible dose and the shortest possible treatment period to control the condition. Treatment for periods longer than three weeks may be associated with an increased risk of toxicity.

HEPATIC COMA
For use as an adjunct in the management of hepatic coma, the recommended dose is 4-12 g per day given in the following regimen:
1. Withdraw protein from diet. Avoid use of diuretic agents.
2. Give supportive therapy including blood products, as indicated.
3. Give Neomycin Sulfate oral solution in doses of 4 to 12 g of Neomycin Sulfate per day in divided doses. Treatment should be continued over a period of five to six days during which time protein should be returned incrementally to the diet.
4. If less potentially toxic drugs cannot be used for chronic hepatic insufficiency, Neomycin in doses of up to 4 g daily may be necessary. The risks for the development of Neomycin-induced toxicity progressively increase when treatment must be extended to preserve the life of a patient with hepatic encephalopathy who has failed to fully respond. Frequent periodic monitoring of these patients to ascertain the presence of drug toxicity is mandatory (see "Precautions"). Also, Neomycin serum concentrations should be monitored to avoid potentially toxic levels. The benefits to the patient should be weighed against the risks of nephrotoxicity, permanent ototoxicity and neuromuscular blockade following the accumulation of Neomycin in the tissues.

PREOPERATIVE PROPHYLAXIS FOR ELECTIVE COLORECTAL SURGERY
Three 1 gm doses of Neomycin are given concomitantly with three 1 gm doses of erythromycin base enteric-coated tablets on the third day of a three-day regimen to prepare the patient for gastrointestinal surgery. In this regimen, bisacodyl is given orally on the first day. On the second day, give 30 ml of a 50% magnesium sulfate solution at three equally spaced intervals and two or more evening enemas until no solid feces are returned. On the third day, two of the oral Neomycin and erythromycin doses should be given in the early afternoon one hour apart and the third dose should be given at bedtime. The rectum should be evacuated on the next day one-half hour before surgery.

For oral administration, Neomycin may be dissolved in suitable diluent. Appropriate buffers, diluents, and excipients may be added.

STORAGE
Store at controlled room temperature 15°-30° C (59°-86° F).

HOW SUPPLIED
SOLUTION: 125 MG/5 ML

BRAND/MANUFACTURER	NDC	SIZE	AWP
◆ **BRAND**			
MYCIFRADIN: Upjohn	00009-0513-02	480 ml	$28.80

For additional alternatives, turn to the section beginning on page 2859.

Neomycin Sulfate and Polymyxin B Sulfate

DESCRIPTION
Neomycin Sulfate/Polymyxin B Sulfate G.U. irrigant is a concentrated sterile antibiotic solution to be diluted for urinary bladder irrigation. Each ml contains Neomycin Sulfate equivalent to 40 mg Neomycin base, 200,000 units Polymyxin B Sulfate and water for injection. Neomycin Sulfate, an antibiotic of the aminoglycoside group, is the Sulfate salt of Neomycin B and C produced by *Streptomyces fradiae*. It has a potency equivalent to not less than 600 µg of Neomycin per mg.

Polymyxin B Sulfate, a polypeptide antibiotic, is the Sulfate salt of Polymyxin B_1 and B_2 produced by the growth of *Bacillus Polymyxa*. It has a potency of not less than 6,000 Polymyxin B units per mg.

CLINICAL PHARMACOLOGY
After prophylactic irrigation of the intact urinary bladder, Neomycin and Polymyxin B are absorbed in clinically insignificant quantities. A Neomycin serum level of 0.1 µg/ml was observed in three of 33 patients receiving the rinse solution. This level is well below that which has been associated with Neomycin-induced toxicity.

When used topically, Polymyxin B Sulfate and Neomycin are rarely irritating.

Microbiology: The prepared Neomycin/Polymyxin G.U. Irrigant Sterile solution is bactericidal. The aminoglycosides act by inhibiting normal protein synthesis in susceptible microorganisms. Polymyxins increase the permeability of bacterial cell wall membranes. The solution is active *in vitro* against
Escherichia coli
Staphylococcus aureus
Haemophilus influenzae
Klebsiella and *Enterobacter* species
Neisseria species, and *Pseudomonas aeruginosa*
It is not active *in vitro* against *Serratia marcescens* and streptococci.

Bacterial resistance may develop following the use of the antibiotics in the catheter-rinse solution.

INDICATIONS AND USAGE
Neomycin/Polymyxin G.U. irrigant is indicated for short-term use (up to 10 days) as a continuous irrigant or rinse in the urinary bladder of abacteriuric patients to help prevent bacteriuria and gram-negative rod septicemia associated with the use of indwelling catheters.

Since organisms gain entrance to the bladder by way of, through, and around the catheter, significant bacteriuria is induced by bacterial multiplication in the bladder urine, in the mucoid film often present between catheter and urethra, and in other sites. Urinary tract infection may result from the repeated presence in the urine of large numbers of pathogenic bacteria. The use of closed systems with indwelling catheters has been shown to reduce the risk of infection. A three-way closed catheter system with constant Neomycin/Polymyxin bladder rinse is indicated to prevent the development of infection while using indwelling catheters.

If uropathogens are isolated, they should be identified and tested for susceptibility so that appropriate antimicrobial therapy for systemic use can be initiated.

CONTRAINDICATIONS
Hypersensitivity to Neomycin, the Polymyxins, or any ingredient in the solution is a contraindication to its use. A history of hypersensitivity or serious toxic reaction to an amino-glycoside may also contraindicate the use of any other aminoglycoside because of the known cross-sensitivity of patients to drugs of this class.

WARNINGS
PROPHYLACTIC BLADDER CARE WITH NEOMYCIN/POLYMYXIN G.U. IRRIGANT STERILE SHOULD NOT BE GIVEN WHERE THERE IS A POSSIBILITY OF SYSTEMIC ABSORPTION. NEOMYCIN/POLYMYXIN G.U. IRRIGANT STERILE SHOULD NOT BE USED FOR IRRIGATION OTHER THAN FOR THE URINARY BLADDER. Systemic absorption after topical application of Neomycin to open wounds, burns, and granulating surfaces is significant and serum concentrations comparable to and often higher than those attained following oral and parenteral therapy have been reported. Absorption of Neomycin from the denuded bladder surface has been reported.

However, the likelihood of toxicity following topical irrigation of the intact urinary bladder with Neomycin/Polymyxin G.U. irrigant sterile is low since no appreciable amounts of these antibiotics enter the systemic circulation by this route if irrigation does not exceed ten days.

Neomycin/Polymyxin G.U. irrigant is intended for continuous prophylactic irrigation of the lumen of the intact urinary bladder of patients with indwelling catheters. Patients should be under constant supervision by a physician. Irrigation

---

◆ RATED THERAPEUTICALLY EQUIVALENT; ◇ THERAPEUTIC EQUIVALENCE UNCONFIRMED; ○ UNRATED

should be avoided in patients with defects in the bladder mucosa or bladder wall, such as vesical rupture, or in association with operative procedures on the bladder wall, because of the risk of toxicity due to systemic absorption following diffusion into absorptive tissues and spaces. When absorbed, Neomycin and Polymyxin B are nephrotoxic antibiotics, and the nephrotoxic potentials are additive. In addition, both antibiotics, when absorbed, are neurotoxins: Neomycin can destroy fibers of the acoustic nerve causing permanent bilateral deafness; Neomycin and Polymyxin B are additive in their neuromuscular blocking effects, not only in terms of potency and duration but also in terms of characteristics of the blocks produced.

Aminoglycosides, when absorbed, can cause fetal harm when administered to a pregnant woman. Aminoglycoside antibiotics cross the placenta and there have been several reports of total, irreversible, bilateral, congenital deafness in children whose mothers received streptomycin during pregnancy. Although serious side effects have not been reported in the treatment of pregnant women with other aminoglycosides, the potential for harm exists. If Neomycin/Polymyxin G.U. irrigant sterile is used during pregnancy, the patient should be apprised of the potential hazard to the fetus (see *"Precautions"*).

PRECAUTIONS

General: Ototoxicity, nephrotoxicity, and neuromuscular blockade may occur if Neomycin/Polymyxin G.U. irrigant ingredients are systemically absorbed (see *"Warnings"*). Absorption of Neomycin from the denuded bladder surface has been reported. Patients with impaired renal function, infants, dehydrated patients, elderly patients, and patients receiving high doses of prolonged treatment are especially at risk for the development of toxicity.

Irrigation of the bladder with Neomycin/Polymyxin G.U. irrigant may result in overgrowth of nonsusceptible organisms, including fungi. Appropriate measures should be taken if this occurs. The safety and effectiveness of the preparation for use in the care of patients with recent lower urinary tract surgery have not been established.

Urine specimens should be collected during prophylactic bladder care for urinalysis, culture, and susceptibility testing. Positive cultures suggest the presence of organisms which are resistant to the bladder rinse antibiotics.

Pregnancy: Teratogenic Effects: Pregnancy Category D. (See *"Warnings"* section.)

ADVERSE REACTIONS

Neomycin occasionally causes skin sensitization when applied topically; however, topical application to mucus membranes rarely results in local or systemic hypersensitivity reactions.

Irritation of the urinary bladder mucosa has been reported. Signs of ototoxicity and nephrotoxicity have been reported following parenteral use of these drugs and following the oral and topical use of Neomycin (see *"Warnings"*).

DOSAGE AND ADMINISTRATION

This preparation is specifically designed for use with "three-way" catheters or with other catheter systems permitting *continuous* irrigation of the urinary bladder. The usual irrigation dose is one 1-ml ampul a day for up to ten days.

Using strict aseptic techniques, the contents of one 1-ml ampul of Neomycin Sulfate/Polymyxin B Sulfate solution for irrigation should be added to a 1,000 ml container of isotonic saline solution. This container should then be connected to the inflow lumen of the "three-way" catheter which has been inserted with full aseptic precautions; use of a sterile lubricant is recommended during insertion of the catheter. The outflow lumen should be connected, via a sterile disposable plastic tube, to a disposable plastic collection bag. Stringent procedures, such as taping the inflow and outflow junction at the catheter, should be observed when necessary to insure the junctional integrity of the system.

For most patients, the inflow rate of the 1,000 ml saline solution of Neomycin and Polymyxin B should be adjusted to a slow drip to deliver about 1,000 ml every twenty-four hours. If the patient's urine output exceeds 2 liters per day, it is recommended that the inflow rate be adjusted to deliver 2,000 ml of the solution in a twenty-four hour period.

It is important that the rinse of the bladder be *continuous*; the inflow or rinse solution should not be interrupted for more than a few minutes.

Preparation of the irrigation solution should be performed with strict aseptic techniques. The prepared solution should be stored at 4°C, and should be used within 48 hours following preparation to reduce the risk of contamination with resistant microorganisms.

Store at 2° to 8°C (36° to 46°F).

HOW SUPPLIED
SOLUTION: 40 MG/ML-200,000 U/ML

AVERAGE UNIT PRICE (AVAILABLE SIZES)

BRAND	$4.82
GENERIC	$2.29

BRAND/MANUFACTURER	NDC	SIZE	AWP
◆ BRAND			
NEOSPORIN G.U. IRRIGANT: Burr Wellcome	00081-0748-93	20 ml	$66.11
	00081-0748-10	1 ml 10s	$56.84
	00081-0748-35	1 ml 50s	$273.90

BRAND/MANUFACTURER	NDC	SIZE	AWP
◆ GENERICS			
Schein	00364-2191-55	20 ml	$36.15
Schein	00364-2190-41	1 ml 25s	$69.50

Neomycin Sulfate / Polymyxin B Sulfate, Irrigant

DESCRIPTION

Neomycin Sulfate/Polymyxin B Sulfate, Irrigant is a concentrated sterile antibiotic solution to be diluted for urinary bladder irrigation. Each mL contains Neomycin Sulfate equivalent to 40 mg Neomycin base, 200,000 units Polymyxin B Sulfate and water for injection. The 20-mL multiple-dose vial contains, in addition to the above, 1 mg methylparaben (0.1%) added as a preservative. Neomycin Sulfate, an antibiotic of the aminoglycoside group, is the Sulfate salt of Neomycin B and C produced by *Streptomyces fradiae*. It has a potency equivalent to not less than 600 µg of Neomycin per mg.

Polymyxin B Sulfate, a polypeptide antibiotic, is the Sulfate salt of Polymyxin B_1 and B_2 produced by the growth of *Bacillus polymyxa*. It has a potency of not less than 6,000 Polymyxin B units per mg.

CLINICAL PHARMACOLOGY

After prophylatic irrigation of the intact urinary bladder, Neomycin and Polymyxin B are absorbed in clinically insignificant quantities. A Neomycin serum level of 0.1 µg/ml was observed in three of 33 patients receiving the rinse solution. This level is well below that which has been associated with Neomycin-induced toxicity.

When used topically, Polymyxin B Sulfate and Neomycin are rarely irritating.

Microbiology: The prepared Neomycin Sulfate/Polymyxin B Sulfate Sterile solution is bactericidal. The aminoglycosides act by inhibiting normal protein synthesis in susceptible microorganisms. Polymyxins increase the permeability of bacterial cell wall membranes. The solution is active *in vitro* against:

Escherichia coli
Staphylococcus aureus
Haemophilus influenzae
Klebsiella and Enterobacter species
Neisseria species, and
Pseudomonas aeruginosa

It is not active *in vitro* against *Serratia marcescens* and streptococci.

Bacterial resistance may develop following the use of the antibiotics in the catheter-rinse solution.

INDICATIONS AND USAGE

Neomycin Sulfate/Polymyxin B Sulfate is indicated for short-term use (up to 10 days) as a continuous irrigant or rinse in the urinary bladder of abacteriuric patients to help prevent bacteriuria and gram-negative rod septicemia associated with the use of indwelling catheters.

Since organisms gain entrance to the bladder by way of, through, and around the catheter, significant bacteriuria is induced by bacterial multiplication in the bladder urine, in the mucoid film often present between catheter and urethra, and in other sites. Urinary tract infection may result from the repeated presence in the urine of large numbers of pathogenic bacteria. The use of closed systems with indwelling catheters has been shown to reduce the risk of infection. A three-way closed catheter system with constant Neomycin-Polymyxin B bladder rinse is indicated to prevent the development of infection while using indwelling catheters.

If uropathogens are isolated, they should be identified and tested for susceptibility so that appropriate antimicrobial therapy for systemic use can be initiated.

CONTRAINDICATIONS

Hypersensitivity to Neomycin, the Polymyxins, or any ingredient in the solution is a contraindication to its use. A history of hypersensitivity or serious toxic reaction to an aminoglycoside may also contraindicate the use of any other aminoglycoside because of the known cross-sensitivity of patients to drugs of this class.

WARNINGS

PROPHYLACTIC BLADDER CARE WITH NEOMYCIN SULFATE/POLYMYXIN B SULFATE STERILE IRRIGANT SHOULD NOT BE GIVEN WHERE THERE IS A POSSIBILITY OF SYSTEMIC ABSORPTION. NEOMYCIN SULFATE/POLYMYXIN B SULFATE STERILE IRRIGANT SHOULD NOT BE USED FOR IRRIGATION OTHER THAN FOR THE URINARY BLADDER. Systemic absorption after topical application of Neomycin to open wounds, burns, and granulating surfaces is significant and serum concentrations comparable to and often higher than those attained following oral and parenteral therapy have been reported. Absorption of Neomycin from the denuded bladder surface has been reported.

However, the likelihood of toxicity following topical irrigation of the intact urinary bladder with Neomycin Sulfate/Polymyxin B Sulfate Sterile is low since no appreciable amounts of these antibiotics enter the systemic circulation by this route if irrigation does not exceed ten days.

➤ SHOWN IN PRODUCT IDENTIFICATION GUIDE

Neomycin Sulfate/Polymyxin B Sulfate Irrigant is intended for continuous prophylactic irrigation of the lumen of the intact urinary bladder of patients with indwelling catheters. Patients should be under constant supervision by a physician. Irrigation should be avoided in patients with defects in the bladder mucosa or bladder wall, such as vesical rupture, or in association with operative procedures on the bladder wall, because of the risk of toxicity due to systemic absorption following diffusion into absorptive tissues and spaces. When absorbed, Neomycin and Polymyxin B are nephrotoxic antibiotics, and the nephrotoxic potentials are additive. In addition, both antibiotics, when absorbed, are neurotoxins: Neomycin can destroy fibers of the acoustic nerve causing permanent bilateral deafness; Neomycin and Polymyxin B are additive in their neuromuscular blocking effects, not only in terms of potency and duration but also in terms of characteristics of the blocks produced.

Aminoglycosides, when absorbed, can cause fetal harm when administered to a pregnant woman. Aminoglycoside antibiotics cross the placenta and there have been several reports of total, irreversible, bilateral, congenital deafness in children whose mothers received streptomycin during pregnancy. Although serious side effects have not been reported in the treatment of pregnant women with other aminoglycosides, the potential for harm exists. If Neomycin Sulfate/Polymyxin B Sulfate Sterile is used during pregnancy, the patient should be apprised of the potential hazard to the fetus (see "Precautions").

PRECAUTIONS

General: Ototoxicity, nephrotoxicity, and neuromuscular blockade may occur if Neomycin Sulfate/Polymyxin B Sulfate ingredients are systemically absorbed (see "Warnings"). Absorption of Neomycin from the denuded bladder surface has been reported. Patients with impaired renal function, infants, dehydrated patients, elderly patients, and patients receiving high doses of prolonged treatment are especially at risk for the development of toxicity.

Irrigation of the bladder with Neomycin Sulfate/Polymyxin B Sulfate may result in overgrowth of nonsusceptible organisms, including fungi. Appropriate measures should be taken if this occurs. The safety and effectiveness of the preparation for use in the care of patients with recent lower urinary tract surgery have not been established.

Urine specimens should be collected during prophylactic bladder care for urinalysis, culture, and susceptibility testing. Positive cultures suggest the presence of organisms which are resistant to the bladder rinse antibiotics.

Pregnancy: Teratogenic Effects: Pregnancy Category D. (See "Warnings" section.)

ADVERSE REACTIONS

Neomycin occasionally causes skin sensitization when applied topically; however, topical application to mucus membranes rarely results in local or systemic hypersensitivity reactions.

Irritation of the urinary bladder mucosa has been reported. Signs of ototoxicity and nephrotoxicity have been reported following parenteral use of these drugs and following the oral and topical use of Neomycin (see "Warnings").

DOSAGE AND ADMINISTRATION

This preparation is specifically designed for use with "three-way" catheters or with other catheter systems permitting *continuous* irrigation of the urinary bladder. The usual irrigation dose is one 1-ml ampul a day for up to ten days.

Using strict aseptic techniques, the contents of one 1-ml ampul of Neomycin Sulfate/Polymyxin B Sulfate Sterile should be added to a 1,000-mL container of isotonic saline solution. This container should then be connected to the inflow lumen of the "three-way" catheter which has been inserted with full aseptic precautions: use of a sterile lubricant is recommended during insertion of the catheter. The outflow lumen should be connected, via a sterile disposable plastic tube, to a disposable plastic collection bag. Stringent procedures, such as taping the inflow and outflow junction at the catheter, should be observed when necessary to insure the junctional integrity of the system.

For most patients, the inflow rate of the 1,000-mL saline solution of Neomycin and Polymyxin B should be adjusted to a slow drip to deliver about 1,000 mL every twenty-four hours. If the patient's urine output exceeds 2 liters per day, it is recommended that the inflow rate be adjusted to deliver 2,000 mL of the solution in a twenty-four hour period.

It is important that the rinse of the bladder be **continuous**; the inflow or rinse solution should not be interrupted for more than a few minutes.

Preparation of the irrigation solution should be performed with strict aseptic techniques. The prepared solution should be stored at 4°C, and should be used within 48 hours following preparation to reduce the risk of contamination with resistant microorganisms.

Store at 2° to 8°C (36° to 46°F).

HOW SUPPLIED
SOLUTION: 40 MG/ML-200,000 U/ML

AVERAGE UNIT PRICE (AVAILABLE SIZES)

BRAND	$4.82
GENERIC	$2.29

BRAND/MANUFACTURER	NDC	SIZE	AWP
◆ **BRAND**			
NEOSPORIN G.U. IRRIGANT: Burr Wellcome	00081-0748-93	20 ml	$66.11
	00081-0748-10	1 ml 10s	$56.84
	00081-0748-35	1 ml 50s	$273.90

BRAND/MANUFACTURER	NDC	SIZE	AWP
◆ **GENERICS**			
Schein	00364-2191-55	20 ml	$36.15
Schein	00364-2190-41	1 ml 25s	$69.50

Neomycin Sulfate/Polymyxin B Sulfate/Prednisolone Acetate

DESCRIPTION

Neomycin Sulfate/Polymyxin B Sulfate/Prednisolone Acetate sterile ophthalmic suspension is a topical anti-inflammatory/anti-infective combination product for ophthalmic use.

Chemical Name: Prednisolone Acetate: 11β, 17, 21-Trihydroxypregna-1, 4-diene-3, 20-dione 21-acetate.

Neomycin Sulfate is the Sulfate salt of Neomycin B and Neomycin C which are produced by the growth of *Streptomyces fradiae* (Fam. *Streptomycetaceae*). It has a potency equivalent to not less than 600 micrograms per milligram of Neomycin base, calculated on an anhydrous basis.

Polymyxin B Sulfate is the Sulfate salt of Polymyxin B_1 and Polymyxin B_2 which are produced by the growth of *Bacillus polymyxa* (Prazmowski) Migula (Fam. *Bacillaceae*). It has a potency of not less than 6,000 Polymyxin B units per milligram, calculated on an anhydrous basis.

Contains:

Neomycin Sulfate	equivalent to 0.35% Neomycin Base
Polymyxin B Sulfate	10,000 units/mL
Prednisolone Acetate (microfine suspension)	0.5%

CLINICAL PHARMACOLOGY

Corticosteroids suppress the inflammatory response to a variety of agents and they probably delay or slow healing. Since corticosteroids may inhibit the body's defense mechanism against infection, a concomitant antimicrobial drug may be used when this inhibition is considered to be clinically significant in a particular case.

The anti-infective components in Neomycin Sulfate/Polymyxin B Sulfate and Prednisolone Acetate are included to provide action against specific organisms susceptible to them. Neomycin Sulfate and Polymyxin B Sulfate are considered active against the following microorganisms: *Staphylococcus aureus; Escherichia coli; Haemophilus influenzae; Klebsiella/Enterobacter* species; *Neisseria* species; and *Pseudomonas aeruginosa.*

When a decision to administer both a corticosteroid and an antimicrobial is made, the administration of such drugs in combination has the advantage of greater patient compliance and convenience, with the added assurance that the appropriate dosage of both drugs is administered. When both types of drugs are in the same formulation, compatibility of ingredients is assured and the correct volume of drug is delivered and retained.

The relative potency of corticosteroids depends on the molecular structure, concentration and release from the vehicle.

INDICATIONS AND USAGE

A steroid/anti-infective combination is indicated for steroid-responsive inflammatory ocular conditions for which a corticosteroid is indicated and where bacterial infection or a risk of bacterial ocular infection exists.

Ocular steroids are indicated in inflammatory conditions of the palpebral and bulbar conjunctiva, cornea, and anterior segment of the globe where the inherent risk of steroid use in certain infective conjunctivitides is accepted to obtain a diminution in edema and inflammation. They are also indicated in chronic anterior uveitis and corneal injury from chemical, radiation or thermal burns or penetration of foreign bodies.

The use of a combination drug with an anti-infective component is indicated where the risk of infection is high or where there is an expectation that potentially dangerous numbers of bacteria will be present in the eye.

The particular anti-infective drugs in this product are active against the following common bacterial eye pathogens: *Staphylococcus aureus; Escherichia coli; Haemophilus influenzae; Klebsiella/Enterobacter* species; *Neisseria* species; and *Pseudomonas aeruginosa.*

The product does not provide adequate coverage against: *Serratia marcescens;* Streptococci, including *Streptococcus pneumoniae.*

CONTRAINDICATIONS

Epithelial herpes simplex keratitis (dendritic keratitis), vaccinia, varicella, and many other viral diseases of the cornea and conjunctiva. Mycobacterial infection of the eye. Fungal diseases of the ocular structures. Hypersensitivity to a component of the medication. (Hypersensitivity to the antibiotic component occurs at a higher rate than for other components.)

The use of these combinations is always contraindicated after uncomplicated removal of a corneal foreign body.

WARNINGS

Prolonged use may result in glaucoma, with damage to the optic nerve, defects in visual acuity and fields of vision, and in posterior subcapsular cataract formation. Prolonged use may suppress the host response and thus increase the hazard of secondary ocular infections. In those diseases causing thinning of the cornea or sclera, perforations have been known to occur with the use of topical steroids. In acute purulent conditions of the eye, steroids may mask infection or enhance existing infection. If these products are used for 10 days or longer, intraocular pressure should be routinely monitored even though it may be difficult in children and uncooperative patients.

Employment of a steroid medication in the treatment of herpes simplex requires great caution.

There exists a potential for Neomycin to cause cutaneous sensitization. The exact incidence of this reaction is unknown.

PRECAUTIONS
The initial prescription and renewal of the medication order beyond 20 milliliters should be made by a physician only after examination of the patient with the aid of magnification, such as slit lamp biomicroscopy and, where appropriate, fluorescein staining. The possibility of persistent fungal infections of the cornea should be considered after prolonged steroid dosing.

ADVERSE REACTIONS
Adverse reactions have occurred with steroid/anti-infective combination drugs which can be attributed to the steroid component, the anti-infective component, or the combination. Exact incidence figures are not available since no denominator of treated patients is available.

Reactions occurring most often from the presence of the anti-infective ingredients are allergic sensitizations. The reactions due to the steroid component in decreasing order of frequency are: elevation of intraocular pressure (IOP) with possible development of glaucoma, and infrequent optic nerve damage; posterior subcapsular cataract formation; and delayed wound healing.

Secondary Infection: The development of secondary infection has occurred after use of combinations containing steroids and antimicrobials. Fungal infections of the cornea are particularly prone to develop coincidentally with long-term applications of steroid. The possibility of fungal invasion must be considered in any persistent corneal ulceration where steroid treatment has been used.

Secondary bacterial ocular infection following suppression of host responses also occurs.

DOSAGE AND ADMINISTRATION
To Treat The Eye: 1 or 2 drops every 3 or 4 hours, or more frequently as required. Acute infections may require administration every 30 minutes, with frequency of administration reduced as the infection is brought under control.

To Treat The Lids: Instill 1 or 2 drops in the eye every 3 to 4 hours, close the eye and rub the excess on the lids and lid margins.

Not more than 20 milliliters should be prescribed initially and the prescription should not be refilled without further evaluation as outlined in the *"Precautions"* section above.

Note: Protect from freezing. Shake well before using.

HOW SUPPLIED
DROP: 0.35%-10,000 U-0.5%

BRAND/MANUFACTURER	NDC	SIZE	AWP
○ **BRAND**			
POLY PRED: Allergan Optical	00023-0028-05	5 ml	$16.18
	00023-0028-10	10 ml	$24.99

Neosar *SEE* CYCLOPHOSPHAMIDE

Neosporin *SEE* BACITRACIN ZINC/NEOMYCIN SULFATE/ POLYMYXIN B SULFATE, OPHTHALMIC *AND* GRAMICIDIN/NEOMYCIN SULFATE/POLYMYXIN B SULFATE, OPHTHALMIC

Neosporin G.U. Irrigant *SEE* NEOMYCIN SULFATE AND POLYMYXIN B SULFATE *AND* NEOMYCIN SULFATE AND POLYMYXIN B SULFATE, IRRIGANT

Neostigmine

DESCRIPTION
Neostigmine Injectable, an anticholinesterase agent, is a sterile aqueous solution intended for intramuscular, intravenous or subcutaneous administration. Neostigmine Injectable is available in the following concentrations:

Neostigmine *1:200 Ampuls*— each ml contains 0.5 Neostigmine Methylsulfate.
Neostigmine *1:4000 Ampuls*— each ml contains 0.25 mg Neostigmine Methylsulfate.
Neostigmine *1:1000 Multiple Dose Vials*— each ml contains 1 mg Neostigmine Methylsulfate.
Neostigmine *1:2000 Multiple Dose Vials*— each ml contains 0.5 mg Neostigmine Methylsulfate.

Neostigmine Bromide is available for oral administration in 15-mg tablets.

Chemically, Neostigmine Bromide Methylsulfate is (*m*-hydroxyphenyl)trimethylammonium methylsulfate dimethylcarbamate. It has a molecular weight of 334.39.

Chemically, Neostigmine Bromide is (*m*-hydroxyphenyl) trimethylammonium bromide dimethylcarbamate. It is a white, crystalline, bitter powder, soluble 1:1 in water, with a molecular weight of 303.20

CLINICAL PHARMACOLOGY
Neostigmine inhibits the hydrolysis of acetylcholine by competing with acetylcholine for attachment to acetylcholinesterase at sites of cholinergic transmission. It enhances cholinergic action by facilitating the transmission of impulses across neuromuscular junctions. It also has a direct cholinomimetic effect on skeletal muscle and possibly on autonomic ganglion cells and neurons of the central nervous system. Neostigmine undergoes hydrolysis by cholinesterase and is also metabolized by microsomal enzymes in the liver. Protein binding to human serum albumin ranges from 15 to 25 percent.

Following intramuscular administration, Neostigmine is rapidly absorbed and eliminated. In a study of five patients with myasthenia gravis, peak plasma levels were observed at 30 minutes, and the half-life ranged from 51 to 90 minutes. Approximately 80 percent of the drug was eliminated in urine within 24 hours; approximately 50% as the unchanged drug, and 30 percent as metabolites. Following intravenous administration, plasma half-life ranges from 47 to 60 minutes have been reported with a mean half-life of 53 minutes.

The clinical effects of Neostigmine usually begin within 20 to 30 minutes after intramuscular injection and last from 2.5 to 4 hours.

Neostigmine Bromide is poorly absorbed from the gastrointestinal tract following oral administration. As a rule, 15 mg of Neostigmine Bromide orally is equivalent to 0.5 mg of Neostigmine Methylsulfate parenterally, due to poor absorption of the tablet from the intestinal tract. In a study in fasting myasthenic patients, the extent of absorption was estimated to be 1 to 2 percent of the ingested 30-mg single oral dose. Peak concentrations in plasma occurred 1 to 2 hours following drug ingestion, with considerable individual variations. The half-life ranged from 42 to 60 minutes with a mean half-life or 52 minutes.

INDICATIONS AND USAGE
Neostigmine Methylsulfate Injectable is indicated for:

—the symptomatic control of myasthenia gravis when oral therapy is impractical.
—the prevention and treatment of postoperative distention and urinary retention after mechanical obstruction has been excluded.
—reversal of effects of nondepolarizing neuromuscular blocking agents (*e.g.*, tubocurarine, metocurine, gallamine, or pancuronium) after surgery.

Oral Neostigmine is indicated for the symptomatic treatment of myasthenia gravis. Its greatest usefulness is in prolonged therapy where no difficulty in swallowing is present. In acute myasthenic crisis where difficulty in breathing and swallowing is present, the parenteral form (Neostigmine Methylsulfate) should be used. The patient can be transferred to the oral form as soon as it can be tolerated.

CONTRAINDICATIONS
Neostigmine is contraindicated in patients with known hypersensitivity to the drug. It is also contraindicated in patients with peritonitis or mechanical obstruction of the intestinal or urinary tract. Because of the presence of the bromide ion, oral Neostigmine should not be used in patients with a previous history of reaction to bromides.

WARNINGS
Neostigmine should be used with caution in patients with epilepsy, bronchial asthma, bradycardia, recent coronary occlusion, vagotonia, hyperthyroidism, cardiac arrhythmias or peptic ulcer. When large doses of Neostigmine Injectable are administered, the prior or simultaneous injection of atropine sulfate may be advisable. Separate syringes should be used for the Neostigmine Injectable and atropine. Because of the possibility of hypersensitivity in an occasional patient, atropine and antishock medication should always be readily available.

Large doses of oral Neostigmine should be avoided in situations where there might be an increased absorption rate from the intestinal tract. It should be used with caution when co-administered with anticholinergic drugs, in order to avoid reduction of intestinal motility.

PRECAUTIONS
General: It is important to differentiate between myasthenic crisis and cholinergic crisis caused by overdosage of Neostigmine. Both conditions result in extreme muscle weakness but require radically different treatment (See *"Overdosage"* section).

Drug Interactions: Neostigmine Injectable does not antagonize, and may in fact prolong, the Phase I block of *deparizing* muscle relaxants such as succinylchline or decamethonium. Certain antibiotics, especially neomycin, streptomycin and kanamycin, have a mild but definite nondepolarizing blocking action which may accentuate neuromuscular block. These antibiotics should be used in the myasthenic patient only where definitely indicated, and then careful adjustment should be made of adjunctive anticholinesterase dosage. Local and some general anesthetics, antiarrhythmic agents and other drugs that interfere with neuromuscular transmission should be used cautiously, if at all, in patients with myasthenia gravis; the dose of Neostigmine may have to be increased accordingly.

Carcinogenesis, Mutagenesis and Impairment of Fertility: There have been no studies with Neostigmine which would permit an evaluation of its carcinogenic or mutagenic potential. Studies on the effect of Neostigmine on fertility and reproduction have not been performed.

Pregnancy: Teratogenic Effects: Pregnancy Category C. There are no adequate or well-controlled studies of Neostigmine in either laboratory animals or in pregnant women. It is not known whether Neostigmine can cause fetal harm when administered to a pregnant woman or can affect reproductive capacity. Neostigmine should be given to a pregnant woman only if clearly needed.

Nonteratogenic Effects: Anticholinesterase drugs may cause uterine irritability and induce premature labor when given intravenously to pregnant women near term.

Nursing Mothers: It is not known whether Neostigmine is excreted in human milk. Because many drugs are excreted in human milk and because of the potential for serious adverse reactions from Neostigmine in nursing infants, a decision should be made whether to discontinue nursing or to discontinue the drug, taking into account the importance of the drug to the mother.

Pediatric Use: Safety and effectiveness in children have not been established.

ADVERSE REACTIONS

Side effects are generally due to an exaggeration of pharmacological effects of which salivation and fasciculation are the most common. Bowel cramps and diarrhea may also occur. The following additional adverse reactions have been reported following the use of either Neostigmine Bromide or Neostigmine Methylsulfate:

Allergic: Allergic reactions and anaphylaxis.

Neurologic: Dizziness, convulsions, loss of consciousness, drowsiness, headache, dysarthria, miosis and visual changes.

Cardiovascular: Cardiac arrhythmias (including bradycardia, tachycardia, A-V block and nodal rhythm) and nonspecific EKG changes have been reported, as well as cardiac arrest, syncope and hypotension. These have been predominantly noted following the use of the injectable form of Prostigmin.

Respiratory: Increased oral, pharyngeal and bronchial secretions, and dyspnea. Respiratory depression, respiratory arrest and bronchospasm have been reported following the use of the injectable form of Neostigmine.

Dermatologic: Rash and urticaria.

Gastrointestinal: Nausea, emesis, flatulence and increased peristalsis.

Genitourinary: Urinary frequency.

Musculoskeletal: Muscle cramps and spasms, arthralgia.

Miscellaneous: Diaphoresis, flushing and weakness.

OVERDOSAGE

Overdosage of Neostigmine can cause cholinergic crisis, which is characterized by increasing muscle weakness, and through involvement of the muscles of respiration, may result in death. Myasthenic crisis, due to an increase in the severity of the disease, is also accompanied by extreme muscle weakness and may be difficult to distinguish from cholinergic crisis on a symptomatic basis. However, such differentiation is extremely important because increases in the dose of Neostigmine or other drugs in this class, in the presence of cholinergic crisis or of a refractory or "insensitive" state, could have grave consequences. The two types of crises may be differentiated by the use of edrophonium chloride as well as by clinical judgment.

Treatment of the two conditions differs radically. Whereas the presence of *myasthenic crisis* requires more intensive anticholinesterase therapy, *cholinergic crisis* calls for the prompt withdrawal of all drugs of this type. The immediate use of atropine in cholinergic crisis is also recommended. Atropine may also be used to abolish or minimize gastrointestinal side effects or other muscarinic reactions; but such use, by masking signs of overdosage, can lead to inadvertent induction of cholinergic crisis.

The LD$_{50}$ of Neostigmine Methylsulfate in mice is 0.3 ± 0.02 mg/kg intravenously, 0.54 ± 0.03 mg/kg subcutaneously, and 0.395 ± 0.025 mg/kg intramuscularly; in rats the LD$_{50}$ is 0.315 ± 0.019 mg/kg intravenously, 0.445 ± 0.032 mg/kg subcutaneously, and 0.423 ± 0.032 mg/kg intramuscularly.

DOSAGE AND ADMINISTRATION

INJECTABLE NEOSTIGMINE

Symptomatic Control of Myasthenia Gravis: One ml of the 1:2000 solution (0.5 mg) subcutaneously or intramuscularly. Subsequent doses should be based on the individual patient's response. In most patients, however, oral treatment with Neostigmine Bromide tablets, 15 mg each, is adequate for control of symptoms.

Prevention of Postoperative Distention and Urinary Retention: One ml of the 1:4000 solution (0.25 mg) subcutaneously or intramuscularly as soon as possible after operation; repeat every 4 to 6 hours for two or three days.

Treatment of Postoperative Distention: One ml of the 1:2000 solution (0.5 mg) subcutaneously or intramuscularly, as required.

Treatment of Urinary Retention: One ml of the 1:2000 solution (0.5 mg) subcutaneously or intramuscularly. If urination does not occur within an hour, the patient should be catheterized. After the patient has voided, or the bladder has been emptied, continue the 0.5 mg injections every three hours for at least 5 injections.

Reversal of Effects of Nondepolarizing Neuromuscular Blocking Agents: When Neostigmine is administered intravenously, it is recommended that atropine sulfate (0.6 to 1.2 mg) also be given intravenously using separate syringes. Some

authorities have recommended that the atropine be injected several minutes before the Neostigmine rather than concomitantly. The usual dose is 0.5 to 2 mg Neostigmine given by *slow* intravenous injection, repeated as required. Only in exceptional cases should the total dose of Neostigmine exceed 5 mg. It is recommended that the patient be well ventilated and a patent airway maintained until complete recovery of normal respiration is assured. The optimum time for administration of the drug is during hyperventilation when the carbon dioxide level of the blood is low. It should never be administered in the presence of high concentrations of halothane or cyclopropane. In cardiac cases and severely ill patients, it is advisable to titrate the exact dose of Neostigmine required, using a peripheral nerve stimulator device. In the presence of bradycardia, the pulse rate should be increased to about 80/minute with atropine before administering Neostigmine.

Parenteral drug products should be inspected visually for particulate matter and discoloration prior to administration, whenever solution and container permit.

The onset of action of Neostigmine given orally is slower than when given parenterally, but the duration of action is longer and the intensity of action more uniform. Dosage requirements for optimal results vary from 15 mg to 375 mg per day. In some instances it may be necessary to exceed these dosages, but the possibility of cholinergic crisis must be recognized. The average dose is 10 tablets (150 mg) administered over a 24-hour period. The interval between doses is of paramount importance. The dosage schedule should be adjusted for each patient and changed as the need arises. Frequently, therapy is required day and night. Larger portions of the total daily dose may be given at times when the patient is more prone to fatigue (afternoon, mealtimes, etc.). The patient should be encouraged to keep a daily record of his or her condition to assist the physician in determining an optimal therapeutic regimen.

J CODES
Up to 0.5 mg IM,IV,SC—J2710

HOW SUPPLIED

NEOSTIGMINE BROMIDE
TABLETS: 15 MG

BRAND/MANUFACTURER	NDC	SIZE	AWP
○ BRAND			
PROSTIGMIN BROMIDE: ICN	00187-3100-10	100s	$38.28

NEOSTIGMINE METHYLSULFATE
INJECTION: 0.25 MG/ML

BRAND/MANUFACTURER	NDC	SIZE	AWP
○ BRAND			
PROSTIGMIN: ICN	00187-3100-40	1 ml 10s	$14.10

INJECTION: 0.5 MG/ML

BRAND/MANUFACTURER	NDC	SIZE	AWP
○ BRAND			
PROSTIGMIN: ICN	00187-3101-30	1 ml 10s	$17.52
	00187-3104-60	10 ml 10s	$121.86
○ GENERICS			
Fujisawa	00469-3820-30	10 ml	$7.86

INJECTION: 1 MG/ML

BRAND/MANUFACTURER	NDC	SIZE	AWP
○ BRAND			
PROSTIGMIN: ICN	00187-3103-50	10 ml 10s	$160.80
○ GENERICS			
Fujisawa	00469-3830-30	10 ml	$10.37

Nephramine *SEE* AMINO ACIDS WITH ELECTROLYTES, INJECTABLE

Neptazane *SEE* METHAZOLAMIDE

Nesacaine *SEE* CHLOROPROCAINE HYDROCHLORIDE

◆ RATED THERAPEUTICALLY EQUIVALENT; ◇ THERAPEUTIC EQUIVALENCE UNCONFIRMED; ○ UNRATED

Netilmicin Sulfate

WARNINGS

PATIENTS TREATED WITH AMINOGLYCOSIDES SHOULD BE UNDER CLOSE CLINICAL OBSERVATION BECAUSE OF THE POTENTIAL TOXICITY ASSOCIATED WITH THE USE OF THESE DRUGS.

NETILMICIN HAS POTENT NEUROMUSCULAR BLOCKING POTENTIAL. NEUROMUSCULAR BLOCKADE AND RESPIRATORY PARALYSIS HAVE BEEN REPORTED IN ANIMALS RECEIVING NETILMICIN. THE POSSIBILITY OF THESE PHENOMENA OCCURRING IN MAN SHOULD BE CONSIDERED IF AMINOGLYCOSIDES ARE ADMINISTERED BY ANY ROUTE TO PATIENTS RECEIVING NEUROMUSCULAR BLOCKING AGENTS, SUCH AS SUCCINYLCHOLINE, TUBOCURARINE, OR DECAMETHONIUM, OR TO PATIENTS RECEIVING MASSIVE TRANSFUSIONS OF CITRATE-ANTICOAGULATED BLOOD. IF NEUROMUSCULAR BLOCKADE OCCURS, CALCIUM SALTS MAY LESSEN IT, BUT MECHANICAL RESPIRATORY ASSISTANCE MAY ALSO BE NECESSARY. AS WITH OTHER AMINOGLYCOSIDES, NETILMICIN SULFATE INJECTION IS POTENTIALLY NEPHROTOXIC. THE RISK IS GREATER IN PATIENTS WITH IMPAIRED RENAL FUNCTION, IN THOSE WHO RECEIVE HIGH DOSAGE OR PROLONGED THERAPY, AND IN THE ELDERLY.

NEUROTOXICITY MANIFESTED BY OTOTOXICITY, BOTH VESTIBULAR AND AUDITORY, CAN OCCUR IN PATIENTS TREATED WITH NETILMICIN, PRIMARILY IN THOSE WITH PREEXISTING RENAL DAMAGE AND IN PATIENTS TREATED WITH HIGHER DOSES AND/OR FOR LONGER PERIODS THAN RECOMMENDED. AMINOGLYCOSIDE-INDUCED OTOTOXICITY IS USUALLY IRREVERSIBLE. OTHER MANIFESTATIONS OF AMINOGLYCOSIDE-INDUCED NEUROTOXICITY INCLUDE NUMBNESS, SKIN TINGLING, MUSCLE TWITCHING, AND CONVULSIONS.

RENAL AND EIGHTH CRANIAL NERVE FUNCTIONS SHOULD BE CLOSELY MONITORED, ESPECIALLY IN PATIENTS WITH KNOWN OR SUSPECTED IMPAIRMENT OF RENAL FUNCTION EITHER AT ONSET OF THERAPY OR DURING THERAPY. URINE SHOULD BE EXAMINED FOR INCREASED EXCRETION OF PROTEIN, THE PRESENCE OF CELLS OR CASTS, AND DECREASED SPECIFIC GRAVITY. SERUM CREATININE CONCENTRATION OR BLOOD UREA NITROGEN SHOULD BE DETERMINED PERIODICALLY. A MORE PRECISE MEASURE OF GLOMERULAR FILTRATION RATE IS A CAREFULLY CONDUCTED DETERMINATION OF CREATININE CLEARANCE RATE OR, OFTEN MORE PRACTICALLY, AN ESTIMATE OF CREATININE CLEARANCE BASED ON PUBLISHED NOMOGRAMS OR EQUATIONS. (SEE *"DOSAGE AND ADMINISTRATION"*). WHEN FEASIBLE IT IS RECOMMENDED THAT SERIAL AUDIOGRAMS BE OBTAINED IN PATIENTS OLD ENOUGH TO BE TESTED, PARTICULARLY IN HIGH-RISK PATIENTS. THE DOSAGE OF NETILMICIN SHOULD BE REDUCED OR ADMINISTRATION DISCONTINUED IF EVIDENCE OF DRUG-INDUCED AUDITORY OR VESTIBULAR TOXICITY (DIZZINESS, VERTIGO, TINNITUS, NYSTAGMUS, OR HEARING LOSS) DEVELOPS DURING THERAPY. IF EVIDENCE OF NEPHROTOXICITY OCCURS, DOSAGE SHOULD BE ADJUSTED. (SEE *"DOSAGE AND ADMINISTRATION," "DOSAGE FOR IMPAIRED RENAL FUNCTION"*). AS WITH THE OTHER AMINOGLYCOSIDES, ON RARE OCCASIONS CHANGES IN RENAL AND EIGHTH CRANIAL NERVE FUNCTIONS MAY NOT BECOME MANIFEST UNTIL SOON AFTER COMPLETION OF THERAPY.

SERUM CONCENTRATIONS OF AMINOGLYCOSIDES SHOULD BE MONITORED WHEN FEASIBLE TO ASSURE ADEQUATE LEVELS AND TO AVOID POTENTIALLY TOXIC LEVELS. AFTER ADMINISTRATION OF AN APPROPRIATE DOSE OF NETILMICIN, PEAK SERUM CONCENTRATIONS OCCUR APPROXIMATELY 30 TO 60 MINUTES AFTER AN INTRAMUSCULAR INJECTION OR AT THE END OF A ONE HOUR INTRAVENOUS INFUSION. DOSAGE SHOULD BE ADJUSTED SO THAT PROLONGED PEAK SERUM CONCENTRATIONS ABOVE 16 MCG/ML ARE AVOIDED.

WHEN MONITORING TROUGH CONCENTRATIONS, DOSAGE SHOULD BE ADJUSTED SO THAT LEVELS ABOVE 4 MCG/ML ARE AVOIDED. EXCESSIVE PEAK AND/OR TROUGH SERUM CONCENTRATIONS OF AMINOGLYCOSIDES MAY INCREASE THE RISK OF RENAL AND EIGHTH CRANIAL NERVE TOXICITY. IN THE EVENT OF OVERDOSE OR TOXIC REACTIONS, HEMODIALYSIS MAY AID IN REMOVAL OF NETILMICIN FROM THE BLOOD, ESPECIALLY IF RENAL FUNCTION IS, OR BECOMES, COMPROMISED. REMOVAL OF NETIMICIN BY PERITONEAL DIALYSIS IS AT A RATE CONSIDERABLY LESS THAN BY HEMODIALYSIS.

CONCURRENT AND/OR SEQUENTIAL SYSTEMIC OR TOPICAL USE OF OTHER POTENTIALLY NEUROTOXIC AND/OR NEPHROTOXIC DRUGS, SUCH AS: CEPHALORIDINE, AMPHOTERICIN B, STREPTOMYCIN, KANAMYCIN, ACYCLOVIR, GENTAMICIN, TOBRAMYCIN, AMIKACIN, NEOMYCIN, VANCOMYCIN, BACITRACIN, POLYMIXIN B, COLISTIN, PAROMOMYCIN, VIOMYCIN, OR CISPLATIN SHOULD BE AVOIDED. THE CONCURRENT USE OF AMINOGLYCOSIDES WITH POTENT DIURETICS, SUCH AS ETHACRYNIC ACID OR FUROSEMIDE, SHOULD BE AVOIDED SINCE CERTAIN DIURETICS BY THEMSELVES MAY CAUSE OTOTOXICITY. IN ADDITION, WHEN ADMINISTERED INTRAVENOUSLY, DIURETICS MAY ENHANCE AMINOGLYCOSIDE TOXICITY BY ALTERING THE ANTIBIOTIC CONCENTRATION IN THE SERUM AND TISSUES. OTHER FACTORS WHICH MAY INCREASE PATIENT RISK OF TOXICITY ARE ADVANCED AGE AND DEHYDRATION.

DESCRIPTION

Netilmicin Sulfate Injection contains Netilmicin Sulfate, USP in clear, sterile aqueous solution with a pH range of 3.5 to 6.0 for intramuscular or intravenous administration. Netilmicin is a semisynthetic, water-soluble antibiotic of the aminoglycoside group, derived from sisomicin. Its chemical name is: O-3-Deoxy-4-C-methyl-3-(methylamino)-β-L-arabinopyranosyl-(1→4)-O-[2,6-diamino-2,3,4,6-tetradeoxy-α-D-*glycero*-hex-4-enopyranosyl-(1→6)]-2-deoxy-N^3-ethyl-L-streptamine sulfate (2:5) (salt).

Each ml of Netilmicin Sulfate Injection contains Netmicin Sulfate, USP equivalent to 100 mg Netilmicin: 10 mg benzyl alcohol as a preservative; 0.1 mg edetate disodium; 2.4 mg sodium metabisulfite; 0.8 mg sodium sulfite; and water for injection, q.s.

Following is its chemical structure:

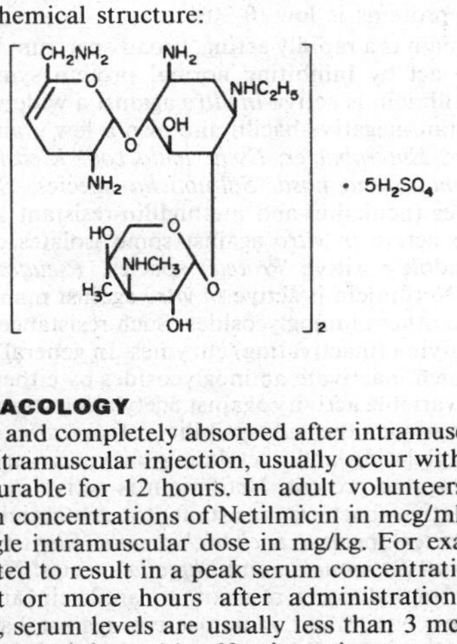

CLINICAL PHARMACOLOGY

Netilmicin is rapidly and completely absorbed after intramuscular injection. Peak serum levels, after intramuscular injection, usually occur within 30 to 60 minutes and levels are measurable for 12 hours. In adult volunteers with normal renal function, peak serum concentrations of Netilmicin in mcg/ml are usually about 3 to 3.5 times the single intramuscular dose in mg/kg. For example, a dose of 2.0 mg/kg may be expected to result in a peak serum concentration of approximately 7 mcg/ml. At eight or more hours after administration of a dose in the recommended range, serum levels are usually less than 3 mcg/ml. When a single dose of Netilmicin is administered by 60-minute intravenous infusion, the peak serum concentrations are similar to those obtained by intramuscular administration. Following a rapid intravenous injection of netilmicin, levels in serum may be transiently 2 to 3 times higher than those of the 60-minute infusion. Netilmicin rapidly distributes to tissues.

The half-life of Netilmicin after single doses is usually 2 to 2.5 hours, a half-life which is very similar to that of gentamicin, and is independent of the route of administration. The half-life increases as the dose increases (e.g., 2.2 hours after a 1 mg/kg dose to 3 hours after a 3 mg/kg dose). Approximately 80% of the administered dose is excreted in the urine within 24 hours; the urine netilmicin concentration after a dose often exceeds 100 mcg/ml. There is no evidence of metabolic transformation of Netilmicin. The drug is excreted principally by glomerular filtration. Probenecid does not affect renal tubular transport of aminoglycosides. The volume of distribution of Netilmicin is approximately 20% of body weight; total body clearance is about 80 ml/min and renal clearance is about 60 ml/min. In multiple-dose studies in volunteers when the drug was administered every 12 hours at doses ranging from 1.0 to 4.0 mg/kg, steady-state levels were obtained by the second day.

The serum levels at steady-state were less than 20% higher than those of the first dose. As with other aminoglycosides, the half-life of Netilmicin increases, and its renal clearance decreases with decreasing renal function.

The endogenous creatinine clearance rate and the serum creatinine level have a high correlation with the half-life of Netilmicin. Results of these tests can serve as a guide for adjusting dosage in patients with renal impairment.

In patients with marked impairment of renal function, there is a decrease in the concentration of aminoglycosides in urine and in their penetration into defective renal parenchyma. This should be considered when treating patients with urinary tract infections. In one study of adults with renal failure undergoing hemodialysis, Netilmicin serum levels were reduced by approximately 63% over an 8-hour dialysis session. Shorter dialysis sessions will remove less drug. No hemodialysis information is available for children. Aminoglycosides are also removed by peritoneal dialysis but at a rate considerably less than by hemodialysis.

Since Netilmicin is distributed in extracellular fluid, peak serum concentrations may be lower than usual in patients whose extracellular fluid volume is expanded (e.g., patients with edema or ascites). Serum concentrations of aminoglycosides in febrile patients may be lower than those in afebrile patients given the same dose. When body temperature returns to normal, serum

➤ SHOWN IN PRODUCT IDENTIFICATION GUIDE

concentrations of the drug may rise. Both febrile and anemic states may be associated with a shorter than usual half-life. (Dosage adjustment is usually not necessary.)

In severely burned patients, the half-life of aminoglycosides may be significantly decreased, and serum concentrations resulting from a particular dose may be lower than anticipated.

The elimination half-life of Netilmicin in neonates during the first week of life is inversely correlated with body weight, ranging from approximately 8 hours for neonates weighing 1.5 to 2.0 kg to approximately 4.5 hours for 3.0 to 4.0 kg neonates. The elimination half-life of infants and children 6 weeks of age and older is 1.5 to 2.0 hours.

Following parenteral administration, aminoglycosides can be detected in serum, tissues, and sputum and in pericardial, pleural, synovial, and peritoneal fluids. A variety of methods are available to measure Netilmicin concentrations in body fluids; these include microbiologic, enzymatic, and radioimmunoassay techniques. Concentrations in renal cortex may be markedly higher than the usual serum levels.

Minute quantities of aminoglycosides have been detected in the urine for up to 30 days after discontinuing administration. Hepatic secretion is minimal. As with all aminoglycosides, Netilmicin diffuses poorly into the subarachnoid space after parenteral administration. Concentrations of Netilmicin in cerebrospinal fluid are often low and dependent upon dose and the degree of meningeal inflammation. Netilmicin crosses the placenta and has been detected in cord blood and in the fetus. Studies in nursing mothers indicate that small amounts of the drug are excreted in breast milk. Netilmicin is poorly absorbed from the intact gastrointestinal tract after oral administration. As with other aminoglycosides, the binding of netilmicin to serum proteins is low (0-30%).

Microbiology: Netilmicin is a rapidly acting, broad-spectrum bactericidal antibiotic which appears to act by inhibiting normal protein synthesis in susceptible microorganisms. Netilmicin is active *in vitro* against a wide variety of pathogenic bacteria, primarily gram-negative bacilli and also a few gram-positive organisms including *Citrobacter, Enterobacter, Escherichia coli, Klebsiella* species, *Proteus mirabilis, Pseudomonas aeruginosa, Salmonella* species, *Shigella* species, and *Staphylococcus* species (penicillin-and methicillin-resistant strains).

Netilmicin is also active *in vitro* against some isolates of *Acinetobacter* and *Neisseria* species, indole-positive *Proteus* species, *Pseudomonas* and *Serratia* species. In addition, Netilmicin is active *in vitro* against many strains which have acquired resistance to other aminoglycosides. Such resistance is usually caused by aminoglycoside modifying (inactivating) enzymes. In general, Netilmicin is active against organisms which inactivate aminoglycosides by either phosphorylation or adenylylation; it has variable activity against acetylating strains, depending on the specific type. For example, the susceptibility of *Serratia* species producing a combination of adenylylating and acetylating enzymes varies according to the level of acetylating enzyme present. Netilmicin is active *in vitro* against certain strains of gram-negative bacteria resistant to gentamicin and tobramycin: *Citrobacter, Enterobacter* species, *Escherichia coli, Klebsiella, Proteus* (indole-positive), *Pseudomonas, Salmonella,* and *Shigella* species. Netilmicin is active *in vitro* against certain staphylococci resistant to amikacin and tobramycin. Like other aminoglycosides, Netilmicin is not active against bacteria with reduced permeability to this class of antibiotics.

Most species of streptococci and anaerobic organisms, such as *Bacteroides* and *Clostridium* species, are resistant to aminoglycosides.

The *in vitro* activity of Netilmicin and of other aminoglycosides is affected by media pH, protein content, divalent cation concentration, and inoculum size.

Netilmicin acts synergistically *in vitro* with members of the penicillin class of antibiotics against *Streptococcus faecalis*. It also acts synergistically with those penicillins which are active alone against many strains of *Pseudomonas*. In addition, many, but not all isolates of *Serratia* which are resistant to multiple antibiotics, are inhibited by synergistic combinations of Netilmicin with carbenicillin, azlocillin, mezlocillin, cefamandole, cefotaxime, or moxalactam. Tests for antibiotic synergy are necessary.

Susceptibility Testing: Quantitative methods that require measurements of zone diameters give the most precise estimates of antibiotic susceptibility. One such procedure has been recommended for use with discs to test susceptibility to Netilmicin. Interpretation involves correlation of the diameters obtained in the disc test with minimal inhibitory concentration (MIC) values for Netilmicin.

Reports from the laboratory giving results of the standardized single disc susceptibility test (Bauer, et al. Am J Clin Path 1966; 45:493 and Federal Register 37:20525-20529, 1972), using a 30 mcg Netilmicin disc should be interpreted according to the following criteria:

Organisms producing zones of 15 mm or greater, or MIC's of 8.0 mcg or less are considered susceptible, indicating that the tested organism is likely to respond to therapy.

Resistant organisms produce zones of 12 mm or less or MIC's of 16 mcg or greater. A report of 'resistant' from the laboratory indicates that the infecting organism is not likely to respond to therapy.

Zones greater than 12 mm and less than 15 mm, or MiC's of greater than 8.0 mcg and less than 16 mcg, indicate intermediate susceptibility. A report of 'intermediate' susceptibility suggests that the organism would be susceptible if the infection is confined to tissues and fluids (e.g., urine), in which high antibiotic levels are attained.

Control organisms are recommended for susceptibility testing. Each time the test is performed one or more of the following organisms should be included: *Escherichia coli* ATCC 25922, *Staphylococcus aureus* ATCC 25923, and *Pseudomonas aeruginosa* ATCC 27853. The control organisms should produce zones of inhibition within the following ranges:

Escherichia coli (ATCC 25922) 22-30 mm
Staphylococcus aureus (ATCC 25923) 22-31 mm
Pseudomonas aeruginosa (ATCC 27853) 17-23 mm

In certain circumstances, particularly with strains of *Pseudomonas aeruginosa*, it may be desirable to do additional susceptibility testing by the tube or agar dilution method. Netilmicin Sulfate powder, a diagnostic reagent, is available for this purpose.

The MIC values of Netilmicin for the control strains are the following:

Escherichia coli (ATCC 25922) 0.25-0.5 mcg/ml
Staphylococcus aureus (ATCC 25923) 0.125-0.25 mcg/ml
Pseudomonas aeruginosa (ATCC 27853) 4-8 mcg/ml in media supplemented with calcium and magnesium.

INDICATIONS AND USAGE

Netilmicin Sulfate injection is indicated for the short-term treatment of patients of all ages, including neonates, infants, and children with serious or life-threatening bacterial infections caused by susceptible strains of the designated microorganisms in the diseases listed below:

Complicated Urinary Tract: infections caused by *Escherichia coli, Klebsiella pneumoniae, Pseudomonas aeruginosa, Enterobacter* species, *Proteus mirabilis, Proteus* species (indole-positive), *Serratia** and *Citrobacter* species, and *Staphylococcus aureus.***

Septicemia: caused by *Escherichia coli, Klebsiella pneumoniae, Pseudomonas aeruginosa, Enterobacter* and *Serratia** species and *Proteus mirabilis.*

Skin and Skin Structure: infections caused by *Escherichia coli, Klebsiella pneumoniae, Pseudomonas aeruginosa, Enterobacter* and *Serratia** species. *Proteus mirabilis, Proteus* (indole-positive), and *Staphylococcus aureus*** (penicillinase- and non-penicillinase-producing strains).

Intra-Abdominal: infections including peritonitis and intra-abdominal abscesss caused by *Escherichia coli, Klebsiella pneumoniae, Pseudomonas aeruginosa, Enterobacter* species, *Proteus mirabilis, Proteus* species (indole-positive), and *Staphylococcus aureus*** (penicillinase- and non-penicillinase- producing strains).

Lower Respiratory Tract: infections caused by *Escherichia coli, Klebsiella pneumoniae, Pseudomonas aeruginosa, Enterobacter* and *Serratia** species, *Proteus mirabilis, Proteus* species (indole-positive), and *Staphylococcus aureus*** (penicillinase- and non-penicillinase- producing strains).

Aminoglycosides are indicated for those infections for which less potentially toxic antimicrobial agents are infective or contraindicated. They are not indicated in the treatment of uncomplicated initial episodes of urinary tract infection unless the causative organisms are resistant to antimicrobial agents having less potential toxicity.

Netilmicin Sulfate injection may be considered as initial therapy in suspected or confirmed gram-negative infections, and therapy may be instituted before obtaining results of susceptibility testing. The decision to continue therapy with Netilmicin should be based on the results of susceptibility tests, the severity of the infection, and the important additional concepts contained in the "Warnings" box above.

If the causative organisms are resistant to Netilmicin, other appropriate therapy should be instituted.

In serious infections when the causative organisms are unknown, Netilmicin may be administered as initial therapy in conjunction with a penicillin-type or cephalosporin-type drug before obtaining results of susceptibility testing. In neonates with suspected sepsis, a penicillin-type drug is also usually indicated as concomitant therapy with netilmicin. If anaerobic organisms are suspected as etiologic agents, other suitable antimicrobial therapy should also be given. Following identification of the organism and its susceptibility, appropriate antibiotic therapy should then be continued. Netilmicin Sulfate injection has been used effectively in combination with carbenicillin or ticarcillin for the treatment of life-threatening infections caused by *Pseudomonas aeruginosa.*

Clinical studies have shown that Netilmicin has been effective in the treatment of serious infections caused by some organisms resistant to other aminoglycosides, *i.e.,* gentamicin, tobramycin, and/or amikacin.

Specimens for bacterial culture should be obtained to isolate and identify causative organisms and to determine their susceptibility to Netilmicin.

CONTRAINDICATION

Hypersensitivity to Netilmicin or to any of the ingredients of the preparation is a contraindication to its use. See "Warnings" if patient is hypersensitive to another aminoglycoside.

WARNINGS

(See "Warnings" box above.) If the patient has a history of hypersensitivity or serious toxic reaction to another aminoglycoside, Netilmicin Sulfate should be used very cautiously, if at all, because cross-sensitivity to drugs in this class has been reported.

---

* (See "Microbiology" section.)
** While not the antibiotic class of first choice, aminoglycosides, including Netilmicin, may be considered for the treatment of serious staphylococcal infections when penicillins or other less potentially toxic drugs are contraindicated and bacterial susceptibility tests and clinical judgment indicate their use. They may also be considered in mixed infections caused by susceptible strains of staphylococci and gram-negative organisms.

Aminoglycosides can cause fetal harm when administered to a pregnant woman. Aminoglycoside antibiotics cross the placenta and there have been several reports of total irreversible bilateral congenital deafness in children whose mothers received streptomycin during pregnancy. Although serious side effects to fetus or newborn have not been reported in the treatment of pregnant women with other aminoglycosides, the potential for harm exists. Reproduction studies in Netilmicin Sulfate have been performed in rats and rabbits using intramuscular and subcutaneous doses approximately 13-15 times the highest adult human dose and have revealed no evidence of impairment of fertility or harm to the fetus. Moreover, there was no evidence of ototoxicity in the offspring of rats treated subcutaneously with netilmicin throughout pregnancy and during the subsequent lactation period. It is not known whether Netilmicin Sulfate can cause fetal harm when administered to a pregnant women or can affect reproduction capacity. However, if this drug is used during pregnancy, or if the patient becomes pregnant while taking this drug, the patient should be apprised of the potential hazard to the fetus.

Netilmicin Sulfate injection contains sodium metabisulfite and sodium sulfite, which may cause allergic-type reactions including anaphylactic symptoms and life-threatening or less severe asthmatic episodes in certain susceptible people. The overall prevalence of sulfite sensitivity in the general population is unknown and probably low. Sulfite sensitivity is seen more frequently in asthmatic than in nonasthmatic people.

PRECAUTIONS

General: Neurotoxic and nephrotoxic antibiotics may be almost completely absorbed from body surfaces (except the urinary bladder) after local irrigation and after topical application during surgical procedures. The potential toxic effects of antibiotics administered in this fashion (neuromuscular blockade, respiratory paralysis, oto- and nephrotoxicity) should be considered. (See *"Warnings"*)

Increased nephrotoxicity has been reported following concomitant administration of aminoglycoside antibiotics with some cephalosporins.

Aminoglycosides should be used with caution in patients with neuromuscular disorders, such as myasthenia gravis, or infant botulism, since these drugs may aggravate muscle weakness because of their potential curare-like effect on the neuromuscular junction.

During or following Netilmicin therapy, parasthesias, tetany, positive Chvostek and Trousseau signs, and mental confusion have been described in patients with hypomagnesemia, hypocalcemia, and hypokalemia. When this has occurred in infants, tetany and muscle weakness has been described. Both adults and infants required appropriate corrective electrolyte therapy.

Elderly patients may have reduced renal function which may not be evident in the results of routine screening tests, such as BUN or serum creatinine levels. Determination of creatinine clearance or an estimate based on published nomograms or equations may be more useful. Monitoring of renal function during treatment with Netilmicin, as with other aminoglycosides, is particularly important in such patients. A Fanconi-like syndrome, with aminoaciduria and metabolic acidosis, has been reported in some adults and infants being given Netilmicin injections.

Patients should be well hydrated during treatment.

Treatment with Netilmicin may result in overgrowth of non-susceptible organisms. If this occurs, appropriate therapy is indicated.

Laboratory Tests: Tests of renal function: Urine should be examined periodically for increased excretion of protein and the presence of cells and casts, keeping in mind the effects of the primary illness on these tests. One or more of the following laboratory measurements should be obtained at the onset of therapy, periodically during therapy, and at, or shortly after, the end of therapy:

- creatinine clearance rate (either carefully measured or estimated from published nomograms or equations based on the patient's age, sex, body weight, and serum creatinine concentration) (preferred over BUN);
- serum creatinine concentration (preferred over BUN);
- blood urea nitrogen (BUN).

More frequent testing is desirable if renal function is changing.

See also *"Precautions, General"* above regarding elderly patients.

Test of Eighth Cranial Nerve Functions: Serial audiometric tests are suggested, particularly when renal function is impaired and/or prolonged aminoglycoside therapy is required; such tests should also be repeated periodically after treatment if there is evidence of a hearing deficit or vestibular abnormality before or during therapy, or when consecutive or concomitant use of other potentially ototoxic drugs is unavoidable.

Drug Interactions: In vitro mixing of an aminoglycoside with beta-lactam-type antibiotics (penicillins or cephalosporins) may result in a significant mutual inactivation. Even when an aminoglycoside and a penicillin-type drug are administered separately by different routes, a reduction in aminoglycoside serum half-life or serum levels has been reported in patients with impaired renal function and in some patients with normal renal function. Usually, such inactivation of the aminoglycoside is clinically significant only in patients with severely impaired renal function. (See also *"Drug/Laboratory Test Interactions"*.) See *"Warnings"* box regarding concurrent use of potent diuretics, concurrent and/or sequential use of other neurotoxic and/or nephrotoxic antibiotics, and for other essential information.

See also *"Precautions, General"*.

Drug/Laboratory Test Interactions: Concomitant cephalosporin therapy may spuriously elevate creatinine determinations.

The inactivation between aminoglycosides and beta-lactam antibiotics described in *"Drug Interactions"* may continue in specimens of body fluids collected for assay, resulting in inaccurate, false low aminoglycoside readings. Such specimens should be properly handled, *i.e.*, assayed promptly, frozen, or treated with beta-lactamase.

Carcinogenesis, Mutagenesis, Impairment of Fertility: Life-time carcinogenicity tests have been undertaken in the mouse and rat and no drug-related tumors were observed. Similarly, mutagenesis tests with Netilmicin have proven negative, and no impairment in fertility has been observed in the rat.

Pregnancy Category D: (See *"Warnings"* Section.)

Nursing Mothers: Clinical studies in nursing mothers indicate that small amounts of Netilmicin are excreted in breast milk. Because of the potential for serious adverse reactions from aminoglycosides in nursing infants, a decision should be made whether to discontinue nursing or to discontinue the drug, taking into account the importance of the drug to the mother.

Pediatric Use: Aminoglycosides should be used with caution in prematures and neonates because of the renal immaturity of these patients and the resulting prolongation of serum half-life of these drugs (also see *"Dosage and Administration"* for use in neonates and children).

ADVERSE REACTIONS

Nephrotoxicity: Adverse renal effects due to Netilmicin were reported in 7 per 100 patients.

They were demonstrated by a rise in serum creatinine and may have been accompanied by oliguria; the presence of casts, cells or protein in the urine; by rising levels of BUN; or by decreasing creatinine clearance rates. These effects occurred more frequently in the elderly, in patients with a history of renal impairment, and in patients treated for longer periods or with larger doses than recommended. While permanent impairment of renal function may occur following aminoglycoside therapy, observed renal impairment associated with Netilmicin was usually mild and reversible after treatment ended while the drug was being excreted.

Neurotoxicity: Adverse effects on both the auditory and vestibular branches of the eighth cranial nerves have been reported.

Audiometric changes associated with Netilmicin occurred in approximately 4 per 100 patients. Subjective Netilmicin-related hearing loss occurred in about 1 per 250 patients. Vestibular abnormalities related to Netilmicin were seen in 1 per 150 patients. Factors which may increase the risk of aminoglycoside-induced ototoxicity include renal impairment (especially if dialysis is required), excessive dosage, dehydration, concomitant administration of ethacrynic acid or furosemide, or previous exposure to other ototoxic drugs. Peripheral neuropathy or encephalopathy including numbness, skin tingling, muscle twitching, convulsions, and myasthenia gravis like syndrome have been reported.

Symptoms include dizziness, vertigo, tinnitus, nystagmus, and hearing loss. Aminoglycoside-induced ototoxicity is usually irreversible. Cochlear damage is usually manifested initially by small changes in audiometric test results at the higher frequencies and may not be associated with subjective hearing loss. Vestibular dysfunction is usually manifested by nystagmus, vertigo, nausea, vomiting, or acute Meniere's syndrome.

The risk of toxic reactions is low in patients with normal renal function who do not receive Netilmicin Sulfate Injection at higher doses or for longer periods of time than recommended. Some patients who have had previous neurotoxic reactions to other aminoglycosides have been treated with netilmicin without further neurotoxicity.

Neuromuscular blockade manifested as acute muscular paralysis and apnea can occur following treatment with aminoglycosides. (See *"Warnings"* box.)

The approximate incidence of other reported adverse reactions to Netilmicin Sulfate Injection follows: increased levels of serum transaminase (SGOT or SGPT), alkaline phosphatase, or bilirubin in 15 patients per 1000; rash or itching in 4 or 5 patients per 1000; eosinophilia in 4 patients per 1000; thrombocytosis in 2 patients per 1000; prolonged prothrombin time in 1 patient per 1000; fever in 1 patient per 1000.

Fewer than one patient per 1000 was reported to have Netilmicin Sulfate-related anemia, leukopenia, thrombocytopenia, leukemoid reaction, immature circulating white blood cells, hyperkalemia, vomiting, diarrhea, palpitations, hypotension, headache, disorientation, blurred vision, or paresthesis.

Local tolerance to intramuscular injection and intravenous infusion of netilmicin is generally excellent, but approximately four patients per 1000 have had severe pain, and similar numbers had induration or hematomas.

OVERDOSAGE

In the event of overdosage or toxic reaction, Netilmicin can be removed from the blood by hemodialysis, and is especially important if renal function is, or becomes, compromised. Although there is no specific information concerning removal of Netilmicin by peritoneal dialysis, other aminoglycosides are known to be removed by this method but at a rate considerably less than by hemodialysis.

DOSAGE AND ADMINISTRATION

Netilmicin injection may be given intramuscularly or intravenously. (See *"Clinical Pharmacology"*.) The recommended dosage for both methods of administration is identical.

The patient's pretreatment body weight should be obtained for calculation of correct dosage. The dosage of aminoglycosides in obese patients should be based on an estimate of the lean body mass.

The status of renal function should be estimated by measurement of the serum creatinine concentration or calculation of the endogenous creatinine clearance rate. The blood urea nitrogen (BUN) level is much less reliable for this purpose. Reassessment of renal function should be made periodically during therapy.

In patients with extensive body surface burns, altered pharmacokinetics may result in reduced serum concentrations of aminoglycosides. Measurement of Netilmicin serum concentrations is particularly important as a basis for dosage adjustment in such patients.

Duration of Treatment: It is desirable to limit the duration of treatment with aminoglycosides to short-term whenever feasible. The usual duration of treatment for all patients is seven to fourteen days. In complicated infections, a longer course of therapy may be necessary. Although prolonged courses of Netilmicin injection have been well tolerated, it is particularly important that patients treated for longer than the usual period be carefully monitored for changes in renal, auditory, and vestibular functions. Dosage should be adjusted if clinically indicated.

Measurement of Serum Concentrations: It is desirable to measure both peak and trough serum concentrations of Netilmicin to determine the adequacy and safety of the administered dosage.

When such measurements are feasible, they should be carried out periodically during therapy. Peak serum concentrations are expected to range from 4 to 12 mcg/ml. Dosage should be adjusted to attain the desired peak and trough concentrations and to avoid prolonged peak serum concentrations above 16 mcg/ml. When monitoring trough concentrations (just prior to the next dose), dosage should be adjusted so that levels above 4 mcg/ml are avoided. Inter-patient variation of aminoglycoside serum concentrations occurs in patients with normal or abnormal renal function. Generally, desirable peak and trough concentrations will be in the range of 6-10 and 0.5-2 mcg/ml, respectively.

Determination of the adequacy of a serum level for a particular patient must take into consideration the susceptibility of the causative organism, the severity of the infection, and the status of the patient's host-defense mechanisms.

The dosage recommendations which follow are not intended as rigid schedules, but are provided as guides for initial therapy, or for when the measurement of Netilmicin Sulfate serum levels during therapy is not feasible.

DOSAGE FOR PATIENTS WITH NORMAL RENAL FUNCTION
Table 1 shows the recommended dosage of Netilmicin Sulfate Injection for patients of various ages with normal renal function.

Table 1
DOSAGE GUIDE FOR ADULTS WITH NORMAL RENAL FUNCTION

Patient's Weight*		For Complicated Urinary Tract Infections. Give 3.0-4.0 mg/kg-day as 1.5-2.0 mg/kg	For Serious Systemic Infections Give 4.0-6.5 mg/kg/day as 1.3-2.2 mg/kg or 2.0-3.25 mg/kg	
kg	(lb)	Every 12 Hours mg/dose	Every 8 Hours mg/dose	Every 12 Hours mg/dose
40	(88)	60-80	52-88	80-130
45	(99)	68-90	59-99	90-146
50	(110)	75-100	65-110	100-163
55	(121)	83-110	72-121	110-179
60	(132)	90-120	78-132	120-195
65	(143)	98-130	85-143	130-211
70	(154)	105-140	91-154	140-228
75	(165)	113-150	98-165	150-244
80	(176)	120-160	104-176	160-260
85	(187)	128-170	111-187	170-276
90	(198)	135-180	117-198	180-293
95	(209)	143-190	124-209	190-309
100	(220)	150-200	130-220	200-325

* *The dosage of aminoglycosides in obese patients should be based on an estimate of the lean body mass.*

Although a causal relationship has not been established, administration of injections preserved with benzyl alcohol has been associated with toxicity in neonates. Caution should be used with Netilmicin Injection (100 mg/ml) is administered to neonates and children.

Neonates (less than 6 weeks): 4.0 to 6.5 mg/kg/day given as 2.0 to 3.25 mg/kg every 12 hours.

Infants and Children (6 weeks through 12 years): 5.5 to 8.0 mg/kg/day given either as 1.8 to 2.7 mg/kg every 8 hours, or as 2.7 to 4.0 mg/kg every 12 hours.

DOSAGE FOR PATIENTS WITH IMPAIRED RENAL FUNCTION
Dosage must be individualized in patients with impaired renal function to ensure therapeutic levels are attained. There are several methods of doing this; however, dosage adjustment based upon the measurement of serum drug concentrations during treatment is the most accurate.

If Netilmicin serum concentrations are not available and renal function is stable, serum creatinine and creatinine clearance values are the most reliable, readily available indicators of the degree of renal impairment for use as a guide for dosage adjustment.

It is also important to recognize that deteriorating renal function may require a greater reduction in dosage than that specified in the guidelines given below for patients with stable renal impairment.

The initial or loading dose is the same as that for a patient with normal renal function. A number of methods are available to adjust the total daily dosage for the degree of renal impairment. Three suggested methods are.

1) Divide the suggested dosage value for patients with normal renal function from Table 1 above by the serum creatinine level to obtain the adjusted size of each dose.

2) If the creatinine clearance rate is known or can be estimated from the serum creatinine levels using the formula given below, the adjusted daily dose of Netilmicin may be determined by multiplying the dose given in Table I by:

$$\frac{\text{Patient's Creatinine Clearance Rate}}{\text{Normal Creatinine Clearance Rate}}$$

3) Alternatively, the following graph may be used to obtain the percentage of the dose selected from Table I, which should be administered at 8-hour intervals:

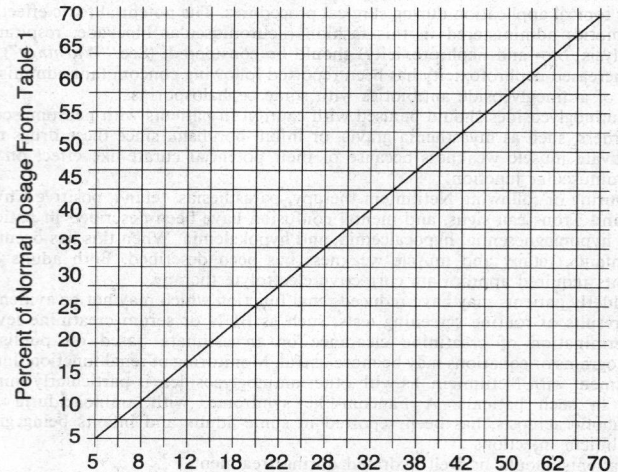

REDUCED DOSAGE GRAPH
PERCENT OF NORMAL DOSAGE FROM TABLE I

Creatinine clearance can be estimated from serum creatinine levels by the following formula for adult males; multiply by 0.85 for adult females (Nephron, 1976; 16:31-41):

$$C_{cr} = \frac{(140 - Age)(Wt.\ Kg)}{72 \times S_{cr}(mg/100\ ml)}$$

The adjusted total daily dose may be administered as one dose at 24-hour intervals, or as 2 or 3 equally divided doses at 12-hour or 8-hour intervals, respectively. Generally, each individual dose should not exceed 3.25 mg/kg. In adults with renal failure who are undergoing hemodialysis, the amount of Netilmicin removed from the blood may vary depending upon the dialysis equipment and methods used. (See *"Clinical Pharmacology".*) In adults, a dose of 2.0 mg/kg at the end of each dialysis period is recommended until the results of tests measuring Netilmicin serum levels become available. Dosage should then be appropriately adjusted based on these tests.

ALTERNATE DOSING METHOD FOR PATIENTS WITH NORMAL OR IMPAIRED RENAL FUNCTION
An alternate method of determining a dosage regimen (dose and dosing interval) applicable to all ages and all states of renal function (both normal and abnormal) is to employ pharmacokinetic parameters derived from measurements of serum concentrations.

Following the administration of an initial dose of Netilmicin and the determination of drug serum concentrations in post-infusion blood samples, the drug's half-life and the patient's elimination rate constant and volume of distribution can be calculated. Desired peak and trough serum levels for a particular patient are then selected by taking into consideration the susceptibility of the causative organism, the severity of infection, and the status of the patient's host-defense mechanisms. The dosage regimen (dose and dosing interval) is then determined using standardized formulae and the appropriate computer program, and the dosage regimen can be adjusted to the nearest practical interval and amount.

ADDITION OF NETILMICIN SULFATE TO VARIOUS INTRAVENOUS PREPARATIONS
In adults, a single dose of Netilmicin injection may be diluted to 50 to 200 ml of one of the parenteral solutions listed below. In infants and children, the volume of

---

diluent should be less according to the fluid requirements of the patient. The solution may be infused over a period of one-half to two hours. Tested at concentrations of 2.1 to 3.0 mg/ml, Netilmicin Sulfate has been shown to be stable in the following large volume parenteral solutions for up to 72 hours when stored in glass containers, both when refrigerated and at room temperature. Use after this time period is not recommended.

Table 2
LARGE VOLUME PARENTERAL SOLUTIONS IN WHICH NETILMICIN SULFATE IS STABLE

Products/Compositions Tested	Other Trade Names and Manufacturers (Solutions of Same Composition)
Sterile Water for injection 0.9% Sodium Chloride Injection alone or with 5% Dextrose 5% or 10% Dextrose Injection in Water, or 5% Dextrose in Polysal Injection, or 5% Dextrose with Electrolyte #48 or #75 Ringer's and Lactated Ringer's, and Lactated Ringer's with 5% Dextrose Injection 10% Injection	
10% Travert with Electrolyte #2 or #3 Injection (Travenol)	Electrolyte #3 (Cooke & Crowley's Solution) with 10% Inverted Sugar Injection (Cutter)
Isolyte E, M, or P with 5% Dextrose Injection 10% Dextran 40 or 6% Dextran 75 in 5% Dextrose Injection	
Plasma-Lyte 56 or 148 Injection with 5% Dextrose (Travenol)	Normal-M or R in D5-W (Abbott), Isolyte H or S with 5% Dextrose (McGaw), Polyonic R-148 or M-56 with 5% Dextrose (Cutter)
Plasma-Lyte M Injection 5% Dextrose (Travenol) Ionosol B in D5-W 5% Amigen Injection alone or with 5% Dextrose	Polysal M with 5% Dextrose (Cutter)
Normosol-R	Polyonic R-148 (Cutter), Isolyte S (McGaw) Plasma-Lyte 148 Injection in Water (Travenol)
Polysal (Plain) Aminosol 5% Injection Fre-Amine II 8.5% Injection Plasma-Lyte 148 Injection (approx. pH 7.4) (Travenol) 10% Fructose Injection	Normosol-R pH 7.4 (Abbott)

Parental drug products should be inspected visually for particulate matter and discoloration prior to administration, whenever solution and container permit.

STORAGE
Store between 2° and 30°C (36° and 86°F).

ANIMAL PHARMACOLOGY AND/OR ANIMAL TOXICOLOGY
Netilmicin Sulfate, administered by the intravenous and intramuscular routes, has been compared to kanamycin, sisomicin, gentamicin, amikacin, and tobramycin in studies ranging in duration from two weeks to three months. Among the aminoglycosides, Netilmicin is one of the more potent neuromuscular-blocking agents; however, in six different species, Netilmicin Sulfate has proven to be the least nephrotoxic and ototoxic of these aminoglycosides, using morphological as well as functional end points. In the clinical trials nephrotoxicity and ototoxicity occurred at about the same frequency in Netilmicin-treated patients as in those treated with other aminoglycosides.

HOW SUPPLIED
INJECTION: 100 MG/ML

BRAND/MANUFACTURER	NDC	SIZE	AWP
○ BRAND NETROMYCIN: Schering	00085-0264-02	1.5 ml 10s	$113.66

Netromycin *SEE* NETILMICIN SULFATE

Neupogen *SEE* FILGRASTIM

Neurontin *SEE* GABAPENTIN

Neut *SEE* SODIUM BICARBONATE

Neutrexin *SEE* TRIMETREXATE GLUCURONATE

Niacin

DESCRIPTION
Niacin or nicotinic acid, a water-soluble B complex vitamin and antihyperlipidemic agent, is 3-pyridinecarboxylic acid. It is a white, crystalline powder, sparingly soluble in water. Each tablet contains 500 mg Niacin (Nicotinic Acid).

Following is its chemical structure:

CLINICAL PHARMACOLOGY
Niacin functions in the body as a component of two hydrogen transporting coenzymes: Coenzyme I (Nicotinamide Adenine Dinucleotide [NAD], sometimes called Diphosphopyridine Nucleotide [DPN]) and Coenzyme II (Nicotinamide Adenine Dinucleotide Phosphate [NADP], sometimes called Triphosphopyridine Nucleotide [TPN]). Niacin, in addition to its functions as a vitamin, exerts several distinctive pharmacological effects which vary according to the dosage level employed. Niacin, in large doses, causes a reduction in serum lipids. The exact mechanism of this action is unknown.

The role of low-density lipoprotein (LDL) cholesterol in atherogenesis is supported by pathological observations, clinical studies and many animal experiments. Observational epidemiological studies have clearly established that high total or LDL (low-density lipoprotein) cholesterol and low HDL (high-density lipoprotein) cholesterol are risk factors for coronary heart disease. The Coronary Drug Project,[1] completed in 1975, was designed to assess the safety and efficacy of Nicotinic Acid and other lipid-altering drugs in men 30 to 64 years old with a history of myocardial infarction. Over an observation period of five (5) years, Nicotinic Acid showed a statistically significant benefit in decreasing nonfatal, recurrent myocardial infarctions. The incidence of definite, nonfatal MI was 8.9% for the 1,119 patients randomized to Nicotinic Acid versus 12.2% for the 2,789 patients who received placebo ($p < 0.004$). Though total mortality was similar in the two groups at five (5) years (24.4%) with Nicotinic Acid versus 25.4% with placebo; $p = N.S.$), in a fifteen (15) year cumulative follow-up there were 11% (69) fewer deaths in the Nicotinic Acid group compared to the placebo cohort (52.0% versus 58.2%; $p = 0.0004$).[2]

The Cholesterol-Lowering Atherosclerosis Study (CLAS) was a randomized, placebo-controlled, angiographic trial testing combined colestipol and Nicotinic Acid therapy in 162 non-smoking males with previous coronary bypass surgery.[3] The primary, persubject cardiac endpoint was global coronary artery change score. After two (2) years, 61% of patients in the placebo group showed disease progression by global change score (N = 82), compared with only 38.8% of drug-treated subjects (N = 80), when both native arteries and grafts were considered ($p < .005$). In a follow-up to this trial in a subgroup of 103 patients treated for four (4) years, again, significantly fewer patients in the drug-treated group demonstrated progression than in the placebo cohort (48% versus 85%, respectively; $p < .0001$).[4]

The Familial Atherosclerosis Treatment Study (FATS) in 146 men ages 62 and younger with apolipoprotein B levels $\geq$ 125 mg/dL, established coronary artery disease, and family histories in vascular disease, assessed change in severity of disease in the proximal coronary arteries by quantitative arteriography.[5] Patients were given dietary counselling and randomized to treatment with either conventional therapy with double placebo (or placebo plus colestipol if the LDL-cholesterol was elevated); lovastatin plus colestipol; or Nicotinic Acid plus colestipol. In the conventional therapy group, 46% of patients had disease progression (and no regression) in at least one of nine proximal coronary segments. In contrast, progression (as the only change) was seen in only 25% in the Nicotinic Acid plus colestipol group. Though not an original endpoint of the trial, clinical events (death, myocardial infarction, or revascularization for worsening angina) occurred in 10 of 52 patients who received conventional therapy, compared with 2 of 48 who received Nicotinic Acid plus colestipol.

Nicotinic Acid (but not nicotinamide) in gram doses produces an average 10-20% reduction in total and LDL-cholesterol, a 30-70% reduction in triglycerides, and an average 20-35% increase in HDL-cholesterol. The magnitude of individual lipid and lipoprotein responses may be influenced by the severity and type of underlying lipid abnormality. The increase in total HDL is associated with a shift in the distribution of HDL subfractions (as defined by ultra-centrifugation) with an increase in the $HDL_2:HDL_3$ ratio; and an increase in apolipoprotein AI content. The mechanism by which Nicotinic Acid exerts these effects is not entirely understood, but may involve several actions, including a decrease in esterification of hepatic triglycerides. Nicotinic Acid treatment also decreases the serum levels of apolipoprotein B-100 (apo B), the major protein component of the VLDL and LDL fractions, and of lipoprotein, Lp(a), a variant form of LDL independently associated with coronary risk. The effect of Nicotinic Acid-induced changes in lipids/lipoproteins on cardiovascular morbidity or mortality in individuals without pre-existing coronary disease has not been established.

PHARMACOKINETICS

Following an oral dose, the pharmacokinetic profile of Nicotinic Acid is characterized by rapid absorption from the gastrointestinal tract and a short plasma elimination half-life. At a 1 gram dose, peak plasma concentrations of 15 to 30 µg/mL are reached within 30 to 60 minutes. Approximately 88% of an oral pharmacologic dose is eliminated by the kidneys as unchanged drug and nicotinuric acid, its primary metabolite. The plasma elimination half-life of Nicotinic Acid ranges from 20 to 45 minutes.

INDICATIONS AND USAGE

1. Therapy with lipid-altering agents should be only one component of multiple risk factor intervention in those individuals at significantly increased risk for atherosclerotic vascular disease due to hypercholesterolemia. Nicotinic Acid, alone or in combination with a bile-acid binding resin, is indicated as an adjunct to diet for the reduction of elevated total and LDL cholesterol levels in patients with primary hypercholesterolemia (Types IIa and IIb), † when the response to a diet restricted in saturated fat and cholesterol and other nonpharmacologic measures alone has been inadequate (see also the N.C.E.P. treatment guidelines[6]). Prior to initiating therapy with Nicotinic Acid, secondary causes for hypercholesterolemia (e.g., poorly controlled diabetes mellitus, hypothyroidism, nephrotic syndrome, dysproteinemias, obstructive liver disease, other drug therapy, alcoholism) should be excluded, and a lipid profile performed to measure total cholesterol, HDL-cholesterol, and triglycerides.

2. Nicotinic acid is also indicated as adjunctive therapy for the treatment of adult patients with very high serum triglyceride levels (Types IV and V hyperlipidemia)† who present a risk of pancreatitis and who do not respond adequately to a determined dietary effort to control them. Such patients typically have serum triglyceride levels over 2000 mg/dL and have elevations of VLDL-cholesterol as well as fasting chylomicrons (Type V hyperlipidemia).† Subjects who consistently have total serum or plasma triglycerides below 1000 mg/dL are unlikely to develop pancreatitis. Therapy with Nicotinic Acid may be considered for those subjects with triglyceride elevations between 1000 and 2000 mg/dL who have a history of pancreatitis or of recurrent abdominal pain typical of pancreatitis. Some Type IV patients with triglycerides under 1000 mg/dL may, through dietary or alcoholic indiscretion, convert to a Type V pattern with massive triglyceride elevations accompanying fasting chylomicronemia, but the influence of Nicotinic Acid therapy on the risk of pancreatitis in such situations has not been adequately studied. Drug therapy is not indicated for patients with Type I hyperlipoproteinemia, who have elevations of chylomicrons and plasma triglycerides, but who have normal levels of very low density lipoprotein (VLDL). Inspection of plasma refrigerated for 14 hours is helpful in distinguishing Types I, IV, and V hyperlipoproteinemia.[7]

Notice: It has not been established whether the drug-induced lowering of serum cholesterol or triglyceride levels has a beneficial effect, no effect, or a detrimental effect on the morbidity or mortality due to atherosclerosis including coronary heart disease. Investigations now in progress may yield an answer to this question.

†CLASSIFICATION OF HYPERLIPOPROTEINEMIAS

Type	Lipoproteins:n1 elevated	Lipid Elevations major	Lipid Elevations minor
I (rare)	chylomicrons	TG	↑→C
IIa	LDL	C	-
IIb	LDL, VLDL	C	TG
III (rare)	IDL	C/TG	-
IV	VLDL	TG	↑→C
V (rare)	chylomicrons, VLDL	TG	↑→C

C = cholesterol,
TG = triglycerides,
LDL = low-density lipoprotein,
VLDL = very-low-density lipoprotein,
IDL = intermediate-density lipoprotein.

CONTRAINDICATIONS

Nicotinic Acid is contraindicated in patients with a known hypersensitivity to any component of this medication; significant or unexplained hepatic dysfunction; active peptic ulcer disease; or arterial bleeding.

WARNINGS

LIVER DYSFUNCTION

Cases of severe hepatic toxicity, including fulminant hepatic necrosis have occurred in patients who have substituted sustained-release (modified-release, timed-release) Nicotinic Acid products for immediate-release (crystalline) Nicotinic Acid at equivalent doses.

Liver function tests should be performed on all patients during therapy with Nicotinic Acid. Serum transaminase levels, including ALT (SGPT), should be monitored before treatment begins, every six weeks to twelve weeks for the first year, and periodically thereafter (e.g., at approximately 6 month intervals). Special attention should be paid to patients who develop elevated serum

transaminase levels, and in these patients, measurements should be repeated promptly and then performed more frequently. If the transaminase levels show evidence of progression, particularly if they rise to three times the upper limit of normal and are persistent, the drug should be discontinued. Liver biopsy should be considered if elevations persist beyond discontinuation of the drug.

Nicotinic Acid should be used with caution in patients who consume substantial quantities of alcohol and/or have a past history of liver disease. Active liver diseases or unexplained transaminase elevations are contraindications to the use of Nicotinic Acid.

SKELETAL MUSCLE

Rare cases of rhabdomyolysis have been associated with concomitant administration of lipid-altering doses ($\geq$ 1 g/day) of Nicotinic Acid and HMG-CoA reductase inhibitors. Physicians contemplating combined therapy with HMG-CoA reductase inhibitors and Nicotinic Acid should carefully weigh the potential benefits and risks and should carefully monitor patients for any signs and symptoms of muscle pain, tenderness, or weakness, particularly during the initial months of therapy and during any periods of upward dosage titration of either drug. Periodic serum creatine phosphokinase (CPK) and potassium determinations should be considered in such situations, but there is no assurance that such monitoring will prevent the occurrence of severe myopathy.

PRECAUTIONS

GENERAL

Before instituting therapy with Nicotinic Acid, an attempt should be made to control hyperlipidemia with appropriate diet, exercise, and weight reduction in obese patients, and to treat other underlying medical problems (see *"Indications and Usage"*).

Great caution must be exercised when Niacin is used in patients with coronary disease or gallbladder disease.

Patients with a past history of jaundice, hepatobiliary disease, or peptic ulcer should be observed closely during Nicotinic Acid therapy. Frequent monitoring of liver function tests and blood glucose should be performed to ascertain that the drug is producing no adverse effects on these organ systems. Diabetic patients may experience a dose-related rise in glucose intolerance, the clinical significance of which is unclear. Diabetic or potentially diabetic patients should be observed closely. Adjustment of diet and/or hypoglycemic therapy may be necessary.

Caution should also be used when Nicotinic Acid is used in patients with unstable angina or in the acute phase of myocardial infarction, particularly when such patients are also receiving vasoactive drugs such as nitrates, calcium channel blockers, or adrenergic blocking agents.

Antihypertensive drugs of the adrenergic-blocking type may have an additive vasodilating effect and produce postural hypotension.

Elevated uric acid levels have occurred with Nicotinic Acid therapy, therefore use with caution in patients predisposed to gout.

Some brands contain FD&C Yellow No. 5 (tartrazine) which may cause allergic-type reactions (including bronchial asthma) in certain susceptible persons. Although the overall incidence of FD&C Yellow No. 5 (tartrazine) sensitivity in the general populations is low, it is frequently seen in patients who also have aspirin hypersensitivity.

DRUG INTERACTIONS

HMG-CoA Reductase Inhibitors: See *"Warnings, Skeletal Muscle:"* Nicotinic Acid may potentiate the effects of ganglionic blocking agents and vasoactive drugs resulting in postural hypotension.

Aspirin: Concomitant aspirin may decrease the metabolic clearance of Nicotinic Acid. The clinical relevance of this finding is unclear.

Other: Concomitant alcohol or hot drinks may increase the side effects of flushing and pruritus and should be avoided at the time of drug ingestion.

CARCINOGENESIS, MUTAGENESIS, IMPAIRMENT OF FERTILITY

Nicotinic Acid administered to mice for a lifetime as a 1% solution in drinking water was not carcinogenic. The mice in this study received approximately 6-8 times a human dose of 3000 milligrams/day as determined on a milligram/square meter basis. Nicotinic acid was negative for mutagenicity in the Ames test. No studies on impairment of fertility have been performed.

PREGNANCY

Pregnancy Category C.

Animal reproduction or teratology studies have not been conducted with Nicotinic Acid. It is also not known whether Nicotinic Acid at doses typically used for lipid disorders can cause fetal harm when administered to pregnant women or whether it can affect reproductive capacity. If a woman receiving Nicotinic Acid for primary hypercholesterolemia (Types IIa or IIb) becomes pregnant, the drug should be discontinued. If a woman being treated with Nicotinic Acid for hypertriglyceridemia (Types IV and V) conceives, the benefits and risks of continued drug therapy should be assessed on an individual basis.

NURSING MOTHERS

It is not known whether this drug is excreted in human milk. Because many drugs are excreted in human milk and because of the potential for serious adverse reactions in nursing infants from lipid-altering doses of nicotinic acid, a decision should be made whether to discontinue nursing or to discontinue the drug, taking into account the importance of the drug to the mother.

PEDIATRIC USE
Safety and effectiveness in children and adolescents have not been established.
KEEP OUT OF REACH OF CHILDREN.

ADVERSE REACTIONS
Cardiovascular: atrial fibrillation and other cardiac arrhythmias; orthostasis; hypotension

Gastrointestinal: dyspepsia; vomiting; diarrhea; peptic ulceration; jaundice; abnormal liver function tests

Skin: mild to severe cutaneous flushing; pruritus; hyperpigmentation; acanthosis nigricans; dry skin

Metabolic: decreased glucose tolerance; hyperuricemia, gout

Eye: toxic amblyopia; cystoid macular edema

Nervous System/Psychiatric: headache

OVERDOSAGE
High doses of Nicotinic Acid may produce temporary flushing, pruritus, and gastrointestinal distress.

Supportive measures should be undertaken in the event of an overdose.

DOSAGE AND ADMINISTRATION
The usual adult dosage of Nicotinic Acid is 1 to 2 grams two or three times a day. Doses should be individualized according to the patient's response. Start with one-half tablet (250 mg) as a single daily dose following the evening meal or with some brands, two tablets (1g) three times a day with food or after meals, taken with cold liquids, if necessary, to facilitate swallowing. The frequency of dosing and total daily dose can be increased every four to seven days until the desired LDL-cholesterol and/or triglyceride level is achieved or the first-level therapeutic dose of 1.5 to 2 grams/day is reached. If the patient's hyperlipidemia is not adequately controlled after 2 months at this level, the dosage can then be increased at two to four week intervals to 3 grams/day (1 gram three times per day). In patients with marked lipid abnormalities, a higher dose is occasionally required, but generally should not exceed 6 grams/day.

Flushing of the skin appears frequently and can be minimized by pretreatment with aspirin or non-steroidal anti-inflammatory drugs. Tolerance to this flushing develops rapidly over the course of several weeks. Flushing, pruritus, and gastrointestinal distress are also greatly reduced by slowly increasing the dose of Nicotinic Acid in increments of 500 mg (1 tablet) while carefully observing the patient and monitoring the plasma cholesterol and/or triglyceride level for therapeutic response and for adverse effects and avoiding administration on an empty stomach. Where the observed adverse reactions or potential hazards exceed the benefits of use, dosage should be reduced to the minimum recommended dosage and, where necessary, discontinued entirely.

Sustained-release (modified-release, timed-release) Nicotinic Acid preparations should *not* be substituted for equivalent doses of immediate-release (crystalline) Nicotinic Acid.

Dispense in a tight container as defined in the USP. Store at controlled room temperature, 15°-30°C (59°-86°F).

REFERENCES
1. The Coronary Drug Project Research Group. Clofibrate and Niacin in Coronary Heart Disease *JAMA* 1975: 231:360-81. 2. Cancer Pl *et al.* Fifteen Year Mortality in Coronary Drug Product Patients: Long-Term Benefit with Niacin. *JACC* 1986; 8(6):1245-55. 3. Blankenhorn DH *et al.* Beneficial Effects of Combined Colestipol-Niacin Therapy on Coronary Atherosclerosis and Coronary Venous Bypass Grafts. *JAMA* 1987; 257 (23):3233-40. 4. Cashin-Hemphill *et al.* Beneficial Effects of Colestipol-Niacin on Coronary Atherosclerosis. *JAMA* 1990, 264 (23):3013-17. 5. Brown G *et al.* Regression of Coronary Artery Diseases as a Result of Intensive Lipid-Lowering Therapy in Men with High Levels of Apolipoprotein B. *NEJM* 1990; 323:1289-98. 6. Report of the National Cholesterol Education Program Expert Panel on Detection, Evaluation, and Treatment of High Blood Cholesterol. *Arch. Int. Med.* 1988; 148:36-69. 7. Nikkila EA: Familial lipoprotein lipase deficiency and related disorders of chylomicron metabolism. In Stabury J.B. *et al.* (ed.): *The Metabolic Basis of Inherited Disease*, 5th ed, McGraw-Hill, 1983, Chap. 30, pp. 622-642.

HOW SUPPLIED
TABLETS: 500 MG
HCFA FUL (100s ea) $0.03

BRAND/MANUFACTURER	NDC	SIZE	AWP
◆ BRAND NICOLAR: RPR	00075-2850-01	100s	$61.80

TABLETS: 500 MG

BRAND/MANUFACTURER	NDC	SIZE	AWP
○ BRAND NIACOR: Upsher-Smith	00245-0066-11	100s	$13.44

Niacor *SEE* NIACIN

Nicardipine Hydrochloride

DESCRIPTION
Nicardipine Hydrochloride is available in capsules or sustained-release capsules for oral administration and in ampuls for intravenous (IV) infusion after dilution.

Each Capsule Contains:
Nicardipine HCl ....20 mg
Nicardipine HCl ....30 mg

Each Sustained Release Capsule Contains:
Nicardipine HCl ....30 mg
Nicardipine HCl ....45 mg
Nicardipine HCl ....60 mg

Each Ampul For Intravenous Injection Contains:
Nicardipine HCl ....2.5 mg/ml

Nicardipine HCL is a dihydropyridine structure with the IUPAC (International Union of Pure and Applied Chemistry) chemical name ± 2-(benzyl-methyl amino) ethyl methyl 1,4-dihydro-2,6-dimethyl-4-(*m*-nitrophenyl)-3,5-pyridinedicarboxylate monohydrochloride.

Nicardipine HCl is a greenish-yellow, odorless, crystalline powder that melts at about 169°C. It is freely soluble in chloroform, methanol, and glacial acetic acid, sparingly soluble in anhydrous ethanol, slightly soluble in n-butanol, water, 0.01 M potassium dihydrogen phosphate, acetone, and dioxane, very slightly soluble in ethyl acetate, and practically insoluble in benzene, ether, and hexane. It has a molecular weight of 515.99.

Following is its chemical structure:

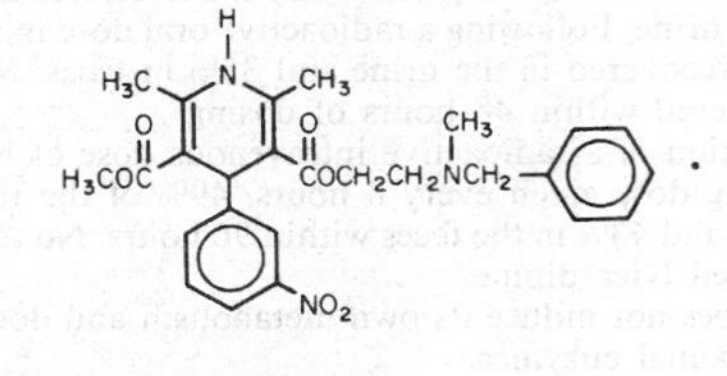

CLINICAL PHARMACOLOGY
MECHANISM OF ACTION
Nicardipine HCl is a calcium entry blocker (slow channel blocker or calcium ion antagonist) which inhibits the transmembrane influx of calcium ions into cardiac muscle and smooth muscle without changing serum calcium concentrations. The contractile processes of cardiac muscle and vascular smooth muscle are dependent upon the movement of extracellular calcium ions into these cells through specific ion channels. The effects of Nicardipine HCl are more selective to vascular smooth muscle than cardiac muscle. In animal models, Nicardipine HCl produces relaxation of coronary vascular smooth muscle at drug levels which cause little or no negative inotropic effect.

PHARMACOKINETICS AND METABOLISM
Nicardipine HCl is completely absorbed following oral doses administered as capsules. Plasma levels are detectable as early as 20 minutes following an oral dose and maximal plasma levels are observed within 30 minutes to two hours (mean T_{max} = 1 hour). While Nicardipine HCl is completely absorbed, it is subject to saturable first pass metabolism and the systemic bioavailability is about 35% following a 30 mg oral dose at steady state.

When Nicardipine HCl was administered one (1) or three (3) hours after a high fat meal, the mean Cmax and mean AUC were lower (20% to 30%) than when Nicardipine HCl was given to fasting subjects. When Nicardipine HCl Sustained Release was administered with a high fat breakfast, mean Cmax was 45% lower, AUC was 25% lower and trough levels were 75% higher than when Nicardipine HCl Sustained Release was given in the fasting state. Thus, taking Nicardipine HCl Sustained Release with the meal reduced the fluctuation in plasma levels. These decreases in plasma levels observed following a meal may be significant but the clinical trials establishing the efficacy and safety of Nicardipine HCl or Nicardipine HCl Sustained Release were done in patients without regard to the timing of meals. Thus the results of these trials reflect the effects of meal-induced variability.

The pharmacokinetics of Nicardipine HCl are nonlinear due to saturable hepatic first pass metabolism. Following oral administration, increasing doses result in a disproportionate increase in plasma levels. Steady state Cmax values following 20, 30, and 40 mg doses every 8 hours averaged 36, 88, and 133 ng/mL, respectively. Hence, increasing the dose from 20 to 30 mg every 8 hours more than doubled Cmax and increasing the dose from 20 to 40 mg every 8 hours increased Cmax more than 3-fold. A similar disproportionate increase in AUC with dose was observed. Considerable inter-subject variability in plasma levels was also observed.

Postabsorption kinetics of Nicardipine HCl are also non-linear, although there is a reproducible terminal plasma half-life that averaged 8.6 hours following 30 and 40 mg doses at steady state (TID). The terminal half-life represents the elimination of less than 5% of the absorbed drug (measured by plasma concentrations). Elimination over the first 8 hours after dosing is much faster with a half-life of 2-4 hours. Steady state plasma levels are achieved after 2 to 3 days of TID dosing (every 8 hours) and are 2-fold higher than after a single dose.

Following oral administration of Nicardipine HCl Sustained Release, levels are detectable as early as 20 minutes and maximal plasma levels are achieved as a broad peak generally between one and four hours. Following oral administration, increasing doses result in disproportionate increases in plasma levels. Steady state Cmax values following 30, 45 and 60 mg doses every 12 hours averaged 13.4, 34.0 and 58.4 ng/ml, respectively. Hence increasing the dose two-fold increases maximum plasma levels 4-5 fold. In comparison with equivalent daily doses of Nicardipine HCl capsules, Nicardipine HCl Sustained Release shows a significant reduction in Cmax. Nicardipine HCl Sustained Release also has somewhat lower bioavailability than Nicardipine HCl except at the highest dose. Minimum plasma levels produced by equivalent daily doses are similar. Nicardipine HCl Sustained Release thus exhibits significantly reduced fluctuation in plasma levels in comparison to Nicardipine HCl capules.

Following infusion, Nicardipine plasma concentrations decline tri-exponentially, with a rapid early distribution phase (α-half-life of 2.7 minutes), an intermediate phase (β-half-life of 44.8 minutes), and a slow terminal phase (γ-half-life of 14.4 hours) that can only be detected after long-term infusions. Total plasma clearance (Cl) is 0.41 L/hr·kg, and the apparent volume of distribution (V_d) using a noncompartment model is 8.3 L/kg. The pharmacokinetics of Nicardipine HCl IV are linear over the dosage range of 0.5 to 40.0 mg/hr. Rapid dose-related increases in Nicardipine plasma concentrations are seen during the first two hours after the start of an infusion of Nicardipine HCl IV. Plasma concentrations increase at a much slower rate after the first few hours, and approach steady state at 24 to 48 hours. On termination of the infusion, Nicardipine concentrations decrease rapidly, with at least a 50% decrease during the first two hours post-infusion. The effects of Nicardipine on blood pressure significantly correlate with plasma concentrations.

Nicardipine HCl is highly protein bound (> 95%) in human plasma over a wide concentration range.

Nicardipine HCl is metabolized extensively by the liver; less than 1% of intact drug is detected in the urine. Following a radioactive oral dose in solution, 60% of the radioactivity was recovered in the urine and 35% in feces. Most of the dose (over 90%) was recovered within 48 hours of dosing.

After coadministration of a radioactive intravenous dose of Nicardipine HCl IV with an oral 30 mg dose given every 8 hours, 49% of the radioactivity was recovered in the urine and 43% in the feces within 96 hours. None of the dose was recovered as unchanged Nicardipine.

Nicardipine HCl does not induce its own metabolism and does not induce or inhibit hepatic microsomal enzymes.

The steady-state pharmacokinetics of Nicardipine HCl and Nicardipine HCl IV in elderly hypertensive patients (≥ 65 years) are similar to those obtained in young normal adults. After one week of Nicardipine HCl dosing at 20 mg three times a day, the Cmax, Tmax, AUC, terminal plasma half-life, and the extent of protein binding of Nicardipine HCl observed in healthy elderly hypertensive patients did not differ significantly from those observed in young normal volunteers.

Nicardipine HCl plasma levels were higher in patients with mild renal impairment (baseline serum creatinine concentration ranged from 1.2 to 5.5 mg/dL) than in normal subjects. After 30 mg Nicardipine HCl TID at steady state, Cmax and AUC were approximately 2-fold higher in these patients.

Because Nicardipine HCl is extensively metabolized by the liver, the plasma levels of the drug are influenced by changes in hepatic function. Nicardipine HCl plasma levels were higher in patients with severe liver disease (hepatic cirrhosis confirmed by liver biopsy or presence of endoscopically-confirmed esophageal varices) than in normal subjects. After 20 mg Nicardipine HCl BID at steady state, Cmax and AUC were 1.8 and 4-fold higher, and the terminal half-life was prolonged to 19 hours in these patients.

The pharmacokinetics of Nicardipine HCl Sustained Release in elderly hypertensive patients (mean age 70 years) were compared to those in younger hypertensive patients (mean age 44 years). After a single dose and after one week of dosing with Nicardipine HCl Sustained Release there were no significant differences in Cmax, Tmax, AUC or clearance between the young and elderly patients. In both groups of patients, steady state plasma levels were significantly higher than following a single dose. In the elderly patients, a disproportional increase in plasma levels with dose was observed similar to that observed in normal subjects.

Nicardipine plasma levels following administration of Nicardipine HCl Sustained Release in hypertensive patients with moderate renal impairment (creatinine clearance 10-55 ml/min) were significantly higher following a single oral dose and at steady state than in hypertensive patients with mildly impaired renal function (creatinine clearance > 55 ml/min). After 45 mg Nicardipine HCl Sustained Release b.i.d. at steady state, Cmax and AUC were 2-3 fold higher in the patients with moderate renal impairment. Plasma levels in patients with mildly impaired renal function were similar to those in normal subjects.

In patients with severe renal impairment undergoing routine hemodialysis, plasma levels following a single dose of Nicardipine HCl Sustained Release were not significantly different from those patients with mildly impaired renal function.

Nicardipine HCl Sustained Release has not been studied in patients with severe liver disease.

HEMODYNAMICS

In man, Nicardipine HCl produces a significant decrease in systemic vascular resistance. The degree of vasodilation and the resultant hypotensive effects are more prominent in hypertensive patients. In hypertensive patients, Nicardipine reduces the blood pressure at rest and during isometric and dynamic exercise. In normotensive patients, a small decrease of about 9 mmHg in systolic and 7 mmHg in diastolic blood pressure may accompany this fall in peripheral resistance. Administration of Nicardipine HCl IV to normotensive volunteers at dosages of 0.25 to 3.0 mg/hr for eight hours produced changes of < 5 mmHg in systolic blood pressure and < 3 mmHg in diastolic blood pressure.

An increase in heart rate may occur in response to the vasodilation and decrease in blood pressure, and in a few patients this heart rate increase may be pronounced. In clinical studies with oral Nicardipine HCl mean heart rate at time of peak plasma levels was usually increased by 5-10 beats per minute compared to placebo, with the greater increases at higher doses, while there was no difference from placebo at the end of the dosing interval. In placebo-controlled trials, the mean increases in heart rate were 7 ± 1 bpm in postoperative patients and 8 ± 1 bpm in patients with severe hypertension at the end of the maintenance period.

Hemodynamic studies following intravenous dosing in patients with coronary artery disease and normal or moderately abnormal left ventricular function have shown significant increases in ejection fraction and cardiac output with no significant change, or a small decrease, in left ventricular end-diastolic pressure (LVEDP). Although there is evidence that Nicardipine HCl increases coronary blood flow, there is no evidence that this property plays any role in its effectiveness in stable angina. In patients with coronary artery disease, intracoronary administration of Nicardipine caused no direct myocardial depression.

Coronary dilatation induced by Nicardipine HCl IV improves perfusion and aerobic metabolism in areas with chronic ischemia, resulting in reduced lactate production and augmented oxygen consumption. In patients with coronary artery disease. Nicardipine HCl IV, administered after beta-blockade, significantly improved systolic and diastolic left ventricular function. In congestive heart failure patients with impaired left ventricular function, Nicardipine HCl IV increased cardiac output both at rest and during exercise. Decreases in left ventricular end-diastolic pressure were also observed. Nicardipine HCl does, however, have a negative inotropic effect in some patients with severe left ventricular dysfunction and could, in patients with very impaired function, lead to worsened failure.

"Coronary Steal", the detrimental redistribution of coronary blood flow in patients with coronary artery disease (diversion of blood from underperfused areas toward better perfused areas), has not been observed during Nicardipine treatment. On the contrary, Nicardipine has been shown to improve systolic shortening in normal and hypokinetic segments of myocardial muscle, and radionuclide angiography has confirmed that wall motion remained improved during an increase in oxygen demand. Nonetheless, occasional patients have developed increased angina upon receiving Nicardipine capsules. Whether this represents steal in those patients, or is the result of increased heart rate and decreased diastolic pressure, is not clear.

In patients with coronary artery disease Nicardipine improves L.V. diastolic distensibility during the early filling phase, probably due to a faster rate of myocardial relaxation in previously underperfused areas. There is little or no effect on normal myocardium, suggesting the improvement is mainly by indirect mechanisms such as afterload reduction, and reduced ischemia. Nicardipine has no negative effect on myocardial relaxation at therapeutic doses. The clinical consequences of these properties are as yet undemonstrated.

ELECTROPHYSIOLOGIC EFFECTS

In general, no detrimental effects on the cardiac conduction system were seen with the use of Nicardipine HCl.

Nicardipine HCl increased the heart rate when given intravenously during acute electrophysiologic studies, and prolonged the corrected QT interval to a minor degree. The sinus node recovery times and SA conduction times were not affected by the drug. The PA. AH, and HV intervals* and the functional and effective refractory periods of the atrium were not prolonged by Nicardipine HCl and the relative and effective refractory periods of the His-Purkinje system were slightly shortened after intravenous Nicardipine HCl.

Because Nicardipine is extensively metabolized by the liver, plasma concentrations are influenced by changes in hepatic function. In a clinical study with Nicardipine HCl capsules in patients with severe liver disease, plasma concentrations were elevated and the half-life was prolonged (see *"Precautions"*). Similar results were obtained in patients with hepatic disease when Nicardipine HCl IV was administered for 24 hours at 0.6 mg/hr.

RENAL FUNCTION

There is a transient increase in electrolyte excretion, including sodium. Nicardipine HCl does not cause generalized fluid retention, as measured by weight changes, although 7-8% of the patients experience pedal edema.

When Nicardipine HCl IV was given to mild to moderate hypertensive patients with moderate degrees of renal impairment, significant reduction in glomerular filtration rate (GFR) and effective renal plasma flow (RPF) was observed. No significant differences in liver blood flow were observed in these patients. A significantly lower systemic clearance and higher area under the curve (AUC) were observed.

When Nicardipine HCl capsules (20 mg or 30 mg TID) were given to hypertensive patients with impaired renal function, mean plasma concentrations. AUC, and Cmax were approximately two-fold higher than in healthy controls. There is a transient increase in electrolyte excretion, including sodium (see *"Precautions"*).

* PA = conduction time from high to low right atrium; AH = conduction time from low right atrium to His bundle deflection, or AV nodal conduction time; HV = conduction time through the His bundle and the bundle branch-Purkinje system.

Acute bolus administration of Nicardipine HCl IV (2.5 mg) in healthy volunteers decreased mean arterial pressure and renal vascular resistance; glomerular filtration rate (GFR), renal plasma flow (RPF), and the filtration fraction were unchanged. In healthy patients undergoing abdominal surgery Nicardipine HCl IV (10 mg over 20 minutes) increased GFR with no change in RPF when compared with placebo. In hypertensive Type II diabetic patients with nephropathy, Nicardipine HCl capsules (20 mg TID) did not change RPF and GFR, but reduced renal vascular resistance.

PULMONARY FUNCTION
In two well-controlled studies of patients with obstructive airway disease treated with Nicardipine HCl IV capsules, no evidence of increased pronchospasm was seen. In one of the studies, Nicardipine HCl capsules improved forced expiratory volume 1 second (FEV 1) and forced vital capacity (FVC) in comparison with metoprolol. Adverse experiences reported in a limited number of patients with asthma, reactive airway disease, or obstructive airway disease are similar to all patients treated with Nicardipine HCl capsules.

EFFECTS IN ANGINA PECTORIS
In controlled clinical trials of up to 12 week's duration in patients with chronic stable angina, Nicardipine HCl increased exercise tolerance and reduced nitroglycerin consumption and the frequency of anginal attacks. The antianginal efficacy of Nicardipine HCl (20-40 mg) has been demonstrated in four placebo-controlled studies involving 258 patients with chronic stable angina. In exercise tolerance testing, Nicardipine HCl significantly increased time to angina, total exercise duration and time to 1 mm ST segment depression. Included among these four studies was a dose-definition study in which dose-related improvements in exercise tolerance at one and four hours post-dosing and reduced frequency of anginal attacks were seen at doses of 10, 20 and 30 mg TID. Effectiveness at 10 mg TID was, however, marginal. In a fifth placebo-controlled study, the antianginal efficacy of Nicardipine HCl was demonstrated at 8 hours post-dose (trough). The sustained efficacy of Nicardipine HCl has been demonstrated over long-term dosing. Blood pressure fell in patients with angina by about 10/8 mmHg at peak blood levels and was little different from placebo at trough blood levels.

EFFECTS IN HYPERTENSION
Nicardipine HCl produced dose-related decreases in both systolic and diastolic blood pressure in clinical trials. The antihypertensive efficacy of Nicardipine HCl administered three times daily has been demonstrated in three placebo-controlled studies involving 517 patients with mild to moderate hypertension. The blood pressure responses in the three studies were statistically significant from placebo at peak (1 hour post-dosing) and trough (8 hours post-dosing) although it is apparent that well over half of the antihypertensive effect is lost by the end of the dosing interval. The results from placebo controlled studies of Nicardipine HCl given three times daily are shown in the following table: (See related table).

The responses are shown as differences from the concurrent placebo control group. The large changes between peak and trough effects were not accompanied by observed side effects at peak response times. In a study using 24 hour intra-arterial blood pressure monitoring, the circadian variation in blood pressure remained unaltered, but the systolic and diastolic blood pressures were reduced throughout the whole 24 hours.

When added to beta-blocker therapy Nicardipine HCl further lowers both systolic and diastolic blood pressure.

Nicardipine HCl Sustained Release produced decreases in both systolic and diastolic blood pressure throughout the dosing interval in clinical trials. The antihypertensive efficacy of Nicardipine HCl Sustained Release administered twice daily has been demonstrated using inclinic blood pressure measures in placebo-controlled trials involving patients with mild to moderate hypertension and in trials using 12 or 24 hour amaulatory blood pressure monitoring.

In patients with mild to moderate chronic stable essential hypertension, Nicardipine HCl IV (0.5. to 4.0 mg/hr) produced dose-dependent decreases in blood pressure, although only the decreases at 4.0 mg/hr were statistically different from placebo. At the end of a 48-hour infusion at 4.0 mg/hr, the decreases were 26.0 mmHg (17%) in systolic blood pressure and 20.7 mmHg (20%) in diastolic blood pressure.

In other settings (e.g., patients with severe or postoperative hypertension), Nicardipine HCl IV (5 to 15 mg/hr) produced dose-dependent decreases in blood pressure. Higher infusion rates produced therapeutic responses more rapidly. The mean time to therapeutic response for severe hypertension, defined as diastolic blood pressure $\leq$ 95 mmHg or $\geq$ 25 mmHg decrease and systolic blood pressure $\leq$ 160 mmHg was 77 $\pm$ 5.2 minutes. The average maintenance dose was 8.0 mg/hr. The mean time to therapeutic response for postoperative hypertension, defined as

$\geq$ 15% reduction in diastolic or systolic blood pressure, was 11.5 $\pm$ 0.8 minutes. The average maintenance dose was 3.0 mg/hr.

INDICATIONS AND USAGE
I. STABLE ANGINA
Nicardipine HCl is indicated for the management of patients with chronic stable angina (effort-associated againa). Nicardipine HCl may be used alone or in combination with beta-blockers.

II. HYPERTENSION
Nicardipine HCl and Nicardipine HCl Sustained Release are indicated for the treatment of hypertension. Nicardipine HCl and Nicardipine HCl Sustained Release may be used alone or in combination with other antihypertensive drugs. In administering Nicardipine it is important to be aware of the relatively large peak to trough differences in blood pressure effect. (See " Dosage and Administration").

Nicardipine HCl IV is indicated for the short-term treatment of hypertension when oral therapy is not feasible or not desirable.

For prolonged control of blood pressure, patients should be transferred to oral medication as soon as their clinical condition permits (see "Dosage and Administration").

UNLABELED USES
Nicardipine HCl is used alone or as an adjunct in the treatment of Raynaud's disease, migraine headache, and cerebral ischemia. It is also used in patients with subarachnoid hemorrhage from ruptured aneurysms to improve neurological outcomes.

CONTRAINDICATIONS
Nicardipine HCl is contraindicated in patients with hypersensitivity to the drug.

Because part of the effect of Nicardipine HCl is secondary to reduced afterload, the drug is also contraindicated in patients with advanced aortic stenosis. Reduction of diastolic pressure in these patients may worsen rather than improve myocardial oxygen balance.

WARNINGS
INCREASED ANGINA
About 7% of patients in short term placebo-controlled angina trials have developed increased frequency, duration or severity of angina on starting Nicardipine HCl or at the time of dosage increases, compared with 4% of patients on placebo. Comparisons with beta-blockers also show a greater frequency of increased angina, 4% vs 1%. The mechanism of this effect has not been established. (See "Adverse Reactions".)

Induction or exacerbation of angina has been seen in less than 1% of coronary artery disease patients treated with Nicardipine HCl IV. The mechanism of this effect has not been established.

USE IN PATIENTS WITH CONGESTIVE HEART FAILURE
Although preliminary hemodynamic studies in patients with congestive heart failure have shown that Nicardipine HCl reduced afterload without impairing myocardial contractility, it has a negative inotropic effect in vitro and in some patients. Caution should be exercised when using the drug in congestive heart failure patients, or in patients with significant left ventricular dysfunction (IV), particularly in combination with a beta blocker.

BETA-BLOCKER WITHDRAWAL
Nicardipine HCl is not a beta-blocker and therefore gives no protection against the dangers of abrupt beta-blocker withdrawal; any such withdrawal should be by gradual reduction of the dose of beta-blocker, preferably over 8-10 days.

RAPID DECREASES IN BLOOD PRESSURE
No clinical events have been reported suggestive of a too rapid decrease in blood pressure with Nicardipine HCl IV. However, as with any antihypertensive agent, blood pressure lowering should be accomplished over as long a time as is compatible with the patient's clinical status.

USE IN PATIENTS WITH PHEOCHROMOCYTOMA
Only limited clinical experience exists in use of Nicardipine HCl IV for patients with hypertension associated with pheochromocytoma. Caution should therefore be exercised when using the drug in these patients.

PERIPHERAL VEIN INFUSION SITE
To minimize the risk of pheripheral venous irritation, it is recommended that the site of infusion of Nicardipine HCl IV be changed every 12 hours.

	Systolic BP (mmHg)					Diastolic BP (mmHg)			
Dose	Number of Patients	Mean Peak Response	Mean Trough Response	Trough Peak	Dose	Number of Patients	Mean Peak Response	Mean Trough Response	Trough/Peak
20 mg	50	—10.3	—4.9	48%	20 mg	50	10.6	—4.6	43%
	52	—17.6	—7.9	45%		52	—9.0	—2.9	32%
30 mg	45	—14.5	—7.2	50%	30 mg	45	—12.8	—4.9	38%
	44	—14.6	—7.5	51%		44	—14.2	—4.3	30%
40 mg	50	—16.3	—9.5	58%	40 mg	50	—15.4	—5.9	38%
	38	—15.9	—6.0	38%		38	—14.8	—3.7	25%

➤ SHOWN IN PRODUCT IDENTIFICATION GUIDE

PRECAUTIONS
GENERAL
Blood Pressure: Because Nicardipine HCl decreases peripheral resistance, careful monitoring of blood pressure during the initial administration and titration of Nicardipine HCl is suggested. Nicardipine HCl, like other calcium channel blockers, may occasionally produce symptomatic hypotension. Caution is advised to avoid systemic hypotension when administering the drug to patients who have sustained an acute cerebral infarction or hemorrhage. Because of prominent effects at the time of peak blood levels, initial titration should be performed with measurements of blood pressure at peak effect (1-2 hours after dosing) and just before the next dose.

Use in Patients with Impaired Hepatic Function: Since the liver is the major site of biotransformation and since Nicardipine HCl is subject to first pass metabolism, the drug should be used with caution in patients having impaired liver function or reduced hepatic blood flow. The use of lower dosage should be considered. Patients with severe liver disease developed elevated blood levels (4-fold increase in AUC) and prolonged half-life (19 hours) of Nicardipine HCl. (See *"Dosage And Administration"*).

Nicardipine administered intravenously has been reported to increase hepatic venous pressure gradient by 4 mmHg in cirrhotic patients at high doses (5 mg/20 min). Nicardipine HCl IV should therefore be used with caution in patients with portal hypertension.

Use in Patients with Impaired Renal Function: When Nicardipine HCl 20 mg or 30 mg TID was given to hypertensive patients with mild renal impairment, mean plasma concentrations. AUC, and Cmax were approximately 2-fold higher in renally impaired patients than in healthy controls. Doses in these patients must be adjusted.

When Nicardipine HCl Sustained Release 45 mg BID was given to hypertensive patients with moderate renal impairment, mean AUC and Cmax values were approximately 2-3 fold higher than in patients with mild renal impairment. Doses in these patients must be adjusted. Mean AUC and Cmax values were similar in patients with mildly impaired renal function and normal volunteers. (See *"Clinical Pharmacology"* and *"Dosage and Administration"*.)

When Nicardipine HCl IV was given to mild to moderate hypertensive patients with moderate renal impairment, a significantly lower systemic clearance and higher AUC was observed. These results are consistent with those seen after oral administration of Nicardipine. Careful dose titration is advised when treating renal impaired patients.

DRUG INTERACTIONS
Since Nicardipine HCl IV may be administered to patients already being treated with other medications, including other antihypertensive agents, careful monitoring of these patients is necessary to detect and promptly treat any undesired effects from concomitant administration.

Beta-Blockers: In controlled clinical studies, adrenergic beta-receptor blockers have been frequently administered concomitantly with Nicardipine HCl. The combination is well tolerated. However, caution should be exercised when using Nicardipine HCl IV in combination with a beta-blocker in congestive heart failure paients (see *"Warnings"*).

Cimetidine: Cimetidine increases Nicardipine HCl plasma levels. Patients receiving the two drugs concomitantly should be carefully monitored. Data with other histamine-2 antagonists are not available.

Digoxin: Some calcium blockers may increase the concentration of digitalis preparations in the blood. Nicardipine HCl usually does not alter the plasma levels of digoxin, however, serum digoxin levels should be evaluated after concomitant therapy with Nicardipine HCl is initiated.

Maalox: Co-administration of Maalox TC had no effect on Nicardipine HCl absorption.

Fentanyl Anesthesia: Severe hypotension has been reported during fentanyl anesthesia with concomitant use of a beta-blocker and a calcium channel blocker. Even though such interactions were not seen during clinical studies with Nicardipine HCl, an increased volume of circulating fluids might be required if such an interaction were to occur.

Cyclosporine: Concomitant administration of Nicardipine and cyclosporine results in elevated plasma cyclosporine levels. Plasma concentrations of cyclosporine should therefore be closely monitored, and its dosage reduced accordingly, in patients treated with Nicardipine.

When therapeutic concentrations of *furosemide, propranolol, dipyridamole, warfarin, quinidine,* or *naproxen* were added to human plasma *(in vitro)*, the plasma protein binding of Nicardipine HCl was not altered.

CARCINOGENESIS, MUTAGENESIS, IMPAIRMENT OF FERTILITY
Rats treated with Nicardipine in the diet (at concentrations calculated to provide daily dosage levels of 5, 15 or 45 mg/kg/day) for two years showed a dose-dependent increase in thyroid hyperplasia and neoplasia (follicular adenoma/carcinoma). One and three month studies in the rat have suggested that these results are linked to a Nicardipine-induced reduction in plasma thyroxine (T4) levels with a consequent increase in plasma levels of thyroid stimulating hormone (TSH). Chronic elevation of TSH is known to cause hyperstimulation of the thyroid. In rats on an iodine deficient diet, Nicardipine administration for one month was associated with thyroid hyperplasia that was prevented by T4 supplementation. Mice treated with Nicardipine in the diet (at concentrations calculated to provide daily dosage levels of up to 100 mg/kg/day) for up to 18 months showed no evidence of neoplasia of any tissue and no evidence of thyroid changes. There was no evidence of thyroid pathology in dogs treated with up to 25 mg Nicardipine/kg/day for one year and no evidence of effects of Nicardipine on thyroid function (plasma T4 and TSH) in man.

There was no evidence of a mutagenic potential of Nicardipine in a battery of genotoxicity tests conducted on microbial indicator organisms, in micronucleus tests in mice and hamsters, or in a sister chromatid exchange study in hamsters. No impairment of fertility was seen in male or female rats administered Nicardipine at oral doses as high as 100 mg/kg/day (50 times the 40 mg TID maximum recommended antianginal or antihypertensive dose in man, assuming a patient weight of 60 kg).

PREGNANCY
Pregnancy Category C: Nicardipine was embryocidal when administered orally to pregnant Japanese White rabbits, during organogenesis, at 150 mg/kg/day (a dose associated with marked body weight gain suppression in the treated doe) but not at 50 mg/kg/day (25 times the maximum recommended antianginal or antihypertensive dose in man). No adverse effects on the fetus were observed when New Zealand albino rabbits were treated, during organogenesis, with up to 100 mg Nicardipine/kg/day (a dose associated with significant mortality in the treated doe). In pregnant rats administered Nicardipine orally at up to 100 mg/kg/day (50 times the maximum recommended human dose) there was no evidence of embryolethality or teratogenicity. However, dystocia, reduced birth weights, reduced neonatal survival and reduced neonatal weight gain were noted. There are no adequate and well-controlled studies in pregnant women. Nicardipine HCl should be used during pregnancy only if the potential benefit justifies the potential risk to the fetus.

Nicardipine HCl IV at doses up to 5 mg/kg/day to pregnant rats and up to 0.5 mg/kg/day to pregnant rabbits produced no embryotoxicity or teratogenicity. Embryotoxicity was seen at 10 mg/kg/day in rats and at 1 mg/kg/day in rabbits, but no teratogenicity was observed at these doses.

NURSING MOTHERS
Studies in rats have shown significant concentrations of Nicardipine HCl in maternal milk following oral or IV administration. For this reason it is recommended that women who wish to breast-feed should not take this drug.

PEDIATRIC USE
Safety and efficacy in patients under the age of 18 have not been established.

USE IN THE ELDERLY
Pharmacokinetic parameters did not differ between elderly hypertensive patients ($\geq$ 65 years) and healthy controls after one week of Nicardipine HCl treatment at 20 mg TID. Plasma Nicardipine HCl concentrations in elderly hypertensive patients were similar to plasma concentrations in healthy young adult subjects when Nicardipine HCl was administered at doses of 10, 20 and 30 mg TID, suggesting that the pharmacokinetics of Nicardipine HCl and Nicardipine HCl Sustained Release are similar in young and elderly hypertensive patients.

Pharmacokinetic parameters did not differ significantly between elderly hypertensive patients (mean age 70 years) and younger hypertensive patients (mean age 44 years) after one week of treatment with Nicardipine HCl Sustained Release. No significant differences in responses to Nicardipine HCl and Nicardipine HCl Sustained Release have been observed in elderly patients and the general adult population of patients who participated in clinical studies.

No significant difference has been observed in the antihypertensive effect of Nifedipine HCl IV in elderly patients ($\geq$ 65 years) compared with other adult patients in clinical studies.

ADVERSE REACTIONS
CAPSULES
In multiple-dose U.S. and foreign controlled short-term (up to three months) studies 1,910 patients received Nicardipine HCl alone or in combination with other drugs. In these studies adverse events were reported spontaneously; adverse experiences were generally not serious but occasionally required dosage adjustment and about 10% of patients left the studies prematurely because of them. Peak responses were not observed to be associated with adverse effects during clinical trials, but physicians should be aware that adverse effects associated with decreases in blood pressure (tachycardia, hypotension, etc.) could occur around the time of the peak effect. Most adverse effects were expected consequences of the vasodilator effects of Nicardipine HCl.

ANGINA
The incidence rates of adverse effects in anginal patients were derived from multicenter, controlled clinical trials. Following are the rates of adverse effects for Nicardipine HCl (N = 520) and placebo (N = 310), respectively, that occurred in 0.4% of patients or more. These represent events considered probably drug-related by the investigator (except for certain cardiovascular events which were recorded in a different category). Where the frequency of adverse effects for Nicardipine HCl and placebo is similar, causal relationship is uncertain. The only dose-related effects were pedal edema and increased angina.

PERCENT OF PATIENTS WITH ADVERSE EFFECTS IN CONTROLLED STUDIES (INCIDENCE OF DISCONTINUATIONS SHOWN IN PARENTHESES)

Adverse Experience	Nicardipine HCl (N = 520)	Placebo (N = 310)
Pedal Edema	7.1 (0)	0.3 (0)

Adverse Experience	Nicardipine HCl (N = 520)	Placebo (N = 310)
Dizziness	6.9 (1.2)	0.6 (0)
Headache	6.4 (0.6)	2.6 (0)
Asthenia	5.8 (0.4)	2.6 (0)
Flushing	5.6 (0.4)	1.0 (0)
Increased Angina	5.6 (3.5)	4.2 (1.9)
Palpitations	3.3 (0.2)	0.3 (0)
Nausea	1.9 (0)	0.3 (0)
Dyspepsia	1.5 (0.6)	0.6 (0.3)
Dry Mouth	1.4 (0)	0.3 (0)
Somnolence	1.4 (0)	1.0 (0)
Rash	1.2 (0.2)	0.3 (0)
Tachycardia	1.2 (0.2)	0.6 (0)
Myalgia	1.0 (0)	0.0 (0)
Other edema	1.0 (0)	0.0 (0)
Paresthesia	1.0 (0.2)	0.3 (0)
Sustained Tachycardia	0.8 (0.6)	0.0 (0)
Syncope	0.8 (0.2)	0.0 (0)
Constipation	0.6 (0.2)	0.6 (0)
Dyspnea	0.6 (0)	0.0 (0)
Abnormal ECG	0.6 (0.6)	0.0 (0)
Malaise	0.6 (0)	0.0 (0)
Nervousness	0.6 (0)	0.3 (0)
Tremor	0.6 (0)	0.0 (0)

In addition, adverse events were observed which are not readily distinguishable from the natural history of the atherosclerotic vascular disease in these patients. Adverse events in this category each occurred in < 0.4% of patients receiving Nicardipine HCl and included myocardial infarction, atrial fibrillation, exertional hypotension, pericarditis, heart block, cerebral ischemia and ventricular tachycardia. It is possible that some of these events were drug-related.

HYPERTENSION

The incidence rates of adverse effects in hypertensive patients were derived from multicenter, controlled clinical trials. Following are the rates of adverse effects for Nicardipine HCl (n = 1390) and placebo (N = 211), respectively, that occurred in 0.4% of patients or more. These represent events considered probably drug-related by the investigator.

Where the frequency of adverse effects for Nicardipine HCl and placebo is similar, causal relationship is uncertain. The only dose-related effect was pedal edema.

PERCENT OF PATIENTS WITH ADVERSE EFFECTS IN CONTROLLED STUDIES (INCIDENCE OF DISCONTINUATIONS SHOWN IN PARENTHESES)

Adverse Experience	Nicardipine HCl (N = 1390)	Placebo (N = 211)
Flushing	9.7 (2.1)	2.8 (0)
Headache	8.2 (2.6)	4.7 (0)
Pedal Edema	8.0 (1.8)	0.9 (0)
Asthenia	4.2 (1.7)	0.5 (0)
Palpitations	4.1 (1.0)	0.0 (0)
Dizziness	4.0 (1.8)	0.0 (0)
Tachycardia	3.4 (1.2)	0.5 (0)
Nausea	2.2 (0.9)	0.9 (0)
Somnolence	1.1 (0.1)	0.0 (0)
Dyspepsia	0.8 (0.3)	0.5 (0)
Insomnia	0.6 (0.1)	0.0 (0)
Malaise	0.6 (0.1)	0.0 (0)
Other edema	0.6 (0.3)	1.4 (0)
Abnormal dreams	0.4 (0)	0.0 (0)
Dry mouth	0.4 (0.1)	0.0 (0)
Nocturia	0.4 (0)	0.0 (0)
Rash	0.4 (0.4)	0.0 (0)
Vomiting	0.4 (0)	0.0 (0)

RARE EVENTS

The following rare adverse events have been reported in clinical trials or the literature:

Body as a Whole: infection, allergic reaction

Cardiovascular: hypotension, postural hypotension, atypical chest pain, peripheral vascular disorder, ventricular extrastoles ventricular tachycardia

Digestive: sore throat, abnormal liver chemistries

Musculoskeletal: arthralgia

Nervous: hot flashes, vertigo, hyperkinesia, impotence, depression, confusion, anxiety

Respiratory: rhinitis, sinusitis

Special Senses: tinnitus, abnormal vision, blurred vision

Urogenital: increased urinary frequency

SUSTAINED-RELEASE CAPSULES

In multiple-dose U.S. and foreign controlled studies, 667 patients received Nicardipine HCl Sustained Release. In these studies adverse events were elicited by nondirected and in some cases directed questioning; adverse events were generally not serious and about 9% of patients withdrew prematurely from the studies because of them.

HYPERTENSION

The incidence rates of adverse events in hypertensive patients were derived from placebo-controlled clinical trials. Following are the rates of adverse events for Nicardipine HCl Sustained Release (N = 322) and placebo (N = 140), respectively, that occurred in 0.6% of patients or more on Nicardipine HCl Sustained Release. These represent events considered probably drug related by the investigator. Where the frequency of adverse events for Nicardipine HCl Sustained Release and placebo is similar, causal relationship is uncertain. The only dose-related effect was pedal edema.

PERCENTAGE OF PATIENTS WITH PROBABLY DRUG RELATED ADVERSE EVENTS IN PLACEBO-CONTROLLED STUDIES

Adverse Event	Nicardipine HCl Sustained Release (N = 322)	Placebo (N = 140)
Headache	6.2	7.1
Pedal Edema	5.9	1.4
Vasodilatation	4.7	1.4
Palpitation	2.8	1.4
Nausea	1.9	0.7
Dizziness	1.6	0.7
Asthenia	0.9	0.7
Postural Hypotension	0.9	0
Increased Urinary Frequency	0.6	0
Pain	0.6	0
Rash	0.6	0
Sweating Increased	0.6	0
Vomiting	0.6	0

INCIDENCE (%) OF DISCONTINUATIONS DUE TO ANY ADVERSE EVENT IN PLACEBO-CONTROLLED STUDIES

Adverse Event	Nicardipine HCl Sustained Release (N = 322)	Placebo (N = 140)
Headache	2.5	1.4
Palpitation	2.2	0.7
Dizziness	1.9	0.7
Asthenia	1.9	0
Pedal Edema	1.2	0
Nausea	1.2	0
Rash	0.9	0.7
Diarrhea	0.9	0
Tachycardia	0.9	0
Blurred Vision	0.6	0
Chest Pain	0.6	0
Face Edema	0.6	0
Myocardial Infarct	0.6	0
Vasodilatation	0.6	0
Vomiting	0.6	0

Uncontrolled experience in over 300 patients with hypertension treated for up to 27.5 months with Nicardipine HCl Sustained Release has shown no unexpected adverse events or increase in incidence of adverse events compared to the controlled clinical trials.

RARE EVENTS

The following rare adverse events have been reported in clinical trials or the literature:

Body as a Whole: infection, allergic reaction

Cardiovascular: hyotension, atypical chest pain, peripheral vascular disorder, ventricular extrasystoles, ventricular tachycardia, angina pectoris

Digestive: sore throat, abnormal liver chemistries

Musculoskeletal: arthralgia

Nervous: hot flashes, vertigo, hyperkinesia, impotence, depression, confusion, anxiety

Respiratory: rhinitis, sinusitis

Special Senses: tinnitus, abnormal vision, blurred vision

ANGINA

Data are available from only 91 patients with chronic stable angina pectoris who received Nicardipine HCl Sustained Release 30-60 mg administered twice daily in open label clinical trials. Fifty-eight of these patients were treated for at least 30 days. The four most frequently reported adverse events thought by the investigators to be probably related to the use of Nicardipine HCl Sustained Release were vasodilatation (5.5%), pedal edema (4.4%), asthenia (4.4%), and dizziness (3.3%).

INTRAVENOUS INFUSION
Two hundred forty-four patients participated in two multicenter, double-blind, placebo controlled trials of Nicardipine HCl IV. Adverse experiences were generally not serious and most were expected consequences of vasodilation. Adverse experiences occasionally required dosage adjustment. Therapy was discontinued in approximately 12% of patients, mainly due to hypotension, headache, and tachycardia.

PERCENT OF PATIENTS WITH ADVERSE EXPERIENCES DURING THE DOUBLE-BLIND PORTION OF CONTROLLED TRIALS

Adverse Experience	Nicardipine HCl IV (n = 144)	Placebo (n = 100)
Body as a Whole		
Headache	14.6	2.0
Asthenia	0.7	0.0
Abdominal pain	0.7	0.0
Chest pain	0.7	0.0
Cardiovascular		
Hypotension	5.6	1.0
Tachycardia	3.5	0.0
ECG abnormality	1.4	0.0
Postural hypotension	1.4	0.0
Ventricular extrasystoles	1.4	0.0
Extrasystoles	0.7	0.0
Hemopericardium	0.7	0.0
Hypertension	0.7	0.0
Supraventricular tachycardia	0.7	0.0
Syncope	0.7	0.0
Vasodilation	0.7	0.0
Ventricular tachycardia	0.7	0.0
Digestive		
Nausea/vomiting	4.9	1.0
Injection Site		
Injection site reaction	1.4	0.0
Injection site pain	0.7	0.0
Metabolic and Nutritional		
Hypokalemia	0.7	0.0
Nervous		
Dizziness	1.4	0.0
Hypesthesia	0.7	0.0
Intracranial hemorrhage	0.7	0.0
Paresthesia	0.7	0.0
Respiratory		
Dyspnea	0.7	0.0
Skin and Appendages		
Sweating	1.4	0.0
Urogenital		
Polyuria	1.4	0.0
Hematuria	0.7	0.0

RARE EVENTS
The following rare events have been reported in clinical trials or in the literature in association with the use of intravenously administered Nicardipine.

Body as a Whole: fever, neck pain

Cardiovascular: angina pectoris, atrioventricular block, ST segment depression, inverted T wave, deep-vein thrombophlebitis

Digestive: dyspepsia

Hemic and Lymphatic: thrombocytopenia

Metabolic and Nutritional: hypophosphatemia, peripheral edema

Nervous: confusion, hypertonia

Respiratory: respiratory disorder

Special Senses: conjunctivitis, ear disorder, tinnitus

Urogenital: urinary frequency

Sinus node dysfunction and myocardial infarction, which may be due to disease progression, have been seen in patients on chronic therapy with orally administered Nicardipine.

OVERDOSAGE
Three overdosages with Nicardipine HCl or Nicardipine HCl Sustained Release have been reported. Two occurred in adults, one of whom ingested 600 mg of Nicardipine HCl and the other 2,160 mg of Nicardipine HCl Sustained Release. Symptoms included marked hypotension, bradycardia, palpitations, flushing, drowsiness, confusion and slurred speech. All symptoms resolved without sequelae. The third overdosage occurred in a one year old child who ingested half of the powder in a 30 mg Nicardipine HCl capsule. The child remained asymptomatic.

Based on results obtained in laboratory animals, overdosage may cause systemic hypotension, bradycardia (following initial tachycardia) and progressive atrioventricular conduction block. Reversible hepatic function abnormalities and sporadic focal hepatic necrosis were noted in some animal species receiving very large doses of Nicardipine.

For treatment of overdose: standard measures (for example, evacuation of gastric contents, elevation of extremities, attention to circulating fluid volume and urine output) including monitoring of cardiac and respiratory functions should be implemented. The patient should be positioned so as to avoid cerebral anoxia. Frequent blood pressure determinations are essential. Vasopressors are clinically indicated for patients exhibiting profound hypotension. Intravenous calcium gluconate may help reverse the effects of calcium entry blockade.

DOSAGE AND ADMINISTRATION
ANGINA
The dose should be individually titrated for each patient beginning with 20 mg three times daily. Doses in the range of 20-40 mg three times a day have been shown to be effective. At least three days should be allowed before increasing the Nicardipine HCl dose to ensure achievement of steady state plasma drug concentrations.

Concomitant Use With Other Antianginal Agents:

1. Sublingual NTG may be taken as required to abort acute anginal attacks during Nicardipine HCl therapy.

2. Prophylactic Nitrate Therapy: Nicardipine HCl may be safely coadministered with short- and long-acting nitrate.

3. Beta blockers: Nicardipine HCl may be safely coadministered with beta blockers. (See *"Drug Interactions".*)

HYPERTENSION
The dose of Nicardipine HCl should be individually adjusted according to the blood pressure response beginning with 20 mg three times daily. The effective doses in clinical trials have ranged from 20 mg to 40 mg three times daily. The maximum blood pressure lowering effect occurs approximately 1-2 hours after dosing. *To assess the adequacy of blood pressure response, the blood pressure should be measured at trough (8 hours after dosing). Because of the prominent peak effects of Nicardipine, blood pressure should be measured 1-2 hours after dosing, particularly during initiation of therapy.*

The dose of Nicardipine HCl Sustained Release should be individually adjusted according to the blood pressure response beginning with 30 mg two times daily. The effective doses in clinical trials have ranged from 30 mg to 60 mg two times daily. The maximum blood pressure lowering effect at steady state is sustained from 2 hours until 6 hours after dosing.

When initiating therapy or upon increasing dose, blood pressure should be measured 2 to 4 hours after the first dose or dose increase, as well as at the end of a dosing interval.

The total daily dose of immediate release Nicardipine may not be a useful guide to judging the effective dose of Nicardipine HCl Sustained Release. Patients currently receiving immediate release Nicardipine may be treated with Nicardipine HCl Sustained Release starting at their current total daily dose of immediate release Nicardipine and then reexamined to assess the adequacy of blood pressure control.

Nicardipine HCl Intravenous is intended for intravenous use. *Dosage Must be Individualized* depending upon the severity of hypertension and the response of the patient during dosing.

Blood pressure should be monitored both during and after the infusion; too rapid or excessive reduction in either systolic or diastolic blood pressure during parenteral treatment should be avoided.

PREPARATION
Warning: Ampuls Must Be Diluted Before Infusion

Dilution: Nicardipine HCl IV, is administered by slow continuous infusion at a CONCENTRATION OF 0.1 MG/ML. Each ampul (25 mg) should be diluted with 240 mL of compatible intravenous fluid (see below), resulting in 250 mL of solution at a concentration of 0.1 mg/mL.

Nicardipine HCl IV has been found to be compatible and stable in glass or polyvinyl chloride containers for 24 hours at controlled room temperature with:
Dextrose (5%) Injection, USP
Dextrose (5%) and Sodium Chloride (0.45%) Injection, USP
Dextrose (5%) and Sodium Chloride (0.9%) Injection, USP
Dextrose (5%) with 40 mEq Potassium, USP
Sodium Chloride (0.45%) Injection, USP
Sodium Chloride (0.9%) Injection, USP
is NOT compatible with Sodium Bicarbonate (5%) Injection, USP, or Lactated Ringer's Injection, USP.

THE DILUTED SOLUTION IS STABLE FOR 24 HOURS AT ROOM TEMPERATURE
Inspection: As with all parenteral drugs, Nicardipine HCl IV, should be inspected visually for particulate matter and discoloration prior to administration, whenever solution and container permit. Nicardipine HCl IV is normally light yellow in color.

AS A SUBSTITUTE FOR ORAL NACARDIPINE THERAPY
The intravenous infusion rate required to produce an average plasma concentration equivalent to a given oral dose at steady state is shown in the following table:

Oral Nicardipine HCl Dose	Equivalent I.V. Infusion Rate
20 mg q8h	0.5 mg/hr
30 mg q8h	1.2 mg/hr
40 mg q8h	2.2 mg/hr

FOR INITIATION OF THERAPY IN A DRUG FREE PATIENT
The time course of blood pressure decrease is dependent on the initial rate of infusion and the frequency of dosage adjustment.

Nicardipine HCl IV is administered by slow continuous infusion at a CONCENTRATION OF 0.1 MG/ML. With constant infusion, blood pressure begins to fall within minutes. It reaches about 50% of its ultimate decrease in about 45 minutes and does not reach final steady state for about 50 hours.

When treating acute hypertensive episodes in patients with chronic hypertension, discontinuation of infusion is followed by a 50% offset of action in 30 ± 7 minutes but plasma levels of drug and gradually decreasing antihypertensive effects exist for about 50 hours.

Titration: For gradual reduction in blood pressure, initiate therapy at 50 mL/hr (5.0 mg/hr). If desired blood pressure reduction is not achieved at this dose, the infusion rate may be increased by 25 mL/hr (2.5 mg/hr) every 15 minutes up to a maximum of 150 mL/hr (15.0 mg/hr), until desired blood pressure reduction is achieved. For more rapid blood pressure reduction, initiate therapy at 50 mL/hr (5.0 mg/hr). If desired blood pressure reduction is not achieved at this dose, the infusion rate may be increased by 25 mL/hr (2.5 mg/hr) every 5 minutes up to a maximum of 150 mL/hr (15.0 mg/hr), until desired blood pressure reduction is achieved. Following achievement of the blood pressure goal, the infusion rate should be decreased to 30 mL/hr (3 mg/hr).

Maintenance: The rate of infusion should be adjusted as needed to maintain desired response.

CONDITIONS REQUIRING INFUSION ADJUSTMENT
Hypotension or Tachycardia: If there is concern of impending hypotension or tachycardia, the infusion should be discontinued. When blood pressure has stabilized, infusion of Nicardipine HCl IV, may be restarted at low doses such as 30-50 mL/hr (3.0-5.0 mg/hr) and adjusted to maintain desired blood pressure.

Infusion Site Changes: Nicardipine HCl IV should be continued as long as blood pressure control is needed. The infusion site should be changed every 12 hours if administered via peripheral vein.

Impaired Cardiac, Hepatic or Renal Function: Caution is advised when titrating Nicardipine HCl IV in patients with congestive heart failure or impaired hepatic or renal function (see "Precautions").

TRANSFER TO ORAL ANTHYPERTENSIVE AGENTS
If treatment includes transfer to an oral antihypertensive agent other than Nicardipine HCl capsules, therapy should generally be initiated upon discontinuation of Nicardipine HCl IV. If Nicardipine HCl capsules are to be used, the first dose of a TID regimen should be administered 1 hour prior to discontinuation of the infusion.

(See "Precautions: Blood Pressures," "Indications" and "Clinical Pharmacology: Peak/Trough Effects in Hypertension".) At least three days should be allowed before increasing the Nicardipine HCl dose to ensure achievement of steady state plasma drug concentrations.

Concomitant use with other Antihypertensive Agents:

1. Diuretics: Nicardipine HCl may be safely coadministered with thiazide diuretics.

2. Beta blockers: Nicardipine HCl may be safely coadministered with beta blockers (See "Drug Interactions".)

SPECIAL PATIENT POPULATIONS
Renal Insufficiency: although there is no evidence that Nicardipine HCl or Nicardipine HCl Sustained Release impairs renal function, careful dose titration beginning with 20 mg TID Nicardipine HCl or 30 mg Nicardipine HCl Sustained Release is advised. (See "Precautions".)

Hepatic Insufficiency: Nicardipine HCl should be administered cautiously in patients with severely impaired hepatic function. A suggested starting dose of 20 mg twice a day is advised with individual titration based on clinical findings maintaining the twice a day schedule. Nicardipine HCl Sustained Release has not been studied in patients with severe liver impairment. (See "Precautions".)

Congestive Heart Failure: Caution is advised when titrating Nicardipine HCl dosage in patients with congestive heart failure. (See "Warnings".)

STORAGE
Store bottles at room temperature and dispense in light-resistant containers.

Store blister packages at room temperature and protect from excessive humidity and light. To protect from light, product should remain in manufacturer's package until consumed.

Store Nicardipine HCl IV at controlled room temperature, 15°-30° C (59°-86°F). Freezing does not adversely affect the product, but exposure to elevated temperatures should be avoided.

Protect from light. Store ampuls in carton until used.

HOW SUPPLIED
CAPSULE: 20 MG

BRAND/MANUFACTURER	NDC	SIZE	AWP
○ BRAND			
▶ CARDENE: Syntex/F.P.	00033-2437-42	100s	$40.71
	00033-2437-53	100s ud	$42.42
	00033-2437-62	500s	$197.46

CAPSULE: 30 MG

BRAND/MANUFACTURER	NDC	SIZE	AWP
○ BRAND			
▶ CARDENE: Syntex/F.P.	00033-2438-42	100s	$64.73
	00033-2438-53	100s ud	$66.46
	00033-2438-62	500s	$313.91

CAPSULE, EXTENDED RELEASE: 30 MG

BRAND/MANUFACTURER	NDC	SIZE	AWP
○ BRAND			
▶ CARDENE SR: Syntex	00033-2440-40	60s	$38.15
	00033-2440-53	100s ud	$63.59
	00033-2440-60	200s	$127.18

CAPSULE, EXTENDED RELEASE: 45 MG

BRAND/MANUFACTURER	NDC	SIZE	AWP
○ BRAND			
▶ CARDENE SR: Syntex	00033-2441-40	60s	$60.60
	00033-2441-53	100s ud	$100.99
	00033-2441-60	200s	$201.98

CAPSULE, EXTENDED RELEASE: 60 MG

BRAND/MANUFACTURER	NDC	SIZE	AWP
○ BRAND			
▶ CARDENE SR: Syntex	00033-2442-40	60s	$72.56
	00033-2442-60	200s	$241.88

INJECTION: 2.5 MG/ML

BRAND/MANUFACTURER	NDC	SIZE	AWP
○ BRAND			
CARDENE IV: Wyeth-Ayerst	00008-0812-02	10 ml 10s	$206.25

Niclocide *SEE* NICLOSAMIDE

Niclosamide

DESCRIPTION
Niclosamide is an anthelmintic provided in chewable tablet form at a strength of 500 mg per tablet. Niclosamide is 2', 5-Dichloro-4'-nitrosalicylanilide.

Following is its chemical structure:

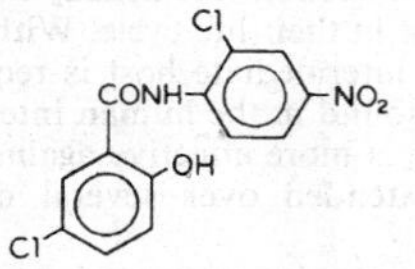

CLINICAL PHARMACOLOGY
Niclosamide inhibits oxidative phosphorylation in the mitochondria of cestodes. Both *in vitro* and *in vivo*, the scolex and proximal segments are killed on contact with the drug. The scolex of the tapeworm, loosened from the gut wall, may be digested in the intestine, and thus may not be identified in the feces even after extensive purging.

The use of Niclosamide has not been associated with the development of anemia, leukopenia or thrombocytopenia nor have there been any effects on normal renal and hepatic functions.

INDICATIONS AND USAGE
Niclosamide is indicated for the treatment of tapeworm infections by *Taenia saginata* (beef tapeworm), *Diphyllobothrium latum* (fish tapeworm) and *Hymenolepis nana* (dwarf tapeworm).

UNLABELED USES
Niclosamide is used alone or as an adjunct in the treatment of dipylidium caninum cestode infections.

CONTRAINDICATIONS
Niclosamide Tablets are contraindicated in individuals who have shown hypersensitivity to any of its components.

▶ SHOWN IN PRODUCT IDENTIFICATION GUIDE

PRECAUTIONS

Niclosamide affects the cestodes of the intestine only. It is without effect in cysticercosis.

Drug Interactions: No data are available regarding interaction of Niclosamide with other drugs.

Carcinogenesis, Mutagesis, Impairment of Fertility: Carcinogenicity Potential: Although carcinogenicity studies on Niclosamide *per se* have not been done, long-term feeding studies on its ethanolamine salt in rats and mice did not show carcinogenicity. Mutagenicity tests have not been performed.

Pregnancy: Pregnancy Category B: Reproduction studies in rabbits and rats at doses of 25 times the human therapeutic dose and in mice at 12 times the human therapeutic dose, have revealed no evidence of impaired fertility or harm to the fetus due to Niclosamide. There are, however, no adequate and well-controlled studies in pregnant women. Because animal studies are not always predictive of human response, the drug should be used during pregnancy only if clearly needed.

Nursing Mothers: No studies are available.

Pediatric Use: In children under 2 years of age, the safety of the drug has not been established.

ADVERSE REACTIONS

The incidence of side effects has been reported as follows: nausea/vomiting 4.1%, abdominal discomfort including loss of appetite 3.4%, diarrhea 1.6%, drowsiness, dizziness, and/or headache 1.4%, and skin rash including pruritus ani 0.3%. Other side effects listed in decreasing order of frequency were: oral irritation, fever, rectal bleeding, weakness, bad taste in mouth, sweating, palpitations, constipation, alopecia, edema of an arm, backache and irritability. There was also one instance of a transient rise in SGOT in an i.v. narcotic addict. Two cases of urticaria reported may be related to the breakdown products of the tapeworm. All side effects were mild or moderate and transitory and did not necessitate discontinuation of the treatment.

OVERDOSAGE

Insufficient data are available. In the event of overdose a fast-acting laxative and enema should be given. Vomiting should not be induced.

DOSAGE AND ADMINISTRATION

1. *Taenia saginata* and *Diphyllobothrium latum*
   a. Adults: 4 tablets (2.0 g) chewed thoroughly in a single dose.
   b. Children weighing more than 34 kg (75 lbs): 3 tablets (1.5 g) chewed thoroughly in a single dose.
   c. Children weighing between 11 and 34 kg (25 to 75 lbs): 2 tablets (1.0 g) chewed thoroughly in a single dose.
2. *Hymenolepis nana*
   a. Adults: 4 tablets (20 g) chewed thoroughly as a single daily dose for 7 days.
   b. Children weighing more than 34 kg (75 lbs): 3 tablets (1.5g) chewed thoroughly on the first day, then 2 tablets (1.0 g) daily for next 6 days.
   c. Children weighing between 11 and 34 kg (25 to 75 lbs): 2 tablets (1.0 g) to be chewed thoroughly on the first day, then one tablet (0.5 g) daily for next 6 days.

T. suginata and *D. latum* infections are usually due to a single adult worm and require an intermediate host in their life cycle. With *Hymenolepis nana* multiple infections are the rule. No intermediate host is required: both larval and adult stages of the worm may be found in the human intestine where the complete life cycle occurs. Since the drug is more effective against the mature than the larval stage, therapy must be extended over several days to cover all stages of maturation.

Patients with *H. nana* must be instructed to observe strict personal and environmental hygiene to avoid autoinfection with this parasite.

3. Niclosamide must be thoroughly chewed and then swallowed with a little water. No special dietary restrictions are necessary before or after treatment. The best time to take the drug is after a light meal (e.g., breakfast). A mild laxative may be desirable in constipated patients to achieve a normal bowel movement. Young children should have the tablets crushed to a fine powder and mixed with a small amount of water to form a paste.

Niclosamide is suitable for administration on an ambulatory or outpatient basis.

4. Follow-up:
As the vermicidal action of Niclosamide renders the tapeworm, especially the scolex and proximal segments, vulnerable to destruction during their passage through the gut, it is not always possible to identify the scolex in stools. The sooner the tapeworm is passed and examined after treatment, the better the chance of identification of the scolex. Segments and/or ova of beef or fish tapeworm may be present in the stool for up to 3 days after therapy. Persistent *T. saginata* or *D. latum* segments and/or ova on the seventh day post therapy indicate failure. A second identical course of treatment may be given at that time.

No patients should be considered cured unless the stool has been negative for a minimum of three months.

Store below 86°F (30°C), avoid freezing.

HOW SUPPLIED
CHEW TABLET: 500 MG

BRAND/MANUFACTURER	NDC	SIZE	AWP
○ BRAND			
NICLOCIDE: Miles Pharm	00026-2721-40	4s	$11.07

Nicoderm *SEE* NICOTINE

Nicolar *SEE* NIACIN

Nicorette *SEE* NICOTINE POLACRILEX

Nicotine

DESCRIPTION

Nicotine is available in a transdermal system that provides systemic delivery of Nicotine following its application to intact skin.

Nicotine is a tertiary amine composed of a pyridine and a pyrrolidine ring. It is a colorless-to-pale yellow, freely water-soluble, strongly alkaline, oily, volatile, hygroscopic liquid obtained from the tobacco plant. Nicotine has a characteristic pungent odor and turns brown on exposure to air or light. Of its two stereoisomers, S(-)-nicotine is the more active and is the more prevalent form in tobacco. The free alkaloid is absorbed rapidly through the skin and respiratory tract.

Chemical Name: S-3-(1-methyl-2-pyrrolidinyl) pyridine

Molecular Formula: $C_{10}H_{14}N_2$

Molecular Weight: 162.23.

Ionization Constants: $pK_{a1} = 7.84$. $pK_{u2} = 3.04$

Octanol-Water Partition Coefficient: 15.1 at pH 7

Nicotine is the active ingredient of the transdermal system; other components of the system are pharmacologically inactive.

The transdermal system delivers Nicotine 29, 31, 40, or 130 mcg/cm² h. Nicotine transdermal systems are labeled as to the dose actually absorbed by the patient. The dose of Nicotine absorbed from a Nicotine transdermal system represents 98% of the amount released from the system in 24 hours or 95% of the amount released in 16 hours.

Dose Absorbed in 24 hours (mg/day)	System Surface Area (cm²)	Total Nicotine Content (mg)
22	7	30
21	22 or 30	114 or 52.5
14	15 or 20	78 or 35.0
11	3.5	15
7	7 or 10	36 or 17.5

	Dose Absorbed in 16 Hours (mg/day)	System Area (cm²)	Total Nicotine Content (mg)
Treatment Dose	15	30	24.9
First Weaning Dose	10	20	16.6
Second Weaning Dose	5	10	8.3

Following is its chemical structure:

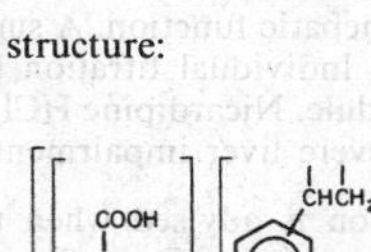

CLINICAL PHARMACOLOGY
PHARMACOLOGIC ACTION

Nicotine, the chief alkaloid in tobacco products, binds stereoselectively to acetylcholine receptors at the autonomic ganglia, in the adrenal medulla, at neuromuscular junctions, and in the brain. Two types of central nervous system effects are believed to be the basis of Nicotine's positively reinforcing properties.

A stimulating effect, exerted mainly in the cortex via the locus ceruleus, produces increased alertness and cognitive performance. A "reward" effect via the "pleasure system" in the brain is exerted in the limbic system. At low doses the stimulant effects predominate while at high doses the reward effects predominate. Intermittent intravenous administration of Nicotine activates neurohormonal pathways, releasing acetylcholine, norepinephrine, dopamine, serotonin, vasopressin, beta-endorphin, growth hormone, and ACTH.

PHARMACODYNAMICS

The cardiovascular effects of Nicotine include peripheral vasoconstriction, tachycardia, and elevated blood pressure. Acute and chronic tolerance to Nicotine develops from smoking tobacco or ingesting Nicotine preparations. Acute tolerance (a reduction in response for a given dose) develops rapidly (less than 1 hour), however, not at the same rate for different physiologic effects (skin temperature, heart rate, subjective effects). Withdrawal symptoms, such as cigarette craving, can be reduced in some individuals by plasma Nicotine levels lower than those from smoking.

Withdrawal from Nicotine in addicted individuals is characterized by craving, nervousness, restlessness, irritability, mood lability, anxiety, drowsiness, sleep disturbances, impaired concentration, increased appetite, minor somatic complaints (headache, myalgia, constipation, fatigue), and weight gain. Nicotine toxicity is characterized by nausea, abdominal pain, vomiting, diarrhea, diaphoresis, flushing, dizziness, disturbed hearing and vision, confusion, weakness, palpitations, altered respirations, and hypotension.

The cardiovascular effects of Nicotine transdermal systems, 14 mg/day, used continuously for 24 hours were compared with smoking every hour during waking hours, for 10 days. A small increase in blood pressure was detectable on the first day but not after 10 days. Heart rate was increased by 3-7% and stroke volume decreased by 5-12% on the 10th day of application. Nicotine transdermal system, 14 mg/day, treatment had no significant influence on cutaneous blood flow or skin temperature.

The cardiovascular effects of Nicotine 22 mg/day systems include slight increase in heart rate and blood pressure. The cardiovascular effects of applying one or two Nicotine 22 mg/day systems used continuously for 24 hours were compared to placebo for 7 days. Changes in heart rate (increased 4 beats/min), systolic blood pressure (increased 4 mmHg) and diastolic blood pressure (increased 3 mmHg) were observed.

The cardiovascular effects of Nicotine transdermal system 21 mg/day used continuously for 24 hours and smoking every 30 minutes during waking hours for 5 days were compared. Both regimens elevated heart rate (about 10 beats/min) and blood pressure (about 5 mm Hg) compared with an abstinence period, and these increases were similar between treatments throughout the 24-hour period, including during sleep.

The circadian pattern and release of plasma cortisol following 5 days of treatment with Nicotine transdermal system 21 mg/day did not differ from that following 5 days of Nicotine abstinence. Urinary excretion of norepinephrine, epinephrine, and dopamine was also similar for Nicotine transdermal system 21 mg/day and abstinence.

Both smoking and Nicotine can increase circulating cortisol and catecholamines, and tolerance does not develop to the catecholamine-releasing effects of Nicotine. Changes in the response to a concomitantly administered adrenergic agonist or antagonist should be watched for when Nicotine intake is altered during Nicotine replacement therapy and/or smoking cessation (see *"Precautions, Drug Interactions"*).

PHARMACOKINETICS

The volume of distribution following IV administration of Nicotine is approximately 2 to 3 L/kg and the half-life ranges from 1 to 2 hours. The major eliminating organ is the liver, and average plasma clearance is about 1.2 L/min; the kidney and lung also metabolize Nicotine. There is no significant skin metabolism of Nicotine. More than 20 metabolites of Nicotine have been identified, all of which are believed to be less active than the parent compound. The primary metabolite of Nicotine in plasma, cotinine, has a half-life of 15 to 20 hours and concentrations that exceed Nicotine by 10-fold.

Plasma-protein binding of Nicotine is < 5%. Therefore, changes in Nicotine binding from use of concomitant drugs or alterations of plasma proteins by disease states would not be expected to have significant effects on Nicotine kinetics.

The primary urinary metabolites are cotinine (15% of the dose) and trans-3-hydroxycotinine (45% of the dose). About 10% of Nicotine is excreted unchanged in the urine. As much as 30% may be excreted unchanged in the urine with high urine flow rates and urine acidification below pH 5.

The pharmacokinetic model which best fits the plasma Nicotine concentrations from Nicotine transdermal systems is an open, two-compartment disposition model with a skin depot through which Nicotine enters the central circulation compartment. The Nicotine is released slowly from the system. Therefore, the decline of plasma Nicotine concentrations is determined primarily by release of Nicotine from the system through the skin.

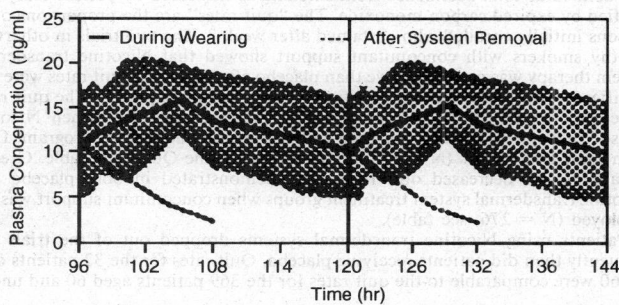

Steady-State Plasma Nicotine Concentrations for Two Consecutive Applications of Habitrol 21 ng/day (Mean ± 2SD, N=9)

Following an initial lag time of 1-2 hours, Nicotine concentrations increase to a broad peak between 4 and 12 hours and then decrease gradually. Steady state for Nicotine is attained within 2 days of initiating Nicotine transdermal system treatment and average plasma Nicotine concentrations are, on average, 0% to 30% higher compared to single dose applications. Upon application of a new system and removal of the old system there is, in some patients, a slight and transient (30-60 min.) increase in Nicotine plasma concentration and its variability. Plasma Nicotine concentrations are proportional to dose (ie, linear kinetics are observed) for the established dosages of Nicotine transdermal systems. Nicotine kinetics are similar for all sites of application.

Plasma Nicotine concentrations from Nicotine transdermal system 21 mg/day are the same as those from simultaneous use of Nicotine transdermal system 14 mg/day and 7 mg/day.

Following removal of Nicotine transdermal systems, plasma Nicotine concentrations decline in an exponential fashion with an apparent mean half-life of 3-4 hours compared with 1-2 hours for IV administration, due to continued absorption from the skin depot. Most nonsmoking patients will have nondetectable Nicotine concentrations in 10 to 12 hours. (See related table).

Half-hourly smoking of cigarettes produces average plasma Nicotine concentrations of approximagely 44 ng/mL. In comparison, average plasma Nicotine concentrations from Nicotine transdermal system 21 mg/day are about 13 or 17 ng/mL.

STEADY STATE NICOTINE PHARMACOKINETIC PARAMETERS FOR NICOTINE TRANSDERMAL SYSTEMS APPLIED FOR 16 HOURS [MEAN ± SD (RANGE), N = 12]

	Delivery Rate (mg/day)		
	15* Mean ± SD (Range)	10 Mean ± SD (Range)	5 Mean ± SD (Range)
C_{max} (ng/mL)	13.0 ± 3.1 (7.8-17.9)	6.9 ± 2.0 (4.8-10.0)	3.5 ± 0.7 (2.7-4.7)
C_{avg} (ng/mL)	9.4 ± 2.4 (5.3-13.3)	4.9 ± 1.2 (3.0-6.8)	2.7 ± 0.5 (2.0-3.6)
C_{avg} 24 (ng/mL)	8.7 ± 2.1 (5.2-11.8)	4.8 ± 1.0 (3.3-6.3)	2.7 ± 0.4 (2.1-3.3)
C_{min} (ng/mL)	2.5 ± 0.8 (1.2-4.1)	1.4 ± 0.5 (0.5-2.4)	0.8 ± 0.3 (0.3-1.2)
T_{max} (hrs)	8 ± 3 (4-16)	9 ± 4 (6-16)	9 ± 4 (3-16)

C_{max}: maximum observed plasma concentration
C_{avg} 16: estimated average plasma concentration during the 0 to 16 hour period, calculated as AUC (0-16)/16
C_{avg} 24: average plasma concentration calculated over 24 hrs
C_{min}: maximum observed plasma concentration
T_{max}: time of maximum plasma concentration
* Data for 15 mg/day system are derived from a different study than the 5 and 10 mg/day systems.

If the 15 mg/day Nicotine transdermal system is left on for 24 hours, as opposed to 16 hours, plasma levels of Nicotine decline from a mean of 7.2 to 5.6 ng/mL over the last 8 hours. The smaller systems may be expected to follow a similar pattern at proportionally lower plasma levels.

There are no differences in nicotine kinetics between men and women using Nicotine transdermal systems. Linear regression of both AUC and C_{max} vs total body weight shows the expected inverse relationship. Obese men using Nicotine transdermal systems had significantly lower AUC and C_{max} values than normal weight men. Men and women having low body weight are expected to have higher AUC and C_{max} values.

CLINICAL STUDIES

The efficacy of Nicotine transdermal system treatment as an aid to smoking cessation was demonstrated in three placebo-controlled, double-blind trials in otherwise healthy patients smoking at least one pack per day (N = 792). In two of these trials, Nicotine transdermal system therapy was combined with concomitant support and in one trial Nicotine transdermal system was used without concomitant support. In all three trials, patients were treated for 7 weeks (3 weeks of titration and 4 weeks of maintenance) followed by 3 weeks of weaning. Quitting was defined as total abstinence from smoking as measured by patient diary and verified by expired carbon monoxide. The "quit rates" are the proportions of all persons initially enrolled who abstained after week 3. The two trials in otherwise healthy smokers with concomitant support showed that Nicotine transdermal system therapy was more effective than placebo after 7 weeks. Quit rates were still significantly different after the additional 3-week weaning period. The quit rates varied approximately 3-fold among clinics for each treatment when Nicotine transdermal system therapy was used with a concomitant support program. Data from these two studies (N = 516) are combined in the Quit Rate table. Greater variability and decreased quit rates were demonstrated in both placebo and Nicotine transdermal system treatment groups when concomitant support was not employed (N = 276, see table).

Patients using Nicotine transdermal system systems dropped out of the trials less frequently than did patients receiving placebo. Quit rates for the 32 patients over age 60 were comparable to the quit rates for the 369 patients aged 60 and under.

QUIT RATES AFTER WEEK 3 BY TREATMENT

Concomitant Support	Treatment	Number of Patients	After 7 Weeks (range)	After Weaning (range)
Yes†	Nicotine transdermal system	260	19-54%	8-43%
	Placebo*	256	9-30%	8-30%
No††	Nicotine transdermal system	141	4-28%	4-20%
	Placebo*	135	0-24%	0-22%

* Sub Therapeutic (ST) Placebo systems contained 13% of the Nicotine found in the respective-sized active system to allow blinding as to color and odor.
† Two trials with 9 clinics, number of patients per treatment ranged from 22 to 39.
†† One trial with 5 clinics, number of patients per treatment ranged from 24 to 40.

The efficacy of Nicotine transdermal system treatment as an aid to smoking cessation was also demonstrated in two placebo-controlled, double-blind trials in otherwise healthy patients smoking at least one pack per day (N = 516). In one of these trials, Nicotine transdermal system therapy was combined with concomitant individual patient counseling (10 minutes each visit), and in the other trial Nicotine transdermal system therapy was used with group counseling (1 hour each visit). In both trials, patients were treated for 8 weeks with a fixed dosage of 22 mg/day or placebo followed by abrupt cessation of Nicotine transdermal system treatment and decrease in support therapy. Patients in these two trials received prestudy counseling at two visits before beginning treatment. Two earlier trials (N = 409) were carried out without prestudy counseling with treatment for 6 weeks and weaning to the 11 mg/day patch in one of them (N = 329). In all four trials quitting was defined as total abstinence from smoking as measured by patient diary and verified by expired carbon monoxide. The "quit rates" are the proportions of all persons initially enrolled who abstained after week 2.

QUIT RATES BY TREATMENT AFTER WEEK 2 (RANGE BY CLINICS)*

Nicotine Treatment	Number of Patients	After 6 Weeks	After 6 Months
Nicotine Transdermal system (22 mg/day)	259	10%-57%	0%-37%
Placebo	257	3%-30%	0%-20%

* Trial involved 7 clinics, number of patients per treatment ranged from 29 to 60.

The two trials with prestudy counseling demonstrated that with concomitant support, fixed-dosage therapy with Nicotine transdermal system therapy was more effective than placebo after 6 weeks and data from these two studies are combined in the quit rate table. At 8 weeks, just prior to abrupt termination of Nicotine transdermal system treatment (no weaning), quit rates were 6% to 50%. At follow-up, 3 to 5 days later, quit rates were 3% to 50%. In the two other studies without prestudy counseling, quit rates of 0% to 46% with Nicotine transdermal system 22 mg/day and 3% to 31% with placebo were observed at 6 weeks. In each of the four studies, there was a large variation in quit rates among clinics for each treatment.

Patients using Nicotine transdermal system systems dropped out of the trials significantly less frequently than did patients receiving placebo (26% vs 3.4%). The quit rate for 30 patients over age 60 was comparable to the quit rate for 486 patients aged 60 and under.

The efficacy of Nicotine transdermal systems as an aid to smoking cessation was also demonstrated in two placebo-controlled, double-blind trials of otherwise healthy patients (n = 756) smoking at least one pack of cigarettes per day. The trials consisted of 6 weeks of active treatment, 6 weeks of weaning off Nicotine transdermal systems, and 12 weeks of follow-up on no medication. Quitting was defined as total abstinence from smoking (as determined by patient diary and verified by expired carbon monoxide). The "quit rates" are the proportion of patients enrolled who abstained after week 2.

The two trials in otherwise healthy smokers showed that all doses were more effective than placebo, and that treatment with Nicotine transdermal system 21 mg/day for 6 weeks provided significantly higher quit rates than the 14 mg/day and placebo treatments at 6 weeks. Data from these two studies are combined in the Quit Rate table. Quit rates were still significantly different after an additional 6-week weaning period and at follow-up 3 months later. All patients were given weekly behavioral supportive care. As shown in the following table, the quit rates on each treatment varied 2- to 3-fold among clinics at 6 weeks.

QUIT RATES AFTER WEEK 2 ACCORDING TO STARTING DOSE (N = 756 SMOKERS IN 9 CLINICS)

Nicotine Delivery Rate (mg/day)	Number of Patients	After 6 Weeks Range*	After Weaning Range*	All 6 Months Range*
21	249	32-92%	18-63%	3-50%
14	254	30-61%	15-52%	0-48%
Placebo	253	15-46%	0-38%	0-35%

* Range for 9 centers, number of patients per treatment ranged from 23-34.

In a study of smokers with coronary artery disease, 77 patients treated with Nicotine transdermal systems (75% on 14 mg/day and 25% on 21 mg/day) had higher quit rates than 78 placebo-treated patients at the end of the 8-week study period (5 weeks of active treatment and 3 weeks of weaning). Nicotine transdermal systems did not affect angina frequency or the appearance of arrhythmias on Holter monitoring in these patients. Symptoms presumed related to Nicotine withdrawal and the stress of smoking cessation caused more patients to terminate the study than symptoms thought to be related to Nicotine substitution. Seven patients on placebo and one on Nicotine transdermal system 14 mg/day dropped out for symptoms (one patient with severe nausea on Nicotine transdermal system 14 mg/day and one with nausea and palpitations on Nicotine transdermal system 21 mg/day).

Patients using Nicotine transdermal systems dropped out of the trials less frequently than patients receiving placebo. Quit rates for the 56 patients over age 60 were comparable to the quit rates for the 821 patients aged 60 and under.

The efficacy of Nicotine transdermal system therapy as an aid to smoking cessation was also demonstrated in two single-center, placebo-controlled double-

STEADY-STATE NICOTINE PHARMACOKINETIC PARAMETERS FOR NICOTINE TRANSDERMAL SYSTEMS APPLIED FOR 24 HOURS (MEAN, STANDARD DEVIATION, RANGE)

Parameter (units)	7 mg/day Mean	SD	Range	14 mg/day (N = 9) Mean	SD	Range	21 mg/day (N = 9) Mean	SD	Range	22 mg/day (N = 22) Mean	SD	Range
C_{max} (ng/mL)	8	2	5-12	12 or 17	4 or 3	6-16 or 10-24	17 or 23	2 or 5	13-19 or 13-32	16	6	7-31
C_{avg} (ng/mL)	6	1	4-10	9 or 12	3	5-12 or 8-17	13 or 17	2 or 4	9-17 or 10-26	11	3	6-17
C_{min} (ng/mL)	4	1	3-6	6 or 7	2	3-10 or 4-11	9 or 11	2 or 3	7-14 or 6-17	5	1	3-9
T_{max} (hrs)	4	4	1-18	5 or 4	3	0-8 or 1-10	6 or 4	3	2-9 or 1-10	9	5	4-24

C_{max}: maximum observed plasma concentration
C_{avg}: average plasma concentration
C_{min}: minimum observed plasma concentration
T_{max}: time of maximum plasma concentration

◆ RATED THERAPEUTICALLY EQUIVALENT; ◇ THERAPEUTIC EQUIVALENCE UNCONFIRMED; ○ UNRATED

blind trials in smokers, smoking ≥ 10 cigarettes per day (n = 509), who were healthy or had diseases as their past medical history such as chronic obstructive pulmonary disease, hypertension, or myocardial infarction.

In both clinics Nicotine transdermal 16-hour systems were applied on awakening and removed at bedtime each day. They were used with only limited behavioral support. Patients in both clinics were treated for 12 weeks followed by a 4 to 6 week weaning period. The subjects were followed for 12 months. Quitting was defined as total abstinence from smoking. The "quit rates" are the proportion of all persons initially enrolled who abstained after week 2.

In both clinics Nicotine transdermal 16-hour therapy was more effective than placebo at 6 weeks, 6 months, and 1 year. Data from both are reported in the quit rate table.

QUIT RATES BY TREATMENT (N = 509 SMOKERS IN 2 CLINICS)*

Treatment Group	Number of Patients	At 6 Weeks	At 6 Months	At 1 Year
Nicotine transdermal 16-hour	258	35-16%	19-35%	12-25%
Placebo	251	7-35%	3-12%	3-9%

* *Trials involved 2 clinics; the number of patients per treatment ranged from 107 to 145.*

Patients using Nicotine transdermal 16-hour systems withdrew from the trials less frequently than the patients receiving placebo. Quit rates for the 79 patients over age 60 were comparable to the quit rates for the 430 patients aged 60 and under.

Patients who used Nicotine transdermal system treatment in clinical trials has a significant reduction in craving for cigarettes, a major nicotine withdrawal symptom, as compared to placebo-treated patients (see graph). Reduction in craving, as with quit rate, is quite variable. This variability is presumed to be due to inherent differences in patient populations, e.g. patient motivation, concomitant illnesses, number of cigarettes smoked per day, number of years smoking, exposure to other smokers, socioeconomic status, etc, as well as differences among the clinics.

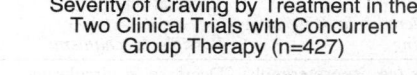

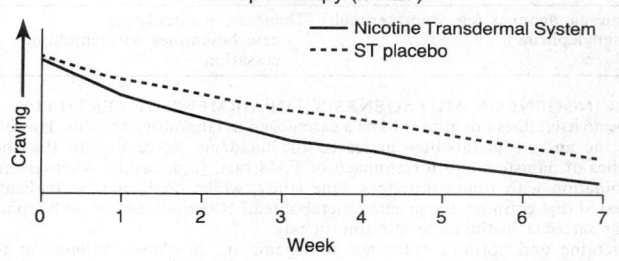

Severity of Craving by Treatment in the Two Clinical Trials with Concurrent Group Therapy (N = 427) — Nicotine transdermal system TTS — ST placebo

INDIVIDUALIZATION OF DOSAGE

It is important to make sure that patients read the instructions made available to them and have their questions answered. They should clearly understand the directions for applying and disposing of Nicotine transdermal systems. They should be instructed to stop smoking completely when the first system is applied.

The success or failure of smoking cessation depends heavily on the quality, intensity, and frequency of supportive care. Patients are more likely to quit smoking if they are seen frequently and participate in formal smoking cessation programs.

The goal of Nicotine transdermal system therapy is complete abstinence. Significant health benefits have not been demonstrated for reduction of smoking. If a patient is unable to stop smoking by the fourth week of therapy, treatment should probably be discontinued. Patients who have not stopped smoking after 4 weeks of Nicotine transdermal system therapy are unlikely to quit on that attempt.

Patients who fail to quit on any attempt may benefit from interventions to improve their chances for success on subsequent attempts. Patients who were unsuccessful should be counseled to determine why they failed. Patients should then probably be given a "therapy holiday" before the next attempt. A new quit attempt should be encouraged when the factors that contributed to failure can be eliminated or reduced, and conditions are more favorable.

Based on the clinical trials, a reasonable approach to assisting patients in their attempt to quit smoking is to assign their initial Nicotine transdermal system dosage using the recommended dosing schedule (see Dosing Schedule below). The need for dose adjustment should be assessed during the first 2 weeks. Patients should continue the dose selected with counseling and support over the following month. Those who have successfully stopped smoking during that time should be supported during 4 to 8 weeks of weaning, after which treatment should be terminated.

DOSING SCHEDULE

	Otherwise Healthy Patients	Other Patients*
Initial/Starting Dose	21 mg/day	14 mg/day
Duration of Treatment	4-8 weeks	4-8 weeks
First Weaning Dose	14 mg/day	7 mg/day
Duration of Treatment	2-4 weeks	2-4 weeks
Second Weaning Dose	7 mg/day	
Duration of Treatment	2-4 weeks	

* *small patient (less than 100 lbs) or light smoker (less than 10 cigarettes/day) or patient with cardiovascular disease*

DOSING SCHEDULE

	Patients ≥ 100 lbs	Patients < 100 lbs
Initial/Starting Dose	22 mg/day	11 mg/day
Duration of Treatment	4-8 weeks	4-8 weeks
Optional Weaning Dose	11 mg/day	off
Duration of Treatment	2-4 weeks	

Initial/Starting Dose	15 mg day
Duration of Treatment	4-12 weeks
First Weaning Dose	1 mg day
Duration of Treatment	2-4 weeks
Second Weaning Dose	5 mg/day
Duration of Treatment	2-4 weeks

The symptoms of Nicotine withdrawal and excess overlap (see "Pharmacodynamics" and "Adverse Reactions"). Since patients using Nicotine transdermal system treatment may also smoke intermittently, it may be difficult to determine if patients are experiencing Nicotine withdrawal or Nicotine excess.

The controlled clinical trials using Nicotine transdermal system therapy suggest that abnormal dreams sweating, rash, dizziness, abdominal pain, and insomnia are more often symptoms of Nicotine excess while flatulence, anxiety, depression, and irritability are more often symptoms of Nicotine withdrawal.

INDICATIONS AND USAGE

Nicotine transdermal system treatment is indicated as an aid to smoking cessation for the relief of Nicotine withdrawal symptoms. Nicotine transdermal system treatment should be used as a part of a comprehensive behavioral smoking cessation program.

The use of Nicotine transdermal systems for longer than 3 months (or 5 months in the case of 16-hour systems) has not been studied.

CONTRAINDICATIONS

Use of Nicotine transdermal systems is contraindicated in patients with hypersensitivity or allergy to Nicotine or to any of the components of the therapeutic system.

WARNINGS

Nicotine from any source can be toxic and addictive. Smoking causes lung cancer, heart disease, emphysema, and may adversely affect the fetus and the pregnant woman. For any smoker, with or without concomitant disease or pregnancy, the risk of Nicotine replacement in a smoking cessation program should be weighed against the hazard of continued smoking while using Nicotine transdermal systems, and the likelihood of achieving cessation of smoking without Nicotine replacement.

PREGNANCY WARNING

Tobacco smoke, which has been shown to be harmful to the fetus, contains Nicotine, hydrogen cyanide, and carbon monoxide. Nicotine has been shown in animal studies to cause fetal harm. It is therefore presumed that Nicotine transdermal system treatment can cause fetal harm when administered to a pregnant woman. The effect of Nicotine delivery by Nicotine transdermal system has not been examined in pregnancy (see "Precautions, Other Effects"). Therefore, pregnant smokers should be encouraged to attempt cessation using educational and behavioral interventions before using pharmacological approaches. If Nicotine transdermal system therapy is used during pregnancy, or if the patient becomes pregnant while using Nicotine transdermal system treatment, the patient should be apprised of the potential hazard to the fetus.

SAFETY NOTE CONCERNING CHILDREN

The amounts of Nicotine that are tolerated by adult smokers can produce symptoms of poisoning and could prove fatal if Nicotine transdermal systems are applied or ingested by children or pets. Used 21 mg/day systems contain about 60% or 73% (32 or 83 mg), used 22 mg/day systems about 27% (8 mg), and used 15 mg/day systems about 40% (10 mg) of their initial drug content. Therefore, patients should be cautioned to keep both used and unused Nicotine transdermal systems out of the reach of children and pets.

PRECAUTIONS

GENERAL

The patient should be urged to stop smoking completely when initiating Nicotine transdermal system therapy (see "Dosage and Administration"). Patients should be informed that if they continue to smoke while using Nicotine transdermal systems, they may experience adverse effects due to peak Nicotine levels higher than those experienced from smoking alone. If there is a clinically significant increase in cardiovascular or other effects attributable to Nicotine, the Nicotine transdermal system dose should be reduced or Nicotine transdermal system treatment discontinued (see *"Warnings"*). Physicians should anticipate that concomitant medications may need dosage adjustment (see *"Drug Interactions"*).The use of Nicotine transdermal systems beyond 3 months (5 months in the case of 16-hour systems) by patients who stop smoking should be discouraged because the chronic consumption of Nicotine by any route can be harmful and addicting.

Allergic Reactions: In a 12-week, open-label dermal irritation and sensitization study of Nicotine transdermal systems, 22 of 223 patients exhibited definite erythema at 24 hours after application. Upon rechallenge, 3 patients exhibited mild-to-moderate contact allergy. Patients with contact sensitization should be cautioned that a serious reaction could occur from exposure to other Nicotine-containing products or smoking. In the efficacy trials, erythema following system removal was typically seen in about 17% of patients, some edema in 4%, and dropouts due to skin reactions occurred in 6% of patients.

In a 3-week open-label dermal irritation and sensitization study of Nicotine transdermal systems, 16 of 205 patients (8%) exhibited definite erythema at 24 hours after system removal. None of those patients exhibited contact allergy. In the first 4 weeks of the efficacy trials, moderate erythema following system removal was seen in 22% of patients, some edema in 8%, and dropouts due to skin reactions occurred in 7% of 459 patients using the 22 mg/day system. Patients who develop contact sensitization should be cautioned that a serious reaction could occur from exposure to other Nicotine-containing products or smoking.

In a 6-week, open-label, dermal irritation and sensitization study of Nicotine transdermal systems, 7 of 230 patients exhibited definite erythema at 24 hours after application. Upon rechallenge, 4 patients exhibited mild to moderate contact allergy. Patients with contact sensitization should be cautioned that a serious reaction could occur from exposure to other Nicotine-containing products or smoking. In the efficacy trials, erythema following system removal was typically seen in about 14% of patients, some edema in 3%, and dropouts due to skin reactions occurred in 2% of patients.

In a 3-week open-label dermal irritation and sensitization study of Nicotine 16-hour transdermal systems applied 23 hours per day, 3 of 215 patients (1.4%) exhibited definite erythema at 24 hours after application. Upon rechallenge, none of the subjects exhibited any contact allergy. In the efficacy trials erythema following system removal was typically seen in 7% of patients, edema was seen in 3%, and dropouts due to skin reactions were reported in 1% of patients. Severe skin reactions were not observed in either of the trials.

Patients who exhibit contact sensitization should be cautioned that a serious reaction could occur from exposure to other Nicotine containing products or smoking.

Patients should be instructed to promptly discontinue the Nicotine transdermal system treatment and contact their physicians if they experience severe or persistent local skin reactions at the site of application (eg. severe erythema, pruritus, or edema) or a generalized skin reaction (eg. urticaria, hives, or generalized rash).

Patients using Nicotine transdermal system therapy concurrently with other transdermal products may exhibit local reactions at both application sites. Reactions were seen in 2 of 7 patients using concomitant estradiol transdermal system in clinical trials. In such patients, use of one or both systems may have to be discontinued.

Skin Disease: Nicotine transdermal systems are usually well tolerated by patients with normal skin, but may be irritating for patients with some skin disorders (psoriasis or atopic or eczematous dermatitis).

Cardiovascular or Peripheral Vascular Diseases: The risks of Nicotine replacement in patients with certain cardiovascular and peripheral vascular diseases should be weighed against the benefits of including Nicotine replacement in a smoking cessation program for them. Specifically, patients with coronary heart disease (history of myocardial infarction and/or angina pectoris), serious cardiac arrhythmias, or vasospastic diseases (Buerger's disease, Prinzmetal's variant angina) should be carefully screened and evaluated before Nicotine replacement is prescribed.

Tachycardia occurring in association with the use of Nicotine transdermal system treatment was reported occasionally. If serious cardiovascular symptoms occur with Nicotine transdermal system treatment, it should be discontinued.

Nicotine transdermal system therapy was as well tolerated as placebo in a controlled trial in patients with coronary artery disease (see *"Clinical Studies"*). One patient on Nicotine transdermal system 21 mg/day, two on Nicotine transdermal system 14 mg/day, and eight on placebo discontinued treatment due to adverse events.

Nicotine transdermal system therapy did not affect angina frequency or the appearance of arrhythmias on Holter monitoring in these patients.

Nicotine transdermal system treatment should generally not be used in patients during the immediate post-myocardial infarction period, patients with serious arrhythmias, and patients with severe or worsening angina pectoris.

Renal or Hepatic Insufficiency: The pharmacokinetics of Nicotine have not been studied in the elderly or in patients with renal or hepatic impairment. However, given that Nicotine is extensively metabolized and that its total system clearance is dependent on liver blood flow, some influence of hepatic impairment on drug kinetics (reduced clearance) should be anticipated. Only severe renal impairment would be expected to affect the clearance of Nicotine or its metabolites from the circulation (see *"Clinical Pharmacology, Pharmacokinetics"*).

Endocrine Diseases: Nicotine transdermal system treatment should be used with caution in patients with hyperthyroidism, pheochromocytoma, or insulin-dependent diabetes since Nicotine causes the release of catecholamines by the adrenal medulla.

Peptic Ulcer Disease: Nicotine delays healing in peptic ulcer disease; therefore, Nicotine transdermal system treatment should be used with caution in patients with active peptic ulcers and only when the benefits of including Nicotine replacement in a smoking cessation program outweigh the risks.

Accelerated Hypertension: Nicotine constitutes a risk factor for development of malignant hypertension in patients with accelerated hypertension; therefore, Nicotine transdermal system treatment should be used with caution in these patients and only when the benefits of including Nicotine replacement in a smoking cessation program outweigh the risks.

Information for Patient: A patient instruction sheet is included in some packages of Nicotine transdermal systems dispensed to the patient. It contains important information and instructions on how to use and dispose of Nicotine transdermal systems properly. Patients should be encouraged to ask questions of the physician and pharmacist.

Patients must be advised to keep both used and unused systems out of the reach of children and pets.

DRUG INTERACTIONS
Smoking cessation, with or without Nicotine replacement, may alter the pharmacokinetics of certain concomitant medications.

May Require a Decrease in Dose at Cessation of Smoking	*Possible Mechanism*
Acetaminophen, caffeine, imipramine, oxazepam, pentazocine, propranolol, theophylline	Deinduction of hepatic enzymes on smoking cessation
Insulin	Increase of subcutaneous insulin absorption with smoking cessation
Adrenergic antagonists (eg, prazosin, labetalol)	Decrease in circulating catecholamines with smoking cessation
May Require an Increase in Dose at Cessation of Smoking	*Possible Mechanism*
Adrenergic agonists (eg, isoproterenol, phenylephrine)	Decrease in circulating catecholamines with smoking cessation

CARCINOGENESIS, MUTAGENESIS, IMPAIRMENT OF FERTILITY
Nicotine itself does not appear to be a carcinogen in laboratory animals. However, Nicotine and its metabolites increased the incidence of tumors in the cheek pouches of hamsters and forestomach of F344 rats, respectively, when given in combination with tumor-initiators. One study, which could not be replicated, suggested that cotinine, the primary metabolite of Nicotine, may cause lymphoreticular sarcoma in the large intestine in rats.

Nicotine and cotinine were not mutagenic in the Ames *Salmonella* test. Nicotine induced repairable DNA damage in an *E. coli* test system. Nicotine was shown to be genotoxic in a test system using Chinese hamster ovary cells. In rats and rabbits, implantation can be delayed or inhibited by a reduction in DNA synthesis that appears to be caused by Nicotine. Studies have shown a decrease in litter size in rats treated with Nicotine during gestation.

PREGNANCY CATEGORY D
(See *"Warnings"*.)

The harmful effects of cigarette smoking on maternal and fetal health are clearly established. These include low birth weight, an increased risk of spontaneous abortion, and increased perinatal mortality. The specific effects of Nicotine transdermal system treatment on fetal development are unknown. Therefore, pregnant smokers should be encouraged to attempt cessation using educational and behavioral interventions before using pharmacological approaches.

Spontaneous abortion during Nicotine replacement therapy has been reported: as with smoking, Nicotine as a contributing factor cannot be excluded.

Nicotine transdermal system treatment should be used during pregnancy only if the likelihood of smoking cessation justifies the potential risk of use of Nicotine replacement by the patient, who may continue to smoke.

TERATOGENICITY
Animal Studies: Nicotine was shown to produce skeletal abnormalities in the offspring of mice when given doses toxic to the dams (25 mg/kg/day IP or SC).

Human Studies: Nicotine teratogenicity has not been studied in humans except as a component of cigarette smoke (each cigarette smoked delivers about 1 mg of Nicotine). It has not been possible to conclude whether cigarette smoking is teratogenic to humans.

OTHER EFFECTS
Animal Studies: A Nicotine bolus (up to 2 mg/kg) to pregnant rhesus monkeys caused acidosis, hypercarbia, and hypotension (fetal and maternal concentrations were about 20 times those achieved after smoking 1 cigarette in 5 minutes). Fetal breathing movements were reduced in the fetal lamb after intravenous injection

of 0.25 mg/kg Nicotine to the ewe (equivalent to smoking 1 cigarette every 20 seconds for 5 minutes). Uterine blood flow was reduced about 30% after infusion of 0.1 mg/kg/min Nicotine for 20 minutes to pregnant rhesus monkeys (equivalent to smoking about six cigarettes every minute for 20 minutes).

Human Experience: Cigarette smoking during pregnancy is associated with an increased risk of spontaneous abortion, low-birth-weight infants and perinatal mortality. Nicotine and carbon monoxide are considered the most likely mediators of these outcomes. The effects of cigarette smoking on fetal cardiovascular parameters have been studied near term. Cigarettes increased fetal aortic blood flow and heart rate and decreased uterine blood flow and fetal breathing movements. Nicotine transdermal system treatment has not been studied in pregnant humans.

LABOR AND DELIVERY
Nicotine transdermal system are not recommended to be left on during labor and delivery. The effects of Nicotine on the mother or the fetus during labor are unknown.

NURSING MOTHERS
Caution should be exercised when Nicotine transdermal system therapy is administered to nursing women. The safety of Nicotine transdermal system treatment in nursing infants has not been examined. Nicotine passes freely into breast milk; the milk-to-plasma ratio averages 2.9. Nicotine is absorbed orally. An infant has the ability to clear Nicotine by hepatic first-pass clearance; however, the efficiency of removal is probably lowest at birth. The Nicotine concentrations in milk can be expected to be lower with Nicotine transdermal system treatment when used as directed than with cigarette smoking, as maternal plasma Nicotine concentrations are generally reduced with Nicotine replacement. The risk of exposure of the infant to Nicotine from Nicotine transdermal systems should be weighed against the risks associated with the infant's exposure to Nicotine from continued smoking by the mother (passive smoke exposure and contamination of breast milk with other components of tobacco smoke) and from Nicotine transdermal systems alone or in combination with continued smoking.

PEDIATRIC USE
Nicotine transdermal systems are not recommended for use in children because the safety and effectiveness of Nicotine transdermal system treatment in children and adolescents who smoke have not been evaluated.

GERIATRIC USE
Thirty to 79 patients over the age of 60 participated in clinical trials of Nicotine transdermal system therapy, Nicotine transdermal system therapy appeared to be as effective in this age group as in younger smokers. However, asthenia, various body aches, and dizziness occurred slightly more often in patients over 60 years of age.

ADVERSE REACTIONS
Assessment of adverse events in the patients who participated in controlled clinical trials is complicated by the occurrence of GI and CNS effects of Nicotine withdrawal as well as Nicotine excess. The actual incidences of both are confounded by concurrent smoking by many of the patients. In the trials, when reporting adverse events, the investigators did not attempt to identify the cause of the symptom. No serious adverse events were reported during the trials.

TOPICAL ADVERSE EVENTS
The most common adverse event associated with topical Nicotine is a short-lived erythema, pruritus, or burning at the application site, which was seen at least once in 35% to 54% of patients on Nicotine transdermal system treatment in the clinical trials. Local erythema after system removal was noted at least once in 7% to 22% of patients and local edema in 3% to 8%. Erythema generally resolved within 24 hours. Cutaneous hypersensitivity (contact sensitization) occurred in 2% to 3% of patients on Nicotine transdermal system treatment (see *"Precautions, Allergic Reactions"*.) About 1% of patients dropped out of clinical trials due to skin reactions.

PROBABLY CAUSALLY RELATED
The following adverse events were reported more frequently in Nicotine transdermal system-treated patients than in placebo-treated patients or exhibited a dose response in clinical trials. The reports of awakening at night were collected as one of the expected withdrawal symptoms.

Digestive System: Abdominal pain*, diarrhea*, dyspepsia*

Mouth/Tooth Disorders: Dry mouth

Musculoskeletal System: Arthralgia*, myalgia*

Nervous System: Abnormal dreams, insomnia (23%), nervousness*, somnolence

Skin: Rash*, sweating†
  Frequencies for 21 and 22 mg/day system
  Unmarked if reported in < 1% of patients.

CAUSAL RELATIONSHIP UNKNOWN
Adverse events reported in Nicotine transdermal system and placebo-treated patients at about the same frequency in clinical trials are listed below. The clinical significance of the association between Nicotine transdermal system treatment

---

*Reported in 3% to 9% of patients.
†Reported in 1% to 3% of patients. Unmarked if reported in < 1% of patients.

---

and these events is unknown, but they are reported as alerting information for the clinician.

Body as a Whole: Allergy†, asthenia*, back pain†, chest pain*

Cardiovascular System: Hypertension

Digestive System: Abdominal pain†, constipation*, dyspepsia†, flatulence†, nausea*, vomiting.†

Nervous System: Dizziness*, concentration impaired†, depression,† headache (11% to 29%), insomnia*, paresthesia*.

Respiratory System: Cough increased*, pharyngitis*, sinusitis*.

Special Senses: Taste perversion*

Urogenital System: Dysmenorrhea*
  Frequencies for 21 or 22 mg/day system

DRUG ABUSE AND DEPENDENCE
Nicotine transdermal systems are likely to have a low abuse potential based on differences between them and cigarettes in four characteristics commonly considered important in contributing to abuse: much slower absorption, much smaller fluctuations in blood levels, lower blood levels of Nicotine, and less frequent use (ie, once daily).

The abuse potential of Nicotine transdermal systems was examined in a prospective, randomized trial of 10 smokers (five drug abusers and five nonabusers). "Liking" scores for either one (22 mg/day) or two systems (44 mg/day) were no different from placebo. No abuse potential was observed in that study.

Dependence on Nicotine polacrilex chewing gum replacement therapy has been reported. Such dependence might also occur from transference to Nicotine transdermal systems of tobacco-based Nicotine dependence. The use of the system beyond 3 months (5 months for 16-hour systems) has not been evaluated and should be discouraged. To minimize the risk of dependence, patients should be encouraged to withdraw gradually from Nicotine transdermal system treatment after 4 to 8 weeks (12 weeks for 16-hours systems) of usage. Recommended dose reduction is to progressively decrease the dose every 2 to 4 weeks (see *"Dosage and Administration"*).

Nicotine transdermal system therapy has been evaluated in both a gradual and abrupt discontinuation of treatment. If gradual withdrawal is desirable, patients using the 22 mg/day Nicotine transdermal system treatment should use the 11 mg/day dosage for 2 to 4 weeks (see *"Individualization of Dosage"* and *"Dosage and Administration"*).

OVERDOSAGE
The effects of applying several Nicotine transdermal systems simultaneously or of swallowing unused Nicotine transdermal systems are unknown (see *"Warnings, Safety Note Concerning Children"*). The oral LD$_{50}$ for Nicotine in rodents varies with species but is in excess of 24 mg/kg; death is due to respiratory paralysis. The oral minimum lethal dose of Nicotine in dogs is greater than 5 mg/kg. The oral minimum acute lethal dose for Nicotine in human adults is reported to be 40 to 60 mg (< 1 mg/kg).

Two or three Nicotine 30 cm^2 transdermal systems in capsules fed to dogs weighing 8-17 kg were emetic, but did not produce any other significant clinical signs. The administration of these patches corresponds to about 6-17 mg/kg of Nicotine. Three dogs, each weighing 11 kg, were fed two damaged Nicotine 14 mg/day transdermal systems. Nicotine plasma concentrations of 32 to 79 ng/mL were observed. No ill effects were apparent.

Nicotine transdermal system gels containing 8 mg of Nicotine were ingested by 12 adult smokers with an average weight of 74 kg (range 62 to 93 kg). Peak Nicotine serum levels were 9.5 ng/mL (range 3 to 18 ng/mL) and occurred at 2 hours (1 to 2 hours) and declined to baseline levels by 8 hours after ingestion. Some gastrointestinal effects (burning on ingestion and nausea) were reported.

Signs and symptoms of an overdose of Nicotine transdermal systems would be expected to be the same as those of acute Nicotine poisoning including; pallor, cold sweat, nausea, salivation, vomiting, abdominal pain, diarrhea, headache, dizziness, disturbed hearing and vision, tremor, mental confusion, and weakness. Prostration, hypotension, and respiratory failure may ensue with large overdoses. Lethal doses produce convulsions quickly and death follows as a result of peripheral or central respiratory paralysis or, less frequently, cardiac failure.

OVERDOSE FROM TOPICAL EXPOSURE
The Nicotine transdermal system should be removed immediately if the patient shows signs of overdosage and the patient should seek immediate medical care. The skin surface may be flushed with water and dried. No soap should be used since it may increase Nicotine absorption. Nicotine will continue to be delivered into the bloodstream for several hours (see *"Clinical Pharmacology, Pharmacokinetics"*) after removal of the system because of a depot of Nicotine in the skin.

OVERDOSE FROM INGESTION
Ingestion of a 22 mg/day Nicotine transdermal system containing 30 mg of Nicotine is potentially more harmful than ingestion of a used system which contains about 8 mg after 24 hours use.

Persons ingesting Nicotine transdermal system should be referred to a health care facility for management. Due to the possibility of Nicotine-induced seizures, activated charcoal should be administered. In unconscious patients with a secure

---

* Reported in 3% to 9% of patients.
† Reported in 1% to 3% of patients. Unmarked if reported in < 1% of patients.

airway, instill activated charcoal via nasogastric tube. A saline cathartic or sorbitol added to the first dose of activated charcoal may speed gastrointestinal passage of the system. Repeated doses of activated charcoal should be administered as long as the system remains in the gastrointestinal tract since it will continue to release Nicotine for many hours.

MANAGEMENT OF NICOTINE POISONING
Other supportive measures include diazepam or barbiturates for seizures, atropine for excessive bronchial secretions or diarrhea, respiratory support for respiratory failure and vigorous fluid support for hypotension and cardiovascular collapse.

DOSAGE AND ADMINISTRATION
Patients must desire to stop smoking and should be instructed to *stop smoking immediately* as they begin using Nicotine transdermal system therapy. The patient should read the patient instruction on Nicotine transdermal system treatment and be encouraged to ask any questions. Treatment should be initiated with Nicotine 22,21, or 14 mg/day transdermal systems, or the 15 mg/day 16-hour system. Patients who weigh less than 100 lb. may start with 11 mg/day instead of 22 mg/day, with the dose increased as appropriate (see *"Clinical Pharmacology, Individualization of Dosage"*).

Once the appropriate dosage is selected the patient should begin 4-8 weeks (4 to 12 weeks for 16-hour systems) of therapy at that dosage. The patient should stop smoking cigarettes completely during this period. If the patient is unable to stop cigarette smoking within 4 weeks, Nicotine transdermal system therapy should probably be stopped, since few additional patients in clinical trials were able to quit after this time. Those who have successfully stopped smoking during that time may have Nicotine transdermal system therapy discontinued. If a gradual reduction is desired, patients may be treated for an additional 2 to 4 weeks, after which treatment should be terminated.

RECOMMENDED DOSING SCHEDULE FOR HEALTHY PATIENTS[a]
SELECTED 24-HOUR SYSTEMS (SEE INDIVIDUALIZATION OF DOSAGE)

Dose	Duration
Nicotine transdermal system 21 mg/day	First 6 Weeks
Nicotine transdermal system 14 mg/day	Next 2 Weeks[b]
Nicotine transdermal system 7 mg/day	Last 2 Weeks[c]

[a] Start with Nicotine transdermal system 14 mg/day for 6 weeks for patients who:
—have cardiovascular disease
—weigh less than 100 pounds
—smoke less than ½ a pack of cigarettes/day
Decrease dose to Nicotine transdermal system 7 mg/day for the final 2-4 weeks.
[b] Patients who have successfully abstained from smoking should have their dose of Nicotine transdermal system reduced after each 2-4 weeks of treatment until the 7 mg/day dose has been used for 2-4 weeks (see "Individualization of Dosage").
[c] The entire course of nicotine substitution and gradual withdrawal should take 6-12 weeks, depending on the size of the initial dose. The use of Nicotine transdermal systems beyond 3 months has not been studied.

RECOMMENDED DOSING SCHEDULE 16-HOUR SYSTEM

Dose	Duration
Nicotine transdermal system 15 mg/day	First 12 weeks
Nicotine transdermal system 10 mg/day	Next 2 weeks[a]
Nicotine transdermal system 5 mg/day	Last 2 weeks[b]

[a] Patients who have successfully abstained from smoking should have their dose of Nicotine reduced after each 2-4 weeks of treatment until the Nicotine transdermal system 5 mg day dose has been used for 2-4 weeks.
[b] The entire course of Nicotine substitution and gradual withdrawal should take 14-20 weeks. The use of Nicotine transdermal system therapy beyond 5 months has not been studied.

A Nicotine transdermal system should be applied promptly upon its removal from the protective pouch to prevent evaporative loss of Nicotine from the system. Nicotine transdermal systems should be used only when the pouch is intact to assure that the product has not been tampered with.

Nicotine transdermal systems should be applied only once a day to a nonhairy, clean, and dry skin site on the trunk or upper, outer arm. After 24 hours, the used Nicotine transdermal system should be removed and a new system applied to an alternate skin site. Skin sites should not be reused for at least a week. Patients should be cautioned not to continue to use the same system for more than 24 hours.

A 16-hour Nicotine transdermal system should be applied only once a day to a nonhairy, clean, and dry skin site on the upper arm or the hip. Each day a 16-hour Nicotine transdermal system should be applied upon waking and removed at bedtime.

SAFETY AND HANDING
Nicotine transdermal systems can be a dermal irritant and can cause contact sensitization. Patients should be instructed in the proper use of Nicotine transdermal systems by using demonstration systems. Although exposure of

health care workers to Nicotine from Nicotine transdermal systems should be minimal, care should be taken to avoid unnecessary contact with active systems. If you do handle active systems, wash with water alone, since soap may increase Nicotine absorption. Do not touch your eyes.

DISPOSAL
When the use system is removed from the skin, it should be folded over and placed in the protective pouch which contained the new system. The used system should be immediately disposed of in such a way as to prevent its access by children or pets. See patient information for further directions for handling and disposal.

HOW TO STORE
Do not store above 86°F (30°C) because Nicotine trandermal systems are sensitive to heat. A slight discoloration of the system is not significant.

Do not store unpouched. Once removed from the protective pouch, Nicotine trandermal systems should be applied promptly since Nicotine is volatile and the system may lose strength.

HOW SUPPLIED
FILM, EXTENDED RELEASE: 7 MG/24 HRS

BRAND/MANUFACTURER	NDC	SIZE	AWP
◆ BRAND			
NICODERM: Marion Merrell Dow	00088-0052-61	14s	$48.60

FILM, EXTENDED RELEASE: 7 MG/24 HRS

BRAND/MANUFACTURER	NDC	SIZE	AWP
○ BRAND			
► HABITROL: Basel	58887-0810-26	30s	$104.37

FILM, EXTENDED RELEASE: 11 MG/24 HRS

BRAND/MANUFACTURER	NDC	SIZE	AWP
○ BRAND			
PROSTEP: Lederle Labs	00005-2401-90	7s	$27.26

FILM, EXTENDED RELEASE: 14 MG/24 HRS

BRAND/MANUFACTURER	NDC	SIZE	AWP
◆ BRAND			
NICODERM: Marion Merrell Dow	00088-0051-61	14s	$52.50

FILM, EXTENDED RELEASE: 14 MG/24 HRS

BRAND/MANUFACTURER	NDC	SIZE	AWP
○ BRAND			
► HABITROL: Basel	58887-0820-26	30s	$110.17

FILM, EXTENDED RELEASE: 21 MG/24 HRS

BRAND/MANUFACTURER	NDC	SIZE	AWP
◆ BRAND			
NICODERM: Marion Merrell Dow	00088-0050-61	14s	$57.18

FILM, EXTENDED RELEASE: 21 MG/24 HRS

BRAND/MANUFACTURER	NDC	SIZE	AWP
○ BRAND			
► HABITROL: Basel	58887-0830-26	30s	$115.96

FILM, EXTENDED RELEASE: 22 MG/24 HRS

BRAND/MANUFACTURER	NDC	SIZE	AWP
○ BRAND			
PROSTEP: Lederle Labs	00005-2402-90	7s	$29.58

Nicotine Polacrilex

DESCRIPTION
Nicotine Polacrilex contains nicotine bound to an ion exchange resin in a sugar-free flavored, chewing gum base that provides systemic delivery of Nicotine following chewing.

Nicotine is a tertiary amine composed of a pyridine and a pyrrolidine ring. It is a colorless to pale yellow, freely water-soluble, strongly alkaline, oily, volatile, hygroscopic liquid obtained from the tobacco plant. Nicotine has a characteristic pungent odor and turns brown on exposure to air or light. Of its two stereoisomers, S(-)nicotine is the more active. It is the prevalent form in tobacco, and is the form in the Nicotine Polacrilex. The free alkaloid is absorbed rapidly through the skin and respiratory tract.

Chemical Name: S-3-(1-methyl-2-pyrrolidinyl) pyridine
Molecular Formula: $C_{10}H_{14}N_2$
Molecular Weight: 162.23
Ionization Constants: $pK_{a1} = 7.84$, $pK_{a2} = 3.04$
Octanol-Water Partition Coefficient: 15:1 at pH 7

◆ RATED THERAPEUTICALLY EQUIVALENT; ◇ THERAPEUTIC EQUIVALENCE UNCONFIRMED; ○ UNRATED

When Nicotine Polacrilex is chewed as directed, nicotine is absorbed primarily through the buccal mucosa. Each piece of gum contains Nicotine Polacrilex equivalent to either 2 or 4 mg nicotine as the active ingredient.

TOTAL AND EXTRACTABLE NICOTINE CONTENT

Nicotine Source	Nicotine Content	Nicotine Extracted
Nicotine Polacrilex		
double strength	4 mg/piece	3.4 mg[a]
Nicotine Polacrilex	2 mg/piece	1.4 mg[a]
American cigarettes	11 mg/cigarette	0.8 mg[b]

[a] Extracted with paced chewing once every other second for 30 minutes (more vigorous than recommended use, see "Patient Instructions").

[b] Nicotine extracted in vitro by smoking machine.

Following is its chemical structure:

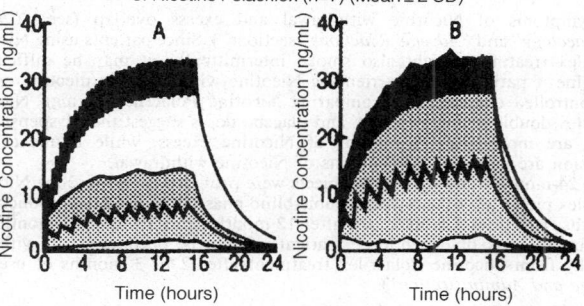

CLINICAL PHARMACOLOGY

PHARMACOLOGIC ACTION

Nicotine, the chief alkaloid in tobacco products, binds stereoselectively to acetylcholine receptors at the autonomic ganglia, in the adrenal medulla, at neuromuscular junctions, and in the brain. Two types of central nervous system effects are believed to be the basis of nicotine's positively reinforcing properties. A stimulating effect, exerted mainly in the cortex via the locus ceruleus, produces increased alertness and cognitive performance. A "reward" effect via the "pleasure system" in the brain is exerted in the limbic system. At low doses the stimulant effects predominate, while at high doses the reward effects predominate. Intermittent intravenous administration of nicotine activites neurohormonal pathways, releasing acetylcholine, norepinephrine, dopamine, serotonin, vasopressin, beta-endorphin, growth hormone, and ACTH.

PHARMACODYNAMICS

The cardiovascular effects of nicotine include peripheral vasoconstriction, tachycardia, and elevated blood pressure. Acute and chronic tolerance to nicotine develops from smoking tobacco or ingesting nicotine preparations. Acute tolerance (a reduction in response for a given dose) develops rapidly (less than 1 hour), however, not at the same rate for different physiologic effects (skin temperature, heart rate, subjective effects). Withdrawal symptoms such as cigarette craving can be reduced in some individuals by plasma nicotine levels lower than those from smoking.

Withdrawal from nicotine in addicted individuals is characterized by craving, nervousness, restlessness, irritability, mood lability, anxiety, drowsiness, sleep disturbances, impaired concentration, increased appetite, minor somatic complaints (headache, myalgia, constipation, fatigue), and weight gain. Nicotine toxicity is characterized by nausea, abdominal pain, vomiting, diarrhea, diaphoresis, flushing, dizziness, disturbed hearing and vision, confusion, weakness, palpitations, altered respirations, and hypotension.

Both smoking and nicotine can increase circulating cortisol and catecholamines, and tolerance does not develop to the catecholamine-releasing effects of nicotine. Changes in the response to a concomitantly administered adrenergic agonist or antagonist should be watched for when nicotine intake is altered during Nicotine Polacrilex therapy and/or smoking cessation (see "Precautions: Drug Interactions").

PHARMACOKINETICS

The volume of distribution following IV administration of nicotine is approximately 2 to 3 L/kg and the half-life ranges from 1 to 2 hours. The major eliminating organ is the liver, and average plasma clearance is about 1.2 L/min; the kidney and lung also metabolize nicotine. More than 20 metabolites of nicotine have been identified, all of which are believed to be less active than the parent compound. The primary metabolite of nicotine is plasma, cotinine, has a half-life of 15 to 20 hours and concentrations that exceed nicotine by 10-fold. Plasma protein binding of nicotine is < 5%. Therefore, changes in nicotine binding from use of concomitant drugs or alterations of plasma proteins by disease states would not be expected to have significant effect on nicotine kinetics.

The primary urinary metabolites are cotinine (15% of the dose) and trans-3-hydroxycotinine (45% of the dose). Usually about 10% of nicotine is excreted unchanged in the urine. As much as 30% may be excreted unchanged in the urine with high urine flow rates and acidification below pH 5.

The amount of nicotine extracted from a Nicotine Polacrilex chewing piece depends on how vigorously it is chewed. The amount of nicotine absorbed depends on the amount extracted and the loss from the buccal cavity due to swallowing or expectoration. Most of the absorption of nicotine from a Nicotine Polacrilex chewing piece occurs directly through the buccal mucosa. The systemic bioavailability of swallowed nicotine is lower due to the amount removed initially by the liver, i.e., the first pass effect. Hence, the high and rapidly rising nicotine concentrations seen after smoking are rarely produced by Nicotine Polacrilex treatment.

The table below presents results from a bioavailability study in which 24 smokers chewed a single Nicotine Polacrilex chewing piece at a vigorous, prescribed rate. The values in this table thus represent maximum plasma nicotine levels (higher than expected upon normal use and recommended chewing).

BIOAVAILABILITY OF SINGLE 2 AND 4 MG DOSES

(N = 24 smokers, vigorous paced chewing)

Labeled Dose (mg)	Number (N)	Extracted Amount (mg)*[a]	Systemically Availability Amount (mg)*[b]
4	16	3.4 (3.1-3.7)	2.5 (1.8-3.2)
2	18	1.4 (1.1-1.6)	1.3 (0.6-1.9)

* Mean, 95% confidence interval.

[a] Determined by measuring amount in the chewing pieces before and after 30 minutes of paced chewing.

[b] Determined by measuring amount in plasma (area-under-the-curve) during and after 30 minutes of paced chewing.

Acidic beverages (e.g. coffee, juices, wine, or soft drinks), interfere with the buccal absorption of nicotine from Nicotine Polacrilex. Eating and drinking should therefore be avoided for 15 minutes before and during chewing of Nicotine Polacrilex.

NICOTINE CONCENTRATIONS IN PLASMA WHILE SMOKING
ad lib (n=14) and Chewing 12 pieces/day
of Nicotine Polacrilex (n=7) (Mean ± 2 SD)

The figure shows simulated Nicotine venous plasma concentrations after multiple dosing of Nicotine Polacrilex 2 mg/piece (plot A), Nicotine Polacrilex mg/piece (plot B), and cigarette smoking (shaded area represents ± SD for the Nicotine Polacrilex products). The dosing regimens and absorbed amounts of Nicotine are idealized from data reported by Benowitz et al. (Clin Pharmacol Ther 1987; 41:467-473). When a single piece was chewed slowly and steadily for 20 minutes every 1.3 hours for 16 hours (12 pieces total), 0.85 mg and 1.22 mg nicotine were absorbed on average from Nicotine Polacrilex and Nicotine Polacrilex double strength respectively. An average of 38 cigarettes of these volunteers' own brands, delivering an average of 1 mg nicotine each, were smoked ad lib over the same time period.

CLINICAL STUDIES

The efficacy of Nicotine Polacrilex treatment as an aid to smoking cessation was demonstrated in four placebo-controlled, double-blind trials in otherwise healthy patients. Two of the trials involved only the 2 mg dose and two used both 2 and 4 mg doses. Quitting was defined as total abstinence from smoking for 4 weeks as measured by patient diary and verified by expired carbon monoxide after an initial two weeks of treatment. The "quit rates" are the proportions of all persons initially enrolled who abstained weeks 2-6.

The two trials using both 2 mg Nicotine Polacrilex and 4 mg Nicotine Polacrilex double strength doses in otherwise healthy smokers with concomitant support (N = 563) showed that Nicotine Polacrilex treatment was more effective than placebo after 6 weeks in the patients (N = 289) using more than 9 pieces per day. These results emphasize the importance of adequate Nicotine doses. The quit rates among clinics varied approximately 2- to 3-fold for each treatment (see table). (See related table).

Patients who used Nicotine Polacrilex in clinical trials had a significant reduction in craving for cigarettes, a major Nicotine withdrawal symptom, as compared to placebo-treated patients. Reduction in craving, as with quit rate, is quite variable. This variability is presumed to be due to inherent differences in patient populations, e.g., patient motivation, concomitant illnesses, number of cigarettes smoked per day, number of years smoking, exposure to other smokers, socioeconomic status, etc, as well as differences among the clinics.

Patients using Nicotine Polacrilex treatment dropped out of the clinical trials less frequently than did patients using placebo.

INDIVIDUALIZATION OF DOSAGE

It is important to make sure that patients read the instructions made available to them and have their questions answered. They should clearly understand the directions for using and disposing of Nicotine Polacrilex. They should be instructed to stop smoking completely when the first Nicotine Polacrilex dose is used. The success or failure of smoking cessation depends heavily on the quality, intensity, and frequency of supportive care. Patients are more likely to quit smoking if they are seen frequently and participate in formal smoking-cessation programs.

The goal of Nicotine Polacrilex therapy is complete abstinence. Significant health benefits have not been demonstrated for reduction of smoking. If a patient is unable to stop smoking by the fourth week of therapy, treatment should probably be discontinued. Patients who have not stopped smoking after 4 weeks of Nicotine Polacrilex therapy are unlikely to quit on that attempt.

Patients who fail to quit on any attempt may benefit from interventions to improve their chances for success on subsequent attempts. Patients who were unsuccessful should be counseled to determine why they failed. Patients should then probably be given a "therapy holiday" before the next attempt. A new quit attempt should be encouraged when the factors that contributed to failure can be eliminated or reduced, and conditions are more favorable.

Based on the clinical trials, a reasonable approach to assisting patients in their attempt to quit smoking is to assign their initial Nicotine Polacrilex dose based on the severity of their dependence (see *"Fagerstrom Tolerance Questionnaire"* below). The need for those adjustment should be assessed during the first 2 weeks. Patients should continue the dose selected with concomitant support and periodic evaluation. Those who have successfully stopped smoking during that time should be supported during 1 to 3 months of weaning, after which treatment should be terminated.

Therapy should generally begin with the Nicotine Polacrilex (4 mg dose) in individuals who score ≥ 7 on the Fagerstrom Tolerance Questionnaire (FTQ) or who are determined to be highly dependent by some other measure (consumption of > 25 cigarettes/day, carbon monoxide, cotinine, et al). (See related table).

The symptoms of Nicotine withdrawal and excess overlap (see *"Clinical Pharmacology"* and *"Adverse Reactions"* sections"). Since patients using Nicotine Polacrilex treatment might also smoke intermittently, it may be difficult to determine if patients are experiencing Nicotine withdrawal or nicotine excess. The controlled clinical trials comparing Nicotine Polacrilex (2 mg), Nicotine Polacrilex double strength (4 mg), and placebo doses suggest that dyspepsia and nausea are more often symptoms of Nicotine excess, while flatulence and depression are more often symptoms of Nicotine withdrawal.

In a 24-month study where all subjects were provided access to 2 mg Nicotine Polacrilex pieces after the 6 week double-blind phase, 54% used the product after 3 months, 16% after 6 months, 6% after 12 months, and 3% after 24 months. To minimize the risk of dependence, patients should be encouraged to withdraw gradually from Nicotine Polacrilex treatment after 2 to 3 months of use (see *"Dosage and Administration"*).

INDICATIONS AND USAGE

Nicotine Polacrilex treatment is indicated as an aid to smoking cessation for the relief of Nicotine withdrawal symptoms. Nicotine Polacrilex treatment should be used as a part of a comprehensive behavioral smoking-cessation program.

The use of Nicotine Polacrilex for longer than 6 months has not been adequately studied.

CONTRAINDICATIONS

Use of Nicotine Polacrilex is contraindicated in patients with hypersensitivity or allergy to Nicotine or to any of the components of Nicotine Polacrilex.

WARNINGS

Nicotine from any source can be toxic and addictive. Smoking causes lung cancer, heart disease, emphysema, and may adversely affect the fetus and the pregnant woman. For any smoker, with or without concomitant disease or pregnancy, the risk of nicotine replacement in a smoking-cessation program should be weighed against the hazard of continued smoking during Nicotine Polacrilex treatment, and the likelihood of achieving cessation of smoking without nicotine replacement.

PREGNANCY WARNING

Tobacco smoke, which has been shown to be harmful to the fetus, contains nicotine, hydrogen cyanide, and carton monoxide. Nicotine has been shown in animal studies to cause fetal harm. It is therefore presumed that Nicotine Polacrilex treatment can cause fetal harm when administered to a pregnant woman. The effect of nicotine delivery by Nicotine Polacrilex has been examined in single dose trials in pregnancy and shown to have less fetal cardiovascular effect than cigarette smoking (see *"Precautions"*).

Pregnant smokers should be encouraged to attempt cessation using educational and behavioral interventions, however, before using pharmacological approaches. If Nicotine Polacrilex therapy is used during pregnancy, or if the patient becomes pregnant while using Nicotine Polacrilex, the patient should be apprised of the potential hazard to the fetus.

SAFETY NOTE CONCERNING CHILDREN

The amounts of nicotine that are tolerated by adult smokers can produce symptoms of poisoning and could prove fatal if Nicotine Polacrilex is chewed or ingested by children or pets. Following recommended use, Nicotine Polacrilex chewing pieces contain about 50% of their initial drug content. Therefore, patients should be cautioned to keep both used and unused Nicotine Polacrilex out of the reach of children and pets.

PRECAUTIONS

The patient should be urged to stop smoking completely when initiating Nicotine Polacrilex therapy (see *"Dosage and Administration"*). Patients should be informed that if they continue to smoke while using Nicotine Polacrilex, they may experience adverse effects due to peak nicotine levels higher than those experienced from smoking alone. If there is a clinically significant increase in cardiovascular or other effects attributable to Nicotine, the Nicotine Polacrilex dose should be reduced or treatment discontinued (see *"Warnings"*). Physicians should anticipate that concomitant medications may need dosage adjustment (see *"Precautions: Drug Interactions"*).

QUIT RATE AFTER WEEK 2 BY STARTING DOSE

(N = 563 smokers in 6 clinics)

| Nicotine Polacrilex (mg/piece) | All patients enrolled | | | | Patients using > 9 pcs/day | | |
	Number of Patients	After 6 Weeks (range)*			Number of Patients	After 6 Weeks (range)†
4	189	17-59%			93	29-74%
2	190	21-47%			104	10-54%
Placebo	184	23-39%			92	20-44%

* Range for 6 clinics, number of patients per treatment ranged from 29-37.
† Range for 6 clinics, number of patients per treatment ranged from 7-23.

THE FAGERSTROM TOLERANCE QUESTIONNAIRE

Questions	Answers	Points
1. How soon after you wake up do you smoke your first cigarette?	Within 30 min.	1
	After 30 min.	0
2. Do you find it difficult to refrain from smoking in places where it is forbidden; e.g. in church, library, cinemas, etc.?	Yes	1
	No	0
3. Which cigarette would you hate the most to give up?	The first one in the morning	1
	Any other	0
4. How many cigarettes a day do you smoke?	≤ 15	0
	16-25	1
	≥ 26	2
5. Do you smoke more frequently during the hours after awakening?	Yes	1
	No	0
6. Do you smoke if you are so ill that you are in bed most of the day?	Yes	1
	No	0
7. What is the nicotine level of your usual brand of cigarette?	≤ 0.6 mg	0
	0.61-1.0 mg	1
	> 1.0 mg	2
8. Do you inhale?	Never	0
	Sometimes	1
	Always	2

Total 0-11. Highly Nicotine dependent smokers ≥ 7 points.

◆ RATED THERAPEUTICALLY EQUIVALENT; ◇ THERAPEUTIC EQUIVALENCE UNCONFIRMED; ○ UNRATED

The sustained use of Nicotine Polacrilex by patients who stop smoking should be discouraged because the chronic consumption of nicotine by any route can be harmful and addicting.

ALLERGIC REACTIONS
Allergic reactions to Nicotine Polacrilex have been reported in post-marketing surveillance. Patients with allergic reactions to Nicotine Polacrilex should be cautioned that a serious reaction could occur from exposure to other Nicotine-containing products or smoking. Patients should be instructed to discontinue the use of Nicotine Polacrilex promptly and contact their physician in the case of severe reactions (e.g., urticaria, hives, or generalized rashes).

ORAL/PHARYNGEAL CONDITIONS
Use with caution in patients with oral or pharyngeal inflammation or a history of esophagitis.

Nicotine Polacrilex has been formulated to minimize its stickiness. As with other chewing gums, it may still adhere to dentures, dental caps, or partial bridges. Patients should be made aware of this, and should be instructed to discontinue use of Nicotine Polacrilex chewing pieces, if stickiness to dental work becomes a problem (see *"Patient Instructions"*).

CARDIOVASCULAR OR PERIPHERAL VASCULAR DISEASES
The risks of Nicotine replacement in patients with certain cardiovascular and peripheral vascular diseases should be weighed against the benefits of including Nicotine replacement in a smoking-cessation program for them. Specifically, patients with coronary heart disease (history of myocardial infarction and/or angina pectoris, serious cardiac arrhythmias, or vasopastic diseases (Buerger's disease, Prinzmetal's variant angina) should be carefully screened and evaluated before Nicotine replacement is prescribed.

Cardiovascular events occurring in association with the use of Nicotine Polacrilex have been reported (see *"Adverse Reactions"*). In postmarketing surveillance of Nicotine Polacrilex 2 mg in the U.S., several deaths have been reported including congestive heart failure, myocardial infarction, cardiac arrest, and cerebrovascular accident. A cause and effect between these events and the use of Nicotine Polacrilex has not been established. If serious cardiovascular symptoms occur with Nicotine Polacrilex therapy, it should be discontinued.

Nicotine Polacrilex should generally not be used in patients during the immediate postmyocardial infarction period, patients with serious arrhythmias, and patients with severe or worsening angina pectoris.

RENAL OR HEPATIC INSUFFICIENCY
The pharmacokinetics of Nicotine have not been studied in the elderly or patients with renal or hepatic impairment. However, given that nicotine is extensively metabolized and that its total systemic clearance is dependent on liver blood flow, some influence of hepatic impairment on drug kinetics (reduced clearance) should be anticipated. Only severe renal impairment would be expected to affect the clearance of Nicotine or its metabolites from the circulation (see *"Clinical Pharmacology: Pharmacokinetics"*).

ENDOCRINE DISEASES
Nicotine Polacrilex treatment should be used with caution in patients with hyperthyroidism, pheochromacytoma, or insulin-dependent diabetes since nicotine causes the release of catecholamines by the adrenal medula.

PEPTIC ULCER DISEASE
Nicotine delays healing in peptic ulcer disease; therefore Nicotine Polacrilex treatment should be used with caution in patients with active peptic ulcers and only when the benefits of including nicotine replacement in a smoking-cessation program outweigh the risks.

ACCELERATED HYPERTENSION
Nicotine constitutes a risk factor for development of malignant hypertension in patients with accelerated hypertension; therefore Nicotine Polacrilex treatment should be used with caution in these patients and only when the benefits of including nicotine replacement in a smoking-cessation program outweigh the risks.

INFORMATION FOR PATIENT
A patient instruction sheet is included in the package of Nicotine Polacrilex dispensed to the patient. It contains important information and instructions on how to properly use and dispose of Nicotine Polacrilex chewing pieces. Patients should be encouraged to ask questions of the physician and pharmacist.

Patients must be advised to keep both used and unused Nicotine Polacrilex out of the reach of children and pets.

DRUG INTERACTIONS
Smoking cessation, with or without Nicotine replacement, may alter the pharmacokinetics of certain concomitant medications. (See related table).

Carcinogenesis, Mutagenesis, Impairment of Fertility: Nicotine itself does not appear to be a carcinogen in laboratory animals. However, nicotine and its metabolites increased the incidences of tumors in the cheek pouches of hamsters and forestomachs of F344 rats, when given in combination with tumor-initiators. One study, which could not be replicated, suggested that cotinine, the primary metabolite of nicotine, may cause lymphoreticular sarcoma in the large intestine in rats. Nicotine and cotinine were not mutagenic in the Ames' *Salmonella* test. Nicotine induced repairable DNA damage in an *E. coli* test system. Nicotine was shown to be genotoxic in a test system using Chinese hamster ovary cells. In rats and rabbits, implantation can be delayed or inhibited by a reduction in DNA synthesis that appears to be caused by nicotine. Studies have shown a decrease in litter size in rats treated with nicotine during gestation.

PREGNANCY
Pregnancy Category C: (see *"Warnings"* section).

The harmful effects of cigarette smoking on maternal and fetal health are clearly established. These include low birth weight, an increased risk of spontaneous abortion, and increased perinatal mortality. Nicotine produced skeletal abnormalities in the offspring of pregnant mice who received toxic doses (25 mg/kg IP or SC, 700 × the 2.5 mg dose absorbed systemically from a single Nicotine Polacrilex double strength in one study. Nicotine, 1.67 mg/kg/day IP on days 6-15 of gestation, caused decreased crown-rump length, fetal weight, and head size and increased rate of cleft palate in the offspring of pregnant mice. There are no adequate and well-controlled multiple dose studies in pregnant women. Therefore, pregnant smokers should be encouraged to attempt cessation using educational and behavioral interventions before using pharmacological approaches. Spontaneous abortion during nicotine replacement therapy has been reported; as with smoking, nicotine as a contributing factor cannot be excluded.

Nicotine Polacrilex treatment should be used during pregnancy only if the potential benefit considering the likelihood of smoking, cessation justifies the potential risk to the fetus of using Nicotine Polacrilex by the patient, who might continue to smoke.

HUMAN STUDIES
Smoking: Cigarette smoking during pregnancy is associated with an increased risk of spontaneous abortion, low birthweight infants, and perinatal mortality. Current thought implicates Nicotine and carbon monoxide as the most likely mediators of these outcomes.

Nicotine: The effect of nicotine, administered as 2 and 4 mg Nicotine gum and cigarette smoking, on fetal cardiovascular parameters, has been studied near term. One or two cigarettes increased fetal aortic blood flow and heart rate, and decreased uterine blood flow and fetal breathing movement. One or two pieces of 2 or 4 mg gum (delivering 1 to 4 mg of nicotine) had less effect on these parameters.

TERATOGENICITY
Animal Studies: Nicotine was shown to produce skelatal abnormalities, cleft palate, and other effects in mice (see *"Pregnancy"*).

Human Studies: Nicotine teratogenicity has not been studied in humans except as a component of cigarette smoke (each cigarette smoked delivers about 1 mg of nicotine). It has not been possible to conclude whether cigarette smoking is teratogenic to humans.

OTHER EFFECTS
Animal Studies: A nicotine bolus (up to 2 mg/kg) to pregnant rhesus monkeys caused acidosis, hypercarbia, and hypotension (fetal and maternal concentrations were about 20 times those achieved after smoking one cigarette in 5 minutes). Fetal breathing movements were reduced in the fetal lamb after intravenous injection of 0.25 mg/kg nicotine to the ewe (equivalent to smoking one cigarette every 20 seconds for 5 minutes). Uterine blood flow was reduced about 30% after infusion of 2 mg/kg nicotine over 20 minutes to pregnant rhesus monkeys (equivalent to smoking about 120 cigarettes over 20 minutes).

LABOR AND DELIVERY
Nicotine Polacrilex treatment is not recommended during labor and delivery. The effects of nicotine on the mother or the fetus during labor are unknown.

USE IN NURSING MOTHERS
Caution should be exercised when Nicotine Polacrilex is administered to nursing women. The safety of Nicotine Polacrilex treatment in nursing infants has not been examined. Nicotine passes freely into breast milk; the milk to plasma ratio averages 2.9. Nicotine is absorbed orally. An infant has the ability to clear nicotine by hepatic first pass clearance; however, the efficiency of removal is probably lowest at birth. The nicotine concentrations in breast milk can be expected to be lower with Nicotine Polacrilex treatment when used as directed than with cigarette smoking, as maternal plasma Nicotine concentrations are

May Require a Decrease in Dose at Cessation of Smoking	*Possible Mechanism*
acetaminophen, caffeine, imipramine, oxazepam, pentazocine, propranolol, theophylline	Deinduction of hepatic enzymes on smoking cessation
insulin	Increase of subcutaneous insulin absorption with smoking cessation
adrenergic antagonists (e.g., prazosin, labetalol)	Decrease in circulating catecholamines with smoking cessation
May Require an Increase in Dose at Cessation of Smoking	*Possible Mechanism*
adrenergic agonists (e.g., isoproterenol, phenylephrine)	Decrease in circulating catecholamines with smoking cessation

➤ SHOWN IN PRODUCT IDENTIFICATION GUIDE

generally reduced with Nicotine replacement. The risk of exposure of the infant to nicotine from Nicotine Polacrilex treatment should be weighed against the risks associated with the infant's exposure to nicotine from continued smoking by the mother (passive smoke exposure and contamination of breast milk with other components of tobacco smoke) or from Nicotine Polacrilex therapy in combination with continued smoking.

PEDIATRIC USE
Nicotine Polacrilex treatment is not recommended for use in children because the safety and effectiveness of Nicotine Polacrilex treatment in children and adolescents who smoke have not been evaluated.

GERIATRIC USE
Review of postmarketing data with Nicotine Polacrilex does not reveal age-related trends in either incidence of character or adverse events.

ADVERSE REACTIONS
Assessment of adverse events in the 519 patients who participated in clinical trials of both 2 mg and 4 mg Nicotine Polacrilex doses is complicated by the occurrence of GI and CNS effects of Nicotine withdrawal as well as nicotine excess. The actual incidences of both are confounded by concurrent smoking by many of the patients. In the trials, when reporting adverse events, the investigators did not attempt to identify the cause of symptom.

ORAL ADVERSE EVENTS
Oral adverse events occurring with a frequency of 1% or greater among 174 patients using Nicotine Polacrilex double strength in clinical trials involving 519 patients were stomatitis (excluding aphthous and ulcerative stomatitis) 5%, aphthous stomatitis 5%, tooth disorder 4%, glossitis 3%, gingival bleeding 1%, tongue ulceration 1%, and ulcerative stomatitis 1%.

PROBABLY CAUSALLY RELATED
The following adverse events were reported more frequently in Nicotine Polacrilex treated patients than in placebo-treated patients or exhibited a dose response in clinical trials.

Digestive System: Diarrhea[†], dyspepsia (12%), hiccups[*], nausea (10%), salivation increased[*]

Mouth/Tooth Disorders: Dry mouth[†]

Musculoskeletal: Myalgia[†]

Nervous System: Paresthesia[*]

Skin and Appendages: Sweating[†]

CAUSAL RELATIONSHIP UNKNOWN
Adverse events reported in Nicotine Polacrilex and placebo-treated patients at about the same frequency in clinical trials are listed below. Selected events from post-marketing surveillance of Nicotine Polacrilex 2 mg treatment are also included. The clinical significance of the association between Nicotine Polacrilex treatment and these events is unknown, but they are reported as alerting information for the clinician.
Italics indicate reports from post-marketing surveillance of Nicotine Polacrilex 2 mg.

Body as a Whole: Allergy[†], back pain[*] chest pain[†], pain[*], *erythemia, pruritus*

Cardiovascular System: Hypertension[†], *edema, flushing, palpitations, tachyarrhythmias, tachycardia*

Digestive System: Abdominal pain[*], *anorexia, alteration of liver function tests,* constipation[*], eructation[†], flatulence[*], *vomiting*

Mouth/Tooth Disorder: Aphthous stomatitis[*], *gingivitis,* glossitis[†], *jaw pain,* stomatitis[*], *taste perception changes,* tooth disorder[*]

Nervous System: Concentration impaired[†], *confusion, convulsions, depression,* dizziness[*], *euphoria,* headache (20%), insomnia[*], *irritability, tinnitus*

Respiratory System: Breathing difficulty, congestion[*], cough increased[*], *hoarseness,* throat irritation[*], *wheezing*

Urogenital System: Dysmenorrhea[*]

DRUG AND DEPENDENCE
Nicotine Polacrilex is likely to have a low abuse potential based on differences between it and cigarettes in four characteristics commonly considered important in contributing to abuse; slower absorption, smaller fluctuations in blood levels, lower blood levels of nicotine, and less frequent use (9-12 pieces/day).
Dependence on Nicotine Polacrilex replacement therapy has been reported. Such dependence may represent transference to Nicotine Polacrilex of tobacco-based nicotine dependence. The use of Nicotine Polacrilex treatment beyond 6 months has not been evaluated in well-controlled studies and should be discouraged.
To minimize the risk of dependence, patients should be encouraged to withdraw gradually from Nicotine Polacrilex therapy after 2 to 3 months of usage. Recommended dose reduction is to progressively decrease the dose every 4 to 7 days (see *"Dosage and Administration"*).

Frequencies for Nicotine Polacrilex.
[†] Reported in 1% to 3% of patients.
[*] Reported in 3% to 9% of patients.
Unmarked if reported in < 1% of patients.

OVERDOSAGE
Overdosage can occur if many pieces are chewed simultaneously or in rapid succession. The polacrilex resin requires chewing to release the nicotine and limits nicotine release from swallowed gum.
The oral LD_{50} for nicotine in rodents varies with species but is in excess of 24 mg/kg: death is due to respiratory paralysis. The oral minimum lethal dose of nicotine in dogs is greater than 5 mg/kg. The oral minimum acute lethal dose for nicotine in human adults is reported to be 40 to 60 mg (< 1 mg/kg).
Signs and symptoms of an overdose of Nicotine Polacrilex would be expected to be the same as those of acute nicotine poisoning including: pallor, cold sweat, nausea, salivation, vomiting, abdominal pain, diarrhea, headache, dizziness, disturbed hearing and vision, tremor, mental confusion, and weakness. Prostration, hypotension, and respiratory failure may ensue with large overdose. Lethal doses produce convulsions quickly and death follows as a result of peripheral or central respiratory paralysis, or less frequently, cardiac failure.

OVERDOSE FROM INGESTION
Review of reported overdoses in children ranging from 20 months to 9 years of age who had chewed or swallowed 1/2-4 pieces of 2 mg Nicotine Polacrilex revealed no fatalities. Symptoms reported include nausea, vomiting, lethargy, abdominal pain, hypotension, agitation, and tachycardia. All symptoms resolved within 24 hours with only supportive treatment and observation. Used Nicotine Polacrilex pieces may contain about 50% of their initial drug content. Therefore, patients should be cautioned to keep both the used and unused Nicotine Polacrilex pieces out of the reach of children and pets.
Due to the slow release of nicotine from the polacrilex resin, activated charcoal alone may be adequate for most ingestions. In unconscious patients with a secure airway, instill activated charcoal. A saline cathartic or sorbitol added to the first dose of activated charcoal may speed gastrointestinal passage of the gum.

MANAGEMENT OF NICOTINE POISONING
Other supportive measures include diazepam or barbiturates for seizures, atropine for excessive bronchial secretions or diarrhea, respiratory support for respiratory failure, and vigorous fluid support for hypotension and cardiovascular collapse.

DOSAGE AND ADMINISTRATION
Patients must desire to stop smoking and should be instructed to *stop smoking immediately.* The patient should read the patient instruction sheet on Nicotine Polacrilex treatment and be encouraged to ask any questions. The initial dosage of Nicotine Polacrilex should be individualized on the basis of each patient's nicotine dependence. Highly dependent smokers (Fagerstrom Tolerance Score ≥ 7, or > 25 cigarettes/day) should receive the 4 mg dosage initially. Other patients should begin treatment with the 2 mg dosage strength. Increasing to the 4 mg dose may be considered for patients who fail to stop smoking with the 2 mg dose, or for those whose nicotine withdrawal symptoms remain so strong as to threaten relapse. (See related table).

It is important for the patients to learn to chew Nicotine Polacrilex slowly and to self-titrate the Nicotine dose, in order to minimize side effects (see *"Patient Instructions"* Sheet at the end of this monograph). Each piece of Nicotine Polacrilex should be chewed intermittently for about 30 minutes. The aim of this chewing procedure is to promote slow buccal absorption of the nicotine released from Nicotine Polacrilex. Chewing too quickly can rapidly release the nicotine which leads to effects similar to oversmoking; nausea, hiccups, or irritation of the throat. Since nicotine is poorly absorbed from the stomach, swallowed nicotine may contribute to gastrointestinal adverse effects without relieving withdrawal. Proper chewing technique (slow paced chewing and intermittent parking) is designed to minimize swallowed nicotine.
Acidic beverages (e.g., coffee, juices, wine, or soft drinks) interfere with the buccal absorption of nicotine from Nicotine Polacrilex. Eating and drinking should therefore be avoided for 15 minutes before and during chewing of Nicotine Polacrilex.
Clinical experience suggests that abstinence (quit) rates may be higher when patients chew Nicotine Polacrilex on a fixed schedule (one piece every 1 to 2 hours) than when allowed to chew it *ad libitum.*
Patients using the 2 mg strength should not exceed 30 pieces per day, whereas those using the 4 mg strength should not exceed 20 pieces per day.
When used for smoking cessation, gradual weaning from Nicotine Polacrilex treatment should be initiated after 2 to 3 months and completed by 4 to 6 months. Some ex-smokers may need Nicotine Polacrilex treatment longer to avoid returning to smoking.

GRADUAL REDUCTION PROCEDURES FOR USE
IN SMOKING CESSATION
Gradual withdrawal of Nicotine Polacrilex treatment should be initiated to avoid the recurrence of symptoms which may lead to a return to smoking. Suggested procedures for gradually reducing Nicotine Polacrilex dosage include:

1. Decrease the total number of pieces of Nicotine Polacrilex used per day by one or more pieces every 4 to 7 days.
2. Decrease the chewing time with each piece of Nicotine Polacrilex from the normal 30 minutes to 10 to 15 minutes for 4 to 7 days. Then gradually decrease the total number of pieces used per day.
3. Others may want to chew each piece for longer than 30 minutes and reduce the number of pieces used per day.

◆ RATED THERAPEUTICALLY EQUIVALENT; ◇ THERAPEUTIC EQUIVALENCE UNCONFIRMED; ○ UNRATED

RECOMMENDED DOSING SCHEDULE FOR HEALTHY PATIENTS

Dose	Patient dependency (FTQ)	Number of pieces to be used per day	Maximum pieces per day
Nicotine Polacrilex double strength	≥ 7	9-12	20
Nicotine Polacrilex 2 mg	< 7	9-12	30

4. Substitute one or more pieces of sugarless gum for an equal number of pieces of Nicotine Polacrilex. Increase the number of pieces of sugarless gum substituted for Nicotine Polacrilex chewing pieces every 4 to 7 days.
5. Replace Nicotine Polacrilex 4 mg with 2 mg and apply any of the above suggested procedures.

Withdrawal of Nicotine Polacrilex treatment may be individualized by modifying or combining the above procedures. Nicotine Polacrilex treatment may be stopped when usage has been reduced to one or two pieces per day.

SAFETY AND HANDLING
Nicotine Polacrilex is dispensed in individual blister packages which pose no known risk to health care workers if given unopened to the patient.

DISPOSAL
Used Nicotine Polacrilex chewing pieces should be placed in a wrapper and disposed of in such a way to prevent its access by children or pets. See patient information for further directions for handling and disposal.

HOW TO STORE
Do not store above 86°F (30°C), because the Nicotine in Nicotine Polacrilex is sensitive to heat. Protect from light.

Do not store out of the blister. Once removed from the protective pack, Nicotine Polacrilex should be used promptly since Nicotine is volatile and it may lose strength.

HOW SUPPLIED
GUM: 2 MG

BRAND/MANUFACTURER	NDC	SIZE	AWP
◆ **BRAND**			
NICORETTE: SK Beecham Cons	00068-0045-55	96s	$36.22

GUM: 4 MG

BRAND/MANUFACTURER	NDC	SIZE	AWP
◆ **BRAND**			
NICORETTE DS: SK Beecham Cons	00068-0047-55	96s	$63.29

Nifedipine

DESCRIPTION
Nifedipine is an antianginal drug belonging to a class of pharmacological agents known as the calcium channel blockers. Nifedipine is 3,5-pyridinedicarboxylic acid, 1,4-dihydro-2,6-dimethyl-4-(2-nitrophenyl)-, dimethyl ester, $C_{17}H_{18}N_2O_6$.

Nifedipine is a yellow crystalline substance, practically insoluble in water but soluble in ethanol. It has a molecular weight of 346.3. Nifedipine Capsules are formulated as soft gelatin capsules for oral administration each containing 10 mg or 20 mg Nifedipine.

Nifedipine Extended Release Tablet is formulated as a once a day controlled release tablet for oral administration designed to deliver 30, 60, or 90 mg of Nifedipine.

Nifedipine Extended Release Tablet is similar in appearance to a conventional tablet. It consists, however, of a semipermeable membrane surrounding an osmotically active drug core. The core itself is divided into two layers: an "active" layer containing the drug, and a "push" layer containing pharmacologically inert (but osmotically active) components. As water from the gastrointestinal tract enters the tablet, pressure increases in the osmotic layer and "pushes" against the drug layer, releasing drug through the precision laser-drilled tablet orifice in the active layer.

Nifedipine Extended Release Tablet is designed to provide Nifedipine at an approximately constant rate over 24 hours. This controlled rate of drug delivery into the gastrointestinal lumen is independent of pH or gastrointestinal motility. Nifedipine depends for its action on the existence of an osmotic gradient between the contents of the bilayer core and fluid in the GI tract. Drug delivery is essentially constant as long as the osmotic gradient remains constant, and then gradually falls to zero. Upon swallowing, the biologically inert components of the tablet remain intact during GI transit and are eliminated in the feces as an insoluble shell.

Following is its chemical structure:

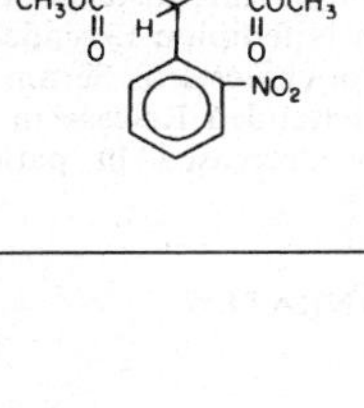

CLINICAL PHARMACOLOGY
Nifedipine is a calcium ion influx inhibitor (slow-channel blocker or calcium ion antagonist) and inhibits the trans-membrane influx of calcium ions into cardiac muscle and smooth muscle. The contractile processes of cardiac muscle and vascular smooth muscle are dependent upon the movement of extracellular calcium ions into these cells through specific ion channels. Nifedipine selectively inhibits calcium ion influx across the cell membrane of cardiac muscle and vascular smooth muscle without altering serum calcium concentrations.

MECHANISM OF ACTION
A) Angina: The precise mechanisms by which inhibition of calcium influx relieves angina has not been fully determined, but includes at least the following two mechanisms:

1) Relaxation and Prevent of Coronary Artery Spasm: Nifedipine dilates the main coronary arteries and coronary arterioles, both in normal and ischemic regions, and is a potent inhibitor of coronary artery spasm, whether spontaneous or ergonovine-induced. This property increases myocardial oxygen delivery in patients with coronary artery spasm, and is responsible for the effectiveness of Nifedipine in vasospastic (Prinzmetal's or variant) angina. Whether this effect plays any role in classical angina is not clear, but studies of exercise tolerance have not shown an increase in the maximum exercise rate-pressure product, a widely accepted measure of oxygen utilization. This suggests that, in general, relief of spasm or dilation of coronary arteries is not an important factor in classical angina.

2) Reduction of Oxygen Utilization: Nifedipine regularly reduces arterial pressure at rest and at a given level of exercise by dilating peripheral arterioles and reducing the total peripheral resistance (afterload) against which the heart works. This unloading of the heart reduces myocardial energy consumption and oxygen requirements, and probably accounts for the effectiveness of Nifedipine in chronic stable angina.

B) Hypertension: The mechanism by which Nifedipine reduces arterial blood pressure involves peripheral arterial vasodilatation and the resulting reduction in peripheral vascular resistance. The increased peripheral vascular resistance that is an underlying cause of hypertension results from an increase in active tension in the vascular smooth muscle. Studies have demonstrated that the increase in active tension reflects an increase in cytosolic free calcium.

Nifedipine is a peripheral arterial vasodilator which acts directly on vascular smooth muscle. The binding of Nifedipine to voltage-dependent and possibly receptor-operated channels in vascular smooth muscle results in an inhibition of calcium influx through these channels. Stores of intracellular calcium in vascular smooth muscle are limited and thus dependent upon the influx of extracellular calcium for contraction to occur. The reduction in calcium influx by Nifedipine causes arterial vasodilation and decreased peripheral vascular resistance which results in reduced arterial blood pressure.

PHARMACOKINETICS AND METABOLISM
Nifedipine is completely absorbed after oral administration. Nifedipine is detectable in serum 10 minutes after oral administration, and peak blood levels occur in approximately 30 minutes. Bioavailability is proportional to dose from 10 to 30 mg; half-life does not change significantly with dose. There is little difference in relative bioavailability when Nifedipine Capsules are given orally and either swallowed whole; bitten and swallowed; or, bitten and held sublingually. However, biting through the capsule prior to swallowing does result in slightly earlier plasma concentrations (27 ng/mL 10 minutes after 10 mg) than if capsules are swallowed intact. Plasma drug concentrations rise at a gradual, controlled rate after a Nifedipine Extended Release Tablet dose and reach a plateau at approximately six hours after the first dose. For subsequent doses, relatively constant plasma concentrations at this plateau are maintained with minimal fluctuations over the 24 hour dosing interval. About a four-fold higher fluctuation index (ratio of peak trough plasma concentration) was observed with the conventional immediate release. Nifedipine Capsule at t.i.d. dosing than with once daily Nifedipine Extended Release Tablet. At steady-state the bioavailability of the Nifedipine Extended Release Tablet is 86% relative to Nifedipine Capsules. Administration of the Nifedipine Extended Release Tablet in the presence of food slightly alters the early rate of drug absorption, but does not influence the extent of drug bioavailability. Markedly reduced GI retention time over prolonged periods (i.e., short bowel syndrome), however, may influence the pharmacokinetic profile of the drug which could potentially result in lower plasma concentrations. Pharmacokinetics of Nifedipine Extended Release Tablet are linear over the dose range of 30 to 180 mg in that plasma drug concentrations are proportional to dose administered. There was no evidence of dose dumping either in the presence or absence of food for over 150 subjects in pharmacokinetic studies.

Nifedipine is extensively metabolized to highly water-soluble, inactive metabolites accounting for 60 to 80% of the dose excreted in the urine. The elimination half-life of Nifedipine is approximately two hours. Only traces (less than 0.1% of the dose) of unchanged form can be detected in the urine. The remainder is excreted in the feces in metabolized form, most likely as a result of biliary excretion. Thus, the pharmacokinetics of Nifedipine are not significantly influenced by the degree of renal impairment. Patients in hemodialysis or chronic ambulatory peritoneal dialysis have not reported significantly altered pharmacokinetics of Nifedipine. Since hepatic biotransformation is the predominant route for the disposition of Nifedipine, the pharmacokinetics may be altered in patients with chronic liver disease. Patients with hepatic impairment (liver cirrhosis) have a longer disposition half-life and higher bioavailability of Nifedipine than healthy volunteers. The degree of serum protein binding of Nifedipine is high (92-98%). Protein binding may be greatly reduced in patients with renal or hepatic impairment.

HEMODYNAMICS

Like other slow-channel blockers, Nifedipine exerts a negative inotropic effect on isolated myocardial tissue. This is rarely, if ever, seen in intact animals or man, probably because of reflex responses to its vasodilating effects. In man, Nifedipine decreases peripheral vascular resistance which leads to a fall in systolic and diastolic pressures, usually minimal in normotensive volunteers (less than 5-10 mm Hg systolic), but sometimes larger. There is usually a small increase in heart rate, a reflex response to vasodilation. With Nifedipine Extended Release Tablets, these decreases in blood pressure are not accompanied by any significant change in heart rate. Hemodynamic studies in patients with normal ventricular function have generally found a small increase in cardiac index without major effects on ejection fraction, left ventricular end diastolic pressure (LVEDP) or volume (LVEDV). In patients with impaired ventricular function, most acute studies have shown some increase in ejection fraction and reduction in left ventricular filling pressure.

ELECTROPHYSIOLOGIC EFFECTS

Although, like other members of its class, Nifedipine causes a slight depression of sinoatrial node function and atrioventricular conduction in isolated myocardial preparations, such effects have not been seen in studies in intact animals or in man. In formal electrophysiologic studies, predominantly in patients with normal conduction systems, Nifedipine has had no tendency to prolong atrioventricular conduction or sinus node recovery time, or to slow sinus rate.

INDICATIONS AND USAGE

I. VASOSPASTIC ANGINA

Nifedipine is indicated for the management of vasospastic angina confirmed by any of the following criteria: 1) classical pattern of angina at rest accompanied by ST segment elevation, 2) angina or coronary artery spasm provoked by ergonovine, or 3) angiographically demonstrated coronary artery spasm. In those patients who have had angiography, the presence of significant fixed obstructive disease is not incompatible with the diagnosis of vasospastic angina, provided that the above criteria are satisfied. Nifedipine may also be used where the clinical presentation suggests a possible vasospastic component but where vasospasm has not been confirmed, e.g., where pain has a variable threshold on exertion or in unstable angina where electrocardiographic findings are compatible with intermittent vasospas, or when angina is refractory to nitrates and/or adequate doses of beta blockers.

II. CHRONIC STABLE ANGINA
(CLASSICAL EFFORT-ASSOCIATED ANGINA)

Nifedipine is indicated for the management of chronic stable angina (effort-associated angina) without evidence of vasospasm in patients who remain symptomatic despite adequate doses of beta blockers and/or organic nitrates, or who cannot tolerate those agents.

In chronic stable angina (effort-associated angina) Nifedipine has been effective in controlled trials of up to eight weeks duration in reducing angina frequency and increasing exercise tolerance, but confirmation of sustained effectiveness and evaluation of long term safety in these patients are incomplete.

Controlled studies in small numbers of patients suggest concomitant use of Nifedipine and beta blocking agents may be beneficial in patients with chronic stable angina, but available information is not sufficient to predict with confidence the effects of concurrent treatment, especially in patients with compromised left ventricular function or cardiac conduction abnormalities. When introducing such concomitant therapy, care must be taken to monitor blood pressure closely since severe hypotension can occur from the combined effects of the drugs. (See "Warnings").

III. HYPERTENSION

Nifedipine Extended Release is indicated for the treatment of hypertension. It may be used alone or in combination with other antihypertensive agents.

UNLABELED USES

Nifedipine is used alone or as an adjunct in the treatment of congestive heart failure and causalgia, and in the relief of postoperative pain. It is also used in migraine headache, and in the symptomatic treatment of esophageal achalasia, biliary colic, and renal colic. In addition, Nifedipine is used to provide protection against cold-water-induced digital vasospasm (Raynaud's disease), as an adjunct in bronchial asthma, and in the management of premature labor and primary dysmenorrhea.

CONTRAINDICATIONS

Known hypersensitivity reaction to Nifedipine.

WARNINGS

EXCESSIVE HYPOTENSION

Although in most angina patients the hypotensive effect of Nifedipine is modest and well tolerated, occasional patients have had excessive and poorly tolerated hypotension. These responses have usually occurred during initial titration or at the time of subsequent upward dosage adjustment, and may be more likely in patients on concomitant beta blockers.

Severe hypotension and/or increased fluid volume requirements have been reported in patients receiving Nifedipine together with a beta-blocking agent who underwent coronary artery bypass surgery using high dose fentanyl anesthesia. The interaction with high dose fentanyl appears to be due to the combination of Nifedipine and a beta blocker, but the possibility that it may occur with Nifedipine alone, with low doses of fentanyl, in other surgical procedures, or with other narcotic analgesics cannot be ruled out. In Nifedipine-treated patients where surgery using high dose fentanyl anesthesia is contemplated, the physician should be aware of these potential problems and if the patient's condition permits, sufficient time (at least 36 hours) should be allowed for Nifedipine to be washed out of the body prior to surgery.

The following information should be taken into account in those patients who are being treated for hypertension as well as angina:

INCREASED ANGINA AND/OR MYOCARDIAL INFARCTION

Rarely, patients, particularly those who have severe obstructive coronary artery disease, have developed well documented increased frequency, duration and/or severity of angina or acute myocardial infarction on starting Nifedipine or at the time of dosage increase. The mechanism of this effect is not established.

BETA BLOCKER WITHDRAWAL

It is important to taper beta blockers if possible, rather than stopping them abruptly before beginning Nifedipine. Patients recently withdrawn from beta blockers may develop a withdrawal syndrome with increased angina, probably related to increased sensitivity to catecholamines. Initiation of Nifedipine treatment will not prevent this occurrence and might be expected to exacerbate it by provoking reflex catecholamine release. There have been occasional reports of increased angina in a setting of beta blocker withdrawal and Nifedipine initiation.

CONGESTIVE HEART FAILURE

Rarely, patients, usually receiving a beta blocker, have developed heart failure after beginning Nifedipine. Patients with tight aortic stenosis may be at greater risk for such an event, as the unloading effect of Nifedipine would be expected to be of less benefit to those patients, owning to their fixed impedance to flow across the aortic valve.

PRECAUTIONS

General—Hypotension: Because Nifedipine decreases peripheral vascular resistance, careful monitoring of blood pressure during the initial administration and titration of Nifedipine is suggested. Close observation is especially recommended for patients already taking medications that are known to lower blood pressure. (See "Warnings").

Peripheral Edema: Mild to moderate peripheral edema typically associated with arterial vasodilation and not due to left ventricular dysfunction, occurs in a dose dependent manner in about one in ten patients treated with Nifedipine or with an incidence ranging from approximately 10% to about 30% at the highest dose studied (180 mg). It is a localized phenomenon thought to be associated with vasodilation of dependent arterioles and small blood vessels and not due to left ventricular dysfunction or generalized fluid retention. It occurs primarily in the lower extremities and usually responds to diuretic therapy. With patients whose angina or hypertension is complicated by congestive heart failure, care should be taken to differentiate this peripheral edema from the effects of increasing left ventricular dysfunction.

Other: As with any other non-deformable material, caution should be used when administering Nifedipine Extended Release in patients with preexisting severe gastrointestinal narrowing (pathologic or iatrogenic). There have been rare reports of obstructive symptoms in patients with known strictures in association with the ingestion of Nifedipine Extended Release.

Information for Patients: Nifedipine Extended Release Tablets should be swallowed whole. Do not chew, divide or crush tablets. Do not be concerned if you occasionally notice in your stool something that looks like a tablet. In Nifedipine Extended Release, the medication is contained within a nonabsorbable shell that has been specially designed to slowly release the drug for your body to absorb. When this process is completed, the empty tablet is eliminated from your body.

Laboratory Tests: Rare, usually transient, but occasionally significant elevations of enzymes such as alkaline phosphatase, CPK, LDH, SGOT and SGPT have been noted. The relationship to Nifedipine therapy is uncertain in most cases, but probable in some. These laboratory abnormalities have rarely been associated with clinical symptoms; however, cholestasis with or without jaundice has been reported. A small (5.4%) increase in mean alkaline phosphatase was noted in patients treated with Nifedipine Extended Release Tablets. This was an isolated finding not associated with clinical symptoms and it rarely resulted in values which fell outside the normal range. Rare instances of allergic hepatitis have been reported. In controlled studies Nifedipine Extended Release did not adversely affect serum uric acid, glucose, or cholesterol. Serum potassium was unchanged in patients receiving Nifedipine Extended Release in the absence of concomitant diuretic therapy, and slightly decreased in patients receiving concomitant diuretics.

◆ RATED THERAPEUTICALLY EQUIVALENT; ◇ THERAPEUTIC EQUIVALENCE UNCONFIRMED; ○ UNRATED

Nifedipine, like other calcium channel blockers, decreases platelet aggregation *in vitro*. Limited clinical studies have demonstrated a moderate but statistically significant decrease in platelet aggregation and increase in bleeding time in some Nifedipine patients. This is thought to be a function of inhibition of calcium transport across the platelet membrane. No clinical significance for these findings has been demonstrated.

Positive direct Coombs test with/without hemolytic anemia has been reported but a causal relationship between Nifedipine administration and positivity of this laboratory test, including hemolysis, could not be determined.

Although Nifedipine has been used safely in patients with renal dysfunction and has been reported to exert a beneficial effect in certain cases, rare reversible elevations in BUN and serum creatinine have been reported in patients with preexisting chronic renal insufficiency. The relationship to Nifedipine therapy is uncertain in most cases but probable in some.

Drug Interactions—Beta-adrenergic blocking agents: (See "Indications" and "Warnings"). Experience in over 1400 patients with capsules in a noncomparative clinical trial has shown that concomitant administration of Nifedipine and beta-blocking agents is usually well tolerated but there have been occasional literature reports suggesting that the combination may increase the likelihood of congestive heart failure, severe hypotension, or exacerbation of angina.

Long Acting Nitrates: Nifedipine may be safely co-administered with nitrates, but there have been no controlled studies to evaluate the antianginal effectiveness of this combination.

Digitalis: Administration of Nifedipine with digoxin increased digoxin levels in nine of twelve normal volunteers. The average increase was 45%. Another investigator found no increase in digoxin levels in thirteen patients with coronary artery disease. In an uncontrolled study of over two hundred patients with congestive heart failure during which digoxin blood levels were not measured, digitalis toxicity was not observed. Since there have been isolated reports of patients with elevated digoxin levels, it is recommended that digoxin levels be monitored when initiating, adjusting, and discontinuing Nifedipine to avoid possible over- or underdigitalization.

Coumarin Anticoagulants: There have been rare reports of increased prothrombin time in patients taking coumarin anticoagulants to whom Nifedipine was administered. However, the relationship to Nifedipine therapy is uncertain.

Cimetidine: A study in six healthy volunteers has shown a significant increase in peak Nifedipine plasma levels (80%) and area-under-the-curve (74%), after a one week course of cimetidine at 1000 mg per day and Nifedipine at 40 mg per day. Ranitidine produced smaller, non-significant increases. The effect may be mediated by the known inhibition of cimetidine on hepatic cytochrome P-450, the enzyme system probably responsible for the first-pass metabolism of Nifedipine. If Nifedipine therapy is initiated in a patient currently receiving cimetidine, cautious titration is advised.

Carcinogenesis, Mutagenesis, Impairment of Fertility: Nifedipine was administered orally to rats for two years and was not shown to be carcinogenic. When given to rats prior to mating, Nifedipine caused reduced fertility at a dose approximately 30 times the maximum recommended human dose. *In vivo* mutagenicity studies were negative.

Pregnancy: Pregnancy Category C. Nifedipine has been shown to be teratogenic in rats when given in doses 30 times the maximum recommended human dose. Nifedipine was embryotoxic (increased fetal resorptions, decreased fetal weight, increased stunted forms, increased fetal deaths, decreased neonatal survival) in rats, mice and rabbits at doses of from 3 to 10 times the maximum recommended human dose. In pregnant monkeys, doses ⅔ and twice the maximum recommended human dose resulted in small placentas and underdeveloped chorionic villi. In rats, doses three times maximum human dose and higher caused prolongation of pregnancy. There are no adequate and well controlled studies in pregnant women. Nifedipine should be used during pregnancy only if the potential benefit justifies the potential risk to the fetus.

ADVERSE EXPERIENCES
In multiple-dose U.S. and foreign controlled studies with Nifedipine capsules in which adverse reactions were reported spontaneously, adverse effects were frequent but generally not serious and rarely required discontinuation of therapy or dosage adjustment. Most were expected consequences of the vasodilator effects of Nifedipine Capsules.

Over 1000 patients from both controlled and open trials with Nifedipine Extended Release Tablets in hypertension and angina were included in the evaluation of adverse experiences. All side effects reported during Nifedipine Extended Release Tablets therapy were tabulated independent of their causal relation to medication. The most common side effect reported with Nifedipine Extended Release was edema which was dose related and ranged in frequency from approximately 10% to about 30% at the highest dose studied (180 mg). Other common adverse experiences reported in placebo-controlled trials include:

Adverse Effect	Nifedipine Extended Release (%) (N = 707)	Placebo (%) (N = 266)
Headache	15.8	9.8
Fatigue	5.9	4.1
Dizziness	4.1	4.5
Constipation	3.3	2.3
Nausea	3.3	1.9

Of these, only edema and headache were more common in Nifedipine Extended Release patients than placebo patients.

The following adverse reactions occurred with an incidence of less than 3.0%. With the exception of leg cramps, the incidence of these side effects was similar to that of placebo alone.

Body as a Whole/Systemic: asthenia, flushing, pain

Cardiovascular: palpitations

Central Nervous System: insomnia, nervousness, paresthesia, somnolence

Dermatologic: pruritus, rash

Gastrointestinal: abdominal pain, diarrhea, dry mouth, dyspepsia, flatulence

Musculoskeletal: arthralgia, leg cramps

Respiratory: chest pain (nonspecific), dyspnea

Urogenital: impotence, polyuria

Other adverse reactions were reported sporadically with an incidence of 1.0% or less. These include:

Body as a Whole/Systemic: face edema, fever, hot flashes, malaise, periorbital edema, rigors

Cardiovascular: arrhythmia, hypotension, increased angina, tachycardia, syncope

Central Nervous System: anxiety, ataxia, decreased libido, depression, hypertonia, hypoesthesia, migraine, paroniria, tremor, vertigo

Dermatologic: alopecia, increased sweating, urticaria, purpura

Gastrointestinal: eructation, gastroesophageal reflux, gum hyperplasia, melena, vomiting, weight increase

Musculoskeletal: back pain, gout, myalgias

Respiratory: coughing, epistaxis, upper respiratory tract infection, respiratory disorder, sinusitis

Special Senses: abnormal lacrimation, abnormal vision, taste perversion, tinnitus

Urogenital/Reproductive: breast pain, dysuria, hematuria, nocturia

Adverse experiences which occurred in less than 1 in 1000 patients cannot be distinguished from concurrent disease states or medications.

The following adverse experiences, reported in less than 1% of patients, occurred under conditions (e.g., open trials, marketing experience) where a causal relationship is uncertain: gastrointestinal irritation, gastrointestinal bleeding.

Adverse Effect	Nifedipine Capsules (%) (N = 226)	Placebo (%) (N = 235)
Dizziness, lightheadedness giddiness	27	15
Flushing, heat sensation	25	8
Headache	23	20
Weakness	12	10
Nausea, heartburn	11	8
Muscle cramps, tremor	8	3
Peripheral edema	7	1
Nervousness, mood changes	7	4
Palpitation	7	5
Dyspnea, cough, wheezing	6	3
Nasal congestion, sore throat	6	8

There is also a large uncontrolled experience in over 2100 patients in the United States. Most of the patients has vasospastic or resistant angina pectoris, and about half had concomitant treatment with beta-adrenergic blocking agents.

The most common adverse events were:

INCIDENCE APPROXIMATELY 10%
Cardiovascular: peripheral edema

Central Nervous System: dizziness or lightheadedness

Gastrointestinal: nausea

Systemic: headache and flushing, weakness

INCIDENCE APPROXIMATELY 5%
Cardiovascular: transient hypotension

INCIDENCE 2% OR LESS
Cardiovascular: palpitation

Respiratory: nasal and chest congestion, shortness of breath

Gastrointestinal: diarrhea, constipation, cramps, flatulence

Musculoskeletal: inflammation, joint stiffness, muscle cramps

Central Nervous System: shakiness, nervousness, jitteriness, sleep disturbances, blurred vision, difficulties in balance

Other: dermatitis, pruritus, urticaria, fever, sweating, chills, sexual difficulties.

INCIDENCE APPROXIMATELY 0.5%
Cardiovascular: syncope. Syncopal episodes did not recur with reduction in the dose of Nifedipine or concomitant antianginal medication.

INCIDENCE LESS THAN 0.5%
Hematologic: thrombocytopenia, anemia, leukopenia, purpura

Gastrointestinal: allergic hepatitis

Oral: gingival hyperplasia

CNS: depression, paranoid syndrome

Special Senses: transient blindness at the peak of plasma level

Other: erythromelalgia, arthritis with ANA (+)

Several of these side effects appear to be dose related. Peripheral edema occurred in about one in 25 patients at doses less than 60 mg per day and in about one patient in eight at 120 mg per day or more. Transient hypotensions, generally of mild to moderate severity and seldom requiring discontinuation of therapy, occurred in one of 50 patients at less than 60 mg per day and in one of 20 patients at 120 mg per day or more. Very rarely, introduction of Nifedipine therapy was associated with an increase in anginal pain, possibly due to associated hypotension.

In addition, more serious adverse events were observed, not readily distinguishable from the natural history of the disease in these patients. It remains possible, however, that some or many of these events were drug related. Myocardial infarction occurred in about 4% of patients and congestive heart failure or pulmonary edema in about 2%. Ventricular arrhythmias or conduction distrubances each occurred in fewer than 0.5% of patients.

In a subgroup of over 1000 patients receiving Nifedipine with concomitant beta blocker therapy, the pattern and incidence of adverse experiences was not different from that of the entire group of Nifedipine treated patients. (See *"Precautions."*)

In a subgroup of approximately 250 patients with a diagnosis of congestive heart failure as well as angina, dizziness or lightheadedness, peripheral edema, headache or flushing each occurred in one in eight patients. Hypotension occurred in about one in 20 patients. Syncope occurred in approximately one patient in 250. Myocardial infarction or symptoms of congestive heart failure each occurred in about one patient in 15. Atrial or ventricular dysrhythmias each occurred in about one patient in 150.

In postmarketing experience, there have been rare reports of exfoliative dermatitis caused by Nifedipine.

OVERDOSAGE
Although there is no well documented experience with Nifedipine overdosage, available data suggest that gross overdosage could result in excessive peripheral vasodilation with subsequent marked and probably prolonged systemic hypotension. Clinically significant hypotension due to Nifedipine overdosage calls for active cardiovascular support including monitoring of cardiovascular and respiratory function, elevation of extremities, judicious use of calcium infusion, pressor agents and fluids, and attention to circulating fluid volume and urine output. A vasoconstrictor (such as norepinephrine) may be helpful in restoring vascular tone and blood pressure, provided that there no contraindication to its use. Clearance of Nifedipine would be expected to be prolonged in patients with impaired liver function. Since Nifedipine is highly protein-bound, dialysis is not likely to be of any benefit.

There has been one reported case of massive overdosage with Nifedipine Extended Release Tablet. The main effect of ingestion of approximately 4800 mg of Nifedipine Extended Release in a young man attempting suicide as a result of cocaine-induced depression was initial dizziness, palpitations, flushing, and nervousness. Within several hours of ingestion, nausea, vomiting, and generalized edema developed. No significant hypotension was apparent at presentation, 18 hours post-ingestion. Electrolyte abnormalities consisted of a mild, transient elevation of serum creatinine, and modest elevations of LDH and CPK, but normal SGOT. Vital signs remained stable, no electrocardiographic abnormalities were noted and renal function returned to normal within 24 to 48 hours with routine supportive measures alone. No prolonged sequelae were observed.

The effect of a single 900 mg ingestion of Nifedipine Capsules in a depressed anginal patient also on tricyclic antidepressants was a loss of consciousness within 30 minutes of ingestion, and profound hypotension, which responded to calcium infusion, pressor agents, and fluid replacement. A variety of ECG abnormalities were seen in this patient with a history of bundle branch block, including sinus bradycardia and varying degrees of AV block. These dictated the prophylactic placement of a temporary ventricular pacemaker, but otherwise resolved spontaneously. Significant hyperglycemia was seen initially in this patient, but plasma glucose levels rapidly normalized without further treatment.

A young hypertensive patient with advanced renal failure ingested 280 mg of Nifedipine Capsules at one time, with resulting marked hypotension responding to calcium infusion and fluids. No AV conduction abnormalities, arrhythmias, or pronounced changes in heart rate were noted, nor was there any further deterioration in renal function.

DOSAGE AND ADMINISTRATION
The dosage of Nifedipine Capsules needed to suppress angina and that can be tolerated by the patient must be established by titration. Excessive doses can result in hypotension.

Therapy should be initiated with the 10 mg capsule. The starting dose is one 10 mg capsule, swallowed whole, 3 times/day. The usual effective dose range is 10-20 mg three times daily. Some patients, especially those with evidence of coronary artery spasm, respond only to higher doses, more frequent administration, or both. In such patients, doses of 20-30 mg three or four times daily may be effective. Doses above 120 mg daily are rarely necessary. More than 180 mg per day is not recommended.

In most cases Nifedipine titration should proceed over a 7-14 day period so that the physician can assess the response to each dose level and monitor the blood pressure before proceeding to higher doses.

If symptoms so warrant, titration may proceed more rapidly, provided that the patient is assessed frequently. Based on the patient's physical activity level, attack frequency, and sublingual nitroglycerin consumption, the dose of Nifedipine may be increased from 10 mg t.i.d. to 20 mg t.i.d. and then to 30 mg t.i.d. over a three-day period.

In hospitalized patients under close observation, the dose may be increased in 10 mg increments over four to six-hour periods as required to control pain and arrhythmias due to ischemia. A single dose should rarely exceed 30 mg.

Dosage of Nifedipine Extended Release Tablets must be adjusted to each patient's needs. Therapy for either hypertension or angina should be initiated with 30 or 60 mg once daily. Nifedipine Extended Release Tablets should be swallowed whole and should not be bitten or divided. In general, titration should proceed over a 7-14 day period so that the physician can fully assess the response to each dose level and monitor blood pressure before proceeding to higher doses. Since steady-state plasma levels are achieved on the second day of dosing, if symptoms so warrant, titration may proceed more rapidly provided the patient is assessed frequently. Titration to doses above 120 mg is not recommended.

Angina patients controlled on Nifedipine Capsules alone or in combination with other antianginal medications may be safely switched to Nifedipine Extended Release Tablets at the nearest equivalent total daily dose (e.g., 30 mg t.i.d. of Nifedipine Capsules may be changed to 90 mg once daily to Nifedipine Extended Release Tablets). Subsequent titration to higher or lower doses may be necessary and should be initiated as clinically warranted. Experience with doses greater than 90 mg in patients with angina is limited. Therefore, doses greater than 90 mg should be used with caution and only when clinically warranted.

No "rebound effect" has been observed upon discontinuation of Nifedipine. However, if discontinuation of Nifedipine is necessary, sound clinical practice suggests that the dosage should be decreased gradually with close physician supervision.

CO-ADMINISTRATION WITH OTHER ANTIANGINAL DRUGS
Sublingual nitroglycerin may be taken as required for the control of acute manifestations of angina, particularly during Nifedipine titration. See *"Precautions, Drug Interactions,"* for information on co-administration of Nifedipine with beta blockers or long acting nitrates.

STORAGE
Store Nifedipine Capsules at controlled room temperature, 59° to 77°F (15° to 25°C); protect from light and moisture.
Store Nifedipine Extended Release Tablets below 86°F (30°C).
Protect from moisture and humidity.

HOW SUPPLIED
CAPSULE: 10 MG

AVERAGE UNIT PRICE (AVAILABLE SIZES)		GENERIC A-RATED AVERAGE PRICE (GAAP)	
		100s	$44.42
BRAND	$0.54	300s	$129.15
GENERIC	$0.44	750s	$354.08
HCFA FUL (100s ea)	$0.13	1000s	$381.33

BRAND/MANUFACTURER	NDC	SIZE	AWP
◆ BRAND			
▶ ADALAT: Miles Pharm	00026-8811-51	100s	$46.51
▶ PROCARDIA: Pfizer Labs	00069-2600-66	100s	$58.25
▶ ADALAT: Miles Pharm	00026-8811-48	100s ud	$51.83
▶ PROCARDIA: Pfizer Labs	00069-2600-41	100s ud	$64.90
▶ ADALAT: Miles Pharm	00026-8811-18	300s	$136.70
▶ PROCARDIA: Pfizer Labs	00069-2600-72	300s	$171.28
◆ GENERICS			
Medirex	57480-0389-06	30s	$13.73
Dixon-Shane	17236-0923-01	100s	$37.50
Amer Generics	58634-0022-01	100s	$39.50
Caraco	57664-0872-08	100s	$39.90
Mason Dist	11845-0410-01	100s	$41.60
Rugby	00536-4065-01	100s	$42.00
Qualitest	00603-4759-21	100s	$42.20
Geneva	00781-2504-01	100s	$42.25
Chase	54429-3227-01	100s	$42.50
Moore,H.L.	00839-7564-06	100s	$43.05
Major	00904-7685-60	100s	$43.25
Caremark	00339-5717-12	100s	$43.34
Major	00904-0407-60	100s	$43.45
Major	00904-0409-60	100s	$43.45
Lemmon	00093-0520-01	100s	$43.50
URL	00677-1398-01	100s	$43.75
Schein	00364-2376-01	100s	$43.75
Goldline	00182-1547-01	100s	$43.75

◆ RATED THERAPEUTICALLY EQUIVALENT; ◇ THERAPEUTIC EQUIVALENCE UNCONFIRMED; ○ UNRATED

BRAND/MANUFACTURER	NDC	SIZE	AWP
Goldline	00182-1562-01	100s	$43.75
Warner Chilcott	00047-0078-24	100s	$43.75
Aligen	00405-4696-01	100s	$44.51
Purepac	00228-2497-10	100s	$44.51
Martec	52555-0126-01	100s	$44.95
Novopharm	55953-0040-40	100s	$48.08
Novopharm	55953-0171-40	100s	$48.08
Parmed	00349-8873-01	100s	$49.50
Raway	00686-0664-20	100s ud	$36.00
U.S. Trading	56126-0449-11	100s ud	$39.39
Major	00904-0407-61	100s ud	$45.86
Major	00904-0409-61	100s ud	$45.86
Schein	00364-2376-90	100s ud	$47.00
UDL	51079-0664-20	100s ud	$47.10
Vangard	00615-0360-13	100s ud	$47.21
Goldline	00182-1547-89	100s ud	$50.40
Novopharm	55953-0040-01	100s	$51.44
Novopharm	55953-0171-41	100s	$51.44
Medirex	57480-0389-01	100s ud	$51.50
Dixon-Shane	17236-0923-30	300s	$109.95
Caraco	57664-0872-11	300s	$110.00
Amer Generics	58634-0022-02	300s	$115.50
Chase	54429-3227-03	300s	$123.63
Mason Dist	11845-0410-00	300s	$124.26
Geneva	00781-2504-03	300s	$125.60
Lemmon	00093-0520-55	300s	$128.25
Schein	00364-2376-29	300s	$128.25
Goldline	00182-1547-96	300s	$128.25
Goldline	00182-1562-96	300s	$128.25
Warner Chilcott	00047-0078-29	300s	$128.25
Martec	52555-0126-03	300s	$129.80
URL	00677-1398-61	300s	$130.35
Moore,H.L.	00839-7564-13	300s	$130.40
Moore,H.L.	00839-7704-13	300s	$130.40
Rugby	00536-4065-03	300s	$130.80
Qualitest	00603-4759-25	300s	$130.88
Major	00904-0407-72	300s	$130.95
Major	00904-0409-72	300s	$130.95
Major	00904-7685-72	300s	$130.95
Aligen	00405-4696-09	300s	$131.54
Purepac	00228-2497-30	300s	$131.54
Balan,J.J.	00304-2294-03	300s	$139.98
Novopharm	55953-0040-60	300s	$142.31
Novopharm	55953-0171-60	300s	$142.31
Parmed	00349-8873-03	300s	$144.50
Glasgow	60809-0300-55	750s ud	$354.08
Glasgow	60809-0300-72	750s ud	$354.08
Caraco	57664-0872-18	1000s	$339.00
Chase	54429-3227-00	1000s	$400.00
Moore,H.L.	00839-7564-16	1000s	$404.99
Novopharm	55953-0171-81	2000s	$690.17

CAPSULE: 20 MG

AVERAGE UNIT PRICE (AVAILABLE SIZES)		GENERIC A-RATED AVERAGE PRICE (GAAP)	
BRAND	$0.97	100s	$81.89
GENERIC	$0.81	300s	$240.28
HCFA FUL (100s ea)	$0.23	750s	$633.68

BRAND/MANUFACTURER	NDC	SIZE	AWP
◆ BRAND			
➤ ADALAT: Miles Pharm	00026-8821-51	100s	$83.70
➤ PROCARDIA: Pfizer Labs	00069-2610-66	100s	$104.83
➤ ADALAT: Miles Pharm	00026-8821-48	100s ud	$93.28
➤ PROCARDIA: Pfizer Labs	00069-2610-41	100s ud	$116.83
➤ ADALAT: Miles Pharm	00026-8821-18	300s	$246.09
➤ PROCARDIA: Pfizer Labs	00069-2610-72	300s	$308.26
◆ GENERICS			
Medirex	57480-0390-06	30s	$22.10
Caraco	57664-0873-08	100s	$59.90
Chase	54429-3453-01	100s	$71.00
Qualitest	00603-4760-21	100s	$71.00
Geneva	00781-2506-01	100s	$78.85
Rugby	00536-4067-01	100s	$80.00
Schein	00364-2377-01	100s	$80.00
Goldline	00182-1548-01	100s	$80.00
Warner Chilcott	00047-0079-24	100s	$80.00
Aligen	00405-4697-01	100s	$80.04
Purepac	00228-2530-10	100s	$80.04
URL	00677-1399-01	100s	$80.13
URL	00677-1434-01	100s	$80.13
Moore,H.L.	00839-7565-06	100s	$80.18
Moore,H.L.	00839-7717-06	100s	$80.18
Lemmon	00093-0521-01	100s	$80.75
Caremark	00339-5718-12	100s	$81.15
Major	00904-0408-60	100s	$84.90
Parmed	00349-8874-01	100s	$86.50
Novopharm	55953-0045-40	100s	$96.15
Martec	52555-0429-01	100s	$99.65
Balan,J.J.	00304-2295-01	100s	$111.98
Raway	00686-0665-20	100s ud	$60.20
U.S. Trading	56126-0453-11	100s ud	$77.70

BRAND/MANUFACTURER	NDC	SIZE	AWP
Goldline	00182-1548-89	100s ud	$80.00
Major	00904-0408-61	100s ud	$81.65
Schein	00364-2377-90	100s ud	$84.00
Vangard	00615-0359-13	100s ud	$84.49
UDL	51079-0665-20	100s ud	$84.80
Medirex	57480-0390-01	100s ud	$99.50
Caraco	57664-0873-11	300s	$167.15
Schein	00364-2377-29	300s	$235.00
URL	00677-1399-61	300s	$236.00
Goldline	00182-1548-96	300s	$236.00
Moore,H.L.	00839-7565-13	300s	$236.10
Rugby	00536-4067-03	300s	$236.14
Major	00904-0408-72	300s	$239.85
Aligen	00405-4697-09	300s	$242.57
Purepac	00228-2530-30	300s	$242.57
Parmed	00349-8874-03	300s	$245.50
Balan,J.J.	00304-2295-03	300s	$279.98
Novopharm	55953-0045-60	300s	$286.54
Glasgow	60809-0301-55	750s ud	$633.68
Glasgow	60809-0301-72	750s ud	$633.68
Caraco	57664-0873-18	1000s	$514.75

TABLET, EXTENDED RELEASE: 30 MG

BRAND/MANUFACTURER	NDC	SIZE	AWP
○ BRAND			
➤ ADALAT CC: Miles Pharm	00026-8841-51	100s	$84.10
➤ PROCARDIA XL: Pfizer Labs	00069-2650-66	100s	$118.45
➤ ADALAT CC: Miles Pharm	00026-8841-48	100s ud	$88.31
➤ PROCARDIA XL: Pfizer Labs	00069-2650-41	100s ud	$131.95
	00069-2650-72	300s	$348.21
	00069-2650-94	5000s	$5803.64

TABLET, EXTENDED RELEASE: 60 MG

BRAND/MANUFACTURER	NDC	SIZE	AWP
○ BRAND			
➤ ADALAT CC: Miles Pharm	00026-8851-51	100s	$145.50
➤ PROCARDIA XL: Pfizer Labs	00069-2660-66	100s	$204.95
➤ ADALAT CC: Miles Pharm	00026-8851-48	100s ud	$152.78
➤ PROCARDIA XL: Pfizer Labs	00069-2660-41	100s ud	$228.39
	00069-2660-72	300s	$602.55
	00069-0266-94	5000s	$10042.46

TABLET, EXTENDED RELEASE: 90 MG

BRAND/MANUFACTURER	NDC	SIZE	AWP
○ BRAND			
➤ ADALAT CC: Miles Pharm	00026-8861-51	100s	$178.23
➤ PROCARDIA XL: Pfizer Labs	00069-2670-66	100s	$245.94
➤ ADALAT CC: Miles Pharm	00026-8861-48	100s ud	$187.14
➤ PROCARDIA XL: Pfizer Labs	00069-2670-41	100s ud	$273.98

Niferex Forte SEE FOLIC ACID/POLYSACCHARIDE-IRON COMPLEX/VITAMIN B$_{12}$

Nimodipine

DESCRIPTION

Nimodipine belongs to the class of pharmacological agents known as calcium channel blockers. Nimodipine is isopropyl (2-methoxyethyl)1,4-dihydro-2,6-dimethyl-4-(3-nitrophenyl)-3,5-pyridine- dicarboxylate. It has a molecular weight of 418.5 and a molecular formula of $C_{21}H_{26}N_2O_7$.

Nimodipine is a yellow crystalline substance, practically insoluble in water.

Following is its chemical structure:

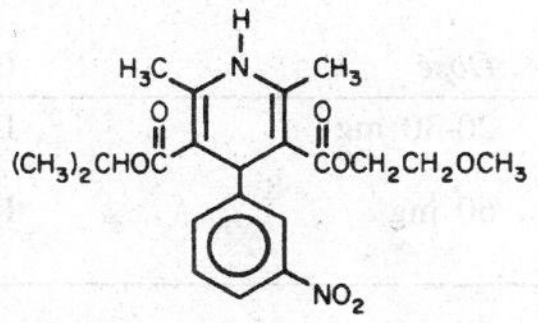

CLINICAL PHARMACOLOGY

Mechanism of Action: Nimodipine is a calcium channel blocker. The contractile processes of smooth muscle cells are dependent upon calcium ions, which enter these cells during depolarization as slow ionic transmembrane currents. Nimodipine inhibits calcium ion transfer into these cells and thus inhibits contractions of vascular smooth muscle. In animal experiments, Nimodipine had a greater effect on cerebral arteries than on arteries elsewhere in the body perhaps because it is highly lipophilic, allowing it to cross the blood-brain barrier; concentrations of Nimodipine as high as 12.5 ng/mL have been detected in the cerebrospinal fluid of Nimodipine treated subarachnoid hemorrhage (SAH) patients.

➤ SHOWN IN PRODUCT IDENTIFICATION GUIDE

Based on animal experiments, it was hoped that Nimodipine would prevent cerebral arterial spasm in SAH patients. While the clinical studies described below demonstrate a favorable effect by Nimodipine on the severity of neurological deficits caused by cerebral vasospasm following SAH, there is no arteriographic evidence that the drug either prevents or relieves the spasm of these arteries. The actual mechanism of action in humans is, therefore, unknown.

Pharmacokinetics and Metabolism: In man, Nimodipine is rapidly absorbed after oral administration, and peak concentrations are generally attained within one hour. The terminal elimination half-life is approximately 8 to 9 hours but earlier elimination rates are much more rapid, equivalent to a half-life of 1-2 hours; a consequence is the need for frequent (every 4 hours) dosing. There were no signs of accumulation when Nimodipine was given three times a day for seven days. Nimodipine is over 95% bound to plasma proteins. The binding was concentration independent over the range of 10 ng/mL to 10 µg/mL. Nimodipine is eliminated almost exclusively in the form of metabolites and less than 1% is recovered in the urine as unchanged drug. Numerous metabolites, all of which are either inactive or considerably less active than the parent compound, have been identified. Because of a high first-pass metabolism, the bioavailability of Nimodipine averages 13% after oral administration. The bioavailability is significantly increased in patients with hepatic cirrhosis, with C_{max} approximately double that in normals which necessitates lowering the dose in this group of patients (see *"Dosage and Administration"*). In a study of 24 healthy male volunteers, administration of Nimodipine capsules following a standard breakfast resulted in a 68% lower peak plasma concentration and 38% lower bioavailability relative to dosing under fasted conditions.

Clinical Trials: Nimodipine has been shown, in 4 randomized, placebo-controlled trials, to reduce the severity of neurological deficits resulting from vasospasm in patients who have had a recent subarachnoid hemorrhage (SAH). The trials used doses ranging from 20-30 mg to 90 mg every 4 hours, with drug given for 21 days in 3 studies, and for at least 18 days in the other. Three of the four trials followed patients for 3-6 months. Three of the trials studied relatively well patients, with all or most patients in Hunt and Hess Grades I-II (essentially free of focal deficits after the initial bleed); the fourth studied much sicker patients, Hunt and Hess Grades III-V. Two studies, one domestic, one French, were similar in design, with relatively unimpaired SAH patients randomized to Nimodipine or placebo. In each, a judgment was made as to whether any late-developing deficit was due to spasm or other causes, and the deficits were graded. Both studies showed significantly fewer severe deficits due to spasm in the Nimodipine group; the second (French) study showed fewer spasm-related deficits of all severities. No effect was seen on deficits not related to spasm. (See related table).

A Canadian study entered much sicker patients, who had a high rate of death and disability, and used a dose of 90 mg every 4 hours, but was otherwise similar to the first two studies. Analysis of delayed ischemic deficits, many of which result from spasm, showed a significant reduction in spasm-related deficits. Among analyzed patients (72 Nimodipine, 82 placebo), there were the following outcomes. (See related table).

A fourth, large, study was performed in the United Kingdom in SAH patients with all grades of severity (but about 90% were in Grades I-III). Outcomes were not defined as spasm related or not but there was a significant reduction in the overall rate of infarction and severely disabling neurological outcome at 3 months:

	Nimodipine	Placebo
Total patients	278	276
Good recovery	199*	169
Moderate disability	24	16
Severe disability	12**	31
Death	43***	60

* *p = 0.0444—good and moderate vs severe and dead*
** *p = 0.001—severe disability*
*** *p = 0.056—death*

A dose-ranging study comparing 30, 60 and 90 mg doses found a generally low rate of spasm-related neurological deficits but no significant relation of response to dose.

The effect of Nimodipine on mortality is not yet clear. The large United Kingdom study showed near-significantly improved survival. The two smaller studies (domestic, French) had too few deaths to contribute to this question. The Canadian study, despite showing markedly decreased spasm-related deficits, showed overall (all patients randomized) greater 90 day mortality, 49/91 (54%) on Nimodipine vs 38/97 (39%) on placebo, a significant difference. Most of the deaths appeared, in this very severely ill group (Hunt and Hess Grades III-V), to be consequences of SAH, but a drug effect cannot be ruled out. In this study 90 mg every 4 hours was the dose used, perhaps too high for the very ill population studied. The 90 mg dose is not recommended nor is treatment of Hunt and Hess Grades IV-V patients.

INDICATIONS AND USAGE

Nimodipine is indicated for the improvement of neurological outcome by reducing the incidence and severity of ischemic deficits in patients with subarachnoid hemorrhage from ruptured congenital aneurysms who are in good neurological condition post-ictus (e.g., Hunt and Hess Grades I-III).

UNLABELED USES
Nimodipine is used alone or as an adjunct in the prophylaxis of common migraine headache and cluster headache, and in the treatment of hypertension. It is also used in acute ischemic stroke, senile dementia, and organic brain syndrome.

CONTRAINDICATIONS
None known.

PRECAUTIONS
General: Blood Pressure: Nimodipine has the hemodynamic effects expected of a calcium channel blocker, although they are generally not marked. In patients with subarachnoid hemorrhage given Nimodipine in clinical studies, about 5% were reported to have had lowering of the blood pressure and about 1% left the study because of this (not all could be attributed to Nimodipine). Nevertheless, blood pressure should be carefully monitored during treatment with Nimodipine based on its known pharmacology and the known effects of calcium channel blockers.

Hepatic Disease: The metabolism of Nimodipine is decreased in patients with impaired hepatic function. Such patients should have their blood pressure and pulse rate monitored closely and should be given a lower dose (see *"Dosage and Administration"*).

Intestinal pseudo-obstruction and ileus have been reported rarely in patients treated with Nimodipine. A causal relationship has not been established. The condition has responded to conservative management.

Laboratory Test Interactions: None known.

Drug Interaction: It is possible that the cardiovascular action of other calcium channel blockers could be enhanced by the addition of Nimodipine.

In Europe Nimodipine was observed to occasionally intensify the effect of antihypertensive compounds taken concomitantly by patients suffering from hypertension; this phenomenon was not observed in North American clinical trials.

A study in eight healthy volunteers has shown a 50% increase in mean peak Nimodipine plasma concentrations and a 90% increase in mean area under the curve, after a one-week course of cimetidine at 1,000 mg/day and Nimodipine at 90 mg/day. This effect may be mediated by the known inhibition of hepatic cytochrome P-450 by cimetidine, which could decrease first-pass metabolism of Nimodipine.

Carcinogenesis, Mutagenesis, Impairment of Fertility: In a two-year study, higher incidences of adenocarcinoma of the uterus and Leydig-cell adenoma of the testes were observed in rats given a diet containing 1800 ppm Nimodipine (equivalent to 91 to 121 mg/kg/day Nimodipine) than in placebo controls. The differences were not statistically significant, however, and the higher rates were well within historical control range for these tumors in the Wistar strain. Nimodipine was

Study	Dose	Grade*	Number Analyzed	Any Deficit Due to Spasm	Numbers With Severe Deficit
1.	20-30 mg	I-III	Nimodipine 56	13	1
			Placebo 60	16	8**
2.	60 mg	I-III	Nimodipine 31	4	2
			Placebo 39	11	10**

* *Hunt and Hess Grade*
** *p = 0.03*

	Delayed Ischemic Deficits (DID)		Permanent Deficits	
	Nimodipine n (%)	Placebo n (%)	Nimodipine n (%)	Placebo n (%)
DID Spasm Alone	8 (11)*	25 (31)	5 (7)*	22 (27)
DID Spasm Contributing	18 (25)	21 (26)	16 (22)	17 (21)
DID Without Spasm	7 (10)	8 (10)	6 (8)	7 (9)
No DID	39 (54)	28 (34)	45 (63)	36 (44)

* *P = 0.001, Nimodipine vs placebo*

DOSE Q4H

Sign/Symptom	Number of Patients (%)					
	Nimodipine					Placebo
	0.35 mg/kg (n = 82)	30 mg (n = 71)	60 mg (n = 494)	90 mg (n = 172)	120 mg (n = 4)	(n = 479)
Decreased Blood Pressure	1 (1.2)	0	19 (3.8)	14 (8.1)	2 (5.0)	6 (1.2)
Abnormal Liver Function Test	1 (1.2)	0	2 (0.4)	1 (0.6)	0	7 (1.5)
Edema	0	0	2 (0.4)	2 (1.2)	0	3 (0.6)
Diarrhea	0	3 (4.2)	0	3 (1.7)	0	3 (0.6)
Rash	2 (2.4)	0	3 (0.6)	2 (1.2)	0	3 (0.6)
Headache	0	1 (1.4)	6 (1.2)	0	0	1 (0.2)
Gastrointestinal Symptoms	2 (2.4)	0	0	2 (1.2)	0	0
Nausea	1 (1.2)	1 (1.4)	6 (1.2)	1 (0.6)	0	0
Dyspnea	1 (1.2)	0	0	0	0	0
EKG Abnormalities	0	1 (1.4)	0	1 (0.6)	0	0
Tachycardia	0	1 (1.4)	0	0	0	0
Bradycardia	0	0	5 (1.0)	1 (0.6)	0	0
Muscle Pain/Cramp	0	1 (1.4)	1 (0.2)	1 (0.6)	0	0
Acne	0	1 (1.4)	0	0	0	0
Depression	0	1 (1.4)	0	0	0	0

found not to be carcinogenic in a 91-week mouse study but the high dose of 1800 ppm Nimodipine-in-feed (546 to 774 mg/kg/day) shortened the life expectancy of the animals. Mutagenicity studies, including the Ames, micronucleus and dominant lethal tests were negative.

Nimodipine did not impair the fertility and general reproductive performance of male and female Wistar rats following oral doses of up to 30 mg/kg/day when administered daily for more than 10 weeks in the males and 3 weeks in the females prior to mating and continued to day 7 of pregnancy. This dose in a rat is about 4 times the equivalent clinical dose of 60 mg q4h in a 50 kg patient.

Pregnancy: Pregnancy Category C. Nimodipine has been shown to have a teratogenic effect in Himalayan rabbits. Incidences of malformations and stunted fetuses were increased at oral doses of 1 and 10 mg/kg/day administered (by gavage) from day 6 through day 18 of pregnancy but not at 3.0 mg/kg/day in one of two identical rabbit studies. In the second study an increased incidence of stunted fetuses was seen at 1.0 mg/kg/day but not at higher doses. Nimodipine was embryotoxic, causing resorption and stunted growth of fetuses, in Long Evans rats at 100 mg/kg/day administered by gavage from day 6 through day 15 of pregnancy. In two other rat studies, doses of 30 mg/kg/day Nimodipine administered by gavage from day 16 of gestation and continued until sacrifice (day 20) of pregnancy or day 21 post partum) were associated with higher incidences of skeletal variation, stunted fetuses and stillbirths but no malformations. There are no adequate and well controlled studies in pregnant women to directly assess the effect on human fetuses. Nimodipine should be used during pregnancy only if the potential benefit justifies the potential risk to the fetus.

Nursing Mothers: Nimodipine and/or its metabolites have been shown to appear in rat milk at concentrations much higher than in maternal plasma. It is not known whether the drug is excreted in human milk. Because many drugs are excreted in human milk, nursing mothers are advised not to breast feed their babies when taking the drug.

Pediatric Use: Safety and effectiveness in children have not been established.

ADVERSE REACTIONS

Adverse experiences were reported by 92 of 823 patients with subarachnoid hemorrhage (11.2%) who were given Nimodipine. The most frequently reported adverse experience was decreased blood pressure in 4.4% of these patients. Twenty-nine of 479 (6.1%) placebo treated patients also reported adverse experiences. The events reported with a frequency greater than 1% are displayed below by dose. (See related table).

There were no other adverse experiences reported by the patients who were given 0.35 mg/kg q4h, 30 mg q4h or 120 mg q4h. Adverse experiences with an incidence rate of less than 1% in the 60 mg q4h dose group were: hepatitis; itching; gastrointestinal hemorrhage; thrombocytopenia; anemia; palpitations; vomiting; flushing; diaphoresis; wheezing; phenytoin toxicity; light-headedness; dizziness; rebound vasospasm; jaundice; hypertension; hematoma.

Adverse experiences with an incidence rate less than 1% in the 90 mg q4h dose group were: itching, gastrointestinal hemorrhage; thrombocytopenia; neurological deterioration; vomiting; diaphoresis; congestive heart failure; hyponatremia; decreasing platelet count; disseminated intravascular coagulation; deep vein thrombosis.

As can be seen from the table, side effects that appear related to Nimodipine use based on increased incidence with higher dose or a higher rate compared to placebo control, included decreased blood pressure, edema and headaches which are known pharmacologic actions of calcium channel blockers. It must be noted, however, that SAH is frequently accompanied by alterations in consciousness which lead to an under reporting of adverse experiences. Patients who received Nimodipine in clinical trials for other indications reported flushing (2.1%), headache (4.1%) and fluid retention (0.3%), typical responses to calcium channel blockers. As a calcium channel blocker, Nimodipine may have the potential to exacerbate heart failure in susceptible patients or to interfere with A-V conduction, but these events were not observed. No clinically significant effects on hematologic factors, renal or hepatic function or carbohydrate metabolism have been causally associated with oral Nimodipine. Isolated cases of non-fasting elevated serum glucose levels (0.8%), elevated LDH levels (0.4%), decreased platelet counts (0.3%), elevated alkaline phosphatase levels (0.2%) and elevated SGPT levels (0.2%) have been reported rarely.

DRUG ABUSE AND DEPENDENCE

There have been no reported instances of drug abuse or dependence with Nimodipine.

OVERDOSAGE

There have been no reports of overdosage from the oral administration of Nimodipine. Symptoms of overdosage would be expected to be related to cardiovascular effects such as excessive peripheral vasodilation with marked systemic hypotension. Clinically significant hypotension due to Nimodipine overdosage may require active cardiovascular support. Norepinephrine or dopamine may be helpful in restoring blood pressure. Since Nimodipine is highly protein-bound, dialysis is not likely to be of benefit.

DOSAGE AND ADMINISTRATION

Nimodipine is given orally in the form of ivory colored, soft gelatin 30 mg capsules for subarachnoid hemorrhage.

The oral dose is 60 mg (two 30 mg capsules) every 4 hours for 21 consecutive days, preferably not less than one hour before or two hours after meals. Oral Nimodipine therapy should commence within 96 hours of the subarachnoid hemorrhage. If the capsule cannot be swallowed, e.g., at the time of surgery, or if the patient is unconscious, a hole should be made in both ends of the capsule with an 18 gauge needle, and the contents of the capsule extracted into a syringe. The contents should then be emptied into the patient's *in situ* naso-gastric tube and washed down the tube with 30 mL of normal saline (0.9%).

Patients with hepatic cirrhosis have substantially reduced clearance and approximately doubled C_{max}. Dosage should be reduced to 30 mg every 4 hours, with close monitoring of blood pressure and heart rate.

The capsules should be stored in the manufacturer's original foil package at a controlled room temperature of 59°F to 86°F (15°C to 30°C).

Capsules should be protected from light and freezing.

HOW SUPPLIED
CAPSULE: 30 MG

BRAND/MANUFACTURER	NDC	SIZE	AWP
○ **BRAND**			
NIMOTOP: Miles Pharm	00026-2855-48	100s ud	$500.84

Nimotop *SEE* NIMODIPINE

Nipent *SEE* PENTOSTATIN

Nitro-Bid *SEE* NITROGLYCERIN

Nitro-Dur *SEE* NITROGLYCERIN

Nitrodisc *SEE* NITROGLYCERIN

Nitrofurantoin

DESCRIPTION

Nitrofurantoin, a synthetic chemical, is a stable, yellow, crystalline compound. Nitrofurantoin is an antibacterial agent for specific urinary tract infections. The chemical name is Nitrofurantoin is available as an oral suspension and as capsules containing larger crystals of controlled size.

Each ml of suspension contains:
Nitrofurantoin ....5 mg

Each capsule contains:
Nitrofurantoin ....25, 50, or 100 mg

The chemical name is 1-[[(5-nitro-2-furanyl)methylene]amino]-2, 4-imidazolidi-nedione. The molecular weight is 238.16.

Following is its chemical structure:

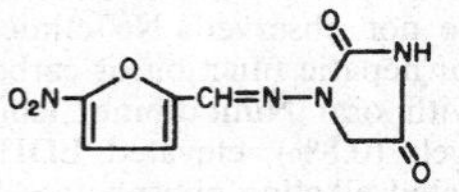

CLINICAL PHARMACOLOGY

Orally administered Nitrofurantoin is readily absorbed and rapidly excreted in urine. Absorption of the capsules is slower, with somewhat less excretion. Blood concentrations at therapeutic dosage are usually low. It is highly soluble in urine, to which it may impart a brown color.

Following a dose regimen of 100 mg q.i.d. for 7 days, average urinary drug recoveries (0-24 hours) on day 1 and day 7 were 42.7% and 43.6% for the oral suspension, 37.9% and 35.0% for the capsules.

One capsule formulation contains two forms of Nitrofurantoin. Twenty-five percent is macrocrystalline Nitrofurantoin, which has slower dissolution and absorption than Nitrofurantoin monohydrate. The remaining 75% is Nitrofurantoin monohydrate contained in a powder blend which, upon exposure to gastric and intestinal fluids, forms a gel matrix that releases Nitrofurantoin over time. Based on urinary pharmacokinetic data, the extent and rate of urinary excretion of Nitrofurantoin from the 100-mg Nitrofurantoin/Nitrofurantoin monohydrate capsule are similar to those of the 50-mg or 100-mg Nitrofurantoin capsule. Approximately 20-25% of a single dose of Nitrofurantoin is recovered from the urine unchanged over 24 hours.

Unlike many drugs, the presence of food or agents delaying gastric emptying can increase the bioavailability of Nitrofurantoin, presumably by allowing better dissolution in gastric juices.

Microbiology: Nitrofurantoin is bactericidal in urine at therapeutic doses. The mechanism of the antimicrobial action of Nitrofurantoin is unusual among antibacterials. Nitrofurantoin is reduced by bacterial flavoproteins to reactive intermediates which inactivate or alter bacterial ribosomal proteins and other macromolecules. As a result of such inactivations, the vital biochemical processes of protein synthesis, aerobic energy metabolism, DNA synthesis, RNA synthesis, and cell wall synthesis are inhibited. The broad-based nature of this mode of action may explain the lack of acquired bacterial resistance to Nitrofurantoin, as the necessary multiple and simultaneous mutations of the target macromolecules would likely be lethal to the bacteria. Development of resistance to Nitrofurantoin has not been a significant problem since its introduction in 1953. Cross-resistance with antibiotics and sulfonamides has not been observed, and transferable resistance is, at most, a very rare phenomenon.

Nitrofurantoin has been shown to be active against most strains of the following bacteria both *in vitro* and in clinical infections: (see *"Indications and Usage."*)

GRAM-POSITIVE AEROBES
Staphylococcus aureus (Nitrofurantoin suspension, Nitrofurantoin capsules)
Enterococci (e.g., *Enterococcus faecalis*) (Nitrofurantoin suspension, Nitrofurantoin capsules)
Staphylococcus saprophyticus (Nitrofurantoin/Nitrofurantoin monohydrate capsules)

GRAM-NEGATIVE AEROBES
Escherichia coli
NOTE: Some strains of *Enterobacter* species and *Klebsiella* species are resistant to Nitrofurantoin.

Nitrofurantoin also demonstrates *in vitro* activity against the following microorganisms, although the clinical significance of these data with respect to treatment with Nitrofurantoin is unknown:

GRAM-POSITIVE AEROBES
Coagulase-negative staphylococci (including *Staphylococcus epidermidis* and *Staphylococcus saprophyticus* Nitrofurantoin suspension, Nitrofurantoin capsules; including Staphylococcus epidermidis—Nitrofurantoin/Nitrofurantoin monohydrate capsules)
Streptococcus agalactiae
Enterococcus faecalis (Nitrofurantoin/Nitrofurantoin monohydrate capsules)
Staphylococcus aureus (Nitrofurantoin/Nitrofurantoin monohydrate capsules)
Group D streptococci
Viridans group streptococci

GRAM-NEGATIVE AEROBES
Citrobacter amalonaticus
Citrobacter diversus
Citrobacter freundi
Klebsiella oxytoca
Klebsiella ozaenae

Nitrofurantoin is not active against most strains of *Proteus* species or *Serratia* species. It has no activity against *Pseudomonas* species.

Antagonism has been demonstrated *in vitro* between Nitrofurantoin and quinolone antimicrobial agents. The clinical significance of this finding is unknown.

SUSCEPTIBILITY TESTS
Diffusion Techniques: Quantitative methods that require measurement of zone diameters give the most precise estimate of the susceptibility of bacteria to antimicrobial agents. One such standard procedure,[1] which has been recommended for use with disks to test susceptibility of organisms to Nitrofurantoin, uses the 300-mcg Nitrofurantoin disk. Interpretation involves the correlation of the diameter obtained in the disk test with the minimum inhibitory concentration (MIC) for Nitrofurantoin.

Reports from the laboratory giving results of the standard single-disk susceptibility test with a 300-mcg Nitrofurantoin disk should be interpreted according to the following criteria:

Zone Diameter (mm)	Interpretation
≥ 17	Susceptible
15-16	Intermediate
≤ 14	Resistant

A report of "susceptible" indicates that the pathogen is likely to be inhibited by generally achievable urinary levels. A report of "intermediate" indicates that the result be considered equivocal and, if the organism is not fully susceptible to alternative clinically feasible drugs, the test should be repeated. This category provides a buffer zone which prevents small uncontrolled technical factors from causing major discrepancies in interpretations. A report of "resistant" indicates that achievable concentrations are unlikely to be inhibitory, and other therapy should be selected.

Standardized procedures require the use of laboratory control organisms. The 300-mcg Nitrofurantoin disk should give the following zone diameters:

Organism	Zone Diameter (mm)
E. coli ATCC 25922	20-25
S. aureus ATCC 25923	18-22

Dilution Techniques: Use a standardized dilution method[2] (broth, agar, microdilution) or equivalent with Nitrofurantoin powder. The MIC values obtained should be interpreted according to the following criteria:

MIC (mcg/mL)	Interpretation
≤ 32	Susceptible
64	Intermediate
≥ 128	Resistant

As with standard diffusion techniques, dilution methods require the use of laboratory control organisms. Standard Nitrofurantoin powder-should provide the following MIC values:

Organism	MIC (mcg/mL)
E. coli ATCC 25922	4-16
S. aureus ATCC 29213	8-32
E. faecalis ATCC 29212	4-16

INDICATIONS AND USAGE
Nitrofurantoin suspension and Nitrofurantoin capsules are specifically indicated for the treatment of urinary tract infections when due to susceptible strains of *Escherichia coli*, enterococci, *Staphylococcus aureus*, and certain susceptible strains of *Klebsiella* and *Enterobacter* species. Nitrofurantoin/Nitrofurantoin monohydrate capsules are indicated only for the treatment of acute uncomplicated urinary tract infections (acute cystitis) caused by susceptible strains of *Escherichia coli* or *Staphylococcus saprophyticus*.

Nitrofurantoin is not indicated for the treatment of pyelonephritis or perinephric abscesses.

◆ RATED THERAPEUTICALLY EQUIVALENT; ◇ THERAPEUTIC EQUIVALENCE UNCONFIRMED; ○ UNRATED

Nitrofurantoins lack the broader tissue distribution of other therapeutic agents approved for urinary tract infections. Consequently, many patients who are treated with Nitrofurantoin are predisposed to persistence or reappearance of bacteriuria. Urine specimens for culture and susceptibility testing should be obtained before and after completion of therapy. If persistence or reappearance of bacteriuria occurs after treatment with Nitrofurantoin, other therapeutic agents with broader tissue distribution should be selected. In considering the use of Nitrofurantoin, lower eradication rates should be balanced against the increased potential for systemic toxicity and for the development of antimicrobial resistance when agents with broader tissue distribution are utilized.

CONTRAINDICATIONS

Anuria, oliguria, or significant impairment of renal function (creatinine clearance under 60 mL per minute or clinically significant elevated serum creatinine) are contraindications. Treatment of this type of patient carries an increased risk of toxicity because of impaired excretion of the drug.

Because of the possibility of hemolytic anemia due to immature erythrocyte enzyme systems (glutathione instability), the drug is contraindicated, in pregnant patients at term (38-42 weeks gestation), during labor and delivery, or when the onset of labor is imminent. For the same reason, the drug is contraindicated in neonates under one month of age.

Nitrofurantoin is also contraindicated in those patients with known hypersensitivity to it.

WARNINGS

ACUTE, SUBACUTE, OR CHRONIC PULMONARY REACTIONS HAVE BEEN OBSERVED IN PATIENTS TREATED WITH NITROFURANTOIN. IF THESE REACTIONS OCCUR, NITROFURANTOIN SHOULD BE DISCONTINUED AND APPROPRIATE MEASURES TAKEN. REPORTS HAVE CITED PULMONARY REACTIONS AS A CONTRIBUTING CAUSE OF DEATH.

CHRONIC PULMONARY REACTIONS (DIFFUSE INTERSTITIAL PNEUMONITIS OR PULMONARY FIBROSIS, OR BOTH) CAN DEVELOP INSIDIOUSLY. THESE REACTIONS OCCUR RARELY AND GENERALLY IN PATIENTS RECEIVING THERAPY FOR SIX MONTHS OR LONGER. CLOSE MONITORING OF THE PULMONARY CONDITION OF PATIENTS RECEIVING LONG-TERM THERAPY IS WARRANTED AND REQUIRES THAT THE BENEFITS OF THERAPY BE WEIGHED AGAINST POTENTIAL RISKS. (SEE "RESPIRATORY REACTIONS".)

Hepatic reactions, including hepatitis, cholestatic jaundice, chronic active hepatitis, and hepatic necrosis, occur rarely. Fatalities have been reported. The onset of chronic active hepatitis may be insidious, and patients should be monitored periodically for changes in liver function. If hepatitis occurs, the drug should be withdrawn immediately and appropriate measures should be taken.

Peripheral neuropathy (including optic neuritis), which may become severe or irreversible, has occurred. Fatalities have been reported. Conditions such as renal impairment (creatinine clearance under 60 mL per minute or clinically significant elevated serum creatinine), anemia, diabetes mellitus, electrolyte imbalance, vitamin B deficiency, and debilitating disease may enhance the occurrence of peripheral neuropathy. Patients receiving long-term therapy should be monitored periodically for changes in renal function.

Cases of hemolytic anemia of the primaquine-sensitivity type have been induced by Nitrofurantoin. Hemolysis appears to be linked to a glucose-6-phosphate dehydrogenase deficiency in the red blood cells of the affected patients. This deficiency is found in 10 percent of Blacks and a small percentage of ethnic groups of Mediterranean and Near-Eastern origin. Hemolysis is an indication for discontinuing Nitrofurantoin; hemolysis ceases when the drug is withdrawn.

PRECAUTIONS

Information for Patients: Patients should be advised to take Nitrofurantoin with food (ideally breakfast and dinner) to further enhance tolerance and improve drug absorption. Patients should be instructed to complete the full course of therapy; however, they should be advised to contact their physician if any unusual symptoms occur during therapy.

Many patients who cannot tolerate small crystal Nitrofurantoin are able to take large crystal Nitrofurantoin without nausea.

Patients should be advised not to use antacid preparations containing magnesium trisilicate while taking Nitrofurantoin.

Drug Interactions: Antacids containing magnesium trisilicate, when administered concomitantly with Nitrofurantoin, reduce both the rate and extent of absorption. The mechanism for this interaction probably is absorption of Nitrofurantoin onto the surface of magnesium trisilicate.

Uricosuric drugs, such as probenecid and sulfinpyrazone, can inhibit renal tubular secretion of Nitrofurantoin. The resulting increase in Nitrofurantoin serum levels may increase toxicity, and the decreased urinary levels could lessen its efficacy as a urinary tract antibacterial.

Drug/Laboratory Test Interactions: As a result of the presence of Nitrofurantoin, a false-positive reaction for glucose in the urine may occur. This has been observed with Benedict's and Fehling's solutions but not with the glucose enzymatic test.

Carcinogenesis, Mutagenesis, Impairment of Fertility: Nitrofurantoin was not carcinogenic when fed to female Holtzman rats for 44.5 weeks or to female Sprague-Dawley rats for 75 weeks. Two chronic rodent bioassays utilizing male and female Sprague-Dawley rats and two chronic bioassays in Swiss mice and in BDF_1 mice revealed no evidence of carcinogenicity.

Nitrofurantoin presented evidence of carcinogenic activity in female $B6C3F_1$ mice as shown by increased incidences of tubular adenomas, benign mixed tumors, and granulosa cell tumors of the ovary. In male F344/N rats, there were increased incidences of uncommon kidney tubular cell neoplasms, osteosarcomas of the bone, and neoplasms of the subcutaneous tissue. In one study involving subcutaneous administration of 75 mg/kg Nitrofurantoin to pregnant female mice, lung papillary adenomas of unknown significance were observed in the F1 generation.

Nitrofurantoin has been shown to induce point mutations in certain strains of *Salmonella typhimurium* and forward mutations in L5178Y mouse lymphoma cells. Nitrofurantoin induced increased numbers of sister chromatid exchanges and chromosomal aberrations in Chinese hamster ovary cells but not in human cells in culture. Results of the sex-linked recessive lethal assay in Drosophila were negative after administration of Nitrofurantoin by feeding or by injection. Nitrofurantoin did not induce heritable mutation in the rodent models examined.

The significance of the carcinogenicity and mutagenicity findings relative to the therapeutic use of Nitrofurantoin in humans is unknown.

The administration of high doses of Nitrofurantoin to rats causes temporary spermatogenic arrest; this is reversible on discontinuing the drug. Doses of 10 mg/kg/day or greater in healthy human males may, in certain unpredictable instances, produce a slight to moderate spermatogenic arrest with a decrease in sperm count.

Pregnancy: Teratogenic effects: Pregnancy Category B. Several reproduction studies have been performed in rabbits and rats at doses up to six times the human dose and have revealed no evidence of impaired fertility or harm to the fetus due to Nitrofurantoin. In a single published study conducted in mice at 68 times the human dose (based on mg/kg administered to the dam), growth retardation and a low incidence of minor and common malformations were observed. However, at 25 times the human dose, fetal malformations were not observed; the relevance of these findings to humans is uncertain. There are, however, no adequate and well-controlled studies in pregnant women. Because animal reproduction studies are not always predictive of human response, this drug should be used during pregnancy only if clearly needed.

Non-teratogenic effects: Nitrofurantoin has been shown in one published transplacental carcinogenicity study to induce lung papillary adenomas in the F1 generation mice at doses 19 times the human dose on a mg/kg basis. The relationship of this finding to potential human carcinogenesis is presently unknown. Because of the uncertainty regarding the human implications of these animal data, this drug should be used during pregnancy only if clearly needed.

Labor and Delivery: See "Contraindications".

Nursing Mothers: Nitrofurantoin has been detected in human breast milk in trace amounts. Because of the potential for serious adverse reactions from Nitrofurantoin in nursing infants under one month of age, a decision should be made whether to discontinue nursing or to discontinue the drug, taking into account the importance of the drug to the mother. (See "Contraindications".)

Pediatric Use: Nitrofurantoin is contraindicated in infants below the age of one month. (See "Contraindications".) Safety and effectiveness of Nitrofurantoin/ Nitrofurantoin monohydrate capsules in children below the age of twelve years have not been established.

ADVERSE REACTIONS

Respiratory: CHRONIC, SUBACUTE, OR ACUTE PULMONARY HYPERSENSITIVITY REACTIONS MAY OCCUR WITH THE USE OF NITROFURANTOIN.

CHRONIC PULMONARY REACTIONS OCCUR GENERALLY IN PATIENTS WHO HAVE RECEIVED CONTINUOUS TREATMENT FOR SIX MONTHS OR LONGER. MALAISE, DYSPNEA ON EXERTION, COUGH, AND ALTERED PULMONARY FUNCTION ARE COMMON MANIFESTATIONS WHICH CAN OCCUR INSIDIOUSLY. RADIOLOGIC AND HISTOLOGIC FINDINGS OF DIFFUSE INTERSTITIAL PNEUMONITIS OR FIBROSIS, OR BOTH, ARE ALSO COMMON MANIFESTATIONS OF THE CHRONIC PULMONARY REACTION. FEVER IS RARELY PROMINENT.

THE SEVERITY OF CHRONIC PULMONARY REACTIONS AND THEIR DEGREE OF RESOLUTION APPEAR TO BE RELATED TO THE DURATION OF THERAPY AFTER THE FIRST CLINICAL SIGNS APPEAR. PULMONARY FUNCTION MAY BE IMPAIRED PERMANENTLY, EVEN AFTER CESSATION OF THERAPY. THE RISK IS GREATER WHEN CHRONIC PULMONARY REACTIONS ARE NOT RECOGNIZED EARLY.

In subacute pulmonary reactions, fever and eosinophilia occur less often than in the acute form. Upon cessation of therapy, recovery may require several months. If the symptoms are not recognized as being drug-related and Nitrofurantoin therapy is not stopped, the symptoms may become more severe.

Acute pulmonary reactions are commonly manifested by fever, chills, cough, chest pain, dyspnea, pulmonary infiltration with consolidation or pleural effusion on x-ray, and eosinophilia. Acute reactions usually occur within the first week of treatment and are reversible with cessation of therapy. Resolution often is dramatic. (See "Warnings".)

Changes in EKG may occur associated with pulmonary reactions.

Collapse and cyanosis have seldom been reported.

Hepatic: Hepatic reactions, including hepatitis, cholestatic jaundice, chronic active hepatitis, and hepatic necrosis, occur rarely. (See "Warnings".)

Neurologic: Peripheral neuropathy (including optic neuritis), which may become severe or irreversible, has occurred. Fatalities have been reported. Conditions such as renal impairment (creatinine clearance under 60 mL per minute or clinically significant elevated serum creatinine), anemia, diabetes mellitus, electrolyte imbalance, vitamin B deficiency, and debilitating diseases may increase the possibility of peripheral neuropathy. (See "Warnings".)

Asthenia, vertigo, nystagmus, dizziness, headache, and drowsiness have also been reported with the use of Nitrofurantoin.

Benign intracranial hypertension has seldom been reported.

Confusion, depression, euphoria, and psychotic reactions have been reported rarely.

Dermatologic: Exfoliative dermatitis and erythema multiforme (including Stevens-Johnson syndrome) have been reported rarely. Transient alopecia also has been reported.

Allergic: A lupus-like syndrome associated with pulmonary reactions to Nitrofurantoin has been reported. Also, angioedema; maculopapular, erythematous, or eczematous eruptions; pruritus; urticaria; anaphylaxis; arthralgia; myalgia; drug fever; and chills have been reported.

Gastrointestinal: Nausea, emesis, and anorexia occur most often. Abdominal pain and diarrhea are less common gastrointestinal reactions. These dose-related reactions can be minimized by reduction of dosage. Sialadenitis and pancreatitis have been reported.

Miscellaneous: As with other antimicrobial agents, superinfections by resistant organisms, *e.g.,* Pseudomonas or Candida species, may occur. However, these are limited to the genitourinary tract because suppression of normal bacterial flora does not occur elsewhere in the body.

In clinical trials of Nitrofurantoin/Nitrofurantoin monohydrate capsules the most frequent clinical adverse events that were reported as possibly or probably drug-related were nausea (8%), headache (6%), and flatulence (1.5%). Additional clinical adverse events reported as possibly or probably drug related occurred in less than 1% of patients studied and are listed below within each body system in order of decreasing frequency:

Gastrointestinal: Diarrhea, dyspepsia, abdominal pain, constipation, emesis
Neurologic: Dizziness, drowsiness, amblyopia
Respiratory: Acute pulmonary hypersensitivity reaction (see *"Warnings"*)
Allergic: Pruritus, urticaria
Dermatologic: Alopecia
Miscellaneous: Fever, chills, malaise.

Laboratory Adverse Events: The following laboratory adverse events have been reported with the use of Nitrofurantoin: increased AST (SGOT), increased ALT (SGPT), decreased hemoglobin, increased serum phosphrus, eosinophilia, glucose-6-phosphate dehydrodenase deficiency anemia (see *"Warnings"*), agranulocytosis, leukopenia, granulocytopenia, hemolytic anemia, thrombocytopenia, megaloblastic anemia. In most cases, these hematologic abnormalities resolved following cessation of therapy. Aplastic anemia has been reported rarely.

OVERDOSAGE

Occasional incidents of acute overdosage of Nitrofurantoin have not resulted in any specific symptoms other than vomiting. Induction of emesis is recommended. There is no specific antidote, but a high fluid intake should be maintained to promote urinary excretion of the drug. It is dialyzable.

DOSAGE AND ADMINISTRATION

Nitrogurantoin should be given with food to improve drug absorption and, in some patients, tolerance.

NITROFURANTOIN SUSPENSION, NITROFURANTOIN CAPSULES
Adults: 50-100 mg four times a day — the lower dosage level is recommended for uncomplicated urinary tract infections.

Children: 5-7 mg/kg of body weight per 24 hours, given in four divided doses (contraindicated under one month of age).

The following table is based on an average weight in each range receiving 5 to 6 mg/kg of body weight per 24 hours, given in four divided doses. It can be used to calculate an average dose of Nitrofurantoin Oral Suspension (5 mg/mL) for children (one 5-mL teaspoon or Nitrofurantoin Oral Suspension contains 25 mg of Nitrofurantoin:

Body Weight		No. Teaspoonfuls
Pounds	Kilograms	4 Times Daily
15 to 26	7 to 11	1/2 (2.5 mL)
27 to 46	12 to 21	1 (5 mL)
47 to 68	22 to 30	1-1/2 (7.5 mL)
69 to 91	31 to 41	2 (10 mL)

Therapy should be continued for one week or for at least 3 days after sterility of the urine is obtained. Continued infection indicates the need for reevaluation.

For long-term suppressive therapy in adults, a reduction of dosage to 50-100 mg at bedtime may be adequate. For long-term suppressive therapy in children, doses as low as 1 mg/kg per 24 hours, given in a single dose or in two divided doses, may be adequate. *See "Warnings" section regarding risks associated with long-term therapy.*

NITROFURANTOIN/NITROFURANTOIN MONOHYDRATE
Adults and Children Over 12 years: One 100-mg capsule every 12 hours for seven days.

Avoid exposure to strong light which may darken the drug. It is stable in storage. It should be dispensed in amber bottles.

Store at controlled room temperature (59° to 86°F or 15° to 30°C).

CLINICAL STUDIES

Controlled clinical trials comparing Nitrofurantoin Monohydrate 100 mg p.o. q12h and Nitrofurantoin 50 mg p.o. q6h in the treatment of acute uncomplicated urinary tract infections demonstrated approximately 75% microbiologic eradication of susceptible pathogens in each treatment group.

REFERENCES

1. National Committee for Clinical Laboratory Standards. Performance Standards for Antimicrobial Disk Susceptibility Tests - Fourth Edition. Approved Standard NCCLS Document MS-A4, Vol. 10, No. 7m NCCLS, Villanova, PA, 1990. 2. National Committee for Clinical Laboratory Standards. Methods for Dilution Antimicrobial Susceptibility Tests for Bacteria that Grow Aerobically - Second Edition. Approved Standard NCCLS Document M7-A2, Vol. 10, No. 8, NCCLS, Villanova, PA, 1990.

HOW SUPPLIED

NITROFURANTOIN
SUSPENSION: 25 MG/5 ML

BRAND/MANUFACTURER	NDC	SIZE	AWP
○ **BRAND**			
FURADANTIN: P&G Pharm	00149-0735-15	60 ml	$19.36
	00149-0735-61	470 ml	$74.98

NITROFURANTOIN, MACROCRYSTALS
CAPSULE: 25 MG

BRAND/MANUFACTURER	NDC	SIZE	AWP
◆ **BRAND**			
► MACRODANTIN: P&G Pharm	00149-0007-05	100s	$54.29
◆ **GENERICS**			
Geneva	00781-2501-01	100s	$41.70

CAPSULE: 50 MG

AVERAGE UNIT PRICE (AVAILABLE SIZES)		GENERIC A-RATED AVERAGE PRICE (GAAP)	
BRAND	$0.72	100s	$60.75
GENERIC	$0.60	500s	$290.45
		1000s	$558.92

BRAND/MANUFACTURER	NDC	SIZE	AWP
◆ **BRAND**			
► MACRODANTIN: P&G Pharm	00149-0008-05	100s	$71.53
	00149-0008-77	100s ud	$77.47
	00149-0008-66	500s	$350.44
	00149-0008-67	1000s	$686.59
◆ **GENERICS**			
Allscrips	54569-0181-06	80s	$46.97
Geneva	00781-2502-01	100s	$58.19
Zenith	00172-2130-60	100s	$58.20
Qualitest	00603-4776-21	100s	$58.20
Moore,H.L.	00839-7518-06	100s	$58.85
Goldline	00182-1944-01	100s	$59.50
Rugby	00536-4831-01	100s	$59.52
Martec	52555-0476-01	100s	$60.55
Aligen	00405-4699-01	100s	$61.24
URL	00677-1224-01	100s	$61.73
Major	00904-7721-60	100s	$66.75
UDL	51079-0584-20	100s ud	$57.98
Goldline	00182-1944-89	100s ud	$64.50
Geneva	00781-2502-13	100s ud	$64.60
Geneva	00781-2502-05	500s	$285.12
Zenith	00172-2130-70	500s	$285.12
Aligen	00405-4699-02	500s	$285.12
Moore,H.L.	00839-7518-12	500s	$288.36
Goldline	00182-1944-05	500s	$291.50
Major	00904-7721-40	500s	$307.45
Zenith	00172-2130-80	1000s	$558.60
Geneva	00781-2502-10	1000s	$559.24

CAPSULE: 100 MG

AVERAGE UNIT PRICE (AVAILABLE SIZES)		GENERIC A-RATED AVERAGE PRICE (GAAP)	
BRAND	$1.24	100s	$103.29
GENERIC	$1.02	500s	$485.39

BRAND/MANUFACTURER	NDC	SIZE	AWP
◆ **BRAND**			
► MACRODANTIN: P&G Pharm	00149-0009-05	100s	$121.42
	00149-0009-77	100s ud	$139.38
	00149-0009-66	500s	$594.95
	00149-0009-67	1000s	$1165.68
◆ **GENERICS**			
Allscrips	54569-1969-02	20s	$20.48
Zenith	00172-2131-60	100s	$98.50
Qualitest	00603-4777-21	100s	$98.50
Geneva	00781-2503-01	100s	$98.79
Moore,H.L.	00839-7519-06	100s	$99.91
Rugby	00536-4832-01	100s	$101.00
Goldline	00182-1945-01	100s	$101.00
Aligen	00405-4700-01	100s	$102.20
Martec	52555-0477-01	100s	$102.40
URL	00677-1225-01	100s	$103.95
Major	00904-7722-60	100s	$108.75
UDL	51079-0585-20	100s ud	$105.39

◆ RATED THERAPEUTICALLY EQUIVALENT; ◇ THERAPEUTIC EQUIVALENCE UNCONFIRMED; ○ UNRATED

BRAND/MANUFACTURER	NDC	SIZE	AWP
Geneva	00781-2503-13	100s ud	$106.38
Goldline	00182-1945-89	100s ud	$116.00
Major	00904-7722-40	500s	$482.65
Zenith	00172-2131-70	500s	$484.00
Moore,H.L.	00839-7519-12	500s	$489.51
Zenith	00172-2131-80	1000s	$948.40

CAPSULE: 100 MG

BRAND/MANUFACTURER	NDC	SIZE	AWP
○ BRAND			
➤ MACROBID: P&G Pharm	00149-0710-01	100s	$122.99

Nitrofurazone, Topical

DESCRIPTION
Chemically, Nitrofurazone is 2-[(5-nitro-2-furanyl) methylene]hydrazine-carboxamide.

Chemically Nitrofurazone is 5 Nitro-2-furaldehyde semicarbazone.

Nitrofurazone Topical Cream, Soluble Dressing and Topical Solution contain 0.2% Nitrofurazone.

Nitrofurazone Topical Cream, Soluble Dressing, and Topical Solution are antibacterial agents for topical use.

Following is its chemical structure:

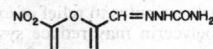

CLINICAL PHARMACOLOGY
Nitrofurazone, Topical is a nitrofuran that is bactericidal for most pathogens commonly causing surface infections, including *Staphylococcus aureus, Streptococcus, Escherichia coli, Clostridium perfringens, Aerobacter aerogenes*, and *Proteus*.

Nitrofurazone, Topical inhibits a number of bacterial enzymes, especially those involved in the aerobic and anaerobic degradation of glucose and pyruvate. The activity appears to involve the pyruvate dehydrogenase system as well as citrate synthetase, malate dehydrogenase, glutathione reductase, and pyruvate decarboxylase. Glutathione reductase inhibition may be caused by control of pentose phosphate metabolism. Although Nitrofurazone, Topical inhibits a variety of enzymes, it is not considered to be a general enzyme inactivator since many enzymes are not inhibited by this compound.

INDICATIONS AND USAGE
Nitrofurazone, Topical is a topical antibacterial agent indicated for adjunctive therapy of patients with second- and third-degree burns when bacterial resistance to other agents is a real or potential problem.

It is also indicated in skin grafting where bacterial contamination may cause graft rejection and/or donor site infection particularly in hospitals with historical resistant-bacteria epidemics.

There is no known evidence of effectiveness of this product in the treatment of minor burns or surface bacterial infections involving wounds, cutaneous ulcers or the various pyodermas.

UNLABELED USES
Nitrofurazone is used as intraoperative vas irrigation to attain azoospermia immediately postvasectomy.

CONTRAINDICATIONS
Known sensitization to any of the components of this preparation is a contraindication for use.

WARNINGS
Nitrofurazone Soluble Dressing and Topical Solution should be used with caution in patients with known or suspected renal impairment. The polyethylene glycols in the base of some brands can be absorbed through denuded skin and may not be excreted normally by the compromised kidney. This may lead to symptoms of progressive renal impairment such as increased BUN, anion gap, and metabolic acidosis. (*Note:* Some brands of Nitrofurazone Topical Cream do not contain polyethylene glycols.)

PRECAUTIONS
General: Use of Nitrofurazone, Topical occasionally allows overgrowth of nonsusceptible organisms including fungi and *Pseudomonas*. If this occurs, or if irritation, sensitization or superinfection develops, treatment with Nitrofurazone, Topical should be discontinued and appropriate therapy instituted.

Information for Patients: Patients should be told to use Nitrofurazone, Topical Cream only as directed by a physician. Patients should be advised to discontinue the drug and contact a physician should rash or irritation occur.

Carcinogenesis, Mutagenesis, and Impairment of Fertility: Nitrofurazone has been shown to produce mammary tumors when fed at high doses to female Sprague-Dawley rats. The relevance of this to topical use in humans in unknown.

Dietary dosage levels of 60 and 30 mg/kg/day shortened the onset time of the typical mammary gland tumors associated with older female rats. These tumors exhibited the same histological characteristics seen in the spontaneously occurring tumors, and were seen only in the female animals. No mammary tumors were seen in rats treated with Nitrofurazone orally in the diet for 1 year at levels of approximately 11 mg/kg/day. Spermatogenic arrest was noted in the male rats in dietary dosage levels of 30 mg/kg/day and above, after one year on test.

Pregnancy: Pregnancy Category C: Nitrofurazone, when administered orally to pregnant rabbits, caused a slight increase in the frequency of still-births when given in doses thirty times the human dose. There are no adequate and well controlled studies in pregnant women. Nitrofurazone, Topical should be used during pregnancy only if the potential benefit justifies the potential risk to the fetus.

Nursing Mothers: It is not known whether this drug is excreted in human milk. Because many drugs are excreted in human milk and because of the potential for tumorigenicity shown for nitrofurazone in animal studies, a decision should be made whether to discontinue nursing or to discontinue the drug, taking into account the importance of the drug to the mother.

Pediatric Use: Safety and effectiveness in children have not been established.

ADVERSE REACTIONS
Instances of clinical skin reactions have been reported for patients treated with Nitrofurazone, Topical formulations. Symptoms appear as varying degrees of contact dermatitides such as rash, pruritus, and local edema. Although the exact incidence of such reactions is difficult to determine, historically, a survey of world literature and clinical trials data indicates an overall incidence of approximately 1%. Allergic reactions to Nitrofurazone, Topical should be treated symptomatically.

DOSAGE AND ADMINISTRATION
Topical cream: Apply Nitrofurazone Topical Cream directly to the lesion, or first place on gauze. Reapply once daily or every few days, depending on the usual dressing technique.

Soluable Dressing: Burns: Apply directly to the lesion with a spatula, or first place on gauze. Impregnated gauze may be used. Reapply depending on the preferred dressing technique. Flushing the dressing with sterile saline facilitates its removal.

Topical Solution: Burns: Apply Nitrofurazone Topical Solution directly to the lesion, or first place on gauze. Impregnated gauze may be used. Reapply depending on the preferred dressing technique. Flushing the dressing with sterile saline facilitates its removal.

PREPARATION OF IMPREGNATED GAUZE
Sterile gauze strips are placed in a tray and covered with Nitrofurazone Soluble Dressing or Topical Solution. Repeat the procedure, adding several layers of gauze for each layer of Nitrofurazone Soluble Dressing or Topical Solution. Sprinkling a little sterile water on each layer of dressing will minimize any color change from autoclaving. Cover the tray very loosely and autoclave at 121°C for 30 minutes at 15 to 20 pounds pressure. To impregnate bandage rolis, place some Nitrofurazone Soluble Dressing or Topical Solution in the bottom of a glass jar. Stand rolls on end. Place more Nitrofurazone Soluble Dressing or Topical Solution on top. Cover top of jar with aluminum foil. Autoclave at 121°C for 45 minutes at 15 to 20 pounds pressure. Do not store impregnated bandage rolls for more than 24 hours. Autoclaving more than once is not recommended.

ANIMAL TOXICOLOGY
The oral administration of Nitrofurazone for 7 days to rats at extremely high dosage levels of 240 mg/kg/day produced severe hepatorenal lesions whereas only renal changes were seen when the dosage level was reduced to 60 mg/kg/day for 60 days. Dogs treated orally with Nitrofurazone for 400 days at levels of 11 mg/kg/day showed no toxic effects related to drug treatment. The single intravenous administration in dogs of 20, 35, or 75 mg/kg Nitrofurazone produced clinical signs of lacrimation, salivation, emesis, diarrhea, excitation, weakness, ataxia, and weight loss, whereas 100 mg/kg/day produced convulsions and death. There was no evidence of toxicosis in rhesus monkeys treated with doses of Nitrofurazone as high as 58 mg/kg/day for 10 weeks and 23 mg/kg/day for 63 weeks. The peroral LD$_{50}$ of Nitrofurazone in mice and rats is 747 and 590 mg/kg respectively.

Avoid exposure to direct sunlight, strong fluorescent lighting, alkaline materials, and excessive heat (over 104°F or 40°C).

HOW SUPPLIED
CREAM: 0.2%

BRAND/MANUFACTURER	NDC	SIZE	AWP
○ BRAND			
FURACIN: Roberts Pharm	54092-0311-28	28 gm	$14.21

OINTMENT: 0.2%

AVERAGE UNIT PRICE (AVAILABLE SIZES)		GENERIC A-RATED AVERAGE PRICE (GAAP)	
BRAND	$0.27	30 gm	$3.96
GENERIC	$0.02	454 gm	$3.96
		454 gm	$7.32

BRAND/MANUFACTURER	NDC	SIZE	AWP
◆ BRAND			
FURACIN: Roberts Pharm	54092-0310-28	28 gm	$10.14
	54092-0310-56	56 gm	$16.32
	54092-0310-16	454 gm	$67.96

BRAND/MANUFACTURER	NDC	SIZE	AWP
◆ **GENERICS**			
Thames	49158-0110-08	30 gm	$1.00
Clay-Park	45802-0030-03	30 gm	$1.51
Thames	49158-0110-16	454 gm	$6.40
Clay-Park	45802-0030-15	454 gm	$6.48
Rugby	00536-9019-98	454 gm	$7.58
URL	00677-1085-44	454 gm	$7.90

SOLUTION: 0.2%

AVERAGE UNIT PRICE (AVAILABLE SIZES)			
GENERIC	$0.01		

BRAND/MANUFACTURER	NDC	SIZE	AWP
◆ **GENERICS**			
Clay-Park	45802-0031-17	480 ml	$6.48
Clay-Park	45802-0031-18	3840 ml	$29.16

SOLUTION: 0.2%

BRAND/MANUFACTURER	NDC	SIZE	AWP
○ **BRAND**			
FURACIN: Roberts Pharm	54092-0312-16	473 ml	$54.31

Nitrogard *SEE* NITROGLYCERIN

Nitroglycerin

DESCRIPTION

Nitroglycerin is 1,2,3-propanetriol trinitrate, an organic nitrate whose empiric formula is $C_3H_5N_3O_9$, and whose molecular weight is 227.09. The organic nitrates are vasodilators, active on both arteries and veins.

Nitroglycerin is available for intravenous use, as a lingual or sublingual spray, as an ointment, as sublingual or buccal tablets, and as a transdermal system.

Nitroglycerin for intravenous use is a clear, practically colorless additive solution for intravenous infusion after dilution. It is not for direct intravenous injection. The solution is sterile, non-pyrogenic, and nonexplosive.

CAUTION

SEVERAL PREPARATIONS OF NITROGLYCERIN FOR INJECTION ARE AVAILABLE. THEY DIFFER IN CONCENTRATION AND/OR VOLUME PER VIAL. WHEN SWITCHING FROM ONE PRODUCT TO ANOTHER ATTENTION MUST BE PAID TO THE DILUTION AND DOSAGE AND ADMINISTRATION INSTRUCTIONS.

Nitroglycerin lingual aerosol is a metered dose aerosol containing Nitroglycerin in propellants. This product delivers Nitroglycerin in the form of spray droplets onto or under the tongue.

Some brands of Nitroglycerin buccal tablets are an extended-release preparation designed to deliver Nitroglycerin through the oral mucosa over a sustained period of time. When a buccal tablet is placed under the lip or in the buccal pouch, it adheres to the mucosa. As the tablet gradually dissolves, it releases Nitroglycerin to the systemic circulation.

The Nitroglycerin transdermal delivery system is a unit designed to provide continuous controlled release of Nitroglycerin through intact skin. The rate of release of Nitroglycerin is linearly dependent upon the area of the applied system.

The remainder of the Nitroglycerin in each system serves as a reservoir and is not delivered in normal use. After 12 hours, for example, each system has delivered 6%, 10%, 14%, or 15% of its original content of Nitroglycerin.

Each mL of injection contains:
Nitroglycerin ....0.5 or 5 mg

Each spray emission of aerosol delivers:
Nitroglycerin ....0.4 mg

Each inch (2.5 cm) of ointment contains:
Nitroglycerin ....approximately 15 mg

Each sublingual or buccal tablet contains:
Nitroglycerin ....0.15, 0.3, 0.4, or 0.6 mg

Each buccal extended-release tablet contains:
Nitroglycerin ....1, 2, 2.5, 3, or 5 mg

Each cm^2 of applied transdermal system delivers:
Nitroglycerin approximately ....0.013, 0.02, 0.026, or 0.03 mg/hour

Following is its chemical structure:

$$CH_2ONO_2 - CHONO_2 - CH_2ONO_2$$

CLINICAL PHARMACOLOGY

The principal pharmacological action of Nitroglycerin is relaxation of vascular smooth muscle and consequent dilatation of peripheral arteries and veins, especially the latter. The mechanism by which Nitroglycerin produces relaxation of smooth muscle is unknown. Dilatation of the post-capillary vessels, including large veins, promotes peripheral pooling of blood and decreases venous return to the heart, thereby reducing left ventricular end-diastolic pressure and pulmonary capillary wedge pressure (preload). Arteriolar relaxation reduces systemic vascular resistance, systolic arterial pressure, and mean arterial pressure (afterload). Dilatation of the coronary arteries also occurs. The relative importance of preload reduction, afterload reduction, and coronary dilatation remains undefined. Myocardial oxygen consumption or demand (as measured by the pressure-rate product, tension-time index and stroke-work index) is decreased by both the arterial and venous effects of Nitroglycerin, and a more favorable supply-demand ratio can be achieved.

Dosing regimens for most chronically used drugs are designed to provide plasma concentrations that are continuously greater than a minimally effective concentration. This strategy is inappropriate for organic nitrates. Several well-controlled clinical trials have used exercise testing to assess the anti-anginal efficacy of continuously-delivered nitrates. In the large majority of these trials, active agents were indistinguishable from placebo after 24 hours (or less) of continuous therapy. Attempts to overcome nitrate tolerance by dose escalation, even to doses far in excess of those used acutely, have consistently failed. Only after nitrates have been absent from the body for several hours has their anti-anginal efficacy been restored.

The mechanism by which Nitroglycerin relieves angina pectoris is not fully understood. Myocardial oxygen consumption or demand (as measured by the pressure-rate product, tension-time index, and stroke-work index) is decreased by both the arterial and venous effects of Nitroglycerin and presumably, a more favorable supply-demand ratio is achieved.

While the large epicardial coronary arteries are also dilated by Nitroglycerin, the extent to which this action contributes to relief of exertional angina is unclear.

Therapeutic doses of Nitroglycerin may reduce systolic, diastolic, and mean arterial blood pressure. Effective coronary perfusion pressure is usually maintained, but can be compromised if blood pressure falls excessively or increased heart rate decreases diastolic filling time.

Elevated central venous and pulmonary capillary wedge pressures, pulmonary vascular resistance and systemic vascular resistance are also reduced by Nitroglycerin therapy. Heart rate is usually slightly increased, presumably a reflex response to the fall in blood pressure. Cardiac index may be increased, decreased, or unchanged. Patients with elevated left ventricular filling pressure and systemic vascular resistance values in conjunction with a depressed cardiac index are likely to experience an improvement in cardiac index.

On the other hand, when filling pressures and cardiac index are normal, cardiac index may be slightly reduced, by intravenous Nitroglycerin.

Pharmacokinetics: The volume of distribution of Nitoglycerin is about 3 L/kg, and Nitroglycerin is cleared from this volume at extremely rapid rates, with a resulting serum half-life of about 3 minutes. The observed clearance rates (close to 1 L/kg/min) greatly exceed hepatic blood flow; known sites of extrahepatic metabolism include red blood cells and vascular walls.

Nitroglycerin is rapidly metabolized *in vivo*, with a liver reductase enzyme having primary importance in the formation of glycerol nitrate metabolites and inorganic nitrate. Two active major metabolites are 1, 2, and 1,3-dinitroglycerols.

The dinitrates are less effective vasodilators than Nitroglycerin, but they are longer-lived in the serum, and their net contribution to the overall effect of chronic Nitroglycerin regimens is not known. The dinitrates are further metabolized to (non-vasoactive) mononitrates and, ultimately, to glycerol and carbon dioxide. At plasma concentrations of between 50 and 500 ng/ml, the binding of Nitroglycerin to plasma proteins is approximately 60%, while that of 1,2 dimitroglycerin and 1,3 dinitroglycerin is 60% and 30% respectively. The activity and half-life of 1,2 dinitroglycerin and 1,3 dinitroglycerin are not well characterized. The mononitrate is not active.

To avoid development of tolerance to Nitroglycerin drug-free intervals of 10-12 hours are known to be sufficient; shorter intervals have not been well studied. In one well-controlled clinical trial, subjects receiving Nitroglycerin appeared to exhibit a rebound or withdrawal effect, so that their exercise tolerance at the end of the daily drug-free interval was *less* than that exhibited by the parallel group receiving placebo.

Reliable assay techniques for plasma Nitroglycerin levels have only recently become available, and studies using these techniques to define the pharmacokinetics of Nitroglycerin ointment or extended-release buccal tablets have not been reported. Published studies using older techniques provide results that often differ, in similar experimental settings, by an order of magnitude. The data are consistent, however, in suggesting that Nitroglycerin levels rise to a steady state within an hour or so of application of ointment, and that after removal of Nitroglycerin ointment, levels wane with a half-life of about half an hour.

The maximal achievable daily duration of antianginal activity provided by Nitroglycerin ointment therapy has not been studied. Recent studies of other formulations of Nitroglycerin suggest that the maximal achievable daily duration of anti-anginal effect from Nitroglycerin ointment will be about 12 hours.

It is reasonable to believe that the rate and extent of Nitroglycerin absorption from ointment may vary with the site and square measure of the skin over which a given dose of ointment is spread, but these relationships have not been adequately studied.

Nitroglycerin is rapidly absorbed following sublingual administration. Its onset of action is approximately one to three minutes. Significant pharmacologic effects are present for 30 to 60 minutes following administration by the above route.

In healthy volunteers, steady-state plasma concentrations of Nitroglycerin are reached by about two hours after application of a transdermal system patch and are maintained for the duration of wearing the system (observations have been limited to 24 hours).

Upon removal of the patch, the plasma concentration declines with a half-life of about an hour.

Clinical Trials: Blinded, placebo-controlled trials of intravenous Nitroglycerin have not been reported, but multiple investigators have reported open-label studies, and there are scattered reports of studies in which intravenous Nitroglycerin was tested in blinded fashion against sodium Nitroprusside.

In each of these studies, therapeutic doses of intravenous Nitroglycerin were found to reduce systolic and diastolic arterial blood pressure. The heart rate was usually increased, presumably as a reflexive response to the fall in blood pressure. Coronary perfusion pressure was usually, but not always, maintained.

Intravenous Nitroglycerin reduced central venous pressure (CVP), right atrial pressure (RAP), pulmonary arterial pressure (PAP), pulmonary-capillary wedge pressure (PCWP), pulmonary vascular resistance (PVR), and systemic vascular resistance (SVR). When these parameters were elevated, reducing them toward normal usually caused a rise in cardiac output. Conversely, intravenous Nitroglycerin usually *reduced* cardiac output when it was given to patients whose CVP, RAP, PAP, PCWP, PVR, and SVR were all normal.

Most clinical trials of intravenous Nitroglycerin have been brief; they have typically followed hemodynamic parameters during a single surgical procedure. In one careful study, one of the few that lasted more than a few hours, continuous intravenous Nitroglycerin had lost almost all of its hemodynamic effect after 48 hours. In the same study, patients who received Nitroglycerin infusions for only 12 hours out of each 24 demonstrated no similar attenuation of effect. These results are consistent with those seen in multiple large, double-blind, placebo-controlled trials of other formulations of Nitroglycerin and other nitrates.

A pharmacokinetic study in 13 healthy men showed no statistically significant differences between the mean values for maximum plasma concentration and time to achieve maximum plasma level with equal doses (0.8 mg) of Nitroglycerin lingual spray and sublingual Nitroglycerin tablets. Peak plasma concentration after 0.8 mg of lingual spray occurred within 4 minutes and the apparent plasma half-life was approximately 5 minutes. In a randomized, double-blind study in patients with exertional angina pectoris dose-related increases in exercise tolerance were seen following doses of 0.2, 0.4, and 0.8 mg delivered by metered spray.

Controlled trials have demonstrated that Nitroglycerin ointment can effectively reduce exercise-related angina for up to 7 hours after a single application. Doses used in clinical trials have ranged from ½ inch (1.3 cm:7.5 mg) to 2 inches (5.1 cm; 30 mg), typically applied to 36 square inches (323 square centimetrs) of truncal skin.

In some controlled trials of other organic nitrate formulations, efficacy has declined with time. Because controlled, long-term trials of Nitroglycerin ointment have not been reported, it is not known how the efficacy of Nitroglycerin ointment may vary during extended therapy.

Controlled single-dose trials in nitrate-free subjects have demonstrated that buccal Nitroglycerin tablets can effectively reduce exercise-related angina for 3-5 hours after a single dose. Anti-anginal activity is present about 3 minutes after dosing. The magnitude and duration of activity of buccal Nitroglycerin appeared to be inversely related: Greater (but shorter-lived) anti-anginal benefit appeared to be achieved by subjects who chewed the buccal tablets, drank hot liquids, moved the tablets about in their mouth, or actively jostled the tablets with their tongues. In general, continuing anti-anginal efect during single-dose trials appeared to correlate with the continuing palpable presence of some portion of a tablet.

Multiple-dose studies of buccal Nitroglycerin have not utilized concurrent placebo controls. For example, subjects in one such study received thrice-daily buccal Nitroglycerin tablets for 14 days. On the last day, these subjects' exercise tolerance (at one hour, three hours, and five hours after dosing) was greater than it had been before dosing or at baseline. The absence of concurrent placebo controls makes these results difficult to interpret; placebo-treated subjects in studies of other Nitroglycerin formulations have sometimes, presumably through a training effect, achieved similar results.

In some controlled trials of other organic nitrate formulations, efficacy has declined with time. Because the multiple-dose trials of buccal Nitroglycerin did not include exercise tests on any day of treatment before the last, it is not known how the efficacy of buccal tablets may vary during extended therapy.

The maximal achievable daily duration of anti-anginal activity provided by buccal Nitroglycerin therapy has not been studied. Recent studies of other formulation of Nitroglycerin suggest that the maximal achievable daily duration of anti-anginal effect from buccal Nitroglycerin will be about 12 hours.

Controlled studies have not directly evaluated the efficacy of buccal Nitroglycerin in aborting an acute episode of angina pectoris. Studies comparing the hemodynamic effects of sublingual and buccal Nitroglycerin suggest that the onset of action of the former is more rapid than that of the latter, but by only a small margin. For example, one trial found that significant reduction of left ventricular end-diastolic pressure took 80 seconds to appear after dosing with sublingual Nitroglycerin, while it took 110 seconds to appear after dosing with buccal Nitroglycerin.

Regimens in which Nitroglycerin transdermal system patches were worn for 12 hours daily have been studied in well-controlled trials up to 4 weeks in duration. Starting about 2 hours after application and continuing until 10-12 hours after application, patches that deliver at least 0.4 mg of Nitroglycerin per hour have consistently demonstrated greater anti-anginal activity than placebo. Lower-dose patches have not been as well studied, but in one large, well-controlled trial in

which higher-dose patches were also studied, patches delivering 0.2 ng/hr had significantly less anti-anginal activity than placebo.

It is reasonable to believe that the rate of Nitroglycerin absorption from patches may vary with the site of application. but this relationship has not been adequately studied.

The onset of action of transdermal Nitroglycerin is not sufficiently rapid for this product to be useful in aborting an acute anginal episode.

INDICATIONS AND USAGE

Intravenous Nitroglycerin is indicated for treatment of perioperative hypertension; for control of congestive heart failure in the setting of acute myocardial infarction; for treatment of angina pectoris in patients who have not responded to sublingual Nitroglycerin and β-blockers; and for induction of intraoperative hypotension.

Nitroglycerin lingual spray is indicated for acute relief of an attack or prophylaxis of angina pectoris due to coronary artery disease.

Nitroglycerin ointment is indicated for the prevention of angina pectoris due to coronary artery disease.

Nitroglycerin sublingual/buccal tablets are indicated for the prophylaxis, treatment and management of patients with angina pectoris.

Nitroglycerin extended-release buccal tablets are indicated for the prevention and treatment of angina pectoris due to coronary artery disease.

Some brands of Nitroglycerin transdermal delivery are indicated for the prevention of angina pectoris due to coronary artery disease and some brands have been conditionally approved by the FDA for this indication. Tolerance to the anti-anginal effects of nitrates (measured by exercise stress testing) has been shown to be a major factor limiting efficacy when transdermal nitrates are used continuously for longer than 12 hours each day. The development of tolerance can be altered (prevented or attenuated) by use of a noncontinuous (intermittent) dosing schedule with a nitrate-free interval of 10-12 hours.

Controlled clinical trial data suggest that the intermittent use of nitrates is associated with decreased exercise tolerance, in comparison to placebo, during the last part of the nitrate-free interval; the clinical relevance of this observation is unknown, but the possibility of increased frequency or severity of angina during the nitrate-free interval should be considered. Further investigations of the tolerance phenomenon and best regimen are ongoing. A final evaluation of the effectiveness of certain products will be announced by the FDA.

UNLABELED USES

Nitroglycerin is used alone or as an adjunct in the treatment of severe ventricular arrhythmias associated with angina, myocardial ischemia, peripheral ischemia, Raynaud's disease, and acetylcholine provocation testing. It is also used in silent myocardial ischemia, achalasia, and biliary tract disorders including biliary colic, pulmonary hypertension, and to relax the uterus to treat retained placenta and to assist intrapartum external cephalic version as a tocolytic agent. Nitroglycerin, in the ointment is also used in the treatment of hypertonic sphincter constipation, esophageal varices to control variceal hemorrhage, pulmonary edema, and thrombophlebitis. It is also used, when applied locally, to increase penile circumference (engorgement or tumescence) in impotent men.

CONTRAINDICATIONS

Allergic reactions to organic nitrates are extremely rare, but they do occur. Nitroglycerin is contraindicated in patients who are allergic to it or who have shown hypersensitivity or idiosyncrasy to it or other nitrates or nitrites.

In patients with pericardial tamponade, restrictive cardiomyopathy, or constrictive pericarditis, cardiac output is dependent upon venous return. Intravenous Nitroglycerin is contraindicated in patients with these conditions.

Sublingual Nitroglycerin therapy is contraindicated in patients with early myocardial infarction, severe anemia, increased intracranial pressure, and those with a known hypersensitivity to Nitroglycerin.

Allergy to the adhesives used in Nitroglycerin patches has also been reported, and it similarly constitutes a contraindication to the use of this product.

WARNINGS

The use of any form of Nitroglycerin during the early days of acute myocardial infarction requires particular attention to hemodynamic monitoring and clinical status.

Nitroglycerin readily migrates into many plastics, including the polyvinyl chloride (PVC) plastics commonly used for intravenous administration sets. Nitroglycerin absorption by PVC tubing is increased when the tubing is long, the flow rates are low, and the Nitroglycerin concentration of the solution is high. The delivered fraction of the solution's original Nitroglycerin content has been 20-60% in published studies using PVC tubing; the fraction varies with time during a single infusion, and no simple correction factor can be used. PVC tubing has been used in most published studies of intravenous Nitroglycerin, but the reported doses have been calculated by simply multiplying the flow rate of the solution by the solution's original concentration of Nitroglycerin. *The actual doses delivered have been less, sometimes much less, than those reported.*

Some in-line intravenous filters also absorb Nitroglycerin; these filters should be avoided.

Because of the absorption problem, the least absorptive tubing available (i.e., non-PVC tubing) should be used for Nitroglycerin infusions.

DOSING INSTRUCTIONS MUST BE FOLLOWED WITH CARE. WHEN THE APPROPRIATE INFUSION SETS ARE USED, THE CALCULATED DOSE WILL BE DELIVERED TO THE PATIENT, BECAUSE THE LOSS OF NITROGLYCERIN SEEN WITH STANDARD PVC TUBING WILL BE AVOIDED. THE DOSAGES REPORTED IN PUBLISHED STUDIES UTI-

LIZED GENERAL-USE PVC ADMINISTRATION SETS, AND RECOMMENDED DOSES BASED ON THIS EXPERIENCE WILL BE TOO HIGH WHEN THE LOW-ABSORBING INFUSION SETS ARE USED.

The benefits of transdermal or buccal Nitroglycerin in patients with acute myocardial infarction or congestive heart failure have not been established. If one elects to use Nitroglycerin in these conditions, careful clinical or hemodynamic monitoring must be used to avoid the hazards of hypotension and tachycardia.

PRECAUTIONS

General: Severe hypotension particularly with upright posture, and shock may occur with even small doses of Nitroglycerin. This drug should therefore be used with caution in patients who may be volume depleted; or who, for whatever reason, are already hypotensive; or who, because of inadequate circulation to the brain or to other vital organs, would be unusually compromised by undue hypotension. Hypotension induced by Nitroglycerin may be accompanied by paradoxical bradycardia and increased angina pectoris.

Nitrate therapy may aggravate the angina caused by hypertrophic cardiomyopathy.

Tolerance to this drug and cross-tolerance to other nitrates and nitrites may occur. Tolerance to the vascular and antianginal effects of nitrates has been demonstrated in clinical trials, experience through occupational exposure, and in isolated tissue experiments in the laboratory.

As tolerance to other forms of Nitroglycerin develops, the effect of sublingual Nitroglycerin on exercise tolerance, although still observable, is somewhat blunted.

In industrial workers who have had long-term exposure to unknown (presumably high) doses of organic nitrates, tolerance clearly occurs. Chest pain, acute myocardial infarction, and even sudden death have occurred during temporary withdrawal of nitrates from these workers, demonstrating the existence of true physical dependence.

Some clinical trials in angina patients have provided Nitroglycerin for about 12 continuous hours of every 24-hour day. During the nitrate-free intervals in some of these trials, anginal attacks have been more easily provoked than before treatment, and patients have demonstrated hemodynamic rebound and *decreased* exercise tolerance. The importance of these observations to the routine, clinical use of Nitroglycerin is not known.

Lower concentrations of Nitroglycerin increase the potential precision of dosing, but these concentrations increase the total fluid volume that must be delivered to the patient. Total fluid load may be a dominant consideration in patients with compromised function of the heart, liver, and/or kidneys.

Nitroglycerin infusions should be administered only via a pump that can maintain a constant infusion rate.

Intracoronary injection of Nitroglycerin infusions has not been studied.

Only the smallest dose of sublingual/buccal tablets required for effective relief of the acute anginal attack should be used. Excessive use may lead to the development of tolerance. Nitroglycerin tablets are intended for sublingual or buccal administration and should not be swallowed. The drug should be discontinued if blurring of vision or drying of the mouth occurs. Excessive dosage of Nitroglycerin may produce severe headaches.

Information for Patients: Daily headaches sometimes accompany treatment with Nitroglycerin. In patients who get these headaches, the headaches are a marker of the activity of the drug. Patients should resist the temptation to avoid headaches by altering the schedule of their treatment with Nitroglycerin, since loss of headache is likely to be associated with simultaneous loss of antianginal efficacy.

Treatment with Nitroglycerin may be associated with lightheadedness on standing, especially just after rising from a recumbent or seated position.

This effect may be more frequent in patients who have also consumed alcohol.

Laboratory Tests: Because of the propylene glycol content of some brands of intravenous Nitroglycerin, serum triglyceride assays that rely on glycerol oxidase may give falsely elevated results in patients receiving this medication.

Drug Interactions: The vasodilating effects of Nitroglycerin may be additive with those of other vasodilators.

Alcohol may enhance sensitivity to the hypotensive effects of nitrates. Nitroglycerin acts directly on vascular muscle. Therefore, any other agents that depend on vascular smooth muscle as the final common path can be expected to have decreased or increased effect depending upon the agent.

Administration of Nitroglycerin infusions through the same infusion set as blood can result in pseudoagglutination and hemolysis. More generally, Nitroglycerin in 5% dextrose or sodium chloride 0.9% should not be mixed with any other medication of any kind.

Intravenous Nitroglycerin interferes, at least in some patients, with the anticoagulant effect of heparin. In patients receiving intravenous Nitroglycerin, concomitant heparin therapy should be guided by frequent measurement of the activated partial thromboplastin time.

Marked symptomatic orthostatic hypotension has been reported when calcium channel blockers and oral controlled-release Nitroglycerin or organic nitrates were used in combination. Dose adjustments of either class of agents may be necessary.

Patients receiving antihypertensive drugs, beta-adrenergic blockers, or phenothiazines and nitrates should be observed for possible additive hypotensive effects.

Drug/Laboratory Test Interactions: Nitrates may interfere with the Zlatkis-Zak color reaction causing a false report of decreased serum cholesterol.

Carcinogenesis, Mutagenesis, and Impairment of Fertility: No long-term studies in animals have been performed to evaluate the carcinogenic potential of Nitroglyc-erin. Studies to evaluate Nitroglycerin's potential for mutagenicity or impairment of fertility have also not been performed.

Pregnancy Category C: Animal reproduction studies have not been conducted with Nitroglycerin. It is also not known whether Nitroglycerin can cause fetal harm when administered to a pregnant woman or whether it can affect reproductive capacity. Nitroglycerin should be given to a pregnant woman only if clearly needed.

Nursing Mothers: It is not known whether Nitroglycerin is excreted in human milk. Because many drugs are excreted in human milk, caution should be exercised when Nitroglycerin is administered to a nursing woman.

Pediatric Use: Safety and effectiveness in children have not been established.

ADVERSE REACTIONS

Adverse reactions to Nitroglycerin are generally dose-related and almost all of these reactions are the result of Nitroglycerin's activity as a vasodilator. Headache, which may be severe, is the most commonly reported side effect. Headache may be recurrent with each daily dose, especially at higher doses. Cutaneous vasodilation with flushing may occur. Transient episodes of dizziness and weakness, as well as other signs of cerebral ischemia associated with postural hypotension, may occasionally develop. An occasional individual may exhibit marked sensitivity to the hypotensive effects of nitrates and severe responses (nausea, vomiting, weakness, restlessness, pallor, perspiration, and collapse) may occur even with therapeutic doses. Drug rash and/or exfoliative dermatitis have been reported in patients receiving nitrate therapy. Nausea and vomiting appear to be uncommon.

Allergic reactions to Nitroglycerin are also uncommon, and the great majority of those reported have been cases of contact dermatitis or fixed drug eruptions in patients receiving Nitroglycerin in ointments or patches. There have been a few reports of genuine anaphylactoid reactions, and these reactions can be probably occur in patients receiving Nitroglycerin by any route.

Hypotension occurs infrequently, but in some patients it may be severe enough to warrant discontinuation of therapy. Syncope, crescendo angina, and rebound hypertension have been reported but are uncommon.

Extremely rarely, ordinary doses of organic nitrates have caused methemoglobinemia in normal-seeming patients. Methemoglobinemia is so infrequent at these doses that further discussion of its diagnosis and treatment is defered (see *"Overdosage"*).

Data are not available to allow estimation of the frequency of adverse reactions during treatment with Nitroglycerin injection, ointment, or buccal tablets.

Application-site irritation may occur with transdermal Nitroglycerin but is rarely severe. In two placebo controlled trials of intermittent therapy with Nitroglycerin patches at 0.2 to 0.8 mg/hr, the most frequent adverse reactions among 307 subjects were as follows:

	placebo	patch
headache	18%	63%
light-headedness	4%	6%
hypotension and/or syncope	0%	4%
increased angina	2%	2%

OVERDOSAGE

Hemodynamic Effects: The ill effects of Nitroglycerin overdose are generally the results of Nitroglycerin's capacity to induce vasodilation, venous pooling, reduced cardiac output, and hypotension. These hemodynamic changes may have protean manifestations, including increased intracranial pressure, with any or all of the following: persistent throbbing headache, confusion, and moderate fever; vertigo; palpitations; visual disturbances; nausea and vomiting (possibly with colic and even bloody diarrhea); syncope (especially in the upright posture); air hunger and dyspnea, later followed by reduced ventilatory effort; diaphoresis, with the skin either flushed or cold and clammy; slow pulse (dicrotic and intermittent); heart block and bradycardia; increased intracranial pressure with cerebral symptoms of confusion and moderate fever, paralysis; coma; seizures; and death.

Laboratory determinations of serum levels of Nitroglycerin and its metabolites are not widely available, and such determinations have, in any event, no established role in the management of Nitroglycerin overdose.

No data are available to suggest physiological maneuvers (e.g., maneuvers to change the pH of the urine) that might accelerate elimination of Nitroglycerin and its active metabolites. Similarly, it is not known which—if any—of these substances can usefully be removed from the body by hemodialysis.

No specific antagonist to the vasodilator effects of Nitroglycerin is known, and no intervention has been subject to controlled study as a therapy of Nitroglycerin overdose. Because the hypotension associated with Nitroglycerin overdose is the result of venodilatation and arterial hypovolemia, prudent therapy in this situation should be directed toward an increase in central fluid volume. Passive elevation of the patient's legs may be sufficient, but intravenous infusion of normal saline or similar fluid may also be necessary.

Keep the patient recumbent in a shock position and comfortably warm. Gastric lavage may be of use if the medication has only recently been swallowed. Passive movement of the extremities may aid venous return. Administer oxygen and artificial ventilation, if necessary.

The use of epinephrine or other arterial vasoconstrictors in this setting is likely to do more harm than good. It and related compunds are contraindicated in this situation.

◆ RATED THERAPEUTICALLY EQUIVALENT; ◇ THERAPEUTIC EQUIVALENCE UNCONFIRMED; ○ UNRATED

In patients with renal disease or congestive heart failure, therapy resulting in central volume expansion is not without hazard. Treatment of Nitroglycerin overdose in these patients may be subtle and difficult, and invasive monitoring may be required.

Methemoglobinemia: Nitrate ions liberated during metabolism of Nitroglycerin can oxidize hemoglobin into methemoglobin. Case reports of clinically significant methemoglobinemia are rare at conventional doses of organic nitrates. The formation of methemoglobin is dose-related and in the case of genetic abnormalities of hemoglobin that favor methemoglobin formation, even conventional doses of organic nitrates could produce harmful concentrations of methemoglobin. Even in patients totally without cytochrome b$_5$ reductase activity, however, and even assuming that the nitrate moieties of Nitroglycerin are quantitatively applied to oxidation of hemoglobin, about 1 mg/kg of Nitroglycerin should be required before any of these patients manifests clinically significant ($\geq$ 10%) methemoglobinemia. In patients with normal reductase function, significant production of methemoglobin should require even larger doses of Nitroglycerin. In one study in which 36 patients received 2-4 weeks of continuous Nitroglycerin therapy at 3.1 to 4.4 mg/hr, the average methemoglobin level measured was 0.2%; this was comparable to that observed in parallel patients who received placebo.

Not withstanding these observations, there are case reports of significant methemoglobinemia in association with moderate overdoses of organic nitrates. None of the affected patients had been thought to be unusually susceptible.

Methemoglobin levels are available from most clinical laboratories. The diagnosis should be suspected in patients who exhibit signs of impaired oxygen delivery despite adequate cardiac output and adequate arterial pO$_2$. Classically, methemoglobinemic blood is described as chocolate brown, without color change on exposure to air.

When methemoglobinemia is diagnosed, the treatment of choice is methylene blue, 1-2 mg/kg intravenously.

DOSAGE AND ADMINISTRATION
INTRAVENOUS NITROGLYCERIN
Not for direct intravenous injection.
NITROGLYCERIN IS A CONCENTRATED, POTENT DRUG WHICH MUST BE DILUTED IN DEXTROSE (5%) INJECTION, USP OR SODIUM CHLORIDE (0.9%) INJECTION, USP PRIOR TO ITS INFUSION. NITROGLYCERIN SHOULD NOT BE MIXED WITH OTHER DRUGS.

1. Initial Dilution:
Aseptically transfer the contents of one Nitroglycerin ampul or vial (containing 25 or 50 mg of Nitroglycerin) into a 500 mL *glass* bottle of either dextrose (5%) injection, USP or sodium chloride injection (0.9%), USP. This yields a final concentration of 50 mcg/mL or 100 mcg/mL. Diluting 5 mg Nitroglycerin into 100 mL will also yield a final concentration of 50 mcg/mL.

2. Maintenance Dilution:
It is important to consider the fluid requirement of the patient as well as the expected duration of infusion in selecting the appropriate dilution of Nitroglycerin. After the initial dosage titration, the concentration of the solution may be increased, if necessary, to limit fluids given to the patient. The Nitroglycerin concentration should not exceed 400 mcg/mL. See chart. (See related table.)

Note: If the concentration is adjusted, it is imperative to flush or replace the infusion set before a new concentration is utilized. If the set is not flushed or replaced, it could take minutes to hours, depending upon the flow rate and the dead space of the set, for the concentration to reach the patient.

Invert the glass parenteral bottle several times to assure uniform dilution of Nitroglycerin. When stored in *glass* containers, the diluted solution is physically and chemically stable for up to 48 hours at room temperature, and up to seven days under refrigeration.

Dosage is affected by the type of container and administration set used. See *"Warnings".*

Although the usual starting adult dose range reported in clinical studies was 25 mcg/min or more, these studies used PVC administration sets. *The use of nonabsorbing tubing will result in the need for reduced doses.*

If a peristaltic action infusion pump is used, an appropriate administration set should be selected, with a drip chamber that delivers approximately 60 microdrops/mL. The dilution and administration table may be used to calculate Nitroglycerin dilution and flow rate in microdrops/minute to achieve the desired Nitroglycerin administration rate.

If a volumetric infusion pump is used, the dilution and administration table may still be used; however, flow rate will be determined directly by the infusion pump, independent of the drop size of the drip chambers. Thus, the reference to "MICRODROPS/MIN" is not applicable, and the corresponding flow rate in mL/hr should be used to determine pump settings.

When using a nonabsorbing infusion set, initial dosage should be 5 mcg/min delivered through an infusion pump capable of exact and constant delivery of the drug. Subsequent titration must be adjusted to the clinical situation, with dose increments becoming more cautious as partial response is seen. Initial titration should be in 5 mcg/min increments, with increases every 3-5 minutes until some response is noted. If no response is seen at 20 mcg/min, increments of 10 and later 20 mcg/min can be used. Once a partial blood pressure response is observed, the dose increase should be reduced and the interval between increases should be lengthened.

Some patients with normal or low left ventricular filling pressures or pulmonary capillary wedge pressure (e.g., angina patients without other complications) may be hypersensitive to the effects of Nitroglycerin and may respond fully to doses as small as 5 mcg/min. These patients require especially careful titration and monitoring.

There is no fixed optimum dose of Nitroglycerin. Due to variations in the responsiveness of individual patients to the drug, each patient must be titrated to the desired level of hemodynamic function. Therefore, continuous monitoring of physiologic parameters (i.e., blood pressure and heart rate in all patients, other measurements such as pulmonary capillary wedge pressure, as appropriate) MUST be performed to achieve the correct dose. Adequate systemic blood pressure and coronary perfusion pressure must be maintained.

As with all parenteral drug products, Nitroglycerin IV should be inspected visually for particulate matter and discoloration prior to administration, whenever solution and container permit.

STORAGE
Protect from freezing.
Store at controlled room temperature 15°-30°C (59°-86°F).

NITROGLYCERIN LINGUAL AEROSOL SPRAY
At the onset of an attack, one or two metered doses should be sprayed onto or under the tongue. No more than three metered doses are recommended within a 15-minute period. If the chest pain persists, prompt medical attention is recommended. Nitroglycerin lingual spray may be used prophylactically five to ten minutes prior to engaging in activities which might precipitate an acute attack.

During application the patient should rest, ideally in the sitting position. The canister should be held vertically with the valve head uppermost and the spray orifice as close to the mouth as possible. The dose should preferably be sprayed onto the tongue by pressing the button firmly and the mouth should be closed immediately after each dose, *The Spray Should Not Be Inhaled.* Patients should be instructed to familiarize themselves with the position of the spray orifice, which can be identified by the finger rest on top of the valve, in order to facilitate orientation for administration at night.

STORAGE
Store at room temperature. Do not expose to temperatures exceeding 50°C (122°F).

Note: The indented statement below is required by the Federal Clean Air Act for all products containing chlorofluorocarbons (CFCs), including products such as this one.
WARNING: Contains CFC-12 substances which harm public health and environment by destroying ozone in the upper atmosphere.

NITROGLYCERIN DILUTION AND ADMINISTRATION TABLE

FLOW RATE MICRODROPS MIN = ML/HR	5 MG NITROGLYCERIN IN 100 ML OR 25 MG NITROGLYCERIN IN 500 ML — 50 MCG/ML	5 MG NITROGLYCERIN IN 50 ML OR 25 MG NITROGLYCERIN IN 250 ML OR 50 MG NITROGLYCERIN IN 500 ML — 100 MCG/ML	DILUTE 10 MG NITROGLYCERIN IN 50 ML OR 50 MG NITROGLYCERIN IN 250 L OR 100 MG NITROGLYCERIN IN 500 ML TO YIELD 200 MCG/ML	100 MG NITROGLYCERIN IN 250 ML 200 MG NITROGLYCERIN IN 500 ML — 400 MCG/ML
	ADMINISTRATION RATE MCG I.V. NITROGLYCERIN/MIN			
3	—	5	10	20
6	5	10	20	40
12	10	20	40	80
24	20	40	80	160
48	40	80	160	320
72	60	120	240	480
96	80	160	320	640

► SHOWN IN PRODUCT IDENTIFICATION GUIDE

NITROGLYCERIN OINTMENT

As noted above ("Clinical Pharmacology"), controlled trials have demonstrated that Nitroglycerin ointment can effectively reduce exercise-related angina for up to 7 hours after a single application. Doses used in clinical trials have ranged from ½ inch (1.3 cm; 7.5 mg) to 2 inches (5.1 cm; 30 mg), typically applied to 36 square inches (232 square centimeters) of truncal skin.

It is reasonable to believe that the rate and extent of Nitroglycerin absorption from ointment may vary with the site and square measure of the skin over which a given dose of ointment is spread, but these relationships have not been adequately studied.

Controlled trials with other formulations of Nitroglycerin have demonstrated that, if plasma levels are maintained continuously, all antianginal efficacy is lost within 24 hours. This tolerance cannot be overcome by increasing the dose of Nitroglycerin. As a result, any regimen of Nitroglycerin ointment administration should include a daily nitrate-free interval. The minimum necessary length of such an interval has not been defined, but studies with other Nitroglycerin formulations have shown that 10 to 12 hours is sufficient. Thus, one appropriate dosing schedule for Nitroglycerin ointment would begin with two daily ½-inch (7.5-mg) doses, one applied on rising in the morning and one applied 6 hours later. The dose could be doubled, and even doubled again, in patients tolerating this dose but failing to respond to it.

Each tube of ointment is supplied with a pad of paper applicators or patches. These applicators or patches allow ointment to be absorbed through a much smaller area of skin than that used in any of the reported clinical trials, and the significance of this difference is not known. To apply the ointment using one of the applicators or patches, place the applicator or patch on a flat surface, printed side down. Squeeze the necessary amount of ointment from the tube onto the applicator or patch, place the applicator or patch (ointment side down) on the desired area of skin, and tape the applicator or patch into place.

Upon removal of the applicator or patch from the skin, be sure to wash the area with soap and water. Note: Nitroglycerin can cause a slight reddening of the skin, especially when applied to an area recently in contact with adhesive tape. The redness is temporary and generally disappears within a few hours.

STORAGE
Keep tube tightly closed and store at controlled room temperature, 15°-30°C (59°-86°F).

NITROGLYCERIN SUBLINGUAL/BUCCAL TABLETS

One tablet should be dissolved under the tongue or in the buccal pouch at the first sign of an acute anginal attack. The dose may be repeated approximately every five minutes until relief is obtained. If the pain persists after a total of 3 tablets in a 15-minute period, the physician should be notified. Sublingual/buccal Nitroglycerin tablets may be used prophylactically five to ten minutes prior to engaging in activities which might precipitate an acute attack.

STORAGE
Store at controlled room temperature, 15°-30°C (59°-86°F).
Protect from moisture.

EXTENDED-RELEASE BUCCAL NITROGLYCERIN TABLETS

As noted above ("Clinical Pharmacology"), careful studies with other formulations of Nitroglycerin have shown that maintenance of continuous 24-hour plasma levels of Nitroglycerin results in tolerance (i.e., loss of clinical response). Every dosing regimen for extended-release buccal tablets should provide a daily nitrate-free interval to avoid the development of this tolerance. The minimum necessary length of such an interval has not been defined, but studies with other Nitroglycerin formulations have shown that 10-12 hours is sufficient. Large controlled studies with other formulations of Nitroglycerin show that no dosing regimen should be expected to provide more than about 12 hours of continuous antianginal efficacy per day.

The pharmacokinetics of Nitroglycerin buccal tablets, and the clinical effects of multiple-dose regimens, have not been well studied. In clinical trials, the initial dose of Nitroglycerin buccal tablets has typically been 1 mg, with subsequent upward dose adjustment guided by symptoms and side effects. The average result of the dose-adjustment process has varied from 1.4 to 3.1 mg. The interval between doses has varied from 4 to 14 hours. Buccal tablets should be placed under the upper lip or in the buccal pouch and permitted to dissolve slowly over a 3-5 hour period. They should not be chewed, swallowed, or placed under the tongue. The rate of dissolution of the tablet, and the short-term anti-anginal efficacy, may be increased by touching the tablet with the tongue or drinking hot liquids. Because of the possibility of aspiration, bedtime use is not recommended.

Buccal Nitroglycerin tablets can be tried as a means of aborting an acute anginal attack. In the even that extended-release buccal tablets fail to provide prompt relief in this setting, sublingual Nitroglycerin is recommended.

STORAGE
Store at controlled room temperature, 15°-30°C (59°-86°F).
Dispense in a tight container as defined in the USP.

NITROGLYCERIN TRANSDERMAL DELIVERY SYSTEM

The suggested starting dose is between 0.2 mg/hr* and 0.4 mg/hr*. Doses between 0.4 mg/hr* and 0.8 mg/hr* have shown continued effectiveness for 10-12 hours

---

* Rated release *in vivo*. Release rates were formerly described in terms of drug delivered per 24 hours. In these terms, the supplied Nitroglycerin systems would be rated at 2.5 mg/24 hours (0.1 mg/hr), 5 mg/24 hours (0.2 mg/hr), 7.5 mg/24 hours (0.3 mg/hour), 10 mg/24 hours (0.4 mg/hr), and 15 mg/24 hours (0.6 mg/hr).

---

daily for at least one month (the longest period studied) of intermittent administration. Although the minimum nitrate-free interval has not been defined, data show that a nitrate-free interval of 10-12 hours is sufficient (see "Clinical Pharmacology"). Thus, an appropriate dosing schedule for Nitroglycerin patches would include a daily patch-on period of 12-14 hours and a daily patch-off period of 10-12 hours.

Although some well-controlled clinical trials using exercise tolerance testing have shown maintenance of effectiveness when patches are worn continuously, the large majority of such controlled trials have shown the development of tolerance (i.e., complete loss of effect) within the first 24 hours after therapy was initiated. Dose adjustment, even to levels much higher than generally used, did not restore efficacy.

STORAGE
Store at controlled room temperature, 15°-25° or 30°C (59°-77° or 86°F). Extremes of temperature and/or humidity should be avoided. Do not refrigerate.

HOW SUPPLIED
CAPSULE, EXTENDED RELEASE: 2.5 MG

BRAND/MANUFACTURER	NDC	SIZE	AWP
○ GENERICS			
Schein	00364-0174-06	60s	$3.47
Moore,H.L.	00839-5146-05	60s	$3.71
Major	00904-0643-52	60s	$4.65
Eon	00185-5174-60	60s	$4.95
Geneva	00781-2718-60	60s	$5.40
NITRO-PAR: Parmed	00349-2102-60	60s	$5.50
Ethex	58177-0004-03	60s	$5.68
NITRO-TIME: Time-Cap	49483-0221-06	60s	$5.70
Schein	00364-0174-01	100s	$3.75
Veratex	17022-5971-02	100s	$3.95
Mason Dist	11845-0305-01	100s	$5.55
Rugby	00536-4083-01	100s	$5.85
Qualitest	00603-4782-21	100s	$5.94
NITROCOT: Truxton	00463-3010-01	100s	$6.00
URL	00677-0485-01	100s	$6.15
Moore,H.L.	00839-5146-06	100s	$6.20
Eon	00185-5174-01	100s	$6.50
Major	00904-0643-60	100s	$6.70
Aligen	00405-4702-01	100s	$6.99
NITROGLYN E-R: Kenwood	00482-1025-01	100s	$7.96
Geneva	00781-2718-01	100s	$8.25
Allscrips	54569-0456-00	100s	$8.25
Ethex	58177-0004-04	100s	$8.83
NITRO-TIME: Time-Cap	49483-0221-10	100s	$8.90
Goldline	00182-0702-01	100s	$8.90
MI-TRATES:	52765-2301-01	100s	$8.95
NITRO-PAR: Parmed	00349-2102-01	100s	$9.10
Southwood	58016-5002-01	100s	$11.45
Vangard	00615-0337-13	100s ud	$11.52
Geneva	00781-2718-13	100s ud	$11.68
Major	00904-0643-61	100s ud	$14.95
Goldline	00182-0702-89	100s ud	$15.00

CAPSULE, EXTENDED RELEASE: 6.5 MG

BRAND/MANUFACTURER	NDC	SIZE	AWP
○ GENERICS			
Major	00904-0644-52	60s	$4.95
Moore,H.L.	00839-5978-05	60s	$5.47
Geneva	00781-2786-60	60s	$6.25
Eon	00185-1235-60	60s	$6.50
► Ethex	58177-0005-03	60s	$7.54
NITRO-TIME: Time-Cap	49483-0222-06	60s	$7.70
NITRO-PAR: Parmed	00349-2097-60	60s	$7.95
Veratex	17022-5992-02	100s	$3.95
Qualitest	00603-4783-21	100s	$6.61
Moore,H.L.	00839-5978-06	100s	$6.74
URL	00677-0486-01	100s	$6.75
Schein	00364-0432-01	100s	$6.75
Rugby	00536-4084-01	100s	$6.77
Mason Dist	11845-0306-01	100s	$7.24
Major	00904-0644-60	100s	$7.35
Geneva	00781-2786-01	100s	$9.15
Allscrips	54569-0459-00	100s	$9.15
NITROGLYN E-R: Kenwood	00482-1065-01	100s	$9.17
Ethex	58177-0005-04	100s	$11.42
NITRO-PAR: Parmed	00349-2097-01	100s	$11.95
Eon	00185-1235-01	100s	$12.95
NITRO-TIME: Time-Cap	49483-0222-10	100s	$13.05
Goldline	00182-0703-01	100s	$13.05
Aligen	00405-4703-01	100s	$13.92
Vangard	00615-0336-13	100s ud	$17.03
Goldline	00182-0703-89	100s ud	$17.10
Major	00904-0644-61	100s ud	$17.45
Geneva	00781-2786-13	100s ud	$17.95

◆ RATED THERAPEUTICALLY EQUIVALENT; ◇ THERAPEUTIC EQUIVALENCE UNCONFIRMED; ○ UNRATED

CAPSULE, EXTENDED RELEASE: 9 MG

BRAND/MANUFACTURER	NDC	SIZE	AWP
○ **GENERICS**			
Schein	00364-0664-06	60s	$5.75
Major	00904-0647-52	60s	$6.40
Goldline	00182-1716-26	60s	$7.45
Moore,H.L.	00839-6724-05	60s	$7.55
Ethex	58177-0006-03	60s	$8.50
Qualitest	00603-4784-20	60s	$9.41
Mason Dist	11845-0307-05	60s	$9.47
NITRO-PAR: Parmed	00349-8756-60	60s	$9.70
Aligen	00405-4704-31	60s	$9.72
URL	00677-0967-06	60s	$9.80
Eon	00185-1217-60	60s	$9.95
Rugby	00536-4090-08	60s	$9.97
NITRO-TIME: Time-Cap	49483-0223-06	60s	$9.99
Goldline	00182-1670-26	60s	$9.99
Geneva	00781-2798-60	60s	$10.55
Allscrips	54569-3317-00	60s	$10.55
Major	00904-0647-60	100s	$8.25
Ethex	58177-0006-04	100s	$13.02
NITRO-PAR: Parmed	00349-8756-01	100s	$13.50
NITROGLYN E-R: Kenwood	00482-1090-01	100s	$14.54
Eon	00185-1217-01	100s	$14.95
Geneva	00781-2798-01	100s	$14.97
NITRO-TIME: Time-Cap	49483-0223-10	100s	$15.05
Major	00904-0647-61	100s ud	$17.95
Goldline	00182-1670-89	100s ud	$18.00

FILM, EXTENDED RELEASE: 0.1 MG/HR

BRAND/MANUFACTURER	NDC	SIZE	AWP
○ **BRAND**			
NITRO-DUR: Key	00085-3305-30	30s	$37.67
	00085-3305-35	30s	$37.67
TRANSDERM-NITRO 2.5: Summit	57267-0902-26	30s	$44.52
	57267-0902-42	30s	$44.52
MINITRAN: 3M Pharm	00089-0301-03	33s	$38.52
TRANSDERM-NITRO 2.5: Summit	57267-0902-30	100s	$148.38

FILM, EXTENDED RELEASE: 0.2 MG/HR

BRAND/MANUFACTURER	NDC	SIZE	AWP
○ **BRAND**			
NITRO-DUR: Key	00085-3310-30	30s	$38.23
	00085-3310-35	30s	$38.23
DEPONIT: Schwarz	00091-4195-01	30s	$40.44
NITRODISC: Roberts Pharm	00025-2058-30	30s	$43.48
TRANSDERM-NITRO 5: Summit	57267-0905-26	30s	$45.57
	57267-0905-42	30s	$45.57
MINITRAN: 3M Pharm	00089-0302-03	33s	$39.00
DEPONIT: Schwarz	00091-4195-11	100s	$134.83
NITRODISC: Roberts Pharm	00025-2058-31	100s	$144.94
TRANSDERM-NITRO 5: Summit	57267-0905-30	100s	$151.87
○ **GENERICS**			
Rugby	00536-4098-07	30s	$32.84
Schein	00364-2501-30	30s	$33.00
Circa	49470-0001-30	30s	$33.06
Goldline	00182-1240-17	30s	$33.06
Warner Chilcott	00047-0835-15	30s	$33.66
Allscrips	54569-3208-00	30s	$35.22
Moore,H.L.	00839-7790-19	30s	$35.78
Qualitest	00603-4725-16	30s	$36.60
Major	00904-0652-46	30s	$37.15
Mylan	00378-9004-93	30s	$43.95

FILM, EXTENDED RELEASE: 0.3 MG/HR

BRAND/MANUFACTURER	NDC	SIZE	AWP
○ **BRAND**			
NITRO-DUR: Key	00085-3315-30	30s	$42.85
	00085-3315-35	30s	$42.85
NITRODISC: Roberts Pharm	00025-2078-30	30s	$45.83
	00025-2078-31	100s	$152.77

FILM, EXTENDED RELEASE: 0.4 MG/HR

BRAND/MANUFACTURER	NDC	SIZE	AWP
○ **BRAND**			
NITRO-DUR: Key	00085-3320-30	30s	$42.85
	00085-3320-35	30s	$42.85
DEPONIT: Schwarz	00091-4196-01	30s	$45.13
NITRODISC: Roberts Pharm	00025-2068-30	30s	$48.17
TRANSDERM-NITRO 10: Summit	57267-0910-26	30s	$52.08
	57267-0910-42	30s	$52.08
MINITRAN: 3M Pharm	00089-0303-03	33s	$43.44
DEPONIT: Schwarz	00091-4196-11	100s	$150.41
NITRODISC: Roberts Pharm	00025-2068-31	100s	$160.52
TRANSDERM-NITRO 10: Summit	57267-0910-30	100s	$173.58

BRAND/MANUFACTURER	NDC	SIZE	AWP
○ **GENERICS**			
Qualitest	00603-4726-16	30s	$38.20
Circa	49470-0004-30	30s	$39.33
Goldline	00182-1267-17	30s	$39.33
Rugby	00536-4111-07	30s	$41.09
Moore,H.L.	00839-7791-19	30s	$41.26
Warner Chilcott	00047-0837-15	30s	$41.66
Allscrips	54569-3209-00	30s	$41.93
Schein	00364-2502-30	30s	$42.00
Major	00904-0653-46	30s	$46.45
Mylan	00378-9012-93	30s	$48.25

FILM, EXTENDED RELEASE: 0.6 MG/HR

BRAND/MANUFACTURER	NDC	SIZE	AWP
○ **BRAND**			
NITRO-DUR: Key	00085-3330-30	30s	$46.46
	00085-3330-35	30s	$46.46
TRANSDERM-NITRO 15: Summit	57267-0915-26	30s	$57.39
	57267-0915-42	30s	$57.39
MINITRAN: 3M Pharm	00089-0304-03	33s	$47.64
TRANSDERM-NITRO 15: Summit	57267-0915-30	100s	$191.25
○ **GENERICS**			
Rugby	00536-4112-07	30s	$46.00
Warner Chilcott	00047-0839-15	30s	$47.50
Qualitest	00603-4727-16	30s	$48.19
Circa	49470-0002-30	30s	$51.30
Mylan	00378-9016-93	30s	$55.10
Major	00904-0654-46	30s	$59.25

FILM, EXTENDED RELEASE: 0.8 MG/HR

BRAND/MANUFACTURER	NDC	SIZE	AWP
○ **BRAND**			
NITRO-DUR: Key	00085-0819-30	30s	$46.46
	00085-0819-35	30s	$46.46

INJECTION: 0.5 MG/ML

BRAND/MANUFACTURER	NDC	SIZE	AWP
○ **GENERICS**			
TRIDIL: Du Pont Multi	00590-0092-10	10 ml 20s	$75.00

For additional alternatives, turn to the section beginning on page 2859.

Nitrol Appli-Kit *SEE* **NITROGLYCERIN**

Nitrolingual *SEE* **NITROGLYCERIN**

Nitrong *SEE* **NITROGLYCERIN**

Nitropress *SEE* **SODIUM NITROPRUSSIDE**

Nitrostat *SEE* **NITROGLYCERIN**

Nizatidine

DESCRIPTION

Nizatidine is a histamine H_2-receptor antagonist. Chemically, it is N-[2-[[[2-[(dimethylamino)-methyl]-4-thiazolyl] methyl]thio]ethyl]-N'-methyl-2-nitro-1,1-ethenediamine.

Nizatidine has the empirical formula $C_{12}H_{21}N_5O_2S_2$ representing a molecular weight of 331.45. It is an off-white to buff crystalline solid that is soluble in water. Nizatidine has a bitter taste and mild sulfur-like odor. Each capsule contains for oral administration gelatin, pregelatinized starch, silicone, starch, titanium dioxide, yellow iron oxide, 150 mg (0.45 mmol) or 300 mg (0.91 mmol) of Nizatidine.

Following is its chemical structure:

CLINICAL PHARMACOLOGY

Nizatidine is a competitive, reversible inhibitor of histamine at the histamine H_2-receptors, particularly those in the gastric parietal cells.

Antisecretory Activity: 1. Effects on Acid Secretion: Nizatidine significantly inhibited nocturnal gastric acid secretion for up to 12 hours. Nizatidine also significantly inhibited gastric acid secretion stimulated by food, caffeine, betazole, and pentagastrin (Table 1).

Table 1
EFFECT OF ORAL NIZATIDINE ON GASTRIC ACID SECRETION

		% Inhibition of Gastric Acid Output by Dose (mg)				
	Time After Dose (h)	20-50	75	100	150	300
Nocturnal	Up to 10	57			73	90
Betazole	Up to 3		93		100	99
Pentagastrin	Up to 6		25		64	67
Meal	Up to 4	41	64		98	97
Caffeine	Up to 3		73		85	96

2. Effects on Other Gastrointestinal Secretions—Pepsin: Oral administration of 75 to 300 mg of Nizatidine did not affect pepsin activity in gastric secretions. Total pepsin output was reduced in proportion to the reduced volume of gastric secretions.

Intrinsic Factor: Oral administration of 75 to 300 mg of Nizatidine increased betazole-stimulated secretion of intrinsic factor.

Serum Gastrin: Nizatidine had no effect on basal serum gastrin. No rebound of gastrin secretion was observed when food was ingested 12 hours after administration of Nizatidine.

3. Other Pharmacologic Actions:
  a. *Hormones:*Nizatidine was not shown to the serum concentrations of gonadotropins, prolactin, growth hormone, antidiuretic hormone, cortisol, triiodothyronine, thyroxin, testosterone, 5α-dihydrotestosterone, androstenedione, or estradiol.
  b. Nizatidine had no demonstrable antiandrogenic action.

4. Pharmacokinetics: The absolute oral bioavailability of Nizatidine exceeds 70%. Peak plasma concentrations (700 to 1,800 µg/L for a 150-mg dose and 1,400 to 3,600 µg/L for a 300-mg dose) occur from 0.5 to 3 hours following the dose. A concentration of 1,000 µg/L is equivalent to 3 µmol/L; a dose of 300 mg is equivalent to 905 µmoles. Plasma concentrations 12 hours after administration are less than 10 µg/L. The elimination half-life is 1 to 2 hours, plasma clearance is 40 to 60 L/h, and the volume of distribution is 0.8 to 1.5 L/kg. Because of the short half-life and rapid clearance of Nizatidine, accumulation of the drug would not be expected in individuals with normal renal function who take either 300 mg once daily at bedtime or 150 mg twice daily. Nizatidine exhibits dose proportionality over the recommended dose range.

The oral bioavailability of Nizatidine is unaffected by concomitant ingestion of propantheline. Antacids consisting of aluminum and magnesium hydroxides with simethicone decrease the absorption of Nizatidine by about 10%. With food, the AUC and C_{max} increase by approximately 10%.

In humans, less than 7% of an oral dose is metabolized as N2-monodesmethyl-nizatidine, an H_2-receptor antagonist, which is the principal metabolite excreted in the urine. Other likely metabolites are the N2-oxide (less than 5% of the dose) and the S-oxide (less than 6% of the dose).

More than 90% of an oral dose of Nizatidine is excreted in the urine within 12 hours. About 60% of an oral dose is excreted as unchanged drug. Renal clearance is about 500 mL/min, which indicates excretion by active tubular secretion. Less than 6% of an administered dose is eliminated in the feces. Moderate to severe renal impairment significantly prolongs the half-life and decreases the clearance of Nizatidine. In individuals who are functionally anephric, the half-life is 3.5 to 11 hours, and the plasma clearance is 7 to 14 L/h. To avoid accumulation of the drug in individuals with clinically significant renal impairment, the amount and/or frequency of doses of Nizatidine should be reduced in proportion to the severity of dysfunction (see "*Dosage and Administration*").

Approximately 35% of Nizatidine is bound to plasma protein, mainly to α₁-acid glycoprotein. Warfarin, diazepam, acetaminophen, propantheline, phenobarbital, and propranolol did not affect plasma protein binding of Nizatidine *in vitro*.

Clinical Trials:
*1. Active Duodenal Ulcer:*In multicenter, double-blind, placebo-controlled studies in the United States, endoscopically diagnosed duodenal ulcers healed more rapidly following administration of Nizatidine 300 mg h.s. or 150 mg b.i.d.,

than with placebo (Table 2). Lower doses, such as 100 mg h.s., had slightly lower effectiveness. (See related table.)

2. Maintenance of Healed Duodenal Ulcer: Treatment with a reduced dose of Nizatidine has been shown to be effective as maintenance therapy following healing of active duodenal ulcers. In multicenter, double-blind, placebo-controlled studies conducted in the United States, 150 mg of Nizatidine taken at bedtime resulted in a significantly lower incidence of duodenal ulcer recurrence in patients treated for up to 1 year (Table 3).

Table 3
PERCENTAGE OF ULCERS RECURRING BY 3, 6, AND 12 MONTHS IN DOUBLE-BLIND STUDIES CONDUCTED IN THE UNITED STATES

Month	Nizatidine 150 mg h.s.	Placebo
3	13% (28/208)*	40% (82/204)
6	24% (45/188)*	57% (106/187)
12	34% (57/166)*	64% (112/175)

* $P < 0.001$ as compared with placebo.

3. Gastroesophageal Reflux Disease (GERD): In 2 multicenter, double-blind, placebo-controlled clinical trials performed in the United States and Canada, Nizatidine was more effective than placebo in improving endoscopically diagnosed esophagitis and in healing erosive and ulcerative esophagitis.

In patients with erosive or ulcerative esophagitis, 150 mg b.i.d. of Nizatidine given to 88 patients compared with placebo in 98 patients in Study 1 yielded a higher healing rate at 3 weeks (16% vs 7%) and at 6 weeks (32% vs 16%, $P < 0.05$). Of 99 patients on Nizatidine and 94 patients on placebo, Study 2 at the same dosage yielded similar results at 6 weeks (21% vs 11%, $P < 0.05$) and at 12 weeks (29% vs 13%, $P < 0.01$).

In addition, relief of associated heartburn was greater in patients treated with Nizatidine. Patients treated with Nizatidine consumed fewer antacids than did patients treated with placebo.

INDICATIONS AND USAGE

Nizatidine is indicated for up to 8 weeks for the treatment of active duodenal ulcer. In most patients, the ulcer will heal within 4 weeks.

Nizatidine is indicated for maintenance therapy for duodenal ulcer patients, at a reduced dosage of 150 mg h.s. after healing of an active duodenal ulcer. The consequences of continuous therapy with Nizatidine for longer than 1 year are not known. Nizatidine is indicated for up to 12 weeks for the treatment of endoscopically diagnosed esophagitis, including erosive and ulcerative esophagitis, and associated heartburn due to GERD.

CONTRAINDICATION

Nizatidine is contraindicated in patients with known hypersensitivity to the drug. Because cross sensitivity in this class of compounds has been observed. H_2-receptor antagonists, including Nizatidine should not be administered to patients with a history of hypersensitivity to other H_2-receptor antagonists.

PRECAUTIONS

General: 1. Symptomatic response to Nizatidine therapy does not preclude the presence of gastric malignancy.
  2. Because Nizatidine is excreted primarily by the kidney, dosage should be reduced in patients with moderate to severe renal insufficiency (see "*Dosage and Administration*").
  3. Pharmacokinetic studies in patients with hepatorenal syndrome have not been done. Part of the dose of Nizatidine is metabolized in the liver. In patients with normal renal function and uncomplicated hepatic dysfunction, the disposition of Nizatidine is similar to that in normal subjects.

Laboratory Tests: False-positive tests for urobilinogen with Multistix® may occur during therapy with Nizatidine.

Drug Interactions: No interactions have been observed between Nizatidine and theophylline, chlordiazepoxide, lorazepam, lidocaine, phenytoin, and warfarin. Nizatidine does not inhibit the cytochrome P-450-linked drug-metabolizing enzyme system; therefore, drug interactions mediated by inhibition of hepatic metabolism are not expected to occur. In patients given very high doses (3,900 mg) of aspirin daily, increases in serum salicylate levels were seen when Nizatidine, 150 mg b.i.d., was administered concurrently.

Carcinogenesis, Mutagenesis, Impairment of Fertility: A 2-year oral carcinogenicity study in rats with doses as high as 500 mg/kg/day (about 80 times the recommended daily therapeutic dose) showed no evidence of a carcinogenic effect. There was a dose-related increase in the density of enterochromaffin-like (ECL) cells in the gastric oxyntic mucosa. In a 2-year study in mice, there was no evidence of a carcinogenic effect in male mice, although hyperplastic nodules of the liver were increased in the high-dose males as compared with placebo. Female mice given the high dose of Nizatidine (2,000 mg/kg/day, about 330 times the human dose) showed marginally statistically significant increases in hepatic carcinoma and hepatic nodular hyperplasia with no numerical increase seen in any of the other dose groups. The rate of hepatic carcinoma in the high-dose animals was within the historical control limits seen for the strain of mice used. The female mice were given a dose larger than the maximum tolerated dose, as indicated by excessive (30%) weight decrement as compared with concurrent controls and evidence of mild liver injury (transaminase elevations). The occurrence of a marginal finding at high dose only in animals given an excessive and somewhat hepatotoxic dose, with no evidence of a carcinogenic effect in rats,

Table 2
HEALING RESPONSE OF ULCERS TO NIZATIDINE

	Nizatidine				Placebo	
	300 mg h.s.		150 mg b.i.d.			
	Number Entered	Healed/ Evaluable	Number Entered	Healed/ Evaluable	Number Entered	Healed/ Evaluable
Study 1						
Week 2			276	93/265 (35%)*	279	55/260 (21%)
Week 4				198/259 (76%)*		95/243 (39%)
Study 2						
Week 2	108	24/103 (23%)*	106	27/101 (27%)*	101	9/93 (10%)
Week 4		65/97 (67%)		66/97 (68%)*		24/84 (29%)
Study 3						
Week 2	92	22/90 (24%)†			98	13/92 (14%)
Week 4		52/85 (61%)*				29/88 (33%)
Week 8		68/83 (82%)*				39/79 (49%)

* P ¢ 0.01 as compared with placebo.
† P < 0.05 as compared with placebo.

male mice, and female mice (given up to 360 mg/kg/day, about 60 times the human dose), and a negative mutagenicity battery are not considered evidence of a carcinogenic potential for Nizatidine.

Nizatidine was not mutagenic in a battery of tests performed to evaluate its potential genetic toxicity, including bacterial mutation tests, unscheduled DNA synthesis, sister chromatid exchange, the mouse lymphoma assay, chromosome aberration tests, and a micronucleus test.

In a 2-generation, perinatal and postnatal fertility study in rats, doses of Nizatidine up to 650 mg/kg/day produced no adverse effects on the reproductive performance of parental animals or their progeny.

Pregnancy—Teratogenic Effects—Pregnancy Category C: Oral reproduction studies in rats at doses up to 300 times the human dose and in Dutch Belted rabbits at doses up to 55 times the human dose revealed no evidence of impaired fertility or teratogenic effect; but, at a dose equivalent to 300 times the human dose, treated rabbits had abortions, decreased number of live fetuses, and depressed fetal weights. On intravenous administration to pregnant New Zealand White rabbits, Nizatidine at 20 mg/kg produced cardiac enlargement, coarctation of the aortic arch, and cutaneous edema in 1 fetus, and at 50 mg/kg, it produced ventricular anomaly, distended abdomen, spina bifida, hydrocephaly, and enlarged heart in 1 fetus. There are, however, no adequate and well-controlled studies in pregnant women. It is also not known whether Nizatidine can cause fetal harm when administered to a pregnant woman or can affect reproduction capacity. Nizatidine should be used during pregnancy only if the potential benefit justifies the potential risk to the fetus.

Nursing Mothers: Studies conducted in lactating women have shown that 0.1% of the administered oral dose of Nizatidine is secreted in human milk in proportion to plasma concentrations. Because of the growth depression in pups reared by lactating rats treated with Nizatidine, a decision should be made whether to discontinue nursing or discontinue the drug, taking into account the importance of the drug to the mother.

Pediatric Use: Safety and effectiveness in children have not been established.

Use in Elderly Patients: Ulcer healing rates in elderly patients are similar to those in younger age groups. The incidence rates of adverse events and laboratory test abnormalities are also similar to those seen in other age groups. Age alone may not be an important factor in the disposition of Nizatidine. Elderly patients may have reduced renal function (see *"Dosage and Administration"*).

ADVERSE REACTIONS
Worldwide, controlled clinical trials of Nizatidine included over 6,000 patients given Nizatidine in studies of varying durations. Placebo-controlled trials in the United States and Canada included over 2,600 patients given Nizatidine and over 1,700 given placebo. Among the adverse events in these placebo-controlled trials, anemia (0.2% vs 0%) and urticaria (0.5% vs 0.1%) were significantly more common in the Nizatidine group.

Incidence in Placebo Controlled Clinical Trials in the United States and Canada: Table 4 lists adverse events that occurred at a frequency of 1% or more among Nizatidine-treated patients who participated in placebo-controlled trials. The cited figures provide some basis for estimating the relative contribution of drug and nondrug factors to the side effect incidence rate in the population studied.

Table 4
INCIDENCE OF TREATMENT-EMERGENT ADVERSE EVENTS IN PLACEBO-CONTROLLED CLINICAL TRIALS IN THE UNITED STATES AND CANADA

Body System/ Adverse Event*	Percentage of Patients Reporting Event	
	Nizatidine (N = 2,694)	Placebo (N = 1,729)
Body as a Whole		
Headache	16.6	15.6
Abdominal pain	7.5	12.5

Body System/ Adverse Event*	Percentage of Patients Reporting Event	
	Nizatidine (N = 2,694)	Placebo (N = 1,729)
Pain	4.2	3.8
Asthenia	3.1	2.9
Back pain	2.4	2.6
Chest pain	2.3	2.1
Infection	1.7	1.1
Fever	1.6	2.3
Surgical procedure	1.4	1.5
Injury; accident	1.2	0.9
Digestive		
Diarrhea	7.2	6.9
Nausea	5.4	7.4
Flatulence	4.9	5.4
Vomiting	3.6	4.4
Dyspepsia	3.6	4.4
Constipation	2.5	3.8
Dry mouth	1.4	1.3
Nausea and vomiting	1.2	1.9
Anorexia	1.2	1.6
Gastrointestinal disorder	1.1	1.2
Tooth disorder	1.0	0.8
Musculoskeletal		
Myalgia	1.7	1.5
Nervous		
Dizziness	4.6	3.8
Insomnia	2.7	3.4
Abnormal dreams	1.9	1.9
Somnolence	1.9	1.6
Anxiety	1.6	1.4
Nervousness	1.1	0.8
Respiratory		
Rhinitis	9.8	9.6
Pharyngitis	3.3	3.1
Sinusitis	2.4	2.1
Cough, increased	2.0	2.0
Skin and Appendages		
Rash	1.9	2.1
Pruritus	1.7	1.3
Special Senses		
Amblyopia	1.0	0.9

* Events reported by at least 1% of Nizatidine-treated patients are included.

A variety of less common events were also reported; it was not possible to determine whether these were caused by Nizatidine.

Hepatic: Hepatocellular injury, evidenced by elevated liver enzyme tests (SGOT [AST], SGPT [ALT], or alkaline phosphatase), occurred in some patients and was possibly or probably related to Nizatidine. In some cases there was marked elevation of SGOT/SGPT enzymes (greater than 500 IU/L) and, in a single instance, SGPT was greater than 2,000 IU/L. The overall rate of occurrences of elevated liver enzymes and elevations to 3 times the upper limit of normal, however, did not significantly differ from the rate of liver enzyme abnormalities in placebo-treated patients. All abnormalities were reversible after discontinuation of Nizatidine. Since market introduction, hepatitis and jaundice have been reported. Rare cases of cholestatic or mixed hepatocellular and cholestatic injury with jaundice have been reported with reversal of the abnormalities after discontinuation of Nizatidine.

➤ SHOWN IN PRODUCT IDENTIFICATION GUIDE

Cardiovascular: In clinical pharmacology studies, short episodes of asymptomatic ventricular tachycardia occurred in 2 individuals administered Nizatidine and in 3 untreated subjects.

CNS: Rare cases of reversible mental confusion have been reported.

Endocrine: Clinical pharmacology studies and controlled clinical trials showed no evidence of antiandrogenic activity due to Nizatidine Impotence and decreased libido were reported with similar frequency by patients who received Nizatidine and by those given placebo. Rare reports of gynecomastia occurred.

Hematologic: Anemia was reported significantly more frequently in Nizatidine- than in placebo-treated patients. Fatal thrombocytopenia was reported in a patient who was treated with Nizatidine and another H_2-receptor antagonist. On previous occasions, this patient had experienced thrombocytopenia while taking other drugs. Rare cases of thrombocytopenic purpura have been reported.

Integumental: Sweating and urticaria were reported significantly more frequently in Nizatidine- than in placebo-treated patients. Rash and exfoliative dermatitis were also reported.

Hypersensitivity: As with other H_2-receptor antagonists, rare cases of anaphylaxis following administration of Nizatidine have been reported. Rare episodes of hypersensitivity reactions (eg, bronchospasm, laryngeal edema, rash, and eosinophilia) have been reported.

Other: Hyperuricemia unassociated with gout or nephrolithiasis was reported. Eosinophilia, fever, and nausea related to Nizatidine administration have been reported.

OVERDOSAGE

Overdoses of Nizatidine have been reported rarely. The following is provided to serve as a guide should such an overdose be encountered.

Signs and Symptoms: There is little clinical experience with overdosage of Nizatidine in humans. Test animals that received large doses of Nizatidine have exhibited cholinergic-type effects, including lacrimation, salivation, emesis, miosis, and diarrhea. Single oral doses of 800 mg/kg in dogs and of 1,200 mg/kg in monkeys were not lethal. Intravenous median lethal doses in the rat and mouse were 301 mg/kg and 232 mg/kg respectively.

Treatment: To obtain up-to-date information about the treatment of overdose, a good resource is your certified Regional Poison Control Center. Telephone numbers of certified poison control centers are listed in the *Physicians' Desk Reference (PDR)*. In managing overdosage, consider the possibility of multiple drug overdoses, interaction among drugs, and unusual drug kinetics in your patient.

If overdosage occurs, use of activated charcoal, emesis, or lavage should be considered along with clinical monitoring and supportive therapy. The ability of hemodialysis to remove Nizatidine from the body has not been conclusively demonstrated; however, due to its large volume of distribution, Nizatidine is not expected to be efficiently removed from the body by this method.

DOSAGE AND ADMINISTRATION

Active Duodenal Ulcer: The recommended oral dosage for adults is 300 mg once daily at bedtime. An alternative dosage regimen is 150 mg twice daily

Maintenance of Healed Duodenal Ulcer: The recommended oral dosage for adults is 150 mg once daily at bedtime.

Gastroesophageal Reflux Disease: The recommended oral dosage in adults for the treatment of erosions, ulcerations, and associated heartburn is 150 mg twice daily.

Dosage Adjustment for Patients With Moderate to Severe Renal Insufficiency: The dose for patients with renal dysfunction should be reduced as follows:

Active Duodenal Ulcer or Gerd	
Ccr	Dose
20-50 mL/min	150 mg daily
< 20 mL/min	150 mg every other day
Maintenance Therapy	
Ccr	Dose
20-50 mL/min	150 mg every other day
< 20 mL/min	150 mg every 3 days

Some elderly patients may have creatinine clearance of less than 50 mL/min, and, based on pharmacokinetic data in patients with renal impairment, the dose for such patients should be reduced accordingly. The clinical effects of this dosage reduction in patients with renal failure have not been evaluated.

Store at controlled room temperature, 59° to 86°F (15° to 30°C).

HOW SUPPLIED
CAPSULE: 150 MG

BRAND/MANUFACTURER	NDC	SIZE	AWP
○ BRAND			
➤ AXID PULVULES: Lilly	00002-3144-60	60s	$90.50
	00002-3144-33	100s ud	$155.20
	00002-3144-82	620s	$950.95

CAPSULE: 300 MG

BRAND/MANUFACTURER	NDC	SIZE	AWP
○ BRAND			
➤ AXID PULVULES: Lilly	00002-3145-30	30s	$87.55

Nizoral *SEE* KETOCONAZOLE, ORAL *AND* KETOCONAZOLE, TOPICAL

Nolamine *SEE* CHLORPHENIRAMINE MALEATE/PHENINDAMINE TARTRATE/PHENYLPROPANOLAMINE HYDROCHLORIDE

Nolvadex *SEE* TAMOXIFEN CITRATE

Norcuron *SEE* VECURONIUM BROMIDE

Nordette *SEE* ETHINYL ESTRADIOL WITH LEVONORGESTREL

Norepinephrine Bitartrate

DESCRIPTION

Norepinephrine (sometimes referred to as *1-arterenol/Levarterenol* or *1-norepinephrine*) is a sympathomimetic amine which differs from epinephrine by the absence of a methyl group on the nitrogen atom.

Norepinephrine Bitartrate is (−)-α-(aminomethyl)-3,4-dihydroxybenzyl alcohol tartrate (1:1) (salt) monohydrate.

Norepinephrine Bitartrate is supplied in sterile aqueous solution in the form of the bitartrate salt to be administered by intravenous infusion following dilution. Norepinephrine is sparingly soluble in water, very slightly soluble in alcohol and ether, and readily soluble in acids. Each mL of Norepinephrine Bitartrate injection contains the equivalent of 1 mg base of Norepinephrine Bitartrate sodium chloride for isotonicity, and not more than 2 mg of sodium metabisulfite as an antioxidant. It has a pH of 3 to 4.5. The air in the ampuls has been displaced by nitrogen gas.

Following is its chemical structure:

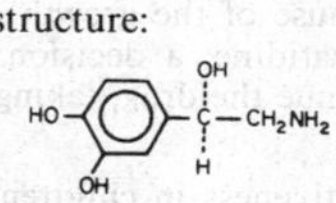

CLINICAL PHARMACOLOGY

Norepinephrine Bitartrate functions as a peripheral vasoconstrictor (alpha-adrenergic action) and as an inotropic stimulator of the heart and dilator of coronary arteries (beta-adrenergic action).

INDICATIONS AND USAGE

For blood pressure control in certain acute hypotensive states (eg. pheochromocytomectomy, sympathectomy, poliomyelitis, spinal anesthesia, myocardial infarction, septicemia, blood transfusion, and drug reactions).

As an adjunct in the treatment of cardiac arrest and profound hypotension.

CONTRAINDICATIONS

Norepinephrine Bitartrate should not be given to patients who are hypotensive from blood volume deficits except as an emergency measure to maintain coronary and cerebral artery perfusion until blood volume replacement therapy can be completed. If Norepinephrine Bitartrate is continuously administered to maintain blood pressure in the absence of blood volume replacement, the following may occur: severe peripheral and visceral vasoconstriction, decreased renal perfusion and urine output, poor systemic blood flow despite "normal" blood pressure, tissue hypoxia, and lactate acidosis.

Norepinephrine Bitartrate should also not be given to patients with mesenteric or peripheral vascular thrombosis (because of the risk of increasing ischemia and extending the area of infarction) unless, in the opinion of the attending physician, the administration of Norepinephrine Bitartrate is necessary as a life-saving procedure.

Cyclopropane and halothane anesthetics increase cardiac autonomic irritability and therefore seem to sensitize the myocardium to the action of intravenously administered epinephrine or norepinephrine. Hence, the use of Norepinephrine Bitartrate during cyclopropane and halothane anesthesia is generally considered contraindicated because of the risk of producing ventricular tachycardia or fibrillation.

◆ RATED THERAPEUTICALLY EQUIVALENT; ◇ THERAPEUTIC EQUIVALENCE UNCONFIRMED; ○ UNRATED

The same type of cardiac arrhythmias may result from the use of Norepinephrine Bitratrate in patients with profound hypoxia or hypercarbia.

WARNINGS

Norepinephrine Bitratrate should be used with extreme caution in patients receiving monoamine oxidase inhibitors (MAOI) or antidepressants of the triptyline or imipramine types, because severe, prolonged hypertension may result.

Norepinephrine Bitartrate Injection contains sodium metabisulfite, a sulfite that may cause allergic-type reactions including anaphylactic symptoms and life-threatening or less severe asthmatic episodes in certain susceptible people. The overall prevalence of sulfite sensitivity in the general population is unknown. Sulfite sensitivity is seen more frequently in asthmatic than in nonasthmatic people.

PRECAUTIONS
GENERAL
Avoid Hypertension: Because of the potency of Norepinephrine Bitartrate and because of varying response to pressor substances, the possibility always exists that dangerously high blood pressure may be produced with overdoses of this pressor agent. It is desirable, therefore, to record the blood pressure every two minutes from the time administration is started until the desired blood pressure is obtained, then every five minutes if administration is to be continued.

The rate of flow must be watched constantly, and the patient should never be left unattended while receiving Norepinephrine Bitartrate. Headache may be a symptom of hypertension due to overdosage.

Site of Infusion: Whenever possible, infusions of Norepinephrine Bitartrate should be given into a large vein, particularly an antecubital vein because, when administered into this vein, the risk of necrosis of the overlying skin from prolonged vasoconstriction is apparently very slight. Some authors have indicated that the femoral vein is also an acceptable route of administration. A catheter tie-in technique should be avoided, if possible, since the obstruction to blood flow around the tubing may cause stasis and increased local concentration of the drug. Occlusive vascular diseases (for example, atherosclerosis, arteriosclerosis, diabetic endarteritis. Buerger's disease) are more likely to occur in the lower than in the upper extremity. Therefore, one should avoid the veins of the leg in elderly patients or in those suffering from such disorders. Gangrene has been reported in a lower extremity when infusions of Norepinephrine Bitartrate were given in an ankle vein.

Extravasation: The infusion site should be checked frequently for free flow. Care should be taken to avoid extravasation of Norepinephrine Bitartrate into the tissues, as local necrosis might ensue due to the vasoconstrictive action of the drug. *Blanching along the course of the infused vein,* sometimes without obvious extravasation, has been attributed to vasa vasorum constriction with increased permeability of the vein wall, permitting some leakage.

This also may progress on rare occasions to superficial slough, particularly during infusion into leg veins in elderly patients or in those suffering from obliterative vascular disease. Hence, if blanching occurs, consideration should be given to the advisability of changing the infusion site at intervals to allow the effects of local vasoconstriction to subside.

IMPORTANT—ANTIDOTE FOR EXTRAVASATION ISCHEMIA: TO PREVENT SLOUGHING AND NECROSIS IN AREAS IN WHICH EXTRAVASATION HAS TAKEN PLACE, THE AREA SHOULD BE INFILTRATED AS SOON AS POSSIBLE WITH 10 ML TO 15 ML OF SALINE SOLUTION CONTAINING FROM 5 MG TO 10 MG OF PHENTOLAMINE, AN ADRENERGIC BLOCKING AGENT. A SYRINGE WITH A FINE HYPODERMIC NEEDLE SHOULD BE USED, WITH THE SOLUTION BEING INFILTRATED LIBERALLY THROUGHOUT THE AREA, WHICH IS EASILY IDENTIFIED BY ITS COLD, HARD, AND PALLID APPEARANCE. SYMPATHETIC BLOCKADE WITH PHENTOLAMINE CAUSES IMMEDIATE AND CONSPICUOUS LOCAL HYPEREMIC CHANGES IF THE AREA IS INFILTRATED WITHIN 12 HOURS. THEREFORE, *PHENTOLAMINE SHOULD BE GIVEN AS SOON AS POSSIBLE* AFTER THE EXTRAVASATION IS NOTED.

Drug Interactions: Cyclopropane and halothane anesthetics increase cardiac automatic irritability and therefore seem to sensitize the myocardium to the action of intravenously administered epinephrine or norepinephrine. Hence, the use of Norepinephrine Bitartrate brand of norepinephrine bitartrate injection, during cyclopropane and halothane anesthesia is generally considered contraindicated because of the risk of producing ventricular tachycardia or fibrillation. The same type of cardiac arrhythmias may result from the use of Norepinephrine Bitartrate in patients with profound hypoxia or hypercarbia.

Norepinephrine Bitratrate should be used with extreme caution in patients receiving monoamine oxidase inhibitors (MAOI) or antidepressants of the triptyline or imipramine types, because severe, prolonged hypertension may result.

Carcinogenesis, Mutagenesis, Impairment of Fertility: Studies have not been performed.

Pregnancy Category C: Animal reproduction studies have not been conducted with Norepinephrine Bitartrate. It is also not known whether Norepinephrine Bitartrate can cause fetal harm when administered to a pregnant woman or can affect reproduction capacity. Norepinephrine Bitartrate should be given to a pregnant woman only if clearly needed.

Nursing Mothers: It is not known whether this drug is excreted in human milk. Because many drugs are excreted in human milk, caution should be exercised when Norepinephrine Bitartrate is administered to a nursing woman.

Pediatric Use: Safety and effectiveness in children have not been established.

ADVERSE REACTIONS
The following reactions can occur:
Body As A Whole: Ischemic injury due to potent vasoconstrictor action and tissue hypoxia.

Cardiovascular System: Bradycardia, probably as a reflex result of a rise in blood pressure, arrhythmias.

Nervous System: Anxiety, transient headache.

Respiratory System: Respiratory difficulty.

Skin and Appendages: Extravasation necrosis at injection site.

Prolonged administration of any potent vasopressor may result in plasma volume depletion which should be continuously corrected by appropriate fluid and electrolyte replacement therapy. If plasma volumes are not corrected hypotension may recur when Norepinephrine Bitartrate is discontinued, or blood pressure may be maintained at the risk of severe peripheral and visceral vasoconstriction (eg, decreased renal perfusion) with diminution in blood flow and tissue perfusion with subsequent tissue hypoxia and lactic acidosis and possible ischemic injury. Gangrene of extremities has been rarely reported.

Overdoses or conventional doses in hypersensitive persons (eg, hyperthyroid patients) cause severe hypertension with violent headache, photophobia, stabbing retrosternal pain, pallor intense sweating, and vomiting.

OVERDOSAGE
Overdosage with Norepinephrine Bitartrate may result in headache, severe hypertension, reflex bradycardia, marked increase in peripheral resistance, and decreased cardiac output. In case of accidental overdosage, as evidenced by excessive blood pressure elevation, discontinue Norepinephrine Bitartrate until the condition of the patient stabilizes.

DOSAGE AND ADMINISTRATION
Norepinephrine Bitartrate Injection is a concentrated, potent drug which must be diluted in dextrose containing solutions prior to infusion. An infusion of Norepinephrine Bitartrate should be given into a large vein (see *"Precautions"*).

RESTORATION OF BLOOD PRESSURE IN ACUTE HYPOTENSIVE STATES
Blood volume depletion should always be corrected as fully as possible before any vasopressor is administered. When, as an emergency measure, intra-aortic pressures must be maintained to prevent cerebral or coronary artery ischemia, Norepinephrine Bitartrate injection can be administered before and concurrently with blood volume replacement.

Diluent: Norepinephrine Bitartrate should be diluted in 5 percent dextrose injection or 5 percent dextrose and sodium chloride injections. These dextrose containing fluids are protection against significant loss of potency due to oxidation. *Administration in saline solution alone is not recommended.* Whole blood or plasma, if indicated to increase blood volume, should be administered separately (for example, by use of a Y-tube and individual containers if given simultaneously).

Average Dosage: Add a 4 mL ampul (4 mg) of Norepinephrine Bitartrate to 1000 mL of a 5 percent dextrose containing solution. Each 1 mL of this dilution contains 4 µg of the base of Norepinephrine Bitartrate. Give this solution by intravenous infusion. Insert a plastic intravenous catheter through a suitable bore needle well advanced centrally into the vein and securely fixed with adhesive tape, avoiding, if possible, a catheter tie-in technique as this promotes stasis. An IV drip chamber or other suitable metering device is essential to permit an accurate estimation of the rate of flow in drops per minute. After observing the response to an initial dose of 2 mL to 3 mL (from 8 µg to 12 µg of base) per minute, adjust the rate of flow to establish and maintain a low normal blood pressure (usually 80 mm Hg to 100 mm Hg systolic) sufficient to maintain the circulation to vital organs. In previously hypertensive patients, it is recommended that the blood pressure should be raised no higher than 40 mm Hg below the preexisting systolic pressure. The average maintenance dose ranges from 0.5 mL to 1 mL per minute (from 2 µg to 4 µg of base).

High Dosage: Great individual variation occurs in the dose required to attain and maintain an adequate blood pressure. In all cases, dosage of Norepinephrine Bitartrate should be titrated according to the response of the patient. Occasionally much larger or even enormous daily doses (as high as 68 mg base or 17 ampuls) may be necessary if the patient remains hypotensive, but occult blood volume depletion should always be suspected and corrected when present. Central venous pressure monitoring is usually helpful in detecting and treating this situation.

Fluid Intake: The degree of dilution depends on clinical fluid volume requirements. If large volumes of fluid (dextrose) are needed at a flow rate that would involve an excessive dose of the pressor agent per unit of time, a solution more dilute than 4 µg per mL should be used. On the other hand, when large volumes of fluid are clinically undesirable, a concentration greater than 4 µg per mL may be necessary.

Duration of Therapy: The infusion should be continued until adequate blood pressure and tissue perfusion are maintained without therapy. Infusions of Norepinephrine Bitartrate should be reduced gradually, avoiding abrupt withdrawal. In some of the reported cases of vascular collapse due to acute myocardial infarction, treatment was required for up to six days.

ADJUNCTIVE TREATMENT IN CARDIAC ARREST
Infusions of Norepinephrine Bitartrate are usually administered intravenously during cardiac resuscitation to restore and maintain an adequate blood pressure after an effective heartbeat and ventilation have been established by other means. [The powerful beta-adrenergic stimulating action of Norepinephrine Bitartrate is also thought to increase the strength and effectiveness of systolic contractions once they occur.]

Average Dosage: To maintain systemic blood pressure during the management of cardiac arrest, Norepinephrine Bitartrate injection is used in the same manner as described under *"Restoration of Blood Pressure in Acute Hypotensive States."*

Parenteral drug products should be inspected visually for particulate matter and discoloration prior to use, whenever solution and container permit.

Store at room temperature. Protect from light.

HOW SUPPLIED
INJECTION: 1 MG/ML

BRAND/MANUFACTURER	NDC	SIZE	AWP
○ **BRAND**			
LEVOPHED BITARTRATE: Sanofi Winthrop	00024-1123-02	4 ml 10s	$109.52
○ **GENERICS**			
Abbott Hosp	00074-7041-01	4 ml 10s	$145.35

Norethindrone

DESCRIPTION
The chemical name for Norethindrone is 17-hydroxy-19-nor-17α-pregn-4-en-20-yn-3-one, for ethinyl estradiol is 19-nor-17α-pregna-1,3,5(10)-trien-20-yne-3,17-diol, and for mestranol is 3-methoxy-19-nor-17α-pregna-1,3,5(10)-trien-20-yn-17-ol.

Following is its chemical structure:

CLINICAL PHARMACOLOGY
The primary mechanism through which Norethindrone prevents conception is not known, but progestogen-only contraceptives are known to alter the cervical mucus, exert a progestational effect on the endometrium, interfering with implantation, and, in some patients, suppress ovulation.

INDICATIONS AND USAGE
Norethindrone is indicated for the prevention of pregnancy in women who elect to use this product as a method of contraception.

Oral contraceptives are highly effective. Table 1 lists the typical accidental pregnancy rates for users of combination oral contraceptives and other methods of contraception. The efficacy of these contraceptive methods, except sterilization, depends upon the reliability with which they are used. Correct and consistent use of methods can result in lower failure rates.

Table 1
LOWEST EXPECTED AND TYPICAL FAILURE RATES DURING THE FIRST YEAR OF CONTINUOUS USE OF A METHOD

% of Women Experiencing an Accidental Pregnancy in the First Year of Continuous Use		
Method	Lowest Expected*	Typical**
(No contraception)	(89)	(89)
Oral contraceptives		3
combined	0.1	N/A***
progestin only	0.5	N/A***
Diaphragm with		
spermicidal	3	18
cream or jelly		
Spermicides alone (foam,		
creams, jellies and		
vaginal suppositories)	3	21
Vaginal sponge		
nulliparous	5	18
multiparous	>8	>28
IUD (medicated)	1	6#
Condom without		
spermicides	2	12
Periodic abstinence		
(all methods)	2-10	20

% of Women Experiencing an Accidental Pregnancy in the First Year of Continuous Use		
Method	Lowest Expected*	Typical**
Female sterilization	0.2	0.4
Male sterilization	0.1	0.15

* *The authors' best guess of the percentage of women expected to experience an accidental pregnancy among couples who initiate a method (not necessarily for the first time) and who use it consistently and correctly during the first year if they do not stop for any other reason.*

** *This term represents "typical" couples who initiate use of a method (not necessarily for the first time), who experience an accidental pregnancy during the first year if they do not stop use for any other reason.*

*** *N/A—Data not available.*

\# *Combined typical rate for both medicated and non-medicated IUD. The rate for medicated IUD alone is not available.*

CONTRAINDICATIONS
Oral contraceptives should not be used in women who currently have the following conditions:
- Thrombophlebitis or thromboembolic disorders
- A past history of deep vein thrombophlebitis or thromboembolic disorders
- Cerebral vascular or coronary artery disease
- Cerebral vascular or coronary artery disease
- Known or suspected carcinoma of the breast
- Carcinoma of the endometrium or other known or suspected estrogen-dependent neoplasia
- Undiagnosed abnormal genital bleeding
- Cholestatic jaundice of pregnancy or jaundice with prior pill use
- Hepatic adenomas or carcinomas
- Known or suspected pregnancy

WARNINGS

CIGARETTE SMOKING INCREASES THE RISK OF SERIOUS CARDIOVASCULAR SIDE EFFECTS FROM ORAL CONTRACEPTIVE USE. THIS RISK INCREASES WITH AGE AND WITH HEAVY SMOKING (15 OR MORE CIGARETTES PER DAY) AND IS QUITE MARKED IN WOMEN OVER 35 YEARS OF AGE. WOMEN WHO USE ORAL CONTRACEPTIVES SHOULD BE STRONGLY ADVISED NOT TO SMOKE.

The use of oral contraceptives is associated with increased risks of several serious conditions including myocardial infarction, thromboembolism, stroke, hepatic neoplasia, and gallbladder disease, although the risk of serious morbidity or mortality is very small in healthy women without underlying risk factors. The risk of morbidity and mortality increases significantly in the presence of other underlying risk factors such as hypertension, hyperlipidemias, obesity and diabetes.

Practitioners prescribing oral contraceptives should be familiar with the following information relating to these risks.

The information contained in this package insert is principally based on studies carried out in patients who used oral contraceptives with higher formulations of estrogens and progestogens than those in common use today. The effect of long term use of the oral contraceptives with lower formulations of both estrogens and progestogens remains to be determined.

Throughout this labeling, epidemiological studies reported are of two types: retrospective or case control studies and prospective or cohort studies. Case control studies provide a measure of the relative risk of a disease, namely, a *ratio* of the incidence of a disease among oral contraceptive users to that among nonusers. The relative risk does not provide information on the actual clinical occurrence of a disease. Cohort studies provide a measure of attributable risk, which is the *difference* in the incidence of disease between oral contraceptive users and nonusers. The attributable risk does provide information about the actual occurrence of a disease in the population (adapted from refs. 2 and 3 with the author's permission). For further information, the reader is referred to a text on epidemiological methods.

1. THROMBOEMBOLIC DISORDERS AND OTHER VASCULAR PROBLEMS
a. Myocardial Infarction
An increased risk of myocardial infarction has been associated with oral contraceptive use. This risk is primarily in smokers or women with other underlying risk factors for coronary artery disease such as hypertension, hypercholesterolemia, morbid obesity, and diabetes. The relative risk of heart attack for current oral contraceptive users has been estimated to be two to six[4-19].

The risk is very low under the age of 30.

Smoking in combination with oral contraceptive use has been shown to contribute substantially to the incidence of myocardial infarctions in women in their mid-thirties or older with smoking accounting for the majority of excess cases[11]. Mortality rates associated with circulatory disease have been shown to increase substantially in smokers, especially in those 35 years of age and older among women who use oral contraceptives.

◆ RATED THERAPEUTICALLY EQUIVALENT; ◇ THERAPEUTIC EQUIVALENCE UNCONFIRMED; ○ UNRATED

CIRCULATORY DISEASE MORTALITY RATES PER 100,000
WOMAN-YEARS BY AGE, SMOKING STATUS
AND ORAL CONTRACEPTIVE USE

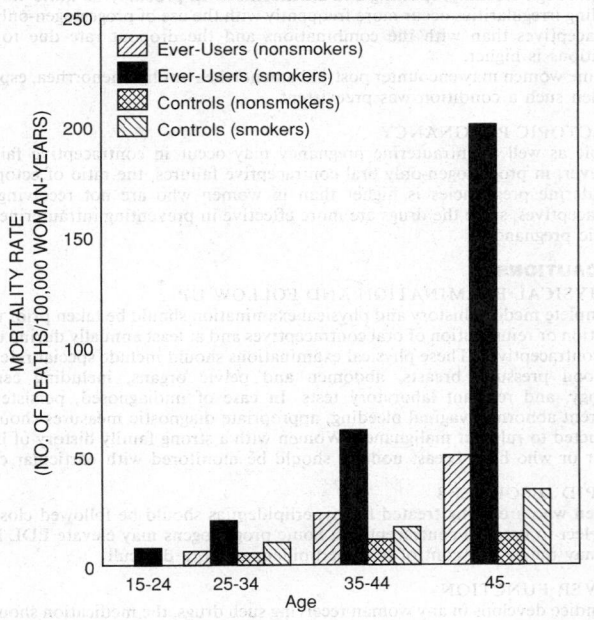

Table 2

(Adapted from P.M. Layde and V. Beral, ref. #12.)

Oral contraceptives may compound the effects of well-known risk factors, such as hypertension, diabetes, hyperlipidemias, age and obesity[13]. In particular, some progestogens are known to decrease HDL cholesterol and cause glucose intolerance, while estrogens may create a state of hyperinsulinism[14-18]. Oral contraceptives have been shown to increase blood pressure among users (see section 9 in "Warnings"). Similar effects on risk factors have been associated with an increased risk of heart disease. Oral contraceptives must be used with caution in women with cardiovascular disease risk factors.

b. Thromboembolism

An increased risk of thromboembolic and thrombotic disease associated with the use of oral contraceptives is well established. Case control studies have found the relative risk of users compared to non-users to be 3 for the first episode of superficial venous thrombosis, 4 to 11 for deep vein thrombosis or pulmonary embolism, and 1.5 to 6 for women with predisposing conditions for venous thromboembolic disease[2,3,18-24]. Cohort studies have shown the relative risk to be somewhat lower, about 3 for new cases and about 4.5 for new cases requiring hospitalization[25]. The risk of thromboembolic disease associated with oral contraceptives is not related to length of use and disappears after pill use is stopped[2].

A two- to four-fold increase in relative risk of post-operative thromboembolic complications has been reported with the use of oral contraceptives[9]. The relative risk of venous thrombosis in women who have predisposing conditions is twice that of women without such medical conditions[26]. If feasible, oral contraceptives should be discontinued at least four weeks prior to and for two weeks after elective surgery of a type associated with an increase in risk of thromboembolism and during and following prolonged immobilization. Since the immediate postpartum period is also associated with an increased risk of thromboembolism, oral contraceptives should be started no earlier than four weeks after delivery in women who elect not to breast feed.

c. Cerebrovascular diseases

Oral contraceptives have been shown to increase both the relative and attributable risks of cerebrovascular events (thrombotic and hemorrhagic strokes), although, in general, the risk is greatest among older (>35 years), hypertensive women who also smoke. Hypertension was found to be a risk factor for both users and non-users, for both types of strokes, and smoking interacted to increase the risk of stroke[27-29].

In a large study, the relative risk of thrombotic strokes has been shown to range from 3 for normotensive users to 14 for users with severe hypertension[30]. The relative risk of hemorrhagic stroke is reported to be 1.2 for non-smokers who used oral contraceptives, 2.6 for smokers who did not use oral contraceptives, 7.6 for smokers who used oral contraceptives, 1.8 for normotensive users and 25.7 for users with severe hypertension[30]. The attributable risk is also greater in older women[3].

d. Dose-related risk of vascular disease from oral contraceptives

A positive association has been observed between the amount of estrogen and progestogen in oral contraceptives and the risk of vascular disease[31-33]. A decline in serum high density lipoproteins (HDL) has been reported with many progestational agents[14-16]. A decline in serum high density lipoproteins has been associated with an increased incidence of ischemic heart disease. Because estrogens increase HDL cholesterol, the net effect of an oral contraceptive depends on a balance achieved between doses of estrogen and progestogen and the activity of the progestogen used in the contraceptive. The activity and amount of both hormones should be considered in the choice of an oral contraceptive.

Minimizing exposure to estrogen and progestogen is in keeping with good principles of therapeutics. For any particular estrogen/progestogen combination, the dosage regimen prescribed should be one which contains the least amount of estrogen and progestogen that is compatible with a low failure rate and the needs of the individual patient. New acceptors of oral contraceptive agents should be started on preparations containing 0.035 mg or less of estrogen.

e. Persistence of risk of vascular disease

There are two studies which have shown persistence of risk of vascular disease for ever-users of oral contraceptives. In a study in the United States, the risk of developing myocardial infarction after discontinuing oral contraceptives persists for at least 9 years for women 40-49 years who had used oral contraceptives for five or more years, but this increased risk was not demonstrated in other age groups[8]. In another study in Great Britain, the risk of developing cerebrovascular disease persisted for at least 6 years after discontinuation of oral contraceptives, although excess risk was very small[34]. However, both studies were performed with oral contraceptive formulations containing 50 micrograms or higher of estrogens.

2. ESTIMATES OF MORTALITY FROM CONTRACEPTIVE USE

One study gathered data from a variety of sources which have estimated the mortality rate associated with different methods of contraception at different ages (Table 3). These estimates include the combined risk of death associated with contraceptive methods plus the risk attributable to pregnancy in the event of method failure. Each method of contraception has its specific benefits and risks. The study concluded that with the exception of oral contraceptive users 35 and older who smoke and 40 and older who do not smoke, mortality associated with all methods of birth control is low and below that associated with childbirth. The observation of an increase in risk of mortality with age for oral contraceptive users is based on data gathered in the 1970's (35). Current clinical recommendation involves the use of lower estrogen dose formulations and a careful consideration of risk factors. In 1989, the Fertility and Maternal Health Drugs Advisory Committee was asked to review the use of oral contraceptives in women 40 years of age and over. The Committee concluded that although cardiovascular disease risks may be increased with oral contraceptive use after age 40 in healthy non-smoking women (even with the newer low-dose formulations), there are also greater potential health risks associated with pregnancy in older women and with the alternative surgical and medical procedures which may be necessary if such women do not have access to effective and acceptable means of contraception. The Committee recommended that the benefits of low-dose oral contraceptive use by healthy non-smoking women over 40 may outweigh the possible risks.

Of course, older women, as all women who take oral contraceptives, should take an oral contraceptive which contains the least amount of estrogen and progestogen that is compatible with a low failure rate and individual patient needs. (See related table).

Adapted from H.W. Ory, ref. #35.

3. CARCINOMA OF THE REPRODUCTIVE ORGANS

Numerous epidemiological studies have been performed on the incidence of breast, endometrial, ovarian and cervical cancer in women using oral contraceptives. While there are conflicting reports, most studies suggest that use of oral contraceptives is not associated with an overall increase in the risk of developing breast cancer. Some studies have reported an increased relative risk of developing breast cancer, particularly at a younger age. This increased relative risk appears to be related to duration of use[36-44, 79-89].

Some studies suggest that oral contraceptive use has been associated with an increase in the risk of cervical intraepithelial neoplasia in some populations of women[45-48]. However, there continues to be controversy about the extent to which such findings may be due to differences in sexual behavior and other factors.

4. HEPATIC NEOPLASIA

Benign hepatic adenomas are associated with oral contraceptive use, although the incidence of benign tumors is rare in the United States. Indirect calculations have estimated the attributable risk to be in the range of 3.3 cases/100,000 for users, a risk that increases after four or more years of use especially with oral contraceptives of higher dose[49]. Rupture of benign, hepatic adenomas may cause death through intra-abdominal hemorrhage[50-51].

Studies from Britain have shown an increased risk of developing hepatocellular carcinoma[52-54] in long-term (> 8 years) oral contraceptive users. However, these cancers are rare in the U.S. and the attributable risk (the excess incidence) of liver cancers in oral contraceptive users approaches less than one per million users.

5. OCULAR LESIONS

There have been clinical case reports of retinal thrombosis associated with the use of oral contraceptives. Oral contraceptives should be discontinued if there is unexplained partial or complete loss of vision; onset of proptosis or diplopia;

papilledema; or retinal vascular lesions. Appropriate diagnostic and therapeutic measures should be undertaken immediately.

6. ORAL CONTRACEPTIVE USE BEFORE OR DURING EARLY PREGNANCY

Extensive epidemiological studies have revealed no increased risk of birth defects in women who have used oral contraceptives prior to pregnancy[56,57]. The majority of recent studies also do not indicate a teratogenic effect, particularly in so far as cardiac anomalies and limb reduction defects are concerned[55,56,58,59], when taken inadvertently during early pregnancy.

The administration of oral contraceptives to induce withdrawal bleeding should not be used as a test for pregnancy. Oral contraceptives should not be used during pregnancy to treat threatened or habitual abortion.

It is recommended that for any patient who has missed two consecutive periods (or after 45 days from the last menstrual period if the progestogen-only oral contraceptives are used), pregnancy should be ruled out before continuing oral contraceptive use. If the patient has not adhered to the prescribed schedule, the possibility of pregnancy should be considered at the time of the first missed period or upon missing one Norethindrone tablet. Oral contraceptive use should be discontinued until pregnancy is ruled out.

7. GALLBLADDER DISEASE

Earlier studies have reported an increased lifetime relative risk of gallbladder surgery in users of oral contraceptives and estrogens[60-61]. More recent studies, however, have shown that the relative risk of developing gallbladder disease among oral contraceptive users may be minimal[62-64]. The recent findings of minimal risk may be related to the use of oral contraceptive formulations containing lower hormonal doses of estrogens and progestogens.

8. CARBOHYDRATE AND LIPID METABOLIC EFFECTS

Oral contraceptives have been shown to cause a decrease in glucose tolerance in a significant percentage of users[17]. This effect has been shown to be directly related to estrogen dose[65]. Progestogens increase insulin secretion and create insulin resistance, this effect varying with different progestational agents[17,66]. However, in the non-diabetic woman, oral contraceptives appear to have no effect on fasting blood glucose[67]. Because of these demonstrated effects, prediabetic and diabetic women in particular should be carefully monitored while taking oral contraceptives.

A small proportion of women will have persistent hypertriglyceridemia while on the pill. As discussed earlier (see "*Warnings*" 1a and 1d), changes in serum triglycerides and lipoprotein levels have been reported in oral contraceptive users.

9. ELEVATED BLOOD PRESSURE

An increase in blood pressure has been reported in women taking oral contraceptives[68] and this increase is more likely in older oral contraceptives users[69] and with extended duration of use[81]. Data from the Royal College of General Practitioners[12] and subsequent randomized trials have shown that the incidence of hypertension increases with increasing progestational activity.

Women with a history of hypertension or hypertension-related diseases, or renal disease[70] should be encouraged to use another method of contraception. If women elect to use oral contraceptives, they should be monitored closely and if significant elevation of blood pressure occurs, oral contraceptives should be discontinued. For most women, elevated blood pressure will return to normal after stopping oral contraceptives, and there is no difference in the occurrence of hypertension between former and never users[66-71].

10. HEADACHE

The onset or exacerbation of migraine or development of headache with a new pattern which is recurrent, persistent or severe requires discontinuation of oral contraceptives and evaluation of the cause.

11. BLEEDING IRREGULARITIES

Breakthrough bleeding and spotting are sometimes encountered in patients on oral contraceptives, especially during the first three months of use. Non-hormonal causes should be considered and adequate diagnostic measures taken to rule out malignancy or pregnancy in the event of breakthrough bleeding, as in the case of any abnormal vaginal bleeding. If pathology has been excluded, time or a change to another formulation may solve the problem. In the event of amenorrhea, pregnancy should be ruled out.

An alteration in menstrual patterns is likely to occur in women using progestogen-only contraceptives. The amount and duration of flow, cycle length, breakthrough bleeding, spotting and amenorrhea will probably be quite variable. Bleeding irregularities occur more frequently with the use of progestogen-only oral contraceptives than with the combinations and the dropout rate due to such conditions is higher.

Some women may encounter post-pill amenorrhea or oligomenorrhea, especially when such a condition was preexistent.

12. ECTOPIC PREGNANCY

Ectopic as well as intrauterine pregnancy may occur in contraceptive failures. However, in progestogen-only oral contraceptive failures, the ratio of ectopic to intrauterine pregnancies is higher than in women who are not receiving oral contraceptives, since the drugs are more effective in preventing intrauterine than ectopic pregnancies.

PRECAUTIONS

1. PHYSICAL EXAMINATION AND FOLLOW UP

A complete medical history and physical examination should be taken prior to the initiation or reinstitution of oral contraceptives and at least annually during use of oral contraceptives. These physical examinations should include special reference to blood pressure, breasts, abdomen and pelvic organs, including cervical cytology, and relevant laboratory tests. In case of undiagnosed, persistent or recurrent abnormal vaginal bleeding, appropriate diagnostic measures should be conducted to rule out malignancy. Women with a strong family history of breast cancer or who have breast nodules should be monitored with particular care.

2. LIPID DISORDERS

Women who are being treated for hyperlipidemias should be followed closely if they elect to use oral contraceptives. Some progestogens may elevate LDL levels and may render the control of hyperlipidemias more difficult.

3. LIVER FUNCTION

If jaundice develops in any woman receiving such drugs, the medication should be discontinued. Steroid hormones may be poorly metabolized in patients with impaired liver function.

4. FLUID RETENTION

Oral contraceptives may cause some degree of fluid retention. They should be prescribed with caution, and only with careful monitoring, in patients with conditions which might be aggravated by fluid retention.

5. EMOTIONAL DISORDERS

Women with a history of depression should be carefully observed and the drug discontinued if depression recurs to a serious degree.

6. CONTACT LENSES

Contact lens wearers who develop visual changes or changes in lens tolerance should be assessed by an ophthalmologist.

7. DRUG INTERACTIONS

Reduced efficacy and increased incidence of breakthrough bleeding and menstrual irregularities have been associated with concomitant use of rifampin. A similar association, though less marked, has been suggested with barbiturates, phenylbutazone, phenytoin sodium, and possibly with griseofulvin, ampicillin and tetracyclines[72].

8. INTERACTIONS WITH LABORATORY TESTS

Certain endocrine and liver function tests and blood components may be affected by oral contraceptives:

a. Increased prothrombin and factors VII, VIII, IX, and X; decreased antithrombin 3; increased norepinephrine-induced platelet aggregability.

b. Increased thyroid binding globulin (TBG) leading to increased circulating total thyroid hormone, as measured by protein-bound iodine (PBI), T4 by column or

Table 3
ANNUAL NUMBER OF BIRTH-RELATED OR METHOD-RELATED DEATHS ASSOCIATED WITH CONTROL OF FERTILITY PER 100,000 NON-STERILE WOMEN, BY FERTILITY CONTROL METHOD ACCORDING TO AGE

Method of control and outcome	15-19	20-24	25-29	30-34	35-39	40-44
No fertility control methods*	7.0	7.4	9.1	14.8	25.7	28.2
Oral contraceptives non-smoker**	0.3	0.5	0.9	1.9	13.8	31.6
Oral contraceptives smoker**	2.2	3.4	6.6	13.5	51.1	117.2
IUD**	0.8	0.8	1.0	1.0	1.4	1.4
Condom*	1.1	1.6	0.7	0.2	0.3	0.4
Diaphragm/ spermicide*	1.9	1.2	1.2	1.3	2.2	2.8
Periodic abstinence*	2.5	1.6	1.6	1.7	2.9	3.6

* *Deaths are birth-related*
** *Deaths are method-related*

by radio-immunoassay. Free T3 resin uptake is decreased, reflecting the elevated TBG, free T4 concentration is unaltered
c. Other binding proteins may be elevated in serum.
d. Sex-binding globulins are increased and result in elevated levels of total circulating sex steroids and corticoids; however, free or biologically active levels remain unchanged.
e. Triglycerides may be increased.
f. Glucose tolerance may be decreased.
g. Serum folate levels may be depressed by oral contraceptive therapy. This may be of clinical significance if a woman becomes pregnant shortly after discontinuing oral contraceptives.

9. CARCINOGENESIS
See *"Warnings"* section.

10. PREGNANCY
Pregnancy Category X. See *"Contraindications"* and *"Warnings"* sections.

11 NURSING MOTHERS
Small amounts of oral contraceptives steroids have been identified in the milk of nursing mothers and a few adverse effects on the child have been reported, including jaundice and breast enlargement. In addition, oral contraceptives given in the postpartum period may interfere with lactation by decreasing the quantity and quality of breast milk. If possible, the nursing mother should be advised not to use oral contraceptives but to use other forms of contraception until she has completely weaned her child.

INFORMATION FOR THE PATIENT
See patient labeling supplied with this product.

ADVERSE REACTIONS
An increased risk of the following serious adverse reactions has been associated with the use of oral contraceptives (see *"Warnings"* section).
- Thrombophlebitis and venous thrombosis with or without embolism
- Arterial thromboembolism
- Pulmonary embolism
- Myocardial infarction
- Cerebral hemorrhage
- Cerebral thrombosis
- Hypertension
- Gallbladder disease
- Hepatic adenomas or benign liver tumors

The following adverse reactions have been reported in patients receiving oral contraceptives and are believed to be drug-related:
- Nausea
- Vomiting
- Gastrointestinal symptoms (such as abdominal cramps and bloating)
- Breakthrough bleeding
- Spotting
- Change in menstrual flow
- Amenorrhea
- Temporary infertility after discontinuation of treatment
- Edema
- Melasma which may persist
- Breast changes: tenderness, enlargement, secretion
- Change in weight (increase or decrease)
- Change in cervical erosion and secretion
- Diminution in lactation when given immediately postpartum
- Cholestatic jaundice
- Migraine
- Rash (allergic)
- Mental depression
- Reduced tolerance to carbohydrates
- Vaginal candidiasis
- Change in corneal curvature (steepening)
- Intolerance to contact lenses

The following adverse reactions have been reported in users of oral contraceptives and the association has been neither confirmed nor refuted:
- Premenstrual syndrome
- Cataracts
- Changes in appetite
- Cystitis-like syndrome
- Headache
- Nervousness
- Dizziness
- Hirsutism
- Loss of scalp hair
- Erythema multiforme
- Erythema nodosum
- Hemorrhagic eruption
- Vaginitis
- Porphyria
- Impaired renal function
- Hemolytic uremic syndrome
- Acne
- Changes in libido
- Colitis

OVERDOSAGE
Serious ill effects have not been reported following acute ingestion of large doses of oral contraceptives by young children. Overdosage may cause nausea, and withdrawal bleeding may occur in females.

DOSAGE AND ADMINISTRATION
To achieve maximum contraceptive effectiveness, Norethindrone must be taken exactly as directed and at intervals not exceeding 24 hours.

Norethindrone is administered on a continuous daily dosage regimen starting on the first day of menstruation, i.e., one tablet each day, every day of the year. Tablets should be taken at the same time each day and continued daily. The patient should be advised that if prolonged bleeding occurs, she should consult her physician.

The use of Norethindrone for contraception may be initiated postpartum (see *"Warnings"* section). When Norethindrone is administered during the postpartum period, the increased risk of thromboembolic disease associated with the postpartum period must be considered. (See *"Contraindications"* and *"Warnings"* concerning thromboembolic disease).

If the patient misses one tablet, Norethindrone should be discontinued immediately and a method of nonhormonal contraception should be used until menses has appeared or pregnancy has been excluded.

Alternatively, if the patient has taken the tablets correctly, and if menses does not appear when expected, a nonhormonal method of contraception should be substituted until an appropriate diagnostic procedure is performed to rule out pregnancy.

ALL ORAL CONTRACEPTIVES
Breakthrough bleeding, spotting, and amenorrhea are frequent reasons for patients discontinuing oral contraceptives. In breakthrough bleeding, as in all cases of irregular bleeding from the vagina, nonfunctional causes should be borne in mind. In undiagnosed persistent or recurrent abnormal bleeding from the vagina, adequate diagnostic measures are indicated to rule out pregnancy or malignancy. If pathology has been excluded, time or a change to another formulation may solve the problem. Changing to an oral contraceptive with a higher estrogen content, while potentially useful in minimizing menstrual irregularity, should be done only if necessary since this may increase the risk of thromboembolic disease.

Use of oral contraceptives in the event of a missed menstrual period:
1. If the patient has not adhered to the prescribed schedule, the possibility of pregnancy should be considered at the time of the first missed period (or upon missing one Norethindrone tablet) and oral contraceptive use should be discontinued until pregnancy is ruled out.
2. If the patient has adhered to the prescribed regimen and misses two consecutive periods (or after 45 days from the last menstrual period if the progestogen-only oral contraceptives are used), pregnancy should be ruled out before continuing oral contraceptive use.

REFERENCES
1. Reproduced with permission of the Population Council from J. Trussell and K. Kost: Contraceptive failure in the United States: A critical review of the literature. Studies in Family Planning, 18 (5), September-October 1987. 2. Stadel BV. Oral contraceptives and cardiovascular disease. (Pt. 1). *N Engl J Med* 1981; 305:612-618. 3. Stadel BV. Oral contraceptives and cardiovascular disease. (Pt. 2). *N Engl J Med* 1981; 305:672-677. 4. Adam SA, Thorogood M. Oral contraception and myocardial infarction revisited: the effects of new preparations and prescribing patterns. *Br J Obstet Gynaecol* 1981; 88:838-845. 5. Mann JI, Inman WH. Oral contraceptives and death from myocardial infarction. *Br Med J* 1975; 2(5965):245-248. 6. Mann JI, Vessey MP, Thorogood M, Doll R. Myocardial infarction in young women with special reference to oral contraceptive practice. *Br Med J* 1975; 2(5956):241-245. 7. Royal College of General Practitioners' Oral Contraception Study: Further analyses of mortality in oral contraceptive users. *Lancet* 1981; 1:541-546. 8. Slone D, Shapiro S, Kaufman DW, Rosenberg L, Miettinen OS, Stolley PD. Risk of myocardial infarction in relation to current and discontinued use of oral contraceptives. *N Engl J Med* 1981; 305:420-424. 9. Vessey MP. Female hormones and vascular disease-an epidemiological overview. *Br J Fam Plann* 1980; 6(Supplement): 1-12. 10. Russell-Briefel RG, Ezzati TM, Fulwood R, Perlman JA, Murphy RS. Cardiovascular risk status and oral contraceptive use, United States, 1976-80. *Prevent Med* 1986; 15:352-362. 11. Goldbaum GM, Kendrick JS, Hogelin GC, Gentry EM. The relative impact of smoking and oral contraceptive use on women in the United States. *JAMA* 1987; 258:1339-1342. 12. Layde PM, Beral V. Further analyses of mortality in oral contraceptive users: Royal College of General Practitioners' Oral Contraception Study. (Table 5) *Lancet* 1981; 1:541-546. 13. Knopp RH. Arteriosclerosis risk: the roles of oral contraceptives and postmenopausal estrogens. *J Reprod Med* 1986; 31(9) (Supplement):913-921. 14. Krauss-RM, Roy S, Mishell DR, Casagrande J. Pike MC. Effects of two low-dose oral contraceptives on serum lipids and lipoproteins: Differential changes in high-density lipoproteins subclasses. *Am J Obstet* 1983; 145:446-452. 15. Wahl P, Walden C, Knopp R, Hoover J, Wallace R, Heiss G, Rifkind B. Effect of estrogen/progestin potency on lipid/lipoprotein cholesterol. *N Engl J Med* 1983; 308:862-867. 16. Wynn V, Niththyananthan R. The effect of progestin in combined oral contraceptives on serum lipids with special reference to high density lipoproteins. *Am J Obstet Gynecol* 1982; 142:766-771. 17. Wynn V, Godsland I. Effects of oral contraceptives on carbohydrate metabolism. *J Reprod Med* 1986; 31(9)(Supplement):892-897. 18. La Rosa JC. Atherosclerotic risk factors in cardiovascular disease. *J Reprod Med* 1986; 31(9) (Supplement):906-912. 19. Inman WH, Vessey MP. Investigation of death from pulmonary, coronary, and cerebral thrombosis and embolism in women of child-bearing age. *Br Med J* 1968; 2(5599):193-199. 20. Maguire MG, Tonascia J, Sartwell PE, Stolley PD, Tockman MS. Increased risk of thrombosis due to oral contraceptives: a further report. *Am J Epidemiol* 1979; 110(2):188-195. 21. Petitti DB, Wingerd J, Pellegrin F, Ramacharan S. Risk of vascular disease in women:

smoking, oral contraceptives, noncontraceptive estrogens, and other factors. *JAMA* 1979;242:1150-1154. 22. Vessey MP, Doll R. Investigation of relation between use of oral contraceptives and thromboembolic disease. *Br Med J* 1968;2(5599):199-205. 23. Vessey MP, Doll R. Investigation of relation between use of oral contraceptives and thromboembolic disease. A further report. *Br Med J* 1969; 2(5658):651-657. 24. Porter JB, Hunter JR, Danielson DA, Jick H, Stergachis A. Oral contraceptives and non-fatal vascular disease-recent experience. *Obstet Gynecol* 1982; 59(3):299-302. 25. Vessey M, Doll R, Peto R, Johnson B, Wiggins P. A longterm follow-up study of women using different methods of contraception: an interim report. *J Biosocial Sci* 1976; 8:375-427. 26. Royal College of General Practitioners: Oral Contraceptives, venous thrombosis, and varicose veins. *J Royal Coll Gen Pract* 1978; 28:393-399. 27. Collaborative Group for the Study of Stroke in Young Women: Oral contraception and increased risk of cerebral ischemia or thrombosis. *N Engl J Med* 1973; 288:871-878. 28. Petitti DB, Wingerd J. Use of oral contraceptives, cigarette smoking, and risk of subarachnoid hemorrhage. *Lancet* 1978; 2:234-236. 29. Inman WH. Oral contraceptives and fatal subsarachnoid hemorrhage. *Br Med J* 1979; 2(6203):1468-1470. 30. Collaborative Group for the Study of Stroke in Young Women: Oral Contraceptives and stroke in young women: associated risk factors. *JAMA* 1975; 231:718-722. 31. Inman WH, Vessey MP, Westerholm B, Engelund A. Thromboembolic disease and the steroidal content of oral contraceptives. A report to the Committee on Safety of Drugs. *Br Med J* 1970; 2:203-209. 32. Meade TW, Greenberg G, Thompson SG. Progestogens and cardiovascular reactions associated with oral contraceptives and a comparison of the safety of 50- and 35-mcg oestrogen preparations. *Br Med J* 1980; 280(6224):1157-1161. 33. Kay CR. Progestogens and arterial disease-evidence from the Royal College of General Practitioners' Study. *Am J Obstet Gynecol* 1982; 142:762-765. 34. Royal College of General Practitioners: Incidence of arterial disease among oral contraceptive users. *J Royal Coll Gen Pract* 1983; 33:75-82. 35. Ory HW. Mortality associated with fertility and fertility control: 1983. *Family Planning Perspectives* 1983; 15:50-56. 36. The Cancer and Steroid Hormone Study of the Centers for Disease Control and the National Institute of Child Health and Human Development: Oral contraceptive use and the risk of breast cancer. *N Engl J Med* 1986; 315:405-411. 37. Pike MC, Henderson BE, Krailo MD, Duke A, Roy S. Breast cancer in young women and use of oral contraceptives: possible modifying effect of formulation and age at use. *Lancet* 1983; 2:926-929. 38. Paul C, Skegg DG, Spears GFS, Kaldor JM. Oral contraceptives and breast cancer: A national study. *Br Med J* 1986; 293:723-725. 39. Miller DR, Rosenberg L, Kaufman DW, Schottenfeld D. Stolley PD, Shapiro S. Breast cancer risk in relation to early oral contraceptive use. *Obstet Gynecol* 1986; 68:863-868. 40. Olson H, Olson KL, Moller TR, Ranstam J, Holm P. Oral contraceptive use and breast cancer in young women in Sweden (letter). *Lancet* 1985; 2:748-749. 41. McPherson K, Vessey M, Neil A, Doll R, Jones L, Roberts M. Early contraceptive use and breast cancer: Results of another case-control study. *Br J Cancer* 1987; 56:653-660. 42. Huggins GR, Zucker PF. Oral contraceptives and neoplasia: 1987 update. *Fertil Steril* 1987; 47:733-761. 43. McPherson K, Drife JO. The pill and breast cancer: why the uncertainty? *Br Med J* 1986; 293:709-710. 44. Shapiro S. Oral contraceptives-time to take stock. *N Engl J Med* 1987; 315:450-451, 45. Ory H, Naib Z, Conger SB, Hatcher RA, Tyler CW. Contraceptive choice and prevalence of cervical dysplasia and carcinoma in situ. *Am J Obstet Gynecol* 1976; 124: 573-577. 46. Vessey MP, Lawless M, McPherson K, Yeates D. Neoplasia of the cervix uteri and contraception: a possible adverse effect of the pill. *Lancet* 1983; 2:930. 47. Brinton LA, Huggins GR, Lehman HF, Malli K, Savitz DA, Trapido E, Rosenthal J, Hoover R. Long term use of oral contraceptives and risk of invasive cervical cancer. *Int J Cancer* 1986; 38:339-344. 48. WHO Collaborative Study of Neoplasia and Steroid Contraceptives: Invasive cervical cancer and combined oral contraceptives. *Br Med J* 1985; 290:961-965. 49. Rooks JB, Ory HW, Ishak KG, Strauss LT, Greenspan JR, Hill AP, Tyler CW. Epidemiology of hepatocellular adenoma: the role of oral contraceptive use. *JAMA* 1979; 242:644-648. 50. Bein NN, Goldsmith HS. Recurrent massive hemorrhage from benign hepatic tumors secondary to oral contraceptives. *Br J Surg* 1977; 64:435. 51. Klatskin G. Hepatic tumors: possible relationship to use of oral contraceptives. *Gastroenterology* 1977; 73:386-394. 52. Henderson BE, Preston-Martin S, Edmondson HA, Peters RL, Pike MC. Hepatocellular carcinoma and oral contraceptives. *Br J Cancer* 1983; 48:437-440. 53. Neuberger J, Forman D, Doll R, Williams R. Oral contraceptives and hepatocellular carcinoma. *Br Med J* 1986; 292:1355-1357. 54. Forman D, Vincent TJ, Doll R. Cancer of the liver and oral contraceptives. *Br Med J* 1986; 292:1357-1361. 55. Harlap S, Eldor J. Births following oral contraceptive failures. *Obstet Gynecol* 1980; 55:447-452. 56. Savolainen E. Saksela E, Saxen L. Teratogenic hazards of oral contraceptives analyzed in a national malformation register. *Am J Obstet Gynecol* 1981: 140:524. 57. Janerich DT, Piper JM, Glebatis DM. Oral contraceptives and birth defects. *Am J Epidemiol* 1980; 112:73-79. 58. Ferencz C, Matanoski GM, Wilson PD, Rubin JD, Neill CA, Gutberlet R. Maternal hormone therapy and congenital heart disease. *Teratology* 1980; 21:225-239. 59. Rothman KJ, Fyler DC, Goldblatt A, Kreidberg MB. Exogenous hormones and other drug exposures of children with congenital heart disease. *Am J Epidemiol* 1979; 109:433-439. 60. Boston Collaborative Drug Surveillance Program: Oral contraceptives and venous thromboembolic disease, surgically confirmed gallbladder disease, and breast tumors. *Lancet* 1973; 1:1399-1404. 61. Royal College of General Practitioners: Oral contraceptives and health. New York, Pittman 1974. 62. Layde PM, Vessey MP, Yeates D. Risk of gallbladder disease: a cohort study of young women attending family planning clinics. *J Epidemiol Community Health* 1982; 36:274-278. 63. Rome Group for Epidemiology and Prevention of Cholelithiasis (GREPCO): Prevalence of gallstone disease in an italian adult female population. *Am J Epidemiol* 1984; 119:796-805. 64. Storm BL, Tamragouri RT, Morse ML, Lazar EL, West SL, Stolley PD, Jones JK, Oral contraceptives and other risk factors for gallbladder disease. *Clin Pharmacol Ther* 1986; 39:335-341. 65. Wynn V, Adams PW, Godsland IF, Melrose J, Niththyananthan R, Oakley NW, Seedj A. Comparison of effects of different combined oral contraceptive formulations on carbohydrate and lipid metabolism. *Lancet* 1979; 1:1045-1049. 66. Wynn V. Effects of progesterone and progestins on carbohydrate metabolism. In: Progesterone and Progestin. Bardin CW, Milgrom E, Mauvis-Jarvis P. eds. New York, Raven Press 1983; pp. 395-410. 67. Perlman JA, Roussell-Briefel RG, Ezzati TM, Lieberknecht G. Oral glucose tolerance and the potency of oral contraceptive progestogens. *J Chronic Dis* 1985;38:857-864. 68. Royal College of General Practitioners' Oral Contraception Study: Effect on hypertension and benign breast disease of progestogen component in combined oral Contraceptives. *Lancet* 1977; 1:624. 69. Fisch IR, Frank J. Oral contraceptives and blood pressure. *JAMA* 1977; 237:2499-2503. 70. Laragh AJ. Oral contraceptive induced hypertension-nine years later. *Am J Obstet Gynecol* 1976; 126:141-147. 71. Ramcharan S, Peritz E, Pellegrin FA, Williams WT. Incidence of hypertension in the Walnut Creek Contraceptive Drug Study cohort: In: Pharmacology of steroid contraceptive drugs. Garattini S, Berendes HW. Eds. New York, Raven Press, 1977; pp. 277-288, (Monographs of the Mario Negri Institute for Pharmacological Research Milan.) 72. Stockley I. Interactions with oral contraceptives. *J Pharm* 1976; 216:140-143. 73. The Cancer and Steroid Hormone Study of the Centers for Disease Control and the National Institute of Child Health and Human Development: Oral contraceptive use and the risk of ovarian cancer. *JAMA* 1983; 249:1596-1599. 74. The Cancer and Steroid Hormone Study of the Centers for Disease Control and the National Institute of Child Health and Human Development: Combination oral contraceptive use and the risk of endometrial cancer. *JAMA* 1987; 257:796-800. 75. Ory HW. Functional ovarian cysts and oral contraceptives: negative association confirmed surgically. *JAMA* 1974; 228:68-69. 76. Ory HW, Cole P, MacMahon B, Hoover R. Oral contraceptives and reduced risk of benign breast disease. *N Engl J Med* 1976; 294:419-422. 77. Ory HW. The noncontraceptive health benefits from oral contraceptive use. *Fam Plann Perspect* 1982; 14:182-184. 78. Ory HW, Forrest JD, Lincoln R. Making choices: Evaluating the health risks and benefits of birth control methods, New York. The Alan Guttmacher Institute, 1983; p.1. 79. Schlesselman J, Stadel BV, Murray P, Lai S. Breast cancer in relation to early use of oral contraceptives. *JAMA* 1988; 259:1828-1833. 80. Hennekens CH, Speizer FE, Lipnick RJ, Rosner B, Bain C, Belanger C, Stampfer MJ, Willett W, Peto R. A case-control study of oral contraceptive use and breast cancer. *JNCI* 1984; 72:39-42. 81. LaVecchia C, Decarli A, Fasoli M, Franceschi S, Gentile A, Negri E, Parazzini F, Tognoni G. Oral contraceptives and cancers of the breast and of the female genital tract. Interim results from a case-control study. *Br J Cancer* 1986; 54:311-317. 82. Meirik O, Lund E, Adami H, Bergstrom R, Christoffersen T, Bergsjo P. Oral contraceptive use and breast cancer in young women. A Joint National Case-control study in Sweden and Norway. *Lancet* 1986; 11:650-654. 83. Kay CR, Hannaford PC. Breast cancer and the pill-A further report from the Royal College of General Practitioners' oral contraception study. *Br J Cancer* 1988; 58:657-680. 84. Stadel BV, Lai S, Schlesselman JJ, Murray P. Oral contraceptives and premenopausal breast cancer in nulliparous women. *Contraception* 1988; 38:287-299. 85. Miller DR, Rosenberg L, Kaufman DW, Stolley P, Warshauer ME, Shapiro S. Breast cancer before age 45 and oral contraceptive use: New Findings. *Am J Epidemiol* 1989; 129:269-280. 86. The UK National Case-Control Study Group, Oral contraceptive use and breast cancer risk in young women. *Lancet* 1989; 1:973-982. 87. Schlesselman JJ. Cancer of the breast and reproductive tract in relation to use of oral contraceptives. *Contraception* 1989; 40:1-38. 88. Vessey MP, McPherson K, Villard-Mackintosh L, Yeates D. Oral contraceptives and breast cancer: latest findings in a large cohort study. *Br J Cancer* 1989; 59:613-617. 89. Jick SS, Walker AM, Stergachis A, Jick H. Oral contraceptives and breast cancer. *Br J Cancer* 1989; 59:618-621.

HOW SUPPLIED
TABLETS: 0.35 MG

BRAND/MANUFACTURER	NDC	SIZE	AWP
○ BRAND			
MICRONOR: Ortho Pharm	00062-1411-01	28s	$27.84
NOR-Q-D: Syntex/F.P.	42987-0107-19	252s	$162.53

Norethindrone Acetate

> **WARNING**
>
> THE USE OF NORETHINDRONE ACETATE DURING THE FIRST FOUR MONTHS OF PREGNANCY IS NOT RECOMMENDED.
>
> PROGESTATIONAL AGENTS HAVE BEEN USED BEGINNING WITH THE FIRST TRIMESTER OF PREGNANCY IN AN ATTEMPT TO PREVENT HABITUAL ABORTION. THERE IS NO ADEQUATE EVIDENCE THAT SUCH USE IS EFFECTIVE WHEN SUCH DRUGS ARE GIVEN DURING THE FIRST FOUR MONTHS OF PREGNANCY. FURTHERMORE, IN THE VAST MAJORITY OF WOMEN, THE CAUSE OF ABORTION IS A DEFECTIVE OVUM, WHICH PROGESTATIONAL AGENTS COULD NOT BE EXPECTED TO INFLUENCE. IN ADDITION, THE USE OF PROGESTATIONAL AGENTS, WITH THEIR UTERINE-RELAXANT PROPERTIES, IN PATIENTS WITH FERTILIZED DEFECTIVE OVA MAY CAUSE A DELAY IN SPONTANEOUS ABORTION. THEREFORE, THE USE OF SUCH DRUGS DURING THE FIRST FOUR MONTHS OF PREGNANCY IS NOT RECOMMENDED.
>
> SEVERAL REPORTS SUGGEST AN ASSOCIATION BETWEEN INTRA-UTERINE EXPOSURE TO PROGESTATIONAL DRUGS IN THE FIRST TRIMESTER OF PREGNANCY AND GENITAL ABNORMALITIES IN MALE AND FEMALE FETUSES. THE RISK OF HYPOSPADIAS, 5 TO 8 PER 1,000 MALE BIRTHS IN THE GENERAL POPULATION, MAY BE APPROXIMATELY DOUBLED WITH EXPOSURE TO THESE DRUGS. THERE ARE INSUFFICIENT DATA TO QUANTIFY THE RISK TO EXPOSED FEMALE FETUSES, BUT INSOFAR AS SOME OF THESE DRUGS INDUCE MILD VIRILIZATION OF THE EXTERNAL GENITALIA OF THE FEMALE FETUS, AND BECAUSE OF THE INCREASED ASSOCIATION OF HYPOSPADIAS IN THE MALE FETUS, IT IS PRUDENT TO AVOID THE USE OF THESE DRUGS DURING THE FIRST TRIMESTER OF PREGNANCY.
>
> IF THE PATIENT IS EXPOSED TO NORETHINDRONE ACETATE TABLETS, USP DURING THE FIRST FOUR MONTHS OF PREGNANCY OR IF SHE BECOMES PREGNANT WHILE TAKING THIS DRUG, SHE SHOULD BE APPRISED OF THE POTENTIAL RISKS TO THE FETUS.

DESCRIPTION
Norethindrone Acetate tablets 5 mg oral tablets Norethindrone Acetate (17-hydroxy-19-nor-17α-pregn-4-en-20-yn-3-one acetate), a synthetic, orally active progestin, is the acetic acid ester of Norethindrone, which is the 17 alpha-ethinyl

---

derivative of 19-nortestosterone. It is a progestational agent for oral administration.

Following is its chemical structure:

CLINICAL PHARMACOLOGY

Norethindrone Acetate induces secretory changes in an estrogen-primed endometrium, i.e., it transforms proliferative endometrium into secretory endometrium. It acts to inhibit the secretion of pituitary gonadotropins which, in turn, prevent follicular maturation and ovulation. On a weight basis, it is twice as potent as Norethindrone.

May also demonstrate some estrogenic, anabolic or androgenic activity but should not be relied upon.

INDICATIONS AND USAGE

Norethindrone Acetate is indicated for the the treatment of secondary amenorrhea, endometriosis, and abnormal uterine bleeding due to hormonal imbalance in the absence of organic pathology, such as submucous fibroids or uterine cancer.

CONTRAINDICATIONS

Thrombophlebitis, thromboembolic disorders, cerebral apoplexy, or a past history of these conditions.

Markedly impaired liver function or liver disease.
Known or suspected carcinoma of the breast or genital organs.
Undiagnosed vaginal bleeding.
Missed abortion.
As a diagnostic test for pregnancy.
Known sensitivity to Norethindrone Acetate.

WARNINGS

1. Discontinue medication pending examination if there is a sudden partial or complete loss of vision or if there is sudden onset of proptosis, diplopia, or migraine. If examination reveals papilledema or retinal vascular lesions, medication should be withdrawn.

2. Because of the occasional occurrence of thrombophlebitis, cerebrovascular disorders, retinal thrombosis, and pulmonary embolism in patients taking progestogens, the physician should be alert to the earliest manifestations of the disease.

3. Masculinization of the female fetus has occurred when progestogens have been used in pregnant women.

PRECAUTIONS

A. GENERAL PRECAUTIONS

1. The pretreatment physical examination should include special reference to breasts and pelvic organs, as well as a Papanicolaou smear.

2. Because this drug may cause some degree of fluid retention, conditions which might be influenced by this factor, such as epilepsy, migraine, asthma, cardiac or renal dysfunctions, require careful observation.

3. In cases of breakthrough bleeding, as in all cases of irregular bleeding per vaginam, nonfunctional causes should be borne in mind. In cases of undiagnosed vaginal bleeding, adequate diagnostic measures are indicated.

4. Patients who have a history of psychic depression should be carefully observed and the drug discontinued if the depression recurs to a serious degree.

5. Any possible influence of prolonged progestogen therapy on pituitary, ovarian, adrenal, hepatic, or uterine functions awaits further study.

6. Concomitant Use in Estrogen Replacement Therapy: In postmenopausal estrogen replacement therapy, studies of the addition of a progestin for 7 or more days of a cycle of estrogen administration have reported a lowered incidence of endometrial hyperplasia. Morphological and biochemical studies of the endometrium suggest that 10 to 13 days of progestin are needed to provide maximal maturation of the endometrium and to eliminate any hyperplastic changes. Whether this will provide protection from endometrial carcinoma has not been clearly established. There are possible additional risks which may be associated with the inclusion of progestin in estrogen replacement regimens. Progestin therapy may have an adverse effect on carbohydrate and lipid metabolism. The dosage used may be important in minimizing these adverse effects.

7. A decrease in glucose tolerance has been observed in a small percentage of patients on estrogen-progestogen combination drugs. The mechanism of this decrease is obscure. For this reason, diabetic patients should be carefully observed while receiving progestogen therapy.

8. The age of the patient constitutes no absolute limiting factor, although treatment with progestogens may mask the onset of the climacteric.

9. The pathologist should be advised of progestogen therapy when relevant specimens are submitted.

B. INFORMATION FOR THE PATIENT
See text which appears at the end of this insert.

C. CARCINOGENESIS, MUTAGENESIS, AND IMPAIRMENT OF FERTILITY
Some beagle dogs treated with medroxyprogesterone acetate developed mammary nodules. Although nodules occasionally appeared in control animals, they were intermittent in nature, whereas nodules in treated animals were larger and more numerous, and persisted. There is no general agreement as to whether the nodules are benign or malignant. Their significance with respect to humans has not been established.

There is no evidence of a carcinogenic effect associated with the oral administration of MPA to rats and mice. Medroxyprogesterone acetate was not mutagenic in a battery of *in vitro* or *in vivo* genetic toxicity assays.

Norethindrone Acetate at high doses is an antifertility drug and high doses would be expected to impair fertility until the cessation of treatment.

D. PREGNANCY CATEGORY X.
See boxed *"Warning."*

E. NURSING MOTHERS
Detectable amounts of progestogens have been identified in the milk of mothers receiving them. The effect of this on the nursing infant has not been determined.

F. PEDIATRIC USE
Safety and effectiveness in children have not been established.

ADVERSE REACTIONS
(See *"Warnings"* for possible adverse effects on the fetus.)

The following adverse reactions have been observed in women taking progestins:

Breakthrough bleeding.
Spotting.
Change in menstrual flow.
Amenorrhea.
Edema.
Changes in weight (decreases, increases).
Changes in cervical erosion and cervical secretions.
Cholestatic jaundice.
Rash (allergic) with and without pruritus.
Melasma or chloasma.
Mental depression.
Breast tenderness and galactorrhea.
Skin sensitivity reactions consisting of urticaria, pruritus, edema and generalized rash.
Acne, alopecia and hirsutism.
Anaphylactoid reactions.
Pyrexia.
Insomnia.
Nausea.
Somnolence.

Progestins may alter the result of pregnanediol determinations. The following laboratory results may be altered by the concomitant use of estrogens with progestins:

Hepatic Function: Coagulation tests—increase in prothrombin, factors VII, VIII, IX, and X.

Increase in PBI, BEI, and a decrease in T^3 uptake.

Reduced Response to Metyrapone Test: A statistically significant association has been demonstrated between use of estrogen-progestogen combination drugs and the following serious adverse reactions: thrombophlebitis, pulmonary embolism, and cerebral thrombosis and embolism. For this reason, patients on progestogen therapy should be carefully observed. Although available evidence is suggestive of an association, such a relationship has been neither confirmed nor refuted for the following serious adverse reactions:

Neuro-ocular Lesions, e.g., Retinal Thrombosis and Optic Neuritis: The following adverse reactions have been observed in patients receiving estrogen-progestogen combination drugs:

1. Rise in blood pressure in susceptible individuals.
2. Premenstrual-like syndrome.
3. Changes in libido.
4. Changes in appetite.
5. Cystitis-like syndrome.
6. Headache.
7. Nervousness.
8. Dizziness.
9. Fatigue.
10. Backache.
11. Hirsutism.
12. Loss of scalp hair.
13. Erythema multiforme.
14. Erythema nodosum.
15. Hemorrhagic eruption.
16. Itching.
17. Dizziness.

In view of these observations, patients on progestogen therapy should be carefully observed.

DOSAGE AND ADMINISTRATION

Therapy with Norethindrome Acetate must be adapted to the specific indications and therapeutic response of the individual patient. This dosage schedule assumes the interval between menses to be 28 days.

Secondary amenorrhea, abnormal uterine bleeding due to hormonal imbalance in the absence of organic pathology: 2.5 to 10 mg Norethindrone Acetate may be given daily for 5 to 10 days during the second half of the theoretical menstrual cycle to produce an optimum secretory transformation of an endometrium that has been adequately primed with either endogenous or exogenous estrogen. Dosage for some brands is 2.5 to 10 mg starting with the fifth day of the menstrual cycle and ending on the 25th day.

Progestin withdrawal bleeding usually occurs within three to seven days after discontinuing Norethindrone Acetate therapy. Patients with a past history of recurrent episodes of abnormal uterine bleeding may benefit from planned menstrual cycling with Norethindrone Acetate.

Endometriosis: Initial daily dosage of 5 mg Norethindrone Acetate for two weeks. Dosage should be increased by 2.5 mg per day every two weeks until 15 mg per day of Norethindrone Acetate is reached. Therapy may be held at this level for six to nine months or until annoying breakthrough bleeding demands temporary termination.

Storage: Store at room temperature (approximately 25° C).
Dispense in a well-closed container as defined in the USP.

INFORMATION FOR THE PATIENT

Your doctor has prescribed Norethindrone Acetate tablets, a progestin or progestational drug, for you. Norethindrone Acetate is similar to the progesterone hormones naturally produced by the body. Progestins are used to treat menstrual disorders and to test if the body is producing certain hormones.

The information below is required by the U.S. Food and Drug Administration to be provided to all patients taking such products. This information relates only to the risk to the unborn child associated with use of progestational drugs during pregnancy. For further information on the use, side effects, and other risks associated with this product, ask your doctor.

Warning: Progesterone or progesterone-like drugs have been used to prevent miscarriage in the first few months of pregnancy. No adequate evidence is available to show that they are effective for this purpose. Furthermore, most cases of early miscarriage are due to causes which could not be helped by these drugs.

There is an increased risk of minor birth defects in children whose mothers take this drug during the first four months of pregnancy. Several reports suggest an association between mothers who take these drugs in the first trimester of pregnancy and genital abnormalities in male and female babies. The risk to the male baby is the possibility of being born with a condition in which the opening of the penis is on the underside rather than the tip of the penis (hypospadias). Hypospadias occurs in about 5 to 8 per 1,000 male births and is about doubled with exposure to these drugs. There is not enough information to quantify the risk to exposed female fetuses, but enlargement of the clitoris and fusion of the labia may occur, although rarely.

Therefore, since drugs of this type may induce mild masculinization of the external genitalia of the female fetus, as well as hypospadias in the male fetus, it is wise to avoid using the drug during the first trimester of pregnancy.

These drugs have been used as a test for pregnancy but such use is no longer considered safe because of possible damage to a developing baby. Also, more rapid methods for testing for pregnancy are now available.

If you take Norethindrone Acetate tablets, and later find you were pregnant when you took it, be sure to discuss this with your doctor as soon as possible.

HOW SUPPLIED
TABLETS: 5 MG

BRAND/MANUFACTURER	NDC	SIZE	AWP
◆ BRAND			
NORLUTATE: Parke-Davis	00071-0918-19	50s	$48.96
◆ GENERICS			
AYGESTIN: Esi Pharma	59911-5894-01	50s	$48.75

Norflex *SEE* ORPHENADRINE CITRATE

Norfloxacin, Ophthalmic

DESCRIPTION

Norfloxacin Ophthalmic Solution is a synthetic broad-spectrum antibacterial agent supplied as a sterile isotonic solution for topical ophthalmic use. Norfloxacin, a fluoroquinolone, is 1-ethyl-6-fluoro-1,4-dihydro-4-oxo-7-(1-piperazinyl)-3-quinoline- carboxylic acid. Its empirical formula is $C_{16}H_{18}FN_3O_3$.

Norfloxacin is a white to pale yellow crystalline powder with a molecular weight of 319.34 and a melting point of about 221°C. It is freely soluble in glacial acetic acid and very slightly soluble in ethanol, methanol and water.

Norfloxacin Ophthalmic Solution 0.3% is supplied as a sterile isotonic solution. Each mL contains 3 mg Norfloxacin.

Norfloxacin, a fluoroquinolone, differs from quinolones by having a fluorine atom at the 6 position and a piperazine moiety at the 7 position.

Following is its chemical structure:

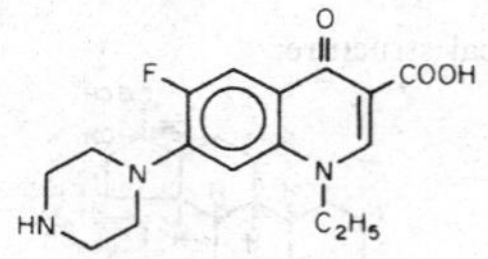

CLINICAL PHARMACOLOGY
MICROBIOLOGY

Norfloxacin has *in vitro* activity against a broad spectrum of gram-positive and gram-negative aerobic bacteria. The fluorine atom at the 6 position provides increased potency against gram-negative organisms and the piperazine moiety at the 7 position is responsible for anti-pseudomonal activity. Norfloxacin inhibits bacterial deoxyribonucleic acid synthesis and is bactericidal. At the molecular level three specific events are attributed to Norfloxacin in *E. coli* cells:

1) inhibition of the ATP-dependent DNA supercoiling reaction catalyzed by DNA gyrase:
2) inhibition of the relaxation of supercoiled DNA;
3) promotion of double-stranded DNA breakage.

There is generally no cross-resistance between Norfloxacin and other classes of antibacterial agents. Therefore Norfloxacin generally demonstrates activity against indicated organisms resistant to some other antimicrobial agents. When such cross-resistance does occur, it is probably due to decreased entry of the drugs into the bacterial cells. Antagonism has been demonstrated *in vitro* between Norfloxacin and nitrofurantoin.

Norfloxacin has been shown to be active against most strains of the following organisms both *in vitro* and clinically in ophthalmic infections (see "Indications and Usage"):

GRAM-POSITIVE BACTERIA including:
Staphylococcus aureus (including both penicillinase-producing and methicillin-resistant strains)
Staphylococcus epidermidis
Staphylococcus warnerii
Streptococcus pneumoniae
Gram-negative bacteria including:
Acinetobacter calcoaceticus
Aeromonas hydrophila
Haemophilus influenzae
Proteus mirabilis
Pseudomonas aeruginosa
Serratia marcescens

Norfloxacin has been shown to be active *in vitro* against most strains of the following organisms: however, *the clinical significance of these data in ophthalmic infections is unknown.*

GRAM-POSITIVE BACTERIA:
Bacillus cereus
Enterococcus faecalis (formerly *Streptococcus faecalis*)
Staphylococcus saprophyticus
Gram-negative bacteria:
Citrobacter diversus
Citrobacter freundii
Edwardsiella tarda
Enterobacter aerogenes
Enterobacter cloacae
Escherichia coli
Hafnia alvei
Haemophilus aegyptius (Koch-Weeks bacillus)
Klebsiella oxytoca
Klebsiella pneumoniae
Klebsiella rhinoscleromatis
Morganella morganii
Neisseria gonorrhoeae
Proteus vulgaris
Providencia alcalifaciens
Providencia rettgeri
Providencia stuartii
Salmonella typhi
Vibrio cholerae
Vibrio parahemolyticus
Yersinia enterocolitica
OTHER
Ureaplasma urealyticum

Norfloxacin is not active against obligate anaerobes.

CLINICAL STUDIES

Clinical studies were conducted comparing Norfloxacin Ophthalmic Solution (n = 152) with ophthalmic solutions of tobramycin, gentamicin, and chloramphenicol (n = 158) in patients with conjunctivitis and positive bacterial cultures. After seven days of therapy with Norfloxacin Ophthalmic Solution, 72 percent of patients were clinically cured. Of those cured, 85 percent had all their pathogens eradicated. Eradication was also achieved in 62 percent (23/37) of patients whose clinical outcome was not completely cured by day seven. These results were similar among all treatment groups.

◆ RATED THERAPEUTICALLY EQUIVALENT; ◇ THERAPEUTIC EQUIVALENCE UNCONFIRMED; ○ UNRATED

Another clinical study compared Norfloxacin Ophthalmic Solution with placebo in patients with conjunctivitis and positive bacterial cultures. Placebo in this study was the liquid vehicle for Norfloxacin Ophthalmic Solution and contained the preservative. After five days of therapy, 64 percent (36/56) of patients on Norfloxacin Ophthalmic Solution were clinically cured compared to 50 percent (23/46) of patients receiving placebo. Of those cured, 78 percent had all their pathogens eradicated. Eradication was also achieved in 50 percent (10/20) of patients whose clinical outcome was not completely cured. The response to Norfloxacin Ophthalmic Solution was statistically significantly better than the response to placebo.

INDICATIONS AND USAGE

Norfloxacin Ophthalmic Solution is indicated for the treatment of conjunctivitis when caused by susceptible strains of the following bacteria:

Acinetobacter calcoaceticus[*]
Aeromonas hydrophila[*]
Haemophilus influenzae
Proteus mirabilis[*]
Pseudemonas aeruginosa[*]
Serratia marcescens[*]
Staphylococcus aureus
Staphylococcus epidermidis
Staphylococcus warnerii[*]
Streptococcus pneumoniae

Appropriate monitoring of bacterial response to topical antibiotic therapy should accompany the use of Norfloxacin Ophthalamic Solution.

CONTRAINDICATIONS

Norfloxacin Ophthalmic Solution is contraindicated in patients with a history of hypersensitivity to Norfloxacin, or the other members of the quinolone group of antibacterial agents or any other component of this medication.

WARNINGS

NOT FOR INJECTION INTO THE EYE.
Serious and occasionally fatal hypersensitivity (anaphylactoid or anaphylactic) reactions, some following the first dose, have been reported in patients receiving systemic quinolone therapy. Some reactions were accompanied by cardiovascular collapse, loss of consciousness, tingling, pharyngeal or facial edema, dyspnea, urticaria, and itching. Only a few patients had a history of hypersensitivity reactions. Serious anaphylactoid or anaphylactic reactions require immediate emergency treatment with epinephrine. Oxygen, intravenous steroids and airway management, including intubation, should be administered as indicated.

PRECAUTIONS

GENERAL

As with other antibiotic preparations, prolonged use may result in overgrowth of nonsusceptible organisms, including fungi. If superinfection occurs, appropriate measures should be initiated. Whenever clinical judgment dictates, the patient should be examined with the aid of magnification, such as slit lamp biomicroscopy and, where appropriate, fluorescein staining.

INFORMATION FOR PATIENTS

Patients should be instructed to avoid allowing the tip of the dispensing container to contact the eye or surrounding structures.

Patients should be advised that Norfloxacin may be associated with hypersensitivity reactions, even following a single dose, and to discontinue the drug at the first sign of a skin rash or other allergic reaction.

Patients being treated for bacterial conjunctivitis generally should not wear contact lenses. However, if the physician considers the use of contact lenses appropriate, patients should be instructed to wait at least 15 minutes after instilling Norfloxacin Ophthalmic Solution before inserting their lenses because the preservative in Norfloxacin Ophthalmic Solution may contain benzalkonium chloride which may be absorbed by contact lenses.

DRUG INTERACTIONS

Specific drug interaction studies have not been conducted with Norfloxacin Ophthalmic solution. However, the systemic administration of some quinolones has been shown to elevate plasma concentrations of theophylline, interfere with the metabolism of caffeine, and enhance the effects of the oral anticoagulant warfarin and its derivatives. Elevated serum levels of cyclosporine have been reported with concomitant use of cyclosporine with Norfloxacin. Therefore, cyclosporine serum levels should be monitored and appropriate cyclosporine dosage adjustments made when these drugs are used concomitantly.

CARCINOGENESIS, MUTAGENESIS, IMPAIRMENT OF FERTILITY

No increase in neoplastic changes was observed with Norfloxacin as compared to controls in a study in rats, lasting up to 96 weeks at doses eight to nine times the usual human oral dose[*].

The usual oral dose of Norfloxacin is 80 mg daily. One drop Norfloxacin Ophthalmic Solution 0.3% containing about 1/6,666 of this dose (0.12 mg).

Norfloxacin was tested for mutagenic activity in a number of *in vivo* and *in vitro* tests. Norfloxacin had no mutagenic effect in the dominant lethal test in mice and did not cause chromosomal aberrations in hamsters or rats at doses 30 to 60 times the usual oral dose[*]. Norfloxacin had no mutagenic activity *in vitro* in

the Ames microbial mutagen test, Chinese hamster fibroblasts and V-79 mammalian cell assay. Although Norfloxacin was weakly positive in the Rec-assay for DNA repair, all other mutagenic assays were negative including a more sensitive test (V-79).

Norfloxacin did not adversely affect the fertility of male and female mice at oral doses up to 33 times the usual human oral dose[*].

PREGNANCY

Pregnancy Category C: Norfloxacin has been shown to produce embryonic loss in monkeys when given in doses 10 times the maximum human oral dose[*] (400 mg b.i.d.), with peak plasma levels that are two to three times those obtained in humans. There has been no evidence of a teratogenic effect in any of the animal species tested (rat, rabbit, mouse, monkey) at 6 to 50 times the human oral dose. There are no adequate and well-controlled studies in pregnant women. Norfloxacin Ophthalmic Solution be used during pregnancy only if the potential benefit justifies the potential risk to the fetus.

NURSING MOTHERS

It is not known whether Nortloxacin is excreted in human milk following ocular administration. Because many drugs are excreted in human milk, and because of the potential for serious adverse reactions in nursing infants from Norfloxacin, a decision should be made to discontinue nursing or to discontinue the drug, taking into account the importance of the drug to the mother (see "Animal Pharmacology").

PEDIATRIC USE

Safety and effectiveness in infants below the age of one year have not been established.

Although quinolones including Norfloxacin have been shown to cause arthropathy in immature animals after oral administration, topical ocular administration of other quinolones to immature animals has not shown any arthropathy and there is no evidence that the ophthalmic dosage form of those quinolones has any effects on the weight-bearing joints.

ADVERSE REACTIONS

In clinical trials, the most frequently reported drug-related adverse reaction was local burning or discomfort. Other drug-related adverse reactions were conjunctival hyperemia, chemosis, photophobia and a bitter taste following instillation.

DOSAGE AND ADMINISTRATION

The recommended dose in adults and pediatric patients (one year and older) is one or two drops of Nortloxacin Ophthalmic Solution applied topically to the affected eye(s) four times daily for up to seven days. Depending on the severity of the infection, the dosage for the first day of therapy may be one or two drops every two hours during the waking hours.

Store Norfloxacin Ophthalmic Solution at room temperature, 15°-30°C (59°-86°F). Protect from light.

ANIMAL PHARMACOLOGY

The oral administration of single doses of Norfloxacin, six times the recommended human oral dose[**], caused lameness in immature dogs. Histologic examination of the weight-bearing joints of these dogs revealed permanent lesions of the cartilage. Related drugs also produced erosions of the cartilage in weight-bearing joints and other signs of arthropathy in immature animals of various species.

ADDITIONAL CAUTIONARY INFORMATION

Norfloxacin is available as an oral dosage form in addition to the ophthalmic dosage form. The following adverse effects, while they have not been reported with the ophthalmic dosage form, have been reported with the oral dosage form. However, it should be noted that the usual dosage of oral Norfloxacin (800 mg/day) contains 6,666 times the amount in one drop of Norfloxacin Ophthalmic Solution 0.3% (0.12 mg).

Convulsions have been reported in patients receiving oral Norfloxacin. Convulsions, increased intracranial pressure, and toxic psychoses have been reported with other drugs in this class. Orally administered quinolones may also cause central nervous system (CNS) stimulation which may lead to tremors, restlessness, light-headedness, confusion and hallucinations. If these reactions occur in patients receiving Norfloxacin, the drug should be discontinued and appropriate measures instituted.

The effects of Norfloxacin on brain function or on the electrical activity of the brain have not been tested. Therefore, as with all quinolones, Norfloxacin should be used with caution in patients with known or suspected CNS disorders, such as severe cerebral arteriosclerosis, epilepsy, and other factors which predispose to seizures.

The following adverse effects have been reported with Norfloxacin tablets.

Hypersensitivity Reactions: Hypersensitivity reactions including anaphylactoid reactions, angioedema, dyspnea, vasculitis, urticaria, arthritis, arthralgia, myalgia.

Gastrointestinal: Pseudomembranous colitis, hepatitis, jaundice, including cholestatic jaundice, pancreatitis.

Hematologic: Neutropenia, leukopenia, thrombocytopenia.

Nervous System/Psychiatric: CNS effects characterized as generalized seizures and myoclonus: neurological changes such as ataxia, diplopia and possible exacerba-

---

[*] Efficacy for this organism was studied in fewer than 10 infections.
[*] All factors are based on a standard patient weight of 50kg.

---

[*] All factors are based on a standard patient weight of 50 kg. The usual oral dose of Norfloxacin is 800 mg daily. One drop of Norfloxacin Ophthalmic Solution 0.3% contains about 1/6.666 of this dose (0.12 mg).

tion of myasthenia gravis: psychic disturbances including psychotic reactions and confusion, depression.

Renal: Interstitial nephritis, renal failure.

Skin: Toxic epidermal necrolysis, Stevens-Johnson syndrome and erythema multiforme, exfoliative dermatitis, rash, photosensitivity.

Special Senses: Transient hearing loss.

Abnormal laboratory values observed with oral Norfloxacin included elevation of ALT (SGPT) and AST (SGOT), alkaline phosphatase, BUN, serum creatinine, and LDH.

Please consult the package circular for Norfloxacin tablets for additional information concerning these and other adverse effects and other cautionary information.

HOW SUPPLIED

DROP: 0.3%

BRAND/MANUFACTURER	NDC	SIZE	AWP
○ **BRAND**			
CHIBROXIN: Merck	00006-3526-03	5 ml	$17.49

Norfloxacin, Oral

DESCRIPTION

Norfloxacin is a synthetic, broad-spectrum antibacterial agent for oral administration. Norfloxacin, a fluoroquinolone, is 1-ethyl-6-fluoro-1,4-dihydro-4-oxo-7-(1-piperazinyl) -3-quinolinecarboxylic acid. Its empirical formula is $C_{16}H_{18}FN_3O_3$.

Norfloxacin is a white to pale yellow crystalline powder with a molecular weight of 319.34 and a melting point of about 221°C. It is freely soluble in glacial acetic acid, and very slightly soluble in ethanol, methanol and water.

Norfloxacin is available in 400-mg tablets.

Norfloxacin, a fluoroquinolone, differs from non-fluorinated quinolones by having a fluorine atom at the 6 position and a piperazine moiety at the 7 position.

Following is its chemical structure:

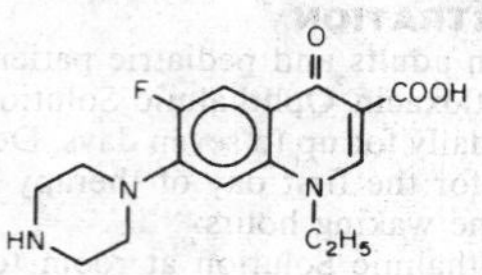

CLINICAL PHARMACOLOGY

In fasting healthy volunteers, at least 30-40% of an oral dose of Norfloxacin is absorbed. Absorption is rapid following single doses of 200 mg, 400 mg and 800 mg. At the respective doses, mean peak serum and plasma concentrations of 0.8, 1.5 and 2.4 mcg/mL are attained approximately one hour after dosing. The presence of food may decrease absorption. The effective half-life of Norfloxacin in serum and plasma is 3-4 hours. Steady-state concentrations of Norfloxacin will be attained within two days of dosing.

In healthy elderly volunteers (65-75 years of age with normal renal function for their age), Norfloxacin is eliminated more slowly because of their slightly decreased renal function. Drug absorption appears unaffected. However, the effective half-life of Norfloxacin in these elderly subjects is 4 hours.

The disposition of Norfloxacin in patients with creatinine clearance rates greater than 30 mL/min/1.73m² is similar to that in healthy volunteers. In patients with creatinine clearance rates equal to or less than 30 mL/min/1.73m², the renal elimination of Norfloxacin decreases so that the effective serum half-life is 6.5 hours. In these patients, alteration of dosage is necessary (see "Dosage and Administration"). Drug absorption appears unaffected by decreasing renal function.

Norfloxacin is eliminated through metabolism, biliary excretion, and renal excretion. After a single 400-mg dose of Norfloxacin, mean antimicrobial activities equivalent to 278, 773, and 82 mcg of Norfloxacin/g of feces were obtained at 12, 24, and 48 hours, respectively. Renal excretion occurs by both glomerular filtration and tubular secretion as evidenced by the high rate of renal clearance (approximately 275 mL/min). Within 24 hours of drug administration, 26 to 32% of the administered dose is recovered in the urine as Norfloxacin with an additional 5-8% being recovered in the urine as six active metabolites of lesser antimicrobial potency. Only a small percentage (less than 1%) of the dose is recovered thereafter. Fecal recovery accounts for another 30% of the administered dose.

Two to three hours after a single 400-mg dose, urinary concentrations of 200 mcg/mL or more are attained in the urine. In healthy volunteers, mean urinary concentrations of Norfloxacin remain above 30 mcg/mL for at least 12 hours following a 400-mg dose. The urinary pH may affect the solubility of Norfloxacin. Norfloxacin is least soluble at urinary pH of 7.5 with greater solubility occurring at pHs above and below this value. The serum protein binding of Norfloxacin is between 10 and 15%.

The following are mean concentrations of Norfloxacin in various fluids and tissues measured 1 to 4 hours post-dose after two 400-mg doses, unless otherwise indicated:

Renal Parenchyma	7.3 µg/g
Prostate	2.5 µg/g
Seminal Fluid	2.7 µg/mL
Testicle	1.6 µg/g
Uterus/Cervix	3.0 µg/g
Vagina	4.3 µg/g
Fallopian Tube	1.9 µg/g
Bile	6.9 µg/mL (after two 200-mg doses)

MICROBIOLOGY

Norfloxacin has in vitro activity a broad range of gram-positive and gram-negative aerobic bacteria. The fluorine atom at the 6 position provides increased potency against gram-negative organisms, and the piperazine moiety at the 7 position is responsible for anti-pseudomonal activity. Norfloxacin inhibits bacterial deoxyribonucleic acid synthesis and is bactericidal. At the molecular level, three specific events are attributed to Norfloxacin in *E. coli* cells:

1) inhibition of the ATP-dependent DNA supercoiling reaction catalyzed by DNA gyrase,
2) inhibition of the relaxation of supercoiled DNA,
3) promotion of double-stranded DNA breakage.

Resistance to Norfloxacin due to spontaneous mutation in vitro is a rare occurrence (range: 10^{-9} to 10^{-12} cells). Resistant organisms have emerged during therapy with Norfloxacin in less than 1% of patients treated. Organisms in which development of resistance is greatest are the following:

Pseudomonas aeruginosa
Klebsiella pneumoniae
Acinetobacter species
Enterococcus species

For this reason, when there is a lack of satisfactory clinical response, repeat culture and susceptibility testing should be done. Nalidixic acid-resistant organisms are generally suspect to Nofloxacin in vitro; however, these organisms may have higher MICs to Norfloxacin than nalidixic acid-susceptible strains. There is generally no cross-resistance between Norfloxacin and other classes of antibacterial agents. Therefore Norfloxacin may demonstrate activity against indicated organisms resistant to some other antimicrobial agents including the aminoglycosides, penicillins, cephalosporins, tetracyclines, macrolides, and sulfonamides, including combinations of sulfamethoxazole and trimethoprim. Antagonism has been demonstrated in vitro between Norfloxacin and nitrofurantoin.

Norfloxacin has been shown to be active against most strains of the following organisms both in vitro and in clinical infections (see "Indications and Usage"):

GRAM-POSITIVE AEROBES
Enterococcus faecalis
Staphylococcus aureus
Staphylococcus epidermidis
Staphylococcus saprophyticus
Streptococcus agalactiae

GRAM-NEGATIVE AEROBES
Citrobacter freundii
Enterobacter aerogenes
Enterobacter cloacae
Escherichia coli
Klebsiella pneumoniae
Neisseria gonorrhoeae
Proteus mirabilis
Proteus vulgaris
Pseudomonas aeruginosa
Serratia marcescens

Norfloxacin has been shown to be active in vitro against most strains of the following organisms: however, *the clinical significance of these data is unknown.*

GRAM-POSITIVE AEROBES
Bacillus cereus

GRAM-NEGATIVE AEROBES
Acinetobacter calcoaceticus
Aeromonas species
Alcaligenes species
Campylobacter species
Citrobacter diversus
Edwardsiella tarda
Flavobacterium species
Hafnia alvei
Klebsiella oxytoca
Klebsiella rhinoscleromatis
Morganella morganii
Providencia alcalifaciens
Providencia rettgeri
Providencia stuartii
Salmonella species
Shigella species
Vibrio cholerae
Vibrio parahemolyticus
Yersinia enterocolitica

◆ RATED THERAPEUTICALLY EQUIVALENT; ◇ THERAPEUTIC EQUIVALENCE UNCONFIRMED; ○ UNRATED

OTHER
Ureaplasma urealyticum

Norfloxacin is not generally active against obligate anaerobes.
Norfloxacin has not been shown to be active against *Treponema pallidum*. (See *"Warnings."*)

SUSCEPTIBILITY TESTS
Diffusion Techniques: Quantitative methods that require measurement of zone diameters give the most precise estimate of the susceptibility of bacteria to antimicrobial agents. One such procedure is the National Committee for Clinical Laboratory Standards (NCCLS) approved procedure (M2-A4-Performance Standards for Antimicrobial Disk Susceptibility Tests 1990). This method has been recommended for use with the 10-mcg Norfloxacin disk to test susceptibility to Norfloxacin. Interpretation involves correlation of the diameters obtained in the disk test with minimum inhibitory concentration (MIC) for Norfloxacin. Reports from the laboratory giving results of the standard single-disk susceptibility test with a 10-mcg Norfloxacin disk should be interpreted according to the following criteria (*these criteria only apply to isolates from urinary tract infections*):

Zone diameter (mm)	Interpretation
≥ 17	(S) Susceptible
13-16	(I) Intermediate
≤ 12	(R) Resistant

A report of "Susceptible" indicates that the pathogen is likely to be inhibited by generally achievable urine levels. A report of "Intermediate" indicates that the test results be considered equivocal or indeterminate. A report of "Resistant" indicates that achievable concentrations of the antibiotic are unlikely to be inhibitory and other therapy should be selected.

Standardized procedures require the use of laboratory control organisms. The 10-mcg Norfloxacin disk should give the following zone diameter:

Organism	Zone diameter (mm)
E. coli ATCC 25922	28-35
P. aeruginosa ATCC 27853	22-29
S. aureus ATCC 25923	17-28

Other quinolone antibacterial disks should not be substituted when performing susceptibility tests for Norfloxacin because of spectrum differences with Norfloxacin. The 10-mcg Norfloxacin disk should be used for all *in vitro* testing of isolates using diffusion techniques.

Dilution Techniques: Broth and agar dilution methods, such as those recommended by the NCCLS (M7-A2—Methods for Dilution Antimicrobial Susceptibility Tests for Bacteria that Grow Aerobically 1990), may be used to determine the minimum inhibitory concentration (MIC) of Norfloxacin. MIC test results should be interpreted according to the following criteria (*these criteria only apply to isolates from urinary tract infections*):

MIC (mcg/mL)	Interpretation
≤ 4	(S) Susceptible
8	(I) Intermediate
≥ 16	(R) Resistant

As with standard diffusion methods, dilution procedures require the use of laboratory control organisms. Standard Norfloxacin powder should give the following MIC values:

Organism	MIC range (mcg/mL)
E. coli ATCC 25922	0.03-0.12
E. faecalis ATCC 29212	2.0-8.0
P. aeruginosa ATCC 27853	1.0-4.0
S. aureus ATCC 29213	0.05-2.0

INDICATIONS AND USAGE
Norfloxacin is indicated for the treatment of adults with the following infections caused by susceptible strains of the designated microorganisms:

Urinary Tract Infections: Uncomplicated urinary tract infections (including cystitis) due to *Enterococcus faecalis, Escherichia coli, Klebsiella pneumoniae, Proteus mirabilis, Pseudomonas aeruginosa, Staphylococcus epidermidis, Staphylococcus saprophyticus, Citrobacter freundii**, *Enterobacter aerogenes** *, Enterobacter cloacae**, *Proteus vulgaris**, Staphylococcus aureus*, or *Streptococcus agalactiae**.

Complicated urinary tract infections due to *Enterococcus faecalis, Escherichia coli, Klebsiella pneumoniae, Proteus mirabilis, Pseudomonas aeruginosa*, or *Serratia marcescens**.

Sexually Transmitted Diseases (see *"Warnings"*):
Uncomplicated urethral and cervical gonorrhea due to *Neisseria gonorrhoeae*. (See *"Dosage and Administration"* for appropriate dosing instructions.)

---

* Efficacy for this organism in this organ system was studied in fewer than 10 infections.

Penicillinase production should have no effect on Norfloxacin activity.
Appropriate culture and susceptibility tests should be performed before treatment in order to isolate and identify organisms causing the infection and to determine their susceptibility to Norfloxacin. Therapy with Norfloxacin may be initiated before results of these tests are known; once results become available, appropriate therapy should be given. Repeat culture and susceptibility testing performed periodically during therapy will provide information not only on the therapeutic effect of the antimicrobial agents but also on the possible emergence of bacterial resistance.

UNLABELED USES
Norfloxacin is used alone or as an adjunct in the prophylactic treatment of serious gram-negative bacillary infections in immunocompromised patients with granulocytopenia. It is also used in prostatitis, salmonella infections, and as prophylaxis against traveler's diarrhea.

CONTRAINDICATIONS
Norfloxacin is contraindicated in patients with a history of hypersensitivity to Norfloxacin or the other members of the quinolone group of antibacterial agents.

WARNINGS
THE SAFETY AND EFFICACY OF ORAL NORFLOXACIN IN CHILDREN, ADOLESCENTS (UNDER THE AGE OF 18), PREGNANT WOMEN, AND NURSING MOTHERS HAVE NOT BEEN ESTABLISHED. (See *"Precautions—Pregnancy, Nursing Mothers and Pediatric Use"*). The oral administration of single doses of Norfloxacin, 6 times[†] the recommended human clinical dose (on a mg/kg basis), caused lameness in immature dogs. Histologic examination of the weight-bearing joints of these dogs revealed permanent lesions of the cartilage. Other quinolones also produced erosions of the cartilage in weight-bearing joints and other signs of arthropathy in immature animals of various species. (See *"Animal Pharmacology."*)

Norfloxacin has not been shown to be effective in the treatment of syphilis. Antimicrobial agents used in high doses for short periods of time to treat gonorrhea may mask or delay the symptoms of incubating syphilis. All patients with gonorrhea should have a serologic test for syphilis at the time of diagnosis. Patients treated with Norfloxacin should have a follow-up serologic test for syphilis after three months.

Serious and occasionally fatal hypersensitivity (anaphylactoid or anaphylactic) reactions, some following the first dose, have been reported in patients receiving quinolone therapy. Some reactions were accompanied by cardiovascular collapse, loss of consciousness, tingling, pharyngeal or facial edema, dyspnea, urticaria and itching. Only a few patients had a history of hypersensitivity reactions. If an allergic reaction to Norfloxacin occurs, discontinue the drug. Serious acute hypersensitivity reactions may require immediate emergency treatment with epinephrine. Oxygen, intravenous fluids, antihistamines, corticosteroids, pressor amines, and airway management, including intubation, should be administered as indicated.

Convulsions have been reported in patients receiving Norfloxacin. Convulsions, increased intracranial pressure, and toxic psychoses have been reported in patients receiving drugs in this class. Quinolones may also cause central nervous system (CNS) stimulation which may lead to tremors, restlessness, lightheadness, confusion, and hallucinations. If these reactions occur in patients receiving Norfloxacin, the drug should be discontinued and appropriate measures instituted.

The effects of Norfloxacin on brain function or on the electrical activity of the brain have not been tested. Therefore, until more information becomes available Norfloxacin, like all other quinolones, should be used with caution in patients with known or suspected CNS disorders, such as severe cerebral arteriosclerosis, epilepsy, and other factors which pre-dispose to seizures. (See *"Adverse Reactions."*)

PRECAUTIONS
GENERAL
Needle-shaped crystals were found in the urine of some volunteers who received either placebo, 800 mg Norfloxacin, or 1600 mg Norfloxacin (at or twice the recommended daily dose, respectively) while participating in a double-blind, crossover study comparing single doses of Norfloxacin with placebo. While crystalluria is not expected to occur under usual conditions with a dosage regimen of 400 mg b.i.d., as a precaution, the daily recommended dosage should not be exceeded and the patient should drink sufficient fluids to ensure a proper state of hydration and adequate urinary output.

Alteration in dosage regimen is necessary for patients with impaired renal function (see *"Dosage and Administration"*).

Moderate to severe phototoxicity reactions have been observed in patients who are exposed to excessive sunlight while receiving some members of this drug class. Excessive sunlight should be avoided. Therapy should be discontinued if phototoxicity occurs.

INFORMATION FOR PATIENTS
Patients should be advised:
—to drink fluids liberally.
—that Norfloxacin should be taken at least one hour before or at least two hours after a meal.
—that multivitamins or other products containing iron or zinc, or antacids should not be taken within the two-hour period before or within the two-hour period after taking Norfloxacin. (See *"Drug Interactions."*)

---

† Based on a patient weight of 50 kg.

—that Norfloxacin can cause dizziness and light-headedness and, therefore, patients should know how they react to Norfloxacin before they operate an automobile or machinery or engage in activities requiring mental alertness and coordination.

—that Norfloxacin may be associated with hypersensitivity reactions, even following the first dose, and to discontinue the drug at the first sign of a skin rash or other allergic reaction.

—to avoid undue exposure to excessive sunlight while receiving Norfloxacin and to discontinue therapy if phototoxicity occurs.

—that some quinolones may increase the effects of theophylline and/or caffeine. (See *"Drug Interactions."*)

DRUG INTERACTIONS

Elevated plasma levels of theophylline have been reported with concomitant quinolone use. There have been reports of theophylline-related side effects in patients on concomitant therapy with Norfloxacin and theophylline. Therefore, monitoring of theophylline plasma levels should be considered and dosage of theophylline adjusted as required.

Elevated serum levels of cyclosporine have been reported with concomitant use of cyclosporine with Norfloxacin. Therefore cyclosporine serum levels should be monitored and appropriate cyclosporine dosage adjustments made when these drugs are used concomitantly.

Quinolones, including Norfloxacin, may enhance the effects of the oral anticoagulant warfarin or its derivatives. When these products are administered concomitantly, prothrombin time or other suitable coagulation tests should be closely monitored.

Diminished urinary excretion of Norfloxacin has been reported during the concomitant administration of probenecid and Norfloxacin.

The concomitant use of nitrofurantoin is not recommended since nitrofurantoin may antagonize the antibacterial effect of Norfloxacin in the urinary tract.

Multivitamins, or other products containing iron or zinc, antacids or sucralfate should not be administered concomitantly with, or within 2 hours of, the administration of Norfloxacin, because they may interfere with absorption resulting in lower serum and urine levels of Norfloxacin.

Some quinolones have also been shown to interfere with the metabolism of caffeine. This may lead to reduced clearance of caffeine and a prolongation of its plasma half-life.

CARCINOGENESIS, MUTAGENESIS, IMPAIRMENT OF FERTILITY

No increase in neoplastic changes was observed with Norfloxacin as compared to controls in a study in rats, lasting up to 96 weeks at doses 8-9 times† the usual human dose (on a mg/kg basis).

Norfloxacin was tested for mutagenic activity in a number of *in vivo* and *in vitro* tests. Norfloxacin had no mutagenic effect in the dominant lethal test in mice and did not cause chromosomal aberrations in hamsters or rats at doses 30-60 times† the usual human dose (on a mg/kg basis). Norfloxacin had no mutagenic activity *in vitro* in the Ames microbial mutagen test. Chinese hamster fibroblasts and V-79 mammalian cell assay. Although Norfloxacin was weakly positive in the Rec-assay for DNA repair, all other mutagenic assays were negative including a more sensitive test (V-79).

Norfloxacin did not adversely affect the fertility of male and female mice at oral doses up to 30 times† the usual human dose (on a mg/kg basis.)

PREGNANCY

Teratogenic Effects. Pregnancy Category C.: Norfloxacin has been shown to produce embryonic loss in monkeys when given in doses 10 times† the maximum daily total human dose (on a mg/kg basis). At this dose, peak plasma levels obtained in monkeys were approximately 2 times those obtained in humans. There has been no evidence of a teratogenic effect in any of the animal species tested (rat, rabbit, mouse, monkey) at 6-50 times† the maximum daily human dose (on a mg/kg basis). There are, however, no adequate and well controlled studies in pregnant women. Norfloxacin should be used during pregnancy only if the potential benefit justifies the potential risk to the fetus.

NURSING MOTHERS

It is not known whether Norfloxacin is excreted in human milk.

When a 200-mg dose of Norfloxacin was administered to nursing mothers, Norfloxacin was not detected in human milk. However, because the dose studied was low, because other drugs in this class are secreted in human milk, and because of the potential for serious adverse reactions from Norfloxacin in nursing infants, a decision should be made to discontinue nursing or to discontinue the drug, taking into account the importance of the drug to the mother.

PEDIATRIC USE

The safety and effectiveness of oral Norfloxacin in children and adolescents below the age of 18 years have not been established. Norfloxacin causes arthropathy in juvenile animals of several animal species. (See *"Warnings"* and *"Animal Pharmacology."*)

ADVERSE REACTIONS

Urinary Tract Infections: In clinical trials involving 1869 patients/subjects, 3.5% reported drug-related adverse experiences. However, the incidence fibures below were calculated without reference to drug relationship.

The most common adverse experiences (> 1%) were: nausea (4.3%), headache (2.9%), dizziness (1.8%), and asthenia (1.1%).

Additional reactions (0.3%-1%) were: rash, abdominal pain, dyspepsia, somnolence, depression, insomnia, constipation, flatulence, heartburn, dry mouth, diarrhea, fever, vomiting, pruritus, loose stools, back pain and hyperhidrosis.

Less frequent reactions included: erythema, anorexia, bitter taste, and asthenia.

Abnormal laboratory values observed in these patient/subjects were: elevation of ALT (SGPT) (1.6%), decreased WBC and neutrophil count (1.6%), elevation of AST (SGOT) (1.4%), eosinophilia (1.4%), and increased alkaline phosphatase (1.2%). Those occurring less frequently included increased BUN, serum creatinine, and LDH, and decreased hematocrit.

Gonorrhea: In clinical trials involving 228 patients who received a single 800-mg dose, 7.0% of patients reported drug-related adverse experiences. However, the following incidence figures were calculated without reference to drug relationship.

The most common adverse experiences (1%-3.5%) were: dizziness (3.5%), nausea (2.2%), abdominal cramping (1.8%), diarrhea (1.3%), anorexia (1.3%), headache (1.3%), and hyperhidrosis (1.3%).

Additional reactions (0.3%-1%) were: vomiting, constipation, dyspepsia, and tingling of the fingers.

Laboratory adverse changes considered drug-related were reported in 2.2% of patients who received a single 800-mg dose of Norfloxacin. These laboratory changes were: decreased hemoglobin and hematocrit (0.9%), decreased platelet count (0.9%), and increased AST (0.4%).

Postmarketing: The most frequently reported adverse reaction in post-marketing experience is rash.

CNS effects characterized as generalized seizures and myoclonus have been reported with Norfloxacin. A causal relationship to Norfloxacin has not been established (see *"Warnings"*). Visual disturbances have been reported with drugs in this class.

The following additional adverse reactions have been reported since the drug was marketed:

Hypersensitivity Reactions: Hypersensitivity reactions have been reported including anaphylactoid reactions, angioedema, dyspnea, vasculitis, urticaria, arthritis, arthralgia and myalgia (see *"Warnings"*).

Skin: Toxic epidermal necrolysis, Stevens-Johnson syndrome and erythema multiforme, exfoliative dermatitis, pruritus, photosensitivity.

Gastrointestinal: Pseudomembranous colitis, hepatitis, jaundice, including cholestatic jaundice, pancreatitis (rare), stomatitis, anorexia.

Renal: Interstitial nephritis, renal failure

Nervous System/Psychiatric: Polyneuropathy including Guillain-Barre Syndrome, ataxia, paresthesia; psychic disturbances including psychotic reactions and confusion

Musculoskeletal: Tendinitis, possible exacerbation of myasthenia gravis

Hematologic: Neutropenia, leukopenia, hemolytic anemia, thrombocytopenia

Special Senses: Transient hearing loss (rare), tinnitus, diplopia

Other adverse events reported with quinolones include: agranulocytosis, albuminuria, candiduria, crystalluria, cylindruria, dysphagia, elevation of blood glucose, elevation of serum cholesterol, elevation of serum potassium, elevation of serum triglycerides, hematuria, hepatic necrosis, symptomatic hypoglycemia, nystagmus, postural hypotension, prolongation of prothrombin time, and vaginal candidiasis.

OVERDOSAGE

No significant lethality was observed in male and female mice and rats at single oral doses up to 4 g/kg.

In the event of acute overdosage, the stomach should be emptied by inducing vomiting or by gastric lavage, and the patient carefully observed and given symptomatic and supportive treatment. Adequate hydration must be maintained.

DOSAGE AND ADMINISTRATION

Tablets Norfloxacin should be taken at least one hour before or at least two hours after a meal with a glass of water. Patients receiving Norfloxacin should be well hydrated (see *"Precautions"*).

NORMAL RENAL FUNCTION

The recommended daily dose of Norfloxacin is as described in the following chart: (See related table).

RENAL IMPAIRMENT

Norfloxacin may be used for the treatment of urinary tract infections in patients with renal insufficiency. In patients with a creatinine clearance rate of 30 mL/min/1.73m^2 or less, the recommended dosage is one 400-mg tablet once daily for the duration given above. At this dosage, the urinary concentration exceeds the MICs for most urinary pathogens susceptible to Norfloxacin, even when the creatinine clearance is less than 10 mL/min/1.73m^2.

When only the serum creatinine level is available, the following formula (based on sex, weight, and age of the patient) may be used to convert this value into creatinine clearance.

The serum creatinine should represent a steady state of renal function.

Males: $= $ (weight in kg) $\times$ $(140 - $ age$)/$
$$(72) \times \text{serum creatinine (mg/100 mL)}$$

Females: $= (0.85) \times$ (above value)

---

† Based on a patient weight of 50 kg.

Infection	Description	Unit Dose	Frequency	Duration	Daily Dose
Urinary Tract	Uncomplicated UTI's (crystitis) due to E. coli K. pneumoniae, or P. mirabilis	400 mg	q12h	3 days	800 mg
	Uncomplicated UTI's due to other indicated organisms	400 mg	q12h	7-10 days	800 mg
	Complicated UTI's	400 mg	q12h	10-21 days	800 mg
Sexually Transmitted Diseases	Uncomplicated Gonorrhea	800 mg	single dose	1 day	800 mg

ELDERLY

Elderly patients being treated for urinary tract infections who have a creatinine clearance of greater than $30 \text{ mL/min}/1.73\text{m}^2$ should receive the dosages recommended under

NORMAL RENAL FUNCTION

Elderly patients being treated for urinary tract infections who have a creatinine clearance of $30 \text{ mL/min}/1.73\text{m}^2$ or less should receive 400 mg once daily as recommended under *"Renal Impairment"*.

Norfloxacin tablets should be stored in a tightly-closed container. Avoid storage at temperatures above 40°C (104°F).

ANIMAL PHARMACOLOGY

Norfloxacin and related drugs have been shown to cause arthropathy in immature animals of most species tested (see *"Warnings"*).

Crystalluria has occurred in laboratory animals tested with Norfloxacin. In dogs, needle-shaped drug crystals were seen in the urine at doses of 50 mg/kg/day. In rats, crystals were reported following doses of 200 mg/kg/day.

Embryo lethality and slight maternotoxicity (vomiting and anorexia) were observed in cynomolgus monkeys at doses of 150 mg/kg/day or higher.

Ocular toxicity, seen with some related drugs, was not observed in any Norfloxacin-treated animals.

HOW SUPPLIED
TABLETS: 400 MG

BRAND/MANUFACTURER	NDC	SIZE	AWP
○ BRAND			
▶ NOROXIN: Merck	00006-0705-20	20s	$49.45
	00006-0705-68	100s	$243.58
	00006-0705-28	100s ud	$243.58

Norgesic *SEE* ASPIRIN/CAFFEINE/ORPHENADRINE CITRATE

Norgestrel

DESCRIPTION

Each tablet contains 0.075 mg of Norgestrel (*dl*-13-beta-ethyl-17-alpha-ethinyl-17-beta-hydroxygon-4-en-3-one), a totally synthetic progestogen. The available data suggest that the d(-)enantiomeric form of Norgestrel is the biologically active portion. This form amounts to 0.0375 mg per Norgestrel tablet.

Following is its chemical structure:

CLINICAL PHARMACOLOGY

The primary mechanism through which Norgestrel prevents conception is not known, but progestogen-only contraceptives are known to alter the cervical mucus, exert a progestational effect on the endometrium, interfering with implantation, and, in some patients, suppress ovulation.

INDICATIONS AND USAGE

Oral contraceptives are indicated for the prevention of pregnancy in women who elect to use this product as a method of contraception.

Oral contraceptives are highly effective. Table 1 lists the typical accidental pregnancy rates for users of combination oral contraceptives and other methods of contraception. The efficacy of these contraceptive methods, except sterilization and the IUD, depends upon the reliability with which they are used. Correct and consistent use of methods can result in lower failure rates.

Table 1

LOWEST EXPECTED AND TYPICAL FAILURE RATES DURING THE FIRST YEAR OF CONTINUOUS USE OF A METHOD

% of Women Experiencing an Accidental Pregnancy in the First Year of Continuous Use

Method	Lowest Expected*	Typical**
(No Contraception)	(89)	(89)
Oral contraceptives		3
combined	0.1	N/A***
progestin only	0.5	N/A***
Diaphragm with spermicidal cream or jelly	3	18
Spermicides alone (foam, creams, jellies and vaginal suppositories)	3	21
Vaginal Sponge		
nulliparous	5	18
multiparous	> 8	>28
IUD (medicated)	1	6#
Condom without spermicides		12
Periodic abstinence (all methods)	2-10	20
Female sterilization	0.2	0.4
Male sterilization	0.1	0.15

Adapted from J. Trussell and K. Kost, Table 11, Studies in Family Planning, 18(5), Sept.-Oct. 1987.

* *The authors' best guess of the percentage of women expected to experience an accidental pregnancy among couples who initiate a method (not necessarily for the first time) and who use it consistently and correctly during the first year if they do not stop for any other reason.*

** *This term represents 'typical' couples who initiate a method (not necessarily for the first time), who experience an accidental pregnancy during the first year if they do not stop use for any other reason.*

*** *N/A—Data not available.*

\# *Combined typical rate for both medicated and nonmedicated IUD. The rate for medicated IUD alone is not available.*

CONTRAINDICATIONS

Oral contraceptives should not be used in women with any of the following conditions:

Thrombophlebitis or thromboembolic disorders.

A past history of deep-vein thrombophlebitis or thromboembolic disorders.

Cerebral-vascular or coronary-artery disease.

Known or suspected carcinoma of the breast.

Carcinoma of the endometrium or other known or suspected estrogen-dependent neoplasia.

Undiagnosed abnormal genital bleeding.

Cholestatic jaundice of pregnancy or jaundice with prior pill use.

Hepatic adenomas or carcinomas.

Known or suspected pregnancy.

WARNINGS

CIGARETTE SMOKING INCREASES THE RISK OF SERIOUS CARDIOVASCULAR SIDE EFFECTS FROM ORAL-CONTRACEPTIVE USE. THIS RISK INCREASES WITH AGE AND WITH HEAVY SMOKING (15 OR MORE CIGARETTES PER DAY) AND IS QUITE MARKED IN WOMEN OVER 35 YEARS OF AGE. WOMEN WHO USE ORAL CONTRACEPTIVES SHOULD BE STRONGLY ADVISED NOT TO SMOKE.

The use of oral contraceptives is associated with increased risks of several serious conditions including myocardial infarction, thromboembolism, stroke, hepatic neoplasia, gallbladder disease, and hypertension, although the risk of serious morbidity or mortality is very small in healthy women without underlying

▶ SHOWN IN PRODUCT IDENTIFICATION GUIDE

risk factors. The risk of morbidity and mortality increases significantly in the presence of other underlying risk factors such as hypertension, hyperlipidemias, obesity, and diabetes.

Practitioners prescribing oral contraceptives should be familiar with the following information relating to these risks.

The information contained in this prescribing information is based principally on studies carried out in patients who used oral contraceptives with higher formulations of estrogens and progestogens than those in common use today. The effect of long-term use of the oral contraceptives with lower formulations of both estrogens and progestogens remains to be determined.

Throughout this labeling, epidemiological studies reported are of two types: retrospective or case control studies and prospective or cohort studies. Case control studies provide a measure of the relative risk of disease, namely, a ratio of the incidence of a disease among oral-contraceptive users to that among nonusers. The relative risk does not provide information on the actual clinical occurrence of a disease. Cohort studies provide a measure of attributable risk, which is the difference in the incidence of disease between oral-contraceptive users and nonusers. The attributable risk does provide information about the actual occurrence of a disease in the population. For further information, the reader is referred to a text on epidemiological methods.

1. THROMBOEMBOLIC DISORDERS AND OTHER VASCULAR PROBLEMS

a. Myocardial Infarction

An increased risk of myocardial infarction has been attributed to oral-contraceptive use. This risk is primarily in smokers or women with other underlying risk factors for coronary-artery disease such as hypertension, hypercholesterolemia, morbid obesity, and diabetes. The relative risk of heart attack for current oral-contraceptive users has been estimated to be two to six. The risk is very low under the age of 30.

Smoking in combination with oral-contraceptive use has been shown to contribute substantially to the incidence of myocardial infarctions in women in their mid-thirties or older with smoking accounting for the majority of excess cases. Mortality rates associated with circulatory disease have been shown to increase substantially in smokers over the age of 35 and nonsmokers over the age of 40 (Table 2) among women who use oral contraceptives.

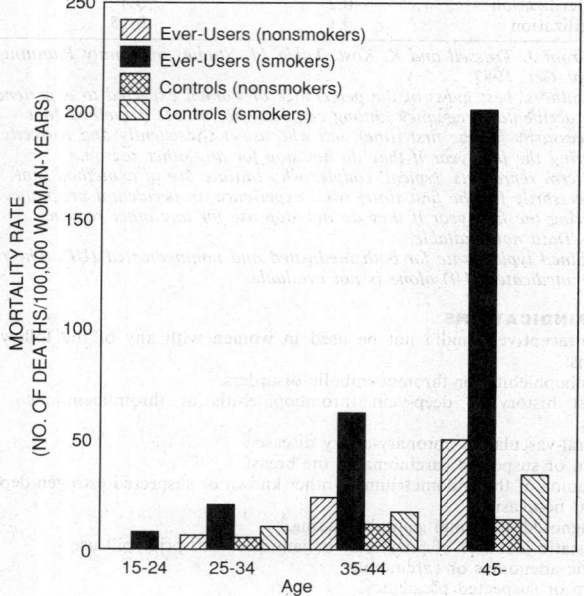

CIRCULATORY DISEASE MORTALITY RATES PER 100,000 WOMAN-YEARS BY AGE, SMOKING STATUS AND ORAL CONTRACEPTIVE USE

Table 2 (Adapted from P.M. Legde and V. Beral, Lancet, *1*:541-546, 1981.)

Oral contraceptives may compound the effects of well-known risk factors, such as hypertension, diabetes, hyperlipidemias, age, and obesity. In particular, some progestogens are known to decrease HDL cholesterol and cause glucose intolerance, while estrogens may create a state of hyperinsulinism. Oral contraceptives have been shown to increase blood pressure among users (see section 9 in "Warnings"). Similar effects on risk factors have been associated with an increased risk of heart disease. Oral contraceptives must be used with caution in women with cardiovascular disease risk factors.

b. Thromboembolism

An increased risk of thromboembolic and thrombotic disease associated with the use of oral contraceptives is well established. Case control studies have found the relative risk of users compared to nonusers to be 3 for the first episode of superficial venous thrombosis, 4 to 11 for deep-vein thrombosis or pulmonary embolism, and 1.5 to 6 for women with predisposing conditions for venous thromboembolic disease. Cohort studies have shown the relative risk to be somewhat lower, about 3 for new cases and about 4.5 for new cases requiring hospitalization. The risk of thromboembolic disease due to oral contraceptives is not related to length of use and disappears after pill use is stopped.

A two- to four-fold increase in relative risk of postoperative thromboembolic complications has been reported with the use of oral contraceptives. The relative risk of venous thrombosis in women who have predisposing conditions is twice that of women without such medical conditions. If feasible, oral contraceptives should be discontinued at least four weeks prior to and for two weeks after elective surgery of a type associated with an increase in risk of thromboembolism and during and following prolonged immobilization. Since the immediate postpartum period is also associated with an increased risk of thromboembolism, oral contraceptives should be started no earlier than four to six weeks after delivery in women who elect not to breast-feed, or a midtrimester pregnancy termination.

c. Cerebrovascular diseases

Oral contraceptives have been shown to increase both the relative and attributable risks of cerebrovascular events (thrombotic and hemorrhagic strokes), although, in general, the risk is greatest among older (> 35 years), hypertensive women who also smoke. Hypertension was found to be a risk factor for both users and nonusers, for both types of strokes, while smoking interacted to increase the risk of hemorrhagic strokes.

In a large study, the relative risk of thrombotic strokes has been shown to range from 3 for normotensive users to 14 for users with severe hypertension. The relative risk of hemorrhagic stroke is reported to be 1.2 for nonsmokers who used oral contraceptives, 2.6 for smokers who did not use oral contraceptives, 7.6 for smokers who used oral contraceptives, 1.8 for normotensive users, and 25.7 for users with severe hypertension. The attributable risk is also greater in older women.

d. Dose-related risk of vascular disease from oral contraceptives

A positive association has been observed between the amount of estrogen and progestogen and the risk of vascular disease. A decline in serum high-density lipoproteins (HDL) has been reported with many progestational agents. A decline in serum high-density lipoproteins has been associated with an increased incidence of ischemic heart disease. Because estrogens increase HDL cholesterol, the net effect of an oral contraceptive depends on a balance achieved between doses of estrogen and progestogen and the nature and absolute amount of progestogen used in the contraceptive. The amount of both hormones should be considered in the choice of an oral contraceptive.

Minimizing exposure to estrogen and progestogen is in keeping with good principles of therapeutics. For any particular estrogen/progestogen combination, the dosage regimen prescribed should be one which contains the least amount of estrogen and progestogen that is compatible with a low failure rate and the needs of the individual patient. New acceptors of oral-contraceptive agents should be started on preparations containing less than 50 mcg of estrogen.

e. Persistence of risk of vascular disease

There are two studies which have shown persistence of risk of vascular disease for ever-users of oral contraceptives. In a study in the United States, the risk of developing myocardial infarction after discontinuing oral contraceptives persists for at least 9 years for women 40 to 49 years who had used oral contraceptives for five or more years, but this increased risk was not demonstrated in other age groups. In another study in Great Britain, the risk of developing cerebrovascular disease persisted for at least 6 years after discontinuation of oral contraceptives, although excess risk was very small. However, both studies were performed with oral-contraceptive formulations containing 50 micrograms or higher of estrogens.

2. ESTIMATES OF MORTALITY FROM CONTRACEPTIVE USE

One study gathered data from a variety of sources which have estimated the mortality rate associated with different methods of contraception at different ages (Table 3). These estimates include the combined risk of death associated with contraceptive methods plus the risk attributable to pregnancy in the event of method failure. Each method of contraception has its specific benefits and risks. The study concluded that with the exception of oral-contraceptive users 35 and older who smoke and 40 and older who do not smoke, mortality associated with all methods of birth control is less than that associated with childbirth. The observation of a possible increase in risk of mortality with age for oral-contraceptive users is based on data gathered in the 1970's—but not reported until 1983. However, current clinical practice involves the use of lower estrogen dose formulations combined with careful restriction of oral-contraceptive use to women who do not have the various risk factors listed in this labeling.

Because of these changes in practice and, also, because of some limited new data which suggest that the risk of cardiovascular disease with the use of oral contraceptives may now be less than previously observed, the Fertility and Maternal Health Drugs Advisory Committee was asked to review the topic in 1989. The Committee concluded that although cardiovascular-disease risks may be increased with oral-contraceptive use after age 40 in healthy nonsmoking women (even with the newer low-dose formulations), there are greater potential health risks associated with pregnancy in older women and with the alternative surgical and medical procedures which may be necessary if such women do not have access to effective and acceptable means of contraception. Therefore, the Committee recommended that the benefits of oral-contraceptive use by healthy nonsmoking women over 40 may outweigh the possible risks. Of course, older women, as all women who take oral contraceptives, should take the lowest possible dose formulation that is effective. (See related table).

3. CARCINOMA OF THE REPRODUCTIVE ORGANS
Numerous epidemiological studies have been performed on the incidence of breast, endometrial, ovarian, and cervical cancer in women using oral contraceptives. The overwhelming evidence in the literature suggests that use of oral contraceptives is not associated with an increase in the risk of developing breast cancer, regardless of the age and parity of first use or with most of the marketed brands and doses. The Cancer and Steroid Hormone (CASH) study also showed no latent effect on the risk of breast cancer for at least a decade following long-term use. A few studies have shown a slightly increased relative risk of developing breast cancer, although the methodology of these studies, which included differences in examination of users and nonusers and differences in age at start of use, has been questioned.

Some studies suggest that oral-contraceptive use has been associated with an increase in the risk of cervical intraepithelial neoplasia in some populations of women. However, there continues to be controversy about the extent to which such findings may be due to differences in sexual behavior and other factors.

In spite of many studies of the relationship between oral-contraceptive use and breast and cervical cancers, a cause-and-effect relationship has not been established.

4. HEPATIC NEOPLASIA
Benign hepatic adenomas are associated with oral-contraceptive use, although the incidence of benign tumors is rare in the United States. Indirect calculations have estimated the attributable risk to be in the range of 3.3 cases/100,000 for users, a risk that increases after four or more years of use. Rupture of rare, benign, hepatic adenomas may cause death through intra-abdominal hemorrhage.

Studies from Britain have shown an increased risk of developing hepatocellular carcinoma in long-term (>8 years) oral-contraceptive users. However, these cancers are extremely rare in the U.S., and the attributable risk (the excess incidence) of liver cancers in oral-contraceptive users approaches less than one per million users.

5. OCULAR LESIONS
There have been clinical case reports of retinal thrombosis associated with the use of oral contraceptives. Oral contraceptives should be discontinued if there is unexplained partial or complete loss of vision; onset of proptosis or diplopia; papilledema; or retinal vascular lesions. Appropriate diagnostic and therapeutic measures should be undertaken immediately.

6. ORAL-CONTRACEPTIVE USE BEFORE OR DURING EARLY PREGNANCY
Extensive epidemiological studies have revealed no increased risk of birth defects in women who have used oral contraceptives prior to pregnancy. Studies also do not suggest a teratogenic effect, particularly insofar as cardiac anomalies and limb-reduction defects are concerned, when taken inadvertently during early pregnancy.

The administration of oral contraceptives to induce withdrawal bleeding should not be used as a test for pregnancy. Oral contraceptives should not be used during pregnancy to treat threatened or habitual abortion.

It is recommended that for any patient who has missed two consecutive periods, pregnancy should be ruled out before continuing oral-contraceptive use. If the patient has not adhered to the prescribed schedule, the possibility of pregnancy should be considered at the time of the first missed period. Oral-contraceptive use should be discontinued if pregnancy is confirmed.

7. GALLBLADDER DISEASE
Earlier studies have reported an increased lifetime relative risk of gallbladder surgery in users of oral contraceptives and estrogens. More recent studies, however, have shown that the relative risk of developing gallbladder disease among oral-contraceptive users may be minimal. The recent findings of minimal risk may be related to the use of oral-contraceptive formulations containing lower hormonal doses of estrogens and progestogens.

8. CARBOHYDRATE AND LIPID METABOLIC EFFECTS
Oral contraceptives have been shown to cause glucose intolerance in a significant percentage of users. Oral contraceptives containing greater than 75 micrograms of estrogens cause hyperinsulinism, while lower doses of estrogen cause less glucose intolerance. Progestogens increase insulin secretion and create insulin resistance, this effect varying with different progestational agents. However, in the nondiabetic woman, oral contraceptives appear to have no effect on fasting blood glucose. Because of these demonstrated effects, prediabetic and diabetic women should be carefully observed while taking oral contraceptives.

A small proportion of women will have persistent hypertriglyceridemia while on the pill. As discussed earlier (see "Warnings, 1a", and "1d".), changes in serum triglycerides and lipoprotein levels have been reported in oral-contraceptive users.

9. ELEVATED BLOOD PRESSURE
An increase in blood pressure has been reported in women taking oral contraceptives, and this increase is more likely in older oral-contraceptive users and with continued use. Data from the Royal College of General Practitioners and subsequent randomized trials have shown that the incidence of hypertension increases with increasing quantities of progestogens.

Women with a history of hypertension or hypertension-related diseases, or renal disease, should be encouraged to use another method of contraception. If women with hypertension elect to use oral contraceptives, they should be monitored closely, and if significant elevation of blood pressure occurs, oral contraceptives should be discontinued. For most women, elevated blood pressure will return to normal after stopping oral contraceptives, and there is no difference in the occurrence of hypertension among ever- and never-users.

10. HEADACHE
The onset or exacerbation of migraine or development of headache with a new pattern that is recurrent, persistent, or severe requires discontinuation of oral contraceptives and evaluation of the cause.

11. BLEEDING IRREGULARITIES
Breakthrough bleeding and spotting are sometimes encountered in patients on oral contraceptives, especially during the first three months of use. The type and dose of progestogen may be important. Non-hormonal causes should be considered and adequate diagnostic measures taken to rule out malignancy or pregnancy in the event of breakthrough bleeding, as in the case of any abnormal vaginal bleeding. If pathology has been excluded, time or a change to another formulation may solve the problem. In the event of amenorrhea, pregnancy should be ruled out.

Some women may encounter post-pill amenorrhea or oligomenorrhea, especially when such a condition was preexistent.

PRECAUTIONS
1. PHYSICAL EXAMINATION AND FOLLOW-UP
A complete medical history and physical examination should be taken prior to the initiation or reinstitution of oral contraceptives and at least annually during use of oral contraceptives. These physical examinations should include special reference to blood pressure, breasts, abdomen and pelvic organs, including cervical cytology, and relevant laboratory tests. In case of undiagnosed, persistent or recurrent abnormal vaginal bleeding, appropriate diagnostic measures should be conducted to rule out malignancy. Women with a strong family history of breast cancer or who have breast nodules should be monitored with particular care.

2. LIPID DISORDERS
Women who are being treated for hyperlipidemias should be followed closely if they elect to use oral contraceptives. Some progestogens may elevate LDL levels and may render the control of hyperlipidemias more difficult. (See "Warnings, 1d".)

3. LIVER FUNCTION
If jaundice develops in any woman receiving such drugs, the medication should be discontinued. Steroid hormones may be poorly metabolized in patients with impaired liver function.

4. FLUID RETENTION
Oral contraceptives may cause some degree of fluid retention. They should be prescribed with caution, and only with careful monitoring, in patients with conditions which might be aggravated by fluid retention.

Table 3
ANNUAL NUMBER OF BIRTH-RELATED OR METHOD-RELATED DEATHS ASSOCIATED WITH CONTROL OF FERTILITY PER 100,000 NONSTERILE WOMEN, BY FERTILITY-CONTROL METHOD ACCORDING TO AGE

Method of control and outcome	15-19	20-24	25-29	30-34	35-39	40-44
No fertility-control methods*	7.0	7.4	9.1	14.8	25.7	28.2
Oral contraceptives nonsmoker**	0.3	0.5	0.9	1.9	13.8	31.6
Oral contraceptives smoker**	2.2	3.4	6.6	13.5	51.1	117.2
IUD**	0.8	0.8	1.0	1.0	1.4	1.4
Condom*	1.1	1.6	0.7	0.2	0.3	0.4
Diaphragm/spermicide*	1.9	1.2	1.2	1.3	2.2	2.8
Periodic abstinence*	2.5	1.6	1.6	1.7	2.9	3.6

*Deaths are birth related
**Deaths are method related

Adapted from H.W. Ory, Family Planning Perspectives, 15:57-63, 1983.

5. EMOTIONAL DISORDERS

Patients becoming significantly depressed while taking oral contraceptives should stop the medication and use an alternate method of contraception in an attempt to determine whether the symptom is drug related. Women with a history of depression should be carefully observed and the drug discontinued if depression recurs to a serious degree.

6. CONTACT LENSES

Contact-lens wearers who develop visual changes or changes in lens tolerance should be assessed by an ophthalmologist.

7. DRUG INTERACTIONS

Reduced efficacy and increased incidence of breakthrough bleeding and menstrual irregularities have been associated with concomitant use of rifampin. A similar association, though less marked, has been suggested with barbiturates, phenylbutazone, phenytoin sodium, and possibly with griseofulvin, ampicillin, and tetracyclines.

8. INTERACTIONS WITH LABORATORY TESTS

Certain endocrine- and liver-function tests and blood components may be affected by oral contraceptives:

a. Increased prothrombin and factors VII, VIII, IX, and X; decreased antithrombin 3; increased norepinephrine-induced platelet aggregability.

b. Increased thyroid-binding globulin (TBG) leading to increased circulating total thyroid hormone, as measured by protein-bound iodine (PBI), T4 by column or by radioimmunoassay. Free T3 resin uptake is decreased, reflecting the elevated TBG; free T4 concentration is unaltered.

c. Other binding proteins may be elevated in serum.

d. Sex-binding globulins are increased and result in elevated levels of total circulating sex steroids and corticoids; however, free or biologically active levels remain unchanged.

e. Triglycerides may be increased.

f. Glucose tolerance may be decreased.

g. Serum folate levels may be depressed by oral-contraceptive therapy. This may be of clinical significance if a woman becomes pregnant shortly after discontinuing oral contraceptives.

9. CARCINOGENESIS

See *"Warnings"* section.

10. PREGNANCY

Pregnancy Category X. See *"Contraindications"* and *"Warnings"* sections.

11. NURSING MOTHERS

Small amounts of oral-contraceptive steroids have been identified in the milk of nursing mothers, and a few adverse effects on the child have been reported, including jaundice and breast enlargement. In addition, oral contraceptives given in the postpartum period may interfere with lactation by decreasing the quantity and quality of breast milk. If possible the nursing mother should be advised not to use oral contraceptives but to use other forms of contraception until she has completely weaned her child.

12. INFORMATION FOR THE PATIENT

See manufacturer's patient information.

ADVERSE REACTIONS

An increased risk of the following serious adverse reactions has been associated with the use of oral contraceptives (see *"Warnings"* section):

Thrombophlebitis.
Arterial thromboembolism.
Pulmonary embolism.
Myocardial infarction.
Cerebral hemorrhage.
Cerebral thrombosis.
Hypertension.
Gallbladder disease.
Hepatic adenomas or benign liver tumors.

There is evidence of an association between the following conditions and the use of oral contraceptives, although additional confirmatory studies are needed:

Mesenteric thrombosis.
Retinal thrombosis.

The following adverse reactions have been reported in patients receiving oral contraceptives and are believed to be drug related:

Nausea.
Vomiting.
Gastrointestinal symptoms (such as abdominal cramps and bloating).
Breakthrough bleeding.
Spotting.
Change in menstrual flow.
Amenorrhea.
Temporary infertility after discontinuation of treatment.
Edema.
Melasma which may persist.
Breast changes: tenderness, enlargement, secretion.
Change in weight (increase or decrease).
Change in cervical erosion and secretion.
Diminution in lactation when given immediately postpartum.

Cholestatic jaundice.
Migraine.
Rash (allergic).
Mental depression.
Reduced tolerance to carbohydrates.
Vaginal candidiasis.
Change in corneal curvature (steepening).
Intolerance to contact lenses.

The following adverse reactions have been reported in users of oral contraceptives, and the association has been neither confirmed nor refuted:

Congenital anomalies.
Premenstrual syndrome.
Cataracts.
Optic neuritis.
Changes in appetite.
Cystitis-like syndrome.
Headache.
Nervousness.
Dizziness.
Hirsutism.
Loss of scalp hair.
Erythema multiforme.
Erythema nodosum.
Hemorrhagic eruption.
Vaginitis.
Porphyria.
Impaired renal function.
Hemolytic uremic syndrome.
Budd-Chiari syndrome.
Acne.
Changes in libido.
Colitis.
Sickle-cell disease.
Cerebral-vascular disease with mitral valve prolapse.
Lupus-like syndromes.

OVERDOSAGE

Serious ill effects have not been reported following acute ingestion of large doses of oral contraceptives by young children. Overdosage may cause nausea, and withdrawal bleeding may occur in females.

NONCONTRACEPTIVE HEALTH BENEFITS

The following noncontraceptive health benefits related to the use of oral contraceptives are supported by epidemiological studies which largely utilized oral-contraceptive formulations containing doses exceeding 0.035 mg of ethinyl estradiol or 0.05 mg of mestranol.

Effects on menses:
Increased menstrual cycle regularity.
Decreased blood loss and decreased incidence of iron-deficiency anemia.
Decreased incidence of dysmenorrhea.

Effects related to inhibition of ovulation:
Decreased incidence of functional ovarian cysts.
Decreased incidence of ectopic pregnancies.

Effects from long-term use:
Decreased incidence of fibroadenomas and fibrocystic disease of the breast.
Decreased incidence of acute pelvic inflammatory disease.
Decreased incidence of endometrial cancer.
Decreased incidence of ovarian cancer.

DOSAGE AND ADMINISTRATION

To achieve maximum contraceptive effectiveness, Norgestrel must be taken exactly as directed and at intervals not exceeding 24 hours.

Norgestrel is administered on a continuous daily dosage regimen starting on the first day of menstruation, i.e., one tablet each day, every day of the year.

Tablets should be taken at the same time each day and continued daily, without interruption, whether bleeding occurs or not. The patient should be advised that, if prolonged bleeding occurs, she should consult her physician. In the nonlactating mother, Norgestrel may be initiated postpartum, for contraception. When the tablets are administered in the postpartum period the increased risk of thromboembolic disease associated with the postpartum period must be considered (see *"Contraindications"*, *"Warnings,"* and *"Precautions"* concerning thromboembolic disease). It is to be noted that early resumption of ovulation may occur if bromocriptine mesylate has been used for the prevention of lactation.

The risk of pregnancy increases with each tablet missed. It the patient misses one tablet, she should be instructed to take it as soon as she remembers and to also take her next tablet at the regular time. If she misses two tablets, she should take one of the missed tablets as soon as she remembers, as well as taking her regular tablet for that day at the proper time. Furthermore, she should use a method of nonhormonal contraception in addition to taking Norgestrel until fourteen tablets have been taken. If more than 2 tablets have been missed, Norgestrel should be discontinued immediately and a method of nonhormonal contraception should be used until menses has appeared or pregnancy has been excluded. If menses does not appear within 45 days from the last period, a method of nonhormonal contraception should be substituted until the start of the next menstrual period or an appropriate diagnostic procedure is performed to rule out pregnancy.

HOW SUPPLIED
TABLETS: 0.075 MG

BRAND/MANUFACTURER	NDC	SIZE	AWP
○ BRAND			
▶ OVRETTE: Wyeth-Ayerst	00008-0062-02	28s	$21.90
	00008-0062-01	168s	$150.69

Norinyl SEE ETHINYL ESTRADIOL AND NORETHINDRONE AND MESTRANOL AND NORETHINDRONE

Norisodrine W/Calcium Iodide SEE CALCIUM IODIDE AND ISOPROTERENOL SULFATE

Norlac Rx SEE VITAMINS, PRENATAL

Norlutate SEE NORETHINDRONE ACETATE

Normodyne SEE LABETALOL HYDROCHLORIDE

Normosol W/5% Dextrose SEE DEXTROSE AND ELECTROLYTES AND DEXTROSE AND ELECTROLYTES, INTRAPERITONEAL

Normosol-R SEE DEXTROSE AND ELECTROLYTES AND ELECTROLYTES, INJECTABLE

Noroxin SEE NORFLOXACIN, ORAL

Norpace SEE DISOPYRAMIDE PHOSPHATE

Norplant System SEE LEVONORGESTREL

Norpramin SEE DESIPRAMINE HYDROCHLORIDE

Nor-QD SEE NORETHINDRONE

Nortriptyline Hydrochloride

DESCRIPTION
Nortriptyline Hydrochloride is 1-Propanamine, 3-(10,11-dihydro-5H-dibenzo[a,d]cyclohepten-5-ylidene)-N- methyl-,hydrochloride.

Its molecular formula is $C_{19}H_{21}N \cdot HCl$ and its molecular weight is 299.8.

Nortriptyline Hydrochloride, USP, is the active ingredient in 10 mg, 25 mg, 50 mg and 75 mg capsules and solution.

Following is its chemical structure:

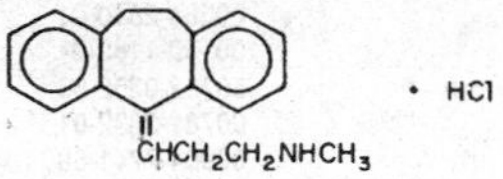

ACTIONS
The mechanism of mood elevation by tricyclic antidepressants is at present unknown. Nortriptyline HCl is not a monoamine oxidase inhibitor. It inhibits the activity of such diverse agents as histamine, 5-hydroxytryptamine, and acetylcho-line. It increases the pressor effect of norepinephrine but blocks the pressor response of phenethylamine. Studies suggest that Nortriptyline HCl interferes with the transport, release, and storage of catecholamines. Operant conditioning techniques in rats and pigeons suggest that Nortriptyline HCl has a combination of stimulant and depressant properties.

INDICATIONS
Nortriptyline HCl is indicated for the relief of symptoms of depression. Endogenous depressions are more likely to be alleviated than are other depressive states.

UNLABELED USES
Nortriptyline is used alone or as an adjunct in the treatment of anorexia nervosa, attention deficit hyperactivity disorder, diabetic neuropathy, and emotionalism. It is also used in enuresis, irritable bowel syndrome, migraine headache, premenstrual syndrome, urinary continence, chronic urticaria, and ventricular arrhythmias.

CONTRAINDICATIONS
The use of Nortriptyline HCl or other tricyclic antidepressants concurrently with a monoamine oxidase (MAO) inhibitor is contraindicated. Hyperpyretic crisis, severe convulsions, and fatalities have occurred when similar tricyclic antidepressants were used in such combinations. It is advisable to have discontinued the MAO inhibitor for at least two weeks before treatment with Nortriptyline HCl is started. Patients hypersensitive to Nortriptyline HCl should not be given the drug.

Cross-sensitivity between Nortriptyline HCl and other dibenzazepines is a possibility.

Nortriptyline HCl is contraindicated during the acute recovery period after myocardial infarction.

WARNINGS
Patients with cardiovascular disease should be given Nortriptyline HCl only under close supervision because of the tendency of the drug to produce sinus tachycardia and to prolong the conduction time. Myocardial infarction, arrhythmia, and stroke have occurred. The antihypertensive action of guanethidine and similar agents may be blocked. Because of its anticholinergic activity, Nortriptyline HCl should be used with great caution in patients who have glaucoma or a history of urinary retention. Patients with a history of seizures should be followed closely when Nortriptyline HCl is administered, inasmuch as this drug is known to lower the convulsive threshold. Great care is required if Nortriptyline HCl is given to hyperthyroid patients or to those receiving thyroid medication, since cardiac arrhythmias may develop.

Nortriptyline HCl may impair the mental and/or physical abilities required for the performance of hazardous tasks, such as operating machinery or driving a car; therefore, the patient should be warned accordingly.

Excessive consumption of alcohol in combination with Nortriptyline therapy may have a potentiating effect, which may lead to the danger of increased suicidal attempts or overdosage, especially in patients with histories of emotional disturbances or suicidal ideation.

The concomitant administration of quinidine and Nortriptyline may result in a significantly longer plasma half-life, higher AUC, and lower clearance of Nortriptyline.

Use in Pregnancy: Safe use of Nortriptyline HCl during pregnancy and lactation has not been established; therefore, when the drug is administered to pregnant patients, nursing mothers, or women of childbearing potential, the potential benefits must be weighed against the possible hazards. Animal reproduction studies have yielded inconclusive results.

Use in Children: This drug is not recommended for use in children, since safety and effectiveness in the pediatric age group have not been established.

PRECAUTIONS
The use of Nortriptyline HCl in schizophrenic patients may result in an exacerbation of the psychosis or may activate latent schizophrenic symptoms. If the drug is given to overactive or agitated patients, increased anxiety and agitation may occur. In manic-depressive patients, Nortriptyline HCl may cause symptoms of the manic phase to emerge.

Administration of reserpine during therapy with a tricyclic antidepressant has been shown to produce a "stimulating" effect in some depressed patients.

Troublesome patient hostility may be aroused by the use of Nortriptyline HCl. Epileptiform seizures may accompany its administration, as is true of other drugs of its class.

Close supervision and careful adjustment of the dosage are required when Nortriptyline HCl is used with other anticholinergic drugs and sympathomimetic drugs.

Concurrent administration of cimetidine and tricyclic antidepressants can produce clinically significant increases in the plasma concentrations of the tricyclic antidepressant. The patient should be informed that the response to alcohol may be exaggerated.

When it is essential, the drug may be administered with electroconvulsive therapy, although the hazards may be increased. Discontinue the drug for several days, if possible, prior to elective surgery.

The possibility of a suicidal attempt by a depressed patient remains after the initiation of treatment; in this regard, it is important that the least possible quantity of drug be dispensed at any given time.

Both elevation and lowering of blood sugar levels have been reported.

▶ SHOWN IN PRODUCT IDENTIFICATION GUIDE

A case of significant hypoglycemia has been reported in a type II diabetic patient maintained on chlorpropamide (250 mg/day), after the addition of Nortriptyline (125 mg/day).

ADVERSE REACTIONS

Note: Included in the following list are a few adverse reactions that have not been reported with this specific drug. However, the pharmacologic similarities among the tricyclic antidepressant drugs require that each of the reactions be considered when Nortriptyline is administered.

Cardiovascular: Hypotension, hypertension, tachycardia, palpitation, myocardial infarction, arrhythmias, heart block, stroke.

Psychiatric: Confusional states (especially in the elderly) with hallucinations, disorientation, delusions; anxiety, restlessness, agitation; insomnia, panic, nightmares; hypomania; exacerbation of psychosis.

Neurologic: Numbness, tingling, paresthesias of extremities; incoordination, ataxia, tremors; peripheral neuropathy; extrapyramidal symptoms; seizures, alteration in EEG patterns; tinnitus.

Anticholinergic: Dry mouth and, rarely, associated sublingual adenitis; blurred vision, distrubance of accommodation, mydriasis: constipation, paralytic ileus; urinary retention delayed micturition, dilation of the urinary tract.

Allergic: Skin rash, petechiae, urticaria, itching, photosensitization (avoid excessive exposure to sunlight); edema (general or of face and tongue), drug fever, cross-sensitivity with other tricyclic drugs.

Hematologic: Bone marrow depression, including agranulocytosis; eosinophilia; purpura; thrombocytopenia.

Gastrointestinal: Nausea and vomiting, anorexia, epigastric distress, diarrhea, peculiar taste, stomatitis, abdominal cramps, blacktongue.

Endocrine: Gynecomastia in the male, breast enlargement and galactorrhea in the female; increased or decreased libido, impotence; testicular swelling; elevation or depression of blood sugar levels; syndrome of inappropriate ADH (antidiuretic hormone) secretion.

Other: Jaundice (simulating obstructive), altered liver function; weight gain or loss; perspiration; flushing; urinary frequency, nocturia; drowsiness, dizziness, weakness, fatigue; headache; parotid swelling; alopecia.

Withdrawal Symptoms: Though these are not indicative of addiction, abrupt cessation of treatment after prolonged therapy may produce nausea, headache, and malaise.

OVERDOSAGE

Toxic overdosage may result in confusion, restlessness, agitation, vomiting, hperpyrexia, muscle rigidity, hyperactive reflexes, tachycardia, ECG evidence of impaired conduction, shock, congestive heart failure, stupor, coma, and CNS stimulation with convulsions followed by respiratory depression. Deaths have occurred following overdosage with drugs of this class.

No specific antidote is known. General supportive measures are indicated, with gastic lavage. Respiratory assistance is apparently the most effective measure when indicated. The use of CNS depressants may worsen the prognosis.

The administration of barbiturates for control of convulsions alleviates an increase in the cardiac work load but should be undertaken with caution to avoid potentiation of respiratory depression.

Intramuscular paraldehyde or diazepam provides anticonvulsant activity with less respiratory depression than do the barbiturates; diazepam seems to be preferred.

The use of digitalis and/or physostigmine may be considered in case of serious cardiovascular abnormalities or cardiac failure.

The value of dialysis has not been established.

DOSAGE AND ADMINISTRATION

Nortriptyline HCl is not recommended for children.

Nortriptyline HCl is administered orally in the form of capsules or liquid. Lower than usual dosages are recommended for elderly patients and adolescents. Lower dosages are also recommended for outpatients than for hospitalized patients who will be under close supervision. The physician should initiate dosage at a low level and increase it gradually, noting carefully the clinical response and any evidence of intolerance. Following remission, maintenance medication may be required for a longer period of time at the lowest dose that will maintain remission.

If a patient develops minor side effects, the dosage should be reduced. The drug should be discontinued promptly if adverse effects of a serious nature or allergic manifestations occur.

Usual Adult Dose: 25 mg three or four times daily; dosage should begin at a low level and be increased as required. As an alternate regimen, the total daily dosage may be given once a day. When doses above 100 mg daily are administered, plasma levels of Nortriptyline should be monitored and maintained in the optimum range of 50-150 ng/mL. Doses above 150 mg/day are not recommended.

Elderly and Adolescent Patients: 30-50 mg/day, in divided doses, or the total daily dosage may be given once a day.

Capsules: Store below 86° F (30° C) and dispense from tight container.

Solution: Store below 86 °F (30 °C) and dispense from tight light-resistant container.

HOW SUPPLIED
CAPSULE: 10 MG

AVERAGE UNIT PRICE (AVAILABLE SIZES)		GENERIC A-RATED AVERAGE PRICE (GAAP)	
BRAND	$0.45	100s	$37.19
GENERIC	$0.37		
HCFA FUL (100s ea)	$0.23		

BRAND/MANUFACTURER	NDC	SIZE	AWP
◆ BRAND			
➤ PAMELOR: Sandoz Pharm	00078-0086-05	100s	$42.96
	00078-0086-06	100s ud	$47.46
◆ GENERICS			
Schein	00364-2508-01	100s	$34.89
Goldline	00182-1190-01	100s	$34.89
Qualitest	00603-4798-21	100s	$35.05
Creighton	50752-0250-05	100s	$35.41
Major	00904-7787-60	100s	$38.15
Major	00904-7795-60	100s	$38.15
Geneva	00781-2630-01	100s	$38.62
Schein	00364-2508-90	100s ud	$38.80
Creighton	50752-0250-06	100s ud	$38.95
UDL	51079-0803-20	100s ud	$39.00
Schein	00364-2508-05	500s	$170.96

CAPSULE: 10 MG

BRAND/MANUFACTURER	NDC	SIZE	AWP
◇ BRAND			
AVENTYL HCL: Lilly	00002-0817-02	100s	$41.69
	00002-0817-33	100s ud	$46.07
	00002-0817-03	500s	$197.66

CAPSULE: 25 MG

AVERAGE UNIT PRICE (AVAILABLE SIZES)		GENERIC A-RATED AVERAGE PRICE (GAAP)	
BRAND	$0.87	100s	$73.34
GENERIC	$0.72	500s	$344.43
HCFA FUL (100s ea)	$0.41		

BRAND/MANUFACTURER	NDC	SIZE	AWP
◆ BRAND			
➤ PAMELOR: Sandoz Pharm	00078-0087-05	100s	$85.86
	00078-0087-08	100s ud	$90.24
	00078-0087-08	500s	$420.24
◆ GENERICS			
Allscrips	54569-3849-00	30s	$21.73
➤ Schein	00364-2509-01	100s	$69.79
Goldline	00182-1191-01	100s	$69.79
Creighton	50752-0251-05	100s	$70.84
Qualitest	00603-4799-21	100s	$70.85
Major	00904-7788-60	100s	$76.35
Major	00904-7796-60	100s	$76.35
Geneva	00781-2631-01	100s	$77.19
➤ Schein	00364-2509-90	100s ud	$73.82
UDL	51079-0804-20	100s ud	$74.00
Creighton	50752-0251-06	100s ud	$74.38
➤ Schein	00364-2509-05	500s	$341.86
Creighton	50752-0251-08	500s	$346.99
➤ Schein	00364-2509-02	1000s	$643.53

CAPSULE: 25 MG

BRAND/MANUFACTURER	NDC	SIZE	AWP
◇ BRAND			
AVENTYL HCL: Lilly	00002-0819-02	100s	$83.24
	00002-0819-33	100s ud	$87.62
	00002-0819-03	500s	$395.55

CAPSULE: 50 MG

AVERAGE UNIT PRICE (AVAILABLE SIZES)		GENERIC A-RATED AVERAGE PRICE (GAAP)	
BRAND	$1.64	100s	$139.45
GENERIC	$1.39		
HCFA FUL (100s ea)	$0.79		

BRAND/MANUFACTURER	NDC	SIZE	AWP
◆ BRAND			
➤ PAMELOR: Sandoz Pharm	00078-0078-05	100s	$161.88
	00078-0078-06	100s ud	$166.02
◆ GENERICS			
Qualitest	00603-4800-21	100s	$131.65
Schein	00364-2510-01	100s	$131.67
Goldline	00182-1192-01	100s	$131.67
Creighton	50752-0252-05	100s	$133.65
Geneva	00781-2632-01	100s	$145.53
Major	00904-7741-60	100s	$149.95
Major	00904-7789-60	100s	$149.95
Major	00904-7797-60	100s	$149.95
Schein	00364-2510-90	100s ud	$135.79
UDL	51079-0805-20	100s ud	$136.50
Creighton	50752-0252-06	100s ud	$137.66
Schein	00364-2510-05	500s	$645.18

◆ RATED THERAPEUTICALLY EQUIVALENT; ◇ THERAPEUTIC EQUIVALENCE UNCONFIRMED; ○ UNRATED

CAPSULE: 75 MG

AVERAGE UNIT PRICE (AVAILABLE SIZES)

		GENERIC A-RATED AVERAGE PRICE (GAAP)	
BRAND	$2.47	100s	$206.69
GENERIC	$2.07		
HCFA FUL (100s ea)	$1.28		

BRAND/MANUFACTURER	NDC	SIZE	AWP
◆ BRAND			
➤ PAMELOR: Sandoz Pharm	00078-0079-05	100s	$246.84
◆ GENERICS			
Schein	00364-2511-01	100s	$200.78
Goldline	00182-1193-01	100s	$200.78
Qualitest	00603-4801-21	100s	$200.97
Creighton	50752-0253-05	100s	$203.79
Major	00904-7742-60	100s	$212.50
Major	00904-7790-60	100s	$212.50
Major	00904-7798-60	100s	$212.50
Schein	00364-2511-90	100s ud	$206.48
Creighton	50752-0253-06	100s ud	$209.90

SOLUTION: 10 MG/5 ML

AVERAGE UNIT PRICE (AVAILABLE SIZES)

BRAND	$0.10

BRAND/MANUFACTURER	NDC	SIZE	AWP
◆ BRAND			
AVENTYL HCL: Lilly	00002-2468-05	480 ml	$44.00
PAMELOR: Sandoz Pharm	00078-0016-33	480 ml	$49.32

Norvasc SEE AMLODIPINE BESYLATE

Notuss SEE CHLORPHENIRAMINE MALEATE/HYDROCODONE BITARTRATE/PSEUDOEPHEDRINE HYDROCHLORIDE

Novacet SEE SULFACETAMIDE SODIUM AND SULFUR

Novafed SEE PSEUDOEPHEDRINE HYDROCHLORIDE

Novafed A SEE CHLORPHENIRAMINE MALEATE AND PSEUDOEPHEDRINE HYDROCHLORIDE

Novahistine Expectorant SEE CODEINE PHOSPHATE/GUAIFENESIN/PSEUDOEPHEDRINE HYDROCHLORIDE

Novahistine-DH SEE CHLORPHENIRAMINE MALEATE/CODEINE PHOSPHATE/PSEUDOEPHEDRINE HYDROCHLORIDE

Novamine SEE AMINO ACIDS, INJECTABLE AND AMINO ACIDS/CALCIUM CHLORIDE/DEXTROSE/ELECTROLYTES

Novantrone SEE MITOXANTRONE HYDROCHLORIDE

Novobiocin Sodium

WARNINGS
NOVOBIOCIN SHOULD BE USED ONLY FOR THOSE SERIOUS INFECTIONS WHERE OTHER LESS TOXIC DRUGS ARE INEFFECTIVE OR CONTRAINDICATED.

NOVOBIOCIN IS ASSOCIATED WITH A HIGH FREQUENCY OF ADVERSE REACTIONS, PRINCIPALLY URTICARIA AND MACULOPAPULAR DERMATITIS. HEPATIC DYSFUNCTION AND BLOOD DYSCRASIAS HAVE OCCURRED LESS FREQUENTLY.

IN ADDITION, NOVOBIOCIN IS ASSOCIATED WITH THE RAPID AND FREQUENT EMERGENCE OF RESISTANT STRAINS, ESPECIALLY STAPHYLOCOCCI.

DESCRIPTION
Novobiocin Sodium Capsules for oral administration contain 250 mg of Novobiocin Sodium which, in the crystalline state, has a light yellow to white color depending upon the state of subdivision. It is odorless or practically odorless. The Sodium salt is freely soluble in water, alcohol, glycerin and propylene glycol. One gram of the calcium salt dissolves in about 250 mL of water, in about 30 mL of alcohol, in about 450 mL of ether and in about 1100 mL of chloroform.

The chemical name is N-[7-[[3-0-(Aminocarbonyl)-5,5-di-C-methyl-4-0-methyl-a-L-lyxopyranosyl]oxy]-4-hydroxy-8-methyl-2-oxo-2H-1- benzopyran-3-yl]-4-hydroxy-3-(3-methyl-2 - butenyl)-benzamide.

Following is its chemical structure:

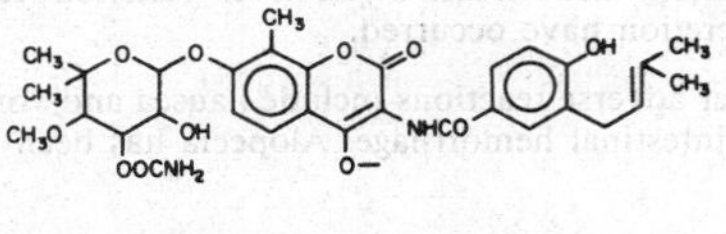

CLINICAL PHARMACOLOGY
Orally administered, Novobiocin is rapidly absorbed, producing peak concentrations in the blood within 2 to 3 hours. It diffuses into pleural and ascitic fluid but does not diffuse into the cerebrospinal fluid. Novobiocin is excreted mainly in the bile. Urinary excretion of active drug is low (approximately 3 percent of the dose administered). *In vitro* Novobiocin shows activity against *Staphylococcus aureus* and against some strains of *Proteus vulgaris*. It shows no cross resistance with penicillin against resistant strains of *S. aureus*; however, *in vitro* studies indicate that *S. aureus* rapidly develops resistance to Novobiocin.

INDICATIONS AND USAGE
Novobiocin is indicated in the treatment of serious infections due to susceptible strains of *Staphylococcus aureus* when other less toxic antibiotics such as the penicillins, cephalosporins, vancomycin, lincomycin, erythromycin, and the tetracyclines cannot be used. Novobiocin may be useful in the few urinary tract infections caused by proteus species sensitive to Novobiocin but resistant to other therapy.

CONTRAINDICATIONS
Novobiocin is contraindicated in patients with a history of hypersensitivity to this antibiotic.

WARNINGS
See boxed *"Warnings"*.

Novobiocin has been shown to affect bilirubin metabolism apparently by inhibiting glucuronyl transferase. Therefore, its use should be avoided in newborn and premature infants.

PRECAUTIONS
1. GENERAL PRECAUTIONS
Novobiocin possesses a high index of sensitization and appropriate precautions should be taken. If allergic reactions develop during treatment and are not readily controlled by the usual measures, the drug should be discontinued. In the case of development of liver dysfunction, the drug should be stopped. If hematologic studies show evidence of the development of leukopenia or other blood dyscrasias, the drug should be stopped. Should new infections appear during therapy, appropriate measures should be taken and consideration given to discontinuance of Novobiocin.

2. INFORMATION FOR PATIENT
Not applicable.

3. LABORATORY TESTS
Hepatic and hematologic studies should be made routinely during treatment.

4. DRUG INTERACTIONS
Novobiocin administration may result in a "pseudojaundice" with yellow discoloration of the skin and plasma. This yellow pigment may interfere with serum bilirubin and icterus index determinations.

Novobiocin may interfere with the hepatic uptake or biliary excretion of sulfobromophthalein in the bromsulphalein (BSP) test.

5. CARCINOGENESIS, MUTAGENESIS, IMPAIRMENT OF FERTILITY
Animal studies have not been performed on carcinogenesis, mutagenesis or impairment of fertility.

6. PREGNANCY
Pregnancy Category C. Animal reproduction studies have not been conducted with Novobiocin. It is also not known whether Novobiocin can cause fetal harm when administered to a pregnant woman or can affect reproductive capacity. Novobiocin should be given to a pregnant woman only if clearly needed.

7. LABOR AND DELIVERY
Not applicable.

➤ SHOWN IN PRODUCT IDENTIFICATION GUIDE

8. NURSING MOTHERS
Novobiocin has been reported to appear in human breast milk in the range of 0.34 to 0.54 mg/100 mL. Caution should be exercised when Novobiocin Sodium Capsules are administered to a nursing woman.

9. PEDIATRIC USE
See "Warnings" section.

ADVERSE REACTIONS

Hypersensitivity Reactions: A relatively high incidence of hypersensitivity reactions has occurred. These have consisted most commonly of skin eruptions, including urticarial, erythematous maculopapular or scarlatiniform rash. Erythema multiforme (Stevens-Johnson Syndrome) has occurred but is rare.

Hematopoietic: Blood dyscrasias including leukopenia, eosinophilia, hemolytic anemia, pancytopenia, agranulocytosis, and thrombocytopenia have occurred.

Hepatic Dysfunction: Liver dysfunction including jaundice, elevation of serum, bilirubin concentration, abnormalities on liver function tests, and impaired bromsulphalein excretion have occurred.

Miscellaneous: Other adverse reactions include nausea and vomiting, loose stools and diarrhea, and intestinal hemorrhage. Alopecia has been reported.

OVERDOSAGE
Oral LD_{50} in the mouse is 1300 mg/kg.
The dialyzability of Novobiocin is not known.

DOSAGE AND ADMINISTRATION
The recommended dose for adults is 250 mg orally every 6 hours or 500 mg every 12 hours, continued for at least 48 hours after the temperature has returned to normal and all evidence of infection has disappeared. In severe or unusually resistant infections 0.5 gram every 6 hours or 1 gram every 12 hours may be employed.
The dosage for children on similar schedules is 15 mg per kilogram of body weight per day for moderate acute infections and may be increased to 30 to 45 mg per kilogram of body weight per day for severe infections.

HOW SUPPLIED
CAPSULE: 250 MG

BRAND/MANUFACTURER	NDC	SIZE	AWP
○ **BRAND**			
ALBAMYCIN: Upjohn	00009-0101-02	100s	$188.70

Novocain SEE PROCAINE HYDROCHLORIDE

Nubain SEE NALBUPHINE HYDROCHLORIDE

Nucofed SEE CODEINE PHOSPHATE WITH PSEUDOEPHEDRINE HYDROCHLORIDE AND CODEINE PHOSPHATE/GUAIFENESIN/PSEUDOEPHEDRINE HYDROCHLORIDE

NuLYTELY SEE ELECTROLYTES AND POLYETHYLENE GLYCOL 3350

Numorphan HCl SEE OXYMORPHONE HYDROCHLORIDE

Nuromax SEE DOXACURIUM CHLORIDE

Nutracort SEE HYDROCORTISONE, TOPICAL

Nutropin SEE SOMATROPIN

Nydrazid SEE ISONIAZID

Nystatin and Triamcinolone Acetonide

DESCRIPTION
Nystatin/Triamcinolone Acetonide cream for dermatologic use contains the antifungal agent Nystatin and the synthetic corticosteroid Triamcinolone Acetonide.
Nystatin is a polyene antimycotic obtained from *Streptomyces noursei*. It is a yellow to light tan powder with a cereal-like odor, very slightly soluble in water, and slightly to sparingly soluble in alcohol.
The empirical formula is $C_{47}H_{75}NO_{17}$ and the molecular weight 926.13.
Triamcinolone Acetonide is designated chemically as 9-fluoro-11β,16α,17,21-tetrahydroxypregna-1,4-diene-3,20-dione cyclic 16,17-acetal with acetone. The white to cream crystalline powder has a slight odor, is practically insoluble in water, and very soluble in alcohol.
The empirical formula is $C_{24}H_{31}FO_6$ and the molecular weight 434.50.
Each gram of Nystatin/Triamcinolone Acetonide cream provides 100,000 units Nystatin and 1.0 mg Triamcinolone Acetonide.

CLINICAL PHARMACOLOGY
NYSTATIN
Nystatin exerts its antifungal activity against a variety of pathogenic and nonpathogenic yeasts and fungi by binding to sterols in the cell membrane. The binding process renders the cell membrane incapable of functioning as a selective barrier. Nystatin provides specific anticandidal activity to *Candida* (Monilia) *albicans* and other Candida species, but is not active against bacteria, protozoa, trichomonads, or viruses.
Nystatin is not absorbed from intact skin or mucous membranes.

TRIAMCINOLONE ACETONIDE
Triamcinolone Acetonide is primarily effective because of its anti-inflammatory, antipruritic and vasoconstrictive actions, characteristic of the topical corticosteroid class of drugs. The pharmacologic effects of the topical corticosteroids are well-known; however, the mechanisms of their dermatologic actions are unclear. Various laboratory methods, including vasoconstrictor assays, are used to compare and predict potencies and/or clinical efficacies of the topical corticosteroids. There is some evidence to suggest that a recognizable correlation exists between vasoconstrictor potency and therapeutic efficacy in man.

PHARMACOKINETICS
The extent of percutaneous absorption of topical corticosteroids is determined by many factors including the vehicle, the integrity of the epidermal barrier, and the use of occlusive dressings (see "Dosage and Administration").
Topical corticosteroids can be absorbed from normal intact skin. Inflammation and/or other disease processes in the skin increase percutaneous absorption. Occlusive dressings substantially increase the percutaneous absorption of topical corticosteroids (see "Dosage and Administration").
Once absorbed through the skin, topical corticosteroids are handled through pharmacokinetic pathways similar to systemically administered corticosteroids. Corticosteroids are bound to plasma proteins in varying degrees. Corticosteroids are metabolized primarily in the liver and are then excreted by the kidneys. Some of the topical corticosteroids and their metabolites are also excreted into the bile.

NYSTATIN AND TRIAMCINOLONE ACETONIDE
During clinical studies of mild to severe manifestations of cutaneous candidiasis, patients treated with Nystatin/Triamcinolone Acetonide cream showed a faster and more pronounced clearing of erythema and pruritus than patients treated with Nystatin or Triamcinolone Acetonide alone.

INDICATIONS AND USAGE
Nystatin/Triamcinolone Acetonide cream is indicated for the treatment of cutaneous candidiasis; it has been demonstrated that the Nystatin-steroid combination provides greater benefit than the Nystatin component alone during the first few days of treatment.

CONTRAINDICATIONS
This preparation is contraindicated in those patients with a history of hypersensitivity to any of its components.

PRECAUTIONS
GENERAL
Systemic absorption of topical corticosteroids has produced reversible hypothalamic-pituitary-adrenal (HPA) axis suppression, manifestations of Cushing's syndrome, hyperglycemia, and glucosuria in some patients.
Conditions that augment systemic absorption include application of the more potent steroids, use over large surface areas, prolonged use, and the addition of occlusive dressings (see "Dosage and Administration").
Therefore, patients receiving a large dose of any potent topical steroid applied to a large surface area should be evaluated periodically for evidence of HPA axis suppression by using the urinary free cortisol and ACTH stimulation tests, and for impairment of thermal homeostasis. If HPA axis suppression or elevation of the body temperature occurs, an attempt should be made to withdraw the drug, to reduce the frequency of application, or to substitute a less potent steroid.

◆ RATED THERAPEUTICALLY EQUIVALENT; ◇ THERAPEUTIC EQUIVALENCE UNCONFIRMED; ○ UNRATED

Recovery of HPA axis function and thermal homeostasis are generally prompt and complete upon discontinuation of the drug. Infrequently, signs and symptoms of steroid withdrawal may occur, requiring supplemental systemic corticosteroids. Children may absorb proportionally larger amounts of topical corticosteroids and thus be more susceptible to systemic toxicity (see *"Precautions, Pediatric Use"*).

If irritation or hypersensitivity develops with the combination Nystatin and Triamcinolone Acetonide, treatment should be discontinued and appropriate therapy instituted.

INFORMATION FOR THE PATIENT

Patients using this medication should receive the following information and instructions:

1. This medication is to be used as directed by the physician. It is for dermatologic use only. Avoid contact with the eyes.

2. Patients should be advised not to use this medication for any disorder other than for which it was prescribed.

3. The treated skin area should not be bandaged or otherwise covered or wrapped as to be occluded (see *"Dosage and Administration"*).

4. Patients should report any signs of local adverse reactions.

5. When using this medication in the inguinal area, patients should be advised to apply the cream sparingly and to wear loosely fitting clothing.

6. Parents of pediatric patients should be advised not to use tight-fitting diapers or plastic pants on a child being treated in the diaper area, as these garments may constitute occlusive dressings.

7. Patients should be advised on preventive measures to avoid reinfection.

LABORATORY TESTS

If there is a lack of therapeutic response, appropriate microbiological studies (e.g., KOH smears and/or cultures) should be repeated to confirm the diagnosis and rule out other pathogens, before instituting another course of therapy.

A urinary free cortisol test and ACTH stimulation test may be helpful in evaluating hypothalamic-pituitary-adrenal (HPA) axis suppression due to corticosteroid.

CARCINOGENESIS, MUTAGENESIS, AND IMPAIRMENT OF FERTIITY

Long-term animal studies have not been performed to evaluate carcinogenic or mutagenic potential, or possible impairment of fertility in males or females.

PREGNANCY CATEGORY C

There are no teratogenic studies with combined Nystatin and Triamcinolone Acetonide. Corticosteroids are generally teratogenic in laboratory animals when administered systemically at relatively low dosage levels. The more potent corticosteroids have been shown to be teratogenic after dermal application in laboratory animals. Therefore, any topical corticosteroid preparation should be used during pregnancy only if the potential benefit justifies the potential risk to the fetus.

Topical preparations containing corticosteroids should not be used extensively on pregnant patients, in large amounts, or for prolonged periods of time.

NURSING MOTHERS

It is not known whether any component of this preparation is excreted in human milk. Because many drugs are excreted in human milk, caution should be exercised during use of this preparation by a nursing woman.

PEDIATRIC USE

In clinical studies of a limited number of pediatric patients ranging in age from two months through 12 years, Nystatin/Triamcinolone Acetonide cream cleared or significantly ameliorated the disease state in most patients.

Pediatric patients may demonstrate greater susceptibility to topical corticosteroid-induced hypothalamic-pituitary-adrenal (HPA) axis suppression and Cushing's syndrome than mature patients because of a larger skin surface area to body weight ratio.

HPA axis suppression, Cushing's syndrome, and intracranial hypertension have been reported in children receiving topical corticosteroids. Manifestations of adrenal suppression in children include linear growth retardation, delayed weight gain, low plasma cortisol levels, and absence of response to ACTH stimulation. Manifestations of intracranial hypertension include bulging fontanelles, headaches, and bilateral papilledema.

Administration of topical corticosteroids to children should be limited to the least amount compatible with an effective therapeutic regimen. Chronic corticosteroid therapy may interfere with the growth and development of children.

ADVERSE REACTIONS

A single case (approximately one percent of patients studied) of acneiform eruption occurred with use of combined Nystatin and Triamcinolone Acetonide in clinical studies.

Nystatin is virtually nontoxic and nonsensitizing and is well tolerated by all age groups, even during prolonged use. Rarely, irritation may occur.

The following local adverse reactions are reported infrequently with topical corticosteroids (reactions are listed in an approximate decreasing order of occurrence): burning, itching, irritation, dryness, folliculitis, hypertrichosis, acneiform eruptions, hypopigmentation, perioral dermatitis, allergic contact dermatitis, maceration of the skin, secondary infection, skin atrophy, striae, and miliaria.

OVERDOSAGE

Topically applied corticosteroids can be absorbed in sufficient amounts to produce systemic effects (see *"Precautions, General"*); however, acute overdosage and serious adverse effects with dermatologic use are unlikely.

DOSAGE AND ADMINISTRATION

Nystatin/Triamcinolone Acetonide cream is usually applied to the affected areas twice daily in the morning and evening by gently and thoroughly massaging the preparation into the skin. The cream should be discontinued if symptoms persist after 25 days of therapy (see *"Precautions, Laboratory Tests"*).

Nystatin/Triamcinolone Acetonide cream should *not* be used with occlusive dressings.

Store at room temperature; avoid freezing.

HOW SUPPLIED
CREAM: 100,000 U/GM-0.1%

AVERAGE UNIT PRICE (AVAILABLE SIZES)		GENERIC A-RATED AVERAGE PRICE (GAAP)	
BRAND	$0.78	15 gm	$3.58
GENERIC	$0.19	30 gm	$6.40
HCFA FUL (15 gm)	$0.13	60 gm	$10.21
HCFA FUL (30 gm)	$0.11	120 gm	$15.53
HCFA FUL (60 gm)	$0.09		
HCFA FUL (120 gm)	$0.13		

BRAND/MANUFACTURER	NDC	SIZE	AWP
◆ BRAND			
MYCOLOG-II: Apothecon	00003-0566-30	15 gm	$13.73
	00003-0566-60	30 gm	$23.19
	00003-0566-65	60 gm	$39.69
◆ GENERICS			
Thames	49158-0214-20	15 gm	$1.90
MYCASONE: Mason Dist	11845-0189-01	15 gm	$2.36
NMC	23317-0150-15	15 gm	$2.40
Taro	51672-1263-01	15 gm	$2.40
MYCO BIOTIC II: Moore,H.L.	00839-7137-47	15 gm	$2.70
MYCO BIOTIC II: Moore,H.L.	00839-7701-47	15 gm	$2.70
MYCO-PAR: Parmed	00349-8477-35	15 gm	$2.80
Schein	00364-0772-72	15 gm	$2.80
N.T.A.: Qualitest	00603-7810-74	15 gm	$2.86
N.T.A.: URL	00677-1063-40	15 gm	$2.90
MYCOGEN II: Goldline	00182-1799-51	15 gm	$3.00
Geneva	00781-7600-27	15 gm	$3.00
MYCO-TRIACET II: Lemmon	00093-0232-15	15 gm	$3.10
Fougera	00168-0081-15	15 gm	$3.20
Major	00904-2574-36	15 gm	$3.25
TRI-STATIN II: Rugby	00536-4910-20	15 gm	$3.29
MYTREX: Savage	00281-0081-15	15 gm	$10.64
Thames	49158-0214-68	30 gm	$3.60
Geneva	00781-7600-03	30 gm	$4.45
MYCASONE: Mason Dist	11845-0189-02	30 gm	$4.48
N.T.A.: Qualitest	00603-7810-98	30 gm	$4.63
MYCO BIOTIC II: Moore,H.L.	00839-7137-49	30 gm	$4.71
MYCO BIOTIC II: Moore,H.L.	00839-7701-49	30 gm	$4.71
NMC	23317-0150-30	30 gm	$4.75
Taro	51672-1263-02	30 gm	$4.75
TRI-STATIN II: Rugby	00536-4910-28	30 gm	$4.80
Major	00904-2574-31	30 gm	$4.95
MYCO-PAR: Parmed	00349-8477-48	30 gm	$5.05
Schein	00364-0772-56	30 gm	$5.10
MYCOGEN II: Goldline	00182-1799-56	30 gm	$5.25
Fougera	00168-0081-30	30 gm	$5.74
MYCO-TRIACET II: Lemmon	00093-0232-30	30 gm	$6.15
N.T.A.: URL	00677-1063-44	30 gm	$8.10
MYTREX: Savage	00281-0081-30	30 gm	$18.07
N.T.A.: URL	00677-1063-45	60 gm	$4.75
Thames	49158-0214-24	60 gm	$5.90
MYCASONE: Mason Dist	11845-0189-03	60 gm	$7.37
Taro	51672-1263-03	60 gm	$7.50
MYCO BIOTIC II: Moore,H.L.	00839-7137-50	60 gm	$7.90
MYCO BIOTIC II: Moore,H.L.	00839-7701-50	60 gm	$7.90
N.T.A.: Qualitest	00603-7810-88	60 gm	$7.94
Geneva	00781-7600-35	60 gm	$7.95
Schein	00364-0772-58	60 gm	$7.95
Major	00904-2574-02	60 gm	$8.20
MYCO-PAR: Parmed	00349-8477-19	60 gm	$8.60
NMC	23317-0150-60	60 gm	$8.60
TRI-STATIN II: Rugby	00536-4910-25	60 gm	$8.75
MYCOGEN II: Goldline	00182-1799-52	60 gm	$8.85
Fougera	00168-0081-60	60 gm	$9.48
MYCO-TRIACET II: Lemmon	00093-0232-92	60 gm	$10.83
MYTREX: Savage	00281-0081-60	60 gm	$31.50
NMC	23317-0150-04	120 gm	$13.90
Major	00904-2574-22	120 gm	$14.40
TRI-STATIN II: Rugby	00536-4910-31	120 gm	$15.15
Thames	49158-0214-12	120 gm	$15.20
MYCOGEN II: Goldline	00182-1799-57	120 gm	$15.90
Thames	49158-0214-16	454 gm	$46.00
TRI-STATIN II: Rugby	00536-4910-98	454 gm	$59.24
MYTREX: Savage	00281-0081-08	1.5 gm 12s	$10.64

OINTMENT: 100,000 U/GM-0.1%

AVERAGE UNIT PRICE (AVAILABLE SIZES)		GENERIC A-RATED AVERAGE PRICE (GAAP)	
BRAND	$0.78	15 gm	$3.93
GENERIC	$0.21	30 gm	$6.95
HCFA FUL (15 gm)	$0.14	60 gm	$12.76
HCFA FUL (30 gm)	$0.10		
HCFA FUL (60 gm)	$0.10		

BRAND/MANUFACTURER	NDC	SIZE	AWP
◆ **BRAND**			
MYCOLOG-II: Apothecon	00003-0466-30	15 gm	$13.73
	00003-0466-60	30 gm	$23.19
	00003-0466-65	60 gm	$39.69
◆ **GENERICS**			
NMC	23317-0155-15	15 gm	$2.40
Taro	51672-1272-01	15 gm	$2.40
MYCO BIOTIC II: Moore,H.L.	00839-7153-47	15 gm	$2.77
NYST-OLONE II: Schein	00364-0784-72	15 gm	$2.80
N.T.A.: URL	00677-1081-40	15 gm	$2.85
MYCO-TRIACET II: Lemmon	00093-0701-15	15 gm	$2.85
N.T.A.: Qualitest	00603-7811-74	15 gm	$3.00
MYCOGEN II: Goldline	00182-1800-51	15 gm	$3.00
Major	00904-2699-36	15 gm	$3.25
Fougera	00168-0089-15	15 gm	$3.35
TRI-STATIN II: Rugby	00536-4920-20	15 gm	$3.53
MYTREX: Savage	00281-0089-15	15 gm	$10.64
MYCO BIOTIC II: Moore,H.L.	00839-7153-49	30 gm	$4.71
NMC	23317-0155-30	30 gm	$4.75
N.T.A.: Qualitest	00603-7811-78	30 gm	$5.10
NYST-OLONE II: Schein	00364-0784-56	30 gm	$5.10
N.T.A.: URL	00677-1081-45	30 gm	$5.20
MYCOGEN II: Goldline	00182-1800-56	30 gm	$5.25
MYCO-TRIACET II: Lemmon	00093-0701-30	30 gm	$5.40
Major	00904-2699-31	30 gm	$5.95
Fougera	00168-0089-30	30 gm	$6.18
Genetco	00302-4232-31	30 gm	$6.41
TRI-STATIN II: Rugby	00536-4920-28	30 gm	$6.75
MYTREX: Savage	00281-0089-30	30 gm	$18.07
Taro	51672-1272-03	60 gm	$7.50
NMC	23317-0155-60	60 gm	$8.60
N.T.A.: URL	00677-1081-43	60 gm	$8.85
MYCOGEN II: Goldline	00182-1800-52	60 gm	$8.85
N.T.A.: Qualitest	00603-7811-88	60 gm	$8.96

Nystatin, Oral

DESCRIPTION

Nystatin is an antimycotic polyene antibiotic that is both fungistatic and fungicidal *in vitro* against a wide variety of yeasts and yeast-like fungi. It is obtained from *Streptomyces noursel.*

The empirical formula is $C_{47}H_{75}NO_{17}$ and the molecular weight is 926.13.

Nystatin, Oral, is available as an oral suspension, tablets, and pastilles that dissolve slowly in the mouth.

Each ml of suspension contains:
Nystatin ....100,000 units

Each tablet contains:
Nystatin ....500,000 units

Each pastille contains:
Nystatin ....200,000 units

Following is its chemical structure:

CLINICAL PHARMACOLOGY

PHARMACOKINETICS

Following oral administation, Nystatin is sparingly absorbed with no detectable blood levels when given in the recommended doses. Most orally administered Nystatin is passed unchanged in the stool. In patients with renal insufficiency receiving oral therapy with conventional dosage forms, significant plasma concentrations of Nystatin may occasionally occur. Mean Nystatin concentrations in excess of those required *in vitro* to inhibit growth of clinically significant *Candida* persisted in saliva for approximately two hours after the start of oral dissolution of two Nystatin pastilles (400,000 units Nystatin) administered simultaneously to 12 healthy volunteers.

MICROBIOLOGY

Nystatin is both fungistatic and fungicidal *in vitro* against a wide variety of yeasts and yeast-like fungi. *Candida albicans* demonstrates no significant resistance to Nystatin *in vitro* on repeated subculture in increasing levels of Nystatin; other *Candida* species become quite resistant. Generally, resistance does not develop *in vivo*. Nystatin acts by binding to sterols in the cell membrane of susceptible fungi with a resultant change in membrane permeability allowing leakage of intracellular components. Nystatin exhibits no appreciable activity against bacteria, protozoa, trichomonads, or viruses.

INDICATIONS AND USAGE

Nystatin, Oral, suspension and pastilles are indicated for the treatment of candidiasis in the oral cavity. Nystatin, Oral, tablets are intended for the treatment of intestinal candidiasis.

UNLABELED USES

Nystatin is used alone or as an adjunct in the treatment of aspergillosis and candida pneumonia. Nystatin is also used to prevent oropharyngeal candidiasis, and acne vulgaris.

CONTRAINDICATION

Nystatin, Oral, preparations are contraindicated in patients with a history of hypersensitivity to any of their components.

PRECAUTIONS

General: Discontinue treatment with Nystatin, Oral, if sensitization or irritation is reported during use.

Nystatin, Oral, pastilles are not to be used for the treatment of systemic mycoses.

In order to achieve maximum effect from the medication, pastilles must be allowed to dissolve slowly in the mouth; therefore, patients for whom the pastille is prescribed, including children and the elderly, must be competent to utilize the dosage form as intended.

Information for the Patient: Patients taking Nystatin, Oral, pastilles should receive the following information and instructions:
1. Use as directed; the medication is not for any disorder other than for which it was prescribed.
2. Allow pastille to dissolve slowly in the mouth; *do not chew or swallow the pastille.*
3. The patient should be advised regarding replacement of any missed doses.
4. There should be no interruption or discontinuation of medication until the prescribed course of treatment is completed even though symptomatic relief may occur within a few days.
5. If symptoms of local irritation develop, the physician should be notified promptly.
6. Good oral hygiene, including proper care of dentures, is particularly important for denture wearers.

Laboratory Tests: If there is a lack of therapeutic response, appropriate microbiological studies (eg, KOH smears and/or cultures) should be repeated to confirm the diagnosis of candidiasis and rule out other pathogens before instituting another course of therapy.

Carcinogenesis, Mutagenesis, Impairment of Fertility: No long-term animal studies have been performed to evaluate carcinogenic potential. There also have been no studies to determine mutagenicity or whether this medication affects fertility in males or females.

Pregnancy: Teratogenic Effects: Category C: Animal reproduction studies have not been conducted with Nystatin, Oral. It is also not known whether Nystatin, Oral, can cause fetal harm when administered to a pregnant woman or can affect reproduction capacity. Nystatin, Oral, should be given to a pregnant woman only if clearly needed.

No adverse effects or complications have been attributed to Nystatin in infants born to women treated with Nystatin.

Nursing Mothers: It is not known whether Nystatin is excreted in human milk. Because many drugs are excreted in human milk, caution should be exercised when Nystatin is administered to a nursing woman.

Pediatric Use: See *"Dosage and Administration".*

ADVERSE REACTIONS

Nystatin is virtually nontoxic and is usually well tolerated by all age groups, including debilitated infants, even with prolonged therapy. Rarely, irritation or sensitization may occur (see *"Precautions, General".*) Nausea has been reported occasionally during therapy. Large oral doses have occasionally produced diarrhea, gastrointestinal distress, nausea and vomiting. Rash, including urticaria, has been reported rarely. Stevens-Johnson syndrome has been reported very rarely.

OVERDOSAGE

Oral doses of Nystatin in excess of five million units daily have caused nausea and gastrointestinal upset. There have been no reports of serious toxic effects or superinfections (see *"Clinical Pharmacology, Pharmacokinetics".*).

◆ RATED THERAPEUTICALLY EQUIVALENT; ◇ THERAPEUTIC EQUIVALENCE UNCONFIRMED; ○ UNRATED

DOSAGE AND ADMINISTRATION

ORAL SUSPENSION

Infants: 2 mL (200,000 USP units Nystatin) four times daily (1 mL in each side of the mouth).

Note: Limited clinical studies in premature and low birth weight infants indicate that 1 mL four times daily is effective.

Children and Adults: 4-6 mL (400,000 to 600,000 units Nystatin) four times daily (one-half of dose in each side of mouth). The preparation should be retained in the mouth as long as possible before swallowing.

Continue treatment for at least 48 hours after perioral symptoms have disappeared and cultures returned to normal.

PASTILLES

Children and Adults: The recommended dose is one or two pastilles (200,000 or 400,000 units Nystatin) four or five times daily for as long as 14 days if necessary. The dosage regimen should be continued for at least 48 hours after disappearance of oral symptoms.

Dosage should be discontinued if symptoms persist after the initial 14 day period of treatment (see *"Precautions, Laboratory Tests"*).

Administration: Pastilles must be allowed to dissolve slowly in the mouth, and should not be chewed or swallowed whole.

TABLETS

The usual therapeutic dosage is one to two tablets (500,000 to 1,000,000 units Nystatin) three times daily. Treatment should generally be continued for at least 48 hours after clinical cure to prevent relapse.

STORAGE

Store suspension at controlled room temperature, 15°—30°C (59°—86°F).

Store tablets at room temperature; avoid excessive heat.

Refrigerate pastilles between 2° and 8°C (36° and 46°F).

Shake suspension well before using.

HOW SUPPLIED

LOZENGE/TROCHE: 200,000 U

BRAND/MANUFACTURER	NDC	SIZE	AWP
○ BRAND			
MYCOSTATIN PASTILLES: Bristol-Myer Onc/Hiv	00003-0543-20	30s	$29.03

SUSPENSION: 100,000 U/ML

AVERAGE UNIT PRICE (AVAILABLE SIZES)		GENERIC A-RATED AVERAGE PRICE (GAAP)	
BRAND	$0.31	480 ml	$42.05
GENERIC	$0.12	60 ml	$6.70
HCFA FUL (60 ml)	$0.05	60 ml	$11.24
HCFA FUL (480 ml)	$0.05	480 ml	$50.71
		5 ml 100s	$105.14

BRAND/MANUFACTURER	NDC	SIZE	AWP
◆ BRAND			
MYCOSTATIN: Apothecon	00003-0588-60	60 ml	$20.96
	00003-0588-10	480 ml	$129.54
◆ GENERICS			
Moore,H.L.	00839-7703-64	60 ml	$3.63
Logen	00820-0116-30	60 ml	$4.00
Thames	49158-0256-48	60 ml	$4.50
Raway	00686-0960-67	60 ml	$4.75
Pennex	00426-8537-60	60 ml	$5.00
Bausch&Lomb Pharm	24208-0960-67	60 ml	$5.40
Warner Chilcott	00047-2922-35	60 ml	$5.69
Lemmon	00093-0366-39	60 ml	$5.70
Qualitest	00603-1480-49	60 ml	$5.71
Goldline	00182-1546-68	60 ml	$5.95
Barre	00472-1320-02	60 ml	$6.25
Rugby	00536-1220-61	60 ml	$6.27
Biocraft	00332-6109-28	60 ml	$6.49
Fougera	00168-0037-60	60 ml	$6.79
Mason Dist	11845-0173-01	60 ml	$6.80
Schein	00364-2075-58	60 ml	$6.95
Moore,H.L.	00839-6698-64	60 ml	$7.36
Major	00904-2761-03	60 ml	$7.50
Aligen	00405-3450-56	60 ml	$7.78
Roxane	00054-3607-46	60 ml	$8.08
URL	00677-0836-25	60 ml	$9.41
Geneva	00781-6105-61	60 ml	$9.46
NYSTEX: Savage	00281-0037-60	60 ml	$14.69
NILSTAT: Lederle Std Prod	00005-5429-18	60 ml	$15.73
Pennex	00426-8537-16	480 ml	$27.25
Moore,H.L.	00839-6698-69	480 ml	$35.76
Qualitest	00603-1480-58	480 ml	$37.52
Rugby	00536-1220-85	480 ml	$39.16
Barre	00472-1320-16	480 ml	$40.03
Biocraft	00332-6109-38	480 ml	$40.03
Warner Chilcott	00047-2922-23	480 ml	$42.73
Schein	00364-2075-16	480 ml	$43.10
Goldline	00182-1546-40	480 ml	$43.45
Major	00904-2761-16	480 ml	$44.50
Lemmon	00093-0366-16	480 ml	$50.00
Aligen	00405-3450-16	480 ml	$52.50

BRAND/MANUFACTURER	NDC	SIZE	AWP
URL	00677-0836-33	480 ml	$77.06
Geneva	00781-6105-16	480 ml	$77.11
NILSTAT: Lederle Std Prod	00005-5429-65	480 ml	$104.61
Bausch&Lomb Pharm	24208-0960-94	480 ml ud	$41.00
Roxane	00054-8607-16	150 ml 40s ud	$46.96
UDL	51079-0307-10	5 ml 50s ud	$56.00
UDL	51079-0732-10	10 ml 50s ud	$66.10
Raway	00686-0307-10	5 ml 100s	$68.00
Fougera	00168-0037-03	5 ml 100s	$120.00
Bausch&Lomb Pharm	24208-0960-60	5 ml 100s ud	$127.42

TABLETS: 500,000 U

AVERAGE UNIT PRICE (AVAILABLE SIZES)		GENERIC A-RATED AVERAGE PRICE (GAAP)	
BRAND	$0.53	100s	$24.26
GENERIC	$0.28		
HCFA FUL (100s ea)	$0.12		

BRAND/MANUFACTURER	NDC	SIZE	AWP
◆ BRAND			
► MYCOSTATIN: Apothecon	00003-0580-53	100s	$53.10
◆ GENERICS			
Aligen	00405-4719-15	15s	$10.63
Aligen	00405-4719-30	30s	$19.63
Majr	00904-0672-60	100s	$15.10
Purepac	00228-2277-10	100s	$17.84
Lemmon	00093-0983-01	100s	$19.65
Moore,H.L.	00839-6282-06	100s	$24.91
Schein	00364-2051-01	100s	$25.20
Goldline	00182-1369-01	100s	$25.45
Qualitest	00603-4830-21	100s	$25.48
Par	49884-0119-01	100s	$25.75
URL	00677-0613-01	100s	$25.90
Mutual	53489-0400-01	100s	$25.90
Geneva	00781-1305-01	100s	$25.95
Martec	52555-0319-01	100s	$25.95
► Rugby	00536-4094-01	100s	$26.93
Aligen	00405-4714-01	100s	$28.27
Eon	00185-0750-01	100s	$31.95
Parmed	00349-8710-01	100s	$32.00
Auro	55829-0396-10	100s ud	$10.20
U.S. Trading	56126-0119-11	100s ud	$12.90
Par	49884-0119-05	500s	$115.87

Nystatin, Topical

DESCRIPTION

Nystatin Cream, Ointment and Powder are for dermatologic use.

Nystatin **Cream** contains the antifungal antibiotic Nystatin at a concentration of 100,000 USP Nystatin units per gram in a cream base.

Nystatin **Topical Powder** provides, in each gram, 100,000 USP Nystatin units dispersed in talc.

Nystatin **Ointment** provides 100,000 USP Nystatin units per gram in a gel base.

Following is its chemical structure:

CLINICAL PHARMACOLOGY

Nystatin is an antifungal antibiotic which is both fungistatic and fungicidal *in vitro* against a wide variety of yeasts and yeast-like fungi. It probably acts by binding to sterols in the cell membrane of the fungus with a resultant change in membrane permeability allowing leakage of intracellular components. Nystatin is a polyene antibiotic of undetermined structural formula that is obtained from *Streptomyces noursei*, and is the first well tolerated antifungal antibiotic of dependable efficacy for the treatment of cutaneous, oral and intestinal infections caused by *Candida* (Monilia) *albicans* and other Candida species. It exhibits no appreciable activity against bacteria.

Nystatin provides specific therapy for all localized forms of candidiasis. Symptomatic relief is rapid, often occurring within 24 to 72 hours after the initiation of treatment. Cure is effected both clinically and mycologically in most cases of localized candidiasis.

INDICATIONS AND USAGE

Nystatin topical preparations are indicated in the treatment of cutaneous or mucocutaneous mycotic infections caused by *Candida* (Monilia) *albicans* and other Candida species.

CONTRAINDICATIONS

Nystatin topical preparations are contraindicated in patients with a history of hypersensitivity to any of their components.

PRECAUTIONS

Should a reaction of hypersensitivity occur the drug should be immediately withdrawn and appropriate measures taken. These preparations are not for ophthalmic use.

ADVERSE REACTIONS

Nystatin is virtually nontoxic and nonsensitizing and is well tolerated by all age groups including debilitated infants, even on prolonged administration. If irritation on topical application should occur, discontinue medication.

DOSAGE AND ADMINISTRATION

The cream and the ointment should be applied liberally to affected areas twice daily or as indicated until healing is complete. The powder should be applied to candidal lesions two or three times daily until lesions have healed. For fungal infection of the feet caused by Candida species, the powder should be dusted freely on the feet as well as in shoes and socks. The cream is usually preferred to the ointment in candidiasis involving intertriginous areas; very moist lesions, however, are best treated with the topical dusting powder. The preparations do not stain skin or mucous membranes and they provide a simple, convenient means of treatment.

STORAGE
Nystatin Cream
  Store at room temperature; avoid freezing.
Nystatin Powder
  Store at room temperature; avoid excessive heat (40°C; 104°F).
  Keep tightly closed.
Nystatin Ointment
  Store at room temperature.

HOW SUPPLIED
CREAM: 100,000 U/GM

AVERAGE UNIT PRICE (AVAILABLE SIZES)		GENERIC A-RATED AVERAGE PRICE (GAAP)	
BRAND	$0.73	15 gm	$2.63
GENERIC	$0.16	30 gm	$4.13
HCFA FUL (15 gm)	$0.10		
HCFA FUL (30 gm)	$0.07		

BRAND/MANUFACTURER	NDC	SIZE	AWP
◆ BRAND			
MYCOSTATIN: Westwood-Squibb	00003-0579-20	15 gm	$11.54
	00003-0579-31	30 gm	$20.86
◆ GENERICS			
Clay-Park	45802-0059-35	15 gm	$1.60
Thames	49158-0149-20	15 gm	$1.80
NMC	23317-0160-15	15 gm	$1.88
Taro	51672-1289-01	15 gm	$2.10
Schein	00364-7210-72	15 gm	$2.10
Geneva	00781-7005-27	15 gm	$2.12
Parmed	00349-9002-35	15 gm	$2.15
Moore,H.L.	00839-7702-47	15 gm	$2.15
Rugby	00536-4830-20	15 gm	$2.19
URL	00677-0733-40	15 gm	$2.20
Major	00904-2706-36	15 gm	$2.20
Qualitest	00603-7820-74	15 gm	$2.20
Moore,H.L.	00839-6130-47	15 gm	$2.23
Fougera	00168-0054-15	15 gm	$2.46
Goldline	00182-0982-51	15 gm	$2.55
UDL	51079-0270-61	15 gm	$5.37
NYSTEX: Savage	00281-3208-44	15 gm	$7.49
Thames	49158-0149-08	30 gm	$2.80
Qualitest	00603-7820-78	30 gm	$2.87
Clay-Park	45802-0059-11	30 gm	$2.94
Schein	00364-7210-56	30 gm	$3.00
NMC	23317-0160-30	30 gm	$3.05
Taro	51672-1289-02	30 gm	$3.20
URL	00677-0733-45	30 gm	$3.55
Moore,H.L.	00839-6130-49	30 gm	$3.58
Parmed	00349-9002-48	30 gm	$3.71
Rugby	00536-4830-28	30 gm	$3.74
Major	00904-2706-31	30 gm	$3.75
Geneva	00781-7005-24	30 gm	$3.75
Goldline	00182-0982-56	30 gm	$3.75
Fougera	00168-0054-30	30 gm	$3.82
UDL	51079-0270-65	30 gm	$5.37
NYSTEX: Savage	00281-3208-45	30 gm	$11.87

OINTMENT: 100,000 U/GM

AVERAGE UNIT PRICE (AVAILABLE SIZES)		GENERIC A-RATED AVERAGE PRICE (GAAP)	
BRAND	$0.73	15 gm	$2.74
GENERIC	$0.16	30 gm	$3.51
HCFA FUL (15 gm)	$0.10		
HCFA FUL (30 gm)	$0.12		

BRAND/MANUFACTURER	NDC	SIZE	AWP
◆ BRAND			
MYCOSTATIN: Westwood-Squibb	00003-0584-40	15 gm	$11.54
	00003-0584-30	30 gm	$20.86

BRAND/MANUFACTURER	NDC	SIZE	AWP
◆ GENERICS			
Clay-Park	45802-0048-35	15 gm	$1.68
NMC	23317-0165-15	15 gm	$1.92
Rugby	00536-4781-20	15 gm	$2.19
Qualitest	00603-7821-74	15 gm	$2.20
Moore,H.L.	00839-7128-47	15 gm	$2.23
URL	00677-1082-40	15 gm	$2.43
Schein	00364-7379-72	15 gm	$2.43
Major	00904-2305-36	15 gm	$2.46
Fougera	00168-0007-15	15 gm	$2.55
Goldline	00182-1678-51	15 gm	$2.55
NYSTEX: Savage	00281-3212-44	15 gm	$7.49
Clay-Park	45802-0048-11	30 gm	$3.02
NMC	23317-0165-30	30 gm	$3.28
Moore,H.L.	00839-7128-49	30 gm	$3.44
URL	00677-1082-45	30 gm	$3.50
Rugby	00536-4781-28	30 gm	$3.6
Major	00904-2305-31	30 gm	$3.60
Goldline	00182-1678-56	30 gm	$3.75
Fougera	00168-0007-30	30 gm	$3.91

POWDER: 100,000 U/GM

BRAND/MANUFACTURER	NDC	SIZE	AWP
○ BRAND			
MYCOSTATIN: Westwood-Squibb	00003-0593-20	15 gm	$21.34
PEDI-DRI TOPICAL POWDER: Pedinol	00884-0394-02	60 gm	$10.00

Octreoscan *SEE* INDIUM IN-111 PENTETREOTIDE

Octreotide Acetate

DESCRIPTION

Octreotide Acetate is a cyclic octapeptide prepared as a clear sterile solution of Octreotide, Acetate salt for administration by deep subcutaneous (intrafat) or intravenous injection. Octreotide Acetate, known chemically as L-Cysteinamide, D-phenylalanyl-L-cysteinyl-L-phenylalanyl -D- tryptophyl-L-lysyl-L-threonyl -N-[2-hydroxy-1-(hydroxymethyl) propyl]-, cyclic (2 → 7)-disulfide; [R-(R*, R*)] acetate salt, is a long-acting octapeptide with pharmacologic actions mimicking those of the natural hormone somatostatin.

Each 1 ml ampule contains:	
Octreotide Acetate	......50, 100, or 500 mcg

Each 5 ml multi-dose vial contains:	
Octreotide Acetate	.....200 or 1000 mcg/ml

The molecular weight of Octreotide Acetate is 1019.3 (free peptide, $C_{49}H_{66}N_{10}O_{10}S_2$).

Following is its chemical structure:

H—D-Phe—Cys—Phe—D-Trp—Lys—Thr—Cys—Thr—ol · xCH₃COOH
       1   2   3   4   5   6   7   8

CLINICAL PHARMACOLOGY

Octreotide Acetate exerts pharmacologic actions similar to the natural hormone, somatostatin. It is an even more potent inhibitor of growth hormone, glucagon, and insulin than somatostatin. Like somatostatin, it also suppresses LH response to GnRH, decreases splanchnic blood flow, and inhibits release of serotonin, gastrin, vasoactive intestinal peptide, secretin, motilin, and pancreatic polypeptide.

By virtue of these pharmacological actions, Octreotide Acetate has been used to treat the symptoms associated with metastatic carcinoid tumors (flushing and diarrhea), and vasoactive intestinal peptide (VIP) secreting adenomas (watery diarrhea).

Octreotide Acetate substantially reduces growth hormone and/or IGF-I (somatomedin C) levels in patients with acromegaly.

Single doses of Octreotide Acetate have been shown to inhibit gallbladder contractility and to decrease bile secretion in normal volunteers. In controlled clinical trials the incidence of gallstone or biliary sludge formation was markedly increased (see *"Warnings"*).

Octreotide Acetate suppresses secretion of thyroid stimulating hormone (TSH).

PHARMACOKINETICS

After subcutaneous injection, Octreotide is absorbed rapidly and completely from the injection site. Peak concentrations of 5.2 ng/mL (100 mcg dose) were reached 0.4 hours after dosing. Using a specific radioimmunoassay, intravenous and subcutaneous doses were found to be bioequivalent. Peak concentrations and area under the curve values were dose proportional after subcutaneous or intravenous single doses up to 400 mcg and with multiple doses of 200 mcg t.i.d. (600 mcg/day). Clearance was reduced by about 66% suggesting non-linear kinetics of the drug at daily doses of 600 mcg/day as compared to 150 mcg/day. The relative decrease in clearance with doses above 600 mcg/day is not defined. In

---

◆ RATED THERAPEUTICALLY EQUIVALENT; ◇ THERAPEUTIC EQUIVALENCE UNCONFIRMED; ○ UNRATED

healthy volunteers the distribution of Octreotide from plasma was rapid (tα ½ = 0.2 h), the volume of distribution (Vdss) was estimated to be 13.6 L, and the total body clearance was 10 L/hr.

In blood, the distribution into the erythrocytes was found to be negligible and about 65% was bound in the plasma in a concentration-independent manner. Binding was mainly to lipoprotein and, to a lesser extent, to albumin.

The elimination of Octreotide from plasma had an apparent half-life of 1.7 hours compared with 1—3 minutes with the natural hormone. The duration of action of Octreotide Acetate is variable but extends up to 12 hours depending upon the type of tumor. About 32% of the dose is excreted unchanged into the urine. In an elderly population, dose adjustments may be necessary due to a significant increase in the half-life (46%) and a significant decrease in the clearance (26%) of the drug.

In patients with acromegaly, the pharmacokinetics differ somewhat from those in healthy volunteers. A mean peak concentration of 2.8 ng/mL (100 mcg dose) was reached in 0.7 hours after subcutaneous dosing. The volume of distribution (Vdss) was estimated to be 21.6 ± 8.5 L and the total body clearance was increased to 18 L/h. The mean percent of the drug bound was 41.2%. The disposition and elimination half-lives were similar to normals.

In patients with severe renal failure requiring dialysis, clearance was reduced to about half that found in normal subjects (from approximately 10 L/h to 4.5 L/h). The effect of hepatic diseases on the disposition of Octreotide is unknown.

INDICATIONS AND USAGE
ACROMEGALY
Octreotide Acetate is indicated to reduce blood levels of growth hormone and IGF-I (somatomedin C) in acromegaly patients who have had inadequate response to or cannot be treated with surgical resection, pituitary irradiation, and bromocriptine mesylate at maximally tolerated doses. The goal is to achieve normalization of growth hormone and IGF-I (somatomedin C) levels (see "Dosage and Administration"). In patients with acromegaly, Octreotide Acetate reduces growth hormone to within normal ranges in 50% of patients and reduces IGF-I (somatomedin C) to within normal ranges in 50%–60% of patients. Since the effects of pituitary irradiation may not become maximal for several years, adjunctive therapy with Octreotide Acetate to reduce blood levels of growth hormone and IGF-I (somatomedin C) offers potential benefit before the effects of irradiation are manifested.

Improvement in clinical signs and symptoms or reduction in tumor size or rate of growth were not shown in clinical trials performed with Octreotide Acetate; these trials were not optimally designed to detect such effects.

CARCINOID TUMORS
Octreotide Acetate is indicated for the symptomatic treatment of patients with metastatic carcinoid tumors where it suppresses or inhibits the severe diarrhea and flushing episodes associated with the disease.

Octreotide Acetate studies were not designed to show an effect on the size, rate of growth or development of metastases.

VASOACTIVE INTESTINAL PEPTIDE TUMORS (VIPOMAS)
Octreotide Acetate is indicated for the treatment of the profuse watery diarrhea associated with VIP-secreting tumors. Octreotide Acetate studies were not designed to show an effect on the size, rate of growth or development of metastases.

CONTRAINDICATIONS
Sensitivity to this drug or any of its components.

WARNINGS
Single doses of Octreotide Acetate have been shown to inhibit gallbladder contractility and decrease bile secretion in normal volunteers. In clinical trials (primarily patients with acromegaly or psoriasis), the incidence of biliary tract abnormalities was 52% (27% gallstones, 22% sludge without stones, 3% biliary duct dilatation). The incidence of stones or sludge in patients who received Octreotide Acetate for 12 months or longer was 48%. Less than 2% of patients treated with Octreotide Acetate for 1 month or less developed gallstones. The incidence of gallstones did not appear related to age, sex or dose. Like patients without gallbladder abnormalities, the majority of patients developing gallbladder abnormalities on ultrasound had gastrointestinal symptoms. The symptoms were not specific for gallbladder disease. A few patients developed acute cholecystitis, ascending cholangitis, biliary obstruction, cholestatic hepatitis, or pancreatitis during Octreotide Acetate therapy or following its withdrawal. One patient developed ascending cholangitis during Octreotide Acetate therapy and died.

PRECAUTIONS
GENERAL
Octreotide Acetate alters the balance between the counterregulatory hormones, insulin, glucagon and growth hormone, which may result in hypoglycemia or hyperglycemia. Octreotide Acetate also suppresses secretion of thyroid stimulating hormone, which may result in hypothyroidism. Cardiac conduction abnormalities have also occurred during treatment with Octreotide Acetate. However, the incidence of these adverse events during long-term therapy was determined vigorously only in acromegaly patients who, due to their underlying disease and/or the subsequent treatment they receive, are at an increased risk for the development of diabetes mellitus, hypothyroidism, and cardiovascular disease. Although the degree to which these abnormalities are related to Octreotide Acetate therapy is not clear, new abnormalities of glycemic control, thyroid

function and ECG developed during Octreotide Acetate therapy as described below.

The hypoglycemia or hyperglycemia which occurs during Octreotide Acetate therapy is usually mild, but may result in overt diabetes mellitus or necessitate dose changes in insulin or other hypoglycemic agents. Hypoglycemia and hyperglycemia occurred on Octreotide Acetate in 3% and 15% of acromegalic patients, respectively. Severe hyperglycemia, subsequent pneumonia, and death following initiation of Octreotide Acetate therapy was reported in one patient with no history of hyperglycemia.

In acromegalic patients, 12% developed biochemical hypothyroidism only, 6% developed goiter, and 4% required initiation of thyroid replacement therapy while receiving Octreotide Acetate. Baseline and periodic assessment of thyroid function (TSH, total and/or free T_4) is recommended during chronic therapy. In acromegalics, bradycardia (< 50 bpm) developed in 21%; conduction abnormalities and arrhythmias each occurred in 9% of patients during Octreotide Acetate therapy. Other EKG changes observed included QT prolongation, axis shifts, early repolarization, low voltage, R/S transition, and early R wave progression. These ECG changes are not uncommon in acromegalic patients. Dose adjustments in drugs such as beta-blockers that have bradycardia effects may be necessary. In one acromegalic patient with severe congestive heart failure, initiation of Octreotide Acetate therapy resulted in worsening of CHF with improvement when drug was discontinued. Confirmation of a drug effect was obtained with a positive rechallenge.

Several cases of pancreatitis have been reported in patients receiving Octreotide Acetate therapy.

Octreotide Acetate may alter absorption of dietary fats in some patients.

In patients with severe renal failure requiring dialysis, the half-life of Octreotide Acetate may be increased, necessitating adjustment of the maintenance dosage.

Depressed vitamin B_{12} levels and abnormal Schilling's tests have been observed in some patients receiving Octreotide Acetate therapy, and monitoring of vitamin B_{12} levels is recommended during chronic Octreotide Acetate therapy.

INFORMATION FOR PATIENTS
Careful instruction in sterile subcutaneous injection technique should be given to the patients and to other persons who may administer Octreotide Acetate injection.

LABORATORY TESTS
Laboratory tests that may be helpful as biochemical markers in determining and following patient response depend on the specific tumor. Based on diagnosis, measurement of the following substances may be useful in monitoring the progress of therapy:

Acromegaly: Growth Hormone, IGF-I (somatomedin C). Responsiveness to Octreotide Acetate may be evaluated by determining growth hormone levels at 1—4 hour intervals for 8—12 hours post dose. Alternatively, a single measurement of IGF-I (somatomedin C) level may be made two weeks after drug initiation or dosage change.

Carcinoid: 5-HIAA (urinary 5-hydroxyindole acetic acid), plasma serotonin, plasma Substance P

VIPoma: VIP (plasma vasoactive intestinal peptide)

Baseline and periodic total and/or free T_4 measurements should be performed during chronic therapy (see "Precautions—General").

DRUG INTERACTIONS
Octreotide Acetate has been associated with alterations in nutrient absorption, so it may have an effect on absorption of orally administered drugs. Concomitant administration of Octreotide Acetate with cyclosporine may decrease blood levels of cyclosporine and result in transplant rejection.

Patients receiving insulin, oral hypoglycemic agents, beta blockers, calcium channel blockers, or agents to control fluid and electrolyte balance, may require dose adjustments of these therapeutic agents.

DRUG LABORATORY TEST INTERACTIONS
No known interference exists with clinical laboratory tests, including amine or peptide determinations.

CARCINOGENESIS/MUTAGENESIS/IMPAIRMENT OF FERTILITY
Studies in laboratory animals have demonstrated no mutagenic potential of Octreotide Acetate.

No carcinogenic potential was demonstrated in mice treated subcutaneously for 85—99 weeks at doses up to 2000 mcg/kg/day. In a 116-week subcutaneous study in rats, a 27% and 12% incidence of injection site sarcomas or squamous cell carcinomas was observed in males and females, respectively, at the highest dose level of 1250 mcg/kg/day compared to an incidence of 8%—10% in the vehicle control groups. The increased incidence of injection site tumors was most probably caused by irritation and the high sensitivity of the rat to repeated subcutaneous injections at the same site. Rotating injection sites would prevent chronic irritation in humans. There have been no reports of injection site tumors in patients treated with Octreotide Acetate for up to 5 years. There was also a 15% incidence of uterine adenocarcinomas in the 1250 mcg/kg/day females compared to 7% in the saline control females and 0% in the vehicle control females. The presence of endometritis coupled with the absence of corpora lutea, the reduction in mammary fibroadenomas, and the presence of uterine dilatation suggest that the uterine tumors were associated with estrogen dominance in the aged female rats which does not occur in humans.

Octreotide Acetate did not impair fertility in rats at doses up to 1000 mcg/kg/day.

PREGNANCY CATEGORY B
Reproduction studies have been performed in rats and rabbits at doses up to 30 times the highest human dose and have revealed no evidence of impaired fertility or harm to the fetus due to Octreotide Acetate. There are, however, no adequate and well-controlled studies in pregnant women. Because animal reproduction studies are not always predictive of human response, this drug should be used during pregnancy only if clearly needed.

NURSING MOTHERS
It is not known whether this drug is excreted in human milk. Because many drugs are excreted in human milk, caution should be exercised when Octreotide Acetate is administered to a nursing woman.

PEDIATRIC USE
Experience with Octreotide Acetate in the pediatric population is limited. The youngest patient to receive the drug was 1 month old. Doses of 1–10 mcg/kg body weight were well tolerated in the young patients. A single case of an infant (nesidioblastosis) was complicated by a seizure thought to be independent of Octreotide Acetate therapy.

ADVERSE REACTIONS
GALLBLADDER ABNORMALITIES
Gallbladder abnormalities, especially stones and/or biliary sludge, frequently develop in patients on chronic Octreotide Acetate therapy (see *"Warnings"*).

CARDIAC
In acromegalics, sinus bradycardia (< 50 bpm) developed in 21%; conduction abnormalities and arrhythmias each developed in 9% of patients during Octreotide Acetate therapy (see *"Precautions— General"*).

GASTROINTESTINAL
Diarrhea, loose stools, nausea and abdominal discomfort were each seen in 30%—58% of acromegalic patients in US studies although only 2% of the patients discontinued therapy due to these symptoms. These symptoms were seen in 5%—10% of patients with other disorders. The frequency of these symptoms was not dose-related, but diarrhea and abdominal discomfort generally resolved more quickly in patients treated with 300 mcg/day than in those treated with 750 mcg/day. Vomiting, flatulence, abnormal stools, abdominal distention, and constipation were each seen in less than 10% of patients.

HYPO/HYPERGLYCEMIA
Hypoglycemia and hyperglycemia occurred in 3% and 15% of acromegalic patients, respectively, but only in about 1.5% of other patients. Symptoms of hypoglycemia were noted in approximately 2% of patients.

HYPOTHYROIDISM
In acromegalics, biochemical hypothyroidism alone occurred in 12% while goiter occurred in 6% during Octreotide Acetate therapy (see *"Precautions—General"*). In patients without acromegaly, hypothyroidism has only been reported in several isolated patients and goiter has not been reported.

OTHER ADVERSE EVENTS
Pain on injection was reported in 7.5% and headache in 6%.

OTHER ADVERSE EVENTS 1%—4%
Other events (relationship to drug not established), each observed in 1%—4% of patients, included dizziness, fatigue, weakness, pruritus, joint pain, backache, urinary tract infection, cold symptoms, flu symptoms, injection site hematoma, bruise, edema, flushing, blurred vision, pollakiuria, fat malabsorption, and hair loss.

OTHER ADVERSE EVENTS < 1%
Events reported in less than 1% of patients and for which relationship to drug is not established are listed:

Gastrointestinal: hepatitis, jaundice, increase in liver enzymes, GI bleeding, hemorrhoids, appendicitis.

Integumentary: rash, cellulitis, petechiae, urticaria.

Musculoskeletal: arthritis, joint effusion, muscle pain, Raynaud's phenomenon.

Cardiovascular: chest pain, shortness of breath, thrombophlebitis, ischemia, congestive heart failure, hypertension, hypertensive reaction, palpitations, orthostatic BP decrease, tachycardia.

CNS: depression, anxiety, libido decrease, syncope, tremor, seizure, vertigo, Bell's Palsy, paranoia, pituitary apoplexy, increased intraocular pressure.

Respiratory: pneumonia, pulmonary nodule, status asthmaticus.

Endocrine: galactorrhea, hypoadrenalism, diabetes insipidus, gynecomastia, amenorrhea, polymenorrhea, vaginitis.

Urogenital: nephrolithiasis, hematuria.

Hematologic: anemia, iron deficiency, epistaxis.

Miscellaneous: otitis, allergic reaction, increased CK, visual disturbance.

Evaluation of 20 patients treated for at least 6 months has failed to demonstrate titers of antibodies exceeding background levels. However antibody titers to Octreotide Acetate were subsequently reported in three patients and

resulted in prolonged duration of drug action in two patients. Anaphylactoid reactions, including anaphylactic shock, have been reported in several patients receiving Octreotide Acetate.

OVERDOSAGE
No frank overdose has occurred in any patient to date. Intravenous bolus doses of 1 mg (1000 mcg) given to healthy volunteers and of 30 mg (30,000 mcg) IV over 20 minutes and of 120 mg (120,000 mcg) IV over 8 hours to research patients have not resulted in serious ill effects. Mortality occurred in mice and rats given 72 mg/kg and 18 mg/kg IV, respectively.

DRUG ABUSE AND DEPENDENCE
There is no indication that Octreotide Acetate has potential for drug abuse or dependence. Octreotide Acetate levels in the central nervous system are negligible, even after doses up to 30,000 mcg.

DOSAGE AND ADMINISTRATION
Octreotide Acetate may be administered subcutaneously or intravenously. Subcutaneous injection is the usual route of administration of Octreotide Acetate for control of symptoms. Pain with subcutaneous administration may be reduced by using the smallest volume that will deliver the desired dose. Multiple subcutaneous injections at the same site within short periods of time should be avoided. Sites should be rotated in a systematic manner.

Parenteral drug products should be inspected visually for particulate matter and discoloration prior to administration. **Do not use if particulates and/or discoloration are observed.** Proper sterile technique should be used in the preparation of parenteral admixtures to minimize the possibility of microbial contamination. **Octreotide acetate is not compatible in Total Parenteral Nutrition (TPN) solutions because of the formation of a glycosyl Octreotide conjugate which may decrease the efficacy of the product.**

Octreotide Acetate is stable in sterile isotonic saline solutions or sterile solutions of dextrose 5% in water for 24 hours. It may be diluted in volumes of 50—200 mL and infused intravenously over 15—30 minutes or administered by IV push over 3 minutes. In emergency situations (e.g.: carcinoid crisis) it may be given by rapid bolus.

The initial dosage is usually 50 mcg administered twice or three times daily. Upward dose titration is frequently required. Dosage information for patients with specific tumors follows.

ACROMEGALY
Dosage may be initiated at 50 mcg t.i.d. Beginning with this low dose may permit adaptation to adverse gastrointestinal effects for patients who will require higher doses. IGF-I (somatomedin C) levels every 2 weeks can be used to guide titration. Alternatively, multiple growth hormone levels at 0–8 hours after Octreotide Acetate administration permit more rapid titration of dose. The goal is to achieve growth hormone levels less than 5 ng/mL or IGF-I (somatomedin C) levels less than 1.9 U/mL in males and less than 2.2 U/mL in females. The dose most commonly found to be effective is 100 mcg t.i.d., but some patients require up to 500 mcg t.i.d. for maximum effectiveness. Doses greater than 300 mcg/day seldom result in additional biochemical benefit, and if an increase in dose fails to provide additional benefit, the dose should be reduced. IGF-I (somatomedin C) or growth hormone levels should be reevaluated at 6 month intervals.

Octreotide Acetate should be withdrawn yearly for approximately 4 weeks from patients who have received irradiation to assess disease activity. If growth hormone or IGF-I (somatomedin C) levels increase and signs and symptoms recur, Octreotide Acetate therapy may be resumed.

CARCINOID TUMORS
The suggested daily dosage of Octreotide Acetate during the first 2 weeks of therapy ranges from 100—600 mcg/day in 2—4 divided doses (mean daily dosage is 300 mcg). In the clinical studies, the median daily maintenance dosage was approximately 450 mcg, but clinical and biochemical benefits were obtained in some patients with as little as 50 mcg, while others required doses up to 1500 mcg/day. However, experience with doses above 750 mcg/day is limited.

VIPOMAS
Daily dosages of 200—300 mcg in 2—4 divided doses are recommended during the initial 2 weeks of therapy (range 150—750 mcg) to control symptoms of the disease. On an individual basis, dosage may be adjusted to achieve a therapeutic response, but usually doses above 450 mcg/day are not required.

STORAGE
For prolonged storage, Octreotide Acetate ampuls and multi-dose vials should be stored at refrigerated temperatures 2°—8°C (36°—46°F) and protected from light. At room temperature, (20°—30°C or 70°—86°F), Octreotide Acetate is stable for 14 days if protected from light. The solution can be allowed to come to room temperature prior to administration. Do not warm artifically. After initial use, multiple dose vials should be discarded within 14 days. Ampuls should be opened just prior to administration and the unused portion discarded.

HOW SUPPLIED
INJECTION: 50 MCG/ML

BRAND/MANUFACTURER	NDC	SIZE	AWP
○ BRAND			
SANDOSTATIN: Sandoz Pharm	00078-0180-03	1 ml 20s	$86.76
	00078-0180-04	1 ml 50s	$214.68

◆ RATED THERAPEUTICALLY EQUIVALENT; ◇ THERAPEUTIC EQUIVALENCE UNCONFIRMED; ○ UNRATED

INJECTION: 100 MCG/ML

BRAND/MANUFACTURER	NDC	SIZE	AWP
○ **BRAND**			
SANDOSTATIN: Sandoz Pharm	00078-0181-03	1 ml 20s	$158.94
	00078-0182-03	1 ml 20s	$727.32
	00078-0181-04	1 ml 50s	$393.36
	00078-0182-04	1 ml 50s	$1800.06

INJECTION: 200 MCG/ML

BRAND/MANUFACTURER	NDC	SIZE	AWP
○ **BRAND**			
SANDOSTATIN: Sandoz Pharm	00078-0183-25	5 ml	$85.50

INJECTION: 1000 MCG/ML

BRAND/MANUFACTURER	NDC	SIZE	AWP
○ **BRAND**			
SANDOSTATIN: Sandoz Pharm	00078-0184-25	5 ml	$421.02

Ocu-Caine SEE PROPARACAINE HYDROCHLORIDE

Ocu-Flur 10 SEE FLUORESCEIN SODIUM

Ocu-Pred SEE PREDNISOLONE ACETATE, OPHTHALMIC AND PREDNISOLONE, SYSTEMIC

Ocu-Tropic SEE TROPICAMIDE

Ocufen SEE FLURBIPROFEN SODIUM, OPHTHALMIC

Ocuflox SEE OFLOXACIN, OPHTHALMIC

Ocupress SEE CARTEOLOL HYDROCHLORIDE, OPHTHALMIC

Ocusert SEE PILOCARPINE, OPHTHALMIC

Ofloxacin, Ophthalmic

DESCRIPTION
Ofloxacin ophthalmic solution 0.3% (3 mg/mL) is a sterile ophthalmic solution. It is a fluorinated carboxyquinolone anti-infective for topical ophthalmic use.

Chemical Name: (±)-9-Fluoro-2,3-dihydro-3-methyl-10-(4-methyl-1-piperazinyl)-7-oxo-7H-pyrido [1,2,3-de]-1,4 benzoxazine-6-carboxylic acid. Its molecular weight is 361.37 and its molecular formula is $C_{18}H_{20}FN_3O_4$.

Ofloxacin is a fluorinated 4-quinolone which differs from other fluorinated 4-quinolones in that there is a six member (pyridobenzoxazine) ring from positions 1 to 8 of the basic ring structure.

Following is its chemical structure:

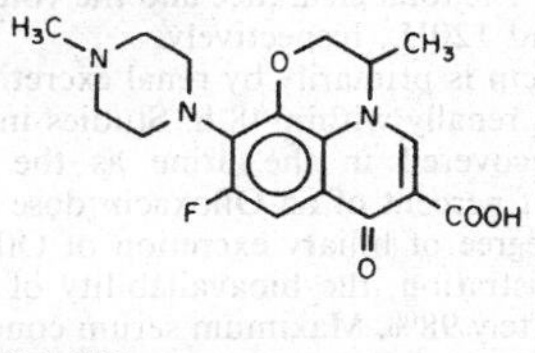

CLINICAL PHARMACOLOGY
Pharmacokinetics: Serum, urine and tear film concentrations of Ofloxacin were measured in 30 healthy women at various time points during a ten-day course of treatment. The mean serum Ofloxacin concentration ranged from 0.4 ng/mL to 1.9 ng/mL. Maximum Ofloxacin concentration increased from 1.1 ng/mL on day one to 1.9 ng/mL on day 11 after q.i.d. dosing for 10 ½ days. Maximum serum Ofloxacin concentrations after ten days of topical ophthalmic dosing were more than 1000 times lower than those reported after standard oral doses of Ofloxacin.

Tear film Ofloxacin concentrations ranged from 5.7 to 31 µg/g during the 40 minute period following the last dose on day 11. Mean tear film levels measured four hours after topical ophthalmic dosing were 9.2 µg/g. Ofloxacin was excreted in the urine primarily unmodified.

Microbiology: Ofloxacin has *in vitro* activity against a broad range of gram-positive and gram-negative aerobic and anaerobic bacteria. Ofloxacin is bactericidal at concentrations equal to or slightly greater than inhibitory concentrations. Ofloxacin is thought to exert a bactericidal effect on susceptible bacterial cells by inhibiting DNA gyrase, an essential bacterial enzyme which is a critical catalyst in the duplication, transcription, and repair of bacterial DNA.

Cross resistance has been observed between Ofloxacin and other fluoroquinolones. There is generally no cross-resistance between Ofloxacin and other classes of antibacterial agents such as beta-lactams or aminoglycosides; therefore organisms resistant to these drugs may be susceptible to Ofloxacin.

Organisms resistant to Ofloxacin may also be susceptible to beta-lactams or aminoglycosides.

Ofloxacin has been shown to be active against most strains of the following organisms both *in vitro* and, clinically, in conjunctival infections as described in the *"Indications and Usage"* section.

AEROBES, GRAM-POSITIVE
Staphylococcus aureus
Staphylococcus epidermidis
Streptococcus pneumoniae

AEROBES, GRAM-NEGATIVE
Enterobacter cloacae
Haemophilus influenzae
Proteus mirabilis
Pseudomonas aeruginosa

The following *in vitro* data are also available: but their clinical significance in ophthalmic infections is unknown.

Ofloxacin exhibits *in vitro* minimal inhibitory concentrations (MIC's) of 2 µg/mL or less against most (90%) strains of the following microorganisms; however, the safety and effectiveness of Ofloxacin in treating ocular infections due to these microorganisms have not been established.

AEROBES, GRAM-POSITIVE
Enterococcus faecalis
Listeria monocytogenes
Streptococcus pyogenes

AEROBES, GRAM-NEGATIVE
Acinetobacter calcoaceticus var. anitratus
Acinetobacter calcoaceticus var. Iwoffi
Citrobacter diversus
Citrobacter freundii
Enterobacter aerogenes
Escherichia coli
Klebsiella oxytoca
Klebsiella pneumoniae
Moraxella (Branhamella) catarrhalis
Morganella morganii
Neisseria gonorrhoeae
Pseudomonas acidovorans
Pseudomonas fluorescens
Serratia marcescens
Shigella sonnei

ANAEROBIC SPECIES
Propionibacterium acnes

OTHER
Chlamydia trachomatis

Clinical Studies: In a randomized, double-masked, multicenter clinical trial, Ofloxacin Ophthalmic solution was superior to its vehicle after 2 days of treatment in patients with conjunctivitis and positive conjunctival cultures. Clinical outcomes for the trial demonstrated a clinical improvement rate of 86% (54/63) for the Ofloxacin treated group versus 72% (48/67) for the placebo treated group after 2 days of therapy. Microbiological outcomes for the same clinical trial demonstrated an eradication rate for causative pathogens of 65% (41/63) for the Ofloxacin treated group versus 25% (17/67) for the vehicle treated group after 2 days of therapy. Please note that microbiologic eradication does not always correlate with clinical outcome in anti-infective trials.

INDICATIONS AND USAGE
Ofloxacin, Ophthalmic, solution is indicated for the treatment of conjunctivitis caused by susceptible strains of the following bacteria:

GRAM-POSITIVE BACTERIA
Staphylococcus aureus
Staphylococcus epidermidis
Streptococcus pneumoniae

GRAM-NEGATIVE BACTERIA
Enterobacter cloacae
Haemophilus influenzae
Proteus mirabilis
Pseudomonas aeruginosa

➤ SHOWN IN PRODUCT IDENTIFICATION GUIDE

UNLABELED USES

Ofloxacin is used alone or as an adjunct in the treatment of bacterial corneal ulcers.

CONTRAINDICATIONS

Ofloxacin, Ophthalmic, solution is contraindicated in patients with a history of hypersensitivity to Ofloxacin, to other quinolones, or to any of the components in this medication.

WARNINGS

NOT FOR INJECTION.

Ofloxacin Ophthalmic solution should not be injected subconjunctivally, nor should it be introduced directly into the anterior chamber of the eye.

Serious and occasionally fatal hypersensitivity (anaphylactic) reactions, some following the first dose, have been reported in patients receiving systemic quinolones, including Ofloxacin. Some reactions were accompanied by cardiovascular collapse, loss of consciousness, angioedema (including laryngeal, pharyngeal or facial edema), airway obstruction, dyspnea, urticaria, and itching. If an allergic reaction to Ofloxacin occurs, discontinue the drug. Serious acute hypersensitivity reactions may require immediate emergency treatment. Oxygen and airway management, including intubation, should be administered as clinically indicated.

PRECAUTIONS

General: As with other anti-infectives, prolonged use may result in overgrowth of nonsusceptible organisms, including fungi. If superinfection occurs or if clinical improvement is not noted within 7 days, discontinue use and institute appropriate therapy. Whenever clinical judgment dictates, the patient should be examined with the aid of magnification, such as slit lamp biomicroscopy and, where appropriate, fluorescein staining.

The systemic administration of quinolones, including Ofloxacin, has led to lesions or erosions of the cartilage in weight-bearing joints and other signs of arthropathy in immature animals of various species. Ofloxacin, administered systemically at 10 mg/kg/day in young dogs (equivalent to 150 times the maximum recommended daily *adult ophthalmic* dose) has been associated with these types of effects.

Information for Patients: Avoid contaminating the applicator tip with material from the eye, fingers or other source.

Systemic quinolones, including Ofloxacin, have been associated with hypersensitivity reactions, even following a single dose. Discontinue use immediately and contact your physician at the first sign of a rash or allergic reaction.

Drug Interactions: Specific drug interaction studies have not been conducted with Ofloxacin Ophthalmic solution.

Carcinogenesis, Mutagenesis, Impairment of Fertility: Long term studies to determine the carcinogenic potential of Ofloxacin have not been conducted.

Ofloxacin was not mutagenic in the Ames test, *in vitro* and *in vivo* cytogenic assay, sister chromatid exchange assay (Chinese hampster and human cell lines), unscheduled DNA synthesis (UDS) assay using human fibroblasts, the dominant lethal assay, or mouse micronucleus assay. Ofloxacin was positive in the UDS test using rat hepatocyte, and in the mouse lymphoma assay.

In fertility studies in rats, Ofloxacin did not affect male or female fertility or morphological or reproductive performance at oral dosing up to 360 mg/kg/day (equivalent to 6000 times the maximum recommended daily ophthalmic dose).

Pregnancy: Teratogenic Effects. Pregnancy Category C: Ofloxacin has been shown to have an embryocidal effect in rats and in rabbits when given in doses of 810 mg/kg/day (equivalent to 13,500 times the maximum recommended daily ophthalmic dose) and 160 mg/kg/day (equivalent to 2600 times the maximum recommended daily ophthalmic dose). These dosages resulted in decreased fetal body weight and increased fetal mortality in rats and rabbits, respectively. Minor fetal skeletal variations were reported in rats receiving doses of 810 mg/kg/day. Ofloxacin has not been shown to be teratogenic at doses as high as 810 mg/kg/day and 160 mg/kg/day when administered to pregnant rats and rabbits, respectively.

Nonteratogenic Effects: Additional studies in rats with doses up to 360 mg/kg/day during late gestation showed no adverse effect on late fetal development, labor, delivery, lactation, neonatal viability, or growth of the newborn.

There are, however, no adequate and well-controlled studies in pregnant women. Ofloxacin, Ophthalmic, solution should be used during pregnancy only if the potential benefit justifies the potential risk to the fetus.

Nursing Mothers: In nursing women a single 200 mg oral dose resulted in concentrations of Ofloxacin in milk which were similar to those found in plasma. It is not known whether Ofloxacin is excreted in human milk following topical ophthalmic administration. Because of the potential for serious adverse reactions from Ofloxacin in nursing infants, a decision should be made whether to discontinue nursing or to discontinue the drug, taking into account the importance of the drug to the mother.

Pediatric Use: Safety and effectiveness in infants below the age of one year have not been established.

Quinolones, including Ofloxacin, have been shown to cause arthropathy in immature animals after oral administration; however, topical ocular administration of Ofloxacin to immature animals has not shown any arthropathy. There is no evidence that the ophthalmic dosage form of Ofloxacin has any effect on weight bearing joints.

ADVERSE REACTIONS

Ophthalmic use: The most frequently reported drug-related adverse reaction was transient ocular burning or discomfort. Other reported reactions were stinging, redness, itching, photophobia, tearing, and dryness. One report of dizziness was also received.

DOSAGE AND ADMINISTRATION

Instill one to two drops every two to four hours for the first two days, and then four times daily in the affected eye(s) for up to five additional days.

Store at 15-25°C (59-77°F).

HOW SUPPLIED

DROP: 0.3%

BRAND/MANUFACTURER	NDC	SIZE	AWP
○ **BRAND** OCUFLOX: Allergan Pharm	11980-0779-05	5 ml	$17.50

Ofloxacin, Systemic

DESCRIPTION

Ofloxacin is a synthetic, broad-spectrum antimicrobial agent available as a solution for intravenous (IV) infusion or as tablets for oral administration.

Each ml of solution for injection contains:	
Ofloxacin ....4, 20, or 40 mg	
Each tablet contains:	
Ofloxacin ....200, 300, or 400 mg	

Chemically, Ofloxacin, a fluorinated carboxyquinolone, is the racemate, (±)-9-fluoro-2,3-dihydro-3-methyl-10-(4-methyl-1-piperazinyl)-7 -oxo-7H-pyrido (1,2,3-de)-1,4-benzoxazine-6-carboxylic acid.

Its empirical formula is $C_{18}H_{20}FN_3O_4$, and its molecular weight is 361.4. Ofloxacin is an off-white to pale yellow crystalline powder. The molecule exists as a zwitterion at the pH conditions in the small intestine. The relative solubility characteristics of Ofloxacin at room temperature, as defined by USP nomenclature, indicate that Ofloxacin is considered to be *soluble* in aqueous solutions with pH between 2 and 5. It is *sparingly* to *slightly soluble* in aqueous solutions with pH 7 and *freely soluble* in aqueous solutions with pH above 9. Ofloxacin has the potential to form stable coordination compounds with many metal ions. This *in vitro* chelation potential has the following formation order: $Fe^{+3} > Al^{+3} > Cu^{+2} > Ni^{+2} > Pb^{+2} > Zn^{+2} > Mg^{+2} > Ca^{+2} > Ba^{+2}$.

Following is its chemical structure:

CLINICAL PHARMACOLOGY

Following a single 60-minute IV infusion of 200 mg or 400 mg of Ofloxacin to normal volunteers, the mean maximum plasma concentrations attained were 2.7 and 4.0 µg/mL, respectively; the concentrations at 12 hours (h) after dosing were 0.3 and 0.7 µg/mL, respectively.

Steady-state concentrations were attained after four doses, and the area under the curve (AUC) was approximately 40% higher than the AUC after a single dose. The mean peak and trough plasma steady-state levels attained following IV administration of 200 mg of Ofloxacin q 12 h for seven days were 2.9 and 0.5 µg/mL, respectively. Following IV doses of 400 mg of Ofloxacin q 12 h, the mean peak and trough plasma steady-state levels ranged, in two different studies, from 5.5 to 7.2 µg/mL and 1.2 to 1.9 µg/mL, respectively.

Following 7 days of IV administration, the elimination half-life of Ofloxacin was 6 h (range 5 to 10 h). The total clearance and the volume of distribution were approximately 15 L/h and 120 L, respectively.

Elimination of Ofloxacin is primarily by renal excretion. Approximately 65% of an IV dose is excreted renally within 48 h. Studies indicate that < 5% of the administered dose is recovered in the urine as the desmethyl or N-oxide metabolites. Four to eight percent of an Ofloxacin dose is excreted in the feces. This indicates a small degree of biliary excretion of Ofloxacin.

Following oral administration, the bioavailability of Ofloxacin in the tablet formulation is approximately 98%. Maximum serum concentrations are achieved one to two hours after an oral dose. Absorption of Ofloxacin after single or multiple doses of 200 to 400 mg is predictable, and the amount of drug absorbed increases proportionally with the dose.

Ofloxacin has biphasic elimination. Following multiple oral doses at steady state administration, the half-lives are approximately 4-5 hours and 20-25 hours. However, the longer half-life represents less than 5% of the total AUC. Accumulation at steady-state can be estimated using a half-life of 9 hours. The total clearance and volume of distribution are approximately similar after single or multiple doses. Elimination is mainly by renal excretion. The following are mean peak serum concentrations in healthy 70-80 kg male volunteers after single oral doses of 200, 300, or 400 mg of Ofloxacin or after multiple oral doses of 400 mg.

Oral Dose	Serum Concentration 2 hours after admin. (μg/mL)	Area Under the Curve $(AUC_{(0-\infty)})$ (μg•h/mL)
200 mg single dose	1.5	14.1
300 mg single dose	2.4	21.2
400 mg single dose	2.9	31.4
400 mg steady state	4.6	61.0

Steady-state concentrations were attained after four oral doses and the area under the curve (AUC) was approximately, 40% higher than the AUC after single doses. Therefore, after multiple-dose administration of 200 mg and 300 mg doses, peak serum levels of 2.2 μg/mL and 3.6 μg/mL, respectively, are predicted at steady-state.

In vitro, approximately 32% of the drug in plasma is protein bound.

The single dose and steady-state plasma profiles of Ofloxacin injection were comparable in extent of exposure (AUC) to those of Ofloxacin tablets when the injectable and tablet formulations of Ofloxacin were administered in equal doses (mg/mg) to the same group of subjects. The mean steady-state $AUC_{(0-12)}$ attained after the IV administration of 400 mg over 60 min was 43.5 μg•h/mL; the mean steady-state $AUC_{(0-12)}$ attained after the oral administration of 400 mg was 41.2 μg•h/ml (two one-sided t-test, 90% confidence interval was 103—109). [See following chart.]

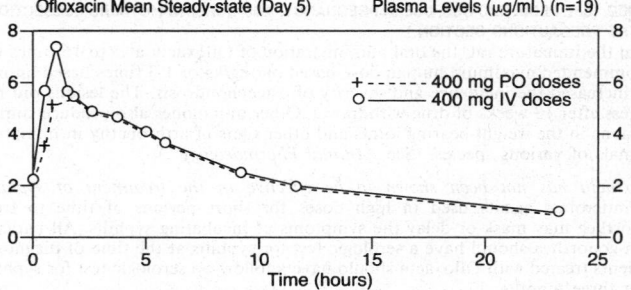

Ofloxacin Mean Steady-state (Day 5)   Plasma Levels (μg/mL) (n=19)

+ - - - - - 400 mg PO doses
o ———— 400 mg IV doses

Between 0 and 6 h following the administration of a single 200 mg oral dose of Ofloxacin to 12 healthy volunteers, the average urine of Ofloxacin concentration was approximately 220 μg/mL. Between 12 and 24 h after administration, the average urine Ofloxacin level was approximately 34 μg/mL. Following oral administration of recommended therapeutic doses, Ofloxacin has been detected in blister fluid, cervix, lung tissue, ovary, prostatic fluid, prostatic tissue, skin, and sputum. The mean concentration of Ofloxacin in each of these various body fluids and tissues after one or more doses was 0.8 to 1.5 times the concurrent plasma level. Inadequate data are presently available on the distribution or levels of Ofloxacin in the cerebrospinal fluid or brain tissue.

Ofloxacin has a pyridobenzoxazine ring that appears to decrease the extent of parent compound metabolism. Between 65% and 80% of the administered oral dose of Ofloxacin is excreted unchanged via the kidneys within 48 hours of dosing. Studies indicate that less than 5% of an administered dose is recovered in the urine as the desmethyl or N-oxide metabolites. Four to eight percent of an Ofloxacin dose is excreted in the feces. This indicates a small degree of biliary excretion of Ofloxacin.

The effect that food has on the absorption of Ofloxacin tablets has not been studied.

Following the administration of oral doses of Ofloxacin to healthy elderly volunteers (64-74 years of age) with normal renal function, the apparent half-life of Ofloxacin was 7 to 8 h, as compared to approximately 6 h in younger adults.

Clearance of Ofloxacin is reduced in patients with impaired renal function (creatinine clearance ≤ 50 ml/min), and dosage adjustment is necessary. (See *"Precautions: General"* and *"Dosage and Administration"*.)

MICROBIOLOGY

Ofloxacin has *in vitro* activity against a broad-spectrum of gram-positive and gram-negative aerobic and anaerobic bacteria. Ofloxacin is often bactericidal at concentrations equal to or slightly greater than inhibitory concentrations. Ofloxacin is thought to exert a bactericidal effect on susceptible micro-organisms by inhibiting DNA gyrase, an essential enzyme that is a critical catalyst in the duplication, transcription, and repair of bacterial DNA.

Ofloxacin has been shown to be active against most strains of the following organisms both *in vitro* and in specific clinical infections: (see *"Indications and Usage"*.)

Chlamydia trachomatis
Citrobacter diversus
Enterobacter aerogenes
Escherichia coli
Haemophilus influenzae
Klebsiella pneumoniae
Neisseria gonorrhoeae

Proteus mirabilis
Pseudomonas aeruginosa
Staphylococcus aureus
Streptococcus aureus (oral only)
Streptococcus pneumoniae
Streptococcus pyogenes

Beta-lactamase production should have no effect on Ofloxacin activity.

The following *in vitro* data are available; *however, their clinical significance is unknown.*

Ofloxacin exhibits *in vitro* minimum inhibitory concentrations of 2 μg/mL or less against most strains of the following organisms; however, the safety and effectiveness of Ofloxacin in treating clinical infections due to these organisms have not been established in adequate and well-controlled trials:

GRAM-POSITIVE AEROBES

Enterococcus faecalis
Staphylococcus epidermidis (including methicillin-resistant strains)
Staphylococcus saprophyticus
Streptococcus agalactiae (Group B)

GRAM-NEGATIVE AEROBES

Acinetobacter calcoaceticus
Aeromonas hydrophila
Bordetella parapertussis
Bordetella pertussis
Campylobacter jejuni
Citrobacter freundii
Enterobacter cloacae
Haemophilus ducreyi
Klebsiella oxytoca
Moraxella (Branhamella) catarrhalis
Morganella morganii
Neisseria meningitidis
Plesiomonas shigelloides
Proteus vulgaris
Providencia rettgeri
Providencia stuartii
Pseudomonas fluorescens
Serratia marcescens

ANAEROBES

Bacteroides fragilis
Bacteroides intermedius
Clostridium perfringens
Clostridium welchii
Eikenella corrodens
Gardnerella vaginalis
Peptococcus niger
Peptostreptococcus species

OTHER ORGANISMS

Chlamydia pneumoniae
Legionella pneumophila
Mycobacterium tuberculosis
Mycoplasma hominis
Mycoplasma pneumoniae
Ureaplasma urealyticum

Many strains of other streptococcal species, *Enterococcus* species, and anaerobes are resistant to Ofloxacin.

Ofloxacin has not been shown to be active against *Treponema pallidum*. (See *"Warnings"*).

Resistance to Ofloxacin due to spontaneous mutation *in vitro* is a rare occurrence (range: 10^{-9} to 10^{-11}). To date, emergence of resistance has been relatively uncommon in clinical practice. With the exception of *Pseudomonas aeruginosa* (10%), less than a 4% rate of resistance emergence has been reported for most other species. Although cross-resistance has been observed between Ofloxacin and other fluoroquinolones, some organisms resistant to other quinolones may be susceptible to Ofloxacin.

SUSCEPTIBILITY TESTS

Diffusion Techniques: Quantitative methods that require measurement of zone diameters give the most precise estimate of the susceptibility of bacteria to antimicrobial agents. One such standardized procedure[1] that has been recommended for use with disks to test the susceptibility of organisms to Ofloxacin uses the 5 μg Ofloxacin disk. Interpretation involves correlation of the diameter obtained in the disk test with the minimum inhibitory concentration (MIC) for Ofloxacin.

Reports from the laboratory giving results of the standard single-disk susceptibility test with a 5 μg Ofloxacin disk should be interpreted according to the following criteria:

Zone diameter (mm)	Interpretation
≥ 16	Susceptible
13-15	Intermediate
≤ 12	Resistant

A report of "Susceptible" indicates that the pathogen is likely to be inhibited by generally achievable drug concentrations. A report of "Intermediate" indicates that the result should be considered equivocal, and, if the organism is not fully susceptible to alternative, clinically feasible drugs, the test should be repeated. This category provides a buffer zone that prevents small uncontrolled technical factors from causing major discrepancies in interpretation. A report of "Resistant" indicates that achievable drug concentrations are unlikely to be inhibitory, and other therapy should be selected.

Standardized susceptibility test procedures require the use of laboratory control organisms. The 5-μg Ofloxacin disk should give the following zone diameters:

Organism	Zone diameter (mm)
E. coli ATCC 25922	29-33
P. aeruginosa ATCC 27853	17-21
S. aureus ATCC 25923	24-28

Dilution Techniques: Use a standardized dilution method[2] (broth, agar, or microdilution) or equivalent with Ofloxacin powder. The MIC values obtained should be interpreted according to the following criteria:

MIC (μg/mL)	Interpretation
≤ 2	(S) Susceptible
4	(I) Intermediate
≥ 8	(R) Resistant

As with standard diffusion methods, dilution procedures require the use of laboratory control organisms. Standard Ofloxacin powder should give the following MIC values:

Organism	MIC range (μg/mL)
E. coli ATCC 25922	0.015-0.120
E. faecalis ATCC 29212	1.000-4.000
P. aeruginosa ATCC 27853	1.000-8.000
S. aureus ATCC 25923	0.120-1.000

INDICATIONS AND USAGE

Ofloxacin injection and tablets are indicated for the treatment of adults with mild to moderate infections caused by susceptible strains of the designated microorganisms in the infections listed below. The injection is used when intravenous administration offers a route of administration advantageous to the patient, (*i.e.*, patient cannot tolerate an oral dosage form, etc.) *The safety and effectiveness of the IV formulation in treating patients with severe infections have not been established.*

Note: IN THE ABSENCE OF VOMITING OR OTHER FACTORS INTERFERING WITH THE ABSORPTION OF ORALLY ADMINISTERED DRUG, PATIENTS RECEIVE ESSENTIALLY THE SAME SYSTEMIC ANTIMICROBIAL THERAPY AFTER EQUIVALENT DOSES OF OFLOXACIN ADMINISTERED BY EITHER THE ORAL OR THE INTRAVENOUS ROUTE. THEREFORE, THE INTRAVENOUS FORMULATION DOES NOT PROVIDE A HIGHER DEGREE OF EFFICACY OR MORE POTENT ANTIMICROBIAL ACTIVITY THAN AN EQUIVALENT DOSE OF THE ORAL FORMULATION OF OFLOXACIN.

LOWER RESPIRATORY TRACT
Acute bacterial exacerbation of chronic bronchitis: due to *Haemophilus influenzae* or *Streptococcus pneumoniae.*

Community-acquired Pneumonia: due to *Haemophilus influenzae* or *Streptococcus pneumoniae.*

SKIN AND SKIN STRUCTURES
Uncomplicated skin and skin structure infections: due to *Staphylococcus aureus, Streptococcus pyogenes,* or *Proteus mirabilis.* *

SEXUALLY TRANSMITTED DISEASES
(See "Warnings".)

Acute, uncomplicated urethral and cervical gonorrhea: due to *Neisseria gonorrhoeae.*

Nongonococcal urethritis and cervicitis: due to *Chlamydia trachomatis.*

Mixed infections of the urethra and cervix: due to *Chlamydia trachomatis* and *Neisseria gonorrhoeae.*

URINARY TRACT
Uncomplicated cystitis: due to *Citrobacter diversus, Enterobacter aerogenes, Escherichia coli, Klebsiella pneumoniae, Proteus mirabilis,* or *Pseudomonas aeruginosa.*

Complicated urinary tract infections: due to *Escherichia coli, Klebsiella pneumoniae, Proteus mirabilis, Citrobacter diversus*, or *Pseudomonas aeruginosa*.

PROSTATE
Prostatitis: due to *Escherichia coli.*

* Although treatment of infections due to this organism in this infection demonstrated a clinically acceptable overall outcome, efficacy was demonstrated in fewer than 10 infections.

Although treatment of infections due to this organism in this infection demonstrated a clinically acceptable overall outcome, efficacy was demonstrated in fewer than 10 infections.

Beta-lactamase production should have no effect on Ofloxacin activity.

Appropriate culture and susceptibility tests should be performed before treatment in order to isolate and identify organisms causing the infection and to determine their susceptibility to Ofloxacin. Therapy with Ofloxacin may be initiated before results of these tests are known; once results become available, appropriate therapy should be continued. As with other drugs in this class, some strains of *Pseudomonas aeruginosa* may develop resistance fairly rapidly during treatment with Ofloxacin. Culture and susceptibility testing performed periodically during therapy will provide information not only on the therapeutic effect of the antimicrobial agent but also on the possible emergence of bacterial resistance.

If anaerobic organisms are suspected of contributing to the infection, appropriate therapy for anaerobic pathogens should be administered.

UNLABELED USES
Ofloxacin is used alone or as an adjunct in the treatment of bone infections including chronic posttraumatic osteitis, *Mycobacterium leprae* infections, otitis media, and Q fever. It is also used in otitis externa, paranasal sinusitis, tonsillitis, salmonella gastroenteritis, and traveler's diarrhea.

CONTRAINDICATIONS

Ofloxacin is contraindicated in persons with a history of hypersensitivity to Ofloxacin or members of the quinolone group of antimicrobial agents.

WARNINGS

THE SAFETY AND EFFICACY OF OFLOXACIN IN CHILDREN, ADOLESCENTS (UNDER THE AGE OF 18 YEARS), PREGNANT WOMEN, AND LACTATING WOMEN HAVE NOT BEEN ESTABLISHED. (SEE PEDIATRIC USE, USE IN PREGNANCY, AND NURSING MOTHERS SUBSECTIONS IN THE PRECAUTIONS SECTION.)

In the immature rat, the oral administration of Ofloxacin at 5 to 16 times the recommended maximum human dose based on mg/kg or 1-3 times based on mg/m^2 increased the incidence and severity of osteochondrosis. The lesions did not regress after 13 weeks of drug withdrawal. Other quinolones also produce similar erosions in the weight-bearing joints and other signs of arthropathy in immature animals of various species. (See *"Animal Pharmacology".*)

Ofloxacin has not been shown to be effective in the treatment of syphilis. Antimicrobial agents used in high doses for short periods of time to treat gonorrhea may mask or delay the symptoms of incubating syphilis. All patients with gonorrhea should have a serologic test for syphilis at the time of diagnosis. Patients treated with Ofloxacin should have a follow-up serologic test for syphilis after three months.

Serious and occasionally fatal hypersensitivity (anaphylactic/anaphylactoid) reactions have been reported in patients receiving therapy with quinolones, including Ofloxacin. These reactions often occur following the first dose. Some reactions were accompanied by cardiovascular collapse, hypotension/shock, seizure, loss of consciousness, tingling, angioedema (including tongue, laryngeal, throat or facial edema/swelling, etc.), airway obstruction (including bronchospasm, shortness of breath and acute respiratory distress), dyspnea, urticaria/hives, itching, and other serious skin reactions. A few patients had a history of hypersensitivity reactions. The drug should be discontinued immediately at the first appearance of a skin rash or any other sign of hypersensitivity. Serious acute hypersensitivity reactions may require treatment with epinephrine and other resuscitative measures, including oxygen, intravenous fluids, antihistamines, corticosteroids, pressor amines, and airway management, as clinically indicated. (See *"Precautions"* and *"Adverse Reactions".*)

Serious and sometimes fatal events of uncertain etiology have been reported in patients receiving therapy with quinolones including, extremely rarely, Ofloxacin. These events may be severe and generally occur following the administration of multiple doses. Clinical manifestations may include one or more of the following: fever, rash or severe dermatologic reactions (e.g., toxic epidermal necrolysis, Stevens-Johnson Syndrome, etc); vasculitis; arthralgia; myalgia; serum sickness; allergic pneumonitis; interstitial nephritis, acute renal insufficiency/failure; hepatitis, jaundice, acute hepatic necrosis/failure; anemia including hemolytic and aplastic, thrombocytopenia, including thrombotic thrombocytopenic purpura, leukopenia, agranulocytosis, pancytopenia, and/or other hematologic abnormalities. The drug should be discontinued immediately at the first appearance of a skin rash or any other sign of hypersensitivity and supportive measures instituted. (See *"Precautions: Information for Patients"* and *"Adverse Reactions".*)

Convulsions, increased intracranial pressure, and toxic psychosis have been reported in patients receiving quinolones, including Ofloxacin. Quinolones, including Ofloxacin, may also cause central nervous system stimulation which may lead to: tremors, restlessness/agitation, nervousness/anxiety, lightheadedness, confusion, hallucinations, paranoia and depression, nightmares, insomnia, and rarely suicidal thoughts or acts. These reactions may occur following the first dose. If these reactions occur in patients receiving Ofloxacin, the drug should be discontinued and appropriate measures instituted. As with all quinolones, Ofloxacin should be used with caution in patients with a known or suspected CNS disorder that may predispose to seizures or lower the seizure threshold (e.g., severe cerebral arteriosclerosis, epilepsy, etc.) or in the presence of other risk factors that may predispose to seizures or lower the seizure threshold (e.g., certain drug therapy, renal dysfunction, etc.). (See *"Precautions: General, Drug Interactions"* and *"Adverse Reactions".*)

Pseudomembranous colitis has been reported with nearly all antibacterial agents, including Ofloxacin, and may range in severity from mild to life-threatening. Therefore, it is important to

---

consider this diagnosis in patients who present with diarrhea subsequent to the administration of any antibacterial agent.

Treatment with antibacterial agents alters the normal flora of the colon and may permit overgrowth of clostridia. Studies indicate a toxin produced by *Clostridium difficile* is one primary cause of "antibiotic-associated colitis".

After the diagnosis of pseudomembranous colitis has been established, therapeutic measures should be initiated. Mild cases of pseudomembranous colitis usually respond to drug discontinuation alone. In moderate to severe cases, consideration should be given to management with fluids and electrolytes, protein supplementation, and treatment with an oral antibacterial drug clinically effective against *C. difficile* colitis. (See *"Adverse Reactions"*.)

PRECAUTIONS
GENERAL
Because a rapid or bolus intravenous injection may result in hypotension, *Ofloxacin Injection should only be administered by slow intravenous infusion over a period of 60 minutes.* (See *"Dosage and Administration"*.)

Adequate hydration of patients receiving Ofloxacin should be maintained to prevent the formation of a highly concentrated urine.

Administer Ofloxacin with caution in the presence of renal or hepatic insufficiency/impairment. In patients with known or suspected renal or hepatic insufficiency/impairment, careful clinical observation and appropriate laboratory studies should be performed prior to and during therapy since elimination of Ofloxacin may be reduced. In patients with impaired renal function (creatinine clearance ≤ 50 mg/mL), alteration of the dosage regimen is necessary. (See *"Clinical Pharmacology"* and *"Dosage and Administration"*.)

Moderate to severe phototoxicity reactions have been observed in patients exposed to direct sunlight while receiving some drugs in this class, including Ofloxacin. Excessive sunlight should be avoided. Therapy should be discontinued if phototoxicity (e.g., a skin eruption, etc.) occurs.

As with all quinolones, Ofloxacin should be used with caution in any patient with a known or suspected CNS disorder that may predispose to seizures or lower the seizure threshold (e.g., severe cerebral arteriosclerosis, epilepsy, etc.) or in the presence of other risk factors that may predispose to seizures or lower the seizure threshold (e.g., certain drug therapy, renal dysfunction, etc.), (See *"Warnings"* and *"Drug Interactions."*)

As with other quinolones, disturbances of blood glucose, including symptomatic hyper- and hypoglycemia, have been reported, usually in diabetic patients receiving concomitant treatment with an oral hypoglycemic agent (e.g., glyburide/glibenclamide, etc.) or with insulin. In these patients careful monitoring of blood glucose is recommended. If a hypoglycemic reaction occurs in a patient being treated with Ofloxacin, discontinue Ofloxacin immediately and consult a physician. (See *"Drug Interactions"* and *"Adverse Reactions"*.) As with any potent drug, periodic assessment of organ system functions, including renal, hepatic, and hematopoietic, is advisable during prolonged therapy. (See *"Warnings"* and *"Adverse Reactions"*.)

INFORMATION FOR PATIENTS
Patients should be advised:
—to drink fluids liberally if able to take fluids by the oral route.
—that Ofloxacin may cause neurologic adverse effects (e.g., dizziness, lightheadedness, etc.) and that patients should know how they react to Ofloxacin before they operate an automobile or machinery or engage in activities requiring mental alertness and coordination. (See *"Warnings"* and *"Adverse Reactions"*.)
—that Ofloxacin may be associated with hypersensitivity reactions, even following the first dose, to discontinue the drug at the first sign of a skin rash, hives or other skin reactions, a rapid heartbeat, difficulty in swallowing or breathing, any swelling suggesting angioedema (e.g., swelling of the lips, tongue, face; tightness of the throat, hoarseness, etc.), or any other symptom of an allergic reaction. (See *"Warnings"* and *"Adverse Reactions"*.)
—to avoid excessive sunlight or artificial ultraviolet light while receiving Ofloxacin and to discontinue therapy if phototoxicity (e.g., skin eruption, etc.) occurs.
—that if they are diabetic and are being treated with insulin or an oral hypoglycemic agent, to discontinue Ofloxacin immediately if a hypoglycemic reaction occurs and consult a physician. (See *"Precautions: General"* and *"Drug Interactions"*.)
—that mineral supplements, vitamins with iron or minerals, calcium-, aluminum- or magnesium-based antacids or sucralfate should not be taken within the two-hour period before or within the two-hour period after taking oral Ofloxacin. (See *"Drug Interactions"*.)
—that Ofloxacin tablets should not be taken with food.

DRUG INTERACTIONS
Antacids, Sucralfate, Metal Cations, Multi-Vitamins: There are no data concerning an interaction of **intravenous** quinolones with **oral** antacids, sucralfate, multi-vitamins, or metal cations. However, no quinolone should be co-administered with any solution containing multivalent cations, e.g., magnesium, through the same intravenous line. (See *"Dosage and Administration"*.)

Quinolones form chelates with alkaline earth and transition metal cations. Administration of oral quinolones with antacids containing calcium, magnesium, or aluminum, with sucralfate, with divalent or trivalent cations such as iron, or with multivitamins containing zinc may substantially interfere with the absorption of quinolones resulting in systemic levels considerably lower than desired. These agents should not be taken within the two-hour period before or within the two-hour period after oral Ofloxacin administration. (See *"Dosage and Administration"*.)

Caffeine: Interactions between Ofloxacin and caffeine have not been detected.

Cimetidine: Cimetidine has demonstrated interference with the elimination of some quinolones. This interference has resulted in significant increases in half-life and AUC of some quinolones. The potential for interaction between Ofloxacin and cimetidine has not been studied.

Cyclosporine: Elevated serum levels of cyclosporine have been reported with concomitant use of cyclosporine with some other quinolones. The potential for interaction between Ofloxacin and cyclosporine has not been studied.

Drug Metabolized by Cytochrome P450 Enzymes: Most quinolone antimicrobial drugs inhibit cytochrome P450 enzyme activity. This may result in a prolonged half-life for some drugs that are also metabolized by this system (e.g., cyclosporine, theophylline/methylxanthines, warfarin, etc.) when co-administered with quinolones. The extent of this inhibition varies among different quinolones. (See other *"Drug Interactions."*)

Nonsteroidal Anti-inflammatory Drugs: The concomitant administration of a nonsteroidal anti-inflammatory drug, with a quinolone, including Ofloxacin, may increase the risk of CNS stimulation and convulsive seizures. (See *"Warnings"* and *"Precautions: General."*)

Probenecid: The concomitant use of probenecid with certain other quinolones has been reported to affect renal tubular secretion. The effect of probenecid on the elimination of Ofloxacin has not been studied.

Theophylline: Although concurrent administration of some quinolones with theophylline may result in impaired elimination of theophylline, the extent of such impairment varies among different quinolones. Steady-state theophylline levels may increase when Ofloxacin and theophylline are administered concurrently. In a pharmacokinetic study involving 15 healthy male subjects, steady-state peak theophylline concentration increased by an average of approximately 9%, and the AUC increased by an average of approximately 13% when oral Ofloxacin and theophylline were administered concurrently. In clinical trials with intravenous Ofloxacin, theophylline concentrations were determined in 41 patients who were treated with both drugs. In 38 patients, no apparent elevation in the serum theophylline was discernible. Marginal increases above the theophylline therapeutic range were reported in three patients; clinical toxicity was, however, not reported in these three patients. Generally, patients receiving theophylline in clinical trials of the intravenous formulation of Ofloxacin reported nausea more frequently than those patients not receiving theophylline. As with some other quinolones, concomitant administration of Ofloxacin may prolong the half-life of theophylline, elevate serum theophylline levels, and may increase the risk of theophylline-related adverse reactions. Theophylline levels should be closely monitored and theophylline dosage adjustments made, if appropriate, when Ofloxacin is co-administered.

Warfarin: Some quinolones have been reported to enhance the effects of the oral anticoagulant warfarin or its derivatives. Therefore, if a quinolone antimicrobial is administered concomitantly with warfarin or its derivatives, the prothrombin time or other suitable coagulation test should be closely monitored.

Antidiabetic Agents (e.g., Insulin, Glyburide/Glibenclamide, etc.): Since disturbances of blood glucose, including hyperglycemia and hypoglycemia, have been reported in patients treated concurrently with quinolones and an antidiabetic agent, careful monitoring of blood glucose is recommended when these agents are used concomitantly (See *"Precautions: General"* and *"Information for Patients"*.)

CARCINOGENESIS, MUTAGENESIS, IMPAIRMENT OF FERTILITY
Long-term studies to determine the carcinogenic potential of Ofloxacin have not been conducted.

Ofloxacin was not mutagenic in the Ames bacterial test, *in vitro* and *in vivo* cytogenetic assay, sister chromatid exchange (Chinese Hamster and Human Cell Lines), unscheduled DNA Repair (UDS) using human fibroblasts, dominant lethal assays, or mouse micronucleus assay. Ofloxacin was positive in the UDS test using rat hepatocytes and Mouse Lymphoma Assay.

PREGNANCY: TERATOGENIC EFFECTS. PREGNANCY CATEGORY C.
Ofloxacin has not been shown to have any teratogenic effects at oral doses as high as 810 mg/kg/day (11 times the recommended maximum human dose based on mg/m^2 or 50 times based on mg/kg) and 160 mg/kg/day (4 times the recommended maximum human dose based on mg/m^2 or 10 times based on mg/kg) when administered to pregnant rats and rabbits, respectively. Additional studies in rats with oral doses up to 360 mg/kg/day (5 times the recommended maximum human dose based on mg/m^2 or 23 times based on mg/kg) demonstrated no adverse effect on late fetal development, labor, delivery, lactation, neonatal viability, or growth of the newborn. Doses equivalent to 50 and 10 times the recommended maximum human dose of Ofloxacin (based on mg/kg) were fetotoxic (i.e., decreased fetal body weight and increased fetal mortality) in rats and rabbits, respectively. Minor skeletal variations were reported in rats receiving doses of 810 mg/kg/day, which is more than 10 times higher than the recommended maximum human dose based on mg/m^2.

There are, however, no adequate and well-controlled studies in pregnant women. Ofloxacin should be used during pregnancy only if the potential benefit justifies the potential risk to the fetus. (See *"Warnings"*.)

NURSING MOTHERS
In lactating females, a single oral 200 mg dose of Ofloxacin resulted in concentrations of Ofloxacin in milk that were similar to those found in plasma. Because of the potential for serious adverse reactions from Ofloxacin in nursing infants, a decision should be made whether to discontinue nursing or to

discontinue the drug, taking into account the importance of the drug to the mother. (See *"Warnings"* and *"Adverse Reactions"*.)

PEDIATRIC USE

Safety and effectiveness in children and adolescents below the age of 18 years have not been established. Ofloxacin causes arthropathy (arthrosis) and osteochondrosis in juvenile animals of several species. (See *"Warnings"*.)

ADVERSE REACTIONS

The following is a compilation of the data for Ofloxacin based on clinical experience with both the oral and intravenous formulations. The incidence of drug-related adverse reactions in patients during Phase 2 and 3 clinical trials was 11%. Among patients receiving multiple-dose therapy, 4% discontinued Ofloxacin due to adverse experiences.

In clinical trials, the following events were considered likely to be drug-related in patients receiving multiple doses of Ofloxacin:

nausea 3%, insomnia 3%, headache 1%, dizziness 1%, diarrhea 1%, vomiting 1%, rash 1%, pruritus 1%, external genital pruritus in women 1%, vaginitis 1%, dysgeusia 1%.

Local injection site reactions (phlebitis, swelling, erythema) were reported in approximately 2% of patients treated with the 3.63 mg/ml final infusion concentration of IV Ofloxacin used in the clinical safety trials. The final infusion concentration of IV Ofloxacin in the commercially available intravenous preparations is 4.0 mg/ml. To date, individuals administered the 4.0 mg/ml concentration of the IV Ofloxacin have demonstrated clinically acceptable rates of local injection site reactions. Due to the small difference in concentration, significant differences in local site reactions are unexpected with the 4.0 mg/ml concentration.

In clinical trials, the most frequently reported adverse events, regardless of relationship to drug, were:

nausea 10%, headache 9%, insomnia 7%, external genital pruritus in women 6%, dizziness 5%, vaginitis 5%, diarrhea 4%, vomiting 4%.

In clinical trials, the following events, regardless of relationship to drug occurred in 1 to 3% of patients:

Abdominal pain and cramps, chest pain, decreased appetite, dry mouth, dysgeusia, fatigue, flatulence, gastrointestinal distress, nervousness, pharyngitis, pruritus, fever, rash, sleep disorders, somnolence, trunk pain, vaginal discharge, visual disturbances, and constipation.

Additional events, occurring in clinical trials at a rate of less than 1%, regardless of relationship to drug, were:

Body as a whole: asthenia, chills, malaise, extremity pain, pain, epistaxis

Cardiovascular System: cardiac arrest, edema, hypertension, hypotension, palpitations, vasodilation

Gastrointestinal System: dyspepsia

Genital/Reproductive System: burning, irritation, pain and rash of the female genitalia; dysmenorrhea; menorrhagia; metrorrhagia

Musculoskeletal System: arthralgia, myalgia

Nervous System: seizures, anxiety, cognitive change, depression, dream abnormality, euphoria, hallucinations, paresthesia, syncope, vertigo, tremor, confusion

Nutritional/Metabolic: thirst, weight loss

Respiratory System: respiratory arrest, cough, rhinorrhea

Skin/Hypersensitivity: angioedema, diaphoresis, urticaria, vasculitis

Special Senses: decreased hearing acuity, tinnitus, photophobia

Urinary System: dysuria, urinary frequency, urinary retention

The following laboratory abnormalities appeared in $\geq$ 1.0% of patients receiving multiple doses of Ofloxacin. It is not known whether these abnormalities were caused by the drug or the underlying conditions being treated.

Hematopoietic: anemia, leukopenia, leukocytosis, neutropenia, neutrophilia, increased band forms, lymphocytopenia, eosinophilia, lymphocytosis, thrombocytopenia, thrombocytosis, elevated ESR

Hepatic: elevated alkaline phosphatase, AST (SGOT), ALT (SGPT)

Serum Chemistry: hyperglycemia, hypoglycemia, elevated creatinine, elevated BUN

Urinary: glucosuria, proteinuria, alkalinuria, hyposthenuria, hematuria, pyuria

POSTMARKETING ADVERSE EVENTS

Additional adverse events, regardless of relationship to drug, reported from worldwide marketing experience with quinolones including Ofloxacin:

Clinical:

Cardiovascular System: cerebral thrombosis, pulmonary edema, tachycardia, hypotension/shock, syncope

Endocrine/Metabolic: hyper- or hypoglycemia, especially in diabetic patients on insulin or oral hypoglycemic agents (See *"Precautions: General"* and *"Drug Interactions"*.)

Gastrointestinal System: hepatic dysfunction including: hepatic necrosis, jaundice (cholestatic or hepatocellular), hepatitis; intestinal perforation; pseudomembranous colitis, GI hemorrhage; hiccough, painful oral mucosa, pyrosis (See *"Warnings"*.)

Genitourinary System: vaginal candidiasis

Hematopoietic: anemia, including hemolytic and aplastic; hemorrhage, pancytopenia, agranuylocytosis, leukopenia, reversible bone marrow depression, thrombocytopenia, thrombotic thrombocytopenic purpura, petechiae, ecchymosis/bruising (see *"Warnings"*.)

Musculoskeletal: tendinitis/rupture: weakness

Nervous System: nightmares, suicidal thoughts or acts, disorientation, psychotic reactions, paranoia: phobia, agitation, restlessness, aggressiveness/hostility, manic reaction, emotional lability; peripheral neuropathy, ataxia, incoordination; possible exacerbation of: myasthenia gravis and extrapyramidal disorders; dysphasia, light-headedness (see *"Warnings"* and *"Precautions"*.)

Respiratory System: dyspnea, bronchospasm, allergic pneumonitis, stridor (see *"Warnings"*.)

Skin/Hypersensitivity: anaphylactic (-toid) reactions/shock; purpura, serum sickness, erythema multiforme/Stevens-Johnson syndrome, erythema nodosum, exfoliative dermatitis, hyperpigmentation, toxic epidermal necrolysis, conjunctivitis, photosensitivity, vesiculobullos eruption (see *"Warnings"* and *"Precautions"*.)

Special Senses: diplopia, nystagmus, blurred vision, disturbances of: taste, smell, hearing and equilibrium, usually reversible following discontinuation

Urinary System: anuria, polyuria, renal calculi, renal failure, interstitial nephritis, hematuria (see *"Warnings"* and *"Precautions"*.)

Laboratory:

Hematopoietic: prolongation of prothrombin time

Serum Chemistry: acidosis, elevation of: serum triglycerides, serum cholesterol, serum potassium, liver function tests including: GGTP, LDH, bilirubin.

Urinary: albuminuria, candiduria

In clinical trials using multiple-dose therapy, ophthalmologic abnormalities, including cataracts and multiple punctate lenticular opacities, have been noted in patients undergoing treatment with other quinolones. The relationship of the drugs to these events is not presently established. *Crystalluria and cylindruria have been reported with other quinolones.*

OVERDOSAGE

Information on overdosage with Ofloxacin is limited. One incident of accidental overdosage has been reported. In this case, an adult female received 3 gm of Ofloxacin intravenously over 45 minutes. A blood sample obtained 15 minutes after the completion of the infusion revealed an Ofloxacin level of 39.3 µg/ml. In 7 h, the level had fallen to 16.2 µg/ml, and by 24 h to 2.7 µg/ml. During the infusion, the patient developed drowsiness, nausea, dizziness, hot and cold flushes, subjective facial swelling and numbness, slurring of speech, and mild to moderate disorientation. All complaints except the dizziness subsided within 1 h after discontinuation of the infusion. The dizziness, most bothersome while standing, resolved in approximately 9 h. Laboratory testing reportedly revealed no clinically significant changes in routine parameters in this patient.

In the event of acute overdose, the stomach should be emptied (oral overdose), and the patient should be observed and appropriate hydration maintained. Ofloxacin is not efficiently removed by hemodialysis or peritoneal dialysis.

DOSAGE AND ADMINISTRATION

Ofloxacin injection should only be administered by *intravenous* infusion. It is not for intramuscular, intrathecal, intraperitoneal, or subcutaneous administration.

Caution: RAPID OR BOLUS IV INFUSION MUST BE AVOIDED. Ofloxacin injection should be infused intravenously slowly over a period of not less than 60 minutes. (See *"Precautions"*.)

The usual dose of Ofloxacin is 200 mg to 400 mg administered by slow infusion over 60 minutes every 12 h, or 200 mg to 400 mg orally every 12 h, as described in the following dosing chart. These recommendations apply to patients with mild to moderate infection and normal renal function (i.e. creatinine clearance > 50 ml/min). For patients with altered renal function (i.e., creatinine clearance $\leq$ 50 ml/min), see the *"Patients with Impaired Renal Function"* subsection.

PATIENTS WITH NORMAL RENAL FUNCTION (SEE RELATED TABLE).

Antacids containing calcium, magnesium, or aluminium; sucralfate; divalent or trivalent cations such as iron; or multivitamins containing zinc should not be taken within the two-hour period before, or within the two-hour period after Ofloxacin administration. (See *"Precautions."*)

PATIENTS WITH IMPAIRED RENAL FUNCTION

Dosage should be adjusted for patients with a creatine clearance $\leq$ 50 mL/min. *After a normal initial dose*, dosage should be adjusted as follows:

Creatinine Clearance	Maintenance Dose	Frequency
10—50 ml/min	the usual recommended unit dose	q24h
<10 ml/min	½ the usual recommended unit dose	q24h

When only the serum creatinine is known, the following formula may be used to estimate creatinine clearance.

Men: Creatinine clearance (mL/min) = $\dfrac{\text{Weight (kg)} \times (140\text{-age})}{72 \times \text{serum creatinine (mg/dL)}}$

Women: 0.85 × the value calculated for men.

The serum creatinine should represent a steady-state of renal function.

Infection	Description*	Unit Dose	Frequency	Duration	Daily Dose
Lower Respiratory Tract	Exacerbation of Chronic Bronchitis	400 mg	q12h	10 days	800 mg
	Com. Acq. Pneumonia	400 mg	q12h	10 days	800 mg
Skin and Skin Structures	Uncomplicated infections	400 mg	q12h	10 days	800 mg
Sexually Transmitted Diseases	Acute, uncomplicated gonorrhea	400 mg	single dose	1 day	400 mg
	Cervicitis/urethritis due to *C. trachomatis*	300 mg	q12h	7 days	600 mg
	Cervicitis/urethritis due to *C. trachomatis* and *N. gonorrhoeae*	300 mg	q12h	7 days	600 mg
Urinary Tract	Cystitis due to *E. coli* or *K. pneumoniae*	200 mg	q12h	3 days	400 mg
	Cystitis due to other approved pathogens	200 mg	q12h	7 days	400 mg
	Complicated UTIs	200 mg	q12h	10 days	400 mg
Prostate	Prostatitis due to *E. coli*	300 mg	q12h	6 weeks**	600 mg

* *DUE TO THE DESIGNAGED PATHOGENS (see "Indications and Usage").*
** *BECAUSE THERE ARE NO SAFETY DATA PRESENTLY AVAILABLE TO SUPPORT THE USE OF THE INTRAVENOUS FORMULATION OF OFLOXACIN FOR MORE THAN 10 DAYS, THERAPY AFTER 10 DAYS SHOULD BE SWITCHED TO THE ORAL TABLET FORMULATION OR OTHER APPROPRIATE THERAPY.*

PATIENTS WITH CIRRHOSIS
The excretion of Ofloxacin may be reduced in patients with severe liver function disorders (e.g., cirrhosis with or without ascites). A maximum dose of 400 mg of Ofloxacin per day should therefore not be exceeded.

Prepare the desired dosage of Ofloxacin for IV infusion according to the following chart.

Desired Dosage Strength	From 10 ml Vial, Withdraw Volume	From 20 ml Vial, Withdraw Volume	Volume of Diluent	Infusion Time
200 mg	5 ml	10 mL	qs 50 mL	60 min
300 mg	7.5 mL	15 mL	qs 75 mL	60 min
400 mg	10 mL	20 mL	qs 100 mL	60 min

For example, to prepare a 200 mg dose using a 10 ml vial (40 mg/ml), withdraw 5 ml and dilute with a compatible intravenous solution to a total volume of 50 ml.

COMPATIBLE INTRAVENOUS SOLUTIONS
Any of the following intravenous solutions may be used to prepare a 4 mg/ml Ofloxacin solution with the approximate pH values.

Intravenous Fluids	pH of 4 mg/ml Ofloxacin IV solution
0.9% Sodium Chloride Injection USP	4.69
5% Dextrose Injection, USP	4.57
5% Dextrose/0.9% NaCl Injection	4.56
5% Dextrose in Lactated Ringers	4.94
5% Sodium Bicarbonate Injection	7.95
Plasma/Lyte® 56/5% Dextrose Injection	5.02
5% Dextrose, 0.45% Sodium Chloride and 0.15% Potassium Chloride Injection	4.64
Sodium Lactate Injection (M/6)	5.64
Water for Injection	4.66

STORAGE
Tablets: Store in well-closed containers below 86°F (30°C).

Vials: Single use: Store at controlled room temperature 59°F—86°F (15°C—30°C). Protect from light.

Premixed containers: Store at or below 77°F (25°C). Avoid excessive heat and protect from freezing and light.

ANIMAL PHARMACOLOGY
Ofloxacin, as well as other drugs of the quinolone class, has been shown to cause arthropathies (arthrosis) in immature dogs and rats. In addition, these drugs are associated with an increased incidence of osteochondrosis in rats as compared to the incidence observed in vehicle-treated rats. (See *"Warnings."*) There is no evidence of arthropathies in fully mature dogs at intravenous doses up to 3 times the recommended maximum human dose (on a mg/m^2 basis or 5 times based on a mg/kg basis) for a one-week exposure period.

Long-term, high-dose systemic use of other quinolones in experimental animals has caused lenticular opacities; however, this finding was not observed in any animal studies with Ofloxacin.

Reduced serum globulin and protein levels were observed in animals treated with other quinolones. In one Ofloxacin study, minor decreases in serum globulin and protein levels were noted in female cynomolgus monkeys dosed orally with 40 mg/kg Ofloxacin daily for one year. These changes, however, were considered to be within normal limits for monkeys.

Crystalluria and ocular toxicity were not observed in any animals treated with Ofloxacin.

REFERENCES
1. National Committee for Clinical Laboratory Standards, Performance Standards for Antimicrobial Disk Susceptibility Tests—Fourth Edition, Approved Standard NCCLS Document M2-A4, Vol. 10, No. 7, NCCLS, Villanova, PA, 1990. 2. National Committee for Clinical Laboratory Standards, Methods for Dilution Antimicrobial Susceptibility Tests for Bacteria that Grow Aerobically—Second Edition. Approved Standard NCCLS Document M7-A2, Vol. 10, No. 8, NCCLS, Villanova, PA, 1990.

HOW SUPPLIED
INJECTION: 20 MG/ML

BRAND/MANUFACTURER	NDC	SIZE	AWP
○ BRAND			
FLOXIN I.V.: Ortho Pharm	00062-1551-01	20 ml	$26.40

INJECTION: 40 MG/ML

BRAND/MANUFACTURER	NDC	SIZE	AWP
○ BRAND			
FLOXIN I.V.: Ortho Pharm	00062-1550-01	10 ml	$26.40

TABLETS: 200 MG

BRAND/MANUFACTURER	NDC	SIZE	AWP
○ BRAND			
▶ FLOXIN: Ortho Pharm	00062-1540-02	50s	$145.72
	00062-1540-05	100s ud	$293.46

TABLETS: 300 MG

BRAND/MANUFACTURER	NDC	SIZE	AWP
○ BRAND			
▶ FLOXIN: Ortho Pharm	00062-1541-02	50s	$173.42
	00062-1541-05	100s ud	$348.98

TABLETS: 400 MG

BRAND/MANUFACTURER	NDC	SIZE	AWP
○ BRAND			
▶ FLOXIN: Ortho Pharm	00062-1542-02	50s	$182.89
	00062-1542-01	100s	$365.78
	00062-1542-05	100s ud	$368.11

Ogen *SEE* ESTROPIPATE

Olsalazine Sodium

DESCRIPTION
The active ingredient in Olsalazine Sodium Capsules is a sodium salt of a salicylate, disodium 3, 3'-azobis (6-hydroxybenzoate) a compound that is effectively bioconverted to 5-aminosalicylic acid (5-ASA), which has anti-inflammatory activity in ulcerative colitis. Its empirical formula is $C_{14}H_8N_2Na_2O_6$ with a molecular weight of 346.21.

Olsalazine Sodium is a yellow crystalline powder which melts with decomposition at 240°C. It is the sodium salt of a weak acid, soluble in water and DMSO, and practically insoluble in ethanol, chloroform and ether. Olsalazine Sodium has acceptable stability under acidic or basic conditions.

Olsalazine Sodium is supplied in hard gelatin capsules for oral administration.

Following is its chemical structure:

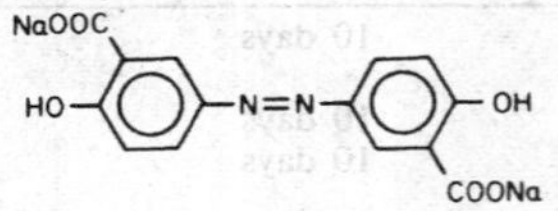

CLINICAL PHARMACOLOGY

After oral administration Olsalazine has limited systemic bioavailability. Based on oral and intravenous dosing studies, approximately 2.4% of a single 1.0 g oral dose is absorbed. Less than 1% of Olsalazine is recovered in the urine. The remaining 98-99% of an oral dose will reach the colon where each molecule is rapidly converted into two molecules of 5-aminosalicylic acid (5-ASA) by colonic bacteria and the low prevailing redox potential found in this environment. The liberated 5-ASA is absorbed slowly resulting in very high local concentrations in the colon.

The conversion of Olsalazine to mesalamine (5-ASA) in the colon is similar to that of sulfasalazine, which is converted into sulfapyridine and mesalamine. It is thought that the mesalamine component is therapeutically active in ulcerative colitis (A.K. Azad-Kahn et al, *Lancet* 2:892-985, 1977). The usual dose of sulfasalazine for maintenance of remission in patients with ulcerative colitis is 2 grams daily, which would provide approximately 0.8 gram of mesalamine to the colon. More than 0.9 gram of mesalamine would usually be made available in the colon from 1 gram of Olsalazine. The mechanism of action of mesalamine (and sulfasalazine) is unknown, but appears to be topical rather than systemic. Mucosal production of arachidonic acid (AA) metabolites, both through the cyclooxygenase pathways, i.e., prostanoids, and through the lipoxygenase pathways, i.e., leukotrienes (LTs) and hydroxyeicosatetraenoic acids (HETEs) is increased in patients with chronic inflammatory bowel disease, and it is possible that mesalamine diminishes inflammation by blocking cyclooxygenase and inhibiting prostaglandin (PG) production in the colon.

PHARMACOKINETICS

The pharmacokinetics of Olsalazine are similar in both healthy volunteers and in patients with ulcerative colitis. Maximum serum concentrations of Olsalazine appear after approximately 1 hour, and even after a 1.0 g single dose are low, e.g., 1.6-6.2 µmol/L. Olsalazine, has a very short serum half-life, approximately 0.9 hours. Olsalazine is more than 99% bound to plasma proteins. It does not interfere with protein binding of warfarin. The urinary recovery of Olsalazine is below 1%. Total recovery of oral 14C labeled Olsalazine in animals and humans ranges from 90 to 97%.

Approximately 0.1% of an oral dose of Olsalazine is metabolized in the liver to olsalazine-O-sulfate (olsalazine-S). Olsalazine-S, in contrast to Olsalazine has a half-life of 7 days. Olsalazine-S accumulates to steady state within 2-3 weeks. Patients on daily doses of 1.0 g Olsalazine for 2-4 years show a stable plasma concentration of Olsalazine-S (3.3-12.4 µmol/L). Olsalazine-S is more than 99% bound to plasma proteins. Its long half-life is mainly due to slow dissociation from the protein binding site. Less than 1% of both Olsalazine and olsalazine-S appears undissociated in plasma.

5-aminosalicylic acid (5-ASA): Serum concentrations of 5-ASA are detected after 4-8 hours. The peak levels of 5-ASA after an oral dose of 1.0 g Olsalazine are low, i.e., 0-4.3 µmol/L. Of the total 5-ASA found in the urine, more than 90% is in the form of N-acetyl-5-ASA (Ac-5-ASA). Only small amounts of 5-ASA are detected.

N-acetyl-5-ASA (Ac-5-ASA), the major metabolite of 5-ASA found in plasma and urine, is acetylated (deactivated) in at least two sites, the colonic epithelium and the liver. Ac-5-ASA is found in the serum, with peak values of 1.7-8.7 µmol/L after a single 1.0 g dose. Approximately 20% of the total 5-ASA is recovered in the urine, where it is found almost exclusively as Ac-5-ASA. The remaining 5-ASA is partially acetylated and is excreted in the feces. From fecal dialysis, the concentration of 5-ASA in the colon following Olsalazine has been calculated to be 18-49 mmol/L.

No accumulation of 5-ASA or Ac-5-ASA in plasma has been detected. 5-ASA and Ac-5-ASA are 74 and 81%, respectively, bound to plasma proteins.

ANIMAL TOXICOLOGY

Preclinical subacute and chronic toxicity studies in rats have shown the kidney to be the major target organ of Olsalazine toxicity. At an oral daily dose of 400 mg/kg or higher, Olsalazine treatment produced nephritis and tubular necrosis in a 4-week study; interstitial nephritis and tubular calcinosis in a 6-month study; and renal fibrosis, mineralization and transitional cell hyperplasia in a 1 year study.

CLINICAL STUDIES

Two controlled studies have demonstrated the efficacy of Olsalazine as maintenance therapy in patients with ulcerative colitis. In the first, ulcerative colitis patients in remission were randomized to Olsalazine 500 mg B.I.D. or placebo, and relapse rates for a six month period of time were compared. For the 52 patients randomized to Olsalazine, 12 relapses occurred, while for the 49 placebo patients, 22 relapses occurred. This difference in relapse rates was significant (p < .02).

In the second study, 164 ulcerative colitis patients in remission were randomized to Olsalazine 500 mg B.I.D. or sulfasalazine 1 gram B.I.D., and relapse rates were compared after six months. The relapse rate for Olsalazine was 19.5% while that for sulfasalazine was 12.2%, a non-significant difference.

INDICATIONS AND USAGE

Olsalazine is indicated for the maintenance of remission of ulcerative colitis in patients who are intolerant of sulfasalazine.

CONTRAINDICATIONS:

Hypersensitivity to salicylates.

PRECAUTIONS

GENERAL

Overall, approximately 17% of subjects receiving Olsalazine in clinical studies reported diarrhea sometime during therapy. This diarrhea resulted in withdrawal of treatment in 6% of patients. This diarrhea appears to be dose related, although it may be difficult to distinguish from the underlying symptoms of the disease.

Exacerbation of the symptoms of colitis thought to have been caused by mesalamine or sulfasalazine has been noted.

Although renal abnormalities were not reported in clinical trials with Olsalazine, the possibility of renal tubular damage due to absorbed mesalamine or its n-acetylated metabolite, as noted in the *Animal Toxicology* section, must be kept in mind, particularly for patients with pre-existing renal disease. In these patients, monitoring with urinalysis, BUN and creatinine determinations is advised.

INFORMATION FOR PATIENTS

Patients should be instructed to take Olsalazine with food. The drug should be taken in evenly divided doses. Patients should be informed that about 17% of subjects receiving Olsalazine during clinical studies reported diarrhea some time during therapy. If diarrhea occurs, patients should contact their physician.

DRUG INTERACTIONS.

Increased prothrombin time in patients taking concomitant warfarin has been reported.

DRUG/LABORATORY TEST INTERACTIONS.

None known.

CARCINOGENESIS, MUTAGENESIS, IMPAIRMENT OF FERTILITY

In a two year oral rat carcinogenicity study, Olsalazine was tested in male and female Wistar rats at daily doses of 200, 400 and 800 mg/kg/day (approximately 10 to 40 times the human maintenance dose, based on a patient weight of 50 kg and a human dose of 1 g). Urinary bladder transitional cell carcinomas were found in three male rats (6%, p = 0.022, exact trend test) receiving 40 times the human dose and were not found in untreated male controls. In the same study, urinary bladder transitional cell carcinoma and papilloma occurred in 2 untreated control female rats (2%). No such tumors were found in any of the female rats treated at doses of 40 times the human dose.

In an eighteen month oral mouse carcinogenicity study, Olsalazine was tested in male and female CD-1 mice at daily doses of 500, 1000 and 2000 mg/kg/day (approximately 25 to 100 times the human maintenance dose). Liver hemangiosarcomata were found in two male mice (4%) receiving Olsalazine at 100 times the human dose, while no such tumor occurred in the other treated male mice groups or any of the treated female mice. The observed incidence of this tumor is within the 4% incidence in historical controls.

Olsalazine was not mutagenic in *in vitro* Ames tests, mouse lymphoma cell mutation assays, human lymphocyte chromosomal aberration tests and the *in vivo* rat bone marrow cell chromosomal aberration test.

Olsalazine in a dose range of 100 to 400 mg/kg/day (approximately 5 to 20 times the human maintenance dose) did not influence the fertility of male or female rats. The oligospermia and infertility in men associated with sulfasalazine have not been reported with Olsalazine.

PREGNANCY: TERATOGENIC EFFECTS. PREGNANCY CATEGORY C

Olsalazine has been shown to produce fetal developmental toxicity as indicated by reduced fetal weights, retarded ossifications and immaturity of the fetal visceral organs when given during organogenesis to pregnant rats in doses 5 to 20 times the human dose (100 to 400 mg/kg). There are no adequate and well-controlled studies in pregnant women. Olsalazine should be used during pregnancy only if the potential benefit justifies the potential risk to the fetus.

NURSING MOTHERS

Oral administration of Olsalazine to lactating rats in doses 5 to 20 times the human dose produced growth retardation in their pups. It is not known whether this drug is excreted in human milk. Because many drugs are excreted in human milk, caution should be exercised when Olsalazine is administered to a nursing woman.

PEDIATRIC USE

Safety and effectiveness in a pediatric population have not been established.

ADVERSE REACTIONS

Olsalazine has been evaluated in ulcerative colitis patients in remission as well as those with acute disease. Both sulfasalazine-tolerant and intolerant patients have been studied in controlled clinical trials. Overall, 10.4% of patients discontinued Olsalazine because of an adverse experience compared with 6.7% of placebo patients. The most commonly reported adverse reactions leading to treatment withdrawal were diarrhea or loose stools (Olsalazine 5.9%; placebo 4.8%), abdominal pain and rash or itching (slightly more than 1% of patients receiving Olsalazine). Other adverse reactions to Olsalazine leading to withdrawal occurred in fewer than 1% of patients (Table 1).

◆ RATED THERAPEUTICALLY EQUIVALENT; ◇ THERAPEUTIC EQUIVALENCE UNCONFIRMED; ○ UNRATED

Table 1
ADVERSE REACTIONS RESULTING IN WITHDRAWAL FROM CONTROLLED STUDIES

	Total	
	Olsalazine (N = 441)	Placebo (N = 208)
Diarrhea/Loose Stools	26 (5.9%)	10 (4.8%)
Nausea	3	2
Abdominal Pain	5 (1.1%)	0
Rash/Itching	5 (1.1%)	0
Headache	3	0
Heartburn	2	0
Rectal Bleeding	1	0
Insomnia	1	0
Dizziness	1	0
Anorexia	1	0
Light-headedness	1	0
Depression	1	0
Miscellaneous	4 (0.9%)	3 (1.4%)
Total Number of Patients Withdrawn	46 (10.4%)	14 (6.7%)

For these controlled studies, the comparative incidences of adverse reactions reported in 1% or more patients treated with Olsalazine or placebo are provided in Table 2.

Table 2
COMPARATIVE INCIDENCE (%) OF ADVERSE EFFECTS REPORTED BY ONE PERCENT OR MORE OF ULCERATIVE COLITIS PATIENTS TREATED WITH OLSALAZINE OR PLACEBO IN DOUBLE BLIND CONTROLLED STUDIES

Adverse Event	Olsalazine (N = 441) %	Placebo (N = 208) %
Digestive System		
Diarrhea	11.1	6.7
Abdominal Pain/Cramps	10.1	7.2
Nausea	5.0	3.9
Dyspepsia	4.0	4.3
Bloating	1.5	1.4
Anorexia	1.3	1.9
Vomiting	1.0	—
Stomatitis	1.0	—
Increased Blood in Stool	—	3.4
CNS/Psychiatric		
Headache	5.0	4.8
Fatigue/Drowsiness/Lethargy	1.8	2.9
Depression	1.5	—
Vertigo/Dizziness	1.0	—
Insomnia	—	2.4
Skin		
Rash	2.3	1.4
Itching	1.3	—
Musculoskeletal		
Arthralgia/Joint Pain	4.0	2.9
Miscellaneous		
Upper Respiratory Infection	1.5	—

Over 2,500 patients have been treated with Olsalazine in various programs. In the uncontrolled studies, Olsalazine was administered mainly to patients intolerant to sulfasalazine. The adverse effects related to Olsalazine in these uncontrolled studies were similar to those seen in the controlled clinical trials. In addition, there were rare reports of the following adverse effects in patients receiving Olsalazine. These were often difficult to distinguish from possible symptoms of the underlying disease and a causal relationship to the drug has not been demonstrated for some of these reactions.

Digestive: Pancreatitis, diarrhea with dehydration, increased blood in stool, rectal bleeding, flare in symptoms, rectal discomfort, epigastric discomfort, vomiting, flatulence.

Rare cases of granulomatous hepatitis and nonspecific, reactive hepatitis have been reported in patients receiving Olsalazine. Additionally, a patient developed mild cholestatic hepatitis during treatment with sulfasalazine and experienced the same symptoms two weeks later after the treatment was changed to Olsalazine. Withdrawal of Olsalazine led to complete recovery in these cases.

Neurologic: Paresthesia, tremors, insomnia, mood swings, irritability, fever, chills.

Dermatologic: Erythema nodosum, photosensitivity, erythema, hot flashes, alopecia.

Musculoskeletal: Muscle cramps.

Cardiovascular/Pulmonary: Pericarditis, second degree heart block, interstitial pulmonary disease, hypertension, orthostatic hypotension, chest pain, tachycardia, palpitations, bronchospasm, shortness of breath. A patient who developed thyroid disease 9 days after starting Olsalazine Sodium was given propranolol and radioactive iodine and subsequently developed shortness of breath and nausea.

The patient died 5 days later with signs and symptoms of acute diffuse myocarditis.

Genitourinary: Frequency, dysuria, hematuria, protein-uria, impotence, menorrhagia.

Hematologic: Leukopenia, neutropenia, lymphopenia, eosinophilia, thrombocytopenia, anemia, reticulocytosis.

Laboratory: ALT (SGPT) or AST (SGOT) elevated beyond the normal range.

Special Senses: Dry mouth, dry eyes, watery eyes, blurred vision.

DRUG ABUSE AND DEPENDENCY
Abuse: None reported.

Dependence: Drug dependence has not been reported with chronic administration of Olsalazine.

OVERDOSAGE
No overdosage has been reported in humans. Maximum single oral doses of 5 g/kg in mice and rats and 2 g/kg in dogs were not lethal. Symptoms of acute toxicity were decreased motor activity and diarrhea in all species tested and in addition, vomiting in dogs.

DOSAGE AND ADMINISTRATION
The usual dosage in adults for maintenance of remission is 1.0 g/day in two divided doses.

Store at controlled room temperature, (15-30°C/59-86°F).

HOW SUPPLIED
CAPSULE: 250 MG

BRAND/MANUFACTURER	NDC	SIZE	AWP
BRAND			
DIPENTUM: Pharmacia	00016-0105-01	100s	$59.50

Omeprazole

DESCRIPTION
The active ingredient in Omeprazole is a substituted benzimidazole. 5-methoxy-2[[(4-methoxy-3,5-dimethyl-2-pyridinyl)methyl] sulfinyl]-1H-benzimidazole, a compound that inhibits gastric acid secretion. Its empirical formula is $C_{17}H_{19}N_3O_3S$, with a molecular weight of 345.42.

Omeprazole is a white to off-white crystalline powder which melts with decomposition at about 155°C. It is a weak base, freely soluble in ethanol and methanol, and slightly soluble in acetone and isopropanol and very slightly soluble in water. The stability of Omeprazole is a function of pH; it is rapidly degraded in acid media, but has acceptable stability under alkaline conditions.

Omeprazole is supplied as delayed-release capsules for oral administration. Each delayed-release capsule contains 20 mg of Omeprazole in the form of enteric-coated granules.

Following is its chemical structure:

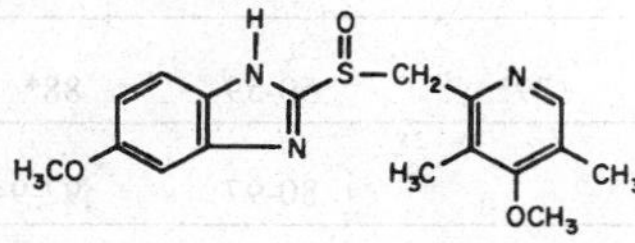

CLINICAL PHARMACOLOGY
PHARMACOKINETICS AND METABOLISM
Omeprazole delayed-release capsules contain an enteric-coated granule formulation (because Omeprazole is acid-labile), so that absorption of Omeprazole begins only after the granules leave the stomach. Absorption is rapid, with peak plasma levels of Omeprazole occurring within 0.5 to 3.5 hours. Peak plasma concentrations of Omeprazole and AUC are approximately proportional to doses up to 40 mg, but because of a saturable first-pass effect, a greater than linear response in peak plasma concentration and AUC occurs with doses greater than 40 mg. Absolute bioavailability (compared to intravenous administration) is about 30-40% at doses of 20-40 mg, due in large part to presystemic metabolism. In healthy subjects the plasma half-life is 0.5 to 1 hour, and the total body clearance is 500-600 mL/min. Protein binding is approximately 95%.

The bioavailability of Omeprazole increases slightly upon repeated administration of Omeprazole delayed-release capsules.

Following single dose oral administration of a buffered solution of Omeprazole, little if any unchanged drug was excreted in urine. The majority of the dose (about 77%) was eliminated in urine as at least six metabolites. Two were identified as hydroxyomeprazole and the corresponding carboxylic acid. The remainder of the dose was recoverable in feces. This implies a significant biliary excretion of the metabolites of Omeprazole. Three metabolites have been identified in plasma—the sulfide and sulfone derivatives of Omeprazole, and hydroxyomeprazole. These metabolites have very little or no antisecretory activity.

In patient with chronic hepatic disease, the bioavailability increased to approximately 100% compared to an I.V. dose, reflecting decreased first-pass effect, and the plasma half-life of the drug increased to nearly 3 hours compared

➤ SHOWN IN PRODUCT IDENTIFICATION GUIDE

to the half-life in normals of 0.5-1 hour. Plasma clearance averaged 70 mL/min, compared to a value of 500-600 mL/min in normal subjects.

In patients with chronic renal impairment, whose creatinine clearance ranged between 10 and 62 mL/min/1.73 m², the disposition of Omeprazole was very similar to that in healthy volunteers, although there was a slight increase in bioavailability. Because urinary excretion is a primary route of excretion of Omeprazole metabolites, their elimination slowed in proportion to the decreased creatinine clearance.

The elimination rate of Omeprazole was somewhat decreased in the elderly, and bioavailability was increased. Omeprazole was 76% bioavailable when a single 40 mg oral dose of Omeprazole (buffered solution) was administered to healthy elderly volunteers, versus 58% in young volunteers given the same dose. Nearly 70% of the dose was recovered in urine as metabolites of Omeprazole and no unchanged drug was detected. The plasma clearance of Omeprazole was 250 mL/min (about half that of young volunteers) and its plasma half-life averaged one hour, about twice that of young healthy volunteers.

PHARMACODYNAMICS

Mechanism of Action: Omeprazole belongs to a new class of antisecretory compounds, the substituted benzimidazoles, that do not exhibit anticholinergic or H_2 histamine antagonist properties, but that suppress gastric acid secretion by specific inhibition of the H^+/K^- ATPase enzyme system at the secretory surface of the gastric parietal cell. Because this enzyme system is regarded as the acid (proton) pump within the gastric mucosa, Omeprazole has been characterized as a gastric acid-pump inhibitor, in that it blocks the final step of acid production. This effect is dose-related and leads to inhibition of both basal and stimulated acid secretion irrespective of the stimulus. Animal studies indicate that after rapid disappearance from plasma, Omeprazole can be found within the gastric mucosa for a day or more.

Antisecretory Activity: After oral administration, the onset of the antisecretory effect of Omeprazole occurs within one hour, with the maximum effect occurring within two hours. Inhibition of secretion is about 50% of maximum at 24 hours and the duration of inhibition lasts up to 72 hours. The antisecretory effect thus lasts far longer than would be expected from the very short (less than one hour) plasma half-life, apparently due to prolonged binding to the parietal H^+/K^- ATPase enzyme. When the drug is discontinued, secretory activity returns gradually, over 3 to 5 days. The inhibitory effect of Omeprazole on acid secretion increases with repeated once-daily dosing, reaching a plateau after four days.

Results from numerous studies of the antisecretory effect of multiple doses of 20 mg and 40 mg of Omeprazole in normal volunteers and patients are shown below. The "max" value represents determinations at a time of maximum effect (2-6 hours after dosing), while "min" values are those 24 hours after the last dose of Omeprazole.

RANGE OF MEAN VALUES FROM MULTIPLE STUDIES OF THE MEAN ANTISECRETORY EFFECTS OF OMEPRAZOLE AFTER MULTIPLE DAILY DOSING

Parameter	Omeprazole 20 mg		Omeprazole 40 mg	
% Decrease in Basal Acid Output	Max	Min	Max	Min
	78	58-80	94*	80-93
% Decrease in Peak Acid Output	79*	50-59	88*	62-68
% Decrease in 24-hr Intragastric Acidity	80-97		92-94	

* Single Studies

Single daily oral doses of Omeprazole ranging from a dose of 10 mg to 40 mg have produced 100% inhibition of 24-hour intragastric acidity in some patients.

Enterochromaffin-like (ECL) Cell Effects: In 24-month carcinogenicity studies in rats, a dose-related significant increase in gastric carcinoid tumors and ECL cell hyperplasia was observed in both male and female animals (see *"Precautions, Carcinogenesis, Mutagenesis, Impairment of Fertility"*). Hypergastrinemia secondary to prolonged and sustained hypochlorhydria has been postulated to be the mechanism by which ECL cell hyperplasia and gastric carcinoid tumors develop. Omeprazole may also affect other cells in the gastrointestinal tract (e.g., G cells), either directly or by inducing sustained hypochlorhydria, but this possibility has not been extensively studied.

Human gastric biopsy specimens from about 200 patients treated continuously with Omeprazole for an average of over 12 months have not detected ECL cell effects of Omeprazole similar to those seen in rats. Longer term data are needed to rule out the possibility of an increased risk for the development of gastric tumors in patients receiving long-term therapy with Omeprazole.

Serum Gastrin Effects: In studies involving more than 200 patients, serum gastrin levels increased during the first 1 to 2 weeks of once-daily administration of therapeutic doses of Omeprazole in parallel with inhibition of acid secretion. No further increase in serum gastrin occurred with continued treatment. In comparison with histamine H_2-receptor antagonists, the median increases produced by 20 mg doses of Omeprazole were higher (1.3 to 3.6 fold vs. 1.1 to 1.8 fold increase). Gastrin values returned to pretreatment levels, usually within 1 to 2 weeks after discontinuation of therapy.

Other Effects: Systemic effects of Omeprazole in the CNS, cardiovascular and respiratory systems have not been found to date. Omeprazole, given in oral doses

of 30 or 40 mg for 2 to 4 weeks, had no effect on thyroid function, carbohydrate metabolism, or circulating levels of parathyroid hormone, cortisol, estradiol, testosterone, prolactin, cholecystokinin or secretin.

No effect on gastric emptying of the solid and liquid components of a test meal was demonstrated after a single dose of Omeprazole 90 mg. In healthy subjects, a single I.V. dose of Omeprazole (0.35 mg/kg) had no effect on intrinsic factor secretion. No systematic dose-dependent effect has been observed on basal or stimulated pepsin output in humans. However, when intragastric pH is maintained at 4.0 or above, basal pepsin output is low, and pepsin activity is decreased.

As do other agents that elevate intragastric pH, Omeprazole administered for 14 days in healthy subjects produced a significant increase in the intragastric concentrations of viable bacteria. The pattern of the bacterial species was unchanged from that commonly found in saliva. All changes resolved within three days of stopping treatment.

CLINICAL STUDIES

Duodenal Ulcer Disease: Active Duodenal Ulcer: In a multicenter, double-blind, placebo-controlled study of 147 patients with endoscopically documented duodenal ulcer, the percentage of patients healed (per protocol) at 2 and 4 weeks was significantly higher with Omeprazole 20 mg once a day than with placebo (p ≤ 0.01).

TREATMENT OF ACTIVE DUODENAL ULCER
% OF PATIENTS HEALED

	Omeprazole 20 mg a.m. (n = 99)	Placebo a.m. (n = 48)
Week 2	41	13
Week 4	*75	27

*(p ≤ 0.01)

Complete daytime and nighttime pain relief occurred significantly faster (p ≤ 0.01) in patients treated with Omeprazole 20 mg than in patients treated with placebo. At the end of the study, significantly more patients who had received Omeprazole had complete relief of daytime pain (p ≤ 0.05) and nighttime pain (p ≤ 0.01).

In a multicenter, double-blind study of 293 patients with endoscopically documented duodenal ulcer, the percentage of patients healed (per protocol) at 4 weeks was significantly higher with Omeprazole 20 mg once a day than with ranitidine 150 mg b.i.d. (p < 0.01).

TREATMENT OF ACTIVE DUODENAL ULCER
% OF PATIENTS HEALED

	Omeprazole 20 mg a.m. (n = 145)	Ranitidine 150 mg b.i.d. (n = 148)
Week 2	42	34
Week 4	*82	63

*(p ≤ 0.01)

Healing occurred significantly faster in patients treated with Omeprazole than in those treated with ranitidine 150 mg b.i.d. (p < 0.01).

In a foreign multinational randomized, double-blind study of 105 patients with endoscopically documented duodenal ulcer, 20 mg and 40 mg of Omeprazole were compared to 150 mg b.i.d. of ranitidine at 2, 4 and 8 weeks. At 2 and 4 weeks both doses of Omeprazole were statistically superior (per protocol) to ranitidine, but 40 mg was not superior to 20 mg of Omeprazole, and at 8 weeks there was no significant difference between any of the active drugs.

TREATMENT OF ACTIVE DUODENAL ULCER
% OF PATIENTS HEALED

	Omeprazole		Ranitidine
	20 mg (n = 34)	40 mg (n = 36)	150 mg b.i.d. (n = 35)
Week 2	*83	*83	53
Week 4	*97	*100	82
Week 8	100	100	94

*(p ≤ 0.01)

Gastroesophageal Reflux Disease (GERD): In a U.S. multicenter double-blind placebo controlled study of 20 mg or 40 mg of Omeprazole delayed-release capsules in patients with symptomatic esophagitis and endoscopically diagnosed erosive esophagitis of grade 2 or above, the percentage healing rates (per protocol) were as follows:

Week	20 mg Omeprazole (n = 83)	40 mg Omeprazole (n = 87)	Placebo (n = 43)
4	39**	45**	7
8	74**	75**	14

**(p < 0.01) Omeprazole versus placebo.

In this study, the 40 mg dose was not superior to the 20 mg dose of Omeprazole in the percentage healing rate. Other controlled clinical trials have also shown that

Omeprazole is effective in severe GERD. In comparisons with histamine H_2-receptor antagonists in patients with erosive esophagitis, grade 2 or above, Omeprazole in a dose of 20 mg was significantly more effective than the active controls. Complete daytime and nighttime heartburn relief occurred significantly faster ($p < 0.01$) in patients treated with Omeprazole than in those taking placebo or histamine H_2-receptor antagonists.

Pathological Hypersecretory Conditions: In open studies of 136 patients with pathological hypersecretory conditions, such as Zollinger-Ellison (ZE) syndrome with or without multiple endocrine adenomas. Omeprazole delayed-release capsules significantly inhibited gastric acid secretion and controlled associated symptoms of diarrhea, anorexia, and pain. Doses ranging from 20 mg every other day to 360 mg per day maintained basal acid secretion below 10 mEq/hr in patients without prior gastric surgery, and below 5 mEq/hr in patients with prior gastric surgery.

Initial doses were titrated to the individual patient need, and adjustments were necessary with time in some patients (*see "Dosage and Administration"*). Omeprazole was well tolerated at these high dose levels for prolonged periods (> 5 years in some patients). In most ZE patients, serum gastrin levels were not modified by Omeprazole. However, in some patients serum gastrin increased to levels greater than those present prior to initiation of Omeprazole therapy. At least 2 patients with ZE syndrome on long-term treatment with Omeprazole developed gastric carcinoids. This finding was believed to be a manifestation of the underlying condition, which is known to be associated with such tumors, rather than the result of the administration of Omeprazole.

INDICATIONS AND USAGE

Short-Term Treatment of Active Duodenal Ulcer: Omeprazole delayed-release capsules are indicated for short-term treatment of active duodenal ulcer. Most patients heal within four weeks. Some patients may require an additional four weeks of therapy.
OMEPRAZOLE SHOULD NOT BE USED AS MAINTENANCE THERAPY FOR TREATMENT OF PATIENTS WITH DUODENAL ULCER DISEASE. (See boxed *"Warning".*)

GASTROESOPHAGEAL REFLUX DISEASE/(GERD)
Severe Erosive Esophagitis: Omeprazole delayed-release capsules are indicated for the short-term treatment (4-8 weeks) of severe erosive esophagitis (grade 2 or above) which has been diagnosed by endoscopy (see *"Clinical Pharmacology, Clinical Studies"*).

Poorly Responsive Symptomatic GERD: Omeprazole delayed-release capsules are also indicated for the short-term treatment (4-8 weeks) of symptomatic gastro-esophageal reflux disease (esophagitis) poorly responsive to customary medical treatment, usually including an adequate course of a histamine H_2-receptor antagonist.

The efficacy of Omeprazole used for longer than 8 weeks in these patients has not been established. In the rare instance of a patient not responding to 8 weeks of treatment, it may be helpful to give up to an additional 4 weeks of treatment. If there is recurrence of severe or symptomatic GERD poorly responsive to customary medical treatment, additional 4-8 week courses of Omeprazole may be considered. THE DRUG SHOULD NOT BE USED AS MAINTENANCE THERAPY. (See boxed *"Warning".*)

Pathological Hypersecretory Conditions: Omeprazole delayed-release capsules are indicated for the long-term treatment of pathological hypersecretory conditions (e.g., Zollinger-Ellison syndrome, multiple endocrine adenomas and systemic mastocytosis).

UNLABELED USES
Omeprazole is used alone or as an adjunct in the treatment of gastric ulcers, esophageal stricture, and ranitidine-resistant peptic ulceration of duodenum. It is also used as an adjunct in patients with duodenitis/non-ulcer dyspepsia and Helicobacter Pylori positive antral histology or culture.

CONTRAINDICATIONS
Omeprazole delayed-release capsules are contraindicated in patients with known hypersensitivity to any component of the formulation.

WARNING

IN LONG-TERM (2 YEAR) STUDIES IN RATS, OMEPRAZOLE PRODUCED A DOSE-RELATED INCREASE IN GASTRIC CARCINOID TUMORS (SEE *"PRECAUTIONS, CARCINOGENESIS, MUTAGENESIS, IMPAIRMENT OF FERTILITY"*). WHILE AVAILABLE ENDOSCOPIC EVALUATIONS AND HISTOLOGIC EXAMINATIONS OF BIOPSY SPECIMENS FROM HUMAN STOMACHS HAVE NOT DETECTED A RISK FROM SHORT-TERM EXPOSURE TO OMEPRAZOLE FURTHER HUMAN DATA ON THE EFFECT OF SUSTAINED HYPOCHLORHYDRIA AND HYPERGASTRINEMIA ARE NEEDED TO RULE OUT THE POSSIBILITY OF AN INCREASED RISK FOR THE DEVELOPMENT OF TUMORS IN HUMANS RECEIVING LONG-TERM THERAPY WITH OMEPRAZOLE. OMEPRAZOLE SHOULD BE PRESCRIBED ONLY FOR THE CONDITIONS, DOSAGE AND DURATION DESCRIBED (SEE *"INDICATIONS AND USAGE AND DOSAGE AND ADMINISTRATION"*).

PRECAUTIONS
General: Symptomatic response to therapy with Omeprazole does not preclude the presence of gastric malignancy.

Information for Patients: Omeprazole delayed-release capsules should be taken before eating. Patients should be cautioned that the Omeprazole delayed-release capsule should not be opened, chewed or crushed, and should be swallowed whole.

Drug Interactions: Omeprazole can prolong the elimination of diazepam, warfarin and phenytoin, drugs that are metabolized by oxidation in the liver. Although in normal subjects no interaction with theophylline or propranolol was found, there have been reports of interaction with other drugs metabolized via the cytochrome P-450 system (e.g., cyclosporine, disulfiram). Patients should be monitored to determine if it is necessary to adjust the dosage of these drugs when taken concomitantly with Omeprazole.

Because of its profound and long lasting inhibition of gastric acid secretion, it is theoretically possible that Omeprazole may interfere with absorption of drugs where gastric pH is an important determinant of their bioavailability (e.g., ketoconazole, ampicillin esters, and iron salts). In the clinical trials, antacids were used concomitantly with the administration of Omeprazole.

Carcinogenesis, Mutagenesis, Impairment of Fertility: In two 24-month carcinogenicity studies in rats, Omeprazole at daily doses of 1.7, 3.4, 13.8, 44.0 and 140.8 mg/kg/day (approximately 4 to 352 times the human dose, based on a patient weight of 50 kg and a human dose of 20 mg) produced gastric ECL cell carcinoids in a dose-related manner in both male and female rats; the incidence of this effect was markedly higher in female rats, which had higher blood levels of Omeprazole. Gastric carcinoids seldom occur in the untreated rat. In addition, ECL cell hyperplasia was present in all treated groups of both sexes. In one of these studies, female rats were treated with 13.8 mg Omeprazole/kg/day (approximately 35 times the human dose) for one year, then followed for an additional year without the drug. No carcinoids were seen in these rats. An increased incidence of treatment-related ECL cell hyperplasia was observed at the end of one year (94% treated vs 10% controls). By the second year the difference between treated and control rats was much smaller (46% vs 26%) but still showed more hyperplasia in the treated group. An unusual primary malignant tumor in the stomach was seen in one rat (2%). No similar tumor was seen in male or female rats treated for two years. For this strain of rat no similar tumor has been noted historically, but a finding involving only one tumor is difficult to interpret. A 78-week mouse carcinogenicity study of Omeprazole did not show increased tumor occurrence, but the study was not conclusive.

Omeprazole was not mutagenic in an *in vitro* Ames *Salmonella typhimurium* assay, an *in vitro* mouse lymphoma cell assay and an *in vivo* rat liver DNA damage assay. A mouse micronucleus test at 625 and 6250 times the human dose gave a borderline result, as did an *in vivo* bone marrow chromosome aberration test. A second mouse micronucleus study at 2000 times the human dose, but with different (suboptimal) sampling times, was negative.

In a rat fertility and general reproductive performance test, Omeprazole in a dose range of 13.8 to 138.0 mg/kg/day (approximately 35 to 345 times the human dose) was not toxic or deleterious to the reproductive performance of parental animals.

PREGNANCY
Pregnancy Category C: Teratology studies conducted in pregnant rats at doses up to 138 mg/kg/day (approximately 345 times the human dose) and in pregnant rabbits at doses up to 69 mg/kg/day (approximately 172 times the human dose) did not disclose any evidence for a teratogenic potential of Omeprazole.

In rabbits, Omeprazole in a dose range of 6.9 to 69.1 mg/kg/day (approximately 17 to 172 times the human dose) produced dose-related increase in embryo-lethality, fetal resorptions and pregnancy disruptions. In rats, dose-related embryo/fetal toxicity and postnatal developmental toxicity were observed in offspring resulting from parents treated with Omeprazole 13.8 to 138.0 mg/kg/day (approximately 35 to 345 times the human dose). There are no adequate or well-controlled studies in pregnant women. Omeprazole should be used during pregnancy only if the potential benefit justifies the potential risk to the fetus.

Nursing Mothers: It is not known whether Omeprazole is excreted in human milk. In rats, Omeprazole administration during late gestation and lactation at doses of 13.8 to 138 mg/kg/day (35 to 345 times the human dose) resulted in decreased weight gain in pups. Because many drugs are excreted in human milk, because of the potential for serious adverse reactions in nursing infants from Omeprazole, and because of the potential for tumorigenicity shown for Omeprazole in rat carcinogenicity studies, a decision should be made whether to discontinue nursing or to discontinue the drug, taking into account the importance of the drug to the mother.

Pediatric Use: Safety and effectiveness in children have not been established.

ADVERSE REACTIONS
Omeprazole delayed-release capsules were generally well tolerated during domestic and international clinical trials in 3096 patients.

In the U.S. clinical trial population of 465 patients (including duodenal ulcer. Zollinger-Ellison syndrome and resistant ulcer patients), the following adverse experiences were reported to occur in 1% or more of patients on therapy with Omeprazole. Numbers in parentheses indicate percentages of the adverse experiences considered by investigators as possibly, probably or definitely related to the drug.

	Omeprazole (n = 465)	Placebo (n = 64)	Ranitidine (n = 195)
Headache	6.9 (2.4)	6.3	7.7 (2.6)
Diarrhea	3.0 (1.9)	3.1 (1.6)	2.1 (0.5)
Abdominal Pain	2.4 (0.4)	3.1	2.1
Nausea	2.2 (0.9)	3.1	4.1 (0.5)
URI	1.9	1.6	2.6
Dizziness	1.5 (0.6)	0.0	2.6 (1.0)
Vomiting	1.5 (0.4)	4.7	1.5 (0.5)
Rash	1.5 (1.1)	0.0	0.0
Constipation	1.1 (0.9)	0.0	0.0
Cough	1.1	0.0	1.5
Asthenia	1.1 (0.2)	1.6 (1.6)	1.5 (1.0)
Back Pain	1.1	0.0	0.5

The following adverse reactions which occurred in 1% or more of Omeprazole-treated patients have been reported in international double-blind, and open-label, clinical trials in which 2.631 patients and subjects received Omeprazole.

INCIDENCE OF ADVERSE EXPERIENCES ≥ 1% CAUSAL RELATIONSHIP

	Omeprazole (n = 2631)	Placebo (n = 120)
Body as a Whole, site unspecified		
Abdominal pain	5.2	3.3
Asthenia	1.3	0.8
Digestive System		
Constipation	1.5	0.8
Diarrhea	3.7	2.5
Flatulence	2.7	5.8
Nausea	4.0	6.7
Vomiting	3.2	10.0
Acid regurgitation	1.9	3.3
Nervous System/Psychiatric		
Headache	2.9	2.5

Additional adverse experiences occurring in < 1% of patients or subjects in domestic and/or international trials, or occurring since the drug was marketed, are shown below within each body system. In many instances, the relationship to Omeprazole was unclear.

Body as a Whole: Fever, pain, fatigue, malaise, abdominal swelling

Cardiovascular: Chest pain or angina, tachycardia, bradycardia, palpitation, elevated blood pressure, peripheral edema.

Digestive: Hepatitis including hepatic failure (rarely), elevated ALT (SGPT), elevated AST (SGOT), elevated γ-glutamyl transpeptidase, elevated alkaline phosphatase, elevated bilirubin (jaundice), anorexia, irritable colon, flatulence, fecal discoloration, esophageal candidiasis, mucosal atrophy of the tongue, dry mouth.

Metabolic/Nutritional: Hypoglycemia, weight gain

Musculoskeletal: Muscle cramps, myalgia, joint pain, leg pain

Nervous System/Psychiatric: Psychic disturbances including depression, aggression, hallucinations, confusion, insomnia, nervousness, tremors, apathy, somnolence, anxiety, dream abnormalities; vertigo; paresthesia; hemifacial dysesthesia.

Respiratory: Epistaxis, pharyngeal pain

Skin: Rash, skin inflammation, urticaria, angioedema. pruritus, alopecia, dry skin, hyperhidrosis

Special Senses: Tinnitus, taste perversion

Urogenital: Urinary tract infection, microscopic pyuria, urinary frequency, elevated serum creatinine, proteinuria, hematuria, glycosuria, testicular pain, gynecomastia

Hematologic: Agranulocytosis has been reported in a 65 year old diabetic male on several drugs in addition to Omeprazole; the relationship of the agranulocytosis to Omeprazole is uncertain. Pancytopenia, thrombocytopenia, neutropenia, anemia, leucocytosis, hemolytic anemia.

The incidence of clinical adverse experiences in patients greater than 65 years of age was similar to that in patients 65 years of age or less.

OVERDOSAGE

There is no experience to date with deliberate overdosage. Dosages of up to 360 mg/day have been well tolerated. No specific antidote is known. Omeprazole is extensively protein bound and is, therefore, not readily dialyzable. In the event of overdosage, treatment should be symptomatic and supportive.

Lethal doses of Omeprazole after single oral administration are about 1500 mg/kg in mice and greater than 4000 mg/kg in rats, and about 100 mg/kg in mice and greater than 40 mg/kg in rats given single intravenous injections. Animals given these doses showed sedation, ptosis, convulsions, and decreased activity, body temperature, and respiratory rate and increased depth of respiration.

DOSAGE AND ADMINISTRATION

Short-Term Treatment of Active Duodenal Ulcer: The recommended adult oral dose is 20 mg once daily. Most patients heal within four weeks. Some patients may require an additional four weeks of therapy (see "Indications and Usage").

Severe Erosive Esophagitis or Poorly Responsive Gastroesophageal Reflux Disease (GERD): The recommended adult oral dose is 20 mg daily for 4 to 8 weeks (see "Indications and Usage").

Pathological Hypersecretory Conditions: The dosage of Omeprazole in patients with pathological hypersecretory conditions varies with the individual patient. The recommended adult oral starting dose is 60 mg once a day. Doses should be adjusted to individual patient needs and should continue for as long as clinically indicated. Doses up to 120 mg t.i.d. have been administered. Daily dosages of greater than 80 mg should be administered in divided doses. Some patients with Zollinger-Ellison syndrome have been treated continuously with Omeprazole for more than 5 years. No dosage adjustment is necessary for patients with renal impairment, hepatic dysfunction or for the elderly Omeprazole delayed-release capsules should be taken before eating. In the clinical trials, antacids were used concomitantly with Omeprazole.

Patients should be cautioned that the Omeprazole delayed-release capsule should not be opened, chewed or crushed, and should be swallowed whole.

Storage: Store Omeprazole delayed-release capsules in a tight container protected from light and moisture. Store between 59°F and 86°F (15°C and 30°C).

HOW SUPPLIED
CAPSULE, EXTENDED RELEASE: 20 MG

BRAND/MANUFACTURER	NDC	SIZE	AWP
○ **BRAND**			
▶ PRILOSEC: Merck	00006-0742-31	30s	$113.44
	00006-0742-28	100s ud	$378.14

OmniHIB *SEE* HAEMOPHILUS B CONJUGATE VACCINE *AND* HEMOPHILUS B CONJUGATE VACCINE (TETANUS TOXOID CONJUGATE)

Omnipaque *SEE* IOHEXOL

Omnipen-N *SEE* AMPICILLIN

Omniscan *SEE* GADODIAMIDE

Oncaspar *SEE* PEGASPARGASE

Oncovin *SEE* VINCRISTINE SULFATE

Ondansetron Hydrochloride

DESCRIPTION

Ondansetron Hydrochloride is the racemic form of Ondansetron and a selective blocking agent of the serotonin 5-HT$_3$ receptor type. Chemically it is (±) 1, 2, 3, 9-tetrahydro-9-methyl-3-[(2-methyl-1H-imidazol-1-yl)methyl]-4H-carbazol-4- one, monohydrochloride, dihydrate.

The empirical formula is $C_{18}H_{19}N_3O \cdot HCl \cdot 2H_2O$, representing a molecular weight of 365.9.

Ondansetron Hydrochloride is a white to off-white powder that is soluble in water and normal saline.

Ondansetron Hydrochloride is available as tablets for oral administration and as nonpyrogenic, sterile solution for intravenous (IV) injection.

Each tablet contains: Ondansetron HCl equivalent to 4 or 8 mg Ondansetron

Each ml of aqueous solution contains: Ondansetron HCl 2 mg

Following is its chemical structure:

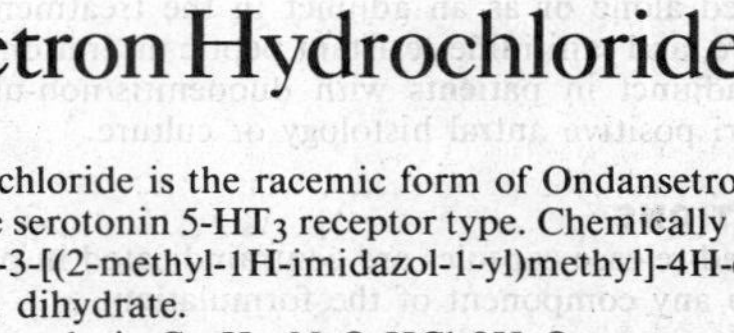

CLINICAL PHARMACOLOGY

Pharmacodynamics: Ondansetron is a selective 5-HT$_3$ receptor antagonist. While Ondansetron's mechanism of action has not been fully characterized, it is not a dopamine-receptor antagonist. Serotonin receptors of the 5-HT$_3$ type are present both peripherally on vagal nerve terminals and centrally in the chemoreceptor trigger zone of the area postrema. It is not certain whether Ondansetron's antiemetic action in chemotherapy-induced emesis is mediated centrally, peripherally, or in both sites. However, cytotoxic chemotherapy appears to be associated with release of serotonin from the enterochromaffin cells of the small intestine. In humans, urinary 5-HIAA (5-hydroxyindoleacetic acid) excretion increases after cisplatin administration in parallel with the onset of emesis. The released serotonin may stimulate the vagal afferents through the 5-HT$_3$ receptors and initiate the vomiting reflex.

In animals, the emetic response to cisplatin can be prevented by pretreatment with an inhibitor of serotonin synthesis, bilateral abdominal vagotomy and greater splanchnic nerve section, or pretreatment with a serotonin 5-HT$_3$ receptor antagonist.

In normal volunteers, single intravenous (IV) doses of 0.15 mg/kg of Ondansetron had no effect on esophageal motility, gastric motility, lower esophageal sphincter pressure, or small intestinal transit time. In another study in six normal male volunteers, a 16-mg dose infused over 5 minutes showed no effect on cardiac output, heart rate, stroke volume, blood pressure, or electrocardiogram (ECG). Multiday administration of Ondansetron has been shown to slow colonic transit in normal volunteers. Ondansetron has no effect on plasma prolactin concentrations.

Ondansetron does not alter the respiratory depressant effects produced by alfentanil or the degree of neuromuscular blockade produced by atracurium. Interactions with general or local anesthetics have not been studied.

Pharmacokinetics: Ondansetron is extensively metabolized in humans, with approximately 5% of a radio-labeled dose recovered as the parent compound from the urine. The primary metabolic pathway is hydroxylation on the indole ring followed by glucuronide or sulfate conjugation.

Although some nonconjugated metabolites have pharmacologic activity, these are not found in plasma concentrations likely to significantly contribute to the biological activity of Ondansetron.

Ondansetron HCl Injection: In normal volunteers, the following mean pharmacokinetic data have been determined following a single 0.15-mg/kg IV dose.

PHARMACOKINETICS IN NORMAL VOLUNTEERS

Age-group	n	Peak Plasma Concentration (ng mL)	Mean Elimination Half-life (h)	Plasma Clearance (L/h/kg)
19-40	11	102	3.5	0.381
61-74	12	106	4.7	0.319
≥ 75	11	170	5.5	0.262

From a single-dose infusion study, patients with severe hepatic impairment showed a five-fold and those with mild-to-moderate liver impairment a two-fold reduction in mean plasma clearance, with increases in the mean apparent volume of distribution of less than two-fold, as compared to normals. The mean half-life of 3.6 hours in normals increased to 9.2 hours in patients with mild-to-moderate hepatic impairment and was prolonged to 20.6 hours in patients with severe hepatic insufficiency.

A reduction in clearance and increase in elimination half-life are seen in patients over 75 years old. In clinical trials with patients with cancer, there was neither a difference in safety nor efficacy between patients over 65 years of age and those under 65 years of age; there was an insufficient number of patients over 75 years of age to permit conclusions in that age group. No adjustment in dosage is recommended in the elderly.

In adult cancer patients, the mean elimination half-life was 4.0 hours, and there was no difference in the multidose pharmacokinetics over a 4-day period. In a study of 21 pediatric cancer patients (aged 4-18 years) who received three IV doses of 0.15 mg/kg of Ondansetron at 4-hour intervals, patients older than 15 years of age exhibited Ondansetron pharmacokinetic parameters similar to those of adults. Patients aged 4-12 years generally showed higher clearance and somewhat larger volume of distribution than adults. Most pediatric patients younger than 15 years of age with cancer had a shorter (2.4 hours) Ondansetron plasma half-life than patients older than 15 years of age. It is not known whether these differences in Ondansetron plasma half-life may result in differences in efficacy between adults and some young children (see "Clinical Trials: Pediatric Studies").

In normal volunteers (19-39 years old, n = 23), the peak plasma concentration was 264 ng/mL following a single 32-mg dose administered as a 15-minute IV infusion. The mean elimination half-life was 4.1 hours. Systemic exposure to 32 mg of Ondansetron was not proportional to dose as measured by comparing dose-normalized AUC values to an 8-mg dose. This is consistent with a small decrease in systemic clearance with increasing plasma concentrations.

Plasma protein binding of Ondansetron as measured *in vitro* was 70%-76%, with binding constant over the pharmacologic concentration range (10-500 ng/mL). Circulating drug also distributes into erythrocytes.

A positive lymphoblast transformation test to Ondansetron has been reported, which suggests immunologic sensitivity to Ondansetron.

Ondansetron HCl tablets: Oral Ondansetron is well absorbed and undergoes limited first-pass metabolism. Following the administration of a single 8-mg Ondansetron tablet to healthy, young, male volunteers and from pooled studies, the time to peak plasma Ondansetron concentration is approximately 1.7 hours, the terminal elimination half-life is approximately 3 hours, and bioavailability is approximately 56%. Gender differences were shown in the disposition of Ondansetron given as a single dose. The extent and rate of Ondansetron's absorption is greater in women than men. Slower clearance in women, a smaller apparent volume of distribution (adjusted for weight) and higher absolute bioavailability resulted in higher plasma Ondansetron levels. These higher plasma levels may in part be explained by differences in body weight between men and women. It is not known whether these gender-related differences were clinically important. More detailed pharmacokinetic information is contained in the following table taken from one study. (See related table).

The administration of oral Ondansetron with food increases significantly (about 17%) the extent of absorption of Ondansetron. The peak plasma concentration and time to peak plasma concentration are not significantly affected. This change in the extent of absorption is not believed to be of any clinical relevance.

There was no significant effect of antacid administration on the pharmacokinetics of orally administered Ondansetron.

Because Ondansetron undergoes extensive metabolism, the modest reduction in clearance in the over 75 age-group was not unexpected. However, since there was neither a difference in safety nor efficacy between patients over 65 years of age and those under 65 years of age, no adjustment in dosage is required in the elderly. Plasma protein binding of Ondansetron as measured *in vitro* was 70%-76% over the concentration range of 10-500 ng/mL. Circulating drug also distributes into erythrocytes.

CLINICAL TRIALS

ONDANSETRON HCL INJECTION

Chemotherapy-Induced Nausea and Vomiting: In a double-blind study of three different dosing regimens of Ondansetron HCl injection, 0.015 mg/kg, 0.15 mg/kg, and 0.30 mg/kg, each given three times during the course of cancer chemotherapy, the 0.15-mg/kg dosing regimen was more effective than the 0.015-mg/kg dosing regimen. The 0.30-mg/kg dosing regimen was not shown to be more effective than the 0.15-mg/kg dosing regimen.

Cisplatin-Based Chemotherapy: In a double-blind study in 28 patients, Ondansetron HCl Injection (three 0.15-mg/kg doses) was significantly more effective than placebo in preventing nausea and vomiting induced by cisplatin-based chemotherapy. Treatment response was as follows:

PREVENTION OF CHEMOTHERAPY-INDUCED NAUSEA AND EMESIS IN SINGLE-DAY CISPLATIN THERAPY*

	Ondansetron Injection	Placebo	p Value†
Number of patients	14	14	
Treatment response			
0 Emetic episodes	2 (14%)	0 (0%)	
1-2 Emetic episodes	8 (57%)	0 (0%)	
3-5 Emetic episodes	2 (14%)	1 (7%)	
More than 5 emetic episodes/rescued	2 (14%)	13 (93%)	0.001
Median number of emetic episodes	1.5	Undefined‡	
Median time to first emetic episode (h)	11.6	2.8	0.001
Median nausea scores (0-100)§	3	59	0.034
Global satisfaction with control of nausea and vomiting (0-100)¹¹	96	10.5	0.009

* Chemotherapy was high dose (100 and 120 mg/m^2: Ondansetron HCl Injection n = 6, placebo n = 5) or moderate dose (50 and 80 mg/m^2; Ondansetron HCl Injection n = 8, Placebo n = 9). Other chemotherapeutic agents included fluorouracil, doxorubicin and cyclophosphamide. There was no difference between treatments in the types of chemotherapy that would account for differences in response.

† Efficacy based on "all patients treated" analysis.

‡ Median undefined since at least 50% of the patients were rescued or had more than five emetic episodes.

§ Visual analog scale assessment of nausea: 0 = no nausea, 100 = nausea as bad as it can be.

¹¹ Visual analog scale assessment of satisfaction: 0 = not at all satisfied, 100 = totally satisfied.

Ondansetron was compared with metoclopramide in a single-blind trial in 307 patients receiving cisplatin ≥ 100 mg/m^2 with or without other chemotherapeutic agents. Patients received the first dose of Ondansetron or metoclopramide 30 minutes before cisplatin. Two additional Ondansetron doses were administered 4 and 8 hours later, or five additional metoclopramide doses were administered 2, 4, 7, 10, and 13 hours later. Cisplatin was administered over a period of 3 hours or less. Episodes of vomiting and retching were tabulated over the period of 24 hours after cisplatin. The results of this study are summarized below:

PREVENTION OF EMESIS
INDUCED BY CISPLATIN (≥ 100 mg/m²) SINGLE-DAY THERAPY*

	Ondansetron Injection	Metoclopramide	p Value
Dose	0.15 mg/kg x 3	2 mg/kg x 6	
Number of patients in efficacy population	136	138	
Treatment response			
0 Emetic episodes	54 (40%)	41 (30%)	
1-2 Emetic episodes	34 (25%)	30 (22%)	
3-5 Emetic episodes	19 (14%)	18 (13%)	
More than 5 emetic episodes/rescued	29 (21%)	49 (36%)	
Comparison of treatments with respect to			
0 Emetic episodes	54/136	41/138	0.083
More than 5 emetic episodes/rescued	29/136	49/138	0.009
Median number of emetic episodes	1	2	0.005
Median time to first emetic episode (h)	20.5	4.3	< 0.001
Global satisfaction with control of nausea and vomiting (0-100)†	85	63	0.001
Acute dystonic reactions	0	8	0.005
Akathisia	0	10	0.002

* In addition to cisplatin, 68% of patients received other chemotherapeutic agents, including cyclophosphamide, etoposide, and fluorouracil. There was no difference between treatments in the types of chemotherapy that would account for differences in response.

† Visual analog scale assessment: 0 = not at all satisfied, 100 = totally satisfied.

Forty-one of the Ondansetron patients were over 65 years of age. The complete response rate (zero emetic episodes) was 41% in this group compared with 40% in those 65 years old or younger.

In a stratified, randomized, double-blind, parallel-group, multicenter study, a single 32-mg dose of Ondansetron was compared with three 0.15-mg/kg doses in patients receiving cisplatin doses of either 50-70 mg/m² or ≥ 100 mg/m². Patients received the first Ondansetron dose 30 minutes before cisplatin. Two additional Ondansetron doses were administered 4 and 8 hours later to the group receiving three 0.15-mg/kg doses. In both strata, significantly fewer patients on the single 32-mg dose than those receiving the three-dose regimen failed.

PREVENTION OF CHEMOTHERAPY-INDUCED NAUSEA AND EMESIS IN SINGLE-DOSE THERAPY

	Ondansetron Dose		
	0.15 mg/kg x3	32 mg x1	p Value
High-dose cisplatin (≥ 100 mg/m²)			
Number of patients	100	102	
Treatment response			
0 Emetic episodes	41 (41%)	49 (48%)	0.315
1-2 Emetic episodes	19 (19%)	25 (25%)	
3-5 Emetic episodes	4 (4%)	8 (8%)	
More than 5 Emetic episodes/rescued	36 (36%)	20 (20%)	0.009
Median time to first emetic episode (h)	21.7	23	0.173
Median nausea scores (0-100)*	28	13	0.004
Medium-dose cisplatin (50-70 mg/m²)			
Number of patients	101	93	
Treatment response			
0 Emetic episodes	62 (61%)	68 (73%)	0.083
1-2 Emetic episodes	11 (11%)	14 (15%)	

	Ondansetron Dose		
	0.15 mg/kg x3	32 mg x1	p Value
3-5 Emetic episodes	6 (6%)	3 (3%)	
More than 5 emetic episodes/rescued	22 (22%)	8 (9%)	0.011
Median time to first emetic episode (h)	Undefined†	Undefined	0.084
Median nausea scores (0-100)*	9	3	0.131

* Visual analog scale assessment: 0 = no nausea, 100 = nausea as bad as it can be.

† Median undefined since at least 50% of patients did not have any emetic episodes.

Cyclophosphamide-Based Chemotherapy: In a double-blind, placebo-controlled study of Ondansetron Injection (three 0.15-mg/kg doses) in 20 patients receiving cyclophosphamide (500-600 mg/m²) chemotherapy, Ondansetron Injection was significantly more effective than placebo in preventing nausea and vomiting. The results are summarized below:

PREVENTION OF CHEMOTHERAPY-INDUCED NAUSEA AND EMESIS IN SINGLE-DAY CYCLOPHOSPHAMIDE THERAPY*

	Ondansetron Injection	Placebo	p Value†
Number of patients	10	10	
Treatment response			
0 Emetic episodes	7 (70%)	0 (0%)	0.001
1-2 Emetic episodes	0 (0%)	2 (20%)	
3-5 Emetic episodes	2 (20%)	4 (40%)	
More than 5 emetic episodes/rescued	1 (10%)	4 (40%)	0.131
Median number of emetic episodes	0	4	0.008
Median time to first emetic episode (h)	Undefined‡	8.79	
Median nausea scores (0-100)§	0	60	0.001
Global satisfaction with control of nausea and vomiting (0-100)Π	100	52	0.008

* Chemotherapy consisted of cyclophosphamide in all patients, plus other agents, including fluorouracil, doxorubicin, methotrexate, and vincristine. There was no difference between treatments in the type of chemotherapy that would account for differences in response.

† Efficacy based on "all patients treated" analysis.

‡ Median undefined since at least 50% of patients did not have any emetic episodes.

§ Visual analog scale assessment of nausea: 0 = no nausea, 100 = nausea as bad as it can be.

Π Visual analog scale assessment of satisfaction: 0 = not at all satisfied, 100 = totally satisfied.

Retreatment: In uncontrolled trials, 127 patients receiving cisplatin (median dose, 100 mg/m²) and Ondansetron who had two or fewer emetic episodes were retreated with Ondansetron and chemotherapy, mainly cisplatin, for a total of 269 retreatment courses (median, 2; range, 1-10). No emetic episodes occurred in 160 (59%), and two or fewer emetic episodes occurred in 217 (81%) retreatment courses.

Pediatric Studies: Four open-label, noncomparative (one US, three foreign) trials have been performed with 209 pediatric cancer patients aged 4-18 years given a variety of cisplatin or noncisplatin regimens. In the three foreign trials, the initial Ondansetron HCl Injection dose ranged from 0.04-0.87 mg/kg for a total dose of 2.16-12 mg. This was followed by the oral administration of Ondansetron ranging from 4-24 mg daily for 3 days. In the US trial, Ondansetron HCl was administered intravenously (only) in three doses of 0.15 mg/kg each for a total daily dose of 7.2-39 mg. In these studies, 58% of the 196 evaluable patients had a complete response (no emetic episodes) on day 1. Thus, prevention of emesis in these

PHARMACOKINETICS IN NORMAL VOLUNTEERS: SINGLE 8-mg ORAL DOSE

Age-group (years)	Mean Weight (kg)	n	Peak Plasma Concentration (ng/mL)	Time of Peak Plasma Concentration (h)	Mean Elimination Half-life (h)	Systematic Plasma Clearance L/h/kg	Absolute Bioavailability
18-40 M	69.0	6	26.2	2.0	3.1	0.403	0.483
F	62.7	5	42.7	1.7	3.5	0.354	0.663
61-74 M	77.5	6	24.1	2.1	4.1	0.384	0.585
F	60.2	6	52.4	1.9	4.9	0.255	0.643
≥ 75 M	78.0	5	37.0	2.2	4.5	0.277	0.619
F	67.6	6	46.1	2.1	6.2	0.249	0.747

◆ RATED THERAPEUTICALLY EQUIVALENT; ◇ THERAPEUTIC EQUIVALENCE UNCONFIRMED; ○ UNRATED

children was essentially the same as for patients older than 18 years of age. Overall, Ondansetron HCl injection was well tolerated in these pediatric patients.

Postoperative Nausea and Vomiting: Prevention of Postoperative Nausea and Vomiting: Surgical patients who received Ondansetron HCl immediately before the induction of general balanced anesthesia (barbiturate: thiopental, methohexital or thiamylal; opioid: alfentanil or fentanyl; nitrous oxide; neuromuscular blockade: succinyl choline/curare and/or vecuronium or atracurium; and supplemental isoflurane) were evaluated in two double-blind US studies involving 554 patients. Ondansetron HCl Injection (4 mg) IV given over 2-5 minutes was significantly more effective than placebo. The results of these studies are summarized below:

PREVENTION OF POSTOPERATIVE NAUSEA AND VOMITING

	Ondansetron 4 mg IV	Placebo	p Value
Study 1			
Emetic episodes:			
Number of patients	136	139	
Treatment response over 24-hr postoperative period			
0 Emetic episodes	103 (76%)	64 (46%)	< 0.001
1 Emetic episode	13 (10%)	17 (12%)	
More than 1 emetic episode/rescued	20 (15%)	58 (42%)	
Nausea assessments:			
Number of patients	134	136	
No nausea over 24-hr postoperative period	56 (42%)	39 (29%)	
Study 2			
Emetic episodes:			
Number of patients	136	143	
Treatment response over 24-hr postoperative period			
0 Emetic episodes	85 (63%)	63 (44%)	0.002
1 Emetic episode	16 (12%)	29 (20%)	
More than 1 emetic episode/rescued	35 (26%)	51 (36%)	
Nausea assessments:			
Number of patients	125	133	
No nausea over 24-hr postoperative period	48 (38%)	42 (32%)	

The study populations in all trials thus far consisted of mainly women undergoing laparoscopic procedures.

While some men were included in some trials with similar results, clearance of the drug is more rapid in men and sufficient numbers of men have not been clinically studied to be certain that efficacy and safety have been established. Few patients undergoing major abdominal surgery have been studied.

Prevention of Further Postoperative Nausea and Vomiting: Surgical patients receiving general balanced anesthesia (barbiturate: thiopental, methohexital or thiamylal; opioid; alfentanil or fentanyl; nitrous oxide, neuromuscular blockade: succinyl choline/curare and/or vecuronium or atracurium; and supplemental isoflurane) who received no prophylactic antiemetics and who experienced nausea and/or vomiting within 2 hours postoperatively were evaluated in two double-blind US studies involving 441 patients. Patients who experienced an episode of postoperative nausea and/or vomiting were given Ondansetron HCl Injection (4 mg) IV over 2-5 minutes, and this was significantly more effective than placebo. The results of these studies are summarized below:

PREVENTION OF FURTHER POSTOPERATIVE NAUSEA AND VOMITING

	Ondansetron 4 mg IV	Placebo	p Value
Study 1			
Emetic episodes:			
Number of patients	104	117	
Treatment response 24 hrs after study drug			
0 Emetic episodes	49 (47%)	19 (16%)	< 0.001
1 Emetic episode	12 (12%)	9 (8%)	
More than 1 emetic episode/rescued	43 (41%)	89 (76%)	
Median time to first emetic episode (min)*	55.0	43.0	
Nausea assessments:			
Number of patients	98	102	
Mean nausea score over 24-hr postoperative period†	1.7	3.1	

	Ondansetron 4 mg IV	Placebo	p Value
Study 2			
Emetic episodes:			
Number of patients	112	108	
Treatment response 24 hrs after study drug			
0 Emetic episodes	49 (44%)	28 (26%)	0.006
1 Emetic episode	14 (13%)	3 (3%)	
More than 1 emetic episode/rescued	49 (44%)	77 (71%)	
Median time to first emetic episode (min)*	60.5	34.0	
Nausea assessments:			
Number of patients	105	85	
Mean nausea score over 24-hr postoperative period†	1.9	2.9	

* After administration of study drug.
† Nausea measured on a scale of 0-10 with 0 = no nausea, 10 = nausea as bad as it can be.

The study populations in all trials thus far consisted of mainly women undergoing laparoscopic procedures.

While some men were included in some trials with similar results, clearance of the drug is more rapid in men and sufficient numbers of men have not been clinically studied to be certain that efficacy and safety have been established. Few patients undergoing major abdominal surgery have been studied.

ONDANSETRON HCL TABLETS

In two double-blind US studies in 304 patients, Ondansetron HCl tablets were significantly more effective than placebo in preventing nausea and vomiting induced by cyclophosphamide-based chemotherapy containing either methotrexate or doxorubicin. Treatment response is based on the total number of emetic episodes over the 3-day study period. The results of these studies are summarized below:

EMETIC EPISODES: TREATMENT RESPONSE*

	Ondansetron 8 mg t.i.d. Oral*	Placebo	p Value
Study 1			
Number of patients	79	81	
Treatment response			
0 Emetic episodes	52 (66%)	15 (19%)	< 0.001
1-2 Emetic episodes	9 (11%)	10 (12%)	
3-5 Emetic episodes	5 (6%)	5 (6%)	
More than 5 emetic episodes/rescued	13 (16%)	51 (63%)	< 0.001
Median number of emetic episodes	0.0	Undefined†	
Median time to first emetic episode (h)	Undefined‡	11.1	
Median nausea scores (0-100)§	5	40	< 0.001
Study 2			
Number of patients	71	73	
Treatment response			
0 Emetic episodes	47 (66%)	9 (12%)	< 0.001
1-2 Emetic episodes	9 (13%)	11 (15%)	
3-5 Emetic episodes	4 (6%)	6 (8%)	
More than 5 emetic episodes/rescued	11 (15%)	47 (64%)	< 0.001
Median number of emetic episodes	0.0	Undefined†	
Median time to first emetic episode (h)	Undefined‡	9.5	
Median nausea scores (0-100)§	5	55	< 0.001

* The first dose was administered 30 minutes before the start of emetogenic chemotherapy, with subsequent doses 4 and 8 hours after the first dose. An 8-mg tablet was administered three times a day for 2 days after completion of chemotherapy. In adults, Ondansetron 4 mg t.i.d. was also studied, with the following results:
Study 1: 0 emetic episodes = 53/81 (65%); more than 5 emetic episodes/rescued = 19/81 (23%).
Study 2: 0 emetic episodes = 48/75 (64%); more than 5 emetic episodes/rescued = 14/75 (19%).
In analyses of patients receiving ≥ 600 mg/m² of cyclophosphamide, there were more failures on the 4-mg dose than on the 8-mg dose, 26% vs. 0% in one study and 14% vs. 4% in the second study.
† Median undefined since at least 50% of the patients were rescued or had more than five emetic episodes.

‡ *Median undefined since at least 50% of patients did not have any emetic episodes.*

§ *Visual analog scale assessment: 0 = no nausea, 100 = nausea as bad as it can be.*

In both studies, the Ondansetron-treated group was statistically significantly ($p < 0.001$) superior to placebo with respect to complete treatment response, treatment failure, the number of emetic episodes, and nausea scores.

Retreatment: In uncontrolled trials, 148 patients receiving cyclophosphamide-based chemotherapy were retreated with 8 mg t.i.d. of oral Ondansetron during subsequent chemotherapy for a total of 396 retreatment courses. No emetic episodes occurred in 314 (79%) of the retreatment courses, and only one to two emetic episodes occurred in 43 (11%) of the retreatment courses.

Pediatric Studies: Three open-label, uncontrolled, foreign trials have been performed with 182 patients 4-18 years old with cancer who were given a variety of cisplatin or noncisplatin regimens. In these foreign trials, the initial dose of Ondansetron Injection ranged from 0.04-0.87 mg/kg for a total dose of 2.16-12 mg. This was followed by the oral administration of Ondansetron ranging from 4-24 mg daily for 3 days. In these studies, 58% of the 170 evaluable patients had a complete response (no emetic episodes) on day 1. Two studies showed the response rates for patients less than 12 years of age who received 4 mg of Ondansetron three times a day to be similar to those in patients 12-18 years of age who received 8 mg of Ondansetron three times daily. Thus, prevention of emesis in these children was essentially the same as for patients older than 18 years of age. Overall, Ondansetron tablets were well tolerated in these pediatric patients.

Elderly Patients: One hundred thirty-seven (137) patients 65 years of age or older have received oral Ondansetron. Prevention of emesis was similar to that in patients younger than 65 years of age and adverse reactions were not seen in increased frequency.

INDICATIONS AND USAGE

ONDANSETRON HCL INJECTION

1. Prevention of nausea and vomiting associated with initial and repeat courses of emetogenic cancer chemotherapy, including high-dose cisplatin. Efficacy of the 32-mg single dose beyond 24 hours in these patients has not been established.

2. Prevention of postoperative nausea and/or vomiting. As with other antiemetics, routine prophylaxis is not recommended for patients in whom there is little expectation that nausea and/or vomiting will occur postoperatively. In patients where nausea and/or vomiting must be avoided postoperatively, Ondansetron HCl Injection is recommended even where the incidence of postoperative nausea and/or vomiting is low. For patients who have nausea and/or vomiting postoperatively, Ondansetron HCl Injection may be given to prevent further episodes (see *"Clinical Trials"*).

ONDANSETRON HCL TABLETS

Ondansetron HCl tablets are indicated for the prevention of nausea and vomiting associated with initial and repeat courses of moderately emetogenic cancer chemotherapy.

UNLABELED USES

Ondansetron Hydrochloride is used alone or as an adjunct in the treatment of radiation-induced nausea and vomiting, psychiatric disorders including schizophrenia, and hallucinations in Parkinson's patients on long-term levodopa therapy.

CONTRAINDICATIONS

Ondansetron HCl is contraindicated for patients known to have hypersensitivity to the drug.

PRECAUTIONS

Ondansetron is not a drug that stimulates gastric or intestinal peristalsis. It should not be used instead of nasogastric suction. As with other antiemetics, the use of Ondansetron in abdominal surgery may mask a progressive ileus and/or gastric distention.

Drug Interactions: Ondansetron does not itself appear to induce or inhibit the cytochrome P-450 drug-metabolizing enzyme system of the liver. Because Ondansetron is metabolized by hepatic cytochrome P-450 drug-metabolizing enzymes, inducers or inhibitors of these enzymes may change the clearance and, hence, the half-life of Ondansetron. On the basis of limited available data, no dosage adjustment is recommended for patients on these drugs. Tumor response to chemotherapy in the P 388 mouse leukemia model is not affected by Ondansetron. In humans, carmustine, etoposide, and cisplatin do not affect the pharmacokinetics of Ondansetron.

Carcinogenesis, Mutagenesis, Impairment of Fertility: Carcinogenic effects were not seen in 2-year studies in rats and mice with oral Ondansetron doses up to 10 and 30 mg/kg per day, respectively. Ondansetron was not mutagenic in standard tests for mutagenicity. Oral administration of Ondansetron up to 15 mg/kg per day did not affect fertility or general reproductive performance of male and female rats.

Pregnancy: Teratogenic Effects: Pregnancy Category B: Reproduction studies have been performed in pregnant rats and rabbits at IV doses up to 4 mg/kg per day and oral doses up to 15 and 30 mg/kg per day, respectively, and have revealed no evidence of impaired fertility or harm to the fetus due to Ondansetron. There are, however, no adequate and well-controlled studies in pregnant women. Because animal reproduction studies are not always predictive of human response, this drug should be used during pregnancy only if clearly needed.

Nursing Mothers: Ondansetron is excreted in the breast milk of rats. It is not known whether Ondansetron is excreted in human milk. Because many drugs are excreted in human milk, caution should be exercised when Ondansetron is administered to a nursing woman.

Pediatric Use: Little information is available about dosage in children 3 years of age or younger for Ondansetron HCl injection, 4 years of age or younger for Ondansetron HCl tablets (see *"Clinical Pharmacology"* and *"Dosage and Administration"* section for use in children 4-18 years of age receiving cancer chemotherapy).

Use Elderly Patients: Dosage adjustment is not needed in patients over the age of 65 (see *"Clinical Pharmacology"*). Prevention of nausea and vomiting in elderly patients was no different than in younger age-groups.

ADVERSE REACTIONS

ONDANSETRON HCL INJECTION

Chemotherapy-Induced Nausea and Vomiting: The following adverse events have been reported in individuals receiving Ondansetron at a dosage of three 0.15-mg/kg doses or as a single 32-mg dose in clinical trials. These patients were receiving concomitant chemotherapy, primarily cisplatin, and IV fluids. Most were receiving a diuretic. (See related table).

The following have been reported during controlled clinical trials or in the routine managment of patients. The percentage figures are based on clinical trial experience.

Gastrointestinal: Constipation has been reported in 11% of chemotherapy patients receiving multiday Ondansetron.

Hepatic: In comparative trials in cisplatin chemotherapy patients with normal baseline values of aspartate transaminase (AST) and alanine transaminase (ALT), these enzymes have been reported to exceed twice the upper limit of normal in approximately 5% of patients. The increases were transient and did not appear to be related to dose or duration of therapy. On repeat exposure, similar transient evaluations in transaminase values occurred in some courses, but symptomatic hepatic disease did not occur.

From a foreign report, one 76-year-old male patient with lymphoma, who was a carrier of hepatitis B, developed liver failure 3 weeks after a second course of Ondansetron (and cyclophosphamide) and subsequently died. The etiology of the liver failure is unclear.

Integumentary: Rash has occurred in approximately 1% of patients receiving Ondansetron.

Central Nervous System: There have been rare reports consistent with, but not diagnostic of, extrapyramidal reactions in patients receiving Ondansetron.

Cardiovascular: Rare instances of tachycardia, angina (chest pain), bradycardia, hypotension, syncope, and electrocardiographic alterations, including second degree heart block. In many cases the relationship Ondansetron HCl injection was unclear.

Special Senses: Transient blurred vision, in some cases associated with abnormalities of accommodation, and transient dizziness during or shortly after IV infusion.

Local Reactions: Pain, redness, and burning at site of injection.

Other: Rare cases of hypokalemia and grand mal seizures have been reported. The relationship to Ondansetron HCl injection was unclear. Rare cases of hypersensitivity reactions, sometimes severe (e.g., anaphylaxis, bronchospasm, shortness of breath, hypotension, shock, angioedema, urticaria), have also been reported.

Postoperative Nausea and Vomiting: The following adverse events have been reported in $\geq 2\%$ of people receiving ondansetron at a dosage of 4 mg IV over 2-5 minutes in clinical trials. Rates of these events were not significantly different in the Ondansetron and placebo groups. These patients were receiving multiple concomitant perioperative and postoperative medications.

	Ondansetron HCl Injection 4 mg IV n = 547 patients	Placebo n = 547 patients
Headache	92 (17%)	77 (14%)
Dizziness	67 (12%)	88 (16%)
Musculoskeletal pain	57 (10%)	59 (11%)
Drowsiness/sedation	44 (8%)	37 (7%)
Shivers	38 (7%)	39 (7%)
Malaise/fatigue	25 (5%)	30 (5%)
Injection site reaction	21 (4%)	18 (3%)
Urinary retention	17 (3%)	15 (3%)
Postoperative CO₂-related pain*	12 (2%)	16 (3%)
Chest pain (unspecified)	12 (2%)	15 (3%)
Anxiety/agitation	11 (2%)	16 (3%)
Dysuria	11 (2%)	9 (2%)
Hypotension	10 (2%)	12 (2%)
Fever	10 (2%)	6 (1%)
Cold sensation	9 (2%)	8 (1%)
Pruritus	9 (2%)	3 (< 1%)
Paresthesia	9 (2%)	2 (< 1%)

* *Sites of pain included abdomen, stomach, joints, rib cage, shoulder.*

◆ RATED THERAPEUTICALLY EQUIVALENT; ◇ THERAPEUTIC EQUIVALENCE UNCONFIRMED; ○ UNRATED

ONDANSETRON HCL TABLETS

The following adverse events have been reported in adults receiving 4 or 8 mg of Ondansetron three times a day for 3 days in two US placebo-controlled trials. These patients were receiving concurrent chemotherapy, primarily cyclophosphamide-based regimens. (See related table).

Central Nervous System: There have been rare reports consistent with, but not diagnostic of, extrapyramidal reactions in patients receiving Ondansetron.

Hepatic: In 723 patients receiving cyclophosphamide-based chemotherapy in US clinical trials, AST and/or ALT values have been reported to exceed twice the upper limit of normal in approximately 1%-2% of patients receiving oral Ondansetron. The increases were transient and did not appear to be related to dose or duration of therapy. On repeat exposure, similar transient elevations in transaminase values occurred in some courses, but symptomatic hepatic disease did not occur. The role of cancer chemotherapy in these biochemical changes cannot be clearly determined.

From a foreign report, one 76-year-old male patient with lymphoma, who was a carrier of hepatitis B, developed liver failure 3 weeks after a second course of Ondansetron (and cyclophosphamide) and subsequently died. The etiology of the liver failure is unclear.

Integumentary: Rash has occurred in approximately 1% of patients receiving Ondansetron.

Other: Rare cases of anaphylaxis, bronchospasm, tachycardia, angina (chest pain), hypokalemia, electrocardiographic alterations, vascular occlusive events, and grand mal seizures have been reported. Except for bronchospasm and anaphylaxis, the relationship to Ondansetron HCl was unclear.

Drug Abuse and Dependence: Animal studies have shown that Ondansetron is not discriminated as a benzodiazepine nor does it substitute for benzodiazepines in direct addiction studies.

OVERDOSAGE

There is no specific antidote for Ondansetron overdose. Patients should be managed with appropriate supportive therapy. Individual doses as large as 145 mg and total daily dosages (three doses) as large as 252 mg have been inadvertently administered intravenously without significant adverse events. These doses are more than 10 times the recommended daily dose.

"Sudden blindness" (amaurosis) of 2-3 minutes' duration plus severe constipation occurred in one patient that was administered 72 mg of Ondansetron intravenously as a single dose. Hypotension (and faintness) occurred in another patient that took 48 mg of oral Ondansetron. Following infusion of 32 mg over only a 4-minute period, a vasovagal episode with transient second degree heart block was observed. In all instances, the events resolved completely.

DOSAGE AND ADMINISTRATION

ONDANSETRON HCL INJECTION

Cancer Chemotherapy: **DILUTE BEFORE USE. Ondansetron HCl Injection should be diluted in 50 mL of 5% dextrose injection or 0.9% sodium chloride injection before administration.** The recommended IV dosage of Ondansetron HCl Injection is a single 32-mg dose or three 0.15-mg/kg doses. A single 32-mg dose is infused over 15 minutes beginning 30 minutes before the start of emetogenic chemotherapy. The recommended infusion rate should not be exceeded (see "*Overdosage*"). With the three-dose (0.15-mg/kg) regimen, the first dose is infused over 15 minutes beginning 30 minutes before the start of emetogenic chemotherapy. Subsequent doses (0.15 mg/kg are administered 4 and 8 hours after the first dose of Ondansetron HCl Injection.

Ondansetron HCl injection should not be mixed with solutions for which physical and chemical compatibility have not been established. In particular, this applies to alkaline solutions as a precipitate may form.

Pediatric Use: **DILUTE BEFORE USE.** On the basis of the limited available information (see "*Clinical Trials: Pediatric Studies*" and "*Clinical Pharmacology:*

Pharmacokinetics"), the dosage in children 4-18 years of age should be three 0.15-mg/kg doses (see above). Little information is available about dosage in children 3 years of age or younger.

Use in the Elderly: **DILUTE BEFORE USE.** The dosage is the same for the general population.

Prevention of Postoperative Nausea and/or Vomiting: **NO DILUTION NECESSARY.** Immediately before induction of anesthesia, or postoperatively if the patient experiences nausea and/or vomiting occurring shortly after surgery, administer 4 mg **undiluted** intravenously in not less than 30 seconds, preferably over 2-5 minutes. Repeat dosing for patients who continue to experience nausea and/or vomiting postoperatively has not been studied. While recommended as a fixed dose for all, few patients above 80 kg or below 40 kg have been studied.

Pediatric Use: There is no experience with the use of Ondansetron HCl Injection in the prevention or treatment of postoperative nausea and vomiting in children.

Use in the Elderly: **NO DILUTION NECESSARY.** The dosage recommendation is the same as for the general population.

Dosage Adjustment for Patients With Impaired Renal Function: No specific studies have been conducted in patients with renal insufficiency.

Dosage Adjustment for Patients With Impaired Hepatic Function: In patients with severe hepatic impairment according to Child-Pugh[1] criteria, a single maximal daily dose of 8 mg to be infused over 15 minutes beginning 30 minutes before the start of the emetogenic chemotherapy is recommended. There is no experience beyond first-day administration of Ondansetron HCl.

Stability: Ondansetron HCl injection is stable at room temperature under normal lighting conditions for 48 hours after dilution with the following IV fluids: 0.9% sodium chloride injection, 5% dextrose injection, 5% dextrose and 0.9% sodium chloride injection, 5% dextrose and 0.45% sodium chloride injection, and 3% sodium chloride injection.

Although Ondansetron HCl injection is chemically and physically stable when diluted as recommended, sterile precautions should be observed because diluents generally do not contain preservative. After dilution, do not use beyond 24 hours.

Note: Parenteral drug products should be inspected visually for particulate matter and discoloration before administration whenever solution and container permit.

Precaution: Occasionally, Ondansetron precipitates at the stopper/vial interface in vials stored upright. Potency and safety are not affected. If a precipitate is observed, resolubilize by shaking the vial vigorously.

ONDANSETRON HCL TABLETS

Prevention of Nausea and Vomiting Associated With Moderately Emetogenic Cancer

Chemotherapy: The recommended oral dosage of Ondansetron HCl Tablets is one 8-mg table given three times a day. The first dose should be administered 30 minutes before the start of emetogenic chemotherapy, with subsequent doses 4 and 8 hours after the first dose. One 8-mg Ondansetron HCl Tablet should be administered three times a day (every 8 hours) for 1-2 days after completion of chemotherapy.

Pediatric Use: For patients 12 years of age and older, the dosage is the same as for adults. For patients 4-12 years of age, the recommended oral dosage is one 4-mg tablet given three times a day. The method and frequency of administration is the same as for adults.

Use in the Elderly: The dosage is the same as for the general population.

Dosage Adjustment for Patients With Impaired Renal Function: No specific studies have been conducted in patients with renal insufficiency.

Dosage Adjustment for Patients With Impaired Hepatic Function: In patients with severe hepatic insufficiency, clearance is reduced, apparent volume of distribution is increased with a resultant increase in plasma half-life, and bioavailability

PRINCIPAL ADVERSE EVENTS IN COMPARATIVE TRIALS

	Number of Patients With Event			
	Ondansetron HCl Injection 0.15 mg/kg × 3 n = 419	Ondansetron HCl Injection 32 mg × 1 n = 220	Metoclopramide n = 156	Placebo n = 34
Diarrhea	16%	8%	44%	18%
Headache	17%	25%	7%	15%
Fever	8%	7%	5%	3%
Akathisia	0%	0%	6%	0%
Acute dystonic reactions*	0%	0%	5%	0%

* *See Central Nervous System below.*

PRINCIPAL ADVERSE EVENTS IN US PLACEBO-CONTROLLED TRIALS: 3 DAYS OF ORAL THERAPY

Event	Ondansetron 8 mg t.i.d. n = 215	Ondansetron 4 mg t.i.d n = 215	Placebo n = 221
Headache	46 (21%)	49 (23%)	24 (11%)
Constipation	15 (7%)	10 (5%)	0 (0%)
Abdominal pain	11 (5%)	7 (4%)	1 (< 1%)
Weakness	7 (3%)	5 (2%)	1 (< 1%)
Xerostomia	4 (2%)	3 (1%)	0 (0%)

▶ SHOWN IN PRODUCT IDENTIFICATION GUIDE

approaches 100%. In such patients, a total daily dose of 8 mg should not be exceeded.

Storage: Store between 2° and 30°C (36° and 86°F). Protect from light.

REFERENCE
1. Pugh RNH, Murray-Lyon IM, Dawson JL, Pietroni MC, Williams R. Transection of the oesophagus for bleeding oesophageal varices *Brit J Surg.* 1973; 60:646-649.

J CODES
Per 1 mg IV—J2405

HOW SUPPLIED
INJECTION: 2 MG/ML

BRAND/MANUFACTURER	NDC	SIZE	AWP
○ **BRAND**			
ZOFRAN: Cerenex	00173-0442-00	20 ml	$214.76
	00173-0442-02	2 ml 5s	$103.75

TABLETS: 4 MG

BRAND/MANUFACTURER	NDC	SIZE	AWP
○ **BRAND**			
▶ ZOFRAN: Cerenex	00173-0446-04	3s	$32.10
	00173-0446-00	30s	$314.70
	00173-0446-02	100s ud	$1070.40

TABLETS: 8 MG

BRAND/MANUFACTURER	NDC	SIZE	AWP
○ **BRAND**			
▶ ZOFRAN: Cerenex	00173-0447-04	3s	$53.50
	00173-0447-00	30s	$524.26
	00173-0447-02	100s ud	$1783.20

Ony-Clear Nail *SEE* MICONAZOLE NITRATE

Ophthaine *SEE* PROPARACAINE HYDROCHLORIDE

Ophthetic *SEE* PROPARACAINE HYDROCHLORIDE

Ophthocort *SEE* CHLORAMPHENICOL/HYDROCORTISONE ACETATE/POLYMYXIN B SULFATE

Opium Tincture

DESCRIPTION
WARNING—MAY BE HABIT-FORMING
Opium Tincture, USP (Deodorized), is for oral administration. It is freed from unpleasant odor or nauseating substances by "denarcotization" with a petroleum distillate. Opium tincture is a clear, reddish-brown hydroalcoholic solution.
Each 100 mL contains 1 g of anhydrous morphine (represents the equivalent of 10 g of powdered opium, USP), alcohol, 19%, and water.
Opium has a very characteristic odor and a very bitter taste. The opiates are the most effective and prompt-acting nonspecific antidiarrheal agents.

CLINICAL PHARMACOLOGY
The opiates act by enhancing tone in the long segments of longitudinal muscle and by inhibiting propulsive contraction of both circular and longitudinal muscles.
Clinical evidence indicates that the analgesic activity of Opium preparations is due to their morphine content. Relatively small doses that do not produce significant analgesia are effective in controlling diarrhea. The papaverine content of the mixed alkaloids is too small to have demonstrable spasmolytic activity.
Following oral administration, morphine is well absorbed from the gastrointestinal tract. It is rapidly metabolized following oral administration, however, and plasma levels of unconjugated morphine are lower than those achieved after parenteral administration. Like other narcotic analgesics, Opium preparations are metabolized in the liver. Morphine undergoes conjugation with glucuronic acid at the 3-hydroxyl group. Secondary conjugation may also occur at the 6-hydroxyl group to form the 3,6-diglucuronide. Morphine is excreted in the urine mainly as morphine-3-glucuronide and smaller amounts of morphine-3,6-diglucuronide and unchanged drug. Approximately 75% of a dose of morphine is excreted in the urine within 48 hours.

INDICATIONS AND USAGE
Opium Tincture is useful for the treatment of diarrhea.

CONTRAINDICATIONS
This preparation is not recommended for use in children.

It should not be used in diarrhea caused by poisoning until the toxic material is eliminated from the gastrointestinal tract.

WARNINGS
Addiction can result from Opium usage. Opium preparations should be given in the smallest effective dose and as infrequently as possible to minimize the development of tolerance and physical dependence.

PRECAUTIONS
General: Opium should be used with caution in the elderly, in debilitated individuals, and in patients with increased intracranial pressure, cerebral arteriosclerosis, hepatic cirrhosis or liver insufficiency, gastrointestinal hemorrhage, myxedema, emphysema, and bronchial asthma.
Drug Interactions: When preparations containing Opium are administered in combination with other drugs, the cautions applicable to each ingredient should be borne in mind. Reduced dosage is indicated in poor-risk patients, in the very young or very old patient, and in those who are receiving other central-nervous-system depressants.
Usage in Pregnancy: Pregnancy Category C: Animal reproduction studies have not been conducted with Opium Tincture, USP (Deodorized). It is also not known whether Opium Tincture, USP (Deodorized), can cause fetal harm when administered to a pregnant woman or can affect reproduction capacity. Opium Tincture, USP (Deodorized), should be given to a pregnant woman only if clearly needed.
Nursing Mothers: Caution should be exercised when Opium Tincture, USP (Deodorized), is administered to a nursing woman.
Usage in Children: Safety and effectiveness in children have not been established. See *"Contraindications"*.

ADVERSE REACTIONS
Constipation, nausea, and vomiting may occur in some patients. Pruritus and urticaria have been observed.

DRUG ABUSE AND DEPENDENCE
Controlled Substance: Opium Tincture, USP (Deodorized), is a Schedule II drug. See *"Warnings"*.

OVERDOSAGE
Signs and Symptoms: Symptoms of toxicity are those of morphine and alcohol, such as nausea, vomiting, miosis, cool and clammy skin, respiratory and CNS depression, bradycardia, hypotension, and skeletal muscle flaccidity. Noncardiogenic pulmonary edema may develop after opioid overdose and monitoring of heart filling pressure may be helpful. Ethanol has been demonstrated to cause hypoglycemia in children or adults with limited glycogen stores. In severe overdosage, apnea, circulatory collapse, cardiac arrest, and death may occur.
Treatment: To obtain up-to-date information about the treatment of overdose, a good resource is your certified Regional Poison Control Center. Telephone numbers of certified poison control centers are listed in the *Physicians' Desk Reference (PDR)*. In managing overdosage, consider the possibility of multiple drug overdoses, interaction among drugs, and unusual drug kinetics in your patient.
Initial management of opioid overdose should emphasize establishment of a secure airway and support of ventilation and perfusion. Meticulously monitor and maintain, within acceptable limits, the patient's vital signs, blood gases, serum electrolytes, blood glucose, etc. Naloxone antagonizes most effects of opioids. Protect the airway as naloxone may induce vomiting. Since naloxone has a shorter duration of action than opioids, repeated doses may be needed. In patients who abuse opioids chronically, a withdrawal syndrome may be manifest on administration of naloxone. This may include yawning, tearing, restlessness, sweating, dilated pupils, piloerection, vomiting, diarrhea, and abdominal cramps. This syndrome usually abates quickly as the effect of naloxone dissipates.
Absorption of drugs from the gastrointestinal tract may be decreased by giving activated charcoal, which, in many cases, is more effective than emesis or lavage; consider charcoal instead of or in addition to gastric emptying. Repeated doses of charcoal over time may hasten elimination of some drugs that have been absorbed. Since Opium Tincture can delay gastric emptying, evacuation of the stomach may be beneficial. Safeguard the patient's airway when employing gastric emptying or charcoal.
Monitor for and treat hypoglycemia.
The use of forced diuresis, peritoneal dialysis, hemodialysis, or charcoal hemoperfusion has not been established to be beneficial.

DOSAGE AND ADMINISTRATION
Usual Adult Dose: 0.6 mL orally 4 times a day.
Storage: Store at controlled room temperature, 59° to 86°F (15° to 30°C).

HOW SUPPLIED
TINCTURE LIQUID (C-II):

BRAND/MANUFACTURER	NDC	SIZE	AWP
○ **GENERICS**			
Lilly	00002-2606-58	120 ml	$42.10
Lilly	00002-2606-05	480 ml	$152.50

Optimine *SEE* AZATADINE MALEATE

◆ RATED THERAPEUTICALLY EQUIVALENT; ◇ THERAPEUTIC EQUIVALENCE UNCONFIRMED; ○ UNRATED

Optipranolol HCl *SEE* METIPRANOLOL

Optiray *SEE* IOVERSOL

Orabase HCA *SEE* HYDROCORTISONE, TOPICAL

Oragrafin *SEE* IPODATE

Oramorph SR *SEE* MORPHINE SULFATE

Orap *SEE* PIMOZIDE

Orasone *SEE* PREDNISONE

Oratrast *SEE* BARIUM SULFATE

Oreticyl *SEE* DESERPIDINE AND HYDROCHLOROTHIAZIDE

Oreton Methyl *SEE* METHYLTESTOSTERONE

Organidin NR *SEE* GUAIFENESIN

Orimune *SEE* POLIO VACCINE

Orinase *SEE* TOLBUTAMIDE *AND* TOLBUTAMIDE SODIUM

Ornade Spansules *SEE* CHLORPHENIRAMINE MALEATE WITH PHENYLPROPANOLAMINE HYDROCHLORIDE

Orphenadrine Citrate

DESCRIPTION
Orphenadrine Citrate is the citrate salt of Orphenadrine (2-dimethylaminoethyl 2-methylbenzhydryl ether citrate). It occurs as a white, crystalline powder having a bitter taste. It is practically odorless; sparingly soluble in water, slightly soluble in alcohol.

Each Orphenadrine Citrate Tablet contains 100 mg Orphenadrine Citrate. Orphenadrine Citrate Injection contains 60mg of Orphenadrine Citrate in aqueous solution.

Following is its chemical structure:

$(CH_3)_2NCH_2CH_2OCH$ · $HO-C-COOH$ with CH_2COOH and CH_2COOH groups

ACTIONS
The mode of therapeutic action has not been clearly identified, but may be related to its analgesic properties. Orphenadrine Citrate also possesses anticholinergic actions.

INDICATIONS
Orphenadrine Citrate is indicated as an adjunct to rest, physical therapy, and other measures for the relief of discomfort associated with acute painful musculoskeletal conditions. The mode of action of the drug has not been clearly identified, but may be related to its analgesic properties. Orphenadrine Citrate does not directly relax tense skeletal muscles in man.

UNLABELED USES
Orphenadrine Citrate is used alone or as an adjunct in the treatment of dyspepsia, drug-induced extrapyramidal reactions, and myalgia.

CONTRAINDICATIONS
Contraindicated in patients with glaucoma, pyloric or duodenal obstruction, stenosing peptic ulcers, prostatic hypertrophy or obstruction of the bladder neck, cardio-spasm (megaesophagus) and myasthenia gravis. Contraindicated in patients who have demonstrated a previous hypersensitivity to the drug.

WARNINGS
Some patients may experience transient episodes of light-headedness, dizziness or syncope. Orphenadrine Citrate may impair the ability of the patient to engage in potentially hazardous activities such as operating machinery or driving a motor vehicle; ambulatory patients should therefore be cautioned accordingly.

Orphenadrine Citrate Injection contains sodium bisulfite, a sulfite that may cause allergic-type reactions including anaphylactic symptoms and life-threatening or less severe asthmatic episodes in certain susceptible people. The overall prevalence of sulfite sensitivity in the general population is unknown and probably low. Sulfite sensitivity is seen more frequently in asthmatic than nonasthmatic people.

PREGNANCY
Pregnancy Category C. Animal reproduction studies have not been conducted with Orphenadrine Citrate. It is also not known whether Orphenadrine Citrate can cause fetal harm when administered to a pregnant woman or can affect reproduction capacity. Orphenadrine Citrate should be given to a pregnant woman only if clearly needed.

USAGE IN CHILDREN
Safety and effectiveness in children have not been established; therefore, this drug is not recommended for use in the pediatric age group.

PRECAUTIONS
Confusion, anxiety and tremors have been reported in a few patients receiving propoxphene and Orphenadrine concomitantly. As these symptoms may be simply due to an additive effect, reduction of dosage and/or discontinuation of one or both agents is recommended in such cases.

Orphenadrine Citrate should be used with caution in patients with tachycardia, cardiac decompensation, coronary insufficiency, cardiac arrhythmias.

Safety of continuous long-term therapy with Orphenadrine has not been established. Therefore, if Orphenadrine is prescribed for prolonged use, periodic monitoring of blood, urine and liver function values is recommended.

ADVERSE REACTIONS
Adverse reactions of Orphenadrine are mainly due to the mild anticholinergic action of Orphenadrine, and are usually associated with higher dosage. Dryness of the mouth is usually the first adverse effect to appear. When the daily dose is increased, possible adverse effects include: tachycardia, palpitation, urinary hesitancy or retention, blurred vision, dilatation of pupils, increased ocular tension, weakness, nausea, vomiting, headache, dizziness, constipation, drowsiness, hypersensitivity reactions, pruritus, hallucinations, agitation, tremor, gastric irritation, and rarely urticaria and other dermatoses. Infrequently, an elderly patient may experience some degree of mental confusion. These adverse reactions can usually be eliminated by reduction in dosage. Very rare cases of aplastic anemia associated with the use of Orphenadrine Tablets have been reported. No causal relationship has been established.

Rare instances of anaphylactic reaction have been reported associated with the intramuscular injection of Orphenadrine Citrate Injection.

DOSAGE AND ADMINISTRATION
Tablets: Adults—Two tablets per day; one in the morning and one in the evening.

Injection: Adults—One 2 mL ampul (60 mg) intravenously or intramuscularly; may be repeated every 12 hours. Relief may be maintained by 1 Orphenadrine Citrate tablet twice daily.

TABLETS AND INJECTION
Store at controlled room temperature, 15°-30°C (59°-86°F).

J CODES
Up to 60 mg IV,IM—J2360

HOW SUPPLIED
INJECTION: 30 MG/ML

AVERAGE UNIT PRICE (AVAILABLE SIZES)		GENERIC A-RATED AVERAGE PRICE (GAAP)	
BRAND	$4.59	10 ml	$12.94
GENERIC	$1.34		

BRAND/MANUFACTURER	NDC	SIZE	AWP
◆ BRAND			
NORFLEX: 3M Pharm	00089-0540-06	2 ml 6s	$55.02

➤ SHOWN IN PRODUCT IDENTIFICATION GUIDE

BRAND/MANUFACTURER	NDC	SIZE	AWP
◆ GENERICS			
Steris	00402-0354-82	2 ml	$2.92
Schein	00364-6747-54	10 ml	$7.65
Steris	00402-0129-10	10 ml	$7.65
ORPHENATE: Hyrex	00314-0549-10	10 ml	$11.90
Rugby	00536-5750-70	10 ml	$15.30
FLEXOJECT: Mayrand	00259-0322-10	10 ml	$22.20
Schein	00364-2182-42	2 ml 25s	$72.90

TABLET, EXTENDED RELEASE: 100 MG

BRAND/MANUFACTURER	NDC	SIZE	AWP
○ BRAND			
▶ NORFLEX: 3M Pharm	00089-0221-10	100s	$142.80
	00089-0221-50	500s	$678.12

Ortho All-Flex SEE DIAPHRAGM

Ortho-Cept SEE DESOGESTREL AND ETHINYL ESTRADIOL

Orthoclone OKT 3 SEE MUROMONAB-CD3

Ortho Cyclen SEE ETHINYL ESTRADIOL AND NORGESTIMATE

Ortho Diaphragm Kit SEE DIAPHRAGM

Ortho Dienestrol SEE DIENESTROL

Ortho-Est SEE ESTROPIPATE

Ortho-Novum SEE ETHINYL ESTRADIOL AND NORETHINDRONE AND MESTRANOL AND NORETHINDRONE

Ortho Tri-Cyclen SEE ETHINYL ESTRADIOL AND NORGESTIMATE

Orudis SEE KETOPROFEN

Oruvail SEE KETOPROFEN

Osmitrol SEE MANNITOL, INJECTABLE

Osmoglyn SEE GLYCERIN

Otic Tridesilon SEE ACETIC ACID AND DESONIDE

Ovcon SEE ETHINYL ESTRADIOL AND NORETHINDRONE

Ovide SEE MALATHION

Ovral SEE ETHINYL ESTRADIOL AND NORGESTREL

Ovrette SEE NORGESTREL

Oxacillin Sodium

DESCRIPTION
Oxacillin Sodium is a semisynthetic antibiotic of the isoxazolyl penicillin series, derived from 6-amino-penicillanic acid. It is the sodium salt in a parenteral dosage form, for intramuscular or intravenous use.

Each Dosage Unit Contains: Oxacillin Sodium equivalent to 250 or 500 mg, or 1, 2, 4, or 10 gm Oxacillin. The chemical name of Oxacillin Sodium is 4-Thia-1-azabicyclo[3.2.0]heptane-2-carboxylic acid, 3.3-dimethyl-6-[[(5-methyl-3-phenyl-4-isoxazolyl) carbonyl] amino]-7-oxo-, monosodium salt, monohydrate, $[2S(2\alpha,5\alpha,6\beta)]$. Its empirical formula is $C_{19}H_{18}N_3NaO_5S \cdot H_2O$ and its molecular weight 441.43.

Following is its chemical structure:

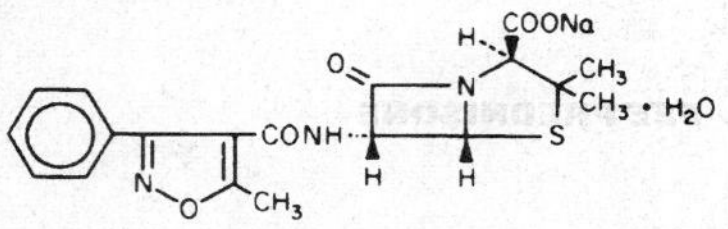

CLINICAL PHARMACOLOGY
Microbiology: Penicillinase-resistant penicillins exert a bactericidal action against penicillin-susceptible microorganisms during the state of active multiplication. All penicillins inhibit the biosynthesis of the bacterial cell wall.

The drugs in this class are highly resistant to inactivation by staphylococcal penicillinase and are active against penicillinase-producing and nonpenicillinase-producing strains of *Staphylococcus aureus.*

The penicillinase-resistant penicillins are active *in vitro* against a variety of other bacteria.

Susceptibility Plate Testing: Quantitative methods of susceptibility testing that require measurement of zone diameters or minimal inhibitory concentrations (MIC's) give the most precise estimates of antibiotic susceptibility. One such procedure has been recommended for use with discs to test susceptibility to this class of drugs. Interpretations correlate diameters on the disc test with MIC values. A penicillinase-resistant class disc may be used to determine microbial susceptibility to cloxacillin, dicloxacillin, methicillin, nafcillin, and Oxacillin. With this procedure, employing a 5 microgram methicillin sodium disc, a report from the laboratory of "susceptible" (zone of at least 14 mm) indicates that the infecting organism is likely to respond to therapy. A report of "resistant" (zone of less than 10 mm) indicates that the infecting organism is not likely to respond to therapy. A report of "intermediate susceptibility" (zone of 10 to 13 mm) suggests that the organism might be susceptible if high doses of the antibiotic are used, or if the infection is confined to tissues and fluids (eg, urine), in which high antibiotic levels are attained.

In general, all staphylococci should be tested against the penicillin G disc and against the methicillin disc. Routine methods of antibiotic susceptibility testing may fail to detect strains of organisms resistant to the penicillinase-resistant penicillins. For this reason, the use of large inocula and 48-hour incubation periods may be necessary to obtain accurate susceptibility studies with these antibiotics. Bacterial strains which are resistant to one of the penicillinase-resistant penicillins should be considered resistant to all of the drugs in the class.

PHARMACOKINETICS
Oxacillin Sodium, with normal doses, has insignificant concentrations in the cerebrospinal and ascitic fluids. It is found in therapeutic concentrations in the pleural, bile, and amniotic fluids. Oxacillin Sodium is rapidly excreted as unchanged drug in the urine by glomerular filtration and active tubular secretion.

Oxacillin Sodium binds to serum protein, mainly albumin. The degree of protein binding reported varies with the method of study and the investigator, but generally has been found to be $94.2 \pm 2.1\%$.

Oxacillin Sodium is resistant to destruction by acid. Intramuscular injections give peak serum levels 30 minutes after injection. A 250 mg dose gives a level of 5.3 µg/ml while a 500 mg dose peaks at 10.9 µg/ml. Intravenous injection gives a peak about 5 minutes after the injection is completed. Slow IV dosing with 500 mg gives a 5-minute peak of 43 µg/ml with a half-life of 20 to 30 minutes.

INDICATIONS AND USAGE
The penicillinase-resistant penicillins are indicated in the treatment of infections caused by penicillinase-producing staphylococci which have demonstrated susceptibility to the drugs. Culture and susceptibility tests should be performed initially to determine the causative organisms and their sensitivity to the drug (see *"Clinical Pharmacology — Susceptibility Plate Testing"*).

The penicillinase-resistant penicillins may be used to initiate therapy in suspected cases of resistant staphylococcal infections prior to the availability of laboratory test results. The penicillinase-resistant penicillins should not be used in infections caused by organisms susceptible to penicillin G. If the susceptibility tests indicate that the infection is due to an organism other than a resistant staphylococcus, therapy should not be continued with a penicillinase-resistant penicillin.

CONTRAINDICATIONS

A history of a hypersensitivity (anaphylactic) reaction to any penicillin is a contraindication.

WARNINGS

Serious and occasionally fatal hypersensitivity (anaphylactic shock with collapse) reactions have occurred in patients receiving penicillin. The incidence of anaphylactic shock in all penicillin-treated patients is between 0.015 and 0.04 percent. Anaphylactic shock resulting in death has occurred in approximately 0.002 percent of the patients treated. Although anaphylaxis is more frequent following parenteral administration, it has occurred in patients receiving oral penicillins.

When penicillin therapy is indicated, it should be initiated only after a comprehensive patient drug and allergy history has been obtained. If an allergic reaction occurs, the drug should be discontinued and the patient should receive supportive treatment, eg, artificial maintenance of ventilation, pressor amines, antihistamines, and corticosteroids. Individuals with a history of penicillin hypersensitivity may also experience allergic reactions when treated with a cephalosporin.

PRECAUTIONS

General: Penicillinase-resistant penicillins should generally not be administered to patients with a history of sensitivity to any penicillin.

Penicillin should be used with caution in individuals with histories of significant allergies and/or asthma. Whenever allergic reactions occur, penicillin should be withdrawn unless, in the opinion of the physician, the condition being treated is life-threatening and amenable only to penicillin therapy.

The oral route of administration should not be relied upon in patients with severe illness, or with nausea, vomiting, gastric dilation, cardiospasm, or intestinal hypermotility. Occasionally patients will not absorb therapeutic amounts of orally administered penicillin.

The use of antibiotics may result in overgrowth of nonsusceptible organisms. If new infections due to bacteria or fungi occur, the drug should be discontinued and appropriate measures taken.

Laboratory Tests: Bacteriologic studies to determine the causative organisms and their susceptibility to the penicillinase-resistant penicillins should be performed (see *"Clinical Pharmacology—Microbiology"*). In the treatment of suspected staphylococcal infections, therapy should be changed to another active agent if culture tests fail to demonstrate the presence of staphylococci.

Periodic assessment of organ system function including renal, hepatic, and hematopoietic should be made during prolonged therapy with the penicillinase-resistant penicillins.

Blood cultures, white blood cell, and differential cell counts should be obtained prior to initiation of therapy and at least weekly during therapy with penicillinase-resistant penicillins.

Periodic urinalysis, blood urea nitrogen, and creatinine determinations should be performed during therapy with the penicillinase-resistant penicillins and dosage alterations should be considered if these values become elevated. If any impairment of renal function is suspected or known to exist, a reduction in the total dosage should be considered and blood levels monitored to avoid possible neurotoxic reactions (see *"Dosage and Administration"*).

SGOT and SGPT values should be obtained periodically during therapy to monitor for possible liver function abnormalities.

Drug Interactions: Tetracycline, a bacteriostatic antibiotic, may antagonize the bactericidal effect of penicillin and concurrent use of these drugs should be avoided.

Carcinogenesis, Mutagenesis, Impairment of Fertility: No long-term animal studies have been conducted with these drugs.

Studies on reproduction (nafcillin) in rats and rabbits reveal no fetal or maternal abnormalities before conception and continuously through weaning (one generation).

Pregnancy Category B: Reproduction studies performed in the mouse, rat, and rabbit have revealed no evidence of impaired fertility or harm to the fetus due to the penicillinase-resistant penicillins. Human experience with the penicillins during pregnancy has not shown any positive evidence of adverse effects on the fetus. There are, however, no adequate or well-controlled studies in pregnant women showing conclusively that harmful effects of these drugs on the fetus can be excluded. Because animal reproduction studies are not always predictive of human response, this drug should be used during pregnancy only if clearly needed.

Nursing Mothers: Penicillins are excreted in breast milk. Caution should be exercised when penicillins are administered to a nursing woman.

Pediatric Use: Because of incompletely developed renal function in newborns, penicillinase-resistant penicillins (especially methicillin) may not be completely excreted, with abnormally high blood levels resulting. Frequent blood levels are advisable in this group with dosage adjustments when necessary. All newborns treated with penicillins should be monitored closely for clinical and laboratory evidence of toxic or adverse effects (see *"Dosage and Administration"*).

ADVERSE REACTIONS

Body as a Whole: The reported incidence of allergic reactions to penicillin ranges from 0.7 to 10 percent (see *"Warnings"*). Sensitization is usually the result of

treatment but some individuals have had immediate reactions to penicillin when first treated. In such cases, it is thought that the patients may have had prior exposure to the drug via trace amounts present in milk and vaccines.

Two types of allergic reactions to penicillin are noted clinically, immediate and delayed.

Immediate reactions usually occur within 20 minutes of administration and range in severity from urticaria and pruritus to angioneurotic edema, laryngospasm, bronchospasm, hypotension, vascular collapse, and death. Such immediate anaphylactic reactions are very rare (see *"Warnings"*) and usually occur after parenteral therapy but have occurred in patients receiving oral therapy. Another type of immediate reaction, an accelerated reaction, may occur between 20 minutes and 48 hours after administration and may include urticaria, pruritus, and fever. Although laryngeal edema, laryngospasm, and hypotension occasionally occur, fatality is uncommon.

Delayed allergic reactions to penicillin therapy usually occur after 48 hours and sometimes as late as 2 to 4 weeks after initiation of therapy. Manifestations of this type of reaction include serum sickness-like symptoms (ie, fever, malaise, urticaria, myalgia, arthralgia, abdominal pain) and various skin rashes. Nausea, vomiting, diarrhea, stomatitis, black or hairy tongue, and other symptoms of gastrointestinal irritation may occur, especially during oral penicillin therapy.

Nervous System Reactions: Neurotoxic reactions similar to those observed with penicillin G may occur with large intravenous doses of the penicillinase-resistant penicillins especially in patients with renal insufficiency.

Urogenital Reactions: Renal tubular damage and interstitial nephritis have been associated with the administration of methicillin sodium and infrequently with the administration of nafcillin and Oxacillin. Manifestations of this reaction may include rash, fever, eosinophilia, hematuria, proteinuria, and renal insufficiency. Methicillin-induced nephropathy does not appear to be dose-related and is generally reversible upon prompt discontinuation of therapy.

Gastrointestinal Reactions: Pseudomembranous colitis has been reported with the use of Oxacillin Sodium (and other broad spectrum antibiotics); therefore, it is important to consider its diagnosis in patients who develop diarrhea in association with antibiotic use.

Treatment with broad spectrum antibiotics alters normal flora of the colon and may permit overgrowth of clostridia. Studies indicate a toxin produced by *Clostridium difficile* is one primary cause of antibiotic-associated colitis. Cholestyramine and colestipol resins have been shown to bind the toxin *in vitro.*

Mild cases of colitis may respond to drug discontinuance alone.

Moderate to severe cases should be managed with fluid, electrolyte and protein supplementation as indicated.

When the colitis is not relieved by drug discontinuance or when it is severe, oral vancomycin is the treatment of choice for antibiotic-associated pseudomembranous colitis produced by *C. difficile.* Other causes of colitis should also be considered.

Metabolic Reactions: Agranulocytosis, neutropenia, and bone marrow depression have been associated with the use of methicillin sodium, nafcillin, Oxacillin, and cloxacillin. Hepatotoxicity, characterized by fever, nausea, and vomiting associated with abnormal liver function tests, mainly elevated SGOT levels, has been associated with the use of Oxacillin and cloxacillin.

DOSAGE AND ADMINISTRATION

The penicillinase-resistant penicillins are available for oral administration and for intramuscular and intravenous injection. The sodium salts of methicillin, Oxacillin, and nafcillin may be administered parenterally and the sodium salts of cloxacillin, dicloxacillin, Oxacillin, and nafcillin are available for oral use.

Bacteriologic studies to determine the causative organisms and their sensitivity to the penicillinase-resistant penicillins should always be performed. Duration of therapy varies with the type and severity of infection as well as the overall condition of the patient, therefore it should be determined by the clinical and bacteriological response of the patient. In severe staphylococcal infections, therapy with penicillinase-resistant penicillins should be continued for at least 14 days. Therapy should be continued for at least 48 hours after the patient has become afebrile, asymptomatic, and cultures are negative. The treatment of endocarditis and osteomyelitis may require a longer term of therapy.

Concurrent administration of the penicillinase-resistant penicillins and probenecid increases and prolongs serum penicillin levels. Probenecid decreases the apparent volume of distribution and slows the rate of excretion by competitively inhibiting renal tubular secretion of penicillin. Penicillin-probenecid therapy is generally limited to those infections where very high serum levels of penicillin are necessary.

Oral preparations of the penicillinase-resistant penicillins should not be used as initial therapy in serious, life-threatening infections (see *"Precautions, General"*). Oral therapy with the penicillinase-resistant penicillins may be used to follow-up the previous use of a parenteral agent as soon as the clinical condition warrants. For intramuscular gluteal injections, care should be taken to avoid sciatic nerve injury. With intravenous administration, particularly in elderly patients, care should be taken because of the possibility of thrombophlebitis. (See related table).

DIRECTIONS FOR USE

For Intramuscular Use: Use sterile water for injection, USP. Add 1.4 ml to 250 mg Oxacillin, 2.7 ml to 500 mg Oxacillin, 5.7 ml to 1 gm Oxacillin, 11.5 ml to 2 gm Oxacillin, and 23 ml to 4 gm Oxacillin. Shake well until a clear solution is obtained. After reconstitution, each 1.5 ml of solution will contain 250 mg of active drug. The reconstituted solution is stable for 3 days at 70°F or for one week under refrigeration (40°F).

For Direct Intravenous Use: Use Sterile Water for Injection or sodium chloride injection. Add 5 mL to 250 mg and 500 mg Oxacillin, 10 mL to 1 gm Oxacillin, 20 ml to 2 gm Oxacillin, and 40 ml to 4 gm Oxacillin. Withdraw the entire contents and administer slowly over a period of approximately 10 minutes.

For Administration by Intravenous Drip: Reconstitute as directed above (For Direct Intravenous Use) prior to diluting with intravenous solution. (See related table).

Stability studies on Oxacillin Sodium at concentrations at 0.5 mg/mL and 2 mg/mL in various intravenous solutions listed below indicate the drug will lose less than 10% activity at room temperature (70°F) during a 6-hour period.

IV Solution: 5% Dextrose in Normal Saline
  10% D-Fructose in Water
  10% D-Fructose in Normal Saline
  Lactated Potassic Saline Injection
  10% Invert Sugar in Normal Saline
  10% Invert Sugar Plus 0.3% Potassium Chloride in Water
  Travert 10% Electrolyte #1
  Travert 10% Electrolyte #2
  Travert 10% Electrolyte #3

Only those solutions listed above should be used for the intravenous infusion of Oxacillin Sodium. The concentration of the antibiotic should fall within the range specified. The drug concentration and the rate and volume of the infusion should be adjusted so that the total dose of Oxacillin is administered before the drug loses its stability in the solution in use.

If another agent is used in conjunction with Oxacillin therapy, *it should not be physically mixed* with Oxacillin but should be administered separately.

Storage: Store sterile powder at controlled room temperature, 15°—30°C (59°—86°F).

J CODES
Up to 250 mg IV,IM—J2700

HOW SUPPLIED
CAPSULE: 250 MG

AVERAGE UNIT PRICE (AVAILABLE SIZES)		GENERIC A-RATED AVERAGE PRICE (GAAP)	
GENERIC	$0.29		
HCFA FUL (100s ea)	$0.22	100s	$28.57

BRAND/MANUFACTURER	NDC	SIZE	AWP
◆ GENERICS			
Raway	00686-3115-09	100s	$20.95
Biocraft	00332-3115-09	100s	$28.40
Qualitest	00603-4927-21	100s	$28.71
Major	00904-2709-60	100s	$28.75
Rugby	00536-1150-01	100s	$28.88
Geneva	00781-2004-01	100s	$29.42
Goldline	00182-1340-01	100s	$30.00
URL	00677-0932-01	100s	$30.05
Schein	00364-2059-01	100s	$30.08
BACTOCILL: SK Beecham Pharm	00029-6010-30	100s	$30.50

CAPSULE: 500 MG

AVERAGE UNIT PRICE (AVAILABLE SIZES)		GENERIC A-RATED AVERAGE PRICE (GAAP)	
GENERIC	$0.53	100s	$53.02
HCFA FUL (100s ea)	$0.42		

BRAND/MANUFACTURER	NDC	SIZE	AWP
◆ GENERICS			
Raway	00686-3117-09	100s	$33.15
Biocraft	00332-3117-09	100s	$52.50
Major	00904-2710-60	100s	$53.20
Moore,H.L.	00839-6413-06	100s	$53.45
Qualitest	00603-4928-21	100s	$54.45
Geneva	00781-2006-01	100s	$54.68
Schein	00364-2060-01	100s	$55.42
Goldline	00182-1341-01	100s	$55.50
BACTOCILL: SK Beecham Pharm	00029-6015-30	100s	$56.85
URL	00677-0933-01	100s	$57.00
Rugby	00536-1160-01	100s	$57.05

POWDER FOR INJECTION: 500 MG

AVERAGE UNIT PRICE (AVAILABLE SIZES)		GENERIC A-RATED AVERAGE PRICE (GAAP)	
GENERIC	$2.43	1s	$2.43

BRAND/MANUFACTURER	NDC	SIZE	AWP
◆ GENERICS			
BACTOCILL: Abbott Hosp	00029-6020-25	1s	$2.05
Apothecon	00015-7979-20	1s	$2.80

POWDER FOR INJECTION: 1 GM

AVERAGE UNIT PRICE (AVAILABLE SIZES)		GENERIC A-RATED AVERAGE PRICE (GAAP)	
GENERIC	$6.93	1s	$4.88
		10s	$130.55

BRAND/MANUFACTURER	NDC	SIZE	AWP
◆ GENERICS			
BACTOCILL: Abbott Hosp	00029-6025-22	1s	$3.10
BACTOCILL: Abbott Hosp	00029-6025-40	1s	$3.40
BACTOCILL: Abbott Hosp	00029-6025-21	1s	$4.35
Apothecon	00015-7981-20	1s	$5.45
Apothecon	00015-7981-18	1s	$5.64
Apothecon	00015-7981-28	1s	$7.36
VHA	00015-7981-22	10s	$111.10
VHA	00015-7981-21	10s	$150.00

POWDER FOR INJECTION: 2 GM

AVERAGE UNIT PRICE (AVAILABLE SIZES)		GENERIC A-RATED AVERAGE PRICE (GAAP)	
GENERIC	$12.09	1s	$8.35
		10s	$233.30

BRAND/MANUFACTURER	NDC	SIZE	AWP
◆ GENERICS			
BACTOCILL: Abbott Hosp	00029-6028-27	1s	$5.00
BACTOCILL: Abbott Hosp	00029-6028-40	1s	$5.30
BACTOCILL: Abbott Hosp	00029-6028-21	1s	$6.25

RECOMMENDED DOSAGES FOR OXACILLIN SODIUM FOR INJECTION, USP

Drug	Adults	Infants and Children < 40 kg (88 lbs)	Other Recommendations
Oxacillin	250 to 500 mg IM or IV every 4 to 6 hours (mild to moderate infections) 1 gram IM or IV every 4 to 6 hours (severe infections)	50 mg/kg/day IM or IV in equally divided doses every 6 hours (mild to moderate infections) 100 mg/kg/day IM or IV in equally divided doses every 4 to 6 hours (severe infections)	Premature and Neonates 25 mg/kg/day IM or IV

STABILITY PERIODS FOR OXACILLIN SODIUM FOR INJECTION, USP

Concentration mg/ml	Sterile H₂O for Injection	Isotonic Sodium Chloride	M/6 Molar Sodium Lactate Solution	5% Dextrose in H₂	5% Dextrose in 0.45% NaCl	10% Invert Sugar	Lactated Ringers Solution
			Room Temperature (25°C)				
10—100	4 Days	4 Days					
10—30			24 Hrs		24 Hrs		
0.5—2				6 Hrs		6 Hrs	6 Hrs
			Refrigeration (4°C)				
10—100	7 Days	7 Days					
10—30			4 Days	4 Days	4 Days	4 Days	4 Days
			Frozen (−15°C)				
50—100	30 Days						
250/1.5 ml	30 Days						
100		30 Days					
10—100			30 Days	30 Days	30 Days	30 Days	30 Days

◆ RATED THERAPEUTICALLY EQUIVALENT; ◇ THERAPEUTIC EQUIVALENCE UNCONFIRMED; ○ UNRATED

BRAND/MANUFACTURER	NDC	SIZE	AWP
Apothecon	00015-7970-20	1s	$10.48
Apothecon	00015-7970-18	1s	$10.66
Apothecon	00015-7970-28	1s	$12.38
VHA	00015-7970-22	10s	$213.80
VHA	00015-7970-21	10s	$252.80

POWDER FOR INJECTION: 4 GM

BRAND/MANUFACTURER	NDC	SIZE	AWP
◆ GENERICS			
BACTOCILL: Abbott Hosp	00029-6030-26	1s	$9.35

POWDER FOR INJECTION: 10 GM

AVERAGE UNIT PRICE (AVAILABLE SIZES)		GENERIC A-RATED AVERAGE PRICE (GAAP)	
GENERIC	$45.56	1s	$45.56

BRAND/MANUFACTURER	NDC	SIZE	AWP
◆ GENERICS			
BACTOCILL: Abbott Hosp	00029-6032-21	1s	$23.75
Apothecon	00015-7103-28	1s	$67.36

POWDER FOR RECONSTITUTION: 250 MG/5 ML

AVERAGE UNIT PRICE (AVAILABLE SIZES)		GENERIC A-RATED AVERAGE PRICE (GAAP)	
GENERIC	$0.07	100 ml	$6.65
HCFA FUL (100 ml)	$0.05		

BRAND/MANUFACTURER	NDC	SIZE	AWP
◆ GENERICS			
Raway	00686-4157-32	100 ml	$3.75
Rugby	00536-1170-82	100 ml	$4.69
Biocraft	00332-4157-32	100 ml	$5.50
Major	00904-1519-04	100 ml	$5.60
Qualitest	00603-6584-64	100 ml	$5.95
Goldline	00182-7069-70	100 ml	$6.45
Apothecon	00015-7985-40	100 ml	$14.58

Oxamniquine

DECRIPTION
Oxamniquine is a tetrahydroquinoline derivative for the oral treatment of *Schistosoma mansoni* infections. It is 1,2,3,4-tetrahydro-2-[[(1-methyle-thyl)amino] - 7 - nitro - 6 - quinolinemethanol. Oxamniquine is a yellow-orange crystalline solid which is sparingly soluble in water, but soluble in methanol, acetone, and chloroform.

The capsules contain 250 mg of Oxamniquine.

Following is its chemical structure:

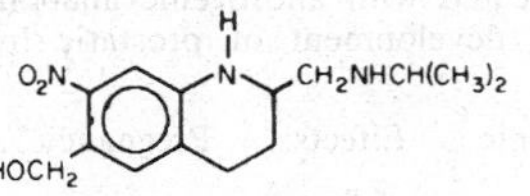

CLINICAL PHARMACOLOGY
Oxamniquine is well absorbed when administered orally. Human plasma concentrations reach a peak at 1 to 1.5 hours after oral administration of therapeutic doses, with a plasma half-life of 1 to 2.5 hours. It is extensively metabolized to inactive acidic metabolites which are largely excreted in the urine.

Male schistosomes are more susceptible than females, but after treatment with Oxamniquine the residual female schistosomes cease to lay eggs thus losing the parasitological aspect of their pathological significance. Animal studies with immature *S. mansoni* infections have demonstrated Oxamniquine to be highly active in the immediate post-infection phase. Oxamniquine significantly reduces the egg load of *S. mansoni*.

INDICATIONS
Oxamniquine is indicated for all stages of *S. mansoni* infection, including the acute phase and the chronic phase with hepatosplenic involvement.

CONTRAINDICATIONS
At present, there are no known contraindications to the administration of Oxamniquine.

WARNINGS
In rare instances epileptiform convulsions have been observed within the first few hours after ingestion of Oxamniquine. When a convulsion occurred, it was mostly in a patient with a previous history of a convulsive condition. Oxamniquine should be used with care in such individuals and they should remain under medical supervision with facilities available to treat a convulsion should it occur.

PRECAUTIONS
Pregnancy Category C: Oxamniquine has been shown to have an embryocidal effect in rabbits and mice when given in doses 10 times the human dose.

There are no adequate and well controlled studies in pregnant women. Oxamniquine should be used during pregnancy only if the potential benefit justifies the potential risk to the fetus.

Nursing Mothers: It is not known whether this drug is excreted in human milk.

Because many drugs are excreted in human milk, caution should be exercised when Oxamniquine is administered to a nursing mother.

ADVERSE EFFECTS
Oxamniquine is generally well tolerated and toleration is improved if the doses are given after food. Transitory dizziness/drowsiness occurred in approximately one-third of the patients assessed. Other effects observed to a lesser degree are headache, nausea, vomiting, abdominal pain and anorexia. Urticaria has also been reported. In rare instances epileptiform convulsions have been observed (see "Warnings").

Minor and transient abnormalities in laboratory data have been observed after treatment with Oxamniquine which were not considered to be drug-related and were of no clinical significance. They included rare instances of mild to moderate liver enzyme elevations but there was no evidence of hepatotoxicity even in patients with severe hepatosplenic involvement. There was evidence, however, of liver abnormalities in animals with the female rat being uniquely sensitive to relatively low doses.

DOSAGE AND ADMINISTRATION
ADULTS
The recommended dosage is 12 to 15 mg per kilogram of body weight given as a single oral dose in patients with Western Hemisphere strains of *S. mansoni*. The recomended capsule dosage according to body weight is as follows:

Body Weight (kg)	No. of Capsules (250 mg)
30- 40	2
41- 60	3
61- 80	4
81-100	5

CHILDREN
The recommended dosage for children under 30 kg in weight is 20 mg/kg of body weight given in two divided doses of 10 mg/kg in one day with an interval of 2 to 8 hours between doses. Toleration is improved if the doses are given after food.

HOW SUPPLIED
CAPSULE: 250 MG

BRAND/MANUFACTURER	NDC	SIZE	AWP
○ BRAND			
VANSIL: Pfizer Labs	00069-6410-24	24s	$117.81

Oxandrolone

DESCRIPTION
Oxandrolone oral tablets contain 2.5 mg of the anabolic steroid Oxandrolone. Oxandrolone is 17β-hydroxy-17α-methyl-2-oxa-5α-androstan-3-one.

Following is its chemical structure:

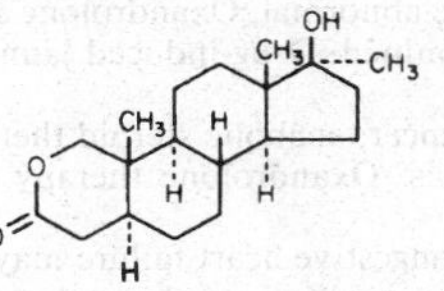

CLINICAL PHARMACOLOGY
Anabolic steroids are synthetic derivatives of testosterone. Certain clinical effects and adverse reactions demonstrate the androgenic properties of this class of drugs. Complete dissociation of anabolic and androgenic effects has not been achieved. The actions of anabolic steroids are therefore similar to those of male sex hormones with the possibility of causing serious disturbances of growth and sexual development if given to young children. Anabolic steroids suppress the gonadotropic functions of the pituitary and may exert a direct effect upon the testes.

During exogenous administration of anabolic androgens, endogenous testosterone release is inhibited through inhibition of pituitary luteinizing hormone (LH). At large doses, spermatogenesis may be suppressed through feedback inhibition of pituitary follicle-stimulating hormone (FSH).

Anabolic steroids have been reported to increase low-density lipoproteins and decrease high-density lipoproteins. These levels revert to normal on discontinuation of treatment.

INDICATIONS AND USAGE
Oxandrolone is indicated as adjunctive therapy to promote weight gain after weight loss following extensive surgery, chronic infections, or severe trauma, and in some patients who without definite pathophysiologic reasons fail to gain or to maintain normal weight, to offset the protein catabolism associated with

➤ SHOWN IN PRODUCT IDENTIFICATION GUIDE

prolonged administration of corticosteroids, and for the relief of the bone pain frequently accompanying osteoporosis. (See "Dosage and Administration".)

UNLABELED USES

Oxandrolone is used alone or as an adjunct in the treatment of wasting associated with human immunodeficiency virus infection (AIDS), alcoholic hepatitis, and inadequate growth hormone secretion. In addition, Oxandrolone is used in the treatment of male hypertriglyceridemia, anemia associated with acute and chronic renal failure, and Turner's syndrome.

DRUG ABUSE AND DEPENDENCE

Oxandrolone is classified as a controlled substance under the Anabolic Steroids Control Act of 1990 and has been assigned to Schedule III (non-narcotic).

CONTRAINDICATIONS

1. Known or suspected carcinoma of the prostate or the male breast.
2. Carcinoma of the breast in females with hypercalcemia (androgenic anabolic steroids may stimulate osteolytic bone resorption).
3. Pregnancy, because of possible masculinization of the fetus. Oxandrolone has been shown to cause embryotoxicity, fetotoxicity, infertility, and masculinization of female animal offspring when given in doses 9 times the human dose.
4. Nephrosis of nephrotic phase of nephritis.
5. Hypercalcemia.

WARNINGS

PELIOSIS HEPATIS, A CONDITION IN WHICH LIVER AND SOMETIMES SPLENIC TISSUE IS REPLACED WITH BLOOD-FILLED CYSTS, HAS BEEN REPORTED IN PATIENTS RECEIVING ANDROGENIC ANABOLIC STEROID THERAPY. THESE CYSTS ARE SOMETIMES PRESENT WITH MINIMAL HEPATIC DYSFUNCTION, BUT AT OTHER TIMES THEY HAVE BEEN ASSOCIATED WITH LIVER FAILURE. THEY ARE OFTEN NOT RECOGNIZED UNTIL LIFE-THREATENING LIVER FAILURE OR INTRA-ABDOMINAL HEMORRHAGE DEVELOPS. WITHDRAWAL OF DRUG USUALLY RESULTS IN COMPLETE DISAPPEARANCE OF LESIONS.

LIVER CELL TUMORS ARE ALSO REPORTED. MOST OFTEN THESE TUMORS ARE BENIGN AND ANDROGEN-DEPENDENT, BUT FATAL MALIGNANT TUMORS HAVE BEEN REPORTED. WITHDRAWAL OF DRUG OFTEN RESULTS IN REGRESSION OR CESSATION OF PROGRESSION OF THE TUMOR. HOWEVER, HEPATIC TUMORS ASSOCIATED WITH ANDROGENS OR ANABOLIC STEROIDS ARE MUCH MORE VASCULAR THAN OTHER HEPATIC TUMORS AND MAY BE SILENT UNTIL LIFE-THREATENING INTRA-ABDOMINAL HEMORRHAGE DEVELOPS. BLOOD LIPID CHANGES THAT ARE KNOWN TO BE ASSOCIATED WITH INCREASED RISK OF ATHEROSCLEROSIS ARE SEEN IN PATIENTS TREATED WITH ANDROGENS OR ANABOLIC STEROIDS. THESE CHANGES INCLUDE DECREASED HIGH-DENSITY LIPOPROTEINS AND SOMETIMES INCREASED LOW-DENSITY LIPOPROTEINS. THE CHANGES MAY BE VERY MARKED AND COULD HAVE A SERIOUS IMPACT ON THE RISK OF ATHEROSCLEROSIS AND CORONARY ARTERY DISEASE.

Cholestatic hepatitis and jaundice may occur with 17-alpha-alkylated androgens at a relatively low dose. If cholestatic hepatitis with jaundice appears or if liver function tests become abnormal, Oxandrolone should be discontinued and the etiology should be determined. Drug-induced jaundice is reversible when the medication is discontinued.

In patients with breast cancer, anabolic steroid therapy may cause hypercalcemia by stimulating osteolysis. Oxandrolone therapy should be discontinued if hypercalcemia occurs.

Edema with or without congestive heart failure may be a serious complication in patients with preexisting cardiac, renal, or hepatic disease. Concomitant administration of adrenal cortical steroid or ACTH may increase the edema.

In children, androgen therapy may accelerate bone maturation without producing compensatory gain in linear growth. This adverse effect results in compromised adult height. The younger the child, the greater the risk of compromising final mature height. The effect on bone maturation should be monitored by assessing bone age of the left wrist and hand every six months. (See "Precautions: Laboratory Tests.")

Geriatric patients treated with androgenic anabolic steroids may be at an increased risk for the development of prostatic hypertrophy and prostatic carcinoma.

ANABOLIC STEROIDS HAVE NOT BEEN SHOWN TO ENHANCE ATHLETIC ABILITY.

PRECAUTIONS

GENERAL

Women should be observed for signs of virilization (deepening of the voice, hirsutism, acne, clitoromegaly). Discontinuation of drug therapy at the time of evidence of mild virilism is necessary to prevent irreversible virilization. Some virilizing changes in women are irreversible even after prompt discontinuance of therapy and are not prevented by concomitant use of estrogens. Menstrual irregularities may also occur.

Anabolic steroids may cause suppression of clotting factors II, V, VII, and X, and an increase in prothombin time.

INFORMATION FOR PATIENTS

The physician should instruct patients to report any of the following side effects of androgens:

Males: Too frequent or persistent erections of the penis, appearance or aggravation of acne.

Females: Hoarseness, acne, changes in menstrual periods, or more facial hair.

All Patients: Nausea, vomiting, changes in skin color, or ankle swelling.

LABORATORY TESTS

Women with disseminated breast carcinoma should have frequent determination of urine and serum calcium levels during the course of therapy (see "Warnings").

Because of the hepatotoxicity associated with the use of 17-alpha-alkylated androgens, liver function tests should be obtained periodically.

Periodic (every 6 months) x-ray examinations of bone age should be made during treatment of children to determine the rate of bone maturation and the effects of androgen therapy on the epiphyseal centers.

Serum lipids and high-density lipoprotein cholesterol determinations should be done periodically as androgenic anabolic steroids have been reported to increase low-density lipoproteins. Serum cholesterol levels may increase during therapy. Therefore, caution is required when administering these agents to patients with a history of myocardial infarction or coronary artery disease. Serial determinations of serum cholesterol should be made and therapy adjusted accordingly.

Hemoglobin and hematocrit should be checked periodically for polycythemia in patients who are receiving high doses of anabolic steroids.

DRUG INTERACTIONS

Anticoagulants: Anabolic steroids may increase sensitivity to oral anticoagulants. Dosage of the anticoagulant may have to be decreased in order to maintain desired prothrombin time. Patients receiving oral anticoagulant therapy require close monitoring, especially whom anabolic steroids are started or stopped.

Oral Hypoglycemic Agents: Oxandrolone may inhibit the metabolism of oral hypoglycemic agents.

Adrenal Steroids or ACTH: In patients with edema, concomitant administration with adrenal cortical steroids or ACTH may increase the edema.

Drug/Laboratory Test Interactions: Anabolic steroids may decrease levels of thyroxine-binding globulin, resulting in decreased total T_4 serum levels and increased resin uptake of T_3 and T_4. Free thyroid hormone levels remain unchanged. In addition, a decrease in PBI and radioactive iodine uptake may occur.

CARCINOGENESIS, MUTAGENESIS, IMPAIRMENT OF FERTILITY

Animal Data: Oxandrolone has not been tested in laboratory animals for carcinogenic or mutagenic effects. In two-year chronic oral rat studies, a dose-related reduction of spermatogenesis and decreased organ weights (testes, prostate, seminal vesicles, ovaries, uterus, adrenals, and pituitary) were shown.

Human Data: Liver cell tumors have been reported in patients receiving long-term therapy with androgenic anabolic steroids in high doses (see "Warnings"). Withdrawal of the drugs did not lead to regression of the tumors in all cases.

Geriatric patients treated with androgenic anabolic steroids may be at an increased risk for the development of prostatic hypertrophy and prostatic carcinoma.

Pregnancy: Teratogenic Effects: Pregnancy Category X. (See "Contraindications".)

Nursing Mothers: It is not known whether anabolic steroids are excreted in human milk. Because of the potential for serious adverse reactions in nursing infants from Oxandrolone, a decision should be made whether to discontinue nursing or to discontinue the drug, taking into account the importance of the drug to the mother.

Pediatric Use: Anabolic agents may accelerate epiphyseal maturation more rapidly than linear growth in children and the effect may continue for six months after the drug has been stopped. Therefore, therapy should be monitored by x-ray studies at six-months intervals in order to avoid the risk of compromising adult height. Androgenic anabolic steroid therapy should be used very cautiously in children and only by specialists who are aware of the effects on bone maturation. (See "Warnings".)

ADVERSE REACTIONS

The following adverse reactions have been associated with use of anabolic steroids:

Hepatic: Cholestatic jaundice with, rarely, hepatic necrosis and death. Hepatocellular neoplasms and peliosis hepatis with long-term therapy (see "Warnings"). Reversible changes in liver function tests also occur including increased bromsulfophthalein (BSP) retention, and increases in serum bilirubin, aspartate aminotransferase (AST, SGOT) and alkaline phosphatase.

In males:

Prepubertal: Phallic enlargement and increased frequency or persistence of erections.

Postpubertal: Inhibition of testicular function, testicular atrophy and oligospermia, impotence, chronic priapism, epididymitis, and bladder irritability.

In females: Clitoral enlargement, menstrual irregularities.

CNS: Habituation, excitation, insomnia, depression, and changes in libido.

◆ RATED THERAPEUTICALLY EQUIVALENT; ◇ THERAPEUTIC EQUIVALENCE UNCONFIRMED; ○ UNRATED

Hematologic: Bleeding in patients on concomitant anticoagulant therapy.

Breast: Gynecomastia.

Larynx: Deepening of the voice in females.

Hair: Hirsutism and male pattern baldness in females.

Skin: Acne (especially in females and prepubertal males).

Skeletal: Premature closure of epiphyses in children (see *"Precautions; Pediatric Use"*).

Fluid and electrolytes: Edema, retention of serum electrolytes (sodium chloride, potassium, phosphate, calcium).

Metabolic/Endocrine: Decreased glucose tolerance (see *"Precautions; Laboratory tests"*), increased creatinine excretion, increased serum levels of creatinine phosphokinase (CPK). Masculinization of the fetus. Inhibition of gonadotropin secretion.

OVERDOSAGE

No symptoms or signs associated with overdosage have been reported. It is possible that sodium and water retention may occur.

The oral LD_{50} of Oxandrolone in mice and dogs is greater than 5,000 mg/kg. No specific antidote is known, but gastric lavage may be used.

DOSAGE AND ADMINISTRATION

Therapy with anabolic steroids is adjunctive to and not a replacement for conventional therapy. The duration of therapy with Oxandrolone will depend on the response of the patient and the possible appearance of adverse reactions. Therapy should be intermittent.

Adults: The usual adult dosage of Oxandrolone is one 2.5-mg tablet two to four times daily. However, the response of individuals to anabolic steroids varies, and a daily dosage of as little as 2.5 mg or as much as 20 mg may be required to achieve the desired response. A course of therapy of two to four weeks is usually adequate. This may be repeated intermittently as indicated.

Children: For children the total daily dosage of Oxandrolone is $\leq$ 0.1 mg per kilogram body weight or $\leq$ 0.045 mg per pound of body weight. This may be repeated intermittently as indicated.

HOW SUPPLIED
TABLETS (C-III): 2.5 MG

BRAND/MANUFACTURER	NDC	SIZE	AWP
○ GENERICS			
OXANDRIN: BTG Pharm Corp	54396-0111-11	100s	$300.00

Oxaprozin

DESCRIPTION

Oxaprozin is a nonsteroidal anti-inflammatory drug (NSAID), chemically designated as 4,5-diphenyl-2-oxazole-propionic acid.

The empirical formula for Oxaprozin is $C_{18}H_{15}NO_3$, and the molecular weight is 293. Oxaprozin is a white to off-white powder with a slight odor and a melting point of 162°C to 163°C. It is slightly soluble in alcohol and insoluble in water, with an octanol/water partition coefficient of 4.8 at physiologic pH (7.4). The pK_a in water is 4.3.

Oxaprozin oral caplets contain 600 mg of Oxaprozin.

Following is its chemical structure:

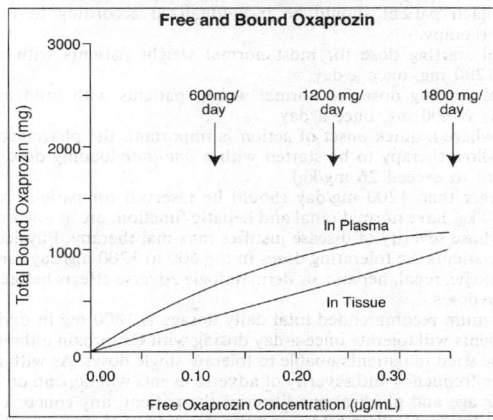

CLINICAL PHARMACOLOGY

Oxaprozin is a nonsteroidal anti-inflammatory drug (NSAID) that has been shown to have anti-inflammatory, analgesic, and antipyretic properties in animal models. As with other nonsteroidal anti-inflammatory agents, all of the modes of action of Oxaprozin are not fully established. Oxaprozin is an inhibitor of several steps along the arachidonic acid pathway of prostaglandin synthesis, and one of its modes of action is presumed to be due to the inhibition of prostaglandin synthesis at the site of inflammation.

Pharmacodynamics: Acute analgesic effects are demonstrable in humans after a single 1200-mg dose of Oxaprozin, but anti-inflammatory effects are not reliably achieved after a single dose. Because of the long half-life of Oxaprozin, it takes several days of dosing to reach steady state (see *"Pharmacokinetics"*).

Pharmacokinetics: The pharmacokinetics of Oxaprozin have been evaluated in approximately 400 individuals, which have included patients with rheumatoid arthritis, osteoarthritis, healthy elderly volunteers, and patients with cardiac, renal, and hepatic disease.

Oxaprozin demonstrates high oral bioavailability (95%), with peak plasma concentrations occurring between 3 and 5 hours after dosing. Food may reduce the rate of absorption of Oxaprozin, but the extent of absorption is unchanged. Antacids have no effect on the rate or extent of Oxaprozin absorption.

As is true for most NSAIDs, approximately 99.9% of the Oxaprozin present in plasma is bound to albumin. The fraction of the drug present in the tissues across the therapeutic dosage range ranges between 40% and 60% of the total drug in the body and is proportional to dose, since the tissue sites are not saturated with the usual clinical doses.

Figure 1 shows the amount of Oxaprozin in the plasma and in the tissue as a function of dose and the concentration of the free drug.

Figure 1
Amount of Oxaprozin in plasma and tissue as a function of dose and free (unbound) Oxaprozin concentration

Unbound Oxaprozin is the pharmacologically active component: it is able to distribute into tissues and to be cleared from the body. The average unbound concentration is a function of the tissue-bound and plasma-bound drug, and it increases proportionally with dose.

As the amount of Oxaprozin in the tissues increases at higher dose, the plasma concentration of Oxaprozin is limited by saturation of plasma protein binding. In addition, the increase in free (unbound) Oxaprozin results in an increase in clearance. Both of these contribute to the total plasma concentration of Oxaprozin increasing less than proportionally with dose.

Oxaprozin kinetics were modeled using a two-compartment model with first-order absorption and protein binding that becomes saturable in the clinical dosage range. As the dose is increased from 600 to 1200 mg daily, the steady state clearance of total Oxaprozin increases from 0.25 to 0.34 L/hr, the steady state apparent volume of distribution increases from 10 to 12.5 L, and the accumulation half-life decreases from 25 to 21 hours. The terminal elimination half-life is approximately twice as long as the accumulation half-life because of the increased binding and decreased clearance at lower concentrations. Steady state concentrations in clinical usage are achieved in 4 to 7 days.

Plasma levels of total Oxaprozin (free and bound drug) in studies of patients taking 600 to 1200 mg/day for several months ranged from 98 to 230 μg/mL, corresponding to estimated levels of free drug ranging from about 0.10 to 0.40 μg/mL.

Oxaprozin is primarily metabolized in the liver, by both microsomal oxidation (65%) and glucuronic acid conjugation (35%). A small amount (< 5%) of active phenolic metabolites is produced, but the contribution to overall activity is minimal. All conjugated metabolites are inactive.

Biliary excretion of unchanged Oxaprozin is a minor elimination pathway, and enterohepatic recycling of Oxaprozin is insignificant. The glucuronide metabolites can be recovered from the urine (65%) and feces (35%), while unchanged Oxaprozin is poorly excreted.

Renal dysfunction appears to alter Oxaprozin binding and to reduce unbound clearance and unbound volume of distribution; dosage reductions should be made (see *"Precautions: General"*).

Age, gender, and well-compensated cardiac failure do not affect the plasma protein binding or the pharmacokinetics of Oxaprozin.

Like other NSAIDs exhibiting a high degree of protein binding and a primarily metabolic route of elimination, Oxaprozin has the potential for drug-drug interactions (see *"Precautions: Drug interactions"*).

CLINICAL STUDIES

Rheumatoid Arthritis: Oxaprozin was evaluated for managing the signs and symptoms of rheumatoid arthritis in placebo and active controlled clinical trials in a total of 646 patients. Oxaprozin was given in single or divided daily doses of 600 to 1800 mg/day and was found to be comparable to 2600 to 3900 mg/day of aspirin. At these doses there was a trend (over all trials) for Oxaprozin to be more effective and cause fewer gastrointestinal side effects than aspirin.

Oxaprozin was given as a once-a-day dose of 1200 mg in most of the clinical trials, but larger doses (up to 26 mg/kg or 1800 mg/day) were used in selected patients. In some patients, Oxaprozin may be better tolerated in divided doses. Due to its long half-life, several days of Oxaprozin therapy were needed for the drug to reach its full effect (see *"Individualization of Dosage"*).

Osteoarthritis: Oxaprozin was evaluated for the management of the signs and symptoms of osteoarthritis in a total of 616 patients in active controlled clinical trials against aspirin (N = 464), piroxicam (N = 102), and other NSAIDs. Oxaprozin was given both in variable (600 to 1200 mg/day) and in fixed (1200 mg/day) dosing schedules in either single or divided doses. In these trials, Oxaprozin was found to be comparable to 2600 to 3200 mg/day doses of aspirin or 20 mg/day doses of piroxicam. Oxaprozin was effective both in once-daily and in divided dosing schedules. In controlled clinical trials several days of Oxaprozin therapy were needed for the drug to reach its full effects (see *"Individualization of Dosage"*).

INDIVIDUALIZATION OF DOSAGE

Oxaprozin like other NSAIDs, shows considerable interindividual differences in both pharmacokinetics and clinical response (pharmacodynamics). Therefore, the dosage for each patient should be individualized according to the patient's response to therapy.

The usual starting dose for most normal weight patients with rheumatoid arthritis is 1200 mg, once a day.

The usual starting dose for normal weight patients with mild to moderate osteoarthritis is 600 mg, once a day.

In cases where a quick onset of action is important, the pharmacokinetics of Oxaprozin allow therapy to be started with a *one-time* loading dose of 1200 to 1800 mg (not to exceed 26 mg/kg).

Doses larger than 1200 mg/day should be reserved for patients who weight more than 50 kg, have normal renal and hepatic function, are at low risk of peptic ulcer, and whose severity of disease justifies maximal therapy. Physicians should ensure that patients are tolerating doses in the 600 to 1200 mg/day range without gastroenterologic, renal, hepatic, or dermatologic adverse effects before advancing to the larger doses.

The maximum recommended total daily dosage is 1800 mg in divided doses.

Most patients will tolerate once-a-day dosing with Oxaprozin although divided doses may be tried in patients unable to tolerate single doses. As with all drugs of this class, the frequency and severity of adverse events will depend on the dose of the drug, the age and physical condition of the patient, any concurrent medical diagnoses, individual vulnerability, and the duration of therapy. In clinical trials of Oxaprozin, no clear dose-response relationship was seen for serious adverse effects, but physicians are cautioned that the reported safety data were developed in patients who had successfully taken lower doses of Oxaprozin before being advanced above 1200 mg/day.

Experience with other NSAIDs has shown that starting therapy with maximal doses in patients at increased risk due to renal or hepatic disease, low body weight, advanced age, a known ulcer diathesis, or known sensitivity to NSAID effects is likely to increase the frequency of adverse events and is not recommended (see *"Precautions"*).

INDICATIONS AND USAGE

Oxaprozin is indicated for acute and long-term use in the management of the signs and symptoms of osteoarthritis and rheumatoid arthritis.

UNLABELED USES

Oxaprozin is used alone or as an adjunct in the treatment of ankylosing spondylitis, juvenile rheumatoid arthritis, Behcet's disease, and acute gout. It is also used to provide more prolonged pain relief in patients with postsurgical oral pain, tendinitis, and bursitis.

CONTRAINDICATIONS

Oxaprozin should not be used in patients with previously demonstrated hypersensitivity to Oxaprozin or any of its components or in individuals with the complete or partial syndrome of nasal polyps, angioedema, and bronchospastic reactivity to aspirin or other nonsteroidal anti-inflammatory drugs (NSAIDs).

Severe and occasionally fatal asthmatic and anaphylactic reactions have been reported in patients receiving NSAIDs, and there have been rare reports of anaphylaxis in patients taking Oxaprozin.

WARNINGS

RISK OF GASTROINTESTINAL (GI) ULCERATION, BLEEDING, AND PERFORATION WITH NONSTEROIDAL ANTI-INFLAMMATORY DRUG THERAPY: Serious gastrointestinal toxicity, such as bleeding, ulceration, and perforation, can occur at any time, with or without warning symptoms, in patients treated with NSAIDs. Although minor upper gastrointestinal problems, such as dyspepsia, are common, and usually develop early in therapy, physicians should remain alert for ulceration and bleeding in patients treated chronically with NSAIDs, even in the absence of previous GI tract symptoms. In patients observed in clinical trials for several months to 2 years, symptomatic upper GI ulcers, gross bleeding, or perforation appear to occur in approximately 1% of patients treated for 3 to 6 months, and in about 2% to 4% of patients treated for 1 year. Physicians should inform patients about the signs and/or symptoms of serious GI toxicity and what steps to take if they occur.

Patients at risk for developing peptic ulceration and bleeding are those with a prior history of serious GI events, alcoholism, smoking, or other factors known to be associated with peptic ulcer disease. Elderly or debilitated patients seem to tolerate ulceration or bleeding less well than other individuals, and most spontaneous reports of fatal GI events are in these populations. Studies to date are inconclusive concerning the relative risk of various nonsteroidal anti-inflammatory drugs (NSAIDs) in causing such reactions. High doses of any NSAID probably carry a greater risk of these reactions, and substantial benefit should be anticipated to patients prior to prescribing maximal doses of Oxaprozin.

PRECAUTIONS

GENERAL

Hepatic Effects: As with other nonsteroidal anti-inflammatory drugs, borderline elevations of one or more liver tests may occur in up to 15% of patients. These abnormalities may progress, remain essentially unchanged, or resolve with continued therapy. The SGPT (ALT) test is probably the most sensitive indicator of liver dysfunction. Meaningful (3 times the upper limit of normal) elevations of SGOT (AST) occurred in controlled clinical trials of Oxaprozin in just under 1% of patients. A patient with symptoms and/or signs suggesting liver dysfunction or in whom an abnormal liver test has occurred should be evaluated for evidence of the development of more severe hepatic reaction while on therapy with this drug. Severe hepatic reactions including jaundice have been reported with Oxaprozin, and there may be a risk of fatal hepatitis with Oxaprozin, such as has been seen with other NSAIDs. Although such reactions are rare, if abnormal liver tests persist or worsen, clinical signs and symptoms consistent with liver disease develop, or systemic manifestations occur (eosinophilia, rash, fever), Oxaprozin should be discontinued.

Well-compensated hepatic cirrhosis does not appear to alter the disposition of unbound Oxaprozin, so dosage adjustment is not necessary. However, the primary route of elimination of Oxaprozin is hepatic metabolism, so caution should be observed in patients with severe hepatic dysfunction.

Renal Effects: Acute interstitial nephritis hematuria, and proteinuria have been reported with Oxaprozin as with other NSAIDs. Long-term administration of some nonsteroidal anti-inflammatory drugs to animals has resulted in renal papillary necrosis and other abnormal renal pathology. This was not observed with Oxaprozin, but the clinical significance of this difference is unknown.

A second form of renal toxicity has been seen in patients with preexisting conditions leading to a reduction in renal blood flow, where the renal prostaglandins have a supportive role in the maintenance of renal perfusion. In these patients administration of a nonsteroidal anti-inflammatory drug may cause a dose-dependent reduction in prostaglandin formation and may precipitate overt renal decompensation. Patients at greatest risk of this reaction are those with previously impaired renal function, heart failure, or liver dysfunction, those taking diuretics, and the elderly. Discontinuation of nonsteroidal anti-inflammatory drug therapy is often followed by recovery to the pretreatment state. Those patients at high risk who chronically take Oxaprozin should have renal function monitored if they have signs or symptoms that may be consistent with mild azotemia, such as malaise, fatigue, or loss of appetite. As with all NSAID therapy, patients may occasionally develop some elevation of serum creatinine and BUN levels without any signs or symptoms. The pharmacokinetics of Oxaprozin may be significantly altered in patients with renal insufficiency or in patients who are undergoing hemodialysis. Such patients should be started on doses of 600 mg/day, with cautious dosage increases if the desired effect is not obtained. Oxaprozin is not dialyzed because of its high degree of protein binding.

Like other NSAIDs, Oxaprozin may worsen fluid retention by the kidneys in patients with uncompensated cardiac failure due to its effect on prostaglandins. It should be used with caution in patients with a history of hypertension, cardiac decompensation, in patients on chronic diuretic therapy, or in those with other conditions predisposing to fluid retention.

Photosensitivity: Oxaprozin has been associated with rash and/or mild photosensitivity in dermatologic testing. An increased incidence of rash on sun-exposed skin was seen in some patients in the clinical trials.

Recommended Laboratory Testing: Because serious GI tract ulceration and bleeding can occur without warning symptoms, physicians should follow chronically treated patients for the signs and symptoms of ulceration and bleeding and should inform them of the importance of this follow-up (see *"Warnings"*).

Anemia may occur in patients receiving Oxaprozin or other NSAIDs. This may be due to fluid retention, gastrointestinal blood loss, or an incompletely described effect upon erythrogenesis. Patients on long-term treatment with Oxaprozin should have their hemoglobin or hematocrit values determined at appropriate intervals as determined by the clinical situation.

Oxaprozin, like other NSAIDs, can affect platelet aggregation and prolong bleeding time. Oxaprozin should be used with caution in patients with underlying hemostatic defects or in those who are undergoing surgical procedures where a high degree of hemostasis is needed.

Information for Patients: Oxaprozin, like other drugs of its class, nonsteroidal anti-inflammatory drugs (NSAIDs), is not free of side effects. The side effects of these drugs can cause discomfort and, rarely, serious side effects, such as gastrointestinal bleeding, which may result in hospitalization and even fatal outcomes.

NSAIDs are often essential agents in the management of arthritis, but they may also be commonly employed for conditions that are less serious.

Physicians may wish to discuss with their patients the potential risks see *"Warnings"*, *"Precautions"* and *"Adverse Reactions"*) and likely benefits of Oxaprozin treatment, particularly in less-serious conditions where treatment without Oxaprozin may represent an acceptable alternative to both the patient and the physician.

Patients receiving Oxaprozin may benefit from physician instruction in the symptoms of the more common or serious gastrointestinal, renal, hepatic, hematologic, and dermatologic adverse effects.

Laboratory Test Interactions: False positive urine drug screening tests for benzodiazepines have been reported in patients taking Oxaprozin. This is due to cross-reactivity. Confirmatory testing is recommended when such screening test results are positive.

◆ RATED THERAPEUTICALLY EQUIVALENT; ◇ THERAPEUTIC EQUIVALENCE UNCONFIRMED; ○ UNRATED

DRUG INTERACTIONS

Aspirin: Concomitant administration of Oxaprozin and aspirin is not recommended because oxaprozin displaces salicylates from plasma protein binding sites. Coadministration would be expected to increase the risk of salicylate toxicity.

Oral Anticoagulants: The anticoagulant effects of warfarin were not affected by the coadministration of 1200 mg/day of Oxaprozin. Nevertheless, caution should be exercised when adding any drug that affects platelet function to the regimen of patients receiving oral anticoagulants.

H₂-receptor Antagonists: The total body clearance of Oxaprozin was reduced by 20% in subjects who concurrently received therapeutic doses of cimetidine or ranitidine; no other pharmacokinetic parameter was affected. A change of clearance of this magnitude lies within the range of normal variation and is unlikely to produce a clinically detectable difference in the outcome of therapy.

Beta-blockers: Subjects receiving 1200 mg Oxaprozin qd with 100 mg metoprolol bid exhibited statistically significant but transient increases in sitting and standing blood pressures after 14 days. Therefore, as with all NSAIDs, routine blood pressure monitoring should be considered in these patients when starting Oxaprozin therapy.

Other drugs: The coadministration of Oxaprozin and antacids, acetaminophen, or conjugated estrogens resulted in no statistically significant changes in pharmacokinetic parameters in single- and/or multiple-dose studies. The interaction of Oxaprozin with lithium and cardiac glycosides has not been studied.

Carcinogenesis, mutagenesis, impairment of fertility: In oncogenicity studies, Oxaprozin administration for 2 years was associated with the exacerbation of liver neoplasms (hepatic adenomas and carcinomas) in male CD mice, but not in female CD mice or rats. The significance of this species-specific finding to man is unknown.

Oxaprozin did not display mutagenic potential. Results from the Ames test, forward mutation in yeast and Chinese hamster ovary (CHO) cells, DNA repair testing in CHO cells, micronucleus testing in mouse bone marrow, chromosomal aberration testing in human lymphocytes, and cell transformation testing in mouse fibroblast all showed no evidence of genetic toxicity or cell-transforming ability.

Oxaprozin administration was not associated with impairment of fertility in male and female rats at oral doses up to 200 mg/kg/day (1180 mg/m^2); the usual human dose is 17 mg/kg/day (629 mg/m^2). However, testicular degeneration was observed in beagle dogs treated with 37.5 to 150 mg/kg/day (750 to 3000 mg/m^2) of Oxaprozin for 6 months, or 37.5 mg/kg/day for 42 days, a finding not confirmed in other species. The clinical relevance of this finding is not known.

Pregnancy: Teratogenic Effects—Pregnancy Category C. There are no adequate or well-controlled studies in pregnant women. Teratology studies with Oxaprozin were performed in mice, rats, and rabbits. In mice and rats, no drug-related developmental abnormalities were observed at 50 to 200 mg/kg/day of Oxaprozin (225 to 900 mg/m^2). However, in rabbits, infrequent malformed fetuses were observed in dams treated with 7.5 to 30 mg/kg/day of Oxaprozin (the usual human dosage range). Oxaprozin should be used during pregnancy only if the potential benefits justify the potential risks to the fetus.

Labor and delivery: The effect of Oxaprozin in pregnant women is unknown. NSAIDs are known to delay parturition, to accelerate closure of the fetal ductus arteriosus, and to be associated with dystocia. Oxaprozin is known to have caused decreases in pup survival in rat studies. Accordingly, the use of Oxaprozin during late pregnancy should be avoided.

Nursing mothers: Studies of Oxaprozin excretion in human milk have not been conducted; however, Oxaprozin was found in the milk of lactating rats. Since the effects of Oxaprozin on infants are not known, caution should be exercised if Oxaprozin is administered to nursing women.

Pediatric use: Safety and effectiveness of Oxaprozin in children have not been established.

Geriatric use: No adjustment of the dose of Oxaprozin is necessary in the elderly for *pharmacokinetic* reasons, although many elderly may need to receive a reduced dose because of low body weight or disorders associated with aging. No significant differences in the pharmacokinetic profile for Oxaprozin were seen in studies in the healthy elderly.

Although selected elderly patients in controlled clinical trials tolerated Oxaprozin as well as younger patients, caution should be exercised in treating the elderly, and extra care should be taken when choosing a dose. As with any NSAID, the elderly are likely to tolerate adverse reactions less well than younger patients.

ADVERSE REACTIONS

Adverse reaction data were derived from patients who received Oxaprozin in multidose, controlled, and open-label clinical trials and from worldwide marketing experience. Rates for events occurring in more than 1% of patients, and for most of the less common events, are based on 2253 patients who took 1200 to 1800 mg Oxaprozin per day in clinical trials. Of these, 1721 were treated for at least 1 month, 971 for at least 3 months, and 366 for more than 1 year. Rates for the rarer events and for events reported from worldwide marketing experience are difficult to estimate accurately and are only listed as less than 1%.

The adverse event rates below refer to the incidence in the first month of use. Most of the events were seen by this time for common adverse reactions. However, the cumulative incidence can be expected to rise with continued therapy, and some events, such as gastrointestinal bleeding (see *"Warnings"*), seem to occur at a constant or possibly increasing rate over time.

The most frequently reported adverse reactions were related to the gastrointestinal tract. They were nausea (8%) and dyspepsia (8%).

INCIDENCE GREATER THAN 1%

In clinical trials the following adverse reactions occurred at an incidence greater than 1% and are probably related to treatment. Reactions occurring in 3% to 9% of patients treated with Oxaprozin are indicated by an asterisk (*); those reactions occurring in less than 3% of patients are unmarked.

Digestive System: abdominal pain distress, anorexia, constipation*, diarrhea*, dyspepsia*, flatulence, nausea*, vomiting.

Nervous System: CNS inhibition (depression, sedation, somnolence, or confusion), disturbance of sleep.

Skin and Appendages: rash*.

Special Senses: tinnitus.

Urogenital System: dysuria or frequency.

INCIDENCE LESS THAN 1%

Probable Causal Relationship: The following adverse reactions were reported in clinical trials or from worldwide marketing experience at an incidence of less than 1%. Those reactions reported only from worldwide marketing experience are in *italics*. The probability of a causal relationship exists between the drug and these adverse reactions.

Body as a Whole: anaphylaxis.

Cardiovascular System: edema, blood pressure changes.

Digestive System: peptic ulceration and/or GI bleeding (see *"Warnings"*), liver function abnormalities including *hepatitis* (see *"Precautions"*), stomatitis, hemorrhoidal or rectal bleeding.

Hematologic System: anemia, thrombocytopenia, leukopenia, ecchymoses.

Metabolic System: weight gain, weight loss.

Nervous System: weakness, malaise.

Respiratory System: symptoms of upper respiratory tract infection.

Skin: pruritus, urticaria, photosensitivity, *exfoliative dermatitis, erythema multiforme, Stevens-Johnson syndrome, toxic epidermal necrolysis (Lyell's syndrome)*.

Special Senses: blurred vision, conjunctivitis.

Urogenital: acute interstitial nephritis, hematuria, renal insufficiency, *acute renal failure,* decreased menstrual flow.

Causal relationship unknown: The following adverse reactions occurred at an incidence of less than 1% in clinical trials, or were suggested from marketing experience, under circumstances where a causal relationship could not be definitely established. They are listed as alerting information for the physician.

Cardiovascular System: palpitations.

Digestive System: alteration in taste.

Respiratory System: sinusitis, pulmonary infections.

Skin and Appendages: alopecia.

Special Senses: hearing decrease.

Urogenital System: increase in menstrual flow.

DRUG ABUSE AND DEPENDENCE

Oxaprozin is a non-narcotic drug. Usually reliable animal studies have indicated that Oxaprozin has no known addiction potential in humans.

OVERDOSAGE

No patient experienced either an accidental or intentional overdosage of Oxaprozin in the clinical trials of the drug. Symptoms following acute overdose with other NSAIDs are usually limited to lethargy, drowsiness, nausea, vomiting, and epigastric pain and are generally reversible with supportive care. Gastrointestinal bleeding and coma have occurred following NSAID overdose. Hypertension, acute renal failure, and respiratory depression are rare.

Patients should be managed by symptomatic and supportive care following an NSAID overdose. There are no specific antidotes. Gut decontamination may be indicated in patients seen within 4 hours of ingestion with symptoms or following a large overdose (5 to 10 times the usual dose). This should be accomplished via emesis and/or activated charcoal (60 to 100 g in adults, 1 to 2 g/kg in children) with an osmotic cathartic. Forced diuresis, alkalization of the urine, or hemoperfusion would probably not be useful due to the high degree of protein binding of Oxaprozin.

DOSAGE AND ADMINISTRATION

Rheumatoid Arthritis: The usual daily dose of Oxaprozin in the management of the signs and symptoms of rheumatoid arthritis is 1200 mg (two 600-mg caplets) once a day. Both smaller and larger doses may be required in individual patients (see *"Individualization of Dosage"*).

Osteoarthritis: The usual daily dose of Oxaprozin for the management of the signs and symptoms of moderate to severe osteoarthritis is 1200 mg (two 600-mg caplets) once a day. For patients of low body weight or with milder disease, an initial dosage of one 600-mg caplet once a day may be appropriate (see *"Individualization of Dosage"*).

Regardless of the indication, the dosage should be individualized to the lowest effective dose of Oxaprozin to minimize adverse effects, and the maximum recommended total daily dose is 1800 mg (or 26 mg/kg, whichever is *lower*) in divided doses.

SAFETY AND HANDLING
Oxaprozin is supplied as a solid dosage form in closed containers, is not known to produce contact dermatitis, and poses no known risk to healthcare workers. it may be disposed of in accordance with applicable local regulations governing the disposal of pharmaceuticals.

Storage: Keep bottles tightly closed and store below 86°F (30°C). Dispense in a tight, light-resistant container with a child-resistant closure. Protect the unit dose from light.

HOW SUPPLIED
TABLETS: 600 MG

BRAND/MANUFACTURER	NDC	SIZE	AWP
○ BRAND			
▶ DAYPRO: Searle	00025-1381-31	100s	$116.68
	00025-1381-34	100s ud	$120.18

Oxazepam

DESCRIPTION
Oxazepam is the first of a chemically new series of compounds, the 3-hydroxybenzodiazepinones. A new therapeutic agent providing versatility and flexibility in control of common emotional disturbances, this product exerts prompt action in a wide variety of disorders associated with anxiety, tension, agitation, and irritability, and anxiety associated with depression. In tolerance and toxicity studies on several animal species, this product reveals significantly greater safety factors than related compounds (chlordiazepoxide and diazepam) and manifests a wide separation of effective doses and doses inducing side effects.

Oxazepam capsules contain 10 mg, 15 mg, or 30 mg Oxazepam.

Oxazepam tablets contain 15 mg Oxazepam.

Oxazepam is 7 chloro- 1,3,-dihydro-3-hydroxy-5-phenyl-2*H*-1,4-benzodiazepin-2-one, a white crystalline powder with a molecular weight of 286.7.

Following is its chemical structure:

CLINICAL PHARMACOLOGY
Pharmacokinetic testing in twelve volunteers demonstrated that when given as a single 30 mg dose, the capsule, tablet, and suspension were equivalent in extent of absorption. For the capsule and tablet, peak plasma levels averaged 450 ng/mL and were observed to occur about 3 hours after dosing. The mean elimination half-life for Oxazepam was approximately 8.2 hours (range 5.7 to 10.9 hours).

This product has a single, major inactive metabolite in man, a glucuronide excreted in the urine.

ANIMAL PHARMACOLOGY AND TOXICOLOGY
In mice, Oxazepam exerts an anticonvulsant activity at 50-percent-effective doses of about 0.6 mg/kg orally. (Such anticonvulsant activity of benzodiazepines correlates with their tranquilizing properties.) To produce ataxia (rotabar test) and sedation (abolition of spontaneous motor activity), the 50 percent effective doses of this product are greater than 5 mg/kg orally. Thus, about ten times the therapeutic (anticonvulsant) dose must be given before ataxia ensues, indicating a wide separation of effective doses and doses inducing side effects.

In evaluation of antianxiety activity of compounds, conflict behavioral tests in rats differentiate continuous response for food in the presence of anxiety-provoking stress (shock) from drug-induced motor incoordination. This product shows significant separation of doses required to relieve anxiety and doses producing sedation or ataxia. Ataxia-producing doses exceed those of related CNS-acting drugs.

Acute oral LD_{50} in mice is greater than 5000 mg/kg, compared to 800 mg/kg for a related compound (chlordiazepoxide).

Subacute toxicity studies in dogs for four weeks at 480 mg/kg daily showed no specific changes; at 960 mg/kg two out of eight died with evidence of circulatory collapse. This wide margin of safety is significant compared to chlordiazepoxide HCl, which showed nonspecific changes in six dogs at 80 mg/kg. On chlordiazepoxide, two out of six died with evidence of circulatory collapse at 127 mg/kg, and six out of six died at 200 mg/kg daily. Chronic toxicity studies of Oxazepam in dogs at 120 mg/kg/day for 52 weeks produced no toxic manifestation.

Fatty metamorphosis of the liver has been noted in six-week toxicity studies in rats given this product at 0.5% of the diet. Such accumulations of fat are considered reversible as there is no liver necrosis or fibrosis.

Breeding studies in rats through two successive litters did not produce fetal abnormality.

Oxazepam has not been adequately evaluated for mutagenic activity.

In a carcinogenicity study Oxazepam was administered with diet to rats for two years. Male rats receiving 30 times the maximum human dose showed a statistical increase, when compared to controls, in benign thyroid follicular cell tumors, testicular interstitial cell adenomas, and prostatic adenomas. An earlier published study reported that mice fed dietary dosages of 35 or 100 times the human daily dose of oxazepam for 9 months developed a dose-related increase in liver adenomas.[1] In an independent analysis of some of the microscopic slides from this mouse study several of these tumors were classified as liver carcinomas. At this time, there is no evidence that clinical use of Oxazepam is associated with tumors.

INDICATIONS
Oxazepam is indicated for the management of anxiety disorders or for the short-term relief of the symptoms of anxiety. Anxiety or tension associated with the stress of everyday life usually does not require treatment with an anxiolytic.

Anxiety associated with depression is also responsive to Oxazepam therapy.

This product has been found particularly useful in the management of anxiety, tension, agitation, and irritability in older patients.

Alcoholics with acute tremulousness, inebriation, or with anxiety associated with alcohol withdrawal are responsive to therapy.

The effectiveness of Oxazepam in long-term use, that is, more than 4 months, has not been assessed by systematic clinical studies. The physician should reassess periodically the usefulness of the drug for the individual patient.

UNLABELED USES
Oxazepam is used in the treatment of insomnia.

CONTRAINDICATIONS
History of previous hypersensitivity reaction to Oxazepam. Oxazepam is not indicated in psychoses.

WARNINGS
As with other CNS-acting drugs, patients should be cautioned against driving automobiles or operating dangerous machinery until it is known that they do not become drowsy or dizzy on Oxazepam therapy.

Patients should be warned that the effects of alcohol or other CNS-depressant drugs may be additive to those of Oxazepam, possibly requiring adjustment of dosage or elimination of such agents.

PHYSICAL AND PSYCHOLOGICAL DEPENDENCE
Withdrawal symptoms, similar in character to those noted with barbiturates and alcohol (convulsions, tremor, abdominal and muscle cramps, vomiting, and sweating), have occurred following abrupt discontinuance of Oxazepam. The more severe withdrawal symptoms have usually been limited to those patients who received excessive doses over an extended period of time. Generally milder withdrawal symptoms (e.g., dysphoria and insomnia) have been reported following abrupt discontinuance of benzodiazepines taken continuously at therapeutic levels for several months. Consequently, after extended therapy, abrupt discontinuation should generally be avoided and a gradual dosage-tapering schedule followed. Addiction-prone individuals (such as drug addicts or alcoholics) should be under careful surveillance when receiving Oxazepam or other psychotropic agents because of the predisposition of such patients to habituation and dependence.

USE IN PREGNANCY
An increased risk of congenital malformations associated with the use of minor tranquilizers (chlordiazepoxide, diazepam, and meprobamate) during the first trimester of pregnancy has been suggested in several studies. Oxazepam, a benzodiazepine derivative, has not been studied adequately to determine whether it, too, may be associated with an increased risk of fetal abnormality. Because use of these drugs is rarely a matter of urgency, their use during this period should almost always be avoided. The possibility that a woman of childbearing potential may be pregnant at the time of institution of therapy should be considered. Patients should be advised that if they become pregnant during therapy or intend to become pregnant they should communicate with their physician about the desirability of discontinuing the drug.

PRECAUTIONS
Although hypotension has occurred only rarely, Oxazepam should be administered with caution to patients in whom a drop in blood pressure might lead to cardiac complications. This is particularly true in the elderly patient.

INFORMATION FOR PATIENTS
To assure the safe and effective use of Oxazepam patients should be informed that, since benzodiazepines may produce psychological and physical dependence, it is advisable that they consult with their physician before either increasing the dose or abruptly discontinuing this drug.

ADVERSE REACTIONS
The necessity for discontinuation of therapy due to undesirable effects has been rare. Transient mild drowsiness is commonly seen in the first few days of therapy. If it persists, the dosage should be reduced. In few instances, dizziness, vertigo, headache, and rarely syncope have occurred either alone or together with drowsiness. Mild paradoxical reactions, i.e., excitement, stimulation of affect, have been reported in psychiatric patients; these reactions may be secondary to relief of anxiety and usually appear in the first two weeks of therapy.

Other side effects occurring during Oxazepam therapy include rare instances of minor diffuse skin rashes—morbilliform, urticarial and maculopapular—nausea, lethargy, edema, slurred speech, tremor, and altered libido. Such side effects have been infrequent and are generally controlled with reduction of dosage.

◆ RATED THERAPEUTICALLY EQUIVALENT; ◇ THERAPEUTIC EQUIVALENCE UNCONFIRMED; ○ UNRATED

Although rare, leukopenia and hepatic dysfunction including jaundice have been reported during therapy. Periodic blood counts and liver-function tests are advisable.

Ataxia with Oxazepam has been reported in rare instances and does not appear to be specifically related to dose or age.

Although the following side reactions have not as yet been reported with Oxazepam, they have occurred with related compounds (chlordiazepoxide and diazepam): paradoxical excitation with severe rage reactions, hallucinations, menstrual irregularities, change in EEG pattern, blood dyscrasias including agranulocytosis, blurred vision, diplopia, incontinence, stupor, disorientation, fever, and euphoria.

Transient amnesia or memory impairment has been reported in association with the use of benzodiazepines.

DOSAGE AND ADMINISTRATION

Because of the flexibility of this product and the range of emotional disturbances responsive to it, dosage should be individualized for maximum beneficial effects.

Oxazepam Usual Dose

Mild-to-moderate anxiety, with associated tension, irritability, agitation, or related symptoms of functional origin or secondary to organic disease.	10 15 mg, 3 or 4 times daily
Severe anxiety syndromes, agitation, or anxiety associated with depression.	15 to 30 mg, 3 or 4 times daily
Older patients with anxiety, tension, irritability, and agitation.	Initial dosage: 10 mg, 3 times daily. If necessary, increase cautiously to 15 mg, 3 or 4 times daily
Alcoholics with acute inebriation, tremulousness, or anxiety on withdrawal	15 to 30 mg, 3 or 4 times daily

This product is not indicated in children under 6 years of age. Absolute dosage for children 6 to 12 years of age is not established.

STORAGE
Keep bottles tightly closed.
Dispense in tight container.
Store at room temperature, approximately 25°C (77°F).

REFERENCE
1. Fox, K.A.; Lahcen, R.B.; Liver-cell Adenomas and Peliosis Hepatis in Mice Associated with Oxazepam. Res. Commun. Chem. Pathol. Pharmacol. 8:481-488, 1974.

HOW SUPPLIED
CAPSULE (C-IV): 10 MG

AVERAGE UNIT PRICE (AVAILABLE SIZES)		GENERIC A-RATED AVERAGE PRICE (GAAP)	
BRAND	$0.65	100s	$24.11
GENERIC	$0.24	500s	$97.89
HCFA FUL (100s ea)	$0.06		

BRAND/MANUFACTURER	NDC	SIZE	AWP
◆ **BRAND**			
SERAX: Wyeth-Ayerst	00008-0051-01	25s	$17.96
	00008-0051-02	100s	$63.15
	00008-0051-03	500s	$297.20
◆ **GENERICS**			
Goldline	00182-1290-01	100s	$16.50
Schein	00364-2154-01	100s	$18.25
Martec	52555-0233-01	100s	$21.10
Qualitest	00603-4950-21	100s	$22.20
Caremark	00339-4023-12	100s	$22.31
Moore,H.L.	00839-7501-06	100s	$23.34
Purepac	00228-2067-10	100s	$23.39
Zenith	00172-4804-60	100s	$23.40
Aligen	00405-0132-01	100s	$24.63
URL	00677-1181-01	100s	$25.95
Parmed	00349-8865-01	100s	$26.00
Goldline	00182-1230-01	100s	$26.00
Warner Chilcott	00047-0690-24	100s	$26.00
Major	00904-1890-60	100s	$26.10
Geneva	00781-2809-01	100s	$26.55
Rugby	00536-4879-01	100s	$26.70
Vangard	00615-0409-13	100s ud	$27.16
Auro	55829-0867-10	100s ud	$28.37
Moore,H.L.	00839-7501-12	500s	$80.93
Purepac	00228-2067-50	500s	$101.59
Zenith	00172-4804-70	500s	$111.15

CAPSULE (C-IV): 15 MG

AVERAGE UNIT PRICE (AVAILABLE SIZES)		GENERIC A-RATED AVERAGE PRICE (GAAP)	
BRAND	$0.81	100s	$31.24
GENERIC	$0.31	500s	$154.62
HCFA FUL (100s ea)	$0.08		

BRAND/MANUFACTURER	NDC	SIZE	AWP
◆ **BRAND**			
SERAX: Wyeth-Ayerst	00008-0006-01	25s	$21.99
	00008-0006-02	100s	$79.38
	00008-0006-04	500s	$378.63
◆ **GENERICS**			
Warner Chilcott	00047-0665-24	100s	$23.59
Schein	00364-2152-01	100s	$24.95
Martec	52555-0234-01	100s	$26.57
Caremark	00339-4025-12	100s	$28.97
Purepac	00228-2069-10	100s	$29.46
Zenith	00172-4805-60	100s	$29.50
Aligen	00405-0133-01	100s	$31.05
UDL	51079-0478-21	100s	$31.71
Goldline	00182-1231-01	100s	$32.00
Qualitest	00603-4951-21	100s	$33.51
Geneva	00781-2810-01	100s	$33.58
Major	00904-1891-60	100s	$33.90
URL	00677-1182-01	100s	$34.11
Moore,H.L.	00839-7502-06	100s	$34.16
Rugby	00536-4877-01	100s	$34.28
Parmed	00349-8866-01	100s	$36.33
Vangard	00615-0410-13	100s ud	$30.86
UDL	51079-0478-20	100s ud	$31.71
Auro	55829-0868-10	100s ud	$33.30
Purepac	00228-2069-50	500s	$139.79
Zenith	00172-4805-70	500s	$140.13
Major	00904-1891-40	500s	$146.90
Aligen	00405-0133-02	500s	$147.50
Moore,H.L.	00839-7502-12	500s	$159.69
Geneva	00781-2810-05	500s	$159.88
Rugby	00536-4877-05	500s	$164.10
Parmed	00349-8866-05	500s	$179.00

CAPSULE (C-IV): 30 MG

AVERAGE UNIT PRICE (AVAILABLE SIZES)		GENERIC A-RATED AVERAGE PRICE (GAAP)	
BRAND	$1.16	100s	$42.16
GENERIC	$0.42	500s	$196.99
HCFA FUL (100s ea)	$0.10		

BRAND/MANUFACTURER	NDC	SIZE	AWP
◆ **BRAND**			
SERAX: Wyeth-Ayerst	00008-0052-01	25s	$30.63
	00008-0052-02	100s	$114.80
	00008-0052-04	500s	$556.48
◆ **GENERICS**			
Goldline	00182-1232-01	100s	$34.50
Goldline	00182-1292-01	100s	$34.50
Warner Chilcott	00047-0667-24	100s	$34.55
Schein	00364-2153-01	100s	$37.75
Martec	52555-0235-01	100s	$38.90
Caremark	00339-4027-12	100s	$40.89
Purepac	00228-2071-10	100s	$41.17
Zenith	00172-4806-60	100s	$41.25
Geneva	00781-2811-01	100s	$41.50
Moore,H.L.	00839-7503-06	100s	$42.78
Qualitest	00603-4952-21	100s	$43.11
Aligen	00405-0134-01	100s	$43.42
Rugby	00536-4878-01	100s	$43.56
URL	00677-1183-01	100s	$43.60
Major	00904-1892-60	100s	$43.90
UDL	51079-0479-21	100s	$47.19
Parmed	00349-8867-01	100s	$49.00
Vangard	00615-0411-13	100s ud	$44.92
UDL	51079-0479-20	100s ud	$47.19
Auro	55829-0869-10	100s ud	$49.55
Major	00904-1892-40	500s	$189.20
Zenith	00172-4806-70	500s	$195.94
Purepac	00228-2073-50	500s	$205.83

TABLETS (C-IV): 15 MG

AVERAGE UNIT PRICE (AVAILABLE SIZES)		GENERIC A-RATED AVERAGE PRICE (GAAP)	
BRAND	$0.79	100s	$28.20
GENERIC	$0.28		
HCFA FUL (100s ea)	$0.28		

BRAND/MANUFACTURER	NDC	SIZE	AWP
◆ **BRAND**			
SERAX: Wyeth-Ayerst	00008-0317-01	100s	$79.38
◆ **GENERICS**			
Major	00904-1894-60	100s	$26.45
URL	00677-1163-01	100s	$29.95

➤ SHOWN IN PRODUCT IDENTIFICATION GUIDE

Oxiconazole Nitrate

DESCRIPTION

Oxiconazole Nitrate Cream and Oxiconazole Nitrate Lotion formulations contain the antifungal active compound, Oxiconazole Nitrate. Both formulations are for topical dermatologic use only.

Chemically, Oxiconazole Nitrate is 2',4'-dichloro-2-imidazol-1-ylacetophenone (Z)-[O-(2,4-dichlorobenzyl)oxime], mononitrate. The compound has the empirical formula $C_{18}H_{13}Cl_4N_3O.HNO_3$, a molecular weight of 492.15.

Oxiconazole Nitrate is a nearly white crystalline powder, soluble in methanol; sparingly soluble in ethanol, chloroform, and acetone, and very slightly soluble in water.

Oxiconazole Nitrate Cream contains 10 mg of Oxiconazole/g of cream in a white to off-white, opaque cream base.

Oxiconazole Nitrate Lotion contains 10 mg of Oxiconazole/g of lotion in a white to off-white, opaque lotion base.

Following is its chemical structure:

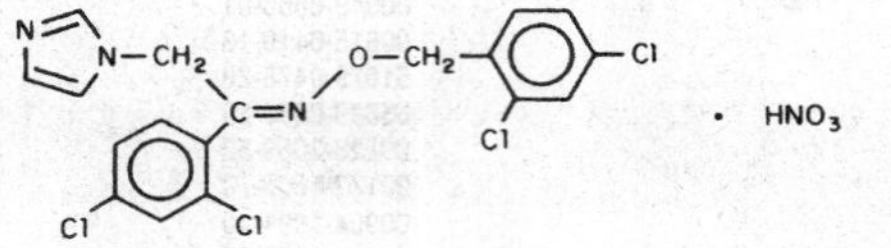

CLINICAL PHARMACOLOGY

Five hours after application of 2.5 mg/cm^2 of Oxiconazole Nitrate Cream onto human skin, the concentration of Oxiconazole Nitrate was demonstrated to be 16.2 µmol in the epidermis, 3.64 µmol in the upper corium, and 1.29 µmol in the deeper corium. Systemic absorption of Oxiconazole Nitrate appears to be low. Less than 0.3% of the applied dose of Oxiconazole Nitrate was recovered in the urine of volunteer subjects up to 5 days after application of the cream formulation.

Neither in vitro nor in vivo studies have been conducted to establish relative activity between the lotion and cream formulations.

MICROBIOLOGY
Oxiconazole Nitrate is an imidazole derivative whose antifungal activity is derived primarily from the inhibition of ergosterol biosynthesis, which is critical for cellular membrane integrity. It has in vitro activity against a wide range of pathogenic fungi.

Oxiconazole has been shown to be active against most strains of the following organisms both in vitro and in clinical infections at indicated body sites: (See "Indications and Usage".)

Epidermophyton floccosum
Trichophyton mentagrophytes
Trichophyton rubrum

The following in vitro data are available: however, their clinical significance is unknown. Oxiconazole Nitrate exhibits satisfactory in vitro MIC's against most strains of the following organisms; however, the safety and efficacy of Oxiconazole Nitrate in treating clinical infections due to these organisms have not been established in adequate and well-controlled clinical trials.

Candida albicans
Malassezia furfur
Microsporum audouini
Microsporum canis
Microsporum gypseum
Trichophyton tonsurans
Trichophyton violaceum.

INDICATIONS AND USAGE

Oxiconazole Nitrate Cream and Oxiconazole Nitrate Lotion are indicated for the topical treatment of the following dermal infections: tinea pedis, tinea cruris, and tinea corporis due to Trichophyton rubrum, Trichophyton mentagrophytes, or Epidermophyton floccosum. (See "Dosage and Administration" and "Clinical Studies".)

UNLABELED USES
Oxiconazole Nitrate has been effective for treating vaginal candidiasis.

CONTRAINDICATIONS

Oxiconazole Nitrate Cream and Oxiconazole Nitrate Lotion are contraindicated in individuals who have shown hypersensitivity to any of their components.

WARNINGS

Oxiconazole Nitrate Cream and Oxiconazole Nitrate Lotion are not for ophthalmic or intravaginal use.

PRECAUTIONS

General: If a reaction suggesting sensitivity or chemical irritation should occur with the use of Oxiconazole Nitrate Cream or Oxiconazole Nitrate Lotion, treatment should be discontinued and appropriate therapy instituted. Oxiconazole Nitrate Cream and Lotion are for external dermal use only. Avoid introduction of Oxiconazole Nitrate Cream or Lotion into the eyes or vagina.

Carcinogenesis, Mutagenesis, Impairment of Fertility: Although no long-term studies in animals have been performed to evaluate carcinogenic potential, no evidence of mutagenic effect was found in two mutation assays (Ames test and Chinese hamster V79 in vitro cell mutation assay) or in two cytogenetic assays (human peripheral blood lymphocyte in vitro chromosome aberration assay and in vivo micronucleus assay in mice).

Reproductive studies revealed no impairment of fertility in rats at oral doses of 3 mg/kg per day in females [1 time the human dose based on mg/m^2] and 15 mg/kg per day in males [4 times the human dose based on mg/m^2]. However, at doses above this level, the following effects were observed: a reduction in the fertility parameters of males and females, a reduction in the number of sperm in vaginal smears, extended estrous cycle, and a decrease in mating frequency.

Pregnancy: Teratogenic Effects: Pregnancy Category B: Reproduction studies have been performed in rabbits, rats, and mice at oral doses up to 100, 150, and 200 mg/kg per day [57, 40, and 27 times the human dose based on mg/m^2], respectively, and revealed no evidence of harm to the fetus due to Oxiconazole Nitrate. There are, however, no adequate and well-controlled studies in pregnant women. Because animal reproduction studies are not always predictive of human response, this drug should be used during pregnancy only if clearly needed.

Nursing Mothers: Because Oxiconazole Nitrate is excreted in human milk, caution should be exercised when the drug is administered to a nursing woman.

ADVERSE REACTIONS

(Numbers in this section include patients treated both once daily and twice daily combined.)

During clinical trials, 41 (4.3%) of 955 patients treated with Oxiconazole Nitrate Cream, 1%, reported adverse reactions thought to be related to drug therapy. These reactions included pruritus (1.6%); burning (1.4%); irritation and allergic contact dermatitis (0.4% each); folliculitis (0.3%); erythema (0.2%); and papules, fissure, maceration, rash, stinging, and nodules (0.1% each).

In a controlled, multicenter clinical trial, 7 (2.6%) of 269 patients treated with Oxiconazole Nitrate Lotion, 1%, reported adverse reactions thought to be related to drug therapy. These reactions included burning and stinging (0.7% each); and pruritus, scaling, tingling, pain, and dyshidrotic eczema (0.4% each).

OVERDOSAGE

When a 5% Oxiconazole Cream was applied at a rate of 1 g/kg to approximately 10% of body surface area of a group of 40 male and female rats for 35 days, 3 deaths and severe dermal inflammation were reported.

DOSAGE AND ADMINISTRATION

Oxiconazole Nitrate Cream or Oxiconazole Nitrate Lotion should be applied to cover affected and immediately surrounding areas once to twice daily in patients with tinea pedis, tinea corporis, or tinea cruris. Tinea corporis and tinea cruris should be treated for 2 weeks and tinea pedis for 1 month to reduce the possibility of recurrence. If a patient shows no clinical improvement after the treatment period, the diagnosis should be reviewed.

Cream/Lotion: Store between 15° and 30°C (59° and 86°fF).

CLINICAL STUDIES

TINEA PEDIS STUDIES
The following definitions were applied to the clinical and microbiological outcomes in patients enrolled in the clinical trials that form the basis for the approvals of Oxiconazole Nitrate Lotion and Oxiconazole Nitrate Cream.

THERE ARE NO HEAD-TO-HEAD COMPARISON TRIALS OF THE OXICONAZOLE NITRATE CREAM AND LOTION FORMULATIONS IN THE TREATMENT OF TINEA PEDIS.

DEFINITIONS
(1) Clinical Improvement: greater than 50% improvement in the clinical signs and symptoms above the baseline assessment.

(2) Clinical Cure: greater than 90% improvement in the clinical signs and symptoms above the baseline assessment.

(3) Mycological Cure: no evidence (culture and KOH preparation) of the baseline (original) pathogen in a specimen from the affected area taken at the two week post-treatment visit.

(4) Overall Cure: both a clinical cure (see above) and a microbiologic eradication (see above) at the two week post-treatment visit.

LOTION FORMULATION
The clinical trial for the lotion formulation line extension involved 332 evaluable patients with clinically and microbiologically established tinea pedis. Of these evaluable patients, 64% were diagnosed with hyperkeratotic plantar tinea pedis and 28% with interdigital tinea pedis, 77% had disease secondary to infection with T. rubrum, 18% had disease secondary to infection with T. mentagrophytes, and 4% had disease secondary to infection with E. floccosum.

The results of this clinical trial at the two-week post-treatment follow-up visit are shown in the following table:

Patient outcome categorized as:	Oxiconazole Nitrate Lotion		
	b.i.d.	q.d	Vehicle
Clinical			
Improvement	82%	80%	50%
Clinical Cure	52%	43%	18%
Mycological Cure	67%	64%	28%
Overall Cure	41%	34%	10%

In this study, the improvement and cure rates of the b.i.d. and q.d. treated groups did not differ significantly (95% CI) from each other but were statistically (95% CI) superior to the vehicle treated group.

CREAM FORMULATION
The two pivotal trials for the cream formulation involved 281 evaluable patients (total from both trials) with clinically and microbiologically established tinea pedis.

The combined results of these two clinical trial at the two-week post-treatment follow-up visit are shown in the following table:

Patient outcome categorized as:	Oxiconazole Nitrate Cream		
	b.i.d.	q.d	Vehicle
Clinical			
Improvement	84%	83%	49%
Mycological Cure	77%	79%	33%
Overall Cure	52%	43%	14%

All the improvement and cure rates of the b.i.d. and q.d. treated groups did not differ significantly (95% CI) from each other but were statistically (95% CI) superior to the vehicle treated group.

HOW SUPPLIED
CREAM: 1%

BRAND/MANUFACTURER	NDC	SIZE	AWP
○ **BRAND**			
OXISTAT: Glaxo Derm	00173-0423-00	15 gm	$12.41
	00173-0423-01	30 gm	$20.72
	00173-0423-04	60 gm	$30.59

LOTION: 1%

BRAND/MANUFACTURER	NDC	SIZE	AWP
○ **BRAND**			
OXISTAT: Glaxo Derm	00173-0448-01	30 ml	$20.72

Oxistat SEE OXICONAZOLE NITRATE

Oxsoralen SEE METHOXSALEN

Oxtriphylline

DESCRIPTION
Oxtriphylline is a xanthine bronchodilator—the choline salt of theophylline. Oxtriphylline is available in extended-release and delayed-release formulations.

Each extended-release tablet contains:

Oxtriphylline ....400 or 600 mg (equivalent to 254 or 382 mg anhydrous theophylline).

Each delayed-release tablet contains:
Oxtriphylline ....100 or 200 mg (equivalent to 64 or 127 mg anhydrous theophylline).

Theophylline occurs as a white, odorless, crystalline powder having a bitter taste. Theophylline anhydrous has the chemical name 1 H-Purine-2,6-dione, 3,7-dihydro-1,3-dimethyl-.
The molecular formula is $C_{12}H_{21}N_5O_3$. The molecular weight is 283.33.

Following is its chemical structure:

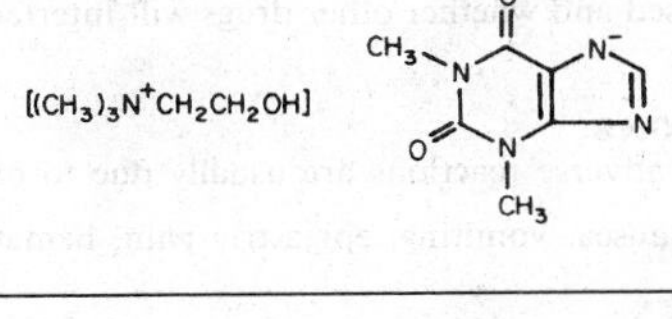

CLINICAL PHARMACOLOGY
Oxtriphylline, the choline salt of theophylline, effects significant improvement in pulmonary function parameters which have been impaired by bronchospasm. It is more soluble than either aminophylline or theophylline. Oxtriphylline extended-release tablets are less irritating to the gastric mucosa than aminophylline.

Oxtriphylline extended-release tablets have been formulated to provide therapeutic serum levels when administered every 12 hours and minimize the peaks and valleys of serum levels commonly found with shorter acting theophylline products.

The sustained action characteristic of Oxtriphylline extended-release tablets has been demonstrated in studies in human subjects. Single and multiple dose studies have shown equivalent steady-state theophylline plasma levels of Oxtriphylline extended-release tablets given every 12 hours when compared with an equal total daily dose of (the nonsustained action) Oxtriphylline elixir given every six hours.

Theophylline directly relaxes the smooth muscle of the bronchial airways and pulmonary blood vessels, thus acting mainly as a bronchodilator, pulmonary vasodilator and smooth muscle relaxant. The drug also possesses other actions typical of the xanthine derivatives: coronary vasodilator, diuretic, cardiac stimulant, cerebral stimulant and skeletal muscle stimulant. It has also been demonstrated that aminophylline has a potent effect on diaphragmatic contractility in normal persons and may then be capable of reducing fatigability and thereby improve contractility in patients with chronic obstructive airways disease. The exact mode of action remains unsettled.

Although theophylline does cause inhibition of phosphodiesterase with a resultant increase in intracellular cyclic AMP, which could mediate smooth muscle relaxation, other agents similarly inhibit the enzyme producing a rise of cyclic AMP but are unassociated with any demonstrable bronchodilation. Other mechanisms proposed include an effect on translocation of intracellular calcium; prostaglandin antagonism; stimulation of catecholamines endogenously; inhibition of cyclic guanosine monophosphate metabolism and adenosine receptor antagonism. None of these mechanisms has been proved, however. At concentrations higher than attained *in vivo*, theophylline also inhibits the release of histamine by mast cells.

Theophylline has been shown to react synergistically with beta agonists that increase intracellular cyclic AMP through the stimulation of adenyl cyclase (isoproterenol).

Apparently, the development of tolerance does not occur with chronic use of theophylline.

The half-life is shortened with cigarette smoking. The half-life is prolonged in alcoholism, reduced hepatic or renal function, congestive heart failure, and in patients receiving antibiotics such as TAO (troleandomycin), erythromycin and clindamycin. High fever for prolonged periods may decrease theophylline elimination.

THEOPHYLLINE ELIMINATION CHARACTERISTICS

	Theophylline Clearance Rates (mean ± S.D.)	Half-Life Average (mean ± S.D.)
Children (over 6 months of age)	1.45 ± .58 ml/kg/min	3.7 ± 1.1 hours
Adult non-smokers with uncomplicated asthma	.65 ± .19 ml/kg/min	8.7 ± 2.2 hours

Newborn infants have extremely slow clearance and half-lives exceeding 24 hours, which approach those seen for older children after about 3—6 months. Older children have rapid clearance rates while most nonsmoking adults have clearance rates between these two extremes. In premature neonates, the decreased clearance is related to oxidative pathways that have yet to be established.

Older adults with chronic obstructive pulmonary disease, and patients with cor pulmonale or other causes of heart failure, and patients with liver pathology may have much lower clearances with half-lives that may exceed 24 hours.

The half-life of theophylline is prolonged in patients with congestive heart failure, in those with reduced hepatic or renal function, and in alcoholism. The half-life of theophylline may also be prolonged by concurrent use of various drugs such as phenobarbital, and certain antibiotics, including troleandomycin, erythromycin, and lincomycin.

In cigarette smokers (1—2 packs/day) the mean half-life is 4—5 hours, much shorter than in nonsmokers. The increase in clearance associated with smoking is presumably due to stimulation of the hepatic metabolic pathway by components of cigarette smoke. The duration of this effect after cessation of smoking is unknown but may require 6 months to 2 years before the rate approaches that of the nonsmoker.

INDICATIONS
Oxtriphylline is indicated for relief and/or prevention of symptoms of acute and chronic bronchial asthma and for reversible bronchospasm associated with chronic bronchitis and emphysema.

UNLABELED USES
Oxtriphylline is used alone or as an adjunct in the treatment of Cheyne-Stokes respiration, cystic fibrosis, essential tremor, and severe headache. It is also used to improve exercise-induced myocardial ischemia in patients with stable angina pectoris, and in treatment of bronchopulmonary dysplasia and cerebral vasospasm.

► SHOWN IN PRODUCT IDENTIFICATION GUIDE

CONTRAINDICATIONS

Oxtriphylline is contraindicated in individuals who have shown hypersensitivity to theophylline or to Oxtriphylline or any of its components. It is also contraindicated in patients with active peptic ulcer disease, and in individuals with underlying seizure disorders (unless receiving appropriate anticonvulsant medication).

WARNINGS

Status asthmaticus is a medical emergency. Optimal therapy frequently requires additional medication including corticosteroids when the patient is not rapidly responsive to bronchodilators.

Excessive theophylline doses may be associated with toxicity, and serum theophylline levels are recommended to assure maximal benefit without excessive risk; incidence of toxicity increases at levels greater than 20 mcg theophylline/ml. Morphine, curare, and stilbamidine should be used with caution in patients with airflow obstruction since they stimulate histamine release and can induce asthmatic attacks. These drugs may also suppress respiration leading to respiratory failure. Alternative drugs should be chosen whenever possible.

Serum levels above 20 µg/mL are rarely found after appropriate administration of the recommended doses. However, in individuals in whom theophylline plasma clearance is reduced *for any reason*, even conventional doses may result in increased serum levels and potential toxicity. Reduced theophylline clearance has been documented in the following readily identifiable groups: 1) patients with impaired liver function; 2) patients over 55 years of age, particularly males and those with chronic lung disease; 3) those with cardiac failure from any cause; 4) patients with sustained high fever; 5) neonates and infants under 1 year of age; and 6) those patients taking certain drugs (see *"Precautions, Drug Interactions"*). Frequently, such patients have markedly prolonged theophylline serum levels following discontinuation of the drug.

Reduction of dosage and laboratory monitoring is especially appropriate in the above individuals.

Serious side effects such as ventricular arrhythmias, convulsions or even death may appear as the first sign of toxicity without any previous warning. Less serious signs of theophylline toxicity (ie, nausea and restlessness) may occur frequently when initiating therapy, but are usually transient; when such signs are persistent during maintenance therapy, they are often associated with serum concentrations above 20 µg/mL. Stated differently; *serious toxicity is not reliably preceded by less severe side effects.* A serum concentration measurement is the only reliable method of predicting potentially life-threatening toxicity.

Many patients who require theophylline exhibit tachycardia due to their underlying disease process so that the cause/effect relationship to elevated serum theophylline concentrations may not be appreciated.

Theophylline products may cause dysrhythmia and/or worsen preexisting arrhythmias and any significant change in rate and/or rhythm warrants monitoring and further investigation.

Studies in laboratory animals (minipigs, rodents, and dogs) recorded the occurrence of cardiac arrhythmias and sudden death (with histologic evidence of myocardial necrosis) when beta-agonists and methylxanthines were administered concurrently. The significance of these findings when applied to humans is currently unknown.

Children have a marked sensitivity to the CNS stimulant action of theophylline. Serious toxic effects, including fatalities have been reported in children as well as adults.

Theophylline products may worsen pre-existing arrhythmias.

CARCINOGENESIS, MUTAGENESIS, AND IMPAIRMENT OF FERTILITY

Long-term carcinogenicity studies have not been performed with theophylline.

Chromosome-breaking activity was detected in human cell cultures at concentrations of theophylline up to 50 times the therapeutic serum concentration in humans. Theophylline was not mutagenic in the dominant lethal assay in male mice given theophylline intraperitoneally in doses up to 30 times the maximum daily dose.

Studies to determine the effect on fertility have not been performed with theophylline.

USAGE IN PREGNANCY

Safe use of Oxtriphylline in pregnancy and lactation has not been established relative to possible adverse effects on fetal or neonatal development. Therefore Oxtriphylline should not be used in patients who are pregnant or who may become pregnant, or during lactation unless, in the judgment of the physician, the potential benefits outweigh the possible hazards.

Theophylline is distributed into breast milk and may cause irritability or other signs of toxicity in nursing infants. Because of the potential for serious adverse reactions in nursing infants from theophylline, a decision should be made whether to discontinue nursing or to discontinue the drug, taking into account the importance of the drug to the mother.

PEDIATRIC USE

Sufficient numbers of infants under the age of 1 year have not been studied in clinical trials to support use in this age group; however, there is evidence recorded that the use of dosage recommendations for older infants and young children (16 mg/kg/24 hours) may result in the development of toxic serum levels. Such findings very probably reflect differences in the metabolic handling of the drug related to absent or undeveloped enzyme systems. Consequently, the use of the drug in this age group should carefully consider the associated benefits and risks.

If used, the maintenance dose must be conservative and in accord with the following guidelines:

Initial Theophylline Maintenance Dosage: Premature Infants:
Up to 24 days postnatal age—1.0 mg/kg q 12h
Beyond 24 days postnatal age—1.5 mg/kg q 12h
Infants 6 to 52 weeks:
$[(0.2 \times$ age in weeks$) + 5.0] \times$ kg body wt = 24 hour dose in mg.
Up to 26 weeks, divide into q 8h dosing intervals.
From 26—52 weeks, divide into q 6h dosing intervals.

Final dosage should be guided by serum concentration after a steady state (no further accumulation of drug) has been achieved.

PRECAUTIONS

Mean half-life in smokers is shorter than nonsmokers, therefore, smokers may require larger doses of theophylline. Theophylline should not be administered concurrently with other xanthine medications or with xanthine-containing beverages or foods. Use with caution in patients with severe cardiac disease, severe hypoxemia, hypertension, hyperthyroidism, acute myocardial injury, cor pulmonale, congestive heart failure, or liver disease, and in the elderly (especially males) and in neonates. Great caution should especially be used in giving theophylline to patients in congestive heart failure. Such patients have shown markedly prolonged theophylline blood level curves with theophylline persisting in serum for long periods following discontinuation of the drug. Use theophylline cautiously in patients with a history of peptic ulcer. Theophylline may occasionally act as a local irritant to the GI tract although gastrointestinal symptoms are more commonly central and associated with serum theophylline concentrations over 20 mcg/ml.

INFORMATION FOR PATIENTS

Tablets should not be chewed, or crushed or dissolved: The importance of taking only the prescribed dose and time interval between doses should be reinforced.

LABORATORY TESTS

Serum levels should be monitored periodically to determine the theophylline level associated with observed clinical response and as the method of predicting toxicity. For such measurements, the serum sample should be obtained at the time of peak concentration, 1 to 2 hours after administration for immediate release products. It is important that the patient will not have missed or taken additional doses during the previous 48 hours and that dosing intervals will have been reasonably equally spaced. DOSAGE ADJUSTMENT BASED ON SERUM THEOPHYLLINE MEASUREMENTS WHEN THESE INSTRUCTIONS HAVE NOT BEEN FOLLOWED MAY RESULT IN RECOMMENDATIONS THAT PRESENT RISK OF TOXICITY TO THE PATIENT.

DRUG INTERACTIONS

Toxic synergism with ephedrine has been documented and may occur with other sympathomimetic bronchodilators. In addition, the following drug interactions have been demonstrated:

Theophylline with:

Drug	Effect
Lithium carbonate	Increased renal excretion of lithium
Propranolol	Antagonism of propranolol effect.
Furosemide	Increased furosemide diuresis.
Hexamethonium	Decreased hexamethonium-induced chronotropic effect
Reserpine	Reserpine-induced tachycardia.
Chlordiazepoxide	Chlordiazepoxide-induced fatty acid mobilization.
Troleandomycin, erythromycin or lincomycin	Increased theophylline plasma levels.
Allopurinol (high-dose)	Increased serum theophylline levels
Cimetidine	Increased serum theophylline levels
Oral Contraceptives	Increased serum theophylline levels
Phenytoin	Decreased theophylline and phenytoin serum levels
Rifampin	Decreased serum theophylline levels

DRUG-LABORATORY TEST INTERACTIONS

Currently available analytical methods, including high pressure liquid chromatography and immunoassay techniques, for measuring serum theophylline levels are specific. Metabolites and other drugs generally do not affect the results. Other new analytic methods are also now in use. The physician should be aware of the laboratory method used and whether other drugs will interfere with the assay for theophylline.

ADVERSE REACTIONS

The most consistent adverse reactions are usually due to overdose and are:

1. *Gastrointestinal:* nausea, vomiting, epigastric pain, hematemesis, diarrhea.

◆ RATED THERAPEUTICALLY EQUIVALENT; ◇ THERAPEUTIC EQUIVALENCE UNCONFIRMED; ○ UNRATED

2. *Central nervous system:* headaches, irritability, restlessness, insomnia, reflex hyperexcitability, muscle twitching, clonic and tonic generalized convulsions.

3. *Cardiovascular:* palpitation, tachycardia, extrasystoles, flushing, hypotension, circulatory failure, life-threatening ventricular arrhythmias.

4. *Respiratory:* tachypnea.

5. *Renal:* albuminuria, increased excretion of renal tubular cells and red blood cells, diuresis, or potentiation of diuresis.

6. *Others:* hyperglycemia and inappropriate antidiuretic hormone (ADH) syndrome alopecia, rash.

OVERDOSAGE

Serious toxic effects due to overdosage may occur suddenly and are not invariably preceded by minor adverse effects. Therefore, careful observation of the patient and prompt institution of appropriate therapeutic measures are essential in all cases of overdosage. All patients suspected of overdosage should be hospitalized.

Signs and symptoms of overdosage are related primarily to the cardiovascular, gastrointestinal, and central nervous systems.

Cardiovascular symptoms include precordial pain, tachycardia, ventricular and other arrhythmias: also varying degrees of hypotension including, in extreme cases, severe shock, cardiovascular collapse and death.

Gastrointestinal symptoms include abdominal pain, nausea, persistent vomiting, and hematemesis.

Central nervous system symptoms include headache, dizziness, restlessness, irritability, tremors, hyperactivity, and agitation followed, in severe cases by convulsions, drowsiness, coma and death.

Treatment of overdosage should be directed toward minimizing absorption and supporting vital functions.

It is suggested that the management principles (consistent with the clinical status of the patient when first seen) outlined below be instituted and that simultaneous contact with a regional poison control center be established. In this way both updated information and individualization regarding required therapy may be provided.

1. When potential oral overdose is established and seizure has not occurred:

a. If patient is alert and seen within the early hours after ingestion, induction of emesis may be of value. Gastric lavage has been demonstrated to be of no value in influencing outcome in patients who present more than 1 hour after ingestion.

b. Administer a cathartic. Sorbitol solution is reported to be of value.

c. Administer repeated doses of activated charcoal and monitor theophylline serum levels.

d. Prophylactic administration of phenobarbital has been shown to increase the seizure threshold in laboratory animals, and administration of this drug can be considered.

2. If patient presents with a seizure:

a. Establish an airway.

b. Administer oxygen.

c. Treat the seizure with intravenous diazepam, 0.1 to 0.3 mg/kg up to 10 mg. If seizures cannot be controlled, the use of general anesthesia should be considered.

d. Monitor vital signs, maintain blood pressure and provide adequate hydration.

3. If postseizure coma is present:

a. Maintain airway and oxygenation.

b. If a result of oral medication, follow above recommendations to prevent absorption of the drug, but intubation and lavage will have to be performed instead of inducing emesis, and the cathartic and charcoal will need to be introduced via large bore gastric lavage tube.

c. Continue to provide full supportive care and adequate hydration until the drug is metabolized. In general, drug metabolism is sufficiently rapid so as not to warrant dialysis. If repeated oral activated charcoal is ineffective (as noted by stable or rising serum levels), charcoal hemoperfusion may be indicated.

In the obtunded patient, the airway should be secured immediately by means of an endotracheal tube with cuff inflated. After the airway has been secured, lavage should be carried out, and activated charcoal slurry and a cathartic should be administered.

CNS stimulation may be controlled with diazepam, 0.1—0.3 mg/kg intravenously in children, and 10 mg intravenously in adults. Respiration should be supported by appropriate means. Hypotension and shock should be treated with appropriate fluid replacement, avoiding the use of vasopressors, if possible. Additional supportive measures should be carried out as required.

Serial serum theophylline levels are of value in following the patient's course and in guiding further management.

Forced diuresis is of no value because of the small amount of theophylline excreted unchanged by the kidney. There has been a single report of survival with the use of an activated charcoal column (hemoperfusion) in massive theophylline overdosage.

DOSAGE AND ADMINISTRATION

Tablets should not be chewed, or crushed or dissolved. Effective use of theophylline (ie, the concentration of drug in the serum associated with optimal benefit and minimal risk of toxicity) is considered to occur when the theophylline concentration is maintained from 10 to 20 µg/ml. The early studies from which these levels were derived were carried out in patients immediately or shortly after recovery from acute exacerbations of their disease (some hospitalized with status asthmaticus).

Although the 20 µg/ml level remains appropriate as a critical value (above which toxicity is more likely to occur) for safety purposes, additional data are now available which indicate that the serum theophylline concentrations required to produce maximum physiologic benefit may, in fact, fluctuate with the degree of bronchospasm present and are variable. Therefore, the physician should individualize the range appropriate to the patient's requirements, based on both symptomatic response and improvement in pulmonary function. It should be stressed that serum theophylline concentrations maintained at the upper level of the 10 to 20 µg/ml range may be associated with potential toxicity when factors known to reduce theophylline clearance are operative. (See *"Warnings"*.)

There is great variation from patient to patient in dosage needed in order to achieve a therapeutic blood level because of variable rates of elimination. Because of this wide variation from patient to patient and the relatively narrow therapeutic blood level range, dosage must be individualized; monitoring of theophylline serum levels is highly recommended. Dosage should be calculated on the basis of lean (ideal) body weight—mg/kg. Theophylline does not distribute into fatty tissue.

Giving Oxtriphylline with food may prevent the rare case of stomach irritation, and although absorption may be slower, it is still complete.

When rapidly absorbed products such as solutions and immediate-release products are used, dosing to maintain "around the clock" blood levels generally requires administration every 6 hours to obtain the greatest efficacy for use in children, dosing intervals up to 8 hours may be satisfactory for adults because of their slower elimination. Children and adults requiring higher than average doses may benefit from products with slower absorption.

This may allow longer dosing intervals and/or less fluctuation in serum concentration over a dosing interval during chronic therapy. In patients receiving concurrent bronchodilator therapy, eg, beta agonists, downward adjustment of Oxtriphylline dosage is necessary.

The following dosage information relates to initiation and titration of daily dosage requirements utilizing a nonsustained action form of Oxtriphylline (eg Oxtriphylline Tabs, Elixir).

Acute symptoms of bronchospasm requiring rapid attainment of theophylline serum levels for bronchodilation.

Note: Status asthmaticus should be considered a medical emergency and is defined as that degree of bronchospasm which is not rapidly responsive to usual doses of conventional bronchodilators. Optimal therapy for such patients frequently requires both *additional medication,* parenterally administered, and *close monitoring,* preferably in an intensive care setting.

A. PATIENTS NOT CURRENTLY RECEIVING THEOPHYLLINE PRODUCTS (SEE RELATED TABLE).

B. THOSE CURRENTLY RECEIVING THEOPHYLLINE PRODUCTS
Determine where possible, the time, amount, route of administration and form of the patient's last dose.

The loading dose for theophylline will be based on the principle that each 0.8 mg/kg of Oxtriphylline (0.5 mg/kg of theophylline) administered as a loading dose

Group	Oral Loading Dose Oxtriphylline	Maintenance Dose for Next 12 Hours Oxtriphylline	Maintenance Dose Beyond 12 Hours Oxtriphylline
1. Children 6 months to 9 years	7.8—9.4 mg/kg *(5—6 mg/kg)	6.2 mg/kg q4 hrs *(4 mg/kg q4 hrs)	6.2 mg/kg q6 hrs *(4 mg/kg q6 hrs)
2. Children age 9—16 and young adult smokers	7.8—9.4 mg/kg *(5—6 mg/kg)	4.7 mg/kg q4 hrs *(3 mg/kg q4 hrs)	4.7 mg/kg q6 hrs *(3 mg/kg q6 hrs)
3. Otherwise healthy nonsmoking adults	7.8—9.4 mg/kg *(5—6 mg/kg)	4.7 mg/kg q6 hrs *(3 mg/kg q6 hrs)	4.7 mg/kg q8 hrs *(3 mg/kg q8 hrs)
4. Older patients and patients with corpulmonale	7.8—9.4 mg/kg *(5—6 mg/kg)	3.1 mg/kg q6 hrs *(2 mg/kg q6 hrs)	3.1 mg/kg q8 hrs *(2 mg/kg q8 hrs)
5. Patients with congestive heart failure, liver failure	7.8—9.4 mg/kg *(5—6 mg/kg)	3.1 mg/kg q8 hrs *(2 mg/kg q8 hrs)	1.6-3.1 mg/kg q12 hrs *(1-2 mg/kg q12 hrs)

*   *Anhydrous theophylline indicated in ( ).*

will result in a 1 mcg/ml increase in serum theophylline concentration. Ideally, then, the loading dose should be deferred if a serum theophylline concentration can be rapidly obtained. If this is not possible, the clinician must exercise judgment in selecting a dose based on the potential for benefit and risk. When there is sufficient respiratory distress to warrant a small risk, 4 mg/kg Oxtriphylline (2.5 mg/kg of theophylline) is likely to increase the serum concentration when administered as a loading dose in rapidly absorbed form by only about 5 mcg/ml. If the patient is not already experiencing theophylline toxicity, this is unlikely to result in dangerous adverse effect.

Following the decision regarding loading dose in this group of patients, the subsequent maintenance dosage recommendations are the same as those described above.

If it is not possible to obtain serum level determinations, restriction of the daily dose (in otherwise healthy adults) to not greater than 13 mg/kg/day (of anhydrous theophylline), to a maximum of 900 mg, in divided doses will result in relatively few patients exceeding serum levels of 20 µg/ml and the resultant greater risk of toxicity.

Patients should be closely monitored for signs of toxicity. The present data suggests that the above dosage recommendations will achieve therapeutic serum concentrations with minimal risk of toxicity for most patients. However, some risk of toxic serum concentrations is still present.

Adverse reactions to theophylline often occur when serum theophylline levels exceed 20 mcg/ml.

CHRONIC ASTHMA

Theophylline is a treatment for the management of reversible bronchospasm (asthma, chronic bronchitis and emphysema) to prevent symptoms and maintain patent airways. A dosage form which allows small incremental doses is desirable for initiating therapy. A liquid preparation should be considered for children to permit both greater ease of and more accurate dosage adjustment. Slow clinical titration is generally preferred to assure acceptance and safety of the medication, and to allow the patient to develop tolerance to transient caffeine-like side effects.

OXTRIPHYLLINE

Initial dose:	25 mg*/kg/day or 625 mg/day (whichever is lower) in 3 to 4 divided doses at 6-8 hour intervals.
Increased dose:	The above dosage may be increased in approximately 25% increments at 2 to 3 day intervals as long as no intolerance is observed until clinical response is satisfactory or the maximum indicated below is reached. The serum concentration may be checked at these intervals, but at a minimum, should be determined at the end of this adjustment period.

* 25 mg Oxtriphylline = 16 mg anhydrous theophylline.

MAXIMUM DOSE OF OXTRIPHYLLINE WITHOUT MEASUREMENT OF SERUM THEOPHYLLINE CONCENTRATION:
Not to exceed the following:
(WARNING, DO NOT ATTEMPT TO MAINTAIN ANY DOSE THAT IS NOT TOLERATED)

Age < 9 years	—37.5 mg/kg/day **(24 mg/kg/day)
Age 9—12 years	—31 mg/kg/day **(20 mg/kg/day)
Age 12—16 years	—28 mg/kg/day **(18 mg/kg/day)
Age > 16 years	—20 mg/kg/day or 1400 mg/day (WHICHEVER IS LESS) **(13 mg/kg/day or 900 mg/day) (WHICHEVER IS LESS)

Note: Use ideal body weight for obese patients.
** Anhydrous theophylline indicated in ( ).

If the total daily maintenance dosage requirement of the Oxtriphylline nonsustained preparation is established at approximately 1200 mg; Oxtriphylline 600 mg Sustained Action Tablets, one every 12 hours, may be substituted to provide smoother steady-state theophylline levels and the convenience of bid dosage. Similarly, if the total daily maintenance dosage is established at approximately 800 mg, Oxtriphylline 400 mg. Sustained Action Tablets, one every 12 hours, may be substituted.

MEASUREMENT OF SERUM THEOPHYLLINE CONCENTRATION DURING CHRONIC THERAPY

If the above maximum dosages are to be maintained or exceeded, serum theophylline measurement is recommended. This should be obtained at the approximate time of peak absorption (1 to 2 hours after dosing) during chronic

therapy. It is important that the patient will have missed *no* doses during the previous 48 hours and that dosing intervals will have been reasonably typical, with no added doses during that period of time.

DOSAGE ADJUSTMENT BASED ON SERUM THEOPHYLLINE MEASUREMENTS IF THE ABOVE INSTRUCTIONS HAVE NOT BEEN FOLLOWED MAY RESULT IN RISK OF TOXICITY TO THE PATIENT.

Caution should be exercised for younger children who cannot complain of minor side effects. Older adults, those with cor pulmonale, congestive heart failure, and/or liver disease, may have unusually low dosage requirements and thus may experience toxicity at the maximal dosage recommended above.

It is important that no patient be maintained on any dosage that is not tolerated. In instructing patients to increase dosage according to the schedule above, they should be instructed to not take a subsequent dose if apparent side effects occur and to resume therapy at a lower dose once adverse effects have disappeared.

FINAL ADJUSTMENT OF DOSAGE
Dosage adjustment after serum theophylline measurement:

If serum theophylline is:		Directions:
Within desired range		Maintain dosage if tolerated.
Too high	20 to 25 µg/mL	Decrease doses by about 10% and recheck serum level after 3 days.
	25 to 30 µg/mL	Skip the next dose and decrease subsequent doses by about 25%. Recheck serum level after 3 days.
	Over 30 µg/mL	Skip next 2 doses and decrease subsequent does by 50%. Recheck serum level after 3 days.
Too low		Increase dosage by 25% at 3-day intervals until either the desired serum concentration and/or clinical response is achieved. The total daily dose may need to be administered at more frequent intervals if symptoms occur repeatedly at the end of a dosing interval.

The serum concentration may be rechecked at appropriate intervals, but at least at the end of any adjustment period. When the patient's condition is otherwise clinically stable and none of the recognized factors which alter elimination are present, measurement of serum levels need to be repeated only every 6 to 12 months.

STORAGE
Store between 15°-30° (59°-86°F).

HOW SUPPLIED
ENTERIC COATED TABLETS: 100 MG

BRAND/MANUFACTURER	NDC	SIZE	AWP
◆ BRAND CHOLEDYL: Parke-Davis	00071-0210-24	100s	$22.67

ENTERIC COATED TABLETS: 200 MG

BRAND/MANUFACTURER	NDC	SIZE	AWP
◆ BRAND CHOLEDYL: Parke-Davis	00071-0211-24	100s	$28.88

TABLET, EXTENDED RELEASE: 400 MG

BRAND/MANUFACTURER	NDC	SIZE	AWP
○ BRAND CHOLEDYL SA: Parke-Davis	00071-0214-24	100s	$34.18

TABLET, EXTENDED RELEASE: 600 MG

BRAND/MANUFACTURER	NDC	SIZE	AWP
○ BRAND CHOLEDYL SA: Parke-Davis	00071-0221-24	100s	$41.00

Oxybutynin Chloride

Each Oxybutynin Chloride Tablet contains 5 mg of Oxybutynin Chloride. Each 5 mL of Oxybutynin Chloride Syrup contains 5 mg of Oxybutynin Chloride. Chemically, Oxybutynin Chloride is d,1 (racemic) 4-diethylamino-2-butynyl phenylcyclohexylglycolate hydrochloride. The empirical formula of Oxybutynin Chloride is $C_{22}H_{31}.HCl$.

Oxybutynin Chloride is a white crystalline solid with a molecular weight of 393.9. It is readily soluble in water and acids, but relatively insoluble in alkalis.

◆ RATED THERAPEUTICALLY EQUIVALENT; ◇ THERAPEUTIC EQUIVALENCE UNCONFIRMED; ○ UNRATED

Therapeutic Category: Antispasmodic, anticholinergic.

Following is its chemical structure:

CLINICAL PHARMACOLOGY

Oxybutynin Chloride exerts direct antispasmodic effect on smooth muscle and inhibits the muscarinic action of acetylcholine on smooth muscle. Oxybutynin Chloride exhibits only one fifth of the anticholinergic activity of atropine on the rabbit detrusor muscle, but four to ten times the antispasmodic activity. No blocking effects occur at skeletal neuromuscular junctions or autonomic ganglia (antinicotinic effects).

Oxybutynin Chloride relaxes bladder smooth muscle. In patients with conditions characterized by involuntary bladder contractions, cystometric studies have demonstrated that Oxybutynin Chloride increases bladder (vesical) capacity, diminishes the frequency of uninhibited contractions of the detrusor muscle, and delays the initial desire to void. Oxybutynin Chloride thus decreases urgency and the frequency of both incontinent episodes and voluntary urination.

Oxybutynin Chloride was well tolerated in patients administered the drug in controlled studies of 30 days' duration and uncontrolled studies in which some of the patients received the drug for 2 years. Pharmacokinetic information is not currently available.

INDICATIONS AND USAGE

Oxybutynin Chloride is indicated for the relief of symptoms of bladder instability associated with voiding in patients with uninhibited neurogenic or reflex neurogenic bladder (ie, urgency, frequency, urinary leakage, urge incontinence, dysuria).

UNLABELED USES

Oxybutynin Chloride is used alone or as an adjunct in the treatment of detrusor hyperreflexia and detrusor instability.

CONTRAINDICATIONS

Oxybutynin Chloride is contraindicated in patients with untreated angle closure glaucoma and in patients with untreated narrow anterior chamber angles since anticholinergic drugs may aggravate these conditions.

It is also contraindicated in partial or complete obstruction of the gastrointestinal tract paralytic ileus, intestinal atony of the elderly or debilitated patient, megacolon, toxic mega-colon complicating ulcerative colitis, severe colitis, and myasthenia gravis. It is contraindicated in patients with obstructive uropathy and in patients with unstable cardiovascular status in acute hemorrhage.

Oxybutynin Chloride is contraindicated in patients who have demonstrated hypersensitivity to the product.

WARNINGS

Oxybutynin Chloride, when administered in the presence of high environmental temperature, can cause heat prostration (fever and heat stroke due to decreased sweating).

Diarrhea may be an early symptom of incomplete intestinal obstruction, especially in patients with ileostomy or colostomy. In this instance treatment with Oxybutynin Chloride would be inappropriate and possibly harmful.

Oxybutynin Chloride may produce drowsiness or blurred vision. The patient should be cautioned regarding activities requiring mental alertness such as operating a motor vehicle or other machinery or performing hazardous work while taking this drug.

Alcohol or other sedative drugs may enhance the drowsiness caused by Oxybutynin Chloride.

PRECAUTIONS

Oxybutynin Chloride should be used with caution in the elderly and in all patients with autonomic neuropathy, hepatic or renal disease. Oxybutynin Chloride may aggravate the symptoms of hyperthyroidism, coronary heart disease, congestive heart failure, cardiac arrhythmias, hiatal hernia, tachycardia, hypertension, and prostatic hypertrophy. Administration of Oxybutynin Chloride to patients with ulcerative colitis may suppress intestinal motility to the point of producing a paralytic ileus and precipitate or aggravate toxic megacolon, a serious complication of the disease.

Carcinogenesis, Mutagenesis, Impairment of Fertility: A 24-month study in rats at dosages up to approximately 400 times the recommended human dosage showed no evidence of carcinogenicity.

Oxybutynin Chloride showed no increase of mutagenic activity when tested in *Schizosaccharomyces pompholiciformis, Saccharomyces cerevisiae* and *Salmonella typhimurium* test systems. Reproduction studies in the hamster, rabbit, rat, and mouse have shown no definite evidence of impaired fertility.

Pregnancy: Category B. Reproduction studies in the hamster, rabbit, rat, and mouse have shown no definite evidence of impaired fertility or harm to the animal fetus. The safety of Oxybutynin Chloride administered to women who are or who may become pregnant has not been established. Therefore, Oxybutynin Chloride should not be given to pregnant women unless, in the judgment of the physician, the probable clinical benefits outweigh the possible hazards.

Nursing Mothers: It is not known whether this drug is excreted in human milk. Because many drugs are excreted in human milk, caution should be exercised when Oxybutynin Chloride is administered to a nursing woman.

Pediatric Use: The safety and efficacy of Oxybutynin Chloride administration have been demonstrated for children 5 years of age and older (see *"Dosage and Administration"*). However, as there is insufficient clinical data for children under age 5, Oxybutynin Chloride is not recommended for this age group.

ADVERSE REACTIONS

Following administration of Oxybutynin Chloride the symptoms that can be associated with the use of other anticholinergic drugs may occur:

Cardiovascular: Palpitations, tachycardia, vasodilation.

Dermatologic: Decreased sweating, rash.

Gastrointestinal/Genitourinary: Constipation, decreased gastrointestinal motility, dry mouth, nausea, urinary hesitance and retention.

Nervous System: Asthenia, dizziness, drowsiness, hallucinations, insomnia, restlessness.

Ophthalmic: Amblyopia, cycloplegia, decreased lacrimation mydriasis.

Other: Impotence, suppression of lactation.

OVERDOSAGE

The symptoms of overdosage with Oxybutynin Chloride may be any of those seen with other anticholinergic agents. Symptoms may include signs of central nervous system excitation (eg, restlessness, tremor, irritability, convulsions, delirium, hallucinations), flushing, fever, nausea, vomiting, tachycardia, hypotension or hypertension, respiratory failure, paralysis, and coma.

In the event of an overdose or exaggerated response, treatment should be symptomatic and supportive. Maintain respiration and induce emesis or perform gastric lavage (emesis is contraindicated in precomatose, convulsive, or psychotic state). Activated charcoal may be administered as well as a cathartic. Physostigmine may be considered to reverse symptoms of anticholinergic intoxication. Hyperpyrexia may be treated symptomatically with ice bags or other cold applications and alcohol sponges.

DOSAGE AND ADMINISTRATION

TABLETS

Adults: The usual dose is one 5-mg tablet two to three times a day. The maximum recommended dose is one 5-mg tablet four times a day.

Children over 5 years of age: The usual dose is one 5-mg tablet two times a day. The maximum recommended dose is one 5-mg tablet three times a day.

SYRUP

Adults: The usual dose is one teaspoon (5 mg/5 mL) syrup two to three times a day. The maximum recommended dose is one teaspoon (5 mg/5 mL) syrup four times a day.

Children over 5 years of age: The usual dose is one teaspoon (5 mg/5 mL) two times a day. The maximum recommended dose is one teaspoon (5 mg/5 mL) three times a day.

Tablets and Syrup: Dispense in tight, light-resistant container as defined in the USP.

Store at controlled room temperature (59°-86°F).

HOW SUPPLIED
SYRUP: 5 MG/5 ML

BRAND/MANUFACTURER	NDC	SIZE	AWP
◆ **BRAND**			
DITROPAN: Marion Merrell Dow	00088-1373-18	480 ml	$48.44

TABLETS: 5 MG

AVERAGE UNIT PRICE (AVAILABLE SIZES)		GENERIC A-RATED AVERAGE PRICE (GAAP)	
BRAND	$0.46	100s	$33.17
GENERIC	$0.31	500s	$142.39
HCFA FUL (100s ea)	$0.16	750s	$211.65
		1000s	$269.78

BRAND/MANUFACTURER	NDC	SIZE	AWP
◆ **BRAND**			
► DITROPAN: Marion Merrell Dow	00088-1375-47	100s	$44.69
	00088-1375-49	100s ud	$48.81
	00088-1375-58	1000s	$435.38
◆ **GENERICS**			
Medirex	57480-0434-06	30s	$13.28
Qualitest	00603-4975-21	100s	$28.15
Rugby	00536-4777-01	100s	$29.95
Major	00904-2821-60	100s	$30.00
URL	00677-1255-01	100s	$30.82
Schein	00364-2310-01	100s	$30.87
Mason Dist	11845-0472-01	100s	$31.16
Moore,H.L.	00839-7504-06	100s	$35.78
Parmed	00349-8827-01	100s	$36.50
Goldline	00182-1289-01	100s	$36.50
Geneva	00781-1629-01	100s	$36.75
► Sidmak	50111-0456-01	100s	$36.75

► SHOWN IN PRODUCT IDENTIFICATION GUIDE

BRAND/MANUFACTURER	NDC	SIZE	AWP
Martec	52555-0105-01	100s	$36.95
Aligen	00405-4735-01	100s	$38.68
U.S. Trading	56126-0404-11	100s ud	$19.31
Auro	55829-0397-10	100s ud	$25.75
Major	00904-2821-61	100s ud	$27.19
Vangard	00615-3512-13	100s ud	$28.22
Raway	00686-0628-20	100s ud	$32.00
Goldline	00182-1289-89	100s ud	$36.50
Medirex	57480-0434-01	100s ud	$44.25
UDL	51079-0628-20	100s ud	$44.59
Rugby	00536-4777-05	500s	$124.43
URL	00677-1255-05	500s	$124.50
Parmed	00349-8827-05	500s	$139.00
▶ Sidmak	50111-0456-02	500s	$144.00
Goldline	00182-1289-05	500s	$180.00
Glasgow	60809-0116-55	750s ud	$211.65
Glasgow	60809-0116-72	750s ud	$211.65
Major	00904-2821-80	1000s	$202.45
Mason Dist	11845-0472-04	1000s	$231.04
Parmed	00349-8827-10	1000s	$250.95
Qualitest	00603-4975-32	1000s	$279.41
▶ Sidmak	50111-0456-03	1000s	$285.00
Martec	52555-0105-10	1000s	$286.50
Aligen	00405-4735-03	1000s	$300.00
Moore, H.L.	00839-7504-16	1000s	$322.91

TABLETS: 5 MG

BRAND/MANUFACTURER	NDC	SIZE	AWP
○ **BRAND**			
UROTROL: Baker Norton	00575-1900-01	100s	$32.81

Oxycodone Hydrochloride

DESCRIPTION

Each tablet contains:

Oxycodone Hydrochloride ....5 mg
(Warning: May be habit forming)

Each 5 mL Oral Solution contains:

Oxycodone Hydrochloride ....5 mg
(WARNING: May be habit forming)

Each mL Concentrated Oral Solution contains:

Oxycodone Hydrochloride ....20 mg
(WARNING: May be habit forming)

Oxycodone is 14-hydroxydihydrocodeinone, a white odorless crystalline powder which is derived from the opium alkaloid, thebaine.

Following is its chemical structure:

ACTIONS

The analgesic ingredient Oxycodone, is a semisynthetic narcotic with multiple actions qualitatively similar to those of morphine; the most prominent of these involve the central nervous system and organs composed of smooth muscle. The principal actions of therapeutic value of Oxycodone are analgesia and sedation.

Oxycodone is similar to codeine and methadone in that it retains at least one half of its analgesic activity when administered orally.

INDICATIONS

For the relief of moderate to moderately severe pain.

CONTRAINDICATIONS

Hypersensitivity to Oxycodone.

WARNINGS

Drug Dependence: Oxycodone can produce drug dependence of the morphine type, and therefore, has the potential for being abused. Psychic dependence, physical dependence and tolerance may develop upon repeated administration of this drug, and it should be prescribed and administered with the same degree of caution appropriate to the use of other oral narcotic-containing medications. Like other narcotic-containing medications, this drug is subject to the Federal Controlled Substances Act.

Usage in Ambulatory Patients: Oxycodone may impair the mental and/or physical abilities required for the performance of potentially hazardous tasks such as driving a car or operating machinery. The patient using this drug should be cautioned accordingly.

Interaction with Other Central Nervous System Depressants: Patients receiving other narcotic analgesics, general anesthetics, phenothiazines, other tranquilizers, sedative-hypnotics or other CNS depressants (including alcohol) concomitantly with Oxycodone hydrochloride may exhibit an additive CNS depression. When such combined therapy is contemplated, the dose of one or both agents should be reduced.

Usage In Pregnancy: Safe use in pregnancy has not been established relative to possible adverse effects on fetal development. Therefore, this drug should not be used in pregnant women unless, in the judgment of the physician, the potential benefits outweigh the possible hazards.

Usage In Children: This drug should not be administered to children.

PRECAUTIONS

Head Injury and Increased Intracranial Pressure: The respiratory depressant effects of narcotics and their capacity to elevate cerebrospinal fluid pressure may be markedly exaggerated in the presence of head injury, other intracranial lesions or a pre-existing increase in intracranial pressure. Furthermore, narcotics produce adverse reactions which may obscure the clinical course of patients with head injuries.

Acute Abdominal Conditions: The administration of this drug or other narcotics may obscure the diagnosis or clinical course in patients with acute abdominal conditions.

Special Risk Patients: This drug should be given with caution to certain patients such as the elderly, or debilitated, and those with severe impairment of hepatic or renal function, hypothyroidism, Addison's disease and prostatic hypertrophy or urethral stricture.

ADVERSE REACTIONS

The most frequently observed adverse reactions include light headedness, dizziness, sedation, nausea and vomiting. These effects seem to be more prominent in ambulatory than in nonambulatory patients, and some of these adverse reactions may be alleviated if the patient lies down.

Other adverse reactions include euphoria, dysphoria, constipation, skin rash and pruritus.

DOSAGE AND ADMINISTRATION

Dosage should be adjusted to the severity of the pain and the response of the patient. It may occasionally be necessary to exceed the usual dosage recommended below in cases of more severe pain or in those patients who have become tolerant to the analgesic effects of narcotics. This drug is given orally. The usual adult dose is one 5 mg tablet or 5 mL every 6 hours as needed for pain.

DRUG INTERACTIONS

The CNS depressant effects of Oxycodone Hydrochloride may be additive with that of other CNS depressants. See *"Warnings"*.

MANAGEMENT OF OVERDOSAGE

Signs and Symptoms: Serious overdose of Oxycodone Hydrochloride is characterized by respiratory depression (a decrease in respiratory rate and/or tidal volume, Cheyne-Stokes respiration, cyanosis), extreme somnolence progressing to stupor or coma, skeletal muscle flaccidity, cold and clammy skin, and sometimes bradycardia and hypotension. In severe overdosage, apnea, circulatory collapse, cardiac arrest and death may occur.

Treatment: Primary attention should be given to the reestablishment of adequate respiratory exchange through provision of a patent airway and the institution of assisted or controlled ventilation. The narcotic antagonist naloxone is a specific antidote against respiratory depression which may result from overdosage or unusual sensitivity to narcotics, including Oxycodone. Therefore, an appropriate dose of naloxone (usual initial adult dose: 0.4 mg) should be administered, preferably by the intravenous route, simultaneously with efforts at respiratory resuscitation. Since the duration of action of Oxycodone may exceed that of the antagonist, the patient should be kept under continued surveillance and repeated doses of the antagonist should be administered as needed to maintain adequate respiration.

An antagonist should not be administered in the absence of clinically significant respiratory or cardiovascular depression.

Oxygen, intravenous fluids, vasopressors and other supportive measures should be employed as indicated.

Gastric emptying may be useful in removing unabsorbed drug.

HOW SUPPLIED
CONCENTRATE (C-II): 20 MG/ML

BRAND/MANUFACTURER	NDC	SIZE	AWP
○ **BRAND**			
ROXICODONE: Roxane	00054-3683-44	30 ml	$35.16

SOLUTION (C-II): 5 MG/5 ML

BRAND/MANUFACTURER	NDC	SIZE	AWP
○ **BRAND**			
ROXICODONE: Roxane	00054-3682-63	500 ml	$36.11
	00054-8782-16	5 ml 40s ud	$48.40

◆ RATED THERAPEUTICALLY EQUIVALENT; ◇ THERAPEUTIC EQUIVALENCE UNCONFIRMED; ○ UNRATED

TABLETS (C-II): 5 MG

BRAND/MANUFACTURER	NDC	SIZE	AWP
○ **BRAND**			
ROXICODONE: Roxane	00054-4657-25	100s	$26.91
	00054-8657-24	100s ud	$36.83

Oxymetholone

DESCRIPTION

Oxymetholone tablets for oral administration each contain 50 mg of the steroid Oxymetholone, a potent anabolic and androgenic drug.

The chemical name for Oxymetholone is 17β-hydroxy-2-(hydroxymethylene)-17-methyl-5α-androstan-3-one .

Following is its chemical structure:

CLINICAL PHARMACOLOGY

Anabolic steroids are synthetic derivatives of testosterone. Nitrogen balance is improved with anabolic agents but only when there is sufficient intake of calories and protein. Whether this positive nitrogen balance is of primary benefit in the utilization of protein-building dietary substances has not been established. Oxymetholone enhances the production and urinary excretion of erythropoietin in patients with anemias due to bone marrow failure and often stimulates erythropoiesis in anemias due to deficient red cell production.

Certain clinical effects and adverse reactions demonstrate the androgenic properties of this class of drugs. Complete dissociation of anabolic and androgenic effects has not been achieved. The actions of anabolic steroids are therefore similar to those of male sex hormones with the possibility of causing serious disturbances of growth and sexual development if given to young children. They suppress the gonadotropic functions of the pituitary and may exert a direct effect upon the testes.

INDICATIONS AND USAGE

Oxymetholone is indicated in the treatment of anemias caused by deficient red cell production. Acquired aplastic anemia, congenital aplastic anemia, myelofibrosis and the hypoplastic anemias due to the administration of myelotoxic drugs often respond.

Oxymetholone should not replace other supportive measures such as transfusion, correction of iron, folic acid, vitamin B₁₂ or pyridoxine deficiency, antibacterial therapy and the appropriate use of corticosteroids.

CONTRAINDICATIONS

1. Carcinoma of the prostate or breast in male patients.
2. Carcinoma of the breast in females with hypercalcemia; androgenic anabolic steroids may stimulate osteolytic resorption of bones.
3. Oxymetholone can cause fetal harm when administered to pregnant women. It is contraindicated in women who are or may become pregnant. If the patient becomes pregnant while taking the drug, she should be apprised of the potential hazard to the fetus.
4. Nephrosis or the nephrotic phase of nephritis.
5. Hypersensitivity to the drug.
6. Severe hepatic dysfunction.

WARNINGS

The following conditions have been reported in patients receiving androgenic anabolic steroids as a general class of drugs:

PELIOSIS HEPATIS, A CONDITION IN WHICH LIVER AND SOMETIMES SPLENIC TISSUE IS REPLACED WITH BLOOD-FILLED CYSTS, HAS BEEN REPORTED IN PATIENTS RECEIVING ANDROGENIC ANABOLIC STEROID THERAPY. THESE CYSTS ARE SOMETIMES PRESENT WITH MINIMAL HEPATIC DYSFUNCTION, BUT AT OTHER TIMES THEY HAVE BEEN ASSOCIATED WITH LIVER FAILURE. THEY ARE OFTEN NOT RECOGNIZED UNTIL LIFE-THREATENING LIVER FAILURE OR INTRA-ABDOMINAL HEMORRHAGE DEVELOPS. WITHDRAWAL OF DRUG USUALLY RESULTS IN COMPLETE DISAPPEARANCE OF LESIONS.

LIVER CELL TUMORS ARE ALSO REPORTED. MOST OFTEN THESE TUMORS ARE BENIGN AND ANDROGEN-DEPENDENT, BUT FATAL MALIGNANT TUMORS HAVE BEEN REPORTED. WITHDRAWAL OF DRUG OFTEN RESULTS IN REGRESSION OR CESSATION OF PROGRESSION OF THE TUMOR. HOWEVER, HEPATIC TUMORS ASSOCIATED WITH ANDROGENS OR ANABOLIC STEROIDS ARE MUCH MORE VASCULAR THAN OTHER HEPATIC TUMORS AND MAY BE SILENT UNTIL LIFE-THREATENING INTRA-ABDOMINAL HEMORRHAGE DEVELOPS. BLOOD LIPID CHANGES THAT ARE KNOWN TO BE ASSOCIATED WITH INCREASED RISK OF ATHEROSCLEROSIS ARE SEEN IN PATIENTS TREATED WITH ANDROGENS AND ANABOLIC STEROIDS. THESE CHANGES INCLUDE DECREASED HIGH DENSITY LIPOPROTEIN AND SOMETIMES INCREASED LOW DENSITY LIPOPROTEIN. THE CHANGES MAY BE VERY MARKED AND COULD HAVE A SERIOUS IMPACT ON THE RISK OF ATHEROSCLEROSIS AND CORONARY ARTERY DISEASE.

Cholestatic hepatitis and jaundice occur with 17-alpha-alkylated androgens at relatively low doses. Clinical jaundice may be painless, with or without pruritus. It may also be associated with acute hepatic enlargement and right upper-quadrant pain, which has been mistaken for acute (surgical) obstruction of the bile duct. Drug-induced jaundice is usually reversible when the medication is discontinued. Continued therapy has been associated with hepatic coma and death. Because of the hepatotoxicity associated with Oxymetholone administration, periodic liver function tests are recommended.

In patients with breast cancer, anabolic steroid therapy may cause hypercalcemia by stimulating osteolysis. In this case, the drug should be discontinued.

Edema with or without congestive heart failure may be a serious complication in patients with pre-existing cardiac, renal or hepatic disease. Concomitant administration with adrenal steroids or ACTH may add to the edema. This is generally controllable with appropriate diuretic and/or digitalis therapy.

Geriatric male patients treated with androgenic anabolic steroids may be at an increased risk for the development of prostate hypertrophy and prostatic carcinoma.

Anabolic steroids have not been shown to enhance athletic ability.

PRECAUTIONS

General: Women should be observed for signs of virilization (deepening of the voice, hirsutism, acne, and clitoromegaly). To prevent irreversible change, drug therapy must be discontinued when mild virilism is first detected. Such virilization is usual following androgenic anabolic steroid use at high doses. Some virilizing changes in women are irreversible even after prompt discontinuance of therapy and are not prevented by concomitant use of estrogens. Menstrual irregularities, including amenorrhea, may also occur.

The insulin or oral hypoglycemic dosage may need adjustment in diabetic patients who receive anabolic steroids.

Anabolic steroids may cause suppression of clotting factors II, V, VII, and X, and an increase in prothrombin time.

Information for the Patient: The physician should instruct patients to report any of the following side effects of androgens.

Adult or Adolescent Males: Too frequent or persistent erections of the penis, appearance or aggravation of acne.

Women: Hoarseness, acne, changes in menstrual periods, or more hair on the face.

All Patients: Any nausea, vomiting, changes in skin color or ankle swelling.

Laboratory Tests: Women with disseminated breast carcinoma should have frequent determination of urine and serum calcium levels during the course of androgenic anabolic steroid therapy (see *"Warnings"*).

Because of the hepatotoxicity associated with the use of 17-alpha-alkylated androgens, liver function tests should be obtained periodically.

Periodic (every 6 months) x-ray examinations of bone age should be made during treatment of prepubertal patients to determine the rate of bone maturation and the effects of androgenic anabolic steroid therapy on the epiphyseal centers. Anabolic steroids have been reported to lower the level of high-density lipoproteins and raise the level of low-density lipoproteins. These changes usually revert to normal on discontinuation of treatment. Increased low-density lipoproteins and decreased high-density lipoproteins are considered cardiovascular risk factors. Serum lipids and high-density lipoprotein cholesterol should be determined periodically.

Hemoglobin and hematocrit should be checked periodically for polycythemia in patients who are receiving high doses of anabolics.

Because iron deficiency anemia has been observed in some patients treated with Oxymetholone, periodic determination of the serum iron and iron binding capacity is recommended. If iron deficiency is detected, it should be appropriately treated with supplementary iron.

Oxymetholone has been shown to decrease 17-ketosteroid excretion.

Drug Interaction: Anabolic steroids may increase sensitivity to anticoagulants; therefore dosage of an anticoagulant may have to be decreased in order to maintain the prothrombin time at the desired therapeutic level.

Drug/Laboratory Test Interferences: Therapy with androgenic anabolic steroids may decrease levels of thyroxine-binding globulin resulting in decreased total T_4 serum levels and increased resin uptake of T_3 and T_4. Free thyroid hormone levels remain unchanged and there is no clinical evidence of thyroid dysfunction. Altered tests usually persist for 2-3 weeks after stopping anabolic therapy.

Anabolic steroids may cause an increase in prothrombin time.

Anabolic steroids have been shown to alter fasting blood sugar and glucose tolerance tests.

Carcinogenesis, Mutagenesis, Impairment of Fertility:

Animal data: Testosterone has been tested by subcutaneous injection and implantation in mice and rats. The implant induced cervical-uterine tumors in mice, which metastasized in some cases. There is suggestive evidence that injection of testosterone into some strains of female mice increases their susceptibility to hepatoma. Testosterone is also known to increase the number of tumors and decrease the degree of differentiation of chemically induced carcinomas of the liver in rats.

Human data: There are rare reports of hepatocellular carcinoma in patients receiving long-term therapy with androgens in high doses. Withdrawal of the drugs did not lead to regression of the tumors in all cases.

Geriatric patients treated with androgens may be at an increased risk of developing prostatic hypertrophy and prostatic carcinoma although conclusive evidence to support this concept is lacking.

This compound has not been tested for mutagenic potential. However, as noted above, carcinogenic effects have been attributed to treatment with androgenic hormones. The potential carcinogenic effects likely occur through a hormonal mechanism rather than by a direct chemical interaction mechanism.

Impairment of fertility was not tested directly in animal species. However, as noted below under *"Adverse Reactions"*, oligospermia in males and amenorrhea in females are potential adverse effects of treatment with Oxymetholone tablets. Therefore, impairment of fertility is a possible outcome of treatment with Oxymetholone.

Pregnancy: Pregnancy Category X. See "Contraindications".

Nursing Mothers: It is not known whether anabolics are excreted in human milk. Because of the potential for serious adverse reactions in nursed infants from anabolics, women who take Oxymetholone should not nurse.

Pediatric Use: Anabolic/androgenic steroids should be used very cautiously in children and only by specialists who are aware of their effects on bone maturation.

Anabolic agents may accelerate epiphyseal maturation more rapidly than linear growth in children, and the effect may continue for 6 months after the drug has been stopped. Therefore, therapy should be monitored by x-ray studies at 6-month intervals in order to avoid the risk of compromising the adult height.

ADVERSE REACTIONS

Hepatic: Cholestatic jaundice with, rarely, hepatic necrosis and death. Hepatocellular neoplasms and peliosis hepatis have been reported in association with long-term androgenic anabolic steroid therapy (see *"Warnings"*).

Genitourinary System:

In Men: Prepubertal: Phallic enlargement and increased frequency of erections.

Postpubertal: Inhibition of testicular function, testicular atrophy and oligospermia, impotence, chronic priapism, epididymitis, bladder irritability, and decrease in seminal volume.

In Women: Clitoral enlargement, menstrual irregularities.

In both sexes: Increased or decreased libido.

CNS: Excitation, insomnia.

Gastrointestinal: Nausea, vomiting, diarrhea.

Hematologic: Bleeding in patients on concomitant anticoagulant therapy, iron-deficiency anemia.

Leukemia has been observed in patients with aplastic anemia treated with Oxymetholone. The role, if any, of Oxymetholone is unclear because malignant transformation has been seen in blood dyscrasias and leukemia has been reported in patients with aplastic anemia who have not been treated with Oxymetholone.

Breast: Gynecomastia.

Larynx: Deepening of the voice in women.

Hair: Hirsutism and male-pattern baldness in women, male-pattern of hair loss in postpubertal males.

Skin: Acne (especially in women and prepubertal boys).

Skeletal: Premature closure of epiphyses in children (see *"Precautions, Pediatric Use"*), muscle cramps.

Body as a Whole: Chills.

Fluid and Electrolytes: Edema, retention of serum electrolytes (sodium, chloride, potassium, phosphate, calcium).

Metabolic/Endocrine: Decreased glucose tolerance (see *"Precautions"*). Increased serum levels of low-density lipoproteins and decreased levels of high-density lipoproteins (see *"Precautions, Laboratory Tests"*), increased creatine and creatinine excretion, increased serum levels of creatinine phosphokinase (CPK). Reversible changes in liver function tests also occur including increased bromsulphalein (BSP) retention and increases in serum bilirubin, glutamic oxaloacetic transaminase (SGOT), and alkaline phosphatase.

DRUG ABUSE AND DEPENDENCE

Controlled Substance: Oxymetholone is considered to be a controlled substance and is listed in Schedule III.

OVERDOSAGE

There have been no reports of acute overdosage with anabolics.

DOSAGE AND ADMINISTRATION

The recommended daily dose in children and adults is 1-5 mg/kg body weight per day. The usual effective dose is 1-2 mg/kg/day but higher doses may be required and the dose should be individualized. Response is not often immediate and a minimum trial of three to six months should be given. Following remission, some patients may be maintained without the drug; others may be maintained on an established lower daily dosage. A continued maintenance dose is usually necessary in patients with congenital aplastic anemia.

HOW SUPPLIED

Current prices are unavailable. Check wholesaler for further information.

Oxymorphone Hydrochloride

DESCRIPTION

Oxymorphone Hydrochloride, a semi-synthetic narcotic substitute for morphine, is a potent analgesic. Oxymorphone Hydrochloride is 4,5α-Epoxy-3,14-dihydroxy-17-methylmorphinan-6-one hydrochloride.

Oxymorphone Hydrochloride occurs as a white or slightly off-white, odorless powder, sparingly soluble in alcohol and ether, but freely soluble in water.

Each ampul for injection contains:
Oxymorphone Hydrochloride 1 mg/ml or Oxymorphone HCl 1.5 mg/ml

Each rectal Suppository contains:
Oxymorphone Hydrochloride 5 mg

Following is its chemical structure:

ACTIONS

Oxymorphone HCl is a potent narcotic analgesic. Administered parenterally, 1 mg of Oxymorphone HCl is approximately equivalent in analgesic activity to 10 mg of morphine sulfate.

The onset of action of parenterally administered Oxymorphone HCl is rapid; initial effects are usually perceived within 5 to 10 minutes. Its duration of action is approximately 3 to 6 hours.

Oxymorphone HCl produces mild sedation and causes little depression of the cough reflex. These properties make it particularly useful in postoperative patients.

INDICATIONS

Oxymorphone HCl is indicated for the relief of moderate to severe pains. This drug is also indicated parenterally for preoperative medication, for support of anesthesia, for obstetrical analgesia, and for relief of anxiety in patients with dyspnea associated with acute left ventricular failure and pulmonary edema.

CONTRAINDICATIONS

Safe use of Oxymorphone HCl in children under 12 years of age has not been established. This drug should not be used in patients known to be hypersensitive to morphine analogs.

WARNINGS

May Be Habit Forming: As with other narcotic drugs, tolerance and addiction may develop. The addicting potential of the drug appears to be about the same as for morphine.

Like other narcotic-containing medications, Oxymorphone HCl is subject to the Federal Controlled Substances Act.

Interaction with Other Central Nervous System Depressants: Patients receiving other narcotic analgesics, general anesthetics, phenothiazines, other tranquilizers, sedatives, hypnotics or other CNS depressants (including alcohol) concomitantly with Oxymorphone HCl may exhibit an additive CNS depression. When such combined therapy is contemplated, the dose of one or both agents should be reduced.

Safe use in pregnancy has not been established (relative to possible adverse effects on fetal development). As with other potent analgesics, the use of Oxymorphone HCl in pregnancy in nursing mothers, or in women of child-bearing potential requires that the possible benefits of the drug be weighed against the possible hazards to the mother and the child.

Sulfites Sensitivity: Some forms of Oxymorphone HCl contain sodium dithionite, a sulfite that may cause allergic-type reactions including anaphylactic symptoms and life-threatening or less severe asthmatic episodes in certain susceptible people. The overall prevalence of sulfite sensitivity in the general population is unknown and probably low. Sulfite sensitivity is seen more frequently in asthmatic than in nonasthmatic people.

PRECAUTIONS

The same care and caution should be taken when administering Oxymorphone HCl as when other potent narcotic analgesics are used. It should be borne in mind that some respiratory depression may occur as with all potent narcotics especially when other analgesic and/or anesthetic drugs with depressant action have been given shortly before administration of Oxymorphone HCl.

The respiratory depressant effects of narcotics and their capacity to elevate cerebrospinal fluid pressure may be markedly exaggerated in the presence of head injury, other intracranial lesions or a pre-existing increase in intracranial pressure. Furthermore narcotics produce adverse reactions which may obscure the clinical course of patients with head injuries.

As with other analgesics, caution must also be exercised in elderly and debilitated patients and in patients who are known to be sensitive to central nervous system depressants, such as those with cardiovascular, pulmonary, or

---

◆ RATED THERAPEUTICALLY EQUIVALENT; ◇ THERAPEUTIC EQUIVALENCE UNCONFIRMED; ○ UNRATED

hepatic disease, in hypothyroidism (myxedema), acute alcoholism, delirium tremens, convulsive disorders, bronchial asthma and kyphoscoliosis. Debilitated and elderly patients and those with severe liver diseases should receive smaller doses of Oxymorphone HCl.

ADVERSE REACTIONS
As with all potent narcotic analgesics, possible side effects include drowsiness, nausea, vomiting, miosis, itching, dysphoria, light-headedness, and headache. Respiratory depression may occur with Oxymorphone as with other narcotics.

DOSAGE AND ADMINISTRATION
Usual Adult Dosage of Oxymorphone HCl Injection: Subcutaneous or intramuscular administration: initially 1 mg to 1.5 mg, repeated every 4 to 6 hours as needed. Intravenous: 0.5 mg initially. In nondebilitated patients the dose can be cautiously increased until satisfactory pain relief is obtained. For analgesia during labor 0.5 mg to 1 mg intramuscularly is recommended.

Usual Adult Dosage of Oxymorphone HCl Rectal Suppositories: One suppository, 5 mg, every 4 to 6 hours. In nondebilitated patients the dose can be cautiously increased until satisfactory pain relief is obtained.

Storage: Store Oxymorphone HCl Injection at controlled room temperature (59°-86°F, 15°-30°C). Protect from light.
   Store Oxymorphone HCl Rectal Suppositories under refrigeration (35°-46°F, 2°-8°C).

MANAGEMENT OF OVERDOSAGE
Signs and Symptoms: Serious overdosage with Oxymorphone HCl is characterized by respiratory depression, (a decrease in respiratory rate and/or tidal volume, Cheyne-Stokes respiration, cyanosis), extreme somnolence progressing to stupor or coma, skeletal muscle flaccidity, cold and clammy skin, and sometimes bradycardia and hypotension. In severe overdosage, apnea, circulatory collapse, cardiac arrest and death may occur.

Treatment: Primary attention should be given to the reestablishment of adequate respiratory exchange through provision of a patent airway and the institution of assisted or controlled ventilation. The narcotic antagonist naloxone HCl is a specific antidote against respiratory depression which may result from overdosage or unusual sensitivity to narcotics including Oxymorphone. Therefore, an appropriate dose of naloxone HCl should be administered (usual initial adult dose 0.4 mg-2 mg) preferably by the intravenous route and simultaneously with efforts at respiratory resuscitation. Since the duration of action of Oxymorphone may exceed that of the antagonist, the patient should be kept under continued surveillance and repeated doses of the antagonist should be administered as needed to maintain adequate respiration.
   Oxygen, intravenous fluids, vasopressors and other supportive measures should be employed as indicated.

J CODES
Up to 1 mg IV,SC,IM—J2410

HOW SUPPLIED
INJECTION (C-II): 1 MG/ML

BRAND/MANUFACTURER	NDC	SIZE	AWP
○ **BRAND**			
NUMORPHAN HCL: Du Pont Multi	00590-0370-10	1 ml 10s	$34.32

INJECTION (C-II): 1.5 MG/ML

BRAND/MANUFACTURER	NDC	SIZE	AWP
○ **BRAND**			
NUMORPHAN HCL: Du Pont Multi	00590-0374-01	10 ml	$43.74
	00590-0373-10	1 ml 10s	$44.88

SUPPOSITORY (C-II): 5 MG

BRAND/MANUFACTURER	NDC	SIZE	AWP
○ **BRAND**			
NUMORPHAN HCL: Du Pont Multi	00590-0761-06	6s	$28.15

Oxytetracycline Hydrochloride

DESCRIPTION
Oxytetracycline is a product of the metabolism of *Streptomyces rimosus* and is one of the family of tetracycline antibiotics. A 1 percent solution in water is acidic (pH about 2.5). Its potency is affected in solutions more acid than pH 2 and it is rapidly destroyed by alkali hydroxides.
   Oxytetracycline diffuses readily through the placenta into the fetal circulation, into the pleural fluid and, under some circumstances, into the cerebrospinal fluid. It appears to be concentrated in the hepatic system and excreted in the bile, so that it appears in the feces, as well as in the urine, in a biologically active form.

Following is its chemical structure:

ACTIONS
Oxytetracycline is primarily bacteriostatic and is thought to exert its antimicrobial effect by the inhibition of protein synthesis. Oxytetracycline is active against a wide range of gram-negative and gram-positive organisms.
   The drugs in the tetracycline class have closely similar antimicrobial spectra, and cross resistance among them is common. Microorganisms may be considered susceptible if the M.I.C. (minimum inhibitory concentration) is not more than 4.0 mcg/ml and intermediate if the M.I.C. is 4.0 to 12.5 mcg/ml.
   Susceptibility plate testing: A tetracycline disc may be used to determine microbial susceptibility to drugs in the tetracycline class. If the Kirby-Bauer method of disc susceptibility testing is used, a 30 mcg tetracycline disc should give a zone of at least 19 mm when tested against a tetracycline-susceptible bacterial strain.
   Tetracyclines are readily absorbed and are bound to plasma proteins in varying degree. They are concentrated by the liver in the bile, and excreted in the urine and feces at high concentrations and in a biologically active form.

INDICATIONS
Oxytetracycline is indicated in infections caused by the following microorganisms:
   Rickettsiae (Rocky Mountain spotted fever, typhus fever and the typhus group, Q fever, rickettsialpox, and tick fevers),
   Mycoplasma pneumoniae (PPLO, Eaton Agent),
   Agents of psittacosis and ornithosis,
   Agents of lymphogranuloma venereum and granuloma inguinale,
   The spirochetal agent of relapsing fever *(Borrelia recurrentis).*
   The following gram-negative micro-organisms:
   Haemophilus ducreyi (chancroid),
   Pasteurella pestis, and *Pasteurella tularensis,*
   Bartonella bacilliformis,
   Bacteroides species,
   Vibrio comma and *Vibrio fetus,*
   Brucella species (in conjunction with streptomycin).
   Because many strains of the following groups of microorganisms have been shown to be resistant to tetracyclines, culture and susceptibility testing are recommended.
   Oxytetracycline is indicated for treatment of infections caused by the following gram-negative microorganisms, when bacteriologic testing indicates appropriate susceptibility to the drug:
   Escherichia coli,
   Enterobacter aerogenes (formerly *Aerobacter aerogenes),*
   Shigella species,
   Mima species and *Herellea* species,
   Haemophilus influenzae (respiratory infections),
   Klebsiella species (respiratory and urinary infections).
   Oxytetracycline is indicated for treatment of infections caused by the following gram-positive microorganisms when bacteriologic testing indicates appropriate susceptibility to the drug:

Streptococcus species: Up to 44 percent of strains of *Streptococcus pyogenes* and 74 percent of *Streptococcus faecalis* have been found to be resistant to tetracycline drugs. Therefore, tetracyclines should not be used for streptococcal disease unless the organism has been demonstrated to be sensitive.
   For upper respiratory infections due to Group A beta-hemolytic streptococci, penicillin is the usual drug of choice, including prophylaxis of rheumatic fever.
   Diplococcus pneumoniae,
   Staphylococcus aureus, skin and soft-tissue infections. Oxytetracycline is not the drug of choice in the treatment of any type of staphylococcal infections.
   When penicillin is contraindicated, tetracyclines are alternative drugs in the treatment of infections due to:
   Neisseria gonorrhoeae,
   Treponema pallidum and *Treponema pertenue*(syphilis and yaws),
   Listeria monocytogenes,
   Clostridium species,
   Bacillus anthracis,
   Fusobacterium fusiforme (Vincent's infection),
   Actinomyces species.
   In acute intestinal amebiasis, the tetracyclines may be a useful adjunct to amebicides.
   In severe acne, the tetracyclines may be useful adjunctive therapy.
   Tetracyclines are indicated in the treatment of trachoma, although the infectious agent is not always eliminated, as judged by immunofluorescence.
   Inclusion conjunctivitis may be treated with oral tetracyclines or with a combination of oral and topical agents.

CONTRAINDICATIONS
This drug is contraindicated in persons who have shown hypersensitivity to any of the tetracyclines.

➤ SHOWN IN PRODUCT IDENTIFICATION GUIDE

WARNINGS

THE USE OF DRUGS OF THE TETRACYCLINE CLASS DURING TOOTH DEVELOPMENT (LAST HALF OF PREGNANCY, INFANCY, AND CHILDHOOD TO THE AGE OF 8 YEARS) MAY CAUSE PERMANENT DISCOLORATION OF THE TEETH (YELLOW-GRAY-BROWN). This adverse reaction is more common during long term use of the drugs but has been observed following repeated short term courses. Enamel hypoplasia has also been reported. *TETRACYCLINE DRUGS, THEREFORE, SHOULD NOT BE USED IN THIS AGE GROUP UNLESS OTHER DRUGS ARE NOT LIKELY TO BE EFFECTIVE OR ARE CONTRAINDICATED.*

If renal impairment exists, even usual oral or parenteral doses may lead to excessive systemic accumulation of the drug and possible liver toxicity. Under such conditions, lower than usual total doses are indicated and, if therapy is prolonged, serum level determinations of the drug may be advisable.

Photosensitivity manifested by an exaggerated sunburn reaction has been observed in some individuals taking tetracyclines. Patients apt to be exposed to direct sunlight or ultraviolet light should be advised that this reaction can occur with tetracycline drugs, and treatment should be discontinued at the first evidence of skin erythema.

The antianabolic action of the tetracyclines may cause an increase in BUN. While this is not a problem in those with normal renal function, in patients with significantly impaired function, higher serum levels of tetracycline may lead to azotemia, hyperphosphatemia, and acidosis.

Usage in Pregnancy: (See above "*Warnings*" about use during tooth development.)

Results of animal studies indicate that tetracyclines cross the placenta, are found in fetal tissues and can have toxic effects on the developing fetus (often related to retardation of skeletal development). Evidence of embryotoxicity has also been noted in animals treated early in pregnancy.

Usage in Newborns, Infants, and Children: (See above "*Warnings*" about use during tooth development.)

All tetracyclines form a stable calcium complex in any bone forming tissue. A decrease in the fibula growth rate has been observed in prematures given oral tetracycline in doses of 25 mg/kg every 6 hours. This reaction was shown to be reversible when the drug was discontinued.

Tetracyclines are present in the milk of lactating women who are taking a drug in this class.

PRECAUTIONS

As with other antibiotic preparations, use of this drug may result in overgrowth of nonsusceptible organisms, including fungi. If superinfection occurs, the antibiotic should be discontinued and appropriate therapy instituted.

In venereal diseases when coexistent syphilis is suspected, a dark field examination should be done before treatment is started and the blood serology repeated monthly for at least 4 months.

Because tetracyclines have been shown to depress plasma prothrombin activity, patients who are on anticoagulant therapy may require downward adjustment of their anticoagulant dosage.

In long term therapy, periodic laboratory evaluation of organ systems, including hematopoietic, renal and hepatic studies should be performed.

All infections due to Group A beta-hemolytic streptococci should be treated for at least 10 days.

Since bacteriostatic drugs may interfere with the bactericidal action of penicillin, it is advisable to avoid giving tetracycline in conjunction with penicillin.

ADVERSE REACTIONS

Gastrointestinal: anorexia, nausea, vomiting, diarrhea, glossitis, dysphagia, enterocolitis, and inflammatory lesions (with monilial overgrowth) in the anogenital region. These reactions have been caused by both the oral and parenteral administration of tetracyclines.

Rare instances of esophagitis and esophageal ulcerations have been reported in patients receiving capsule and tablet forms of drugs in the tetracycline class. Most of these patients took medications immediately before going to bed. (See "*Dosage and Administration*".)

Skin: maculopapular and erythematous rashes. Exfoliative dermatitis has been reported but is uncommon. Photosensitivity is discussed above. (See "*Warnings*".)

Renal toxicity: Rise in BUN has been reported and is apparently dose related. (See "*Warnings*".)

Hypersensitivity reactions: Urticaria, angioneurotic edema, anaphylaxis, anaphylactoid purpura, pericarditis and exacerbation of systemic lupus erythematosus.

Bulging fontanels in infants and benign intracranial hypertension in adults have been reported in individuals receiving full therapeutic dosages. These conditions disappeared rapidly when the drug was discontinued.

Blood: Hemolytic anemia, thrombocytopenia, neutropenia and eosinophilia have been reported.

When given over prolonged periods, tetracyclines have been reported to produce brown-black microscopic discoloration of thyroid glands. No abnormalities of thyroid function studies are known to occur.

DOSAGE AND ADMINISTRATION

Adults: Usual daily dose, 1-2 g divided in four equal doses, depending on the severity of the infection.

For children above eight years of age: Usual daily dose, 10-20 mg per pound (25-50 mg/kg) of body weight divided in four equal doses.

Therapy should be continued for at least 24-48 hours after symptoms and fever have subsided.

For treatment of brucellosis, 500 mg Oxytetracycline four times daily for 3 weeks should be accompanied by streptomycin, 1 gram intramuscularly twice daily the first week, and once daily the second week.

For treatment of uncomplicated gonorrhea, when penicillin is contraindicated, tetracycline may be used for the treatment of both males and females in the following divided dosage schedule: 1.5 grams initially followed by 0.5 gram q.i.d. for a total of 9.0 grams.

For treatment of syphilis, a total of 30-40 grams in equally divided doses over a period of 10-15 days should be given. Close follow-up, including laboratory tests, is recommended.

Administration of adequate amounts of fluid along with capsule and tablet forms of drugs in the tetracycline class is recommended to wash down the drugs and reduce the risk of esophageal irritation and ulceration. (See "*Adverse Reactions*".)

Concomitant therapy: Antacids containing aluminum, calcium, or magnesium impair absorption and should not be given to patients taking oral tetracyclines.

Food and some dairy products also interfere with absorption. Oral forms of tetracyclines should be given 1 hour before or 2 hours after meals. Pediatric oral dosage forms should not be given with milk formulas and should be given at least 1 hour prior to feeding.

In patients with renal impairment (See "*Warnings*".) Total dosage should be decreased by reduction of recommended individual doses and/or by extending time intervals between doses.

In the treatment of streptococcal infections, a therapeutic dose of Oxytetracycline should be administered for at least 10 days.

J CODES

Up to 50 mg IM—J2460

HOW SUPPLIED

CAPSULE: 250 MG

BRAND/MANUFACTURER	NDC	SIZE	AWP
◆ BRAND			
TERRAMYCIN: Pfizer Labs	00069-0730-66	100s	$75.10

Oxytetracycline Hydrochloride with Polymyxin B Sulfate

DESCRIPTION

Each gram of sterile ointment contains Oxytetracycline HCl equivalent to 5 mg Oxytetracycline, and 10,000 units of Polymyxin B Sulfate.

ACTIONS

Oxytetracycline HCl with Polymyxin B Sulfate is a widely used antibiotic with clinically proved activity against gram-positive and gram-negative bacteria, rickettsiae, spirochetes, large viruses, and certain protozoa.

Polymyxin B Sulfate, one of a group of related antibiotics derived from *Bacillus polymyxa*, is rapidly bactericidal. This action is exclusively against gram-negative organisms. It is particularly effective against *Pseudomonas aeruginosa (B. pyocyaneus)* and Koch-Weeks bacillus, frequently found in local infections of the eye.

There is thus made available a particularly effective antimicrobial combination of the broad-spectrum antibiotic Oxytetracycline HCl with Polymyxin B Sulfate as well as Polymyxin B Sulfate against primarily causative or secondarily infecting organisms.

INDICATIONS

The sterile preparation, Oxytetracycline with Polymyxin B Sulfate Ophthalmic Ointment, is indicated for the treatment of superficial ocular infections involving the conjunctiva and/or cornea caused by Oxytetracycline with Polymyxin B Sulfate susceptible organisms.

It may be administered topically alone, or as an adjunct to systemic therapy.

It is effective in infections caused by susceptible strains of staphylococci, streptococci, pneumococci, *Hemophilus influenzae, Pseudomonas aeruginosa,* Koch-Weeks bacillus, and *Proteus.*

CONTRAINDICATIONS

This drug is contraindicated in individuals who have shown hypersensitivity to any of its components.

PRECAUTIONS

As with all antibiotic preparations, use of this drug may result in overgrowth of nonsusceptible organisms, including fungi. If superinfection occurs, the antibiotic should be discontinued and appropriate specific therapy should be instituted.

ADVERSE REACTIONS

Oxytetracycline with Polymyxin B Sulfate Ophthalmic Ointment is well tolerated by the epithelial membranes and other tissues of the eye. Allergic or inflammatory reactions due to individual hypersensitivity are rare.

◆ RATED THERAPEUTICALLY EQUIVALENT; ◇ THERAPEUTIC EQUIVALENCE UNCONFIRMED; ○ UNRATED

DOSAGE AND ADMINISTRATION

Approximately 1/2 inch of the ointment is squeezed from the tube onto the lower lid of the affected eye two to four times daily.

The patient should be instructed to avoid contamination of the tip of the tube when applying the ointment.

J CODES

Up to 50 mg IM—J2460

HOW SUPPLIED

OINTMENT: 5 MG-10,000 U/GM

BRAND/MANUFACTURER	NDC	SIZE	AWP
○ **BRAND**			
TERRAMYCIN: Roerig	00049-0801-08	3.75 gm	$8.23
○ **GENERICS**			
AKTETRA: Akorn	17478-0230-35	3.5 gm	$8.75

Oxytetracycline Hydrochloride/ Phenazopyridine/Sulfamethizole

DESCRIPTION

Each capsule contains:

Oxytetracycline Hydrochloride equivalent to 250 mg. oxytetracycline
Sulfamethizole ....250 mg.
Phenazopyridine Hydrochloride ....50 mg.

ACTIONS

Oxytetracycline Hydrochloride/Phenazopyridine Hydrochloride/Sulfamethizole is a product designed for use specifically in urinary tract infections. Oxytetracycline Hydrochloride is a widely used antibiotic with clinically proved activity against gram-positive and gram-negative bacteria, rickettsiae, spirochetes, large viruses, and certain protozoa. Oxytetracycline Hydrochloride is well tolerated and well absorbed after oral administration. It diffuses readily through the placenta and is present in the fetal circulation. It diffuses into the pleural fluid, and under some circumstances, into the cerebrospinal fluid. Oxytetracycline Hydrochloride appears to be concentrated in the hepatic system and is excreted in the bile. It is excreted in the urine and in the feces, in high concentrations, in a biologically active form.

Sulfamethizole is a chemotherapeutic agent active against a number of important gram-positive and gram-negative bacteria. This sulfonamide is well absorbed, has a low degree of acetylation, and is extremely soluble. Because of these features and its rapid renal excretion, Sulfamethizole has a low order of toxicity and provides prompt and high concentrations of the active drug in the urinary tract.

Phenazopyridine is an orally absorbed agent which produces prompt and effective local analgesia and relief of urinary symptoms by virtue of its rapid excretion in the urinary tract. These effects are confined to the genitourinary system and are not accompanied by generalized sedation or narcosis.

INDICATIONS

BASED ON A REVIEW OF THIS DRUG BY THE NATIONAL ACADEMY OF SCIENCES-NATIONAL RESEARCH COUNCIL AND/OR OTHER INFORMATION, FDA HAS CLASSIFIED THE INDICATIONS AS FOLLOWS:

"LACKING SUBSTANTIAL EVIDENCE OF EFFECTIVENESS AS A FIXED COMBINATION":

THIS COMBINATION IS INDICATED IN THE THERAPY OF A NUMBER OF GENITOURINARY INFECTIONS CAUSED BY SUSCEPTIBLE ORGANISMS. THESE INFECTIONS INCLUDE THE FOLLOWING: PYELONEPHRITIS, PYELITIS, URETERITIS, CYSTITIS, PROSTATITIS, AND URETHRITIS.

SINCE BOTH OXYTETRACYCLINE HYDROCHLORIDE AND SULFAMETHIZOLE PROVIDE EFFECTIVE LEVELS IN BLOOD, TISSUE, AND URINE, THE COMBINATION PROVIDES A MULTIPLE ANTIMICROBIAL APPROACH AT THE SITE OF INFECTION. BOTH ANTIBACTERIAL COMPONENTS ARE ACTIVE AGAINST THE MOST COMMON URINARY PATHOGENS, INCLUDING *ESCHERICHIA COLI, PSEUDOMONAS AERUGINOSA, AEROBACTER AEROGENES, STREPTOCOCCUS FAECALIS, STREPTOCOCCUS HEMOLYTICUS, AND MICROCOCCUS PYOGENES.* THE COMBINATION IS PARTICULARLY USEFUL IN THE TREATMENT OF INFECTIONS CAUSED BY BACTERIA MORE SENSITIVE TO THE COMBINATION THAN TO EITHER COMPONENT ALONE. THE COMBINATION IS ALSO OF VALUE IN THOSE CASES WITH MIXED INFECTIONS, AND IN THOSE INSTANCES WHERE THE CAUSATIVE ORGANISM IS UNKNOWN PENDING LABORATORY ISOLATION.

FINAL CLASSIFICATION OF THE LESS THAN EFFECTIVE INDICATIONS REQUIRE FURTHER INVESTIGATION. CLINICAL STUDIES TO SUBSTANTIATE THE EFFICACY OF THIS COMBINATION ARE ONGOING. COMPLETION OF THESE ONGOING STUDIES WILL PROVIDE DATA FOR FINAL CLASSIFICATION OF THESE INDICATIONS.

CONTRAINDICATIONS

This drug is contraindicated in individuals who have shown hypersensitivity to any of its components.

This drug, because of the sulfonamide component, should not be used in patients with a history of sulfonamide sensitivities, and in pregnant females at term.

WARNINGS

If renal impairment exists, even usual oral or parenteral doses may lead to excessive systemic accumulation of the drug and possible liver toxicity. Under such conditions, lower than usual doses are indicated and if therapy is prolonged, tetracycline serum level determinations may be advisable.

Oxytetracycline Hydrochloride, which is one of the ingredients of this combination, may form a stable calcium complex in any bone-forming tissue with no serious harmful effects reported thus far in humans. However, use of Oxytetracycline during tooth development (last trimester of pregnancy, neonatal period and early childhood) may cause discoloration of the teeth (yellow-grey-brownish). This effect occurs mostly during long term use of the drug but it also has been observed in usual short treatment courses.

Because of its sulfonamide content, this drug should be used only after critical appraisal in patients with liver damage, renal damage, urinary obstruction, or blood dyscrasias. Deaths have been reported from hypersensitivity reactions, agranulocytosis, aplastic anemia, and other blood dyscrasias associated with sulfonamide administration. When used intermittently, or for a prolonged period, blood counts and liver and kidney function tests should be performed.

Certain hypersensitive individuals may develop a photodynamic reaction precipitated by exposure to direct sunlight during the use of this drug. This reaction is usually of the photoallergic type which may also be produced by other tetracycline derivatives. Individuals with a history of photosensitivity reactions should be instructed to avoid exposure to direct sunlight while under treatment with this or other tetracycline drugs, and treatment should be discontinued at first evidence of skin discomfort.

Note: Reactions of a photoallergic nature are exceedingly rare with Oxytetracycline Hydrochloride. Phototoxic reactions are not believed to occur with Oxytetracycline Hydrochloride.

PRECAUTIONS

As with all antibiotic preparations, use of this drug may result in overgrowth of nonsusceptible organisms, including fungi. If superinfection occurs, the antibiotic should be discontinued and appropriate specific therapy should be instituted. This drug should be used with caution in persons having histories of significant allergies and/or asthma.

ADVERSE REACTIONS

Glossitis, stomatitis, proctitis, nausea, diarrhea, vaginitis, and dermatitis, as well as reactions of an allergic nature, may occur during Oxytetracycline Hydrochloride therapy, but are rare. If adverse reactions, individual idiosyncrasy, or allergy occur, discontinue medication. Rare instances of esophagitis and esophageal ulcerations have been reported in patients receiving capsule forms of drugs in the tetracycline class. Most of these patients took medications immediately before going to bed. (See *"Dosage and Administration."*)

With Oxytetracycline therapy bulging fontanels in infants and benign intracranial hypertension in adults have been reported in individuals receiving full therapeutic dosages. These conditions disappeared rapidly when the drug was discontinued.

As in all sulfonamide therapy, the following reactions may occur: nausea, vomiting, diarrhea, hepatitis, pancreatitis, blood dyscrasias, neuropathy, drug fever, skin rash, infection of the conjunctiva and sclera, petechiae, purpura, hematuria and crystalluria. The dosage should be decreased or the drug withdrawn, depending upon the severity of the reaction.

DOSAGE AND ADMINISTRATION

This combination is recommended in adults only. A dose of 1 capsule four times daily is suggested. In refractory cases 2 capsules four times a day may be used.

Therapy should be continued for a minimum of seven days or until bacteriologic cure in acute urinary tract infections. Administration of adequate amounts of fluid along with capsule forms of drugs in the tetracycline class is recommended to wash down the drugs and reduce the risk of esophageal irritation and ulceration. (See *"Adverse Reaction."*)

To aid absorption of the drug, it should be given at least one hour before or two hours after eating. Aluminum hydroxide gel given with antibiotics has been shown to decrease their absorption and is contraindicated.

HOW SUPPLIED

CAPSULE: 250 MG-50 MG-250 MG

BRAND/MANUFACTURER	NDC	SIZE	AWP
○ **BRAND**			
UROBIOTIC-250: Roerig,J.B.	00049-0920-50	50s	$72.09

► SHOWN IN PRODUCT IDENTIFICATION GUIDE

Oxytocin

DESCRIPTION

Oxytocin is a synthetic, (1-6) cyclic nonapeptide available as an injection for intravenous (IV) or intramuscular (IM) use and as a nasal spray.

Each mL of solution for injection contains:

Oxytocin ....10 units
(oxytocic activity equivalent to 10 posterior pituitary units)

Each mL of nasal spray contains:
Oxytocin ....40 units

Oxytocin occurs as a white powder and is soluble in water.

Chemically, Oxytocin is designated as Glycinamide, L-cysteinyl-L-tyrosyl-L-isoleucyl-L-glutaminyl-L-asparaginyl-L-cysteinyl-L-prolyl-L-leucyl-, cyclic (1-6)-disulfide.

Its empirical formula is: $C_{43}H_{66}N_{12}O_{12}S_2$ and its molecular weight is 1007-19.

Oxytocin is one of the polypeptide hormones of the posterior lobe of the pituitary gland.

Since Oxytocin, a polypeptide, is subject to inactivation by the proteolytic enzymes of the alimentary tract, it is **not absorbed from the gastrointestinal tract.**

The hormone is prepared synthetically to avoid possible contamination with vasopressin (ADH) and other small polypeptides with biologic activity.

CLINICAL PHARMACOLOGY

The pharmacologic and clinical properties of Oxytocin are identical with those of the naturally occurring Oxytocin principle of the posterior lobe of the pituitary. Oxytocin injection does not contain the amino acids characteristic of vasopressin, and therefore has fewer and less severe cardiovascular effects. Oxytocin exerts a selective action on the smooth musculature of the uterus, particularly toward the end of pregnancy, during labor, and immediately following delivery. Oxytocin stimulates rhythmic contractions of the uterus, increases the frequency of existing contractions, and raises the tone of the uterine musculature.

Uterine motility depends on the formation of the contractile protein actomyosin under the influence of the Ca^{2-}-dependent phosphorylating enzyme myosin light-chain kinase. Oxytocin promotes contractions by increasing the intracellular Ca^{2-}. Oxytocin has specific receptors in the myometrium.

When given in appropriate doses during pregnancy, Oxytocin is capable of eliciting graded increases in uterine motility from a moderate increase in the rate and force of spontaneous motor activity to sustained tetanic contraction. The response to a given dose of Oxytocin is very individualized and depends on the sensitivity of the uterus, which is determined by the Oxytocin receptor concentration and increases progressively throughout pregnancy until term when it is maximal. However, the physician should be aware of the fact that Oxytocin even in its pure form has inherent pressor and antidiuretic properties which may become manifest when large doses are administered. These properties are thought to be due to the fact that Oxytocin and vasopressin differ in regard to only two of the eight amino acids. (See *"Precautions".*) Oxytocin is distributed throughout the extracellular fluid. Small amounts of this drug probably reach the fetal circulation. Oxytocin has a plasma half-life of about 1 to 6 minutes which is decreased in late pregnancy and during lactation. Following intravenous administration of Oxytocin, uterine response occurs almost immediately and subsides within 1 hour. Following intramuscular injection of the drug, uterine response occurs within 3 to 5 minutes and persists for 2 to 3 hours. Its rapid removal from plasma is accomplished largely by the kidney and the liver. Only small amounts of Oxytocin are excreted in the urine unchanged.

Oxytocin nasal spray acts specifically on the myoepithelial elements surrounding the alveoli of the breast, and making up the walls of the lactiferous ducts, causing their smooth muscle fibers to contract and thus force milk into the large ducts or sinuses where it is more readily available to the baby. Oxytocin does not possess galactopoietic properties and its use is intended only for the purpose of milk ejection.

PHARMACOKINETICS

Oxytocin nasal spray is promptly absorbed by the nasal mucosa to enter the systemic circulation. Intranasal application of the spray preparation, however, is a practical and effective method of administration. Half-life is extremely short—less than 10 minutes—and Oxytocin is then rapidly removed from plasma by the kidney, liver, and lactating mammary gland. The enzyme oxytocinase is believed to be elaborated by placental and uterine tissues. This enzyme inactivates the hormone by cleavage of the cysteine-tyrosine peptide bond. Excretion is mainly urinary following inactivation of metabolites.[1]

Following is its chemical structure:

$$H-Cys-Tyr-Ile-Glu(NH_2)-Asp(NH_2)-Cys-Pro-Leu-Gly-NH_2$$
$$123456789$$

INDICATIONS AND USAGE
PARENTERAL

> **IMPORTANT NOTICE**
> OXYTOCIN IS INDICATED FOR THE MEDICAL RATHER THAN THE ELECTIVE INDUCTION OF LABOR. AVAILABLE DATA AND INFORMATION ARE INADEQUATE TO DEFINE THE BENEFITS-TO-RISKS CONSIDERATIONS IN THE USE OF THE DRUG PRODUCT FOR ELECTIVE INDUCTION. ELECTIVE INDUCTION OF LABOR IS DEFINED AS THE INITIATION OF LABOR FOR CONVENIENCE IN AN INDIVIDUAL WITH A TERM PREGNANCY WHO IS FREE OF MEDICAL INDICATIONS.

Antepartum: Parenteral Oxytocin is indicated for the initiation or improvement of uterine contractions, where this is desirable and considered suitable for reasons of fetal or maternal concern, in order to achieve early vaginal delivery. It is indicated for (1) induction of labor in patients with a medical indication for the initiation of labor, such as Rh problems, maternal diabetes, preeclampsia at or near term, when delivery is in the best interest of mother and fetus or when membranes are prematurely ruptured and delivery is indicated; (2) stimulation or reinforcement of labor, as in selected cases of uterine inertia; (3) as adjunctive therapy in the management of incomplete or inevitable abortion. In the first trimester, curettage is generally considered primary therapy. In second trimester abortion, Oxytocin infusion will often be successful in emptying the uterus. Other means of therapy, however, may be required in such cases.

Postpartum: Parenteral Oxytocin is indicated to produce uterine contractions during the third stage of labor and to control postpartum bleeding or hemorrhage.

Oxytocin nasal spray is indicated to assist initial postpartum milk ejection from the breasts once milk formation has commenced.

UNLABELED USES
Oxytocin is used alone or as an adjunct to induce abortion.

CONTRAINDICATIONS

Parenteral: Oxytocin is contraindicated in any of the following conditions:
significant cephalopelvic disproportion;
unfavorable fetal positions or presentations which are undeliverable without conversion prior to delivery, e.g., transverse lies;
in obstetrical emergencies where the benefit-to-risk ratio for either the fetus or the mother favors surgical intervention; in cases of fetal distress where delivery is not imminent; hypertonic uterine patterns;
hypersensitivity to the drug.
Prolonged use in uterine inertia or severe toxemia is contraindicated.

Oxytocin should not be used in cases where vaginal delivery is not indicated, such as invasive cervical carcinoma, active herpes genitalis, cord presentation or prolapse, total placenta previa, and vasa previa.

Pregnancy and hypersensitivity are the only known contraindications to the use of Oxytocin nasal spray.

WARNINGS

Oxytocin, when given for induction or stimulation of labor, must be administered only by intravenous infusion (drip method) and with adequate medical supervision in a hospital.

PRECAUTIONS
PARENTERAL
General:

1. All patients receiving intravenous infusions of Oxytocin must be under continuous observation by trained personnel with a thorough knowledge of the drug and qualified to identify complications. A physician qualified to manage any complications should be immediately available. Electronic fetal monitoring provides the best means for early detection of overdosage (see *"Overdosage"* section). However, it must be borne in mind that only intrauterine pressure recording can accurately measure the intrauterine pressure during contractions. A fetal scalp electrode provides a more dependable recording of the fetal heart rate than any external monitoring system.

2. When properly administered, Oxytocin should stimulate uterine contractions similar to those seen in normal labor. Overstimulation of the uterus by improper administration can be hazardous to both mother and fetus. Even with proper administration and adequate supervision, hypertonic contractions can occur in patients whose uteri are hypersensitive to Oxytocin. This fact must be considered by the physician in exercising his judgment regarding patient selection.

3. Except in unusual circumstances, Oxytocin should not be administered in the following conditions: fetal distress, partial placenta previa, prematurity, borderline cephalopelvic disproportion, any condition in which there is a predisposition for uterine rupture, such as previous major surgery on the cervix or uterus, including cesarean section, overdistention of the uterus, grand multiparity, or past history of uterine sepsis or traumatic delivery, or invasive cervical carcinoma. Because of the variability of the combinations of factors which may be present in the conditions listed above, the definition of "unusual circumstances" must be left to the judgment of the physician. The decision can only be made by carefully weighing the potential benefits which Oxytocin can provide in a given case against the rare occurrence of hypertonicity or tetanic spasm with this drug.

4. Maternal deaths due to hypertensive episodes, subarachnoid hemorrhage, rupture of the uterus, fetal deaths and permanent CNS or brain damage of the infant due to various causes have been reported to be associated with the use of

parenteral oxytocic drugs for induction of labor or for augmentation in the first and second stages of labor.

5. Oxytocin has been shown to have an intrinsic antidiuretic effect, acting to increase water reabsorption from the glomerular filtrate. Consideration should, therefore, be given to the possibility of water intoxication, particularly when Oxytocin is administered continuously by infusion and the patient is receiving fluids by mouth.

6. When Oxytocin is used for induction or reinforcement of already existent labor, patients should be carefully selected. Pelvic adequacy must be considered and maternal and fetal conditions thoroughly evaluated before use of the drug.

NASAL SPRAY
No particular information regarding any special care to be exercised by the practitioner for safe and effective use of Oxytocin nasal spray is known at this time.

Information for Patients: The squeeze bottle should be held in an upright position when administering the drug to the nose and the patient should be in a sitting position rather than lying down. If preferred, the solution can be instilled in drop form by inverting the squeeze bottle and exerting very gentle pressure on its walls.

DRUG INTERACTIONS
Severe hypertension has been reported when Oxytocin was given 3 to 4 hours following prophylactic administration of a vasoconstrictor in conjunction with caudal-block anesthesia. Cyclopropane anesthesia may modify Oxytocin's cardiovascular effects, so as to produce unexpected results such as hypotension. Maternal sinus bradycardia with abnormal atrioventricular rhythms has also been noted when Oxytocin was used concomitantly with cyclopropane anesthesia.

CARCINOGENESIS, MUTAGENESIS, IMPAIRMENT OF FERTILITY
There are no animal or human studies on the carcinogenicity and mutagenicity of this drug, nor is there any information on its effect on fertility.

PREGNANCY
Category X. See *"Indications and Usage"* and *"Contraindications"*.

Oxytocin nasal spray is contraindicated during pregnancy since it may provoke a uterotonic effect to precipitate contractions and abortion. Its proper use is during the first week postpartum, as needed.

Teratogenic Effects: Animal reproduction studies have not been conducted with Oxytocin. There are no known indications for use in the first trimester of pregnancy other than in relation to spontaneous or induced abortion. Based on the wide experience with this drug and its chemical structure and pharmacological properties, it would not be expected to present a risk of fetal abnormalities when used as indicated.

Nonteratogenic Effects: See *"Adverse Reaction"* in the fetus or infant.

LABOR AND DELIVERY
See *"Indications and Usage"*.

Nursing Mothers: Oxytocin may be found in small quantities in mother's milk. If a patient requires the drug postpartum to control severe bleeding, she should not commence nursing until the day after Oxytocin has been discontinued.

While harmful effects on the newborn have not been reported it should be noted that Oxytocin nasal spray is intended to be used only for initial milk propulsion and ejection during the first week postpartum, and not for continued use. Caution shall be exercised when Oxytocin nasal spray is administered to a nursing mother.

Pediatric Use: Oxytocin is not intended for use in children.

ADVERSE REACTIONS
Parenteral: The following adverse reactions have been reported in the mother:
Anaphylactic reaction
Postpartum hemorrhage
Cardiac arrhythmia
Fatal afibrinogenemia
Nausea
Vomiting
Premature ventricular contractions
Pelvic hematoma
Excessive dosage or hypersensitivity to the drug may result in uterine hypertonicity, spasm, tetanic contraction, or rupture of the uterus.

The possibility of increased blood loss and afibrinogenemia should be kept in mind when administering the drug.

Severe water intoxication with convulsions and coma has occurred, associated with a slow Oxytocin infusion over a 24-hour hour period. Maternal death due to Oxytocin-induced water intoxication has been reported.

The following adverse reactions have been reported in the fetus or infant:
Due to induced uterine motility
Bradycardia
Premature ventricular contractions and other arrhythmias
Permanent CNS or brain damage
Fetal death
Due to use of Oxytocin in the mother
Low Apgar scores at five minutes
Neonatal jaundice
Neonatal retinal hemorrhage

Nasal Spray: Lack of efficacy has been the most frequent adverse effect (seven cases), followed by nasal irritation and/or rhinorrhea, uterine bleeding, excessive uterine contractions, and lacrimation.

One case each of seizure and "psychotic state" are the most severe reactions reported. No other reactions have been described.[2]

DRUG ABUSE AND DEPENDENCE
There is no evidence that Oxytocin has been abused or has provoked drug dependence. These problems have not been encountered with Oxytocin nasal spray. This may be due to the fact that synthetic Oxytocin acts like the natural posterior pituitary hormone. Also, its clinical use is limited to the first week following delivery, to assist in initial milk letdown.

OVERDOSAGE
Overdosage with Oxytocin depends essentially on uterine hyperactivity whether or not due to hypersensitivity to this agent. Hyperstimulation with strong (hypertonic) or prolonged (tetanic) contractions, or a resting tone of 15 to 20 mmH$_2$O or more between contractions can lead to tumultuous labor, uterine rupture, cervical and vaginal lacerations, postpartum hemorrhage, utero-placental hypoperfusion, and variable deceleration of fetal heart, fetal hypoxia, hypercapnia, or death. Water intoxication with convulsions, which is caused by the inherent antidiuretic effect of Oxytocin, is a serious complication that may occur if large doses (40 to 50 milliunits/minute) are infused for long periods. Management consists of immediate discontinuation of Oxytocin, restriction of fluid intake, diuresis, IV hypertonic saline solution, correction of electrolyte imbalance, control of convulsions with judicious use of a barbiturate, and special nursing care for the comatose patient.

No case of overdosage with Oxytocin nasal spray has been reported since the preparation became commercially available in 1961. It is theoretically possible for very large doses to be self-administered depending on the topical tolerance of the nasal mucosa. With such massive use, painful uterine contractions could be induced, although these effects persist for only about 15 minutes.[3] Also, an antidiuretic effect could occur resulting in water intoxification. Should this ensue, diuresis, should be forced with appropriate agents such as furosemide.[4]

DOSAGE AND ADMINISTRATION
PARENTERAL
Parenteral drug products should be inspected visually for particulate matter and discoloration prior to administration, whenever solution and container permit.

Dosage of Oxytocin is determined by uterine response and must therefore be individualized and initiated at a very low level. The following dosage information is based upon the various regimens and indications in general use.

A. Induction or Stimulation of Labor: Intravenous infusion (drip method) is the only acceptable method of administration for the induction or stimulation of labor.

Accurate control of the rate of infusion flow is essential. An infusion pump or other such device and frequent monitoring of strength of contractions and fetal heart rate are necessary for the safe administration of Oxytocin for the induction or stimulation of labor. If uterine contractions become too powerful, the infusion can be abruptly stopped, and oxytocic stimulation of the uterine musculature will soon wane.

1. An intravenous infusion of nonoxytocin-containing solution should be started. Physiologic electrolyte solution should be used except under unusual circumstances.

2. To prepare the usual solution for infusion, the contents of one 1-mL container (10 units) are combined aseptically with 1,000 mL of nonhydrating diluent (physiologic electrolyte solution). The same concentration can be obtained by mixing the contents of one 0.5-mL container, containing 5 units of Oxytocin, with 500 mL of electrolyte solution. The combined solution, rotated in the infusion bottle to insure thorough mixing, contains 10 mU/mL. Add the container with dilute oxytocic solution to the system through use of a constant infusion pump or other such device, to control accurately the rate of infusion.

3. The initial dose should be no more than 1 to 2 mU/min. The dose may be gradually increased at 30- to 60-minute intervals in increments of no more than 1 to 2 mU/min. until a contraction pattern has been established which is similar to normal labor.

Studies of the concentrations of Oxytocin in the maternal plasma during Oxytocin infusion have shown that infusion rates up to 6 mU/min give the same Oxytocin levels that are found in spontaneous labor. At term, higher infusion rates should be given with great care, and rates exceeding 9-10 mU/min are rarely required. Before term, when the sensitivity of the uterus is lower because of a lower concentration of Oxytocin receptors, a higher infusion rate may be required.

4. The fetal heart rate, resting uterine tone, and the frequency, duration, and force of contractions should be monitored. Attention should be given to tonus, amplitude and frequency of contractions and to the fetal heart rate in relation to uterine contractions.

5. The Oxytocin infusion should be discontinued immediately in the event of uterine hyperactivity or fetal distress. Oxygen should be administered to the mother, who should preferably be in a lateral position. The mother and the fetus must be evaluated by the responsible physician.

B. Control of Postpartum Uterine Bleeding:
1. Intravenous Infusion (Drip Method):
To control postpartum bleeding, 10 to 40 units of Oxytocin may be added to 1,000 mL of a nonhydrating diluent (physiologic electrolyte solution) and run at a rate necessary to sustain uterine contraction and control uterine atony.

2. Intramuscular Administration:
1 mL (10 units) of Oxytocin can be given after delivery of the placenta.

C. Treatment of Incomplete or Inevitable Abortion: Intravenous infusion of 10 units of Oxytocin added to 500 mL of a physiologic saline solution or 5% dextrose-in-water or physiologic saline solution may help the uterus contract after a suction or sharp curettage for an incomplete, inevitable or elective abortion. Subsequent to intra-amniotic injection of hypertonic saline, prostaglandins, urea, etc., for midtrimester elective abortion, the injection-to-abortion time may be shortened by infusion of Oxytocin at the rate of 10 to 20 milliunits (20 to 40 drops) per minute. The total dose should not exceed 30 units in a 12-hour period due to the risk of water intoxication.

Nasal Spray: One spray into one or both nostrils two to three minutes before nursing or pumping of breasts.

STORAGE
Store in a refrigerator or between 59° and 77° F (15° and 25° C).
Do not freeze.
Do not use if solution is discolored or contains a precipitate. When stored out of refrigeration this product has exhibited acceptable data for a period not exceeding three (3) months.
Store nasal spray below 77° F.

REFERENCES
1. Goodman and Gilman: The Pharmacological Basis of Therapeutics. Sixth Ed., 937-8. 2. Data collected by the Medical Services Department, Sandoz Pharmaceuticals Corporation. 3. Borglin, N.E.: The use of intranasal oxytocin for the induction of labor. *Zbl. Gynak.* **85**: 193-199 (Feb. 9) 1963. 4. Sandoz Overdosage Manual, 1984, Syntocinon® Injection. 5. Seitchik J. Castillo M: Oxytocin augmentation of dysfunctional labor. I. Clinical data. *Am J Obstet Gynecol* 1982; 144:899-905. 6. Seitchik J. Castillo M: Oxytocin augmentation of dysfunctional labor. II. Multiparous patients. *Am J Obstet Gynecol* 1983; 145:777-780. 7. Fuchs A. Goeschen K, Husslein P, et al: Oxytocin and the initiation of human parturition. III. Plasma concentrations of oxytocin and 13, 14-dihydro-15-keto-prostaglandin $F_{2\alpha}$ in spontaneous and oxytocin-induced labor at term. *Am J Obstet Gynecol* 1983; 145:497-502. 8. Seitchik J, Amico J, et al: Oxytocin augmentation of dysfunctional labor. IV. Oxytocin Pharmacokinetics. *Am J Obstet Gynecol.* 1984; 150:225-228. 9. American College of Obstetricians and Gynecologists: ACOG Technical Bulletin Number 110. November 1987: Induction and augmentation of labor.

J CODES
Up to 10 units IV,IM—J2590

HOW SUPPLIED
INJECTION: 10 U/ML

AVERAGE UNIT PRICE (AVAILABLE SIZES)

BRAND	$1.09
GENERIC	$1.32

BRAND/MANUFACTURER	NDC	SIZE	AWP
◆ BRAND			
PITOCIN: Parke-Davis	00071-4160-10	10 ml	$6.13
	00071-4160-03	1 ml 10s	$9.49
	00071-4160-40	1 ml 10s ud	$18.30
	00071-4160-45	1 ml 25s	$23.74
◆ GENERICS			
Fujisawa	00469-1012-15	1 ml	$1.22
Fujisawa	00469-0012-25	10 ml	$5.92
Wyeth-Ayerst	00008-0406-01	1 ml 10s	$21.34

INJECTION: 10 IU/ML

BRAND/MANUFACTURER	NDC	SIZE	AWP
◆ BRAND			
SYNTOCINON: Sandoz Pharm	00078-0060-04	1 ml 50s	$128.70

SPRAY: 40 IU/ML

BRAND/MANUFACTURER	NDC	SIZE	AWP
○ BRAND			
SYNTOCINON NASAL SPRAY: Sandoz Pharm	00078-0061-23	2 ml	$31.68
	00078-0061-25	5 ml	$60.00

P1E1 *SEE EPINEPHRINE BITARTRATE AND PILOCARPINE HYDROCHLORIDE*

Pacaps *SEE ACETAMINOPHEN/BUTALBITAL/CAFFEINE*

Paclitaxel

WARNING
PACLITAXEL SHOULD BE ADMINISTERED UNDER THE SUPERVISION OF A PHYSICIAN EXPERIENCED IN THE USE OF CANCER CHEMOTHERAPEUTIC AGENTS. APPROPRIATE MANAGEMENT OF COMPLICATIONS IS POSSIBLE ONLY WHEN ADEQUATE DIAGNOSTIC AND TREATMENT FACILITIES ARE READILY AVAILABLE.

SEVERE HYPERSENSITIVITY REACTIONS CHARACTERIZED BY DYSPNEA AND HYPOTENSION REQUIRING TREATMENT, ANGIOEDEMA, AND GENERALIZED URTICARIA HAVE OCCURRED IN 2% OF PATIENTS RECEIVING PACLITAXEL. ONE OF THESE REACTIONS WAS FATAL IN A PATIENT TREATED WITHOUT PREMEDICATION IN A PHASE 1 STUDY. PATIENTS RECEIVING PACLITAXEL SHOULD BE PRETREATED WITH CORTICOSTEROIDS, DIPHENHYDRAMINE, AND H_2 ANTAGONISTS TO PREVENT THESE REACTIONS. (SEE *"DOSAGE AND ADMINISTRATION"* SECTION.) PATIENTS WHO EXPERIENCE SEVERE HYPERSENSITIVITY REACTIONS TO PACLITAXEL SHOULD NOT BE RECHALLENGED WITH THE DRUG.

PACLITAXEL THERAPY SHOULD NOT BE GIVEN TO PATIENTS WITH BASELINE NEUTROPHIL COUNTS OF LESS THAN 1.500 CELLS/MM³. IN ORDER TO MONITOR THE OCCURRENCE OF BONE MARROW SUPPRESSION, PRIMARILY NEUTROPENIA, WHICH MAY BE SEVERE AND RESULT IN INFECTION, IT IS RECOMMENDED THAT FREQUENT PERIPHERAL BLOOD CELL COUNTS BE PERFORMED ON ALL PATIENTS RECEIVING PACLITAXEL.

DESCRIPTION
Paclitaxel for Injection Concentrate is a clear colorless to slightly yellow viscous solution. It is supplied as a nonaqueous solution intended for dilution with a suitable parenteral fluid prior to intravenous infusion. Paclitaxel is available in 30 mg (5 mL) single-dose vials. Each mL of sterile nonpyrogenic solution contains 6 mg Paclitaxel

Paclitaxel is a natural product with antitumor activity. The chemical name for Paclitaxel is 5β3,20-Epoxy-1,2α,4,7β,10β, 13α-hexhydroxytax-11-en-9-one 4,10-diacetate, 2-benzoate 13-ester with (2R,3S)-N-benzoyl-3-phenylisosenine.

Paclitaxel is a white to off-white crystalline powder with the empirical formula $C_{14}H_{51}NO_{14}$ and a molecular weight 853.9. It is highly lipophilic, insoluble in water, and melts at around 216-217°C.

Following is its chemical structure:

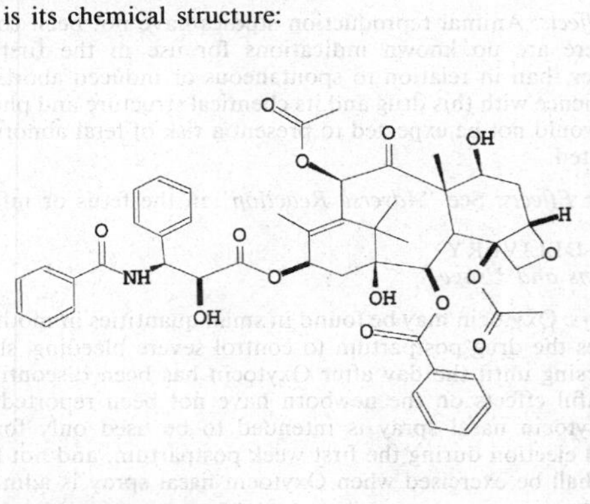

CLINICAL PHARMACOLOGY
Paclitaxel is a novel antimicrotubule agent that promotes the assembly of microtubules from tubulin dimers and stabilizes microtubules by preventing depolymerization. This stability results in the inhibition of the normal dynamic reorganization of the microtubule network that is essential for vital interphase and mitotic cellular functions. In addition, Paclitaxel induces abnormal arrays or "bundles" of microtubules throughout the cell cycle and multiple asters of microtubules during mitosis.

The pharmacokinetics of Paclitaxel have been evaluated in adult cancer patients who received single doses of 15-135 mg/m² given by 1-hour infusions (n = 15), 30-275 mg/m² given by 6-hour infusions (n = 36), and 135-275 mg/m² given by 24-hour infusions (n = 54).

Following intravenous administration of Paclitaxel, the drug exhibited a biphasic decline in plasma concentrations. The initial rapid decline represents distribution to the peripheral compartment and significant elimination of the drug. The later phase is due, in part, to a relatively slow efflux of Paclitaxel from the peripheral compartment. Values for mean terminal phase half-life, total body clearance, and apparent volume of distribution at steady state were determined following 1-hour and 6-hour infusions at dosing levels of 15-275 mg/m². Mean (standard deviation) terminal half-life was estimated to range from 5.3 (4.6) to 17.4 (4.7) hours. Mean (SD) values for total body clearance ranged from 5.8 (2.3) to 16.3 (2.3) L/h/m². The mean (SD) steady state volume of distribution ranged from 42 (15) to 162 (133) L/m², indicating extensive extravascular distribution and/or tissue binding of Paclitaxel. Mean (SD) values for total body clearance ranged from 14.2 (2.3) to 17.2 (2.8) L/h/m² following 24-hour infusions of 200-275 mg/m².

In vitro studies of binding to human serum proteins, using Paclitaxel concentrations ranging from 0.1 to 50 μg/mL, indicate that between 89-98% of drug is bound; the presence of cimetidine, ranitidine, dexamethasone, or diphenhydramine did not affect protien binding of Paclitaxel.

◆ RATED THERAPEUTICALLY EQUIVALENT; ◇ THERAPEUTIC EQUIVALENCE UNCONFIRMED; ○ UNRATED

Mean (SD) C_{MAX} values ranged from 435 (111) to 802 (260) ng/mL following 24-hour infusions at doses of 200 to 275 mg/m^2, and were approximately 10-30% of those following 6-hour infusions of equivalent doses. After administration of doses of Paclitaxel of 170 mg/m^2 or higher by infusion lasting 6 or 24 hours, plasma concentrations above 85 ng/mL, the level shown to be pharmacologically active *in vitro*, were regularly observed for at least 6 to 12 hours.

The disposition of Paclitaxel has not been fully elucidated in humans. After intravenous administration of 15-275 mg/m^2 doses of Paclitaxel as 1,6, 24-hour infusions, mean (SD) values for cumulative urinary recovery of unchanged drug ranged from 1.3% (0.5%) to 12.6% (16.2%) of the dose, indicating extensive non-renal clearance. Paclitaxel has been demonstrated to be metabolized in the liver in animals and there is evidence suggesting hepatic metabolism in humans. High Paclitaxel concentrations have been reported in the bile of patients treated with Paclitaxel. The effect of renal or hepatic dysfunction on the disposition of Paclitaxel has not been investigated.

Possible interactions of Paclitaxel with concomitantly administered medications have not been formally investigated.

Clinical Studies: Data from five clinical studies (189 patients) as well as an interim analysis of data from more than 300 patients enrolled in a Treatment Referral Center program were used in support of the use of Paclitaxel in patients with metastatic carcinoma of the ovary. Two of the studies (92 patients) utilized an initial dose of 135 to 170 mg/m^2 in most patients (> 90%) administered over 24 hours by continuous infusion. Response rates in these two studies were 22% (95% Cl = 11-37%) and 30% (95% Cl = 18-46%) with a total of six complete and 18 partial responses in 92 patients. The median duration of overall response in these two studies measured from the first day of treatment was 7.2 months (range: 3.5 - 15.8 months) and 7.5 months (range: 5.3 - 17.4 months), respectively. The median survival was 8.1 months (range: 0.2 - 36.7 months) and 15.9 months (range: 1.8 - 34.5+ months).

In general, the results of the studies performed at initial Paclitaxel doses of 135-170 mg/m^2 were similar to results from three other studies in patients with ovarian carcinoma using higher initial doses of Paclitaxel and, in two of the studies, concomitant administration of G-CSF.

The effect of Paclitaxel was similar in the subset of patients who had developed resistance to platinum-containing therapy (defined as tumor progression while on, or tumor relapse within 6 months from completion of, a platinum-containing regimen) to the effect in patients overall.

INDICATIONS
Paclitaxel is indicated, after failure of first-line or subsequent chemotherapy for the treatment of metastatic carcinoma of the ovary.

UNLABELED USES
Paclitaxel is used alone or as an adjunct in the treatment of metastatic breast cancer and acute lymphocytic and nonlymphocytic leukemia.

CONTRAINDICATIONS
Paclitaxel is contraindicated in patients who have a history of hypersensitivity reactions to Paclitaxel or other drugs formulated in polyoxyethylated castor oil. Paclitaxel should not be used in patients with baseline neutropenia of < 1,500 cells/mm^3.

WARNINGS
Patients should be pretreated with corticosteroids (such as dexamethasone), diphenhydramine and H$_2$ antagonists (such as cimetidine or ranitidine) before receiving Paclitaxel. (See *"Dosage and Administration"* section.) Severe hypersensitivity reactions characterized by dyspnea and hypotension requiring treatment, angioedema, and generalized urticaria have occurred in 2% of patients receiving Paclitaxel. These reactions are probably histamine-mediated. One of these reactions was fatal in a patient with pulmonary metastases who was a participant in a Phase I trial. This patient received no premedication; the first course of Paclitaxel, which was uneventful, was administered at 190 mg/m^2 infused over three hours. Within a few minutes from the beginning of a second course of Paclitaxel, the patient developed severe hypotension and died. Patients who experience severe hypersensitivity reactions to Paclitaxel should not be rechallenged with the drug.

Bone marrow suppression (primarily neutropenia) is dose-dependent and is the dose-limiting toxicity. Neutrophil nadirs occurred at a median of 11 days. Paclitaxel should not be administered in patients with baseline neutrophil counts of less than 1,500 cells/mm^3. Frequent monitoring of blood counts should be instituted during Paclitaxel treatment. Patients should not be re-treated with subsequent cycles of Paclitaxel until neutrophils recover to a level > 1,500 cells/mm^3 and platelets recover to a level > 100,000 cells/mm^3. Severe conduction abnormalities have been documented in two (< 1%) patients during Paclitaxel therapy. In one case insertion of a pacemaker was required due to the recurrence of atrioventricular block. In the second case, Paclitaxel infusion was completed despite the occurrence of asymptomatic recurrent atrioventricular block and a pacemaker was subsequently placed to allow further Paclitaxel treatment. If patients develop significant conduction abnormalities during Paclitaxel administration, appropriate therapy should be administered and continuous cardiac monitoring should be performed during subsequent therapy with Paclitaxel.

Paclitaxel may cause fetal harm when administered to a pregnant woman. Paclitaxel has been shown to be embryo- and feto-toxic in rats and rabbits and to decrease fertility in rats. In these studies, Paclitaxel was shown to result in abortions, decreased corpora lutea, a decrease in implantations and live fetuses, and increased resorptions and embryo-fetal deaths. No gross external, soft tissue or skeletal alterations occurred. There are no studies in pregnant women. If

Paclitaxel is used during pregnancy, or if the patient becomes pregnant while receiving this drug, the patient should be apprised of the potential hazard. Women of childbearing potential should be advised to avoid becoming pregnant during therapy with Paclitaxel.

PRECAUTIONS
Contact of the undiluted concentrate with plasticized polyvinyl chloride (PVC) equipment or devices used to prepare solutions for infusion is not recommended. In order to minimize patient exposure to the plasticizer DEHP [di-(2-ethylhexyl)phthalate], which may be leached from PVC infusion bags or sets, diluted Paclitaxel solutions should preferably be stored in bottles (glass, polypropylene) or plastic bags (polypropylene, polyolefin) and administered through polyethylene-lined administration sets.

Paclitaxel should be administered through an in-line filter with a microporous membrane not greater than 0.22 microns. Use of filter devices such as IVEX-2® filters which incorporate short inlet and outlet PVC-coated tubing has not resulted in significant leaching of DEHP.

Drug Interaction: In a Phase I trial[1] using escalating doses of Paclitaxel (110-200 mg/m^2) and cisplatin (50 or 75 mg/m^2) given as sequential infusions, myelosuppression was more profound when Paclitaxel was given after cisplatin than with the alternate sequence (i.e., Paclitaxel before cisplatin). Pharmacokinetic data from these patients demonstrated a decrease in Paclitaxel clearance of approximately 33% when Paclitaxel was administered following cisplatin.

Based on *in vitro* data, there is the possibility of an inhibition of Paclitaxel metabolism in patients treated with ketoconazole. As a result, caution should be exercised when treating patients with Paclitaxel when they are receiving ketoconazole as concomitant therapy.

Hematology: Paclitaxel therapy should not be administered to patients with baseline neutrophil counts of less than 1,500 cells/mm^3. In order to monitor the occurrence of myelotoxicity, it is recommended that frequent peripheral blood cell counts be performed on all patients receiving Paclitaxel. Patients should not be re-treated with subsequent cycles of Paclitaxel until neutrophils recover to a level > 1,500 cells/mm^3 and platelets recover to a level > 100,000 cells/mm^3. In the case of severe neutropenia (< 500 cells/mm^3 for seven days or more) during a course of Paclitaxel therapy, a 20% reduction in dose for subsequent courses of therapy is recommended. Patients who have received previous radiation therapy have experienced more myelosuppression. There is little experience in such patients at doses above 135 mg/m^2.

Hypersensitivity Reactions: Patients with a history of severe hypersensitivity reactions to products containing polyoxyethylated castor oil (e.g., cyclosporin for injection concentrate and teniposide for injection concentrate) should not be treated with Paclitaxel. In order to avoid the occurrence of severe hypersensitivity reactions, all patients treated with Paclitaxel should be premedicated with corticosteroids (such as dexamethasone), diphenhydramine and H$_2$ antagonists (such as cimetidine or ranitidine). Minor symptoms such as flushing, skin reactions, dyspnea, hypotension or tachycardia do not require interruption of therapy. However, severe reactions, such as hypotension requiring treatment, dyspnea requiring bronchodilators, angiodema or generalized urticaria require immediate discontinuation of Paclitaxel and aggressive symptomatic therapy. Patients who have developed severe hypersensitivity reactions should not be rechallenged with Paclitaxel.

Cardiovascular: Hypotension and bradycardia have been observed during administration of Paclitaxel, but generally do not require treatment. Frequent vital sign monitoring, particularly during the first hour of Paclitaxel infusion, is recommended. Continuous cardiac monitoring is not required except for patients with serious conduction abnormalities (See *"Warnings"* section.)

Nervous System: Although, the occurrence of peripheral neuropathy is frequent, the development of severe symptomatology is unusual and requires a dose reduction of 20% for all subsequent courses of Paclitaxel.

Hepatic: There is no evidence that the toxicity of Paclitaxel is enhanced in patients with elevated liver enzymes, but no data are available for patients with severe baseline cholestasis. However, evidence suggests that the liver plays an important role in the metabolism of Paclitaxel. As a result, since there are no data available from patients with severe liver disease, caution should be exercised when administering Paclitaxel to patients with severe hepatic impairment.

Carcinogenesis, Mutagenesis, Impairment of Fertility: The carcinogenic potential of Paclitaxel has not been studied. Paclitaxel has been shown to be mutagenic *in vitro* (chromosome aberrations in human lymphocytes) and *in vivo* (micro-nucleus test in mice) mammalian test systems, however, it did not induce mutagenicity in the Ames test or the CHO/HGPRT gene mutation assay. Paclitaxel at an I.V. dose of 1 mg/kg (6 mg/m^2) produced low fertility and fetal toxicity in rats. Paclitaxel has also been shown to be maternal and embryo-fetal toxic in rabbits receiving the drug at an I.V. dose of 3 mg/kg (33 mg/m^2) during organogenesis. (See *"Warnings"* section.)

Pregnancy: Pregnancy "Category D." (See *"Warnings"* section.)

Nursing Mothers: It is not known whether the drug is excreted in human milk. Because many drugs are excreted in human milk and because of the potential for serious adverse reactions in nursing infants, it is recommended that nursing be discontinued when receiving Paclitaxel therapy.

Pediatric Use: The safety and effectiveness of Paclitaxel in children have not been established.

ADVERSE REACTIONS

Data in the following table are based on the experience of 402 patients enrolled in eight studies in carcinoma of the ovary and of the breast. Four studies (three in ovarian carcinoma, one in breast carcinoma) were single agent trials with increasing entry dose levels of Paclitaxel ranging from 135-250 mg/m^2 administered over 24 hours. Three studies (two in ovarian carcinoma, one in breast carcinoma) utilized Paclitaxel doses of 170-300 mg/m^2 administered over 24 hours and incorporated G-CSF as hematopoietic support. The eighth study was a randomized trial in patients with ovarian carcinoma comparing two doses of Paclitaxel (135 or 175 mg/m^2) and two dose schedules (3 or 24 hours).

SUMMARY OF ADVERSE EVENTS IN 402 PATIENTS RECEIVING PACLITAXEL

	% Incidence
■ Bone Marrow	
Neutropenia	
<2,000/mm^3	92
< 500/mm^3	67
Leukopenia	
< 4,000/mm^3	93
< 1,000/mm^3	26
Thrombocytopenia	
< 100,000/mm^3	27
< 50,000/mm^3	10
Anemia	
< 11 g/dL	90
< 8 g/dL	24
Infections	35
Bleeding	19
Packed Cell Transfusions	34
Platelet Transfusions	3
■ Hypersensitivity Reactions*	
All	41
Severe	2
■ Cardiovascular	
Bradycardia during infusion	10
Hypotension during infusion	23
Severe cardiovascular events	1
■ Abnormal ECG	
All Pts (N = 402)	30
Pts with normal baseline	
(N = 236)	19
■ Peripheral Neuropathy	
Any symptoms	62
Severe symptoms	4
■ Myalgia/Arthralgia	
Any symptoms	55
Severe symptoms	4
■ Gastrointestinal	
Nausea and vomiting	59
Diarrhea	43
Mucositis	39
■ Alopecia	82
■ Hepatic (Pts with normal baseline and on study data)	
Bilirubin elevations (N = 370)	8
Alkaline phosphatase elevations (N = 293)	23
AST (SGOT) elevations (N = 287)	16

* *All patients received premedication*
None of the observed toxicities were clearly influenced by age.

Hematologic: Bone marrow suppression was the major dose limiting toxicity of Paclitaxel. Neutropenia was dose related and generally rapidly reversible. During the first course of treatment, severe neutropenia (< 500 cells/mm^3) occurred in 52% of the patients. During the entire treatment period, severe neutropenia was reported in 67% of the patients. At the recommended dose severe neutropenia occurred in 47% of patients. Although frequent, severe neutropenia was of short duration, with only 7% of the patients having a neutrophil count below 500/mm^3 for 7 days or more. Neutrophil nadirs occurred at a median of 11 days after Paclitaxel administration. Myelosuppression seemed to be more frequent and more severe for patients who had received prior radiation therapy.

Fever was frequent (19% of all treatment courses) and was associated with severe neutropenia in 5% of the courses. Thirty-five percent of all patients reported at least one infection and 13% of all courses were associated with an infectious episode. Urinary tract infections, upper respiratory tract infections and sepsis were the most frequently reported infectious complications. Five septic episodes (approximately 1% of patients), which were associated with severe neutropenia attributable to Paclitaxel administration, were fatal.

Thrombocytopenia was less frequent and less pronounced than neutropenia. Seventy-three percent of the patients maintained a platelet count greater than 100,000/mm^3 throughout the treatment period and only 10% (5% at the recommended dose) had a platelet nadir count below 50,000/mm^3. Day 8 or 9 was consistently the median day of nadir for platelets. Nineteen percent of patients

had bleeding episodes, but most of the hemorrhagic episodes were localized and appeared disease related. Six patients had severe hemorrhage but only in one case was severe thrombocytopenia (< 25,000/mm^3) present. Fourteen patients (3%) received platelet transfusions.

Anemia (Hb less than 11 g/dL) has been observed in 90% of the patients. Incidence and severity of anemia seemed to increase with increasing exposure to Paclitaxel. Severe anemia (Hb < 8 g/dL) occurred in 24% of the patients overall, in 13% of those with baseline Hb ≥ 11 g/dL, and in 40% of those with anemia at study entry. Thirty-four percent of all patients received packed cell transfusions: 18% of those with Hb ≥ 11 g/dL at entry versus 58% of the patients with baseline anemia.

Hypersensitivity Reactions (HSRs): Overall 19% of all courses were associated with HSRs. Ten patients (2%) developed severe HSRs requiring therapeutic intervention and/or discontinuation of Paclitaxel infusion during the first or second course of treatment despite premedication. Severe symptoms occurred generally within the first hour of Paclitaxel infusion. Dyspnea and hypotension requiring treatment and chest pains were the most frequent manifestations. In three cases, interruption of the infusion was the only treatment required. Bronchodilators (albuterol or theophylline), epinephrine, antihistamines and corticosteroids were utilized as single agents, or in combination, for the treatment of the 7 remaining patients. Five of these ten patients tolerated Paclitaxel therapy subsequently.

Besides these 10 patients with severe HSRs, 156 (39%) patients experienced minor manifestations compatible with HSR. The most frequent minor manifestations were flushing, rash and dyspnea and were observed in 32%, 9%, and 4% of all patients, respectively. The proportion of patients developing a first reaction decreased from 25% during course 1, to 10% during course 2, and to less than 5% after course 2. None of the minor reactions required interruption of Paclitaxel infusion nor prevented completion of treatment.

Cardiovascular: Hypotension or bradycardia occurred in 101 (25%) and 47 (12%) of all patients, respectively. Among the 47 patients who experienced bradycardia, 42 (10%) were bradycardic during Paclitaxel infusion. None of these episodes required specific treatment. Among the 101 patients with hypotension, 91 (23%) were hypotensive during Paclitaxel infusion. Bradycardia and hypotension did not usually occur during the same course. The majority of episodes were asymptomatic and did not require treatment, except 2 cases of hypotension associated with severe HSRs.

Six severe cardiovascular events, possibly related to Paclitaxel administration, were identified in the 402 patients (approximately 1.5% of patients) treated with Paclitaxel in studies. Four patients experienced arrhythmias (asymptomatic ventricular tachycardia, bigeminy, two syncopal episodes) and there were two cases of complete AV block requiring pacemaker placement. It was not clear in all cases that the events were caused by Paclitaxel infusion.

Thirty percent of all patients had an abnormal ECG on study. Nineteen percent of the patients with normal ECG prior to study entry developed an abnormal tracing while on study as compared to 57% in the subset with abnormal baseline. The most frequently reported ECG modifications were non-specific repolarization abnormalities (20%), sinus tachycardia (19%) and premature beats (7%). Because there was no monitored control group for comparison, the relationship between Paclitaxel administration and ECG alterations was not clear. Of the 119 patients experiencing ECG alterations, only two required therapeutic intervention.

Neurologic: Peripheral neuropathy was observed in 62% of all patients, with mild paresthesia occurring most frequently. Four percent of all patients experienced severe neurologic symptoms. Peripheral neuropathy was dose dependent with 42% of the patients affected at the recommended dose versus 69% at higher doses. Severity of the symptoms also increased with dose, with no patients experiencing severe symptoms at the recommended dose versus 6% at higher doses. Thirty-one percent of patients at the recommended dose and 49% at higher doses experienced neurologic symptoms following the first course and symptoms tended to worsen with increasing expposure to Paclitaxel. The incidence of neurologic symptoms was comparable in the subsets of patients previously treated with cisplatin (57%). Peripheral neuropathy was rarely the cause of Paclitaxel discontinuation (2%). Sensory symptoms have usually improved or resolved within several months of Paclitaxel discontinuation. Pre-existing neuropathies resulting from prior therapies are not a contraindication for Paclitaxel therapy. Besides peripheral neuropathy, the only severe neurologic manifestation was a grand mal seizure experienced by one patient during Paclitaxel infusion, with recurrence at time of Paclitaxel rechallenge.

Arthralgia/Myalgia: Arthralgia/myalgia usually consisting of pain in the large joints of the arms and legs occurred in 55% of patients and were usually mild. The symptoms were usually transient occurring two or three days after Paclitaxel administration and resolving within a few days. The incidence and severity of arthralgia/myalgia was clearly dose-dependent and somewhat more frequent in patients receiving G-CSF.

Hepatic: Modifications of the liver function tests on study showed some dose relationships consistent with Paclitaxel contribution. Analysis restricted to patients with normal baseline liver function, showed that 8% of the patients had elevated bilirubin on study, 23% elevated alkaline phosphatase, 16% elevated AST (SGOT) and 33% elevated ALT (SGPT). A dose effect was suggested by all tests except for ALT.

Other Clinical Events: Alopecia has been observed in almost all of the patients. Gastrointestinal side effects such as nausea/vomiting, diarrhea and mucositis were reported by 59%, 43% and 39% of the patients, respectively. These manifestations were usually mild to moderate at the recommended dose.

OVERDOSAGE

There is no known antidote for Paclitaxel overdosage. The primary anticipated complications of overdosage would consist of bone marrow suppression, peripheral neurotoxicity and mucositis.

DOSAGE AND ADMINISTRATION

Note: Contact of the undiluted concentrate with plasticized PVC equipment or devices used to prepare solutions for infusion is not recommended. In order to minimize patient exposure to the plasticizer DEHP[di-(2-ethylhexyl)phthalate], which may be leached from PVC infusion bags or sets, diluted Paclitaxel solutions should be stored in bottles (glass, polypropylene) or plastic bags (polypropylene, polyolefin) and administered through polyethylene-lined administration sets.

All patients should be premedicated prior to Paclitaxel administration in order to prevent severe hypersensitivity reactions. Such premedication may consist of dexamethasone 20 mg PO administered approximately 12 and 6 hours before Paclitaxel, diphenhydramine (or its equivalent) 50 mg I.V. 30 to 60 minutes prior to Paclitaxel, and cimetidine (300 mg) or ranitidine (50 mg) I.V. 30 to 60 minutes before Paclitaxel.

Adequate trials of dose-response have not been completed. Paclitaxel at a dose of 135 mg/m^2 administered intravenously over 24 hours every three weeks has been shown to be effective in patients with metastatic carcinoma of the ovary after failure of first-line or subsequent chemotherapy. Larger doses, with or without G-CSF, have so far produced responses similar to 135 mg/m^2. Courses of Paclitaxel should not be repeated until the neutrophil count is at least 1,500 cells/mm^3 and the platelet count is at least 100,000 cells/mm^3. Patients who experience severe neutropenia (neutrophil < 500 cells/mm^3 for a week or longer) or severe peripheral neuropathy during Paclitaxel therapy should have dosage reduced by 20% for subsequent courses of Paclitaxel. The incidence and severity of neurotoxicity and hematologic toxicity increase with dose, especially above 190 mg/m^2.

Preparation and Administration Precautions: Paclitaxel is a cytotoxic anticancer drug and, as with other potentially toxic compounds, caution should be exercised in handling Paclitaxel. The use of gloves is recommended. If Paclitaxel solution contacts the skin, wash the skin immediately and thoroughly with soap and water. If Paclitaxel contact mucous membranes, the membranes should be flushed thoroughly with water.

Preparation for Intravenous Administration: Paclitaxel for Injection Concentrate must be diluted prior to infusion. Paclitaxel should be diluted in 0.9% Sodium Chloride Injection, USP, 5% Dextrose Injection, USP, 5% Dextrose and 0.9% Sodium Chloride Injection, USP or 5% Dextrose in Ringer's Injection to a final concentration of 0.3 to 1.2 mg/mL. The solutions are physically and chemically stable for up to 27 hours at ambient temperature (approximately 25°C) and room lighting conditions. Parenteral drug products should be inspected visually for particulate matter and discoloration prior to administration whenever solution and container permit.

Upon preparation, solutions may show haziness, which is attributed to the formulation vehicle. No significant losses in potency have been noted following simulated delivery of the solution through I.V. tubing containing an in-line (0.22 micron) filter.

Data collected for the presence of the extractable plasticizer DEHP [di-(2-ethylhexyl)phthalate] show that levels increase with time and concentration when dilutions are prepared in PVC containers. Consequently, the use of plasticized PVC containers and administration sets is not recommended. Solutions for infusion should be prepared and stored in glass, polypropylene or polyolefin containers. Non-PVC containing administration sets, such as those which are polyethylene-lined, should be used.

Paclitaxel should be administered through an in-line filter with a microporous membrane not greater than 0.22 microns. Use of filter devices such as IVEX-2 filters which incorporate short inlet and outlet PVC-coated tubing has not resulted in significant leaching of DEHP.

Stability: Unopened vials of Paclitaxel for injection Concentrate are stable until the date indicated on the package when stored under refrigeration, 2°-8° C (36°-46° F), in the original package. Freezing does not adversely affect the product. Upon refrigeration components in the Paclitaxel vial may precipitate, but will redissolve upon reaching room temperature with little or no agitation. There is no impact on product quality under these circumstances. If the solution remains cloudy or if an insoluble precipitate is noted, the vial should be discarded. Solutions for infusion prepared as recommended are stable at ambient temperature (approximately 25°C) and lighting conditions for up to 27 hours.

Handling and Disposal: Procedures for proper handling and disposal of anticancer drugs should be considered. Several guidelines on this subject have been published.[2-8] There is no general agreement that all of the procedures recommended in the guidelines are necessary or appropriate.

Storage: Store the vials in original cartons under refrigeration, 2°-8°C (36°-46°F). Retain in the original package to protect from light.

REFERENCES

1. Rowinsky EK, et al: Sequences of Taxol and Cisplatin: A Phase I and Pharmacologic Study. J Clin Oncol 1991; 9(9):1692-1703. 2. Recommendations for the safe handling of parenteral antineoplastic drugs. NIH Publication No. 83-2621. For sale by the Superintendent of Documents, US Government Printing Office, Washington, DC 20402. 3. AMA Council Report. Guidelines for handling parenteral antineoplastics. JAMA 1985; 253(11):1590-1592. 4. National Study Commission on Cytotoxic

Exposure—Recommendations for handling cytotoxic agents. Available from Louis P. Jeffrey, Chairman, National Study Commission on Cytotoxic Exposure. Massachusetts College of Pharmacy and Allied Health Sciences. 179 Longwood Avenue, Boston, Massachusetts, 02115. 5. Clinical Oncological Society of Australia. Guidelines and recommendations for safe handling of antineoplastic agents. Med J Australia 1983; 1:426-428. 6. Jones RB, et al: Safe handling of chemotherapeutic agents: a report from the Mount Sinai Medical Center. CA-A Cancer Journal for Clinicians 1983; Sept./Oct. 258-263. 7. American Society of Hospital Pharmacists Technical Assistance Bulletin on Handling Cytotoxic and Hazardous Drugs. Am J Hosp Phar 1990; 47:1033-1049. 8. OSHA Work-Practice guidelines for personnel dealing with cytotoxic (antineoplastic) drugs. Am J Hosp Pharm 1986; 43:1193-1204.

J CODES
30 mg IV—J9265

HOW SUPPLIED
INJECTION: 6 MG/ML

BRAND/MANUFACTURER	NDC	SIZE	AWP
○ **BRAND**			
TAXOL: Bristol-Myer Onc/Hiv	00015-3456-20	5 ml	$182.63

Pamelor *SEE* NORTRIPTYLINE HYDROCHLORIDE

Pamidronate Disodium

DESCRIPTION

Pamidronate Disodium is a bone-resorption inhibitor for intravenous administration. The pH of a 1% solution of Pamidronate Disodium in distilled water is approximately 8.3. Pamidronate Disodium, a member of the group of chemical compounds known as bisphosphonates, is an analog of pyrophosphate. Pamidronate Disodium is designated chemically as phosphonic acid (3-amino-1-hydroxypropylidene) bis-, disodium salt, pentahydrate.

Pamidronate Disodium is a white-to-practically-white powder. It is soluble in water and in 2N sodium hydroxide, sparingly soluble in 0.1N hydrochloric acid and in 0.1N acetic acid, and practically insoluble in organic solvents. Its molecular formula is $C_3H_9NO_7P_2Na_2.5H_2O$ and its molecular weight is 369.1.

Following is its chemical structure:

CLINICAL PHARMACOLOGY

The principal pharmacologic action of Pamidronate Disodium is inhibition of bone resorption. Although the mechanism of antiresorptive action is not completely understood, several factors are thought to contribute to this action. Pamidronate Disodium adsorbs to calcium phosphate (hydroxyapatite) crystals in bone and may directly block dissolution of this mineral component of bone. *In vitro* studies also suggest that inhibition of osteoclast activity contributes to inhibition of bone resorption. In animal studies, at doses recommended for the treatment of hypercalcemia, Pamidronate Disodium inhibits bone resorption apparently without inhibiting bone formation and mineralization. Of relevance to the treatment of hypercalcemia of malignancy is the finding that Pamidronate Disodium inhibits the accelerated bone resorption that results from osteoclast hyperactivity induced by various tumors in animal studies.

In cancer patients who had minimal or no bony involvement who were given an intravenous infusion of 60 mg of Pamidronate Disodium over 4 or 24 hours, a mean of 51% (32-80%) of the drug was excreted unchanged in the urine within 72 hours. Body retention during this period was calculated to be a mean of 49% (range 20-68%) of the dose, or 29.3 mg (12-41 mg). The urinary excretion-rate profile after administration of 60 mg of Pamidronate Disodium over 4 hours exhibited biphasic disposition characteristics with an alpha half-life of 1.6 hours and a beta half-life of 27.2 hours. There are no human pharmacokinetic data for Pamidronate Disodium on the 90-mg dose or in patients who have either renal or hepatic insufficiency. The rate of elimination of Pamidronate Disodium from bone has not been determined.

After intravenous administration of radiolabeled Pamidronate Disodium in rats, approximately 50-60% of the compound was rapidly adsorbed by bone and slowly eliminated from the body by the kidneys. In rats given 10 mg/kg bolus injections of radiolabeled Pamidronate Disodium, approximately 30% of the compound was found in the liver shortly after administration and was then redistributed to bone or eliminated by the kidneys over 24-48 hours. Studies in rats injected with radiolabeled Pamidronate Disodium showed that the compound was rapidly cleared from the circulation and taken up mainly by bones, liver, spleen, teeth, and tracheal cartilage. Radioactivity was eliminated from most soft tissues within 1-4 days; was detectable in liver and spleen for 1 and 3 months, respectively; and remained high in bones, trachea, and teeth for 6 months after dosing. Bone uptake occurred preferentially in areas of high bone turnover. The terminal phase of elimination half-life in bone was estimated to be approximately 300 days.

➤ SHOWN IN PRODUCT IDENTIFICATION GUIDE

Serum phosphate levels have been noted to decrease after administration of Pamidronate Disodium, presumably because of decreased release of phosphate from bone and increased renal excretion as parathyroid hormone levels, which are usually suppressed in hypercalcemia associated with malignancy, return towards normal. Phosphate therapy was administered in 30% of the patients in response to a decrease in serum phosphate levels. Phosphate levels usually returned towards normal within 7-10 days.

Urinary calcium/creatinine and urinary hydroxyproline/creatinine ratios decrease and usually return to within or below normal after treatment with Pamidronate Disodium. These changes occur within the first week after treatment, as do decreases in serum calcium levels, and are consistent with an antiresorptive pharmacologic action.

HYPERCALCEMIA OF MALIGNANCY

Osteoclastic hyperactivity resulting in excessive bone resorption is the underlying pathophysiologic derangement in metastatic bone disease and hypercalcemia of malignancy. Excessive release of calcium into the blood as bone is resorbed results in polyuria and gastrointestinal disturbances, with progressive dehydration and decreasing glomerular filtration rate. This, in turn, results in increased renal resorption of calcium, setting up a cycle of worsening systemic hypercalcemia. Correction of excessive bone resorption and adequate fluid administration to correct volume deficits are therefore essential to the management of hypercalcemia.

Most cases of hypercalcemia associated with malignancy occur in patients who have breast cancer, squamous-cell tumors of the lung or head and neck; renal-cell carcinoma; and certain hematologic malignancies, such as multiple myeloma and some types of lymphomas. A few less-common malignancies, including vasoactive intestinal-peptide-producing tumors and cholangiocarcinoma, have a high incidence of hypercalcemia as a metabolic complication. Patients who have hypercalcemia of malignancy can generally be divided into two groups, according to the pathophysiologic mechanism involved.

In humoral hypercalcemia, osteoclasts are activated and bone resorption is stimulated by factors such as parathyroid-hormone-related protein, which are elaborated by the tumor and circulate systemically. Humoral hypercalcemia usually occurs in squamous-cell malignancies of the lung or head and neck or in genitourinary tumors such as renal-cell carcinoma or ovarian cancer. Skeletal metastases may be absent or minimal in these patients.

Extensive invasion of bone by tumor cells can also result in hypercalcemia due to local tumor products that stimulate bone resorption by osteoclasts. Tumors commonly associated with locally mediated hypercalcemia include breast cancer and multiple myeloma.

Total serum calcium levels in patients who have hypercalcemia of malignancy may not reflect the severity of hypercalcemia, since concomitant hypoalbuminemia is commonly present. Ideally, ionized calcium levels should be used to diagnose and follow hypercalcemic conditions; however, these are not commonly or rapidly available in many clinical situations. Therefore, adjustment of the total serum calcium value for differences in albumin levels is often used in place of measurement of ionized calcium; several nomograms are in use for this type of calculation (see *"Dosage and Administration"*).

CLINICAL TRIALS

In one double-blind clinical trial, 52 patients who had hypercalcemia of malignancy were enrolled to receive 30 mg, 60 mg, or 90 mg of Pamidronate Disodium as a single 24-hour intravenous infusion if their corrected serum calcium levels were $\geq$ 12.0 mg/dL after 48 hours of saline hydration.

The mean baseline corrected serum calcium for the 30 mg, 60 mg and 90 mg groups were 13.8 mg/dL, 13.8 mg/dL and 13.3 mg/dL, respectively.

The majority of the patients (64%) had decreases in albumin-corrected serum calcium levels by 24 hours after initiation of treatment. Mean-corrected serum calcium levels at days 2-7 after initiation of treatment with Pamidronate Disodium were significantly reduced from baseline in all three dosage groups. As a result, by 7 days after initiation of treatment of Pamidronate Disodium 40%, 61%, and 100% of the patients receiving 30 mg, 60 mg, and 90 mg of Pamidronate Disodium, respectively, had normal corrected serum calcium levels. Many patients (33-53%) in the 60-mg and 90-mg dosage groups continued to have normal-corrected serum calcium levels, or a partial response ($\geq$ 15% decrease of corrected serum calcium from baseline), at day 14.

In a second double-blind, controlled clinical trial, 65 cancer patients who had corrected serum calcium levels of $\geq$ 12.0 mg/dL after at least 24 hours of saline hydration were randomized to receive either 60 mg of Pamidronate Disodium as a single 24-hour intravenous infusion or 7.5 mg/kg of etidronate disodium as a 2-hour intravenous infusion daily for 3 days. Thirty patients were randomized to receive Pamidronate Disodium and 35 to receive etidronate disodium.

The mean baseline corrected serum calcium for the Pamidronate Disodium 60 mg and etidronate disodium groups were 14.6 mg/dL and 13.8 mg/dL, respectively.

By day 7, 70% of the patients in the Pamidronate Disodium group and 41% of the patients in the etidronate disodium group had normal corrected serum calcium levels (P < 0.05). When partial responders ($\geq$ 15% decrease of serum calcium from baseline) were also included, the response rates were 97% for the Pamidronate Disodium group and 65% for the etidronate disodium group (P < 0.01). Mean corrected serum calcium for the Pamidronate Disodium and etidronate disodium groups decreased from baseline values to 10.4 and 11.2 mg/dL, respectively, on day 7. At day 14, 43% of patients in the Pamidronate Disodium group and 18% of patients in the etidronate disodium group still had normal corrected serum calcium levels, or maintenance of a partial response. For

responders in the Pamidronate Disodium and etidronate disodium groups, the median duration of response was similar (7 and 5 days, respectively). The time course of effect on corrected serum calcium is summarized in the following table.

CHANGE IN CORRECTED SERUM CALCIUM BY TIME FROM INITIATION OF TREATMENT

Time (hr)	Mean Change from Baseline in Corrected Serum Calcium (mg/dL)		
	Pamidronate Disodium	*etidronate disodium*	*p Value*[1]
Baseline	*14.6*	*13.8*	
24	— 0.3	— 0.5	
48	— 1.5	— 1.1	
72	— 2.6	— 2.0	
96	— 3.5	— 2.0	<0.01
168	— 4.1	— 2.5	<0.01

1   Comparison between treatment groups

In both trials, patients treated with Pamidronate Disodium had similar response rates in the presence or absence of bone metastases. Concomitant administration of furosemide did not affect response rates.

Twenty-five patients who had recurrent or refractory hypercalcemia of malignancy were given a second course of 60 mg of Pamidronate Disodium. Of these, 40% showed a complete response and 20% showed a partial response to the retreatment, and these responders had about a 3 mg/dL fall in mean corrected serum calcium levels 7 days after treatment.

INDICATIONS AND USAGE

Pamidronate Disodium in conjunction with adequate hydration, is indicated for the treatment of moderate or severe hypercalcemia associated with malignancy, with or without bone metastases. Patients who have either epidermoid or non-epidermoid tumors respond to treatment with Pamidronate Disodium. Vigorous saline hydration, an integral part of hypercalcemia therapy, should be initiated promptly and an attempt should be made to restore the urine output to about 2 L/day throughout treatment. Mild or asymptomatic hypercalemia may be treated with conservative measures (i.e., saline hydration, with or without loop diuretics). Patients should be hydrated adequately throughout the treatment, but overhydration, especially in those patients who have cardiac failure, must be avoided. Diuretic therapy should not be employed prior to correction of hypovolemia. The safety and efficacy of Pamidronate Disodium in the treatment of hypercalcemia associated with hyperparathyroidism or with other nontumor-related conditions has not been established.

UNLABELED USES

Pamidronate Disodium is used alone or as an adjunct in the treatment of Paget's Disease of bone and of osteoporosis.

CONTRAINDICATIONS

Pamidronate Disodium is contraindicated in patients with clinically significant hypersensitivity to Pamidronate Disodium or other bisphosphonates.

WARNINGS

In both rats and dogs, nephropathy has been associated with intravenous, bolus administration of Pamidronate Disodium. A 3-month study in rats found cortical tubular changes including epithelial degeneration with intravenous doses $\geq$ 5 mg/kg, given once every two weeks. Following a recovery period (1 month), the degenerative changes were completely reversed. Focal fibrosis of renal tubules was partially reversed.

In two studies conducted in dogs, Pamidronate Disodium was given as a bolus intravenous injection either daily for 1 month or once a week for 3 months. In the 1-month study, tubulointerstitial nephritis, tubular degeneration and dilation occurred at 2 mg/kg. At recovery (1 month) the severity of these lesions was minimal or trace. Similar lesions (slight to marked severity) were noted in the 3-month study at 3 mg/kg and higher. However, no improvement of the lesions was observed following the 1-month recovery period.

Patients with hypercalcemia who receive an intravenous infusion of Pamidronate Disodium should have periodic evaluations of standard laboratory and clinical parameters of renal function. Studies conducted in young rats have reported the disruption of dental enamel formation with single-dose administration of bisphosphonates. The clinical significance of these findings is unknown.

PRECAUTIONS

GENERAL

Standard hypercalcemia-related metabolic parameters, such as serum levels of calcium, phosphate, magnesium, and potassium should be carefully monitored following initiation of therapy with Pamidronate Disodium. Cases of asymptomatic hypophosphatemia (16%), hypokalemia (9%), hypomagnesemia (12%), and hypocalcemia (6-12%), were reported in Pamidronate Disodium treated patients. Rare cases of symptomatic hypocalcemia (including tetany) have been reported in association with Pamidronate Disodium therapy. If hypocalcemia occurs, short-term calcium therapy may be necessary.

Pamidronate Disodium has not been tested in patients who have class Dc renal impairment (creatinine > 5.0 mg/dL). Clinical judgment should determine whether the potential benefit outweighs the potential risk in such patients.

◆ RATED THERAPEUTICALLY EQUIVALENT; ◇ THERAPEUTIC EQUIVALENCE UNCONFIRMED; ○ UNRATED

LABORATORY TESTS

Serum calcium, electrolytes, phosphate, magnesium and creatinine, and CBC, differential, and hematocrit/hemoglobin must be closely monitored in patients treated with Pamidronate Disodium. Patients who have preexisting anemia, leukopenia, or thrombocytopenia should be monitored carefully in the first 2 weeks following treatment.

DRUG INTERACTIONS

Concomitant administration of a loop diuretic had no effect on the calcium-lowering action of Pamidronate Disodium.

CARCINOGENESIS, MUTAGENESIS, IMPAIRMENT OF FERTILITY

In a 104-week carcinogenicity study (daily oral administration) in rats, there was a positive dose response relationship for benign adrenal pheochromocytoma in males (p > 0.00001). Although this condition was also observed in females, the incidence was not statistically significant. When the dose calculations were adjusted to account for the limited oral bioavailability of Pamidronate Disodium in rats, the lowest daily dose associated with adrenal pheochromocytoma was similar to the intended clinical dose. Pamidronate Disodium (daily oral administration) was not carcinogenic in an 80-week study in mice.

Pamidronate Disodium was nonmutagenic in four mutagenicity assays: Ames test, nucleus-anomaly test, sister-chromatid-exchange study, and point-mutation test.

In rats, decreased fertility occurred in first-generation off-spring of parents who had received 150 mg/kg of Pamidronate Disodium orally; however, this occurred only when animals were mated with members of the same dose group. Pamidronate Disodium has not been administered intravenously in such a study.

PREGNANCY CATEGORY C

Pamidronate Disodium has been shown to increase the length of gestation and parturition in rats resulting in an increasing pup mortality when given orally at daily doses of 60 and 150 mg/kg/day from before pregnancy until after parturition. When corrected for oral bioavailability, each daily dose is approximately 0.7 to 1.7 times the highest recommended human dose for a single intravenous infusion. Oral doses of 25 to 150 mg/kg/day during the period of gestation failed to demonstrate any teratogenic, fetotoxic, or embryotoxic effects in rats or rabbits. Animal reproduction studies have not been conducted with intravenously administered Pamidronate Disodium. It is not known if intravenous Pamidronate Disodium can cause fetal harm when administered to pregnant women or if it can affect reproduction capacity. There are no adequate and well-controlled studies in pregnant women. Pamidronate Disodium should be used during pregnancy only if the potential benefit justifies the potential risk to the fetus.

NURSING MOTHERS

It is not known whether Pamidronate Disodium is excreted in human milk. Because many drugs are excreted in human milk, caution should be exercised when Pamidronate Disodium is administered to a nursing woman.

PEDIATRIC USE

Safety and effectiveness of Pamidronate Disodium in children have not been established.

ADVERSE REACTIONS

Transient mild elevation of temperature by at least 1°C was noted 24-48 hours after administration of Pamidronate Disodium in 27% of the patients in clinical trials.

Drug-related local soft-tissue symptoms (redness, swelling or induration and pain on palpation) at the site of catheter insertion were most common (18%) in patients treated with 90 mg of Pamidronate Disodium. When all on-therapy events are considered, that rate rises to 41%. Symptomatic treatment resulted in rapid resolution in all patients.

Uveitis was reported in 1 patient who had hypercalcemia of malignancy; another patient who had Paget's disease of bone developed mild iritis that was responsive to indomethacin and topical steroid. Both of these patients received Pamidronate Disodium in uncontrolled studies.

Four of 82 patients (4.9%) who received Pamidronate Disodium during the 2 U.S. controlled hypercalcemia clinical studies were reported to have had seizures, 2 of whom had preexisting seizure disorders. None of the seizures were considered to be drug-related by the investigators. However, a possible relationship between the drug and the occurrence of seizures cannot be ruled out.

At least 15% of patients treated with Pamidronate Disodium for hypercalcemia of malignancy also experienced the following adverse events during a clinical trial:

General: Fluid overload, generalized pain

Cardiovascular: Hypertension

Gestrointestinal: Abdominal pain, anorexia, constipation, nausea, vomiting

Genitourinary: Urinary tract infection

Musculoskeletal: Bone pain

Laboratory abnormality: Anemia, hypokalemia, hypomagnesemia, hypophosphatemia

Many of these adverse experiences may have been related to the underlying disease state.

The following table lists the adverse experiences considered to be related to treatment with bisphosphonates during comparative, controlled U.S. trials.

BISPHOSPHONATE-RELATED ADVERSE EXPERIENCES IN TWO U.S. CONTROLLED CLINICAL TRAILS

	Percent of Patients		
	Pamidronate Disodium (N = 67)		etidronate disodium (N = 35)
	60 mg	90 mg	7.5 mg/kg × 3 days
General			
Fatigue	0	12	0
Fever	20	18	9
Fluid overload	0	0	6
Infusion-site reaction	6	18	0
Moniliasis	0	6	0
Gastrointestinal			
Abdominal pain	2	0	0
Anorexia	2	12	0
Constipation	0	6	3
Gastrointestinal hemorrhage	0	6	0
Nausea	0	18	6
Ulcerative stomatitis	0	0	3
Respiratory System			
Dyspnea	0	0	3
Rales	0	6	0
Rhinitis	0	6	0
Upper respiratory infection	2	0	0
CNS			
Convulsions	0	0	3
Insomnia	2	0	0
Somnolence	2	6	0
Taste perversion	0	0	3
Abnormal vision	2	0	0
Cardiovascular			
Atrial fibrillation	0	6	0
Hypertension	0	6	0
Syncope	0	6	0
Tachycardia	0	6	0
Endocrine System			
Hypothyroidism	0	6	0
Hemic and Lymphatic System			
Anemia	0	6	0
Laboratory Abnormality			
Hypocalcemia	2	12	0
Hypokalemia	4	18	0
Hypomagnesemia	8	6	0
Hypophosphatemia	14	18	3
Abnormal hepatic function	0	0	3

OVERDOSAGE

One obese woman (95 kg) who was treated with 285 mg of Pamidronate Disodium/day for 3 days, experienced high fever (39.5°C), hypotension (from 170/90 mmHg to 90/60 mmHg), and transient taste perversion, noted about 6 hours after the first infusion. The fever and hypotension were rapidly corrected with steroids.

If overdosage occurs, symptomatic hypocalcemia could also result; such patients should be treated with short-term intravenous calcium.

DOSAGE AND ADMINISTRATION

Consideration should be given to the severity of as well as the symptoms of hypercalcemia. The recommended dose of Pamidronate Disodium in moderate hypercalcemia (corrected serum calcium of approximately 12-13.5 mg/dL) is 60-90 mg, and in severe hypercalcemia (corrected serum calcium, > 13.5 mg/dL), is 90 mg, given as an initial, single-dose, intravenous infusion over 24 hours. Albumin-corrected serum calcium (CCa, mg/dL) = serum calcium, mg/dL + 0.8 (4.0 − serum albumin, g/dL).

Vigorous saline hydration alone may be sufficient for treating mild, asymptomatic hypercalcemia. Overhydration should be avoided in patients who have potential for cardiac failure. In hypercalcemia associated with hematologic malignancies, the use of glucocorticoid therapy may be helpful. A limited number of patients have received more than one treatment with Pamidronate Disodium for hypercalcemia. Retreatment with Pamidronate Disodium may be considered if hypercalcemia recurs. It is recommended that a minimum of 7 days elapse before retreatment, to allow for full response to the initial dose. The dose and manner of retreatment is identical to that of the initial therapy.

PREPARATION OF SOLUTION

Pamidronate Disodium is reconstituted by adding 10 mL of Sterile Water for Injection, USP, to each vial, resulting in a solution of 30 mg/10 mL, 60 mg/10 mL, or 90 mg/10 mL. The pH of the reconstituted solution is 6.0-7.4. The drug should be completely dissolved before the solution is withdrawn. The daily dose must be administered as an intravenous infusion over 24 hours. The recommended dose should be diluted in 1000 mL of sterile 0.45% or 0.9% Sodium Chloride, USP, or 5% Dextrose Injection, USP. This infusion is stable for up to 24 hours at

➤ SHOWN IN PRODUCT IDENTIFICATION GUIDE

room temperature. *Pamidronate Disodium must not be mixed with calcium-containing infusion solutions, such as Ringer's solution.*

Note: **Parenteral drug products should be inspected visually for particulate matter and discoloration prior to administration, whenever solution and container permit.**

Pamidronate Disodium reconstituted with Sterile Water for Injection may be stored under refrigeration at 36-46°F (2-8°C) for up to 24 hours.

Do not store above 86°F (30°C).

HOW SUPPLIED
POWDER FOR INJECTION: 30 MG

BRAND/MANUFACTURER	NDC	SIZE	AWP
○ **BRAND**			
AREDIA: Ciba Pharm	00083-2601-04	4s	$681.68

Pamine *SEE* METHSCOPOLAMINE BROMIDE

Panacet 5/500 *SEE* ACETAMINOPHEN WITH HYDROCODONE BITARTRATE

Panafil *SEE* CHLOROPHYLLIN COPPER COMPLEX/PAPAIN/UREA

Panasal 5/500 *SEE* ASPIRIN WITH HYDROCODONE BITARTRATE

Pancof HC *SEE* CHLORPHENIRAMINE MALEATE/HYDROCODONE BITARTRATE/PSEUDOEPHEDRINE HYDROCHLORIDE

Pancof XP *SEE* GUAIFENESIN/HYDROCODONE BITARTRATE/PSEUDOEPHEDRINE HYDROCHLORIDE

Pancrease *SEE* PANCRELIPASE

Pancreatin and Pepsin

DESCRIPTION
Pancreatin/Pepsin tablets are available for oral administration.

Each tablet contains:

Pancreatin	300	mg
Pepsin	250	mg

CONSTRUCTION
Pancreatin/Pepsin is a specially constructed tablet. The outer layer dissolves in the stomach and releases pepsin. The "inner tablet" is protected by an enteric coating that disintegrates in the alkaline medium of the small intestine and releases pancreatin, thus preserving the digestive potency of the pancreatin as it passes through the stomach.

CLINICAL PHARMACOLOGY
The special Pancreatin/Pepsin coating permits release of pepsin in acid gastric contents (where, as a protease, it participates in digestion of protein) and of the other ingredients in the relatively alkaline intestinal contents. Pancreatin's protease, amylase, and lipase components thus subsequently participate in digestion of protein, starch, and fat, respectively.

INDICATIONS AND USAGE
Digestant supplement where secretion of certain natural digestive enzymes and aids is considered deficient.

CONTRAINDICATIONS
Significant cholelithiasis; presence of jaundice; marked hepatic insufficiency; complete obstruction of the common or hepatic bile ducts or of the G.I. or G.U. tracts; hypersensitivity to any of the ingredients.

WARNINGS
No data supporting a recommended pediatric dose are available. Thus, this drug should not be used in children under 12 years of age. Do not administer to patients who are allergic to pork products.

PRECAUTIONS
Carcinogenesis, Mutagenesis: Long-term studies in animals have not been performed to evaluate carcinogenic potential.

Pregnancy Category C: Animal reproduction studies have not been conducted with Pancreatin/Pepsin. It is not known whether Pancreatin/Pepsin can cause fetal harm when administered to a pregnant woman or can affect reproduction capacity. Pancreatin/Pepsin should be given to a pregnant woman only if clearly needed.

Nursing Mothers: It is not known whether this drug is excreted in human milk. Because many drugs are excreted in human milk, caution should be exercised when Pancreatin/Pepsin is administered to a nursing woman.

Pediatric Use: Safety and effectiveness in children have not been established.

ADVERSE REACTIONS
Skin rash is the most frequently reported adverse reaction to Pancreatin/Pepsin, and appears to be associated with hypersensitivity to pork protein in the pancreatin.

DOSAGE AND ADMINISTRATION
Do not crush or chew Pancreatin/Pepsin
Usual adult dosage: 1 or 2 tablets three times daily—with, or immediately after, meals. Initial and subsequent dosage should be adjusted to the individual patient's needs.

Store at controlled room temperature, 15°-30°C (59°-86°F).

Dispense in a tight, light-resistant container as defined in the USP, with a child-resistant closure, as required.

HOW SUPPLIED
TABLETS:

BRAND/MANUFACTURER	NDC	SIZE	AWP
○ **GENERICS**			
DIGESTOZYME II: Richlyn	00115-3252-01	100s	$9.32
DIGESTOZYME II: Richlyn	00115-3252-03	1000s	$71.70

Pancrelipase

DESCRIPTION
Orally administered Pancrelipase capsules, tablets, and powder and Pancreatin (high lipase concentrate) capsules contain porcine pancreatic enzyme concentrate, predominately steapsin (pancreatic lipase), amylase and protease), for digestive enzyme replacement therapy.

Pancrelipase capsules are available in the following strengths:

Lipase	4,000 U.S.P. Units
Amylase	20,000 U.S.P. Units
Protease	25,000 U.S.P. Units
Lipase	4,000 U.S.P. Units
Amylase	12,000 U.S.P. Units
Protease	12,000 U.S.P. Units
Lipase	8,000 USP Units
Protease	30,000 USP Units
Amylase	30,000 USP Units
Lipase	10,000 U.S.P. Units
Amylase	30,000 U.S.P. Units
Protease	30,000 U.S.P. Units
Lipase	16,000 U.S.P. Units
Amylase	48,000 U.S.P. Units
Protease	48,000 U.S.P. Units
Lipase	25,000 U.S.P. Units
Amylase	70,000 U.S.P. Units
Protease	55,000 U.S.P. Units
Lipase	32,000 USP Units
Amylase	90,000 USP Units
Protease	70,000 USP Units

Each Pancrelipase tablet contains:	*Each 0.7g Pancrelipase powder (¼ teaspoonful) contains*

Lipase	8,000 USP Units
Protease	30,000 USP Units
Amylase	30,000 USP Units
Lipase	16,800 USP Units
Protease	70,000 USP Units
Amylase	70,000 USP Units

Pancreatin capsules are available in the following strengths:

Lipase	10,000 Units
Amylase	33,200 Units
Protease	37,500 Units
Lipase	25,000 Units
Amylase	74,700 Units
Protease	62,500 Units

◆ RATED THERAPEUTICALLY EQUIVALENT; ◇ THERAPEUTIC EQUIVALENCE UNCONFIRMED; ○ UNRATED

CLINICAL PHARMACOLOGY

Pancrelipase and Pancreatin are pancreatic enzyme concentrates which hydrolyzes fats to glycerol and fatty acids, changes protein into proteases and derived substances, and converts starch into dextrins and sugars. The administration of pancreatic enzymes reduces the fat and nitrogen content in the stool. Pancreatic enzymes are normally secreted in great excess. Generally, steatorrhea and malabsorption occur only after a 90 percent or greater reduction in secretion of lipase and proteolytic enzymes. It has been estimated that approximately 8,000 units of lipase per hour should be delivered into the duodenum postprandially. Even if all the enzymes taken orally reached the proximal intestine in active form, ingestion of 24,000 units of lipase (8,000 units per hour) for 3 postprandial hours would be required. If one could deliver sufficient pancreatic enzymes to the small intestine, malabsorption could be corrected. It is rarely possible to achieve complete relief of steatorrhea although major improvement in fat absorption can be achieved in most patients.

Under conditions of the USP test method (*in vitro*) Pancrelipase has the following total digestive capacity:

	Each Tablet	Each 0.7g powder
Dietary fat, grams	28	59
Dietary protein, grams	30	70
Dietary starch, grams	30	70

The digestive capacity of a pancreatic enzyme concentrate depends on the amount that passes through the stomach unchanged and is available at the site of action in the small intestine.

Pancrelipase and Pancreatin capsules resist gastric inactivation and deliver predictable, high levels of biologically active enzymes into the duodenum.

INDICATIONS AND USAGE

Pancrelipase and Pancreatin capsules are indicated for patients with exocrine pancreatic enzyme deficiency such as:

- cystic fibrosis
- chronic pancreatitis
- post-pancreatectomy
- post-gastrointestinal bypass surgery (e.g. Billroth II gastroenterostomy)
- ductal obstruction from neoplasm (e.g. of the pancreas or common bile duct)

Pancrelipase may be used in pancreatic insufficiency and for steatorrhea of malabsorption syndrome. May also be used as a presumptive test for pancreatic function, especially in pancreatic insufficiency due to chronic pancreatitis.

CONTRAINDICATIONS

Pancrelipase and Pancreatin capsules are contraindicated in patients known to be hypersensitive to pork protein.

Pancrelipase and Pancreatin capsules are contraindicated in patients with acute pancreatitis or with acute exacerbations of chronic pancreatic diseases.

WARNINGS

Should hypersensitivity occur, discontinue medication and treat symptomatically. Pancreatic exocrine replacement therapy should not delay or supplant treatment of the primary disorder. Use with caution in patients known to be hypersensitive to enzymes.

PRECAUTIONS

GENERAL

Where swallowing of capsules is difficult, they may be opened and the contents shaken onto a small quantity of a soft food (e.g. applesauce, gelatin, etc.), which does not require chewing, and swallowed immediately and followed with a glass of water or juice to swallowing.

In the event that capsules are opened for any reason care should be taken so that powder is not inhaled or spilled on hands since it may prove irritating to the skin or mucous membranes.

General: Individuals previously sensitized to trypsin, pancreatin or pancrelipase may have allergic manifestations.

INFORMATION FOR PATIENTS

If capsules are opened, avoid inhalation of the powder. Sensitive individuals may experience allergic reactions. Pancrelipase should not be held in the mouth as the proteolytic action may cause irriation of the mucosa.

DRUG INTERACTIONS

The serum iron response to oral iron may be decreased by concomitant administration of pancreatic extracts.

CARCINOGENESIS, MUTAGENESIS, AND IMPAIRMENT OF FERTILITY

Long-term studies in animals have not been performed to evaluate the carcinogenic, mutagenic or impairment of fertility potential of Pancrelipase or Pancreatin.

Pregnancy Category C. Animal reproduction studies have not been conducted with Pancrelipase or Pancreatin capsules. It is also not known whether Pancrelipase or Pancreatin can cause fetal harm when administered to a pregnant woman or can affect reproduction capacity. Pancrelipase or Pancreatin should be given to a pregnant woman only if clearly needed. Certain brands of Pancrelipase contain Diethyl phthalate, an enteric coating component of the capsules, which has been shown with high intraperitoneal dosing to be tetratogenic in rats. However, when this coating was administered orally to rats up to 100 times the human dose, no teratogenic or embryocidal effects were observed. There were no adequate and well-controlled studies in pregnant women.

NURSING MOTHERS

It is not known whether Pancrelipase or Pancreatin is excreted in human milk. Because many drugs are excreted in human milk, caution should be exercised when Pancrelipase or Pancreatin is administered to a nursing woman.

ADVERSE REACTIONS

The most frequently reported adverse reactions to pancreatic enzyme containing products are gastrointestinal in nature. High doses may cause nausea, bloating, abdominal cramps and/or diarrhea in certain patients. Less frequently, allergic-type reactions have also been observed. Finely powdered pancreatic enzyme concentrate may be irritating to the mucous membranes and respiratory tract. Inhalation of the airborne powder may precipitate an asthma attack in sensitive individuals. The literature also contains several references to asthma due to inhalation in patients sensitized to pancreatic enzyme concentrates. Extremely high doses of exogenous pancreatic enzymes have been associated with hyperuricosuria and hyperuricemia when the preparations given were pancrelipase in powdered or capsule form, or pancreatin in tablet form.

OVERDOSAGE

Acute toxicity determinations in animals have not been possible since the maximum dose that could be given orally produced no toxic reaction. In chronic feeding tests, rats developed swollen salivary glands. This is believed due to the proteolytic activity and the mucosal irritation caused by tissue digestion.

No acute toxic reactions have been reported.

DOSAGE AND ADMINISTRATION

Dosage should be adjusted according to the severity of the exocrine pancreatic enzyme deficiency. The number of capsules or capsule strength given with meals and/or snacks should be estimated by assessing which dose minimizes steatorrhea and maintains good nutritional status.

In some patients with pancreatic enzyme deficiency, satisfactory responses have been achieved with dosages (expressed in U.S.P. units of lipase) similar to the ones stated below.

However, dosages should be adjusted according to the response of the patient. In severe deficiencies the dose may be increased or the frequency of administration may increase to hourly intervals if nausea, cramps and/or diarrhea do not occur.

Children 7 to 12 years: 4,000 to 12,000 units (more if necessary) with each meal and with snacks.

Children 1 to 6 years: 4,000 to 8,000 units with each meal and 4,000 units with snacks.

Children under 1 year: Dosage for children under 6 months of age has not been established. Children 6 months to 1 year have responded to 2,000 units of lipase per meal.

The assessment of the end points in children is aided by charting growth curves.

Adults: 4,000 to 32,000 units (more if necessary) with each meal and with snacks.

Storage: Keep bottle tightly closed. Store at controlled room temperature (15°-30°C, 59°-86°F), in a dry place. Do not refrigerate. Dispense in tight container as defined in the official compendium.

Store in tightly closed container in a dry place at a temperature not exceeding 25°C (77°F).

Dispense tablets and powder in tight container, preferably with a desiccant.

CLINICAL STUDIES

The effectiveness of Pancrelipase as a digestive aid in the treatment of patients with exocrine pancreatic insufficiency has been documented in the literature as follows:

1. Regan, PT, Malagelada J-R, DiMagno EP, Glanzman SL, Go VLW: Comparative effects of antacids, cimetidine and enteric coating on the therapeutic response to oral enzymes in severe pancreatic insufficiency. *N. Engl. J. Med.* 297:854-8, 1977.

2. Graham DY: Enzyme replacement therapy of exocrine pancreatic insufficiency in man. *N. Engl. J. Med.* 296:1314-7, 1977.

HOW SUPPLIED

PANCREATIN
CAPSULE:

BRAND/MANUFACTURER	NDC	SIZE	AWP
○ GENERICS			
ENCRON-10: Rugby	00536-5694-10	100s	$36.84

ENTERIC COATED CAPSULES:

BRAND/MANUFACTURER	NDC	SIZE	AWP
○ GENERICS			
ENCRON 10: Econolab	55053-0880-01	100s	$33.95
ENCRON 10: Econolab	55053-0880-02	250s	$81.95

➤ SHOWN IN PRODUCT IDENTIFICATION GUIDE

TABLETS:

BRAND/MANUFACTURER	NDC	SIZE	AWP
○ **BRAND**			
DONNAZYME: Wyeth-Ayerst	00031-4650-63	100s	$29.99

PANCRELIPASE

CAPSULE:

BRAND/MANUFACTURER	NDC	SIZE	AWP
○ **BRAND**			
COTAZYM: Organon	00052-0381-91	100s	$19.18
PANCREASE MT 4: McNeil Pharm	00045-0341-60	100s	$25.84
ULTRASE: Scandipharm	58914-0001-10	100s	$27.60
PANCREASE: McNeil Pharm	00045-0095-60	100s	$32.80
ULTRASE: Scandipharm	58914-0002-10	100s	$47.88
	58914-0018-10	100s	$71.82
	58914-0004-10	100s	$79.38
PANCREASE MT 16: McNeil Pharm	00045-0343-60	100s	$103.70
PANCREASE MT 20: McNeil Pharm	00045-0346-60	100s	$129.17
PANCREASE: McNeil Pharm	00045-0095-69	250s	$78.12
COTAZYM: Organon	00052-0381-95	500s	$90.85
ULTRASE: Scandipharm	58914-0004-50	500s	$379.20
○ **GENERICS**			
PANCOTE: Parmed	00349-8840-01	100s	$17.95
PANASE: Qualitest	00603-5021-21	100s	$25.30
Alphagen	59743-0025-01	100s	$25.40
PROTILASE: Rugby	00536-4929-01	100s	$28.24
Goldline	00182-1554-01	100s	$29.50
URL	00677-1322-01	100s	$29.94
KU-ZYME HP: Schwarz	00091-3525-01	100s	$35.19
Goldline	00182-1390-01	100s	$73.50
ENZYMASE-16: Econolab	55053-0790-01	100s	$74.00
PANCRELIPASE MST-16: Pecos	59879-0122-01	100s	$89.95
Major	00904-3470-70	250s	$52.45
PANASE: Qualitest	00603-5021-24	250s	$58.00
Alphagen	59743-0025-25	250s	$58.10
Moore,H.L.	00839-7526-09	250s	$67.49

CAPSULE: 30,000-30,000-10,000 U

BRAND/MANUFACTURER	NDC	SIZE	AWP
○ **BRAND**			
PANCREASE MT 10: McNeil Pharm	00045-0342-60	100s	$64.58

CAPSULE, COATED PELLETS:

BRAND/MANUFACTURER	NDC	SIZE	AWP
○ **GENERICS**			
PANCRELIPASE: Jones Medical	52604-2000-01	100s	$23.69

CAPSULE, EXTENDED RELEASE:

BRAND/MANUFACTURER	NDC	SIZE	AWP
○ **BRAND**			
ZYMASE: Organon	00052-0393-91	100s	$54.00
CREON 20: Solvay	00032-1220-01	100s	$81.88
	00032-1220-07	250s	$197.55
○ **GENERICS**			
COTAZYM-S: Organon	00052-0388-91	100s	$25.96
COTAZYM-S: Organon	00052-0388-95	500s	$122.16

ENTERIC COATED CAPSULES:

BRAND/MANUFACTURER	NDC	SIZE	AWP
○ **BRAND**			
CREON 10: Solvay	00032-1210-01	100s	$40.94
	00032-1210-07	250s	$98.78
○ **GENERICS**			
PANCOTE: Econolab	55053-0400-01	100s	$16.90
Geneva	00781-2219-01	100s	$23.54
PANCOTE: Econolab	55053-0323-01	100s	$26.75
Geneva	00781-2219-25	250s	$56.07
PANCOTE: Econolab	55053-0323-02	250s	$60.00

POWDER:

BRAND/MANUFACTURER	NDC	SIZE	AWP
○ **BRAND**			
VIOKASE: Robins Pharm	00031-9115-12	120 gm	$54.13
	00031-9115-25	240 gm	$92.15

TABLETS:

BRAND/MANUFACTURER	NDC	SIZE	AWP
○ **BRAND**			
VIOKASE: Robins Pharm	00031-9111-63	100s	$22.24
	00031-9111-70	500s	$100.10

BRAND/MANUFACTURER	NDC	SIZE	AWP
○ **GENERICS**			
VIO-MOORE: Moore,H.L.	00839-7618-06	100s	$12.81
PANOKASE: Major	00904-3472-60	100s	$15.70
PANOKASE: Rugby	00536-4395-01	100s	$16.58
Goldline	00182-1741-01	100s	$17.00
PANOKASE: Econolab	55053-0320-01	100s	$17.22
ILOZYME: Savage	00281-2001-19	250s	$108.22
PANOKASE: Major	00904-3472-40	500s	$71.50
PANOKASE: Econolab	55053-0320-05	500s	$77.55

Pancuronium Bromide

> THIS DRUG SHOULD BE ADMINISTERED BY ADEQUATELY TRAINED INDIVIDUALS FAMILIAR WITH ITS ACTIONS, CHARACTERISTICS, AND HAZARDS.

DESCRIPTION

Pancuronium Bromide injection is a nondepolarizing neuro-muscular blocking agent chemically designated as the aminosteroid 2 β, 16 β - dipiperidino-5α-androstane-3α, 17-β diol diacetate dimethobromide.

Pancuronium Bromide is supplied as a sterile, isotonic, nonpyrogenic solution for injection. Each mL contains 1 mg or 2 mg Pancuronium Bromide, 2 mg sodium acetate and 1% benzyl alcohol as preservative. The solution is adjusted to isotonicity with sodium chloride and to a pH of 4 with acetic acid and/or sodium hydroxide; water is used as the solvent.

Following is its chemical structure:

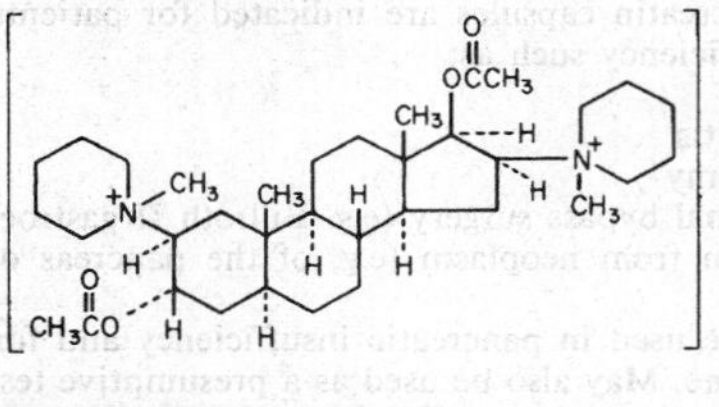

CLINICAL PHARMACOLOGY

Pancuronium Bromide is a nondepolarizing neuromuscular blocking agent possessing all of the characteristic pharmacological actions of this class of drugs (curariform). It acts by competing for cholinergic receptors at the motor end-plate. The antagonism to acetylcholine is inhibited and neuromuscular block is reversed by anticholinesterase agents such as pyridostigmine, neostigmine, and edrophonium. Pancuronium Bromide is approximately 1/3 less potent than vecuronium and approximately 5 times as potent as d-tubocurarine; the duration of neuromuscular blockade produced by Pancuronium Bromide is longer than that of vecuronium at initially equipotent doses.

The ED_{95} (dose required to produce 95% suppression of muscle twitch response) is approximately 0.05 mg/kg under balanced anesthesia and 0.03 mg/kg under halothane anesthesia. These doses produce effective skeletal muscle relaxation (as judged by time from maximum effect to 25% recovery of control twitch height) for approximately 22 minutes; the duration from injection to 90% recovery of control twitch height is approximately 65 minutes. The intubating dose of 0.1 mg/kg (balanced anesthesia) will effectively abolish twitch response within approximately 4 minutes; time from injection to 25% recovery from this dose is approximately 100 minutes.

Supplemental doses to maintain muscle relaxation slightly increase the magnitude of block and significantly increase the duration of block. The use of a peripheral nerve stimulator is of benefit in assessing the degree of neuromuscular blockade.

The most characteristic circulatory effects of Pancuronium Bromide, studied under halothane anesthesia, are a moderate rise in heart rate, mean arterial pressure and cardiac output; systemic vascular resistance is not changed significantly and central venous pressure may fall slightly. The heart rate rise is inversely related to the rate immediately before administration of Pancuronium Bromide, is blocked by prior administration of atropine, and appears unrelated to the concentration of halothane or dose of Pancuronium Bromide.

Data on histamine assays and available clinical experience indicate that hypersensitivity reactions such as bronchospasm, flushing, redness, hypotension, tachycardia, and other reactions commonly associated with histamine release are rare. (See *"Adverse Reactions"*).

Pharmacokinetics: The elimination half-life of Pancuronium Bromide has been reported to range between 89-161 minutes. The volume of distribution ranges from 241-280 mL/kg and plasma clearance is approximately 1.1-1.9 mL/minute/kg. Approximately 40% of the total dose of Pancuronium Bromide has been recovered in urine as unchanged Pancuronium Bromide and its metabolites while approximately 11% has been recovered in bile. As much as 25% of an injected dose may be recovered as 3-hydroxy metabolite, which is half as potent a blocking agent as Pancuronium Bromide. Less than 5% of the injected dose is recovered as 17-hydroxy metabolite and 3.17-dihydroxy metabolite, which have been judged to be approximately 50 times less potent than Pancuronium Bromide. Pancuronium

Bromide exhibits strong binding to gamma globulin and moderate binding to albumin. Approximately 13% is unbound to plasma protein. In patients with cirrhosis the volume of distribution is increased by approximately 50%, the plasma clearance is decreased by approximately 22% and the elimination half-life is doubled. Similar results were noted in patients with biliary obstruction, except that plasma clearance was less than half the normal rate. The initial total dose to achieve adequate relaxation may thus be high in patients with hepatic and/or biliary tract dysfunction, while the duration of action is greater than usual.

The elimination half-life is doubled and the plasma clearance is reduced by approximately 60% in patients with renal failure. The volume of distribution is variable, and in some cases elevated. The rate of recovery of neuromuscular blockade, as determined by peripheral nerve stimulation is variable and sometimes very much slower than normal.

INDICATIONS AND USAGE

Pancuronium Bromide injection is indicated as an adjunct to general anesthesia, to facilitate tracheal intubation and to provide skeletal muscle relaxation during surgery or mechanical ventilation.

UNLABELED USES

Pancuronium Bromide is used alone or as an adjunct in the treatment of tetanus and torticollis.

CONTRAINDICATIONS

Pancuronium Bromide is contraindicated in patients known to be hypersensitive to the drug.

WARNINGS

PANCURONIUM BROMIDE SHOULD BE ADMINISTERED IN CAREFULLY ADJUSTED DOSES BY OR UNDER THE SUPERVISION OF EXPERIENCED CLINICIANS WHO ARE FAMILIAR WITH ITS ACTIONS AND THE POSSIBLE COMPLICATIONS THAT MIGHT OCCUR FOLLOWING ITS USE. THE DRUG SHOULD NOT BE ADMINISTERED UNLESS FACILITIES FOR INTUBATION, ARTIFICIAL RESPIRATION, OXYGEN THERAPY, AND REVERSAL AGENTS ARE IMMEDIATELY AVAILABLE. THE CLINICIAN MUST BE PREPARED TO ASSIST OR CONTROL RESPIRATION.

In patients who are known to have myasthenia gravis or the myasthenic (Eaton-Lambert) syndrome, small doses of Pancuronium Bromide may have profound effects. In such patients, a peripheral nerve stimulator and use of a small test dose may be of value in monitoring the response to administration of muscle relaxants.

PRECAUTIONS

USE OF A PERIPHERAL NERVE STIMULATOR WILL USUALLY BE OF VALUE FOR MONITORING OF NEUROMUSCULAR BLOCKING EFFECT, AVOIDING OVERDOSAGE AND ASSISTING IN EVALUATION OF RECOVERY.

General: Although Pancuronium Bromide has been used successfully in many patients with pre-existing pulmonary, hepatic, or renal disease, caution should be exercised in these situations.

Renal Failure: A major portion of Pancuronium Bromide, as well as an active metabolite, are recovered in urine. The elimination half-life is doubled and the plasma clearance is reduced in patients with renal failure; at the same time, the rate of recovery of neuromuscular blockade is variable and sometimes very much slower than normal (see "Pharmacokinetics"). This information should be taken into consideration if Pancuronium Bromide is selected, for other reasons, to be used in a patient with renal failure.

Altered Circulation Time: Conditions associated with slower circulation time in cardiovascular disease, old age, edematous states resulting in increased volume of distribution may contribute to a delay in onset time; therefore, dosage should not be increased.

Hepatic and/or Biliary Tract Disease: The doubled elimination half-life and reduced plasma clearance determined in patients with hepatic and/or biliary tract disease, as well as limited data showing that recovery time is prolonged an average of 65% in patients with biliary tract obstruction, suggests that prolongation of neuromuscular blockade may occur. At the same time, these conditions are characterized by an approximately 50% increase in volume of distribution of Pancuronium Bromide, suggesting that the total initial dose to achieve adequate relaxation may in some cases be high. The possibility of slower onset, higher total dosage and prolongation of neuromuscular blockade must be taken into consideration when Pancuronium Bromide is used in these patients (see also "Pharmacokinetics").

Long-term Use in I.C.U.: In the intensive care unit, in rare cases, long-term use of neuromuscular blocking drugs to facilitate mechanical ventilation may be associated with prolonged paralysis and/or skeletal muscle weakness, that may be first noted during attempts to wean such patients from the ventilator. Typically, such patients receive other drugs such as broad spectrum antibiotics, narcotics and/or steroids and may have electrolyte imbalance and diseases which lead to electrolyte imbalance, hypoxic episodes of varying duration, acid-base imbalance and extreme debilitation, any of which may enhance the actions of a neuromuscular blocking agent. Additionally, patients immobilized for extended periods frequently develop symptoms consistent with disuse muscle atrophy. Therefore, when there is a need for long-term mechanical ventilation, the benefits-to-risk ratio of neuromuscular blockade must be considered.

Continuous infusion or intermittent bolus dosing to support mechanical ventilation, has not been studied sufficiently to support dosage recommendations.

UNDER THE ABOVE CONDITIONS, APPROPRIATE MONITORING, SUCH AS USE OF A PERIPHERAL NERVE STIMULATOR, TO ASSESS THE DEGREE OF NEUROMUSCULAR BLOCKADE, MAY PRECLUDE INADVERTANT EXCESS DOSING.

Severe Obesity or Neuromuscular Disease: Patients with severe obesity or neuromuscular disease may pose airway and/or ventilatory problems requiring special care before, during and after the use of neuromuscular blocking agents such as Pancuronium Bromide.

C.N.S.: Pancuronium Bromide has no known effect on consciousness, the pain threshold or cerebration. Administration should be accompanied by adequate anesthesia or sedation.

Drug Interactions: Prior administration of succinylcholine may enhance the neuromuscular blocking effect of Pancuronium Bromide and increase its duration of action. If succinylcholine is used before Pancuronium Bromide, the administration of Pancuronium Bromide should be delayed until the patient starts recovering from succinylcholine-induced neuromuscular blockade.

If a small dose of Pancuronium Bromide is given at least 3 minutes prior to the administration of succinylcholine, in order to reduce the incidence and intensity of succinylcholine-induced fasiculations, this dose may induce a degree of neuromuscular block sufficient to cause respiratory depression in some patients.

Other nondepolarizing neuromuscular blocking agents (vecuronium, atracurium, d-tubocurarine, metocurine, and gallamine) behave in a clinically similar fashion to Pancuronium Bromide. The combinations of Pancuronium Bromide-metocurine and Pancuronium Bromide-d-tubocurarine are significantly more potent than the additive effects of each of the individual drugs given alone; however, the duration of blockade of these combinations is not prolonged. There are insufficient data to support concomitant use of Pancuronium Bromide and the other three above mentioned muscle relaxants in the same patients.

Inhalational Anesthetics: Use of volatile inhalational anesthetics such as enflurane, insoflurane, and halothane with Pancuronium Bromide will enhance neuromuscular blockade. Potentiation is most prominent with use of enflurane and isoflurane.

With the above agents, the intubating dose of Pancuronium Bromide may be the same as with balanced anesthesia unless the inhalational anesthetic has been administered for a sufficient time at a sufficient dose to have reached clinical equilibrium. The relatively long duration of action of Pancuronium Bromide should be taken into consideration when the drug is selected for intubation in these circumstances.

Clinical experience and animal experiments suggest that Pancuronium Bromide should be given with caution to patients receiving chronic tricyclic antidepressant therapy who are anesthetized with halothane because severe ventricular arrhythmias may result from this combination. The severity of the arrhythmias appears in part related to the dose of Pancuronium Bromide.

Antibiotics: Parenteral/intraperitoneal administration of high doses of certain antibiotics may intensify or produce neuromuscular block on their own. The following antibiotics have been associated with various degrees of paralysis: aminoglycosides (such as neomycin, streptomycin, kanamycin, gentamicin, and dihydrostreptomycin); tetracyclines; bacitracin; polymyxin B; colistin; and sodium colistimethate. If these or other newly introduced antibiotics are used preoperatively or in conjunction with Pancuronium Bromide, unexpected prolongation of neuromuscular block should be considered a possibility.

Other: Experience concerning injection of quinidine during recovery from use of other muscle relaxants suggests that recurrent paralysis may occur. This possibility must also be considered for Pancuronium Bromide injection.

Electrolyte imbalance and diseases which lead to electrolyte imbalance, such as adrenal cortical insufficiency, have been shown to alter neuromuscular blockade. Depending on the nature of the imbalance, either enhancement or inhibition may be expected. Magnesium salts, administered for the management of toxemia of pregnancy, may enhance the neuromuscular blockade.

Drug/Laboratory Test Interactions: None known.

Carcinogenesis, Mutagenesis, Impairment of Fertility: Long-term studies in animals have not been performed to evaluate carcinogenic or mutagenic potential or impairment of fertility.

Pregnancy: Pregnancy Category C: Animal reproduction studies have not been performed. It is not known whether Pancuronium Bromide can cause fetal harm when administered to a pregnant woman or can affect reproduction capacity. Pancuronium Bromide should be given to a pregnant woman only if the administering clinician decides that the benefits outweigh the risks.

Pancuronium Bromide may be used in operative obstetrics (Cesarean section), but reversal of Pancuronium Bromide may be unsatisfactory in patients receiving magnesium sulfate for toxemia of pregnancy, because magnesium salts enhance neuromuscular blockade. Dosage should usually be reduced, as indicated, in such cases. It is also recommended that the interval between use of Pancuronium Bromide and delivery be reasonably short to avoid clinically significant placental transfer.

Pediatric Use: Dose response studies in children indicate that, with the exception of neonates, dosage requirements are the same as for adults. Neonates are especially sensitive to nondepolarizing neuromuscular blocking agents, such as Pancuronium Bromide during the first month of life. It is recommended that a test dose of 0.02 mg/kg be given first in this group to measure responsiveness.

The prolonged use of Pancuronium Bromide for the management of neonates undergoing mechanical ventilation has been associated in rare cases with severe skeletal muscle weakness that may first be noted during attempts to wean such patients from the ventilator; such patients usually receive other drugs such as antibiotics which may enhance neuromuscular blockade. Microscopic changes consistent with disuse atrophy have been noted at autopsy. Although a cause-and-effect relationship has not been established, the benefits-to-risk ratio must be considered when there is a need for neuromuscular blockade to facilitate long-term mechanical ventilation of neonates.

Rare cases of unexplained, clinically significant methemoglobinemia have been reported in premature neonates undergoing emergency anesthesia and surgery which included combined use of Pancuronium Bromide, fentanyl, and atropine. A direct cause-and-effect relationship between the combined use of these drugs and the reported cases of methemoglobinemia has not been established.

ADVERSE REACTIONS

Neuromuscular: The most frequent adverse reaction to nondepolarizing blocking agents as a class consists of an extension of drug's pharmacological action beyond the time period needed. This may vary from skeletal muscle weakness to profound and prolonged skeletal muscle paralysis resulting in respiratory insufficiency or apnea. (see *"Precautions: Pediatric Use"*).

Inadequate reversal of the neuromuscular blockade is possible with Pancuronium Bromide as with all curariform drugs. These adverse experiences are managed by manual or mechanical ventilation until recovery is judged adequate.

Prolonged paralysis and/or skeletal muscle weakness have been reported after long-term use to support mechanical ventilation in the intensive care unit.

Cardiovascular: See discussion of circulatory effects in *"Clinical Pharmacology"*.

Gastrointestinal: Salivation is sometimes noted during very light anesthesia, especially if no anticholinergic premedication is used.

Skin: An occasional transient rash is noted accompanying the use of Pancuronium Bromide.

Other: Although histamine release is not a characteristic action of Pancuronium Bromide rare hypersensitivity reactions such as bronchospasm, flushing, redness, hypotension, tachycardia, and other reactions possibly mediated by histamine release have been reported.

OVERDOSAGE

The possibility of iatrogenic overdosage can be minimized by carefully monitoring the muscle twitch response to peripheral nerve stimulation.

Excessive doses of Pancuronium Bromide produce enhanced pharmacological effects. Residual neuromuscular blockade beyond the time period needed may occur with Pancuronium Bromide as with other neuromuscular blockers. This may be manifested by skeletal muscle weakness, decreased respiratory reserve, low tidal volume, or apnea. A peripheral nerve stimulator may be used to assess the degree of residual neuromuscular blockade and help to differentiate residual neuromuscular blockade from other causes of decreased respiratory reserve.

Regonol injection, neostigmine, or edrophonium, in conjunction with atropine or glycopyrrolate, will usually antagonize the skeletal muscle relaxant action of Pancuronium Bromide. Satisfactory reversal can be judged by adequacy of skeletal muscle tone and by adequacy of respiration. A peripheral nerve stimulator may also be used to monitor restoration of twitch response.

Failure of prompt reversal (within 30 minutes) may occur in the presence of extreme debilitation, carcinomatosis, and with concomitant use of certain broad spectrum antibiotics, or anesthetic agents and other drugs which enhance neuromuscular blockade or cause respiratory depression of their own. Under such circumstances, the management is the same as that of prolonged neuromuscular blockade. Ventilation must be supported by artificial means until the patient has resumed control of his respiration. Prior to the use of reversal agents, reference should be made to the specific package insert of the reversal agent.

DOSAGE AND ADMINISTRATION

Pancuronium Bromide injection is for intravenous use only. This drug should be administered by or under the supervision of experienced clinicians familiar with the use of neuromuscular blocking agents. DOSAGE MUST BE INDIVIDUALIZED IN EACH CASE. The dosage information which follows is derived from studies based upon units of drug per unit of body weight and is intended to serve as a guide only. Since potent inhalational anesthetics or prior use of succinylcholine may enhance the intensity and duration of Pancuronium Bromide (see *"Precautions: Drug Interactions"*), the lower end of the recommended initial dosage range may suffice when Pancuronium Bromide is first used after intubation with succinylcholine and/or after maintenance doses of volatile liquid inhalational anesthetics are started. To obtain maximum clinical benefits of Pancuronium Bromide and to minimize the possibility of overdosage, the monitoring of muscle twitch response to a peripheral nerve stimulator is advised.

In adults under balanced anesthesia the initial intravenous dosage range is 0.04 to 0.1 mg/kg. Later incremental doses starting at 0.01 mg/kg may be used. These increments slightly increase the magnitude of the blockade and significantly increase the duration of blockade, because a significant number of myoneural junctions are still blocked when there is clinical need for more drug.

If Pancuronium Bromide is used to provide skeletal muscle relaxation for endotracheal intubation, a bolus dose of 0.06 to 0.1 mg/kg are recommended. Conditions satisfactory in intubation are usually present within 2 to 3 minutes, (see *"Precautions"*).

Dosage in Children: Dose response studies in children indicate that, with the exception of neonates, dosage requirements are the same as for adults. Neonates are especially sensitive to nondepolarizing neuromuscular blocking agents, such as

Pancuronium Bromide during the first month of life. It is recommended that a test dose of 0.02 mg/kg be given first in this group to measure responsiveness.

Cesarean Section: The dosage to provide relaxation for intubation and operation is the same as for general surgical procedures. The dosage to provide relaxation following usage of succinylcholine for intubation (see *"Precautions: Drug Interactions"*), is the same as for general surgical procedures.

Compatibility: Pancuronium Bromide is compatible in solution with:
0.9% sodium chloride injection
5% dextrose and sodium chloride injection
5% dextrose injection
Lactated Ringer's injection

Parenteral drug products should be inspected visually for particulate matter and discoloration prior to administration, whenever solution and container permit.

When mixed with the above solutions in glass or plastic containers, Pancuronium Bromide will remain stable in solution for 48 hours with no alteration in potency or pH; no decomposition is observed and there is no absorption to either the glass or plastic container.

Storage: Both concentrations of Pancuronium Bromide will maintain full clinical potency for six months if kept at a room temperature of 18° to 22°C (65° to 72°F); or for 3 years when refrigerated at 2° to 8°C (36° to 46°F).

HOW SUPPLIED
INJECTION: 1 MG/ML

AVERAGE UNIT PRICE (AVAILABLE SIZES)		GENERIC A-RATED AVERAGE PRICE (GAAP)	
BRAND	$1.41	10 ml 25s	$429.57
GENERIC	$1.52		

BRAND/MANUFACTURER	NDC	SIZE	AWP
◆ **BRAND**			
PAVULON: Organon	00052-0443-25	10 ml 25s	$353.20
◆ **GENERICS**			
Astra	00186-1322-12	10 ml 5s	$63.75
Gensia	00703-2804-03	10 ml 10s	$138.63
Elkins-Sinn	00641-2547-45	10 ml 25s	$350.00
Abbott Hosp	00074-4646-01	10 ml 25s	$509.14

INJECTION: 2 MG/ML

AVERAGE UNIT PRICE (AVAILABLE SIZES)		GENERIC A-RATED AVERAGE PRICE (GAAP)	
BRAND	$2.86	2 ml 10s	$52.47
GENERIC	$3.02	5 ml 10s	$121.13
		2 ml 25s	$179.34
		5 ml 25s	$404.39

BRAND/MANUFACTURER	NDC	SIZE	AWP
◆ **BRAND**			
PAVULON: Organon	00052-0444-26	2 ml 25s	$151.60
	00052-0444-25	5 ml 25s	$334.90
◆ **GENERICS**			
Astra	00186-1334-03	2 ml 10s	$48.00
Astra	00186-1336-23	2 ml 10s	$49.06
Astra	00186-1331-13	2 ml 10s	$54.00
Astra	00186-1333-23	2 ml 10s	$58.81
Astra	00186-0692-01	5 ml 10s	$112.50
Astra	00186-1335-03	5 ml 10s	$112.50
Astra	00186-1332-13	5 ml 10s	$125.63
Astra	00186-0676-01	5 ml 10s	$133.88
Raway	00686-2812-04	2 ml 25s	$60.00
Gensia	00703-2812-04	2 ml 25s	$147.19
Elkins-Sinn	00641-1475-35	2 ml 25s	$150.00
Elkins-Sinn	00641-0469-25	2 ml 25s	$156.25
Abbott Hosp	00074-4645-01	2 ml 25s	$383.27
Raway	00686-2823-04	5 ml 25s	$72.00
Gensia	00703-2823-04	5 ml 25s	$324.38
Elkins-Sinn	00641-1476-35	5 ml 25s	$331.25
Elkins-Sinn	00641-2546-45	5 ml 25s	$337.81
Abbott Hosp	00074-4645-02	5 ml 25s	$956.53

Panhematin *SEE* HEMIN

Panmycin *SEE* TETRACYCLINE HYDROCHLORIDE, ORAL

PanOxyl *SEE* BENZOYL PEROXIDE

Papaverine Hydrochloride

COMPOSITION

Each capsule contains:

Papaverine Hydrochloride . . . . 150 mg

◆ RATED THERAPEUTICALLY EQUIVALENT; ◇ THERAPEUTIC EQUIVALENCE UNCONFIRMED; ○ UNRATED

in a specially prepared base to provide prolonged activity.

Following is its chemical structure:

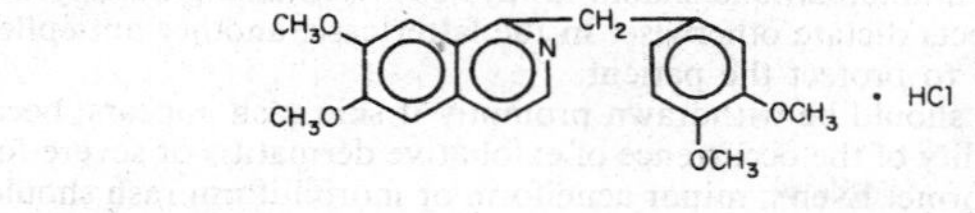

ACTION AND USES

The main actions of Papaverine HCl are exerted on cardiac and smooth muscle. Like quinidine, Papaverine HCl acts directly on the heart muscle to depress conduction and prolong the refractory period. Papaverine HCl relaxes various smooth muscles. This relaxation may be prominent if spasm exists. The muscle cell is not paralyzed by Papaverine HCl, and still responds to drugs and other stimuli causing contraction. The antispasmodic effect is a direct one, and unrelated to muscle innervation. Papaverine HCl is practically devoid of effects on the central nervous system.

Papaverine HCl relaxes the smooth musculature of the larger blood vessels, especially coronary, systemic peripheral, and pulmonary arteries. Perhaps by its direct vasodilating action on cerebral blood vessels, Papaverine HCl increases cerebral blood flow and decreases cerebral vascular resistance in normal subjects; oxygen consumption is unaltered. These effects may explain the benefit reported from the drug in cerebral vascular encephalopathy.

The direct actions of Papaverine HCl on the heart to depress conduction and irritability and to prolong the refractory period of the myocardium provide the basis for its clinical trial in abrogating atrial and ventricular premature systoles and ominous ventricular arrhythmias. The coronary vasodilator action could be an additional factor of therapeutic value when such rhythms are secondary to insufficiency or occlusion of the coronary arteries.

In patients with acute coronary thrombosis, the occurrence of ventricular rhythms is serious and requires measures designed to decrease myocardial irritability. Papaverine HCl may have advantages over quinidine, used for a similar purpose, in that it may be given in an emergency by the intravenous route, does not depress myocardial contraction or cause cinchonism, and produces coronary vasodilation.

INDICATIONS

For the relief of cerebral and peripheral ischemia associated with arterial spasm and myocardial ischemia complicated by arrhythmias.

UNLABELED USES
Papaverine HCl is used alone or as an adjunct in the treatment of erectile impotence.

PRECAUTIONS

Use with caution in patients with glaucoma. Hepatic hypersensitivity has been reported with gastrointestinal symptoms, jaundice, eosinophilia, and altered liver function tests. Discontinue medication if these occur.

ADVERSE REACTIONS

Although occurring rarely, the reported side effects of Papaverine HCl include nausea, abdominal distress, anorexia, constipation, malaise, drowsiness, vertigo, sweating, headache, diarrhea, and skin rash.

DOSAGE AND ADMINISTRATION

One capsule every 12 hours. In difficult cases administration may be increased to one capsule every 8 hours or two capsules every 12 hours.

J CODES

Up to 60 mg IV,IM—J2440

INJECTION: 30 MG/ML

BRAND/MANUFACTURER	NDC	SIZE	AWP
○ GENERICS			
YorPharm Inc	61147-8009-01	2 ml	$2.73
Allscrips	54569-2360-00	10 ml	$3.72
YorPharm Inc	61147-8009-03	10 ml	$6.28
Lilly	00002-1676-01	10 ml	$3.72
Lilly	00002-1676-25	10 ml 25s	$83.58

For additional alternatives, turn to the section beginning on page 2859.

Paradione *SEE* PARAMETHADIONE

Paraflex *SEE* CHLORZOXAZONE

Parafon Forte DSC *SEE* CHLORZOXAZONE

Paraldehyde

DESCRIPTION

Paraldehyde 2,4,6-trimethyl-1,3,5-trioxane, is a colorless, transparent liquid having a characteristic aromatic odor and warm, but disagreeable taste.

Following is its chemical structure:

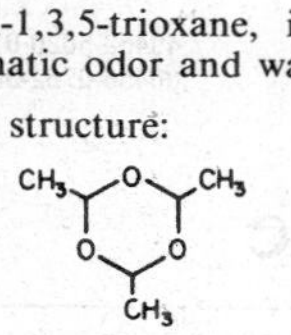

INDICATIONS AND USAGE

The indications for the use of Paraldehyde as a hypnotic are the same as for chloral hydrate. Because of its odor, Paraldehyde cannot often be employed for the purpose of mild sedation in ambulatory patients. In delirium tremens and in other psychiatric states characterized by excitement, Paraldehyde has special value. It is administered to quiet the patient and to produce sleep. Quite large doses (15 to 30 ml or more) may be needed for this purpose.

UNLABELED USES
Paraldehyde is used alone or as an adjunct in the treatment of acute symptomatic relief of alcohol withdrawal.

CONTRAINDICATIONS AND DISADVANTAGES

In bronchopulmonary disease, Paraldehyde at times may be contraindicated because of the excretion of the drug by the lungs. Hepatic insufficiency also constitutes a contraindication to the use of Paraldehyde inasmuch as approximately 80 per cent of the drug is destroyed in the body, presumably by the liver. In patients with gastroenteritis, especially if ulceration is present, Paraldehyde may cause considerable irritation. One of the chief disadvantages of Paraldehyde arises from the odor it imparts to the exhaled air for as long as 24 hours after ingestion. The entire room may be "perfumed" by a patient who has received the drug, and in the summertime swarms of flies may be attracted. However, the patient is unaware of the odor. A second disadvantage of Paraldehyde is the unpleasant taste and the irritation of the throat and gastric mucosa which may ensue if the drug is not given well diluted in a proper vehicle. The belief that Paraldehyde is quite toxic when combined with morphine apparently is unfounded and the depressant actions of the two drugs are probably only summative.

PRECAUTIONS

Pregnancy Category C: Annual reproduction studies have not been conducted with Paraldehyde. It is also not known whether Paraldehyde can cause fetal harm when administered to a pregnant woman or can affect reproduction capacity. Paraldehyde should be given to a pregnant woman only if clearly needed.

Pediatric Use: Safety and effectiveness in children have not been established.

CAUTION: Paraldehyde may oxidize to form acetic acid. UNDER NO CIRCUMSTANCES use material that has a brownish color or a sharp, penetrating odor of acetic acid. Oxidation occurs more rapidly in opened, partially filled containers. Discard any unused portion remaining in an opened container.

OVERDOSAGE

The acute toxicity of Paraldehyde taken by mouth is low, and the drug possesses a wide margin of safety. Even very large doses usually cause only prolonged sleep or stupor. Although rare, fatalities have occurred, death being due to respiratory depression and cardiovascular collapse. Most of the reported cases of poisoning or death are in patients given the drug intravenously or rectally, but on occasion Paraldehyde given by mouth has resulted in death. (See Kotz et al., 1938; Shoor, 1941; Burstein, 1943; Hemphill and Heller, 1944; and others.)

So-called hypersusceptibility to Paraldehyde may be due in some cases to the presence of liver damage. It is not known whether Paraldehyde can cause liver damage or aggravate pre-existing liver injury.

The symptoms and treatment of acute Paraldehyde poisoning are much the same as those for chloral hydrate. Respiration is usually very rapid and labored, the pulse feeble and fast, and the blood pressure very low. The diagnosis is facilitated by the characteristic odor of the drug on the breath. Data obtained in animals and in man indicate that pentyienetetrazol is superior to picrotoxin as an analeptic in Paraldehyde intoxication (Bodansky et al., 1941).

DOSAGE

Paraldehyde may be given orally or rectally.

The usual hypnotic dose is 4 to 8 ml, given orally in capsule form or in milk or iced fruit juice to mask the taste and odor. In delirium tremens 10 to 35 ml may be necessary. It may also be given rectally dissolved in oil or isotonic sodium chloride solution to avoid rectal irritation.

REFERENCES
1. Pharmacological Basis of Therapeutics by Goodman and Gilman, Second Edition 2. American Hospital Formulary

J CODES
Up to 5 ml OTH—J2490

▶ SHOWN IN PRODUCT IDENTIFICATION GUIDE

HOW SUPPLIED
LIQUID (C-IV):

BRAND/MANUFACTURER	NDC	SIZE	AWP
○ GENERICS	49452-5020-01	30 ml	$24.50
PARAL: Forest Pharm	00456-0762-30	30 ml 25s	$192.44

Paramethadione

> BECAUSE OF ITS POTENTIAL TO PRODUCE FETAL MALFORMATIONS AND SERIOUS SIDE EFFECTS, PARAMETHADIONE SHOULD ONLY BE UTILIZED WHEN OTHER LESS TOXIC DRUGS HAVE BEEN FOUND INEFFECTIVE IN CONTROLLING ABSENCE (PETIT MAL) SEIZURES.

DESCRIPTION

Paramethadione is an antiepileptic agent. An oxazolidinedione compound, it is chemically identified as 5-Ethyl-3,5-dimethyl-2,4-oxazolidinedione. Paramethadione is a synthetic, oily, slightly water-soluble liquid. It is supplied in capsule form for oral use only. The capsules are available in two dosage strengths. One strength contains 150 mg, the other 300 mg of Paramethadione per capsule.

Following is its chemical structure:

CLINICAL PHARMACOLOGY

Paramethadione has been shown to prevent pentylenetetrazol-induced and thujone-induced seizures in experimental animals; the drug has a less marked effect on seizures induced by picrotoxin, procaine, cocaine, or strychnine. Unlike the hydantoins and antiepileptic barbiturates, Paramethadione does not modify the maximal seizure pattern in patients undergoing electroconvulsive therapy. Paramethadione has a sedative effect that may increase to the point of ataxia when excessive doses are used. A toxic dose of the drug in animals (approximately 1 g/kg) produced sleep, unconsciousness, and respiratory depression.

Paramethadione is rapidly absorbed from the gastrointestinal tract. It is demethylated by liver microsomes to an active N-demethylated metabolite, and is excreted slowly in this form by the kidney; almost no unmetabolized Paramethadione is excreted.

INDICATIONS AND USAGE

Paramethadione is indicated for the control of absence (petit mal) seizures that are refractory to treatment with other drugs.

CONTRAINDICATIONS

Paramethadione is contraindicated in patients with a known hypersensitivity to the drug.

WARNINGS

Paramethadione may cause serious side effects. Strict medical supervision of the patient is mandatory, especially during the initial year of therapy.

Usage During Pregnancy: THERE ARE MULTIPLE REPORTS IN THE CLINICAL LITERATURE WHICH INDICATE THAT THE USE OF ANTIEPILEPTIC DRUGS DURING PREGNANCY RESULTS IN AN INCREASED INCIDENCE OF BIRTH DEFECTS IN THE OFFSPRING. DATA ARE MORE EXTENSIVE WITH RESPECT TO TRIMETHADIONE, PARAMETHADIONE, PHENYTOIN AND PHENOBARBITAL THAN WITH OTHER ANTIEPILEPTIC DRUGS.

THEREFORE, ANTIEPILEPTIC DRUGS SUCH AS PARAMETHADIONE SHOULD BE ADMINISTERED TO WOMEN OF CHILDBEARING POTENTIAL ONLY IF THEY ARE CLEARLY SHOWN TO BE ESSENTIAL IN THE MANAGEMENT OF THEIR SEIZURES. EFFECTIVE MEANS OF CONTRACEPTION SHOULD ACCOMPANY THE USE OF PARAMETHADIONE IN SUCH PATIENTS. IF A PATIENT BECOMES PREGNANT WHILE TAKING PARAMETHADIONE, TERMINATION OF THE PREGNANCY SHOULD BE CONSIDERED. A PATIENT WHO REQUIRES THERAPY WITH PARAMETHADIONE AND WHO WISHES TO BECOME PREGNANT SHOULD BE ADVISED OF THE RISKS.

REPORTS HAVE SUGGESTED THAT THE MATERNAL INGESTION OF ANTIEPILEPTIC DRUGS, PARTICULARLY BARBITURATES, IS ASSOCIATED WITH A NEONATAL COAGULATION DEFECT THAT MAY CAUSE BLEEDING DURING THE EARLY (USUALLY WITHIN 24 HOURS OF BIRTH) NEONATAL PERIOD. THE POSSIBILITY OF THE OCCURRENCE OF THIS DEFECT WITH THE USE OF PARAMETHADIONE SHOULD BE KEPT IN MIND. THE DEFECT IS CHARACTERIZED BY DECREASED LEVELS OF VITAMIN K-DEPENDENT CLOTTING FACTORS, AND PROLONGATION OF EITHER THE PROTHROMBIN TIME OR THE PARTIAL THROMBOPLASTIN TIME, OR BOTH. IT HAS BEEN SUGGESTED THAT PROPHYLACTIC VITAMIN K BE GIVEN TO THE MOTHER ONE MONTH PRIOR TO, AND DURING DELIVERY, AND TO THE INFANT, INTRAVENOUSLY, IMMEDIATELY AFTER BIRTH.

PRECAUTIONS

General: Abrupt discontinuation of Paramethadione may precipitate absence (petit mal) status. Paramethadione should always be withdrawn gradually unless serious adverse effects dictate otherwise. In the latter case, another antiepileptic may be substituted to protect the patient.

Paramethadione should be withdrawn promptly if skin rash appears, because of the grave possibility of the occurrence of exfoliative dermatitis or severe forms of erythema multiforme. Even a minor acneiform or morbilliform rash should be allowed to clear completely before treatment with Paramethadione is resumed; reinstitute therapy cautiously. Paramethadione should ordinarily not be used in patients with severe blood dyscrasias.

Hepatitis has been associated rarely with the use of oxazolidinediones. Jaundice or other signs of liver dysfunction are an indication for withdrawal of Paramethadione. Paramethadione should ordinarily not be used in patients with severe hepatic impairment.

Fatal nephrosis has been reported with the use of oxazolidinediones. Persistent or increasing albuminuria, or the development of any other significant renal abnormality, is an indication for withdrawal of the drug. Paramethadione should ordinarily not be used in patients with severe renal dysfunction.

Hemeralopia has occurred with the use of oxazolidinedione compounds; this appears to be an effect of the drugs on the neural layers of the retina, and usually can be reversed by a reduction in dosage. Scotomata are an indication for withdrawal of the drug. Caution should be observed when treating patients who have diseases of the retina or optic nerve. Manifestations of systemic lupus erythematosus have been associated with the use of the oxazolidinediones, as they have with the use of certain other antiepileptics. Lymphadenopathies simulating malignant lymphoma have also occurred. Lupus-like manifestations or lymph node enlargement are indications for withdrawal of Paramethadione. Signs and symptoms may disappear after discontinuation of therapy, and specific treatment may be unnecessary.

A myasthenia gravis-like syndrome has been associated with the chronic use of the oxazolidinediones. Symptoms suggestive of this condition are indications for withdrawal of Paramethadione.

The 300 mg capsule of Paramethadione contains FD&C Yellow No. 5 (tartrazine) which may cause allergic-type reactions (including bronchial asthma) in certain susceptible individuals. Although the overall incidence of FD&C Yellow No. 5 (tartrazine) sensitivity in the general population is low, it is frequently seen in patients who also have aspirin hypersensitivity.

Information for Patients: Patients should be advised to report immediately such signs and symptoms as sore throat, fever, malaise, easy-bruising, petechiae, or epistaxis, or others that may be indicative of an infection or bleeding tendency.

Laboratory Tests: A complete blood count should be done prior to initiating therapy with Paramethadione and at monthly intervals thereafter. A marked depression of the blood count is an indication for withdrawal of the drug. If no abnormality appears within 12 months, the interval between blood counts may be extended. A moderate degree of neutropenia, with or without a corresponding drop in the leukocyte count, is not uncommon. Therapy need not be withdrawn unless the neutrophil count is 2500 or less; more frequent blood examinations should be done when the count is less than 3,000. Other blood dyscrasias, including leukopenia, eosinophilia, thrombocytopenia, pancytopenia, agranulocytosis, hypoplastic anemia, and fatal aplastic anemia, have occurred with the use of oxazolidinediones.

Liver function tests should be done prior to initiating therapy with Paramethadione and at monthly intervals thereafter. A urinalysis should be done prior to initiating therapy with Paramethadione and at monthly intervals thereafter.

Drug Interactions: Drugs known to cause toxic effects similar to those of the oxazolidinediones should be avoided or used only with extreme caution during therapy with Paramethadione.

Carcinogenesis: No data are available on long-term potential for carcinogenicity in animals or humans.

Pregnancy: Pregnancy Category D. See *"Warnings"* section.

Nursing Mothers: It is not known whether this drug is excreted in human milk. Because many drugs are excreted in human milk and because of the potential for serious adverse reactions in nursing infants from Paramethadione a decision should be made whether to discontinue nursing or to discontinue the drug, taking into account the importance of the drug to the mother.

ADVERSE REACTIONS

The following side effects, in decreasing order of severity, have been associated with the use of oxazolidinedione compounds. Although not all of them have been reported with the use of Paramethadione the possibility of their occurrence should be kept in mind when the drug is prescribed.

Renal: Fatal nephrosis has occurred. Albuminuria.

Hematologic: Fatal aplastic anemia, hypoplastic anemia, pancytopenia, agranulocytosis, leukopenia, neutropenia, thrombocytopenia, eosinophilia, retinal and petechial hemorrhages, vaginal bleeding, epistaxis, and bleeding gums.

Hepatic: Hepatitis has been reported rarely.

Dermatologic: Acneiform or morbilliform skin rash that may progress to severe forms of erythema multiforme or to exfoliative dermatitis. Hair loss.

CNS/Neurologic: A myasthenia gravis-like syndrome has been reported. Precipitation of tonic-clonic (grand mal) seizures, vertigo, personality changes, increased irritability, drowsiness, headache, parasthesias, fatigue, malaise, and insomnia.

◆ RATED THERAPEUTICALLY EQUIVALENT; ◇ THERAPEUTIC EQUIVALENCE UNCONFIRMED; ○ UNRATED

Drowsiness usually subsides with continued therapy. If it persists, a reduction in dosage is indicated.

Ophthalmologic: Diplopia, hemeralopia, and photophobia.

Cardiovascular: Changes in blood pressure.

Gastrointestinal: Vomiting, abdominal pain, gastric distress, nausea, anorexia, weight loss, and hiccups.

Other: Lupus erythematosus, and lymphadenopathies simulating malignant lymphoma, have been reported. Pruritus associated with lymphadenopathy and hepatosplenomegaly has occurred in hypersensitive individuals.

OVERDOSAGE
Symptoms of acute Paramethadione overdosage include drowsiness, nausea, dizziness, ataxia, visual disturbances. Coma may follow massive overdosage.

Gastric evacuation, either by induced emesis, or by lavage, or both, should be done immediately. General supportive care, including frequent monitoring of the vital signs and close observation of the patient, are required.

It has been reported that alkalinization of the urine may be expected to increase the excretion of the N-demethylated metabolite of Paramethadione.

A blood count and a careful evaluation of hepatic and renal function should be done following recovery.

DOSAGE AND ADMINISTRATION
Paramethadione is administered orally.

Usual Adult Dosage: 0.9-2.4 g daily in 3 or 4 equally divided doses (i.e., 300-600 mg 3 or 4 times daily).

Initially, give 0.9 g daily; increase this dose by 300 mg at weekly intervals until therapeutic results are seen or until toxic symptoms appear.

Maintenance dosage should be the least amount of drug required to maintain control.

Children's Dosage: Usually 0.3-0.9 g daily in 3 or 4 equally divided doses.

Recommended Storage: 59°-77°F (15°-25°C).

HOW SUPPLIED
CAPSULE: 150 MG

BRAND/MANUFACTURER	NDC	SIZE	AWP
BRAND			
PARADIONE: Abbott Pharm	00074-3976-01	100s	$41.06

CAPSULE: 300 MG

BRAND/MANUFACTURER	NDC	SIZE	AWP
BRAND			
PARADIONE: Abbott Pharm	00074-3838-01	100s	$74.20

Paraplatin SEE CARBOPLATIN

Parathar SEE TERIPARATIDE ACETATE

Paregoric

DESCRIPTION
Each 5 mL (one teaspoonful) contains:

Anhydrous Morphine (from Opium) ....2 mg
WARNING: May be habit forming.

CLINICAL PHARMACOLOGY
Morphine produces its major effects on the central nervous system (CNS) and on the bowel.

INDICATIONS AND USAGE
Paregoric is useful for the treatment of diarrhea.

CONTRAINDICATIONS
Hypersensitivity to Morphine. Because of its stimulating effect on the spinal cord, Morphine should not be used in convulsive states, such as those occurring in status epilepticus, tetanus, and strychnine poisoning.

This preparation should not be used in diarrhea caused by poisoning until the toxic material is eliminated from the gastrointestinal tract.

PRECAUTIONS
General: Head Injury and Increased Intracranial Pressure—The respiratory depressant effects of narcotics and their capacity to elevate cerebrospinal-fluid pressure may be markedly exaggerated in the presence of head injury, other intracranial lesions, or a preexisting increase in intracranial pressure. Furthermore, narcotics produce additional effects that may obscure the clinical course in patients with head injuries.

Acute Abdominal Conditions: The administration of Morphine or other narcotics may obscure the diagnosis or clinical course in patients with acute abdominal conditions.

Special-Risk Patients: Morphine should be given with caution to certain patients, such as the elderly or debilitated and those with severe impairment of hepatic or renal function, hypothyroidism, Addison's disease, and prostatic hypertrophy or urethral stricture.

Morphine should be used with extreme caution in patients with disorders characterized by hypoxia, since even usual therapeutic doses of narcotics may decrease respiratory drive to the point of apnea while simultaneously increasing airway resistance.

Hypotensive Effect: The administration of Morphine may result in severe hypotension in the postoperative patient or any individual whose ability to maintain blood pressure has been compromised by a depleted blood volume or the administration of such drugs as the phenothiazines or certain anesthetics.

Supraventricular Tachycardias: Because of a possible vagolytic action that may produce a significant increase in the ventricular response rate, Morphine should be used with caution in patients with atrial flutter and other supraventricular tachycardias.

Convulsions: Morphine may aggravate preexisting convulsions in patients with convulsive disorders. If dosage is escalated substantially above recommended levels because of tolerance development, convulsions may occur in individuals without a history of convulsive disorders.

Information for Patients: Morphine may impair the mental and/or physical abilities required for the performance of potentially hazardous tasks, such as driving a car or operating machinery.

Drug Interactions: Morphine in combination with other narcotic analgesics, general anesthetics, phenothiazines, tranquilizers, sedative/hypnotics or other CNS depressants (including alcohol) has additive depressant effects, and the patient should be so advised. When such combination therapy is contemplated, the dosage of one or both agents should be reduced.

Carcinogenesis, Mutagenesis, Impairment of Fertility: Paregoric has no known carcinogenic or mutagenic potential. However no long-term animal studies are available to support this observation.

Usage in Pregnancy: Pregnancy Category C — Animal reproduction studies have not been conducted with Morphine. It is not known whether Morphine can cause fetal harm when administered to a pregnant woman or can affect reproduction capacity. Paregoric should be given to a pregnant woman only if clearly needed.

Nursing Mothers: Morphine appears in the milk of nursing mothers. Caution should be exercised when Paregoric is administered to a nursing woman.

ADVERSE REACTIONS
The most frequent adverse reactions include light-headedness, dizziness, sedation, nausea, and vomiting. These effects seem to be more prominent in ambulatory than in non-ambulatory patients, and some of these adverse reactions may be alleviated if the patient lies down.

Other adverse reactions include euphoria, dysphoria, constipation, and pruritus.

DRUG ABUSE AND DEPENDENCE
Controlled Substance: Paregoric is a Schedule III narcotic.

Dependence: Morphine can produce drug dependence and therefore has the potential for being abused. Patients receiving therapeutic dosage regimens of 10 mg every 4 hours for 1 to 2 weeks have exhibited mild withdrawal symptoms. Development of the dependent state is recognizable by an increased tolerance to the analgesic effect and the appearance of purposive phenomena (complaints, pleas, demands, or manipulative actions) shortly before the time of the next scheduled dose. A patient in withdrawal should be treated in a hospital environment. Usually, it is necessary only to provide supportive care with administration of a tranquilizer to suppress anxiety. Severe symptoms of withdrawal may require administration of a replacement narcotic.

OVERDOSAGE
Signs and Symptoms: Serious overdosage of Morphine is characterized by respiratory depression (a decrease in respiratory rate and/or tidal volume, Cheyne-Stokes respiration, cyanosis), extreme somnolence progressing to stupor or coma, skeletal muscle flaccidity, cold and clammy skin and sometimes bradycardia and hypotension. In severe overdosage apnea, circulatory collapse, cardiac arrest and death may occur.

Treatment: Primary attention should be given to the reestablishment of adequate respiratory exchange through provision of a patent airway and institution of assisted or controlled ventilation. The narcotic antagonist naloxone hydrochloride is a specific antidote against the respiratory depression that may result from overdosage or unusual sensitivity to narcotics. Therefore, an appropriate dose of the antagonist should be administered, preferably by the intravenous route, simultaneously with efforts at respiratory resuscitation. Since the duration of action of Morphine may exceed that of the antagonist, the patient should be kept under continued surveillance and repeated doses of the antagonist should be administered as needed to maintain adequate respiration.

Oxygen, intravenous fluids, vasopressors and other supportive measures should be employed as indicated.

DOSAGE AND ADMINISTRATION

Usual Pediatric Dosage: 0.25 to 0.5 mL/kg of body weight 1 to 4 times a day.

Usual Adult Dosage: 5 to 10 mL (1 to 2 teaspoonfuls) 1 to 4 times a day.

Storage: Store at controlled room temperature 15°-30°C (59°-86°F). Protect from light.

NOTE: This product may deposit a sediment if exposed to low temperatures. Filter if necessary.

Dispense in a tight, light-resistant container as defined in the USP.

HOW SUPPLIED
LIQUID (C-III):

AVERAGE UNIT PRICE (AVAILABLE SIZES)			
GENERIC			$0.01
BRAND/MANUFACTURER	NDC	SIZE	AWP
◆ GENERICS			
Cenci,H.R.	00556-0257-16	480 ml	$7.30
Cenci,H.R.	00556-0257-28	3840 ml	$35.90

Paremyd *SEE* HYDROXYAMPHETAMINE HYDROBROMIDE
WITH
TROPICAMIDE

Parlodel *SEE* BROMOCRIPTINE MESYLATE

Parnate *SEE* TRANYLCYPROMINE SULFATE

Paromomycin Sulfate

DESCRIPTION

Paromomycin Sulfate is a broad spectrum antibiotic produced by *Streptomyces rimosus* var. *paromomycinus*. It is a white, amorphous, stable, water-soluble product supplied as capsules containing the equivalent of 250 mg Paromomycin.

Following is its chemical structure:

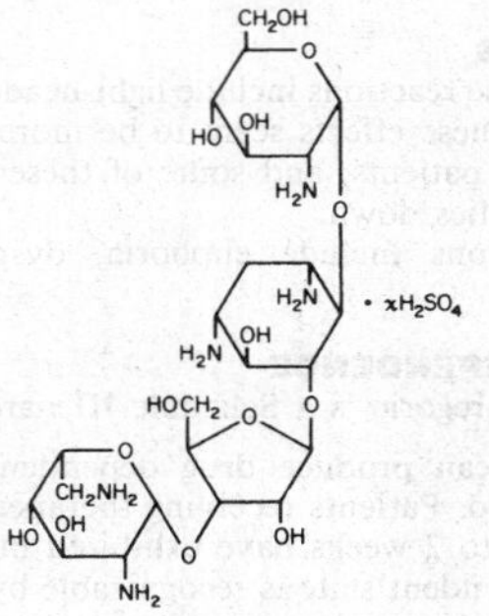

ACTION

The *in vitro* and *in vivo* antibacterial action of Paromomycin closely parallels that of neomycin. It is poorly absorbed after oral administration, with almost 100% of the drug recoverable in the stool.

INDICATIONS

Paromomycin Sulfate is indicated for intestinal amebiasis: acute and chronic.

Note: It is not effective in extraintestinal amebiasis); management of hepatic coma: as adjunctive therapy.

UNLABELED USES

Paromomycin Sulfate is used alone or as an adjunct in the treatment of infectious diarrhea, Leishmaniasis, and Giardiasis. Paromomycin Sulfate is also used in the treatment of tapeworm infections secondary to Hymenolepis nana, Taenia Saginata, and Diphyllobothrium latum infections.

CONTRAINDICATIONS

Paromomycin Sulfate is contraindicated in individuals with a history of previous hypersensitivity reactions to it. It is also contraindicated in intestinal obstruction.

PRECAUTIONS

The use of this antibiotic, as with other antibiotics, may result in an overgrowth of nonsusceptible organisms, including fungi. Constant observation of the patient is essential. If new infections caused by nonsusceptible organisms appear during therapy, appropriate measures should be taken.

The drug should be used with caution in individuals with ulcerative lesions of the bowel to avoid renal toxicity through inadvertent absorption.

ADVERSE REACTIONS

Nausea, abdominal cramps, and diarrhea have been reported in patients on doses over 3 g daily.

DOSAGE AND ADMINISTRATION

Intestinal amebiasis: Adults and Children: Usual dose—25 to 35 mg/kg body weight daily, administered in three doses with meals, for five to ten days.

Management of Hepatic Coma: Adults: Usual dose—4 g daily in divided doses, given at regular intervals for five to six days.

Store at controlled room temperature, 15°-30°C (59°-86°F).

Protect from moisture.

HOW SUPPLIED
CAPSULE: 250 MG

BRAND/MANUFACTURER	NDC	SIZE	AWP
○ BRAND			
HUMATIN: Parke-Davis	00071-0529-24	100s	$188.45

Paroxetine Hydrochloride

DESCRIPTION

Paroxetine Hydrochloride is an orally administered antidepressant with a chemical structure unrelated to other selective serotonin reuptake inhibitors or to tricyclic, tetracyclic or other available antidepressant agents. It is the hydrochloride salt of a phenylpiperidine compound identified chemically as (-)- *trans-4-R-*(4'-fluorophenyl)-3 *S*-[(3',4'- methylenedioxyphenoxy) methyl] piperidine hydrochloride hemihydrate and has the empirical formula of $C_{19}H_{20}FNO_3 \cdot HCl \cdot \frac{1}{2}H_2O$. The molecular weight is 374.8 (329.4 as free base).

Paroxetine Hydrochloride is an odorless, off-white powder, having a melting point range of 120° to 138°C and a solubility of 5.4 mg/mL in water.

Following is its chemical structure:

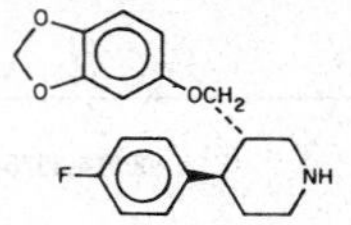

CLINICAL PHARMACOLOGY
PHARMACODYNAMICS

The antidepressant action of Paroxetine HCl is presumed to be linked to potentiation of serotonergic activity in the central nervous system resulting from inhibition of neuronal reuptake of serotonin (5-hydroxy-tryptamine, 5-HT). Studies at clinically relevant doses in humans have demonstrated that Paroxetine blocks the uptake of serotonin into human platelets. *In vitro* studies in animals also suggest that Paroxetine is a potent and highly selective inhibitor of neuronal serotonin reuptake and has only very weak effects on norepinephrine and dopamine neuronal reuptake. *In vitro* radioligand binding studies indicate that Paroxetine HCl has little affinity for muscarinic, alpha$_1$-, alpha$_2$-, beta-adrenergic-, dopamine (D$_2$)-, 5-HT$_1$-, 5-HT$_2$- and histamine (H$_1$)-receptors; antagonism of muscarinic, histaminergic and alpha$_1$-adrenergic receptors has been associated with various anticholinergic, sedative and cardiovascular effects for other psychotropic drugs. Because the relative potencies of Paroxetine HCl's major metabolites are at most 1/50 of the parent compound, they are essentially inactive.

PHARMACOKINETICS

Paroxetine Hydrochloride is completely absorbed after oral dosing of a solution of the Hydrochloride salt. In a study in which normal male subjects (n = 15) received 30 mg tablets daily for 30 days, steady-state Paroxetine HCl concentrations were achieved by approximately 10 days for most subjects, although it may take substantially longer in an occasional patient. At steady state, mean values of C_{max}, T_{max}, C_{min} and $T_{\frac{1}{2}}$ were 61.7 ng/mL (CV 45%), 5.2 hr. (CV 10%), 30.7 ng/mL (CV 67%) and 21.0 hr. (CV 32%), respectively.

The steady-state C_{max} and C_{min} values were about 6 and 14 times what would be predicted from single-dose studies. Steady-state drug exposure based on AUC_{0-24} was about 8 times greater than would have been predicted from single-dose data in these subjects. The excess accumulation is a consequence of the fact that one of the enzymes that metabolizes Paroxetine HCl is readily saturable.

In steady-state dose proportionality studies involving elderly and nonelderly patients, at doses of 20 to 40 mg daily for the elderly and 20 to 50 mg daily for the nonelderly, some nonlinerity was observed in both populations, again reflecting a saturable metabolic pathway. In comparison to C_{min} values after 20 mg daily, values after 40 mg daily were only about 2 to 3 times greater than doubled.

Paroxetine HCl is extensively metabolized after oral administration. The principal metabolites are polar and conjugated products of oxidation and methylation, which are readily cleared. Conjugates with glucuronic acid and sulfate predominate, and major metabolites have been isolated and identified. Data indicate that the metabolites have no more than 1/50 the potency of the parent compound at inhibiting serotonin uptake. The metabolism of Paroxetine HCl is accomplished in part by cytochrome $P_{450}IID_6$. Saturation of this enzyme

---

at clinical doses appears to account for the nonlinearity of Paroxetine HCl kinetics with increasing dose and increasing duration of treatment. The role of this enzyme in Paroxetine metabolism also suggests potential drug-drug interactions (see *"Precautions"*).

Approximately 64% of a 30 mg oral solution dose of Paroxetine was excreted in the urine with 2% as the parent compound and 62% as metabolites over a 10-day post-dosing period. About 36% was excreted in the feces (probably via the bile), mostly as metabolites and less than 1% as the parent compound over the 10-day post-dosing period.

Distribution: Paroxetine HCl distributes throughout the body, including the CNS, with only 1% remaining in the plasma.

Protein Binding: Approximately 95% and 93% of Paroxetine HCl is bound to plasma protein at 100 ng/mL and 400 ng/mL, respectively. Under clinical conditions, Paroxetine HCl concentrations would normally be less than 400 ng/mL. Paroxetine HCl does not alter the *in vitro* protein binding of phenytoin or warfarin.

Renal and Liver Disease: Increased plasma concentrations of Paroxetine HCl occur in subjects with renal and hepatic impairment. The mean plasma concentrations in patients with creatinine clearance below 30 mL/min was approximately 4 times greater than seen in normal volunteers. Patients with creatinine clearance of 30 to 60 mL/min and patients with hepatic functional impairment had about a 2-fold increase in plasma concentrations (AUC, C_{max}).

The initial dosage should therefore be reduced in patients with severe renal or hepatic impairment, and upward titration, if necessary, should be at increased intervals (see *"Dosage and Administration"*).

Elderly Patients: In a multiple-dose study in the elderly at daily Paroxetine HCl doses of 20, 30 and 40 mg, C_{min} concentrations were about 70% to 80% greater than the respective C_{min} concentrations in nonelderly subjects. Therefore the initial dosage in the elderly should be reduced. (See *"Dosage and Administration"*.)

CLINICAL TRIALS

The efficacy of Paroxetine HCl as a treatment for depression has been established in 6 placebo-controlled studies of patients with depression (ages 18 to 73). In these studies Paroxetine HCl was shown to be significantly more effective than placebo in treating depression by at least 2 of the following measures: Hamilton Depression Rating Scale (HDRS), the Hamilton depressed mood item, and the Clinical Global Impression (CGI)-Severity of Illness. Paroxetine HCl was significantly better than placebo in improvement of the HDRS sub-factor scores, including the depressed mood item, sleep disturbance factor and anxiety factor.

A study of depressed outpatients who had responded to Paroxetine HCl (HDRS total score < 8) during an initial 8-week open-treatment phase and were then randomized to continuation on Paroxetine HCl or placebo for 1 year demonstrated a significantly lower relapse rate for patients taking Paroxetine HCl (15%) compared to those on placebo (39%). Effectiveness was similar for male and female patients.

INDICATIONS AND USAGE

Paroxetine HCl is indicated for the treatment of depression.

The efficacy of Paroxetine HCl in the treatment of a major depressive episode was established in 6-week controlled trials of out-patients whose diagnoses corresponded most closely to the DSM-III category of major depressive disorder (see *"Clinical Pharmacology"*).

A major depressive episode implies a prominent and relatively persistent depressed or dysphoric mood that usually interferes with daily functioning (nearly every day for at least 2 weeks); it should include at least 4 of the following 8 symptoms; change in appetite, change in sleep, psychomotor agitation or retardation, loss of interest in usual activities or decrease in sexual drive, increased fatigue, feelings of guilt or worthlessness, slowed thinking or impaired concentration, and a suicide attempt or suicidal ideation.

The antidepressant action of Paroxetine HCl in hospitalized depressed patients has not been adequately studied.

The efficacy of Paroxetine HCl in maintaining an antidepressant response for up to 1 year was demonstrated in a placebo-controlled trial (see *"Clinical Pharmacology"*). Nevertheless, the physician who elects to use Paroxetine HCl for extended periods should periodically re-evaluate the long-term usefulness of the drug for the individual patient.

UNLABELED USES

Paroxetine Hydrochloride is used alone or as an adjunct in the treatment of diabetic neuropathy and chronic tension headache.

CONTRAINDICATIONS

Concomitant use in patients taking monoamine oxidase inhibitors (MAOIs) is contraindicated (see *"Warnings"*).

WARNINGS

Potential for Interaction with Monoamine Oxidase Inhibitors:

In patients receiving another serotonin reuptake inhibitor drug in combination with a monoamine oxidase inhibitor (MAOI), there have been reports of serious, sometimes fatal, reactions including hyperthermia, rigidity, myoclonus, autonomic instability with possible rapid fluctuations of vital signs, and mental status changes that include extreme agitation progressing to delirium and coma. These reactions have also been reported in patients who have recently discontinued that drug and have been started on a MAOI. Some cases presented with features resembling neuroleptic malignant syndrome. While there are no human data showing such an interaction with Paroxetine HCl limited animal data on the effects of combined use of paroxetine

and MAOIs suggest that these drugs may act synergistically to elevate blood pressure and evoke behavioral excitation. Therefore, it is recommended that Paroxetine HCl not be used in combination with a MAOI, or within 14 days of discontinuing treatment with a MAOI. At least 2 weeks should be allowed after stopping Paroxetine HCl before starting a MAOI.

PRECAUTIONS

GENERAL

Activation of Mania/Hypomania: During premarketing testing, hypomania or mania occurred in approximately 1.0% of Paroxetine HCl treated unipolar patients compared to 1.1% of active-control and 0.3% of placebo-treated unipolar patients. In a subset of patients classified as bipolar, the rate of manic episodes was 2.2% for Paroxetine HCl and 11.6% for the combined active-control groups. As with all antidepressants, Paroxetine HCl should be used cautiously in patients with a history of mania.

Seizures: During premarketing testing, seizures occurred in 0.1% of Paroxetine HCl treated patients, a rate similar to that associated with other antidepressants. Paroxetine HCl should be used cautiously in patients with a history of seizures. It should be discontinued in any patient who develops seizures.

Suicide: The possibility of a suicide attempt is inherent in depression and may persist until significant remission occurs. Close supervision of high-risk patients should accompany initial drug therapy. Prescriptions for Paroxetine HCl should be written for the smallest quantity of tablets consistent with good patient management, in order to reduce the risk of overdose.

Hyponatremia: Several cases of hyponatremia have been reported. The hyponatremia appeared to be reversible when Paroxetine HCl was discontinued. The majority of these occurrences have been in elderly individuals, some in patients taking diuretics or who were otherwise volume depleted.

Use in Patients with Concomitant Illness: Clinical experience with Paroxetine HCl in patients with certain concomitant systemic illness is limited. Caution is advisable in using Paroxetine HCl in patients with diseases or conditions that could affect metabolism or hemodynamic responses.

Paroxetine HCl has not been evaluated or used to any appreciable extent in patients with a recent history of myocardial infarction or unstable heart disease. Patients with these diagnoses were excluded from clinical studies during the product's premarket testing. Evaluation of electrocardiograms of 682 patients who received Paroxetine HCl in double-blind, placebo-controlled trials, however, did not indicate that Paroxetine HCl is associated with the development of significant ECG abnormalities. Similarly, Paroxetine HCl does not cause any clinically important changes in heart rate or blood pressure.

Increased plasma concentrations of paroxetine occur in patients with severe renal impairment (creatinine clearance < 30 mL/min.) or severe hepatic impairment. A lower starting dose should be used in such patients (see *"Dosage and Administration"*).

INFORMATION FOR PATIENTS

Physicians are advised to discuss the following issues with patients for whom they prescribe Paroxetine HCl.

Interference with Cognitive and Motor Performance: Any psychoactive drug may impair judgment, thinking or motor skills. Although in controlled studies Paroxetine HCl has not been shown to impair psychomotor performance, patients should be cautioned about operating hazardous machinery, including automobiles, until they are reasonably certain that Paroxetine HCl therapy does not affect their ability to engage in such activities.

Completing Course of Therapy: While patients may notice improvement with Paroxetine HCl therapy in 1 to 4 weeks, they should be advised to continue therapy as directed.

Concomitant Medication: Patients should be advised to inform their physician if they are taking, or plan to take, any prescription or over-the-counter drugs, since there is a potential for interactions.

Alcohol: Although Paroxetine HCl has not been shown to increase the impairment of mental and motor skills caused by alcohol, patients should be advised to avoid alcohol while taking Paroxetine HCl.

Pregnancy: Patients should be advised to notify their physician if they become pregnant or intend to become pregnant during therapy.

Nursing: Patients should be advised to notify their physician if they are breast-feeding an infant. (See *"Precautions—Nursing Mothers"*).

LABORATORY TESTS

There are no specific laboratory tests recommended.

DRUG INTERACTIONS

Tryptophan: As with other serotonin reuptake inhibitors, an interaction between Paroxetine HCl and tryptophan may occur when they are co-administered. Adverse experiences, consisting primarily of headache, nausea, sweating and dizziness, have been reported when tryptophan was administered to patients taking Paroxetine HCl. Consequently, concomitant use of Paroxetine HCl with tryptophan is not recommended.

Monoamine Oxidase Inhibitors: See *"Contraindications"* and *"Warnings"*.

Warfarin: Preliminary data suggest that there may be a pharmacodynamic interaction (that causes an increased bleeding diathesis in the face of unaltered prothrombin time) between Paroxetine HCl and warfarin. Since there is little clinical experience, the concomitant administration of Paroxetine HCl and warfarin should be undertaken with caution.

Drugs Affecting Hepatic Metabolism: The metabolism and pharmacokinetics of Paroxetine HCl may be affected by the induction or inhibition of drug-metabolizing enzymes.

Cimetidine: Cimetidine inhibits many cytochrome P_{450} (oxidative) enzymes. In a study where Paroxetine HCl (30 mg q.d.) was dosed orally for 4 weeks, steady-state plasma concentrations of paroxetine were increased by approximately 50% during co-administration with oral cimetidine (300 mg t.i.d.) for the final week. Therefore, when these drugs are administered concurrently, dosage adjustment of Paroxetine HCl after the 20 mg starting dose should be guided by clinical effect. The effect of Paroxetine HCl on cimetidine's pharmacokinetics was not studied.

Phenobarbital: Phenobarbital induces many cytochrome P_{450} (oxidative) enzymes. When a single oral 30 mg dose of Paroxetine HCl was administered at phenobarbital steady state (100 mg q.d. for 14 days), Paroxetine AUC and $T\frac{1}{2}$ were reduced (by an average of 25% and 38%, respectively) compared to Paroxetine HCl administered alone. The effect of Paroxetine HCl on phenobarbital pharmacokinetics was not studied. Since Paroxetine HCl exhibits nonlinear pharmacokinetics, the results of this study may not address the case where the 2 drugs are both being chronically dosed. No initial Paroxetine HCl dosage adjustment is considered necessary when co-administered with phenobarbital; any subsequent adjustment should be guided by clinical effect.

Phenytoin: When a single oral 30 mg dose of Paroxetine HCl was administered at phenytoin steady state (300 mg q.d. for 14 days), Paroxetine AUC and $T\frac{1}{2}$ were reduced (by an average of 50% and 35%, respectively) compared to Paroxetine HCl administered alone. In a separate study, when a single oral 300 mg dose of phenytoin was administered at Paroxetine steady state (30 mg q.d. for 14 days), phenytoin AUC was slightly reduced (12% on average) compared to phenytoin administered alone. Since both drugs exhibit nonlinear pharmacokinetics, the above studies may not address the case where the 2 drugs are both being chronically dosed. No initial dosage adjustments are considered necessary when these drugs are co-administered; any subsequent adjustments should be guided by clinical effect.

Drugs Metabolized by Cytochrome $P_{450}IID_6$: Concomitant use of Paroxetine HCl with drugs metabolized by cytochrome $P_{450}IID_6$ has not been formally studied but may require lower doses than usually prescribed for either Paroxetine HCl or the other drug. Many drugs, including most antidepressants (Paroxetine, other SSRIs and many tricyclics), are metabolized by the cytochrome P_{450} isozyme $P_{450}IID_6$. In most patients (> 90%), this $P_{450}IID_6$ isozyme is saturated early during Paroxetine HCl dosing. Like other agents that are metabolized by $P_{450}IID_6$, Paroxetine HCl may significantly inhibit the activity of this isozyme.

Therefore, co-administration of Paroxetine HCl with other drugs that are metabolized by this isozyme, including certain antidepressants (e.g., nortriptyline, amitriptyline, imipramine, desipramine and fluoxetine), phenothiazines (e.g., thioridazine) and Type 1C antiarrhythmics (e.g., propafenone, flecainide and encainide), or that inhibit this enzyme (e.g., quinidine), should be approached with caution.

At steady state, when the $P_{450}IID_6$ pathway is essentially saturated, Paroxetine HCl clearance is governed by alternative P_{450} isozymes which, unlike $P_{450}IID_6$, show no evidence of saturation.

Drugs Highly Bound to Plasma Protein: Because Paroxetine HCl is highly bound to plasma protein, administration of Paroxetine HCl to a patient taking another drug that is highly protein bound may cause increased free concentrations of the other drug, potentially resulting in adverse events. Conversely, adverse effects could result from displacement of Paroxetine HCl by other highly bound drugs.

Alcohol: Although Paroxetine HCl does not increase the impairment of mental and motor skills caused by alcohol, patients should be advised to avoid alcohol while taking Paroxetine HCl.

Lithium: A multiple-dose study has shown that there is no pharmacokinetic interaction between Paroxetine HCl and lithium carbonate. However, since there is little clinical experience, the concurrent administration of Paroxetine and lithium should be undertaken with caution.

Digoxin: The steady-state pharmacokinetics of Paroxetine was not altered when administered with digoxin at steady state. Mean digoxin AUC at steady state decreased by 15% in the presence of Paroxetine. Since there is little clinical experience, the concurrent administration of Paroxetine HCl and digoxin should be undertaken with caution.

Diazepam: Under steady-state conditions, diazepam does not appear to affect Paroxetine HCl kinetics. The effects of Paroxetine HCl on diazepam were not evaluated.

Procyclidine: Daily oral dosing of Paroxetine HCl (30 mg q.d.) increased steady-state $AUC_{0.24}$, C_{max} and C_{min} values of procyclidine (5 mg oral q.d.) by 35%, 37% and 67%, respectively, compared to procyclidine alone at steady state. If anticholinergic effects are seen, the dose of procyclidine should be reduced.

Propranolol: In a study where propranolol (80 mg b.i.d.) was dosed orally for 18 days, the established steady-state plasma concentrations of propranolol were unaltered during co-administration with Paroxetine HCl (30 mg q.d.) for the final 10 days. The effects of propranolol on Paroxetine HCl have not been evaluated.

Electroconvulsive Therapy (ECT): There are no clinical studies of the combined use of ECT and Paroxetine HCl.

CARCINOGENESIS, MUTAGENESIS, IMPAIRMENT OF FERTILITY

Carcinogenesis: Two-year carcinogenicity studies were conducted in mice and rats given Paroxetine HCl in the diet at 1, 5 and 25 mg/kg/day (mice) and 1, 5 and 20 mg/kg/day (rats). The maximum doses in these studies were approximately 25 (mouse) and 20 (rat) times the maximum dose recommended for human use on a mg/kg basis or 2.5 (mouse) and 5.8 (rat) times the maximum recommended human dose on a mg/m^2 basis. There was a significantly greater number of male rats in the high-dose group with reticulum cell sarcomas (1/100, 0/50, 0/50 and 4/50 for control, low-, middle- and high-dose groups, respectively) and a significantly increased linear trend across dose groups for the occurrence of lymphoreticular tumors in male rats. Female rats were not affected. Although there was a dose-related increae in the number of tumors in mice, there was no drug-related increase in the number of mice with tumors. The relevance of these findings to humans is unknown.

Mutagenesis: Paroxetine HCl produced no genotoxic effects in a battery of 5 *in vitro* and 2 *in vivo* assays that included the following: bacterial mutation assay, mouse lymphoma mutation assay, unscheduled DNA synthesis assay, and tests for cytogenetic aberrations *in vivo* in mouse bone marrow and *in vitro* in human lymphocytes and in a dominant lethal test in rats.

Impairment of Fertility: Serotonergic compounds are known to affect reproductive function in animals. Impaired reproductive function (i.e., reduced pregnancy rate, increased pre- and post-implantation losses, decreased viability of pups) was found in reproduction studies in rats at doses of Paroxetine which were 15 or more times the highest recommended human dose on 2 mg/kg basis, or 4.4 times on a mg/m^2 basis. Irreversible lesions occurred in the reproductive tract of male rats after dosing in toxicity studies for 2 to 52 weeks. These lesions, which consisted of vacuolation of epididymal tubular epithelium and atrophic changes in the seminiferous tubules of the testes with arrested spermatogenesis occurred at doses which were 25 times the highest recommended human dose on a mg/kg basis or 7.3 times on a mg/m^2 basis.

PREGNANCY

Teratogenic Effects—Pregnancy Category B: Reproduction studies performed in rats and rabbits at doses up to 50 and 6 times the maximum recommended human dose on a mg/kg basis or 10 and 2 times on a mg/m^2 basis, respectively, have revealed no evidence of teratogenic effects. There are no adequate and well-controlled studies in pregnant women. Because animal reproduction studies are not always predictive of human response, this drug should be used during pregnancy only if clearly needed.

LABOR AND DELIVERY

The effect of Paroxetine HCl on labor and delivery in humans is unknown.

NURSING MOTHERS

Like many other drugs, Paroxetine HCl is secreted in human milk, and caution should be exercised when Paroxetine HCl is administered to a nursing woman.

USAGE IN CHILDREN

Safety and effectiveness in children have not been established.

GERIATRIC USE

In worldwide Paroxetine HCl clinical trials, 17% of Paroxetine HCl treated patients (approximately 700) were 65 years of age or older Pharmacokinetic studies revealed a decreased clearance in the elderly, and a lower starting dose is recommended; there were, however, no overall differences in the adverse event profile between elderly and younger patients, and effectiveness was similar in younger and older patients. (See *"Clinical Pharmacology"* and *"Dosage and Administration"*).

ADVERSE REACTIONS

ASSOCIATED WITH DISCONTINUATION OF TREATMENT

Twenty-one percent (881/4,126) of Paroxetine HCl patients in worldwide clinical trials discontinued treatment due to an adverse event. The most common events ($\geq$ 1%) associated with discontinuation and considered to be drug related (i.e., those events associated with dropout at a rate approximately twice or greater for Paroxetine HCl compared to placebo) included:

CNS	
Somnolence	2.3%
Insomnia	1.9%
Agitation	1.3%
Tremor	1.3%
Anxiety	1.1%
Gastrointestinal	
Nausea	3.4%
Diarrhea	1.0%
Dry mouth	1.0%
Vomiting	1.0%
Other	
Asthenia	1.7%
Abnormal ejaculation	1.6%
Sweating	1.1%

INCIDENCE IN CONTROLLED TRIALS

Commonly Observed Adverse Events in Controlled Clinical Trials: The most commonly observed adverse events associated with the use of Paroxetine HCl (incidence of 5% or greater and incidence for Paroxetine HCl at least twice that for placebo, derived from 1% table below) were: asthenia, sweating, nausea, decreased appetite, somnolence, dizziness, insomnia, tremor, nervousness, ejaculatory disturbance and other male genital disorders.

Adverse Events Occurring at an Incidence of 1% or More Among Paroxetine HCl-Treated Patients: The table that follows enumerates adverse events that occurred at an incidence of 1% or more among Paroxetine HCl-treated patients who participated in short-term (6-week) placebo-controlled trials in which patients were dosed in a range of 20 to 50 mg/day. Reported adverse events were classified using a standard COSTART-based Dictionary terminology.

The prescriber should be aware that these figures cannot be used to predict the incidence of side effects in the course of usual medical practice where patient characteristics and other factors differ from those which prevailed in the clinical trials. Similarly, the cited frequencies cannot be compared with figures obtained from other clinical investigations involving different treatments, uses and investigators. The cited figures, however, do provide the prescribing physician with some basis for estimating the relative contribution of drug and nondrug factors to the side effect incidence rate in the population studied.

Table 1.
TREATMENT-EMERGENT ADVERSE EXPERIENCE INCIDENCE IN PLACEBO-CONTROLLED CLINICAL TRIALS[1]

Body System	Preferred Term	Paroxetine HCl (n = 421)	Placebo (n = 421)
Body as a Whole	Headache	17.6%	17.3%
	Asthenia	15.0%	5.9%
	Abdominal Pain	3.1%	4.0%
	Fever	1.7%	1.7%
	Chest Pain	1.4%	2.1%
	Trauma	1.4%	0.5%
	Back Pain	1.2%	2.4%
Cardiovascular	Palpitation	2.9%	1.4%
	Vasodilation	2.6%	0.7%
	Postural Hypotension	1.2%	0.5%
Dermatologic	Sweating	11.2%	2.4%
	Rash	1.7%	0.7%
Gastrointestinal	Nausea	25.7%	9.3%
	Dry Mouth	18.1%	12.1%
	Constipation	13.8%	8.6%
	Diarrhea	11.6%	7.6%
	Decreased Appetite	6.4%	1.9%
	Flatulence	4.0%	1.7%
	Vomiting	2.4%	1.7%
	Oropharynx Disorder[2]	2.1%	0.0%
	Dyspepsia	1.9%	1.0%
	Increased Appetite	1.4%	0.5%
Musculoskeletal	Myopathy	2.4%	1.4%
	Myalgia	1.7%	0.7%
	Myasthenia	1.4%	0.2%
Nervous System	Somnolence	23.3%	9.0%
	Dizziness	13.3%	5.5%
	Insomnia	13.3%	6.2%
	Tremor	8.3%	1.9%
	Nervousness	5.2%	2.6%
	Anxiety	5.0%	2.9%
	Parethesia	3.8%	1.7%
	Libido Decreased	3.3%	0.0%
	Agitation	2.1%	1.9%
	Drugged Feeling	1.7%	0.7%
	Myoclonus	1.4%	0.7%
	CNS Stimulation	1.2%	3.6%
	Confusion	1.2%	0.2%
Respiration	Respiratory Disorder[3]	5.9%	6.4%
	Yawn	3.8%	0.0%
	Pharyngitis	2.1%	2.9%
Special Senses	Blurred Vision	3.6%	1.4%
	Taste Perversion	2.4%	0.2%
Urogenital System	Ejaculatory Disturbance[4,5]	12.9%	0.0%
	Other Male Genital Disorders[4,6]	10.0%	0.0%
	Urinary Frequency	3.1%	0.7%
	Urinary Disorder[7]	2.9%	0.2%
	Female Genital Disorders[4,8]	1.8%	0.0%

1. *Events reported by at least 1% of patients treated with Paroxetine HCl are included.*

2. *Includes mostly "lump in throat" and "tightness in throat."*
3. *Includes mostly "cold symptoms" or "URI."*
4. *Percentage corrected for gender.*
5. *Mostly "ejaculatory delay."*
6. *Includes "anorgasmia," "erectile difficulties", "delayed ejaculation/orgasm," and "sexual dysfunction," and "impotence."*
7. *Includes mostly "difficulty with micturition" and "urinary hesitancy."*
8. *Includes mostly "anorgasmia" and "difficulty reaching climax/organism."*

Dose Dependency of Adverse Events: A comparison of adverse event rates in a fixed-dose study comparing Paroxetine HCl 10, 20, 30 and 40 mg/day with placebo revealed a clear dose dependency for some of the more common adverse events associated with Paroxetine HCl use, as shown in the following table: (See related table).

Adaptation to Certain Adverse Events: Over a 4-to 6-week period, there was evidence of adaptation to some adverse events with continued therapy (e.g., nausea and dizziness), but less to other effects (e.g., dry mouth, somnolence and asthenia).

Weight and Vital Sign Changes: Significant weight loss may be an undesirable result of treatment with Paroxetine HCl for some patients but, on average, patients in controlled trials had minimal (about 1 pound) weight loss vs. smaller changes on placebo and active control. No significant changes in vital signs (systolic and diastolic blood pressure, pulse and temperature) were observed in patients treated with Paroxetine HCl in controlled clinical trials.

ECG Changes: In an analysis of ECGs obtained in 682 patients treated with Paroxetine HCl and 415 patients treated with placebo in controlled clinical trials, no clinically significant changes were seen in the ECGs of either group.

Liver Function Tests: In placebo-controlled clinical trials, patients treated with Paroxetine HCl exhibited abnormal values on liver function tests at no greater rate than that seen in placebo-treated patients. In particular, the Paroxetine HCl-vs.-placebo comparison for alkaline phosphatase was 0% vs. 0%, SGOT 0.3% vs. 0.3% SGPT 1% vs. 0.3% and bilirubin 0% vs. 0.8%.

OTHER EVENTS OBSERVED DURING THE PREMARKETING EVALUATION OF PAROXETINE HCL
During its premarketing assessment, multiple doses of Paroxetine HCl were administered to 4, 126 patients in phase 2 and 3 studies. The conditions and duration of exposure to Paroxetine HCl varied greatly and included (in overlapping categories) open and double-blind studies, uncontrolled and controlled studies, inpatient and outpatient studies, and fixed-dose and titration studies. Untoward events associated with this exposure were recorded by clinical investigators using terminology of their own choosing. Consequently, it is not possible to provide a meaningful estimate of the proportion of individuals experiencing adverse events without first grouping similar types of untoward events into a smaller number of standardized event categories.

In the tabulations that follow, reported adverse events were classified using a standard COSTART-based Dictionary terminology. The frequencies presented, therefore, represent the proportion of the 4,126 patients exposed to multiple doses of Paroxetine HCl who experienced an event of the type cited on at least one occasion while receiving Paroxetine HCl. All reported events are included except those already listed in Table 1, those reported in terms so general as to be uninformative and those events where a drug cause was remote. It is important to emphasize that although the events reported occurred during treatment with Paroxetine HCl, they were not necessarily caused by it.

Events are further categorized by body system and listed in order of decreasing frequency according to the following definitions: frequent adverse events are those occurring on one or more occasions in at least 1/100 patients (only those not already listed in the tabulated results from placebo-controlled trials appear in this listing); infrequent adverse events are those occurring in 1/100 to 1/1000 patients; rare events are those occurring in fewer than 1/1000 patients. Events of major clinical importance are also described in the *"Precautions"* section.

Body as a Whole: frequent: chills, malaise; *infrequent:* allergic reaction, carcinoma, face edema, moniliasis, neck pain; *rare:* abscess, adrenergic syndrome, cellulitis, neck rigidity, pelvic pain, peritonitis, ulcer.

Cardiovascular System: frequent: hypertension, syncope, tachycardia; *infrequent:* bradycardia, conduction abnormalities, electrocardiogram abnormal, hypotension, migraine, peripheral vascular disorder; *rare:* angina pectoris, arrhythmia, atrial fibrillation, bundle branch block, cerebral ischemia, cerebrovascular accident, congestive heart failure, low cardiac output, myocardial infarct, myocardial ischemia, pallor, phlebitis, pulmonary embolus, supraventricular extrasystoles, thrombosis, varicose vein, vascular headache, ventricular extrasystoles.

Digestive System: infrequent: bruxism, dysphagia, eructation, gastritis, glossitis, increased salivation, liver function tests abnormal, mouth ulceration, rectal hemorrhage: *rare:* aphthous stomatitis, bloody diarrhea, bulimia, colitis, duodenitis, esophagitis, fecal impactions, fecal incontinence, gastritis, gastroenteritis, gingivitis, hematemesis, hepatitis, ileus, jaundice, melena, peptic ulcer, salivary gland enlargement, stomach ulcer, stomatitis, tongue edema, tooth caries.

Endocrine System: rare: diabetes mellitus, hyperthyroidism, hypothyroidism, thyroiditis.

Hemic and Lymphatic Systems: infrequent: anemia, leukopenia, lymphadenopathy, purpura: *rare:* abnormal erythrocytes, eosinophilia, leukocytosis, lymphedema, abnormal lymphocytes, lymphocytosis, microcytic anemia, monocytosis, normocytic anemia.

Metabolic and Nutritional: frequent: edema, weight gain, weight loss: *infrequent*: hyperglycemia, peripheral edema, thirst; *rare*: alkaline phosphatase increased, bilirubinemia, dehydration, gout, hypercholesteremia, hypocalcemia, hypoglycemia, hypokalemia, hyponatremia, SGOT increased, SGPT increased.

Musculoskeletal System: infrequent: arthralgia, arthritis; *rare*: arthrosis, bursitis, myositis, osteoporosis, tetany.

Nervous System: frequent: amnesia, CNS stimulation, concentration impaired, depression, emotional lability, vertigo; *infrequent*: abnormal thinking, akinesia, alcohol abuse, ataxia, convulsion, depersonalization, hallucinations, hyperkinesia, hypertonia, incoordination, lack of emotion, manic reaction, paranoid reaction; *rare*: abnormal electroencephalogram, abnormal gait, antisocial reaction, choreoathetosis, delirium, delusions, diplopia, drug dependence, dysarthria, dyskinesia, dystonia, euophoria, fasciculations, grand mal convulsion, hostility, hyperalgesia, hypokinesia, hysteria, libido increased, manic-depressive reaction, meningitis, myelitis, neuralgia, neuropathy, nystagmus, paralysis, psychosis, psychotic depression, reflexes increased, stupor, withdrawal syndrome.

Respiratory System: frequent: cough increased, rhinitis; *infrequent*: asthma, bronchitis, dyspnea, epistaxis, hyperventilation, pneumonia, respiratory flu, sinusitis; *rare*: carcinoma of lung, hiccups, lung fibrosis, sputum increased.

Skin and Appendages: frequent: pruritus; *infrequent*: acne, alopecia, dry skin, ecchymosis, eczema, furunculosis, urticaria: *rare*: angioedema, contact dermatitis, erythema nodosum, maculopapular rash, photosensitivity, skin discoloration, skin melanoma.

Special Senses: infrequent: abnormality of accommodation, ear pain, eye pain, mydriasis, otitis media, taste loss, tinnitus; *rare*: amblyopia, cataract, conjunctivitis, corneal ulcer, exophthalmos, eye hemorrhage, glaucoma, hyperacusis, otitis externa, photophobia.

Urogenital System: infrequent: abortion, amenorrhea, breast pain, cystitis, dysmenorrhea, dysuria, menorrhagia, nocturia, polyuria, urethritis, urinary incontinence, urinary retention, urinary urgency, vaginitis: *rare*: breast atrophy, breast carcinoma, breast neoplasm, female lactation, hematuria, kidney calculus, kidney function abnormal, kidney pain, mastitis, nephritis, oliguria, prostatic carcinoma, vaginal moniliasis.

NON-U.S. POSTMARKETING REPORTS

Voluntary reports of adverse events in patients taking *Paxil* that have been received since market introduction and may have no causal relationship with the drug include elevated liver function tests (the most severe case was a death due to liver necrosis, and one other case involved grossly elevated transaminases associated with severe liver dysfunction).

DRUG ABUSE AND DEPENDENCE

Controlled Substance Class: Paroxetine HCl is not a controlled substance.

Physical and Psychologic Dependence: Paroxetine HCl has not been systematically studied in animals or humans for its potential for abuse, tolerance or physical dependence. While the clinical trials did not reveal any tendency for any drug-seeking behavior, these observations were not systematic and it is not possible to predict on the basis of this limited experience the extent to which a CNS-active drug will be misused, diverted and/or abused once marketed. Consequently, patients should be evaluated carefully for history of drug abuse, and such patients should be observed closely for signs of Paroxetine HCl misuse or abuse (e.g., development of tolerance, incrementations of dose, drug-seeking behavior).

OVERDOSAGE

Human Experience: No deaths were reported following acute overdose with Paroxetine HCl alone or in combination with other drugs and/or alcohol (18 cases, with doses up to 850 mg) during premarketing clinical trials. Signs and symptoms of overdose with Paroxetine HCl included: nausea, vomiting, drowsiness, sinus tachycardia and dilated pupils. There were no reports of ECG abnormalities, coma or convulsions following overdosage with Paroxetine HCl alone.

Overdosage Management: Treatment should consist of those general measures employed in the management of overdosage with any antidepressant. There are no specific antidotes for Paroxetine HCl. Establish and maintain an airway, ensure adequate oxygenation and ventilation. Gastric evacuation either by the induction of emesis or lavage or both should be performed. In most cases, following evacuation, 20 to 30 grams of activated charcoal may be administered every 4 to 6 hours during the first 24 to 48 hours after ingestion. An ECG should be taken and monitoring of cardiac function instituted if there is any evidence of abnormality. Supportive care with frequent monitoring of vital signs and careful observation is indicated. Due to the large volume of distribution of Paroxetine HCl forced diuresis, dialysis, hemoperfusion and exchange transfusion are unlikely to be of benefit.

A specific caution involves patients taking or recently having taken paroxetine who might ingest by accident or intent excessive quantities of a tricyclic antidepressant. In such a case, accumulation of the parent tricyclic and its active metabolite may increase the possibility of clinically significant sequelae and extend the time needed for close medical observation.

In managing overdosage, consider the possibility of multiple-drug involvement. The physician should consider contacting a poison control center for additional information on the treatment of any overdose.

DOSAGE AND ADMINISTRATION

DEPRESSION

Usual Initial Dosage: Paroxetine HCl should be administered as a single daily dose, usually in the morning. The recommended initial dose is 20 mg/day. Patients were dosed in a range of 20 to 50 mg/day in the clinical trials demonstrating the antidepressant effectiveness of Paroxetine HCl. As with all antidepressants, the full antidepressant effect may be delayed. Some patients not responding to a 20 mg dose may benefit from dose increases, in 10 mg/day increments, up to a maximum of 50 mg/day. Dose changes should occur at intervals of at least 1 week.

Dosage for Elderly or Debilitated, and Patients with Severe Renal or Hepatic Impairment: The recommended initial dose is 10 mg/day for elderly, debilitated

Table 2.

TREATMENT-EMERGENT ADVERSE EXPERIENCE INCIDENCE IN A DOSE-COMPARISON TRIAL*

Body System/ Preferred Term	Placebo n = 51	Paroxetine HCl			
		10 mg n = 102	20 mg n = 104	30 mg n = 101	40 mg n = 102
Body as a Whole					
Asthenia	0.0%	2.9%	10.6%	13.9%	12.7%
Dermatology					
Sweating	2.0%	1.0%	6.7%	8.9%	11.8%
Gastrointestinal					
Constipation	5.9%	4.9%	7.7%	9.9%	12.7%
Decreased Appetite	2.0%	2.0%	5.8%	4.0%	4.9%
Diarrhea	7.8%	9.8%	19.2%	7.9%	14.7%
Dry Mouth	2.0%	10.8%	18.3%	15.8%	20.6%
Nausea	13.7%	14.7%	26.9%	34.7%	36.3%
Nervous System					
Anxiety	0.0%	2.0%	5.8%	5.9%	5.9%
Dizziness	3.9%	6.9%	6.7%	8.9%	12.7%
Nervousness	0.0%	5.9%	5.8%	4.0%	2.9%
Paresthesia	0.0%	2.0%	1.0%	5.0%	5.9%
Somnolence	7.8%	12.7%	18.3%	20.8%	21.6%
Tremor	0.0%	0.0%	7.7%	7.9%	14.7%
Special Senses					
Blurred Vision	2.0%	2.9%	2.9%	2.0%	7.8%
Urogenital					
Abnormal Ejaculation	0.0%	5.8%	6.5%	10.6%	13.0%
Impotence	0.0%	1.9%	4.3%	6.4%	1.9%
Male Genital Disorders	0.0%	3.8%	8.7%	6.4%	3.7%

* *Rule for including adverse events in table: incidence at least 5% for one of Paroxetine HCl groups and ≥ twice the placebo incidence for at least one paroxetine group.*

◆ RATED THERAPEUTICALLY EQUIVALENT; ◇ THERAPEUTIC EQUIVALENCE UNCONFIRMED; ○ UNRATED

patients, and/or patients with severe renal or hepatic impairment. Increases may be made if indicated. Dosage should not exceed 40 mg/day.

Maintenance Therapy: There is no body of evidence available to answer the question of how long the patient treated with Paroxetine HCl should remain on it. It is generally agreed that acute episodes of depression require several months or longer of sustained pharmacologic therapy. Whether the dose of an antidepressant needed to induce remission is identical to the dose needed to maintain and/or sustain euthymia is unknown.

Systematic evaluation of the efficacy of Paroxetine HCl has shown that efficacy is maintained for periods of up to 1 year with doses that averaged about 30 mg.

Switching Patients to or from a Monoamine Oxidase Inhibitor: At least 14 days should elapse between discontinuation of a MAOI and initiation of Paroxetine HCl therapy. Similarly at least 14 days should be allowed after stopping Paroxetine HCl before starting a MAOI.

Storage: Store at controlled room temperature (15° to 30° C; 59° to 86° F).

HOW SUPPLIED
TABLETS: 20 MG

BRAND/MANUFACTURER	NDC	SIZE	AWP
○ **BRAND**			
▶ PAXIL: SK Beecham Pharm	00029-3211-13	30s	$54.60
	00029-3211-20	100s	$181.90
	00029-3211-21	100s	$185.65

TABLETS: 30 MG

BRAND/MANUFACTURER	NDC	SIZE	AWP
○ **BRAND**			
▶ PAXIL: SK Beecham Pharm	00029-3212-13	30s	$56.20

Pavabid Plateau *SEE* PAPAVERINE HYDROCHLORIDE

Pavulon *SEE* PANCURONIUM BROMIDE

Paxil *SEE* PAROXETINE HYDROCHLORIDE

Paxipam *SEE* HALAZEPAM

PBZ *SEE* TRIPELENNAMINE HYDROCHLORIDE

PCE Dispertab *SEE* ERYTHROMYCIN, ORAL

Pedameth *SEE* RACEMETHIONINE

Pediacof *SEE* CHLORPHENIRAMINE MALEATE/CODEINE PHOSPHATE/PHENYLEPHRINE HYDROCHLORIDE/POTASSIUM IODIDE

Pediaflor *SEE* SODIUM FLUORIDE

Pediapred *SEE* PREDNISOLONE, SYSTEMIC

Pediazole *SEE* ERYTHROMYCIN ETHYLSUCCINATE WITH SULFISOXAZOLE ACETYL

Pedvax HIB *SEE* HAEMOPHILUS B CONJUGATE VACCINE *AND* HEMOPHILUS B CONJUGATE VACCINE (TETANUS TOXOID CONJUGATE)

Pegademase Bovine

DESCRIPTION
Pegademase Bovine Injection is a modified enzyme used for enzyme replacement therapy for the treatment of severe combined immunodeficiency disease (SCID) associated with a deficiency of adenosine deaminase.

Pegademase Bovine Injection is supplied in an isotonic, pyrogen-free, sterile solution, pH 7.2-7.4, for intramuscular injection only. The solution is clear and colorless.

The chemical name for Pegademase Bovine Injection is (monomethoxypolyethylene glycol succinimidyl)$_{11-17}$-adenosine deaminase. It is a conjugate of numerous strands of monomethoxypolyethylene glycol (PEG), molecular weight 5,000, covalently attached to the enzyme adenosine deaminase (ADA). ADA (adenosine deaminase EC 3.5.4.4) used in the manufacture of Pegademase Bovine Injection is derived from bovine intestine.

Each milliliter of Pegademase Bovine Injection contains 250 units of Pegademase Bovine. (One unit of activity is defined as the amount of ADA that converts 1 μM of adenosine to inosine per minute at 25°C and pH 7.3.)

Following is its chemical structure:

$$\left[CH_3(OCH_2CH_2)_x - O - CCH_2CH_2 - C - NH \right]_y - adenosine\ deaminase$$
$$\qquad\qquad\qquad\qquad\quad \overset{\|}{O} \qquad\qquad \overset{\|}{O}$$

x = 114 oxyethylene groups per PEG strand
y = 11-17 primary amino groups of lysine onto which succinyl PEG is attached

CLINICAL PHARMACOLOGY
SEVERE COMBINED IMMUNODEFICIENCY DISEASE ASSOCIATED WITH ADA DEFICIENCY
Severe combined immunodeficiency disease (SCID) associated with a deficiency of ADA is a rare, inherited, and often fatal disease. In the absence of the ADA enzyme, the purine substrates adenosine and 2'-deoxyadenosine accumulate, causing metabolic abnormalities that are directly toxic to lymphocytes.

The immune deficiency can be cured by bone marrow transplantation. When a suitable bone marrow donor is unavailable or when bone marrow transplantation fails, non-selective replacement of the ADA enzyme has been provided by periodic irradiated red blood cell transfusions. However, transmission of viral infections and iron overload are serious risks associated with irradiated red blood cell transfusions, and relatively few ADA deficient patients have benefitted from chronic transfusion therapy.

Pegademase Bovine Injection provides specific and direct replacement of the deficient enzyme, but will not benefit patients with immunodeficiency due to other causes. In patients with ADA deficiency, rigorous adherence to a schedule of Pegademase Bovine Injection administration can eliminate the toxic metabolites of ADA deficiency and result in improved immune function. It is imperative that treatment with Pegademase Bovine Injection be carefully monitored by measurement of the level of ADA activity in plasma. Monitoring of the level of deoxyadenosine triphosphate (dATP) in erythrocytes is also helpful in determining that the dose of Pegademase Bovine Injection is adequate.

ACTIONS
Pegademase Bovine Injection provides specific replacement of the deficient enzyme.

In the absence of the enzyme ADA, the purine substrates adenosine, 2'-deoxyadenosine and their metabolites are toxic to lymphocytes. The direct action of Pegademase Bovine Injection is the correction of these metabolic abnormalities. Improvement in immune function and diminished frequency of opportunistic infections compared with the natural history of combined immunodeficiency due to ADA deficiency only occurs after metabolic abnormalities are corrected. There is a lag between the correction of the metabolic abnormalities and improved immune function. This period of time is variable, and has been reported to be from a few weeks to as long as 6 months. In contrast to the natural history of combined immunodeficiency disease due to ADA deficiency, a trend toward diminished frequency of opportunistic infections and fewer complications of infections has occurred in patients receiving Pegademase Bovine Injection.

PHARMACOKINETICS
The pharmacokinetics and biochemical effects of Pegademase Bovine Injection have been studied in six children ranging in age from 6 weeks to 12 years with SCID associated with ADA deficiency.

After the intramuscular injection of Pegademase Bovine Injection, peak plasma levels of ADA activity were reached 2 to 3 days following administration. The plasma elimination half-life of ADA following the administration of Pegademase Bovine Injection was variable, even for the same child. The range was 3 to > 6 days. Following weekly injections of Pegademase Bovine Injection at 15 U/kg, the average trough level of ADA activity in plasma was between 20 and 25 μmol/hr/mL.

BIOCHEMICAL EFFECTS
The changes in red blood cell deoxyadenosine nucleotide (dATP) and S-adenosylhomocysteine hydrolase (SAHase) have been evaluated. In patients with ADA deficiency, inadequate elimination of 2'-deoxyadenosine caused a marked elevation in dATP and a decrease in SAHase level in red blood cells. Prior to treatment with Pegademase Bovine Injection, the levels of dATP in the red blood cells ranged from 0.056 to 0.899 μmol/mL of erythrocytes. After 2 months of

maintenance treatment with Pegademase Bovine Injection, the levels decreased to a range of 0.007 to 0.0015 µmol/mL. The normal value of dATP is below 0.001 µmol/mL. In the same period of time, the levels of SAHase increased from the pretreatment range of 0.09 to 0.22 nmol/hr/mg protein to a range of 2.37 to 5.16 nmol/hr/mg protein. The normal value for SAHase is 4.18 ± 1.9 nmol/hr/mg protein.

The optimal dosage and schedule of administration of Pegademase Bovine Injection should be established for each patient, based on monitoring of plasma ADA activity levels (trough levels before maintenance injection), biochemical markers of ADA deficiency (primarily red cell dATP content), and parameters of immune function. Since improvement in immune function follows correction of metabolic abnormalities, maintenance dosage in individual patients should be aimed at achieving the following biochemical goals: 1) maintain plasma ADA activity (trough levels) in the range of 15-35 µmol/hr/mL (assayed at 37°C); and 2) decline in erythrocytes dATP to ≤ 0.005-0.015 µmol/mL packed erythrocytes, or ≤ 1% of the total erythrocytes adenine nucleotide (ATP + dATP) content, with a normal ATP level, as measured in a pre-injection sample.

In vitro immunologic data (lymphocyte response to mitrogens and lymphocyte surface antigens) were obtained, but their clinical significance is unknown. Prior to treatment with Pegademase Bovine Injection, immune status was significantly below normal, as indicated by < 10% of normal mitogen responses and circulating mononuclear cells bearing T-cell surface antigens. These parameters improved, though not always to normal, within 2 to 6 months of therapy.

INDICATIONS AND USAGE

Pegademase Bovine Injection is indicated for enzyme replacement therapy for adenosine deaminase (ADA) deficiency in patients with severe combined immunodeficiency disease (SCID) who are not suitable candidates for—or who have failed—bone marrow transplantation. Pegademase Bovine Injection is recommended for use in infants from birth or in children of any age at the time of diagnosis. Pegademase Bovine Injection is not intended as a replacement for HLA indentical bone marrow transplant therapy. Pegademase Bovine Injection is also not intended to replace continued close medical supervision and the initiation of appropriate diagnostic tests and therapy (e.g., antibiotics, nutrition, oxygen, gammaglobulin) as indicated for intercurrent illnesses.

CONTRAINDICATIONS

There is no evidence to support the safety and efficacy of Pegademase Bovine Injection as preparatory or support therapy for bone marrow transplantation. Since Pegademase Bovine Injection is administered by intramuscular injection, it should be used with caution in patients with thrombocytopenia and should not be used if thrombocytopenia is severe.

PRECAUTIONS

WARNINGS

At present, testing prior to distribution may not assure the initial and continuing potency of each new lot of Pegademase Bovine Injection. Any laboratory or clinical indication of a decrease in potency of Pegademase Bovine Injection should be reported immediately by telephone to ENZON, Inc. Telephone 908-980-4500. Fax 908-980-5911.

GENERAL

There have been no reports of hypersensitivity reactions in patients who have been treated with Pegademase Bovine Injection.

One of 12 patients showed an enhanced rate of clearance of plasma ADA activity after 5 months of therapy at 15 U/kg/week. Enhanced clearance was correlated with the appearance of an antibody that directly inhibited both unmodified ADA and Pegademase Bovine Injection. Subsequently, the patient was treated with twice weekly intramuscular injections at an increased dose of 20 U/kg, or a total weekly dose of 40 U/kg. No adverse effects were observed at the higher dose and effective levels of plasma ADA were restored. After 4 months, the patient returned to a weekly dosage schedule of 20 U/kg and effective plasma levels have been maintained.

Appropriate care to protect immune deficient patients should be maintained until improvement in immune function has been documented. The degree of immune function improvement may vary from patient to patient and, therefore, each patient will require appropriate care consistent with immunologic status.

LABORATORY TESTS

The treatment of SCID associated with ADA deficiency with Pegademase Bovine Injection should be monitored by measuring plasma ADA activity and red blood cell dATP levels.

Plasma ADA activity and red cell dATP should be determined prior to treatment. Once treatment with Pegademase Bovine Injection has been initiated, a desirable range of plasma ADA activity (trough level before maintenance injection) should be 15-35 µmol/hr/mL. This minimum trough level will ensure that plasma ADA activity from injection to injection is maintained above the level of total erythrocyte ADA activity in the blood of normal individuals.

Plasma ADA activity (pre-injection) should be determined every 1-2 weeks during the first 8-12 weeks of treatment in order to establish an effective dose of Pegademase Bovine Injection. After two months of maintenance treatment with Pegademase Bovine Injection, red cell dATP levels should decrease to a range of ≤ 0.005 to 0.015 µmol/mL. The normal value of dATP is below 0.001 µmol/mL. Once the level of dATP has fallen adequately, it should be measured 2-4 times a year during the remainder of the first year and 2-3 times a year thereafter, assuming no interruption in therapy.

Between 3 and 9 months, plasma ADA should be determined twice a month, then monthly until after 18-24 months of treatment with Pegademase Bovine Injection. Patients who have successfully been maintained on therapy for two years should continue to have plasma ADA measured every 2-4 months and red cell dATP measured twice yearly. More frequent monitoring would be necessary if therapy were interrupted or if an enhanced rate of clearance of plasma ADA activity develops.

Once effective ADA plasma levels have been established, should a patient's plasma ADA activity level fall below 10 µmol/hr/mL (which cannot be attributed to improper dosing, sample handling or antibody development) then all patients receiving this lot of Pegademase Bovine Injection will be required to have a blood sample for plasma ADA determination taken prior to their next injection of Pegademase Bovine Injection. The index patient will require re-testing for determination of plasma ADA activity prior to his/her next injection of Pegademase Bovine Injection. If this value, as well as the value from one of the other patients from a different site, is less than 10 µmol/hr/mL then the lot in use will be recalled and replaced with a new clinical lot.

Immune function, including the ability to produce antibodies, generally improves after 2-6 months of therapy, and matures over a longer period. Compared with the natural history of combined immunodeficiency disease due to ADA deficiency, a trend toward diminished frequency of opportunistic infections and fewer complications of infections has occurred in patients receiving Pegademase Bovine Injection. However, the lag between the correction of the metabolic abnormalities and improved immune function with a trend toward diminished frequency of infections and complications of infection is variable, and has ranged from a few weeks to approximately 6 months. Improvement in the general clinical status of the patient may be gradual (as evidenced by improvement in various clinical parameters) but should be apparent by the end of the first year of therapy. Antibody to Pegademase Bovine Injection may develop in patients and may result in more rapid clearance of Pegademase Bovine Injection. Antibody to Pegademase Bovine Injection should be suspected if a persistent fall in pre-injection levels of plasma ADA to ≤ 10 µmol/hr/mL occurs. If other causes for a decline in plasma ADA levels can be ruled out [such as improper storage of Pegademase Bovine Injection vials (freezing or prolonged storage at temperatures above 8°C), or improper handling of plasma samples (e.g., repeated freezing and thawing during transport to laboratory)], then a specific assay for antibody to ADA and Pegademase Bovine Injection (ELISA, enzyme inhibition) should be performed.

In patients undergoing treatment with Pegademase Bovine Injection, a decline in immune function, with increased risk of opportunistic infections and complications of infection, will result from failure to maintain adequate levels of plasma ADA activity [whether due to the development of antibody to Pegademase Bovine Injection, to improper calculation of Pegademase Bovine Injection dosage, to interruption of treatment or to improper storage of Pegademase Bovine Injection with subsequent loss of activity]. If a persistent decline in plasma ADA activity occurs, immune function and clinical status should be monitored closely and precautions should be taken to minimize the risk of infection. If antibody to ADA or Pegademase Bovine Injection is found to be the cause of a persistent fall in plasma ADA activity, then adjustment in the dosage of Pegademase Bovine Injection and other measures may be taken to induce tolerance and restore adequate ADA activity.

DRUG INTERACTIONS

There are no known drug interactions with Pegademase Bovine Injection. However, vidarabine is a substrate for ADA and 2'-deoxycoformycin is a potent inhibitor of ADA. Thus, the activities of these drugs and Pegademase Bovine Injection could be substantially altered if they are used in combination with one another.

CARCINOGENESIS, MUTAGENESIS, IMPAIRMENT OF FERTILITY

Long-term carcinogenic studies in animals have not been performed with Pegademase Bovine Infection nor have studies been performed on impairment of fertility. Pegademase Bovine Injection did not exhibit a mutagenic effect when tested against *Salmonella typhimurium* strains in the Ames assay.

PREGNANCY

Pregnancy Category C. Animal reproduction studies have not been conducted with Pegademase Bovine Injection. It is also not known whether Pegademase Bovine Injection can cause fetal harm when administered to a pregnant woman or can affect reproduction capacity. Pegademase Bovine Injection should be given to a pregnant woman only if clearly needed.

NURSING MOTHERS

It is not known whether Pegademase Bovine Injection is excreted in human milk. Because many drugs are excreted in human milk, caution should be exercised when Pegademase Bovine Injection is administered to a nursing woman.

ADVERSE REACTIONS

Clinical experience with Pegademase Bovine Injection has been limited. The following adverse reactions have been reported: headache in one patient and pain at the injection site in two patients.

OVERDOSAGE

There is no documented experience with Pegademase Bovine Injection overdosage. An intraperitoneal dose of 50,000 U/kg of Pegademase Bovine Injection in mice resulted in weight loss up to 9%.

DOSAGE AND ADMINISTRATION

Before prescribing Pegademase Bovine Injection, the physician should be thoroughly familiar with the details of this prescribing information. For further information concerning the essential monitoring of Pegademase Bovine Injection therapy, the prescribing physican should contact ENZON, Inc., 40 Kingsbridge Road, Piscataway, NJ 08854. Telephone 908-980-4500. Fax 908-980-5911.

Pegademase Bovine Injection is recommended for use in infants from birth or in children of any age at the time of diagnosis.

Parenteral drug products should be inspected visually for particulate matter and discoloration prior to administration, whenever solution and container permits.

Pegademase Bovine Injection should not be diluted nor mixed with any other drug prior to administration.

Pegademase Bovine Injection should be administered every 7 days as an intramuscular injection. The dosage of Pegademase Bovine Injection should be individualized. The recommended dosing schedule is 10 U/kg for the first dose, 15 U/kg for the second dose, and 20 U/kg for the third dose. The usual maintenance dose is 20 U/kg per week. Further increases of 5 U/kg/week may be necessary, but a maximum single dose of 30 U/kg should not be exceeded. Plasma levels of ADA more than twice the upper limit of 35 μmol/hr/mL have occurred on occasion in several patients, and have been maintained for several weeks in one patient who received twice weekly injections (20 U/kg per dose) of Pegademase Bovine Injection. No adverse effects have been observed at these higher levels; there is no evidence that maintaining pre-injection plasma ADA above 35 μmol/hr/mL produces any additional clinical benefits.

Dose proportionality has not been established and patients should be closely monitored when the dosage is increased.

Pegademase Bovine Injection is not recommended for intravenous administration. The optimal dosage and schedule of administration should be established for each patient based on monitoring of plasma ADA activity levels (through levels before maintenance injection) and biochemical markers of ADA deficiency (primarily red cell dATP content). Since improvement in immune function follows correction of metabolic abnormalities, maintenance dosage in individual patients should be aimed at achieving the following biochemical goals: 1) maintain plasma ADA activity (trough levels before maintenance injection) in the range of 15-35 μmol/hr/mL (assayed at 37°C); and 2) decline in erythrocyte dATP to ≤ 0.005-0.015 μmol/mL packed erythrocytes, or ≤ 1% of the total erythrocyte adenine nucleotide (ATP - dATP) content, with a normal ATP level, as measured in a pre-injection sample. In addition, continued monitoring of immune function and clinical status is essential in any patient with a primary immunodeficiency disease and should be continued in patients undergoing treatment with Pegademase Bovine Injection.

Refrigerate. Store between 2°C and 8°C (36°F and 46°F). DO NOT FREEZE. Pegademase Bovine Injection should not be stored at room temperature. This product should not be used if there are any indications that it may have been frozen.

REFERENCES

1. Hershfield MS, Buckley RH, Greenberg ML, et al. Treatment of adenosine deaminase deficiency with polyethylene glycol-modified adenosine deaminase. N Engl J Med 1987; 316:589-96. 2. Levy Y, Hershfield MS, Fernandez-Mejia C, Polmar ST, Scudiery D, Berger M, Sorensen RU. Adenosine deaminase deficiency with late onset of recurrent infections; response to treatment with polyethylene glycol-modified adenosine deaminase, J. Pediatr 1988; 113:312-17. 3. Kredich NM, Hershfield MS. Immunodeficiency diseases caused by adenosine deaminase deficiency and purine nucleoside phosphorylase deficiency. 6th ed. In: Scriver CR, Beaudet AL, Sly WS, Valle D, eds. The metabolic basis of inherited disease. New York: McGraw Hill, 1989; 1045-75. 4. Hirschhorn R. Inherited enzyme deficiencies and immunodeficiency adenosine deaminase (ADA) and purine nucleoside phosphorylase (PNP) deficiencies. Clin Immunol Immunopathol 1986; 40:157-65. 5. Hirschhorn R, Roegner-Maniscalco V, Kuritsky L, Rosen FS. Bone marrow transplantation only partially restores purine metabolites to normal adenosine deaminase-deficient patients, J Clin Invest 1981; 68:1387-93. 6. Polmar AH, Stern RC, Schwartz AL, Wetzler EM, Chase PA, Hirschhorn R. Enzyme replacement therapy for adenosine deaminase deficiency and severe combined immunodeficiency. N Engl J Med 1976; 295:1337-43. 7. Rubinstein A, Hirschhorn R, Sicklick M, Murphy RA. In vivo and in vitro effects of thymosin and adenosine deaminase on adenosine-deaminase-deficient lymphocytes. N Engl J Med 1979; 300:387-92. 8. Hirschhorn R, Papageorgiou PS, Kesarwala HH, Taft LT. Amelioration of neurologic abnormalities after 'enzyme replacement' in adenosine deaminase deficiency. N Engl J Med 1980; 303:377-80. 9. Hirshhorn R, Ratech H, Rubinstein A, et al. Increased excretion of modified adenine nucleosides by children with adenosine deaminase deficiency. Pediatr Res 1982; 16:362-9. 10. Polmar SH. Enzyme replacement and other biochemical approaches to the therapy of adenosine deaminase deficiency. In: Elliott K, Whelan J, eds. Enzyme defects and immune dysfunction. Amsterdam: Excerpta Medica, 1979; 213-30.

HOW SUPPLIED
INJECTION: 250 U/ML

BRAND/MANUFACTURER	NDC	SIZE	AWP
○ **BRAND**			
ADAGEN — Enzon	57665-0001-01	1.5 ml	$2200.00

Peganone SEE ETHOTOIN

Pegaspargase

DESCRIPTION

Pegaspargase is a modified version of the enzyme L-asparginase. It is an oncolytic agent used in combination chemotherapy for the treatment of patients with acute lymphoblastic leukemia who are hypersensitive to native forms of L-asparaginase (as described in *"Clinical Pharmacology"*).

The chemical name is monomethoxypolyethylene glycol succinimidyl L-asparaginase. L-asparaginase is modified by covalently conjugating units of monomethoxypolyethylene glycol (PEG), molecular weight of 5,000, to the enzyme, forming the active ingredient PEG-L-asparaginase. The L-asparaginase (L-asparagine amidohydrolase, type EC-2, EC 3.5.1.1) used in the manufacture of Pegaspargase is derived from *Escherichia coli*.

Pegaspargase is supplied as an isotonic sterile solution in phosphate buffered saline, pH 7.3, for intramuscular or intravenous administration only. The solution is clear, colorless and contains no preservatives. It is supplied in 5 mL single-dose vials. Use only one dose per vial; do not re-enter the vial. Discard unused portions. Do not save unused drug for later administration.

Pegaspargase activity is expressed in International Units (IU) according to the recommendation of the International Union of Biochemistry. One IU of L-asparaginase is defined as that amount of enzyme required to generate 1 μmol of ammonia per minute at pH 7.3 and 37°C.

Each milliliter of Pegaspargase contains:

PEG-L-asparaginase ....750 IU ± 20 %

The specific activity of Pegaspargase is at least 85 IU per milligram protein.

Following is its chemical structure:

$$\left[H_3C-(O-CH_2-CH_2)_n-O-\overset{\displaystyle O}{\overset{\|}{C}}-CH_2-CH_2-\overset{\displaystyle O}{\overset{\|}{C}}-NH \right]_{n'} - \text{asparaginase}$$

$n=114$ $n'=74$

CLINICAL PHARMACOLOGY

Leukemic cells are unable to synthesize asparagine due to a lack of asparagine synthetase and are dependent on an exogenous source of asparagine for survival. Rapid depletion of asparagine which results from treatment with the enzyme L-asparaginase, kills the leukemic cells. Normal cells, however, are less affected by the rapid depletion due to their ability to synthesize asparagine. This is an approach to therapy based on a specific metabolic defect in some leukemic cells which do not produce asparagine synthetase.[1]

In a study in predominately L-asparaginase naive adult patients with leukemia and lymphoma, initial plasma levels of L-asparaginase following intravenous administration were determined. Plasma half-life did not appear to be influenced by dose levels, and it could not be correlated with age, sex, surface area, renal or hepatic function, diagnosis or extent of disease. Apparent volume of distribution was equal to estimated plasma volume. L-asparaginase was measurable for at least 15 days following the initial treatment with Pegaspargase. The enzyme could not be detected in the urine.[2]

In a study of newly diagnosed pediatric patients with acute lymphoblastic leukemia (ALL) who received either a single intramuscular injection of Pegaspargase (2,500 IU/m²), *E. coli* L-asparaginase (25,000 IU/m²), or *Erwinia* L-asparaginase (25,000 IU/m²), the plasma half-lives for the three forms of L-asparaginase were:[3]

PLASMA HALF-LIVES OF THREE FORMS OF L-ASPARAGINASE

Treatment Group	No. of Patients	Mean (Days)	Standard Deviation
Pegaspargase	10	5.73	3.24
E. coli L-asparaginase	17	1.24	0.17
Erwinia L-asparaginase	10	0.65	0.13

In this same study of newly diagnosed pediatric ALL patients, the *in vivo* early leukemic cell kill after a single intramuscular injection of native *E. coli* L-asparaginase (25,000 IU/m²), *Erwinia* L-asparaginase (25,000 IU/m²), and Pegaspargase (2,500 IU/m²) during a five day "investigational window" was studied.[4] Bone marrow aspirates were taken before and five days after a single dose of one of the three different forms of L-asparaginase. Rhodamine-123 (RH-123), a selectively incorporated fluorescent mitochondrial dye, was used in an *in vitro* assay on the bone marrow aspirates to ascertain cell viability. The percent reduction of viable lymphoblasts at day five for each group is presented in the following table:[4]

RHODAMINE-123 (*IN VIVO* CELL KILL)

Treatment Group	No. of Patients	Percent Reduction of Viable Lymphoblasts at Day 5 Mean ± S.D.
Pegaspargase	21	55.7 ± 10.2
E. coli L-asparaginase	28	57.8 ± 10.1
Erwinia L-asparaginase	19	57.9 ± 13.8

➤ SHOWN IN PRODUCT IDENTIFICATION GUIDE

In three pharmacokinetic studies, 37 relapsed ALL patients received Pegaspargase at 2,500 IU/m^2 every two weeks. The plasma half-life of Pegaspargase was 3.24 ± 1.83 days in nine patients who were previously hypersensitive to native L-asparaginase and 5.69 ± 3.25 days in 28 nonhypersensitive patients. The area under the curve was 9.50 ± 3.95 IU/mL/day in the previously hypersensitive patients, and 9.83 ± 5.94 IU/mL/day in the nonhypersensitive patients.

HYPERSENSITIVITY REACTIONS

Hypersensitivity reactions to *E. coli* L-asparaginase have been reported in the literature in 3% to 73% of patients.[1] Patients in Pegaspargase clinical studies were considered to be previously hypersensitive if they experienced a systemic rash, urticaria, bronchospasm, laryngeal edema, or hypotension following administration of any form of native L-asparaginase. Patients were also considered to be previously hypersensitive if they experienced local erythema, urticaria, or swelling, greater than two centimeters, for at least ten minutes following administration of any form of native L-asparaginase. The National Cancer Institute Common Toxicity Criteria (CTC) were used to classify the severity of the hypersensitivity reactions. These are: grade 1 — transient rash (mild); grade 2 — mild bronchospasm (moderate); grade 3 — moderate bronchospasm and/or serum sickness (severe); grade 4 — hypotension and/or anaphylaxis (life-threatening). Additionally, most transient local urticaria were considered grade 2 hypersensitivity reactions, while most sustained urticaria distant from the injection site were considered grade 3 hypersensitivity reactions. In general, the moderate to life-threatening hypersensitivity reactions were considered dose-limiting; that is, they required L-asparaginase treatment to be discontinued.

In separate studies, Pegaspargase was administered intravenously to 48 patients and intramuscularly to 126 patients. The incidence of hypersensitivity reactions when Pegaspargase was administered intramuscularly was 30% in patients who were previously hypersensitive to native L-asparaginase and 11% in non-hypersensitive patients (p-value of 0.007). The incidence of hypersensitivity reactions when Pegaspargase was administered intravenously was 60% in patients who were previously hypersensitive to native L-asparaginase and 12% in non-hypersensitive patients. Since only five previously hypersensitive patients received Pegaspargase intravenously, no meaningful analysis of the incidence of hypersensitivity reactions was possible between either the previously hypersensitive and nonhypersensitive patients, or between the intravenous and intramuscular routes of administration.

The overall incidence of hypersensitivity reactions in 174 patients who received Pegaspargase in five clinical studies is shown in the table below:

INCIDENCE OF PEGASPARGASE HYPERSENSITIVITY REACTIONS

| Patient Status | N | CTC Grade of Hypersensitivity Reaction | | | | Total |
		1	2	3	4	
Previously Hypersensitive Patients	62	7	8	4	1	20 (32%)
Non-Hypersensitive Patients	112	5	4	1	1	11 (10%)
Total Patients	174	12	12	5	2	31 (18%)

The probability of a previously hypersensitive or non-hypersensitive patient completing 8 doses of Pegaspargase therapy without developing a dose-limiting hypersensitivity reaction was 77% and 95%, respectively.

All of the 62 hypersensitive patients treated with Pegaspargase in five clinical studies had previous hypersensitivity reactions to one or more of the native forms of L-asparaginase. Of the 35 patients who had previous hypersensitivity reactions to *E. coli* L-asparaginase only, 5 (14%) had Pegaspargase dose-limiting hypersensitivity reactions. Of the 27 patients who had hypersensitivity reactions to both *E. coli* and *Erwinia* L-asparaginase, 7 (26%) had Pegaspargase dose-limiting hypersensitivity reactions. The overall incidence of dose-limiting hypersensitivity reactions in 174 patients treated with Pegaspargase was 9% (19% in 62 hypersensitive and 3% in 112 non-hypersensitive patients). Of the total of 9% dose-limiting hypersensitivity reactions, 1% were anaphylactic (CTC grade 4) and the other 8% were ≤ CTC grade 3.

CLINICAL ACTIVITY

Pegaspargase was evaluated as part of combination therapy in four open label studies comprising 42 multiply-relapsed, previously hypersensitive acute leukemia patients [39 (93%) with ALL] at a dose of 2,000 or 2,500 IU/m^2 administered intramuscularly or intravenously every 14 days during induction combination chemotherapy. The reinduction response rate was 50% (36% complete remissions and 14% partial remissions), with a 95% confidence interval of 35% to 65%. This response rate is comparable to that reported in the literature for relapsed patients treated with native L-asparaginase as part of combination chemotherapy.[1]

Pegaspargase was also shown to have some activity as a single agent in multiply-relapsed hypersensitive ALL patients, the majority of whom were pediatric. Treatment with Pegaspargase resulted in three responses (one complete remission and two partial remissions) in nine previously hypersensitive patients who would not have been able to receive any further L-asparaginase treatment.

Pegaspargase was also studied in non-hypersensitive, relapsed ALL patients who were randomized to receive two doses of Pegaspargase at 2,500 IU/m^2 every 14 days or twelve doses of *E. coli* L-asparaginase at 10,000 IU/m^2 three times a week during a 28 day induction combination chemotherapy regimen (which included vincristine and prednisone). Although the enrollment in this study was too small to be conclusive, the data showed that for 20 patients there was no

significant difference between the overall response rates of 60% and 50%, respectively, or the complete remission rates of 50% and 50%, respectively.

Pegaspargase was administered during maintenance therapy regimens to 33 previously hypersensitive patients. The average number of doses received during maintenance therapy was 5.8 (range of 1 to 24) and the average duration of maintenance therapy was 126 (range of 1 to 513) days for this patient population.

INDICATIONS AND USAGE

Pegaspargase is indicated for patients with acute lymphoblastic leukemia who require L-asparaginase in their treatment regimen, but have developed hypersensitivity to the native forms of L-asparaginase (See *"Clinical Pharmacology"*). Pegaspargase, like native L-asparaginase, is generally used in combination with other chemotherapeutic agents, such as vincristine, methotrexate, cytarabine, daunorubicin, and doxorubicin.[1,5] Use of Pegaspargase as a single agent should only be undertaken when multi-agent chemotherapy is judged to be inappropriate for the patient.

UNLABELED USES

Pegaspargase is used alone or as an adjunct in the treatment of refractory non-Hodgkin's lymphoma.

CONTRAINDICATIONS

Pegaspargase is contraindicated in patients with pancreatitis or a history of pancreatitis. Pegaspargase is contraindicated in patients who have had significant hemorrhagic events associated with prior L-asparaginase therapy. Pegaspargase is also contraindicated in patients who have had previous serious allergic reactions, such as generalized urticaria, bronchospasm, laryngeal edema, hypotension, or other unacceptable adverse reactions to Pegaspargase.

WARNINGS

It is recommended that Pegaspargase be given under the supervision of an individual who is qualified by training and experience to administer cancer chemotherapeutic agents.

Especially in patients with known hypersensitivity to the other forms of L-asparaginase, hypersensitivity reactions to Pegaspargase, including life-threatening anaphylaxis, may occur during therapy. As a routine precaution, patients should be kept under observation for one hour with resuscitation equipment and other agents necessary to treat anaphylaxis (epinephrine, oxygen, intravenous steroids, etc.) available.

PRECAUTIONS

GENERAL

This drug may be a contact irritant, and the solution must be handled and administered with care. Gloves are recommended. Inhalation of vapors and contact with skin or mucous membranes, especially those of the eyes, must be avoided. In case of contact, wash with copious amounts of water for at least 15 minutes. Anaphylactic reactions require the immediate use of epinephrine, oxygen, intravenous steroids, and antihistamines. Patients taking Pegaspargase are at higher than usual risk for bleeding problems, especially with simultaneous use of other drugs that have anticoagulant properties, such as aspirin, and non-steroidal anti-inflammatories (see *"Drug Interactions"*). Pegaspargase may have immunosuppressive activity. Therefore, it is possible that use of the drug in patients may predispose the patient to infection. Severe hepatic and central nervous system toxicity following multi-agent chemotherapy that includes Pegaspargase may occur. Caution appears warranted when treating patients with Pegaspargase given in combination with hepatotoxic agents, particularly when liver dysfunction is present.

Patients undergoing Pegaspargase therapy must be carefully monitored and the therapeutic regimen adjusted according to response and toxicity. Physicians using a given treatment regimen incorporating Pegaspargase should be thoroughly familiar with its benefits and risks.

INFORMATION FOR PATIENTS

Patients should be informed of the possibility of hypersensitivity reactions, including immediate anaphylaxis, to Pegaspargase. Patients taking Pegaspargase are at higher than usual risk for bleeding problems. Patients should be instructed that the simultaneous use of Pegaspargase with other drugs that may increase the risk of bleeding should be avoided (see *"Drug Interactions"*). Pegaspargase may affect the ability of the liver to function normally in some patients. Therapy with Pegaspargase may increase the toxicity of other medications (see *"Drug Interactions"*). Pegaspargase may have immunosuppressive activity. Therefore, it is possible that use of the drug in patients may predispose the patient to infection. Patients should notify their physicians of any adverse reactions that occur.

LABORATORY TESTS

A fall in circulating lymphoblasts is often noted after initiating therapy. This may be accompanied by a marked rise in serum uric acid. As a guide to the effects of therapy, the patient's peripheral blood count and bone marrow should be monitored.

Frequent serum amylase determinations should be obtained to detect early evidence of pancreatitis (see *"Contraindications"*). Blood sugar should be monitored during therapy with Pegaspargase because hyperglycemia may occur. When using Pegaspargase in conjunction with hepatotoxic chemotherapy, patients should be monitored for liver dysfunction.

Pegaspargase may affect a number of plasma proteins; therefore, monitoring of fibrinogen, PT, and PTT may be indicated.

◆ RATED THERAPEUTICALLY EQUIVALENT; ◇ THERAPEUTIC EQUIVALENCE UNCONFIRMED; ○ UNRATED

DRUG INTERACTIONS

Unfavorable interactions of L-asparaginase with some antitumor agents have been demonstrated.[1] It is recommended, therefore, that Pegaspargase be used in combination regimens only by physicians familiar with the benefits and risks of a given regimen. Depletion of serum proteins by Pegaspargase may increase the toxicity of other drugs which are protein bound. Additionally, during the period of its inhibition of protein synthesis and cell replication, Pegaspargase may interfere with the action of drugs such as methotrexate, which require cell replication for their lethal effects. Pegaspargase may interfere with the enzymatic detoxification of other drugs, particularly in the liver. Physicians using a given treatment regimen should be thoroughly familiar with its benefits and risks.

Imbalances in coagulation factors have been noted with the use of Pegaspargase predisposing to bleeding and/or thrombosis. Caution should be used when administering any concurrent anticoagulant therapy, such as coumadin, heparin, dipyridamole, aspirin, or non-steroidal anti-inflammatories.

CARCINOGENESIS, MUTAGENESIS, IMPAIRMENT OF FERTILITY

Long-term carcinogenic studies in animals have not been performed with Pegaspargase nor have studies been performed on impairment of fertility. Pegaspargase did not exhibit a mutagenic effect when tested against *Salmonella typhimurium* strains in the Ames assay.

PREGNANCY

Pregnancy Category C. Animal reproduction studies have not been conducted with Pegaspargase. It is also not known whether Pegaspargase can cause fetal harm when administered to a pregnant woman or can affect reproduction capacity. Pegaspargase should be given to a pregnant woman only if clearly needed.

NURSING MOTHERS

It is not known whether Pegaspargase is excreted in human milk. Because many drugs are excreted in human milk and because of the potential for serious adverse reactions due to Pegaspargase in nursing infants, a decision should be made to discontinue nursing or discontinue the drug, taking into account the importance of the drug to the mother.

ADVERSE REACTIONS

Adverse reactions have been reported in adults and pediatric patients. Overall, the adult patients treated with Pegaspargase had a somewhat higher incidence of known L-asparaginase toxicities, except for hypersensitivity reactions, than the pediatric patients treated with Pegaspargase.

Excluding hypersensitivity reactions, the most frequently occurring known L-asparaginase related toxicities and adverse experiences reported for the 174 patients in clinical studies were chemical hepatotoxicities and coagulopathies, the majority of which did not result in any significant clinical events. The incidence of significant clinical events included clinical pancreatitis (1%), hyperglycemia requiring insulin therapy (3%), and thrombosis (4%).

The following adverse reactions related to Pegaspargase were reported for 174 patients in five clinical studies.

The adverse reactions reported most frequently (greater than 5%) were allergic reactions (which may have included rash, erythema, edema, pain, fever, chills, urticaria, dyspnea, or bronchospasm), SGPT increase, nausea and/or vomiting, fever, and malaise.

The adverse reactions reported occasionally (greater than 1% but less than 5%) were anaphylactic reactions, dyspnea, injection site hypersensitivity, lip edema, rash, urticaria, abdominal pain, chills, pain in the extremities, hypotension, tachycardia, thrombosis, anorexia, diarrhea, jaundice, abnormal liver function test, decreased anticoagulant effect, disseminated intravascular coagulation, decreased fibrinogen, hemolytic anemia, leukopenia, pancytopenia, thrombocytopenia, increased thromboplastin, injection site pain, injection site reaction, bilirubinemia, hyperglycemia, hyperuricemia, hypoglycemia, hypoproteinemia, peripheral edema, increased SGOT, arthralgia, myalgia, convulsion, headache, night sweats, and paresthesia.

The adverse reactions reported rarely (less than 1%) were bronchospasm, petechial rash, face edema, lesional edema, sepsis, septic shock, chest pain, endocarditis, hypertension, constipation, flatulence, gastrointestinal pain, hepatomegaly, increased appetite, liver fatty deposits, coagulation disorder, increased coagulation time, decreased platelet count, purpura, increased amylase, edema, excessive thirst, hyperammonemia, hyponatremia, weight loss, bone pain, joint disorder, confusion, dizziness, emotional lability, somnolence, increased cough, epistaxis, upper respiratory infection, erythema simplex, pruritus, hematuria, increased urinary frequency, and abnormal kidney function.

The following Pegaspargase related adverse reactions have been observed in patients with hematologic malignancies, primarily acute lymphoblastic leukemia (approximately 75%), non-Hodgkins lymphoma (approximately 13%), acute myelogenous leukemia (approximately 3%), and a variety of solid tumors (approximately 9%):

Hypersensitivity Reactions: a variety of hypersensitivity reactions have occurred. These reactions may be acute or delayed, and include acute anaphylaxis, bronchospasm, dyspnea, urticaria, arthralgia, erythema, induration, edema, pain, tenderness, hives, swelling, lip edema, chills, fever, and skin rashes (see "*Warnings*" and "*Contraindications*").

Pancreatic Function: pancreatitis, sometimes fulminant and fatal, has occurred. Increased serum amylase and lipase have also occurred.

Liver Function: a variety of liver function abnormalities have been observed, including elevations of SGOT, SGPT, and bilirubin (direct and indirect).

Jaundice, ascites, and hypoalbuminemia, which may be associated with peripheral edema, have been observed. These abnormalities usually are reversible on discontinuance of therapy, and some reversal may occur during the course of therapy. Fatty changes in the liver and liver failure have occurred.

Hematologic: hypofibrinogenemia, prolonged prothrombin times, prolonged partial thromboplastin times, and decreased antithrombin III have been observed. Superficial and deep venous thrombosis, sagittal sinus thrombosis, venous catheter thrombosis, and atrial thrombosis have occurred. Leukopenia, agranulocytosis, pancytopenia, thrombocytopenia, disseminated intravascular coagulation, severe hemolytic anemia, and anemia have been observed. Clinical hemorrhage, which may be fatal; easy bruisability, and ecchymosis have also been observed.

Metabolic: mild to severe hyperglycemia have been observed in low incidence, and usually responds to discontinuation of Pegaspargase and the judicious use of intravenous fluid and insulin. Hypoglycemia, increased thirst and hyponatremia, uric acid nephropathy, hyperuricemia, hypoproteinemia, and peripheral edema have also been observed. Hypoalbuminemia, proteinuria, weight loss, and metabolic acidosis have occurred. Therapy with Pegaspargase is associated with an increase in blood ammonia during the conversion of L-asparagine to aspartic acid by the enzyme.

Neurologic: status epilepticus and temporal lobe seizures, somnolence, coma, malaise, mental status changes, dizziness, emotional lability, headache, lip numbness, finger paresthesia, mood changes, night sweats, and a Parkinson-like syndrome have occurred. Mild to severe confusion, disorientation, and paresthesia have also occurred. These side effects usually have reversed spontaneously after treatment was stopped.

Renal: increased BUN, increased creatinine, increased urinary frequency, hematuria due to thrombopenia, severe hemorrhagic cystitis, renal dysfunction, and renal failure have been observed.

Cardiovascular: chest pain, subacute bacterial endocarditis, hypertension, severe hypotension, and tachycardia have occurred.

Digestive: anorexia, constipation, decreased appetite, diarrhea, indigestion, flatulence, gas, gastrointestinal pain, mucositis, hepatomegaly, elevated gamma-glutamyltranspeptidase, increased appetite, mouth tenderness, severe colitis, and nausea and/or vomiting have been observed.

Musculoskeletal: diffuse and local musculoskeletal pain, arthralgia, joint stiffness, and cramps have occurred.

Respiratory: cough, epistaxis, severe bronchospasm, and upper respiratory infection have been observed.

Skin/Appendages: itching, alopecia, fever blister, purpura, hand whiteness and fungal changes, nail whiteness and ridging, erythema simplex, jaundice, and petechial rash have occurred.

General: localized edema, injection site reactions (including pain, swelling, or redness), malaise, infection, sepsis, fatigue, and septic shock may occur.

OVERDOSAGE

Three patients received 10,000 IU/m^2 of Pegaspargase as an intravenous infusion. One patient experienced a slight increase in liver enzymes. A second patient developed a rash ten minutes after the start of the infusion, which was controlled with the administration of an antihistamine and by slowing down the infusion rate. A third patient did not experience any adverse reactions.

DOSAGE AND ADMINISTRATION

As a component of selected multiple agent regimens, the recommended dose of Pegaspargase is 2,500 IU/m^2 every 14 days by either the intramuscular or intravenous route of administration.

The preferred route of administration, however, is the intramuscular route because of the lower incidence of hepatotoxicity, coagulopathy, and gastrointestinal and renal disorders compared to the intravenous route of administration.

The safety and effectiveness of Pegaspargase have been established in patients with known previous hypersensitivity to L-asparaginase whose ages ranged from 1 to 21 years old. The recommended dose of Pegaspargase for children with a body surface area $\geq$ 0.6 m^2 is 2,500 IU/m^2 administered every 14 days. The recommended dose of Pegaspargase for children with a body surface area < 0.6 m^2 is 82.5 IU/kg administered every 14 days.

Do not administer Pegaspargase if there is any indication that the drug has been frozen. Although there may not be an apparent change in the appearance of the drug, Pegaspargase's activity is destroyed after freezing.

When administering Pegaspargase intramuscularly, the volume at a single injection site should be limited to 2 mL. If the volume to be administered is greater than 2 mL, multiple injection sites should be used.

When administered intravenously, Pegaspargase should be given over a period of 1 to 2 hours in 100 mL of sodium chloride or dextrose injection 5%, through an infusion that is already running.

Anaphylactic reactions require the immediate use of antihistamines, epinephrine, oxygen, and intravenous steroids.

Use of Pegaspargase as the sole induction agent should be undertaken only in an unusual situation when a combined regimen, which uses other chemotherapeutic agents such as vincristine, methotrexate, cytarabine, daunorubicin, or doxorubicin, is inappropriate because of toxicity or other specific patient-related factors, or in patients refractory to other therapy. When Pegaspargase is to be used as the sole induction agent, the recommended dosage regimen is also 2,500 IU/m^2 every 14 days.

➤ SHOWN IN PRODUCT IDENTIFICATION GUIDE

When a remission is obtained, appropriate maintenance therapy may be instituted. Pegaspargase may be used as part of a maintenance regimen.

Parenteral drug products should be inspected visually for particulate matter, cloudiness or discoloration prior to administration, whenever solution and container permit.

Avoid excessive agitation. DO NOT SHAKE.

Keep refrigerated at 2°C to 8°C (36°F to 46°F).

Do not use if cloudy or if precipitate is present.

Do not use if stored at room temperature for more than 48 hours.

DO NOT FREEZE. Do not use product if it is known to have been frozen. Freezing destroys activity, which cannot be detected visually.

REFERENCES

1. Capizzi, RL and Holcenberg, JS. Asparaginase. In: Holland and Frei (eds). *Cancer Med* third edition, Lea and Febiger, Phila. PA, 1993. 2. Ho, DH, et al. Clinical pharmacology of polyethylene glycol-L-asparaginase. *Drug Metab Dispos* 14 (3): 349-352, 1986. 3. Asselin, BL, et al. Comparative Pharmacokinetic Studies of Three L-asparaginase Preparations. *J Clin Oncology* (11): 1780-1786, 1993. 4. Data on File at ENZON. 5. Clavell, LA, et al. Four-agent induction and intensive asparaginase therapy for treatment of childhood acute lymphoblastic leukemia. *N Engl J Med* 315 (11): 657-663, 1986.

HOW SUPPLIED
INJECTION: 750 IU/ML

BRAND/MANUFACTURER	NDC	SIZE	AWP
○ BRAND			
ONCASPAR: RPR	00075-0640-05	5 ml	$1225.00

Pemoline

DESCRIPTION

Pemoline is a central nervous system stimulant. Pemoline is structurally dissimilar to the amphetamines and methylphenidate.

It is an oxazolidine compound and is chemically identified as 2-amino-5-phenyl-2-oxazolin-4-one.

Pemoline is a white, tasteless, odorless powder, relatively insoluble (less than 1 mg/mL) in water, chloroform, ether, acetone, and benzene; its solubility in 95% ethyl alcohol is 2.2 mg/mL.

Following is its chemical structure:

CLINICAL PHARMACOLOGY

Pemoline has a pharmacological activity similar to that of other known central nervous system stimulants; however, it has minimal sympathomimetic effects. Although studies indicate that Pemoline may act in animals through dopaminergic mechanisms, the exact mechanism and site of action of the drug in man is not known.

There is neither specific evidence which clearly establishes the mechanism whereby Pemoline produces its mental and behavioral effects in children, nor conclusive evidence regarding how these effects relate to the condition of the central nervous system.

Pemoline is rapidly absorbed from the gastrointestinal tract. Approximately 50% is bound to plasma proteins. The serum half-life of Pemoline is approximately 12 hours. Peak serum levels of the drug occur within 2 to 4 hours after ingestion of a single dose. Multiple dose studies in adults at several dose levels indicate that steady state is reached in approximately 2 to 3 days. In animals given radiolabeled Pemoline, the drug was widely and uniformly distributed throughout the tissues, including the brain.

Pemoline is metabolized by the liver. Metabolites of Pemoline include Pemoline conjugate, Pemoline dione, mandelic acid, and unidentified polar compounds. Pemoline is excreted primarily by the kidneys with approximately 50% excreted unchanged and only minor fractions present as metabolites. Pemoline has a gradual onset of action. Using the recommended schedule of dosage titration, significant clinical benefit may not be evident until the third or fourth week of drug administration.

INDICATIONS AND USAGE

Pemoline is indicated in Attention Deficit Disorder (ADD) with hyperactivity as an integral part of a total treatment program which typically includes other remedial measures (psychological, educational, social) for a stabilizing effect in children with a behavioral syndrome characterized by the following group of developmentally inappropriate symptoms: moderate to severe distractibility, short attention span, hyperactivity, emotional lability, and impulsivity. The diagnosis of this syndrome should not be made with finality when these symptoms are only of comparatively recent origin. Nonlocalizing (soft) neurological signs, learning disability, and abnormal EEG may or may not be present, and a diagnosis of central nervous system dysfunction may or may not be warranted.

UNLABELED USES

Pemoline is used alone or as an adjunct in the treatment of narcolepsy.

CONTRAINDICATIONS

Pemoline is contraindicated in patients with known hypersensitivity or idiosyncrasy to the drug. Pemoline should not be administered to patients with impaired hepatic function. (See "Adverse Reactions" section.)

WARNINGS

Decrements in the predicted growth (i.e., weight gain and/or height) rate have been reported with the long-term use of stimulants in children. Therefore, patients requiring long-term therapy should be carefully monitored.

PRECAUTIONS

General: Clinical experience suggests that in psychotic children, administration of Pemoline may exacerbate symptoms of behavior disturbance and thought disorder.

Pemoline should be administered with caution to patients with significantly impaired renal function.

Laboratory Tests: Liver function tests should be performed prior to and periodically during therapy with Pemoline. The drug should be discontinued if abnormalities are revealed and confirmed by follow-up tests. (See "Adverse Reactions" section regarding reports of abnormal liver functin tests, hepatitis and jaundice.)

Drug Interactions: The interaction of Pemoline with other drugs has not been studied in humans. Patients who are receiving Pemoline concurrently with other drugs, especially drugs with CNS activity, should be monitored carefully.

Decreased seizure threshold has been reported in patients receiving Pemoline concomitantly with *antiepileptic medications.*

Carcinogenesis: Long-term studies have been conducted in rats with doses as high as 150 mg/kg/day for eighteen months. There was no significant difference in the incidence of any neoplasm between treated and control animals.

Mutagenesis: Data are not available concerning long-term effects on mutagenicity in animals or humans.

Impairment of Fertility: The results of studies in which rats were given 18.75 and 37.5 mg/kg/day indicated that Pemoline line did not affect fertility in males or females at those doses.

Pregnancy: Teratogenic effects: Pregnancy Category B. Reproduction studies have been performed in rats and rabbits at doses of 18.75 and 37.5 mg/kg/day and have revealed no evidence of impaired fertility or harm to the fetus. There are, however, no adequate and well-controlled studies in pregnant women. Because animal reproduction studies are not always predictive of human response, this drug should be used during pregnancy only if clearly needed.

Nonteratogenic effects: Studies in rats have shown an increased incidence of stillbirths and cannibalization when Pemoline was administered at a dose of 37.5 mg/kg/day. Postnatal survival of offspring was reduced at doses of 18.75 and 37.5 mg/kg/day.

Nursing Mothers: It is not known whether this drug is excreted in human milk. Because many drugs are excreted in human milk, caution should be exercised when Pemoline is administered to a nursing woman.

Pediatric Use: Safety and effectiveness in children below the age of 6 years have not been established.

Long-term effects of Pemoline in children have not been established (see "Warnings" section).

CNS stimulants, including Pemoline, have been reported to precipitate motor and phonic tics and Tourette's syndrome. Therefore, clinical evaluation for tics and Tourette's syndrome in children and their families should precede use of stimulant medications.

Drug treatment is not indicated in all cases of ADD with hyperactivity and should be considered only in light of complete history and evaluation of the child. The decision to prescribe Pemoline should depend on the physician's assessment of the chronicity and severity of the child's symptoms and their appropriateness for his/her age. Prescription should not depend solely on the presence of one or more of the behavioral characteristics.

ADVERSE REACTIONS

The following are adverse reactions in decreasing order of severity within each category associated with Pemoline.

Hepatic: There have been reports of hepatic dysfunction including elevated liver enzymes, hepatitis and jaundice in patients taking Pemoline. The occurrence of elevated liver enzymes is not rare and these reactions appear to be reversible upon drug discontinuance. Most patients with elevated liver enzymes were asymptomatic. Although no causal relationship has been established, there have been rare reports of hepatic-related fatalities involving patients taking Pemoline.

Hematopoietic: There have been isolated reports of aplastic anemia.

Central Nervous System: The following CNS effects have been reported with the use of Pemoline convulsive seizures; literature reports indicate that Pemoline may precipitate attacks of Gilles de la Tourette syndrome; hallucinations; dyskinetic movements of the tongue, lips, face and extremities; abnormal oculomotor function including nystagmus and oculogyric crisis; mild depression; dizziness; increased irritability; headache; and drowsiness.

Insomnia is the most frequently reported side effect of Pemoline; it usually occurs early in therapy prior to an optimum therapeutic response. In the majority of cases it is transient in nature or responds to a reduction in dosage.

◆ RATED THERAPEUTICALLY EQUIVALENT; ◇ THERAPEUTIC EQUIVALENCE UNCONFIRMED; ○ UNRATED

Gastrointestinal: Anorexia and weight loss may occur during the first weeks of therapy. In the majority of cases it is transient in nature; weight gain usually resumes within three to six months.

Nausea and stomach ache have also been reported.

Genitourinary: A case of elevated acid phosphatase in association with prostatic enlargement has been reported in a 63-year-old male who was treated with Pemoline for sleepiness. The acid phosphatase normalized with discontinuation of Pemoline and was again elevated with rechallenge.

Miscellaneous: Suppression of growth has been reported with the long-term use of stimulants in children. (See *"Warnings"* section.) Skin rash has been reported with Pemoline.

Mild adverse reactions appearing early during the course of treatment with Pemoline often remit with continuing therapy. If adverse reactions are of a significant or protracted nature, dosage should be reduced or the drug discontinued.

DRUG ABUSE AND DEPENDENCE

Controlled Substance: Pemoline is subject to control under DEA schedule IV.

Abuse: Pemoline failed to demonstrate a potential for self-administration in primates. However, the pharmacologic similarity of Pemoline to other psychostimulants with known dependence liability suggests that psychological and/or physical dependence might also occur with Pemoline. There have been isolated reports of transient psychotic symptoms occurring in adults following the long-term misuse of excessive oral doses of Pemoline. Pemoline should be given with caution to emotionally unstable patients who may increase the dosage on their own initiative.

OVERDOSAGE

Signs and symptoms of acute overdosage, resulting principally from overstimulation of the central nervous system and from excessive sympathomimetic effects, may include the following; vomiting, agitation, tremors, hyperreflexia, muscle twitching, convulsions (may be followed by coma), euphoria, confusion, hallucinations, delirium, sweating, flushing, headache, hyperpyrexia, tachycardia, hypertension and mydriasis. Treatment consists of appropriate supportive measures. The patient must be protected agaisnt self-injury and against external stimuli that would aggravate overstimulation already present. If signs and symptoms are not too severe and the patient is conscious, gastric contents may be evacuated. Chlorpromazine has been reported in the literature to be useful in decreasing CNS stimulation and sympathomimetic effects.

Efficacy of peritoneal dialysis or extracorporeal hemodialysis for Pemoline overdosage has not been established.

DOSAGE AND ADMINISTRATION

Pemoline is administered as a single oral dose each morning. The recommended starting dose is 37.5 mg/day. This daily dose should be gradually increased by 18.75 mg at one week intervals until the desired clinical response is obtained. The effective daily dose for most patients will range from 56.25 to 75 mg. The maximum recommended daily dose of Pemoline is 112.5 mg.

Clinical improvement with Pemoline is gradual. Using the recommended schedule of dosage titration, significant benefit may not be evident until the third or fourth week of drug administration.

Where possible, drug administration should be interrupted occasionally to determine if there is a recurrence of behavioral symptoms sufficient to require continued therapy.

Store below 86°F (30°C).

HOW SUPPLIED
CHEW TABLET (C-IV): 37.5 MG

BRAND/MANUFACTURER	NDC	SIZE	AWP
○ BRAND CYLERT: Abbott Pharm	00074-6088-13	100s	$124.13

TABLETS (C-IV): 18.75 MG

BRAND/MANUFACTURER	NDC	SIZE	AWP
○ BRAND CYLERT: Abbott Pharm	00074-6025-13	100s	$72.45

TABLETS (C-IV): 37.5 MG

BRAND/MANUFACTURER	NDC	SIZE	AWP
○ BRAND CYLERT: Abbott Pharm	00074-6057-13	100s	$113.88

TABLETS (C-IV): 75 MG

BRAND/MANUFACTURER	NDC	SIZE	AWP
○ BRAND CYLERT: Abbott Pharm	00074-6073-13	100s	$196.64

Penbutolol Sulfate

DESCRIPTION

Penbutolol Sulfate is a synthetic β-receptor antagonist for oral administration. The chemical name of Penbutolol Sulfate is (S)-1-tert-butylamino-3-(o-cyclopen-tylphenoxy)-2-propanol sulfate. It is provided as the levorotatory isomer. The empirical formula for Penbutolol Sulfate is $C_{36}H_{60}N_2O_8S$. Its molecular weight is 680.94. A dose of 20 mg is equivalent to 29.4 μmol.

Penbutolol Sulfate is a white, odorless, crystalline powder. Each tablet contains 20 mg of Penbutolol Sulfate.

Following is its chemical structure:

CLINICAL PHARMACOLOGY

Penbutolol Sulfate is a β-1, β-2 (nonselective) adrenergic receptor antagonist. Experimental studies showed a dose-dependent increase in heart rate in reserpinized (norepinephrine-depleted) rats given Penbutolol Sulfate intravenously at doses of 0.25 to 1.0 mg/kg, suggesting that Penbutolol Sulfate has some intrinsic sympathomimetic activity. In human studies, however, heart rate decreases have been similar to those seen with propranolol.

Penbutolol Sulfate antagonizes the heart rate effects of exercise and infused isoproterenol. The β-blocking potency of Penbutolol Sulfate is approximately 4 times that of propranolol. An oral dose of less than 10 mg will reduce exercise-induced tachycardia to one-half its usual level; maximum antagonism follows doses of 10 to 20 mg. The peak effect is between 1.5 and 3 hours after oral administration. The duration of effect exceeds 20 hours during a once-daily dosing regimen. During chronic administration of Penbutolol Sulfate, the duration of antihypertensive effects permits a once-daily dosage schedule.

Acute hemodynamic effects of Penbutolol Sulfate have been studied following single intravenous doses between 0.1 and 4 mg. The cardiovascular responses included significant reductions in heart rate, left ventricular maximum dP/dt, cardiac output, stroke volume index, stroke work, and stroke work index. Systolic pressure and mean arterial pressure were reduced, and total peripheral resistance was increased.

Chronic administration of Penbutolol Sulfate to hypertensive patients results in the hemodynamic pattern typical of β-adrenergic blocking drugs: a reduction in cardiac index, heart rate, systolic and diastolic blood pressures, and the product of heart rate and mean arterial pressure both at rest and with all levels of exercise, without significant change in total peripheral resistance. Penbutolol Sulfate causes a reduction in left ventricular contractility. Penbutolol Sulfate decreases glomerular filtration rate, but not significantly.

Clinical trial doses of 10 to 80 mg per day in single daily doses have reduced supine and standing systolic and diastolic blood pressures. In most studies, effects were small, generally a change in blood pressure 5 to +8/3 to 5 mm Hg greater than seen with a placebo measured 24 hours after dosing. It is not clear whether this relatively small effect reflects a characteristic of Penbutolol Sulfate or the particular population studied (the population had relatively mild hypertension but did not appear unusual in others respects). In a direct comparison of Penbutolol Sulfate with adequate doses of twice daily propranolol, no difference in blood pressure effect was seen. In a comparison of placebo and 10-, 20- and 40-mg single daily doses of Penbutolol Sulfate, no significant dose-related difference was seen in response to active drug at 6 weeks, but compared to the 10-mg dose, the two larger doses showed greater effects at 2 and 4 weeks and reached their maximum effect at 2 weeks. In several studies, dose increases from 40 to 80 mg were without additional effect on blood pressure. Response rates to Penbutolol Sulfate are unaffected by sex or age but are greater in caucasians than blacks.

Penbutolol Sulfate decreases plasma renin activity in normal subjects and in patients with essential and renovascular hypertension. The mechanisms of the antihypertensive actions of β-receptor antagonists have not been established. However, factors that may be involved are: (1) competitive antagonism of catecholamines at peripheral adrenergic receptor sites (especially cardiac) that leads to decreased cardiac output; (2) a central-nervous-system (CNS) action that results in a decrease in tonic sympathetic neural outflow to the periphery; and (3) a reduction of renin secretion through blockade of β-receptors involved in release of renin from the kidneys.

Penbutolol Sulfate dose dependently increases the RR and QT intervals. There is no influence on the PR, QRS or QT c (corrected) intervals.

Pharmacokinetics: Following oral administration, Penbutolol Sulfate is rapidly and completely absorbed. Peak plasma concentrations of Penbutolol Sulfate occur between 2 and 3 hours after oral administration and are proportional to single and multiple doses between 10 and 40 mg once a day. The average plasma elimination half-life of Penbutolol Sulfate is approximately 5 hours in normal subjects. There is no significant difference in the plasma half-life of Penbutolol Sulfate in healthy elderly persons or patients on renal dialysis. Twelve to 24 hours after oral administration of doses up to 120 mg, plasma concentrations of parent drug are 0% to 10% of the peak level. No accumulation of Penbutolol Sulfate is observed in hypertensive patients after 8 days of therapy at doses of 40 mg daily or 20 mg twice a day. Penbutolol Sulfate is approximately 80% to 98% bound to plasma proteins.

The metabolism of Penbutolol Sulfate in humans involves conjugation and oxidation. The metabolites are excreted principally in the urine. When radiolabeled Penbutolol was adminstered to humans, approximately 90% of the radioactivity was excreted in the urine. Approximately +1/6 of the dose of Penbutolol Sulfate was recovered as Penbutolol Sulfate conjugate, while the remaining fraction was not identified. Conjugated Penbutolol Sulfate has a plasma elimination half-life of approximately 20 hours in healthy persons, 25 hours in healthy elderly persons and 100 hours in patients on renal dialysis. Thus, accumulation of Penbutolol Sulfate conjugate may be expected upon multiple-dosing in renal insufficiency. An oxidative metabolite of Penbutolol Sulfate, 4-hydroxy penbutolol, has been identified in small quantities in plasma and urine. It is ⅛ to +1/15 times as active as the parent compound in blocking isoproterenol-induced β-adrenergic receptor responses in isolated guinea-pig trachea and is 1/8 to 1 times as potent in anesthetized dogs.

INDICATIONS AND USAGE

Penbutolol Sulfate is indicated in the treatment of mild to moderate arterial hypertension. It may be used alone or in combination with other antihypertensive agents, especially thiazide-type diuretics.

CONTRAINDICATIONS

Penbutolol Sulfate is contraindicated in patients with cardiogenic shock, sinus bradycardia, second and third degree atrioventricular conduction block, bronchial asthma, and those with known hypersensitivity to this product (see "Warnings").

WARNINGS

Cardiac Failure: Sympathetic stimulation may be essential for supporting circulatory function in patients with heart failure, and its inhibition by β-adrenergic receptor blockade may precipitate more severe failure. Although β-blockers should be avoided in overt congestive heart failure, Penbutolol Sulfate can, if necessary, be used with caution in patients with a history of cardiac failure who are well compensated, on treatment with vasodilators, digitalis and/or diuretics. Both digitalis and Penbutolol Sulfate slow AV conduction. Beta-adrenergic receptor antagonists do not inhibit the inotropic action of digitalis on heart muscle. If cardiac failure persists, treatment with Penbutolol Sulfate should be discontinued.

Patients Without History of Cardiac Failure: Penbutolol Sulfate Continued depression of the myocardium with β-blocking agents over a period of time can. in some cases, lead to cardiac failure. At the first evidence of heart failure, patients receiving Penbutolol Sulfate should be given appropriate treatment, and the response should be closely observed. If cardiac failure continues despite adequate intervention with appropriate drugs, Penbutolol Sulfate should be withdrawn (gradually, if possible).

Exacerbation of Ischemic Heart Disease Following Abrupt Withdrawal: Hypersensitivity to catecholamines has been observed in patients who were withdrawn from therapy with β-blocking agents; exacerbation of angina, and in some cases, myocardial infarction have occurred after abrupt discontinuation of such therapy. When discontinuing Penbutolol Sulfate, particularly in patients with ischemic heart disease, the dosage should be reduced gradually over a period of 1 to 2 weeks and the patient should be monitored carefully. If angina becomes more pronounced or acute coronary insufficiency develops, administration of Penbutolol Sulfate should be reinstated promptly, at least on a temporary basis, and appropriate measures should be taken for the management of unstable angina. Patients should be warned against interruption or discontinuation of therapy without the physician's advice. Because coronary artery disease is common and may not be recognized, it may not be prudent to discontinue Penbutolol Sulfate abruptly, even in patients who are being treated only for hypertension.

Nonallergic Bronchospasm (e.g. Chronic Bronchitis, Emphysema): Penbutolol Sulfate is contraindicated in bronchial asthma. In general, patients with bronchospastic diseases should not receive β-blockers Penbutolol Sulfate should be administered with caution because it may block bronchodilation produced by endogenous catecholamine stimulation of β-2 receptors.

Anesthesia and Major Surgery: The necessity, or desirability, of withdrawal of a β-blocking therapy prior to major surgery is controversial. Beta-adrenergic receptor blockade impairs the ability of the heart to respond to β-adrenergically mediated reflex stimuli. Although this might be of benefit in preventing arrhythmic response, the risk of excessive myocardial depression during general anesthesia may be enhanced and difficulty in restarting and maintaining the heartbeat has been reported with β-blockers. If treatment is continued, particular care should be taken when using anesthetic agents that depress the myocardium, such as ether, cyclopropane, and trichloroethylene, and it is prudent to use the lowest possible dose of Penbutolol Sulfate. Penbutolol Sulfate like other β-blockers, is a competitive inhibitor of β-receptor agonists, and its effect on the heart can be reversed by cautious administration of such agents (e.g., dobutamine or isoproterenol—see "Overdosage"). Manifestations of excessive vagal tone (e.g., profound bradycardia, hypotension) may be corrected with atropine 1 to 3 mg IV in divided doses.

Diabetes Mellitus and Hypoglycemia: Beta-adrenergic receptor blockade may prevent the appearance of signs and symptoms of acute hypoglycemia, such as tachycardia and blood pressure changes. This is especially important in patients with labile diabetes. Beta-blockade also reduces the release of insulin in response to hyperglycemia; therefore, it may be necessary to adjust the dose of hypoglycemic drugs. Beta-adrenergic blockade may also impair the homeostatic recovery from hypoglycemia may be delayed during treatment with β-adrenergic receptor antagonists.

Thyrotozicosis: Beta-adrenergic blockade may mask certain clinical signs (e.g., tachycardia) of hyperthyrodism. Patients suspected of developing thyrotoxicosis should be managed carefully to avoid abrupt withdrawal of β-adrenergic receptor blockers that might precipitate a thyroid storm.

PRECAUTIONS

Information for Patients: Patients, especially those with evidence of coronary artery insufficiency, should be warned against interruption or discontinuation of Penbutolol Sulfate without the physician's advice. Although cardiac failure rarely occurs in properly selected patients, those being treated with β-adrenergic receptor antagonists should be advised of the symptoms of heart failure and to report such symptoms immediately, should they develop.

Drug Interactions: Penbutolol Sulfate has been used in combination with hydrochlorothiazide in at least 100 patients without unexpected adverse reactions.

In one study, the combination of Penbutolol Sulfate and alcohol increased the number of errors in the eye-hand psychomotor function test.

Penbutolol Sulfate increases the volume of distribution of lidocaine in normal subjects. This could result in a requirement for higher loading doses of lidocaine.

Cimetidine has no effect on the clearance of Penbutolol Sulfate. The major metabolite of Penbutolol Sulfate is a glucuronide, and it has been shown that cimetidine does not inhibit glucoronidation. Synergistic hypotensive effects, bradycardia, and arrhythmias have been reported in some patients receiving β-adrenergic blocking agents when an oral calcium antagonist was added to the treatment regimen.

Generally, Penbutolol Sulfate should not be used in patients receiving catecholamine-depleting drugs.

Risk of Anaphylactic Reaction: While taking beta-blockers, patients with a history of severe anaphylactic reaction to a variety of allergens may be more reactive to repeated challenge, either accidental, diagnostic, or therapeutic. Such patients may be unresponsive to the usual doses of epinephrine used to treat allergic reaction.

Carcinogenesis, Mutagenesis, and Impairment of Fertility: There was no evidence of carcinogenicity observed in a 21-month study in mice or a 2-year study in rats. Mice were given Penbutolol Sulfate in the diet for 18 months at doses up to 395 mg/kg/day (about 500 times the maximum recommended dose of 40 mg in a 50 kg person). Rats were given 141 mg/kg/day for the same length of time. Mice were observed for 3 months and rats for 5.5 to 7 months after termination of treatment before necropsy was performed.

No evidence of mutagenic activity of Penbutolol Sulfate was seen in the *Salmonella* mutagenicity test (Ames test), the point mutation induction test (*Saccharomyces*), and the micronucleus test.

Penbutolol Sulfate had no adverse effects on fertility or general reproductive performance in mice and rats at oral doses up to 172 mg/kg/day.

Pregnancy—Teratogenic Effects: Pregnancy Category C: Teratology studies in rats and rabbits revealed no teratogenic effects related to treatment with Penbutolol Sulfate at oral doses up to 200 mg/kg/day (250 times the maximum recommended human dose). In rabbits, a slight increase in the intrauterine fetal mortality and a reduced 24-hour offspring survival rate were observed in the groups treated with 125 mg/kg/day (156 times the maximum recommended dose) but not in the groups treated with 0.2 and 5 mg (0.25 to 6 times the maximum recommended dose).

There are no adequate and well-controlled studies in pregnant women. Penbutolol Sulfate should be used during pregnancy only if the potential benefit justifies the potential risk to the fetus.

Nonteratogenic Effects: In a perinatal and postnatal study in rats, the pup body weight and pup survival rate were reduced at the highest dose level of 160 mg/kg/day (200 times the maximum recommended dose).

Nursing Mothers: It is not known whether Penbutolol Sulfate is excreted in human milk. Because many drugs are excreted in human milk, caution should be exercised when Penbutolol Sulfate is administered to a nursing woman.

Usage in Children: Safety and effectiveness of Penbutolol Sulfate in children have not been established.

ADVERSE REACTIONS

Penbutolol Sulfate is usually well tolerated in properly selected patients. Most adverse effects observed during clinical trials have been mild and reversible.

Table 1 lists the adverse reactions reported from 4 controlled studies conducted in the United States involving once-a-day administration of Penbutolol Sulfate (at doses ranging from 10 to 120 mg) as monotherapy or in combination with hydrochlorothiazide. Penbutolol Sulfate doses above 40 mg/day are not, however, recommended. The table includes only those events where the prevalence rate in the Penbutolol Sulfate group was at least 1.5%, or where the reaction is of particular interest.

Over a dose range from 10 to 40 mg, once a day, fatigue, nausea, and sexual impotence occurred at a greater frequency as the dose was increased. (See related table).

In a double-blind clinical trial comparing Penbutolol Sulfate (40 mg and greater once a day) and propranolol (40 mg or more twice a day), heart rates of less than 60 beats/min were recorded at least once in 25% of the patients in the group receiving Penbutaolol Sulfate and in 37% of the patients in the propranolol group. Corresponding figures for heart rates of less than 50 beats/min were 1.2% and 6%, respectively. No symptoms associated with bradycardia were reported.

Discontinuations of Penbutolol Sulfate because of adverse reactions have ranged between 2.4% and 6.9% of patients in double-blind, parallel, controlled clinical trials, as compared to 1.8% to 4.1% in the corresponding control groups that were given placebo. The frequency and severity of adverse reactions have not increased during long-term administration of Penbutolol Sulfate. The prevalence

---

◆ RATED THERAPEUTICALLY EQUIVALENT; ◇ THERAPEUTIC EQUIVALENCE UNCONFIRMED; ○ UNRATED

of adverse reactions reported from 4 controlled clinical trials (referred to in Table 1) as reasons for discontinuation of therapy by ≥ 0.5% of the Penbutolol Sulfate group is listed in Table 2. (See related table).

Potential Adverse Effects: In addition, certain adverse effects not listed above have been reported with other β-blocking agents and should also be considered as potential adverse effects of Penbutolol Sulfate.

Central Nervous System: Reversible mental depression progressing to catatonia (an acute syndrome characterized by disorientation for time and place), short-term memory loss, emotional lability, slightly clouded sensorium, and decreased performance (neuropsychometrics).

Cardiovascular: Intensification of AV block (see *"Contraindications"*).

Allergic: Erythematous rash, fever combined with aching and sore throat, laryngospasm, and respiratory distress.

Hematologic: Agranulocytosis, nonthrombocytopenic, and thrombocytopenic purpura.

Gastrointestinal: Mesenteric arterial thrombosis and ischemic colitis.

Miscellaneous: Reversible alopecia and Peyronie's disease. The oculomucocutaneous syndrome associated with the β-blocker practolol has not been reported with Penbutolol Sulfate during investigational use and extensive foreign clinical experience.

OVERDOSAGE

There is no actual experience with Penbutolol Sulfate overdose. The signs and symptoms that would be expected with overdosage of β-adrenergic receptor antagonists are symptomatic bradycardia, hypotension, bronchospasm, and acute cardiac failure. In addition to discontinuation of Penbutolol Sulfate, gastric emptying, and close observation of the patient, the following measures might be considered as appropriate.

Excessive Bradycardia: Administer atropine sulfate to induce vagal blockade. If bradycardia persists, intravenous insoprterenol hydrochloride may be administered cautiously; larger than usual doses may be needed. In refractory cases, the use of a transvenous cardiac pacemaker may be necessary.

Hypotension: Sympathomimetic drug therapy, such as dopamine, dobutamine, or levarterenol, may be considered if hypotension persists despite correction of bradycardia. In refractory cases, administration of glucagon hydrochloride has been reported to be useful.

Bronchospasm: A β-2-agonist or isoproterenol hydrochloride may be administered. Additional therapy with aminophylline may be considered.

Acute Cardiac Failure: Institute conventional therapy immediately. Intravenous administration of dobutamine and glucagon hydrochloride has been reported to be useful.

Heart Block (Second or Third Degree): Isoproterenol hydrochloride or a transvenous cardiac pacemaker may be used.

DOSAGE AND ADMINISTRATION

The usual starting and maintenance dose of Penbutolol Sulfate used alone or in combination with other antihypertensive agents, such as thiazide-type diuretics, is 20 mg given once daily.

Doses of 40 mg and 80 mg have been well-tolerated but have not been shown to give a greater antihypertensive effect. The full effect of a 20- or 40-mg dose is seen by the end of 2 weeks. A dose of 10 mg also lowers blood pressure, but the full effect is not seen for 4 to 6 weeks.

Store at controlled room temperature 15°-30°C (59°-86°F). Keep tightly closed and protect from light.

ANIMAL TOXICOLOGY

Studies in rats indicated that the combination of Penbutolol Sulfate, triamterene, and hydrochlorothiazide (up to 40, 50 and 25 mg/kg, respectively) increased the incidence and severity of renal tubular dilation and regeneration when compared to that in rats treated only with triamterene and hydrochlorothiazide. Dogs administered the same doses of triamterene and hydrochlorothiazide alone and in combination with Penbutolol Sulfate had an increase in serum alkaline phosphatase and serum alanine transferase, but there were no gross or microscopic abnormalities observed. No significant toxicologic findings were observed in rats and dogs treated with a combination of Penbutolol Sulfate and hydrochlorothiazide.

HOW SUPPLIED
TABLETS: 20 MG

BRAND/MANUFACTURER	NDC	SIZE	AWP
○ **BRAND**			
LEVATOL: Reed & Carnrick	00021-4500-15	100s	$92.66

Table 1
ADVERSE REACTIONS DURING CONTROLLED U.S. STUDIES

Body System Experience	Penbutolol Sulfate (N = 628) %	Placebo (N = 212) %	Propranolol (N = 266) %
Body as a Whole			
Asthenia	1.6	0.9	4.9
Pain, chest	2.4	2.8	2.3
Pain, limb	2.4	1.4	1.5
Digestive System			
Diarrhea	3.3	1.9	2.6
Nausea	4.3	0.9	2.3
Dyspepsia	2.7	1.4	5.3
Nervous System			
Dizziness	4.9	2.4	4.2
Fatigue	4.4	1.9	2.6
Headache	7.8	6.1	7.5
Insomnia	1.9	0.9	2.6
Respiratory System			
Cough	2.1	0.5	1.1
Dyspnea	2.1	1.4	3.4
Upper respiratory infection	2.5	3.3	4.9
Skin and Appendages			
Sweating, excessive	1.6	0.5	2.3
Urogenital System			
Impotence, sexual	0.5	0.0	0.8

Table 2
DISCONTINUATIONS DURING CONTROLLED U.S. STUDIES

Body System Experience	Penbutolol Sulfate (N = 628) %	Placebo (N = 212) %	Propranolol (N = 266) %
Body as a Whole			
Asthenia	0.6	0.0	0.4
Pain, chest	0.6	1.4	0.4
Digestive System			
Nausea	0.8	0.0	0.8
Nervous System			
Depression	0.6	0.5	0.8
Dizziness	0.6	0.5	0.8
Fatigue	0.6	0.5	0.0
Headache	0.6	0.5	0.4

➤ SHOWN IN PRODUCT IDENTIFICATION GUIDE

Penetrex SEE ENOXACIN

Penicillamine

PHYSICIANS PLANNING TO USE PENICILLAMINE SHOULD THOROUGHLY FAMILIARIZE THEMSELVES WITH ITS TOXICITY, SPECIAL DOSAGE CONSIDERATIONS, AND THERAPEUTIC BENEFITS. PENICILLAMINE SHOULD NEVER BE USED CASUALLY. EACH PATIENT SHOULD REMAIN CONSTANTLY UNDER THE CLOSE SUPERVISION OF THE PHYSICIAN. PATIENTS SHOULD BE WARNED TO REPORT PROMPTLY ANY SYMPTOMS SUGGESTING TOXICITY.

DESCRIPTION

Penicillamine is a chelating agent used in the treatment of Wilson's disease. It is also used to reduce cystine excretion in cystinuria and to treat patients with severe, active rheumatoid arthritis unresponsive to conventional therapy (see "Indications"). It is 3-mercapto-D-valine. It is a white or practically white, crystalline powder, freely soluble in water, slightly soluble in alcohol, and insoluble in ether, acetone, benzene, and carbon tetrachloride. Although its configuration is D, it is levorotatory as usually measured:

$$[\alpha]25° = -62.5° ± 2° (c = 1, 1N \text{ NaOH}),$$

calculated on a dried basis.

The empirical formula is $C_5H_{11}NO_2S$, giving it a molecular weight of 149.21. It reacts readily with formaldehyde or acetone to form a thiazolidine-carboxylic acid.

Penicillamine for oral administration contains either 125 mg or 250 mg of Penicillamine.

Following is its chemical structure:

$$HS-\overset{\overset{\displaystyle CH_3}{|}}{\underset{\underset{\displaystyle CH_3}{|}}{C}}-\overset{\overset{\displaystyle H}{|}}{\underset{\underset{\displaystyle NH_2}{|}}{C}}-COOH$$

CLINICAL PHARMACOLOGY

Penicillamine is a chelating agent recommended for the removal of excess copper in patients with Wilson's disease. From in vitro studies which indicate that one atom of copper combines with two molecules of Penicillamine, it would appear that one gram of Penicillamine should be followed by the excretion of about 200 milligrams of copper; however, the actual amount excreted is about one percent of this.

Penicillamine also reduces excess cystine excretion in cystinuria. This is done, at least in part, by disulfide interchange between Penicillamine and cystine, resulting in formation of penicillamine-cysteine disulfide, a substance that is much more soluble than cystine and is excreted readily. Penicillamine interferes with the formation of cross-links between tropocollagen molecules and cleaves them when newly formed.

The mechanism of action of Penicillamine in rheumatoid arthritis is unknown although it appears to suppress disease activity. Unlike cytotoxic immunosuppressants, Penicillamine markedly lowers IgM rheumatoid factor but produces no significant depression in absolute levels of serum immunoglobulins. Also unlike cytotoxic immunosuppressants which act on both, Penicillamine in vitro depresses T-cell activity but not B-cell activity.

In vitro Penicillamine dissociates macroglobulins (rheumatoid factor) although the relationship of the activity to its effect in rheumatoid arthritis is not known.

In rheumatoid arthritis, the onset of therapeutic response to Penicillamine may not be seen for two or three months. In those patients who respond, however, the first evidence of suppression of symptoms such as pain, tenderness, and swelling is generally apparent within three months. The optimum duration of therapy has not been determined. If remissions occur, they may last from months to years, but usually require continued treatment (see "Dosage and Administration").

In all patients receiving Penicillamine, it is important that Penicillamine be given on an empty stomach, at least one hour before meals or two hours after meals, and at least one hour apart from any other drug, food, or milk. This permits maximum absorption and reduces the likelihood of inactivation by metal binding in the gastrointestinal tract.

Methodology for determining the bioavailability of Penicillamine is not available; however, Penicillamine is known to be a very soluble substance.

INDICATIONS

Penicillamine is indicated in the treatment of Wilson's disease, cystinuria, and in patients with severe, active rheumatoid arthritis who have failed to respond to an adequate trial of conventional therapy. Available evidence suggests that Penicillamine is not of value in ankylosing spondylitis.

Wilson's Disease: Wilson's disease (hepatolenticular degeneration) results from the interaction of an inherited defect and an abnormality in copper metabolism. The metabolic defect, which is the consequence of the autosomal inheritance of one abnormal gene from each parent, manifests itself in a greater positive copper balance than normal. As a result, copper is deposited in several organs and appears eventually to produce pathologic effects most prominently seen in the brain, where degeneration is widespread; in the liver, where fatty infiltration, inflammation, and hepatocellular damage progress to postnecrotic cirrhosis; in the kidney, where tubular and glomerular dysfunction results; and in the eye, where characteristic corneal copper deposits are known as Kayser-Fleischer rings.

Two types of patients require treatment for Wilson's disease: (1) the symptomatic, and (2) the asymptomatic in whom it can be assumed the disease will develop in the future if the patient is not treated.

Diagnosis, suspected on the basis of family or individual history, physical examination, or a low serum concentration of ceruloplasmin,* is confirmed by the demonstration of Kayser-Fleischer rings or, particularly in the asymptomatic patient, by the quantitative demonstration in a liver biopsy specimen of a concentration of copper in excess of 250 mcg/g dry weight.

Treatment has two objectives:
(1) to minimize dietary intake and absorption of copper.
(2) to promote excretion of copper deposited in tissues.

The first objective is attained by a daily diet that contains no more than one or two milligrams of copper. Such a diet should exclude, most importantly, chocolate, nuts, shellfish, mushrooms, liver, molasses, broccoli, and cereals enriched with copper, and be composed to as great an extent as possible of foods with a low copper content. Distilled or demineralized water should be used if the patient's drinking water contains more than 0.1 mg of copper per liter.

For the second objective, a copper chelating agent is used. In symptomatic patients this treatment usually produces marked neurologic improvement, fading of Kayser-Fleischer rings, and gradual amelioration of hepatic dysfunction and psychic disturbances.

Clinical experience to date suggests that life is prolonged with the above regimen.

Noticeable improvement may not occur for one to three months. Occasionally, neurologic symptoms become worse during initiation of therapy with Penicillamine. Despite this, the drug should not be discontinued permanently, although temporary interruption may result in clinical improvement of the neurological symptoms but it carries an increased risk of developing a sensitivity reaction upon resumption of therapy (see "Warnings").

Treatment of asymptomatic patients has been carried out for over ten years. Symptoms and signs of the disease appear to be prevented indefinitely if daily treatment with Penicillamine can be continued.

Cystinuria: Cystinuria is characterized by excessive urinary excretion of the dibasic amino acids, arginine, lysine, ornithine, and cystine, and the mixed disulfide of cysteine and homocysteine. The metabolic defect that leads to cystinuria is inherited as an autosomal, recessive trait. Metabolism of the affected amino acids is influenced by at least two abnormal factors: (1) defective gastrointestinal absorption and (2) renal tubular dysfunction.

Arginine, lysine, ornithine, and cysteine are soluble substances, readily excreted. There is no apparent pathology connected with their excretion in excessive quantities.

Cystine, however, is so slightly soluble at the usual range of urinary pH that it is not excreted readily, and so crystallizes and forms stones in the urinary tract. Stone formation is the only known pathology in cystinuria.

Normal daily output of cystine is 40 to 80 mg. In cystinuria, output is greatly increased and may exceed 1 g/day. At 500 to 600 mg/day, stone formation is almost certain. When it is more than 300 mg/day, treatment is indicated.

Conventional treatment is directed at keeping urinary cystine diluted enough to prevent stone formation, keeping the urine alkaline enough to dissolve as much cystine as possible, and minimizing cystine production by a diet low in methionine (the major dietary precursor of cystine). Patients must drink enough fluid to keep urine specific gravity below 1.010, take enough alkali to keep urinary pH at 7.5 to 8, and maintain a diet low in methionine. This diet is not recommended in growing children and probably is contraindicated in pregnancy because of its low protein content (see "Precautions").

When these measures are inadequate to control recurrent stone formation Penicillamine may be used as additional therapy. When patients refuse to adhere to conventional treatment, Penicillamine may be a useful substitute. It is capable of keeping cystine excretion to near normal values, thereby hindering stone formation and the serious consequences of pyelonephritis and impaired renal function that develop in some patients.

Bartter and colleagues depict the process by which Penicillamine interacts with cystine to form Penicillamine-cysteine mixed disulfide as:

$$CSSC + PS' \rightleftharpoons CS' + CSSP$$
$$PSSP + CS' \rightleftharpoons PS' + CSSP$$
$$CSSC + PSSP \rightleftharpoons 2 CSSP$$

CSSC = cysteine
CS' = deprotonated cysteine
PSSP = penicillamine
PS' = deprotonated penicillamine sulfhydryl
CSSP = penicillamine-cysteine mixed disulfide

In this process, it is assumed that the deprotonated form of Penicillamine, PS', is the active factor in bringing about the disulfide interchange.

---

* For quantitative test for serum ceruloplasmin see: Morell, A.G.; Windsor, J.; Sternlieb, I.; Scheinberg, I.H.: Measurement of the concentration of ceruloplasmin in serum by determination of its oxidase activity, in *Laboratory Diagnosis of Liver Disease*, F.W. Sunderman; F.W. Sunderman, Jr. (eds.), St. Louis, Warren H. Green, Inc., 1968, pp. 193-195.

Rheumatoid Arthritis: Because Penicillamine can cause severe adverse reactions, its use in rheumatoid arthritis should be restricted to patients who have severe, active disease and who have failed to respond to an adequate trial of conventional therapy. Even then, benefit-to-risk ratio should be carefully considered. Other measures, such as rest, physiotherapy, salicylates, and corticosteroids should be used, when indicated, in conjunction with Penicillamine (see *"Precautions"*).

CONTRAINDICATIONS

Except for the treatment of Wilson's disease or certain cases of cystinuria, use of Penicillamine during pregnancy is contraindicated (see *"Warnings"*).

Although breast milk studies have not been reported in animals or humans, mothers on therapy with Penicillamine should not nurse their infants.

Patients with a history of Penicillamine-related aplastic anemia or agranulocytosis should not be restarted on Penicillamine (see *"Warnings"* and *"Adverse Reactions"*). Because of its potential for causing renal damage, Penicillamine should not be administered to rheumatoid arthritis patients with a history or other evidence of renal insufficiency.

WARNINGS

The use of Penicillamine has been associated with fatalities due to certain diseases such as aplastic anemia, agranulocytosis, thrombocytopenia, Goodpasture's syndrome, and myasthenia gravis.

Because of the potential for serious hematological and renal adverse reactions to occur at any time, routine urinalysis, white and differential blood cell count, hemoglobin determination, and direct platelet count must be done every two weeks for at least the first six months of penicillamine therapy and monthly thereafter. Patients should be instructed to report promptly the development of signs and symptoms of granulocytopenia and/or thrombocytopenia such as fever, sore throat, chills, brusing or bleeding. The above laboratory studies should then be promptly repeated.

Leukopenia and thrombocytopenia have been reported to occur in up to five percent of patients during Penicillamine therapy. Leukopenia is of the granulocytic series and may or may not be associated with an increase in eosinophils. A confirmed reduction in WBC below 3500/mm^3 mandates discontinuance of penicillamine therapy. Thrombocytopenia may be on an idiosyncratic basis, with decreased or absent megakaryocytes in the marrow, when it is part of an aplastic anemia. In other cases the thrombocytopenia is presumably on an immune basis since the number of megakaryocytes in the marrow has been reported to be normal or sometimes increased. The development of a platelet count below 100,000/mm^3 3, even in the absence of clinical bleeding, requires at least temporary cessation of Penicillamine therapy. A progressive fall in either platelet count or WBC in three successive determinations, even though values are still within the normal range, likewise requires at least temporary cessation.

Proteinuria and/or hematuria may develop during therapy and may be warning signs of membranous glomerulopathy which can progress to a nephrotic syndrome. Close observation of these patients is essential. In some patients the proteinuria disappears with continued therapy; in others Penicillamine must be discontinued. When a patient develops proteinuria or hematuria the physician must ascertain whether it is a sign of drug-induced glomerulopathy or is unrelated to penicillamine.

Rheumatoid arthritis patients who develop moderate degrees of proteinuria may be continued cautiously on Penicillamine therapy, provided that quantitative 24-hour urinary protein determinations are obtained at intervals of one to two weeks. Penicillamine dosage should not be increased under these circumstances. Proteinuria which exceeds 1 g/24 hours, or proteinuria which is progressively increasing, requires either discontinuance of the drug or a reduction in the dosage. In some patients, proteinuria has been reported to clear following reduction in dosage.

In rheumatoid arthritis patients, Penicillamine should be discontinued if unexplained gross hematuria or persistent microscopic hematuria develops.

In patients with Wilson's disease or cystinuria the risks of continued Penicillamine therapy in patients manifesting potentially serious urinary abnormalities must be weighed against the expected therapeutic benefits.

When Penicillamine is used in cystinuria, an annual x-ray for renal stones is advised. Cystine stones form rapidly, sometimes in six months.

Up to one year or more may be required for any urinary abnormalities to disappear after Penicillamine has been discontinued.

Because of rare reports of intrahepatic cholestasis and toxic hepatitis, liver function tests are recommended every six months for the duration of therapy.

Goodpasture's syndrome has occurred rarely. The development of abnormal urinary findings associated with hemoptysis and pulmonary infiltrates on x-ray requires immediate cessation of Penicillamine.

Obliterative bronchiolitis has been reported rarely. The patient should be cautioned to report immediately pulmonary symptoms such as exertional dyspnea, unexplained cough or wheezing. Pulmonary function studies should be considered at that time.

Myasthenic syndrome sometimes progressing to myasthenia gravis has been reported. Ptosis and diplopia, with weakness of the extraocular muscles, are often early signs of myasthenia. In the majority of cases, symptoms of myasthenia have receded after withdrawal of penicillamine.

Most of the various forms of pemphigus have occurred during treatment with Penicillamine. Pemphigus vulgaris and pemphigus foliaceus are reported most frequently, usually as a late complication of therapy. The seborrhea-like characteristics of pemphigus foliaceus may obscure an early diagnosis. When pemphigus is suspected, Penicillamine should be discontinued. Treatment has consisted of high doses of corticosteroids alone or, in some cases, concomitantly with an immuno-

suppressant. Treatment may be required for only a few weeks or months, but may need to be continued for more than a year.

Once instituted for Wilson's disease or cystinuria, treatment with Penicillamine should, as a rule, be continued on a daily basis. Interruptions for even a few days have been followed by sensitivity reactions after reinstitution of therapy.

Use in Pregnancy: Penicillamine has been shown to be teratogenic in rats when given in doses 6 times higher than the highest dose recommended for human use. Skeletal defects, cleft palates and fetal toxicity (resorptions) have been reported.

There are no controlled studies on the use of Penicillamine in pregnant women. Although normal outcomes have been reported, characteristic congenital cutis laxa and associated birth defects have been reported in infants born of mothers who received therapy with Penicillamine during pregnancy. Penicillamine should be used in women of childbearing potential only when the expected benefits outweigh the possible hazards. Women on therapy with Penicillamine who are of childbearing potential should be apprised of this risk, advised to report promptly any missed menstrual periods or other indications of possible pregnancy, and followed closely for early recognition of pregnancy.

Wilson's Disease: Reported experience[*] shows that continued treatment with Penicillamine throughout pregnancy protects the mother against relapse of the Wilson's disease, and that discontinuation of Penicillamine has deleterious effects on the mother.

If Penicillamine is administered during pregnancy to patients with Wilson's disease, it is recommended that the daily dosage be limited to 1 g. If cesarean section is planned, the daily dosage should be limited to 250 mg during the last six weeks of pregnancy and postoperatively until wound healing is complete.

Cystinuria: If possible, Penicillamine should not be given during pregnancy to women with cystinuria (see *"Contraindications"*). There are reports of women with cystinuria on therapy with Penicillamine who gave birth to infants with generalized connective tissue defects who died following abdominal surgery. If stones continue to form in these patients, the benefits of therapy to the mother must be evaluated against the risk to the fetus.

Rheumatoid Arthritis: Penicillamine should not be administered to rheumatoid arthritis patients who are pregnant (see *"Contraindications"*) and should be discontinued promptly in patients in whom pregnancy is suspected or diagnosed.

There is a report that a woman with rheumatoid arthritis treated with less than one gram a day of Penicillamine during pregnancy gave birth (cesarean delivery) to an infant with growth retardation, flattened face with broad nasal bridge, low set ears, short neck with loose skin folds, and unusually lax body skin.

PRECAUTIONS

Some patients may experience drug fever, a marked febrile response to Penicillamine, usually in the second to third week following initiation of therapy. Drug fever may sometimes be accompanied by a macular cutaneous eruption.

In the case of drug fever in patients with Wilson's disease or cystinuria, Penicillamine should be temporarily discontinued until the reaction subsides. Then Penicillamine should be reinstituted with a small dose that is gradually increased until the desired dosage is attained. Systemic steroid therapy may be necessary, and is usually helpful, in such patients in whom toxic reactions develop a second or third time.

In the case of drug fever in rheumatoid arthritis patients, because other treatments are available, Penicillamine should be discontinued and another therapeutic alternative tried since experience indicates that the febrile reaction will recur in a very high percentage of patients upon readministration of Penicillamine.

The skin and mucous membranes should be observed for allergic reactions. Early and late rashes have occurred. Early rash occurs during the first few months of treatment and is more common. It is usually a generalized pruritic, erythematous, maculopapular or morbilliform rash and resembles the allergic rash seen with other drugs. Early rash usually disappears within days after stopping Penicillamine and seldom recurs when the drug is restarted at a lower dosage. Pruritus and early rash may often be controlled by the concomitant administration of antihistamines. Less commonly, a late rash may be seen, usually after six months or more of treatment, and requires discontinuation of Penicillamine. It is usually on the trunk, is accompanied by intense pruritus, and is usually unresponsive to topical corticosteroid therapy. Late rash may take weeks to disappear after Penicillamine is stopped and usually recurs if the drug is restarted.

The appearance of a drug eruption accompanied by fever, arthralgia, lymphadenopathy or other allergic manifestations usually requires discontinuation of Penicillamine.

Certain patients will develop a positive antinuclear antibody (ANA) test and some of these may show a lupus erythematosus-like syndrome similar to drug-induced lupus associated with other drugs. The lupus erythematosus-like syndrome is not associated with hypocomplementemia and may be present without nephropathy. The development of a positive ANA test does not mandate discontinuance of the drug; however, the physician should be alerted to the possibility that a lupus erythematosus-like syndrome may develop in the future.

Some patients may develop oral ulcerations which in some cases have the appearance of aphthous stomatitis. The stomatitis usually recurs on rechallenge but often clears on a lower dosage. Although rare, cheilosis, glossitis and gingivostomatitis have also been reported. These oral lesions are frequently dose-related and may preclude further increase in Penicillamine dosage or require discontinuation of the drug.

* Scheinberg, I.H., Sternlieb, I.: N. Engl. J. Med. 293: 1300-1302, Dec. 18, 1975.

Hypogeusia (a blunting or diminution in taste perception) has occurred in some patients. This may last two to three months or more and may develop into a total loss of taste; however, it is usually self-limited despite continued Penicillamine treatment. Such taste impairment is rare in patients with Wilson's disease.

Penicillamine should not be used in patients who are receiving concurrently gold therapy, antimalarial or cytotoxic drugs, oxyphenbutazone or phenylbutazone because these drugs are also associated with similar serious hematologic and renal adverse reactions. Patients who have had gold salt therapy discontinued due to a major toxic reaction may be at greater risk of serious adverse reactions with Penicillamine but not necessarily of the same type.

Patients who are allergic to penicillin may theoretically have cross-sensitivity to Penicillamine. The possibility of reactions from contamination of Penicillamine by trace amounts of penicillin has been eliminated now that Penicillamine is being produced synthetically rather than as a degradation product of penicillin.

Because of their dietary restrictions, patients with Wilson's disease and cystinuria should be given 25 mg/day of pyridoxine during therapy, since Penicillamine increases the requirement for this vitamin. Patients also may receive benefit from a multivitamin preparation, although there is no evidence that deficiency of any vitamin other than pyridoxine is associated with Penicillamine. In Wilson's disease, multivitamin preparations must be copper-free.

Rheumatoid arthritis patients whose nutrition is impaired should also be given a daily supplement of pyridoxine. Mineral supplements should not be given, since they may block the response to Penicillamine.

Iron deficiency may develop, especially in children and in menstruating women. In Wilson's disease, this may be a result of adding the effects of the low copper diet, which is probably also low in iron, and the Penicillamine to the effects of blood loss or growth. In cystinuria, a low methionine diet may contribute to iron deficiency, since it is necessarily low in protein. If necessary, iron may be given in short courses, but a period of two hours should elapse between administration of Penicillamine and iron, since orally administered iron has been shown to reduce the effects of Penicillamine.

Penicillamine causes an increase in the amount of soluble collagen. In the rat this results in inhibition of normal healing and also a decrease in tensile strength of intact skin. In man this may be the cause of increased skin friability at sites especially subject to pressure or trauma, such as shoulders, elbows, knees, toes, and buttocks. Extravasations of blood may occur and may appear as purpuric areas, with external bleeding if the skin is broken, or as vesicles containing dark blood. Neither type is progressive. There is no apparent association with bleeding elsewhere in the body and no associated coagulation defect has been found. Therapy with Penicillamine may be continued in the presence of these lesions. They may not recur if dosage is reduced. Other reported effects probably due to the action of Penicillamine on collagen are excessive wrinkling of the skin and development of small, white papules at venipuncture and surgical sites.

The effects of Penicillamine on collagen and elastin make it advisable to consider a reduction in dosage to 250 mg/day, when surgery is contemplated. Reinstitution of full therapy should be delayed until wound healing is complete.

Carcinogenesis: Long-term animal carcinogenicity studies have not been done with Penicillamine. There is a report that five of ten autoimmune disease-prone NZB hybrid mice developed lymphocytic leukemia after 6 months' intraperitoneal treatment with a dose of 400 mg/kg Penicillamine 5 days per week.

Nursing Mothers: See *"Contraindications"*.

Usage in Children: The efficacy of Penicillamine in juvenile rheumatoid arthritis has not been established.

ADVERSE REACTIONS

Penicillamine is a drug with a high incidence of untoward reactions, some of which are potentially fatal. Therefore, it is mandatory that patients receiving Penicillamine therapy remain under close medical supervision throughout the period of drug administration (see *"Warnings"* and *"Precautions"*).

Reported incidences (%) for the most commonly occurring adverse reactions in rheumatoid arthritis patients are noted, based on 17 representative clinical trials reported in the literature (1270 patients).

Allergic: Generalized pruritus, early and late rashes (5%), pemphigus (see *"Warnings"*), and drug eruptions which may be accompanied by fever, arthralgia, or lymphadenopathy have occurred (see *"Warnings"* and *"Precautions"*). Some patients may show a lupus erythematosus like syndrome similar to drug-induced lupus produced by other pharmacological agents (see *"Precautions"*).

Urticaria and exfoliative dermatitis have occurred.

Thyroiditis has been reported; hypoglycemia in association with anti-insulin antibodies has been reported. These reactions are extremely rare.

Some patients may develop a migratory polyarthralgia, often with objective synovitis (see *"Dosage and Administration"*).

Gastrointestinal: Anorexia, epigastric pain, nausea, vomiting, or occasional diarrhea may occur (17%).

Isolated cases of reactivated peptic ulcer have occurred, as have hepatic dysfunction and pancreatitis. Intrahepatic cholestasis and toxic hepatitis have been reported rarely. There have been a few reports of increased serum alkaline phosphatase, lactic dehydrogenase, and positive cephalin flocculation and thymol turbidity tests.

Some patients may report a blunting, diminution, or total loss of taste perception (12%); or may develop oral ulcerations. Although rare, cheilosis, glossitis, and gingivostomatitis have been reported (see *"Precautions"*).

Gastrointestinal side effects are usually reversible following cessation of therapy.

Hematological: Penicillamine can cause bone marrow depression (see *"Warnings"*). Leukopenia (2%) and thrombocytopenia (4%) have occurred. Fatalities have been reported as a result of thrombocytopenia, agranulocytosis, aplastic anemia, and sideroblastic anemia.

Thrombotic thrombocytopenic purpura, hemolytic anemia, red cell aplasia, monocytosis, leukocytosis, eosinophilia, and thrombocytosis have also been reported.

Renal: Patients on Penicillamine therapy may develop proteinuria (6%) and/or hematuria which, in some, may progress to the development of the nephrotic syndrome as a result of an immune complex membraneous glomerulopathy (see *"Warnings"*).

Central Nervous System: Tinnitus, optic neuritis and peripheral sensory and motor neuropathies (including polyradiculoneuropathy, i.e., Guillain-Barre syndrome) have been reported. Muscular weakness may or may not occur with the peripheral neuropathies. Visual and psychic disturbances have been reported.

Neuromuscular: Myasthenia gravis (see *"Warnings"*).

Other: Adverse reactions that have been reported rarely include thrombophlebitis; hyperpyrexia (see *"Precautions"*); falling hair or alopecia; lichen planus; polymyositis; dermatomyositis; mammary hyperplasia; elastosis perforans serpiginosa; toxic epidermal necrolysis; anetoderma (cutaneous macular atrophy); and Goodpasture's syndrome, a severe and ultimately fatal glomerulonephritis associated with intra-alveolar hemorrhage (see *"Warnings"*). Fatal renal vasculitis has also been reported. Allergic alveolitis, obliterative bronchiolitis, interstitial pneumonitis and pulmonary fibrosis have been reported in patients with severe rheumatoid arthritis, some of whom were receiving penicillamine. Bronchial asthma also has been reported.

Increased skin friability, excessive wrinkling of skin, and development of small white papules at venipuncture and surgical sites have been reported (see *"Precautions"*).

The chelating action of the drug may cause increased excretion of other heavy metals such as zinc, mercury and lead. There have been reports associating Penicillamine with leukemia. However, circumstances involved in these reports are such that a cause and effect relationship to the drug has not been established.

DOSAGE AND ADMINISTRATION

In all patients receiving penicillamine, it is important that Penicillamine be given on an empty stomach, at least one hour before meals or two hours after meals, and at least one hour apart from any other drug, food, or milk. Because Penicillamine increases the requirement for pyridoxine, patients may require a daily supplement of pyridoxine (see *"Precautions"*).

Wilson's Disease: Optimal dosage can be determined by measurement of urinary copper excretion and the determination of free copper in the serum. The urine must be collected in copper-free glassware, and should be quantitatively analyzed for copper before and soon after initiation of therapy with Penicillamine.

Determination of 24-hour urinary copper excretion is of greatest value in the first week of therapy with Penicillamine. In the absence of any drug reaction, a dose between 0.75 and 1.5 g that results in an initial 24-hour cupriuresis of over 2 mg should be continued for about three months, by which time the most reliable method of monitoring maintenance treatment is the determination of free copper in the serum. This equals the difference between quantitatively determined total copper and ceruloplasmin-copper. Adequately treated patients will usually have less than 10 mcg free copper/dL of serum. It is seldom necessary to exceed a dosage of 2 g/day. If the patient is intolerant to therapy with Penicillamine alternative treatment is trientine hydrochloride.

In patients who cannot tolerate as much as 1 g/day initially, initiating dosage with 250 mg/day, and increasing gradually to the requisite amount, gives closer control of the effects of the drug and may help to reduce the incidence of adverse reactions.

Cystinuria: It is recommended that Penicillamine be used along with conventional therapy. By reducing urinary cystine, it decreases crystalluria and stone formation. In some instances, it has been reported to decrease the size of, and even to dissolve, stones already formed.

The usual dosage of Penicillamine in the treatment of cystinuria is 2 g/day for adults, with a range of 1 to 4 g/day. For children, dosage can be based on 30 mg/kg/day. The total daily amount should be divided into four doses. If four equal doses are not feasible, give the larger portion at bedtime. If adverse reactions necessitate a reduction in dosage, it is important to retain the bedtime dose.

Initiating dosage with 250 mg/day, and increasing gradually to the requisite amount, gives closer control of the effects of the drug and may help to reduce the incidence of adverse reactions.

In addition to taking Penicillamine patients should drink copiously. It is especially important to drink about a pint of fluid at bedtime and another pint once during the night when urine is more concentrated and more acid than during the day. The greater the fluid intake, the lower the required dosage of Penicillamine.

Dosage must be individualized to an amount that limits cystine excretion to 100-200 mg/day in those with no history of stones, and below 100 mg/day in those who have had stone formation and/or pain. Thus, in determining dosage, the inherent tubular defect, the patient's size, age, and rate of growth, and his diet and water intake all must be taken into consideration.

◆ RATED THERAPEUTICALLY EQUIVALENT; ◇ THERAPEUTIC EQUIVALENCE UNCONFIRMED; ○ UNRATED

The standard nitroprusside cyanide test has been reported useful as a qualitative measure of the effective dose[*] Add 2 mL of freshly prepared 5 percent sodium cyanide to 5 mL of a 24-hour aliquot of protein-free urine and let stand ten minutes. Add 5 drops of freshly prepared 5 percent sodium nitroprusside and mix. Cystine will turn the mixture magneta. If the result is negative, it can be assumed that cystine excretion is less than 100 mg/g creatinine.

Although Penicillamine is rarely excreted unchanged, it also will turn the mixture magneta. If there is any question as to which substance is causing the reaction, a ferric chloride test can be done to eliminate doubt: Add 3 percent ferric chloride dropwise to the urine. Penicillamine will turn the urine an immediate and quickly fading blue. Cystine will not produce any change in appearance.

Rheumatoid Arthritis: The principal rule of treatment with Penicillamine in rheumatoid arthritis is patience. The onset of therapeutic response is typically delayed. Two or three months may be required before the first evidence of a clinical response is noted (see *"Clinical Pharmacology"*).

When treatment with Penicillamine has been interrupted because of adverse reactions or other reasons, the drug should be reintroduced cautiously by starting with a lower dosage and increasing slowly.

Initial Therapy: The currently recommended dosage regimen in rheumatoid arthritis begins with a single daily dose of 125 mg or 250 mg which is thereafter increased at one to three month intervals, by 125 mg or 250 mg/day, as patient response and tolerance indicate. If a satisfactory remission of symptoms is achieved, the dose associated with the remission should be continued (see *"Maintenance Therapy"*). If there is no improvement and there are no signs of potentially serious toxicity after two to three months of treatment with doses of 500-750 mg/day, increases of 250 mg/day at two to three month intervals may be continued until a satisfactory remission occurs (see *"Maintenance Therapy"*) or signs of toxicity develop (see *"Warnings"* and *"Precautions"*). If there is no discernible improvement after three to four months of treatment with 1000 to 1500 mg of Penicillamine/day, it may be assumed the patient will not respond and Penicillamine should be discontinued.

Maintenance Therapy: The maintenance dosage of Penicillamine must be individualized, and may require adjustment during the course of treatment. Many patients respond satisfactorily to a dosage within the 500-750 mg/day range. Some need less.

Changes in maintenance dosage levels may not be reflected clinically or in the erythrocyte sedimentation rate for two to three months after each dosage adjustment.

Some patients will subsequently require an increase in the maintenance dosage to achieve maximal disease suppression. In those patients who do respond, but who evidence incomplete suppression of their disease after the first six to nine months of treatment, the daily dosage of Penicillamine may be increased by 125 mg or 250 mg/day at three-month intervals. It is unusual in current practice to employ a dosage in excess of 1 g/day, but up to 1.5 g/day has sometimes been required.

Management of Exacerbations: During the course of treatment some patients may experience an exacerbation of disease activity following an initial good response. These may be self-limited and can subside within twelve weeks. They are usually controlled by the addition of non-steroidal anti-inflammatory drugs, and only if the patient has demonstrated a true "escape" phenomenon (as evidenced by failure of the flare to subside within this time period) should an increase in the maintenance dose ordinarily be considered.

In the rheumatoid patient, migratory polyarthralgia due to penicillamine is extremely difficult to differentiate from an exacerbation of the rheumatoid arthritis. Discontinuance or a substantial reduction in dosage of Penicillamine for up to several weeks will usually determine which of these processes is responsible for the arthralgia.

Duration of Therapy: The optimum duration of therapy with Penicillamine in rheumatoid arthritis has not been determined. If the patient has been in remission for six months or more, a gradual, stepwise dosage reduction in decrements of 125 mg or 250 mg/day at approximately three month intervals may be attempted.

Concomitant Drug Therapy: Penicillamine should not be used in patients who are receiving gold therapy, antimalarial or cytotoxic drugs, oxyphenbutazone, or phenylbutazone (see *"Precautions"*). Other measures, such as salicylates, other non-steroidal anti-inflammatory drugs, or systemic corticosteroids, may be continued when Penicillamine is initiated. After improvement commences, analgesic and anti-inflammatory drugs may be slowly discontinued as symptoms permit. Steroid withdrawal must be done gradually, and many months of treatment with Penicillamine may be required before steroids can be completely eliminated.

Dosage Frequency: Based on clinical experience dosages up to 500 mg/day can be given as a single daily dose. Dosages in excess of 500 mg/day should be administered in divided doses.

Storage: Keep container tightly closed.

---

[*] Lotz., M., Potts, J.T. and Bartter, F.C.: Brit. Med. J. 2:521, Aug. 28, 1965 (in Medical Memoranda).

HOW SUPPLIED
CAPSULE: 125 MG

BRAND/MANUFACTURER	NDC	SIZE	AWP
BRAND			
CUPRIMINE: Merck	00006-0672-68	100s	$62.88

CAPSULE: 250 MG

BRAND/MANUFACTURER	NDC	SIZE	AWP
BRAND			
CUPRIMINE: Merck	00006-0602-68	100s	$89.76

TABLETS: 250 MG

BRAND/MANUFACTURER	NDC	SIZE	AWP
BRAND			
DEPEN: Wallace	00037-4401-01	100s	$135.74

Penicillin G Benzathine

DESCRIPTION

Sterile Penicillin G Benzathine suspension is prepared by the reaction of dibenzylethylene diamine with two molecules of Penicillin G. It is chemically designated as 3,3-dimethyl-7-oxo-6- (2-phenylacetamido)-4-thia-1-azabicyclo [3.2.0]heptane-2-carboxylic acid compound with N,N'-dibenzylethylenediamine (2:1), tetrahydrate.

It is available for deep, intramuscular injection. It contains sterile Penicillin G Benzathine in aqueous suspension with sodium citrate buffer and, as w/v, approximately 0.5% lecithin, 0.6% carboxymethylcellulose, 0.6% povidone, 0.1% methylparaben, and 0.01% propylparaben. It occurs as a white, crystalline powder and is very slightly soluble in water and sparingly soluble in alcohol.

Penicillin G Benzathine in the multiple-dose vial formulation, disposable syringe formulation and TUBEX formulation is viscous and opaque. The multiple-dose vial formulation contains the equivalent of 300,000 units per mL of Penicillin G as the Benzathine salt. The disposable syringe formulation is available in a 4 mL size containing the equivalent of 2,400,000 units of Penicillin G as the Benzathine salt. The TUBEX formulation is available in 1 mL and 2 mL TUBEX Sterile Cartridge-Needle Units containing the equivalent of 600,000 units and 1,200,000 units respectively of Penicillin G as the Benzathine salt. Read *"Contraindications," "Warnings," "Precautions"* and *"Dosage and Administration"* sections prior to use.

Following is its chemical structure:

CLINICAL PHARMACOLOGY
GENERAL

Penicillin G Benzathine has an extremely low solubility and, thus, the drug is slowly released from intramuscular injection sites. The drug is hydrolyzed to Penicillin G. This combination of hydrolysis and slow absorption results in blood serum levels much lower but much more prolonged than other parenteral penicillins.

Intramuscular administration of 300,000 units of Penicillin G Benzathine in adults results in blood levels of 0.03 to 0.05 units per mL, which are maintained for 4 to 5 days. Similar blood levels may persist for 10 days following administration of 600,000 units and for 14 days following administration of 1,200,000 units. Blood concentrations of 0.003 units per mL may still be detectable 4 weeks following administration of 1,200,000 units.

Approximately 60% of Penicillin G is bound to serum protein. The drug is distributed throughout the body tissues in widely varying amounts. Highest levels are found in the kidneys with lesser amounts in the liver, skin, and intestines. Penicillin G penetrates into all other tissues and the spinal fluid to a lesser degree. With normal kidney function, the drug is excreted rapidly by tubular excretion. In neonates and young infants and in individuals with impaired kidney function, excretion is considerably delayed.

MICROBIOLOGY

Penicillin G exerts a bactericidal action against Penicillin-susceptible microorganisms during the stage of active multiplication. It acts through the inhibition of biosynthesis of cell-wall mucopeptide. It is not active against the Penicillinase-producing bacteria, which include many strains of staphylococci.

The following *in vitro* data are available, but their clinical significance is unknown. Penicillin G exerts high *in vitro* activity against staphylococci (except penicillinase-producing strains), streptococci (Groups A, C, G, H, L, and M), and pneumococci. Other organisms susceptible to Penicillin G are *Neisseria gonorrhoeae, Corynebacterium diphtheriae, Bacillus anthracis,* Clostridia species, *Actinomyces bovis, Streptobacillus moniliformis, Listeria monocytogenes,* and Leptospira species. *Treponema pallidum* is extremely susceptible to the bactericidal action of Penicillin G.

Susceptibility Test: If the Kirby-Bauer method of disc susceptibility is used, a 20-unit Penicillin disc should give a zone greater than 28 mm when tested against a Penicillin-susceptibile bacterial strain.

INDICATIONS AND USAGE

Intramuscular Penicillin G Benzathine is indicated in the treatment of infections due to Penicillin-G-sensitive microorganisms that are susceptible to the low and very prolonged serum levels common to this particular dosage form. Therapy should be guided by bacteriological studies (including sensitivity tests) and by clinical response.

The following infections will usually respond to adequate dosage of intramuscular Penicillin G Benzathine:

Mild-to-moderate infections of the upper respiratory tract due to susceptible streptococci.

Venereal Infections: Syphilis, yaws, bejel, and pinta.

Medical Conditions in Which Penicillin G Benzathine Therapy Is Indicated as Prophylaxis:

Rheumatic Fever and/or Chorea: Prophylaxis with Penicillin G Benzathine has proven effective in preventing recurrence of these conditions. It has also been used as follow-up prophylactic therapy for rheumatic heart disease and acute glomerulonephritis.

UNLABELED USES

Penicillin G Benzathine is used alone or as an adjunct in the treatment of Lyme arthritis (Borreli burgdorger infections).

CONTRAINDICATIONS

A history of a previous hypersensitivity reaction to any of the penicillins is a contraindication.

Do not inject into or near an artery or nerve.

WARNINGS

Penicillin G Benzathine should only be prescribed for the indications listed in this insert.

Serious and occasionally fatal hypersensitivity (anaphylactoid) reactions have been reported in patients receiving Penicillin. Although anaphylaxis is more frequent following parenteral administration, it has occurred in patients on oral penicillins. These reactions are more apt to occur in individuals with a history of sensitivity to multiple allergens.

There are reports of patients with a history of Penicillin hypersensitivity reactions who experienced severe hypersensitivity reactions when treated with a cephalosporin. Before therapy with a Penicillin, careful inquiry should be made about previous hypersensitivity reactions to Penicillins, cephalosporins, and other allergens. If an allergic reaction occurs, the drug should be discontinued and appropriate therapy should be instituted. Serious anaphylactoid reactions require immediate emergency treatment with epinephrine. Oxygen, intravenous steroids, airway management, including intubation, should also be administered as indicated.

Inadvertent intravascular administration, including inadvertent direct intra-arterial injection or injection immediately adjacent to arteries, of Penicillin G Benzathine and other Penicillin preparations has resulted in severe neurovascular damage, including transverse myelitis with permanent paralysis, gangrene requiring amputation of digits and more proximal portions of extremities, and necrosis and sloughing at and surrounding the injection site. Such severe effects have been reported following injections into the buttock, thigh, and deltoid areas. Other serious complications of suspected intravascular administration which have been reported include immediate pallor, mottling, or cyanosis of the extremity both distal and proximal to the injection site, followed by bleb formation; severe edema requiring anterior and/or posterior compartment fasciotomy in the lower extremity. The above-described severe effects and complications have most often occurred in infants and small children. Prompt consultation with an appropriate specialist is indicated if any evidence of compromise of the blood supply occurs at, proximal to, or distal to the site of injection.[1-9] See *"Contraindications," "Precautions,"* and *"Dosage and Administration"* sections. Quadriceps femoris fibrosis and atrophy have been reported following repeated intramuscular injections of Penicillin preparations into the anterolateral thigh.

Injection into or near a nerve may result in permanent neurological damage.

PRECAUTIONS

GENERAL

Penicillin should be used with caution in individuals with histories of significant allergies and/or asthma.

Care should be taken to avoid intravenous or intra-arterial administration, or injection into or near major peripheral nerves or blood vessels, since such injection may produce neurovascular damage. See *"Contraindications", "Warnings,"* and *"Dosage and Administration"* sections.

Prolonged use of antibiotics may promote the overgrowth of nonsusceptible organisms, including fungi. Should superinfection occur, appropriate measures should be taken.

LABORATORY TESTS

In streptococcal infections, therapy must be sufficient to eliminate the organism; otherwise, the sequelae of streptococcal disease may occur. Cultures should be taken following completion of treatment to determine whether streptococci have been eradicated.

DRUG INTERACTIONS

Tetracycline, a bacteriostatic antibiotic, may antagonize the bactericidal effect of Penicillin, and concurrent use of these drugs should be avoided.

Concurrent administration of Penicillin and probenecid increases and prolongs serum Penicillin levels by decreasing the apparent volume of distribution and slowing the rate of excretion by competitively inhibiting renal tubular secretion of Penicillin.

PREGNANCY CATEGORY B

Reproduction studies performed in the mouse, rat, and rabbit have revealed no evidence of impaired fertility or harm to the fetus due to Penicillin G. Human experience with the Penicillins during pregnancy has not shown any positive evidence of adverse effects on the fetus. There are, however, no adequate and well-controlled studies in pregnant women showing conclusively that harmful effects of these drugs on the fetus can be excluded. Because animal reproduction studies are not always predictive of human response, this drug should be used during pregnancy only if clearly needed.

NURSING MOTHERS

Soluble Penicillin G is excreted in breast milk. Caution should be exercised when Penicillin G Benzathine is administered to a nursing woman.

CARCINOGENESIS, MUTAGENESIS, IMPAIRMENT OF FERTILITY

No long-term animal studies have been conducted with this drug.

PEDIATRIC USE

See *"Indications and Usage"* and *"Dosage and Administration".*

ADVERSE REACTIONS

As with other Penicillins, untoward reactions of the sensitivity phenomena are likely to occur, particularly in individuals who have previously demonstrated hypersensitivity to Penicillins or in those with a history of allergy, asthma, hay fever, or urticaria.

As with other treatments for syphilis, the Jarisch-Herxheimer reaction has been reported.

The following have been reported with parenteral Penicillin G:

General: Hypersensitivity reactions including the following: skin eruptions (maculopapular to exfoliative dermatitis), urticaria, laryngeal edema, fever, eosinophilia; other serum-sicknesslike reactions (including chills, fever, edema, arthralgia, and prostration); anaphylaxis. Note: Urticaria, other skin rashes, and serum-sicknesslike reactions may be controlled with antihistamines and, if necessary, systemic corticosteroids.

Whenever such reactions occur, Penicillin G should be discontinued unless, in the opinion of the physician, the condition being treated is life-threatening and amenable only to therapy with Penicillin G.

Serious anaphylactic reactions require the immediate use of epinephrine, oxygen, and intravenous steroids.

Hematologic: Hemolytic anemia, leukopenia, thrombocytopenia.

Neurologic: Neuropathy.

Urogenital: Nephropathy.

OVERDOSAGE

Penicillin in overdosage has the potential to cause neuromuscular hyperirritability or convulsive seizures.

DOSAGE AND ADMINISTRATION

STREPTOCOCCAL (GROUP A) UPPER-RESPIRATORY INFECTIONS (For example, pharyngitis)

Adults—a single injection of 1,200,000 units; older children—a single injection of 900,000 units; infants and children (under 60 lbs.)—300,000 to 600,000 units.

SYPHILIS

Primary, secondary, and latent—2,400,000 (1 dose). Late (tertiary and neurosyphilis)—2,400,000 at 7-day intervals for three doses.

Congenital—under 2 years of age: 50,000 units/kg/body weight; ages 2-12 years: adjust dosage based on adult dosage schedule.

—1,200,000 (1 injection).

Following an acute attack Penicillin G Benzathine (parenteral) may be given in doses of 1,200,000 units once a month or 600,000 units every 2 weeks.

Administer by DEEP INTRAMUSCULAR INJECTION in the upper, outer quadrant of the buttock. In infants and small children, the midlateral aspect of the thigh may be preferable. When doses are repeated, vary the injection site. When using the multiple-dose vial:

After selection of the proper site and insertion of the needle into the selected muscle, aspirate by pulling back on the plunger. While maintaining negative pressure for 2-3 seconds, carefully observe the barrel of the syringe immediately proximal to the needle hub for appearance of blood or any discoloration. Blood or "typical blood color" may *not* be seen if a blood vessel has been entered—only a mixture of blood and Penicillin G Benzathine. The appearance of any discoloration is reason to withdraw the needle and discard the syringe. If it is elected to inject at another site, a new syringe and needle should be used. If no blood or discoloration appears, inject the contents of the syringe slowly. Discontinue delivery of the dose if the subject complains of severe immediate pain at the injection site or if in infants and young children symptoms or signs occur suggesting onset of severe pain.

When using the TUBEX cartridge:

The TUBEX cartridge for this product incorporates several features that are designed to facilitate the visualization of blood on aspiration if a blood vessel is inadvertently entered.

The design of this cartridge is such that blood which enters its needle will be quickly visualized as a red or dark-colored "spot." This "spot" will appear on the barrel of the glass cartridge immediately proximal to the blue hub. The TUBEX is designed with two orientation marks, in order to determine where the 'spot' can be seen. First insert and secure the cartridge in the TUBEX injector in the usual fashion. Locate the yellow rectangle at the base of the blue hub. This yellow rectangle is aligned with the blood visualization "spot." An imaginary straight line, drawn from this yellow rectangle to the shoulder of the glass cartridge, will point to the area on the cartridge where the "spot" can be visualized. When the needle cover is removed, a second yellow rectangle will be visible. The second yellow rectangle is also aligned with the blood visualization "spot" to assist the operator in locating this "spot." If the 2mL metal or plastic syringe is used, the glass cartridge should be rotated by turning the plunger of the syringe clockwise until the yellow rectangle is visualized. If the 1 mL metal syringe is used, it will not be possible to continue to rotate the glass cartridge clockwise once it is properly engaged and fully threaded; it can, however, then be rotated counter-clockwise as far as necessary to properly orient the yellow rectangles and locate the observation area. (In this same area in some cartridges, a dark spot may sometimes be visualized prior to injection. This is the proximal end of the needle and does not represent a foreign body in, or other abnormality of, the suspension.)

Thus, before the needle is inserted into the selected muscle, it is important for the operator to orient the yellow rectangle so that any blood which may enter after needle insertion and during aspiration can be visualized in the area on the cartridge where it will appear and not be obscured by any obstructions.

After selection of the proper site and insertion of the needle into the selected muscle, aspirate by pulling back on the plunger. While maintaining negative pressure for 2 to 3 seconds, carefully observe the barrel of the cartridge in the area previously identified (see above) for the appearance of a red or dark-colored "spot."

Blood or "typical blood color" may *not* be seen if a blood vessel has been entered—only a mixture of blood and Penicillin G Benzathine. The appearance of any discoloration is reason to withdraw the needle and discard the glass TUBEX cartridge. If it is elected to inject at another site, a new cartridge should be used. If no blood or discoloration appears, inject the contents of the cartridge slowly. Discontinue delivery of the dose if the subject complains of severe immediate pain at the injection site or if, especially in infants and young children, symptoms or signs occur suggesting onset of severe pain.

Some TUBEX cartridges may contain a small air bubble which may be disregarded, since it does not affect administration of the product.

Because of the high concentration of suspended material in this product, the needle may be blocked if the injection is not made at a slow, steady rate.

When using the disposable syringe:

The disposable syringe for this product incorporates several new features that are designed to facilitate its use.

A single small indentation, or "dot," has been punched into the metal or plastic ring that surrounds the neck of the syringe near the base of the needle. It is important that this "dot" be placed in a position so that it can be easily visualized by the operator following the intramuscular insertion of the syringe needle.

After selection of the proper site and insertion of the needle into the selected muscle, aspirate by pulling back on the plunger. While maintaining negative pressure for 2 to 3 seconds, carefully observe the barrel of the syringe immediately proximal to the location of the "dot" for appearance of blood or any discoloration. Blood or "typical blood color" may *not* be seen if a blood vessel has been entered—only a mixture of blood and Penicillin G Benzathine. The appearance of any discoloration is reason to withdraw the needle and discard the syringe. If it is elected to inject at another site, a new syringe should be used. If no blood or discoloration appears, inject the contents of the syringe slowly. Discontinue delivery of the dose if the subject complains of severe immediate pain at the injection site or if in infants and young children symptoms or signs occur suggesting onset of severe pain.

Some disposable syringes may contain a small air bubble which may be disregarded, since it does not affect administration of the product.

Because of the high concentration of suspended material in this product, the needle may be blocked if the injection is not made at a slow, steady rate.

Parenteral drug products should be inspected visually for particulate matter and discoloration prior to administration whenever solution and container permit.

STORAGE
Store in a refrigerator.
Keep from freezing.
Shake multiple-dose vials well before using.

REFERENCES
1. SHAW, E.: Transverse myelitis from injection of penicillin. *Am J. Dis. Child.*, 111: 548, 1966. 2. KNOWLES, J.: Accidental intra-arterial injection of penicillin, *Am. J. Dis. Child.*, 111: 552, 1966. 3. DARBY, C., et al: Ischemia following an intragluteal injection of benzathine-procaine penicillin G mixture in a one-year-old boy. *Clin. Pediatrics,* 12: 485, 1973. 4. BROWN, L. & NELSON, A.: Postinfectious intravascular thrombosis with gangrene. *Arch. Surg,* 94: 652, 1967. 5. BORENSTINE, J.: Transverse myelitis and penicillin (Correspondence), *Am. J. Dis. Child.,* 112: 166, 1966. 6. ATKINSON, J.: Transverse myelopathy secondary to penicillin injection. *J. Pediatrics,* 75: 867, 1969. 7. TALBERT, J. et al: Gangrene of the foot following intramuscular injection in the lateral thigh: A case report with recommendations for prevention. *J. Pediatrics,* 70: 110, 1967. 8. FISHER, T.: Medicolegal affairs. *Canad. Med. Assoc. J.,*
112: 395, 1975. 9. SCHANZER, H. et al: Accidental intra-arterial injection of penicillin G. *JAMA*, 242: 1289, 1979.

J CODES
Up to 2,400,000 units IM—J0580
Up to 1,200,000 units IM—J0570
Up to 600,000 units IM—J0560

HOW SUPPLIED
INJECTION: 300,000 U/ML

BRAND/MANUFACTURER	NDC	SIZE	AWP
○ **BRAND**			
BICILLIN L-A: Wyeth-Ayerst	00008-0163-01	10 ml	$19.96

INJECTION: 600,000 U/ML

BRAND/MANUFACTURER	NDC	SIZE	AWP
◇ **BRAND**			
BICILLIN L-A: Wyeth-Ayerst	00008-0021-08	1 ml 10s	$67.79
PERMAPEN: Roerig	00049-0210-35	2 ml 10s	$59.50
BICILLIN L-A: Wyeth-Ayerst	00008-0021-07	2 ml 10s	$117.39
	00008-0021-12	4 ml 10s	$240.56

Penicillin G Benzathine and Penicillin G Procaine

DESCRIPTION
Penicillin G Benzathine/Penicillin G Procaine suspension contains equal amounts of the Benzathine and Procaine salts of Penicillin G or the equivalent of 900,000 units of penicillin G as the Benzathine and 300,000 units of penicillin G as the Procaine salts. It is available for deep intramuscular injection.

Penicillin G Benzathine is prepared by the reaction of dibenzylethylene diamine with two molecules of Penicillin G. It is chemically designated as 3,3-dimethyl-7-oxo-6-(2-phenylacetamido)-4-thia-1-azabicyclo [3.2.0] heptane-2-carboxylic acid compound with *N,N*-dibenzylethylenediamine (2:1), tetrahydrate. It occurs as a white, crystalline powder and is very slightly soluble in water and sparingly soluble in alcohol.

Penicillin G Procaine, 3,3-dimethyl-7-oxo-6-(2-phenylacetamido)-4-thia-1-azabicyclo [3.2.0] heptane-2-carboxylic acid compound with 2-(diethylamino)ethyl p-aminobenzoate compound (1:1) monohydrate, is an equimolar salt of Procaine and Penicillin G. It occurs as white crystals or a white, microcrystalline powder and is slightly soluble in water.

Penicillin G Benzathine/Penicillin G Procaine suspension contains: in each mL the equivalent of 150,000 units of Penicillin G as the Benzathine salt and 150,000 units of Penicillin G as the Procaine salt, in a stabilized aqueous suspension.

Each disposable syringe (2 mL size) contains the equivalent of 1,200,000 units of Penicillin G comprising: the equivalent of 600,000 units Penicillin G as the Benzathine salt and the equivalent of 600,000 units Penicillin G as the Procaine salt in a stabilized aqueous suspension.

Each disposable syringe (4 mL size) contains the equivalent of 2,400,000 units of Penicillin G comprising: the equivalent of 1,200,000 units of Penicillin G as the Benzathine salt and the equivalent of 1,200,000 units of Penicillin G as the Procaine salt in a stabilized aqueous suspension.

Each cartridge (1 mL size) contains the equivalent of 600,000 units of Penicillin G comprising: the equivalent of 300,000 units Penicillin G as the Benzathine salt and the equivalent of 300,000 units Penicillin G as the Procaine salt in a stabilized aqueous suspension.

Each cartridge (2 mL size) contains the equivalent of 1,200,000 units of Penicillin G comprising: the equivalent of 600,000 units of Penicillin G as the Benzathine salt and the equivalent of 600,000 units of Penicillin G as the Procaine salt, or the equivalent to 1,200,000 units of Penicillin G as follows: Penicillin G Benzathine equivalent to 900,000 units of Penicillin G and Penicillin G Procaine equivalent to 300,000 units of Penicillin G in a stabilized aqueous suspension, in a stabilized aqueous suspension.

CLINICAL PHARMACOLOGY
GENERAL
Penicillin G Benzathine/Penicillin G Procaine have a low solubility and, thus, the drugs are slowly released from intramuscular injection sites. The drugs are hydrolyzed to Penicillin G. This combination of hydrolysis and slow absorption results in blood serum levels much lower but more prolonged than other parenteral penicillins. Intramuscular administration of 600,000 units Penicillin G Benzathine/Penicillin G Procaine in adults usually produces peak blood levels of 1.0 to 1.3 units per mL within 3 hours: this level falls to an average concentration of 0.32 units per mL at 12 hours, 0.19 units per mL at 24 hours, and 0.03 units per mL at seven days.

Intramuscular administration of 1,200,000 units of Penicillin G Benzathine/Penicillin G Procaine in adults usually produces peak blood levels of 2.1 to 2.6 units per mL within 3 hours: this level falls to an average concentration of 0.75 units per mL at 12 hours, 0.28 units per mL at 24 hours, and 0.04 units per mL at seven days. Intramuscular administration of 1,200,000 units of Penicillin G Benzathine/Penicillin G Procaine 900/300 in patients weighing 100 to 140 lbs. usually produces average blood levels of 0.24 units/mL at 24 hours, 0.039 units/mL at 7 days, and 0.024 units/mL at 10 days.

Approximately 60% of Penicillin G is bound to serum protein. The drug is distributed throughout the body tissues in widely varying amounts. Highest levels are found in the kidneys with lesser amounts in the liver, skin, and intestines. Penicillin G penetrates into all other tissues and the spinal fluid to a lesser degree. With normal kidney function, the drug is excreted rapidly by tubuler excretion. In neonates and young infants and in individuals with impaired kidney function, excretion is considerably delayed.

MICROBIOLOGY

Penicillin G exerts a bactericidal action against penicillin-susceptible microorganisms during the stage of active multiplication. It acts through the inhibition of biosynthesis of cell-wall mucopeptide. It is not active against the penicillinase-producing bacteria, which include many strains of staphylococci. The following in-vitro data are available, but their clinical significance is unknown. Penicillin G exerts high in-vitro activity against staphylococci (except penicillinase-producing strains), streptococci (Groups A, C, G, H, L, and M), and pneumococci. Other organisms susceptible to Penicillin G are *Neisseria gonorrhoeae*, *Corynebacterium diphtheriae*, *Bacillus anthracis*, Clostridia species, *Actinomyces bovis*, *Streptobacillus moniliformis*, *Listeria monocytogenes*, and Leptospira species, *Treponema pallidum* is extremely susceptible to the bactericidal action of Penicillin G.

Susceptibility Test: If the Kirby-Bauer method of disc susceptibility is used, a 10-unit penicillin disc should give a zone greater than 28 mm when tested against a penicillin sensitive bacterial strain.

INDICATIONS AND USAGE

This drug is indicated in the treatment of moderately severe infections due to penicillin-G-susceptible microorganisms that are susceptible to serum levels common to this particular dosage form. Therapy should be guided by bacteriological studies (including susceptibility testing) and by clinical response.

Penicillin G Benzathine/Penicillin G Procaine is indicated in the treatment of the following in children of all ages:

Moderately severe to severe infections of the upper-respiratory tract, scarlet fever, erysipelas, and skin and soft-tissue infections due to susceptible streptococci.

Note: Streptococci in Groups A, C, G, H, L, and M are very sensitive to Penicillin G. Other groups, including Group D (enterococci), are resistant. Penicillin G sodium or potassium is recommended for streptococcal infections with bacteremia.

Moderately severe pneumonia and otitis media due to susceptible pneumococci.

Note: Severe pneumonia, empyema, bacteremia, pericarditis, meningitis, peritonitis, and arthritis of pneumococcal etiology are better treated with Penicillin G sodium or potassium during the acute stage.

When high, sustained serum levels are required, Penicillin G sodium or potassium, either IM or IV, should be used. This drug should not be used in the treatment of venereal diseases, including syphilis, gonorrhea, yaws, bejel, and pinta.

CONTRAINDICATIONS

A previous hypersensitivity reaction to any penicillin or to procaine is a contraindication.

Do not inject into or near an artery or nerve.

WARNINGS

The combination of Penicillin G Benzathine/Penicillin G Procaine should only be prescribed for the indications listed in this insert.

Serious and occasionally fatal hypersensitivity (anaphylactoid) reactions have been reported in patients on penicillin therapy. Although anaphylaxis is more frequent following parenteral therapy, it has occurred in patients on oral penicillins. These reactions are more apt to occur in individuals with a history of sensitivity to multiple allergens.

There are reports of patients with a history of penicillin hypersensitivity reactions who experienced severe hypersensitivity reactions when treated with a cephalosporin. Before therapy with a penicillin, careful inquiry should be made about previous hypersensitivity reactions to Penicillins, cephalosporins, and other allergens. If an allergic reaction occurs, the drug should be discontinued and appropriate therapy should be instituted. Serious anaphylactoid reactions require immediate emergency treatment with epinephrine. Oxygen, intravenous steroids, airway management, including intubation, should also be administered as indicated.

Inadvertent intravascular administration, including inadvertent direct intra-arterial injection or injection immediately adjacent to arteries, of Penicillin G Benzathine/Penicillin G Procaine and other penicillin preparations has resulted in severe neurovascular damage, including transverse myelitis with permanent paralysis, gangrene requiring amputation of digits and more proximal portions of extremities, and necrosis and sloughing at and surrounding the injection site. Such severe effects have been reported following injections into the buttock, thigh, and deltoid areas. Other serious complications of suspected intravascular administration which have been reported include immediate pallor, mottling or cyanosis of the extremity both distal and proximal to the injection site followed by bleb formation; severe edema requiring anterior and/or posterior compartment fasciotomy in the lower extremity. The above-described severe effects and complications have most often occurred in infants and small children. Prompt consultation with an appropriate specialist is indicated if any evidence of compromise of the blood supply occurs at, proximal to, or distal to the site of injection.[1-9] See *"Contraindications"*, *"Precautions"*, and *"Dosage and Administration"* sections.

Quadriceps femoris fibrosis and atrophy have been reported following repeated intramuscular injections of penicillin preparations into the anterolateral thigh.

Injection into or near a nerve may result in permanent neurological damage.

PRECAUTIONS

GENERAL

Penicillin should be used with caution in individuals with histories of significant allergies and/or asthma.

Care should be taken to avoid intravenous or intra-arterial administration, or injection into or near major peripheral nerves or blood vessels, since such injections may produce neurovascular damage. See *"Contraindications"*, *"Warnings"*, and *"Dosage and Administration"* sections.

A small percentage of patients are sensitive to procaine. If there is a history of sensitivity make the usual test: Inject intradermally 0.1 mL of a 1 to 2 percent procaine solution. Development of an erythema, wheal, flare, or eruption indicates procaine sensitivity. Sensitivity should be treated by the usual methods, including barbiturates, and procaine penicillin preparations should not be used. Antihistaminics appear beneficial in treatment of procaine reactions.

The use of antibiotics may result in overgrowth of nonsusceptible organisms. Constant observation of the patient is essential. If new infections due to bacteria or fungi appear during therapy, the drug should be discontinued and appropriate measures taken.

Whenever allergic reactions occur, penicillin should be withdrawn unless, in the opinion of the physician, the condition being treated is life-threatening and amenable only to penicillin therapy.

In prolonged therapy with penicillin, and particularly with high-dosage schedules, periodic evaluation of the renal and hematopoietic systems is recommended.

LABORATORY TESTS

In streptococcal infections, therapy must be sufficient to eliminate the organism: otherwise, the sequelae of streptococcal disease may occur. Cultures should be taken following completion of treatment to determine whether streptococci have been eradicated.

DRUG INTERACTIONS

Tetracycline, a bacteriostatic antibiotic, may antagonize the bactericidal effect of penicillin, and concurrent use of these drugs should be avoided.

Concurrent administration of penicillin and probenecid increases and prolongs serum penicillin levels by decreasing the apparent volume of distribution and slowing the rate of excretion by competitively inhibiting renal tubular secretion of penicillin.

PREGNANCY CATEGORY B

Reproduction studies performed in the mouse, rat, and rabbit have revealed no evidence of impaired fertility or harm to the fetus due to penicillin G. Human experience with the penicillins during pregnancy has not shown any positive evidence of adverse effects on the fetus. There are, however, no adequate and well-controlled studies in pregnant women showing conclusively that harmful effects of these drugs on the fetus can be excluded. Because animal reproduction studies are not always predictive of human response, this drug should be used during pregnancy only if clearly needed.

NURSING MOTHERS

Soluble Penicillin G is excreted in breast milk. Caution should be exercised when Penicillin G Benzathine/Penicillin G Procaine is administered to a nursing woman.

CARCINOGENESIS, MUTAGENESIS, IMPAIRMENT OF FERTILITY

No long-term animal studies have been conducted with these drugs.

PEDIATRIC USE

See *"Indications and Usage"* and *"Dosage and Administration"*.

ADVERSE REACTIONS

As with other penicillins, untoward reactions of the sensitivity phenomena are likely to occur, particularly in individuals who have previously demonstrated hypersensitivity to penicillins or in those with a history of allergy, asthma, hay fever, or urticaria.

The following have been reported with parenteral Penicillin G:

General: Hypersensitivity reactions including the following: skin eruptions (maculopapular to exfoliative dermatitis), urticaria, laryngeal edema, fever, eosinophilia; other serum-sicknesslike reactions (including chills, fever, edema, arthralgia, and prostration); anaphylaxis. Note: Urticaria, other skin rashes, and serum-sicknesslike reactions may be controlled with antihistamines and, if necessary, systemic corticosteroids. Whenever such reactions occur, Penicillin G should be discontinued unless, in the opinion of the physician, the condition being treated is life-threatening and amenable only to therapy with Penicillin G. Serious anaphylactic reactions require the immediate use of epinephrine, oxygen, and intravenous steroids.

Hematologic: Hemolytic anemia, leukopenia, thrombocytopenia.

Neurologic: Neuropathy

Urogenital: Nephropathy.

OVERDOSAGE
Penicillin in overdosage has the potential to cause neuromuscular hyperirritability or convulsive seizures.

DOSAGE AND ADMINISTRATION
Shake multiple-dose vial vigorously before withdrawing the desired dose.

Administer by DEEP, INTRAMUSCULAR INJECTION in the upper, outer quadrant of the buttock. In infants and small children, the midlateral aspect of the thigh may be preferable. When doses are repeated, vary the injection site.

WHEN USING MULTIPLE-DOSE VIAL
After selection of the proper site and insertion of the needle into the selected muscle, aspirate by pulling back on the plunger. While maintaining negative pressure for 2 to 3 seconds, carefully observe the neck of the syringe immediately proximal to the needle hub for appearance of blood or any discoloration. Blood or "typical blood color" may *not* be seen if a blood vessel has been entered—only a mixture of blood and Penicillin G Benzathine/Penicillin G Procaine. The appearance of any discoloration is reason to withdraw the needle and discard the syringe. If it is elected to inject at another site, a new syringe and needle should be used. If no blood or discoloration appears, inject the contents of the syringe slowly. Discontinue delivery of the dose if the subject complains of severe immediate pain at the injection site or if in infants and young children symptoms or signs occur suggesting onset of severe pain.

WHEN USING A CARTRIDGE
After selection of the proper site and insertion of the needle into the selected muscle, aspirate by pulling back on the plunger. While maintaining negative pressure for 2 to 3 seconds, carefully observe the neck of the glass cartridge immediately proximal to the plastic needle hub for appearance of blood or any discoloration.

Blood or "typical blood color" may *not* be seen if a blood vessel has been entered—only a mixture of blood and Penicillin G Benzathine/Penicillin G Procaine. The appearance of *any* discloration is reason to withdraw the needle and discard the cartridge. If it is elected to inject at another site, a new cartridge should be used. If no blood or discloration appears, inject the contents of the cartridge slowly. Discontinue delivery of the dose if the subject complains of severe immediate pain at the injection site or if in infants and young children symptoms or signs occur suggesting onset of severe pain.

Some cartridges may contain a small air bubble which may be disregarded since it does not affect administration of the product.

Because of the high concentration of suspended material in this product, the needle may be blocked if the injection is not made at a slow, steady rate.

WHEN USING A DISPOSABLE SYRINGE
After selection of the proper site and insertion of the needle into the selected muscle, aspirate by pulling back on the plunger. While maintaining negative pressure for 2 to 3 seconds, carefully observed the barrel of the syringe appearance of blood or any discoloration. Blood or "typical blood color" may *not* be seen if a blood vessel has been entered—only a mixture of blood and Penicillin G Benzathine/Penicillin G Procaine. The appearance of any discoloration is reason to withdraw the needle and discard the syringe. If it is elected to inject at another site, a new syringe should be used. If no blood or discoloration appears, inject the contents of the syringe slowly. Discontinue delivery of the dose if the subject complains of severe immediate pain at the injection site or if in infants and young children symptoms or signs occur suggesting onset of severe pain.

Some disposable syringes may contain a small air bubble which may be disregarded since it does not affect administration of the product.

Because of the high concentration of suspended material in this product, the needle may be blocked if the injection is not made at a slow, steady rate.

Streptococcal Infections Groups A: Infections of the upper-respiratory tract, skin and soft-tissue infections, scarlet fever, and erysipelas.

The following doses are recommended:

Adults and children over 60 lbs. in weight: 2,400,000 units. Children from 30 to 60 lbs.: 900,000 units to 1,200,000 units. Infants and children under 30 lbs.: 600,000 units.

Note: Treatment with the recommended dosage is usually given at a single session using multiple IM sites when indicated. An alternative dosage schedule may be used, giving one-half (½) the total dose on day 1 and one-half (½) on day 3. This will also insure the penicillinemia required over a 10-day period; however, this alternate schedule should be used only when the physician can be assured of the patient's cooperation.

Streptococcal Infections: A single injection of Penicillin G Benzathine/Penicillin G Procaine 900/300 is usually sufficient for the treatment of Group A streptococcal infections in children of all ages.

Pneumococcal Infections (except Pneumococcal meningitis): 600,000 units in children and 1,200,000 units in adults or one cartridge of Penicillin G Benzathine/Penicillin G Procaine 900/300, repeated every 2 or 3 days until the temperature is normal for 48 hours. Other forms of Penicillin may be necessary for severe cases.

Parenteral drug products should be inspected visually for particulate matter and discoloration prior to administration whenever solution and container permit.

STORAGE
Store in a refrigerator.
Keep from freezing.

REFERENCES
1. SHAW, E.: Transverse myelitis from injection of penicillin. *Am. J. Dis. Child,* 111:548, 1966. 2. KNOWLES, J.: Accidental intra-arterial injection of penicillin. *Am. J. Dis. Child.,* 111:552, 1966. 3. DARBY, C., et al: Ischemia following an intragluteal injection of benzathine-procaine penicillin G mixture in a one-year-old boy. *Clin. Pediatrics,* 12:485, 1973. 4. BROWN, L. & NELSON, A.: Postinfectious intravascular thrombosis with gangrene. *Arch. Surg,* 94:652, 1967. 5. BORENSTINE, J.: Transverse myelitis and penicillin (Correspondence), *Am. J. Dis. Child.,* 112:166, 1966. 6. ATKINSON, J.: Transverse myelopathy secondary to penicillin injection. *J. Pediatrics,* 75:867, 1969. 7. TALBERT, J. et al: Gangrene of the foot following intramuscular injection in the lateral thigh: A case report with recommendations for prevention. *J. Pediatrics,* 70:110, 1967. 8. FISHER, T.: Medicolegal affairs. *Canad. Med. Assoc. J.,* 112:395, 1975. 9. SCHANZER, H, et al: Accidental intraarterial injection of penicillin G. *JAMA,* 242;1289, 1979

HOW SUPPLIED
INJECTION: 300,000 U/ML

BRAND/MANUFACTURER	NDC	SIZE	AWP
BRAND			
BICILLIN C-R: Wyeth-Ayerst	00008-0176-01	10 ml	$13.50

INJECTION: 600,000 U/ML

BRAND/MANUFACTURER	NDC	SIZE	AWP
BRAND			
BICILLIN C-R: Wyeth-Ayerst	00008-0026-17	1 ml 10s	$47.68
	00008-0026-16	2 ml 10s	$93.61
BICILLIN C-R 900/300: Wyeth-Ayerst	00008-0079-01	2 ml 10s	$97.40
BICILLIN C-R: Wyeth-Ayerst	00008-0026-22	4 ml 10s	$200.46

Penicillin G Potassium

DESCRIPTION
Penicillin G Potassium is a sterile, pyrogen-free powder for reconstitution. Penicillin G Potassium for injection is an antibacterial agent for intramuscular, continuous intravenous drip, intrapleural or other local infusion, and intrathecal administration.

Each million units of Penicillin contains approximately 6.8 mg of sodium (0.3 mEq) and 65.6 mg of Potassium (1.68 mEq).

Chemically, Penicillin G Potassium is monopotassium 3,3-dimethyl-7oxo-6-(2-phenylacetamido)-4-thia-1-azabicyclo (3.2.0) heptane-2-carboxylate. It has a molecular weight of 372.48 and the empirical formula is $C_{16}H_{17}KN_2O_4S$. Penicillin G Potassium is a colorless or white crystal, or a white crystalline powder which is odorless, or practically so, and moderately hygroscopic. Penicillin G Potassium is very soluble in water. The pH of the reconstituted product is between 6.0-8.5.

Following is its chemical structure:

CLINICAL PHARMACOLOGY
Aqueous Penicillin G is rapidly absorbed following both intramuscular and subcutaneous injection. Initial blood levels following parenteral administration are high but transient. Penicillins bind to serum proteins, mainly albumin. Therapeutic levels of the Penicillins are easily achieved under normal circumstances in extracellular fluid and most other body tissues. Penicillins are distributed in varying degrees into pleural, pericardial, peritoneal, ascitic, synovial, and interstitial fluids. Penicillins are excreted in breast milk. Penetration into the cerebrospinal fluid, eyes, and prostate is poor. Penicillins are rapidly excreted in the urine by glomerular filtration and active tubular secretion, primarily as unchanged drug. Approximately 60 percent of the total dose of 300,000 units is excreted in the urine within a 5 hour period. For this reason high and frequent doses are required to maintain the elevated serum levels desirable in treating certain severe infections in individuals with normal kidney function. In neonates and young infants, and in individuals with impaired kidney function, excretion is considerably delayed.

MICROBIOLOGY
Penicillin G exerts a bactericidal action against Penicillin-susceptible microorganisms during the stage of active multiplication. It acts through the inhibition of biosynthesis of cell wall mucopeptide rendering the cell wall osmotically unstable. It is not active against the penicillinase-producing bacteria, which include many strains of staphylococci. While *in vitro* studies have demonstrated the susceptibility of most strains of the following organisms, clinical efficacy for infections other than those included in the *"Indications and Usage"* section has not been documented. Penicillin G exerts high *in vitro* activity against staphylococci (except penicillinase-producing strains), streptococci (groups A, C, G, H, L, and M), and pneumococci. Other organisms susceptible to Penicillin G are *N. gonorrhoeae, Corynebacterium diphtheriae, Bacillus anthracis, Clostridia, Antinomyces bovis, Streptobacillus moniliformis, Listeria monocytogenes* and *Leptospira. Treponema pallidum* is extremely sensitive to the bactericidal action of Penicillin G. Some species of gram-negative bacilli are sensitive to moderate to high concentrations of the drug obtained with intravenous administration. These

include most strains of *Escherichia coli*; all strains of *Proteus mirabilis*, Salmonella and Shigella; and some strains of *Enterobacter aerogenes (*formerly *Aerobacter aerogenes)* and *Alacaligenes faecalis*.

Penicillin acts synergistically with gentamicin or tobramycin against many strains of enterococci.

Susceptiblity Testing: Penicillin G Suceptibility Powder or 10 units Penicillin G Susceptibility Discs may be used to determine microbial susceptibility of Penicillin G using one of the following standard methods recommended by the National Committee for Laboratory Standards.

M2-A3, "Performance Standards for Antimicrobial Disk Susceptibility Tests"
M7-A, "Methods for Dilution Antimicrobial Susceptibilty Tests for Bacteria that Grow Aerobically"
M11-A, "Reference Agar Dilution Procedure for Antimicrobial Susceptibilty Testing of Anaerobic Bacteria"
M-17-P, "Alternative Methods for Antimicrobial Susceptibility Testing of Anaerobic Bacteria"

Tests should be interpreted by the following criteria:

Zone Diameter, nearest whole mm

	Susceptible	Moderately Susceptible	Resistant
Staphylococci	≥29	-	≤28
N. gonorrhoeae	≥20	-	≤19
Enterococci	-	≥15	≤14
Non-enterococcal streptococci and *L. monocytogenes*	≥28	20-27	≤19

Approximate MIC Correlates

	Susceptible	Resistant
Staphylococci	≤0.1 μg/mL	β-lactamase
N. gonorrhoeae	≤0.1 μg/mL	β-lactamase
Enterococci	-	≥16 μg/mL
Non-enterococcal streptococci and *L. monocytogenes*	≤0.12 μg/mL	≥ 4 μg/mL

Interpretations of susceptible, intermediate, and resistant correlate zone size diameters with MIC values. A laboratory report of "suceptible" indicates that the suspected causative microorganism most likely will respond to therapy with Penicillin G. A laboratory report of "resistant" indicates that the infecting microorganism most likely will not respond to therapy. A laboratory report of "moderately susceptible" indicates that the microorganism is most likely susceptible if a high dosage of Penicillin G is used, or if the infection is such that high levels of Penicillin G may be attained, as in urine. A report of "intermediate" using the disk diffusion method may be considered an equivocal result, and dilution tests may be indicated.

Control organisms are recommended for susceptibility testing. Each time the test is performed the following organisms should be included. The range for zones of inhibition is shown below:

Control Organism	Zone of Inhibition Range
Staphylococcus aureus (ATCC 25923)	27-35

If the Kirby-Bauer method of disc susceptibility is used, a 10 U Penicillin disc should give a zone greater than 28 mm when tested against a Penicillin-susceptible bacterial strain.

INDICATIONS AND USAGE

Aqueous Penicillin G (parenteral) is indicated in the therapy of severe infections caused by Penicillin G-susceptible microorganisms when rapid and high Penicillin levels are required in the conditions listed below. Therapy should be guided by bacteriological studies (including susceptibility tests) and by clinical response.

The following infections will usually respond to adequate dosage of aqueous Penicillin G (parenteral):

Streptococcal infections.
Note: Streptococci in groups A, C, H, G, L, and M are very sensitive to Penicillin G. Some group D organisms are sensitive to the high serum levels obtained with aqueous Penicillin G.

Aqueous Penicillin G Potassium is the Penicillin dosage form of choice for bacteremia, empyema, severe pneumonia, pericarditis, endocarditis, meningitis, and other severe infections caused by sensitive strains of the gram-positive species listed above.

Pneumococcal infections.
Staphylococcal infections—Penicillin G sensitive.

Other infections:
Anthrax.
Actinomycosis.
Clostridial infections (including tetanus).
Diphtheria (to prevent carrier state).
Erysipeloid (*Erysipelothrix insidiosa*) endocarditis.

Fusospirochetal infections—severe infections of the oropharynx (Vincent's gingivitis and pharyngitis. *Note:* necessary dental care should be accomplished in infections involving gum tissue) lower respiratory tract and genital area due to *Fusobacterium fusiformisans* spirochetes.

Gram-negative bacillary infections (bacteremias)—(*E. coli, E. aerogenes, A. faecalis,* Salmonella, Shigella and *P. mirabilis*).
Listeria infections (*Listeria monocytogenes*).
Meningitis and endocarditis.
Pasteurella infections (*Pasteurella multocida*).
Bacteremia and meningitis.
Rat-bite fever (*Spirillum minus* or *Streptobacillus moniliformis*).
Gonorrheal endocarditis and arthritis (*N. gonorrhoeae*).
Syphilis (*T. pallidum*) including congenital syphilis.
Meningococcic meningitis.

Although no controlled clinical efficacy studies have been conducted, in patients unable to take oral antibiotics, aqueous crystalline Penicillin G for injection (except Penicillin G procaine suspension) has been suggested by the American Heart Association and the American Dental Association for prophylaxis against bacterial endocarditis in patients with congenital heart disease or rheumatic, or other acquired valvular heart disease when they undergo dental procedures and surgical procedures of the upper respiratory tract.[1] Since it may happen that *alpha* hemolytic streptococci relatively resistant to Penicillin may be found when patients are receiving continuous oral Penicillin for secondary prevention of rheumatic fever, prophylactic agents other than Penicillin may be chosen for these patients and prescribed in addition to their continuous rheumatic fever prophylactic regimen.

Note: When selecting antibiotics for the prevention of bacterial endocarditis, the physician or dentist should read the full joint statement of the American Heart Association and the American Dental Association.[1]

CONTRAINDICATIONS

A history of a previous hypersensitivity reaction to any Penicillin is a contraindication.

WARNINGS

Serious and occasionally fatal hypersensitivity (anaphylactoid) reactions have been reported in patients on Penicillin therapy. Although anaphylaxis is more frequent following parenteral administration, it has occurred in patients on oral Penicillins. These reactions are more likely to occur in individuals with a history of Penicillin hypersensitivity and/or a history of sensitivity to multiple allergens. There have been reports of individuals with a history of Penicillin hypersensitivity who have experienced severe reactions when treated with cephalosporins. Before initiating therapy with any Penicillin, careful inquiry should be made concerning previous hypersensitivity reactions to Penicillin, cephalosporins, or other allergens. If an allergic reaction occurs, the drug should be discontinued and the appropriate therapy instituted, e.g., pressor amines, antihistamines, and corticosteroids. Serious anaphylactoid reactions are not controlled by antihistamines alone and require immediate emergency treatment with epinephrine. Oxygen, aminophylline, intravenous steroids, and airway management including intubation, should also be administered as indicated.

PRECAUTIONS

General: Penicillin should be used with caution in individuals with histories of significant allergies and/or asthma.

Intramuscular Therapy: Care should be taken to avoid intravenous or accidental intra-arterial administration, or injection into or near major peripheral nerves or blood vessels, since such injections may produce neurovascular damage. Particular care should be taken with IV administration because of the possibility of thrombophlebitis.

In streptococcal infections, therapy must be sufficient to eliminate the organism (10 days minimum); otherwise, the sequelae of streptococcal disease may occur. Cultures should be taken following the completion of treatment to determine whether streptococci have been eradicated.

The use of antibiotics may result in overgrowth of nonsusceptible organisms, including fungi. Constant observation of the patient is essential. Should superinfection occur, appropriate measures should be taken. Indwelling intravenous catheters encourage superinfections and should be avoided whenever possible. If new infections due to bacteria or fungi appear during therapy, the drug should be discontinued and appropriate measures taken. Whenever allergic reactions occur, Penicillin should be withdrawn unless, in the opinion of the physician, the condition being treated is life threatening and amenable only to Penicillin therapy.

Therapy of susceptible infections should be accompanied by any indicated surgical procedures.

Aqueous Penicillin G by the intravenous route in high doses (above 10 million units) should be administered slowly because of the adverse effects of electrolyte imbalance from either the Potassium or sodium content of the Penicillin. Penicillin G Potassium contains 1.7 mEq Potassium and 0.3 mEq sodium per million units. The patient's renal, cardiac, and vascular status should be evaluated and if impairment of function is suspected or known to exist a reduction in the total dosage should be considered. Frequent evaluation of electrolyte balance, renal and hematopoietic function is recommended during therapy when high doses of intravenous aqueous Penicillin G Potassium are used.

Any entry into the container to effect solution of the powder or withdrawal of contents must be accomplished with strict aseptic technique and sterile equipment.

Laboratory Tests: In prolonged therapy with Penicillin, periodic evaluation of the renal, hepatic, and hematopoietic systems is recommended for organ system dysfunction. This is particularly important in prematures, neonates and other infants, and when high doses are used.

Positive Coomb's tests have been reported after large intravenous doses.

Monitor serum Potassium and implement corrective measures when necessary.

When treating gonococcal infections in which primary and secondary syphilis are suspected, proper diagnostic procedures, including dark field examinations, should be done before receiving Penicillin and monthly serological tests made for at least four months. All cases of Penicillin treated syphilis should receive clinical and serological examinations every six months for two to three years.

In suspected staphylococcal infections, proper laboratory studies, including susceptibility tests, should be performed. In streptococcal infections, cultures should be taken following completion of treatment to determine whether streptococci have been eradicated. Therapy must be sufficient to eliminate the organism (a minimum of 10 days), otherwise the sequelae of streptococcal disease (e.g., endocarditis, rheumatic fever) may occur.

Drug Interactions: Concurrent administration of bacteriostatic antibiotics (e.g., erythromycin, tetracycline) may diminish the bactericidal effects of Penicillins by slowing the rate of bacterial growth. Bactericidal agents work most effectively against the immature cell wall of rapidly proliferating microorganisms. This has been demonstrated *in vitro*; however, the clinical significance of this interaction is not well documented. There are few clinical situations in which the concurrent use of "static" and "cidal" antibiotics are indicated. However, in selected circumstances in which such therapy is appropriate, using adequate doses of antibacterial agents and beginning Penicillin therapy first, should minimize the potential for interaction.

Penicillin blood levels may be prolonged by concurrent administration of prebenecid which blocks the renal tubular secretion of Penicillins.

Displacement of Penicillin from plasma protein binding sites will elevate the level of free Penicillin in the serum.

Carcinogenesis, Mutagenesis, Impairment of Fertility: No information on long-term studies are available on the carcinogenesis, mutagenesis, or the impairment of fertility with the use of Pencillins.

Pregnancy Category B: Teratogenic Effects: Reproduction studies performed in the mouse, rat, and rabbit have revealed no evidence of impaired fertility or harm to the fetus due to Penicillin G. Human experience with the Penicillins during pregnancy has not shown any positive evidence of adverse effects on the fetus. There are, however, no adequate and well controlled studies in pregnant women showing conclusively that harmful effects of these drugs on the fetus can be excluded. Because animal reproduction studies are not always predictive of human response, this drug should be used during pregnancy only if clearly needed.

Nursing Mothers: Penicillins are excreted in human milk. Caution should be exercised when Penicillin G is administered to a nursing woman.

Pediatric Use: Penicillins are excreted largely unchanged by the kidney. Because of incompletely developed renal function in infants, the rate of elimination will be slow. Use caution in administering to newborns and evaluate organ system function frequently.

ADVERSE REACTIONS

Penicillin is a substance of low toxicity but does have a significant index of sensitization. The following hypersensitivity reactions have been reported: skin rashes ranging from maculopapular eruptions to exfoliative dermatitis; urticaria; and reactions resembling serum sickness, including chills, fever, edema, arthralgia and prostration. Severe and occasionally fatal anaphylaxis has occurred (see *"Warnings"*).

Hemolytic anemia, leukopenia, thrombocytopenia, nephropathy, and neuropathy are rarely observed adverse reactions and are usually associated with high intravenous dosage. Urticaria, other skin rashes, and serum sickness-like reactions may be controlled by antihistamines and, if necessary, corticosteroids. Whenever such reactions occur, Penicillin should be discontinued unless, in the opinion of the physician, the condition being treated is life-threatening and amenable only to Penicillin therapy. Patients given continuous intravenous therapy with Penicillin G Potassium in high dosage (10 million to 100 million units daily) may suffer severe or even fatal Potassium poisoning, particularly if renal insufficiency is present. Hyperreflexia, convulsions and coma may be indicative of this syndrome.

Cardiac arrhythmias and cardiac arrest may also occur. (High dosage of Penicillin G sodium may result in congestive heart failure due to high sodium intake).

The Jarisch-Herxheimer reaction has been reported in patients treated for syphilis.

OVERDOSAGE

Neurological adverse reactions, including convulsions, may occur with the attainment of high CSF levels of beta-lactams. In case of overdosage, discontinue medication, treat symptomatically, and institute supportive measures as required. Penicillin G Potassium is hemodialyzable.

DOSAGE AND ADMINISTRATION

Severe infections due to Susceptible Strains of Streptococci, Pneumococci and Staphylococci: bacteremia, pneumonia, endocarditis, pericarditis, empyema, meningitis and other severe infections—a minimum of 5 million units daily.

Syphilis: Aqueous Penicillin G Potassium may be used in the treatment of acquired and congenital syphilis, but because of the necessity of frequent dosage, hospitalization is recommended. Dosage and duration of therapy will be determined by age of patient and stage of the disease.

Gonorrheal endocarditis and arthritis: a minimum of 5 millions unit daily.

Meningococcic meningitis: 1-2 million units intramuscularly every 2 hours, or continuous IV drip of 20-30 million units/day.

Actinomycosis: 1-6 million units/day for cervicofacial cases; 10-20 million units/day for thoracic and abdominal disease.

Clostridial infections: 20 million units/day; penicillin is adjunctive therapy to antitoxin.

Fusospirochetal infections: severe infections of oropharynx, lower respiratory tract and genital area—5–10 million units/day.

Rat bite fever (Spirillum minus or Streptobacillus moniliformis): 12-15 million units/day for 3-4 weeks.

Listeria infections (Listeria monocytogenes).

Neonates: 500,000 to 1 million units/day.

Adults with meningitis: 15-20 million units/day for 2 weeks.

Adults with endocarditis: 15-20 million units/day for 4 weeks.

Pasteurella infections (Pasteurella multocida): Bacteremia and meningitis: 4-6 million units/day for 2 weeks.

Erysipeloid (Erysipelothrix insidiosa).

Endocarditis: 2-20 million units/day for 4-6 weeks.

Gram-negative, bacillary infections (E. coli, Enterobacter aerogenes, A. faecalis, Salmonella, Shigella and Proteus mirabilis).

Bacteremia: 20-80 million units/day.

Diphtheria (carrier state or as adjunctive therapy for prevention of the carrier state): 300,000-400,000 units of Penicillin/day in divided doses for 10-12 days.

Anthrax: A minimum of 5 million units of Penicillin/day in divided doses until cure is effected.

Prevention of bacterial endocarditis (patients unable to take oral antibiotics: For prophylaxis against bacterial endocarditis[1] in patients with congenital heart disease or rheumatic, or other acquired valvular heart disease when undergoing dental procedures or surgical procedures of the upper respiratory tract, administer 2 million units (50,000 units/kg for children) Aqueous Penicillin G, *except* Penicillin G procaine suspension, intravenously or intramuscularly 30 to 60 minutes before the procedure and 1 million units (25,000 units/kg for children) six hours later.

Doses for children should not exceed recommendations for adults for a single dose or for a 24 hour period.

RECONSTITUTION

The following table shows the amount of solvent required for solution of various concentrations.

Approx. Desired Concentration (Units/ml)	Approx. Volume (ml) 100,000,000 units	Solvent for Vial of 5,000,000 units	Infusion Only 10,000,000 units	Infusion Only 20,000 units
50,000	20.0	-	-	-
100,000	9.6-10.0	-	-	-
200,000	4.6	23	-	-
250,000	3.6-4.0	18-18.2	-	75.0
500,000	1.8	8-8.2	15.5	31.6-33.0
750,000	-	4.8	-	-
1,000,000	-	3 ml 3.2	5.4	11.5

Solutions of Penicillin should be prepared as follows: Loosen powder. Hold vial horizontally and rotate it while *slowly* directing the stream of diluent against the wall of the vial. Shake vial vigorously after all the diluent has been added. Depending on the route of administration, use sterile water for injection, isotonic sodium chloride injection, or dextrose injection. *Note:* Penicillins are rapidly inactivated in the presence of carbohydrate are rapidly inactivated in the presence of carbohydrate solutions at alkaline pH.

When the required volume of solvent is greater than the capacity of the vial, the Penicillin can be dissolved by first injecting only a portion of the solvent into the vial, then withdrawing the resultant solution and combining it with the remainder of the solvent in a larger sterile container. Penicillin G Potassium for injection is highly water soluble. All solutions should be stored in a refrigerator. When refrigerated, Penicillin solutions may be stored for seven days without significant loss of potency. Penicillin G Potassium may be given intramuscularly or by continuous intravenous drip for dosages of 500,000, 1,000,000 or 5,000,000 units. It is also suitable for intrapleural, intraarticular, and other local instillations. THE 10,000,000 AND 20,000,000 UNIT DOSAGES MAY BE ADMINISTERED BY INTRAVENOUS INFUSION ONLY.

(1) Intramuscular Injection: Keep total volume of injection small. The intramuscular route is the preferred route of administration. Solutions containing up to 100,000 units of Penicillin per ml of diluent may be used with a minimum of discomfort. Greater concentration of Penicillin G per ml is physically possible and may be employed where therapy demands. When large dosages are required,

it may be advisable to administer aqueous solutions of Penicillin by means of continuous intravenous drip.

(2) Continuous Intravenous Drip: Determine the volume of fluid and rate of its administration required by the patient in a 24-hour period in the usual manner for fluid therapy, and add the appropriate daily dosage of Penicillin to this fluid. For example, if an adult patient requires 2 liters of fluid in 24 hours and a daily dosage of 10 million units of Penicillin, add 5 million units to 1 liter and adjust the rate of flow so that the liter will be infused in 12 hours.

(3) Intrapleural or Other Local Infusion: If fluid is aspirated, give infusion in a volume equal to 1/4 or 1/2 the amount of fluid aspirated, otherwise, prepare as for intramuscular injection.

(4) Intrathecal Use: The intrathecal use of Penicillin in meningitis must be highly individualized. It should be employed only with full consideration of the possible irritating effects of Penicillin when used by this route. The preferred route of therapy in bacterial meningitides is intravenous, supplemented by intramuscular injection.

Parenteral drug products should be inspected visually for particulate matter and discoloration prior to administration, whenever solution and container permit.

STORAGE
The dry powder is relatively stable and may be stored at room temperature without significant loss of potency. Sterile solutions may be kept in the refrigerator one week without significant loss of potency. Solutions prepared for intravenous infusion are stable at room temperature for at least 24 hours.

REFERENCE
1. American Heart Association: Prevention of bacterial endocarditis. Circulation 70: 1123A-1127A, 1984

J CODES
Up to 600,00 units IM,IV—J2540

HOW SUPPLIED
POWDER FOR INJECTION: 1 MILLION U

BRAND/MANUFACTURER	NDC	SIZE	AWP
◆ GENERICS			
Apothecon	00003-0634-41	1s	$1.27

POWDER FOR INJECTION: 5 MILLION U

BRAND/MANUFACTURER	NDC	SIZE	AWP
◆ BRAND			
PFIZERPEN: Roerig	00049-0520-83	10s	$34.44
◆ GENERICS			
Apothecon	00003-0673-71	1s	$2.63

POWDER FOR INJECTION: 10 MILLION U

BRAND/MANUFACTURER	NDC	SIZE	AWP
◆ GENERICS			
Apothecon	00003-0734-11	1s	$6.40

POWDER FOR INJECTION: 20 MILLION U

AVERAGE UNIT PRICE (AVAILABLE SIZES)	
BRAND	$10.21

BRAND/MANUFACTURER	NDC	SIZE	AWP
◆ BRAND			
PFIZERPEN: Roerig	00049-0530-28	1s	$10.09
	00049-0530-83	10s	$103.19
◆ GENERICS			
Apothecon	00003-0735-31	1s	$7.27

TABLETS: 250,000 U

BRAND/MANUFACTURER	NDC	SIZE	AWP
◆ GENERICS			
URL	00677-0097-01	100s	$6.95

TABLETS: 400,000 U

AVERAGE UNIT PRICE (AVAILABLE SIZES)		GENERIC A-RATED AVERAGE PRICE (GAAP)	
GENERIC	$0.09	100s	$9.19

BRAND/MANUFACTURER	NDC	SIZE	AWP
◆ GENERICS			
Moore,H.L.	00839-5142-06	100s	$8.78
PEN-G: Goldline	00182-0107-01	100s	$9.60

Penicillin G Procaine

DESCRIPTION
Penicillin G Procaine is a highly potent antibacterial agent effective against a wide variety of pathogenic organisms. It is an equimolecular compound of Procaine and Penicillin G in aqueous suspension for intramuscular administration.

Chemically, Penicillin G Procaine is: 3,3-Dimethyl-7-oxo-6-(2-phenylacetamido)-4-thia-1-azabicyclo [3.2.0] heptane-2-carboxylic acid compound with 2-(diethylamino) ethyl-p-amino-benzoate (1:1) monohydrate.

It has a molecular weight of 588.72 and the molecular formula is $C_{16}H_{18}N_2O_4S \cdot C_{13}H_{20}N_2O_2 \cdot H_2O$. Penicillin G Procaine is a white, fine crystal, or a white, very fine microcrystalline powder. Penicillin G Procaine is odorless or practically so and 1 gram is soluble in 250 ml water. The pH of the aqueous suspension is between 5.0-7.5.

Following is its chemical structure:

CLINICAL PHARMACOLOGY
Penicillin G Procaine is an equimolecular compound of procaine and penicillin G administered intramuscularly as a suspension. It dissolves slowly at the site of injection, giving a plateau type of blood level at about 4 hours, which falls slowly over a period of the next 15-20 hours.

Approximately 60% of Penicillin G is bound to serum protein. The drug is distributed throughout the body tissues in widely varying amounts. Highest levels are found in the kidneys with lesser amounts in the liver, skin, and intestines. Penicillin G penetrates into all other tissues to a lesser degree with a very small level found in the cerobrospinal fluid. With normal kidney function the drug is excreted rapidly by tubular excretion. In neonates and young infants, and in individuals with impaired kidney function, excretion is considerably delayed. Approximately 60%-90% of a dose of parenteral Penicillin G is excreted in the urine within 24-36 hours. Penicillin G crosses the placental barrier and is found in the amniotic fluid and cord serum.

MICROBIOLOGY
Penicillin G exerts a bactericidal action against Penicillin-susceptible microorganisms during the stage of active multiplication. It acts through the inhibition of biosynthesis of cell wall mucopeptide. It is not active against the penicillinase-producing bacteria, which include many strains of staphylococci. While *in vitro* studies have demonstrated the susceptibility of most strains of the following organisms, clinical efficacy for infections other than those included in the *"Indications and Usage"* section has not been documented. Penicillin G exerts high *in vitro* activity against staphylococci (except penicillinase-producing strains), streptococci (groups A, C, G, H, L, and M), and pneumococci. Other organisms sensitive to Penicillin G are *N. gonorrhoeae, Corynebacterium diphtheriae, Bacillus anthracis,* Clostridia, *Actinomyces bovis. Streptobacillus moniliformis, Listeria monocytogenes,* and Leptospira. *Treponema pallidum* is extremely sensitive to the bactericidal action of Penicillin G.

Penicillin acts synergistically with gentamicin or tobramycin against many strains of enterococci.

Susceptibility Testing: Penicillin G Susceptibility Powder or 10 units Penicillin G Susceptibility Discs may be used to determine microbial susceptibility to Penicillin G using one of the following standard methods recommended by the National Committee for Laboratory Standards:

M2-A3, "Performance Standards for Antimicrobial Disk Susceptibility Tests"

M7-A, "Methods for Dilution Antimicrobial Susceptibility Tests for Bacteria that Grow Aerobically"

M11-A, "Reference Agar Dilution Procedure for Antimicrobial Susceptibility Testing of Anaerobic Bacteria"

M17-P, "Alternative Methods for Antimicrobial Susceptibility Testing of Anaerobic Bacteria"

Tests should be interpreted by the following criteria:

ZONE DIAMETER, NEAREST WHOLE MM

	Susceptible	Moderately Susceptible	Resistant
Staphylococci	≥ 29	—	≥ 28
N. *gonorrhoeae*	≥ 20	—	≤ 19
Enterococci	—	≥ 15	≤ 14
Nonenterococcal streptococci and *L. monocytogenes*	≥ 28	20-27	≤ 19

APPROXIMATE MIC CORRELATES

	Susceptible	Resistant
Staphylococci	≤ 0.1 µg/mL	β-lactamase
N. *gonorrhoeae*	≤ 0.1 µg/mL	β-lactamase
Enterococci	—	≥ 16 µ/mL
Non-enterococcal streptococci and *L. monocytogenes*	≤ 0.12 µg/mL	≥ 4 µg/mL

Interpretations of susceptible, intermediate, and resistant correlate zone size diameters with MIC values. A laboratory report of "susceptible" indicates that the suspected causative microorganism most likely will respond to therapy with Penicillin G. A laboratory report of "resistant" indicates that the infecting microorganism most likely will not respond to therapy. A laboratory report of "moderately susceptible" indicates that the microorganism is most likely susceptible if a high dosage of Penicillin G is used, or if the infection is such that high levels of Penicillin G may be attained as in urine. A report of "intermediate" using the disk diffusion method may be considered an equivocal result, and dilution tests may be indicated.

Control organisms are recommended for susceptibility testing. Each time the test is performed the following organisms should be included. The range for zones of inhibition is shown below:

Control Organism	Zone of Inhibition Range
Staphylococcus aureus (ACTT 25923)	27-35

INDICATIONS AND USAGE

Penicillin G Procaine is indicated in the treatment of moderately severe infections in both adults and children due to Penicillin G-susceptible microorganisms that are susceptible to the low and persistent serum levels common to this particular dosage form in the indications listed below. Therapy should be guided by bacteriological studies (including susceptibility tests) and by clinical response.

Note: When high sustained serum levels are required, aqueous Penicillin G either IM or IV should be used.

The following infections will usually respond to adequate dosages of intramuscular Penicillin G Procaine.

Streptococcal infections Group A (without bacteremia): Moderately severe to severe infections of the upper respiratory tract (including middle ear infections-otitis media), skin and soft tissue infections, scarlet fever, and erysipelas.

Note: Streptococci in groups A, C, H, G, L, and M are very sensitive to Penicillin G. Other groups, including group D (enterococcus), are resistant. Aqueous penicillin is recommended for streptococcal infections with bacteremia.

Pneumococcal infections: Moderately severe infections of the respiratory tract (including middle ear infections-otitis media).

Note: Severe pneumonia, empyema, bacteremia, pericarditis, meningitis, peritonitis, and purulent or septic arthritis of pneumococcal etiology are better treated with aqueous Penicillin G during the acute stage.

Staphylococcal infections: Penicillin G-sensitive. Moderately severe infections of the skin and soft tissues.

Note: Reports indicate an increasing number of strains of staphylococci resistant to Penicillin G emphasizing the need for culture and sensitivity studies in treating suspected staphylococcal infections.

Indicated surgical procedures should be performed.

Fusospirochetosis (Vincent's gingivitis and pharyngitis): Moderately severe infections of the oropharynx respond to therapy with Penicillin G Procaine.

Note: Necessary dental care should be accomplished in infections involving the gum tissue.

Treponema pallidum (syphilis): all stages.

N. gonorrhoeae: acute and chronic (without bacteremia). Yaws, Bejel, Pinta.

C. diphtheriae: Penicillin G Procaine as an adjunct to antitoxin for prevention of the carrier stage.

Anthrax.

Streptobacillus moniliformis and Spirillum minus infections (rat bite fever). Erysipeloid.

Subacute bacterial endocarditis (group A streptococcus): only in extremely sensitive infections.

Prophylaxis Against Bacterial Endocarditis: Although no controlled clinical efficacy studies have been conducted, aqueous crystalline Penicillin G for injection and Penicillin G Procaine suspension have been suggested by the American Heart Association and the American Dental Association for use as part of a combined parenteral-oral regimen for prophylaxis against bacterial endocarditis in patients with congenital heart disease or rheumatic, or other acquired valvular heart disease or rheumatic, or other acquired valvular heart disease when they undergo dental procedures and surgical procedures of the upper respiratory tract.[1] Since it may happen that alpha hemolytic streptococci relatively resistant to pencillin may be found when patients are receiving continuous oral Penicillin for secondary prevention of rheumatic fever, prophylactic agents other than Penicillin may be chosen for these patients and prescribed in addition to their continuous rheumatic fever prophylactic regimen.

Note: When selecting antibiotics for the prevention of bacterial endocarditis the physician or dentist should read the full joint statement of the American Heart Association and the American Dental Association.[1]

CONTRAINDICATIONS

A previous hypersensitivity reaction to any Penicillin or Procaine is a contraindication.

WARNINGS

Serious and occasionally fatal hypersensitivity (anaphylactoid) reactions have been reported in patients on Penicillin therapy. These reactions are more likely to occur in individuals with a history of Penicillin hypersensitivity and/or a history of sensitivity to multiple allergens. There have been reports of individuals with a history of Penicillin hypersensitivity who have experienced severe reactions when treated with cephalosporins. Before initiating therapy with any Penicillin, careful inquiry should be made concerning previous hypersensitivity reactions to Penicillin, cephalosporins, or other allergens. If an allergic reaction occurs, the drug should be discontinued and the appropriate therapy instituted. Serious anaphylactoid reactions require immediate emergency treatment with epinephrine. Oxygen, intravenous steroids, and airway management—including intubation, should be administered as indicated.

Immediate toxic reactions to Procaine may occur in some individuals, particularly when a large single dose is administered in the treatment of gonorrhea (4.8 million units). These reactions may be manifested by mental disturbances including anxiety, confusion, agitation, depression, weakness, seizures, hallucinations, combativeness, and expressed "fear of impending death." The reactions noted in carefully controlled studies occurred in approximately one in 500 patients treated for gonorrhea. Reactions are transient, lasting from 15-30 minutes.

PRECAUTIONS

General: Penicillin should be used with caution in individuals with histories of significant allergies and/or asthma.

Intramuscular Therapy: Care should be taken to avoid intravenous or accidental intra-arterial administration, or injection into or near major peripheral nerves or blood vessels, since such injections may produce neurovascular damage.

As with all intramuscular preparations, Penicillin G Procaine should be injected well within the body of a relatively large muscle. ADULTS: The preferred site is the upper quadrant of the buttock (i.e., gluteus maximus), or the mid-lateral thigh. CHILDREN: It is recommended that intramuscular injections be given preferably in the mid-lateral muscles of the thigh. In infants and small children the periphery of the upper outer quadrant of the gluteal region should only be used when necessary, such as in burn patients, in order to minimize the possibility of damage to the sciatic nerve.

The deltoid area should be used only if well developed, such as in certain adults and older children, and then only with caution to avoid radial nerve injury. Intramuscular injections should not be made into the lower and mid-third of the upper arm. As with all intramuscular injections, aspiration is necessary to help avoid inadvertent injection into a blood vessel.

In streptococcal infections, therapy must be sufficient to eliminate the organism (10 days minimum), otherwise the sequelae of streptococcal disease may occur. Cultures should be taken following completion of treatment to determine whether streptococci have been eradicated.

The use of antibiotics may result in overgrowth of nonsusceptible organisms. Constant observation of the patient is essential. If new infections due to bacteria or fungi appear during therapy, the drug should be discontinued and appropriate measures taken. Whenever allergic reactions occur, Penicillin should be withdrawn unless, in the opinion of the physician, the condition being treated is life threatening and amenable only to Penicillin therapy.

A small percentage of patients are sensitive to Procaine. If there is a history of sensitivity make the usual test: Inject intradermally 0.1 ml of a 1 to 2 percent solution. Development of an erythema, wheal, flare, or eruption indicates Procaine sensitivity. Sensitivity should be treated by the usual methods, including barbiturates, and Penicillin G Procaine preparations should not be used. Antihistamines appear beneficial in treatment of Procaine reactions.

Laboratory Tests: In prolonged therapy with Penicillin, periodic evaluation of the renal, hepatic, and hematopoietic systems is recommended. This is particularly important in prematures, neonates and other infants, and when high doses are used.

When treating gonococcal infections in which primary or secondary syphilis may be suspected, proper diagnostic procedures, including dark field examinations, should be done. In all cases in which concomitant syphilis is suspected, monthly serological tests should be made for at least four months. All cases of Penicillin treated syphilis should receive clinical and serological examinations every six months for two to three years.

In suspected staphylococcal infections, proper laboratory studies, including susceptibility tests, should be performed. In streptococcal infections, cultures should be taken following completion of treatment to determine whether streptococci have been eradicated.

Drug Interactions: Concurrent administration of bacteriostatic antibiotics (e.g., erythromycin, tetracycline) may diminish the bactericidal effects of penicillins by slowing the rate of bacterial growth. Bactericidal agents work most effectively against the immature cell wall of rapidly proliferating microorganisms. This has been demonstrated in vitro; however, the clinical significance of this interaction is not well documented. There are few clinical situations in which the concurrent use of "static" and "cidal" antibiotics are indicated. However, in selected circumstances in which such therapy is appropriate, using adequate doses of antibacterial agents and beginning Penicillin therapy first, should minimize the potential for interaction.

Penicillin blood levels may be prolonged by concurrent administration of probenecid, which blocks the renal tubular secretion of Penicillins.

Displacement of Penicillins from plasma protein binding sites will elevate the level of free Penicillin in the serum.

Carcinogenesis, Mutagenesis, Impairment of Fertility: No information or long-term studies are available on the carcinogenesis, mutagenesis, or the impairment of fertility with the use of Penicillin.

Pregnancy Category B: Teratogenic Effects: Reproduction studies performed in the mouse, rat, and rabbit have revealed no evidence of impaired fertility or harm to the fetus due to Penicillin G. Human experience with the Penicillins during pregnancy has not shown any positive evidence of adverse effects on the fetus.

There are, however, no adequate and well controlled studies in pregnant women showing conclusively that harmful effects of these drugs on the fetus can be excluded. Because animal reproduction studies are not always predictive of human response, this drug should be used during pregnancy only if clearly needed.

Nursing Mothers: Penicillin G Procaine has been reported in milk. Caution should be exercised when Penicillin G is administered to a nursing woman.

Pediatric Use: Penicillins are excreted largely unchanged by the kidney. Because of incompletely developed renal function in infants, the rate of elimination will be slow. Use caution in administering to newborns and evaluate organ system function frequently.

ADVERSE REACTIONS

Penicillin is a substance of low toxicity, but does possess a significant index of sensitization. The following hypersensitivity reactions associated with use of Penicillin have been reported: skin rashes, ranging from maculopapular eruptions to exfoliative dermatitis; urticaria, serum sickness-like reactions, including chills, fever, edema, arthralgia, and prostration. Severe and often fatal anaphylaxis has been reported (see *"Warnings"*). As with other treatments for syphilis, the Jarisch Herxheimer reaction has been reported. Procaine toxicity manifestations have been reported (see *"Warnings"*). Procaine hypersensitivity reactions have not been reported with this drug.

OVERDOSAGE

In case of overdosage, discontinue medication, treat symptomatically, and institute supportive measures as required. Convulsions have been reported in individuals receiving 4.8 million units.

Penicillin is hemodialyzable.

DOSAGE AND ADMINISTRATION

Pediatric Dosage Schedule: In children under 3 months of age, the absorption of aqueous Penicillin G produces such high and sustained levels that Penicillin G Procaine dosage forms offer no advantages and are usually unnecessary.

In children under 12 years of age, dosage should be adjusted in accordance with the age and weight of the child, and the severity of the infection.

Under 2 years of age, the dose may be divided between the two buttocks if necessary.

Penicillin G Procaine (aqueous) is for intramuscular injection only.

RECOMMENDED DOSAGE FOR PENICILLIN G PROCAINE AQUEOUS

Pneumonia: (pneumococcal), moderately severe (uncomplicated): 600,000-1,000,000 units daily.

Streptococcal Infections: (group A), moderately severe to severe tonsillitis, erysipelas, scarlet fever, upper respiratory tract, skin and soft tissue: 600,000-1,000,000 units daily for a minimum of 10 days.

Staphylococcal Infections: moderately severe to severe: 600,000-1,000,000 units daily.

Bacterial Endocarditis (group A streptococci), only in extremely sensitive infections: 600,000-1,000,000 units daily.

For prophylaxis against bacterial endocarditis[1] in patients with congenital heart disease or rheumatic or other acquired valvular heart disease, when undergoing dental procedures or surgical procedures of the upper respiratory tract, use a combined parenteral-oral regimen. One million units of aqueous crystalline Penicillin G (30,000 units/kg in children) intramuscularly, mixed with 600,000 units Penicillin G (600,000 units for children) should be given one-half to one hour before the procedure. Oral Penicillin V (phenoxymethyl Penicillin), 500 mg for adults or 250 mg for children less than 60 lb. should be given every six hours for 8 doses. Doses for children should not exceed recommendations for adults for a single dose or for a 24-hour period.

Syphilis: Primary, secondary and latent with a negative spinal fluid in adults and children over 12 years of age: 600,000 units daily for 8 days, total 4,800,000 units.

Late (tertiary neurosyphilis and latent syphilis with positive spinal fluid examination or no spinal fluid examination): 600,000 units daily for 10-15 days, total 6-9 million units.

Congenital Syphilis (early and late): 50,000 units/kg per day for a minimum of 10 days.

Yaws, Bejel, and Pinta: Treatment as syphilis in corresponding stage of disease.

Gonorrheal Infections (uncomplicated): Men or women—4.8 million units intramuscularly divided into at least two doses and injected at different sites at one visit, together with 1 gram of oral probenecid, preferably given at least 30 minutes prior to the injection.

Note: Gonorrheal endocarditis should be treated intensively with aqueous Penicillin G.

Diphtheria: adjunctive therapy with antitoxin: 300,000-600,000 units daily.

Diphtheria: carrier state: 300,000 units daily for 10 days.

Anthrax: cutaneous: 600,000-1,000,000 units/day.

Vincent's Infection: (fusospirochetosis): 600,000-1,000,000 units/day.

Erysipeloid: 600,000-1,000,000 units/day.

Streptobacillus moniliformis and *Spirillum minus* (rat bite fever): 600,000-1,000,000 units/day.

Parenteral drug products should be inspected visually for particulate matter and discoloration prior to administration, whenever solution and container permit.

STORAGE
The product should be stored between 2°-8°C (36°-46°F).

REFERENCE
1. American Heart Association, 1977. Prevention of Bacterial Endocarditis. Circulation 56:139A-143A.

J CODES
Up to 600,000 units IM,IV—J2510

HOW SUPPLIED
INJECTION: 600,000 U/ML

AVERAGE UNIT PRICE (AVAILABLE SIZES)

BRAND $2.63

BRAND/MANUFACTURER	NDC	SIZE	AWP
◆ **BRAND**			
WYCILLIN: Wyeth-Ayerst	00008-0018-10	1 ml 10s	$28.96
	00008-0018-08	2 ml 10s	$48.21
	00008-0018-12	4 ml 10s	$102.69

Penicillin G Sodium

DESCRIPTION
Penicillin G Sodium is crystalline Penicillin G Sodium as a sterile powder for use by intravenous or intramuscular administration. The preparation contains approximately 28 mg citrate buffer (composed of sodium citrate and not more than 0.92 mg citric acid) and 2.0 mEq Sodium per million units of Penicillin.

Following is its chemical structure:

CLINICAL PHARMACOLOGY
Penicillin G Sodium is bactericidal against penicillin-susceptible microorganisms during the stage of active multiplication. It acts by inhibiting biosynthesis of cell-wall mucopeptide. It is not active against the penicillinase-producing bacteria, which include many strains of staphylococci. Penicillin G Sodium is highly active *in vitro* against staphylococci (except penicillinase-producing strains), streptococci (groups A, C, G, H, L, and M) and pneumococci. Other organisms susceptible *in vitro* to Penicillin G are *Neisseria gonorrhoeae, Corynebacterium diphtheriae, Bacillus anthracis,* Clostridia, *Actinomyces bovis, Streptobacillus moniliformis, Listeria monocytogenes,* and Leptospira; *Treponema pallidum* is extremely susceptible. Some species of gram-negative bacilli are susceptible to moderate to high concentrations of Penicillin G Sodium obtained with intravenous administration. These include most strains of *Escherichia coli;* all strains of *Proteus mirabilis,* Salmonella, and Shigella; and some strains of *Enterobacter aerogenes* (formerly *Aerobacter aerogenes*) and *Alcaligenes faecalis.*

Susceptibility plate testing: If the Kirby-Bauer method of disc susceptibility is used, a 10 unit Penicillin disc should give a zone greater than 28 mm when tested against a penicillin-susceptible bacterial strain.

Aqueous Penicillin G Sodium is rapidly absorbed following both intramuscular and subcutaneous injection. Approximately 60 percent of the total dose of 300,000 units is excreted in the urine within this five-hour period. Therefore, high and frequent doses are required to maintain the elevated serum levels desirable in treating certain severe infections in individuals with normal kidney function. In neonates and young infants and in individuals with impaired kidney function, excretion is considerably delayed.

INDICATIONS AND USAGE
Penicillin G Sodium is indicated in the treatment of severe infections caused by Penicillin G-susceptible microorganisms when rapid and high penicillinemia is required. Therapy should be guided by bacteriological studies, including susceptibility tests, and by clinical response.

The following infections will usually respond to adequate dosage:

Streptococcal infections. Note: Streptococci in groups A, C, G, H, L, and M are very susceptible to Penicillin G. Some group D organisms are susceptible to the high serum levels obtained with aqueous Penicillin G. Aqueous Penicillin G is the Penicillin dosage form of choice for bacteremia, empyema, severe pneumonia, pericarditis, endocarditis, meningitis, and other severe infections caused by susceptible strains of the gram-positive species listed above.

Pneumococcal infections, Staphylococcal infections: Penicillin G-susceptible

Anthrax

Actinomycosis

Clostridial infections (including tetanus)

Diphtheria (to prevent the carrier state)

Erysipeloid endocarditis (Erysipelothrix insidiosa)

Vincent's gingivitis and pharyngitis (fusospirochetosis)—Severe infections of the oropharynx (Note: Necessary dental care should be accomplished in infections involving gum tissue.) and:

Lower respiratory tract and genital area infections due to *F. fusiformisans* spirochetes

Gram-negative bacillary infections (bacteremias)—(*E. coli, E. aerogenes, A. faecalis*, Salmonella, Shigella, and *P. mirabilis*)

Listeria infections (*L. monocytogenes*)

Meningitis and endocarditis

Pasteurella infections (*P. multocida*) bacteremia and meningitis

Rat-bite fever (*S. minus* or *S. moniliformis*)

Gonorrheal endocarditis and arthritis (*N. gonorrhoeae*)

Syphilis (*T. pallidum*) including congenital syphilis

Meningococcic meningitis

Prevention of bacterial endocarditis: (Patients unable to take oral antibiotics): Although no controlled clinical efficacy studies have been conducted, aqueous crystalline Penicillin G for injection (**except** Penicillin G procaine suspension) has been suggested by the American Heart Association and the American Dental Association for prophylaxis against bacterial endocarditis in patients with congenital heart disease or rheumatic or other acquired valvular heart disease when they undergo dental procedures and surgical procedures of the upper respiratory tract.[1] Since it may happen that *alpha* hemolytic streptococci relatively resistant to penicillin may be found when patients are receiving continuous oral Penicillin for secondary prevention of rheumatic fever, prophylactic agents other than penicillin may be chosen for these patients and prescribed in addition to their continuous rheumatic fever prophylactic regimen. **NOTE: When selecting antibiotics for the prevention of bacterial endocarditis, the physician or dentist should read the full joint statement of the American Heart Association and the American Dental Association.**[1]

CONTRAINDICATIONS
Contraindicated in patients with a history of hypersensitivity to any penicillin.

WARNINGS
Serious and occasional fatal hypersensitivity (anaphylactoid) reactions have been reported in patients on Penicillin therapy. Although anaphylaxis is more frequent following parenteral administration, it has occurred in patients on oral penicillins. These reactions are more apt to occur in individuals with a history of sensitivity to multiple allergens.

There have been well-documented reports of individuals with a history of Penicillin hypersensitivity who have experienced severe hypersensitivity reactions when treated with cephalosporins. Before therapy with a Penicillin, careful inquiry should be made concerning previous hypersensitivity reactions to Penicillins, cephalosporins, and other allergens. If an allergic reaction occurs, the drug should be discontinued and the patient treated with the usual agents, e.g., pressor amines, antihistamines, and corticosteroids. Serious anaphylactoid reactions are not controlled by antihistamines alone, and require such emergency measures as the immediate use of epinephrine, aminophylline, oxygen, and intravenous corticosteroids.

PRECAUTIONS
Penicillin G Sodium should be used with caution in individuals with histories of significant allergies and/or asthma.

In prolonged therapy with Penicillin G Sodium and particularly with high dosage schedules, periodic evaluation of the renal and hematopoietic systems is recommended.

In streptococcal infections, therapy must be sufficient to eliminate the organism (ten days minimum); otherwise, the sequelae of streptococcal disease may occur. Cultures should be taken following the completion of treatment to determine whether streptococci have been eradicated.

In high doses (above 10 million units), intravenous aqueous Penicillin G Sodium should be administered slowly because of the adverse effects of electrolyte imbalance from the sodium content of the penicillin. The patient's renal, cardiac, and vascular status should be evaluated and if impairment of function is suspected or known to exist, a reduction in the total dosage should be considered. Frequent evaluation of electrolyte balance, and renal and hematopoietic function is recommended during therapy when high doses of intravenous aqueous Penicillin G Sodium are used.

Prolonged use of antibiotics may promote overgrowth of nonsusceptible organisms, including fungi. Should superinfection occur, appropriate measures should be taken. Indwelling intravenous catheters encourage superinfections and should be avoided whenever possible.

Therapy of susceptible infections should be accompanied by any indicated surgical procedures. In suspected staphylococcal infections, proper laboratory studies, including susceptibility tests, should be performed.

When treating gonococcal infections in which primary or secondary syphilis may be suspected, proper diagnostic procedures, including darkfield examinations, should be done. In all cases in which concomitant syphilis is suspected, monthly serological tests should be made for at least four months. All cases of penicillin-treated syphilis should receive clinical and serological examinations every six months for at least two or three years.

Any entry into the container to effect solution of the powder or withdrawal of contents must be accomplished with strict aseptic technique and sterile equipment.

ADVERSE REACTIONS
Penicillin G Sodium is a substance of low toxicity but does possess a significant index of sensitization.

The hypersensitivity reactions reported are skin rashes ranging from maculopapular eruptions to exfoliative dermatitis; urticaria; and serum sickness-like reactions including chills, fever, edema, arthralgia, and prostration. Severe and occasionally fatal anaphylaxis has occurred (see *"Warnings"*).

Hemolytic anemia, leukopenia, thrombocytopenia, neuropathy, and nephropathy are rarely observed adverse reactions and are usually associated with high intravenous dosage. Urticaria, other skin rashes, and serum sickness-like reactions may be controlled by antihistamines and, if necessary, corticosteroids. Whenever such reactions occur, penicillin should be discontinued unless, in the opinion of the physician, the condition being treated is life-threatening and amenable only to penicillin therapy. High dosage of Penicillin G Sodium may result in congestive heart failure due to high sodium intake.

The Jarisch-Herxheimer reaction has been reported in patients treated for syphilis.

DOSAGE AND ADMINISTRATION
Penicillin G Sodium may be given intramuscularly or by continuous intravenous drip.

The usual dose recommendation is as follows:

Severe infections due to susceptible strains of streptococci, pneumococci, and staphylococci; bacteremia, pneumonia, endocarditis, pericarditis, empyema, meningitis, and other severe infections: a minimum of 5 million units daily.

Anthrax: a minimum of 5 million units/day in divided doses until cure is effected.

Actinomycosis: 1 to 6 million units/day for cervicofacial cases; 10 to 20 million units/day for thoracic and abdominal disease.

Clostridal infections (as adjunctive therapy to antitoxin): 20 million units/day.

Diphtheria: adjunctive therapy to antitoxin for prevention of the carrier state: 300,000 to 400,000 units/day in divided doses for 10 to 12 days.

Erysipeloid endocarditis: 2 to 20 million units/day for four to six weeks.

Fusospirochetal infections: (fusospirochetosis)—severe infections of the oropharynx, lower respiratory tract and genital area: 5 to 10 million units/day.

Gram-negative bacillary infections: (*E. coli, E. aerogenes, A. faecalis,* Salmonella, Shigella, and *P. mirabilis); Bacteremia:* 20 to 80 million units/day.

Listeria infections (*L. monocytogenes): Neonates:* 500,000 to 1 million units/day; *Adults with meningitis:* 15 to 20 million units/day for two weeks; *Adults with endocarditis:* 15 to 20 million units/day for four weeks.

Pasteurella infections (*P. multocida): Bacteremia and meningitis:* 4 to 6 million units/day for two weeks.

Rat-bite fever (*S. minus* or *S. moniliformis):* 12 to 15 million units/day for three to four weeks.

Gonorrheal endocarditis and arthritis: a minimum of 5 million units daily.

Syphilis: aqueous Penicillin G Sodium may be used in the treatment of acquired and congenital syphilis but, because of the necessity of frequent dosage, hospitalization is recommended. Dosage and duration of therapy are determined by the age of the patient and the stage of the disease.

Meningococcic meningitis: 1 to 2 million units IM every two hours or continuous IV drip of 20 to 30 million units/day.

Prevention of bacterial endocarditis (Patients unable to take oral antibiotics: For prophylaxis against bacterial endocarditis[1] in patients with congenital heart disease or rheumatic or other acquired valvular heart disease when undergoing dental procedures or surgical procedures of the upper respiratory tract, administer 2 million units (50,000 units/kg for children) aqueous Penicillin G Sodium, intravenously or intramuscularly 30 to 60 minutes before the procedure and 1 million units (25,000 units/kg for children) six hours later. Doses for children should not exceed recommendations for adults for a single dose or for a 24-hour period.

PREPARATION OF SOLUTIONS
Solutions of Penicillin G Sodium should be prepared as follows: Loosen powder. Hold vial horizontally and rotate it while *slowly* directing the stream of diluent against the wall of the vial. Shake vial vigorously after all the diluent has been added. Depending on the route of administration, use Sterile Water for Injection, USP, 0.9% Sodium Chloride Injection, USP, or Dextrose Injection, USP. *Note*: Penicillins are rapidly inactivated in the presence of carbohydrate solutions at alkaline pH.

Constitute with 23 mL, 18 mL, 8 mL, or 3 mL diluent to provide concentrations of 200,000 units, 250,000 units, 500,000 units, or 1,000,000 units per mL, respectively.

STORAGE
The dry powder is relatively stable and may be stored at room temperature without significant loss of potency. Sterile solutions may be kept in the refrigerator one week without significant loss of potency. Solutions prepared for intravenous infusion are stable at room temperature for at least 24 hours.

REFERENCE
1. American Heart Association: Prevention of bacterial endocarditis. Circulation 70:1123A-1127A, 1984.

HOW SUPPLIED
POWDER FOR INJECTION: 5 MILLION U

BRAND/MANUFACTURER	NDC	SIZE	AWP
○ GENERICS			
Apothecon	00003-0668-05	1s	$6.34
Marsam	00209-8586-22	10s	$67.50

Penicillin V Potassium

DESCRIPTION
Penicillin V is the phenoxymethyl analog of penicillin G. Penicillin V Potassium is the potassium salt of Penicillin V. Pencillin V Potassium tablets contain Penicillin V Potassium equivalent to 250 mg (400,000 units) or 500 mg (800,000 units) Penicillin V.

Pencillin V Potassium for oral solution is a powder which when reconstituted as directed yields a suspension of Pencillin V Potassium equivalent to 125 mg (200,000 units) or 250 mg (400,000 units) Penicillin V per 5 mL.

Following is its chemical structure:

ACTION AND PHARMACOLOGY
Penicillin V exerts a bactericidal action against Penicillin-sensitive microorganisms during the stage of active multiplication. It acts through the inhibition of biosynthesis of cell-wall mucopeptide. It is not active against the penicillinase-producing bacteria, which include many strains of staphylococci. The drug exerts high *in vitro* activity against staphylococci (except penicillinase-producing strains), streptococci (groups A, C, G, H, L, and M), and pneumococci. Other organisms sensitive *in vitro* to Penicillin V are *Corynebacterium diphtheriae, Bacillus anthracis,* Clostridia, *Actinomyces bovis, Streptobacillus moniliformis, Listeria monocytogenes,* Leptospira, and *Neisseria gonorrhoeae. Treponema pallidum* is extremely sensitive.

The potassium salt of Penicillin V has the distinct advantage over penicillin G in resistance to inactivation by gastric acid. It may be given with meals; however, blood levels are slightly higher when the drug is given on an empty stomach. Average blood levels are two to five times higher than the levels following the same dose of oral penicillin G and also shown much less individual variation.

Once absorbed, Penicillin V is about 80% bound to serum protein. Tissue levels are highest in the kidneys, with lesser amounts in the liver, skin, and intestines. Small amounts are found in all other body tissues and the cerebrospinal fluid. The drug is excreted as rapidly as it is absorbed in individuals with normal kidney function; however, recovery of the drug from the urine indicates that only about 25% of the dose given is absorbed. In neonates, young infants, and individuals with impaired kidney function, excretion is considerably delayed.

INDICATIONS
Penicillin V Potassium is indicated in the treatment of mild to moderately severe infections due to penicillin G-sensitive microorganisms. Therapy should be guided by bacteriological studies (including sensitivity tests) and by clinical response.

Note: Severe pneumonia, empyema, bacteremia, pericarditis, meningitis, and arthritis should not be treated with Penicillin V during the acute stage.
   Indicated surgical procedures should be performed.
   The following infections will usually respond to adequate dosage of Penicillin V.

Streptococcal infections (without bacteremia). Mild-to-moderate infections of the upper respiratory tract, scarlet fever, and mild erysipelas.
   Note: Streptococci in groups A, C, G, H, L, and M are very sensitive to Penicillin. Other groups, including group D (enterococcus), are resistant.

Pneumococcal infections. Mild to moderately severe infections of the respiratory tract.

Staphylococcal infections: penicillin-G-sensitive. Mild infections of the skin and soft tissues.
   Note: Reports indicate an increasing number of strains of staphylococci resistant to penicillin G, emphasizing the need for culture and sensitivity studies in treating suspected staphylococcal infections.

Fusospirochetosis (Vincent's gingivitis and pharyngitis)—Mild to moderately severe infections of the oropharynx usually respond to therapy with oral Penicillin.
   Note: Necessary dental care should be accomplished in infections involving the gum tissue.
   Medical conditions in which oral Penicillin therapy is indicated as prophylaxis:

For the prevention of recurrence following rheumatic fever and/or chorea: Prophylaxis with oral Penicillin on a continuing basis has proven effective in preventing recurrence of these conditions.

Although no controlled clinical efficacy studies have been conducted, Penicillin V has been suggested by the American Heart Association and the American Dental Association for use as an oral regimen for prophylaxis against bacterial endocarditis in patients who have congenital heart disease or rheumatic or other acquired valvular heart disease when they undergo dental procedures and surgical procedures of the upper respiratory tract.[1] Oral Penicillin should not be used in those patients at particularly high risk for endocarditis (e.g., those with prosthetic heart valves or surgically constructed systemic-pulmonary shunts). Penicillin V should not be used as adjunctive prophylaxis for genitourinary instrumentation or surgery, lower-intestinal-tract surgery, sigmoidoscopy, and childbirth. Since it may happen that *alpha* hemolytic streptococci relatively resistant to Penicillin may be found when patients are receiving continuous oral Penicillin for secondary prevention of rheumatic fever, prophylactic agents other than Penicillin may be chosen for these patients and prescribed in addition to their continuous rheumatic fever prophylactic regimen.

Note: When selecting antibiotics for the prevention of bacterial endocarditis, the physician or dentist should read the full joint statement of the American Heart Association and the American Dental Association.[1]

CONTRAINDICATIONS
A previous hypersensitivity reaction to any Penicillin is a contraindication.

WARNINGS
Serious and occasionally fatal hypersensitivity (anaphylactoid) reactions have been reported in patients on Penicillin therapy. Although anaphylaxis is more frequent following parenteral therapy, it has occurred in patients on oral Penicillins. These reactions are more apt to occur in individuals with a history of sensitivity to multiple allergens.

There have been well-documented reports of individuals with a history of Penicillin hypersensitivity reactions who have experienced severe hypersensitivity reactions when treated with a cephalosporin.

Before therapy with a Penicillin, careful inquiry should be made concerning previous hypersensitivity reactions to penicillins, cephalosporins, and other allergens. If an allergic reaction occurs, the drug should be discontinued and the patient treated with the usual agents, e.g., pressor amines, antihistamines, and corticosteroids.

PRECAUTIONS
Penicillin should be used with caution in individuals with histories of significant allergies and/or asthma.

The oral route of administration should not be relied upon in patients with severe illness, or with nausea, vomiting, gastric dilatation, cardiospasm, or intestinal hypermotility. Occasional patients will not absorb therapeutic amounts of orally administered Penicillin.

In streptococcal infections, therapy must be sufficient to eliminate the organism (10-day minimum); otherwise the sequelae of streptococcal disease may occur. Cultures should be taken following completion of treatment to determine whether streptococci have been eradicated.

Prolonged use of antibiotics may promote the overgrowth of nonsusceptible organisms, including fungi. Should superinfection occur, appropriate measures should be taken.

ADVERSE REACTIONS
Although the incidence of reactions to oral Penicillins has been reported with much less frequency than following parenteral therapy, it should be remembered that all degrees of hypersensitivity, including fatal anaphylaxis, have been reported with oral Penicillin.

The most common reactions to oral Penicillins are nausea, vomiting, epigastric distress, diarrhea, and black hairy tongue. The hypersensitivity reactions reported are skin eruptions (maculopapular to exfoliative dermatitis), urticaria and other serum-sicknesslike reactions, laryngeal edema, and anaphylaxis. Fever and eosinophilia may frequently be the only reaction observed. Hemolytic anemia, leukopenia, thrombocytopenia, neuropathy, and nephropathy are infrequent reactions and usually associated with high doses of parenteral Penicillin.

DOSAGE AND ADMINISTRATION
The dosage of Penicillin V should be determined according to the sensitivity of the causative microorganisms and the severity of infection, and adjusted to the clinical response of the patient.

The usual dosage recommendations for adults and children 12 years and over are as follows:

Streptococcal infections: Mild to moderately severe of the upper respiratory tract and including scarlet fever and erysipelas: 125 to 250 mg (200,000 to 400,000 units) every 6 to 8 hours for 10 days.

Pneumococcal infections: Mild to moderately severe of the respiratory tract, including otitis media: 250 to 500 mg (400,000 to 800,000 units) every 6 hours until the patient has been afebrile for at least 2 days.

Staphylococcal infections: Mild infections of skin and soft tissue (culture and sensitivity tests should be performed): 250 to 500 mg (400,000 to 800,000 units) every 6 to 8 hours.

Fusospirochetosis (Vincent's infection) of the oropharynx: Mild to moderately severe infections: 250 to 500 mg (400,000 to 800,000 units) every 6 to 8 hours.

◆ RATED THERAPEUTICALLY EQUIVALENT; ◇ THERAPEUTIC EQUIVALENCE UNCONFIRMED; ○ UNRATED

For the prevention of recurrence following rheumatic fever and/or chorea: 125 to 250 mg (200,000 to 400,000 units) twice daily on a continuing basis.

For prophylaxis against bacterial endocarditis[1] in patients with congenital heart disease or rheumatic or other acquired valvular heart disease when undergoing dental procedures or surgical procedures of the upper respiratory tract: 2.0 gram of Penicillin V (1.0 gram for children under 60 lbs.) 1 hour before the procedure, and then, 1.0 gram (500 mg for children under 60 lbs.) 6 hours later.

Keep tightly closed.

Dispense in tight container.

After reconstitution, solution must be stored in a refrigerator.

Discard any unused portion after 14 days.

REFERENCE
1. American Heart Association, 1984. Prevention of bacterial endocarditis, Circulation 70(6);1123A-1127A.

HOW SUPPLIED
POWDER FOR RECONSTITUTION: 125 MG/5 ML

AVERAGE UNIT PRICE (AVAILABLE SIZES)		GENERIC A-RATED AVERAGE PRICE (GAAP)	
GENERIC	$0.02	100 ml	$2.02
HCFA FUL (100 ml)	$0.02	200 ml	$3.10

BRAND/MANUFACTURER	NDC	SIZE	AWP
◆ GENERICS			
Rugby	00536-2540-82	100 ml	$1.56
VEETIDS: Apothecon	00003-0681-44	100 ml	$1.67
Moore,H.L.	00839-5189-73	100 ml	$1.74
PEN-VEE K: Wyeth-Ayerst	00008-0004-06	100 ml	$1.81
LEDERCILLIN VK: Lederle Std Prod	00005-3874-46	100 ml	$1.91
Schein	00364-2023-61	100 ml	$2.00
BEEPEN-VK: SK Beecham Pharm	00029-6165-23	100 ml	$2.00
URL	00677-0109-27	100 ml	$2.04
Goldline	00182-0276-70	100 ml	$2.05
Major	00904-4001-04	100 ml	$2.16
Biocraft	00332-4125-32	100 ml	$2.16
Qualitest	00603-6605-64	100 ml	$2.28
Warner Chilcott	00047-2449-17	100 ml	$2.38
Aligen	00405-3500-60	100 ml	$2.51
LEDERCILLIN VK: Lederle Std Prod	00005-3874-49	150 ml	$2.40
Rugby	00536-2540-84	200 ml	$2.25
Moore,H.L.	00839-5189-78	200 ml	$2.36
VEETIDS: Apothecon	00003-0681-54	200 ml	$2.87
Goldline	00182-0276-73	200 ml	$3.00
URL	00677-0109-29	200 ml	$3.03
BEEPEN-VK: SK Beecham Pharm	00029-6165-24	200 ml	$3.05
PEN-VEE K: Wyeth-Ayerst	00008-0004-07	200 ml	$3.14
LEDERCILLIN VK: Lederle Std Prod	00005-3874-60	200 ml	$3.18
Major	00904-4001-08	200 ml	$3.34
Biocraft	00332-4125-36	200 ml	$3.34
Qualitest	00603-6605-68	200 ml	$3.34
Warner Chilcott	00047-2449-20	200 ml	$3.47
Aligen	00405-3500-70	200 ml	$3.92

POWDER FOR RECONSTITUTION: 250 MG/5 ML

AVERAGE UNIT PRICE (AVAILABLE SIZES)		GENERIC A-RATED AVERAGE PRICE (GAAP)	
BRAND	$0.04	100 ml	$2.61
GENERIC	$0.02	150 ml	$3.47
HCFA FUL (100 ml)	$0.02	200 ml	$4.26

BRAND/MANUFACTURER	NDC	SIZE	AWP
◆ BRAND			
V-CILLIN K: Lilly	00002-2316-48	100 ml	$4.46
	00002-2316-68	150 ml	$6.72
	00002-2316-89	200 ml	$7.65
◆ GENERICS			
Rugby	00536-2560-82	100 ml	$1.94
Moore,H.L.	00839-5190-73	100 ml	$2.15
VEETIDS: Apothecon	00003-0682-44	100 ml	$2.16
LEDERCILLIN VK: Lederle Std Prod	00005-3875-46	100 ml	$2.18
Schein	00364-2024-61	100 ml	$2.48
URL	00677-0110-27	100 ml	$2.50
Goldline	00182-0308-70	100 ml	$2.55
BEEPEN-VK: SK Beecham Pharm	00029-6170-23	100 ml	$2.60
PEN-VEE K: Wyeth-Ayerst	00008-0036-04	100 ml	$2.73
Major	00904-4004-04	100 ml	$2.95
Biocraft	00332-4127-32	100 ml	$2.95
Aligen	00405-3525-60	100 ml	$3.03
Qualitest	00603-6606-64	100 ml	$3.08
Warner Chilcott	00047-2506-17	100 ml	$3.24
LEDERCILLIN VK: Lederle Std Prod	00005-3875-49	150 ml	$3.15
PEN-VEE K: Wyeth-Ayerst	00008-0036-03	150 ml	$3.79
Moore,H.L.	00839-5190-78	200 ml	$3.09
Rugby	00536-2560-84	200 ml	$3.12
VEETIDS: Apothecon	00003-0682-54	200 ml	$3.64
Goldline	00182-0308-73	200 ml	$4.05
Schein	00364-2024-63	200 ml	$4.06
PEN-VEE K: Wyeth-Ayerst	00008-0036-05	200 ml	$4.06
LEDERCILLIN VK: Lederle Std Prod	00005-3875-60	200 ml	$4.16
URL	00677-0110-29	200 ml	$4.30

BRAND/MANUFACTURER	NDC	SIZE	AWP
BEEPEN-VK: SK Beecham Pharm	00029-6170-24	200 ml	$4.35
Major	00904-4004-08	200 ml	$5.07
Biocraft	00332-4127-36	200 ml	$5.07
Qualitest	00603-6606-68	200 ml	$5.07
Warner Chilcott	00047-2506-20	200 ml	$5.31

POWDER FOR RECONSTITUTION: 250 MG

BRAND/MANUFACTURER	NDC	SIZE	AWP
◆ GENERICS			
Aligen	00405-3525-70	200 ml	$5.42

TABLETS: 250 MG

AVERAGE UNIT PRICE (AVAILABLE SIZES)		GENERIC A-RATED AVERAGE PRICE (GAAP)	
BRAND	$0.21	100s	$7.28
GENERIC	$0.06	1000s	$50.71
HCFA FUL (100s ea)	$0.06		

BRAND/MANUFACTURER	NDC	SIZE	AWP
◆ BRAND			
V-CILLIN K: Lilly	00002-0329-02	100s	$21.46
	00002-0329-03	500s	$101.27
◆ GENERICS			
Biocraft	00332-1171-09	100s	$5.34
➤ Biocraft	00332-1172-09	100s	$5.34
Major	00904-2449-60	100s	$5.50
Major	00904-2450-60	100s	$5.50
Rugby	00536-2520-01	100s	$5.78
Rugby	00536-2527-01	100s	$5.78
Schein	00364-2021-01	100s	$5.78
PEN-V: Goldline	00182-0869-01	100s	$6.00
Mylan	00378-0111-01	100s	$6.26
Mylan	00378-0195-01	100s	$6.26
Geneva	00781-1205-01	100s	$6.35
➤ LEDERCILLIN VK: Lederle Std Prod	00005-3865-23	100s	$6.69
➤ VEETIDS: Apothecon	00003-0115-50	100s	$6.84
Aligen	00405-4762-01	100s	$7.20
Aligen	00405-4768-01	100s	$7.20
URL	00677-0107-01	100s	$7.31
URL	00677-0411-01	100s	$7.31
Moore,H.L.	00839-5187-06	100s	$7.36
Moore,H.L.	00839-5188-06	100s	$7.36
➤ Warner Chilcott	00047-0648-24	100s	$8.12
➤ PEN-VEE K: Wyeth-Ayerst	00008-0059-02	100s	$12.24
UDL	51079-0615-20	100s ud	$12.60
PEN-VEE K: Wyeth-Ayerst	00008-0059-10	100s ud	$13.34
➤ LEDERCILLIN VK: Lederle Std Prod	00005-3865-61	480s	$37.78
➤ PEN-VEE K: Wyeth-Ayerst	00008-0059-04	500s	$48.13
Rugby	00536-2520-10	1000s	$39.60
Rugby	00536-2527-10	1000s	$39.60
Biocraft	00332-1171-15	1000s	$42.79
➤ Biocraft	00332-1172-15	1000s	$42.79
Major	00904-2450-80	1000s	$43.00
Mason Dist	11845-0463-04	1000s	$45.36
Mason Dist	11845-0465-04	1000s	$45.36
Schein	00364-2021-02	1000s	$45.78
PEN-V: Goldline	00182-0116-10	1000s	$45.90
PEN-V: Goldline	00182-0869-10	1000s	$45.90
Mylan	00378-0111-10	1000s	$48.62
Mylan	00378-0195-10	1000s	$48.62
Aligen	00405-4762-03	1000s	$51.47
Aligen	00405-4768-03	1000s	$51.47
Moore,H.L.	00839-5187-16	1000s	$53.45
Moore,H.L.	00839-5188-16	1000s	$53.45
VEETIDS: Apothecon	00003-0115-75	1000s	$57.44
URL	00677-0107-10	1000s	$58.75
URL	00677-0411-10	1000s	$58.75
Geneva	00781-1205-10	1000s	$58.80
Qualitest	00603-5067-32	1000s	$59.10
➤ Warner Chilcott	00047-0648-32	1000s	$59.47
➤ BEEPEN-VK: SK Beecham Pharm	00029-6150-33	1000s	$59.70
➤ LEDERCILLIN VK: Lederle Std Prod	00005-3865-34	1000s	$61.94

TABLETS: 500 MG

AVERAGE UNIT PRICE (AVAILABLE SIZES)		GENERIC A-RATED AVERAGE PRICE (GAAP)	
BRAND	$0.39	100s	$12.83
GENERIC	$0.11	500s	$67.55
HCFA FUL (100s ea)	$0.07	1000s	$85.55

BRAND/MANUFACTURER	NDC	SIZE	AWP
◆ BRAND			
➤ V-CILLIN K: Lilly	00002-0346-02	100s	$40.60
	00002-0346-03	500s	$190.07
◆ GENERICS			
Geneva	00781-1655-01	100s	$7.50
Biocraft	00332-1174-09	100s	$9.24
➤ Biocraft	00332-1173-09	100s	$9.24
Rugby	00536-2530-01	100s	$9.50
Rugby	00536-2537-01	100s	$9.50
Schein	00364-2058-01	100s	$9.63

➤ SHOWN IN PRODUCT IDENTIFICATION GUIDE

BRAND/MANUFACTURER	NDC	SIZE	AWP
Major	00904-2451-60	100s	$9.90
Major	00904-2452-60	100s	$9.90
Mylan	00378-0112-01	100s	$10.62
▶ Mylan	00378-0198-01	100s	$10.62
PEN-V: Goldline	00182-0115-01	100s	$11.40
PEN-V: Goldline	00182-1537-01	100s	$11.40
Moore,H.L.	00839-1766-06	100s	$11.68
Moore,H.L.	00839-6393-06	100s	$11.68
Aligen	00405-4763-01	100s	$12.25
Aligen	00405-4769-01	100s	$12.25
URL	00677-0108-01	100s	$12.38
URL	00677-0576-01	100s	$12.38
▶ LEDERCILLIN VK: Lederle Std Prod	00005-3866-23	100s	$12.81
▶ VEETIDS: Apothecon	00003-0116-50	100s	$13.01
▶ Warner Chilcott	00047-0673-24	100s	$14.91
Qualitest	00603-5068-21	100s	$15.33
▶ PEN-VEE K: Wyeth-Ayerst	00008-0390-01	100s	$23.01
UDL	51079-0616-20	100s ud	$24.60
▶ PEN-VEE K: Wyeth-Ayerst	00008-0390-04	100s ud	$26.13
▶ Warner Chilcott	00047-0673-30	500s	$59.52
▶ BEEPEN-VK: SK Beecham Pharm	00029-6160-32	500s	$61.25
▶ LEDERCILLIN VK: Lederle Std Prod	00005-3866-31	500s	$62.44
▶ PEN-VEE K: Wyeth-Ayerst	00008-0390-05	500s	$86.98
Rugby	00536-2530-10	1000s	$63.69
Rugby	00536-2537-10	1000s	$63.69
Moore,H.L.	00839-1766-16	1000s	$67.76
Major	00904-2452-80	1000s	$81.00
Schein	00364-2022-02	1000s	$82.50
Mason Dist	11845-0464-04	1000s	$84.33
Mason Dist	11845-0466-04	1000s	$84.33
Major	00904-2451-80	1000s	$84.54
Biocraft	00332-1174-15	1000s	$84.54
▶ Biocraft	00332-1173-15	1000s	$84.54
URL	00677-0108-10	1000s	$87.95
URL	00677-0576-10	1000s	$87.95
PEN-V: Goldline	00182-0115-10	1000s	$88.00
PEN-V: Goldline	00182-1537-10	1000s	$88.00
Schein	00364-2058-02	1000s	$89.93
▶ VEETIDS: Apothecon	00003-0116-75	1000s	$92.95
Mylan	00378-0112-10	1000s	$96.26
▶ Mylan	00378-0198-10	1000s	$96.26
Aligen	00405-4769-03	1000s	$99.47
Aligen	00405-4763-03	1000s	$103.37

Pentagastrin

DESCRIPTION

Pentagastrin is a diagnostic agent for evaluation of gastric acid secretory function.

Chemical name: N-t-butyloxycarbonyl-B-alanyl-L-tryptophyl-L-methionyl-L-aspartyl-L-phenylalanyl amide.

Pentagastrin is a synthetic pentapeptide containing the carboxyl terminal tetrapeptide, the active portion found in all natural gastrins. Pentagastrin is a colorless crystalline solid. It is soluble in dimethylformamide and dimethylsulfoxide; it is almost insoluble in water, ethanol, ether, benzene, chloroform, and ethyl acetate. Pentagastrin is sterile and nonpyrogenic.

Each mL of injection contains 0.25 mg (250 mcg) Pentagastrin.

Following is its chemical structure:

$$N-(CH_3)_3COC-\beta Ala-Trp-Met-Asp-Phe-NH_2$$

CLINICAL PHARMACOLOGY

Pentagastrin contains the C-terminal tetrapeptide responsible for the actions of the natural gastrins and, therefore, acts as a physiologic gastric acid secretagogue. The recommended dose of 6 mcg/kg subcutaneously produces a peak acid output which is reproducible when used in the same individual.

Pentagastrin stimulates gastric acid secretion approximately ten minutes after subcutaneous injection, with peak responses occurring in most cases twenty to thirty minutes after administration. Duration of activity is usually between sixty and eighty minutes.

In amounts in excess of recommended dose, Pentagastrin may cause inhibition of gastric acid secretion.

In clinical studies of gastric acid secretion, peak gastric output in mEq/hr resulting from the subcutaneous injection of 6 mcg/kg Pentagastrin does not differ significantly from that caused by the standard subcutaneous injection of the histamine acid phosphate dose used in the augmented histamine test (40 mcg/kg). For example, in 25 normal volunteers, Pentagastrin produced an average peak acid output of 28.4 mEq/hr, compared with 24.7 mEq/hr by histamine. In 45 patients with duodenal ulcer, or suspected duodenal ulcer, Pentagastrin produced an average peak gastric acid output of 39.7 mEq/hr, compared with 33.7 mEq/hr by histamine. In 18 patients with gastric ulcer, or suspected gastric ulcer, Pentagastrin produced an average peak acid output of 17.4 mEq/hr, compared with 19.4 mEq/hr by histamine. The overall mean for peak acid secretion by Pentagastrin was 24.8 mEq/hr, compared with 22.6 mEq/hr by histamine. No biochemical abnormality which might indicate specific organ toxicity has been encountered following the administration of Pentagastrin.

INDICATIONS AND USAGE

Pentagastrin is used as a diagnostic agent to evaluate gastric acid secretory function. It is useful in testing for:

Anacidity: as a diagnostic aid in patients with suspected pernicious anemia, atrophic gastritis, or gastric carcinoma.

Hypersecretion: as a diagnostic aid in patients with suspected duodenal ulcer or postoperative stomal ulcer, and for the diagnosis of Zollinger-Ellison tumor.

Pentagastrin is also useful in determining the adequacy of acid-reducing operations for peptic ulcer.

CONTRAINDICATIONS

Hypersensitivity or idiosyncrasy to Pentagastrin.

WARNINGS

In amounts in excess of the recommended dose, Pentagastrin may cause inhibition of gastric acid secretion.

PRECAUTIONS

Use with caution in patients with pancreatic, hepatic, or biliary disease. Like gastrin, Pentagastrin could, in some cases, have the physiologic effect of stimulating pancreatic enzyme and bicarbonate secretion, as well as biliary flow.

CARCINOGENESIS, MUTAGENESIS, IMPAIRMENT OF FERTILITY

Long-term studies in animals to evaluate carcinogenic potential and studies to evaluate the mutagenic potential or effect on fertility have not been conducted.

PREGNANCY: TERATOGENIC EFFECTS

Pregnancy Category C: Animal reproduction studies have not been conducted with Pentagastrin. It is also not known whether Pentagastrin can cause fetal harm when administered to a pregnant woman or can affect reproduction capacity. Pentagastrin should be given to a pregnant woman only if clearly needed.

NURSING MOTHERS

It is not known whether this drug is excreted in human milk. Because many drugs are excreted in human milk, caution should be exercised when Pentagastrin is administered to a nursing woman.

PEDIATRIC USE

Safety and effectiveness in children have not been established.

ADVERSE REACTIONS

Pentagastrin causes fewer and less severe cardiovascular and other adverse reactions than histamine or betazole. The majority of reactions to Pentagastrin are related to the gastrointestinal tract.

The following reactions associated with the use of Pentagastrin have been reported.

Gastrointestinal: Abdominal pain, desire to defecate, nausea, vomiting, borborygmi, blood-tinged mucus.

Cardiovascular: Flushing, tachycardia.

Central Nervous System: Dizziness, faintness or light-headedness, drowsiness, sinking feeling, transient blurring of vision, tiredness, headache.

Allergic and Hypersensitivity Reactions: May occur in some patients.

Miscellaneous: Shortness of breath, heavy sensation in arms and legs, tingling in fingers, chills, sweating, generalized burning sensation, warmth, pain at site of injection, bile in collected specimens.

OVERDOSAGE

In case of overdosage or idiosyncrasy, symptomatic treatment should be administered as required.

DOSAGE AND ADMINISTRATION

Adults: 6 mcg/kg subcutaneously. Effect begins in about ten minutes; peak response usually occurs in twenty to thirty minutes. (For discussion of the test and explicit directions, consult Baron, JH; Gastric Function Tests, in Wastell, C: *Chronic Duodenal Ulcer,* New York, Appleton-Century-Crofts, 1972, pp 82-114.)

Parenteral drug products should be inspected visually for particulate matter and discoloration prior to administration, whenever solution and container permit.

Refrigerate, 2°C to 8°C (36°F to 46°F), and protect from light. Do not use if discolored.

HOW SUPPLIED

INJECTION: 0.25 MG/ML

BRAND/MANUFACTURER	NDC	SIZE	AWP
○ **BRAND**			
PEPTAVLON: Wyeth-Ayerst	00046-3290-10	2 ml 10s	$318.83

Pentam 300 *SEE* PENTAMIDINE ISETHIONATE

◆ RATED THERAPEUTICALLY EQUIVALENT; ◇ THERAPEUTIC EQUIVALENCE UNCONFIRMED; ○ UNRATED

Pentamidine Isethionate

DESCRIPTION

Pentamidine Isethionate, an anti-protozoal agent, is a sterile and nonpyrogenic lyophilized product.

Pentamidine Isethionate, 4,4'-diamidinodiphenoxypentane di-(β-hydroxyethanesulfonate), is a white crystalline powder soluble in water and glycerin and insoluble in ether, acetone, and chloroform. The molecular formula is $C_{23}H_{36}N_4O_{10}S_2$ and the molecular weight 592.68.

Pentamidine Isethionate is available for inhalation and for intravenous (IV) or intramuscular (IM) injection.

Each vial contains 300 mg sterile Pentamidine Isethionate.

Following is its chemical structure:

CLINICAL PHARMACOLOGY

MICROBIOLOGY

Pentamidine Isethionate, an aromatic diamidine, is known to have activity against *Pneumocystis carinii*. The mode of action is not fully understood. *In vitro* studies with mammalian tissues and the protozoan *Crithidia oncopelti* indicate that the drug interferes with protozoal nuclear metabolism by inhibition of DNA, RNA, phospholipid and protein synthesis.

PHARMACOKINETICS

In 5 AIDS patients with suspected *Pneumocystis carinii* pneumonia (PCP), the mean concentrations of Pentamidine Isethionate determined 18 to 24 hours after inhalation therapy were 23.2 ng/mL (range 5.1 to 43.0 ng/mL) in bronchoalveolar lavage fluid and 705 ng/mL (range 140 to 1336 ng/mL) in sediment after administration of a 300 mg single dose via nebulizer. In 3 AIDS patients with suspected PCP, the mean concentrations of Pentamidine Isethionate determined 18 to 24 hours after a 4 mg/kg intravenous dose were 2.6 ng/mL (range 1.5 to 4.0 ng/mL) in bronchoalveolar lavage fluid and 9.3 ng/mL (range 6.9 to 12.8 ng/mL) in sediment. In the patients who received aerosolized Pentamidine Isethionate the peak plasma levels of Pentamidine Isethionate were at or below the lower limit of detection of the assay (2.3 ng/mL).

Following a single 2-hour intravenous infusion of 4 mg/kg of Pentamidine Isethionate to 6 AIDS patients, the mean plasma Cmax, T½, and clearance were 612 ± 371 ng/mL, 6.4 ± 1.3 hr, and 248 ± 91 L/hr, respectively. In another study of aerosolized Pentamidine Isethionate in 13 AIDS patients with acute PCP who received 4 mg/kg/day, peak plasma levels of Pentamidine Isethionate averaged 18.8 ± 11.9 ng/mL after the first dose. During the next 14 days of repeated dosing, the highest observed Cmax averaged 20.5 ± 21.2 ng/mL. In a third study, following daily administration of 600 mg of inhaled Pentamidine Isethionate for 21 days in 11 patients with acute PCP, mean plasma levels measured shortly after the 21st dose averaged 11.8 ± 10.0 ng/mL.

Plasma concentrations after aerosol administration are substantially lower than those observed after a comparable intravenous dose. The extent of Pentamidine Isethionate accumulation and distribution following chronic inhalation therapy are not known.

Preliminary studies have shown that in seven patients treated with daily IM doses of Pentamidine at 4 mg/kg for 10 to 12 days, plasma concentrations were between 0.3 and 0.5 mcg/mL. The levels did not appreciably change with time after injection or from day to day. Higher plasma levels were encountered in patients with an elevated BUN. The patients continued to excrete decreasing amounts of Pentamidine in urine up to six to eight weeks after cessation of the treatment.

Tissue distribution has been studied in mice given a single intraperitoneal injection of Pentamidine at 10 mg/kg. The concentration in the kidneys was the highest followed by that in the liver. In mice, Pentamidine was excreted unchanged, primarily via the kidneys with some elimination in the feces. The ratio of amounts excreted in the urine and feces (4:1) was constant over the period of study.

In rats, intravenous administration of a 5 mg/kg dose resulted in concentrations of Pentamidine Isethionate in the liver and kidney that were 87.5- and 62.3-fold higher, respectively, than levels in those organs following 5 mg/kg administered as an aerosol.

No pharmacokinetic data are available following aerosol administration of Pentamidine Isethionate in humans with impaired hepatic or renal function.

INDICATIONS AND USAGE

Pentamidine Isethionate is indicated for the prevention of *Pneumocystis carinii* pneumonia (PCP) in high-risk, HIV-infected patients defined by one or both of the following criteria.

i. A history of one or more episodes of PCP

ii. A peripheral CD4+ (T4 helper/inducer) lymphocyte count less than or equal to 200/mm³.

These indications are based on the results of an 18-month randomized, dose-response trial in high-risk, HIV-infected patients and on existing epidemiological data from natural history studies.

The patient population of the controlled trial consisted of 408 patients, 237 of whom had a history of one or more episodes of PCP. The remaining patients without a history of PCP included 55 patients with Kaposi's sarcoma and 116

patients with other AIDS diagnoses, ARC or asymptomatic HIV infection. Patients were randomly assigned to receive Pentamidine Isethionate inhalation at one of the following three doses: 30 mg every two weeks (n = 135), 150 mg every two weeks (n = 134), or 300 mg every four weeks (n = 139). The results of the trial demonstrated a significant protective effect (p < 0.01) against PCP with the 300 mg every four week dosage regimen compared to the 30 mg every two week dosage regimen. The 300 mg dose regimen reduced the risk of developing PCP by 50 to 70% compared to the 30 mg regimen. A total of 293 patients (72% of all patients) also received zidovudine at sometime during the trial. The analysis of the data demonstrated the efficacy of the 300 mg dose even after adjusting for the effect of zidovudine.

The results of the trial further demonstrate that the dose and frequency of dosing are important to the efficacy of aerosolized Pentamidine Isethionate prophylaxis in that multiple analyses consistently demonstrated a trend toward greater efficacy with 300 mg every four weeks as compared to 150 mg every two weeks.

No dose-response was observed for reduction in overall mortality; however, mortality from PCP was low in all three dosage groups.

UNLABELED USES

Pentamidine is used alone or as an adjunct in the treatment of clinical manifestations of babesiosis, leishmaniasis, and trypanosomiasis.

CONTRAINDICATIONS

Pentamidine Isethionate inhalation is contraindicated in patients with a history of an anaphylactic reaction to inhaled or parenteral Pentamidine Isethionate. Once the diagnosis of *Pheumocystis carinii* pneumonia has been firmly established, there are no absolute contraindications to the use of parenteral Pentamidine Isethionate.

WARNINGS

The potential for development of acute PCP still exists in patients receiving aerosolized Pentamidine Isethionate prophylaxis. Therefore, any patient with symptoms suggestive of the presence of a pulmonary infection, including but not limited to dyspnea, fever or cough, should receive a thorough medical evaluation and appropriate diagnostic tests for possible acute PCP as well as for other opportunistic and nonopportunistic pathogens. The use of aerosolized Pentamidine Isethionate may alter the clinical and radiographic features of PCP and could result in an atypical presentation, including but not limited to mild disease or focal infection. Prior to initiating aerosolized Pentamidine Isethionate prophylaxis, symptomatic patients should be evaluated appropriately to exclude the presence of PCP. The recommended dose of aerosolized Pentamidine Isethionate for the prevention of PCP is insufficient to treat acute PCP.

Fatalities due to severe hypotension, hypoglycemia, and cardiac arrhythmias have been reported in patients treated with Pentamidine Isethionate, both by the IM and IV routes. Severe hypotension may result after a single dose (see *"Precautions"*). The administration of the drug should, therefore, be limited to the patients in whom *Pneumocystis carinii* has been demonstrated. Patients should be closely monitored for the development of serious adverse reactions (see *"Precautions"* and *"Adverse Reactions"*).

PRECAUTIONS

IMPORTANT: DO NOT MIX THE PENTAMIDINE ISETHIONATE SOLUTION FOR INHALATION WITH ANY OTHER DRUGS.

PULMONARY

Inhalation of Pentamidine Isethionate may induce bronchospasm or cough. This has been noted particularly in some patients who have a history of smoking or asthma. In clinical trials, cough and bronchospasm were the most frequently reported adverse experiences associated with aerosolized Pentamidine Isethionate administration (38% and 15%, respectively, of patients receiving the 300 mg dose); however, less than 1% of the doses were interrupted or terminated due to these effects. For the majority of patients, cough and bronchospasm were controlled by administration of an aerosolized bronchodilator (only 1% of patients withdrew from the study due to treatment-associated cough or bronchospasm). In patients who experience bronchospasm or cough, administration of an inhaled bronchodilator prior to giving each aerosolized Pentamidine Isethionate dose may minimize recurrence of the symptoms.

GENERAL

The extent and consequence of Pentamidine Isethionate accumulation following chronic inhalation therapy are not known. As a result, patients receiving aerosolized Pentamidine Isethionate should be closely monitored for the development of serious adverse reactions that have occurred in patients receiving parenteral Pentamidine, including hypotension, hypoglycemia, hyperglycemia, hypocalcemia, anemia, thrombocytopenia, leukopenia, hepatic or renal dysfunction, ventricular tachycardia, pancreatitis, and Stevens-Johnson syndrome.

Extrapulmonary infection with *P. carinii* has been reported infrequently. Most, but not all, of the cases have been reported in patients who have a history of PCP. The presence of extrapulmonary pneumocystosis should be considered when evaluating patients with unexplained signs and symptoms.

Cases of acute pancreatitis have been reported in patients receiving aerosolized Pentamidine Isethionate. Pentamidine Isethionate should be discontinued if signs or symptoms of acute pancreatitis develop.

Pentamidine Isethionate should be used with caution in patients with hypertension, hypotension, hypoglycemia, hyperglycemia, hypocalcemia, leukopenia, thrombocytopenia, anemia, and hepatic or renal dysfunction.

► SHOWN IN PRODUCT IDENTIFICATION GUIDE

Patients may develop sudden, severe hypotension after a single dose of Pentamidine Isethionate, whether given IV or IM. Therefore, patients receiving the drug should be lying down and the blood pressure should be monitored closely during administration of the drug and several times thereafter until the blood pressure is stable. Equipment for emergency resuscitation should be readily available. If Pentamidine Isethionate is administered IV, it should be infused over a period of 60 minutes.

Pentamidine Isethionate-induced hypoglycemia has been associated with pancreatic islet cell necrosis and inappropriately high plasma insulin concentrations. Hyperglycemia and diabetes mellitus, with or without preceding hypoglycemia, have also occurred, sometimes several months after therapy with Pentamidine Isethionate. Therefore, blood glucose levels should be monitored daily during therapy with Pentamidine Isethionate, and several times thereafter.

LABORATORY TESTS
The following tests should be carried out before, during and after therapy.
   a) Daily blood urea nitrogen and serum creatinine determinations
   b) Daily blood glucose determinations
   c) Complete blood count and platelet count
   d) Liver function test, including bilirubin, alkaline phosphatase, AST (SGOT), and ALT (SGPT)
   e) Serum calcium determinations
   f) Electrocardiograms at regular intervals

DRUG INTERACTIONS
While specific studies on drug interactions with Pentamidine Isethionate have not been conducted, the majority of patients in clinical trials received concomitant medications, including zidovudine, with no reported interactions.

CARCINOGENESIS, MUTAGENESIS AND IMPAIRMENT OF FERTILITY
No studies have been conducted to evaluate the potential of Pentamidine Isethionate as a carcinogen or mutagen or to determine its effects on fertility.

PREGNANCY, PREGNANCY CATEGORY C
Animal reproduction studies have not been conducted with Pentamidine Isethionate. It is also not known whether Pentamidine Isethionate can cause fetal harm when administered to a pregnant woman or can affect reproduction capacity. Pentamidine Isethionate should be given to a pregnant woman only if clearly needed. Pentamidine Isethionate should not be given to a pregnant woman unless the potential benefits are judged to outweigh the unknown risk.

NURSING MOTHERS
It is not known whether Pentamidine Isethionate is excreted in human milk. Because of the potential for serious adverse reactions in nursing infants from Pentamidine Isethionate, a decision should be made whether to discontinue nursing or to discontinue the drug, taking into account the importance of the drug to the mother. Because many drugs are excreted in human milk, Pentamidine Isethionate should not be given to a nursing mother unless the potential benefits are judged to outweigh the unknown risk.

PEDIATRIC USE
The safety and effectiveness of Pentamidine Isethionate in children have not been established.

ADVERSE REACTIONS
INHALATION
The most frequent adverse effects attributable to aerosolized Pentamidine Isethionate administration are cough and bronchospasm (reported by 38% and 15%, respectively, of patients receiving 300 mg every four weeks).

The most frequently reported adverse experiences in the controlled clinical trials in which 607 patients were treated with aerosolized Pentamidine Isethionate (139 patients at 300 mg every four weeks, 232 at 150 mg every two weeks, 101 at 100 mg every two weeks and 135 at 30 mg every two weeks) were as follows:

53-72% Fatigue, bad (metallic) taste, shortness of breath and decreased appetite

31-47% Dizziness and rash

10-23% Nausea, pharyngitis, chest pain or congestion, night sweats, chills and vomiting

In nearly all cases, neither the relationship to treatment or underlying disease nor the severity of adverse experiences was recorded.

Other less frequently occurring adverse experiences (reported by greater than 1% and up to 5% of patients in two clinical trials) were pneumothorax, diarrhea, headache, anemia (generally associated with zidovudine use), myalgia, abdominal pain and edema.

From a total experience with 1130 patients, adverse events reported with a frequency of 1% or less were as follows. No causal relationship to treatment has been established for these adverse events.

General: Allergic reaction and extrapulmonary pneumocytosis

Cardiovascular: Tachycardia, hypotension, hypertension, palpitations, syncope, cerebrovascular accident, vasodilatation, and vasculitis

Metabolic: Hypoglycemia, hyperglycemia, and hypocalcemia

Gastrointestinal: Gingivitis, dyspepsia, oral ulcer/abscess, gastritis, gastric ulcer, hypersalivation, dry mouth, splenomegaly, melena, hematochezia, esophagitis, colitis, and pancreatitis.

Hematological: Pancytopenia, neutropenia, eosinophilia and thrombocytopenia

Hepatorenal: Hepatitis, hepatomegaly, hepatic dysfunction, renal failure, flank pain, and nephritis

Musculoskeletal: Arthralgia

Neurological: Tremors, confusion, anxiety, memory loss, seizure, neuropathy, paresthesia, insomnia, hypesthesia, drowsiness, emotional lability, vertigo, paranoia, neuralgia, hallucination, depression, and unsteady gait

Respiratory: Rhinitis, laryngitis, laryngospasm, hyperventilation, hemoptysis, gagging, eosinophilic or interstitial pneumonitis, pleuritis, cyanosis, tachypnea, and rales

Skin: Pruritis, erythema, dry skin, desquamation and urticaria

Special Senses: Eye discomfort, conjunctivitis, blurred vision, blepharitis and loss of taste and smell

Urogenital: Incontinence

Reproductive: Miscarriage

INJECTION
Caution: Fatalities due to severe hypotension, hypoglycemia, and cardiac arrhythmias have been reported in patients treated with Pentamidine Isethionate, both by the IM and IV routes. The administration of the drug should, therefore, be limited to the patients in whom *Pneumocystis carinii* has been demonstrated.

Of 424 patients treated with parenteral Pentamidine Isethionate, 244 (57.5%) developed some adverse reaction. Most of the patients had the acquired immunodeficiency syndrome (AIDS). In the following table, "Severe" refers to life-threatening reactions or reactions that required immediate corrective measures and led to discontinuation of Pentamidine Isethionate.

Adverse Reactions	Number	%
Severe		
Leukopenia (< 1000/mm³)	12	2.8
Hypoglycemia (< 25 mg/dL)	10	2.4
Thrombocytopenia (< 20,000/mm³)	7	1.7
Hypotension (< 60 mm Hg systolic)	4	0.9
Acute renal failure (serum creatinine > 6 mg/dL)	2	0.5
Hypocalcemia	1	0.2
Stevens-Johnson syndrome	1	0.2
Ventricular tachycardia	1	0.2
Total number of patients with severe effects*	37	8.7
Moderate		
Elevated serum creatinine (2.4 to 6.0 mg/dL)	98	23.1
Sterile abscess, pain, or induration at the site of IM injection	47	11.1
Elevated liver function tests	37	8.7
Leukopenia	32	7.5
Nausea, anorexia	25	5.9
Hypotension	17	4.0
Fever	15	3.5
Hypoglycemia	15	3.5
Rash	14	3.3
Bad taste in mouth	7	1.7
Confusion/hallucinations	7	1.7
Anemia	5	1.2
Neuralgia	4	0.9
Thrombocytopenia	4	0.9
Hyperkalemia	3	0.7
Phlebitis	3	0.7
Dizziness (without hypotension)	2	0.5
Other moderate adverse reactions**	5	1.2
Total number of patients with moderate adverse reactions*	207	48.8

* *Patient total may not equal sum of reactions, since some patients had more than one reaction.*

** *Each of the following moderate adverse reactions was reported in one patient: hypocalcemia, abnormal ST segment of electrocardiogram, bronchospasm, diarrhea, and hyperglycemia.*

OVERDOSAGE
Overdosage has not been reported with Pentamidine Isethionate. The symptoms and signs of overdosage are not known.

A serious overdosage, to the point of producing systemic drug levels similar to those following parenteral administration, would have the potential of producing similar types of serious systemic toxicity (see *"Precautions"*).

Available clinical pharmacology data (see *"Clinical Pharmacology"*) suggest that a dose up to 40 times the recommended Pentamidine Isethionate dosage would be required to produce systemic levels similar to a single 4 mg/kg intravenous dose.

◆ RATED THERAPEUTICALLY EQUIVALENT; ◇ THERAPEUTIC EQUIVALENCE UNCONFIRMED; ○ UNRATED

DOSAGE AND ADMINISTRATION

INHALATION:

IMPORTANT: PENTAMIDINE ISETHIONATE MUST BE DISSOLVED ONLY IN STERILE WATER FOR INJECTION, USP. DO NOT USE SALINE SOLUTION FOR RECONSTITUTION BECAUSE THE DRUG WILL PRECIPITATE. DO NOT MIX THE PENTAMIDINE ISETHIONATE SOLUTION WITH ANY OTHER DRUGS.

RECONSTITUTION

The contents of one vial (300 mg) must be dissolved in 6 mL sterile water for injection. Place the entire reconstituted contents of the vial into the nebulizer reservoir for administration.

DOSAGE

The recommended adult dosage of Pentamidine Isethionate for the prevention of *Pneumocystis carinii* pneumonia is 300 mg once every four weeks.

The dose should be delivered until the nebulizer chamber is empty (approximately 30 to 45 minutes). The flow rate should be 5 to 7 liters per minute from a 40 to 50 pounds per square inch (PSI) air or oxygen source. Alternatively, a 40 to 50 PSI air compressor can be used with flow limited by setting the flowmeter at 5 to 7 liters per minute or by setting the pressure at 22 to 25 PSI. Low pressure (less than 20 PSI) compressors should not be used.

STABILITY

Freshly prepared solutions for aerosol use are recommended. After reconstitution with sterile water, the Pentamidine Isethionate solution is stable for 48 hours in the original vial at room temperature if protected from light.

Injection: Pentamidine Isethionate should be administered IM or IV only. The recommended regimen for adults and children is 4 mg/kg once a day for 14 days. The benefits and risks of therapy with Pentamidine Isethionate for more than 14 days are not well defined.

INTRAMUSCULAR INJECTION

The contents of one vial (300 mg) should be dissolved in 3 mL of sterile water for injection. The calculated daily dose should then be withdrawn and administered by deep IM injection.

INTRAVENOUS INJECTION

The contents of one vial should first be dissolved in 3 to 5 mL of sterile water for injection or 5% dextrose injection. The calculated dose of Pentamidine Isethionate should then be withdrawn and diluted further in 50 to 250 mL of 5% dextrose injection. **The diluted IV solutions containing Pentamidine Isethionate should be infused over a period of 60 minutes.**

Aseptic technique should be employed in preparation of all solutions. Parenteral drug products should be inspected visually for particulate matter and discoloration prior to administration.

Stability: Intravenous infusion solutions of Pentamidine Isethionate at 1 mg and 2.5 mg/mL prepared in 5% dextrose injection are stable at room temperature for up to 24 hours.

STORAGE

Store the dry product at controlled room temperature 15-30°C (59°-86°F).

Protect the dry product and the reconstituted solution from light.

J CODES

INH—J2545

HOW SUPPLIED

AEROSOL LIQUID: 300 MG

BRAND/MANUFACTURER	NDC	SIZE	AWP
○ BRAND NEBUPENT: Fujisawa	57317-0210-06	15 ml	$98.75

POWDER FOR INJECTION: 300 MG

BRAND/MANUFACTURER	NDC	SIZE	AWP
◆ GENERICS Abbott Hosp	00074-4548-01	1s	$109.17

POWDER FOR INJECTION: 300 MG

BRAND/MANUFACTURER	NDC	SIZE	AWP
○ BRAND PENTAM 300: Fujisawa	57317-0211-03	1s	$98.75

Pentasa *SEE* MESALAMINE

Pentaspan *SEE* PENTASTARCH

Pentastarch

DESCRIPTION

Pentastarch (10% Pentastarch in 0.9% sodium chloride injection) is a sterile, nonpyrogenic solution. The composition of each 100 mL is as follows:

Pentastarch	10.0 g
Sodium Chloride USP	0.9 g
Water for Injection USP	qs

Concentration of Electrolytes (mEq/Liter): Sodium 154, Chloride 154
pH: Approx. 5.0; Calculated Osmolarity: Approx. 326 mOsM

Pentastarch is an artificial colloid derived from a waxy starch composed almost entirely of amylopectin. Hydroxyethyl ether groups are introduced into the glucose units of the starch and the resultant material is hydrolyzed to yield a product with a molecular weight suitable for use as an erythrocyte sedimenting agent. Pentastarch is characterized by its molar substitution, and also by its molecular weight. The degree of substitution is 0.45 which means Pentastarch has 45 hydroxyethyl groups for every 100 glucose units. The weight average molecular weight of Pentastarch is approximately 264,000 with a range of 150,000 to 350,000 and with 80% of the polymers falling between 10,000 and 2,000,000. Hydroxyethyl groups are attached by an ether linkage primarily at C-2 of the glucose unit and to a lesser extent at C-3 and C-6. The polymer resembles glycogen, and the polymerized glucose units are joined primarily by 1-4 linkages with occasional 1-6 branching linkages. The degree of branching is approximately 1:20 which means that there is one 1-6 branch for every 20 glucose monomer units.

The chemical name for Pentastarch is hydroxyethyl starch.

Amylopectin derivative in which R_2, R_3, and R_6 are H or CH_2CH_2OH, or R_6 is a branching point in the starch polymer connected through a 1-6 linkage to additional α-D-glucopyranosyl units.

Pentastarch is a clear, pale yellow to amber solution. Exposure to prolonged adverse storage conditions may result in a change to a turbid deep brown or the formation of a crystalline precipitate. Do not use the solution if these conditions are evident.

CLINICAL PHARMACOLOGY

The addition of Pentastarch to whole blood increases the erythrocyte sedimentation rate. Therefore, 10% pentastarch in 0.9% sodium chloride injection is used to improve the efficiency of leukocyte collection by centrifugal means.

Pentastarch molecules below 50,000 molecular weight are rapidly eliminated by renal excretion. A single dose of approximately 500 mL of Pentastarch (approximately 50 g) results in elimination in the urine of approximately 70% of the dose within 24 hours, and approximately 80% of the dose within one week. An additional 5-6% of the Pentastarch dose is recovered in the leukapheresis collection bag. The remaining 12-15% (approximately 6.8 g) of an administered dose is presumed to undergo slower elimination. This is a variable process but generally results in an intravascular Pentastarch concentration below the level of detection by one week. The hydroxyethyl group is not cleaved by the body, but remains intact and attached to glucose units when excreted.

The colloidal properties of the related product hetastarch (6% hetastarch in 0.9% sodium chloride injection) approximate those of 5% human albumin. Intravenous infusion of hetastarch results in expansion of plasma volume that decreases over the succeeding 24 to 36 hours. Similar, although reduced duration, volume expansion may be expected to occur following use of Pentastarch (10% pentastarch in 0.9% sodium chloride injection) in leukapheresis procedures.

INDICATIONS AND USAGE

10% Pentastarch in 0.9% sodium chloride injection is indicated as an adjunct in leukapheresis, to improve the harvesting and increase the yield of leukocytes by centrifugal means.

CONTRAINDICATIONS

Pentastarch is contraindicated in donors with known hypersensitivity to hydroxyethyl starch, or with bleeding disorders, or with congestive heart failure where volume overload is a potential problem. Pentastarch should not be used in renal disease with oliguria or anuria.

WARNINGS

Slight declines in platelet counts and hemoglobin levels have been observed in donors undergoing repeated leukapheresis procedures using hetastarch due to the volume expanding effects of hetastarch and to the collection of platelets and erythrocytes. Hemoglobin levels usually return to normal within 24 hours. Similar effects may be expected with Pentastarch. Hemodilution by Pentastarch and saline may also result in 24 hour declines of total protein, albumin, calcium and fibrinogen values. None of these decreases are to a degree recognized to be clinically significant risks to healthy donors.

Large volumes of Pentastarch may slightly alter the coagulation mechanism; *i.e.*, transient prolongation of prothrombin, partial thromboplastin and clotting times. The physician should also be alert to the possibility of transient prolongation of bleeding time.

PRECAUTIONS

General: Regular and frequent clinical evaluation and complete blood counts (CBC) are necessary for proper monitoring of Pentastarch use during leukapheresis. If the frequency of leukapheresis is to exceed the guidelines for whole blood donation, you may wish to consider the following additional studies: total leukocyte and platelet counts, leukocyte differential count, hemoglobin and hematocrit, prothrombin time (PT), and partial thromboplastin time (PTT) tests.

The possibility of circulatory overload should be kept in mind. Caution should be used when the risk of pulmonary edema and/or congestive heart failure is increased. Special care should be exercised in patients who have impaired renal clearance since this is the principal way in which Pentastarch is eliminated.

The serum chemistries of sixteen normal volunteers who were given 500 to 2000 mL infusions of Pentastarch were essentially unchanged pre- and post-infusion, except for dilutional effects. However, indirect bilirubin levels of 8.3 mg/L (normal 0-7 mg/L) have been reported in 2 out of 20 normal subjects who received multiple Hetastarch infusions. Total bilirubin was within normal limits at all times; indirect bilirubin returned to normal by 96 hours following the final infusion. The significance, if any, of these elevations is not known; however, caution should be observed before administering Pentastarch to patients with a history of liver disease.

Pentastarch has been reported to produce hypersensitivity reactions such as wheezing and urticaria. However, Pentastarch has not been observed to stimulate antibody formation. If hypersensitivity effects occur, they are readily controlled by discontinuation of the drug and, if necessary, administration of an antihista-minic agent.

Elevated serum amylase levels may be observed temporarily following administration of Pentastarch, although no association with pancreatitis has been demonstrated.

Carcinogenesis, mutagenesis, impairment of fertility: Long-term studies in animals have not been performed to evaluate the carcinogenic potential of Pentastarch.

Teratogenic Effects: Pregnancy Category C. Pentastarch has been shown to be embryocidal in New Zealand rabbits and in Swiss Mice when given in doses 5 times the human dose. There are no adequate and well-controlled clinical studies using Pentastarch in pregnant women. Pentastarch should be used during pregnancy only if the potential benefits justify the potential risk to the fetus.

Pentastarch was administered to mated New Zealand rabbits and Swiss Mice with intravenous doses of 10, 20, and 40 mL/kg/day during the period of gestation. The results demonstrated that at 10 and 20 mL/kg/day Pentastarch produced no higher incidence of teratogenicity or embryotoxicity in either species than normal saline did in control animals. At 40 mL/kg/day, however, Pentastarch increased the number of resorptions and minor visceral anomalies (diffuse edema of the trunk and extremities and diffuse whitish color of the heart, lungs, liver, and kidneys) in rabbits and reduced nidation in the mouse.

Nursing mothers: It is not known whether pentastarch is excreted in human milk. Because many drugs are excreted in human milk, caution should be exercised when Pentastarch is administered to a nursing woman.

Pediatric use: The safety and effectiveness of Pentastarch in children have not been established.

ADVERSE REACTIONS

The following have been reported in association with the use of Pentastarch in leukapheresis: headache, diarrhea, nausea, weakness, temporary weight gain, insomnia, fatigue, fever, edema, paresthesia, acne, malaise, shakiness, dizziness, chest pain, chills, nasal congestion, anxiety, and increased heart rate. It is uncertain whether they are attributable to the drug, the procedure, additional adjunctive medication, or some combination of these factors.

DOSAGE AND ADMINISTRATION

250 to 700 mL Pentastarch to which citrate anticoagulant has been added is typically administered by aseptic addition to the input line of the centrifugation apparatus at a ratio of 1:8 to 1:13 to venous whole blood. The bottle containing Pentastarch and citrate should be thoroughly mixed to assure effective anticoagulation of blood as it flows through the leukapheresis machine.

Parenteral drug products should be inspected visually for particulate matter and discoloration prior to administration whenever solution and container permit.

The safety and compatibility of other additives have not been established.

DIRECTIONS FOR USE

Caution: Before administering to patient, perform the following checks: 1. Each container should be inspected before use. Read the label. Insure solution is the one ordered, is within the expiration date, and that label name agrees with the abbreviated name stamped on closure. Check the security of bail and band.

2. Invert container and carefully inspect the solution in good light for cloudiness, haze, or particulate matter; check the bottle for cracks or other damage. In checking for cracks, do not be confused by normal surface mold marks and seams on bottom and sides of bottle. These are not flaws. Look instead for bright reflections that have depth and penetrate into the wall of the bottle. Reject any such bottle.

3. Check for vacuum, first by confirming the presence of depressions in the latex disk and then by audible hiss when the disk is removed. Reject any container that does not meet these criteria.

4. After admixtures and during administration, reinspect solution as frequently as possible. If any evidence of solution contamination or instability is found or if the patient exhibits any signs of fever or chills or other reaction not readily explainable, discontinue administration immediately and notify physician.

HOW SUPPLIED
INJECTION: 10%

BRAND/MANUFACTURER	NDC	SIZE	AWP
○ BRAND			
PENTASPAN: Du Pont Pharma	00056-0081-95	500 ml 12s	$878.40

Pentazocine Lactate

DESCRIPTION

Pentazocine Lactate injection is a member of the benzazocine series (also known as the benzomorphan series). Chemically, pentazocine lactate is 1, 2, 3, 4, 5, 6-hexahydro-6, 11-dimethyl-3-(3-methyl-2-butenyl)-2-6-methano-3-benzazocin-8-ol lactate, a white, crystalline substance soluble in acidic aqueous solutions.

Following is its chemical structure:

CLINICAL PHARMACOLOGY

Pentazocine Lactate is a potent analgesic and 30 mg is usually as effective an analgesic as morphine 10 mg or meperidine 75 mg to 100 mg; however, a few studies suggest the Pentazocine Lactate to morphine ratio may range from 20 mg to 40 mg Pentazocine Lactate to 10 mg morphine. The duration of analgesia may sometimes be less than that of morphine. Analgesia usually occurs within 15 to 20 minutes after intramuscular or subcutaneous injection and within 2 to 3 minutes after intravenous injection. Pentazocine Lactate weakly antagonizes the analgesic effects of morphine, meperidine, and phenazocine, in addition, it produces incomplete reversal of cardiovascular, respiratory, and behavioral depression induced by morphine and meperidine. Pentazocine Lactatate has about 1/50 the antagonistic activity of nalorphine. It also has sedative activity.

INDICATIONS AND USAGE

For the relief of moderate to severe pain. Pentazocine Lactate may also be used for preoperative or preanesthetic medication and as a supplement to surgical anesthesia.

CONTRAINDICATION

Pentazocine Lactate should not be administered to patients who are hypersensitive to it.

WARNINGS

Drug Dependence: Special care should be exercised in prescribing Pentazocine Lactate for emotionally unstable patients and for those with a history of drug misuse. Such patients should be closely supervised when greater than 4 or 5 days of therapy is contemplated. There have been instances of psychological and physical dependence on Pentazocine Lactate in patients with such a history and, rarely, in patients without such a history. Extended use of parenteral Pentazocine Lactate may lead to physical or psychological dependence in some patients. When Pentazocine Lactate is abruptly discontinued, withdrawal symptoms such as abdominal cramps, elevated temperature, rhinorrhea, restlessness, anxiety, and lacrimation may occur. However, even when these have occurred, discontinuance has been accomplished with minimal difficulty. In the rare patient in whom more than minor difficulty has been encountered, reinstitution of parenteral Pentazocine Lactate with gradual withdrawal has ameliorated the patient's symptoms. Substituting methadone or other narcotics for Pentazocine Lactate in the treatment of the Pentazocine Lactate abstinence syndrome should be avoided. There have been rare reports of possible abstinence syndromes in newborns after prolonged use of Pentazocine Lactate during pregnancy.

In prescribing parenteral Pentazocine Lactate for chronic use, particularly if the drug is to be self-administered, the physician should take precautions to avoid increases in dose and frequency of injection by the patient.

Just as with all medication, the oral form of Pentazocine Lactate is preferable for chronic administration.

Tissue Damage at Injection Sites: Severe sclerosis of the skin, subcutaneous tissues, and underlying muscle have occurred at the injection sites of patients who have received multiple doses of Pentazocine Lactate. Constant rotation of injection sites is, therefore, essential. In addition, animal studies have demonstrated that Pentazocine Lactate is tolerated less well subcutaneously than intramuscularly. (See *"Dosage and Administration".*)

Head Injury and Increased Intracranial Pressure: As in the case of other potent analgesics, the potential of Pentazocine Lactate injection for elevating cerebrospinal fluid pressure may be attributed to CO_2 retention due to the respiratory depressant effects of the drug. These effects may be markedly exaggerated in the presence of head injury, other intracranial lesions, or a preexisting increase in intracranial pressure. Furthermore, Pentazocine Lactate can produce effects which may obscure the clinical course of patients with head injuries. In such patients, Pentazocine Lactate must be used with extreme caution and only if its use is deemed essential.

◆ RATED THERAPEUTICALLY EQUIVALENT; ◇ THERAPEUTIC EQUIVALENCE UNCONFIRMED; ○ UNRATED

Usage in Pregnancy: Safe use of Pentazocine Lactate during pregnancy (other than labor) has not been established. Animal reproduction studies have not demonstrated teratogenic or embryotoxic effects. However, Pentazocine Lactate should be administered to pregnant patients (other than labor) only when, in the judgment of the physician, the potential benefits outweigh the possible hazards. Patients receiving Pentazocine Lactate during labor have experienced no adverse effects other than those that occur with commonly used analgesics. Pentazocine Lactate should be used with caution in women delivering premature infants.

Acute CNS Manifestations: Patients receiving therapeutic doses of Pentazocine Lactate have experienced hallucinations (usually visual), disorientation, and confusion which have cleared spontaneously within a period of hours. The mechanism of this reaction is not known. Such patients should be closely observed and vital signs checked. If the drug is reinstituted, it should be done with caution since these acute CNS manifestations may recur.

Due to the potential for increased CNS depressant effects, alcohol should be used with caution in patients who are currently receiving Pentazocine.

Usage in Children: Because clinical experience in children under twelve years of age is limited, the use of Pentazocine Lactate in this age group is not recommended.

Ambulatory Patients: Since sedation, dizziness, and occasional euphoria have been noted, ambulatory patients should be warned not to operate machinery, drive cars, or unnecessarily expose themselves to hazards.

Myocardial Infarction: Caution should be exercised in the intravenous use of Pentazocine Lactate for patients with acute myocardial infarction accompanied by hypertension or left ventricular failure. Data suggest that intravenous administration of Pentazocine Lactate increases systemic and pulmonary arterial pressure and systemic vascular resistance in patients with acute myocardial infarction.

Note: Certain dosage forms of Pentazocine Lactate contain acetone sodium bisulfite, a sulfite that may cause allergic-type reactions including anaphylactic symptoms and life-threatening or less severe asthmatic episodes in certain susceptible people. The overall prevalence of sulfite sensitivity in the general population is unknown and probably low. Sulfite sensitivity is seen more frequently in asthmatic than in nonasthmatic people.

PRECAUTIONS

Certain Respiratory Conditions: The possibility that Pentazocine Lactate may cause respiratory depression should be considered in treatment of patients with bronchial asthma. Pentazocine Lactate injection, brand of Pentazocine Lactate injection, should be administered only with caution and in low dosage to patients with respiratory depression (eg, from other medication, uremia, or severe infection), severely limited respiratory reserve, obstructive respiratory conditions, or cyanosis.

Impaired Renal or Hepatic Function: Although laboratory tests have not indicated that Pentazocine Lactate causes or increases renal or hepatic impairment, the drug should be administered with caution to patients with such impairment. Extensive liver disease appears to predispose to greater side effects (eg, marked apprehension, anxiety, dizziness, sleepiness) from the usual clinical dose, and may be the result of decreased metabolism of the drug by the liver.

Biliary Surgery: Narcotic drug products are generally considered to elevate biliary tract pressure for varying periods following their administration. Some evidence suggests that Pentazocine Lactate may differ from other marketed narcotics in this respect (ie, it causes little or no elevation in biliary tract pressures). The clinical significance of these findings, however, is not yet known.

Patients Receiving Narcotics: Pentazocine Lactate is a mild narcotic antagonist. Some patients previously given narcotics, including methadone for the daily treatment of narcotic dependence, have experienced withdrawal symptoms after receiving Pentazocine Lactate.

CNS Effect. Caution should be used when Pentazocine Lactate is administered to patients prone to seizures; seizures have occurred in a few such patients in association with the use of Pentazocine Lactate although no cause and effect relationship has been established.

Use in Anesthesia: Concomitant use of CNS depressants with parenteral Pentazocine Lactate may produce additive CNS depression. Adequate equipment and facilities should be available to identify and treat systemic emergencies should they occur.

ADVERSE REACTIONS
The most commonly occurring reactions are: nausea, dizziness or lightheadedness, vomiting, euphoria.

Dermatologic Reactions: Soft tissue induration, nodules, and cutaneous depression can occur at injection sites. Ulceration (sloughing) and severe sclerosis of the skin and subcutaneous tissues (and, rarely, underlying muscle) have been reported after multiple doses. Other reported dermatologic reactions include diaphoresis, sting on injection, flushed skin including plethora, dermatitis including pruritus.

Infrequently occurring reactions are respiratory: respiratory depression, dyspnea, transient apnea in a small number of newborn infants whose mothers received Pentazocine Lactate during labor.

Cardiovascular: circulatory depression, shock, hypertension.

CNS Effects: dizziness, lightheadedness, hallucinations, sedation, euphoria, headache, confusion, disorientation; infrequently weakness, disturbed dreams, insomnia, syncope, visual blurring and focusing difficulty, depression; and rarely tremor, irritability, excitement, tinnitus.

Gastrointestinal: constipation, dry mouth.

Other: Urinary retention, headache, paresthesia, alterations in rate or strength of uterine contractions during labor.
Rarely reported reactions include.

Neuromuscular and psychiatric: muscle tremor, insomnia, disorientation, hallucinations.

Gastrointestinal: taste alteration, diarrhea and cramps.

Ophthalmic: blurred vision, nystagmus, diplopia, miosis.

Hematologic: depression of white blood cells (especially granulocytes), which is usually reversible, moderate transient eosinophilia.

Other: tachycardia, weakness or faintness, chills, allergic reactions including edema of the face, toxic epidermal necrolysis.
See *"Acute CNS Manifestations"* and *"Drug Dependence"* under *"Warnings"*.

DOSAGE AND ADMINISTRATION
Adults, Excluding Patients in Labor. The recommended single parenteral dose is 30 mg by intramuscular, subcutaneous, or intravenous route. This may be repeated every 3 to 4 hours. Doses in excess of 30 mg intravenously or 60 mg intramuscularly or subcutaneously are not recommended. Total daily dosage should not exceed 360 mg.

The subcutaneous route of administration should be used only when necessary because of possible severe tissue damage at injection sites (see *"Warnings"*). When frequent injections are needed, the drug should be administered intramuscularly. In addition, constant rotation of injection sites (eg, the upper outer quadrants of the buttocks, mid-lateral aspects of the thighs, and the deltoid areas) is essential.

Patients in Labor. A single, intramuscular 30 mg dose has been most commonly administered. An intravenous 20 mg dose has given adequate pain relief to some patients in labor when contractions become regular, and this dose may be given two or three times at two-to three-hour intervals, as needed.

Children Under 12 Years of Age. Since clinical experience in children under twelve years of age is limited, the use of Pentazocine Lactate in this age group is not recommended.

Caution: Pentazocine Lactate should not be mixed in the same syringe with soluble barbiturates because precipitation will occur.

OVERDOSAGE
Manifestations: Clinical experience with Pentazocine Lactate overdosage has been insufficient to define the signs of this condition.

Treatment: Oxygen, intravenous fluids, vasopressors, and other supportive measures should be employed as indicated. Assisted or controlled ventilation should also be considered. For respiratory depression due to overdosage or unusual sensitivity to Pentazocine Lactate injection, parenteral naloxone is a specific and effective antagonist.

J CODES
Up to 30 mg IM,SC,IV—J3070

HOW SUPPLIED
INJECTION (C-IV): 30 MG/ML

BRAND/MANUFACTURER	NDC	SIZE	AWP
○ **BRAND**			
TALWIN LACTATE: Sanofi Winthrop	00024-1916-01	10 ml	$30.58
	00024-1917-02	2 ml 10s	$19.52
	00024-1918-02	2 ml 10s	$21.91
	00024-1919-02	2 ml 10s	$25.33
	00024-1924-04	1 ml 25s ud	$95.85
	00024-1924-14	1 ml 25s ud	$95.85
	00024-1925-04	1.5 ml 25s ud	$110.20
	00024-1926-14	2 ml 25s	$129.62
	00024-1926-04	2 ml 25s ud	$129.62

Penthrane *SEE* METHOXYFLURANE

Pentobarbital Sodium

DESCRIPTION
The barbiturates are nonselective central nervous system depressants which are primarily used as sedative hypnotics and also anticonvulsants in subhypnotic doses. The barbiturates and their sodium salts are subject to control under the Federal Controlled Substances Act (see *"Drug Abuse and Dependence"* section).

Barbiturates are substituted pyrimidine derivatives in which the basic structure common to these drugs is barbituric acid, a substance which has no central nervous system (CNS) activity. CNS activity is obtained by substituting alkyl, alkenyl, or aryl groups on the pyrimidine ring. Pentobarbital Sodium is chemically represented by sodium 5-ethyl-5-(1-methylbutyl) barbiturate.

The sodium salt of Pentobarbital occurs as a white, slightly bitter powder which is freely soluble in water and alcohol but practically insoluble in benzene and ether.

It is available as capsules for oral administration, solution for intravenous (IV) or intramuscular (IM) injection, and as rectal suppositories.

Each capsule contains:
Pentobarbital Sodium ....50 or 100 mg

Each ml of solution contains:
Pentobarbital Sodium ....50 mg

Each suppository contains:
Pentobarbital Sodium ....30, 60, 120, or 200 mg

Following is its chemical structure:

CLINICAL PHARMACOLOGY

Barbiturates are capable of producing all levels of CNS mood alteration from excitation to mild sedation, to hypnosis, and deep coma. Overdosage can produce death. In high enough therapeutic doses barbiturates induce anesthesia.

Barbiturates depress the sensory cortex, decrease motor activity, alter cerebellar function, and produce drowsiness, sedation, and hypnosis.

Barbiturate-induced sleep differs from physiological sleep. Sleep laboratory studies have demonstrated that barbiturates reduce the amount of time spent in the rapid eye movement (REM) phase of sleep or dreaming stage. Also, Stages III and IV sleep are decreased. Following abrupt cessation of barbiturates used regularly, patients may experience markedly increased dreaming, nightmares, and/or insomnia. Therefore, withdrawal of a single therapeutic dose over 5 or 6 days has been recommended to lessen the REM rebound and disturbed sleep which contribute to drug withdrawal syndrome (for example, decrease the dose from 3 to 2 doses a day for 1 week).

In studies, secobarbital sodium and Pentobarbital Sodium have been found to lose most of their effectiveness for both inducing and maintaining sleep by the end of 2 weeks of continued drug administration at fixed doses. The short-, intermediate-, and, to a lesser degree, long-acting barbiturates have been widely prescribed for treating insomnia. Although the clinical literature abounds with claims that the short-acting barbiturates are superior for producing sleep while the intermediate-acting compounds are more effective in maintaining sleep, controlled studies have failed to demonstrate these differential effects. Therefore, as sleep medications, the barbiturates are of limited value beyond short-term use.

Barbiturates have little analgesic action at subanesthetic doses. Rather, in subanesthetic doses these drugs may increase the reaction to painful stimuli. All barbiturates exhibit anticonvulsant activity in anesthetic doses. However, of the drugs in this class, only Phenobarbital, mephobarbital, and metharbital have been clinically demonstrated to be effective as oral anticonvulsants in subhypnotic doses.

Barbiturates are respiratory depressants. The degree of respiratory depression is dependent upon dose. With hypnotic doses, respiratory depression produced by barbiturates is similar to that which occurs during physiologic sleep with slight decrease in blood pressure and heart rate.

Studies in laboratory animals have shown that barbiturates cause reduction in the tone and contractility of the uterus, ureters, and urinary bladder. However, concentrations of the drugs required to produce this effect in humans are not reached with sedative-hypnotic doses.

Barbiturates do not impair normal hepatic function, but have been shown to induce liver microsomal enzymes, thus increasing and/or altering the metabolism of barbiturates and other drugs. (See *"Precautions— Drug Interactions"* section.)

Pharmacokinetics: Barbiturates are absorbed in varying degrees following oral, rectal, or parenteral administration. The salts are more rapidly absorbed than are the acids. The rate of absorption is increased if the sodium salt is ingested as a dilute solution or taken on an empty stomach.

The onset of action for oral or rectal administration varies from 20 to 60 minutes. For IM administration, the onset of action is slightly faster. Following IV administration, the onset of action ranges from almost immediately for Pentobarbital Sodium to 5 minutes for phenobarbital sodium. Maximal CNS depression may not occur until 15 minutes or more after IV administration for phenobarbital sodium.

Duration of action, which is related to the rate at which the barbiturates are redistributed throughout the body, varies among persons and in the same person from time to time. In Table 1, the barbiturates are classified according to their duration of action. This classification should not be used to predict the exact duration of effect, but the grouping of drugs should be used as a guide in the selection of barbiturates. No studies have demonstrated that the different routes of administration are equivalent with respect to bioavailability.

[See Table 1.]

Table 1

CLASSIFICATION, ONSET, AND DURATION OF ACTION OF COMMONLY USED BARBITURATES TAKEN ORALLY

Classification	Onset of action	Duration of action
Long-acting		
Phenobarbital	1 hour or longer	10 to 12 hours
Intermediate		
Amobarbital		
Butabarbital	¾ to 1 hour	6 to 8 hours
Short-acting		
Pentobarbital		
Secobarbital	10 to 15 minutes	3 to 4 hours

Barbiturates are weak acids that are absorbed and rapidly distributed to all tissues and fluids with high concentrations in the brain, liver, and kidneys. Lipid solubility of the barbiturates is the dominant factor in their distribution within the body. The more lipid soluble the barbiturate, the more rapidly it penetrates all tissues of the body. Barbiturates are bound to plasma and tissue proteins to a varying degree with the degree of binding increasing directly as a function of lipid solubility.

Phenobarbital has the lowest lipid solubility, lowest plasma binding, lowest brain protein binding, the longest delay in onset of activity, and the longest duration of action. At the opposite extreme is secobarbital which has the highest lipid solubility, plasma protein binding, brain protein binding, the shortest delay in onset of activity, and the shortest duration of action. Butabarbital is classified as an intermediate barbiturate.

The plasma half-life for Pentobarbital in adults is 15 to 50 hours and appears to be dose dependent.

Barbiturates are metabolized primarily by the hepatic microsomal enzyme system, and the metabolic products are excreted in the urine, and less commonly, in the feces. Approximately 25 to 50 percent of a dose of aprobarbital or phenobarbital is eliminated unchanged in the urine, whereas the amount of other barbiturates excreted unchanged in the urine is negligible. The excretion of unmetabolized barbiturate is one feature that distinguishes the long-acting category from those belonging to other categories which are almost entirely metabolized. The inactive metabolites of the barbiturates are excreted as conjugates of glucuronic acid.

INDICATIONS AND USAGE

Sedatives

Hypnotics, for the short-term treatment of insomnia, since they appear to lose their effectiveness for sleep induction and sleep maintenance after 2 weeks (See *"Clinical Pharmacology"* section).

Pentobarbital Sodium capsules and injection are also indicated for use as preanesthetics.

Pentobarbital Sodium injection is also indicated as an anticonvulsant, in anesthetic doses, in the emergency control of certain acute convulsive episodes, e.g., those associated with status epilepticus, cholera, eclampsia, meningitis, tetanus, and toxic reactions to strychnine or local anesthetics. Barbiturates administered rectally are absorbed from the colon and are used when oral or parenteral administration may be undesirable.

UNLABELED USES

Pentobarbital is used alone or as an adjunct in the treatment of intracranial hypertension including intracranial pressure associated with Reye's syndrome.

CONTRAINDICATIONS

Barbiturates are contraindicated in patients with known barbiturate sensitivity. Barbiturates are also contraindicated in patients with a history of manifest or latent porphyria.

WARNINGS

1. Habit forming: Barbiturates may be habit forming. Tolerance, psychological and physical dependence may occur with continued use. (See *"Drug Abuse and Dependence"* and *"Pharmacokinetics"* sections.) Patients who have psychological dependence on barbiturates may increase the dosage or decrease the dosage interval without consulting a physician and may subsequently develop a physical dependence on barbiturates. To minimize the possibility of overdosage or the development of dependence, the prescribing and dispensing of sedative-hypnotic barbiturates should be limited to the amount required for the interval until the next appointment. Abrupt cessation after prolonged use in the dependent person may result in withdrawal symptoms, including delirium, convulsions, and possibly death. Barbiturates should be withdrawn gradually from any patient known to be taking excessive dosage over long periods of time. (See *"Drug Abuse and Dependence"* section.)

Acute or chronic pain: Caution should be exercised when barbiturates are administered to patients with acute or chronic pain, because paradoxical excitement could be induced or important symptoms could be masked. However, the use of barbiturates as sedatives in the postoperative surgical period and as adjuncts to cancer chemotherapy is well established.

3. Use in pregnancy: Barbiturates can cause fetal damage when administered to a pregnant woman. Retrospective, case-controlled studies have suggested a connection between the maternal consumption of barbiturates and a higher than expected incidence of fetal abnormalities. Following oral or parenteral administration, barbiturates readily cross the placental barrier and are distributed throughout fetal tissues with highest concentrations found in the placenta, fetal liver, and brain. It is presumed that this effect will also be seen following rectal administration. Fetal blood levels approach maternal blood levels following parenteral administration.

Withdrawal symptoms occur in infants born to mothers who receive barbiturates throughout the last trimester of pregnancy. (See *"Drug Abuse and Dependence"* section.) If this drug is used during pregnancy, or if the patient becomes pregnant while taking this drug, the patient should be apprised of the potential hazard to the fetus.

4. Synergistic effects: The concomitant use of alcohol or other CNS depressants may produce additive CNS depressant effects.

5. IV administration: Too rapid administration may cause respiratory depression, apnea, laryngospasm, or vasodilation with fall in blood pressure.

PRECAUTIONS

General: Barbiturates may be habit forming. Tolerance and psychological and physical dependence may occur with continuing use. (See *"Drug Abuse and Dependence"* section.) Barbiturates should be administered with caution, if at all, to patients who are mentally depressed, have suicidal tendencies, or a history of drug abuse.

Elderly or debilitated patients may react to barbiturates with marked excitement, depression, and confusion. In some persons, barbiturates repeatedly produce excitement rather than depression.

In patients with hepatic damage, barbiturates should be administered with caution and initially in reduced doses. Barbiturates should not be administered to patients showing the premonitory signs of hepatic coma.

Certain brands of Pentobarbital Sodium contain FD&C Yellow No. 5 (tartrazine) which may cause allergic-type reactions (including bronchial asthma) in certain susceptible individuals. Although the overall incidence of FD&C Yellow No. 5 (tartrazine) sensitivity in the general population is low, it is frequently seen in patients who also have aspirin hypersensitivity.

Parenteral solutions of barbiturates are highly alkaline. Therefore, extreme care should be taken to avoid perivascular extravasation or intra-arterial injection. Extravascular injection may cause local tissue damage with subsequent necrosis; consequences of intra-arterial injection may vary from transient pain to gangrene of the limb. Any complaint of pain in the limb warrants stopping the injection.

Information for the Patient: Practitioners should give the following information and instructions to patients receiving barbiturates.

1. The use of barbiturates carries with it an associated risk of psychological and/or physical dependence. The patient should be warned against increasing the dose of the drug without consulting a physician.

2. Barbiturates may impair mental and/or physical abilities required for the performance of potentially hazardous tasks (e.g., driving, operating machinery, etc.).

3. Alcohol should not be consumed while taking barbiturates. Concurrent use of the barbiturates with other CNS depressants (e.g., alcohol, narcotics, tranquilizers, and antihistamines) may result in additional CNS depressant effects.

Laboratory Tests: Prolonged therapy with barbiturates should be accompanied by periodic laboratory evaluation of organ systems, including hematopoietic, renal, and hepatic systems. (See *"Precautions—General"* and *"Adverse Reactions"* sections.)

Drug Interactions: Most reports of clinically significant drug interactions occurring with the barbiturates have involved phenobarbital. However, the application of these data to other barbiturates appears valid and warrants serial blood level determinations of the relevant drugs when there are multiple therapies.

1. Anticoagulants: Phenobarbital lowers the plasma levels of dicumarol (name previously used: bishydroxycoumarin) and causes a decrease in anticoagulant activity as measured by the prothrombin time. Barbiturates can induce hepatic microsomal enzymes resulting in increased metabolism and decreased anticoagulant response of oral anticoagulants (e.g., warfarin, acenocoumarol, dicumarol, and phenprocoumon). Patients stabilized on anticoagulant therapy may require dosage adjustments if barbiturates are added to or withdrawn from their dosage regimen.

2. Corticosteroids: Barbiturates appear to enhance the metabolism of exogenous corticosteroids probably through the induction of hepatic microsomal enzymes. Patients stabilized on corticosteroid therapy may require dosage adjustments if barbiturates are added to or withdrawn from their dosage regimen.

3. Griseofulvin: Phenobarbital appears to interfere with the absorption of orally administered griseofulvin, thus decreasing its blood level. The effect of the resultant decreased blood levels of griseofulvin on therapeutic response has not been established. However, it would be preferable to avoid concomitant administration of these drugs.

4. Doxycycline: Phenobarbital has been shown to shorten the half-life of doxycycline for as long as 2 weeks after barbiturate therapy is discontinued. This mechanism is probably through the induction of hepatic microsomal enzymes that metabolize the antibiotic. If phenobarbital and doxycycline are administered concurrently, the clinical response to doxycycline should be monitored closely.

5. Phenytoin, sodium valproate, valproic acid: The effect of barbiturates on the metabolism of phenytoin appears to be variable. Some investigators report an accelerating effect, while others report no effect. Because the effect of barbiturates on the metabolism of phenytoin is not predictable, phenytoin and barbiturate

blood levels should be monitored more frequently if these drugs are given concurrently. Sodium valproate and valproic acid appear to decrease barbiturate metabolism; therefore, barbiturate blood levels should be monitored and appropriate dosage adjustments made as indicated.

6. Central nervous system depressants: The concomitant use of other central nervous system depressants including other sedatives or hypnotics, antihistamines, tranquilizers, or alcohol, may produce additive depressant effects.

7. Monoamine oxidase inhibitors: (MAOI): MAOI prolong the effects of barbiturates probably because metabolism of the barbiturate is inhibited.

8. Estradiol, estrone, progesterone and other steroidal hormones: Pretreatment with or concurrent administration of phenobarbital may decrease the effect of estradiol by increasing its metabolism. There have been reports of patients treated with antiepileptic drugs (e.g., phenobarbital) who became pregnant while taking oral contraceptives. An alternate contraceptive method might be suggested to women taking phenobarbital.

Carcinogenesis:

1. Animal data. Phenobarbital sodium is carcinogenic in mice and rats after lifetime administration. In mice, it produced benign and malignant liver cell tumors. In rats, benign liver cell tumors were observed very late in life.

2. Human Data. In a 29-year epidemiological study of 9,136 patients who were treated on an anticonvulsant protocol that included phenobarbital, results indicated a higher than normal incidence of hepatic carcinoma. Previously, some of these patients were treated with thorotrast, a drug that is known to produce hepatic carcinomas. Thus, this study did not provide sufficient evidence that phenobarbital sodium is carcinogenic in humans.

Data from one retrospective study of 235 children in which one types of barbiturates are not identified suggested an association between exposure to barbiturates prenatally and an increased incidence of brain tumor. (Gold, E., et al., "Increased Risk of Brain Tumors in Children Exposed to Barbiturates," Journal of National Cancer Institute, 61:1031-1034, 1978).

Pregnancy:

1. *Teratogenic effects*: Pregnancy Category D— See *"Warnings—Use in Pregnancy"* section.

2. *Nonteratogenic effects:* Reports of infants suffering from long-term barbiturate exposure in utero included the acute withdrawal syndrome of seizures and hyperirritability from birth to a delayed onset of up to 14 days. (See *"Drug Abuse and Dependence"* section.)

Labor and Delivery: Hypnotic doses of these barbiturates do not appear to significantly impair uterine activity during labor. Full anesthetic doses of barbiturates decrease the force and frequency of uterine contractions. Administration of sedative-hypnotic barbiturates to the mother during labor may result in respiratory depression in the newborn. Premature infants are particularly susceptible to the depressant effects of barbiturates. If barbiturates are used during labor and delivery, resuscitation equipment should be available. Data are currently not available to evaluate the effect of these barbiturates when forceps delivery or other intervention is necessary. Also, data are not available to determine the effect of these barbiturates on the later growth, development, and functional maturation of the child.

Nursing Mothers: Caution should be exercised when a barbiturate is administered to a nursing woman since small amounts of barbiturates are excreted in the milk.

ADVERSE REACTIONS

The following adverse reactions and their incidence were compiled from surveillance of thousands of hospitalized patients. Because such patients may be less aware of certain of the milder adverse effects of barbiturates, the incidence of these reactions may be somewhat higher in fully ambulatory patients.

More than 1 in 100 Patients: The most common adverse reaction estimated to occur at a rate of 1 to 3 patients per 100 is:

Nervous System: Somnolence.

Less than 1 in 100 Patients: Adverse reactions estimated to occur at a rate of less than 1 in 100 patients listed below, grouped by organ system, and by decreasing order of occurrence are:

Nervous System: Agitation, confusion, hyperkinesia, ataxia, CNS depression, nightmares, nervousness, psychiatric disturbance, hallucinations, insomnia, anxiety, dizziness, thinking abnormality.

Respiratory System: Hypoventilation, apnea.

Cardiovascular System: Bradycardia, hypotension, syncope.

Digestive System: Nausea, vomiting, constipation.

Other Reported Reactions: Headache, injection site reactions, hypersensitivity reactions (angioedema, skin rashes, exfoliative dermatitis), fever, liver damage, megaloblastic anemia following chronic phenobarbital use.

DRUG ABUSE AND DEPENDENCE

Pentobarbital Sodium is subject to control by the Federal Controlled Substances Act under DEA schedule II (schedule III for rectal suppositories). Barbiturates may be habit forming. Tolerance, psychological dependence, and physical dependence may occur especially following prolonged use of high doses of barbiturates. Daily administration in excess of 400 mg of Pentobarbital or secobarbital for approximately 90 days is likely to produce some degree of physical dependence. A dosage of from 600 to 800 mg taken for at least 35 days is sufficient to produce withdrawal seizures. The average daily dose for the barbiturate addict is usually about 1.5 gm. As tolerance to barbiturates develops, the amount needed to maintain the same level of intoxication increases; tolerance to a fatal dosage, however, does not increase more than two-fold. As this occurs, the margin between an intoxicating dosage and fatal dosage becomes smaller.

Symptoms of acute intoxication with barbiturates include unsteady gait, slurred speech, and sustained nystagmus. Mental signs of chronic intoxication include confusion, poor judgment, irritability, insomnia, and somatic complaints.

Symptoms of barbiturate dependence are similar to those of chronic alcoholism. If an individual appears to be intoxicated with alcohol to a degree that is radically disproportionate to the amount of alcohol in his or her blood the use of barbiturates should be suspected. The lethal dose of a barbiturate is far less if alcohol is also ingested.

The symptoms of barbiturate withdrawal can be severe and may cause death. Minor withdrawal symptoms may appear 8 to 12 hours after the last dose of a barbiturate. These symptoms usually appear in the following order: anxiety, muscle twitching, tremor of hands and fingers, progressive weakness, dizziness, distortion in visual perception, nausea, vomiting, insomnia, and orthostatic hypotension. Major withdrawal symptoms (convulsions and delirium) may occur within 16 hours and last up to 5 days after abrupt cessation of these drugs. Intensity of withdrawal symptoms gradually declines over a period of approximately 15 days. Individuals susceptible to barbiturate abuse and dependence include alcoholics and opiate abusers, as well as other sedative-hypnotic and amphetamine abusers.

Drug dependence to barbiturates arises from repeated administration of a barbiturate or agent with barbiturate-like effect on a continuous basis, generally in amounts exceeding therapeutic dose levels. The characteristics of drug dependence to barbiturates include: (a) a strong desire or need to continue taking the drug; (b) a tendency to increase the dose; (c) a psychic dependence on the effects of the drug related to subjective and individual appreciation of those effects; and (d) a physical dependence on the effects of the drug requiring its presence for maintenance of homeostasis and resulting in a definite, characteristic, and self-limited abstinence syndrome when the drug is withdrawn.

Treatment of barbiturate dependence consists of cautious and gradual withdrawal of the drug. Barbiturate-dependent patients can be withdrawn by using a number of different withdrawal regimens. In all cases withdrawal takes an extended period of time. One method involves substituting a 30 mg dose of phenobarbital for each 100 to 200 mg dose of barbiturate that the patient has been taking. The total daily amount of phenobarbital is then administered in 3 to 4 divided doses, not to exceed 600 mg daily. Should signs of withdrawal occur on the first day of treatment, a loading dose of 100 to 200 mg of phenobarbital may be administered IM in addition to the oral dose. After stabilization on phenobarbital, the total daily dose is decreased by 30 mg a day as long as withdrawal is proceeding smoothly. A modification of this regimen involves initiating treatment at the patient's regular dosage level and decreasing the daily dosage by 10 percent if tolerated by the patient.

Infants physically dependent on barbiturates may be given phenobarbital 3 to 10 mg/kg/day. After withdrawal symptoms (hyperactivity, disturbed sleep, tremors, hyperreflexia) are relieved, the dosage of phenobarbital should be gradually decreased and completely withdrawn over a 2 week period.

OVERDOSAGE

The toxic dose of barbiturates varies considerably. In general, an oral dose of 1 gm of most barbiturates produces serious poisoning in an adult. Death commonly occurs after 2 to 10 gm of ingested barbiturate. Barbiturate intoxication may be confused with alcoholism, bromide intoxication, and with various neurological disorders.

Acute overdosage with barbiturates is manifested by CNS and respiratory depression which may progress to Cheyne-Stokes respiration, areflexia, constriction of the pupils to a slight degree (though in severe poisoning they may show paralytic dilation), oliguria, tachycardia, hypotension, lowered body temperature, and coma. Typical shock syndrome (apnea, circulatory collapse, respiratory arrest, and death) may occur.

In extreme overdose, all electrical activity in the brain may cease, in which case a "flat" EEG normally equated with clinical death cannot be accepted. This effect is fully reversible unless hypoxic damage occurs. Consideration should be given to the possibility of barbiturate intoxication even in situations that appear to involve trauma.

Complications such as pneumonia, pulmonary edema, cardiac arrhythmias, congestive heart failure, and renal failure may occur. Uremia may increase CNS sensitivity to barbiturates. Differential diagnosis should include hypoglycemia, head trauma, cerebrovascular accidents, convulsive states, and diabetic coma. Blood levels from acute overdosage for some barbiturates are listed in Table 2. (See related table).

Treatment of overdosage is mainly supportive and consists of the following:

1. Maintenance of an adequate airway, with assisted respiration and oxygen administration as necessary.
2. Monitoring of vital signs and fluid balance.
3. After oral ingestion, if the patient is conscious and has not lost the gag reflex, emesis may be induced with ipecac. Care should be taken to prevent pulmonary aspiration of vomitus. After completion of vomiting, 30 gm activated charcoal in a glass of water may be administered.
4. If emesis is contraindicated, gastric lavage may be performed with a cuffed endotracheal tube in place with the patient in the face down position. Activated charcoal may be left in the emptied stomach and a saline cathartic administered.

5. Fluid therapy and other standard treatment for shock, if needed.
6. If renal function is normal, forced diuresis may aid in the elimination of the barbiturate. Alkalinization of the urine increases renal excretion of some barbiturates, especially phenobarbital, also aprobarbital, and mephobarbital (which is metabolized to phenobarbital).
7. Although not recommended as a routine procedure, hemodialysis may be used in severe barbiturate intoxications or if the patient is anuric or in shock.
8. Patient should be rolled from side to side every 30 minutes.
9. Antibiotics should be given if pneumonia is suspected.
10. Appropriate nursing care to prevent hypostatic pneumonia, decubiti, aspiration, and other complications of patients with altered states of consciousness.

DOSAGE AND ADMINISTRATION

Dosages of barbiturates must be individualized with full knowledge of their particular characteristics and recommended rate of administration. Factors of consideration are the patient's age, weight, and condition. Parenteral routes should be used only when oral administration is impossible or impractical.

PENTOBARBITAL SODIUM CAPSULES

Adults: The usual hypnotic dose consists of 100 mg at bedtime.

Children: The preoperative dose is 2 to 6 mg/kg/24 hours (maximum 100 mg), depending on age, weight, and the desired degree of sedation.

The proper hypnotic dose for children must be judged on the basis of individual age and weight.

Special Patient Population: Dosage should be reduced in the elderly or debilitated because these patients may be more sensitive to barbiturates. Dosage should be reduced for patients with impaired renal function or hepatic disease.

PENTOBARBITAL SODIUM INJECTION

Intramuscular Administration: IM injection of the sodium salts of barbiturates should be made deeply into a large muscle, and a volume of 5 ml should not be exceeded at any one site because of possible tissue irritation. After IM injection of a hypnotic dose, the patient's vital signs should be monitored. The usual adult dosage of Pentobarbital Sodium solution is 150 to 200 mg as a single IM injection; the recommended pediatric dosage ranges from 2 to 6 mg/kg as a single IM injection not to exceed 100 mg.

Intravenous Administration: Pentobarbital Sodium solution should not be admixed with any other medication or solution. IV injection is restricted to conditions in which other routes are not feasible, either because the patient is unconscious (as in cerebral hemorrhage, eclampsia, or status epilepticus), or because the patient resists (as in delirium), or because prompt action is imperative. Slow IV injection is essential and patients should be carefully observed during administration. This requires that blood pressure, respiration, and cardiac function be maintained, vital signs be recorded, and equipment for resuscitation and artificial ventilation be available. The rate of IV injection should not exceed 50 mg/min for Pentobarbital Sodium.

There is no average intravenous dose of Pentobarbital Sodium solution that can be relied on to produce similar effects in different patients. The possibility of overdose and respiratory depression is remote when the drug is injected slowly in fractional doses.

A commonly used initial dose for the 70 kg adult is 100 mg. Proportional reduction in dosage should be made for pediatric or debilitated patients. At least one minute is necessary to determine the full effect of intravenous Pentobarbital. If necessary, additional small increments of the drug may be given up to a total of from 200 to 500 mg for normal adults.

Anticonvulsant Use: In convulsive states, dosage of Pentobarbital Sodium solution should be kept to a minimum to avoid compounding the depression which may follow convulsions. The injection must be made slowly with due regard to the time required for the drug to penetrate the blood-brain barrier.

Special Patient Population: Dosage should be reduced in the elderly or debilitated because these patients may be more sensitive to barbiturates. Dosage should be reduced for patients with impaired renal function or hepatic disease.

Inspection: Parenteral drug products should be inspected visually for particulate matter and discoloration prior to administration, whenever solution containers permit. Solutions for injection showing evidence of precipitation should not be used.

PENTOBARBITAL SODIUM SUPPOSITORIES

Typical hypnotic doses for adults and children are given below. These are intended only as a guide, and administration should be adjusted to the individual needs of each patient. For sedation, in children 5—14 years and in adults, reduce dose appropriately.

Adults (average to above average weight): one 120 mg or one 200 mg suppository.

Children:	
12-14 years .... (80-110 lbs)	one 60 mg or one 120 mg suppository
5-12 years .... (40-80 lbs)	one 60 mg suppository
1-4 years .... (20-40 lbs)	one 30 mg or one 60 mg suppository
2 months-1 year .... (10-20 lbs)	one 30 mg suppository

Suppositories should not be divided.

◆ RATED THERAPEUTICALLY EQUIVALENT; ◇ THERAPEUTIC EQUIVALENCE UNCONFIRMED; ○ UNRATED

Table 2.
CONCENTRATION OF BARBITURATE IN THE BLOOD VERSUS DEGREE OF CNS DEPRESSION

Barbiturate	Onset/ duration	Blood barbiturate level in ppm (µg/ml) Degree of depression in nontolerant persons*				
		1	2	3	4	5
Pentobarbital	Fast/short	≤ 2	0.5 to 3	10 to 15	12 to 25	15 to 40
Secobarbital	Fast/short	≤ 2	0.5 to 5	10 to 15	15 to 25	15 to 40
Amobarbital	Intermediate/ intermediate	≤ 3	2 to 10	30 to 40	30 to 60	40 to 80
Butabarbital	Intermediate/ intermediate	≤ 5	3 to 25	40 to 60	50 to 80	60 to 100
Phenobarbital	Slow/long	≤ 10	5 to 40	50 to 80	70 to 120	100 to 200

* Categories of degree of depression in nontolerant persons.
1. Under the influence and appreciably impaired for purposes of driving a motor vehicle or performing tasks requiring alertness and unimpaired judgment and reaction time.
2. Sedated, therapeutic range, calm, relaxed, and easily aroused.
3. Comatose, difficult to arouse, significant depression of respiration.
4. Compatible with death in aged or ill persons or in presence of obstructed airway, other toxic agents, or exposure to cold.
5. Usual lethal level, the upper end of the range includes those who received some supportive treatment.

Special Patient Population: Dosage should be reduced in the elderly or debilitated because these patients may be more sensitive to barbiturates. Dosage should be reduced for patients with impaired renal function or hepatic disease.

RECOMMENDED STORAGE
Store capsules below 86°F (30°C). Store solution at 86°F. Brief exposure up to 104°F (40°C) does not adversely affect the solution. Avoid excessive heat. Protect from freezing. Store rectal suppositories in a refrigerator (36°–46°F).

J CODES
IM,IV,OTH—J2515

HOW SUPPLIED
CAPSULE (C-II): 50 MG

BRAND/MANUFACTURER	NDC	SIZE	AWP
◆ BRAND NEMBUTAL SODIUM: Abbott Pharm	00074-3150-11	100s	$32.06

CAPSULE (C-II): 100 MG

AVERAGE UNIT PRICE (AVAILABLE SIZES)			
BRAND			$0.51

BRAND/MANUFACTURER	NDC	SIZE	AWP
◆ BRAND NEMBUTAL SODIUM: Abbott Pharm	00074-3114-01	100s	$50.20
	00074-3114-21	100s ud	$54.71
	00074-3114-02	500s	$243.45

ELIXIR (C-II): 18.2 MG/5 ML

BRAND/MANUFACTURER	NDC	SIZE	AWP
○ BRAND NEMBUTAL: Abbott Pharm	00074-3142-01	480 ml	$62.31

INJECTION (C-II): 50 MG/ML

AVERAGE UNIT PRICE (AVAILABLE SIZES)			
BRAND			$0.74

BRAND/MANUFACTURER	NDC	SIZE	AWP
◆ BRAND NEMBUTAL SODIUM: Abbott Pharm	00074-3778-04	20 ml	$11.73
	00074-3778-05	50 ml	$21.86
	00074-6899-04	2 ml 25s	$59.21
◆ GENERICS Wyeth-Ayerst	00008-0303-02	2 ml 10s	$22.14

SUPPOSITORY (C-III): 30 MG

BRAND/MANUFACTURER	NDC	SIZE	AWP
○ BRAND NEMBUTAL SODIUM: Abbott Pharm	00074-3272-01	12s	$39.90

SUPPOSITORY (C-III): 60 MG

BRAND/MANUFACTURER	NDC	SIZE	AWP
○ BRAND NEMBUTAL SODIUM: Abbott Pharm	00074-3148-01	12s	$46.83

SUPPOSITORY (C-III): 120 MG

BRAND/MANUFACTURER	NDC	SIZE	AWP
○ BRAND NEMBUTAL SODIUM: Abbott Pharm	00074-3145-01	12s	$52.21

SUPPOSITORY (C-III): 200 MG

BRAND/MANUFACTURER	NDC	SIZE	AWP
○ BRAND NEMBUTAL SODIUM: Abbott Pharm	00074-3164-01	12s	$64.19

Pentostatin

> **WARNING**
> PENTOSTATIN SHOULD BE ADMINISTERED UNDER THE SUPERVISION OF A PHYSICIAN QUALIFIED AND EXPERIENCED IN THE USE OF CANCER CHEMOTHERAPEUTIC AGENTS. THE USE OF HIGHER DOSES THAN THOSE SPECIFIED (SEE *"DOSAGE AND ADMINISTRATION"*) IS NOT RECOMMENDED. DOSE-LIMITING SEVERE RENAL, LIVER, PULMONARY, AND CNS TOXICITIES OCCURRED IN PHASE 1 STUDIES THAT USED PENTOSTATIN AT HIGHER DOSES (20-50 MG/M^2 IN DIVIDED DOSES OVER 5 DAYS) THAN RECOMMENDED.
> IN A CLINICAL INVESTIGATION IN PATIENTS WITH REFRACTORY CHRONIC LYMPHOCYTIC LEUKEMIA USING PENTOSTATIN AT THE RECOMMENDED DOSE IN COMBINATION WITH FLUDARABINE PHOSPHATE, 4 OF 6 PATIENTS ENTERED IN THE STUDY HAD SEVERE OR FATAL PULMONARY TOXICITY. THE USE OF PENTOSTATIN IN COMBINATION WITH FLUDARABINE PHOSPHATE IS NOT RECOMMENDED.

DESCRIPTION
Each vial of Pentostatin contains 10 mg of Pentostatin.

Pentostatin, also known as 2′-deoxycoformycin (DCF), is a potent inhibitor of the enzyme adenosine deaminase and is isolated from fermentation cultures of *Streptomyces antibioticus*. Pentostatin is known chemically as (R)-3-(2-deoxy-β-D-*erythro*-pentofuranosyl)-3, 6, 7, 8-tetrahydroimidazo[4,5-d] [1,3]diazepin-8-ol with a molecular formula of $C_{11}H_{16}N_4O_4$ and a molecular weight of 268.27. Pentostatin is a white to off-white solid, freely soluble in distilled water.

Following is its chemical structure:

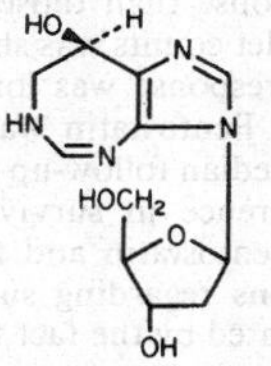

CLINICAL PHARMACOLOGY
MECHANISM OF ACTION
Pentostatin is a potent transition state inhibitor of the enzyme adenosine deaminase (ADA). The greatest activity of ADA is found in cells of the lymphoid system with T-cells having higher activity than B-cells and T-cell malignancies

higher ADA activity than B-cell malignancies. Pentostatin inhibition of ADA, particularly in the presence of adenosine or deoxyadenosine, leads to cytotoxicity, and this is believed to be due to elevated intracellular levels of dATP which can block DNA synthesis through inhibition of ribonucleotide reductase. Pentostatin can also inhibit RNA synthesis as well as cause increased DNA damage. In addition to elevated dATP, these mechanisms may contribute to the overall cytotoxic effect of Pentostatin. The precise mechanism of Pentostatin's antitumor effect, however, in hairy cell leukemia is not known.

PHARMACOKINETICS/DRUG METABOLISM

A tissue distribution and whole-body autoradiography study in the rat revealed that radioactivity concentrations were highest in the kidneys with very little central nervous system penetration.

In man, following a single dose of 4 mg/m^2 of Pentostatin infused over 5 minutes, the distribution half-life was 11 minutes, the mean terminal half-life was 5.7 hours, the mean plasma clearance was 68 mL/min/m^2, and approximately 90% of the dose was excreted in the urine as unchanged Pentostatin and/or metabolites as measured by adenosine deaminase inhibitory activity. The plasma protein binding of Pentostatin is low, approximately 4%.

A positive correlation was observed between Pentostatin clearance and creatinine clearance (CrCl) in patients with creatinine clearance values ranging from 60 mL/min to 130 mL/min.[1] Pentostatin half-life in patients with renal impairment (CrCl < 50 mL/min, n = 2) was 18 hours, which was much longer than that observed in patients with normal renal function (CrCl > mL/min, n = 14), about 6 hours.

CLINICAL STUDIES

The following table provides efficacy results for 4 groups (columns) of patients with hairy cell leukemia: patients who initially received Pentostatin, patients who initially received alpha-interferon (IFN), and 2 different groups of patients who received Pentostatin after proving to be refractory to, or intolerant of IFN therapy. The first 2 groups represent treatment results from the SWOG 8691 study, a large multicenter study comparing Pentostatin and IFN in untreated (frontline) patients with confirmed hairy cell leukemia. The third group represents evaluable patients from the SWOG study who crossed over to Pentostatin after initially receiving IFN. The fourth group, labeled NCI Phase 2 studies, displays pooled results of 2 noncomparative studies (MD Anderson and CALGB), in which Pentostatin was used to treat patients with confirmed IFN-refractory disease.

In the SWOG 8691 study, Pentostatin was administered at a dose of 4 mg/m^2 every 2 weeks. After 6 months of treatment, patients were evaluated for response. If a complete response was achieved, 2 additional doses of Pentostatin were administered and then discontinued. If a partial response was achieved, Pentostatin was continued for up to an additional 6 months. Pentostatin was discontinued for stable disease after 6 months or progressive disease after 2 months of therapy. IFN was administered 3 million units subcutaneously 3 times per week. Patients who achieved a complete or partial response after 6 months of treatment continued on IFN for another 6 months. IFN was discontinued if patients did not achieve a complete or partial response after 6 months of initial treatment and progressed after 2 months. This study allowed cross-over of patients intolerant of, or refractory to initial treatment.

Interferon-refractory patients enrolled into the MD Anderson study received Pentostatin at a dose of 4 mg/m^2 every other week for 3 months and responding patients received 3 additional months. CALGB patients received 4 mg/m of Pentostatin every other week for 3 months and responding patients were treated monthly for up to 9 additional months. Almost all patients had a PS of 0 to 2 in the Phase 2 and 3 studies.

For each study, a complete response (CR) required clearing of the peripheral blood and bone marrow of all hairy cells, normalization of organomegaly and lymphadenopathy by physical examination, and recovery of hemoglobin to at least 12 g/dL, platelet count to at least 100,000/mm^3, and granulocyte count to at least 1500/mm^3. A partial response (PR) required that the percentage of hairy cells in the blood and bone marrow decrease by more than 50%, enlarged organs and lymph nodes decreased by more than 50% by physical examination, and hematologic parameters had to meet the same criteria as for complete response. The table below reports the response rate for 2 groups of patients: (1) Evaluable, ie, patients who could be evaluated for response and (2) Intent-to-Treat, ie, patients diagnosed with hairy cell leukemia. (See related table).

The results show that frontline patients treated with Pentostatin achieved a significantly higher rate of response than those treated with IFN. The time to recovery of neutrophil and platelet counts was shorter with Pentostatin treatment and the estimated duration of response was longer. The response rate in IFN-refractory patients treated with Pentostatin was similar to that in Pentostatin treated frontline patients. At a median follow-up duration of 46 months, there was no statistically significant difference in survival between hairy cell leukemia patients initially treated with Pentostatin and those initially treated with IFN. However, no definite conclusions regarding survival can be made from these results because they are complicated by the fact that the majority of IFN patients crossed over to Pentostatin treatment.

In the Phase 3 SWOG study, 25 patients with hairy cell leukemia died during treatment or follow-up: 18 patients had last received Pentostatin (3 of whom had crossed over from IFN), and 7 patients had last received IFN (1 of whom crossed over from Pentostatin). Eleven of the 25 deaths occurred within 60 days of the last dose of treatment. Of these, hairy cell leukemia was cited by the investigators as a contributory cause for 1 death in the Pentostatin group and 3 deaths in the IFN group. Additionally, infection contributed to the deaths of 3 patients in the

Pentostatin group and 2 patients in the IFN group. Approximately 4% of hairy cell leukemia patients, in each arm, died more than 60 days after the last dose of either treatment and there was no outstanding cause of death among these patients.

INDICATIONS AND USAGE

Pentostatin is indicated as single-agent treatment for both untreated and alpha-interferon-refractory hairy cell leukemia patients with active disease as defined by clinically significant anemia, neutropenia, thrombocytopenia, or disease-related symptoms.

UNLABELED USES

Pentostatin is used in the treatment of Chronic Lymphocytic Leukemia and Mycosis Fungoides/Sezary Syndrome.

CONTRAINDICATIONS

Pentostatin is contraindicated in patients who have demonstrated hypersensitivity to Pentostatin.

WARNINGS

See boxed Warning.

Patients with hairy cell leukemia may experience myelosuppression primarily during the first few courses of treatment. Patients with infections prior to Pentostatin treatment have in some cases developed worsening of their condition leading to death, whereas others have achieved complete response. Patients with infection should be treated only when the potential benefit of treatment justifies the potential risk to the patient. Efforts should be made to control the infection before treatment is initiated or resumed.

In patients with progressive hairy cell leukemia, the initial courses of Pentostatin treatment were associated with worsening of neutropenia. Therefore, frequent monitoring of complete blood counts during this time is necessary. If severe neutropenia continues beyond the initial cycles, patients should be evaluated for disease status, including a bone marrow examination.

Elevations in liver function tests occurred during treatment with Pentostatin and were generally reversible.

Renal toxicity was observed at higher doses in early studies; however, in patients treated at the recommended dose, elevations in serum creatinine were usually minor and reversible. There were some patients who began treatment with normal renal function who had evidence of mild to moderate toxicity at a final assessment. (See "Dosage and Administration".)

Rashes, occasionally severe, were commonly reported and may worsen with continued treatment. Withholding of treatment may be required. (See "Dosage and Administration".)

PREGNANCY CATEGORY D

Pentostatin can cause fetal harm when administered to a pregnant woman. Pentostatin was administered intravenously at doses of 0, 0.01, 0.1, or 0.75 mg/kg/day (0, 0.06, 0.6, and 4.5 mg/m^2) to pregnant rats on days 6 through 15 of gestation. Drug-related maternal toxicity occurred at doses of 0.1 and 0.75 mg/kg/day (0.6 and 4.5 mg/m^2). Teratogenic effects were observed at 0.75 mg/kg/day (4.5 mg/m^2) manifested by increased incidence of various skeletal malformations. In a dose range-finding study, Pentostatin was administered intravenously to rats at doses of 0, 0.05, 0.1, 0.5, 0.75, or 1 mg/kg/day (0, 0.3, 0.6, 3, 4.5, 6 mg/m^2) on days 6 through 15 of gestation. Fetal malformations that were observed were an omphalocele at 0.05 mg/kg (0.3 mg/m^2), gastroschisis at 0.75 mg/kg and 1 mg/kg (4.5 and 6 mg/m^2), and a flexure defect of the hindlimbs at 0.75 mg/kg (4.5 mg/m^2). Pentostatin was also shown to be teratogenic in mice when administered as a single 2 mg/kg (6 mg/m^2) intraperitoneal injection on day 7 of gestation. Pentostatin was not teratogenic in rabbits when administered intravenously on days 6 through 18 of gestation at doses of 0, 0.005, 0.01, or 0.02 mg/kg/day (0, 0.015, 0.03, or 0.06 mg/m^2); however maternal toxicity, abortions, early deliveries, and deaths occurred in all drug-treated groups. There are no adequate and well-controlled studies in pregnant women. If Pentostatin is used during pregnancy, or if the patient becomes pregnant while taking (receiving) this drug, the patient should be apprised of the potential hazard to the fetus. Women of childbearing potential receiving Pentostatin should be advised to avoid becoming pregnant.

PRECAUTIONS

GENERAL

Therapy with Pentostatin requires regular patient observation and monitoring of hematologic parameters and blood chemistry values. If severe adverse reactions occur, the drug should be withheld (see "Dosage and Administration"), and appropriate corrective measures should be taken according to the clinical judgment of the physician.

Pentostatin treatment should be withheld or discontinued in patients showing evidence of nervous system toxicity.

INFORMATION FOR PATIENTS

Patients should be advised of the signs and symptoms of adverse events associated with Pentostatin therapy. (See "Adverse Reactions".)

LABORATORY TESTS

Prior to initiating therapy with Pentostatin renal function should be assessed with a serum creatinine and/or a creatinine clearance assay. (See "Clinical Pharmacology" and "Dosage and Administration".) Complete blood counts and serum-creatinine should be performed before each dose of Pentostatin and at other appropriate periods during therapy (see "Dosage and Administration"). Severe

Parameter	Frontline		IFN-Refractory[a]	
	Evaluable Pentostatin N = 138	Evaluable IFN N = 130	SWOG 8691[b] Crossover N = 79	NCI Phase 2 Studies N = 44
Response Rates (%)				
Evaluable CR	84	18	85	58
PR	6	24	4	28
Intent-to-Treat	N = 170	N = 170		
CR	68	14		
PR	5	18		
Median Time to Response (months)				
CR	6.6	11.5	6.0	4.2
PR	4.0	6.2	5.8	—
Median Duration of Response (months)				
CR	NR	8.3	NR	7.7[c] (CALGB)
				> 15.2[c] (MDA)
PR	NR	15.2	NR	—
% Estimated to be in Response After 24 Months				
CR	76	16	85	
PR	50	21		
Median Time to Recovery (days)				
ANC (1500/m^3)	70	106	—	—
Platelets (100,000/m^3)	22	36	—	—

NR = Not reached by Kaplan-Meier method; ANC = Absolute neutrophil count.
[a] Evaluable patients
[b] Patients either refractory to, or intolerant of IFN
[c] Kaplan-Meier estimate

neutropenia has been observed following the early courses of treatment with Pentostatin and therefore frequent monitoring of complete blood counts is recommended during this time. If hematologic parameters do not improve with subsequent courses, patients should be evaluated for disease status, including a bone marrow examination. Periodic monitoring of the peripheral blood for hairy cells should be performed to assess the response to treatment.

In addition, bone marrow aspirates and biopsies may be required at 2 to 3 month intervals to assess the response to treatment.

DRUG INTERACTIONS
Allopurinol and Pentostatin are both associated with skin rashes. Based on clinical studies in 25 refractory patients who received both Pentostatin and allopurinol, the combined use of Pentostatin and allopurinol did not appear to produce a higher incidence of skin rashes than observed with Pentostatin alone. There has been a report of one patient who received both drugs and experienced a hypersensitivity vasculitis that resulted in death. It was unclear whether this adverse event and subsequent death resulted from the drug combination.

Biochemical studies have demonstrated that Pentostatin enhances the effects of vidarabine, a purine nucleoside with antiviral activity. The combined use of vidarabine and Pentostatin may result in an increase in adverse reactions associated with each drug. The therapeutic benefit of the drug combination has not been established.

The combined use of Pentostatin and fludarabine phosphate is not recommended because it may be associated with an increased risk of fatal pulmonary toxicity (see "Warnings").

CARCINOGENESIS, MUTAGENESIS, IMPAIRMENT OF FERTILITY
Carcinogenesis: No animal carcinogenicity studies have been conducted with Pentostatin.

Mutagenesis: Pentostatin was nonmutagenic when tested in *Salmonella typhimurium* strains TA-98, TA-1535, TA-1537, and TA-1538. When tested with strain TA-100, a repeatable statistically significant response trend was observed with and without metabolic activation. The response was 2.1 to 2.2 fold higher than the background at 10 mg/plate, the maximum possible drug concentration. Formulated Pentostatin was clastogenic in the *in vivo* mouse bone marrow micronucleus assay at 20, 120, and 240 mg/kg. Pentostatin was not mutagenic to V79 Chinese hamster lung cells at the HGPRT locus exposed 3 hours to concentrations of 1 to 3 mg/mL with or without metabolic activation. Pentostatin did not significantly increase chromosomal aberrations in V79 Chinese hamster lung cells exposed 3 hours to 1 to 3 mg/mL in the presence or absence of metabolic activation.

Impairment of Fertility: No fertility studies have been conducted in animals; however, in a 5-day intravenous toxicity study in dogs, mild seminiferous tubular degeneration was observed with doses of 1 and 4 mg/kg. The possible adverse effects on fertility in humans have not been determined.

PREGNANCY
Pregnancy Category D: See "Warnings"

NURSING MOTHERS
It is not known whether Pentostatin is excreted in human milk. Because many drugs are excreted in human milk, and because of the potential for serious adverse reactions in nursing infants from Pentostatin, a decision should be made whether to discontinue nursing or discontinue the drug, taking into account the importance of Pentostatin to the mother.

PEDIATRIC USE
Safety and effectiveness in children or adolescents have not been established.

ADVERSE REACTIONS
Most patients treated for hairy cell leukemia in the five NCI-sponsored Phase 2 studies and the Phase 3 SWOG study experienced an adverse event. The following table lists the most frequently occurring adverse events in patients treated with Pentostatin (both frontline and IFN-refractory patients) compared with IFN (frontline only), regardless of drug association. The drug association of some adverse events is uncertain as they may be associated with the disease itself (eg, infection, hematologic suppression), but other events, such as the gastrointestinal symptoms, rashes, and abnormal liver function tests, can in many cases be attributed to the drug. Most adverse events that were assessed for severity were either mild or moderate, and diminished in frequency with continued therapy.

	Percent of Patients		
All Adverse Events[a]	Frontline, Treated With Pentostatin N = 180	Frontline, Treated With IFN N = 176	IFN-Refractory, Treated With Pentostatin N = 197
Nausea and/or Vomiting	63	22	53[b]
Fever	46	59	42
Rash	43	30	26
Fatigue	42	55	29
Leukopenia	22	15	60
Pruritus	21	6	10
Coughing/Increased Cough	20	15	17
Myalgia	19	36	11
Chills	19	34	11
Headache	17	29	13
Diarrhea	17	17	15
Abdominal Pain	16	15	4
Anoxeria	13	10	16
Upper Respiratory Infection	13	8	16
Asthenia	12	13	10
Stomatitis	12	7	5
Rhinitis	11	15	10
Dyspnea	11	13	8
Anemia	8	5	35
Pain	8	19	20
Pharyngitis	8	11	10
Sweating Increased/Sweating	8	21	10
Viral Infection	8	17	NR
Infection	7[c]	2[c]	36
Arthralgia	6	14	3
Thrombocytopenia	6	6	32
Skin Disorder	4	5	17
Allergic Reaction	2	1	11

All Adverse Events[a]	Percent of Patients		
	Frontline, Treated With Pentostatin N = 180	Frontline, Treated With IFN N = 176	IFN-Refractory, Treated With Pentostatin N = 197
Hepatic Disorder/Elevated Liver Function Tests[d]	2	2	19
Neurologic Disorder, CNS/ CNS Toxicity	1	NR	11
Lung Disorder/Disease	NR	1	12
Nausea	NR	NR	22
Genitourinary Disorder	NR	NR	15

NR = Not Reported.
[a] Occurring in more than 10% of patients, in any group, regardless of drug association.
[b] Includes only nausea with vomiting.
[c] These figures represent only unspecified infections. Refer to Infection table.
[d] Elevated liver enzymes and liver disorder for SWOG

The total incidence for all types of infections is considerably higher for both treatment groups in the SWOG 8691 study than is listed in the table above. An intent-to-treat analysis of infections found that 38% of patients treated with Pentostatin and 34% of patients treated with IFN averaged 2.4 and 1.9 documented infections during treatment, respectively, The following table lists the different types of infections that were reported as adverse events during the initial phase of the SWOG study.

There were no apparent differences in the types of infection between the 2 treatment groups, with the possible exception of herpes, zoster which was reported more frequently for Pentostatin (8%) than for IFN (1%).

Type of Infection	Percent of Patients	
	Frontline, Treated With Pentostatin N = 180	Frontline, Treated With IFN N = 176
Upper Respiratory Infection	13	8
Rhinitis	11	15
Herpes Zoster	8	1
Pharyngitis	8	11
Viral Infection	8	17
Infection (Unspecified)	7	6
Sinusitis	6	4
Cellulitis	6	4
Bacterial Infection	6	4
Pneumonia	5	7
Conjunctivitis	4	2
Furunculosis	4	<1
Herpes Simplex	4	1
Bronchitis	3	2
Sepsis	3	2
Urinary Tract Infection	3	3
Abscess, Skin	2	4
Moniliasis, Oral	2	<1
Mycotic Infection, Skin	<1	3
Osteomyelitis	1	0

The drug relatedness of the adverse events listed below cannot be excluded. The following adverse events occurred in 3% to 10% of Pentostatin-treated patients in the initial phase of the SWOG study.

Body as a Whole: Chest Pain, Death, Face Edema, Peripheral Edema

Cardiovascular System: Hemorrhage, Hypotension

Digestive System: Dental Abnormalities, Dyspepsia, Flatulence, Gingivitis

Hemic and Lymphatic System: Agranulocytosis

Laboratory Deviations: Elevated Creatinine

Musculoskeletal System: Arthralgia

Nervous System: Confusion, Dizziness, Insomnia, Paresthesia, Somnolence

Psychobiologic Function: Anxiety, Depression, Nervousness

Respiratory System: Asthma

Skin & Appendages: Skin Dry, Urticaria

The remaining adverse events which occurred in less than 3% of Pentostatin treated patients during the initial phase of the SWOG study:

Body as a Whole: Flu-like Symptoms, Hangover Effect, Neoplasm

Cardiovascular System: Angina Pectoris, Arrhythmia, A-V Block, Bradycardia, Extrasystoles Ventricular, Heart Arrest, Heart Failure, Hypertension, Pericardial Effusion, Phlebitis, Pulmonary Embolus, Sinus Arrest, Tachycardia, Thrombophlebitis Deep, Vasculitis

Digestive System: Constipation, Dysphagia, Glossitis, Ileus

Hemic and Lymphatic System: Acute Leukemia, Anemia-Hemolytic, Aplastic Anemia

Laboratory Deviations: Hypercalcemia, Hyponatremia

Musculoskeletal System: Arthritis, Gout

Nervous System: Amnesia, Ataxia, Convulsions, Dreaming Abnormal, Dysarthria, Encephalitis, Hyperkinesia, Meningism, Neuralgia, Neuritis, Neuropathy, Paralysis, Syncope, Twitching, Vertigo

Psychobiologic Function: Decrease/Loss Libido, Emotional Lability, Hallucination, Hostility, Neurosis, Thinking Abnormal

Respiratory System: Bronchospasm, Larynx Edema

Skin and Appendages: Acne, Alopecia, Eczema, Petechial Rash, Photosensitivity Reaction

Special Senses: Amblyopia, Deafness, Earache, Eyes Dry, Labyrinthitis, Lacrimation Disorder, Nonreactive Eye, Photophobia, Retinopathy, Tinnitus, Unusual Taste, Vision Abnormal, Watery Eyes

Urogenital System: Amenorrhea, Breast Lump, Impotence, Kidney Function Abnormal, Nephropathy, Renal Failure, Renal Insufficiency, Renal Stone

One patient with hairy cell leukemia treated with Pentostatin during another clinical study developed unilateral uveitis with vision loss.

Nineteen (5%) patients withdrew from the Phase 3 SWOG 8691 study because of adverse events: 9 during initial Pentostatin treatment, 4 during Pentostatin crossover, 5 during initial IFN treatment, and 1 during both initial IFN treatment and Pentostatin crossover. In the Phase 2 studies in IFN-refractory hairy cell leukemia, 11% of patients withdrew from treatment with Pentostatin due to an adverse event.

OVERDOSAGE
No specific antidote for Pentostatin overdose is known. Pentostatin administered at higher doses (20-50 mg/m^2 in divided doses over 5 days) than recommended was associated with deaths due to severe renal, hepatic, pulmonary, and CNS toxicity. In case of overdose, management would include general supportive measures through any period of toxicity that occurs.

DOSAGE AND ADMINISTRATION
It is recommended that patients receive hydration with 500 to 1,000 mL of 5% Dextrose in 0.5 Normal Saline or equivalent before Pentostatin administration. An additional 500 mL of 5% Dextrose or equivalent should be administered after Pentostatin is given.

The recommended dosage of Pentostatin for the treatment of hairy cell leukemia is 4 mg/m^2 every other week. Pentostatin may be administered intravenously by bolus injection or diluted in a larger volume and given over 20 to 30 minutes. (See *"Preparation of Intravenous Solution"*.)

Higher doses are not recommended.

No extravasation injuries were reported in clinical studies. The optimal duration of treatment has not been determined. In the absence of major toxicity and with observed continuing improvement, the patient should be treated until a complete response has been achieved. Although not established as required, the administration of two additional doses has been recommended following the achievement of a complete response.

All patients receiving Pentostatin at 6 months should be assessed for response to treatment. If the patient has not achieved a complete or partial response, treatment with Pentostatin should be discontinued.

If the patient has achieved a partial response, Pentostatin treatment should be continued in an effort to achieve a complete response. At any time thereafter that a complete response is achieved, two additional doses of Pentostatin are recommended. Pentostatin treatment should then be stopped. If the best response to treatment at the end of 12 months is a partial response, it is recommended that treatment with Pentostatin be stopped.

Withholding or discontinuation of individual doses may be needed when severe adverse reactions occur. Drug treatment should be withheld in patients with severe rash, and withheld or discontinued in patients showing evidence of nervous system toxicity.

Pentostatin treatment should be withheld in patients with active infection occurring during the treatment but may be resumed when the infection is controlled.

Patients who have elevated serum creatinine should have their dose withheld and a creatinine clearance determined. There are insufficient data to recommend a starting or a subsequent dose for patients with impaired renal function (creatinine clearance < 60 mL/min).

Patients with impaired renal function should be treated only when the potential benefit justifies the potential risk. Two patients with impaired renal function (creatinine clearances 50 to 60 mL/min) achieved complete response without unusual adverse events when treated with 2 mg/m^2.

No dosage reduction is recommended at the start of therapy with Pentostatin in patients with anemia, neutropenia, or thrombocytopenia. In addition, dosage reductions are not recommended during treatment in patients with anemia and thrombocytopenia if patients can be otherwise supported hematologically. Pentostatin should be temporarily withheld if the absolute neutrophil count falls during treatment below 200 cells/mm^3 in a patient who had an initial neutrophil count greater than 500 cells/mm^3 and may be resumed when the count returns to predose levels.

PREPARATION OF INTRAVENOUS SOLUTION

1. Procedures for proper handling and disposal of anticancer drugs should be followed. Several guidelines on this subject have been published.[2-7] There is no general agreement that all of the procedures recommended in the guidelines are necessary or appropriate. Spills and wastes should be treated with a 5% sodium hypochlorite solution prior to disposal.
2. Protective clothing including polyethylene gloves must be worn.
3. Transfer 5 mL of Sterile Water for Injection USP to the vial containing Pentostatin and mix thoroughly to obtain complete dissolution of a solution yielding 2 mg/mL. Parenteral drug products should be inspected visually for particulate matter and discoloration prior to administration.
4. Pentostatin may be given intravenously by bolus injection or diluted in a larger volume (25 to 50 mL) with 5% Dextrose Injection USP or 0.9% Sodium Chloride Injection USP. Dilution of the entire contents of a reconstituted vial with 25 mL or 50 mL provides a Pentostatin concentration of 0.33 mg/mL or 0.18 mg/mL, respectively, for the diluted solutions.
5. Pentostatin solution when diluted for infusion with 5% Dextrose Injection USP or 0.9% Sodium Chloride Injection USP does not interact with PVC infusion containers or administration sets at concentrations of 0.18 mg/mL to 0.33 mg/mL.

STABILITY
Pentostatin vials are stable at refrigerated storage temperature 2° to 8°C (36° to 46°F) for the period stated on the package. Vials reconstituted or reconstituted and further diluted as directed may be stored at room temperature and ambient light but should be used within 8 hours because Pentostatin contains no preservatives.

STORAGE
Store Pentostatin vials under refrigerated storage conditions 2° to 8° C (36° to 46°F).

REFERENCES
1. Malspeis L. et. al. Clinical Pharmacokinetics of 2'-Deoxycoformycin. Cancer Treatment Symposia 2:7-15, 1984. 2. Recommendations for the safe handling of parenteral antineoplastic drugs. NIH publication 83-2621. For sale by the Superintendent of Documents. US Government Printing Office, Washington, DC 20402. 3. AMA council report. Guidelines for handling parenteral antineoplastics. JAMA 25:590-2, 1985. 4. National Study Commission on Cytotoxic Exposure—Recommendations for handling cytotoxic agents. Director of Pharmacy Services, Rhode Island Hospital, 593 Eddy Street, Providence, RI 02902. 5. Clinical Oncological Society of Australia: Guidelines and recommendations for safe handling of antineoplastic agents. Med J Australia 1:426-8, 1983. 6. Jones RB, et. al. Safe handling of chemotherapeutic agents: A report from the Mount Sinai Medical Center, CA: A Cancer Journal for Clinicians 33:258-63, 1983. 7. American Society of Hospital Pharmacists technical assistance bulletin on handling cytotoxic and hazardous drugs. Am J Hosp Pharm 47:1033-49, 1990.

J CODES
Per 10 mg IV—J9268

HOW SUPPLIED
POWDER FOR INJECTION: 10 MG

BRAND/MANUFACTURER	NDC	SIZE	AWP
○ BRAND			
NIPENT: Parke-Davis	00071-4243-01	1s	$1440.00

Pentothal *SEE* THIOPENTAL SODIUM

Pentoxifylline

DESCRIPTION
Pentoxifylline tablets contain 400 mg Pentoxifylline. Pentoxifylline is a trisubstituted xanthine derivative designated chemically as 1-(5-oxohexyl)-3, 7-dimethylxanthine that, unlike theophylline, is a hemorheologic agent, i.e. an agent that affects blood viscosity. Pentoxifylline is soluble in water and ethanol, and sparingly soluble in toluene. The CAS Registry Number is 6493-05-6.

Following is its chemical structure:

CLINICAL PHARMACOLOGY
MODE OF ACTION
Pentoxifylline and its metabolites improve the flow properties of blood by decreasing its viscosity. In patients with chronic peripheral arterial disease, this increases blood flow to the affected microcirculation and enhances tissue oxygenation. The precise mode of action of pentoxifylline and the sequence of events leading to clinical improvement are still to be defined. Pentoxifylline administration has been shown to produce dose related hemorheologic effects, lowering blood viscosity, and improving erythrocyte flexibility. Leukocyte properties of hemorheologic importance have been modified in animal and in vitro human studies. Pentoxifylline has been shown to increase leukocyte deformability and to inhibit neutrophil adhesion and activation. Tissue oxygen levels have been shown to be significantly increased by therapeutic doses of Pentoxifylline in patients with peripheral arterial disease.

PHARMACOKINETICS AND METABOLISM
After oral administration in aqueous solution Pentoxifylline is almost completely absorbed. It undergoes a first pass effect and the various metabolites appear in plasma very soon after dosing. Peak plasma levels of the parent compound and its metabolites are reached within 1 hour. The major metabolites are Metabolite 1 (1-[5-hydroxyhexyl]-3,7-dimethylxanthine) and Metabolite V (1-[3-carboxypropyl]-3, 7-dimethylxanthine), and plasma levels of these metabolites are 5 and 8 times greater, respectively, than Pentoxifylline.

Following oral administration of aqueous solutions containing 100 to 400 mg of Pentoxifylline, the pharmacokinetics of the parent compound and Metabolite I are dose-related and not proportional (non-linear), with half-life and area under the blood-level time curve (AUC) increasing with dose. The elimination kinetics of Metabolite V are not dose-dependent. The apparent plasma half-life of Pentoxifylline varies from 0.4 to 0.8 hours and the apparent plasma half-lives of its metabolites vary from 1 to 1.6 hours. There is no evidence of accumulation or enzyme induction (Cytochrome P_{450}) following multiple oral doses.

Excretion is almost totally urinary; the main biotransformation product is Metabolite V. Essentially no parent drug is found in the urine. Despite large variations in plasma levels of parent compound and its metabolites, the urinary recovery of Metabolite V is consistent and shows dose proportionality. Less than 4% of the administered dose is recovered in feces. Food intake shortly before dosing delays absorption of an immediate release dosage form but does not affect total absorption. The pharmacokinetics and metabolism of Pentoxifylline have not been studied in patients with renal and/or hepatic dysfunction, but AUC was increased and elimination rate decreased in an older population (60-68 years) compared to younger individuals (22-30 years).

After administration of the 400 mg controlled-release Pentoxifylline tablet, plasma levels of the parent compound and its metabolites reach their maximum within 2 to 4 hours and remain constant over an extended period of time. The controlled release of Pentoxifylline from the tablet eliminates peaks and troughs in plasma levels for improved gastrointestinal tolerance.

INDICATIONS AND USAGE
Pentoxifylline is indicated for the treatment of patients with intermittent claudication on the basis of chronic occlusive arterial disease of the limbs. Pentoxifylline can improve function and symptoms but is not intended to replace more definitive therapy, such as surgical bypass, or removal of arterial obstructions when treating peripheral vascular disease.

UNLABELED USES
Pentoxifylline is used alone or as an adjunct in the treatment of human immunodeficiency virus infections, to improve cerebral blood flow in patients with cerebrovascular accidents and cerebrovascular disease. It is also used in patients with primary dementia (senile dementia and multi-infarct dementia), transient ischemic attacks, chronic obstructive pulmonary disease, diabetic atherosclerosis, and peripheral diabetic neuropathy. Pentoxifylline is also prescribed to reduce the incidence of arteriovenous shunt thrombosis, to treat vascular impotence, pityriasis lichenoides *et* varioliformis, Raynaud's syndrome, and to increase sperm motility in infertile men.

CONTRAINDICATIONS
Pentoxifylline should not be used in patients with recent cerebral and/or retinal hemorrhage or in patients who have previously exhibited intolerance to this product or methylxanthines such as caffeine theophylline, and theobromine.

PRECAUTIONS
General: Patients with chronic occlusive arterial disease of the limbs frequently show other manifestations of arteriosclerotic disease. Pentoxifylline has been used safely for treatment of peripheral arterial disease in patients with concurrent coronary artery and cerebrovascular diseases, but there have been occasional reports of angina, hypotension, and arrhythmia. Controlled trials do not show that Pentoxifylline causes such adverse effects more often than placebo, but, as it is a methylxanthine derivative, it is possible some individuals will experience such responses. Patients on Warfarin should have more frequent monitoring of prothrombin times, while patients with other risk factors complicated by hemorrhage (e.g. recent surgery, peptic ulceration, cerebral and/or retinal bleeding) should have periodic examinations for bleeding including hematocrit and/or hemoglobin.

Drug Interactions: Although a causal relationship has not been established, there have been reports of bleeding and/or prolonged prothrombin time in patients treated with Pentoxifylline with and without anticoagulants or platelet aggregation inhibitors. Patients on Warfarin should have more frequent monitoring of prothrombin times, while patients with other risk factors complicated by hemorrhage (e.g., recent surgery, peptic ulceration) should have periodic examinations for bleeding including hematocrit and/or hemoglobin. Pentoxifylline has been used concurrently with antihypertensive drugs, beta blockers, digitalis, diuretics, antidiabetic agents, and antiarrhythmics, without observed problems. Small decreases in blood pressure have been observed in some patients treated with Pentoxifylline; periodic systemic blood pressure monitoring is recommended for patients receiving concomitant antihypertensive therapy. If indicated, dosage of the antihypertensive agents should be reduced.

INCIDENCE (%) OF SIDE EFFECTS

	Controlled-Release Tablets Commercially Available		Immediate-Release Capsules Used only for Controlled Clinical Trials	
	Pentoxifylline	Placebo	Pentoxifylline	Placebo
(Numbers of Patients at Risk)	(321)	(128)	(177)	(138)
Discontinued for Side Effect	3.1	0	9.6	7.2
Cardiovascular System				
Angina/Chest pain	0.3	-	1.1	2.2
Arrhythmia/Palpitation	-	-	1.7	0.7
Flushing	-	-	2.3	0.7
Digestive System				
Abdominal Discomfort	-	-	4.0	1.4
Belching/Flatus/Bloating	0.6	-	9.0	3.6
Diarrhea	-	-	3.4	2.9
Dyspepsia	2.8	4.7	9.6	2.9
Nausea	2.2	0.8	28.8	8.7
Vomiting	1.2	-	4.5	0.7
Nervous System				
Agitation/Nervousness	-	-	1.7	0.7
Dizziness	1.9	3.1	11.9	4.3
Drowsiness	-	-	1.1	5.8
Headache	1.2	1.6	6.2	5.8
Insomnia	-	-	2.3	2.2
Tremor	0.3	0.8	-	-
Blurred Vision	-	-	2.3	1.4

Carcinogenesis, Mutagenesis and Impairment of Fertility: Long-term studies of the carcinogenic potential of Pentoxifylline were conducted in mice and rats by dietary administration of the drug at doses up to approximately 24 times (570 mg/kg) the maximum recommended human daily dose (MRHD) of 24 mg/kg for 18 months in mice and 18 months in rats with an additional 6 months without drug exposure in the latter. No carcinogenic potential for Pentoxifylline was noted in the mouse study. In the rat study, there was a statistically significant increase in benign mammary fibroadenomas in females in the high dose group (24 × MRHD). The relevance of this finding to human use is uncertain since this was only a marginal statistically significant increase for a tumor that is common in aged rats. Pentoxifylline was devoid of mutagenic activity in various strains of *Salmonella* (Ames test) when tested in the presence and absence of metabolic activation.

Pregnancy: Category C. Teratogenic studies have been performed in rats and rabbits at oral doses up to about 25 and 10 times the maximum recommended human daily dose (MRHD) of 24 mg/kg, respectively. No evidence of fetal malformation was observed. Increased resorption was seen in rats at 25 times MRHD. There are, however, no adequate and well controlled studies in pregnant women. Because animal reproduction studies are not always predictive of human response. Pentoxifylline should be used during pregnancy only if clearly needed.

Nursing Mothers: Pentoxifylline and its metabolites are excreted in human milk. Because of the potential for tumorigenicity shown for Pentoxifylline in rats, a decision should be made whether to discontinue nursing or discontinue the drug, taking into account the importance of the drug to the mother.

Pediatric Use: Safety and effectiveness in children below the age of 18 years have not been established.

ADVERSE REACTIONS
Clinical trials were conducted using either controlled-release Pentoxifylline tablets for up to 60 weeks or immediate release Pentoxifylline capsules for up to 24 weeks. Dosage ranges in the tablet studies were 400 mg bid to tid and in the capsule studies, 200-400 mg tid.

The table summarizes the incidence (in percent) of adverse reactions considered drug related, as well as the numbers of patients who received controlled-release Pentoxifylline tablets, immediate-release Pentoxifylline capsules, or the corresponding placebos. The incidence of adverse reactions was higher in the capsule studies (where dose related increases were seen in digestive and nervous system side effects) than in the tablet studies. Studies with the capsule include domestic experience, whereas studies with the controlled-release tablets were conducted outside the U.S. The table indicates that in the tablet studies few patients discontinued because of adverse effects. (See related table).

Pentoxifylline has been marketed in Europe and elsewhere since 1972. In addition to the above symptoms, the following have been reported spontaneously since marketing or occurred in other clinical trials with an incidence of less than 1%; the causal relationship was uncertain:

Cardiovascular: dyspnea, edema, hypotension.

Digestive: anorexia, cholecystitis, constipation, dry mouth/thirst.

Nervous: anxiety, confusion, depression, seizure.

Respiratory: epistaxis, flu-like symptoms, laryngitis, nasal congestion.

Skin and Appendages: brittle fingernails, pruritus, rash, urticaria, angiodema.

Special Senses: blurred vision, conjunctivitis, earache, scotoma.

Miscellaneous: bad taste, excessive salivation, leukopenia, malaise, sore throat/swollen neck glands, weight change.

A few rare events have been reported spontaneously worldwide since marketing in 1972. Although they occurred under circumstances in which a causal relationship with Pentoxifylline could not be established, they are listed to serve as information for physicians: "Cardiovascular-angina, arrhythmia, tachycardia anaphylactoid reactions."

Digestive: hepatitis, jaundice, increased liver enzymes; and

Hemic and Lymphatic: decreased serum fibrinogen, pancytopenia, aplastic anemia, leukemia, purpura, thrombocytopenia.

OVERDOSAGE
Overdosage with Pentoxifylline has been reported in children and adults. Symptoms appear to be dose related. A report from a poison control center on 44 patients taking overdoses of enteric-coated Pentoxifylline tablets noted that symptoms usually occurred 4-5 hours after ingestion and lasted about 12 hours. The highest amount ingested was 80 mg/kg; flushing, hypotension, convulsions, somnolence, loss of consciousness, fever, and agitation occurred. All patients recovered.

In addition to symptomatic treatment and gastric lavage, special attention must be given to supporting respiration, maintaining systemic blood pressure, and controlling convulsions. Activated charcoal has been used to absorb Pentoxifylline in patients who have overdosed.

DOSAGE AND ADMINISTRATION
The usual dosage Pentoxifylline in controlled-release tablet form is one tablet (400 mg) three times a day with meals.

While the effect of Pentoxifylline may be seen within 2 to 4 weeks, it is recommended that treatment be continued for at least 8 weeks. Efficacy has been demonstrated in double-blind clinical studies of 6 months duration. Digestive and central nervous system side effects are dose related. If patients develop these side effects it is recommended that the dosage be lowered to one tablet twice a day (800 mg/day). If side effects persist at this lower dosage, the administration of Pentoxifylline should be discontinued.

Store at controlled room temperature (59° - 86°F).

Dispense in well closed, light resistant containers.

HOW SUPPLIED
TABLET, EXTENDED RELEASE: 400 MG

BRAND/MANUFACTURER	NDC	SIZE	AWP
○ BRAND			
▶ TRENTAL: Hoechst	00039-0078-10	100s	$53.40
	00039-0078-11	100s ud	$55.75

Pepcid *SEE* FAMOTIDINE

Peptavlon *SEE* PENTAGASTRIN

Percocet *SEE* ACETAMINOPHEN AND OXYCODONE HYDROCHLORIDE

◆ RATED THERAPEUTICALLY EQUIVALENT; ◇ THERAPEUTIC EQUIVALENCE UNCONFIRMED; ○ UNRATED

Percodan SEE ASPIRIN/OXYCODONE HYDROCHLORIDE/ OXYCODONE TEREPHTHALATE

Perfect Choice SEE STANNOUS FLUORIDE

Pergolide Mesylate

DESCRIPTION

Pergolide Mesylate is an ergot derivative dopamine receptor agonist at both D_1 and D_2 receptor sites. Pergolide Mesylate is chemically designated as 8β-[(Methylthio)methyl-6-propylergoline monomethanesulfonate.

The formula weight of the base is 314.5; 1 mg of base corresponds to 3.18 μmol.

Pergolide Mesylate is provided for oral administration in tablets containing 0.05 mg (0.159 μmol), 0.25 mg (0.795 μmol), or 1 mg (3.18 μmol) Pergolide as the base.

Following is its chemical structure:

CLINICAL PHARMACOLOGY

Pharmacodynamic Information: Pergolide Mesylate is a potent dopamine receptor agonist. Pergolide is 10 to 1,000 times more potent than bromocriptine on a milligram per milligram basis in various *in vitro* and *in vivo* test systems. Pergolide Mesylate inhibits the secretion of prolactin in humans; it causes a transient rise in serum concentrations of growth hormone and a decrease in serum concentrations of luteinizing hormone. In Parkinson's disease, Pergolide Mesylate is believed to exert its therapeutic effect by directly stimulating postsynaptic dopamine receptors in the nigrostriatal system.

Pharmacokinetic Information (Absorption, Distribution, Metabolism, and Elimination): Information on oral systemic bioavailability of Pergolide Mesylate is unavailable because of the lack of a sufficiently sensitive assay to detect the drug after the administration of a single dose. However, following oral administration of ^{14}C radiolabeled Pergolide Mesylate, approximately 55% of the administered radioactivity can be recovered from the urine and 5% from expired CO_2, suggesting that a significant fraction is absorbed. Nothing can be concluded about the extent of presystemic clearance, if any. Data on postabsorption distribution of Pergolide are unavailable.

At least 10 metabolites have been detected, including N-despropylpergolide, Pergolide sulfoxide, and Pergolide sulfone. Pergolide sulfoxide and Pergolide sulfone are dopamine agonists in animals. The other detected metabolites have not been identified, and it is not known whether any other metabolites are active pharmacologically.

The major route of excretion is the kidney.

Pergolide is approximately 90% bound to plasma proteins. This extent of protein binding may be important to consider when Pergolide Mesylate is coadministered with other drugs known to affect protein binding.

INDICATIONS AND USAGE

Pergolide Mesylate is indicated as adjunctive treatment to levodopa/carbidopa in the management of the signs and symptoms of Parkinson's disease.

Evidence to support the efficacy of Pergolide Mesylate as an antiparkinsonian adjunct was obtained in a multicenter study enrolling 376 patients with mild to moderate Parkinson's disease who were intolerant to *l*-dopa/carbidopa as manifested by moderate to severe dyskinesia and/or on-off phenomena. On average, the patients evaluated had been on *l*-dopa/carbidopa for 3.9 years (range, 2 days to 16.8 years).

The administration of Pergolide Mesylate permitted a 5% to 30% reduction in the daily dose of *l*-dopa. On average these patients treated with Pergolide Mesylate maintained an equivalent or better clinical status than they exhibited at baseline.

UNLABELED USES

Pergolide Mesylate is used alone or as an adjunct in the treatment of cocaine withdrawal, acromegaly, hyperprolactinemia, and in progressive supranuclear palsy.

CONTRAINDICATIONS

Pergolide Mesylate is contraindicated in patients who are hypersensitive to this drug or other ergot derivatives.

WARNINGS

Symptomatic Hypotension: In clinical trials, approximately 10% of patients taking Pergolide Mesylate with *l*-dopa versus 7% taking placebo with *l*-dopa experienced symptomatic orthostatic and/or sustained hypotension, especially during initial treatment. With gradual dosage titration, tolerance to the hypotension usually develops. It is therefore important to warn patients of the risk, to begin therapy with low doses, and to increase the dosage in carefully adjusted increments over a period of 3 to 4 weeks (see *"Dosage and Administration"*).

Hallucinosis: In controlled trials, Pergolide Mesylate with *l*-dopa caused hallucinosis in about 14% of patients as opposed to 3% taking placebo with *l*-dopa. This was of sufficient severity to cause discontinuation of treatment in about 3% of those enrolled; tolerance to this untoward effect was not observed.

Fatalities: In the placebo-controlled trial, 2 of 187 patients treated with placebo died as compared with 1 of 189 patients treated with Pergolide Mesylate. Of the 2.299 patients treated with Pergolide Mesylate in premarketing studies evaluated as of October 1988, 143 died while on the drug or shortly after discontinuing it. Because the patient population under evaluation was elderly, ill, and at high risk for death, it seems unlikely that Pergolide Mesylate played any role in these deaths, but the possibility that Pergolide shortens survival of patients cannot be excluded with absolute certainty.

In particular, a case-by-case review of the clinical course of the patients who died failed to disclose any unique set of signs, symptoms, or laboratory results that would suggest that treatment with Pergolide caused their deaths. Sixty-eight percent (68%) of the patients who died were 65 years of age or older. No death (other than a suicide) occurred within the first month of treatment; most of the patients who died had been on Pergolide for years. A relative frequency of the causes of death by organ system are: Pulmonary failure/Pneumonia, 35%; Cardiovascular, 30%; Cancer, 11%; Unknown, 8.4%; Infection, 3.5%; Extrapyramidal syndrome, 3.5%; Stroke, 2.1%; Dysphagia, 2.1%; Injury, 1.4%; Suicide, 1.4%; Dehydration, 0.7%; Glomerulonephritis, 0.7%.

PRECAUTIONS

General: Caution should be exercised when administering Pergolide Mesylate to patients prone to cardiac dysrhythmias.

In a study comparing Pergolide Mesylate and placebo, patients taking Pergolide Mesylate were found to have significantly more episodes of atrial premature contractions (APCs) and sinus tachycardia.

The use of Pergolide Mesylate in patients on *l*-dopa may cause and/or exacerbate preexisting states of confusion and hallucinations (see *"Warnings"*) and preexisting dyskinesia. Also, the abrupt discontinuation of Pergolide Mesylate in patients receiving it chronically as an adjunct to *l*-dopa may precipitate the onset of hallucinations and confusion; these may occur within a span of several days. Discontinuation of Pergolide should be undertaken gradually whenever possible, even if the patient is to remain on *l*-dopa.

Information for Patients: Patients and their families should be informed of the common adverse consequences of the use of Pergolide Mesylate (see *"Adverse Reations"*) and the risk of hypotension (see *"Warnings"*).

Patients should be advised to notify their physician if they become pregnant or intend to become pregnant during therapy.

Patients should be advised to notify their physician if they are breast-feeding an infant.

Laboratory Tests: No specific laboratory tests are deemed essential for the management of patients on Pergolide Mesylate. Periodic routine evaluation of all patients, however, is appropriate.

Drug Interactions: Dopamine antagonists, such as the neuroleptics (phenothiazines, butyrophenones, thioxanthines) or metoclopramide, ordinarily should not be administered concurrently with Pergolide Mesylate (a dopamine agonist); these agents may diminish the effectiveness of Pergolide Mesylate.

Because Pergolide Mesylate is approximately 90% bound to plasma proteins, caution should be exercised if Pergolide Mesylate is coadministered with other drugs known to affect protein binding.

Carcinogenesis, Mutagenesis, and Impairment of Fertility: A 2-year carcinogenicity study was conducted in mice using dietary levels of Pergolide Mesylate equivalent to oral doses of 0.6, 3.7, and 36.4 mg/kg/day in males and 0.6, 4.4, and 40.8 mg/kg/day in females. A 2-year study in rats was conducted using dietary levels equivalent to oral doses of 0.04, 0.18, and 0.88 mg/kg/day in males and 0.05, 0.28, and 1.42 mg/kg/day in females. The highest doses tested in the mice and rats were approximately 340 and 12 times the maximum human male dose administered in controlled clinical trials (6 mg/day equivalent to 0.12 mg/kg/day).

A low incidence of uterine neoplasms occurred in both rats and mice. Endometrial adenomas and carcinomas were observed in rats. Endometrial sarcomas were observed in mice. The occurrence of these neoplasms is probably attributable to the high estrogen/progesterone ratio that would occur in rodents as a result of the prolactin-inhibiting action of Pergolide Mesylate. The endocrine mechanisms believed to be involved in the rodents are not present in humans. However, even though there is no known correlation between uterine malignancies occurring in Pergolide-treated rodents and human risk, there are no human data to substantiate this conclusion.

Pergolide Mesylate was evaluated for mutagenic potential in a battery of tests that included an Ames bacterial mutation assay, a DNA repair assay in cultured rat hepatocytes, an *in vitro* mammalian cell-point-mutation assay in cultured L5178Y cells, and a determination of chromosome alteration in bone marrow cells of Chinese hamsters. A weak mutagenic response was noted in the mammalian cell-point-mutation assay only after metabolic activation with rat liver microsomes. No mutagenic effects were obtained in the 2 other *in vitro* assays and in the *in vivo* assay. The relevance of these findings in humans is unknown.

► SHOWN IN PRODUCT IDENTIFICATION GUIDE

A fertility study in male and female mice showed that fertility was maintained at 0.6 and 1.7 mg/kg/day but decreased at 5.6 mg/kg/day. Prolactin has been reported to be involved in stimulating and maintaining progesterone levels required for implantation in mice, and, therefore, the impaired fertility at the high dose may have occurred because of depressed prolactin levels.

Usage in Pregnancy: Pregnancy Category B: Reproduction studies were conducted in mice at doses of 5, 16, and 45 mg/kg/day and in rabbits at doses of 2, 6, and 16 mg/kg/day. The highest doses tested in mice and rabbits were 375 and 133 times the 6 mg/kg/day maximum human dose administered in controlled clinical trials. In these studies, there was no evidence of harm to the fetus due to Pergolide Mesylate.

There are, however, no adequate and well-controlled studies in pregnant women. Among women who received Pergolide Mesylate for endocrine disorders in premarketing studies, there were 33 pregnancies that resulted in healthy babies and 5 pregnancies that resulted in congenital abnormalities (2 major, 3 minor); a causal relationship has not been established. Because human data are limited and because animal reproduction studies are not always predictive of human response, this drug should be used during pregnancy only if clearly needed.

Nursing Mothers: It is not known whether this drug is excreted in human milk. The pharmacologic action of Pergolide Mesylate suggests that it may interfere with lactation. Because many drugs are excreted in human milk and because of the potential for serious adverse reactions to Pergolide Mesylate in nursing infants, a decision should be made whether to discontinue nursing or to discontinue the drug, taking into account the importance of the drug to the mother.

Pediatric Use: Safety and effectiveness in children have not been established.

ADVERSE REACTIONS

Commonly Observed: In premarketing clinical trials, the most commonly observed adverse events associated with use of Pergolide Mesylate which were not seen at an equivalent incidence among placebo-treated patients were: nervous system complaints, including dyskinesia, hallucinations, somnolence, insomnia; digestive complaints, including nausea, constipation, diarrhea, dyspepsia; and respiratory system complaints, including rhinitis.

Associated With Discontinuation of Treatment: Twenty-seven percent (27%) of approximately 1,200 patients receiving Pergolide Mesylate for treatment of Parkinson's disease in premarketing clinical trials in the US and Canada discontinued treatment due to adverse reactions. The events most commonly causing discontinuation were related to the nervous system (15.5%), primarily hallucinations (7.8%) and confusion (1.8%).

Fatalities: See "Warnings."

Incidence in Controlled Clinical Trials: The table that follows enumerates adverse events that occurred at a frequency of 1% or more among patients taking Pergolide Mesylate who participated in the premarketing controlled clinical trials comparing Pergolide Mesylate with placebo. In a double-blind, controlled study of 6 months' duration, patients with Parkinson's disease were continued on *l*-dopa/carbidopa and were randomly assigned to receive either Pergolide Mesylate or placebo as additional therapy.

The prescriber should be aware that these figures cannot be used to predict the incidence of side effects in the course of usual medical practice where patient characteristics and other factors differ from those which prevailed in the clinical trials. Similarly, the cited frequencies cannot be compared with figures obtained from other clinical investigations involving different treatments, uses, and investigators. The cited figures, however, do provide the prescribing physician with some basis for estimating the relative contribution of drug and nondrug factors to the side-effect incidence rate in the population studied.

INCIDENCE OF TREATMENT-EMERGENT ADVERSE EXPERIENCES IN THE PLACEBO-CONTROLLED CLINICAL TRIAL

Body System/ Adverse Event*	Percentage of Patients Reporting Events	
	Pergolide Mesylate N = 189	Placebo N = 187
Body as a Whole		
Pain	7.0	2.1
Abdominal pain	5.8	2.1
Injury, accident	5.8	7.0
Headache	5.3	6.4
Asthenia	4.2	4.8
Chest pain	3.7	2.1
Flu syndrome	3.2	2.1
Neck pain	2.7	1.6
Back pain	1.6	2.1
Surgical procedure	1.6	< 1
Chills	1.1	0
Face edema	1.1	0
Infection	1.1	< 1
Cardiovascular		
Postural hypotension	9.0	7.0
Vasodilatation	3.2	< 1
Palpitation	2.1	< 1
Hypotension	2.1	< 1
Syncope	2.1	1.1
Hypertension	1.6	1.1

Body System/ Adverse Event*	Percentage of Patients Reporting Events	
	Pergolide Mesylate N = 189	Placebo N = 187
Arrhythmia	1.1	< 1
Myocardial infarction	1.1	< 1
Digestive		
Nausea	24.3	12.8
Constipation	10.6	5.9
Diarrhea	6.4	2.7
Dyspepsia	6.4	2.1
Anorexia	4.8	2.7
Dry mouth	3.7	< 1
Vomiting	2.7	1.6
Hemic and Lymphatic		
Anemia	1.1	< 1
Metabolic and Nutritional		
Peripheral edema	7.4	4.3
Edema	1.6	0
Weight gain	1.6	0
Musculoskeletal		
Arthralgia	1.6	2.1
Bursitis	1.6	< 1
Myalgia	1.1	< 1
Twitching	1.1	0
Nervous System		
Dyskinesia	62.4	24.6
Dizziness	19.1	13.9
Hallucinations	13.8	3.2
Dystonia	11.6	8.0
Confusion	11.1	9.6
Somnolence	10.1	3.7
Insomnia	7.9	3.2
Anxiety	6.4	4.3
Tremor	4.2	7.5
Depression	3.2	5.4
Abnormal dreams	2.7	4.3
Personality disorder	2.1	< 1
Psychosis	2.1	0
Abnormal gait	1.6	1.6
Akathisia	1.6	< 1
Extrapyramidal syndrome	1.6	1.1
Incoordination	1.6	< 1
Paresthesia	1.6	3.2
Akinesia	1.1	1.1
Hypertonia	1.1	1.1
Neuralgia	1.1	< 1
Speech disorder	1.1	1.6
Respiratory System		
Rhinitis	12.2	5.4
Dyspnea	4.8	1.1
Epistaxis	1.6	< 1
Hiccup	1.1	0
Skin and Appendages		
Rash	3.2	2.1
Sweating	2.1	2.7
Special Senses		
Abnormal vision	5.8	5.4
Diplopia	2.1	0
Taste perversion	1.6	0
Eye disorder	1.1	0
Urogenital System		
Urinary frequency	2.7	6.4
Urinary tract infection	2.7	3.7
Hematuria	1.1	< 1

* *Events reported by at least 1% of patients receiving Pergolide Mesylate are included.*

Events Observed During the Premarketing Evaluation of Pergolide Mesylate: This section reports event frequencies evaluated as of October 1988 for adverse events occurring in a group of approximately 1,800 patients who took multiple doses of Pergolide Mesylate. The conditions and duration of exposure to Pergolide Mesylate varied greatly, involving well-controlled studies as well as experience in open and uncontrolled clinical settings. In the absence of appropriate controls in some of the studies, a causal relationship between these events and treatment with Pergolide Mesylate cannot be determined.

The following enumeration by organ system describes events in terms of their relative frequency of reporting in the data base. Events of major clinical importance are also described in the "Warnings" and "Precautions" sections.

The following definitions of frequency are used: frequent adverse events are defined as those occurring in at least 1/100 patients; infrequent adverse events are those occurring in 1/100 to 1/1,000 patients; rare events are those occurring in fewer than 1/1,000 patients.

Body as a Whole: Frequent: headache, asthenia, accidental injury, abdominal pain, chest pain, back pain, flu syndrome, neck pain, fever; *Infrequent*: facial edema, chills, enlarged abdomen, malaise, neoplasm, hernia, pelvic pain, sepsis, cellulitis, moniliasis, abscess, jaw pain, hypothermia; *Rare*: acute abdominal syndrome, LE syndrome

Cardiovascular System: Frequent: postural hypotension, syncope, hypertension, palpitations, vasodilatations, congestive heart failure; *Infrequent*: myocardial infarction, tachycardia, heart arrest, abnormal electrocardiogram, angina pectoris, thrombophlebitis, bradycardia, ventricular extrasystoles, cerebrovascular accident, ventricular tachycardia, cerebral ischemia, atrial fibrillation, varicose vein, pulmonary embolus, AV block, shock; *Rare*: vasculitis, pulmonary hypertension, pericarditis, migraine, heart block, cerebral hemorrhage

Digestive System: Frequent: nausea, vomiting, dyspepsia, diarrhea, constipation, dry mouth, dysphagia; *Infrequent*: flatulence, abnormal liver function tests, increased appetite, salivary gland enlargement, thirst, gastroenteritis, gastritis, periodontal abscess, intestinal obstruction, nausea and vomiting, gingivitis, esophagitis, cholelithiasis, tooth caries, hepatitis, stomach ulcer, melena, hepatomegaly, hematemesis, eructation; *Rare*: sialadenitis, peptic ulcer, pancreatitis, jaundice, glossitis, fecal incontinence, duodenitis, colitis, cholecystitis, aphthous stomatitis, esophageal ulcer

Endocrine System: Infrequent: hypothyroidism, adenoma, diabetes mellitus, ADH inappropriate; *Rare*: endocrine disorder, thyroid adenoma

Hemic and Lymphatic System: Frequent: anemia; *Infrequent*: leukopenia, lymphadenopathy, leukocytosis, thrombocytopenia, petechia, megaloblastic anemia, cyanosis; *Rare*: purpura, lymphocytosis, eosinophilia, thrombocythemia, acute lymphoblastic leukemia, polycythemia, splenomegaly

Metabolic and Nutritional System: Frequent: peripheral edema, weight loss, weight gain; *Infrequent*: dehydration, hypokalemia, hypoglycemia, iron deficiency anemia, hyperglycemia, gout, hypercholesteremia; *Rare*: electrolyte imbalance, cachexia, acidosis, hyperuricemia

Musculoskeletal System: Frequent: twitching, myalgia, arthralgia; *Infrequent*: bone pain, tenosynovitis, myositis, bone sarcoma, arthritis; *Rare*: osteoporosis, muscle atrophy, osteomyelitis

Nervous System: Frequent: dyskinesia, dizziness, hallucinations, confusion, somnolence, insomnia, dystonia, paresthesia, depression, anxiety, tremor, akinesia, extrapyramidal syndrome, abnormal gait, abnormal dreams, incoordination, psychosis, personality disorder, nervousness, choreoathetosis, amnesia, paranoid reaction, abnormal thinking; *Infrequent*: akathisia, neuropathy, neuralgia, hypertonia, delusions, convulsion, libido increased, euphoria, emotional lability, libido decreased, vertigo, myoclonus, coma, apathy, paralysis, neurosis, hyperkinesia, ataxia, acute brain syndrome, torticollis, meningitis, manic reaction, hypokinesia, hostility, agitation, hypotonia; *Rare*: stupor, neuritis, intracranial hypertension, hemiplegia, facial paralysis, brain edema, myelitis, hallucinations and confusion after abrupt discontinuation

Respiratory System: Frequent: rhinitis, dyspnea, pneumonia, pharyngitis, cough increased; *Infrequent*: epistaxis, hiccup, sinusitis, bronchitis, voice alteration, hemoptysis, asthma, lung edema, pleural effusion, laryngitis, emphysema, apnea, hyperventilation; *Rare*: pneumothorax, lung fibrosis, larynx edema, hypoxia hypoventilation, hemothorax, carcinoma of lung

Skin and Appendages System: Frequent: sweating, rash; *Infrequent*: skin discoloration, pruritus, acne, skin ulcer, alopecia, dry skin, skin carcinoma, seborrhea, hirsutism, herpes simplex, eczema, fungal dermatitis, herpes zoster; *Rare*: vesiculobullous rash, subcutaneous nodule, skin nodule, skin benign neoplasm, lichenoid dermatitis

Special Senses System: Frequent: diplopia; *Infrequent*: otitis media, conjunctivitis, tinnitus, deafness, taste perversion, ear pain, eye pain, glaucoma, eye hemorrhage, photophobia, visual field defect; *Rare*: blindness, cataract, retinal detachment, retinal vascular disorder

Urogenital System: Frequent: urinary tract infection, urinary frequency, urinary incontinence, hematuria, dysmenorrhea; *Infrequent*: dysuria, breast pain, menorrhagia, impotence, cystitis, urinary retention, abortion, vaginal hemorrhage, vaginitis, priapism, kidney calculus, fibrocystic breast, lactation, uterine hemorrhage, urolithiasis, salpingitis, pyuria, metrorrhagia, menopause, kidney failure, breast carcinoma, cervical carcinoma; *Rare*: amenorrhea, bladder carcinoma, breast engorgement, epididymitis, hypogonadism, leukorrhea, nephrosis, pyelonephritis, urethral pain, uricaciduria, withdrawal bleeding

OVERDOSAGE
There is no clinical experience with massive overdosage. The largest overdose involved a young hospitalized adult patient who was not being treated with Pergolide Mesylate but who intentionally took 60 mg of the drug. He experienced vomiting, hypotension, and agitation. Another patient receiving a daily dosage of 7 mg of Pergolide Mesylate unintentionally took 19 mg/day for 3 days, after which his vital signs were normal but he experienced severe hallucinations. Within 36 hours of resumption of the prescribed dosage level, the hallucinations stopped. One patient unintentionally took 14 mg/day for 23 days instead of her prescribed 1.4 mg/day dosage. She experienced severe involuntary movements and tingling in her arms and legs. Another patient who inadvertently received 7 mg instead of the prescribed 0.7 mg experienced palpitations, hypotension, and ventricular extrasystoles. The highest total daily dose (prescribed for several patients with refractory Parkinson's disease) has exceeded 30 mg.

Symptoms: Animal studies indicate that the manifestations of overdosage in man might include nausea, vomiting, convulsions, decreased blood pressure, and CNS stimulation. The oral median lethal doses in mice and rats were 54 and 15 mg/kg respectively.

Treatment: To obtain up-to-date information about the treatment of overdose, a good resource is your certified Regional Poison Control Center. Telephone numbers of certified poison control centers are listed in the *Physicians' Desk Reference (PDR)*. In managing overdosage, consider the possibility of multiple drug overdoses, interaction among drugs, and unusual drug kinetics in your patient.

Management of overdosage may require supportive measures to maintain arterial blood pressure. Cardiac function should be monitored; an antiarrhythmic agent may be necessary. If signs of CNS stimulation are present, a phenothiazine or other butyrophenone neuroleptic agent may be indicated; the efficacy of such drugs in reversing the effects of overdose has not been assessed.

Protect the patient's airway and support ventilation and perfusion. Meticulously monitor and maintain, within acceptable limits, the patient's vital signs, blood gases, serum electrolytes, etc. Absorption of drugs from the gastrointestinal tract may be decreased by giving activated charcoal, which, in many cases, is more effective than emesis or lavage; consider charcoal instead of or in addition to gastric emptying. Repeated doses of charcoal over time may hasten elimination of some drugs that have been absorbed. Safeguard the patient's airway when employing gastric emptying or charcoal.

There is no experience with dialysis or hemoperfusion, and these procedures are unlikely to be of benefit.

DOSAGE AND ADMINISTRATION
Administration of Pergolide Mesylate should be initiated with a daily dosage of 0.05 mg for the first 2 days. The dosage should then be gradually increased by 0.1 or 0.15 mg/day every third day over the next 12 days of therapy. The dosage may then be increased by 0.25 mg/day every third day until an optimal therapeutic dosage is achieved.

Pergolide Mesylate is usually administered in divided doses 3 times per day. During dosage titration, the dosage of concurrent *l*-dopa/carbidopa may be cautiously decreased.

In clinical studies, the mean therapeutic daily dosage of Pergolide Mesylate was 3 mg/day. The average concurrent daily dosage of *l*-dopa/carbidopa (expressed as *l*-dopa) was approximately 650 mg/day. The efficacy of Pergolide Mesylate at doses above 5 mg/day has not been systematically evaluated.

Store at controlled room temperature, 59° to 86°F (15° to 30°C).

HOW SUPPLIED
TABLETS: 0.05 MG

BRAND/MANUFACTURER	NDC	SIZE	AWP
BRAND			
PERMAX: Athena	59075-0615-30	30s	$11.04

TABLETS: 0.25 MG

BRAND/MANUFACTURER	NDC	SIZE	AWP
BRAND			
PERMAX: Athena	59075-0625-10	100s	$76.46

TABLETS: 1 MG

BRAND/MANUFACTURER	NDC	SIZE	AWP
BRAND			
PERMAX: Athena	59075-0630-10	100s	$253.86

Pergonal *SEE* MENOTROPINS

Periactin *SEE* CYPROHEPTADINE HYDROCHLORIDE

Peridex *SEE* CHLORHEXIDINE GLUCONATE

Periogard *SEE* CHLORHEXIDINE GLUCONATE

Permapen *SEE* PENICILLIN G BENZATHINE

Permax *SEE* PERGOLIDE MESYLATE

Permethrin

DESCRIPTION

Permethrin 5% Cream is a topical scabicidal agent for the treatment of infestation with *Sarcoptes scabiei* (scabies). It is available in an off-white, vanishing cream base. Permethrin Cream is for topical use only. Each gram contains Permethrin 50 mg (5%).

Chemical Name: The Permethrin used is an approximate 1:3 mixture of the cis and trans isomers of the pyrethroid (±)-3-phenoxybenzyl 3-(2,2-dichlorovinyl)-2,2-dimethylcyclopropanecarboxylate. Permethrin has a molecular formula of $C_{21}H_{20}Cl_2O_3$ and a molecular weight of 391.29. It is a yellow to light orange-brown, low melting solid or viscous liquid.

Following is its chemical structure:

CLINICAL PHARMACOLOGY

Permethrin, a pyrethroid, is active against a broad range of pests including lice, ticks, fleas, mites, and other arthropods. It acts on the nerve cell membrane to disrupt the sodium channel current by which the polarization of the membrane is regulated. Delayed repolarization and paralysis of the pests are the consequences of this disturbance.

Permethrin is rapidly metabolized by ester hydrolysis to inactive metabolites which are excreted primarily in the urine. Although the amount of Permethrin absorbed after a single application of the 5% cream has not been determined precisely, data from studies with ^{14}C-labeled Permethrin and absorption studies of the cream applied to patients with moderate to severe scabies indicate it is 2% or less of the amount applied.

INDICATIONS AND USAGE

Permethrin 5% Cream is indicated for the treatment of infestation with *Sarcoptes Scabiei* (scabies).

CONTRAINDICATIONS

Permethrin is contraindicated in patients with known hypersensitivity to any of its components, to any synthetic pyrethroid or pyrethrin.

WARNINGS

If hypersensitivity to Permethrin occurs, discontinue use.

PRECAUTIONS

General: Scabies infestation is often accompanied by pruritus, edema and erythema. Treatment with Permethrin may temporarily exacerbate these conditions.

Information for Patients: Patients with scabies should be advised that itching, mild burning and/or stinging may occur after application of Permethrin. In clinical trials approximately 75% of patients treated with Permethrin who continued to manifest pruritus at 2 weeks had cessation by 4 weeks. If irritation persists, they should consult their physician. Permethrin may be very mildly irritating to the eyes. Patients should be advised to avoid contact with eyes during application and to flush with water immediately if Permethrin gets in the eyes.

Carcinogenesis, Mutagenesis, Impairment of Fertility: Six carcinogenicity bioassays were evaluated with Permethrin, three each in rats and mice. No tumorigenicity was seen in the rat studies. However, species-specific increases in pulmonary adenomas, a common benign tumor of mice of high spontaneous background incidence, were seen in the three mouse studies. In one of these studies there was an increased incidence of pulmonary alveolar-cell carcinomas and benign liver adenomas only in female mice when Permethrin was given in their food at a concentration of 5000 ppm. Mutagenicity assays, which give useful correlative data for interpreting results from carcinogenicity bioassays in rodents, were negative. Permethrin showed no evidence of mutagenic potential in a battery of *in vitro* and *in vivo* genetic toxicity studies.

Permethrin did not have any adverse effect on reproductive function at a dose of 180 mg/kg/day orally in a three-generation rat study.

Pregnancy: Teratogenic Effects: Pregnancy Category B: Reproduction studies have been performed in mice, rats, and rabbits (200 to 400 mg/kg/day orally) and have revealed no evidence of impaired fertility or harm to the fetus due to Permethrin. There are, however, no adequate and well-controlled studies in pregnant women. Because animal reproduction studies are not always predictive of human response, this drug should be used during pregnancy only if clearly needed.

Nursing Mothers: It is not known whether this drug is excreted in human milk. Because many drugs are excreted in human milk and because of the evidence for tumorigenic potential of Permethrin in animal studies, consideration should be given to discontinuing nursing temporarily or withholding the drug while the mother is nursing.

Pediatric Use: Permethrin is safe and effective in children two months of age and older. Safety and effectiveness in children less than two months of age have not been established.

ADVERSE REACTIONS

In clinical trials, generally mild and transient burning and stinging followed application with Permethrin in 10% of patients and was associated with the severity of infestation. Pruritus was reported in 7% of patients at various times post-application. Erythema, numbness, tingling, and rash were reported in 1 to 2% or less of patients (see *"Precautions: General"*).

OVERDOSAGE

No instance of accidental ingestion of Permethrin has been reported. If ingested, gastric lavage and general supportive measures should be employed.

DOSAGE AND ADMINISTRATION

Adults and children: Thoroughly massage Permethrin into the skin from the head to the soles of the feet. Scabies rarely infests the scalp of adults, although the hairline, neck, temple, and forehead may be infested in infants and geriatric patients. Usually 30 grams is sufficient for an average adult. The cream should be removed by washing (shower or bath) after 8 to 14 hours. Infants should be treated on the scalp, temple and forehead. *One application is generally curative.*

Patients may experience persistent pruritus after treatment. This is rarely a sign of treatment failure and is not an indication for retreatment. Demonstrable living mites after 14 days indicate that retreatment is necessary.

Store at 15° to 25°C (59° to 77°F).

HOW SUPPLIED

CREAM: 5%

BRAND/MANUFACTURER	NDC	SIZE	AWP
○ **BRAND**			
ELIMITE: Allergan Herbert	00023-7915-60	60 gm	$16.36

Permitil *SEE* FLUPHENAZINE

Perphenazine

DESCRIPTION

Perphenazine, USP (4-[3-(2-chlorophenothiazin-10-yl)propyl]-1-piperazineethanol), is a piperazinyl phenothiazine having the chemical formula, $C_{21}H_{26}ClN_3OS$. They are available as *Tablets*, 2, 4, 8 and 16 mg; *Concentrate*, 16 mg Perphenazine per 5 mL and *Injection*, Perphenazine 5 mg per 1 mL.

Following is its chemical structure:

ACTIONS

Perphenazine has actions at all levels of the central nervous system, particularly the hypothalamus. However, the site and mechanism of action of therapeutic effect are not known.

INDICATIONS

Perphenazine is indicated for use in the management of the manifestations of psychotic disorders; and for the control of severe nausea and vomiting in adults.

Perphenazine has not been shown effective for the management of behavioral complications in patients with mental retardation.

CONTRAINDICATIONS

Perphenazine products are contraindicated in comatose or greatly obtunded patients and in patients receiving large doses of central nervous system depressants (barbiturates, alcohol, narcotics, analgesics, or antihistamines); in the presence of existing blood dyscrasias, bone marrow depression, or liver damage; and in patients who have shown hypersensitivity to Perphenazine products, their components, or related compounds.

Perphenazine products are also contraindicated in patients with suspected or established subcortical brain damage, with or without hypothalamic damage, since a hyperthermic reaction with temperatures in excess of 104°F may occur in such patients, sometimes not until 14 to 16 hours after drug administration. Total body ice-packing is recommended for such a reaction; antipyretics may also be useful.

WARNINGS

Tardive dyskinesia, a syndrome consisting of potentially irreversible, involuntary, dyskinetic movements, may develop in patients treated with neuroleptic (antipsychotic) drugs. Although the prevalence of the syndrome appears to be highest among the elderly, especially elderly women, it is impossible to rely upon prevalence estimates to predict, at the inception of neuroleptic treatment, which patients are likely to develop the syndrome. Whether neuroleptic drug products differ in their potential to cause tardive dyskinesia is unknown.

Both the risk of developing the syndrome and the likelihood that it will become irreversible are believed to increase as the duration of treatment and the total cumulative dose of neuroleptic drugs administered to the patient increase.

However, the syndrome can develop, although much less commonly, after relatively brief treatment periods at low doses. There is no known treatment for established cases of tardive dyskinesia, although the syndrome may remit, partially or completely, if neuroleptic treatment is withdrawn. Neuroleptic treatment itself, however, may suppress (or partially suppress) the signs and symptoms of the syndrome, and thereby may possibly mask the underlying disease process. The effect that symptomatic suppression has upon the long-term course of the syndrome is unknown.

Given these considerations, neuroleptics should be prescribed in a manner that is most likely to minimize the occurrence of tardive dyskinesia. Chronic neuroleptic treatment should generally be reserved for patients who suffer from a chronic illness that, 1) is known to respond to neuroleptic drugs, and 2) for whom alternative, equally effective, but potentially less harmful treatments are *not* available or appropriate. In patients who do require chronic treatment, the smallest dose and the shortest duration of treatment producing a satisfactory clinical response should be sought. The need for continued treatment should be reassessed periodically.

If signs and symptoms of tardive dyskinesia appear in a patient on neuroleptics, drug discontinuation should be considered. However, some patients may require treatment despite the presence of the syndrome.

(For further information about the description of tardive dyskinesia and its clinical detection, please refer to *"Information for Patients"* and *"Adverse Reactions".*)

Perphenazine Injection contains sodium bisulfite, a sulfite that may cause allergic-type reactions including anaphylactic symptoms and life-threatening or less severe asthmatic episodes in certain susceptible people. The overall prevalence of sulfite sensitivity is seen more frequently in asthmatic than in non-asthmatic people.

NEUROLEPTIC MALIGNANT SYNDROME (NMS)
A potentially fatal symptom complex sometimes referred to as Neuroleptic Malignant Syndrome (NMS) has been reported in association with antipsychotic drugs. Clinical manifestations of NMS are hyperpyrexia, muscle rigidity, altered mental status and evidence of autonomic instability (irregular pulse or blood pressure, tachycardia, diaphoresis, and cardiac dysrhythmias).

The diagnostic evaluation of patients with this syndrome is complicated. In arriving at a diagnosis, it is important to identify cases where the clinical presentation includes both serious medical illness (e.g., pneumonia, systemic infection, etc.) and untreated or inadequately treated extrapyramidal signs and symptoms (EPS). Other important considerations in the differential diagnosis include central anticholinergic toxicity, heat stroke, drug fever and primary central nervous system (CNS) pathology.

The management of NMS should include 1) immediate discontinuation of antipsychotic drugs and other drugs not essential to concurrent therapy, 2) intensive symptomatic treatment and medical monitoring, and 3) treatment of any concomitant serious medical problems for which specific treatments are available. There is no general agreement about specific pharmacological treatment regimens for uncomplicated NMS.

If a patient requires antipsychotic drug treatment after recovery from NMS, the potential reintroduction of drug therapy should be carefully considered. The patient should be carfully monitored, since recurrences of NMS have been reported.

If hypotension develops, epinephrine should not be administered since its action is blocked and partially reversed by Perphenazine. If a vasopressor is needed, norepinephrine may be used. Severe, acute hypotension has occurred with the use of phenothiazines and is particularly likely to occur in patients with mitral insufficiency or pheochromocytoma. Rebound hypertension may occur in pheochromocytoma patients.

Perphenazine products can lower the convulsive threshold in susceptible individuals; they should be used with caution in alcohol withdrawal and in patients with convulsive disorders. If the patients is being treated with an anticonvulsant agent, increased dosage of that agent may be required when Perphenazine products are used concomitantly.

Perphenazine products should be used with caution in patients with psychic depression.

Perphenzaine may impair the mental and/or physical abilities required for the performance of hazardous tasks such as driving a car or operating machinery; therefore, the patient should be warned accordingly.

Perphenazine products are not recommended for children under 12 years of age.

Usage in Pregnancy: Safe use of Perphenazine during pregnancy and lactation has not been established; therefore, in administering the drug to pregnant patients, nursing mothers, or women who may become pregnant, the possible benefits must be weighed against the possible hazards to mother and child.

PRECAUTIONS
The possibility of suicide in depressed patients remains during treatment and until significant remission occurs. This type of patient should not have access to large quantities of this drug.

As with all phenothiazine compounds, Perphenazine should not be used indiscriminately. Caution should be observed in giving it to patients who have previously exhibited severe adverse reactions to other phenothiazines. Some of the untoward actions of Perphenazine tend to appear more frequently when high doses are used. However, as with other phenothiazine compounds, patients receiving Perphenazine products in any dosage should be kept under close supervision.

Neuroleptic drugs elevate prolactin levels; the elevation persists during chronic administration. Tissue culture experiments indicate that approximately one-third of human breast cancers are prolactin dependent *in vitro*, a factor of potential importance if the prescription of these drugs is contemplated in a patient with a previously detected breast cancer. Although disturbances such as galactorrhea, amenorrhea, gynecomastia, and impotence have been reported, the clinical significance of elevated serum prolactin levels is unknown for most patients. An increase in mammary neoplasma has been found in rodents after chronic administration of neuroleptic drugs. Neither clinical studies nor epidemiologic studies conducted to date, however, have shown an association between chronic administration of these drugs and mammary tumorigenesis; the available evidence is considered too limited to be conclusive at this time.

The antiemetic effect of Perphenazine may obscure signs of toxicity due to overdosage or other drugs, or render more difficult the diagnosis of disorders such as brain tumors or intestinal obstruction.

A significant, not otherwise explained, rise in body temperature may suggest individual intolerance to Perphenazine, in which case it should be discontinued.

Patients on large doses of a phenothiazine drug who are undergoing surgery should be watched carefully for possible hypotensive phenomena. Moreover, reduced amounts of anesthetics or central nervous system depressants may be necessary.

Since phenothiazines and central nervous system depressants (opiates, analgesics, antihistamines, barbiturates) can potentiate each other, less than the usual dosage of the added drug is recommended, and caution is advised, when they are administered concomitantly.

Use with caution in patients who are receiving atropine or related drugs because of additive anticholinergic effects and also in patients who will be exposed to extreme heat or phosphorus insecticides.

The use of alcohol should be avoided, since additive effects and hypotension may occur. Patients should be cautioned that their response to alcohol may be increased while they are being treated with Perphenazine products. The risk of suicide and the danger of overdose may be increased in patients who use alcohol excessively due to its potentiation of the drug's effect.

Blood counts and hepatic and renal functions should be checked periodically. The appearance of signs of blood dyscrasias requires the discontinuance of the drug and institution of appropriate therapy. If abnormalities in hepatic tests occur, phenothiazine treatment should be discontinued. Renal function in patients on long-term therapy should be monitored; if blood urea nitrogen (BUN) becomes abnormal, treatment with the drug should be discontinued.

The use of phenothiazine derivatives in patients with diminished renal function should be undertaken with caution.

Use with caution in patients suffering from respiratory impairment due to acute pulmonary infections, or in chronic respiratory disorders such as severe asthma or emphysema. In general, phenothiazines, including Perphenazine, do not produce psychic dependence. Gastritis, nausea and vomiting, dizziness, and tremulousness have been reported following abrupt cessation of high-dose therapy. Reports suggest that these symptoms can be reduced by continuing concomitant antiparkinson agents for several weeks after the phenothiazine is withdrawn.

The possibility of liver damage, corneal and lenticular deposits, and irreversible dyskinesias should be kept in mind when patients are on long-term therapy.

Because photosensitivity has been reported, undue exposure to the sun should be avoided during phenothiazine treatment.

Information for Patients: This information is intended to aid in the safe and effective use of this medication. It is not a disclosure of all possible adverse or intended effects.

Given the likelihood that a substantial proportion of patients exposed chronically to neuroleptics will develop tardive dyskinesia, it is advised that all patients in whom chronic use is contemplated be given, if possible, full information about this risk. The decision to inform patients and/or their guardians must obviously take into account the clinical circumstances and the competency of the patient to understand the information provided.

ADVERSE REACTIONS
Not all of the following adverse reactions have been reported with this specific drug; however, pharmacological similarities among various phenothiazine derivatives require that each be considered. With the piperazine group (of which Perphenazine is an example) the extrapyramidal symptoms are more common, and others (e.g., sedative effects, jaundice, and blood dyscrasias) are less frequently seen.

CNS Effects: Extrapyramidal Reactions: opisthotonus, trismus, torticollis, retrocollis, aching and numbness of the limbs, motor restlessness, oculogyric crisis, hyperreflexia, dystonia, including protrusion, discoloration, aching and rounding of the tongue, tonic spasm of the masticatory muscles, tight feeling in the throat, slurred speech, dysphagia, akathisia, dyskinesia, parkinsonism, and ataxia. Their incidence and severity usually increase with an increase in dosage, but there is considerable individual variation in the tendency to develop such symptoms. Extrapyramidal symptoms can usually be controlled by the concomitant use of effective antiparkinsonian drugs, such as benztropine mesylate, and/or by reduction in dosage. In some instances, however, these extrapyramidal reactions may persist after discontinuation of treatment with Perphenazine.

Persistent Tardive Dyskinesia: As with all antipsychotic agents, tardive dyskinesia may appear in some patients on long-term therapy or may appear after drug therapy has been discontinued. Although the risk appears to be greater in elderly patients on high-dose therapy, especially females, it may occur in either sex and in children. The symptoms are persistent and in some patients appear to be irreversible. The syndrome is characterized by rhythmical, involuntary movements of the tongue, face, mouth, or jaw (e.g. protrusion of tongue, puffing of cheeks, puckering of mouth, chewing movements). Sometimes these may be accompanied by involuntary movements of the extremities. There is no known effective treatment for tardive dyskinesia; antiparkinsonism agents usually do not alleviate the symptoms of this syndrome. It is suggested that all antipsychotic agents be discontinued if these symptoms appear. Should it be necessary to reinstitute treatment, or increase the dosage of the agent, or switch to a different antipsychotic agent, the syndrome may be masked. It has been reported that fine, vermicular movements of the tongue may be an early sign of the syndrome, and if the medication is stopped at that time the syndrome may not develop.

Other CNS effects include cerebral edema; abnormality of cerebrospinal fluid proteins; convulsive seizures, particularly in patients with EEG abnormalities or a history of such disorders, and headaches.

Neuroleptic malignant syndrome has been reported in patients treated with neuroleptic drugs (see *"Warnings"* for further information).

Drowsiness may occur, particularly during the first or second week, after which it generally disappears. If troublesome, lower the dosage. Hypnotic effects appear to be minimal, especially in patients who are permitted to remain active.

Adverse behavioral effects include paradoxical exacerbation of psychotic symptoms, catatonic-like states, paranoid reactions, lethargy, paradoxical excitement, restlessness, hyperactivity, nocturnal confusion, bizarre dreams, and insomnia. Hyperreflexia has been reported in the newborn when a phenothiazine was used during pregnancy.

Autonomic Effects: dry mouth or salivation, nausea, vomiting, diarrhea, anorexia, constipation, obstipation, fecal impaction, urinary retention, frequency or incontinence, bladder paralysis, polyuria, nasal congestion, pallor, myosis, mydriasis, blurred vision, glaucoma, perspiration, hypertension, hypotension, and change in pulse rate occasionally may occur. Significant autonomic effects have been infrequent in patients receiving less than 24 mg Perphenazine daily.

Adynamic ileus occasionally occurs with phenothiazine therapy and if severe can result in complications and death. It is of particular concern in psychiatric patients, who may fail to seek treatment of this condition.

Allergic Effects: urticaria, erythema, eczema, exfoliative dermatitis, pruritus, photosensitivity, asthma, fever, anaphylactoid reactions, laryngeal edema, and angioneurotic edema; contact dermatitis in nursing personnel administering the drug, and in extremely rare instances, individual idiosyncrasy or hypersensitivity to phenothiazines has resulted in cerebral edema, circulatory collapse, and death.

Endocrine Effects: lactation, galactorrhea, moderate breast enlargement in females and gynecomastia in males on large doses, disturbances in the menstrual cycle, amenorrhea, changes in libido, inhibition of ejaculation, syndrome of inappropriate ADH (antidiuretic hormone) secretion, false positive pregnancy tests, hyperglycemia, hypoglycemia, glycosuria.

Cardiovascular Effects: postural hypotension, tachycardia (especially with sudden marked increase in dosage), bradycardia, cardiac arrest, faintness, and dizziness. Occasionally the hypotensive effect may produce a shock-like condition. ECG changes, nonspecific, (quinidine-like effect) usually reversible, have been observed in some patients receiving phenothiazine tranquilizers.

Sudden death has occasionally been reported in patients who have received phenothiazines. In some cases the death was apparently due to cardiac arrest, in others, the cause appeared to be asphyxia due to failure of the cough reflex. In some patients, the cause could not be determined nor could it be established that the death was due to the phenothiazine.

Hematological Effects: agranulocytosis, eosinophilia, leukopenia, hemolytic anemia, thrombocytopenic purpura, and pancytopenia. Most cases of agranulocytosis have occurred between the fourth and tenth weeks of therapy. Patients should be watched closely especially during that period for the sudden appearance of sore throat or signs of infection. If white blood cell and differential cell counts show significant cellular depression, discontinue the drug and start appropriate therapy. However, a slightly lowered white count is not in itself an indication to discontinue the drug.

Other Effects: Special considerations in long-term therapy include pigmentation of the skin, occurring chiefly in the exposed areas, ocular changes consisting of deposition of fine particulate matter in the cornea and lens, progressing in more severe cases to star-shaped lenticular opacities; epithelial keratopathies; and pigmentary retinopathy. Also noted: peripheral edema, reversed epinephrine effect, increase in PBI not attributable to an increase in thyroxine, parotid swelling (rare), hyperpyrexia, systemic lupus erythematosus-like syndrome, increases in appetite and weight, polyphagia, photophobia, and muscle weakness.

Liver damage (biliary stasis) may occur. Jaundice may occur, usually between the second and fourth weeks of treatment and is regarded as a hypersensitivity reaction. Incidence is low. The clinical picture resembles infectious hepatitis but with laboratory features of obstructive jaundice. It is usually reversible; however, chronic jaundice has been reported.

Side effects with intramuscular Perphenazine Injection have been infrequent and transient. Dizziness or significant hypotension after treatment with Perphenazine Injection is a rare occurrence.

OVERDOSAGE

In the event of overdosage, emergency treatment should be started immediately. All patients suspected of having taken an overdose should be hospitalized as soon as possible.

Manifestations: Overdosage of Perphenazine primarily involves the extrapyramidal mechanism and produces the same side effects described under *"Adverse Reactions"*, but to a more marked degree. It is usually evidenced by stupor or coma; children may have convulsive seizures.

Treatment: Treatment is symptomatic and supportive. There is no specific antidote. The patient should be induced to vomit even if emesis has occurred spontaneously. Pharmacologic vomiting by the administration of ipecac syrup is a preferred method. It should be noted that ipecac has a central mode of action in addition to its local gastric irritant properties, and the central mode of action may be blocked by the antiemetic effect of Perphenazine products. Vomiting should not be induced in patients with impaired consciousness. The action of ipecac is facilitated by physical activity and by the administration of 8 to 12 fluid ounces of water. If emesis does not occur within 15 minutes, the dose of ipecac should be repeated. Precautions against aspiration must be taken, especially in infants and children. Following emesis, any drug remaining in the stomach may be absorbed by activated charcoal administered as a slurry with water. If vomiting is unsuccessful or contraindicated, gastric lavage should be performed. Isotonic and one-half isotonic saline are the lavage solutions of choice. Saline cathartics, such as milk of magnesia, draw water into the bowel by osmosis and therefore may be valuable for their action in rapid dilution of bowel content.

Standard measures (oxygen, intravenous fluids, corticosteroids) should be used to manage circulatory shock or metabolic acidosis. An open airway and adequate fluid intake should be maintained. Body temperature should be regulated. Hypothermia is expected, but severe hyperthermia may occur and must be treated vigorously. (See *"Contraindications"*.)

An electrocardiogram should be taken and close monitoring of cardiac function instituted if there is any sign of abnormality. Cardiac arrhythmias may be treated with neostigmine, pyridostigmine, or propranolol. Digitalis should be considered for cadiac failure. Close monitoring of cardiac function is advisable for not less than five days. Vasopressors such as norepinephrine may be used to treat hypotension, but epinephrine should NOT be used.

Anticonvulsants (an inhalation anesthetic, diazepam, or paraldehyde) are recommended for control of convulsions, since Perphenazine increases the central nervous system depressant action, but not the anticonvulsant action of barbiturates.

If acute parkinson-like symptoms result from Perphenazine intoxication, benztropine mesylate or diphenydramine may be administered.

Central nervous system depression may be treated with nonconvulsant doses of CNS stimulants. Avoid stimulants that may cause convulsions (e.g., picrotoxin and pentylenetetrazol).

Signs of arousal may not occur for 48 hours.

Dialysis is of no value because of low plasma concentrations of the drug.

Since overdosage is often deliberate, patients may attempt suicide by other means during the recovery phase. Deaths by deliberate or accidental overdosage have occurred with this class of drugs.

DOSAGE AND ADMINISTRATION

Dosage must be individualized and adjusted according to the severity of the condition and the response obtained. As with all potent drugs, the best dose is the lowest dose that will produce the desired clinical effect. Since extrapyramidal symptoms increase in frequency and severity with increased dosage, it is important to employ the lowest effective dose. These symptoms have disappeared upon reduction of dosage, withdrawal of the drug or administration of an antiparkinsonian agent.

Prolonged administration of doses exceeding 24 mg daily should be reserved for hospitalized patients or patients under continued observation for early detection and management of adverse reactions. An antiparkinsonian agent, such as trihexyphenidyl hydrochloride or benztropine mesylate, is valuable in controlling drug-induced, extrapyramidal symptoms.

PERPHENAZINE TABLETS
Suggested dosages for Tablets for various conditions follow:

Moderately disturbed non-hospitalized psychotic patients: Tablets 4 to 8 mg t.i.d., initially; reduce as soon as possible to minimum effective dosage.

Hospitalized psychotic patients: Tablets 8 to 16 mg b.i.d. to q.i.d.; avoid dosages in excess of 64 mg daily.

Severe nausea and vomiting in adults: Tablets 8 to 16 mg daily in divided doses; 24 mg occasionally may be necessary; early dosage reduction is desirable.

PERPHENAZINE INJECTION
Intramuscular Administration

The injection is used when rapid effect and prompt control of acute or intractable conditions is required or when oral administration is not feasible. Perphenazine Injection, administered by deep intramuscular injection, is well tolerated. The injection should be given with the patient seated or recumbent, and the patient should be observed for a short period after administration.

Therapeutic effect is usually evidenced in 10 minutes and is maximal in 1 to 2 hours. The average duration of effective action is 6 hours, occasionally 12 to 24 hours.

Pediatric dosage has not yet been established. Children over 12 years may receive the lowest limit of adult dosage.

The usual initial dose is 5 mg (1 mL). This may be repeated every 6 hours. Ordinarily, the total daily dosage should not exceed 15 mg in ambulatory patients or 30 mg in hospitalized patients. When required for satisfactory control of symptoms in severe conditions, an initial 10 mg intramuscular dose may be given.

◆ RATED THERAPEUTICALLY EQUIVALENT; ◇ THERAPEUTIC EQUIVALENCE UNCONFIRMED; ○ UNRATED

Patients should be placed on oral therapy as soon as practicable. Generally, this may be achieved within 24 hours. In some instances, however, patients have been maintained on injectable therapy for several months. It has been established that Perphenazine Injection is more potent than Perphenazine Tablets. Therefore, equal or higher dosage should be used when the patient is transferred to oral therapy after receiving the injection.

Psychotic Conditions: While 5 mg of the Injection has a definite tranquilizing effect, it may be necessary to use 10 mg doses to initiate therapy in severely agitated states. Most patients will be controlled and amendable to oral therapy within a maximum of 24 to 48 hours. Acute conditions (hysteria, panic reaction) often respond well to a single dose whereas in chronic conditions, several injections may be required. When transferring patients to oral therapy, it is suggested that increased dosage be employed to maintain adequate clinical control. This should be followed by gradual reduction to the minimal maintenance dose which is effective.

Severe Nausea and Vomiting in Adults: To obtain rapid control of vomiting, administer 5 mg (1 mL): in rare instances it may be necessary to increase the dose to 10 mg, in general, higher doses should be given only to hospitalized patients. Perphenazine Injection—Intravenous Administration.

The intravenous administration of Perphenazine Injection is seldom required. This route of administration should be used with particular caution and care and only when absolutely necessary to control severe vomiting, intractable hiccoughs, or acute conditions, such as violent retching during surgery. Its use should be limited to recumbent, hospitalized adults in doses not exceeding 5 mg. When employed in this manner, intravenous injection ordinarily should be given as a diluted solution by either fractional injection or a slow drip infusion. In the surgical patient, slow infusion of no more than 5 mg is preferred. When administered in divided doses, Perphenazine Injection should be diluted to 0.5 mg/mL (1 mL mixed with 9 mL of physiologic saline solution), and not more than 1 mg per injection given at not less than one-to two-minute intervals. Intravenous injection should be discontinued as soon as symptoms are controlled and should not exceed 5 mg. The possibility of hypotensive and extrapyramidal side effects should be considered and appropriate means for management kept available. Blood pressure and pulse should be monitored continuously during intravenous administration. Pharmacologic and clinical studies indicate that intravenous administration of norepinephrine should be useful in alleviating the hypotensive effect.

PERPHENAZINE CONCENTRATE

In hospitalized psychotic patients, the usual dosage range is 3 to 16 mg b.i.d. to q.i.d., depending on the severity of symptoms and individual response. Although a number of investigators have employed higher dosages, a total daily dose of more than 64 mg ordinarily is not required. The Concentrate should be diluted only with water, saline, Seven-Up, homogenized milk, carbonated orange drink and pineapple, apricot, prune, orange, V-8, tomato, and grapefruit juices. Perphenazine Concentrate should not be mixed with beverages containing caffeine (coffee, cola) tannics (tea), or pectinates (apple juice) since physical incompatibility may result. Suggested dilution is approximately two fluid ounces of diluent for each 5 mL (16 mg) teaspoonful of Perphenazine Concentrate. For convenience in measuring smaller doses, a graduated dropper marked to measure 8 mg or 4 mg is supplied with each bottle.

STORAGE

Tablets: Store between 2° and 25° C (36° and 77° F).

Concentrate Liquid: Store between 2° and 30° C (36° and 86° F).
Protect from light. Shake well before using.

Injection: Keep package closed to protect from light. Exposure may cause discoloration. Slight yellowish discoloration will not alter potency or therapeutic efficacy; if markedly discolored, ampul should be discarded. Protect from light. Store in carton until contents are used.

J CODES
Up to 5 mg IM,IV—J3310

HOW SUPPLIED
CONCENTRATE: 16 MG/5 ML

BRAND/MANUFACTURER	NDC	SIZE	AWP
○ **BRAND**			
TRILAFON: Schering	00085-0363-02	120 ml	$32.30

INJECTION: 5 MG/ML

BRAND/MANUFACTURER	NDC	SIZE	AWP
○ **BRAND**			
TRILAFON: Schering	00085-0012-04	1 ml 100s	$480.70

TABLETS: 2 MG

AVERAGE UNIT PRICE (AVAILABLE SIZES)		GENERIC A-RATED AVERAGE PRICE (GAAP)	
BRAND	$0.57	100s	$41.60
GENERIC	$0.41	500s	$176.44
HCFA FUL (100s ea)	$0.34		

BRAND/MANUFACTURER	NDC	SIZE	AWP
◆ **BRAND**			
TRILAFON: Schering	00085-0705-04	100s	$56.71

BRAND/MANUFACTURER	NDC	SIZE	AWP
◆ **GENERICS**			
Mason Dist	11845-0169-01	100s	$26.92
Warrick	59930-1600-01	100s	$36.00
Lemmon	00093-0789-01	100s	$39.85
Zenith	00172-3667-60	100s	$40.30
Goldline	00182-1865-01	100s	$40.50
URL	00677-1385-01	100s	$40.51
Qualitest	00603-5090-21	100s	$40.55
Rugby	00536-4131-01	100s	$40.56
Geneva	00781-1046-01	100s	$40.83
Major	00904-1872-60	100s	$40.90
Moore,H.L.	00839-7423-06	100s	$40.97
Parmed	00349-8773-01	100s	$44.30
Martec	52555-0380-01	100s	$45.50
Major	00904-1872-61	100s ud	$36.04
Geneva	00781-1046-13	100s ud	$47.81
UDL	51079-0738-20	100s ud	$51.76
Medirex	57480-0442-01	100s ud	$53.89
Moore,H.L.	00839-7423-12	500s	$160.37
Major	00904-1872-40	500s	$178.15
Zenith	00172-3667-70	500s	$190.80

TABLETS: 4 MG

AVERAGE UNIT PRICE (AVAILABLE SIZES)		GENERIC A-RATED AVERAGE PRICE (GAAP)	
BRAND	$0.78	100s	$56.27
GENERIC	$0.55	500s	$246.71
HCFA FUL (100s ea)	$0.47		

BRAND/MANUFACTURER	NDC	SIZE	AWP
◆ **BRAND**			
TRILAFON: Schering	00085-0940-05	100s	$77.58
◆ **GENERICS**			
Warrick	59930-1603-01	100s	$49.50
Moore,H.L.	00839-7424-06	100s	$51.50
Mason Dist	11845-0170-01	100s	$51.90
Lemmon	00093-0790-01	100s	$52.95
Rugby	00536-4132-01	100s	$54.63
URL	00677-1386-01	100s	$54.65
Qualitest	00603-5091-21	100s	$54.70
Major	00904-1873-60	100s	$54.85
Goldline	00182-1866-01	100s	$55.00
Zenith	00172-3668-60	100s	$55.15
Aligen	00405-4780-01	100s	$55.22
Geneva	00781-1047-01	100s	$55.86
Parmed	00349-8774-01	100s	$60.65
Martec	52555-0381-01	100s	$64.90
Major	00904-1873-61	100s ud	$46.51
UDL	51079-0739-20	100s ud	$64.15
Medirex	57480-0443-01	100s ud	$64.15
Geneva	00781-1047-13	100s ud	$66.63
Moore,H.L.	00839-7424-12	500s	$222.74
Major	00904-1873-40	500s	$239.25
Goldline	00182-1866-05	500s	$260.00
Zenith	00172-3668-70	500s	$264.85

TABLETS: 8 MG

AVERAGE UNIT PRICE (AVAILABLE SIZES)		GENERIC A-RATED AVERAGE PRICE (GAAP)	
BRAND	$0.94	100s	$69.92
GENERIC	$0.68	500s	$290.93
HCFA FUL (100s ea)	$0.57		

BRAND/MANUFACTURER	NDC	SIZE	AWP
◆ **BRAND**			
TRILAFON: Schering	00085-0313-05	100s	$94.14
◆ **GENERICS**			
Warrick	59930-1605-01	100s	$59.80
Mason Dist	11845-0171-01	100s	$61.75
Moore,H.L.	00839-7425-06	100s	$62.90
Lemmon	00093-0791-01	100s	$64.25
URL	00677-1388-01	100s	$64.95
Qualitest	00603-5092-21	100s	$64.95
Rugby	00536-4133-01	100s	$65.00
Major	00904-1874-60	100s	$65.60
Goldline	00182-1867-01	100s	$66.00
Zenith	00172-3669-60	100s	$66.90
Aligen	00405-4781-01	100s	$67.30
Geneva	00781-1048-01	100s	$67.78
Parmed	00349-8775-01	100s	$73.60
Martec	52555-0382-01	100s	$77.85
Major	00904-1874-61	100s ud	$57.46
Geneva	00781-1048-13	100s ud	$75.72
Medirex	57480-0444-01	100s ud	$98.00
UDL	51079-0740-20	100s ud	$98.82
Rugby	00536-4133-02	250s	$154.63
Moore,H.L.	00839-7425-12	500s	$261.48
Major	00904-1874-40	500s	$273.25
Goldline	00182-1867-05	500s	$310.00
Zenith	00172-3669-70	500s	$319.00

➤ SHOWN IN PRODUCT IDENTIFICATION GUIDE

TABLETS: 16 MG

AVERAGE UNIT PRICE (AVAILABLE SIZES)		GENERIC A-RATED AVERAGE PRICE (GAAP)	
BRAND	$1.27	100s	$91.33
GENERIC	$0.91	500s	$423.38
HCFA FUL (100s ea)	$0.76		

BRAND/MANUFACTURER	NDC	SIZE	AWP
◆ **BRAND**			
TRILAFON: Schering	00085-0077-05	100s	$126.67
◆ **GENERICS**			
Warrick	59930-1610-01	100s	$80.60
Mason Dist	11845-0172-01	100s	$84.44
Lemmon	00093-0792-01	100s	$86.75
Goldline	00182-1868-01	100s	$88.00
URL	00677-1389-01	100s	$88.83
Rugby	00536-4134-01	100s	$88.88
Major	00904-1875-60	100s	$89.25
Zenith	00172-3670-60	100s	$90.05
Aligen	00405-4782-01	100s	$90.82
Geneva	00781-1049-01	100s	$91.20
Moore,H.L.	00839-7426-06	100s	$91.46
Martec	52555-0383-01	100s	$107.55
Major	00904-1875-61	100s ud	$71.52
Geneva	00781-1049-13	100s ud	$106.57
UDL	51079-0823-20	100s ud	$114.10
Major	00904-1875-40	500s	$411.75
Zenith	00172-3670-70	500s	$435.00

Persa-Gel SEE BENZOYL PEROXIDE

Persantine SEE DIPYRIDAMOLE, INJECTABLE AND DIPYRIDAMOLE, ORAL

Petameth SEE RACEMETHIONINE

Pfizerpen SEE PENICILLIN G POTASSIUM

Phenacemide

DESCRIPTION

Phenacemide is a valuable antiepileptic drug for use in selected patients with epilepsy. Since therapy with Phenacemide involves certain risks, *physicians should thoroughly familiarize themselves with the undesirable side effects which may occur and the precautions to be observed.* Phenacemide is a substituted acetylurea derivative. Chemically Phenacemide is identified as N-(aminocarbonyl)-benzeneacetamide. Tablets contain 500 mg Phenacemide for oral administration.

Following is its chemical structure:

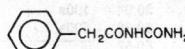

CLINICAL PHARMACOLOGY

In experimental animals, Phenacemide in doses well below those causing neurological signs, elevates the threshold for minimal electroshock convulsions and abolishes the tonic phase of maximal electroshock seizures. The drug prevents or modifies seizures induced by pentylenetetrazol or other convulsants. In comparative tests, Phenacemide was found to be equal to or more effective than other commonly used antiepileptics against complex partial (psychomotor) seizures which were induced in mice by low frequency stimulation of the cerebral cortex. Studies in mice have shown that Phenacemide exerts a synergistic antiepileptic effect with mephenytoin, phenobarbital, or trimethadione.

Given orally to laboratory animals, Phenacemide has a low acute toxicity. In mice, slight ataxia appears at 400 mg/kg and light sleep occurs at 800 mg/kg. In high doses the drug causes marked ataxia and coma, the fatal dose being in the range of 3 to 5 g/kg for mice, rats, and cats.

Phenacemide is metabolized by the liver; however, further definition of human pharmacokinetics has not been determined.

INDICATIONS AND USAGE

Phenacemide is indicated for the control of severe epilepsy, particularly mixed forms of complex partial (psychomotor) seizures, refractory to other drugs.

CONTRAINDICATIONS

Phenacemide should not be administered unless other available antiepileptics have been found to be ineffective in satisfactorily controlling seizures.

WARNINGS

Phenacemide can produce serious side effects as well as direct organ toxicity. As a consequence its use entails the assumption of certain risks which must be weighed against the benefit to the patient. *Ordinarily* Phenacemide *should not be administered unless other available antiepileptics have been found to be ineffective in controlling seizures.* Death attributable to liver damage during therapy with Phenacemide has been reported. Phenacemide should be used with caution in patients with a history of previous liver dysfunction. If jaundice or other signs of hepatitis appear, the drug should be discontinued.

Aplastic anemia has occurred in association with Phenacemide therapy and death from this condition has been reported. Phenacemide should ordinarily not be used in patients with severe blood dyscrasias. Marked depression of the blood count is an indication for withdrawal of the drug.

Usage During Pregnancy: Phenacemide can cause fetal harm when administered to a pregnant woman. There are multiple reports in the clinical literature which indicate that the use of antiepileptic drugs during pregnancy results in an increased incidence of birth defects in the offspring. Reports have also suggested that the maternal ingestion of antiepileptic drugs, particularly barbiturates, is associated with a neonatal coagulation defect that may cause bleeding during the early (usually within 24 hours of birth) neonatal period. The possibility of the occurrence of this defect with the use of Phenacemide should be kept in mind. The defect is characterized by decreased levels of vitamin K-dependent clotting factors, and prolongation of either the prothrombin time or the partial thromboplastin time, or both. It has been suggested that vitamin K be given prophylactically to the mother one month prior to and during delivery, and to the infant, intravenously, immediately after birth. If this drug is used during pregnancy, or if the patient becomes pregnant while taking this drug, the patient should be apprised of the potential hazard to the fetus.

PRECAUTIONS

General: Extreme caution must be exercised in treating patients who previously have shown personality disorders. It may be advisable to hospitalize such patients during the first week of treatment. Personality changes, including attempts at suicide and the occurrence of psychoses requiring hospitalization, have been reported during therapy with Phenacemide. Severe or exacerbated personality changes are an indication for withdrawal of the drug.

Phenacemide should be used with caution in patients with a history of previous liver dysfunction.

Phenacemide should be administered with caution to patients with a history of allergy, particularly in association with the administration of other antiepileptics. The drug should be discontinued at the first sign of a skin rash or other allergic manifestation.

Information for Patients: The patient and his family should be aware of the possibility of personality changes so the family can watch for changes in the behavior of the patient such as decreased interest in surroundings, depression, or aggressiveness.

The patient should be told to report immediately any symptoms indicative of a developing blood dyscrasia such as malaise, sore throat, or fever.

Laboratory Tests: Liver function tests should be performed before and during therapy. Death attributable to liver damage during therapy with Phenacemide has been reported. If jaundice or other signs of hepatitis appear, the drug should be discontinued.

Complete blood counts should be made before instituting Phenacemide and at monthly intervals thereafter. If no abnormality appears within 12 months, the interval between blood counts may be extended. Blood changes have been reported with leukopenia (leukocyte count of 4,000 or less per cubic millimeter of blood) as the most commonly observed effect. However, aplastic anemia has occurred in association with Phenacemide therapy, and death from this condition has been reported. *The total number of each cellular element per cubic millimeter is a better index of possible blood dyscrasia than the percentage of cells.* Marked depression of the blood count is an indication for withdrawal of the drug.

Similarly, as nephritis has occasionally occurred in patients on Phenacemide, the urine should be examined at regular intervals. Abnormal urinary findings are an indication for discontinuance of therapy.

Drug Interactions: Extreme caution is essential if Phenacemide is administered with any other antiepileptic which is known to cause similar toxic effects.

Considerable caution should be exercised if Phenacemide is administered concurrently with ethotoin since paranoid symptoms have been reported during therapy with this combination.

Carcinogenesis: No data are available on long-term potential for carcinogenicity in animals or humans.

Pregnancy: Pregnancy Category D. See "Warnings" section.

Nursing Mothers: It is not known whether this drug is excreted in human milk. Because many drugs are excreted in human milk and because of the potential for serious adverse reactions in nursing infants from Phenacemide, a decision should be made whether to discontinue nursing or to discontinue the drug, taking into account the importance of the drug to the mother.

Pediatric Use: Safety and effectiveness in children below the age of 5 years have not been established.

ADVERSE REACTIONS

The following adverse effects associated with Phenacemide are listed by decreasing order of frequency based on data from one large clinical study.[1]

Psychiatric: Psychic changes (17 in 100 patients).

Gastrointestinal: Gastrointestinal disturbances (8 in 100 patients), including anorexia (5 in 100 patients) and weight loss (less than 1 in 100 patients).

Dermatologic: Skin rash (5 in 100 patients). Stevens-Johnson Syndrome with epidermal necrolysis has been reported in one non-fatal case.

CNS: Drowsiness (4 in 100 patients), headache (2 in 100 patients), insomnia (1 in 100 patients), dizziness and paresthesias (less than 1 in 100 patients).

Hematopoietic: Blood dyscrasias (primarily leukopenia), including fatal aplastic anemia (2 in 100 patients).

Hepatic: Hepatitis, including fatalities (2 in 100 patients)

Renal: Abnormal urinary findings, including a rise in serum creatinine[2], and nephritis (1 in 100 patients or less).

Other: Fatigue, fever, muscle pain and palpitation (less than 1 in 100 patients).

OVERDOSAGE

Symptoms of acute overdosage include excitement or mania, followed by drowsiness, ataxia and coma. In one case of acute overdosage, dizziness was followed by coma which lasted nearly 24 hours. Treatment should be started by inducing emesis; gastric lavage may be considered as an alternative or adjunct. General supportive measures will be necessary. A careful evaluation of liver and kidney function, mental state, and the blood-forming organs should be made following recovery.

DOSAGE AND ADMINISTRATION

Phenacemide is administered orally.

Since Phenacemide may produce serious toxic effects, it is strongly recommended that the dosage be held to the minimum amount necessary to achieve an adequate therapeutic effect.

For adults the usual starting dose is 1.5 g daily, administered in three divided doses of 500 mg each. After the first week, if seizures are not controlled and the drug is well tolerated, an additional 500 mg tablet may be taken upon arising. In the third week, if necessary, the dosage may be further increased by another 500 mg at bedtime. Satisfactory results have been noted in some patients on an initial dose of 250 mg three times per day. The effective total daily dose for adults usually ranges from 2 to 3 g, although some patients have required as much as 5 g daily.

For the pediatric patient from 5 to 10 years of age, approximately one-half the adult dose is recommended. It should be given at the same intervals as for adults.

Phenacemide may be administered alone or in conjunction with other antiepileptics. However, extreme caution must be exercised if other antiepileptics cause toxic effects similar to Phenacemide.

When Phenacemide is to replace other antiepileptic medication, the latter should be withdrawn gradually as the dosage of Phenacemide is increased to maintain seizure control.

REFERENCES

1. Tyler, M. W., King, E. Q.: "Phenacemide in Treatment of Epilepsy," *JAMA* 147: 17-21 (1951). 2. Richards, R.K., Bjornsson, T.D. Waterbury, L. D.: Rise in Serum and Urine Creatinine After Phenacemide, *Clin. Pharmacol. Ther.* 23: 430-437 (1978).

HOW SUPPLIED
TABLETS: 500 MG

BRAND/MANUFACTURER	NDC	SIZE	AWP
○ **BRAND**			
PHENURONE: Abbott Pharm	00074-3971-05	100s	$50.38

Phenaphen with Codeine *SEE*
ACETAMINOPHEN WITH CODEINE PHOSPHATE

Phenazopyridine Hydrochloride

DESCRIPTION

Phenazopyridine Hydrochloride is chemically designated 2,6-Pyridinediamine, 3-(phenylazo), monohydrochloride. It is a urinary tract analgesic agent for oral administration. Phenazopyridine Hydrochloride tablets contain 100 mg or 200 mg Phenazopyridine Hydrochloride.

Following is its chemical structure:

CLINICAL PHARMACOLOGY

Phenazopyridine Hydrochloride is excerted in the urine where it exerts a topical analgesic effect on the mucosa of the urinary tract. This action helps to relieve pain, burning, urgency and frequency. The precise mechanism of action is not known.

The pharmacokinetic properties of Phenazopyridine Hydrochloride have not been determined. Phenazopyridine is rapidly excreted by the kidneys, with as much as 65% of an oral dose being excreted unchanged in the urine.

INDICATIONS AND USAGE

Phenazopyridine Hydrochloride is indicated for the symptomatic relief of pain, burning, urgency, frequency, and other discomforts arising from irritation of the lower urinary tract mucosa caused by infection, trauma, surgery, endoscopic procedures, or the passage of sounds or catheters. The use of Phenazopyridine Hydrochloride for relief of symptoms should not delay definitive diagnosis and treatment of causative conditions. Because it provides only symptomatic relief, prompt appropriate treatment of the cause of pain must be instituted and Phenazopyridine Hydrochloride should be discontinued when symptoms are controlled.

The analgesic action may reduce or eliminate the need for systemic analgesics or narcotics. It is, however, compatible with antibacterial therapy and can help to relieve pain and discomfort during the interval before antibacterial therapy controls the infection. Treatment of a urinary tract infection with Phenazopyridine Hydrochloride should not exceed 2 days because there is a lack of evidence that the combined administration of Phenazopyridine Hydrochloride and an antibacterial provides greater benefit than administration of the antibacterial alone after 2 days. (See *"Dosage and Administration"* Section.)

CONTRAINDICATIONS

Phenazopyridine Hydrochloride should not be used in patients who have previously exhibited hypersensitivity to it. The use of Phenazopyridine Hydrochloride is contraindicated in patients with renal insufficiency.

PRECAUTIONS

General: A yellowish tinge of the skin or sclera may indicate accumulation due to impaired renal excretion and the need to discontinue therapy.

The decline in renal function associated with advanced age should be kept in mind.

Information for Patients: Phenazopyridine Hydrochloride produces an orange to red color in the urine and may stain fabric. Staining of contact lenses has been reported.

Laboratory Test Interactions: Due to its properties as an azo dye, Phenazopyridine HCl may interfere with urinalysis based on spectrometry or color reactions.

Carcinogenesis, Mutagenesis, Impairment of Fertility: Long-term administration of phenazopyridine hydrochloride has induced neoplasia in rats (large intestine) and mice (liver). Although no association between Phenazopyridine Hydrochloride and human neoplasia has been reported, adequate epidemiological studies along these lines have not been conducted.

Pregnancy Category B: Reproduction studies have been performed in rats at doses up to 50 mg/kg/day and have revealed no evidence of impaired fertility or harm to the fetus due to Phenazopyridine Hydrochloride. There are, however, no adequate and well controlled studies in pregnant women. Because animal reproduction studies are not always predictive of human response, this drug should be used during pregnancy only if clearly needed.

Nursing Mothers: No information is available on the appearance of Phenazopyridine Hydrochloride or its metabolites in human milk.

ADVERSE REACTIONS

Headache, rash, pruritus and occasional gastrointestinal disturbance. An anaphylactoid-like reaction has been described. Methemoglobinemia, hemolytic anemia, renal and hepatic toxicity have been described, usually at overdose levels (see *"Overdosage"* section). Staining of contact lenses has been reported.

OVERDOSAGE

Exceeding the recommended dose in patients with good renal function or administering the usual dose to patients with impaired renal function (common in elderly patients), may lead to increased serum levels and toxic reactions. Methemoglobinemia generally follows a massive, acute overdose. Methylene blue, 1 to 2 mg/kg body weight intravenously, or ascorbic acid 100 to 200 mg given orally should cause prompt reduction of the methemoglobinemia and disappearance of the cyanosis which is an aid in diagnosis. Oxidative Heinz body hemolytic anemia may also occur, and "bite cells" (degmacytes) may be present in a chronic overdosage situation. Red blood cell G-6-PD deficiency may predispose to hemolysis. Renal and hepatic impairment and occasional failure, usually due to hypersensitivity, may also occur.

DOSAGE AND ADMINISTRATION

100 mg tablets: Adult dosage is two tablets 3 times a day after meals, 200 mg tablets: Adult dosage is one tablet 3 times a day after meals.

When used concomitantly with an antibacterial agent for the treatment of a urinary tract infection, the administration of Phenazopyridine Hydrochloride should not exceed 2 days.

Store tablets at controlled room temperature, 15° to 30°C (59° to 86° F).

HOW SUPPLIED
TABLETS: 95 MG

BRAND/MANUFACTURER	NDC	SIZE	AWP
○ **GENERICS**			
Mfg Chemists	00148-9125-03	30s	$4.35
Mfg Chemists	00148-9125-01	100s	$5.80

► SHOWN IN PRODUCT IDENTIFICATION GUIDE

TABLETS: 100 MG

BRAND/MANUFACTURER	NDC	SIZE	AWP
○ BRAND			
PYRIDIUM: Parke-Davis	00071-0180-24	100s	$50.25
○ GENERICS			
Allscrips	54569-0199-06	4s	$0.47
Southwood	58016-0151-06	6s	$2.85
Allscrips	54569-0199-03	8s	$0.95
Southwood	58016-0151-08	8s	$2.94
Southwood	58016-0151-09	9s	$3.32
Pharm Corp/America	51655-0153-53	10s	$1.95
Allscrips	54569-0199-00	10s	$1.99
Southwood	58016-0151-10	10s	$3.69
Allscrips	54569-5064-00	10s	$4.95
Allscrips	54569-0199-05	12s	$1.42
Southwood	58016-0151-12	12s	$3.57
Cheshire	55175-4080-02	12s	$4.00
Allscrips	54569-0199-04	15s	$1.78
Cheshire	55175-4080-05	15s	$4.50
Southwood	58016-0151-15	15s	$4.64
Southwood	58016-0151-16	16s	$3.71
Allscrips	54569-0199-07	18s	$2.13
Allscrips	54569-0199-02	20s	$2.37
Southwood	58016-0151-20	20s	$5.15
Southwood	58016-0151-24	24s	$6.16
Allscrips	54569-0199-01	30s	$3.56
Mfg Chemists	00148-9130-03	30s	$4.40
Cheshire	55175-4080-03	30s	$5.50
Southwood	58016-0151-30	30s	$5.69
ERIDIUM: Mallard	59441-0163-32	32s	$2.99
Southwood	58016-0151-40	40s	$7.76
PHENAZODINE: Lannett	00527-1211-01	100s	$2.00
PYRIDIATE: Richlyn	00115-4334-01	100s	$4.66
Mfg Chemists	00148-9130-01	100s	$5.85
Pharmacist's Choice	54979-0146-01	100s	$8.15
UDL	51079-0098-40	100s	$8.96
Schein	00364-0286-01	100s	$9.72
URL	00677-0575-01	100s	$10.24
Major	00904-0191-60	100s	$10.25
Geneva	00781-1510-01	100s	$10.25
Vintage	00254-4971-28	100s	$10.50
Qualitest	00603-5141-21	100s	$10.50
PYRIDIATE: Rugby	00536-4388-01	100s	$11.25
Moore,H.L.	00839-1503-06	100s	$12.15
Goldline	00182-0138-01	100s	$14.00
Parmed	00349-8975-01	100s	$16.95
Alphagen	59743-0013-01	100s	$30.95
Barre	00472-0196-10	100s	$41.42
U.S. Trading	56126-0278-11	100s ud	$6.08
Major	00904-0191-61	100s ud	$6.50
UDL	51079-0098-20	100s ud	$10.04
Major	00904-0191-70	250s	$10.60
PYRIDIATE: Veratex	17022-7567-06	1000s	$15.90
PYRIDIATE: Truxton	00463-6162-10	1000s	$31.20
Parmed	00349-8741-10	1000s	$31.99
PYRIDIATE: Richlyn	00115-4334-03	1000s	$35.85
Mfg Chemists	00148-9130-02	1000s	$36.00
Major	00904-0191-80	1000s	$73.35
Pharmacist's Choice	54979-0146-10	1000s	$73.35
Vintage	00254-4971-38	1000s	$79.63
Qualitest	00603-5141-32	1000s	$79.63
PYRIDIATE: Rugby	00536-4388-10	1000s	$79.75
Moore,H.L.	00839-1503-16	1000s	$91.94
Goldline	00182-0138-10	1000s	$94.00
Able	53265-0196-11	1000s	$95.05
Alphagen	59743-0013-10	1000s	$283.50

TABLETS: 200 MG

BRAND/MANUFACTURER	NDC	SIZE	AWP
○ BRAND			
VIRIDIUM: Vita Elixir	00181-0530-00	100s	$14.50
PYRIDIUM: Parke-Davis	00071-0181-24	100s	$96.84
○ GENERICS			
Allscrips	54569-0197-04	6s	$1.52
Phys Formlry	53261-0072-06	6s	$1.88
Cheshire	55175-4178-06	6s	$3.00
Southwood	58016-0152-06	6s	$3.06
Southwood	58016-0152-08	8s	$3.41
Allscrips	54569-7101-00	9s	$1.73
Pharm Corp/America	51655-0175-85	9s	$1.95
Allscrips	54569-0197-07	9s	$2.27
Cheshire	55175-4178-09	9s	$3.20
Southwood	58016-0152-09	9s	$3.84
Allscrips	54569-5065-01	10s	$1.92
Phys Formlry	53261-0072-10	10s	$2.00
Cheshire	55175-4178-00	10s	$3.30
Southwood	58016-0152-10	10s	$4.17
Allscrips	54569-0197-06	12s	$3.03
Cheshire	55175-4178-02	12s	$3.50
Southwood	58016-0152-12	12s	$4.72
Pharm Corp/America	51655-0175-54	15s	$2.30
Phys Formlry	53261-0072-15	15s	$2.85
Allscrips	54569-0197-01	15s	$3.79
Cheshire	55175-4178-05	15s	$3.90

BRAND/MANUFACTURER	NDC	SIZE	AWP
Southwood	58016-0152-15	15s	$5.17
Allscrips	54569-5065-00	20s	$3.84
Cheshire	55175-4178-03	20s	$5.10
Southwood	58016-0152-20	20s	$5.75
Allscrips	54569-0197-08	21s	$5.30
Southwood	58016-0152-24	24s	$6.63
Mfg Chemists	00148-9135-03	30s	$4.80
Allscrips	54569-0197-03	30s	$7.58
Southwood	58016-0152-50	50s	$11.37
Allscrips	54569-0197-05	60s	$15.15
PHENAZODINE: Lannett	00527-1163-01	100s	$4.05
Mfg Chemists	00148-9135-01	100s	$6.55
PYRIDIATE: Richlyn	00115-4336-01	100s	$7.39
Pharmacist's Choice	54979-0147-01	100s	$11.25
UDL	51079-0099-40	100s	$13.41
Moore,H.L.	00839-1556-06	100s	$14.92
Schein	00364-0321-01	100s	$17.72
Major	00904-0192-60	100s	$18.90
URL	00677-0804-01	100s	$19.35
Goldline	00182-0904-01	100s	$22.00
Vintage	00254-4972-28	100s	$23.13
Qualitest	00603-5142-21	100s	$23.13
PYRIDIATE: Rugby	00536-4392-01	100s	$23.95

Phenazopyridine Hydrochloride and Sulfamethoxazole

DESCRIPTION

Phenazopyridine Hydrochloride/Sulfamethoxazole tablets combine the antibacterial effectiveness of Sulfamethoxazole with the local urinary analgestic activity of Phenazopyridine Hydrochloride. Each tablet contains 0.5 gm Sulfamethoxazole and 100 mg Phenazopyridine Hydrochloride.

Sulfamethoxazole is an intermediate-dosage sulfonamide. Sulfamethoxazole is an almost white, odorless, tasteless compound. Chemically, it is N_1-(5-methyl-3-isoxazolyl) sulfanilamide.

Phenazopyridine Hydrochloride is a urinary analgestic. Chemically, it is 3-phenylazo-2,6-diaminopyridine hydrochloride.

Sulfonamides exist in the blood as free, conjugated (acetylated and possibly other forms) and protein-bound forms. The "free" form is considered to be the therapeutically active form. It has been shown that approximately 70 per cent of Sulfamethoxazole is protein bound in the blood;[1] of the unbound portion 80 to 90 per cent is in the nonacetylated form.[2,3] Excretion of sulfonamides is chiefly by the kidneys with glomerular filtration as the primary mechanism.

ACTIONS

The systemic sulfonamides are bacteriostatic agents. The spectrum of activity is similar for all. Sulfonamides competitively inhibit bacterial synthesis of folic acid (pteroylglutamic acid) from para-aminobenzoic acid. Resistant strains are capable of utilizing folic acid precursors or preformed folic acid.

Phenazopyridine Hydrochloride has a specific analgesic effect in the urinary tract, promptly relieving pain and burning.

INDICATIONS

For the initial treatment of uncomplicated urinary tract infections caused by susceptible strains of the following microorganisms: *Escherichia coli*, *Klebsiella* species, *Enterobacter* species, *Proteus mirabilis*, *Proteus vulgaris* and *Staphylococcus aureus* when relief of symptoms of pain, burning or urgency is needed during the first 2 days of therapy. Treatment with Phenazopyridine HCl/Sulfamethoxazole should not exceed 2 days. There is a lack of evidence that the combination of Sulfamethoxazole and Phenazopyridine Hydrochloride provides greater benefit than Sulfamethoxazole alone after 2 days. Treatment beyond 2 days should only be continued with Sulfamethoxazole. (See "*Dosage and Administration*" section.)

Important note: In vitro sulfonamide sensitivity tests are not always reliable. The test must be carefully coordinated with bacteriologic and clinical response. When the patient is already taking sulfonamides, follow-up cultures should have aminobenzoic acid added to the culture media.

Currently, the increasing frequency of resistant organisms is a limitation of the usefulness of antibacterial agents including the sulfonamides.

Wide variation in blood levels may result with identical doses. Blood levels should be measured in patients receiving sulfonamides for serious infections. Free sulfonamide blood levels of 5 to 15 mg per 100 ml may be considered therapeutically effective for most infections, with blood levels of 12 to 15 mg per 100 ml optimal for serious infections; 20 mg per 100 ml should be the maximum total sulfonamide level, as adverse reactions occur more frequently above this level.

CONTRAINDICATIONS

Children below age 12. Hypersensitivity to sulfonamides. Pregnancy at term and during the nursing period, because sulfonamides pass the placenta and are excreted in the milk and may cause kernicterus.

Because Phenazopyridine HCl/Sulfamethoxazole contains Phenazopyridine Hydrochloride, it is contraindicated in glomerulonephritis, severe hepatitis, uremia, and pyelonephritis of pregnancy with gastrointestinal disturbances.

◆ RATED THERAPEUTICALLY EQUIVALENT; ◇ THERAPEUTIC EQUIVALENCE UNCONFIRMED; ○ UNRATED

WARNINGS

Usage in Pregnancy: The safe use of sulfonamides in pregnancy has not been established. The teratogenicity potential of most sulfonamides has not been thoroughly investigated in either animals or humans. However, a significant increase in the incidence of cleft palate and other bony abnormalities of offspring has been observed when certain sulfonamides of the short, intermediate and long-acting types were given to pregnant rats and mice at high oral doses (7 to 25 times the human therapeutic dose).

Deaths associated with the administration of sulfonamides have been reported from hypersensitivity reactions, hepatocellular necrosis, agranulocytosis, aplastic anemia and other blood dyscrasias.

The presence of clinical signs such as sore throat, fever, arthralgia, cough, shortness of breath, pallor, purpura or jaundice may be early indications of serious reactions, including serious blood disorders. Complete blood counts should be done frequently in patients receiving sulfonamides.

The frequency of renal complications is considerably lower in patients receiving the more soluble sulfonamides. Urinalysis with careful microscopic examination should be obtained frequently in patients receiving sulfonamides.

PRECAUTIONS

Sulfonamides should be given with caution to patients with impaired renal or hepatic function and to those with severe allergy or bronchial asthma. In glucose-6-phosphate dehydrogenase-deficient individuals, hemolysis may occur. This reaction is frequently dose-related. Adequate fluid intake must be maintained in order to prevent crystalluria and stone formation.

Carcinogenesis: Phenazopyridine HCl/Sulfamethoxazole has not undergone adequate trials relating to carcinogenicity; each component, however, has been evaluated separately. Rats appear to be especially susceptible to the goitrogenic effects of sulfonamides, and long-term administration of sulfonamides has resulted in thyroid malignancies in this species. Long term administration of Phenazopyridine Hydrochloride has induced neoplasia in rats (large intestine) and mice (liver). Although no association between Phenazopyridine Hydrochloride and human neoplasia has been reported, adequate epidemiological studies have not been conducted.

ADVERSE REACTIONS

Blood Dyscrasias: Agranulocytosis, aplastic anemia, thrombocytopenia, leukopenia, hemolytic anemia, purpura, hypoprothrombinemia, methemoglobinemia, and eosinophilia.

Allergic Reactions: Erythema multiforme (Stevens-Johnson syndrome), generalized skin eruptions, epidermal necrolysis, urticaria, serum sickness, pruritus, exfoliative dermatitis, anaphylactoid reactions, periorbital edema, conjunctival and scleral injection, photosensitization, arthralgia and allergic myocarditis.

Gastrointestinal Reactions: Nausea, emesis, abdominal pains, hepatitis, hepatocellular necrosis, diarrhea, anorexia, pancreatitis and stomatitis.

CNS Reactions: Headache, peripheral neuritis, mental depression, convulsions, ataxia, hallucinations, tinnitus, vertigo and insomnia.

Miscellaneous Reactions: Drug fever, chills, and toxic nephrosis with oliguria and anuria. Polyarteritis nodosa and L.E. phenomenon have occurred.

Respiratory Reactions: Pulmonary infiltrates.

The sulfonamides bear certain chemical similarities to some goitrogens, diuretics (acetazolamide and the thiazides) and oral hypoglycemia agents. Goiter production, diuresis and hypoglycemia have occurred rarely in patients receiving sulfonamides. Cross-sensitivity may exist with these agents.

DOSAGE AND ADMINISTRATION

Phenazopyridine HCl/Sulfamethoxazole is intended for the acute, painful phase of urinary tract infections. The usual dosage in adults is 4 tablets initially followed by 2 tablets morning and evening for up to 2 days. Treatment with Phenazopyridine HCl/Sulfamethoxazole should not exceed 2 days. Treatment beyond 2 days should only be continued with Sulfamethoxazole.

Note: Patients should be told that the orange-red dye Phenazopyridine Hydrochloride will color the urine soon after ingestion of the medication.

REFERENCES

1. Struller, T.: *Antibiot, Chemother.*, 14:179, 1968. 2. Boger, W. P., and Gavin, J. J.: *Antibiotics and Chemother.*, 10:572. 1960. 3. Brandman, O., and Engelberg, R.: *Curr. Therap. Res.*, 2:364, 1960.

HOW SUPPLIED

TABLETS: 100 MG-500 MG

BRAND/MANUFACTURER	NDC	SIZE	AWP
○ **BRAND**			
▶ AZO GANTANOL: Roche Labs	00004-0011-01	100s	$71.57

Phenazopyridine Hydrochloride and Sulfisoxazole

DESCRIPTION

Phenazopyridine Hydrochloride/Sulfisoxazole is a combination drug containing 500 mg of the antibacterial Sulfisoxazole and 50 mg of the urinary analgesic Phenazopyridine Hydrochloride per tablet for oral administration.

Sulfisoxazole, an antibacterial sulfonamide, is N^1-(3,4-dimethyl-5-isoxazoyl) sulfanilamide. It is a white to slightly yellowish, odorless, slightly bitter, crystalline powder which is soluble in alcohol and very slightly soluble in water. Sulfisoxazole has an empirical formula of $C_{11}H_{13}N_3O_3S$, a molecular weight of 267.30.

Phenazopyridine Hydrochloride, a local urinary analgesic, is 2,6-diamino-3-(phenylazo) pyridine monohydrochloride. It is a light or dark red to dark violet, odorless, slightly bitter, crystalline powder with an empirical formula of $C_{11}H_{11}N_5$.HCl, a molecular weight of 249.70.

CLINICAL PHARMACOLOGY

Following oral administration, Sulfisoxazole is rapidly and completely absorbed: the small intestine is the major site of absorption, but some of the drug is absorbed from the stomach. Sulfonamides are present in the blood as "free", conjugated (acetylated and possibly other forms) and protein-bound forms. The amount present as "free" drug is considered to be the therapeutically active form. Approximately 85% of a dose of Sulfisoxazole is bound to plasma proteins, primarily to albumin; 65% to 72% of the unbound portion is in the nonacetylated form.

Maximum plasma concentrations of intact Sulfisoxazole following a single 2-Gm oral dose to healthy adult volunteers ranged from 127 to 211 mcg/mL (mean 169 mcg/mL), and the time of peak plasma concentration ranged from 1 to 4 hours (mean 2.5 hours). The elimination half-life of Sulfisoxazole ranged from 4.6 to 7.8 hours after oral administration. The elimination of Sulfisoxazole has been shown to be slower in elderly subjects (63 to 75 years) with diminished renal function (creatinine clearance 37 to 68 mL/min).[1] After multiple-dose oral administration of 500 mg q.i.d. to healthy volunteers, the average steady-state plasma concentrations of intact Sulfisoxazole ranged from 49.9 to 88.8 mcg/mL (mean 63.4 mcg/mL).[2]

Wide variation in blood levels may result following identical doses of a sulfonamide. Blood levels should be measured in patients receiving sulfonamides at the higher recommended doses or being treated for serious infections. Free sulfonamide blood levels of 50 to 150 mcg/mL may be considered therapeutically effective for most infections, with blood levels of 120 to 150 mcg/mL being optimal for serious infections. The maximum sulfonamide level should not exceed 200 mcg/mL, since adverse reactions occur more frequently above this concentration.

Sulfisoxazole and its acetylated metabolites are excreted primarily by the kidneys through glomerular filtration. Concentrations of Sulfisoxazole are considerably higher in the urine than in the blood. The mean urinary recovery following oral administration of Sulfisoxazole is 97% within 48 hours; 52% of this is intact drug, and the remaining is the N^4-acetylated metabolite.

Sulfisoxazole is distributed only in extracellular body fluid. It is excreted in human milk. It readily crosses the placental barrier and enters into fetal circulation and also crosses the blood-brain barrier. In healthy subjects, cerebrospinal fluid concentrations of Sulfisoxazole vary: in patients with meningitis, however, concentrations of free drug in cerebrospinal fluid as high as 94 mcg/mL have been reported.

Phenazopyridine Hydrochloride has a specific local analgesic effect in the urinary tract, promptly relieving pain and burning. In six healthy subjects, 90% of a 600 mg oral dose of Phenazopyridine Hydrochloride was eliminated in the urine in 24 hours, 41% as unchanged drug and 49% as metabolites. No additional pharmacokinetic data are available on this drug.

Microbiology: The sulfonamides are bacteriostatic agents and the spectrum of activity is similar for all. Sulfonamides inhibit bacterial synthesis of dihydrofolic acid by preventing the condensation of the pteridine with aminobenzoic acid through competitive inhibition of the enzyme dihydropteroate synthetase. Resistant strains have altered dihydropteroate synthetase with reduced affinity for sulfonamides or produce increased quantities of aminobenzoic acid.

INDICATIONS AND USAGE

Phenazopyridine/Sulfisoxazole is indicated for the initial treatment of uncomplicated urinary tract infections caused by susceptible strains of the following microorganisms: *Escherichia coli, Klebiella species, Enterobacter species, Proteus mirabilis, Proteus vulgaris* and *Staphylococcus aureus* when relief of symptoms of pain, burning or urgency is needed during the first 2 days of therapy. There is a lack of evidence that the combination of Sulfisoxazole and Phenazopyridine Hydrochloride provides greater benefit than Sulfisoxazole alone after 2 days. Therefore, treatment with Phenazopyridine/Sulfisoxazole should not exceed 2 days, and the remaining therapeutic course should be completed with sulfisoxazole alone. (See *"Dosage and Administration"* section.)

The frequency of resistant organisms limits the usefulness of sulfonamides as sole therapy in the treatment of urinary tract infections.

Important Note: In vitro susceptibility tests for sulfonamides are not always reliable. When the patient is already taking sulfonamides, follow-up cultures should have aminobenzoic acid added to the culture media.

CONTRAINDICATIONS

Phenazopyridine/Sulfisoxazole is contraindicated in the following patient populations:

Patients with a known sensitivity to either of its components;
Children younger than 2 months;
Pregnant women *at term;* and
Mothers nursing infants less than 2 months of age.
Use in pregnant women at term, in children less than 2 months of age and in mothers nursing infants less than 2 months of age is contraindicated because

sulfonamides may promote kernicterus in the newborn by displacing bilirubin from plasma proteins.

Because Phenazopyridine/Sulfisoxazole contains Phenazopyridine Hydrochloride, it is also contraindicated in patients with glomerulonephritis, severe hepatitis, uremia, and pyelonephritis of pregnancy with gastrointestinal disturbances.

WARNINGS: FATALITIES ASSOCIATED WITH THE ADMINISTRATION OF SULFONAMIDES, ALTHOUGH RARE, HAVE OCCURRED DUE TO SEVERE REACTIONS, INCLUDING STEVENS-JOHNSON SYNDROME, TOXIC EPIDERMAL NECROLYSIS, FULMINANT HEPATIC NECROSIS, AGRANULOCYTOSIS, APLASTIC ANEMIA AND OTHER BLOOD DYSCRASIAS.

SULFONAMIDES, INCLUDING PHENAZOPYRIDINE/SULFISOXAZOLE, SHOULD BE DISCONTINUED AT THE FIRST APPEARANCE OF SKIN RASH OR ANY SIGN OF ADVERSE REACTION. In rare instances a skin rash may be followed by a more severe reaction, such as Stevens-Johnson syndrome, toxic epidermal necrolysis, hepatic necrosis and serious blood disorders. (See "Precautions".)

Clinical signs such as rash, sore throat, fever, arthralgia, pallor, purpura or jaundice may be early indications of serious reactions.

Cough, shortness of breath and pulmonary infiltrates are hypersensitivity reactions of the respiratory tract that have been reported in association with Sulfonamide treatment.

The sulfonamides should not be used for the treatment of group A beta-hemolytic streptococcal infections. In the established infection, they will not eradicate the streptococcus and, therefore, will not prevent sequelae such as rheumatic fever.

Pseudomembranous coilitis has been reported with nearly all antibacterial agents, including Sulfisoxazole, and may range in severity from mild to life-threatening. Therefore, it is important to consider this diagnosis in patients who present with diarrhea subsequent to the administration of antibacterial agents.

Treatment with antibacterial agents alters the normal flora of the colon and may permit overgrowth of clostridia. Studies indicate that a toxin product by *Clostridium difficile* is one primary cause of "antibiotic-associated colitis".

After the diagnosis of pseudomembranous colitis has been established, therapeutic measures should be initiated. Mild cases of pseudomembranous colitis usually respond to drug discontinuation alone. In moderate to severe cases, consideration should be given to management with fluids and electrolytes, protein supplementation, and treatment with an oral antibacterial drug effective against *C. difficile*.

PRECAUTIONS

GENERAL
Sulfonamides should be given with caution to patients with impaired renal or hepatic function and to those with severe allergy or bronchial asthma. In glucose-6-phosphate dehydrogenase-deficient individuals, hemolysis may occur; this reaction is frequently dose-related.

The frequency of resistant organisms limits the usefulness of sulfonamides as sole therapy in the treatment of urinary tract infections. Since sulfonamides are bacteriostatic and not bacteriocidal, a complete course is needed to prevent immediate regrowth and the development of resistant uropathogens.

INFORMATION FOR PATIENTS
Patients should maintain an adequate fluid intake to prevent crystalluria and stone formation. Patients should also be told that soon after ingestion of this medication, the Phenazopyridine Hydrochloride component will produce a reddish-orange discoloration of the urine.

LABORATORY TESTS
Complete blood counts should be done frequently in patients receiving sulfonamides. If a significant reduction in the count of any formed blood element is noted, sulfonamide therapy should be discontinued. Urinalysis with careful microscopic examination and renal function tests should be performed during therapy, particularly for those patients with impaired renal function. Blood levels should be measured in patients receiving a sulfonamide for serious infections. (See "Indications and Usage".)

DRUG INTERACTIONS
It has been reported that Sulfisoxazole may prolong the prothrombin time in patients who are receiving anticoagulants, including warfarin. This interaction should be kept in mind when Phenazopyridine/Sulfisoxazole is given to patients already on anticoagulant therapy, and the coagulation time should be reassessed.

It has been proposed that Sulfisoxazole competes with thiopental for plasma protein binding. In one study involving 48 patients, intravenous Sulfisoxazole resulted in a decrease in the amount of thiopental required for anesthesia and in a shortening of the awakening time. It is not known whether chronic oral doses of Sulfisoxazole have a similar effect. Until more is known about this interaction, physicians should be aware that patients receiving Sulfisoxazole might require less thiopental for anesthesia.

Sulfonamides can displace methotrexate from plasma protein-binding sites, thus increasing free methotrexate concentrations. Studies in man have shown Sulfisoxazole infusions to decrease plasma protein-bound methotrexate by one-fourth.

Sulfisoxazole can also potentiate the blood sugar-lowering activity of sulfonylureas.

CARCINOGENESIS, MUTAGENESIS, IMPAIRMENT OF FERTILITY
Carcinogenesis: Phenazopyridine/Sulfisoxazole has not undergone adequate trials relating to carcinogenicity; each component, however, has been evaluated separately. Sulfisoxazole was not carcinogenic in either sex when administered to

mice by gavage for 103 weeks at dosages up to approximately 36 times the recommended human dose or to rats at 7 times the human dose. Rats appear to be especially susceptible to the goitrogenic effects of sulfonamides, and long-term administration of sulfonamides has resulted in thyroid malignancies in this species. Long-term administration of Phenazopyridine Hydrochloride has induced neoplasia in rats (large intestine) and mice (liver). Although no association between Phenazopyridine Hydrochloride and human neoplasia has been reported, adequate epidemiological studies have not been conducted.

Mutagenesis: There are no studies available that adequately evaluate the mutagenic potential of Phenazopyridine/Sulfisoxazole or either of its components. However, Sulfisoxazole was not observed to be mutagenic in *E. coli* Sd-4-73 when tested in the absence of a metabolic activating system.

Impairment of Fertility: Phenazopyridine/Sulfisoxazole has not undergone adequate trials relating to impairment of fertility. In a reproduction study in rats given 14 times the human dose per day of Sulfisoxazole, no effects were observed regarding mating behavior, conception rate or fertility index (percent pregnant). In a single 2-litter reproductive study of rats given 10 times the recommended human dose, Phenazopyridine demonstrated no adverse effect on fertility.

PREGNANCY
Teratogenic Effects: Pregnancy Category C. At dosages 14 times the human daily dose, Sulfisoxazole was not teratogenic in either rats or rabbits. However, in two other teratogenicity studies, cleft palates developed in both rats and mice after administration of 9 to 18 times the human therapeutic dose of Sulfisoxazole. Phenazopyridine has not been adequately tested in animals for teratogenicity; however, data from a single study demonstrated no congenital malformations in rats given 10 times the human daily dose.

There are no adequate or well-controlled studies of Phenazopyridine/Sulfisoxazole in either laboratory animals or in pregnant women. It is not known whether Phenazopyridine/Sulfisoxazole can cause fetal harm when administered to a pregnant woman prior to term or can affect reproduction capacity. Phenazopyridine/Sulfisoxazole should be used during pregnancy only if the potential benefit justifies the potential risk to the fetus.

Nonteratogenic Effects: Kernicterus may occur in the newborn as a result of treatment of a pregnant woman *at term* with sulfonamides. (See "Contraindications".)

NURSING MOTHERS
Phenazopyridine/Sulfisoxazole is excreted in human milk. Because of the potential for the development of kernicterus in neonates due to the displacement of bilirubin from plasma proteins by Sulfisoxazole, a decision should be made whether to discontinue nursing or discontinue the drug taking into account the importance of the drug to the mother. (See "Contraindications".)

PEDIATRIC USE
Safety and effectiveness in children have not been established. Not for use in children under 2 months of age. (See "Contraindications".)

ADVERSE REACTIONS
Included in the listing that follows are adverse reactions that have been reported with other sulfonamide products; pharmacologic similarities require that each of the reactions be considered with Phenazopyridine/Sulfisoxazole administration.

Allergic/Dermatologic: Anaphylaxis, erythema multiforme (Stevens-Johnson syndrome), toxic epidermal necrolysis, exfoliative dermatitis, angioedema, arteritis and vasculitis, allergic myocoarditis, serum sickness, rash, urticaria, pruritus, photosensitivity, and conjunctival and scleral injection. In addition, periarteritis nodosa and systemic lupus erythematosus have been reported. (See "Warnings".)

Cardiovascular: Tachycardia, palpitations, syncope and cyanosis.

Endocrine: The sulfonamides bear certain chemical similarities to some goitrogens, diuretics (acetazolamide and the thiazides) and oral hypoglycemic agents. Cross-sensitivity may exist with these agents. Development of goiter, diuresis and hypoglycemia have occurred rarely in patients receiving sulfonamides.

Gastrointestinal: Hepatitis, hepatocellular necrosis, jaundice, pseudomembranous colitis, nausea, emesis, anorexia, abdominal pain, diarrhea, gastrointestinal hemorrhage, melena, flatulence, glessitis, stomatitis, salivary gland enlargement and pancreatitis.

Onset of pseudomembranous colitis symptoms may occur during or after treatment with Sulfisoxazole, a component of Phenazopyridine/Sulfisoxazole. (See "Warnings".)

Both components of Phenazopyridine/Sulfisoxazole have been reported to cause increased elevation of liver-associated enzymes in patients with hepatitis.

Genitourinary: Crystalluria, hematuria, BUN and creatinine elevations, nephritis and toxic nephrosis with oliguria and anuria. Acute renal failure and uirinary retention have also been reported. The frequency of renal complications, commonly associated with some sulfonamides, is lower in patients receiving the more soluble sulfonamides such as Sulfisoxazole.

Hematologic: Leukopenia, agranulocytosis, aplastic anemia, thrombocytopenia, purpura, hemolytic anemia, anemia, eosinophilia, clotting disorders including hypoprothrombinemia and hypofibrinogenemia, sulfhemoglobinemia and methemoglobinemia.

Musculoskeletal: Arthralgia and myalgia.

Neurologic: Headache, dizziness, peripheral neuritis, paresthesia, convulsions, tinnitus, vertigo, ataxia and intracranial hypertension.

Psychiatric: Psychosis, hallucinations, disorentation, depression and anxiety.

Respiratory: Cough, shortness of breath and pulmonary infiltrates. (See *"Warnings".*)

Vascular: Angioedema, arteritis and vasculitis.

Miscellaneous: Edema (including periorbital), pyrexia, drowsiness, weakness, fatigue, lassitude, rigors, flushing, hearing loss, insomnia and pneumonitis.

OVERDOSAGE

The amount of a single dose that is associated with symptoms of overdosage or is likely to be life-threatening has not been reported. Signs and symptoms of overdosage with Phenazopyridine/Sulfisoxazole include anorexia, colic, nausea, vomiting, headache, dizziness, drowsiness, and unconsciousness. Pyrexia, hematuria and crystalluria may be noted. Blood dyscrasias and jaundice are potential late manifestations of overdosage.

General principles of treatment include the immediate discontinuation of the drug, instituting gastric lavage or emesis, forcing oral fluids, and administering intravenous fluids if urine output is low and renal function is normal. The patient should be monitored with blood counts and appropriate blood chemistries, including electrolytes. If the patient becomes cyanotic, the possibility of methemoglobinemia should be considered and, if present, the condition should be treated appropriately with intravenous 1% methylene blue. If a significant blood dyscrasia or jaundice occurs, specific therapy should be instituted for these complications.

Peritoneal dialysis is not effective, and hemodialysis is only moderately effective in removing sulfonamides.

DOSAGE AND ADMINISTRATION

The recommended dosage in adults is 4 tablets initially, followed by 2 tablets four times daily for up to two days. *Treatment with Phenazopyridine/Sulfisoxazole should not exceed 2 days.* A full course of therapy for an uncomplicated urinary tract infection should be completed with Sulfisoxazole alone.

REFERENCES

1. Boivert A, Barbeau G, Belanger PM: Pharmacokinetics of Sulfisoxazole in young and elderly subjects. *Gerontology 30:* 125-131, 1984.   2. Oie S, Gambertoglio JG, Fleckenstein L: Comparison of the disposition of total and unbound Sulfisoxazole after single and multiple dosing *J Pharmacokinet Biopharm 10:* 157-172, 1982.

HOW SUPPLIED
TABLETS: 50 MG-500 MG

BRAND/MANUFACTURER	NDC	SIZE	AWP
○ **BRAND**			
➤ AZO GANTRISIN: Roche Labs	00004-0012-01	100s	$30.92
	00004-0012-14	500s	$153.46
○ **GENERICS**			
Cheshire	55175-3254-00	40s	$17.55
Mfg Chemists	00148-9410-01	100s	$9.75
AZO-TRUXAZOLE: Truxton	00463-6036-10	1000s	$76.00
Mfg Chemists	00148-9410-02	1000s	$84.80

Phendimetrazine Tartrate

DESCRIPTION

Chemical name: Phendimetrazine Tartrate (+)3,4 dimethyl-2-phenylmorpholine Tartrate. Phendimetrazine Tartrate is a white, odorless powder with a bitter taste. It is soluble in water, methanol and ethanol. It has a molecular weight of 341.

Each tablet contains:
Phendimetrazine Tartrate 35mg

Each timed or slow release capsule contains:
Phendimetrazine Tartrate 105mg

Following is its chemical structure:

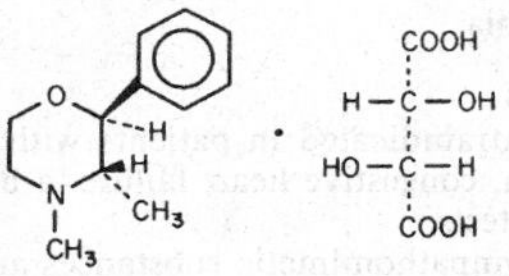

CLINICAL PHARMACOLOGY

Phendimetrazine Tartrate is a sympathomimetic amine with pharmacologic activity similar to the prototype drugs of this class used in obesity, the amphetamines. Actions include central nervous system stimulation and elevation of blood pressure. Tachyphylaxis and tolerance have been demonstrated with all drugs of this class in which these phenomena have been looked for.

Drugs of this class used in obesity are commonly known as "anorectics" or "anorexigenics". It has not been established, however, that the action of such drugs in treating obesity is primarily one of appetite suppression. Other central nervous system actions, or metabolic effects, may be involved, for example.

Adult obese subjects instructed in dietary management and treated with "anorectic" drugs lose more weight on the average than those treated with placebo and diet, as determined in relatively short-term clinical trials.

The magnitude of increased weight loss of drug-treated patients over placebo-treated patients is only a fraction of a pound a week. The rate of weight loss is greatest in the first weeks of therapy for both drug and placebo subjects and tends to decrease in succeeding weeks. The possible origins of the increased weight loss due to the various drug effects are not established. The amount of weight loss associated with the use of an "anorectic" drug varies from trial to trial, and the increased weight loss appears to be related in part to variables other than the drug prescribed, such as the physician-investigator, the population treated, and the diet prescribed. Studies do not permit conclusions as to the relative importance of the drug and nondrug factors on weight loss.

The natural history of obesity is measured in years, whereas the studies cited are restricted to a few weeks' duration; thus, the total impact of drug-induced weight loss over that of diet alone must be considered clinically limited.

The active drug, 105 mg of Phendimetrazine Tartrate in each capsule of the special timed or slow release dosage form, approximates the action of three 25 mg non-timed doses taken at four-hour intervals.

The major route of elimination is via the kidneys where most of the drug and metabolites are excreted. Some of the drug is metabolized to phenmetrazine and also phendimetrazine-N-oxide.

The average half-life of elimination when studied under controlled conditions is about 3.7 hours for both the timed and nontimed forms. Others have shown the average half-life of elimination when studied under controlled conditions is about 1.9 hours for the nontimed and 9.8 hours for the slow-released dosage form. The absorption half-life of the drug from conventional nontimed 35 mg Phendimetrazine Tartrate tablets is appreciably more rapid than the absorption rate of the drug from the timed release formulation.

The absorption half-life of the drug from conventional nontimed 25 mg Phendimetrazine tablets is approximately the same. These data indicate that the slow-release product has a similar onset of action to the conventional nontime-release product and, in addition, has a prolonged therapeutic effect.

INDICATIONS AND USAGE

Phendimetrazine Tartrate is indicated in the management of exogenous obesity as a short-term adjunct (a few weeks) in a regimen of weight reduction based on caloric restriction. The limited usefulness of agents of this class (see *"Clinical Pharmacology"*) should be measured against possible risk factors inherent in their use such as those described below.

CONTRAINDICATIONS

Advanced arteriosclerosis, symptomatic cardiovascular disease, moderate to severe hypertension, hyperthyroidism, known hypersensitivity or idiosyncrasy to the sympathomimetic amines, glaucoma.

Agitated states.

Patients with a history of drug abuse.

Patients taking other CNS stimulants.

During or within 14 days following the administration of monoamine oxidase inhibitors (hypertensive crises may result).

WARNINGS

Tolerance to the anorectic effect usually develops within a few weeks. When this occurs, the recommended dose should not be exceeded in an attempt to increase the effect; rather, the drug should be discontinued.

Abrupt cessation of administration following prolonged high dosage results in extreme fatigue and depression.

Phendimetrazine Tartrate may impair the ability of the patient to engage in potentially hazardous activities such as operating machinery or driving a motor vehicle; the patient should therefore be cautioned accordingly.

DRUG DEPENDENCE

Phendimetrazine Tartrate is related chemically and pharmacologically to the amphetamines. Amphetamines and related stimulant drugs have been extensively abused, and the possibility of abuse of Phendimetrazine Tartrate should be kept in mind when evaluating the desirability of including a drug as part of a weight reduction program. Abuse of amphetamines and related drugs may be associated with intense psychological dependence and severe social dysfunction. There are reports of patients who have increased the dosage to many times that recommended. Abrupt cessation following prolonged high dosage administration results in extreme fatigue and mental depression; changes are also noted on the sleep EEG. Manifestations of chronic intoxication with anorectic drugs include severe dermatoses, marked insomnia, irritability, hyperactivity, and personality changes. The most severe manifestation of chronic intoxication is psychosis, often clinically indistinguishable from schizophrenia.

Usage in Pregnancy: The safety of Phendimetrazine Tartrate in pregnancy and lactation has not been established. Therefore Phendimetrazine Tartrate should not be taken by women who are or may become pregnant unless, in the opinion of the physician, the potential benefits outweight the possible hazards.

Usage in Children: Phendimetrazine Tartrate is not recommended for use in children under 12 years of age.

PRECAUTIONS

Caution is to be exercised in prescribing Phendimetrazine Tartrate for patients with even mild hypertension.

Insulin requirements in diabetes mellitus may be altered in association with the use of Phendimetrazine Tartrate and the concomitant dietary regimen.

Phendimetrazine Tartrate may decrease the hypotensive effect of guanethidine.

The least amount feasible should be prescribed or dispensed at one time in order to minimize the possibility of overdosage.

ADVERSE REACTIONS

Cardiovascular: Palpitation, tachycardia, elevation of blood pressure.

Central Nervous System: Overstimulation, restlessness, dizziness, insomnia, euphoria, dysphoria, tremor, headache; rarely psychotic episodes at recommended doses, agitation, flushing, sweating, blurring of vision.

Gastrointestinal: Dryness of the mouth, unpleasant taste, diarrhea, constipation, nausea, stomach pain, other gastrointestinal disturbances.

Allergic: Urticaria.

Endocrine: Impotence, changes in libido, urinary frequency, dysuria.

OVERDOSAGE

Manifestations of acute overdosage with Phendimetrazine Tartrate include restlessness, tremor, hyperreflexia, rapid respiration, confusion, assaultiveness, hallucinations, panic states.

Fatigue and depression usually follow the central stimulation.

Cardiovascular effects include arrhythmias, hypertension or hypotension and circulatory collapse. Gastrointestinal symptoms include nausea, vomiting, diarrhea, and abdominal cramps. Poisoning may result in convulsions, coma, and death. Management of acute Phendimetrazine Tartrate intoxication is largely symptomatic and includes lavage and sedation with a barbiturate. Experience with hemodialysis or peritoneal dialysis is inadequate to permit recommendation in this regard. Acidification of the urine increases Phendimetrazine Tartrate excretion. Intravenous phentolamine has been suggested for possible acute, severe hypertension, if this complicates Phendimetrazine Tartrate overdosage.

DOSAGE AND ADMINISTRATION

1 tablet (35 mg) b.i.d. or t.i.d., one hour before meals.

Dosage should be individualized to obtain an adequate response with the lowest effective dosage. In some cases, ½ tablet per dose may be adequate; dosage should not exceed 2 tablets t.i.d.. Limit to one timed release capsule (105 mg Phendimetrazine Tartrate) in the morning, or one slow-release capsule taken 30 to 60 minutes before the morning meal.

Phendimetrazine Tartrate is not recommended for use in children under 12 years of age.

Store at controlled room temperature, 15°-30°C (59°-86°F).

HOW SUPPLIED
CAPSULE, EXTENDED RELEASE (C-III): 105 MG

BRAND/MANUFACTURER	NDC	SIZE	AWP
◇ **BRAND**			
BONTRIL SLOW-RELEASE: Carnrick	00086-0047-10	100s	$24.75
PRELU-2: Boehr Ingelheim	00597-0064-01	100s	$95.16
◇ **GENERICS**			
Allscrips	54569-2198-02	7s	$3.32
Allscrips	54569-2198-00	14s	$6.65
Allscrips	54569-2198-10	30s	$14.94
Rexar	00478-5462-01	100s	$20.75
ANOREX-SR: Dunhall	00217-2819-01	100s	$29.00
Rexar	00478-5462-02	250s	$45.60
Rexar	00478-5462-05	500s	$76.42
Rexar	00478-5462-10	1000s	$128.20

CAPSULE, EXTENDED RELEASE (C-III): 105 MG

BRAND/MANUFACTURER	NDC	SIZE	AWP
○ **BRAND**			
APPECON: Lunsco	10892-0117-10	100s	$59.88

TABLETS (C-III): 35 MG

AVERAGE UNIT PRICE (AVAILABLE SIZES)		GENERIC A-RATED AVERAGE PRICE (GAAP)	
BRAND	$0.26	100s	$6.61
GENERIC	$0.04	1000s	$32.29
HCFA FUL (100s ea)	$0.07	1008s	$25.86
		5000s	$198.55

BRAND/MANUFACTURER	NDC	SIZE	AWP
◆ **BRAND**			
BONTRIL PDM: Carnrick	00086-0048-10	100s	$10.35
PLEGINE: Wyeth-Ayerst	00046-0755-81	100s	$62.55
BONTRIL PDM: Carnrick	00086-0048-90	1000s	$61.25
◆ **GENERICS**			
Eon	00185-4057-01	100s	$5.10
Camall	00147-0107-10	100s	$5.73
Rexar	00478-5460-01	100s	$9.00
Eon	00185-4057-10	1000s	$21.40
Eon	00185-4095-10	1000s	$21.40
Parmed	00349-8039-10	1000s	$21.99
Eon	00185-4057-10	1000s	$23.05
Rosemont	00832-0202-10	1000s	$25.25
Rugby	00536-5617-10	1000s	$25.58
Major	00904-4270-80	1000s	$26.80
Moore,H.L.	00839-5108-16	1000s	$28.34
Moore,H.L.	00839-5955-16	1000s	$28.34
Moore,H.L.	00839-5955-16	1000s	$28.34
Camall	00147-0107-20	1000s	$30.30
PHENDIMET: Parmed	00349-8648-10	1000s	$33.80

BRAND/MANUFACTURER	NDC	SIZE	AWP
Camall	00147-0103-20	1000s	$33.91
Camall	00147-0105-20	1000s	$33.91
Camall	00147-0106-20	1000s	$33.91
Camall	00147-0135-20	1000s	$38.77
Rexar	00478-5458-10	1000s	$52.80
Rexar	00478-5459-10	1000s	$52.80
Rexar	00478-5460-10	1000s	$52.80
OBEZINE: Jones-Western	52604-9143-08	1008s	$25.86
OBEZINE: Jones-Western	52604-9145-08	1008s	$25.86
OBEZINE: Jones-Western	52604-9146-08	1008s	$25.86
OBEZINE: Jones-Western	52604-9147-08	1008s	$25.86
Camall	00147-0107-30	5000s	$112.66
Rexar	00478-5460-50	5000s	$226.80
Rexar	00478-5458-50	5000s	$256.20

TABLETS (C-III): 105 MG

BRAND/MANUFACTURER	NDC	SIZE	AWP
○ **BRAND**			
MELFIAT: Numark	00032-1082-01	100s	$82.20

Phenelzine Sulfate

DESCRIPTION

Phenelzine Sulfate belongs to the class of drugs known as monoamine oxidase (MAO) inhibitors.

Chemically it is phenethylhydrazine sulfate, a hydrazine derivative.

Its molecular weight: 234.27

Each Phenelzine Sulfate tablet for oral administration contains Phenelzine Sulfate equivalent to 15 mg of Phenelzine base.

Following is its chemical structure:

$CH_2CH_2NHNH_2$ · H_2SO_4

ACTIONS

Monoamine oxidase is a complex enzyme system, widely distributed throughout the body. Drugs that inhibit monoamine oxidase in the laboratory are associated with a number of clinical effects. Thus, it is unknown whether MAO inhibition *per se*, other pharmacologic actions, or an interaction of both is responsible for the clinical effects observed. Therefore, the physician should become familiar with all the effects produced by drugs of this class.

All the currently employed MAO inhibitors are readily absorbed when given by mouth. They are not given parenterally. These drugs produce maximal inhibition of MAO in biopsy samples from man within 5 to 10 days. There is little information on their pharmacokinetics. However, their biological activity is prolonged due to the characteristics of their interaction with the enzyme.

INDICATIONS

Phenelzine Sulfate has been found to be effective in depressed patients clinically characterized as "atypical," "nonendogenous," or "neurotic." These patients often have mixed anxiety and depression and phobic or hypochondriacal features. There is less conclusive evidence of its usefulness with severely depressed patients with endogenous features.

Phenelzine Sulfate should rarely be the first antidepressant drug used. Rather, it is more suitable for use with patients who have failed to respond to the drugs more commonly used for these conditions.

UNLABELED USES

Phenelzine Sulfate is used alone or as an adjunct in the treatment of bulimia nervosa, agoraphobia with panic attacks, globus hystericus syndrome, and chronic headache. It is also used in orthostatic hypotension, refractory migraine headache, narcolepsy, obsessive-compulsive disorder, panic attacks, posttraumatic stress disorder, and social phobia.

CONTRAINDICATIONS

Phenelzine Sulfate is contraindicated in patients with known sensitivity to the drug, pheochromocytoma, congestive heart failure, a history of liver disease, or abnormal liver function tests.

The potentiation of sympathomimetic substances and related compounds by MAO inhibitors may result in hypertensive crises. (See *"Warnings".*) Therefore, patients being treated with Phenelzine Sulfate should not take *sympathomimetic drugs* (including amphetamines, cocaine, methylphenidate, dopamine, epinephrine and norepinephrine) or related compounds (including methyldopa, L-dopa, L-tryptophan, L-tyrosine, and phenylalanine). Hypertensive crises during Phenelzine therapy may also be caused by the ingestion of foods with a high concentration of tyramine or dopamine. Therefore, patients being treated with Phenelzine should avoid high protein food that has undergone protein breakdown by aging, fermentation, pickling, smoking, or bacterial contamination; patients should also avoid cheeses (especially aged varieties), pickled herring, beer, wine, liver, yeast extract (including brewer's yeast in large quantities), dry sausage (including Genoa salami, hard salami, pepperoni, and Lebanon bologna), pods of broad beans (Fava beans), and yogurt. Excessive amounts of caffeine and chocolate may also cause hypertensive reactions.

◆ RATED THERAPEUTICALLY EQUIVALENT; ◇ THERAPEUTIC EQUIVALENCE UNCONFIRMED; ○ UNRATED

Phenelzine should not be used in combination with dextromethorphan or with CNS depressants such as alcohol and certain narcotics. Excitation, seizures, delirium, hyperpyrexia, circulatory collapse, coma, and death have been reported in patients receiving MAOI therapy who have been given a single dose of meperidine. Phenelzine should not be administered together with or in rapid succession to other MAO inhibitors because *Hypertensive Crises* and convulsive seizures, fever, marked sweating, excitation, delirium, tremor, coma, and circulatory collapse may occur.

List of MAO Inhibitors
(Generic Name):
pargyline hydrochloride
pargyline hydrochloride and methyclothiazide furazolidone
isocarboxazid
procarbazine
tranylcypromine

Phenelzine should also not be used in combination with buspirone HCl, since several cases of elevated blood pressure have been reported in patients taking MAO inhibitors who were then given buspirone HCl. At least 10 days should elapse between the discontinuation of Phenelzine Sulfate and the institution of another antidepressant or buspirone HCl, or the discontinuation of another MAO inhibitor and the institution of Phenelzine.

There have been reports of serious reactions (including hyperthermia, rigidity, myoclonic movements and death) when fluoxetine has been combined with an MAO inhibitor. Therefore, Phenelzine should not be used in combination with fluoxetine. Allow at least five weeks between discontinuation of fluoxetine and initiation of Phenelzine and at least 10 days between discontinuation of Phenelzine and initiation of fluoxetine. The combination of MAO inhibitors and tryptophan has been reported to cause behavioral and neurologic syndromes including disorientation, confusion, amnesia, delirium, agitation, hypomanic signs, ataxia, myoclonus, hyperreflexia, shivering, ocular oscillations and Babinski signs.

The concurrent administration of an MAO inhibitor and bupropion hydrochloride is contraindicated. At least 14 days should elapse between discontinuation of an MAO inhibitor and initiation of treatment with bupropion hydrochloride.

Patients taking Phenelzine should not undergo elective surgery requiring general anesthesia. Also, they should not be given cocaine or local anesthesia containing sympathomimetic vasoconstrictors. The possible combined hypotensive effects of Phenelzine and spinal anesthesia should be kept in mind. Phenelzine Sulfate should be discontinued at least 10 days prior to elective surgery.

MAO inhibitors including Phenelzine are contraindicated in patients receiving guanethidine.

WARNINGS

The most serious reactions to Phenelzine involve changes in blood pressure.

Hypertensive Crises: The most important reaction associated with Phenelzine administration is the occurrence of hypertensive crises, which have sometimes been fatal.

These crises are characterized by some or all of the following symptoms: occipital headache which may radiate frontally, palpitation, neck stiffness or soreness, nausea, vomiting, sweating (sometimes with fever and sometimes with cold, clammy skin), dilated pupils, and photophobia. Either tachycardia or bradycardia may be present and can be associated with constricting chest pain.

Note: Intracranial bleeding has been reported in association with the increase in blood pressure.

Blood pressure should be observed frequently to detect evidence of any pressor response in all patients receiving Phenelzine. Therapy should be discontinued immediately upon the occurrence of palpitation or frequent headaches during therapy.

Recommended Treatment in Hypertensive Crisis: If a hypertensive crisis occurs Phenelzine should be discontinued immediately and therapy to lower blood pressure should be instituted immediately. On the basis of present evidence, phentolamine is recommended. (The dosage reported for phentolamine is 5 mg intravenously.) Care should be taken to administer this drug slowly in order to avoid producing an excessive hypotensive effect. Fever should be managed by means of external cooling.

Warning to the Patient: All patients should be warned that the following foods, beverages and medications must be avoided while taking Phenelzine, and for two weeks after discontinuing use.

FOODS AND BEVERAGES TO AVOID
Meat and Fish
Pickled herring
Liver
Dry sausage (including Genoa salami, hard salami, pepperoni, and Lebanon bologna)

Vegetables
Broad bean pods (fava bean pods)
Sauerkraut

Dairy Products
Cheese (cottage cheese and cream cheese are allowed)
Yogurt

Beverages
Beer and wine
Alcohol-free and reduced-alcohol beer and wine products
Miscellaneous
Yeast extract (including brewer's yeast in large quantities)
Meat extract
Excessive amounts of chocolate and caffeine

Also, any spoiled or improperly refrigerated, handled or stored protein-rich foods such as meats, fish, and dairy products, including foods that may have undergone protein changes by aging, pickling, fermentation, or smoking to improve flavor should be avoided.

OTC MEDICATIONS TO AVOID
Cold and cough preparations (including those containing dextromethorphan)
Nasal decongestants (tablets, drops or spray)
Hay-fever medications
Sinus medications
Asthma inhalant medications
Antiappetite medicines
Weight-reducing preparations
"Pep" pills
L-tryptophan containing preparations
Also, certain prescription drugs should be avoided. Therefore, patients under the care of another physician or dentist, should inform him/her they are taking Phenelzine.

Patients should be warned that the use of the above foods, beverages or medications may cause a reaction characterized by headache and other serious symptoms due to a rise in blood pressure, with the exception of dextromethorphan which may cause reactions similar to those seen with meperidine. Also, there has been a report of an interaction between Phenelzine and dextromethorphan (ingested as a lozenge) causing drowsiness and bizarre behavior.

Patients should be instructed to report promptly the occurrence of headache or other unusual symptoms.

PRECAUTIONS

General: In depressed patients, the possibility of suicide should always be considered and adequate precautions taken. It is recommended that careful observations of patients undergoing Phenelzine treatment be maintained until control of depression is achieved. If necessary, additional measures (ECT, hospitalization, etc.) should be instituted.

All patients undergoing treatment with Phenelzine should be closely followed for symptoms of postural hypotension. Hypotensive side effects have occurred in hypertensive as well as normal and hypotensive patients. Blood pressure usually returns to pretreatment levels rapidly when the drug is discontinued or the dosage is reduced.

Because the effect of Phenelzine on the convulsive threshold may be variable, adequate precautions should be taken when treating epileptic patients.

Of the more severe side effects that have been reported with any consistency, hypomania has been the most common. This reaction has been largely limited to patients in whom disorders characterized by hyperkinetic symptoms coexist with, but are obscured by, depressive affect; hypomania usually appeared as depression improved. If agitation is present, it may be increased with Phenelzine. Hypomania and agitation have also been reported at higher than recommended doses, or following long-term therapy.

Phenelzine may cause excessive stimulation in schizophrenic patients; in manic-depressive states it may result in a swing from a depressive to a manic phase.

MAO inhibitors, including Phenelzine potentiate hexobarbital hypnosis in animals. Therefore, barbiturates should be given at a reduced dose with Phenelzine.

MAO inhibitors inhibit the destruction of serotonin and norepinephrine, which are believed to be released from tissue stores by rauwolfia alkaloids. Accordingly, caution should be exercised when rauwolfia is used concomitantly with an MAO inhibitor, including Phenelzine.

There is conflicting evidence as to whether or not MAO inhibitors affect glucose metabolism or potentiate hypoglycemic agents. This should be kept in mind if Phenelzine is administered to diabetics.

Phenelzine, as with other hydrazine derivatives, has been reported to induce pulmonary and vascular tumors in an uncontrolled lifetime study in mice.

Information for Patients: See "To the Patients" in the "Warning" section.

Drug Interactions: See "Contraindications" and "Warnings" sections for additional drug interactions.

Phenelzine Sulfate should be used with caution in combination with antihypertensive drugs, including thiazide diuretics and β-blockers, since exaggerated hypotensive effects may result.

Concomitant Use with Dibenzazepine Derivative Drugs: If the decision is made to administer Phenelzine Sulfate concurrently with other antidepressant drugs, or within less than 10 days after discontinuation of antidepressant therapy, the patient should be cautioned by the physician regarding the possibility of adverse drug interaction.

List of Dibenzazepine Derivative Drugs:
nortriptyline hydrochloride,
amitriptyline hydrochloride,
perphenazine and amitriptyline hydrochloride,
clomipramine hydrochloride,

➤ SHOWN IN PRODUCT IDENTIFICATION GUIDE

desipramine hydrochloride,
imipramine hydrochloride,
doxepin,
carbamazepine,
cyclobenzaprine hydrochloride,
amoxapine,
maprotiline hydrochloride,
trimipramine maleate,
protriptyline hydrochloride

Pregnancy Category C: Phenelzine has been shown to have an adverse effect in mice when given in doses well exceeding the maximum recommended human dose. There are no adequate and well-controlled studies in pregnant women. Phenelzine should be used during pregnancy only if the potential benefit justifies the potential risk to the fetus.

Doses of Phenelzine in pregnant mice well exceeding the maximum recommended human dose have caused a significant decrease in the number of viable offspring per mouse. In addition, the growth of young dogs and rats has been retarded by doses exceeding the maximum human dose.

Nursing Mothers: It is not known whether this drug is excreted in human milk. Because many drugs are excreted in human milk and because of the potential for serious adverse reactions in nursing infants from Phenelzine, a decision should be made whether to discontinue the drug, taking into account the importance of the drug to the mother.

Pediatric Use: Phenelzine is not recommended for patients under 16 years of age, since there are no controlled studies of safety in this age group.

ADVERSE REACTIONS

Phenelzine is a potent inhibitor of monoamine oxidase. Because this enzyme is widely distributed throughout the body, diverse pharmacologic effects can be expected to occur. When they occur, such effects tend to be mild or moderate in severity (see below), often subside as treatment continues, and can be minimized by adjusting dosage; rarely is it necessary to institute counteracting measures or to discontinue Phenelzine.

Common side effects include:

Nervous System: Dizziness, headache, drowsiness, sleep disturbances (including insomnia and hypersomnia), fatigue, weakness, tremors, twitching, myoclonic movements, hyperreflexia.

Gastrointestinal: Constipation, dry mouth, gastrointestinal disturbances, elevated serum transaminases (without accompanying signs and symptoms).

Metabolic: Weight gain.

Cardiovascular: Postural hypotension, edema.

Genitourinary: Sexual disturbances, ie, anorgasmia and ejaculatory disturbances:

Less common mild to moderate side effects (some of which have been reported in a single patient or by a single physician) include:

Nervous System: Jitteriness, palilalia, euphoria, nystagmus, paresthesias.

Genitourinary: Urinary retention.

Metabolic: Hypernatremia.

Dermatologic: Skin rash, sweating.

Special senses: Blurred vision, glaucoma.

Although reported less frequently, and sometimes only once, additional severe side effects include:

Nervous System: Ataxia, shock-like coma, toxic delirium, manic reaction, convulsions, acute anxiety reaction, precipitation of schizophrenia, transient respiratory and cardiovascular depression following ECT.

Gastrointestinal: To date, fatal progressive necrotizing hepatocellular damage has been reported in a very few patients. Reversible jaundice.

Hematologic: Leukopenia.

Metabolic: Hypermetabolic syndrome (which may include, but is not limited to, hyperpyrexia, tachycardia, tachypnea, muscular rigidity, elevated CK levels, metabolic acidosis, hypoxia, coma and may resemble an overdose).

Respiratory: Edema of the glottis.
Withdrawal may be associated with nausea, vomiting and malaise.

General: Fever associated with increased muscle tone.

An uncommon withdrawal syndrome following abrupt withdrawal of Phenelzine has been infrequently reported. Signs and symptoms of this syndrome generally commence 24 to 72 hours after drug discontinuation and may range from vivid nightmares with agitation to frank psychosis and convulsions. This syndrome generally responds to reinstitution of low-dose Phenelzine therapy followed by cautious downward titration and discontinuation.

OVERDOSAGE

Note: For management of *hypertensive crises* see "Warnings" section.

Accidental or intentional overdosage may be more common in patients who are depressed. It should be remembered that multiple drugs and/or alcohol may have been ingested.

Depending on the amount of overdosage with Phenelzine a varying and mixed clinical picture may develop, involving signs and symptoms of central nervous system and cardiovascular stimulation and/or depression. Signs and symptoms may be absent or minimal during the initial 12-hour period following ingestion and may develop slowly thereafter, reaching a maximum in 24-48 hours. Death has been reported following overdosage. Therefore, immediate hospitalization, with continuous patient observation and monitoring throughout this period, is essential.

Signs and symptoms of overdosage may include, alone or in combination, any of the following: drowsiness, dizziness, faintness, irritability, hyperactivity, agitation, severe headache, hallucinations, trismus, opisthotonus, convulsions and coma; rapid and irregular pulse, hypertension, hypotension and vascular collapse; precordial pain, respiratory depression and failure, hyperpyrexia, diaphoresis, and cool, clammy skin.

Intensive symptomatic and supportive treatment may be required. Induction of emesis or gastric lavage with instillation of charcoal slurry may be helpful in early poisoning, provided the airway has been protected against aspiration. Signs and symptoms of central nervous system stimulation, including convulsions, should be treated with diazepam, given slowly intravenously. Phenothiazine derivatives and central nervous system stimulants should be avoided. Hypotension and vascular collapse should be treated with intravenous fluids and, if necessary, blood pressure titration with an intravenous infusion of dilute pressor agent. It should be noted that adrenergic agents may produce a markedly increased pressor response.

Respiration should be supported by appropriate measures, including management of the airway, use of supplemental oxygen, and mechanical ventilatory assistance, as required. Body temperature should be monitored closely. Intensive management of hyperpyrexia may be required. Maintenance of fluid and electrolyte balance is essential.

There are no data on the lethal dose in man. The pathophysiologic effects of massive overdosage may persist for several days, since the drug acts by inhibiting physiologic enzyme systems. With symptomatic and supportive measures, recovery from *mild* overdosage may be expected within 3 to 4 days. Hemodialysis, peritoneal dialysis, and charcoal hemoperfusion may be of value in massive overdosage, but sufficient data are not available to recommend their routine use in these cases.

Toxic blood levels of Phenelzine have not been established, and assay methods are not practical for clinical or toxicological use.

DOSAGE AND ADMINISTRATION

Initial Dose: the usual starting dose of Phenelzine is one tablet (15 mg) three times a day.

Early Phase Treatment: Dosage should be increased to at least 60 mg per day at a fairly rapid pace consistent with patient tolerance. It may be necessary to increase dosage up to 90 mg per day to obtain sufficient MAO inhibition. Many patients do not show a clinical response until treatment at 60 mg has been continued for at least 4 weeks.

Maintenance Dose: After maximum benefit from Phenelzine is achieved, dosage should be reduced slowly over several weeks. Maintenance dose may be as low as 1 tablet, 15 mg, a day or every other day, and should be continued for as long as is required.

Storage: Store tablets between 15°-30°C (59°-86°F).

HOW SUPPLIED
TABLETS: 15 MG

BRAND/MANUFACTURER	NDC	SIZE	AWP
○ BRAND			
NARDIL: Parke-Davis	00071-0270-24	100s	$38.32

Phenergan *SEE* PROMETHAZINE HYDROCHLORIDE

Phenergan VC *SEE* PHENYLEPHRINE HYDROCHLORIDE AND PROMETHAZINE HYDROCHLORIDE

Phenergan VC with Codeine
SEE CODEINE PHOSPHATE/PHENYLEPHRINE HYDROCHLORIDE/ PROMETHAZINE HYDROCHLORIDE

Phenergan with Codeine *SEE* CODEINE PHOSPHATE AND PROMETHAZINE HYDROCHLORIDE

Phenergan with DM *SEE* DEXTROMETHORPHAN HYDROBROMIDE AND PROMETHAZINE HYDROCHLORIDE

◆ RATED THERAPEUTICALLY EQUIVALENT; ◇ THERAPEUTIC EQUIVALENCE UNCONFIRMED; ○ UNRATED

Pheniramine Maleate/ Phenylpropanolamine Hydrochloride/Phenyltoloxamine Citrate/Pyrilamine Citrate

DESCRIPTION

Each teaspoonful (5 ml) contains:

Phenylpropanolamine HCl ....12.5 mg
Phenyltoloxamine Citrate ....4.0 mg
Pyrilamine Maleate ....4.0 mg
Pheniramine Maleate ....4.0 mg
Alcohol 4%

Antihistamine/Decongestant.

INDICATIONS

Pheniramine Maleate/Phenylpropanolamine Hydrochloride/Phenyltoloxamine Citrate/Pyrilamine Maleate (Pheniramine/PPA/Phenyltoloxamine/Pyrilamine) is indicated for the relief of respiratory congestion accompanying allergic rhinitis, or sinusitis.

CONTRAINDICATIONS

Generally contraindicated for individuals who are sensitive or allergic to any of the components.

PRECAUTIONS

Use with caution in patients with hyperthyroidism, hypertension, cardiovascular disease, diabetes mellitus or urinary retention. Drowsiness may occur due to the antihistaminic components. Patients should be cautioned against driving or operating machinery if this occurs.

ADVERSE REACTIONS

Adverse reactions to Pheniramine/PPA/Phenyltoloxamine/Pyrilamine may include nervousness, dry mouth and throat, headache, dizziness, paresthesia and nausea.

DOSAGE AND ADMINISTRATION

Adults - 2 teaspoonful every 4 hours. Children 6 to 12 years - 1 teaspoonful every 4 hours. Children 2 to 6 years - 1/2 teaspoonful every 4 hours. Children under 2 years - as directed by a physician.

Keep this and all drugs out of the reach of children.

Store between 59°-86°F (15°-30°C). Dispense in tight, light resistant containers as defined in the USP/NF.

HOW SUPPLIED
CAPSULE:

BRAND/MANUFACTURER	NDC	SIZE	AWP
○ GENERICS			
POLY-HISTINE-D: Bock	00563-1658-01	100s	$43.33
➤ POLY-HISTINE-D: Bock	00563-1656-01	100s	$62.28

ELIXIR:

BRAND/MANUFACTURER	NDC	SIZE	AWP
○ GENERICS			
POLY-D: Alphagen	59743-0107-16	480 ml	$16.40
METAHISTINE D: Moore,H.L.	00839-7846-69	480 ml	$18.89
POLY D: Qualitest	00603-1528-58	480 ml	$18.91
UNI-MULTIHIST D: URL	00677-1489-33	480 ml	$19.04
DELHISTINE D: Rugby	00536-2702-85	480 ml	$19.71
METAHISTINE D: Econolab	55053-0830-16	480 ml	$19.95
POLY-HISTINE-D: Bock	00563-1662-16	480 ml	$22.57
TRIHIST-D: Aligen	00405-3878-16	480 ml	$22.94

Pheniramine Maleate/ Phenylpropanolamine Hydrochloride/Pyrilamine Maleate

DESCRIPTION

Each mL of Pheniramine Maleate/Phenylpropanolamine Hydrochloride/Pyrilamine Maleate Oral Infant Drops contains: Phenylpropanolamine Hydrochloride 20 mg, Pheniramine Maleate 10 mg, and Pyrilamine Maleate 10 mg.

This product combines the nasal decongestant properties of Phenylpropanolamine Hydrochloride with the antihistaminic activities of Pheniramine Maleate and Pyrilamine Maleate.

Phenylpropanolamine Hydrochloride, a sympathomimetic drug, is structurally related to ephedrine and amphetamine. Pheniramine Maleate is an anthistamine of the alkylamine class while Pyrilamine Maleate belongs to the ethylenediamine class.

CLINICAL PHARMACOLOGY

Phenylpropanolamine presumably acts on α-adrenergic receptors in the mucosa of the respiratory tract producing vasoconstriction which results in shrinkage of swollen mucous membranes, reduction of tissue hyperemia, edema and nasal congestion, and an increase in nasal airway patency. Antihistamines competitively act as H_1 receptor antagonists of histamine. They exhibit anticholinergic (drying) and sedative side effects. There are several classes of antihistamines which vary with respect to potency, dosage and the relative incidence of side effects. Antihistamines inhibit the effects of histamine on capillary permeability and on vascular, bronchial and many other types of smooth muscle.

INDICATIONS AND USAGE

For relief from such symptoms as nasal congestion and postnasal drip associated with colds, allergies, sinusitis and rhinitis. Also for relief of symptoms associated with allergic rhinitis such as sneezing, rhinorrhea, pruritus and lacrimation.

CONTRAINDICATIONS

Pheniramine Maleate/Phenylpropanolamine Hydrochloride/Pyrilamine Maleate Oral Infant Drops are contraindicated in patients exhibiting hypersensitivity to any of the ingredients. Antihistamines are contraindicated in patients receiving monoamine oxidase inhibitors since these agents may prolong and intensify the anticholinergic and CNS depressant effects of antihistamines (see *"Drug Interactions"*). Antihistamines *should not* be used to treat lower respiratory tract symptoms or be given to premature or newborn infants. Sympathomimetic agents such as phenylpropanolamine are contraindicated in patients with severe hypertension, severe coronary artery disease and in those taking monoamine oxidase inhibitors.

WARNINGS

Rare fatalities have occurred with overdoses in children under six months of age.

Sympathomimetic agents should be used with caution in patients with hypertension, hyperthyroidism, diabetes mellitus and cardiovascular disease. Antihistamines should be used with caution in patients with narrow angle glaucoma, stenosing peptic ulcer, pyloroduodenal obstruction, symptomatic prostatic hypertrophy, bladder neck obstruction or chronic pulmonary disease.

PRECAUTIONS

General: see "Warnings".

Information For Patients: Antihistamines have additive effects with other CNS depressants (hypnotics, sedatives, tranquilizers, alcohol, etc.) Mothers should be informed of the potential for sedation or drowsiness when prescribing antihistamine preparations. Tell patient to adhere to dosing information. Patients should be cautioned against mechanical activity requiring alertness.

Drug Interactions:

(1) Monoamine oxidase inhibitors: MAO inhibitors prolong and intensify the anticholinergic effects of antihistamines and potentiate the pressor effects of sympathomimetics.

(2) Alcohol and CNS depressants: These agents potentiate the sedative effects of antihistamines.

(3) Certain antihypertensives: Sympathomimetics may reduce the antihypertensive effects of methyldopa, mecamylamine, reserpine and veratrum alkaloids.

Carcinogenesis, Mutagenesis, Impairment Of Fertility: No data are available on the long-term potential for carcinogenicity, mutagenicity or impairment of fertility in animals or humans.

Pediatric Use: Pheniramine Maleate/Phenylpropanolamine Hydrochloride/Pyrilamine Maleate Oral Infant Drops have been formulated to provide safe and effective symptomatic relief for infants and small children. Precise dosage (on a body weight basis) is facilitated through the use of the plastic squeeze bottle with attached dropper tip (see *"Dosage and Administration"*). It is important to note the variability of response infants and small children exhibit to antihistamines and sympathomimetics. As in adults, the combination of an antihistamine and sympathomimetic can elicit either mild stimulation or mild sedation in children. In the young child, mild stimulation is the response most frequently seen. In infants and children, overdosage of antihistamines may cause hallucinations, convulsions or death.

ADVERSE REACTIONS

The most frequent adverse reactions are italicized.

(1) General: urticaria, drug rash, anaphylactic shock, photosensitivity, excessive perspiration, chills, *dryness of mouth, nose, and throat.*

(2) Cardiovascular System: hypotension, headache, palpitations, tachycardia, extrasystoles.

(3) Hematologic System: hemolytic anemia, thrombocytopenia, agranulocytosis.

(4) Nervous System: sedation, sleepiness, dizziness, disturbed coordination, fatigue, confusion, restlessness, excitation, nervousness, tremor, irritability, insomnia, euphoria, paresthesias, blurred vision, diplopia, vertigo, tinnitus, acute labyrinthitis, hysteria, neuritis, convulsions, CNS depression, hallucinations.

(5) GI System: epigastric distress, anorexia, nausea, vomiting, diarrhea, constipation.

➤ SHOWN IN PRODUCT IDENTIFICATION GUIDE

(6) GU System: urinary frequency, difficult urination, urinary retention.

(7) Respiratory System: thickening of bronchial secretions, tightness of chest and wheezing, nasal stuffiness.

OVERDOSAGE

Pheniramine Maleate/Phenylpropanolamine Hydrochloride/Pyrilamine Maleate product overdosage reactions may vary from central nervous system depression to stimulation. Stimulation is particularly likely in children. Atropine-like signs and symptoms—dry mouth; fixed, dilated pupils; flushing —and gastrointestinal symptoms may also occur.

If vomiting has not occurred spontaneously, the conscious patient should be induced to vomit. This is best done by having the patient drink a glass of water or milk after which they should be made to gag. Precautions against aspiration must be taken, especially in infants and children.

If vomiting is unsuccessful, gastric lavage is indicated within 3 hours after ingestion, and even later if large amounts of milk or cream were given beforehand. Isotonic and ½ isotonic saline is the lavage solution of choice.

Saline cathartics, such as milk of magnesia, draw water by osmosis into the bowel and therefore are valuable for their action in rapid dilution of bowel content.

Stimulants should *not* be used. Vasopressors may be used to treat hypotension.

DOSAGE AND ADMINISTRATION

1 drop per 2 pounds of body weight administered orally 4 times daily. The prescribed number of drops may be put directly into child's mouth or on a spoon for administration.

Store Pheniramine Maleate/Phenylpropanolamine Hydrochloride/Pyrilamine Maleate Oral Infant Drops at room temperature.

HOW SUPPLIED
DROP: 20 MG-10 MG-10 MG/ML

BRAND/MANUFACTURER	NDC	SIZE	AWP
○ **BRAND**			
TRIAMINIC INFANT: Sandoz Consumer	00043-0506-15	15 ml	$10.84
GENERICS			
Aligen	00405-3530-61	15 ml	$6.95
LIQUI-MINIC: Liquipharm	54198-0139-15	15 ml	$7.75

TABLET, EXTENDED RELEASE: 20 MG-10 MG-10 MG

BRAND/MANUFACTURER	NDC	SIZE	AWP
○ **BRAND**			
TRIAMINIC TR: Sandoz Consumer	00043-0020-51	100s	$40.44

Pheniramine Maleate/ Phenyltoloxamine Citrate/ Pyrilamine Maleate

DESCRIPTION

Each teaspoonful (5 ml) contains:

Phenyltoloxamine Citrate	4.0 mg
Pyrilamine Maleate	4.0 mg
Pheniramine Maleate	4.0 mg
Alcohol	4%

INDICATIONS

Perennial and seasonal allergic rhinitis. Vasomotor rhinitis. Allergic conjunctivitis due to inhalant allergens and food. Mild, uncomplicated allergic skin manifestations of urticaria.

PRECAUTIONS

Patients should be cautioned against mechanical activities requiring alertness such as driving an automobile or working with machinery.

ADVERSE REACTIONS

Drowsiness, nervousness, dry mouth and throat, headaches, dizziness, paresthesia and nausea.

Keep this and all drugs out of the reach of children.

DOSAGE AND ADMINISTRATION

Adults—2 teaspoonsful every 4 hours. Children 6 to 12 years—1 teaspoonful every 4 hours. Children 2 to 6 years—½ teaspoonful every 4 hours. Children under 2 years—as directed by a physician.

Store between 59°-86° F (15°-30° C)

Dispense in tight, light-resistant containers as defined in the USP/NF.

HOW SUPPLIED
ELIXIR:

BRAND/MANUFACTURER	NDC	SIZE	AWP
○ **BRAND**			
POLY-HISTINE: Bock	00563-1647-16	480 ml	$22.57

Phenobarbital

DESCRIPTION

The barbiturates are nonselective central nervous system (CNS) depressants that are primarily used as sedative-hypnotics. In subhypnotic doses, they are also used as anticonvulsants. The barbiturates and their sodium salts are subject to control under the Federal Controlled Substances Act.

Phenobarbital is a barbituric acid derivative and occurs as white, odorless, small crystals or crystalline powder that is very slightly soluble in water; soluble in alcohol, in ether, and in solutions of fixed alkali hydroxides and carbonates; sparingly soluble in chloroform. The sodium salt of Phenobarbital which is available as an injection occurs as a white, slightly bitter powder crystalline granules or flaky crystals; it is soluble in alcohol and practically insoluble in ether or chloroform. Phenobarbital is 5-ethyl-5-phenylbarbituric acid and has the empirical formula $C_{12}H_{12}N_2O_3$. Its molecular weight is 232.24. Phenobarbital sodium has the empirical formula $C_{12}H_{11}N_2NaO_3$ and the molecular weight 254.22.

Phenobarbital is a substituted pyrimidine derivative in which the basic structure is barbituric acid, a substance that has no CNS activity. CNS activity is obtained by substituting alkyl, alkenyl, or aryl groups on the pyrimidine ring. Phenobarbital is available as an elixir and tablets, Phenobarbital sodium as a sterile solution for intramuscular (IM) or slow intravenous (IV) administration as a long-acting barbiturate.

Each 5 ml of the elixir contains:
Phenobarbital ....20 mg (0.086 mmol)

The tablets contain:
Phenobarbital ....15 mg (0.064 mmol), 30 mg (0.129 mmol), 60 mg (0.258 mmol), or 100 mg (0.431 mmol)

Each ml of solution for injection contains:
Phenobarbital Sodium ....65 or 130 mg

Following is its chemical structure:

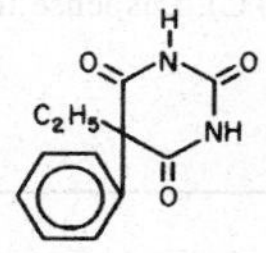

CLINICAL PHARMACOLOGY

Barbiturates are capable of producing all levels of CNS mood alteration, from excitation to mild sedation, hypnosis, and deep coma. Overdosage can produce death. In high enough therapeutic doses, barbiturates induce anesthesia.

Barbiturates depress the sensory cortex, decrease motor activity, alter cerebellar function, and produce drowsiness, sedation, and hypnosis.

Barbiturate-induced sleep differs from physiologic sleep. Sleep laboratory studies have demonstrated that barbiturates reduce the amount of time spent in the rapid eye movement (REM) phase of sleep or the dreaming stage. Also, Stages III and IV sleep are decreased. Following abrupt cessation of barbiturates used regularly, patients may experience markedly increased dreaming, nightmares, and/or insomnia. Therefore, withdrawal of a single therapeutic dose over 5 or 6 days has been recommended to lessen the REM rebound and disturbed sleep that contribute to drug-withdrawal syndrome (for example, the dose should be decreased from 3 to 2 doses/day for 1 week).

In studies, secobarbital sodium and pentobarbital sodium have been found to lose most of their effectiveness for both inducing and maintaining sleep by the end of 2 weeks of continued drug administration even with the use of multiple doses. As with secobarbital sodium and pentobarbital sodium, other barbiturates (including amobarbital) might be expected to lose their effectiveness for inducing and maintaining sleep after about 2 weeks. The short-, intermediate-, and to a lesser degree, long-acting barbiturates have been widely prescribed for treating insomnia. Although the clinical literature abounds with claims that the short-acting barbiturates are superior for producing sleep whereas the intermediate-acting compounds are more effective in maintaining sleep, controlled studies have failed to demonstrate these differential effects. Therefore, as sleep medications, the barbiturates are of limited value beyond short-term use.

Barbiturates have little analgesic action at subanesthetic doses. Rather, in subanesthetic doses, these drugs may increase the reaction to painful stimuli. All barbiturates exhibit anticonvulsant activity in anesthetic doses. However, of the

---

◆ RATED THERAPEUTICALLY EQUIVALENT; ◇ THERAPEUTIC EQUIVALENCE UNCONFIRMED; ○ UNRATED

drugs in this class, only Phenobarbital, mephobarbital, and metharbital are effective as oral anticonvulsants in subhypnotic doses.

Barbiturates are respiratory depressants by virtue of their direct effect on the medullary respiratory center. They diminish and, in high doses, may abolish the sensitivity of the respiratory center to its normal stimulus, carbon dioxide.

Ordinary hypnotic doses of barbiturates have no significant effect on the cardiovascular system. The barbiturates tend to decrease the tonus of the gastrointestinal musculature. They have no direct injurious effect on the normal kidney. Severe oliguria or anuria may occur in acute barbiturate poisoning, largely as a result of the marked hypotension.

Hypnotic doses tend to reduce slightly the metabolic rate in man. Body temperature is reduced slightly, owing to lessened activity and to depression of the central temperature-regulatory mechanisms.

While anesthetic doses of all barbiturates exert an anticonvulsant effect, Phenobarbital has a selective anticonvulsant activity independent of the degree of sedation produced. Phenobarbital limits the spread of seizures and raises the seizure threshold in grand mal (generalized tonic-clonic) epilepsy.

The degree of respiratory depression is dependent upon the dose. With hypnotic doses, respiratory depression produced by barbiturates is similar to that which occurs during physiologic sleep and is accompanied by a slight decrease in blood pressure and heart rate.

Studies in laboratory animals have shown that barbiturates cause reduction in the tone and contractility of the uterus, ureters, and urinary bladder. However, concentrations of the drugs required to produce this effect in humans are not reached with sedative-hypnotic doses.

Barbiturates do not impair normal hepatic function but have been shown to induce liver microsomal enzymes, thus increasing and/or altering the metabolism of barbiturates and other drugs (see *"Drug Interactions"* under *"Precautions"*).

Pharmacokinetics: Barbiturates are absorbed in varying degrees following oral or parenteral administration. Following IV administration, the onset of action is 5 minutes for Phenobarbital sodium. For IM administration, the onset of action is slightly slower. Maximal CNS depression may not occur until 15 minutes or more after IV administration. The salts are more rapidly absorbed than are the acids. The rate of absorption is increased if the sodium salt is ingested as a dilute solution or taken on an empty stomach.

Duration of action, which is related to the rate at which the barbiturates are redistributed throughout the body, varies among persons and in the same person from time to time. No studies have demonstrated that the different routes of administration are equivalent with respect to bioavailability. Phenobarbital is classified as a long-acting barbiturate when taken orally. Its onset of action is 1 hour or longer, and its duration of action ranges from 10 to 12 hours.

Barbiturates are weak acids that are absorbed and rapidly distributed to all tissues and fluids, with high concentrations in the brain, liver, and kidneys. Lipid solubility of the barbiturates is the dominant factor in their distribution within the body. The more lipid soluble the barbiturate, the more rapidly it penetrates all tissues of the body. Barbiturates are bound to plasma and tissue proteins to a varying degree with the degree of binding increasing directly as a function of lipid solubility.

Phenobarbital has the lowest lipid solubility, lowest plasma binding, lowest brain protein binding, the longest delay in onset activity, and the longest duration of action. Its diffusion across the blood-brain barrier and its distribution into other tissues occurs more slowly than with other short-acting barbiturates. Fifteen minutes or more may be required for maximal central depression following intravenous administration of Phenobarbital. However, with time, Phenobarbital distributes into all tissues and fluids. Barbiturates are known to cross the placenta. Phenobarbital is 20-45% protein bound. The plasma half-life for Phenobarbital in adults ranges between 53 and 118 hours with a mean of 79 hours. The plasma half-life for Phenobarbital in children and newborns (less than 48 hours old) ranges between 60 to 180 hours with a mean of 110 hours.

Barbiturates are metabolized primarily by the hepatic microsomal enzyme system, and the metabolic products are excreted in the urine and, less commonly in the feces.

Approximately 25% to 50% of a dose of Phenobarbital is eliminated unchanged in the urine, whereas the amount of other barbiturates excreted unchanged in the urine is negligible. Urinary pH and rate of urine flow affect the renal circulation of unchanged Phenobarbital, a greater quantity being eliminated in alkaline urine and at increased flow rates. The excretion of unmetabolized barbiturate is one feature that distinguishes the long-acting category from those belonging to other categories, which are almost entirely metabolized. The inactive metabolites of the barbiturates are excreted as conjugates of glucuronic acid.

INDICATIONS AND USAGE

a. Sedative, for the relief of anxiety, tension, and apprehension.

b. Hypnotic, for the short-term treatment of insomnia, since it appears to lose its effectiveness for sleep induction and sleep maintenance after 2 weeks (see *"Clinical Pharmacology"*).

c. Preanesthetic (IV or IM only).

d. For the treatment of generalized tonic-clonic and cortical focal seizures. In the emergency control of certain acute convulsive episodes, e.g., those associated with status epilepticus, cholera, eclampsia, cerebral hemorrhage, meningitis, tetanus and toxic reactions to strychnine or local anesthetics. Phenobarbital sodium may be administered intramuscularly or intravenously as an anticonvulsant for emergency use (see *"Warnings"*). When administered IV, it may require 15 or more minutes before reaching peak concentrations in the brain. Therefore, injecting Phenobarbital Sodium until the convulsions stop may cause the brain

level to exceed that required to control the convulsions and lead to severe barbiturate-induced depression.

UNLABELED USES

Phenobarbital is used alone or as an adjunct in the treatment of alcohol withdrawal, diabetes mellitus (noninsulin-dependent), in patients with severe encephalitis due to measles, varicella, influenza, rubella, mononucleosis, and pertussis. It is also used in essential tremor, febrile seizure, to reduce neonatal intraventricular hemorrhage, and seizures due to head injury, malaria, and neonatal seizures. Phenobarbital is also prescribed in the treatment of tetanus and status epilepticus.

CONTRAINDICATIONS

Barbiturates are contraindicated in patients with known barbiturate sensitivity. Barbiturates are also contraindicated in patients with a history of manifest or latent porphyria, marked impairment of liver functions or with severe respiratory distress where dyspnea or obstruction is evident. Large doses are contraindicated in nephritic subjects.

Barbiturates should not be administered to persons with known previous addiction to the sedative-hypnotic group since ordinary doses may be ineffectual and may contribute to further addiction.

Intra-arterial administration is contraindicated. Its consequences vary from transient pain to gangrene. Subcutaneous administration produces tissue irritation, ranging from tenderness and redness to necrosis and is not recommended. (See *"Dosage and Administration"* — *Treatment of Adverse Effects Due to Inadvertent Error in Adminstration.*)

WARNINGS

1. Habit Forming: Phenobarbital may be habit forming. Tolerance and psychological and physical dependence may occur with continued use (see *"Drug Abuse and Dependence"* and *"Pharmacokinetics"* under *"Clinical Pharmacology"*). Patients who have psychologic dependence on barbiturates may increase the dosage or decrease the dosage interval without consulting a physician and may subsequently develop a physical dependence on barbiturates. In order to minimize the possibility of overdosage or the development of dependence, the prescribing and dispensing of sedative-hypnotic barbiturates should be limited to be the amount required for the interval until the next appointment. Abrupt cessation after prolonged use in a person who is dependent on the drug may result in withdrawal symptoms, including delirium, convulsions, and possibly death. Barbiturates should be withdrawn gradually from any patient known to be taking excessive doses over long periods of time (see *"Drug Abuse and Dependence"*).

2. Dermatologic Reactions: Exfoliative dermatitis and Stevens-Johnson syndrome, possibly fatal, are rare hypersentivity reactions to Phenobarbital. Physicians should be alert to signs which may precede the onset of barbiturate-induced cutaneous lesions, and the drug should be discontinued whenever dermatological reactions below.

3. Intravenous Administration: Too rapid administration may cause severe respiratory depression, apnea, laryngospasm, hypertension or vasodilation with fall in blood pressure.

When administered intravenously, it may require 15 or more minutes before reaching peak concentrations in the brain. Therefore, injecting Phenobarbital Sodium until the convulsions stop may cause brain levels to exceed that required to control the convulsions and lead to severe barbiturate-induced depression.

4. Acute or Chronic Pain: Caution should be exercised when barbiturates are administered to patients with acute or chronic pain, because paradoxical excitement could be induced or important symptoms could be masked. However, the use of barbiturates as sedatives in the postoperative surgical period and as adjuncts to cancer chemotherapy is well established.

5. Usage in Pregnancy: Barbiturates can cause fetal damage when administered to a pregnant woman. Retrospective, case-controlled studies have suggested a connection between the maternal consumption of barbiturates and a higher-than-expected incidence of fetal abnormalities, following oral or parenteral administration. Barbiturates readily cross the placental barrier and are distributed throughout fetal tissues; the highest concentrations are found in the placenta, fetal liver, and brain. Fetal blood levels approach maternal blood levels following parenteral administration.

Withdrawal symptoms occur in infants born to women who receive barbiturates throughout the last trimester of pregnancy (see *"Drug Abuse and Dependence"*).

Phenobarbital should be used during pregnancy only when clearly indicated. If Phenobarbital is used during pregnancy or if the patient becomes pregnant while taking this drug, the patient should be apprised of the potential hazard to the fetus.

6. Usage in Children: Phenobarbital has been reported to be associated with cognitive deficits in children taking it for complicated febrile seizures.

7. Synergistic Effects: The concomitant use of alcohol or other CNS depressants may produce additive CNS depressant effects.

PRECAUTIONS

General: Barbiturates may be habit forming. Tolerance and psychological and physical dependence may occur with continued use (see *"Drug Abuse and Dependence"*).

Barbiturates should be administered with caution, if at all, to patients who are mentally depressed, have suicidal tendencies, or have a history of drug abuse.

Elderly or debilitated patients may react to barbiturates with marked excitement, depression, or confusion. In some persons, especially children, barbiturates repeatedly produce excitement rather than depression.

In patients with hepatic damage, barbiturates should be administered with caution and initially in reduced doses. Barbiturates should not be administered to patients showing the premonitory signs of hepatic coma.

The systemic effects of exogenous and endogenous corticosteroids may be diminished by Phenobarbital. Thus, this product should be administered with caution to patients with borderline hypoadrenal function, regardless of whether it is of pituitary or of primary adrenal origin.

Untoward reactions may occur in the presence of fever, hyperthyroidism, diabetes mellitus and severe anemia. In cases of great debility, severely impaired liver function, pulmonary or cardiac disease, status asthmaticus, shock or uremia, Phenobarbital Sodium should be used with extreme caution. Intramuscular injection should be confined to a total volume of 5 ml and made in a large muscle in order to avoid possible tissue irritation.

Parenteral solutions of barbiturates are highly alkaline. Therefore, extreme care should be taken to avoid perivascular extravasation or intra-arterial injection. Extravascular injection may cause local tissue damage with subsequent necrosis; consequences of intra-arterial injection may vary from transient pain to gangrene of the limb. Any complaint of pain in the limb warrants stopping the injection.

Information for Patients: The following information and instructions should be given to patients receiving barbiturates.

1. The use of barbiturates carries with it an associated risk of psychological and/or physical dependence. The patient should be warned against increasing the dose of the drug without consulting a physician.

2. Barbiturates may impair the mental and/or physical abilities required for the performance of potentially hazardous tasks, such as driving a car or operating machinery. The patient should be cautioned accordingly.

3. Alcohol should not be consumed while taking barbiturates. The concurrent use of the barbiturates with other CNS depressants (eg, alcohol, narcotics, tranquilizers, and antihistamines) may result in additional CNS-depressant effects.

4. If Phenobarbital is used during pregnancy, the patient should be apprised of the potential hazard to the fetus (see *"Warnings"*).

Laboratory Tests: Prolonged therapy with barbiturates should be accompanied by periodic laboratory evaluation of organ systems, including hematopoietic, renal, and hepatic systems (see *"General"* under *"Precautions"* and *"Adverse Reactions"*).

Drug Interactions: Most reports of clinically significant drug interactions occurring with the barbiturates have involved Phenobarbital. However, the application of these data to other barbiturates appears valid and warrants serial blood level determinations of the relevant drugs when there are multiple therapies.

1. Anticoagulants: Phenobarbital lowers the plasma levels of dicumarol (bishydroxycoumarin) and causes a decrease in anticoagulant activity as measured by the prothrombin time. Barbiturates can induce hepatic microsomal enzymes resulting in increased metabolism and decreased anticoagulant response of oral anticoagulants (eg, warfarin, acenocoumarol, dicumarol, and phenprocoumon). Patients stabilized on anticoagulant therapy may require dosage adjustments if barbiturates are added to or withdrawn from their dosage regimen.

2. Corticosteroids: Barbiturates appear to enhance the metabolism of exogenous corticosteroids, probably through the induction of hepatic microsomal enzymes. Patients stablized on corticosteroid therapy may require dosage adjustments if barbiturates are added to or withdrawn from their dosage regimen.

3. Griseofulvin: Phenobarbital appears to interfere with the absorption of orally administered griseofulvin, thus decreasing its blood level. The effect of the resultant decreased blood levels of griseofulvin on therapeutic response has not been established. However, it would be preferable to avoid concomitant administration of these drugs.

4. Doxycycline: Phenobarbital has been shown to shorten the half-life of doxycycline for as long as 2 weeks after barbiturate therapy is discontinued. This mechanism is probably through the induction of hepatic microsomal enzymes that metabolize the antibiotic. If Phenobarbital and doxycycline are administered concurrently, the clinical response to doxycycline should be monitored closely.

5. Phenytoin, Sodium Valproate, Valproic Acid: The effect of barbiturates on the metabolism of phenytoin appears to be variable. Some investigators report an accelerating effect, whereas others report no effect. Because the effect of barbiturates on the metabolism of phenytoin is not predicatable, phenytoin and barbiturate blood levels should be monitored more frequently if these drugs are given concurrently. Sodium valproate and valproic acid increase the Phenobarbital serum levels; therefore, Phenobarbital blood levels should be closely monitored and appropriate dosage adjustments made as clinically indicated.

6. CNS Depressants: The concurrent use of other CNS depressants, including other sedatives or hypnotics, antihistamines, tranquilizers, or alcohol, may produce additive depressant effects.

7. Monoamine Oxidase Inhibitors (MAOIs): MAOIs prolong the effects of barbiturates, probably because metabolism of the barbiturate is inhibited.

8. Estradiol, Estrone, Progesterone; and Other Steroidal Hormones: Pretreatment with or concurrent administration of Phenobarbital may decrease the effect of estradiol by increasing its metabolism. There have been reports of patients treated with antiepileptic drugs (eg, Phenobarbital) who become pregnant while taking oral contraceptives. An alternate contraceptive method might be suggested to women taking phenobarbital.

Other drugs reported to interact with the barbiturates include digitoxin and disulfiram.

Carcinogenesis: 1. Animal Data: Phenobarbital sodium is carcinogenic in mice and rats after lifetime administration. In mice, it produced benign and malignant liver cell tumors. In rats, benign liver cell tumors were observed very late in life.

2. Human Data: In a 29-year epidemiologic study of 9,136 patients who were treated on an anticonvulsant protocol that included Phenobarbital, results indicated a higher than normal incidence of hepatic carcinoma. Previously, some of these patients had been treated with thorotrast, a drug which is known to produce hepatic carcinomas. Thus, this study did not provide sufficient evidence that Phenobarbital is carcinogenic in humans.

A retrospective study of 84 children with brain tumors matched to 73 normal controls and 78 cancer controls (malignant disease other than brain tumors) suggested an association between exposure to barbiturates prenatally and an increased incidence of brain tumors.

Usage in Pregnancy: 1. Teratogenic Effects. Pregnancy Category D: See *"Usage in Pregnancy"* under *'Warnings"*.

2. Nonteratogenic Effects: Reports of infants suffering from long-term barbiturate exposure in utero included the acute withdrawal syndrome of seizures and hyperirritability from birth to a delayed onset of up to 14 days (See *"Drug Abuse and Dependence"*).

Labor and Delivery: Hypnotic doses of barbiturates do not appear to impair uterine activity significantly during labor. Full anesthetic doses of barbiturates decrease the force and frequency of uterine contractions. Administration of sedative-hypnotic barbiturates to the mother during labor may result in respiratory depression in the newborn. Premature infants are particularly susceptible to the depressant effects of barbiturates. If barbiturates are used during labor and delivery, resuscitation equipment should be available.

Barbiturates are additive with other CNS depressants admininistered during labor and delivery.

Data are not available to evaluate the effect of barbiturates when forceps delivery or other intervention is necessary or to determine the long-term effects of obstetrically administered barbiturates on the later growth development, and functional maturation of the child.

While barbiturates are usually reported to have a minimal effect on neonatal behavior, a delayed interest in breast-feeding and a depressed response to auditory and visual stimuli have been noted.

Nursing Mothers: Caution should be exercised when Phenobarbital is administered to a nursing woman, because small amounts of barbiturates are excreted in the milk.

ADVERSE REACTIONS

The following adverse reactions have been reported:

CNS Depression: Residual sedation or "hangover," drowsiness, lethargy, and vertigo. Emotional disturbances and phobias may be accentuated. In some persons, barbiturates such as Phenobarbital repeatedly produce excitement rather than depression, and the patient may appear to be inebriated. Irritability and hyperactivity can occur in children. Like other nonanalgesic hypnotic drugs, barbiturates such as Phenobarbital, when given in the presence of pain, may cause restlessness, excitement, and even delirium. Rarely, the use of barbiturates results in localized or diffuse myalgic, neuralgic, or arthritic pain, especially in psychoneurotic patients with insomnia. The pain may appear in paroxysms, is most intense in the early morning hours, and is most frequently located in the region of the neck, shoulder girdle, and upper limbs. Symptoms may last for days after the drug is discontinued.

Respiratory/Circulatory: Respiratory depression, apnea, circulatory collapse.

Allergic: Acquired hypersonsitivity to barbiturates consists chiefly in allergic reactions that occur especially in persons who tend to have asthma, urticaria, angioedema, and similar conditions. Hypersensitivity reactions in this category include localized swelling, particularly of the eyelids, cheeks, or lips, and erythematous dermatitis. Rarely, exfoliative dermatitis (eg. Stevens-Johnson syndrome and toxic epidermal necrolysis) may be caused by Phenobarbital and can prove fatal. The skin eruption may be associated with fever, delirium, and marked degenerative changes in the liver and other parenchymatous organs. In a few cases, megaloblastic anemia has been associated with the chronic use of Phenobarbital.

Other: Nausea and vomiting; headache, osteomalacia.

The following adverse reactions and their incidence were compiled from surveillance of thousands of hospitalized patients who received barbiturates. Because such patients may be less aware of the milder adverse effects of barbiturates, the incidence of these reactions may be somewhat higher in fully ambulatory patients.

MORE THAN 1 IN 100 PATIENTS
The most common adverse reaction, estimated to occur at a rate of 1 to 3 patients per 100, is:

Nervous System: Somnolence.

LESS THAN 1 IN 100 PATIENTS
Adverse reactions estimated to occur at a rate of less than 1 in 100 patients are listed below, grouped by organ, system and by decreasing order of occurrence:

Nervous System: Agitation, confusion, hyperkinesia, ataxia, CNS depression, nightmares, nervousness, psychiatric disturbance, hallucinations, insomnia, anxiety, dizziness, abnormality in thinking.

Respiratory System: Hypoventilation, apnea

Cardiovascular System: Bradycardia, hypotension, syncope

Digestive System: Nausea, vomiting, constipation

Other Reported Reactions: Headache, injection site reactions, hypersensitivity reactions (angioedema, skin rashes, exfoliative dermatitis), Stevens-Johnson syndrome, toxic epidermal necrolysis, fever, liver damage, megaloblastic anemia following chronic Phenobarbital use.

DRUG ABUSE AND DEPENDENCE

Controlled Substance: Phenobarbital is a Schedule IV drug.

Dependence: Barbiturates may be habit forming. Tolerance, psychological dependence, and physical dependence may occur, especially following prolonged use of high doses of barbiturates. Daily administration in excess of 400 mg of pentobarbital or secobarbital for approximately 90 days is likely to produce some degree of physical dependence. A dosage of 600 to 800 mg taken for at least 35 days is sufficient to produce withdrawal seizures. Plasma levels greater than 30 μg/ml may be toxic. Levels between 65 μg/ml to 117 μg/ml may be lethal. The average daily dose for the barbiturate addict is usually about 1.5 g. As tolerance to barbiturates develops, the amount needed to maintain the same level of intoxication increases; tolerance to a fatal dosage, however, does not increase more than twofold. As this occurs, the margin between intoxicating dosage and fatal dosage becomes smaller.

Symptoms of acute intoxication with barbiturates include unsteady gait, slurred speech, and sustained nystagmus. Mental signs of chronic intoxication include confusion, poor judgment, irritability, insomnia, and somatic complaints.

Symptoms of barbiturate dependence are similar to those of chronic alcoholism. If an individual appears to be intoxicated with alcohol to a degree that is radically disproportionate to the amount of alcohol in his or her blood, the use of barbiturates should be suspected. The lethal dose of a barbiturate is far less if alcohol is also ingested.

The symptoms of barbiturate withdrawal can be severe and may cause death. Minor withdrawal symptoms may appear 8 to 12 hours after the last dose of a barbiturate. These symptoms usually appear in the following order: anxiety, muscle twitching, tremor of hands and fingers, progressive weakness, dizziness, distortion in visual perception, nausea, vomiting, insomnia, and orthostatic hypotension. Major withdrawal symptoms (convulsions and delirium) may occur within 16 hours and last up to 5 days after abrupt cessation of barbiturates. The intensity of withdrawal symptoms gradually declines over a period of approximately 15 days. Individuals susceptible to barbiturate abuse and dependence include alcoholics and opiate abusers as well as other sedative-hypnotic and amphetamine abusers.

Drug dependence on barbiturates arises from repeated administration of a barbiturate or agent with barbiturate-like effect on a continuous basis, generally in amounts exceeding therapeutic dose levels. The characteristics of drug dependence on barbiturates include: (a) a strong desire or need to continue taking the drug; (b) a tendency to increase the dose; (c) a psychic dependence on the effects of the drug related to subjective and individual appreciation of those effects; and (d) a physical dependence on the effects of the drug, requiring its presence for maintenance of homeostasis and resulting in a definite, characteristic, and self-limited abstinence syndrome when the drug is withdrawn. Individuals subject to barbiturate abuse and dependence include alcoholics and opiate abusers as well as other sedative-hypnotics and amphetamine abusers.

Treatment of barbiturate dependence consists of cautious and gradual withdrawal of the drug. Barbiturate-dependent patients can be withdrawn by using a number of different withdrawal regimens. In all cases, withdrawal requires an extended period of time. One method involves substituting a 30-mg dose of Phenobarbital for each 100- to 200-mg dose of barbiturate that the patient has been taking. The total daily amount of Phenobarbital is then administered in 3 or 4 divided doses, not to exceed 600 mg daily. If signs of withdrawal occur on the first day of treatment, a loading dose of 100 to 200 mg of Phenobarbital may be administered IM in addition to the oral dose. After stabilization on Phenobarbital, the total daily dose is decreased by 30 mg/day as long as withdrawal is proceeding smoothly. If withdrawal symptoms appear, dosage is maintained at that level or increased slightly until symptoms disappear. A modification of this regimen involves initiating treatment at the patient's regular dosage level and decreasing the daily dosage by 10% if tolerated by the patient.

Infants who are physically dependent on barbiturates may be given Phenobarbital, 3 to 10 mg/kg/day. After withdrawal symptoms (hyperactivity, disturbed sleep, tremors, and hyperreflexia) are relieved, the dosage of Phenobarbital should be gradually decreased and completely withdrawn over a 2-week period.

OVERDOSAGE

Signs and Symptoms: The onset of symptoms following a toxic oral exposure to Phenobarbital may not occur until several hours following ingestion. The toxic dose of barbiturates varies considerably. In general, an oral dose of 1 g of most barbiturates produces serious poisoning in an adult. Death commonly occurs after 2 to 10 g of ingested barbiturate. The sedated, therapeutic blood levels of Phenobarbital range between 5 to 40 μg/mL; the usual lethal blood level ranges from 100 to 200 μg/mL. Barbiturate intoxication may be confused with alcoholism, bromide intoxication, and various neurologic disorders. Potential tolerance must be considered when evaluating significance of dose and plasma concentration.

The manifestations of a long-acting barbiturate in overdose include nystagmus, ataxia, CNS depression, drowsiness, confusion, excitation, ataxia, vertigo, headache, respiratory depression that may progress to Cheyne-Stokes respiration, hypothermia, hypotension, and coma. Other findings may include absent or depressed reflexes, constriction of the pupils to a slight degree (though in severe poisoning they may show paralytic dilation), oliguria, tachycardia, cyanosis, weak, rapid pulse, cold and clammy skin, and erythematous or hemorrhagic blisters (primarily at pressure points). Following massive exposure to Phenobarbital, pulmonary edema, circulatory collapse with loss of peripheral vascular tone, apnea, respiratory arrest, cardiac arrest, and death may occur.

In extreme overdose, all electrical activity in the brain may cease, in which case a "flat" EEG normally equated with clinical death should not be accepted. This effect is fully reversible unless hypoxic damage occurs.

Consideration should be given to the possibility of barbiturate intoxication even in situations that appear to involve trauma.

Complications such as pneumonia, pulmonary edema, cardiac arrhythmias, congestive heart failure, and renal failure may occur. Uremia may increase CNS sensitivity to barbiturates if renal function is impaired. Differential diagnosis should include hypoglycemia, head trauma, cerebrovascular accidents, convulsive states, and diabetic coma.

Treatment: To obtain up-to-date information about the treatment of overdose, a good resource is your certified Regional Poison Control Center. Telephone numbers of certified poison control centers are listed in the *Physicians' Desk Reference (PDR)*. In managing overdosage, consider the possibility of multiple drug overdoses, interaction among drugs, and unusual drug kinetics in your patient.

Treatment of overdosage is mainly supportive and consists of the following:
1. Protect the patient's airway and support ventilation and perfusion.
2. Meticulously monitor and maintain, within acceptable limits, the patient's vital signs, blood gases, serum electrolytes, etc.
Maintenance of an adequate airway, with assisted respiration and oxygen administration as necessary.
Monitoring of vital signs and fluid balance.
3. If the patient is conscious and has not lost the gag reflex, emesis may be included with ipecac. Care should be taken to prevent pulmonary aspiration of vomitus. After completion of vomiting, 30 grams activated charcoal in a glass of water may be administered.
4. If emesis is contraindicated, gastric lavage may be performed with a cuffed endotracheal tube in place with the patient in the face down position. Activated charcoal may be left in the emptied stomach and a saline cathartic administered.
5. Fluid therapy and other standard treatment for shock, if needed.
6. If renal function is normal, forced diuresis may aid in the elimination of the barbiturate. Alkalinization of the urine increases renal excretion of Phenobarbital.
7. Although not recommended as a routine procedure, hemodialysis may be used in severe barbiturate intoxication or if the patient is anuric or in shock. Hemoperfusion through an anion-exchange resin or activated charcoal has been successful. Peritoneal dialysis is significantly less effective in removing barbiturates.
8. Patient should be rolled from side to side every 30 minutes.
9. Antibiotics should be given if pneumonia is suspected.
10. Appropriate nursing care to prevent hypostatic pneumonia, decubiti, aspiration and other complications of patients with altered states of consciousness.
11. The use of analeptic agents is not recommended.
Absorption of drugs from the gastrointestinal tract may be decreased by activated charcoal, which, in many cases, is more effective than emesis or lavage. Repeated doses of charcoal over time may hasten elimination of some drugs that have been absorbed. Safeguard the patient's airway when employing gastric emptying or charcoal.
If the patient has chronically abused sedatives, withdrawal reactions may be manifest following acute overdose.

DOSAGE AND ADMINISTRATION

The dose of Phenobarbital must be individualized with full knowledge of its particular characteristics and recommended rate of administration. Factors of consideration are the patient's age, weight, and condition.

ORAL ADMINISTRATION

Oral Sedation: For sedation the drug may be administered in single doses of 30 to 120 mg repeated at intervals: frequency will be determined by the patient's response. It is generally considered that no more than 400 mg of phenobarbital should be administered during a 24-hour period.

Adults: Daytime Sedation: 30 to 120 mg daily in 2 to 3 divided doses.
Oral Hypnotic: 100 to 200 mg.

Anticonvulsant Use: Clinical laboratory reference values should be used to determine the therapeutic anticonvulsant level of Phenobarbital in the serum. To achieve the blood levels considered therapeutic in children, higher per-kilogram dosages are generally necessary for Phenobarbital and most other anticonvulsants. In children and infants, Phenobarbital at a loading dose of 15 to 20 mg/kg produces blood levels of about 20 μg/mL shortly after administration.

Phenobarbital has been used in the treatment and prophylaxis of febrile seizures. However, it has not been established that prevention of febrile seizure influences the subsequent development of epilepsy.

Adults: 60 to 200 mg/day.
Children: 3 to 6 mg/kg/day.

► SHOWN IN PRODUCT IDENTIFICATION GUIDE

Special Patient Population: Dosage should be reduced in the elderly or debilitated because these patients may be more sensitive to barbiturates. Dosage should be reduced for patients with impaired renal function or hepatic disease.

PARENTERAL

Pediatric Dosage: Recommended by the American Academy of Pediatrics (intended as a guide)

Preoperative Sedation: 1 to 3 mg/kg IM or IV

Anticonvulsion: 4 to 6 mg/kg/day for 7 to 10 days to blood level of 10 to 15 mcg/mL or 10 to 15 mg/kg/day IM or IV

Status Epilepticus: 15 to 20 mg/kg over 10 to 15 minutes IV

Adult Dosage: (intended as a guide)

Daytime Sedation: 30 to 120 mg daily in 2 to 9 divided doses IM or IV

Bedtime Hypnosis: 100 to 320 mg IM or IV

Preoperative Sedation: IM only — 100 to 200 mg 60 to 90 minutes before surgery

Acute Convulsions: 20 to 320 mg IM or IV, repeated in 6 hours as necessary

Parenteral routes should be used only when oral administration is impossible or impractical.

Intramuscular injection of the sodium salts of barbiturates should be made deeply into a large muscle and a volume of 5 mL should not be exceeded at any one site because of possible tissue irritation, injection into or near peripheral nerves may result in permanent neurological deficit. After intramuscular injection of a hypnotic dose, the patient's vital signs should be monitored.

Subcutaneous administration is not recommended (see *"Contraindications"*).

INTRAVENOUS ADMINISTRATION

Intravenous injection is restricted to conditions in which other routes are not feasible, either because the patient is unconscious (as in cerebral hemorrhage, eclampsia or status epilepticus), or because the patient resists (as in delirium) or because prompt action is imperative. Slow IV injection is essential, and patients should be carefully observed during administration. This requires that blood pressure, respiration and cardiac function be maintained, vital signs be recorded and equipment for resuscitation and artificial ventilation be available. Larger doses may occasionally be necessary in persons with status epilepticus, psychoses, and pronounced excitement, and in mental patients with insomnia.

The effect of large doses must be closely watched. Alkalis should be given and the bowels regulated during prolonged use. The rate of intravenous injection for adults should not exceed 60 mg/min for Phenobarbital Sodium, or a total dose of 600 mg in 24 hours.

When given intravenously, do not use small veins, such as those on the dorsum of the hand or wrist. Preference should be given to a larger vein to minimize the risk of irritation with the possibility of resultant thrombosis. Avoid administration into varicose veins because circulation there is retarded. Inadvertent injection into or adjacent to an artery has resulted in gangrene requiring amputation of an extremity or a portion thereof. Careful technique, including aspiration, is necessary to avoid inadvertent intra-arterial injection. (See below.)

TREATMENT OF ADVERSE EFFECTS DUE TO INADVERTENT ERROR IN ADMINISTRATION

Extravasation into subcutaneous tissues causes tissue irritation. This may vary from slight tenderness and redness to necrosis. Recommended treatment includes the application of moist heat and the injection of 0.5% procaine solution into the affected area.

Intra-arterial injection of any barbiturate must be avoided. The accidental intra-arterial injection of a small amount of the solution may cause spasm and severe pain along the course of the artery. The injection should be terminated if the patient complains of pain or if other indications of accidental intra-arterial injection occur, such as a white hand with cyanosed skin or patches of discolored skin and delayed onset of hypnosis.

The consequences of intra-arterial injection of Phenobarbital can vary from transient pain to gangrene. It is not possible to formulate strict rules for management of such accidents. The following procedures have been suggested: 1) release of the tourniquet or restrictive garments to permit dilution of injected drug, 2) relief of arterial spasm by injecting 10 mL of a 1% procaine solution into the artery and, if considered necessary, brachial plexus block, 3) prevention of thrombosis by early anticoagulant therapy and 4) supportive treatment.

ANTICONVULSANT USE

A therapeutic anticonvulsant level of Phenobarbital in the serum is 10 to 25 μg/mL. To achieve the blood levels considered therapeutic in children, higher per-kilogram dosages are generally necessary for Phenobarbital and most other anticonvulsants. In children and infants, Phenobarbital at loading doses of 15 to 20 mg/kg produces blood levels of about 20 μg/mL shortly after administration.

In status epilepticus, it is imperative to achieve therapeutic blood levels of a barbiturate (or other anticonvulsants) as rapidly as possible. When administered intravenously, Phenobarbital Sodium may require 15 minutes or more to attain peak concentrations in the brain. If Phenobarbital Sodium is injected continuously until the convulsions stop, the brain concentration will continue to rise and can eventually exceed that required to control the seizures. Because a barbiturate-induced depression may occur along with a postictal depression once the seizures are controlled, it is important, therefore, to use the minimal amount required and to wait for the anticonvulsant effect to develop before administering a second dose.

Phenobarbital has been used in the treatment and prophylaxis of febrile seizures. However, it has not been established that prevention of febrile seizures influences the subsequent development of epilepsy.

Parenteral drug products should be inspected visually for particulate matter and discoloration prior to administration, whenever solution and container permit.

Do not use if solution is discolored or contains a precipitate.

SPECIAL PATIENT POPULATION

Dosage should be reduced in the elderly or debilitated because these patients may be more sensitive to barbiturates. Dosage should be reduced for patients with impaired renal function or hepatic disease.

STORAGE

Keep tightly closed. Store at controlled room temperature, 59° to 86°F (15° to 30°C).

J CODES

Up to 120 mg IM,IV—J2560

HOW SUPPLIED

PHENOBARBITAL
CAPSULE (C-IV): 16 MG

BRAND/MANUFACTURER	NDC	SIZE	AWP
○ BRAND			
SOLFOTON: Poythress	00095-0025-01	100s	$10.50

ELIXIR (C-IV): 15 MG/5 ML

BRAND/MANUFACTURER	NDC	SIZE	AWP
○ GENERICS			
UDL	51079-0365-30	3.75 ml 100s ud	$29.12
Pharm Assoc	00121-0518-05	5 ml 100s ud	$33.20
Pharm Assoc	00121-0518-10	10 ml 100s ud	$34.30
Pharm Assoc	00121-0518-20	20 ml 100s ud	$38.19

ELIXIR (C-IV): 20 MG/5 ML

BRAND/MANUFACTURER	NDC	SIZE	AWP
○ GENERICS			
Bio-Pharm	59741-0136-16	480 ml	$3.65
Century	00436-0585-16	480 ml	$4.00
Moore,H.L.	00839-5398-69	480 ml	$4.17
Purepac	00228-2024-16	480 ml	$4.40
Liquipharm	54198-0130-16	480 ml	$4.50
Aligen	00405-0155-16	480 ml	$4.95
Halsey Pharm	00879-0049-16	480 ml	$4.95
Schein	00364-7046-16	480 ml	$5.00
Cenci,H.R.	00556-0112-16	480 ml	$5.00
Barre	00472-1015-16	480 ml	$5.13
Major	00904-1015-16	480 ml	$5.25
Qualitest	00603-1508-58	480 ml	$5.31
Morton Grove	60432-0026-16	480 ml	$5.50
URL	00677-0805-33	480 ml	$5.95
Allscrips	54569-2031-00	480 ml	$5.95
Pharm Assoc	00121-0518-16	480 ml	$5.95
Goldline	00182-0314-40	480 ml	$6.00
Rugby	00536-1590-85	480 ml	$6.53
Lilly	00002-2438-05	480 ml	$11.13
Century	00436-0585-32	960 ml	$6.25
Century	00436-0585-28	3840 ml	$25.00
Rugby	00536-1590-90	3840 ml	$25.69
Liquipharm	54198-0130-28	3840 ml	$27.50
Morton Grove	60432-0026-28	3840 ml	$29.10
Major	00904-1015-28	3840 ml	$29.25
Truxton	00463-9018-28	3840 ml	$30.00
Cenci,H.R.	00556-0112-28	3840 ml	$31.00
Halsey Pharm	00879-0049-28	3840 ml	$31.55
Barre	00472-1015-28	3840 ml	$31.57
Goldline	00182-0314-41	3840 ml	$35.85
UDL	51079-0366-30	5 ml 100s ud	$33.50
Pharm Assoc	00121-0531-05	5 ml 100s ud	$41.50
Roxane	00054-8704-04	5 ml 100s ud	$45.77
Pharm Assoc	00121-0531-07	7.5 ml 100s ud	$42.21
Roxane	00054-8701-04	7.5 ml 100s ud	$47.99
Pharm Assoc	00121-0531-15	15 ml 100s ud	$45.10

ELIXIR (C-IV): 30 MG/5 ML

BRAND/MANUFACTURER	NDC	SIZE	AWP
○ GENERICS			
UDL	51079-0367-30	7.5 ml 100s ud	$35.00

INJECTION (C-IV): 60 MG/ML

BRAND/MANUFACTURER	NDC	SIZE	AWP
○ GENERICS			
Allscrips	54569-3282-00	1 ml 10s	$25.54

INJECTION (C-IV): 130 MG/ML

BRAND/MANUFACTURER	NDC	SIZE	AWP
○ BRAND			
LUMINAL SODIUM: Sanofi Winthrop	00024-1171-06	1 ml 100s	$318.16

◆ RATED THERAPEUTICALLY EQUIVALENT; ◇ THERAPEUTIC EQUIVALENCE UNCONFIRMED; ○ UNRATED

POWDER (C-IV):

BRAND/MANUFACTURER	NDC	SIZE	AWP
○ GENERICS			
Amend	17137-0519-02	30 gm	$15.05
Amend	17137-0519-04	125 gm	$49.00

For additional alternatives, turn to the section beginning on page 2859.

Phenoxybenzamine Hydrochloride

DESCRIPTION

Phenoxybenzamine Hydrochloride is N-(2-Chloroethyl)-N-(1-methyl-2-phenoxyethyl)benzylamine hydrochloride.

Phenoxybenzamine Hydrochloride is a colorless, crystalline powder with a molecular weight of 340.3 which melts between 136° and 141°C. It is soluble in water, alcohol and chloroform; insoluble in ether.

Each tablet contains:

Phenoxybenzamine 10mg

Following is its chemical structure:

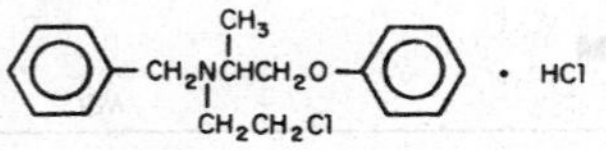

CLINICAL PHARMACOLOGY

Phenoxybenzamine HCl is a long-acting, adrenergic, *alpha*-receptor blocking agent which can produce and maintain "chemical sympathectomy" by oral administration. It increases blood flow to the skin, mucosa and abdominal viscera, and lowers both supine and erect blood pressures. It has no effect on the parasympathetic system.

Twenty to 30 percent of orally administered Phenoxybenzamine appears to be absorbed in the active form.[1]

The half-life of orally administered Phenoxybenzamine Hydrochloride is not known; however, the half-life of intravenously administered drug is approximately 24 hours. Demonstrable effects with intravenous administration persist for at least 3 to 4 days, and the effects of daily administration are cumulative for nearly a week.[1]

INDICATION AND USAGE

Pheochromocytoma, to control episodes of hypertension and sweating. If tachycardia is excessive, it may be necessary to use a beta-blocking agent concomitantly.

UNLABELED USES

Phenoxybenzamine is used alone or as an adjunct in the treatment of bladder instability, including postoperative urinary retention and neurogenic bladder. It is used as a male contraceptive to inhibit sperm upon orgasm, and is prescribed to induce erection in impotent men, to inhibit premature ejaculation, and to relieve urinary obstruction secondary to benign prostatic hyperplasia. It is also used in the treatment of hyperhidrosis in spinal cord injury, and in Raynaud's disease.

CONTRAINDICATIONS

Conditions where a fall in blood pressure may be undesirable.

WARNING

Phenoxybenzamine HCl induced *alpha*-adrenergic blockade leaves *beta*-adrenergic receptors unopposed. Compounds that stimulate both types of receptors may therefore produce an exaggerated hypotension response and tachycardia.

PRECAUTIONS

General: Administer with caution in patients with marked cerebral or coronary arteriosclerosis or renal damage. Adrenergic blocking effect may aggravate symptoms of respiratory infections.

Drug Interactions[2]: Phenoxybenzamine HCl may interact with compounds that stimulate both *alpha*- and *beta*-adrenergic receptors (i.e., epinephrine) to produce an exaggerated hypotensive response and tachycardia. (See *"Warning".*)

Phenoxybenzamine HCl blocks hyperthermia production by levarterenol and blocks hypothermia production by reserpine.

Carcinogenesis, Mutagenesis, Impairment of Fertility: Phenoxybenzamine HCl has shown *in vitro* mutagenic activity in the Ames test and in the mouse lymphoma assay; it has not shown mutagenic activity in the micronucleus test in mice. In rats and mice repeated intraperitoneal administration of Phenoxybenzamine HCl resulted in peritoneal sarcomas. Chronic oral dosing in rats has produced malignant tumors in the gastrointestinal tract. The majority of these tumors were found in the nonglandular stomach of the rats.

In chronic oral studies in rats, ulcerative and/or erosive gastritis of the glandular stomach occurred which was probably drug related.

Pregnancy–Teratogenic Effects: Pregnancy Category C.: Adequate reproductive studies have not been performed with Phenoxybenzamine HCl. It is also not known whether Phenoxybenzamine HCl can cause fetal harm when administered to a pregnant woman. Phenoxybenzamine HCl should be given to a pregnant woman only if clearly needed.

Nursing Mothers: It is not known whether this drug is excreted in human milk. Because many drugs are excreted in human milk, and because of the potential for serious adverse reactions from Phenoxybenzamine HCl, a decision should be made whether to discontinue nursing or to discontinue the drug, taking into account the importance of the drug to the mother.

Pediatric Use: Safety and effectiveness in children have not been established.

ADVERSE REACTIONS

The following adverse reactions have been observed, but there are insufficient data to support an estimate of their frequency:

Autonomic Nervous System*: Postural hypotension, tachycardia, inhibition of ejaculation, nasal congestion, miosis.

Miscellaneous: Gastrointestinal irritation, drowsiness, fatigue.

OVERDOSAGE

Symptoms: These are largely the result of block of the sympathetic nervous system and of the circulating epinephrine. They may include postural hypotension resulting in dizziness or fainting; tachycardia, particularly postural; vomiting; lethargy; shock.

Treatment: When symptoms and signs of overdosage exist, discontinue the drug. Treatment of circulatory failure, if present, is a prime consideration. In cases of mild overdosage, recumbent position with legs elevated usually restores cerebral circulation. In the more severe cases, the usual measures to combat shock should be instituted. Usual pressor agents are *not* effective. Epinephrine is contraindicated because it stimulates both *alpha* and *beta* receptors; since *alpha* receptors are blocked, the net effect of epinephrine administration is vasodilation and a further drop in blood pressure (epinephrine reversal).

The patient may have to be kept flat for 24 hours or more in the case of overdose, as the effect of the drug is prolonged. Leg bandages and an abdominal binder may shorten the period of disability.

I.V. infusion of levarterenol bitartrate may be used to combat severe hypotensive reactions, because it stimulates *alpha* receptors primarily. Although Phenoxybenzamine HCl is an *alpha*-adrenergic blocking agent, a sufficient dose of levarterenol bitartrate will overcome this effect.

The oral LD_{50} for Phenoxybenzamine HCl is approximately 2000 mg/kg in rats and approximately 500 mg/kg in guinea pigs.

DOSAGE AND ADMINISTRATION

The dosage should be adjusted to fit the needs of each patient. Small initial doses should be *slowly* increased until the desired effect is obtained or the side effects from blockade become troublesome. *After each increase, the patient should be observed on that level before instituting another increase.*The dosage should be carried to a point where symptomatic relief and/or objective improvement are obtained, but not so high that the side effects from blockade become troublesome. Initially, 10 mg of Phenoxybenzamine HCl twice a day. Dosage should be increased every other day, usually to 20 to 40 mg 2 or 3 times a day, until an optimal dosage is obtained, as judged by blood pressure control.

REFERENCES

1. Weiner, N.: Drugs That Inhibit Adrenergic Nerves and Block Adrenergic Receptors, in Goodman, L., and Gilman, A. *The Pharmacological Basis of Therapeutics*, ed. 6, New York, Macmillan Publishing Co., 1980, p. 179; p. 182. 2. Martin E.W.: *Drug Interactions Index 1978/1979*, Philadelphia, J.B. Lippincott Co., 1978, pp. 209-210.

HOW SUPPLIED
CAPSULE: 10 MG

BRAND/MANUFACTURER	NDC	SIZE	AWP
○ BRAND			
DIBENZYLINE: SK Beecham Pharm	00007-3533-20	100s	$59.50

Phensuximide

DESCRIPTION

Phensuximide is an anticonvulsant succinimide, chemically designated as N-methyl-2-phenylsuccinimide. Each capsule contains 500 mg Phensuximide USP.

Following is its chemical structure:

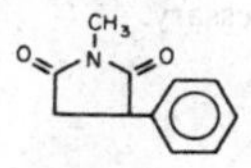

CLINICAL PHARMACOLOGY

Phensuximide suppresses the paroxysmal three-cycle-per-second spike and wave activity associated with lapses of consciousness which is common in absence (petit mal) seizures. The frequency of epileptiform attacks is reduced, apparently by depression of the motor cortex and elevation of the threshold of the central nervous system to convulsive stimuli.

INDICATIONS AND USAGE

Phensuximide is indicated for the control of absence (petit mal) seizures.

---

* These so-called "side effects" are actually evidence of adrenergic blockade and vary according to the degree of blockade.

➤ SHOWN IN PRODUCT IDENTIFICATION GUIDE

CONTRAINDICATION

Phensuximide should not be used in patients with a history of hypersensitivity to succinimides.

WARNINGS

Blood dyscrasias, including some with fatal outcome, have been reported to be associated with the use of succinimides; therefore, periodic blood counts should be performed. Should signs and/or symptoms of infection (eg sore throat, fever) develop, blood counts should be considered at that point.

It has been reported that succinimides have produced morphological and functional changes in animal liver. For this reason, Phensuximide should be administered with extreme caution to patients with known liver or renal diseases. Periodic urinalysis and liver function studies are advised for all patients receiving the drug.

Cases of systemic lupus erythematosus have been reported with the use of succinimides. The physician should be alert to this possibility.

Usage in Pregnancy: The effects of Phensuximide in human pregnancy and nursing infants are unknown.

Recent reports suggest an association between the use of anticonvulsant drugs by women with epilepsy and an elevated incidence of birth defects in children born to these women. Data is more extensive with respect to phenytoin and phenobarbital, but these are also the most commonly prescribed anticonvulsants; less systematic or anecdotal reports suggest a possible similar association with the use of all known anticonvulsant drugs.

The reports suggesting an elevated incidence of birth defects in children of drug-treated epileptic women cannot be regarded as adequate to prove a definite cause-and-effect relationship. There are intrinsic methodologic problems in obtaining adequate data on drug teratogenicity in humans; the possibility also exists that other factors, eg, genetic factors or the epileptic condition itself, may be more important than drug therapy in leading to birth defects. The great majority of mothers on anticonvulsant medication deliver normal infants. It is important to note that anticonvulsant drugs should not be discontinued in patients in whom the drug is administered to prevent major seizures because of the strong possibility of precipitating status epilepticus with attendant hypoxia and threat to life. In individual cases where the severity and frequency of the seizure disorder are such that the removal of medication does not pose a serious threat to the patient, discontinuation of the drug may be considered prior to and during pregnancy, although it cannot be said with any confidence that even minor seizures do not pose some hazard to the developing embryo or fetus.

The prescribing physician will wish to weigh these considerations in treating or counseling epileptic women of childbearing potential.

Hazardous Activities: Phensuximide may impair the mental and/or physical abilities required for the performance of potentially hazardous tasks, such as driving a motor vehicle or other such activity requiring alertness; therefore, the patient should be cautioned accordingly.

PRECAUTIONS

GENERAL

Phensuximide, when used alone in mixed types of epilepsy, may increase the frequency of grand mal seizures in some patients.

As with other anticonvulsants, it is important to proceed slowly when increasing or decreasing dosage, as well as when adding or eliminating other medication. Abrupt withdrawal of anticonvulsant medication may precipitate absence (petit mal) status.

INFORMATION FOR PATIENTS

Phensuximide may impair the mental and/or physical abilities required for the performance of potentially hazardous tasks, such as driving a motor vehicle or other such activity requiring alertness, therefore, the patient should be cautioned accordingly.

Patients taking Phensuximide should be advised of the importance of adhering strictly to the prescribed regimen.

Patients should be instructed to promptly contact their physician if they develop signs and/or symptoms suggesting an infection (eg sore throat, fever).

DRUG INTERACTIONS

Since Phensuximide, as a member of the succinimide class, may interact with concurrently administered antiepileptic drugs, periodic serum level determinations of these drugs may be necessary.

PREGNANCY

See "Warnings".

ADVERSE REACTIONS

Gastrointestinal System: Gastrointestinal symptoms, such as nausea, vomiting, and anorexia, occur frequently, but may be the result of overdosage.

Nervous System: Neurologic and sensory reactions reported during therapy with Phensuximide have included drowsiness, dizziness, ataxia, headache, dreamlike state, and lethargy. Side effects, such as drowsiness and dizziness, may be relieved by a reduction in total dosage.

Integumentary System: Dermatologic manifestations reported to be associated with the administration of Phensuximide have included pruritus, skin eruptions, erythema multiforme, erythematous rashes, Stevens-Johnson syndrome, and alopecia.

Genitourinary System: Genitourinary complications which have been reported include urinary frequency, renal damage, and hematuria.

Hemopoietic System: Hemopoietic complications associated with the administration of Phensuximide include granulocytopenia, transient leukopenia, and pancytopenia with or without bone marrow suppression.

Musculoskeletal System: Muscular weakness.

OVERDOSAGE

Acute overdoses may produce nausea, vomiting, and CNS depression including coma with respiratory depression.

TREATMENT

Treatment should include emesis (unless the patient is, or could rapidly become, obtunded, comatose, or convulsing) or gastric lavage, activated charcoal, cathartics and general supportive measures. Forced diuresis and exchange transfusions are ineffective.

DOSAGE AND ADMINISTRATION

Phensuximide is administered by the oral route in doses of 500 mg to 1 g two or three times daily. As with other anticonvulsant medication, the dosage should be adjusted to suit individual requirements. The total dosage, irrespective of age, may, therefore, vary between 1 and 3 g per day, the average being 1.5 g.

Phensuximide may be administered in combination with other anticonvulsants when other forms of epilepsy coexist with absence (petit mal).

HOW SUPPLIED
CAPSULE: 0.5 GM

BRAND/MANUFACTURER	NDC	SIZE	AWP
○ BRAND MILONTIN: Parke-Davis	00071-0393-24	100s	$68.78

Phentermine

DESCRIPTION

Phentermine capsules are available in formulations of Phentermine Resin and Phentermine Hydrochloride.

Each capsule contains:

Phentermine as the cationic exchange resin complex ....15 or 30 mg
or
Phentermine HCl ....30 mg (equivalent to 24 mg Phentermine)

Phentermine HCl, is a white crystalline powder very soluble in water and alcohol, Chemically, the product is phenyl-tertiary-butylamine hydrochloride.

Following is its chemical structure:

ACTIONS

Phentermine is a sympathomimetic amine with pharmacologic activity similar to the prototype drug of this class used in obesity, amphetamine (d- and d *l*-amphetamine). Actions include central nervous system stimulation and elevation of blood pressure. Tachyphylaxis and tolerance have been demonstrated with all drugs of this class in which these phenomena have been looked for.

Drugs of this class used in obesity are commonly known as "anorectics" or "anorexigenics." It has not been established, however, that the action of such drugs in treating obesity is primarily one of appetite suppression. Other central nervous system actions, or metabolic effects may be involved.

Adult obese subjects instructed in dietary management and treated with "anorectic" drugs, lose more weight on the average than those treated with placebo and diet, as determined in relatively short-term clinical trials.

The magnitude of increased weight loss of drug-treated patients over placebo-treated patients is only a fraction of a pound a week. The rate of weight loss is greatest in the first weeks of therapy for both drug and placebo subjects and tends to decrease in succeeding weeks. The possible origins of the increased weight loss due to the various drug effects are not established. The amount of weight loss associated with the use of an "anorectic" drug varies from trial to trial, and the increased weight loss appears to be related in part to variables other than the drugs prescribed, such as the physician-investigator, the population treated, and the diet prescribed. Studies do not permit conclusions as to the relative importance of the drug and non-drug factors on weight loss. The natural history of obesity is measured in years, whereas the studies cited are restricted to a few weeks' or months' duration; thus, the total impact of drug-induced weight loss over that of diet alone must be considered clinically limited. The bioavailability of Phentermine has been studied in humans in which blood levels of Phentermine were measured by a gas chromatography method. Blood levels obtained with the 15 mg and 30 mg resin complex formulations indicated slower absorption with a reduced but prolonged peak concentration and without a significant difference in prolongation of blood levels when compared with the same doses of Phentermine HCl. The clinical significance of these differences is not known. In clinical trials establishing the efficacy of Phentermine Resin, a single daily dose produced an effect comparable to that produced by other regimens of "anorectic" drug therapy.

INDICATION

Phentermine is indicated in the management of exogenous obesity as a short-term (a few weeks) adjunct in a regimen of weight reduction based on caloric restriction. The limited usefulness of agents of this class (see *"Actions"*) should be measured against possible risk factors inherent in their use such as those described below.

CONTRAINDICATIONS

Advanced arteriosclerosis, symptomatic cardiovascular disease, moderate to severe hypertension, hyperthyroidism, known hypersensitivity, or idiosyncrasy to the sympathomimetic amines, glaucoma.

Agitated states.

Patients with a history of drug abuse.

During or within 14 days following the administration of monoamine oxidase inhibitors (hypertensive crises may result).

WARNINGS

Tolerance to the anorectic effect usually develops within a few weeks. When this occurs, the recommended dose should not be exceeded in an attempt to increase the effect; rather, the drug should be discontinued. Phentermine may impair the ability of the patient to engage in potentially hazardous activities such as operating machinery or driving a motor vehicle; the patient should therefore be cautioned accordingly.

When using CNS active agents, consideration must always be given to the possibility of adverse interactions with alcohol.

Drug Dependence: Phentermine is related chemically and pharmacologically to amphetamine (d- and d *l*-amphetamine) and other stimulant drugs that have been extensively abused. The possibility of abuse of Phentermine in should be kept in mind when evaluating the desirability of including a drug as part of a weight reduction program. Abuse of amphetamine (d- and d *l*-amphetamine) and related drugs may be associated with intense psychological dependence and severe social dysfunction. There are reports of patients who have increased the dosage of some of these drugs to many times that recommended. Abrupt cessation following prolonged high dosage administration results in extreme fatigue and mental depression; changes are also noted on the sleep EEG. Manifestations of chronic intoxication with anorectic drugs include severe dermatoses, marked insomnia, irritability, hyperactivity, and personality changes. The most severe manifestation of chronic intoxications is psychosis, often clinically indistinguishable from schizophrenia.

Usage in Pregnancy: Safe use in pregnancy has not been established. Use of Phentermine by women who are or may become pregnant, and those in the first trimester of pregnancy, requires that the potential benefit be weighed against the possible hazard to mother and infant.

Usage in Children: Phentermine is not recommended for use in children under 12 years of age.

PRECAUTIONS

Caution is to be exercised in prescribing Phentermine for patients with even mild hypertension. Insulin requirements in diabetes mellitus may be altered in association with the use of Phentermine and the concomitant dietary regimen.

Phentermine may decrease the hypotensive effect of adrenergic neuron blocking drugs such as guanethidine.

The least amount feasible should be prescribed or dispensed at one time in order to minimize the possibility of overdosage.

ADVERSE REACTIONS

Cardiovascular: Palpitation, tachycardia, elevation of blood pressure.

Central Nervous System: Overstimulation, restlessness, dizziness, insomnia, euphoria, dysphoria, tremor, headache; rarely psychotic episodes at recommended doses with some drugs in this class.

Gastrointestinal: Dryness of the mouth, unpleasant taste, diarrhea, constipation, other gastrointestinal disturbances.

Allergic: Urticaria.

Endocrine: Impotence, changes in libido.

OVERDOSAGE

Manifestations of acute overdosage with Phentermine may include restlessness, tremor, hyperreflexia, rapid respiration, confusion, assaultiveness, hallucinations, panic states.

Fatigue and depression usually follow the central stimulation.

Cardiovascular effects include arrhythmias, hypertension or hypotension, and circulatory collapse. Gastrointestinal symptoms include nausea, vomiting, diarrhea, and abdominal cramps. Overdosage of pharmacologically similar compounds has resulted in fatal poisoning, usually terminating in convulsions and coma.

Management of acute Phentermine intoxication is largely symptomatic and includes lavage and sedation with a barbiturate. Experience with hemodialysis or peritoneal dialysis is inadequate to permit recommendation in this regard. Acidification of the urine increases Phentermine excretion. Intravenous phentolamine has been suggested on pharmacologic grounds for possible acute, severe hypertension, if this complicates Phentermine overdosage.

DOSAGE AND ADMINISTRATION

Phentermine Resin: One capsule daily, before breakfast or 10-14 hours before retiring. For individuals exhibiting greater drug responsiveness, the 15-mg capsule will usually suffice. The 30-mg capsule is recommended for less responsive patients. Phentermine Resin is not recommended for use in children under 12 years of age. Phentermine Resin capsules should be swallowed whole.

Phentermine HCl: One capsule at approximately 2 hours after breakfast for appetite control. Late evening medication should be avoided because of the possibility of resulting insomnia.

Administration of one capsule (30 mg) daily has been found to be adequate in depression of the appetite for twelve to fourteen hours.

Phentermine HCl is not recommended for use in children under 12 years of age.

HOW SUPPLIED

PHENTERMINE HYDROCHLORIDE
CAPSULE: 37.5 MG

AVERAGE UNIT PRICE (AVAILABLE SIZES)		GENERIC A-RATED AVERAGE PRICE (GAAP)	
BRAND	$0.97	100s	$19.72
GENERIC	$0.12	1000s	$61.35
HCFA FUL (100s ea)	$0.14		

BRAND/MANUFACTURER	NDC	SIZE	AWP
◆ BRAND			
ADIPEX-P: Gate	57844-0019-01	100s	$96.76
◆ GENERICS			
Camall	00147-0254-10	100s	$9.35
Camall	00147-0231-10	100s	$9.35
Camall	00147-0234-10	100s	$9.35
Camall	00147-0235-10	100s	$9.35
OBENIX: Abana	12463-0217-01	100s	$61.20
Camall	00147-0231-20	1000s	$61.35
Camall	00147-0234-20	1000s	$61.35
Camall	00147-0235-20	1000s	$61.35
Camall	00147-0251-20	1000s	$61.35
Camall	00147-0253-20	1000s	$61.35
Camall	00147-0254-20	1000s	$61.35

CAPSULE (C-IV): 15 MG

AVERAGE UNIT PRICE (AVAILABLE SIZES)	
GENERIC	$0.03

BRAND/MANUFACTURER	NDC	SIZE	AWP
◆ GENERICS			
Eon	00185-0644-01	100s	$3.74
Eon	00185-0644-10	1000s	$24.22

CAPSULE (C-IV): 18.75 MG

AVERAGE UNIT PRICE (AVAILABLE SIZES)	
GENERIC	$0.06

BRAND/MANUFACTURER	NDC	SIZE	AWP
◆ GENERICS			
Camall	00147-0249-10	100s	$7.33
Camall	00147-0249-20	1000s	$38.60

CAPSULE (C-IV): 30 MG

AVERAGE UNIT PRICE (AVAILABLE SIZES)		GENERIC A-RATED AVERAGE PRICE (GAAP)	
BRAND	$0.93	100s	$7.96
GENERIC	$0.07	1000s	$44.97
HCFA FUL (100s ea)	$0.04		

BRAND/MANUFACTURER	NDC	SIZE	AWP
◆ BRAND			
FASTIN: SK Beecham Pharm	00029-2205-30	100s	$94.30
	00029-2205-39	450s	$410.35
◆ GENERICS			
Allscrips	54569-3069-05	7s	$1.05
Allscrips	54569-3069-03	14s	$2.10
Allscrips	54569-3069-02	15s	$2.25
Allscrips	54569-3069-06	28s	$4.19
Allscrips	54569-3069-00	30s	$4.49
Allscrips	54569-3069-04	60s	$8.99
Eon	00185-0647-01	100s	$4.55
Eon	00185-5000-01	100s	$5.95
Major	00904-3921-60	100s	$6.15
Qualitest	00603-5190-21	100s	$6.63
Rexar	00478-5469-01	100s	$7.35
Camall	00147-0201-10	100s	$7.37
Camall	00147-0202-10	100s	$7.37
Camall	00147-0198-10	100s	$7.46
Geneva	00781-2415-01	100s	$7.64
URL	00677-0460-01	100s	$8.38
Rosemont	00832-0204-00	100s	$8.54
Goldline	00182-1026-01	100s	$8.85
OBY-CAP: Richwood	58521-0333-01	100s	$8.98
Major	00904-0614-60	100s	$9.90
Rugby	00536-4236-01	100s	$10.03

➤ SHOWN IN PRODUCT IDENTIFICATION GUIDE

BRAND/MANUFACTURER	NDC	SIZE	AWP
Rugby	00536-4235-01	100s	$10.05
Aligen	00405-4796-01	100s	$10.05
OBY-CAP: Richwood	58521-0333-05	500s	$35.98
Moore,H.L.	00839-6298-16	1000s	$29.69
Eon	00185-0647-10	1000s	$31.88
Moore,H.L.	00839-5099-16	1000s	$35.09
Camall	00147-0201-20	1000s	$38.89
Camall	00147-0202-20	1000s	$38.89
Camall	00147-0198-20	1000s	$39.24
Major	00904-3921-80	1000s	$39.30
Rexar	00478-5465-10	1000s	$40.45
Rexar	00478-5468-10	1000s	$40.45
Rexar	00478-5469-10	1000s	$40.45
Rexar	00478-5474-10	1000s	$40.45
Qualitest	00603-5190-32	1000s	$40.94
Rosemont	00832-0204-10	1000s	$43.84
Major	00904-0614-80	1000s	$48.75
URL	00677-0460-10	1000s	$49.50
Rugby	00536-4235-10	1000s	$49.59
Rugby	00536-4236-10	1000s	$49.59
Eon	00185-5000-10	1000s	$49.95
Goldline	00182-1026-10	1000s	$57.15
Parmed	00349-2165-10	1000s	$95.23

CAPSULE (C-IV): 30 MG

BRAND/MANUFACTURER	NDC	SIZE	AWP
○ BRAND			
T-DIET: Jones Medical	52604-0010-01	100s	$61.55

CAPSULE (C-IV): 37.5 MG

AVERAGE UNIT PRICE (AVAILABLE SIZES)		GENERIC A-RATED AVERAGE PRICE (GAAP)	
BRAND	$0.97	100s	$19.72
GENERIC	$0.12	1000s	$61.35
HCFA FUL (100s ea)	$0.14		

BRAND/MANUFACTURER	NDC	SIZE	AWP
◆ BRAND			
ADIPEX-P: Gate	57844-0019-01	100s	$96.76
◆ GENERICS			
Camall	00147-0254-10	100s	$9.35
Camall	00147-0231-10	100s	$9.35
Camall	00147-0234-10	100s	$9.35
Camall	00147-0235-10	100s	$9.35
OBENIX: Abana	12463-0217-01	100s	$61.20
Camall	00147-0231-20	1000s	$61.35
Camall	00147-0234-20	1000s	$61.35
Camall	00147-0235-20	1000s	$61.35
Camall	00147-0251-20	1000s	$61.35
Camall	00147-0253-20	1000s	$61.35
Camall	00147-0254-20	1000s	$61.35

TABLETS (C-IV): 8 MG

AVERAGE UNIT PRICE (AVAILABLE SIZES)		GENERIC A-RATED AVERAGE PRICE (GAAP)	
GENERIC	$0.02	1000s	$18.91

BRAND/MANUFACTURER	NDC	SIZE	AWP
◆ GENERICS			
Camall	00147-0102-20	1000s	$15.72
Camall	00147-0136-20	1000s	$15.72
Rugby	00536-4288-10	1000s	$21.71
Goldline	00182-0204-10	1000s	$22.50

TABLETS (C-IV): 37.5 MG

AVERAGE UNIT PRICE (AVAILABLE SIZES)		GENERIC A-RATED AVERAGE PRICE (GAAP)	
BRAND	$0.88	100s	$9.38
GENERIC	$0.08	1000s	$54.36
HCFA FUL (100s ea)	$0.07		

BRAND/MANUFACTURER	NDC	SIZE	AWP
◆ BRAND			
ADIPEX-P: Gate	57844-0009-01	100s	$95.06
	57844-0009-26	400s	$361.32
ADIPEX-P: Gate	57844-0009-10	1000s	$777.90
◆ GENERICS			
Qualitest	00603-5191-21	100s	$8.90
URL	00677-0829-01	100s	$9.10
Goldline	00182-0205-01	100s	$9.15
Camall	00147-022-10	100s	$9.35
Camall	00147-0248-10	100s	$9.35
Rugby	00536-4237-01	100s	$10.43
Rugby	00536-4237-10	1000s	$47.25
Goldline	00182-0205-10	1000s	$47.50
Camall	00147-0232-20	1000s	$61.35
Camall	00147-0248-20	1000s	$61.35

PHENTERMINE RESIN
CAPSULE, EXTENDED RELEASE (C-IV): 15 MG

BRAND/MANUFACTURER	NDC	SIZE	AWP
○ BRAND			
IONAMIN: Fisons Presc	00585-0903-71	100s	$98.38
	00585-0903-84	400s	$374.82

CAPSULE, EXTENDED RELEASE (C-IV): 30 MG

BRAND/MANUFACTURER	NDC	SIZE	AWP
○ BRAND			
IONAMIN: Fisons Presc	00585-0904-71	100s	$112.74
	00585-0904-84	400s	$429.19

Phentolamine Mesylate

DESCRIPTION

Phentolamine Mesylate USP is an antihypertensive, available in vials for intravenous and intramuscular administration. Each vial contains Phentolamine Mesylate USP, 5 mg.

Phentolamine Mesylate is 4,5-dihydro-2-[N-(m-hydroxyphenyl)-N-(p-methyl-phenyl) aminomethyl]-1H-imidazole 1:1 methanesulfonate.

Phentolamine Mesylate USP is a white or off-white, odorless crystalline powder with a molecular weight of 377.46. Its solutions are acid to litmus. It is freely soluble in water and in alcohol, and slightly soluble in chloroform. It melts at about 178°C.

Following is its chemical structure:

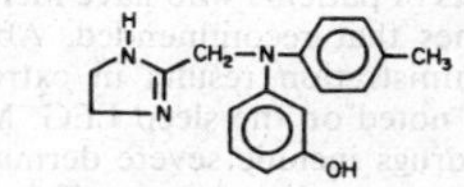

CLINICAL PHARMACOLOGY

Phentolamine Mesylate produces an alpha-adrenergic block of relatively short duration. It also has direct, but less marked, positive inotropic and chronotropic effects on cardiac muscle and vasodilator effects on vascular smooth muscle.

Phentolamine Mesylate has a half-life in the blood of 19 minutes following intravenous administration. Approximately 13% of a single intravenous dose appears in the urine as unchanged drug.

INDICATIONS AND USAGE

Phentolamine Mesylate is indicated for the prevention or control of hypertensive episodes that may occur in a patient with pheochromocytoma as a result of stress or manipulation during preoperative preparation and surgical excision.

Phentolamine Mesylate is indicated for the prevention or treatment of dermal necrosis and sloughing following intravenous administration or extravasation of norepinephrine.

Phentolamine Mesylate is also indicated for the diagnosis of pheochromocytoma by the Phentolamine Mesylate blocking test.

UNLABELED USES

Phentolamine is used alone or as an adjunct in the treatment of cardiac arrhythmias including ventricular premature complexes, premature atrial contraction, supraventricular premature contractions, and conduction defects. It is also used to improve exercise-induced bronchospasm in asthmatic patients, in cardiac diseases, including congestive heart failure, cocaine-induced myocardial ischemia, alcoholic cardiomyopathy, juvenile diabetes mellitus, idiopathic hypertrophic subaortic stenosis, and acute myocardial infarction. Phentolamine is also prescribed for the treatment of erectile impotence and Raynaud's phenomenon.

CONTRAINDICATIONS

Myocardial infarction, history of myocardial infarction, coronary insufficiency, angina, or other evidence suggestive of coronary artery disease; hypersensitivity to Phentolamine or related compounds.

WARNINGS

Myocardial infarction, cerebrovascular spasm, and cerebrovascular occlusion have been reported to occur following the administration of Phentolamine Mesylate, usually in association with marked hypotensive episodes.

For screening tests in patients with hypertension, the generally available urinary assays of catecholamines or other biochemical assays have largely replaced the Phentolamine Mesylate and other pharmacological tests for reasons of accuracy and safety. None of the chemical or pharmacological tests is infallible in the diagnosis of pheochromocytoma. The Phentolamine Mesylate blocking test is not the procedure of choice and should be reserved for cases in which additional confirmatory evidence is necessary and the relative risks involved in conducting the test have been considered.

◆ RATED THERAPEUTICALLY EQUIVALENT; ◇ THERAPEUTIC EQUIVALENCE UNCONFIRMED; ○ UNRATED

PRECAUTIONS

GENERAL
Tachycardia and cardiac arrhythmias may occur with the use of Phentolamine Mesylate or other alpha-adrenergic blocking agents. When possible, administration of cardiac glycosides should be deferred until cardiac rhythm returns to normal

DRUG INTERACTIONS
See "Dosage and Administration, Diagnosis of pheochromocytoma, Preparation".

CARCINOGENESIS, MUTAGENESIS, IMPAIRMENT OF FERTILITY
Long-term carcinogenicity studies, mutagenicity studies and fertility studies have not been conducted with Phentolamine Mesylate

PREGNANCY CATEGORY C
Administration of Phentolamine Mesylate to pregnant rats and mice at oral doses 24-30 times the usual daily human dose (based on a 60-kg human) resulted in slightly decreased growth and slight skeletal immaturity of the fetuses. Immaturity was manifested by increased incidence of incomplete or unossified calcanei and phalangeal nuclei of the hind limb and of incompletely ossified sternebrae. At oral doses 60 times the usual daily human dose (based on a 60-kg human), a slightly lower rate of implantation was found in the rat. Phentolamine Mesylate did not affect embryonic or fetal development in the rabbit at oral doses 20 times the usual daily human dose (based on a 60-kg human). No teratogenic or embryotoxic effects were observed in the rat, mouse, or rabbit studies.

There are no adequate and well-controlled studies in pregnant women. Phentolamine Mesylate should be used during pregnancy only if the potential benefit justifies the potential risk to the fetus.

NURSING MOTHERS
It is not known whether this drug is excreted in human milk. Because many drugs are excreted in human milk and because of the potential for serious adverse reactions in nursing infants from Phentolamine Mesylate, a decision should be made whether to discontinue nursing or to discontinue the drug, taking into account the importance of the drug to the mother.

PEDIATRIC USE
See "Dosage and Administration".

ADVERSE REACTIONS
Acute and prolonged hypotensive episodes, tachycardia, and cardiac arrhythmias have been reported. In addition, weakness, dizziness, flushing, orthostatic hypotension, nasal stuffiness, nausea, vomiting, and diarrhea may occur.

OVERDOSAGE

ACUTE TOXICITY
No deaths due to acute poisoning with Phentolamine Mesylate have been reported.
Oral LD_{50}'s (mg/kg): mice, 1000; rats, 1250.

SIGNS AND SYMPTOMS
Overdosage with Phentolamine Mesylate is characterized chiefly by cardiovascular disturbances, such as arrhythmias, tachycardia, hypotension, and possibly shock. In addition, the following might occur: excitation, headache, sweating, pupillary contraction, visual disturbances; nausea, vomiting, diarrhea; hypoglycemia.

TREATMENT
There is no specific antidote.
A decrease in blood pressure to dangerous levels or other evidence of shocklike conditions should be treated vigorously and promptly. The patient's legs should be kept raised and a plasma expander should be administered. If necessary, intravenous infusion of norepinephrine, titrated to maintain blood pressure at the normotensive level, and all available supportive measures should be included. Epinephrine should not be used, since it may cause a paradoxical reduction in blood pressure.

DOSAGE AND ADMINISTRATION
The reconstituted solution should be used upon preparation and should not be stored.

Note: Parenteral drug products should be inspected visually for particulate matter and discoloration prior to administration, whenever solution and container permit.

1. PREVENTION OR CONTROL OF HYPERTENSIVE EPISODES IN THE PATIENT WITH PHEOCHROMOCYTOMA.
For preoperative reduction of elevated blood pressure, 5 mg of Phentolamine Mesylate (1 mg for children) is injected intravenously or intramuscularly 1 or 2 hours before surgery, and repeated if necessary.

During surgery, Phentolamine Mesylate (5 mg for adults, 1 mg for children) is administered intravenously as indicated, to help prevent or control paroxysms of hypertension, tachycardia, respiratory depression, convulsions, or other effects of epinephrine intoxication. (Postoperatively, norepinephrine may be given to control the hypotension that commonly follows complete removal of a pheochromocytoma.)

2. PREVENTION OR TREATMENT OF DERMAL NECROSIS AND SLOUGHING FOLLOWING INTRAVENOUS ADMINISTRATION OR EXTRAVASATION OF NOREPINEPHRINE.
For Prevention: 10 mg of Phentolamine Mesylate is added to each liter of solution containing norepinephrine. The pressor effect of norepinephrine is not affected.

For Treatment: 5-10 mg of Phentolamine Mesylate in 10 ml of saline is injected into the area of extravasation within 12 hours.

3. DIAGNOSIS OF PHEOCHROMOCYTOMA—PHENTOLAMINE MESYLATE BLOCKING TEST.
The test is most reliable in detecting pheochromocytoma in patients with sustained hypertension and least reliable in those with paroxysmal hypertension. False-positive tests may occur in patients with hypertension without pheochromocytoma.

a. Intravenous
Preparation: The "Contraindications", "Warnings", and "Precautions" sections should be reviewed. Sedatives, analgesics, and all other medications except those that might be deemed essential (such as digitalis and insulin) are withheld for at least 24 hours, as preferably 48-72 hours, prior to the test. Antihypertensive drugs are withheld until blood pressure returns to the untreated, hypertensive level. This test is not performed on a patient who is normotensive.

Procedure: The patient is kept at rest in the supine position throughout the test, preferably in a quiet, darkened room. Injection of Phentolamine Mesylate is delayed until blood pressure is stabilized, as evidenced by blood pressure readings taken every 10 minutes for at least 30 minutes.

Five milligrams of Phentolamine Mesylate is dissolved in 1 ml of Sterile Water for Injection. The dose for adults is 5 mg; for children, 1 mg.

The syringe needle is inserted into the vein, and injection is delayed until pressor response to venipuncture has subsided. Phentolamine Mesylate is injected rapidly. Blood pressure is recorded immediately after injection, at 30-second intervals for the first 3 minutes, and at 60-second intervals for the next 7 minutes.

Interpretation: A positive response, suggestive of pheochromocytoma, is indicated when the blood pressure is reduced more than 35 mm Hg systolic and 25 mm Hg diastolic. A typical positive response is a reduction in pressure of 60 mm Hg systolic and 25 mm Hg diastolic. Usually, maximal effect is evident within 2 minutes after injection. A return to preinjection pressure commonly occurs within 15-30 minutes but may occur more rapidly.

If blood pressure decreases to a dangerous level, the patient should be treated as outlined under "Overdosage".

A positive response should always be confirmed by other diagnostic procedures, preferably by measurement of urinary catecholamines or their metabolites.

A negative response is indicated when the blood pressure is elevated, unchanged, or reduced less than 35 mm Hg systolic and 25 mm Hg diastolic after injection of Phentolamine Mesylate. A negative response to this test does not exclude the diagnosis of pheochromocytoma, especially in patients with paroxysmal hypertension in whom the incidence of false-negative responses is high.

b. Intramuscular
If the intramuscular test for pheochromocytoma is preferred, preparation is the same as for the intravenous test. Five milligrams of Phentolamine Mesylate is then dissolved in 1 ml of Sterile Water for Injection. The dose for adults is 5 mg intramuscularly; for children, 3 mg. Blood pressure is recorded every 5 minutes for 30-45 minutes following injection. A positive response is indicated when the blood pressure is reduced 35 mm Hg systolic and 25 mm Hg diastolic, or more, within 20 minutes following injection.

Storage: Store between 59° and 86°F.

J CODES
Up to 5 ml IM,IV—J2760

HOW SUPPLIED
INJECTION: 5 MG

BRAND/MANUFACTURER	NDC	SIZE	AWP
○ BRAND REGITINE: Ciba Pharm	00083-6830-02	1 ml 2s	$56.28

Phenurone *SEE* PHENACEMIDE

Phenylephrine Hydrochloride and Sulfacetamide Sodium

DESCRIPTION
Phenylephrine Hydrochloride/Sulfacetamide Sodium ophthalmic solution is a sterile solution for ophthalmic administration having the following composition:

Phenylephrine HCl ....1.25 mg/mL
  (sympathomimetic)
Sulfacetamide Sodium ....150 mg/mL
  (bacteriostatic antibacterial)

The chemical name for Phenylephrine Hydrochloride is Benzenemethanol, 3-hydroxy-α-[(methylamino)-methyl]-, hydrochloride (R)-.

The chemical name for Sulfacetamide Sodium is Acetamide, N-[(4-aminophenyl)sulfonyl]-, monosodium salt, monohydrate.

CLINICAL PHARMACOLOGY

Phenylephrine HCl is an alpha sympathetic receptor agonist producing vasoconstriction.

Sulfacetamide Sodium exerts a bacteriostatic effect against a wide range of gram-positive and gram-negative microorganisms by restricting through competition with p-aminobenzoic acid, the synthesis of folic acid which bacteria require for growth.

INDICATIONS AND USAGE

Phenylephrine HCl/Sulfacetamide Sodium ophthalmic solution is indicated for the treatment of conjunctivitis, corneal ulcer, and other superficial ocular infections due to susceptible microorganisms, and an adjunctive in systemic sulfonamide therapy of trachoma.

CONTRAINDICATIONS

Contraindicated in persons hypersensitive to one or more of the components of the preparation.

PRECAUTIONS

The solutions are incompatible with silver preparations. Local anesthetics related to p-aminobenzoic acid may antagonize the action of the sulfonamides. Bacteria initially sensitive to sulfonamides may acquire resistance to the drug. Nonsusceptible organisms, including fungi, may proliferate with the use of this preparation. Sulfonamides are inactivated by the p-aminobenzoic acid present in purulent exudates.

If signs of hypersensitivity or other untoward reactions occur, discontinue use of the preparation.

To prevent contaminating the dropper tip and solution, care should be taken not to touch the eyelids or surrounding area with the dropper tip of the bottle. Keep bottle tightly closed when not in use and protect from light. Do not use if the solution has darkened or contains a precipitate.

For topical use only.

Carcinogenesis, Mutagenesis, Impairment of Fertility: There have been no long-term studies done using Sulfacetamide and/or Phenylephrine in animals to evaluate carcinogenic potential.

Pregnancy: Pregnancy Category C. Animal reproduction studies have not been conducted with Sulfacetamide and/or Phenylephrine. It is also not known whether Sulfacetamide and/or Phenylephrine can cause fetal harm when administered to a pregnant woman or can affect reproduction capacity. Sulfacetamide and/or Phenylephrine should be given to a pregnant woman only if clearly needed.

Nursing Mothers: It is not known whether these drugs are excreted in human milk. Because many drugs are excreted in human milk, caution should be exercised when Sulfacetamide and/or Phenylephrine is administered to a nursing woman.

Pediatric Use: Safety and effectiveness in children have not been established.

ADVERSE REACTIONS

Headache or browache, blurred vision, local irritation, burning, transient stinging, transient epithelial keratitis, and reactive hyperemia. Sensitization reactions to Sulfacetamide Sodium may occur, although rarely. Reactions occurring most often from the presence of the anti-infective ingredient are allergic sensitizations. Although hypersensitivity reactions to Sulfacetamide Sodium are rare, instances of Stevens-Johnson syndrome, systemic lupus erythematosus (in one case producing a fatal outcome), exfoliative dermatitis, toxic epidermal necrolysis, and photosensitivity have been reported following the use of sulfonamide preparations.

DOSAGE AND ADMINISTRATION

Instill one or two drops into lower conjunctival sac every two or three hours during the day, less often at night.

Keep tightly closed when not in use. Protect from light.

Store at 15° to 30°C (59° to 86°F).

HOW SUPPLIED
DROP: 0.125%-15%

BRAND/MANUFACTURER	NDC	SIZE	AWP
○ BRAND			
VASOSULF: Iolab	00058-2883-05	5 ml	$8.88
	00058-2883-15	15 ml	$12.00

Phenylephrine Hydrochloride

DESCRIPTION

Phenylephrine Hydrochloride is a vasoconstrictor and pressor drug chemically related to epinephrine and ephedrine.

Phenylephrine Hydrochloride is a synthetic sympathomimetic agent in sterile form for parenteral injection. Chemically, Phenylephrine Hydrochloride is (−)-*m*-Hydroxy-α-[(methylamino)methyl]benzyl alcohol Hydrochloride.

Following is its chemical structure:

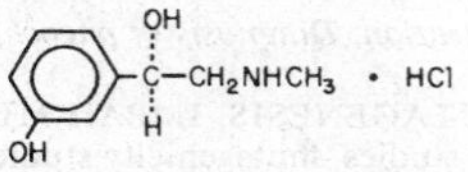

CLINICAL PHARMACOLOGY

Phenylephrine Hydrochloride produces vasoconstriction that lasts longer than that of epinephrine and ephedrine. Responses are more sustained than those to epinephrine, lasting 20 minutes after intravenous and as long as 50 minutes after subcutaneous injection. Its action on the heart contrasts sharply with that of epinephrine and ephedrine, in that it slows the heart rate and increases the stroke output, producing no disturbance in the rhythm of the pulse.

Phenylephrine is a powerful postsynaptic alpha-receptor stimulant with little effect on the beta receptors of the heart. In therapeutic doses, it produces little if any stimulation of either the spinal cord or cerebrum. A singular advantage of this drug is the fact that repeated injections produce comparable effects.

The predominant actions of Phenylephrine are on the cardiovascular system. Parenteral administration causes a rise in systolic and diastolic pressures in man and other species. Accompanying the pressor response to Phenylephrine is a marked reflex bradycardia that can be blocked by atropine; after atropine, large doses of the drug increase the heart rate only slightly. In man, cardiac output is slightly decreased and peripheral resistance is considerably increased. Circulation time is slightly prolonged, and venous pressure is slightly increased; venous constriction is not marked. Most vascular beds are constricted; renal splanchnic, cutaneous, and limb blood flows are reduced but coronary blood flow is increased. Pulmonary vessels are constricted, and pulmonary arterial pressure is raised.

The drug is a powerful vasoconstrictor, with properties very similar to those of norepinephrine but almost completely lacking the chronotropic and inotropic actions on the heart. Cardiac irregularities are seen only very rarely even with large doses.

INDICATIONS AND USAGE

Phenylephrine Hydrochloride is intended for the maintenance of an adequate level of blood pressure during spinal and inhalation anesthesia and for the treatment of vascular failure in shock, shocklike states, and drug-induced hypotension, or hypersensitivity. It is also employed to overcome paroxysmal supraventricular tachycardia, to prolong spinal anesthesia, and as a vasoconstrictor in regional analgesia.

UNLABELED USES
Phenylephrine Hydrochloride is used alone or as an adjunct in the treatment of orthostatic hypotension and papaverine-induced penile erection in priapism.

CONTRAINDICATIONS

Phenylephrine Hydrochloride should not be used in patients with severe hypertension, ventricular tachycardia, or in patients who are hypersensitive to it.

WARNINGS

If used in conjunction with oxytocic drugs, the pressor effect of sympathomimetic pressor amines is potentiated (see Drug Interaction). The obstetrician should be warned that some oxytocic drugs may cause severe persistent hypertension and that even a rupture of a cerebral blood vessel may occur during the postpartum period.

Contains sodium metabisulfite, a sulfite that may cause allergic-type reactions including anaphylactic symptoms and life-threatening or less severe asthmatic episodes in certain susceptible people. The overall prevalence of sulfite sensitivity in the general population is unknown and probably low. Sulfite sensitivity is seen more frequently in asthmatic than in nonasthmatic people.

PRECAUTIONS

Phenylephrine Hydrochloride should be employed only with extreme caution in elderly patients or in patients with hyperthyroidism, bradycardia, partial heart block, myocardial disease, or severe arteriosclerosis.

Drug Interactions: Vasopressors, particularly metaraminol, may cause serious cardiac arrhythmias during halothane anesthesia and therefore should be used only with great caution or not at all.

MAO Inhibitors: The pressor effect of sympathomimetic pressor amines is markedly potentiated in patients receiving monoamine oxidase inhibitors (MAOI). Therefore, when initiating pressor therapy in these patients, the initial dose should be small and used with due caution. The pressor response of adrenergic agents may also be potentiated by tricyclic antidepressants.

Carcinogenesis, Mutagenesis, Impairment of Fertility: No long-term animal studies have been done to evaluate the potential of Phenylephrine in these areas.

Pregnancy Category C: Animal reproduction studies have not been conducted with Phenylephrine. It is also not known whether Phenylephrine can cause fetal harm when administered to a pregnant woman or can affect reproduction capacity. Phenylephrine should be given to a pregnant woman only if clearly needed.

Labor and Delivery: If vasopressor drugs are either used to correct hypotension or added to the local anesthetic solution, the obstetrician should be cautioned that some oxytocic drugs may cause severe persistent hypertension and that even a rupture of a cerebral blood vessel may occur during the postpartum period (see "Warnings").

Nursing Mother: It is not known whether this drug is excreted in human milk. Because many are excreted in human milk, caution should be exercised when Phenylephrine Hydrochloride injection, is administered to a nursing woman.

Pediatric Use: To combat hypotension during spinal anesthesia in children, a dose of 0.5 mg to 1 mg per 25 pounds body weight, administered subcutaneously or intramuscularly, is recommended.

ADVERSE REACTIONS
Headache, reflex bradycardia, excitability, restlessness, and rarely arrhythmias.

OVERDOSAGE
Overdosage may induce ventricular extrasystoles and short paroxysms of ventricular tachycardia, a sensation of fullness in the head and tingling of the extremities.

Should an excessive elevation of blood pressure occur, it may be immediately relieved by an α-adrenergic blocking agent, eg, phentolamine.

The oral LD_{50} in the rat is 350 mg/kg, in the mouse 120 mg/kg.

DOSAGE AND ADMINISTRATION
Phenylephrine is generally injected subcutaneously, intramuscularly, slowly intravenously, or in dilute solution as a continuous intravenous infusion. In patients with paroxysmal supraventricular tachycardia and, if indicated, in case of emergency. Phenylephrine is administered directly intravenously. The dose should be adjusted according to the pressor response.

DOSAGE CALCULATIONS

Dose Required	Use Phenylephrine 1%
10 mg	1 mL
5 mg	0.5 mL
1 mg	0.1 mL

For convenience in intermittent intravenous administration, dilute 1 mL Phenylephrine 1% with 9 mL Sterile Water for Injection, USP, to yield 0.1% Phenylephrine.

Dose Required	Use Diluted Phenylephrine (0.1%)
0.1 mg	0.1 mL
0.2 mg	0.2 mL
0.5 mg	0.5 mL

MILD OR MODERATE HYPOTENSION
Subcutaneously or Intramuscularly: Usual dose, from 2 mg to 5 mg. Range, from 1 mg to 10 mg. Initial dose should not exceed 5 mg.

Intravenously: Usual dose, 0.2 mg. Range, from 0.1 mg to 0.5 mg. Initial dose should not exceed 0.5 mg.

Injections should not be repeated more often than every 10 to 15 minutes. A 5 mg intramuscular dose should raise blood pressure for one to two hours. A 0.5 mg intravenous dose should elevate the pressure for about 15 minutes.

SEVERE HYPOTENSION AND SHOCK—INCLUDING DRUG-RELATED HYPOTENSION
Blood volume depletion should always be corrected as fully as possible before any vasopressor is administered. When, as an emergency measure, intraaortic pressures must be maintained to prevent cerebral or coronary artery ischemia, Phenylephrine Hydrochloride, brand of Phenylephrine Hydrochloride injection, can be administered before and concurrently with blood volume replacement.

Hypotension and occasionally severe shock may result from overdosage or idiosyncrasy following the administration of certain drugs, especially adrenergic and ganglionic blocking agents, rauwolfia and veratrum alkaloids, and phenothiazine tranquilizers. Patients who receive a phenothiazine derivative as preoperative medication are especially susceptible to these reactions. As an adjunct in the management of such episodes Phenylephrine Hydrochloride is a suitable agent for restoring blood pressure.

Higher initial and maintenance doses of Phenylephrine are required in patients with persistent or untreated severe hypotension or shock. Hypotension produced by powerful peripheral adrenergic blocking agents, chlorpromazine, or pheochromocytomy may also require more intensive therapy.

Continuous Infusion: Add 10 mg of the drug (1 mL of 1 percent solution) to 500 mL of Dextrose Injection, USP, or Sodium Chloride Injection, USP (providing a 1:50,000 solution). To raise the blood pressure rapidly, start the infusion at about 100 µg to 180 µg per minute (based on 20 drops per mL this would be 100 to 180 drops per minute). When the blood pressure is stabilized (at a low normal level for the individual), a maintenance rate of 40 µg to 60 µg per minute usually suffices (based on 20 drops per mL this would be 40 to 60 drops per minute). If the drop size of the infusion system varies from the 20 drops per mL, the dose must be adjusted accordingly.

If a prompt initial pressor response is not obtained, additional increments of Phenylephrine (10 mg or more) are added to the infusion bottle. The rate of flow

is then adjusted until the desired blood pressure level is obtained. (In some cases, a more potent vasopressor, such as norepinephrine bitartrate, may be required.) Hypertension should be avoided. The blood pressure should be checked frequently. Headache and/or bradycardia may indicate hypertension. Arrhythmias are rare.

SPINAL ANESTHESIA—HYPOTENSION
Routine parenteral use of Phenylephrine has been recommended for the prophylaxis and treatment of hypotension during spinal anesthesia. It is best administered subcutaneously or intramuscularly three or four minutes before injection of the spinal anesthetic. The total requirement for high anesthetic levels is usually 3 mg, and for lower levels, 2 mg. For hypotensive emergencies during spinal anesthesia, Phenylephrine may be injected intravenously, using an initial dose of 0.2 mg. Any subsequent dose should not exceed the previous dose by more than 0.1 mg to 0.2 mg and no more than 0.5 mg should be administered in a single dose. To combat hypotension during spinal anesthesia in children, a dose of 0.5 mg to 1 mg per 25 pounds body weight, administered subcutaneously or intramuscularly, is recommended.

PROLONGATION OF SPINAL ANESTHESIA
The addition of 2 mg to 5 mg of Phenylephrine Hydrochloride to the anesthetic solution increases the duration of motor block by as much as approximately 50 percent without any increase in the incidence of complications such as nausea, vomiting, or blood pressure disturbances.

VASOCONSTRICTOR FOR REGIONAL ANALGESIA
Concentrations about ten times those employed when epinephrine is used as a vasoconstrictor are recommended. The optimum strength is 1:20,000 (made by adding 1 mg of Phenylephrine Hydrochloride to every 20 mL of local anesthetic solution). Some pressor responses can be expected when 2 mg or more are injected.

PAROXYSMAL SUPRAVENTRICULAR TACHYCARDIA
Rapid intravenous injection (within 20 to 30 seconds) is recommended; the initial dose should not exceed 0.5 mg, and subsequent doses, which are determined by the initial blood pressure response, should not exceed the preceding dose by more than 0.1 mg to 0.2 mg, and should never exceed 1 mg.

STORAGE
Protect from light if removed from carton or dispensing bin.

J CODES
Up to 1 ml SC,IM,IV—J2370

HOW SUPPLIED
INJECTION: 10 MG/ML

BRAND/MANUFACTURER	NDC	SIZE	AWP
○ **BRAND**			
NEO-SYNEPHRINE: Sanofi Winthrop	00024-1342-04	1 ml 25s	$187.33
	00024-1340-02	2 ml 50s	$104.19
○ **GENERICS**			
Elkins-Sinn	00641-0482-25	1 ml 25s	$76.88
Amer Regent	00517-0299-25	1 ml 25s	$78.13
Schein	00364-2426-46	1 ml 25s	$80.00

Phenylephrine Hydrochloride and Promethazine Hydrochloride

DESCRIPTION
Each teaspoon (5 mL) Phenylephrine Hydrochloride/Promethazine Hydrochloride (Phenylephrine/Promethazine) contains 6.25 mg Promethazine Hydrochloride and 5 mg Phenylephrine Hydrochloride in a flavored syrup base with a pH between 4.7 and 5.2. Alcohol 7 %.

Promethazine Hydrochloride is a racemic compound; the empirical formula is $C_{17}H_{20}N_2S.HCl$ and its molecular weight is 320.88.

Promethazine Hydrochloride, a phenothiazine derivative, is designated chemically as N,N,α-trimethyl-10H-phenothiazine-10-ethanamine monohydrochloride.

Promethazine Hydrochloride occurs as white to faint yellow, practically odorless, crystalline powder which slowly oxidizes and turns blue on prolonged exposure to air. It is soluble in water and freely soluble in alcohol.

Phenylephrine Hydrochloride is a sympathomimetic amine salt. It may be chemically named as 3-hydroxy-α-[(methyl-amino)methyl]-benzenemethanol hydrochloride.

Phenylephrine Hydrochloride occurs as white or nearly white crystals, having a bitter taste. It is freely soluble in water and alcohol, with a molecular weight of 203.67. The empirical formula is $C_9H_{13}NO_2.HCl$, and the stereochemistry is R-isomer as indicated in the structure; Specific Rotation—between -42° and -47.5°. Phenylephrine Hydrochloride is subject to oxidation and must be protected from light and air.

CLINICAL PHARMACOLOGY
PROMETHAZINE
Promethazine is a phenothiazine derivative which differs structurally from the antipsychotic phenothiazines by the presence of a branched side chain and no ring

substitution. It is thought that this configuration is responsible for its relative lack (1/10 that of chlorpromazine) of dopaminergic (CNS) action.

Promethazine is an H_1 receptor blocking agent. In addition to its antihistaminic action, it provides clinically useful sedative and antiemetic effects. In therapeutic dosages Promethazine produces no significant effects on the cardiovascular system.

Promethazine is well absorbed from the gastrointestinal tract. Clinical effects are apparent within 20 minutes after oral administration and generally last four to six hours, although they may persist as long as 12 hours. Promethazine is metabolized by the liver to a variety of compounds; the sulfoxides of Promethazine and N-demethylpromethazine are the predominant metabolites appearing in the urine.

PHENYLEPHRINE

Phenylephrine is a potent postsynaptic α-receptor agonist with little effect on β receptors of the heart. Phenylephrine has no effect on β-adrenergic receptors of the bronchi or peripheral blood vessels. A direct action at receptors accounts for the greater part of its effects, only a small part being due to its ability to release norepinephrine.

Therapeutic doses of Phenylephrine mainly cause vasoconstriction. Phenylephrine increases resistance and, to a lesser extent, decreases capacitance of blood vessels. Total peripheral resistance is increased, resulting in increased systolic and diastolic blood pressure. Pulmonary arterial pressure is usually increased, and renal blood flow is usually decreased. Local vasoconstriction and hemostasis occur following topical application or infiltration of Phenylephrine into tissues. The main effect of phenylephrine on the heart is bradycardia; it produces a positive inotropic effect on the myocardium in doses greater than those usually used therapeutically. Rarely, the drug may increase the irritability of the heart, causing arrhythmias. Cardiac output is decreased slightly. Phenylephrine increases the work of the heart by increasing peripheral arterial resistance.

Phenylephrine has a mild central stimulant effect.

Following oral administration or topical application of Phenylephrine to the mucosa, constriction of blood vessels in the nasal mucosa relieves nasal congestion associated with allergy or head colds. Following oral administration, nasal decongestion may occur within 15 or 20 minutes and may persist for up to 4 hours.

Phenylephrine is irregularly absorbed from and readily metabolized in the gastrointestinal tract. Phenylephrine is metabolized in the liver and intestine by monoamine oxidase. The metabolites and their route and rate of excretion have not been identified. The pharmacologic action of Phenylephrine is terminated at least partially by uptake of the drug into tissues.

INDICATIONS AND USAGE

Phenylephrine/Promethazine indicated for the temporary relief of upper respiratory symptoms, including nasal congestion, associated with allergy or the common cold.

CONTRAINDICATIONS

Promethazine is contraindicated in individuals known to be hypersensitive or to have had an idiosyncratic reaction to Promethazine or to other phenothiazines.

Antihistamines are contraindicated for use in the treatment of lower respiratory tract symptoms or asthma.

Phenylephrine is contraindicated in patients with hypertension or with peripheral vascular insufficiency (ischemia may result with risk of gangrene or thrombosis of compromised vascular beds). Phenylephrine should not be used in patients known to be hypersensitive to the drug or in those receiving a monoamine oxidase inhibitor (MAOI).

WARNINGS

PROMETHAZINE

Promethazine may cause marked drowsiness. Ambulatory patients should be cautioned against such activities as driving or operating dangerous machinery until it is known that they do not become drowsy or dizzy from Promethazine therapy.

The sedative action of Promethazine Hydrochloride is additive to the sedative effects of central nervous system depressants; therefore, agents such as alcohol, narcotic analgesics, sedatives, hypnotics, and tranquilizers should either be eliminated or given in reduced dosage in the presence of Promethazine Hydrochloride. When given concomitantly with Promethazine Hydrochloride, the dose of barbiturates should be reduced by at least one-half, and the dose of analgesic depressants, such as morphine or meperidine, should be reduced by one-quarter to one-half.

Promethazine may lower seizure threshold. This should be taken into consideration when administering to persons with known seizure disorders or when giving in combination with narcotics or local anesthetics which may also affect seizure threshold.

Sedative drugs or CNS depressants should be avoided in patients with a history of sleep apnea.

Antihistamines should be used with caution in patients with narrow-angle glaucoma, stenosing peptic ulcer, pyloroduodenal obstruction, and urinary bladder obstruction due to symptomatic prostatic hypertrophy and narrowing of the bladder neck.

Administration of Promethazine has been associated with reported cholestatic jaundice.

PHENYLEPHRINE

Because Phenylephrine is an adrenergic agent, it should be given with caution to patients with thyroid diseases, diabetes mellitus, and heart diseases or those receiving tricyclic anti-depressants.

Men with symptomatic, benign prostatic hypertrophy can experience urinary retention when given oral nasal decongestants.

Phenylephrine can cause a decrease in cardiac output, and extreme caution should be used when administering the drug, parenterally or orally, to patients with arteriosclerosis, to elderly individuals, and/or to patients with initially poor cerebral or coronary circulation.

Phenylephrine should be used with caution in patients taking diet preparations, such as amphetamines or phenylpropanolamine, because synergistic adrenergic effects could result in serious hypertensive response and possible stroke.

PRECAUTIONS

Animal reproduction studies have not been conducted with the drug combination—Promethazine and Phenylephrine. It is not known whether this drug combination can cause fetal harm when administered to a pregnant woman or can affect reproduction capacity. Phenylephrine/Promethazine should be given to a pregnant woman only if clearly needed.

GENERAL

Promethazine should be used cautiously in persons with cardiovascular disease or impairment of liver function.

Phenylephrine should be used with caution in patients with cardiovascular disease, particularly hypertension.

INFORMATION FOR PATIENTS

Phenylephrine/Promethazine may cause marked drowsiness or impair the mental and/or physical abilities required for the performance of potentially hazardous tasks, such as driving a vehicle or operating machinery. Ambulatory patients should be told to avoid engaging in such activities until it is known that they do not become drowsy or dizzy from Phenylephrine/Promethazine therapy. Children should be supervised to avoid potential harm in bike riding or other hazardous activities.

The concomitant use of alcohol or other central nervous system depressants, including narcotic analgesics, sedatives, hypnotics, and tranquilizers, may have an additive effect and should be avoided or their dosage reduced.

Patients should be advised to report any involuntary muscle movements or unusual sensitivity to sunlight.

DRUG INTERACTIONS
PROMETHAZINE

The sedative action of Promethazine is additive to the sedative effects of other central nervous system depressants, including alcohol, narcotic analgesics, sedatives, hypnotics, tricyclic antidepressants, and tranquilizers; therefore, these agents should be avoided or administered in reduced dosage to patients receiving Promethazine.

PHENYLEPHRINE

Drug	Effect
Phenylephrine with prior administration of monoamine oxidase inhibitors (MAOI).	Cardiac pressor response potentiated. May cause acute hypertensive crisis.
Phenylephrine with tricyclic antidepressants.	Pressor response increased.
Phenylephrine with ergot alkaloids.	Excessive rise in blood pressure.
Phenylephrine with bronchodilator sympathomimetic agents and with epinephrine or other sympathomimetics.	Tachycardia or other arrhythmias may occur
Phenylephrine with prior administration of propranolol or other β-adrenergic blockers.	Cardiostimulating effects blocked.
Phenylephrine with atropine sulfate.	Reflex bradycardia blocked; pressor response enhanced.
Phenylephrine with prior administration of phentolamine or other α-adrenergic blockers.	Pressor response decreased.
Phenylephrine with diet preparations, such as amphetamines or phenylpropanolamine.	Synergistic adrenergic response.

DRUG/LABORATORY TEST INTERACTIONS

The following laboratory tests may be affected in patients who are receiving therapy with Promethazine Hydrochloride:

Pregnancy Tests: Diagnostic pregnancy tests based on immunological reactions between HCG and anti-HCG may result in false-negative or false-positive interpretations.

Glucose Tolerance Test: An increase in blood glucose has been reported in patients receiving Promethazine.

CARCINOGENESIS, MUTAGENESIS, IMPAIRMENT OF FERTILITY

Promethazine: Long-term animal studies have not been performed to assess the carcinogenic potential of Promethazine, nor are there other animal or human data concerning carcinogenicity, mutagenicity, or impairment of fertility with this drug. Promethazine was nonmutagenic in the *Salmonella* test system of Ames.

Phenylephrine: A study which followed the development of cancer in 143,574 patients over a four-year period indicated that in 11,981 patients who received Phenylephrine (systemic or topical), there was no statistically significant association between the drug and cancer at any or all sites.

Long-term animal studies have not been performed to assess the carcinogenic potential of Phenylephrine, nor are there other animal or human data concerning mutagenicity.

A study of the effects of adrenergic drugs on ovum transport in rabbits indicated that treatment with Phenylephrine did not alter incidence of pregnancy; the number of implantations was significantly reduced when high doses of the drug were used.

PREGNANCY

Teratogenic Effects—Pregnancy Category C:

Promethazine: Teratogenic effects have not been demonstrated in rat-feeding studies at doses of 6.25 and 12.5 mg/kg of Promethazine. These doses are 8.3 and 16.7 times the maximum recommended total daily dose of Promethazine for a 50-kg subject. Specific studies to test the action of the drug on parturition, lactation, and development of the animal neonate were not done, but a general preliminary study in rats indicated no effect on these parameters. Although antihistamines, including Promethazine, have been found to produce fetal mortality in rodents, the pharmacological effects of histamine in the rodent do not parallel those in man. There are no adequate and well-controlled studies of Promethazine in pregnant women.

Phenylephrine: A study in rabbits indicated that continued moderate overexposure to Phenylephrine (3 mg/day) during the second half of pregnancy (22nd day of gestation to delivery) may contribute to perinatal wastage, prematurity, premature labor, and possibly fetal anomalies; when Phenylephrine (3 mg/day) was given to rabbits during the first half of pregnancy (3rd day after mating for seven days), a significant number gave birth to litters of low birth weight. Another study showed that Phenylephrine was associated with anomalies of aortic arch and with ventricular septal defect in the chick embryo. Phenylephrine/Promethazine should be used during pregnancy only if the potential benefit justifies the potential risk to the fetus.

Nonteratogenic Effects: Promethazine taken within two weeks of delivery may inhibit platelet aggregation in the newborn.

LABOR AND DELIVERY

Administration of Phenylephrine to patients in late pregnancy or labor may cause fetal anoxia or bradycardia by increasing contractility of the uterus and decreasing uterine blood flow. See also *"Nonteratogenic Effects."*

NURSING MOTHERS

It is not known whether Promethazine or Phenylephrine is excreted in human milk.

Caution should be exercised when Phenylephrine/Promethazine is administered to a nursing woman.

PEDIATRIC USE

This product should not be used in children under 2 years of age because safety for such use has not been established.

ADVERSE REACTIONS

PROMETHAZINE

Nervous System: Sedation, sleepiness, occasional blurred vision, dryness of mouth, dizziness; rarely confusion, disorientation, and extrapyramidal symptoms such as oculogyric crisis, torticollis, and tongue protrusion (usually in association with parenteral injection or excessive dosage).

Cardiovascular: Increased or decreased blood pressure.

Dermatologic: Rash, rarely photosensitivity.

Hematologic: Rarely leukopenia, thrombocytopenia; agranulocytosis (1 case).

Gastrointestinal: Nausea and vomiting.

PHENYLEPHRINE

Nervous System: Restlessness, anxiety, nervousness, and dizziness.

Cardiovascular: Hypertension (see *"Warnings"*).

Other: Precordial pain, respiratory distress, tremor, and weakness.

OVERDOSAGE

PROMETHAZINE

Signs and symptoms of overdosage with Promethazine range from mild depression of the central nervous system and cardiovascular system to profound hypotension, respiratory depression, and unconsciousness.

Stimulation may be evident, especially in children and geriatric patients. Convulsions may rarely occur. A paradoxical reaction has been reported in children receiving single doses of 75 mg to 125 mg orally, characterized by hyperexcitability and nightmares.

Atropine-like signs and symptoms—dry mouth, fixed, dilated pupils, flushing as well as gastrointestinal symptoms, may occur.

PHENYLEPHRINE

Signs and symptoms of overdosage with Phenylephrine include hypertension, headache, convulsions, cerebral hemorrhage, and vomiting. Ventricular premature beats and short paroxysms of ventricular tachycardia may also occur. Headache may be a symptom of hypertension. Bradycardia may also be seen early in Phenylephrine overdosage through stimulation of baroreceptors.

TREATMENT

Treatment of overdosage with Phenylephrine/Promethazine is essentially symptomatic and supportive. Only in cases of extreme over-dosage or individual sensitivity do vital signs including respiration, pulse, blood pressure, temperature, and EKG need to be monitored. Activated charcoal orally or by lavage may be given, or sodium or magnesium sulfate orally as a cathartic. Attention should be given to the reestablishment of adequate respiratory exchange through provision of a patent airway and institution of assisted or controlled ventilation. Diazepam may be used to control convulsions. Acidosis and electrolyte losses should be corrected. Note that any depressant effects of Promethazine are not reversed by naloxone. Avoid analeptics which may cause convulsions.

Severe hypotension usually responds to the administration of norepinephrine or Phenylephrine. EPINEPHRINE SHOULD NOT BE USED, since its use in patients with partial adrenergic blockade may further lower the blood pressure.

Limited experience with dialysis indicates that it is not helpful.

DOSAGE AND ADMINISTRATION

The recommended adult dose is one teaspoon (5 mL) every 4 to 6 hours, not to exceed 30.0 mL in 24 hours. For children 6 years to under 12 years of age, the dose is one-half to one teaspoon (2.5 to 5.0 mL) repeated at 4- to 6-hour intervals, not to exceed 30.0 mL in 24 hours. For children 2 years to under 6 years of age, the dose is one-quarter to one-half teaspoon (1.25 to 2.5 mL) every 4 to 6 hours.

Phenylephrine/Promethazine is not recommended for children under 2 years of age.

Keep bottles tightly closed and store at room temperature between 15° and 25°C (59° and 77°F).

Protect from light.

Dispense in light-resistant, glass, tight containers.

HOW SUPPLIED
SYRUP: 5 MG-6.25 MG/5 ML

AVERAGE UNIT PRICE (AVAILABLE SIZES)		GENERIC A-RATED AVERAGE PRICE (GAAP)	
BRAND	$0.03	480 ml	$16.73
GENERIC	$0.01	3840 ml	$16.73
HCFA FUL (480 ml)	$0.01	120 ml	$2.27
		120 ml	$2.15
		480 ml	$5.40
		3840 ml	$29.75

BRAND/MANUFACTURER	NDC	SIZE	AWP
◆ **BRAND**			
PHENERGAN VC: Wyeth-Ayerst	00008-0551-01	120 ml	$2.89
	00008-0551-03	480 ml	$17.80
	00008-0551-02	120 ml 24s	$118.33
◆ **GENERICS**			
PHENAMETH VC: Major	00904-1512-20	120 ml	$1.65
Moore,H.L.	00839-7060-65	120 ml	$1.89
Cenci,H.R.	00556-0346-04	120 ml	$2.00
Rugby	00536-1785-97	120 ml	$2.10
Mason Dist	11845-0439-04	120 ml	$2.11
Major	00904-1512-00	120 ml	$2.15
Qualitest	00603-1582-54	120 ml	$2.16
Aligen	00405-3625-76	120 ml	$2.33
Barre	00472-1628-04	120 ml	$2.34
Halsey Pharm	00879-0514-04	120 ml	$2.40
Geneva	00781-6635-04	120 ml	$3.10
Qualitest	00603-1582-58	480 ml	$4.70
Cenci,H.R.	00556-0346-16	480 ml	$5.20
Moore,H.L.	00839-7060-69	480 ml	$5.20
Schein	00364-0860-16	480 ml	$5.25
Rugby	00536-1785-85	480 ml	$5.40
Major	00904-1512-16	480 ml	$5.40
Aligen	00405-3625-16	480 ml	$5.64
URL	00677-0964-33	480 ml	$5.65
Goldline	00182-1711-40	480 ml	$5.70
Barre	00472-1628-16	480 ml	$6.24
Geneva	00781-6635-16	480 ml	$6.25
Halsey Pharm	00879-0514-16	480 ml	$6.30
Major	00904-1512-28	3840 ml	$27.15
Moore,H.L.	00839-7060-70	3840 ml	$28.96
Rugby	00536-1785-90	3840 ml	$31.20
Cenci,H.R.	00556-0346-28	3840 ml	$31.40
Goldline	00182-1711-41	3840 ml	$31.50
Barre	00472-1628-28	3840 ml	$36.39
Halsey Pharm	00879-0514-28	3840 ml	$36.45

► SHOWN IN PRODUCT IDENTIFICATION GUIDE

Phenylephrine Hydrochloride and Scopolamine Hydrobromide

DESCRIPTION
Each mL contains: Phenylephrine Hydrochloride 100 mg (10%); Scopolamine Hydrobromide 3 mg (0.3% as trihydrate).

Established Name: Phenylephrine Hydrochloride
The molecular formula of Phenylephrine Hydrochloride is $C_9H_{13}NO_2 \cdot HCl$. Its molecular weight is 203.67.

Chemical Name: Benzenemethanol, 3-hydroxy-α-[(methylamino)methyl]-, hydrochloride(R).

Established Name: Scopolamine Hydrobromide

Chemical Name: Benzeneacetic acid, (α)-(hydroxymethyl)-, 9-methyl-3-oxa-9-aza-tricyclo [3.3.1.0^{2,4}]non-7-yl ester, hydrobromide, trihydrate, [7(S)-(1α, 2β, 4β, 5α, 7β)]-. Its molecular formula is $C_{17}H_{21}NO_4 \cdot HBr \cdot 3H_2O$ and its molecular weight is 438.31.

CLINICAL PHARMACOLOGY
Phenylephrine produces pupil dilation and vasoconstriction (alpha adrenergic effects). Scopolamine produces dilation of the pupil and paralysis of accommodation (anticholinergic effects).

INDICATIONS AND USAGE
Phenylephrine Hydrochloride/Scopolamine Hydrobromide is indicated for mydriasis, cycloplegia and treatment of iritis to prevent formation of posterior synechiae.

CONTRAINDICATIONS
Narrow angle glaucoma, a tendency toward glaucoma or hypersensitivity to any ingredient.

WARNINGS
For topical ophthalmic use only. This product may increase IOP in the normal eye. Do not use in children under 6 years of age. Contains sodium metabisulfite, a sulfite that may cause allergic-type reactions including anaphylactic symptoms and life-threatening or less severe asthmatic episodes in certain susceptible people. The overall prevalence of sulfite sensitivity in the general population is unknown and probably low. Sulfite sensitivity is seen more frequently in asthmatic than in nonasthmatic people.

PRECAUTIONS
Phenylephrine Hydrochloride/Scopolamine Hydrobromide should be used with caution in patients with marked hypertension or advanced arteriosclerotic changes and insulin dependent diabetics. To avoid excessive absorption, the lacrimal puncta should be occluded with digital pressure for 1 to 2 minutes after instillation.

To avoid inducing angular closure glaucoma, an estimation of the depth of the angle of the anterior chamber should be made.

DRUG INTERACTIONS
The pressor effect of sympathomimetic amines is markedly potentiated by monoamine oxidase (MAO) inhibitors. Excessive elevation of blood pressure and hypertensive crisis may occur if used concomitantly.

PATIENT WARNING
Patients should be advised not to drive or engage in other hazardous activities when drowsy or while pupils are dilated. Patients may experience sensitivity to light and should protect eyes in bright illumination during dilation. Patients should be warned not to get this preparation in their child's mouth and to wash their hands and the child's hands following administration.

ADVERSE REACTIONS
Transitory stinging on initial instillation may be expected. Redness usually occurs which is a normal therapeutic response. Headache or browache frequently occurs but will usually diminish on continued treatment. Conjunctival allergy rarely occurs. Pigmentary deposits in the lids, conjunctiva or cornea may occur after prolonged use. Systemic effects have occasionally been reported such as anxiety, fear, palpitation, tachycardia, extrasystoles, cardiac arrythmia, hypertension, trembling, sweating and pallor.

DOSAGE AND ADMINISTRATION
Mydriasis: Initially, instill 1 or 2 drops in eye[s]. Repeat in 5 minutes if necessary to produce mydriasis in highly pigmented irides. Post-op: instill 1 or 2 drops in eye(s) 3 to 4 times a day when desirable to maintain dilation and rest ciliary body.
FOR OPHTHALMIC USE ONLY
DO NOT USE IF IMPRINTED NECKBAND IS NOT INTACT.

Note: DO NOT USE IF BROWNISH COLOR APPEARS.
Store between 15° - 30°C (59° - 86°F).

Protect from light.
Keep tightly closed.
Keep out of reach of children.

HOW SUPPLIED
DROP:

BRAND/MANUFACTURER	NDC	SIZE	AWP
○ GENERICS			
MUROCOLL 2: Bausch&Lomb Pharm	24208-0278-05	5 ml	$11.25

Phenytoin

DESCRIPTION
Phenytoin is an antiepileptic drug. Phenytoin Sodium is related to the barbiturates in chemical structure, but has a five-membered ring. The chemical name is 5,5-diphenyl-2,4-imidazolidinedione. It is available as tablets, extended-absorption capsules, oral suspension, and injection.

Each tablet contains:
Phenytoin ....50 mg

Each extended capsule contains:
Phenytoin Sodium ....30 or 100 mg

Each teaspoonful of suspension contains:
Phenytoin ....30 or 125 mg

Each ml of solution for injection
Phenytoin Sodium ....50 mg

Phenytoin Sodium extended is characterized by a slow and extended rate of absorption with peak blood concentrations expected in 4 to 12 hours.

Following is its chemical structure:

CLINICAL PHARMACOLOGY
Phenytoin is an antiepileptic (anticonvulsant) drug which can be useful in the treatment of status epilepticus of the grand mal type. The primary, size activity is inhibited. Possibly by promoting sodium efflux from neurons, Phenytoin tends to *stabilize* the threshold against hyperexcitability caused by excessive stimulation or environmental changes capable of reducing membrane sodium gradient. This includes the reduction of posttetanic potentiation at synapses. Loss of posttetanic potentiation prevents cortical seizure foci from detonating adjacent cortical areas. Phenytoin reduces the maximal activity of brain stem centers responsible for the tonic phase of tonic-colonic (grand mal) seizures.

The plasma half-life in man after oral administration of Phenytoin extended capsules or oral suspension averages 22 hours, with a range of 7 to 42 hours, after administration of tablets, 14 hours with a range of 7 to 29 hours. Steady-state therapeutic levels are achieved 7 to 10 days (5 to 7 half-lives) after initiation of therapy with recommended doses of 300 mg/day. The plasma half-life in man after intravenous administration ranges from 10 to 15 hours.

When serum level determinations are necessary, they should be obtained at least 5-7 half-lives after treatment initiation, dosage change, or addition or subtraction of another drug to the regimen so that equilibrium or steady-state will have been achieved. Trough levels provide information about clinically effective serum level range and confirm patient compliance and are obtained just prior to the patient's next scheduled dose. Peak levels indicate an individual's threshold for emergence of dose-related side effects and are obtained at the time of expected peak concentration. For Phenytoin tablets and oral suspension, peak serum levels occur 1 ½-3 hours after administration; for Phenytoin Sodium extended capsules peak serum levels occur 4-12 hours after administration.

Optimum control without clinical signs of toxicity occurs more often with serum levels between 10 and 20 mcg/ml, although some mild cases of tonic-clonic (grand mal) epilepsy may be controlled with lower-serum levels of Phenytoin. In most patients maintained at a steady dosage, stable Phenytoin serum levels are achieved. There may be wide interpatient variability in Phenytoin serum levels with equivalent dosages. Patients with unusually low levels may be noncompliant or hypermetabolizers of Phenytoin. Unusually high levels result from liver disease, congenital enzyme deficiency or drug interactions which result in metabolic interference. The patient with large variations in Phenytoin plasma levels, despite standard doses, presents a difficult clinical problem. Serum level determinations in such patients may be particularly helpful. As Phenytoin is highly protein bound, free Phenytoin levels may be altered in patients whose protein binding characteristics differ from normal.

Most of the drug is excreted in the bile as inactive metabolites which are then reabsorbed from the intestinal tract and excreted in the urine. Urinary excretion of Phenytoin and its metabolites occurs partly with glomerular filtration but more importantly, by tubular secretion. Because Phenytoin is hydroxylated in the liver by an enzyme system which is saturable at high plasma levels, small incremental doses may increase the half-life and produce very substantial increases in serum levels, when these are in the upper range. The steady-state level may be disproportionately increased, with resultant intoxication, from an increase in dosage of 10% or more.

A fall in plasma levels may occur when patients are changed from oral to intramuscular administration. The drop is caused by slower absorption, as compared to oral administration, due to the poor water solubility of Phenytoin. Intravenous administration is the preferred route for producing rapid therapeutic serum levels.

There are occasions when intramuscular administration may be required, ie, postoperatively, in comatose patients, for GI upsets. During these periods, a sufficient dose must be administered intramuscularly to maintain the plasma level within the therapeutic range. Where oral dosage is resumed following intramuscular usage, the oral dose should be properly adjusted to compensate for the slow, continuing IM absorption to avoid toxic symptoms.

Patients stabilized on a daily oral regimen of Phenytoin experience a drop in peak blood levels to 50-60 percent of stable levels if crossed over to an equal dose administered intramuscularly. However, the intramuscular depot of poorly soluble material is eventually absorbed, as determined by urinary excretion of 5-(p-hydroxyphenyl)-5-phenylhydantoin (HPPH), the principal metabolite, as well as the total amount of drug eventually appearing in the blood.

A short-term (one week) study indicates that patients do not experience the expected drop in blood levels when crossed over to the intramuscular (IM) route if the Phenytoin Sodium IM dose is increased by 50 percent over the previously established oral dose. To avoid drug accumulation due to absorption from the muscle depots, it is recommended that for the first week back on oral Phenytoin, the dose be reduced to half of the original oral dose (one third of the IM dose). Experience for periods greater than one week is lacking and blood level monitoring is recommended. For administration of Phenytoin in patients who cannot take oral medication for periods greater than a week, gastric intubation may be considered.

Clinical studies show that chewed and unchewed Phenytoin tablets are bioequivalent, yield approximately equivalent plasma levels, and are more rapidly absorbed than 100-mg Phenytoin Sodium extended capsules.

INDICATIONS AND USAGE
Phenytoin is indicated for the control of tonic-clonic and psychomotor (grand mal and temporal lobe) seizures and prevention and treatment of seizures occurring during or following neurosurgery.

Phenytoin serum level determinations may be necessary for optimal dosage adjustments (see *"Dosage and Administration"*).

UNLABELED USES
Phenytoin is used alone or as an adjunct in the treatment of spacticity and neuropathy due to thiamine deficiency. It is used in the treatment of cardiovascular complications due to tricyclic antidepressant overdose and for prophylaxis of migraine headaches. It is also used in trigeminal neuraligia and in the short-term treatment of syndrome of inappropriate antidiuretic hormone (SIADH) secondary to increased hypothalamic release of antidiuretic hormone. Phenytoin is also prescribed for cardiac arrhythmias including atrial and ventricular arrhythmias, and arrhythmias secondary to digitalis intoxication and mild hypertension.

CONTRAINDICATIONS
Phenytoin is contraindicated in those patients who are hypersensitive to Phenytoin or other hydantoins.

Because of its effect on ventricular automaticity, Phenytoin is contraindicated in sinus bradycardia, sino-atrial block, second and third degree A-V block, and patients with Adams-Stokes syndrome.

WARNINGS

IMPORTANT NOTE

PHENYTOIN SODIUM INJECTION MUST BE ADMINISTERED SLOWLY. IN ADULTS DO NOT EXCEED 50 MG PER MINUTE INTRAVENOUSLY. IN NEONATES, THE DRUG SHOULD BE ADMINISTERED AT A RATE NOT EXCEEDING 1-3 MG/KG/MIN.

Abrupt withdrawal of Phenytoin in epileptic patients may precipitate status epilepticus. When, in the judgment of the clinician, the need for dosage reduction, discontinuation, or substitution of alternative antiepileptic medication arises, this should be done gradually. However, in the event of an allergic or hypersensitivity reaction, rapid substitution of alternative therapy may be necessary. In this case, alternative therapy should be an antiepileptic drug not belonging to the hydantoin chemical class.

There have been a number of reports suggesting a relationship between Phenytoin and the development of lymphadenopathy (local or generalized) including benign lymph node hyperplasia, pseudolymphoma, lymphoma, and Hodgkin's Disease.

Although a cause and effect relationship has not been established, the occurrence of lymphadenopathy indicates the need to differentiate such a condition from other types of lymph node pathology. Lymph node involvement may occur with or without symptoms and signs resembling serum sickness, eg, fever, rash and liver involvement.

In all cases of lymphadenopathy, follow-up observation for an extended period is indicated and every effort should be made to achieve seizure control using alternative antiepileptic drugs.

Acute alcoholic intake may increase phenytoin serum levels while chronic alcoholic use may decrease serum levels.

In view of isolated reports associating Phenytoin with exacerbation of porphyria, caution should be exercised in using this medication in patients suffering from this disease.

Intravenous administration should not exceed 50 mg per minute in adults. In neonates, the drug should be administered at a rate not exceeding 1-3mg/kg/min.

Severe cardiotoxic reactions and fatalities have been reported with atrial and ventricular conduction depression and ventricular fibrillation. Severe complications are most commonly encountered in elderly or gravely ill patients.

Parenteral Phenytoin should be used with caution in patients with hypotension and severe myocardial insufficiency.

Hypotension usually occurs when the drug is administered rapidly by the intravenous route.

The intramuscular route is not recommended for the treatment of status epilepticus since blood levels of Phenytoin in the therapeutic range cannot be readily achieved with doses and methods of administration ordinarily employed.

USAGE IN PREGNANCY
A number of reports suggest an association between the use of antiepileptic drugs by women with epilepsy and a higher incidence of birth defects in children born to these women. Data are more extensive with respect to Phenytoin and phenobarbital, but these are also the most commonly prescribed antiepileptic drugs; less systematic or anecdotal reports suggest a possible similar association with the use of all known antiepileptic drugs.

The reports suggesting a higher incidence of birth defects in children of drug-treated epileptic women cannot be regarded as adequate to prove a definite cause and effect relationship. There are intrinsic methodologic problems in obtaining adequate data on drug teratogenicity in humans; genetic factors or the epileptic condition itself may be more important than drug therapy in leading to birth defects. The great majority of mothers on antiepileptic medication deliver normal infants. It is important to note that antiepileptic drugs should not be discontinued in patients in whom the drug is administered to prevent major seizures, because of the strong possibility of precipitating status epilepticus with attendant hypoxia and threat to life. In individual cases where the severity and frequency of the seizure disorder are such that the removal of medication does not pose a serious threat to the patient, discontinuation of the drug may be considered prior to and during pregnancy, although it cannot be said with any confidence that even minor seizures do not pose some hazard to the developing embryo or fetus. The prescribing physician will wish to weigh these considerations in treating and counseling epileptic women of childbearing potential.

In addition to the reports of increased incidence of congenital malformations, such as cleft lip/palate and heart malformations in children of women receiving Phenytoin and other antiepileptic drugs, there have more recently been reports of a fetal hydantoin syndrome. This consists of prenatal growth deficiency, microcephaly and mental deficiency in children born to mothers who have received Phenytoin, barbiturates, alcohol, or trimethadione. However, these features are all interrelated and are frequently associated with intrauterine growth retardation from other causes.

There have been isolated reports of malignancies, including neuroblastoma, in children whose mothers received Phenytoin during pregnancy.

An increase in seizure frequency during pregnancy occurs in a high proportion of patients, because of altered Phenytoin absorption of metabolism. Periodic measurement of serum Phenytoin levels is particularly valuable in the management of a pregnant epileptic patients as a guide to an appropriate adjustment of dosage. However, postpartum restoration of the original dosage will probably be indicated.

Neonatal coagulation defects have been reported within the first 24 hours in babies born to epileptic mothers receiving phenobarbital and/or Phenytoin. Vitamin K has been shown to prevent or correct this defect and has been recommended to be given to the mother before delivery and the neonate after birth.

PRECAUTIONS
GENERAL
The liver is the chief site of biotransformation of Phenytoin; patients with impaired liver function, elderly patients, or those who are gravely ill may show early signs of toxicity.

A small percentage of individuals who have been treated with Phenytoin have been shown to metabolize the drug slowly. Slow metabolism may be due to limited enzyme availability and lack of induction; it appears to be genetically determined.

Phenytoin should be discontinued if a skin rash appears (see *"Warnings"* section regarding drug discontinuation). If the rash is exfoliative, purpuric, or bullous or if lupus erythematosus, Stevens-Johnson syndrome, or toxic epidermal necrolysis is suspected, use of the drugs should not be resumed, and alternative therapy should be considered. (See *"Adverse Reactions"*.) If the rash is of a milder type (measles-like or scarlatiniform), therapy may be resumed after the rash has completely disappeared. If the rash recurs upon reinstitution of therapy, further Phenytoin medication is contraindicated.

Phenytoin and other hydantoins are contraindicated in patients who have experienced Phenytoin hypersensitivity. Additionally, caution should be exercised if using structurally similar compounds (eg, barbiturates, succinimides, oxazolidinediones and other related compounds) in these same patients.

Hyperglycemia, resulting from the drug's inhibitory effects on insulin release, has been reported. Phenytoin may also raise the serum glucose level in diabetic patients.

Osteomalacia has been associated with Phenytoin therapy and is considered to be due to Phenytoin's interference with Vitamin D metabolism.

Phenytoin is not indicated for seizures due to hypoglycemic or other metabolic causes. Appropriate diagnostic procedures should be performed as indicated.

Phenytoin is not effective for absence (petit mal) seizures. If tonic-clonic (grand-mal) and absence (petit mal) seizures are present, combined drug therapy is needed.

Serum levels of Phenytoin sustained above the optimal range may produce confusional states referred to as "delirium," "psychosis", or "encephalopathy," or rarely irreversible cerebellar dysfunction. Accordingly, at the first sign of acute toxicity, plasma levels are recommended. Dose reduction of Phenytoin therapy is indicated if plasma levels are excessive; if symptoms persist, termination is recommended. (See *"Warnings".*)

The addition of Phenytoin Sodium solution for injection solution to intravenous infusion is not recommended due to lack of solubility and resultant precipitation.

Parenteral Phenytoin Sodium should be injected slowly (not exceeding 50 mg per minute in adults), directly into a large vein through a large-gauge needle or intravenous catheter. Each injection of intravenous Phenytoin Sodium should be followed by an injection of sterile saline through the same needle or intravenous catheter to avoid local venous irritation due to the alkalinity of the solution. Continuous infusion should be avoided.

Soft tissue irritation and inflammation has occurred at the site of injection with and without extravasation of intravenous Phenytoin. Soft tissue irritation may vary from slight tenderness to extensive necrosis, sloughing, and in rare instances has led to amputation. Improper administration including subcutaneous or perivascular injection should be avoided to help prevent possibility of the above.

INFORMATION FOR PATIENTS
Patients taking Phenytoin should be advised of the importance of adhering strictly to the prescribed dosage regimen, and of informing the physician of any clinical condition in which it is not possible to take the drug orally as prescribed, eg, surgery, etc.

Patients should also be cautioned on the use of other drugs or alcoholic beverages without first seeking the physician's advice.

Patients should be instructed to call their physician if skin rash develops.

The importance of good dental hygiene should be stressed in order to minimize the development of gingival hyperplasia and its complications.

LABORATORY TESTS
Phenytoin serum level determinations may be necessary to achieve optimal dosage adjustments.

DRUG INTERACTIONS
There are many drugs which may increase or decrease Phenytoin levels or which Phenytoin may affect. Serum level determinations for Phenytoin are especially helpful when possible drug interactions are suspected. The most commonly occurring drug interactions are listed below.

1. Drugs which may increase Phenytoin serum levels include: acute alcohol intake, amiodarone, chloramphenicol, chlordiazepoxide, cimetidine, diazepam, dicumarol, disulfiram, estrogens, ethosuximide, H$_2$-antagonists, halothane, isoniazid, methylphenidate, phenothiazines, phenylbutazone, salicylates, succinimides, sulfonamides, tolbutamide, trazodone.
2. Drugs which may decrease Phenytoin levels include: carbamazepine, chronic alcohol abuse, reserpine, and sucralfate. One brand of molindone hydrochloride contains calcium ions which interfere with the absorption of Phenytoin. Ingestion times of Phenytoin and antacid preparations containing calcium should be staggered in patients with low serum Phenytoin levels to prevent absorption problems.
3. Drugs which may either increase or decrease Phenytoin serum levels include: phenobarbital, sodium valproate, and valproic acid. Similarly, the effect of Phenytoin on phenobarbital, valproic acid and sodium valproate serum levels is unpredictable.
4. Although not a true drug interaction, tricyclic antidepressants may precipitate seizures in susceptible patients and Phenytoin dosage may need to be adjusted.
5. Drugs whose efficacy is impaired by Phenytoin include: corticosteroids, coumarin anticoagulants, digitoxin, doxycycline, estrogens, furosemide, oral contraceptives, quinidine, rifampin, theophylline, vitamin D.

DRUG/LABORATORY TEST INTERACTIONS
Phenytoin may cause decreased serum levels of protein-bound iodine (PBI). It may also produce lower than normal values for dexamethasone or metyrapone tests. Phenytoin may cause raised serum levels of glucose, alkaline phosphatase, and gamma glutamyl transpeptidase (GGT).

CARCINOGENESIS
See *"Warnings"* section for information on carcinogenesis.

PREGNANCY
See *"Warnings."*

NURSING MOTHERS
Infant breast feeding is not recommended for women taking this drug because Phenytoin appears to be secreted in low concentrations in human milk.

ADVERSE REACTIONS
Central Nervous System: The most common manifestations encountered with Phenytoin therapy are referable to this system and are usually dose-related. These include nystagmus, ataxia, slurred speech, decreased coordination, and mental confusion. Dizziness, insomnia, transient nervousness, motor twitchings, and headaches have also been observed. There have also been rare reports of Phenytoin-induced dyskinesias, including chorea, dystonia, tremor and asterixis, similar to those induced by phenothiazine and other neuroleptic drugs.

A predominantly sensory peripheral polyneuropathy has been observed in patients receiving long-term Phenytoin therapy.

GASTROINTESTINAL SYSTEM
Nausea, vomiting, constipation, toxic hepatitis and liver damage.

INTEGUMENTARY SYSTEM
Dermatological manifestations sometimes accompanied by fever have included scarlatiniform or morbilliform rashes. A morbilliform rash (measles-like) is the most common; other types of dermatitis are seen more rarely. Other more serious forms which may be fatal have included bullous, exfoliative or purpuric dermatitis, lupus erythematosus, Steven-Johnson syndrome, and toxic epidermal necrolysis (see *"Precautions"*).

HEMOPOIETIC SYSTEM
Hemopoietic complications, some fatal, have occasionally been reported in association with administration of Phenytoin. These have included thrombocytopenia, leukopenia, granulocytopenia, agranulocytosis, and pancytopenia with or without bone marrow suppression. While macrocytosis and megaloblastic anemia have occurred, these conditions usually respond to folic acid therapy. Lymphadenopathy including benign lymph node hyperplasia, pseudolymphoma, lymphoma, and Hodgkin's Disease have been reported (see *"Warnings"*).

CONNECTIVE TISSUE SYSTEM
Coarsening of the facial features, enlargement of the lips, gingival hyperplasia, hirsutism, and Peyronie's Disease.

CARDIOVASCULAR
Periarteritis nodosa with parenteral Phenytoin Sodium, severe cardiotoxic reactions and fatalities have been reported with atrial and ventricular conduction depression and ventricular fibrillation. Severe complications are most commonly encountered in elderly or gravely ill patients.

IMMUNOLOGIC
Hypersensitivity syndrome (which may include, eosinophilia, fever, liver dysfunction, periarteritis nodosa, toxic hepatitis, lymphadenopathy or rash), systemic lupus erythematosus, and immunoglobulin abnormalities.

Injection Site: Local irritation, inflammation, tenderness, necrosis, and sloughing have been reported with or without extravasation of intravenous Phenytoin.

The most notable signs of toxicity associated with the intravenous use of this drug are cardiovascular collapse and/or central nervous system depression. Hypotension does occur when the drug is administered rapidly by the intravenous route. The *rate* of administration is very important; it should not exceed 50 mg per minute in adults, and 1-3 mg/kg/min in neonates. At this rate, toxicity should be minimized.

OVERDOSAGE
The lethal dose in children is not known. The lethal dose in adults is estimated to be 2 to 5 grams. The initial symptoms are nystagmus, ataxia, and dysarthria. Other signs are tremor, hyperreflexia, lethargy, slurred speech, nausea, vomiting. The patient may become comatose and hypotensive. Death is due to respiratory and circulatory depression.

There are marked variations among individuals with respect to Phenytoin plasma levels where toxicity may occur. Nystagmus, on lateral gaze, usually appears at 20 mcg/ml, ataxia at 30 mcg/ml, dysarthria and lethargy appear when the plasma concentration is over 40 mcg/ml, but as high a concentration as 50 mcg/ml has been reported without evidence of toxicity. As much as 25 times the therapeutic dose has been taken to result in a serum concentration over 100 mcg/ml with complete recovery.

TREATMENT
Treatment is nonspecific since there is no known antidote. The adequacy of the respiratory and circulatory systems should be carefully observed and appropriate supportive measures employed. Hemodialysis can be considered since Phenytoin is not completely bound to plasma proteins. Total exchange transfusion has been used in the treatment of severe intoxication in children.

In acute overdosage the possibility of other CNS depressants, including alcohol, should be borne in mind.

DOSAGE AND ADMINISTRATION
Serum concentrations should be monitored in changing from the sodium salt to the free acid form. Because there is approximately an 8% increase in drug content with the free acid form over that of the sodium salt, dosage adjustments and serum level monitoring may be necessary when switching from a product formulated with the acid to a product formulated with the sodium salt and vice versa. When given in equal doses, for example, Phenytoin tablets yield higher plasma levels than Phenytoin Sodium, extended, capsules.

GENERAL
Dosage should be individualized to provide maximum benefit. In some cases serum blood level determinations may be necessary for optimal dosage adjustments—the clinically effective serum level is usually 10-20 mcg/ml. With recommended dosage, a period of seven to ten days may be required to achieve

steady-state blood levels with Phenytoin and changes in dosage (increase or decrease) should not be carried out at intervals shorter than seven to ten days.

PHENYTOIN TABLETS

Phenytoin tablets are not for once a day dosing. They can be either chewed thoroughly before being swallowed or swallowed whole.

Adult Dosage: Patients who have received no previous treatment may be started on two Phenytoin tablets three times daily, and the dose is then adjusted to suit individual requirements. For most adults, the satisfactory maintenance dosage will be six to eight Phenytoin tablets daily: an increase to twelve Phenytoin tablets daily may be made, if necessary.

PHENYTOIN SODIUM EXTENDED CAPSULES
Adult Dosage:

Divided Daily Dosage: Patients who have received no previous treatment may be started on one 100 mg Phenytoin Sodium extended capsule three times daily and the dosage then adjusted to suit individual requirements. For most adults, the satisfactory maintenance dosage will be one capsule three to four times a day. An increase up to two capsules three times a day may be made, if necessary.

Once-a-Day Dosage: In adults, if seizure control is established with divided doses of three 100 mg Phenytoin Sodium extended capsules daily, once-a-day dosage with 300 mg of Phenytoin Sodium extended capsules may be considered. Studies comparing divided doses of 300 mg with a single daily dose of this quantity indicated absorption, peak plasma levels, biologic half-life, difference between peak and minimum values, and urinary recovery were equivalent. Once-a-day dosage offers a convenience to the individual patient or to nursing personnel for institutionalized patients and is intended to be used only for patients requiring this amount of drug daily. A major problem in motivating non-compliant patients may also be lessened when the patient can take this drug once a day. However, patients should be cautioned not to miss a dose, inadvertently.

Only Phenytoin Sodium extended capsules are recommended for once-a-day dosing. Inherent differences in dissolution characteristics and resultant absorption rates of Phenytoin due to different manufacturing procedures and/or dosage forms preclude such recommendation for other Phenytoin products. When a change in the dosage form or brand is prescribed, careful monitoring of Phenytoin serum levels should be carried out.

Loading Dose: Some authorities have advocated use of an oral loading dose of Phenytoin in adults who require rapid steady-state serum levels and where intravenous administration is not desirable This dosing regimen should be reserved for patients in a clinic or hospital setting where Phenytoin serum levels can be closely monitored. Patients with a history of renal or liver disease should not receive the oral loading regimen.

Initially, one gram of Phenytoin capsules is divided into 3 doses (400 mg, 300 mg, 300 mg) and administered at two-hourly intervals. Normal maintenance dosage is then instituted 24 hours after the loading dose, with frequent serum level determinations.

PHENYTOIN ORAL SUSPENSION

Patients who have received no previous treatment may be started on one teaspoonful (5 mL) of Phenytoin suspension three times daily, and the dose is then adjusted to suit individual requirements. An increase to five teaspoonfuls daily may be made, if necessary.

Pediatric Dosage (all oral forms): Initially, 5 mg/kg day in two or three equally divided doses, with subsequent dosage individualized to a maximum of 300 mg daily. A recommended daily maintenance dosage is usually 4 to 8 mg/kg. Children over 6 years old may require the minimum adult dose (300 mg/day). If the daily dosage cannot be divided equally, the larger dose should be given before retiring.

PARENTERAL PHENYTOIN SODIUM

The addition of parenteral Phenytoin solution to intravenous infusion is not recommended due to lack of solubility and resultant precipitation.

Not to exceed 50 mg per minute, intravenously in adults, and not exceeding 1-3 mg/kg/min in neonates. There is a relatively small margin between full therapeutic effect and minimally toxic doses of this drug.

The solution is suitable for use as long as it remains free of haziness and precipitate. Upon refrigeration or freezing, a precipitate might form; this will dissolve again after the solution is allowed to stand at room temperature. The product is still suitable for use. Only a clear solution should be used. A faint yellow coloration may develop; however, this has no effect on the potency of the solution.

In the treatment of status epilepticus, the intravenous route is preferred because of the delay in absorption of Phenytoin when administered intramuscularly.

Status Epilepticus: In adults, a loading dose of 10 to 15 mg/kg should be administered slowly intravenously, at a rate not exceeding 50 mg per minute (this will require approximately 20 minutes in a 70-kg patient). The loading dose should be followed by maintenance doses of 100 mg orally or intravenously every 6-8 hours.

Recent work in neonates and children has shown that absorption of Phenytoin is unreliable after oral administration, but a loading dose of 15-20 mg/kg of Phenytoin Sodium intravenously will usually produce plasma concentrations of Phenytoin within the generally accepted therapeutic range (10-20 mcg/mL). The drug should be injected slowly intravenously at a rate not exceeding 1-3 mg/kg/ min.

Parenteral Phenytoin Sodium should be injected *slowly* and directly into a large vein through a large-gauge needle or intravenous catheter. Each injection of intravenous Phenytoin Sodium should be followed by an injection of sterile saline through the same needle or catheter to avoid local venous irritation due to alkalinity of the solution. Continuous infusion should be avoided; the addition of parenteral Phenytoin Sodium to intravenous infusion fluids is not recommended because of the likelihood of precipitation.

Continuous monitoring of the electrocardiogram and blood pressure is essential. The patient should be observed for signs of respiratory depression. Determination of Phenytoin plasma levels is advised when using parenteral Phenytoin Sodium in the management of status epilepticus and in the subsequent establishment of maintenance dosage.

Other measures, including concomitant administration of an intravenous benzodiazepine such as diazepam, or an intravenous short-acting barbiturate, will usually be necessary for rapid control of seizures because of the required slow rate of administration of parenteral Phenytoin Sodium.

If administration of parenteral Phenytoin Sodium does not terminate seizures, the use of other anticonvulsants, intravenous barbiturates, general anesthesia, and other appropriate measures should be considered.

Intramuscular administration should not be used in the treatment of status epilepticus because the attainment of peak plasma levels may require up to 24 hours.

Neurosurgery: Prophylactic dosage—100 to 200 mg (2 to 4 mL) intramuscularly at approximately 4-hour intervals during surgery and continued during the postoperative period. When intramuscular administration is required for a patient previously stabilized orally, compensating dosage adjustments are necessary to maintain therapeutic plasma levels. An intramuscular dose 50% greater than the oral dose is necessary to maintain these levels. When returned to oral administration, the dose should be reduced by 50% of the original oral dose for one week to prevent excessive plasma levels due to sustained release from intramuscular tissue sites.

If the patient requires more than a week of IM Phenytoin Sodium, alternative routes should be explored, such as gastric intubation. For time periods less than one week, the patient shifted back from IM administration should receive one half the original oral dose for the same period of time the patient received IM Phenytoin Sodium. Monitoring plasma levels would help prevent a fall into the subtherapeutic range. Serum blood level determinations are especially helpful when possible drug interactions are suspected.

May be manufactured with CFC-12, a substance which harms public health and environment by destroying ozone in the upper atmosphere.

Storage: Store below 30°C (86°F). Protect from light and moisture. Protect suspension from freezing.

J CODES
IM,IV—J1165

HOW SUPPLIED

PHENYTOIN
CHEW TABLET: 50 MG

BRAND/MANUFACTURER	NDC	SIZE	AWP
○ **BRAND**			
▶ DILANTIN INFATABS: Parke-Davis	00071-0007-24	100s	$19.48
	00071-0007-40	100s ud	$27.62

SUSPENSION: 125 MG/5 ML

BRAND/MANUFACTURER	NDC	SIZE	AWP
○ **BRAND**			
DILANTIN-125: Parke-Davis	00071-2214-40	100s ud	$75.09
	00071-2214-20	237 ml	$28.25

PHENYTOIN SODIUM, PROMPT
CAPSULE: 100 MG

BRAND/MANUFACTURER	NDC	SIZE	AWP
◇ **GENERICS**			
Zenith	00172-2057-60	100s	$6.80
Rugby	00536-3764-10	1000s	$54.53
Goldline	00182-0197-10	1000s	$58.50
Major	00904-2057-80	1000s	$60.00
Zenith	00172-2057-80	1000s	$63.20

CAPSULE, EXTENDED RELEASE: 100 MG

AVERAGE UNIT PRICE (AVAILABLE SIZES)		GENERIC A-RATED AVERAGE PRICE (GAAP)	
GENERIC	$0.09	100s	$10.45

BRAND/MANUFACTURER	NDC	SIZE	AWP
◆ **GENERICS**			
Major	00904-2067-60	100s	$8.95
Major	00904-2067-61	100s ud	$11.95
Major	00904-2067-80	1000s	$69.60

INJECTION: 50 MG/ML

AVERAGE UNIT PRICE (AVAILABLE SIZES)		GENERIC A-RATED AVERAGE PRICE (GAAP)	
BRAND	$1.17	2 ml 25s	$47.71
GENERIC	$0.63	5 ml 25s	$53.65

BRAND/MANUFACTURER	NDC	SIZE	AWP
◆ BRAND			
DILANTIN: Parke-Davis	00071-4488-41	2 ml 10s	$49.33
	00071-4488-45	2 ml 25s	$36.00
	00071-4475-45	5 ml 25s	$42.00
◆ GENERICS			
Sanofi Winthrop	00024-1549-01	2 ml 10s	$12.94
Sanofi Winthrop	00024-1549-05	5 ml 10s	$20.71
Elkins-Sinn	00641-1465-35	2 ml 25s	$25.00
Elkins-Sinn	00641-0493-25	2 ml 25s	$40.00
Solo Pak	39769-0034-02	2 ml 25s	$78.13
Elkins-Sinn	00641-1466-35	5 ml 25s	$31.25
Elkins-Sinn	00641-2555-45	5 ml 25s	$47.50
Sanofi Winthrop	00024-1549-25	5 ml 25s	$51.46
Solo Pak	39769-0034-05	5 ml 25s	$84.38

INJECTION: 50 MG/ML

BRAND/MANUFACTURER	NDC	SIZE	AWP
◇ GENERICS			
Abbott Hosp	00074-1317-01	2 ml 25s	$58.48
Abbott Hosp	00074-1317-02	5 ml 25s	$68.58

PHENYTOIN SODIUM, EXTENDED
CAPSULE, EXTENDED RELEASE: 30 MG

BRAND/MANUFACTURER	NDC	SIZE	AWP
○ BRAND			
▷ DILANTIN KAPSEALS: Parke-Davis	00071-0365-24	100s	$18.78

CAPSULE, EXTENDED RELEASE: 100 MG

BRAND/MANUFACTURER	NDC	SIZE	AWP
○ BRAND			
▷ DILANTIN KAPSEALS: Parke-Davis	00071-0362-24	100s	$18.88
	00071-0362-40	100s ud	$20.84

pHisoHex *SEE* HEXACHLOROPHENE

Phos-Flur *SEE* SODIUM FLUORIDE

PhosLo *SEE* CALCIUM ACETATE

Phospholine Iodide *SEE* ECHOTHIOPHATE IODIDE

Phrenilin *SEE* ACETAMINOPHEN WITH BUTALBITAL

Phyllocontin *SEE* AMINOPHYLLINE

Physiosol *SEE* DEXTROSE AND ELECTROLYTES

Physostigmine Salicylate

DESCRIPTION

Physostigmine Salicylate is a derivative of the Calabar bean, and its active moiety, Physostigmine, is also known as eserine.

It is soluble in water and a 0.5% aqueous solution has a pH of 5.8.

Physostigmine Salicylate Injection is available in 2 mL ampuls, each mL containing 1 mg of Physostigmine Salicylate.

Following is its chemical structure:

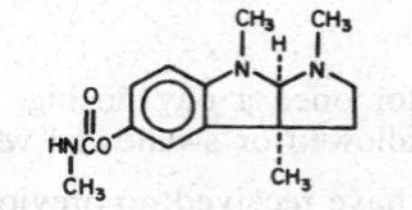

CLINICAL PHARMACOLOGY

Physostigmine Salicylate is a reversible anticholinesterase which effectively increases the concentration of acetylcholine at the sites of cholinergic transmission. The action of acetylcholine is normally very transient because of its hydrolysis by the enzyme, acetylcholinesterase. Physostigmine Salicylate inhibits the destructive action of acetylcholinesterase and thereby prolongs and exaggerates the effect of the acetylcholine.

Physostigmine Salicylate contains a tertiary amine and easily penetrates the blood brain barrier, while an anticholinesterase, such as neostigmine, which has a quaternary ammonium ion is not capable of crossing the barrier. Physostigmine Salicylate can reverse both central and peripheral anticholinergia. The anticholinergic syndrome has both central and peripheral signs and symptoms. Central toxic effects include anxiety, delirium, disorientation, hallucinations, hyperactivity and seizures. Severe poisoning may produce coma, medullary paralysis and death. Peripheral toxicity is characterized by tachycardia, hyperpyrexia, mydriasis, vasodilatation, urinary retention, diminution of gastrointestinal motility, decrease of secretion in salivary and sweat glands, and loss of secretions in the pharynx, bronchi, and nasal passages.

Dramatic reversal of the effects of anticholinergic symptoms can be expected in minutes after the intravenous administration of Physostigmine Salicylate if the diagnosis is correct and the patient has not suffered anoxia or other insult. The duration of action of Physostigmine Salicylate is relatively short, approximately 45 to 60 minutes.

Numerous drugs and some plants produce the anticholinergic syndrome either directly or as a side effect; this undesirable or potentially dangerous phenomenon may be brought about by either therapeutic doses or overdoses of the drugs. Such drugs include among others, atropine, other derivatives of the belladonna alkaloids, tricyclic antidepressants, phenothiazines, and antihistamines.

INDICATIONS AND USAGES

To reverse the effect upon the central nervous system, caused by clinical or toxic dosages of drugs capable of producing the anticholinergic syndrome.

CONTRAINDICATIONS

Physostigmine Salicylate should not be used in the presence of asthma, gangrene, diabetes, cardiovascular disease, mechanical obstruction of the intestine or urogenital tract or any vagotonic state, and in patients receiving choline esters or depolarizing neuromuscular blocking agents (decamethonium succinylcholine).

For postanesthesia, the concomitant use of atropine with the Physostigmine Salicylate is not recommended, since the atropine antagonizes the action of Physostigmine.

WARNINGS

Contains sodium bisulfite, a sulfite that may cause allergic-type reactions including anaphylactic symptoms and life-threatening or less severe asthmatic episodes in certain susceptible people. The overall prevalence of sulfite sensitivity in the general population is unknown and probably low. Sulfite sensitivity is seen more frequently in asthmatic than in nonasthmatic people.

If excessive symptoms of salivation, emesis, urination and defecation occur, the use of Physostigmine Salicylate should be terminated. If excessive sweating or nausea occur, the dosage should be reduced.

Intravenous administration should be a slow, controlled rate, no more than 1 mg per minute (see *"Dosage"*). Rapid administration can cause bradycardia, hypersalivation leading to respiratory difficulties and possible convulsions.

An overdosage of Physostigmine Salicylate can cause a cholinergic crisis.

PRECAUTIONS

Because of the possibility of hypersensitivity in an occasional patient, atropine sulfate injection should always be at hand since it is an antagonist and antidote for Physostigmine.

USAGE IN PREGNANCY

Safe use in pregnancy and lactation has not been established; therefore, use in pregnant women, nursing mothers or women who may become pregnant requires that possible benefits be weighed against possible hazards to mother and child.

ADVERSE REACTIONS

Nausea, vomiting and salivation, can be offset by reducing dosage. Bradycardia and convulsions, if intravenous administration is too rapid. (See *"Dosage and Administration"*.)

OVERDOSAGE

Can cause a cholinergic crisis. Appropriate antidote is atropine sulfate.

DOSAGE AND ADMINISTRATION

Post Anesthesia Care: 0.5 to 1.0 mg intramuscularly or intravenously. INTRAVENOUS ADMINISTRATION SHOULD BE AT A SLOW CONTROLLED RATE OF NO MORE THAN 1 MG PER MINUTE. Dosage may be repeated at intervals of 10 to 30 minutes if desired patient response is not obtained.

◆ RATED THERAPEUTICALLY EQUIVALENT; ◇ THERAPEUTIC EQUIVALENCE UNCONFIRMED; ○ UNRATED

Overdosages of Drugs That Cause Anticholinergia: 2.0 mg intramuscularly or INTRAVENOUSLY AT SLOW CONTROLLED RATE (SEE ABOVE). Dosage may be repeated if life threatening signs, such as arrhythmia, convulsions or coma occurs.

Pediatric Dosage: Recommended dosage is 0.02 mg/kg, intramuscularly or by slow intravenous injection, no more than 0.5 mg per minute. If the toxic effects persist, and there is no sign of cholinergic effects, the dosage may be repeated at 5 to 10 minute intervals until a therapeutic effect is obtained or a maximum dose of 2 mg is attained.

IN ALL CASES OF POISONING, THE USUAL SUPPORTIVE MEASURES SHOULD BE UNDERTAKEN.

SOME DRUGS WHICH PRODUCE
THE ANTICHOLINERGIC SYNDROME
Amitriptyline, Amoxapine, Anisotropine, Atropine, Benztropine, Biperiden, Carbinoxamine, Clidinium, Cyclobenzaprine, Desipramine, Doxepin, Homatropine, Hyoscine, Hyoscyamine, Hyoscyamus, Imipramine, Lorazepam, Maprotiline, Mepenzolate, Nortriptyline, Propantheline, Protriptyline, Scopolamine, Trimipramine.

SOME PLANTS THAT PRODUCE
THE ANTICHOLINERGIC SYNDROME
Black Henbane, Deadly Night Shade, Devil's Apple, Jimson Weed, Loco Seeds or Weeds, Matrimony Vine, Night Blooming Jessamine, Stinkweed.

HOW SUPPLIED
INJECTION: 1 MG/ML

BRAND/MANUFACTURER	NDC	SIZE	AWP
○ **BRAND**			
ANTILIRIUM: Forest Pharm	00456-1037-12	2 ml 12s	$111.16
○ **GENERICS**			
Hope	60267-0600-66	2 ml 10s	$73.25

Physostigmine Sulfate

DESCRIPTION
Physostigmine Sulfate ophthalmic ointment is a sterile ointment for ophthalmic administration having the following composition:

Physostigmine Sulfate ....2.5 mg/g (cholinesterase inhibitor)

The chemical name is pyrrolo(2,3-b)indol-5-ol,1,2,3,3a,8,8a-hexahydro-1,3a,8-trimethyl-, methylcarbamate (ester), (3aS-cis)-, sulfate (2:1)

Following is its chemical structure:

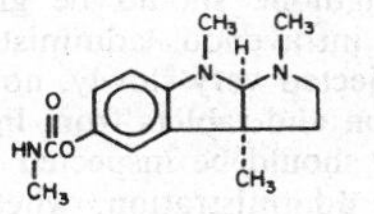

CLINICAL PHARMACOLOGY
Physostigmine is an anticholinesterase agent which temporarily inactivates cholinesterase and potentiates the action of acetylcholine on the parasympathetic end organs. It produces miosis in 30 minutes, persisting for 12-36 hours.

INDICATIONS AND USAGE
Physostigmine Sulfate is indicated for the treatment of primary glaucoma by causing a reduction of intraocular pressure. It may be used in conjunction with adrenergic agents, beta adrenergic blocking agents, carbonic anhydrase inhibitors, or hyperosmotic agents.

CONTRAINDICATIONS
In any inflammatory disease of the iris or ciliary body and in those individuals showing hypersensitivity to any of the components in this preparation.

WARNINGS
Overdosage may produce systemic gastrointestinal disturbances (see *"Adverse Reactions"* section).

Precautions: Ophthalmic ointments may retard corneal healing.
The miosis usually causes difficulty in dark adaptation. The patient should be cautioned when involved in night driving and other hazardous occupations in poor light.

Carcinogenesis, Mutagenesis, Impairment of Fertility: There have been no long-term studies done in animals with Physostigmine to evaluate carcinogenic potential.

Pregnancy: Pregnancy Category C. Animal reproduction studies have not been done with Physostigmine. It is also not known whether Physostigmine can cause fetal harm when administered to a pregnant woman or can affect reproduction capacity. Physostigmine should be given to a pregnant woman only if clearly needed.

Nursing Mothers: It is not known whether this drug is excreted in human milk. Because many drugs are excreted in human milk, caution should be exercised when Physostigmine is administered to a nursing woman.

Pediatric Use: Safety and effectiveness in children have not been established.

ADVERSE REACTIONS
Ocular: Allergic follicular conjunctivitis, eczematoid dermatitis, accommodative spasm, browache especially when medication is first started, and lid twitching may occur.
Retinal detachment has been reported following use of miotics in predisposed individuals.

Systemic: Systemic reactions are infrequently seen but may include gastrointestinal disturbances, faintness, and sweating.

DOSAGE AND ADMINISTRATION
Apply a small quantity to lower fornix up to three times a day.
Protect from heat. Keep tightly closed.

HOW SUPPLIED
OINTMENT: 0.25%

BRAND/MANUFACTURER	NDC	SIZE	AWP
○ **BRAND**			
PHYSOSTIGMINE SULFATE	54569-1661-01	3.5 gm	$1.62
	00168-0068-38	3.5 gm	$4.14
	00686-0068-38	3.75 gm	$3.25
○ **GENERICS**			
Allscrips	54569-1661-01	3.5 gm	$1.62
ESERINE SULFATE OPTH PREP.: CMC-Cons	00223-4122-03	3.5 gm	$2.75
Fougera	00168-0068-38	3.5 gm	$4.14
ESERINE SULFATE OPTH PREP.: Iolab	00058-3085-01	3.5 gm	$12.84
Raway	00686-0068-38	3.75 gm	$3.25

Phytonadione

WARNING—INTRAVENOUS USE
SEVERE REACTIONS, INCLUDING FATALITIES, HAVE OCCURRED DURING AND IMMEDIATELY AFTER INTRAVENOUS INJECTION OF PHYTONADIONE EVEN WHEN PRECAUTIONS HAVE BEEN TAKEN TO DILUTE THE PHYTONADIONE AND TO AVOID RAPID INFUSION. TYPICALLY THESE SEVERE REACTIONS HAVE RESEMBLED HYPERSENSITIVITY OR ANAPHYLAXIS, INCLUDING SHOCK AND CARDIAC AND/OR RESPIRATORY ARREST. SOME PATIENTS HAVE EXHIBITED THESE SEVERE REACTIONS ON RECEIVING PHYTONADIONE FOR THE FIRST TIME. THEREFORE THE *INTRAVENOUS* ROUTE SHOULD BE RESTRICTED TO THOSE SITUATIONS WHERE OTHER ROUTES ARE NOT FEASIBLE AND THE SERIOUS RISK INVOLVED IS CONSIDERED JUSTIFIED.

DESCRIPTION
Phytonadione is a vitamin, which is a clear, yellow to amber, viscous, odorless or nearly odorless liquid. It is insoluble in water, soluble in chloroform and slightly soluble in ethanol. It has a molecular weight of 450.70.
Phytonadione is 2-methyl-3-phytyl-1,4-naphthoquinone. Its empirical formula is $C_{31}H_{46}O_2$.
Phytonadione injection is a yellow, sterile, aqueous colloidal solution of vitamin K_1, with a pH of 5.0 to 7.0, available for injection by the intravenous, intramuscular, and subcutaneous routes.

Each milliliter contains:

Phytonadione ....2 mg or 10 mg

Each tablet contains:

Phytonadione ....5 mg

Following is its chemical structure:

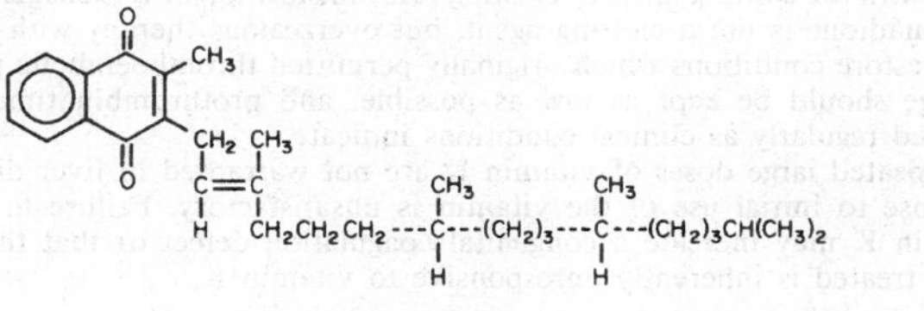

E component

CLINICAL PHARMACOLOGY
Phytonadione aqueous colloidal solution of vitamin K_1 for parenteral injection and tablets possesses the same type and degree of activity as does naturally-occurring vitamin K, which is necessary for the production via the liver of active prothrombin (factor II), proconvertin (factor VII), plasma thromboplastin

component (factor IX), and Stuart factor (factor X). The prothrombin test is sensitive to the levels of three of these four factors—II, VII, and X. Vitamin K is an essential cofactor for a microsomal enzyme that catalyzes the post-translational carboxylation of multiple, specific, peptide-bound glutamic acid residues in inactive hepatic precursors of factors II, VII, IX, and X. The resulting gamma-carboxyglutamic acid residues convert the precursors into active coagulation factors that are subsequently secreted by liver cells into the blood.

Phytonadione is readily absorbed following intramuscular administration; oral Phytonadione is adequately absorbed from the gastrointestinal tract only if bile salts are present. After absorption, Phytonadione is initially concentrated in the liver, but the concentration declines rapidly. Very little vitamin K accumulates in tissues. Little is known about the metabolic fate of vitamin K. Almost no free unmetabolized vitamin K appears in bile or urine.

In normal animals and humans, Phytonadione is virtually devoid of pharmacodynamic activity. However, in animals and humans deficient in vitamin K, the pharmacological action of vitamin K is related to its normal physiological function, that is, to promote the hepatic biosynthesis of vitamin K dependent clotting factors.

The action of the aqueous colloidal solution, when administered intravenously, is generally detectable within an hour or two and hemorrhage is usually controlled within 3 to 6 hours. A normal prothrombin level may often be obtained in 12 to 14 hours.

In the prophylaxis and treatment of hemorrhagic disease of the newborn, parenteral Phytonadione has demonstrated a greater margin of safety than that of the water-soluble vitamin K analogues.

Phytonadione tablets generally exert their effect within 6 to 10 hours.

INDICATIONS AND USAGE

Phytonadione is indicated in the following coagulation disorders which are due to faulty formation of factors II, VII, IX and X when caused by vitamin K deficiency or interference with vitamin K activity.

Phytonadione injection is indicated in:

— anticoagulant-induced prothrombin deficiency caused by coumarin or indanedione derivatives;
— prophylaxis and therapy of hemorrhagic disease of the newborn;
— hypoprothrombinemia due to antibacterial therapy;
— hypoprothrombinemia secondary to factors limiting absorption or synthesis of vitamin K, e.g., obstructive jaundice, biliary fistula, sprue, ulcerative colitis, celiac disease, intestinal resection, cystic fibrosis of the pancreas, and regional enteritis;
— other drug-induced hypoprothrombinemia where it is definitely shown that the result is due to interference with vitamin K metabolism, e.g., salicylates.

Phytonadione tablets are indicated in:

— anticoagulant-induced prothrombin deficiency caused by coumarin or indanedione derivatives;
— hypoprothrombinemia secondary to antibacterial therapy;
— hypoprothrombinemia secondary to administration of salicylates;
— hypoprothrombinemia secondary to obstructive jaundice or biliary fistulas but only if bile salts are administered concurrently, since otherwise the oral vitamin K will not be absorbed.

CONTRAINDICATION

Hypersensitivity to any component of this medication.

WARNINGS

Benzyl alcohol as a preservative in Bacteriostatic Sodium Chloride Injection has been associated with toxicity in newborns. Data are unavailable on the toxicity of other preservatives in this age group. There is no evidence to suggest that the small amount of benzyl alcohol contained in Phytonadione, when used as recommended, is associated with toxicity.

An immediate coagulant effect should not be expected after administration of Phytonadione. It takes a minimum of 1 to 2 hours for measurable improvement in the prothrombin time. Whole blood or component therapy may also be necessary if bleeding is severe.

Phytonadione will not counteract the anticoagulant action of heparin.

When vitamin K₁ is used to correct excessive anticoagulant-induced hypoprothrombinemia, anticoagulant therapy still being indicated, the patient is again faced with the clotting hazards existing prior to starting the anticoagulant therapy. Phytonadione is not a clotting agent, but overzealous therapy with vitamin K₁ may restore conditions which originally permitted thromboembolic phenomena. Dosage should be kept as low as possible, and prothrombin time should be checked regularly as clinical conditions indicate.

Repeated large doses of vitamin K are not warranted in liver disease if the response to initial use of the vitamin is unsatisfactory. Failure to respond to vitamin K may indicate a congenital coagulation defect or that the condition being treated is inherently unresponsive to vitamin K.

PRECAUTIONS

DRUG INTERACTIONS
Temporary resistance to prothrombin-depressing anticoagulants may result, especially when larger doses of Phytonadione are used. If relatively large doses have been employed, it may be necessary when reinstituting anticoagulant therapy to use somewhat larger doses of the prothrombin-depressing anticoagulant, or to use one which acts on a different principle, such as heparin sodium.

LABORATORY TESTS
Prothrombin time should be checked regularly as clinical conditions indicate.

CARCINOGENESIS, MUTAGENESIS, IMPAIRMENT OF FERTILITY
Studies of carcinogenicity or impairment of fertility have not been conducted with Phytonadione. Phytonadione at concentrations up to 2000 mcg/plate with or without metabolic activation was negative in the Ames microbial mutagen test.

PREGNANCY: PREGNANCY CATEGORY C
Animal reproduction studies have not been conducted with Phytonadione. It is also not known whether Phytonadione can cause fetal harm when administered to a pregnant woman or can affect reproduction capacity. Phytonadione should be given to a pregnant woman only if clearly needed.

NURSING MOTHERS
It is not known whether this drug is excreted in human milk. Because many drugs are excreted in human milk, caution should be exercised when Phytonadione is administered to a nursing woman.

PEDIATRIC USE
Hemolysis, jaundice, and hyperbilirubinemia in newborns, particularly in premature infants, have been reported with vitamin K and may be related to the dose of Phytonadione. Therefore, the recommended dose should not be exceeded (see "Adverse Reactions" and "Dosage and Administration"). Safety and effectiveness in children have not been established with oral Phytonadione.

ADVERSE REACTIONS
Deaths have occurred after intravenous administration. (See "Warning" at beginning of circular.)

Transient "flushing sensations" and "peculiar" sensations of taste have been observed with parenteral Phytonadione, as well as rare instances of dizziness, rapid and weak pulse, profuse sweating, brief hypotension, dyspnea, and cyanosis.

Pain, swelling, and tenderness at the injection site may occur.

The possibility of allergic sensitivity, including an anaphylactoid reaction, should be kept in mind.

Infrequently, usually after repeated injection, erythematous, indurated, pruritic plaques have occurred; rarely, these have progressed to sclerodermalike lesions that have persisted for long periods. In other cases, these lesions have resembled erythema perstans.

Hyperbilirubinemia has been observed in the newborn following administration of parenteral Phytonadione. This has occurred rarely and primarily with doses above those recommended. (See "Precautions, Pediatric Use".)

OVERDOSAGE
The intravenous and oral LD₅₀ of Phytonadione in the mouse are approximately 1.17 g/kg and greater than 24.18 g/kg, respectively.

DOSAGE AND ADMINISTRATION
Whenever possible, Phytonadione should be given by the subcutaneous or intramuscular route. When intravenous administration is considered unavoidable, the drug should be injected very slowly, not exceeding 1 mg per minute.

Protect parenteral solution and tablets from light at all times.

Parenteral drug products should be inspected visually for particulate matter and discoloration prior to administration, whenever solution and container permit.

DIRECTIONS FOR DILUTION
Phytonadione may be diluted with 0.9% Sodium Chloride Injection, 5% Dextrose Injection, or 5% Dextrose and Sodium Chloride Injection. Benzyl alcohol as a preservative has been associated with toxicity in newborns. *Therefore, all of the above diluents should be preservative-free* (see "Warnings"). *Other diluents should not be used.* When dilutions are indicated, administration should be started immediately after mixture with the diluent, and unused portions of the dilution should be discarded, as well as unused contents of the ampul.

PROPHYLAXIS OF HEMORRHAGIC DISEASE OF THE NEWBORN
The American Academy of Pediatrics recommends that vitamin K₁ be given to the newborn. A single intramuscular dose of Phytonadione 0.5 to 1 mg within one hour of birth is recommended.

TREATMENT OF HEMORRHAGIC DISEASE OF THE NEWBORN
Empiric administration of vitamin K₁ should not replace proper laboratory evaluation of the coagulation mechanism.

A prompt response (shortening of the prothrombin time in 2 to 4 hours) following administration of vitamin K₁ is usually diagnostic of hemorrhagic disease of the newborn, and failure to respond indicates another diagnosis or coagulation disorder.

Phytonadione 1 mg should be given either subcutaneously or intramuscularly. Higher doses may be necessary if the mother has been receiving oral anticoagulants.

PHYTONADIONE SUMMARY OF DOSAGE GUIDELINES (SEE CIRCULAR TEXT FOR DETAILS)

Newborns (Parenteral)	*Dosage*
Hemorrhagic Disease of the Newborn	
Prophylaxis	0.5-1 mg IM within 1 hour of birth

Newborns (Parenteral)	Dosage
Treatment	1 mg SC or IM (Higher doses may be necessary if the mother has been receiving oral anticoagulants)

Adults (Oral and Parenteral)	Initial Dosage
Anticoagulant-Induced Prothrombin Deficiency (caused by coumarin or indanedione derivatives)	2.5 mg-10 mg or up to 25 mg (rarely 50 mg)
Hypoprothrombinemia due to other causes (Antibiotics: Salicylates or other drugs; Factors limiting absorption or synthesis)	2.5 mg-25 mg or more (rarely up to 50 mg)

Whole blood or component therapy may be indicated if bleeding is excessive. This therapy, however, does not correct the underlying disorder and Phytonadione should be given concurrently.

ANTICOAGULANT-INDUCED PROTHROMBIN DEFICIENCY IN ADULTS

To correct excessively prolonged prothrombin time caused by oral anticoagulant therapy—2.5 to 10 mg or up to 25 mg initially is recommended. In rare instances 50 mg may be required. Frequency and amount of subsequent doses should be determined by prothrombin time response or clinical condition (see *"Warnings"*). If in 6 to 8 hours after parenteral administration, or 12 to 48 hours after oral administration, the prothrombin time has not been shortened satisfactorily, the dose should be repeated.

In the event of shock or excessive blood loss, the use of whole blood or component therapy is indicated.

HYPOPROTHROMBINEMIA DUE TO OTHER CAUSES IN ADULTS

A dosage of 2.5 to 25 mg or more (rarely up to 50 mg) is recommended, the amount and route of administration depending upon the severity of the condition and response obtained.

The oral route should be avoided when the clinical disorder would prevent proper absorption. Bile salts must be given with the tablets when the endogenous supply of bile to the gastrointestinal tract is deficient.

If possible, discontinuation or reduction of the dosage of drugs interfering with coagulation mechanisms (such as salicylates, antibiotics) is suggested as an alternative to administering concurrent Phytonadione. The severity of the coagulation disorder should determine whether the immediate administration of Phytonadione is required in addition to discontinuation or reduction of interfering drugs.

HOW SUPPLIED
INJECTION: 1 MG/0.5 ML

BRAND/MANUFACTURER	NDC	SIZE	AWP
◇ **BRAND**			
KONAKION: Roche Labs	00004-1907-06	1 ml 10s	$27.39
AQUAMEPHYTON: Merck	00006-7784-33	0.5 ml 25s	$56.19

INJECTION: 10 MG/ML

BRAND/MANUFACTURER	NDC	SIZE	AWP
◇ **BRAND**			
AQUAMEPHYTON: Merck	00006-7782-30	2.5 ml	$11.55
	00006-7782-03	5 ml	$22.91
	00006-7780-64	1 ml 6s	$27.50
KONAKION: Roche Labs	00004-1908-06	1 ml 10s	$56.48
AQUAMEPHYTON: Merck	00006-7780-66	1 ml 25s	$109.65

TABLETS: 5 MG

BRAND/MANUFACTURER	NDC	SIZE	AWP
○ **BRAND**			
MEPHYTON: Merck	00006-0043-68	100s	$52.20

Pilagan with C Cap *SEE* PILOCARPINE, OPHTHALMIC

Pilocar *SEE* PILOCARPINE, OPHTHALMIC

Pilocarpine Hydrochloride, Oral

DESCRIPTION

Pilocarpine Hydrochloride is a cholinergic agonist for oral use. Pilocarpine Hydrochloride is a hygroscopic, odorless, bitter tasting white crystal or powder which is soluble in water and alcohol and virtually insoluble in most nonpolar solvents. Pilocarpine Hydrochloride, with a chemical name of 2(3H)-Furanone, 3-ethyldihydro-4-[(1-methyl-1H-imidazol-5-yl)methyl] -monohydrochloride, (3S-cis), has a molecular weight of 244.72.

Each Pilocarpine Hydrochloride tablet for oral administration contains 5 mg of Pilocarpine Hydrochloride.

Following is its chemical structure:

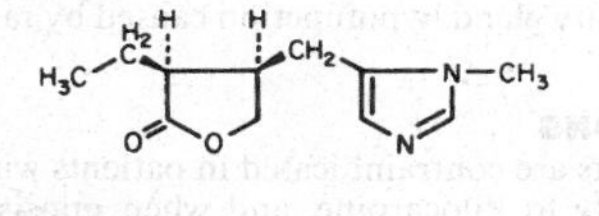

CLINICAL PHARMACOLOGY

Pharmacodynamics: Pilocarpine is a cholinergic parasympathomimetic agent exerting a broad spectrum of pharmacologic effects with predominant muscarinic action. Pilocarpine, in appropriate dosage, can increase secretion by the exocrine glands. The sweat, salivary, lacrimal, gastric, pancreatic, and intestinal glands and the mucous cells of the respiratory tract may be stimulated. When applied topically to the eye as a single dose it causes miosis, spasm of accommodation, and may cause a transitory rise in intraocular pressure followed by a more persistent fall. Dose-related smooth muscle stimulation of the intestinal tract may cause increased tone, increased motility, spasm, and tenesmus. Bronchial smooth muscle tone may increase. The tone and motility of urinary tract, gallbladder, and biliary duct smooth muscle may be enhanced. Pilocarpine may have paradoxical effects on the cardiovascular system. The expected effect of a muscarinic agonist is vasodepression, but administration of Pilocarpine may produce hypertension after a brief episode of hypotension. Bradycardia and tachycardia have both been reported with use of Pilocarpine.

In a study in 12 healthy male volunteers there was a dose-related increase in unstimulated salivary flow following single 5 and 10 mg oral doses of Pilocarpine HCl tablets. The stimulatory effect was time-related with an onset at 20 minutes and peak at 1 hour with a duration of 3 to 5 hours. (See *"Pharmacokinetics"* section.)

In a 12 week randomized, double-blind, placebo-controlled study in 207 patients (placebo, N = 65; 5 mg, N = 73; 10 mg, N = 69), increases from baseline (means 0.072 and 0.112 mL/min, ranges −0.690 to 0.728 and −0.380 to 1.689) of whole saliva flow for the 5 mg (63%) and 10 mg (90%) tablet, respectively, were seen 1 hour after the first dose of Pilocarpine HCl tablets. Increases in unstimulated parotid flow were seen following the first dose (means 0.025 and 0.046 mL/min, ranges 0 to 0.414 and −0.070 to 1.002 mL/min for the 5 and 10 mg dose, respectively). In this study, no correlation existed between the amount of increase in salivary flow and the degree of symptomatic relief. (See *"Clinical Studies"* section for details.)

Pharmacokinetics: In a multiple-dose pharmacokinetic study in male volunteers following 2 days of 5 or 10 mg of oral Pilocarpine HCl tablets given at 8 a.m., noontime, and 6 p.m., the mean elimination half-life was 0.76 hours for the 5 mg dose and 1.35 hours for the 10 mg dose. T_{max} values were 1.25 hours and 0.85 hours. C_{max} values were 15 ng/mL and 41 ng/mL. The AUC trapezoidal values were 33 h (ng/mL) and 108 h(ng/mL), respectively, for the 5 and 10 mg doses following the last 6 hour dose.

Pharmacokinetics in elderly male volunteers (n = 11) were comparable to those in younger men. In five healthy elderly female volunteers, the mean C_{max} and AUC were approximately twice that of elderly males and young male volunteers.

When taken with a high fat meal by 12 healthy male volunteers, there was a decrease in the rate of absorption of Pilocarpine from Pilocarpine HCl tablets. Mean T_{max}'s were 1.47 and 0.87 hours, and mean C_{max}'s were 51.8 and 59.2 ng/mL for fed and fasted, respectively.

Limited information is available about the metabolism and elimination of Pilocarpine in humans. Inactivation of Pilocarpine is thought to occur at neuronal synapses and probably in plasma. Pilocarpine and its minimally active or inactive degradation products, including pilocarpic acid, are excreted in the urine.

Clinical Studies: A 12 week randomized, double-blind, placebo-controlled study in 207 patients (142 men, 65 women) was conducted in patients whose mean age was 58.5 years with a range of 19 to 77; the racial distribution was Caucasian 95%, Black 4%, and other 1%. In this population, a statistically significant improvement in mouth dryness occurred in the 5 and 10 mg Pilocarpine HCl tablet treated patients compared to placebo treated patients. The 5 and 10 mg treated patients could not be distinguished. (See *"Pharmacodynamics"* section for flow study details.)

Another 12 week, double-blind, randomized, placebo-controlled study was conducted in 162 patients whose mean age was 57.8 years with a range of 27 to 80; the racial distribution was Caucasian 88%, Black 10%, and other 2%. The effects of placebo were compared to 2.5 mg three times a day of Pilocarpine HCl tablets for 4 weeks followed by titration to 5 mg three times a day and 10 mg three times a day. Lowering of the dose was necessary because of adverse events in 3 of 67 patients treated with 5 mg of Pilocarpine HCl tablets and in 7 of 66 patients treated with 10 mg of Pilocarpine HCl tablets. After 4 weeks of treatment, 2.5 mg of Pilocarpine HCl tablets three times a day was comparable to placebo in relieving dryness. In patients treated with 5 mg and 10 mg of Pilocarpine HCl tablets, the greatest improvement in dryness was noted in patients with no measurable salivary flow at baseline.

In both studies, some patients noted improvement in the global assessment of their xerostomia, speaking without liquids, and a reduced need for supplemental oral comfort agents.

In the two placebo-controlled clinical trials, the most common adverse events related to drug, and increasing in rate as dose increases, were sweating, nausea, rhinitis, chills, flushing, urinary frequency, dizziness, and asthenia. The most common adverse experience causing withdrawal from treatment was sweating (5 mg = < 1%; 10 mg = 12%).

INDICATIONS AND USAGE

Pilocarpine HCl tablets are indicated for the treatment of symptoms of xerostomia from salivary gland hypofunction caused by radiotherapy for cancer of the head and neck.

CONTRAINDICATIONS

Pilocarpine HCl tablets are contraindicated in patients with uncontrolled asthma, known hypersensitivity to Pilocarpine, and when miosis is undesirable, e.g., in acute iritis and in narrow-angle (angle closure) glaucoma.

WARNINGS

Cardiovascular Diseases: Patients with significant cardiovascular disease may be unable to compensate for transient changes in hemodynamics or rhythm induced by Pilocarpine. Pulmonary edema has been reported as a complication of Pilocarpine toxicity from high ocular doses given for acute angle-closure glaucoma. Pilocarpine should be administered with caution in and under close medical supervision of patients with cardiovascular disease.

Ocular: Careful examination of the fundus should be carried out prior to initiating therapy with Pilocarpine. An association of ocular Pilocarpine use and retinal detachment in patients with preexisting retinal disease has been reported. The systemic blood level that is associated with this finding is not known.

Ocular formulations of Pilocarpine have been reported to cause visual blurring which may result in decreased visual acuity, especially at night and in patients with central lens changes, and to cause impairment of depth perception. Caution should be advised while driving at night or performing hazardous activities in reduced lighting.

Pulmonary Disease: Pilocarpine has been reported to increase airway resistance, bronchial smooth muscle tone, and bronchial secretions. Pilocarpine HCl should be administered with caution to and under close medical supervision in patients with controlled asthma, chronic bronchitis, or chronic obstructive pulmonary disease.

PRECAUTIONS

General: Pilocarpine toxicity is characterized by an exaggeration of its parasympathomimetic effects. These may include: headache, visual disturbance, lacrimation, sweating, respiratory distress, gastrointestinal spasm, nausea, vomiting, diarrhea, atrioventricular block, tachycardia, bradycardia, hypotension, hypertension, shock, mental confusion, cardiac arrhythmia, and tremors.

The dose-related cardiovascular pharmacologic effects of Pilocarpine include hypotension, hypertension, bradycardia, and tachycardia.

Pilocarpine should be administered with caution to patients with known or suspected cholelithiasis or biliary tract disease. Contractions of the gallbladder or biliary smooth muscle could precipitate complications including cholecystitis, cholangitis, and biliary obstruction.

Pilocarpine may increase ureteral smooth muscle tone and could theoretically precipitate renal colic (or "ureteral reflux"), particularly in patients with nephrolithiasis.

Cholinergic agonists may have dose-related central nervous system effects. This should be considered when treating patients with underlying cognitive or psychiatric disturbances.

Renal Insufficiency: The pharmacokinetics of orally administered Pilocarpine in patients with renal and hepatic disease is not known.

Information for Patients: Patients should be informed that Pilocarpine may cause visual disturbances, especially at night, that could impair their ability to drive safely.

If a patient sweats excessively while taking Pilocarpine HCl and cannot drink enough liquid, the patient should consult a physician. Dehydration may develop.

Drug Interactions: Pilocarpine should be administered with caution to patients taking beta adrenergic antagonists because of the possibility of conduction disturbances. Drugs with parasympathomimetic effects administered concurrently with Pilocarpine would be expected to result in additive pharmacologic effects. Pilocarpine might antagonize the anticholinergic effects of drugs used concomitantly. These effects should be considered when anticholinergic properties may be contributing to the therapeutic effect of concomitant medication (e.g., atropine, inhaled ipratropium).

Carcinogenesis, Mutagenesis, Impairment of Fertility: No definitive long term animal studies have evaluated the carcinogenic potential of Pilocarpine HCl.

No evidence that Pilocarpine HCl has the potential to cause genetic toxicity was obtained in a series of studies that included: 1) bacterial assays (Salmonella and E. coli) for reverse gene mutations; 2) an *in vitro* chromosome aberration assay in a Chinese hamster ovary cell line; 3) an *in vivo* chromosome aberration assay (micronucleus test) in mice; and 4) a primary DNA damage assay (unscheduled DNA synthesis) in rat hepatocyte primary cultures. In a published report, male rats who received Pilocarpine at a dosage of 39 mg/kg/day (approximately 11 times the maximum recommended dose for a 60 kg human based upon body surface area [mg/m^2] estimates) exhibited morphologic evidence of reduced spermatogenesis. The possibility that Pilocarpine may impair male fertility in humans cannot be excluded. The effects of Pilocarpine on male and female fertility in humans have not been systematically studied.

Pregnancy Category C: Pilocarpine HCl was associated with a reduction in the mean fetal body weight and an increase in the incidence of skeletal variations when given to pregnant rats at a dosage of 90 mg/kg/day (approximately 26 times the maximum recommended dose for a 60 kg human based upon body surface area [mg/m^2] estimates). These effects may have been secondary to maternal toxicity. There are no adequate and well-controlled studies in pregnant women. Pilocarpine HCl tablets should be used during pregnancy only if the potential benefit justifies the potential risk to the fetus.

Nursing Mothers: It is not known whether this drug is excreted in human milk. Because many drugs are excreted in human milk and because of the potential for serious adverse reactions in nursing infants from Pilocarpine HCl tablets, a decision should be made whether to discontinue nursing or to discontinue the drug, taking into account the importance of the drug to the mother.

Pediatrics: Safety and effectiveness of this drug in children have not been established.

Geriatric Use: In the placebo-controlled clinical trials (see "Clinical Studies" section) the mean age of patients was approximately 58 years (range 19 to 80). Of these patients, 97/369 (61/217 receiving Pilocarpine) were over the age of 65 years. In the healthy volunteer studies, 15/150 subjects were over the age of 65 years. In both study populations, the adverse events reported by those over 65 years and those 65 years and younger were comparable. Of the 15 elderly volunteers (5 women, 10 men), the 5 women had higher C$_{max's}$ and AUC's than the men. (See "Pharmacokinetics" section.)

ADVERSE REACTIONS

In controlled studies, 217 patients received Pilocarpine, of whom 68% were men and 32% were women. Race distribution was 91% Caucasian, 8% Black, and 1% of other origin. Mean age was approximately 58 years. The majority of patients were between 50 and 64 years (51%), 33% were 65 years and older and 16% were younger than 50 years of age. The most frequent adverse experiences associated with Pilocarpine HCl tablets were a consequence of the expected pharmacologic effects of Pilocarpine.

Adverse Event	Placebo t.i.d. n = 152	5 mg t.i.d. n = 141	10 mg t.i.d. n = 121
Sweating	9%	29%	68%
Nausea	4	6	15
Rhinitis	7	5	14
Chills	< 1	3	14
Flushing	3	8	13
Urinary Frequency	7	9	12
Dizziness	4	5	12
Asthenia	3	6	12

In addition, the following adverse events (≥ 1% incidence) were reported at doses of 5 and 10 mg in the controlled clinical trials:

Adverse Event	Placebo t.i.d. n = 152	Pilocarpine HCl t.i.d. n = 212
Headache	8%	11%
Dyspepsia	5	7
Lacrimation	8	6
Diarrhea	5	6
Edema	4	5
Abdominal Pain	4	4
Amblyopia	2	4
Vomiting	1	4
Pharyngitis	8	3
Hypertension	1	3
Conjunctivitis	4	2
Tachycardia	1	2
Epistaxis	1	2
Tremor	0	2
Dysphagia	< 1	2
Voice Alteration	0	2
Rash	4	1
Taste Perversion	2	1
Sinusitis	2	1
Abnormal Vision	1	1
Myalgias	1	1
Pruritus	< 1	1

The following events were reported rarely in treated patients (< 1%): Causal relation is unknown.

Body as a whole: body odor, hypothermia, mucous membrane abnormality

Cardiovascular: bradycardia ECG abnormality, palpitations, syncope

Digestive: anorexia, increased appetite, esophagitis, gastrointestinal disorder, tongue disorder

Hematologic: leukopenia, lymphadenopathy

Nervous: anxiety, confusion, depression, abnormal dreams, hyperkinesia, hypesthesia, nervousness, paresthesias, speech disorder, twitching

◆ RATED THERAPEUTICALLY EQUIVALENT; ◇ THERAPEUTIC EQUIVALENCE UNCONFIRMED; ○ UNRATED

Respiratory: increased sputum, stridor, yawning

Skin: seborrhea

Special Senses: deafness, eye pain, glaucoma

Urogenital: dysuria, metrorrhagia, urinary impairment

In long-term treatment were two patients with underlying cardiovascular disease of whom one experienced a myocardial infarct and another an episode of syncope. The association with drug is uncertain.

The following adverse experiences have been reported rarely with ocular Pilocarpine: malignant glaucoma, macular hole, shock, middle ear disturbance, A-V block, depression, delusion, eyelid twitching, visual hallucination, confusion, agitation, dermatitis, ciliary congestion, and iris cysts.

OVERDOSE

Pilocarpine fatal overdosage resulting from poisoning has been reported in the scientific literature at doses presumed to be greater than 100 mg in two hospitalized patients. 100 mg of Pilocarpine is considered potentially fatal. Overdosage should be treated with atropine titration (0.5 mg to 1.0 mg given subcutaneously or intravenously) and supportive measures to maintain respiration and circulation. Epinephrine (0.3 mg to 1.0 mg, subcutaneously or intramuscularly) may also be of value in the presence of severe cardiovascular depression or bronchoconstriction. It is not known if Pilocarpine is dialyzable.

DOSAGE AND ADMINISTRATION

The recommended oral dose of Pilocarpine HCl tablets for the initiation of treatment is 5 mg three times a day. Titration up to 10 mg three times a day may be considered for patients who have not responded adequately and who can tolerate lower doses. The incidence of the most common adverse events increases with dose. The lowest dose that is tolerated and effective should be used for maintenance.

Store at controlled room temperature, 15°-30°C (59°-86°F).

HOW SUPPLIED
TABLETS: 5 MG

BRAND/MANUFACTURER	NDC	SIZE	AWP
○ BRAND SALAGEN: MGI	58063-0705-10	100s	$107.40

Pilocarpine, Ophthalmic

DESCRIPTION

Pilocarpine, Ophthalmic, is a cholinergic available as an ophthalmic solution, an ophthalmic gel, and a continuous-release system.

Each ml of solution contains:
Pilocarpine Hydrochloride ....0.25%, 0.5%, 1%, 2%, 3%, 4%, 5%, 6%, 8%, or 10%
or
Pilocarpine Nitrate ....1%, 2%, or 4%

Each gm of gel contains:
Pilocarpine Hydrochloride ....4% (40 mg)

The continuous-release system contains:
Pilocarpine 5 or 11 mg, to release, respectively, 20 or 40 mcg/hr over the period of a week

---

Pilocarpine is designated chemically as 2(3H)-Furanone,3-ethyldihydro-4[(1-methyl-1H-imidazol-5-yl) methyl]-, methyl], (CS-cis)- Pilocarpine Hydrochloride 2(3H)-Furanone, 3-ethyldihydro-4-[(1-methyl-1H-imidazol-5-yl)-methyl]-, monohydrochloride, (3S-cis), and Pilocarpine Nitrate as 2(3H)-Furanone, 3-ethyldihydro-4-[(1-methyl-1H-imidazol-5-yl)methyl]-, (3S-cis)-,mononitrate.

During the first few hours of the seven day time course, the release rate is higher than that prevailing over the remainder of the one-week period. The system releases drug at three times the rated value in the first hours and drops to the rated value in approximately six hours. A total of 0.3 mg to 0.7 mg Pilocarpine (Pilo-20 or Pilo-40, respectively) is released during this initial six-hour period (one drop of 2% Pilocarpine ophthalmic solution contains 1 mg Pilocarpine). During the remainder of the seven day period the release rate is within ± 20% of the rated value.

CLINICAL PHARMACOLOGY

Pilocarpine is a direct acting cholinergic parasympathomimetic agent which duplicates the moscarinic effects of acetylcholine but has no nicotinic effects. It acts through direct stimulation of muscarinic neuro receptors and smooth muscle such as the iris and secretory glands Pilocarpine and has no effect on striated muscle stimulates the ciliary muscle and produces miosis through contraction of the iris sphincter, causing increased tension on the scleral spur and opening of the trabecular mesh work spaces to facilitate outflow of aqueous humor and decrease aqueous secretion. Outflow resistance is thereby reduced, lowering intraocular pressure. Pilocarpine is released from the Pilocarpine continuous-release system as soon as it is placed in contact with the conjunctival surfaces.

Preclinical Results: The levels of ^{14}C-pilocarpine in the ocular tissues of rabbits following Pilocarpine continuous-release system and eyedrop administration have been determined. The Pilocarpine continuous-release system produces constant low Pilocarpine levels in the ciliary body and iris. Following ^{14}C-pilocarpine eyedrop treatment, the initial levels of Pilocarpine in the cornea, aqueous humor, ciliary body and iris are 3 to 5 times higher than the corresponding levels with the Pilocarpine continuous-release system, declining over the next six hours to approximately the tissue concentrations maintained by the Pilocarpine continuous-release system. In contrast, in the conjunctiva, lens, and vitreous the ^{14}C-pilocarpine concentrations remain consistently high from eyedrops and do not return to the constant low levels maintained by the Pilocarpine continuous-release system. Pilocarpine does not accumulate in ocular tissues during Pilocarpine continuous-release system use. These studies in rabbits have not been done in humans.

Clinical Results: The ocular hypotensive effect of the Pilocarpine continuous-release systems is fully developed within 1 ½ to 2 hours after placement in the cul-de-sac of the eye. A satisfactory ocular hypotensive response is maintained around-the-clock. Intraocular pressure reduction for an entire week is achieved with the Pilocarpine continuous-release system from either 3.4 mg or 6.7 mg Pilocarpine (20 or 40 µg/hour times 24 hours/day times 7 days, respectively), as compared with 28 mg administered as a 2% ophthalmic solution four times a day.

During the first several hours after insertion of Pilocarpine continuous-release system into the conjunctival cul-de-sac, induced myopia may occur. In contrast to the fluctuating and high levels of induced myopia typical of Pilocarpine administration by eyedrop, the amount of induced myopia with Pilocarpine continuous-release systems decreases after the first several hours to a low baseline level, approximately 0.5 diopters or less, which persists for the therapeutic life of the Pilocarpine continuous-release system. Pilocarpine-induced miosis approximately parallels the induced myopia.

Of the 302 patients who used the Pilocarpine continuous-release system in clinical studies for more than two weeks, 229 (75%) preferred it to previously used Pilocarpine eyedrops. This percentage increased with further wearing experience.

INDICATIONS AND USAGE

Pilocarpine is a miotic (parasympathomimetic) indicated for control of elevated intraocular pressure in Pilocarpine-response patients. Clinical studies have demonstrated Pilocarpine continuous-release system efficacy in certain glaucomatous patients. Pilocarpine Nitrate solution is also indicated for emergency relief of mydriasis in an acutely glaucomatous situation and to reverse mydriasis caused by cycloplegic agents.

The patient should be instructed on the use of the Pilocarpine continuous-release system and should demonstrate to the ophthalmologist his or her ability to place, adjust and remove the units.

Concurrent Therapy: Pilocarpine Hydrochloride may be used in combination with other miotics, beta blockers, carbonic anhydrase inhibitors, sympathomimetics, or hyperosmotic agents. Continuous-release systems have been used concomitantly with various ophthalmic medications. The release rate of Pilocarpine from the system is not influenced by carbonic anhydrase inhibitors, epinephrine or timolol ophthalmic solutions, fluorescein, or anesthetic, antibiotic, or anti-inflammatory steroid ophthalmic solutions. Systemic reactions consistent with an increased rate of absorption from the eye of an autonomic drug, such as epinephrine, have been observed. The occurrence of mild bulbar conjunctival edema, which is frequently present with epinephrine ophthalmic solutions, is not influenced by the continuous-release Pilocarpine system.

CONTRAINDICATIONS

Miotics are contraindicated where pupillary constriction is undesirable, such as in acute iritis, for glaucomas associated with acute inflammatory disease of the anterior segment of the eye, and glaucomas occurring or persisting after extracapsular cataract extraction where posterior synechiae may occur. They are also contraindicated in those persons showing hypersensitivity to any of their components, and in pupillary block glaucoma.

WARNINGS

Pilocarpine HCl solution and gel are for topical use only, NOT FOR INJECTION. Pilocarpine is readily absorbed systemically through the conjunctiva. Excessive application (instillation) may elicit systemic toxicity symptoms in some individuals.

Patients with acute infectious conjunctivitis or keratitis should be given special consideration and evaluation prior to the use of the Pilocarpine continuous-release system.

Damaged or deformed systems should not be placed or retained in the eye. Systems believed to be associated with an unexpected increase in drug action should be removed and replaced with a new system.

PRECAUTIONS
GENERAL

Pilocarpine has been reported to elicit retinal detachment in individuals with pre-existing retinal disease or predisposed to retinal tears. Fundus examination is advised for all patients prior to initiation of Pilocarpine therapy.

Pilocarpine continuous-release system safety in retinal detachment patients and in patients with filtration blebs has not been established. The conjunctival erythema and edema associated with epinephrine ophthalmic solutions are not substantially altered by concomitant Pilocarpine continuous-release system therapy. The use of Pilocarpine drops should be considered when intense miosis is desired in certain ocular conditions.

► SHOWN IN PRODUCT IDENTIFICATION GUIDE

DRUG INTERACTIONS

Although ophthalmic solutions have been used effectively in conjunction with the Pilocarpine continuous-release system, systemic reactions consistent with an increased rate of absorption from the eye of an autonomic drug, such as epinephrine, have been observed. In rare instances, reactions of this type can be severe.

Information for Patients: Do not touch dropper or tube tip to any surface, as this may contaminate the solution or gel. The miosis usually causes difficulty in dark adaptation. Patient should be advised to exercise caution in night driving and other hazardous occupations in poor illumination.

CARCINOGENESIS, MUTAGENESIS, IMPAIRMENT OF FERTILITY

No long-term carcinogenicity and reproduction studies in animals have been conducted with Pilocarpine.

PREGNANCY CATEGORY C

Animal reproduction studies have not been conducted with Pilocarpine. It is also not known whether Pilocarpine can cause fetal harm when administered to a pregnant woman or can affect reproduction capacity. Pilocarpine should be given to a pregnant woman only if clearly needed.

Although the use of the Pilocarpine continuous-release system has not been reported to have adverse effect on pregnancy, the safety of its use in pregnant women has not been absolutely established. While systemic absorption of Pilocarpine from the Pilocarpine continuous-release system is highly unlikely, pregnant women should use it only if clearly needed.

NURSING MOTHERS

It is not known whether Pilocarpine is excreted in human milk. Because many drugs are excreted in human milk, caution should be exercised when Pilocarpine is administered to a nursing woman.

PEDIATRIC USE

Safety and effectiveness in children have not been established.

ADVERSE REACTIONS

Adverse reactions associated with topical Pilocarpine Nitrate solution is also indicated for therapy include: visual blurring due to miosis and accommodative spasm, poor dark adaptation caused by the failure of the pupil to dilate in reduced illumination, and conjunctival hyperemia.

The following additional adverse experiences associated with Pilocarpine therapy have been reported: lacrimation, burning or discomfort, temporal or periorbital headache, ciliary spasm, conjunctival vascular congestion, superficial keratitis and induced myopia.

Ciliary spasm is not a contraindication to continued therapy unless the induced myopia is debilitating to the patient. Irritation from Pilocarpine has been infrequently encountered and may require cessation of therapy depending on the judgement of the physician. True allergic reactions are uncommon but require discontinuation of therapy should they occur. Corneal abrasion and visual impairment have been reported with use of the Pilocarpine continuous-release system. Systemic reactions following topical administration are extremely rare, but occasional patients are peculiarly sensitive to develop sweating and gastrointestinal overactivity following suggested dosage and administration. Ocular reactions usually occur during initiation of therapy and often will not persist with continued therapy. Reduced visual acuity in poor illumination is frequently experienced by older individuals and in those with lens opacity. A subtle corneal granularity was observed in about 10% of patients treated with Pilocarpine HCl gel. Cases of retinal detachment have been reported during treatment with miotic agents, especially in young myopic patients. Lens opacity may occur with prolonged use of Pilocarpine.

Although withdrawal of the peripheral iris from the anterior chamber angle by miosis may reduce the tendency for narrow angle closure, miotics can occasionally precipitate angle closure by increasing the resistance to aqueous flow from posterior to anterior chamber.

Some patients may notice signs of conjunctival irritation, including mild erythema with or without a slight increase in mucous secretion when they first use Pilocarpine continuous-release systems. These symptoms tend to lessen or disappear after the first week of therapy. In rare instances a sudden increase in Pilocarpine effects has been reported during system use.

OVERDOSAGE

Systemic toxicity following topical ocular administration of Pilocarpine is rare, but occasional patients are peculiarly sensitive and develop sweating and gastrointestinal overactivity following suggested dosage and administration. Overdosage can produce sweating, salivation, nausea, lacrimation, vomiting, diarrhea, tremors and slowing of the pulse and a decrease in blood pressure. Bronchial constriction may develop in asthmatic patients. In moderate overdosage, spontaneous recovery is to be expected and is aided by intravenous fluids to compensate for dehydration. For cases demonstrating severe poisoning, atropine is the pharmacologic antagonist to Pilocarpine.

A topical ocular overdose of an ophthalmic product containing Pilocarpine may be flushed from the eye(s) with warm tap water or normal saline.

If accidentally ingested, induce emesis or perform gastric lavage.

DOSAGE AND ADMINISTRATION

Pilocarpine HCl Solution: Two drops topically in the eye(s) one to two to four times daily as directed by a physician. Under selected conditions, more frequent instillations may be indicated. Individuals with heavily pigmented irides may require higher strengths. To aid in emergency miosis, 1 to 2 drops of one of the higher concentrations should be used. The dosage and strength required to reverse mydriasis depends on the cycloplegic used.

Pilocarpine HCl Gel: Apply a one-half inch ribbon in the lower conjunctival sac of the affected eye(s) once a day at bedtime.

PILOCARPINE CONTINUOUS-RELEASE SYSTEM

Initiation of Therapy: A patient whose introcular pressure has been controlled by 1% or 2% Pilocarpine eyedrop solution has a higher probability of pressure control with the 20-mcg system than a patient who has used a higher strength Pilocarpine solution and might require 40-mcg therapy. However, there is no direct correlation between the Pilocarpine continuous-release system and the strength of Pilocarpine eyedrop solutions required to achieve a given level of pressure lowering. The Pilocarpine continuous-release system reduces the amount of drug necessary to achieve adequate medical control; therefore, therapy may be started with the Pilocarpine continuous-release 20-mcg system irrespective of the strength of Pilocarpine solution the patient previously required. Because of the patient's age, family history, and disease status or progression, however, the ophthamologist may elect to begin therapy with the 40-mcg system. The patient should then return during the first week of therapy for evaluation of his intraocular pressure, and as often thereafter as the ophthalmologist deems necessary.

If the pressure is satisfactorily reduced with the Pilocarpine continuous-release 20-mcg system the patient should continue its use, replacing each unit every 7 days. If the physician desires intraocular pressure reduction greater than that achieved by the Pilocarpine continuous-release 20-mcg system, the patient should be transferred to the Pilocarpine continuous-release 40-mcg system. If necessary, an epinephrine ophthalamic solution or a carbonic anhydrase inhibitor may be used concurrently with Pilocarpine continuous-release system.

After a satisfactory therapeutic regimen has been established with the Pilocarpine continuous-release system, the frequency of follow-up should be determined by the ophthalmologist according to the status of the patient's disease process.

Placement and Removal of the Pilocarpine Continuous-Release System: The Pilocarpine continuous-release system is readily placed in the eye by the patient. It is strongly recommended that the patient's ability to manage the placement and removal of the system be reviewed at the first patient visit after initiation of therapy.

Since the Pilocarpine-induced myopia from the continuous-release systems may occur during the first several hours of therapy (average of 1.4 diopters in a group of young subjects), the patient should be advised to place the system into the conjunctival cul-de-sac at bedtime. By morning the induced myopia is at a stable level (about 0.5 diopters or less in young subjects).

Sanitary Handling: Patients should be instructed to wash their hands thoroughly with soap and water before touching or manipulating the Pilocarpine continuous-release system. In the event a displaced unit contacts unclean surfaces, rinsing with cool tap water before replacing is advisable. Obviously bacteriologically contaminated units should be discarded and replaced with a fresh unit.

System Retention in the Eye: During the initial adaptation period, the Pilocarpine continuous-release unit may slip out of the conjunctival cul-de-sac onto the cheek. The patient is usually aware of such movement and can replace the unit without difficulty.

In those patients in whom retention of the continuous-release unit is a problem, superior cul-de-sac placement is often more desirable. The continuous-release unit can be manipulated from the lower to the upper conjunctival cul-de-sac by a gentle digital massage through the lid, a technique readily learned by the patient. If possible the unit should be moved before sleep to the upper conjunctival cul-de-sac for best retention. Should the unit slip out of the conjunctival cul-de-sac during sleep, its ocular hypotensive effect following loss continues for a period of time comparable to that following instillation of eyedrops. The patient should be instructed to check for the presence of the continuous-release unit before retiring at night and upon arising.

STORAGE AND HANDLING

Store solution at 46°-80°F; protect from freezing. Shake well before use.
    Store gel at 36°-80°F; avoid excessive heat; do not freeze.
    Store continuous-release system under refrigeration (36°-46°F).

HOW SUPPLIED

PILOCARPINE HYROCHLORIDE
DEVICE: 20 MCG/HR

BRAND/MANUFACTURER	NDC	SIZE	AWP
○ BRAND			
OCUSERT: Alza	17314-4064-03	8s	$35.06

DEVICE: 40 MCG/HR

BRAND/MANUFACTURER	NDC	SIZE	AWP
○ BRAND			
OCUSERT: Alza	17314-4086-03	8s	$35.06

◆ RATED THERAPEUTICALLY EQUIVALENT; ◇ THERAPEUTIC EQUIVALENCE UNCONFIRMED; ○ UNRATED

DROP: 0.25%

BRAND/MANUFACTURER	NDC	SIZE	AWP
○ BRAND			
ISOPTO CARPINE: Alcon Ophthalmic	00998-0201-15	15 ml	$12.13

DROP: 0.5%

BRAND/MANUFACTURER	NDC	SIZE	AWP
◆ GENERICS			
PILOSOL: Ocusoft	54799-0521-15	15 ml	$4.70

DROP: 0.5%

BRAND/MANUFACTURER	NDC	SIZE	AWP
○ BRAND			
PILOCAR: Iolab	00058-2514-15	15 ml	$10.02
ISOPTO CARPINE: Alcon Ophthalmic	00998-0202-15	15 ml	$12.13
PILOCAR: Iolab	00058-2514-34	15 ml 2s	$15.30

DROP: 1%

AVERAGE UNIT PRICE (AVAILABLE SIZES)		GENERIC A-RATED AVERAGE PRICE (GAAP)	
GENERIC	$0.35	15 ml	$5.25

BRAND/MANUFACTURER	NDC	SIZE	AWP
◆ GENERICS			
PILOSOL: Ocusoft	54799-0522-15	15 ml	$4.95
Fougera	00168-0173-15	15 ml	$5.55

DROP: 1%

BRAND/MANUFACTURER	NDC	SIZE	AWP
○ BRAND			
PILOCAR: Iolab	00058-2515-15	15 ml	$10.32
ADSORBOCARPINE: Alcon Ophthalmic	00998-0212-15	15 ml	$12.13
ISOPTO CARPINE: Alcon Ophthalmic	00998-0203-15	15 ml	$12.13
	00998-0203-30	30 ml	$18.75
PILOCAR: Iolab	00058-2515-34	15 ml 2s	$15.78
	00058-0781-12	1 ml 12s	$24.96

DROP: 2%

AVERAGE UNIT PRICE (AVAILABLE SIZES)		GENERIC A-RATED AVERAGE PRICE (GAAP)	
GENERIC	$0.41	15 ml	$6.08

BRAND/MANUFACTURER	NDC	SIZE	AWP
◆ GENERICS			
PILOSOL: Ocusoft	54799-0523-15	15 ml	$5.30
Fougera	00168-0174-15	15 ml	$6.85

DROP: 2%

BRAND/MANUFACTURER	NDC	SIZE	AWP
○ BRAND			
PILOCAR: Iolab	00058-2516-15	15 ml	$10.32
ADSORBOCARPINE: Alcon Ophthalmic	00998-0213-15	15 ml	$12.31
ISOPTO CARPINE: Alcon Ophthalmic	00998-0204-15	15 ml	$12.31
	00998-0204-30	30 ml	$18.75
PILOCAR: Iolab	00058-2516-34	15 ml 2s	$15.90
	00058-0782-12	1 ml 12s	$24.96

DROP: 3%

BRAND/MANUFACTURER	NDC	SIZE	AWP
◆ GENERICS			
Aligen	00405-6122-15	15 ml	$8.13

DROP: 3%

BRAND/MANUFACTURER	NDC	SIZE	AWP
○ BRAND			
PILOCAR: Iolab	00058-2517-15	15 ml	$11.10
ISOPTO CARPINE: Alcon Ophthalmic	00998-0205-15	15 ml	$13.38
	00998-0205-30	30 ml	$20.38
PILOCAR: Iolab	00058-2517-34	15 ml 2s	$17.64

DROP: 4%

AVERAGE UNIT PRICE (AVAILABLE SIZES)		GENERIC A-RATED AVERAGE PRICE (GAAP)	
GENERIC	$0.48	15 ml	$7.20

BRAND/MANUFACTURER	NDC	SIZE	AWP
◆ GENERICS			
PILOSOL: Ocusoft	54799-0524-15	15 ml	$6.55
Fougera	00168-0175-15	15 ml	$7.85

DROP: 4%

BRAND/MANUFACTURER	NDC	SIZE	AWP
○ BRAND			
PILOCAR: Iolab	00058-2518-15	15 ml	$11.10
ADSORBOCARPINE: Alcon Ophthalmic	00998-0214-15	15 ml	$13.38
ISOPTO CARPINE: Alcon Ophthalmic	00998-0206-15	15 ml	$13.38
	00998-0206-30	30 ml	$20.38
PILOCAR: Iolab	00058-2518-34	15 ml 2s	$17.82
	00058-0783-12	1 ml 12s	$24.96

DROP: 5%

BRAND/MANUFACTURER	NDC	SIZE	AWP
○ BRAND			
ISOPTO CARPINE: Alcon Ophthalmic	00998-0207-15	15 ml	$11.88

DROP: 6%

BRAND/MANUFACTURER	NDC	SIZE	AWP
◆ GENERICS			
Aligen	00405-6124-15	15 ml	$12.46

DROP: 6%

BRAND/MANUFACTURER	NDC	SIZE	AWP
○ BRAND			
PILOCAR: Iolab	00058-2519-15	15 ml	$12.00
ISOPTO CARPINE: Alcon Ophthalmic	00998-0208-15	15 ml	$14.69
	00998-0208-30	30 ml	$22.38
PILOCAR: Iolab	00058-2519-34	15 ml 2s	$19.80

DROP: 8%

BRAND/MANUFACTURER	NDC	SIZE	AWP
○ BRAND			
ISOPTO CARPINE: Alcon Ophthalmic	00998-0209-15	15 ml	$16.31

DROP: 10%

BRAND/MANUFACTURER	NDC	SIZE	AWP
○ BRAND			
ISOPTO CARPINE: Alcon Ophthalmic	00998-0211-15	15 ml	$18.75

GEL: 4%

BRAND/MANUFACTURER	NDC	SIZE	AWP
○ BRAND			
PILOPINE-HS: Alcon Ophthalmic	00065-0215-35	3.5 gm	$22.00

PILOCARPINE NITRATE
DROP: 1%

BRAND/MANUFACTURER	NDC	SIZE	AWP
○ BRAND			
PILAGAN WITH C CAP: Allergan Pharm	11980-0879-45	15 ml	$9.55
◆ GENERICS			
Southwood	58016-6103-01	15 ml	$17.06

DROP: 2%

BRAND/MANUFACTURER	NDC	SIZE	AWP
○ BRAND			
PILAGAN WITH C CAP: Allergan Pharm	11980-0878-45	15 ml	$9.91

DROP: 4%

BRAND/MANUFACTURER	NDC	SIZE	AWP
○ BRAND			
PILAGAN WITH C CAP: Allergan Pharm	11980-0877-45	15 ml	$10.29

Pilopine HS SEE PILOCARPINE, OPHTHALMIC

Pimozide

DESCRIPTION
Pimozide is an orally active antipsychotic agent of the diphenyl-butylpiperidine series. Chemically, Pimozide is 1-(1-(4,4- bis(4-fluorophenyl)butyl)-4-piperidinyl) -1,3-dihydro-2 H-benzimidazol-2-one.

The solubility of Pimozide in water is less than 0.01 mg/ml; it is slightly soluble in most organic solvents.

Each tablet contains 2 mg of Pimozide.

➤ SHOWN IN PRODUCT IDENTIFICATION GUIDE

Following is its chemical structure:

CLINICAL PHARMACOLOGY

PHARMACODYNAMIC ACTIONS

Pimozide is an orally active antipsychotic drug product which shares with other antipsychotics the ability to blockade dopaminergic receptors on neurons in the central nervous system. Although its exact mode of action has not been established, the ability of Pimozide to suppress motor and phonictics in Tourette's Disorder is thought to be a function of its dopaminergic-blocking activity. However, receptor blockade is often accompanied by a series of secondary alterations in central dopamine metabolism and function which may contribute to both Pimozide's therapeutic and untoward effects. In addition, Pimozide, in common with other antipsychotic drugs, has various effects on other central nervous system receptor systems which are not fully characterized.

METABOLISM AND PHARMACOKINETICS

More than 50% of a dose of Pimozide is absorbed after oral administration. Based on the pharmacokinetic and metabolic profile, Pimozide appears to undergo significant first pass metabolism. Peak serum levels occur generally six to eight hours (range 4-12 hours) after dosing. Pimozide is extensively metabolized, primarily by N-dealkylation in the liver. Two major metabolites have been identified, 1-(4-piperidyl)-2-benzimidazolinone and 4,4-bis(4-fluorophenyl) butyric acid. The antipsychotic activity of these metabolites is undetermined. The major route of elimination of Pimozide and its metabolites is through the kidney.

The mean serum elimination half-life of Pimozide in schizophrenic patients was approximately 55 hours. There was a 13-fold interindividual difference in the area under the serum Pimozide level-time curve and an equivalent degree of variation in peak serum levels among patients studied. The significance of this is unclear since there are few correlations between plasma levels and clinical findings.

Effects of food, disease or concomitant medication upon the absorption, distribution, metabolism and elimination of Pimozide are not known.

INDICATIONS AND USAGE

Pimozide is indicated for the suppression of motor and phonictics in patients with Tourette's Disorder who have failed to respond satisfactorily to standard treatment.

Pimozide is not intended as a treatment of first choice, nor is it intended for the treatment for tics that are merely annoying or cosmetically troublesome. Pimozide should be reserved for use in Tourette's Disorder patients whose development and/or daily life function is severely compromised by the presence of motor and phonic tics.

Evidence supporting approval of Pimozide for use in Tourette's Disorder was obtained in two controlled clinical investigations which enrolled patients between the ages of 8 and 53 years. Most subjects in the two trials were 12 or older.

UNLABELED USES

Pimozide is used alone or as an adjunct in the treatment of schizophrenia, to alleviate psychopathology in senile dementia, Huntington's chorea, postherpetic neuralgia, and onychotillomania.

CONTRAINDICATIONS

1. Pimozide is contraindicated in the treatment of simple tics or tics other than those associated with Tourette's Disorder.

2. Pimozide should not be used in patients taking drugs that may, themselves, cause motor and phonic tics (e.g., pemoline, methylphenidate and amphetamines) until such patients have been withdrawn from these drugs to determine whether or not the drugs, rather than Tourette's Disorder, are responsible for the tics.

3. Because Pimozide prolongs the QT interval of the electrocardiogram it is contraindicated in patients with congenital long QT syndrome, patients with a history of cardiac arrhythmias, or patients taking other drugs which prolong the QT interval of the electrocardiogram (see *"Drug Interactions"*).

4. Pimozide is contraindicated in patients with severe toxic central nervous system depression or comatose states from any cause.

5. Pimozide is contraindicated in patients with hypersensitivity to it. As it is not known whether cross-sensitivity exists among the antipsychotics, Pimozide should be used with appropriate caution in patients who have demonstrated hypersensitivity to other antipsychotic drugs.

WARNINGS

The use of Pimozide in the treatment of Tourette's Disorder involves different risk/benefit considerations than when antipsychotic drugs are used to treat other conditions. Consequently, a decision to use Pimozide should take into consideration the following (see *"Precaution — Information for Patients"*).

TARDIVE DYSKINESIA

A syndrome consisting of potentially irreversible, involuntary, dyskinetic movements may develop in patients treated with antipsychotic drugs. Although the prevalence of the syndrome appears to be highest among the elderly, especially elderly women, it is impossible to rely upon prevalence estimates to predict, at the inception of antipsychotic treatment, which patients are likely to develop the syndrome. Whether antipsychotic drug products differ in their potential to cause tardive dyskinesia is unknown.

Both the risk of developing tardive dyskinesia and the likelihood that it will become irreversible are believed to increase as the duration of treatment and the total cumulative dose of antipsychotic drugs administered to the patient increase.

However, the syndrome can develop, although much less commonly, after relatively brief treatment periods at low doses.

There is no known treatment for established cases of tardive dyskinesia, although the syndrome may remit, partially or completely, if antipsychotic treatment is withdrawn. Antipsychotic treatment, itself, however, may suppress (or partially suppress) the signs and symptoms of the syndrome and thereby may possibly mask the underlying process. The effect that symptomatic suppression has upon the long-term course of the syndrome is unknown.

Given these considerations, antipsychotic drugs should be prescribed in a manner that is most likely to minimize the occurrence of tardive dyskinesia. Chronic antipsychotic treatment should generally be reserved for patients who suffer from a chronic illness that, 1) is known to respond to antipsychotic drugs, and 2) for whom alternative, equally effective, but potentially less harmful treatments are not available or appropriate. In patients who do require chronic treatment, the smallest dose and the shortest duration of treatment producing a satisfactory clinical response should be sought. The need for continued treatment should be reassessed periodically.

If signs and symptoms of tardive dyskinesia appear in a patient on antipsychotics, drug discontinuation should be considered. However, some patients may require treatment despite the presence of the syndrome.

(For further information about the description of tardive dyskinesia and its clinical detection, please refer to *"Adverse Reactions"* and *"Precautions — Information for Patients"*.)

NEUROLEPTIC MALIGNANT SYNDROME (NMS)

A potentially fatal symptom complex sometimes referred to as Neuroleptic Malignant Syndrome (NMS) has been reported in association with antipsychotic drugs. Clinical manifestations of NMS are hyperpyrexia, muscle rigidity, altered mental status (including catatonic signs) and evidence of autonomic instability (irregular pulse or blood pressure, tachycardia, diaphoresis, and cardiac dysrhythmias).

Additional signs may include elevated creatine phosphokinase, myoglobinuria (rhabdomyolysis) and acute renal failure.

The diagnostic evaluation of patients with this syndrome is complicated. In arriving at a diagnosis, it is important to identify cases where the clinical presentation includes both serious medical illness (e.g., pneumonia, systemic infection, etc.) and untreated or inadequately treated extrapyramidal signs and symptoms (EPS). Other important considerations in the differential diagnosis include central anticholinergic toxicity, heat stroke, drug fever and primary central nervous system (CNS) pathology.

The management of NMS should include 1) immediate discontinuation of antipsychotic drugs and other drugs not essential to concurrent therapy, 2) intensive symptomatic treatment and medical monitoring, and 3) treatment of any concomitant serious medical problems for which specific treatments are available. There is no general agreement about specific pharmacological treatment regimens for uncomplicated NMS.

If a patient requires antipsychotic drug treatment after recovery from NMS, the potential reintroduction of drug therapy should be carefully considered. The patient should be carefully monitored, since recurrences of NMS have been reported.

Hyperpyrexia, not associated with the above symptom complex, has been reported with other antipsychotic drugs.

OTHER

Sudden, unexpected deaths have occurred in experimental studies of conditions other than Tourette's Disorder. These deaths occurred while patients were receiving dosages in the range of 1 mg per kg. One possible mechanism for such deaths is prolongation of the QT interval predisposing patients to ventricular arrhythmia. An electrocardiogram should be performed before Pimozide treatment is initiated and periodically thereafter, especially during the period of dose adjustment.

Pimozide may have a tumorigenic potential. Based on studies conducted in mice, it is known that Pimozide can produce a dose-related increase in pituitary tumors. The full significance of this finding is not known, but should be taken into consideration in the physician's and patient's decisions to use this drug product. This finding should be given special consideration when the patient is young and chronic use of Pimozide is anticipated. (see *"Precautions — Carcinogenesis, Mutagenesis, Impairment of Fertility"*)

PRECAUTIONS

GENERAL

Pimozide may impair the mental and/or physical abilities required for the performance of potentially hazardous tasks, such as driving a car or operating machinery, especially during the first few days of therapy.

Pimozide produces anticholinergic side effects and should be used with caution in individuals whose conditions may be aggravated by anticholinergic activity.

Pimozide should be administered cautiously to patients with impairment of liver or kidney function, because it is metabolized by the liver and excreted by the kidneys.

Antipsychotics should be administered with caution to patients receiving anticonvulsant medication, with a history of seizures, or with EEG abnormalities, because they may lower the convulsive threshold. If indicated, adequate anticonvulsant therapy should be maintained concomitantly.

INFORMATION FOR PATIENTS

Treatment with Pimozide exposes the patient to serious risks. A decision to use Pimozide chronically in Tourette's Disorder is one that deserves full consideration by the patient (or patient's family) as well as by the treating physician. Because the goal of treatment is symptomatic improvement, the patient's view of the need for treatment and assessment of response are critical in evaluating the impact of therapy and weighing its benefits against the risks. Since the physician is the primary source of information about the use of a drug in any disease, it is recommended that the following information be discussed with patients and/or their families.

Pimozide is intended only for use in patients with Tourette's Disorder whose symptoms are severe and who cannot tolerate, or who do not respond to haloperidol.

Given the likelihood that a proportion of patients exposed chronically to antipsychotics will develop tardive dyskinesia, it is advised that all patients in whom chronic use is contemplated be given, if possible, full information about this risk.

The decision to inform patients and/or their guardians must obviously take into account the clinical circumstances and the competency of the patient to understand the information provided.

There is *very* little information available on the use of Pimozide in children under 12 years of age.

The information available on Pimozide from foreign marketing experience and from U.S. clinical trials indicate that Pimozide has a side effect profile similar to that of other antipsychotic drugs. Patients should be informed that all types of side effects associated with the use of antipsychotics may be associated with the use of Pimozide.

In addition, sudden, unexpected deaths have occurred in patients taking high doses of Pimozide for conditions other than Tourette's Disorder. These deaths may have been the result of an effect of Pimozide upon the heart. Therefore, patients should be instructed not to exceed the prescribed dose of Pimozide and they should realize the need for the initial ECG and for follow-up ECGs during treatment.

Also, Pimozide, at a dose about 15 times that given humans, caused an increase in the number of benign tumors of the pituitary gland in female mice. It is not possible to say how important this is. Similar tumors were not seen in rats given Pimozide, nor at lower doses in mice, which is reassuring. However, any such finding must be considered to suggest a possible risk of long-term use of the drug.

LABORATORY TESTS

An ECG should be done at baseline and periodically thereafter throughout the period of dose adjustment. Any indication of prolongation of the QT_c interval beyond an absolute limit of 0.47 seconds (children) or 0.52 seconds (adults), or more than 25% above the patient's original baseline should be considered a basis for stopping further dose increase (see "Contraindications") and considering a lower dose.

Since hypokalemia has been associated with ventricular arrhythmias, potassium insufficiency, secondary to diuretics, diarrhea, or other cause, should be corrected before Pimozide therapy is initiated and normal potassium maintained during therapy.

DRUG INTERACTIONS

Because Pimozide prolongs the QT interval of the electrocardiogram, an additive effect on QT interval would be anticipated if administered with other drugs, such as phenothiazines, tricyclic antidepressants or antiarrhythmic agents, which prolong the QT interval. Such concomitant administration should not be undertaken (see "Contraindications").

Pimozide may be capable of potentiating CNS depressants, including analgesics, sedatives, anxiolytics, and alcohol.

CARCINOGENESIS, MUTAGENESIS, IMPAIRMENT OF FERTILITY

Carcinogenicity studies were conducted in mice and rats. In mice, Pimozide causes a dose-related increase in pituitary and mammary tumors.

When mice were treated for up to 18 months with Pimozide, pituitary gland changes developed in females only. These changes were characterized as hyperplasia at doses approximating the human dose and adenoma at doses about fifteen times the maximum recommended human dose on a mg per kg basis. The mechanism for the induction of pituitary tumors in mice is not known.

Mammary gland tumors in female mice were also increased, but these tumors are expected in rodents treated with antipsychotic drugs which elevate prolactin levels. Chronic administration of an antipsychotic also causes elevated prolactin levels in humans. Tissue culture experiments indicate that approximately one-third of human breast cancers are prolactin-dependent *in vitro*, a factor of potential importance if the prescription of these drugs is contemplated in a patient with a previously detected breast cancer. Although disturbances such as galactorrhea, amenorrhea, gynecomastia, and impotence have been reported with antipsychotic drugs, the clinical significance of elevated serum prolactin levels is unknown for most patients. Neither clinical studies nor epidemiologic studies conducted to date have shown an association between chronic administration of these drugs and mammary tumorigenesis. The available evidence, however, is considered too limited to be conclusive at this time.

In a 24-month carcinogenicity study in rats, animals received up to 50 times the maximum recommended human dose. No increased incidence of overall tumors or tumors at any site was observed in either sex. Because of the limited number of animals surviving this study, the meaning of these results is unclear.

Pimozide did not have mutagenic activity in the Ames test with four bacterial test strains, in the mouse-dominant lethal test or in the micronucleus test in rats.

Reproduction studies in animals were not adequate to assess all aspects of fertility. Nevertheless, female rats administered Pimozide had prolonged estrus cycles, an effect also produced by other antipsychotic drugs.

PREGNANCY

Category C: Reproduction studies performed in rats and rabbits at oral doses up to 8 times the maximum human dose did not reveal evidence of teratogenicity. In the rat, however, this multiple of the human dose resulted in decreased pregnancies and in the retarded development of fetuses. These effects are thought to be due to an inhibition or delay in implantation which is also observed in rodents administered other antipsychotic drugs. In the rabbit, maternal toxicity, mortality, decreased weight gain, and embryotoxicity including increased resorptions were dose related. Because animal reproduction studies are not always predictive of human response, Pimozide should be given to a pregnant woman only if the potential benefits of treatment clearly outweigh the potential risks.

LABOR AND DELIVERY

This drug has no recognized use in labor or delivery.

NURSING MOTHERS

It is not known whether Pimozide is excreted in human milk. Because many drugs are excreted in human milk and because of the potential for tumorigenicity and unknown cardiovascular effects in the infant, a decision should be made whether to discontinue nursing or to discontinue the drug, taking into account the importance of the drug to the mother.

PEDIATRIC USE

Although Tourette's Disorder most often has its onset between the ages of 2 and 15 years, information on the use and efficacy of Pimozide in patients less than 12 years of age is limited.

Because it use and safety have not been evaluated in other childhood disorders, Pimozide is not recommended for use in any condition other than Tourette's Disorder.

ADVERSE REACTIONS

GENERAL

Extrapyramidal Reactions: Neuromuscular (extrapyramidal) reactions during the administration of Pimozide have been reported frequently, often during the first few days of treatment. In most patients, these reactions involved Parkinson-like symptoms which, when first observed, were usually mild to moderately severe and usually reversible. Other type of neuromuscular reactions (motor restlessness, dystonia, akathisia, hyperreflexia, opisthotonos, oculogyric crises) have been reported far less frequently. Severe extra-pyramidal reactions have been reported to occur at relatively low doses. Generally the occurrence and severity of most extrapyramidal symptoms are dose related since they occur at relatively high doses and have been shown to disappear or become less severe when the dose is reduced. Administration of antiparkinson drugs such as benztropine mesylate or trihexyphenidyl hydrochloride may be required for control of such reactions. It should be noted that persistent extrapyramidal reactions have been reported and that the drug may have to be discontinued in such cases.

Withdrawal Emergent Neurological Signs: Generally, patients receiving short-term therapy experience no problems with abrupt discontinuation of antipsychotic drugs. However, some patients on maintenance treatment experience transient dyskinetic signs after abrupt withdrawal. In certain of these cases, the dyskinetic movements are indistinguishable from the syndrome described below under "Tardive Dyskinesia" except for duration. It is not known whether gradual withdrawal of antipsychotic drugs will reduce the rate of occurrence of withdrawal emergent neurological signs but until further evidence becomes available, it seems reasonable to gradually withdraw use of Pimozide.

Tardive Dyskinesia: Pimozide may be associated with persistent dyskinesias. Tardive dyskinesia, a syndrome consisting of potentially irreversible, involuntary, dyskinetic movements, may appear in some patients on long-term therapy or may occur after drug therapy has been discontinued. The risk appears to be greater in elderly patients on high-dose therapy, especially females. The symptoms are persistent and in some patients appear irreversible. The syndrome is characterized by rhythmical involuntary movements of tongue, face mouth or jaw (e.g., protrusion of tongue, puffing of cheeks, puckering of mouth, chewing movements). Sometimes these may be accompanied by involuntary movements of extremities and the trunk.

There is no known effective treatment for tardive dyskinesia; antiparkinson agents usually do not alleviate the symptoms of this syndrome. It is suggested that all antipsychotic agents be discontinued if these symptoms appear. Should it be necessary to reinstitute treatment, or increase the dosage of the agent, or switch to a different antipsychotic agent, this syndrome may be masked.

It has been reported that fine vermicular movement of the tongue may be an early sign of tardive dyskinesia, and if the medication is stopped at that time the syndrome may not develop.

Electrocardiographic Changes: Electrocardiographic changes have been observed in clinical trials of Pimozide in Tourette's Disorder and schizophrenia. These have included prolongation of the QT interval, flattening, notching and inversion of the T wave and the appearance of U waves. Sudden, unexpected deaths and grand mal seizure have occurred at doses above 20 mg/day.

Neuroleptic Malignant Syndrome: Neuroleptic malignant syndrome (NMS) has been reported with Pimozide (See *"Warnings"* for further information concerning NMS).

Hyperpyrexia: Hyperpyrexia has been reported with other anti-psychotic drugs.

CLINICAL TRIALS
The following adverse reaction tabulation was derived from 20 patients in a 6-week-long placebo-controlled clinical trial of Pimozide in Tourette's Disorder.

Body System/Adverse Reaction	Pimozide (N = 20)	Placebo (N = 20)
Body as Whole		
Headache	1	2
Gastrointestinal		
Dry mouth	5	1
Diarrhea	1	0
Nausea	0	2
Vomiting	0	1
Constipation	4	2
Eructations	0	1
Thirsty	1	0
Appetite increase	1	0
Endocrine		
Menstrual disorder	0	1
Breast secretions	0	1
Musculoskeletal		
Muscle cramps	0	1
Muscle tightness	3	0
Stooped posture	2	0
CNS		
Drowsiness	7	3
Sedation	14	5
Insomnia	2	1
Dizziness	0	1
Akathisia	8	0
Rigidity	2	0
Speech disorder	2	0
Handwriting change	1	0
Akinesia	8	0
Psychiatric		
Depression	2	3
Excitement	0	1
Nervous	1	0
Adverse behavior effect	5	0
Special Senses		
Visual disturbance	4	0
Taste change	1	0
Sensitivity of eyes to light	0	1
Decreased accommodation	4	0
Spots before eyes	0	1
Urogenital		
Impotence	3	0

Because clinical investigational experience with Pimozide in Tourette's Disorder is limited, uncommon adverse reactions may not have been detected. The physician should consider that other adverse reactions associated with antipsychotics may occur.

OTHER ADVERSE REACTIONS
In addition to the adverse reactions listed above, those listed below have been reported in U.S. clinical trials of Pimozide in conditions other than Tourette's Disorder.

Body as a Whole: Asthenia, chest pain, periorbital edema.

Cardiovascular/Respiratory: Postural hypotension, hypotension, hypertension, tachycardia, palpitations.

Gastrointestinal: Increased salivation, nausea, vomiting, anorexis, GI distress.

Endocrine: Loss of libido.

Metabolic/Nutritional: Weight gain, weight loss.

Central Nervous System: Dizziness, tremor, parkinsonism, fainting, dyskinesia.

Psychiatric: Excitement.

Skin: Rash, sweating, skin irritation.

Special Senses: Blurred vision, cataracts.

Urogenital: Nocturia, urinary frequency.

POSTMARKETING REPORTS
The following experiences were described in spontaneous postmarketing reports. These reports do not provide sufficient information to establish a clear causal relationship with the use of Pimozide.

Hematologic: Hemolytic anemia.

Other: Seizure has been reported in one patient.

OVERDOSAGE
In general, the signs and symptoms of overdosage with Pimozide would be an exaggeration of known pharmacologic effects and adverse reactions, the most prominent of which would be: 1) electrocardiographic abnormalities, 2) severe extrapyramidal reactions, 3) hypotension, 4) a comatose state with respiratory depression.

In the event of overdosage, gastric lavage, establishment of a patent airway and, if necessary, mechanically-assisted respiration are advised. Electrocardiographic monitoring should commence immediately and continue until the ECG parameters are within the normal range. Hypotension and circlatory collapse may be counteracted by use of intravenous fluids, plasma, or concentrated albumin, and vasopressor agents such as metaraminol, phenylephrine and norepinephrine. Epinephrine should not be used. In case of severe extrapyramidal reactions, antiparkinson medication should be administered. Because of the long half-life of Pimozide, patients who take an overdose should be observed for at least 4 days. As with all drugs, the physician should consider contacting a poison control center for additional information on the treatment of overdose.

DOSAGE AND ADMINISTRATION
Reliable dose response data for the effects of Pimozide on tic manifestations in Tourette's Disorder patients below the age of twelve are not available. Consequently, the suppression of tics by Pimozide requires a slow and gradual introduction of the drug. The patient's dose should be carefully adjusted to a point where the suppression of tics and the relief afforded is balanced against the untoward side effects of the drug.

An ECG should be done at baseline and periodically thereafter especially during the period of dose adjustment (see *"Warnings"* and *"Precautions-Laboratory Tests"*).

In general, treatment with Pimozide should be initiated with a dose of 1 to 2 mg a day in divided doses. The dose may be increased thereafter every other day. Most patients are maintained at less than 0.2 mg/kg per day, or 10 mg/day, whichever is less. Doses greater than 0.2 mg/kg/day or 10 mg/day are not recommended.

Periodic attempts should be made to reduce the dosage of Pimozide to see whether or not tics persist at the level and extent first identified. In attempts to reduce the dosage of Pimozide consideration should be given to the possibility that increases of tic intensity and frequency may represent a transient, withdrawal-related phenomenon rather than a return of disease symptoms. Specifically, one to two weeks should be allowed to elapse before one concludes that an increase in tic manifestations is a function of the underlying disease syndrome rather than a response to drug withdrawal. A gradual withdrawal is recommended in any case.

Dispense in a tight, light-resistant container as defined in the official compendium.

ANIMAL PHARMACOLOGY
A chronic study in dogs indicated that Pimozide caused gingival hyperplasia when administered for several months at about 5 times the maximum recommended human dose. This condition was reversible after withdrawal. This condition has not been observed following chronic administration of Pimozide to man.

HOW SUPPLIED
TABLETS: 2 MG

BRAND/MANUFACTURER	NDC	SIZE	AWP
○ **BRAND**			
ORAP: Gate	57844-0187-01	100s	$66.32

Pindolol

DESCRIPTION
Pindolol, a synthetic beta-adrenergic receptor blocking agent with intrinsic sympathomimetic activity is 4-(2-hydroxy-3-isopropylamino-propoxy)-indole.

Pindolol is a white to off-white odorless powder soluble in organic solvents and aqueous acids. Pindolol is intended for oral administration.

Active Ingredient: Pindolol, available in 5 mg and 10 mg tablets.

Following is its chemical structure:

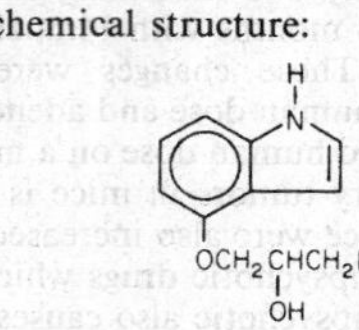

CLINICAL PHARMACOLOGY
Pindolol is a nonselective beta-adrenergic antagonist (beta-blocker) which possesses intrinsic sympathomimetic activity (ISA) in therapeutic dosage ranges but does not possess quinidine-like membrane stabilizing activity.

PHARMACODYNAMICS
In standard pharmacologic tests in man and animals, Pindolol attenuates increases in heart rate, systolic blood pressure, and cardiac output resulting from exercise and isoproterenol administration, thus confirming its beta-blocking

properties. The ISA or partial agonist activity of Pindolol is mediated directly at the adrenergic receptor sites and may be blocked by other beta-blockers. In catecholamine depleted animal experiments, ISA is manifested as an increase in the inotropic and chronotropic activity of the myocardium. In man, ISA is manifested by a smaller reduction in the resting heart rate (4-8 beats/min) than is seen with drugs lacking ISA. There is also a smaller reduction in resting cardiac output. The clinical significance of this observation has not been evaluated and there is no evidence, or reason to believe, that exercise cardiac output is less affected by Pindolol.

Pindolol has been shown in controlled, double-blind clinical studies to be an effective antihypertensive agent when used as monotherapy, or when added to therapy with thiazide-type diuretics. Divided dosages in the range of 10-60 mg daily have been shown to be effective. As monotherapy, Pindolol is as effective as propranolol, α-methyldopa, hydrochlorothiazide, and chlorthalidone in reducing systolic and diastolic blood pressure. The effect on blood pressure is not orthostatic, i.e. Pindolol was equally effective in reducing the supine and standing blood pressure.

In open, long-term studies up to 4 years, no evidence of diminution of the blood pressure lowering response was observed. An average 3-pound increase in body weight has been noted in patients treated with Pindolol alone, a larger increase than was observed with propranolol or placebo. The weight gain appeared unrelated to blood pressure response and was not associated with an increased risk of heart failure, although edema was more common than in control patients. Pindolol does not have a consistent effect on plasma renin activity.

The mechanism of the antihypertensive effects of beta-blocking agents has not been established, but several mechanisms have been postulated: 1) an effect on the central nervous system resulting in a reduced sympathetic outflow to the periphery, 2) competitive antagonism of catecholamines at peripheral (especially cardiac) adrenergic receptor sites, leading to decreased cardiac output, 3) an inhibition of renin release. These mechanisms appear less likely for Pindolol than other beta-blockers in view of the modest effect on resting cardiac output and renin.

Beta-blockade therapy is useful when it is necessary to suppress the effects of beta-adrenergic agonists in order to achieve therapeutic goals. However, in certain clinical situations, (e.g., cardiac failure, heart block, bronchospasm), the preservation of an adequate sympathetic tone may be necessary to maintain vital functions. Although a beta-antagonist with ISA such as Pindolol does not eliminate sympathetic tone entirely, there is no controlled evidence that it is safer than other beta-blockers in such conditions as heart failure, heart block, or bronchospasm or is less likely to cause those conditions. In single dose studies of the effects of beta-blockers on FEV_1, Pindolol was indistinguishable from other non-cardioselective agents in its reduction of FEV_1, and its reduction in the effectiveness of an exogenous beta agonist.

Exacerbation of angina and, in some cases, myocardial infarction and ventricular dysrhythmias have been reported after abrupt discontinuation of therapy with beta-adrenergic blocking agents in patients with coronary artery disease. Abrupt withdrawal of these agents in patients without coronary artery disease has resulted in transient symptoms, including tremulousness, sweating, palpitation, headache, and malaise. Several mechanisms have been proposed to explain these phenomena, among them increased sensitivity to catecholamines because of increased numbers of beta receptors.

PHARMACOKINETICS AND METABOLISM
Pindolol is rapidly and reproducibly absorbed (greater than 95%), achieving peak plasma concentrations within 1 hour of drug administration. Pindolol has no significant first-pass effect. The blood concentrations are proportional in a linear manner to the administered dose in the range of 5-20 mg. Upon repeated administration to the same subject, variation is minimal. After a single dose, intersubject variation for peak plasma concentrations was about 4-fold (e.g., 45-167 ng/mL for a 20 mg dose). Upon multiple dosing, intersubject variation decreased to 2-2.5 fold. Pindolol is only 40% bound to plasma proteins and is evenly distributed between plasma and red cells. The volume of distribution in healthy subjects is about 2 L/kg. Pindolol undergoes extensive metabolism in animals and man. In man, 35%-40% is excreted unchanged in the urine and 60%-65% is metabolized primarily to hydroxy-metabolites which are excreted as glucuronides and ethereal sulfates. The polar metabolites are excreted with a half-life of approximately 8 hours and thus multiple dosing therapy (q.8H) results in a less than 50% accumulation in plasma. About 6%-9% of an administered intravenous dose is excreted by the bile into the feces.

The disposition of Pindolol after oral administration is monophasic with a half-life in healthy subjects or hypertensive patients with normal renal function of approximately 3-4 hours. Following t.i.d. administration (q.8H), no significant accumulation of Pindolol is observed. In elderly hypertensive patients with normal renal function, the half-life of Pindolol is more variable, averaging about 7 hours, but with values as high as 15 hours.

In hypertensive patients with renal diseases, the half-life is within the range expected for healthy subjects. However, a significant decrease (50%) in volume of distribution (V_D) is observed in uremic patients and V_D appears to be directly correlated to creatinine clearance. Therefore, renal drug clearance is significantly reduced in uremic patients, resulting in a significant decrease in urinary excretion of unchanged drug. Uremic patients with a creatinine clearance of less than 20 mL/min generally excreted less than 15% of the administered dose unchanged in the urine.

In patients with histologically diagnosed cirrhosis of the liver, the elimination of Pindolol was more variable in rate and generally significantly slower than in healthy subjects. The total body clearance of Pindolol in cirrhotic patients ranged from about 50-300 mL/min and was directly correlated to antipyrine clearance. The half-life ranges from 2.5 hours to greater than 30 hours. These findings strongly suggest that caution should be exercised in dosage adjustments of Pindolol in such patients.

The bioavailability of Pindolol is not significantly affected by co-administration of food, hydralazine, hydrochlorothiazide or aspirin. Pindolol has no effect on warfarin activity or the clinical effectiveness of digoxin, although small transient decreases in plasma digoxin concentrations were noted.

INDICATIONS AND USAGE
Pindolol is indicated in the management of hypertension It may be use alone or concomitantly with other antihypertensive agents, particularly with a thiazide-type diuretic.

UNLABELED USES
Pindolol is used alone or as an adjunct in the treatment of aggressive behavior, angina pectoris, hyperthroidism, and supraventricular arrhythmias. Pindolol in the ophthalmic solution is used in open-angle glaucoma.

CONTRAINDICATIONS
Pindolol is contraindicated in: 1) bronchial asthma; 2) overt cardiac failure; 3) cardiogenic shock; 4) second- and third-degree heart block; 5) severe bradycardia. (See "Warnings".)

WARNINGS
CARDIAC FAILURE
Sympathetic stimulation may be a vital component supporting circulatory function in patients with congestive heart failure, and its inhibition by beta-blockade may precipitate more severe failure. Although beta-blockers should be avoided in overt congestive heart failure, if necessary, Pindolol can be used with caution in patients with a history of failure who are well-compensated, usually with digitalis and diuretics. Beta-adrenergic blocking agents do not abolish the inotropic action of digitalis on heart muscle.

IN PATIENTS WITHOUT HISTORY OF CARDIAC FAILURE
In patients with latent cardiac insufficiency, continued depression of the myocardium with beta-blocking agents over a period of time can, in some cases, lead to cardiac failure. At the first sign or symptom of impending cardiac failure, patients should be fully digitalized and/or be given a diuretic, and the response observed closely. If cardiac failure continues, despite adequate digitalization and diuretic, Pindolol therapy should be withdrawn (gradually if possible).

EXACERBATION OF ISCHEMIC HEART DISEASE FOLLOWING ABRUPT WITHDRAWAL
Hypersensitivity to catecholamines has been observed in patients withdrawn from beta-blocker therapy; exacerbation of angina and, in some cases, myocardial infarction have occurred after *abrupt* discontinuation of such therapy. When discontinuing chronically administered Pindolol, particularly in patients with ischemic heart disease, the dosage should be gradually reduced over a period of 1-2 weeks and the patient should be carefully monitored. If angina markedly worsens or acute coronary insufficiency develops, Pindolol administration should be reinstituted promptly, at least temporarily, and other measures appropriate for the management of unstable angina should be taken. Patients should be warned against interruption or discontinuation of therapy without the physician's advice. Because coronary artery disease is common and may be unrecognized, it may be prudent not to discontinue Pindolol therapy abruptly even in patients treated only for hypertension.

NONALLERGIC BRONCHOSPASM (E.G., CHRONIC BRONCHITIS, EMPHYSEMA)—PATIENTS WITH BRONCHOSPASTIS DISEASES SHOULD IN GENERAL NOT RECEIVE BETA-BLOCKERS
Pindolol should be administered with caution since it may block bronchodilation produced by endogenous or exogenous catecholamine stimulation of $beta_2$ receptors.

MAJOR SURGERY
Because beta blockade impairs the ability of the heart to respond to reflex stimuli and may increase the risks of general anesthesia and surgical procedures, resulting in protracted hypotension or low cardiac output, it has generally been suggested that such therapy should be gradually withdrawn several days prior to surgery. Recognition of the increased sensitivity to catecholamines of patients recently withdrawn from beta-blocker therapy, however, has made this recommendation controversial. If possible, beta-blockers should be withdrawn well before surgery takes place. In the event of emergency surgery, the anesthesiologist should be informed that the patient is on beta-blocker therapy.

The effects of Pindolol can be reversed by administration of beta-receptor agonists such as isoproterenol, dopamine, dobutamine, or levarterenol. Difficulty in restarting and maintaining the heart beat has also been reported with beta-adrenergic receptor blocking agents.

DIABETES AND HYPOGLYCEMIA
Beta-adrenergic blockade may prevent the appearance of premonitory signs and symptoms (e.g., tachycardia and blood pressure changes) of acute hypoglycemia. This is especially important with labile diabetics. Beta-blockade also reduces the release of insulin in response to hyperglycemia; therefore, it may be necessary to adjust the dose of antidiabetic drugs.

THYROTOXICOSIS

Beta-adrenergic blockade may mask certain clinical signs (e.g., tachycardia) of hyperthyroidism. Patients suspected of developing throtoxicosis should be managed carefully to avoid abrupt withdrawal of beta-blockade which might precipitate a thyroid crisis.

PRECAUTIONS

IMPAIRED RENAL OR HEPATIC FUNCTION

Beta-blocking agents should be used with caution in patients with impaired hepatic or renal function. Poor renal function has only minor effects on Pindolol clearance, but poor hepatic function may cause blood levels of Pindolol to increase substantially.

INFORMATION FOR PATIENTS

Patients, especially those with evidence of coronary artery insufficiency, should be warned against interruption or discontinuation of Pindolol therapy without the physician's advice. Although cardiac failure rarely occurs in properly selected patients, patients being treated with beta-adrenergic blocking agents should be advised to consult the physician at the first sign or symptom of impending failure.

DRUG INTERACTIONS

Catecholamine-depleting drugs (e.g., reserpine) may have an additive effect when given with beta-blocking agents. Patients receiving Pindolol plus a catecholamine-depleting agent should, therefore, be closely observed for evidence of hypotension and/or marked bradycardia which may produce vertigo, syncope, or postural hypotension.

Pindolol has been used with a variety of antihypertensive agents, including hydrochlorothiazide, hydralazine, and guanethidine without unexpected adverse interactions.

Pindolol has been shown to increase serum thioridazine levels when both drugs are co-administered. Pindolol levels may also be increased with this combination.

Risk of Anaphylactic Reaction: While taking beta blockers, patients with a history of severe anaphylactic reaction to a variety of allergens may be more reactive to repeated challenge, either accidental, diagnostic, or therapeutic. Such patients may be unresponsive to the usual doses of epinephrine used to treat allergic reaction.

CARCINOGENESIS, MUTAGENESIS, IMPAIRMENT OF FERTILITY

In chronic oral toxicologic studies (1-2 years) in mice, rats, and dogs, Pindolol did not produce any significant toxic effects. In 2-year oral carcinogenicity studies in rats and mice in doses as high as 59 mg/kg/day and 124 mg/kg/day (50 and 100 times the maximum recommended human dose), respectively, Pindolol did not produce any neoplastic, preneoplastic, or nonneoplastic pathologic lesions. In fertility and general reproductive performance studies in rats, Pindolol caused no adverse effects at a dose of 10 mg/kg.

In the male fertility and general reproductive performance test in rats, definite toxicity characterized by mortality and decreased weight gain was observed in the group given 100 mg/kg/day. At 30 mg/kg/day, decreased mating was associated with testicular atrophy and/or decreased spermatogenesis. This response is not clearly drug related, however, as there was no dose response relationship within this experiment and no similar effect on tests of rats administered Pindolol as a dietary admixture for 104 weeks. There appeared to be an increase in prenatal mortality in males given 100 mg/kg but development of offspring was not impaired.

In females administered Pindolol prior to mating through day 21 of lactation, mating behavior was decreased at 100 mg/kg and 30 mg/kg. At these dosages there also was increased mortality of offspring. Prenatal mortality was increased at 10 mg/kg but there was not a clear dose response relationship in this experiment. There was an increased resorption rate at 100 mg/kg observed in females necropsied on the 15th day of gestation.

PREGNANCY

Category B: Studies in rats and rabbits exceeding 100 times the maximum recommended human doses, revealed no embryotoxicity or teratogenicity. Since there are no adequate and well-controlled studies in pregnant women, and since animal reproduction studies are not always predictive of human response, Pindolol, as with any drug, should be employed during pregnancy only if the potential benefit justifies the potential risk to the fetus.

NURSING MOTHERS

Since Pindolol is secreted in human milk, nursing should not be undertaken by mothers receiving the drug.

PEDIATRIC USE

Safety and effectiveness in children have not been established.

CLINICAL LABORATORY

Minor persistent elevations in serum transaminases (SGOT, SGPT) have been noted in 7% of patients during Pindolol administration, but progressive elevations were not observed. These elevations were not associated with any other abnormalities that would suggest hepatic impairment, such as decreased serum albumin and total proteins. During more than a decade of worldwide marketing, there have been no reports in the medical literature of overt hepatic injury. Alkaline phosphatase, lactic acid dehydrogenase (LDH), and uric acid are also elevated on rare occasions. The significance of these findings is unknown.

ADVERSE REACTIONS

Most adverse reactions have been mild. The incidences listed in the following table are derived from 12-week comparative double-blind, parallel design trails in hypertensive patients given Pindolol as monotherapy, given various active control drugs as monotherapy, or given placebo. Data for Pindolol and the positive controls were pooled from several trials because no striking differences were seen in the individual studies, with one exception. When considering all adverse reactions reported, the frequency of edema was noticeably higher in positive control trials [16% Pindolol vs. 9% positive control] than in placebo-controlled trials [6% Pindolol vs. 3% placebo]. The table includes adverse reactions either volunteered or elicited, and at least possibly drug related, which were reported in greater than 2% of Pindolol patients and other selected important reactions.

ADVERSE REACTIONS WHICH WERE VOLUNTEERED OR ELICITED (AND AT LEAST POSSIBLY DRUG-RELATED)

Body System/Adverse Reactions	Pindolol (N = 322) %	Active Controls* (N = 188) %	Placebo (N = 78) %
Central Nervous System			
Bizarre or Many Dreams	5	0	6
Dizziness	9	11	1
Fatigue	8	4	4
Hallucinations	< 1	0	0
Insomnia	10	3	10
Nervousness	7	3	5
Weakness	4	2	1
Autonomic Nervous System			
Paresthesia	3	1	6
Cardiovascular			
Dyspnea	5	4	6
Edema	6	3	1
Heart Failure	< 1	< 1	0
Palpitations	< 1	1	0
Musculoskeletal			
Chest Pain	3	1	3
Joint Pain	7	4	4
Muscle Cramps	3	1	0
Muscle Pain	10	9	8
Gastrointestinal			
Abdominal Discomfort	4	4	5
Nausea	5	2	1
Skin			
Pruritus	1	< 1	0
Rash	< 1	< 1	1

* *Active Controls: Patients received either propranolol, α-methyldopa or a diuretic (hydrochlorothiazide or chlorthalidone).*

The following selected (potentially important) adverse reactions were seen in 2% or fewer patients and their relationship to Pindolol is uncertain.

Central Nervous System: anxiety, lethargy;

Autonomic Nervous System: visual disturbances, hyperhidrosis;

Cardiovascular: bradycardia, claudication, cold extremities, heart block, hypotension, syncope, tachycardia, weight gain;

Gastrointestinal: diarrhea, vomiting;

Respiratory: wheezing;

Urogenital: impotence, pollakiuria;

Miscellaneous: eye discomfort or burning eyes.

POTENTIAL ADVERSE EFFECTS

In addition, other adverse effects not aforementioned have been reported with other beta-adrenergic blocking agents and should be considered potential adverse effects of Pindolol.

CENTRAL NERVOUS SYSTEM

Reversible mental depression progressing to catatonia; an acute reversible syndrome characterized by disorientation for time and place, short-term memory loss, emotional lability, slightly clouded sensorium, and decreased performance on neuropsychometrics.

Cardiovascular: Intensification of AV block. (See *"Contraindications".*)

Allergic: Erythematous rash; fever combined with aching and sore throat; laryngospasm; respiratory distress.

Hematologic: Agranulocytosis; thrombocytopenic and nonthrombocytopenic purpura.

Gastrointestinal: Mesenteric arterial thrombosis; ischemic colitis.

Miscellaneous: Reversible alopecia; Peyronie's disease.

The oculomucocutaneous syndrome associated with the beta-blocker practolol has not been reported with Pindolol during investigational use and extensive foreign experience amounting to over 4-million patient-years.

◆ RATED THERAPEUTICALLY EQUIVALENT; ◇ THERAPEUTIC EQUIVALENCE UNCONFIRMED; ○ UNRATED

OVERDOSAGE

No specific information on emergency treatment of overdosage is available. Therefore, on the basis of the pharmacologic actions of Pindolol, the following general measures should be employed as appropriate in addition to gastric lavage:

Excessive Bradycardia: administer atropine; if there is no response to vagal blockade, adminster isoproterenol cautiously.

Cardiac Failure: digitalize the patient and/or administer diuretic. It has been reported that glucagon may be useful in this situation.

Hypotension: administer vasopressors, e.g., epinephrine or levarterenol, with serial monitoring of blood pressure. (There is evidence that epinephrine may be the drug of choice.)

Bronchospasm: administer a beta$_2$ stimulating agent such as isoproterenol and/or a theophylline derivative.

A case of an acute overdosage has been reported with an intake of 500 mg of Pindolol by a hypertensive patient. Blood pressure increased and heart rate was $\geq$ 80 beats/min. Recovery was uneventful. In another case, 250 mg of Pindolol was taken with 150 mg diazepam and 50 mg nitrazepam, producing coma and hypotension. The patient recovered in 24 hours.

DOSAGE AND ADMINISTRATION

The dosage of Pindolol should be individualized. The recommended initial dose of Pindolol is 5 mg b.i.d. alone or in combination with other antihypertensive agents. An antihypertensive response usually occurs within the first week of treatment. Maximal response, however, may take as long as or occasionally longer than 2 weeks. If a satisfactory reduction in blood pressure does not occur within 3-4 weeks, the dose may be adjusted in increments of 10 mg/day at these intervals up to a maximum of 60 mg/day.

Store and Dispense: Below 86°F (30°C); tight, light-resistant container.

HOW SUPPLIED
TABLETS: 5 MG

AVERAGE UNIT PRICE (AVAILABLE SIZES)

BRAND	$0.73	GENERIC A-RATED AVERAGE PRICE (GAAP)	
GENERIC	$0.60	100s	$61.10
HCFA FUL (100s ea)	$0.46	500s	$286.38

BRAND/MANUFACTURER	NDC	SIZE	AWP
◆ BRAND			
➤ VISKEN: Sandoz Pharm	00078-0111-05	100s	$72.54
◆ GENERICS			
Medirex	57480-0810-06	30s	$15.59
Par	49884-0442-01	100s	$58.00
Goldline	00182-1946-01	100s	$59.75
Martec	52555-0545-01	100s	$59.80
Zenith	00172-4217-60	100s	$59.95
Qualitest	00603-5220-21	100s	$59.98
Mutual	53489-0430-01	100s	$60.45
Schein	00364-2547-01	100s	$60.50
Rugby	00536-4243-01	100s	$60.64
Novopharm	55953-0088-40	100s	$60.65
URL	00677-1457-01	100s	$61.11
Moore,H.L.	00839-7761-06	100s	$62.09
Mylan	00378-0052-01	100s	$65.25
Major	00904-7893-60	100s	$65.25
Medirex	57480-0810-01	100s ud	$61.95
Zenith	00172-4217-70	500s	$284.75
Novopharm	55953-0088-70	500s	$288.00

TABLETS: 10 MG

AVERAGE UNIT PRICE (AVAILABLE SIZES)

BRAND	$0.96	GENERIC A-RATED AVERAGE PRICE (GAAP)	
GENERIC	$0.81	100s	$81.16
HCFA FUL (100s ea)	$0.64	500s	$379.88

BRAND/MANUFACTURER	NDC	SIZE	AWP
◆ BRAND			
➤ VISKEN: Sandoz Pharm	00078-0073-05	100s	$96.12
◆ GENERICS			
Medirex	57480-0811-06	30s	$24.53
Martec	52555-0546-01	100s	$79.28
Zenith	00172-4218-60	100s	$79.50
Goldline	00182-1947-01	100s	$79.50
Qualitest	00603-5221-21	100s	$79.51
Par	49884-0443-01	100s	$79.90
Schein	00364-2548-01	100s	$80.25
Mutual	53489-0431-01	100s	$80.30
Rugby	00536-4244-01	100s	$80.41
Novopharm	55953-0093-40	100s	$80.45
URL	00677-1458-01	100s	$81.20
Moore,H.L.	00839-7762-06	100s	$81.26
Mylan	00378-0127-01	100s	$86.45
Major	00904-7894-60	100s	$86.50
Medirex	57480-0811-01	100s ud	$81.75

BRAND/MANUFACTURER	NDC	SIZE	AWP
Zenith	00172-4218-70	500s	$377.60
Novopharm	55953-0093-70	500s	$382.15

Pipecuronium Bromide

> THIS DRUG SHOULD BE ADMINISTERED BY ADEQUATELY-TRAINED INDIVIDUALS FAMILIAR WITH ITS ACTIONS, CHARACTERISTICS, AND HAZARDS.

DESCRIPTION

Pipecuronium Bromide for injection is a long-acting nondepolarizing neuromuscular blocking agent, chemically designated as piperazinium, 4, 4′-[(2β, 3α, 5α, 16β, 17β)-3, 17-bis(acetyloxy) androstane-2, 16-diyl] bis [1, 1-dimethyl]-, dibromide, dihydrate.

The chemical formula is $C_{35}H_{62}N_4O_4Br_2 \cdot 2H_2O$ with a molecular weight of 798.74. At normal physiological states, the compound exists primarily in the ionized form and is poorly soluble in fat.

Pipecuronium Bromide is supplied as a sterile nonpyrogenic freeze-dried cake, for intravenous injection only. Each 10 mL vial contains 10 mg Pipecuronium Bromide and 380 mg mannitol, USP (to adjust tonicity). When necessary, pH is adjusted with sodium hydroxide and/or hydrochloric acid (pH6).

Bacteriostatic water for injection, USP, when supplied contains 0.9% w/v Benzyl Alcohol, *which is not for use in newborns*.

Following is its chemical structure:

CLINICAL PHARMACOLOGY

Pipecuronium Bromide for injection is a long-acting nondepolarizing neuromuscular blocking agent possessing all of the characteristic pharmacological actions of this class of drugs (curariform). It acts by competing for cholinergic receptors at the motor end-plate. This action is antagonized by acetylcholinesterase inhibitors, such as neostigmine.

Pharmacodynamics: The individual cumulative ED$_{95}$ (dose required to produce 95% suppression of T$_1$ of the train-of-four or 95% suppression of single twitch response) during balanced anesthesia has averaged 41 μg/kg actual body weight (ABW) (range 20-91 μg/kg). Maximum blockade is achieved in approximately 5 minutes following single doses of 70 to 85 μg/kg ABW. Under balanced anesthesia, following single doses of 70 μg/kg ABW in 4 clinical trials (n = 65), the mean times to recovery to 25% of control (clinical duration) were 47-98 minutes (range 30-175 min.). The mean times to recovery following 80-85 μg/kg ABW single doses in 4 clinical trials (n = 69) were 80-124 minutes (range 40-211 min.). Pipecuronium Bromide was shown to have an onset time and clinical duration (range and variability) similar to those of pancuronium bromide at comparable doses (historic data and limited comparisons).

An analysis of 282 cases in U.S. clinical trials utilizing a variety of premedications, varying lengths of surgery, and various anesthetic agents, indicates that two-thirds of the patients had clinical durations within 30 minutes of the duration predicted by the dose adjusted by ideal body weight (IBW) and calculated creatinine clearance (there is an inverse relationship between renal function and clinical duration such that the mean clinical duration more than doubles when the calculated creatinine clearance goes from 100 to 40 mL/min.).

The likelihood of prolonged clinical duration may be decreased by calculating creatinine clearance based on serum creatinine and ideal body weight based on height, or by using doses at the lower end of the recommended dosage range for intubation in patients with moderate decreases in renal function. In patients with renal failure the drug should be used with caution (see Table 2, *"Individualization of Dosage"* subsection of *"Clinical Pharmacology"*, and *"Precautions"*).

In 333 of nearly 600 cases in U.S. clinical trials with evaluable clinical duration data, clinical durations greater than 120 minutes for the dose of 70 μg/kg ABW or greater than 150 minutes for doses of 80 μg/kg ABW or more were reported in approximately 8% (27/333) of cases. In about one-third (10/27) of such cases, dosage was administered to obese patients (defined as 30% or more above ideal body weight for height) based on actual body weight. Prolonged clinical duration was approximately 2 times more common in obese patients (10/73 cases) than among non-obese (17/260 cases) patients. Therefore, in calculating dosage on a mg/kg basis, ideal body weight can also be used to decrease the variability in clinical duration and to reduce the possibility of overdosage in the obese population (see *"Individualization of Dosage"* subsection of *"Clinical Pharmacology"*).

Limited data (3 studies, n = 29) are available on the administration of single doses of 100 μg/kg ABW of Pipecuronium Bromide. No significant differences were observed in mean clinical duration compared to that seen with doses of 80-

➤ SHOWN IN PRODUCT IDENTIFICATION GUIDE

85 µg/kg ABW. Doses above 100 µg/kg based on actual or ideal body weight are not recommended because of the possibility of even longer duration of action for individual patients.

The mean time for spontaneous recovery from 25% to 50% of control T_1, based on 90 patients in 6 studies in whom the final dose produced a T_1 less than 25% of control, is approximately 24 minutes (range 8-131 minutes). Because of the use of antagonism following surgery, there are insufficient data to report the time required for greater than 50% spontaneous recovery of T_1.

Pipecuronium Bromide can be administered following recovery from succinylcholine, when the latter is used to facilitate endotracheal intubation. Preliminary data (from 1 study in 25 patients) suggest that, if a single dose of 50 µg/kg ABW Pipecuronium Bromide is administered under these conditions, prolongation in clinical duration may be noted (range of 23-95 minutes following succinylcholine versus 8-50 minutes without it). Prior use of succinylcholine has not been shown to alter the clinical duration of larger doses of Pipecuranium Bromide (80 or more µg/kg ABW administered after recovery from succinylcholine, n = 53).

Initial Pipecuronium Bromide doses of 70 to 85 µg/kg ABW, used without succinylcholine (from 3 studies, in 43 patients), have produced good to excellent intubation conditions within 2.5 to 3.0 minutes of injection (which is before maximum blockade). Review of the time (range from 2-6 minutes) to intubation and any comments about the quality of intubation in patients receiving up to 100 µg/kg ABW indicated no reports of problems in intubating such patients.

The mean clinical duration of first maintenace doses of 10-15 µg/kg ABW Pipecuronium Bromide administered at 25% recovery of control T_1 is approximately 50 minutes (range 17-175 minutes; 6 studies, 148 patients).

Hemodynamics: Administration of Pipecuronium Bromide doses up to and including 100 µg/kg (= 2.5 × ED95) as a rapid bolus over 5 sec. to healthy patients during stable state balanced anesthesia produced no dose-related effects on heart-rate or blood pressure.

In patients undergoing surgery for coronary artery bypass grafting, hemodynamic studies were performed using higher than currently recommended Pipecuronium Bromide doses, i.e., 100 µg/kg ABW and 200 µg/kg ABW. Pipecuronium Bromide was administered during induction of anesthesia with a narcotic or etomidate/narcotic combination, respectively. Observed hemodynamic effects were small and included reductions in mean systolic and mean arterial pressures (↓ 10-14%), ventricular stroke-work index (↓ 8-25%) and cardiac output (↓ 20%); sustained increases in pulmonary capillary wedge and central venous pressures and changes in mean heart rate were not observed. Pipecuronium Bromide has not been studied in patients with hemodynamic dysfunction secondary to cardiac valvular disease.

Pipecuronium Bromide has not been found to influence the cardiovascular depression or stimulations associated with other drugs administered during anesthesia or with surgical stimulation. The most common observations, comparing vital signs immediately prior to initial dosage with Pipecuronium Bromide and two minutes after injection, are a slight decrease in heart rate, systolic blood pressure and diastolic blood pressure.

Human plasma histamine concentrations, following effective initial doses of Pipecuronium Bromide, have not been studied. However, clinical experience with more than 1000 patients indicates hypersensitivity reactions such as bronchospasm, tachycardia, and other reactions commonly associated with histamine release are unlikely to occur.

Pharmacokinetics: Only limited information is available, at the present time, regarding the pharmacokinetics of Pipecuronium Bromide in humans. Preliminary pharmacokinetic results from 4 normal subjects and 7 subjects undergoing cadaver renal transplant is reproduced in Table 1. These results tend to indicate that some prolongation of plasma levels can be expected in patients with severe impairment of renal function which may in turn significantly extend recovery time. A clear relationship between plasma levels and the degree or extent of muscle twitch suppression has not been determined at this time.

Table 1
PRELIMINARY[1] PHARMACOKINETIC PARAMETERS OF PIPECURONIUM BROMIDE

	Mean (range)[2]	
	Normal Renal and Hepatic Function n = 4	*Renal Transplant* n = 7
Clearance (L/hr/kg)	0.12 (0.10-0.14)	0.08 (0.02-0.12)
Volume of Distribution at Steady State (L/kg)	0.25 (0.12-0.37)	0.37 (0.28-0.51)
$t_{1/2}$ distribution (min)	6.22 (1.34-10.66)	4.33 (1.69-6.17)
$t_{1/2}$ elimination (hr)	1.7 (0.9-2.7)	4.0 (2.0-8.2)

[1] *Due to the small number of subjects represented by these data, and the interpatient variation seen with Pipecuronium Bromide, this information is being provided to the clinician as a general guide only. Definitive concentration-effect and pharmacokinetic relationships have not yet been established for Pipecuronium Bromide.*

[2] *Determined following rapid administration of a single bolus dose of 70 µg/kg ABW, in patients with normal renal and hepatic function, or with renal failure undergoing cadaver renal transplant surgery under halothane anesthesia, who have been adequately dialyzed prior to surgery.*

Studies of distribution, metabolism, and excretion in animals (rats, dogs, and cats), indicate that Pipecuronium Bromide is eliminated primarily by the kidneys (more than 75% of drug recovered in the urine, primarily as the unchanged drug). The 3-deacetyl, 17-deacetyl, and 3,17-dideacetyl derivatives of Pipecuronium Bromide have been identified in urine collected from dogs; these metabolites account for approximately 20% of the administered dose. The 3-deacetyl derivative is the only metabolite with substantial neuromuscular blocking activity, manifesting approximately 40-50% of the activity of the parent drug in the cat and the dog. On the basis of experience gained with other agents in this category it is most probable that similar metabolites exist in other animal species and in humans.

At the present time only the 3-deacetyl metabolite of Pipecuronium Bromide has been detected in the urine of humans undergoing coronary artery bypass surgery. Following administration of 200 µg/kg ABW, 56% of the administered dose was recovered in the urine, of which 41% was unchanged drug and the remaining 15% was the 3-deacetyl metabolite of Pipecuronium Bromide. In the same study no metabolites of Pipecuronium Bromide were found in the plasma.

Individualization of Dosage: Pipecuronium Bromide like other long-acting neuromuscular blocking agents, displays a great deal of variability in the clinical duration of its effect. With experience, anesthesiologists will determine when and how to modify dosage on individual patients based on clinical factors like age, sex, weight/degree of obesity, renal, hepatic and/or other diseases, etc., much as they do with pancuronium. Tables 2 and 3 are included in this prescribing information to assist those physicians who may wish to adjust dosage based on ideal body weight and renal function, two factors which were identified in controlled clinical trials that may warrant dosage adjustment. Although the tables differ in approach and thus appear different, i.e., one derives the total dose in mg and the other presents it as µg/kg IBW, they ultimately suggest the same dose for patients with the same height, weight, age and serum creatinine level.

It should be noted from the tables that for small patients with decreased renal function the suggested initial dose is less than 70 to 85 µg/kg IBW, i.e., less than 2× the average ED95 dose which is generally the recommended intubating dose for neuromuscular blocking agents. A review of 80 patients who received initial doses < 70 µg/kg IBW compared with 202 who received > 70 µg/kg doses in controlled clinical trials showed neither longer mean time to intubation nor any problems during intubation. HOWEVER, PHYSICIANS SHOULD USE EXTRA CARE DURING INTUBATION OF ANY PATIENT IN WHOM, IN ORDER TO DECREASE THE POSSIBILITY OF PROLONGED CLINICAL DURATION, THEY ELECT TO USE LESS THAN 70 µG/KG IBW FOR INTUBATION.

Dosing in accordance with the following tables may reduce the variability in clinical duration to bring approximately 20% more patients to within ± 30 minutes of the duration predicted by the dose adjusted by IBW and calculated creatinine clearance. It should be emphasized, however, that it will not entirely eliminate the variability associated with the use of long acting neuromuscular blocking agents and physicians must be prepared to monitor patients carefully during surgery and recovery to support them until they have adequate return of muscular function. (See related table).

Table 3
CALCULATED DOSE IN µG/KG

Ideal Body Weight* *Adjusted for Renal Function (Estimated Creatinine Clearance**)*				
Creatinine Clearance in mL/min ≥				
< 40	60	80	100	> 100
(50)	55	70	85	[100]
— µg/kg ideal body wt. —				

( ) *Minimum calculated dose for adequate intubation - in these patients prolonged clinical blockade should be anticipated.*

[ ] *Maximum calculated dose for intubation - in these patients use of maintenance doses should be anticipated.*

* *IBW men in kg = [106 + (6 lbs./inch in ht > 5 feet)]/2.2*
  IBW women in kg = [100 + (5 lbs./inch in ht > 5 feet)]/2.2

Note: Use actual body weight in the calculation if it is less than ideal body weight.

** Est CRcl = $\dfrac{(140 - age\ in\ years) \times IBW\ (kg)^* \times 0.85\ for\ females\ only}{72 \times serum\ creatinine\ in\ mg/100\ mL}$

INDICATIONS AND USAGE

Pipecuronium Bromide for injection is a long-acting neuromuscular blocking agent, indicated as an adjunct to general anesthesia, to provide skeletal muscle relaxation during surgery. Pipecuronium Bromide can also be used to provide skeletal muscle relaxation for endotracheal intubation.

CONTRAINDICATIONS

None known.

◆ RATED THERAPEUTICALLY EQUIVALENT; ◇ THERAPEUTIC EQUIVALENCE UNCONFIRMED; ○ UNRATED

WARNINGS

PIPECURONIUM BROMIDE FOR INJECTION SHOULD BE ADMINISTERED IN CAREFULLY ADJUSTED DOSAGE BY OR UNDER THE SUPERVISION OF EXPERIENCED CLINICIANS WHO ARE FAMILIAR WITH THE DRUG'S ACTIONS AND THE POSSIBLE COMPLICATIONS OF ITS USE. THE DRUG SHOULD NOT BE ADMINISTERED UNLESS FACILITIES FOR INTUBATION, ARTIFICIAL RESPIRATION, OXYGEN THERAPY, AND AN ANTAGONIST ARE WITHIN IMMEDIATE REACH. IT IS RECOMMENDED THAT CLINICIANS ADMINISTERING LONG-ACTING NEUROMUSCULAR BLOCKING AGENTS SUCH AS PIPECURONIUM BROMIDE EMPLOY A PERIPHERAL NERVE STIMULATOR TO MONITOR DRUG RESPONSE, NEED FOR ADDITIONAL RELAXANT, AND ADEQUACY OF SPONTANEOUS RECOVERY OR ANTAGONISM.

In patients with myasthenia gravis or myasthenic (Eaton-Lambert) syndrome, small doses of nondepolarizing neuromuscular blocking agents may have profound effects. Shorter acting muscle relaxants than Pipecuronium Bromide may be more suitable for these patients.

PRECAUTIONS

General: Since Pipecuronium Bromide for injection has little or no effect on the heart rate, the drug will not counteract the bradycardia produced by many opioid anesthetic agents or vagal stimulation.

Renal Failure: Pipecuronium Bromide in the dose of 70 μg/kg ABW, has been studied in a limited number of patients (n = 20) undergoing renal transplant surgery, recently dialyzed in preparation for cadaver renal transplant. The mean clinical duration (injection to 25% recovery) of 103 minutes was not judged prolonged, however, there was wide individual variation (30 to 267 minutes). Pipecuronium Bromide has not otherwise been studied in patients with renal failure (for elective or emergency non-renal surgery. Because it is primarily excreted by the kidney, Pipecuronium Bromide should be used with caution in patients with renal failure (see Table 2, "Individualization of Dosage" subsection of "Clinical Pharmacology").

Increased Volume of Distribution: Conditions associated with an increased volume of distribution, e.g., slower circulation time in cardiovascular disease, old age or edematous states, may be associated with a delay in onset time. Because higher doses of Pipecuronium Bromide may produce a longer duration of action, the initial dosage should not usually be increased in these patients to enhance onset time; instead, more time should be allowed for the drug to achieve maximum effect.

Hepatic Disease: There are no data on dosage requirements, onset, duration or pharmacokinetics in patients with moderate or severe hepatic dysfunction and/or biliary obstruction. This should be considered in selection of muscle relaxants for use in these patients.

Obesity: The most common patient condition associated with prolonged clinical duration was obesity, defined as 30% or more over ideal body weight (see "Clinical Pharmacology"). Clinical study subjects were dosed on the basis of actual body weight, which may have contributed to the higher incidence of prolonged duration. It is therefore recommended that dosage be based upon ideal body weight for height in obese patients (see "Dosage and Administration").

Malignant Hyperthermia (MH): Human malignant hyperthermia has not been reported with the administration of Pipecuronium Bromide. Because Pipecuronium Bromide is never used alone, and because the occurrence of malignant hyperthermia during anesthesia is possible even in the absence of known triggering agents, clinicians should be familiar with early signs, confirmatory diagnosis and treatment of malignant hyperthermia prior to the start of any anesthetic. In an animal study in MH-susceptible swine (n = 7), the administration of Pipecuronium Bromide was not associated with the development of malignant hyperthermia.

Long-Term Use in the Intensive Care Unit (ICU): No data are available on the long-term use of Pipecuronium Bromide in patients undergoing mechanical ventilation in the I.C.U.

Central Nervous System: Pipecuronium Bromide has no known effect on consciousness, the pain threshold or cerebration. Therefore, administration must be accompanied by adequate anesthesia.

Drug Interactions: Pipecuronium Bromide can be administered following recovery from succinylcholine when the latter is used to facilitate endotracheal intubation (see "Dosage and Administration" and "Clinical Pharmacology").

The use of Pipecuronium Bromide before succinylcholine, in order to attenuate some of the side effects of succinylcholine is not recommended because it has not been studied.

There are no clinical data on concomitant use of Pipecuronium Bromide and other nondepolarizing neuromuscular blocking agents.

Inhalational Anesthetics: Use of volatile inhalation anesthetics have been shown to enhance the activity of other neuromuscular blocking agents on the order of enflurane > isoflurane > halothane.

Since the neuromuscular blocking agents are routinely administered before or shortly after the administration of the inhalation anesthetic, minimal effects are generally observed on onset time and peak effect. In routine use of neuromuscular blocking agents, only clinical duration is generally affected (prolonged). No definite interaction between Pipecuronium Bromide and halothane, as used clinically, has been demonstrated. Use of isoflurane in one study of 25 patients resulted in an increase in mean clinical duration by 12%. In another study of 25 patients first anesthetized with enflurane for 5 minutes or more, the mean clinical duration was increased by 50%. Therefore, a prolonged clinical duration following initial or maintenance doses and prolonged recovery from neuromuscular blocking effect of Pipecuronium Bromide should generally be anticipated, with enflurane > isoflurane > halothane.

Antibiotics: Parenteral/intraperitoneal administration of high doses of certain antibiotics may intensify or produce neuromuscular block on their own.

The following antibiotics have been associated with various degrees of paralysis: aminoglycosides (such as neomycin, streptomycin, kanamycin, gentamicin, and dihydrostreptomycin); tetracyclines; bacitracin; polymyxin B; colistin; and sodium colistimethate. If these or other newly introduced antibiotics are used in conjunction with Pipecuronium Bromide during surgery, prolongation of neuromuscular block should be considered a possibility.

Other: Experience concerning injection of quinidine during recovery from use of other muscle relaxants suggests that recurrent paralysis may occur. This possibility must also be considered for Pipecuronium Bromide.

Pipecuronium Bromide induced neuromuscular blockade has been counteracted by alkalosis and enhanced by acidosis in experimental animals (cat). In addition, experience with other drugs has suggested that acute (e.g., diarrhea) or chronic (e.g., adrenocortical insufficiency) electrolyte imbalance may alter neuromuscular blockade. Since electrolyte imbalance and acid-base imbalance are usually mixed, either enhancement or inhibition may occur. Magnesium salts, administered for the management of toxemia of pregnancy, may enhance neuromuscular blockade.

Drug/Laboratory Test Interactions: None known.

Carcinogenesis, Mutagenesis, Impairment of Fertility: Studies in animals have not been performed to evaluate carcinogenic potential or impairment of fertility. Mutagenicity studies (Ames test, Sister Chromatid Exchange) conducted with Pipecuronium Bromide revealed no mutagenic potential

Pregnancy Category C: A teratogenicity study has been conducted in rats using intravenously administered doses of Pipecuronium Bromide approximating the clinical dose in humans (50 μg/kg). No teratogenic effects were observed in this study. An embryotoxic effect (secondary to maternal toxicity) was observed at the highest dose administered (50 μg/kg) as demonstrated by an increase in earlier fetal resorptions. There are no adequate and well-controlled studies in pregnant women. Pipecuronium Bromide should be used during pregnancy only if the potential benefit justifies the potential risk to the fetus.

Use in Obstetrics (Caesarean section): There are insufficient data on placental transfer of Pipecuronium Bromide and possible related effect(s) upon the neonate following Caesarean section delivery. In addition, the duration of action of Pipecuronium Bromide exceeds the duration of operative obstetrics (Caesarean section). Therefore Pipecuronium Bromide is not recommended for use in patients undergoing C-section.

Pediatric Use: Infants (3 months to 1 year) under balanced anesthesia (2 studies in 52 infants), or halothane anesthesia (1 study in 29 infants), manifest similar dose response to Pipecuronium Bromide as do adults on a μg/kg ABW basis. Children (1 to 14 years) under balanced anesthesia (4 studies in 57 children), or halothane anesthesia (2 studies in 29 children), may be less sensitive than adults. These conclusions come from studies involving titrating patient response, by the incremental method, to approximately 1.2 times ED95. There are no data on either onset time or clinical duration of larger doses in infants or children. There are no data on maintenance dosing in infants and children.

Pharmacokinetic studies in infants and children have not been performed, therefore, no pharmacokinetic modeling of incremental dosing can be attempted. The use of Pipecuronium Bromide in neonates and infants below 3 months of age has not been investigated. Antagonism has not been systematically studied in infants or children, however, usual clinical doses of neostigmine administered following significant levels of spontaneous recovery (recovery of T_1 to more than 50% of control) produced complete antagonism of residual neuromuscular block in less than 10 minutes in the majority of cases.

Table 2
CALCULATED DOSE IN MG

| | *Based on Ideal Body Weight in kg* and Estimated Creatinine Clearance** (mg = mL if 10 mg vial is reconstituted with 10 mL)* | | | | | | |
mL/min	kg IBW	50	60	70	80	90	100	kg IBW
				Creatinine Clearance				
< = 40		(2.5)	(3.0)	(3.5)	(4.0)	(4.5)	(5.0)	
60		(2.5)	(3.0)	3.8	4.9	6.2	7.7	
80		2.6	3.7	5.0	6.5	8.3	[10.0]	
> = 100 mL/min		3.2	4.6	6.3	8.2	[9.0]	[10.0]	

► SHOWN IN PRODUCT IDENTIFICATION GUIDE

ADVERSE REACTIONS

The most frequent side effect of nondepolarizing blocking agents, as a class, is an extension of the drug's pharmacological action beyond the time period needed for surgery and anesthesia (see *"Clinical Pharmacology"*). Clinical signs may vary from skeletal muscle weakness to profound and prolonged skeletal muscle paralysis resulting in respiratory insufficiency or apnea. This may be due to the drug's effect or inadequate antagonism.

The following listings are based upon U.S. clinical studies involving nearly 600 patients, utilizing a variety of premedications, varying lengths of surgical procedures and various anesthetic agents.

Adverse experiences in greater than 1% of cases and judged by the investigator to have a possible causal relationship:
  Clinically significant hypotension (2.5% of cases).
  Clinically significant bradycardia (1.4% of cases).
Adverse experiences in less than 1% of cases and judged by the investigator to have a possible causal relationship:

Cardiovascular: hypertension, myocardial ischemia, cerebrovascular accident, thrombosis, atrial fibrillation, ventricular extrasystole.

Metabolic and Nutritional: increased creatinine, hypoglycemia, hyperkalemia.

Musculoskeletal: muscle atrophy, difficult intubation.

Nervous: hypesthesia, CNS depression.

Respiratory: dyspnea, respiratory depression, laryngismus, atelectasis.

Skin and Appendages: rash, urticaria.

Urogenital system: anuria.

OVERDOSAGE

No cases of significant accidental or intentional gross overdose have been reported. In foreign clinical studies with doses up to 200 µg/kg ABW, no non-musculoskeletal effects were seen than could be attributed to the higher dosage.

In case of relative or absolute overdosage ventilation must be supported by artificial means until no longer required. Intensified monitoring of vital organ function is required for the period of paralysis and during an extended period post recovery.

ANTAGONISM OF NEUROMUSCULAR BLOCKADE

ANTAGONISTS (SUCH AS NEOSTIGMINE) SHOULD NOT BE ADMINISTERED PRIOR TO THE DEMONSTRATION OF SOME SPONTANEOUS RECOVERY FROM NEUROMUSCULAR BLOCK-ADE. THE USE OF A NERVE STIMULATOR TO DOCUMENT RECOVERY AND ANTAGONISM OF NEUROMUSCULAR BLOCKADE IS RECOMMENDED.

In an analysis (across U.S. studies) of different degrees of spontaneous recovery prior to antagonism among patients antagonized by neostigmine (usual dose 0.04 mg/kg ABW), approximately 75% of patients antagonized at a T_1 of approximately 25% and approximately 42% of patients antagonized at a T_1 of approximately 10% manifested a T_4/T_1 of 0.7 or greater within 10 minutes. When T_1 had recovered to at least 10 or 25% of the preblock value, T_4/T_1 was often zero; antagonism with neostigmine 0.04 mg/kg ABW was usually inadequate 10 minutes after intravenous dosing in these cases. If train-of-four monitoring is available, T_4/T_1 should be > zero before antagonism with neostigmine is attempted. However, if T_1 has recovered to at least 10% of the preblock value, additional time (more than 10 minutes) or additional neostigmine dosing usually resulted in adequate antagonism.

Patients should be evaluated for adequate clinical evidence of antagonism, e.g., 5 second head lift, adequate phonation, ventilation and upper airway maintenance. Ventilation must be supported until no longer required. As with other neuromuscular blocking agents, physicians should be alert to the possibility that the action of the drugs used to antagonize neuromuscular blockade may wear off before plasma levels of Pipecuronium Bromide for injection have declined sufficiently.

Antagonism may be delayed in the presence of debilitation, carcinomatosis, and concomitant use of certain broad spectrum antibiotics, or anesthetic agents and other drugs which which enhance neuromuscular blockade or separately cause respiratory depression. Under such circumstances the management is the same as that of prolonged neuromuscular blockade.

In clinical trials, edrophonium doses of 0.5 mg/kg ABW were not as effective as neostigmine doses of 0.04 mg/kg ABW in antagonizing Pipecuronium Bromide induced neuromuscular block, and were often inadequate. Therefore, the use of edrophonium 0.5 mg/kg ABW is not recommended to antagonize Pipecuronium Bromide induced neuromuscular blockade. The use of greater (1.0 mg/kg ABW) doses of edrophonium or of pyridostigmine has not been investigated.

DOSAGE AND ADMINISTRATION

PIPECURONIUM BROMIDE FOR INJECTION IS FOR INTRAVENOUS USE ONLY. THIS DRUG SHOULD BE ADMINISTERED BY OR UNDER THE SUPERVISION OF EXPERIENCED CLINICIANS FAMILIAR WITH THE USE OF NEUROMUSCULAR BLOCKING AGENTS. DOSAGE MUST BE INDIVIDUALIZED IN EACH CASE.

The dosage information which follows is derived from studies based upon units of drug per unit of body weight. It is expressed in this section in units of mg/kg (instead of µg/kg) to assist the clinician in calculating individual patient dosage requirements relative to the product as supplied for clinical use. It is intended to serve as an initial guide to clinicians familiar with other neuromuscular blocking agents to acquire experience with Pipecuronium Bromide. The monitoring of twitch response is recommended to evaluate recovery from Pipecuronium Bromide and decrease the hazards of overdosage if additional doses are administered (see *"Clinical Pharmacology"*, and *"Maintenance Dosing"* below).

It is recommended that the clinicians administering long-acting neuromuscular blocking agents such as Pipecuronium Bromide employ a peripheral nerve stimulator to monitor drug response, need for additional relaxant and adequacy of spontaneous recovery or antagonism.

Dose for Endotracheal Intubation: The recommended initial dose of Pipecuronium Bromide for injection under balanced anesthesia, halothane, isoflurane, or enflurane anesthesia in patients with normal renal function who were not obese is 0.07-0.085 mg/kg (70-85 µg/kg) (see *"Clinical Pharmacology"*). Good to excellent intubating conditions are generally provided within 2.5 to 3 minutes. Maximum blockade, usually > 95%, is achieved in approximately 5 minutes. Doses in this range provide approximately 1-2 hours of clinical relaxation under balanced anesthesia (range 47-124 minutes). Under halothane, isoflurane and enflurane anesthesia, extension of the period of clinical relaxation should be expected (see *"Inhalational Anesthetics"* subsection of *"Precautions"*).

For obese patients (30% or more above ideal body weight for height) it is particularly important that a dosage adjustment be considered and the dosage administered according to ideal body weight (see *"Individualization of Dosage"* subsection of *"Clinical Pharmocology"*).

Use Following Succinylcholine: If succinylcholine is used to facilitate endotracheal intubation, Pipecuronium Bromide may be administered after recovery from succinylcholine paralysis. In patients with normal renal function who are not obese starting doses of 0.05 mg/kg (50 µg/kg) of Pipecuronium Bromide are recommended and will provide approximately 45 minutes of clinical relaxation (see *"Clinical Pharmacology"*). In patients with normal renal function who are not obese higher Pipecuronium Bromide doses of 0.07-0.085 mg/kg (70-85µg/kg), if administered after recovery from succinylcholine, are associated with approximately the same clinical duration as Pipecuronium Bromide without prior administration of succinylcholine.

Maintenance Dosing: Maintenance doses of 0.010-0.015 mg/kg (10-15 µg/kg), Pipecuronium Bromide administered at 25% recovery of control T_1, provide approximately 50 minutes (range 17 to 175 minutes) clinical duration under balanced anesthesia (see *"Clinical Pharmacology"*). A lower dose should be considered in patients receiving inhalation anesthetics (see *"Drug Interactions"* subsection of *"Precautions"*). In all cases, dosing should be guided based on the clinical duration following initial dose or prior maintenance dose and not administered until signs of neuromuscular function are evident.

Use in Pediatrics: Infants (3 months to 1 year) under balanced anesthesia (2 studies in 52 infants), or halothane anesthesia (1 study in 20 infants), manifest similar dose response to Pipecuronium Bromide as do adults on a µg/kg ABW basis, children (1 to 14 years) under balanced anesthesia (4 studies in 57 children), or halothane anesthesia (2 studies in 29 children), may be less sensitive than adults. The clinical duration of doses averaging 0.04 mg/kg ABW (40 µg/kg) in infants, and 0.057 mg/kg ABW, (57 µg/kg) in children, ranged from 10 to 44 minutes, and from 18 to 52 minutes, respectively. These doses were approximately 1.2 times ED$_{95}$. There are no data on either onset time or clinical duration of larger doses used to facilitate intubation in infants or children, therefore, no specific dosage recommendations above the approximate ED$_{95}$ can be made. There are no data on maintenance dosing in infants or children. The use of Pipecuronium Bromide in neonates and infants below 3 months of age has not been investigated.

Compatibility: Pipecuronium Bromide is compatible with, and can be reconstituted using the following commonly used I.V. solutions:

0.9% NaCl solution
5% glucose in saline
5% glucose in water
lactated ringer's
sterile water for injection
bacteriostatic water for injection

Pipecuronium Bromide is not recommended for dilution into and/or administration from large volume I.V. solutions.
  Use within 24 hours of mixing with the above solutions.
  Parenteral drug products should be inspected visually for particulate matter and discoloration prior to administration, whenever solution and container permit.

Storage: 2°-30°C (35°-86°F). Protect from light.

After Reconstitution: When reconstituted with bacteriostatic water for injection, USP: Contains Benzyl Alcohol, WHICH IS NOT INTENDED FOR USE IN NEWBORNS. Use within 5 days. May be stored at room temperature or refrigerated.

When reconstituted with sterile water for injection or other compatible I.V. solutions: Refrigerate vial. Use within 24 hours. Single use only. Discard unused portion.

HOW SUPPLIED
POWDER FOR INJECTION: 10 MG/ML

BRAND/MANUFACTURER	NDC	SIZE	AWP
○ **BRAND**			
ARDUAN: Organon	00052-0446-36	6s	$257.03

◆ RATED THERAPEUTICALLY EQUIVALENT; ◇ THERAPEUTIC EQUIVALENCE UNCONFIRMED; ○ UNRATED

Piperacillin Sodium

DESCRIPTION

Piperacillin Sodium is a semisynthetic broad-spectrum penicillin for parenteral use derived from D(-)α-aminobenzylpenicillin. The chemical name of Piperacillin Sodium is 4-Thia-1-azabicyclo [3.2.0] heptane-2-carboxylic acid, 6-[[[[(4-ethyl-2,3-dioxo-1-piperazinyl) carbonyl]amino]phenylacetyl]amino] 3,3-dimethyl-7-oxo-, monosodium salt, [2S-[2α,5α,6β(S*)]]. Piperacillin Sodium is a white to off-white solid having the characteristic appearance of products prepared by freeze-drying. Freely soluble in water and in alcohol. The pH of the aqueous solution is 5.5 to 7.5. One g contains 1.85 mEq (42.5 mg) of sodium (Na+).

Following is its chemical structure:

CLINICAL PHARMACOLOGY

Intravenous Administration: In healthy adult volunteers, mean serum levels immediately after a two- to three-minute intravenous injection of 2, 4, or 6 g were 305, 412, and 775 mcg/mL. Serum levels lack dose proportionality. (See related tables).

A 30-minute infusion of 6 g every 6 h gave, on the fourth day, a mean peak serum concentration of 420 mcg/mL.

Intramuscular Administration: Piperacillin Sodium is rapidly absorbed after intramuscular injection. In healthy volunteers, the mean peak serum concentration occurs approximately 30 minutes after a single dose of 2 g and is about 36 mcg/mL. The oral administration of 1 g probenecid before injection produces an increase in piperacillin peak serum level of about 30%. The area under the curve (AUC) is increased by approximately 60%.

General: Piperacillin Sodium is not absorbed when given orally. Peak serum concentrations are attained approximately 30 minutes after intramuscular injections and immediately after completion of intravenous injection or infusion. The serum half-life in healthy volunteers ranges from 36 minutes to 1 hour and 12 minutes. The mean elimination half-life of Piperacillin Sodium in healthy adult volunteers is 54 minutes following administration of 2 g and 63 minutes following 6 g. As with other penicillins, Piperacillin Sodium is eliminated primarily by glomerular filtration and tubular secretion; it is excreted rapidly as unchanged drug in high concentrations in the urine. Approximately 60% to 80% of the administered dose is excreted in the urine in the first 24 hours. Piperacillin urine concentrations, determined by microbioassay, were as high as 14,100 mcg/mL following a 6 g intravenous dose and 8,500 mcg/mL following a 4 g intravenous dose. These urine drug concentrations remained well above 1,000 mcg/mL throughout the dosing interval. The elimination half-life is increased twofold in mild to moderate renal impairment and fivefold to sixfold in severe impairment.

Piperacillin Sodium binding to human serum proteins is 16%. The drug is widely distributed in human tissues and body fluids, including bone, prostate, and heart, and reaches high concentrations in bile. After a 4 g bolus, maximum biliary concentrations averaged 3,205 mcg/mL. It penetrates into the cerebrospinal fluid in the presence of inflamed meninges. Because Piperacillin Sodium is excreted by the biliary route as well as by the renal route, it can be used safely in appropriate dosage (see *"Dosage And Administration"*) in patients with severely restricted kidney function, and can be used effectively in treatment of hepatobiliary infections.

Microbiology: Piperacillin Sodium is an antibiotic which exerts its bactericidal activity by inhibiting both septum and cell wall synthesis. It is active against a variety of gram-positive and gram-negative aerobic and anaerobic bacteria. *In vitro*, piperacillin is active against most strains of clinical isolates of the following microorganisms:

Aerobic and facultatively anaerobic organisms: Gram-negative bacteria:
  Escherichia coli
  Proteus mirabilis
  Proteus vulgaris
  Morganella morganii (formerly *Proteus morganii*)
  Providencia rettgeri (formerly *Proteus rettgeri*)
  Serratia species including *S marcescens* and *S liquefaciens*
  Klebsiella pneumoniae
  Klebsiella species
  Enterobacter species including *E aerogenes* and *E cloacae*
  Citrobacter species including *C freundii* and *C diversus*
  Salmonella species*
  Shigella species*
  Pseudomonas aeruginosa
  Pseudomonas species including *P cepacia,* *P maltophilia,* and *P fluorescens*
  Acinetobacter species (formerly *Mima-Herellea*)
  Haemophilus influenzae (non-β-lactamase-producing strains)
  Neisseria gonorrhoeae
  *Neisseria meningitidis**
  Moraxella species*
  Yersinia species* (formerly *Pasteurella*)

Gram-positive bacteria:
  Group D streptococci including
  Enterococci (*Streptococcus faecalis, S faecium*)
  Non-enterococci*
  β-hemolytic streptococci including
  Group A *Streptococcus* (*S pyogenes*)
  Group B *Streptococcus* (*S agalactiae*)
  Streptococcus pneumoniae
  Streptococcus viridans
  Staphylococcus aureus (non-penicillinase-producing)*
  Staphylococcus epidermidis (non-penicillinase-producing)*

Anaerobic bacteria:
  Actinomyces species*
  Bacteriodes species including
  B fragilis group (*B fragilis, B vulgatus*)
  Non-*B fragilis* group (*B melaninogenicus*)
  *B asaccharolyticus**
  Clostridium species including
  C perfringens and *C difficile**
  Eubacterium species
  Fusobacterium species including
  F nucleatum and *F necrophorum*
  Peptococcus species
  Peptostreptococcus species
  Veillonella species

In vitro, Piperacillin Sodium is inactivated by staphylococcal β-lactamases, and β-lactamases produced by gram-negative bacteria. However, it is active against β-lactamase-producing gonococci.

Many strains of gram-negative organisms resistant to certain antibiotics have been found to be susceptible to Piperacillin Sodium.

Piperacillin Sodium has excellent activity against gram-positive organisms, including enterococci (*S faecalis*). It is active against obligate anaerobes such as *Bacteroides* species and also against *C difficile* (which has been associated with pseudomembranous colitis).

Piperacillin is active against many gram-negative bacteria including *Enterobacteriaceae, Klebsiella, Serratia, Pseudomonas, E coli, Proteus,* and *Citrobacter,* and, in addition, it is active against anaerobes and enterococci.

---

* Piperacillin has been shown to be active *in vitro* against these organisms; however, clinical efficacy has not yet been established.

PIPERACILLIN SERUM LEVELS IN ADULTS (mcg/mL) AFTER A TWO- TO THREE-MINUTE IV INJECTION

Dose	0	10 min	20 min	30 min	1 h	1.5 h	2 h	3 h	4 h	6 h	8 h
2	305 (159-615)	202 (164-225)	156 (52-165)	67 (41-88)	40 (25-57)	24 (18-31)	20 (14-24)	8 (3-11)	3 (2-4)	2 (< 0.6-3)	
4	412 (389-484)	344 (315-379)	295 (269-330)	117 (98-138)	93 (78-110)	60 (50-67)	36 (26-51)	20 (17-24)	8 (7-11)	4 (3.7-4.1)	0.9 (0.7-1)
6	775 (695-849)	609 (530-670)	563 (492-630)	325 (292-363)	208 (180-239)	138 (115-175)	90 (71-113)	38 (29-53)	33 (25-44)	8 (3-19)	3.2 (< 2-6)

PIPERACILLIN SERUM LEVELS IN ADULTS (mcg/mL) AFTER A 30-MINUTE IV INFUSION

Dose	0	5 min	10 min	15 min	30 min	45 min	1 h	1.5 h	2 h	4 h	6 h	7.5 h
4	244 (155-298)	215 (169-247)	186 (140-209)	177 (142-213)	141 (122-156)	146 (110-265)	105 (85-133)	72 (53-105)	53 (36-69)	15 (6-24)	4 (1-9)	2 (0.5-3)
6	353 (324-371)	298 (242-339)	298 (232-331)	272 (219-314)	229 (185-249)	180 (144-209)	149 (117-171)	104 (89-113)	73 (66-94)	22 (12-39)	16 (5-49)	—

➤ SHOWN IN PRODUCT IDENTIFICATION GUIDE

In vitro tests show piperacillin to act synergistically with aminoglycoside antibiotics against most isolates of *P aerugisoa*.

Susceptibility Testing: The use of a 100 mcg piperacillin antibiotic disk with susceptibility test methods which measure zone diameter gives an accurate estimation of susceptibility of organisms to Piperacillin Sodium. The following standard procedure† has been recommended for use with disks for testing antimicrobials.

With this type of procedure, a report of "susceptible" from the laboratory indicates that the infecting organism is likely to respond to therapy. A report of "intermediate susceptibility" suggests that the organism would be susceptible if high dosage is used or if the infection is confined to tissue and fluids (eg, urine) in which high antibiotic levels are obtained. A report of "resistant" indicates that the infecting organism is not likely to respond to therapy. With the piperacillin disk, a zone of 18 mm or greater indicates susceptibility, zone sizes of 14 mm or less indicate resistance, and zone sizes of 15 to 17 mm indicate intermediate susceptibility.

Haemophilus and *Neisseria* species which give zones of $\geq$ 29 mm are susceptible; resistant strains give zones of $\leq$ 28 mm. The above interpretive criteria are based on the use of the standardized procedure. Antibiotic susceptibility testing requires carefully prescribed procedures. Susceptibility tests are biased to a considerable degree when different methods are used.

The standardized procedure requires the use of control organisms. The 100 mcg piperacillin disk should give zone diameters between 24 and 30 mm for *E coli* ATCC No. 25922 and between 25 and 33 mm for *Pseudomonas aeruginosa* ATCC No. 27853.

Dilution methods such as those described in the International Collaborative Study‡ have been used to determine susceptibility of organisms to Piperacillin Sodium.

Enterobacteriaceae, Pseudomonas species and *Acinetobacter* sp are considered susceptible if the minimal inhibitory concentration (MIC) of piperacillin is no greater than 64 mcg/mL and are considered resistant if the MIC is greater than 128 mcg/mL.

Haemophilus and *Neisseria* species are considered susceptible if the MIC of piperacillin is $\leq$ 1 mcg/mL.

When anaerobic organisms are isolated from infection sites, it is recommended that other tests such as the modified Broth-Disk Method§ be used to determine the antibiotic susceptibility of these slowly growing organisms.

INDICATIONS AND USAGE

Therapeutic: Piperacillin Sodium is indicated for the treatment of serious infections caused by susceptible strains of the designated organisms in the conditions as listed below.

Intra-abdominal Infections: Including hepatobiliary and surgical infections caused by *E coli, P aeruginosa,* enterococci, *Clostridium* sp, anaerobic cocci, and *Bacteroides* sp, including *B fragilis.*

Urinary Tract Infections: caused by *E coli, Klebsiella* sp, *P aeruginosa, Proteus* sp, including *P mirabilis,* and enterococci.

Gynecologic Infections: including endometritis, pelvic inflammatory disease, pelvic cellulitis caused by *Bacteroides* sp including *B fragilis,* anaerobic cocci, *Neisseria gonorrhoeae,* and enterococci (*S faecalis*).

Septicemia: including bacteremia caused by *E coli, Klebsiella* sp, *Enterobacter* sp, *Serratia* sp, *P mirabilis S pneumoniae,* enterococci, *P aeruginosa, Bacteroides* sp, and anaerobic cocci.

Lower Respiratory Tract Infections: caused by *E coli, Klebsiella* sp, *Enterobacter* sp, *Pseudomonas aeruginosa, Seratia* sp, *H influenzae, Bacteroides* sp, and anaerobic cocci. Although improvement has been noted in patients with cystic fibrosis, lasting bacterial eradication may not necessarily be achieved.

Skin and Skin Structure Infections: caused by *E coli, Klebsiella* sp, *Serratia* sp, *Acinetobacter* sp, *Enterobacter* sp, *Pseudomonas aeruginosa,* indole-positive *Proteus* sp, *Proteus mirabilis, Bacteroides* sp, including *B fragilis,* anaerobic cocci, and enterococci.

Bone and Joint Infections: caused by *P aeruginosa,* enterococci, *Bacteroides* sp, and anaerobic cocci.

Gonococcal Infections: Piperacillin Sodium has been effective in the treatment of uncomplicated gonococcal urethritis.

Piperacillin Sodium *sterile piperacillin sodium* has also been shown to be clinically effective for the treatment of infections at various sites caused by *Streptococcus* species including Group A beta-hemolytic *Streptococcus* and *S pneumoniae;* however, infections caused by these organisms are ordinarily treated with more narrow spectrum penicillins. Because of its broad spectrum of bactericidal activity against gram-positive and gram-negative aerobic and anaerobic bacteria, Piperacillin Sodium is particularly useful for the treatment of mixed infections and presumptive therapy prior to the identification of the causative organisms.

† NCCLS Approved Standard; M2-A2 (Formerly ASM-2) Performance Standards for Antimicrobic Disk Susceptibility Tests, Second Edition, available from the National Committee of Clinical Laboratory Standards.
‡ *Acta Pathol Microbiol Scand* (B) 1971; suppl 217.
§ Wilkins TD and Thiel T. *Antimicrob Agents Chemother* 1973;3:350-356.

Also Piperacillin Sodium may be administered as single drug therapy in some situations where normally two antibiotics might be employed.

Piperacillin has been successfully used with aminoglycosides, especially in patients with impaired host defenses. Both drugs should be used in full therapeutic doses.

Appropriate cultures should be made for susceptibility testing before initiating therapy and therapy adjusted, if appropriate, once the results are known.

Prophylaxis: Piperacillin Sodium is indicated for prophylactic use in surgery including intra-abdominal (gastrointestinal and biliary) procedures, vaginal hysterectomy, abdominal hysterectomy, and cesarean section. Effective prophylactic use depends on the time of administration, and Piperacillin Sodium should be given one-half to 1 hour before the operation so that effective levels can be achieved in the site prior to the procedure.

The prophylactic use of piperacillin should be stopped within 24 hours, since continuing administration of any antibiotic increases the possibility of adverse reactions, but in the majority of surgical procedures, does not reduce the incidence of subsequent infections. If there are signs of infection, specimens for culture should be obtained for identification of the causative organism so that appropriate therapy can be instituted.

CONTRAINDICATIONS

A history of allergic reactions to any of the penicillins and/or cephalosporins.

WARNINGS

Serious and occasionally fatal hypersensitivity (anaphylactic) reactions have been reported in patients receiving therapy with penicillins. These reactions are more apt to occur in persons with a history of sensitivity to multiple allergens. There have been reports of patients with a history of penicillin hypersensitivity who have experienced severe hypersensitivity reactions when treated with a cephalosporin. Before initiating therapy with Piperacillin Sodium, careful inquiry should be made concerning previous hypersensitivity reactions to penicillins, cephalosporins, and other allergens. If an allergic reaction occurs during therapy with Piperacillin Sodium, the antibiotic should be discontinued. The usual agents (antihistamines, pressor amines, and corticosteroids) should be readily available. SERIOUS ANAPHYLACTOID REACTIONS REQUIRE IMMEDIATE EMERGENCY TREATMENT WITH EPINEPHRINE. OXYGEN AND INTRAVENOUS CORTICOSTEROIDS AND AIRWAY MANAGEMENT INCLUDING INTUBATION SHOULD ALSO BE ADMINISTERED AS NECESSARY.

PRECAUTIONS

General: While piperacillin possesses the characteristic low toxicity of the penicillin group of antibiotics, periodic assessment of organ system functions, including renal, hepatic, and hematopoietic, during prolonged therapy is advisable. Bleeding manifestations have occurred in some patients receiving beta-lactam antibiotics, including piperacillin. These reactions have sometimes been associated with abnormalities of coagulation tests such as clotting time, platelet aggregation and prothrombin time and are more likely to occur in patients with renal failure.

If bleeding manifestations occur, the antibiotic should be discontinued and appropriate therapy instituted.

The possibility of the emergence of resistant organisms which might cause superinfections should be kept in mind, particularly during prolonged treatment. If this occurs, appropriate measures should be taken.

As with other penicillins, patients may experience neuromuscular excitability or convulsions if higher than recommended doses are given intravenously.

Piperacillin Sodium is a monosodium salt containing 1.85 mEq of Na+ per g. This should be considered when treating patients requiring restricted salt intake. Periodic electrolyte determinations should be made in patients with low potassium reserves, and the possibility of hypokalemia should be kept in mind with patients who have potentially low potassium reserves and who are receiving cytotoxic therapy or diuretics.

Antimicrobials used in high doses for short periods to treat gonorrhea may mask or delay the symptoms of incubating syphilis. Therefore, prior to treatment, patients with gonorrhea should also be evaluated for syphilis. Specimens for darkfield examination should be obtained from patients with any suspected primary lesion, and serologic tests should be performed. In all cases where concomitant syphilis is suspected, monthly serological tests should be made for a minimum of 4 months.

As with other semisynthetic penicillins, Piperacillin Sodium therapy has been associated with an increased incidence of fever and rash in cystic fibrosis patients.

Drug Interactions: The mixing of piperacillin with an aminoglycoside *in vitro* an result in substantial inactivation of the aminoglycosides.

Pregnancy: Pregnancy Category B: Although reproduction studies in mice and rats performed at doses up to four times the human dose have shown no evidence of impaired fertility or harm to the fetus, safety of Piperacillin Sodium use in pregnant women has not been determined by adequate and well-controlled studies. Because animal reproduction studies are not always predictive of human response, this drug should be used during pregnancy only if clearly needed. It has been found to cross the placenta in rats.

Nursing Mothers: Caution should be exercised when Piperacillin Sodium is administered to nursing mothers. It is excreted in low concentrations in milk.

Pediatric Use: Dosages for children under the age of 12 have not been established. The safety of Piperacillin Sodium in neonates is not known. In dog neonates, dilated renal tubules and peritubular hyalinization occurred following administration of Piperacillin Sodium.

ADVERSE EFFECTS

Piperacillin Sodium is generally well tolerated. The most common adverse reactions have been local in nature, following intravenous or intramuscular injection. The following adverse reactions may occur.

Local Reactions: In clinical trials thrombophlebitis was noted in 4% of patients. Pain, erythema, and/or induration at the injection site occurred in 2% of patients. Less frequent reactions including ecchymosis, deep vein thrombosis, and hematomas have also occurred.

Gastrointestinal: Diarrhea and loose stools were noted in 2% of patients. Other less frequent reactions included vomiting, nausea, increases in liver enzymes (LDH, SGOT, SGPT), hyperbilirubinemia, cholestatic hepatitis, bloody diarrhea, and, rarely, pseudomembranous colitis.

Hypersensitivity Reactions: Anaphylactoid reactions, (see *"Warnings"*).
Rash was noted in 1% of patients. Other less frequent findings included pruritus, vesicular eruptions, positive Coombs tests.
Other dermatologic manifestations such as erythema multiforme and Stevens-Johnson syndrome have been reported rarely.

Renal: Elevations of creatinine or BUN, and, rarely, interstitial nephritis.

Central Nervous System: Headache, dizziness, fatigue.

Hemic and Lymphatic: Reversible leukopenia, neutropenia, thrombocytopenia, and/or eosinophilia have been reported. As with other beta-lactam antibiotics, reversible leukopenia (neutropenia) is more apt to occur in patients receiving prolonged therapy at high dosages or in association with drugs known to cause this reaction.

Serum Electrolytes: Individuals with liver disease or individuals receiving cytotoxic therapy or diuretics were reported rarely to demonstrate a decrease in serum potassium concentrations with high doses of piperacillin.

Skeletal: Rarely, prolonged muscle relaxation.

Other: Superinfection, including candidiasis. Hemorrhagic manifestations.

DOSAGE AND ADMINISTRATION

Piperacillin Sodium may be administered by the intramuscular route (see *"Note"*) or intravenously or given in a 3- to 5-minute intravenous injection. The usual dosage of Piperacillin Sodium for serious infections is 3 to 4 g given every 4 to 6 hours as a 20- to 30-minute infusion. For serious infections, the intravenous route should be used.
Piperacillin Sodium should not be mixed with an aminoglycoside in a syringe or infusion bottle since this can result in inactivation of the aminoglycoside.
The maximum daily dose for adults is usually 24 g/day, although higher doses have been used.
Intramuscular injections (see *"Note"*) should be limited to 2 g per injection site. This route of administration has been used primarily in the treatment of patients with uncomplicated gonorrhea and urinary tract infections.

DOSAGE RECOMMENDATIONS

Type of Infection	Usual Total Daily Dose
Serious infections such as septicemia, nosocomial pneumonia, intra-abdominal infections, aerobic and anaerobic gynecologic infections, and skin and soft tissue infections	12 to 18 g/d IV (200 to 300 mg/kg/d) in divided doses every 4 to 6 h
Complicated urinary tract infections	8 to 16 g/d IV (125 to 200 mg/kg/d) in divided doses every 6 to 8 h
Uncomplicated urinary tract infections and most community-acquired pneumonia	6 to 8 g/d IM or IV (100 to 125 mg/kg/d) in divided doses every 6 to 12 h
Uncomplicated gonorrhea infections	2 g IM'' as a one-time dose

One g of probenecid given orally one-half hour prior to injections.

The average duration of Piperacillin Sodium treatment is from 7 to 10 days, except in the treatment of gynecologic infections, in which it is from 3 to 10 days; the duration should be guided by the patient's clinical and bacteriological progress. For most acute infections, treatment should be continued for at least 48 to 72 hours after the patient becomes asymptomatic. Antibiotic therapy for Group A beta-hemolytic streptococcal infections should be maintained for at least 10 days to reduce the risk of rheumatic fever or glomerulonephritis.
When Piperacillin Sodium is given concurrently with aminoglycosides, both drugs should be used in full therapeutic doses.

Renal Impairment:

DOSAGE IN RENAL IMPAIRMENT

Creatinine Clearance mL/min	Urinary Tract Infection (uncomplicated)	Urinary Tract Infection (complicated)	Serious Systemic Infection
> 40	No dosage adjustment necessary		
20 to 40	No dosage adjustment necessary	9 g/day 3 g every 8 h	12 g/day 4 g every 8 h
< 20	6 g/day 3 g every 12 h	6 g/day 3 g every 12 h	8 g/day 4 g every 12 h

For patients on hemodialysis, the maximum daily dose is 6 g/day (2 g every 8 hours). In addition, because hemodialysis removes 30% to 50% of piperacillin in 4 hours, 1 g additional dose should be administered following each dialysis period. For patients with renal failure and hepatic insufficiency, measurement of serum levels of Piperacillin Sodium will provide additional guidance for adjusting dosage.

Prophylaxis: When possible, Piperacillin Sodium should be administered as a 20- to 30-minute infusion just prior to anesthesia. Administration while the patient is awake will facilitate identification of possible adverse reactions during drug infusion.

Indication	1st Dose	2nd Dose	3rd Dose
Intra-abdominal Surgery	2 g IV just prior to surgery	2 g during surgery	2 g every 6 h postop for no more than 24h
Vaginal Hysterectomy	2 g IV just prior to surgery	2 g 6 h after 1st dose	2 g 12 h after 1st dose
Cesarean Section	2 g IV after cord is clamped	2 g 4 h after 1st dose	2 g 8 h after 1st dose
Abdominal Hysterectomy	2 g IV just prior to surgery	2 g on return to recovery room	2 g after 6 h

Infants and Children: Dosages in infants and children under 12 years of age have not been established.

PRODUCT RECONSTITUTION/DOSAGE PREPARATION

Conventional Vials:
　Diluents for Reconstitution
　　Sterile Water for Injection
　　Bacteriostatic$^{\sharp}$ Water for Injection
　　Sodium Chloride Injection
　　Bacteriostatic$^{\sharp}$ Sodium Chloride Injection
　　Dextrose 5% in Water
　　Dextrose 5% and 0.9% Sodium Chloride
　　Lidocaine HCl 0.5% to 1% (without epinephrine)[#]
　　$^{\sharp}$ Either Parabens or Benzyl Alcohol

Conventional Vials:
　Intravenous Solutions
　　Dextrose 5% in Water
　　0.9% Sodium Chloride
　　Dextrose 5% and 0.9% Sodium Chloride
　　Lactated Ringer's Injection
　　Dextran 6% in 0.9% Sodium Chloride

Intravenous Admixtures
　　Normal Saline (+ KCl 40 mEq)
　　5% Dextrose in Water (+ KCl 40 mEq)
　　5% Dextrose/Normal Saline (+ KCl 40 mEq)
　　Ringer's Injection (+ KCl 40 mEq)
　　Lactated Ringer's Injection (+ KCl 40 mEq)

INTRAVENOUS ADMINISTRATION

Reconstitution Directions for Conventional Vials: Reconstitute each gram of Piperacillin Sodium with at least 5 mL of a suitable diluent (except Lidocaine HCl 0.5% to 1% without epinephrine) listed above. Shake well until dissolved. Reconstituted solution may be further diluted to the desired volume (eg. 50 or 100 mL) in the above listed intravenous solutions and admixtures.

Reconstitution Directions for Pharmacy Bulk Vial: Reconstitute the 40 g vial with 172 mL of a suitable diluent (except Lidocaine HCl 0.5% to 1% without epinephrine) listed above to achieve a concentration of 1 g per 5 mL.

Directions for Administration: Intermittent IV Infusion. Infuse diluted solution over period of about 30 minutes. During infusion it is desirable to discontinue the primary intravenous solution.

Intravenous Injection (Bolus): Reconstituted solution should be injected slowly over a 3- to 5-minute period to help avoid vein irritation.

INTRAMUSCULAR ADMINISTRATION (CONVENTIONAL VIALS ONLY)

Reconstitution Directions: Reconstitute each gram of Piperacillin Sodium with 2 mL of a suitable diluent listed above to achieve a concentration of 1 g per 2.5 mL. Shake well until dissolved.

For Intramuscular Use Only. Lidocaine is contraindicated in patients with a known history of hypersensitivity to local anesthetics of the amide type.

➤ SHOWN IN PRODUCT IDENTIFICATION GUIDE

Directions for Administration: When indicated by clinical and bacteriological findings, intramuscular administration of 6 to 8 g daily of Piperacillin Sodium, in divided doses, may be utilized for initiation of therapy. In addition, intramuscular administration of the drug may be considered for maintenance therapy after clinical and bacteriologic improvement has been obtained with intravenous piperacillin sodium treatment. Intramuscular administration should not exceed 2 g per injection at any one site.

The preferred site is the upper outer quadrant of the buttock (ie, gluteus maximus).

The deltoid area should be used only if well-developed, and then only with caution to avoid radial nerve injury. Intramuscular injections should not be made into the lower or mid-third of the upper arm.

STABILITY OF PIPERACILLIN FOLLOWING RECONSTITUTION
Piperacillin Sodium is stable in both glass and plastic containers when reconstituted with recommended diluents and when diluted with the intravenous solutions and intravenous admixtures indicated above.

Extensive stability studies have demonstrated chemical stability (potency, pH, and clarity) through 24 hours at room temperature, up to 1 week refrigerated, and up to 1 month frozen ($-10°$ to $-20°$C). (Note: The 40 g Pharmacy Bulk Vial should not be frozen after reconstitution.) Appropriate consideration of aseptic technique and individual hospital policy, however, may recommend discarding unused portions after storage for 48 hours under refrigeration and discarding after 24 hours storage at room temperature.

STORAGE
Vials: This product should be stored at controlled room temperature, 15°-30°C (59°-86°F).

HOW SUPPLIED
POWDER FOR INJECTION: 2 GM

BRAND/MANUFACTURER	NDC	SIZE	AWP
○ **BRAND**			
PIPRACIL: Lederle Labs	00206-3879-16	10s	$110.15
	00206-3879-27	10s	$113.11
	00206-3879-47	10s	$117.59

POWDER FOR INJECTION: 3 GM

BRAND/MANUFACTURER	NDC	SIZE	AWP
○ **BRAND**			
PIPRACIL: Lederle Labs	00206-3882-55	10s	$165.20
	00206-3882-28	10s	$169.68
	00206-3882-65	10s	$176.36

POWDER FOR INJECTION: 4 GM

BRAND/MANUFACTURER	NDC	SIZE	AWP
○ **BRAND**			
PIPRACIL: Lederle Labs	00206-3880-25	10s	$220.28
	00206-3880-29	10s	$226.24
	00206-3880-66	10s	$235.16

POWDER FOR INJECTION: 40 GM

BRAND/MANUFACTURER	NDC	SIZE	AWP
○ **BRAND**			
PIPRACIL: Lederle Labs	00206-3877-60	1s	$190.51

Piperacillin Sodium and Tazobactam Sodium

DESCRIPTION
Piperacillin Sodium/Tazobactam Sodium is an injectable antibacterial combination product consisting of the semisynthetic antibiotic Piperacillin Sodium and the beta-lactamase inhibitor Tazobactam Sodium for intravenous administration.

Piperacillin Sodium is derived from D(-)-α- aminobenzyl-penicillin. The chemical name of Piperacillin Sodium is sodium (2S, 5R, 6R)-6-[(R)-2-(4-ethyl-2, 3-dioxo-1-piperazine-carboxyamido)-3, 3-dimethyl -7- oxo-4-thia-1-azabicyclo [3.2.0]-heptane-2-carboxylate. The chemical formula is $C_{23}H_{26}N_5NaO_7S$ and the molecular weight is 539.5.

Tazobactam Sodium, a derivative of the penicillin nucleus, is a penicillinic acid sulfone. Its chemical name is sodium (2S, 3S, 5R)-3-methyl-7-oxo-3-(1H-1, 2, 3-triazol-1-ylmethyl)- 4-thia-1-azabicyclo-[3.2.0]heptane-2-carboxylate-4, 4-dioxide. The chemical formula is $C_{10}H_{11}N_4NaO_5S$ and the molecular weight is 322.3.

Piperacillin Sodium/Tazobactam Sodium parenteral combination, is a white to off-white sterile, cryodesiccated powder consisting of Piperacillin and Tazobactam as their sodium salts packaged in glass vials. The product does not contain excipients or preservatives.

Each Piperacillin Sodium/Tazobactam Sodium 2.25 g single dose vial contains an amount of drug sufficient for withdrawal of Piperacillin Sodium equivalent to 2 grams of Piperacillin and Tazobactam Sodium equivalent to 0.25 g of Tazobactam.

Each Piperacillin Sodium/Tazobactam Sodium 3.375 g single dose vial contains an amount of drug sufficient for withdrawal of Piperacillin Sodium

equivalent to 3 grams of Piperacillin and Tazobactam Sodium equivalent to 0.375 g of Tazobactam.

Each Piperacillin Sodium/Tazobactam Sodium 4.5 g single dose vial contains an amount of drug sufficient for withdrawal of Piperacillin Sodium equivalent to 4 grams of Piperacillin and Tazobactam Sodium equivalent to 0.5 g of Tazobactam.

Piperacillin Sodium/Tazobactam Sodium is a monosodium salt of Piperacillin and a monosodium salt of Tazobactam containing a total of 2.35 mEq (54 mg) of Na^+ per gram of Piperacillin in the combination product.

CLINICAL PHARMACOLOGY
Peak plasma concentrations of Piperacillin and Tazobactam are attained immediately after completion of an intravenous infusion of Piperacillin Sodium/Tazobactam Sodium. Piperacillin plasma concentrations, following a 30-minute infusion of Piperacillin Sodium/Tazobactam Sodium, were similar to those attained when equivalent doses of Piperacillin were administered alone, with mean peak plasma concentrations of approximately 134, 242, and 298 μg/mL for the 2.25 g, 3.375 g, and 4.5 g Piperacillin Sodium/Tazobactam Sodium doses, respectively. The corresponding mean peak plasma concentrations of Tazobactam were 15, 24, and 34 μg/mL, respectively.

Following a 30-minute I.V. infusion of 3.375 g Piperacillin Sodium/Tazobactam Sodium every 6 hours, steady-state plasma concentrations of Piperacillin and Tazobactam were similar to those attained after the first dose. In like manner, steady-state plasma concentrations were not different from those attained after the first dose when 2.25 g or 4.5 g doses of Piperacillin Sodium/Tazobactam Sodium were administered via 30-minute infusions every 6 hours.

Steady-state plasma concentrations after 30-minute infusions every 6 hours are provided in Table 1.

Following single or multiple Piperacillin Sodium/Tazobactam Sodium doses to healthy subjects, the plasma half-life of Piperacillin and of Tazobactam ranged from 0.7 to 1.2 hours and were unaffected by dose or duration of infusion.

Piperacillin is metabolized to a minor microbiologically active desethyl metabolite. Tazobactam is metabolized to a single metabolite that lacks pharmacological and antibactarial activities. Both Piperacillin and Tazobactam are eliminated via the kidney by glomerular filtration and tubular secretion. Piperacillin is excreted rapidly as unchanged drug with 68% of the administered dose excreted in the urine. Tazobactam and its metabolite are eliminated primarily by renal excretion with 80% of the administered dose excreted as unchanged drug and the remainder as the single metabolite. Piperacillin, Tazobactam, and desethyl piperacillin are also secreted into the bile.

Both Piperacillin and Tazobactam are approximately 30% bound to plasma proteins. The protein binding of either Piperacillin or Tazobactam is unaffected by the presence of the other compound. Protein binding of the Tazobactam metabolite is negligible.

Piperacillin and Tazobactam are widely distributed into tissues and body fluids including intestinal mucosa, gallbladder, lung, female reproductive tissues (uterus, ovary, and fallopian tube), interstitial fluid, and bile. Mean tissue concentrations are generally 50-100% of those in plasma. Distribution of Piperacillin and Tazobactam into cerebrospinal fluid is low in subjects with noninflamed meninges, as with other penicillins.

After the administration of single doses of Piperacillin/Tazobactam to subjects with renal impairment, the half-life of Piperacillin and of Tazobactam increases with decreasing creatinine clearance. At creatinine clearance below 20 mL/min, the increase in half-life is twofold for Piperacillin and fourfold for Tazobactam compared to subjects with normal renal function. Dosage adjustments for Piperacillin Sodium/Tazobactam Sodium *sterile Piperacillin Sodium and Tazobactam Sodium* are recommended when creatinine clearance is below 40 mL/min in patients receiving the usual recommended daily dose of Piperacillin Sodium/Tazobactam Sodium. (See *"Dosage and Administration"* section for specific recommendations for the treatment of patients with renal insufficiency.)

Hemodialysis removes 30-40% of Piperacillin/Tazobactam dose with an additional 5% of the Tazobactam dose removed as the Tazobactam metabolite. Peritoneal dialysis removes approximately 6% and 21% of the Piperacillin and Tazobactam doses, respectively, with up to 16% of the Tazobactam dose removed as the Tazobactam metabolite. For dosage recommendations for patients undergoing hemodialysis, see *"Dosage and Administration"* section.

The half-life of Piperacillin and of Tazobactam increases by approximately 25% and 18%, respectively, in patients with hepatic cirrhosis compared to healthy subjects. However, this difference does not warrant dosage adjustment of Piperacillin Sodium/Tazobactam Sodium due to hepatic cirrhosis. (See related tables).

Microbiology: Piperacillin Sodium exerts bactericidal activity by inhibiting septum formation and cell wall synthesis. *In vitro,* Piperacillin is active against a variety of gram-positive and gram-negative aerobic and anaerobic bacteria. Tazobactam Sodium, which has very little intrinsic microbiologic activity due to its very low level of binding to penicillin-binding proteins, is a β-lactamase inhibitor of the Richmond-Sykes class III (Bush class 2b & 2b′) penicillinases and cephalosporinases. It varies in its ability to inhibit class II and IV (2a & 4) penicillinases. Tazobactam does not induce chromosomally-mediated β-lactamases at Tazobactam levels achieved with the recommended dosing regimen.

Piperacillin/Tazobactam has been shown to be active against most strains of the following Piperacillin resistant β-lactamase producing microorganisms both *in vitro* and in clinical infections as described in the *"Indications and Usage"* section.

GRAM-POSITIVE AEROBES
Staphylococcus aureus (Not methicillin/oxacillin-resistant strains)

GRAM-NEGATIVE AEROBES
Escherichia coli:

Haemophilus influenzae (NOT ampicillin-resistant β-lactamase negative strains)

GRAM-NEGATIVE ANAEROBES
Bacteroides fragilis group (*B. fragilis, B. ovatus, B. thetaiotaomicron* or *B. vulgatus*)

The following *in vitro* data are available; *but their clinical significance is unknown.*

Piperacillin/Tazobactam exhibits *in vitro* minimum inhibitory concentrations (MICs) of 16 μg/mL or less against most (≥ 90%) strains of the following microorganisms (or MICs of 1 μg/mL or less against *Haemophilus* species or *Neisseria* species of MICs of 8 μg/mL or less against *Staphylococcus* species); however, the safety and effectiveness of Piperacillin/Tazobactam in treating clinical infections due to these microorganisms have not been established in adequate and well-controlled clinical trials.

GRAM-POSITIVE AEROBES
Enterococcus faecalis[†]
Staphylococcus epidermidis (NOT methicillin/oxacillin-resistant strains)
Streptococcus agalactiae[†]
Streptococcus pneumoniae[†]
Streptococcus pyogenes[†]
Viridans group streptococci[†]

GRAM-NEGATIVE AEROBES
Klebsiella oxytoca
Klebsiella pneumoniae
Moraxella catarrhalis
Morganella morganii
Neisseria gonorrhoeae
Neisseria meningitidis[†]
Proteus mirabilis
Proteus vulgaris
Serratia marcescens

GRAM-POSITIVE ANAEROBES
Clostridium perfringens

GRAM-NEGATIVE ANAEROBES
Bacteroides distasonis
Fusobacterium nucleatum
Prevotella melaninogenica (formerly *Bacteroides melaninogenicus*)
[†]These are not beta-lactamase producing strains and, therefore, are susceptible to Piperacillin alone.

Susceptibility Tests: Measurement of MIC or MBC and achieved antimicrobial compound concentrations may be appropriate to guide therapy in some infections.

(See *"Clinical Pharmacology"* section for further information on drug concentrations achieved in infected body sites and other pharmacokinetic properties of this antimicrobial drug product.)

Diffusion Techniques: Quantitative methods that require measurement of zone diameters provide reproducible estimates of the susceptibility of bacteria to antimicrobial compounds. One such standardized procedure[1] that has been recommended for use with disks to test the susceptibility of microorganisms to Piperacillin/Tazobactam uses the 100 μg/10 μg Piperacillin/Tazobactam disk. Interpretation involves correlation of the diameter obtained in the disk test with the MIC for Piperacillin/Tazobactam.

Reports from the laboratory giving results of the standard single-disk susceptibility test with a 100 μg/10 μg Piperacillin/Tazobactam disk should be interpreted according to the following criteria:

For Enterobacteriaceae:

Zone Diameter (mm)	Interpretation
≥ 21	Susceptible (S)
18-20	Intermediate (I)
≤ 17	Resistant (R)

For *Haemophilus* species:

Zone Diameter (mm)	Interpretation
≥ 27	Susceptible (S)
≤ 26	Resistant (R)

For *Staphylococcus* species:

Zone Diameter (mm)	Interpretation
≥ 20	Susceptible (S)
≤ 19	Resistant (R)

A report of "Susceptible" indicates that the pathogen is likely to be inhibited by usually achievable concentrations of the antimicrobial compound in the blood. A report of "Intermediate" indicates that the result should be considered equivocal, and, if the microorganism is not fully susceptible to alternative, clinically feasible drugs, the test should be repeated. This category implies clinical applicability in body sites where the drug is physiologically concentrated or in situations where high dosage of drug can be used. This category also provides a buffer zone that prevents small uncontrolled technical factors from causing major discrepancies in interpretation. A report of "Resistant" indicates that usually achievable concentrations of the antimicrobial compound in the blood are unlikely to be inhibitory and other therapy should be selected.

Standardized susceptibility test procedures require the use of laboratory control microorganisms. The 100 μg/10 μg Piperacillin/Tazobactam disk should give the following zone diameters in these laboratory test quality control strains:

Microorganism	Zone Diameter (mm)
Escherichia coli ATCC 25922	24-30
Escherichia coli ATCC 35218	25-31
Haemophilus influenzae ATCC 49247	32-36

Table 1
STEADY STATE MEAN PLASMA CONCENTRATIONS IN ADULTS AFTER 30-MINUTE INTRAVENOUS INFUSION OF PIPERACILLIN/TAZOBACTAM EVERY 6 HOURS
PIPERACILLIN

Piperacillin/ Tazobactam Dose	No. of Evaluable Subjects	Plasma Concentrations (mcg/mL)						AUC (mcg•hr/mL)
		30 min	1 hr	2 hr	3 hr	4 hr	6 hr	AUC$_{0-6}$
2.25 g	24	134 (14)	57 (14)	17.1 (23)	5.2 (32)	2.5 (35)	0.9 (14)[a]	131 (14)
3.375 g	22	242 (12)	106 (8)	34.6 (20)	11.5 (19)	5.1 (22)	1.0 (10)	242 (10)
4.5 g	24	298 (14)	141 (19)	46.6 (28)	16.4 (29)	6.9 (29)	1.4 (30)	322 (16)

a N = 4

TAZOBACTAM

Piperacillin/ Tazobactam Dose	No. of Evaluable Subjects	Plasma Concentrations (mcg/mL)						AUC (mcg•hr/mL)
		30 min	1 hr	2 hr	3 hr	4 hr	6 hr	AUC$_{0-6}$
2.25 g	24	14.8 (14)	7.2 (22)	2.6 (30)	1.1 (35)	0.7 (6)[b]	< 0.5	16.0 (21)
3.375 g	22	24.2 (14)	10.7 (7)	4.0 (18)	1.4 (21)	0.7 (16)[a]	< 0.5	25.0 (8)
4.5 g	24	33.8 (15)	17.3 (16)	6.8 (24)	2.8 (25)	1.3 (30)	< 0.5	39.8 (15)

a N = 4
b N = 3
c Piperacillin and Tazobactam were given in combination.
Twenty-four (2.25 g and 4.5 g) and 22 (3.375 g) subjects were enrolled in the study and all were evaluable for pharmacokinetic analysis.

Dilution Techniques: Quantitative methods that are used to determine minimum inhibitory concentrations provide reproducible estimates of the susceptibility of bacteria to antimicrobial compounds. One such standardized procedure uses a dilution method[2,4] (broth, agar, or microdilution) or equivalent with Piperacillin/Tazobactam powder. The MIC values obtained should be interpreted according to the following criteria:

For *Enterobacteriaceae*:

MIC (μg/mL)	Interpretation
≤ 16	Susceptible (S)
32-64	Intermediate (I)
≥ 128	Resistant (R)

For *Haemophilus* species:

MIC (μg/mL)	Interpretation
≤ 1	Susceptible (S)
≥ 2	Resistant (R)

For *Staphylococcus* species:

MIC (μg/mL)	Interpretation
≤ 8	Susceptible (S)
≥ 16	Resistant (R)

Interpretation is as stated above for results using diffusion techniques.

As with standard diffusion techniques, dilution methods require the use of laboratory control microorganisms.

Standard Pipercillin/Tazobactam (8:1) powder should provide the following MIC values:

Microorganism	MIC (μg/mL)
Escherichia coli ATCC 25922	1-4
Escherichia coli ATCC 35218	2-8
Staphylococcus aureus ATCC 29213	1-4
Haemophilus influenzae ATCC 49247	0.06-0.25

Anaerobic Techniques: For anaerobic bacteria, the susceptibility to Piperacillin/Tazobactam can be determined by the reference agar dilution method or by alternate standardized test methods.[3,4]

For *Bacteroides* species, the dilution and zone diameters should be interpreted as follows:

MIC (μg/mL)	Zone Diameter (mm)	Interpretation
≤ 16	≥ 21	Susceptible (S)
≥ 32	≤ 20	Resistant (R)

As with standard diffusion techniques, dilution methods require the use of laboratory control microorganisms. Standard Piperacillin/Tazobactam powder should provide the following MIC values:

Microorganism	MIC (μg/mL)
Bacteroides fragilis ATCC 25285	1-4

INDICATIONS AND USAGE

Piperacillin Sodium/Tazobactam Sodium is indicated for the treatment of patients with moderate to severe infections caused by Piperacillin resistant, Piperacillin/Tazobactam susceptible, β-lactamase producing strains of the designated microorganisms in the specific conditions listed below:

Appendicitis (complicated by rupture or abscess) and peritonitis caused by Piperacillin resistant, β-lactamase producing strains of *Eschericha coli* or the following members of the *Bacteroides fragilis* group: *B. fragilis, B. ovatus, B. thetaiotaomicron,* or *B. vulgatus.* The individual members of this group were studied in less than 10 cases.

Uncomplicated and complicated skin and skin structure infections, including cellulitis, cutaneous abscesses, and ischemic/diabetic foot infections caused by Piperacillin resistant, β-lactamase producing strains of *Staphylococcus aureus.*

Postpartum endometritis or pelvic inflammatory disease caused by Piperacillin resistant, β-lactamase producing strains of *Escherichia coli.*

Community-acquired pneumonia (moderate severity only) caused by Piperacillin resistant, β-lactamase producing strains of *Haemophilus influenzae.*

Clinical trial data for the treatment of complicated urinary tract infections demonstrated inadequate efficacy at the dosage regimen of Piperacillin Sodium/Tazobactam Sodium studied (i.e., 3.375 g every 8 hours). There are no other adequate and well controlled trial data to support the use of this product in the treatment of complicated urinary tract infections.

As a combination product, Piperacillin Sodium/Tazobactam Sodium is indicated only for the specified conditions listed above. Infections caused by Piperacillin susceptible organisms for which Piperacillin has been shown to be effective are also amendable to Piperacillin Sodium/Tazobactam Sodium treatment due to its Piperacillin content. The Tazobactam component of this combination product does not decrease the activity of the Piperacillin component against Piperacillin susceptible organisms. Therefore, the treatment of mixed infections caused by Piperacillin susceptible organisms and Piperacillin resistant, β-lactamase producing organisms susceptible to Piperacillin Sodium/Tazobactam Sodium should not require the addition of another antibiotic.

Piperacillin Sodium/Tazobactam Sodium is useful as presumptive therapy in the indicated conditions prior to the identification of causative organisms because of its broad spectrum of bactericidal activity against gram-positive and gram-negative aerobic and anaerobic organisms.

Appropriate cultures should usually be performed before initiating antimicrobial treatment in order to isolate and identify the organisms causing infection and to determine their susceptibility to Piperacillin Sodium/Tazobactam Sodium. Antimicrobial therapy should be adjusted, if appropriate, once the results of culture(s) and antimicrobial susceptibility testing are known.

CONTRAINDICATIONS

Piperacillin Sodium/Tazobactam Sodium is contraindicated in patients with a history of allergic reactions to any of the penicillins, cephalosporins, or β-lactamase inhibitors.

WARNINGS

SERIOUS AND OCCASIONALLY FATAL HYPERSENSITIVITY (ANAPHYLACTIC) REACTIONS HAVE BEEN REPORTED IN PATIENTS ON PENICILLIN THERAPY. THESE REACTIONS ARE MORE LIKELY TO OCCUR IN INDIVIDUALS WITH A HISTORY OF PENICILLIN HYPERSENSITIVITY OR A HISTORY OF SENSITIVITY TO MULTIPLE ALLERGENS. THERE HAVE BEEN REPORTS OF INDIVIDUALS WITH A HISTORY OF PENICILLIN HYPERSENSITIVITY WHO HAVE EXPERIENCED SEVERE REACTIONS WHEN TREATED WITH CEPHALOSPORINS. BEFORE INITIATING THERAPY WITH PIPERACILLIN SODIUM/TAZOBACTAM SODIUM, CAREFUL INQUIRY SHOULD BE MADE CONCERNING PREVIOUS HYPERSENSITIVITY REACTIONS TO PENICILLINS, CEPHALOSPORINS, OR OTHER ALLERGENS. IF AN ALLERGIC REACTION OCCURS, PIPERACILLIN SODIUM/TAZOBACTAM SODIUM SHOULD BE DISCONTINUED AND APPROPRIATE THERAPY INSTITUTED. SERIOUS ANAPHYLACTIC REACTIONS REQUIRE IMMEDIATE EMERGENCY TREATMENT WITH EPINEPHRINE. OXYGEN, INTRAVENOUS STEROIDS, AND AIRWAY MANAGEMENT, INCLUDING INTUBATION, SHOULD ALSO BE ADMINISTERED AS INDICATED.

Pseudomembranous colitis has been reported with nearly all antibacterial agents, including Piperacillin/Tazobactam, and may range in severity from mild to life-threatening. Therefore, it is important to consider this diagnosis in patients who present with diarrhea subsequent to the administration of antibacterial agents.

Treatment with antibacterial agents alters the normal flora of the colon and may permit overgrowth of clostridia. Studies indicate that a toxin produced by *Clostridium difficile* is one primary cause of "antibiotic-associated colitis."

After the diagnosis of pseudomembranous colitis has been established, therapeutic measures should be initiated. Mild cases of pseudomembranous colitis usually respond to drug discontinuation alone. In moderate to severe cases, consideration should be given to management with fluids and electrolytes, protein supplementation, and treatment with an antibacterial drug clinically effective against *Clostridium difficile* colitis.

PRECAUTIONS

General: Bleeding manifestations have occurred in some patients receiving β-lactam antibiotics, including Piperacillin. These reactions have sometimes been associated with abnormalities of coagulation tests such as clotting time, platelet aggregation, and prothrombin time and are more likely to occur in patients with renal failure. If bleeding manifestations occur, Piperacillin Sodium/Tazobactam Sodium should be discontinued and appropriate therapy instituted.

The possibility of the emergence of resistant organisms that might cause superinfections should be kept in mind. If this occurs, appropriate measures should be taken.

As with other penicillins, patients may experience neuromuscular excitability or convulsions if higher than recommended doses are given intravenously (particularly in the presence of renal failure).

Piperacillin Sodium/Tazobactam Sodium is a monosodium salt of Piperacillin and a monosodium salt of Tazobactam and contains a total of 2.35 mEq (54 mg) of Na$^+$ per gram of Piperacillin in the combination product. This should be considered when treating patients requiring restricted salt intake. Periodic electrolyte determinations should be performed in patients with low potassium reserves, and the possibility of hypokalemia should be kept in mind with patients who have potentially low potassium reserves and who are receiving cytotoxic therapy or diuretics.

As with other semisynthetic penicillins, Piperacillin therapy has been associated with an increased incidence of fever and rash in cystic fibrosis patients.

Laboratory Tests: Periodic assessment of hematopoietic function should be performed, especially with prolonged therapy, i.e., ≥ 21 days. (See *"Adverse Reactions—Adverse Laboratory Events".*)

Drug Interactions: Aminoglycosides: The mixing of Piperacillin Sodium/Tazobactam Sodium with an aminoglycoside *in vitro* can result in substantial inactivation

---

◆ RATED THERAPEUTICALLY EQUIVALENT; ◇ THERAPEUTIC EQUIVALENCE UNCONFIRMED; ○ UNRATED

of the aminoglycoside. (See *"Compatible Intravenous Diluents, Dosage and Administration"*.)

When Piperacillin Sodium/Tazobactam Sodium is co-administered with tobramycin, the area under the curve, renal clearance, and urinary recovery of tobramycin were decreased by 11%, 32%, and 38%, respectively. The alterations in the pharmacokinetics of tobramycin when administered in combination with Piperacillin/Tazobactam may be due to *in vivo* and *in vitro* inactivation of tobramycin in the presence of Piperacillin/Tazobactam. The inactivation of aminoglycosides in the presence of penicillin class drugs has been recognized. It has been postulated that penicillin-aminoglycoside complexes form; these complexes are microbiologically inactive and of unknown toxicity. In patients with severe renal dysfunction (i.e., chronic hemodialysis patients), the pharmacokinetics of tobramycin are significantly altered when tobramycin is administered in combination with Piperacillin.[5] The alteration of tobramycin pharmacokinetics and the potential toxicity of the penicillin-aminoglycoside complexes in patients with mild to moderate renal dysfunction who are administered an aminoglycoside in combination with Piperacillin/Tazobactam is unknown.

Probenecid: Probenecid administered concomitantly with Piperacillin Sodium/Tazobactam Sodium prolongs the half-life of Piperacillin by 21% and of Tazobactam by 71%.

Vancomycin: No pharmacokinetic interactions have been noted between Piperacillin Sodium/Tazobactam Sodium and vancomycin.

Heparin: Coagulation parameters should be tested more frequently and monitored regularly during simultaneous administration of high doses of heparin, oral anticoagulants, or other drugs that may affect the blood coagulation system or the thrombocyte function.

Vecuronium: Piperacillin when used concomitantly with vecuronium has been implicated in the prolongation of the neuromuscular blockade of vecuronium. Piperacillin Sodium/Tazobactam Sodium could produce the same phenomenon if given along with vecuronium. Due to their similar mechanism of action, it is expected that the neuromuscular blockade produced by any of the non-depolarizing muscle relaxants could be prolonged in the presence of Piperacillin. (See package insert for vecuronium bromide.)

Drug/Laboratory Test Interactions: As with other penicillins, the administration of Piperacillin Sodium/Tazobactam Sodium may result in a false-positive reaction for glucose in the urine using a copper-reduction method. It is recommended that glucose tests based on enzymatic glucose oxidase reactions be used.

Carcinogenesis, Mutagenesis, Impairment of Fertility: Longterm carcinogenicity studies in animals have not been conducted with Piperacillin/Tazobactam, Piperacillin, or Tazobactam.

Piperacillin/Tazobactam was negative in microbial mutagenicity assays at concentrations up to 14.81/1.86 μg/plate. Piperacillin/Tazobactam was negative in the unscheduled DNA synthesis (UDS) test at concentrations up to 5689/711 μg/mL. Piperacillin/Tazobactam was negative in a mammalian point mutation (Chinese hamster ovary cell HPRT) assay at concentrations up to 8000/1000 μg/mL. Piperacillin/Tazobactam was negative in a mammalian cell (BALB/c-3T3) transformation assay at concentrations up to 8/1 μg/mL. *In vivo*, Piperacillin/Tazobactam did not induce chromosomal aberrations in rats dosed I.V. with 1500/187.5 mg/kg; this dose is similar to the maximum recommended human daily dose on a body-surface-area basis (mg/m^2).

Piperacillin was negative in microbial mutagenicity assays at concentrations up to 50 μg/plate. There was no DNA damage in bacteria (Rec assay) exposed to Piperacillin at concentrations up to 200 μg/disk. Piperacillin was negative in the UDS test at concentrations up to 10,000 μg/mL. In a mammalian point mutation (mouse lymphoma cells) assay, Piperacillin was positive at concentrations ≥ 2500 μg/mL. Piperacillin was negative in a cell (BALB/c-3T3) transformation assay at concentrations up to 3000 μg/mL. *In vivo*, Piperacillin did not induce chromosomal abberations in mice at I.V. doses up to 2000 mg/kg/day or rats at I.V. doses up to 1500 mg/kg/day. These doses are half (mice) or similar (rats) to the maximum recommended human daily dose based on body-surface area (mg/m^2). In another *in vivo* test, there was no dominant lethal effect when Piperacillin was administered to rats at I.V. doses up to 2000 mg/kg/day, which is similar to the maximum recommended human daily dose based on body-surface area (mg/m^2). When mice were administered Piperacillin at I.V. doses up to 2000 mg/kg/day, which is half the maximum recommended human daily dose based on body-surface area (mg/m^2), urine from these animals was not mutagenic when tested in a microbial mutagenicity assay. Bacteria injected into the peritoneal cavity of mice administered Piperacillin at I.V. doses up to 2000 mg/kg/day did not show increased mutation frequencies.

Tazobactam was negative in microbial mutagenicity assays at concentrations up to 333 μg/plate. Tazobactam was negative in the UDS test at concentrations up to 2000 μg/mL. Tazobactam was negative in a mammalian point mutation (Chinese hamster ovary cell HPRT) assay at concentrations up to 5000 μg/mL. In another mammalian point mutation (mouse lymphoma cells) assay, Tazobactam was positive at concentrations ≥ 3000 μg/mL. Tazobactam was negative in a cell (BALB/c-3T3) transformation assay at concentrations up to 900 μg/mL. In an *in vitro* cytogenetics (Chinese hamster lung cells) assay, Tazobactam was negative at concentrations up to 3000 μg/mL. *In vivo*, Tazobactam did not induce chromosomal aberrations in rats at I.V. doses up to 5000 mg/kg, which is 23 times the maximum recommended human daily dose based on body-surface area (mg/m^2).

Pregnancy: Teratogenic Effects. Pregnancy Category B:

Piperacillin/Tazobactam: Reproduction studies have been performed in rats and have revealed no evidence of impaired fertility due to Piperacillin/Tazobactam administered up to a dose which is similar to the maximum recommended human daily dose based on body-surface area (mg/m^2).

Teratology studies have been performed in mice and rats and have revealed no evidence of harm to the fetus due to Piperacillin/Tazobactam administered up to a dose which is 1 to 2 times and 2 to 3 times the human dose of Piperacillin and Tazobactam, respectively, based on body-surface area (mg/m^2).

Piperacillin: Reproduction and teratology studies have been performed in mice and rats and have revealed no evidence of impaired fertility or harm to the fetus due to Piperacillin administered up to a dose which is half (mice) or similar (rats) to the maximum recommended human daily dose based on body-surface area (mg/m^2).

Tazobactam: Reproduction studies have been performed in rats and have revealed no evidence of impaired fertility due to Tazobactam administered at doses up to 3 times the maximum recommended human daily dose based on body-surface area (mg/m^2).

Teratology studies have been performed in mice and rats and have revealed no evidence of harm to the fetus due to Tazobactam administered at doses up to 6 and 14 times, respectively, the human dose based on body-surface area (mg/m^2). In rats, Tazobactam crosses the placenta. Concentrations in the fetus are less than or equal to 10% of that found in maternal plasma.

There are, however, no adequate and well-controlled studies with the Piperacillin/Tazobactam combination or with Piperacillin or Tazobactam alone in pregnant women. Because animal reproduction studies are not always predictive of the human response, this drug should be used during pregnancy only if clearly needed.

Nursing Mothers: Piperacillin is excreted in low concentrations in human milk; Tazobactam concentrations in human milk have not been studied. Caution should be exercised when Piperacillin Sodium/Tazobactam Sodium is administered to a nursing woman.

Pediatric Use: Safety and efficacy in children below the age of 12 years have not been established.

Geriatric Use: Patients over 65 years are not at an increased risk of developing adverse effects solely because of age. However, dosage should be adjusted in the presence of renal insufficiency. (See *"Dosage and Administration"*.)

ADVERSE REACTIONS

During the clinical investigation, 2621 patients worldwide were treated with Piperacillin Sodium/Tazobactam Sodium in phase 3 trials. In the key North American clinical trials (n = 830 patients), 90% of the adverse events reported were mild to moderate in severity and transient in nature. However, in 3.2% of the patients treated worldwide, Piperacillin Sodium/Tazobactam Sodium was discontinued because of adverse events primarily involving the skin (1.3%), including rash and pruritus; the gastrointestinal system (0.9%), including diarrhea, nausea, and vomiting; and allergic reactions (0.5%).

Adverse local reactions that were reported, irrespective of relationship to therapy with Piperacillin Sodium/Tazobactam Sodium, were phlebitis (1.3%), injection site reaction (0.5%), pain (0.2%), inflammation (0.2%), thrombophlebitis (0.2%), and edema (0.1%).

Adverse Clinical Events: Based on patients from the North American trials (n = 1063), the events with the highest incidence in patients, irrespective of relationship to Piperacillin Sodium/Tazobactam Sodium therapy, were diarrhea (11.3%); headache (7.7%); constipation (7.7%); nausea (6.9%); insomnia (6.6%); rash (4.2%), including maculopapular, bullous, urticarial, and eczematoid; vomiting (3.3%); dyspepsia (3.3%); pruritus (3.1%); stool changes (2.4%); fever (2.4%); agitation (2.1%); pain (1.7%); moniliasis (1.6%); hypertension (1.6%); dizziness (1.4%); abdominal pain (1.3%); chest pain (1.3%); edema (1.2%); anxiety (1.2%); rhinitis (1.2%); and dyspnea (1.1%).

Additional adverse systemic clinical events reported in 1.0% or less of the patients are listed below within each body system:

Autonomic Nervous System: hypotension, ileus, syncope

Body as a Whole: rigors, back pain, malaise

Cardiovascular: tachycardia, including supraventricular and ventricular; bradycardia; arrhythmia, including atrial fibrillation, ventricular fibrillation, cardiac arrest, cardiac failure, circulatory failure, myocardial infarction.

Central Nervous System: tremor, convulsions, vertigo

Gastrointestinal: melena, flatulence, hemorrhage, gastritis, hiccough, ulcerative stomatitis

Pseudomembranous colitis was reported in one patient during the clinical trials. The onset of pseudomembranous colitis symptoms may occur during or after antibacterial treatment. (See *"Warnings"*.)

Hearing: tinnitus

Hypersensitivity: anaphylaxis

Metabolic and Nutritional: symptomatic hypoglycemia, thirst

Musculoskeletal: myalgia, arthralgia

Platelet, Bleeding, Clotting: mesenteric embolism, purpura, epistaxis, pulmonary embolism (See *"Precautions—General"*.)

Psychiatric: confusion, hallucination, depression

Reproductive, Female: Leukorrhea, vaginitis

Respiratory: pharyngitis, pulmonary edema, bronchospasm, coughing

Skin and Appendages: genital pruritus, diaphoresis

Special Senses: taste perversion

Urinary: retention, dysuria, oliguria, hematuria, incontinence

Vision: photophobia

Vascular (extracardiac): flushing

Adverse Laboratory Events: Changes in laboratory parameters, without regard to drug relationship, including:

Hematologic: Decreases in hemoglobin and hematocrit, thrombocytopenia, increases in platelet count, eosinophilia, leukopenia, neutropenia. The leukopenia/neutropenia associated with Piperacillin Sodium/Tazobactam Sodium administration appears to be reversible and most frequently associated with prolonged administration, i.e., ≥ 21 days of therapy. These patients were withdrawn from therapy; some had accompanying systemic symptoms (e.g., fever, rigors, chills).

Coagulation: Positive direct Coombs' test, prolonged prothrombin time, prolonged partial thromboplastin time

Hepatic: Transient elevations of AST (SGOT), ALT (SGPT), alkaline phosphatase, bilirubin

Renal: Increases in serum creatinine, blood urea nitrogen

Urinalysis: Proteinuria, hematuria, pyuria

Additional laboratory events include abnormalities in electrolytes (i.e., increases and decreases in sodium, potassium, and calcium), hyperglycemia, decreases in total protein or albumin

The following adverse reactions have also been reported for Piperacillin Sodium.

Skin and Appendages: Erythema multiforme and Stevens-Johnson syndrome, rarely reported.

Gastrointestinal: Cholestatic hepatitis

Renal: Rarely, interstitial nephritis

Skeletal: Prolonged muscle relaxation (See *"Precautions—Drug Interactions"*.)

OVERDOSAGE

Information on overdosage of Piperacillin Sodium/Tazobactam Sodium in humans is not available. Excessive serum levels of either Piperacillin or Tazobactam may be reduced by hemodialysis. (See *"Clinical Pharmacology"*.) No specific antidote is known. As with other penicillins, neuromuscular excitability or convulsions have occurred following large intravenous doses, primarily in patients with impaired renal function.

In the case of motor excitability or convulsions, general supportive measures, including administration of anticonvulsive agents (e.g., diazepam or barbiturates) may be considered.

DOSAGE AND ADMINISTRATION

Piperacillin Sodium/Tazobactam Sodium should be administered by intravenous infusion over 30 minutes.

The usual total daily dose of Piperacillin Sodium/Tazobactam Sodium for adults is 12 g/1.5 g, given as 3.375 g every six hours.

Renal Insufficiency: In patients with renal insufficiency, the intravenous dose should be adjusted to the degree of actual renal function impairment. The recommended daily doses are as follows:

PIPERACILLIN SODIUM/TAZOBACTAM SODIUM
DOSAGE RECOMMENDATIONS

Creatinine Clearance (mL/min)	Recommended Dosage Regimen
> 40	12 g/1.5 g/day in divided doses of 3.375 g q6h
20-40	8 g/1.0 g/day in divided doses of 2.25 g q6h
< 20	6 g/0.75 g/day in divided doses of 2.25 g q8h

For patients on hemodialysis, the maximum dose is 2.25 g Piperacillin Sodium/Tazobactam Sodium q8h. In addition, because hemodialysis removes 30%-40% of a Piperacillin Sodium/Tazobactam Sodium dose in four hours, one additional dose of 0.75 g Piperacillin Sodium/Tazobactam Sodium should be administered following each dialysis period. For patients with renal failure, measurement of serum levels of Piperacillin and Tazobactam will provide additional guidance for adjusting dosage.

Duration of Therapy: The usual duration of Piperacillin Sodium/Tazobactam Sodium treatment is from seven to ten days. The duration should be guided by the severity of the infection and the patient's clinical and bacteriological progress.

Intravenous Administration: Reconstitute Piperacillin Sodium/Tazobactam Sodium per gram of Piperacillin with 5 mL of a suitable diluent from the list provided below. Shake well until dissolved. Single dose vials should be used immediately after reconstitution. Discard any unused portion after 24 hours if stored at room temperature, or after 48 hours if stored at refrigerated temperature [2 to 8°C (36 to 46°F)]. It may be further diluted to the desired final volume with the diluent.

Compatible Intravenous Diluents:
0.9% Sodium Chloride for Injection
Sterile Water for Injection
Dextran 6% in Saline

Dextrose 5%
Potassium Chloride 40 mEq
Bacteriostatic Saline/Parabens
Bacteriostatic Water/Parabens
Bacteriostatic Saline/Benzyl Alcohol
Bacteriostatic Water/Benzyl Alcohol

Lactated Ringers Solution Is Not Compatible With Piperacillin Sodium/Tazobactam Sodium.

Intermittent Intravenous Infusion—Reconstitute as previously described with 5 mL of an acceptable diluent per 1 gram of Piperacillin and then further dilute in the desired volume (at least 50 mL). Administer by infusion over a period of at least 30 minutes. During the infusion it is desirable to discontinue the primary infusion solution.

When concomitant therapy with aminoglycosides is indicated, Piperacillin Sodium/Tazobactam Sodium and the aminoglycoside should be reconstituted and administered separately, due to the *in vitro* inactivation of the aminoglycoside by the penicillin. (See *"Precautions"—Drug Interactions*.)

Piperacillin Sodium/Tazobactam Sodium can be used in ambulatory intravenous infusion pumps.

Stability of Piperacillin Sodium/Tazobactam Sodium Following Reconstitution: Piperacillin Sodium/Tazobactam Sodium is stable in glass and plastic containers (plastic syringes, I.V. bags, and tubing) when reconstituted with acceptable diluents.

Stability studies in the I.V. bags have demonstrated chemical stability (potency, pH of reconstituted solution, and clarity of solution) for up to 24 hours at room temperature and up to one week at refrigerated temperature. Piperacillin Sodium/Tazobactam Sodium contains no preservatives. Appropriate consideration of aseptic technique should be used.

Stability of Piperacillin Sodium/Tazobactam Sodium in an ambulatory intravenous infusion pump has been demonstrated for a period of 12 hours at room temperature. Each dose was reconstituted and diluted to a volume of 37.5 mL or 25 mL. One-day supplies of dosing solution were aseptically transferred into the medication reservoir (I.V. bags or cartridge). The reservoir was fitted to a preprogrammed ambulatory intravenous infusion pump per the manufacturer's instructions. Stability of Piperacillin Sodium/Tazobactam Sodium is not affected when administered using an ambulatory intravenous infusion pump.

Parenteral drug products should be inspected visually for particulate matter and discoloration prior to administration, whenever solution and container permit.

Piperacillin Sodium/Tazobactam Sodium vials should be stored at controlled room temperature 15° to 30°C (59° to 86°F) prior to reconstitution.

REFERENCES

1. National Committee for Clinical Laboratory Standards, Performance Standard for Antimicrobial Disk Susceptibility Tests—Fourth Edition. Approved Standard NCCLS Document M2-A4, Vol. 10, No. 7, NCCLS, Villanova, PA, April, 1990. 2. National Committee for Clinical Laboratory Standards, Methods for Dilution Antimicrobial Susceptibility Tests for Bacteria that Grow Aerobically—Second Edition. Approved Standard NCCLS Document M7-A2, Vol. 10, No. 8, NCCLS, Villanova, PA, April, 1990. 3. National Committee for Clinical Laboratory Standards, Methods for Antimicrobial Susceptibility Testing for Anaerobic Bacteria—Second Edition. Approved Standard NCCLS Document M11-A2, Vol. 10, No. 15, NCCLS, Villanova, PA, December, 1990. 4. National Committee For Clinical Laboratory Standards, Performance Standard for Antimicrobial Susceptibility Testing; Fourth Informational Supplement, Approved Standard NCCLS Document M100-S4 (ISBN 1-56238-136-9), NCCLS, Villanova, PA, 1992. 5. Halstenson CE, Hirata CAI, Heim-Duthoy KL, Abraham PA, and Matzke GR. Effect of concomitant administration of piperacillin on the dispositions of netilmicin and tobramycin in patients with end-stage renal disease. Antimicrob Agents Chemother. 34(1):128-133, 1990.

HOW SUPPLIED
POWDER FOR INJECTION: 2 GM-0.25 GM

BRAND/MANUFACTURER	NDC	SIZE	AWP
◇ BRAND			
ZOSYN: Lederle Labs	00206-8452-16	10s	$98.71

POWDER FOR INJECTION: 3 GM-0.375 GM

BRAND/MANUFACTURER	NDC	SIZE	AWP
◇ BRAND			
ZOSYN: Lederle Labs	00206-8454-55	10s	$148.06

POWDER FOR INJECTION: 4 GM-0.5 GM

BRAND/MANUFACTURER	NDC	SIZE	AWP
◇ BRAND			
ZOSYN: Lederle Labs	00206-8455-25	10s	$197.43

POWDER FOR INJECTION: 36 GM-4.5 GM

BRAND/MANUFACTURER	NDC	SIZE	AWP
◇ BRAND			
ZOSYN: Lederle Labs	00206-8620-11	1s	$177.70

◆ RATED THERAPEUTICALLY EQUIVALENT; ◇ THERAPEUTIC EQUIVALENCE UNCONFIRMED; ○ UNRATED

Pipobroman

DESCRIPTION

Pipobroman is a neutral amide chemically designated as 1,4-bis (3-bromopropionyl) piperazine.

Pipobroman is an oral antineoplastic agent available as tablets containing 25 mg of Pipobroman.

Following is its chemical structure:

$$BrCH_2CH_2C-N \qquad N-CCH_2CH_2Br$$

CLINICAL PHARMACOLOGY

The mechanism of action of Pipobroman is not known; however, it has been classified as an alkylating agent. Pipobroman is readily absorbed from the gastrointestinal tract following oral administration. The metabolic fate and route of excretion are unknown.

INDICATIONS AND USAGE

Pipobroman is indicated primarily in the treatment of polycythemia vera. Pipobroman has also been found to be useful in the treatment of chronic granulocytic leukemia. Because of wider experience with its use, busulfan is the preferred agent in chemotherapy of chronic granulocytic leukemia. However, Pipobroman may be especially helpful in patients who are refractory to busulfan.

CONTRAINDICATIONS

Since it frequently causes bone marrow depression, Pipobroman should not be administered to patients with bone marrow depression resulting from x-ray or cytotoxic chemotherapy.

WARNINGS

Depression of the bone marrow may not occur for four weeks, or more, after treatment is initiated. The most reliable guide to the activity of the bone marrow is provided by the leukocyte count, but the platelet count also provides a good index to bone marrow activity. If the leukocyte count falls to 3000 or less, or if the platelet count is reduced to 150,000 or less, the drug should be temporarily discontinued. Therapy may be cautiously reinstated when the leukocyte or platelet count has risen.

A dose dependent anemia, which usually responds to blood transfusions and reduction dosage, frequently develops. However, a rapid drop in hemoglobin, increased bilirubin levels, and reticulocytosis suggest a hemolytic process, in which case the drug should be discontinued.

Usage in Pregancy: Pregnancy Category D. Alkylating agents may cause fetal harm when administered to a pregnant woman. Pipobroman has been shown to be teratogenic in mice at doses of 60 mg/kg and in rats at doses of 30 mg/kg when administered during the organogenetic period. There are no adequate and well-controlled studies in pregnant women. If this drug is used during pregnancy, or if the patient becomes pregnant while taking this drug, the patient should be apprised of the potential hazard to the fetus. Women of childbearing potential should be advised to avoid becoming pregnant.

PRECAUTIONS

General: It is advisable to initiate therapy in the hospital where patients can be more closely observed, especially during the initial course of treatment.

Information for Patients: Patients should be instructed to report promptly the development of fever, sore throat, signs of local infection, easy bruising, bleeding from any site or symptoms suggestive of anemia.

Laboratory Test: Bone marrow study should be performed prior to therapy and again at the time of maximal hematologic response. Complete blood counts once or twice weekly, and leukocyte counts every other day, should be done until the desired response is obtained or until significant toxic effects intervene.

Ancillary laboratory determinations, including liver and kidney function tests, should be performed prior to therapy and periodically thereafter.

Drug Interactions: Although specific drug interactions have not been reported with Pipobroman, drug interactions should be considered whenever antineoplastic agents are used.

Caution should be observed when Pipobroman and *other antineoplastic agents* are used concomitantly since the risk of bone marrow damage is increased.

Carcinogenesis, Mutagenesis, Impairment of Fertility: Studies have not been conducted with Pipobroman to determine long-term potential for carcinogenicity in animals or humans. Other alkylating agents have been shown to be carcinogenic in animals and have been associated with an increased risk of development of secondary malignant neoplasms, especially leukemia, in humans.

Alkylating agents have been reported to cause alterations in sperm cells which could result in mutagenicity and teratogenicity.

Pregnancy: Pregnancy Category D. See *"Warnings"* section.

Nursing Mothers: It is not known whether this drug is excreted in human milk. Because many drugs are excreted in human milk and because of the potential for serious adverse reactions in nursing infants from Pipobroman, a decision should be made whether to discontinue nursing or to discontinue the drug, taking into account the importance of the drug to the mother.

Pediatric Use: Safety and effectiveness in children below the age of 15 years have not been established.

ADVERSE REACTIONS

The adverse reactions that have been reported in decreasing order of severity are: bone marrow depression resulting in leukopenia, thrombocytopenia and anemia (see *"Warnings"* section); vomiting, diarrhea, nausea, abdominal cramping and skin rash.

OVERDOSAGE

There is no known antidote to Pipobroman. No reports of overdose with this compound have been received. The principal toxic effect is on the bone marrow; however, hematologic toxicity is likely to be more profound with chronic overdosage. The hematologic status should be closely monitored and vigorous supportive measures instituted if necessary.

DOSAGE AND ADMINISTRATION

Pipobroman is administered orally in divided daily doses. Maintenance doses should be adjusted to the response of the patient.

Polycythemia Vera: For the treatment of polycythemia vera the recommended initial dose is 1 mg/kg/day. Larger doses (1.5 to 3 mg/kg/day) may be required in patients who have been refractory to other treatment, but such doses should not be used until a dose of 1 mg/kg/day has been given for at least 30 days without improvement. Maintenance therapy is usually initiated when the hematocrit has been reduced to 50-55%. Maintenance dosage in patients with polycythemia vera ranges from 0.1 to 0.2 mg/kg/day.

Chronic Granulocytic Leukemia: For the treatment of chronic granulocytic leukemia the recommended initial dose ranges from 1.5 to 2.5 mg/kg/day. This dosage is generally continued until a maximal clinical or hematologic response is obtained. If the leukocyte count falls too rapidly, the drug should be discontinued until the rate of decrease levels off. Maintenance therapy is usually started as the leukocyte count approaches 10,000. If relapse is rapid (doubling of leukocyte count within 70 days), continuous treatment is indicated. Intermittent therapy is generally adequate if more than 70 days are required to double the leukocyte count. The maintenance dose ranges from about 7 mg daily (50 mg weekly) to 175 mg daily.

Therapy of the foregoing conditions should be continued as long as needed to maintain satisfactory clinical response.

Procedures for proper handling and disposal of anticancer drugs should be considered. Several guidelines on this subject have been published.[1-6] There is no general agreement that all of the procedures recommended in the guidelines are necessary or appropriate.

Storage: Store below 86°F (30°C).

REFERENCES

1. Recommendations for the Safe Handling of Parenteral Antineoplastic Drugs, NIH Publication No. 83-2621. For sale by the Superintendent of Documents, U.S. Government Printing Office, Washington, D.C. 20402. 2. AMA Council Report, Guidelines for Handling Parenteral Antineoplastics, *JAMA* 253(11): 1590-1592, March 15, 1985. 3. National Study Commission on Cytotoxic Exposure—Recommendations for Handling Cytotoxic Agents. Available from Louis P. Jeffrey, Sc. D., Director of Pharmacy Services, Rhode Island Hospital, 593 Eddy Street, Providence, RI 02902. 4. Clinical Oncological Society of Australia: Guidelines and Recommendations for Safe Handling of Antineoplastic Agents, *Med J Aust* 1(9):426-428, April 30, 1983. 5. Jones, R. B., *et al.*, Safe Handling of Chemotherapeutic Agents: A Report From the Mount Sinai Medical Center, *Ca-A Cancer Journal for Clinicians*, 258-263, Sept/Oct 1983. 6. American Society of Hospital Pharmacists Technical Assistance Bulletin on Handling cytotoxic Drugs in Hospital, *Am J Hosp Pharm* 42(1):131-137, January 1985.

HOW SUPPLIED
TABLETS: 25 MG

BRAND/MANUFACTURER	NDC	SIZE	AWP
○ BRAND			
VERCYTE: Abbott Pharm	00074-7363-01	100s	$57.98

Pipracil SEE PIPERACILLIN SODIUM

Pirbuterol Acetate

DESCRIPTION

The active component of Pirbuterol Acetate Inhaler is α^6-{[(1,1-dimethylethyl)amino]methyl}-3-hydroxy-2,6-pyridine- dimethanol monoacetate salt, a beta-2 adrenergic bronchodilator.

Pirbuterol Acetate is a white, crystalline, racemic mixture of two optically active isomers. It is a powder, freely soluble in water, with a molecular weight of 300.3 and empirical formula of $C_{12}H_{20}N_2O_3 \cdot C_2H_4O_2$.

Pirbuterol Acetate inhaler is a metered dose aerosol unit for oral inhalation. It provides a fine-particle suspension of Pirbuterol Acetate in a propellant.

Each actuation delivers from the mouthpiece Pirbuterol Acetate equivalent to 0.2 mg of Pirbuterol.

Some units are breath-actuated so that the medication is delivered automatically during inspiration without the need for the patient to coordinate actuation with inspiration.

Following is its chemical structure:

CLINICAL PHARMACOLOGY

In vitro studies and *in vivo* pharmacologic studies have demonstrated that Pirbuterol Acetate has a preferential effect on beta-2 adrenergic receptors compared with isoproterenol. While it is recognized that beta-2 adrenergic receptors are the predominant receptors in bronchial smooth mucle, recent data indicate that there is a population of beta-2 receptors in the human heart, existing in a concentration between 10-50%. The precise function of these, however, is not yet established (see WARNINGS section).

The pharmacologic effects of beta adrenergic agonist drugs, including Pirbuterol Acetate, are at least in part attributable to stimulation through beta adrenergic receptors of intracellular adenyl cyclase, the enzyme which catalyzes the conversion of adenosine triphosphate (ATP) to cyclic-3',5'-adenosine monophosphate (c-AMP). Increased c-AMP levels are associated with relaxation of bronchial smooth muscle and inhibition of release of mediators of immediate hypersensitivity from cells, especially from mast cells.

Bronchodilator activity of Pirbuterol Acetate was manifested clinically by an improvement in various pulmonary function parameters (FEV_1, MMF, PEFR, airway resistance [RAW] and conductance [GA/V_{tg}]).

In controlled double-blind single dose clinical trials, the onset of improvement in pulmonary function occurred within 5 minutes in most patients as determined by forced expiratory volume in one second (FEV_1). FEV_1 and MMF measurements also showed that maximum improvement in pulmonary function generally occurred 30-60 minutes following one (1) or two (2) inhalations of Pirbuterol (0.2-0.4 mg).

The duration of action of Pirbuterol Acetate is maintained for 5 hours (the time at which the last observations were made) in a substantial number of patients, based on a 15% or greater increase in FEV_1. In controlled repetitive dose studies of 12 weeks duration, 74% of 156 patients on Pirbuterol and 62% of 141 patients on metaproterenol showed a clinically significant improvement based on a 15% or greater increase in FEV_1 on at least half of the days. Onset and duration were equivalent to that seen in single dose studies. Continued effectiveness was demonstrated over the 12-week period in the majority (94%) of responding patients; however, chronic dosing was associated with the development of tachyphylaxis (tolerance) to the bronchodilator effect in some patients in both treatment groups.

A placebo-controlled double-blind single dose study (24 patients per treatment group), utilizing continuous Holter monitoring for 5 hours after drug administration, showed no significant difference in ectopic activity between the placebo control group and Pirbuterol Acetate at the recommended dose (0.2-0.4 mg), and twice the recommended dose (0.8 mg). As with other inhaled beta adrenergic agonists, supraventrieular and ventricular ectopic beats have been seen with Pirbuterol Acetate (see *"Warnings"*).

Recent studies in laboratory animals (minipigs, rodents, and dogs) recorded the occurrence of cardiac arrhythmias and sudden death (with histologic evidence of myocardial necrosis) when beta agonists and methylxanthines were administered concurrently. The significance of these findings when applied to humans is currently unknown.

Two randomized, double-blind, cross-over studies in a total of 97 patients, have compared the clinical effects of either one inhalation or two inhalations of the Pirbuterol formulations in the breath-actuated inhaler and the conventional inhaler and demonstrated no significant difference between the formulations for the means of peak changes in FEV_1, time to peak FEV_1, onset, duration, or area under the FEV_1 curve.

PHARMACOKINETICS

As expected by extrapolation from oral data, systemic blood levels of Pirbuterol are below the limit of assay sensitivity (2-5 ng/ml) following inhalation of doses up to 0.8 mg (twice the maximum recommended dose). A mean of 51% of the dose is recovered in urine as Pirbuterol plus its sulfate conjugate following administration by aerosol. Pirbuterol is not metabolized by catechol-O-methyltransferase. The percent of administered dose recovered as Pirbuterol plus its sulfate conjugate does not change significantly over the dose range of 0.4 mg to 0.8 mg and is not significantly different from that after oral administration of Pirbuterol. The plasma half-life measured after oral administration is about two hours.

INDICATIONS AND USAGE

Pirbuterol Acetate inhaler is indicated for the prevention and reversal of bronchospasm in patients with reversible bronchospasm including asthma. It may be used with or without concurrent theophylline and/or steroid therapy.

CONTRAINDICATIONS

Pirbuterol Acetate is contraindicated in patients with a history of hypersensitivity to any of its ingredients.

WARNINGS

As with other beta adrenergic aerosols, Pirbuterol Acetate should not be used in excess. Controlled clinical studies and other clinical experience have shown that Pirbuterol Acetate like other inhaled beta adrenergic agonists, can produce a significant cardiovascular effect in some patients, as measured by pulse rate, blood pressure, symptoms, and/or ECG changes. As with other beta adrenergic aerosols, the potential for paradoxical bronchospasm (which can be life threatening) should be kept in mind. If it occurs, the preparation should be discontinued immediately and alternative therapy instituted.

Fatalities have been reported in association with excessive use of inhaled sympathomimetic drugs.

The contents of Pirbuterol Acetate inhaler are under pressure. Do not puncture. Do not use or store near heat or open flame. Exposure to temperature above 120° F may cause bursting. Never throw container into fire or incinerator. Keep out of reach of children.

PRECAUTIONS

GENERAL

Since Pirbuterol is a sympathomimetic amine, it should be used with caution in patients with cardiovascular disorders, including ischemic heart disease, hypertension, or cardiac arrhythmias, in patients with hyperthyroidism or diabetes mellitus, and in patients who are unusually responsive to sympathomimetic amines or who have convulsive disorders. Significant changes in systolic and diastolic blood pressure could be expected to occur in some patients after use of any beta adrenergic aerosol bronchodilator.

INFORMATION FOR PATIENTS

Pirbuterol Acetate effects may last up to five hours or longer. It should not be used more often than recommended and the patient should not increase the number of inhalations or frequency of use without first asking the physician. If symptoms of asthma get worse, adverse reactions occur, or the patient does not respond to the usual dose, the patient should be instructed to contact the physician immediately.

The breath-actuated inhaler should not be used with any other inhalation aerosol canister. In addition, canisters for use with the breath-actuated inhaler should not be utilized with any other actuator.

DRUG INTERACTIONS

Other beta adrenergic aerosol bronchodilators should not be used concomitantly with Pirbuterol Acetate because they may have additive effects. Beta adrenergic agonists should be administered with caution to patients being treated with monoamine oxidase inhibitors or tricyclic antidepressants, since the action of beta adrenergic agonists on the vascular system may be potentiated.

CARCINOGENESIS, MUTAGENESIS AND IMPAIRMENT OF FERTILITY

Pirbuterol hydrochloride administered in the diet to rats for 24 months and to mice for 18 months was free of carcinogenic activity at doses corresponding to 200 times the maximum human inhalation dose. In addition, the intragastric intubation of the drug at doses corresponding to 6250 times the maximum recommended human daily inhalation dose resulted in no increase in tumors in a 12-month rat study. Studies with Pirbuterol revealed no evidence of mutagenesis. Reproduction studies in rats revealed no evidence of impaired fertility.

TERATOGENIC EFFECTS—PREGNANCY CATEGORY C

Reproduction studies have been performed in rats and rabbits by the inhalation route at doses up to 12 times (rat) and 16 times (rabbit) the maximum human inhalation dose and have revealed no significant findings. Animal reproduction studies in rats at *oral doses* up to 300 mg/kg and in rabbits at oral doses up to 100 mg/kg have shown no adverse effect on reproductive behavior, fertility, litter size, peri- and postnatal viability or fetal development. In rabbits at the highest dose level given, 300 mg/kg, abortions and fetal mortality were observed. There are no adequate and well controlled studies in pregnant women and Pirbuterol Acetate should be used during pregnancy only if the potential benefit justifies the potential risk to the fetus.

NURSING MOTHERS

It is not known whether Pirbuterol Acetate is excreted in human milk. Therefore, Pirbuterol Acetate should be used during nursing only if the potential benefit justifies the possible risk to the newborn.

PEDIATRIC USE

Pirbuterol Acetate inhaler is not recommended for patients under the age of 12 years because of insufficient clinical data to establish safety and effectiveness.

ADVERSE REACTIONS

The following rates of adverse reactions to Pirbuterol are based on single and multiple dose clinical trials involving 761 patients, 400 of whom received multiple doses (mean duration of treatment was 2.5 months and maximum was 19 months).

The following were the adverse reactions reported more frequently than 1 in 100 patients:

CNS: nervousness (6.9%), tremor (6.0%), headache (2.0%), dizziness (1.2%).

Cardiovascular: palpitations (1.7%), tachycardia (1.2%).

Respiratory: cough (1.2%).

Gastrointestinal: nausea (1.7%).

The following adverse reactions occurred less frequently than 1 in 100 patients and there may be a causal relationship with Pirbuterol:

CNS: depression, anxiety, confusion, insomnia, weakness, hyperkinesia, syncope.

Cardiovascular: hypotension, skipped beats, chest pain.

◆ RATED THERAPEUTICALLY EQUIVALENT; ◇ THERAPEUTIC EQUIVALENCE UNCONFIRMED; ○ UNRATED

Gastrointestinal: dry mouth, glossitis, abdominal pain/cramps, anorexia, diarrhea, stomatitis, nausea and vomiting.

Ear, Nose and Throat: smell/taste changes, sore throat.

Dermatological: rash, pruritus.

Other: numbness in extremities, alopecia, bruising, fatigue, edema, weight gain, flushing.

Other adverse reactions were reported with a frequency of less than 1 in 100 patients but a causal relationship between Pirbuterol and the reaction could not be determined: migraine, productive cough, wheezing, and dermatitis.

The following rates of adverse reactions during three-month controlled clinical trials involving 310 patients are noted. The table does not include mild reactions.

PERCENT OF PATIENTS WITH MODERATE TO SEVERE ADVERSE REACTIONS

Reaction	Pirbuterol N = 157	Metaproterenol N = 153
Central Nervous System		
tremors	1.3%	3.3%
nervousness	4.5%	2.6%
headache	1.3%	2.0%
weakness	.0%	1.3%
drowsiness	.0%	0.7%
dizziness	0.6%	.0%
Cardiovascular		
palpitations	1.3%	1.3%
tachycardia	1.3%	2.0%
Respiratory		
chest pain/tightness	1.3%	.0%
cough	.0%	0.7%
Gastrointestinal		
nausea	1.3%	2.0%
diarrhea	1.3%	0.7%
dry mouth	1.3%	1.3%
vomiting	.0%	0.7%
Dermatological		
skin reaction	.0%	0.7%
rash	.0%	1.3%
Other		
bruising	0.6%	.0%
smell/taste change	0.6%	.0%
backache	.0%	0.7%
fatigue	.0%	0.7%
hoarseness	.0%	0.7%
nasal congestion	.0%	0.7%

OVERDOSAGE

The expected symptoms with overdosage are those of excessive beta-stimulation and/or any of the symptoms listed under adverse reactions, e.g., angina, hypertension or hypotension, arrhythmias, nervousness, headache, tremor, dry mouth, palpitation, nausea, dizziness, fatigue, malaise, and insomnia.

Treatment consists of discontinuation of Pirbuterol together with appropriate symptomatic therapy.

The oral acute lethal dose in male and female rats and mice was greater than 2000 mg base/kg. The aerosol acute lethal dose was not determined.

DOSAGE AND ADMINISTRATION

The usual dose for adults and children 12 years and older is two inhalations (0.4 mg), repeated every 4-6 hours. One inhalation (0.2 mg), repeated every 4-6 hours may be sufficient for some patients.

A total daily dose of 12 inhalations should not be exceeded. If a previously effective dosage regimen fails to provide the usual relief, medical advice should be sought immediately, as this is often a sign of seriously worsening asthma which would require reassessment of therapy.

Store between 15° and 30°C (59° to 86°F).

HOW SUPPLIED
AEROSOL SOLID W/ADAPTER: 0.2 MG/INH

BRAND/MANUFACTURER	NDC	SIZE	AWP
○ **BRAND**			
MAXAIR AUTOHALER: 3M Pharm	00089-0817-10	2.8 gm	$9.24
	00089-0815-21	14 gm	$32.82
MAXAIR: 3M Pharm	00089-0790-21	25.6 gm	$23.04

Piroxicam

DESCRIPTION

Piroxicam is 4-Hydroxy-2-methyl-N-2-pyridinyl-2H-1,2-benzothiazine-3-carboxamide 1,1-dioxide, an oxicam. Members of the oxicam family are not carboxylic acids, but they are acidic by virtue of the enolic 4-hydroxy substituent. Piroxicam occurs as a white crystalline solid, sparingly soluble in water, dilute acid and most organic solvents. It is slightly soluble in alcohols and in aqueous alkaline solution.

It exhibits a weakly acidic 4-hydroxy proton (pKa 5.1) and a weakly basic pyridyl nitrogen (pKa 1.8).

Following is its chemical structure:

CLINICAL PHARMACOLOGY

Piroxicam has shown anti-inflammatory, analgesic and antipyretic properties in animals. Edema, erythema, tissue proliferation, fever, and pain can all be inhibited in laboratory animals by the administration of Piroxicam. It is effective regardless of the etiology of the inflammation. The mode of action of Piroxicam is not fully established at this time. However, a common mechanism for the above effects may exist in the ability of Piroxicam to inhibit the biosynthesis of prostaglandins, known mediators of inflammation.

It is established that Piroxicam does not act by stimulating the pituitary-adrenal axis.

Piroxicam is well absorbed following oral administration. Drug plasma concentrations are proportional for 10 and 20 mg doses, generally peak within three to five hours after medication, and subsequently decline with a mean half-life of 50 hours (range of 30 to 86 hours, although values outside of this range have been encountered).

This prolonged half-life results in the maintenance of relatively stable plasma concentrations throughout the day on once daily doses and to significant drug accumulation upon multiple dosing. A single 20 mg dose generally produces peak Piroxicam plasma levels of 1.5 to 2 mcg/mL, while maximum drug plasma concentrations, after repeated daily ingestion of 20 mg Piroxicam, usually stabilize at 3-8 mcg/mL. Most patients approximate steady state plasma levels within 7 to 12 days. Higher levels, which approximate steady state at two to three weeks, have been observed in patients in whom longer plasma half-lives of Piroxicam occurred.

Piroxicam and its biotransformation products are excreted in urine and feces, with about twice as much appearing in the urine as the feces. Metabolism occurs by hydroxylation at the 5 position of the pyridyl side chain and conjugation of this product; by cyclodehydration; and by a sequence of reactions involving hydrolysis of the amide linkage, decarboxylation, ring contraction, and N-demethylation. Less than 5% of the daily dose is excreted unchanged.

Concurrent administration of aspirin (3900 mg/day) and Piroxicam (20 mg/day) resulted in a reduction of plasma levels of Piroxicam to about 80% of their normal values. The use of Piroxicam in conjunction with aspirin is not recommended because data are inadequate to demonstrate that the combination produces greater improvement than that achieved with aspirin alone and the potential for adverse reactions is increased. Concomitant administration of antacids had no effect on Piroxicam plasma levels. The effects of impaired renal function or hepatic disease on plasma levels have not been established.

Piroxicam, like salicylates and other nonsteroidal anti-inflammatory agents, is associated with symptoms of gastrointestinal tract irritation (see *"Adverse Reactions"*). However, in a study utilizing ^{51}Cr-tagged red blood cells, 20 mg of Piroxicam administered as a single dose for four days did not result in a significant increase in fecal blood loss and did not detectably affect the gastric mucosa. In the same study a total daily dose of 3900 mg of aspirin, i.e., 972 mg q.i.d., caused a significant increase in fecal blood loss and mucosal lesions as demonstrated by gastroscopy.

In controlled clinical trials, the effectiveness of Piroxicam has been established for both acute exacerbations and long-term management of rheumatoid arthritis and osteoarthritis.

The therapeutic effects of Piroxicam are evident early in the treatment of both diseases with a progressive increase in response over several (8-12) weeks. Efficacy is seen in terms of pain relief and, when present, subsidence of inflammation. Doses of 20 mg/day Piroxicam display a therapeutic effect comparable to therapeutic doses of aspirin, with a lower incidence of minor gastrointestinal effects and tinnitus.

Piroxicam has been administered concomitantly with fixed doses of gold and corticosteroids. The existence of a "steroid-sparing" effect has not been adequately studied to date.

INDICATIONS AND USAGE

Piroxicam is indicated for acute or long-term use in the relief of signs and symptoms of the following:

1. osteoarthritis
2. rheumatoid arthritis

Dosage recommendations for use in children have not been established.

UNLABELED USES
Piroxicam is used alone or as an adjunct in the treatment of ankylosing spondylitis, dysmenorrhea, gout, and pain.

CONTRAINDICATIONS

Piroxicam should not be used in patients who have previously exhibited hypersensitivity to it, or in individuals with the syndrome comprised of bronchospasm, nasal polyps, and angioedema precipitated by aspirin or other nonsteroidal anti-inflammatory drugs.

➤ SHOWN IN PRODUCT IDENTIFICATION GUIDE

WARNINGS

RISK OF GI ULCERATION, BLEEDING AND PERFORATION WITH NSAID THERAPY

Serious gastrointestinal toxicity such as bleeding, ulceration, and perforation can occur at any time, with or without warning symptoms, in patients treated chronically with NSAID therapy. Although minor upper gastrointestinal problems, such as dyspepsia, are common, usually developing early in therapy, physician should remain alert for ulceration and bleeding in patients treated chronically with NSAIDs even in the absence of previous GI tract symptoms. In patients observed in clinical trials of several months to two years duration, symptomatic upper GI ulcers, gross bleeding or perforation appear to occur in approximately 1% of patients treated for 3-6 months, and in about 2-4% of patients treated for one year. Physicians should inform patients about the signs and/or symptoms of serious GI toxicity and what steps to take if they occur.

Studies to date have not identified any subset of patients not at risk of developing peptic ulceration and bleeding. Except for a prior history of serious GI events and other risk factors known to be associated with peptic ulcer disease, such as alcoholism, smoking, etc., no risk factors (e.g., age, sex) have been associated with increased risk. Elderly or debilitated patients seem to tolerate ulceration or bleeding less well than other individuals and most spontaneous reports of fatal GI events are in this population. Studies to date are inconclusive concerning the relative risk of various NSAIDs in causing such reactions. High doses of any NSAID probably carry a greater risk of these reactions, although controlled clinical trials showing this do not exist in most cases. In considering the use of relatively large doses (within the recommended dosage range), sufficient benefit should be anticipated to offset the potential increased risk of GI toxicity.

PRECAUTIONS

Renal Effects: As with other nonsteroidal anti-inflammatory drugs, long-term administration of Piroxicam to animals has resulted in renal papillary necrosis and other abnormal renal pathology. In humans, there have been reports of acute interstitial nephritis with hematuria, proteinuria, and occasionally nephrotic syndrome.

A second form of renal toxicity has been seen in patients with prerenal conditions leading to a reduction in renal blood flow or blood volume, where the renal prostaglandins have a supportive role in the maintenance of renal perfusion. In these patients administration of an NSAID may cause a dose-dependent reduction in prostaglandin formation and may precipitate overt renal decompensation. Patients at greatest risk of this reaction are those with impaired renal function, heart failure, liver dysfunction, those taking diuretics, and the elderly. Discontinuation of NSAID therapy is typically followed by recovery to the pretreatment state. Because of extensive renal excretion of Piroxicam and its biotransformation products (less than 5% of the daily dose excreted unchanged, see *"Clinical Pharmacology"*), lower doses of Piroxicam should be anticipated in patients with impaired renal function, and they should be carefully monitored.

Although other nonsteroidal anti-inflammatory drugs do not have the same direct effects on platelets that aspirin does, all drugs inhibiting prostaglandin biosynthesis do interfere with platelet function to some degree; therefore, patients who may be adversely affected by such an action should be carefully observed when Piroxicam is administered.

Because of reports of adverse eye findings with nonsteroidal anti-inflammatory agents, it is recommended that patients who develop visual complaints during treatment with Piroxicam have ophthalmic evaluation.

As with other nonsteroidal anti-inflammatory drugs, borderline elevations of one or more liver tests may occur in up to 15% of patients. These abnormalities may progress, may remain essentially unchanged, or may be transient with continued therapy. The SGPT (ALT) test is probably the most sensitive indicator of liver dysfunction. Meaningful (3 times the upper limit of normal) elevations of SGPT or SGOT (AST) occurred in controlled clinical trials in less than 1% of patients. A patient with symptoms and/or signs suggesting liver dysfunction, or in whom an abnormal liver test has occurred, should be evaluated for evidence of the development of more severe hepatic reaction while on therapy with Piroxicam. Severe hepatic reactions, including jaundice and cases of fatal hepatitis, have been reported with Piroxicam. Although such reactions are rare, if abnormal liver tests persist or worsen, if clinical signs and symptoms consistent with liver disease develop, or if systemic manifestations occur (e.g., eosinophilia, rash, etc.), Piroxicam should be discontinued. (See also *"Adverse Reactions"*.)

Although at the recommended dose of 20 mg/day of Piroxicam increased fecal blood loss due to gastrointestinal irritation did not occur (see *"Clinical Pharmacology"*), in about 4% of the patients treated with Piroxicam alone or concomitantly with aspirin, reductions in hemoglobin and hematocrit values were observed. Therefore, these values should be determined if signs or symptoms of anemia occur. Peripheral edema has been observed in approximately 2% of the patients treated with Piroxicam. Therefore, as with othernonsteroidal anti-inflammatory drugs, Piroxicam should be used with caution in patients with heart failure, hypertension or other conditions predisposing to fluid retention, since its usage may be associated with a worsening of these conditions.

A combination of dermatological and/or allergic signs and symptoms suggestive of serum sickness have occasionally occurred in conjunction with the use of Piroxicam. These include arthralgias, pruritus, fever, fatigue, and rash including vesiculo bullous reactions and exfoliative dermatitis.

INFORMATION FOR PATIENTS

Piroxicam, like other drugs of its class, is not free of side effects. The side effects of these drug can cause discomfort and, rarely, there are more serious side effects, such as gastrointestinal bleeding, which may result in hospitalization and even fatal outcomes.

NSAIDs (Nonsteroidal Anti-Inflammatory Drugs) are often essential agents in the management of arthritis, but they also may be commonly employed for conditions which are less serious.

Physicians may wish to discuss with their patients the potential risks (see *"Warnings," "Precautions,"* and *"Adverse Reactions"* sections) and likely benefits of NSAID treatment, particularly when the drugs are used for less serious conditions where treatment without NSAIDs may represent an acceptable alternative to both the patient and physician.

LABORATORY TESTS

Because serious GI tract ulceration and bleeding can occur without warning symptoms, physicians should follow chronically treated patients for the signs and symptoms of ulceration and bleeding and should inform them of the importance of this follow-up (see *"Risk of GI Ulceration, Bleeding and Perforation with NSAID Therapy"*).

DRUG INTERACTIONS

Piroxicam is highly protein bound, and, therefore, might be expected to displace other protein-bound drugs. Although this has not occurred in *in vitro* studies with coumarin-type anticoagulants, interactions with coumarin-type anticoagulants have been reported with Piroxicam since marketing, therefore, physicians should closely monitor patients for a change in dosage requirements when administering Piroxicam to patients on coumarin-type anticoagulants and other highly protein-bound drugs.

Plasma levels of Piroxicam are depressed to approximately 80% of their normal values when Piroxicam is administered in conjunction with aspirin (3900 mg/day), but concomitant administration of antacids has no effect on piroxicam plasma levels (see *"Clinical Pharmacology"*).

Nonsteroidal anti-inflammatory agents, including Piroxicam, have been reported to increase steady state plasma lithium levels. It is recommended that plasma lithium levels be monitored when initiating, adjusting and discontinuing Piroxicam.

CARCINOGENESIS, CHRONIC ANIMAL TOXICITY AND IMPAIRMENT OF FERTILITY

Subacute and chronic toxicity studies have been carried out in rats, mice, dogs, and monkeys.

The pathology most often seen was that characteristically associated with the animal toxicology of anti-inflammatory agents: renal papillary necrosis (see *"Precautions"*) and gastrointestinal lesions.

In classical studies in laboratory animals Piroxicam did not show any teratogenic potential.

Reproductive studies revealed no impairment of fertility in animals.

PREGNANCY AND NURSING MOTHERS

Like other drugs which inhibit the synthesis and release of prostaglandins, Piroxicam increased the incidence of dystocia and delayed parturition in pregnant animals when Piroxicam administration was continued late into pregnancy. Gastrointestinal tract toxicity was increased in pregnant females in the last trimester of pregnancy compared to non-pregnant females or females in earlier trimesters of pregnancy.

Piroxicam is not recommended for use in nursing mothers or in pregnant women because of the animal findings and since safety for such use has not been established in humans.

USE IN CHILDREN

Dosage recommendations and indications for use in children have not been established.

ADVERSE REACTIONS

The incidence of adverse reactions to Piroxicam is based on clinical trials involving approximately 2300 patients, about 400 of whom were treated for more than one year and 170 for more than two years. About 30% of all patients receiving daily doses of 20 mg of Piroxicam experienced side effects. Gastrointestinal symptoms were the most prominent side effects—occurring in approximately 20% of the patients, which in most instances did not interfere with the course of therapy. Of the patients experiencing gastrointestinal side effects, approximately 5% discontinued therapy with an overall incidence of peptic ulceration of about 1%.

Other than the gastrointestinal symptoms, edema, dizziness, headache, changes in hematological parameters, and rash have been reported in a small percentage of patients. Routine ophthalmoscopy and slit-lamp examinations have revealed no evidence of ocular changes in 205 patients followed from 3 to 24 months while on therapy.

INCIDENCE GREATER THAN 1%

The following adverse reactions occurred more frequently than 1 in 100.

Gastrointestinal: stomatitis, anorexia, epigastric distress* nausea*, constipation, abdominal discomfort, flatulence, diarrhea, abdominal pain, indigestion.

Hematological: decreases in hemoglobin* (see *"Precautions"*), anemia, leucopenia, eosinophilia

Dermatologic: pruritus, rash

Central Nervous System: dizziness, somnolence, vertigo

---

* Reactions occurring in 3% to 9% of patients treated with Piroxicam. Reactions occurring in 1-3% of patients are unmarked.

◆ RATED THERAPEUTICALLY EQUIVALENT; ◇ THERAPEUTIC EQUIVALENCE UNCONFIRMED; ○ UNRATED

Urogenital: BUN and creatinine elevations (see *"Precautions"*)

Body as a Whole: headache, malaise

Special Senses: tinnitus

Cardiovascular/Respiratory: edema (see *"Precautions"*)

INCIDENCE LESS THAN 1% (CAUSAL RELATIONSHIP PROBABLE)
The following adverse reactions occurred less frequently than 1 in 100. The probability exists that there is a causal relationship between Piroxicam and these reactions.

Gastrointestinal: liver function abnormalities, jaundice, hepatitis (see *"Precautions"*), vomiting, hematemesis, melena, gastrointestinal bleeding, perforation, and ulceration (see *"Warnings"*), dry mouth

Hematological: thrombocytopenia, petechial rash, ecchymosis, bone marrow depression including aplastic anemia, epistaxis

Dermatologic: sweating, erythema, bruising, desquamation, exfoliative dermatitis, erythema multiforme, toxic epidermal necrolysis, Stevens-Johnson syndrome, vesiculo bullous reaction, photoallergic skin reactions

Central Nervous System: depression, insomnia, nervousness

Urogenital: hematuria, proteinuria, interstitial nephritis, renal failure, hyperkalemia, glomerulitis, papillary necrosis, nephrotic syndrome (see *"Precautions"*)

Body as a Whole: pain (colic), fever, flu-like syndrome (see *"Precautions"*)

Special Senses: swollen eyes, blurred vision, eye irritations

Cardiovascular/Respiratory: hypertension, worsening of congestive heart failure (see *"Precautions"*), exacerbation of angina

Metabolic: hypoglycemia, hyperglycemia, weight increase, weight decrease

Hypersensitivity: anaphylaxis, bronchospasm, urticaria/angioedema, vasculitis, "serum sickness" (see *"Precautions"*)

INCIDENCE LESS THAN 1% (CAUSAL RELATIONSHIP UNKNOWN)
Other adverse reactions were reported with a frequency of less than 1 in 100, but a causal relationship between Piroxicam and the reaction could not be determined.

Gastrointestinal: pancreatitis

Dermatologic: onycholysis, loss of hair

Central Nervous System: akathisia, hallucinations, mood alterations, dream abnormalities, mental confusion, paresthesias

Urogenital System: dysuria

Body as a Whole: weakness

Cardiovascular/Respiratory: palpitations, dyspnea

Hypersensitivity: positive ANA

Special Senses: transient hearing loss

Hematological: hemolytic anemia

OVERDOSAGE
In the event treatment for overdosage is required the long plasma half-life (see *"Clinical Pharmacology"*) of Piroxicam should be considered. The absence of experience with acute overdosage precludes characterization of sequelae and recommendation of specific antidotal efficacy at this time. It is reasonable to assume, however, that the standard measures of gastric evacuation and general supportive therapy would apply. In addition to supportive measures, the use of activated charcoal may effectively reduce the absorption and reabsorption of Piroxicam. Experiments in dogs have demonstrated that the use of multiple-dose treatments with activated charcoal could reduce the half-life of Piroxicam elimination from 27 hours (without charcoal) to 11 hours and reduce the systemic bioavailability of Piroxicam by as much as 37% when activated charcoal is given as late as 6 hours after administration of Piroxicam.

ADMINISTRATION AND DOSAGE
RHEUMATOID ARTHRITIS, OSTEOARTHRITIS
It is recommended that Piroxicam therapy be initiated and maintained at a single daily dose of 20 mg. If desired the daily dose may be divided. Because of the long half-life of Piroxicam, steady-state blood levels are not reached for 7-12 days. Therefore, although the therapeutic effects of Piroxicam are evident early in treatment, there is a progressive increase in response over several weeks and the effect of therapy should not be assessed for two weeks.

Dosage recommendations and indications for use in children have not been established.

HOW SUPPLIED
CAPSULE: 10 MG

AVERAGE UNIT PRICE (AVAILABLE SIZES)		GENERIC A-RATED AVERAGE PRICE (GAAP)	
GENERIC	$1.21	100s	$121.49
HCFA FUL (100s ea)	$0.36		

BRAND/MANUFACTURER	NDC	SIZE	AWP
◆ GENERICS			
Roxane	00054-2660-25	100s	$86.39
Qualitest	00603-5222-21	100s	$118.77
URL	00677-1430-01	100s	$119.00

BRAND/MANUFACTURER	NDC	SIZE	AWP
Mutual	53489-0441-01	100s	$119.00
Goldline	00182-1933-01	100s	$119.00
➤ SCS Pharm	00905-5752-31	100s	$119.36
West Point	59591-0617-68	100s	$119.36
Moore,H.L.	00839-7734-06	100s	$120.15
Rugby	00536-5558-01	100s	$120.28
Lemmon	00093-0756-01	100s	$120.28
Schein	00364-2545-01	100s	$120.28
Royce	51875-0335-01	100s	$120.94
Martec	52555-0972-01	100s	$122.30
Sidmak	50111-0853-01	100s	$124.00
Par	49884-0440-01	100s	$125.75
Aligen	00405-4807-01	100s	$125.75
Major	00904-7697-60	100s	$127.00
Major	00904-7845-60	100s	$127.00
Novopharm	55953-0617-40	100s	$127.00
Mylan	00378-1010-01	100s	$128.64
Lederle Std Prod	00005-3327-43	100s	$130.93
Moore,H.L.	00839-7773-06	100s	$132.03
UDL	51079-0742-20	100s ud	$120.98
Martec	52555-0972-05	500s	$599.27

CAPSULE: 10 MG

BRAND/MANUFACTURER	NDC	SIZE	AWP
○ BRAND			
➤ FELDENE: Pfizer Labs	00069-3220-66	100s	$144.54

CAPSULE: 20 MG

AVERAGE UNIT PRICE (AVAILABLE SIZES)		GENERIC A-RATED AVERAGE PRICE (GAAP)	
GENERIC	$2.03	100s	$204.13
HCFA FUL (100s ea)	$0.71	500s	$1006.34
		1000s	$2024.15

BRAND/MANUFACTURER	NDC	SIZE	AWP
◆ GENERICS			
Allscrips	54569-8521-00	90s	$188.75
Roxane	00054-2661-25	100s	$140.43
Qualitest	00603-5223-21	100s	$203.92
URL	00677-1431-01	100s	$204.00
Mutual	53489-0442-01	100s	$204.00
Goldline	00182-1934-01	100s	$204.00
West Point	59591-0640-68	100s	$204.21
➤ SCS Pharm	00905-5762-31	100s	$204.24
Rugby	00536-5559-01	100s	$205.82
Lemmon	00093-0757-01	100s	$205.82
Schein	00364-2546-01	100s	$205.82
Du Pont Multi	00056-0260-70	100s	$207.00
Royce	51875-0336-01	100s	$207.87
Martec	52555-0973-01	100s	$209.83
Sidmak	50111-0854-01	100s	$210.00
Par	49884-0441-01	100s	$215.19
Aligen	00405-4808-01	100s	$215.19
Major	00904-7698-60	100s	$217.50
Major	00904-7812-60	100s	$217.50
Novopharm	55953-0640-40	100s	$217.50
➤ Mylan	00378-2020-01	100s	$220.14
Lederle Std Prod	00005-3328-43	100s	$224.23
Moore,H.L.	00839-7774-06	100s	$225.57
Moore,H.L.	00839-7735-06	100s	$241.37
Vangard	00615-0389-13	100s ud	$78.17
UDL	51079-0743-20	100s ud	$213.89
Roxane	00054-2661-29	500s	$723.59
Schein	00364-2546-05	500s	$977.64
Goldline	00182-1934-05	500s	$999.00
Qualitest	00603-5223-28	500s	$999.21
URL	00677-1431-05	500s	$999.50
Mutual	53489-0442-05	500s	$999.50
Du Pont Multi	00056-0260-85	500s	$999.60
➤ SCS Pharm	00905-5762-51	500s	$999.91
Royce	51875-0336-02	500s	$999.99
Major	00904-7698-40	500s	$1022.65
Major	00904-7812-40	500s	$1022.65
Lemmon	00093-0757-05	500s	$1024.10
Martec	52555-0973-05	500s	$1028.20
Sidmak	50111-0854-02	500s	$1030.00
Novopharm	55953-0640-70	500s	$1033.10
Par	49884-0441-05	500s	$1053.47
Lederle Std Prod	00005-3328-31	500s	$1054.28
Moore,H.L.	00839-7735-12	500s	$1076.42
➤ Mylan	00378-2020-05	500s	$1077.69
Novopharm	55953-0640-80	1000s	$1962.95
Moore,H.L.	00839-7774-04	1000s	$2009.49
Par	49884-0441-10	1000s	$2100.00

CAPSULE: 20 MG

BRAND/MANUFACTURER	NDC	SIZE	AWP
○ BRAND			
➤ FELDENE: Pfizer Labs	00069-3230-66	100s	$247.35
	00069-3230-41	100s ud	$256.96
	00069-3230-73	500s	$1210.89

➤ SHOWN IN PRODUCT IDENTIFICATION GUIDE

Pitocin *SEE* OXYTOCIN

Pitressin *SEE* VASOPRESSIN

Placidyl *SEE* ETHCHLORVYNOL

Plaquenil Sulfate *SEE* HYDROXYCHLOROQUINE SULFATE

Plasma Protein Fraction (Human)

DESCRIPTION

Plasma Protein Fraction Human 5% is a sterile solution of protein consisting of Albumin and Globulin derived from Human venous plasma that was non reactive when tested for hepatitis B surface antigen (HBsAg) by FDA required test. Each 100 ml contains 5.0 g selected plasma proteins. The plasma proteins, as determined by electrophoresis are at least 83% Albumin and no more than 17% Globulins: no more than 1% of the proteins are Gamma Globulins. The solution is iso-osmotic with normal human plasma. Approximate concentrations of significant electrolytes are: Sodium 130-160 mEq per liter; and Potassium not more than 2mEq per liter.

Plasma Protein Fraction, Human is stabilized with 0.004 molar Sodium Acetyltryptophanate and 0.004 molar Sodium Caprylate, and contains no preservative. It is heat treated at 60°C, for 10 hours. This product has been prepared in accordance with the requirements established by the Food and Drug Administration and is in compliance with the standards of the United States Pharmacopeia.

Plasma Protein Fraction (Human) 5% is to be administered by the intravenous route.

Each bottle contains:

Selected Plasma Proteins 2.5g	....	50 mL
Selected Plasma Proteins 12.5g	....	250 mL
Selected Plasma Proteins 25g	....	500 mL

CLINICAL PHARMACOLOGY

Plasma Protein Fraction (Human) is effective in the maintenance of a normal blood volume but has not been proved effective in the maintenance of oncotic pressure. When the circulating blood volume has been depleted, the hemodilution following albumin administration persists for many hours. In individuals with normal blood volume, it usually lasts only a few hours.

Unlike whole blood plasma, Plasma Protein Fraction (Human) 5% is considered free of the danger of homologous serum hepatitis. No cross-matching is required and the absence of cellular elements removes the risk of sensitization with repeated infusions.

INDICATIONS AND USAGE

Shock: Plasma Protein Fraction, Human is indicated in the emergency treatment of shock due to burns, trauma, surgery, infections, in the treatment of injuries of such severity that shock, although not immediately present, is likely to ensue, and in other similar conditions where the restoration of blood volume is urgent. It supplies additional fluid for adequate plasma volume expansion in dehydrated patients. Blood transfusion may be indicated if there has been considerable loss of red blood cells.

Burns: Plasma Protein Fraction, Human is indicated to prevent marked hemoconcentration and to maintain appropriate electrolyte balance.

Hypoproteinemia: Plasma Protein Fraction (Human) 5% may be used in hypoproteinemic patients, providing sodium restriction is not a problem. If sodium restriction is imperative, the use of 25% Normal Serum Albumin (Human) is recommended.

CONTRAINDICATIONS

Plasma Protein Fraction, Human may be contraindicated in patients with severe anemia or cardiac failure. Do not use in patients on cardiopulmonary bypass.

WARNINGS

Do not use if the solution is turbid, or if there is a sediment in the bottle. Since the product contains no preservative, do not begin administration more than 4 hours after opening the bottle. Unused portions should be discarded.

PRECAUTIONS

GENERAL

Administration of large quantities of Plasma Protein Fraction, Human should be supplemented with or replaced by whole blood to combat the relative anemia which would follow such use. Rapid infusion (greater than 10 ml/minute) may produce hypotension. Blood pressure should be monitored during use and infusion slowed or ceased if sudden hypotension occurs.

When used to reverse shock or hypotension, careful observation of the patient is necessary to detect bleeding points which failed to bleed at lower pressure.

Dehydrated patients require administration of additional fluids to replace fluid withdrawn from tissues by osmotic action of Plasma Protein Fraction, Human.

Administer with caution to patients with low cardiac reserve or with no albumin deficiency because a rapid increase in plasma volume may cause circulatory embarrassment or pulmonary edema.

This product cannot be used for correction of defects of the coagulation mechanism. Administration should be by intravenous route only.

PREGNANCY CATEGORY C

Animal reproduction studies have not been conducted with Plasma Protein Fraction (Human) 5 %. It is also not known whether Plasma Protein Fraction, Human can cause fetal harm when administered to a pregnant woman or can affect reproduction capacity. Plasma Protein Fraction, Human should be given to a pregnant woman only if clearly needed.

ADVERSE REACTIONS

Incidence of untoward reactions is low. Nausea may occur, but should be evaluated with respect to the nature of the present illness. Hypotension, particularly following rapid infusion or intraarterial administration to patients on cardiopulmonary bypass.

DOSAGE AND ADMINISTRATION

Plasma Protein Fraction (Human) 5% is given intravenously without further dilution. This concentration is iso-osmotic with normal human plasma. When it is administered to patients with normal blood volume, the rate of infusion should be slow enough (1 mL per minute) to present too rapid expansion of plasma volume.

Treatment of Shock: Dosage is based almost entirely on the nature of the individual case and the response to therapy. The usual minimum effective dose if 250-500 ml.

The rate of administration for the emergency treatment of shock in adults in dependent on the response to therapy and the flow should be adjusted as the patient improves. Administration rates of 10 ml per minute should not be exceeded.

In infants and small children, Plasma Protein Fraction, Human has been found to be very useful in the initial therapy of shock due to dehydration and infection. A dose of 15 ml per pound of body weight infused intravenously at a rate up to 5 to 10 ml per minute for the treatment of acute shock states in infants is desirable. As with any plasma expander the rate should be adjusted or slowed according to the clinical response and rising blood pressure.

Treatment of Burns: The dosage is dependent on the extent and severity of the burn. An optimal regimen for use of Plasma Protein Fraction (Human), crystalloids, electrolytes and water in the treatment of burns has not been established.

Treatment of Hypoproteinemia: The adult dose of Plasma Protein Fraction (Human) 5% is 1000 to 1500 ml daily to yield 50 to 75 g of plasma protein. Since blood volume in these patients may be normal, doses of more than 500 ml should not be given faster than 500 ml in 30 to 45 minutes to avoid circulatory embarrassment. If slower administration is desired, 1000 ml may be given by continuous drip at a rate of 100 ml per hour. If sodium restriction is imperative, 25% Normal Serum Albumin (Human) is recommended.

Parenteral drug products should be inspected visually for particulate matter and discoloration prior to administration whenever solution and container permit.

Storage: Store at controlled room temperature—between 15°-30°C (59°-86°F). Do not allow to freeze.

REFERENCES

1. Bertrand, J.J.; Feichtmeir, T.V.; Kolomeyer, N.; Beatty, J.O.; Murphy, P.L.; Waldschmidt, W.D.; and McLean, E.B.; Clinical Investigations with a Heat-Treated Plasma Protein Fraction, Vox. Sang. 4:385—402, 1959. 2. Cock, T.C.; Binger, D.C.; and Dennis, J.L.; A New Plasma Substitute for Pediatric Therapy, Calif. Med. 89:257, 1958. 3. Hink, J.H. Jr.; Hidalgo, J.; Seeberg, V.P.; and Johnson, F.F.; Preparation and Properties of a Heat-Treated Human Plasma Protein Fraction, Vox Sanguinis 2:174, 1957. 4. Bland, J.H.; Laver, M.B.; and Lowenstein, E.; Vasodilator Effect of Commercial 5% Plasma Protein Fraction Solutions, JAMA 224:172114 1724, 1973.

HOW SUPPLIED
INJECTION: 5%

BRAND/MANUFACTURER	NDC	SIZE	AWP
○ GENERICS			
PLASMANATE: Miles Biol	00192-0613-20	50 ml	$23.75
PLASMA-PLEX: Armour	00053-7753-03	50 ml	$36.00
PROTENATE: Baxter Biotech	00944-0450-01	250 ml	$56.00
PLASMANATE: Miles Biol	00192-0613-25	250 ml	$58.88
Amer Red Cross	52769-0430-25	250 ml	$65.00
PLASMATEIN: Alpha Therapeutic	49669-5721-01	250 ml	$75.00
PLASMA-PLEX: Armour	00053-7753-01	250 ml	$90.00
PROTENATE: Baxter Biotech	00944-0450-02	500 ml	$112.00
PLASMANATE: Miles Biol	00192-0613-27	500 ml	$118.50

◆ RATED THERAPEUTICALLY EQUIVALENT; ◇ THERAPEUTIC EQUIVALENCE UNCONFIRMED; ○ UNRATED

BRAND/MANUFACTURER	NDC	SIZE	AWP
Amer Red Cross	52769-0430-50	500 ml	$130.00
PLASMATEIN: Alpha Therapeutic	49669-5721-02	500 ml	$150.00
PLASMA-PLEX: Armour	00053-7753-02	500 ml	$180.00

Plasma-Lyte *SEE* DEXTROSE AND ELECTROLYTES, DEXTROSE AND ELECTROLYTES, INTRAPERITONEAL *AND* ELECTROLYTES, INJECTABLE

Platinol *SEE* CISPLATIN

Plegine *SEE* PHENDIMETRAZINE TARTRATE

Plegisol *SEE* CARDIOPLEGIC SOLUTION

Plendil *SEE* FELODIPINE

Plicamycin

WARNING
IT IS RECOMMENDED THAT PLICAMYCIN BE ADMINISTERED ONLY TO HOSPITALIZED PATIENTS BY OR UNDER THE SUPERVISION OF A QUALIFIED PHYSICIAN WHO IS EXPERIENCED IN THE USE OF CANCER CHEMOTHERAPEUTIC AGENTS, BECAUSE OF THE POSSIBILITY OF SEVERE REACTIONS. FACILITIES FOR THE DETERMINATION OF NECESSARY LABORATORY STUDIES MUST BE AVAILABLE.

SEVERE THROMBOCYTOPENIA, A HEMORRHAGIC TENDENCY AND EVEN DEATH MAY RESULT FROM THE USE OF MITHRACIN. ALTHOUGH SEVERE TOXICITY IS MORE APT TO OCCUR IN PATIENTS WHO HAVE FAR-ADVANCED DISEASE OR ARE OTHERWISE CONSIDERED POOR RISKS FOR THERAPY, SERIOUS TOXICITY MAY ALSO OCCASIONALLY OCCUR EVEN IN PATIENTS WHO ARE IN RELATIVELY GOOD CONDITION.

IN THE TREATMENT OF EACH PATIENT, THE PHYSICIAN MUST WEIGH CAREFULLY THE POSSIBILITY OF ACHIEVING THERAPEUTIC BENEFIT VERSUS THE RISK OF TOXICITY WHICH MAY OCCUR WITH MITHRACIN THERAPY. THE FOLLOWING DATA CONCERNING THE USE OF MITHRACIN IN THE TREATMENT OF TESTICULAR TUMORS, HYPERCALCEMIC AND/OR HYPERCALCIURIC CONDITIONS ASSOCIATED WITH VARIOUS ADVANCED MALIGNANCIES, SHOULD BE THOROUGHLY REVIEWED BEFORE ADMINISTERING THIS COMPOUND.

DESCRIPTION
Plicamycin is a yellow crystalline compound which is produced by a microorganism, *Streptomyces plicatus*. Plicamycin is available in vials as a freeze-dried, sterile preparation for intravenous administration. Each vial contains 2500 meg (2.5 mg) of Plicamycin with 100 mg of mannitol and sufficient disodium phosphate to adjust to pH 7. After reconstitution with sterile water for injection, the solution has a pH of 7. The drug is unstable in acid solutions with a pH below 4. Plicamycin is an antineoplastic agent. It has an empirical formula of $C_{52}H_{76}O_{24}$.

Following is its chemical structure:

CLINICAL PHARMACOLOGY
Although the exact mechanism by which Plicamycin causes tumor inhibition is not yet known, studies have indicated that this compound forms a complex with deoxyribonucleic acid (DNA) and inhibits cellular ribonucleic acid (RNA) and enzymic RNA synthesis. The binding of Plicamycin to DNA in the presence of Mg^{++} (or other divalent cations) is responsible for the inhibition of DNA-dependent or DNA-directed RNA synthesis. This action presumably accounts for the biological properties of Plicamycin.

Plicamycin shows potent cytotoxicity against malignant cells of human origin (Hela cells) growing in tissue culture. Plicamycin is lethal to Hela cells in 48 hours at concentrations as low as 0.5 micrograms per milliliter of tissue culture medium.

Plicamycin has shown significant anti-tumor activity against experimental leukemia in mice when administered intraperitoneally.

Plicamycin may lower serum calcium levels; the exact mechanism (or mechanisms) by which the drug exerts this effect is unknown. It appears that Plicamycin may block the hypercalcemic action of pharmacologic doses of vitamin D. It has also been suggested that Plicamycin may lower calcium serum levels by inhibiting the effect of parathyroid hormone upon osteoclasts. Plicamycin's inhibition of DNA-dependent RNA synthesis appears to render osteoclasts unable to fully respond to parathyroid hormone with the biosynthesis necessary for osteolysis. Decreases in serum phosphate levels and urinary calcium excretion accompany the lowering of serum calcium concentrations.

Radioautography studies[1] with ^{3}H-labeled Plicamycin in C3H mice show that the greatest concentrations of the isotope are in the Kupffer cells of the liver and cells of the renal tubules. Plicamycin is rapidly cleared from the blood within the first 2 hours and excretion is also rapid. Sixty-seven percent of measured excretion occurs within 4 hours, 75% within 8 hours, and 90% is recovered in the first 24 hours after injection. There is no evidence of protein binding, nor is there any evidence of metabolism of the carbohydrate moiety of the drug to carbon dioxide and water with loss through respiration. Plicamycin crosses the blood-brain barrier; the concentration found in brain tissue is low but it persists longer than in other tissues. The experimental results in animals correlate closely with results achieved in man.[2]

INDICATIONS
Plicamycin is a potent antineoplastic agent which has been shown to be useful in the treatment of carefully selected hospitalized patients with malignant tumors of the testis in whom successful treatment by surgery and/or irradiation is impossible. Also, on the basis of limited clinical experience to date, it may be considered in the treatment of certain symptomatic patients with hypercalcemia and hypercalciuria associated with a variety of advanced neoplasms.

The use of Plicamycin in other types of neoplastic disease is not recommended at the present time.

UNLABELED USES
Plicamycin is used alone or as an adjunct in the treatment of Paget's Disease.

CONTRAINDICATIONS
Plicamycin is contraindicated in patients with thrombocytopenia, thrombocytopathy, coagulation disorder or an increased susceptibility to bleeding due to other causes. Plicamycin should not be administered to any patient with impairment of bone marrow function.

Plicamycin may cause fetal harm when administered to a pregnant woman. Plicamycin is contraindicated in women who are or may become pregnant. If this drug is used during pregnancy or if the patient becomes pregnant while taking this drug, the patient should be apprised of the potential hazard to the fetus.

PRECAUTIONS
General: Plicamycin should be administered only to patients who are hospitalized and who can be observed carefully and frequently during and after therapy.

Severe thrombocytopenia, a hemorrhagic tendency and even death may result from the use of Plicamycin. Although severe toxicity is more apt to occur in patients who have far-advanced disease or are otherwise considered poor risks for therapy, serious toxicity may also occasionally occur even in patients who are in relatively good condition.

Electrolyte imbalance, especially hypocalcemia, hypokalemia, and hypophosphatemia, should be corrected with appropriate electrolyte therapy prior to treatment with Plicamycin.

Plicamycin should be used with extreme caution in patients with significant impairment of renal or hepatic function.

Plicamycin should not normally be administered to patients who are pregnant or to mothers who are breast feeding.

In the treatment of each patient, the physician must weigh carefully the possibility of achieving therapeutic benefit versus the risk of toxicity which may occur with Plicamycin therapy.

Laboratory Tests: The following laboratory studies should be obtained frequently during therapy and for several days following the last dose: platelet count, prothrombin time, bleeding time. The occurrence of thrombocytopenia or a significant prolongation of prothrombin time or bleeding time is an indication for the termination of therapy.

Carcinogenesis, Mutagenesis, Impairment of Fertility: No long-term studies in animals have been performed to evaluate the carcinogenic potential of Plicamycin Histologic evidence of inhibition of spermatogenesis was observed in a substantial number of male rats receiving doses of 0.6 mg/kg/day and above.

Pregnancy Category X: See "Contraindications" section.

Nursing Mothers: It is not known whether this drug is excreted in human milk. Because many drugs are excreted in human milk and because of the potential for serious adverse reactions in nursing infants from Plicamycin, a decision should be made whether to discontinue nursing or to discontinue the drug, taking into account the importance of the drug to the mother.

ADVERSE REACTIONS
THE MOST IMPORTANT FORM OF TOXICITY ASSOCIATED WITH THE USE OF PLICAMYCIN CONSISTS OF A BLEEDING SYNDROME WHICH USUALLY BEGINS WITH AN EPISODE OF EPISTAXIS. This bleeding tendency may only consist of a single or several episodes of epistaxis and progress no further. However, in some cases, this hemorrhagic syndrome can start with an

➤ SHOWN IN PRODUCT IDENTIFICATION GUIDE

episode of hematemesis which may progress to more wide-spread hemorrhage in the gastrointestinal tract or to a more generalized bleeding tendency. This hemorrhagic diathesis is most likely due to abnormalities in multiple clotting factors.

A detailed analysis of the clinical data in 1,160 patients treated with Plicamycin indicates that the hemorrhagic syndrome is dose related. With doses of 30 mcg/kg/day or less for 10 or fewer doses, the incidence of bleeding episodes has been 5.4% with an associated drug-related mortality rate of 1.6%. With doses greater than 30 mcg/kg/day and/or for more than 10 doses, a significantly larger number of bleeding episodes occurred (11.9%) and the associated drug-related mortality rate was also significantly higher (5.7%).

The most common side effects reported with the use of Plicamycin consist of gastrointestinal symptoms: anorexia, nausea, vomiting, diarrhea, and stomatitis. Other less frequently reported side effects include fever, drowsiness, weakness, lethargy, malaise, headache, depression, phlebitis, facial flushing, and skin rash.

The following laboratory abnormalities have been reported during therapy with Plicamycin and in most instances were reversible following cessation of treatment:

Hematologic Abnormalities: Depression of platelet count, white count, hemoglobin and prothrombin content; elevation of clotting time and bleeding time; abnormal clot retraction. Thrombocytopenia may be rapid in onset and may occur at any time during therapy or within several days following the last dose. With the occurrence of severe thrombocytopenia, the infusion of platelet concentrates of platelet-rich plasma may be helpful in elevating the platelet count.

The occurrence of leukopenia with the use of Plicamycin is relatively uncommon, occurring only in approximately 6% of patients.

It has been uncommon for abnormalities in clotting time or clot retraction to be demonstrated prior to the onset of an overt bleeding episode noted in some patients treated with Plicamycin. Nevertheless, the performance of these tests periodically is recommended because in a few instances, an abnormality in one of these studies may have served as a warning to terminate therapy because of impeding serious toxicity.

Abnormal Liver Function Tests: Increased levels of serum glutamic oxalacetic transaminase, serum glutamic pyruvic transaminase, lactic dehydrogenase, alkaline phosphatase, serum bilirubin, ornithine carbamyl transferase, isocitric dehydrogenase, and increased retention of bromsulphalein.

Abnormal Renal Function Tests: Increased blood urea nitrogen and serum creatinine: proteinuria.

Abnormalities in Electrolyte Concentrations: Depression of serum calcium, phosphorus, and potassium.

OVERDOSAGE

Generally, adverse effects following the use of Plicamycin especially the hemorrhagic syndrome, are dose related. Therefore, following administration of an overdose, patients can be expected to experience an exaggeration of the usual adverse effects. Close monitoring of the hematologic picture, including factors involved in the clotting mechanism, hepatic and renal functions, and serum electrolytes, is necessary. No specific antidote for Plicamycin is known. Management of overdosage would include general supportive measures to sustain the patient through the period of toxicity.

DOSAGE

The daily dose of Plicamycin is based on the patient's body weight. If a patient has abnormal fluid retention such as edema, hydrothorax or ascites, the patient's ideal weight rather than actual body weight should be used to calculate the dose.

Treatment of Testicular Tumors: In the treatment of patients with testicular tumors the recommended daily dose of Plicamycin is 25 to 30 mcg (0.025-0.030 mg) per kilogram of body weight. Therapy should be continued for a period of 8 to 10 days unless significant side effects or toxicity occur during therapy. A course of therapy consisting of more than 10 daily doses is not recommended. Individual daily doses should not exceed 30 mcg (0.030 mg) per kilogram of body weight.

In those patients with responsive tumors, some degree of tumor regression is usually evident within 3 or 4 weeks following the initial course of therapy. If tumor masses remain unchanged following an initial course of therapy, additional courses of therapy at monthly intervals are warranted.

When a significant tumor regression is obtained, it is suggested that additional courses of therapy be given at monthly intervals until a complete regression of tumor masses is achieved or until definite tumor progression or new tumor masses occur in spite of continued courses of therapy.

Treatment of Hypercalcemia and Hypercalciuria: Reversal of hypercalcemia and hypercalciuria can usually be achieved with Plicamycin at doses considerably lower than those recommended for use in the treatment of testicular tumors. In hypercalcemia and hypercalciuria associated with advanced malignancy the recommended course of treatment with Plicamycin is 25 mcg (0.025 mg) per kilogram of body weight per day for 3 or 4 days.

If the desired degree of reversal of hypercalcemia or hypercalciuria is not achieved with the initial course of therapy, additional courses of therapy may then be administered at intervals of one week or more to achieve the desired result or to maintain serum calcium and urinary calcium excretion at normal levels. It may be possible to maintain normal calcium balance with single, weekly doses or with a schedule of 2 or 3 doses per week.

Note: BECAUSE OF THE DRUG'S TOXICITY AND THE LIMITED CLINICAL EXPERIENCE TO DATE IN THESE INDICATIONS, THE FOLLOWING RECOMMENDATIONS SHOULD BE KEPT IN MIND BY THE PHYSICIAN.

1. CONSIDER CASES OF HYPERCALCEMIA AND HYPERCALCIURIA NOT RESPONSIVE TO CONVENTIONAL TREATMENT.

2. APPLY SAME CONTRAINDICATIONS AND PRECAUTIONARY MEASURES AS IN ANTITUMOR TREATMENT.

3. RENAL FUNCTION SHOULD BE CAREFULLY MONITORED BEFORE, DURING, AND AFTER TREATMENT.

4. BENEFITS OF USE DURING PREGNANCY OR IN WOMEN OF CHILD-BEARING AGE SHOULD BE WEIGHED AGAINST POTENTIAL TOXICITY TO EMBRYO OR FETUS.

ADMINISTRATION

By IV administration only. The appropriate daily dose of Plicamycin should be diluted in one liter of 5% Dextrose Injection, USP or Sodium Chloride Injection, USP and administered by slow intravenous infusion over a period of 4 to 6 hours. Rapid direct intravenous injection of Plicamycin should be avoided as it may be associated with a higher incidence and greater severity of gastrointestinal side effects. Extravasation of solutions of Plicamycin may cause local irritation and cellulitis at injection sites. Should thrombophlebitis or perivascular cellulitis occur, the infusion should be terminated and reinstituted at another site. The application of moderate heat to the site of extravasation may help to disperse the compound and minimize discomfort and local tissue irritation. The use of antiemetic compounds prior to and during treatment with Plicamycin may be helpful in relieving nausea and vomiting.

Procedures for proper handling and disposal of anti-cancer drugs should be considered. Several guidelines on this subject have been published.[3-8] There is no general agreement that all of the procedures recommended in the guidelines are necessary or appropriate.

ANIMAL PHARMACOLOGY AND TOXICOLOGY

In mice the average intravenous LD50 of Plicamycin is 2,000 meg/kg of body weight. When administered orally, it is not toxic to mice even at doses 100 times greater than the intravenous LD_{50}. In rats the average intravenous LD_{50} of Plicamycin is 1,700 mcg/kg of body weight. It is not toxic to rats when administered orally at doses 17 times greater than the intravenous LD50. In dogs and monkeys Plicamycin is essentially non-toxic when administered intravenously for 24 days at daily doses as high as 50 and 24 mcg/kg of body weight, respectively. However, at higher doses of 100 mcg/kg/day intravenously it is lethal to dogs and monkeys. Signs of toxicity in dogs and monkeys included anorexia, vomiting, listlessness, nelena, anemia, lymphopenia, elevated alkaline phosphatase, serum glutamic oxalacetic transaminase, serum glutamic pyruvic transaminase values, hypochloremia, and azotemia. Dogs also showed marked thrombocytopenia, hyponatremia, hypokalemia, hypocalcemia, and decreased prothrombin consumption. Necropsy findings consisted of necrosis of lymphoid tissue and multiple generalized hemorrhages. Plicamycin was only mildly irritating when injected intramuscularly in rabbits and subcutaneously in guinea pigs. Histologic evidence of inhibition of spermatogenesis was observed in a substantial number of male rats receiving doses of 0.6 mg/kg/day and above. This preclinical finding of selective drug effect constituted the scientific rationale for clinical trials in testicular tumors.

CLINICAL REPORTS

Treatment of Patients with Inoperable Testicular Tumors: In a combined series of 305 patients with inoperable testicular tumors treated with Plicamycin, 33 patients (10.8%) showed a complete disappearance of tumor masses and an additional 80 patients (26.2%) responded with significant partial regression of tumor masses. The longest duration of a continuing complete response is now over 8 1/2 years. The therapeutic responses in this series of patients have been summarized by type of testicular tumor in the accompanying table. (See related table).

Plicamycin may be useful in the treatment of patients with testicular tumors which are resistant to other chemotherapeutic agents. Prior radiation therapy or prior chemotherapy did not alter the response rate with Plicamycin. This suggests that there is no significant cross resistance between Plicamycin and other chemotherapeutic agents.

Treatment of Patients with Hypercalcemia and Hypercalciuria: A limited number of patients with hypercalcemia (range: 12.0-25.8 mg%) and patients with hypercalciuria (range 215-492 mg/day) associated with malignant disease were treated with Plicamycin. Hypercalcemia and hypercalciuria were promptly reversed in all patients. In some patients, the primary malignancy was of non-testicular origin.

REFERENCES

1. Kennedy, B.D., et al: Cancer Res.27:1534, 1967. 2. Ransohoff, J., et al: Cancer Chemother. Rep. 49:51, 1965. 3. Recommendations for the Safe Handling of Parenteral Antieoplastic Drugs. NIH Publication No. 83-2621. For sale by the Superintendent of Documents, U.S. Government Printing Office, Washington, D.C. 20402. 4. AMA Council Report. Guidelines for Handling Parenteral Antineoplastics. JAMA, March 15, 1985. 5. National Study Commission on Cytotoxic Exposure—Recommendations for Handling Cytotoxic Agents. Available from Louis P. Jeffrey, Sc.D., Director of Pharmacy Services, Rhode Island Hospital, 593 Eddy Street, Providence, Rhode Island 02902. 6. Clinical Oncological Society of Australia: Guidelines and recommendations for safe handling of antineoplastic agents. Med J Australia 1:426-428, 1983. 7. Jones, R.B., et al: Safe handling of chemotherapeutic agents: A report from the Mount Sinai Medical Center. Ca—A Cancer Journal for Clinicians, Sept/Oct. 258-263, 1983. 8. American Society of Hospital Pharmacists technical assistance bulletin on handling cytotoxic drugs in hospitals. Am J Hosp Pharm 42:131-137, 1985.

◆ RATED THERAPEUTICALLY EQUIVALENT; ◇ THERAPEUTIC EQUIVALENCE UNCONFIRMED; ○ UNRATED

RESULTS IN 305 TESTICULAR TUMOR CASES BY TUMOR TYPE

Type of Testicular Tumor	Total	Complete Response	Partial Response	No Response
Embryonal Cell	173	26	42	105
Teratoma	5	0	1	4
Teratocarcinoma	23	0	5	18
Seminoma	18	0	7	11
Choriocarcinoma	13	1	6	6
Mixed Tumor	73	6	19	48
Totals	305	33	80	192

HOW SUPPLIED

POWDER FOR INJECTION: 2.5 MG

BRAND/MANUFACTURER	NDC	SIZE	AWP
BRAND			
MITHRACIN: Miles Pharm	00026-8161-15	10s	$783.53

PMB *SEE* ESTROGENS, CONJUGATED AND MEPROBAMATE

Pneumococcal Vaccine, Polyvalent

DESCRIPTION

Pneumococcal Vaccine, Polyvalent, is a sterile, liquid vaccine for intramuscular or subcutaneous injection. It consists of a mixture of highly purified capsular polysaccharides from the 23 most prevalent or invasive pneumococcal types accounting for at least 90% of pneumococcal blood isolates and at least 85% of all pneumococcal isolates from sites which are generally sterile as determined by ongoing surveillance of U.S. data.

Each 0.5 mL dose of vaccine contains 25 μg of each polysaccharide type dissolved in isotonic saline solution containing 0.25% phenol as preservative.

Type 6B pneumococcal polysaccharide exhibits somewhat greater stability in purified form than does Type 6A. A high degree of cross-reactivity between the two types has been demonstrated in adult volunteers. Therefore, Type 6B has replaced Type 6A, which had been used in the 14-valent vaccine. Although contained in the 14-valent vaccine, Type 25 is not included in Pneumococcal Vaccine, Polyvalent, because it has recently become a rare isolate in many parts of the world including the United States, Canada and Europe. (See related table).

CLINICAL PHARMACOLOGY

Pneumococcal infection is a leading cause of death throughout the world and a major cause of pneumonia, meningitis, and otitis media. The emergence of strains of pneumococci with increased resistance to one or more of the common antibiotics and recent isolations of pneumococci with multiple antibiotic resistance emphasize the importance of vaccine prophylaxis against pneumococcal disease. Based on projection from limited observations in the United States, it has been estimated that 400,000 to 500,000 cases of pneumococcal pneumonia may occur annually. The overall case fatality rate ranges from 5-10%. Populations at high risk are the elderly; individuals with immune deficiencies; patients with asplenia or splenic deficiencies, including sickle cell anemia and other severe hemoglobinopathies; alcoholics; and patients with the following diseases: Hodgkin's disease, multiple myeloma and nephrotic syndrome. About 25% of all persons with pneumococcal pneumonia develop bacteremia.

Death occurs in about 28% of these bacteremic patients over 50 years of age. Of all patients with pneumococcal bacteremia who died despite treatment with penicillin or tetracycline, as many as 60% died within five days of onset of the illness.

The annual incidence of pneumococcal meningitis is approximately 1.5 to 2.5 per 100,000 population. One-half of the cases occur in children, in whom the fatality rate is about 40%. Children with sickle cell disease have been estimated to have a risk of pneumococcal meningitis nearly 600 times greater than normal children. Other illnesses caused by pneumococci include acute exacerbations of chronic bronchitis, sinusitis, arthritis and conjunctivitis.

Invasive pneumococcal disease causes high morbidity and mortality in spite of effective antimicrobial control by antibiotics. These effects of pneumococcal disease appear due to irreversible physiologic damage caused by the bacteria during the first 5 days following onset of illness, and occur irrespective of antimicrobial therapy. Vaccination offers an effective means of further reducing the mortality and morbidity of this disease.

At present, there are 83 known pneumococcal capsular types. However, the preponderance of pneumococcal diseases is caused by only some capsular types. For example, a 10-year (1952-1962) surveillance at a New York medical center, showed that 56% of all deaths due to pneumococcal pneumonia were caused by 6 capsular types and that approximately 78% of all pneumococcal pneumonias were caused by 12 capsular types. Such unequal distribution of pneumococcal capsular types causing disease has been shown throughout the world. It is on the basis of this information that the Pneumococcal Vaccine is composed of 23 capsular types, designed to provide coverage of approximately 90% of the most frequently reported types.

It has been established that the purified pneumococcal capsular polysaccharides induce antibody production and that such antibody is effective in preventing pneumococcal disease. Studies in humans have demonstrated the immunogenicity (antibody-stimulating capability) of each of the 23 capsular types when tested in polyvalent vaccines. Adults of all ages responded immunologically to the vaccines. Earlier studies with 12- and 14-valent Pneumococcal Vaccines in children two years of age and older and in adults showed immunogenic responses. Protective capsular type-specific antibody levels develop by the third week following vaccination.

The protective efficacy of Pneumococcal Vaccines containing 6 and 12 capsular polysaccharides was investigated in controlled studies of gold miners in South Africa, in whom there is a high attack rates for pneumococcal pneumonia. Capsular type-specific attack rates for pneumococcal pneumonia were observed for the period from 2 weeks through about 1 year after vaccination. The rates for pneumonia caused by the same capsular types represented in the vaccines are given in the table. Protective efficacy was 76% and 92%, respectively, in the two studies for the capsular types represented.

PNEUMOCOCCAL VACCINE, POLYVALENT

Number of Capsular Types in Pneumococcal Vaccine	Rate/1000 for Pneumonia Caused by Homologous Capsular Types		Protective Efficacy
	Vaccinated Group	Control Group	
6	9.2	38.3	76%
12	1.8	22.0	92%

In similar studies carried out by Dr. R. Austrian and associates using similar Pneumococcal Vaccines prepared for the National Institute of Allergy and Infectious Diseases, the reduction in pneumonias caused by the capsular types contained in the vaccines was 79%. Reduction in type-specific pneumococcal bacteremia was 82%. A preliminary report suggests that in patients with sickle cell anemia and/or anatomical or functional asplenia, the vaccine was highly effective in persons over two years of age in preventing severe pneumococcal disease and bacteremia.

The duration of protective effect of Pneumococcal Vaccine, Polyvalent is presently unknown, but it has been shown in previous studies with other Pneumococcal Vaccines that antibody induced by the vaccine may persist for as long as 5 years. Type-specific antibody levels induced by Pneumococcal Vaccine, Polyvalent (14-valent) have been observed to decline over a 42-month period of observation, but remain significantly above prevaccination levels in almost all recipients who manifest an initial response.

INDICATIONS AND USAGE

Pneumococcal Vaccine, Polyvalent is indicated for immunization against pneumococcal disease caused by those pneumococcal types included in the vaccine. Effectiveness of the vaccine in the prevention of pneumococcal pneumonia and pneumococcal bacteremia has been demonstrated in controlled trials.

Pneumococcal Vaccine, Polyvalent, will not immunize against capsular types of pneumococcus other than those contained in the vaccine.

Use in Selected Individuals over 2 Years of Age as Follows: (1) patients who have anatomical asplenia or who have splenic dysfunction due to sickle cell disease or other causes; (2) persons with chronic illnesses in which there is an increased risk of pneumococcal disease, such as functional impairment of cardiorespiratory, hepatic and renal systems; (3) persons 50 years of age or older; (4) patients with other chronic illnesses who may be at greater risk of developing pneumococcal infection or experiencing more severe pneumococcal illness as a result of alcohol abuse or coexisting diseases including diabetes mellitus, chronic cerebrospinal fluid leakage, or conditions associated with immunosuppression; (5) patients with

23 PNEUMOCOCCAL CAPSULAR TYPES INCLUDED IN PNEUMOCOCCAL VACCINE, POLYVALENT

Nomenclature	Pneumococcal Types							
Danish	1 2 3 4 5 6B	7F 8 9N 9V	10A 11A 12F	14 15B 17F	18C 19F 19A	20 22F 23F 33F
U.S.	1 2 3 4 5 26	51 8 9 68	34 43 12	14 54 17	56 19 57	20 22 23 70

➤ SHOWN IN PRODUCT IDENTIFICATION GUIDE

Hodgkin's disease if immunization can be given at least 10 days prior to treatment. For maximal antibody response immunization should be given at least 14 days prior to the start of treatment with radiation or chemotherapy. Immunization of patients less than 10 days prior to or during treatment is not recommended. (See *"Contraindications".*)

Use in Communities: Persons over 2 years of age as follows (1) closed groups such as those in residential schools, nursing homes and other institutions. (To decrease the likelihood of acute outbreaks of pneumococcal disease in closed institutional populations where there is increased risk that the disease may be severe, vaccination of the entire closed population should be considered where there are no other contraindications.); (2) groups epidemiologically at risk in the community when there is a generalized outbreak in the population due to a single pneumococcal type included in the vaccine; (3) patients at high risk of influenza complications, particularly pneumonia.

Pneumococcal Vaccine, Polyvalent may not be effective in preventing infection resulting from basilar skull fracture or from external communication with cerebrospinal fluid.

Simultaneous administration of pneumococcal polysaccharide vaccine and whole-virus influenza vaccine gives satisfactory antibody response without increasing the occurrence of adverse reactions. Simultaneous administration of the Pneumococcal Vaccine and split-virus influenza vaccine may also be expected to yield satisfactory results.

REVACCINATION
Routine revaccination of adults previously vaccinated with Pneumococcal Vaccine, Polyvalent is not recommended because an increased incidence and severity of adverse reactions have been reported among healthy adults revaccinated with Pneumococcal Vaccines at intervals under three years. This was probably due to sustained high antibody levels.

Based on a clinical study, revaccination with Pneumococcal Vaccine, Polyvalent is recommended for adults at highest risk of fatal pneumococcal infection who were initially vaccinated with Pneumococcal Vaccine, Polyvalent (14-valent) without serious or severe reaction four or more years previously.*

Children at highest risk for pneumococcal infection (e.g., children with asplenia, sickle cell disease or nephrotic syndrome) may have lower peak antibody levels and/or more rapid antibody decline than do healthy adults. There is evidence that some of these high-risk children, (e.g., asplenic children) benefit from revaccination with vaccine containing antigen types 7F, 8, 19F. The Immunization Practices Advisory Committee (ACIP) recommends that revaccination after three to five years should be considered for children at highest risk for pneumococcal infection (e.g., children with asplenia, sickle cell disease or nephrotic syndrome) who would be ten years old or younger at revaccination.

CONTRAINDICATIONS
Hypersensitivity to any component of the vaccine. Epinephrine injection (1:1000) must be immediately available should an acute anaphylactoid reaction occur due to any component of the vaccine.

Revaccination of adults with Pneumococcal Vaccine, Polyvalent is contraindicated except as described under *"Indications and Usage".*

Patients with Hodgkin's disease immunized less than 7 to 10 days prior to immunosuppressive therapy have in some instances been found to have postimmunization antibody levels below their pre-immunization levels. Because of these results, immunization less than 10 days prior to or during treatment is contraindicated.

Patients with Hodgkin's disease who have received extensive chemotherapy and/or nodal irradiation have been shown to have an impaired antibody response to a 12-valent Pneumococcal Vaccine. Because, in some intensively treated patients, administration of that vaccine depressed pre-existing levels of antibody to some pneumococcal types Pneumococcal Vaccine, Polyvalent, is not recommended at this time for patients who have received these forms of therapy for Hodgkin's disease.

WARNINGS
If the vaccine is used in persons receiving immunosuppressive therapy, the expected serum antibody response may not be obtained.

Intradermal administration may cause severe local reactions.

PRECAUTIONS
GENERAL
Caution and appropriate care should be exercised in administering Pneumococcal Vaccine, Polyvalent to individuals with severely compromised cardiac and/or pulmonary function in whom a systemic reaction would pose a significant risk.

Any febrile respiratory illness or other active infection is reason for delaying use of Pneumococcal Vaccine, Polyvalent, except when, in the opinion of the physician, withholding the agent entails even greater risk.

---

* NOTE: The Immunization Practices Advisory Committee (ACIP) has stated that, without more information: persons who received the 14-valent Pneumococcal Vaccine should not be routinely revaccinated with the 23-valent vaccine, as increased coverage is modest and duration of protection is not well defined. However, revaccination with the 23-valent vaccine should be strongly considered for persons who received the 14-valent vaccine if they are at highest risk of fatal pneumococcal infection (e.g., asplenic patients). Revaccination should also be considered for adults at highest risk who received the 23-valent vaccine ≥ 6 years before and for those shown to have rapid decline in pneumococcal antibody levels (e.g., patients with nephrotic syndrome, renal failure, or transplant recipients).

In patients who require penicillin (or other antibiotic) prophylaxis against pneumococcal infection, such prophylaxis should not be discontinued after vaccination with Pneumococcal Vaccine, Polyvalent.

PREGNANCY
Pregnancy Category C: Animal reproduction studies have not been conducted with Pneumococcal Vaccine, Polyvalent. It is also not known whether Pneumococcal Vaccine, Polyvalent can cause fetal harm when administered to a pregnant woman or can affect reproduction capacity Pneumococcal Vaccine, Polyvalent should be given to a pregnant woman only if clearly needed.

NURSING MOTHERS
It is not known whether this drug is excreted in human milk. Because many drugs are excreted in human milk, caution should be exercised when Pneumococcal Vaccine, Polyvalent is administered to a nursing woman.

PEDIATRIC USE
Children less than 2 years of age do not respond satisfactorily to the capsular types of Pneumococcal Vaccine, Polyvalent, that are most often the cause of pneumococcal disease in this age group. Safety and effectiveness in children below the age of 2 years have not been established. Accordingly Pneumococcal Vaccine, Polyvalent, is not recommended in this age group.

ADVERSE REACTIONS
Local reactions including local injection site soreness, erythema and swelling, usually of less than 48 hours duration, occurs commonly; local induration occurs less commonly. In a study of Pneumococcol Vaccine, Polyvalent, (containing 22 capsular types) in 29 adults, 21 (71%) showed local reaction characterized principally by local soreness and/or induration at the injection site within 2 days after vaccination.

Rash, urticaria, arthritis, arthralgia, serum sickness, and adenitis have been reported rarely.

Low grade fever (less than 100.9°F) occurs ocassionally and is usually confined to the 24-hour period following vaccination. Although rare, fever over 102°F has been reported. Malaise, myalgia, headache, and asthenia also have been reported.

Patients with otherwise stabilized idiopathic thrombocytopenic purpura have, on rare occasions, experienced a relapse in their thrombocytopenia, occurring 2 to 14 days after vaccination, and lasting up to 2 weeks.

Reactions of greater severity, duration, or extent are unusual. Neurological disorders such as paresthesias and acute radiculoneuropathy including Guillain-Barré syndrome have been rarely reported in temporal association with administration of Pneumococcal Vaccine. No cause and effect relationship has been established. Rarely, anaphylactoid reactions have been reported.

DOSAGE AND ADMINISTRATION
Do not inject intravenously. Intradermal administration should be avoided.

Parenteral drug products should be inspected visually for particulate matter and discoloration prior to administration, whenever solution and container permit Pneumococcal Vaccine, Polyvalent, is a clear, colorless solution.

Administer a single 0.5 mL dose of Pneumococcal Vaccine, Polyvalent, subcutaneously or intramuscularly (preferably in the deltoid muscle or lateral mid-thigh), with appropriate precautions to avoid intravascular administration.

SINGLE-DOSE AND 5-DOSE VIALS
For Syringe Use Only: Withdraw 0.5 mL from the vial using a sterile needle and syringe free of preservatives, antiseptics and detergents.

It is important to use a separate sterile syringe and needle for each individual patient to prevent transmission of hepatitis B and other infectious agents from one person to another. Store unopened and opened vials at 2-8°C (36-46°F). The vaccine is used directly as supplied. No dilution or reconstitution is necessary. Phenol 0.25% added as preservative. All vaccine must be discarded after the expiration date.

HOW SUPPLIED
INJECTION:

BRAND/MANUFACTURER	NDC	SIZE	AWP
○ BRAND			
PNEUMOVAX 23: Merck	00006-4739-00	2.5 ml	$51.05
PNU-IMUNE 23: Lederle Labs	00005-2309-31	2.5 ml	$67.79
PNEUMOVAX 23: Merck	00006-4741-00	0.5 ml 5s	$57.28
PNU-IMUNE 23: Lederle Labs	00005-2309-33	0.5 ml 5s	$76.03

Pneumomist *SEE* GUAIFENESIN

Pneumotussin Hc *SEE* GUAIFENESIN AND
HYDROCODONE BITARTRATE

Pneumovax 23 *SEE* PNEUMOCOCCAL VACCINE,
POLYVALENT

Pnu-Imune 23 SEE PNEUMOCOCCAL VACCINE, POLYVALENT

Podofilox

DESCRIPTION

Podofilox is an antimitotic drug which can be chemically synthesized or purified from the plant families Coniferae and Berberidaceae (e.g. species of Juniperus and Podophyllum). Podofilox 0.5% solution is formulated for topical administration. Each milliliter of solution contains 5 mg of Podofilox, in a vehicle containing lactic acid and sodium lactate in alcohol 95%, USP.

Podofilox has a molecular weight of 414.4 daltons, and is soluble in alcohol and sparingly soluble in water. Its chemical name is 5,8,8a,9-Tetrahydro-9-hydroxy-5- (3,4,5-trimethoxylphenyl)furo [3′,4′:6,7] naphtho [2,3,d] -1,3-dioxol-6(5aH)-one.

Following is its chemical structure:

CLINICAL PHARMACOLOGY

MECHANISM OF ACTION

Treatment of genital warts with Podofilox results in necrosis of visible wart tissue. The exact mechanism of action is unknown.

PHARMACOKINETICS

In systemic absorption studies in 52 patients, topical applications of 0.05 mL of 0.5% Podofilox solution to external genitalia did not result in detectable serum levels. Applications of 0.1 to 1.5 mL resulted in peak serum levels of 1 to 17 ng/mL one to two hours after application. The elimination half-life ranged from 1.0 to 4.5 hours. The drug was not found to accumulate after multiple treatments.

CLINICAL STUDIES

In clinical studies with Podofilox Solution, the test product and its vehicle were applied in a double-blind fashion to comparable patient groups. Patients were treated for two to four weeks, and reevaluated at a two-week follow-up examination. Although the number of patients and warts evaluated at each time period varied, the results among investigators were relatively consistent.

The following table represents the responses noted in terms of frequency of response by lesions treated and the overall response by patients. Data are presented for the 2-week follow-up only for those patients evaluated at that time point.

RESPONSES IN TREATED PATIENTS

	Initially Cleared*	Recurred after Clearing*	Cleared at 2-Week Follow-Up*
% Warts (n = 524)	79% (412/524)	35% (146/412)	60% (269/449)
% Patients (n = 70)	50% (35/70)	60% (21/35)	25% (14/57)

* Cleared and clearing mean no visible wart tissue remained at the treated sites

INDICATIONS AND USAGE

Podofilox solution is indicated for the topical treatment of external genital warts (Condyloma acuminatum). This products is not indicated in the treatment of perianal or mucous membrane warts (see "Precautions").

DIAGNOSIS

Although genital warts have a characteristic appearance, histopathologic confirmation should be obtained if there is any doubt of the diagnosis. Differentiating warts from squamous cell carcinoma (so-called "Bowenoid papulosis") is of particular concern. Squamous cell carcinoma may also be associated with human papillomavirus but should not be treated with Podofilox solution.

CONTRAINDICATIONS

Podofilox solution is contraindicated for patients who develop hypersensitivity or intolerance to any component of the formulation.

WARNINGS

Correct diagnosis of the lesions to be treated is essential. See the "Diagnosis" subsection of the "Indications and Usage" statement.

Podofilox solution is intended for cutaneous use only.

Avoid contact with the eye. If eye contact occurs, patients should immediately flush the eye with copious quantities of water and seek medical advice.

PRECAUTIONS

GENERAL

Data are not available on the safe and effective use of this product for treatment of warts occurring in the perianal area or mucous membranes of the genital area (including the urethra, rectum and vagina). The recommended method of application, frequency of application, and duration of usage should not be exceeded (see "Dosage And Administration").

INFORMATION FOR PATIENTS

The patient should be provided with a Patient Information leaflet when Podofilox prescription is filled.

CARCINOGENESIS, MUTAGENESIS AND IMPAIRMENT OF FERTILITY

Reports of lifetime carcinogenicity studies in mice are not available. Published animal studies, in general, have not shown the drug substance, Podofilox, to be carinogenic.[1,2,3,4,5]. There are published reports that, in mouse studies, crude podophyllin resin (containing Podofilox) applied topically to the cervix produced changes resembling carcinoma in situ.[6] These changes were reversible at five weeks after cessation of treatment. In one reported experiment, epidermal carcinoma of the vagina and cervix was found in 1 out of 18 mice after 120 applications of podophyllin[7] (the drug was applied twice weekly over a 15-month period).

Podofilox was not mutagenic in the Ames plate reverse mutation assay at concentrations up to 5 mg/plate, with and without metabolic activation. No cell transformation related to potential oncogenicity was observed in BALB/3T3 cells after exposure to Podofilox at concentrations up to 0.008 µg/mL without metabolic activation and 12 µg/mL Podofilox with metabolic activation. Results from the mouse micronucleus in vivo assay using podofilox 0.5% solution in concentrations up to 25 mg/kg, indicate that Podofilox should be considered a potential clastogen (a chemical that induces disruption and breakage of chromosomes).

Daily topical applications of Podofilox Solution at doses up to the equivalent of 0.2 mg/kg (5 times the recommended maximum human dose) to rats throughout gametogenesis, mating, gestation, parturition and lactation for two generations demonstrated no impairment of fertility.

PREGNANCY

Pregnancy Category C: Podofilox was not teratogenic in the rabbit following topical application of up to 0.21 mg/kg (5 times the maximum human dose) once daily for 13 days. The scientific literature contains references that Podofilox is embryotoxic in rats when administered systemically in a dose approximately 250 times the recommended maximum human dose.[8,9] Teratogenicity and embryotoxicity have not been studied with intravaginal application. Many antimitotic drug products are known to be embryotoxic. There are no adequate and well-controlled studies in pregnant women. Podofilox should be used in pregnancy only if the potential benefit justifies the potential risk to the fetus.

NURSING MOTHERS

It is not known whether this drug is excreted in human milk. Because of the potential for serious adverse reactions in nursing infants from Podofilox, a decision should be made whether to discontinue nursing or to discontinue the drug, taking into account the importance of the drug to the mother.

PEDIATRIC USE

Safety and effectiveness in children have not been established.

ADVERSE REACTIONS

In clinical trials, the following local adverse reactions were reported at some point during treatment.

Adverse Experience	Males	Females
Burning	64%	78%
Pain	50%	72%
Inflammation	71%	63%
Erosion	67%	67%
Itching	50%	65%

Reports of burning and pain were more frequent and of greater severity in women than in men.

Adverse effects reported in less than 5% of the patients included pain with intercourse, insomnia, tingling, bleeding, tenderness, chafing, malodor, dizziness, scarring, vesicle formation, crusting, edema, dryness/peeling, foreskin irretraction, hematuria, vomiting and ulceration.

OVERDOSAGE

Topically applied Podofilox may be absorbed systemically (see "Clinical Pharmacology" section). Toxicity reported following systemic administration of Podofilox in investigational use for cancer treatment included: nausea, vomiting, fever, diarrhea, bone marrow depression, and oral ulcers. Following 5 to 10 daily intravenous doses of 0.5 to 1 mg/kg/day, significant hematological toxicity occurred but was reversible. Other toxicities occurred at lower doses. Toxicity reported following systemic administration of podophyllum resin included: nausea, vomiting, fever, diarrhea, peripheral neuropathy, altered mental status, lethargy, coma, tachypnea, respiratory failure, leukocytosis, pancytosis, hematuria, renal failure, and seizures. Treatment of topical overdosage should include washing the skin free of any remaining drug and symptomatic and supportive therapy.

DOSAGE AND ADMINISTRATION

In order to ensure that the patient is fully aware of the correct method of therapy and to identify which specific warts should be treated, the technique for initial application of the medication should be demonstrated by the prescriber.

Apply twice daily morning and evening (every 12 hours), for 3 consecutive days, then withhold use for 4 consecutive days. This one week cycle of treatment may be repeated up to four times until there is no visible wart tissue. **If there is incomplete response after four treatment weeks, alternative treatments should be considered. Safety and effectiveness of more than four treatment weeks have not been established.**

Podofilox solution is applied to the warts with a cotton-tipped applicator supplied with the drug. The drug-dampened applicator should be touched to the wart to be treated, applying the minimum amount of solution necessary to cover the lesion. **Treatment should be limited to less than 10 cm^2 of wart tissue and to no more than 0.5 mL of the solution per day.** There is no evidence to suggest that more frequent application will increase efficacy, but additional applications would be expected to increase the rate of local adverse reactions and systemic absorption.

Care should be taken to allow the solution to dry before allowing the return of opposing skin surfaces to their normal positions. After each treatment, the used applicator should be carefully disposed of and the patient should wash his or her hands.

Store at controlled room temperature between 15 and 30°C (59° and 86°F). *Avoid excessive heat. Do not freeze.*

REFERENCES

1. Berenblum, 1951. *J. Natl. Cancer Inst.* 11:839-841   2. H.A. Kaminetsky and M. Swerdlow, 1965. *Am. J. Obst. Gyn.* 93:486-490   3. E.A. McGrew and H.A. Kaminetsky. 1961. *Am J. Clin. Pathol.* 35:538-545   4. F.J.C. Roe and M.H. Salaman, 1955. *Brit. J. Cancer.* 9:177-203   5. H.S. Taper, 1977. Z. Kerbsforsch, 90:197-210   6. H.A. Kaminetsky and E.A. McGrew, and R.L. Phillips, 1959. *Am. J. Obst. Gyn.* 14. 1-3   7. H.A. Kaminetsky and E.A. McGrew, 1963. *Arch. Path.*73:481-485   8. K. Didcock, D. Jackson, and J.M. Robson, 1956. *Brit. J. Pharmacol.* 11:437-441   9. J. Thiersch, 1963. *Soc. Exptl. Biol. Med. Proc.* 113:124-127

HOW SUPPLIED
SOLUTION: 0.5%

BRAND/MANUFACTURER	NDC	SIZE	AWP
○ BRAND			
CONDYLOX: Oclassen	55515-0101-01	3.5 ml	$50.40

Point-Two SEE SODIUM FLUORIDE

Polaramine SEE DEXCHLORPHENIRAMINE MALEATE

Polaramine Expectorant SEE
DEXCHLORPHENIRAMINE MALEATE/GUAIFENESIN/
PSEUDOEPHEDRINE SULFATE

Polio Vaccine

DESCRIPTION
POLIO VACCINE, ORAL LIVE

Manufacture and Composition: Polio Vaccine, Oral Live is a mixture of three types of attenuated polioviruses that have been propagated in monkey kidney cell culture. The cells are grown in the presence of Eagle's basal medium consisting of Earle's balanced salt solution containing amino acids, antibiotics, and calf serum. After cell growth, the medium is removed and replaced with fresh medium containing the inoculating virus but no calf serum. The final vaccine is diluted with a modified cell-culture maintenance medium containing sorbitol. Each dose (0.5 mL) contains less than 25 micrograms of each of the antibiotics, streptomycin and neomycin.

Potency of the vaccine is expressed in terms of the amount of virus ($\log_{10}$) contained in the recommended dose as tissue culture infective doses ($TCID_{50}$). The human dose of vaccine containing all three virus types shall be constituted to have infectivity titers in the final container material of $10^{5.4}$ to $10^{6.4}$ for Type 1, $10^{4.5}$ to $10^{5.5}$ for Type 2, and $10^{5.2}$ to $10^{6.2}$ for Type 3, when the primary monkey kidney tube titration method is used.[1] If the more sensitive Hep-2 microtitration procedure is employed to determine the infectivity titers in each human dose, then equivalent vaccine is achieved with numerical infectivity titers of $10^{6.0}$ to $10^{7.0}$ for Type 1, $10^{5.1}$ to $10^{6.1}$ for Type 2, and $10^{5.8}$ to $10^{6.8}$ for Type 3.[2]

POLIO VACCINE, INACTIVATED

Polio Vaccine, Inactivated, is a sterile suspension of three types of poliovirus: Type 1 (Mahoney), Type 2 (MEF-1), and Type 3 (Saukett). The viruses are grown in cultures of VERO cells, a continuous line of monkey kidney cells, by the microcarrier technique. The viruses are concentrated, purified, and made noninfectious by inactivation with formaldehyde. Each sterile immunizing dose (0.5 ml) of trivalent vaccine is formulated to contain 40 D antigen units of Type 1, 8 D antigen units of Type 2, and 32 D antigen units of Type 3 poliovirus, determined by comparison to a reference preparation. The Polio Vaccine is dissolved in phosphate buffered saline. Also present are 0.5% of 2-phenoxyethanol and a maximum of 0.02% of formaldehyde per dose as preservatives. Neomycin, streptomycin, and polymyxin B are used in vaccine production, and although purification procedures eliminate measurable amounts, less than 5 ng neomycin, 200 ng streptomycin, and 25 ng polymyxin B per dose may still be present. The vaccine is clear and colorless and should be administered subcutaneously.

CLINICAL PHARMACOLOGY
POLIO VACCAINE, ORAL LIVE

Administration of attenuated, Live Oral Poliovirus Vaccine (OPV) simulates natural infection, inducing active mucosal and systemic immunity without producing symptoms of disease. For optimal mucosal immunity to occur, it is necessary for the viruses to multiply in the intestinal tract. A primary series of trivalent vaccine is designed to produce an antibody response to poliovirus Types 1, 2, and 3. This response is comparable to the immunity induced by the natural disease. The antibodies thus formed help protect the individual against clinical poliomyelitis infection by any of the three types of poliovirus. Multiple sequential doses of OPV are administered to ensure that immunity to all three types of poliovirus has been achieved.[3] When used in the prescribed manner for immunization, type-specific neutralizing antibodies will be induced in 95% or more of susceptibles.[4]

POLIO VACCINE, INACTIVATED

Polio Vaccine, Inactivated is a highly purified, Inactivated Poliovirus Vaccine produced by microcarrier culture.[5,6] This culture technique and improvements in purification, concentration and standardization of poliovirus antigen have resulted in a more potent and more consistently immunogenic vaccine than the Polio Vaccine Inactivated which was available in the U.S. prior to 1988. These new methods allow for the production of vaccine that induces antibody responses in most children after administering fewer doses[7] than with vaccine available prior to 1988.

Studies in developed[7] and developing[8,9] countries with a similar Inactivated Poliovirus Vaccine produced by the same technology have shown that a direct relationship exists between the antigenic content of the vaccine, the frequency of seroconversion, and resulting antibody titer.

A study in the U.S. was carried out, which involved 219 two-month old infants who had received three doses of a Polio Vaccine, Inactivated. Seroconversion to all three types of poliovirus was demonstrated in 99% of these infants after two doses of vaccine. Following a third dose of vaccine at 18 months of age, high titers of neutralizing antibody were present in 99.1% of children to Type 1 and 100% of children to Types 2 and 3 polioviruses.[10]

Additional studies were carried out in the U.S. with Polio Vaccine, Inactivated. Results were reported for 120 infants who received two doses of Polio Vaccine, Inactivated at 2 and 4 months of age. Of these 120 children, detectable serum neutralizing antibody was induced after two doses of vaccine in 98.3% (Type 1), 100% (Type 2) and 97.5% (Type 3) of the children. In 83 children receiving three doses at 2, 4, and 12 months of age detectable serum neutralizing antibodies were detected in 97.6% (Type 1) and 100% (Types 2 and 3) of the children.[11,12]

Polio Vaccine, Inactivated reduces pharyngeal excretion of poliovirus[13-16]. Field studies in Europe have demonstrated immunity in populations thoroughly immunized with another IPV[17-21]. A survey of Swedish children and young adults given a Swedish IPV demonstrated persistence of circulating antibodies for at least 10 years to all three types of poliovirus[17].

Paralytic polio has not been reported in association with administration of Poliovirus Vaccine Inactivated.

INDICATIONS AND USAGE
POLIOVIRUS VACCINE, ORAL LIVE

This vaccine is indicated for use in the prevention of poliomyelitis caused by poliovirus Types 1, 2, and 3.

Infants from 6 to 12 weeks of age, *all unimmunized children,* and *adolescents* up to age 18 are the usual candidates for routine prophylaxis.

Polio Vaccine, Inactivated is indicated for active immunization of infants, children, and adults for the prevention of poliomyelitis.

The Immunization Practices Advisory Committee (ACIP) of the Public Health Service states that trivalent Oral Poliovirus Vaccine (OPV) and Inactivated Poliovirus Vaccine (IPV) are both effective in preventing poliomyelitis.

It is recommended that all infants, unimmunized children and adolescents not previously immunized be vaccinated routinely against paralytic poliomyelitis.[22] Polio Vaccine, Inactivated should be offered to individuals who have refused Polio Vaccine Live Oral or in whom OPV is contraindicated. Parents should be adequately informed of the risks and benefits of both inactivated and oral polio vaccines so that they can make an informed choice (Report of An Evaluation of Poliomyelitis Vaccine Policy Options, Institute of Medicine, National Academy of Sciences, Washington, D.C., 1988).

The choice of OPV as the preferred Poliovirus Vaccine for primary administration to children in the United States has been made by the ACIP, the Committee on Infectious Diseases of the American Academy of Pediatrics, and a special expert committee of the Institute of Medicine, National Academy of Science.[3,4,22,23] OPV is preferred because it induces intestinal immunity, is simple

---

◆ RATED THERAPEUTICALLY EQUIVALENT; ◇ THERAPEUTIC EQUIVALENCE UNCONFIRMED; ○ UNRATED

to administer, is well accepted by patients, results in immunization of some contacts of vaccinated persons, and has a record of having essentially eliminated disease associated with wild poliovirus in this country.[4] OPV is also recommended for control of epidemic poliomyelitis.[3,23]

IPV is specifically indicated for use in immunodeficient individuals, their household contacts, or in certain adults (see *"Contraindications"* and *"Indications and Usage: Use in Adults"* for details).[22]

OPV should not be used in households with immunodeficient individuals because OPV is excreted in the stool by healthy vaccines and can infect an immunocompromised household member, which may result in paralytic disease. In a household with an immunocompromised member, only Poliovirus Vaccine, Inactivated should be used for all those requiring poliovirus immunization.[3]

Children of all ages should have their immunization status reviewed and be considered for supplemental immunization as follows for adults. Time intervals between doses longer than those recommended for routine primary immunization do not necessitate additional doses as long as a final total of four doses is reached (see *Dosage and Administration"*).

Prior to immunization, the parent, guardian, or adult patient should be informed of the two types of poliovirus vaccines available, the risks and benefits of each to the individual and to the community, and the reasons why recommendations are made for giving specific vaccines under certain circumstances.

Past history of clinical poliomyelitis or prior vaccination with IPV in otherwise healthy individuals does not preclude the administration of OPV when otherwise indicated. Similarly, previous clinical poliomyelitis (usually due to only a single poliovirus type) or incomplete immunization with OPV are not contraindications to completing the primary series of immunization with Polio Vaccine, Inactivated.

The simultaneous administration of OPV, diphtheria and tetanus toxoids and pertussis vaccine (DTP), and/or measles-mumps-rubella vaccine (MMR), has resulted in seroconversion rates and rates of side effects similar to those observed when the vaccines are administered separately.[24]

Administration of Immune Globulin (IG), if necessary, within 7 days prior to immunization with OPV does not reduce the antibody response to OPV based on a study conducted in Peace Corps volunteers.[25]

Use in Adults: Routine primary poliovirus immunization of adults (generally those 18 years of age or older), residing in the United States, is not recommended by the Immunization Practices Advisory Committee (ACIP). Immunization *is* recommended by the ACIP for certain adults who are at greater risk of exposure to either vaccine or to wild polioviruses than the general population, including travelers to areas where poliomyelitis is endemic or epidemic, members of communities or specific population groups with disease caused by wild polioviruses, laboratory workers handling specimens that may contain polioviruses, and health care workers in close contact with patients who might be excreting polioviruses as follows:

Unimmunized adults: primary immunization with enhanced-potency IPV is recommended. However, if less than 1 month is available before protection is needed, a single dose of either OPV or enhanced-potency IPV is recommended, with the remaining doses given later if the person remains at increased risk. *Incompletely immunized adults* who have had (1) at least one dose of OPV, (2) fewer than three doses of conventional IPV, or (3) a combination of conventional IPV and OPV totaling fewer than three doses, should receive at least one dose of OPV or enhanced-potency IPV. Additional doses needed to complete a primary series should be given prior to exposure, if time permits. *Adults who have completed a primary series* with any one or a combination of polio vaccines may be given a dose of OPV or enhanced-potency IPV.[22]

Immunization with IPV may be undertaken in unimmunized or inadequately immunized adults in households in which children are to be given OPV (see *"Adverse Reactions"*),[3,22] provided that the immunization of the child can be assured and not unduly delayed. The adult should be informed of the small OPV related risk to the contact.

Epidemic Control: Polio Vaccine, Oral Live has been recommended for epidemic control. Within an epidemic area, OPV should be provided for all persons over 6 weeks of age who have not been completely immunized or whose immunization status is unknown, with the exceptions noted under immunodeficiency.[3,23] (See *"Contraindications"*).

In certain tropical endemic areas, where poliomyelitis has been increasing in recent years, the physician may wish to administer OPV to the infant at birth. Because successful immunization is less likely in newborn infants, a complete series of OPV should follow the neonatal dose beginning when the infants are 2 months old.[3] If the physician elects to immunize the infant at birth, it may be prudent to wait until the child is 3 days old, and to recommend abstention from breast-feeding for 2 to 3 hours before and after oral immunization to minimize exposure of the vaccine viruses to colostrum and to permit the establishment of the vaccine viruses in the gut.

CONTRAINDICATIONS
POLIO VACCINE, ORAL LIVE
Under no circumstances should Polio Vaccine, Oral Live be administered parenterally.

Patients with recognized immunodeficiency are at greater risk of developing paralysis when exposed to live poliovirus than persons with a normal immune system.

Polio Vaccine, Oral Live must not be administered to patients with immune deficiency diseases such as combined immunodeficiency, hypogammaglobulinemia and agammaglobulin-

emia. Further, **Polio Vaccine, Oral Live *must not* be administered to patients with altered immune states, such as those occurring in human immunodeficiency virus (HIV) infection, thymic abnormalities, leukemia, lymphoma, generalized malignancy, or advanced debilitating conditions, or by lowered resistance from therapy with corticosteroids, alkylating drugs, antimetabolites, or radiation. Because vaccine viruses are excreted by the vaccinee, and may spread to contacts, Polio Vaccine, Oral Live should not be used in families with immunodeficient members.[3,4]**

Recipients of the vaccine should avoid close household-type contact with all persons with altered immune status for at least 6 to 8 weeks.

Because of the possibility of immunodeficiency in other children born to a family in which there has been one such case, OPV should not be given to a member of a household in which there is a family history of immunodeficiency until the immune status of the intended recipient and other children in the family is determined to be normal.[4]

Immunization of all persons in the above described circumstances should be with IPV. Patients with an altered immune state may or may not develop a protective response against paralytic poliomyelitis after administration of Polio Vaccine, Inactivated.[27]

POLIO VACCINE, INACTIVATED
Polio Vaccine, Inactivated is contraindicated in persons with a history of hypersensitivity to any component of the vaccine, including neomycin, streptomycin and polymyxin B.

If anaphylaxis or anaphylactic shock occurs within 24 hours of administration of a dose of vaccine, no further doses should be given.

Vaccination of persons with any acute, febrile illness should be deferred until after recovery; however, minor illnesses such as mild upper respiratory infections, are not in themselves reasons for postponing vaccine administration.

WARNINGS
Under no circumstances should Polio Vaccine, Oral Live be administered parenterally.

Immunization with Polio Vaccine, Oral Live should be deferred during the course of any febrile illness or acute infection. In addition, immunization should be deferred in the presence of persistent vomiting or diarrhea, or suspected gastroenteritis infection. Other viruses (including poliovirus and other enteroviruses) may compromise the desired response to Polio Vaccine, Oral Live, since their presence in the intestinal tract may interfere with replication of the attenuated strains of poliovirus.

Neomycin, streptomycin, and polymyxin B are used in the production of Polio Vaccine, Inactivated. Although purification procedures eliminate measurable amounts of these substances, traces may be present (see *"Description"*) and allergic reactions may occur in persons sensitive to these substances.

PRECAUTIONS
Polio Vaccine, Oral Live is not effective in modifying or preventing cases of existing and/or incubating poliomyelitis.

Records Required by the National Childhood Vaccine Injury Act: This Act requires that the manufacturer and lot number of the vaccine administered be recorded by the health care provider in the vaccine recipient's permanent record, along with the date of administration of the vaccine and the name, address, and title of the person administering the vaccine.

The Act further requires that the health care provider report to a health department or to the FDA the occurrence, following immunization, of any event set forth in the Vaccine Injury Table including: paralytic poliomyelitis—in a nonimmunodeficient recipient within 30 days of vaccination,—in an immunodeficient recipient within 6 months of vaccination; any vaccine-associated community case of paralytic poliomyelitis; or any acute complication or sequela (including death) of above events.[28]

Before injection of the vaccine, the physician should carefully review the recommendations for product use and the patient's medical history including possible hypersensitivities and side effects that may have occurred following previous doses of the vaccine.

Epinephrine hydrochloride (1:1000) and other appropriate agents should be available to control immediate allergic reactions.

Concerns have been raised about whether stimulation of the immune system of a patient with HIV infection by immunization with inactivated vaccines might cause deterioration in immunologic function. However, such effects have not been noted thus far among children with AIDS or among immunosuppressed individuals after immunizations with inactivated vaccines. The potential benefits of immunization of these children outweigh the undocumented risk of such adverse events.[22]

Drug Interactions: There are no known interactions of Poliovirus Vaccine, Inactivated with drugs or foods. Simultaneous administration of other parenteral vaccines is not contraindicated.

Carcinogenesis, Mutagenesis, Impairment of Fertility: Long term studies in animals to evaluate carcinogenic potential or impairment of fertility have not been conducted.

Pediatric Use: Safety and efficacy of Polio Vaccine, Inactivated have been shown in children 6 weeks of age and older[10,12] (see *"Dosage and Administration"*).

Use in Pregnancy: Pregnancy Category C: Animal reproduction studies have not been conducted with Polio Vaccine, Oral Live or Polio Vaccine, Inactivated. It is also not known whether OPV or IPV can cause fetal harm when administered to a pregnant woman or can affect reproduction capacity.

Although there is no convincing evidence documenting adverse effects of either OPV or IPV on the developing fetus or pregnant women, it is prudent on theoretical grounds to avoid vaccinating pregnant women. However, if immediate protection against poliomyelitis is needed, OPV is recommended[3,22] (See "Contraindications" and "Adverse Reactions".) IPV should be given to a pregnant woman only if clearly needed.

ADVERSE REACTIONS
POLIO VACCINE, ORAL LIVE
Paralytic disease following the ingestion of live poliovirus vaccines has been, on rare occasion, reported in individuals receiving the vaccine, and in persons who were in close contact with vaccinees.[3,4,29,30] The vaccine viruses are shed in the vaccinee's stools up to 6 to 8 weeks as well as via the pharyngeal route. Most reports of paralytic disease following ingestion of the vaccine or contact with a recent vaccinee are based on epidemiological analysis and temporal association between vaccination or contact and the onset of symptoms and most authorities believe that a causal relationship exists.[2,23,28,29,30]

A retrospective study of a large population given OPV suggests that this vaccine may also be temporally associated with Guillain-Barré syndrome.[31] **A causal relationship has not been established.**

Prior to administration of the vaccine, the attending physician should warn or specifically direct personnel acting under his/her authority to convey the warnings to the vaccinee, parent, guardian, or other responsible person of the possibility of vaccine-associated paralysis, particularly to the recipient, susceptible family members, and other close personal contacts.[3,4]

The Centers for Disease Control report that during the years 1973 through 1984 approximately 274.1 million OPV doses were distributed in the United States. During this same period, 105 vaccine-associated cases were reported (1 case per 2.6 million doses distributed). Of these 105 cases, 35 occurred in vaccine recipients (1 case per 7.8 million doses distributed), 50 occurred in household and nonhousehold contacts of vaccinees (1 case per 5.5 million doses distributed), 14 occurred in immunodeficient recipients or contacts, and 6 occurred in persons with no history of vaccine exposure, from whom vaccine-like viruses were isolated.[29] Thirty-three (94%) of the recipient cases, 41 (82%) of the contact cases, and 5 (36%) of the immune deficient cases were associated with the recipient's first dose of OPV. Because most cases of vaccine-associated paralysis have occurred in association with the first dose, the CDC has estimated the likelihood of paralysis in association with first v subsequent doses of OPV, using the number of births during 1973-1984 to estimate the number of first doses distributed, and subtracting this from the total distribution to estimate the number of subsequent doses distributed. This method estimates a frequency of paralysis for recipients of one case per 1.2 million first doses v one case per 116.5 million subsequent doses; for contacts, one case per 1 million first doses v one case per 25.9 million subsequent doses; with an overall frequency of 1 case per 520,000 first doses v one case per 12.3 million subsequent doses.[29]

Other methods of estimating the likelihood of paralysis in association with OPV have been described. Because the number of susceptible vaccine recipients or contacts of recipients is not known, the true risk of vaccine-associated poliomyelitis is impossible to determine precisely.[28]

When the attenuated vaccine strains are to be introduced into a household with adults who are unimmunized or whose immune status cannot be determined, the risk of vaccine-associated paralysis can be reduced by giving these adults two doses of enhanced potency IPV a month apart before the children receive Polio Vaccine, Oral Live. The children may receive the first dose of Polio Vaccine, Oral Live at the same visit that the adults receive the second dose of enhanced potency IPV. For partially immunized adult contacts, a booster dose of enhanced potency IPV can be given at the same visit that the first dose of OPV is given to the child.[3]

The responsible adult should also be informed of precautions to be taken such as handwashing after diaper changes.[32] The ACIP states: "Because of the overriding importance of ensuring prompt and complete immunization of the child and the extreme rarity of OPV-associated disease in contacts, the Committee recommends the administration of OPV to a child regardless of the poliovirus-vaccine status of adult household contacts. This is the usual practice in the United States. The responsible adult should be informed of the small risk involved. An acceptable alternative, if there is a strong assurance that ultimate, full immunization of the child will not be jeopardized or unduly delayed, is to immunize adults...[with IPV]... before giving OPV to the child."[4]

The American Academy of Pediatrics and the American College of Physicians have made similar recommendations.[3,32]

POLIO VACCINE, INACTIVATED
In earlier studies with the vaccine grown in primary monkey kidney cells, transient local reactions at the site of injection were observed during a clinical trial.[10] Erythema, induration and pain occurred in 3.2%, 1%, and 13%, respectively, of vaccinees within 48 hours post-vaccination. Temperatures $\geq 39°C$ ($\geq 102°F$) were reported in up to 38% of vaccinees. Other symptoms noted included sleepiness, fussiness, crying, decreased appetite, and spitting up of feedings. Because Polio Vaccine, Inactivated was given in a different site but concurrently with diphtheria and tetanus toxoids and pertussis vaccine adsorbed (DTP), systemic reactions could not be attributed to a specific vaccine. However, these systemic reactions were comparable in frequency and severity to that reported for DTP given without IPV.

In another study using Polio Vaccine, Inactivated in the United States, there were no significant local or systemic reactions following injection of the vaccine. There were 7% (6/86), 12% (8/65), and 4% (2/45) of children with temperatures over 100.6°F, following the first, second, and third doses respectively. Most of the children received DTP at the same time as IPV and therefore it was not possible to attribute reactions to a particular vaccine; however, such reactions were not significantly different than when DTP is given alone.

Guillain-Barre Syndrome (GBS) has been temporally related to administration of Polio Vaccine, Inactivated.

DOSAGE AND ADMINISTRATION
POLIO VACCINE, ORAL LIVE
Polio Vaccine, Oral Live is to be administered *orally, under the supervision of a physician. Under no circumstances should this vaccine be administered parenterally.* For convenience, the vaccine is supplied in a disposable pipette containing a single dose of 0.5 mL which should be administered directly into the mouth of the vaccine. Breast feeding does not interfere with successful immunization when OPV is administered according to the following schedule.[4]

Primary Series: The primary series consists of three doses.

Infants: The ACIP and AAP recommend that the first dose of OPV be administered when the infant is approximately 2 months (6 to 12 weeks) of age. The second dose should be given not less than 6 and preferably 8 weeks later, commonly at 4 months of age. A third dose of OPV should be given when the child is approximately 15 to 18 months of age to complete the primary series, but may be given at any time between 12 and 24 months of age.[3] In endemic areas an additional dose administered 2 months after the second dose is desirable.[3,4]

Older Children and Adolescents (up to 18 years of age): Unimmunized children and adolescents should receive two doses given not less than 6 and preferably 8 weeks apart, followed by a third dose 6 to 12 months after the second dose. If there is substantial risk of exposure to polio, the third dose should be given 6 to 8 weeks after the second dose.[3,4]

Children at any age who are unimmunized or partially immunized should receive the number of doses necessary to complete the required series of three doses. If the schedule has been interrupted, the series does not need to be reinitiated.[3,24]

Adults: See "Indications" and "Adverse Reactions". Where OPV is given to unimmunized adults the dosage regimen is as indicated for older children and adolescents.

Supplemental Doses: School Entry: On entering elementary school, all children who have completed the primary series should be given a single follow-up dose of OPV[3,4] (all others should complete the primary series). The fourth supplemental dose is not required in those who received the third primary dose on or after their fourth birthday.[3,4] The ACIP and AAP do not recommend routine booster doses of vaccine beyond that given at the time of entering school.[3,4] It has been shown that over 95% of children studied 5 years after full immunization with oral polio vaccine had protective antibodies to all three types of poliovirus.[33]

Increased Risk: If an individual who has completed a primary series is subjected to a substantially increased risk because of personal contact, travel, or occupation, a single dose of OPV may be given.[3,4]

SIMULTANEOUS ADMINISTRATION WITH OTHER VACCINES
The simultaneous administration of OPV, diphtheria and tetanus toxoids and pertussis vaccine (DTP) and/or measles-mumps-rubella vaccine (MMR), has resulted in seroconversion rates and rates of side effects similar to those observed when the vaccines are administered separately.[24] The AAP states that OPV, DTP, MMR and/or Haemophilus b conjugate vaccines may be given concomitantly.[3,34]

STORAGE
To maintain the potency of *Polio Vaccine, Oral Live,* it is necessary to store this vaccine at a temperature which will maintain ice continuously in a solid state (below 0°C or 32°F). However, since some brands contain sorbitol, they may remain fluid at temperatures above —14°C (+ 7°F). Ice cubes that remain frozen continuously when stored in the same freezer compartment will confirm that the temperature is appropriate for storage of Polio Vaccine, Oral Live. If frozen, the vaccine must be completely thawed prior to use. A container of vaccine that has been frozen and then is thawed may be carried through a maximum of 10 freeze-thaw cycles, provided the temperature does not exceed 8°C (46°F) during the periods of thaw, and provided the total cumulative duration of thaw does not exceed 24 hours. If the 24-hour period is exceeded, the vaccine must then be used within 30 days, during which time it must be stored at a temperature between 2°C to 8°C (36°F to 46°F). Ideally, Polio vaccine, Oral Live should be removed from the freezer and thawed immediately prior to use.

Color Change: This vaccine contains phenol red as a pH indicator. The usual color of the vaccine is pink, although some containers of vaccine, shipped or stored in dry ice, may exhibit a yellow coloration due to the very low temperature or possible absorption of carbon dioxide. The color of the vaccine prior to use (red-pink-yellow) has no effect on the virus or efficacy of the vaccine.

VACCINE, INACTIVATED
Parenteral drug products should be inspected visually for particulate matter and/or discoloration prior to administration. If these conditions exist, vaccine should not be administered.

After preparation of the injection site, immediately administer the vaccine subcutaneously. In infants and small children, the mid-lateral aspect of the thigh is the preferred site. In adults the vaccine should be administered in the deltoid area.

Care should be taken to avoid administering the injection into or near blood vessels and nerves. After aspiration, if blood or any suspicious discoloration appears in the syringe, do not inject but discard contents and repeat procedures using a new dose of vaccine administered at a different site.

Do not administer vaccine intravenously.

CHILDREN

Primary Immunization: A primary series of Polio Vaccine, Inactivated consists of three 0.5-ml doses administered subcutaneously. The interval between the first two doses should be at least four weeks, but preferably eight weeks. The first two doses are usually administered with DTP immunization and are given at two and four months of age. The third dose should follow at least six months but preferably 12 months after the second dose. It may be desirable to administer this dose with MMR and other vaccines, but at a different site, in children 15-18 months of age. All children who received a primary series of Polio Vaccine, Inactivated, or a combination of IPV and OPV, should be given a booster dose of OPV or IPV before entering school, unless the final (third dose) of the primary series was administered on or after the fourth birthday.[22]

The need to routinely administer additional doses is unknown at this time.[22]

A final total of four doses is necessary to complete a series of primary and booster doses. Children and adolescents with a previously incomplete series of IPV should receive sufficient additional doses to reach this number.

ADULTS

Unvaccinated Adults: For unvaccinated adults at increased risk of exposure to poliovirus, a primary series of Polio Vaccine, Inactivated is recommended. While the responses of adults to primary series have not been studied, the recommended schedule for adults is two doses given at a 1-to-2 month interval and a third dose given 6 to 12 months later. If less than 3 months but more than 2 months are available before protection is needed, 3 doses of Polio Vaccine, Inactivated should be given at least 1 month apart. Likewise, if only 1 or 2 months are available, two doses of Polio Vaccine, Inactivated should be given at least 1 month apart. If less than 1 month is available, a single dose of either OPV or IPV is recommended.

Incompletely Vaccinated Adults: Adults who are at an increased risk of exposure to poliovirus and who have had at least one dose of OPV, fewer than 3 doses of conventional IPV, or a combination of conventional IPV or OPV totalling fewer than 3 doses should receive at least 1 dose of OPV or Polio Vaccine, Inactivated. Additional doses needed to complete a primary series should be given if time permits.

Completely Vaccinated Adults: Adults who are at an increased risk of exposure to poliovirus and who have previously completed a primary series with one or a combination of polio vaccines can be given a dose of either OPV or IPV.[4]

STORAGE

The vaccine is stable if stored in the refrigerator between 2°C and 8°C (35°F and 46°F). *The vaccine must not be frozen.*

REFERENCES

1. *Code of Federal Regulations.* 21 CFR:630.17[c], page 94, Revised April 1, 1989. 2. Albrecht P, Enterline JC, Boone EJ, et al. Poliovirus and polio antibody assay in Hep-2 and Vero cell cultures. *J Biol Stand.* 1983 11:91-97. 3. *Report of the Committee on Infectious Diseases, American Academy of Pediatrics.* 21st Edition, 1988; 334-342. Elk Grove Village, IL 4. Recommendations of the Immunization Practices Advisory Committee [ACIP], Poliomyelitis Prevention. *MMWR.* 1982; 31[3]:22-34. 5. van Wezel, A.L., et al: Inactivated poliovirus vaccine. Current production methods and new developments. Rev Infect Dis 6 (Suppl 2): S335-S340, 1984 6. Montagnon, B.J., et al: Industrial scale production of inactivated poliovirus vaccine prepared by culture of Vero cells on microcarrier. Rev Infect Dis 6 (Suppl 2): S341-S344, 1984 7. Salk, J., et al: Antigen content of inactivated poliovirus vaccine for use in a one- or two-dose regimen. Ann Clin Res 14: 204-212, 1982 8. Salk, J., et al: Killed poliovirus antigen titration in humans. Develop Biol Standard 41: 110-132, 1978 9. Salk, J., et al: Theoretical and practical considerations in the application of killed poliovirus vaccine for the control of paralytic poliomyelitis. Develop Biol Standard 47: 181-198, 1981 10. McBean, A.M., et al: Serologic response to oral polio vaccine and enhanced-potency inactivated polio vaccines. Am J Epidemiol 128: 615-628, 1988 11. Unpublished data available from Pasteur Merieux Serums & Vaccins S.A. 12. Faden, H., et al: Comparative evaluation of immunization with live attenuated and enhanced potency inactivated trivalent poliovirus vaccines in childhood: Systemic and local immune responses. J Infect Dis 162: 1291-1297, 1990 13. Marine, W.M., et al: Limitation of fecal and pharyngeal poliovirus excretion in Salk-vaccinated children. A family study during a Type 1 poliomyelitis epidemic. Amer J Hyg 76: 173-175, 1962 14. Bottiger, M., et al: Vaccination with attenuated Type 1 poliovirus, the Chat strain, II. Transmission of virus in relation to age. Acta Paed Scand 55: 416-421, 1966 15. Dick, G.W.A., et al: Vaccination against poliomyelitis with live virus vaccines. Effect of previous Salk vaccination on virus excretion. Brit Med J 2: 266-269, 1961 16. Wehrle, P.F., et al: Transmission of poliovirus; III. Prevalence of polioviruses in pharyngeal secretions of infected household contacts of patients with clinical disease. Pediatrics 27: 762-764, 1961 17. Bottiger, M.: Long-term immunity following vaccination with killed poliovirus vaccine in Sweden, a country with no circulating polivirus. Rev Infect Dis 6 (Suppl 2); S545-551, 1984 18. Chin, T.D.Y.: Immunity induced by inactivated poliovirus vaccine and excretion of virus. Rev Infect Dis 6 (Suppl 2): S369-S370, 1984 19. Salk, D.: Herd effect and virus eradication with use of killed poliovirus vaccine. Develop Biol Standard 47: 247-255, 1981 20. Bijerk, H.: Surveillance and control of poliomyelitis in the Netherlands. Rev Infect Dis 6 (Suppl 2): S451-S456, 1984 21. Lapinleimu, K.: Elimination of poliomyelitis in Finland. Rev Infect Dis 6 (Suppl 2): S457-S460, 1984 22 ACIP. Poliomyelitis prevention: Enhanced-Potency Inactivated Poliomyelitis Vaccine—Supplementary Statement. *MMWR.* 1987; 36[48]:795-798. 23. An evaluation of poliomyelitis vaccine policy options. Institute of Medicine, National Academy of Sciences, 1988, Publication No. 10M 88-04. 24. ACIP. General recommendations on immunization. *MMWR.* 1989; 38[13]:206-227. 25. Kaplan JE, Nelson DB, Schonberger LB, et al. The effect of immune globulin on the response to trivalent oral poliovirus and yellow fever vaccinations. *Bull WHO.* 1984; 62[4]:585-590. 26. Welsh JH, et al. Anti-infective properties of breast milk. *J Pediatr.* 1979; 94[1]:1-9. 27. ACIP: Immunization of children infected with human T-lymphotropic virus type III/lymphadenopathy-associated virus. MMWR 35: 595-606, 1986 28. National Childhood Injury Act: Requirements for permanent vaccination records and for reporting of selected events after vaccination. *MMWR.* 1988; 37[13]; 197-200. 29. Nkowane BM, Wassilak SGF, Orenstein WA, et al. Vaccine-associated paralytic poliomyelitis. United States 1973 through 1984. *JAMA.* 1987; 257[10]:1335-1340. 30. Esteves K. Safety of oral poliomyelitis vaccine: results of a WHO enquiry. *Bull WHO.* 1988; 66[6]:739-746. 31. Kinnunen E, Farkkila M, Hovi T, et al. Incidence of Guillain-Barre syndrome during a nationwide oral poliovirus vaccine campaign. *Neurology.* 1989; 39:1034-1036. 32. Guide for Adult Immunization. American College of Physicians, 2nd Edition, 25, 1990. Philadelphia, PA. 33. Krugman RD, et al. Antibody persistence after primary immunization with trivalent oral poliovirus vaccine. *Pediatrics.* 1977; 60[1]:80-82. 34. American Academy of Pediatrics, Haemophilus Influenzae Type B Conjugate Vaccines. Immunization of children 2 to 15 months of age. *PED COMM: AAP MEMBER ALERT,* October 1990.

HOW SUPPLIED

POLIO VACCINE, INACTIVATED
INJECTION:

BRAND/MANUFACTURER	NDC	SIZE	AWP
○ **BRAND**			
IPOL: Connaught	49281-8605-01	0.5 ml	$24.24
	49281-8605-02	0.5 ml 10s	$231.00

POLIO VACCINE, ORAL LIVE
SOLUTION:

BRAND/MANUFACTURER	NDC	SIZE	AWP
○ **BRAND**			
ORIMUNE: Lederle Labs	00005-2084-08	0.5 ml 10s	$148.04
	00005-2084-12	0.5 ml 50s	$689.91

Polocaine SEE MEPIVACAINE HYDROCHLORIDE

PolyHistForte SEE CHLORPHENIRAMINE MALEATE/ PHENYLEPHRINE HYDROCHLORIDE/PHENYLPROPANOLAMINE HYDROCHLORIDE/PYRILAMINE MALEATE

PolyPred SEE NEOMYCIN SULFATE/POLYMYXIN B SULFATE/PREDNISOLONE ACETATE

Poly-Vi-Flor SEE SODIUM FLUORIDE AND VITAMINS, MULTI

Poly-Vi-Flor with Iron SEE FERROUS SULFATE/SODIUM FLUORIDE/VITAMINS, MULTI

Polycitra SEE CITRIC ACID/POTASSIUM CITRATE/SODIUM CITRATE

Polycitra-K SEE CITRIC ACID AND POTASSIUM CITRATE

Polymyxin B Sulfate

> **WARNING**
>
> *CAUTION: WHEN THIS DRUG IS GIVEN INTRAMUSCULARLY AND/OR INTRATHECALLY, IT SHOULD BE GIVEN ONLY TO HOSPITALIZED PATIENTS, SO AS TO PROVIDE CONSTANT SUPERVISION BY A PHYSICIAN.*
>
> RENAL FUNCTION SHOULD BE CAREFULLY DETERMINED AND PATIENTS WITH RENAL DAMAGE AND NITROGEN RETENTION SHOULD HAVE REDUCED DOSAGE. PATIENTS WITH NEPHROTOXICITY DUE TO POLYMYXIN B SULFATE USUALLY SHOW ALBUMINURIA, CELLULAR CASTS, AND AZOTEMIA. DIMINISHING URINE OUTPUT AND A RISING BUN ARE INDICATIONS FOR DISCONTINUING THERAPY WITH THIS DRUG.
>
> NEUROTOXIC REACTIONS MAY BE MANIFESTED BY IRRITABILITY, WEAKNESS, DROWSINESS, ATAXIA, PERIORAL PARESTHESIA, NUMBNESS OF THE EXTREMITIES, AND BLURRING OF VISION. THESE ARE USUALLY ASSOCIATED WITH HIGH SERUM LEVELS FOUND IN PATIENTS WITH IMPAIRED RENAL FUNCTION AND/OR NEPHROTOXICITY. THE

CONCURRENT USE OF OTHER NEPHROTOXIC AND NEUROTOXIC DRUGS, PARTICULARLY KANAMYCIN, STREPTOMYCIN, CEPHALORIDINE, PAROMOMYCIN, TOBRAMYCIN, POLYMYXIN E (COLISTIN), NEOMYCIN, GENTAMICIN, AND VIOMYCIN, SHOULD BE AVOIDED.

THE NEUROTOXICITY OF POLYMYXIN B SULFATE CAN RESULT IN RESPIRATORY PARALYSIS FROM NEUROMUSCULAR BLOCKADE, ESPECIALLY WHEN THE DRUG IS GIVEN SOON AFTER ANESTHESIA AND/OR MUSCLE RELAXANTS.

USAGE IN PREGNANCY: THE SAFETY OF THIS DRUG IN HUMAN PREGNANCY HAS NOT BEEN ESTABLISHED.

DESCRIPTION

Polymyxin B Sulfate is one of a group of basic polypeptide antibiotics derived from *B polymyxa* (*B aerosporous*).

Polymyxin B Sulfate is available in powder form suitable for preparation of sterile solutions for intramuscular, intravenous drip, intrathecal, or ophthalmic use.

In the medical literature, dosages have frequently been given in terms of equivalent weight of pure Polymyxin B base. Each milligram of pure Polymyxin B base is equivalent to 10,000 units of Polymyxin B and each microgram of pure Polymyxin B base is equivalent to 10 units of Polymyxin B.

Aqueous solutions of Polymyxin B Sulfate may be stored up to 12 months without significant loss of potency if kept under refrigeration. In the interest of safety, solutions for parenteral use should be stored under refrigeration and any unused portion should be discarded after 72 hours. Polymyxin B Sulfate should not be stored in alkaline solutions since they are less stable.

Following is its chemical structure:

$$\left[-CH_2-N-\overset{\displaystyle CH_2OH}{\underset{\displaystyle \underset{O}{\overset{\displaystyle \|}{C}}}{}}-N- \right]_x$$

ACTIONS

Polymyxin B Sulfate has a bactericidal action against almost all gram-negative bacilli except the Proteus group. Polymyxins increase the permeability of bacterial cell wall membranes. All gram-positive bacteria, fungi, and the gram-negative cocci, *N gonorrhoeae* and *N meningitidis*, are resistant. Susceptibility plate testing: If the Kirby-Bauer method of disc susceptibility testing is used, a 300-unit Polymyxin B disc should give a zone of over 11 mm when tested against a Polymyxin B-susceptible bacterial strain.

Polymyxin B Sulfate is not absorbed from the normal alimentary tract. Since the drug loses 50 percent of its activity in the presence of serum, active blood levels are low. Repeated injections may give a cumulative effect. Levels tend to be higher in infants and children. The drug is excreted slowly by the kidneys. Tissue diffusion is poor and the drug does not pass the blood brain barrier into the cerebrospinal fluid. In therapeutic dosage, Polymyxin B Sulfate causes some nephrotoxicity with tubule damage to a slight degree.

INDICATIONS

Acute infections caused by susceptible strains of *Pseudomonas aeruginosa*. Polymyxin B Sulfate is a drug of choice in the treatment of infections of the urinary tract, meninges, and bloodstream caused by susceptible strains of *Ps aeruginosa*. It may also be used topically and subconjunctivally in the treatment of infections of the eye caused by susceptible strains of *Ps aeruginosa*.

It may be indicated in serious infections caused by susceptible strains of the following organisms, when less potentially toxic drugs are ineffective or contraindicated:

H influenzae, specifically meningeal infections.
Escherichia coli, specifically urinary tract infections.
Aerobacter aerogenes, specifically bacteremia.
Klebsiella pneumoniae, specifically bacteremia.

Note: In meningeal infections, Polymyxin B Sulfate should be administered only by the intrathecal route.

CONTRAINDICATIONS

This drug is contraindicated in persons with a prior history of hypersensitivity reactions to the Polymyxins.

PRECAUTIONS

See "*Warning*" box.

Baseline renal function should be done prior to therapy, with frequent monitoring of renal function and blood levels of the drug during parenteral therapy.

Avoid concurrent use of curariform muscle relaxant and other neurotoxic drugs (ether, tubocurarine, succinylcholine, gallamine, decamethonium and sodium citrate) which may precipitate respiratory depression. If signs of respiratory paralysis appear, respiration should be assisted as required, and the drug discontinued.

As with other antibiotics, use of this drug may result in overgrowth of nonsusceptible organisms, including fungi. If superinfection occurs, appropriate therapy should be instituted.

ADVERSE REACTIONS

See "*Warning*" box.

Nephrotoxic Reactions: Albuminuria, cylinduria, azotemia, and rising blood levels without any increase in dosage.

Neurotoxic Reactions: Facial flushing, dizziness progressing to ataxia, drowsiness, peripheral paresthesias (circumoral and stocking-glove), apnea due to concurrent use of curariform muscle relaxants and other neurotoxic drugs or inadvertent overdosage, and signs of meningeal irritation with intrathecal administration, e.g., fever, headache, stiff neck, and increased cell count and protein cerebrospinal fluid.

Other Reactions Occasionally Reported: Drug fever, urticarial rash, pain (severe) at intramuscular injection sites, and thrombophlebitis at intravenous injection sites.

DOSAGE AND ADMINISTRATION

PARENTERAL

Intravenous: Dissolve 500,000 units Polymyxin B sulfate in 300-500 cc of 5 percent dextrose in water for continuous intravenous drip.

Adults and Children: 15,000-25,000 units/kg body weight/day in individuals with normal kidney function. This amount should be reduced from 15,000 units/kg downward for individuals with kidney impairment. Infusions may be given every 12 hours; however, the total daily dose must not exceed 25,000 units/kg/day.

Infants: Infants with normal kidney function may receive up to 40,000 units/kg/day without adverse effects.

Intramuscular: Not recommended routinely because of severe pain at injection sites, particularly in infants and children. Dissolve 500,000 units Polymyxin B Sulfate in 2 cc sterile distilled water (Water for Injection, U.S.P.) or sterile physiologic saline (Sodium Chloride Injection, U.S.P.) or 1 percent procaine hydrochloride solution.

Adults and Children: 25,000-30,000 units/kg/day. This should be reduced in the presence of renal impairment. The dosage may be divided and given at either 4- or 6-hour intervals.

Infants: Infants with normal kidney function may receive up to 40,000 units/kg/day without adverse effects.

Note: Doses as high as 45,000 units/kg/day have been used in limited clinical studies in treating prematures and newborn infants for sepsis caused by *Ps aeruginosa*.

Intrathecal: A treatment of choice for *Ps aeruginosa* meningitis. Dissolve 500,000 units Polymyxin B Sulfate in 10 cc of sterile physiologic saline (Sodium Chloride Injection, U.S.P.) for 50,000 units per ml dosage unit.

Adults and Children over 2 years of age: Dosage is 50,000 units once daily intrathecally for 3-4 days, then 50,000 units once every other day for at least 2 weeks after cultures of the cerebrospinal fluid are negative and sugar content has returned to normal.

Children under 2 years of age: 20,000 units once daily, intrathecally for 3-4 days or 25,000 units once every other day. Continue with a dose of 25,000 units once every other day for at least 2 weeks after cultures of the cerebrospinal fluid are negative and sugar content has returned to normal.

In the interest of safety, solutions for parenteral use should be stored under refrigeration, and any unused portions should be discarded after 72 hours.

TOPICAL

Ophthalmic: Dissolve 500,000 units Polymyxin B Sulfate in 20-50 cc sterile distilled water (Water for Injection, U.S.P.) or sterile physiologic saline (Sodium Chloride Injection, U.S.P.) for a 10,000-25,000 units per cc concentration.

For the treatment of *Ps aeruginosa* infections of the eye, a concentration of 0.1 percent to 0.25 percent (10,000 units to 25,000 units per cc) is administered 1-3 drops every hour, increasing the intervals as response indicates.

Subconjunctival injection of up to 10,000 units/day may be used for the treatment of *Ps aeruginosa* infections of the cornea and conjunctiva.

Note: Avoid total systemic and ophthalmic instillation over 25,000 units/kg/day.

STORAGE

Store at 15° to 25°C (59° to 77°F).

HOW SUPPLIED
POWDER FOR INJECTION: 500,000 U

AVERAGE UNIT PRICE (AVAILABLE SIZES)

GENERIC	$14.76

BRAND/MANUFACTURER	NDC	SIZE	AWP
◆ GENERICS			
Roerig	00049-0500-28	1s	$5.33
Burr Wellcome	00081-0035-10	10s	$241.94

Polymyxin B Sulfate and Trimethoprim Sulfate

DESCRIPTION

Polymyxin B Sulfate/Trimethoprin Sulfate is a sterile antimicrobial solution for topical ophthalmic use. Each mL contains Trimethoprim Sulfate equivalent to 1 mg Trimethoprim and Polymyxin B Sulfate 10,000 units.

Trimethoprim Sulfate, 2,4-diamino-5-(3,4,5-trimethoxy-benzyl)pyrimidine sulfate (2:1), is a white, odorless, crystalline powder with a molecular weight of 678.72.

Polymyxin B Sulfate is the sulfate salt of Polymyxin B$_1$ and B$_2$ which are produced by the growth of *Bacillus polymyxa* (Prazmowski) Migula (Fam. Bacillaceae). It has a potency of not less than 6,000 Polymyxin B units per mg, calculated on an anhydrous basis.

CLINICAL PHARMACOLOGY

Trimethoprim is a synthetic antibacterial drug active against a wide variety of aerobic gram-positive and gram-negative ophthalmic pathogens. Trimethoprim blocks the production of tetrahydrofolic acid from dihydrofolic acid by binding to and reversibly inhibiting the enzyme dihydrofolate reductase. This binding is very much stronger for the bacterial enzyme than for the corresponding mammalian enzyme. For that reason Trimethoprim selectively interferes with bacterial biosynthesis of nucleic acids and proteins.

Polymyxin B, a cyclic lipopeptide antibiotic, is rapidly bactericidal for a variety of gram-negative organisms, especially *Pseudomonas aeruginosa*. It increases the permeability of the bacterial cell membrane by interacting with the phospholipid components of the membrane.

When used topically, Trimethoprim and Polymyxin B absorption through intact skin and mucous membranes is insignificant.

Blood samples were obtained from 11 human volunteers at 20 minutes, 1 hour and 3 hours following instillation in the eye of 2 drops of ophthalmic solution containing 1 mg Trimethoprim and 10,000 units Polymyxin B per mL. Peak serum concentrations were approximately 0.03 μL/mL Trimethoprim and 1 unit/mL Polymyxin B.

Microbiology: In vitro studies have demonstrated that the anti-infective components of Polymyxin B Sulfate/Trimethoprim Sulfate are active against the following bacterial pathogens that are capable of causing external infections of the eye:

Trimethoprim: Staphylococcus aureus and *Staphylococcus epidermidis, Streptococcus pyogenes, Streptococcus faecalis, Streptococcus pneumoniae, Haemophilus influenzae, Haemophilus aegyptius, Escherichia coli, Klebsiella pneumoniae, Proteus mirabilis* (indole-negative), *Proteus vulgaris* (indole-positive), *Enterobacter aerogenes,* and *Serratia marcescens.*

Polymyxin B: Pseudomonas aeruginosa, Escherichia coli, Klebsiella pneumoniae, Enterobacter aerogenes and *Haemophilus influenzae.*

INDICATIONS AND USAGE

Polymyxin B Sulfate/Trimethoprim Sulfate Ophthalmic Solution is indicated in the treatment of surface ocular bacterial infections, including acute bacterial conjunctivitis, and blepharoconjunctivitis, caused by susceptible strains of the following microorganisms: *Staphylococcus aureus, Staphylococcus epidermidis, Streptococcus pneumoniae, Streptococcus viridans, Haemophilus influenzae* and *Pseudomonas aeruginosa.*[*]

   [*] Efficacy for this organism in this organ system was studied in fewer than 10 infections.

CONTRAINDICATIONS

Polymyxin B Sulfate/Trimethoprim Sulfate Ophthalmic Solution is contraindicated in patients with known hypersensitivity to any of its components.

WARNINGS

NOT FOR INJECTION INTO THE EYE. If a sensitivity reaction to Polymyxin B Sulfate/Trimethoprim Sulfate occurs, discontinue use. Polymyxin B Sulfate/Trimethoprim Sulfate Ophthalmic Solution is not indicated for the prophylaxis or treatment of ophthalmia neonatorum.

PRECAUTIONS

General: As with other antimicrobial preparations, prolonged use may result in overgrowth of nonsusceptible organisms, including fungi. If superinfection occurs, appropriate therapy should be initiated.

Information for Patients: Avoid contaminating the applicator tip with material from the eye, fingers, or other source. This precaution is necessary if the sterility of the drops is to be maintained.

If redness, irritation, swelling or pain persists or increases, discontinue use immediately and contact your physician.

Carcinogenesis, Mutagenesis, Impairment of Fertility:

Carcinogenesis: Long-term studies in animals to evaluate carcinogenic potential have not been conducted with Polymyxin B Sulfate or Trimethoprim.

Mutagenesis: Trimethoprim was demonstrated to be non-mutagenic in the Ames assay. In studies at two laboratories no chromosomal damage was detected in cultured Chinese hamster ovary cells at concentrations approximately 500 times human plasma levels after oral administration; at concentrations approximately 1000 times human plasma levels after oral administration in these same cells a low level of chromosomal damage was induced at one of the laboratories. Studies to evaluate mutagenic potential have not been conducted with Polymyxin B Sulfate.

Impairment of Fertility: Polymyxin B Sulfate has been reported to impair the motility of equine sperm, but its effects on male or female fertility are unknown.

No adverse effects on fertility or general reproductive performance were observed in rats given Trimethoprim in oral dosages as high as 70 mg/kg/day for males and 14 mg/kg/day for females.

Pregnancy: Teratogenic Effects: Pregnancy Category C. Animal reproduction studies have not been conducted with Polymyxin B Sulfate. It is not known whether Polymyxin B Sulfate can cause fetal harm when administered to a pregnant woman or can affect reproduction capacity.

Trimethoprim has been shown to be teratogenic in the rat when given in oral doses 40 times the human dose. In some rabbit studies, the overall increase in fetal loss (dead and resorbed and malformed conceptuses) was associated with oral doses 6 times the human therapeutic dose.

While there are no large well-controlled studies on the use of Trimethoprim in pregnant women, Brumfitt and Pursell, in a retrospective study, reported the outcome of 186 pregnancies during which the mother received either placebo or oral Trimethoprim in combination with sulfamethoxazole. The incidence of congenital abnormalities was 4.5% (3 of 66) in those who received placebo and 3.3% (4 of 120) in those receiving Trimethoprim and sulfamethoxazole. There were no abnormalities in the 10 children whose mothers received the drug during the first trimester. In a separate survey, Brumfitt and Pursell also found no congenital abnormalities in 35 children whose mothers had received oral Trimethoprim and sulfamethoxazole at the time of conception or shortly thereafter.

Because Trimethoprim may interfere with folic acid metabolism, Trimethoprim should be used during pregnancy only if the potential benefit justifies the potential risk to the fetus.

Nonteratogenic Effects: The oral administration of Trimethoprim to rats at a dose of 70 mg/kg/day commencing with the last third of gestation and continuing through parturition and lactation caused no deleterious effects on gestation or pup growth and survival.

Nursing Mothers: It is not known whether this drug is excreted in human milk. Because many drugs are excreted in human milk, caution should be exercised when Polymyxin B Sulfate/Trimethoprim Sulfate Ophthalmic Solution is administered to a nursing woman.

Pediatric Use: Safety and effectiveness in children below the age of 2 months have not been established (see "Warnings").

ADVERSE REACTIONS

The most frequent adverse reaction to Polymyxin B Sulfate/Trimethoprim Sulfate Ophthalmic Solution is local irritation consisting of increased redness, burning, stinging, and/or itching. This may occur on insillation, within 48 hours, or at any time with extended use. There are also multiple reports of hypersensitivity reactions consisting of lid edema, itching, increased redness, tearing, and/or circumocular rash.

Photosensitivity has been reported in patients taking oral trimethoprim.

DOSAGE AND ADMINISTRATION

Adults: In mild to moderate infections, instill one drop in the affected eye(s) every three hours (maximum of 6 doses per day) for a period of 7 to 10 days.

Pediatric Use: Clinical studies have shown Polymyxin B Sulfate/Trimethoprim Sulfate to be safe and effective for use in children over two months of age. The dosage regimen is the same as for adults.

Store at 15°-25°C (59°-77°F) and protect from light.

HOW SUPPLIED
DROP: 10,000 U-1 MG/ML

BRAND/MANUFACTURER	NDC	SIZE	AWP
○ **BRAND**			
POLYTRIM: Allergan Optical	00023-7824-10	10 ml	$15.79

Polysporin *SEE* BACITRACIN AND POLYMYXIN, OPHTHALMIC

Polythiazide

DESCRIPTION

Polythiazide is designated chemically as 2H-1,2,4-Benzothiadiazine-7-sulfonamide, 6-chloro-3,4-dihydro-2-methyl-3-[[(2,2,2-trifluoroethyl) thio]methyl]-, 1,1-dioxide. It is a white crystalline substance, insoluble in water but readily soluble in alkaline solution.

Following is its chemical structure:

ACTION

The mechanism of action results in an interference with the renal tubular mechanism of electrolyte reabsorption. At maximal therapeutic dosage all thiazides are approximately equal in their diuretic potency. The mechanism whereby thiazides function in the control of hypertension is unknown.

INDICATIONS

Polythiazide is indicated as adjunctive therapy in edema associated with congestive heart failure, hepatic cirrhosis, and corticosteroid and estrogen therapy.

Polythiazide has also been found useful in edema due to various forms of renal dysfunction such as: nephrotic syndrome; acute glomerulonephritis; and chronic renal failure.

Polythiazide is indicated in the management of hypertension either as the sole therapeutic agent or to enhance the effectiveness of other antihypertensive drugs in the more severe forms of hypertension.

Usage in Pregnancy: The routine use of diuretics in an otherwise healthy woman is inappropriate and exposes mother and fetus to unnecessary hazard. Diuretics do not prevent development of toxemia of pregnancy, and there is no satisfactory evidence that they are useful in the treatment of developed toxemia.

Edema during pregnancy may arise from pathological causes or from the physiologic and mechanical consequences of pregnancy. Thiazides are indicated in pregnancy when edema is due to pathologic causes, just as they are in the absence of pregnancy (however, see *"Warnings"* below). Dependent edema in pregnancy, resulting from restriction of venous return by the expanded uterus, is properly treated through elevation of the lower extremities and use of support hose; use of diuretics to lower intravascular volume in this case is illogical and unnecessary. There is hypervolemia during normal pregnancy which is harmful to neither the fetus nor the mother (in the absence of cardiovascular disease), but which is associated with edema, including generalized edema, in the majority of pregnant women. If this edema produces discomfort, increased recumbency will often provide relief. In rare instances, this edema may cause extreme discomfort which is not relieved by rest. In these cases, a short course of diuretics may provide relief and may be appropriate.

CONTRAINDICATIONS

Anuria. Hypersensitivity to this or other sulfonamide derived drugs.

WARNINGS

Thiazides should be used with caution in severe renal disease. In patients with renal disease, thiazides may precipitate azotemia. Cumulative effects of the drug may develop in patients with impaired renal function.

Thiazides should be used with caution in patients with impaired hepatic function or progressive liver disease, since minor alterations of fluid and electrolyte balance may precipitate hepatic coma.

Thiazides may add to or potentiate the action of other antihypertensive drugs. Potentiation occurs with ganglionic or peripheral adrenergic blocking drugs.

Sensitivity reactions may occur in patients with a history of allergy or bronchial asthma.

The possibility of exacerbation or activation of systemic lupus erythematosus has been reported.

Usage in Pregnancy: Thiazides cross the placental barrier and appear in cord blood. The use of thiazides in pregnant women requires that the anticipated benefit be weighed against possible hazards to the fetus. These hazards include fetal or neonatal jaundice, thrombocytopenia, and possibly other adverse reactions which have occurred in the adult.

Nursing Mothers: Thiazides appear in breast milk. If use of the drug is deemed essential, the patient should stop nursing.

PRECAUTIONS

Periodic determination of serum electrolytes to detect possible electrolyte imbalance should be performed at appropriate intervals.

All patients receiving thiazide therapy should be observed for clinical signs of fluid or electrolyte imbalance; namely, hyponatremia, hypochloremic alkalosis, and hypokalemia. Serum and urine electrolyte determinations are particularly important when the patient is vomiting excessively or receiving parenteral fluids. Medication such as digitalis may also influence serum electrolytes. Warning signs, irrespective of cause, are: dryness of mouth, thirst, weakness, lethargy, drowsiness, restlessness, muscle pains or cramps, muscular fatigue, hypotension, oliguria, tachycardia, and gastrointestinal disturbances such as nausea and vomiting.

Hypokalemia may develop with thiazides as with any other potent diuretic, especially with brisk diuresis, when severe cirrhosis is present, or during concomitant use of corticosteroids or ACTH.

Interference with adequate oral electrolyte intake will also contribute to hypokalemia. Digitalis therapy may exaggerate metabolic effects of hypokalemia especially with reference to myocardial activity.

Any chloride deficit is generally mild and usually does not require specific treatment except under extraordinary circumstances (as in liver disease or renal disease). Dilutional hyponatremia may occur in edematous patients in hot weather; appropriate therapy is water restriction, rather than administration of salt except in rare instances when the hyponatremia is life threatening. In actual salt depletion, appropriate replacement is the therapy of choice.

Hyperuricemia may occur or frank gout may be precipitated in certain patients receiving thiazide therapy.

Insulin requirements in diabetic patients may be increased, decreased, or unchanged. Latent diabetes mellitus may become manifest during thiazide administration.

Thiazide drugs may increase the responsiveness to tubocurarine.

The antihypertensive effects of the drug may be enhanced in the postsympathectomy patient.

Thiazides may decrease arterial responsiveness to norepinephrine. This diminution is not sufficient to preclude effectiveness of the pressor agent for therapeutic use.

If progressive renal impairment becomes evident, as indicated by a rising nonprotein nitrogen or blood urea nitrogen, a careful reappraisal of therapy is necessary with consideration given to withholding or discontinuing diuretic therapy.

Thiazides may decrease serum PBI levels without signs of thyroid disturbance.

ADVERSE REACTIONS

A. GASTROINTESTINAL SYSTEM REACTIONS
1. anorexia
2. gastric irritation
3. nausea
4. vomiting
5. cramping
6. diarrhea
7. constipation
8. jaundice (intrahepatic cholestatic jaundice)
9. pancreatitis

B. CENTRAL NERVOUS SYSTEM REACTIONS
1. dizziness
2. vertigo
3. paresthesias
4. headache
5. xanthopsia

C. HEMATOLOGIC REACTIONS
1. leukopenia
2. agranulocytosis
3. thrombocytopenia
4. aplastic anemia

D. DERMATOLOGIC—HYPERSENSITIVITY REACTIONS
1. purpura
2. photosensitivity
3. rash
4. urticaria
5. necrotizing angiitis (vasculitis) (cutaneous vasculitis)

E. CARDIOVASCULAR REACTION
Orthostatic hypotension may occur and may be aggravated by alcohol, barbiturates or narcotics.

F. OTHER
1. hyperglycemia
2. glycosuria
3. hyperuricemia
4. muscle spasm
5. weakness
6. restlessness

Whenever adverse reactions are moderate or severe, thiazide dosage should be reduced or therapy withdrawn.

DOSAGE AND ADMINISTRATION

Therapy should be individualized according to patient response. This therapy should be titrated to gain maximal therapeutic response as well as the minimal dose possible to maintain that therapeutic response. The usual dosage of Polythiazide tablets for diuretic therapy is 1 to 4 mg daily, and for antihypertensive therapy is 2 to 4 mg daily.

HOW SUPPLIED
TABLETS: 1 MG

BRAND/MANUFACTURER	NDC	SIZE	AWP
○ BRAND			
RENESE: Pfizer Labs	00069-3750-66	100s	$39.65

TABLETS: 2 MG

BRAND/MANUFACTURER	NDC	SIZE	AWP
○ BRAND			
RENESE: Pfizer Labs	00069-3760-66	100s	$51.89

TABLETS: 4 MG

BRAND/MANUFACTURER	NDC	SIZE	AWP
○ BRAND			
RENESE: Pfizer Labs	00069-3770-66	100s	$86.75

◆ RATED THERAPEUTICALLY EQUIVALENT; ◇ THERAPEUTIC EQUIVALENCE UNCONFIRMED; ○ UNRATED

Polythiazide and Prazosin Hydrochloride

THIS FIXED COMBINATION DRUG IS NOT INDICATED FOR INITIAL THERAPY OF HYPERTENSION. HYPERTENSION REQUIRES THERAPY TITRATED TO THE INDIVIDUAL PATIENT. IF THE FIXED COMBINATION REPRESENTS THE DOSE SO DETERMINED, ITS USE MAY BE MORE CONVENIENT IN PATIENT MANAGEMENT. THE TREATMENT OF HYPERTENSION IS NOT STATIC, BUT MUST BE RE-EVALUATED AS CONDITIONS IN EACH PATIENT WARRANT.

DESCRIPTION

Prazosin Hydrochloride, a quinazoline derivative, is the first of a new chemical class of antihypertensives. It is the hydrochloride salt of 1-(4-amino-6, 7-dimethoxy-2-quinazolinyl)-4-(2-furoyl) piperazine.

It is a white, crystalline substance, slightly soluble in water and isotonic saline, and has a molecular weight of 419.87. Each 1 mg capsule of Prazosin HCl contains drug equivalent to 1 mg free base.

Polythiazide is an orally effective, nonmercurial diuretic, saluretic, and antihypertensive agent.

It is designated chemically as 2H-1,2,4-Benzothiadiazine-7-sulfonamide,6-chloro-3,4-dihydro -2- methyl -3-[[(2,2,2-trifluoroethyl) thio]methyl]-,1,1-dioxide.

It is a white, crystalline substance insoluble in water, but readily soluble in alkaline solution.

POLYTHIAZIDE/PRAZOSIN HCL IS AVAILABLE AS

Strength	Components
Polythiazide/Prazosin HCl 1	1 mg prazosin - 0.5 mg polythiazide
Polythiazide/Prazosin HCl 2	2 mg prazosin - 0.5 mg polythiazide
Polythiazide/Prazosin HCl 5	5 mg prazosin - 0.5 mg polythiazide

CLINICAL PHARMACOLOGY

POLYTHIAZIDE/PRAZOSIN HCL

Polythiazide/Prazosin HCl produces a more pronounced antihypertensive response than occurs after either Prazosin Hydrochloride or Polythiazide alone in equivalent doses.

PRAZOSIN HCL

The exact mechanism of the hypotensive action of Prazosin is unknown. Prazosin causes a decrease in total peripheral resistance and was originally thought to have a direct relaxant action on vascular smooth muscle. Recent animal studies, however, have suggested that the vasodilator effect of Prazosin is also related to blockade of postsynaptic *alpha*-adrenoceptors. The results of dog forelimb experiments demonstrate that the peripheral vasodilator effect of Prazosin is confined mainly to the level of the resistance vessels (arterioles). Unlike conventional *alpha*-blockers, the antihypertensive action of Prazosin is usually not accompanied by a reflex tachycardia. Tolerance has not been observed to develop in long term therapy.

Hemodynamic studies have been carried out in man following acute single dose administration and during the course of long term maintenance therapy. The results confirm that the therapeutic effect is a fall in blood pressure unaccompanied by a clinically significant change in cardiac output, heart rate, renal blood flow, and glomerular filtration rate. There is no measurable negative chronotropic effect.

In clinical studies to date, Prazosin HCl has not increased plasma renin activity.

In man, blood pressure is lowered in both the supine and standing positions. This effect is most pronounced on the diastolic blood pressure.

Following oral administration, human plasma concentrations reach a peak at about three hours with a plasma half-life of two to three hours. The drug is highly bound to plasma protein. Bioavailability studies have demonstrated that the total absorption relative to the drug in a 20% alcoholic solution is 90%, resulting in peak levels approximately 65% of that of the drug in solution. Animal studies indicate that Prazosin HCl is extensively metabolized, primarily by demethylation and conjugation, and excreted mainly via bile and feces. Less extensive human studies suggest similar metabolism and excretion in man.

Prazosin HCl has been administered without any adverse drug interaction in limited clinical experience to date with the following: (1) cardiac glycosides—digitalis and digoxin; (2) hypoglycemics—insulin, chlorpropamide, phenformin, tolazamide, and tolbutamide; (3) tranquilizers and sedatives—chlordiazepoxide, diazepam, and phenobarbital; (4) antigout—allopurinol, colchicine, and probenecid; (5) antiarrhythmics—procainamide, propranolol (see *"Warnings"* however), and quinidine; and (6) analgesics, antipyretics and anti-inflammatories—propoxyphene, aspirin indomethacin, and phenylbutazone.

POLYTHIAZIDE

Polythiazide is a member of the benzothiadiazine (thiazide) family of diuretic/antihypertensive agents. Its mechanism of action results in an interference with the renal tubular mechanism of electrolyte reabsorption. At maximal therapeutic dosage all thiazides are approximately equal in their diuretic potency. The mechanism whereby thiazides function in the control of hypertension is unknown. Polythiazide is well absorbed, giving peak human plasma concentrations about 5 hours after oral administration. Drug is removed slowly thereafter with a plasma elimination half-life of approximately 27 hours. One fifth of the drug is recovered unchanged in human urine; the remainder is cleared via feces and as metabolites. Animal studies indicate metabolism occurs by rupture of the thiadiazine ring and loss of the side chain.

INDICATIONS AND USAGE

Polythiazide/Prazosin HCl is indicated in the treatment of hypertension. (See *"Box Warning"*.)

CONTRAINDICATIONS

Polythiazide/Prazosin HCl is contraindicated in patients with anuria, and in patients known to be sensitive to thiazides or to other sulfonamide derivatives.

WARNINGS

PRAZOSIN HCL

Prazosin HCl may cause syncope with sudden loss of consciousness. In most cases this is believed to be due to an excessive postural hypotensive effect, although occasionally the syncopal episode has been preceded by a bout of severe tachycardia with heart rates of 120-160 beats per minute. Syncopal episodes have usually occurred within 30 to 90 minutes of the initial dose of the drug; occasionally they have been reported in association with rapid dosage increases or the introduction of another antihypertensive drug into the regimen of a patient taking high doses of Prazosin HCl. The incidence of syncopal episodes is approximately 1% in patients given an initial dose of 2 mg or greater. Clinical trials conducted during the investigational phase of this drug suggest that syncopal episodes can be minimized by limiting the initial dose of the drug to 1 mg, by subsequently increasing the dosage slowly, and by introducing any additional antihypertensive drugs into the patient's regimen with caution (see *"Dosage And Administration"*). Hypotension may develop in patients given Prazosin HCl who are also receiving a beta-blocker such as propanolol.

If syncope occurs, the patient should be placed in the recumbent position and treated supportively as necessary. This adverse effect is self-limiting and in most cases does not recur after the initial period of therapy or during subsequent dose titration.

Patients should always be started on the 1 mg capsules of Prazosin HCl. The 2 and 5 mg capsules are not indicated for initial therapy.

More common than loss of consciousness are the symptoms often associated with lowering of the blood pressure, namely, dizziness and light-headedness. The patient should be cautioned about these possible adverse effects and advised what measures to take should they develop. The patient should also be cautioned to avoid situations where injury could result should syncope occur during the initiation of Prazosin HCl therapy.

POLYTHIAZIDE

Polythiazide should be used with caution in severe renal disease. In patients with renal disease, thiazides may precipitate azotemia. Cumulative effects of the drug may develop in patients with impaired renal function.

Thiazides should be used with caution in patients with impaired hepatic function or progressive liver disease, since minor alterations of fluid and electrolyte balance may precipitate hepatic coma.

Sensitivity reactions may occur in patients with a history of allergy or bronchial asthma.

The possibility of exacerbation or activation of systemic lupus erythematosus has been reported.

Thiazides may be additive or potentiative of the action of other antihypertensive drugs.

Potentiation occurs with ganglionic or peripheral adrenergic blocking drugs.

Periodic determinations of serum electrolytes to detect possible electrolyte imbalance should be performed at appropriate intervals.

All patients receiving thiazide therapy should be observed for clinical signs of fluid or electrolyte imbalance, namely, hyponatremia, hypochloremic alkalosis, and hypokalemia. Serum and urine electrolyte determinations are particularly important when the patient is vomiting excessively or receiving parenteral fluids. Medications such as digitalis may also influence serum electrolytes. Warning signs, irrespective of cause, are: dryness of mouth, thirst, weakness, lethargy, drowsiness, restlessness, muscle pains or cramps, muscular fatigue, hypotension, oliguria, tachycardia, and gastrointestinal disturbances such as nausea and vomiting.

Hypokalemia may develop with thiazides as with any potent diuretic, especially with brisk diuresis, when severe cirrhosis is present, or during concomitant use of corticosteroids or ACTH.

Interference with adequate oral electrolyte intake will also contribute to hypokalemia. Digitalis therapy may exaggerate the metabolic effects of hypokalemia, especially with reference to myocardial activity.

Any chloride deficit is generally mild and usually does not require specific treatment except under extraordinary circumstances (as in hepatic or renal disease. Dilutional hyponatremia may occur in edematous patients in hot weather; appropriate therapy is water restriction rather than administration of salt, except in rare instances when the hyponatremia is life-threatening. In actual salt depletion, appropriate replacement is the therapy of choice.

Hyperuricemia may occur or frank gout may be precipitated in certain patients receiving thiazide therapy.

Insulin requirements in diabetic patients may be either increased, decreased, or unchanged. Latent diabetes mellitus may become manifest during thiazide administration.

Thiazide drugs may increase responsiveness to tubocurarine. The antihypertensive effects of the drug may be enhanced in the post-sympathectomy patient.

Thiazides may decrease arterial responsiveness to norepinephrine. This diminution is not sufficient to preclude effectiveness of the pressor agent for therapeutic use.

If progressive renal impairment becomes evident, as indicated by a rising nonprotein nitrogen or blood urea nitrogen, a careful reappraisal of therapy is necessary with consideration given to withholding or discontinuing diuretic therapy. Thiazides may decrease serum protein-bound iodine levels without signs of thyroid disturbance.

PRECAUTIONS

Drug/Laboratory Test Interactions: In a study on five patients given from 12 to 24 mg of Prazosin per day for 10 to 14 days, there was an average increase of 42% in the urinary metabolite of norepinephrine and an average increase in urinary VMA of 17%. Therefore, false positive results may occur in screening tests for pheochromocytoma in patients who are being treated with Prazosin. If an elevated VMA is found, Prazosin should be discontinued and the patient retested after a month.

Carcinogenesis, Mutagenesis, Impairment of Fertility: No carcinogenic or mutagenic studies have been conducted with Prazosin HCl. However, no carcinogenic potential was demonstrated in 18 month studies in rats with either Prazosin HCl or Polythiazide at dose levels more than 100 times the usual maximum human doses. Prazosin HCl was not mutagenic in *in vivo* genetic toxicology studies.

Prazosin HCl produced no impairment of fertility in male or female rats at 50 and 25 mg/kg/day of Prazosin HCl and Polythiazide respectively. In chronic studies (one year or more) of Prazosin HCl in rats and dogs, testicular changes consisting of atrophy and necrosis occurred at 25 mg/kg/day (60 times the usual maximum recommended human dose). No testicular changes were seen in rats or dogs at 10 mg/kg/day (24 times the usual maximum recommended human dose). In view of the testicular changes observed in animals, 105 patients on long term Prazosin HCl therapy were monitored for 17-ketosteroid excretion and no changes indicating a drug effect were observed. In addition, 27 males on Prazosin HCl alone for up to 51 months did not have changes in sperm morphology suggestive of drug effect.

Use in Pregnancy: Pregnancy Category C. Polythiazide was not teratogenic in either rats or rabbits when administered in oral doses more than 100 times the usual maximum human dose. Studies in rats indicated that the combination of Polythiazide (40 times the usual maximum recommended human dose) and Prazosin HCl (8 times the usual maximum recommended human dose) caused a greater number of still-births, a more prolonged gestation, and a decreased survival of pups to weaning than that caused by Prazosin HCl alone. There are no adequate and well controlled studies in pregnant women. Therefore, Polythiazide should be used in pregnancy only if the potential-benefit justifies the potential risk to the fetus.

Nursing Mothers: It is not known whether Prazosin HCl or Polythiazide are excreted in human milk. Thiazides appear in breast milk. Thus, if use of the drug is deemed essential the patient should stop nursing.

Pediatric Use: Safety and effectiveness in children has not been established.

ADVERSE REACTIONS
PRAZOSIN HCL

The most common reactions associated with Prazosin HCl therapy are: dizziness 10.3%, headache 7.8%, drowsiness 7.6%, lack of energy 6.9%, weakness 6.5%, palpitations 5.3%, and nausea 4.9%. In most instances side effects have disappeared with continued therapy or have been tolerated with no decrease in dose of drug.

The following reactions have been associated with Prazosin HCl, some of them rarely. (In some instances exact causal relationships have not been established.)

Gastrointestinal: vomiting, diarrhea, constipation, abdominal discomfort and/or pain, liver function abnormalities, pancreatitis.

Cardiovascular: edema, dyspnea, syncope, tachycardia.

Central Nervous System: nervousness, vertigo, depression, paresthesia, hallucinations.

Dermatologic: rash, pruritus, alopecia, lichen planus.

Genitourinary: urinary frequency, incontinence, impotence, priapism.

EENT: blurred vision, reddened sclera, epistaxis, tinnitus, dry mouth, nasal congestion.

Other: diaphoresis, fever.

Single reports of pigmentary mottling and serous retinopathy, and a few reports of cataract development or disappearance have been reported. In these instances, the exact causal relationship has not been established because the baseline observations were frequently inadequate.

In more specific slit-lamp and funduscopic studies, which included adequate baseline examinations, no drug-related abnormal ophthalmological findings have been reported.

Literature reports exist associating Prazosin HCl therapy with a worsening of pre-existing narcolepsy. A causal relationship is uncertain in these cases.

POLYTHIAZIDE

Gastrointestinal: anorexia, gastric irritation, nausea, vomiting, cramping, diarrhea, constipation, jaundice (intrahepatic cholestatic jaundice), pancreatitis.

Central Nervous System: dizziness, vertigo, paresthesia, headache, xanthopsia.

Hematologic: leukopenia, agranulocytosis, thrombocytopenia, aplastic anemia.

Dermatologic: purpura, photosensitivity, rash, urticaria, necrotizing angiitis, (vasculitis) (cutaneous vasculitis).

Cardiovascular: Orthostatic hypotension may occur and be aggravated by alcohol, barbiturates, or narcotics.

Other: hyperglycemia, glycosuria, hyperuricemia, muscle spasm, weakness, restlessness.

OVERDOSAGE
PRAZOSIN HCL

Accidental ingestion of at least 50 mg of Prazosin HCl in a two year old child resulted in profound drowsiness and depressed reflexes. No decrease in blood pressure was noted. Recovery was uneventful.

Should overdosage lead to hypotension, support of the cardiovascular system is of first importance. Restoration of blood pressure and normalization of heart rate may be accomplished by keeping the patient in the supine position. If this measure is inadequate, shock should first be treated with volume expanders. If necessary, vasopressors should then be used. Renal function should be monitored and supported as needed. Laboratory data indicated that Prazosin HCl is not dialyzable because it is protein bound.

POLYTHIAZIDE

Should overdosage with Polythiazide occur, electrolyte balance and adequate hydration should be maintained. Gastric lavage is recommended, followed by supportive treatment. Where necessary, this may include intravenous dextrose and saline with potassium and other electrolyte therapy, administered with caution as indicated by laboratory testing at appropriate intervals.

DOSAGE AND ADMINISTRATION
PRAZOSIN HCL

Dosage: as determined by individual titration of Prazosin HCl and Polythiazide. (See "Box Warning".)

Usual Prazosin HCl dosage is one capsule two or three times daily, the strength depending upon individual requirement following titration.

The following is a general guide to the administration of the individual components of Prazosin HCl.

PRAZOSIN HCL

Initial Dose: 1 mg two or three times a day. (See "Warnings".)

Maintenance Dose: Dosage may be slowly increased to a total daily dose of 20 mg given in divided doses. The therapeutic dosages most commonly employed have ranged from 6 mg to 15 mg daily given in divided doses. Doses higher than 20 mg usually do not increase efficacy, however a few patients may benefit from further increases up to a daily dose of 40 mg given in divided doses. After initial titration some patients can be maintained adequately on a twice daily dosage regimen.

Use With Other Drugs: When adding a diuretic or other antihypertensive agent, the dose of Prazosin HCl should be reduced to 1 mg or 2 mg three times a day and retitration then carried out.

POLYTHIAZIDE

The usual dose of Polythiazide for antihypertensive therapy is 2 to 4 mg daily.

HOW SUPPLIED
CAPSULE: 0.5 MG-1 MG

BRAND/MANUFACTURER	NDC	SIZE	AWP
○ BRAND			
▶ MINIZIDE: Pfizer Labs	00663-4300-66	100s	$59.12

CAPSULE: 0.5 MG-2 MG

BRAND/MANUFACTURER	NDC	SIZE	AWP
○ BRAND			
▶ MINIZIDE: Pfizer Labs	00663-4320-66	100s	$74.43

CAPSULE: 0.5 MG-5 MG

BRAND/MANUFACTURER	NDC	SIZE	AWP
○ BRAND			
▶ MINIZIDE: Pfizer Labs	00663-4360-66	100s	$112.91

Polythiazide and Reserpine

WARNINGS

THIS FIXED COMBINATION DRUG IS NOT INDICATED FOR INITIAL THERAPY OF HYPERTENSION. HYPERTENSION REQUIRES THERAPY TITRATED TO THE INDIVIDUAL PATIENT. IF THE FIXED COMBINATION REPRESENTS THE DOSAGE SO DETERMINED, ITS USE MAY BE MORE CONVENIENT IN PATIENT MANAGEMENT. THE TREATMENT OF HYPERTENSION IS NOT STATIC, BUT MUST BE REEVALUATED AS CONDITIONS IN EACH PATIENT WARRANT.

◆ RATED THERAPEUTICALLY EQUIVALENT; ◇ THERAPEUTIC EQUIVALENCE UNCONFIRMED; ○ UNRATED

DESCRIPTION

Polythiazide/Reserpine tablets combine two antihypertensive agents with complementary properties.

Each tablet contains:

Polythiazide	2.0 mg
Reserpine	0.25 mg

Polythiazide is a member of the benzothiazide (thiazide) family of diuretic/antihypertensive agents. It is designated chemically as 2H-1,2,4-Benzothiadiazine-7-sulfonamide,6-chloro3,4-dihydro-2-methyl-3-[[2,2,2-trifluoroethyl)thio]methyl]-,1,1-dioxide with a molecular formula of $C_{11}H_{13}C1F_3N_3O_4S_3$ and a molecular weight of 439.87.

Polythiazide is a white crystalline substance insoluble in water, but readily soluble in alkaline solution. Reserpine is one of the alkaloids of *Rauwolfia serpentina*.

Reserpine, which is administered orally, is insoluble in water, very slightly soluble in ether, 1 g in about 1800 mL alcohol and about 6 mL chloroform, slightly soluble in benzene, freely soluble in acetic acid.

It has a molecular weight of 608.69 and its molecular formula is $C_{33}H_{40}N_2O_9$. Reserpine is chemically designated as Yohimban-16-carboxylic acid, 11,17-dimethoxy-18-[(3,4,5-trimethoxybenzoyl)oxy]-, methyl ester, (3β, 16β, 17α, 18β, 20α)-. It is a white or pale buff to slightly yellowish crystalline powder that is insoluble in water.

CLINICAL PHARMACOLOGY

Polythiazide: Polythiazide alone has demonstrated clinical effectiveness in lowering elevated blood pressure in patients without visible edema as well as in edematous hypertensive patients. Its mechanism of action results in an interference with the renal tubular mechanism of electrolyte reabsorption. At maximal therapeutic dosage all thiazides are approximately equal in their diuretic potency. The mechanism whereby thiazides function in the control of hypertension is unknown. Polythiazide is well absorbed following oral administration with diuresis beginning approximately 2 hours later. Peak human plasma concentrations occur about 5 hours after ingestion. Polythiazide is removed slowly thereafter with a plasma elimination half-life of approximately 27 hours. One-fifth of the drug is recovered unchanged in human urine; the remainder is cleared via feces and as metabolites. Animal studies indicate metabolism occurs by rupture of the thiadiazine ring and loss of the side chain.

Reserpine: Reserpine has several complementary actions of benefit to the hypertensive patient, including a calming effect and a slowing of the pulse rate.

Depletion of norepinephrine from tissue receptor sites is thought to be responsible for the decrease in peripheral vascular resistance and subsequent fall in blood pressure. Bradycardia is usually associated with this effect.

The tranquilizing effect of Reserpine is apparently due to serotonin and catecholamine depletion in the brain.

Sympathetic inhibition produced by Reserpine also may result in vasodilation and increased cutaneous blood flow with resulting flushing, feeling of warmth, or nasal congestion. Increased parasympathomimetic activity may produce increased gastrointestinal motility, increased gastric acid secretion and miosis.

Reserpine is absorbed orally and is widely distributed in body tissues, especially adipose tissue. A study in a small number of normal subjects who received a radioactively labeled 0.25 mg dose of Reserpine showed a biphasic half-life of 4.5 hours during the first phase, and 11.3 days during the second phase. The full therapeutic effects of Reserpine may not be seen for 2-3 weeks.

Reserpine is extensively metabolized to inactive compounds. It is slowly excreted via the urine and feces.

Reserpine crosses the blood-brain barrier and the placenta, and appears in cord blood.

Since Polythiazide reduces or eliminates the sodium and fluid retention frequently associated with hypertension, it enhances the efficacy of Reserpine in lowering elevated blood pressure. Polythiazide/Reserpine often has been found to be more effective than equivalent doses of either agent alone. Both the cardiovascular and central nervous system effects may persist following withdrawal of the drug.

INDICATIONS AND USAGE

Hypertension (see box *"Warning"*).

Usage in Pregnancy: The routine use of diuretics in an otherwise healthy woman is inappropriate and exposes mother and fetus to unnecessary hazard. Diuretics do not prevent development of toxemia of pregnancy, and there is no satisfactory evidence that they are useful in the treatment of developed toxemia.

Edema during pregnancy may arise from pathological causes or from the physiologic and mechanical consequences of pregnancy. Thiazides are indicated in pregnancy when edema is due to pathologic causes, just as they are in the absence of pregnancy (however, see *"Precautions/Pregnancy"* section). Dependent edema in pregnancy, resulting from restriction of venous return by the expanded uterus, is properly treated through elevation of the lower extremities and use of support hose; use of diuretics to lower intravascular volume in this case is illogical and unnecessary. There is hypervolemia during normal pregnancy which is harmful to neither the fetus nor the mother (in the absence of cardiovascular disease), but which is associated with edema—including generalized edema, in the majority of pregnant women. If this edema produces discomfort, increased recumbency will often provide relief. In rare instances, this edema may cause extreme discomfort which is not relieved by rest. In these cases, a short course of diuretics may provide relief and may be appropriate.

CONTRAINDICATIONS

A. Related to Polythiazide
  1. Advanced renal or hepatic failure.
  2. Hypersensitivity to this or other sulfonamide derivatives.
B. Related to Reserpine
  1. Demonstrated hypersensitivity.
  2. Patients with a history of mental depression.
  3. Demonstrated peptic ulcer or ulcerative colitis.

WARNINGS

Serum electrolyte determinations are especially indicated for patients with severe derangement of metabolic processes, e.g., surgery, vomiting, or parenteral fluid therapy. Electrolyte imbalance may be caused by certain diseases such as cirrhosis, or it may result from drug therapy, such as therapy with corticosteroids. Patients with cirrhosis who are continually receiving Polythiazide/Reserpine should be observed carefully for the development of hepatic precoma or coma. Indications of impending hepatic failure are tremor, confusion, drowsiness, and hepatic fetor.

Thiazides may precipitate kidney failure and uremia in patients with pre-existing renal pathology and impaired renal function.

Available information tends to implicate all oral dosage forms of potassium salts ingested in solid form with or without thiazides in the etiology of nonspecific, small bowel lesions consisting of ulceration with or without stenosis, causing obstruction, hemorrhage and perforation, and frequently requiring surgery. Deaths due to these complications have been reported. All oral dosage forms of potassium salts ingested in solid form should be used only when adequate dietary supplementation is not practical, and should be discontinued immediately if abdominal pain, distention, nausea, vomiting, or gastrointestinal bleeding occur. Polythiazide/Reserpine does not itself contain enteric-coated potassium.

Electroshock therapy should not be given within one week of cessation of Reserpine.

Reserpine may cause mental depression. Recognition of depression may be difficult because this condition may often be disguised by somatic complaints (Masked Depression). The drug should be discontinued at first signs of depression such as despondency, early morning insomnia, loss of appetite, impotence, or self-deprecation. Drug-induced depression may persist for several months after drug withdrawal and may be severe enough to result in suicide.

PRECAUTIONS

GENERAL

Polythiazide: Since all diuretic agents may reduce serum levels of sodium, chloride, and potassium—especially with brisk diuresis or when used concurrently with steroids—patients should be observed regularly for early signs of fluid or electrolyte imbalance, and serum electrolyte studies should be performed periodically. Warning signs of possible electrolyte imbalance, irrespective of cause, include fatigue, muscle cramps, gastrointestinal disturbances, lethargy, oliguria, and tachycardia. In extreme cases, hypotension, shock, and coma may develop. Frequently, serum electrolyte levels do not correlate with signs or symptoms of electrolyte imbalance. Unduly restricted salt intake as well as concurrent administration of digitalis may exaggerate metabolic effects of hypokalemia. A favorable ratio of potassium to sodium excretion lessens the possibility of hypokalemia. However, should this occur or be suspected, foods with a high potassium content (bananas, apricots, citrus fruits, prune juice, etc.) should be given. When necessary, oral potassium supplements may be administered. If other antihypertensive agents are used concurrently, lower than usual doses of Polythiazide/Reserpine and of the other agents should be considered.

The antihypertensive effects of the drug may be enhanced in the postsympathectomy patient.

Reserpine: Since Reserpine may increase gastric acid secretion, it should be used cautiously in patients with a history of peptic ulcer or ulcerative colitis. Extreme caution is needed in patients with a history of mental depression, and Reserpine should be discontinued at the first sign of depressive symptoms. Parkinsonism and confusion have been encountered, particularly in psychiatric patients, and constitute an indication for withdrawal of the drug. Caution should be exercised when treating patients with impairment of renal function, as lowered blood pressure may result in further decompensation and embarrassment of function.

Discontinue the drug one to two weeks prior to elective surgery since an unexpected degree of hypotension and bradycardia have been reported in patients receiving anesthetic agents concurrently with Reserpine, probably due to a reduced responsiveness to norepinephrine. For emergency surgical procedures vagal blocking agents may be given parenterally to prevent or reverse hypotension and/or bradycardia. Reserpine may cause increased appetite and weight gain in some patients.

Information for Patients: Since Polythiazide/Reserpine may increase urination, it is advisable to take it early during the day. If stomach upset occurs, take the drug with food or milk.

Notify your physician if muscle weakness, cramps, nausea, or dizziness occur as these may indicate the loss of too much potassium from your body.

A few people who take this medicine may be more sensitive to sunlight than they are normally. Avoid too much sun or use of a sunlamp until you see how you react.

Polythiazide/Reserpine may cause drowsiness. Make sure you know how you react before driving, using machinery, or performing tasks that require alertness.

Notify your physician if changes in mood or sleep patterns occur. Dizziness or light-headedness may occur when getting up from a sitting or lying position. Getting up slowly may help. Notify your physician if the problem worsens.

Laboratory Tests: Determination of serum electrolytes to detect possible electrolyte imbalance should be performed at appropriate intervals.

DRUG INTERACTIONS

Polythiazide: Thiazides may add to or potentiate the action of other antihypertensive drugs. Potentiation occurs with ganglionic or peripheral adrenergic blocking drugs.

Hypokalemia may be more likely to develop during concomitant use of corticosteroids or ACTH. Diuretic-induced hypokalemia may precipitate digitalis toxicity.

Thiazide drugs may augment the paralyzing actions of tubocurarine, and may decrease the arterial responsiveness to norepinephrine. Extra precautions may be necessary in patients who may require these drugs or their derivatives, as in surgery.

Dosage adjustment of antidiabetic agents is frequently indicated during thiazide administration. Indomethacin may partially antagonize the hypotensive effect of the thiazide diuretics. Generally, do not give lithium with diuretics because they reduce lithium's renal clearance and add a high risk of lithium toxicity.

Quinidine, a weak base, may have its half-life prolonged by concomitant administration of thiazide diuretics which alkalinize the urine.

Sulfonamides may potentiate the action of the thiazide diuretics, possibly by displacement from binding sites on plasma albumin.

Orthostatic hypotension may be aggravated by the use of alcohol, barbiturates, or narcotics with thiazide diuretics.

Reserpine: Reserpine should be used cautiously with digitalis or quinidine as the concurrent use may enhance the appearance of arrhythmias.

Additive CNS depressant effects may occur when Reserpine is administered concomitantly with other CNS depressants such as barbiturates and alcohol.

Concomitant administration of Reserpine and levodopa has been reported to reduce the patient's response to levodopa. Reserpine should be avoided in patients receiving levodopa.

The effects of indirect-acting sympathomimetic amines such as ephedrine may be decreased.

Patients who are receiving monoamine oxidase inhibitors may experience excitation and hypertension when Reserpine is added. The combination should be avoided.

Reserpine may add to the pharmacologic effects of beta-adrenegic blocking agents (i.e., CNS depression and cardiovascular effects).

DRUG/LABORATORY TEST INTERACTIONS

Polythiazide: The thiazides may alter various laboratory test results. These include all electrolytes, particularly potassium, BUN, glucose, and PBI. Thiazides may decrease serum PBI levels without signs of thyroid disturbance.

Like other thiazide diuretics, Polythiazide may cause a rise in serum uric acid levels with or without overt symptoms of gout.

Reserpine: Chronic administration results in a decrease in urinary catecholamines and vanillylmandelic acid excretion.

Interference with colorimetric assay procedures for the determination of urinary 17-hydroxycorticosteroids by the Glenn-Nelson technique and 17-ketosteroids by the Holtorff Koch modification of the Zimmerman reaction have been reported.

Animal Tumorigenicity: Although long-term studies in animals have not been conducted with Polythiazide/Reserpine, rodent studies have shown that Reserpine is an animal tumorigen, causing an increased incidence of mammary fibroadenomas in female mice, malignant tumors of the seminal vesicles in male mice, and malignant adrenal medullary tumors in male rats. These findings arose in 2 year studies in which the drug was administered in the feed at concentrations of 5 and 10 ppm—about 100 to 300 times the usual human dose. The breast neoplasms are thought to be related to Reserpine's prolactin-elevating effect.

Several other prolactin-elevating drugs have also been associated with an increased incidence of mammary neoplasia in rodents.

The extent to which these findings indicate a risk to humans is uncertain. Tissue culture experiments show that about one-third of human breast tumors are prolactin-dependent *in vitro,* a factor of considerable importance if the use of the drug is contemplated in a patient with previously detected breast cancer. The possibility of an increased risk of breast cancer in Reserpine users has been studied extensively; however, no firm conclusion has emerged. Although a few epidemiologic studies have suggested a slightly increased risk (less than twofold in all studies except one) in women who have used Reserpine, other studies of generally similar design have not confirmed this. Epidemiologic studies conducted using other drugs (neuroleptic agents) that, like Reserpine, increase prolactin levels and therefore would be considered rodent mammary carcinogens, have not shown an association between chronic administration of the drug and human mammary tumorigenesis. While long-term clinical observation has not suggested such an association, the available evidence is considered too limited to be conclusive at this time. An association of Reserpine intake with pheochromocytoma or tumors of the seminal vesicles has not been explored.

Pregnancy - Teratogenic Effects: Pregnancy Category C. Animal reproduction studies have not been conducted with Polythiazide/Reserpine. There are no adequate and well controlled studies in pregnant women. It is also not known whether Polythiazide/Reserpine can cause fetal harm when administered to a pregnant woman or can affect reproduction capacity. Polythiazide/Reserpine should be given to a pregnant woman only if clearly needed.

Nonteratogenic Effects: Thiazides cross the placental barrier and appear in cord blood. When Polythiazide and Reserpine are used in women of childbearing age, the potential benefits of this drug combination should be weighed against the possible hazards to the fetus. The hazards include fetal or neonatal jaundice, thrombocytopenia, and possible other adverse reactions which have occurred in the adult.

Nursing Mothers: Thiazides and Reserpine appear in breast milk. Because of the potential for serious adverse reactions in nursing infants from Polythiazide/Reserpine a decision should be made whether to discontinue nursing or to discontinue the drug, taking into account the importance of the drug to the mother.

Pediatric Use: Safety and effectiveness in children have not been established.

ADVERSE REACTIONS

The following adverse reactions have been observed, but there is not enough systemic collection of data to support an estimate of their frequency.

Polythiazide: The most common reactions associated with Polythiazide therapy are weakness and dizziness, but seldom require cessation of therapy. Weakness is reported in less than 3% of patients receiving the drug, and dizziness is reported in less than 2% of patients. These can be overcome by reducing the dose or taking measures to improve electrolytic balance.

Other reactions, reported to occur in less than 1% of patients, are:

Gastrointestinal: nausea, gastrointestinal disturbances, reversible cholestatic jaundice, necrotizing angiitis, pancreatitis.

Dermatological: maculopapular skin rash, photosensitivity.

Central Nervous System: vertigo, paresthesia, fatigue, headache.

Cardiovascular: orthostatic hypotension.

EENT: xanthopsia.

Hematological: Leukopenia (neutropenia), agranulocytosis, and aplastic anemia have been reported with the older thiazides but not with the newer compounds such as Polythiazide. Purpura (with or without thrombocytopenia) has been reported with Polythiazide.

Reserpine: The most common reactions associated with Reserpine therapy, dizziness and drowsiness, are reported in less than 2% of patients. Reactions to Reserpine are usually reversible and disappear when the drug is discontinued.

Other reactions, occurring in less than 1% of patients on Reserpine are:

Gastrointestinal: hypersecretion, nausea, vomiting, diarrhea, anorexia, dry mouth.

Dermatological: rash, pruritus, purpura.

Central Nervous System: depression, nervousness, paradoxical anxiety, nightmares, headache, and rare Parkinsonian syndrome to CNS sensitization manifested by deafness, glaucoma, uveitis, and optic atrophy.

Cardiovascular: angina-like symptoms, arrhythmias—particularly when used concurrently with digitalis or quinidine, flushing of the skin, and bradycardia.

EENT: nasal congestion, miosis.

Sexual Difficulties: Impotence or decreased libido.

OVERDOSAGE

One case of Polythiazide/Reserpine overdosage is reported after ingestion of an unknown number of tablets. Electrolyte replacement therapy was successful in treating the symptoms.

Polythiazide: An overdose of Polythiazide may cause electrolyte imbalance, manifested by fatigue, muscle weakness, cramps, gastrointestinal disturbances, lethargy, tachycardia, and/or other arrhythmias, and hypotension.

Should overdosage with Polythiazide occur, electrolyte balance and adequate hydration should be maintained. Gastric lavage is recommended followed by supportive treatment. Where necessary, this may include intravenous dextrose and saline with potassium and other electrolyte therapy, administered with caution as indicated by laboratory testing at appropriate intervals.

Reserpine: Signs of overdosage include CNS depression ranging from drowsiness to coma, bradycardia and hypotension, respiratory depression, hypothermia, diarrhea, vomiting, mental depression, skin flushing, miosis, and extrapyramidal signs such as stiffness and tremors. Emesis or gastric lavage to remove unabsorbed drug is of benefit in conscious patients, even if several hours have elapsed since ingestion. Treatment is symptomatic and supportive.

Parasympathomimetic side effects usually can be controlled with small doses of atropine or other anticholinergics. Evidence of motor dysfunction often can be controlled by drugs useful for parkinsonism. Avoid vasopressor drugs (except in cases of extreme hypotension) and rapid intravenous infusions because of the uncertain cardiac status.

It is not known whether dialysis would be of benefit in treating cases of overdosage of Polythiazide/Reserpine.

DOSAGE AND ADMINISTRATION

As determined by individual titration (see box "*Warning*").

Initial dosages of the combination should conform to those dosages of the individual components established during titration.

◆ RATED THERAPEUTICALLY EQUIVALENT; ◇ THERAPEUTIC EQUIVALENCE UNCONFIRMED; ○ UNRATED

Maintenance dosages range from ½ tablet to 2 tablets daily. Dosage of other antihypertensive agents, particularly ganglionic blockers, that are used concomitantly should be reduced.

Polythiazide/Reserpine should be stored at room temperature. Dispense in tight, light-resistant container.

HOW SUPPLIED
TABLETS:

BRAND/MANUFACTURER	NDC	SIZE	AWP
○ BRAND			
RENESE-R: Pfizer Labs	00069-4460-66	100s	$75.26

Polytrim SEE POLYMYXIN B SULFATE AND TRIMETHOPRIM SULFATE

Pondimin SEE FENFLURAMINE HYDROCHLORIDE

Ponstel SEE MEFENAMIC ACID

Pontocaine HCl SEE TETRACAINE HYDROCHLORIDE, INJECTABLE AND TETRACAINE HYDROCHLORIDE, OPHTHALMIC

Potaba SEE AMINOBENZOATE POTASSIUM

Potassium Acetate

DESCRIPTION
Potassium Acetate for Injection, is a sterile, non-pyrogenic, concentrated solution of Potassium Acetate ($C_2H_3KO_2$) in Water for Injection. It must be diluted prior to administration.

Each 20 ml vial contains:
Potassium Acetate (anhydrous) ....3.92 gm

Each 50 ml vial contains:
Potassium Acetate (anhydrous) ....9.8 gm or 19.6 gm

Each 100 ml vial (Pharmacy Bulk Package) contains:
Potassium Acetate (anhydrous) ....19.6 gm or 39.2 gm

The solution is intended as an alternative to Potassium Chloride to provide potassium (K^+) for addition to large volume infusion fluids for intravenous use. Unused portion should be discarded.

CLINICAL PHARMACOLOGY
Potassium is found in low concentration in plasma and extracellular fluids. It is the chief cation of body cells, and is concerned with the maintenance of body fluid composition and electrolyte balance. The major amount of Potassium is excreted in the urine. Therefore, the kidney normally determines Potassium balance.

The acetate ion is completely metabolized in the body, providing a source of hydrogen ion acceptors.

INDICATIONS AND USAGE
Potassium Acetate is indicated in the treatment of Potassium deficiency states when oral replacement therapy is not feasible.

CONTRAINDICATIONS
Potassium administration is contraindicated in diseases where high Potassium levels may be encountered.

WARNINGS
Potassium Acetate injection must be diluted before use. To avoid Potassium intoxication, infuse Potassium containing solutions slowly. Potassium replacement therapy should be monitored whenever possible by continuous or serial electrocardiography.

Solutions containing Potassium ions should be used with great care, if at all, in patients with hyperkalemia, severe renal failure and in conditions in which Potassium retention is present.

In patients with diminished renal function, oradrenal insufficiency, administration of solutions containing Potassium ions may result in Potassium retention or intoxication.

Solutions containing acetate ion should be used with great care in patients with metabolic or respiratory alkalosis. Acetate should be administered with great care in those conditions in which there is an increased level or an impaired utilization of this ion, such as severe hepatic insufficiency.

PRECAUTIONS
Potassium replacement therapy should be guided primarily by serial electrocardiograms. Plasma Potassium levels are not necessarily indicative of tissue Potassium levels.

High plasma concentrations of Potassium may cause death through cardiac depression, arrhythmias or arrest. Potassium Acetate should be used with caution in the presence of cardiac disease, particularly in digitalized patients or in the presence of renal disease, metabolic acidosis, Addison's disease, acute dehydration, prolonged or severe diarrhea, familial periodic paralysis, hypoadrenalism, hyperkalemia, hyponatremia and myotonia congenita.

ADVERSE REACTIONS
Nausea, vomiting, abdominal pain and diarrhea have been reported. The signs and symptoms of Potassium intoxication include paresthesias of the extremities, flaccid paralysis, listlessness, mental confusion, weakness and heaviness of the legs, hypotension, cardiac arrhythmias, heart block, electrocardiographic abnormalities such as disappearance of p waves, spreading and slurring of the QRS complex with development of a biphasic curve, and cardiac arrest. See *"Warnings"* and *"Precautions"*.

USE IN PREGNANCY
Teratogenic effects. Pregnancy Category C. Safety for use in pregnancy has not been established. Use of Potassium Acetate in women of childbearing potential requires that anticipated benefits be weighted against possible hazards.

OVERDOSAGE
In the event of overdosage, discontinue the infusion immediately, and institute intensive corrective therapy to reduce the serum Potassium levels and restore acid-base balance if necessary. (See *"Warnings," "Precautions"*, and *"Adverse Reactions"*)

DOSAGE AND ADMINISTRATION
Potassium Acetate must be diluted before administration. The dose and rate of injection are dependent upon the individual condition of each patient. ECG and serum Potassium should be monitored as a guide to dosage. Withdraw the calculated volume aseptically and transfer to appropriate intravenous fluids to provide the desired number of milliequivalents of Potassium (K^+) with an equal number of milliequivalents of Acetate (CH_3COO-).

DIRECTIONS FOR DISPENSING FROM 100 ML VIALS—PHARMACY BULK PACKAGE—NOT FOR DIRECT INFUSION
The 100 mL vial or Pharmacy Bulk Package is for use in a Pharmacy Admixture Service only. The 100 mL vial or Pharmacy Bulk Package should be inserted into the plastic hanging device provided and suspended as a unit in the laminar flow hood. Prior to entering a vial or Pharmacy Bulk Package, remove the flip-off seal and cleanse the rubber closure with a suitable antiseptic agent. Entry into the vial or Pharmacy Bulk Package must be made with a sterile transfer set or other sterile dispensing device and the contents dispensed in aliquots using aseptic technique. Use of a syringe needle is not recommended as it may cause leakage. *Any unused portion must be discarded within 4 hours after initial entry.* The date and the time the vial or Pharmacy Bulk Package was initially opened should be recorded in the space provided on the label.

Directions for using the Plastic Hanging Device with 100 ml vials or Pharmacy Bulk Package:

1) Remove the flip-off seal from the 100 ml vial or Pharmacy Bulk Package.
2) Place the center hole of the plastic hanging device over the top of the 100 ml vial or Pharmacy Bulk Package.
3) Pull the plastic hanging device down as far as possible and attach the transfer set using aseptic technique.
4) Invert the 100 ml vial or Pharmacy Bulk Package, grasp the outer ring of the plastic hanging device and hang in the laminar flow hood.

Parenteral drug products should be inspected visually for particulate matter and discoloration, whenever solution and container permit.

STORAGE
Store at controlled room temperature between 15°-30°C (59°-86°F).

HOW SUPPLIED
INJECTION: 2 MEQ/ML

AVERAGE UNIT PRICE (AVAILABLE SIZES)

GENERIC		$0.14	

BRAND/MANUFACTURER	NDC	SIZE	AWP
◆ GENERICS			
Fujisawa	00469-7600-40	20 ml	$2.01
Fujisawa	00469-7600-60	50 ml	$3.90
Fujisawa	00469-7601-00	100 ml	$10.45
Abbott Hosp	00074-8183-01	20 ml 25s	$115.19
Abbott Hosp	00074-3294-51	50 ml 25s	$227.11
Abbott Hosp	00074-3294-06	100 ml 25s	$380.59

➤ SHOWN IN PRODUCT IDENTIFICATION GUIDE

INJECTION: 4 MEQ/ML

BRAND/MANUFACTURER	NDC	SIZE	AWP
◆ GENERICS			
Fujisawa	00469-3300-60	50 ml	$6.46

Potassium Acid Phosphate

DESCRIPTION
Each tablet contains Potassium Acid Phosphate 500 mg. Each tablet yields approximately 114 mg of phosphorus and 144 mg of Potassium or 3.7 mEq.
Potassium Acid Phosphate is a highly effective urinary acidifier.

INDICATIONS
For use in patients with elevated urinary pH. Helps keep calcium soluble and reduces odor and rash caused by ammoniacal urine. Also, by acidifying the urine, it increases the antibacterial activity of methenamine mandelate and methenamine hippurate.

CONTRAINDICATIONS
This product is contraindicated in patients with infected Phosphate stones; in patients with severely impaired renal function (less than 30% of normal) and in the presence of hyperphosphatemia and hyperkalemia.

PRECAUTIONS
General: This product contains Potassium and should be used with caution if regulation of this element is desired. Occasionally, some individuals may experience a mild laxative effect during the first few days of Phosphate therapy. If laxation persists to an unpleasant degree, reduce the daily dosage until this effect subsides or, if necessary, discontinue the use of this product.
Caution should be exercised when prescribing this product in the following conditions: Cardiac disease (particularly in digitalized patients); severe adrenal insufficiency (Addison's disease); acute dehydration; severe renal insufficiency or chronic renal disease; extensive tissue breakdown (such as severe burns); myotonia congenita; hypoparathyroidism; and acute pancreatitis. Rickets may benefit from Phosphate therapy, but caution should be exercised. High serum Phosphate levels may increase the incidence of extraskeletal calcification.

Information for Patients: Patients with kidney stones may pass old stones when Phosphate therapy is started and should be warned of this possibility. Patients should be advised to avoid the use of antacids containing aluminum, calcium, or magnesium which may prevent the absorption of Phosphate. To assure against gastrointestinal injury associated with oral ingestion of concentrated Potassium salt preparations, patients should be instructed to dissolve tablets completely in an appropriate amount of water before taking.

Laboratory Tests: Careful monitoring of renal function and serum electrolytes (calcium, phosphorous, Potassium) may be required at periodic intervals during Phosphate therapy. Other tests may be warranted in some patients, depending on conditions.

Drug Interactions: The use of antacids containing magnesium, calcium, or aluminium in conjunction with Phosphate preparations may bind the Phosphate and prevent its absorption. Potassium-containing medications or Potassium-sparing diuretics may cause hyperkalemia when used concurrently with Potassium salts. Patients should have serum Potassium level determinations at periodic intervals. Concurrent use of salicylates may lead to increased serum salicylate levels since excretion of salicylates is reduced in acidified urine. Serum salicylate levels should be closely monitored to avoid toxicity.

Carcincogenesis, Mutagenesis, Impairment of Fertility: There have been no studies in animals or humans to evaluate the carcinogenesis, mutagenesis, or impairment of fertility for this product.

Pregnancy: Pregnancy Category C. Animal reproduction studies have not been conducted with this product. It is also not known whether this product can cause fetal harm when administered to a pregnant woman or can affect reproduction capacity. This product should be given to a pregnant woman only if clearly needed.

Nursing Mothers: It is not known whether this drug is excreted in human milk. Because many drugs are excreted in human milk, caution should be exercised when this product is administered to a nursing woman.

ADVERSE REACTIONS
Gastrointestinal upset (diarrhea, nausea, stomach pain, and vomiting) may occur with the use of Potassium Phosphates. Also, bone and joint pain (possible Phosphate-induced osteomalacia) could occur. The following adverse effects may be observed with Potassium administration: irregular heartbeat; dizziness; mental confusion; weakness or heaviness of legs; unusual tiredness; muscle cramps; numbness, tingling, pain, or weakness in hands or feet; numbness or tingling around lips; shortness of breath or troubled breathing.

DIRECTIONS
Two tablets dissolved in 6-8 oz. of water 4 times daily with meals and at bedtime. For best results, let the tablets soak in water for 2 to 5 minutes, or more if necessary, and stir. If any tablet particles remain undissolved, they may be crushed and stirred vigorously to speed dissolution.

HOW SUPPLIED TABLETS:

BRAND/MANUFACTURER	NDC	SIZE	AWP
○ BRAND			
K-PHOS ORIGINAL: Beach	00486-1111-01	100s	$8.15
	00486-1111-05	500s	$39.10

Potassium Acid Phosphate and Sodium Acid Phosphate

DESCRIPTION
Each single strength Potassium Acid Phosphate/Sodium Acid Phosphate tablet contains Potassium Acid Phosphate 155 mg and Sodium Acid Phosphate, anhydrous 350 mg. Each tablet yields approximately 125.6 mg of phosphorus, 44.5 mg of Potassium or 1.1 mEq and 67 mg of Sodium or 2.9 mEq. Each double strength Potassium Acid Phosphate/Sodium Acid Phosphate tablet contains Potassium Acid Phosphate 305 mg and Sodium Acid Phosphate, anhydrous, 700 mg. Each tablet yields approximately 250 mg of phosphorus, 88 mg of Potassium or 2.3 mEq and 134 mg of Sodium or 5.8 mEq.

ACTIONS
These products are highly effective urinary acidifiers.

INDICATIONS
For use in patients with elevated urinary pH. These products help keep calcium soluble and reduce odor and rash caused by ammoniacal urine. Also, by acidifying the urine they increase the antibacterial activity of methenamine mandelate and methenamine hippurate.

CONTRAINDICATIONS
These products are contraindicated in patients with infected Phosphate stones; in patients with severely impaired renal function (less than 30% of normal) and in the presence of hyperPhosphatemia.

PRECAUTIONS
Drug Interactions: Use of antacids containing magnesium, aluminum or calcium in conjuction with Phosphate preparations may bind the Phosphate and prevent its absorption. Concurrent use of antihypertensives, especially diazoxide, guanethidine, hydralazine, methyldopa or rauwolfia alkaloids; or corticosteroids, especially mineralocorticoids or corticotropin, with Sodium Phosphate may result in hypernatremia. Potassium-containing medications or Potassium-sparing diuretics may cause hyperkalemia when used with Potassium Phosphates. Patients should have serum Potassium level determinations at periodic intervals. Plasma levels of salicylates may be increased since salicylate excretion is decreased in acidified urine; administration of monobasic Phosphates to patients stabilized on salicylates may lead to toxic salicylate levels.

General: Contains Potassium and Sodium and should be used with caution if regulation of these elements is desired. Occasionally, some individuals may experience a mild laxative effect during the first few days of Phosphate therapy. If laxation persists to an unpleasant degree, reduce the daily dosage until this effect subsides or, if necessary, discontinue the use of this product. Use of this medication should be carefully considered when the following medical problems exist: Cardiac disease (particularly in digitalized patients), Addison's disease, acute dehydration, extensive tissue break-down, myotonia congenita, cardiac failure, cirrhosis of the liver or severe hepatic disease, peripheral and pulmonary edema, hypernatremia, hypertension, toxemia of pregnancy, hypoparathyroidism, and acute pancreatitis. Rickets may benefit from Phosphate therapy but caution should be observed. High serum Phosphate levels increase the risk of extraskeletal calcification.

Information for Patients: Patients with kidney stones may pass old stones when Phosphate therapy is started and should be warned of this possibility. Patients should be advised to avoid the use of antacids containing aluminum, magnesium or calcium which may prevent the absorption of Phosphate.

Laboratory Tests: Careful monitoring of renal function and serum electrolytes (calcium, phosphorus, Potassium, Sodium) may be required at periodic intervals. Other tests may be warranted in some patients, depending on conditions.

Carcinogenesis, Mutagenesis, Impairment of Fertility: Long term animal studies to evaluate the carcinogenic, mutagenic, or teratogenic potential of these products have not been performed.

Pregnancy: Pregnancy Category C. Animal reproduction studies have not been conducted with these products. It is also not known whether these products can cause fetal harm when administered to a pregnant woman or can affect reproduction capacity. These products should be given to a pregnant woman only if clearly needed.

Nursing Mothers: It is not known whether these drugs are excreted in human milk. Because many drugs are excreted in human milk, caution should be exercised when these products are administered to a nursing woman.

ADVERSE REACTIONS
Gastrointestinal upset (diarrhea, nausea, stomach pain and vomiting) may occur with Phosphate therapy. Also, bone and joint pain (possible Phosphate-induced

---

◆ RATED THERAPEUTICALLY EQUIVALENT; ◇ THERAPEUTIC EQUIVALENCE UNCONFIRMED; ○ UNRATED

osteomalacia) could occur. The following adverse effects may be observed (primarily from Sodium or Potassium): headaches; dizziness; mental confusion; seizures; weakness or heaviness of legs; unusual tiredness or weakness; muscle cramps; numbness, tingling, pain, or weakness of hands or feet; numbness or tingling around lips; fast or irregular heartbeat; shortness of breath or troubled breathing; swelling of feet or lower legs; unusual weight gain; low urine output unusual thirst.

DIRECTIONS

Single strength Potassium Acid Phosphate/Sodium Acid Phosphate: Two tablets four times daily with a full glass of water.

Double strength Potassium Acid Phosphate/Sodium Acid Phosphate: One tablets four times daily with a full glass of water. When the urine is difficult to acidify administer one tablet every two hours not to exceed eight tablets in a 24-hour period.

HOW SUPPLIED
TABLETS: 155 MG-350 MG

BRAND/MANUFACTURER	NDC	SIZE	AWP
○ BRAND			
K-PHOS M.F.: Beach	00486-1135-01	100s	$8.15
	00486-1135-05	500s	$39.10

TABLETS: 305 MG-700 MG

BRAND/MANUFACTURER	NDC	SIZE	AWP
○ BRAND			
K-PHOS NO. 2: Beach	00486-1134-01	100s	$12.40
	00486-1134-05	500s	$59.50

Potassium Bicarbonate

DESCRIPTION
Potassium Bicarbonate effervescent tablets for oral solution, are an oral Potassium supplement offered as an effervescent tablet for dissolution. Each tablet in solution provides 25 or 50 mEq (978 or 1955 mg) Potassium as bicarbonate and citrate, or the equivalent of 25 or 50 mEq (1865 or 3730 mg) Potassium Chloride.

CLINICAL PHARMACOLOGY
The Potassium ion is the principal intracellular cation of most body tissues. Potassium ions participate in a number of essential physiological processes including numerous enzymatic reactions in intermediary metabolism, the maintenance of intracellular tonicity, the transmission of nerve impulses, the contraction of cardiac, skeletal, and smooth muscle, and the maintenance of normal renal function. Disturbances in Potassium metabolism may, therefore elicit a broad range of clinical disorders. The normal serum potassium level is maintained principally by close renal regulation of Potassium balance.

The intracellular concentration of Potassium is approximately 150 to 160 mEq per liter. The normal adult plasma concentration is 3.5 to 5 mEq per liter. An active ion transport system maintains this gradient across the plasma membrane.

Potassium is a normal dietary constituent and under steady state conditions the amount of Potassium absorbed from the gastrointestinal tract is equal to the amount excreted in the urine. The usual dietary intake of Potassium is 50 to 100 mEq per day.

Potassium depletion will occur whenever the rate of Potassium loss through renal excretion and/or loss from the gastrointestinal tract exceeds the rate of Potassium intake. Such depletion usually develops as a consequence of therapy with diuretics, primary or secondary hyperaldosteronism, diabetic ketoacidosis, severe vomiting and diarrhea or inadequate replacement of Potassium in patients on prolonged parenteral nutrition. Depletion can develop rapidly with severe diarrhea, especially if associated with vomiting. Potassium depletion due to these causes is usually accompanied by a concomitant loss of chloride and is manifested by hypokalemia and metabolic alkalosis.

Potassium deficiency may be manifested by generalized weakness, fatigue, drowsiness, anorexia, and nausea; oliguria, edema, and chronic ileus with distention; shallow and infrequent respirations; low blood pressure, altered cardiac rhythms (primarily ectopic beats), and systolic murmurs; hypokalemia and such ECG changes as prominent U wave, lengthening of the Q-T interval, depression of the S-T segment, and depression or inversion of the T-wave, and, in advanced cases, flaccid paralysis and/or impaired ability to concentrate urine.

If Potassium depletion associated with metabolic alkalosis cannot be managed by correcting the fundamental cause of the deficiency, e.g., where the patient requires long term diuretic therapy, supplemental Potassium in the form of high Potassium food or Potassium salts may be able to restore normal Potassium levels.

In rare circumstances (e.g., patients with renal tubular acidosis) Potassium depletion may be associated with metabolic acidosis and hyperchloremia. In such patients Potassium replacement should be accomplished with potassium salts such as Potassium Bicarbonate, Potassium citrate, Potassium acetate, or Potassium gluconate.

INDICATIONS AND USAGE
1. For the treatment of patients with hypokalemia, with or without metabolic alkalosis; in digitalis intoxication; and in patients with hypokalemic familial periodic paralysis. If hypokalemia is the result of diuretic therapy, consideration should be given to the use of a lower dose of diuretic, which may be sufficient without leading to hypokalemia.

2. For the prevention of hypokalemia in patients who would be at particular risk if hypokalemia were to develop, e.g., digitalized patients or patients with significant cardiac arrhythmias.

Potassium Bicarbonate is useful when thiazide diuretics, corticosteroids, or vomiting and diarrhea cause excessive potassium loss; and when dietary potassium is low. Potassium Bicarbonate with chloride is recommended in the management of hypokalemia accompanied by metabolic alkalosis and hypochloremia, eg, as induced by vomiting.

The use of Potassium salts in patients receiving diuretics for uncomplicated essential hypertension is often unnecessary when such patients have a normal dietary pattern and when low doses of the diuretic are used Serum Potassium should be checked periodically, however, and if hypokalemia occurs, dietary supplementation with Potassium-containing foods may be adequate to control milder cases. In more severe cases, and if dose adjustment of the diuretic is ineffective or unwarranted, supplementation with Potassium salts may be indicated.

UNLABELED USES
Potassium Bicarbonate is used alone or as an adjunct in the treatment of atrial tachycardia, ventricular arrhythmias, hypertension, and for inducing peripheral insulin levels and improving glucose utilization in obese patients. It is also used to lower the risk of myocardial infarction.

CONTRAINDICATIONS
Potassium supplements are contraindicated in patients with hyperkalemia since a further increase in serum Potassium concentration in such patients can produce cardiac arrest. Hyperkalemia may complicate any of the following conditions: chronic renal failure, systemic acidosis such as diabetic acidosis, acute dehydration, extensive tissue breakdown as in severe burns, adrenal insufficiency, or the administration of a Potassium-sparing diuretic (e.g., spironolactone, triamterene, or amiloride) (see *"Overdosage"*).

WARNINGS
Hyperkalemia (see "Overdosage"): In patients with impaired mechanisms for excreting Potassium, the administration of Potassium salts can produce hyperkalemia and cardiac arrest. This occurs most commonly in patients given Potassium by the intravenous route but may also occur in patients given Potassium orally. Potentially fatal hyperkalemia can develop rapidly and be asymptomatic. The use of Potassium salts in patients with chronic renal disease, or any other condition which impairs Potassium excretion, requires particularly careful monitoring of the serum Potassium concentration and appropriate dosage adjustment.

Interaction with Potassium-Sparing Diuretics: Hypokalemia should not be treated by the concomitant administration of Potassium salts and a Potassium-sparing diuretic (e.g., spironolactone, triamterene, or amiloride), since the simultaneous administration of these agents can produce severe hyperkalemia.

Interaction with Angiotensin Converting Enzyme Inhibitors: Angiotensin converting enzyme (ACE) inhibitors (e.g., captopril, enalapril) will produce some Potassium retention by inhibiting aldosterone production. Potassium supplements should be given to patients receiving ACE inhibitors only with close monitoring.

Metabolic Acidosis: Hypokalemia in patients with metabolic acidosis should be treated with an alkalinizing Potassium salt such as Potassium Bicarbonate, Potassium citrate, Potassium acetate, or Potassium gluconate.

PRECAUTIONS
General: The diagnosis of Potassium depletion is ordinarily made by demonstrating hypokalemia in a patient with a clinical history suggesting some cause for Potassium depletion. In interpreting the serum Potassium level, the physician should bear in mind that acute alkalosis per se can produce hypokalemia in the absence of a deficit in total body Potassium while acute acidosis per se can increase the serum Potassium concentration into the normal range even in the presence of a reduced total body Potassium. The treatment of Potassium depletion, particularly in the presence of cardiac disease, renal disease, or acidosis requires careful attention to acid-base balance and appropriate monitoring of serum electrolytes, the electrocardiogram, and the clinical status of the patient.

Information for Patients: Physicians should consider reminding the patient to take this medicine following the frequency and amount prescribed by the physician. This is especially important if the patient is also taking diuretics and/or digitalis preparations.

To minimize the possibility of gastrointestinal irritation associated with the oral ingestion of concentrated Potassium salt preparations, patients should be carefully directed to dissolve each dose completely in the stated amount of water.

Laboratory Tests: When blood is drawn for analysis of plasma potassium it is important to recognize that artifactual elevations can occur after improper venipuncture technique or as a result of *in vitro* hemolysis of the sample.

Frequent clinical evaluation of the patient should include ECG and serum Potassium determinations.

Drug Interactions: Potassium-sparing diuretic, angiotensin converting enzyme inhibitors: see *"Warnings"*.

The simultaneous administration of potassium supplements and a Potassium-sparing diuretic can produce severe hyperkalemia. Potassium supplements should be used cautiously in patients who are using salt substitutes because most of the latter contain substantial amounts of Potassium. Such concomitant use could result in hyperkalemia.

Carcinogenesis, Mutagenesis, Impairment of Fertility: Carcinogenicity, mutagenicity, and fertility studies in animals have not been performed. Potassium is a normal dietary constituent.

Pregnancy Category C: Animal reproduction studies have not been conducted with Potassium salts. It is also not known whether Potassium salts can cause fetal harm when administered to a pregnant woman or can affect reproduction capacity. Potassium supplements should be given to a pregnant woman only if clearly needed.

Nursing Mothers: Many drugs are excreted in human milk and because of the potential for serious adverse reactions in nursing infants from oral Potassium supplements, a decision should be made whether to discontinue nursing or discontinue the drug, taking into account the importance of the drug to the mother.

Pediatric Use: Safety and effectiveness in children have not been established.

ADVERSE REACTIONS

One of the most severe adverse effects is hyperkalemia.

Hyperkalemia occurs only rarely in patients with normal renal function receiving Potassium supplements orally. Signs and symptoms of hyperkalemia are cardiac arrhythmias, mental confusion, unexplained anxiety, numbness or tingling in hands, feet or lips, shortness of breath or difficult breathing, unusual tiredness or weakness and weakness or heaviness of legs (see *"Contraindications", "Warnings"* and *"Overdosage"*).

The most common adverse reactions to the oral Potassium salts are nausea, vomiting, flatulence, abdominal pain/discomfort, and diarrhea. These symptoms are due to irritation of the gastrointestinal tract and are best managed by diluting the preparation further, ensuring that the tablet is dissolved completely, taking the dose with meals, or reducing dose.

OVERDOSAGE

The administration of oral Potassium salts to persons with normal excretory mechanisms for Potassium rarely causes serious hyperkalemia. However, if excretory mechanisms are impaired or if Potassium is administered too rapidly intravenously, potentially fatal hyperkalemia can result (see *"Contraindications"* and *"Warnings"*). It is important to recognize that hyperkalemia is usually asymptomatic and may be manifested only by an increased serum Potassium concentration (6.5-8.0 mEq/L) and characteristic electrocardiographic changes (peaking of T-waves, loss of P-wave, depression of S-T segment, and prolongation of the QT interval). Late manifestations include muscle paralysis and cardiovascular collapse from cardiac arrest (9-12 mEq/L).

The treatment of severe hyperkalemia should focus on reducing the serum Potassium concentration by promoting the transfer of Potassium from the extracellular to the intracellular space. The measures taken may include the following: a) intravenous administration of 1 liter of a 10% glucose solution containing 30 to 40 units of insulin or 300 to 500 ml/hr of 10% dextrose solution containing 10 to 20 units of insulin per 1,000 ml; b) in the acidotic patient, intravenous administration of 150 mEq to 300 mEq of sodium bicarbonate. Other measures should include the elimination of Potassium-containing medications and Potassium-sparing diuretics and frequently the oral administration of a cation exchange resin (such as sodium polystyrene sulfonate) to remove gastrointestinal Potassium. To assure rapid movement of the resin through the gastrointestinal tract, a nonabsorbable polyhydric alcohol (eg, sorbitol) should be given in quantities sufficient to induce a soft to semiliquid bowel movement every few hours.

Hemodialysis is an effective alternative means of removing excess Potassium.

In treating hyperkalemia, it should be recalled that in patients who have been stabilized on digitalis, too rapid a lowering of the serum Potassium concentration can produce digitalis toxicity.

DOSAGE AND ADMINISTRATION

The usual dietary Potassium intake by the average adult is 50 to 100 mEq per day. Potassium depletion sufficient to cause hypokalemia usually requires the loss of 200 or more mEq of Potassium from the total body store.

Dosage must be adjusted to the individual needs of each patient. The dose for the prevention of hypokalemia is typically in the range of 25 mEq per day. Doses of 50-100 mEq per day or more are used for the treatment of Potassium depletion. Dosage should be divided if more than 25 mEq per day is given such that no more than 25 mEq is given in a single dose.

The usual adult dose is 25-100 mEq of Potassium per day.

This can be given as: One (1) Potassium Bicarbonate 50 mEq with chloride tablet or one (1) Potassium Bicarbonate 50 mEq tablet completely dissolved in 6 to 8 ounces of cold or ice water, 1 to 2 times daily, depending on the requirements of the patient; one (1) Potassium Bicarbonate 25 mEq with chloride tablet or one (1) Potassium Bicarbonate 25 mEq tablet completely dissolved in 3 to 4 ounces of cold or ice water, 2 to 4 times daily, depending on the requirements of the patient.

Note: It is suggested that all Potassium Bicarbonate products be taken with meals and sipped slowly over a 5 to 10 minute period.

These preparations, like other Potassium supplements, must be properly diluted to avoid the possibility of gastrointestinal irritation.

Store at controlled room temperature, 59°-86°F (15°-30°C).

HOW SUPPLIED
TABLET, EFFERVESCENT: 25 MEQ

BRAND/MANUFACTURER	NDC	SIZE	AWP
○ **GENERICS**			
Moore,H.L.	00839-6619-19	30s	$5.74
K-ELECTROLYTE: Copley	38245-0205-03	30s	$6.69
Bajamar	44184-0016-02	30s	$6.95
Bajamar	44184-0024-02	30s	$6.95
Moore,H.L.	00839-7278-19	30s	$7.09
Allscrips	54569-3542-00	30s	$7.25
Geneva	00781-1525-31	30s	$7.25
URL	00677-0819-07	30s	$7.43
Qualitest	00603-4170-16	30s	$7.46

For additional alternatives, turn to the section beginning on page 2859.

Potassium Chloride and Potassium Gluconate

DESCRIPTION

Potassium Chloride/Potassium Gluconate Liquid is an oral Potassium supplement. Each table-spoonful (15 mL) provides 20 mEq Potassium ion and 3.4 mEq Chloride ion. These mEq quantities are derived from the presence of Potassium Gluconate 3.9 g and Potassium Chloride 0.25 g. Potassium Chloride/Potassium Gluconate Liquid is an electrolyte replenisher.

CLINICAL PHARMACOLOGY

The Potassium ion is the principal intracellular cation of most body tissues. Potassium ions participate in a number of essential physiological processes including the maintenance of intracellular tonicity, the transmission of nerve impulses, the contraction of cardiac, skeletal and smooth muscle and the maintenance of normal renal function.

The intracellular concentration of Potassium is approximately 150 to 160 mEq per liter. The normal adult plasma concentration is 3.5 to 5.0 mEq per liter. An active ion transport system maintains this gradient across the plasma membrane.

Potassium is a normal dietary constituent and under steady state conditions the amount of Potassium absorbed from the gastrointestinal tract is equal to the amount excreted in the urine. The usual dietary intake of Potassium is 50 to 100 mEq per day.

Potassium depletion will occur whenever the rate of Potassium loss through renal excretion and/or loss from the gastrointestinal tract exceeds the rate of Potassium intake. Such depletion usually develops as a consequence of therapy with diuretics, primary or secondary hyperaldosteronism, diabetic ketoacidosis or inadequate replacement of Potassium in patients on prolonged parenteral nutrition. Depletion can develop rapidly with severe diarrhea, especially if associated with vomiting. Potassium depletion due to these causes is usually accompanied by a concomitant loss of chloride and is manifested by hypokalemia and metabolic alkalosis. Potassium depletion may produce weakness, fatigue, disturbances of cardiac rhythm (primarily ectopic beats), prominent U-waves in the electrocardiogram, and, in advanced cases, flaccid paralysis and/or impaired ability to concentrate urine.

If Potassium depletion associated with metabolic alkalosis cannot be managed by correcting the fundamental cause of the deficiency, e.g., where the patient requires long term diuretic therapy, supplemental Potassium in the form of high Potassium food or Potassium Chloride may be able to restore normal Potassium levels.

In rare circumstances (e.g., patients with renal tubular acidosis) Potassium depletion may be associated with metabolic acidosis and hyperchloremia. In such patients Potassium replacement should be accomplished with Potassium salts other than the Chloride, such as Potassium bicarbonate, Potassium citrate, Potassium acetate or Potassium Gluconate.

INDICATIONS AND USAGE

1. For the treatment of patients with hypokalemia, with or without metabolic alkalosis; in digitalis intoxication; and in patients with hypokalemic familial periodic paralysis. If hypokalemia is the result of diuretic therapy, consideration should be given to the use of a lower dose of diuretic, which may be sufficient without leading to hypokalemia.

2. For the prevention of hypokalemia in patients who would be at particular risk if hypokalemia were to develop, e.g., digitalized patients or patients with significant cardiac arrhythmias.

The use of Potassium salts in patients receiving diuretics for uncomplicated essential hypertension is often unnecessary when such patients have a normal dietary pattern and when low doses of the diuretic are used. Serum Potassium should be checked periodically, however, and if hypokalemia occurs, dietary supplementation with Potassium-containing foods may be adequate to control milder cases. In more severe cases, and if dose adjustment of the diuretic is ineffective or unwarranted, supplementation with Potassium salts may be indicated.

CONTRAINDICATIONS

Potassium supplements are contraindicated in patients with hyperkalemia since a further increase in serum Potassium concentration in such patients can produce cardiac arrest. Hyperkalemia may complicate any of the following conditions: chronic renal failure, systemic acidosis such as diabetic acidosis, acute dehydration, extensive tissue breakdown as in severe burns, adrenal insufficiency or the administration of a Potassium-sparing diuretic (e.g., spironolactone, triamterene, amiloride) (see *"Overdosage"*). Potassium Chloride/Potassium Gluconate Liquid is contraindicated in patients with known hypersensitivity to any ingredient in this product.

WARNINGS

HYPERKALEMIA (see *"Overdosage"*)
In patients with impaired mechanisms for excreting Potassium, the administration of Potassium salts can produce hyperkalemia and cardiac arrest. This occurs most commonly in patients given Potassium by the intravenous route but may also occur in patients given Potassium orally. Potentially fatal hyperkalemia can develop rapidly and be asymptomatic.

The use of Potassium salts in patients with chronic renal disease, or any other condition which impairs Potassium excretion, requires particularly careful monitoring of the serum Potassium concentration and appropriate dosage adjustment.

DIGITALIS TOXICITY
Both hypokalemia and hyperkalemia are undesirable in the presence of digitalis toxicity. Potassium salts should not be administered to patients who have second degree or complete A-V block unless an electronic pacemaker is in place, as they may further depress A-V conduction and ventricular responsiveness.

INTERACTION WITH POTASSIUM-SPARING DIURETICS
Hypolkalemia should not be treated by the concomitant administration of Potassium salts and a Potassium-sparing diuretic (e.g., spironolactone, triameterene or amiloride) since the simultaneous administration of these agents can produce severe hyperkalemia.

INTERACTION WITH ANGIOTENSIN CONVERTING ENZYME INHIBITORS
Angiotensin converting enzyme (ACE) inhibitors (e.g., captopril, enalapril) will produce some Potassium retention by inhibiting aldosterone production. Potassium supplements should be given to patients receiving ACE inhibitors only with close monitoring.

METABOLIC ACIDOSIS
Hypokalemia in patients with metabolic acidosis should be treated with an alkalinizing Potassium salt such as Potassium bicarbonate, Potassium citrate, Potassium acetate or Potassium Gluconate.

PRECAUTIONS

GENERAL
The diagnosis of Potassium depletion is ordinarily made by demonstrating hypokalemia in a patient with a clinical history suggesting some cause for Potassium depletion. In interpreting the serum Potassium level, the physician should bear in mind that acute alkalosis per se can produce hypokalemia in the absence of a deficit in total body Potassium while acute acidosis per se can increase the serum Potassium concentration into the normal range even in the presence of a reduced total body Potassium. The treatment of Potassium depletion, particularly in the presence of cardiac disease, renal disease or acidosis requires careful attention to acid-base balance and appropriate monitoring of serum electrolytes, the electrocardiogram and the clinical status of the patient.

INFORMATION FOR PATIENTS
Physicians should consider reminding the patient of the following:

■ To take each dose with meals and in 30 mL (one fluid ounce) or more of water.
■ To take this medicine following the frequency and amount prescribed by the physician. This is especially important if the patient is also taking diuretics and/or digitalis preparations.
■ To check with the physician at once if tarry stools or other evidence of gastrointestinal bleeding is noticed.

LABORATORY TESTS
When blood is drawn for analysis of plasma Potassium it is important to recognize that artifactual elevations can occur after improper venipuncture technique or as a result of *in vitro* hemolysis of the sample.

DRUG INTERACTIONS
Potassium-sparing diuretic, angiotensin converting enzyme inhibitors (see *"Warnings"*).

CARCINOGENESIS, MUTAGENESIS, IMPAIRMENT OF FERTILITY
Carcinogenicity, mutagenicity and fertility studies in animals have not been performed. Potassium is a normal dietary constituent.

PREGNANCY: TERATOGENIC EFFECTS—PREGNANCY CATEGORY C
Animal reproduction studies have not been conducted with Potassium Chloride/ Potassium Gluconate Liquid. It is also not know whether Potassium Chloride/ Potassium Gluconate Liquid can cause fetal harm when administered to a pregnant woman or can affect reproduction capacity. Potassium Chloride/Potassium Gluconate should be given to a pregnant woman only if clearly needed.

NURSING MOTHERS
The normal Potassium ion content of human milk is about 13 mEq per liter. Since oral Potassium becomes part of the body Potassium pool, so long as body Potassium is not excessive, the contribution of Potassium Chloride supplementation should have little or no effect on the level in human milk.

PEDIATRIC USE
Safety and effectiveness in children have not been established.

ADVERSE REACTIONS
One of the most severe adverse effects is hyperkalemia (see *"Contraindications," "Warnings"* and *"Overdosage"*).

The most common adverse reactions to the oral Potassium salts are nausea, vomiting, flatulence, abdominal pain/discomfort and diarrhea. These symptoms are due to irritation of the gastrointestinal tract and are best managed by diluting the preparation further, taking the dose with meals, or reducing the amount taken at one time.

OVERDOSAGE
The administration of oral Potassium salts to persons with normal excretory mechanisms for Potassium rarely causes serious hyperkalemia. However, if excretory mechanisms are impaired, or if Potassium is administered too rapidly intravenously, potentially fatal hyperkalemia can result (see *"Contraindications"* and *"Warnings"*). It is important to recognize that hyperkalemia is usually asymptomatic and may be manifested only by an increased serum Potassium concentration (6.5-8.0 mEq/L) and characteristic electrocardiographic changes (peaking of T-waves, loss of P-wave, depression of S-T segment and prolongation of the QT interval). Late manifestations include muscle paralysis and cardiovascular collapse from cardiac arrest (9-12 mEq/L).

Treatment measures for hyperkalemia include the following:

1. Elimination of foods and medications containing Potassium and of any agents with Potassium-sparing properties;
2. Intravenous administration of 300 to 500 mL/hr of 10% dextrose solution containing 10-20 units of crystalline insulin per 1,000 mL;
3. Correction of acidosis, if present, with intravenous sodium bicarbonate;
4. Use of cation exchange resins, hemodialysis or peritoneal dialysis.

In treating hyperkalemia it should be recalled that in patients who have been stabilized on digitalis, too rapid a lowering of the serum Potassium concentration can produce digitalis toxicity.

DOSAGE AND ADMINISTRATION
The usual dietary Potassium intake by the average adult is 50 to 100 mEq per day. Potassium depletion sufficient to cause hypokalemia usually requires the loss of 200 or more mEq of Potassium from the total body store.

Dosage must be adjusted to the individual needs of each patient. The dose for the prevention of hypokalemia is typically in the range of 20 mEq per day. Doses of 40-100 mEq per day or more are used for the treatment of Potassium depletion. The usual adult dose of Potassium Chloride/Potassium Gluconate Liquid is one tablespoonful (15 mL) in 30 mL (one fluid ounce) or more of water twice daily. This daily dose of Potassium Chloride/Potassium Gluconate Liquid supplies 40 mEq of Potassium ion, as well as 6.7 mEq of Chloride ion. Potassium Chloride/ Potassium Gluconate Liquid should be taken with meals. Deviations from this recommendation may be indicated; as no average total daily dose can be defined, the response of the patient to the dose of the drug must be assessed clinically. Larger doses may be required, but should be administered under close supervision because of the possibility of Potassium intoxication.

Dispense in a light-resistant container. Store at room temperature.

HOW SUPPLIED
ELIXIR: 20 MEQ/15 ML

BRAND/MANUFACTURER	NDC	SIZE	AWP
○ **BRAND**			
KAON: Savage	00281-3203-51	480 ml	$27.34
○ **GENERICS**			
Qualitest	00603-1537-58	480 ml	$5.49
Goldline	00182-0245-40	480 ml	$6.00
Barre	00472-1459-16	480 ml	$7.43
Norton,HN	50732-0628-16	480 ml	$8.69
Norton,HN	50732-0628-28	3840 ml	$47.72

LIQUID: 20 MEQ/15 ML

BRAND/MANUFACTURER	NDC	SIZE	AWP
○ **GENERICS**			
KAYLIXIR: Lannett	00527-0827-27	480 ml	$3.60
CMC-Cons	00223-6295-01	480 ml	$5.25
Rugby	00536-1710-85	480 ml	$6.75
Major	00904-1459-16	480 ml	$7.45
KAYLIXIR: Lannett	00527-0827-28	3840 ml	$23.20
CMC-Cons	00223-6295-02	3840 ml	$32.50

TABLETS: 99 MG

BRAND/MANUFACTURER	NDC	SIZE	AWP
○ **GENERICS**			
Moore,H.L.	00839-7310-06	100s	$2.15
Mission	00178-1970-01	100s	$2.49

► SHOWN IN PRODUCT IDENTIFICATION GUIDE

TABLETS: 500 MG

BRAND/MANUFACTURER	NDC	SIZE	AWP
○ GENERICS			
Allscrips	54569-2747-01	30s	$5.05
Camall	00147-0238-10	100s	$3.53
Rugby	00536-4317-01	100s	$3.60
Goldline	00182-1024-01	100s	$4.95
Allscrips	54569-2747-00	100s	$6.80
Camall	00147-0238-20	1000s	$19.38
Rugby	00536-4317-10	1000s	$20.92
GLU-K: Jones-Western	52604-5750-02	1000s	$23.76
Goldline	00182-1024-10	1000s	$24.75
GLU-K: Jones-Western	52604-5750-08	1008s	$24.42
Camall	00147-0238-30	5000s	$76.75

TABLETS: 595 MG

BRAND/MANUFACTURER	NDC	SIZE	AWP
○ GENERICS			
Southwood	58016-0982-30	30s	$4.88

Potassium Chloride and Sodium Chloride

DESCRIPTION

Intravenous solutions with Potassium Chloride (IV solutions with KCl) are sterile and nonpyrogenic solutions in water for injection. They are for administration by intravenous infusion only.

See table for summary of content and characteristics of these solutions. (See related table).

The solutions contain no bacteriostat, antimicrobial agent or added buffer and each is intended only for use as a single-dose injection. When smaller doses are required the unused portion should be discarded.

These solutions are parenteral fluid and/or electrolyte replenishers.

Potassium Chloride, USP is chemically designated KCl, a white granular powder freely soluble in water.

Sodium Chloride, USP is chemically designated NaCl, a white crystalline powder freely soluble in water.

Water for Injection, USP is chemically designated H_2O.

CLINICAL PHARMACOLOGY

When administered intravenously, these solutions provide a source of water and Potassium Chloride with 0.9% sodium chloride.

Intravenous solutions containing potassium chloride are particularly intended to provide needed potassium cation (K^+). Potassium is the chief cation of body cells (160 mEq/liter of intracellular water). It is found in low concentration in plasma and extracellular fluids (3.5 to 5.0 mEq/liter in a healthy adult). Potassium plays an important role in electrolyte balance. Normally about 80 to 90% of the potassium intake is excreted in the urine; the remainder in the stools, and to a small extent, in the perspiration. The kidney does not conserve potassium well so that during fasting or in patients on a potassium-free diet, potassium loss from the body continues resulting in potassium depletion. A deficiency of either potassium or chloride will lead to a deficit of the other.

Sodium Chloride in water dissociates to provide sodium (Na^+) and chloride (Cl^-) ions. Sodium (Na^+) is the principal cation of the extracellular fluid and plays a large part in the therapy of fluid and electrolyte disturbances. Chloride (Cl^-) has an integral role in buffering action when oxygen and carbon dioxide exchange occurs in the red blood cells. The distribution and excretion of sodium (Na^+) and chloride (Cl^-) are largely under the control of the kidney which maintains a balance between intake and output.

Water is an essential constituent of all body tissues and accounts for approximately 70% of total body weight. Average normal adult daily requirement ranges from two to three liters (1.0 to 1.5 liters each for insensible water loss by perspiration and urine production).

Water balance is maintained by various regulatory mechanisms. Water distribution depends primarily on the concentration of electrolytes in the body compartments and sodium (Na^+) plays a major role in maintaining physiologic equilibrium.

INDICATIONS AND USAGE

These solutions are indicated in patients requiring parenteral administration of Potassium Chloride and Sodium Chloride.

CONTRAINDICATIONS

Solutions containing Potassium Chloride are contraindicated in diseases where high Potassium levels may be encountered.

WARNINGS

Solutions which contain potassium ions should be used with great care, if at all, in patients with hyperkalemia, severe renal failure and in conditions in which potassium retention is present.

To avoid potassium intoxication, do not infuse these solutions rapidly. In patients with severe renal insufficiency or adrenal insufficiency, administration of Potassium Chloride may cause potassium intoxication.

Solutions containing sodium ions should be used with great care, if at all, in patients with congestive heart failure, severe renal insufficiency and in clinical states in which there exists edema with sodium retention.

In patients with diminished renal function, administration of solutions containing sodium or potassium ions may result in sodium or potassium retention.

The intravenous administration of these solutions can cause fluid and/or solute overloading resulting in dilution of serum electrolyte concentrations, overhydration, congested states or pulmonary edema.

The risk of dilutional states is inversely proportional to the electrolyte concentration of administered parenteral solutions. The risk of solute overload causing congested states with peripheral and pulmonary edema is directly proportional to the electrolyte concentrations of such solutions.

PRECAUTIONS

Clinical evaluation and periodic laboratory determinations are necessary to monitor changes in fluid balance, electrolyte concentrations and acid-base balance during prolonged parenteral therapy or whenever the condition of the patient warrants such evaluation.

Caution must be exercised in the administration of parenteral fluids, especially those containing sodium ions, to patients receiving corticosteroids or corticotropin.

Potassium replacement therapy should be guided primarily by serial electrocardiograms. Plasma potassium levels are not necessarily indicative of tissue potassium levels.

High plasma concentrations of potassium may cause death through cardiac depression, arrhythmias or arrest.

Potassium-containing solutions should be used with caution in the presence of cardiac disease, particularly in digitalized patients or in the presence of renal disease.

Care should be exercised to insure that the needle (or catheter) is well within the lumen of the vein and that extravasation does not occur.

Do not administer unless solution is clear and container is undamaged. Discard unused portion.

Pregnancy Category C: Animal reproduction studies have not been conducted with Potassium Chloride or Sodium Chloride. It is also not known whether Potassium Chloride or Sodium Chloride can cause fetal harm when administered to a pregnant woman or can affect reproduction capacity. Potassium Chloride or Sodium Chloride should be given to a pregnant woman only if clearly needed.

ADVERSE REACTIONS

Reactions which may occur because of the solutions or technique of administration include febrile response, infection at the site of injection, venous thrombosis or phlebitis extending from the site of injection, extravasation and hypervolemia.

If an adverse reaction does occur, discontinue the infusion, evaluate the patient, institute appropriate therapeutic countermeasures and save the remainder of the fluid for examination if deemed necessary.

Nausea, vomiting, abdominal pain and diarrhea have been reported with potassium therapy. The signs and symptoms of potassium intoxication include paresthesias of the extremities, flaccid paralysis, listlessness, mental confusion, weakness and heaviness of the legs, hypotension, cardiac arrhythmias, heart block, electrocardiographic abnormalities such as disappearance of P waves, spreading and slurring of the QRS complex with development of a biphasic curve and cardiac arrest.

Potassium-containing solutions are intrinsically irritating to tissues. Therefore, extreme care should be taken to avoid perivascular infiltration. Local tissue necrosis and subsequent sloughing may result if extravasation occurs. Chemical phlebitis and venospasm have also been reported.

Should perivascular infiltration occur, IV administration at that site should be discontinued at once. Local infiltration of the affected area with procaine hydrochloride, 1%, to which hyaluronidase may be added, will often reduce venospasm and dilute the potassium remaining in the tissues locally. Local application of heat may also be helpful.

Potassium Chloride in 0.9% Sodium Chloride Inj.		Composition (g/L)				Approx. Ionic Concentrations (mEq/L)			
mEq Potassium	Size (mL)	Sodium Chloride	Potassium Chloride	Calculated Osmolarity (mOsm/L)	pH (range)	Sodium (Na^+)	Potassium (K^+)	Chloride (Cl^-)	approximate kcal/L
20 mEq	1000	9	1.49	348	4.8 (3.5 - 6.5)	154	20	174	0
40 mEq	1000	9	2.98	388	4.8 (3.5 - 6.5)	154	40	194	0

◆ RATED THERAPEUTICALLY EQUIVALENT; ◇ THERAPEUTIC EQUIVALENCE UNCONFIRMED; ○ UNRATED

OVERDOSAGE

In the event of potassium overdosage, discontinue the infusion immediately and institute intensive corrective therapy to reduce serum potassium levels. See *"Warnings"* and *"Precautions"*.

DOSAGE AND ADMINISTRATION

These solutions should be administered only by intravenous infusion and as directed by the physician. The dose and rate of injection are dependent upon the age, weight and clinical condition of the patient. If the serum potassium level is greater than 2.5 mEq/liter, potassium should be given at a rate not to exceed 10 mEq/hour in a concentration less than 30 mEq/liter. Somewhat faster rates and greater concentrations (usually up to 40 mEq/liter) of potassium may be indicated in patients with more severe potassium deficiency. The total 24-hour dose should not generally exceed 200 mEq of potassium.

DRUG INTERACTIONS

Additives may be incompatible. Consult with pharmacist, if available. When introducing additives, use aseptic technique, mix thoroughly and do not store.

Parenteral drug products should be inspected visually for particulate matter and discoloration prior to administration, whenever solution and container permit. See *"Precautions"*.

To Add Medication:
1. Prepare additive port.
2. Using aseptic technique and an additive delivery needle of appropriate length, puncture resealable additive port at target area, inner diaphragm and inject. Withdraw needle after injecting medication.
3. The additive port may be protected by covering with an additive cap.
4. Mix container contents thoroughly.

Preparation for Administration

(Use aseptic technique):
1. Close flow control clamp of administration set.
2. Remove cover from outlet port at bottom of container.
3. Insert piercing pin of administration set into port with a twisting motion until the set is firmly seated. *Note:* See full directions on administration set carton.
4. Suspend container from hanger.
5. Squeeze and release drip chamber to establish proper fluid level in chamber.
6. Open flow control clamp and clear air from set. Close clamp.
7. Attach set to venipuncture device. If device is not indwelling, prime and make venipuncture.
8. Regulate rate of administration with flow control clamp.
   WARNING: Do not use flexible container in series connections.

Storage: Exposure of pharmaceutical products to heat should be minimized. Avoid excessive heat. Protect from freezing. It is recommended that the product be stored at room temperature (25°C); however, brief exposure up to 40°C does not adversely affect the product.

HOW SUPPLIED
INJECTION: 0.3%

BRAND/MANUFACTURER	NDC	SIZE	AWP
◆ GENERICS			
Baxter	00338-0695-04	1000 ml 12s	$201.46

INJECTION: 20 MEQ

AVERAGE UNIT PRICE (AVAILABLE SIZES)		GENERIC A-RATED AVERAGE PRICE (GAAP)	
GENERIC	$0.02	1000 ml 12s	$246.08

BRAND/MANUFACTURER	NDC	SIZE	AWP
◆ GENERICS			
Baxter	00338-0691-03	500 ml 12s	$79.92
Baxter	00338-0691-04	1000 ml 12s	$201.46
Abbott Hosp	00074-7115-09	1000 ml 12s	$290.70

INJECTION: 40 MEQ

BRAND/MANUFACTURER	NDC	SIZE	AWP
◆ GENERICS			
Abbott Hosp	00074-7116-09	1000 ml 12s	$293.41

Potassium Chloride, Injectable

DESCRIPTION

Potassium Chloride, Injectable, is a sterile, nonpyrogenic, concentrated solution of Potassium Chloride in water for injection to be administered by intravenous infusion only after dilution in a larger volume of fluid. It is available in single-dose and multiple-dose units and in pharmacy bulk packages.

Each ml provides:

Potassium Chloride 112 or 149 mg ....(1.5 or 2 mEq/ml Potassium)

Potassium Chloride, Injectable, (appropriately diluted) is a parenteral fluid and electrolyte replenisher.

Potassium Chloride, is chemically designated KCl, a white granular powder freely soluble in water. The pH range is 4.0-8.0 and the osmolarity is 3000 to 4000 mOsmol/ml calculated. The molecular weight is 74.55.

CLINICAL PHARMACOLOGY

Potassium is the chief cation of body cells (160 mEq/liter of intracellular water) and is concerned with the maintenance of body fluid composition and electrolyte balance. Potassium participates in carbohydrate utilization and protein synthesis, and is critical in the regulation of nerve conduction and muscle contraction, particularly in the heart. Chloride, the major extracellular anion, closely follows the metabolism of sodium, and changes in the acid-base balance of the body are reflected by changes in the Chloride concentration.

Normally about 80 to 90% of the Potassium intake is excreted in the urine, the remainder in the stools and, to a small extent, in perspiration. The kidney does not conserve Potassium well so that during fasting, or in patients on a Potassium-free diet, Potassium loss from the body continues, resulting in Potassium depletion. A deficiency of either Potassium or Chloride will lead to a deficit of the other.

INDICATIONS AND USAGE

Potassium Cl, Injectable, is indicated in the treatment of potassium deficiency states when oral replacement is not feasible.

UNLABELED USES

Potassium Cl is used alone or as an adjunct in the treatment of supraventricular and ventricular arrhythmias, hypertension, and myocardial infarction. In addition, Potassium Cl is used for myocardial protection during cardiac surgery.

CONTRAINDICATIONS

Potassium Cl, Injectable, is contraindicated in diseases where high Potassium levels may be encountered, and in patients with hyperkalemia, renal failure and in conditions in which Potassium retention is present.

WARNINGS

To avoid Potassium intoxication, do not infuse solutions rapidly. In patients with severe renal insufficiency, administration of Potassium Cl may cause Potassium intoxication and life-threatening hyperkalemia.

The administration of intravenous solutions can cause fluid and/or solute overload resulting in dilution of serum electrolyte concentrations, overhydration, congested states or pulmonary edema.

The risk of dilutional states is inversely proportional to the electrolyte concentration. The risk of solute overload causing congested states with peripheral and pulmonary edema is directly proportional to the electrolyte concentration.

PRECAUTIONS
GENERAL

Clinical evaluation and periodic laboratory determinations are necessary to monitor changes in fluid balance, electrolyte concentrations, and acid-base balance during prolonged parenteral therapy or whenever the condition of the patient warrants such evaluation. Significant deviations from normal concentrations may require the use of additional electrolyte supplements, or the use of electrolyte-free dextrose solutions to which individualized electrolyte supplements may be added.

Potassium therapy should be guided primarily by serial electrocardiograms, especially in patients receiving digitalis. Serum Potassium levels are not necessarily indicative of tissue Potassium levels. Solutions containing Potassium should be used with caution in the presence of cardiac disease, particularly in the presence of renal disease, and in such instances, cardiac monitoring is recommended.

Solutions containing dextrose should be used with caution in patients with overt or known subclinical diabetes mellitus, or carbohydrate intolerance for any reason.

If the administration is controlled by a pumping device, care must be taken to discontinue pumping action before the container runs dry or air embolism may result.

PREGNANCY

Teratogenic Effects: Pregnancy category C. Animal reproduction studies have not been conducted with Potassium Cl. It is also not known whether Potassium Cl can cause fetal harm when administered to a pregnant woman or can affect reproduction capacity. Potassium Cl should be given to a pregnant woman only if clearly needed.

ADVERSE REACTIONS

Reactions which may occur because of the solution or the technique of administration include febrile response, infection at the site of injection, venous thrombosis, or phlebitis extending from the site of injection, extravasation, hypervolemia, and hyperkalemia.

Too rapid infusion of hypertonic solutions may cause local pain, and rarely, vein irritation. Rate of administration should be adjusted according to tolerance.

Reactions reported with the use of Potassium-containing solutions include nausea, vomiting, abdominal pain, and diarrhea. The signs and symptoms of Potassium intoxication include paresthesias of the extremities, areflexia, muscular or respiratory paralysis, mental confusion, weakness, hypotension, cardiac arrhythmias, heart block, electrocardiographic abnormalities, and cardiac arrest. Potassium deficits result in disruption of neuromuscular function, and intestinal ileus and dilatation.

If an adverse reaction does occur, discontinue the infusion, evaluate the patient, institute appropriate therapeutic countermeasures, and save the remainder of the fluid for examination if deemed necessary.

OVERDOSAGE

In the event of fluid overload during parenteral therapy, re-evaluate the patient's condition, and institute appropriate corrective treatment.

In the event of overdosage with Potassium-containing solutions, discontinue the infusion immediately and institute corrective therapy to reduce serum Potassium levels.

Treatment of hyperkalemia includes the following:

1. Dextrose Injection USP, 10% or 25%, containing 10 units of crystalline insulin per 20 grams of dextrose administered intravenously, at a rate of 300 to 500 mL per hour.

2. Absorption and exchange of Potassium using sodium or ammonium cycle cation exchange resin, orally and as retention enema.

3. Hemodialysis and peritoneal dialysis. The use of Potassium-containing foods or medications must be eliminated. However, in cases of digitalization, too rapid a lowering of plasma Potassium concentration can cause digitalis toxicity.

DOSAGE AND ADMINISTRATION

Potassium Cl, Injectable, must be diluted before administration. Care must be taken to ensure there is complete mixing of the Potassium Cl with the large volume fluid, particularly if soft or bag type containers are used.

The dose and rate of administration are dependent upon the specific condition or individual needs of each patient.

If the serum potassium level is greater than 2.5 mEq/liter, Potassium can be given at a rate not to exceed 10 mEq/hour in a concentration of up to 40 mEq/liter. The 24-hour total dose should not exceed 200 mEq.

If urgent treatment is indicated (serum Potassium level less than 2.0 mEq/liter with electrocardiographic changes and/or muscle paralysis) Potassium Cl may be infused very cautiously at a rate of up to 40 mEq/hour. In such cases, continuous cardiac monitoring is essential. As much as 400 mEq may be administered in a 24-hour period. In critical conditions, Potassium Cl may be administered in saline (unless contraindicated), rather than in dextrose-containing fluids, as dextrose may lower serum Potassium levels.

Prior to entering a vial, remove the seal and cleanse the rubber closure with a suitable antiseptic agent.

Parenteral drug products should be inspected visually for particulate matter and discoloration prior to administration, whenever solution and container permit.

Do not administer unless solution is clear and seal intact. Discard unused portion.

TO PREVENT NEEDLE-STICK INJURIES, NEEDLES SHOULD NOT BE RECAPPED, PURPOSELY BENT, OR BROKEN BY HAND.

DIRECTIONS FOR PROPER USE OF PHARMACY BULK PACKAGE

The pharmacy bulk package is for use in a Pharmacy Admixture service only. It should be inserted into the plastic hanging device provided and suspended as a unit in the laminar flow hood. A single entry through the vial closure should be made with a sterile dispensing set which allows measured dispensing of the contents. Transfer individual dose(s) to appropriate intravenous infusion solutions without delay. Use of a syringe with needle is not recommended. Multiple entries will also increase the potential of microbial and particulate contamination. The above process should be carried out under a laminar flow hood using aseptic technique. ANY UNUSED PORTION MUST BE DISCARDED WITHIN 4 HOURS.

STORAGE

Store at controlled room temperature 15° to 30°C (59° to 86°F). Avoid excessive heat. Protect from freezing. Brief exposure up to 40°C does not adversely affect the product.

HOW SUPPLIED
INJECTION: 1.5 MEQ/ML

BRAND/MANUFACTURER	NDC	SIZE	AWP
◆ GENERICS			
Abbott Hosp	00074-4993-01	20 ml 25s	$191.48

INJECTION: 2 MEQ/ML

AVERAGE UNIT PRICE (AVAILABLE SIZES)		GENERIC A-RATED AVERAGE PRICE (GAAP)	
GENERIC	$0.23	250 ml 12s	$489.74
		5 ml 25s	$107.57
		10 ml 25s	$85.53
		15 ml 25s	$100.94
		20 ml 25s	$95.06
		10 ml 100s	$112.50
		20 ml 100s	$113.33

BRAND/MANUFACTURER	NDC	SIZE	AWP
◆ GENERICS			
Fujisawa	00469-6505-15	5 ml	$1.18
Fujisawa	00469-6510-15	10 ml	$1.42
Fujisawa	00469-6515-15	15 ml	$1.56
Fujisawa	00469-6520-15	20 ml	$1.65
Fujisawa	00469-0067-15	30 ml	$1.73
Intl Med Sys	00548-6557-00	200 ml 12s	$90.00

BRAND/MANUFACTURER	NDC	SIZE	AWP
McGaw	00264-1940-20	250 ml 12s	$473.47
Abbott Hosp	00074-1513-02	250 ml 12s	$506.02
McGaw	00264-1940-10	500 ml 12s	$473.47
Abbott Hosp	00074-6635-01	5 ml 25s	$63.53
Abbott Hosp	00074-4931-01	5 ml 25s	$81.64
Abbott Hosp	00074-4991-01	5 ml 25s	$177.53
Amer Regent	00517-2110-25	10 ml 25s	$19.69
Amer Regent	00517-2210-25	10 ml 25s	$22.19
Abbott Hosp	00074-6651-06	10 ml 25s	$65.91
Abbott Hosp	00074-3907-03	10 ml 25s	$77.19
Abbott Hosp	00074-4932-01	10 ml 25s	$87.58
Intl Med Sys	00548-6056-00	10 ml 25s	$104.70
Abbott Hosp	00074-1497-01	10 ml 25s	$124.69
Abbott Hosp	00074-4992-01	10 ml 25s	$182.28
Abbott Hosp	00074-6636-01	15 ml 25s	$71.55
Abbott Hosp	00074-1498-01	15 ml 25s	$130.33
Amer Regent	00517-2120-25	20 ml 25s	$24.69
Amer Regent	00517-2220-25	20 ml 25s	$30.94
Abbott Hosp	00074-6653-05	20 ml 25s	$72.73
Abbott Hosp	00074-4939-01	20 ml 25s	$89.06
Abbott Hosp	00074-3934-02	20 ml 25s	$93.81
Abbott Hosp	00074-1499-01	20 ml 25s	$142.50
Abbott Hosp	00074-4994-01	20 ml 25s	$211.67
Amer Regent	00517-2130-25	30 ml 25s	$27.19
Raway	00686-2110-25	10 ml 100s	$99.00
Baxter	00338-0655-61	10 ml 100s	$126.00
Raway	00686-2210-25	20 ml 100s	$99.00
Raway	00686-2120-25	20 ml 100s	$100.00
Baxter	00338-0655-62	20 ml 100s	$141.00
Raway	00686-2130-25	30 ml 100s	$165.00

INJECTION: 3 MEQ/ML

BRAND/MANUFACTURER	NDC	SIZE	AWP
◆ GENERICS			
Fujisawa	00469-6830-25	30 ml	$1.88

Potassium Chloride, Oral

DESCRIPTION

Potassium Chloride, Oral, is an electrolyte replenisher.

It is available as extended-release tablets and capsules, effervescent granules, and liquid. The extended-release forms provide a slow release of Potassium to minimize the likelihood of producing high, localized concentrations of Potassium within the gastrointestinal tract, with resultant mucosal ulceration.

Each extended-release tablet contains:
Potassium Chloride ....600, 750, or 1500 mg
(equivalent to 8, 10, or 20 mEq of Potassium, respectively)

Each extended-release capsule contains:
Potassium Chloride ....600 or 750 mg
(equivalent to 8 or 10 mEq)

Each 2.8 gm of effervescent granules contains:
Lysine Hydrochloride ....0.913 gm
Potassium Bicarbonate ....0.5 gm
Potassium Chloride ....1.125 gm

Each tablespoonful (15 ml) of liquid contains:
Potassium Chloride ....1.5 gm (20 mEq)

Potassium Chloride is a white, granular powder or colorless crystals. It is odorless and has a saline taste. Its solutions are neutral to litmus. It is freely soluble in water and insoluble in alcohol.

The solid oral dosage forms may be in a wax matrix, microencapsulated, or enteric-coated.

CLINICAL PHARMACOLOGY

The Potassium ion is the principal intracellular cation of most body tissues. Potassium ions participate in a number of essential physiological processes, including the maintenance of intracellular tonicity, the transmission of nerve impulses, the contraction of cardiac, skeletal, and smooth muscle, and the maintenance of normal renal function.

The intracellular concentration of Potassium is approximately 150 to 160 mEq per liter.

In adults normal plasma potassium concentration is 3.5-5.0 mEq/L. An active ion transport system maintains this gradient across the plasma membrane.

Potassium is a normal dietary constituent and under steady state conditions the amount of Potassium absorbed from the gastrointestinal tract is equal to the amount excreted in the urine. The usual dietary intake of Potassium is 50 to 100 mEq per day.

Potassium depletion may occur whenever the rate of potassium loss through renal excretion and/or loss from the gastrointestinal tract exceeds the rate of Potassium intake. Such depletion usually develops slowly as a consequence of prolonged therapy with oral diuretics, primary or secondary hyperaldosteronism, diabetic ketoacidosis, severe diarrhea, or inadequate replacement of Potassium in patients on prolonged parenteral nutrition. Depletion can develop rapidly with

---

◆ RATED THERAPEUTICALLY EQUIVALENT; ◇ THERAPEUTIC EQUIVALENCE UNCONFIRMED; ○ UNRATED

severe diarrhea, especially if associated with vomiting. Potassium depletion due to these causes is usually accompanied by a concomitant deficiency of chloride and is manifested by hypokalemia and metabolic alkalosis. Potassium depletion may produce weakness, fatigue, disturbances of cardiac rhythm (primarily ectopic beats), prominent U-waves in the electrocardiogram, and in advanced cases flaccid paralysis and/or impaired ability to concentrate urine.

If Potassium depletion associated with metabolic alkalosis cannot be managed by correcting the fundamental cause of the deficiency, e.g., where the patient requires long term diuretic therapy, supplemental Potassium in the form of high Potassium food or Potassium Chloride may be able to restore normal Potassium levels.

In rare circumstances (e.g., patients with renal tubular acidosis) potassium depletion may be associated with metabolic acidosis and hyperchloremia. In such patients Potassium replacement should be accomplished with Potassium salts other than the Chloride, such as Potassium bicarbonate, Potassium citrate, Potassium acetate, or potassium gluconate.

INDICATIONS AND USAGE

Solid Oral Dosage Forms: BECAUSE OF REPORTS OF INTESTINAL AND GASTRIC ULCERATION AND BLEEDING WITH EXTENDED-RELEASE POTASSIUM CHLORIDE PREPARATIONS, THESE DRUGS SHOULD BE RESERVED FOR THOSE PATIENTS WHO CANNOT TOLERATE OR REFUSE TO TAKE LIQUID OR EFFERVESCENT POTASSIUM PREPARATIONS OR FOR PATIENTS IN WHOM THERE IS A PROBLEM OF COMPLIANCE WITH THESE PREPARATIONS.

1. For therapeutic use in patients with hypokalemia with or without metabolic alkalosis; in digitalis intoxication and in patients with hypokalemic familial periodic paralysis. If hypokalemia is the result of diuretic therapy, consideration should be given to the use of a lower dose of diuretic therapy, which may be sufficient without leading to hypokalemia.

2. For prevention of Potassium depletion when the dietary intake of potassium is inadequate in the following conditions and/or in patients who would be at particular risk if hypokalemia were to develop: patients receiving digitalis and diuretics for congestive heart failure; patients with significant cardiac arrhythmias; hepatic cirrhosis with ascites; states of aldosterone excess with normal renal function; potassium-losing nephropathy, and certain diarrheal states.

3. The use of Potassium salts in patients receiving diuretics for uncomplicated essential hypertension is often unnecessary when such patients have a normal dietary pattern. Serum Potassium should be checked periodically, however, and, if hypokalemia occurs, dietary supplementation with potassium-containing foods may be adequate to control milder cases. In more severe cases, and if dose adjustment of the diuretic is ineffective or unwarranted, supplementation with Potassium salts may be indicated.

Effervescent Granules and Liquid: For the prevention and treatment of Potassium depletion and hypokalemic-hypochloremic alkalosis. Deficits of body Potassium and Chloride can occur as a consequence of therapy with potent diuretic agents and adrenal corticosteroids.

UNLABELED USES

Potassium Chloride is used alone or as an adjunct in the treatment of atrial tachycardia, ventricular arrhythmias, hypertension, and for inducing peripheral insulin levels and improving glucose utilization in obese patients. It is also used to lower the risk of myocardial infarction.

CONTRAINDICATIONS

Solid Oral Dosage Forms: Potassium supplements are contraindicated in patients with hyperkalemia, since a further increase in serum Potassium concentration in such patients can produce cardiac arrest. Hyperkalemia may complicate any of the following conditions: chronic renal failure, systemic acidosis such as diabetic acidosis, acute dehydration, heat cramps, extensive tissue breakdown as in severe burns, adrenal insufficiency, or the administration of a potassium-sparing diuretic (e.g., spironolactone, triamterene, amiloride) (see *"Overdosage"*).

All solid oral dosage forms of Potassium supplements are contraindicated in any patient in whom there is structural, pathological (e.g., diabetic gastroparesis) or pharmacologic (use of anticholinergic agents or other agents with anticholinergic properties at sufficient doses to exert anticholinergic effects) cause for arrest or delay in tablet or capsule passage through the gastrointestinal tract. In these instances, Potassium supplementation should be with a liquid preparation. Wax-matrix and controlled-release Potassium Chloride preparations have produced esophageal ulceration in certain cardiac patients with esophageal compression due to an enlarged left atrium. Potassium supplementation, when indicated in such patients, should be given as a liquid preparation or as an aqueous (water) suspension.

Effervescent Granules and Liquid: Severe renal impairment characterized by azotemia or oliguria, untreated Addison's disease, familial periodic paralysis, acute dehydration, heat cramps, patients receiving aldosterone-inhibiting or Potassium-sparing diuretic agents or hyperkalemia from any cause.

WARNINGS

HYPERKALEMIA
(See *"Overdosage"*.)

In patients with impaired mechanisms for excreting potassium, the administration of potassium salts can produce hyperkalemia and cardiac arrest. This occurs most commonly in patients given potassium by the intravenous route but may also occur in patients given Potassium orally. Potentially fatal hyperkalemia can develop rapidly and be asymptomatic.

The use of potassium salts in patients with chronic renal disease, or any other condition which impairs Potassium excretion, requires particularly careful monitoring of the serum Potassium concentration and appropriate dosage adjustment.

INTERACTION WITH POTASSIUM-SPARING DIURETICS
Hypokalemia should not be treated by the concomitant administration of potassium salts and a potassium-sparing diuretic (e.g., spironolactone, triamterene, or amiloride), since the simultaneous administration of these agents can produce severe hyperkalemia.

INTERACTION WITH ANGIOTENSIN CONVERTING ENZYME INHIBITORS
Angiotensin converting enzyme (ACE) inhibitors (e.g., captopril, enalapril) will produce some Potassium retention by inhibiting aldosterone production. Potassium supplements should be given to patients receiving ACE inhibitors only with close monitoring.

GASTROINTESTINAL LESIONS
Solid oral dosage forms of Potassium Chloride have produced stenotic and/or ulcerative lesions of the small bowel and deaths, in addition to upper gastrointestinal bleeding. These lesions are caused by a high localized concentration of potassium ion in the region of a rapidly dissolving tablet, which injures the bowel wall and thereby produces obstruction, hemorrhage, or perforation. Extended-release tablets and capsules are formulated to provide a slow rate of release of Potassium Chloride and thus to minimize the possibility of a high local concentration of potassium ion near the bowel wall. While the reported frequency of small-bowel lesions is much less with wax-matrix tablets (less than one per 100,000 patient-years) than with enteric-coated Potassium Chloride tablets (40-50 per 100,000 patient-years) cases associated with wax-matrix tablets have been reported both in foreign countries and in the United States. In addition, perhaps because the wax-matrix preparations are not enteric-coated and release potassium in the stomach, there have been reports of upper gastrointestinal bleeding associated with these products. The total number of gastrointestinal lesions remains approximately one per 100,000 patient-years. Because of the lack of extensive marketing experience with microencapsulated products, a comparison between such products and wax matrix or enteric coated products is not available.

Prospective trials have been conducted in normal human volunteers in which the upper gastrointestinal tract was evaluated by endoscopic inspection before and after one week of solid oral Potassium Chloride therapy. The ability of this model to predict events occurring in usual clinical practice is unknown. Trials which approximated usual clinical practice did not reveal any clear differences between the wax matrix and microencapsulated dosage forms. In contrast, there was a higher incidence of gastric and duodenal lesions in subjects receiving a high dose of a wax matrix controlled-release formulation under conditions which did not resemble usual or recommended clinical practice (i.e., 96 mEq per day in divided doses of Potassium Chloride administered to fasted patients, in the presence of an anticholinergic drug to delay gastric emptying). The upper gastrointestinal lesions observed by endoscopy were asymptomatic and were not accompanied by evidence of bleeding (hemoccult testing). The relevance of these findings to the usual conditions (i.e., nonfasting, no anticholinergic agent, smaller doses) under which controlled-release Potassium Chloride products are used is uncertain; epidemiologic studies have not identified an elevated risk, compared to microencapsulated products, for upper gastrointestinal lesions in patients receiving wax matrix formulations.

The ulcerogenic potential of microencapsulated Potassium Chloride was studied in anesthetized cats by direct applications on exteriorized gastric mucosa. The microcapsules of Potassium Chloride were found to be non-ulcerogenic and significantly less irritating than wax-matrix tablets and 20% solution of Potassium Chloride.

In groups of monkeys (up to 8 monkeys per group) receiving different formulations of Potassium Chloride at equivalent daily dosage (2400 mg Potassium Chloride) for four and one-half days, Microencapsulated Potassium Chloride showed no tendency to cause intestinal ulceration (similar to liquid Potassium Chloride and a wax-matrix preparation but in contrast to an enteric-coated Potassium Chloride tablet) and minimal gastric irritation (less than a wax-matrix preparation).

Potassium Chloride tablets or capsules should be discontinued immediately and the possibility of ulceration, bowel obstruction or perforation considered if severe vomiting, abdominal pain, distention, or gastrointestinal bleeding occurs.

METABOLIC ACIDOSIS
Hypokalemia in patients with metabolic *acidosis* should be treated with an alkalinizing potassium salt such as potassium bicarbonate, potassium citrate, potassium acetate, or potassium gluconate.

PRECAUTIONS

General: In response to a rise in the concentration of body Potassium, renal excretion of the ion is increased. In the presence of normal renal function and hydration, it is difficult to produce potassium intoxication by oral Potassium salt supplements.

Since the extent of Potassium deficiency cannot be accurately determined, it is prudent to proceed cautiously in undertaking Potassium replacement.

The diagnosis of Potassium depletion is ordinarily made by demonstrating hypokalemia in a patient with a clinical history suggesting some cause for Potassium depletion. In interpreting the serum Potassium level, the physician should bear in mind that acute alkalosis *per se* can produce hypokalemia in the absence of a deficit in total body Potassium, while acute acidosis *per se* can increase the serum Potassium concentration into the normal range even in the presence of a reduced total body Potassium.

Regular serum Potassium determinations are recommended. The treatment of Potassium depletion, particularly in the presence of cardiac disease, renal disease, or acidosis requires careful attention to acid-base balance and appropriate monitoring of serum electrolytes, the electrocardiogram, and the clinical status of the patient. Potassium should generally not be given in the immediate postoperative period until urine flow is established.

INFORMATION FOR PATIENTS
Physicians should consider reminding the patient of the following:

To take each dose without crushing, chewing, or sucking the tablets.

If patients are having difficulty swallowing whole tablets, they may try one of the following alternate methods of administration, when feasible:

    a. Break the tablet in half, and take each half separately with a glass of water.
    b. Prepare an aqueous (water) suspension as follows:

1. Place the whole tablet(s) in approximately one-half glass of water (4 fluid ounces).
2. Allow approximately 2 minutes for the tablet(s) to disintegrate.
3. Stir for about half a minute after the tablet(s) has disintegrated.
4. Swirl the suspension and consume the entire contents of the glass immediately by drinking or by the use of a straw.
5. Add another one fluid ounce of water, swirl, and consume immediately.
6. Then, add an additional one fluid ounce of water, swirl, and consume immediately.

Aqueous suspension of Potassium Chloride tablets that is not taken immediately should be discarded. The use of other liquids for suspending Potassium Chloride tablets is not recommended.

To take each dose with meals and with a full glass of water or other liquid.

To take this medicine only as directed. This is especially important if the patient is also taking diuretics and/or digitalis preparations.

To check with the physician if there is trouble swallowing tablets or capsules or if the tablets or capsules seem to stick in the throat.

To check with the doctor at once if tarry stools or other evidence of gastrointestinal bleeding is noticed.

To be aware that the expended matrix in wax matrix formulations is not absorbed and may be excreted intact in the stool.

To minimize gastrointestinal irritation associated with Potassium Chloride preparations, patients should dissolve the Potassium Chloride Effervescent granules in 3 to 4 ounces of cold water, fruit juice or other liquid, or dilute each tablespoonful of Potassium Chloride liquid in 3 to 4 ounces of cold water. Both of these solutions should be ingested slowly with or immediately after meals.

LABORATORY TESTS
Regular serum Potassium determinations are recommended, especially in patients with renal insufficiency or diabetic nephropathy. In addition, during the treatment of Potassium depletion, careful attention should be paid to acid-base balance, other serum electrolyte levels, the electrocardiogram, and the clinical status of the patient, particularly in the presence of cardiac disease, renal disease, or acidosis.

When blood is drawn for analysis of plasma Potassium it is important to recognize that artifactual elevations can occur after improper venipuncture technique or as a result of *in vitro* hemolysis of the sample. See *"Precautions; General."*

DRUG INTERACTIONS
Potassium-sparing diuretics, angiotensin converting enzyme inhibitors; see *"Warnings"*.

CARCINOGENESIS, MUTAGENESIS, IMPAIRMENT OF FERTILITY
Carcinogenicity, mutagenicity and fertility studies in animals have not been performed. Potassium is a normal dietary constituent.

PREGNANCY CATEGORY C
Animal reproduction studies have not been conducted with Potassium Chloride preparations. It is also not known whether Potassium Chloride preparations can cause fetal harm when administered to a pregnant woman or can affect reproduction capacity. Although it is unlikely that Potassium supplementation that does not lead to hyperkalemia would have an adverse effect on the fetus or would affect reproductive capacity, Potassium Chloride should be given to a pregnant woman only if clearly needed.

NURSING MOTHERS
The normal Potassium ion content of human milk is about 13 mEq/L. Since oral Potassium becomes part of the body Potassium pool, so long as body Potassium is not excessive, the contribution of Potassium Chloride supplementation should have little or no effect on the level in human milk. Caution should be exercised when Potassium Chloride is administered to a nursing woman.

PEDIATRIC USE
Safety and effectiveness in children have not been established.

ADVERSE REACTIONS
One of the most severe adverse effects is hyperkalemia (see *"Contraindications"*, *"Warnings"* and *"Overdosage"*). There have also been reports of upper and lower gastrointestinal conditions including obstruction, bleeding, ulceration, and perforation in patients treated with solid oral dosage forms of Potassium salts (see

"Contraindications" and *"Warnings"*); other factors known to be associated with such conditions were present in many of these patients.

The most common adverse reactions to oral Potassium salts are nausea, vomiting, flatulence, abdominal/pain discomfort, and diarrhea. These symptoms are due to irritation of the gastrointestinal tract and are best managed by diluting the preparation further, taking the dose with meals, or reducing the amount taken at one time.

Skin rash has been reported rarely.

The symptoms and signs of Potassium intoxication include paresthesias, heaviness, muscle weakness and flaccid paralysis of the extremities. Potassium intoxication can produce listlessness, mental confusion, a fall in blood pressure, shock, cardiac arrhythmias, heart block and cardiac arrest.

The EKG picture of hyperkalemia is characterized by the early appearance of tall, peaked T waves. The R wave is decreased in amplitude and the S wave deepens; the QRS complex widens progressively. The P wave widens and decreases in amplitude until it disappears. Occasionally, an apparent elevation of the RS-T junction and a cove plane RS-T segment and T wave will be noted in AVL.

OVERDOSAGE
The administration of oral Potassium salts to persons with normal excretory mechanisms for Potassium rarely causes serious hyperkalemia. However, if excretory mechanisms are impaired or if Potassium is administered too rapidly intravenously, potentially fatal hyperkalemia can result (see *"Contraindications"* and *"Warnings"*). It is important to recognize that hyperkalemia is usually asymptomatic and may be manifested only by an increased serum Potassium concentration (6.5-8.0 mEq/L) and characteristic electrocardiographic changes (peaking of T waves, loss of P wave, depression of S-T segment, and prolongation of the Q-T interval), and widening and slurring of the QRS complex. Late manifestations include muscle paralysis and cardiovascular collapse from cardiac arrest (9-12 mEq/L).

Treatment measures for hyperkalemia include the following: (1) elimination of foods and medications containing Potassium and of any agents with Potassium-sparing properties; (2) intravenous administration of 300-500 ml/hr of 10% dextrose solution containing 10-20 units of insulin per 1,000 ml; (3) correction of acidosis, if present, with intravenous sodium bicarbonate; (4) hemodialysis, or peritoneal dialysis; (5) adsorption and exchange of Potassium using sodium or ammonium cycle cation exchange resins, orally and as a retention enema.

(Caution: Ammonium compounds should not be used in patients with hepatic cirrhosis.)

In treating hyperkalemia in patients who have been stabilized on digitalis, too rapid a lowering of the serum Potassium concentration can produce digitalis toxicity.

DOSAGE AND ADMINISTRATION
Solid Oral Dosage Forms: The usual dietary intake of Potassium by the average adult ranges from 40-80 to 50-100 mEq per day. Potassium depletion sufficient to cause hypokalemia usually requires the loss of 200 or more mEq of Potassium from the total body store. Dosage must be adjusted to the individual needs of each patient but is typically in the range of 20-30 mEq per day for the prevention of hypokalemia to 40-100 mEq or more per day for the treatment of Potassium depletion. Dosage should be divided if more than 20 mEq per day is given such that no more than 20 mEq is given in a single dose.

Note: Most Potassium Chloride extended-release tablets must be swallowed whole and never crushed, chewed, or sucked. Some tablets can be broken in half or crushed, without an unpleasant taste.

Those patients having difficulty swallowing capsules may be advised to sprinkle the contents onto a spoonful of soft food to facilitate ingestion.

Patients having difficulty swallowing whole tablets may try one of the following alternate methods of administration when feasible:

    a. Break the tablet in half, and take each half separately with a glass of water.
    b. Prepare an aqueous (water) suspension as follows:

1. Place the whole tablet(s) in approximately one-half glass of water (4 fluid ounces).
2. Allow approximately 2 minutes for the tablet(s) to disintegrate.
3. Stir for about half a minute after the tablet(s) has disintegrated.
4. Swirl the suspension and consume the entire contents of the glass immediately by drinking or by the use of a straw.
5. Add another one fluid ounce of water, swirl, and consume immediately.
6. Then, add an additional one fluid ounce of water, swirl, and consume immediately.

Aqueous suspension of Potassium Chloride tablets that is not taken immediately should be discarded. The use of other liquids for suspending Potassium Chloride tablets is not recommended.

Effervescent Granules: Adults—(20 mEq each of Potassium and Chloride completely dissolved in 3 to 4 ounces of cold water, fruit juice or other liquid 2 to 4 times daily depending upon the requirements of the patients.

Liquid: Adults—One tablespoonful (15 mL) (20 mEq of Potassium Chloride) completely diluted in 3 to 4 ounces of cold water 2 to 4 times daily depending upon the requirements of the patient.

Both of these solutions should be ingested slowly with meals or immediately after eating. Deviations from these recommended dosages may be indicated in certain cases of hypokalemia based upon the patient's status. The average total daily dosage must be governed by the patient's response as determined by frequent evaluation of serum electrolytes, EKG and clinical status.

Storage: Store at controlled room temperature 15°-30°C (59°-86°F). Protect from moisture. Protect from light.

Dispense in tight, light-resistant container (USP).

HOW SUPPLIED
CAPSULE, EXTENDED RELEASE: 8 MEQ

AVERAGE UNIT PRICE (AVAILABLE SIZES)		GENERIC A-RATED AVERAGE PRICE (GAAP)	
BRAND	$0.15	100s	$10.33
GENERIC	$0.10	1000s	$99.53

BRAND/MANUFACTURER	NDC	SIZE	AWP
◆ BRAND			
➤ MICRO-K: Robins Pharm	00031-5720-63	100s	$14.60
	00031-5720-64	100s ud	$17.21
	00031-5720-70	500s	$65.46
◆ GENERICS			
Warner Chilcott	00047-0951-24	100s	$10.05
URL	00677-1096-01	100s	$10.60
URL	00677-1096-10	1000s	$99.00
Warner Chilcott	00047-0951-32	1000s	$100.05

CAPSULE, EXTENDED RELEASE: 10 MEQ

AVERAGE UNIT PRICE (AVAILABLE SIZES)	
BRAND	$0.16
GENERIC	$0.12

BRAND/MANUFACTURER	NDC	SIZE	AWP
◆ BRAND			
K-NORM: Fisons Presc	00585-0010-71	100s	$15.68
➤ MICRO-K 10: Robins Pharm	00031-5730-63	100s	$16.05
	00031-5730-68	100s	$16.10
	00031-5730-64	100s ud	$18.10
K-NORM: Fisons Presc	00585-0010-85	500s	$70.92
MICRO-K 10: Robins Pharm	00031-5730-70	500s	$72.44
◆ GENERICS			
Allscrips	54569-8548-01	90s	$11.67
➤ Ethex	58177-0001-04	100s	$10.71
Allscrips	54569-8548-00	180s	$23.35
➤ Ethex	58177-0001-08	500s	$48.42

CAPSULE, EXTENDED RELEASE: 10 MEQ

BRAND/MANUFACTURER	NDC	SIZE	AWP
◇ GENERICS			
URL	00677-1097-01	100s	$11.23
URL	00677-1097-10	1000s	$89.00

LIQUID: 20 MEQ/15 ML

AVERAGE UNIT PRICE (AVAILABLE SIZES)		GENERIC A-RATED AVERAGE PRICE (GAAP)	
GENERIC	$0.004	480 ml	$2.48
		3840 ml	$12.79

BRAND/MANUFACTURER	NDC	SIZE	AWP
◆ GENERICS			
Cenci,H.R.	00556-0150-16	480 ml	$2.20
Cenci,H.R.	00556-0317-16	480 ml	$2.48
Cenci,H.R.	00556-0434-16	480 ml	$2.76
Cenci,H.R.	00556-0150-28	3840 ml	$11.80
Cenci,H.R.	00556-0317-28	3840 ml	$12.00
Cenci,H.R.	00556-0434-28	3840 ml	$14.56

LIQUID: 20 MEQ/15 ML

BRAND/MANUFACTURER	NDC	SIZE	AWP
◇ BRAND			
KAY CIEL: Forest Pharm	00456-0661-04	120 ml	$11.17
KAOCHLOR S-F: Savage	00281-3093-51	480 ml	$2.52
KLORVESS: Sandoz Pharm	00078-0207-33	480 ml	$20.22
KAOCHLOR LIQUID: Savage	00281-3103-51	480 ml	$21.17
KAY CIEL: Forest Pharm	00456-0661-16	480 ml	$44.40
	00456-0661-28	3840 ml	$337.14

LIQUID: 40 MEQ/15 ML

AVERAGE UNIT PRICE (AVAILABLE SIZES)		GENERIC A-RATED AVERAGE PRICE (GAAP)	
GENERIC	$0.005	480 ml	$2.97
		3840 ml	$14.30

BRAND/MANUFACTURER	NDC	SIZE	AWP
◆ GENERICS			
Cenci,H.R.	00556-0103-16	480 ml	$2.60
Cenci,H.R.	00556-0442-16	480 ml	$2.80
Major	00904-1001-16	480 ml	$3.50
Cenci,H.R.	00556-0103-28	3840 ml	$13.90
Cenci,H.R.	00556-0442-28	3840 ml	$14.70

LIQUID: 40 MEQ/15 ML

BRAND/MANUFACTURER	NDC	SIZE	AWP
◇ BRAND			
KAON-CL 20 %: Savage	00281-3113-51	480 ml	$26.94

POWDER FOR RECONSTITUTION: 15 MEQ

AVERAGE UNIT PRICE (AVAILABLE SIZES)		GENERIC A-RATED AVERAGE PRICE (GAAP)	
GENERIC	$0.12	30s	$4.44

BRAND/MANUFACTURER	NDC	SIZE	AWP
◆ GENERICS			
K+CARE: Alra	51641-0121-03	30s	$3.55
K+CARE: Alra	51641-0140-03	30s	$5.32
K+CARE: Alra	51641-0121-01	100s	$10.10
K+CARE: Alra	51641-0121-99	2500s	$230.00

POWDER FOR RECONSTITUTION: 20 MEQ

AVERAGE UNIT PRICE (AVAILABLE SIZES)		GENERIC A-RATED AVERAGE PRICE (GAAP)	
BRAND	$0.68	100s	$17.06
GENERIC	$0.16	2500s	$354.09

BRAND/MANUFACTURER	NDC	SIZE	AWP
◆ BRAND			
MICRO-K LS: Robins Pharm	00031-5760-56	30s	$20.89
	00031-5760-63	100s	$66.28
◆ GENERICS			
K+CARE: Alra	51641-0120-03	30s	$5.32
K+CARE: Alra	51641-0120-01	100s	$17.06
K+CARE: Alra	51641-0140-01	100s	$17.06
K+CARE: Alra	51641-0120-99	2500s	$354.09
K+CARE: Alra	51641-0140-99	2500s	$354.09

POWDER FOR RECONSTITUTION: 20 MEQ

BRAND/MANUFACTURER	NDC	SIZE	AWP
◇ BRAND			
➤ K-LOR: Abbott Pharm	00074-3611-01	30s	$29.89
	00074-7349-30	30s	$29.89
KAY CIEL: Forest Pharm	00456-0662-70	30s	$48.30
KATO: ICN	00187-0112-03	30s ud	$16.86
➤ K-LOR: Abbott Pharm	00074-3611-02	100s	$96.64
	00074-7349-11	100s	$96.64
KAY CIEL: Forest Pharm	00456-0662-71	100s	$118.64
KATO: ICN	00187-0112-12	120s ud	$63.90

TABLET, EXTENDED RELEASE: 6.7 MEQ

BRAND/MANUFACTURER	NDC	SIZE	AWP
◇ BRAND			
KAON-CL: Savage	00281-3071-17	100s	$24.34
	00281-3071-19	250s	$58.82
	00281-3071-23	1000s	$230.86

TABLET, EXTENDED RELEASE: 8 MEQ

AVERAGE UNIT PRICE (AVAILABLE SIZES)		GENERIC A-RATED AVERAGE PRICE (GAAP)	
GENERIC	$0.11	100s	$12.95
HCFA FUL (100s ea)	$0.08	500s	$34.55
		1000s	$94.87

BRAND/MANUFACTURER	NDC	SIZE	AWP
◆ BRAND			
➤ SLOW-K: Summit	57267-0165-30	100s	$16.31
	57267-0165-40	1000s	$161.32
	57267-0165-65	1200s	$197.57
◆ GENERICS			
Allscrips	54569-8566-01	90s	$9.40
Qualitest	00603-5237-21	100s	$7.28
➤ Copley	38245-0225-10	100s	$9.50
Aligen	00405-4810-01	100s	$9.79
Martec	52555-0481-01	100s	$10.05
K-8: Alra	51641-0175-01	100s	$10.10
Moore,H.L.	00839-7193-06	100s	$10.25
Geneva	00781-1516-01	100s	$10.44
Schein	00364-0861-01	100s	$10.60
Major	00904-2300-60	100s	$10.85
Goldline	00182-1319-01	100s	$11.40
Rugby	00536-4322-01	100s	$12.39
UDL	51079-0744-20	100s ud	$15.15
Goldline	00182-1839-89	100s ud	$15.50
K-8: Alra	51641-0175-11	100s ud	$21.20
Allscrips	54569-8566-00	180s	$18.79
Qualitest	00603-5237-28	500s	$32.70
K-8: Alra	51641-0175-05	500s	$33.50
Major	00904-3360-40	500s	$37.45
K-8: Alra	51641-0175-10	1000s	$78.50
➤ Copley	38245-0225-20	1000s	$90.26
Moore,H.L.	00839-7193-16	1000s	$94.89
Major	00904-2300-80	1000s	$95.90
Rugby	00536-4322-10	1000s	$95.93

➤ SHOWN IN PRODUCT IDENTIFICATION GUIDE

BRAND/MANUFACTURER	NDC	SIZE	AWP
Geneva	00781-1516-10	1000s	$99.12
Aligen	00405-4810-03	1000s	$100.10
Schein	00364-0861-02	1000s	$100.70
Parmed	00349-8777-10	1000s	$113.80

TABLET, EXTENDED RELEASE: 8 MEQ

BRAND/MANUFACTURER	NDC	SIZE	AWP
◇ **GENERICS**			
► KLOR-CON 8: Upsher-Smith	00245-0040-11	100s	$7.57
Abbott Pharm	00074-7767-13	100s	$9.63
Moore,H.L.	00839-7736-06	100s	$10.25
Goldline	00182-1839-01	100s	$10.50
► KLOR-CON 8: Upsher-Smith	00245-0040-01	100s ud	$8.90
► KLOR-CON 8: Upsher-Smith	00245-0040-15	500s	$34.00
Moore,H.L.	00839-7736-12	500s	$37.79
Goldline	00182-1839-05	500s	$43.50
Abbott Pharm	00074-7767-19	1000s	$82.54

TABLET, EXTENDED RELEASE: 10 MEQ

AVERAGE UNIT PRICE (AVAILABLE SIZES)	
GENERIC	$0.13

BRAND/MANUFACTURER	NDC	SIZE	AWP
◆ **GENERICS**			
Caremark	00339-5646-12	100s	$12.97
Major	00904-2295-61	100s ud	$11.43

TABLET, EXTENDED RELEASE: 10 MEQ

BRAND/MANUFACTURER	NDC	SIZE	AWP
◇ **BRAND**			
► TEN-K: Summit	57267-0146-30	100s	$13.18
► K-DUR 10: Key	00085-0263-01	100s	$19.60
KLOTRIX: Apothecon	00087-0770-41	100s	$22.08
► K-TAB: Abbott Pharm	00074-7804-13	100s	$32.48
► TEN-K: Summit	57267-0146-32	100s ud	$15.10
► K-DUR 10: Key	00085-0263-81	100s ud	$20.31
KLOTRIX: Apothecon	00087-0770-43	100s ud	$26.66
► K-TAB: Abbott Pharm	00074-7804-11	100s ud	$36.00
KLOTRIX: Apothecon	00087-0770-42	1000s	$214.06
► K-TAB: Abbott Pharm	00074-7804-19	1000s	$308.55
	00074-7804-59	5000s	$1496.46
	00074-7804-25	25000s	$7257.84
◇ **GENERICS**			
► KLOR-CON 10: Upsher-Smith	00245-0041-11	100s	$9.86
Moore,H.L.	00839-7194-06	100s	$9.92
Moore,H.L.	00839-7737-06	100s	$10.25
Qualitest	00603-5241-21	100s	$11.08
Goldline	00182-1840-01	100s	$11.25
Rugby	00536-4311-01	100s	$13.04
K-10: Alra	51641-0177-01	100s	$13.50
Abbott Pharm	00074-7763-13	100s	$32.48
► KLOR-CON 10: Upsher-Smith	00245-0041-01	100s ud	$11.45
Goldline	00182-1840-89	100s ud	$17.00
K-10: Alra	51641-0177-11	100s ud	$21.20
Abbott Pharm	00074-7763-11	100s ud	$36.06
Moore,H.L.	00839-7194-12	500s	$32.39
K-10: Alra	51641-0177-05	500s	$35.05
Qualitest	00603-5241-28	500s	$36.11
► KLOR-CON 10: Upsher-Smith	00245-0041-15	500s	$44.28
Parmed	00349-8545-05	500s	$44.98
Moore,H.L.	00839-7737-12	500s	$45.89
Major	00904-3361-40	500s	$47.25
Goldline	00182-1840-05	500s	$47.40
Abbott Pharm	00074-7763-53	500s	$148.46
K-10: Alra	51641-0177-10	1000s	$78.50
Parmed	00349-8545-10	1000s	$82.98
Rugby	00536-4311-10	1000s	$98.40

TABLET, EXTENDED RELEASE: 10 MEQ

BRAND/MANUFACTURER	NDC	SIZE	AWP
○ **BRAND**			
► KAON-CL 10: Savage	00281-3131-17	100s	$24.15
	00281-3131-18	100s ud	$26.83
	00281-3131-21	500s	$116.96
	00281-3131-23	1000s	$229.23

TABLET, EXTENDED RELEASE: 20 MEQ

BRAND/MANUFACTURER	NDC	SIZE	AWP
◇ **BRAND**			
► K-DUR 20: Key	00085-0787-01	100s	$36.47
	00085-0787-81	100s ud	$39.16
	00085-0787-06	500s	$175.99
	00085-0787-10	1000s	$344.39

TABLETS: 8 MEQ

AVERAGE UNIT PRICE (AVAILABLE SIZES)		GENERIC A-RATED AVERAGE PRICE (GAAP)	
GENERIC	$0.09	100s	$8.82

BRAND/MANUFACTURER	NDC	SIZE	AWP
◆ **GENERICS**			
Qualitest	00603-5238-21	100s	$10.36
Qualitest	00603-5238-32	1000s	$89.40

Potassium Citrate

DESCRIPTION
Potassium Citrate is a Citrate salt of Potassium. Its empirical formula is $K_3C_6H_5O_7 \cdot H_2O$.

Potassium Citrate is a white granular powder that is soluble in water at 154 g/100 ml, almost insoluble in alcohol, and insoluble in organic solvents.

Potassium Citrate is supplied as wax matrix tablets, containing 5 mEq (540 mg) Potassium Citrate and 10 mEq (1080 mg) Potassium Citrate each, for oral administration.

CLINICAL PHARMACOLOGY
When Potassium Citrate is given orally, the metabolism of absorbed citrate produces an alkaline load. The induced alkaline load in turn increases urinary pH and raises urinary citrate by augmenting citrate clearance without measurably altering ultraliterable serum citrate. Thus, Potassium Citrate therapy appears to increase urinary citrate principally by modifying the renal handling of citrate, rather than by increasing the filtered load of citrate. The increased filtered load of citrate may play some role, however, as in small comparisons of oral citrate and oral bicarbonate, citrate had a greater effect on urinary citrate.

In addition to raising urinary pH and citrate, Potassium Citrate increases urinary potassium by approximately the amount contained in the medication. In some patients, Potassium Citrate causes a transient reduction in urinary calcium.

The changes induced by Potassium Citrate produce a urine that is less conductive to the crystallization of stone-forming salts (calcium oxalate, calcium phosphate and uric acid): Increased citrate in the urine, by complexing with calcium, decreases calcium ion activity and thus the saturation of calcium oxalate. Citrate also inhibits the spontaneous nucleation of calcium oxalate and calcium phosphate (brushes).

The increase in urinary pH also decreases calcium ion activity by increasing calcium complexation to dissociated anions. The rise in urinary pH also increases the ionization of uric acid to more soluble urate ion.

Potassium Citrate therapy does not alter the urinary saturation of calcium phosphate, since the effect of increased citrate complexation of calcium is opposed by the rise in pH-dependent dissociation of phosphate. Calcium phosphate stones are more stable in alkaline urine.

In the setting of normal renal function, the rise in urinary citrate following a single dose begins by the first hour and lasts for 12 hours. With multiple doses the rise in citrate excretion reaches its peak by the third day and averts the normally wide circadian fluctuation in urinary citrate, thus maintaining urinary citrate at a higher, more constant level throughout the day. When the treatment is withdrawn, urinary citrate begins to decline toward the pre-treatment level on the first day.

The rise in citrate excretion is directly dependent on the Potassium Citrate dosage. Following long-term treatment, Potassium Citrate at a dosage of 60 mEq/day, raises urinary citrates by approximately 400 mg/day and increases urinary pH by approximately 0.7 units.

In patients with severe renal tubular acidosis or chronic diarrheal syndrome where urinary citrate may be very low (< 100 mg/day), Potassium Citrate may be relatively ineffective in raising urinary citrate. A higher dose of Potassium Citrate may therefore be required to produce a satisfactory citraturic response. In patients with renal tubular acidosis in whom urinary pH may be high, Potassium Citrate produces a relatively small rise in urinary pH.

INDICATIONS AND USAGE
Potassium Citrate is indicated for the management of renal tubular acidosis (RTA) with calcium stones, hypocitraturic calcium oxalate nephrolithiasis of any etiology, and uric acid nephrolithiasis with or without calcium stones.

CONTRAINDICATIONS
Potassium Citrate is contraindicated in patients with hyperkalemia (or who have conditions predisposing them to hyperkalemia), as a further rise in serum Potassium concentration may produce cardiac arrest. Such conditions include: chronic renal failure, uncontrolled diabetes mellitus, acute dehydration, strenuous physical exercise in unconditioned individuals, adrenal insufficiency, extensive tissue breakdown, or the administration of a Potassium-sparing agent (such as triamterene, spironolectone or amiloride).

Potassium Citrate is contraindicated in patients in whom there is cause for arrest or delay in tablet passage through the gastrointestinal tract, such as those suffering from delayed gastric emptying, esophageal compression, intestinal obstruction or stricture, or those taking anticholinergic medication. Because of its ulcerogenic potential, Potassium Citrate should not be given to patients with peptic ulcer disease.

Potassium Citrate is contraindicated in patients with active urinary tract infection (with either urea-splitting or other organisms, in association with either calcium or struvite stones). The ability of Potassium Citrate to increase urinary

---

◆ **RATED THERAPEUTICALLY EQUIVALENT;** ◇ **THERAPEUTIC EQUIVALENCE UNCONFIRMED;** ○ **UNRATED**

citrate may be attenuated by bacterial enzymatic degradation of citrate. Moreover, the rise in urinary pH resulting from Potassium Citrate therapy might promote further bacterial growth.

Potassium Citrate is contraindicated in patients with renal insufficiency (glomerular filtration rate of less than 0.7 ml/kg/min), because of the danger of soft tissue calcification and increased risk for the development of hyperkalemia.

WARNINGS

Hyperkalemia: In patients with impaired mechanisms for excreting potassium, Potassium Citrate administration can produce hyperkalemia and cardiac arrest. Potentially fatal hyperkalemia can develop rapidly and be asymptomatic. The use of Potassium Citrate in patients with chronic renal failure, or any other condition which impairs potassium excretion such as severe myocardial damage of heart failure, should be avoided.

Interaction with Potassium-Sparing Diuretics: Concomitant administration of Potassium Citrate and a Potassium-sparing diuretic (such as triamterene, spironolactone or amiloride) should be avoided, since the simultaneous administration of these agents can produce severe hyperkalemia.

Gastrointestinal Lesions: Because of reports of upper gastrointestinal mucosal lesions following administration of Potassium chloride (wax-matrix), an endoscopic examination of the upper gastrointestinal mucosa was performed in 30 normal volunteers after they had taken glycopyrrolate 2 mg. p.o. t.i.d., Potassium Citrate 96 mEq/day, wax-matrix potassium chloride 96 mEq/day or wax matrix placebo, in thrice daily schedule in the fasting state for one week. Potassium Citrate and the wax-matrix formulation of Potassium chloride were indistinguishable but both were significantly more irritating than the wax-matrix placebo. In a subsequent similar study, lesions were less severe when glycopyrrolate was omitted.

Solid dosage forms of Potassium chloride have produced stenotic and/or ulcerative lesions of the small bowel and deaths. These lesions are caused by a high local concentration of Potassium ions in the region of the dissolving tablets, which injured the bowel. In addition, perhaps because wax-matrix preparations are not enteric-coaled and release some of their Potassium content in the stomach, there have been reports of upper gastrointestinal bleeding associated with these products. The frequency of gastrointestinal lesions with wax-matrix Potassium chloride products is estimated at one per 100,000 patient-years. Experience with Potassium Citrate is limited, but a similar frequency of gastrointestinal lesions should be anticipated.

If there is severe vomiting, abdominal pain or gastro-intestinal bleeding, Potassium Citrate should be discontinued immediately and the possibility of bowel perforation or obstruction investigated.

PRECAUTIONS

INFORMATION FOR PATIENTS

Physicians should consider reminding the patient of the following:

To take each dose without crushing, chewing or sucking the tablet.

To take this medicine only as directed. This is especially important if the patient is also taking both diuretics and digitalis preparations.

To check with physician if there is trouble swallowing tablets or if the tablet seems to stick in the throat.

To check with the doctor at once if tarry stools or other evidence of gastrointestinal bleeding is noticed.

Laboratory tests: Regular serum Potassium determinations are recommended. Careful attention should be paid to acid-base balance, other serum electrolyta levels, the electrocardiogram, and the clinical status of the patient, particularly in the presence of cardiac disease, renal disease or acidosis.

Drug Interactions: Potassium-sparing Diuretics: see "Warnings" section.

Drugs That Slow Gastrointestinal Transit Time: (such as anticholinergics) can be expected to increase the gastrointestinal irritation produced by Potassium salts. (See "Contraindications" section).

Carcinogenesis, Mutagenesis, Impairment of Fertility: Long-term carcinogenicity studies in animals have not been performed.

Pregnancy Category C: Animal reproduction studies have not been conducted with Potassium Citrate. It is also not known whether Potassium Citrate can cause fetal harm when administered to a pregnant woman or can affect reproduction capacity. Potassium Citrate should be given in a pregnant women only if clearly needed.

Nursing Mothers: The normal Potassium ion content of human milk is about 13 meq/l. If it is not known if Potassium Citrate has an affect on this content. Caution should be exercised when Potassium Citrate is administered to a nursing woman.

Pediatric Use: Safety and effectiveness in children have not been established.

ADVERSE REACTIONS

Some patients may develop minor gastrointestinal complaints during Potassium Citrate therapy, such as abdominal discomfort, vomiting, diarrhea, loose bowel movements or nausea. Those symptoms are due to the irritation of the gastrointestinal tract, and may be alleviated by taking the dose with meals or snack, or by reducing the dosage. Patients may find intact matrices in feces. (See also "Contraindications, Warnings".)

OVERDOSAGE

The administration of Potassium salts to persons without predisposing conditions for hyperkalemia (see "Contraindications") rarely causes serious hyperkalemia at recommended dosages. It is important to recognize that hyperkalemia is usually asymptomatic and may be manifested only by an increased serum Potassium concentration and characteristic electrocardiographic changes (peaking of T-wave, loss of P-wave, depression of S-T segment and prolongation of the QT interval). Late manifestations include muscle paralysis and cardiovascular collapse from cardiac arrest.

Treatment measures for hyperkalemia include the following: (1) elimination of Potassium-rich foods, medications containing Potassium, and of Potassium-sparing diuretics, (2) intravenous administration of 300-500 ml/hr of 10% dextrose solution containing 10-20 units of insulin/1000 ml, (3) correction of acidosis, if present, with intravenous sodium bicarbonate, and (4) use of exchange resins, hemodialysis or peritoneal dialysis.

In treating hyperkalemia, it should be recalled that in patients who have been stabilized on digitalis, too rapid a lowering of the serum Potassium concentration can produce digitalis toxicity.

DOSAGE AND ADMINISTRATION

Treatment with Potassium Citrate should be added to regimen that limits salt intake (avoidance of foods with high salt content and of added salt at the table) and encourages high fluid intake (urine volume should be at least two liters per day). The objective of treatment with Potassium Citrate is to provide Potassium Citrate in sufficient dosage to restore normal urinary citrate (greater than 320 mg/day and as close to the normal mean of 640 mg/day as possible), and to increase urinary pH to a level of 8.0 to 7.0.

In patients with severe hypocitraturia (urinary citrate of less than 150 mg/day), therapy should be initiated at a dosage of 60 mEq/day (20 mEq three times/day or 15 mEq four times/day with meals or within 30 minutes after meals or bedtime snack). In patients with mild-moderate hypocitraturia (> 150 mg/day). Potassium Citrate should be initiated at a dosage of 30 mEq/day (10 mEq three times/day with meals). Twenty-four hour urinary citrate and/or urinary pH measurements should be used to determine the adequacy of the initial dosage and to evaluate the effectiveness of any dosage change. In addition, urinary citrate and/or pH should be measured every four months.

Doses of Potassium Citrate greater than 100 mEq/day have not been studied and should be avoided.

Serum electrolytes (sodium, potassium, chloride and carbon dioxide), serum creatinine, and compound blood count should be monitored every four months. Treatment should be discontinued if there is hyperkalemia, a significant rise in serum creatinine, or a significant fall in blood hematocrit or hemoglobin.

Store in a cool, dry place.

HOW SUPPLIED
TABLETS: 5 MEQ

BRAND/MANUFACTURER	NDC	SIZE	AWP
○ GENERICS			
UROCIT-K: Mission	00178-0600-01	100s	$14.44

TABLETS: 10 MEQ

BRAND/MANUFACTURER	NDC	SIZE	AWP
○ GENERICS			
UROCIT-K: Mission	00178-0610-01	100s	$18.38

Potassium Citrate and Potassium Gluconate

DESCRIPTION

Each 15 mL (one tablespoonful) Potassium Citrate/Potassium Gluconate supplies 20 mEq of potassium ions as a combination of Potassium Gluconate and Potassium Citrate in a sorbitol and saccharin solution.

INDICATIONS AND USAGE

For use as oral potassium therapy in the prevention or treatment of hypokalemia which may occur secondary to diuretic or corticosteroids administration. It may be used in the treatment of cardiac arrhythmias due to digitalis intoxication.

CONTRAINDICATIONS

Severe renal impairment with oliguria or azotemia untreated Addison's disease, adynamia episodica hereditaria, acute dehydration, heat cramps and hyperkalemia from any cause. This product should not be used in patients receiving aldosterone antagonists or triamterene.

WARNINGS

Potassium Citrate/Potassium Gluconate is a palatable oral potassium replacement. It appears that little if any Potassium Gluconate-Citrate is transported to the jejunum or ileum where enteric coated Potassium chloride lesions have been noted. Excessive, undiluted doses may cause a saline laxative effect.

PRECAUTIONS

Potassium is a major intracellular cation which plays a significant role in body physiology. The serum level of Potassium is normally 3.8 • 5.0 mEq/liter. While the serum or plasma level is a poor indicator of total body stores, a plasma or serum level below 3.5 mEq/liter is considered to be indicative of hypokalemia.

The most common cause of hypokalemia is excessive loss of Potassium in the urine. However, hypokalemia can also occur with vomiting gastric drainage and diarrhea.

Usually a Potassium deficiency can be corrected by oral administration of Potassium supplements. With normal kidney function, it is difficult to produce Potassium intoxication by oral administration. However, Potassium supplements must be administered with caution since, usually, the exact amount of the deficiency is not accurately known. Checks on the patient's clinical status and serum Potassium levels should be made. High serum Potassium levels may cause death by cardiac depression, arrhythmias or arrest.

In patients with hypokalemia who also have alkalosis and a chloride deficiency (hypokalemic-hypochloremic alkalosis), there will be a requirement for chloride ions. This product is not recommended for use in these patients.

ADVERSE REACTIONS

Symptoms of Potassium intoxication include paresthesias of the extremities, flaccid paralysis, listlessness, mental confusion, weakness and heaviness of the legs, fall in blood pressure, cardiac arrhythmias and heart block. Hyperkalemia may exhibit the following electrocardiographic abnormalities: disappearance of the P wave, widening and slurring of the QRS complex changes of the ST segment and tall peaked T waves.

Potassium Citrate/Potassium Gluconate taken on an empty stomach in undiluted doses larger than 30 mL (two tablespoons) can produce gastric irritation with nausea, vomiting, diarrhea and abdominal discomfort.

OVERDOSAGE

The administration of oral Potassium supplements to persons with normal kidney function rarely causes serious hyperkalemia. However, if the renal excretory function is impaired, potentially fatal hyperkalemia can result. It is important to note that hyperkalemia is usually asymptomatic and may be manifested only by an increased serum Potassium concentration and characteristic E.K.G. changes.

Treatment measures include:
1. Elimination of Potassium-containing drugs or foods.
2. Elimination of Potassium-sparing diuretics.
3. Intravenous administration of 300 to 500 mL/hr of a 10% dextrose solution containing 10-20 units of crystalline insulin per 1,000 milliliters.
4. Correction of acidosis, if present with intravenous sodium bicarbonate.
5. Use of exchange resins, hemodialysis, or peritoneal dialysis. In treating hyperkalemia, it should be noted that patients stabilized on digitalis can develop digitalis toxicity when the serum Potassium concentration is lowered too rapidly.

DOSAGE AND ADMINISTRATION

The usual adult dosage is one tablespoonful (15 mL) in 8 fluid ounces of water or fruit juice, two to four times a day. This will supply 40 to 80 mEq of Potassium ions. The usual maintenance dose of Potassium is 20 mEq per day while replacement doses range from 30 mEq to 100 mEq per day. Because of the potential for gastrointestinal irritation, undiluted large single doses (more than a tablespoonful or 15 mL) of Potassium Citrate/Potassium Gluconate are to be avoided.

To minimize gastrointestinal irritation, it is recommended that Potassium Citrate/Potassium Gluconate be taken with meals or diluted with water or fruit juice. A tablespoonful (15 mL) in 8 ounces of water is approximately isotonic. More than a single tablespoonful should not be taken without prior dilution.

Deviations from this schedule may be indicated, since no average total daily dose can be defined, but must be governed by close observation for clinical effects.

Store at controlled room temperature, 15°-30°C (59°-86°F).

HOW SUPPLIED
LIQUID:

BRAND/MANUFACTURER	NDC	SIZE	AWP
○ **BRAND**			
TWIN-K: Boots Pharm	00048-0021-16	480 ml	$22.45
○ **GENERICS**			
KEM-K: Norton, HN	50732-0105-16	480 ml	$17.31

Potassium Citrate and Sodium Citrate

DESCRIPTION

Each tablet contains Potassium Citrate, anhydrous 50 mg, and Sodium Citrate, anhydrous 950 mg.

INDICATIONS

Potassium Citrate/Sodium Citrate is an effective urinary alkalinizing agent.

CONTRAINDICATIONS

Patients with renal insufficiency should not take Potassium Citrate/Sodium Citrate with compounds containing aluminium. Severe renal impairment with oliguria or azotemia, untreated Addison's disease or severe myocardial damage.

PRECAUTIONS

General: Use caution when taken concurrently with products containing aluminum. Should be used with caution by patients with low urinary output. Sodium salts should be used cautiously in patients with cardiac failure, hypertension, peripheral and pulmonary edema and toxemia of pregnancy. Concurrent administration of potassium-containing medication, potassium-sparing diuretics, or cardiac glycosides may lead to toxicity. Periodic examination and determinations of serum electrolytes, particularly serum bicarbonate level, should be carried out in those patients with renal disease in order to avoid these complications.

Carcinogenesis, Mutagenesis, Impairment of Fertility: Long term animal studies to evaluate the carcinogenic, mutagenic, or impairment of fertility potential of this product have not been performed.

PREGNANCY

Teratogenic effects: Pregnancy Category C: Animal reproduction studies have not been conducted with this product. It is also not known whether this product can cause fetal harm when administered to a pregnant woman or can affect reproductive capacity. This product should be given to a pregnant woman only if clearly needed.

Nursing Mothers: It is not known whether this drug is excreted in human milk. Because many drugs are excreted in human milk, caution should be exercised when this product is administered to a nursing woman.

ADVERSE REACTIONS

As with any alkalinizing agent, caution must be used in certain patients with abnormal renal mechanisms to avoid development of hyperkalemia or alkalosis, especially in the presence of hypocalcemia. Potassium intoxication causes listlessness, weakness, mental confusion and tingling of extremities.

OVERDOSAGE

Overdosage with sodium salts may cause diarrhea, nausea and vomiting, hypernatremia, and convulsions. Overdosage with potassium salts may cause hyperkalemia and alkalosis, especially in the presence of renal disease.

ADVANTAGES

Potassium Citrate/Sodium Citrate offers the advantages of citrates (Shohl's Solution type) in tablet form and effectively alkalizes the urine on a 24 hour basis. The unpleasant taste of liquid alkalizers is eliminated by the tablet dosage form.

DOSAGE AND ADMINISTRATION

Directions: 1 to 4 tablets, with a full glass of water, after meals and at bedtime. Dosage is regulated by frequent urinary pH determinations.

Storage: Tablets Keep tightly closed. Store at controlled room temperature 15°-30°C (59°-86°F). Dispense in tight, light-resistant containers.

HOW SUPPLIED
TABLETS:

BRAND/MANUFACTURER	NDC	SIZE	AWP
○ **BRAND**			
CITROLITH: Beach	00486-1136-01	100s	$8.30

Potassium Iodide

DESCRIPTION

Potassium Iodide Oral Solution is a saturated solution of Potassium Iodide.

Oral solution contains:
Potassium Iodide 1g/mL

Syrup contains:
Potassium Iodide ....5 grs./tsp.

CLINICAL PHARMACOLOGY

Potassium Iodide is thought to act as an expectorant by increasing respiratory tract secretions and thereby decreasing the viscosity of mucus.

INDICATIONS AND USAGE

For use as an expectorant in the symptomatic treatment of chronic pulmonary diseases where tenacious mucus complicates the problem, including bronchial asthma, bronchitis and pulmonary emphysema.

CONTRAINDICATIONS

Contraindicated in patients with hyperthyroidism or known sensitivity to iodides.

WARNINGS

Potassium Iodide can cause fetal harm, abnormal thyroid function, and goiter when administered to a pregnant woman. Because of the possible development of fetal goiter, if the drug is used during pregnancy or if the patient becomes pregnant during therapy, apprise the patient of the potential hazard.

PRECAUTIONS

General: In some patients prolonged use of iodide can lead to hyperthyroidism.

In patients sensitive to Iodides, in hyperthyroidism, and in rare cases iodine-induced goiter may occur.

Drug Interactions: Concurrent use with lithium and other antithyroid drugs may potentiate the hypothyroid and goitrogenic effect of these medications. Concurrent use with potassium-containing medications and potassium-sparing diuretics may result in hyperkalemia and cardiac arrhythmias or cardiac arrest.

◆ RATED THERAPEUTICALLY EQUIVALENT; ◇ THERAPEUTIC EQUIVALENCE UNCONFIRMED; ○ UNRATED

Drug/Laboratory Test Interactions: Thyroid function tests may be altered by iodide.

Pregnancy Category D: see *"Warnings"* section.

Nursing Mothers: It is not known if Potassium Iodide is excreted in breast milk. Exercise caution when administering to a nursing mother.

Pediatric Use: Safety and effectiveness in children have not been established.

ADVERSE REACTIONS

The most frequent adverse reactions to Potassium Iodide are skin rash and salivary gland swelling or tenderness. Less frequent adverse reactions include gastrointestinal bleeding or upset, confusion, irregular heartbeat, numbness, tingling, pain or weakness in hands or feet, unusual tiredness, weakness or heaviness of legs, fever and swelling of neck or throat. Other adverse reactions which may occur with prolonged use are burning of mouth or throat, severe headache, metallic taste, soreness of teeth and gums, symptoms of head cold, and unusual increase in salivation. These adverse reactions may require medical attention. The following side effects require medical attention only if they continue or are bothersome: diarrhea, nausea, vomiting, skin eruptions, and stomach pain.

OVERDOSAGE

Acute toxicity from Potassium Iodide is relatively rare. An occasional individual may show marked sensitivity and the onset can occur immediately or hours after administration. Angioedema, laryngeal edema and cutaneous hemorrhages may occur. Symptoms disappear soon after discontinuation of the drug. Abundant fluid and salt intake aids in iodide elimination.

DOSAGE AND ADMINISTRATION

Oral Solution: Adults— 0.3 mL (300 mg) or 0.6 mL (600 mg) diluted in one glassful of water, fruit juice or milk 3 to 4 times daily.

Syrup: Children—one half to one tsp. and adults one or two tsp. every 4-6 hours.

Storage of Oral Solution: Keep tightly closed and protected from light.

Oxidation of Potassium Iodide may occur causing the solution to turn brownish yellow in color. If this occurs, the solution should be discarded.

Notice: When exposed to cold temperatures, crystallization may occur, but on warming and shaking the crystals will redissolve.

Dispense in tight, light resistant containers with child resistant closures.
Store at controlled room temperature 59°-96° F (15°-20° C).

HOW SUPPLIED
SOLUTION:

BRAND/MANUFACTURER	NDC	SIZE	AWP
○ GENERICS			
Century	00436-0542-08	240 ml	$14.24

For additional alternatives, turn to the section beginning on page 2859.

Potassium Iodide and Theophylline

DESCRIPTION

Potassium Iodide is either colorless or white cubical crystals, or a white power. Theophylline is a bronchodilator structurally classified as a xanthine derivative. It occurs as a white odorless, crystalline powder having a bitter taste. Theophylline anhydrous has the chemical name, 1H-Purine-2, 6-dione, 3, 7-dihydro-1, 3-dimethyl.

Potassium Iodide/Theophylline Elixir is available as a liquid intended for oral administration, containing 130 mg Potassium Iodide, 80 mg of Theophylline anhydrous and 10% alcohol in each 15 mL (tablespoonful).

CLINICAL PHARMACOLOGY

Theophylline directly relaxes the smooth muscle of the bronchial airways and pulmonary blood vessels, thus acting as a bronchodilator and smooth muscle relaxant. It has been demonstrated that aminophylline has a potent effect on diaphragmatic contractility in normal persons and may then be capable of reducing fatigability and thereby improve contractility in patients with chronic obstructive airways disease. The exact mode of action remains unsettled. Although Theophylline does cause inhibition of phosphodiesterase with a resultant increase in intracellular cyclic AMP, other agents similarly inhibit the enzyme producing a rise of cyclic AMP, but are unassociated with any demonstrable bronchodilation. Other mechanisms proposed include an effect on translocation of intracellular calcium, prostaglandin antagonism, stimulation of catecholamines endogenously, inhibition of cyclic guanosine monophosphate metabolism and adenosine receptor antagonism. None of these mechanisms has been proved, however.

In vitro, Theophylline has been shown to act synergistically with beta agonists and there are now available data which do demonstrate an additive effect *in vivo* with combined use. Potassium Iodide acts as an expectorant by liquifying tenacious bronchial secretions.

PHARMACOKINETICS

The half-life of Theophylline is influenced by a number of known variables. It may be prolonged in chronic alcoholics, particularly those with liver disease (cirrhosis or alcoholic liver disease). In patients with congestive heart failure, and in those patients taking certain other drugs (see *"Precautions, Drug Interactions"*). Newborns and neonates have extremely slow clearance rate compared to older infants and children, i.e., those over 1 year. Older children have rapid clearance rates while most non-smoking adults have clearance rates between these two extremes. In premature neonates the decreased clearance is related to oxidative pathways that have yet to be established.

THEOPHYLLINE ELIMINATION CHARACTERISTICS

	Half-Life (in hours)	
	Range	*Mean*
Children	1 - 9	37
Adults	3 - 15	77

In cigarette smokers (1-2 packs/day) the mean half-life is 4 to 5 hours, much shorter than in nonsmokers. The increase in clearance associated with smoking is presumably due to stimulation of the hepatic metabolic pathway by components of cigarette smoke. The duration of this effect after cessation of smoking is unknown but may require 6 months to 2 years before the rate approaches that of the nonsmoker.

INDICATIONS AND USAGE

For excessive tenacious mucus and for relief and/or prevention of symptoms from asthma and reversible bronchospasm associated with chronic bronchitis and emphysema.

CONTRAINDICATIONS

This product is contraindicated in individuals who have shown hypersensitivity to its components. It is also contraindicated in patients with active peptic ulcer disease and in individuals with underlying seizure disorders (unless receiving appropriate anticonvulsant medication).

WARNINGS

Serum levels above 20 mcg/mL are rarely found after appropriate administration of the recommended doses. However, in individuals in whom Theophylline plasma clearance is reduced *for any reason,* even conventional doses may result in increased serum levels and potential toxicity. Reduced Theophylline clearance has been documented in the following readily identifiable groups:

1) patients with impaired renal or liver function;
2) patients over 55 years of age, particularly males and those with chronic lung disease;
3) those with cardiac failure from any cause;
4) patients with sustained high fever;
5) neonates and infants under 1 year of age;
6) those patients taking certain drugs (see *"Precautions, Drug Interactions"*). Frequently, such patients have markedly prolonged theophylline serum levels following discontinuation of the drug.

Reduction of dosage and laboratory monitoring is especially appropriate in the above individuals.

Serious side effects such as ventricular arrhythmias convulsions or even death may appear as the first sign of toxicity without any previous warning. Less serious signs of Theophylline toxicity (i.e., nausea and restlessness) may occur frequently when initiating therapy, but are usually transient. When such signs are persistent during maintenance therapy, they are often associated with serum concentrations above 20 mcg/mL. Stated differently: *serious toxicity is not reliably preceded by less severe side effects.* A serum concentration measurement is the only reliably method of predicting potentially life-threatening toxicity.

Many patients who require Theophylline exhibit tachycardia due to their underlying disease process so that the cause/effect relationship to elevated serum Theophylline concentrations may not be appreciated.

Theophylline products may cause or worsen arrhythmias and any significant change in rate and/or rhythm warrants monitoring and further investigation.

Studies in laboratory animals (minipigs, rodents, and dogs) recorded the occurrence of cardiac arrhythmias and sudden death (with histologic evidence of myocardia necrosis) when beta-agonists and methylxanthines were administered concurrently. The significance of these findings when applied to humans is currently unknown

Potassium Iodide can cause fetal harm when administered to a pregnant woman. Because of the possible development of fetal goiter if this drug is used during pregnancy, or if the patient becomes pregnant while taking it, the patient should be apprised of the potential hazard to the fetus.

Potassium Iodide/Theophylline Elixir contains sodium bisulfite, a sulfite that may cause allergic-type reactions including anaphylactic symptoms and life-threatening or less severe asthmatic episodes in certain susceptible people. The overall prevalence of sulfite sensitivity in the general population is unknown and probably low. Sulfite sensitivity is seen more frequently in asthmatic than in nonasthmatic people.

PRECAUTIONS

GENERAL
Occasionally, persons are markedly sensitive to iodides and care should be used in administering Potassium Iodide/Theophylline Elixir for the first time. Caution is recommended in patients sensitive to iodides and in patients receiving potassium-sparing diuretics or potassium supplements.

On the average, Theophylline half-life is shorter in cigarette and marijuana smokers than in nonsmokers, but smokers can have half-lives as long as non-smokers. Potassium Iodide/Theophylline Elixir should not be administered concurrently with other xanthine medications. Use with caution in patients with hypoxemia, hypertension or those with a history of peptic ulcer. Theophylline preparations should be used cautiously in patients with a history of peptic ulcer, since they may occasionally act as a local irritant to the GI tract. Gastrointestinal symptoms, however, are more commonly centrally mediated and associated with serum drug concentrations over 20 mcg/mL.

INFORMATION FOR PATIENTS

The importance of taking only the prescribed dose and time interval between doses should be reinforced.

LABORATORY TESTS

Serum levels should be monitored periodically to determine the Theophylline level associated with observed clinical response and as the method of predicting toxicity. For such measurements, the serum sample should be obtained at the time of peak concentration, 1 to 2 hours after administration. It is important that the patient will not have missed or taken additional doses during the previous 48 hours and that dosing intervals will have been reasonably equally spaced. DOSAGE ADJUSTMENT BASED ON SERUM THEOPHYLLINE MEASUREMENTS WHEN THESE INSTRUCTIONS HAVE NOT BEEN FOLLOWED MAY RESULT IN RECOMMENDATIONS THAT PRESENT RISK OF TOXICITY TO THE PATIENT.

DRUG INTERACTIONS

Drug-Drug: Toxic synergism with ephedrine has been documented and may occur with other sympathomimetic bronchodilators. In addition the following drug interactions have been demonstrated:

Theophylline with

Allopurinal (high dose)	Increased serum Theophylline levels
Cimetidine	Increased serum Theophylline levels
Ciprofloxacin	Increased serum Theophylline levels
Erythromycin Troleandoycin	Increased serum Theophylline levels
Lithium carbonate	Increased renal excretion of lithium
Oral Contraceptives	Increased serum Theophylline levels
Phenytoin	Decreased Theophylline and phenytoin serum levels
Propranolol	Increased serum Theophylline levels
Rifampin	Decreased serum Theophylline levels
Potassium iodide with lithium carbonate	Increased hypothyroid and goitrogenic effect

Drug-Laboratory Test Interactions: Currently available analytical methods, including high pressure liquid chromatography and immunoassay techniques, for measuring serum Theophylline levels are specific. Metabolites and other drugs generally do not affect the results. Other new analytic methods are also now in use. The physician should be aware of the laboratory method used and whether other drugs will interfere with the assay for Theophylline.

Potassium Iodide-Thyroid function tests may be altered by iodides. As with any potassium-containing medication, the potential for developing hyperkalemia is increased.

Carcinogenesis, Mutagenesis, and Impairment of Fertility: Long-term carcinogenicity studies have not been performed with Theophylline.

Chromosome-breaking activity was detected in human cell cultures at concentrations of Theophylline up to 50 times the therapeutic serum concentration in humans. Theophylline was not mutagenic in the dominant lethal assay in male mice given Theophylline intraperitoneally in doses up to 30 times the maximum daily human oral dose.

Studies to determine the effect on fertility have not been performed with Theophylline.

Pregnancy: Teratogenic Effects:

Pregnancy Category C: Animal reproduction studies have not been conducted with Theophylline. It is also not known whether Theophylline can cause fetal harm when administered to a pregnant woman or can affect reproduction capacity. Xanthines should be given to a pregnant woman only if clearly needed.

Nursing Mothers: Iodides are secreted in human milk. Theophylline is also distributed into breast milk and may cause irritability or other signs of toxicity in nursing infants. Because of the potential for serious adverse reactions in nursing infants, a decision should be made whether to discontinue nursing or to discontinue the drug, taking into account the importance of the drug to the mother.

Pediatric Use: Since safety and effectiveness in children have not been established, it is recommended that Potassium Iodide/Theophylline Elixir not be used in children under 12 years of age.

ADVERSE REACTIONS

The following adverse reactions have been observed, but there has not been enough systematic collection of data to support an estimate of their frequency. The most consistent adverse reactions are usually due to overdosage.

1. Gastrointestinal: nausea, vomiting, epigastric pain, hematemesis, diarrhea.

2. Central Nervous System: headaches, irritability, restlessness, insomnia, reflex hyperexcitability, muscle twitching, clonic and tonic generalized convulsions.

3. Cardiovascular: palpitation, tachycardia, extrasystoles, flushing, hypotension, circulatory failure, ventricular arrhythmias.

4. Respiratory: tachypnea.

5. Renal: potentiation of diuresis.

6. Others: alopecia, hyperglycemia, inappropriate ADH syndrome, rash.

Potassium Iodide-Thyroid adenoma, goiter and myxedema are possible side effects of Potassium Iodide.

Hypersensitivity to iodides may be manifested by angioneurotic edema, cutaneous and mucosal hemorrhages, and symptoms resembling serum sickness, such as fever, arthralgia, lymph node enlargement and eosinophilia.

Iodism or chronic iodine poisoning may occur during prolonged treatment. The symptoms of iodism include a metallic taste, soreness of the mouth, increased salivation, coryza, sneezing, and swelling of the eyelids. There may be a severe headache, productive cough, pulmonary edema and swelling and tenderness of the salivary glands. Acneform skin lesions are seen in the seborrheic areas. Severe and sometimes fatal skin eruptions may develop. Gastric disturbance and diarrhea are common. If iodism appears, the drug should be withdrawn and the patient given appropriate supportive therapy.

OVERDOSAGE

MANAGEMENT

It is suggested that the management principles (consistent with the clinical status of the patient when first seen) outlined below be instituted and that simultaneously, contact with a regional poison control center be established. In this way both updated information and individualization regarding required therapy may be provided.

1. When potential oral overdose is established and seizure has not occurred:
a) If patient is alert and seen within the early hours after ingestion, induction of emesis may be of value. Gastric lavage has been demonstrated to be of no value in influencing outcome in patients who present more than 1 hour after ingestion.
b) Administer a cathartic. Sorbitol solution is reported to be of value.
c) Administer repeated doses of activated charcoal and monitor Theophylline serum levels.
d) Prophylactic administration of phenobarbital has been shown to increase the seizure threshold in laboratory animals, and administration of this drug can be considered.
2. If patient presents with a seizure:
a) Establish an airway.
b) Administer oxygen.
c) Treat the seizure with intravenous diazepam, 0.1 to 0.3 mg/kg up to 10 mg. If seizures cannot be controlled, the use of general anesthesia should be considered.
d) Monitor vital signs, maintain blood pressure and provide adequate hydration.
3. If post-seizure coma is present:
a) Maintain airway and oxygenation.
b) If a result of oral medication, follow above recommendations to prevent absorption of the drug; but intubation and lavage will have to be performed instead of inducing emesis, and the cathartic and charcoal will need to be introduced via a large bore gastric lavage tube.
d) Continue to provide full supportive care and adequate hydration until the drug is metabolized. In general, drug metabolism is sufficiently rapid so as not to warrant dialysis. If repeated oral activated charcoal is ineffective (as noted by stable or rising serum levels), charcoal hemoperfusion may be indicated.

DOSAGE AND ADMINISTRATION

Effective use of Theophylline (i.e. the concentration of drug in the serum associated with optimal benefit and minimal risk of toxicity) is considered to occur when the Theophylline concentration is maintained from 10 to 20 mcg/mL. The early studies from which these levels are derived were carried out in patients immediately or shortly after recovery from acute exacerbations of their disease (some hospitalized with status asthmaticus).

Although the 20 mcg/mL level remains appropriate as a critical value (above which toxicity is more likely to occur) for safety purposes, additional data are now available which indicate that the serum Theophylline concentrations required to produce maximum physiologic benefit may, in fact, fluctuate with the degree of bronchospasm present and are variable. Therefore, the physician should individualize the range appropriate to the patients requirements based on both symptomatic response and improvement in pulmonary function. It should be stressed that serum Theophylline concentrations maintained at the upper level of the 10 to 20 mcg/mL range may be associated with potential toxicity when factors known to reduce Theophylline clearance are operative (see *"Warnings"*).

If it is not possible to obtain serum level determinations restrictions of the daily dose (in otherwise healthy adults) to not greater than 13 mg/kg/day, to a maximum of 900 mg of Theophylline in divided doses, will result in relatively few patients exceeding serum levels of 20 mcg/mL and the resultant greater risk of toxicity.

Caution should be exercised for younger children who cannot complain of minor side effects. Older adults, those with cor pulmonale, congestive heart failure, and/or liver disease, may have unusually low dosage requirements and thus may experience toxicity at the maximal dosage recommended below.

Theophylline does not distribute into fatty tissue. Dosage should be calculated on the basis of lean (ideal) body weight where mg/kg doses are presented.

Frequency of Dosing: When immediate release products with rapid absorption are used, dosing to maintain serum levels generally requires administration every 6 hours. This is particularly true in children, but dosing intervals up to 8 hours may

---

◆ RATED THERAPEUTICALLY EQUIVALENT; ◇ THERAPEUTIC EQUIVALENCE UNCONFIRMED; ○ UNRATED

be satisfactory in adults since they eliminate the drug at a slower rate. Some children, and adults requiring higher than average doses (those having rapid rates of clearance, e.g., half-lives of under 6 hours) may benefit and be more effectively controlled during chronic therapy when given products with sustained-release characteristics since these provide longer dosing intervals and/or less fluctuation in serum concentration between dosing.

Dosage guidelines are approximations only and the wide range of Theophylline clearance between individuals (particularly those with concomitant disease) makes indiscriminate usage hazardous.

DOSAGE GUIDELINES

I. Acute Symptoms

Note: Status asthmaticus should be considered a medical emergency and is defined as that degree of bronchospasm which is not rapidly responsive to usual doses of conventional bronchodilators. Optimal therapy for such patients frequently requires both *additional medication*, parenterally administered, and *close monitoring*, preferably in an intensive care setting.

A. Patients not currently receiving Theophylline products:

	Theophylline Dosage	
	Oral Loading	Maintenance
Children age 9 to under 16 years; and smokers	5mg/kg	3mg/kg q 6 hours
Otherwise healthy non-smoking adults	5mg/kg	3mg/kg q 8 hours
Older patients and patients with cor pulmonale	5mg/kg	2mg/kg q 8 hours
Patients with congestive heart failure	5mg/kg	1-2mg/kg q 12 hours

B. Patients currently receiving Theophylline products:

Determine, where possible, the time, amount dosage form and route of administration of the last dose the patient received.

The loading dose for Theophylline is based on the principle that each 0.5 mg/kg of Theophylline administered as a loading dose will result in a 1.0 mcg/mL increase in serum Theophylline concentration. Ideally, the loading dose should be deferred if a serum Theophylline concentration can be obtained rapidly.

If this is not possible, the clinician must exercise judgment in selecting a dose based on the potential for benefit and risk. When there is sufficient respiratory distress to warrant a small risk, then 2.5 mg/kg of Theophylline administered in rapidly absorbed form is likely to increase serum concentration by approximately 5 mcg/mL. If the patient is not experiencing Theophylline toxicity this is unlikely to result in dangerous adverse effects.

Subsequent to the decision regarding use of a loading dose for this group of patients, the maintenance dosage recommendations are the same as those described above.

II. Chronic Therapy

Theophylline is a treatment for the management of reversible bronchospasm (asthma, chronic bronchitis and emphysema) to prevent symptoms and maintain patent airways. A dosage form which allows small incremental doses is desirable for initiating therapy. A liquid preparation should be considered for children to permit easier and more accurate dosage adjustment. Slow clinical titration is generally preferred to help assure acceptance and safety of the medication and to allow the patient to develop tolerance to transient caffeine-like side effects.

Initial Dose: 16 mg/kg/24 hours or 400 mg/24 hours (whichever is less) of Theophylline in divided doses at 6 or 8 hour intervals.

Increasing Dose: The above dosage may be increased in approximately 25 percent increments at 3 day intervals so long as the drug is tolerated: until clinical response is satisfactory or the maximum dose as indicated in section III (below) is reached. The serum concentration may be checked at these intervals, but at a minimum, should be determined at the end of this adjustment period.

It is important that no patient be maintained on any dosage that is not tolerated. When instructing patients to increase dosage according to the schedule above, they should be told not to take a subsequent dose if apparent side effects occur and to resume therapy at a lower dose once adverse effects have disappeared.

III. Maximum Dose of Theophylline Where the Serum Concentration is not Measured

WARNING: DO NOT ATTEMPT TO MAINTAIN ANY DOSE THAT IS NOT TOLERATED.
Not to exceed the following (or 900 mg, whichever is less):

Age 1 - under 9 years	24 mg/kg/day
Age 9 - under 12 years	20 mg/kg/day
Age 12 - under 16 years	18 mg/kg/day
Age 16 years and older	13 mg/kg/day

IV. Measurement of Serum Theophylline Concentrations During Chronic Therapy

If the above maximum doses are to be maintained or exceeded, serum Theophylline measurement is essential (see "Precautions, Laboratory Tests," for guidance).

V. Final Adjustment of Dosage

Dosage adjustment after serum Theophylline measurement:

If Serum Theophylline is:	Directions:
Within desired range	Maintain dosage if tolerated
Too high 20 to 25 mcg/mL	Decrease doses by about 10% and recheck serum level after 3 days.
25 to 30 mcg/mL	Skip the next dose and decrease subsequent doses by about 25%. Recheck serum level after 3 days.
Over 30 mcg/mL	Skip next 2 doses and decrease subsequent doses by 50%. Recheck serum level after 3 days.
Too low	Increase dosage by 25% at 3 day intervals until either the desired serum concentration and/or clinical response is achieved. The total daily dose may need to be administered at more frequent intervals if symptoms occur repeatedly at the end of a dosing interval.

The serum concentration may be rechecked at appropriate intervals, but at least at the end of any adjustment period. When the patient's condition is otherwise clinically stable and none of the recognized factors which after elimination are present, measurement of serum levels need be repeated only every 6 to 12 months.

Store at controlled room temperature 15°-30°C (59°-86°F).
Dispense in tight containers.

HOW SUPPLIED

ELIXIR:

BRAND/MANUFACTURER	NDC	SIZE	AWP
○ **BRAND**			
ELIXOPHYLLIN KI: Forest Pharm	00456-0645-08	240 ml	$69.49
○ **GENERICS**			
Major	00904-1445-16	480 ml	$4.90
CMC-Cons	00223-6623-01	480 ml	$5.50

Potassium Nitrate and Silver Nitrate

DESCRIPTION

Potassium Nitrate/Silver Nitrate applicators provide a simple and convenient means of treating small lesions of the skin and mucous membranes. On contact with living tissue, Silver Nitrate acts as an escharotic. Deep action is avoided by the formation of a dense surface film of coagulated albumin.

Silver Nitrate is a powerful chemical germicide. Despite precipitation, it retains substantial germicidal potency even in the presence of large quantities of albuminous material, possibly by gradually redissolving the silver.

SPECIAL PROPERTIES

The combination of Silver Nitrate with Potassium Nitrate has been called *toughened Silver Nitrate*, also *lunar caustic*. When the tip of the applicator is impregnated with this compound, as in Potassium Nitrate/Silver Nitrate, the Silver Nitrate can be applied quickly and conveniently to the precise area to be treated without spread of the escharotic to adjacent healthy tissues.

Exposure to light causes the silver in the tip to oxidize and turn brown in color. This discoloration does not affect the therapeutic action of the tip and the oxidized film readily dissolves when dipped in water.

Moisture has a deteriorating effect on the tip. It may cause it to break or loosen from the applicator; therefore the applicators should be kept in a dry place.

INDICATIONS

On the skin: applications of Silver Nitrate are recommended for cauterization of wounds and sluggish ulcers, also for removal of granulation tissue and warts.

On mucous membranes: Silver Nitrate may be applied to small ulcers and aphthae in the mouth resulting from injury or stomatitis, to infected tonsils, to rectal fissures and fistulae, and to vaginal or cervical ulcerations or erosions. Epistaxis may be controlled by direct application to the site of hemorrhage within the nostrils.

DOSAGE AND ADMINISTRATION

APPLICATION

Potassium Nitrate/Silver Nitrate may be applied to mucous membranes and other moist surfaces. In the case of dry skin, the applicator tip should be dipped in water immediately before use. Apply carefully to the area to be treated. **DO NOT USE ON THE EYES.**

SIDE EFFECTS

Silver Nitrate blackens the tissues to which it is applied but this discoloration gradually disappears. In the case of applicators, poisoning from ingestion is rare.

ANTIDOTE

In case of accidental poisoning, follow these directions:

External:

Eye Exposure—

First: Wash out the eye with lukewarm water for at least fifteen (15) minutes *then* call your physician or go to your nearest Emergency Room.

Skin Exposure—

First: Wash the area very thoroughly with soap and water *then* call your physician.

Internal:

First: Give one (1) glass of milk or water *then* call your physician or go to your nearest Emergency Room.

HAZARDS

Long continued applications to large areas may produce argyria, a slate-blue discoloration of the skin and mucous membranes.

HOW SUPPLIED

SWAB:

BRAND/MANUFACTURER	NDC	SIZE	AWP
○ GENERICS			
Arzol	12870-0001-02	100s	$6.84
Arzol	12870-0001-01	100s	$7.32

Potassium Phosphate

DESCRIPTION

CAUTION: FOR INTRAVENOUS USE ONLY MUST BE DILUTED PRIOR TO ADMINISTRATION.

Potassium Phosphates Injection, USP, is a sterile, nonpyrogenic, concentrated solution containing a mixture of monobasic and dibasic Potassium Phosphate in Water for Injection. It must be diluted prior to administration.

Each mL of the solution consists of two phosphate salts provided as follows:

Ingredient(s)	Phosphate	Potassium
Monobasic Potassium Phosphate - 224 mg	285.0 mg	170.0 mg
	or	or
Dibasic Potassium Phosphate - 236 mg	3 mM	4.4 mEq

The solution contains no bacteriostatic agent or other preservative.

The solution is intended to provide Phosphate ion, (PO_4^{-3}), for addition to large volume infusion fluids for intravenous use. Unused portions should be discarded.

CLINICAL PHARMACOLOGY

Phosphorus in the form of organic and inorganic Phosphate has a variety of important biochemical functions in the body and is involved in many significant metabolic and enzyme reactions in almost all organs and tissues. It exerts a modifying influence on the steady state of calcium levels, a buffering effect on acidbase equilibrium and a primary role in the renal excretion of hydrogen ion.

Phosphorus is present in plasma and other extracellular fluid, in cell membranes and intra-cellular fluid, as well as in collagen and bone tissues. Phosphate in the extracellular fluid is primarily in inorganic form, and plasma-levels may vary somewhat with age. The ratio of disodium phosphate and monosodium phosphate in the extracellular fluid is 4:1 (80% : 20%) at the normal pH of 7.4. This buffer ratio varies with the pH, but owing to its relatively low concentration, it contributes little to the buffering-capacity of the extracellular fluids.

Phosphate, present in large amounts in erythrocytes and other tissue cells, plays a significant intracellular role in the synthesis of high energy organic Phosphates.

Hypophosphatemia should be avoided during periods of total parenteral nutrition, or other lengthy periods of intravenous infusions. Serum Phosphate levels should be regularly monitored, and appropriate amounts of Phosphate should be added to the infusions to maintain normal serum Phosphate levels. Intravenous infusion of inorganic Phosphate may be accompanied by a decrease in the serum level and urinary excretion of calcium. Intravenously infused phosphate not taken up by the tissues is excreted almost entirely in the urine.

INDICATIONS AND USAGE

Potassium Phosphates Injection, USP is indicated as a source of Phosphate, for addition to large volume intravenous fluids, to prevent or correct hypophospha-temia in patients with restricted or no oral intake. It is also useful as an additive for preparing specific intravenous fluid formulas when the needs of the patient cannot be met by standard electrolyte or nutrient solutions.

CONTRAINDICATIONS

Potassium Phosphates Injection, USP is contraindicated in diseases where high potassium, high phosphate or low calcium levels may be encountered.

WARNINGS

Potassium Phosphates Injection, USP must be diluted before use.

To avoid Potassium or Phosphate intoxication, infuse solutions containing Potassium Phosphates slowly. In patients with severe renal or adrenal insufficien-cy, administration of Potassium Phosphates Injection may cause Potassium Phosphates intoxication. Infusing high concentrations of Phosphate may cause hypocalcemia, and calcium levels should be monitored.

PRECAUTIONS

Phosphate replacement therapy with Potassium Phosphates should be guided primarily by the serum inorganic phosphate level and the limits imposed by the accompanying potassium (K^+) ion.

High plasma concentrations of potassium may cause death through cardiac depression, arrhythmias or arrest.

Use with caution in the presence of cardiac disease, particularly in digitalized patients or in the presence of renal disease.

Pregnancy: Teratogenic Effects. Pregnancy Category C. Animal reproduction studies have not been conducted with Potassium Phosphates Injection, USP. It is also not known whether Potassium Phosphates Injection, USP can cause fetal harm when administered to a pregnant woman or can affect reproduction capacity. Potassium Phosphates Injection, USP should be given to a pregnant woman only if clearly needed.

ADVERSE REACTIONS

Adverse reactions involve the possibility of combined potassium and phosphate intoxication from overdosage. The signs and symptoms of potassium intoxication include paresthesias of the extremities, flaccid paralysis, listlessness, mental confusion, weakness and heaviness of the legs, hypotension, cardiac arrhythmias, heart block, electrocardiographic abnormalities such as disappearance of P waves, spreading and slurring of the QRS complex with development of a biphasic curve and cardiac arrest. Phosphate intoxication results in a reduction of serum calcium, and the symptoms are those of hypocalcemic tetany. See *"Warnings"*.

OVERDOSAGE

In the event of overdosage, discontinue infusions containing Potassium Phos-phates immediately, and institute corrective therapy to restore depressed serum calcium and to reduce elevated serum potassium levels.

DOSAGE AND ADMINISTRATION

Potassium Phosphates Injection, USP is administered intravenously only after dilution in a larger volume of fluid. The dose and rate of administration are dependent upon the individual needs of the patient. Serum Potassium, inorganic phosphorus and calcium levels should be monitored as a guide to dosage.

Withdraw the calculated volume aseptically and transfer to appropriate intravenous fluid to provide the desired number of millimoles (mM) of Phosphate and milliequivalent (mEq) of Potassium (K^+).

Parental drug products should be inspected visually for particulate matter and discoloration, whenever solution and container permit.

Store at controlled room temperature 15°-30°C (59°-86°F).

The products do not contain a bacteriostatic agent or other preservatives. Any unused portion should be discarded.

HOW SUPPLIED

INJECTION: 3 mM/ML-4.4 MEQ/ML

AVERAGE UNIT PRICE (AVAILABLE SIZES)			
GENERIC	$0.32		

BRAND/MANUFACTURER	NDC	SIZE	AWP
◆ GENERICS			
Fujisawa	00469-8600-30	5 ml	$1.28
Fujisawa	00469-8600-50	15 ml	$1.77
Fujisawa	00469-8600-60	50 ml	$6.57
Abbott Hosp	00074-7296-01	5 ml 25s	$84.91
Abbott Hosp	00074-7295-01	15 ml 25s	$135.38
Abbott Hosp	00074-4201-01	50 ml 25s	$429.28

Potassium Phosphate, Monobasic and Sodium Phosphate, Dibasic

DESCRIPTION

Each tablet contains 852 mg Dibasic Sodium Phosphate anhydrous, 155 mg Monobasic Potassium Phosphate, and 130 mg Monobasic Sodium Phosphate monohydrate. Each tablet yields approximately 250 mg of Phosphorus, 298 mg of Sodium (13.0 mEq) and 45 mg of Potassium (1.1 mEq).

INDICATIONS

Potassium Phosphate, Monobasic/Sodium Phosphate, Dibasic increases urinary Phosphate and pyrophosphate. As a phosphorus supplement, each tablet supplies 25% of the U.S. Recommended Daily Allowance (U.S.RDA) of Phosphorus for adults.

CONTRAINDICATIONS

This product is contraindicated in patients with infected Phosphate stones, in patients with severely impaired renal function (less than 30% of normal) and in the presence of hyperphosphatemia.

PRECAUTIONS

General: This product contains Potassium and Sodium and should be used with caution if regulation of these elements is desired. Occasionally, some individuals may experience a mild laxative effect during the first few days of Phosphate therapy. If laxation persists to an unpleasant degree, reduce the daily dosage until this effect subsides or, if necessary, discontinue the use of this product.

Caution should be exercised when prescribing this product in the following conditions: Cardiac disease (particularly in digitalized patients); severe adrenal insufficiency (Addison's disease); acute dehydration; severe renal insufficiency; renal function impairment or chronic renal disease; extensive tissue breakdown (such as severe burns); myotonia congenita; cardiac failure; cirrhosis of the liver or severe hepatic disease; peripheral or pulmonary edema; hypernathremia; hypertension; toxemia of pregnancy; hypoparathyroidism; and acute pancreatitis. Rickets may benefit from Phosphate therapy, but caution should be exercised. High serum Phosphate may increase the incidence of extra-skeletal calcification.

Information For Patients: Patients with kidney stones may pass old stones when Phosphate therapy is started and should be warned of this possibility. Patients should be advised to avoid the use of antacids containing aluminum, magnesium or calcium which may prevent the absorption of Phosphate.

Laboratory Tests: Careful monitoring of renal function and serum electrolytes (calcium, phosphorus, potassium, sodium) may be required at periodic intervals during Phosphate therapy. Other tests may be warranted in some patients, depending on conditions.

Drug Interactions: The use of antacids containing magnesium, aluminum or calcium in conjunction with Phosphate preparations may bind the phosphate and prevent its absorption. Concurrent use of antihypertensives, especially diazoxide, guanethidine, hydralazine, methyldopa, or rauwolfia alkaloids; or corticosteroids, especially mineralocorticoids or corticotropin, with Sodium Phosphate may result in hypernatremia. Calcium-containing preparations and/or vitamin D may antagonize the effects of Phosphates in the treatment of hypercalcemia. Potassium-containing medications or potassium-sparing diuretics may cause hyperkalemia. Patients should have serum potassium level determinations at periodic intervals.

Carcinogenesis, Mutagenesis, Impairment of Fertility: There have been no studies in animals or humans to evaluate the carcinogenesis, mutagenesis, or impairment of fertility for this product.

Pregnancy: Pregnancy Category C. Animal reproduction studies have not been conducted with this product. It is also not known whether this product can cause fetal harm when administered to a pregnant woman or can affect reproduction capacity. This product should be given to a pregnant woman only if clearly needed.

Nursing Mothers: It is known whether this drug is excreted in human milk. Because many drugs are excreted in human milk, caution should be exercised when this product is administered to a nursing woman.

ADVERSE REACTIONS
Gastrointestinal upset (diarrhea, nausea, stomach pain, and vomiting) may occur with Phosphate therapy. Also, bone and joint pain (possible Phosphate-induced osteomalacia) could occur. The following adverse effects may be observed (primarily from Sodium or Potassium); headaches; dizziness; mental confusion; seizures; weakness or heaviness of legs; unusual tiredness or weakness; muscle cramps; numbness, tingling, pain, or weakness of hands or feet; numbness or tingling around lips; fast or irregular heartbeat; shortness of breath or troubled breathing; swelling of feet or lower legs; unusual weight gain; low urine output; unusual thirst.

DOSAGE AND ADMINISTRATION
Adults: One or two tablets four times a day with a full glass of water.

HOW SUPPLIED
TABLETS:

BRAND/MANUFACTURER	NDC	SIZE	AWP
○ **BRAND**			
K-PHOS NEUTRAL: Beach	00486-1125-01	100s	$10.90
	00486-1125-05	500s	$52.30
○ **GENERICS**			
URO-KP-NEUTRAL: Star	00076-0109-03	100s	$19.80

Povidone-Iodine

DESCRIPTION
Povidone-Iodine is a broad-spectrum microbicide with the chemical formulas: 2-pyrrolidinone, 1-ethenyl-, homopolymer, compound with Iodine; 1-vinyl-2-pyrrolidinone polymer, compound with Iodine.

Povidone-Iodine sterile ophthalmic prep solution contains 5% Povidone-Iodine (0.5% available Iodine) as a sterile solution stabilized by glycerin.

CLINICAL PHARMACOLOGY
A placebo-controlled study in 38 normal volunteers yielded data for 36 subjects who showed a mean $\log_{10}$ units in total aerobes at 10 minutes following prepping the skin with Povidone-Iodine sterile ophthalmic prep solution compared with reduction of 1.58 $\log_{10}$ units after prepping with vehicle free of the Iodine complex. This placebo-controlled study indicates a mean $\log_{10}$ reduction by the Iodine complex compared with the control solution of 1.47 $\log_{10}$ reduction at 10 minutes and 1.79 $\log_{10}$ units at 45 minutes. The base-line mean aerobic bacterial count was 7,586 organisms per square cm.

INDICATIONS AND USAGE
Povidone-Iodine sterile ophthalmic prep solution for the eye is indicated for prepping of the periocular region (lids, brow, and cheek) and irrigation of the ocular surface (cornea, conjunctiva, and palpebral fornices).

CONTRAINDICATIONS
Do not use on individuals known to be sensitive to Iodine.

WARNINGS
For external use only. NOT for intraocular injection or irrigation.

PRECAUTIONS
General: No studies are available in patients with thyroid disorders; therefore, caution is advised in using Povidone-Iodine sterile ophthalmic prep solution in these patients due to the possibility of Iodine absorption.

Carcinogenesis, Mutagenesis, Impairment of Fertility: No long term studies in animals have been performed to evaluate the carcinogenic or mutagenic potential of Povidone-Iodine.

One report of the mutagenic potential of Povidone-Iodine indicated that it was positive in a modification of the Ames *S. typhimurium* model, but these results could not be reproduced by another researcher. Another test using mouse lymphoma and Balb/3T3 cells showed that Povidone-Iodine has no significant mutagenic or transformation capabilities. Other data indicated that it does not produce mutagenic effects in mice or hamsters according to the dominant lethal test, micronucleus test, and chromosome analysis.

Pregnancy Category C: Animal reproduction studies have not been conducted with Povidone-Iodine sterile ophthalmic prep solution. It is also not known whether Povidone-Iodine sterile ophthalmic prep solution can cause fetal harm when administered to a pregnant woman or can affect reproductive capacity. Povidone-Iodine sterile ophthalmic prep solution should only be used on a pregnant woman if clearly needed.

Nursing Mothers: Because of the potential for serious adverse reactions in nursing infants from Povidone-Iodine sterile ophthalmic prep solution, a decision should be made to discontinue nursing or discontinue the drug, taking into account the importance of the drug to the mother.

Pediatric Use: Safety and effectiveness in children have not been established.

ADVERSE REACTIONS
There have been no reports from clinical trials of adverse reactions to Povidone-Iodine sterile ophthalmic prep solution; however, in occasional instances, local sensitivity has been exhibited by some individuals to Povidone-Iodine solution (Povidone-Iodine, 10%).

DOSAGE AND ADMINISTRATION
While the inner surface and contents of the immediate container (i.e. bottle) are sterile, the outer surface of the bottle is not sterile. The use of the bottle in a sterile field should be avoided.

Povidone-Iodine sterile ophthalmic prep solution is used as follows:
1. Twist clear overcap, piercing the blue container. Remove the overcap and gently squeeze entire contents of bottle into a sterile prep cup.
2. Saturate sterile cotton-tipped applicator to prep lashes and lid margins using one or more applicators per lid; repeat once.
3. Saturate sterile prep sponge or other suitable material to prep lids, brow and cheek in a circular ever-expanding fashion until the entire field is covered; repeat prep three (3) times.
4. While separating the lids, irrigate the cornea, conjunctiva and palpebral fornicas with Povidone-Iodine sterile ophthalmic prep solution using a sterile bulb syringe.
5. After the Povidone-Iodine sterile ophthalmic prep solution has been left in contact for two minutes, sterile saline solution in a bulb syringe should be used to flush the residual prep solution from the cornea, conjunctiva, and the palpebral fornices.
Store at controlled room temperature 15-30°C (59-86°F).

HOW SUPPLIED
SOLUTION: 5%

BRAND/MANUFACTURER	NDC	SIZE	AWP
○ **BRAND**			
BETADINE 5%: Purdue Frederick	00034-0410-20	50 ml	$8.44

Pralidoxime Chloride

DESCRIPTION
Chemical name: 2-formyl-1-methylpyridinium chloride oxime. Available in the United States as Pralidoxime Chloride, is frequently referred to as 2-PAM Chloride.

Pralidoxime Chloride occurs as an odorless, white, nonhygroscopic, crystalline powder which is soluble in water to the extent of 1 g in less than 1 mL. Stable in air, it melts between 215° and 225°C, with decomposition.

The specific activity of the drug resides in the 2-formyl-1-methylpyridinium ion and is independent of the particular salt employed. The chloride is preferred because of physiologic compatibility, excellent water solubility at all temperatures, and high potency per gram, due to its low (173) molecular weight.

Pralidoxime Chloride is a cholinesterase reactivator.

► SHOWN IN PRODUCT IDENTIFICATION GUIDE

Pralidoxime Chloride for intravenous injection or infusion is prepared by cryodesiccation. Each vial contains 1 g of sterile Pralidoxime Chloride, to be reconstituted with 20 mL of Sterile Water for Injection, USP. The pH of the reconstituted solution is 3.5 to 4.5. Intramuscular or subcutaneous injection may be used when intravenous injection is not feasible.

Following is its chemical structure:

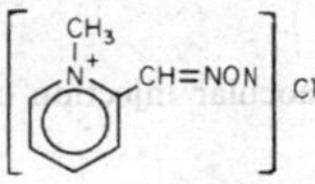

CLINICAL PHARMACOLOGY

The principal action of Pralidoxime is to reactivate cholinesterase (mainly outside of the central nervous system) which has been inactivated by phosphorylation due to an organophosphate pesticide or related compound. The destruction of accumulated acetylcholine can then proceed, and neuromuscular junctions will again function normally. Pralidoxime also slows the process of "aging" of phosphorylated cholinesterase to a nonreactivatable form, and detoxifies certain organophosphates by direct chemical reaction. The drug has its most critical effect in relieving paralysis of the muscles of respiration. Because Pralidoxime is less effective in relieving depression of the respiratory center, atropine is always required concomitantly to block the effect of accumulated acetylcholine at this site. Pralidoxime relieves muscarinic signs and symptoms, salivation, broncho-spasm, etc., but this action is relatively unimportant since atropine is adequate for this purpose.

Pralidoxime is distributed throughout the extracellular water; it is not bound to plasma protein. The drug is rapidly excreted in the urine partly unchanged, and partly as a metabolite produced by the liver. Consequently, Pralidoxime is relatively short acting, and repeated doses may be needed, especially where there is any evidence of continuing absorption of the poison.

The minimum therapeutic concentration of Pralidoxime in plasma is 4 μg/mL; this level is reached in about 16 minutes after a single injection of 600 mg Pralidoxime Chloride. The apparent half-life of Pralidoxime Chloride is 74 to 77 minutes. It has been reported[1] that the supplemental use of oxime cholinesterase reactivators (such as Pralidoxime) reduces the incidence and severity of developmental defects in chick embryos exposed to such known teratogens as parathion, bidrin, carbachol, and neostigmine. This protective effect of the oximes was shown to be dose related.

INDICATIONS AND USAGE

Pralidoxime Chloride is indicated as an antidote: (1) in the treatment of poisoning due to those pesticides and chemicals of the organophosphate class which have anticholinesterase activity. and (2) in the control of overdosage by anticholinesterase drugs used in the treatment of myasthenia gravis.

The principal indications for the use of Pralidoxime are muscle weakness and respiratory depression. In severe poisoning, respiratory depression may be due to muscle weakness.

CONTRAINDICATIONS

There are no known absolute contraindications for the use of Pralidoxime Chloride. Relative contraindications include known hypersensitivity to the drug and other situations in which the risk of its use clearly outweighs possible benefit (see "Precautions").

WARNINGS

Pralidoxime Chloride is not effective in the treatment of poisoning due to phosphorus, inorganic phosphates, or organophosphates not having anticholinesterase activity.

Pralidoxime Chloride is not indicated as an antidote for intoxication by pesticides of the carbamate class since it may increase the toxicity of carbaryl.

PRECAUTIONS

GENERAL

Pralidoxime has been very well tolerated in most cases, but it must be remembered that the desperate condition of the organophosphate-poisoned patient will generally mask such minor signs and symptoms as have been noted in normal subjects.

Intravenous administration of Pralidoxime Chloride should be carried out slowly and, preferably, by infusion, since certain side effects, such as tachycardia, laryngospasm, and muscle rigidity, have been attributed in a few cases to a too-rapid rate of injection. (See "Dosage and Administration".)

Pralidoxime Chloride should be used with great caution in treating organophosphate overdosage in cases of myasthenia gravis since it may precipitate a myasthenic crisis.

Because Pralidoxime is excreted in the urine, a decrease in renal function will result in increased blood levels of the drug. Thus, the dosage of Pralidoxime should be reduced in the presence of renal insufficiency.

LABORATORY TESTS

Treatment of organophosphate poisoning should be instituted without waiting for the results of laboratory tests. Red blood cell, plasma cholinesterase, and urinary paranitrophenol measurements (in the case of parathion exposure) may be helpful in confirming the diagnosis and following the course of the illness. A reduction in red blood cell cholinesterase concentration to below 50% of normal has been seen only with organophosphate ester poisoning.

DRUG INTERACTIONS

When atropine and Pralidoxime are used together, the signs of atropinization (flushing, mydriasis, tachycardia, dryness of the mouth and nose) may occur earlier than might be expected when atropine is used alone. This is especially true if the total dose of atropine has been large and the administration of Pralidoxime has been delayed.[2-4]

The following precautions should be kept in mind in the treatment of anticholinesterase poisoning, although they do not bear directly on the use of Pralidoxime: since barbiturates are potentiated by the anticholinesterases, they should be used cautiously in the treatment of convulsions: morphine, theophylline, aminophylline, succinylcholine, reserpine, and phenothiazine-type tranquilizers should be avoided in patients with organophosphate poisoning.

CARCINOGENESIS, MUTAGENESIS, IMPAIRMENT OF FERTILITY

Since Pralidoxime Chloride is indicated for short-term emergency use only, no investigations of its potential for carcinogenesis, mutagenesis, or impairment of fertility have been conducted by the manufacturer, or reported in the literature.

PREGNANCY

Teratogenic Effects—Pregnancy Category C: Animal reproduction studies have not been conducted with Pralidoxime. It is also not known whether Pralidoxime can cause fetal harm when administered to a pregnant woman or can affect reproduction capacity. Pralidoxime should be given to a pregnant woman only if clearly needed.

NURSING MOTHERS

It is not known whether this drug is excreted in human milk. Because many drugs are excreted in human milk, caution should be exercised when Pralidoxime is administered to a nursing woman.

PEDIATRIC USE

Safety and effectiveness in children have not been established.

ADVERSE REACTIONS

Forty to 60 minutes after intramuscular injection, mild to moderate pain may be experienced at the site of injection. Pralidoxime may cause blurred vision, diplopia and impaired accommodation, dizziness, headache, drowsiness, nausea, tachycardia, increased systolic and diastolic blood pressure, hyperventilation, and muscular weakness when given parenterally to normal volunteers who have not been exposed to anticholinesterase poisons. In patients, it is very difficult to differentiate the toxic effects produced by atropine or the organophosphate compounds from those of the drug.

Elevations in SGOT and/or SGPT enzyme levels were observed in 1 of 6 normal volunteers given 1200 mg of Pralidoxime Chloride intramuscularly, and in 4 of 6 volunteers given 1800 mg intramuscularly. Levels returned to normal in about 2 weeks. Transient elevations in creatine phosphokinase were observed in all normal volunteers given the drug. A single intramuscular injection of 330 mg in 1 mL in rabbits caused myonecrosis, inflammation, and hemorrhage.

When atropine and Pralidoxime are used together, the signs of atropinization may occur earlier than might be expected when atropine is used alone. This is especially true if the total dose of atropine has been large and the administration of Pralidoxime has been delayed.[2-4] Excitement and manic behavior immediately following recovery of consciousness have been reported in several cases. However, similar behavior has occurred in cases of organophosphate poisoning that were not treated with Pralidoxime.[3,5,6]

DRUG ABUSE AND DEPENDENCE

Pralidoxime Chloride is not subject to abuse and possesses no known potential for dependence.

OVERDOSAGE

MANIFESTATIONS OF OVERDOSAGE

Observed in normal subjects only: dizziness, blurred vision, diplopia, headache, impaired accommodation, nausea, slight tachycardia. In therapy it has been difficult to differentiate side effects due to the drug from those due to the effects of the poison.

TREATMENT OF OVERDOSAGE

Artificial respiration and other supportive therapy should be administered as needed.

ACUTE TOXICITY

IV—man TDLo: 14 mg/kg (toxic effects: CNS)
IV—rat LD50: 96 mg/kg
IM—rat LD50: 150 mg/kg
ORAL—mouse LD50: 4100 mg/kg
IP—mouse LD50: 155 mg/kg
IV—mouse LD50: 90 mg/kg
IM—mouse LD50: 180 mg/kg
IV—rabbit LD50: 95 mg/kg
IM—guinea pig LD50: 168 mg/kg

DOSAGE AND ADMINISTRATION

ORGANOPHOSPHATE POISONING

"Pralidoxime is most effective if administered immediately after poisoning. Generally, little is accomplished if the drug is given more than 36 hours after termination of exposure. When the poison has been ingested, however, exposure may continue for some time due to slow absorption from the lower bowel, and fatal relapses have been reported after initial improvement. Continued administration for several days may be useful in such patients. Close supervision of the patient is indicated for at least 48 to 72 hours. If dermal exposure has occurred, clothing should be removed and the hair and skin washed thoroughly with sodium bicarbonate or alcohol as soon as possible. Diazepam may be given cautiously if convulsions are not controlled by atropine."[7] Severe poisoning (coma, cyanosis, respiratory depression) requires intensive management. This includes the removal of secretions, airway management, the correction of acidosis, and hypoxemia.

Atropine should be given as soon as possible after hypoxemia is improved. Atropine should not be given in the presence of significant hypoxia due to the risk of atropine-induced ventricular fibrillation. In adults, atropine may be given intravenously in doses of 2 to 4 mg. This should be repeated at 5- to 10-minute intervals until full atropinization (secretions are inhibited) or signs of atropine toxicity appear (delirium, hyperthermia, muscle twitching).

The dosage of atropine for children, 0.05 to 0.10 mg/kg, should be given on a similar schedule.

Some degree of atropinization should be maintained for at least 48 hours, and until any depressed blood cholinesterase activity is reversed.

Morphine, theophylline, aminophylline, and succinylcholine are contraindicated. Tranquilizers of the reserpine or phenothiazine type are to be avoided.

After the effects of atropine become apparent Pralidoxime Chloride may be administered.

PRALIDOXIME CHLORIDE INJECTION
Parenteral drug products should be inspected visually for particulate matter and discoloration prior to administration, whenever solution and container permit.

Discard unused solution after a dose has been withdrawn.

In adults, inject an initial dose of 1 to 2 g of Pralidoxime Chloride, preferably as an infusion in 100 mL of saline, over a 15- to 30-minute period. If this is not practical or if pulmonary edema is present, the dose should be given slowly by intravenous injection as a 5 percent solution in water over not less than five minutes. After about an hour, a second dose of 1 to 2 g will be indicated if muscle weakness has not been relieved. Additional doses may be given cautiously if muscle weakness persists. Too-rapid administration may result in temporary worsening of cholinergic manifestations. Injection rate should not exceed 200 mg/minute. If intravenous administration is not feasible, intramuscular or subcutaneous injection should be used.

In children, the dose should be 20 to 40 mg/kg body weight using the same procedure.

In severe cases, especially after ingestion of the poison, it may be desirable to monitor the effect of therapy electrocardiographically because of the possibility of heart block due to the anticholinesterase. Where the poison has been ingested, it is particularly important to take into account the likelihood of continuing absorption from the lower bowel since this constitutes new exposure. In such cases, additional doses of Pralidoxime may be needed every three to eight hours. In effect, the patient should be "titrated" with Pralidoxime Chloride as long as signs of poisoning recur. As in all cases of organophosphate poisoning, care should be taken to keep the patient under observation for at least 24 hours.

If convulsions interfere with respiration, they may be controlled by the slow intravenous injection of diazepam, up to 20 mg in adults and at 0.1 to 0.2 mg/kg in children.

ANTICHOLINESTERASE OVERDOSAGE
As an antagonist to such anticholinesterase as neostigmine, pyridostigmine, and ambenonium, which are used in the treatment of myasthenia gravis, Pralidoxime Chloride may be given in a dosage of 1 to 2 g intravenously followed by increments of 250 mg every five minutes.

ANIMAL PHARMACOLOGY AND TOXICOLOGY
The following table lists chemical and trade or generic names of pesticides, chemicals, and drugs against which Pralidoxime Chloride (usually administered in conjunction with atropine) has been found to have antidotal activity on the basis of animal experiments. All compounds listed are organophosphates having anticholinesterase activity. A great many additional substances are in industrial use but have been omitted because of lack of special information.

AAT—see PARATHION
AFLIX—see FORMOTHION
ALKRON®—See PARATHION
AMERICAN CYANAMID 3422—see PARATHION
AMITON—diethyl-S-(2-diethylaminoethyl)phosphorothiolate
ANTHIO®—see FORMOTHION
APHAMITE—see PARATHION
ARMIN—ethyl-4-nitrophenylethylphosphonate
AZINPHOS-METHYL—dimethyl-S-(4-oxo-1,2,3,-benzotriazin-3 (4H)-ylmethyl) phosphorodithioate
MORPHOTHION—dimethyl-S-2-keto-2-(N-morpholy)ethyl-phosphorodithioate
NEGUVON®—see TRICHLOROFON
NIRAN®—see PARATHION
NITROSTIGMINE—see PARATHION
O,O-DIETHYL-O-p-NITROPHENYL PHOSPHOROTHIOATE— see PARATHION
O,O-DIETHYL-O-p-NITROPHENYLTHIO PHOSPHATE— see PARATHION
OR 1191—see PHOSPHAMIDON
OS 1836—see VINYLPHOS

OXYDEMETONMETHYL—dimethyl-S-2-(ethylsulfinyl) ethyl phosphorothiolate
PARAOXON—diethyl (4-nitrophenyl) phosphate
PARATHION—diethyl (4-nitrophenyl) phosphorothionate
PENPHOS—see PARATHION
PHENCAPTON—diethyl-S-(2,5-dichlorophenylmercaptomethyl) phosphorodithioate
PHOSDRIN®—see MEVINPHOS
PHOS-KIL—see PARTHION
PHOSPHAMIDON—1-chloro-1-diethylcarbamoyl-1-propen-2-yl-dimethylphosphate
PHOSPHOLINE IODIDE®—see echothiophate iodide
PHOSPHOROTHIOIC ACID, O,O-DIETHYL-O-p-NI-TROPHE-NYL ESTER—see PARATHION
PLANTHION—see PARATHION
QUELETOX—see FENTHION
RHODIATOX®—see PARATHION
RUELENE®—4-tert-butyl-2-chlorophenylmethyl-N-methylphosphoroamidate
SARIN—isopropyl-methylphosphonofluoridate
SHELL OS 1836—see VINYLPHOS
SHELL 2046—see MEVINPHOS
SNP—see PARATHION
SOMAN—pinacolyl-methylphosphonofluoridate
SYSTOX®—diethyl-(2-ethylmercaptoethyl) phosphorothionate
TEP—see TEPP
TEPP—tetraethylpyro phosphate
THIOPHOS®—see PARATHION
TIGUVON—see FENTHION
TRICHLOROFON—dimethyl-1-hydroxy-2,2,2-trichloroethylphosphonate
VAPONA®—see DICHLORVOS
VAPOPHOS—see PARATHION
VINYLPHOS—diethyl-2-chloro-vinylphosphate

Pralidoxime Chloride appears to be ineffective, or marginally effective, against poisoning by:
CIODRIN® (alpha-methylbenzyl-3[dimethoxyphosphinyloxy]-ciscrotonate)
DIMEFOX (tetramethylphosphorodimidic fluoride)
DIMETHOATE (dimethyl-S-[N-methylcarbamoylmethyl]-phosphorodithioate)
METHYL DIAZINON (dimethyl-[2-isopropyl-4-methyl-pyrimidyl]-phosphorothionate)
METHYL PHENCAPTON (dimethyl-S-[2,5-dichlorophenyl-mer-captomethyl] phosphorodithioate)
PHORATE (diethyl-S-ethylmercaptomethylphosphorodithioate)
SCHRADAN (octamethylpyrophosphoramide)
WEPSYN® (5-amino-1-[bis-(dimethylamino) phosphinyl]-3-phenyl-1,2,4-triazole)

The use of Pralidoxime Chloride should, nevertheless, be considered in any life-threatening situation resulting from poisoning by these compounds, since the limited and arbitrary conditions of pharmacologic screening do not always accurately reflect the usefulness of Pralidoxime Chloride in the clinical situation.

CLINICAL STUDIES
The use of Pralidoxime Chloride has been reported in the treatment of human cases of poisoning by the following substances:

Azodrin
Diazinon
Dichlorvos (DDVP) with chlordane
Disulfoton
EPN
Isoflurophate
Malathion
Metasystox I® and Fenthion
Methyldemeton
Methylparathion
Mevinphos
Parathion
Parathion and Mevinphos
Phosphamidon
Sarin
Systox®
TEPP

Of these cases, over 100 were due to parathion, about a dozen each to malathion, diazinon, and mevinphos, and a few to each of the other compounds.

REFERENCES
1. LANDAUER, W.: Cholinomimetic teratogens. V. The effect of oximes and related cholinesterase reactivators, *Teratology* 15:33 (Feb) 1977. 2. MOLLER, K.O., JENSEN-HOLM, J., and LAUSEN, H.H.: *Ugeskr. Laeg.* 123:501, 1961. 3. NAMBA, T., NOLTE, C.T., JACKREL, J. and GROB, D.: Poisoning due to organophosphate insecticides. Acute and chronic manifestations, *Amer. J. Med.* 50:475 (Apr), 1971. 4. ARENA, J.M.:

Poisoning, Toxicology Symptoms, Treatments, ed. 4, Springfield, IL. Charles C. Thomas, 1979, p. 133. 5. BRACHFELD, J., and ZAVON, M.R.: Organic phosphate (Phosdrin®) intoxication. Report of a case and the results of treatment with 2 PAM, *Arch. Environ. Health 11*:859, 1965. 6. HAYES, W.J., Jr.: Toxicology of Pesticides, Baltimore, The Williams & Wilkins Company, 1975, p. 416. 7. AMA Department of Drugs: AMA Drug Evaluations, ed. 4, Chicago, American Medical Association, 1980, p. 1455.

J CODES
Up to 1 g IV,IM,SC—J2730

HOW SUPPLIED
INJECTION: 1 GM/20 ML

BRAND/MANUFACTURER	NDC	SIZE	AWP
◆ **BRAND**			
PROTOPAM CHLORIDE: Wyeth-Ayerst	00046-0374-06	20 ml 6s	$173.14

Pramilet Fa *SEE* VITAMINS, PRENATAL

Pramosone *SEE* HYDROCORTISONE ACETATE AND PRAMOXINE HYDROCHLORIDE

Pravachol *SEE* PRAVASTATIN SODIUM

Pravastatin Sodium

DESCRIPTION
Pravastatin Sodium is one of a new class of lipid-lowering compounds, the HMG-CoA reductase inhibitors, which reduce cholesterol biosynthesis. These agents are competitive inhibitors of 3-hydroxy-3-methylglutaryl-coenzyme A (HMG-CoA) reductase, the enzyme catalyzing the early rate-limiting step in cholesterol biosynthesis, conversion of HMG-CoA to mevalonate.

Pravastatin Sodium is designated chemically as 1-Naphthalene-heptanoic acid, 1,2,6,7,8,8a-hexahydro-β, 6-trihydroxy-2-methyl-8-(2-methyl-1-oxobutoxy)-, monosodium salt, [1S-[1α(βS*,S*),2α,6α, 8β(R*),8aα]]-.

Pravastatin Sodium is an odorless, white to off-white, fine or crystalline powder. It is a relatively polar hydrophilic compound with a partition coefficient (octanol/water) of 0.59 at a pH of 7.0. It is soluble in methanol and water (>300 mg/mL), slightly soluble in isopropanol, and practically insoluble in acetone, acetonitrile, chloroform, and ether.

Pravastatin Sodium is available for oral administration as 10 mg, 20 mg and 40 mg tablets.

Following is its chemical structure:

CLINICAL PHARMACOLOGY
MECHANISM OF ACTION
Cholesterol and triglycerides in the bloodstream circulate as part of lipoprotein complexes. These complexes can be separated by density ultracentrifugation into high (HDL), intermediate (IDL), low (LDL), and very low (VLDL) density lipoprotein fractions. Triglycerides (TG) and cholesterol synthesized in the liver are incorporated into very low density lipoproteins (VLDLs) and released into the plasma for delivery to peripheral tissues. In a series of subsequent steps, VLDLs are transformed into intermediate density lipoproteins (IDLs), and cholesterol-rich low density lipoproteins (LDLs). High density lipoproteins (HDLs), containing apolipoprotein A, are hypothesized to participate in the reverse transport of cholesterol from tissues back to the liver.

Pravastatin Sodium produces its lipid-lowering effect in two ways. First, as a consequence of its reversible inhibition of HMG-CoA reductase activity, it effects modest reductions in intracellular pools of cholesterol. This results in an increase in the number of LDL-receptors on cell surfaces and enhanced receptor-mediated catabolism and clearance of circulating LDL. Second, Pravastatin inhibits LDL production by inhibiting hepatic synthesis of VLDL, the LDL precursor.

Clinical and pathologic studies have shown that elevated levels of total cholesterol (Total-C), low density lipoprotein cholesterol (LDL-C), and apolipoprotein B (a membrane transport complex for LDL) promote human atherosclerosis. Similarly, decreased levels of HDL-cholesterol (HDL-C) and its transport complex, apolipoprotein A, are associated with the development of atherosclerosis. Epidemiologic investigations have established that cardiovascular morbidity and mortality vary directly with the level of Total-C and LDL-C and inversely with the level of HDL-C. In multicenter clinical trials, those pharmacologic and/or non-pharmacologic interventions that simultaneously lowered LDL-C and increased HDL-C reduced the rate of cardiovascular events (both fatal and nonfatal myocardial infarctions). In both normal volunteers and patients with hypercholesterolemia, treatment with Pravastatin Sodium reduced Total-C, LDL-C, and apolipoprotein B. Pravastatin Sodium also modestly reduced VLDL-C and TG while producing increases of variable magnitude in HDL-C and apolipoprotein A. The effects of Pravastatin on Lp(a), fibrinogen, and certain other independent biochemical risk markers for coronary heart disease are unknown. The effect of Pravastatin-induced changes in lipoprotein levels on the evolution of atherosclerosis is also unknown. Although Pravastatin is relatively more hydrophilic than other HMG-CoA reductase inhibitors, the effect of relative hydrophilicity, if any, on either efficacy or safety has not been established.

PHARMACOKINETICS/METABOLISM
Pravastatin Sodium is administered orally in the active form. In clinical pharmacology studies in man, Pravastatin is rapidly absorbed, with peak plasma levels of parent compound attained 1 to 1.5 hours following ingestion. Based on urinary recovery of radiolabeled drug, the average oral absorption of Pravastatin is 34% and absolute bioavailability is 17%. While the presence of food in the gastrointestinal tract reduces systemic bioavailability, the lipid-lowering effects of the drug are similar whether taken with, or 1 hour prior, to meals.

Pravastatin undergoes extensive first-pass extraction in the liver (extraction ratio 0.66), which is its primary site of action, and the primary site of cholesterol synthesis and of LDL-C clearance. *In vitro* studies demonstrated that Pravastatin Sodium is transported into hepatocytes with substantially less uptake into other cells. In view of Pravastatin's apparently extensive first-pass hepatic metabolism, plasma levels may not necessarily correlate perfectly with lipid-lowering efficacy. Pravastatin plasma concentrations [including: area under the concentration-time curve (AUC), peak (Cmax), and steady-state minimum (Cmin)] are directly proportional to administered dose. Systemic bioavailability of Pravastatin administered following a bedtime dose was decreased 60% compared to that following an AM dose. Despite this decrease in systemic bioavailability, the efficacy of Pravastatin administered once daily in the evening, although not statistically significant, was marginally more effective than that after a morning dose. This finding of lower systemic bioavailability suggests greater hepatic extraction of the drug following the evening dose. Steady-state AUCs, Cmax and Cmin plasma concentrations showed no evidence of Pravastatin accumulation following once or twice daily administered of Pravastatin Sodium tablets. Approximately 50% of the circulating drug is bound to plasma proteins. Following single dose administration of ^{14}C-Pravastatin, the elimination half-life (t½) for total radioactivity (Pravastatin plus metabolites) in humans is 77 hours.

Pravastatin, like other HMG-CoA reductase inhibitors, has variable bioavailability. The coefficient of variation, based on between-subject variability, was 50% to 60% for AUC. Approximately 20% of a radiolabeled oral dose is excreted in urine and 70% in the feces. After intravenous administration of radiolabeled Pravastatin to normal volunteers, approximately 47% of total body clearance was via renal excretion and 53% by non-renal routes (i.e., biliary excretion and biotransformation). Since there are dual routes of elimination, the potential exists both for compensatory excretion by the alternate route as well as for accumulation of drug and/or metabolites in patients with renal or hepatic insufficiency.

In a study comparing the kinetics of Pravastatin in patients with biopsy confirmed cirrhosis (N = 7) and normal subjects (N = 7), the mean AUC varied 18-fold in cirrhotic patients and 5-fold in healthy subjects. Similarly, the peak Pravastatin values varied 47-fold for cirrhotic patients compared to 6-fold for healthy subjects.

Biotransformation pathways elucidated for Pravastatin include: (a) isomerization to 6-epi Pravastatin and the 3α-hydroxyisomer of Pravastatin (SQ 31,906), (b) enzymatic ring hydroxylation to SQ 31,945, (c) -1 oxidation of the ester side chain, (d) β-oxidation of the carboxy side chain, (e) ring oxidation followed by aromatization, (f) oxidation of a hydroxyl group to a keto group, and (g) conjugation. The major degradation product is the 3α-hydroxy isomeric metabolite, which has one-tenth to one-fortieth the HMG-CoA reductase inhibitory activity of the parent compound.

CLINICAL STUDIES
Pravastatin Sodium is highly effective in reducing Total-C and LDL-C in patients with heterozygous familial, presumed familial combined, and non-familial (non-FH) forms of primary hypercholesterolemia. A therapeutic response is seen within 1 week, and the maximum response usually is achieved within 4 weeks. This response is maintained during extended periods of therapy.

A single daily dose administered in the evening (the recommended dosing) is as effective as the same total daily dose given twice a day. Once daily administration in the evening appears to be marginally more effective than once daily administration in the morning, perhaps because hepatic cholesterol is synthesized mainly at night. In multicenter, double-blind, placebo-controlled studies of patients with primary hypercholesterolemia, treatment with pravastatin in daily doses ranging from 10 mg to 40 mg consistently and significantly decreased Total-C, LDL-C, and Total-C/HDL-C and LDL-C/HDL-C ratios: modestly decreased VLDL-C and plasma TG levels; and produced increases in HDL-C of variable magnitude.

◆ RATED THERAPEUTICALLY EQUIVALENT; ◇ THERAPEUTIC EQUIVALENCE UNCONFIRMED; ○ UNRATED

**PRIMARY HYPERCHOLESTEROLEMIA STUDY
DOSE RESPONSE OF PRAVASTATIN SODIUM
ONCE DAILY ADMINISTRATION AT BEDTIME**

Dose	Total-C	LDL-C	HDL-C	TG
10 mg	-16%	-22%	+7%	-15%
20 mg	-24%	-32%	+2%	-11%
40 mg	-25%	-34%	+12%	-24%

In another clinical trial, patients treated with Pravastatin in combination with cholestyramine (70% of patients were taking cholestyramine 20 or 24 g per day) had reductions equal to or greater than 50% in LDL-C. Furthermore, Pravastatin attenuated cholestyramine-induced increases in TG levels (which are themselves of uncertain clinical significance).

INDICATIONS AND USAGE

Therapy with lipid-altering agents should be considered a component of multiple risk factor intervention in those individuals at increased risk for atherosclerotic vascular disease due to hypercholesterolemia. Pravastatin Sodium is indicated as an adjunct to diet for the reduction of elevated total and LDL-cholesterol levels in patients with primary hypercholesterolemia (Type IIa and IIb)[1] when the response to a diet restricted in saturated fat and cholesterol has not been adequate.

Prior to initiating therapy with Pravastatin, secondary causes for hypercholesterolemia (e.g., poorly controlled diabetes mellitus, hypothyroidism, nephrotic syndrome, dysproteinemias, obstructive liver disease, other drug therapy, alcoholism) should be excluded, and a lipid profile performed to measure Total-C, HDL-C, and TG. For patients with triglycerides (TG) < 400 mg/dL (< 4.5 mmol/L), LDL-C can be estimated using the following equation:

LDL-C = Total-C − HDL-C − 1/5 TG

For TG levels > 400 mg/dL (> 4.5 mmol/L), this equation is less accurate and LDL-C concentrations should be determined by ultracentrifugation. In many hypertriglyceridemic patients, LDL-C may be low or normal despite elevated Total-C. In such cases, HMG-CoA reductase inhibitors are not indicated.

Lipid determinations should be performed at intervals of no less than four weeks and dosage adjusted according to the patient's response to therapy.

The National Cholesterol Education Program's Treatment Guidelines[†] are summarized below:

	LDL-Cholesterol mg/dL (mmol/L)		Total-Cholesterol mg/dL (mmol/L)
	Initiation Level	Minimum Goal	Minimum Goal
Without Definite CHD or Two Other Risk Factors[*]	≥ 190 (≥ 4.9)	< 160 (< 4.1)	< 240 (< 6.2)
With Definite CHD or Two Other Risk Factors[*]	≥ 160 (≥ 4.1)	< 130 (< 3.4)	< 200 (< 5.2)

[*] *Other risk factors for coronary heart disease (CHD) include: male sex, family history of premature CHD, cigarette smoking, hypertension, confirmed HDL-C < 35 mg/dL (< 0.91 mmol/L), diabetes mellitus, definite cerebrovascular or peripheral vascular disease, or severe obesity.*

[†] *For adult diabetic subjects, a modification of these guidelines is recommended—see: American Diabetes Association Consensus Statement: Role of Cardiovascular Risk Factors in Prevention and Treatment of Macrovascular Disease in Diabetes. Diabetes Care 12(8):573-579, 1989.*

[1] CLASSIFICATION OF HYPERLIPOPROTEINEMIAS

Type	Lipoproteins Elevated	Lipid Elevations major	minor
I (rare)	chylomicrons	TG	→C
IIa	LDL	C	—
IIb	LDL, VLDL	C	TG
III (rare)	IDL	C/TG	→C
IV	VLDL	TG	→C
V (rare)	chylomicrons, VLDL	TG	→C

C = cholesterol, TG = triglycerides,
LDL = low density lipoprotein,
VLDL = very low density lipoprotein,
IDL = intermediate density lipoprotein.

1 Fredrickson classification: Type IIa—elevation of LDL; Type IIb—elevation of LDL and VLDL. Type III (familial dysbetalipoproteinemia)-elevation of IDL. Fredrickson, DS, Fat transport in lipoproteins—an integrated approach to mechanism and disorders, N Eng J Med 276:34, 1967.

Since the goal of treatment is to lower LDL-C, the NCEP recommends that LDL-C levels be used to initiate and assess treatment response. Only if LDL-C levels are not available, should the Total-C be used to monitor therapy.

As with other lipid-lowering therapy, Pravastatin Sodium is not indicated when hypercholesterolemia is due to hyperalphalipoproteinemia (elevated HDL-C). The efficacy of Pravastatin has not been evaluated in patients with combined elevated Total-C and hypertriglyceridemia [> 500 mg/dL (> 5.7 mmol/L) or in patients with elevated intermediate density lipoproteins as their primary lipid abnormality.

CONTRAINDICATIONS

Hypersensitivity to any component of this medication.

Active liver disease or unexplained, persistent elevations in liver function tests (see *"Warnings"*).

Pregnancy and Lactation: Atherosclerosis is a chronic process and discontinuation of lipid-lowering drugs during pregnancy should have little impact on the outcome of long-term therapy of primary hypercholesterolemia. Cholesterol and other products of cholesterol biosynthesis are essential components for feal development (including synthesis of steroids and cell membranes). Since HMG-CoA reductase inhibitors decrease cholesterol synthesis and possibly the synthesis of other biologically active substances derived from cholesterol, they may cause fetal harm when administered to pregnant women. Therefore, HMG-CoA reductase inhibitors are contraindicated during pregnancy and in nursing mothers. *Pravastatin should be administered to women of childbearing age only when such patients are highly unlikely to conceive and have been informed of the potential hazards.* If the patient becomes pregnant while taking this class of drug, therapy should be discontinued and the patient apprised of the potential hazard to the fetus.

WARNINGS

LIVER ENZYMES

HMG-CoA reductase inhibitors, like some other lipid-lowering therapies, have been associated with biochemical abnormalities of liver function. Increases of serum transaminase (ALT, AST) values to more than 3 times the upper limit of normal occurring on 2 or more (not necessarily sequential) occasions have been reported in 1.3% of patients treated with Pravastatin in the US over an average period of 18 months. These abnormalities were not associated with cholestasis and did not appear to be related to treatment duration. In those patients in whom these abnormalities were believed to be related to Pravastatin and who were discontinued from therapy, the transaminase levels usually fell slowly to pretreatment levels. These biochemical findings are usually asymptomatic although worldwide experience indicates that anorexia, weakness, and/or abdominal pain may also be present in rare patients.

As with other lipid-lowering agents, liver function tests should be performed during therapy with Pravastatin. *Serum aminotransferases, including ALT (SGPT), should be monitored before treatment begins, every six weeks for the first three months, every eight weeks during the remainder of the first year, and periodically thereafter (e.g., at about six-month intervals).* Special attention should be given to patients who develop increased transaminase levels. Liver function tests should be repeated to confirm an elevation and subsequently monitored at more frequent intervals. If increases in AST and ALT equal or exceed three times the upper limit of normal and persist, then therapy should be discontinued. Persistence of significant aminotransferase elevations following discontinuation of therapy may warrant consideration of liver biopsy.

Active liver disease or unexplained transaminase elevations are contraindications to the use of Pravastatin (see *"Contraindications"*). Caution should be exercised when Pravastatin is administered to patients with a history of liver disease or heavy alcohol ingestion (see *"Clinical Pharmacology; Pharmacokinetics/Metabolism"*). Such patients should be closely monitored, started at the lower end of the recommended dosing range, and titrated to the desired therapeutic effect.

SKELETAL MUSCLE

Rhabdomyolysis with renal dysfunction secondary to myoglobinuria has been reported with Pravastatin and other drugs in this class. Uncomplicated myalgia has been reported in Pravastatin-treated patients (see *"Adverse Reactions"*). Myopathy, defined as muscle aching or muscle weakness in conjunction with increases in creatine phosphokinase (CPK) values to greater than 10 times the upper limit of normal was reported to be possibly due to Pravastatin in only one patient in clinical trials (≥ 0.1%). Myopathy should be considered in any patient with diffuse myalgias, muscle tenderness or weakness, and/or marked elevation of CPK. Patients should be advised to report promptly unexplained muscle pain, tenderness or weakness, particularly if accompanied by malaise or fever. *Pravastatin therapy should be discontinued if markedly elevated CPK levels occur or myopathy is diagnosed or suspected. Pravastatin therapy should also be temporarily withheld in any patient experiencing an acute or serious condition predisposing to the development of renal failure secondary to rhabdomyolysis, e.g., sepsis; hypotension; major surgery; trauma; severe metabolic, endocrine, or electrolyte disorders; or uncontrolled epilepsy.*

The risk of myopathy during treatment with another HMG-CoA reductase inhibitor is increased if therapy with either cyclosporine gemfibrozil, erythromycin, or riacin is administered concurrently. There is no experience with the use of Pravastatin together with cyclosporine. Myopathy has not been observed in clinical trials involving small numbers of patients who were treated with Pravastatin together with niacin. One trial of limited size involving combined therapy with Pravastatin and gemfibrozil showed a trend toward more frequent CPK elevations and patient withdrawals due to musculoskeletal symptoms in the group receiving combined treatment as compared with the groups receiving placebo, gemfibrozil, or Pravastatin monotherapy. Myopathy was not reported in this trial (see "*Precautions: Drug Interactions*"). One patient developed myopathy when clofibrate was added to a previously well tolerated regimen of Pravastatin; the myopathy resolved when clofibrate therapy was stopped and Pravastatin treatment continued. *The use of fibrates alone may occasionally be associated with myopathy. The combined use of Pravastatin Sodium and fibrates should generally be avoided.*

PRECAUTIONS

GENERAL

Pravastatin may elevate creatine phosphokinase and transaminase levels (see "*Adverse Reactions*"). This should be considered in the differential diagnosis of chest pain in a patient on therapy with Pravastatin.

Homozygous Familial Hypercholesterolemia: Pravastatin has not been evaluated in patients with rare homozygous familial hypercholesterolemia. In this group of patients, it has been reported that HMG-CoA reductase inhibitors are less effective because the patients lack functional LDL receptors.

Renal Insufficiency: A single 20 mg oral dose of Pravastatin was administered to 24 patients with varying degrees of renal impairment (as determined by creatinine clearance). No effect was observed on the pharmacokinetics of Pravastatin or its 3α-hydroxy isomeric metabolite (SQ 31,908). A small increase was seen in mean AUC values and half-life (t½) for the inactive enzymatic ring hydroxylation metabolite (SQ 31,945). Given this small sample size, the dosage administered, and the degree of individual variability, patients with renal impairment who are receiving Pravastatin should be closely monitored.

INFORMATION FOR PATIENTS

Patients should be advised to report promptly unexplained muscle pain, tenderness or weakness, particularly if accompanied by malaise or fever.

DRUG INTERACTIONS

Immunosuppressive Drugs, Genfibrozil, Niacin (Nicotinic Acid), Erythromycin: See "*Warnings: Skeletal Muscle.*"

Antipyrine: Since concomitant administration of Pravastatin had no effect on the clearance of antipyrine, interactions with other drugs metabolized via the same hepatic cytochrome isozymes are not expected.

Cholestyramine/Colestipol: Concomitant administration resulted in an approximately 40 to 50% decrease in the mean AUC of Pravastatin. However, when Pravastatin was administered 1 hour before or 4 hours after cholestyramine or 1 hour before colestipol and a standard meal, there was no clinically significant decrease in bioavailability or therapeutic effect. (See "*Dosage and Administration: Concomitant Therapy*".)

Warfarin: In a study involving 10 healthy male subjects given Pravastatin and warfarin concomitantly for 6 days, bioavailability parameters at steady state for Pravastatin (parent compound) were not altered. Pravastatin did not alter the plasma protein-binding of warfarin. Concomitant dosing did increase the AUC and Cmax of warfarin but did not produce any changes in its anticoagulant action (i.e., no increase was seen in mean prothrombin time after 6 days of concomitant therapy). However, bleeding and extreme prolongation of prothrombin time has been reported with another drug in this class. Patients receiving warfarin-type anticoagulants should have their prothrombin times closely monitored when Pravastatin is initiated or the dosage of Pravastatin is changed.

Cimetidine: The AUC$_{0-12hr}$ for Pravastatin when given with cimetidine was not significantly different from the AUC for Pravastatin when given alone. A significant difference was observed between the AUC's for Pravastatin when given with cimetidine compared to when administered with antacid.

Digoxin: In a crossover trial involving 18 healthy male subjects given pravastatin and digoxin concurrently for 9 days, the bioavailability parameters of digoxin were not affected. The AUC of Pravastatin tended to increase, but the overall bioavailability of pravastatin plus its metabolites SQ 31,906 and SQ 31,945 was not altered.

Gemfibrozil: In a crossover study in 20 healthy male volunteers given concomitant single doses of Pravastatin and gemfibrozil, there was a significant decrease in urinary excretion and protein binding of Pravastatin. In addition, there was a significant increase in AUC, Cmax, and Tmax for the Pravastatin metabolite SQ 31,906. Combination therapy with Pravastatin and gemfibrozil is generally not recommended. In interaction studies with *aspirin, antacids* (1 hour prior to Pravastatin Sodium) *cimetidine, nicotinic acid,* or *Probucol,* no statistically significant differences in bioavailability were seen when Pravastatin Sodium was administered.

Other Drugs: During clinical trials, no noticeable drug interactions were reported when Pravastatin Sodium was added to: diuretics, antihypertensives, digitalis, converting-enzyme inhibitors, calcium channel blockers, beta-blockers, or nitroglycerin.

ENDOCRINE FUNCTION

HMG-CoA reductase inhibitors interfere with cholesterol synthesis and lower circulating cholesterol levels and, as such, might theoretically blunt adrenal or gonadal steroid hormone production. Results of clinical trials with Pravastatin in males and post-menopausal females were inconsistent with regard to possible effects of the drug on basal steroid hormone levels. In a study of 21 males, the mean testosterone response to human chorionic gonadotropin was significantly reduced (p < 0.004) after 16 weeks of treatment with 40 mg of Pravastatin.

However, the percentage of patients showing a ≥ 50% rise in plasma testosterone after human chorionic gonadotropin stimulation did not change significantly after therapy in these patients. The effects of HMG-CoA reductase inhibitors on spermatogenesis and fertility have not been studied in adequate numbers of patients. The effects, if any, of Pravastatin Sodium on the pituitary-gonadal axis in pre-menopausal females are unknown. Patients treated with Pravastatin who display clinical evidence of endocrine dysfunction should be evaluated appropriately. Caution should be exercised if an HMG-CoA reductase inhibitor or other agent used to lower cholesterol levels is administered to patients also receiving other drugs (e.g., ketoconazole spironolactone, cimetidine) that may diminish the levels or activity of steroid hormones.

CNS TOXICITY

CNS vascular lesions, characterized by perivascular hemorrhage and edema and mononuclear cell infiltration of perivascular spaces, were seen in dogs treated with Pravastatin at a dose of 25 mg/kg/day, a dose that produced a plasma drug level about 50 times higher than the mean drug level in humans taking 40 mg/day. Similar CNS vascular lesions have been observed with several other drugs in this class.

A chemically similar drug in this class produced optic nerve degeneration (Wallerian degeneration of retinogeniculate fibers) in clinically normal dogs in a dose-dependent fashion starting at 60 mg/kg/day, a dose that produced mean plasma drug levels about 30 times higher than the mean drug level in humans taking the highest recommended dose (as measured by total enzyme inhibitory activity). This same drug also produced vestibulocochlear Wallerian-like degeneration and retinal ganglion cell chromatolysis in dogs treated for 14 weeks at 180 mg/kg/day, a dose which resulted in a mean plasma drug level similar to that seen with the 60 mg/kg/day dose.

CARCINOGENESIS, MUTAGENESIS, IMPAIRMENT OF FERTILITY

In a 2-year study in rats fed Pravastatin at doses of 10, 30, or 100 mg/kg body weight, there was an increased incidence of hepatocellular carcinomas in males at the highest dose (p < 0.01). Although rats were given up to 125 times the human dose (HD) on a mg/kg body weight basis, serum drug levels were only 6 to 10 times higher than those measured in humans given 40 mg Pravastatin as measured by AUC.

The oral administration of 10, 30, or 100 mg/kg (producing plasma drug levels approximately 0.5 to 5.0 times the human drug levels at 40 mg) of Pravastatin to mice for 22 months resulted in a statistically significant increase in the incidence of malignant lymphomas in treated females when all treatment groups were pooled and compared to controls (p < 0.05). The incidence was not dose-related and male mice were not affected.

A chemically similar drug in this class was administered to mice for 72 weeks at 25, 100, and 400 mg/kg body weight, which resulted in mean serum drug levels approximately 3, 15, and 33 times higher than the mean human serum drug concentration (as total inhibitory activity) after a 40 mg oral dose. Liver carcinomas were significantly increased in high-dose females and mid- and high-dose males, with a maximum incidence of 90 percent in males. The incidence of adenomas of the liver was significantly increased in mid- and high-dose females. Drug treatment also significantly increased the incidence of lung adenomas in mid- and high-dose males and females. Adenomas of the eye Harderian gland (a gland of the eye of rodents) were significantly higher in high-dose mice than in controls.

No evidence of mutagenicity was observed *in vitro*, with or without rat-liver metabolic activation, in the following studies: microbial mutagen tests, using mutant strains of *Salmonella typhimurium* or *Escherichia coli*; a forward mutation assay in L5178YTK +/- mouse lymphoma cells; a chromosomal aberration test in hamster cells; and a gene conversion assay using *Saccharomyces cerevisiae*. In addition, there was no evidence of mutagenicity in either a dominant lethal test in mice or a micronucleus test in mice.

In a study in rats, with daily doses up to 500 mg/kg, Pravastatin did not produce any adverse effects on fertility or general reproductive performance. However, in a study with another HMG-CoA reductase inhibitor, there was decreased fertility in male rats treated for 34 weeks at 25 mg/kg body weight, although this effect was not observed in a subsequent fertility study when this same dose was administered for 11 weeks (the entire cycle of spermatogenesis, including epididymal maturation). In rats treated with this same reductase inhibitor at 180 mg/kg/day, seminiferous tubule degeneration (necrosis and loss of spermatogenic epithelium) was observed. Although not seen with Pravastatin, two similar drugs in this class caused drug-related testicular atrophy, decreased spermatogenesis, spermatocytic degeneration, and giant cell formation in dogs. The clinical significance of these findings is unclear.

PREGNANCY

Pregnancy Category X: See "*Contraindications*". Safety in pregnant women has not been established. Pravastatin was not teratogenic in rats at doses up to 1000 mg/kg daily or in rabbits at doses of up to 50 mg/kg daily. These doses resulted in 20 x (rabbit) or 240 x (rat) the human exposure based on surface area (mg/meter^2). However, in studies with another HMG-CoA reductase inhibitor, skeletal malformations were observed in rats and mice. There has been one report of severe congenital bony deformity, tracheoesophageal fistula, and anal atresia (Vater association) in a baby born to a women who took another HMG-CoA reductase inhibitor with dextroamphetamine sulfate during the first trimester of pregnancy. Pravastatin Sodium should be administered to women of childbearing potential only when such patients are highly unlikely to conceive and have been informed of the potential hazards. If the woman becomes pregnant while

---

taking Pravastatin Sodium it should be discontinued and the patient advised again as to the potential hazards to the fetus.

NURSING MOTHERS
A small amount of Pravastatin is excreted in human breast milk. Because of the potential for serious adverse reactions in nursing infants, women taking Pravastatin Sodium should not nurse (see "Contraindications").

PEDIATRIC USE
Safety and effectiveness in individuals less than 18 years old have not been established. Hence, treatment in patients less than 18 years old is not recommended at this time.

ADVERSE REACTIONS
Pravastatin is generally well tolerated: adverse reactions have usually been mild and transient. In 4-month long placebo-controlled trials, 1.7% of Pravastatin-treated patients and 1.2% of placebo-treated patients were discontinued from treatment because of adverse experiences attributed to study drug therapy; this difference was not statistically significant. In long-term studies, the most common reasons for discontinuation were asymptomatic serum transaminase increases and mild, non-specific gastrointestinal complaints. During clinical trials the overall incidence of adverse events in the elderly was not different than the incidence observed in younger patients.

ADVERSE CLINICAL EVENTS
All adverse clinical events (regardless of attribution) reported in more than 2% of Pravastatin-treated patients in the placebo-controlled trials are identified in the table below; also shown are the percentages of patients in whom these medical events were believed to be related or possibly related to the drug. (See related table).

The following effects have been reported with drugs in this class; not all the effects listed below have necessarily been associated with Pravastatin therapy:

Skeletal: myopathy, rhabdomyolysis, arthralgia.

Neurological: dysfunction of certain cranial nerves (including alteration of taste, impairment of extra-ocular movement, facial parasis), tremor, vertigo, memory loss, paresthesia, peripheral neuropathy, peripheral nerve palsy, anxiety, insomnia, depression.

Hypersensitivity Reactions: An apparent hypersensitivity syndrome has been reported rarely which has included one or more of the following features: anaphylaxis, angioedema, lupus erythematous-like syndrome, polymyalgia rheumatica, vasculitis, purpura, thrombocytopenia, leukopenia, hemolytic anemia, positive ANA, ESR increase, arthritis, arthralgia, urticaria, asthenia, photosensitivity, fever, chills, flushing, malaise, dyspnea, toxic epidermal necrolysis, erythema multiforme, including Stevens-Johnson syndrome.

Gastrointestinal: pancreatitis, hepatitis, including chronic active hepatitis, cholestatic jaundice, fatty change in liver, and, rarely, cirrhosis, fulminant hepatic necrosis, and hepatoma; anorexia, vomiting.

Skin: alopecia.

Reproductive: gynecomastia, loss of libido, erectile dysfunction.

Eye: progression of cataracts (lens opacities), ophthalmoplegia.

Laboratory Abnormalities: elevated transaminases, alkaline phosphatase, and bilirubin; thyroid function abnormalities.

LABORATORY TEST ABNORMALITIES
Increases in serum transaminase (ALT, AST) values and CPK have been observed (see "Warnings").

Transient, asymptomatic epsinophilia has been reported. Eosinophil counts usually returned to normal despite continued therapy. Anemia, thrombocytopenia, and leukopenia have been reported with other HMG-CoA reductase inhibitors.

CONCOMITANT THERAPY
Pravastatin has been administered concurrently with cholestyramine, colestipol, nicotinic acid, probucol and gemfibrozil. Preliminary data suggest that the addition of either probucol or gemfibrozil to therapy with lovastatin or Pravastatin is **not** associated with greater reduction in LDL-cholesterol than that achieved with lovastatin or Pravastatin alone. No adverse reactions unique to the combination or in addition to those previously reported for each drug alone have been reported. Myopathy and rhabdomyolysis (with or without acute renal failure) have been reported when another HMG-CoA reductase inhibitor was used in combination with immunosuppressive drugs, gemfibrozil, erythromycin, or lipid-lowering doses of nicotinic acid. Concomitant therapy with HMG-CoA reductase inhibitors and these agents is generally not recommended. (See "Warning: Skeletal Muscle" and "Precautions: Drug Interactions".)

OVERDOSAGE
There have been no reports of overdoses with Pravastatin. Should an accidental overdose occur, treat symptomatically and institute supportive measures as required.

DOSAGE AND ADMINISTRATION
Prior to initiating Pravastatin Sodium, the patient should be placed on a standard cholesterol-lowering diet (AHA Phase I or NCEP Step 1) for a minimum of 3 to 6 months, depending upon the severity of the lipid elevation. Dietary therapy should be continued during treatment.

The recommended starting dose is 10 or 20 mg once daily at bedtime. In primary hypercholesterolemic patients with a history of significant renal or hepatic dysfunction, and in the elderly, a starting dose of 10 mg daily at bedtime is recommended. Pravastatin Sodium may be taken without regard to meals.

Since the maximal effect of a given dose is seen within 4 weeks, periodic lipid determinations should be performed at this time and dosage adjusted according to the patient's response to therapy and established treatment guidelines. The recommended dosage range is generally 10 to 40 mg administered once a day at bedtime. In the elderly, maximum reductions in LDL-cholesterol may be achieved with daily doses of 20 mg or less.

Body System/Event	All Events Pravastatin (N = 900%)	All Events Placebo (N = 411%)	Events Attributed to Study Drug (Pravastatin (N = 900%)	Events Attributed to Study Drug Placebo (N = 411%)
Cardiovascular				
Cardiac Chest				
Pain	4.0	3.4	0.1	0.0
Dermatologic				
Rash	4.0*	1.1	1.3	0.9
Gastrointestinal				
Nausea/Vomiting	7.3	7.1	2.9	3.4
Diarrhea	6.2	5.6	2.0	1.9
Abdominal Pain	5.4	6.9	2.0	3.9
Constipation	4.0	7.1	2.4	5.1
Flatulence	3.3	3.6	2.7	3.4
Heartburn	2.9	1.9	2.0	0.7
General				
Fatigue	3.8	3.4	1.9	1.0
Chest Pain	3.7	1.9	0.3	0.2
Influenza	2.4*	0.7	0.0	0.0
Musculoskeletal				
Localized Pain	10.0	9.0	1.4	1.5
Myalgia	2.7	1.0	0.6	0.0
Nervous System				
Headache	6.2	3.9	1.7*	0.2
Dizziness	3.3	3.2	1.0	0.5
Renal/Genitourinary				
Urinary				
Abnormality	2.4	2.9	0.7	1.2
Respiratory				
Common Cold	7.0	6.3	0.0	0.0
Rhinitis	4.0	4.1	0.1	0.0
Cough	2.6	1.7	0.1	0.0

* *Statistically significantly different from placebo.*

► SHOWN IN PRODUCT IDENTIFICATION GUIDE

CONCOMITANT THERAPY

The lipid-lowering effects of Pravastatin Sodium on total and LDL cholesterol are enhanced when combined with a bile-acid-binding resin. When administering a bile-acid-binding resin (e.g., cholestyramine, colestipol) and Pravastatin, Pravastatin Sodium should be given either 1 hour or more before or at least 4 hours following the resin. See also "*Adverse Reactions: Concomitant Therapy.*"

STORAGE

Do not store above 86°F (30°C). Keep tightly closed (protect from moisture). Protect from light.

HOW SUPPLIED
TABLETS: 10 MG

BRAND/MANUFACTURER	NDC	SIZE	AWP
○ BRAND			
▶ PRAVACHOL: Squibb, E.R.	00003-0154-50	100s	$170.49
	00003-0154-51	100s ud	$173.53

TABLETS: 20 MG

BRAND/MANUFACTURER	NDC	SIZE	AWP
○ BRAND			
▶ PRAVACHOL: Squibb, E.R.	00003-0178-50	100s	$179.95
	00003-0178-51	100s ud	$183.18

TABLETS: 40 MG

BRAND/MANUFACTURER	NDC	SIZE	AWP
○ BRAND			
▶ PRAVACHOL: Squibb, E.R.	00003-0194-50	100s	$304.20

Prazepam

DESCRIPTION

Prazepam is a benzodiazepine derivative. Chemically, Prazepam is 7-chloro-1-(cyclopropylmethyl)-1,3-dihydro-5-phenyl-2H-1,4-benzodiazepin-2-one, and has a molecular weight of 324.8.

Each Prazepam capsule contains 5 mg, 10 mg, or 20 mg Prazepam, USP.

Following is its chemical structure:

CLINICAL PHARMACOLOGY

Studies in normal subjects have shown that Prazepam has depressant effects on the central nervous system. Oral administration of single doses as high as 60 mg and of divided doses up to 100 mg three times a day (300 mg total daily dosage) were without toxic effects.

Single, oral doses of Prazepam in normal subjects produced average peak blood levels of the major metabolite norprazepam at 6 hours postadministration, with significant amounts still present after 48 hours. Prazepam was slowly absorbed over a prolonged period; rather constant blood levels were maintained on multiple-dose schedules; and excretion was prolonged. The mean half-life of norprazepam measured in subjects given 10 mg Prazepam three times a day for one week was 63 (± 15 SD) hours before and 70 (± 10 SD) hours after multiple dosing—a nonsignificant difference. Human metabolism studies showed that prior to elimination from the body, Prazepam is metabolized in large part to 3-hydroxyprazepam and oxazepam.

INDICATIONS

Prazepam is indicated for the management of anxiety disorders or for the short-term relief of the symptoms of anxiety. Anxiety or tension associated with the stress of everyday life usually does not require treatment with an anxiolytic.

The effectiveness of Prazepam in long-term use, that is, more than 4 months, has not been assessed by systematic clinical studies. The physician should periodically reassess the usefulness of the drug for the individual patient.

CONTRAINDICATIONS

Prazepam is contraindicated in patients with a known hypersensitivity to the drug and in those with acute narrow-angle glaucoma.

WARNINGS

Prazepam is not recommended in psychotic states and in those psychiatric disorders in which anxiety is not a prominent feature.

Patients taking Prazepam should be cautioned against engaging in hazardous occupations requiring mental alertness, such as operating dangerous machinery including motor vehicles.

Since Prazepam has a central nervous system depressant effect, patients should be advised against the simultaneous ingestion of alcohol and other CNS-depressant drugs during Prazepam therapy.

Physical and Psychological Dependence: Withdrawal symptoms, similar in character to those noted with barbiturates and alcohol (convulsions, tremor, abdominal and muscle cramps, vomiting and sweating), have occurred following abrupt discontinuance of benzodiazepines. The more severe withdrawal symptoms have usually been limited to those patients who received excessive doses over an extended period of time. Generally milder withdrawal symptoms (e.g., dysphoria and insomnia) have been reported following abrupt discontinuance of benzodiazepines taken continuously at therapeutic levels for several months. Consequently, after extended therapy, abrupt discontinuation should generally be avoided and a gradual dosage tapering schedule followed. Addiction-prone individuals (such as drug addicts or alcoholics) should be under careful surveillance when receiving Prazepam or other psychotropic agents because of the predisposition of such patients to habituation and dependence.

PRECAUTIONS
INFORMATION FOR PATIENTS

To assure the safe and effective use of benzodiazepines, patients should be informed that since benzodiazepines may produce psychological and physical dependence, it is advisable that they consult with their physician before either increasing the dose or abruptly discontinuing this drug. Patients should also be advised to inform their physician if they are nursing, pregnant, planning to become pregnant or become pregnant while on this medication and about any alcohol consumption or medication they are taking. In addition, as with all CNS-acting agents, patients should be cautioned against driving or engaging in hazardous activities requiring mental alertness until they experience how this medication affects them.

Usage in Pregnancy and Lactation: An increased risk of congenital malformations associated with the use of minor tranquilizers (chlordiazepoxide, diazepam, and meprobamate) during the first trimester of pregnancy has been suggested in several studies. Prazepam, a benzodiazepine derivative, has not been studied adequately to determine whether it, too, may be associated with an increased risk of fetal abnormality. Because use of these drugs is rarely a matter of urgency, their use during this period should almost always be avoided. The possibility that a woman of childbearing potential may be pregnant at the time of institution of therapy should be considered. Patients should be advised that if they become pregnant during therapy or intend to become pregnant, they should communicate with their physicians about the desirability of discontinuing the drug. In view of their molecular size, Prazepam and its metabolites are probably excreted in human milk. Therefore, this drug should not be given to nursing mothers.

In those patients in whom a degree of depression accompanies the anxiety, suicidal tendencies may be present and protective measures may be required. The least amount of drug that is feasible should be available to the patient at any one time.

Patients taking Prazepam for prolonged periods should have blood counts and liver function tests periodically. The usual precautions in treating patients with impaired renal or hepatic functions should also be observed. Hepatomegaly and cholestasis were observed in chronic toxicity studies in rats and dogs.

In elderly or debilitated patients, the initial dose should be small, and increments should be made gradually, in accordance with the response of the patient, to preclude ataxia or excessive sedation.

If Prazepam is to be combined with other psychotropic agents or anticonvulsant drugs, careful consideration should be given to the pharmacology of the agents to be employed—particularly with known compounds which may potentiate the action of Prazepam, such as phenothiazines, narcotics, barbiturates, MAO inhibitors and other antidepressants.

Pediatric Use: Safety and effectiveness in patients below the age of 18 have not been established.

DRUG INTERACTIONS

If Prazepam is to be combined with other drugs acting on the central nervous system, careful consideration should be given to the pharmacology of the agents to be employed. The actions of the benzodiazepines may be potentiated by barbiturates, narcotics, phenothiazines, monoamine oxidase inhibitors, or other antidepressants.

If Prazepam is used to treat anxiety associated with somatic disease states, careful attention must be paid to possible drug interaction with concomitant medication.

ADVERSE REACTIONS

The side effects most frequently reported during double-blind, placebo-controlled trials employing a typical 30 mg divided total daily dosage and the percent incidence in the Prazepam group were fatigue (11.6%), dizziness (8.7%), weakness (7.7%), drowsiness (6.8%), lightheadedness (6.8%), and ataxia (5.0%). Less frequently reported were headache, confusion, tremor, vivid dreams, slurred speech, palpitation, stimulation, dry mouth, diaphoresis, and various gastrointestinal complaints. Other side effects included pruritus, transient skin rashes, swelling of feet, joint pains, various genitourinary complaints, blurred vision, and syncope. Single, nightly dose, controlled trials of variable dosages showed a dose-related incidence of these same side effects. Transient and reversible aberrations of liver function tests have been reported, as have been slight decreases in blood pressure and increases in body weight.

These findings are characteristic of benzodiazepine drugs.

OVERDOSAGE

As in the management of overdosage with any drug, it should be borne in mind that multiple agents may have been taken. Vomiting should be induced if it has not occurred spontaneously. Immediate gastric lavage is also recommended. General supportive care, including frequent monitoring of vital signs and close observation of the patient, is indicated. Hypotension, though unlikely, may be controlled with levarterenol bitartrate, or metaraminol bitartrate.

Flumazenil, a specific benzodiazepine receptor antagonist, is indicated for the complete or partial reversal of the sedative effects of benzodiazepines and may be used in situations when an overdose with a benzodiazepine is known or suspected. Flumazenil is intended as an adjunct to, not as a substitute for, proper management of benzodiazepine overdose. Patients treated with flumazenil should be monitored for re-sedation, respiratory depression, and other residual benzodiazepine effects for an appropriate period after treatment. The prescriber should be aware of a risk of seizure in association with flumazenil treatment, particularly in long-term benzodiazepine users and in cyclic antidepressant overdose. The complete flumazenil package insert including "Contraindications", "Warnings", and "Precautions" should be consulted prior to use.

DOSAGE AND ADMINISTRATION

Prazepam is administered orally in divided doses. The usual daily dose is 30 mg. The dose should be adjusted gradually within the range of 20 mg to 60 mg daily in accordance with the response of the patient. In elderly or debilitated patients it is advisable to initiate treatment at a divided daily dose of 10 mg to 15 mg (see "Precautions").

Prazepam may also be administered as a single, daily dose at bedtime. The recommended starting nightly dose is 20 mg. The response of the patient to several days' treatment will permit the physician to adjust the dose upwards or, occasionally, downwards to maximize antianxiety effect with a minimum of daytime drowsiness. The optimum dosage will usually range from 20 mg to 40 mg.

Store between 15° and 25° C (59° and 77° F). Protect from moisture.

HOW SUPPLIED
CAPSULE (C-IV): 10 MG

BRAND/MANUFACTURER	NDC	SIZE	AWP
○ GENERICS			
Allscrips	54569-2802-01	30s	$12.50
Allscrips	54569-2802-00	100s	$30.05

Praziquantel

DESCRIPTION

Praziquantel is a trematodicide provided in tablet form for the oral treatment of schistosome infections and infections due to liver fluke.

Praziquantel is 2-(cyclohexylcarbonyl)-1,2,3,6,7, 11b-hexahydro-4H-pyrazino [2, 1-a] isoquinolin-4-one with the molecular formula; $C_{19}H_{24}N_2O_2$.

Praziquantel is a white to nearly white crystalline powder of bitter taste. The compound is stable under normal conditions and melts at 136-140°C with decomposition. The active substance is hygroscopic. Praziquantel is easily soluble in chloroform and dimethylsulfoxide, soluble in ethanol and very slightly soluble in water.

Praziquantel tablets contain 600 mg of Praziquantel.

Following is its chemical structure:

CLINICAL PHARMACOLOGY

Praziquantel induces a rapid contraction of schistosomes by a specific effect on the permeability of the cell membrane. The drug further causes vacuolization and disintegration of the schistosome tegument.

After oral administration Praziquantel is rapidly absorbed (80%), subjected to a first pass effect, metabolized and eliminated by the kidneys. Maximal serum concentration is achieved 1-3 hours after dosing. The half-life of Praziquantel in serum is 0.8-1.5 hours.

INDICATIONS AND USAGE

Praziquantel is indicated for the treatment of infections due to: all species of schistosoma (eg. *Schistosoma mekongi, Schistosoma japonicum, Schistosoma mansoni and Schistosoma hernatobium)*, and infections due to the liver flukes, *Clonorchis sinensis/Opisthorchis viverrini* (approval of this indication was based on studies in which the two species were not differentiated).

UNLABELED USES

Praziquantel is used alone or as an adjunct in the treatment of paragonimiasis, neurocysticercosis, and cysticercosis. It is also used in Hymenolepis nana and Fasciolopsis buski infections.

CONTRAINDICATIONS

Praziquantel should not be given to patients who previously have shown hypersensitivity to the drug. Since parasite destruction within the eye may cause irreparable lesions, ocular cysticercosis should not be treated with this compound.

PRECAUTIONS

Information for the Patient: Patients should be warned not to drive a car and not to operate machinery on the day of Praziquantel treatment and the following day.

Minimal increases in liver enzymes have been reported in some patients.

When schistosomiasis or fluke infection is found to be associated with cerebral cysticercosis it is advised to hospitalize the patient for the duration of treatment.

Drug Interactions: No data are available regarding interaction of Praziquantel with other drugs.

Mutagenesis, Carcinogenesis: Mutagenic effects in Salmonella tests found by one laboratory have not been confirmed in the same tested strain by other laboratories. Long term carcinogenicity studies in rats and golden hamsters did not reveal any carcinogenic effect.

Pregnancy Category B: Reproduction studies have been performed in rats and rabbits at doses up to 40 times the human dose and have revealed no evidence of impaired fertility or harm to the fetus due to Praziquantel. There are, however, no adequate and well-controlled studies in pregnant women. An increase of the abortion rate was found in rats at three times the single human therapeutic dose. While animal reproduction studies are not always predictive of human response, this drug should be used during pregnancy only if clearly needed.

Nursing Mothers: Praziquantel appeared in the milk of nursing women at a concentration of about ¼ that of maternal serum. Women should not nurse on the day of Praziquantel treatment and during the subsequent 72 hours.

Pediatric Use: Safety in children under 4 years of age has not been established.

ADVERSE EFFECTS

In general Praziquantel is very well tolerated. Side effects are usually mild and transient and do not require treatment. The following side effects were observed generally in order of severity: malaise, headache, dizziness, abdominal discomfort with or without nausea, rise in temperature and, rarely, urticaria. Such symptoms can, however, also result from the infection itself. Such side effects may be more frequent and/or serious in patients with a heavy worm burden. In patients with liver impairment caused by the infection, no adverse effects of Praziquantel have occurred which would necessitate restriction in use.

OVERDOSAGE

In rats and mice the acute LD_{50} was about 2,500 mg/kg. No data are available in humans. In the event of overdose a fast-acting laxative should be given.

DOSAGE AND ADMINISTRATION

The dosage recommended for the treatment of schistosomiasis is: 3×20 mg/kg bodyweight as a one day treatment. The recommended dose for clonorchiasis and opisthorchiasis is: 3×25 mg/kg as a one day treatment. The tablets should be washed down unchewed with some liquid during meals. Keeping the tablets or segments thereof in the mouth can reveal a bitter taste which can promote gagging or vomiting. The interval between the individual doses should not be less than 4 and not more than 6 hours.

Tablets: When broken each of the four segments contain 150 mg of active ingredient so that the dosage can be easily adjusted to the patient's bodyweight.

Segments are broken off by pressing the score (notch) with thumbnails. If ¼ of a tablet is required, this is best achieved by breaking the segment from the outer end.

Storage: Store below 86°F (30°C).

HOW SUPPLIED
TABLETS: 600 MG

BRAND/MANUFACTURER	NDC	SIZE	AWP
○ BRAND			
BILTRICIDE: Miles Pharm	00026-2521-06	6s	$61.88

Prazosin Hydrochloride

DESCRIPTION

Prazosin Hydrochloride, a quinazoline derivative, is the first of a new chemical class of antihypertensives. It is the Hydrochloride salt of 1-(4-amino-6,7-dimethoxy-2-quinazolinyl)-4-(2-furoyl) piperazine.

It is a white, crystalline substance, slightly soluble in water and isotonic saline, and has a molecular weight of 419.87. Each 1 mg capsule of Prazosin Hydrochloride for oral use contains drug equivalent to 1 mg free base.

Prazosin HCl is available as a 1 mg, 2 mg, and 5 mg capsule for oral administration.

Following is its chemical structure:

CLINICAL PHARMACOLOGY

The exact mechanism of the hypotensive action of Prazosin is unknown. Prazosin causes a decrease in total peripheral resistance and was originally thought to have a direct relaxant action on vascular smooth muscle. Recent animal studies, however, have suggested that the vasodilator effect of Prazosin is also related to blockade of postsynaptic *alpha*-adrenoceptors. The results of dog forelimb experiments demonstrate that the peripheral vasodilator effect of Prazosin is confined mainly to the level of the resistance vessels (arterioles). Unlike conventional *alpha*-blockers, the antihypertensive action of Prazosin is usually not accompanied by a reflex tachycardia. Tolerance has not been observed to develop in long term therapy.

Hemodynamic studies have been carried out in man following acute single dose administration and during the course of long term maintenance therapy. The results confirm that the therapeutic effect is a fall in blood pressure unaccompanied by a clinically significant change in cardiac output, heart rate, renal blood flow and glomerular filtration rate. There is no measurable negative chronotropic effect.

In clinical studies to date, Prazosin HCl has not increased plasma renin activity.

In man, blood pressure is lowered in both the supine and standing positions. This effect is most pronounced on the diastolic blood pressure.

Following oral administration, human plasma concentrations reach a peak at about three hours with a plasma half-life of two to three hours. The drug is highly bound to plasma protein. Bioavailability studies have demonstrated that the total absorption relative to the drug in a 20% alcoholic solution is 90%, resulting in peak levels approximately 65% of that of the drug in solution. Animal studies indicate that Prazosin HCl is extensively metabolized, primarily by demethylation and conjugation, and excreted mainly via bile and feces. Less extensive human studies suggest similar metabolism and excretion in man.

In clinical studies in which lipid profiles were followed, there were generally no adverse changes noted between pre- and posttreatment lipid levels.

INDICATIONS AND USAGE

Prazosin HCl is indicated in the treatment of hypertension. It can be used alone or in combination with other antihypertensive drugs such as diuretics or beta-adrenergic blocking agents.

UNLABELED USES

Prazosin is used alone or as an adjunct in the treatment of congestive heart failure and Raynaud's disease, and in the symptomatic treatment of benign prostatic hyperplasia.

CONTRAINDICATIONS

None known.

WARNINGS

Prazosin HCl may cause syncope with sudden loss of consciousness. In most cases this is believed to be due to an excessive postural hypotensive effect, although occasionally the syncopal episode has been preceded by a bout of severe tachycardia with heart rates of 120-160 beats per minute. Syncopal episodes have usually occurred within 30 to 90 minutes of the initial dose of the drug; occasionally they have been reported in association with rapid dosage increases or the introduction of another antihypertensive drug into the regimen of a patient taking high doses of Prazosin HCl. The incidence of syncopal episodes is approximately 1% in patients given an initial dose of 2 mg or greater. Clinical trials conducted during the investigational phase of this drug suggest that syncopal episodes can be minimized by limiting the initial dose of the drug to 1 mg, by subsequently increasing the dosage slowly, and by introducing any additional antihypertensive drugs into the patient's regimen with caution (see "Dosage and Administration"). Hypotension may develop in patients given Prazosin HCl who are also receiving a beta-blocker such as Propranolol.

If syncope occurs, the patient should be placed in the recumbent position and treated supportively as necessary. This adverse effect is self-limiting and in most cases does not recur after the initial period of therapy or during subsequent dose titration.

Patients should always be started on the 1 mg capsules of Prazosin HCl. The 2 and 5 mg capsules are not indicated for initial therapy.

More common than loss of consciousness are the symptoms often associated with lowering of the blood pressure, namely, dizziness and lightheadedness. The patient should be cautioned about these possible adverse effects and advised what measures to take should they develop. The patient should also be cautioned to avoid situations where injury could result should syncope occur during the initiation of Prazosin HCl therapy.

PRECAUTIONS

Information for Patients: Dizziness or drowsiness may occur after the first dose of this medicine. Avoid driving or performing hazardous tasks for the first 24 hours after taking this medicine or when the dose is increased. Dizziness, lightheadedness or fainting may occur, especially when rising from a lying or sitting position. Getting up slowly may help lessen the problem. These effects may also occur if you drink alcohol, stand for long periods of time, exercise, or if the weather is hot. While taking Prazosin HCl, be careful in the amount of alcohol you drink. Also, use extra care during exercise or hot weather, or if standing for long periods. Check with your physician if you have any questions.

Drug Interactions: Prazosin HCl has been administered without any adverse drug interaction in limited clinical experience to date with the following: (1) cardiac glycosides—digitalis and digoxin; (2) hypoglycemics—insulin, chlorpropamide, phenformin, tolazamide, and tolbutamide; (3) tranquilizers and sedatives—chlordiazepoxide, diazepam, and phenobarbital; (4) antigout—allopurinol, colchicine, and probenecid; (5) antiarrhythmics—procainamide, propranolol (see "Warnings" however), and quinidine; and (6) analgesics, antipyretics and anti-inflammatories—propoxyphene, aspirin, indomethacin, and phenylbutazone.

Addition of a diuretic or other antihypertensive agent to Prazosin HCl has been shown to cause an additive hypotensive effect. This effect can be minimized by reducing the Prazosin HCl dose to 1 to 2 mg three times a day, by introducing additional antihypertensive drugs cautiously and then by retitrating Prazosin HCl based on clinical response.

Drug/Laboratory Test Interactions: In a study on five patients given from 12 to 24 mg of Prazosin per day for 10 to 14 days, there was an average increase of 42% in the urinary metabolite of norepinephrine and an average increase in urinary VMA of 17%. Therefore, false positive results may occur in screening tests for pheochromocytoma in patients who are being treated with Prazosin. If an elevated VMA is found, Prazosin should be discontinued and the patient retested after a month.

Laboratory Tests: In clinical studies in which lipid profiles were followed, there were generally no adverse changes noted between pre- and post-treatment lipid levels.

Carcinogenesis, Mutagenesis, Impairment of Fertility: No carcinogenic potential was demonstrated in an 18 month study in rats with Prazosin HCl at dose levels more than 225 times the usual maximum recommended human dose of 20 mg per day. Prazosin HCl was not mutagenic in *in vivo* genetic toxicology studies. In a fertility and general reproductive performance study in rats, both males and females, treated with 75 mg/kg (225 times the usual maximum recommended human dose), demonstrated decreased fertility while those treated with 25 mg/kg (75 times the usual maximum recommended human dose) did not.

In chronic studies (one year or more) of Prazosin HCl in rats and dogs, testicular changes consisting of atrophy and necrosis occurred at 25 mg/kg/day (75 times the usual maximum recommended human dose). No testicular changes were seen in rats or dogs at 10 mg/kg/day (30 times the usual maximum recommended human dose). In view of the testicular changes observed in animals, 105 patients on long term Prazosin HCl therapy were monitored for 17-ketosteroid excretion and no changes indicating a drug effect were observed. In addition, 27 males on Prazosin HCl for up to 51 months did not have changes in sperm morphology suggestive of drug effect.

Usage in Pregnancy: Pregnancy Category C. Prazosin HCl has been shown to be associated with decreased litter size at birth, 1, 4, and 21 days of age in rats when given doses more than 225 times the usual maximum recommended human dose. No evidence of drug-related external, visceral, or skeletal fetal abnormalities were observed. No drug-related external, visceral, or skeletal abnormalities were observed in fetuses of pregnant rabbits and pregnant monkeys at doses more than 225 times and 12 times the usual maximum recommended human dose respectively.

The use of Prazosin and a beta-blocker for the control of severe hypertension in 44 pregnant women revealed no drug-related fetal abnormalities or adverse effects. Therapy with Prazosin was continued for as long as 14 weeks.[1]

Prazosin has also been used alone or in combination with other hypotensive agents in severe hypertension of pregnancy by other investigators. No fetal or neonatal abnormalities have been reported with the use of Prazosin.[2]

There are no adequate and well controlled studies which establish the safety of Prazosin HCl in pregnant women. Prazosin HCl should be used during pregnancy only if the potential benefit justifies the potential risk to the mother and fetus.

Nursing Mothers: Prazosin HCl has been shown to be excreted in small amounts in human milk. Caution should be exercised when Prazosin HCl is administered to a nursing woman.

Usage in Children: Safety and effectiveness in children have not been established.

ADVERSE REACTIONS

Clinical trials were conducted on more than 900 patients. During these trials and subsequent marketing experience the most frequent reactions associated with Prazosin HCl therapy are: dizziness 10.3%, headache 7.8%, drowsiness 7.6%, lack of energy 6.9%, weakness 6.5%, palpitations 5.3%, and nausea 4.9%. In most instances side effects have disappeared with continued therapy or have been tolerated with no decrease in dose of drug.

Less frequent adverse reactions which are reported to occur in 1-4% of patients are:

Gastrointestinal: vomiting, diarrhea, constipation.

Cardiovascular: edema, orthostatic hypotension, dyspnea, syncope.

Central Nervous System: vertigo, depression, nervousness.

Dermatologic: rash.

Genitourinary: urinary frequency.

EENT: blurred vision, reddened sclera, epistaxis, dry mouth, nasal congestion.

In addition, fewer than 1% of patients have reported the following (in some instances, exact causal relationships have not been established).

Gastrointestinal: abdominal discomfort and/or pain, liver function abnormalities, pancreatitis.

Cardiovascular: tachycardia.

Central Nervous System: paresthesia, hallucinations.

Dermatologic: pruritus, alopecia, lichen planus.

Genitourinary: incontinence, impotence, priapism.

EENT: tinnitus.

Other: diaphoresis, fever, positive ANA titer, arthralgia.

◆ **RATED THERAPEUTICALLY EQUIVALENT;** ◇ **THERAPEUTIC EQUIVALENCE UNCONFIRMED;** ○ **UNRATED**

Single reports of pigmentary motting and serous retinopathy, and a few reports of cataract development or disappearance have been reported. In these instances, the exact causal relationship has not been established because the baseline observations were frequently inadequate.

In more specific slit-lamp and funduscopic studies, which included adequate baseline examinations, no drug-related abnormal ophthalmological findings have been reported.

Literature reports exist associating Prazosin HCl therapy with a worsening of pre-existing narcolepsy. A causal relationship is uncertain in these cases.

OVERDOSAGE

Accidental ingestion of at least 50 mg of Prazosin HCl in a two year old child resulted in profound drowsiness and depressed reflexes. No decrease in blood pressure was noted. Recovery was uneventful.

Should overdosage lead to hypotension, support of the cardiovascular system is of first importance. Restoration of blood pressure and normalization of heart rate may be accomplished by keeping the patient in the supine position. If this measure is inadequate, shock should first be treated with volume expanders. If necessary, vasopressors should then be used. Renal function should be monitored and supported as needed. Laboratory data indicate Prazosin HCl is not dialysable because it is protein bound.

DOSAGE AND ADMINISTRATION

The dose of Prazosin HCl should be adjusted according to the patient's individual blood pressure response. The following is a guide to its administration:

INITIAL DOSE
1 mg two or three times a day. (See *"Warnings"*).

MAINTENANCE DOSE
Dosage may be slowly increased to a total daily dose of 20 mg given in divided doses. The therapeutic dosages most commonly employed have ranged from 6 mg to 15 mg daily given in divided doses. Doses higher than 20 mg usually do not increase efficacy, however a few patients may benefit from further increases up to a daily dose of 40 mg given in divided doses. After initial titration some patients can be maintained adequately on a twice daily dosage regimen.

USE WITH OTHER DRUGS
When adding a diuretic or other antihypertensive agent, the dose of Prazosin HCl should be reduced to 1 mg or 2 mg three times a day and retitration then carried out.

REFERENCES
1. Lubbe, WF, and Hodge, JV: *New Zealand Med J* **94**(691) 169-172, 1981. 2. Davey, DA, and Dommisse, J: *S.A. Med J*, Oct 4, 1980 (551-556). 69-2318-37-2

HOW SUPPLIED
CAPSULE: 1 MG

AVERAGE UNIT PRICE (AVAILABLE SIZES)		GENERIC A-RATED AVERAGE PRICE (GAAP)	
BRAND	$0.43	60s	$18.18
GENERIC	$0.25	100s	$27.10
HCFA FUL (100s ea)	$0.06	250s	$56.50
		1000s	$218.20

BRAND/MANUFACTURER	NDC	SIZE	AWP
◆ BRAND			
➤ MINIPRESS: Pfizer Labs	00663-4310-41	100s ud	$48.04
	00069-4310-71	250s	$103.54
	00663-4310-71	250s	$103.54
	00663-4310-82	1000s	$405.99
◆ GENERICS			
Schein	00364-2389-06	60s	$13.95
Major	00904-1040-52	60s	$22.40
Schein	00364-2389-01	100s	$22.35
➤ Goldline	00182-1920-01	100s	$22.50
Moore,H.L.	00839-7554-06	100s	$23.34
Lederle Std Prod	00005-3473-43	100s	$23.51
Qualitest	00603-5286-21	100s	$23.80
Parmed	00349-8694-01	100s	$24.11
Geneva	00781-2211-01	100s	$24.11
URL	00677-1368-01	100s	$24.72
Purepac	00228-2500-10	100s	$24.77
Aligen	00405-4816-01	100s	$24.80
Zenith	00172-4067-60	100s	$26.05
➤ Goldline	00182-1255-01	100s	$26.05
Mylan	00378-1101-01	100s	$26.21
Martec	52555-0279-01	100s	$26.85
U.S. Trading	56126-0463-11	100s ud	$10.04
Schein	00364-2389-90	100s ud	$24.60
Vangard	00615-0386-13	100s ud	$26.04
➤ Goldline	00182-1920-89	100s ud	$41.55
Medirex	57480-0384-01	100s ud	$48.25
UDL	51079-0630-20	100s ud	$48.28
Rugby	00536-4845-02	250s	$34.88
Qualitest	00603-5286-24	250s	$48.11
Goldline	00182-1920-02	250s	$52.50
Schein	00364-2389-04	250s	$52.80
Moore,H.L.	00839-7554-09	250s	$52.92

BRAND/MANUFACTURER	NDC	SIZE	AWP
Purepac	00228-2500-25	250s	$52.93
Lederle Std Prod	00005-3473-27	250s	$55.99
URL	00677-1368-03	250s	$57.35
Geneva	00781-2211-25	250s	$57.40
Major	00904-1040-70	250s	$59.70
Zenith	00172-4067-65	250s	$63.10
➤ Goldline	00182-1255-02	250s	$63.10
Aligen	00405-4816-04	250s	$63.20
Mylan	00378-1101-25	250s	$63.60
Parmed	00349-8694-25	250s	$69.96
Schein	00364-2389-05	500s	$100.58
Lederle Std Prod	00005-3473-34	1000s	$168.95
Moore,H.L.	00839-7554-16	1000s	$203.11
Geneva	00781-2211-10	1000s	$211.23
Purepac	00228-2500-96	1000s	$216.49
Parmed	00349-8694-10	1000s	$217.79
Major	00904-1040-80	1000s	$234.15
Zenith	00172-4067-80	1000s	$246.90
Mylan	00378-1101-10	1000s	$247.00

CAPSULE: 2 MG

AVERAGE UNIT PRICE (AVAILABLE SIZES)		GENERIC A-RATED AVERAGE PRICE (GAAP)	
BRAND	$0.60	100s	$36.22
GENERIC	$0.33	250s	$76.09
HCFA FUL (100s ea)	$0.07	1000s	$294.91

BRAND/MANUFACTURER	NDC	SIZE	AWP
◆ BRAND			
➤ MINIPRESS: Pfizer Labs	00663-4370-41	100s ud	$66.53
	00663-4370-71	250s	$144.15
	00663-4370-82	1000s	$565.10
◆ GENERICS			
Major	00904-1041-52	60s	$31.20
Moore,H.L.	00839-7555-06	100s	$29.96
Schein	00364-2390-01	100s	$31.13
Lederle Std Prod	00005-3474-43	100s	$31.18
Purepac	00228-2501-10	100s	$32.17
Aligen	00405-4817-01	100s	$32.80
Geneva	00781-2212-01	100s	$33.58
Qualitest	00603-5287-21	100s	$33.95
Parmed	00349-8695-01	100s	$33.98
URL	00677-1369-01	100s	$34.00
Zenith	00172-4068-60	100s	$34.30
Goldline	00182-1256-01	100s	$34.30
Mylan	00378-2302-01	100s	$34.50
Goldline	00182-1921-01	100s	$34.50
Martec	52555-0280-01	100s	$34.98
U.S. Trading	56126-0464-11	100s ud	$12.92
Schein	00364-2390-90	100s ud	$34.10
Vangard	00615-0387-13	100s ud	$36.16
Goldline	00182-1921-89	100s ud	$57.55
Medirex	57480-0385-01	100s ud	$59.15
UDL	51079-0631-20	100s ud	$59.17
Rugby	00536-4846-02	250s	$46.00
Moore,H.L.	00839-7555-09	250s	$49.88
Purepac	00228-2501-25	250s	$72.13
Schein	00364-2390-04	250s	$73.56
Qualitest	00603-5287-24	250s	$73.96
Goldline	00182-1921-02	250s	$75.00
Lederle Std Prod	00005-3474-27	250s	$77.96
Aligen	00405-4817-04	250s	$78.03
URL	00677-1369-03	250s	$79.00
Major	00904-1041-70	250s	$83.15
Zenith	00172-4068-65	250s	$83.65
Geneva	00781-2212-25	250s	$83.65
Goldline	00182-1256-02	250s	$83.65
Mylan	00378-2302-25	250s	$83.95
Martec	52555-0280-02	250s	$85.35
Parmed	00349-8695-25	250s	$88.45
Schein	00364-2390-05	500s	$140.10
Moore,H.L.	00839-7555-16	1000s	$224.36
Lederle Std Prod	00005-3474-34	1000s	$225.48
Purepac	00228-2501-96	1000s	$294.35
Parmed	00349-8695-10	1000s	$303.95
Major	00904-1041-80	1000s	$325.90
Geneva	00781-2212-10	1000s	$326.00
Zenith	00172-4068-80	1000s	$329.20
Mylan	00378-2302-10	1000s	$330.00

For additional alternatives, turn to the section beginning on page 2859.

For additional alternatives, turn to the section beginning on page 2859.

Pre-Pen SEE BENZYLPENICILLOYL POLYLYSINE

Pred Forte SEE PREDNISOLONE ACETATE, OPHTHALMIC AND PREDNISOLONE, SYSTEMIC

➤ SHOWN IN PRODUCT IDENTIFICATION GUIDE

Pred Mild SEE PREDNISOLONE ACETATE, OPHTHALMIC AND PREDNISOLONE, SYSTEMIC

Pred-G SEE GENTAMICIN SULFATE AND PREDNISOLONE ACETATE

Prednicarbate

DESCRIPTION

FOR DERMATOLOGIC USE ONLY. NOT FOR USE IN EYES.

Prednicarbate emollient cream 0.1% contains the nonhalogenated prednisolone derivative, Prednicarbate. Topical corticosteroids constitute a class of primarily synthetic steroids used topically as anti-inflammatory and antipruritic agents. Each gram of Prednicarbate emollient cream 0.1% contains 1.0 mg of Prednicarbate in a base consisting of white petrolatum USP, purified water USP, isopropyl myristate NF, lanolin alcohols NF, mineral oil USP, cetostearyl alcohol NF, aluminum stearate, edetate disodium USP, lactic acid USP, and magnesium stearate DAB 9.

The chemical name of Prednicarbate is 11β, 17, 21-trihydroxypregna-1,4-diene-3,20-dione 17-(ethyl carbonate) 21-propionate. Prednicarbate has the empirical formula $C_{27}H_{36}O_8$ and a molecular weight of 488.58.

The CAS Registry Number is 73771-04-7.

Following is its chemical structure:

CLINICAL PHARMACOLOGY

In common with other topical corticosteroids, Prednicarbate has anti-inflammatory, antipruritic, and vasoconstrictive properties. In general, the mechanism of the anti-inflammatory activity of topical steroids is unclear. However, corticosteroids are thought to act by the induction of phospholipase A_2 inhibitory proteins, collectively called lipocortins. It is postulated that these proteins control the biosynthesis of potent mediators of inflammation such as prostaglandins and leukotrienes by inhibiting the release of their common precursor arachidonic acid. Arachidonic acid is released from membrane phospholipids by phospholipase A_2.

PHARMACOKINETICS

The extent of percutaneous absorption of topical corticosteroids is determined by many factors, including the vehicle and the integrity of the epidermal barrier. Use of occlusive dressings with hydrocortisone for up to 24 hours has not been shown to increase penetration; however, occlusion of hydrocortisone for 96 hours does markedly enhance penetration. Topical corticosteroids can be absorbed from normal intact skin, whereas inflammation and/or other disease processes in the skin increase percutaneous absorption.

Studies performed with Prednicarbate emollient cream 0.1% indicate that the drug is in the medium range of potency compared with other topical corticosteroids.

INDICATIONS AND USAGE

Prednicarbate emollient cream 0.1% is a medium-potency corticosteroid indicated for the relief of the inflammatory and pruritic manifestations of corticosteroid-responsive dermatoses.

CONTRAINDICATIONS

Prednicarbate emollient cream 0.1% is contraindicated in those patients with a history of hypersensitivity to any of the components of the preparations.

PRECAUTIONS

GENERAL

Systemic absorption of topical corticosteroids can produce reversible hypothalamic-pituitary-adrenal (HPA) axis suppression with the potential for glucocorticosteroid insufficiency after withdrawal of treatment. Manifestations of Cushing's syndrome, hyperglycemia, and glucosuria can also be produced in some patients by systemic absorption of topical corticosteroids while on treatment.

Patients receiving a large dose of a higher-potency topical steroid applied to a large surface area or under occlusion should be evaluated periodically for evidence of HPA-axis suppression. This may be done by using the ACTH stimulation, AM plasma cortisol, and urinary free cortisol tests.

Prednicarbate emollient cream 0.1% did not produce significant HPA-axis suppression when used at a dose of 30 g/day for a week in 10 patients with extensive psoriasis or atopic dermatitis.

If HPA-axis suppression is noted, an attempt should be made to withdraw the drug, to reduce the frequency of application, or to substitute a less potent corticosteroid. Recovery of HPA-axis function is generally prompt and complete upon discontinuation of topical corticosteroids. Infrequently, signs and symptoms of glucocorticosteroid insufficiency may occur, requiring supplemental systemic corticosteroids. For information on systemic supplementation, see prescribing information for those products.

Children may be more susceptible to systemic toxicity from equivalent doses due to their larger skin surface to body mass ratios. (See "Precautions—Pediatric Use".)

If irritation develops, Prednicarbate emollient cream 0.1% should be discontinued and appropriate therapy instituted. Allergic contact dermatitis with corticosteroids is usually diagnosed by observing failure to heal rather than noting a clinical exacerbation, as observed with most topical products not containing corticosteroids. Such an observation should be corroborated with appropriate diagnostic patch testing.

If concomitant skin infections are present or develop, an appropriate antifungal or antibacterial agent should be used. If a favorable response does not occur promptly, use of Prednicarbate emollient cream 0.1% should be discontinued until the infection has been adequately controlled.

INFORMATION FOR PATIENTS

Patients using topical corticosteroids should receive the following information and instructions:

1. This medication is to be used as directed by the physician. It is for external use only. Avoid contact with the eyes.

2. This medication should not be used for any disorder other than that for which it was prescribed.

3. The treated skin area should not be bandaged or otherwise covered or wrapped so as to be occlusive, unless directed by the physician.

4. Patients should report any signs of local adverse reactions to their physician.

LABORATORY TESTS

The following tests may be helpful in evaluating patients for HPA-axis suppression:

ACTH stimulation test
AM plasma cortisol test
Urinary free cortisol test

CARCINOGENESIS, MUTAGENESIS, AND IMPAIRMENT OF FERTILITY

In a study of the effect of Prednicarbate on fertility, pregnancy, and postnatal development in rats, no effect was noted on the fertility or pregnancy of the parent animals or postnatal development of the off-spring after administration of up to 0.80 mg/kg of Prednicarbate subcutaneously.

Prednicarbate has been evaluated in the Salmonella reversion test (Ames test) over a wide range of concentrations in the presence and absence of an S-9 liver microsomal fraction, and did not demonstrate mutagenic activity. Similarly, Prednicarbate did not produce any significant changes in the numbers of micronuclei seen in erythrocytes when mice were given doses ranging from 1 to 160 mg/kg of the drug.

PREGNANCY: TERATOGENIC EFFECTS: PREGNANCY CATEGORY C

Corticosteroids have been shown to be teratogenic in laboratory animals when administered systemically at relatively low dosage levels. Some corticosteroids have been shown to be teratogenic after dermal application in laboratory animals.

Prednicarbate has been shown to be teratogenic and embryotoxic in Wistar rats and Himalayan rabbits when given subcutaneously during gestation at doses 1900 × and 45 × the recommended topical human dose, assuming a percutaneous absorption of approximately 3%.

In the rats, slightly retarded fetal development and an incidence of thickened and wavy ribs higher than the spontaneous rate were noted.

In rabbits, increased liver weights and slight increase in the fetal intrauterine death rate were observed. The fetuses that were delivered exhibited reduced placental weight, increased frequency of cleft palate, ossification disorders in the sternum, omphalocele, and anomalous posture of the forelimbs.

There are no adequate and well-controlled studies in pregnant women on teratogenic effects of Prednicarbate. Therefore, Prednicarbate emollient cream 0.1% should be used during pregnancy only if the potential benefit justifies the potential risk to the fetus.

NURSING MOTHERS

Systemically administered corticosteroids appear in human milk and could suppress growth, interfere with endogenous corticosteroid production, or cause other untoward effects. It is not known whether topical administration of corticosteroids could result in sufficient systemic absorption to produce detectable quantities in human milk. Because many drugs are excreted in human milk, caution should be exercised when Prednicarbate emollient cream 0.1% is administered to a nursing woman.

PEDIATRIC USE

Safety and effectiveness of Prednicarbate Emollient Cream 0.1% in persons below the age of 18 years have not been established. Because of a higher ratio of skin surface area to body mass, children are at a greater risk than adults of HPA-axis suppression when they are treated with topical corticosteroids. They are therefore also at greater risk of glucocorticosteroid insufficiency after withdrawal of treatment and at greater risk of Cushing's syndrome while on treatment. Adverse effects including striae have been reported with inappropriate use of topical corticosteroids in infants and children (see "Precautions").

HPA-axis suppression, Cushing's syndrome, and intracranial hypertension have been reported in children receiving topical corticosteroids. Manifestations of adrenal suppression in children include linear growth retardation, delayed weight

---

◆ RATED THERAPEUTICALLY EQUIVALENT; ◇ THERAPEUTIC EQUIVALENCE UNCONFIRMED; ○ UNRATED

gain, low plasma cortisol levels, and absence of response to ACTH stimulation. Manifestations of intracranial hypertension include bulging fontanelles, headaches, and bilateral papilledema.

ADVERSE REACTIONS
In controlled clinical studies, the incidence of adverse reactions probably or possibly associated with the use of Prednicarbate emollient cream 0.1%, was approximately 4%. Reported reactions included mild signs of skin atrophy in 1% of treated patients, as well as the following reactions which were reported in less than 1% of patients: pruritus, edema, paresthesia, urticaria, burning, allergic contact dermatitis and rash.

The following additional local adverse reactions are reported infrequently with topical corticosteroids, but may occur more frequently with the use of occlusive dressings and especially with higher-potency corticosteroids. These reactions are listed in an approximate decreasing order of occurrence: dryness, folliculitis, acneiform eruptions, hypopigmentation, perioral dermatitis, secondary infection, striae, and miliaria.

OVERDOSAGE
Topically applied corticosteroids can be absorbed in sufficient amounts to produce systemic effects (see *"Precautions"*).

DOSAGE AND ADMINISTRATION
Apply a thin film of Prednicarbate emollient cream 0.1% to the affected skin areas twice daily. Rub in gently.
Store between 41° and 77°F (5° and 25°C).

CLINICAL STUDIES
Prednicarbate emollient cream 0.1% was studied in vehicle controlled clinical trials in psoriasis and atopic dermatitis. In both studies, patients were to be treated twice daily for 21 days. Improvement in erythema, induration and scaling were studied in the psoriasis protocol. At Endpoint (i.e., patient's last visit), the mean total sign scores for patients had decreased from baseline (i.e., improved) by 37% and were significantly better than vehicle (p< 0.001).

Improvement in erythema, induration and pruritus were studied in the atopic dermatitis protocol. At Endpoint (i.e., patient's last visit), the mean total sign/symptom scores for patients had decreased from baseline (i.e., improved) by 76% and were significantly better than vehicle (p< 0.001).

The evaluations were performed in separate protocols by different panels of investigators. Different sets of signs/symptoms were evaluated in each protocol. These data are presented for comparison purposes only.

OVERALL IMPROVEMENT OF DISEASE AT ENDPOINT — % OF PATIENTS

	Scale Number					
Indication	0	1	2	3	4	5
Psoriasis (n=105)	1%	16%	17%	51%	13%	1%
Atopic Dermatitis (n=98)	31%	42%	9%	12%	2%	4%

Scale:
0 = Cleared; 100% clearance of signs except for residual discoloration
1 = Excellent improvement; at least 75%, but less than 100% clearance of signs monitored
2 = Moderate improvement; at least 50%, but less than 75% clearance of signs monitored
3 = Slight improvement; less than 50% clearance of signs monitored
4 = No change; no detectable improvement from baseline condition
5 = Exacerbation; flare of sites under study

HOW SUPPLIED
CREAM: 0.1%

BRAND/MANUFACTURER	NDC	SIZE	AWP
○ BRAND			
DERMATOP: Hoechst Derm	00039-0088-15	15 gm	$10.75
	00039-0088-60	60 gm	$28.30

Prednisolone and Sulfacetamide Sodium

DESCRIPTION
Prednisolone/Sulfacetamide Sodium is a topical anti-inflammatory/anti-infective combination product for ophthalmic use.

Prednisolone/Sulfacetamide Sodium is available as a sterile ophthalmic suspension, ointment, and solution.

The suspension contains:
Prednisolone Acetate 0.2%
Sulfacetamide Sodium 10.0%

The ointment contains:
Prednisolone Acetate ....0.2% or 5 mg/gm
Sulfacetamide Sodium ....10.0% or 100 mg/gm

The solution contains:
Prednisolone Sodium Phosphate ....2.5 mg/ml
(equivalent to Prednisolone Phosphate 2.3 mg/ml)
Sulfacetamide Sodium ....100 mg/ml

The anti-inflammatory components, Prednisolone Acetate and Prednisolone Sodium Phosphate, both corticosteroids, are known chemically, respectively, as:
11β, 17, 21-trihydroxypregna-1, 4-diene-3, 20-dione 21-acetate
and
11β, 17, 21-trihydroxypregna-1, 4-diene-3, 20-dione, 21-(disodium phosphate)
The anti-infective component, Sulfacetamide Sodium, a bacteriostatic antibacterial, is known chemically as: N-sulfanilyl acetamide monosodium salt monohydrate.

CLINICAL PHARMACOLOGY
Corticosteroids suppress the inflammatory response to a variety of agents and they probably delay or slow healing. Since corticosteroids may inhibit the body's defense mechanism against infection, a concomitant antimicrobial drug may be used when this inhibition is considered to be clinically significant in a particular case.

Microbiology: Sulfacetamide Sodium exerts a bacteriostatic effect against susceptible bacteria by restricting the synthesis of folic acid required for growth through competition with p-aminobenzoic acid.

Some strains of these bacteria may be resistant to Sulfacetamide or resistant strains may emerge *in vivo*.

The anti-infective component in Prednisolone Sulfacetamide Sodium is included to provide action against specific organisms susceptible to it. Sulfacetamide Sodium is considered active against the following microorganisms: *Escherichia coli, Staphylococcus aureus, Streptococcus pneumoniae, Streptococcus (viridans group), Pseudomonas* species, *Haemophilus influenzae, Klebsiella* species, and *Enterobacter* species.

When a decision to administer both a corticosteroid and an antimicrobial is made, the administration of such drugs in combination has the advantage of greater patient compliance and convenience, with the added assurance that the appropriate dosage of both drugs is administered. When both types of drugs are in the same formulation, compatibility of ingredients is assured and the correct volume of drug is delivered and retained. The relative potency of corticosteroids depends on the molecular structure, concentration, and release from the vehicle.

INDICATIONS AND USAGE
A steroid/anti-infective combination is indicated for steroid-responsive inflammatory ocular conditions for which a corticosteroid is indicated and where superficial bacterial ocular infection or a risk of bacterial ocular infection exists.

Ocular steroids are indicated in inflammatory conditions of the palpebral and bulbar conjunctiva, cornea, and anterior segment of the globe where the inherent risk of steroid use in certain infective conjunctivitides is accepted to obtain a diminution in edema and inflammation. They are also indicated in chronic anterior uveitis and corneal injury from chemical, radiation, or thermal burns or penetration of foreign bodies. The use of a combination drug with an anti-infective component is indicated where the risk of superficial ocular infection is high or where there is an expectation that potentially dangerous numbers of bacteria will be present in the eye.

The particular anti-infective drug in this product is active against the following common bacterial eye pathogens: *Escherichia coli, Staphyloccus aureus, Streptococcus pneumoniae, Streptococcus (viridans group), Pseudomonas* species, *Haemophilus influenzae, Klebsiella* species, and *Enterobacter* species. This product does not provide adequate coverage against *Neisseria* species and *Serratia marcescens*.

A significant percentage of staphylococcal isolates are completely resistant to sulfa drugs.

CONTRAINDICATIONS
Epithelial herpes simplex keratitis (dendritic keratitis) vaccinia, varicella, and many other viral diseases of the cornea and conjunctiva. Mycobacterial infection of the eye. Fungal diseases of the ocular structures. Hypersensitivity to a component of the medication. (Hypersensitivity to the anti-microbial component occurs at a higher rate than for other components.)

The use of these combinations is always contraindicated after uncomplicated removal of a corneal foreign body.

WARNINGS
Prednisolone/Sulfacetamide Sodium solution is not for injection into the eye.

Prolonged use of corticosteroids may result in ocular hypertension glucoma, with damage to the optic nerve, defects in visual acuity and fields of vision, and in posterior subcapsular cataract formation. Prolonged use may suppress the host response and thus increase the hazard of secondary ocular infections. In those diseases causing thinning of the cornea or sclera, perforations have been known to occur with the use of topical steroids. In acute purulent conditions of the eye, steroids may mask infection or enhance existing infection. If these products are used for 10 days or longer, intraocular pressure should be routinely monitored even though it may be difficult in children and uncooperative patients. Corticosteroids should be used with caution in the presence of glaucoma. Intraocular pressure should be checked frequently.

The use of ocular corticosteroids may prolong the course and may exacerbate the severity of many viral infections of the eye (including herpes simplex).

Employment of a steroid medication in the treatment of herpes simplex requires great caution.

A significant percentage of staphylococcal isolates are completely resistant to sulfa drugs.

Acute anterior uveitis may occur in susceptible individuals, primarily Blacks.

The use of steroids after cataract surgery may delay healing and increase the incidence of filtering blebs.

Topical steroids are not effective in mustard gas keratitis and Sjögren's keratoconjunctivitis.

Fatalities have occurred, although rarely, due to severe reactions to sulfonamides including Stevens-Johnson syndrome, toxic epidermal necrolysis, fulminant hepatic necrosis, agranulocytosis, aplastic anemia, and other blood dyscrasias. Sensitizations may recur when a sulfonamide is readministered, irrespective of the route of administration. If signs of hypersensitivity or other serious reactions occur, discontinue use of this preparation.

Cross-sensitivity among corticosteroids has been demonstrated (see "Adverse Reactions").

Some brands contain thimerosal as a preservative. Do not administer to patients who are sensitive/allergic to thimerosal or any other mercury-containing ingredient.

PRECAUTIONS

The initial prescription and renewal of the medication order beyond 20 ml of the suspension or solution or 8 g of the ointment should be made by a physician only after examination of the patient with the aid of magnification, such as slit lamp biomicroscopy and, where appropriate, fluorescein staining. If signs and symptoms fail to improve after two days, the patient should be re-evaluated.

The possibility of fungal infections of the cornea should be considered after prolonged steroid dosing.

Ophthalmic ointments may retard corneal healing.

Use with caution in patients with severe dry eye. Fungal cultures should be taken when appropriate.

The p-aminobenzoic acid present in purulent exudates competes with sulfonamides and can reduce their effectiveness.

Sulfonamide solutions darken on prolonged standing and exposure to heat and light. Do not use if solution has darkened. Yellowing does not affect activity.

Information for Patients: If inflammation or pain persists longer than 18 hours or becomes aggravated, the patient should be advised to discontinue use of the medication and consult a physician (see "Warning").

This product is sterile when packaged. To prevent contamination, care should be taken to avoid touching the container tip to eyelids or to any other surface. The use of this container by more than one person may spread infection. Keep container tightly closed when not in use. Protect from light. Sulfonamide solutions darken on prolonged standing and exposure to heat and light. Do not use if solution has darkened. Yellowing does not affect activity. Keep out of the reach of children.

Laboratory Tests: Eyelid cultures and tests to determine the susceptibility of organisms to Sulfacetamide may be indicated if signs and symptoms persist or recur in spite of the recommended course of treatment with Prednisolone/Sulfacetamide Sodium Ophthalmic suspension, ointment, or solution.

Drug Interactions: The ointment and solution are incompatible with silver preparations. Local anesthetics related to p-aminobenzoic acid may antagonize the action of the sulfonamides.

Carcinogenesis, Mutagenesis, Impairment of Fertility: Prednisolone has been reported to be noncarcinogenic. Long-term animal studies for carcinogenic potential have not been performed with Prednisolone or Sulfacetamide.

One author detected chromosomal nondisjunction in the yeast *Saccharomyces cerevisiae* following application of Sulfacetamide Sodium. The significance of this finding to topical ophthalmic use of Sulfacetamide Sodium in the human is unknown.

Mutagenic studies with Prednisolone have been negative. Studies on reproduction and fertility have not been performed with Sulfacetamide. A long-term chronic toxicity study in dogs showed that high oral doses of Prednisolone prevented estrus. A decrease in fertility was seen in male and female rats that were mated following oral dosing with another glucocorticosteroid.

Pregnancy: Teratogenic Effects: Pregnancy Category C: Animal reproduction studies have not been conducted with Sulfacetamide Sodium. Prednisolone has been shown to be teratogenic in rabbits, hamsters, and mice. In mice, Prednisolone has been shown to be teratogenic when given in doses 1 to 10 times the human ocular dose. Dexamethasone, hydrocortisone, and Prednisolone were ocularly applied to both eyes of pregnant mice five times per day on days 10 through 13 of gestation. A significant increase in the incidence of cleft palate was observed in the fetuses of the treated mice. There are no adequate well-controlled studies in pregnant women dosed with corticosteroids.

Kernicterus may be precipitated in infants by sulfonamides being given systemically during the third trimester of pregnancy. It is not known whether Sulfacetamide Sodium can cause fetal harm when administered to a pregnant woman or whether it can affect reproductive capacity.

Prednisolone/Sulfacetamide Sodium should be used during pregnancy only if the potential benefit justifies the potential risk to the fetus.

Nursing Mothers: It is not known whether topical administration of corticosteroids could result in sufficient systemic absorption to produce detectable quantities in human milk. Systemically administered corticosteroids appear in human milk and could suppress growth, interfere with endogenous corticosteroid production, or cause other untoward effects. Systemically administered sulfonamides are capable of producing kernicterus in infants of lactating women. Because of the potential for serious adverse reactions in nursing infants from Prednisolone/Sulfacetamide Sodium, a decision should be made whether to discontinue nursing or to discontinue the medication.

Pediatric Use: Safety and effectiveness in children below the age of six have not been established.

ADVERSE REACTIONS

Adverse reactions have occurred with steroid/anti-infective combination drugs which can be attributed to the steroid component, the anti-infective component, or the combination. Exact incidence figures are not available since no denominator of treated patients is available.

Reactions occurring most often from the presence of the anti-infective ingredient are allergic sensitizations. Fatalities have occurred, although rarely, due to severe reactions to sulfonamides including Stevens-Johnson syndrome, toxic epidermal necrolysis, fulminant hepatic necrosis, agranulocytosis, aplastic anemia, and other blood dyscrasias (see "Warnings").

Sulfacetamide Sodium may cause local irritation. The reactions due to the steroid component in decreasing order of frequency are: elevation of intraocular pressure (IOP) with possible development of glaucoma, and infrequent optic nerve damage; posterior subcapsular cataract formation; and delayed wound healing.

Although systemic effects are extremely uncommon, there have been rare occurrences of systemic hypercorticoidism after use of topical steroids.

Corticosteroid-containing preparations can also cause acute anterior uveitis or perforation of the globe. Mydriasis, loss of accommodation and ptosis have occasionally been reported following local use of corticosteroids.

Secondary infection: The development of secondary infection has occurred after use of combinations containing steroids and antimicrobials. Fungal and viral infections of the cornea are particularly prone to develop coincidentally with long-term applications of steroid. The possibility of fungal invasion must be considered in any persistent corneal ulceration where steroid treatment has been used.

Secondary bacterial ocular infection following suppression of host responses also occurs.

DOSAGE AND ADMINISTRATION

THE SUSPENSION

Optimal dosage is 1 drop two to four times daily, depending upon the severity of the condition.

In general, during early or acute stages of blepharitis, the suspension produces results most rapidly—and most efficiently—with installation directly into the eye, with the excess spread on the lid (Method I). When the condition is confined to the lid, however, the suspension may be applied directly to the site of the lesions (Method II).

Method I: In the Eye and On the Lid:
1. Wash hands carefully. Tilt head back and drop **1 drop** into the eye.
2. Close the eye and spread the excess medication present after closing the eye on the full length of the upper and lower lids.
3. Do not wipe any of the medication off the lids. It will dry completely in 4 or 5 minutes to a clear film that remains on the lids for several hours—it cannot be seen by others, nor will it interfere with vision.
4. The medication should be washed off the lids once or twice a day. **However, it should be reapplied after each washing.**

Method II: On the Lid:
1. Wash hands carefully. With head tilted back and **eye closed**, drop 1 drop onto the lid—preferably at the corner of the eye close to the nose.
2. Spread the medication over the full length of the upper and lower lids.
3. Do not wipe away any medication—it will dry in 4 to 5 minutes to a clear, invisible film which will remain on the lids for several hours.
4. The medication should be washed off the lids once or twice a day. **However, it should be reapplied after each washing.**

Not more than 20 ml should be prescribed initially and the prescription should not be refilled without further evaluation as outlined in "Precautions" above.

THE OINTMENT

(Approximately ½ inch ribbon of ointment). A small amount should be applied in the conjunctival sac three or four times daily and once or twice at night. Not more than 8 gm should be prescribed initially and the prescription should not be refilled without further evaluation as outlined in "Precautions" above.

THE SOLUTION

Instill two drops topically in the eye(s) every four hours.

Not more than 20 ml should be prescribed initially.

The dosing of Prednisolone/Sulfacetamide Sodium may be reduced, but care should be taken not to discontinue therapy prematurely. In chronic conditions, withdrawal of treatment should be carried out by gradually decreasing the frequency of application.

If signs and symptoms fail to improve after two days, the patient should be re-evaluated (see "Precautions").

Note: Store ointment and solution away from heat at controlled room temperature, 15°-30°C (59°-86°F). Protect suspension and solution from freezing. Shake suspension well before using.

◆ RATED THERAPEUTICALLY EQUIVALENT; ◇ THERAPEUTIC EQUIVALENCE UNCONFIRMED; ○ UNRATED

HOW SUPPLIED
DROP: 10%-0.2%

AVERAGE UNIT PRICE (AVAILABLE SIZES)

BRAND	$2.47
GENERIC	$1.33

BRAND/MANUFACTURER	NDC	SIZE	AWP
◆ **BRAND**			
BLEPHAMIDE: Allergan Inc	11980-0022-05	5 ml	$14.39
	11980-0022-10	10 ml	$20.56
◆ **GENERICS**			
SULPRED: Bausch&Lomb Pharm	24208-0915-60	5 ml	$9.29
SULPRED: Bausch&Lomb Pharm	24208-0915-62	10 ml	$7.92

DROP: 0.5%-10%

AVERAGE UNIT PRICE (AVAILABLE SIZES)

BRAND	$4.76
GENERIC	$0.38

BRAND/MANUFACTURER	NDC	SIZE	AWP
◆ **BRAND**			
METIMYD: Schering	00085-0074-05	5 ml	$23.81
◆ **GENERICS**			
PREDSULFAIR: Bausch&Lomb Pharm	24208-0775-60	5 ml	$1.60
PREDSULFAIR: Bausch&Lomb Pharm	24208-0775-64	15 ml	$6.67

DROP: 0.25%-10%

BRAND/MANUFACTURER	NDC	SIZE	AWP
○ **BRAND**			
ISOPTO CETAPRED: Alcon Ophthalmic	00998-0613-05	5 ml	$15.31
	00998-0613-15	15 ml	$26.25

DROP: 5 MG-100 MG/5 ML

BRAND/MANUFACTURER	NDC	SIZE	AWP
◆ **GENERICS**			
AK-CIDE: Akorn	17478-0275-10	5 ml	$6.88

DROP: 100 MG-2.5 MG/ML

AVERAGE UNIT PRICE (AVAILABLE SIZES)

GENERIC	$1.15

BRAND/MANUFACTURER	NDC	SIZE	AWP
◆ **GENERICS**			
SUPRED: Ocusoft	54799-0517-10	5 ml	$7.75
SUPRED: Ocusoft	54799-0517-12	15 ml	$11.30

OINTMENT: 0.5%-10%

AVERAGE UNIT PRICE (AVAILABLE SIZES)

BRAND	$4.59

BRAND/MANUFACTURER	NDC	SIZE	AWP
◆ **BRAND**			
VASOCIDIN: Iolab	00058-3095-01	3.5 gm	$11.22
METIMYD: Schering	00085-0695-05	3.5 gm	$20.93
◆ **GENERICS**			
AK-CIDE: Akorn	17478-0276-35	3.5 gm	$6.88

OINTMENT: 10%-0.2%

BRAND/MANUFACTURER	NDC	SIZE	AWP
○ **BRAND**			
BLEPHAMIDE S.O.P.: Allergan Inc	00023-0313-04	3.5 gm	$13.81

OINTMENT: 0.25%-10%

BRAND/MANUFACTURER	NDC	SIZE	AWP
○ **BRAND**			
CETAPRED: Alcon Ophthalmic	00065-0607-35	3.5 gm	$15.31

OINTMENT: 100 MG-2.5 MG/GM

BRAND/MANUFACTURER	NDC	SIZE	AWP
◆ **GENERICS**			
SUPRED: Ocusoft	54799-0517-35	3.5 gm	$7.05

Prednisolone Acetate, Ophthalmic

DESCRIPTION
Prednisolone Acetate, Ophthalmic, sterile ophthalmic suspension is a topical anti-inflammatory agent for ophthalmic use.

Chemical Name:
11β,17,21-Trihydroxypregna-1,4-diene-3,20-dione 21-acetate.

Contains:
Prednisolone Acetate (microfine suspension) . . . . .0.12% or 1.0%

Following is its chemical structure:

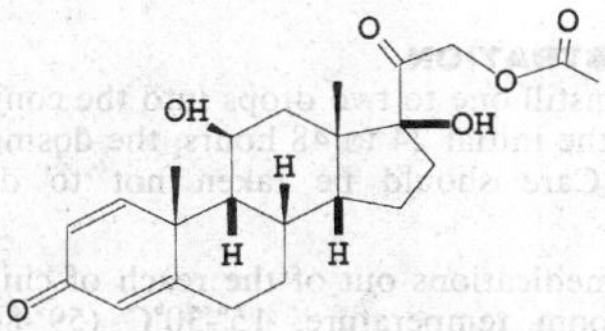

CLINICAL PHARMACOLOGY
Prednisolone Acetate is a glucocorticoid that, on the basis of weight, has 3 to 5 times the anti-inflammatory potency of hydrocortisone. Glucocorticoids inhibit the edema, fibrin deposition, capillary dilation and phagocytic migration of the acute inflammatory response as well as capillary proliferation, deposition of collagen and scar formation.

INDICATIONS AND USAGE
Prednisolone Acetate, Ophthalmic, 0.12% is indicated for the treatment of mild to moderate allergic and inflammatory disorders of the lid, conjunctiva, cornea and sclera (including chemical and thermal burns). Prednisolone Acetate, Ophthalmic, 1.0% is indicated for the treatment of steroid responsive inflammation of the palpebral and bulbar conjunctiva, cornea and anterior segment of the globe.

CONTRAINDICATIONS
Prednisolone Acetate, Ophthalmic, is contraindicated in acute untreated purulent ocular infections, acute superficial herpes simplex (dendritic keratitis), vaccinia, varicella, and most other viral diseases of the cornea and conjunctiva, ocular tuberculosis, and fungal diseases of the eye. It is also contraindicated for individuals sensitive to any component of the formulation.

WARNINGS
In those diseases causing thinning of the cornea, perforation has been reported with the use of topical steroids. Since some brands of Prednisolone Acetate, Ophthalmic, contain no antimicrobial, if infection is present, appropriate measures must be taken to counteract the organisms involved when applicable. Acute purulent infections of the eye may be masked or enhanced by the use of topical steroids. Use of steroid medication in the presence of stromal herpes simplex requires caution and should be followed by frequent mandatory slit-lamp microscopy. As fungal infections of the cornea have been reported coincidentally with long-term local steroid applications, fungal invasion may be suspected in any persistent corneal ulceration where a steroid has been used, or is in use.

Use of topical corticosteroids may cause increased intraocular pressure in certain individuals. This may result in damage to the optic nerve with defects in the visual fields. It is advisable that the intraocular pressure be checked frequently. Posterior subcapsular cataract formation has been reported after heavy or protracted use of topical ophthalmic corticosteroids.

Some brands contain sodium bisulfite, a sulfite that may cause allergic-type reactions including anaphylactic symptoms and life-threatening or less severe asthmatic episodes in certain susceptible people. The overall prevalence of sulfite sensitivity in the general population is unknown and probably low. Sulfite sensitivity is seen more frequently in asthmatic than in nonasthmatic people.

PRECAUTIONS
General: Patients with histories of herpes simplex keratitis should be treated with caution.

Carcinogenesis, Mutagenesis, Impairment of Fertility: No studies have been conducted in animals or in humans to evaluate the potential of these effects.

Pregnancy Category C: Prednisolone has been shown to be teratogenic in mice when given in doses 1-10 times the human dose. There are no adequate well-controlled studies in pregnant women. Prednisolone should be used during pregnancy only if the potential benefit justifies the potential risk to the fetus.

Dexamethasone, hydrocortisone and Prednisolone were ocularly applied to both eyes of pregnant mice five times per day on days 10 through 13 of gestation. A significant increase in the incidence of cleft palate was observed in the fetuses of the treated mice.

Nursing Mothers: It is not known whether topical administration of corticosteroids could result in sufficient systemic absorption to produce detectable quantities in breast milk. Systemically administered corticosteroids are secreted into breast milk in quantities not likely to have a deleterious effect on the infant. Nevertheless, caution should be exercised when topical corticosteroids are administered to a nursing woman.

Pediatric Use: Safety and effectiveness in children have not been established.

ADVERSE REACTIONS
Adverse reactions include increased intraocular pressure which may be associated with optic nerve damage and defects in the visual fields; posterior subcapsular cataract formation; secondary ocular infections from fungi or viruses liberated from ocular tissues; and perforation of the globe when used in conditions where

there is thinning of the cornea or sclera. Systemic side effects may occur rarely with extensive use of topical steroids.

OVERDOSAGE
Overdosage will not ordinarily cause acute problems. If accidentally ingested, drink fluids to dilute.

DOSAGE AND ADMINISTRATION
Shake well before using: Instill one to two drops into the conjunctival sac two to four times daily. During the initial 24 to 48 hours, the dosing frequency may be increased if necessary. Care should be taken not to discontinue therapy prematurely.

Note: Keep this and all medications out of the reach of children.
Store at controlled room temperature, 15°-30°C (59°-86°F). Protect from freezing.

HOW SUPPLIED
DROP: 0.12%

BRAND/MANUFACTURER	NDC	SIZE	AWP
○ **BRAND**			
PRED MILD: Allergan Optical	11980-0174-05	5 ml	$13.25
	11980-0174-10	10 ml	$18.88

DROP: 0.125%

BRAND/MANUFACTURER	NDC	SIZE	AWP
○ **BRAND**			
ECONOPRED: Alcon Ophthalmic	00998-0635-05	5 ml	$13.25
	00998-0635-10	10 ml	$20.00

DROP: 1%

AVERAGE UNIT PRICE (AVAILABLE SIZES)	
BRAND	$2.82

BRAND/MANUFACTURER	NDC	SIZE	AWP
◆ **BRAND**			
PRED FORTE: Allergan Optical	11980-0180-01	1 ml	$4.69
	11980-0180-05	5 ml	$13.15
ECONOPRED PLUS: Alcon Ophthalmic	00998-0637-05	5 ml	$14.88
	00998-0637-10	10 ml	$21.88
PRED FORTE: Allergan Optical	11980-0180-10	10 ml	$22.51
	11980-0180-15	15 ml	$32.60

DROP: 1%

BRAND/MANUFACTURER	NDC	SIZE	AWP
○ **BRAND**			
OCU-PRED-A: Ocumed	51944-5440-35	5 ml	$1.80
	51944-5440-40	10 ml	$2.25

Prednisolone Tebutate

> *FOR INTRA-ARTICULAR, INTRALESIONAL, AND SOFT TISSUE INJECTION ONLY.*

NOT FOR INTRAVENOUS USE

DESCRIPTION
Prednisolone Tebutate, a synthetic adrenocortical steroid, is a white to slightly yellow powder sparingly soluble in alcohol, freely soluble in chloroform, and very slightly soluble in water. The molecular weight is 476.61 (monohydrate). It is designated chemically as 11β,17-dihydroxy-21-[(3,3-dimethyl-1-oxobutyl) oxy]pregna-1,4-diene-3,20-dione. The empirical formula is $C_{27}H_{38}O_6$.

Prednisolone Tebutate sterile suspension is a white to slightly yellow suspension (pH 6.0 to 8.0) that settles upon standing. Each mL contains Prednisolone Tebutate, 20 mg.

Following is its chemical structure:

ACTIONS
Prednisolone Tebutate has a slow onset but long duration of action when compared with more soluble preparations. Because of its slight solubility, it is suitable for intra-articular, intralesional, and soft tissue injection where its anti-inflammatory effects are confined mainly to the area in which it has been injected, although it is capable of producing systemic hormonal effects.

Naturally occurring glucocorticoids (hydrocortisone and cortisone), which also have salt-retaining properties, are used as replacement therapy in adrenocortical deficiency states. Their synthetic analogs, including prednisolone, are primarily used for their potent anti-inflammatory effects in disorders of many organ systems.

Glucocorticoids cause profound and varied metabolic effects. In addition, they modify the body's immune responses to diverse stimuli.

INDICATIONS
A. By intra-articular or soft tissue injection: As adjunctive therapy for short-term administration (to tide the patient over an acute episode or exacerbation) in:

Synovitis of osteoarthritis
Rheumatoid arthritis
Acute and subacute bursitis
Acute gouty arthritis
Epicondylitis
Acute nonspecific tenosynovitis
Posttraumatic osteoarthritis

B. By intralesional injection: May be useful in cystic tumors of an aponeurosis or tendon (ganglia).

CONTRAINDICATIONS
Systemic fungal infections
Hypersensitivity to any component of this product.

WARNINGS
Because rare instances of anaphylactoid reactions have occurred in patients receiving parenteral corticosteroid therapy, appropriate precautionary measures should be taken prior to administration, especially when the patient has a history of allergy to any drug. Anaphylactoid and hypersensitivity reactions have been reported for Sterile Suspension Prednisolone Tebutate, (see *"Adverse Reactions"*).

In patients on corticosteroid therapy subjected to any unusual stress, increased dosage of rapidly acting corticosteroids before, during, and after the stressful situation is indicated.

Drug-induced secondary adrenocortical insufficiency may result from too rapid withdrawal of corticosteroids and may be minimized by gradual reduction of dosage. This type of relative insufficiency may persist for months after discontinuation of therapy; therefore, in any situation of stress occurring during that period, hormone therapy should be reinstituted. If the patient is receiving steroids already, dosage may have to be increased. Since mineralocorticoid secretion may be impaired, salt and/or a mineralocorticoid should be administered concurrently.

Corticosteroids may mask some signs of infection, and new infections may appear during their use. There may be decreased resistance and inability to localize infection when corticosteroids are used. Moreover, corticosteroids may affect the nitroblue-tetrazolium test for bacterial infection and produce false negative results.

In cerebral malaria, a double-blind trial has shown that the use of corticosteroids is associated with prolongation of coma and a higher incidence of pneumonia and gastrointestinal bleeding.

Corticosteroids may activate latent amebiasis. Therefore, it is recommended that latent or active amebiasis be ruled out before initiating corticosteroid therapy in any patient who has spent time in the tropics or any patient with unexplained diarrhea.

Prolonged use of corticosteroids may produce posterior subcapsular cataracts, glaucoma with possible damage to the optic nerves, and may enhance the establishment of secondary ocular infections due to fungi or viruses.

Usage in Pregnancy: Since adequate human reproduction studies have not been done with corticosteroids, use of these drugs in pregnancy or in women of childbearing potential requires that the anticipated benefits be weighed against the possible hazards to the mother and embryo or fetus. Infants born of mothers who have received substantial doses of corticosteroids during pregnancy should be carefully observed for signs of hypoadrenalism.

Corticosteroids appear in breast milk and could suppress growth, interfere with endogenous corticosteroid production, or cause other unwanted effects. Mothers taking pharmacologic doses of corticosteroids should be advised not to nurse. Average and large doses of cortisone or hydrocortisone can cause elevation of blood pressure, salt and water retention, and increased excretion of potassium. These effects are less likely to occur with the synthetic derivatives except when used in large doses. Dietary salt restriction and potassium supplementation may be necessary. All corticosteroids increase calcium excretion.

Administration of live virus vaccines, including smallpox, is contraindicated in individuals receiving immunosuppressive doses of corticosteroids. If inactivated viral or bacterial vaccines are administered to individuals receiving immunosuppressive doses of corticosteroids, the expected serum antibody response may not be obtained.

Patients who are on drugs which suppress the immune system are more susceptible to infections than healthy individuals. Chickenpox and measles, for example, can have a more serious or even fatal course in non-immune children or adults on corticosteroids. In such children or adults who have not had these diseases, particular care should be taken to avoid exposure. The risk of developing a disseminated infection varies among individuals and can be related to the dose, route and duration of corticosteroid administration as well as to the underlying disease. If exposed to chickenpox, prophylaxis with varicella zoster immune globulin (VZIG) may be indicated. If chickenpox develops, treatment with antiviral agents may be considered. If exposed to measles, prophylaxis with immune globulin (IG) may be indicated. (See the respective package inserts for VZIG and IG for complete prescribing information.)

◆ RATED THERAPEUTICALLY EQUIVALENT; ◇ THERAPEUTIC EQUIVALENCE UNCONFIRMED; ○ UNRATED

If corticosteroids are indicated in patients with latent tuberculosis or tuberculin reactivity, close observation is necessary as reactivation of the disease may occur. During prolonged corticosteroid therapy, these patients should receive chemoprophylaxis.

Literature reports suggest an apparent association between use of corticosteroids and left ventricular free wall rupture after a recent myocardial infarction; therefore, therapy with corticosteroids should be used with great caution in these patients.

PRECAUTIONS

This product, like many other steroid formulations, is sensitive to heat. Therefore, it should not be autoclaved when it is desirable to sterilize the exterior of the vial.

Following prolonged therapy, withdrawal of corticosteroids may result in symptoms of the corticosteroid withdrawal syndrome including fever, myalgia, arthralgia, and malaise. This may occur in patients even without evidence of adrenal insufficiency.

There is an enhanced effect of corticosteroids in patients with hypothyroidism and in those with cirrhosis. Corticosteroids should be used cautiously in patients with ocular herpes simplex for fear of corneal perforation. Psychic derangements may appear when corticosteroids are used, ranging from euphoria, insomnia, mood swings, personality changes, and severe depression to frank psychotic manifestations. Also, existing emotional instability or psychotic tendencies may be aggravated by corticosteroids. Aspirin should be used cautiously in conjunction with corticosteroids in hypoprothrombinemia.

Steroids should be used with caution in nonspecific ulcerative colitis, if there is a probability of impending perforation, abscess, or other pyogenic infection, also in diverticulitis, fresh intestinal anastomoses, active or latent peptic ulcer, renal insufficiency, hypertension, osteoporosis, and myasthenia gravis. Signs of peritoneal irritation following gastrointestinal perforation in patients receiving large doses of corticosteroids may be minimal or absent. Fat embolism has been reported as a possible complication of hypercortisonism.

When large doses are given, some authorities advise that antacids be administered between meals to help to prevent peptic ulcer.

Growth and development of infants and children on prolonged corticosteroid therapy should be carefully followed. Steroids may increase or decrease motility and number of spermatozoa in some patients.

Phenytoin, phenobarbital, ephedrine, and rifampin may enhance the metabolic clearance of corticosteroids, resulting in decreased blood levels and lessened physiologic activity, thus requiring adjustment in corticosteroid dosage. The prothrombin time should be checked frequently in patients who are receiving corticosteroids and coumarin anticoagulants at the same time because of reports that corticosteroids have altered the response to these anticoagulants. Studies have shown that the usual effect produced by adding corticosteroids is inhibition of response to coumarins, although there have been some conflicting reports of potentiation not substantiated by studies.

When corticosteroids are administered concomitantly with potassium-depleting diuretics, patients should be observed closely for development of hypokalemia.

Intra-articular injection of a corticosteroid may produce systemic as well as local effects.

Appropriate examination of any joint fluid present is necessary to exclude a septic process.

A marked increase in pain accompanied by local swelling, further restriction of joint motion, fever, and malaise is suggestive of septic arthritis. If this complication occurs and the diagnosis of sepsis is confirmed, appropriate antimicrobial therapy should be instituted.

Injection of a steroid into an infected site is to be avoided. Corticosteroids should not be injected into unstable joints. Patients should be impressed strongly with the importance of not overusing joints in which symptomatic benefit has been obtained as long as the inflammatory process remains active.

Frequent intra-articular injection may result in damage to joint tissues.

INFORMATION FOR PATIENTS
Susceptible patients who are on immunosuppressant doses of corticosteroids should be warned to avoid exposure to chickenpox or measles. Patients should also be advised that if they are exposed, medical advice should be sought without delay.

ADVERSE REACTIONS
Fluid and Electrolyte Disturbances
Sodium retention
Fluid retention
Congestive heart failure in susceptible patients
Potassium loss
Hypokalemic alkalosis
Hypertension

Musculoskeletal
Muscle weakness
Steroid myopathy
Loss of muscle mass
Osteoporosis
Vertebral compression fractures
Aseptic necrosis of femoral and humeral heads
Pathologic fracture of long bones
Tendon rupture

Gastrointestinal
Peptic ulcer with possible subsequent perforation and hemorrhage
Perforation of the small and large bowel, particularly in patients with inflammatory bowel disease
Pancreatitis
Abdominal distention
Ulcerative esophagitis

Dermatologic
Impaired wound healing
Thin fragile skin
Petechiae and ecchymoses
Erythema
Increased sweating
May suppress reactions to skin tests
Other cutaneous reactions, such as allergic dermatitis, urticaria, angioneurotic edema

Neurologic
Convulsions
Increased intracranial pressure with papilledema (pseudo-tumor cerebri) usually after treatment
Vertigo
Headache
Psychic disturbances

Endocrine
Menstrual irregularities
Development of cushingoid state
Suppression of growth in children
Secondary adrenocortical and pituitary unresponsiveness, particularly in times of stress, as in trauma, surgery, or illness
Decreased carbohydrate tolerance
Manifestations of latent diabetes mellitus
Increased requirements for insulin or oral hypoglycemic agents in diabetics
Hirsutism

Ophthalmic
Posterior subcapsular cataracts
Increased intraocular pressure
Glaucoma
Exophthalmos

Metabolic
Negative nitrogen balance due to protein catabolism

Cardiovascular
Myocardial rupture following recent myocardial infarction (see "Warnings").

Other
Anaphylactoid or hypersensitivity reactions
Thromboembolism
Weight gain
Increased appetite
Nausea
Malaise

Foreign body granulomatous reactions involving the synovium have been reported with repeated injections of Prednisolone Tebutate.

Localized pain and swelling, sometimes distal to the site of injection and persisting for several days, have been reported. The following *additional* adverse reactions are related to injection of corticosteroids:

Rare instances of blindness associated with intralesional therapy around the face and head
Hyperpigmentation or hypopigmentation
Subcutaneous and cutaneous atrophy
Sterile abscess
Postinjection flare (following intra-articular use)
Charcot-like arthropathy

DOSAGE AND ADMINISTRATION

> *FOR INTRA-ARTICULAR, INTRALESIONAL, AND SOFT TISSUE INJECTION ONLY.*

NOT FOR INTRAVENOUS USE

DOSAGE AND FREQUENCY OF INJECTION ARE VARIABLE AND MUST BE INDIVIDUALIZED ON THE BASIS OF THE DISEASE AND THE RESPONSE OF THE PATIENT.

The initial dose varies from 4 to 40 mg depending on the disease being treated and the size of the area to be injected. Frequency of injection depends on symptomatic response, and usually is once every two or three weeks. Severe conditions may require injection once a week. Frequent intra-articular injection may result in damage to joint tissues. If satisfactory clinical response does not occur after a reasonable period of time, discontinue Prednisolone Tebutate sterile suspension and transfer the patient to other therapy.

Patients should be observed closely for signs that might require dosage adjustment, including changes in clinical status resulting from remissions or exacerbations of the disease, and individual drug responsiveness.

➤ SHOWN IN PRODUCT IDENTIFICATION GUIDE

For rapid onset of action, a soluble adrenocortical hormone preparation, such as dexamethasone sodium phosphate injection or prednisolone sodium phosphate injection, may be given with Prednisolone Tebutate.

If desired, a local anesthetic may be used, and may be injected before Prednisolone Tebutate, or mixed in a syringe with Prednisolone Tebutate and given simultaneously.

If used prior to intra-articular injection of the steroid, inject most of the anesthetic into the soft tissues of the surrounding area and instill a small amount into the joint.

If given together, mixing should be done in the injection syringe by drawing the steroid in *first*, then the anesthetic. In this way, the anesthetic will not be introduced inadvertently into the vial of steroid. *The mixture must be used immediately and any unused portion discarded.*

Some of the usual single doses are:

Large Joints (e.g., Knee)	20 mg (1mL), occasionally 30 mg (1.5 mL). Doses over 40 mg (2mL) not recommended.
Small Joints (e.g., Interphalangeal, Temporomandibular)	8 to 10 mg (0.4 to 0.5 mL).
Bursae	20 to 30 mg (1 to 1.5 mL).
Tendon Sheaths	4 to 10 mg (0.2 to 0.5 mL).
Ganglia	10 to 20 mg (0.5 to 1 mL).

Sensitive to heat. Do not autoclave.
Protect from freezing.
Protect from light. Store container in carton until contents have been used.

J CODES
Up to 20 mg VAR—J1690

HOW SUPPLIED
INJECTION: 20 MG/ML

BRAND/MANUFACTURER	NDC	SIZE	AWP
◇ **BRAND**			
HYDELTRA-T.B.A.: Merck	00006-7572-01	1 ml	$5.18
	00006-7572-03	5 ml	$19.84

Prednisolone, Systemic

DESCRIPTION
Prednisolone is a glucocorticoid. Glucocorticoids are adrenocortical steroids, both naturally occurring and synthetic, which are readily absorbed from the gastrointestinal tract. Prednisolone. IIβ, 17, 21-Trihydroxy-pregna-1, 4-diene-3, 20-dione, is a synthetic dehydrogenated analogue of cortisone. It is approximately three to five times more potent on a milligram basis than cortisone or hydrocortisone. Prednisolone is a white to practically white, odorless, crystalline powder. It is very slightly soluble in water, slightly soluble in alcohol, in chloroform, in dioxane, and in methanol.

Its molecular formula is $C_{21}H_{28}O_5$ and its molecular weight is 360.45 (anhydrous).

Prednisolone acetate is 11β,17,21-Trihydroxypregna-1,4-diene-3,20-dione 21-Acetate, with the molecular formula $C_{23}H_{30}O_6$

Prednisolone is available as tablets and syrup for oral administration; Prednisolone acetate is available as a suspension for intramuscular and intra-articular injection; Prednisolone sodium phosphate is available as an oral liquid and a solution for intravenous, intramuscular, intra-articular, intralesional, and soft-tissue administration.

Each tablets contains:
Prednisolone ....5 mg

Each 5 ml of syrup contains:
Prednisolone ....15 mg

Each ml of suspension contains:
Prednisolone acetate ....25 mg, 40 mg, or 50 mg

Each 5 ml (teaspoonful) of Oral liquid contains:
Prednisolone sodium phosphate ....6.7 mg (5 mg Prednisolone base)

Each ml of solution contains:
Prednisolone sodium phosphate equivalent to 20 mg Prednisolone phosphate

It is freely soluble in water, soluble in methanol; slightly soluble in alcohol and in chloroform; and very slightly soluble in acetone and in dioxane. The chemical name of Prednisolone sodium phosphate is pregna-1,4-diene-3,20-dione, 11,17-dihydroxy-21-(phosphonooxyl)-, disodium salt, (11β)-. The empirical formula is $C_{21}H_{27}Na_2O_8P$; the molecular weight is 484.39.

CLINICAL PHARMACOLOGY OR ACTIONS
Naturally occurring glucocorticoids (hydrocortisone and cortisone), which also have salt-retaining properties, are used as replacement therapy in adrenocortical deficiency states. Their synthetic analogs, such as Prednisolone, are primarily used for their potent anti-inflammatory effects in disorders of many organ systems.

Some of Prednisolone's glucocorticoid properties reproduce the physiological actions of endogenous glucocorticosteroids, but others do not necessarily reflect any of the adrenal hormones' normal functions; they are seen only after administration of large therapeutic doses of the drug. The pharmacological effects of Prednisolone which are due to its glucocorticoid properties include: promotion of gluconeogenesis; increased deposition of glycogen in the liver; inhibition of the utilization of glucose; anti-insulin activity; increased catabolism of protein; increased lipolysis; stimulation of fat synthesis and storage; increased glomerular filtration rate and resulting increase in urinary excretion of urate (creatinine excretion remains unchanged); and increased calcium excretion.

Depressed production of eosinophils and lymphocytes occurs, but erythropoiesis and production of polymorphonuclear leukocytes are stimulated. Anti-inflammatory processes (edema, fibrin deposition, capillary dilatation, migration of leukocytes and phagocytosis) and the later stages of wound healing (capillary proliferation, deposition of collagen, cicatrization) are inhibited. Prednisolone can stimulate secretion of various components of gastric juice. Stimulation of the production of corticotropin may lead to suppression of endogenous corticosteroids. Prednisolone has slight mineralocorticoid activity, whereby entry of sodium into cells and loss of intracellular potassium is stimulated. This is particularly evident in the kidney, where rapid ion exchange leads to sodium retention and hypertension. At equipotent anti-inflammatory doses, Prednisolone has less tendency to cause salt and water retention than either hydrocortisone or cortisone.

Glucocorticoids also modify the body's immune responses to diverse stimuli.

Prednisolone is 70-90% protein-bound in the plasma and it is eliminated from the plasma with a half-life of 2 to 4 hours. It is metabolized mainly in the liver and excreted in the urine as sulfate and glucuronide conjugates.

Prednisolone is rapidly and well absorbed from the gastrointestinal tract following oral administration. Prednisolone sodium phosphate oral liquid produces a 20% higher peak plasma level of Prednisolone which occurs approximately 15 minutes earlier than the peak seen with tablet formulations.

Prednisolone sodium phosphate injection has a rapid onset but short duration of action when compared with less soluble preparations. Because of this, it is suitable for the treatment of acute disorders responsive to adrenocortical steroid therapy.

INDICATIONS
Prednisolone tablets, syrup, oral liquid and when oral therapy is not feasible and the strength, dosage form and route of administration of the drug lend the preparation to the treatment of the condition, intramuscular Prednisolone acetate suspension and intramuscular or intravenous Prednisolone sodium phosphate solution, are indicated as follows:

1. Endocrine Disorders. Primary or secondary adrenocortical insufficiency (hydrocortisone or cortisone is the first choice. Prednisolone and other synthetic analogues may be used in conjunction with mineralocorticoids where applicable in infancy mineralocorticoid supplementation is of particular importance). Congenital adrenal hyperplasia. Nonsuppurative thyroiditis. Hypercalcemia associated with cancer.

2. Prednisolone acetate suspension (IM) and Prednisolone sodium phosphate solution (IM and IV) are also indicated for acute adrenocortical insufficiency (hydrocortisone or cortisone is the drug of choice, mineralocorticoid supplementation may be necessary, particularly when synthetic analogs are used). Preoperatively and in the event of serious trauma or illness, in patients with known adrenal insufficiency or when adrenocortical reserve is doubtful. Prednisolone acetate suspension is also indicated in shock unresponsive to conventional therapy if adrenocortical insufficiency exists or is suspected.

Rheumatic Disorders. As adjunctive therapy for short-term administration (to tide the patient over an acute episode or exacerbation) in:
Psoriatic arthritis.
Rheumatoid arthritis, including juvenile rheumatoid arthritis (selected cases may require low-dose maintenance therapy).
Ankylosing spondylitis.
Acute and subacute bursitis.
Acute nonspecific tenosynovitis (tablets and syrup).
Acute gouty arthritis.
Post-traumatic osteoarthritis.
Synovitis of esteoarthritis.
Epicondylitis.

3. Collagen Diseases. During an exacerbation or as maintenance therapy in selected cases of: Systemic lupus erythematosus, Acute rheumatic carditis.

4. Dermatologic Diseases. Pemphigus, Bollous dermatitis herpetiforms, Severe erythema multiforme (Stevens-Johnson syndrome), Exfoliative dermatitis, Mycosis fungoides, Severe psoriasis, Severe seborrheic dermatitis, Systemic dermatomyositis (polymyositis).

5. Allergic States. Control of severe or incapacitating allergic conditions intractable to adequate trials of conventional treatment Seasonal or perennial allergic rhinitis, Bronchial asthma, Contact dermatitis, Atopic dermatitis, Serum sickness, Drug hypersensitivity reactions.

Prednisolone acetate suspension (IM) and prednisolone sodium phosphate solution (IM and IV) are also indicated in: Orticarial transfusion reaction, Acute noninfectious laryngeal edema (epinephrine is the drug of first choice).

6. Ophthalmic Diseases. Severe acute and chronic allergic and inflammatory processes involving the eye and its adnexa such as Allergic conjunctivitis, Keratitis (tablets, syrup, oral liquid, and solution), Allergic corneal marginal ulcer, Herpes zoster ophthalmicus, tritis and iridocyclitis, Chorioretinitis, Anterior

---

◆ RATED THERAPEUTICALLY EQUIVALENT; ◇ THERAPEUTIC EQUIVALENCE UNCONFIRMED; ○ UNRATED

segment inflammation. Diffuse posterior uveitis and choroiditis, Optic neuritis, Sympathetic ophthalmia.

7. Respiratory Diseases. Symptomatic sarcoidosis, Loeffler's syndrome not manageable by other means, Berylliosis, Fulminating or disseminated pulmonary tuberculosis when used concurrently with appropriate antituberculous chemotherapy, Aspiration pneumonitis.

8. Hematologic Disorders. Idiopathic thrombocytopenic purpura in adults (IM administration is contraindicated), Secondary thrombocytopenia in adults, Acquired (autoimmune) hemolytic anemia, Erythroblastopenia (RBC anemia), Congenital (erythroid) hypoplastic anemia.

9. Neoplastic Diseases. For palliative management of: Leukemias and lymphomas in adults, Acute leukemia of childhood.

10. Edematous States. To induce diuresis or remission of proteinuria in the nephrotic syndrome, without uremia, of the idiopathic type or that due to lupus erythematosus.

11. Gastrointestinal Diseases. To tide the patient over a critical period of the disease in: Ulcerative colitis (systemic therapy), Regional enteritis (Systemic therapy).

12. Nervous System. Acute exacerbations of multiple sclerosis (tablets, suspension, oral liquid).

13 Miscellaneous. Tuberculous meningitis with subarachnoid block or impending block when concurrently accompanied by appropriate antituberculous chemotherapy, Trichinosis with neurologic or myocardial involvement.

Intra-Articular or Soft Tissue Administration: When the strength and dosage of the drug lend the preparation to the treatment of the condition, sterile Prednisolone acetate suspension and Prednisolone sodium phosphate solution for "intra-articular or soft tissue administration" are indicated:

As adjunctive therapy for short-term administration (to tide the patient over an acute episode or exacerbation) in:
Synovitis of osteoarthritis.
Rheumatoid arthritis.
Acute and subacute bursitis.
Acute gouty arthritis.
Epicondylitis.
Acute nonspecific tenosynovitis.
Post-traumatic osteoarthritis.

Intralesional Administration: When the strength and dosage form of the drug lend the preparation to the treatment of the condition, sterile Prednisolone acetate suspension for 'intralesional administration' are indicated for:
Keloids.
Localized hypertrophic infiltrated inflammatory lesions of: lichen planus, psoriatic plaques, granuloma annulare and lichen simplex chronicus (neurodermatitis).
Discoid lupus erythematosus.
Necrobiosis lipoidica diabeticorum.
Alopecia areata.
Prednisolone Acetate suspension may also be useful in cystic tumors of an aponeurosis or tendon (ganglia).

UNLABELED USES
Prednisolone is used alone or as an adjunct in the treatment of reflex sympathetic dystrophy and Bell's palsy, and as an adjunctive therapy in breast cancer. It is also used in biopsy-proven myocarditis and to reduce morbidity and progression of pulmonary disease in cystic fibrosis patients. It is prescribed for temporal arteritis or giant cell arteritis, and for Cogan's syndrome. In addition, it is used as an adjunct in chronic active hepatitis B, Hodgkin's disease, male infertility, Duchenne muscular dystrophy, fever, myasthenia gravis, chronic erosive gastritis, and kidney transplantation.

CONTRAINDICATIONS
Systemic fungal injections.
Prednisolone acetate suspension and Prednisolone sodium phosphate solution are also contraindicated in those persons who have shown hypersensitivity to any component of this preparation.

WARNINGS
In patients on corticosteroid therapy subjected to unusual stress, increased dosage of rapidly acting corticosteroids before, during, and after the stressful situation is indicated.

Corticosteroids may mask some signs of infection, and new infections may appear during their use. There may be decreased resistance and inability to localize infection when corticosteroids are used. Moreover, corticosteroids may affect the nitroblue-tetrazolium test for bacterial infection and produce false negative results.

Corticosteroids may exacerbate systemic fungal infections and therefore should not be used in the presence of such infections unless they are needed to control drug reactions due to amphotericin B. Moreover, there have been cases reported in which concomitant use of amphotericin B and hydrocortisone was followed by cardiac enlargement and congestive failure.

Prolonged use of corticosteroids may produce posterior subcapsular cataracts, glucoma with possible damage to the optic nerves, and may enhance the establishment of secondary ocular infections due to fungi or viruses.

Note: Some brands of Prednisolone acetate contain benzyl alcohol. Benzyl alcohol has been associated with a fatal "Gasping Syndrome" in premature infants and infants of low birth weight.

Some brands of injectable Prednisolone sodium phosphate contain sodium bisulfite, a sulfite that may cause allergic-type reactions including anaphylactic symptoms and life-threatening or less severe asthmatic episodes in certain susceptible people. The overall prevalence of sulfite sensitivity in the general population is unknown and probably low. Sulfite sensitivity is seen more frequently in asthmatic than in nonasthmatic people.

Drug Interactions: Drugs such as barbiturates which induce hepatic microsomal drug metabolizing enzyme activity may enhance metabolism of Prednisolone and require that the dosage of Prednisolone be increased. Phenytoin, Phenobarbital, Ephedrine, and rifampin may enhance the metabolic clearance of corticosteroids, resulting in decreased blood levels and lessened physiologic activity, thus requiring adjustment in corticosteroid dosage.

The prothrombin time should be checked frequently in patients who are receiving corticosteroids and coumarin anticoagulants at the same time because of reports that corticosteroids have altered the response to these anticoagulants. Studies have shown that the usual effect produced by adding corticosteroids is inhibition of response to coumarins, although there have been some conflicting reports of potention not substantiated by studies.

When corticosteroids are administered concomitantly with potassium-depleting diuretics, patients should be observed closely for development of hypokalemia.

Pregnancy: Pregnancy Category C—Prednisolone has been shown to be teratogenic in many species when given in doses equivalent to the human dose. Animal studies in which prednisolone has been given to pregnant mice, rats and rabbits have yielded an increased incidence of cleft palate in the offspring.

Since adequate human reproduction studies have not been done with corticosteroids, the use of these drugs in pregnancy, or women of childbearing potential requires that the possible benefits of the drugs be weighed against the potential hazards to the mother and embryo or fetus. Infants born of mothers who have received substantial doses of corticosteroids during pregnancy should be carefully observed for signs of hypoadrenalism.

Nursing Mothers: Corticosteroids appear in breast milk and could suppress growth, interfere with endogenous corticosteroid production, or cause other unwanted effects. Mothers taking pharmacologic doses of corticosteroids should be advised not to nurse.

Average and large doses of hydrocortisone or cortisone can cause elevation of blood pressure, salt and water retention, and increased excretion of potassium. These effects are less likely to occur with the synthetic derivatives except when used in large doses. Dietary salt restriction and potassium supplementation may be necessary. All corticosteroids increase calcium excretion.

While on corticosteroid therapy patients should not be vaccinated against smallpox. Other immunization procedures should not be undertaken in patients who are on corticosteroids, especially in high doses, because of possible hazards of neurological complications and lack of antibody response. However, immunization procedures may be undertaken in patients who are receiving corticosteroids as replacement therapy, e.g., for Addison's disease.

Patients who are on drugs which suppress the immune system are more susceptible to infections than healthy individuals. Chickenpox and measles, for example, can have a more serious or even fatal course in non-immune children or adults on corticosteroids. In such children or adults who have not had these diseases, particular care should be taken to avoid exposure. How the dose, route and duration of corticosteroid administration affects the risk of developing a disseminated infection is not known. The contribution of the underlying disease and/or prior corticosteroid treatment to the risk is also not known. If exposed to chickenpox, prophylaxis with varicella zoster immune globulin (VZIG) may be indicated. If exposed to measles, prophylaxis with pooled intravenous immunoglobulin (IVIG) or pooled intramuscular immunoglobulin (IG) may be indicated. (See the respective package inserts for complete VZIG and IVIG or IG prescribing information.) If chickenpox develops, treatment with antiviral agents may be considered.

The use of Prednisolone, Prednisolone acetate, or Prednisolone sodium phosphate in active tuberculosis should be restricted to those cases of fulminating or disseminated tuberculosis in which the corticosteroid is used for the management of the disease in conjunction with an appropriate antituberculous regimen.

If corticosteroids are indicated in patients with latent, tuberculosis or tuberculin reactivity, close observation is necessary as reactivation of the disease may occur. During prolonged corticosteroid therapy, these patients should receive chemoprophylaxis.

Because rare instances of anaphylactoid reactions have occurred in patients receiving parenteral corticosteroid therapy, appropriate precautionary measures should be taken prior to administration, especially when the patient has a history of allergy to any drug. Anaphylactoid and hypersensitivity reactions have been reported for some brands of injectable Prednisolone sodium phosphate (see "Adverse Reactions").

Literature reports suggest an apparent association between use of corticosteroids and left ventricular free wall rupture after a recent myocardial infarction; therefore, therapy with corticosteroids should be used with great caution in these patients.

In cerebral malaria, a double-blind trial has shown that the use of corticosteroids is associated with prolongation of coma and a higher incidence of pneumonia and gastrointestinal bleeding.

Corticosteroids may activate latent amebiasis. Therefore, it is recommended that latent or active amebiasis be ruled out before initiating corticosteroid therapy in any patient who has spent time in the tropics or any patient with unexplained diarrhea.

PRECAUTIONS

Drug-induced secondary adrenocortical insufficiency may result from too rapid withdrawal of corticosteroids and may be minimized by gradual reduction of dosage. This type of relative insufficiency may persist for months after discontinuation of therapy, therefore, in any situation of stress occurring during that period, hormone therapy should be reinstituted. Since mineralocorticoid secretion may be impaired, salt and/or a mineralocorticoid should be administered concurrently.

Following prolonged therapy, withdrawal of corticosteroids may result in symptoms of the corticosteroid withdrawal syndrome including fever, myalgia, arthralgia, and malaise. This may occur in patients even without evidence of adrenal insufficiency.

There is an enhanced effect of corticosteroids in patients with hypothyroidism and in those with cirrhosis.

Corticosteroids should be used cautiously in patients with ocular herpes simplex because of possible corneal perforation.

The lowest possible dose of corticosteroid should be used to control the condition under treatment, and when reduction in dosage is possible, the reduction should be gradual.

Psychic derangements may appear when corticosteroids are used, ranging from euphoria, insomnia, mood swings, personality changes, and severe depression, to frank psychotic manifestations. Also, existing emotional instability or psychotic tendencies may be aggravated by corticosteroids.

Aspirin should be used cautiously in conjunction with corticosteroids in hypoprothrombinemia.

Steroids should be used with caution in nonspecific ulcerative colitis, if there is a probability of impending perforation, abscess or other pyogenic infection: diverticulitis; fresh intestinal anastomoses; active or latent peptic ulcer; renal insufficiency, hypertension; osteoporosis; and myasthenia gravis. Signs of peritoneal irritation following gastrointestinal perforation in patients receiving large doses of corticosteroids may be minimal or absent. Fat embolism has been reported as a possible complication of hypercortisonism.

When large doses are given, some authorities advise that antacids be administered between meals to help to prevent peptic ulcer.

Growth and development of infants and children on prolonged corticosteroid therapy should be carefully observed.

Steroids may increase or decrease motility and number of spermatozoa in some patients.

Although controlled clinical trials have shown corticosteroids to be effective in speeding the resolution of acute exacerbations of multiple sclerosis they do not show that they affect the ultimate outcome or natural history of the disease. The studies do show that relatively high doses of corticosteroids are necessary to demonstrate a significant effect. (See "Dosage and Administration" section).

Since complications of treatment with glucocorticoids are dependent on the size of the dose and the duration of treatment, a risk/benefit decision must be made in each individual case as to dose, duration of treatment and as to whether daily or intermittent therapy should be used.

Information for Patients: Patients should be warned not to discontinue the use of Prednisolone abruptly or without medical supervision to advice any medical attendants that they are taking Prednisolone and to seek medical advice at once should they develop fever or other signs of infection. Patients who are on immunosuppressant doses of corticosteroids should be warned to avoid exposure to chickenpox or measles. Patients should also be advised that if they are exposed, medical advice should be sought without delay.

The following additional precautions apply for parenteral corticosterids: Intraarticular injection of a corticosteroid may produce systemic as well as local effects.

Appropriate examination of any joint fluid present is necessary to exclude a septic process.

A marked increase in pain accompanied by local swelling, further restriction of joint motion, fever, and malaise is suggestive of septic arthritis. If this complication occurs and the diagnosis of sepsis is confirmed, appropriate antimicrobial therapy should be instituted.

Local injection of a steroid into a previously infected site or joint is to be avoided.

Corticosteroids should not be injected into unstable joints.

Patients should be impressed strongly with the importance of not overusing joints in which symptomatic benefit has been obtained as long as the inflammatory process remains active.

Frequent intra-articular injection may result in damage to joint tissues.

The slower rate of absorption by intramuscular administration should be recognized.

Prednisolone sodium phosphate solution, like many other steroid formulations, is sensitive to heat. Therefore, it should not be autoclaved when it is desirable to sterilize the exterior of the vial.

ADVERSE REACTIONS

Fluid and Electrolyte Disturbances: Sodium retention, fluid retention, congestive heart failure in susceptible patients, potassium loss, hypokalemic alkalosis, hypertension.

Musculoskeletal: Muscle weakness, steroid myopathy, loss of muscle mass, osteoporosis, vertebral compression fractures, aseptic necrosis of femoral and humeral heads, pathologic fracture of long bones, Prednisolone sodium phosphate solution is also associated with tendon rupture.

Gastrointestinal: Peptic ulcer with possible perforation and hemorrhage, pancreatitis, abdominal distention, ulcerative esophagitis, Prednisolone sodium phosphate solution is also associated with perforation of the small and large bowel, particularly in patients with inflammatory bowel disease.

Dermatologic: Impaired wound healing, thin fragile skin, petechiae and ecchymoses, facial erythema, increased sweating. May suppress reactions to skin tests. Prednisolone soldium phosphate solution is also associate with burning or tingling, especially in the perineal area (after I.V. injection) and other cutaneous reactions, such as allergic dermatitis, urticaria, angioneurotic edema.

Metabolic: Negative nitrogen balance due to protein catabolism.

Neurological: Convulsions, increased intracranial pressure with papilledema (pseudotumor cerebri) usually after treatment, vertigo, headache. Prednisolone sodium phosphate solution is also associated with psychic disturbances.

Endocrine: Menstrual irregularities, development of Cushingoid state, suppression of growth in children, secondary adrenocortical and pituitary unresponsiveness particularly in time of stress, as in trauma, surgery or illness, decreased carbohydrate tolerance, manifestations latent diabetes mellitus, increased requirements for insulin or oral hypoglycemic agents in diabetics. Prednisolone sodium phosphate solution is also associated with hirsutism.

Ophthalmic: Posterior subcapsular cataracts, increased intraocular pressure, glaucoma, exophthalmos.

Cardiovascular: Myocardial rupture following recent myocardial infarction (see "Warnings"). Prednisolone Acetate suspension and Prednisolone Sodium Phosphate solution).

Others: Urticaria and other allergic anaphylactic or hypersensitivity reactions. Prednisolone sodium phosphate solution is also associated with thromboembolism, weight gain, increased appetite, nausea, malaise.

The following *additional* adverse reactions are related to parenteral corticosteroid therapy:

Rare instances of blindness associated with intralesional therapy around the face and head.

Hyperpigmentation or hypopigmentation.

Subcutaneous and cutaneous atrophy.

Sterile abscess.

Post injection flare, (following intra-articular use).

Charcot-like arthropathy.

OVERDOSAGE

Reports of acute toxicity and/or death following overdosage of glucocorticoids are rare. The effects of accidental ingestion of large quantities of Prednisolone over a very short period of time have not been reported, but prolonged use of the drug can produce mental symptoms, moon face, abnormal fat deposits, fluid retention, excessive appetite, weight gain, hypertrichosis, acne, striae, ecchymosis, increased sweating, pigmentation, dry scaly skin, thinning scalp hair, increased blood pressure, tachycardia, thrombophlebitis, decreased resistance to infection, negative nitrogen balance with delayed bone and wound healing, headache, weakness, menstrual disorders, accentuated menopausal symptoms, neuropathy, fractures, osteoporosis, peptic ulcer, decreased glucose tolerance, hypokalemia, and adrenal insufficiency. Hepatomegaly and abdominal distention have been observed in children.

Treatment of acute overdosage is by immediate gastric lavage or emesis; no specific antidote is available. For chronic overdosage in the face of severe disease requiring continuous steroid therapy the dosage of Prednisolone may be reduced only temporarily, or alternate day treatment may be introduced.

The intraperitoneal LD_{50} of Prednisolone phosphate disodium in female mice was 1190 mg/kg.

DOSAGE AND ADMINISTRATION

Dosage of Prednisolone should be individualized according to the severity of the disease and the response of the patient. For infants and children, the recommended dosage should be governed by the same considerations rather than strict adherence to the ratio indicated by age or body weight.

Hormone therapy is an adjunct to and not a replacement for conventional therapy.

Dosage should be decreased or discontinued gradually when the drug has been administered for more than a few days.

The severity, prognosis, expected duration of the disease, and the reaction of the patient to medication are primary factors in determining dosage.

If a period of spontaneous remission occurs in a chronic condition, treatment should be discontinued.

Blood pressure, body weight, routine laboratory studies, including two-hour postprandial blood glucose and serum potassium, and a chest X-ray should be obtained at regular intervals during prolonged therapy. Upper GI X-rays are desirable in patients with known or suspected peptic ulcer disease.

The initial dosage of Prednisolone may vary from 5 mg to 60 mg per day, of Prednisolone acetate or sodium phosphate from 4 mg to 60 mg per day, and of Prednisolone sodium phosphate oral liquid 5 ml to 60 ml (5 to 60 mg Prednisotone base) per day, depending on the specific disease entity being treated. In situations of less severity lower doses will generally suffice, while in selected patients higher initial doses may be required. Usually, the parenteral dosage ranges are one-third to one-half the oral dose given every 12 hours. However, in certain overwhelming, acute, life-threatening situations, administration in dosages exceeding the usual dosages may be justified and may be in multiples of the oral dosages. Usually the daily parenteral dose of Prednisolone sodium phosphate

---

◆ RATED THERAPEUTICALLY EQUIVALENT; ◇ THERAPEUTIC EQUIVALENCE UNCONFIRMED; ○ UNRATED

(IV and IM) injection is the same as the daily oral dose of Prednisolone and the dosage interval is every 4 to 8 hours.

Prednisolone sodium phosphate (IV and IM) injection can be given directly from the vial, or it can be added to sodium chloride injection or dextrose injection and given by intravenous drip. Benzyl alcohol as a preservative has been associated with toxicity in premature infants. Solutions used for intravenous administration or further dilution of this product should be preservative-free when used in the neonate, especially the premature infant.

When it is mixed with an infusion solution, sterile precautions should be observed. Since infusion solutions generally do not contain preservatives, mixtures should be used within 24 hours. The initial dosage should be maintained or adjusted until a satisfactory response is noted. If after a reasonable period of time there is a lack of satisfactory clinical response. Prednisolone or Prednisolone acetate should be discontinued and the patient transferred to other appropriate therapy. *It should be emphasized that dosage requirements are variable and must be individualized on the basis of the disease under treatment and the response of the patient.*

After a favorable response is noted, the proper maintenance dosage should be determined by decreasing the initial dosage in small decrements at appropriate time intervals until the lowest dosage which will maintain an adequate clinical response is reached. It should be kept in mind that constant monitoring is needed in regard to drug dosage. Included in the situations which may make dosage adjustments necessary are changes in clinical status secondary to remissions of exacerbations in the disease process, the patient's individual drug responsiveness, and the effect of patient exposure to stressful situations not directly related to the disease entity under treatment; in this latter situation it may be necessary to increase the dosage of Prednisolone for a period of time consistent with the patient's condition. If after long-term therapy the drug is to be stopped, it is recommended that it be withdrawn gradually rather than abruptly.

Multiple Sclerosis: In the treatment of acute exacerbations of multiple sclerosis daily doses of 200 mg of Prednisolone for a week followed by 80 mg every other day or 4 to 8 mg dexamethasone every other day for 1 month have shown to be effective. For the purpose of comparison, the following is the equivalent milligram dosage of the various glucocorticoids: cortisone, 25; hydrocortisone, 20; Prednisolone, 5; Prednisone, 5; methylprednisolone, 4; triamcinolone, 4; paramethasone, 2; betamethasone, 0.75; dexamethasone, 0.75. These dose relationships apply only to oral or intravenous administration of these compounds. When these substances or their derivatives are injected intramuscularly or into joint spaces, their relative properties may be greatly altered.

Intra-articular, Intralesional, and Soft Tissue Injection: Intra-articular, intralesional, and soft tissue injections are generally employed when the affected joints or areas are limited to one or two sites. Dosage and frequency of injection vary depending on the condition being treated and the site of injection. The usual dose is from 2 to 30 mg. The frequency usually ranges from once every three to five days to once every two to three weeks. Frequent intra-articular injection may result in damage to joint tissues.

Some of the usual single doses are:

	Doses	
Site of Injection	*Amount of Injection (ml)*	*Amount of Prednisolone Phosphate (mg)*
Large Joints (e.g., Knee)	0.5 to 1	10 to 20
Small Joints (e.g., Interphalangeal, Temporomandibular)	0.2 to 0.25	4 to 5
Bursae	0.5 to 0.75	10 to 15
Tendon Sheaths	0.1 to 0.25	2 to 5
Soft Tissue Infiltration	0.5 to 1.5	10 to 30
Ganglia	0.25 to 0.5	5 to 10

Prednisolone sodium phosphate injection is particularly recommended for use in conjunction with one of the less soluble, longer-acting steroids, such as Prednisolone tebutate suspension or Hydrocortisone acetate sterile suspension, available for intra-articular and soft tissue injection.

Alternate-Day Therapy: Alternate-day therapy is a corticosteroid dosing regimen in which twice the usual daily dose of corticoid is administered every other morning. The purpose of this mode of therapy is to provide the patient requiring long-term pharmacologic dose treatment with the beneficial effects of corticoids while minimizing certain undesirable effects, including pituitary adrenal suppression, the Cushingoid state, corticoid withdrawal symptoms, and growth suppression in children.

The rationale for this treatment schedule is based on two major premises: (a) the anti-inflammatory or therapeutic effect of corticoids persists longer than their physical presence and metabolic effects and (b) administration of the corticosteroid every other morning allows for reestablishment of more nearly normal hypothalamic-pituitary-adrenal (HPA) activity on the offsteroid day.

A brief review of the HPA physiology may be helpful in understanding this rational. Actin primarily through the hypothalamus a fall in free cortisol stimulates the pituitary gland to produce increasing amounts of corticortropin (ACTH) while a rise in free cortisol inhibits ACTH secretion. Normally, the HPA system is characterized by diurnal (circadian) rhythm. Serum levels of ACTH rise from a low point about 10 p.m. to a peak level about 6 a.m. Increasing levels of ATH stimulate adrenocortical activity resulting in a rise in plasma cortisol with maximal levels occurring between 2 a.m. and 8 a.m. This rise in cortisol dampens ACTH production and in turn adrenocortical activity. There is a gradual fall in plasma corticoids during the day with lowest levels occurring about midnight.

The diurnal rhythm of the HPA axis is lost in Cushing's disease, a syndrome of adrenocortical hyperfunction characterized by obesity with centripetal fat distribution, thinning of the skin with easy bruisability, muscle wasting with weakness, hypertension, latent diabetes, osteoporosis, electrolyte imbalance, etc. The same clinical findings of hyperadrenocorticism may be noted during long-term pharmacologic dose corticoid therapy administered in conventional daily divided doses. It would appear, then, that a disturbance in the diurnal cycle with maintenance of elevated corticoid values during the night may play a significant role in the development of undesirable corticoid effects. Escape from these constantly elevated plasma levels for even short periods of time may be instrumental in protecting against undesirable pharmacologic effects.

During conventional pharmacologic dose corticosteroid therapy, ACTH production is inhibited with subsequent suppression of cortisol production by the adrenal cortex. Recovery time for normal HPA activity is variable depending upon the dose and duration of treatment. During this time the patient is vulnerable to any stressful situation. Although it has been shown that there is considerably less adrenal suppression following a single morning dose of prednisolone (10 mg) as opposed to a quarter of that dose administered every 6 hours, there is evidence that some suppressive effect on adrenal activity may be carried over into the following day when pharmacologic doses are used. Further, it has been shown that a single dose of certain corticosteroids will produce adrenocortical suppression for two or more days. Other corticoids, including methylprednisolone, hydrocortisone, prednisone, and prednisolone, are considered to be short acting (producing adrenocortical suppression for 1-1 ¼ to 1-1 ½ days following a single dose) and thus are recommended for alternate-day therapy.

The following should be kept in mind when considering alternate-day therapy:

1) Basic principles and indications for corticosteroids therapy should apply. The benefits of alternate-day therapy should not encourage the indiscriminate use of steroids.

2) Alternate-day therapy is a therapeutic technique primarily designed for patients in whom long term pharmacologic corticoid therapy is anticipated.

3) In less severe disease processes in which corticoid therapy is indicated, it may be possible to initiate treatment with alternate-day therapy. More severe disease states usually will require daily divided high dose therapy for initial control of the disease process. The initial suppressive dose level should be continued until satisfactory clinical response is obtained, usually four to ten days in the case of many allergic and collagen diseases. It is important to keep the period of initial suppressive dose as brief as possible particularly when subsequent use of alternate-day therapy is intended.

Once control has been established, two courses are available: (a) change to alternate-day therapy and then gradually reduce amount of corticoid given every other day, or (b) following control of the disease process, reduce the daily dose of corticoid to the lowest effective level as rapidly as possible and then change over to an alternate-day schedule. Theoretically, course (a) may be preferable.

4) Because of the advantages of alternate-day therapy, it may be desirable to try patients on this form of therapy who have been on daily corticoids for long periods of time (e.g., patients with rheumatoid arthritis). Since these patients may already have suppressed HPA axis establishing them on alternate-day therapy may be difficult and not always successful. However, it is recommended that regular attempts be made to change them over. It may be helpful to triple or even quadruple the daily maintenance dose and administer this every other day rather than just doubling the daily dose if difficulty is encountered. Once the patient is again controlled, an attempt should be made to reduce this dose to a minimum.

5) As indicated above, certain corticosteroids, because of their prolonged suppressive effect on adrenal activity, are not recommended for alternate-day therapy (e.g., dexamethasone and betamethasone).

6) The maximal activity of the adrenal cortex is between 2 a.m. and 8 a.m., and it is minimal between 4 p.m. and midnight. Exogenous corticosteroids suppress adrenocortical activity the least, when given at the time of maximal activity (a.m.).

7) In using alternate-day therapy it is important, as in all therapeutic situations, to individualize and tailor the therapy to each patient. Complete control of symptoms will not be possible in all patients. An explanation of the benefits of alternate-day therapy will help the patient to understand and tolerate the possible flare-up in symptoms which may occur in the latter part of the off-steroid day. Other symptomatic therapy may be added or increased at this time if needed.

8) In the event of an acute flare-up of the disease process, it may be necessary to return to a full suppressive daily divided corticoid dose for control. Once control is again established alternate-day therapy may be reinstituted.

9) Although many of the undesirable features of corticosteroid therapy can be minimized by alternate-day therapy, as in any therapeutic situation, the physician must carefully weigh the benefit-risk ratio for each patient in whom corticoid therapy is being considered.

Parenteral drug products should be inspected visually for particulate matter and discoloration prior to administration whenever the solution and container permit.

Storage: Store at controlled room temperature, 15°-30°C (59°-86°F). Do not refrigerate syrup. Do not freeze suspension; shake well before using. Dispense in a well-closed light-resistant container as defined in USP/NF.

Store oral liquid at 4°-25° C (39°-77° F). May be refrigerated. Keep tightly closed and out of the reach of children.

Prednisolone sodium phosphate solution is sensitive to heat. Do not autoclave. Protect from light. Store container in carton until contents have been used.

Pharmacist: Dispense Prednisolone Syrup with a suitable calibrated measuring device to assure proper measuring of dose.

Dose/Volume Chart
15 mg Prednisolone = 1 teaspoon
10 mg Prednisolone = ⅔ teaspoon
7.5 mg Prednisolone = ½ teaspoon
5 mg Prednisolone = ⅓ teaspoon

J CODES
5 mg ORAL K0167
Up to 1 ml IM—J2650
Up to 20 mg IM,IV—J2640

HOW SUPPLIED

PREDNISOLONE
SYRUP: 15 MG/5 ML

BRAND/MANUFACTURER	NDC	SIZE	AWP
○ BRAND			
PRELONE: Muro	00451-1500-08	240 ml	$40.28
	00451-1500-16	480 ml	$64.46

TABLET: 5 MG

BRAND/MANUFACTURER	NDC	SIZE	AWP
◆ GENERICS			
Major	00904-2155-80	1000s	$26.50

TABLET: 5 MG

BRAND/MANUFACTURER	NDC	SIZE	AWP
◇ GENERICS			
Moore,H.L.	00839-5076-06	100s	$4.04
Richlyn	00115-4280-01	100s	$4.27
Schein	00364-0217-01	100s	$4.37
Aligen	00405-4823-01	100s	$4.60
Major	00904-2155-60	100s	$4.95
Moore,H.L.	00839-5076-16	1000s	$21.59
Rugby	00536-4346-10	1000s	$25.58
Schein	00364-0217-02	1000s	$28.71
Aligen	00405-4823-03	1000s	$30.22
Richlyn	00115-4280-03	1000s	$32.85

TABLET: 5 MG

BRAND/MANUFACTURER	NDC	SIZE	AWP
○ GENERICS			
CMC-Cons	00223-1512-01	100s	$3.25
COTOLONE: Truxton	00463-6071-10	1000s	$20.50
CMC-Cons	00223-1512-02	1000s	$23.95

PREDNISOLONE ACETATE
INJECTION: 25 MG/ML

BRAND/MANUFACTURER	NDC	SIZE	AWP
◇ GENERICS			
Schein	00364-6626-54	10 ml	$5.03
KEY-PRED: Hyrex	00314-0695-70	10 ml	$6.90
Rugby	00536-6400-75	30 ml	$8.62
URL	00677-0294-23	30 ml	$9.00
Moore,H.L.	00839-5617-36	30 ml	$9.03
Schein	00364-6626-56	30 ml	$9.15
Steris	00402-0073-30	30 ml	$9.15
KEY-PRED: Hyrex	00314-0695-30	30 ml	$12.50

INJECTION: 25 MG/ML

BRAND/MANUFACTURER	NDC	SIZE	AWP
○ GENERICS			
CMC-Cons	00223-8345-01	10 ml	$6.00
Veratex	17022-2638-07	30 ml	$6.45
CMC-Cons	00223-8345-30	30 ml	$7.50
COTOLONE: Truxton	00463-1019-30	30 ml	$9.30
Interstate	00814-6255-46	30 ml	$12.46

INJECTION: 40 MG/ML

BRAND/MANUFACTURER	NDC	SIZE	AWP
○ GENERICS			
DEPO-PREDATE: Legere	25332-0121-03	10 ml	$14.95

INJECTION: 50 MG/ML

BRAND/MANUFACTURER	NDC	SIZE	AWP
◇ GENERICS			
Schein	00364-6627-54	10 ml	$6.60
Steris	00402-0249-10	10 ml	$6.60
KEY-PRED: Hyrex	00314-0697-70	10 ml	$9.90
Rugby	00536-6405-70	10 ml	$11.85
PREDAJECT-50: Mayrand	00259-0310-10	10 ml	$17.65
Schein	00364-6627-56	30 ml	$9.98
Steris	00402-0249-30	30 ml	$9.98
Moore,H.L.	00839-5126-30	30 ml	$11.73
Rugby	00536-6405-75	30 ml	$17.25
Goldline	00182-0939-66	30 ml	$18.45

INJECTION: 50 MG/ML

BRAND/MANUFACTURER	NDC	SIZE	AWP
○ GENERICS			
Veratex	17022-2659-03	10 ml	$4.60
Keene	00588-5352-70	10 ml	$5.75
PREDICORT-50: Dunhall	00217-8404-08	10 ml	$6.00
PREDCOR-50: Roberts/Hauck	59441-0606-10	10 ml	$6.25
COTOLONE: Truxton	00463-1020-10	10 ml	$6.50
PREDACORT 50: Clint	55553-0249-10	10 ml	$7.50
CMC-Cons	00223-8346-02	10 ml	$7.50
PREDALONE 50: Forest Pharm	00456-0924-10	10 ml	$7.75
PREDATE-50: Legere	25332-0031-10	10 ml	$10.95
Veratex	17022-2659-07	30 ml	$6.95
PRED-JECT-50: Hauser,A.F.	52637-0325-10	30 ml	$6.98
CMC-Cons	00223-8346-30	30 ml	$11.50
Allscrips	54569-2161-00	30 ml	$12.59

INJECTION: 80 MG/ML

BRAND/MANUFACTURER	NDC	SIZE	AWP
○ GENERICS			
DEPO-PREDATE: Legere	25332-0062-05	5 ml	$14.95

INJECTION: 20 MG/ML

AVERAGE UNIT PRICE (AVAILABLE SIZES)

BRAND	$7.63		

BRAND/MANUFACTURER	NDC	SIZE	AWP
◆ BRAND			
HYDELTRASOL: Merck	00006-7577-02	2 ml	$16.25
	00006-7577-03	5 ml	$35.64
◆ GENERICS			
KEY-PRED SP: Hyrex	00314-0696-70	10 ml	$9.90

INJECTION: 20 MG/ML

BRAND/MANUFACTURER	NDC	SIZE	AWP
○ GENERICS			
CMC-Cons	00223-8347-00	10 ml	$8.00

INJECTION: 22 MG/ML

BRAND/MANUFACTURER	NDC	SIZE	AWP
○ GENERICS			
PREDICORT-RP: Dunhall	00217-8410-08	10 ml	$7.50

LIQUID: 5 MG/5 ML

BRAND/MANUFACTURER	NDC	SIZE	AWP
○ BRAND			
PEDIAPRED: Fisons Presc	00585-2250-01	120 ml	$14.89

Prednisone

DESCRIPTION
Prednisone Tablets contain a glucocorticoid. Glucocorticoids are adrenocortical steroids, both naturally occurring and synthetic, which are readily absorbed from the gastrointestinal tract. Prednisone is a white to practically white, odorless, crystalline powder. It is very slightly soluble in water; slightly soluble in alcohol, in chloroform, in dioxane, and in methanol.

The chemical name for Prednisone is pregna-1,4-diene-3,11,20-trione, 17,21-dihydroxy- and its molecular weight is 358.43.

◆ RATED THERAPEUTICALLY EQUIVALENT; ◇ THERAPEUTIC EQUIVALENCE UNCONFIRMED; ○ UNRATED

Prednisone Tablets are available in 5 strengths: 2.5 mg, 5 mg, 10 mg, 20 mg and 50 mg.

Following is its chemical structure:

ACTIONS

Naturally occurring glucocorticoids (hydrocortisone and cortisone), which also have salt-retaining properties, are used as replacement therapy in adrenocortical deficiency states. Their synthetic analogs are primarily used for their potent anti-inflammatory effects in disorders of many organ systems.

Glucocorticoids cause profound and varied metabolic effects. In addition, they modify the body's immune responses to diverse stimuli.

INDICATIONS

Prednisone Tablets are indicated in the following conditions:

1. *Endocrine Disorders:* Primary or secondary adrenocortical insufficiency (hydrocortisone or cortisone is the first choice; synthetic analogs may be used in conjunction with mineralocorticoids where applicable; in infancy mineralocorticoid supplementation is of particular importance)
   Congenital adrenal hyperplasia
   Hypercalcemia associated with cancer
   Nonsuppurative thyroiditis

2. *Rheumatic Disorders:* As adjunctive therapy for short-term administration (to tide the patient over an acute episode or exacerbation) in:
   Psoriatic arthritis
   Rheumatoid arthritis, including juvenile rheumatoid arthritis (selected cases may require low-dose maintenance therapy)
   Ankylosing spondylitis
   Acute and subacute bursitis
   Acute nonspecific tenosynovitis
   Acute gouty arthritis
   Post-traumatic osteoarthritis
   Synovitis of osteoarthritis
   Epicondylitis

3. *Collagen Diseases:* During an exacerbation or as maintenance therapy in selected cases of:
   Systemic lupus erythematosus
   Systemic dermatomyositis (polymyositis)
   Acute rheumatic carditis

4. *Dermatologic Diseases:* Pemphigus
   Bullous dermatitis herpetiformis
   Severe erythema multiforme
   (Stevens-Johnson syndrome)
   Exfoliative dermatitis
   Mycosis fungoides
   Severe psoriasis
   Severe seborrheic dermatitis

5. *Allergic States:* Control of severe or incapacitating allergic conditions intractable to adequate trials of conventional treatment:
   Seasonal or perennial allergic rhinitis
   Bronchial asthma
   Contact dermatitis
   Atopic dermatitis
   Serum sickness
   Drug hypersensitivity reactions

6. *Ophthalmic Diseases:* Severe acute and chronic allergic and inflammatory processes involving the eye and its adnexa such as:
   Allergic corneal marginal ulcers
   Herpes zoster ophthalmicus
   Anterior segment inflammation
   Diffuse posterior uveitis and choroiditis
   Sympathetic ophthalmia
   Allergic conjunctivitis
   Keratitis
   Chorioretinitis
   Optic neuritis
   Iritis and iridocyclitis

7. *Respiratory Diseases:* Symptomatic sarcoidosis
   Loeffler's syndrome not manageable by other means
   Berylliosis
   Fulminating or disseminated pulmonary tuberculosis when used concurrently with appropriate antituberculous chemotherapy
   Aspiration pneumonitis

8. *Hematologic Disorders:* Idiopathic thrombocytopenic purpura in adults
   Secondary thrombocytopenia in adults
   Acquired (autoimmune) hemolytic anemia

Erythroblastopenia (RBC anemia)
Congenital (erythroid) hypoplastic anemia

9. *Neoplastic Diseases:* For palliative management of:
   Leukemias and lymphomas in adults
   Acute leukemia of childhood

10. *Edematous States:* To induce a diuresis or remission of proteinuria in the nephrotic syndrome, without uremia, of the idiopathic type or that due to lupus erythematosus

11. *Gastrointestinal Diseases:* To tide the patient over a critical period of the disease in:
    Ulcerative colitis
    Regional enteritis

12. *Nervous System:* Acute exacerbations of multiple sclerosis

13. *Miscellaneous:* Tuberculous meningitis with subarachnoid block or impending block when used concurrently with appropriate antituberculous chemotherapy Trichinosis with neurologic or myocardial involvement.

UNLABELED USES

Prednisone is used alone or as an adjunct in treatment to prevent respiratory deterioration in children with Pneumocystis carinii pneumonia and acquired immunodeficiency syndrome. It is also used in the treatment of alcoholic hepatitis, Bell's palsy, causalgia, cluster headache, and Crohn's disease.

Prednisone is prescribed as an adjunctive therapy in breast cancer and in biopsy-proven myocarditis. It is used to reduce morbidity and progression of pulmonary disease in cystic fibrosis patients and is prescribed for temporal arteritis or giant cell arteritis, Graves' ophthalmopathy, and Cogan's syndrome. In addition, it is used in acute otitis media, chronic active hepatitis B, Hodgkin's disease, hyphema, infantile spasms, male infertility, Duchenne muscular dystrophy, postherpetic neuralgia, fever, and myasthenia gravis. It is also prescribed to help prevent rejection after heart transplantation.

CONTRAINDICATIONS

Systemic fungal infections and known hypersensitivity to components.

WARNINGS

In patients on corticosteroid therapy subjected to unusual stress, increased dosage of rapidly acting corticosteroids before, during, and after the stressful situation is indicated.

Corticosteroids may mask some signs of infection, and new infections may appear during their use. There may be decreased resistance and inability to localize infection when corticosteroids are used.

Prolonged use of corticosteroids may produce posterior subcapsular cataracts, glaucoma with possible damage to the optic nerves, and may enhance the establishment of secondary ocular infections due to fungi or viruses.

Usage in Pregnancy: Since adequate human reproduction studies have not been done with corticosteroids, the use of these drugs in pregnancy, nursing mothers, or women of childbearing potential requires that the possible benefits of the drug be weighed against the potential hazards to the mother and embryo or fetus. Infants born of mothers who have received substantial doses of corticosteroids during pregnancy, should be carefully observed for signs of hypo-adrenalism.

Average and large doses of hydrocortisone or cortisone can cause elevation of blood pressure, salt and water retention, and increased excretion of potassium. These effects are less likely to occur with the synthetic derivatives except when used in large doses. Dietary salt restriction and potassium supplementation may be necessary. All corticosteroids increase calcium excretion.

While on corticosteroid therapy patients should not be vaccinated against smallpox. Other immunization procedures should not be undertaken in patients who are on corticosteroids, especially on high dose, because of possible hazards of neurological complications and a lack of antibody response.

The use of Prednisone Tablets in active tuberculosis should be restricted to those cases of fulminating or disseminated tuberculosis in which the corticosteroid is used for the management of the disease in conjunction with an appropriate anti-tuberculous regimen.

If corticosteroids are indicated in patients with latent tuberculosis or tuberculin reactivity, close observation is necessary as reactivation of the disease may occur. During prolonged corticosteroid therapy, these patients should receive chemoprophylaxis.

Persons who are on drugs which suppress the immune system are more susceptible to infections than healthy individuals. Chicken pox and measles, for example, can have a more serious or even fatal course in non-immune children or adults on corticosteroids. In such children or adults who have not had these diseases, particular care should be taken to avoid exposure. How the dose, route and duration of corticosteroid administration affects the risk of developing a disseminated infection is not known. The contribution of the underlying disease and/or prior corticosteroid treatment to the risk is also not known. If exposed to chicken pox, prophylaxis with varicella zoster immune globulin (VZIG) may be indicated. If exposed to measles, prophylaxis with pooled intramuscular immunoglobulin (IG) may be indicated. (See the respective package inserts for complete VZIG and IG prescribing information.) If chicken pox develops, treatment with antiviral agents may be considered.

PRECAUTIONS

Drug-induced secondary adrenocortical insufficiency may be minimized by gradual reduction of dosage. This type of relative insufficiency may persist for months after discontinuation of therapy; therefore, in any situation of stress occurring during that period, hormone therapy should be reinstituted. Since mineralocorticoid secretion may be impaired, salt and/or a mineralocorticoid should be administered concurrently.

There is an enhanced effect of corticosteroids on patients with hypothyroidism and in those with cirrhosis.

Corticosteroids should be used cautiously in patients with ocular herpes simplex because of possible corneal perforation.

The lowest possible dose of corticosteroid should be used to control the condition under treatment, and when reduction in dosage is possible, the reduction should be gradual.

Psychic derangements may appear when corticosteroids are used, ranging from euphoria, insomnia, mood swings, personality changes, and severe depression, to frank psychotic manifestations. Also, existing emotional instability or psychotic tendencies may be aggravated by corticosteroids.

Steroids should be used with caution in nonspecific ulcerative colitis, if there is a probability of impending perforation, abscess or other pyogenic infection; diverticulitis; fresh intestinal anastomoses; active or latent peptic ulcer; renal insufficiency; hypertension; osteoporosis; and myasthenia gravis.

Growth and development of infants and children on prolonged corticosteroid therapy should be carefully observed.

Although controlled clinical trials have shown corticosteroids to be effective in speeding the resolution of acute exacerbations of multiple sclerosis, they do not show that corticosteroids affect the ultimate outcome or natural history of the disease. The studies do show that relatively high doses of corticosteroids are necessary to demonstrate a significant effect. (See *"Dosage and Administration"*.)

Since complications of treatment with glucocorticoids are dependent on the size of the dose and the duration of treatment, a risk/benefit decision must be made in each individual case as to dose and duration of treatment and as to whether daily or intermittent therapy should be used.

Convulsions have been reported with concurrent use of methylprednisolone and cyclosporin. Since concurrent use of these agents results in a mutual inhibition of metabolism, it is possible that adverse events associated with the individual use of either drug may be more apt to occur.

DRUG INTERACTIONS

The pharmacokinetic interactions listed below are potentially clinically important. Drugs that induce hepatic enzymes such as phenobarbital, phenytoin and rifampin may increase the clearance of corticosteroids and may require increases in the corticosteroid dose to achieve the desired response. Drugs such as troleandomycin and ketoconazole may inhibit the metabolism of corticosteroids and thus decrease their clearance. Therefore, the dose of corticosteroid should be titrated to avoid steroid toxicity. Corticosteroids may increase the clearance of chronic high dose aspirin. This could lead to decreased salicylate serum levels or increase the risk of salicylate toxicity when corticosteroid is withdrawn. Aspirin should be used cautiously in conjunction with corticosteroids in patients suffering from hypoprothrombinemia. The effect of corticosteroids on oral anticoagulants is variable. There are reports of enhanced as well as diminished effects of anticoagulants when given concurrently with corticosteroids. Therefore, coagulation indices should be monitored to maintain the desired anticoagulant effect.

INFORMATION FOR THE PATIENT

Persons who are on immunosuppressant doses of corticosteroids should be warned to avoid exposure to chicken pox or measles. Patients should also be advised that if they are exposed, medical advice should be sought without delay.

ADVERSE REACTIONS

Fluid and Electrolyte Disturbances:
Sodium retention
Fluid retention
Congestive heart failure in susceptible patients
Potassium loss
Hypokalemic alkalosis
Hypertension
Musculoskeletal:
Muscle weakness
Steroid myopathy
Loss of muscle mass
Osteoporosis
Vertebral compression fractures
Aseptic necrosis of femoral and humeral heads
Pathologic fracture of long bones
Gastrointestinal:
Peptic ulcer with possible perforation and hemorrhage
Pancreatitis
Abdominal distention
Ulcerative esophagitis
Increases in alanine transaminase (ALT, SGPT), aspartate transaminase (AST, SGOT) and alkaline phosphatase have been observed following corticosteroid treatment. These changes are usually small, not associated with any clinical syndrome and are reversible upon discontinuation.
Dermatologic:
Impaired wound healing
Thin fragile skin
Petechiae and ecchymoses
Facial erythema
Increased sweating
May suppress reactions to skin tests

Metabolic:
Negative nitrogen balance due to protein catabolism
Neurological:
Increased intracranial pressure with papilledema (pseudo-tumor cerebri) usually after treatment
Convulsions
Vertigo
Headache
Endocrine:
Menstrual irregularities
Development of Cushingoid state
Secondary adrenocortical and pituitary unresponsiveness, particularly in times of stress, as in trauma, surgery or illness.
Suppression of growth in children
Decreased carbohydrate tolerance
Manifestations of latent diabetes mellitus
Increased requirements for insulin or oral hypoglycemic agents in diabetics
Ophthalmic:
Posterior subcapsular cataracts
Increased intraocular pressure
Glaucoma
Exophthalmos

Additional Reactions: Urticaria and other allergic, anaphylactic or hypersensitivity reactions

DOSAGE AND ADMINISTRATION

The initial dosage of Prednisone Tablets may vary from 5 mg to 60 mg of Prednisone per day depending on the specific disease entity being treated. In situations of less severity, lower doses will generally suffice, while in selected patients higher initial doses may be required. The initial dosage should be maintained or adjusted until a satisfactory response is noted. If after a reasonable period of time there is a lack of satisfactory clinical response, Prednisone should be discontinued and the patient transferred to other appropriate therapy. IT SHOULD BE EMPHASIZED THAT DOSAGE REQUIREMENTS ARE VARIABLE AND MUST BE INDIVIDUALIZED ON THE BASIS OF THE DISEASE UNDER TREATMENT AND THE RESPONSE OF THE PATIENT.

After a favorable response is noted, the proper maintenance dosage should be determined by decreasing the initial drug dosage in small decrements at appropriate time intervals until the lowest dosage which will maintain an adequate clinical response is reached. It should be kept in mind that constant monitoring is needed in regard to drug dosage. Included in the situations which may make dosage adjustments necessary are changes in clinical status secondary to remissions or exacerbations in the disease process, the patient's individual drug responsiveness, and the effect of patient exposure to stressful situations not directly related to the disease entity under treatment; in this latter situation, it may be necessary to increase the dosage of Prednisone for a period of time consistent with the patient's condition. If after long-term therapy the drug is to be stopped, it is recommended that it be withdrawn gradually rather than abruptly.

MULTIPLE SCLEROSIS

In the treatment of acute exacerbations of multiple sclerosis, daily doses of 200 mg of prednisolone for a week followed by 80 mg every other day for 1 month have been shown to be effective. (Dosage range is the same for Prednisone and prednisolone).

ADT (ALTERNATE DAY THERAPY)

ADT is a corticosteroid dosing regimen in which twice the usual daily dose of corticoid is administered every other morning. The purpose of this mode of therapy is to provide the patient requiring long-term pharmacologic dose treatment with the beneficial effects of corticoids while minimizing certain undesirable effects, including pituitary-adrenal suppression, the Cushingoid state, corticoid withdrawal symptoms, and growth suppression in children.

The rationale for this treatment schedule is based on two major premises: (a) the anti-inflammatory or therapeutic effect of corticoids persists longer than their physical presence and metabolic effects and (b) administration of the corticosteroid every other morning allows for re-establishment of more nearly normal hypothalamic-pituitary-adrenal (HPA) activity on the off-steroid day.

A brief review of the HPA physiology may be helpful in understanding this rationale. Acting primarily through the hypothalamus, a fall in free cortisol stimulates the pituitary gland to produce increasing amounts of corticotropin (ACTH) while a rise in free cortisol inhibits ACTH secretion. Normally the HPA system is characterized by diurnal (circadian) rhythm. Serum levels of ACTH rise from a low point about 10 pm to a peak level about 6 am. Increasing levels of ACTH stimulate adrenocortical activity resulting in a rise in plasma cortisol with maximal levels occurring between 2 am and 8 am. This rise in cortisol dampens ACTH production and in turn adrenocortical activity. There is a gradual fall in plasma corticoids during the day with lowest levels occurring about midnight.

The diurnal rhythm of the HPA axis is lost in Cushing's disease, a syndrome of adrenocortical hyperfunction characterized by obesity with centripetal fat distribution, thinning of the skin with easy bruisability, muscle wasting with weakness, hypertension, latent diabetes, osteoporosis, electrolyte imbalance, etc. The same clinical findings of hyperadrenocorticism may be noted during long-term pharmacologic dose corticoid therapy administered in conventional daily divided doses. It would appear, then, that a disturbance in the diurnal cycle with maintenance of elevated corticoid values during the night may play a significant role in the development of undesirable corticoid effects. Escape from these constantly elevated plasma levels for even short periods of time may be instrumental in protecting against undesirable pharmacologic effects.

During conventional pharmacologic dose corticosteroid therapy. ACTH production is inhibited with subsequent suppression of cortisol production by the adrenal cortex. Recovery time for normal HPA activity is variable depending upon the dose and duration of treatment. During this time the patient is vulnerable to any stressful situation. Although it has been shown that there is considerably less adrenal suppression following a single morning dose of prednisolone (10 mg) as opposed to a quarter of that dose administered every 6 hours, there is evidence that some suppressive effect on adrenal activity may be carried over into the following day when pharmacologic doses are used. Further, it has been shown that a single dose of certain corticosteroids will produce adrenocortical suppression for two or more days. Other corticoids, including methylprednisolone, hydrocortisone, Prednisone and prednisolone, are considered to be short acting (producing adrenocortical suppression for 1 ¼ to 1 ½ days following a single dose) and thus are recommended for alternate day therapy.

The following should be kept in mind when considering alternate day therapy:

1) Basic principles and indications for corticosteroid therapy should apply. The benefits of ADT should not encourage the indiscriminate use of steroids.

2) ADT is a therapeutic technique primarily designed for patients in whom long-term pharmacologic corticoid therapy is anticipated.

3) In less severe disease processes in which corticoid therapy is indicated, it may be possible to initiate treatment with ADT. More severe disease states usually will require daily divided high dose therapy for initial control of the disease process. The initial suppressive dose level should be continued until satisfactory clinical response is obtained, usually four to ten days in the case of many allergic and collagen diseases. It is important to keep the period of initial suppressive dose as brief as possible particularly when subsequent use of alternate day therapy is intended.

Once control has been established, two courses are available: (a) change to ADT and then gradually reduce the amount of corticoid given every other day or (b) following control of the disease process, reduce the daily dose of corticoid to the lowest effective level as rapidly as possible and then change over to an alternate day schedule. Theoretically, course (a) may be preferable.

4) Because of the advantages of ADT, it may be desirable to try patients on this form of therapy who have been on daily corticoids for long periods of time (eg, patients with rheumatoid arthritis). Since these patients may already have a suppressed HPA axis, establishing them on ADT may be difficult and not always successful. However, it is recommended that regular attempts be made to change them over. It may be helpful to triple or even quadruple the daily maintenance dose and administer this every other day rather than just doubling the daily dose if difficulty is encountered. Once the patient is again controlled, an attempt should be made to reduce this dose to a minimum.

5) As indicated above, certain corticosteroids, because of their prolonged suppressive effect on adrenal activity, are not recommended for alternate day therapy (eg, dexamethasone and betamethasone).

6) The maximal activity of the adrenal cortex is between 2 am and 8 am, and it is minimal between 4 pm and midnight. Exogenous corticosteroids suppress adrenocortical activity the least, when given at the time of maximal activity (am).

7) In using ADT it is important, as in all therapeutic situations to individualize and tailor the therapy to each patient. Complete control of symptoms will not be possible in all patients. An explanation of the benefits of ADT will help the patient to understand and tolerate the possible flare-up in symptoms which may occur in the later part of the off-steroid day. Other symptomatic therapy may be added or increased at this time if needed.

8) In the event of an acute flare-up of the disease process, it may be necessary to return to a full suppressive daily corticoid dose for control. Once control is again established alternate day therapy may be re-instituted.

9) Although many of the undesirable features of corticosteroid therapy can be minimized by ADT, as in any therapeutic situation, the physician must carefully weigh the benefit-risk ratio for each patient in whom corticoid therapy is being considered.

J CODES
Tab, 5 mg ORAL K0125
Any dose, 100 tablet ORAL—J7506

HOW SUPPLIED
SOLUTION: 5 MG/5 ML

AVERAGE UNIT PRICE (AVAILABLE SIZES)			
GENERIC	$0.07		

BRAND/MANUFACTURER	NDC	SIZE	AWP
◆ GENERICS			
Roxane	00054-3722-63	500 ml	$17.22
Roxane	00054-8722-16	5 ml 40s ud	$20.87

SYRUP: 5 MG/5 ML

BRAND/MANUFACTURER	NDC	SIZE	AWP
◇ BRAND			
LIQUID PRED: Muro	00451-1201-04	120 ml	$11.55
	00451-1201-08	240 ml	$22.58

TABLETS: 1 MG

AVERAGE UNIT PRICE (AVAILABLE SIZES)		GENERIC A-RATED AVERAGE PRICE (GAAP)	
BRAND	$0.02	100s	$4.08
GENERIC	$0.04		

BRAND/MANUFACTURER	NDC	SIZE	AWP
◆ BRAND			
▶ ORASONE: Solvay	00032-2808-01	100s	$2.51
	00032-2808-10	1000s	$22.37
◆ GENERICS			
Caremark	00339-5775-12	100s	$2.51
▶ Roxane	00054-4741-25	100s	$3.25
▶ Roxane	00054-8739-25	100s ud	$6.47
▶ Roxane	00054-4741-31	1000s	$23.81

TABLETS: 1 MG

BRAND/MANUFACTURER	NDC	SIZE	AWP
◇ BRAND			
METICORTEN: Schering	00085-0843-03	100s	$14.20

TABLETS: 2.5 MG

AVERAGE UNIT PRICE (AVAILABLE SIZES)		GENERIC A-RATED AVERAGE PRICE (GAAP)	
GENERIC	$0.07	100s	$6.61

BRAND/MANUFACTURER	NDC	SIZE	AWP
◆ GENERICS			
▶ Roxane	00054-4742-25	100s	$5.02
▶ Roxane	00054-8740-25	100s ud	$8.19

TABLETS: 2.5 MG

BRAND/MANUFACTURER	NDC	SIZE	AWP
◇ GENERICS			
▶ DELTASONE: Upjohn	00009-0032-01	100s	$2.73

TABLETS: 5 MG

AVERAGE UNIT PRICE (AVAILABLE SIZES)		GENERIC A-RATED AVERAGE PRICE (GAAP)	
BRAND	$0.03	21s	$4.30
GENERIC	$0.06	100s	$5.17
HCFA FUL (100s ea)	$0.03	1000s	$22.77
		5000s	$79.19

BRAND/MANUFACTURER	NDC	SIZE	AWP
◆ BRAND			
ORASONE: Solvay	00032-2810-01	100s	$3.03
	00032-2810-10	1000s	$21.16
◆ GENERICS			
▶ DELTASONE: Upjohn	00009-0045-04	21s	$3.05
Horizon Pharm Inc	60904-0286-20	21s	$3.25
Moore, H.L.	00839-5143-58	21s	$3.36
Major	00904-2157-19	21s	$3.90
Qualitest	00603-5332-15	21s	$3.95
STERAPRED: Mayrand	00259-0284-01	21s	$5.85
PREDNICEN-M: Central	00131-2228-81	21s	$6.75
Major	00904-2157-46	30s	$1.95
Major	00904-2157-52	60s	$2.55
Parmed	00349-2162-01	100s	$2.13
Caremark	00339-5293-12	100s	$3.03
▶ DELTASONE: Upjohn	00009-0045-01	100s	$3.05
Qualitest	00603-5332-21	100s	$3.40
Major	00904-2157-60	100s	$3.50
West-Ward	00143-1475-01	100s	$3.50
Schein	00364-0218-01	100s	$3.91
▶ URL	00677-0117-01	100s	$4.10
▶ Mutual	53489-0138-01	100s	$4.10
Aligen	00405-4828-01	100s	$4.20
▶ Roxane	00054-4728-25	100s	$4.23
Moore, H.L.	00839-5143-06	100s	$4.59
Geneva	00781-1495-01	100s	$5.08
▶ DELTASONE: Upjohn	00009-0045-05	100s ud	$3.45
Raway	00686-0032-20	100s ud	$6.00
Auro	55829-0422-10	100s ud	$6.06
UDL	51079-0032-20	100s ud	$6.37
Major	00904-2157-61	100s ud	$6.74
Goldline	00182-0201-89	100s ud	$7.00
Vangard	00615-0536-13	100s ud	$7.08
Roxane	00054-8724-25	100s ud	$7.21
Schein	00364-0218-90	100s ud	$7.50
West-Ward	00143-1475-25	100s ud	$7.50
Geneva	00781-1495-13	100s ud	$7.75
Medirex	57480-0351-01	100s ud	$7.75
▶ DELTASONE: Upjohn	00009-0045-02	500s	$7.68
▶ DELTASONE: Upjohn	00009-0045-01	1000s	$14.56
Mason Dist	11845-0178-04	1000s	$18.46
West-Ward	00143-1475-10	1000s	$19.25
▶ Rugby	00536-4324-10	1000s	$19.43
Major	00904-2157-80	1000s	$20.00
Goldline	00182-0201-10	1000s	$20.00
Schein	00364-0218-02	1000s	$21.09

▶ SHOWN IN PRODUCT IDENTIFICATION GUIDE

BRAND/MANUFACTURER	NDC	SIZE	AWP
Purepac	00228-2336-96	1000s	$22.46
Parmed	00349-8933-10	1000s	$22.58
Qualitest	00603-5332-32	1000s	$23.08
➤ URL	00677-0117-10	1000s	$24.00
➤ Mutual	53489-0138-10	1000s	$24.00
➤ Roxane	00054-4728-31	1000s	$25.99
Aligen	00405-4828-03	1000s	$29.50
Moore,H.L.	00839-5143-16	1000s	$29.97
Geneva	00781-1495-10	1000s	$29.98
➤ Mutual	53489-0138-50	5000s	$71.00
➤ Rugby	00536-4324-50	5000s	$87.38

TABLETS: 5 MG

BRAND/MANUFACTURER	NDC	SIZE	AWP
◇ GENERICS			
Richlyn	00115-4294-01	100s	$3.00
Halsey Pharm	00879-0129-01	100s	$3.25
Halsey Pharm	0879-0129-10	1000s	$18.50
Richlyn	00115-4294-03	1000s	$23.10

TABLETS: 10 MG

AVERAGE UNIT PRICE (AVAILABLE SIZES)		GENERIC A-RATED AVERAGE PRICE (GAAP)	
BRAND	$0.04	100s	$7.29
GENERIC	$0.08	500s	$24.36
HCFA FUL (100s ea)	$0.05	1000s	$43.64

BRAND/MANUFACTURER	NDC	SIZE	AWP
◆ BRAND			
ORASONE: Solvay	00032-2812-01	100s	$4.58
	00032-2812-10	1000s	$41.01
◆ GENERICS			
STERAPRED DS: Mayrand	00259-0364-21	21s	$10.25
Allscrips	54569-3302-02	45s	$3.17
STERAPRED DS: Mayrand	00259-0364-48	48s	$14.95
➤ DELTASONE: Upjohn	00009-0193-01	100s	$3.84
Caremark	00339-5295-12	100s	$4.58
Rugby	00536-4325-01	100s	$4.90
Major	00904-2141-60	100s	$5.25
Qualitest	00603-5333-21	100s	$5.30
Parmed	00349-8934-01	100s	$5.35
➤ Purepac	00228-2338-01	100s	$5.37
➤ Mutual	53489-0139-01	100s	$5.75
West-Ward	00143-1473-01	100s	$5.75
Schein	00364-0461-01	100s	$5.77
URL	00677-0698-01	100s	$6.01
Roxane	00054-4730-25	100s	$6.09
Moore,H.L.	00839-1520-06	100s	$6.62
Geneva	00781-1500-01	100s	$7.05
Goldline	00182-1334-01	100s	$7.05
Aligen	00405-4829-01	100s	$7.76
➤ DELTASONE: Upjohn	00009-0193-03	100s ud	$4.43
Goldline	00182-1334-89	100s ud	$7.10
Roxane	00054-8725-25	100s ud	$8.85
UDL	51079-0033-20	100s ud	$9.94
Major	00904-2141-61	100s ud	$11.10
Schein	00364-0461-90	100s ud	$11.50
Medirex	57480-0352-01	100s ud	$11.75
Auro	55829-0423-10	100s ud	$12.15
West-Ward	00143-1473-25	100s ud	$13.00
➤ DELTASONE: Upjohn	00009-0193-02	500s	$13.39
Aligen	00405-4829-02	500s	$22.20
➤ Mutual	53489-0139-05	500s	$22.75
Schein	00364-0461-05	500s	$25.94
Parmed	00349-8934-05	500s	$26.75
➤ Purepac	00228-2338-50	500s	$26.85
➤ Roxane	00054-4730-29	500s	$28.09
Moore,H.L.	00839-1520-12	500s	$28.89
Schein	00364-0461-02	1000s	$34.50
Mason Dist	11845-0179-04	1000s	$35.84
Major	00904-2141-80	1000s	$37.75
West-Ward	00143-1473-10	1000s	$38.00
Rugby	00536-4325-10	1000s	$39.83
Qualitest	00603-5333-32	1000s	$43.02
➤ Mutual	53489-0139-10	1000s	$43.50
URL	00677-0698-10	1000s	$46.86
Aligen	00405-4829-03	1000s	$47.38
Goldline	00182-1334-10	1000s	$48.75
Geneva	00781-1500-10	1000s	$48.85
Moore,H.L.	00839-1520-16	1000s	$51.57

TABLETS: 20 MG

AVERAGE UNIT PRICE (AVAILABLE SIZES)		GENERIC A-RATED AVERAGE PRICE (GAAP)	
BRAND	$0.08	100s	$11.54
GENERIC	$0.10	500s	$41.50
HCFA FUL (100s ea)	$0.06	1000s	$70.35

BRAND/MANUFACTURER	NDC	SIZE	AWP
◆ BRAND			
ORASONE: Solvay	00032-2814-01	100s	$8.56
	00032-2814-10	1000s	$75.60

BRAND/MANUFACTURER	NDC	SIZE	AWP
◆ GENERICS			
➤ DELTASONE: Upjohn	00009-0165-01	100s	$6.70
Mason Dist	11845-0180-01	100s	$7.55
➤ Rugby	00536-4326-01	100s	$7.95
Major	00904-2140-60	100s	$8.25
West-Ward	00143-1477-01	100s	$8.25
Caremark	00339-5777-12	100s	$8.56
Parmed	00349-8935-01	100s	$8.95
Purepac	00228-2337-01	100s	$9.23
Qualitest	00603-5334-21	100s	$9.48
Schein	00364-0442-01	100s	$9.57
URL	00677-0427-01	100s	$10.50
➤ Mutual	53489-0140-01	100s	$10.50
Goldline	00182-1086-01	100s	$10.50
Aligen	00405-4830-01	100s	$10.88
Geneva	00781-1485-01	100s	$11.75
➤ Roxane	00054-4729-31	100s	$11.77
Moore,H.L.	00839-1517-06	100s	$12.89
Raway	00686-0022-20	100s ud	$7.00
➤ DELTASONE: Upjohn	00009-0165-03	100s ud	$7.41
Goldline	00182-1086-89	100s ud	$11.90
Geneva	00781-1485-13	100s ud	$12.25
➤ Roxane	00054-8726-25	100s ud	$13.17
UDL	51079-0022-20	100s ud	$15.89
Schein	00364-0442-90	100s ud	$17.00
Medirex	57480-0472-01	100s ud	$17.20
Auro	55829-0424-10	100s ud	$17.61
West-Ward	00143-1477-25	100s ud	$18.00
Major	00904-2140-61	100s ud	$18.53
➤ DELTASONE: Upjohn	00009-0165-02	500s	$25.09
Schein	00364-0442-05	500s	$31.80
West-Ward	00143-1477-05	500s	$34.00
➤ Rugby	00536-4326-05	500s	$34.95
➤ Mutual	53489-0140-05	500s	$39.50
Aligen	00405-4830-02	500s	$40.86
Purepac	00228-2337-50	500s	$46.15
➤ Roxane	00054-4729-29	500s	$57.72
Moore,H.L.	00839-1517-12	500s	$63.45
Schein	00364-0442-02	1000s	$51.75
West-Ward	00143-1477-10	1000s	$61.75
Mason Dist	11845-0180-04	1000s	$61.99
➤ Rugby	00536-4326-10	1000s	$67.12
Qualitest	00603-5334-32	1000s	$72.12
Major	00904-2140-80	1000s	$74.55
URL	00677-0427-10	1000s	$75.00
➤ Mutual	53489-0140-10	1000s	$75.00
Goldline	00182-1086-10	1000s	$85.50

TABLETS: 20 MG

BRAND/MANUFACTURER	NDC	SIZE	AWP
◇ GENERICS			
Halsey Pharm	00879-0438-01	100s	$9.95
Halsey Pharm	00879-0438-05	500s	$43.25
Halsey Pharm	00879-0438-10	1000s	$79.95

TABLETS: 50 MG

AVERAGE UNIT PRICE (AVAILABLE SIZES)		GENERIC A-RATED AVERAGE PRICE (GAAP)	
BRAND	$0.17	100s	$24.26
GENERIC	$0.24		
HCFA FUL (100s ea)	$0.18		

BRAND/MANUFACTURER	NDC	SIZE	AWP
◆ BRAND			
ORASONE: Solvay	00032-2816-01	100s	$17.41
◆ GENERICS			
➤ Rugby	00536-4328-01	100s	$14.00
➤ DELTASONE: Upjohn	00009-0388-01	100s	$15.28
Caremark	00339-5296-12	100s	$17.41
Geneva	00781-1450-01	100s	$22.67
➤ Roxane	00054-4733-25	100s	$25.88
Major	00904-0527-60	100s	$26.95
➤ Roxane	00054-8729-25	100s ud	$29.27
West-Ward	00143-1481-25	100s ud	$32.00
Geneva	00781-1450-13	100s ud	$34.92

Pregnyl SEE GONADOTROPIN, CHORIONIC

Prelone SEE PREDNISOLONE, SYSTEMIC

Prelu-2 SEE PHENDIMETRAZINE TARTRATE

◆ RATED THERAPEUTICALLY EQUIVALENT; ◇ THERAPEUTIC EQUIVALENCE UNCONFIRMED; ○ UNRATED

Premarin *SEE* ESTROGENS, CONJUGATED

Premarin W/Methyltestosterone *SEE* ESTROGENS, CONJUGATED AND METHYLTESTOSTERONE

Prepidil *SEE* DINOPROSTONE, CERVICAL

Prevident *SEE* SODIUM FLUORIDE

Prilocaine Hydrochloride and Prilocaine with Epinephrine

DESCRIPTION

Prilocaine Hydrochloride Injection is a sterile, nonpyrogenic isotonic solution that contains a local anesthetic agent with or without Epinephrine (as bitartrate) and is administered parenterally by injection. See *"Indications and Usage"* for specific uses. The quantitative composition of each available injection is shown in Table 1.

Prilocaine Hydrochloride is chemically designated as propanamide, N-(2-methyl-phenyl)-2-(propylamino)-, monohydrochloride. Epinephrine is (−)-3,4-Dihydroxy-α-[(methylamino)methyl] benzyl alcohol.

Prilocaine has the chemical formula $C_{13}H_{20}N_2O \cdot HCl$ and molecular weight of 256.77. Epinephrine has the chemical formula $C_9H_{13}NO_3$ and molecular weight of 183.21.

Parenteral drug products should be inspected visually for particulate matter and discoloration prior to administration. The specific quantitative composition of each available injection is shown in Table 1. (See related table).

Note: Sodium hydroxide and/or hydrochloric acid may be used to adjust the pH of Prilocaine Injections. Filled under nitrogen.

CLINICAL PHARMACOLOGY

Mechanism of Action: Prilocaine stabilizes the neuronal membrane by inhibiting the ionic fluxes required for the initiation and conduction of impulses, thereby effecting local anesthetic action.

Onset and Duration of Action: When used for infiltration injection in dental patients, the time of onset of anesthesia with Prilocaine Injection and Prilocaine with Epinephrine Injection averages less than 2 minutes with an average duration of soft tissue anesthesia of approximately 2 hours with Prilocaine Injection and approximately 2¼ hours with Prilocaine with Epinephrine Injection.

Based on electrical stimulation studies, Prilocaine Injection provides a duration of pulpal anesthesia of approximately 10 minutes in maxillary infiltration injections. In clinical studies, this has been found to provide complete anesthesia for procedures lasting an average of 20 minutes.

When used for inferior alveolar nerve block, the time of onset of Prilocaine Injection and Prilocaine with Epinephrine Injection averages less than three minutes with an average duration of soft tissue anesthesia of approximately 2 1/2 hours with Prilocaine Injection and approximately 3 hours with Prilocaine with Epinephrine Injection.

Hemodynamics: Excessive blood levels may cause changes in cardiac output, total peripheral resistance, and mean arterial pressure. These changes may be attributable to a direct depressant effect of the local anesthetic agent on various components of the cardiovascular system and/or the beta-adrenergic receptor stimulating action of Epinephrine when present.

Pharmacokinetics and Metabolism: Information derived from diverse formulations, concentrations and usages reveals that Prilocaine is completely absorbed following parenteral administration, its rate of absorption depending, for example, upon such factors as the site of administration and the presence or absence of a vasoconstrictor agent. Prilocaine is metabolized in both the liver and the kidney and excreted via the kidney. It is not metabolized by plasma esterases. Hydrolysis of Prilocaine by amidases yields ortho-toluidine and N-propylalanine. Both of these compounds may undergo ring hydroxylation.

O-toluidine has been found to produce methemoglobin, both *in vitro* and *in vivo* (see *"Adverse Reactions"*).

Because Prilocaine is metabolized in both the liver and kidneys, hepatic and renal dysfunction may alter Prilocaine kinetics.

As with other local anesthetic agents, the plasma binding of Prilocaine may be dependent on drug concentration. At 0.5-1.0 µg/mL it is 55% protein bound.

Prilocaine crosses the blood-brain and placental barriers, presumably by passive diffusion.

Factors such as acidosis and the use of CNS stimulants and depressants affect the CNS levels of Prilocaine required to produce overt systemic effects. In the rhesus monkey, arterial blood levels of 20 µg/mL have been shown to be the threshold for convulsive activity.

INDICATIONS AND USAGE

Prilocaine Hydrochloride 4% Plain and 4% Prilocaine with Epinephrine Injections are indicated for the production of local anesthesia in denistry by nerve block or infiltration techniques. Only accepted procedures for these techniques as described in standard textbooks are recommended.

CONTRAINDICATIONS

Prilocaine is contraindicated in patients with a known history of hypersensitivity to local anesthetics of the amide type and in those rare patients with congenital or idiopathic methemoglobinemia.

WARNINGS

DENTAL PRACTITIONERS WHO EMPLOY LOCAL ANESTHETIC AGENTS SHOULD BE WELL VERSED IN DIAGNOSIS AND MANAGEMENT OF EMERGENCIES THAT MAY ARISE FROM THEIR USE. RESUSCIATIVE EQUIPMENT, OXYGEN AND OTHER RESUSCITATIVE DRUGS SHOULD BE AVAILABLE FOR IMMEDIATE USE.

To minimize the likelihood of intravascular injection, aspiration should be performed before the local anesthetic solution is injected. If blood is aspirated, the needle must be repositioned until no return of blood can be elicited by aspiration. Note, however, that the absence of blood in the syringe does not assure that intravascular injection will be avoided.

Certain brands of Prilocaine with Epinephrine Injections contain sodium metabisulfite, a sulfite that may cause allergic-type reactions including anaphylactic symptoms and life-threatening or less severe asthmatic episodes in certain susceptible people. The overall prevalence of sulfite sensitivity in the general population is unknown and probably low. Sulfite sensitivity is seen more frequently in asthmatic than in nonasthmatic people.

PRECAUTIONS

General: The safety and effectiveness of Prilocaine depend on proper dosage, correct technique, adequate precautions, and readiness for emergencies. Standard textbooks should be consulted for specific techniques and precautions for various regional anesthetic procedures. Resuscitative equipment, oxygen, and other resuscitative drugs should be available for immediate use. (See *"Warnings"* and *"Adverse Reactions"*.) The lowest dosage that results in effective anesthesia should be used to avoid high plasma levels and serious adverse effects. Repeated doses of Prilocaine may cause significant increases in blood levels with each repeated dose because of slow accumulation of the drug or its metabolites. Tolerance to elevated blood levels varies with the status of the patient. Debilitated, elderly patients, acutely ill patients, and children should be given reduced doses commensurate with their age and physical status. Prilocaine should also be used with caution in patients with severe shock or heart block.

Local anesthetic injections containing a vasoconstrictor should be used cautiously in areas of the body supplied by end arteries or having otherwise compromised blood supply. Patients with peripheral vascular disease and those with hypertensive vascular disease may exhibit exaggerated vasoconstrictor response. Ischemic injury or necrosis may result. Preparations containing a vasoconstrictor should be used with caution in patients during or following the administration of potent general anesthetic agents, since cardiac arrhythmias may occur under such conditions.

Cardiovascular and respiratory (adequacy of ventilation) vital signs and the patient's state of consciousness should be monitored after each local anesthetic injection. Restlessness, anxiety, tinnitus, dizziness, blurred vision, tremors, depression or drowsiness should alert the practitioner to the possibility of central nervous system toxicity. Signs and symptoms of depressed cardiovascular function may commonly result from a vasovagal reaction, particularly if the patient is in an upright position. (See *"Adverse Reactions, Cardiovascular System"*.)

Since amide-type local anesthetics are metabolized by the liver, Prilocaine should be used with caution in patients with hepatic disease.

Table 1
COMPOSITION OF AVAILABLE INJECTIONS

Product Identification	Formula (mg/mL)				
	Prilocaine HCl	Epinephrine (as the Bitartrate)	Citric Acid	Sodium Metabisulfite	pH
Prilocaine Injection	40.0	None	None	None	6.0-7.0
Prilocaine Injection with Epinephrine	40.0	0.005	0.2	0.5	3.3-5.5

➤ SHOWN IN PRODUCT IDENTIFICATION GUIDE

Patients with severe hepatic disease, because of their inability to metabolize local anesthetics normally, are at greater risk of developing toxic plasma concentrations. Prilocaine should also be used with caution in patients with impaired cardiovascular function since they may be less able to compensate for functional changes associated with the prolongation of A-V conduction produced by these drugs.

Many drugs used during the conduct of anesthesia are considered potential triggering agents for familial malignant hyperthermia. Since it is not known whether amide-type local anesthetics may trigger this reaction and since the need for supplemental general anesthesia cannot be predicted in advance, it is suggested that a standard protocol for the management of malignant hyperthermia should be available. Early unexplained signs of tachycardia, tachypnea, labile blood pressure and metabolic acidosis may precede temperature elevation. Successful outcome is dependent on early diagnosis, prompt discontinuance of the suspect triggering agent(s) and institution of treatment, including oxygen therapy, indicated supportive measures and dantrolene (consult dantrolene sodium intravenous package insert before using).

Prilocaine should be used with caution in persons with known drug sensitivities. Patients allergic to para-aminobenzoic acid derivatives (procaine, tetracaine, benzocaine, etc.) have not shown cross sensitivity to Prilocaine.

Use in the Head and Neck Area: Small doses of local anesthetics injected into the head and neck area, including retrobulbar, dental and stellate ganglion blocks, may produce adverse reactions similar to systemic toxicity seen with unintentional intravascular injections of larger doses. Confusion, convulsions, respiratory depression and/or respiratory arrest, and cardiovascular stimulation or depression have been reported. These reactions may be due to intra-arterial injection of the local anesthetic with retrograde flow to the cerebral circulation. Patients receiving these blocks should have their circulation and respiration monitored and be constantly observed. Resuscitative equipment and personnel for treating adverse reactions should be immediately available. Dosage recommendations should not be exceeded. (See *"Dosage and Administration"*.)

Information for Patients: The patient should be informed of the possibility of temporary loss of sensation and muscle function following infiltration or nerve block injections.

The patient should be advised to exert caution to avoid inadvertent trauma to the lips, tongue, cheek mucosae or soft palate when these structures are anesthetized. The ingestion of food should therefore be postponed until normal function returns.

The patient should be advised to consult the dentist if anesthesia persists, of if a rash develops.

Clinically Significant Drug Interactions: The administration of local anesthetic injections containing Epinephrine or norepinephrine to patients receiving monoamine oxidase inhibitors, tricyclic antidepressants or phenothiazines may produce severe, prolonged hypotension or hypertension. Concurrent use of these agents should generally be avoided. In situations when concurrent therapy is necessary, careful patient monitoring is essential.

Concurrent administration of vasopressor drugs and ergot-type oxytocic drugs may cause severe, persistent hypertension or cerebrovascular accidents.

Drug/Laboratory Test Interactions: The intramuscular injection of Prilocaine may result in an increase in creatine phosphokinase levels. Thus, the use of this enzyme determination, without isoenzyme separation, as a diagnostic test for the presence of acute myocardial infarction may be compromised by the intramuscular injection of Prilocaine.

Carcinogenesis, Mutagenesis, Impairment of Fertility: Studies of Prilocaine in animals to evaluate the carcinogenic and mutagenic potential or the effect on fertility have not been conducted.

Chronic oral toxicity studies of ortho-toluidine, a metabolite of Prilocaine, in mice (150-4800 mg/kg) and rats (150-800 mg/kg) have shown that ortho-toluidine is a carcinogen in both species. The lowest dose corresponds to approximately 50 times the maximum amount or ortho-toluidine to which a 50 kg subject would be expected to be exposed following a single injection (8 mg/kg) of Prilocaine.

Ortho-toluidine (0.5 µg/mL) showed positive results in *Escherichia coli* DNA repair and phage-induction assays. Urine concentrates from rats treated with ortho-toluidine (300 mg/kg, orally) were mutagenic for *Salmonella typhimurium* with metabolic activation. Several other tests, including reverse mutations in five different *Salmonella typhimurium* strains with or without metabolic activation and single strand breaks in DNA of V79 Chinese hamster cells, were negative.

Use in Pregnancy: Teratogenic Effects. Pregnancy Category B. Reproduction studies have been performed in rats at doses up to 30 times the human dose and revealed no evidence of impaired fertility or harm to the fetus due to Prilocaine. There are, however, no adequate and well-controlled studies in pregnant women. Animal reproduction studies are not always predictive of human response. General consideration should be given to this fact before administering Prilocaine to women of childbearing potential, especially during early pregnancy when maximum organogenesis takes place.

Nursing Mothers: It is not known whether this drug is excreted in human milk. Because many drugs are excreted in human milk, caution should be exercised Prilocaine is administered to a nursing woman.

Pediatric Use: Dosages in children should be reduced, commensurate with age, body weight, and physical condition. (See *"Dosage and Administration"*.)

ADVERSE REACTIONS

Swelling and persistent paresthesia of the lips and oral tissues may occur. Persistent paresthesia lasting weeks to months, and in rare instances paresthesia lasting greater than one year have been reported.

Adverse experiences following the administration of Prilocaine are similar in nature to those observed with other amide local anesthetic agents. These adverse experiences are, in general, dose-related and may result from high plasma levels caused by excessive dosage, rapid absorption or unintentional intravascular injection, or may result from a hypersensitivity, idiosyncrasy or diminished tolerance on the part of the patient. Serious adverse experiences are generally systemic in nature. The following types are those most commonly reported:

Central Nervous System: CNS manifestations are excitatory and/or depressant and may be characterized by light-headedness, nervousness, apprehension, euphoria, confusion, dizziness, drowsiness, tinnitus, blurred or double vision, vomiting, sensations of heat, cold or numbness, twitching, tremors, convulsions, unconsciousness, respiratory depression, and arrest. The excitatory manifestations may be very brief or may not occur at all, in which case the first manifestation of toxicity may be drowsiness merging into unconsciousness and respiratory arrest.

Drowsiness following the administration of Prilocaine is usually an early sign of a high blood level of the drug and may occur as a consequence of rapid absorption.

Cardiovascular System: Cardiovascular manifestations are usually depressant and are characterized by bradycardia, hypotension, and cardiovascular collapse, which may lead to cardiac arrest.

Signs and symptoms of depressed cardiovascular function may commonly result from a vasovagal reaction, particularly if the patient is in an upright position. Less commonly, they may result from a direct effect of the drug. Failure to recognize the premonitory signs such as sweating, a feeling of faintness, changes in pulse or sensorium may result in progressive cerebral hypoxia and seizure or serious cardiovascular catastrophe. Management consists of placing the patient in the recumbent position and ventilation with oxygen. Supportive treatment of circulatory depression may require the administration of intravenous fluids, and, when appropriate, a vasopressor (e.g., ephedrine) as directed by the clinical situation.

Allergic: Allergic reactions are characterized by cutaneous lesions, urticaria, edema or anaphylactoid reactions. Allergic reactions as a result of sensitivity to Prilocaine are extremely rare and, if they occur, should be managed by conventional means. The detection of sensitivity by skin testing is of doubtful value.

Neurologic: The incidences of adverse reactions (e.g., persistent neurologic deficit) associated with the use of local anesthetics may be related to the technique employed, the total dose of local anesthetic administered, the particular drug used, the route of administration, and the physical condition of the patient.

OVERDOSAGE

Acute emergencies from local anesthetics are generally related to high plasma levels encountered during therapeutic use of local anesthetics (see *"Adverse Reactions," "Warnings,"* and *"Precautions"*).

Management of Local Anesthetic Emergencies: The first consideration is prevention, best accomplished by careful and constant monitoring of cardiovascular and respiratory vital signs and the patient's state of consciousness after each local anesthetic injection. At the first sign of change, oxygen should be administered.

The first step in the management of convulsions consists of immediate attention to the maintenance of a patent airway and assisted or controlled ventilation with oxygen and a delivery system capable of permitting immediate positive airway pressure by mask. Immediately after the institution of these ventilatory measures, the adequacy of the circulation should be evaluated, keeping in mind that drugs used to treat convulsions sometimes depress the circulation when administered intravenously. Should convulsions persist despite adequate respiratory support, and if the status of the circulation permits, small increments of an ultra-short acting barbiturate (such as thiopental or thiamylal) or a benzodiazepine (such as diazepam) may be administered intravenously. The clinician should be familiar, prior to use of local anesthetics, with these anticonvulsant drugs. Supportive treatment of circulatory depression may require administration of intravenous fluids and, when appropriate, a vasopressor as directed by the clinical situation (e.g., ephedrine).

If not treated immediately, both convulsions and cardiovascular depression can result in hypoxia, acidosis, bradycardia, arrhythmias and cardiac arrest. If cardiac arrest should occur, standard cardiopulmonary resuscitative measures should be instituted.

Endotracheal intubation, employing drugs and techniques familiar to the clinician, may be indicated, after initial administration of oxygen by mask, if difficulty is encountered in the maintenance of a patent airway or if prolonged ventilatory support (assisted or controlled) is indicated.

Dialysis is of negligible value in the treatment of acute overdosage with Prilocaine.

Administration of Prilocaine in doses exceeding 400 mg has been associated with methemoglobinemia in adult patients and with proportionately lower doses in children. While methemoglobin values of less than 20% do not generally produce any clinical symptoms, the appearance of cyanosis at 2-4 hours following administration should be evaluated in terms of the general health status of the patient.

◆ RATED THERAPEUTICALLY EQUIVALENT; ◇ THERAPEUTIC EQUIVALENCE UNCONFIRMED; ○ UNRATED

Methemoglobinemia can be reversed when indicated by intravenous administration of methylene blue at a dosage of 1-2 mg/kg given over a five minute period.

The subcutaneous LD$_{50}$ of Prilocaine HCl in female mice is 550 (359-905) mg/kg.

DOSAGE AND ADMINISTRATION

The dosage of Prilocaine Injection and Prilocaine with Epinephrine Injection varies and depends on the physical status of the patient, the area of the oral cavity to be anesthetized, the vascularity of the oral tissues, and the technique of anesthesia. The least volume of injection that results in effective local anesthesia should be administered. For specific techniques and procedures of local anesthesia in the oral cavity, refer to standard textbooks.

Inferior Alveolar Block: There are no practical clinical differences between Prilocaine with and without Epinephrine when used for inferior alveolar blocks.

Maxillary Infiltration: Prilocaine is recommended for use in maxillary infiltration anesthesia for procedures in which the painful aspects can be completed within 15 minutes after the injection. Prilocaine is therefore especially suited to short procedures in the maxillary anterior teeth. For long procedures, or those involving maxillary posterior teeth where soft tissue numbness is not troublesome to the patient, Prilocaine with Epinephrine is recommended.

For most routine procedures, initial dosages of 1 to 2 mL of Prilocaine Injection or Prilocaine with Epinephrine Injection will usually provide adequate infiltration or major nerve block anesthesia. No more than 600 mg (15 mL; 8 cartridges) should ever be administered within a two hour period in normal healthy adults.

In children under 10 years of age it is rarely necessary to administer more than one-half cartridge (40 mg) of Prilocaine Injection or Prilocaine with Epinephrine Injection per procedure to achieve local anesthesia for a procedure involving a single tooth. In maxillary infiltration, this amount will often suffice to the treatment of two or even three teeth. In the mandibular block, however, satisfactory anesthesia achieved with this amount of drug will allow treatment of the teeth in an entire quadrant.

Aspiration Prior to Injection is Recommended: since it reduces the possibility of intravascular injection, thereby keeping the incidence of side effects and anesthetic failure to a minimum.

Note: Parenteral drug products should be inspected visually for particulate matter and discoloration prior to administration whenever the solution and container permit. Solutions that are discolored and/or contain particulate matter should not be used.

Any unused portion of a cartridge of Prilocaine or Prilocaine with Epinephrine Injection should be discarded.

Maximum Recommended Dosages: Normal Healthy Adults: No more than 600 mg (8 mg/kg or 4 mg/lb) of Prilocaine HCl should be administered as a single injection.

Children: It is difficult to recommend a maximum dose of any drug for children since this varies as a function of age and weight. For children of less than ten years who have a normal lean body mass and normal body development, the maximum dose may be determined by the application of one the standard pediatric drug formulas (e.g., Clark's rule). For example, in a child of five years weighing 50 lbs., the dose of Prilocaine Hydrochloride should not exceed 150-200 mg (6.6-8.8 mg/kg or 3-4 mg/lb of body weight) when calculated according to Clark's rule.

STERILIZATION, STORAGE AND TECHNICAL PROCEDURES

1. Cartridges of Prilocaine Injection and Prilocaine with Epinephrine Injection should not be autoclaved, because solutions of Epinephrine and the closures employed in cartridges cannot withstand autoclaving temperatures and pressures.

2. If chemical disinfection of anesthetic cartridges is desired, either 91% isopropyl alcohol or 70% ethyl alcohol is recommended. Many commercially available brands of rubbing alcohol, as well as solutions of ethyl alcohol not of U.S.P. grade, contain denaturants that are injurious to rubber and, therefore, are not to be used. It is recommended that chemical disinfection be accomplished by wiping the cartridge cap thoroughly with a pledget of cotton that has been moistened with the recommended alcohol just prior to use. *Immersion Is Not Recommended.*

3. Certain metallic ions (mercury, zinc, copper, etc.) have been related to swelling and edema after local anesthesia in dentistry. Therefore, chemical disinfectants containing or releasing these ions are not recommended. Antirust tablets usually contain metal ions. Accordingly, aluminum sealed cartridges should not be kept in such solutions.

4. Quaternary ammonium salts, such as benzalkonium chloride, are electrolytically incompatible with aluminum. Cartridges of Prilocaine Injection and Prilocaine with Epinephrine Injection are sealed with aluminum caps and therefore should not be immersed in any solution containing these salts.

5. To avoid leakage of solutions during injection, be sure to penetrate the center of the rubber diaphragm when loading the syringe. An off-center penetration produces an oval shaped puncture that allows leakage around the needle.

Other causes of leakage and breakage include badly worn syringes, aspirating syringes with bent harpoons, the use of syringes not designed to take 1.8 mL cartridges, and inadvertent freezing.

6. Cracking of glass cartridges is most often the result of an attempt to use a cartridge with an extruded plunger. An extruded plunger loses its lubrication and can be forced back into the cartridge only with difficulty. Cartridges with extruded plungers should be discarded.

7. Store at room temperature, approximately 25°C (77°F).

8. Solutions containing Epinephrine should be protected from light.

HOW SUPPLIED
INJECTION: 4%

BRAND/MANUFACTURER	NDC	SIZE	AWP
○ **BRAND**			
CITANEST HCL FORTE: Astra	00186-0540-14	1.8 ml 100s	$35.00
CITANEST HCL PLAIN: Astra	00186-0520-14	1.8 ml 100s	$35.00

Prilosec SEE OMEPRAZOLE

Primacor I.V. SEE MILRINONE LACTATE

Primaplex SEE VITAMINS, MULTI, INJECTABLE

Primaquine Phosphate

> **WARNING**
> PHYSICIANS SHOULD COMPLETELY FAMILIARIZE THEMSELVES WITH THE COMPLETE CONTENTS OF THIS LEAFLET BEFORE PRESCRIBING PRIMAQUINE PHOSPHATE.

DESCRIPTION

Primaquine Phosphate is 8-[(4-Amino-1-methylbutyl) amino]-6-methoxyquinoline phosphate, a synthetic compound with potent antimalarial activity. The dosage is customarily expressed in terms of the base.

Following is its chemical structure:

$$CH(CH_3) - CH_2CH_2CH_2 - NH_2$$

$$\cdot \; 2H_3PO_4$$

ACTION

Primaquine is an 8-amino-quinoline compound which eliminates tissue (exo-erythrocytic) infection. Thereby, it prevents the development of the blood (erythrocytic) forms of the parasite which are responsible for relapses in vivax malaria. Primaquine Phosphate is also active against gametocytes of *Plasmodium falciparum.*

INDICATION

Primaquine is indicated for the radical cure (prevention of relapse) of vivax malaria.

CONTRAINDICATIONS

Primaquine is contraindicated in acutely ill patients suffering from systemic disease manifested by tendency to granulocytopenia, such as rheumatoid arthritis and lupus erythematosus. The drug is also contraindicated in patients receiving concurrently other potentially hemolytic drugs or depressants of myeloid elements of the bone marrow.

Because quinacrine hydrochloride appears to potentiate the toxicity of antimalarial compounds which are structurally related to Primaquine the use of quinacrine in patients receiving Primaquine is contraindicated. Similarly Primaquine should not be administered to patients who have received quinacrine recently, as toxicity is increased.

WARNINGS

Discontinue the use of Primaquine promptly if signs suggestive of hemolytic anemia occur (darkening of the urine, marked fall of hemoglobin or erythrocytic count).

Hemolytic reactions (moderate to severe) may occur in glucose-6-phosphate dehydrogenase (G-6-PD) deficient Caucasians (particularly in Sardinians and in individuals with a family or personal history of favism). Dark-skinned persons Negroes, for example) have a great tendency to develop hemolytic anemia (due to congenital deficiency of erythrocytic glucose-6-phosphate dehydrogenase) while receiving Primaquine and related drugs.

Usage in Pregnancy: Safe usage of this preparation in pregnancy has not been established. Therefore, use of it during pregnancy should be avoided except when in the judgment of the physician the benefit outweighs the possible hazard.

PRECAUTIONS

Since anemia, methemoglobinemia, and leukopenia have been observed following administration of large doses of Primaquine the adult dosage of 1 tablet (=15 mg base) daily for fourteen days should not be exceeded. It is also advisable to make routine blood examinations (particularly blood cell counts and hemoglobin determinations) during therapy.

If Primaquine is prescribed for (1) an individual who has shown a previous idiosyncrasy to Primaquine (as manifested by hemolytic anemia, methemoglobinemia, or leukopenia), (2) an individual with a family or personal history of favism, or (3) an individual with erythrocytic glucose-6-phosphate dehydrogenase (G-6-PD) deficiency or nicotinamide adenine dinucleotide (NADH) methemoglobin reductase deficiency, the person should be observed closely for tolerance. The drug should be discontinued immediately if marked darkening of the urine or sudden decrease in hemoglobin concentration or leukocyte count occurs.

ADVERSE REACTIONS

Gastrointestinal: nausea, vomiting, epigastric distress, and abdominal cramps.

Hematologic: leukopenia, hemolytic anemia in glucose-6-phosphate dehydrogenase (G-6-PD) deficient individuals, and methemoglobinemia in nicotinamide adenine dinucleotide (NADH) methemoglobin reductase deficient individuals.

DOSAGE AND ADMINISTRATION

Primaquine is recommended only for the radical cure of vivax malaria, the prevention of relapse in vivax malaria, or following the termination of chloroquine phosphate suppressive therapy in an area where vivax malaria is endemic. Patients suffering from an attack of vivax malaria or having parasitized red blood cells should receive a course of chloroquine phosphate, which quickly destroys the erythrocytic parasites and terminates the paroxysm. Primaquine should be administered concurrently in order to eradicate the exo-erytrocytic parasites in a dosage of 1 tablet (equivalent to 15 mg base) daily for 14 days.

OVERDOSAGE

Symptoms of overdosage of Primaquine are similar to those seen after overdosage of pamaquine. They include abdominal cramps, vomiting, burning epigastric distress, central nervous system and cardiovascular disturbances, cyanosis, methemoglobinemia, moderate leukocytosis or leukopenia, and anemia. The most striking symptoms are granulocytopenia and acute hemolytic anemia in sensitive persons. Acute hemolysis occurs, but patients recover completely if the dosage is discontinued.

CLINICAL STUDIES

Malariologists agree that malaria produced by *Plasmodium vivax* is the most difficult form to treat. This is ascribed to the ability of the parasite to develop extremely resistant tissue forms which are not eradicated by ordinary antimalarial compounds.

Thus, persons with acute attacks of vivax malaria, provoked by the release of erythrocytic forms of the parasite, respond readily to therapy, particularly to chloroquine phosphate. However, prior to the discovery of Primaquine no antimalarial drug was available that could be relied on to eliminate tissue (exo-erythrocytic) infection and to prevent relapses. The various investigations made with Primaquine PO₄ in experimentally induced vivax malaria in human volunteers and in persons with naturally occurring infections have demonstrated that the drug is a valuable adjunct to conventional therapy in this refractory form of the disease.

HOW SUPPLIED
TABLETS: 26.3 MG

BRAND/MANUFACTURER	NDC	SIZE	AWP
○ BRAND			
PRIMAQUINE PHOSPHATE: Sanofi Winthrop	00024-1597-04	100s	$62.94

Primaquine Phosphate *SEE PRIMAQUINE*
PHOSPHATE

Primaxin *SEE* CILASTATIN SODIUM AND IMIPENEM

Primidone

Primidone is a white, crystalline, highly stable substance, M.P. 279-284°C. It is poorly soluble in water (60 mg per 100 mL at 37°C) and in most organic solvents. It possesses no acidic properties, in contrast to its barbiturate analog.

DESCRIPTION
Chemical name: 5-ethyldihydro-5-phenyl-4,6 (1H, 5H) Pyrimidinedione.

Following is its chemical structure:

ACTIONS

Primidone raises electro- or chemoshock seizure thresholds or alters seizure patterns in experimental animals. The mechanism(s) of Primidone's antiepilptic action is not known.

Primidone *per se* has anticonvulsant activity as do its two metabolites, phenobarbital and phenylethylamalonamide (PEMA). In addition to its anticonvulsant activity, PEMA potentiates the anticonvulsant activity of phenobarbital in experimental animals.

INDICATIONS

Primidone used alone or concomitantly with other anticonvulsants, is indicated in the control of grand mal, psychomotor, and focal epileptic seizures. It may control grand mal seizures refractory to other anticonvulsant therapy.

UNLABELED USES
Primidone is used alone or as an adjunct in the treatment of essential tremor.

CONTRAINDICATIONS

Primidone is contraindicated in: 1) patients with porphyria and 2) patients who are hypersensitive to phenobarbital (see *"Actions"*).

WARNINGS

The abrupt withdrawal of antiepileptic medication may precipitate status epilepticus.

The therapeutic efficacy of a dosage regimen takes several weeks before it can be assessed.

USAGE IN PREGNANCY

The effects of Primidone in human pregnancy and nursing infants are unknown.

Recent reports suggest an association between the use of anticonvulsant drugs by women with epilepsy and an elevated incidence of birth defects in children born to these women. Data are more extensive with respect to diphenylhydantoin and phenobarbital, but these are also the most commonly prescribed anticonvulsants; less systematic or anecdotal reports suggest a possible similar association with the use of all known anticonvulsant drugs.

The reports suggesting an elevated incidence of birth defects in children of drug-treated epileptic women cannot be regarded as adequate to prove a definite cause and effect relationship. There are intrinsic methodologic problems in obtaining adequate data on drug teratogenicity in humans; the possibility also exists that other factors leading to birth defects, *e.g.*, genetic factors or the epileptic condition itself, may be more important than drug therapy. The majority of mothers on anticonvulsant medication deliver normal infants. It is important to note that anticonvulsant drugs should not be discontinued in patients in whom the drug is administered to prevent major seizures because of the strong possibility of precipitating status epilepticus with attendant hypoxia and threat to life. In individual cases where the severity and frequency of the seizure disorders are such that the removal of medication does not pose a serious threat to the patient, discontinuation of the drug may be considered prior to and during pregnancy, although it cannot be said with any confidence that even minor seizures do not pose some hazard to the developing embryo or fetus.

The prescribing physician will wish to weigh these considerations in treating or counseling epileptic women of childbearing potential.

Neonatal hemorrhage, with a coagulation defect resembling vitamin K deficiency, has been described in newborns whose mothers were taking Primidone and other anticonvulsants. Pregnant women under anticonvulsant therapy should receive prophylactic vitamin K₁ therapy for one month prior to, and during, delivery.

PRECAUTIONS

The total daily dosage should not exceed 2 g. Since Primidone therapy generally extends over prolonged periods, a complete blood count and a sequential multiple analysis-12 (SMA-12) test should be made every six months.

IN NURSING MOTHERS

There is evidence that in mothers treated with Primidone, the drug appears in the milk in substantial quantities. Since tests for the presence of Primidone in biological fluids are too complex to be carried out in the average clinical laboratory, it is suggested that the presence of undue somnolence and drowsiness in nursing newborns of Primidone-treated mothers be taken as an indication that nursing should be discontinued.

ADVERSE REACTIONS

The most frequently occurring early side effects are ataxia and vertigo. These tend to disappear with continued therapy, or with reduction of initial dosage. Occasionally, the following have been reported: nausea, anorexia, vomiting, fatigue, hyperirritability, emotional disturbances, sexual impotency, diplopia, nystagmus, drowsiness, and morbilliform skin eruptions. Granulocytopenia, and red-cell hypoplasia and aplasia, have been reported rarely. These and, occasionally, other persistent or severe side effects may necessitate withdrawal of the drug.

◆ RATED THERAPEUTICALLY EQUIVALENT; ◇ THERAPEUTIC EQUIVALENCE UNCONFIRMED; ○ UNRATED

Megaloblastic anemia may occur as a rare idiosyncrasy to Primidone and to other anticonvulsants. The anemia responds to folic acid without necessity of discontinuing medication.

DOSAGE AND ADMINISTRATION

ADULT DOSAGE

Patients 8 years of age and older who have received no previous treatment may be started on Primidone according to the following regimen using either 50 mg or scored 250 mg Primidone tablets.

Days 1 to 3: 100 to 125 mg at bedtime
Days 4 to 6: 100 to 125 mg b.i.d.
Days 7 to 9: 100 to 125 mg t.i.d.
Day 10 to maintenance: 250 mg t.i.d.

For most adults and children 8 years of age and over, the usual maintenance dosage is three to four 250 mg Primidone tablets daily in divided doses (250 mg t.i.d. or q.i.d.). If required, an increase to five or six 250 mg tablets daily may be made by daily doses should not exceed 500 mg q.i.d.

INITIAL ADULTS AND CHILDREN OVER 8

Key: ·· = 50 mg tablet			■ = 250 mg tablet		
Day	1	2	3	4	5	6
AM						
NOON						
PM	··	··	··	··		

Day	7	8	9	10	11	12
AM				■		
NOON	··	··	··	■		Adjust to
PM	··	··	··	■		Maintenance

Dosage should be individualized to provide maximum benefit. In some cases, serum blood level determinations of Primidone may be necessary for optimal dosage adjustment. The clinically effective serum level for Primidone is between 5 to 12μg/mL.

IN PATIENTS ALREADY RECEIVING OTHER ANTICONVULSANTS

Primidone should be started at 100 to 125 mg at bedtime and gradually increased to maintenance level as the other drug is gradually decreased. This regimen should be continued until satisfactory dosage level is achieved for the combination, or the other medication is completely withdrawn. When therapy with Primidone alone is the objective, the transition from concomitant therapy should not be completed in less than two weeks.

PEDIATRIC DOSAGE

For children under 8 years of age, the following regimen may be used:

Days 1 to 3: 50 mg at bedtime
Days 4 to 6: 50 mg b.i.d.
Days 7 to 9: 100 mg b.i.d.
Day 10 to maintenance: 125 mg t.i.d. to 250 mg t.i.d.

For children under 8 years of age, the usual maintenance dosage is 125 to 250 mg three times daily or, 10 to 25 mg/kg/day in divided doses.

STORAGE

Store at room temperature, approximately 25° C (77° F).
Dispense in a tight, light-resistant container as defined in the U.S.P.

HOW SUPPLIED

SUSPENSION: 250 MG/5 ML

BRAND/MANUFACTURER	NDC	SIZE	AWP
○ BRAND			
MYSOLINE: Wyeth-Ayerst	00046-3850-08	240 ml	$34.90

TABLETS: 50 MG

AVERAGE UNIT PRICE (AVAILABLE SIZES)			
BRAND	$0.15		

BRAND/MANUFACTURER	NDC	SIZE	AWP
◆ BRAND			
MYSOLINE: Wyeth-Ayerst	00046-0431-81	100s	$15.31
	00046-0431-85	500s	$72.86

TABLETS: 250 MG

AVERAGE UNIT PRICE (AVAILABLE SIZES)		GENERIC A-RATED AVERAGE PRICE (GAAP)	
BRAND	$0.45	100s	$33.62
GENERIC	$0.33	1000s	$327.29

BRAND/MANUFACTURER	NDC	SIZE	AWP
◆ BRAND			
MYSOLINE: Wyeth-Ayerst	00046-0430-81	100s	$44.58
	00046-0430-99	100s ud	$47.71
	00046-0430-91	1000s	$424.40
◆ GENERICS			
Caremark	00339-5659-12	100s	$29.15
Qualitest	00603-5370-21	100s	$29.36
Schein	00364-0366-01	100s	$32.34

BRAND/MANUFACTURER	NDC	SIZE	AWP
Lannett	00527-1231-01	100s	$33.00
Major	00904-0560-60	100s	$35.85
URL	00677-0354-01	100s	$35.98
Moore,H.L.	00839-1552-06	100s	$36.03
Rugby	00536-4373-01	100s	$38.28
Goldline	00182-0701-01	100s	$38.50
Aligen	00405-4836-01	100s	$41.25
U.S. Trading	56126-0289-11	100s ud	$15.00
Major	00904-0560-61	100s ud	$34.88
Medirex	57480-0361-01	100s ud	$37.50
Schein	00364-0366-02	1000s	$295.57
Moore,H.L.	00839-1552-16	1000s	$307.38
Lannett	00527-1231-10	1000s	$310.00
Major	00904-0560-80	1000s	$320.70
URL	00677-0354-10	1000s	$330.40
Rugby	00536-4373-10	1000s	$351.95
Goldline	00182-0701-10	1000s	$375.00

Prinivil SEE LISINOPRIL

Prinzide SEE HYDROCHLOROTHIAZIDE AND LISINOPRIL

Priscoline Hydrochloride SEE TOLAZOLINE HYDROCHLORIDE

Pro-Banthine SEE PROPANTHELINE BROMIDE

Probenecid

DESCRIPTION

Probenecid is a uricosuric and renal tubular transport blocking agent.

Probenecid is the generic name for 4-[(dipropylamino) sulfonyl] benzoic acid (molecular weight 285.36).

Probenecid is a white or nearly white, fine, crystalline powder. Probenecid is soluble in dilute alkali, in alcohol, in chloroform, and in acetone; it is practically insoluble in water and in dilute acids.

Each tablet contains 0.5 g Probenecid.

Following is its chemical structure:

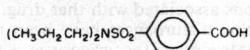

$(CH_3CH_2CH_2)_2NSO_2 -\bigcirc\!\!\!- COOH$

ACTIONS

Probenecid is a uricosuric and renal tubular blocking agent. It inhibits the tubular reabsorption of urate, thus increasing the urinary excretion of uric acid and decreasing serum urate levels. Effective uricosuria reduces the miscible urate pool, retards urate deposition, and promotes resorption of urate deposits.

Probenecid inhibits the tubular secretion of penicillin and usually increaases penicillin plasma levels by any route the antibiotic is given. A 2-fold to 4-fold elevation has been demonstrated for various penicillins.

Probenecid also has been reported to inhibit the renal transport of many other compounds including aminohippuric acid (PAH), aminosalicylic acid (PAS), indomethacin, sodium iodomethamate and related iodinated organic acids, 17-keto-steroids, pantothenic acid, phenolsulfonphthalein (PSP), sulfonamides, and sulfonylureas. (See also "Drug Interactions".)

Probenecid decreases both hepatic and renal excretion of sulfobromophthalein (BSP). The tubular reabsorption of phosphorus is inhibited in hypoparathyroid but not in euparathyroid individuals.

Probenecid does not influence plasma concentrations of salicylates, nor the excretion of streptomycin, chloramphenicol, chlortetracycline, oxytetracycline, or neomycin.

INDICATIONS

For treatment of the hyperuricemia associated with gout and gouty arthritis.

As an adjuvant to therapy with penicillin or with ampicillin, methicillin, oxacillin, cloxacillin, or nafcillin, for elevation and prolongation of plasma levels by whatever route the antibiotic is given.

UNLABELED USES

Probenecid is used as an adjunct in the treatment of gonorrhea, including anorectal gonorrhea. It is also used to aid in the diagnosis and differentiation of parkinsonism and depressive syndromes.

CONTRAINDICATIONS

Hypersensitivity to this product.
Children under 2 years of age.

Not recommended in persons with known blood dyscrasias or uric acid kidney stones.

Therapy with Probenecid should not be started until an acute gouty attack has subsided.

WARNINGS

Exacerbation of gout following therapy with Probenecid may occur; in such cases colchicine or other appropriate therapy is advisable.

Probenecid increases plasma concentrations of methotrexate in both animals and humans. In animal studies, increased methotrexate toxicity has been reported. If Probenecid is given with methotrexate, the dosage of methotrexate should be reduced and serum levels may need to be monitored.

In patients on Probenecid, the use of salicylates in either small or large doses is contraindicated because it antagonizes the uricosuric action of Probenecid. The biphasic action of salicylates in the renal tubules accounts for the so-called 'paradoxical effect' of uricosuric agents. In patients on Probenecid who require a mild analgesic agent, the use of acetaminophen rather than small doses of salicylates would be preferred.

Rarely, severe allergic reactions and anaphylaxis have been reported with the use of Probenecid. Most of these have been reported to occur within several hours after readministration following prior usage of the drug.

The appearance of hypersensitivity reactions requires cessation of therapy with Probenecid.

Use in Pregnancy: Probenecid crosses the placental barrier and appears in cord blood. The use of any drug in women of childbearing potential requires that the anticipated benefit be weighed against possible hazards.

PRECAUTIONS
GENERAL

Hematuria, renal colic, costovertebral pain, and formation of uric acid stones associated with the use of Probenecid in gouty patients may be prevented by alkalization of the urine and a liberal fluid intake (see *"Dosage and Administration"*). In these cases when alkali is administered, the acidbase balance of the patient should be watched.

Use with caution in patients with a history of peptic ulcer. Probenecid has been used in patients with some renal impairment but dosage requirements may be increased. Probenecid may not be effective in chronic renal insufficiency particularly when the glomerular filtration rate is 30 mL/minute or less. Because of its mechanism of action, Probenecid is not recommended in conjunction with a penicillin in the presence of *known* renal impairment.

A reducing substance may appear in the urine of patients receiving Probenecid. This disappears with discontinuance of therapy. Suspected glycosuria should be confirmed by using a test specific for glucose.

DRUG INTERACTIONS

When Probenecid is used to elevate plasma concentrations of penicillin or other beta-lactams, or when such drugs are given to patients taking Probenecid therapeutically, high plasma concentrations of the other drug may increase the incidence of adverse reactions associated with that drug. In the case of penicillin or other beta-lactams, psychic disturbances have been reported.

The use of salicylates antagonizes the uricosuric action of Probenecid (see *"Warnings"*). The uricosuric action of Probenecid is also antagonized by pyrazinamide.

Probenecid produces an insignificant increase in free sulfonamide plasma concentrations but a significant increase in total sulfonamide plasma levels. Since Probenecid decreases the renal excretion of conjugated sulfonamides, plasma concentrations of the latter should be determined from time to time when a sulfonamide and Probenecid are coadministered for prolonged periods. Probenecid may prolong or enhance the action of oral sulfonylureas and thereby increase the risk of hypoglycemia.

It has been reported that patients receiving Probenecid require significantly less thiopental for induction of anesthesia. In addition, ketamine and thiopental anesthesia were significantly prolonged in rats receiving Probenecid.

The concomitant administration of Probenecid increases the mean plasma elimination half-life of a number of drugs which can lead to increased plasma concentrations. These include agents such as indomethacin, acetaminophen, natproxen, ketoprofen, meclofenamate, lorazepam, and rifampin. Although the clinical significance of this observation has not been established, a lower dosage of the drug may be required to produce a therapeutic effect, and increases in dosage of the drug in question should be made cautiously and in small increments when Probenecid is being co-administered. Although specific instances of toxicity due to this potential interaction have not been observed to date, physicians should be alert to this possibility.

Probenecid given concomitantly with sulindac had only a slight effect on plasma sulfide levels, while plasma levels of sulindac and sulfone were increased. Sulindac was shown to produce a modest reduction in the uricosuric action of Probenecid, which probably is not significant under most circumstances.

In animals and in humans, Probenecid has been reported to increase plasma concentrations of methotrexate (see *"Warnings"*).

Falsely high readings for theophylline have been reported in an *in vitro* study, using the Schack and Waxler technic, when therapeutic concentrations of theophylline and Probenecid were added to human plasma.

ADVERSE REACTIONS

The following adverse reactions have been observed and within each category are listed in order of decreasing severity.

Central Nervous System: headache, dizziness.

Metabolic: precipitation of acute gouty arthritis.

Gastrointestinal: hepatic necrosis, vomiting, nausea, anorexia, sore gums.

Genitourinary: nephrotic syndrome, uric acid stones with or without hematuria, renal colic, costovertebral pain, urinary frequency.

Hypersensitivity: anaphylaxis, fever, urticaria, pruritus.

Hematologic: aplastic anemia, leukopenia, hemolytic anemia which in some patients could be related to genetic deficiency of glucose -6- phosphate dehydrogenase in red blood cells, anemia.

Integumentary: dermatitis, alopecia, flushing.

DOSAGE AND ADMINISTRATION
GOUT

Therapy with Probenecid should not be *started* until an acute gouty attack has subsided. However, if an acute attack is precipitated *during* therapy, Probenecid may be continued without changing the dosage, and full therapeutic dosage of colchicine or other appropriate therapy should be given to control the acute attack.

The recommended adult dosage is 0.25 g (½ tablet of Probenecid twice a day for one week, followed by 0.5 g (1 tablet) twice a day thereafter.

Some degree of renal impairment may be present in patients with gout. A daily dosage of 1 g may be adequate. However, if necessary, the daily dosage may be increased by 0.5 g increments every 4 weeks within tolerance (and usually not above 2 g per day) if symptoms of gouty arthritis are not controlled or the 24 hour uric acid excretion is not above 700 mg. As noted, Probenecid may not be effective in chronic renal insufficiency particularly when the glomerular filtration rate is 30 mL/minute or less.

Gastric intolerance may be indicative of overdosage, and may be corrected by decreasing the dosage.

As uric acid tends to crystallize out of an acid urine, a liberal fluid intake is recommended, as well as sufficient sodium bicarbonate (3 to 7.5 g daily) or potassium citrate (7.5 g daily) to maintain an alkaline urine (see *"Precautions"*).

Alkalization of the urine is recommended until the serum urate level returns to normal limits and tophaceous deposits disappear, i.e., during the period when urinary excretion of uric acid is at a high level. Thereafter, alkalization of the urine and the usual restriction of purine-producing foods may be somewhat relaxed.

Probenecid should be continued at the dosage that will maintain normal serum urate levels. When acute attacks have been absent for 6 months or more and serum urate levels remain within normal limits, the daily dosage may be decreased by 0.5 g every 6 months. The maintenance dosage should not be reduced to the point where serum urate levels tend to rise.

PROBENECID AND PENICILLIN THERAPY (GENERAL)
Adults: The recommended dosage is 2 g (4 tablets of Probenecid) daily in divided doses. This dosage should be reduced in older patients in whom renal impairment may be present.

Children 2-14 years of age: Initial dose: 25 mg/kg body weight (or 0.7 g/square meter body surface).

Maintenance dose: 40 mg/kg body weight (*or* 1.2 g/square meter body surface) per day, divided into 4 doses.

For children weighing more than 50 kg (110 lb) the adult dosage is recommended.

Probenecid is contraindicated in children under 2 years of age.

The PSP excretion test may be used to determine the effectiveness of Probenecid in retarding penicillin excretion and maintaining therapeutic levels. The renal clearance of PSP is reduced to about one-fifth the normal rate when dosage of Probenecid is adequate.

PENICILLIN THERAPY (GONORRHEA) (SEE RELATED TABLE).

HOW SUPPLIED
TABLETS: 500 MG

AVERAGE UNIT PRICE (AVAILABLE SIZES)		GENERIC A-RATED AVERAGE PRICE (GAAP)	
BRAND	$0.32	100s	$16.01
GENERIC	$0.16	1000s	$142.32
HCFA FUL (100s ea)	$0.11		

BRAND/MANUFACTURER	NDC	SIZE	AWP
◆ BRAND			
BENEMID: Merck	00006-0501-68	100s	$30.60
	00006-0501-28	100s ud	$34.84
	00006-0501-82	1000s	$290.45
◆ GENERICS			
Mylan	00378-0156-01	100s	$12.76
Moore,H.L.	00839-5081-06	100s	$13.97
Rugby	00536-4366-01	100s	$15.36
Schein	00364-0314-01	100s	$15.75
Zenith	00172-2190-60	100s	$15.85
Aligen	00405-4841-01	100s	$15.85
Goldline	00182-0600-01	100s	$15.90
Major	00904-2190-60	100s	$15.95
Geneva	00781-1021-01	100s	$15.95

◆ RATED THERAPEUTICALLY EQUIVALENT; ◇ THERAPEUTIC EQUIVALENCE UNCONFIRMED; ○ UNRATED

PROBENECID PENICILLIN THERAPY (GONORRHEA)*

	Recommended Regimens**	Remarks
Uncomplicated gonococcal infection in men and women (urethral, cervical, rectal)	4.8 million units of aqueous procaine penicillin G† I.M., in at least 2 doses injected at different sites at one visit + 1 g of Probenecid orally just before injections *or* 3.5 g of ampicillin† orally + 1 g of Probenecid orally given simultaneously.	Follow-up: Obtain urethral and other appropriate cultures from men, and cervical, anal, and other appropriate cultures from women, 7 to 14 days after completion of treatment. Treatment of sexual partners: Persons with known recent exposure to gonorrhea should receive same treatment as those known to have gonorrhea. Examination and treatment of male sex partners of persons with gonorrhea are essential because of high prevalence of nonsymptomatic urethral gonococcal infection in such men.
Pharyngeal gonococcal infection in men and women	4.8 million units of aqueous procaine penicillin G† I.M., in at least 2 doses injected at different sites at one visit + 1 g of Probenecid orally just before injections	Pharyngeal gonococcal infections may be more difficult to treat than anogenital gonorrhea. Posttreatment cultures are essential.
Uncomplicated gonorrhea in pregnant patients	4.8 million units of aqueous procaine Penicillin G† I.M., in at least 2 doses injected at different sites at one visit *or* 3.5 g of ampicillin† orally + 1 g of Probenecid orally given simultaneously	
Acute gonococcal salpingitis	*Outpatients:* Aqueous procaine penicillin G† or ampicillin† with Probenecid as for gonorrhea in pregnancy, followed by 500 mg of ampicillin 4 times a day for 10 days. *Hospitalized patients:* See details in CDC recommendations	Follow-up of patients with acute salpingitis is essential. All patients should receive repeat pelvic examinations and cultures for *Neisseria gonorrhoeae* after treatment. Examination and appropriate treatment of male sex partners are essential because of high prevalence of nonsymptomatic urethral gonorrhea in such men.
Disseminated gonococcal infection (arthritis-dermatitis syndrome)	10 million units of aqueous crystalline penicillin G† I.V. a day for 3 days or till significant clinical improvement occurs. May be followed with 500 mg of ampicillin† 4 times a day orally to complete 7 days of treatment *or* 3.5 g ampicillin† orally with 1g of Probenecid followed by 500 mg of ampicillin† 4 times a day for at least 7 days	
Gonococcal infection in children	For postpubertal children and/or those weighing over 45 kg (100 lb) use the dosage regimens given above for adults. Uncomplicated vulvovaginitis and urethritis: aqueous procaine G† 75,000—100,000 units/kg I.M., with Probenecid 23 mg/kg orally	See CDC recommendations for detailed information about prevention and treatment of neonatal gonococcal infection and gonococcal ophthalmia.

Note: Before treating gonococcal infections in patients with suspected primary or secondary syphilis, perform proper diagnostic procedures including darkfield examinations. If concomitant syphilis is suspected, perform monthly serological tests for at least 4 months.
* *Recommended by Venereal Disease Control Advisory Committee, Center for Disease Control, U.S. Department of Health, Education, and Welfare, Public Health Service (Morbidity and Mortality Weekly Report, Vol. 23: 341, 342, 347, 348, Oct. 11, 1974).*
** *See CDC recommendations for definition of regimens of choice, alternative regimens, treatment of hypersensitive patients, and other aspects of therapy.*
† *See package circulars of manufacturers for detailed information about contraindications, warnings, precautions, and adverse reactions.*

BRAND/MANUFACTURER	NDC	SIZE	AWP
Martec	52555-0336-01	100s	$15.95
Qualitest	00603-5381-21	100s	$16.30
U.S. Trading	56126-0383-11	100s ud	$22.58
Rugby	00536-4366-10	1000s	$137.21
Major	00904-2190-80	1000s	$140.30
Zenith	00172-2190-80	1000s	$144.30
Goldline	00182-0600-10	1000s	$144.75
Schein	00364-0314-02	1000s	$145.06

Probucol

DESCRIPTION

Probucol film-coated tablets for oral administration contain 250 mg or 500 mg of Probucol per tablet. Probucol is an agent for the reduction of elevated serum cholesterol. The chemical name is 4,4'-[(1-methylethylidene)bis(thio)]bis[2,6-bis(1,1-dimethylethyl)phenol]. Its chemical structure does not resemble that of any other available cholesterol-lowering agent. It is lipophilic.

Following is its chemical structure:

CLINICAL PHARMACOLOGY

Probucol lowers total serum cholesterol and has relatively little effect on serum triglycerides. Patients responding to Probucol exhibit a decrease in low-density lipoprotein (LDL) cholesterol. Cholesterol is reduced not only in the LDL fraction, but also in the high-density lipoprotein (HDL) fraction with proportionately greater effect on the high-density portion. Epidemiologic studies have shown that both low HDL-cholesterol and high LDL-cholesterol are independent risk factors for coronary heart disease. The risk of lowering HDL-cholesterol while lowering LDL-cholesterol remains unknown. There is little or no effect reported on very low-density lipoprotein (VLDL).

Studies on the mode of action of Probucol indicate that it increases the fractional rate of LDL catabolism. This effect may be linked to the observed increased excretion of fecal bile acids, a final metabolic pathway for the elimination of cholesterol from the body. Probucol also exhibits inhibition of early stages of cholesterol biosynthesis and slight inhibition of absorption of dietary cholesterol. There is no increase in the cyclic precursors of cholesterol, namely desmosterol and 7-dehydrocholesterol. On this basis, it is concluded that Probucol does not affect the later stages of cholesterol biosynthesis.

Absorption of Probucol from the gastrointestinal tract is limited and variable. When it is administered with food, peak blood levels are higher and less variable. With continuous administration in a dosage of 500 mg b.i.d., the blood levels of an individual gradually increase over the first three to four months and thereafter remain fairly constant. In 116 patients treated with Probucol for periods of three months to one year, the mean blood level was 23.6 ± 17.2 mcg/mL (± S.D.) ranging to 78.3 mcg/mL. Levels observed after seven years of treatment in 40 patients yielded an average value of 21.5 ± 16.5 mcg/mL (± S.D.) ranging to 62.0 mcg/mL. In a separate study in eight patients, blood levels averaged 19.0 mcg/mL at the end of 12 months of treatment. Six weeks after cessation of therapy, the average had fallen by 60%. After six months, the average had fallen by 80%.

In December 1984, a National Institutes of Health Consensus Development Conference Panel[1] concluded that lowering definitely elevated blood cholesterol levels (specifically blood levels of LDL-cholesterol) will reduce the risk of heart attacks due to coronary heart disease. The effect of Probucol-induced reduction of serum cholesterol or triglyceride levels, or reduction of HDL-cholesterol levels on morbidity or mortality due to coronary heart disease has not been established.

INDICATIONS AND USAGE

Serious animal toxicity has been encountered with Probucol. See *"Warnings"* and *"Animal Pharmacology and Toxicology"* sections. Probucol is not an innocuous drug and strict attention should be paid to the *"Indications," "Contraindications,"* and *"Warnings".*

Drug therapy should not be used for the routine treatment of elevated blood lipids for the prevention of coronary heart disease. Dietary therapy specific for the type of hyperlipidemia is the initial treatment of choice. Excess body weight may be an important factor and should be addressed prior to any drug therapy. Physical exercise can be an important ancillary measure. Contributory disease such as hypothyroidism or diabetes mellitus should be looked for and adequately treated. The use of drugs should be considered only when reasonable attempts have been made to obtain satisfactory results with nondrug methods. If the decision ultimately is to use drugs, the patient should be instructed that this does not reduce the importance of adhering to diet.

➤ SHOWN IN PRODUCT IDENTIFICATION GUIDE

The selection of patients for cholesterol-lowering drug therapy should take into account other important coronary risk factors such as smoking, hypertension, and diabetes mellitus. Consideration should be given to the efficacy, safety, and compliance factors for each of the cholesterol-lowering drugs prior to selecting the one most appropriate for an individual patient.

Probucol may be indicated for the reduction of elevated serum cholesterol in patients with primary hypercholesterolemia (Types IIa and IIb hyperlipoproteinemia),[2] whose elevated LDL-cholesterol has not responded adequately to diet, weight reduction and control of diabetes mellitus. Probucol may be useful to lower elevated LDL-cholesterol that occurs in those patients with combined hypercholesterolemia and hypertriglyceridemia (Type IIb) due to elevation of both LDL and VLDL, but it is not indicated where hypertriglyceridemia is the abnormality of most concern. After establishing that the elevation in serum total cholesterol represents a primary lipid disorder, it should be determined that patients being considered for treatment with Probucol have an elevated LDL-cholesterol as the cause for an elevated total serum cholesterol. This may be particularly relevant for patients with elevated triglycerides or with markedly elevated HDL-cholesterol values, where non-LDL fractions may contribute significantly to total cholesterol levels without apparent increase in cardiovascular risk. In most patients, LDL-cholesterol may be estimated according to the following equation:

LDL-cholesterol = Total cholesterol - [(0.16 × triglycerides) + HDL-cholesterol]

When total triglycerides are greater than 400 mg/dL, this equation is less accurate. In such patients, LDL-cholesterol may be obtained by ultracentrifugation.

It is not always possible to predict from the lipoprotein type or other factors which patients will exhibit favorable results. Lipid level, including HDL-cholesterol, should be periodically assessed.

The effect of Probucol-induced reduction of serum cholesterol or triglyceride levels, or reduction of HDL-cholesterol levels on morbidity or mortality due to coronary heart disease has not been established.

CONTRAINDICATIONS

(See also *"Warnings"* and *"Precautions."*) Probucol is contraindicated in patients who are known to have a hypersensitivity to it. Probucol is contraindicated in patients with evidence of recent or progressive myocardial damage or findings suggestive of serious ventricular arrhythmias or with unexplained syncope or syncope of cardiovascular origin. **Probucol is contraindicated in patients with an abnormally long QT interval.**

WARNINGS

Serious Animal Toxicity Has Been Encountered With Probucol in Rhesus Monkey Fed an Atherogenic Diet and in Beagle Dogs. (See "Animal Pharmacology" and "Toxicology Section".)

Prolongation of the QT interval can occur in patients on Probucol. Serious arrhythmias have been seen in association with an abnormally long QT interval in patients on Probucol alone and in patients on Probucol and a concomitant antiarrhythmic drug. The following precautions are deemed prudent:

1. Patients should be advised to adhere to a low cholesterol, low fat diet at the start of treatment with Probucol and throughout the treatment period.

2. An ECG should be done prior to starting treatment and repeated at appropriate intervals during treatment. If an abnormally long QT interval is observed, the possible benefits and risks should be carefully considered before making a decision to continue Probucol.

Probucol therapy should be discontinued or not started if the QT interval at an observed heart rate on a resting ECG is persistently more than one of the values listed below:

Observed Heart Rate (beats/min)	QT Interval in sec (15% above the upper limit of normal)*	
	Males	Females
40	0.56	0.58
50	0.52	0.53
60	0.49	0.50
70	0.45	0.47
80	0.43	0.44
86	0.42	0.43
92	0.40	0.41
100	0.39	0.40
109	0.37	0.38
120	0.36	0.36
133	0.34	0.35

* *Values calculated from Burch GE, Winsor T. A primer of electrocardiography. Philadelphia, PA: Lea and Febiger; 1958; p. 272 (Table 6).*

3. Patients developing unexplained syncope or syncope of cardiovascular origin should have Probucol therapy discontinued and should have ECG surveillance.

4. Drugs that prolong the QT interval are more likely to be associated with ventricular tachycardia after:
a. An increase in the dose of the drug.

b. Addition of a second drug that prolongs the QT interval (including tricyclic antidepressants, class I and III antiarrhythmics, and phenothiazines).

c. Hypokalemia or hypomagnesemia.

d. Severe bradycardia due to intrinsic heart disease or drug effects on the atrial rate (beta-blockers) or AV block (digoxin).

e. Development of recent or acute myocardial infarction, ischemia, or inflammation.

The use of Probucol in patients receiving any of these drugs should be based on the conclusion that alternate methods of hypocholesterolemic therapy are either ineffective or not tolerated, and the potential benefits of cholesterol lowering outweigh the risk of serious arrhythmia.

The following conditions should be resolved or corrected prior to initiation of therapy with Probucol:
a. Hypokalemia
b. Hypomagnesemia
c. Severe bradycardia due to intrinsic heart disease or drug effects on the atrial rate (beta-blockers) or AV block (digoxin).
d. Recent or acute myocardial infarction, ischemia, or inflammation.

PRECAUTIONS

General: Before instituting therapy with Probucol, adequate baseline studies should be performed to determine that the patient has persistently elevated total and LDL-cholesterol levels representing a primary lipid disorder, and that the increased cholesterol is not due to secondary conditions such as hypothyroidism, poorly controlled diabetes mellitus, obstructive liver disease, nephrotic syndrome, or dysproteinemias. Serum lipid levels, including HDL-cholesterol, should be determined after an overnight fast before treatment, during an adequate trial of diet and weight reduction therapy prior to addition of drug therapy, and periodically during combined diet and drug treatment, including assessment during the first several months of drug treatment. A favorable trend in lipid levels should be evident during the first three to four months of administration of Probucol, and if satisfactory lipid alteration is not achieved, the drug should be discontinued. Probucol lowers serum total and LDL-cholesterol, and also lowers HDL-cholesterol in most patients with elevated LDL-cholesterol. Epidemiologic studies within hypercholesterolemic populations have shown that serum HDL-cholesterol is an independent, inversely correlated, risk factor for coronary heart disease (see *"Clinical Pharmacology"*). Human studies which will attempt to confirm or deny the hypothesis that drug-induced alteration in HDL-cholesterol affects cardiovascular risk are currently under evaluation. It is not known whether Probucol-induced reduction of serum HDL-cholesterol will affect cardiovascular risk since no long-term, controlled clinical trials of Probucol for the prevention of coronary heart disease, similar to the LRC-CPPT (see *"Clinical Studies"*), have been performed. The probable benefits obtained from LDL-cholesterol reduction must be weighed against the possible risk of a reduction in HDL-cholesterol when assessing the response of each patient receiving Probucol treatment. If satisfactory lipid alteration is not achieved, the drug should be discontinued.

Information for Patients: The patient should be instructed to adhere to a prudent diet. Females should be cautioned against becoming pregnant for at least six months after discontinuing Probucol and should not breast-feed their infants during therapy with Probucol.

Laboratory Tests: The physician should schedule periodic blood lipid determinations and periodic ECGs. (See *"Warnings".*)

Elevations of the serum transaminases (SGOT, SGPT), bilirubin, alkaline phosphatase, creatine phosphokinase, uric acid, blood urea nitrogen and blood glucose above the normal range were observed on one or more occasions in various patients treated with Probucol. Most often these were transient and/or could have been related to the patient's clinical state or other modes of therapy. Although the basis for the relationship between Probucol and these abnormalities is not firm, the possibility that some of these are drug related cannot be excluded. In the controlled trials, the incidence of abnormal laboratory values was no higher in the patients treated with Probucol than in the patients who received placebo. If abnormal laboratory tests persist or worsen, if clinical signs consistent with the abnormal laboratory tests develop, or if systemic manifestations occur, Probucol should be discontinued.

Drug Interactions: The addition of clofibrate to Probucol is not recommended, since the lowering effect on mean serum levels of either LDL or total cholesterol is generally not significantly additive and, in some patients, there may be a pronounced lowering of HDL-cholesterol.

Neither oral hypoglycemic agents nor oral anticoagulants alter the effect of Probucol serum cholesterol. The dosage of these agents is not usually modified when given with Probucol.

Monkeys fed a high fat, high cholesterol diet admixed with Probucol exhibited serious toxicity. (See *"Warnings"* and *"Animal Pharmacology and Toxicology"* sections.) Prolongation of the QT interval can occur in patients on Probucol and serious arrhythmias have been seen in association with an abnormally long QT interval in patients on Probucol. The addition of a second drug that prolongs the QT interval (including tricyclic antidepressants, class I and III antiarrhythmics, and phenothiazines) may increase the risk of serious arrhythmia. (See *"Contraindications"* and *"Warnings".*)

Carcinogenesis, Mutagenesis, Impairment of Fertility: In chronic studies of two years' duration in rats, no toxicity or carcinogenicity was observed. These results are consistent with the lack of any adverse effect on fertility and the negative findings in tests for mutagenic activity in rats.

Pregnancy: Teratogenic Effects: Pregnancy—Category B: Reproduction studies have been performed in rats and rabbits at doses up to 50 times the human dose, and have revealed no evidence of impaired fertility or harm to the fetus due to Probucol. There are, however, no adequate and well-controlled studies in pregnant women. Because animal reproduction studies are not always predictive of human response, this drug should be used during pregnancy only if clearly needed. Furthermore, if a patient wishes to become pregnant, it is recommended that the drug be withdrawn and birth control procedures be used for at least six months because of persistence of the drug in the body for prolonged periods. (See *"Clinical Pharmacology".*)

Labor and Delivery: The effect of Probucol on human labor and delivery is unknown.

Nursing Mothers: It is not known whether this drug is excreted in human milk, but it is likely, since such excretion has been shown in animals. It is recommended that nursing not be undertaken while a patient is on Probucol.

Pediatric Use: Safety and effectiveness in children have not been established.

ADVERSE REACTIONS
Gastrointestinal: diarrhea or loose stools, flatulence, abdominal pain, nausea, vomiting, indigestion, gastrointestinal bleeding

Cardiovascular: prolongation of the QT interval on ECG, syncope, ventricular arrhythmias (ventricular tachycardia, torsades de pointes, ventricular fibrillation), sudden death

Neurologic: headache, dizziness, paresthesia, insomnia, tinnitus, peripheral neuritis

Hematologic: eosinophilia, low hemoglobin and/or hematocrit, thrombocytopenia.

Dermatologic: rash, pruritus, ecchymosis, petechiae, perhidrosis, fetid sweat

Genitourinary: impotence, nocturia

Ophthalmic: conjunctivitis, tearing, blurred vision

Endocrine: enlargement of multinodular goiter

Idiosyncrasies: observed with initiation of therapy and characterized by dizziness, palpitations, syncope, nausea, vomiting and chest pain

Other: diminished sense of taste and smell, anorexia, angioneurotic edema

DRUG ABUSE AND DEPENDENCE
No evidence of abuse potential has been associated with Probucol nor is there evidence of psychological or physical dependence in humans.

OVERDOSAGE
There is a single report of a 15-kg, three-year-old, male child who ingested 5 g of Probucol. Emesis was induced by ipecac. The child remained well, apart from a brief episode of loose stools and flatulence. No specific information is available on the treatment of overdosage with Probucol and no specific antidote is available. Probucol is not dialyzable. Treatment is symptomatic and supportive. Probucol has shown no identifiable acute toxicity in mice and rats. In these animals, the LD_{50} (oral) is in excess of 5 g/kg of body weight.

DOSAGE AND ADMINISTRATION
For adult use only. The recommended and maximal dose is 1000 mg daily given in two divided doses of 500 mg each (two 250 mg tablets or one 500 mg tablet) with the morning and evening meals.

Keep well closed. Store in a dry place. Avoid excessive heat. Dispense in well-closed light-resistant containers with child-resistant closures.

ANIMAL PHARMACOLOGY AND TOXICOLOGY
In rhesus monkeys, administration of Probucol in diets containing unusually high amounts of cholesterol and saturated fat resulted in the death of four of eight animals after several weeks. Premonitory syncope was frequently observed and was associated with a pronounced prolongation of the QT intervals (30 to 50% longer than that observed in untreated monkeys). Serum levels of Probucol greater than 20 mcg/mL were generally associated with some prolongation in the QT interval in the cholesterol-fed monkey. A 75 msec or greater increase in QT interval from control values was usually seen at 40 mcg/mL and above. Blood levels in humans receiving Probucol average approximately 20 mcg/mL and not uncommonly reach levels of 40 mcg/mL and higher. Rhesus monkeys fed normal (low fat) chow and receiving Probucol three to thirty times the human dose equivalent achieved blood levels only one-third those of many human subjects. No adverse effects were detected in these monkeys over an eight-year period of continuous drug administration. In another study in rhesus monkeys, an atherogenic diet was fed for two years and daily treatment with Probucol, separated in time from the atherogenic meal, was carried out during the second year. Serum Probucol levels ranged 20 to 50 mcg/mL in five of ten monkeys, and less in the remaining animals. Marked prolongation of the QT_c interval in the ECG or syncopal behavior was never observed over the entire one-year treatment period. Regression of gross aortic lesions comparable to that observed in a parallel group of monkeys receiving cholestyramine was seen in animals receiving Probucol. It should be emphasized that both HDL-cholesterol and LDL-cholesterol were markedly reduced in this regression study. During the performance of a two-year chronic study involving 32 Probucol-treated dogs (beagles), there were 12 fatalities.

Subsequent experiments have indicated that Probucol sensitizes the canine myocardium to epinephrine, resulting in ventricular fibrillation in many dogs.

Among the animal species in which Probucol has been studied, the dog is peculiar with respect to the phenomenon of sudden death due to the sensitization of the myocardium to epinephrine. In contrast to findings in the dog, injections of epinephrine to Probucol-treated monkeys did not induce ventricular fibrillation.

In other studies, monkeys were given Probucol either before and after, or only after myocardial infarction induced by coronary artery ligation. In these studies, there was no difference between Probucol- and placebo-treated groups with respect to either survival or detailed blind quantitation of myocardial changes (gross and histopathologic).

Probucol has shown no identifiable toxicity in mice and rats. In these animals, the LD_{50} (oral) is in excess of 5 g/kg of body weight. In chronic studies of two years' duration in rats, no toxicity or carcinogenicity was observed.

From studies in rats, dogs, and monkeys, it is known that Probucol accumulates slowly in adipose tissue. Approximately 90% of Probucol administered orally is unabsorbed. For that which is absorbed, the biliary tract is the major pathway for clearance from the body and very little is excreted by way of the kidneys.

Myocardial injury was produced in various groups of rats by one of the following procedures: aortic coarctation, coronary ligation, or cobalt or isoproterenol injection. After Probucol administration, no deleterious effects related to treatment occurred as measured by survival and microscopic examination of myocardial damage.

Probucol was administered to minipigs beginning ten days before ligation of coronary artery and continued for 60 days after surgery. Challenge with epinephrine at the end of 60 days failed to induce ventricular fibrillation in any of the coronary-ligated Probucol-treated minipigs.

CLINICAL STUDIES
In a multicenter, randomized double-blind study, the LRC-CPPT[3], hypercholesterolemic patients treated with an oral bile acid sequestrant (cholestyramine) and a cholesterol-lowering diet experienced average total and LDL-cholesterol reductions greater than those obtained in the placebo group treated with diet alone. The cumulative seven-year incidence of the primary end point—combined incidence of definite CHD death and/or definite nonfatal myocardial infarction—was 7% in the cholestyramine group and 8.6% in the placebo group. This was a 19% reduction in risk (P less than 0.05, single-tail test) of the primary end point reflecting a 24% reduction in definite CHD death and a 19% reduction in nonfatal myocardial infarction.

The subjects included in the study were middle-aged men (35-59 years old) with serum cholesterol levels at least 265 mg/dL and no previous history of heart disease. It is not clear to what extent these findings can be extrapolated to other segments of the hypercholesterolemic population not studied.

The bile acid sequestrant, cholestyramine, was used in the above trial. Caution should be exercised in extrapolating these results to Probucol since it differs from cholestyramine with regard to its mode of action, spectrum of cholesterol-lowering potency, effect on HDL-cholesterol, and possible toxicity. The effect of Probucol-induced reduction of serum cholesterol levels on morbidity or mortality due to coronary heart disease has not been established.

REFERENCES
1. Consensus Development Panel. Lowering blood cholesterol to prevent heart disease. *JAMA.* 1985; 253:2080-2086. 2. Fredrickson DS, Levy RI, Lees RS. Fat transport in lipoproteins—an integrated approach to mechanisms and disorders. *N. Engl J Med.* 1967; 276:34-44. 3. The Lipid Research Clinics Program. The Lipid Research Clinics coronary primary prevention trial results: I. Reduction in incidence of coronary heart disease. *JAMA.* 1984; 251:351-364.

HOW SUPPLIED
TABLETS: 250 MG

BRAND/MANUFACTURER	NDC	SIZE	AWP
○ **BRAND**			
▶ LORELCO: Marion Merrell Dow	00068-0051-52	120s	$80.46

TABLETS: 500 MG

BRAND/MANUFACTURER	NDC	SIZE	AWP
○ **BRAND**			
▶ LORELCO: Marion Merrell Dow	00068-0053-61	100s	$116.04

Procainamide Hydrochloride

WARNING

POSITIVE ANA TITER: THE PROLONGED ADMINISTRATION OF PROCAINAMIDE OFTEN LEADS TO THE DEVELOPMENT OF A POSITVE ANTINUCLEAR ANTIBODY (ANA) TEST, WITH OR WITHOUT SYMPTOMS OF A LUPUS ERYTHEMATOSUS-LIKE SYNDROME. IF A POSITIVE ANA TITER DEVELOPS, THE BENEFITS VERSUS RISKS OF CONTINUED PROCAINAMIDE THERAPY SHOULD BE ASSESSED.

DESCRIPTION
Procainamide Hydrochloride, a Group 1A cardiac antiarrhythmic drug, is p-amino-N-2-(diethylamino)-ethyl)-benzamide monohydrochloride, molecular weight 271.79; empirical formula $C_{13}H_{21}N_2O$•HCl.

▶ SHOWN IN PRODUCT IDENTIFICATION GUIDE

Procainamide Hydrochloride differs from procaine which is the p-aminobenzoyl ester of 2-(diethylamino)-ethanol. Procainamide as the free base has a pk_a of 9.23; the monohydrochloride is very soluble in water.

Procainamide Hydrochloride is available as Extended Release (ER) tablets, capsules, and injection.

Procainamide Hydrochloride is a white to tan odorless, crystalline salt that is readily soluble in water.

Procainamide Hydrochloride Injection is a sterile, nonpyrogenic solution of Procainamide Hydrochloride in water for injection.

Procainamide Hydrochloride Injection is intended for intravenous or intramuscular administration.

Procainamide HCl ER tablets contain:
Procainamide HCl ....250 mg, 500 mg, 750 mg, or 1000 mg

Procainamide HCl injection 2 mL vial contains:
Procainamide HCl ....500 mg/mL

Procainamide HCl injection 10 mL vial contains:
Procainamide HCl ....100 mg/mL

Procainamide HCl capsules contain:
Procainamide HCl ....250 mg, 375 mg, or 500 mg

Following is its chemical structure:

$$NH_2 - \bigcirc - CONHCH_2CH_2N(C_2H_5)_2 \cdot HCl$$

CLINICAL PHARMACOLOGY

Procainamide increases the effective refractory period of the atria, and to a lesser extent the bundle of His-Purkinje system and ventricles of the heart. It reduces impulse conduction velocity in the atria, His-Purkinje fibers, and ventricular muscle, but has variable effects on the atrioventricular (A-V) node, a direct slowing action and a weaker vagolytic effect which may speed A-V conduction slightly. Myocardial excitability is reduced in the atria, Purkinje fibers, papillary muscles, and ventricles by an increase in the threshold for excitation, combined with inhibition of ectopic pacemaker activity by retardation of the slow phase of diastolic depolarization, thus decreasing automaticity especially in ectopic sites. Contractility of the undamaged heart is usually not affected by therapeutic concentrations, although slight reduction of cardiac output may occur, and may be significant in the presence of myocardial damage. Therapeutic levels of Procainamide may exert vagolytic effects and produce slight acceleration of heart rate, while high or toxic concentrations may prolong A-V conduction time or induce A-V block, or even cause abnormal automaticity and spontaneous firing, by unknown mechanisms.

Procainamide HCl ER tablets are designed to provide the biopharmaceutic characteristics of an extended and relatively constant rate of release and absorption, independent of dose, primarily from the small intestine.

The electrocardiogram may reflect these effects by showing slight sinus tachycardia (due to the anticholinergic action) and widened QRS complexes and, less regularly, prolonged Q-T and P-R intervals (due to longer systole and slower conduction), as well as some decrease in QRS and T wave amplitude. These direct effects of Procainamide on electrical activity, conduction, responsiveness, excitability and automaticity are characteristic of a Group 1A antiarrhythmic agent, the prototype for which is quinidine-Procainamide effects are very similar. However, Procainamide has weaker vagal blocking action than does quinidine, does not induce alpha-adrenergic blockade, and is less depressing to cardiac contractility.

Ingested Procainamide is resistant to digestive hydrolysis, and the drug is well absorbed from the entire small intestinal surface, but individual patients vary in their completeness of absorption of Procainamide. Following oral administration every six hours Procainamide HCl ER tablets achieve a mean steady state of Procainamide (as well as plus N-acetylprocainamide) serum concentrations approximately equivalent to those from a comparable dose of an immediate-release dosage form given every three hours. Procainamide HCl ER tablets have a half-life which is significantly longer than that of Procainamide HCl ER immediate-release dosage forms. Following intramuscular injection, Procainamide is rapidly absorbed into the bloodstream, and plasma levels peak in 15 to 60 minutes, considerably faster than orally administered Procainamide HCl tablets or capsules which produce peak plasma levels in 90 to 120 minutes. Intravenous administration of Procainamide HCl injection can produce therapeutic Procainamide levels within minutes after infusion is started. Following oral administration of Procainamide HCl, plasma Procainamide levels peak in approximately 45 to 120 minutes. About 15 to 20 percent of Procainamide is reversibly bound to plasma proteins, and considerable amounts are more slowly and reversibly bound to tissues of the heart, liver, lung, and kidney. The apparent volume of distribution eventually reaches about 2 liters per kilogram body weight with a half-time of approximately five minutes. While Procainamide has been shown in the dog to cross the blood-brain barrier, it did not concentrate in the brain at levels higher than in plasma. It is not known if Procainamide crosses the placenta. Plasma esterases are far less active in hydrolysis of Procainamide than of procaine. The half-time for elimination is three to four hours in patients with normal renal function, but reduced creatinine clearance and advancing age each prolong the half-time of elimination of Procainamide.

A significant fraction of the circulating Procainamide may be metabolized in hepatocytes to N-acetylprocainamide (NAPA), ranging from 16 to 21 percent of an administered dose in 'slow acetylators' to 24 to 33 percent in "fast acetylators."

Since NAPA also has significant antiarrhythmic activity and somewhat slower renal clearance than Procainamide, both hepatic acetylation rate capability and renal function, as well as age, have significant effects on the effective biologic half-time of therapeutic action of administered Procainamide and the NAPA derivative. Trace amounts may be excreted in the urine as free and conjugated p-aminobenzoic acid, 30 to 60 percent as unchanged Procainamide, and 6 to 52 percent as the NAPA derivative. Both Procainamide and NAPA are eliminated by active tubular secretion as well as by glomerular filtration. Action of Procainamide on the central nervous system is not prominent, but high plasma concentrations may cause tremors. While therapeutic plasma levels for Procainamide have been reported to be 3 to 10 μg/mL, certain patients such as those with sustained ventricular tachycardia, may need higher levels for adequate control. This may justify the increased risk of toxicity (see "Overdosage"). Where programmed ventricular stimulation has been used to evaluate efficacy of Procainamide in preventing recurrent ventricular tachyarrhythmias, higher plasma levels (mean, 13.6 μg/mL) of Procainamide were found necessary for adequate control.

INDICATIONS AND USAGE

Procainamide HCl is indicated for the treatment of documented ventricular arrhythmias, such as sustained ventricular tachycardia, that, in the judgment of the physician, are life-threatening. Because of the proarrhythmic effects of Procainamide HCl its use with lesser arrhythmias is generally not recommended. Treatment of patients with asymptomatic ventricular premature contractions should be avoided. Initiation of Procainamide HCl treatment, as with other antiarrhythmic agents used to treat life-threatening arrhythmias, should be carried out in the hospital.

Antiarrhythmic drugs have not been shown to enhance survival in patients with ventricular arrhythmias.

Because Procainamide HCl has the potential to produce serious hematological disorders (0.5 percent), particularly leukopenia or agranulocytosis (sometimes fatal), its use should be reserved for patients in whom, in the opinion of the physician, the benefits of treatment clearly outweigh the risks. (See "Warnings" and boxed "Warning".)

UNLABELED USES
Procainamide is used alone or as an adjunct in the treatment of atrial fibrillation and in determination of acetylator status.

CONTRAINDICATIONS

Complete Heart Block: Procainamide should not be administered to patients with complete heart block because of its effects in suppressing nodal or ventricular pacemakers and the hazard of asystole. It may be difficult to recognize complete heart block in patients with ventricular tachycardia, but if significant slowing of ventricular rate occurs during Procainamide treatment without evidence of A-V conduction appearing, Procainamide should be stopped. In cases of second degree A-V block or various types of hemiblock, Procainamide should be avoided or discontinued because of the possibility of increased severity of block, unless the ventricular rate is controlled by an electrical pacemaker.

Idiosyncratic Hypersensitivity: In patients sensitive to procaine or other ester-type local anesthetics, cross sensitivity to Procainamide is unlikely; however, it should be borne in mind, and Procainamide should not be used if it produces acute allergic dermatitis, asthma, or anaphylactic symptoms.

Lupus Erythematosus: An established diagnosis of systemic lupus erythematosus is a contraindication to Procainamide therapy, since aggravation of symptoms is highly likely.

Torsades de Pointes: In the unusual ventricular arrhythmia called "les torsades de pointes" (twistings of the points), characterized by alternation of one or more ventricular premature beats in the directions of the QRS complexes on ECG in persons with prolonged Q-T and often enhanced U waves, Group 1A antiarrhythmic drugs are contraindicated. Administration of Procainamide in such cases may aggravate this special type of ventricular extrasystole or tachycardia instead of suppressing it.

WARNINGS

Mortality: In the National Heart, Lung and Blood Institute's Cardiac Arrhythmia Suppression Trial (CAST), a long-term, multicentered, randomized, double-blind study in patients with asymptomatic non-life-threatening ventricular arrhythmias who had had myocardial infarctions more than six days but less than two years previously, an excessive mortality or non-fatal cardiac arrest rate was seen in patients treated with encainide or flecainide (56/730) compared with that seen in patients assigned to matched, placebo-treated groups (22/725). The average duration of treatment with encainide or flecainide in this study was ten months.

The applicability of these results to other populations (e.g., those without recent myocardial infarctions) or to other antiarrhythmic drugs is uncertain, but at present it is prudent to consider any antiarrhythmic agent to have a significant risk in patients with structural heart disease.

BLOOD DYSCRASIAS: AGRANULOCYTOSIS, BONE MARROW DEPRESSION, NEUTROPENIA, HYPOPLASTIC ANEMIA AND THROMBOCYTOPENIA HAVE BEEN REPORTED AT A RATE OF APPROXIMATELY 0.5% IN PATIENTS RECEIVING PROCAINAMIDE HCL. MOST OF THESE PATIENTS RECEIVED PROCAINAMIDE HCL WITHIN THE RECOMMENDED DOSAGE RANGE. FATALITIES HAVE OCCURRED (WITH APPROXIMATELY 20-25 PERCENT MORTALITY IN REPORTED CASES OF AGRANULOCYTOSIS).

SINCE MOST OF THESE EVENTS HAVE BEEN NOTED DURING THE FIRST 12 WEEKS OF THERAPY, IT IS RECOMMENDED THAT COMPLETE BLOOD COUNTS INCLUDING WHITE CELL, DIFFERENTIAL AND PLATELET COUNTS BE PERFORMED AT WEEKLY INTERVALS FOR THE FIRST THREE MONTHS OF THERAPY; AND PERIODICALLY THEREAFTER. COMPLETE BLOOD COUNTS SHOULD BE PERFORMED PROMPTLY IF THE PATIENT DEVELOPS ANY SIGNS OF INFECTION (SUCH AS FEVER, CHILLS, SORE THROAT, OR STOMATITIS), BRUISING, OR BLEEDING. IF ANY OF THESE HEMATOLOGIC DISORDERS ARE IDENTIFIED, PROCAINAMIDE THERAPY SHOULD BE DISCONTINUED. BLOOD COUNTS USUALLY RETURN TO NORMAL WITHIN ONE MONTH OF DISCONTINUATION. CAUTION SHOULD BE USED IN PATIENTS WITH PREEXISTING MARROW FAILURE OR CYTOPENIA OF ANY TYPE (SEE "ADVERSE REACTIONS").

Digitalis Intoxication: Caution should be exercised in the use of Procainamide in arrhythmias associated with digitalis intoxication. Procainamide can suppress digitalis-induced arrhythmias; however, if there is concomitant marked disturbance of atrioventricular conduction, additional depression of conduction and ventricular asystole or fibrillation may result. Therefore use of Procainamide should be considered only if discontinuation of digitalis, and therapy with potassium, lidocaine, or phenytoin are ineffective.

First Degree Heart Block: Caution should be exercised also if the patient exhibits or develops first degree heart block while taking Procainamide, and dosage reduction is advised in such cases. If the block persists despite dosage reduction, continuation of Procainamide administration must be evaluated on the basis of current benefit versus risk of increased heart block.

Predigitalization for Atrial Flutter or Fibrillation: Patients with atrial flutter or fibrillation should be cardioverted or digitalized prior to Procainamide administration to avoid enhancement of A-V conduction which may result in ventricular rate acceleration beyond tolerable limits. Adequate digitalization reduces but does not eliminate the possibility of sudden increase in ventricular rate as the atrial rate is slowed by Procainamide in these arrhythmias.

Congestive Heart Failure: For patients in congestive heart failure, and those with acute ischemic heart disease or cardiomyopathy, caution should be used in Procainamide therapy, since even slight depression of myocardial contractility may further reduce the cardiac output of the damaged heart.

Concurrent Other Antiarrhythmic Agents: Concurrent use of Procainamide with other Group 1A antiarrhythmic agents such as quinidine or disopyramide may produce enhanced prolongation of conduction or depression of contractility and hypotension, especially in patients with cardiac decompensation. Such use should be reserved for patients with serious arrhythmias unresponsive to a single drug and employed only if close observation is possible.

Renal Insufficiency: Renal insufficiency may lead to accumulation of high plasma levels from conventional doses of Procainamide, with effects similar to those of overdosage (see "Overdosage"), unless dosage is adjusted for the individual patient.

Myasthenia Gravis: Patients with myasthenia gravis may show worsening of symptoms from Procainamide due to its procaine-like effect on diminishing acetylcholine release at skeletal muscle motor nerve endings, so that Procainamide administration may be hazardous without optimal adjustment of anticholinesterase medications and other precautions.

Sulfite Sensitivity: Some brands of Procainamide HCl injection contains sodium metabisulfite, a sulfite that may cause allergic-type reactions including anaphylactic symptoms and life-threatening or less severe asthmatic episodes in certain susceptible people. The overall prevalence of sulfite sensitivity in the general population is unknown and probably low. Sulfite sensitivity is seen more frequently in asthmatic than in nonasthmatic people.

PRECAUTIONS

General: Immediately after initiation of Procainamide therapy, patients should be closely observed for possible hypersensitivity reactions, especially if procaine or local anesthetic sensitivity is suspected, and for muscular weakness if myasthenia gravis is a possibility.

In conversion of atrial fibrillation to normal sinus rhythm by any means, dislodgment of mural thrombi may lead to embolization, which should be kept in mind.

After approximately two days for the extended release form and a day or so for the immediate release form, steady state plasma Procainamide levels are produced following regular oral administration of a given dose of Procainamide HCl tablets or capsules at set intervals, with peak plasma concentrations at about 45 to 120 minutes after each dose of immediate release Procainamide HCl. After achieving and maintaining therapeutic plasma concentrations and satisfactory electrocardiographic and clinical responses, continued frequent periodic monitoring of vital signs and electrocardiograms is advised. If evidence of QRS widening of more than 25 percent or marked prolongation of the Q-T interval occurs, concern for overdosage is appropriate, and reduction in dosage or interruption of the Procainamide infusion is advisable if a 50 percent increase occurs. Elevated serum creatinine or urea nitrogen, reduced creatinine clearance, or history of renal insufficiency, as well as use in older patients (over age 50), provide grounds to anticipate that less than the usual dosage or infusion rate and longer time intervals between doses may suffice, since the urinary elimination of Procain-

amide and NAPA may be reduced, leading to gradual accumulation beyond normally predicted amounts. If facilities are available for measurement of plasma Procainamide and NAPA, or acetylation capability, individual dose adjustment for optimal therapeutic levels may be easier, but close observation of clinical effectiveness is the most important criterion. In the longer term, periodic complete blood counts are useful to detect possible idiosyncratic hematologic effects of Procainamide on neutrophil, platelet or red cell homeostasis; agranulocytosis has been reported to occur occasionally in patients on long-term Procainamide therapy. A rising titer of serum ANA may precede clinical symptoms of the lupoid syndrome (see boxed "Warnings" and "Adverse Reactions"). If the lupus erythematosus-like syndrome develops in a patient with recurrent life-threatening arrhythmias not controlled by other agents, corticosteroid suppressive therapy may be used concomitantly with Procainamide. Since the Procainamide-induced lupoid syndrome rarely includes the dangerous pathologic renal changes, Procainamide therapy may not necessarily have to be stopped unless the symptoms of serositis and the possibility of further lupoid effects are of greater risk than the benefit of Procainamide in controlling arrhythmias. Patients with rapid acetylation capability are less likely to develop the lupoid syndrome after prolonged Procainamide therapy.

Blood-Pressure and ECG Monitoring: Blood pressure should be monitored with the patient supine during parenteral, especially intravenous, administration of Procainamide (see "Dosage and Administration"). There is a possibility that relatively high although transient plasma levels of Procainamide may be attained and cause hypotension before the Procainamide can be distributed from the plasma volume to its full apparent volume of distribution which is approximately 50 times greater. Therefore, caution should be exercised to avoid overly rapid administration of Procainamide. If the blood pressure falls 15 mm Hg or more, Procainamide administration should be temporarily discontinued. Electrocardiographic (ECG) monitoring is advisable as well, both for observation of the progress and response of the arrhythmia under treatment, and for early detection of any tendency to excessive widening of the QRS complex, prolongation of the P-R interval, or any signs of heart block (see "Overdosage"). Parenteral therapy with Procainamide should be limited to use in hospitals in which monitoring and intensive supportive care are available, or to emergency situations in which equivalent observation and treatment can be provided.

Information for Patients: The physician is advised to explain to the patient that close cooperation in adhering to the prescribed dosage schedule is of great importance in controlling the cardiac arrhythmia safely. The patient should understand clearly that more medication is not necessarily better and may be dangerous, that skipping doses or increasing intervals between doses to suit personal convenience may lead to loss of control of the heart problem, and that "making up" missed doses by doubling up later may be hazardous.

The patient should be encouraged to disclose any past history of drug sensitivity, especially to procaine or other local anesthetic agents, or aspirin, and to report any history of kidney disease, congestive heart failure, myasthenia gravis, liver disease, or lupus erythematosus.

The patient should be counseled to report promptly any symptoms of arthralgia, myalgia, fever, chills, skin rash, easy bruising, sore throat or sore mouth, infections, dark urine or icterus, wheezing, muscular weakness, chest or abdominal pain, palpitations, nausea, vomiting, anorexia, diarrhea, hallucinations, dizziness, or depression.

The patient should be advised not to break or chew the tablet as this would interfere with designed dissolution characteristics. The tablet matrix of Procainamide HCl ER may be seen in the stool since it does not disintegrate following release of Procainamide HCl ER.

Laboratory Tests: Laboratory tests such as complete blood count (CBC), electrocardiogram, and serum creatinine or urea nitrogen may be indicated, depending on the clinical situation, and periodic rechecking of the CBC and ANA may be helpful in early detection of untoward reactions.

Drug Interactions: If other antiarrhythmic drugs are being used, additive effects on the heart may occur with Procainamide administration and dosage reduction may be necessary (see "Warnings").

Anticholinergic drugs administered concurrently with Procainamide may produce additive antivagal effects on A-V nodal conduction, although this is not as well documented for Procainamide as for quinidine.

Patients taking Procainamide who require neuromuscular blocking agents such as succinylcholine may require less than usual doses of the latter, due to Procainamide effects on reducing acetylcholine release.

Of 10,867 patients treated with mexiletine in a compassionate use program, six cases of agranulocytosis were reported. Five of the six cases involved patients who were concomitantly receiving Procainamide.

Drug/Laboratory Test Interactions: Suprapharmacologic concentrations of lidocaine and meprobamate may inhibit fluorescence of Procainamide and NAPA and propranolol shows a native fluorescence close to the Procainamide NAPA peak wavelengths, so that tests which depend on fluorescence measurement may be affected.

Carcinogenesis, Mutagenesis, Impairment of Fertility: Long term studies in animals have not been performed.

Pregnancy: Teratogenic Effects: Pregnancy Category C: Animal reproduction studies have not been conducted with Procainamide. It also is not known whether Procainamide can cause fetal harm when administered to a pregnant woman or can affect reproduction capacity. Procainamide should be given to a pregnant woman only if clearly needed.

Nursing Mothers: Both Procainamide and NAPA are excreted in human milk, and absorbed by the nursing infant. Because of the potential for serious adverse reactions in nursing infants, a decision to discontinue nursing or the drug should be made, taking into account the importance of the drug to the mother.

Pediatric Use: Safety and effectiveness in children have not been established.

ADVERSE REACTIONS

Cardiovascular System: Hypotension following oral Procainamide administration is rare. Hypotension and serious disturbances of cardiorhythm such as ventricular asystole or fibrillation are more common after intravenous administration of Procainamide than with intramuscular administration. Because Procainamide is a peripheral vasodilator in concentrations higher than the usual therapeutic range, transient high plasma levels which may occur especially during intravenous administration may produce temporary but at times severe lowering of blood pressure. (see *"Overdosage," "Warnings"*). Second degree heart block has been reported in 2 of almost 500 patients taking Procainamide orally.

Multisystem Effects: A lupus erythematosus-like syndrome of arthralgia, pleural or abdominal pain, and sometimes arthritis, pleural effusion, pericarditis, fever, chills, myalgia, and possibly related hematologic or skin lesions (see below) is fairly common after prolonged Procainamide administration, perhaps more often in patients who are slow acetylators (see boxed *"Warnings"* and *"Precautions"*). While some series have reported less than 1 in 500, others have reported the syndrome in up to 30 percent of patients on long term oral Procainamide therapy. If discontinuation of Procainamide does not reverse the lupoid symptoms, corticosteroid treatment may be effective.

Hematologic System: Neutropenia, thrombocytopenia, or hemolytic anemia may rarely be encountered. Agranulocytosis has occurred after repeated use of Procainamide, and deaths have been reported (see *"Warnings"* and boxed *"Warnings"*).

Skin: Angioneurotic edema, urticaria, pruritus, flushing, and maculopapular rash have also occurred.

Gastrointestinal System: Anorexia, nausea, vomiting, abdominal pain, bitter taste, or diarrhea may occur in 3 to 4 percent of patients taking oral Procainamide or after single parenteral doses of Procainamide. Hepatomegaly with increased serum aminotransferase activity has been reported after a single oral or parenteral dose.

Nervous System: Dizziness or giddiness, weakness, mental depression, and psychosis with hallucinations have been reported.

OVERDOSAGE

Progressive widening of the QRS complex, prolonged Q-T and P-R intervals, lowering of the R and T waves, as well as increasing A-V block, may be seen with doses which are excessive for a given patient. Increased ventricular extrasystoles, or even ventricular tachycardia or fibrillation may occur. After intravenous administration but seldom after oral therapy, transient high plasma levels of Procainamide may induce hypotension, affecting systolic more than diastolic pressures, especially in hypertensive patients. Such high levels may also produce central nervous depression, tremor, and even respiratory depression.

Plasma levels above 10 µg/mL are increasingly associated with toxic findings, which are seen occasionally in the 10 to 12 µg/mL range, more often in the 12 to 15 µg/mL range, and commonly in patients with plasma levels greater than 15 µg/mL. A single may produce overdosage symptoms, while 3 g may be dangerous, especially if the patient is a slow acetylator, has decreased renal function, or underlying organic heart disease.

Treatment of overdosage or toxic manifestations includes general supportive measures, close observation, monitoring of vital signs and possibly intravenous pressor agents and mechanical cardiorespiratory support. If available Procainamide and NAPA plasma levels may be helpful in assessing the potential degree of toxicity and response to therapy. Both Procainamide and NAPA are removed from the circulation by hemodialysis but not peritoneal dialysis. No specific antidote for Procainamide is known.

DOSAGE AND ADMINISTRATION

The oral dose and interval of administration should be adjusted for the individual patient, based on clinical assessment of the degree of underlying myocardial disease, the patient's age, and renal function.

As a general guide, for younger patients with normal renal function, an initial total daily oral dose of up to 50 mg/kg of body weight of Procainamide HCl ER tablets or Procainamide HCl capsules may be used, given in divided doses, every six hours for the ER tablets, every three hours for the capsules, to maintain therapeutic blood levels. For older patients, especially those over 50 years of age, or for patients with renal, hepatic or cardiac insufficiency, lesser amounts or longer intervals may produce adequate blood levels, and decrease the probability of occurrence of dose related adverse reactions. The initial total daily dose of Procainamide HCl capsules should be divided for administration at three, four, or six hour intervals as estimated for the patient's needs; then, the dose and interval should be adjusted for the individual.

TO PROVIDE UP TO 50 MG PER KG OF BODY WEIGHT PER DAY*

Patients weighing	Procainamide HCl ER	Procainamide HCl Capsules
88-100 lb (40-50 kg)	500 mg q6 hrs	250 mg q3h to 500 mg q6h
132-154 lb (60-70 kg)	750 mg q6 hrs	375 mg q3h to 750 mg q6h
176-198 lb (80-90 kg)	1 g q6 hrs	500 mg q3h to 1 g q6h
> 220 lb (> 100 kg)	1.25 g q6 hrs	625 mg q3h to 1.25 g q6h

*Initial dosage schedule guide only, to be adjusted for each patient individually, based on age, cardiorenal function, blood level (if available), and clinical response.

Procainamide HCl injection is useful for arrhythmias which require immediate suppression and for maintenance of arrhythmia control. Intravenous therapy allows most rapid control of serious arrhythmias, including those following myocardial infarction; it should be carried out in circumstances where close observation and monitoring of the patient are possible, such as in hospital or emergency facilities. Intramuscular administration is less apt to produce temporary high plasma levels but therapeutic plasma levels are not obtained as rapidly as with intravenous administration. Oral Procainamide HCl dosage forms are preferable for less urgent arrhythmias as well as for long-term maintenance after initial parenteral Procainamide HCl therapy.

Intramuscular administration may be used as an alternative to the oral route for patients with less threatening arrhythmias but who are nauseated or vomiting, who are ordered to receive nothing by mouth preoperatively, or who may have malabsorptive problems. An initial daily dose of 50 mg per kg body weight may be estimated. This amount should be divided into fractional doses of one-eighth to one-quarter to be injected intramuscularly every three to six hours until oral therapy is possible. If more than three injections are given, the physician may wish to assess patient factors such as age and renal function (see below), clinical response and, if available, blood levels of Procainamide HCl and NAPA in adjusting further doses for that individual. For treatment of arrhythmias associated with anesthesia or surgical operation, the suggested dose is 100 to 500 mg by intramuscular injection.

Intravenous administration of Procainamide HCl injection should be done cautiously to avoid a possible hypotensive response (see *"Precautions"* and *"Overdosage"*). Initial arrhythmia control, under ECG monitoring, may usually be accomplished safely within a half-hour by either of the two methods which follow:

a) Direct injection into a vein or into tubing of an established infusion line should be done slowly at a rate not to exceed 50 mg per minute. It is advisable to dilute either the 100 mg/mL or the 500 mg/mL concentrations of Procainamide HCl prior to intravenous injection to facilitate control of dosage rate. Doses of 100 mg may be administered every 5 minutes at this rate until the arrhythmia is suppressed or until 500 mg has been administered, after which it is advisable to wait 10 minutes or longer to allow for more distribution into tissues before resuming.

b) Alternatively, a loading infusion containing 20 mg of Procainamide HCl per mL (1 g diluted to 50 mL with 5% Dextrose Injection, USP) may be administered at a constant rate of 1 mL per minute for 25 to 30 minutes to deliver 500 to 600 mg of Procainamide HCl. Some effects may be seen after infusion of the first 100 or 200 mg; it is unusual to require more than 600 mg to achieve satisfactory antiarrhythmic effects.

The maximum advisable dosage to be given either by repeated bolus injections or such loading infusion is 1 g.

To maintain therapeutic levels, a more dilute intravenous infusion at a concentration of 2 mg/mL is convenient (1000 mg Procainamide HCl in 500 mL of 5% Dextrose Injection, USP), and may be administered at 1 to 3 mL/minute. If daily total fluid intake must be limited a 4 mg/mL concentration (1 g of Procainamide HCl injection in 250 mL of 5% Dextrose Injection, USP) administered at 0.5 to 1.5 mL/minute will deliver an equivalent 2 to 6 mg per minute. The amount needed in a given patient to maintain the therapeutic level should be assessed principally from the clinical response, and will depend upon the patient's weight and age, renal elimination, hepatic acetylation rate, and cardiac status, but should be adjusted for each patient based upon close observation. A maintenance infusion rate of 50 µg/min/kg body weight to a person with a normal renal Procainamide HCl elimination half-time of three hours may be expected to produce a plasma level of approximately 6.5 µg/mL.

Since the principal route for elimination of Procainamide HCl and NAPA is renal excretion, reduced excretion will prolong the half-life of elimination and lower the dose rate needed to maintain therapeutic levels. Advancing age reduces the renal excretion of Procainamide HCl and NAPA independently of reductions in creatinine clearance; compared to normal young adults, there is approximately 25 percent reduction at age 50 and 50 percent at age 75.

Intravenous therapy should be terminated if persistent conduction disturbances or hypotension develop. As soon as the patient's basic cardiac rhythm appears to be stabilized, oral antiarrhythmic maintenance therapy is preferable, if indicated and possible. A period of about three to four hours (one half-time for renal elimination, ordinarily) should elapse after the last intravenous dose before administering the first dose of Procainamide HCl tablets or capsules.

Parenteral drug products should be examined visually for particulate matter and discoloration prior to administration. (See related table).

Store Procainamide HCl ER tablets below 30°C (86°F); protect from moisture.

Store Procainamide HCl capsules and injection at controlled room temperature, 15°-30°C (59°-86°F).

◆ RATED THERAPEUTICALLY EQUIVALENT; ◇ THERAPEUTIC EQUIVALENCE UNCONFIRMED; ○ UNRATED

DILUTIONS AND RATES FOR INTRAVENOUS INFUSIONS*
Procainamide HCl Injection, USP

	Final Concentration	Infusion Volume†	Procainamide HCl To Be Added	Infusion Rate
Initial Loading Infusion	20 mg/mL	50 mL	1000 mg	1 mL/min (for up to 25-30 min*)
Maintenance Infusion	2 mg/mL	500 mL	1000 mg	1 to 3 mL/min
	or			
	4 mg/mL	250 mL	1000 mg	0.5 to 1.5 mL/min

The maintenance infusion rates are calculated to deliver 2 to 6 mg per minute, depending on body weight, renal elimination rate, and steady-state plasma level needed to maintain control of the arrhythmia*. The 4 mg/mL maintenance concentration may be preferred if total infused volume must be limited.

† *(All infusions should be made up to final volume with 5% Dextrose Injection, USP.)*
* *Please see text under "Dosage and Administration" for further details. The flow rate of any intravenous Procainamide infusion must be monitored closely to avoid transiently high plasma levels and possible hypotension (see "Precautions").*

J CODES
Up to 1g IM,IV—J2690

HOW SUPPLIED
CAPSULE: 250 MG

AVERAGE UNIT PRICE (AVAILABLE SIZES)		GENERIC A-RATED AVERAGE PRICE (GAAP)	
BRAND	$0.49		
GENERIC	$0.08	100s	$8.77
HCFA FUL (100s ea)	$0.07	1000s	$60.60

BRAND/MANUFACTURER	NDC	SIZE	AWP
◆ BRAND			
PRONESTYL: Apothecon	00003-0758-50	100s	$49.07
◆ GENERICS			
Moore,H.L.	00839-5224-06	100s	$6.74
Schein	00364-0219-01	100s	$7.00
URL	00677-0450-01	100s	$7.20
Qualitest	00603-5404-21	100s	$7.30
Major	00904-2345-60	100s	$7.50
Zenith	00172-2345-60	100s	$8.30
Aligen	00405-4851-01	100s	$8.35
Goldline	00182-0705-01	100s	$9.00
Rugby	00536-4367-01	100s	$9.10
Parmed	00349-2179-01	100s	$9.15
Vangard	00615-0342-13	100s ud	$9.02
UDL	51079-0101-20	100s ud	$9.10
Raway	00686-0101-20	100s ud	$9.50
Schein	00364-0219-90	100s ud	$15.50
Major	00904-2345-70	250s	$17.80
Parmed	00349-2179-10	1000s	$39.52
Schein	00364-0219-02	1000s	$51.85
Major	00904-2345-80	1000s	$64.15
Rugby	00536-4367-10	1000s	$72.50
Zenith	00172-2345-80	1000s	$75.00

CAPSULE: 375 MG

AVERAGE UNIT PRICE (AVAILABLE SIZES)		GENERIC A-RATED AVERAGE PRICE (GAAP)	
BRAND	$0.68	100s	$10.72
GENERIC	$0.10	1000s	$70.00
HCFA FUL (100s ea)	$0.07		

BRAND/MANUFACTURER	NDC	SIZE	AWP
◆ BRAND			
PRONESTYL: Apothecon	00003-0756-50	100s	$68.05
◆ GENERICS			
Schein	00364-0343-01	100s	$8.50
Qualitest	00603-5405-21	100s	$8.88
Major	00904-2346-60	100s	$9.30
URL	00677-0667-01	100s	$9.74
Goldline	00182-0925-01	100s	$9.75
Moore,H.L.	00839-1563-06	100s	$9.79
Rugby	00536-4377-01	100s	$9.90
Zenith	00172-2346-60	100s	$9.90
U.S. Trading	56126-0291-11	100s ud	$11.70
UDL	51079-0125-20	100s ud	$12.50
Schein	00364-0343-90	100s ud	$18.00
Major	00904-2346-70	250s	$21.40
Major	00904-2346-40	500s	$34.25
Parmed	00349-2181-10	1000s	$60.10
Major	00904-2346-80	1000s	$65.20
Zenith	00172-2346-80	1000s	$84.70

CAPSULE: 500 MG

AVERAGE UNIT PRICE (AVAILABLE SIZES)		GENERIC A-RATED AVERAGE PRICE (GAAP)	
BRAND	$0.88	100s	$12.91
GENERIC	$0.12	1000s	$87.47

BRAND/MANUFACTURER	NDC	SIZE	AWP
◆ BRAND			
PRONESTYL: Apothecon	00003-0757-50	100s	$88.36

BRAND/MANUFACTURER	NDC	SIZE	AWP
◆ GENERICS			
Major	00904-2347-60	100s	$9.20
Moore,H.L.	00839-5050-06	100s	$9.44
Schein	00364-0344-01	100s	$9.65
URL	00677-0470-01	100s	$9.70
Qualitest	00603-5406-21	100s	$9.72
Goldline	00182-0521-01	100s	$10.50
Zenith	00172-2347-60	100s	$11.00
Parmed	00349-2180-01	100s	$12.10
Rugby	00536-4368-01	100s	$12.70
Raway	00686-0102-20	100s ud	$15.50
Vangard	00615-0343-13	100s ud	$15.56
UDL	51079-0102-20	100s ud	$16.00
Vangard	00615-2577-13	100s ud	$19.70
Major	00904-2347-61	100s ud	$17.64
Schein	00364-0344-90	100s ud	$22.00
Major	00904-2347-70	250s	$21.40
Parmed	00349-2180-10	1000s	$71.17
Schein	00364-0344-02	1000s	$89.85
Major	00904-2347-80	1000s	$93.00
Zenith	00172-2347-80	1000s	$95.85

INJECTION: 100 MG/ML

AVERAGE UNIT PRICE (AVAILABLE SIZES)		GENERIC A-RATED AVERAGE PRICE (GAAP)	
BRAND	$3.32	10 ml	$11.06
GENERIC	$1.43	10 ml 25s	$438.66

BRAND/MANUFACTURER	NDC	SIZE	AWP
◆ BRAND			
PRONESTYL: Apothecon	00003-0759-20	10 ml	$33.16
◆ GENERICS			
Schein	00364-2452-54	10 ml	$10.50
Elkins-Sinn	00641-2587-41	10 ml	$11.61
Intl Med Sys	00548-1199-00	10 ml 25s	$346.50
Abbott Hosp	00074-1902-01	10 ml 25s	$530.81

INJECTION: 500 MG/ML

AVERAGE UNIT PRICE (AVAILABLE SIZES)		GENERIC A-RATED AVERAGE PRICE (GAAP)	
BRAND	$16.58	2 ml 10s	$30.55
GENERIC	$5.20		

BRAND/MANUFACTURER	NDC	SIZE	AWP
◆ BRAND			
PRONESTYL: Apothecon	00003-1443-04	2 ml	$33.16
◆ GENERICS			
Elkins-Sinn	00641-0489-21	2 ml	$11.61
Schein	00364-2453-47	2 ml 10s	$10.50
Sanofi Winthrop	00024-1526-02	2 ml 10s	$50.59
Abbott Hosp	00074-1903-01	2 ml 25s	$530.81
Intl Med Sys	00548-6201-00	4 ml 25s	$652.50

TABLET, EXTENDED RELEASE: 250 MG

AVERAGE UNIT PRICE (AVAILABLE SIZES)		GENERIC A-RATED AVERAGE PRICE (GAAP)	
GENERIC	$0.15	100s	$15.85
HCFA FUL (100s ea)	$0.11	500s	$67.41

BRAND/MANUFACTURER	NDC	SIZE	AWP
◆ GENERICS			
Major	00904-2367-60	100s	$13.70
Major	00904-7736-60	100s	$13.70
Sidmak	50111-0339-01	100s	$13.75
Schein	00364-0715-01	100s	$14.75
Moore,H.L.	00839-7027-06	100s	$14.76
Goldline	00182-1707-01	100s	$15.00

► SHOWN IN PRODUCT IDENTIFICATION GUIDE

BRAND/MANUFACTURER	NDC	SIZE	AWP
Rugby	00536-4355-01	100s	$15.74
Geneva	00781-1147-01	100s	$16.99
Parmed	00349-8394-01	100s	$18.18
Aligen	00405-4858-01	100s	$26.31
U.S. Trading	56126-0332-11	100s ud	$8.37
Medirex	57480-0353-01	100s ud	$13.67
Geneva	00781-1147-13	100s ud	$16.80
Major	00904-2367-61	100s ud	$17.72
Schein	00364-0715-90	100s ud	$18.25
Major	00904-2367-70	250s	$29.20
Sidmak	50111-0339-02	500s	$67.32
Rugby	00536-4355-05	500s	$67.50

TABLET, EXTENDED RELEASE: 500 MG

AVERAGE UNIT PRICE (AVAILABLE SIZES)		GENERIC A-RATED AVERAGE PRICE (GAAP)	
BRAND	$0.62	100s	$26.03
GENERIC	$0.24	500s	$113.78
HCFA FUL (100s ea)	$0.14		

BRAND/MANUFACTURER	NDC	SIZE	AWP
◆ **BRAND**			
➤ PROCAN SR: Parke-Davis	00071-0204-24	100s	$60.69
	00071-0204-40	100s ud	$63.65
◆ **GENERICS**			
Copley	38245-0188-10	100s	$20.43
Sidmak	50111-0340-01	100s	$22.44
Major	00904-2368-60	100s	$22.85
Goldline	00182-1708-01	100s	$22.90
Rugby	00536-5576-01	100s	$23.70
Martec	52555-0480-01	100s	$23.80
Qualitest	00603-5411-21	100s	$24.30
URL	00677-0987-01	100s	$26.88
Geneva	00781-1157-01	100s	$26.92
Invamed	52189-0201-24	100s	$26.95
Moore,H.L.	00839-7028-06	100s	$28.28
Schein	00364-0716-01	100s	$29.09
Parmed	00349-8395-01	100s	$29.75
Parmed	00349-8978-01	100s	$29.95
Aligen	00405-4859-01	100s	$37.40
U.S. Trading	56126-0333-11	100s ud	$10.70
Goldline	00182-1708-89	100s ud	$25.00
Major	00904-2368-61	100s ud	$27.03
Auro	55829-0444-10	100s ud	$28.35
Medirex	57480-0354-01	100s ud	$28.40
Schein	00364-0716-90	100s ud	$31.61
Major	00904-2368-70	250s	$51.40
Rugby	00536-4357-05	500s	$79.98
Major	00904-2368-40	500s	$92.50
Copley	38245-0188-50	500s	$99.25
Goldline	00182-1708-05	500s	$100.45
Qualitest	00603-5411-28	500s	$106.45
Rugby	00536-5576-05	500s	$106.60
Sidmak	50111-0340-02	500s	$107.25
URL	00677-0987-05	500s	$111.95
Schein	00364-0716-05	500s	$112.00
Martec	52555-0480-05	500s	$112.95
Parmed	00349-8395-05	500s	$117.98
Geneva	00781-1157-05	500s	$130.71
Invamed	52189-0201-29	500s	$130.75
Parmed	00349-8978-05	500s	$139.95
Aligen	00405-4859-02	500s	$158.00
Major	00904-2368-80	1000s	$112.65

TABLET, EXTENDED RELEASE: 500 MG

BRAND/MANUFACTURER	NDC	SIZE	AWP
◇ **BRAND**			
PRONESTYL-SR: Apothecon	00003-0775-50	100s	$58.68

TABLET, EXTENDED RELEASE: 750 MG

AVERAGE UNIT PRICE (AVAILABLE SIZES)		GENERIC A-RATED AVERAGE PRICE (GAAP)	
BRAND	$0.92	100s	$35.17
GENERIC	$0.35	500s	$161.95
HCFA FUL (100s ea)	$0.21		

BRAND/MANUFACTURER	NDC	SIZE	AWP
◆ **BRAND**			
➤ PROCAN SR: Parke-Davis	00071-0205-24	100s	$90.09
	00071-0205-40	100s ud	$93.05
◆ **GENERICS**			
Copley	38245-0114-10	100s	$31.35
Goldline	00182-1709-01	100s	$31.45
Schein	00364-0717-01	100s	$31.90
Martec	52555-0456-01	100s	$33.35
URL	00677-0988-01	100s	$34.00
Qualitest	00603-5412-21	100s	$34.70
Rugby	00536-4358-01	100s	$34.75
Moore,H.L.	00839-7029-06	100s	$37.40
Aligen	00405-4860-01	100s	$40.57

BRAND/MANUFACTURER	NDC	SIZE	AWP
Parmed	00349-8396-01	100s	$44.95
Schein	00364-0717-90	100s ud	$32.50
Copley	38245-0114-50	500s	$153.90
Rugby	00536-4358-05	500s	$170.00

TABLET, EXTENDED RELEASE: 1000 MG

BRAND/MANUFACTURER	NDC	SIZE	AWP
◆ **BRAND**			
➤ PROCAN SR: Parke-Davis	00071-0207-24	100s	$115.28

TABLETS: 250 MG

BRAND/MANUFACTURER	NDC	SIZE	AWP
◆ **BRAND**			
PRONESTYL: Apothecon	00003-0431-50	100s	$49.07

TABLETS: 375 MG

BRAND/MANUFACTURER	NDC	SIZE	AWP
◆ **BRAND**			
PRONESTYL: Apothecon	00003-0434-50	100s	$68.05
◆ **GENERICS**			
Aligen	00405-4852-01	100s	$9.60

TABLETS: 500 MG

BRAND/MANUFACTURER	NDC	SIZE	AWP
◆ **BRAND**			
PRONESTYL: Apothecon	00003-0438-50	100s	$88.36
◆ **GENERICS**			
Aligen	00405-4853-01	100s	$11.20

Procaine Hydrochloride

DESCRIPTION

Procaine Hydrochloride is benzoic acid, 4-amino-, 2-(diethylamino) ethyl ester, monohydrochloride, the ester of diethylaminoethanol and aminobenzoic acid or para-aminobenzoic acid.

It is a white crystalline, odorless powder that is freely soluble in water, but less soluble in alcohol and has a molecular weight of 272.77.

Each mL contains:	
Procaine Hydrochloride 1%	10 mg
Procaine Hydrochloride 2%	20 mg
Procaine Hydrochloride 10%	100 mg

Procaine is related chemically and pharmacologically to the ester-type local anesthetics. It contains an ester linkage between the aromatic nucleus and the amino group.

Procaine Hydrochloride is available as sterile solutions for injection.

DO NOT USE SOLUTIONS IF CRYSTALS, CLOUDINESS, OR DISCOLORATION IS OBSERVED. EXAMINE SOLUTIONS CAREFULLY BEFORE USE. REAUTOCLAVING INCREASES LIKELIHOOD OF CRYSTAL FORMATION.

Following is its chemical structure:

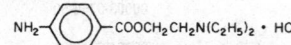

$$NH_2 - \bigcirc - COOCH_2CH_2N(C_2H_5)_2 \cdot HCl$$

CLINICAL PHARMACOLOGY

Local anesthetics block the generation and the conduction of nerve impulses, presumably by increasing the threshold for electrical excitation in the nerve, by slowing the propagation of the nerve impulse, and by reducing the rate of rise of the action potential. In general, the progression of anesthesia is related to the diameter, myelination, and conduction velocity of affected nerve fibers. Clinically, the order of loss of nerve function is as follows: pain, temperature, touch, proprioception, and skeletal muscle tone. Procaine lacks topical anesthetic activity.

Systemic absorption of local anesthetics produces effects on the cardiovascular and central nervous systems. At blood concentrations achieved with normal therapeutic doses, changes in cardiac conduction, excitability, refractoriness, contractility, and peripheral vascular resistance are minimal. However, toxic blood concentrations depress cardiac conduction and excitability, which may lead to atrioventricular block and ultimately to cardiac arrest. In addition, myocardial contractility is depressed and peripheral vasodilation occurs, leading to decreased cardiac output and arterial blood pressure.

Following systemic absorption, local anesthetics can produce central nervous system stimulation, depression, or both. Apparent central stimulation is manifested as restlessness, tremors and shivering, progressing to convulsions, followed by depression, and coma progressing ultimately to respiratory arrest. However, the local anesthetics have a primary depressant effect on the medulla and on higher centers. The depressed stage may occur without a prior excited stage.

◆ RATED THERAPEUTICALLY EQUIVALENT; ◇ THERAPEUTIC EQUIVALENCE UNCONFIRMED; ○ UNRATED

PHARMACOKINETICS

The rate of systemic absorption of local anesthetics is dependent upon the total dose and concentration of drug administered, the route of administration, the vascularity of the administration site, and the presence or absence of epinephrine in the anesthetic solution. A dilute concentration of epinephrine (1:200,000 or 5 μg/mL) usually reduces the rate of absorption and plasma concentration of Procaine HCl. It also will promote local hemostasis and increase the duration of anesthesia.

Onset of anesthesia with Procaine HCl is rapid, the time of onset for sensory block ranging from about two to five minutes depending upon such factors as the anesthetic technique, the type of block, the concentration of the solution, and the individual patient. The degree of motor blockade produced is dependent on the concentration of the solution.

The duration of anesthesia also varies depending upon the technique and type of block, the concentration, and the individual. Procaine HCl will normally provide anesthesia which is adequate for one to one and a half hours.

Local anesthetics are bound to plasma proteins in varying degrees. Generally, the lower the plasma concentration of drug, the higher the percentage of drug bound to plasma.

Local anesthetics appear to cross the placenta by passive diffusion. The rate and degree of diffusion is governed by the degree of plasma protein binding, the degree of ionization, and the degree at lipid solubility. Fetal/maternal ratios of local anesthetics appear to be inversely related to the degree of plasma protein binding, because only the free, unbound drug is available for placental transfer. The extent of placental transfer is also determined by the degree of ionization and lipid solubility of the drug. Lipid-soluble, nonionized drugs readily enter the fetal blood from the maternal circulation.

Depending upon the route of administration, local anesthetics are distributed to some extent to all body tissues, with high concentrations found in highly perfused organs such as the liver, lungs, heart, and brain.

Various pharmacokinetic parameters of the local anesthetics can be significantly altered by the presence of hepatic or renal disease, addition of epinephrine, factors affecting urinary pH, renal blood flow, the route of drug administration, and the age of the patient. The *in vitro* plasma half-life of Procaine HCl in adults is 40 ± 9 seconds and in neonates 84 ± 30 seconds.

Procaine HCl is readily absorbed following parenteral administration and is rapidly hydrolyzed by plasma cholinesterase to aminobenzoic acid or (10%) para-aminobenzoic acid (1% and 2%) and diethylaminoethanol.

The para-aminobenzoic acid metabolite inhibits the action of the sulfonamides. (See *"Precautions"*.)

For Procaine HCl, approximately 90% of the para-aminobenzoic acid metabolite and its conjugates and 33% of the diethylaminoethanol metabolite are recovered in the urine, while less than 2% of the administered dose is recovered unchanged in the urine.

A vasoconstrictor may be added to the solution of Procaine HCl, to promote local hemostasis, delay systemic absorption, and increase duration of anesthesia.

INDICATIONS AND USAGE

Procaine HCl is indicated for the production of local or regional analgesia and anesthesia by local infiltration and peripheral nerve block techniques.

The routes of administration and concentrations are: for local infiltration use 0.25% to 0.5% (via dilution) and for peripheral nerve blocks use 0.5% (via dilution), 1%, and 2%. (See *"Dosage and Administration"* for additional information.)

Some brands are indicated for spinal anesthesia, some are not intended for spinal or epidural anesthesia or for dental use.

Standard textbooks should be consulted to determine the accepted procedures and techniques for the administration of Procaine HCl.

CONTRAINDICATIONS

Procaine HCl is contraindicated in patients with a known hypersensitivity to Procaine, drugs of a similar chemical configuration, or para-aminobenzoic acid or its derivatives.

It is also contraindicated in patients with a known hypersensitivity to other components of solutions of Procaine HCl.

Spinal anesthesia with Procaine HCl is contraindicated in patients with generalized septicemia: sepsis at the proposed injection site; certain diseases of the cerebrospinal system, eg, meningitis, syphilis; and a known hypersensitivity to the drug, drugs of a similar chemical configuration, or aminobenzoic acid or its derivatives.

The decision as to whether or not spinal anesthesia should be used in an individual case should be made by the physician after weighing the advantages with the risks and possible complications.

WARNINGS

Some brands contain acetone sodium bisulfite, a sulfite that may cause allergic-type reactions including anaphylactic symptoms and life-threatening or less severe asthmatic episodes in certain susceptible people. The overall prevalence of sulfite sensitivity in the general population is unknown and probably low. Sulfite sensitivity is seen more frequently in asthmatic than in nonasthmatic people.

LOCAL ANESTHETICS SHOULD ONLY BE EMPLOYED BY CLINICIANS WHO ARE WELL VERSED IN DIAGNOSIS AND MANAGEMENT OF DOSE-RELATED TOXICITY AND OTHER ACUTE EMERGENCIES WHICH MIGHT ARISE FROM THE BLOCK TO BE EMPLOYED, AND THEN ONLY AFTER INSURING THE *IMMEDIATE* AVAILABILITY OF OXYGEN, OTHER RESUSCITATIVE DRUGS, CARDIOPULMONARY RESUSCITATIVE EQUIPMENT, AND THE PERSONNEL RESOURCES NEEDED FOR PROPER MANAGEMENT OF TOXIC REACTIONS AND RELATED EMERGENCIES. (SEE ALSO *"ADVERSE REACTIONS"* AND *"PRECAUTIONS"*.) DELAY IN

PROPER MANAGEMENT OF DOSE-RELATED TOXICITY, UNDERVENTILATION FROM ANY CAUSE, AND/OR ALTERED SENSITIVITY MAY LEAD TO THE DEVELOPMENT OF ACIDOSIS, CARDIAC ARREST, AND, POSSIBLY, DEATH.

Spinal anesthesia should only be administered by those qualified to do so.

It is essential that aspiration for blood or cerebrospinal fluid, where applicable, be done prior to injecting any local anesthetic, both the original dose and all subsequent doses, to avoid intravascular or subarachnoid injection. However, a negative aspiration does not ensure against an intravascular or subarachnoid injection.

Reactions resulting in fatality have occurred on rare occasions with the use of local anesthetics, even in the absence of a history of hypersensitivity. Large doses of local anesthetics should not be used in patients with heartblock.

Vasopressor agents such as epinephrine (administered for the treatment of hypotension or added to the anesthetic solution for vasoconstriction) should be used with extreme caution in the presence of oxytocic drugs as they may produce severe, persistent hypertension with possible rupture of a cerebral blood vessel. Likewise, solutions of Procaine HCl containing a vasoconstrictor, such as epinephrine, should be used with extreme caution in patients receiving monoamine oxidase inhibitors (MAOI) or antidepressants of the triptyline or imipramine types, because severe prolonged hypertension or hypotension or disturbances of cardiac rhythm may occur.

Local anesthetic procedures should be used with caution when there is inflammation and/or sepsis in the region of the proposed injection.

Mixing or the prior or intercurrent use of any local anesthetic with Procaine HCl cannot be recommended because of insufficient data on the clinical use of such mixtures.

PRECAUTIONS

Standard textbooks should be consulted for specific techniques and precautions for various spinal anesthetic procedures.

GENERAL

The safety and effectiveness of local anesthetics, including spinal, depend on proper dosage, correct technique, adequate precautions, and readiness for emergencies. Resuscitative equipment, oxygen, and other resuscitative drugs should be available for immediate use. (See *"Warnings"* and *"Adverse Reactions"*.) During major regional nerve blocks, the patient should have IV fluids running via an indwelling catheter to assure a functioning intravenous pathway. The lowest dosage of local anesthetic that results in effective anesthesia should be used to avoid high plasma levels and serious adverse effects. Injections should be made slowly, with frequent aspirations before and during the injection to avoid intravascular injection. Current opinion favors fractional administration with constant attention to the patient, rather than rapid bolus injection. Syringe aspirations should also be performed before and during each supplemental injection in continuous (intermittent) catheter techniques. An intravascular injection is still possible even if aspirations for blood are negative.

Injection of repeated doses of local anesthetics may cause significant increases in plasma levels with each repeated dose due to slow accumulation of the drug or its metabolites or to slow metabolic degradation. Tolerance to elevated blood levels varies with the status of the patient. Debilitated, elderly patients and acutely ill patients should be given reduced doses commensurate with their age, weight, and physical status. Reduced dosages are also indicated for patients with increased intra-abdominal pressure. Local anesthetics should also be used with caution in patients with severe disturbances of cardiac rhythm, shock, heartblock, or hypotension.

Careful and constant monitoring of cardiovascular and respiratory (adequacy of ventilation) vital signs and the patient's state of consciousness should be performed after each local anesthetic injection. It should be kept in mind at such times that restlessness, anxiety, incoherent speech, light-headedness, numbness, and tingling of the mouth and lips, metallic taste, tinnitus, dizziness, blurred vision, tremors, twitching, depression, or drowsiness may be early warning signs of central nervous system toxicity.

The decision whether or not to use spinal anesthesia in the following disease states depends on the physician's appraisal of the advantages as opposed to the risk: cardiovascular disease (ie, shock, hypertension, anemia, etc), pulmonary disease, renal impairment, metabolic or endocrine disorders, gastrointestinal disorders (ie, intestinal obstruction, peritonitis, etc), or complicated obstrical deliveries.

Local anesthetic solutions containing a vasoconstrictor should be used cautiously and in carefully circumscribed quantities in areas of the body supplied by end arteries, or those areas having otherwise compromised blood supply such as digits, nose, external ear, penis. Patients with peripheral vascular disease and hypertensive vascular disease may exhibit an exaggerated vasoconstrictor response. Ischemic injury or necrosis may result.

Procaine HCl should be used with caution in patients with known allergies and sensitivities. A thorough history of the patient's prior experience with Procaine HCl or other local anesthetics as well as concomitant or recent drug use should be taken. (See *"Contraindications"* and *"Warnings"*.)

Because ester-type local anesthetics such as Procaine HCl are hydrolyzed by plasma cholinesterase produced by the liver and excreted by the kidneys, these drugs, especially repeat doses, should be used cautiously in patients with hepatic disease. Because of their inability to metabolize local anesthetics normally, patients with severe hepatic disease are at a greater risk of developing toxic plasma concentrations. Local anesthetics should also be used with caution in patients with impaired cardiovascular function because they may be less able to compensate for functional changes associated with the prolongation of AV conduction produced by these drugs.

Serious dose-related cardiac arrhythmias may occur if preparations containing a vasoconstrictor such as epinephrine are employed in patients during or following the administration of potent inhalation anesthetics. In deciding whether to use these products concurrently in the same patient, the combined action of both agents upon the myocardium, the concentration and volume of vasoconstrictor used, and the time since injection, when applicable, should be taken into account.

Many drugs used during the conduction of anesthesia are considered potential triggering agents for familial malignant hyperthermia. Because it is not known whether ester-type local anesthetics may trigger this reaction and because the need for supplemental general anesthesia cannot be predicted in advance, it is suggested that a standard protocol for management should be available. Early unexplained signs of tachycardia, tachypnea, labile blood pressure, and metabolic acidosis may precede temperature elevation. Successful outcome is dependent on early diagnosis, prompt discontinuance of the suspect triggering agent(s), and institution of treatment, including oxygen therapy, indicated supportive measures, and dantrolene. (Consult dantrolene sodium intravenous package insert before using.)

USE IN HEAD AND NECK AREA
Small doses of local anesthetics injected into the head and neck area may produce adverse reactions similar to systemic toxicity seen with unintentional intravascular injections of larger doses. Confusion, convulsions, respiratory depression and/or respiratory arrest, and cardiovascular stimulation or depression have been reported.

These reactions may be due to intra-arterial injection of the local anesthetic with retrograde flow to the cerebral circulation. Patients receiving these blocks should have their circulation and respiration monitored and be constantly observed. Resuscitative equipment and personnel for treating adverse reactions should be immediately available. Dosage recommendations should not be exceeded.

INFORMATION FOR PATIENTS
When appropriate, patients should be informed, in advance, that they may experience temporary loss of sensation and motor activity following proper administration of regional anesthesia. Also, when appropriate, the physician should discuss other information including adverse reactions in the package insert.

CLINICALLY SIGNIFICANT DRUG INTERACTIONS
The administration of local anesthetic solutions containing epinephrine or norepinephrine to patients receiving monoamine oxidase inhibitors or tricyclic antidepressants may produce severe, prolonged hypertension. Concurrent use of these agents should generally be avoided. In situations when concurrent therapy is necessary, careful patient monitoring is essential.

Concurrent administration of vasopressor drugs and of ergot-type oxytocic drugs may cause severe, persistent hypertension or cerebrovascular accidents. Solutions containing a vasopressor should be used with caution in the presence of diseases which may adversely affect the cardiovascular system.

Phenothiazines and butyrophenones may reduce or reverse the pressor effect of epinephrine.

The clinical observation has been made that despite adequate sulfonamide therapy, local infections have occurred in areas infiltrated with Procaine HCl prior to diagnostic punctures and drainage procedures. Therefore, Procaine HCl should not be used in any condition in which a sulfonamide drug is being employed since aminobenzoic acid and para-aminobenzoic acid inhibit the action of the sulfonamide.

CARCINOGENESIS, MUTAGENESIS, AND IMPAIRMENT OF FERTILITY
Long-term studies in animals of most local anesthetics, including Procaine HCl, to evaluate the carcinogenic potential have not been conducted. Mutagenic potential or the effect on fertility have not been determined. There is no evidence from human data that Procaine HCl may be carcinogenic, or mutagenic, or that it impairs fertility.

PREGNANCY CATEGORY C
Animal reproduction studies have not been conducted with Procaine HCl. It is not known whether Procaine can cause fetal harm when administered to a pregnant woman or can affect reproduction capacity. Procaine HCl should be given to a pregnant woman only if clearly needed and the potential benefits outweigh the risk, particularly during early pregnancy. This does not exclude the use of Procaine HCl at term for obstetrical anesthesia or analgesia. (See "Labor and Delivery".)

LABOR AND DELIVERY
Local anesthetics rapidly cross the placenta, and when used for paracervical or pudendal block anesthesia, can cause varying degrees of maternal, fetal, and neonatal toxicity. (see "Clinical Pharmacology".) The incidence and degree of toxicity depend upon the procedure performed, the type and amount of drug used, and the technique of drug administration. Adverse reactions in the parturient, fetus, and neonate involve alterations of the central nervous system, peripheral vascular tone, and cardiac function.

Maternal hypotension has resulted from regional anesthesia. Local anesthetics produce vasodilation by blocking sympathetic nerves. Elevating the patient's legs and positioning her on her left side will help prevent decreases in blood pressure. The fetal heart rate also should be monitored continuously and electronic fetal monitoring is highly advisable.

Paracervical or pudendal anesthesia may alter the forces at parturition through changes in uterine contractility or maternal expulsive efforts. In one study, paracervical block anesthesia was associated with a decrease in the mean duration of first stage labor and facilitation of cervical dilation. The use of obstetrical anesthesia may increase the need for forceps assistance.

The use of some local anesthetic drug products during labor and delivery may be followed by diminished muscle strength and tone for the first day or two of life. The long-term significance of these observations is unknown.

Fetal bradycardia which frequently follows paracervical block may be indicative of high fetal blood concentrations of Procaine with resultant fetal acidosis. Fetal heart rate should be monitored prior to and during paracervical block. Added risk appears to be present in prematurity, toxemia of pregnancy, and fetal distress. The physician should weigh considering paracervical block in these conditions. Careful adherence to recommended dosage is of the utmost importance in paracervical block. Failure to achieve adequate analgesia with these doses should arouse suspicion of intravascular or fetal injection.

Cases compatible with unintended fetal intracranial injection of local anesthetic solution have been reported following intended paracervical or pudendal block or both. Babies so affected present with unexplained neonatal depression at birth, which correlates with high local anesthetic serum levels, and usually manifest seizures within six hours. Prompt use of supportive measures combined with forced urinary excretion of the local anesthetic has been used successfully to manage this complication.

Case reports of maternal convulsions and cardiovascular collapse following use of some local anesthetics for paracervical block in early pregnancy (as anesthesia for elective abortion) suggest that systemic absorption under these circumstances may be rapid. The recommended maximum dose of the local anesthetic should not be exceeded. Injection should be made slowly and with frequent aspiration. Allow a five-minute interval between sides.

It is extremely important to avoid aortocaval compression by the gravid uterus during administration of regional block to parturients. To do this, the patient must be maintained in the left lateral decubitus position or a blanket roll or sandbag may be placed beneath the right hip and the gravid uterus displaced to the left.

NURSING MOTHERS
It is not known whether local anesthetic drugs are excreted in human milk. Because many drugs are excreted in human milk, caution should be exercised when local anesthetics are administered to a nursing women.

PEDIATRIC USE
(See "Dosage and Administration".)

ADVERSE REACTIONS
Reactions to Procaine are characteristic of those associated with other ester-type local anesthetics. A major cause of adverse reactions to this group of drugs is excessive plamsa levels which may be due to overdosage, rapid absorption, inadvertent intravascular injection, or slow metabolic degradation.

A small number of reactions may result from hypersensitivity, idiosyncrasy, or diminished tolerance to normal dosage.

SYSTEMIC
The most commonly encountered acute adverse experiences which demand immediate countermeasures are related to the central nervous system and the cardiovascular system. These adverse experiences are generally dose related and due to high plasma levels which may result from overdosage, rapid absorption from the injection site, diminished tolerance, or from unintentional intravascular injection of the local anesthetic solution. In addition to systemic dose-related toxicity, unintentional subarachnoid injection of drug during the intended performance of nerve blocks near the vertebral column (especially in the head and neck region), may result in underventilation or apnea ("Total or High Spinal"). Also use of inappropriate doses or techniques in spinal anesthesia may result in extensive spinal blockade leading to hypotension and respiratory arrest.

A small number of reactions may result from hypersensitivity, idiosyncrasy, or diminished tolerance to normal dosage. Factors influencing plasma protein binding, such as acidosis, systemic diseases which alter protein production, or competition of other drugs for protein binding sites may diminish individual tolerance.

Plasma cholinesterase deficiency may also account for diminished tolerance to ester-type local anesthetics.

CENTRAL NERVOUS SYSTEM REACTIONS
These are characterized by excitation and/or depression. Restlessness, anxiety, dizziness, tinnitus, blurred vision, or tremors may occur, possibly proceeding to convulsions. However, excitement may be transient or absent, with depression being the first manifestation of an adverse reaction. This may quickly be followed by drowsiness merging into unconsciousness and respiratory arrest.

The incidence of convulsions associated with the use of local anesthetics varies with the procedure used and the total dose administered.

CARDIOVASCULAR REACTIONS
High doses or inadvertent intravascular injection may lead to high plasma levels and related depression of the myocardium, decreased cardiac output, heartblock, hypotension (or sometimes hypertension), bradycardia, ventricular arrhythmias, and cardiac arrest. (See "Warnings, Precautions" and "Overdosage" sections.)

ALLERGIC

Allergic-type reactions are rare and may occur as a result of sensitivity to the local anesthetic or to other formulation ingredients. These reactions are characterized by signs such as cutaneous lesions of delayed onset, urticaria, pruritus, erythema, angioneurotic edema (including laryngeal edema), tachycardia, sneezing, nausea, vomiting, dizziness, syncope, excessive sweating, elevated temperature, and, possibly, anaphylactoid-like symptomatology (including severe hypotension). The reaction may be abrupt and severe and is not usually dose related. Cross sensitivity among members of the ester-type local anesthetic group has been reported. The usefulness of screening for sensitivity has not been definitely established.

NEUROLOGIC

The incidences of adverse neurologic reactions associated with the use of local anesthetics may be related to the total dose of local anesthetic administered, and are also dependent upon the particular drug used, the route of administration, and the physical status of the patient. Many of these effects may be related to local anesthetic techniques, with or without a contribution from the drug.

The following adverse reactions may occur with spinal anesthesia.

Central Nervous System: postspinal headache, meningismus, arachnoiditis, palsies, or spinal nerve paralysis.

Cardiovascular: hypotension due to vasomotor paralysis and pooling of the blood in the venous bed.

Respiratory: respiratory impairment or paralysis due to the level of anesthesia extending to the upper thoracic and cervical segments.

Gastrointestinal: nausea and vomiting.

Treatment of Reactions: Toxic effects of local anesthetics require symptomatic treatment; there is no specific cure. The physician should be prepared to maintain an airway and to support ventilation with oxygen and assisted or controlled respiration as required. Supportive treatment of the cardiovascular system includes intravenous fluids and, when appropriate, vasopressors (preferably those that stimulate the myocardium, such as ephedrine). Convulsions may be controlled with oxygen and by the intravenous administration of diazepam or ultrashort-acting barbiturates or a short-acting muscle relaxant (succinylcholine). Intravenous anticonvulsant agents and muscle relaxants should only be administered by those familiar with their use and only when ventilation and oxygenation are assured. (See "Overdosage".) In spinal and epidural anesthesia, sympathetic blockade also occurs as a pharmacological reaction, resulting in peripheral vasodilation and often *hypotension*. The extent of the hypotension will usually depend on the number of dermatomes blocked. The blood pressure should therefore be monitored in the early phases of anesthesia. If hypotension occurs, it is readily controlled by vasoconstrictors administered either by the intramuscular or the intravenous route, the dosage of which would depend on the severity of the hypotension and the response to treatment.

OVERDOSAGE

Acute emergencies from local anesthetics are generally related to high plasma levels encountered during therapeutic use of local anesthetics or to unintended subarachnoid injection of local anesthetic solution. (See "Adverse Reactions," "Warnings," and "Precautions".)

MANAGEMENT OF LOCAL ANESTHETIC EMERGENCIES

The first consideration is prevention, best accomplished by careful and constant monitoring of cardiovascular and respiratory vital signs and the patient's state of consciousness after each local anesthetic injection. At the first sign of change, oxygen should be administered.

The first step in the management of systemic toxic reactions, as well as underventilation or apnea due to unintentional subarachnoid injection of drug solution, consists of immediate attention to the establishment and maintenance of a patent airway, and effective assisted or controlled ventilation with 100% oxygen with a delivery system capable of permitting immediate positive airway pressure by mask. This may prevent convulsions if they have not already occurred.

If necessary, use drugs to control the convulsions. A 50 mg to 100 mg bolus IV injection of succinylcholine will paralyze the patient without depressing the central nervous or cardiovascular systems and facilitate ventilation. A bolus IV dose of 5 mg to 10 mg of diazepam or 50 mg to 100 mg of thiopental will permit ventilation and counteract central nervous system stimulation, but these drugs also depress central nervous system, respiratory and cardiac function, add to postictal depression, and may result in apnea. Intravenous barbiturates, anticonvulsant agents, or muscle relaxants should only be administered by those familiar with their use. Immediately after the institution of these ventilatory measures, the adequacy of the circulation should be evaluated. Supportive treatment of circulatory depression may require administration of intravenous fluids and, when appropriate, a vasopressor dictated by the clinical situation (such as ephedrine or epinephrine to enhance myocardial contractile force).

Endotracheal intubation, employing drugs and techniques familiar to the clinician, may be indicated, after initial administration of oxygen by mask, if difficulty is encountered in the maintenance of a patent airway or if prolonged ventilatory support (assisted or controlled) is indicated.

Recent clinical data from patients experiencing local anesthetic-induced convulsions demonstrated rapid development of hypoxia, hypercarbia, and acidosis within a minute of the onset of convulsions. These observations suggest that oxygen consumption and carbon dioxide production are greatly increased during local anesthetic convulsions, and emphasize the importance of immediate and effective ventilation with oxygen which may avoid cardiac arrest.

If not treated immediately, convulsions with simultaneous hypoxia, hypercarbia, and acidosis plus myocardial depression, from the direct effects of the local anesthetic, may result in cardiac arrhythmias, bradycardia, asystole, ventricular fibrillation, or cardiac arrest. Respiratory abnormalities, including apnea, may occur. Underventilation or apnea due to unintentional subarachnoid injection of local anesthetic solution may produce these same signs and also lead to cardiac arrest if ventilatory support is not instituted. If cardiac arrest should occur, standard cardiopulmonary resuscitative measures should be instituted and maintained for a prolonged period if necessary. Recovery has been reported after prolonged resuscitative efforts.

The supine position is dangerous in pregnant women at term because of aortocaval compression by the gravid uterus. Therefore, during treatment of systemic toxicity, maternal hypotension, or fetal bradycardia following regional block, the parturient should be maintained in the left lateral decubitus position if possible, or manual displacement of the uterus off the great vessels be accomplished.

The intravenous and subcutaneous and intraperitoneal LD$_{50}$ of Procaine HCl in mice is 46 mg/kg to 80 mg/kg and 400 mg/kg and 200 mg/kg respectively.

DOSAGE AND ADMINISTRATION

The dose of any local anesthetic administered varies with the anesthetic procedure, the area to be anesthetized, the vascularity of the tissues, the number of neuronal segments to be blocked, the depth of anesthesia and degree of muscle relaxation required, the duration of anesthesia desired, individual tolerance, and the physical condition of the patient. The smallest dose and concentration required to produce the desired result should be administered. Dosages of Procaine HCl should be reduced for elderly and debilitated patients and patients with cardiac and/or liver disease. The rapid injection of a large volume of local anesthetic solution should be avoided and fractional doses should be used when feasible.

For specific techniques and procedures, refer to standard textbooks.

For infiltration anesthesia, 0.25% or 0.5% solution; 350 mg to 600 mg is generally considered to be a single safe total dose. To prepare 60 mL of a 0.5% solution (5 mg/mL), dilute 30 mL of the 1% solution with 30 mL sodium chloride injection 0.9%. To prepare 60 mL of a 0.25% solution (2.5 mg/mL), dilute 15 mL of the 1% solution with 45 mL sodium chloride injection 0.9%. An anesthetic solution of 0.5 mL. to 1 mL of epinephrine 1:1,000 per 100 mL may be added for vasoconstrictive effect (1:200,000 to 1:100,000). (See "Warnings" and "Precautions".)

For peripheral nerve block, 0.5% solution (up to 200 mL), 1% solution (up to 100 mL), or 2% solution (up to 50 mL). The use of the 2% solution should usually be limited to cases requiring a small volume of anesthetic solution (10 mL to 25 mL). An anesthetic solution of 0.5 mL to 1 mL of epinephrine 1:1,000 per 100 mL may be added for vasoconstrictive effect (1:200,000 to 1:100,000). (See "Warnings" and "Precautions".)

THE USUAL TOTAL DOSE DURING ONE TREATMENT SHOULD NOT EXCEED 1,000 MG.

This product should be inspected visually for particulate matter and discoloration prior to administration whenever solution and container permit. Do not use solutions if crystals, cloudiness, or discoloration is observed. Examine solution carefully before use. Reautoclaving increases likelihood of crystal formation. Solutions which are discolored or which contain particulate matter should not be administered.

Unused portions of solutions not containing preservatives should be discarded.

PEDIATRIC USE

In children, 15 mg/kg of a 0.5% solution for local infiltration is the maximum recommended dose.

RECOMMENDED DOSAGE FOR SPINAL ANESTHESIA

	Procaine HCl 10% Solution			
Extent of Anesthesia	Volume of 10% Solution (mL)	Volume of Diluent (mL)	Total Dose (mg)	Site of Injection (lumbar interspace)
Perineum	0.5	0.5	50	4th
Perineum and lower extremities	1	1	100	3rd or 4th
Up to costal margin	2	1	200	2nd, 3rd or 4th

The diluent may be sterile normal saline, sterile distilled water, spinal fluid; and for hyperbaric technique, sterile dextrose solution.

The usual rate of injection is 1 mL per 5 seconds. Full anesthesia and fixation usually occur in 5 minutes.

STERILIZATION

The drug in intact ampuls is sterile. The preferred method of destroying bacteria on the exterior of ampuls before opening is heat sterilization (autoclaving). Immersion in antiseptic solution is not recommended.

Autoclave at 15-pound pressure, at 121°C (250°F), for 15 minutes. The diluent dextrose may show some brown discoloration due to caramelization.

HOW SUPPLIED
INJECTION: 1%

AVERAGE UNIT PRICE (AVAILABLE SIZES)

BRAND	$0.97

BRAND/MANUFACTURER	NDC	SIZE	AWP
◆ **BRAND**			
NOVOCAIN: Sanofi Winthrop	00024-1385-01	30 ml	$13.72
	00024-1381-25	2 ml 25s	$74.65
	00024-1381-05	6 ml 50s	$284.47
◆ **GENERICS**			
Abbott Hosp	00074-1923-04	30 ml 25s	$84.31

INJECTION: 2%

AVERAGE UNIT PRICE (AVAILABLE SIZES)

		GENERIC A-RATED AVERAGE PRICE (GAAP)	
BRAND	$0.46	30 ml	$3.87
GENERIC	$0.13		

BRAND/MANUFACTURER	NDC	SIZE	AWP
◆ **BRAND**			
NOVOCAIN: Sanofi Winthrop	00024-1386-01	30 ml	$13.72
◆ **GENERICS**			
Torrance	00389-0527-30	30 ml	$2.69
Schein	00364-2371-56	30 ml	$4.13
Truxton	00463-1052-30	30 ml	$4.80
Abbott Hosp	00074-1953-04	30 ml 25s	$84.31

INJECTION: 10%

BRAND/MANUFACTURER	NDC	SIZE	AWP
○ **BRAND**			
NOVOCAIN: Sanofi Winthrop	00024-1384-25	2 ml 25s	$166.81

INJECTION: 20 MG/ML

BRAND/MANUFACTURER	NDC	SIZE	AWP
◆ **GENERICS**			
Steris	00402-0527-30	30 ml	$4.13

Procalamine *SEE* AMINO ACIDS WITH ELECTROLYTES, INJECTABLE

Procan SR *SEE* PROCAINAMIDE HYDROCHLORIDE

Procarbazine Hydrochloride

> **WARNING**
>
> IT IS RECOMMENDED THAT PROCARBAZINE HYDROCHLORIDE BE GIVEN ONLY BY OR UNDER THE SUPERVISION OF A PHYSICIAN EXPERIENCED IN THE USE OF POTENT ANTINEOPLASTIC DRUGS. ADEQUATE CLINICAL AND LABORATORY FACILITIES SHOULD BE AVAILABLE TO PATIENTS FOR PROPER MONITORING OF TREATMENT.

DESCRIPTION

Procarbazine Hydrochloride (Procarbazine HCl) a hydrazine derivative antineoplastic agent, is available as capsules containing the equivalent of 50 mg Procarbazine as the Hydrochloride.

Chemically, Procarbazine Hydrochloride is *N*-isopropyl-α-(2-methylhydrazino)-p-toluamide monohydrochloride. It is a white to pale yellow crystalline powder which is soluble but unstable in water or aqueous solutions. The molecular weight of Procarbazine Hydrochloride is 257.76.

Following is its chemical structure:

$$(CH_3)_2CHNHC \underset{\text{(benzene ring)}}{\overset{O}{\parallel}} CH_2NHNHCH_3 \cdot HCl$$

CLINICAL PHARMACOLOGY

The precise mode of cytotoxic action of Procarbazine has not been clearly defined. There is evidence that the drug may act by inhibition of protein, RNA and DNA synthesis. Studies have suggested that Procarbazine may inhibit transmethylation of methyl groups of methionine into t-RNA. The absence of functional t-RNA could cause the cessation of protein synthesis and consequently DNA and RNA synthesis. In addition, Procarbazine may directly damage DNA. Hydrogen peroxide, formed during the auto-oxidation of the drug, may attack protein sulfhydryl groups contained in residual protein which is tightly bound to DNA.

Procarbazine is metabolized primarily in the liver and kidneys. The drug appears to be auto-oxidized to the azo derivative with the release of hydrogen peroxide. The azo derivative isomerizes to the hydrazone, and following hydrolysis splits into a benzyladehyde derivative and methylhydrazine. The methylhydrazine is further degraded to CO_2 and CH_4 and possibly hydrazine, whereas the aldehyde is oxidized to N-isopropylterephthalamic acid, which is excreted in the urine.

Procarbazine is rapidly and completely absorbed. Following oral administration of 30 mg of ^{14}C-labeled Procarbazine maximum peak plasma radioactive concentrations were reached within 60 minutes.

After intravenous injection, the plasma half-life of Procarbazine is approximately 10 minutes. Approximately 70% of the radioactivity is excreted in the urine as *N*-isopropylterephthalamic acid within 24 hours following both oral and intravenous administration of ^{14}C-labeled Procarbazine. Procarbazine crosses the blood-brain barrier and rapidly equilibrates between plasma and cerebrospinal fluid after oral administration.

INDICATIONS AND USAGE

Procarbazine Hydrochloride is indicated for use in combination with other anti-cancer drugs for the treatment of Stage III and IV Hodgkin's disease. Procarbazine Hydrochloride is used as part of the MOPP (nitrogen mustard, vincristine, Procarbazine, prednisone) regimen.

UNLABELED USES

Procarbazine Hydrochloride is used alone or as an adjunct in the treatment of brainstem glioma, glioblastoma, and non-Hodgkin's lymphoma. It is also used in malignant melanoma and Peyronie's disease.

CONTRAINDICATIONS

Procarbazine Hydrochloride is contraindicated in patients with known hypersensitivity to the drug or inadequate marrow reserve as demonstrated by bone marrow aspiration. Due consideration of this possible state should be given to each patient who has leukopenia, thrombocytopenia or anemia.

WARNINGS

To minimize CNS depression and possible potentiation, barbiturates, antihistamines, narcotics, hypotensive agents or phenothiazines should be used with caution. Ethyl alcohol should not be used since there may be an Antabuse (disulfiram)-like reaction. Because Procarbazine Hydrochloride exhibits some monoamine oxidase inhibitory activity, sympathomimetic drugs, tricyclic antidepressant drugs (e.g., amitriptyline HCl, imipramine HCl) and other drugs and foods with known high tyramine content, such as wine, yogurt, ripe cheese and bananas, should be avoided. A further phenomenon of toxicity common to many hydrazine derivatives is hemolysis and the appearance of Heinz-Ehrlich inclusion bodies in erythrocytes.

Pregnancy: Teratogenic effects: Pregnancy Category D. Procarbazine Hydrochloride can cause fetal harm when administered to a pregnant woman. While there are no adequate and well-controlled studies with Procarbazine Hydrochloride in pregnant women, there are case reports of malformations in the offspring of women who were exposed to Procarbazine Hydrochloride in combination with other anti-neoplastic agents during pregnancy. Procarbazine Hydrochloride should be used during pregnancy only if the potential benefit justifies the potential risk to the fetus. If this drug is used during pregnancy, or if the patient becomes pregnant while taking this drug, the patient should be apprised of the potential hazard to the fetus. Women of childbearing potential should be advised to avoid becoming pregnant. Procarbazine Hydrochloride is teratogenic in the rat when given at doses approximately 4 to 13 times the maximum recommended human therapeutic dose of 6 mg/kg/day.

Nonteratogenic effects: Procarbazine Hydrochloride has not been adequately studied in animals for its effects on peri- and postnatal development. However, neurogenic tumors were noted in the offspring of rats given intravenous injections of 125 mg/kg of Procarbazine Hydrochloride on day 22 of gestation. Compounds which inhibit DNA, RNA and protein synthesis might be expected to have adverse effects on peri- and postnatal development.

Carcinogenesis, Mutagenesis and Impairment of Fertility Carcinogenesis: The carcinogenicity of Procarbazine Hydrochloride in mice, rats and monkeys has been reported in a considerable number of studies. Instances of a second non-lymphoid malignancy, including acute myelocytic leukemia, have been reported in patients with Hodgkin's disease. treated with Procarbazine in combination with other chemotherapy and/or radiation. The International Agency for Research on Cancer (IARC) considers that there is "sufficient evidence" for the human carcinogenicity of Procarbazine Hydrochloride when it is given in intensive regimens which include other antineoplastic agents, but that there is inadequate evidence of carcinogenicity in humans given Procarbazine Hydrochloride alone.

Mutagenesis: Procarbazine Hydrochloride has been shown to be mutagenic in a variety of bacterial and mammalian test systems.

Impairment of fertility: Azoospermia and antifertility effects associated with Procarbazine Hydrochloride administration in combination with other chemotherapeutic agents for treating Hodgkin's disease have been reported in human clinical studies. Since these patients received multicombination therapy, it is difficult to determine to what extent Procarbazine Hydrochloride alone was involved in the male germ-cell damage. The usual Segment 1 fertility/reproduction studies in laboratory animals have not been carried out with Procarbazine Hydrochloride. However, compounds which inhibit DNA, RNA and/or protein

---

◆ RATED THERAPEUTICALLY EQUIVALENT; ◇ THERAPEUTIC EQUIVALENCE UNCONFIRMED; ○ UNRATED

synthesis might be expected to have adverse effects on gametogenesis. Unscheduled DNA synthesis in the testis of rabbits and decreased fertility in male mice treated with Procarbazine Hydrochloride have been reported.

PRECAUTIONS

General: Undue toxicity may occur if Procarbazine Hydrochloride is used in patients with impairment of renal and/or hepatic function. When appropriate, hospitalization for the initial course of treatment should be considered.

If radiation or a chemotherapeutic agent known to have marrow-depressant activity has been used, an interval of one month or longer without such therapy is recommended before starting treatment with Procarbazine Hydrochloride. The length of this interval may also be determined by evidence of bone marrow recovery based on successive bone marrow studies.

Prompt cessation of therapy is recommended if any one of the following occurs:

Central nervous system signs or symptoms such as paresthesias, neuropathies or confusion.

Leukopenia (white blood count under 4000).

Thrombocytopenia (platelets under 100,000).

Hypersensitivity reaction.

Stomatitis—The first small ulceration or persistent spot soreness around the oral cavity is a signal for cessation of therapy.

Diarrhea—Frequent bowel movements or watery stools.

Hemorrhage or bleeding tendencies.

Bone marrow depression often occurs 2 to 8 weeks after the start of treatment. If leukopenia occurs, hospitalization of the patient may be needed for appropriate treatment to prevent systemic infection.

Information for Patients: Patients should be warned not to drink alcoholic beverages while on Procarbazine Hydrochloride therapy since there may be an Antabuse (disulfiram)-like reaction. They should also be cautioned to avoid foods with known high tyramine content such as wine, yogurt, ripe cheese and bananas. Over the counter drug preparations which contain antihistamines or sympathomimetic drugs should also be avoided. Patients taking Procarbazine Hydrochloride should also be warned against the use of prescription drugs without the knowledge and consent of their physician.

Laboratory tests: Baseline laboratory data should be obtained prior to initiation of therapy. The hematologic status as indicated by hemoglobin, hematocrit, white blood count (WBC), differential, reticulocytes and platelets should be monitored closely—at least every 3 or 4 days.

Hepatic and renal evaluation are indicated prior to beginning therapy. Urinalysis, transaminase, alkaline phosphatase and blood urea nitrogen tests should be repeated at least weekly.

Drug interactions: See "Warnings" section.

No cross-reference with other chemotherapeutic agents, radiotherapy or steroids has been demonstrated.

Carcinogenesis, Mutagenesis and Impairment of Fertility: See "Warnings" section.

Pregnancy: Pregnancy Category D. See "Warnings" section.

Nursing mothers: It is not known whether Procarbazine Hydrochloride is excreted in human milk. Because of the potential for tumorigenicity shown for Procarbazine Hydrochloride in animal studies, mothers should not nurse while receiving this drug.

ADVERSE REACTIONS

Leukopenia, anemia and thrombopenia occur frequently.

Nausea and vomiting are the most commonly reported side effects. Other adverse reactions are:

Hematologic: Pancytopenia; eosinophilia; hemolytic anemia; bleeding tendencies such as petechiae, purpura, epistaxis and hemoptysis.

Gastrointestinal: Hepatic dysfunction, jaundice, stomatitis, hematemesis, melena, diarrhea, dysphagia, anorexia, abdominal pain, constipation, dry mouth.

Neurologic: Coma, convulsions, neuropathy, ataxia, paresthesia, nystagmus, diminished reflexes, falling, foot drop, headache, dizziness, unsteadiness.

Cardiovascular: Hypotension, tachycardia, syncope.

Ophthalmic: Retinal hemorrhage, papilledema, photophobia, diplopia, inability to focus.

Respiratory: Pneumonitis, pleural effusion, cough.

Dermatologic: Herpes, dermatitis, pruritis, alopecia, hyperpigmentation, rash, urticaria, flushing.

Allergic: Generalized allergic reactions.

Genitourinary: Hematuria, urinary frequency, nocturia.

Musculoskeletal: Pain, including myalgia and arthralgia; tremors.

Psychiatric: Hallucinations, depression, apprehension, nervousness, confusion, nightmares.

Endocrine: Gynecomastia in prepubertal and early pubertal boys.

Miscellaneous: Intercurrent infections, hearing loss, pyrexia, diaphoresis, lethargy, weakness, fatigue, edema, chills, insomnia, slurred speech, hoarseness, drowsiness.

Second nonlymphoid malignancies, including acute myelocytic leukemia and malignant myelosclerosis, and azoospermia have been reported in patients with Hodgkin's disease treated with Procarbazine in combination with other chemotherapy and/or radiation.

OVERDOSAGE

The major manifestations of overdosage with Procarbazine Hydrochloride would be anticipated to be nausea, vomiting, enteritis, diarrhea, hypotension, tremors, convulsions and coma. Treatment should consist of either the administration of an emetic or gastric lavage. General supportive measures such as intravenous fluids are advised. Since the major toxicity of Procarbazine Hydrochloride is hematologic and hepatic, patients should have frequent complete blood counts and liver function tests throughout their period of recovery and for a minimum of two weeks thereafter. Should abnormalities appear in any of these determinations, appropriate measures for correction and stabilization should be immediately undertaken.

The estimated mean lethal dose of Procarbazine Hydrochloride in laboratory animals varied from approximately 150 mg/kg in rabbits to 1300 mg/kg in mice.

DOSAGE AND ADMINISTRATION

The following doses are for administration of the drug as a single agent. When used in combination with other anticancer drugs, the Procarbazine Hydrochloride dose should be appropriately reduced, *e.g.*, in the MOPP regimen, the Procarbazine Hydrochloride dose is 100 mg/m^2 daily for 14 days. All dosages are based on the patient's actual weight. However, the estimated lean body mass (dry weight) is used if the patient is obese or if there has been a spurious weight gain due to edema, ascites or other forms of abnormal fluid retention.

Adults: To minimize the nausea and vomiting experienced by a high percentage of patients beginning Procarbazine Hydrochloride therapy, single or divided doses of 2 to 4 mg/kg/day for the first week are recommended. Daily dosage should then be maintained at 4 to 6 mg/kg/day until maximum response is obtained or until the white blood count falls below 4000/cmm or the platelets fall below 100,000/cmm. When maximum response is obtained, the dose may be maintained at 1 to 2 mg/kg/day. Upon evidence of hematologic or other toxicity (see "Precautions" section), the drug should be discontinued until there has been satisfactory recovery. After toxic side effects have subsided, therapy may then be resumed at the discretion of the physician, based on clinical evaluation and appropriate laboratory studies, at a dosage of 1 to 2 mg/kg/day.

Children: Very close clinical monitoring is mandatory. Undue toxicity, evidenced by tremors, coma and convulsions, has occurred in a few cases. Dosage, therefore, should be individualized. The following dosage schedule is provided as a guideline only.

Fifty (50) mg per square meter of body surface per day is recommended for the first week. Dosage should then be maintained at 100 mg per square meter of body surface per day until maximum response is obtained or until leukopenia or thrombocytopenia occurs. When maximum response is attained, the dose may be maintained at 50 mg per square meter of body surface per day. Upon evidence of hematologic or other toxicity (see "Precautions" section), the drug should be discontinued until there has been satisfactory recovery, based on clinical evaluation and appropriate laboratory tests. After toxic side effects have subsided, therapy may then be resumed.

Procedures for proper handling and disposal of anticancer drugs should be considered. Several guidelines on this subject have been published.[1-6] There is no general agreement that all of the procedures recommended in the guidelines are necessary or appropriate.

REFERENCES

1. Recommendations for the safe handling of parenteral antineoplastic drugs. Washington, DC, U.S. Government Printing Office (NIH Publication No. 83-2621). 2. AMA Council Report. Guidelines for handling parenteral antineoplastics. *JAMA* 253:1590-1592. Mar 15, 1985. 3. National Study Commission on Cytoxic Exposure: Recommendations for handling cytotoxic agents. Available from Louis P. Jeffrey, ScD, Director of Pharmacy Services, Rhode Island Hospital, 593 Eddy Street, Providence, Rhode Island 02902. 4. Clinical Oncological Society of Australia: Guidelines and recommendations for safe handling of antineoplastic agents. *Med. J. Aust* 1:426-428, Apr 30, 1983. 5. Jones RB, Frank R. Mass T: Safe handling of chemotherapeutic agents: a report from the Mount Sinai Medical Center. *CA* 33:258-263, Sept-Oct 1983. 6. ASHP technical assistance bulletin on handling cytotoxic drugs in hospitals. *Am J Hosp Pharm* 42: 131-137, Jan 1985.

HOW SUPPLIED
CAPSULE: 50 MG

BRAND/MANUFACTURER	NDC	SIZE	AWP
○ **BRAND**			
MATULANE: Roche Labs	00004-0053-01	100s	$66.89

Procardia SEE NIFEDIPINE

Prochlorperazine

DESCRIPTION

Prochlorperazine is available as tablets, sustained-release capsules, and syrup, for oral administration; suppositories; and injection.

Each capsule contains:
Prochlorperazine Maleate equiv. to Prochlorperazine ....10 or 15 mg

Each suppository contains:
Prochlorperazine ....2.5, 5, or 25 mg

Each 5 ml of syrup contains:
Prochlorperazine Edisylate ....5 mg

Each tablet contains:
Prochlorperazine Maleate equiv. to Prochlorperazine ....10, or 25 mg

Each ml of solution for injection contains:
Prochlorperazine Edisylate ....5 mg

Chemically, Prochlorperazine Edisylate is 2-Chloro-10-[3-(4-methyl-1-piperazinyl) propyl] phenothiazine 1,2-ethanedisulfonate (1:1). It has a molecular weight of 564.13.

CLINICAL PHARMACOLOGY

Prochlorperazine is a propylpiperazine derivative of phenothiazine. Like other phenothiazines, it exerts an antiemetic effect through a depressant action on the chemoreceptor trigger zone. It also has a clinically useful anti-psychotic effect. Following intramuscular administration of Prochlorperazine Edisylate, the drug has an onset of action within ten to twenty minutes and a duration of action of three to four hours.

Following is its chemical structure:

INDICATIONS

For control of severe nausea and vomiting. For management of the manifestations of psychotic disorders.

Prochlorperazine is effective for the short-term treatment of generalized non-psychotic anxiety. However, Prochlorperazine is not the first drug to be used in therapy for most patients with non-psychotic anxiety, because certain risks associated with its use are not shared by common alternative treatments (e.g., benzodiazepines).

When used in the treatment of non-psychotic anxiety, Prochlorperazine should not be administered at doses of more than 20 mg per day or for longer than 12 weeks, because the use of Prochlorperazine at higher doses or for longer intervals may cause persistent tardive dyskinesia that may prove irreversible (see *"Warnings"*).

The effectiveness of Prochlorperazine as treatment for non-psychotic anxiety was established in 4-week clinical studies of outpatients with generalized anxiety disorder. This evidence does not predict that Prochlorperazine will be useful in patients with other non-psychotic conditions in which anxiety, or signs that mimic anxiety, are found (e.g., physical illness, organic mental conditions, agitated depression, character pathologies, etc.).

Prochlorperazine has not been shown effective in the management of behavioral complications in patients with mental retardation.

UNLABELED USES
Prochlorperazine is used alone or as an adjunct in the treatment of migraine headache, tension headache, and Ménière's disease. Prochlorperazine is also used as an adjunct to general anesthesia.

CONTRAINDICATIONS

Do not use in patients with known hypersensitivity to phenothiazines.

Do not use in comatose states or in the presence of large amounts of central nervous system depressants (alcohol, barbiturates, narcotics, etc.).

Do not use in pediatric surgery.

Do not use in children under 2 years of age or under 20 lbs.

Do not use in children for conditions for which dosage has not been established.

WARNINGS

The extrapyramidal symptoms which can occur secondary to Prochlorperazine may be confused with the central nervous system signs of an undiagnosed primary disease responsible for the vomiting, e.g., Reye's syndrome or other encephalopathy. The use of Prochlorperazine and other potential hepatotoxins should be avoided in children and adolescents whose signs and symptoms suggest Reye's syndrome.

Tardive Dyskinesia: Tardive dyskinesia, a syndrome consisting of potentially irreversible, involuntary, dyskinetic movements, may develop in patients treated with neuroleptic (antipsychotic) drugs. Although the prevalence of the syndrome appears to be highest among the elderly, especially elderly women, it is impossible to rely upon prevalence estimates to predict, at the inception of neuroleptic treatment, which patients are likely to develop the syndrome. Whether neuroleptic drug products differ in their potential to cause tardive dyskinesia is unknown.

Both the risk of developing the syndrome and the likelihood that it will become irreversible are believed to increase as the duration of treatment and the total cumulative dose of neuroleptic drugs administered to the patient increase. However, the syndrome can develop, although much less commonly, after relatively brief treatment periods at low doses. There is no known treatment for established cases of tardive dyskinesia, although the syndrome may remit, partially or completely, if neuroleptic treatment is withdrawn. Neuroleptic treatment itself, however, may suppress (or partially suppress) the signs and symptoms of the syndrome and thereby may possibly mask the underlying disease process. The effect that symptomatic suppression has upon the long-term course of the syndrome is unknown.

Given these considerations, neuroleptics should be prescribed in a manner that is most likely to minimize the occurrence of tardive dyskinesia. Chronic neuroleptic treatment should generally be reserved for patients who suffer from a chronic illness that, 1) is known to respond to neuroleptic drugs, and 2) for whom alternative, equally effective, but potentially less harmful treatments are *not* available or appropriate. In patients who do require chronic treatment, the smallest dose and the shortest duration of treatment producing a satisfactory clinical response should be sought. The need for continued treatment should be reassessed periodically.

If signs and symptoms of tardive dyskinesia appear in a patient on neuroleptics, drug discontinuation should be considered. However, some patients may require treatment despite the presence of the syndrome.

For further information about the description of tardive dyskinesia and its clinical detection, please refer to the sections on *"Precautions"* and *"Adverse Reactions"*.

Neuroleptic Malignant Syndrome (NMS): A potentially fatal symptom complex sometimes referred to as Neuroleptic Malignant Syndrome (NMS) has been reported in association with antipsychotic drugs. Clinical manifestations of NMS are hyperpyrexia, muscle rigidity, altered mental status and evidence of autonomic instability (irregular pulse or blood pressure, tachycardia, diaphoresis, and cardiac dysrhythmias).

The diagnostic evaluation of patients with this syndrome is complicated. In arriving at a diagnosis, it is important to identify cases where the clinical presentation includes both serious medical illness (e.g., pneumonia, systemic infection, etc.) and untreated or inadequately treated extrapyramidal signs and symptoms (EPS). Other important considerations in the differential diagnosis include central anticholinergic toxicity, heat stroke, drug fever and primary central nervous system (CNS) pathology.

The management of NMS should include 1) immediate discontinuation of antipsychotic drugs and other drugs not essential to concurrent therapy, 2) intensive symptomatic treatment and medical monitoring, and 3) treatment of any concomitant serious medical problems for which specific treatments are available. There is no general agreement about specific pharmacological treatment regimens for uncomplicated NMS.

If a patient requires antipsychotic drug treatment after recovery from NMS, the potential reintroduction of drug therapy should be carefully considered. The patient should be carefully monitored, since recurrences of NMS have been reported.

General: Patients with bone marrow depression or who have previously demonstrated a hypersensitivity reaction (e.g., blood dyscrasias, jaundice) with a phenothiazine should not receive any phenothiazine, including Prochlorperazine, unless in the judgment of the physician the potential benefits of treatment outweigh the possible hazards.

Prochlorperazine may impair mental and/or physical abilities, especially during the first few days of therapy. Therefore, caution patients about activities requiring alertness (e.g., operating vehicles or machinery).

Phenothiazines may intensify or prolong the action of central nervous system depressants (e.g., alcohol, anesthetics, narcotics).

Usage in Pregnancy: Safety for the use of Prochlorperazine during pregnancy has not been established. Therefore, Prochlorperazine is not recommended for use in pregnant patients except in cases of severe nausea and vomiting that are so serious and intractable that, in the judgment of the physician, drug intervention is required and potential benefits outweigh possible hazards.

There have been reported instances of prolonged jaundice, extrapyramidal signs, hyperreflexia or hyporeflexia in newborn infants whose mothers received phenothiazines.

Nursing Mothers: There is evidence that phenothiazines are excreted in the breast milk of nursing mothers. Caution should be exercised when Prochlarperazine is administered to a nursing woman.

PRECAUTIONS

The antiemetic action of Prochlorperazine may mask the signs and symptoms of overdosage of other drugs and may obscure the diagnosis and treatment of other conditions such as intestinal obstruction, brain tumor and Reye's syndrome (see *"Warnings"*).

When Prochlorperazine is used with cancer chemotherapeutic drugs, vomiting as a sign of the toxicity of these agents may be obscured by the antiemetic effect of Prochlorperazine.

Because hypotension may occur, large doses and parenteral administration should be used cautiously in patients with impaired cardiovascular systems. To minimize the occurrence of hypotension after injection, keep patient lying down and observe for at least ½ hour. If hypotension occurs after parenteral or oral dosing, place patient in head-low position with legs raised. If a vasoconstrictor is required, norepinephrine bitartrate and phenylephrine hydrochloride are suitable.

◆ RATED THERAPEUTICALLY EQUIVALENT; ◇ THERAPEUTIC EQUIVALENCE UNCONFIRMED; ○ UNRATED

Other pressor agents, including epinephrine, should not be used because they may cause a paradoxical further lowering of blood pressure.

Aspiration of vomitus has occurred in a few postsurgical patients who have received Prochlorperazine as an antiemetic. Although no causal relationship has been established, this possibility should be borne in mind during surgical aftercare. Deep sleep, from which patients can be aroused, and coma have been reported, usually with overdosage.

Neuroleptic drugs elevate prolactin levels; the elevation persists during chronic administration. Tissue culture experiments indicate that approximately ⅓ of human breast cancers are prolactin-dependent *in vitro*, a factor of potential importance if the prescribing of these drugs is contemplated in a patient with a previously detected breast cancer. Although disturbances such as galactorrhea, amenorrhea, gynecomastia and impotence have been reported, the clinical significance of elevated serum prolactin levels is unknown for most patients. An increase in mammary neoplasms has been found in rodents after chronic administration of neuroleptic drugs. Neither clinical nor epidemiologic studies conducted to date, however, have shown an association between chronic administration of these drugs and mammary tumorigenesis; the available evidence is considered too limited to be conclusive at this time.

Chromosomal aberrations in spermatocytes and abnormal sperm have been demonstrated in rodents treated with certain neuroleptics.

As with all drugs which exert an anticholinergic effect, and/or cause mydriasis, Prochlorperazine should be used with caution in patients with glaucoma.

Because phenothiazines may interfere with thermoregulatory mechanisms, use with caution in persons who will be exposed to extreme heat.

Phenothiazines can diminish the effect of oral anticoagulants.

Phenothiazines can produce alpha-adrenergic blockade. Thiazide diuretics may accentuate the orthostatic hypotension that may occur with phenothiazines.

Antihypertensive effects of guanethidine and related compounds may be counteracted when phenothiazines are used concomitantly.

Concomitant administration of propranolol with phenothiazines results in increased plasma levels of both drugs.

Phenothiazines may lower the convulsive threshold: dosage adjustments of anticonvulsants may be necessary. Potentiation of anticonvulsant effects does not occur. However, it has been reported that phenothiazines may interfere with the metabolism of Phenytoin and thus precipitate Phenytoin toxicity.

The presence of phenothiazines may produce false positive phenylketonuria (PKU) test results.

Long-Term Therapy: Given the likelihood that some patients exposed chronically to neuroleptics will develop tardive dyskinesia, it is advised that all patients in whom chronic use is contemplated be given, if possible, full information about this risk. The decision to inform patients and/or their guardians must obviously take into account the clinical circumstances and the competency of the patient to understand the information provided.

To lessen the likelihood of adverse reactions related to cumulative drug effect, patients with a history of long-term therapy with Prochlorperazine and/or other neuroleptics should be evaluated periodically to decide whether the maintenance dosage could be lowered or drug therapy discontinued.

Children with acute illnesses (e.g., chickenpox, C.N.S. infections, measles, gastroenteritis) or dehydration seem to be much more susceptible to neuromuscular reactions, particularly dystonias, than are adults. In such patients, the drug should be used only under close supervision.

Drugs which lower the seizure threshold, including phenothiazine derivatives, should not be used with Metrizamide. As with other phenothiazine derivatives, Prochlorperazine should be discontinued at least 48 hours before myelography, should not be resumed for at least 24 hours postprocedure, and should not be used for the control of nausea and vomiting occurring either prior to myelography with metrizamide or postprocedure.

ADVERSE REACTIONS

Drowsiness, dizziness, amenorrhea, blurred vision, skin reactions and hypotension may occur. Neuroleptic Malignant Syndrome (NMS) has been reported in association with antipsychotic drugs (see *"Warnings"*).

Cholestatic jaundice has occurred. If fever with grippe-like symptoms occurs, appropriate liver studies should be conducted. If tests indicate an abnormality, stop treatment. There have been a few observations of fatty changes in the livers of patients who have died while receiving the drug. No causal relationship has been established.

Leukopenia and agranulocytosis have occurred. Warn patients to report the sudden appearance of sore throat or other signs of infection. If white blood cell and differential counts indicate leukocyte depression, stop treatment and start antibiotic and other suitable therapy.

Neuromuscular (Extrapyramidal) Reactions: These symptoms are seen in a significant number of hospitalized mental patients. They may be characterized by motor restlessness, be of the dystonic type, or they may resemble Parkinsonism.

Depending on the severity of symptoms, dosage should be reduced or discontinued. If therapy is reinstituted, it should be at a lower dosage. Should these symptoms occur in children or pregnant patients, the drug should be stopped and not reinstituted. In most cases barbiturates by suitable route of administration will suffice. (Or, injectable diphenhydramine hydrochloride may be useful.) In more severe cases, the administration of an anti-parkinsonism agent, except levodopa, usually produces rapid reversal of symptoms. Suitable supportive measures such as maintaining a clear airway and adequate hydration should be employed.

Motor Restlessness: Symptoms may include agitation or jitteriness and sometimes insomnia. These symptoms often disappear spontaneously. At times these symptoms may be similar to the original neurotic or psychotic symptoms. Dosage should not be increased until these side effects have subsided.

If these symptoms become too troublesome, they can usually be controlled by a reduction of dosage; change of drug or concomitant administration of a barbiturate. Treatment with anti-parkinsonian agents, benzodiazepines or propranolol may be helpful.

Dystonias: Symptoms may include: spasm of the neck muscles, sometimes progressing to torticollis; extensor rigidity of back muscles, sometimes progressing to opisthotonos; carpopedal spasm, trismus, swallowing difficulty, oculogyric crisis and protrusion of the tongue.

These usually subside within a few hours, and almost always within 24 to 48 hours, after the drug has been discontinued. *In mild cases*, reassurance or a barbiturate is often sufficient. *In moderate cases*, barbiturates will usually bring rapid relief. *In more severe adult cases*, the administration of an anti-parkinsonism agent, except levodopa, usually produces rapid reversal of symptoms. *In children*, reassurance and barbiturates will usually control symptoms. (Or, injectable diphenydramine hydrochloride may be useful. *Note*: See diphenhydramine hydrochloride prescribing information for appropriate *children's* dosage.) If appropriate treatment with anti-parkinsonism agents or diphenhydramine hydrochloride fails to reverse the signs and symptoms, the diagnosis should be reevaluated.

Pseudo-Parkinsonism: Symptoms may include: mask-like facies; drooling; tremors; pillrolling motion; cogwheel rigidity; and shuffling gait. Reassurance and sedation are important. In most cases these symptoms are readily controlled when an anti-parkinsonism agent is administered concomitantly. Anti-parkinsonism agents should be used only when required. Generally, therapy of a few weeks to 2 or 3 months will suffice. After this time patients should be evaluated to determine their need for continued treatment. (*Note:* Levodopa has not been found effective in pseudo-parkinsonism). Occasionally it is necessary to lower the dosage of Prochlorperazine or to discontinue the drug.

Tardive Dyskinesia: As with all antipsychotic agents, tardive dyskinesia may appear in some patients on long-term therapy or may appear after drug therapy has been discontinued. The syndrome can also develop, although much less frequently, after relatively brief treatment periods at low doses. This syndrome appears in all age groups. Although its prevalence appears to be highest among elderly patients, especially elderly women, it is impossible to rely upon prevalence estimates to predict at the inception of neuroleptic treatment which patients are likely to develop the syndrome. The symptoms are persistent and in some patients appear to be irreversible. The syndrome is characterized by rhythmical involuntary movements of the tongue, face, mouth or jaw (e.g., protrusion of tongue, puffing of cheeks, puckering of mouth, chewing movements). Sometimes these may be accompanied by involuntary movements of extremities. In rare instances, these involuntary movements of the extremities are the only manifestations of tardive dyskinesia. A variant of tardive dyskinesia, tardive dystonia, has also been described.

There is no known effective treatment for tardive dyskinesia; antiparkinsonism agents do not alleviate the symptoms of this syndrome. It is suggested that all antipsychotic agents be discontinued if these symptoms appear.

Should it be necessary to reinstitute treatment, or increase the dosage of the agent, or switch to a different antipsychotic agent, the syndrome may be masked.

It has been reported that fine vermicular movements of the tongue may be an early sign of the syndrome and if the medication is stopped at that time the syndrome may not develop.

Contact Dermatitis: Avoid getting the injection solution on hands or clothing because of the possibility of contact dermatitis.

Adverse Reactions Reported with Prochlorperazine or Other Phenothiazine Derivatives: Adverse reactions with different phenothiazines vary in type, frequency, and mechanism of occurrence, i.e., some are dose-related, while others involve individual patient sensitivity. Some adverse reactions may be more likely to occur, or occur with greater intensity, in patients with special medical problems; e.g., patients with mitral insufficiency or pheochromocytoma have experienced severe hypotension following recommended doses of certain phenothiazines.

Not all of the following adverse reactions have been observed with every phenothiazine derivative, but they have been reported with 1 or more and should be borne in mind when drugs of this class are administered: extrapyramidal symptoms (opisthotonos, oculogyric crisis, hyperreflexia, dystonia, akathisia, dyskinesia, parkinsonism) some of which have lasted months and even years—particularly in elderly patients with previous brain damage; grand mal and petit mal convulsions, particularly in patients with EEG abnormalities or history of such disorders; altered cerebrospinal fluid proteins; cerebral edema; intensification and prolongation of the action of central nervous system depressants (opiates, analgesics, antihistamines, barbiturates, alcohol), atropine, heat, organophosphorus insecticides; autonomic reactions (dryness of mouth, nasal congestion, headache, nausea, constipation, obstipation, adynamic ileus, ejaculatory disorders/impotence, priapism, atonic colon, urinary retention, miosis and mydriasis); reactivation of psychotic processes, catatonic-like states; hypotension (sometimes fatal); cardiac arrest; blood dyscrasias (pancytopenia, thrombocytopenic purpura, leukopenia, agranulocytosis, eosinophilia, hemolytic anemia, aplastic anemia); liver damage (jaundice, biliary stasis); endocrine disturbances (hyperglycemia, hypoglycemia, glycosuria, lactation, galactorrhea, gynecomastia, menstrual irregularities, false positive pregnancy tests); skin disorders (photosensitivity, itching, erythema, urticaria, eczema up to exfoliative dermatitis); other allergic reactions (asthma, laryngeal edema, angioneurotic edema, anaphylactoid reactions); peripheral edema; reversed epinephrine effect; hyperpyrexia; mild fever after large I.M. doses; increased appetite; increased weight; a systemic lupus erythematosus-like syndrome; pigmentary retinopathy; with prolonged administration of substantial doses, skin pigmentation, epithelial keratopathy, and lenticular and corneal deposits.

EKG changes—particularly nonspecific, usually reversible Q and T wave distortions—have been observed in some patients receiving phenothiazine tranquilizers.

Although phenothiazines cause neither psychic nor physical dependence, sudden discontinuance in long-term psychiatric patients may cause temporary symptoms, e.g., nausea and vomiting, dizziness, tremulousness.

Note: There have been occasional reports of sudden death in patients receiving phenothiazines. In some cases, the cause appeared to be cardiac arrest or asphyxia due to failure of the cough reflex.

OVERDOSAGE
(See also *"Adverse Reactions"*.)

Symptoms: Primarily involvement of the extrapyramidal mechanism producing some of the dystonic reactions described above.

Symptoms of central nervous system depression to the point of somnolence or coma. Agitation and restlessness may also occur. Other possible manifestations include convulsions, EKG changes and cardiac arrhythmias, fever and autonomic reactions such as hypotension, dry mouth and ileus.

Treatment: It is important to determine other medications taken by the patient since multiple-drug therapy is common in overdosage situations. Treatment is essentially symptomatic and supportive. Early gastric lavage is helpful following oral overdose. Keep patient under observation and maintain an open airway, since involvement of the extrapyramidal mechanism may produce dysphagia and respiratory difficulty in severe overdosage. **Do not attempt to induce emesis because a dystonic reaction of the head or neck may develop that could result in aspiration of vomitus.** Extrapyramidal symptoms may be treated with antiparkinsonism drugs, barbiturates, or diphenhydramine hydrochloride. See prescribing information for these products. Care should be taken to avoid increasing respiratory depression.

If administration of a stimulant is desirable, amphetamine, dextroamphetamine or caffeine with sodium benzoate is recommended.

Stimulants that may cause convulsions (e.g., picrotoxin or pentylenetetrazol) should be avoided.

If hypotension occurs, the standard measures for managing circulatory shock should be initiated. If it is desirable to administer a vasoconstrictor, norepinephrine bitartrate and phenylephrine hydrochloride are most suitable. Other pressor agents, including epinephrine, are not recommended because phenothiazine derivatives may reverse the usual elevating action of these agents and cause a further lowering of blood pressure.

Limited experience indicates that phenothiazine are *not* dialyzable.

Special Note on Spansule capsules: Since much of the Spansule capsule medication is coated for gradual release, therapy directed at reversing the effects of the ingested drug and at supporting the patient should be continued for as long as overdosage symptoms remain. Saline cathartics are useful for hastening evacuation of pellets that have not already released medication.

DOSAGE AND ADMINISTRATION
NOTES ON INJECTION
Stability: This solution should be protected from light. This is a clear, colorless to pale yellow solution; a slight yellowish discoloration will not alter potency. If markedly discolored, solution should be discarded.

Compatibility: It is recommended that Prochlarperazine injection not be mixed with other agents in the syringe.

DOSAGE AND ADMINISTRATION: ADULTS
(For children's dosage and administration, see below.) Dosage should be increased more gradually in debilitated or emaciated patients.

Elderly Patients: In general, dosages in the lower range are sufficient for most elderly patients. Since they appear to be more susceptible to hypotension and neuromuscular reactions, such patients should be observed closely. Dosage should be tailored to the individual, response carefully monitored, and dosage adjusted accordingly. Dosage should be increased more gradually in elderly patients.

1. To Control Severe Nausea and Vomiting: Adjust dosage to the response of the individual. Begin with the lowest recommended dosage.

Oral Dosage: Tablets: Usually one 5 mg or 10 mg tablet 3 or 4 times daily. Daily dosages above 40 mg should be used only in resistant cases.

Sustained-release Capsules: Initially, usually one 15 mg capsule on arising or one 10 mg capsule q12h. Some patients may subsequently require one 30 mg capsule in the morning. Daily doses above 40 mg should be used only in resistant cases.

Rectal Dosage: 25 mg twice daily.

IM Dosage: Initially 5 to 10 mg (1 to 2 mL) injcted *deeply* into the upper outer quadrant of the buttock. If necessary, repeat every 3 or 4 hours. Total IM dosage should not exceed 40 mg per day.

IV Dosage: 2½ to 10 mg (½ to 2 ml) by slow IV injection or infusion at a rate not to exceed 5 mg per minute. Prochlorperazine injection may be administered either undiluted or diluted in isotonic solution. A single dose of the drug should not exceed 10 mg; total IV dosage should not exceed 40 mg per day. When

administered IV do not use bolus injection. Hypotension is a possibility if the drug is given by IV injection or infusion.
Subcutaneous administration is not advisable because of local irritation.

2. Adult Surgery (for severe nausea and vomiting): Total parenteral dosage should not exceed 40 mg per day. Hypotension is a possibility if the drug is given by I.V. injection or infusion.

IM Dosage: 5 to 10 mg (1 to 2 ml) 1 to 2 hours before induction of anesthesia (repeat once in 30 minutes, if necessary), or to control acute symptoms during and after surgery (repeat once if necessary).

IV Dosage: 5 to 10 mg (1 to 2 ml) as a slow IV injection or infusion 15 to 30 minutes before induction of anesthesia, or to control acute symptoms during or after surgery. Repeat once if necessary. Prochlarperazine may be administered either undiluted or diluted in isotonic solution, but a single dose of the drug should not exceed 10 mg. The rate of administration should not exceed 5 mg/ml per minute. When administered IV do not use bolus injection.

3. In Adult Psychiatric Disorders: Adjust dosage to the response of the individual and according to the severity of the condition. Begin with the lowest recommended dose. Although response ordinarily is seen within a day or 2, longer treatment is usually required before maximal improvement is seen.

Oral Dosage: Non-Psychotic Anxiety: Usual dosage is 5 mg 3 or 4 times daily: by sustained-release capsule, usually one 15 mg capsule on arising or one 10 mg capsule q12h. Do not administer in doses of more than 20 mg per day or for longer than 12 weeks.

Psychotic Disorders: In relatively mild conditions, as seen in private psychiatric practice or in outpatient clinics, dosage is 5 or 10 mg 3 or 4 times daily.

In moderate to severe conditions: for hospitalized or adequately supervised patients, usual starting dosage is 10 mg 3 or 4 times daily. Increase dosage gradually until symptoms are controlled or side effects become bothersome. When dosage is increased by small increments every 2 or 3 days, side effects either do not occur or are easily controlled. Some patients respond satisfactorily on 50 to 75 mg daily.

In more severe disturbances optimum dosage is usually 100 to 150 mg daily.

IM Dosage: For immediate control of severely disturbed adults, inject an initial dose of 10 to 20 mg (2 to 4 ml) *deeply* into the upper outer quadrant of the buttock. Many patients respond shortly after the first injection. If necessary, however, repeat the initial dose every 2 to 4 hours (or, in resistant cases, every hour) to gain control of the patient. More than 3 or 4 doses are seldom necessary. After control is achieved, switch patient to an oral form of the drug at the same dosage level or higher. If, in rare cases, parenteral therapy is needed for a prolonged period, give 10 to 20 mg (2 to 4 ml) every 4 to 6 hours. Pain and irritation at the site of injection have seldom occurred.
Subcutaneous administration is not advisable because of local irritation.

DOSAGE AND ADMINISTRATION: CHILDREN
Do not use in pediatric surgery.

Children seem more prone to develop extrapyramidal reactions, even on moderate doses. Therefore, use lowest effective dosage. Tell parents not to exceed prescribed dosage, since the possibility of adverse reactions increases as dosage rises. Occasionally, the patient may react to the drug with signs of restlessness and excitement; if this occurs, do not administer additional doses. Take particular precaution in administering the drug to children with acute illnesses or dehydration (see under *"Dystonias"*).

When writing a prescription for the 2½ mg size suppository, write "2 ½" not "2.5"; this will help avoid confusion with the 25 mg adult size.

1. Severe Nausea and Vomiting in Children: Prochlorperazine should not be used in children under 20 pounds in weight or 2 years of age. It should not be used in conditions for which children's dosages have not been established. Dosage and frequency of administration should be adjusted according to the severity of the symptoms and the response of the patient. The duration of activity following intramuscular administration may last up to 12 hours. Subsequent doses may be given by the same route if necessary.

Oral or Rectal Dosage: More than 1 day's therapy is seldom necessary.

Weight	Usual Dosage	Not to Exceed
under 20 lbs	not recommended	
20 to 29 lbs	2½ mg 1 or 2 times a day	7.5 mg per day
30 to 39 lbs	2½ mg 2 or 3 times a day	10 mg per day
40 to 85 lbs	2½ mg 3 times a day or 5 mg 2 times a day	15 mg per day

IM Dosage: Calculate each dose on the basis of 0.06 mg of the drug per lb of body weight; give by deep IM injection.
Control is usually obtained with 1 dose.

2. In Psychotic Children: Oral or Rectal Dosage: For children 2 to 12 years, starting dosage is 2½ mg 2 or 3 times daily. Do not give more than 10 mg the first day. Then increase dosage according to patient's response.

For Ages 2 to 5, total daily dosage usually does not exceed 20 mg.

◆ RATED THERAPEUTICALLY EQUIVALENT; ◇ THERAPEUTIC EQUIVALENCE UNCONFIRMED; ○ UNRATED

For Ages 6 to 12, total daily dosage usually does not exceed 25 mg.

IM Dosage: For ages under 12, calculate each dose on the basis of 0.06 mg of Prochlorperazine per lb of body weight; give by deep IM injection. Control is usually obtained with 1 dose. After control is achieved, switch the patient to an oral form of the drug at the same dosage level or higher.

Parenteral drug products should be inspected visually for particulate matter and discoloration prior to administration, whenever solution and container permit.

J CODES
Up to 10 mg IM,IV—J0780

HOW SUPPLIED

PROCHLORPERAZINE
INJECTION: 5 MG/ML

AVERAGE UNIT PRICE (AVAILABLE SIZES)		GENERIC A-RATED AVERAGE PRICE (GAAP)	
BRAND	$4.54	10 ml	$10.89
GENERIC	$1.84		

BRAND/MANUFACTURER	NDC	SIZE	AWP
◆ BRAND			
COMPAZINE: SK Beecham Pharm	00007-3343-01	10 ml	$33.05
	00007-3351-01	2 ml	$13.80
	00007-3352-16	2 ml 25s	$170.30
◆ GENERICS			
Moore, H.L.	00839-7409-30	10 ml	$9.03
Rugby	00536-2152-70	10 ml	$12.75
Wyeth-Ayerst	00008-0542-01	1 ml 10s	$31.45
Wyeth-Ayerst	00008-0542-02	2 ml 10s	$41.09

INJECTION: 5 MG/5 ML

BRAND/MANUFACTURER	NDC	SIZE	AWP
◆ BRAND			
COMPAZINE: SK Beecham Pharm	00007-3352-09	2 ml 15s	$102.20

INJECTION: 5 MG/10 ML

BRAND/MANUFACTURER	NDC	SIZE	AWP
◆ GENERICS			
Major	00904-0087-10	10 ml	$17.00

INJECTION: 10 MG/2 ML

BRAND/MANUFACTURER	NDC	SIZE	AWP
◆ GENERICS			
VHA	00007-3342-76	2 ml 100s	$507.00

SUPPOSITORY: 2.5 MG

BRAND/MANUFACTURER	NDC	SIZE	AWP
○ BRAND			
COMPAZINE: SK Beecham Pharm	00007-3360-03	12s	$23.75

SUPPOSITORY: 5 MG

BRAND/MANUFACTURER	NDC	SIZE	AWP
○ BRAND			
COMPAZINE: SK Beecham Pharm	00007-3361-03	12s	$26.40

SUPPOSITORY: 25 MG

BRAND/MANUFACTURER	NDC	SIZE	AWP
◆ BRAND			
COMPAZINE: SK Beecham Pharm	00007-3362-03	12s	$32.70

SYRUP: 5 MG/5 ML

BRAND/MANUFACTURER	NDC	SIZE	AWP
◆ BRAND			
COMPAZINE: SK Beecham Pharm	00007-3363-44	120 ml	$18.05

TABLETS: 5 MG

AVERAGE UNIT PRICE (AVAILABLE SIZES)	
GENERIC	$0.22

BRAND/MANUFACTURER	NDC	SIZE	AWP
◆ GENERICS			
Moore, H.L.	00839-6301-06	100s	$34.43
Parmed	00349-7017-10	1000s	$92.66

TABLETS: 25 MG

BRAND/MANUFACTURER	NDC	SIZE	AWP
◆ GENERICS			
Parmed	00349-7021-10	1000s	$140.31

PROCHLORPERAZINE EDISYLATE
INJECTION: 5 MG/ML

AVERAGE UNIT PRICE (AVAILABLE SIZES)		GENERIC A-RATED AVERAGE PRICE (GAAP)	
GENERIC	$1.50	10 ml	$10.35
		2 ml 25s	$85.85

BRAND/MANUFACTURER	NDC	SIZE	AWP
◆ GENERICS			
Steris	00402-0831-82	2 ml	$5.06
Schein	00364-2231-54	10 ml	$8.40
Steris	00402-0830-10	10 ml	$8.40
Goldline	00182-3049-63	10 ml	$14.25
Solo Pak	39769-0076-02	2 ml 25s	$65.00
Schein	00364-2231-48	2 ml 25s	$66.00
Schein	00364-2231-42	2 ml 25s	$126.55
Solo Pak	39769-0076-10	10 ml 25s	$309.38

INJECTION: 10 MG/ML

BRAND/MANUFACTURER	NDC	SIZE	AWP
◆ GENERICS			
Elkins-Sinn	00641-0491-25	2 ml 25s	$54.69

INJECTION: 10 MG

BRAND/MANUFACTURER	NDC	SIZE	AWP
◆ GENERICS			
Sanofi Winthrop	00024-1598-01	2 ml 10s	$25.88

PROCHLORPERAZINE MALEATE
CAPSULE, EXTENDED RELEASE: 10 MG

BRAND/MANUFACTURER	NDC	SIZE	AWP
○ BRAND			
➤ COMPAZINE SPANSULE: SK Beecham Pharm	00007-3344-15	50s	$50.55

CAPSULE, EXTENDED RELEASE: 15 MG

BRAND/MANUFACTURER	NDC	SIZE	AWP
○ BRAND			
➤ COMPAZINE SPANSULE: SK Beecham Pharm	00007-3346-15	50s	$75.15

POWDER:

BRAND/MANUFACTURER	NDC	SIZE	AWP
○ GENERICS			
Gallipot	51552-0074-20	20 gm	$54.40

TABLETS: 5 MG

BRAND/MANUFACTURER	NDC	SIZE	AWP
○ BRAND			
➤ COMPAZINE TABLETS: SK Beecham Pharm	00007-3366-20	100s	$55.20
	00007-3366-21	100s ud	$57.55

TABLETS: 10 MG

BRAND/MANUFACTURER	NDC	SIZE	AWP
○ BRAND			
➤ COMPAZINE TABLETS: SK Beecham Pharm	00007-3367-20	100s	$82.90
	00007-3367-21	100s ud	$85.25

Procrit *SEE* EPOETIN ALFA

Procto-HC *SEE* HYDROCORTISONE, RECTAL

Proctocort *SEE* HYDROCORTISONE, RECTAL

proctoFoam HC *SEE* HYDROCORTISONE ACETATE AND PRAMOXINE HYDROCHLORIDE

➤ SHOWN IN PRODUCT IDENTIFICATION GUIDE

Procyclidine Hydrochloride

DESCRIPTION

Procyclidine Hydrochloride is a synthetic antispasmodic compound of relatively low toxicity. It has been shown to be useful for the symptomatic treatment of parkinsonism (paralysis agitans) and extrapyramidal dysfunction caused by tranquilizer therapy. Procyclidine Hydrochloride was developed.

Procyclidine Hydrochloride is a white crystalline substance which is soluble in water and almost tasteless. It is known chemically as α-cyclohexyl-α-phenyl-1-pyrrolidinepropanol hydrochloride.

Procyclidine Hydrochloride is available in tablet form for oral administration. Each scored tablet contains 5 mg Procyclidine Hydrochloride.

Following is its chemical structure:

CLINICAL PHARMACOLOGY

Pharmacologic tests have shown that Procyclidine Hydrochloride has an atropine-like action and exerts an antispasmodic effect on smooth muscle. It is a potent mydriatic and inhibits salivation. It has no sympathetic ganglion-blocking activity in doses as high as 4 mg/kg, as measured by the lack of inhibition of the response of the nictitating membrane to preganglionic electrical stimulation.

The intravenous LD_{50} in mice was about 60 mg/kg. Subcutaneously, doses of 300 mg/kg were not toxic. In dogs the intraperitoneal administration of Procyclidine Hydrochloride in doses of 5 mg/kg caused maximal dilation of the pupil and inhibition of salivation, but had no toxic action. When the dose was increased to 20 mg/kg the same symptoms occurred, and in addition there were tremors and ataxia lasting 4 to 5 hours. In one animal convulsions occurred which were controlled by pentobarbital. In all animals behavior returned to normal within 24 hours.

Chronic toxicity tests in rats showed that the compound caused only a very slight retardation in growth, and no change in the erythrocyte count or the histological appearance of the lungs, liver, spleen, and kidney when as much as 10 mg/kg body weight was given subcutaneously daily for 9 weeks.

INDICATIONS

Procyclidine Hydrochloride is indicated in the treatment of parkinsonism including the postencephalitic, arteriosclerotic and idiopathic types. Partial control of the parkinsonism symptoms is the usual therapeutic accomplishment. Procyclidine Hydrochloride is usually more efficacious in the relief of rigidity than tremor; but tremor, fatigue, weakness, and sluggishness are frequently beneficially influenced. It can be substituted for all the previous medications in mild and moderate cases. For the control of more severe cases, other drugs may be added to Procyclidine therapy as indications warrant.

Clinical reports indicate that Procyclidine often successfully relieves the symptoms of extrapyramidal dysfunction (dystonia, dyskinesia, akathisia, and parkinsonism) which accompany the therapy of mental disorders with phenothiazine and rauwolfia compounds. In addition to minimizing the symptoms induced by tranquilizing drugs, the drug effectively controls sialorrhea resulting from neuroleptic medication. At the same time, freedom from the side effects induced by tranquilizer drugs, as provided by the administration of Procyclidine, permits a more sustained treatment of the patient's mental disorder.

Clinical results in the treatment of parkinsonism indicate that most patients experience subjective improvement characterized by a feeling of well-being and increased alertness, together with dimished salivation and a marked improvement in muscular coordination as demonstrated by objective tests of manual dexterity and by increased ability to carry out ordinary self-care activities. While the drug exerts a mild atropine-like action and therefore causes mydriasis, this may be kept minimal by careful adjustment of the daily dosage.

CONTRAINDICATIONS

Procyclidine Hydrochloride should not be used in angle-closure glaucoma although simple type glaucomas do not appear to be adversely affected.

WARNINGS

Use in Children: Safety and efficacy have not been established in the pediatric age group; therefore, the use of Procyclidine Hydrochloride in this age group requires that the potential benefits be weighted against the possible hazards to the child.

Pregnancy Warning: The safe use of this drug in pregnancy has not been established; therefore, the use of Procyclidine Hydrochloride in pregnancy, lactation, or in women of childbearing age requires that the potential benefits be weighed against the possible hazards to the mother and child.

PRECAUTIONS

Conditions in which inhibition of the parasympathetic nervous system is undesirable, such as tachycardia and urinary retention (such as may occur with marked prostatic hypertrophy), require special care in the administration of the drug. Hypotensive patients who receive the drug should be observed closely. Occasionally, particularly in older patients, mental confusion and disorientation may occur with the development of agitation, hallucinations, and psychotic-like symptoms.

Patients with mental disorders occasionally experience a precipitation of a psychotic episode when the dosage of antiparkinsonism drugs is increased to treat the extrapyramidal side effects of phenothiazine and rauwolfia derivatives.

ADVERSE REACTIONS

Anticholinergic effects can be produced by therapeutic doses although these can frequently be minimized or eliminated by careful dosage. They include: dryness of the mouth, mydriasis, blurring of vision, giddiness, light-headedness, and gastrointestinal disturbances such as nausea, vomiting, epigastric distress, and constipation. Occasionally an allergic reaction such as a skin rash may be encountered. Feelings of muscular weakness may occur. Acute suppurative parotitis as a complication of dry mouth has been reported.

DOSAGE AND ADMINISTRATION

For Parkinsonism: The dosage of the drug for the treatment of parkinsonism depends upon the age of the patient, the etiology of the disease, and individual responsiveness. Therefore, the dosage must remain flexible to permit adjustment to the individual tolerance and requirements of each patient. In general, younger and postencephalitic patients require and tolerate a somewhat higher dosage than older patients and those with arteriosclerosis.

For Patients Who Have Received No Other Therapy: The usual dose of Procyclidine Hydrochloride for initial treatment is 2.5 mg administered three times daily after meals. If well tolerated, this dose may be gradually increased to 5 mg three times a day and occasionally 5 mg given before retiring. In some cases smaller doses may be employed with good therapeutic results.

Occasionally a patient is encountered who cannot tolerate a bedtime dose of the drug. In such cases it may be desirable to adjust dosage so that the bedtime dose is omitted and the total daily requirement is administered in three equal daytime doses. It is best administered during or after meals to minimize the development of side reactions.

To Transfer Patients to Procydidine Hydrochloride from Other Therapy: Patients who have been receiving other drugs may be transferred to Procyclidine Hydrochloride. This is accomplished gradually by substituting 2.5 mg three times a day for all or part of the original drug. The dose of Procyclidine is then increased as required while that of the other drug is correspondingly omitted or decreased until complete replacement is achieved. The total daily dosage may then be adjusted to the level which produces maximum benefit.

For Drug-Induced Extrapyramidal Symptoms: For treatment of symptoms of extrapyramidal dysfunction induced by tranquilizer drugs during the therapy of mental disorders, the dosage of Procyclidine Hydrochloride will depend on the severity of side effects associated with tranquilizer administration. In general the larger the dosage of the tranquilizer the more severe will be the associated symptoms, including rigidity and tremors. Accordingly, the drug dosage should be adjusted to suit the needs of the individual patient and to provide maximum relief of the induced symptoms. A convenient method to establish the daily dosage of Procyclidine is to begin with the administration of 2.5 mg three times daily. This may be increased by 2.5 mg daily increments until the patient obtains relief of symptoms. In most cases excellent results will be obtained with 10 to 20 mg daily.

Store at 15° to 30°C (59° to 86°F) in a dry place.

HOW SUPPLIED
TABLETS: 5 MG

BRAND/MANUFACTURER	NDC	SIZE	AWP
○ **BRAND**			
KEMADRIN: Burr Wellcome	00081-0604-55	100s	$40.06

Profasi *SEE* GONADOTROPIN, CHORIONIC

Profenal *SEE* SUPROFEN

Profilate Osd *SEE* ANTIHEMOPHILIC FACTOR, HUMAN

Progest *SEE* PROGESTERONE

Progestasert System *SEE* PROGESTERONE

◆ RATED THERAPEUTICALLY EQUIVALENT; ◇ THERAPEUTIC EQUIVALENCE UNCONFIRMED; ○ UNRATED

Progesterone

THE USE OF PROGESTATIONAL AGENTS DURING THE FIRST 4 MONTHS OF PREGNANCY IS NOT RECOMMENDED

PROGESTATIONAL AGENTS HAVE BEEN USED, BEGINNING WITH THE FIRST TRIMESTER OF PREGNANCY, IN AN ATTEMPT TO PREVENT HABITUAL ABORTION OR TO TREAT THREATENED ABORTION. THERE IS NO ADEQUATE EVIDENCE THAT SUCH USE IS EFFECTIVE, AND THERE IS EVIDENCE OF POTENTIAL HARM TO THE FETUS WHEN SUCH DRUGS ARE GIVEN DURING THE FIRST 4 MONTHS OF PREGNANCY. FURTHERMORE, IN THE VAST MAJORITY OF WOMEN, THE CAUSE OF ABORTION IS A DEFECTIVE OVUM, WHICH PROGESTATIONAL AGENTS COULD NOT BE EXPECTED TO INFLUENCE. IN ADDITION, THE USE OF PROGESTATIONAL AGENTS, WITH THEIR UTERINE-RELAXANT PROPERTIES, MAY CAUSE A DELAY IN SPONTANEOUS ABORTION IN PATIENTS WITH FERTILIZED DEFECTIVE OVA. THEREFORE, THE USE OF SUCH DRUGS DURING THE FIRST 4 MONTHS OF PREGNANCY IS NOT RECOMMENDED.

SEVERAL REPORTS SUGGEST THAT THERE IS AN ASSOCIATION BETWEEN INTRAUTERINE EXPOSURE TO FEMALE SEX HORMONES AND CONGENITAL ANOMALIES, INCLUDING CONGENITAL HEART DEFECTS AND LIMB-REDUCTION DEFECTS.[1-5] ONE STUDY[4] ESTIMATED THAT THERE IS A 4.7-FOLD INCREASED RISK OF LIMB-REDUCTION DEFECTS IN INFANTS EXPOSED *IN UTERO* TO SEX HORMONES (I.E., ORAL CONTRACEPTIVES, HORMONE WITHDRAWAL TEST FOR PREGNANCY, OR ATTEMPTED TREATMENT FOR THREATENED ABORTION). SOME OF THESE EXPOSURES WERE VERY SHORT AND INVOLVED ONLY A FEW DAYS OF TREATMENT. THE DATA SUGGEST THAT THE RISK OF LIMB-REDUCTION DEFECTS IN EXPOSED FETUSES IS SOMEWHAT LESS THAN 1 IN 1,000.

IF THE PATIENT IS EXPOSED TO PROGESTERONE DURING THE FIRST 4 MONTHS OF PREGNANCY OR IF SHE BECOMES PREGNANT WHILE TAKING THIS DRUG, SHE SHOULD BE APPRISED OF THE POTENTIAL RISKS TO THE FETUS.

DESCRIPTION

Progesterone (pregn-4-ene-3,20-dione) is the characteristic crystalline progestational steroid of the corpus luteum. Prepared synthetically, it occurs as a white or off-white crystalline powder that is odorless, stable in air, and practically insoluble in water.

The empirical formula is $C_{21}H_{30}O_2$; the molecular weight is 314.47. It is available as an injection and as an intrauterine contraceptive system. Progesterone injection is administered intramuscularly. Each ml contains Progesterone 50 mg.

The Progesterone Intrauterine System contains a reservoir of 38 mg of Progesterone.

Progesterone is released from the system *in situ* at an average rate of 65 µg/day for one year by membrane-controlled diffusion from the reservoir.

Following is its chemical structure:

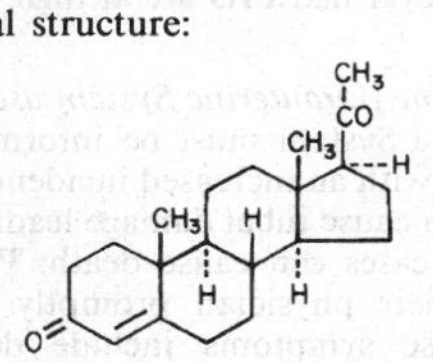

CLINICAL PHARMACOLOGY

Progesterone inhibits the release of pituitary gonadotropin and thereby prevents follicular maturation and ovulation. It also inhibits uterine contractility and induces secretory changes in the endometrium. Unreliable estrogenic or androgenic activity can sometimes be observed.

The natural progestational substance acts on target genital tissues and endocrine glands and also has general systemic effects. Parenteral preparations in oil are used primarily to treat menstrual disorders; responsiveness to Progesterone in the target organ depends on the priming action of estrogen. Progesterone injected in oily solution is readily absorbed but at a rate that is too rapid for optimum therapeutic efficiency. In animal tests, several doses per day are more effective than the same dose one daily, and less frequent dosage is quite inefficient. Inactivation takes place largely in the liver. Many pregnane derivatives and isomers conjugated with glucuronide or sulfate are found in the urine. One of the major urinary products is the glucuronide of pregnane-3α, 20α-diol. The rate of turnover of endogenous Progesterone is unusually rapid, the half-life in blood being a few minutes, and exogenous material is undoubtedly handled in the same way. A small amount of Progesterone is stored in body fat, but this is generally regarded as quantitatively unimportant. Although it is quickly disposed of, Progesterone given at daily intervals in a sufficient dose is thoroughly effective; its actions on tissue continue after it has disappeared from the plasma.

When Progesterone is given by mouth, it is much less effective, but a similar proportion is eliminated in the urine as pregnanediol. Absorption from the intestinal tract is prompt, but the compound is rapidly transformed during passage through the liver and possibly also during absorption through the intestinal mucosa.

About 50% to 60% of administered radioactive Progesterone appears in the urine and about 10% in the feces. Pregnanediol in urine accounts for 12% to 15% of the Progesterone metabolized.

Available data indicate that the contraceptive effectiveness of the Progesterone Intrauterine System is enhanced by its continuous release of Progesterone into the uterine cavity. The mechanism by which Progesterone enhances the contraceptive effectiveness of the system is local, not systemic. The concentrations of luteinizing hormone, estradiol, and Progesterone in systemic venous plasma follow regular cyclic patterns indicative of ovulation during use of the Progesterone Intrauterine System. Blood chemistry studies related to liver, kidney, and thyroid function also reveal no clinically meaningful changes.

During use of the Progesterone Intrauterine System, the endometrium shows progestational influence. Progesterone released from the system at an average rate of 65 µg/day suppresses endometrial proliferation (an antiestrogenic effect). Following system removal, the cyclic endometrial pattern rapidly returns to normal. The local mechanism by which continuously released Progesterone enhances the contraceptive effectiveness of the system has not been conclusively demonstrated. Two hypotheses have been offered: Progesterone-induced inhibition of sperm capacitation or survival; and alteration of the uterine milieu so as to prevent nidation.

INDICATIONS AND USAGE

Progesterone Injection is indicated in amenorrhea and in abnormal uterine bleeding due to hormonal imbalance in the absence of organic pathology, such as submucous fibroids or uterine cancer.

The Progesterone Intrauterine System is indicated for intrauterine contraception in women who have had at least one child, are in a stable, mutually monogamous relationship, and have no history of pelvic inflammatory disease. The Progesterone Intrauterine System must be replaced every 12 months for continued contraceptive effect.

UNLABELED USES

Progesterone is used alone or as an adjunct in the treatment of menorrhagia, to increase ventilatory capacity in patients with Pickwickian syndrome, preterm labor, endometriosis, premenstrual syndrome, and in women without ovaries, to prepare the uterus for receiving an *in vitro* fertilized egg.

CONTRAINDICATIONS

Progesterone injection is contraindicated for patients with a history of thromboembolic disorders, carcinoma of the breast, undiagnosed vaginal bleeding, and missed abortion. It is contraindicated as a diagnostic test for pregnancy.

The Progesterone Intrauterine System is contraindicated when one or more of the following conditions exist:

1. Pregnancy or suspected pregnancy.
2. History of ectopic pregnancy or a condition that predisposes to ectopic pregnancy (see *"Warnings—Ectopic Pregnancy"*).
3. Presence of—or a history of—pelvic inflammatory disease (PID) or factors that predispose to PID (see *"Warnings—Pelvic Infection"*).
4. Patient or her partner has multiple sexual partners.
5. Presence of—or a history of—sexually transmitted disease (one or more episodes), including but not limited to gonorrhea or chlamydial infections of the genital tract.
6. Postpartum endometritis or infected abortion.
7. Incomplete involution of the uterus following abortion or childbirth.
8. A previously inserted IUD is still in place.
9. History of pelvic surgery that may be associated with an increased risk of ectopic pregnancy, such as surgery of the fallopian tubes or surgery for pelvic adhesions or endometriosis.
10. Abnormalities of the uterus resulting in distortion of the uterine cavity or uteri that measure less than 6 cm or greater than 10 cm by sounding.
11. Known or suspected uterine or cervical malignancy including an unresolved, abnormal Pap smear.
12. Genital bleeding of unknown etiology.
13. Vaginitis or cervicitis unless and until infection has been eradicated and has been shown to be non-gonococcal and non-chlamydial.
14. Genital actinomycosis.
15. Conditions or treatments associated with increased susceptibility to infections with microorganisms. Such conditions include, but are not limited to, leukemia, diabetes, a history of endocarditis or certain types of heart disease that are associated with an increased risk of endocarditis, acquired immune deficiency syndrome (AIDS), and conditions requiring chronic corticosteroid therapy.
16. IV drug abuse.

WARNINGS

PROGESTERONE INJECTION

Progesterone injection should be discontinued pending an examination if there is a sudden loss of vision or if there is a sudden onset of proptosis, diplopia, or migraine. If the examination reveals papilledema or retinal vascular lesions, Progesterone therapy should be stopped.

The physician should be alert to the earliest manifestations of thrombotic disorders (eg, thrombophlebitis, cerebrovascular disorders, pulmonary embolism, and retinal thrombosis). If these occur or are suspected, the drug should be discontinued immediately.

Masculinization of the female fetus has occurred when progestogens have been used in pregnant women.

PROGESTERONE INTRAUTERINE SYSTEM

1. Ectopic Pregnancy: The Progesterone Intrauterine System is contraindicated in patients who, in the physician's judgment, are at special risk of having an ectopic pregnancy. Ectopic pregnancy is potentially fatal and appears to occur more frequently with Progesterone Intrauterine System use than with other IUDs and other contraceptives. Therefore, the possibility of ectopic pregnancy must always be considered in Progesterone Intrauterine System users-including those lacking the specific risk factors described below.

The material that follows is intended to aid the physician in the following:

- Understanding the risks of ectopic pregnancy in Progesterone Intrauterine System users (Section 1a).
- Proper selection of women for Progesterone Intrauterine System use by identifying and excluding those at special risk to ectopic pregnancy (Section 1b).
- Diagnosing and managing ectopic pregnancy in IUD users (Sections 1c and 1d).
- Informing patients of ectopic pregnancy risks (Section 1e).

a. Risks of ectopic pregnancy with Progesterone Intrauterine system use: Should a woman become pregnant while using the Progesterone Intrauterine System, the pregnancy is more likely to be ectopic than a pregnancy in a woman using no contraception, ovulation-suppressing oral contraception, or barrier methods.[6,7] This is because the Progesterone Intrauterine System acts in the uterus to prevent uterine pregnancy, but it does not prevent either ovulation of ectopic pregnancy. Thus, each month that the Progesterone intrauterine System is used, there is protection against uterine pregnancy but not against ectopic pregnancy. In clinical trials of the Progesterone Intrauterine System, 1 of 3.6 pregnancies in parous women and 1 of 6.2 pregnancies in nulliparous women were ectopic.

The per-year risk of ectopic pregnancy in Progesterone intrauterine System users is approximately 5 per 1,000 or 1 ectopic pregnancy in 200 users per year. This risk is approximately the same as in noncontracepting, sexually active women. In contrast, barrier contraceptives, which prevent fertilization, or oral contraceptives that prevent ovulation, reduce the risk of ectopic pregnancy to a few percent of the risk in noncontracepting, sexually active women.

Two clinical studies conducted by the World Health Organization compared the risk of ectopic pregnancies among 2,239 women wearing a Progesterone-releasing IUD similar to the Progesterone Intrauterine System with the risk in 3,303 women wearing a copper-releasing IUD. For the first year the risk of ecotopic pregnancy was approximately 6 times higher among women using Progesterone systems than among women using copper systems. Over the two years that the studies ran, the risk of an ectopic pregnancy with the Progesterone-releasing IUD was about 10 times higher than that with copper-releasing IUDs.

b. Women at special risk to ectopic pregnancy: Several factors have been identified as placing a woman at special risk to ectopic pregnancy. The presence of any of these factors contraindicates use of the Progesterone Intrauterine System. Factors indicating high risk to ectopic pregnancy include a history of ectopic pregnancy or a history or presence of a condition predisposing to ectopic pregnancy such as PID. A prospective clinical study was conducted over 9.5 years in 415 women who had had verified PID and 100 healthy control subjects. The ratio between ectopic and intrauterine pregnancies after PID was 1/24. In contrast, the ratio in the controls was 1/147. Further analysis of these data suggests that women who have had PID subsequently have an 8- to 10-fold greater risk of ectopic pregnancy than sexually active noncontracepting women who have never had PID.

Factors other than PID may also indicate a high risk to ectopic pregnancy. These factors include multiple sexual partners or a partner with multiple sexual partners, pelvic surgery of certain types, retrograde menstruation, endometritis, and endometriosis.

c. Diagnosis of ectopic pregnancy: The absence of risk factors for ectopic pregnancy described above does not rule out ectopic pregnancy. In every instance of pregnancy occurring in a Progesterone Intrauterine System user it is essential that proper measures be taken to determine if the pregnancy is ectopic.

To determine whether ectopic pregnancy has occurred, special attention should be directed to patients with any of the following symptoms or conditions: unusual, abnormal, or irregular vaginal bleeding; delayed or missed menses; pelvic pain, usually unilateral, which may be associated with fainting or the urge to defecate; unexplained pain in the shoulder; or pain associated with bleeding if not part of the usual menstrual cycle. Ectopic pregnancy test or elevated B-HCG values but who lack ultrasonographic or other evidence of intrauterine pregnancy.

d. Management of diagnosed or suspected ectopic pregnancy: When ectopic pregnancy is suspected, diagnostic uncertainty should be resolved as quickly as possible, in view of the life-threatening risk of ruptured ectopic pregnancy. When ectopic pregnancy is diagnosed, immediate surgery is often required because a ruptured ectopic pregnancy may occur at any time.

e. Ectopic pregnancy warning to Progesterone Intrauterine System users: All women who choose the Progesterone Intrauterine System must be informed before insertion that a pregnancy occurring in a Progesterone Intrauterine System user is more likely to be ectopic than one occurring in users of ovulation-preventing oral contraceptives, barrier modes or other IUDs. They should be taught to recognize and report to their physician promptly any symptoms of ectopic pregnancy. Women should also be informed that ectopic pregnancy has been associated with complications leading to loss of fertility.

2. Intrauterine Pregnancy: Intrauterine pregnancy can occur during use of the Progesterone Intrauterine System (see *"Clinical Studies"* section for pregnancy rates).

a. Long-term effects and congenital anomalies: When pregnancy occurs or proceeds with the Progesterone Intrauterine System in place, long-term effects on the offspring are unknown. Congenital anomalies have occurred under such conditions. Their relationship to the Progesterone Intrauterine System has not been established. Systemically administered sex steroids, including progestational agents, have been associated with an increased risk of congenital anomalies. It is not known whether an increased risk of such anomalies exists when pregnancy continues with a Progesterone Intrauterine System in place. The decision to continue or terminate pregnancy should take into account this unknown risk.

b. Septic abortion: Reports have indicated an increased incidence of septic abortion—with septicemia, septic shock, and death—in patients becoming pregnant with an IUD in place. Most of these reports have been associated with, but are not limited to, the mid-trimester of pregnancy. In some cases, the initial symptoms have been insidious and not easily recognized. If pregnancy should occur with a Progesterone Intrauterine System *in situ,* the system should be removed if removal is easily accomplished.

Removal or manipulation of the Progesterone Intrauterine System may precipitate abortion. If removal would be or proves to be difficult, termination of the pregnancy should be considered and offered to the patient as an option, bearing in mind that the risks associated with an elective abortion increase with gestational age.

c. Continuation of pregnancy: If the patient chooses to continue the pregnancy with the system in place, she must be warned that this increases the risk of spontaneous abortion and sepsis, which may cause death. In addition, she is at increased risk of premature labor and delivery. As a consequence of premature birth, the fetus is at increased risk of damage. She should be followed more closely than the usual obstetrical patient. She must be advise to report immediately all symptoms such as flu-like syndrome, fever, chills, abdominal cramping and pain, bleeding, or vaginal discharge, because generalized symptoms of septicema may be insidious.

3. Pelvic Infection (Pelvic Inflammatory Disease): The Progesterone intrauterine System is contraindicated in the presence of PID or suspected PID or in women with a history of PID. Use of all IUDs, including the Progesterone intrauterine System, has been associated with an increased incidence of PID. In a hospital-based, case-control study done in the United States in 1976-1978, women using IUD's had a relative risk of PID of 1.6 compared with women using no method.[8] Therefore a decision to use the Progesterone intrauterine system must include consideration of the risk of PID. The highest rate of PID occurs shortly after insertion and up to four months thereafter. Administration of prophylactic antibiotics may be useful, but the utility of this treatment is still under consideration (see *"Insertion Precautions"*). PID can necessitate hysterectomy; can lead to tubo-ovarian abscesses, tubal occlusion and infertility and tubal damage that predisposes to ectopic pregnancy; can result in peritonitis; and can cause death in infrequent cases. The effect of PID on fertility is especially important for women who may wish to have children at a later date.

a. Women at special risk to PID: PID is usually a sexually transmitted disease, and the Progesterone intrauterine system does not protect against sexually transmitted disease. The risk of PID appears to be greater for women who have multiple sexual partners and also for women whose sexual partner(s) have multiple sexual partners. Women who have ever had PID are at high risk for a recurrence or re-infection.

b. PID warning to Progesterone intrauterine System users: All women who choose the Progesterone intrauterine System must be informed prior to insertion that IUD use has been associated with an increased incidence of PID and that PID can necessitate hysterectomy, can cause tubal damage leading to ectopic pregnancy or infertility, or in infrequent cases can cause death. Patients must be taught to recognize and report to their physician promptly any symptoms of pelvic inflammatory disease. These symptoms include development of menstrual disorders (prolonged or heavy bleeding), unusual vaginal discharge, abdominal or pelvic pain or tenderness, dyspareunia, chills, and fever.

c. Asymptomatic PID: PID may be asymptomatic but still result in tubal damage and its sequelae.[9,10]

d. Treatment of PID: Following diagnosis of PID, or suspected PID, bacteriologic specimens should be obtained and antibiotic therapy should be initiated promptly. Removal of the Progesterone Intrauterine Contraceptive System after initiation of antibiotic therapy is required.

Guidelines for PID treatment are available from the Centers for Disease Control (CDC), Atlanta, Georgia. The guidelines were established after deliberation by a group of experts and staff of the CDC but they should not be construed as rules suitable for use in all patients. Adequate PD treatment requires the application of current standards of therapy prevailing at the time of occurrence of the infection with reference to the specific antibiotics' prescription labeling.

Genital actinomycosis has been associated primarily with long-term IUD use. If it occurs, promptly institute appropriate antibiotic therapy and remove the Progesterone intrauterine system.

4. Embedment: Partial penetration or embedment of the Progesterone Intrauterine System in the endometrium or myometrium may decrease contraceptive effectiveness and can result in difficult removals. In some cases, this can result in fragmentation of the IUD, necessitating surgical removal.

5. *Fragmentation:* If fragmentation of the Progesterone intrauterine System occurs, all pieces should be removed if possible.

6. *Perforation:* Partial or total perforation of the uterine wall or cervix may occur with use of a uterine sound or the Progesterone intrauterine System. It is generally believed that perforations, if they occur, happen at the time of insertion, although the perforation may not be detected until some time later. The possibility of perforation must be kept in mind during insertion and at the time of any subsequent examination. It is recommended that the Progesterone intrauterine System insertion be postponed postpartum, or post abortion until involution of the uterus is complete since the incidence of perforation and expulsion is greater if involution is not complete. Involution may be delayed in nursing mothers; there is an increased risk of perforation in women who are lactating. If perforation occurs, the Progesterone intrauterine System should be removed. A surgical procedure may be required. Adhesions, foreign body reactions, peritonitis, cystic masses in the pelvis, intestinal penetrations, intestinal obstruction and local inflammatory reaction with abscess formation and erosion of adjacent viscera may result if an IUD is left in the peritoneal cavity.

7. *Risks of Mortality:* The available data from a variety of sources have been analyzed to estimate the risk of death associated with various methods of contraception. The estimates of risk of death include the combined risk of the contraceptive method plus the risk of pregnancy or abortion in the event of method failure. The findings of the analysis are shown in Table 1.[11]

Table 1
ANNUAL NUMBER OF BIRTH-RELATED OR METHOD-RELATED DEATHS ASSOCIATED WITH CONTROL OF FERTILITY PER 100,000 NONSTERILE WOMEN, BY FERTILITY CONTROL METHOD ACCORDING TO AGE

Method of control and outcome	15-19	20-24	25-29	30-34	35-39	40-44
No fertility control methods*	7.0	7.4	9.1	14.8	25.7	28.2
Oral contraceptives/ nonsmokers**	0.3	0.5	0.9	1.9	13.8	31.6
Oral contraceptives/ smokers**	2.2	3.4	6.6	13.5	51.1	117.2
IUD**	0.8	0.8	1.0	1.0	1.4	1.4
Condom*	1.1	1.6	0.7	0.2	0.3	0.4
Diaphragm/ spermicide*	1.9	1.2	1.2	1.3	2.2	2.8
Periodic abstinence*	2.5	1.6	1.6	1.7	2.9	3.6

* *Deaths are birth related*
** *Deaths are method related*

PRECAUTIONS
PROGESTERONE INJECTION
General: The pretreatment physical examination should include special reference to the breasts and pelvic organs as well as a Papanicolaou smear.

Because Progesterone may cause some degree of fluid retention, conditions that might be influenced by this factor (eg, epilepsy, migraine, asthma, and cardiac or renal dysfunction) require careful observation.

In breakthrough bleeding, as in all instances of irregular bleeding *per vaginam*, nonfunctional causes should be considered. In cases of undiagnosed vaginal bleeding, adequate diagnostic measures are indicated.

Patients who have a history of psychic depression should be carefully observed, and the drug should be discontinued if the depression recurs to a serious degree.

Any possible influence of prolonged progestogen therapy on pituitary, ovarian, adrenal, hepatic, or uterine functions awaits further study.

A decrease in glucose tolerance has been noted in a small percentage of patients on estrogen-progestogen combination drugs. The mechanism of such a decrease is obscure. For this reason, diabetic patients should be carefully observed while receiving progestogen therapy.

The age of the patient constitutes no absolute limiting factor, although treatment with progestogens may mask the onset of the climacteric.

The pathologist should be advised of progesterone therapy when relevant specimens are submitted.

Laboratory Tests: The following laboratory results may be altered by the concomitant use of an estrogen and a progestogen:
Hepatic function: increased sulfobromophthalein retention and other tests
Coagulation tests: increase in prothrombin, Factors VII, VIII, IX and X
Thyroid function: increase in PBI and BEI and a decrease in T_3-uptake values
Metyrapone test

Carcinogenesis, Mutagenesis, Impairment of Fertility: In dogs, the experimental administration of the progestational agent medroxyprogesterone acetate increased the frequency of mammary nodules. Although nodules occasionally appeared in control animals, they were intermittent in nature, whereas nodules in treated animals were larger, more numerous, and persistent. There is no general agreement as to whether the nodules are benign or malignant. Their significance with respect to humans has not been established.

Pregnancy—Pregnancy Category D: See "Warnings" and information in the box at the beginning of this prescribing information.

Nursing Mothers: Detectable amounts of Progesterone have been identified in the milk of mothers receiving the steroid. Its effect on the nursing infant has not been determined.

Because of the potential for tumorigenicity shown for Progesterone in animal studies, a decision should be made either to discontinue nursing or to discontinue the drug, taking into account the importance of the drug to the mother.

Usage in Children: Safety and effectiveness in children have not been established.

PROGESTERONE INTRAUTERINE SYSTEM
1. Patient Counseling: a. Patients should be counseled that this product does not protect against HIV infection (AIDS) and other sexually transmitted diseases.

b. Patients must be informed of the availability, effectiveness, and risks of the Progesterone intrauterine System and other forms of contraception. They should also be informed of the health risks associated with pregnancy resulting from failure to use any contraception.

c. Prior to insertion of the Progesterone intrauterine System, the physician, nurse, or other trained health professional must provide the patient with a patient information leaflet. The patient must read the leaflet in its entirety and discuss fully any questions she has concerning the Progesterone intrauterine System and other methods of contraception. She must then initial and sign the leaflet, including an informed choice statement, if applicable.

2. Patient Evaluation and Clinical Considerations: a. A complete medical and social history should be obtained to determine conditions that might influence the selection of the Progesterone intrauterine System or contraindicate its use (see "Contraindications"). Physical examination should include a pelvic examination, Pap smear, N. gonorrhea and Chlamydia culture (or other specific tests for these organisms) and, if indicated, appropriate tests for other forms of venereal disease. **Special attention must be given to ascertaining whether the woman is at increased risk of ectopic pregnancy or PID. The Progesterone intrauterine System is contraindicated in these women.**

b. The Progesterone intrauterine System is not intended for immediate postabortion or postpartum insertion. It should not be inserted until involution of the uterus is complete. (Involution may be delayed in nursing mothers.) The incidence of perforation and expulsion is greater if involution is not completed. Data also suggest there may be an increased risk of perforation and expulsion if the woman is lactating[12,13].

c. The physician should determine that the patient is not pregnant. possibility of insertion in the presence of an existing undetermined pregnancy is reduced if insertion is performed during or shortly following a menstrual period.

d. Patients with certain types of valvular heart disease and surgically constructed systemic-pulmonary shunts have an increased risk of infective endocarditis. Use of a Progesterone intrauterine System in these patients may represent a potential source of septic emboli and is contraindicated. Other conditions predisposing to infection (see "Contraindications") are also contraindications to Progesterone intrauterine System insertion.

e. IUDs should be used with caution in those patients who have an anemia or a history of menorrhagia or hypermenorrhea. Patients experiencing menorrhagia and/or metrorrhagia following IUD insertion may be at risk for the development of hypochromic microcytic anemia. Also, IUDs should be used with caution in patients who have a coagulopathy or are receiving anticoagulants.

f. Use of the Progesterone intrauterine System in patients with vaginitis or cervicitis should be postponed until proper treatment has eradicated the infection and until the cervicitis has been shown not to be due to gonorrhea or chlamydia (see "Contraindications").

3. Insertion Precautions: a. Because the presence of organisms capable of establishing PID cannot be determined by apperance, and because IUD insertion may be associated with introduction of vaginal bacteria into the uterus, administration of prophylactic antibiotics may be considered, but the utility of this treatment is still under evaluation. Regimens include doxycycline 200 mg orally 1 hour before insertion or erythromycin 500 mg orally 1 hour before insertion and 500 mg orally 6 hours after insertion. The use of antibiotics in nursing mothers is not recommended. Before prescribing the above mentioned antibiotics, refer to their prescription drug labeling, and make certain that the patient is a suitable candidate for the drug.

b. The uterus should be carefully sounded prior to insertion to determine the degree of patency of the endocervical canal and the internal os, and the direction and depth of the uterine cavity. In occasional cases, severe cervical stenosis may be encountered. Do not use excessive force to overcome this resistance.

c. The uterus should sound to a depth of 6 to 10 centimeters (cm). Insertion of the Progesterone intrauterine system into a uterine cavity measuring less than 6.5 cm by sounding may increase the incidence of expulsion, bleeding, and pain.

d. Syncope, bradycardia, or other neurovascular episodes may occur during insertion or removal of the Progesterone intrauterine system, especially in patients with a previous disposition of these conditions or cervical stenosis. If decreased pulse, perspiration, or pallor are observed, the patient should remain supine until these signs have disappeared.

e. The patient should be told that some bleeding and/or cramps may occur during the first few weeks after insertion. If her symptoms continue or are severe she should report them to her physician. She should also be given instructions on what other symptoms require her to call her physician. She should be instructed on how to check after her menstrual period to make certain that the thread, if there is one, still protrudes from the cervix and cautioned not to pull on the thread and displace the Progesterone intrauterine System. She should be informed that there is no contraceptive protection if the Progesterone intrauterine System is displaced or expelled. If a partial expulsion occurs, removal is indicated.

f. The patient must be told to return within 3 months for a checkup and at 12 months after insertion for removal of the Progesterone intrauterine system. Patient reminder cards should be properly completed and given to the patient.

4. Requirements for Continuation and Removal:
a. The Progesterone intrauterine system must be replaced every 12 months. There is no evidence of decreasing contraceptive efficacy with time before 12 months, but contraceptive effectiveness after 12 months decreases; therefore, the patient should be informed of the known duration of contraceptive efficacy and be advised to return in 12 months for removal and possible insertion of a new Progesterone intrauterine System.

b. The Progesterone intrauterine System should be removed for the following medical reasons: menorrhagia- and/or metrorrhagia-producing anemia; acquired immune deficiency syndrome (AIDS); sexually transmitted disease; pelvic infection; endometritis; genital actinomycosis; intractable pelvic pain; dyspareunia; pregnancy; endometrial or cervical malignancy; uterine or cervical perforation; increase in length of the threads, if there are any, extending from the cervix, or any other indication of partial expulsion.

c. If the retrieval threads, if there are any, are not visible, they may have retracted into the uterus or have been broken, or the Progesterone intrauterine System may have been broken, perforated the uterus, or have been expelled. Location may be determined by feeling with a probe, X-ray, or sonography.

5. Continuing Care of Patients Using the Progesterone interauterine system: a. Any inquires regarding pain, odorous discharge, bleeding, fever, genital lesions or sores, or a missed period should be promptly responded to and prompt examination recommended.

b. If examination during visits subsequent to insertion reveals that the length of the threads, if any, has visibly or palpably changed from the length at time of insertion, the system should be considered displaced and should be removed. A new system may be inserted at that time or during the next menses if it is certain that conception has not occurred. When the thread, if there is one, cannot be seen by the physician, further investigation is necessary.

c. Since the Progesterone intrauterine System may be expelled or displaced, patients should be reexamined and evaluated shortly after the first postinsertion menses, but definitely within 3 months after insertion. **The Progesterone intrauterine System must be removed every 12 months because of diminished contraceptive effectiveness thereafter.** At the time of reinsertion, appropriate medical and laboratory examinations should be carried out.

d. In the event a pregnancy is confirmed during Progesterone intrauterine System use, the following steps should be taken:

■ Determine whether pregnancy is ectopic and take appropriate measures if it is.

■ Inform patient of the risks of leaving an IUD *in situ* or removing it during pregnancy and of the lack of data on the Progesterone intrauterine System's long-term effects on the offspring of women who have had it *in utero* during conception or gestation (see *"Warnings"*).

■ If possible the Progesterone intrauterine System should be removed after the patient has been warned of the risks of removal. If removal is difficult, the patient should be counseled about and offered pregnancy termination.

■ If the Progesterone intrauterine System is left in place, the patient's course should be followed closely.

e. Should be patient's relationship cease to be mutually monogamous, or should her partner become HIV positive, or acquire a sexually transmitted disease, she should be instructed to report this change and see her physician immediately.

ADVERSE REACTIONS

Administration of Progesterone is only rarely accompanied by side effects, and these effects are usually mild. The following adverse reactions have been observed in women taking progestogens: break-through bleeding, spotting, change in menstrual flow, amenorrhea, edema, change in weight (increase or decrease), changes in cervical erosion and cervical secretions, cholestatic jaundice, rash (allergic) with and without pruritus, melasma or chloasma, and mental depression. A small percentage of patients have local reactions at the site of injection.

The administration of large doses of Progesterone (50 to 100 mg daily) may result in a moderate catabolic effect and a transient increase in sodium and chloride excretion.

The result of a pregnanediol determination may be altered if the patient is being treated with a progestogen.

A statistically significant association has been demonstrated between use of estrogen-progestogen combination drugs and the following serious adverse reactions: thrombophlebitis, pulmonary embolism, and cerebral thrombosis and embolism. For this reason, patients on progestogen therapy should be carefully observed.

Although available evidence is suggestive of an association, such a relationship has been neither confirmed nor refuted for the following serious adverse reactions:

Neuro-ocular lesions, eg, retinal thrombosis and optic neuritis

The following adverse reactions have been observed in patients receiving estrogen-progestogen combination drugs: rise in blood pressure in susceptible individuals, premenstrual-like syndrome, changes in libido, changes in appetite, cystitis-like syndrome, headache, nervousness, dizziness, fatigue, backache, hirsutism, loss of hair, erythema multiforme, erythema nodosum, hemorrhagic eruption, and itching.

In view of these observations, patients on progestogen therapy should be carefully observed for the occurrence of these adverse reactions.

Reported adverse reactions with intrauterine contraceptives include: endometritis; spontaneous abortion; septic abortion; septicemia; perforation of the uterus and cervix; embedment; fragmentation of the IUD; pelvic infection; tubo-ovarian abscess; tubal damage; vaginitis; leukorrhea; cervical erosion; pregnancy; ectopic pregnancy; fetal damage and congenital anomalies; difficult removal; complete or partial expulsion of the IUD; intermenstrual spotting; prolongation of menstrual flow; anemia; amenorrhea or delayed menses; pain and cramping; dysmenorrhea; backaches; dyspareunia; neurovascular episodes, including bradycardia and syncope secondary to insertion. Uterine perforation and IUD displacement into the abdomen have been followed by peritonitis, abdominal adhesions, intestinal penetration, intestinal obstruction, local inflammatory reaction with abscess formation and erosion of adjacent viscera, and cystic masses in the pelvis. Certain of these adverse reactions can lead to loss of fertility, partial or total removal of reproductive organs, hormonal imbalance, or death.

OVERDOSAGE

To obtain up-to-date information about the treatment of overdose, a good resource is your certified regional poison control center. Telephone numbers of certified poison control centers are listed in the *Physicians' Desk Reference (PDR)*. In managing overdosage, consider the possibility of multiple drug overdoses, interaction among drugs, and unusual drug kinetics in your patient.

DOSAGE AND ADMINISTRATION

PROGESTERONE INJECTION
Progesterone is administered by intramuscular injection. It differs from other commonly used steroids in that it is irritating at the place of injection. This is true whether the preparation is in an oil or an aqueous vehicle. The latter is particularly painful.

Secondary Amenorrhea: 5 to 10 mg given for 6 to 8 consecutive days. If there has been sufficient ovarian activity to produce a proliferative endometrium, one can expect withdrawal bleeding 48 to 72 hours after the last injection. This may be followed by spontaneous normal cycles.

Functional Uterine Bleeding: 5 to 10 mg given *daily* for 6 doses. Bleeding may be expected to cease within 6 days. When estrogen is given as well, the administration of Progesterone should begin after 2 weeks of estrogen therapy. If menstrual flow begins during the course of injections of Progesterone, injections should be discontinued.

Prior to administration, parenteral drug products should be inspected visually for particulate matter and discoloration. Slight discoloration does not alter potency. If cloudiness occurs, warm the vial gently to effect a clear solution.

Directions for Use: A single Progesterone Intrauterine System is to be inserted into the uterine cavity (see *"Precautions"*). The system must be removed 12 months after insertion and replaced for continued contraceptive effectiveness. See *"Insertion and Removal Instructions"*.

PROGESTERONE INTRAUTERINE SYSTEM
Insertion and Removal Instructions:

Note: Physicians are cautioned to become thoroughly familiar with the insertion instructions in their entirety before attempting placement of the Progesterone intrauterine Contraceptive System.

There is debate as to how many IUD insertions constitute adequate training for a clinician. It is probably wise to have done 15-25 insertions under supervision prior to inserting an IUD unsupervised. A practitioner with only 4-6 insertions would probably not have had adequate experience with difficult insertions.

The usual time of insertion is during the latter part of the menstrual period, or one or two days thereafter.

The Progesterone Intrauterine System retains its efficacy for 12 months. Therefore, it must be removed and a new one inserted no more than 12 months after insertion for continued contraceptive efficacy.

Preliminary Preparation:
1. Before insertion, the patient must read and initial each section of a patient information leaflet; the medical and social history and counseling of the patient must be completed; and an informed choice statement must be signed by the patient and by the doctor.
2. Refer to *"Contraindications"*, *"Warnings"*, and *"Precautions"*.
3. Prior to insertion of the Progesterone intrauterine System, a cervical Pap smear, N. gonorrhea and Chlamydia cultures (or other specific tests for these organisms), and pelvic examination are to be performed.
4. If appropriate, commence antibiotic prophylaxis one hour before insertion.
5. Use of aseptic technique during insertion is essential.
6. The cervix should be cleansed with an antiseptic solution and a tenaculum applied to the cervix with downward traction for stabilization of the cervix and correction of angulation.
7. Prior to insertion, determine by uterine sounding the depth and position of the uterus and the patency of the cervical canal. Insertion into a uterus that sounds less than 6 cm or more than 10 cm is contraindicated.

Great care must be exercised during the preinsertion sounding and subsequent insertion. No attempt should be made to force the insertion.

Note: Any intrauterine procedure can result in severe pain, bradycardia, and syncope.

System Insertion: 1. Place the pouch on a hard, flat surface. Peel the clear cover back completely. Inspect the inserter to make sure the thread-retaining plug is secure at the end of the inserter with 2.5-5.0 cm. of the long "retainer" thread protruding. Do not insert the system if the plug cannot be easily secured.

Remove the system and inserter by grasping the inserter at a point between the two sets of graduations. DO NOT CONTAMINATE THE END CONTAINING THE SYSTEM.

2. IMMEDIATELY PRIOR TO INSERTION, cock the arms of the Progesterone Intrauterine System by holding the inserter vertically with the arm cocker flat on the sterile interior of the pouch. Press down firmly to cock the arms. This will cause the arms to fold against the sides of the inserter.

Note: To avoid alteration of system shape, do not leave the system cocked for more than five minutes.

3. *Examine the curvature of the inserter.* Make any necessary adjustments to the curvature of the inserter to fit the flexion of the uterus, maintaining aseptic technique. For an anteverted uterus, the black numbers on the inserter should face up; they should face down for a retroverted uterus. Be certain that the thread-retaining plug is still secure in the end of the inserter, then introduce the inserter into the cervical canal. The feet of the arm-cocker will rest centered on the cervical os as you push the inserter gently but steadily through the cervical canal.

4. When the fundus is reached, the number on the inserter at the base of the arm-cocker should equal the previously sounded uterine depth.

5. DO NOT PULL BACK ON THE ARMCOCKER OR INSERTER. Release the Progesterone intrauterine contraceptive system by squeezing the wings of the thread-retaining plug and removing it.

6. Slowly withdraw the inserter. The Progesterone intrauterine system remains in the uterus as the inserter is withdrawn. After insertion is complete, check to make certain that no components of the inserter are in the uterus. Dispose of the inserter shaft with attached armcocker, as well as the thread-retaining plug.

To be fully effective the Progesterone intrauterine system must be placed at the fundus. To confirm the correct position of the Progesterone intrauterine system, measure the length of the short "indicator" thread against the graduations on the thread-retaining end of the inserter. The length of this short thread should be the difference between 9 cm, and the uterine depth.

For example, if the uterus was sounded to 7 cm., the short "indicator" thread should extend out of the cervix 9 cm − 7 cm = 2 cm.

Cut the long "retainer" thread to a standard length of your choice—at least 3 cm. from the cervix. This can be used for future reference in determining if fundal placement is being maintained. (If pregnancy, displacement, or perforation occurs, the thread may be drawn up through the cervix.) Record the uterine depth and length of cut "retainer" thread in the patient's chart.

System Removal: To remove the Progesterone intrauterine system, pull gently on the exposed threads. The arms of the system will fold upward as it is withdrawn from the uterus. Even if removal proves difficult, the system should not remain in the uterus after one year.

Storage and Handling: Store Progesterone intrauterine system and Progesterone injection at room temperature, (15-30°C; 59-86°F).

CLINICAL STUDIES
Different event rates have been reported with the use of different IUDs. Inasmuch as these rates are usually derived from separate studies conducted by different investigators in several population groups, they cannot be compared with precision. Clinical trials of the Progesterone Intrauterine System were conducted by the World Health Organization from 1970 to 1981; use-effectiveness was determined from combined data as tabulated by the life table method. (Rates are expressed as events per 100 women through 12 months of use.) This experience is based on 5104 women who completed 12 months of use.

	Parous*	12 Months Nulliparous*
Pregnancy		
Intrauterine	1.3	2.1
Extrauterine (ectopic)	0.5	0.4
Total	1.8	2.5
Expulsion	2.7	7.6
Medical Removals	9.3	12.0
Continuation Rate	81.2	73.4

* *Columns do not total 100 because rates are not included for the following scheduled removals, removals for planned pregnancy, release from studies, and lost-to-follow-up.*

The lowest expected and typical failure rates during the first year of continuous use of all contraceptive methods are listed in Table 2.[9]

Table 2
PERCENTAGE OF WOMEN EXPERIENCING AN ACCIDENTAL PREGNANCY IN THE FIRST YEAR OF CONTINUOUS USE

Method	Lowest Expected*	Typical**
No Contraception	85.0	85.0
Oral Contraceptives		3.0
combined	0.1	N/A***
progestin only	0.5	N/A***
Diaphragm with spermicidal cream or jelly	6.0	18.0
Spermicides alone (foam, creams, jellies and vaginal suppositories)	3.0	21.0
Vaginal Sponge		
nulliparous	6.0	18.0
multiparous	9.0	28.0
IUD Progesterone Intrauterine System)	2.0	3.0 †
Condom without spermicides	2.0	12.0
Periodic abstinence (all methods)	1.0 - 9.0	20.0
Female sterilization	0.2	0.4
Male sterilization	0.1	0.15
Norplant	0.04	0.04

* *The author's best guess of the percentage of women expected to experience an accidental pregnancy among couples who initiate a method (not necessarily for the first time) and use it consistently and correctly during the first year if they do not stop for any other reason.*

** *This term represents "typical" couples who initiate use of a method (not necessary for the first time), who experience an accidental pregnancy during the first year if they do not stop use for any other reason.*

*** *N/A — Data not available.*

† *Combined typical rate for both the Progesterone Intrauterine System and Copper T 380A. The typical rate for the Progesterone intrauterine System alone is not available.*

REFERENCES
1. Gal I, Kirman B, Stern J: Hormonal pregnancy tests and congenital malformation. *Nature* 1967; 216:83. 2. Levy EP, Cohen A, Fraser FC: Hormone treatment during pregnancy and congenital heart defects. *Lancet* 1973;1:611. 3. Nora J, Nora A: Birth defects and oral contraceptives. *Lancet*1973;1:941. 4. Janerich DT, Piper JM, Glebatis DM: Oral contraceptives and congenital limb-reduction defects. *N Engl J Med* 1974;291:697. 5. Heinonen OP, Slone D, Monson RR, Hook EB, Shapiro S: Cardiovascular birth defects and antenatal exposure to female sex hormones. *N Engl J Med* 1977;296:67. 6. World Health Organization's Special Programme of Research, Development and Research Training in Human Reproduction: A multi-national case-control study of ectopic pregnancy. *Clin. Reprod. Fertil.* 1985; 3:131-143. 7. Ory, H.W.: Women's Health Study: Ectopic pregnancy and intrauterine contraceptive devices: New perspectives. *Obstet. Gynecol.* 1981; 57:137-144.Y 8. Lee, N.C., Rubin, G.L., and Borucki, R.: The Intrauterine Device and Pelvic Inflammatory Disease Revisited: New Results From the Women's Health Study. *Obstet. Gynecol.* 1988; 72:1-6. 9. Cramer, D.W. et al: Tubal infertility and the intrauterine device. *N. Engl. J. Med.* 1985; 312:941-947. 10. Daling, J.R. et al: Primary tubal infertility in relation to the use of an intrauterine device. *N. Engl. J. Med.* 1985;312:937-941. 11. Ory, H.W.: Mortality associated with fertility and fertility control. *Family Planning Perspectives* 1983; 15:57-63. 12. Heartwell, S.F., Schlesselman, S.: Risk of uterine perforation among users of intrauterine devices. *Obstet. Gynecol.* 1983; 61:31-36. 13. Chi, I.C., Kelly, E.: Is lactation a risk factor of IUD and sterilisation-related uterine perforations? A hypothesis. *Int. J. Gynaecol. Obstet.* 1984; 22:315-317. 14. Trussel, J, Kost, K.: Contraceptive failure in the United States: A critical review of the literature. *Studies in Family Planning* 1990; 21:51-54.

J CODES
IM—J2675

HOW SUPPLIED
DEVICE:

BRAND/MANUFACTURER	NDC	SIZE	AWP
○ BRAND			
PROGESTASERT SYSTEM: Alza	17314-4231-01	6s	$656.82

INJECTION: 50 MG/ML

AVERAGE UNIT PRICE (AVAILABLE SIZES)		GENERIC A-RATED AVERAGE PRICE (GAAP)		
GENERIC	$1.63	10 ml		$16.30

BRAND/MANUFACTURER	NDC	SIZE	AWP
◆ GENERICS			
Schein	00364-6683-54	10 ml	$8.70
Steris	00402-0379-10	10 ml	$8.70
	00574-0704-10	10 ml	$11.65
Major	00904-1050-10	10 ml	$13.45
Moore,H.L.	00839-5165-30	10 ml	$14.84
URL	00677-0301-21	10 ml	$14.95
Goldline	00182-0862-63	10 ml	$18.60
Rugby	00536-7400-70	10 ml	$19.50
Lilly	00002-1438-01	10 ml	$36.30

INJECTION: 50 MG/ML

BRAND/MANUFACTURER	NDC	SIZE	AWP
○ BRAND			
PROGEST: Truxton	00463-1056-10	10 ml	$10.20

Proglycem SEE DIAZOXIDE

Prograf SEE TACROLIMUS

Prohance SEE GADOTERIDOL

ProHIBiT SEE HAEMOPHILUS B CONJUGATE VACCINE AND HEMOPHILUS B CONJUGATE VACCINE (TETANUS TOXOID CONJUGATE)

Prohim SEE YOHIMBINE HYDROCHLORIDE

Prolastin SEE PROTEINASE INHIBITOR (HUMAN), ALPHA₁

Proleukin SEE ALDESLEUKIN

Prolex DH SEE GUAIFENESIN AND HYDROCODONE BITARTRATE

Prolixin SEE FLUPHENAZINE

Proloprim SEE TRIMETHOPRIM

Promazine Hydrochloride

With any compound it is good to review carefully not only its therapeutic efficacy but also the possibilities of the occurrence of undesirable side effects. The physician, therefore, should be thoroughly familiar with the data presented in this prescribing information prior to prescribing Promazine Hydrochloride.

DESCRIPTION
Promazine Hydrochloride is a member of the group of phenothiazines containing an acyclic aliphatic moiety at the 10 position.

Each mL contains 50 mg Promazine Hydrochloride.

Following is its chemical structure:

$$CH_2CH_2CH_2N(CH_3)_2 \cdot HCl$$

ACTIONS
Promazine has actions at all levels of the central nervous system as well as on multiple-organ systems. The mechanism whereby its therapeutic action takes place is not known.

INDICATIONS
Promazine is effective in the management of manifestations of psychotic disorders.

Promazine Hydrochloride has not been shown effective in the management of behavioral complications in patients with mental retardation.

CONTRAINDICATIONS
Promazine should not be used in comatose states due to central nervous system depressants (alcohol, barbiturates, opiates, etc.). In patients with cerebral arteriosclerosis, coronary heart disease, severe hypotension, or other conditions where a drop in blood pressure may be undesirable, Promazine should be used with caution. Intra-arterial injection of Promazine is contraindicated.

Promazine is contraindicated in patients known to be sensitive to Promazine. Bone marrow depression is also a contraindication.

WARNINGS
The drug is not recommended for use in children under 12 years of age.

The use of alcohol should be avoided since there may be additive effects and hypotension. The sedative effect of Promazine is a desirable action under most circumstances; however, in certain cases the drug may cause undesirable drowsiness. Drowsiness will usually disappear on continued therapy or can be controlled by decreasing the dose.

Promazine may impair the mental and/or physical abilities required for the performance of potentially hazardous tasks, such as driving a car or operating machinery, especially during the first few days of therapy.

The recommended parenteral route of administration is by intramuscular injection. Promazine Hydrochloride 50 mg/mL, is not recommended for use by the intravenous route. Under no circumstances should intra-arterial injections be given.

TARDIVE DYSKINESIA
Tardive dyskinesia, a syndrome consisting of potentially irreversible, involuntary, dyskinetic movements, may develop in patients treated with neuroleptic (antipsychotic) drugs. Although the prevalence of the syndrome appears to be highest among the elderly, especially elderly women, it is impossible to rely upon prevalence estimates to predict, at the inception of neuroleptic treatment, which patients are likely to develop the syndrome. Whether neuroleptic drug products differ in their potential to cause tardive dyskinesia is unknown.

Both the risk of developing the syndrome and the likelihood that it will become irreversible are believed to increase as the duration of treatment and the total cumulative dose of neuroleptic drugs administered to the patient increase. However, the syndrome can develop, although much less commonly, after relatively brief treatment periods at low doses.

There is no known treatment for established cases of tardive dyskinesia, although the syndrome may remit, partially or completely, if neuroleptic treatment is withdrawn. Neuroleptic treatment, itself, however, may suppress (or partially suppress) the signs and symptoms of the syndrome and thereby may possibly mask the underlying disease process. The effect that symptomatic suppression has upon the long-term course of the syndrome is unknown. Given these considerations, neuroleptics should be prescribed in a manner that is most likely to minimize the occurrence of tardive dyskinesia. Chronic neuroleptic treatment should generally be reserved for patients who suffer from a chronic illness that 1) is known to respond to neuroleptic drugs and 2) for whom alternative, equally effective, but potentially less harmful treatments are *not* available or appropriate. In patients who do require chronic treatment, the smallest dose and the shortest duration of treatment producing a satisfactory clinical response should be sought. The need for continued treatment should be reassessed periodically.

If signs and symptoms of tardive dyskinesia appear in a patient on neuroleptics, drug discontinuation should be considered. However, some patients may require treatment despite the presence of the syndrome.

(For further information about the description of tardive dyskinesia and its clinical detection, please refer to the section on "Adverse Reactions".)

NEUROLEPTIC MALIGNANT SYNDROME (NMS)
A potentially fatal symptom complex sometimes referred to as Neuroleptic Malignant Syndrome (NMS) has been reported in association with antipsychotic drugs. Clinical manifestations of NMS are hyperpyrexia, muscle rigidity, altered mental status, and evidence of autonomic instability (irregular pulse or blood pressure, tachycardia, diaphoresis, and cardiac dysrhythmias).

The diagnostic evaluation of patients with this syndrome is complicated. In arriving at a diagnosis, it is important to identify cases where the clinical presentation includes both serious medical illness (e.g., pneumonia, systemic infection, etc.) and untreated or inadequately treated extrapyramidal signs and symptoms (EPS). Other important considerations in the differential diagnosis include central anticholinergic toxicity, heat stroke, drug fever, and primary central nervous system (CNS) pathology.

The management of NMS should include 1) immediate discontinuation of antipsychotic drugs and other drugs not essential to concurrent therapy, 2) intensive symptomatic treatment and medical monitoring, and 3) treatment of any concomitant serious medical problems for which specific treatments are available. There is no general agreement about specific pharmacological treatment regimens for uncomplicated NMS.

If a patient requires antipsychotic drug treatment after recovery from NMS, the potential reintroduction of drug therapy should be carefully considered. The patient should be carefully monitored, since recurrences of NMS have been reported.

USAGE IN PREGNANCY
Safe use of Promazine in pregnancy has not been established; therefore, it should be given to pregnant patients, nursing mothers, or women of childbearing potential only when the expected benefits outweigh the possible hazards to mother and child. Adequate animal-reproduction studies have not been done.

PRECAUTIONS
Patients with history of epilepsy should be treated with phenothiazine compounds only when such therapy is absolutely necessary. In such cases adequate anticonvulsant therapy should be given concomitantly.

Promazine may potentiate the effects of organic phosphates found in certain insecticides.

Promazine must be used with caution in persons exposed to extreme heat and administered cautiously to persons with cardiovascular or liver disease.

It should be kept in mind that the antiemetic effect may mask toxicity of other drugs or obscure other diagnoses, such as gastrointestinal obstruction. Promazine should be given with caution to patients who are suffering from respiratory impairment due to acute pulmonary infections or chronic respiratory disorders, such as severe asthma or emphysema.

ADDITIVE EFFECT
Promazine prolongs and intensifies the central nervous system depressant action of anesthetic barbiturates and narcotics; ¼ to ½ the usual dose of these drugs is required when Promazine is administered concomitantly. When the additive effect is not desired, such depressants should be discontinued before starting Promazine therapy.

◆ RATED THERAPEUTICALLY EQUIVALENT; ◇ THERAPEUTIC EQUIVALENCE UNCONFIRMED; ○ UNRATED

Promazine should also be used with caution in persons receiving atropine or related drugs, since phenothiazine have occasionally been shown to potentiate anticholinergic drugs.

ABRUPT WITHDRAWAL
In general, phenothiazines (including Promazine) do not produce psychic dependence.

However, gastritis, nausea and vomiting, dizziness, and tremulousness have been reported following abrupt cessation of high-dose therapy. Reports suggest that these symptoms can be reduced if concomitant antiparkinson agents are continued for several weeks after the phenothiazine is withdrawn.

ADVERSE REACTIONS
Note: Not all of the following adverse reactions have occurred with this specific drug, but pharmacological similarities among the various phenothiazine derivatives require that each be considered when Promazine is administered.

Note: Sudden death has occasionally been reported in patients who have received phenothiazines. In some cases, death was apparently due to cardiac arrest. In others, the cause appeared to be asphyxia due to the failure of the cough reflex. In others, the cause could not be determined, nor could it be established that death was due to the administration of the phenothiazine.

DROWSINESS
The sedative effect of Promazine is a desirable action under most circumstances; however, in certain cases the drug may cause undesirable drowsiness. Drowsiness will usually disappear on continued therapy or can be controlled by decreasing the dose.

JAUNDICE
Overall incidence is low. This is generally regarded as a sensitivity reaction and usually occurs during the early weeks of therapy. The clinical picture resembles infectious hepatitis, but the liver-function-test results mimic those of hepatic obstruction. There is no conclusive evidence that preexisting liver disease makes patients more susceptible to jaundice. It is usually reversible on withdrawal of the phenothiazine, though chronic jaundice has been reported.

HEMATOLOGIC DISORDERS
Include agranulocytosis, eosinophilia, leukopenia, hemolytic anemia, thrombocytopenic purpura, and pancytopenia; though rare, have been reported.

AGRANULOCYTOSIS
Most cases have occurred between the 4th and 10th week of therapy. Patients should be watched closely during that period for the sudden appearance of signs of infection, such as sore throat. If white-blood-cell count and differential smears give an indication of significant cellular depression, discontinue the drug and start appropriate therapy. However, a slightly lowered white count in itself is not necessarily an indication for immediate discontinuance of the drug.

CARDIOVASCULAR
TRANSITORY POSTURAL HYPOTENSION HAS BEEN NOTED IN A FEW PATIENTS, USUALLY FOLLOWING THE FIRST PARENTERAL DOSE, PARTICULARLY WHEN GIVEN INTRAVENOUSLY AND RELATED TO THE RATE OF ADMINISTRATION. WHEN THIS HAPPENED, RECOVERY WAS SPONTANEOUS AND THE SYMPTOMS OF WEAKNESS AND DIZZINESS DISAPPEARED. RARELY, PARTICULARLY IN ALCOHOLICS, THE DOSAGE HAD TO BE DECREASED OR THE DRUG DISCONTINUED. IT IS DESIRABLE TO KEEP PATIENTS UNDER OBSERVATION (PREFERABLY IN BED) FOR A SHORT TIME AFTER THE INITIAL DOSE.

Should hypotension occur, it can usually be controlled by placing the patient in a recumbent position with head lowered and legs elevated. Administration of oxygen may also be advisable. Occasionally, the effects are severe and prolonged, producing a shocklike condition.

IF IT IS DESIRABLE TO ADMINISTER A VASOPRESSOR DRUG, NOREPINEPHRINE APPEARS TO BE THE MOST SUITABLE. EPINEPHRINE SHOULD NOT BE USED, BECAUSE PROMAZINE HYDROCHLORIDE MAY REVERSE ITS ACTION, CAUSING A FURTHER LOWERING OF BLOOD PRESSURE INSTEAD OF ITS USUAL ELEVATING EFFECT.

EKG changes, nonspecific, usually reversible, have been observed in some patients receiving phenothiazines. The relationship to myocardial damage has not been confirmed. When the patient's blood pressure has returned to normal, Promazine therapy may be resumed at a lower dosage level.

CNS EFFECT
Extrapyramidal symptoms, including pseudoparkinsonism, dysarthria, and dyskinetic disturbances, have been reported following the use of large doses of Promazine, as in hospitalized mental patients. These symptoms are reversible and may be managed by reducing the dose or the addition of antiparkinsonism drugs; if severe, Promazine therapy should be discontinued.

In rare instances, persistent dyskinesia, usually involving the face, tongue, and jaw, has been reported to be irreversible, particularly in elderly patients with previous brain damage. Hyperreflexia has been reported in the newborn when a phenothiazine was used during pregnancy.

ADVERSE BEHAVIORAL EFFECTS
Paradoxical exacerbation of psychotic symptoms.

OTHER CNS EFFECTS
Cerebral edema, abnormality of CSF protein, convulsive seizures, particularly in patients with EEG abnormalities or a history of seizures.

ALLERGIC REACTION
Allergic skin reactions, including dermatitis, dry skin, and edema, have been reported in rare instances during the use of Promazine. The incidence is considerably lower than that reported for chlorpromazine.

Mild urticaria and photosensitivity are seen. To minimize, avoid undue exposure to sunlight. Nursing personnel sensitive to phenothiazines should exercise caution when handling these compounds and thus avoid contact dermatitis.

Evidence has become available to indicate a relationship between phenothiazine therapy and the occurrence of systemic lupus erythematosuslike syndrome.

ENDOCRINE DISORDERS
Lactation, moderate breast engorgement, and amenorrhea in females and gynecomastia in males may necessitate a lower dosage or withdrawal of the drug. False-positive pregnancy tests have been reported but are less likely to occur when a serum test is used. Hyperglycemia, hypoglycemia, and glycosuria have been reported.

AUTONOMIC REACTIONS
Autonomic reactions, such as dryness of the mouth, may occur, particularly when large oral doses are administered over prolonged periods of time.

Nasal congestion, constipation, adynamic ileus, miosis, and mydriasis have been reported with other phenothiazines.

PERSISTENT TARDIVE DYSKINESIA
As with all antipsychotic agents, tardive dyskinesia may appear in some patients on long-term therapy or may occur after drug therapy has been discontinued. However, the syndrome can develop, although much less commonly, after relatively brief treatment periods at low doses. The risk appears to be greater in elderly patients on high-dose therapy, especially females. The symptoms are persistent and in some patients appear irreversible. The syndrome is characterized by rhythmical involuntary movements of the tongue, face, mouth, or jaw (e.g., protrusion of tongue, puffing of cheeks, puckering of mouth, chewing movements). Sometimes these may be accompanied by involuntary movements of extremities. There is no known effective treatment for tardive dyskinesia; antiparkinsonism agents usually do not alleviate the symptoms of the syndrome. It is suggested that all antipsychotic agents be discontinued, if clinically feasible, if these symptoms appear. Should it be necessary to reinstitute treatment, or increase the dosage of the agent, or switch to a different antipsychotic agent, this syndrome may be masked.

It has been reported that fine, vermicular movements of the tongue may be an early sign of the syndrome, and if the medication is stopped at that time the syndrome may not develop.

OTHER ADVERSE REACTIONS
Mild fever may occur after large intramuscular doses. Increase in appetite and weight sometimes occurs. Reactions occurring with other phenothiazines have included ocular changes and changes related to skin pigmentation; such reactions should be kept in mind during the administration of Promazine even though they have not been noted with this agent to date. The etiology of these reactions is not clear, but exposure to light, along with dosage/duration of therapy, appears to be the most significant factor. If any of these reactions is observed, the physician should weigh the benefits of continued therapy against the possible risks and, on the merits of the individual case, determine whether or not to continue present therapy, lower the dosage, or withdraw the drug.

NEUROLEPTIC MALIGNANT SYNDROME (NMS)
(See *"Warnings"* section.)

OVERDOSAGE
One of three clinical pictures may be seen—

1. Extreme somnolence; patient can usually be roused with prodding, but if permitted will fall asleep. General condition is usually satisfactory. The skin, though pale, is warm and dry.

Slight blood pressure, respiratory, and pulse changes may occur but are not problems.

2. Mild-to-moderate drop in blood pressure (whether the patient is conscious or unconscious). Skin is markedly gray but warm and dry. Nail beds are pink. Respiration is slow and regular. Pulse is strong but rate slightly increased.

3. Severe hypotension, possibly accompanied by weakness, cyanosis, perspiration, rapid thready pulse, and respiratory depression.

Treatment is essentially symptomatic and supportive. Early gastric lavage and intestinal purges may help. Centrally acting emetics will not help because of the antiemetic effect of Promazine. Give hot coffee or tea.

Severe hypotension usually responds to measures described under hypotensive effects.

Additional measures include pressure bandages to lower limbs, oxygen, and IV fluids.

Avoid stimulants that may cause convulsion (e.g., picrotoxin and pentylenetetrazol).

Limited experience with dialysis indicates that it is not helpful.

DOSAGE AND ADMINISTRATION
Parenteral drug products should be inspected visually for particulate matter and discoloration prior to administration, whenever solution and container permit.

The amount, route of administration, and frequency of dose should be governed by the severity of the condition treated and the response of the patient. For maximal therapeutic benefit, dosage must be individualized for the patient.

The oral route of administration should be used whenever possible, but when it is thought that the effect obtained by oral dosage would not produce a sufficient response, it may be given parenterally, as for instance when nausea, vomiting, or lack of cooperation is evident.

The recommended parenteral route of administration is by intramuscular injection. Promazine Hydrochloride, 50 mg/mL, is not recommended for use by the intravenous route. Under no circumstances should intra-arterial injections be given. In general, intramuscular administration should be reserved for bedfast patients, although acute states in ambulatory patients may also be treated by intramuscular injection, provided proper precautions are taken to eliminate the possibility of postural hypotension. It is important to make sure that intramuscular injections are given deeply into large muscle masses, i.e., gluteal region.

MENTAL AND EMOTIONAL DISTURBANCES
The dosage of Promazine Hydrochloride for either acute or chronic mental disease will vary with the severity of the condition.

In the management of severely agitated patients, it is recommended that Promazine Hydrochloride be given intramuscularly in initial doses of 50 mg to 150 mg, depending on the degree of excitation. In general, these doses are sufficient, but if the desired calming effect is not apparent within 30 minutes, additional doses up to a total of 300 mg may be given. Once the desired control is obtained, Promazine Hydrochloride may then be given orally. The oral or intramuscular dose is 10 mg to 200 mg at 4- to 6-hour intervals, depending upon the response of the patient.

In less severe disturbances, dosage should be adjusted downward. Maintenance dosage may range from 10 mg to 200 mg, given at 4- to 6-hour intervals. The degree of central nervous system depression induced by Promazine Hydrochloride has not been great; however, in the acutely inebriated patient the initial dose should not exceed 50 mg, to be sure that the depressant effect of alcohol is not enhanced.

Note: THE PERCENTAGE OF EFFECTIVE RESULTS DOES NOT APPEAR TO BE MATERIALLY AFFECTED BY THE ADMINISTRATION OF DOSES IN EXCESS OF 800 MG TO 1,000 MG PER DAY. IT IS THEREFORE RECOMMENDED THAT THE TOTAL DAILY DOSE OF PROMAZINE HYDROCHLORIDE NOT EXCEED ONE (1) GRAM (1,000 MG).

DOSAGE IN CHILDREN
In acute episodes of chronic psychotic disease in children over 12, 10 to 25 mg every 4 to 6 hours.

Storage: Store at room temperature, approximately 25° C (77°F).
Protect from light.
Do not use if solution is discolored or contains a precipitate.

J CODES
Up to 25 mg IM—J2950

HOW SUPPLIED
INJECTION: 50 MG/ML

AVERAGE UNIT PRICE (AVAILABLE SIZES)

BRAND			$3.06

BRAND/MANUFACTURER	NDC	SIZE	AWP
◆ **BRAND**			
SPARINE: Wyeth-Ayerst	00008-0040-01	2 ml	$6.71
	00008-0040-02	10 ml	$27.66
◆ **GENERICS**			
Schein	00364-6668-54	10 ml	$4.13

TABLETS: 25 MG

BRAND/MANUFACTURER	NDC	SIZE	AWP
○ **BRAND**			
SPARINE: Wyeth-Ayerst	00008-0029-01	50s	$18.45

TABLETS: 50 MG

BRAND/MANUFACTURER	NDC	SIZE	AWP
○ **BRAND**			
SPARINE: Wyeth-Ayerst	00008-0028-01	50s	$22.43

Promethazine Hydrochloride

DESCRIPTION
Promethazine Hydrochloride is available as tablets, suppositories, syrup, and injection.

Each tablet contains:
Promethazine HCl ....12.5, 25, or 50 mg

Each rectal suppository contains:
Promethazine HCl ....12.5, 25, or 50 mg

Each teaspoonful (5 ml) of syrup contains:
Promethazine HCl ....6.25 or 25 mg

Each ml for injection contains:
Promethazine HCl ....25 or 50 mg

Promethazine hydrochloride is a racemic compound; the empirical formula is $C_{17}H_{20}N_2S \cdot HCl$ and its molecular weight is 320.88.

Promethazine HCl, a phenothiazine derivative, is designated chemically as N,N,α-trimethyl-10H-phenothiazine-10-ethanamine monohydrochloride.

Promethazine HCl occurs as a white to faint yellow, practically odorless, crystalline powder which slowly oxidizes and turns blue on prolonged exposure to air. It is soluble in water and freely soluble in alcohol.

Following is its chemical structure:

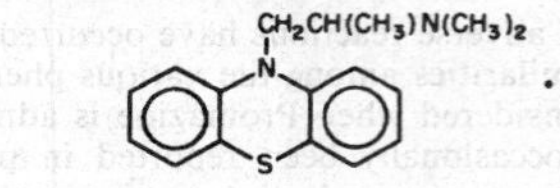

CLINICAL PHARMACOLOGY
Promethazine HCl is a phenothiazine derivative which differs structurally from the antipsychotic phenothiazines by the presence of a branched side chain and no ring substitution. It is thought that this configuration is responsible for its relative lack (1/10 that of chlorpromazine) of dopaminergic (CNS) action.

Promethazine HCl is an H_1 receptor blocking agent. As an antihistamine, it acts by competitive antagonism but does not block the release of histamine. It antagonizes in varying degrees most but not all of the pharmacological effects of histamine. In addition to its antihistaminic action, it provides clinically useful sedative, antimotion sickness, anticholinergic, and antiemetic effects. In therapeutic dosage, Promethazine produces no significant effects on the cardiovascular system.

Promethazine HCl is well absorbed from the gastrointestinal tract. Clinical effects are apparent within 20 minutes after oral administration and generally last four to six hours, although they may persist as long as 12 hours. The duration of action after injection is generally from four to six hours. Promethazine HCl is metabolized by the liver to a variety of compounds; the sulfoxides of Promethazine HCl and N-demethylpromethazine are the predominant metabolites appearing in the urine.

INDICATIONS AND USAGE
Promethazine HCl, is useful for: Perennial and seasonal allergic rhinitis (oral/rectal).

Vasomotor rhinitis (oral/rectal).

Allergic conjunctivitis due to inhalant allergens and foods (oral/rectal).

Mild, uncomplicated allergic skin manifestations of urticaria and angioedema (oral/rectal).

Amelioration of allergic reactions to blood or plasma.

Dermographism (oral/rectal).

Anaphylactic reactions, as adjunctive therapy to epinephrine and other standard measures, after the acute manifestations have been controlled.

For other uncomplicated allergic conditions of the immediate type when oral therapy is impossible or contraindicated.

Preoperative, postoperative, or obstetric sedation.

Prevention and control of nausea and vomiting associated with certain types of anesthesia and surgery.

Therapy adjunctive to meperidine or other analgesics for control of postoperative pain.

Sedation in both children and adults, as well as relief of apprehension and production of light sleep from which the patient can be easily aroused.

Active and prophylactic treatment of motion sickness (oral/rectal); active treatment of motion sickness (injection).

Antiemetic therapy in postoperative patients.

Intravenously in special surgical situations, such as repeated bronchoscopy, ophthalmic surgery, and poor-risk patients, with reduced amounts of meperidine or other narcotic analgesic as an adjunct to anesthesia and analgesia.

UNLABELED USES
Promethazine Hydrochloride is used alone or as an adjunct with intrauterine transfusions in the treatment of erythroblastosis fetalis. It is also used in the prevention of graft rejection, to increase sleep time in patients with insomnia, and to control levodopa-induced dyskinesia and nausea and vomiting.

CONTRAINDICATIONS
Promethazine HCl is contraindicated in individuals known to be hypersensitive or to have had an idiosyncratic reaction to Promethazine or to other phenothiazines.

Promethazine is contraindicated in comatose states, in patients who have received large amounts of central-nervous-system depressants (alcohol, sedative hypnotics, including barbiturates, general anesthetics, narcotics, narcotic analgesics, tranquilizers, etc.).

Antihistamines are contraindicated for use in the treatment of lower respiratory tract symptoms including asthma.

Under no circumstances should Promethazine be given by intra-arterial injection due to the likelihood of severe arteriospasm and the possibility of resultant gangrene (see *"Warnings"*).

Promethazine HCl injection should not be given by the subcutaneous route: evidence of chemical irritation has been noted, and necrotic lesions have resulted

---

◆ RATED THERAPEUTICALLY EQUIVALENT; ◇ THERAPEUTIC EQUIVALENCE UNCONFIRMED; ○ UNRATED

on rare occasions following subcutaneous injection. The preferred parenteral route of administration is by deep intramuscular injection.

WARNINGS

Promethazine may cause marked drowsiness. Ambulatory patients should be cautioned against such activities as driving or operating dangerous machinery until it is known that they do not become drowsy or dizzy from Promethazine therapy.

The sedative action of Promethazine Hydrochloride is additive to the sedative effects of central nervous system depressants; therefore, agents such as alcohol, narcotics, narcotic analgesics, sedatives, hypnotics (including barbiturates), general anesthetics, and tranquilizers should either be eliminated or given in reduced dosage in the presence of Promethazine Hydrochloride. When given concomitantly with Promethazine Hydrochloride, the dose of barbiturates should be reduced by at least one-half, and the dose of analgesic depressants, such as morphine or meperidine, should be reduced by one-quarter to one-half. Dosage must be individualized. Excessive amounts of Promethazine relative to a narcotic may lead to restlessness and motor hyperactivity in the patient with pain; these symptoms usually disappear with adequate control of the pain.

Promethazine HCl may lower seizure threshold. This should be taken into consideration when administering to persons with known seizure disorders or when giving in combination with narcotics and local anesthetics which may also affect seizure threshold.

Sedative drugs or CNS depressants should be avoided in patients with a history of sleep apnea.

Antihistamines should be used with caution in patients with narrow-angle glaucoma, stenosing peptic ulcer, pyloroduodenal obstruction, and urinary bladder obstruction due to symptomatic prostatic hypertrophy and narrowing of the bladder neck.

Administration of Promethazine has been associated with reported cholestatic jaundice.

Some brands of Promethazine HCl contain sodium metabisulfite, a sulfite that may cause allergic-type reactions, including anaphylactic symptoms and life-threatening or less severe asthmatic episodes, in certain susceptible people. The overall prevalence of sulfite sensitivity in the general population is unknown and probably low. Sulfite sensitivity is seen more frequently in asthmatic than in nonasthmatic people.

INADVERTENT INTRA-ARTERIAL INJECTION

Due to the close proximity of arteries and veins in the areas most commonly used for intravenous injection, extreme care should be exercised to avoid perivascular extravasation or inadvertent intra-arterial injection. Reports compatible with inadvertent intra-arterial injection of Promethazine usually in conjunction with other drugs intended for intravenous use, suggest that pain, severe chemical irritation, severe spasm of distal vessels, and resultant gangrene requiring amputation are likely under such circumstances. Intravenous injection was intended in all the cases reported, but perivascular extravasation or arterial placement of the needle is now suspect. There is no proven successful management of this condition after it occurs, although sympathetic block and heparinization are commonly employed during the acute management because of the results of animal experiments with other known arteriolar irritants. Aspiration of dark blood does not preclude intra-arterial needle placement, because blood is discolored upon contact with Promethazine HCl. Use of syringes with rigid plungers or of small bore needles might obscure typical arterial backflow if this is relied upon alone.

When used intravenously, Promethazine HCl should be given in a concentration no greater than 25 mg per mL and at a rate not to exceed 25 mg per minute. When administering any irritant drug intravenously, it is usually preferable to inject it through the tubing of an intravenous infusion set that is known to be functioning satisfactorily. In the event that a patient complains of pain during intended intravenous injection of Promethazine HCl the injection should immediately be stopped to provide for evaluation of possible arterial placement or perivascular extravasation.

PRECAUTIONS

GENERAL

Promethazine HCl should be used cautiously in persons with cardiovascular disease or with impairment of liver function.

Drugs having anticholinergic properties should be used with caution in patients with asthmatic attack, narrow-angle glaucoma, prostatic hypertrophy, stenosing peptic ulcer, pyloroduodenal obstruction, and bladder-neck obstruction. Promethazine HCl should be used with caution in patients with bone-marrow depression. Leukopenia and agranulocytosis have been reported, usually when Promethazine HCl has been used in association with other known toxic agents.

INFORMATION FOR PATIENTS

Promethazine HCl may cause marked drowsiness or impair the mental and/or physical abilities required for the performance of potentially hazardous tasks, such as driving a vehicle or operating machinery. Ambulatory patients should be told to avoid engaging in such activities until it is known that they do not become drowsy or dizzy from Promethazine HCl therapy. Children should be supervised to avoid potential harm in bike riding or in other hazardous activities.

The concomitant use of alcohol or other central nervous system depressants, including narcotic analgesics, sedatives, hypnotics, and tranquilizers, may have an additive effect and should be avoided or their dosage reduced.

Patients should be advised to report any involuntary muscle movements or unusual sensitivity to sunlight.

DRUG INTERACTIONS

The sedative action of Promethazine is additive to the sedative effects of other central nervous system depressants, including alcohol, narcotic analgesics, sedatives, hypnotics, tricyclic antidepressants, and tranquilizers; therefore, these agents should be avoided or administered in reduced dosage to patients receiving Promethazine.

Drug interactions, including an increased incidence of extrapyramidal effects, have been reported when some MAOI and phenothiazines are used concomitantly. Although such a reaction has not been reported with Promethazine HCl, the possibility should be considered.

DRUG/LABORATORY TEST INTERACTIONS

The following laboratory tests may be affected in patients who are receiving therapy with Promethazine:

Pregnancy Tests: Diagnostic pregnancy tests based on immunological reactions between HCG and anti-HCG may result in false-negative or false-positive interpretations.

Glucose Tolerance Test: An increase in blood glucose has been reported in patients receiving Promethazine.

CARCINOGENESIS, MUTAGENESIS, IMPAIRMENT OF FERTILITY

Long-term animal studies have not been performed to assess the carcinogenic potential of Promethazine, nor are there other animal or human data concerning carcinogenicity, mutagenicity, or impairment of fertility with this drug. Promethazine was nonmutagenic in the *Salmonella* test system of Ames.

PREGNANCY

Teratogenic Effects—Pregnancy Category C: Teratogenic effects have not been demonstrated in rat-feeding studies at doses of 6.25 and 12.5 mg/kg of Promethazine. These doses are from approximately 2.1 to 4.2 times the maximum recommended total daily dose of Promethazine for a 50-kg subject, depending upon the indication for which the drug is prescribed. Specific studies to test the action of the drug on parturition, lactation, and development of the animal neonate were not done, but a general preliminary study in rats indicated no effect on these parameters. Although antihistamines, including Promethazine, have been found to produce fetal mortality in rodents, the pharmacological effects of histamine in the rodent do not parallel those in man. There are no adequate and well-controlled studies of Promethazine in pregnant women. Promethazine HCl should be used during pregnancy only if the potential benefit justifies the potential risk to the fetus.

Nonteratogenic Effects: Promethazine taken within two weeks of delivery may inhibit platelet aggregation in the newborn.

LABOR AND DELIVERY

Promethazine HCl, in appropriate dosage form, may be used alone or as an adjunct to narcotic analgesics during labor and delivery. (See *"Indications and Usage"* and *"Dosage and Administration"*.)

See also *"Nonteratogenic Effects"*.

NURSING MOTHERS

It is not known whether Promethazine is excreted in human milk. Caution should be exercised when Promethazine is administered to a nursing woman.

PEDIATRIC USE

This product should not be used in children under 2 years of age because safety for such use has not been established.

Excessively large dosages of antihistamines, including Promethazine HCl in children may cause hallucinations, convulsions, and sudden death. In children who are acutely ill associated with dehydration, there is an increased susceptibility to dystonias with the use of Promethazine injection.

ADVERSE REACTIONS

TABLETS, SUPPOSITORIES, SYRUP

Nervous System: Sedation, sleepiness, occasional blurred vision, dryness of mouth, dizziness; rarely confusion, disorientation, and extrapyramidal symptoms such as oculogyric crisis, torticollis, and tongue protrusion (usually in association with parenteral injection or excessive dosage).

Cardiovascular: Increased or decreased blood pressure.

Dermatologic: Rash, rarely photosensitivity.

Hematologic: Rarely leukopenia, thrombocytopenia; agranulocytosis (1 case).

Gastrointestinal: Nausea and vomiting.

INJECTION

CNS Effects: Drowsiness is the most prominent CNS effect of this drug.

Extrapyramidal reactions may occur with high doses; this is almost always responsive to a reduction in dosage. Other reported reactions include dizziness, lassitude, tinnitus, incoordination, fatigue, blurred vision, euphoria, diplopia, nervousness, insomnia, tremors, convulsive seizures, oculogyric crises, excitation, catatonic-like states, and hysteria.

Cardiovascular Effects: Tachycardia, bradycardia, faintness, dizziness, and increases and decreases in blood pressure have been reported following the use of Promethazine Hydrochloride injection. Venous thrombosis at the injection site has been reported. INTRA-ARTERIAL INJECTION MAY RESULT IN GANGRENE OF THE AFFECTED EXTREMITY (see *"Warnings"*).

Gastrointestinal: Nausea and vomiting have been reported, usually in association with surgical procedures and combination drug therapy.

Allergic Reactions: These include urticaria, dermatitis, asthma, and photosensitivity. Angioneurotic edema has been reported.

Other Reported Reactions: Leukopenia and agranulocytosis, usually when Promethazine HCl has been used in association with other known toxic agents, have been reported. Thrombocytopenic purpura and jaundice of the obstructive type have been associated with the use of Promethazine. The jaundice is usually reversible on discontinuation of the drug. Subcutaneous injection has resulted in tissue necrosis. Nasal stuffiness may occur. Dry mouth has been reported.

OVERDOSAGE

Signs and symptoms of overdosage with Promethazine range from mild depression of the central nervous system and cardiovascular system to profound hypotension, respiratory depression, and unconsciousness.

Stimulation may be evident, especially in children and geriatric patients. Convulsions may rarely occur. A paradoxical reaction has been reported in children receiving single doses of 75 mg to 125 mg orally, characterized by hyperexcitability, abnormal movements, delirium, agitated behavior, and nightmares. Consideration should be given to discontinuing Promethazine and using other drugs.

Atropinelike signs and symptoms—dry mouth, fixed, dilated pupils, flushing, as well as gastrointestinal symptoms, may occur.

TREATMENT

Treatment of overdosage is essentially symptomatic and supportive. Early gastric lavage may be beneficial if Promethazine has been taken orally. Centrally acting emetics are of little use. Only in cases of extreme overdosage or individual sensitivity do vital signs, including respiration, pulse, blood pressure, temperature, and EKG, need to be monitored. Activated charcoal orally or by lavage may be given, or sodium or magnesium sulfate orally as a cathartic. Attention should be given to the reestablishment of adequate respiratory exchange through provision of a patent airway and institution of assisted or controlled ventilation. Diazepam may be used to control convulsions. Acidosis and electrolyte losses should be corrected. Note that any depressant effects of Promethazine are not reversed by naloxone. Avoid analeptics which may cause convulsions.

Severe hypotension usually responds to the administration of norepinephrine or phenylephrine. *Epinephrine Should Not Be Used*, since its use in patients with partial adrenergic blockade may further lower the blood pressure. Extrapyramidal reactions may be treated with anticholinergic antiparkinson agents, diphenhydramine, or barbiturates. Additional measures include oxygen and intravenous fluids.

Limited experience with dialysis indicates that it is not helpful.

DOSAGE AND ADMINISTRATION

TABLETS, SUPPOSITORIES, SYRUP

Allergy: The average oral dose is 25 mg taken before retiring; however, 12.5 mg may be taken before meals and on retiring, if necessary. Children tolerate this product well. Single 25-mg doses at bedtime or 6.25 to 12.5 mg taken three times daily will usually suffice. After initiation of treatment in children or adults, dosage should be adjusted to the smallest amount adequate to relieve symptoms. Promethazine HCl suppositories may be used if the oral route is not feasible, but oral therapy should be resumed as soon as possible if continued therapy is indicated. The administration of Promethazine HCl in 25-mg doses will control minor transfusion reactions of an allergic nature.

Motion Sickness: The average adult dose is 25 mg taken twice daily. The initial dose should be taken one-half to one hour before anticipated travel and be repeated 8 to 12 hours later, if necessary. On succeeding days of travel, it is recommended that 25 mg be given on arising and again before the evening meal. For children, Promethazine HCl tablets, syrup, or rectal suppositories, 12.5 to 25 mg, twice daily, may be administered.

Nausea and Vomiting: The average effective dose of Promethazine HCl for the active therapy of nausea and vomiting in children or adults is 25 mg. When oral medication cannot be tolerated, the dose should be given parenterally or by rectal suppository. 12.5- to 25-mg doses may be repeated as necessary at 4- to 6-hour intervals.

For nausea and vomiting in children, the usual dose is 0.5 mg per pound of body weight, and the dose should be adjusted to the age and weight of the patient and the severity of the condition being treated.

For prophylaxis of nausea and vomiting, as during surgery and the postoperative period, the average dose is 25 mg repeated at 4- to 6-hour intervals, as necessary.

Sedation: This product relieves apprehension and induces a quiet sleep from which the patient can be easily aroused. Administration of 12.5 to 25 mg Promethazine HCl by the oral route or by rectal suppository at bedtime will provide sedation in children. Adults usually require 25 to 50 mg for nighttime, presurgical, or obstetrical sedation.

Pre- and Postoperative Use: Promethazine HCl in 12.5- to 25-mg doses for children and 50-mg doses for adults the night before surgery relieves apprehension and produces a quiet sleep.

For preoperative medication children require doses of 0.5 mg per pound of body weight in combination with an equal dose of meperidine and the appropriate dose of an atropinelike drug.

Usual adult dosage is 50 mg Promethazine HCl with an equal amount of meperidine and the required amount of a bella-donna alkaloid.

Postoperative sedation and adjunctive use with analgesics may be obtained by the administration of 12.5 to 25 mg in children and 25- to 50-mg doses in adults.

Promethazine HCl tablets, suppositories, and syrup are not recommended for children under 2 years of age.

INJECTION

The preferred parenteral route of administration for Promethazine HCl is by deep intramuscular injection. The proper intravenous administration of this product is well tolerated, but use of this route is not without some hazard.

INADVERTENT INTRA-ARTERIAL INJECTION CAN RESULT IN GANGRENE OF THE AFFECTED EXTREMITY (see *"Warnings"*). SUBCUTANEOUS INJECTION IS CONTRAINDICATED, AS IT MAY RESULT IN TISSUE NECROSIS (see *"Contraindications"*). When used intravenously, Promethazine HCl should be given in concentration no greater than 25 mg/mL at a rate not to exceed 25 mg per minute; it is preferable to inject through the tubing of an intravenous infusion set that is known to be functioning satisfactorily.

Allergic Conditions: The average adult parenteral dose is 25 mg. This dose may be repeated within two hours if necessary, but continued therapy, if indicated, should be via the oral route as soon as existing circumstances permit. After initiation of treatment, dosage should be adjusted to the smallest amount adequate to relieve symptoms. The average adult dose for amelioration of allergic reactions to blood or plasma is 25 mg.

Sedation: In hospitalized adult patients, nighttime sedation may be achieved by a dose of 25 to 50 mg of Promethazine HCl.

Pre- and Postoperative Use: As an adjunct to pre- or postoperative medication, 25 to 50 mg of Promethazine HCl in adults may be combined with appropriately reduced doses of analgesics and atropine-like drugs as desired. Dosage of concomitant analgesic or hypnotic medication should be reduced accordingly.

Nausea and Vomiting: For control of nausea and vomiting, the usual adult dose is 12.5 to 25 mg, not to be repeated more frequently than every four hours. When used for control of postoperative nausea and vomiting, the medication may be administered either intramuscularly or intravenously and dosage of analgesics and barbiturates reduced accordingly.

Obstetrics: Promethazine HCl in doses of 50 mg will provide sedation and relieve apprehension in the early stages of labor. When labor is definitely established, 25 to 75 mg (average dose, 50 mg Promethazine HCl may be given intramuscularly or intravenously with an appropriately reduced dose of any desired narcotic. Amnesic agents may be administered as necessary. If necessary, Promethazine HCl with a reduced dose of analgesic may be repeated once or twice at four-hour intervals in the course of a normal labor. A maximum total dose of 100 mg of Promethazine HCl may be administered during a 24-hour period to patients in labor.

Children: In children under the age of 12 years, the dosage should not exceed half that of the suggested adult dose. As an adjunct to premedication, the suggested dose is 0.5 mg per lb. of body weight in combination with an equal dose of narcotic or barbiturate and the appropriate dose of an atropine-like drug. Antiemetics should not be used in vomiting of unknown etiology in children.

Parenteral drug products should be inspected visually for particulate matter and discoloration prior to administration, whenever solution and container permit.

STORAGE

Tablets: Keep tablets in tightly closed bottles.
  Store at room temperature, between 15°C and 25°C (59°F and 77°F).
  Protect from light.
  Dispense in light-resistant, tight container.
  Use carton to protect contents from light.

Suppositories: Store refrigerated 2°-8°C (36°-46°F).
  Dispense in well-closed container.

Syrup: Keep bottles tightly closed.
  Store at room temperature, between 15° C and 25° C (59° F and 77° F).
  Protect from light.
  Dispense in light-resistant, glass, tight containers.

Injection: Store at room temperature between 15°C-25°C (59°F-77°F).
  Protect from light.
  Do not use if solution is discolored or contains a precipitate.

J CODES

Up to 50 mg IM,IV—J2550

HOW SUPPLIED
INJECTION: 25 MG/ML

AVERAGE UNIT PRICE (AVAILABLE SIZES)		GENERIC A-RATED AVERAGE PRICE (GAAP)	
BRAND	$1.16	10 ml	$7.50
GENERIC	$0.71		

BRAND/MANUFACTURER	NDC	SIZE	AWP
◆ BRAND			
PHENERGAN: Wyeth-Ayerst	00008-0416-01	1 ml 10s	$15.53
	00008-0063-01	1 ml 25s	$19.24

◆ RATED THERAPEUTICALLY EQUIVALENT; ◇ THERAPEUTIC EQUIVALENCE UNCONFIRMED; ○ UNRATED

BRAND/MANUFACTURER	NDC	SIZE	AWP
◆ GENERICS			
Schein	00364-6570-54	10 ml	$5.17
Steris	00402-0258-10	10 ml	$5.17
PROREX: Hyrex	00314-0684-70	10 ml	$6.90
Rugby	00536-8451-70	10 ml	$9.75
Goldline	00182-0774-63	10 ml	$10.50
Elkins-Sinn	00641-1495-35	1 ml 25s	$12.74

INJECTION: 50 MG/ML

AVERAGE UNIT PRICE (AVAILABLE SIZES)		GENERIC A-RATED AVERAGE PRICE (GAAP)	
BRAND	$1.41	10 ml	$8.53
GENERIC	$0.83		

BRAND/MANUFACTURER	NDC	SIZE	AWP
◆ BRAND			
PHENERGAN: Wyeth-Ayerst	00008-0417-01	1 ml 10s	$18.68
	00008-0746-01	1 ml 25s	$23.79
◆ GENERICS			
Schein	00364-6571-54	10 ml	$5.55
Steris	00402-0259-10	10 ml	$5.55
Genl Inject	52584-0259-10	10 ml	$6.57
Insource	58441-1114-01	10 ml	$6.57
PROREX: Hyrex	00314-0685-70	10 ml	$7.10
Moore,H.L.	00839-5158-30	10 ml	$7.41
Goldline	00182-0501-63	10 ml	$11.55
Rugby	00536-8460-70	10 ml	$11.85
PHENOJECT-50: Mayrand	00259-0308-10	10 ml	$14.65
Elkins-Sinn	00641-1496-35	1 ml 25s	$16.00

SUPPOSITORY: 12.5 MG

BRAND/MANUFACTURER	NDC	SIZE	AWP
◇ BRAND			
▶ PHENERGAN: Wyeth-Ayerst	00008-0498-01	12s	$25.94

SUPPOSITORY: 25 MG

BRAND/MANUFACTURER	NDC	SIZE	AWP
◇ BRAND			
▶ PHENERGAN: Wyeth-Ayerst	00008-0212-01	12s	$29.76

SUPPOSITORY: 50 MG

BRAND/MANUFACTURER	NDC	SIZE	AWP
◇ BRAND			
PROMETHEGAN: G&W	00713-0132-12	12s	$35.00
▶ PHENERGAN: Wyeth-Ayerst	00008-0229-01	12s	$38.11
◇ GENERICS			
Cheshire	55175-0242-04	4s	$14.64
Cheshire	55175-0242-06	6s	$17.15
Rugby	00536-7405-12	12s	$28.00
Major	00904-1290-12	12s	$37.45

SYRUP: 6.25 MG/5 ML

AVERAGE UNIT PRICE (AVAILABLE SIZES)		GENERIC A-RATED AVERAGE PRICE (GAAP)	
BRAND	$0.04	480 ml	$16.30
GENERIC	$0.01	3840 ml	$16.30
HCFA FUL (480 ml)	$0.01	120 ml	$2.41
		480 ml	$5.14
		3840 ml	$32.05

BRAND/MANUFACTURER	NDC	SIZE	AWP
◆ BRAND			
PHENERGAN: Wyeth-Ayerst	00008-0549-01	120 ml	$2.48
	00008-0549-03	480 ml	$20.81
	00008-0549-02	120 ml 24s	$133.95
◆ GENERICS			
Cenci,H.R.	00556-0365-04	120 ml	$2.10
Moore,H.L.	00839-6314-65	120 ml	$2.16
Morton Grove	60432-0608-04	120 ml	$2.20
Barre	00472-1504-04	120 ml	$2.25
Aligen	00405-3600-76	120 ml	$2.35
Rugby	00536-1745-97	120 ml	$2.40

BRAND/MANUFACTURER	NDC	SIZE	AWP
Major	00904-1508-00	120 ml	$2.40
Major	00904-1508-20	120 ml	$2.40
Geneva	00781-6575-04	120 ml	$3.44
Schein	00364-0733-16	480 ml	$4.50
Cenci,H.R.	00556-0365-16	480 ml	$4.50
Qualitest	00603-1580-58	480 ml	$4.56
Moore,H.L.	00839-6314-69	480 ml	$4.79
Morton Grove	60432-0608-16	480 ml	$4.80
Rugby	00536-1745-85	480 ml	$4.88
Major	00904-1508-16	480 ml	$4.95
Aligen	00405-3600-16	480 ml	$5.43
Goldline	00182-1737-40	480 ml	$5.70
Barre	00472-1504-16	480 ml	$5.85
Geneva	00781-6575-16	480 ml	$6.30
Moore,H.L.	00839-6314-70	3840 ml	$24.96
Rugby	00536-1745-90	3840 ml	$27.71
Cenci,H.R.	00556-0365-28	3840 ml	$28.80
Major	00904-1508-28	3840 ml	$29.20
Goldline	00182-1737-41	3840 ml	$31.50
Barre	00472-1504-28	3840 ml	$35.90
Geneva	00781-6575-28	3840 ml	$41.93

SYRUP: 25 MG/5 ML

BRAND/MANUFACTURER	NDC	SIZE	AWP
◆ BRAND			
PHENERGAN: Wyeth-Ayerst	00008-0231-01	480 ml	$43.35

TABLET: 12.5 MG

BRAND/MANUFACTURER	NDC	SIZE	AWP
◇ BRAND			
▶ PHENERGAN: Wyeth-Ayerst	00008-0019-01	100s	$17.26

TABLET: 25 MG

BRAND/MANUFACTURER	NDC	SIZE	AWP
◇ BRAND			
▶ PHENERGAN: Wyeth-Ayerst	00008-0027-02	100s	$30.49
	00008-0027-07	100s	$31.00
◇ GENERICS			
Moore,H.L.	00839-1535-06	100s	$2.55
Richlyn	00115-4306-01	100s	$3.02
Schein	00364-0222-01	100s	$3.69
Geneva	00781-1830-01	100s	$3.96
Raway	00686-1540-13	100s ud	$6.15
Vangard	00615-1540-13	100s ud	$9.49
Moore,H.L.	00839-1535-16	1000s	$14.43
Richlyn	00115-4306-03	1000s	$23.25
Schein	00364-0222-02	1000s	$24.72
Geneva	00781-1830-10	1000s	$28.80

TABLET: 50 MG

BRAND/MANUFACTURER	NDC	SIZE	AWP
◇ BRAND			
▶ PHENERGAN: Wyeth-Ayerst	00008-0227-01	100s	$46.74
◇ GENERICS			
Schein	00364-0345-01	100s	$5.96
Geneva	00781-1832-01	100s	$5.98

Promethegan SEE PROMETHAZINE HYDROCHLORIDE

Pronestyl SEE PROCAINAMIDE HYDROCHLORIDE

Propafenone Hydrochloride

DESCRIPTION
Propafenone Hydrochloride is an antiarrhythmic drug. Propafenone has some structural similarities to beta-blocking agents.

The structural formula of Propafenone Hydrochloride is given below:

Propafenone Hydrochloride occurs as colorless crystals or white crystalline powder with a very bitter taste and has a molecular weight of 377.92. It is slightly soluble in water (20°C), chloroform and ethanol.

▶ SHOWN IN PRODUCT IDENTIFICATION GUIDE

Following is its chemical structure:

CLINICAL PHARMACOLOGY

MECHANISM OF ACTION

Propafenone HCl is a Class IC antiarrhythmic drug with local anesthetic effects, and a direct stabilizing action on myocardial membranes. The electrophysiological effect of Propafenone HCl manifests itself in a reduction of upstroke velocity (Phase 0) of the monophasic action potential. In Purkinje fibers, and to a lesser extent myocardial fibers, Propafenone HCl reduces the fast inward current carried by sodium ions. Diastolic excitability threshold is increased and effective refractory period prolonged. Propafenone HCl reduces spontaneous automaticity and depresses triggered activity. Studies in anesthetized dogs and isolated organ preparations show that Propafenone HCl has beta-sympatholytic activity at about 1/50 the potency of propranolol. Clinical studies employing isoproterenol challenge and exercise testing after single doses of Propafenone indicate a beta-adrenergic blocking potency (per mg) about 1/40 that of propranolol in man. In clinical trials, resting heart rate decreases of about 8% were noted at the higher end of the therapeutic plasma concentration range. At very high concentrations *in vitro*, Propafenone HCl can inhibit the slow inward current carried by calcium but this calcium antagonist effect probably does not contribute to antiarrhythmic efficacy. Propafenone HCl has local anesthetic activity approximately equal to procaine.

ELECTROPHYSIOLOGY

Electrophysiology studies in patients with ventricular tachycardia have shown that Propafenone HCl prolongs atrioventricular conduction while having little or no effect on sinus node function. Both AV nodal conduction time (AH interval) and His-Purkinje conduction time (HV interval) are prolonged. Propafenone has little or no effect on the atrial functional refractory period, but AV nodal functional and effective refractory periods are prolonged. In patients with WPW, Propafenone HCl reduces conduction and increases the effect refractory period of the accessory pathway in both directions. Propafenone HCl slows conduction and consequently produces dose-related changes in the PR interval and QRS duration. QT_c interval, does not change. (See related table).

In any individual patient, the above ECG changes cannot be readily used to predict either efficacy or plasma concentration.

Propafenone HCl causes a dose-related and concentration-related decrease in the rate of single and multiple PVCs and can suppress recurrence of ventricular tachycardia. Based on the percent of patients attaining substantial (80-90%) suppression of ventricular ectopic activity, it appears that trough plasma levels of 0.2 to 1.5 μg/mL can provide good suppression, with higher concentrations giving a greater rate of good response.

HEMODYNAMICS

Sympathetic stimulation may be a vital component supporting circulatory function in patients with congestive heart failure and its inhibition by the beta blockade produced by Propafenone HCl may in itself aggravate congestive heart failure. Additionally, like other Class IC antiarrhythmic drugs, studies in humans have shown that Propafenone HCl exerts a negative inotropic effect on the myocardium. Cardiac catheterization studies in patients with moderately impaired ventricular function (mean C.I. = 2.61 L/min/m2) utilizing intravenous Propafenone infusions (2 mg/kg over 10 min + 2 mg/min for 30 min) that gave mean plasma concentrations of 3.0 μ/mL (well above the therapeutic range of 0.2-1.5 μ/mL) showed significant increases in pulmonary capillary wedge pressure, systemic and pulmonary vascular resistances and depression of cardiac output and cardiac index.

PHARMACOKINETICS AND METABOLISM

Propafenone HCl is nearly completely absorbed after oral administration with peak plasma levels occurring approximately 3.5 hours after administration in most individuals. Propafenone HCl exhibits extensive saturable presystemic biotransformation (first pass effect) resulting in a dose dependent and dosage form dependent absolute bioavailability; e.g., a 150 mg tablet had absolute bioavailability of 3.4%, while a 300 mg tablet had absolute bioavailability of 10.6%. A 300 mg solution which was rapidly absorbed, had absolute bioavailability of 21.4%. At still larger doses, above those recommended, bioavailability increases still further. Decreased liver function also increases bioavailability;

bioavailability is inversely related to indocyanine green clearance reaching 60-70% at clearances of 7 mL/min and below. The clearance of Propafenone HCl is reduced and the elimination half-life increased in patients with significant hepatic dysfunction (see "*Precautions*").

Propafenone HCl follows a nonlinear pharmacokinetic disposition presumably due to saturation of first pass hepatic metabolism as the liver is exposed to higher concentrations of Propafenone HCl and shows a very high degree of interindividual variability. For example, for a three-fold increase in daily dose from 300 to 900 mg/day there is a ten-fold increase in steady-state plasma concentration. The top 25% of patients given 375 mg/day, however, had a mean concentration of Propafenone HCl larger than the bottom 25%, and about equal to the second 25%, of patients given a dose of 900 mg. Although food increased peak blood level and bioavailability in a single dose study, during multiple dose administration of Propafenone HCl to healthy volunteers food did not change bioavailability significantly.

There are two genetically determined patterns of Propafenone HCl metabolism. In over 90% of patients, the drug is rapidly and extensively metabolized with an elimination half-life from 2-10 hours. These patients metabolize Propafenone HCl into two active metabolites: 5-hydroxypropafenone and N-depropylpropafenone. *In vitro* preparations have shown these two metabolites to have antiarrhythmic activity comparable to Propafenone HCl, but in man they both are usually present in concentrations less than 20% of Propafenone HCl. Nine additional metabolites have been identified, most in only trace amounts. It is the saturable hydroxylation pathway that is responsible for the nonlinear pharmacokinetic disposition. In less than 10% of patients (and in any patient also receiving quinidine, see "*Precautions*") metabolism of Propafenone HCl is slower because the 5-hydroxy metabolite is not formed or is minimally formed. The estimated Propafenone HCl elimination half-life ranges from 10-32 hours. Decreased ability to form the 5-hydroxy metabolite of Propafenone HCl is associated with a diminished ability to metabolize debrisoquine and a variety of other drugs (encainide, metoprolol, dextromethorphan). In these patients, the N-depropyl-propafenone occurs in quantities comparable to the levels occurring in extensive metabolizers. In slow metabolizers Propafenone HCl pharmacokinetics are linear.

There are significant differences in plasma concentrations of Propafenone HCl in slow and extensive metabolizers, the former achieving concentrations 1.5 to 2.0 times those of the extensive metabolizers at daily doses of 675-900 mg/day. At low doses the differences are greater, with slow metabolizers attaining concentrations more than five times that of extensive metabolizers. Because the difference decreases at high doses and is mitigated by the lack of the active 5-hydroxy metabolite in the slow metabolizers, and because steady-state conditions are achieved after 4-5 days of dosing in all patients, the recommended dosing regimen is the same for all patients. The greater variability in blood levels requires that the drug be titrated carefully in all patients with close attention to clinical and ECG evidence of toxicity (see "*Dosage and Administration*").

INDICATIONS AND USAGE

Propafenone HCl is indicated for the treatment of documented ventricular arrhythmias, such as sustained ventricular tachycardia, that, in the judgment of the physician are life-threatening. Because of the proarrhythmic effects of Propafenone HCl, its use with lesser arrhythmias is generally not recommended. Treatment of patients with asymptomatic ventricular premature contractions should be avoided.

Initiation of Propafenone HCl treatment, as with other antiarrhythmic agents used to treat life-threatening arrhythmias, should be carried out in the hospital. Antiarrhythmic drugs have not been shown to enhance survival in patients with ventricular arrhythmias.

UNLABELED USES

Propafenone HCl is used in the treatment of atrial fibrillation.

CONTRAINDICATIONS

Propafenone HCl is contraindicated in the presence of uncontrolled congestive heart failure, cardiogenic shock, sinoatrial, atrioventricular and intraventricular disorders of impulse generation and/or conduction (e.g., sick sinus node syndrome, atrioventricular block) in the absence of an artificial pacemaker, bradycardia, marked hypotension, bronchospastic disorders, manifest electrolyte imbalance, and known hypersensitivity to the drug.

WARNINGS

MORTALITY

In the National Heart, Lung and Blood Institute's Cardiac Arrhythmia Suppression Trial (CAST), a long-term, multicentered, randomized, double-blind study in patients with asymptomatic non-life-threatening arrhythmias who had had myocardial infarctions more than six days but less than two years previously, an excessive mortality or non-fatal cardiac arrest rate was seen in patients treated

MEAN CHANGES IN ECG INTERVALS* TOTAL DAILY DOSE (MG)

Interval	337.5 mg		450 mg		675 mg		900 mg	
	msec	(%)	msec	(%)	msec	(%)	msec	(%)
RR	−14.5	−1.8	30.6	3.8	31.5	3.9	41.7	5.1
PR	3.6	2.1	19.1	11.6	28.9	17.8	35.6	21.9
QRS	5.6	6.4	5.5	6.1	7.7	8.4	15.6	17.3
QT_c	2.7	0.7	−7.5	−1.8	5.0	1.2	14.7	3.7

* *Change and percent change based on mean baseline values for each treatment group.*

♦ RATED THERAPEUTICALLY EQUIVALENT; ◇ THERAPEUTIC EQUIVALENCE UNCONFIRMED; ○ UNRATED

with encainide or flecainide (56/730) compared with that seen in patients assigned to matched placebo-treated groups (22/725). The average duration of treatment with encainide or flecainide in this study was ten months.

The applicability of these results to other populations (e.g., those without recent myocardial infarctions) or to other antiarrhythmic drugs is uncertain, but at present it is prudent to consider any antiarrhythmic agent to have a significant risk in patients with structural heart disease.

PROARRHYTHMIC EFFECTS
Propafenone HCl, like other antiarrhythmic agents, may cause new or worsened arrhythmias. Such proarrhythmic effects range from an increase in frequency of PVCs to the development of more severe ventricular tachycardia, ventricular fibrillation or torsade de pointes: i.e., tachycardia that is more sustained or more rapid which may lead to fatal consequences. It is therefore essential that each patient given Propafenone HCl be evaluated electrocardiographically and clinically prior to, and during therapy to determine whether the response to Propafenone HCl supports continued treatment.

Overall in clinical trials with Propafenone HCl, 4.7% of all patients had new or worsened ventricular arrhythmia possibly representing a proarrhythmic event (0.7% was an increase in PVCs; 4.0% a worsening, or new appearance, of VT or VF). Of the patients who had a worsening of VT (4%), 92% had a history of VT and/or VT/VF, 71% had coronary artery disease, and 68% had a prior myocardial infarction. The incidence of proarrhythmia in patients with less serious or benign arrhythmias, which include patients with an increase in frequency of PVCs, was 1.6%. Although most proarrhythmic events occurred during the first week of therapy, late events also were seen and the CAST study (see above) suggests that an increased risk is present throughout treatment.

NONALLERGIC BRONCHOSPASM (E.G., CHRONIC BRONCHITIS, EMPHYSEMA)
Patients with bronchospastic disease should in general not receive Propafenone HCl or other agents with beta-adrenergic-blocking activity.

CONGESTIVE HEART FAILURE
During treatment with oral Propafenone HCl in patients with depressed baseline function (mean EF = 33.5%), no significant decreases in ejection fraction were seen. In clinical trial experience, new or worsened CHF has been reported in 3.7% of patients; of those, 0.9% were considered probably or definitely related to Propafenone HCl. Of the patients with congestive heart failure probably related to Propafenone HCl, 80% had preexisting heart failure and 85% had coronary artery disease. CHF attributable to Propafenone HCl developed rarely (< 0.2%) in patients who had no previous history of CHF. As Propafenone HCl exerts both beta blockade and a (dose-related) negative inotropic effect on cardiac muscle, patients with congestive heart failure should be fully compensated before receiving Propafenone HCl. If congestive heart failure worsens, Propafenone HCl should be discontinued (unless congestive heart failure is due to the cardiac arrhythmia) and, if indicated, restarted at a lower dosage only after adequate cardiac compensation has been established.

CONDUCTION DISTURBANCES
Propafenone HCl slows atrioventricular conduction and also causes first degree AV block. Average PR interval prolongation and increases in QRS duration are closely correlated with dosage increases and concomitant increases in Propafenone HCl plasma concentrations. The incidence of first degree, second degree, and third degree AV block observed in 2,127 patients was 2.5%, 0.6%, and 0.2%, respectively. Development of second or third degree AV block requires a reduction in dosage or discontinuation of Propafenone HCl. Bundle branch block (1.2%) and intraventricular conduction delay (1.1%) have been reported in patients receiving Propafenone HCl. Bradycardia has also been reported (1.5%). Experience in patients with sick sinus node syndrome is limited and these patients should not be treated with Propafenone HCl.

EFFECTS ON PACEMAKER THRESHOLD
Propafenone HCl may alter both pacing and sensing thresholds of artificial pacemakers. Pacemakers should be monitored and programmed accordingly during therapy.

HEMATOLOGIC DISTURBANCES
One case of agranulocytosis with fever and sepsis, probably related to the use of Propafenone HCl, was seen in U.S. clinical trials. The agranulocytosis appeared after 8 weeks of therapy. Propafenone HCl therapy was stopped and the white count had normalized by 14 days. The patient recovered. In the course of over 800,000 patient years of exposure during marketing outside the U.S. since 1978, seven additional cases have been reported. In one of these, concomitant captopril, a drug known to cause agranulocytosis, was used. Unexplained fever and/or decrease in white cell count, particularly during the first three months of therapy, warrant consideration of possible agranulocytosis/granulocytopenia. Patients should be instructed to promptly report the development of any signs of infection such as fever, sore throat, or chills.

PRECAUTIONS
HEPATIC DYSFUNCTION
Propafenone HCl is highly metabolized by the liver and should, therefore, be administered cautiously to patients with impaired hepatic function. Severe liver dysfunction increases the bioavailability of Propafenone HCl to approximately 70% compared to 3-40% for patients with normal liver function. In eight patients with moderate to severe liver disease, the mean half-life was approximately 9 hours. As a result, the dose of Propafenone HCl given to patients with impaired

hepatic function should be approximately 20-30% of the dose given to patients with normal hepatic function (see *"Dosage and Administration"*). Careful monitoring for excessive pharmacological effects (see *"Overdosage"*) should be carried out.

RENAL DYSFUNCTION
A considerable percentage of Propafenone HCl metabolites (18.5%-38% of the dose/48 hours) are excreted in the urine. Until further data are available, Propafenone HCl should be administered cautiously to patients with impaired renal function. These patients should be carefully monitored for signs of overdosage (see *"Overdosage"*).

ELEVATED ANA TITERS
Positive ANA titers have been reported in patients receiving Propafenone HCl. They have been reversible upon cessation of treatment and may disappear even in the face of continued Propafenone HCl therapy. These laboratory findings were usually not associated with clinical symptoms, but there is one published case of drug-induced lupus erythematosus (positive rechallenge); it resolved completely upon discontinuation of therapy. Patients who develop an abnormal ANA test should be carefully evaluated and, if persistent or worsening elevation of ANA titers is detected, consideration should be given to discontinuing therapy.

IMPAIRED SPERMATOGENESIS
Reversible disorders of spermatogenesis have been demonstrated in monkeys, dogs and rabbits after high dose intravenous administration. Evaluation of the effects of short-term Propafenone HCl administration on spermatogenesis in 11 normal subjects suggests that Propafenone HCl produced a reversible, short-term drop (within normal range) in sperm count. Subsequent evaluation in 11 patients receiving Propafenone HCl chronically have suggested no effect of Propafenone HCl on sperm count.

DRUG INTERACTIONS
Quinidine: Small doses of quinidine completely inhibit the hydroxylation metabolic pathway, making all patients, in effect, slow metabolizers (see *"Clinical Pharmacology"*). There is, as yet, too little information to recommend concomitant use of Propafenone HCl and quinidine.

Local Anesthetics: Concomitant use of local anesthetics (i.e., during pacemaker implantations, surgery, or dental use) may increase the risks of central nervous system side effects.

Digitalis: Propafenone HCl produces dose-related increases in serum digoxin levels ranging from about 35% at 450 mg/day to 85% at 900 mg/day of Propafenone HCl without affecting digoxin renal clearance. These elevations of digoxin levels were maintained for up to 16 months during concomitant administration. Plasma digoxin levels of patients on concomitant therapy should be measured, and digoxin dosage should ordinarily be reduced when Propafenone HCl is started, especially if a relatively large digoxin dose is used or if plasma concentrations are relatively high.

Beta-Antagonists: In a study involving healthy subjects, concomitant administration of Propafenone HCl and propranolol has resulted in substantial increases in propranolol plasma concentration and elimination half-life with no change in Propafenone HCl plasma levels from control values. Similar observations have been reported with metoprolol. Propafenone HCl appears to inhibit the hydroxylation pathway for the two beta-antagonists (just as quinidine inhibits Propafenone HCl metabolism). Increased plasma concentrations of metoprolol could overcome its relative cardioselectivity. In Propafenone HCl clinical trials, patients who were receiving beta-blockers concurrently did not experience an increased incidence of side effects. While the therapeutic range for beta-blockers is wide, a reduction in dosage may be necessary during concomitant administration with Propafenone HCl.

Warfarin: In a study of eight healthy subjects receiving Propafenone HCl and warfarin concomitantly, mean steady-state warfarin plasma concentrations increased 39% with a corresponding increase in prothrombin times of approximately 25%. It is therefore recommended that prothrombin times be routinely monitored and the dose of warfarin be adjusted if necessary.

Cimetidine: Concomitant administration of Propafenone HCl and cimetidine in 12 healthy subjects resulted in a 20% increase in steady-state plasma concentrations of Propafenone HCl with no detectable changes in electrocardiographic parameters beyond that measured on Propafenone HCl alone.

Other: Limited experience with Propafenone HCl combined with calcium antagonists and diuretics has been reported without evidence of clinically significant adverse reactions.

Carcinogenesis, Mutagenesis, Impairment of Fertility: Lifetime maximally tolerated oral dose studies in mice (up to 360 mg/kg/day) and rats (up to 270 mg/kg/day) provided no evidence of a carcinogenic potential for Propafenone HCl. Propafenone HCl was not mutagenic when assayed for genotoxicity in 1) mouse Dominant Lethal test, 2) rat bone marrow Chromosome Analysis, 3) Chinese hamster bone marrow and spermatogonia chromosome analysis, 4) Chinese hamster micronucleus test, and 5) Ames bacterial test.

Propafenone HCl administered intravenously to rabbits, dogs, and monkeys has been shown to decrease spermatogenesis. These effects were reversible, were not found following oral dosing of Propafenone HCl, were seen only at lethal or sublethal dose levels and were not seen in rats treated either orally or intravenously (see *"Precautions, Impaired Spermatogenesis"*). Propafenone HCl did not affect either male or female fertility rates when administered intravenously to rats and rabbits at dose levels up to 18 times the maximum recommended daily human dose of 900 mg (based on 60 kg human body weight).

Pregnancy-Teratogenic Effects: Pregnancy Category C: Propafenone HCl has has been shown to be embryotoxic in rabbits and rats when given in doses 10 and 40 times, respectively, the maximum recommended human dose. No teratogenic potential was apparent in either species. There are no adequate and well-controlled studies in pregnant women. Propafenone HCl should be used during pregnancy only if the potential benefit justifies the potential risk to the fetus.

Pregnancy-Nonteratogenic Effects: In a perinatal and postnatal study in rats, Propafenone HCl, at dose levels of 6 or more times the maximum recommended human dose, produced dose dependent increases in maternal and neonatal mortality, decreased maternal and pup body weight gain and reduced neonatal physiologic development.

Labor and Delivery: It is not known whether the use of Propafenone HCl during labor or delivery has immediate or delayed adverse effects on the fetus, or whether it prolongs the duration of labor or increases the need for forceps delivery or other obstetrical intervention.

Nursing Mothers: It is not known whether this drug is excreted in human milk. Because many drugs are excreted in human milk and because of the potential for serious adverse reactions in nursing infants from Propafenone HCl, a decision should be made whether to discontinue nursing or to discontinue the drug, taking into account the importance of the drug to the mother.

Pediatric Use: The safety and efficacy of Propafenone HCl in children has not been established.

Geriatric Use: There do not appear to be any age-related differences in adverse reaction rates in the most commonly reported adverse reactions. Because of the possible increased risk of impaired hepatic or renal function in this age group, Propafenone HCl should be used with caution. The effective dose may be lower in these patients.

Animal Toxicology: Renal changes have been observed in the rat following 6 months of oral administration of Propafenone HCl at doses of 180 and 360 mg/kg/day (12-24 times the maximum recommended human dose) but not 90 mg/kg/day. Both inflammatory and noninflammatory changes in the renal tubules with accompanying interstitial nephritis were observed. These lesions were reversible in that they were not found in rats treated at these dosage levels and allowed to recover for 6 weeks. Fatty degenerative changes of the liver were found in rats following chronic administration of Propafenone HCl at dose levels 19 times the maximum recommended human dose.

ADVERSE REACTIONS

Adverse reactions associated with Propafenone HCl occur most frequently in the gastrointestinal, cardiovascular, and central nervous systems. About 20% of patients discontinued due to adverse reactions. Results of controlled trials comparing adverse reaction rates on Propafenone HCl and placebo, and on Propafenone HCl and quinidine are shown in the following table. Adverse reactions appearing in the table were reported for ≥ 1% of the patients receiving Propafenone HCl. The most common events were dizziness, unusual taste, first degree AV block, intraventricular conduction delay, nausea and/or vomiting, and constipation. Headache was relatively common also, but was not increased compared to placebo. (See related table).

Adverse reactions reported for ≥ 1% of 2127 patients who received Propafenone HCl in U.S. clinical trials are presented in the following table by Propafenone HCl daily dose. The most common adverse reactions in controlled clinical trials appeared dose related (but note that most patients spent more time at the larger doses), especially dizziness, unusual taste, nausea and/or vomiting, constipation, and blurred vision. Some less common reactions may also have been dose related such as first degree AV block, congestive heart failure, dyspepsia, and weakness. The principal causes of discontinuation were the most common events and are shown in the table. (See related tables.)

In addition, the following adverse reactions were reported less frequently than 1% either in clinical trials or in marketing experience (*adverse events for marketing experience are given in italics*). Causality and relationship to Propafenone HCl therapy cannot necessarily be judged from these events.

Cardiovascular System: Atrial flutter, AV dissociation, cardiac arrest, flushing, hot flashes, sick sinus syndrome, sinus pause or arrest, supraventricular tachycardia.

Nervous System: Abnormal dreams, abnormal speech, abnormal vision, *apnea, coma,* confusion, depression, memory loss, numbness, paresthesias, psychosis/mania, seizures (0.3%), tinnitus, unusual smell sensation, vertigo.

Gastrointestinal: A number of patients with liver abnormalities associated with Propafenone HCl therapy have been reported in foreign post-marketing experience. Some appeared due to hepatocellular injury, some were cholestatic and some showed a mixed picture. Some of these reports were simply discovered through clinical chemistries, others because of clinical symptoms. One case was rechallenged with a positive outcome.
  Cholestasis (0.2%), elevated liver enzymes (alkaline phosphatase, serum transaminases) (0.2%), gastroenteritis, hepatitis (0.03%)

Hematologic: Agranulocytosis, anemia, bruising, granulocytopenia, *increased bleeding time,* leukopenia, purpura, thrombocytopenia

Other: Alopecia, eye irritation, *hyponatremia/inappropriate ADH secretion,* impotence, increased glucose, *kidney failure,* positive ANA (0.7%), *lupus erythematosus,* muscle cramps, muscle weakness, nephrotic syndrome, pain, pruritus.

OVERDOSAGE

The symptoms of overdosage, which are usually most severe within 3 hours of ingestion, may include hypotension, somnolence, bradycardia, intra-atrial and intraventricular conduction disturbances, and rarely convulsions and high grade ventricular arrhythmias. Defibrillation as well as infusion of dopamine and isoproterenol have been effective in controlling rhythm and blood pressure. Convulsions have been alleviated with intravenous diazepam. General supportive measures such as mechanical respiratory assistance and external cardiac message may be necessary.

ADVERSE REACTIONS REPORTED FOR ≥ 1% OF THE PATIENTS

	Prop./Placebo Trials		Prop./Quinidine Trial	
	Prop. (N = 247)	Placebo (N = 111)	Prop. (N = 53)	Quinidine (N = 52)
Unusual Taste	7.3%	0.9%	22.6%	0.0%
Dizziness	6.5%	5.4%	15.1%	9.6%
First Degree AV Block	4.5%	0.9%	1.9%	0.0%
Headache(s)	4.5%	4.5%	1.9%	7.7%
Constipation	4.0%	0.0%	5.7%	1.9%
Intraventricular Conduction Delay	4.0%	0.0%	—	—
Nausea and/or Vomiting	2.8%	0.9%	5.7%	15.4%
Fatigue	—	—	3.8%	1.9%
Palpitations	2.4%	0.9%	—	—
Blurred Vision	2.0%	0.9%	5.7%	1.9%
Dry Mouth	2.0%	0.9%	5.7%	5.8%
Dyspnea	2.0%	2.7%	3.8%	0.0%
Abdominal Pain/Cramps	—	—	1.9%	7.7%
Dyspepsia	—	—	1.9%	7.7%
Congestive Heart Failure	—	—	1.9%	1.9%
Fever	—	—	1.9%	9.6%
Tinnitus	—	—	1.9%	1.9%
Vision Abnormal	—	—	1.9%	1.9%
Esophagitis	—	—	1.9%	0.0%
Gastroenteritis	—	—	1.9%	0.0%
Anxiety	2.0%	1.8%	—	—
Anorexia	1.6%	0.9%	—	1.9%
Proarrhythmia	1.2%	0.0%	1.9%	0.0%
Flatulence	1.2%	0.0%	1.9%	0.0%
Angina	1.2%	0.0%	1.9%	3.8%
Second Degree AV Block	1.2%	0.0%	—	—
Bundle Branch Block	1.2%	0.0%	1.9%	1.9%
Loss of Balance	1.2%	0.0%	—	—
Diarrhea	1.2%	0.9%	5.7%	38.5%

◆ RATED THERAPEUTICALLY EQUIVALENT; ◇ THERAPEUTIC EQUIVALENCE UNCONFIRMED; ○ UNRATED

ADVERSE REACTIONS REPORTED FOR ≥ 1% OF THE PATIENTS N = 2127

Incidence by Total Daily Dose

	450 mg (N = 1430)	600 mg (N = 1337)	≥ 900 mg (N = 1333)	Total Incidence (N = 2127)	% of Pts. Who Discont.
Dizziness	3.6%	6.6%	11.0%	12.5%	2.4%
Nausea and/or Vomiting	2.4%	6.1%	8.9%	10.7%	3.4%
Unusual Taste	2.5%	4.9%	6.3%	8.8%	0.7%
Constipation	2.0%	4.1%	5.3%	7.2%	0.5%
Fatigue	1.8%	2.8%	4.1%	6.0%	1.0%
Dyspnea	2.2%	2.3%	3.6%	5.3%	1.6%
Proarrhythmia	2.0%	2.1%	2.9%	4.7%	4.7%
Angina	1.7%	2.1%	3.2%	4.6%	0.5%
Headache(s)	1.5%	2.5%	2.8%	4.5%	1.0%
Blurred Vision	0.6%	2.4%	3.1%	3.8%	0.8%
CHF	0.8%	2.2%	2.6%	3.7%	1.4%
Ventricular Tachycardia	1.4%	1.6%	2.9%	3.4%	1.2%
Dyspepsia	1.3%	1.7%	2.5%	3.4%	0.9%
Palpitations	0.6%	1.6%	2.6%	3.4%	0.5%
Rash	0.6%	1.4%	1.9%	2.6%	0.8%
AV Block, First Degree	0.8%	1.2%	2.1%	2.5%	0.3%
Diarrhea	0.5%	1.6%	1.7%	2.5%	0.6%
Weakness	0.6%	1.6%	1.7%	2.4%	0.7%
Dry Mouth	0.9%	1.0%	1.4%	2.4%	0.2%
Syncope/Near Syncope	0.8%	1.3%	1.4%	2.2%	0.7%
QRS Duration, Increased	0.5%	0.9%	1.7%	1.9%	0.5%
Chest Pain	0.5%	0.7%	1.4%	1.8%	0.2%

ADVERSE REACTIONS REPORTED FOR ≥ 1% OF THE PATIENTS

N = 2127
Incidence by Total Daily Dose

	450 mg (N = 1430)	600 mg (N = 1337)	≥ 900 mg (N = 1333)	Total Incidence (N = 2127)	% of Pts. Who Discont.
Anorexia	0.5%	0.7%	1.6%	1.7%	0.4%
Abdominal Pain/Cramps	0.8%	0.9%	1.1%	1.7%	0.4%
Ataxia	0.3%	0.6%	1.5%	1.6%	0.2%
Insomnia	0.3%	1.3%	0.7%	1.5%	0.3%
Premature Ventricular Contraction(s)	0.6%	0.6%	1.1%	1.5%	0.1%
Bradycardia	0.5%	0.8%	1.1%	1.5%	0.5%
Anxiety	0.7%	0.5%	0.9%	1.5%	0.6%
Edema	0.6%	0.4%	1.0%	1.4%	0.2%
Tremor(s)	0.3%	0.8%	1.1%	1.4%	0.3%
Diaphoresis	0.6%	0.4%	1.1%	1.4%	0.3%
Bundle Branch Block	0.3%	0.7%	1.0%	1.2%	0.5%
Drowsiness	0.6%	0.5%	0.7%	1.2%	0.2%
Atrial Fibrillation	0.7%	0.7%	0.5%	1.2%	0.4%
Flatulence	0.3%	0.7%	0.9%	1.2%	0.1%
Hypotension	0.1%	0.5%	1.0%	1.1%	0.4%
Intraventricular Conduction Delay	0.2%	0.7%	0.9%	1.1%	0.1%
Pain, Joint(s)	0.2%	0.4%	0.9%	1.0%	0.1%

DOSAGE AND ADMINISTRATION

The dose of Propafenone HCl must be individually titrated on the basis of response and tolerance. It is recommended that therapy be initiated with 150 mg Propafenone HCl given every eight hours (450 mg/day). Dosage may be increased at a minimum of 3 to 4 day intervals to 225 mg every 8 hours (675 mg/day) and, if necessary, to 300 mg every 8 hours (900 mg/day). The usefulness and safety of dosages exceeding 900 mg per day have not been established. In those patients in whom significant widening of the QRS complex or second or third degree AV block occurs, dose reduction should be considered.

As with other antiarrhythmic agents, in the elderly or in patients with marked previous myocardial damage, the dose of Propafenone HCl should be increased more gradually during the initial phase of treatment.

Store at controlled room temperature, 59° to 86°F (15°-30°C). Dispense in tight, light-resistant container as defined in U.S.P.

HOW SUPPLIED
TABLETS: 150 MG

BRAND/MANUFACTURER	NDC	SIZE	AWP
○ **BRAND** RYTHMOL: Knoll	00044-5022-02	100s	$80.21
	00044-5022-10	100s ud	$84.20

TABLETS: 225 MG

BRAND/MANUFACTURER	NDC	SIZE	AWP
○ **BRAND** RYTHMOL: Knoll			
	00044-5024-02	100s	$114.34
	00044-5024-10	100s ud	$120.01

TABLETS: 300 MG

BRAND/MANUFACTURER	NDC	SIZE	AWP
○ **BRAND** RYTHMOL: Knoll			
	00044-5023-02	100s	$145.52
	00044-5023-10	100s ud	$152.81

Propantheline Bromide

DESCRIPTION

Propantheline Bromide oral tablets contain 15 mg or 7 ½ mg of the anticholinergic Propantheline Bromide, (2-hydroxyethyl)-diisopropylmethylammonium bromide xanthene-9-carboxylate.

Propantheline Bromide is very soluble in water, alcohol, and chloroform, but it is practically insoluble in ether and in benzene. Its molecular weight is 448.40.

Following is its chemical structure:

CLINICAL PHARMACOLOGY

Propantheline Bromide inhibits gastrointestinal motility and diminishes gastric acid secretion. The drug also inhibits the action of acetylcholine at the postganglionic nerve endings of the parasympathetic nervous system.

Propantheline Bromide is extensively metabolized in man primarily by hydrolysis to the inactive materials xanthene-9-carboxylic acid and (2-hydroxyethyl) diisopropylmethyl-ammonium bromide. After a single 30-mg oral dose given as two 15-mg tablets the mean peak plasma concentration of Propantheline Bromide was 21 ng/ml at one hour in six healthy subjects.

The plasma elimination half-life of Propantheline is about 1.6 hours. Approximately 70% of the dose is excreted in the urine, mostly as metabolites. The urinary excretion of Propantheline is about 3% after oral tablet administration.

INDICATIONS AND USAGE

Propantheline Bromide is effective as adjunctive therapy in the treatment of peptic ulcer.

UNLABELED USES
Propantheline is used alone or as an adjunct in the treatment of bladder instability, including detrusor hyperreflexia and detrusor instability causing urinary incontinence.

CONTRAINDICATIONS

Propantheline Bromide is contraindicated in patients with:

1. Glaucoma, since mydriasis is to be avoided.
2. Obstructive disease of the gastrointestinal tract (pyloroduodenal stenosis, achalasia, paralytic ileus, etc).
3. Obstructive uropathy (eg, bladder-neck obstruction due to prostatic hypertrophy).
4. Intestinal atony of elderly or debilitated patients.
5. Severe ulcerative colitis or toxic megacolon complicating ulcerative colitis.
6. Unstable cardiovascular adjustment in acute hemorrhage.
7. Myasthenia gravis.

WARNINGS

In the presence of a high environmental temperature, heat prostration (fever and heat stroke due to decreased sweating) can occur with the use of Propantheline Bromide.

Diarrhea may be an early symptom of incomplete intestinal obstruction, especially in patients with ileostomy or colostomy. In this instance treatment with Propantheline Bromide would be inappropriate and possibly harmful.

With overdosage, a curare-like action may occur (ie, neuromuscular blockade leading to muscular weakness and possible paralysis).

Propantheline Bromide may cause increased heart rate and, therefore, should be used with caution in patients with heart disease.

PRECAUTIONS

General: Propantheline Bromide should be used with caution in the elderly and in all patients with autonomic neuropathy, hepatic or renal disease, hyperthyroidism, coronary heart disease, congestive heart failure, cardiac tachyarrhythmias, hypertension, or hiatal hernia associated with reflux esophagitis, since anticholinergics may aggravate this condition.

In patients with ulcerative colitis, large doses of Propantheline Bromide may suppress intestinal motility to the point of producing paralytic ileus and, for this reason, may precipitate or aggravate toxic megacolon, a serious complication of the disease.

Information for Patients: Propantheline Bromide may produce drowsiness or blurred vision. The patient should be cautioned regarding activities requiring mental alertness, such as operating a motor vehicle or other machinery or performing hazardous work, while taking this drug.

Drug Interactions: Anticholinergics may delay absorption of other medication given concomitantly.

Excessive cholinergic blockade may occur if Propantheline Bromide is given concomitantly with belladonna alkaloids, synthetic or semisynthetic anticholinergic agents, narcotic analgesics such as meperidine, Type 1 antiarrhythmic drugs (eg, disopyramide, procainamide, or quinidine), antihistamines, phenothiazines, tricyclic antidepressants, or other psychoactive drugs. Propantheline Bromide may also potentiate the sedative effect of phenothiazines. Increased intraocular pressure may result from concurrent administration of anticholinergics and corticosteroids.

Concurrent use of Propantheline Bromide with slow-dissolving tablets of digoxin may cause increased serum digoxin levels. This interaction can be avoided by using only those digoxin tablets that rapidly dissolve by USP standards.

Carcinogenesis, Mutagenesis, Impairment of Fertility: No long-term fertility, carcinogenicity, or mutagenicity studies have been done with Propantheline Bromide.

Pregnancy: Pregnancy Category C. Animal reproduction studies have not been conducted with Propantheline Bromide. It is also not known whether Propantheline Bromide can cause fetal harm when administered to a pregnant woman or can affect reproduction capacity. Propantheline Bromide should be given to a pregnant woman only if clearly needed.

Nursing mothers: It is not known whether this drug is excreted in human milk. Because many drugs are excreted in human milk, caution should be exercised when Propantheline Bromide is administered to a nursing woman. Suppression of lactation may occur with anticholinergic drugs.

Pediatric use: Safety and effectiveness in children have not been established.

ADVERSE REACTIONS

Varying degrees of drying of salivary secretions may occur as well as decreased sweating. Ophthalmic side effects include blurred vision, mydriasis, cycloplegia, and increased ocular tension. Other reported adverse reactions include urinary hesitancy and retention, tachycardia, palpitations, loss of the sense of taste, headache, nervousness, mental confusion, drowsiness, weakness, dizziness, insomnia, nausea, vomiting, constipation, bloated feeling, impotence, suppression of lactation, and allergic reactions or drug idiosyncrasies, including anaphylaxis, urticaria, and other dermal manifestations.

OVERDOSAGE

The symptoms of overdosage with Propantheline Bromide progress from an intensification of the usual side effects to CNS disturbances (from restlessness and excitement to psychotic behavior), circulatory changes (flushing, fall in blood pressure, circulatory failure), respiratory failure; paralysis, and coma.

Measures to be taken are (1) immediate induction of emesis or lavage of the stomach, (2) injection of physostigmine 0.5 to 2 mg intravenously, repeated as necessary up to a total of 5 mg, and (3) monitoring of vital signs and managing as necessary.

Fever may be treated symptomatically (cooling blanket or alcohol sponging). Excitement of a degree which demands attention may be managed with thiopental sodium 2% solution given slowly intravenously, or diazepam, 5 to 10 mg intravenously or 10 mg intramuscularly. In the event of progression of the curare-like effect to paralysis of the respiratory muscles, mechanical respiration should be instituted and maintained until effective respiratory action returns. The oral LD_{50} of Propantheline Bromide is 780 mg/kg in the mouse and 370 mg/kg in the rat.

DOSAGE AND ADMINISTRATION

The usual initial adult dosage of Propantheline Bromide tablets is 15 mg taken 30 minutes before each meal and 30 mg at bedtime (a total of 75 mg daily). Subsequent dosage adjustment should be made according to the patient's individual response and tolerance. The administration of one 7½-mg tablet three times a day is convenient for patients with mild manifestations, for geriatric patients, and for those of small stature.

Store below 86°F (30°C).

HOW SUPPLIED
CAPSULE: 15 MG

BRAND/MANUFACTURER	NDC	SIZE	AWP
◆ **GENERICS**			
U.S. Trading	56126-0393-11	100s ud	$15.55

TABLETS: 7.5 MG

BRAND/MANUFACTURER	NDC	SIZE	AWP
○ **BRAND**			
PRO-BANTHINE: Roberts Pharm	54092-0073-01	100s	$40.28

TABLETS: 15 MG

AVERAGE UNIT PRICE (AVAILABLE SIZES)		GENERIC A-RATED AVERAGE PRICE (GAAP)	
GENERIC	$0.20	100s	$21.03
HCFA FUL (100s ea)	$0.17	500s	$97.79
		1000s	$130.58

BRAND/MANUFACTURER	NDC	SIZE	AWP
◆ **GENERICS**			
Richlyn	00115-4308-01	100s	$12.93
Rugby	00536-4338-01	100s	$19.62
Major	00904-2344-60	100s	$20.25
Roxane	00054-4721-25	100s	$21.53
URL	00677-1207-01	100s	$22.18
Goldline	00182-1858-01	100s	$22.45
Par	49884-0118-01	100s	$22.95
Aligen	00405-4879-01	100s	$23.38
Martec	52555-0118-01	100s	$23.40
Moore,H.L.	00839-1545-06	100s	$24.10
Roxane	00054-8737-25	100s ud	$18.51
Rugby	00536-4338-05	500s	$86.00
Major	00904-2344-40	500s	$96.40
Aligen	00405-4879-02	500s	$100.76
Par	49884-0118-05	500s	$108.00
Richlyn	00115-4308-03	1000s	$99.45
Roxane	00054-4721-31	1000s	$161.70

◆ RATED THERAPEUTICALLY EQUIVALENT; ◇ THERAPEUTIC EQUIVALENCE UNCONFIRMED; ○ UNRATED

TABLETS: 15 MG

BRAND/MANUFACTURER	NDC	SIZE	AWP
○ BRAND			
PRO-BANTHINE: Roberts Pharm	54092-0074-01	100s	$61.37
	54092-0074-52	100s ud	$66.54
	54092-0074-05	500s	$288.03

Proparacaine Hydrochloride

DESCRIPTION

Proparacaine Hydrochloride is a topical anesthetic prepared as a sterile aqueous ophthalmic solution.

The chemical name is Benzoic acid, 3-amino-4-propoxy-,2-(diethylamino) ethyl ester, monohydrochloride.

Each mL contains: Proparacaine Hydrochloride 0.5% (5 mg).

Following is its chemical structure:

$$CH_3CH_2CH_2O - \bigotimes - COOCH_2CH_2N(C_2H_5)_2 \cdot HCl$$
$$NH_2$$

CLINICAL PHARMACOLOGY

Proparacaine HCl solution is a rapid acting local anesthetic suitable for ophthalmic use. The onset of anesthesia usually begins within 30 seconds and persists for 15 minutes or longer.

The main site of anesthetic action is the nerve cell membrane where Proparacaine interferes with the large transient increase in the membrane permeability to sodium ions that is normally produced by a slight depolarization of the membrane. As the anesthetic action progressively develops in a nerve, the threshold for electrical stimulation gradually increases and the safety factor for conduction decreases; when this action is sufficiently well developed, block of conduction is produced.

The exact mechanism whereby Proparacaine and other local anesthetics influence the permeability of the cell membrane is unknown; however, several studies indicate that local anesthetics may limit sodium ion permeability through the lipid layer of the nerve cell membrane. This limitation prevents the fundamental change necessary for the generation of the action potential.

INDICATIONS AND USAGE

Proparacaine HCl solution is indicated for topical anesthesia in ophthalmic practice. Representative ophthalmic procedures in which the preparation provides good local anesthesia include measurement of intraocular pressure (tonometry), removal of foreign bodies and sutures from the cornea, conjunctival scraping in diagnosis and gonioscopic examination; it is also indicated for use as a topical anesthetic prior to surgical opertions such as cataract extraction.

CONTRAINDICATIONS

This preparation is contraindicated in patients with known hypersensitivity to any component of the solution. This product should never be prescribed for the patient's own use.

WARNINGS

For topical ophthalmic use only. Prolonged use of a topical ocular anesthetic may produce permanent corneal opacification with accompanying loss of vision.

PRECAUTIONS

General: Proparacaine HCL should be used cautiously and sparingly in patients with known allergies, cardiac disease, or hyperthyroidism. The long-term toxicity of Proparacaine is unknown, prolonged use may possibly delay wound healing. Although exceedingly rare with ophthalmic application of local anesthetics, it should be borne in mind that systemic toxicity (manifested by central nervous system stimulation followed by depression) may occur.

Protection of the eye from irritating chemicals, foreign bodies and rubbing during the period of anesthesia is very important. Tonometers soaked in sterilizing or detergent solutions should be thoroughly rinsed with sterile distilled water prior to use. Patients should be advised to avoid touching the eye until the anesthesia has worn off. Do not touch dropper tip to any surface as this may contaminate the solution.

Carcinogenesis, Mutagenesis, Impairment of Fertility: Long-term studies in animals have not been performed to evaluate carcinogenic potential, mutagencity, or possible impairment of fertility in males or females.

Pregnancy Category C: Animal reproduction studies have not been conducted with Proparacaine HCl solution. It is also not known whether Proparacaine HCl can cause fetal harm when adminstered to a pregnant woman or can affect reproduction capacity. Proparacaine HCl should be administered to a pregnant woman only if clearly needed.

Nursing Mothers: It is not known whether this drug is excreted in human milk. Because many drugs are execreted in human milk, caution should be exercised when Proparacaine HCl is administered to a nursing woman.

Pediatric Use: Controlled clinical studies have not been performed with Proparacaine HCl solution to establish safety and effectiveness in children; however, the literature cites the use of Proparacaine HCl as a topical ophthalmic anesthetic agent in children.

ADVERSE REACTIONS

Pupillary dilation or cycloplegic effects have rarely been observed with Proparacaine HCl. The drug appears to be safe for use in patients sensitive to other local anesthetics, but local or systemic sensitivity occasionally occurs. Instillation of Proparacaine in the eye at recommended concentration and dosage usually produces little or no initial irritation, stinging, burning, conjunctival redness, lacrimation or increased winking. However, some local irritation and stinging may occur several hours after the instillation.

Rarely, a severe, immediate-type, apparently hyperallergic corneal reaction may occur which includes acute, intense and diffuse epithelial keratitis; a gray, ground-glass appearance; sloughing of large areas of necrotic epithelium; corneal filaments and sometimes, iritis with descemetitis.

Allergic contact dermatitis with drying and fissuring of the fingertips has been reported. Softening and erosion of the corneal epithelium and conjunctival congestion and hemorrhage have been reported.

DOSAGE AND ADMINISTRATION

Deep anesthesia as in cataract extraction:
Instill 1 drop every 5 to 10 minutes for 5 to 7 doses.
Removal of sutures:
Instill 1 or 2 drops 2 or 3 minutes before removal of stitches.
Removal of foreign bodies:
Instill 1 or 2 drops prior to operating.
Tonometry:
Instill 1 or 2 drops immediately before measurement.
Store at 8°-24°C (46°—75°F) before opening. Store at 2°—8°C (35°—46°F) after opening to retard discoloration of solution. Do not use a discolored solution.

HOW SUPPLIED
DROP: 0.5%

AVERAGE UNIT PRICE (AVAILABLE SIZES)		GENERIC A-RATED AVERAGE PRICE (GAAP)	
BRAND	$0.88	15 ml	$6.99
GENERIC	$1.15		

BRAND/MANUFACTURER	NDC	SIZE	AWP
◆ BRAND			
OPHTHETIC: Allergan Optical	11980-0048-15	15 ml	$11.89
ALCAINE: Alcon Ophthalmic	00998-0016-15	15 ml	$12.44
OPHTHAINE: Apothecon	00003-0646-30	15 ml	$15.25
◆ GENERICS			
Raway	00686-0730-01	2 ml	$4.00
Moore,H.L.	00839-6686-31	15 ml	$6.74
Bausch&Lomb Pharm	24208-0730-06	15 ml	$7.23
Bausch&Lomb Pharm	24208-0730-01	2 ml 12s	$39.60

DROP: 0.5%

BRAND/MANUFACTURER	NDC	SIZE	AWP
○ BRAND			
OCU-CAINE: Ocumed	51944-4460-32	2 ml	$1.73
	51944-4460-42	15 ml	$3.00

Propine *SEE* DIPIVEFRIN HYDROCHLORIDE

Propofol

DESCRIPTION

Propofol Injection is a sterile, nonpyrogenic emulsion containing 10 mg/mL of Propofol suitable for intravenous administration. Propofol is chemically described as 2,6-diisopropylphenol and has a molecular weight of 178.27. The empirical formulas is $C_{12}H_{18}O$.

Propofol is very slightly soluble in water and, thus, is formulated in a white, oil-in-water emulsion. The pKa is 11.03. The octanol/water partition coefficient for Propofol is 5012:1 The emulsion is isotonic and has a pH of 7.0-8.5.

Propofol Injection is a single-use parenteral product and contains no antimicrobial preservatives. THE VEHICLE IS CAPABLE OF SUPPORTING RAPID GROWTH OF MICRO-ORGANISMS. (See *"Dosage and Administration, Handling Procedures".*)

Following is its chemical structure:

$$(CH_3)_2CH - \bigotimes^{OH} - CH(CH_3)_2$$

CLINICAL PHARMACOLOGY
GENERAL

Propofol Injection is an intravenous sedative hypnotic agent for use in the induction and maintenance of anesthesia or sedation. Intravenous injection of a therapeutic dose of Propofol produces hypnosis rapidly and smoothly with minimal excitation, usually within 40 seconds from the start of an injection (the time for one arm-brain circulation). As with other rapidly acting intravenous anesthetic agents, the half-time of the blood-brain equilibration is approximately 1 to 3 minutes, and this accounts for the rapid induction of anesthesia.

PHARMACODYNAMICS

Pharmacodynamic properties of Propofol are dependent upon the therapeutic blood Propofol concentrations. Steady state Propofol blood concentrations are generally proportional to infusion rates, especially within an individual patient. Undesirable side effects such as cardiorespiratory depression are likely to occur at higher blood levels which result from bolus dosing or rapid increase in infusion rate. An adequate interval (3 to 5 minutes) must be allowed between clinical dosage adjustments in order to assess drug effects. Table 1 presents these data for adults. No comparable data are available for children.

Table 1
PLASMA CONCENTRATION-EFFECT RELATIONSHIPS IN ADULTS

Technique	Plasma Propofol Range (µg/mL)
Monitored Anesthesia Care Sedation	0.5-1
Light Intensive Care Unit Sedation	0.5-1
Deep Intensive Care Unit Sedation	1-1.5
Light General Anesthesia, with nitrous oxide	3-5
Deep General Anesthesia, with nitrous oxide	4-7
Total Intravenous Anesthesia	
Propofol/opioid/oxygen	4-7
Propofol/oxygen	8-16

The hemodynamic effects of Propofol Injection during induction of anesthesia vary. If spontaneous ventilation is maintained, the major cardiovascular effects are arterial hypotension (sometimes greater than a 30% decrease) with little or no change in heart rate and no appreciable decrease in cardiac output. If ventilation is assisted or controlled (positive pressure ventilation), the degree and incidence of decrease in cardiac output are accentuated. Addition of a potent opioid (eg, fentanyl) when used as a premedicant further decreases cardiac output and respiratory drive.

If anesthesia is continued by infusion of Propofol Injection, the stimulation of endotracheal intubation and surgery may return arterial pressure towards normal. However, cardiac output may remain depressed. Comparative clinical studies have shown that the hemodynamic effects of Propofol Injection during induction of anesthesia are generally more pronounced than with other IV induction agents traditionally used for this purpose.

Insufficient data are available regarding the cardiovascular effects of Propofol Injection when used for induction and/or maintenance of anesthesia or sedation in elderly, hypotensive, debilitated patients, patients with severe cardiac disease (ejection fraction < 50%) or other ASA III/IV patients. However, limited information suggests that these patients may have more profound adverse cardiovascular responses. It is recommended that if Propofol Injection is used in these patients, a lower induction dose and a slower maintenance rate of administration of the drug be used. (See *"Dosage and Administration".*)

Clinical and preclinical studies suggest that Propofol Injection is rarely associated with elevation of plasma histamine levels.

Induction of anesthesia with Propofol Injection is frequently associated with apnea in both adults and children. In 1573 adult patients who received Propofol Injection (2.0 to 2.5 mg/kg), apnea lasted less than 30 seconds in 7% of patients, 30-60 seconds in 24% of patients, and more than 60 seconds in 12% of patients. In the 213 pediatric patients between the ages of 3 and 12 years assessable for apnea who received Propofol Injection (1.0 to 3.6 mg/kg), apnea lasted less than 30 seconds in 12% of patients, 30-60 seconds in 10% of patients, and more than 60 seconds in 5% of patients.

During maintenance Propofol Injection causes a decrease in ventilation usually associated with an increase in carbon dioxide tension which may be marked depending upon the rate of administration and other concurrent medications (eg, opioids, sedatives, etc.).

During monitored anesthesia care (MAC) sedation, attention must be given to the cardiorespiratory effects of Propofol Injection. Hypotension, oxyhemoglobin desaturation, apnea, airway obstruction, and/or oxygen desaturation can occur, especially following a rapid bolus of Propofol Injection. During initiation of MAC sedation, slow infusion or slow injection techniques are preferable over rapid bolus administration, and during maintenance of MAC sedation, a variable rate infusion is preferable over intermittent bolus administration in order to minimize undesirable cardiorespiratory effects. In the elderly, debilitated and ASA III or IV patients, rapid (single or repeated) bolus dose administration should not be used for MAC sedation. (See *"Warnings".*) Propofol Injection is not recommended for MAC sedation in children because safety and effectiveness have not been established.

Clinical studies in humans and studies in animals show that Propofol Injection does not suppress the adrenal response to ACTH.

Preliminary findings in patients with normal intraocular pressure indicate that Propofol Injection anesthesia produces a decrease in intraocular pressure which may be associated with a concomitant decrease in systemic vascular resistance.

Animal studies and limited experience in susceptible patients have not indicated any propensity of Propofol Injection to induce malignant hyperthermia.

Studies to date indicate that Propofol Injection when used in combination with hypocarbia increases cerebrovascular resistance and decreases cerebral blood flow, cerebral metabolic oxygen consumption, and intracranial pressure. Propofol Injection does not effect cerebrovascular reactivity to changes in arterial carbon dioxide tension. (See *"Clinical Trials—Neuroanesthesia".*)

PHARMACOKINETICS

The proper use Propofol Injection requires an understanding of the disposition and elimination characteristics of Propofol.

The pharmacokinetics of Propofol are well described by a three compartment linear model with compartments representing the plasma, radidly equilibrating tissues, and slowly equilibrating tissues. Following an IV bolus dose, plasma levels initially decline rapidly due to both high metabolic clearance and rapid drug distribution into tissues. Distribution accounts for about half of this decline following a bolus of Propofol. After longer infusions, the return to the plasma of the drug accumulated in the tissues causes plasma levels to fall more slowly. Plasma levels fall to about 50% of peak levels in about 5 minutes following a 1 hour infusion and in about 7 minutes following a 10 hour infusion. Titration of infusion to clinical response in MAC or ICU sedation corresponds to a plasma level of about 1 µg/mL. A fall in plasma level of about 50% (0.5 µg/mL) generally corresponds to patient awakening. The figure illustrates the fall in plasma levels following a one hour and a 10 hour infusion.

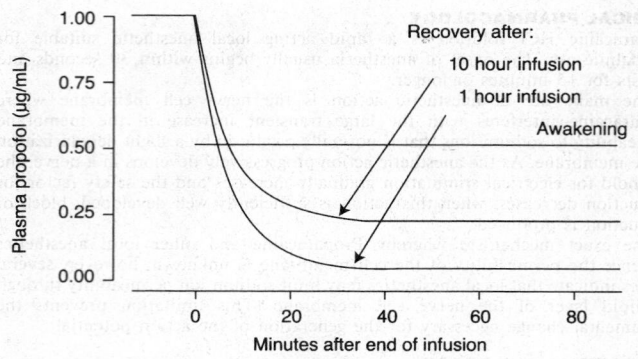

The large contribution of distribution (about 50%) to the fall of Propofol plasma levels following brief infusions means that after very long infusions (at steady state), about half the initial rate will maintain the same plasma levels. Thus, titration to clinical response and daily evaluation of sedation levels are important during use of Propofol Injection infusion for ICU sedation, especially of long duration.

Adults: Propofol clearance ranges from 23-50 mL/kg/min (1.6 to 3.4 L/min in 70 kg adults). It is chiefly eliminated by hepatic conjugation to inactive metabolites which are excreted by the kidney. A glucuronide conjugate accounts for about 50% of the administered dose. Propofol has a steady state volume of distribution (10 day infusion) approaching 60L/kg in healthy adults. A difference in pharmacokinetics due to gender has not been observed. The terminal half-life of Propofol after a 10 day infusion is 1 to 3 days.

Geriatrics: With increasing age, the dose of Propofol needed to achieve a defined anesthetic endpoint (dose-requirement) decreases. This dose not appear to be an age-related change of pharmacodynamics or brain sensitivity, as measured by EEG burst suppression. With increasing age pharmacokinetic changes are such that for a given IV bolus dose, higher peak plasma concentrations occur, which can explain the decreased dose requirement. These higher peak plasma concentrations in the elderly can predispose patients to cardiorespiratory effects including hypotension, apnea, airway obstruction and/or oxygen desaturation. The higher plasma levels reflect an age-related decrease in volume of distribution and reduced intercompartmental clearance. Lower doses are thus recommended for initiation and maintenance of seadtion/anesthesia in elderly patients. (See *"Clinical Pharmacology"—Individualization of Dosage.*)

Pediatrics: The pharmacokinetics of Propofol in children between the ages of 3 and 12 years are also best described as a three-compartment pharmacokinetic model. A study of 53 children undergoing general surgeries lasting approximately 1 to 2 hours, with less than 8 hours of plasma sampling, showed an elimination half-life of 250-400 minutes, steady state distributional volumes of 7-10 L/kg, and clearances of approximately 35 mL/kg/min. These estimates are consistent with the known high clearance and high lipid solubility of Propofol Injection. The observed differences between pediatric patients and adults in terms of elimination phase and distributional volume are related to the much longer duration of Propofol administration in adults.

Organ Failure: The pharmacokinetics of Propofol do not appear to be different in people with chronic hepatic cirrhosis or chronic renal impairment compared to adults with normal hepatic and renal function. The effects of acute hepatic or renal failure on the pharmacokinetics of Propofol have not been studied.

CLINICAL TRIALS
ANESTHESIA AND MONITORED ANESTHESIA CARE (MAC) SEDATION
Propofol Injection was compared to intravenous and inhalational anesthetic or sedative agents in 91 trials involving a total of 5,135 patients. Of these 3,354 received Propofol Injection and comprised the overall safety database for anesthesia and MAC sedation. Fifty-five of these trials, 20 for anesthesia induction and 35 for induction and maintenance of anesthesia or MAC sedation, were carried out in the US or Canada and provided the basis for dosage recommendations and the adverse event profile during anesthesia or MAC sedation.

PEDIATRIC ANESTHESIA
Propofol Injection was compared to standard anesthetic agents in 12 clinical trials involving 534 patients receiving Propofol Injection. Of these, 349 were from US/Canadian clinial trials and comprised the overall safety database for Pediatric Anesthesia.

Table 2
PEDIATRIC ANESTHESIA CLINICAL TRIALS

| | Patients Receiving Propofol Injection Median and (Range) | |
	Induction Only	Induction and Maintenance
Number of Patients*	243	105
Induction Bolus Dosages (mg/kg)	2.5 (1.0-3.5)	3.0 (2.0-3.6)
Injection Duration (sec)	20 (6-45)	-
Maintenance Dosage (µg/kg/min)	-	181 (107-418)
Maintenance Duration (min)	-	78 (29-268)

* Body weight recorded for one patient.

NEUROANESTHESIA
Propofol Injection was studied in 50 patients undergoing craniotomy for supratentorial tumors in two clinical trials. The mean lesion size (anterior/posterior and lateral) was 31 and 32 mm in one trial and 55 and 42 mm in the other trial respectively.

Table 3
NEUROANESTHESIA CLINICAL TRIALS

| | | Patients Receiving Propofol Injection Median and (Range) | | |
Patient Type	No. of Patients	Induction Bolus Dosages (mg/kg)	Maintenance Dosage (µg/kg/min)	Maintenance Duration (min)
Craniotomy patients	50	1.36 (0.9-6.9)	146 (68-425)	285 (48-622)

In ten of these patients, Propofol Injection was administered by infusion in a controlled clinical trial to evaluate the effect of Propofol Injection on cerebrospinal fluid pressure (CSFP). The mean arterial pressure was maintained relatively constant over 25 minutes with a change from baseline of -4% ± 17% (mean ± SD), whereas the percent change in cerebrospinal fluid pressure (CSFP) was -46% ± 14%. As CSFP is an indirect measure of intracranial pressure (ICP), when given by infusion or slow bolus, Propofol Injection, in combination with hypocarbia, is capable of decreasing ICP independent of changes in arterial pressure.

INTENSIVE CARE UNIT (ICU) SEDATION
Propofol Injection was compared to benzodiazepines and/or opioids in 14 clinical trials involving a total of 550 ICU patients. Of these, 302 received Propofol Injection and comprise the overall safety database for ICU sedation. Six of these studies were carried out in the US or Canada and provide the basis for dosage recommendations and the adverse event profile.

Information from 193 literature reports of Propofol Injection used for ICU sedation in over 950 patients and information from the clinical trials are summarized below. (See related table).

INDIVIDUALIZATION OF DOSAGE
General: Propofol blood concentrations at steady state are generally proportional to infusion rates, especially within an individual patient. Undesirable effects such as cardiorespiratory depression are likely to occur at higher blood levels which result from bolus dosing or rapid increases in the infusion rate. An adequate interval (3 to 5 minutes) must be allowed between clinical dosage adjustments in order to assess drug effects.

When administering Propofol Injection by infusion, syringe pumps or volumetric pumps are recommended to provide controlled infusion rates. When infusing Propofol Injection to patients undergoing magnetic resonance imaging, metered control devices may be utilized if mechanical pumps are impractical.

Changes in vital signs (increases in pulse rate, blood pressure, sweating and/or tearing) that indicate a response to surgical stimulation or lightening of anesthesia may be controlled by the administration of Propofol Injection 25 mg (2.5 mL) to 50 mg (5.0 mL) incremental boluses and/or by increasing the infusion rate.

For minor surgical procedures (eg. body surface) nitrous oxide (60%-70%) can be combined with a variable rate Propofol Injection infusion to provide satisfactory anesthesia. With more stimulating surgical procedures (eg. intra-abdominal), or if supplementation with nitrous oxide is not provided, administration rate(s) of Propofol Injection and/or opioids should be increased in order to provide adequate anesthesia.

Infusion rates should always be titrated downward in the absence of clinical signs of light anesthesia until a mild response to surgical stimulation is obtained in order to avoid administration of Propofol Injection at rates higher than are clinically necessary. Generally, rates of 50 to 100µg/kg/min in adults, should be achieved during maintenance in order to optimize recovery times.

Other drugs that cause CNS depression (hypnotics/sedatives, inhalational anesthetics and opioids) can increase CNS depression induced by Propofol. Morphine premedication (0.15 mg/kg) with nitrous oxide 67% in oxygen has been shown to decrease the necessary Propofol injection maintenance infusion rate and therapeutic blood concentrations when compared to non-narcotic (lorazepam) premedication.

INDUCTION OF ANESTHESIA
Adult Patients: Most adult patients under 55 years of age and classified ASA I or II require 2.0 to 2.5 mg/kg of Propofol Injection for induction when unpremedicated or when premedicated with oral benzodiazepines or intramuscular opioids. For induction, Propofol Injection should be titrated (approximately 40 mg every 10 seconds) against the response of the patient until the clinical signs show the onset of anesthesia. As with other sedative hypnotic agents, the amount of intravenous opioid and/or benzodiazepine premedication will influence the response of the patient to an induction dose of Propofol Injection.

Geriatric Patients: It is important to be familiar and experienced with the intravenous use of Propofol Injection before treating elderly, debilitated and ASA III or IV patients. Due to the reduced clearance and higher blood levels, most elderly patients require approximately 1.0 to 1.5 mg/kg (approximately 20 mg every 10 seconds of Propofol Injection for induction of anesthesia according to their condition and responses. A rapid bolus should not be used as this will increase the likelihood of undesirable cardiorespiratory depression including hypotension, apnea, airway obstruction and/or oxygen desaturation. (See "Dosage and Administration").

Neurosurgical Patients: Slower induction is recommended using boluses of 20 mg every 10 seconds. Slower boluses or infusions of Propofol Injection for induction of anesthesia, titrated to clinical responses, will generally result in reduced induction dosage requirements (1.0 to 2.0 mg/kg). (See "Precautions" and "Dosage and Administration".)

MAINTENANCE OF ANESTHESIA
In adults, anesthesia can be maintained by administering Propofol Injection by infusion or intermittent IV bolus injection. The patient's clinical response will determine the infusion rate or the amount and frequency of incremental injections.

Continuous Infusion: Propofol Injection 100 to 200 µg/kg/min administered in a variable rate infusion with 60%-70% nitrous oxide and oxygen provides anesthesia for patients undergoing general surgery. Maintenance by infusion of Propofol Injection should immediately follow the induction dose in order to provide satisfactory or continuous anesthesia during the induction phase. During this initial period following the induction dose higher rates of infusion are generally required (150 to 200 µg/kg/min) for the first 10 to 15 minutes. Infusion rates should subsequently be decreased 30%-50% during the first half-hour of maintenance.

Other drugs that cause CNS depression (hypnotics/sedatives, inhalational anesthetics and opioids) can increase the CNS depression induced by Propofol. Morphine premedication (0.15 mg/kg) with nitrous oxide 67% in oxygen has been shown to decrease the necessary Propofol Injection maintenance infusion rate and therapeutic blood concentrations when compared to non-narcotic (lorazepam) premedication.

Intermittent Bolus: Increments of Propofol Injection 25 mg (2.5 mL) to 50 mg (5.0 mL) may be administered with nitrous oxide in adult patients undergoing general surgery. The incremental boluses should be administered when changes in vital signs indicate a response to surgical stimulation or light anesthesia.

Propofol Injection has been used with a variety of agents commonly used in anesthesia such as atropine, scopolamine, glycopyrrolate, diazepam, depolarizing and nondepolarizing muscle relaxants, and opioid analgesics, as well as with inhalational and regional anesthetic agents.

In the elderly, rapid bolus doses should not be used as this will increase cardiorespiratory effects including hypotension, apnea, airway obstruction and/or oxygen desaturation.

PEDIATRIC ANESTHESIA
Induction of Anesthesia: Most pediatric patients over the age of 3 years and classified ASA I or II require 2.5 to 3.5 mg/kg of Propofol Injection for induction when unpremedicated or when lightly premedicated with oral benzodiazepines or intramuscular opioids. Within this dosage range, younger children may require larger induction doses than older children. As with other sedative hypnotic agents, the amount of intravenous opioid and/or benzodiazepine premedication will influence the response of the patient to an induction dose of Propofol Injection. In addition, a lower dosage is recommended for children ASA III or IV. Attention should be paid to minimize pain on injection when administering Propofol Injection to pediatric patients. Rapid boluses of Propofol Injection may be

administered if small veins are pretreated with lidocaine or when antecubital or larger veins are utilized (See "Precautions—General").

Propofol Injection administered in a variable rate infusion with nitrous oxide 60-70% provides satisfactory anesthesia for most pediatric patients aged 3 years or older, ASA I or II, undergoing general anesthesia.

Maintenance of Anesthesia: Maintenance by infusion of Propofol Injection at a rate of 200-300 µg/kg/min should immediately follow the induction dose. Following the first half hour of maintenance, if clinical signs of light anesthesia are not present, the infusion rate should be decreased: during this period, infusion rates of 125-150 µg/kg/min are typically needed. However, younger children (5 years or less) may require larger maintenance infusion rates than older children.

MONITORED ANESTHESIA CARE (MAC) SEDATION IN ADULTS

When Propofol Injection is administered for MAC sedation, rates of administration should be individualized and titrated to clinical response. In most patients the rates of Propofol Injection administration will be in the range of 25-75 µg/kg/min.

During initiation of MAC sedation, slow infusion or slow injection techniques are preferable over rapid bolus administration. During maintenance of MAC sedation, a variable rate infusion is preferable over intermittent bolus dose administration. In the elderly, debilitated and ASA III or IV patients, rapid (single or repeated) bolus dose administration should not be used for MAC sedation. (See *"Warnings"*.) **A rapid bolus injection can result in undesirable cardiorespiratory depression including hypotension, apnea, airway obstruction and/or oxygen desaturation.**

Initiation of MAC Sedation: For initiation of MAC sedation, either an infusion or a slow injection method may be utilized while closely monitoring cardiorespiratory function. With the infusion method, sedation may be initiated by infusing Propofol Injection at 100 to 150 µg/kg/min (6 to 9 mg/kg/h) for a period of 3 to 5 minutes and titrating to the desired level of sedation while closely monitoring respiratory function. With the slow injection method for initiation, patients will require approximately 0.5 mg/kg administered over 3 to 5 minutes and titrated to clinical responses. When Propofol Injection is administered slowly over 3 to 5 minutes, most patients will be adequately sedated and the peak drug effect can be achieved while minimizing undesirable cardiorespiratory effects occurring at high plasma levels.

In the elderly, debilitated, and ASA III or IV patients, rapid (single or repeated) bolus dose administration should not be used for MAC sedation. (See *"Warnings"*.) The rate of administration should be over 3-5 minutes and the dosage of Propofol Injection should be reduced to approximately 80% of the adult dosage in these patients according to their condition, responses, and changes in vital signs. (See *"Dosage and Administration"*.)

Maintenance of MAC Sedation: For maintenance of sedation, a variable rate infusion method is preferable over an intermittent bolus dose method. With the variable rate infusion method, patients will generally require maintenance rates of 25 to 75 µg/kg/min (1.5 to 4.5 mg/kg/h) during the first 10 to 15 minutes of sedation maintenance. Infusion rates should subsequently be decreased over time to 25 to 50 µg/kg/min and adjusted to clinical responses. In titrating to clinical effect, allow approximately 2 minutes for onset of peak drug effect.

Infusion rates should always be titrated downward in the absence of clinical signs of light sedation until mild responses to stimulation and obtained in order to avoid sedative administration of Propofol Injection at rates higher than are clinically necessary.

If the intermittent bolus dose method is used, increments of Propofol Injection 10 mg (1.0 mL) or 20 mg (2.0 mL) can be administered and titrated to desired level of sedation. With the intermittent bolus method of sedation maintenance there is the potential for respiratory depression, transient increases in sedation depth, and/or prolongation of recovery. In the elderly, debilitated, and ASA III or IV patients, rapid (single or repeated) bolus dose administration should not be used for MAC sedation. (See *"Warnings"*.) The rate of administration and the

dosage of Propofol Injection should be reduced to approximately 80% of the adult dosage in these patients according to their condition, responses, and changes in vital signs (See *"Dosage and Administration"*.)

Propofol Injection can be administered as the sole agent for maintenance of MAC sedation during surgical/diagnostic procedures. When Propofol Injection sedation is supplemented with opioid and/or benzodiazepine medications, these agents increase the sedative and respiratory effects of Propofol Injection and may also result in a slower recovery profile. (See *"Precautions, Drug Interactions"*.)

ICU SEDATION

Strict aseptic techniques must be followed when handling Propofol Injection as the vehicle is capable of supporting rapid growth of microorganisms. (See *"Dosage and Administration, Handling Procedures"*.) For intubated mechanically ventilated adult patients, Intensive Care Unit (ICU) sedation should be initiated slowly with a continuous infusion in order to titrate to desired clinical effect and minimize hypotension. (See *"Dosage and Administration"*.)

Across all 6 US/Canadian clinical studies, the mean infusion maintenance rate for all Propofol Injection patients was 27 ± 21 µg/kg/min. The maintenance infusion rates required to maintain adequate sedation ranged from 0.3 µg/kg/min, to 130 µg/kg/min. The infusion rate was lower in patients over 55 years of age (approximately 20 µg/kg/min) compared to patients under 55 years of age (approximately 38 µg/kg/min). In these studies, morphine or fentanyl was used as needed for analgesia.

Most adult ICU patients recovering from the effects of general anesthesia or deep sedation will require maintenance rates of 5 to 50 µg/kg/min (0.3 to 3.0 mg/kg/h) individualized and titrated to clinical response. (See *"Dosage and Administration"*.) With medical ICU patients or patients who have recovered from the effects of general anesthesia or deep sedation, the rate of administration of 50 µg/kg/min or higher may be required to achieve adequate sedation. These higher rates of administration may increase the likelihood of patients developing hypotension.

Although there are reports of reduced analgesic requirements, most patients received opioids for analgesia during maintenance of ICU sedation. Some patients also received benzodiazepines and/or neuromuscular blocking agents. During long term maintenance of sedation, some ICU patients were awakened once or twice every 24 hours for assessment of neurologic or respiratory function. (See *"Clinical Trials"*, Table 4.)

In post-CABG (coronary artery bypass graft) patients, the maintenance rate of Propofol administration was usually low (median 11 µg/kg/min) due to the intraoperative administration of high opioid doses. Patients receiving Propofol Injection required 35% less nitroprusside than midazolam patients; this difference was statistically significant ($P < 0.05$). During initiation of sedation in Post-CABG patients, a 15% to 20% decrease in blood pressure was seen in the first 60 minutes. It was not possible to determine cardiovascular effects in patients with severe cardiac compromise. (See *"Clinical Trials"*, Table 4).

In Medical or Postsurgical ICU studies comparing Propofol Injection to benzodiazepine infusion or bolus, there were no apparent differences in maintenance of adequate sedation, mean arterial pressure, or laboratory findings. Like the comparators, Propofol Injection reduced blood cortisol during sedation while maintaining responsivity to challenge with adrenocorticotropic hormone (ACTH). Two case reports from the literature of patients with a history of porphyria or malignant hyperthermia were without adverse consequences.

In hemodynamically stable head trauma patients ranging in age from 19-43 years, adequate sedation was maintained with Propofol Injection or morphine (N = 7 in each group). There were no apparent differences in adequacy of sedation, intracranial pressure, cerebral perfusion pressure, or neurologic recovery between the treatment groups. In literature reports from Neurosurgical ICU and severely head injured patients Propofol Injection infusion with or without diuretics and hyperventilation controlled intracranial pressure while maintaining cerebral perfusion pressure. In some patients bolus doses resulted in decreased blood

Table 4
ICU SEDATION CLINICAL TRIALS AND LITERATURE

			Patients receiving Propofol Injection Median and (Range)		
	Number of Patients		**Sedation Dose**		
ICU Patient Type	Trials	Literature	µg/kg/min	mg/kg/h	Sedation Duration Hours
Post-CABG	41	-	11 (0.1-30)	.66 (.006-1.8)	10 (2-14)
	-	334	(5-100)	(0.3-6.0)	(4-24)
Post-Surgical	60	-	20 (6-53)	1.2 (0.4-3.2)	18 (0.3-187)
	-	142	(23-82)	(1.4-4.9)	(6-96)
Neuro/Head Trauma	7	-	25 (13-37)	1.5 (0.8-2.2)	168 (112-282)
	-	184	(8.3-87)	(0.5-5.2)	(8 hr-5 days)
Medical	49	-	41 (9-131)	2.5 (0.5-7.9)	72 (0.4-337)
	-	76	(3.3-62)	(0.2-3.7)	(4-96)
Special Patients					
ARDS/Resp. Failure		56	(10-142)	(0.6-8.5)	(1.0 hrs-8 days)
COPD/Asthma		49	(17-75)	(1.0-4.5)	(1-8 days)
Status Epilepticus		15	(25-167)	(1.5-10)	(1-21 days)
Tetanus		11	(5-100)	(0.3-6.0)	(1-25 days)

Trials (individual patients from clinical studies)
Literature (individual patients from published reports)
CABG (Coronary Artery Bypass Graft)
ARDS (Adult Respiratory/Distress Syndrome)

---

pressure and compromised cerebral perfusion pressure. (See *"Clinical Trials"*, Table 4.)

Propofol Injection was found to be effective in status epilepticus which was refractory to the standard anticonvulsant therapies. For these patients as well as for ARDS/respiratory failure and tetanus patients sedation maintenance dosages were generally higher than those for other critically ill patient populations. (See *"Clinical Trials"*, Table 4.)

Abrupt discontinuation of Propofol Injection prior to weaning or for daily evaluation of sedation levels should be avoided. This may result in rapid awakening with associated anxiety, agitation and resistance to mechanical ventilation. Infusions of Propofol Injection should be adjusted to maintain a light level of sedation through the weaning process or evaluation of sedation level (See *"Precautions"*.)

INDICATIONS AND USAGE

Propofol Injection is an IV anesthetic agent that can be used for both induction and/or maintenance of anesthesia as part of a balanced anesthetic technique for inpatient and outpatient surgery in adults and in children age 3 years or older.

Propofol Injection, when administered intravenously as directed, can be used to initiate and maintain monitored anesthesia care (MAC) sedation during diagnostic procedures in adults. Propofol Injection may also be used for MAC sedation in conjunction with local/regional anesthesia in patients undergoing surgical procedures. (See *"Precautions"*.)

Propofol Injection should only be administered to intubated, mechanically ventilated adult patients in the Intensive Care Unit (ICU) to provide continuous sedation and control of stress responses. In this setting, Propofol Injection should be administered only by persons skilled in the medical management of critically ill patients and trained in cardiovascular resuscitation and airway managment.

Propofol Injection is not recommended for obstetrics, including cesarean section deliveries. Propofol Injection crosses the placenta, and as with other general anesthetic agents, the administration of Propofol Injection may be associated with neonatal depression. (See *"Precautions"*.) Propofol Injection is not recommended for use in nursing mothers because Propofol Injection has been reported to be excreted in human milk and the effects of oral absorption of small amounts of Propofol are not known. (See *"Precautions"*.)

Propofol Injection is not recommended for anesthesia in children below the age of 3 years because safety and effectiveness have not been established. Propofol Injection is not recommended for MAC sedation in children because safety and effectiveness have not been established. Propofol Injection is not recommended for pediatric ICU sedation because safety and effectiveness have not been established.

UNLABELED USES

Propofol is used alone or as an adjunct in the treatment of nausea and vomiting, morphine-induced pruritus, and endotracheal intubation.

CONTRAINDICATIONS

Propofol Injection is contraindicated in patients with a known hypersensitivity to Propofol Injection or its components, or when general anesthesia or sedation are contraindicated.

WARNINGS

For general anesthesia or monitored anesthesia care (MAC) sedation Propofol Injection should be administered only by persons trained in the administration of general anesthesia and not involved in the conduct of the surgical/diagnostic procedure. Patients should be continuously monitored and facilities for maintenance of a patient airway, artificial ventilation, and oxygen enrichment and circulatory resuscitation must be immediately available.

For sedation of intubated, mechanically ventilated adult patients in the Intensive Care Unit (ICU), Propofol Injection should be administered only by persons skilled in the management of critically ill patients and trained in cardiovascular resuscitation and airway management.

In the elderly, debilitated and ASA III or IV patients, rapid (single or repeated) bolus administration should not be used during general anesthesia or MAC sedation in order to minimize undesirable cardiorespiratory depression including hypotension, apnea, airway obstruction and/or oxygen desaturation.

MAC sedation patients should be continuously monitored by persons not involved in the conduct of the surgical or diagnostic procedure; oxygen supplementation should be immediately available and provided where clinically indicated; and oxygen saturation should be monitored in all patients. Patients should be continuously monitored for early signs of hypotension, apnea, airway obstruction and/or oxygen desaturation. These cardiorespiratory effects are more likely to occur following rapid initiation (loading) boluses or during supplemental maintenance boluses, especially in the elderly, debilitated and ASA III or IV patients.

Propofol Injection should not be coadministered through the same IV catheter with blood or plasma because compatibility has not been established. *In vitro* tests have shown that aggregates of the globular component of the emulsion vehicle have occurred with blood/plasma/serum from humans and animals. The clinical significance is not known.

Strict aseptic techniques must always be maintained during handling as Propofol Injection is a single-use parenteral product and contains no antimicrobial preservatives. THE VEHICLE IS CAPABLE OF SUPPORTING RAPID GROWTH OF MICROORGANISMS. (See *"Dosage and Administration, Handling Procedures"*.)

Failure to follow aseptic handling procedures may result in microbial contamination causing fever, infection/sepsis and/or other adverse consequences which could lead to life-threatening illness.

PRECAUTIONS

General: A lower induction dose and a slower maintenance rate of administration should be used in elderly, debilitated and ASA III or IV patients. (See *"Clinical Pharmacology—Individualization of Dosage"*.) Patients should be continuously monitored for early signs of significant hypotension and/or bradycardia. Treatment may include increasing the rate of intravenous fluid, elevation of lower extremities, use of pressor agents, or administration of atropine. Apnea often occurs during induction and may persist for more than 60 seconds. Ventilatory support may be required. Because Propofol Injection is an emulsion, caution should be exercised in patients with disorders of lipid metabolism such as primary hyperlipoproteinemia, diabetic hyperlipemia, and pancreatitis.

The clinical criteria for discharge from the recovery/day surgery area established for each institution should be satisfied before discharge of the patient from the care of the anesthesiologist.

When Propofol Injection is administered to an epileptic patient, there may be a risk of seizure during the recovery phase.

In adults and children, attention should be paid to minimize pain on administration of Propofol Injection. Transient local pain during intravenous injection may be reduced by prior injection of IV lidocaine (1.0 mL of a 1% solution). Pain on injection occurred in 10% of 349 Pediatric patients. Forty-five percent of these patients reported pain in the hand, forearm, and wrist, 5% in the hand (used with lidocaine), and 9% in the antecubital fossa.

Venous sequelae (phlebitis or thrombosis) have been reported rarely (< 1%). In two well-controlled clinical studies using dedicated intravenous catheters, no instances of venous sequelae were reported up to 14 days following induction. Accidental clinical extravasation and intentional injection into subcutaneous or perivascular tissues of animals caused minimal tissue reaction. Intra-arterial injection in animals did not induce local tissue effects. Accidental intra-arterial injection has been reported in patients, and other than pain, there were no major sequelae.

Perioperative myoclonia, rarely including convulsions and opisthotones, has occurred in temporal relationship in cases in which Propofol Injection has been administered.

Clinical features of anaphylaxis, which may include bronchospasm, erythema and hypotension, occur rarely following Propofol Injection administration, although use of other drugs in most instances makes the relationship to Propofol Injection unclear.

There have been rare reports of pulmonary edema in temporal relationship to the administration of Propofol Injection, although a causal relationship is unknown.

Propofol Injection has no vagolytic activity and has been associated with reports of bradycardia, occasionally profound, and/or asystole. The intravenous administration of anticholinergic agents (eg, atropine or glycopyrrolate) should be considered to modify potential increases in vagal tone due to concomitant agents (eg, succinylcholine) or surgical stimuli.

There have been rare reports of cardiac arrest in temporal relationship to the administration of Propofol Injection.

Intensive Care Unit Sedation: **Strict aseptic techniques must be followed when handling Propofol Injection as the vehicle is capable of supporting rapid growth of microorganisms.** (See *"Dosage and Administration, Handling Procedures"*.) The administration of Propofol Injection should be initiated as a continuous infusion and changes in the rate of administration made slowly (> 5 min) in order to minimize hypotension and avoid acute overdosage. (See *"Clinical Pharmacology—Individualization of Dosage"*.)

Patients should be monitored for early signs of significant hypotension and/or cardiovascular depression, which may be profound. These effects are responsive to discontinuation of Propofol Injection, IV fluid administration, and/or vasopressor therapy.

As with other sedative medications there is wide interpatient variability in Propofol Injection dosage requirements, and these requirements may change with time.

Opiods and paralytic agents should be discontinued and respiratory function optimized prior to weaning patients from mechanical ventilation. Infusions of Propofol Injection should be adjusted to maintain a light level of sedation prior to weaning patients from mechanical ventilatory support. Throughout the weaning process this level of sedation may be maintained in the absence of respiratory depression. Because of the rapid clearance of Propofol Injection, abrupt discontinuation of a patient's infusion may result in rapid awakening of the patient with associated anxiety, agitation, and resistance to mechanical ventilation, making weaning from mechanical ventilation difficult. It is therefore recommended that administration of Propofol Injection be continued in order to maintain a light level of sedation throughout the weaning process until 10-15 minutes prior to extubation at which time the infusion can be discontinued.

Since Propofol Injection is formulated in an oil-in-water emulsion elevations in serum triglycerides may occur when Propofol Injection is administered for extended periods of time. Patients at risk of hyperlipidemia should be monitored for increases in serum triglycerides or serum turbidity. Administration of Propofol Injection should be adjusted if fat is being inadequately cleared from the body. A reduction in the quantity of concurrently administered lipids is indicated to compensate for the amount of lipid infused as part of the Propofol Injection formulation: 1.0 mL of Propofol Injection contains approximately 0.1 g of fat (1.1 kcal).

The long term administration of Propofol Injection to patients with renal failure and/or hepatic insufficiency has not been evaluated.

Neurosurgical Anesthesia: When Propofol Injection is used in patients with increased intracranial pressure or impaired cerebral circulation, significant decreases in mean arterial pressure should be avoided because of the resultant decreases in cerebral perfusion pressure. To avoid significant hypotension and decreases in cerebral perfusion pressure, an infusion or slow bolus of approximately 20 mg every 10 seconds should be utilized instead of rapid and large boluses of Propofol Injection. Slower induction titrated to clinical responses, will generally result in reduced induction dosage requirements (1.0 to 2.0 mg/kg). When increased ICP is suspected, hyperventilation and hypocarbia should accompany the administration of Propofol Injection. (See *"Dosage and Administration".*)

Information for Patients: Patients should be advised that performance of activities requiring mental alertness, such as operating a motor vehicle, or hazardous machinery or signing legal documents may be impaired for some time after general anesthesia or sedation.

Drug Interactions: The induction dose requirements of Propofol Injection may be reduced in patients with intramuscular or intravenous premedication, particularly with narcotics (eg. morphine, meperidine, and fentanyl, etc.) and combinations of opioids and sedatives (eg. benzodiazepines, barbiturates, chloral hydrate, droperidol, etc.). These agents may increase the anesthetic or sedative effects of Propofol Injection and may also result in more pronounced decreases in systolic, diastolic, and mean arterial pressures and cardiac output.

During maintenance of anesthesia or sedation, the rate of Propofol Injection administration should be adjusted according to the desired level of anesthesia or sedation and may be reduced in the presence of supplemental analgesic agents (e.g. nitrous oxide or opioids). The concurrent administration of potent inhalational agents (e.g. isoflurane, enflurane, and halothane) during maintenance with Propofol Injection has not been extensively evaluated. These inhalational agents can also be expected to increase the anesthetic or sedative and cardiorespiratory effects of Propofol Injection.

Propofol Injection does not cause a clinically significant change in onset, intensity or duration of action of the commonly used neuromuscular blocking agents (e.g. succinylcholine and nondepolarizing muscle relaxants).

No significant adverse interactions with commonly used premedications or drugs used during anesthesia or sedation (including a range of muscle relaxants, inhalational agents, analgesic agents, and local anesthetic agents) have been observed.

Carcinogenesis, Mutagenesis, Impairment of Fertility: Animal carcinogenicity studies have not been performed with Propofol.

In vitro and *in vivo* animal tests failed to show any potential for mutagenicity by Propofol. Tests for mutagenicity included the Ames (using *Salmonella* sp) mutation test, gene mutation/gene conversion using *Saccharomyces cerevisiae, in vitro* cytogenetic studies in Chinese hamsters and a mouse micronucleus test.

Studies in female rats at intravenous doses up to 15 mg/kg/day (6 times the maximum recommended human induction dose) for 2 weeks before pregnancy to day 7 of gestation did not show impaired fertility. Male fertility in rats was not affected in a dominant lethal study at intravenous doses up to 15 mg/kg/day for 5 days.

Pregnancy Category B: Reproduction studies have been performed in rats and rabbits at intravenous doses of 15 mg/kg/day (6 times the recommended human induction dose) and have revealed no evidence of impaired fertility or harm to the fetus due to Propofol. Propofol, however, has been shown to cause maternal deaths in rats and rabbits and decreased pup survival during the lactating period in dams treated with 15 mg/kg/day (or 6 times the recommended human induction dose). The pharmacological activity (anesthesia) of the drug on the mother is probably responsible for the adverse effects seen in the offspring. There are, however, no adequate and well-controlled studies in pregnant women. Because animal reproduction studies are not always predictive of human responses, this drug should be used during pregnancy only if clearly needed.

Labor and Delivery: Propofol Injection is not recommended for obstetrics, including cesarean section deliveries. Propofol Injection crosses the placenta, and as with other general anesthetic agents, the administration of Propofol Injection may be associated with neonatal depression.

Nursing Mothers: Propofol Injection is not recommended for use in nursing mothers because Propofol Injection has been reported to be excreted in human milk and the effects of oral absorption of small amounts of Propofol are not known.

Pediatrics: Propofol Injection for anesthesia is not recommended for use in children below the age of 3 years because safety and effectiveness have not been established. Propofol Injection for ICU Sedation use or MAC sedation is not recommended for use in children because safety and effectiveness have not been established.

Although no causal relationship has been established, serious adverse events (including fatalities) have been reported in children given Propofol Injection for ICU sedation. These events were seen most often in children with respiratory tract infections given doses in excess of those recommended for adults.

ADVERSE REACTIONS

GENERAL

Adverse event information is derived from controlled clinical trials and worldwide marketing experience. In the description below, rates of the more common events represent US/Canadian clinical study results. Less frequent events are derived principally from publications and marketing experience in over 8 million patients; there are insufficient data to support an accurate estimate of their incidence rates. These studies were conducted using a variety of premedicants, varying lengths of surgical/diagnostic procedures and various other anesthetic/ sedative agents. Most adverse events were mild and transient.

ANESTHESIA AND MAC SEDATION IN ADULTS

The following estimates of adverse events for Propofol Injection are derived from clinical trials in general anesthesia/MAC sedation (N=2889 adult patients). The adverse events listed below as probably causally related are those events in which the actual incidence rate in patients treated with Propofol injection was greater than the comparator incident rate in these trials. Therefore, incidence rates for anesthesia and MAC sedation in adults generally represent estimates of the percentage of clinical trial patients which appeared to have probable causal relationship.

The adverse experience profile from reports of 150 patients in the MAC sedation clinical trials is similar to the profile established with Propofol Injection during anesthesia (see below). During MAC sedation clinical trials, significant respiratory events included cough, upper airway obstruction, apnea, hypoventilation, and dyspnea.

ANESTHESIA IN CHILDREN

Generally the adverse experience profile from reports of 349 Propofol Injection pediatric patients between the ages of 3 and 12 years in the US/Canadian anesthesia clinical trials is similar to the profile established with Propofol Injection during anesthesia in adults [see Pediatric percentages (Peds%) below]. Although not reported as an adverse event in clinical trials, apnea is frequently observed in pediatric patients.

ICU SEDATION IN ADULTS

The following estimates of adverse events are derived from clinical trials in ICU sedation (N = 159) patients. Probable related incidence rates for ICU sedation were determined by individual case report form review. Probable causality was based upon an apparent dose response relationship and/or positive responses to rechallenge. In many instances the presence of concomitant disease and concomitant therapy made the causal relationship unknown. Therefore, incidence rates for ICU sedation generally represent estimates of the percentage of clinical trial patients which appeared to have a probable causal relationship.

INCIDENCE GREATER THAN 1%—PROBABLY CAUSALLY RELATED

Events from ICU sedation only are indicated in parentheses. Events from ICU sedation and anesthesia/MAC sedation are indicated by *italicization.* Pediatric adverse events occurring in greater than 5% of patients are indicated by brackets. Events occurring only in anesthesia/MAC sedation are unmarked. Peds: refers to frequency in pediatric clinical trials.

Cardiovascular: Bradycardia, (Decreased Cardiac Output). *Hypotension*[*] (ICU: 26%) [Peds: 17%], [Hypertension Peds: 8%] [See also *"Clinical Pharmacology"*]

Central Nervous System: Movement[*] [Peds: 17%]

Injection Site: Burning/Stinging or Pain, 17.6%, [Peds: 10%]

Metabolic/Nutritional: (Hyperlipemia[*])

Respiratory: Apnea [see also *"Clinical Pharmacology"*] (Respiratory Acidosis During Weaning[*])

Skin and Appendages: Rash [Peds: 5%]
   [*] Incidence of events 3% to 10%

INCIDENCE LESS THAN 1%—PROBABLY CAUSALLY RELATED

Events occurring in ICU patients are indicated in parentheses. Events from both ICU sedation and anesthesia/MAC sedation are indicated by underscore. Events from post-marketing surveillance or literature are listed in italics. Events occurring in anesthesia/MAC sedation patients are unmarked.

Body as a Whole: Anaphylaxis/Anaphylactoid, Reaction, Perinatal Disorder.

Cardiovascular: Premature Atrial Contractions, Syncope.

Central Nervous System: (Agitation), Hypertonia/Dystonia, Paresthesia.

Digestive: Hypersalivation.

Musculoskeletal: Myalgia.

Respiratory: (Decreased Lung Function), Wheezing.

Skin and Appendages: Flushing, Pruritus

Special Senses: Amblyopia.

Urogenital: Cloudy Urine, (*Green Urine*)

INCIDENCE LESS THAN 1%—CAUSAL RELATIONSHIP UNKNOWN

Events from ICU sedation only are indicated in parentheses. Events from both ICU sedation and anesthesia/MAC sedation are indicated by underscore. Events from postmarketing surveillance or literature are listed in italics. Events occurring in only anesthesia/MAC sedation patients are presumably rarer and are unmarked. The clinical significance of the association of these events with Propofol Injection is unknown, but they are reported as altering information for the clinician.

Body as a Whole: Asthenia, Awareness, Chest Pain, Extremities Pain, Fever, Increased Drug Effect, Neck Rigidity/Stiffness, (Sepsis), Trunk Pain, (Whole Body Weakness).

Cardiovascular: <u>Arrhythmia</u>, <u>Atrial Fibrillation</u>. Atrioventricular Heart Block, <u>Bigeminy</u>, Bleeding, Bundle Branch Block, <u>Cardiac Arrest</u>, ECG Abnormal, Edema, <u>Extrasystole</u>, Heart Block, Hypertension, Myocardial Infarction, *Myocardial Ischemia*, Premature Ventricular Contractions, Premature Ventricular Contractions, (Right Heart Failure), ST Segment Depression, Supraventricular Tachycardia, Tachycardia, Ventricular Fibrillation, (Ventricular Tachycardia).

Central Nervous System: Abnormal Dreams, Agitation, *Amorous Behavior*, Anxiety, Bucking/Jerking/Thrashing, <u>Chills/Shivering</u>, Clonic/Myoclonic Movement, Combativeness, Confusion, Delirium, Depression, Dizziness, Emotional Lability, Euphoria, Fatigue, *Hallucinations*, Headache, *Hypotonia*, Hysteria, Insomnia, (Intracranial Hypertension), Moaning, *Neuropathy, Opisthotonos*, Rigidity, <u>Seizures</u>, <u>Somnolence</u>, (Thinking Abnormal), Tremor, Twitching

Digestive: Cramping, Diarrhea, Dry Mouth, Enlarged Parotid, (Ileus), (Liver Function Abnormal), Nausea, Swallowing, Vomiting.

Hematologic/Lymphatic: Coagulation Disorder, Leukocytosis

Injection Site: Hives/Itching, Phlebitis, Redness/Discoloration

Metabolic/Nutritional: (BUN Increased), (Creatinine Increased), (Dehydration), (Hyperglycemia), Hyperkalemia, Hyperlipemia, (Metabolic Acidosis), (Osmolality Increased)

Respiratory: Bronchospasm, Burning in Throat, Cough, Dyspnea, Hiccough, Hyperventilation, Hypoventilation, <u>Hypoxia</u>, Laryngospasm, Pharyngitis, Sneezing, Tachypnea, Upper Airway Obstruction

Skin and Appendages: Conjunctival Hyperemia, Diaphoresis, (Rash), Urticaria

Special Senses: Diplopia, Ear Pain, Eye Pain, *Nystagmus*, Taste Perversion, Tinnitus

Urogenital: (Kidney Failure), Oliguria, Urine Retention

DRUG ABUSE AND DEPENDENCE

Rare cases of self administration of Propofol Injection by health care professionals have been reported, including some fatalities. Propofol Injection should be managed to prevent the risk of diversion including restriction of access and accounting procedures as appropriate to the clinical setting.

OVERDOSAGE

If overdosage occurs Propofol Injection administration should be discontinued immediately. Overdosage is likely to cause cardiorespiratory depression. Respiratory depression should be treated by artificial ventilation with oxygen. Cardiovascular depression may require repositioning of the patient by raising the patient's legs, increasing the flow rate of intravenous fluids and administering pressor agents and/or anticholinergic agents.

DOSAGE AND ADMINISTRATION

Dosage and rate of administration should be individualized and titrated to the desired effect according to clinically relevant factors including preinduction and concomitant medications, age, ASA physical classification and level of debilitation of the patient.

The following is abbreviated dosage and administration information which is only intended as a general guide in the use of Propofol Injection. Prior to administering Propofol Injection, it is imperative that the physician review and be completely familiar with the specific dosage and administration information detailed in the "Clinical Pharmacology — Individualization of Dosage" section.

In the elderly, debilitated and ASA III or IV patients, rapid bolus doses should not be used in the methods of administration described below. (See "Warnings".)

INTENSIVE CARE UNIT SEDATION
Strict aseptic techniques must be followed when handling Propofol Injection as the vehicle is capable of supporting rapid growth of microorganisms. (See *"Dosage and Administration"*, Handling Procedures Propofol Injection should be individualized according to the patient's condition and response, blood lipid profile, and vital signs. (See *"Precautions—ICU sedation."*) For intubated, mechanically ventilated adult patients. Intensive Care Unit (ICU) sedation should be initiated slowly with a continuous infusion in order to titrate to desired clinical effect and minimize hypotension. When indicated, initiation of sedation should begin at 5 µg/kg/min (0.3 mg/kg/h). The infusion rate should be increased by increments of 5 to 10 µg/kg/min (0.3 to 0.6 mg/kg/h) until the desired level of sedation is achieved. A minimum period of 5 minutes between adjustments should be allowed for onset of peak drug effect. Most adult patients require maintenance rates of 5 to 50 µg/kg/min (0.3 to 3.0 mg/kg/h) or higher. Dosage of Propofol Injection should be reduced in patients who have received large dosages of narcotics. As with other sedative medications, there is interpatient variability in dosage requirements and these requirements may change with time. (see *"Dosage Guide"*) EVALUATION OF LEVEL OF SEDATION AND ASSESSMENT OF CNS FUNCTION SHOULD BE CARRIED OUT DAILY THROUGHOUT MAINTENANCE TO DETERMINE THE MINIMUM DOSE OF PROPOFOL INJECTION REQUIRED FOR SEDATION (See *"Clinical Trials, ICU Sedation"*). Bolus administration of 10 or 20 mg should only be used to rapidly increase depth of sedation in patients where hypotension is not likely to occur. Patients with compromised myocardial function, intravascular volume depletion or abnormally low vascular tone (eg, sepsis) may be more susceptible to hypotension. (See *"Precautions"*.)

Summary of Dosage Guidelines: Dosages and rates of administration in the following table should be individualized and titrated to clinical response. Safety

and dosage requirements in Pediatric patients have only been established for induction and maintenance of anesthesia.

For complete dosage information, see *"Clinical Pharmacology-Individualization of Dosage"*.

Indication	Dosage and Administration
Induction of Anesthesia	
	Healthy Adults Less Than 55 Years of Age: 40 mg every 10 seconds until induction onset (2.0 to 2.5 mg/kg).
	Elderly, Debilitated and ASA III or IV Patients: 20 mg every 10 seconds until induction onset (1.0 to 1.5 mg/kg).
	Neurosurgical Patients: 20 mg every 10 seconds until induction onset (1.0 to 2.0 mg/kg).
	Pediatric—healthy, 3 years or older: 2.5 to 3.5 mg/kg administered over 20-30 seconds.
Maintenance of Anesthesia: Infusion	
	Healthy Adults Less Than 55 Years of Age: 100 to 200 µg/kg/min (6 to 12 mg/kg/h).
	Elderly, Debilitated, ASA III or IV Patients: 50 to 100 µg/kg/min (3 to 6 mg/kg/h).
	Neurosurgical Patients: 100 to 200 µg/kg/min (6 to 12 mg/kg/h).
	Pediatric-healthy, 3 years or older: 125 to 300 µg/kg/min (7.5 to 18 mg/kg/h)
Maintenance of Anesthesia: Intermittent Bolus	
	Adults: Increments of 25 to 50 mg as needed.
Initiation of MAC Sedation	
	Adults: Slow infusion or slow injection techniques are recommended to avoid apnea or hypotension. Most patients require an infusion of 100 to 150 µ/kg/min (6 to 9 mg/kg/h) for 3 to 5 minutes or a slow injection of 0.5 mg/kg over 3 to 5 minutes followed immediately by a maintenance infusion.
	Elderly, Debilitated, Neurosurgical, ASA III or IV Patients: Most patients require dosage similar to healthy adults. Rapid boluses are to be avoided (see *"Warnings"*).
Maintenance of MAC Sedation	
	Adults: A variable rate infusion technique is preferable over an intermittent bolus technique. Most patients require an infusion of 25 to 75 µg/kg/min (1.5 to 4.5 mg/kg/h) or incremental bolus doses of 10 mg or 20 mg. **Elderly, Debilitated, Neurosurgical, and ASA III or IV Patients:** Most patients require a 20% reduction of the adult dose. A rapid (single or repeated) bolus dose should not be used. (See *"Warnings".*)
Initiation and Maintenance of ICU Sedation in Intubated, Mechanically Ventilated	
	Adult Patients: Because of the lingering effects of previous anesthetic or sedative agents, most patients require an infusion of 5 µg/kg/min (0.3 mg/kg/h) for at least 5 minutes. Subsequent increments of 5 to 10 µg/kg/min (0.3 to 0.6 mg/kg/h) over 5 to 10 minutes may be used until desired level of sedation is achieved. Maintenance rates of 5 to 50 µg/kg/min (0.3 to 3.0 mg/kg/h) or higher may be required. Evaluation of level of sedation and assessment of CNS function should be carried out daily throughout maintenance to determine the minimum dose of Propofol Injection required for sedation. The tubing and any unused portions of Propofol Injection should be discarded after 12 hours because Propofol Injection contains no preservatives and is capable of supporting rapid growth of microorganisms.

Compatibility and Stability: Propofol Injection should not be mixed with other therapeutic agents prior to administration.

Dilution Prior to Administration: When Propofol Injection is diluted prior to administration, it should only be diluted with 5% Dextrose Injection, USP, and it should not be diluted to a concentration less than 2 mg/mL because it is an emulsion. In diluted form it has been shown to be more stable when in contact with glass than with plastic (95% potency after 2 hours of running infusion in plastic).

Administration with Other Fluids: Compatibility of Propofol Injection with the coadministration of blood/serum/plasma has not been established (See *"Warnings"*.) Propofol Injection has been shown to be compatible when administered with the following intravenous fluids.
—5% Dextrose Injection, USP
—Lactated Ringers Injection, USP
—Lactated Ringers and 5% Dextrose Injection
—5% Dextrose and 0.45% Sodium Chloride Injection, USP
—5% Dextrose and 0.2% Sodium Chloride Injection, USP

► SHOWN IN PRODUCT IDENTIFICATION GUIDE

HANDLING PROCEDURES

General: Parenteral drug products should be inspected visually for particulate matter and discoloration prior to administration whenever solution and container permit. Propofol Injection must not be administered through filters with a pore size less than 5 µm because this could restrict the flow of Propofol Injection and/or cause the breakdown of the emulsion.

Do not use if there is evidence of separation of the phases of the emulsion.

Strict aseptic techniques must always be maintained during handling as Propofol Injection is a single-use parenteral product and contains no antimicrobial preservatives. THE VEHICLE IS CAPABLE OF SUPPORTING RAPID GROWTH OF MICROORGANISMS.

Failure to follow aseptic handling procedures may result in microbial contamination causing fever, infection/sepsis and/or other adverse consequences which could lead to life-threatening illness.

Rare cases of self administration of Propofol Injection by health care professionals have been reported, including some fatalities (see *"Drug Abuse and Dependence"*).

GENERAL ANESTHESIA/MAC SEDATION

Propofol Injection should be prepared for use just prior to initiation of each individual anesthetic/sedative procedure. The ampule neck surface or vial rubber stopper should be disinfected using 70% isopropyl alcohol. Propofol Injection should be drawn into sterile syringes immediately after ampules or vials are opened. When withdrawing Propofol Injection from vials, a sterile vent spike should be used. The syringe(s) should be labeled with appropriate information including the date and time the ampule or vial was opened. Administration should commence promptly and be completed within 6 hours after the ampules or vials have been opened.

Propofol Injection should be prepared for single patient use only. Any unused portions of Propofol Injection, reservoirs, dedicated administration tubing and/or solutions containing Propofol Injection must be discarded at the end of the anesthetic procedure or at 6 hours, whichever occurs sooner. The IV line should be flushed every 6 hours and at the end of the anesthetic procedure to remove residual Propofol Injection.

ICU SEDATION

When Propofol Injection is administered directly from the vial, strict aseptic techniques must be followed. The vial rubber stopper should be disinfected using 70% isopropyl alcohol. A sterile vent spike and sterile tubing must be used for administration of Propofol Injection. As with other lipid emulsions the number of IV line manipulations should be minimized. Administration should commence promptly and must be completed within 12 hours after the vial has been spiked. The tubing and any unused portions of Propofol Injection must be discarded after 12 hours.

If Propofol Injection is transferred to a syringe or other container prior to administration, the handling procedures for General anesthesia/MAC sedation should be followed and the product should be discarded and administration lines changed after 6 hours.

STORAGE

Store below 22°C (72°F). Do not store below 4°C (40°F). Refrigeration is not recommended. Protect from light. Shake well before use.

HOW SUPPLIED

INJECTION: 10 MG/ML

BRAND/MANUFACTURER	NDC	SIZE	AWP
○ **BRAND**			
DIPRIVAN: Stuart	00038-0290-50	50 ml	$30.89
	00038-0290-11	100 ml	$61.78
	00038-0290-20	20 ml 5s	$61.78

Propoxyphene Hydrochloride

DESCRIPTION

Propoxyphene Hydrochloride, USP is an odorless, white crystalline powder with a bitter taste. It is freely soluble in water. Chemically, it is (2S, 3R)-(-)-4-(Dimethylamino)-3-methyl- 1,2-diphenyl-2-butanol propionate (ester) hydrochloride. Its molecular weight is 375.94.

Each capsule of Propoxyphene Hydrochloride contains 65 mg (172.9 µmol) (No. 365) Propoxyphene Hydrochloride.

Following is its chemical structure:

$$(CH_3)_2NCH_2 - \underset{\underset{H}{|}}{C} - \underset{\underset{\phi}{|}}{\overset{\overset{OCC_2H_5}{|}}{C}} - CH_2 \phi \cdot HCl$$

CLINICAL PHARMACOLOGY

Propoxyphene is a centrally acting narcotic analgesic agent. Equimolar doses of Propoxyphene Hydrochloride or napsylate provide similar plasma concentrations. Following administration of 65, 130, or 195 mg of Propoxyphene Hydrochloride, the bioavailability of Propoxyphene is equivalent to that of 100, 200, or 300 mg

respectively of Propoxyphene napsylate. Peak plasma concentrations of Propoxyphene are reached in 2 to 2 ½ hours. After a 65-mg oral dose of Propoxyphene Hydrochloride, peak plasma levels of 0.05 to 0.1 µg/mL are achieved.

Repeated doses of Propoxyphene at 6-hour intervals lead to increasing plasma concentrations, with a plateau after the ninth dose at 48 hours.

Propoxyphene is metabolized in the liver to yield norpropoxyphene. Propoxyphene has a half-life of 6 to 12 hours, whereas that of norpropoxyphene is 30 to 36 hours.

Norpropoxyphene has substantially less central-nervous-system-depressant effect than Propoxyphene but a greater local anesthetic effect, which is similar to that of amitriptyline and antiarrhythmic agents, such as lidocaine and quinidine.

In animal studies in which Propoxyphene and norpropoxyphene were continuously infused in large amounts, intracardiac conduction time (PR and QRS intervals) was prolonged. Any intracardiac conduction delay attributable to high concentrations of norpropoxyphene may be of relatively long duration.

ACTIONS

Propoxyphene is a mild narcotic analgesic structurally related to methadone. The potency of Propoxyphene Hydrochloride is from two-thirds to equal that of codeine.

INDICATIONS

Propoxyphene Hydrochloride is indicated for the relief of mild to moderate pain.

UNLABELED USES

Propoxyphene is used alone or as an adjunct in the treatment of rheumatoid arthritis and restless leg syndrome.

CONTRAINDICATION

Hypersensitivity to Propoxyphene, aspirin, or caffeine.

WARNINGS

> ■ **DO NOT PRESCRIBE PROPOXYPHENE FOR PATIENTS WHO ARE SUICIDAL OR ADDICTION-PRONE.**
>
> ■ **PRESCRIBE PROPOXYPHENE WITH CAUTION FOR PATIENTS TAKING TRANQUILIZERS OR ANTIDEPRESSANT DRUGS AND PATIENTS WHO USE ALCOHOL IN EXCESS.**
>
> ■ **TELL YOUR PATIENTS NOT TO EXCEED THE RECOMMENDED DOSE AND TO LIMIT THEIR INTAKE OF ALCOHOL.**
>
> PROPOXYPHENE PRODUCTS IN EXCESSIVE DOSES, EITHER ALONE OR IN COMBINATION WITH OTHER CNS DEPRESSANTS, INCLUDING ALCOHOL, ARE A MAJOR CAUSE OF DRUG-RELATED DEATHS. FATALITIES WITHIN THE FIRST HOUR OF OVERDOSAGE ARE NOT UNCOMMON. IN A SURVEY OF DEATHS DUE TO OVERDOSAGE CONDUCTED IN 1975, IN APPROXIMATELY 20% OF THE FATAL CASES, DEATH OCCURRED WITHIN THE FIRST HOUR (5% OCCURRED WITHIN 15 MINUTES). PROPOXYPHENE SHOULD NOT BE TAKEN IN DOSES HIGHER THAN THOSE RECOMMENDED BY THE PHYSICIAN. THE JUDICIOUS PRESCRIBING OF PROPOXYPHENE IS ESSENTIAL TO THE SAFE USE OF THIS DRUG. WITH PATIENTS WHO ARE DEPRESSED OR SUICIDAL, CONSIDERATION SHOULD BE GIVEN TO THE USE OF NON-NARCOTIC ANALGESICS. PATIENTS SHOULD BE CAUTIONED ABOUT THE CONCOMITANT USE OF PROPOXYPHENE PRODUCTS AND ALCOHOL BECAUSE OF POTENTIALLY SERIOUS CNS-ADDITIVE EFFECTS OF THESE AGENTS. BECAUSE OF ITS ADDED DEPRESSANT EFFECTS, PROPOXYPHENE SHOULD BE PRESCRIBED WITH CAUTION FOR THOSE PATIENTS WHOSE MEDICAL CONDITION REQUIRES THE CONCOMITANT ADMINISTRATION OF SEDATIVES, TRANQUILIZERS, MUSCLE RELAXANTS, ANTIDEPRESSANTS, *OR* OTHER CNS-DEPRESSANT DRUGS. PATIENTS SHOULD BE ADVISED OF THE ADDITIVE DEPRESSANT EFFECTS OF THESE COMBINATIONS.
>
> MANY OF THE PROPOXYPHENE-RELATED DEATHS HAVE OCCURRED IN PATIENTS WITH PREVIOUS HISTORIES OF EMOTIONAL DISTURBANCES OR SUICIDAL IDEATION OR ATTEMPTS AS WELL AS HISTORIES OF MISUSE OF TRANQUILIZERS, ALCOHOL, AND OTHER CNS-ACTIVE DRUGS. SOME DEATHS HAVE OCCURRED AS A CONSEQUENCE OF THE ACCIDENTAL INGESTION OF EXCESSIVE QUANTITIES OF PROPOXYPHENE ALONE OR IN COMBINATION WITH OTHER DRUGS. PATIENTS TAKING PROPOXYPHENE SHOULD BE WARNED NOT TO EXCEED THE DOSAGE RECOMMENDED BY THE PHYSICIAN.

Drug Dependence: Propoxyphene, when taken in higher-than-recommended doses over long periods of time, can produce drug dependence characterized by psychic dependence and, less frequently, physical dependence and tolerance. Propoxyphene will only partially suppress the withdrawal syndrome in individuals physically dependent on morphine or other narcotics. The abuse liability of Propoxyphene is qualitatively similar to that of codeine although quantitatively less, and Propoxyphene should be prescribed with the same degree of caution appropriate to the use of codeine.

Usage in Ambulatory Patients: Propoxyphene may impair the mental and/or physical abilities required for the performance of potentially hazardous tasks, such as driving a car or operating machinery. The patient should be cautioned accordingly.

Warning: Reye syndrome is a rare but serious disease which can follow flu or chickenpox in children and teenagers. Although the cause of Reye syndrome is unknown, some reports claim aspirin (or salicylates) may increase the risk of developing this disease.

PRECAUTIONS

General: Salicylates should be used with extreme caution in the presence of peptic ulcer or coagulation abnormalities. Propoxyphene should be administered with caution to patients with hepatic or renal impairment since higher serum concentrations or delayed elimination may occur.

Drug Interactions: The CNS-depressant effect of Propoxyphene is additive with that of other CNS depressants, including alcohol.

Salicylates may enhance the effect of anticoagulants and inhibit the uricosuric effect of uricosuric agents.

As is the case with medicinal agents, Propoxyphene may slow the metabolism of a concomitantly administered drug. Should this occur, the higher serum concentrations of that drug may result in increased pharmacologic or adverse effects of that drug. Such occurrences have been reported when Propoxyphene was administered to patients on antidepressants, anticonvulsants, or warfarin-like drugs. Severe neurologic signs, including coma, have occurred with concurrent use of carbamazepine.

Usage in Pregnancy: Safe use in pregnancy has not been established relative to possible adverse effects on fetal development. Instances of withdrawal symptoms in the neonate have been reported following usage during pregnancy. Therefore, Propoxyphene should not be used in pregnant women unless, in the judgment of the physician, the potential benefits outweigh the possible hazards. Aspirin does not appear to have teratogenic effects. However, prolonged pregnancy and labor with increased bleeding before and after delivery, decreased birth weight, and increased rate of stillbirth were reported with high blood salicylate levels. Because of possible adverse effects on the neonate and the potential for increased maternal blood loss, aspirin should be avoided during the last 3 months of pregnancy.

Usage in Nursing Mothers: Low levels of Propoxyphene have been detected in human milk. In postpartum studies involving nursing mothers who were given Propoxyphene, no adverse effects were noted in infants receiving mother's milk.

Usage in Children: Propoxyphene is not recommended for use in children, because documented clinical experience has been insufficient to establish safety and a suitable dosage regimen in the pediatric age group.

Usage in the Elderly: The rate of Propoxyphene metabolism may be reduced in some patients. Increased dosing interval should be considered.

A Patient Information Sheet is available for this product.

ADVERSE REACTIONS

In a survey conducted in hospitalized patients, less than 1% of patients taking Propoxyphene Hydrochloride at recommended doses experienced side effects. The most frequently reported were dizziness, sedation, nausea, and vomiting. Some of these adverse reactions may be alleviated if the patient lies down.

Other adverse reactions include constipation, abdominal pain, skin rashes, light-headedness, headache, weakness, euphoria, dysphoria, hallucinations, and minor visual disturbances.

Propoxyphene therapy has been associated with abnormal liver function tests and, more rarely, with instances of reversible jaundice (including cholestatic jaundice).

Renal papillary necrosis may result from chronic aspirin use, particularly when the dosage is greater than recommended and when combined with acetaminophen.

Subacute painful myopathy has occurred following chronic Propoxyphene overdosage.

MANAGEMENT OF OVERDOSAGE

In all cases of suspected overdosage, call your regional poison control center to obtain the most up-to-date information about the treatment of overdose. This recommendation is made because, in general, information regarding the treatment of overdosage may change more rapidly than do package inserts.

Initial consideration should be given to the management of the CNS effects of Propoxyphene overdosage. Resuscitative measures should be initiated promptly.

Symptoms of Propoxyphene Overdosage: The manifestations of acute overdosage with Propoxyphene are those of narcotic overdosage. The patient is usually somnolent but may be stuporous or comatose and convulsing. Respiratory depression is characteristic. The ventilatory rate and/or tidal volume is decreased, which results in cyanosis and hypoxia. Pupils, initially pinpoint, may become dilated as hypoxia increases. Cheyne-Stokes respiration and apnea may occur. Blood pressure and heart rate are usually normal initially, but blood pressure falls and cardiac performance deteriorates, which ultimately results in pulmonary edema and circulatory collapse, unless the respiratory depression is corrected and adequate ventilation is restored promptly. Cardiac arrhythmias and conduction delay may be present. A combined respiratory-metabolic acidosis occurs owing to retained CO_2 (hypercapnia) and to lactic acid formed during anaerobic glycolysis. Acidosis may be severe if large amounts of salicylates have also been ingested. Death may occur.

Treatment of Propoxyphene Overdosage: Attention should be directed first to establishing a patent airway and to restoring ventilation. Mechanically assisted ventilation, with or without oxygen, may be required, and positive pressure respiration may be desirable if pulmonary edema is present. The narcotic antagonist naloxone will markedly reduce the degree of respiratory depression, and 0.4 to 2 mg should be administered promptly, preferably intravenously. If the desired degree of counteraction with improvement in respiratory functions is not obtained, naloxone should be repeated at 2- to 3-minute intervals. The duration of action of the antagonist may be brief. If no response is observed after 10 mg of naloxone have been administered, the diagnosis of Propoxyphene toxicity should be questioned. Naloxone may also be administered by continuous intravenous infusion.

Treatment of Propoxyphene Overdosage in Children: The usual initial dose of naloxone in children is 0.01 mg/kg body weight given intravenously. If this dose does not result in the desired degree of clinical improvement, a subsequent increased dose of 0.1 mg/kg body weight may be administered. If an IV route of administration is not available, naloxone may be administered IM or subcutaneously in divided doses. If necessary, naloxone can be diluted with Sterile Water for Injection.

Blood gases, pH, and electrolytes should be monitored in order that acidosis and any electrolyte disturbance present may be corrected promptly. Acidosis, hypoxia, and generalized CNS depression predispose to the development of cardiac arrhythmias. Ventricular fibrillation or cardiac arrest may occur and necessitate the full complement of cardiopulmonary resuscitation (CPR) measures. Respiratory acidosis rapidly subsides as ventilation is restored and hypercapnia eliminated, but lactic acidosis may require intravenous bicarbonate for prompt correction.

Electrocardiographic monitoring is essential. Prompt correction of hypoxia, acidosis, and electrolyte disturbance (when present) will help prevent these cardiac complications and will increase the effectiveness of agents administered to restore normal cardiac function.

In addition to the use of a narcotic antagonist, the patient may require careful titration with an anticonvulsant to control convulsions. Analeptic drugs (for example, caffeine or amphetamine) should not be used because of their tendency to precipitate convulsions.

General supportive measures, in addition to oxygen, include, when necessary, intravenous fluids, vasopressor-inotropic compounds, and, when infection is likely, anti-infective agents. Gastric lavage may be useful and activated charcoal can adsorb a significant amount of ingested Propoxyphene. Dialysis is of little value in poisoning due to Propoxyphene. Efforts should be made to determine whether other agents, such as alcohol, barbiturates, tranquilizers, or other CNS depressants, were also ingested, since these increase CNS depression as well as cause specific toxic effects.

Symptoms of Salicylate Overdosage: Such symptoms include central nausea and vomiting, tinnitus and deafness, vertigo and headaches, mental dullness and confusion, diaphoresis, rapid pulse, and increased respiration and respiratory alkalosis.

Treatment of Salicylate Overdosage: When aspirin/caffeine/propoxyphene/hydrochloride has been ingested, the clinical picture may be complicated by salicylism.

The treatment of acute salicylate intoxication includes minimizing drug absorption, promoting elimination through the kidneys, and correcting metabolic derangements affecting body temperature, hydration, acid-base balance, and electrolyte balance. The technique to be employed for eliminating salicylate from the bloodstream depends on the degree of drug intoxication.

If the patient is seen within 4 hours of ingestion, the stomach should be emptied by inducing vomiting or by gastric lavage as soon as possible.

The nomogram of Done is a useful prognostic guide in which the expected severity of salicylate intoxication is based on serum salicylate levels and the time interval between ingestion and taking the blood sample.

Exchange transfusion is most feasible for a small infant. Intermittent peritoneal dialysis is useful for cases of moderate severity in adults. Intravenous fluids alkalinized by the addition of sodium bicarbonate or potassium citrate are helpful. Hemodialysis with the artificial kidney is the most effective means of removing salicylate and is indicated for the very severe cases of salicylate intoxication.

DOSAGE AND ADMINISTRATION

These products are given orally. The usual dosage of Propoxyphene Hydrochloride is 65 mg every 4 hours as needed for pain.

The maximum recommended dose of Propoxyphene Hydrochloride is 390 mg/day.

Consideration should be given to a reduced total daily dosage in patients with hepatic or renal impairment.

Store at controlled room temperature, 59° to 86°F (15° to 30°C).

HOW SUPPLIED
CAPSULE (C-IV): 65 MG

AVERAGE UNIT PRICE (AVAILABLE SIZES)		GENERIC A-RATED AVERAGE PRICE (GAAP)	
BRAND	$0.34	100s	$9.31
GENERIC	$0.07	500s	$25.60
HCFA FUL (100s ea)	$0.05	1000s	$43.49

BRAND/MANUFACTURER	NDC	SIZE	AWP
◆ BRAND			
▶ DARVON: Lilly	00002-0803-02	100s	$32.74
	00002-0803-33	100s ud	$37.12
	00002-0803-03	500s	$156.38

▶ SHOWN IN PRODUCT IDENTIFICATION GUIDE

BRAND/MANUFACTURER	NDC	SIZE	AWP
◆ GENERICS			
West-Ward	00143-3235-01	100s	$5.21
➤ Lemmon	00093-0741-01	100s	$5.25
Geneva	00781-2140-01	100s	$5.48
PP-CAP: Alra	51641-0321-01	100s	$5.80
Moore,H.L.	00839-5098-06	100s	$5.93
Zenith	00172-2186-60	100s	$6.00
Goldline	00182-0698-01	100s	$6.60
Qualitest	00603-5459-21	100s	$6.61
Major	00904-7700-60	100s	$6.65
Parmed	00349-2285-01	100s	$7.17
URL	00677-0356-01	100s	$7.35
Purepac	00228-2082-10	100s	$7.40
Aligen	00405-0175-01	100s	$7.48
Rugby	00536-4382-01	100s	$7.90
Schein	00364-0312-01	100s	$7.95
Mylan	00378-0129-01	100s	$8.45
West-Ward	00143-3235-52	100s	$25.00
Major	00904-7700-61	100s	$27.65
Auro	55829-0864-01	100s ud	$8.57
Vangard	00615-0439-13	100s ud	$9.30
PP-CAP: Alra	51641-0321-11	100s ud	$12.08
West-Ward	00143-3235-25	100s ud	$15.00
➤ Lemmon	00093-0741-05	500s	$18.75
West-Ward	00143-3235-05	500s	$20.39
Major	00904-7700-40	500s	$21.75
URL	00677-0356-05	500s	$22.80
Moore,H.L.	00839-5098-12	500s	$22.94
Qualitest	00603-5459-28	500s	$23.11
PP-CAP: Alra	51641-0321-05	500s	$23.90
Goldline	00182-0698-05	500s	$24.30
Rugby	00536-4382-05	500s	$24.75
Mylan	00378-0129-05	500s	$24.95
Zenith	00172-2186-70	500s	$25.60
Schein	00364-0312-05	500s	$33.40
Aligen	00405-0175-02	500s	$34.78
Purepac	00228-2082-50	500s	$37.00
➤ Lemmon	00093-0741-10	1000s	$37.50
West-Ward	00143-3235-10	1000s	$38.08
Major	00904-7700-20	1000s	$39.75
Goldline	00182-0698-10	1000s	$41.55
PP-CAP: Alra	51641-0321-10	1000s	$43.50
Moore,H.L.	00839-5098-16	1000s	$43.88
URL	00677-0356-10	1000s	$44.00
Rugby	00536-4382-10	1000s	$44.85
Geneva	00781-2140-10	1000s	$46.56
Zenith	00172-2186-80	1000s	$48.90
Parmed	00349-2285-10	1000s	$49.82

Propoxyphene Napsylate

DESCRIPTION

Propoxyphene Napsylate, USP is an odorless, white crystalline powder with a bitter taste. It is very slightly soluble in water and soluble in methanol, ethanol, chloroform, and acetone. Chemically, it is (α S, 1 R)-α-[2-(Dimethylamino)-1-methylethyl]- α -phenylphenethyl propionate compound with 2-naphthalenesulfonic acid (1:1) monohydrate. Its molecular weight is 565.72.

Propoxyphene Napsylate differs from propoxyphene hydrochloride in that it allows more stable liquid dosage forms and tablet formulations. Because of differences in molecular weight, a dose of 100 mg (176.8 μmol) of propoxyphene napsylate is required to supply an amount of Propoxyphene equivalent to that present in 65 mg (172.9 μmol) of propoxyphene hydrochloride.

Each tablet of Propoxyphene Napsylate contains 100 mg (176.8 μmol) Propoxyphene Napsylate.

Each 5 mL of Propoxyphene Napsylate suspension contains 50 mg (88.4 μmol) Propoxyphene Napsylate.

Following is its chemical structure:

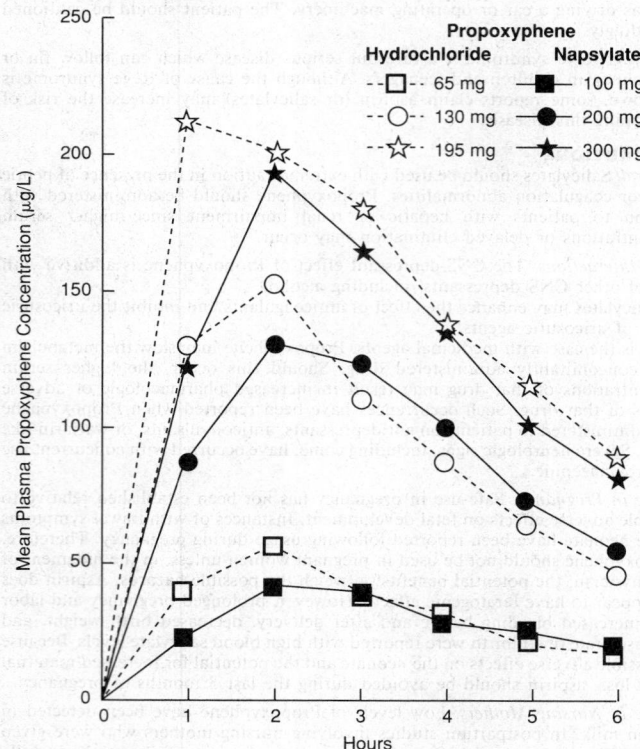

CLINICAL PHARMACOLOGY

Propoxyphene is a centrally acting narcotic analgesic agent. Equimolar doses of propoxyphene hydrochloride or napsylate provide similar plasma concentrations. Following administration of 65, 130, or 195 mg of propoxyphene hydrochloride, the bioavailability of Propoxyphene is equivalent to that of 100, 200, or 300 mg respectively of Propoxyphene Napsylate. Peak plasma concentrations of Propoxyphene are reached in 2 to 2 ½ hours. After a 100-mg oral dose of Propoxyphene Napsylate, peak plasma levels of 0.05 to 0.1 μg/ml are achieved. As shown in Figure 1, the Napsylate salt tends to be absorbed more slowly than the hydrochloride. At or near therapeutic doses, this absorption difference is small when compared with that among subjects and among doses. (See figure 1.)

Figure 1. Mean plasma concentrations of Propoxyphene in 8 human subjects following oral administration of 65 and 130 mg of the hydrochloride salt and 100 and 200 mg of the napsylate salt and in 7 given 195 mg of the hydrochloride and 300 mg of the napsylate salt

Because of this several hundredfold difference in solubility, the absorption rate of very large doses of the Napsylate salt is significantly lower than that of equimolar doses of the hydrochloride.

Repeated doses of Propoxyphene at 6-hour intervals lead to increasing plasma concentrations, with a plateau after the ninth dose at 48 hours.

Propoxyphene is metabolized in the liver to yield norpropoxyphene. Propoxyphene has a half-life of 6 to 12 hours, whereas that of norpropoxyphene is 30 to 36 hours.

Norpropoxyphene has substantially less central-nervous-system-depressant effect than propoxyphene but a greater local anesthetic effect, which is similar to that of amitriptyline and antiarrhythmic agents, such as lidocaine and quinidine.

In animal studies in which propoxyphene and norpropoxyphene were continuously infused in large amounts, intracardiac conduction time (PR and QRS intervals) was prolonged. Any intracardiac conduction delay attributable to high concentrations of norpropoxyphene may be of relatively long duration.

ACTIONS

Propoxyphene is a mild narcotic analgesic structurally related to methadone. The potency of Propoxyphene Napsylate is from two-thirds to equal that of codeine.

INDICATIONS

Propoxyphene Napsylate is indicated for the relief of mild to moderate pain.

UNLABELED USES

Propoxyphene Napsylate is used alone or as an adjunct in the treatment of rheumatoid arthritis and restless leg syndrome, and for detoxification and maintenance treatment of narcotic addicts.

CONTRAINDICATIONS

Hypersensitivity to Propoxyphene or acetaminophen.

WARNINGS

▪ DO NOT PRESCRIBE PROPOXYPHENE FOR PATIENTS WHO ARE SUICIDAL OR ADDICTION-PRONE.

▪ PRESCRIBE PROPOXYPHENE WITH CAUTION FOR PATIENTS TAKING TRANQUILIZERS OR ANTIDEPRESSANT DRUGS AND PATIENTS WHO USE ALCOHOL IN EXCESS.

▪ TELL YOUR PATIENTS NOT TO EXCEED THE RECOMMENDED DOSE AND TO LIMIT THEIR INTAKE OF ALCOHOL.

PROPOXYPHENE PRODUCTS IN EXCESSIVE DOSES, EITHER ALONE OR IN COMBINATION WITH OTHER CNS DEPRESSANTS, INCLUDING ALCOHOL, ARE A MAJOR CAUSE OF DRUG-RELATED DEATHS. FATALITIES WITHIN THE FIRST HOUR OF OVERDOSAGE ARE NOT

UNCOMMON. IN A SURVEY OF DEATHS DUE TO OVERDOSAGE CONDUCTED IN 1975. IN APPROXIMATELY 20% OF THE FATAL CASES, DEATH OCCURRED WITHIN THE FIRST HOUR (5% OCCURRED WITHIN 15 MINUTES). PROPOXYPHENE SHOULD NOT BE TAKEN IN DOSES HIGHER THAN THOSE RECOMMENDED BY THE PHYSICIAN. THE JUDICIOUS PRESCRIBING OF PROPOXYPHENE IS ESSENTIAL TO THE SAFE USE OF THIS DRUG. WITH PATIENTS WHO ARE DEPRESSED OR SUICIDAL, CONSIDERATION SHOULD BE GIVEN TO THE USE OF NON-NARCOTIC ANALGESICS. PATIENTS SHOULD BE CAUTIONED ABOUT THE CONCOMITANT USE OF PROPOXYPHENE PRODUCTS AND ALCOHOL BECAUSE OF POTENTIALLY SERIOUS CNS-ADDITIVE EFFECTS OF THESE AGENTS. BECAUSE OF ITS ADDED DEPRESSANT EFFECTS, PROPOXYPHENE SHOULD BE PRESCRIBED WITH CAUTION FOR THOSE PATIENTS WHOSE MEDICAL CONDITION REQUIRES THE CONCOMITANT ADMINISTRATION OF SEDATIVES, TRANQUILIZERS, MUSCLE RELAXANTS. ANTIDEPRESSANTS, OR OTHER CNS-DEPRESSANT DRUGS. PATIENTS SHOULD BE ADVISED OF THE ADDITIVE DEPRESSANT EFFECTS OF THESE COMBINATIONS.

MANY OF THE PROPOXYPHENE-RELATED DEATHS HAVE OCCURRED IN PATIENTS WITH PREVIOUS HISTORIES OF EMOTIONAL DISTURBANCES OR SUICIDAL IDEATION OR ATTEMPTS AS WELL AS HISTORIES OF MISUSE OF TRANQUILIZERS, ALCOHOL, AND OTHER CNS-ACTIVE DRUGS. SOME DEATHS HAVE OCCURRED AS A CONSEQUENCE OF THE ACCIDENTAL INGESTION OF EXCESSIVE QUANTITIES OF PROPOXYPHENE ALONE OR IN COMBINATION WITH OTHER DRUGS. PATIENTS TAKING PROPOXYPHENE SHOULD BE WARNED NOT TO EXCEED THE DOSAGE RECOMMENDED BY THE PHYSICIAN.

Drug Dependence: Propoxyphene, when taken in higher-than-recommended doses over long periods of time, can produce drug dependence characterized by psychic dependence and, less frequently, physical dependence and tolerance. Propoxyphene will only partially suppress the withdrawal syndrome in individuals physically dependent on morphine or other narcotics. The abuse liability of Propoxyphene is qualitatively similar to that of codeine although quantitatively less, and Propoxyphene should be prescribed with the same degree of caution appropriate to the use of codeine.

Usage in Ambulatory Patients: Propoxyphene may impair the mental and/or physical abilities required for the performance of potentially hazardous tasks, such as driving a car or operating machinery. The patient should be cautioned accordingly.

PRECAUTIONS

General: Propoxyphene should be administered with caution to patients with hepatic or renal impairment, since higher serum concentrations or delayed elimination may occur.

Drug Interactions: The CNS-depressant effect of Propoxyphene is additive with that of other CNS depressants, including alcohol.

As is the case with many medicinal agents, Propoxyphene may slow the metabolism of a concomitantly administered drug. Should this occur, the higher serum concentrations of that drug may result in increased phamacologic or adverse effects of that drug. Such occurrences have been reported when Propoxyphene was administered to patients on antidepressants, anticonvulsants, or warfarin-like drugs. Severe neurologic signs, including coma, have occurred with concurrent use of carbamazepine.

Usage in Pregnancy: Safe use in pregnancy has not been established relative to possible adverse effects on fetal development. Instances of withdrawal symptoms in the neonate have been reported following usage during pregnancy. Therefore, Propoxyphene should not be used in pregnant women unless, in the judgment of the physician, the potential benefits outweigh the possible hazards.

Usage in Nursing Mothers: Low levels of Propoxyphene have been detected in human milk. In postpartum studies involving nursing mothers who were given Propoxyphene, no adverse effects were noted in infants receiving mother's milk.

Usage in Children: Propoxyphene is not recommended for use in children, because documented clinical experience has been insufficient to establish safety and a suitable dosage regimen in the pediatric age group.

Usage in the Elderly: The rate of Propoxyphene metabolism may be reduced in some patients. Increased dosing interval should be considered.

ADVERSE REACTIONS

In a survey conducted in hospitalized patients, less than 1% of patients taking Propoxyphene Hydrochloride at recommended doses experienced side effects. The most frequently reported were dizziness, sedation, nausea, and vomiting. Some of these adverse reactions may be alleviated if the patient lies down.

Other adverse reactions include constipation, abdominal pain, skin rashes, light-headedness, headache, weakness, euphoria, dysphoria, hallucinations, and minor visual disturbances.

Liver dysfunction has been reported in association with both active components of (Propoxyphene Napsylate and acetaminophen tablets, USP).

Propoxyphene therapy has been associated with abnormal liver function tests and more rarely, with instances of reversible jaundice (including cholestatic jaundice). Hepatic necrosis may result from acute overdose of acetaminophen (see "*Management of Overdosage*"). In chronic ethanol abusers, this has been reported rarely with short-term use of acetaminophen doses of 2.5 to 10 g/day. Fatalities have occurred. Renal papillary necrosis may result from chronic acetaminophen use, particularly when the dosage is greater than recommended and when combined with aspirin.

Subacute painful myopathy has occurred following chronic Propoxyphene overdosage.

MANAGEMENT OF OVERDOSAGE

In all cases of suspected overdosage, call your regional poison control center to obtain the most up-to-date information about the treatment of overdose. This recommendation is made because, in general, information regarding the treatment of overdosage may change more rapidly than do package inserts.

Initial consideration should be given to the management of the CNS effects of Propoxyphene overdosage. Resuscitative measures should be initiated promptly.

Symptoms of Propoxyphene Overdosage: The manifestations of acute overdosage with Propoxyphene are those of narcotic overdosage. The patient is usually somnolent but may be stuporous or comatose and convulsing. Respiratory depression is characteristic. The ventilatory rate and/or tidal volume is decreased, which results in cyanosis and hypoxia. Pupils, initially pinpoint, may become dilated as hypoxia increases. Cheyne-Stokes respiration and apnea may occur. Blood pressure and heart rate are usually normal initially, but blood pressure falls and cardiac performance deteriorates, which ultimately results in pulmonary edema and circulatory collapse, unless the respiratory depression is corrected and adequate ventilation is restored promptly. Cardiac arrhythmias and conduction delay may be present. A combined respiratory-metabolic acidosis occurs owing to retained CO_2 (hypercapnia) and to lactic acid formed during anaerobic glycolysis. Acidosis may be severe if large amounts of salicylates have also been ingested. Death may occur.

Treatment of Propoxyphene Overdosage: Attention should be directed first to establishing a patent airway and to restoring ventilation. Mechanically assisted ventilation, with or without oxygen, may be required, and positive pressure respiration may be desirable if pulmonary edema is present. The narcotic antagonist naloxone will markedly reduce the degree of respiratory depression, and 0.4 to 2 mg should be administered promptly, preferably intravenously. If the desired degree of counteraction with improvement in respiratory functions is not obtained, naloxone should be repeated at 2- to 3-minute intervals. The duration of action of the antagonist may be brief. If no response is observed after 10 mg of naloxone have been administered, the diagnosis of Propoxyphene toxicity should be questioned. Naloxone may also be administered by continuous intravenous infusion.

Treatment of Propoxyphene Overdosage in Children: The usual initial dose of naloxone in children is 0.01 mg/kg body weight given intravenously. If this dose does not result in the desired degree of clinical improvement, a subsequent increased dose of 0.1 mg/kg body weight may be administered. If an IV route of administration is not available, naloxone may be administered IM or subcutaneously in divided doses. If necessary, naloxone can be diluted with Sterile Water for Injection.

Blood gases, pH, and electrolytes should be monitored in order that acidosis and any electrolyte disturbance present may be corrected promptly. Acidosis, hypoxia, and generalized CNS depression predispose to the development of cardiac arrhythmias. Ventricular fibrillation or cardiac arrest may occur and necessitate the full complement of cardiopulmonary resuscitation (CPR) measures. Respiratory acidosis rapidly subsides as ventilation is restored and hypercapnia eliminated, but lactic acidosis may require intravenous bicarbonate for prompt correction.

Electrocardiographic monitoring is essential. Prompt correction of hypoxia, acidosis, and electrolyte disturbance (when present) will help prevent these cardiac complications and will increase the effectiveness of agents administered to restore normal cardiac function.

In addition to the use of a narcotic antagonist, the patient may require careful titration with an anticonvulsant to control convulsions. Analeptic drugs (for example, caffeine or amphetamine) should not be used because of their tendency to precipitate convulsions.

General supportive measures, in addition to oxygen, include, when necessary, intravenous fluids, vasopressor-inotropic compounds, and, when infection is likely, anti-infective agents. Gastric lavage may be useful, and activated charcoal can adsorb a significant amount of ingested Propoxyphene. Dialysis is of little value in poisoning due to Propoxyphene. Efforts should be made to determine whether other agents, such as alcohol, barbiturates, tranquilizers, or other CNS depressants, were also ingested, since these increase CNS depression as well as cause specific toxic effects.

Symptoms of Acetaminophen Overdosage: Shortly after oral ingestion of an overdose of acetaminophen and for the next 24 hours, anorexia, nausea, vomiting, diaphoresis, general malaise, and abdominal pain have been noted. The patient may then present no symptoms, but evidence of liver dysfunction may become apparent up to 72 hours after ingestion, with elevated serum transaminase and lactic dehydrogenase levels, an increase in serum bilirubin concentrations, and a prolonged prothrombin time. Death from hepatic failure may result 3 to 7 days after overdosage.

Acute renal failure may accompany the hepatic dysfunction and has been noted in patients who do not exhibit signs of fulminant hepatic failure. Typically, renal impairment is more apparent 6 to 9 days after ingestion of the overdose.

Treatment of Acetaminophen Overdosage: Acetaminophen in massive overdosage may cause hepatic toxicity in some patients. *In all cases of suspected overdose, immediately call your regional poison center or the Rocky Mountain Poison Center's toll-free number* (800-525-6115) for assistance in diagnosis and for directions in the use of N-acetylcysteine as an antidote.

In adults, hepatic toxicity has rarely been reported with acute overdoses of less than 10 g and fatalities with less than 15 g. Importantly, young children seem to be more resistant than adults to the hepatotoxic effect of an acetaminophen overdose. Despite this, the measures outlined below should be initiated in any adult or child suspected of having ingested an acetaminophen overdose.

Because clinical and laboratory evidence of hepatic toxicity may not be apparent until 48 to 72 hours postingestion, liver function studies should be obtained initially and repeated at 24-hour intervals.

Consider emptying the stomach promptly by lavage or by induction of emesis with syrup of ipecac. Patients' estimates of the quantity of a drug ingested are notoriously unreliable. Therefore, if an acetaminophen overdose is suspected, a serum acetaminophen assay should be obtained as early as possible, but no sooner than 4 hours following ingestion. The antidote, N-acetylcysteine, should be administered as early as possible, and within 16 hours of the overdose ingestion for optimal results. Following recovery, there are no residual, structural, or functional hepatic abnormalities.

DOSAGE AND ADMINISTRATION
These products are given orally. The usual dosage of Propoxyphene Napsylate tablets, USP is 100 mg Propoxyphene Napsylate every 4 hours as needed for pain.

The maximum recommended dose of Propoxyphene Napsylate is 600 mg/day.

Consideration should be given to a reduced total daily dosage in patients with hepatic or renal impairment.

Suspension: Shake well before using. Avoid freezing. Keep tightly closed.

Store at controlled room temperature, 59° to 86°F (15° to 30°C).

ANIMAL TOXICOLOGY
The acute lethal doses of the hydrochloride and napsylate salts of propoxyphene were determined in 4 species. The results shown in Figure 2 indicate that, on a molar basis, the Napsylate salt is less toxic than the hydrochloride. This may be due to the relative insolubility and retarded absorption of Propoxyphene Napsylate.

Figure 2
ACUTE ORAL TOXICITY OF PROPOXYPHENE

Species	LD_{50} (mg/kg) ± SE LD_{50} (mmol/kg) Propoxyphene Hydrochloride	Propoxyphene Napsylate
Mouse	282 ± 39 0.75	915 ± 163 1.62
Rat	230 ± 44 0.61	647 ± 95 1.14
Rabbit	ca. 82 0.22	≥ 183 > 0.32
Dog	ca. 100 0.27	≥ 183 > 0.32

Some indication of the relative insolubility and retarded absorption of Propoxyphene Napsylate was obtained by measuring plasma propoxyphene levels in 2 groups of 4 dogs following oral administration of equimolar doses of the 2 salts. As shown in Figure 3, the peak plasma concentration observed with propoxyphene hydrochloride was much higher than that obtained after administration of the Napsylate salt.

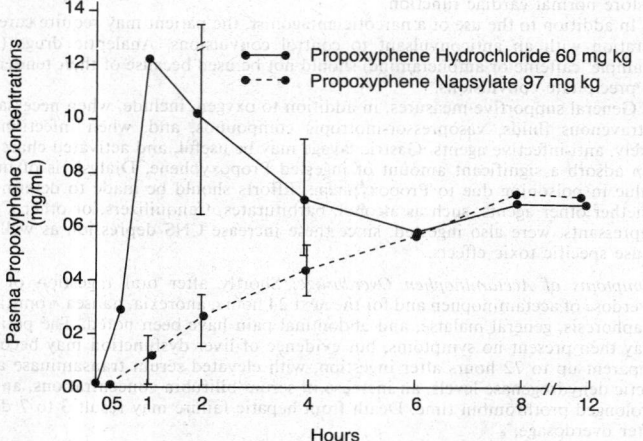

Figure 3. Plasma propoxyphene concentrations in dogs following large doses of the hydrochloride and nasylate salts

Although none of the animals in this experiment died, 3 of the 4 dogs given propoxyphene hydrochloride exhibited convulsive seizures during the time interval corresponding to the peak plasma levels. The 4 animals receiving the napsylate salt were mildly ataxic but not acutely ill.

HOW SUPPLIED
TABLETS (C-IV): 100 MG

BRAND/MANUFACTURER	NDC	SIZE	AWP
○ **BRAND**			
▶ DARVON-N: Lilly	00002-0353-02	100s	$47.65
	00002-0353-33	100s ud	$52.03
	00002-0353-03	500s	$225.24

Propranolol Hydrochloride

DESCRIPTION
Propranolol Hydrochloride is a synthetic beta-adrenergic receptor blocking agent chemically described as 1-(Isopropylamino)-3-(1-naphthyloxy)-2-propanol hydrochloride.

Propranolol HCl is a stable, white, crystalline solid which is readily soluble in water and ethanol. Its molecular weight is 295.81.

Propranolol HCl Long Acting is formulated to provide a sustained release of Propranolol HCl. Propranolol HCl Long Acting is available as 60 mg, 80 mg, 120 mg, and 160 mg capsules.

Following is its chemical structure:

$$OCH_2CHCH_2NHCH(CH_3)_2$$

· HCl

CLINICAL PHARMACOLOGY
Propranolol HCl is a nonselective beta-adrenergic receptor blocking agent possessing no other autonomic nervous system activity. It specifically competes with beta-adrenergic receptor stimulating agents for available receptor sites. When access to beta-receptor sites is blocked by Propranolol HCl the chronotropic, inotropic, and vasodilator responses to beta-adrenergic stimulation are decreased proportionally.

Propranolol is almost completely absorbed from the gastro-intestinal tract, but a portion is immediately bound by the liver. Peak effect occurs in one to one and one-half hours. The biologic half-life is approximately four hours.

There is no simple correlation between dose or plasma level and therapeutic effect, and the dose-sensitivity range as observed in clinical practice is wide. The principal reason for this is that sympathetic tone varies widely between individuals. Since there is no reliable test to estimate sympathetic tone or to determine whether total beta blockade has been achieved proper dosage requires titration.

Propranolol HCl Long Acting Capsules (60, 80, 120, and 160 mg) release Propranolol HCl at a controlled and predictable rate. Peak blood levels following dosing with Propranolol HCl Long Acting occur at about 6 hours, and the apparent plasma half-life is about 10 hours. When measured at steady state over a 24-hour period the areas under the Propranolol plasma concentration-time curve (AUCs) for the capsules are approximately 60% to 65% of the AUCs for a comparable divided daily dose of Propranolol HCl Tablets. The lower AUCs for the capsules are due to greater hepatic metabolism of Propranolol, resulting from the slower rate of absorption of Propranolol. Over a twenty-four (24) hour period, blood levels are fairly constant for about twelve (12) hours, then decline exponentially.

Propranolol HCl Long Acting should not be considered a simple mg-for-mg substitute for conventional Propranolol and the blood levels achieved do not match (are lower than) those of two to four times daily dosing with the same dose. When changing to Propranolol HCl Long Acting from conventional Propranolol, a possible need for retitration upwards should be considered, especially to maintain effectiveness at the end of the dosing interval. In most clinical settings, however, such as hypertension or angina where there is little correlation between plasma levels and clinical effect. Propranolol HCl Long Acting has been therapeutically equivalent to the same mg dose of conventional Propranolol HCl as assessed by 24-hour effects on blood pressure and on 24-hour exercise responses of heart rate, systolic pressure, and rate pressure product. Propranolol HCl Long Acting can provide effective beta blockade for a 24-hour period.

The mechanism of the antihypertensive effect of Propranolol HCl has not been established. Among the factors that may be involved in contributing to the antihypertensive action are (1) decreased cardiac output, (2) inhibition of renin release by the kidneys, and (3) diminution of tonic sympathetic nerve outflow from vasomotor centers in the brain. Although total peripheral resistance may increase initially, it readjusts to or below the pretreatment level with chronic use. Effects on plasma volume appear to be minor and somewhat variable, Propranolol HCl has been shown to cause a small increase in serum potassium concentration when used in the treatment of hypertensive patients.

In angina pectoris, Propranolol generally reduces the oxygen requirement of the heart at any given level of effort by blocking the catecholamine-induced increases in the heart rate, systolic blood pressure, and the velocity and extent of myocardial contraction. Propranolol may increase oxygen requirements by increasing left ventricular fiber length, end diastolic pressure, and systolic ejection period. The net physiologic effect of beta-adrenergic blockade is usually advantageous and is manifested during exercise by delayed onset of pain and increased work capacity.

Propranolol exerts its antiarrhythmic effects in concentrations associated with beta-adrenergic blockade and this appears to be its principal antiarrhythmic mechanism of action. In dosages greater than required for beta blockade, Propranolol HCl also exerts a quinidine-like or anesthetic-like membrane action, which affects the cardiac action potential. The significance of the membrane action in the treatment of arrhythmias is uncertain.

The mechanism of the antimigraine effect of Propranolol has not been established. Beta-adrenergic receptors have been demonstrated in the pial vessels of the brain.

The specific mechanism of Propranolol HCl's antitremor effects has not been established, but beta-2 (noncardiac) receptors may be involved. A central effect is also possible. Clinical studies have demonstrated that Propranolol HCl is of benefit in exaggerated physiological and essential (familial) tremor.

Beta receptor blockade can be useful in conditions in which, because of pathologic or functional changes, sympathetic activity is detrimental to the patient. But there are also situations in which sympathetic stimulation is vital. For example, in patients with severely damaged hearts, adequate ventricular function is maintained by virtue of sympathetic drive, which should be preserved. In the presence of AV block greater than first degree, beta blockade may prevent the necessary facilitating effect of sympathetic activity on conduction. Beta blockade results in bronchial constriction by interfering with adrenergic bronchodilator activity, which should be preserved in patients subject to bronchospasm.

Propranolol is not significantly dialyzable.

The Beta-Blocker Heart Attack Trial (BHAT) was a National Heart, Lung and Blood Institute-sponsored multicenter, randomized, double-blind, placebo-controlled trial conducted in 31 U.S. centers (plus one in Canada) in 3,837 persons without history of severe congestive heart failure or presence of recent heart failure; certain conduction defects; angina since infarction, who had survived the acute phase of myocardial infarction. Propranolol was administered at either 60 or 80 mg t.i.d. based on blood levels achieved during an initial trial of 40 mg. t.i.d. Therapy with Propranolol HCl begun 5 to 21 days following infarction, was shown to reduce overall mortality up to 39 months, the longest period of follow-up. This was primarily attributable to a reduction in cardiovascular mortality. The protective effect of Propranolol HCl was consistent regardless of age, sex, or site of infarction. Compared with placebo, total mortality was reduced 39% at 12 months and 26% over an average follow-up period of 25 months. The Norwegian Multicenter Trial in which Propranolol was administered at 40 mg q.i.d. gave overall results which support the findings in the BHAT.

Although the clinical trials used either t.i.d. or q.i.d. dosing, clinical, pharmacologic, and pharmacokinetic data provide a reasonable basis for concluding that b.i.d. dosing with Propranolol should be adequate in the treatment of postinfarction patients.

CLINICAL

In the BHAT, patients on Propranolol HCl were prescribed either 180 mg/day (82% of patients) or 240 mg/day (18% of patients). Patients were instructed to take the medication 3 times a day at mealtimes. This dosing schedule would result in an overnight dosing interval of 12 to 14 hours which is similar to the dosing interval for a b.i.d. regimen. In addition, blood samples were drawn at various times and analyzed for Propranolol. When the patients were grouped into tertiles based on the blood levels observed and the mortality in the upper and lower tertiles was compared, there was no evidence that blood levels affected mortality.

PHARMACOLOGIC

Studies in normal volunteers have shown that a 90 mg b.i.d. regimen maintains beta blockade at, or above, the minimum for 60 mg t.i.d. dosing for 24 hours even though differences occurred at two time intervals. At 10 to 12 hours after the first dose of the day, t.i.d. dosing gave more beta blockade than b.i.d. dosing; at 20 to 24 hours the trend of the relationship was reversed. These relationships were similar in direction to those observed for plasma Propranolol levels. (See "Pharmacokinetic".)

PHARMACOKINETIC

A bioavailability study in normal volunteers showed that the blood levels produced by 180 mg/day given b.i.d. are below those provided by the same daily dosage given t.i.d. at 10 to 12 hours after the first dose of the day, but above those of a t.i.d. regimen at 20 to 24 hours. However, the blood levels produced by b.i.d. dosing were always equivalent to or above the minimum for t.i.d. dosing throughout the 24 hours. In addition, the mean AUC on the fourth day for the b.i.d. regimen was about 17% greater than for the t.i.d. regimen (1,194 vs. 1,024 ng/mL.hr).

INDICATIONS AND USAGE

HYPERTENSION

Propranolol HCl and Propranolol HCl Long Acting are indicated in the management of hypertension. It may be used alone or used in combination with other antihypertensive agents, particularly a thiazide diuretic. Propranolol HCl and Propranolol HCl Long Acting is not indicated in the management of hypertensive emergencies.

ANGINA PECTORIS DUE TO CORONARY ATHEROSCLEROSIS

Propranolol HCl and Propranolol HCl Long Acting are indicated for the long-term management of patients with angina pectoris.

CARDIAC ARRHYTHMIAS (PROPRANOLOL HCL)

1.) Supraventricular arrhythmias

a) Paroxysmal atrial tachycardias, particularly those arrhythmias induced by catecholamines or digitalis or associated with the Wolff-Parkinson-White syndrome. (See "W-P-W" under "Warnings".)

b) Persistent sinus tachycardia which is noncompensatory and impairs the well-being of the patient.

c) Tachycardias and arrhythmias due to thyrotoxicosis when causing distress or increased hazard and when immediate effect is necessary as adjunctive, short-term (2 to 4 weeks) therapy.

May be used with, but not in place of, specific therapy. (See "Thyrotoxicosis" under "Warnings".)

d) Persistent atrial extrasystoles which impair the well-being of the patient and do not respond to conventional measures.

e) Atrial flutter and fibrillation when ventricular rate cannot be controlled by digitalis alone, or when digitalis is contraindicated.

2.) Ventricular tachycardias

Ventricular arrhythmias do not respond to Propranolol as predictably as do the supraventricular arrhythmias.

a) Ventricular tachycardias

With the exception of those induced by catecholamines or digitalis, Propranolol HCl is not the drug of first choice. In critical situations when cardioversion techniques or other drugs are not indicated or are not effective, Propranolol HCl may be considered. If, after consideration of the risks involved, Propranolol HCl is used, it should be given intravenously in low dosage and very slowly. (See "Dosage and Administration".) *Care in the administration of Propranolol HCl with constant electrocardiographic monitoring is essential as the failing heart requires some sympathetic drive for maintenance of myocardial tone.*

b) Persistent premature ventricular extrasystoles which do not respond to conventional measures and impair the well-being of the patient.

3.) Tachyarrhythmias of digitalis intoxication

If digitalis-induced tachyarrhythmias persist following discontinuance of digitalis and correction of electrolyte abnormalities, they are usually reversible with *oral* Propranolol HCl. Severe bradycardia may occur. (See "Overdosage".)

Intravenous Propranolol HCl is reserved for life-threatening arrhythmias. Temporary maintenance with oral therapy may be indicated. (See "Dosage and Administration".)

4.) Resistant tachyarrhythmias due to excessive catecholamine action during anesthesia

Tachyarrhythmias due to excessive catecholamine action during anesthesia may sometimes arise because of release of endogenous catecholamines or administration of catecholamines. When usual measures fail in such arrhythmias, Propranolol HCl may be given intravenously to abolish them. All general inhalation anesthetics produce some degree of myocardial depression. Therefore, when Propranolol HCl is used to treat arrhythmias during anesthesia, it should be used with extreme caution and constant ECG and central venous pressure monitoring. (See "Warnings".)

MYOCARDIAL INFARCTION

Propranolol HCl is indicated to reduce cardiovascular mortality in patients who have survived the acute phase of myocardial infarction and are clinically stable.

MIGRAINE

Propranolol HCl and Propranolol HCl Long Acting are indicated for the prophylaxis of common migraine headache. The efficacy of Propranolol in the treatment of a migraine attack that has started has not been established and Propranolol is not indicated for such use.

ESSENTIAL TREMOR

Propranolol HCl is indicated in the management of familial or hereditary essential tremor. Familial or essential tremor consists of involuntary, rhythmic, oscillatory movements, usually limited to the upper limbs. It is absent at rest but occurs when the limb is held in a fixed posture or position against gravity and during active movement. Propranolol HCl causes a reduction in the tremor amplitude but not in the tremor frequency. Propranolol HCl is not indicated for the treatment of tremor associated with Parkinsonism.

HYPERTROPHIC SUBAORTIC STENOSIS

Propranolol HCl and Propranolol HCl Long Acting are useful in the management of hypertrophic subaortic stenosis, especially for treatment of exertional or other stress-induced angina, palpitations, and syncope. Propranolol HCl and Propranolol HCl Long Acting also improve exercise performance. The effectiveness of Propranolol HCl in this disease appears to be due to a reduction of the elevated outflow pressure gradient, which is exacerbated by beta-receptor stimulation. Clinical improvement may be temporary.

PHEOCHROMOCYTOMA

After primary treatment with an alpha-adrenergic blocking agent has been instituted, Propranolol HCl may be useful as *adjunctive* therapy if the control of tachycardia becomes necessary before or during surgery.

It is hazardous to use Propranolol HCl unless alpha-adrenergic blocking drugs are already in use, since this would predispose to serious blood pressure elevation. Blocking only the peripheral dilator (beta) action of epinephrine leaves its constrictor (alpha) action unopposed.

In the event of hemorrhage or shock, there is a disadvantage in having both beta and alpha blockade since the combination prevents the increase in heart rate and peripheral vasoconstriction needed to maintain blood pressure.

With inoperable or metastatic pheochromocytoma, Propranolol HCl may be useful as an adjunct to the management of symptoms due to excessive beta-receptor stimulation.

UNLABELED USES
Propranolol is used alone or as an adjunct in the treatment of alcohol withdrawal, ascites, and to control aggressive and assaultive behavior in psychiatric patients. It is also used in causalgia, mixed migraine and muscle contraction headache, cyclosporine-induced headache, and hyperparathyroidism. It is also used as an alternative to exogenous estrogens in the treatment of menopausal vasomotor symptoms. Propranolol is used in patients with panic attacks, diazepam withdrawal, Huntington's disease to control aggressive behavior, and in the treatment of thyrotoxicosis in hyperthyroidism. It is also used as a vaginal contraceptive, in neuroleptic-induced akathisia, to control rage and violent behavior in patients with organic brain dysfunction, in Shy-Drager syndrome to control orthostatic hypotension, parkinsonian tremor, posttraumatic stress disorder, priapism, chronic schizophrenia, in the prevention of variceal hemorrhage in alcoholic cirrhotic patients, bladder instability, and to reduce the risk of gastrointestinal bleeding in patients with cirrhosis.

CONTRAINDICATIONS
Propranolol HCl is contraindicated in 1) cardiogenic shock, 2) sinus bradycardia and greater than first degree block, 3) bronchial asthma, 4) congestive heart failure (see *"Warnings"*) unless the failure is secondary to a tachyarrhythmia treatable with Propranolol HCl.

WARNINGS
CARDIAC FAILURE
Sympathetic stimulation may be a vital component supporting circulatory function in patients with congestive heart failure, and its inhibition by beta blockade may precipitate more severe failure. Although beta blockers should be avoided in overt congestive heart failure, if necessary, they can be used with close follow-up in patients with a history of failure who are well compensated and are receiving digitalis and diuretics. Beta-adrenergic blocking agents do not abolish the inotropic action of digitalis on heart muscle.

In Patients without a History of Heart Failure: continued use of beta blockers can, in some cases, lead to cardiac failure. Therefore, at the first sign or symptom of heart failure, the patient should be digitalized and/or treated with diuretics, and the response observed closely, or Propranolol HCl should be discontinued (gradually, if possible).

> IN PATIENTS WITH ANGINA PECTORIS, THERE HAVE BEEN REPORTS OF EXACERBATION OF ANGINA AND, IN SOME CASES, MYOCARDIAL INFARCTION, FOLLOWING *ABRUPT* DISCONTINUANCE OF PROPRANOLOL HCL THERAPY. THEREFORE, WHEN DISCONTINUANCE OF PROPRANOLOL HCL IS PLANNED, THE DOSAGE SHOULD BE GRADUALLY REDUCED OVER AT LEAST A FEW WEEKS AND THE PATIENT SHOULD BE CAUTIONED AGAINST INTERRUPTION OR CESSATION OF THERAPY WITHOUT THE PHYSICIAN'S ADVICE. IF PROPRANOLOL HCL THERAPY IS INTERRUPTED AND EXACERBATION OF ANGINA OCCURS, IT USUALLY IS ADVISABLE TO REINSTITUTE PROPRANOLOL HCL THERAPY AND TAKE OTHER MEASURES APPROPRIATE FOR THE MANAGEMENT OF UNSTABLE ANGINA PECTORIS. SINCE CORONARY ARTERY DISEASE MAY BE UNRECOGNIZED, IT MAY BE PRUDENT TO FOLLOW THE ABOVE ADVICE IN PATIENTS CONSIDERED AT RISK OF HAVING OCCULT ATHEROSCLEROTIC HEART DISEASE WHO ARE GIVEN PROPRANOLOL FOR OTHER INDICATIONS.

NONALLERGIC BRONCHOSPASM (E.G., CHRONIC BRONCHITIS, EMPHYSEMA)
Patients with bronchospastic diseases should in general not receive beta blockers. Propranolol HCl should be administered with caution since it may block bronchodilation produced by endogenous and exogenous catecholamine stimulation of beta receptors.

MAJOR SURGERY
The necessity or desirability of withdrawal of beta-blocking therapy prior to major surgery is controversial. It should be noted, however, that the impaired ability of the heart to respond to reflex adrenergic stimuli may augment the risks of general anesthesia and surgical procedures.

Propranolol HCl like other beta blockers, is a competitive inhibitor of beta-receptor agonists and its effects can be reversed by administration of such agents, e.g., dobutamine or isoproterenol. However, such patients may be subject to protracted severe hypotension. Difficulty in starting and maintaining the heartbeat has also been reported with beta blockers.

DIABETES AND HYPOGLYCEMIA
Beta blockers should be used with caution in diabetic patients if a beta-blocking agent is required. Beta blockers may mask tachycardia occurring with hypoglycemia, but other manifestations such as dizziness and sweating may not be significantly affected. Following insulin-induced hypoglycemia, Propranolol may cause a delay in the recovery of blood glucose to normal levels.

THYROTOXICOSIS
Beta blockade may mask certain clinical signs of hyperthyroidism. Therefore, abrupt withdrawal of Propranolol may be followed by an exacerbation of symptoms of hyperthyroidism, including thyroid storm. Propranolol may change thyroid-function tests, increasing T_4 and reverse T_3 and decreasing T_3

In patients with Wolff-Parkinson-White Syndrome, several cases have been reported in which, after Propranolol, the tachycardia was replaced by a severe bradycardia requiring a demand pacemaker. In one case this resulted after an initial dose of 5 mg Propranolol.

PRECAUTIONS
GENERAL
Propranolol should be used with caution in patients with impaired hepatic or renal function. Propranolol HCl is not indicated for the treatment of hypertensive emergencies.

Beta-adrenoreceptor blockade can cause reduction of intraocular pressure. Patients should be told that Propranolol HCl may interfere with the glaucoma screening test. Withdrawal may lead to a return of increased intraocular pressure.

CLINICAL LABORATORY TESTS
Elevated blood urea levels in patients with severe heart disease, elevated serum transaminase, alkaline phosphatase, lactate dehydrogenase.

DRUG INTERACTIONS
Patients receiving catecholamine-depleting drugs such as reserpine should be closely observed if Propranolol HCl is administered. The added catecholamine-blocking action may produce an excessive reduction of resting sympathetic nervous activity, which may result in hypotension, marked bradycardia, vertigo, syncopal attacks, or orthostatic hypotension.

Caution should be exercised when patients receiving a beta blocker are administered a calcium-channel blocking drug, especially intravenous verapamil, for both agents may depress myocardial contractility or atrioventricular conduction. On rare occasions, the concomitant intravenous use of a beta blocker and verapamil has resulted in serious adverse reactions, especially in patients with severe cardiomyopathy, congestive heart failure or recent myocardial infarction. Blunting of the antihypertensive effect of beta-adrenoceptor blocking agents by nonsteridal anti-inflammatory drugs has been reported.

Hypotension and cardiac arrest have been reported with the concomitant use of Propranolol and haloperidol.

Aluminum hydroxide gel greatly reduces intestinal absorption of Propranolol.
Ethanol shows the rate of absorption of Propranolol.
Phenytoin, phenobarbitone, and *rifampin* accelerate Propranolol clearance.
Chlorpromazine, when used concomitantly with Propranolol, results in increased plasma levels of both drugs.
Antipyrine and *lidocaine* have reduced clearance when used concomitantly with Propranolol.
Thyroxine may result in a lower than expected T_3 concentration when used concomitantly with Propranolol.
Cimetidine decreases the hepatic metabolism of Propranolol, delaying elimination and increasing blood levels.
Theophylline clearance is reduced when used concomitantly with Propranolol.

CARCINOGENESIS, MUTAGENESIS, IMPAIRMENT OF FERTILITY
Long-term studies in animals have been conducted to evaluate toxic effects and carcinogenic potential. In 18-month studies, in both rats and mice, employing doses up to 150 mg/kg/day, there was no evidence of significant drug-induced toxicity. There were no drug-related tumorigenic effects at any of the dosage levels. Reproductive studies in animals did not show any impairment of fertility that was attributable to the drug.

PREGNANCY
Pregnancy Category C: Propranolol HCl has been shown to be embryotoxic in animal studies at doses about 10 times greater than the maximum recommended human dose.

There are no adequate and well-controlled studies in pregnant women. Propranolol HCl should be used during pregnancy only if the potential benefit justifies the potential risk to the fetus.

NURSING MOTHERS
Propranolol HCl is excreted in human milk. Caution should be exercised when Propranolol HCl is administered to a nursing woman.

PEDIATRIC USE
High serum Propranolol levels have been noted in patients with Down's syndrome (trisomy 21), suggesting that the bioavailability of Propranolol may be increased in patients with this condition.

Evaluation of the effects of Propranolol in children, relative to the drug's efficacy and safety, has not been as systematically performed as in adults. Information is available in the medical literature to allow fair estimates, and specific dosing information has been reasonably studied.

Cardiovascular diseases that are common to adults and children are generally as responsive to Propranolol intervention in children as they are in adults. Adverse reactions are also similar; for example, bronchospasm and congestive heart failure related to Propranolol therapy have been reported in children and occur through the same mechanisms as previously described in adults.

The normal echocardiogram evolves through a series of changes as the heart matures during growth and development in children. Should echocardiography be

---

◆ RATED THERAPEUTICALLY EQUIVALENT; ◇ THERAPEUTIC EQUIVALENCE UNCONFIRMED; ○ UNRATED

used to monitor Propranolol therapy in children, the age-related changes in the echocardiogram need to be borne in mind.

Safety and effectiveness of Propranolol HCl Long Acting in children have not been established.

ADVERSE REACTIONS

Most adverse effects have been mild and transient and have rarely required the withdrawal of therapy.

Cardiovascular: Bradycardia; congestive heart failure; intensification of AV block; hypotension; paresthesia of hands; thrombocytopenic purpura; arterial insufficiency, usually of the Raynaud type.

Central Nervous System: Light-headedness: mental depression manifested by insomnia, lassitude, weakness, fatigue; reversible mental depression progressing to catatonia; visual disturbances; hallucinations, vivid dreams, an acute reversible syndrome characterized by disorientation for time and place, short-term memory loss, emotional lability, slightly clouded sensorium, and decreased performance on neuropsychometrics. For immediate formulations, total daily doses above 160 mg (when administered as divided doses of greater than 80 mg each) may be associated with an increased incidence of fatigue, lethargy, and vivid dreams.

Gastrointestinal: Nausea, vomiting epigastric distress, abdominal cramping, diarrhea, constipation, mesenteric arterial thrombosis, ischemic colitis.

Allergic: Pharyngitis and agranulocytosis, erythematous rash, fever combined with aching and sore throat, laryngospasm, and respiratory distress.

Respiratory: Bronchospasm.

Hematologic: Agranulocytosis, nonthrombocytopenic purpura, thrombocytopenic purpura.

Autoimmune: In extremely rare instances, systemic lupus erythematosus has been reported.

Miscellaneous: Alopecia, LE-like reactions, psoriasiform rashes, dry eyes, male impotence, and Peyronie's disease have been reported rarely. Oculomucocutaneous reactions involving the skin, serous membranes and conjunctivae reported for a beta blocker (practolol) have not been associated with Propranolol.

OVERDOSAGE

Propranolol HCl is not significantly dialyzable. In the event of overdosage or exaggerated response, the following measures should be employed:

General: If ingestion is or may have been recent, evacuate gastric contents, taking care to prevent pulmonary aspiration.

Bradycardia: Administer atropine (0.25 mg to 1.0 mg). If there is no response to vagal blockade, administer isoproterenol cautiously.

Cardiac Failure: Digitalization and diuretics.

Hypotension: Vasopressors, e.g. levarterenol or epinephrine (there is evidence that epinephrine is the drug of choice).

Bronchospasm: Administer isoproterenol and aminophylline.

DOSAGE AND ADMINISTRATION

The dosage range for Propranolol HCl is different for each indication.

ORAL

Propranolol HCl Long Acting provides Propranolol HCl in a sustained-release capsule for administration once daily. If patients are switched from Tablets to Propranolol HCl Capsules, care should be taken to assure that the desired therapeutic effect is maintained. Propranolol HCl Long Acting should not be considered a simple mg-for-mg substitute for Propranolol HCl. Propranolol HCl Long Acting has different kinetics and produces lower blood levels. Retitration may be necessary, especially to maintain effectiveness at the end of the 24-hour dosing interval.

Hypertension: Dosage must be individualized: The usual initial dosage is 40 mg Propranolol HCl twice daily, whether used alone or added to a diuretic. Dosage may be increased gradually until adequate blood pressure control is achieved. The usual maintenance dosage is 120 mg to 240 mg per day. In some instances a dosage of 640 mg a day may be required. The time needed for full antihypertensive response to a given dosage is variable and may range from a few days to several weeks.

While twice-daily dosing is effective and can maintain a reduction in blood pressure throughout the day, some patients, especially when lower doses are used, may experience a modest rise in blood pressure toward the end of the 12-hour dosing interval. This can be evaluated by measuring blood pressure near the end of the dosing interval to determine whether satisfactory control is being maintained throughout the day. If control is not adequate, a larger dose, or 3-times-daily therapy may achieve better control.

The usual initial dosage is 80 mg Propranolol HCl Long Acting once daily, whether used alone or added to a diuretic. The dosage may be increased to 120 mg once daily or higher until adequate blood pressure control is achieved. The usual maintenance dosage is 120 to 160 mg once daily. In some instances a dosage of 640 mg may be required. The time needed for full hypertensive response to a given dosage is variable and may range from a few days to several weeks.

Angina Pectoris: Dosage must be individualized: Total daily doses of 80 mg to 320 mg, when administered orally, twice a day, three times a day, or four times a day, have been shown to increase exercise tolerance and to reduce ischemic changes in the ECG.

Starting with 80 mg Propranolol HCl Long Acting once daily, dosage should be gradually increased at three- to seven-day intervals until optimal response is obtained. Although individual patients may respond at any dosage level, the average optimal dosage appears to be 160 mg once daily. In angina pectoris, the value and safety of dosage exceeding 320 mg per day have not been established.

If treatment is to be discontinued, reduce dosage gradually over a period of several weeks. (See *"Warnings"*.)

Arrhythmias: 10 mg to 30 mg three or four times daily, before meals and at bedtime.

Myocardial Infarction: The recommended daily dosage is 180 mg to 240 mg per day in divided doses. Although a t.i.d. regimen was used in the Beta-Blocker Heart Attack Trial and a q.i.d. regimen in the Norwegian Multicenter Trial, there is a reasonable basis for the use of either a t.i.d. or b.i.d. regimen (see *"Clinical Pharmacology"*). The effectiveness and safety of daily dosages greater than 240 mg for prevention of cardiac mortality have not been established. However, higher dosages may be needed to effectively treat coexisting diseases such as angina or hypertension (see above).

Migraine: Dosage must be individualized: The initial oral dose is 80 mg Propranolol HCl daily in divided doses or once daily if using Propranolol HCl Long Acting. The usual effective dose range is 160 mg to 240 mg per day. The dosage may be increased gradually to achieve optimum migraine prophylaxis.

If a satisfactory response is not obtained within four to six weeks after reaching the maximum dose, Propranolol HCl therapy should be discontinued. It may be advisable to withdraw the drug gradually over a period of several weeks.

Essential Tremor: Dosage must be individualized: The initial dosage is 40 mg Propranolol HCl twice daily. Optimum reduction of essential tremor is usually achieved with a dose of 120 mg per day. Occasionally, it may be necessary to administer 240 mg to 320 mg per day.

Hypertrophic Subaortic Stenosis: 20 mg to 40 mg three or four times daily, before meals and at bedtime. 80 to 160 mg Propranolol HCl Long Lasting once daily.

Pheochromocytoma: Preoperatively: 60 mg daily in divided doses for three days prior to surgery, concomitantly with an alpha-adrenergic blocking agent.

Management of Inoperable Tumor: 30 mg daily in divided doses.

Use In Children: Intravenous administration of Propranolol HCl is not recommended in children. Oral dosage for treating hypertension requires individual titration, beginning with a 1.0 mg per kg (body weight) per day dosage regimen (i.e., 0.5 mg per kg b.i.d.).

The usual pediatric dosage range is 2 mg to 4 mg per kg per day in two equally divided doses (i.e., 1.0 mg per kg b.i.d. to 2.0 mg per kg b.i.d.). Pediatric dosage calculated by weight (recommended) generally produces Propranolol plasma levels in a therapeutic range similar to that in adults. On the other hand, pediatric doses calculated on the basis of body surface area (*not* recommended) usually result in plasma levels above the mean adult therapeutic range. Doses above 16 mg per kg per day should not be used in children.

At this time the data on the use of Propranolol HCl Long Acting in this age group are too limited to permit adequate directions for use.

If treatment with Propranolol HCl is to be discontinued, a gradually decreasing dose titration over a 7- to 14-day period is necessary.

INTRAVENOUS

Parenteral drug products should be inspected visually for particulate matter and discoloration prior to administration, whenever solution and container permit.

Intravenous administration is reserved for life-threatening arrhythmias or those occurring under anesthesia. The usual dose is from 1 mg to 3 mg administered under careful monitoring, e.g., electrocardiographic, central venous pressure. The rate of administration should not exceed 1 mg (1 mL) per minute to diminish the possibility of lowering blood pressure and causing cardiac standstill. Sufficient time should be allowed for the drug to reach the site of action even when a slow circulation is present. If necessary, a second dose may be given after two minutes. Thereafter, additional drug should not be given in less than four hours. Additional Propranolol HCl should not be given when the desired alteration in rate and/or rhythm is achieved.

Transference to oral therapy should be made as soon as possible.

The intravenous administration of Propranolol HCl has not been evaluated adequately in the management of hypertensive emergencies.

STORAGE

Store at room temperature (approximately 25° C). Dispense in a well-closed, light-resistant container as defined in the USP.

Protect from light, moisture, freezing, and excessive heat.

Use carton to protect contents from light.

J CODES

Up to 1 mg IV—J1800

HOW SUPPLIED
CAPSULE, EXTENDED RELEASE: 60 MG

AVERAGE UNIT PRICE (AVAILABLE SIZES)		GENERIC A-RATED AVERAGE PRICE (GAAP)	
BRAND	$0.75	100s	$64.23
GENERIC	$0.64		
HCFA FUL (100s ea)	$0.60		

BRAND/MANUFACTURER	NDC	SIZE	AWP
◆ **BRAND**			
➤ INDERAL LA: Wyeth-Ayerst	00046-0470-81	100s	$76.74
	00046-0470-91	1000s	$736.68
◆ **GENERICS**			
Qualitest	00603-5497-21	100s	$61.12
Caremark	00339-5753-12	100s	$62.47
Rugby	00536-4911-01	100s	$62.54
Major	00904-0421-60	100s	$62.55
URL	00677-1363-01	100s	$63.45
Schein	00364-2413-01	100s	$63.50
Inwood	00258-3609-01	100s	$63.99
Geneva	00781-2061-01	100s	$64.20
Goldline	00182-1926-01	100s	$64.90
Moore,H.L.	00839-7572-06	100s	$64.92
Lemmon	00093-0691-01	100s	$66.85
Parmed	00349-8699-01	100s	$67.19
Aligen	00405-4890-01	100s	$67.36

CAPSULE, EXTENDED RELEASE: 80 MG

AVERAGE UNIT PRICE (AVAILABLE SIZES)		GENERIC A-RATED AVERAGE PRICE (GAAP)	
BRAND	$0.89	100s	$75.64
GENERIC	$0.75		
HCFA FUL (100s ea)	$0.73		

BRAND/MANUFACTURER	NDC	SIZE	AWP
◆ **BRAND**			
➤ INDERAL LA: Wyeth-Ayerst	00046-0471-81	100s	$89.71
	00046-0471-99	100s ud	$91.26
	00046-0471-91	1000s	$861.41
◆ **GENERICS**			
Allscrips	54569-8594-00	90s	$67.54
Qualitest	00603-5498-21	100s	$72.90
Rugby	00536-4912-01	100s	$73.10
Schein	00364-2414-01	100s	$73.50
Major	00904-0422-60	100s	$73.55
Caremark	00339-5755-12	100s	$73.80
URL	00677-1364-01	100s	$74.16
Geneva	00781-2062-01	100s	$75.04
Goldline	00182-1927-01	100s	$75.80
Inwood	00258-3610-01	100s	$77.30
Moore,H.L.	00839-7573-06	100s	$77.34
Lemmon	00093-0692-01	100s	$77.52
Parmed	00349-8700-01	100s	$77.90
Aligen	00405-4891-01	100s	$81.36
Rugby	00536-4912-02	250s	$182.75

CAPSULE, EXTENDED RELEASE: 120 MG

AVERAGE UNIT PRICE (AVAILABLE SIZES)		GENERIC A-RATED AVERAGE PRICE (GAAP)	
BRAND	$1.10	100s	$96.35
GENERIC	$0.96		
HCFA FUL (100s ea)	$0.90		

BRAND/MANUFACTURER	NDC	SIZE	AWP
◆ **BRAND**			
➤ INDERAL LA: Wyeth-Ayerst	00046-0473-81	100s	$111.21
	00046-0473-99	100s ud	$112.34
	00046-0473-91	1000s	$1067.66
◆ **GENERICS**			
Qualitest	00603-5499-21	100s	$89.88
Schein	00364-2415-01	100s	$90.50
Rugby	00536-4913-01	100s	$90.63
Major	00904-0423-60	100s	$90.90
URL	00677-1365-01	100s	$92.60
Geneva	00781-2063-01	100s	$93.03
Caremark	00339-5757-12	100s	$93.92
Goldline	00182-1928-01	100s	$94.04
Lemmon	00093-0693-01	100s	$95.50
Inwood	00258-3611-01	100s	$96.24
Moore,H.L.	00839-7574-06	100s	$96.24
Parmed	00349-8701-01	100s	$96.50
Aligen	00405-4892-01	100s	$132.63

CAPSULE, EXTENDED RELEASE: 160 MG

AVERAGE UNIT PRICE (AVAILABLE SIZES)		GENERIC A-RATED AVERAGE PRICE (GAAP)	
BRAND	$1.44	100s	$124.18
GENERIC	$1.24		
HCFA FUL (100s ea)	$1.18		

BRAND/MANUFACTURER	NDC	SIZE	AWP
◆ **BRAND**			
➤ INDERAL LA: Wyeth-Ayerst	00046-0479-81	100s	$145.61
	00046-0479-99	100s ud	$146.11
	00046-0479-91	1000s	$1397.91
◆ **GENERICS**			
Rugby	00536-4914-01	100s	$118.66
Major	00904-0424-60	100s	$118.90
Qualitest	00603-5500-21	100s	$119.25
Schein	00364-2416-01	100s	$119.50
URL	00677-1366-01	100s	$120.02
Caremark	00339-5759-12	100s	$120.17
Geneva	00781-2064-01	100s	$121.80
Goldline	00182-1929-01	100s	$123.16
Lemmon	00093-0694-01	100s	$125.83
Inwood	00258-3612-01	100s	$126.00
Moore,H.L.	00839-7575-06	100s	$126.02
Parmed	00349-8707-01	100s	$137.34
Aligen	00405-4893-01	100s	$137.63

INJECTION: 1 MG/ML

BRAND/MANUFACTURER	NDC	SIZE	AWP
◆ **BRAND**			
➤ INDERAL: Wyeth-Ayerst	00046-3265-10	1 ml 10s	$43.14
◆ **GENERICS**			
Solo Pak	39769-0075-02	1 ml 25s	$156.25

SOLUTION: 20 MG/5 ML

AVERAGE UNIT PRICE (AVAILABLE SIZES)	
GENERIC	$0.16

BRAND/MANUFACTURER	NDC	SIZE	AWP
◆ **GENERICS**			
Roxane	00054-3727-63	500 ml	$31.50
Roxane	00054-8764-16	5 ml 40s ud	$50.74

SOLUTION: 40 MG/5 ML

AVERAGE UNIT PRICE (AVAILABLE SIZES)	
GENERIC	$0.23

BRAND/MANUFACTURER	NDC	SIZE	AWP
◆ **GENERICS**			
Roxane	00054-3730-63	500 ml	$45.01
Roxane	00054-8765-16	5 ml 40s ud	$72.57

For additional alternatives, turn to the section beginning on page 2859.

Propulsid SEE CISAPRIDE

Propylthiouracil

DESCRIPTION

Propylthiouracil (6-propyl-2-thiouracil) is one of the thiocarbamide compounds. It is a white, crystalline substance that has a bitter taste and is very slightly soluble in water.

Propylthiouracil is an antithyroid drug administered orally.

Each tablet contains Propylthiouracil 50 mg. $C_7H_{10}N_2OS$.

Following is its chemical structure:

CLINICAL PHARMACOLOGY

Propylthiouracil inhibits the synthesis of thyroid hormones and thus is effective in the treatment of hyperthyroidism. The drug does not inactivate existing thyroxine and triiodothyronine that are stored in the thyroid or circulating in the blood, nor does it interfere with the effectiveness of thyroid hormones given by mouth or by injection.

Propylthiouracil is readily absorbed from the gastrointestinal tract. It is metabolized rapidly and requires frequent administration. Approximately 35% of the drug is excreted in the urine, in intact and in conjugated forms, within 24 hours.

In laboratory animals, various interventions, including Propylthiouracil administration, that continuously suppress thyroid function and thereby increase TSH secretion result in thyroid tissue hypertrophy.

INDICATIONS AND USAGE

Propylthiouracil is indicated in the medical treatment of hyperthyroidism. Long-term therapy may lead to remission of the disease. Propylthiouracil may also be used to ameliorate hyperthyroidism in preparation for subtotal thyroidectomy or radioactive iodine therapy. Propylthiouracil is also used when thyroidectomy is contraindicated or not advisable.

UNLABELED USES

Propylthiouracil is used alone or as an adjunct to reduce mortality secondary to alcoholic liver disease.

CONTRAINDICATIONS

Propylthiouracil is contraindicated in the presence of hypersensitivity to the drug and in nursing mothers because the drug is excreted in milk.

WARNINGS

Agranulocytosis is potentially the most serious side effect of propylthiouracil therapy. Patients should be instructed to report any symptoms of agranulocytosis, such as fever or sore throat. Leukopenia, thrombocytopenia, and aplastic anemia (pancytopenia) may also occur. The drug should be discontinued in the presence of agranulocytosis, aplastic anemia (pancytopenia), hepatitis, fever, or exfoliative dermatitis. The patient's bone marrow function should be monitored.

Propylthiouracil can cause fetal harm when administered to a pregnant woman. Because the drug readily crosses placental membranes and can induce goiter and even cretinism in the developing fetus, it is important that a sufficient, but not excessive, dose be given. In many pregnant women, the thyroid dysfunction diminishes as the pregnancy proceeds; consequently a reduction of dosage may be possible. In some instances, Propylthiouracil can be withdrawn 2 or 3 weeks before delivery.

If this drug is used during pregnancy, or if the patient becomes pregnant while taking this drug, the patient should be warned of the potential hazard to the fetus.

Postpartum patients receiving Propylthiouracil should not nurse their babies.

Rare reports exist of severe hepatic reactions including encephalopathy, fulminant hepatic necrosis, and death in patients receiving Propylthiouracil. Symptoms suggestive of hepatic dysfunction (anorexia, pruritus, right upper quadrant pain, etc.) should prompt evaluation of liver function. Treatment with Propylthiouracil should be discontinued promptly in the event of clinically significant evidence of liver abnormality, including hepatic transaminases in excess of 3 times the upper limit of normal.

PRECAUTIONS

General: Patients who receive Propylthiouracil should be under close surveillance and should be impressed with the necessity of reporting immediately any evidence of illness, particularly sore throat, skin eruptions, fever, headache, or general malaise. In such cases, white blood cell and differential counts should be made to determine whether agranulocytosis has developed. Particular care should be exercised with patients who are receiving additional drugs known to cause agranulocytosis.

Laboratory Tests: Because Propylthiouracil may cause hypoprothrombinemia and bleeding, prothrombin time should be monitored during therapy with the drug, especially before surgical procedures. Thyroid function tests should be monitored periodically during therapy. Once clinical evidence of hyperthyroidism has resolved, the finding of an elevated serum TSH indicates that a lower maintenance dose of Propylthiouracil should be employed.

Drug Interactions: The activity of anticoagulants may be potentiated by anti-vitamin-K activity attributed to Propylthiouracil.

Carcinogenesis, Mutagenesis, Impairment of Fertility: Laboratory animals treated with Propylthiouracil for > 1 year have demonstrated thyroid hyperplasia and carcinoma formation[1]. Such animal findings are seen with continuous suppression of thyroid function by sufficient doses of a variety of antithyroid agents, as well as in dietary iodine deficiency, subtotal thyroidectomy, and implantation of autonomous thyrotropic hormone-secreting pituitary tumors. Pituitary adenomas have also been described.

Usage in Pregnancy - Pregnancy Category D: See "Warnings".

Nursing Mothers: The drug appears in human milk and is contraindicated in nursing mothers. See "Warnings".

Usage in Children: See "Dosage & Administration".

ADVERSE REACTIONS

Major adverse reactions (much less common than the minor adverse reactions) include inhibition of myelopoiesis (agranulocytosis, granulopenia, and thrombo-cytopenia), aplastic anemia, drug fever, a lupus-like syndrome including splenomegaly, hepatitis, periarteritis, and hypoprothrombinemia and bleeding. Nephritis, interstitial pneumonitis, and erythema nodosum have been reported.

Minor adverse reactions include skin rash, urticaria, nausea, vomiting, epigastric distress, arthralgia, paresthesias, loss of taste, abnormal loss of hair, myalgia, headache, pruritus, drowsiness, neuritis, edema, vertigo, skin pigmentation, jaundice, sialadenopathy, and lymphadenopathy.

It should be noted that about 10% of patients with untreated hyperthyroidism have leukopenia (white blood cell count of less than 4,000/mm³), often with relative granulopenia.

OVERDOSAGE

Signs and Symptoms: Nausea, vomiting, epigastric distress, headache, fever, arthralgia, pruritus, edema, and pancytopenia. Agranulocytosis is the most serious effect. Rarely, exfoliative dermatitis, hepatitis, neuropathies, or CNS stimulation or depression may occur. No information is available on the following: LD_{50}; concentration of Propylthiouracil in biologic fluids associated with toxicity and/or death; the amount of drug in a single dose usually associated with symptoms of overdosage; or the amount of Propylthiouracil in a single dose likely to be life-threatening.

Treatment: To obtain up-to-date information about the treatment of overdose, a good resource is the certified Regional Poison Control Center. Telephone numbers of certified poison control centers are listed in the *Physicians' Desk Reference* (PDR). In managing overdosage, consider the possibility of multiple drug overdoses, interaction among drugs, and unusual drug kinetics in the patient.

Protect the patient's airway and support ventilation and perfusion. Meticulously monitor and maintain, within acceptable limits, the patient's vital signs, blood gases, serum electrolytes, etc. The patient's bone marrow function should be monitored. Absorption of drugs from the gastrointestinal tract may be decreased by giving activated charcoal, which, in many cases, is more effective than emesis or lavage; consider charcoal instead of or in addition to gastric emptying. Repeated doses of charcoal over time may hasten elimination of some drugs that have been absorbed. Safeguard the patient's airway when employing gastric emptying or charcoal.

Forced diuresis, peritoneal dialysis, hemodialysis, or charcoal hemoperfusion have not been established as beneficial for an overdose of Propylthiouracil.

DOSAGE AND ADMINISTRATION

Propylthiouracil is administered orally. The total daily dosage is usually given in 3 equal doses at approximately 8-hour intervals. *Adult* - The initial dose is 300 mg daily. In patients with severe hyperthyroidism, very large goiters, or both, the beginning dosage usually should be 400 mg daily; an occasional patient will require 600 to 900 mg/day initially. The usual maintenance dosage is 100 to 150 mg daily.

Pediatric: For children 6 to 10 years of age, the initial dosage is 50 to 150 mg daily. For children 10 years and over, the initial dosage is 150 to 300 mg daily. The maintenance dosage is determined by the response of the patient.

Storage: Store at controlled room temperature 15°-30°C (59°-86°F).

REFERENCE:
1. International Agency for Research on Cancer. IARC Monographs on the Evaluation of the Carcinogenic Risk of Chemicals to Man. 1974; 7; 67-76.

HOW SUPPLIED
TABLETS: 50 MG

BRAND/MANUFACTURER	NDC	SIZE	AWP
◆ GENERICS			
U.S. Trading	56126-0441-11	100s ud	$9.51

TABLETS: 50 MG

BRAND/MANUFACTURER	NDC	SIZE	AWP
◇ GENERICS			
Lederle Std Prod	00005-4609-23	100s	$5.26
Purepac	00228-2348-10	100s	$5.33
Richlyn	00115-4322-01	100s	$5.81
Major	00904-2173-60	100s	$7.05
West-Ward	00143-1480-25	100s ud	$13.50
Moore, H.L.	00839-5093-16	1000s	$32.39
Lederle Std Prod	00005-4609-34	1000s	$33.40
West-Ward	00143-1480-10	1000s	$35.00
Goldline	00182-0598-10	1000s	$43.50
Richlyn	00115-4322-03	1000s	$44.70
Major	00904-2173-80	1000s	$46.90

Proscar *SEE* FINASTERIDE

ProSom *SEE* ESTAZOLAM

ProStep *SEE* NICOTINE

► SHOWN IN PRODUCT IDENTIFICATION GUIDE

Prostigmin *SEE* NEOSTIGMINE

Prostin E2 *SEE* DINOPROSTONE, CERVICAL *AND* DINOPROSTONE, VAGINAL

Prostin VR Pediatric *SEE* ALPROSTADIL

Protamine Sulfate

DESCRIPTION

Protamines are simple proteins of low molecular weight that are rich in arginine and strongly basic. They occur in the sperm of salmon and certain other species of fish.

Protamine Sulfate occurs as fine white or off-white amorphous or crystalline powder. It is sparingly soluble in water. The pH is between 6 and 7. The cationic hydrogenated Protamine at a pH of 6.8 to 7.1 reacts with anionic heparin at a pH of 5.0 to 7.5 to form an inactive complex.

Protamine Sulfate Injection, USP, is a sterile, isotonic solution of Protamine Sulfate. It acts as a heparin antagonist. It is also a weak anticoagulant.

Each 5 mL ampoule of Protamine Sulfate Injection contains Protamine Sulfate equivalent to 50 mg of activity, and each 25 mL vial contains Protamine Sulfate equivalent to 250 mg of activity. Both products also contain 0.9% Sodium Chloride Reagent in Water for Injection, USP. Sodium phosphate and/or sulfuric acid may have been added during manufacture to adjust the pH. Contains no preservative. Protamine Sulfate is administered intravenously.

CLINICAL PHARMACOLOGY

When administered alone, Protamine has an anticoagulant effect. However, when it is given in the presence of heparin (which is strongly acidic), a stable salt is formed and the anticoagulant activity of both drugs is lost.

Protamine Sulfate has a rapid onset of action. Neutralization of heparin occurs within 5 minutes after intravenous administration of an appropriate dose of Protamine Sulfate. Although the metabolic fate of the heparin-protamine complex has not been elucidated, it has been postulated that Protamine Sulfate in the heparin-protamine complex may be partially metabolized or may be attacked by fibrinolysin, thus freeing heparin.

INDICATIONS AND USAGE

Protamine Sulfate is indicated in the treatment of heparin overdosage.

CONTRAINDICATION

Protamine Sulfate is contraindicated in patients who have shown previous intolerance to the drug.

WARNINGS

Hyperheparinemia or bleeding has been reported in experimental animals and in some patients 30 minutes to 18 hours after cardiac surgery (under cardiopulmonary bypass) in spite of complete neutralization of heparin by adequate doses of Protamine Sulfate at the end of the operation. It is important to keep the patient under close observation after cardiac surgery. Additional doses of Protamine Sulfate should be administered if indicated by coagulation studies, such as the heparin titration test with Protamine and the determination of plasma thrombin time.

Too-rapid administration of Protamine Sulfate can cause severe hypotensive and anaphylactoid reactions (see "Dosage and Administration"). Facilities to treat shock should be available.

PRECAUTIONS

General: **Because of the anticoagulant effect of protamine, it is unwise to give more than 50 mg over a short period unless a larger dose is clearly needed.**

Patients with a history of allergy to fish may develop hypersensitivity reactions to Protamine, although to date no relationship has been established between allergic reactions to Protamine and fish allergy.

Previous exposure to Protamine through use of protamine-containing insulins or during heparin neutralization may predispose susceptible individuals to the development of untoward reactions from the subsequent use of this drug. Reports of the presence of antiprotamine antibodies in the serums of infertile or vasectomized men suggest that some of these individuals may react to use of Protamine Sulfate.

Fatal anaphylaxis has been reported in one patient with no prior history of allergies.

Drug Interactions: Protamine Sulfate has been shown to be incompatible with certain antibiotics, including several of the cephalosporins and penicillins (see *"Dosage and Administration"*).

Carcinogenesis, Mutagenesis, Impairment of Fertility: Studies have not been performed to determine potential for carcinogenicity, mutagenicity, or impairment of fertility.

Usage in Pregnancy—Pregnancy Category C: Animal reproduction studies have not been conducted with Protamine Sulfate. It is also not known whether Protamine Sulfate can cause fetal harm when administered to a pregnant woman or can affect reproduction capacity. Protamine Sulfate should be given to a pregnant woman only if clearly needed.

Nursing Mothers: It is not known whether this drug is excreted in human milk. Because many drugs are excreted in human milk, caution should be exercised when Protamine Sulfate is administered to a nursing woman.

Pediatric Use: Safety and effectiveness in children have not been established.

ADVERSE REACTIONS

The intravenous administration of Protamine Sulfate may cause a sudden fall in blood pressure and bradycardia. Other reactions include transitory flushing and feeling of warmth, dyspnea, nausea, vomiting, and lassitude. Back pain has been reported in conscious patients undergoing such procedures as cardiac catheterization.

Severe adverse reactions have been reported including: (1) Anaphylaxis that resulted in severe respiratory distress, circulatory collapse, and capillary leak (see *"Precautions"*). Fatal anaphylaxis has been reported in one patient with no prior history of allergies; (2) Anaphylactoid reactions with circulatory collapse, capillary leak, and noncardiogenic pulmonary edema; acute pulmonary hypertension.

Complement activation by the heparin-protamine complexes, release of lysosomal enzymes from neutrophils, and prostaglandin and thromboxane generation have been associated with the development of anaphylactoid reactions.

Severe and potentially irreversible circulatory collapse associated with myocardial failure and reduced cardiac output can also occur. The mechanism(s) of this reaction and the role played by concurrent factors are unclear.

High-protein, noncardiogenic pulmonary edema associated with the use of Protamine has been reported in patients on cardiopulmonary bypass who are undergoing cardiovascular surgery. The etiologic role of Protamine in the pathogenesis of this condition is uncertain, and multiple factors have been present in most cases. The condition has been reported in association with administration of certain blood products, other drugs, cardiopulmonary bypass alone, and other etiologic factors. It is difficult to treat, and it can be life threatening. Because fatal anaphylactic and anaphylactoid reactions have been reported after the administration of Protamine Sulfate, the drug should be given only when resuscitation techniques and treatment of anaphylactic and anaphylactoid shock are readily available.

OVERDOSAGE

Signs and Symptoms: Overdose of Protamine Sulfate may cause bleeding. Protamine has a weak anticoagulant effect due to an interaction with platelets and with many proteins including fibrinogen. This effect should be distinguished from the rebound anticoagulation that may occur 30 minutes to 18 hours following the reversal of heparin with Protamine.

Rapid administration of Protamine is more likely to result in bradycardia, dyspnea, a sensation of warmth, flushing, and severe hypotension. Hypertension has also occurred.

The median lethal intravenous dose of Protamine Sulfate is 50 mg/kg in mice. Serum concentrations of Protamine Sulfate are not clinically useful. Information is not available on the amount of drug in a single dose that is associated with overdosage or is likely to be life threatening.

Treatment: To obtain up-to-date information about the treatment of overdose, a good resource is your certified Regional Poison Control Center. Telephone numbers of certified poison control centers are listed in the *Physicians' Desk Reference (PDR)*. In managing overdosage, consider the possibility of multiple drug overdoses, interaction among drugs, and unusual drug kinetics in your patient.

Replace blood loss with blood transfusions or fresh frozen plasma.

If the patient is hypotensive, consider fluids, epinephrine, dobutamine, or dopamine.

DOSAGE AND ADMINISTRATION

Each mg of Protamine Sulfate neutralizes approximately 90 USP units of heparin activity derived from lung tissue or about 115 USP units of heparin activity derived from intestinal mucosa.

Protamine Sulfate Injection should be given by very slow intravenous injection over a 10-minute period in doses not to exceed 50 mg (see *"Warnings"*).

Protamine Sulfate is intended for injection without further dilution; however, if further dilution is desired, D5-W or normal saline may be used. Diluted solutions should not be stored since they contain no preservative.

Protamine Sulfate should not be mixed with other drugs without knowledge of their compatibility, because Protamine Sulfate has been shown to be incompatible with certain antibiotics, including several of the cephalosporins and penicillins.

Because heparin disappears rapidly from the circulation, the dose of Protamine Sulfate required also decreases rapidly with the time elapsed following intravenous injection of heparin. For example, if the Protamine Sulfate is administered 30 minutes after the heparin, one half the usual dose may be sufficient.

The dosage of Protamine Sulfate should be guided by blood coagulation studies (see *"Warnings"*).

Parenteral drug products should be inspected visually for particulate matter and discoloration prior to administration whenever solution and container permit.

Ampoules and vials should be stored in the refrigerator between 2° and 8°C (35.6° and 46.4°F).

J CODES

Up to 5 ml IV—J2720

◆ RATED THERAPEUTICALLY EQUIVALENT; ◇ THERAPEUTIC EQUIVALENCE UNCONFIRMED; ○ UNRATED

HOW SUPPLIED
INJECTION: 10 MG/ML

AVERAGE UNIT PRICE (AVAILABLE SIZES)		GENERIC A-RATED AVERAGE PRICE (GAAP)		
GENERIC	$0.80	25 ml		$17.15
BRAND/MANUFACTURER		NDC	SIZE	AWP
◆ GENERICS				
Fujisawa		00469-2290-20	5 ml	$5.32
Elkins-Sinn		00641-2554-41	25 ml	$17.01
Fujisawa		00469-2290-50	25 ml	$17.28
Lilly		00002-1462-01	25 ml	$19.25
Elkins-Sinn		00641-1494-35	5 ml 25s	$101.56

Proteinase Inhibitor (Human), Alpha₁

DESCRIPTION

Proteinase Inhibitor (Human), Alpha₁, is a sterile, stable, lyophilized preparation of purified human Alpha₁-Proteinase Inhibitor (alpha₁-PI) also known as alpha₁-antitrypsin. Proteinase Inhibitor (Human), Alpha₁, is intended for use in therapy of congenital alpha₁-antitrypsin deficiency.

Proteinase Inhibitor (Human), Alpha₁, is prepared from pooled human plasma of normal donors by modification and refinements of the cold ethanol method of Cohn.[1] Part of the fractionation may be performed by another licensed manufacturer. In order to reduce the potential risk of transmission of infectious agents, Proteinase Inhibitor (Human), Alpha₁, has been heat-treated in solution at $60\pm0.5°C$ for not less than 10 hours. However, no procedure has been found to be totally effective in removing viral infectivity from plasma fractionation products.

The specific activity of Proteinase Inhibitor (Human), Alpha₁, is ≥ 0.35 mg functional alpha₁-PI/mg protein and when reconstituted as directed, the concentration of alpha₁-PI is ≥ 20 mg/mL. Proteinase Inhibitor (Human), Alpha₁ contains small amounts of other plasma proteins including alpha₂-plasmin inhibitor, alpha₁-antichymotrypsin, C₁-esterase inhibitor, haptoglobin, antithrombin III, alpha₁-lipoprotein, albumin, and IgA.[1]

Each vial of Proteinase Inhibitor (Human), Alpha₁, contains the labeled amount of functionally active alpha₁-PI in milligrams per vial (mg/vial), as determined by capacity to neutralize porcine pancreatic elastase.[1] Proteinase Inhibitor (Human), Alpha₁ contains no preservative and must be administered by the intravenous route.

CLINICAL PHARMACOLOGY

Alpha₁-antitrypsin deficiency is a chronic hereditary, usually fatal, autosomal recessive disorder in which a low concentration of alpha₁-PI (alpha₁-antitrypsin) is associated with slowly progressive, severe, panacinar emphysema that most often manifests itself in the third to fourth decades of life.[2-9] [Although the terms "Alpha₁-Proteinase Inhibitor" and "alpha₁-antitrypsin" are used interchangeably in the scientific literature, the hereditary disorder associated with a reduction in the serum level of alpha₁-PI is conventionally referred to as "alpha₁-antitrypsin deficiency" while the deficient protein is referred to as "Alpha₁-Proteinase Inhibitor"[10]]. The emphysema is typically worse in the lower lung zones.[4,8,9] The pathogenesis of development of emphysema in alpha₁-antitrypsin deficiency is not well understood at this time. It is believed, however, to be due to a chronic biochemical imbalance between elastase (an enzyme capable of degrading elastin tissues, released by inflammatory cells, primarily neutrophils, in the lower respiratory tract) and alpha₁-PI (the principal inhibitor of neutrophil elastase) which is deficient in alpha₁-antitrypsin disease.[11-15] As a result, it is believed that alveolar structures are unprotected from chronic exposure to elastase released from a chronic, low level burden of neutrophils in the lower respiratory tract, resulting in progressive degradation of elastin tissues.[11-15]

The eventual outcome is the development of emphysema. Neonatal hepatitis with cholestatic jaundice appears in approximately 10% of newborns with alpha₁-antitrypsin deficiency.[15] In some adults, alpha₁-antitrypsin deficiency is complicated by cirrhosis.[15]

A large number of phenotypic variants of alpha₁-antitrypsin deficiency exists.[15] The most severely affected individuals are those with the PiZZ variant, typically characterized by alpha₁-PI serum levels <35% normal.[15] Epidemiologic studies of individuals with various phenotypes of alpha₁-antitrypsin deficiency have demonstrated that individuals with endogenous serum levels of alpha₁-PI ≤ 50 mg/dL (based on commercial standards) have a risk of > 80% of developing emphysema over a lifetime.[3-6,8,9,16] However, individuals with endogenous alpha₁-PI levels > 80 mg/dL, in general, do not manifest an increased risk for development of emphysema above the general population background risk.[5,15] From these observations, it is believed that the "threshold" level of alpha₁-PI in the serum required to provide adequate anti-elastase activity in the lung of individuals with alpha₁-antitrypsin deficiency is about 80 mg/dL (based on commercial standards for immunologic assay of alpha₁-PI).[12,15,17] In clinical studies of Proteinase Inhibitor (Human), Alpha₁, 23 subjects with the PiZZ variant of congenital deficiency of alpha₁-antitrypsin deficiency and documented destructive lung disease participated in a study of acute and/or chronic replacement therapy with Proteinase Inhibitor (Human), Alpha₁.[18] The mean *in vivo* recovery of alpha₁-PI was 4.2 mg (immunologic) dL per mg (functional)/kg body weight administered.[18,19] The half-life of alpha₁-PI *in vivo* was approxi-

mately 4.5 days.[18,19] Based on these observations, a program of chronic replacement therapy was developed. Nineteen of the subjects in these studies received Proteinase Inhibitor (Human), Alpha₁, replacement therapy, 60 mg/kg body weight, once weekly for up to 26 weeks (average 24 weeks of therapy). With this schedule of replacement therapy, blood levels of alpha₁-PI were maintained above 80 mg/dL (based on the commercial standards for alpha₁-PI immunologic assay).[18-20] Within a few weeks of commencing this program, bronchoalveolar lavage studies demonstrated significantly increased levels of alpha₁-PI and functional antineutrophil elastase capacity in the epithelial lining fluid of the lower respiratory tract of the lung, as compared to levels prior to commencing the program of chronic replacement therapy with Proteinase Inhibitor (Human), Alpha₁.[18-20]

All 23 individuals who participated in the investigations were immunized with Hepatitis B Vaccine and received a single dose of Hepatitis B Immune Globulin (Human) on entry into the investigation. Although no other steps were taken to prevent hepatitis, neither hepatitis B nor non-A, non-B hepatitis occurred in any of the subjects.[18,19] All subjects remained seronegative for HIV antibody. None of the subjects developed any detectable antibody to alpha₁-PI or other serum protein.

Long-term controlled clinical trials to evaluate the effect of chronic replacement therapy with Proteinase Inhibitor (Human), Alpha₁, on the development of or progression of emphysema in patients with congenital alpha₁-antitrypsin deficiency have not been performed. Estimates of the sample size required of this rare disorder and the slow progressive nature of the clinical course have been considered impediments in the ability to conduct such a trial.[21] Studies to monitor the long-term effects will continue as part of the postapproval process.

INDICATIONS AND USAGE

CONGENITAL ALPHA₁-ANTITRYPSIN DEFICIENCY

Proteinase Inhibitor (Human), Alpha₁, is indicated for chronic replacement therapy of individuals having congenital deficiency of alpha₁-PI (alpha₁-antitrypsin deficiency) with clinically demonstrable panacinar emphysema. Clinical and biochemical studies have demonstrated that with such therapy, it is possible to increase plasma levels of alpha₁-PI, and that levels of functionally active alpha₁-PI in the lung epithelial lining fluid are increased proportionately.[18-20] As some individuals with alpha₁-antitrypsin deficiency will not go on to develop panacinar emphysema, only those with early evidence of such disease should be considered for chronic replacement therapy with Proteinase Inhibitor (Human), Alpha₁.[22] Subjects with the PiMZ or PiMS phenotypes of alpha₁-antitrypsin deficiency should not be considered for such treatment as they appear to be at small risk for panacinar emphysema.[22] Clinical data are not available as to the long-term effects derived from chronic replacement therapy of individuals with alpha₁-antitrypsin deficiency with Proteinase Inhibitor (Human), Alpha₁, to date. Only adult subjects have received Proteinase Inhibitor (Human), Alpha₁, to date.

Proteinase Inhibitor (Human), Alpha₁, is not indicated for use in patients other than those with PiZZ, PiZ(null), or Pi(null) (null) phenotypes.

CONTRAINDICATIONS

Individuals with selective IgA deficiencies who have known antibody against IgA (anti-IgA antibody) should not receive Proteinase Inhibitor (Human), Alpha₁, since these patients may experience severe reactions, including anaphylaxis, to IgA which may be present.

WARNINGS

This product is prepared from pooled human plasma which may contain the causative agents of hepatitis and other viral diseases. Prescribed manufacturing procedures utilized at the plasma collection centers, plasma testing laboratories, and the fractionation facilities are designed to reduce the risk of transmitting viral infection. However, the risk of viral infectivity from this product cannot be totally eliminated.

Individuals who receive infusions of blood or plasma products may develop signs and/or symptoms of some viral infections, particularly non-A, non-B hepatitis.

Proteinase Inhibitor (Human), Alpha₁, has been heat-treated in solution at 60°C for 10 hours in order to reduce the potential for transmission of infectious agents.[1] No cases of hepatitis, either hepatitis B or non-A, non-B hepatitis have been recorded to date in individuals receiving Proteinase Inhibitor (Human), Alpha₁.[18] However, as all individuals received prophylaxis against hepatitis B, no conclusion can be drawn at this time regarding potential transmission of hepatitis B virus.

PRECAUTIONS

GENERAL

1. Administer within 3 hours after reconstitution. Do not refrigerate after reconstitution.
2. Administer only by the intravenous route.
3. As with any colloid solution there will be an increase in plasma volume following intravenous administration of Proteinase Inhibitor (Human), Alpha₁.[23] Caution should therefore be used in patients at risk for circulatory overload.
4. It is recommended that in preparation for receiving Proteinase Inhibitor (Human), Alpha₁, recipients be immunized against hepatitis B using a licensed Hepatitis B Vaccine according to the manufacturer's recommendations. Should it become necessary to treat an individual with Proteinase Inhibitor (Human), Alpha₁, and time is insufficient for adequate antibody response to vaccination, individuals should receive a single dose of Hepatitis B Immune Globulin (Human), 0.06 mL/kg body weight, intramuscularly, at the time of administration of the initial dose of Hepatitis B Vaccine.

➤ SHOWN IN PRODUCT IDENTIFICATION GUIDE

5. Proteinase Inhibitor (Human), Alpha₁, should be given alone, without mixing with other agents or diluting solutions.

6. Administration equipment and any reconstituted Proteinase Inhibitor (Human), Alpha₁, not used should be appropriately discarded.

CARCINOGENESIS, MUTAGENESIS, IMPAIRMENT OF FERTILITY
Long-Term studies in animals to evaluate carcinogenesis, mutagenesis or impairment of fertility have not been conducted.

PREGNANCY CATEGORY C
Animal reproduction studies have not been conducted with Proteinase Inhibitor (Human), Alpha₁. It is also not known whether Proteinase Inhibitor (Human), Alpha₁, can cause fetal harm when administered to a pregnant woman or can affect reproduction capacity Proteinase Inhibitor (Human), Alpha₁, should be given to a pregnant woman only if clearly needed.

NURSING MOTHERS
It is not known whether Proteinase Inhibitor (Human), Alpha₁, is excreted in human milk. Because many drugs are excreted in human milk, caution should be exercised when Proteinase Inhibitor (Human), Alpha₁, is administered to a nursing woman.

PEDIATRIC USE
Safety and effectiveness in children have not been established.

ADVERSE REACTIONS
Therapeutic administration of Proteinase Inhibitor (Human), Alpha₁, 60 mg/kg weekly, has been demonstrated to be well-tolerated. In clinical studies, six reactions were observed with 517 infusions of Proteinase Inhibitor (Human), Alpha₁, or 1.16%. None of the reactions was severe.[18] The adverse reactions reported included delayed fever (maximum temperature rise was 38.9°C, resolving spontaneously over 24 hours) occurring up to 12 hours following treatment (0.77%), light-headedness, (0.19%), and dizziness (0.19%).[18] Mild transient leukocytosis and dilutional anemia several hours after infusion have also been noted.[18] Since market entry, occasional reports of other flu-like symptoms, allergic-like reactions, chills, dyspnea, rash, tachycardia, and, rarely, hypotension have also been received.

DOSAGE AND ADMINISTRATION
Each bottle of Proteinase Inhibitor (Human), Alpha₁, has the functional activity, as determined by inhibition of porcine pancreatic elastase,[1] stated on the label of the bottle. The "threshold" level of alpha₁-PI in the serum believed to provide adequate anti-elastase activity in the lung of individuals with alpha₁-antitrypsin deficiency is 80 mg/dL (based on commercial standards for alpha₁-PI immunologic assay).[12,15,17] However, assays of alpha₁-PI based on commercial standards measure antigenic activity of alpha₁-PI whereas the labeled potency value of alpha₁-PI is expressed as actual functional activity, i.e., actual capacity to neutralize porcine pancreatic elastase. As functional activity may be less than antigenic activity, serum levels of alpha₁-PI determined using commercial immunologic assays may not accurately reflect actual functional alpha₁-PI levels. Therefore, although it may be helpful to monitor serum levels of alpha₁-PI in individuals receiving Proteinase Inhibitor (Human), Alpha₁, using currently available commercial assays of antigenic activity, results of these assays should not be used to determine the required therapeutic dosage.

The recommended dosage of Proteinase Inhibitor (Human), Alpha is 60 mg/kg body weight administered once weekly. This dose is intended to increase and maintain a level of functional alpha₁-PI in the epithelial lining of the lower respiratory tract providing adequate anti-elastase activity in the lung of individuals with alpha₁-antitrypsin deficiency. Proteinase Inhibitor (Human), Alpha₁, may be given at a rate of 0.08 mL/kg/min or greater and must be administered intravenously. The recommended dosage of 60 mg/kg takes approximately 30 minutes to infuse.

Parenteral drug products should be inspected visually for particulate matter and discoloration prior to administration, whenever solution and container permit.

1. Warm the unopened diluent and concentrate to room temperature (NMT 37°C, 99°F).
2. After removing the plastic flip-top caps, aseptically cleanse rubber stoppers of both bottles.
3. Remove the protective cover from the plastic transfer needle cartridge with tamper-proof seal and penetrate the stopper of the diluent bottle.
4. Remove the remaining portion of the plastic cartridge. Invert the diluent bottle and penetrate the rubber seal on the concentrate bottle with the needle at an angle.
5. The vacuum will draw the diluent into the concentrate bottle. For best results, and to avoid foaming, hold the diluent bottle at an angle to the concentrate bottle in order to direct the jet of diluent against the wall of the concentrate bottle.
6. After removing the diluent bottle and transfer needle (Fig. D), gently swirl the concentrate bottle until the powder is completely dissolved.
7. Swab top of reconstituted bottle of Alpha₁-Proteinase Inhibitor (Human), again.
8. Attach the sterile filter needle provided to syringe. With filter needle in place, insert syringe into reconstituted bottle of Proteinase Inhibitor (Human), Alpha₁, and withdraw Proteinase Inhibitor (Human), Alpha₁, solution into syringe.
9. To administer Proteinase Inhibitor (Human), Alpha₁, replace filter needle with appropriate injection needle and follow procedure for I.V. administration.
10. The contents of more than one bottle of Proteinase Inhibitor (Human), Alpha₁, may be drawn into the same syringe before administration. If more than

one bottle of Proteinase Inhibitor (Human), Alpha₁ is used, withdraw contents from bottles using aseptic technique. Place contents into an admnistration container (plastic minibag or glass bottle) using a syringe.* Avoid pushing an I.V. administration set spike into the product container stopper as this has been known to force the stopper into the vial, with a resulting loss of sterility.

Proteinase Inhibitor (Human), Alpha₁, should be stored under refrigeration (2°-8°C; 35°-46°F). Freezing should be avoided as breakage of the diluent bottle might occur.

REFERENCES
1. Coan MH, Brockway WJ, Eguizabal H, et al: Preparation and properties of alpha₁-proteinase inhibitor concentrate from human plasma. *Vox Sang* 48(6):333-42, 1985. 2. Laurell CB, Eriksson S: The electrophoretic alpha₁-globulin pattern of serum in alpha₁-antitrypsin deficiency. *Scand J Clin Lab Invest* 15:132-40, 1963. 3. Eriksson S: Pulmonary emphysema and alpha₁-antitrypsin deficiency. *Acta Med Scand* 175(2):197-205, 1964. 4. Eriksson S: Studies in alpha₁-antitrypsin deficiency. *Acta Med Scand* Suppl 432:1-85, 1965. 5. Kueppers F, Black LF: Alpha₁-antitrypsin and its deficiency. *Am Rev Respir Dis* 110(2):176-94, 1974. 6. Morse JO: Alpha₁-antitrypsin deficiency. *N Engl J Med* 299:1045-8; 1099-105, 1978. 7. Black LF, Kueppers F: Alpha₁-antitrypsin deficiency in nonsmokers. *Am Rev Respir Dis* 117(3):421-8, 1978. 8. Tobin JM, Cook PJ, Hutchison DC: Alpha₁-antitrypsin deficiency: the clinical and physiological features of pulmonary emphysema in subjects homozygous for Pi type Z. A survey by the British Thoracic Association. *Br J Dis Chest* 77(1): 14-27, 1983. 9. Larsson C. Natural history and life expectancy in severe alpha₁-antitrypsin deficiency, Pi Z. *Acta Med Scand* 204(5):345-51, 1978. 10. Pannell R. Johnson D, Travis J: Isolation and properties of human plasma alpha₁-proteinase inhibitor. *Biochemistry* 13(26):5439-45, 1974. 11. Lieberman J; Elastase, collagenase, emphysema, and alpha₁-antitrypsin deficiency. *Chest* 70(1):62-7, 1976. 12. Gadek JE, Fells GA, Zimmerman RL, et al: Antielastases of the human alveolar structures: implications for the protease-antiprotease theory of emphysema. *J Clin Invest* 68(4):889-98, 1981. 13. Beatty K, Bieth J, Travis J: Kinetics of association of serine proteinases with native and oxidized alpha-1-proteinase inhibitor and alpha-1-antichymotrypsin. *J Biol Chem* 255(9):3931-4, 1980. 14. Janoff A, White R, Carp H, et al: Lung injury induced by leukocytic proteases. *Am J Pathol* 97(1):111-36, 1979. 15. Gadek JE, Crystal RG: Alpha₁-antitrypsin deficiency. In: Stanbury JB, Wyngaarden JB, Frederickson DS, et al. eds.: *The Metabolic Basis of Inherited Disease* 5th ed. New York, McGraw-Hill, 1983, p. 1450-67. 16. Larsson C, Dirksen H, Sundstrom G, et al: Lung function studies in asymptomatic individuals with moderately (Pi SZ) and severely (PiZ) reduced levels of alpha₁-antitrypsin. *Scand J Respir Dis* 57(6):267-80, 1976. 17. Gadek JE, Klein HG, Holland PV, et al: Replacement therapy of alpha₁-antitrypsin deficiency: reversal of protease-antiprotease imbalance within the alveolar structures of PiZ subjects. *J Clin Invest* 68(5):1158-65, 1981. 18. Data on file, Miles Inc., Cutter Biological. 19. Wewers MD, Casolaro MA, Sellers SE, et al: Replacement therapy for alpha₁-antitrypsin deficiency associated with emphysema. *N Engl J Med* 316(17):1055-62, 1987. 20. Wewers MD, Casolaro MA, Crystal RG: Comparison of alpha-1-antitrypsin levels and antineutrophil elastase capacity of blood and lung in a patient with the alpha-1-antitrypsin phenotype null-null before and during alpha-1-antitrypsin augmentation therapy. *Am Rev Respir Dis* 135(3):539-43, 1987. 21. Burrows B: A clinical trial of efficacy of antiproteolytic therapy: can it be done? *Am Rev Respir Dis* 127(2:2):S42-3, 1983. 22. Cohen AB: Unraveling the mysteries of alpha₁-antitrypsin deficiency. *N Engl J Med* 314(12):778-9, 1986. 23. Finlayson JS: Albumin products. *Semin Thromb Hemost* 6(2):85-120, 1980.

J CODES
IV—J0256

HOW SUPPLIED
POWDER FOR INJECTION:

BRAND/MANUFACTURER	NDC	SIZE	AWP
○ BRAND			
PROLASTIN: Miles Biol	00192-0601-30	1s	$0.19
	00192-0601-35	1s	$0.19

Protirelin

DESCRIPTION
Chemically, Protirelin is identified as 5-oxo-L-prolyl-L-histidyl-L-proline amide. It is a synthetic tripeptide which is believed to be structurally identical with the naturally-occurring thyrotropin-releasing hormone produced by the hypothalamus. The CAS Registry Number is 24305-27-9.

Protirelin is supplied as 1 mL ampuls. Each ampul contains 500 µg Protirelin in a sterile nonpyrogenic isotonic saline solution having a pH of approximately 6.5. In addition, each ampul contains sodium chloride 9.0 mg, Water for Injection, hydrochloric acid and sodium hydroxide as needed to adjust pH. Protirelin is intended for intravenous administration.

---

* For a patient of average weight (about 70 kg), the volume needed will exceed the limit of one syringe.

Following is its chemical structure:

CLINICAL PHARMACOLOGY

Pharmacologically, Protirelin increases the release of the thyroid stimulating hormone (TSH) from the anterior pituitary. Prolactin release is also increased. It has recently been observed that approximately 65% of acromegalic patients tested respond with a rise in circulating growth hormone levels; the clinical significance is as yet not clear. Following intravenous administration, the mean plasma half-life of Protirelin in normal subjects is approximately five minutes. TSH levels rise rapidly and reach a peak at 20 to 30 minutes. The decline in TSH levels takes place more slowly, approaching baseline levels after approximately three hours.

INDICATIONS AND USAGE

Protirelin is indicated as an adjunctive agent in the diagnostic assessment of thyroid function. As an adjunct to other diagnostic procedures, testing Protirelin may yield useful information in patients with pituitary or hypothalamic dysfunction.

Protirelin is indicated as an adjunct to evaluate the effectiveness of thyrotropin suppression with a particular dose of T4 in patients with nodular or diffuse goitre. A normal TSH baseline value and a minimal difference between the 30 minute and baseline response to Protirelin injection would indicate adequate suppression of the pituitary secretion of TSH. Protirelin may be used, adjunctively, for adjustment of thyroid hormone dosage given to patients with primary hypothyroidism. A normal or slightly blunted TSH response, thirty minutes following Protirelin injection, would indicate adequate replacement therapy.

CONTRAINDICATIONS

Protirelin is contraindicated in patients with a known hypersensitivity to the drug.

WARNINGS

Transient changes in blood pressure, either increases or decreases, frequently occur immediately following administration of Protirelin. Blood pressure should therefore be measured before Protirelin is administered and at frequent intervals during the first 15 minutes after its administration.

Increases in systolic pressure (usually less than 30 mm Hg) and/or increases in diastolic pressure (usually less than 20 mm Hg) have been observed more frequently than decreases in pressure. These changes have not ordinarily persisted for more than 15 minutes nor have they required therapy. More severe degrees of hypertension or hypotension with or without syncope have been reported in a few patients. To minimize the incidence and/or severity of hypotension, the patient should be supine before, during, and after Protirelin administration. If a clinically important change in blood pressure occurs, monitoring of blood pressure should be continued until it returns to baseline levels. Protirelin should not be administered to patients in whom marked, rapid changes in blood pressure would be dangerous unless the potential benefit clearly outweighs the potential risk.

PRECAUTIONS

Thyroid hormones reduce the TSH response to Protirelin. Accordingly, patients in whom Protirelin is to be used diagnostically should be taken off liothyronine (T3) approximately seven days prior to testing and should be taken off thyroid medications containing levothyroxine (T4), e.g., desiccated thyroid, thyroglobulin, or liotrix, at least 14 days before testing. Hormone therapy is NOT to be discontinued when the test is used to evaluate the effectiveness of thyroid suppression with a particular dose of T4 in patients with nodular or diffuse goitre, or for adjustment of thyroid hormone dosage given to patients with primary hypothyroidism.

Chronic administration of levodopa has been reported to inhibit the TSH response to Protirelin.

It is not advisable to withdraw maintenance doses of adrenocortical drugs used in the therapy of known hypopituitarism. Several published reports have shown that prolonged treatment with glucocorticoids at physiologic doses has no significant effect on the TSH response to thyrotropin releasing hormone, but that the administration of pharmacologic doses of steroids reduces the TSH response. Therapeutic doses of acetylsalicylic acid (2 to 3.6 g/day) have been reported to inhibit the TSH response to Protirelin. The ingestion of acetylsalicylic acid caused the peak level of TSH to decrease approximately 30% as compared to values obtained without acetylsalicylic acid administration. In both cases, the TSH peak occurred 30 minutes post administration of Protirelin.

CARCINOGENESIS, MUTAGENESIS, IMPAIRMENT OF FERTILITY

Long-term animal studies have not been performed to evaluate the carcinogenic potential of Protirelin. Studies to determine potential effects concerning mutagenesis or impairment of fertility have also not been performed.

PREGNANCY (CATEGORY C)

Protirelin has been shown to increase the number of resorptions in rabbits, but not in rats, when given in doses 1½ and 6 times the human dose. There are no adequate and well-controlled studies in pregnant women. Protirelin should be used during pregnancy only if the potential benefit justifies the potential risk to the fetus.

NURSING MOTHERS

It is not known whether this drug is excreted in human milk. Because many drugs are excreted in human milk, caution should be exercised when Protirelin is administered to a nursing woman.

ADVERSE REACTIONS

Side effects have been reported in about 50% of the patients tested with Protirelin. Generally, the side effects are minor, have occurred promptly, and have persisted for only a few minutes following injection.

CARDIOVASCULAR REACTIONS

Marked changes in blood pressure, including both hypertension and hypotension with or without syncope, have been reported in a small number of patients.

ENDOCRINE REACTION

Breast enlargement and leakage in lactating women for up to two or three days.

OTHER REACTIONS

Headaches, sometimes severe, and transient amaurosis in patients with pituitary tumors. Rarely, convulsions may occur in patients with predisposing conditions, e.g. epilepsy, brain damage. Nausea; urge to urinate; flushed sensation; lightheadedness; bad taste; abdominal discomfort; and dry mouth. Less frequently reported were: anxiety; sweating; tightness in the throat; pressure in the chest; tingling sensation; drowsiness; and allergic reactions.

Pituitary apoplexy requiring acute neurosurgical intervention has been reported infrequently for patients with pituitary macroadenomas following the acute administration of Protirelin (TRH) injection in the setting of combined anterior pituitary function testing in conjunction with LHRH and insulin.

DOSAGE AND ADMINISTRATION

Protirelin is intended for intravenous administration with the patient in the supine position. The drug is administered as a bolus over a period of 15 to 30 seconds, with the patient remaining supine until all scheduled postinjection blood samples have been taken. Blood pressure should be measured before Protirelin is administered and at frequent intervals during the first 15 minutes thereafter (see "Warnings"). Have the patient urinate before injecting Protirelin.

DOSAGE:

Adults: 500 µg. Doses between 200 and 500 µg have been used. 500 µg is considered the optimum dose to give the maximum response in the greatest number of patients. Doses greater than 500 µg are unlikely to elicit a greater TSH response.

Children Age 6 to 16 Years: 7 µg/kg body weight up to a dose of 500 µg.

Infants and Children Up to 6 Years: Experience is limited in this age group; doses of 7 µg/kg have been administered.

One blood sample for TSH assay should be drawn immediately prior to the injection of Protirelin, and a second sample should be obtained 30 minutes after injection.

The TSH response to Protirelin is reduced by repetitive administration of the drug. Accordingly, if the Protirelin test is repeated, an interval of seven days before testing is recommended. Elevated serum lipids may interfere with the TSH assay. Thus, fasting (except in patients with hypopituitarism) or a low-fat meal is recommended prior to the test.

INTERPRETATION OF TEST RESULTS

Interpretation of the TSH response to Protirelin requires an understanding of thyroid-pituitary-hypothalamic physiology and knowledge of the clinical status of the individual patient.

Because the TSH test results may vary with the laboratory, the physician should be familiar with the TSH assay method used and the normal range for the laboratory performing the assay. TSH response 30 minutes after Protirelin administration in normal subjects and in patients with hyperthyroidism and hypothyroidism are presented in Figure 1. The diagnoses were established prior to the administration of Protirelin on the basis of the clinical history, physical examination, and the results of other thyroid and/or pituitary function tests.

➤ SHOWN IN PRODUCT IDENTIFICATION GUIDE

Figure 1

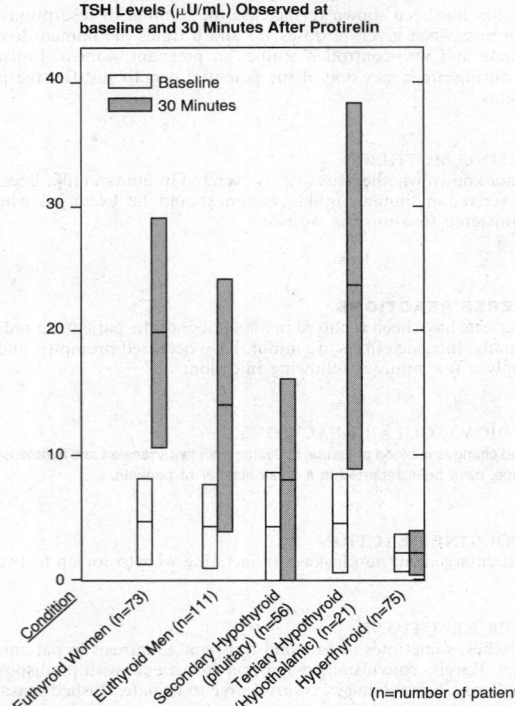

Mean ± One Standard Deviation of TSH Levels (μU/mL) Observed at baseline and 30 Minutes After Protirelin

□ Baseline
▨ 30 Minutes

Condition: Euthyroid Women (n=73), Euthyroid Men (n=111), Secondary Hypothyroid (pituitary) (n=56), Tertiary Hypothyroid (Hypothalamic) (n=21), Hyperthyroid (n=75)

(n=number of patients)

Among the normal euthyroid subjects, women and children were found to have higher levels of TSH at 30 minutes than men. Among the patients with hyperthyroidism or primary (thyroidal), secondary (pituitary), or tertiary (hypothalamic) hypothyroidism, no significant differences in TSH levels by age or sex were found.

Normal: Baseline TSH levels of less than 10 microunits/mL (μU/mL) were observed in 97% of euthyroid normal subjects tested. Thirty minutes after Protirelin, the serum TSH increased by 2.0 μU/mL or more in 95% of euthyroid subjects.

Hyperthyroidism: All hyperthyroid patients tested had baseline TSH levels of less than 10 μU/mL and a rise of less than 2 μU/mL 30 minutes after Protirelin. Primary (thyroidal) hypothyroidism: The diagnosis of primary hypothyroidism is frequently supported by finding clearly elevated baseline TSH levels: 93% of patients tested had levels above 10 μU/mL. Protirelin administration to these patients generally would not be expected to yield additional useful information. Ninety-four percent of patients with primary hypothyroidism given Protirelin in clinical trials responded with a rise in TSH of 2.0 μU/mL or greater, since this response is also found in normal subjects. Protirelin testing does not differentiate primary hypothyroidism from normal.

Table 1

CHARACTERIZATION BASED ON SERUM TSH LEVELS AT BASELINE AND 30 MINUTES AFTER PROTIRELIN

	Baseline (Serum TSH (μU/mL)	Change of Serum TSH (μU/mL) at 30 minutes
Euthyroidism (normal thyroid function)	10 or less (usually 6 or less; 20% have <1.5 μU/mL)	2 or more (usually 6 to 30)
Hyperthyroidism	10 or less (usually 4 or less)	less than 2
Primary Hypothyroidism (thyroidal)	more than 10 (usually 15 to 100)	2 or more (usually 20 or more)
Secondary Hypothyroidism (pituitary)	10 or less (usually 6 or less)	less than 2 (59%) 2 to 50 (41%)
Tertiary Hypothyroidism (hypothalamic)	10 or less (often less than 2)	2 or more

Secondary (pituitary) and tertiary (hypothalamic) hypothyroidism: In the presence of clinical and other laboratory evidence of hypothyroidism, the finding of a baseline TSH level less than 10 μU/mL should suggest secondary or tertiary hypothyroidism. In this situation, a response to Protirelin of less than 2 μU/mL suggests secondary hypothyroidism since this response was observed in about 60% of patients with secondary hypothyroidism and only approximately 5% of patients with tertiary hypothyroidism. A TSH response to Protirelin greater than 2 μU/mL

is not helpful in differentiating between secondary and tertiary hypothyroidism since this response was noted in about 40% of the former and about 95% in the latter.

Establishing the diagnosis of secondary or tertiary hypothyroidism requires a careful history and physical examination along with appropriate test of anterior pituitary and/or target gland function. The Protirelin test should not be used as the only laboratory determinant for establishing these diagnoses.

STORAGE
Store at controlled room temperatures (59-86°F).

HOW SUPPLIED
INJECTION: 500 MCG/ML

BRAND/MANUFACTURER	NDC	SIZE	AWP
◆ BRAND THYREL TRH: Ferring	55566-0081-05	1 ml 5s	$113.40

Protopam Chloride *SEE* PRALIDOXIME CHLORIDE

Protriptyline Hydrochloride

DESCRIPTION
Protriptyline Hydrochloride is N-methyl-5H-dibenzo[a,d]-cycloheptene-5-propanamine hydrochloride. Its empirical formula is $C_{19}H_{21}N.HCl$.

Protriptyline Hydrochloride, a dibenzocycloheptene derivative, has a molecular weight of 299.84. It is a white to yellowish powder that is freely soluble in water and soluble in dilute Hydrochloride. Protriptyline Hydrochloride is supplied as 5 mg and 10 mg film coated tablets.

Following is its chemical structure:

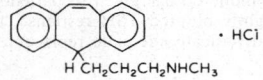

ACTIONS
Protriptyline Hydrochloride is an antidepressant agent. The mechanism of its antidepressant action in man is not known. It is not a monoamine oxidase inhibitor, and it does not act primarily by stimulation of the central nervous system.

Protriptyline HCl has been found in some studies to have a more rapid onset of action than imipramine or amitriptyline. The initial clinical effect may occur within one week. Sedative and tranquilizing properties are lacking. The rate of excretion is slow.

METABOLISM
Metabolic studies indicate that Protriptyline HCl is well absorbed from the gastrointestinal tract and is rapidly sequestered in tissues. Relatively low plasma levels are found after administration, and only a small amount of unchanged drug is excreted in the urine of dogs and rabbits. Preliminary studies indicate that demethylation of the secondary amine moiety occurs to a significant extent, and that metabolic transformation probably takes place in the liver. It penetrates the brain rapidly in mice and rats, and moreover that which is present in the brain is almost all unchanged drug.

Studies on the disposition of radioactive Protriptyline HCl in human test subjects showed significant plasma levels within 2 hours, peaking at 8 to 12 hours, then declining gradually. Urinary excretion studies in the same subjects showed significant amounts of radioactivity in 2 hours. The rate of excretion was slow. Cumulative urinary excretion during 16 days accounted for approximately 50% of the drug. The fecal route of excretion did not seem to be important.

INDICATIONS
Protriptyline HCl is indicated for the treatment of symptoms of mental depression in patients who are under close medical supervision. Its activating properties make it particularly suitable for withdrawn and anergic patients.

UNLABELED USES
Protriptyline HCl is used alone or as an adjunct in the treatment of narcolepsy and sleep apnea.

CONTRAINDICATIONS
Protriptyline HCl is contraindicated in patients who have shown prior hypersensitivity to it.

It should not be given concomitantly with a monoamine oxidase inhibiting compound. Hyperpyretic crises, severe convulsions, and deaths have occurred in patients receiving tricyclic antidepressant and monoamine oxidase inhibiting drugs simultaneously. When it is desired to substitute Protriptyline HCl for a monoamine oxidase inhibitor, a minimum of 14 days should be allowed to elapse after the latter is discontinued. Protriptyline HCl should then be initiated cautiously with gradual increase in dosage until optimum response is achieved.

This drug should not be used during the acute recovery phase following myocardial infarction.

WARNINGS

Protriptyline HCl may block the antihypertensive effect of guanethidine or similarly acting compounds.

Protriptyline HCl should be used with caution in patients with a history of seizures, and, because of its autonomic activity, in patients with a tendency to urinary retention, or increased intraocular tension.

Tachycardia and postural hypotension may occur more frequently with Protriptyline HCl than with other antidepressant drugs. Protriptyline HCl should be used with caution in elderly patients and patients with cardiovascular disorders; such patients should be observed closely because of the tendency of the drug to produce tachycardia, hypotension, arrhythmias, and prolongation of the conduction time. Myocardial infarction and stroke have occurred with drugs of this class.

On rare occasions, hyperthyroid patients or those receiving thyroid medication may develop arrhythmias when this drug is given.

In patients who may use alcohol excessively, it should be borne in mind that the potentiation may increase the danger inherent in any suicide attempt or overdosage.

USAGE IN CHILDREN

This drug is not recommended for use in children because safety and effectiveness in the pediatric age group have not been established.

USAGE IN PREGNANCY

Safe use in pregnancy and lactation has not been established; therefore, use in pregnant women, nursing mothers or women who may become pregnant requires that possible benefits be weighed against possible hazards to mother and child.

In mice, rats and rabbits, doses about ten times greater than the recommended human doses had no apparent adverse effects on reproduction.

PRECAUTIONS

When Protriptyline HCl is used to treat the depressive component of schizophrenia, psychotic symptoms may be aggravated. Likewise, in manic-depressive psychosis, depressed patients may experience a shift toward the manic phase if they are treated with an antidepressant drug. Paranoid delusions, with or without associated hostility, may be exaggerated. In any of these circumstances, it may be advisable to reduce the dose of Protriptyline HCl or to use a major tranquilizing drug concurrently.

Symptoms, such as anxiety or agitation, may be aggravated in overactive or agitated patients.

When Protriptyline HCl is given with anticholinergic agents or sympathomimetic drugs, including epinephrine combined with local anesthetics, close supervision and careful adjustment of dosages are required.

Hyperpyrexia has been reported when tricyclic antidepressants are administered with anticholinergic agents or with neuroleptic drugs, particularly during hot weather.

Cimetidine is reported to reduce hepatic metabolism of certain tricyclic antidepressants, thereby delaying elimination and increasing steady-state concentrations of these drugs. Clinically significant effects have been reported with the tricyclic antidepressants when used concomitantly with cimetidine. Increases in plasma levels of tricyclic antidepressants, and in the frequency and severity of side effects, particularly anticholinergic, have been reported when cimetidine was added to the drug regimen. Discontinuation of cimetidine in well-controlled patients receiving tricyclic antidepressants and cimetidine may decrease the plasma levels and efficacy of the antidepressants.

It may enhance the response to alcohol and the effects of barbiturates and other CNS depressants.

The possibility of suicide in depressed patients remains during treatment and until significant remission occurs. This type of patient should not have access to large quantities of the drug.

Concurrent administration of Protriptyline HCl and electroshock therapy may increase the hazards of therapy. Such treatment should be limited to patients for whom it is essential. Discontinue the drug several days before elective surgery, if possible.

Both elevation and lowering of blood sugar levels have been reported.

Information for Patients: While on therapy with Protriptyline HCl, patients should be advised as to the possible impairment of mental and/or physical abilities required for performance of hazardous tasks, such as operating machinery or driving a motor vehicle.

ADVERSE REACTIONS

Within each category the following adverse reactions are listed in order of decreasing severity. Included in the listing are a few adverse reactions which have not been reported with this specific drug. However, the pharmacological similarities among the tricyclic antidepressant drugs require that each of the reactions be considered when Protriptyline is administered. Protriptyline HCl is more likely to aggravate agitation and anxiety and produce cardiovascular reactions such as tachycardia and hypotension.

Cardiovascular: Myocardial infarction; stroke; heart block; arrhythmias; hypotension, particularly orthostatic hypotension; hypertension; tachycardia; palpitation.

Psychiatric: Confusional states (especially in the elderly) with hallucinations, disorientation, delusions, anxiety, restlessness, agitation; hypomania; exacerbation of psychosis; insomnia, panic, and nightmares.

Neurological: Seizures; incoordination; ataxia; tremors; peripheral neuropathy; numbness, tingling, and paresthesias of extremities; extrapyramidal symptoms; drowsiness; dizziness; weakness and fatigue; headache; syndrome of inappropriate ADH (antidiuretic hormone) secretion; tinnitus; alteration in EEG patterns.

Anticholinergic: Paralytic ileus; hyperpyrexia; urinary retention, delayed micturition, dilatation of the urinary tract; constipation; blurred vision, disturbance of accomodation, increased intraocular pressure, mydriasis; dry mouth and rarely associated sublingual adenitis.

Allergic: Drug fever; petechiae, skin rash, urticaria, itching, photosensitization (avoid excessive exposure to sunlight); edema (general, or of face and tongue).

Hematologic: Agranulocytosis; bone marrow depression; leukopenia; thrombocytopenia; purpura; eosinophilia.

Gastrointestinal: Nausea and vomiting; anorexia; epigastric distress; diarrhea; peculiar taste; stomatitis; abdominal cramps; black tongue.

Endocrine: Impotence, increased or decreased libido; gynecomastia in the male; breast enlargement and galactorrhea in the female; testicular swelling; elevation or depression of blood sugar levels.

Other: Jaundice (simulating obstructive); altered liver function; parotid swelling; alopecia; flushing; weight gain or loss, urinary frequency, nocturia; perspiration.

Withdrawal Symptoms: Though not indicative of addiction, abrupt cessation of treatment after prolonged therapy may produce nausea, headache, and malaise.

OVERDOSAGE

Manifestations: High doses may cause temporary confusion, disturbed concentration, or transient visual hallucinations. Overdosage may cause drowsiness; hypothermia; tachycardia and other arrhythmic abnormalities, for example, bundle branch block; ECG evidence of impaired conduction; congestive heart failure; dilated pupils; convulsions; severe hypotension; stupor; and coma. Other symptoms may be agitation, hyperactive reflexes, muscle rigidity, vomiting, hyperpyrexia, or any of those listed under *"Adverse Reactions"*.

Experience in the management of overdosage with Protriptyline is limited. The following recommendations are based on the management of overdosage with other tricyclic antidepressants.

All patients suspected of having taken an overdosage should be admitted to a hospital as soon as possible. *Treatment* is symptomatic and supportive. Empty the stomach as quickly as possible by emesis followed by gastric lavage upon arrival at the hospital. Following gastric lavage, activated charcoal may be administered. Twenty to 30 g of activated charcoal may be given every four to six hours during the first 24 to 48 hours after ingestion. An ECG should be taken and close monitoring of cardiac function instituted if there is any sign of abnormality. Maintain an open airway and adequate fluid intake; regulate body temperature.

The intravenous administration of 1-3 mg of physostigmine salicylate is reported to reverse the symptoms of other tricyclic antidepressnat poisoning in humans. Because physostigmine is rapidly metabolized, the dosage of physostigmine should be repeated as required particularly if life threatening signs such as arrhythmias, convulsions, and deep coma recur or persist after the initial dosage of physostigmine. Because physostigmine itself may be toxic, it is not recommended for routine use.

Standard measures should be used to manage circulatory shock and metabolic acidosis. Cardiac arrhythmias may be treated with neostigmine, pyridostigmine, or propranolol. Should cardiac failure occur, the use of digitalis should be considered. Close monitoring of cardiac function for not less than five days is advisable.

Anticonvulsants may be given to control convulsions.

Dialysis is of no value because of low plasma concentrations of the drug.

Since overdosage is often deliberate, patients may attempt suicide by other means during the recovery phase.

Deaths by deliberate or accidental overdosage have occurred with this class of drugs.

DOSAGE AND ADMINISTRATION

Dosage should be initiated at a low level and increased gradually, noting carefully the clinical response and any evidence of intolerance.

Usual Adult Dosage: Fifteen to 40 mg a day divided into 3 or 4 doses. If necessary, dosage may be increased to 60 mg a day. Dosages above this amount are not recommended. Increases should be made in the morning dose.

Adolescent and Elderly Patients: In general, lower dosages are recommended for these patients. Five mg 3 times a day may be given initially, and increased gradually if necessary. In elderly patients, the cardiovascular system must be monitored closely if the daily dose exceeds 20 mg. When satisfactory improvement has been reached, dosage should be reduced to the smallest amount that will maintain relief of symptoms.

Minor adverse reactions require reduction in dosage. Major adverse reactions or evidence of hypersensitivity require prompt discontinuation of the drug.

Usage in Children: This drug is not recommended for use in children because safety and effectiveness in the pediatric age group have not been established.

STORAGE

Store Protriptyline HCl Tablets in a tightly closed container. Avoid storage at temperatures above 40°C (104°F).

HOW SUPPLIED
TABLES: 5 MG

BRAND/MANUFACTURER	NDC	SIZE	AWP
○ **BRAND**			
VIVACTIL: Merck	00006-0026-68	100s	$45.05

TABLETS: 10 MG

BRAND/MANUFACTURER	NDC	SIZE	AWP
○ **BRAND**			
VIVACTIL: Merck	00006-0047-68	100s	$65.28
	00006-0047-28	100s ud	$70.13

Protropin SEE SOMATREM

Proventil SEE ALBUTEROL

Provera SEE MEDROXYPROGESTERONE ACETATE, ORAL

Provocholine SEE METHACHOLINE CHLORIDE

Prozac SEE FLUOXETINE HYDROCHLORIDE

Pseudoephedrine Hydrochloride

DESCRIPTION
Each capsule contains 120 mg of Pseudoephedrine Hydrochloride in specially formulated pellets designed to provide continuous therapeutic effect for 12 hours. About one-half of the active ingredient is released soon after administration and the rest slowly over the remaining time period.

Following is its chemical structure:

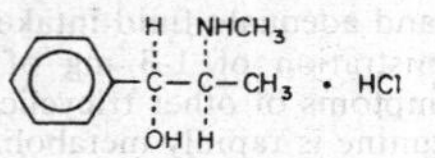

ACTIONS
Pseudoephedrine (a sympathomimetic) is an orally effective nasal decongestant with peripheral effects similar to epinephrine and central effects similar to, but less intense than, amphetamines. It has the potential for excitatory side effects. At the recommended oral dosage, it has little or no pressor effect in normotensive adults. Patients have not been reported to experience the rebound congestion sometimes experienced with frequent, repeated use of topical decongestants.

INDICATIONS
Relief of nasal congestion or eustachian tube congestion. May be given concomitantly with analgesics, antihistamines, expectorants and antibiotics.

UNLABELED USES
Pseudoephedrine Hydrochloride is used alone or as an adjunct in the treatment of urinary incontinence and osthostatic hypotension.

CONTRAINDICATIONS
Patients with severe hypertension, severe coronary artery disease, and patients on MAO inhibitor therapy. Also contraindicated in patients with hypersensitivity or idiosyncrasy to sympathomimetic amines which may be manifested by insomnia, dizziness, weakness, tremor or arrhythmias.

Children under 12: Should not be used by children under 12 years.

Nursing Mothers: Contraindicated because of the higher than usual risk for infants from sympathomimetic amines.

WARNINGS
Use judiciously and sparingly in patients with hypertension, diabetes mellitus, ischemic heart disease, increased intraocular pressure, hyperthyroidism, or prostatic hypertrophy. (See, however, *"Contraindications"*). Sympathomimetics may produce central nervous stimulation with convulsions or cardiovascular collapse with accompanying hypotension. Do not exceed recommended dosage.

Use in Pregnancy: Safety in pregnancy has not been established.

Use in Elderly: The elderly (60 years and older) are more likely to have adverse reactions to sympathomimetics. Overdosage of sympathomimetics in the elderly may cause hallucinations, convulsions, CNS depression, and death. Safe use of a short-acting sympathomimetic should be demonstrated in the individual elderly patient before considering the use of a sustained-action formulation.

PRECAUTIONS
Patients with diabetes, hypertension, cardiovascular disease and hyper-reactivity to ephedrine.

ADVERSE REACTIONS
Hyper-reactive individuals may display ephedrine-like reactions such as tachycardia, palpitations, headache, dizziness or nausea. Sympathomimetics have been associated with certain untoward reactions including fear, anxiety, tenseness, restlessness, tremor, weakness, pallor, respiratory difficulty, dysuria, insomnia, hallucinations, convulsions, CNS depression, arrhythmias, and cardiovascular collapse with hypotension.

DRUG INTERACTIONS
MAO inhibitors and beta adrenergic blockers increase the effects of pseudoephedrine. Sympathomimetics may reduce the antihypertensive effects of methylodpa, mecamylamine, reserpine and veratrum alkaloids.

DOSAGE AND ADMINISTRATION
One capsule every 12 hours. Do not give to children under 12 years of age.

HOW SUPPLIED
CAPSULE, EXTENDED RELEASE:

BRAND/MANUFACTURER	NDC	SIZE	AWP
○ **BRAND**			
NOVAFED: Marion Merrell Dow	00068-0104-61	100s	$42.42

TABLETS: 30 MG

BRAND/MANUFACTURER	NDC	SIZE	AWP
○ **GENERICS**			
Medirex	57480-0210-01	100s ud	$4.77

TABLETS: 60 MG

BRAND/MANUFACTURER	NDC	SIZE	AWP
○ **GENERICS**			
Raway	00686-0012-20	100s ud	$5.50

Pseudoephedrine Hydrochloride and Terfenadine

> **WARNING**
> **QT INTERVAL PROLONGATION/VENTRICULAR ARRHYTHMIA**
> RARE CASES OF SERIOUS CARDIOVASCULAR ADVERSE EVENTS, INCLUDING DEATH, CARDIAC ARREST, TORSADES DE POINTES, AND OTHER VENTRICULAR ARRHYTHMIAS, HAVE BEEN OBSERVED IN THE FOLLOWING CLINICAL SETTINGS, FREQUENTLY IN ASSOCIATION WITH INCREASED TERFENADINE LEVELS WHICH LEAD TO ELECTROCARDIOGRAPHIC QT PROLONGATION:
> 1. CONCOMITANT ADMINISTRATION OF KETOCONAZOLE OR ITRACONAZOLE
> 2. OVERDOSE, INCLUDING SINGLE TERFENADINE DOSES AS LOW AS 360 MG
> 3. CONCOMITANT ADMINISTRATION OF CLARITHROMYCIN, ERYTHROMYCIN, OR TROLEANDOMYCIN
> 4. SIGNIFICANT HEPATIC DYSFUNCTION
> TERFENADINE IS CONTRAINDICATED IN PATIENTS TAKING KETOCONAZOLE, ITRACONAZOLE, ERYTHROMYCIN, CLARITHROMYCIN, OR TROLEANDOMYCIN, AND IN PATIENTS WITH SIGNIFICANT HEPATIC DYSFUNCTION.
> DO NOT EXCEED RECOMMENDED DOSE.
> IN SOME CASES, SEVERE ARRHYTHMIAS HAVE BEEN PRECEDED BY EPISODES OF SYNCOPE. SYNCOPE IN PATIENTS RECEIVING TERFENADINE SHOULD LEAD TO DISCONTINUATION OF TREATMENT AND FULL EVALUATION OF POTENTIAL ARRHYTHMIAS.
> (SEE *"CONTRAINDICATIONS," "WARNINGS," "CLINICAL PHARMACOLOGY,"* AND *"PRECAUTIONS: DRUG INTERACTIONS".*)

DESCRIPTION
Pseudoephedrine Hydrochloride/Terfenadine extended-release tablets are available for oral administration.

Each tablet contains 60 mg Terfenadine and 10 mg of Pseudoephedrine Hydrochloride in an outer press-coat for immediate release and 110 mg Pseudoephedrine Hydrochloride in an extended-release core.

Terfenadine is a histamine H_1-receptor antagonist with the chemical name α-[4-(1,1-Dimethylethyl)phenyl]-4-(hydroxydiphenylmethyl)-1-piperidinebutanol(±).

The molecular weight is 471.68. The molecular formula is $C_{32}H_{41}NO_2$.

◆ RATED THERAPEUTICALLY EQUIVALENT; ◇ THERAPEUTIC EQUIVALENCE UNCONFIRMED; ○ UNRATED

Terfenadine occurs as a white to off-white crystalline powder. It is freely soluble in chloroform, soluble in ethanol, and very slightly soluble in water.

Pseudoephedrine Hydrochloride is an adrenergic (vasoconstrictor) agent with the chemical name $[S-(R^*,R^*)]-\alpha-[1-(methylamino)ethyl]$-benzenemethanol hydrochloride.

The molecular weight is 201.70. The molecular formula is $C_{10}H_{15}NO \cdot HCl$.

Pseudoephedrine Hydrochloride occurs as fine, white to off-white crystals or powder, having a faint characteristic odor. It is very soluble in water, freely soluble in alcohol, and sparingly soluble in chloroform.

CLINICAL PHARMACOLOGY

Terfenadine, a histamine H_1-receptor antagonist, is chemically distinct from other antihistamines.

Histamine skin wheal studies have shown that Terfenadine in single and repeated doses of 60 mg in 64 subjects has an antihistaminic effect beginning at 1-2 hours, reaching its maximum at 3-4 hours, and lasting in excess of 12 hours. The correlation between response on skin wheal testing and clinical efficacy is unclear.

The four best controlled and largest clinical trials each lasted 7 days and involved about 1,000 total patients in comparisons of Terfenadine (60 mg b.i.d.) with an active drug (chlorpheniramine, 4 mg t.i.d.; dexchlorpheniramine, 2 mg t.i.d.; or clemastine 1 mg b.i.d.). About 50-70% of Terfenadine or other antihistamine recipients had moderate to complete relief of symptoms, compared with 30-50% of placebo recipients. The frequency of drowsiness with Terfenadine was similar to the frequency with placebo and less than with other antihistamines. In studies which included 52 subjects in whom EEG assessments were made, no depressant effects have been observed. Pseudoephedrine/Terfenadine has not been studied for effectiveness in relieving the symptoms of the common cold.

Animal studies have demonstrated that Terfenadine is a histamine H_1-receptor antagonist. In these animal studies, no sedative or anticholinergic effects were observed at effective antihistamine doses. Radioactive disposition and autoradiographic studies in rats and radioligand binding studies with guinea pig brain H_1-receptors indicate that, at effective antihistamine doses, neither Terfenadine nor its metabolites penetrate the blood brain barrier well.

On the basis of a mass balance study using ^{14}C labeled Terfenadine the oral absorption of Terfenadine was estimated to be at least 70%. Terfenadine itself undergoes extensive (99%) first pass metabolism to two primary metabolites, an active acid metabolite and an inactive dealkylated metabolite. Therefore, systemic availability of Terfenadine is low under normal conditions, and parent Terfenadine is not normally detectable in plasma at levels > 10 ng/mL. Although in rare cases there was measurable plasma Terfenadine in apparently normal individuals without identifiable risk factors, the implications of this finding with respect to the variability of Terfenadine metabolism in the normal population cannot be assessed without further study. Further studies of Terfenadine metabolism in the general population are pending. From information gained in the ^{14}C study it appears that approximately forty percent of the total dose is eliminated renally (40% as acid metabolite, 30% dealkyl metabolite, and 30% minor unidentified metabolites). Sixty percent of the dose is eliminated in the feces (50% as the acid metabolite, 2% unchanged Terfenadine, and the remainder as minor unidentified metabolites). Studies investigating the effect of hepatic and renal insufficiency on the metabolism and excretion of Terfenadine are incomplete. Preliminary information indicates that in cases of hepatic impairment, significant concentrations of unchanged Terfenadine can be detected with the rate of acid metabolite formation being decreased. A single-dose study in patients with hepatic impairment revealed increased parent Terfenadine and impaired metabolism, suggesting that additional drug accumulation may occur after repetitive dosing in such patients. Terfenadine is contraindicated for use in patients with significant hepatic dysfunction. (See "Contraindications" and "Warnings".) In subjects with normal hepatic function, unchanged Terfenadine plasma concentrations have not been detected. *Elevated levels of parent Terfenadine, whether due to significant hepatic dysfunction, concomitant medications, or overdose, have been associated with QT interval prolongation and serious cardiac adverse events. (See "Contraindications" and "Warnings".)* In controlled clinical trials in otherwise normal patients with rhinitis, small increases QTc interval were observed at doses of 60 mg b.i.d. In studies at 300 mg b.i.d. a mean increase in QTc of 10% (range − 4% to +30%) (mean increase of 46 msec) was observed.

Data have been reported demonstrating that compared to young subjects, elderly subjects experience a 25% reduction in clearance of the acid metabolite after single-dose oral administration of 120 mg. Further studies are necessary to fully characterize pharmacokinetics in the elderly.

In vitro studies demonstrate that Terfenadine is extensively (97%) bound to human serum protein while the acid metabolite is approximately 70% bound to human serum protein. Based on data gathered from *in vitro* models of antihistaminic activity, the acid metabolite of Terfenadine has approximately 30% of the H_1-blocking activity of Terfenadine. The relative contribution of Terfenadine and the acid metabolite to the pharmacodynamic effects have not been clearly defined. Since unchanged Terfenadine is usually not detected in plasma and active acid metabolite concentrations are relatively high, the acid metabolite may be the entity responsible for the majority of efficacy after oral administration of Terfenadine.

In a study involving the administration of a single 60 mg Terfenadine tablet to 24 subjects, mean peak plasma levels of the acid metabolite were 263 ng/mL (range 133-423 ng/mL) and occurred approximately 2.5 hours after dosing. Plasma concentrations of unchanged Terfenadine were not detected. The elimination profile of the acid metabolite was biphasic in nature with an initial mean plasma half-life of 3.5 hours followed by a mean plasma half-life of 6 hours. Ninety percent of the plasma level time curve was associated with these half-lives.

Although the elimination profile is somewhat complex, the effective pharmacokinetic half-life can be estimated at approximately 8.5 hours. However, receptor binding and pharmacologic effects, both therapeutic and adverse, may persist well beyond that time.

Pseudoephedrine is an orally active sympathomimetic amine and exerts a decongestant action on the nasal mucosa. It is recognized as an effective agent for the relief of nasal congestion due to allergic rhinitis. Pseudoephedrine produces peripheral effects similar to those of epinephrine and central effects similar to, but less intense than, amphetamines. It has the potential for excitatory side effects. At the recommended oral dose it has little or no pressor effect in normotensive adults. The serum half-life of Pseudoephedrine is approximately 4 to 6 hours. The serum half-life is decreased with increased excretion of drug at urine pH lower than 6 and may be increased with decreased excretion at urine pH higher than 8.

Ingestion of food was found not to affect the absorption of Pseudoephedrine from Pseudoephedrine/Terfenadine. The effect of food on the absorption of Terfenadine from Pseudoephedrine/Terfenadine is not known; however, plasma levels of active metabolite do not appear to be affected by food administered with Pseudoephedrine/Terfenadine.

A bioavailability study comparing Pseudoephedrine/Terfenadine to immediate-release Terfenadine and immediate-release Pseudoephedrine showed that Pseudoephedrine is slowly released from Pseudo- ephedrine/Terfenadine to permit twice daily dosage.

INDICATIONS AND USAGE

Pseudoephedrine/Terfenadine is indicated for the relief of symptoms associated with seasonal allergic rhinitis such as sneezing, rhinorrhea, pruritus, lacrimation, and nasal congestion. It should be administered when both the antihistaminic properties of Terfenadine and the nasal decongestant activity of Pseudoephedrine hydrochloride are desired (see "Clinical Pharmacology").

Pseudoephedrine/Terfenadine has not been studied for effectiveness in relieving the symptoms of the common cold.

CONTRAINDICATIONS

CONCOMITANT ADMINISTRATION OF PSEUDOEPHEDRINE/TERFENADINE WITH KETOCONAZOLE OR ITRACONAZOLE IS CONTRAINDICATED. PSEUDOEPHEDRINE/TERFENADINE IS ALSO CONTRAINDICATED IN PATIENTS WITH DISEASE STATES OR OTHER CONCOMITANT MEDICATIONS KNOWN TO IMPAIR ITS METABOLISM, INCLUDING SIGNIFICANT HEPATIC DYSFUNCTION, AND CONCURRENT USE OF CLARITHROMYCIN, ERYTHROMYCIN, OR TROLEANDOMYCIN. QT PROLONGATION HAS BEEN DEMONSTRATED IN SOME PATIENTS TAKING TERFENADINE IN THESE SETTINGS, AND RARE CASES OF SERIOUS CARDIOVASCULAR EVENTS, INCLUDING DEATH, CARDIAC ARREST, AND TORSADES DE POINTES, HAVE BEEN REPORTED IN THESE PATIENT POP- ULATIONS. (See "Warnings and Precautions: Drug Interactions".)

Pseudoephedrine/Terfenadine is contraindicated in nursing mothers, patients with severe hypertension or severe coronary artery disease, patients receiving monoamine oxidase (MAO) inhibitor therapy, and in patients with a known hypersensitivity to any of its ingredients (see "Description" section).

WARNINGS

Terfenadine undergoes extensive metabolism in the liver by a specific cytochrome P450 isoenzyme. This metabolic pathway may be impaired in patients with hepatic dysfunction (alcoholic cirrhosis, hepatitis) or who are taking drugs such as ketoconazole, itraconazole, or clarithromycin, erythromycin, or troleandomycin (macrolide antibiotics), or other potent inhibitors of this isoenzyme. Interference with this metabolism can lead to elevated Terfenadine plasma levels associated with QT prolongation and increased risk of ventricular tachyarrhythmias (such as torsades de pointes, ventricular tachycardia, and ventricular fibrillation) at the recommended dose. Pseudoephedrine/Terfenadine is contraindicated for use by patients with these conditions (see "Warning Box," "Contraindications," and "Precautions: Drug Interactions").

Other patients who may be at risk for these adverse cardiovascular events include patients who may experience new or increased QT prolongation while receiving certain drugs or having conditions which lead to QT prolongation. These include patients taking certain antiarrhythmics, bepridil, certain psychotropics, probucol, or astemizole; patients with electrolyte abnormalities such as hypokalemia or hypomagnesemia, or taking diuretics with potential for inducing electrolyte abnormalities; and patients with congenital QT syndrome. Pseudoephedrine/Terfenadine is not recommended for use by patients with these conditions.

The relationship of underlying cardiac disease to the development of ventricular tachyarrhythmias while on Pseudoephedrine/Terfenadine therapy is unclear; nonetheless, Pseudoephedrine/Terfenadine should also be used with caution in these patients.

Sympathomimetic amines should be used judiciously and sparingly in patients with hypertension, diabetes mellitus, ischemic heart disease, increased intraocular pressure, hyperthyroidism, or prostatic hypertrophy (see "Contraindications"). Sympathomimetic amines may produce CNS stimulation with convulsions or cardiovascular collapse with accompanying hypotension.

Use in Elderly: The elderly are more likely to have adverse reactions to sympathomimetic amines.

PRECAUTIONS

General: Pseudoephedrine/Terfenadine should be used with caution in patients with diabetes, hypertension, cardiovascular disease, and hyper-reactivity to ephedrine.

Information for Patients: Patients taking Pseudoephedrine/Terfenadine should receive the following information and instructions. Patients should be advised to take Pseudoephedrine/Terfenadine only as needed and NOT TO EXCEED THE PRESCRIBED DOSE. Patients should be questioned about use of any other prescription or over-the-counter medication, and should be cautioned regarding the potential for life-threatening arrhythmias with concurrent use of ketoconazole, itraconazole, clarithromycin, erythromycin, or troleandomycin. Patients should be advised to consult the physician before concurrent use of other medications with Terfenadine. Patients should be questioned about pregnancy or lactation before starting Pseudoephedrine/Terfenadine therapy, since the drug is contraindicated in nursing women and should be used in pregnancy only if the potential benefit justifies the potential risk to the fetus. Patients should be directed to swallow the tablet whole. Patients should also be instructed to store this medication in a tightly closed container in a cool, dry place, away from heat moisture, or direct sunlight, and away from children.

Drug Interaction: (see *"Contraindications"*): Monoamine oxidase (MAO) inhibitors and beta-adrenergic agonists increase the effect of sympathomimetic amines. Sympathomimetic amines may reduce the antihypertensive effects of methyldopa, mecamylamine, and reserpine. MAO inhibitors may prolong and intensify the effects of antihistamines.

Care should be taken in the administration of Pseudoephedrine/Terfenadine concomitantly with other sympathomimetic amines because combined effects on the cardiovascular system may be harmful to the patient.

KETOCONAZOLE

Spontaneous adverse reaction reports of patients taking concomitant ketoconazole with recommended dose of Terfenadine demonstrate QT interval prolongation and rare serious cardiac events, e.g. death, cardiac arrest, and ventricular arrhythmia including torsades de pointes. Pharmacokinetic data indicate that ketoconazole markedly inhibits the metabolism of Terfenadine, resulting in elevated plasma Terfenadine levels. Presence of unchanged Terfenadine is associated with statistically significant prolongation of the QT and QTc intervals. Concomitant administration of ketoconazole and Pseudoephedrine/Terfenadine is contraindicated (see *"Contraindications," "Warnings," and "Adverse Reactions"*).

ITRACONAZOLE

Torsades de pointes and elevated parent Terfenadine levels have been reported during concomitant use of Terfenadine and itraconazole in clinical trials of itraconazole and from foreign post-marketing sources. One death has also been reported from foreign post-marketing sources. Concomitant administration of itraconazole and Pseudoephedrine/Terfenadine is contraindicated (see *"Contraindications," "Warnings" and "Adverse Reactions"*).

Due to the chemical similarity of other azole-type antifungal agents (including fluconazole, metronidazole, and miconazole) to ketoconazole and itraconazole, concomitant use of these products with Pseudoephedrine/Terfenadine is not recommended pending full examination of potential interactions.

MACROLIDES

Clinical drug interactions studies indicate that erythromycin and clarithromcin can exert an effect on Terfenadine metabolism by a mechanism which may be similar to that of ketoconazole, but to a lesser extent. Although erythromycin measurably decreases the clearance of the Terfenadine acid metabolite, its influence on Terfenadine plasma levels is still under investigation. A few spontaneous accounts of QT interval prolongation with ventricular arrhythmia including torsades de pointes have been reported in patients receiving erythromycin or troleandomycin.

Concomitant administration of Pseudoephedrine/Terfenadine with clarithromycin, erythromycin, or troleandomycin is contraindicated (see *"Contraindications," "Warnings," and "Adverse Reactions"*). Pending full characterization of potential interactions, concomitant administration of Pseudoephedrine/Terfenadine with other macrolide antibiotics, including azithromycin, is not recommended. Studies to evaluate the potential interaction of Terfenadine with azithromycin are in progress.

Carcinogenesis, Mutagenesis, Impairment of Fertility: No studies have been conducted to evaluate the carcinogenic potential of Pseudoephedrine/Terfenadine.

Oral doses of Terfenadine, corresponding to 63 times the recommended human daily dose, in mice for 18 months or in rats for 24 months, revealed no evidence of tumorigenicity. Microbial and micronucleus test assays with Terfenadine have revealed no evidence of mutagenesis.

Reproduction and fertility studies with Terfenadine in rats showed no effects on male or female fertility at oral doses of up to 21 times the human daily dose. At 63 times the human daily dose there was a small but significant reduction in implants and at 125 times the human daily dose reduced implants and increased post-implantation losses were observed, which were judged to be secondary to maternal toxicity. Animal reproduction studies have not been carried out with Pseudoephedrine.

Pregnancy Category C: The combination of Terfenadine and Pseudoephedrine Hydrochloride (in a ratio of 1:2 by weight) has been shown to produce reduced fetal weight in rats and rabbits at 42 times the human dose, and delayed ossification with wavy ribs in few fetus when given to rats at a dose of 45 times the human daily dose. There are no adequate and well-controlled studies in pregnant women. Pseudoephedrine/Terfenadine should be used during pregnancy only if the potential benefit justifies the potential risk to the fetus.

Nursing Mothers: (see *"Contraindications"*): Terfenadine has caused decreased pup weight gain and survival in rats given doses 63 times and 125 times the human daily dose throughout pregnancy and lactation.

Pediatric Use: Safety and effectiveness of Pseudoephedrine/Terfenadine in children below the age of 12 years have not been established.

ADVERSE REACTIONS

Cardiovascular Adverse Events: With Terfenadine, rare reports of severe cardiovascular adverse effects have been received which include ventricular tachyarrhythmias (torsades de pointes, ventricular tachycardia, ventricular fibrillation, and cardiac arrest), hypotension, palpitations, syncope, and dizziness. Rare reports of deaths resulting from ventricular tachyarrhythmias have been received (see *"Contraindications," "Warnings"*, and *"Precautions, Drug Interactions"*). Hypotension, palpitations, syncope, and dizziness could reflect undetected ventricular arrhythmia. IN SOME PATIENTS, DEATH, CARDIAC ARREST, OR TORSADES DE POINTES HAVE BEEN PRECEDED BY EPISODES OF SYNCOPE (See *"Warning Box"*). Rare reports of serious cardiovascular adverse events have been received, some involving QT prolongation and torsades de pointes, in apparently normal individuals without identifiable risk factors; there is not conclusive evidence of a causal relationship of these events with Terfenadine. Although in rare cases there was measurable plasma Terfenadine, the implications of this finding with respect to the variability of Terfenadine metabolism in the normal population cannot be assessed without further study. In controlled clinical trials in otherwise normal patients with rhinitis, small increases in QTc interval were observed at doses of 60 mg b.i.d. In studies at 300 mg b.i.d. a mean increase in QTc of 10% (range −4% to +30%) (mean increase of 46 msec) was observed.

General Adverse Events: In double-blind, parallel, controlled studies in over 300 patients in which Pseudoephedrine/Terfenadine was compared to extended-release Pseudoephedrine, adverse reactions reported for greater than 1% of the patients receiving Pseudoephedrine/Terfenadine were not clinically different from those reported for patients receiving Pseudoephedrine (see Table below).

FREQUENTLY (> 1%) REPORTED ADVERSE EVENTS FOR PSEUDOEPHEDRINE/TERFENADINE IN DOUBLE-BLIND, PARALLEL, CONTROLLED CLINICAL TRIALS*

Adverse Event	Pseudo-ephedrine/ Terfenadine (n=374)	Pseudo-ephedrine (n=287)	Placebo (n=193)
Central Nervous System			
Insomnia	25.9	26.8	6.2
Headache	17.4	17.1	22.3
Drowsiness/Sedation	7.2	4.9	11.4
Nervousness	6.7	8.4	1.6
Anorexia	3.7	3.8	0.0
Fatigue	2.1	1.4	2.1
Restlessness	2.1	1.0	0.0
Irritability	1.1	0.0	1.0
Disorientation	1.1	0.0	0.5
Increased Energy	1.1	0.0	0.0
Hyperkinesia	1.1	1.0	0.0
Autonomic			
Dry Mouth/Nose/ Throat	21.7	21.3	11.4
Blurring of Vision	1.1	0.3	0.5
Gastrointestinal			
Nausea	4.5	6.6	5.2
Skin			
Rash	1.1	0.0	0.0
Cardiovascular			
Palpitations	2.4	3.8	0.5
Allergy Symptoms			
Sore Throat			
Cough	1.9	1.7	1.0
Other	1.6	0.3	1.0
Infection, Upper Respiratory	1.3	2.4	0.5
Taste Alterations	1.1	1.0	1.0

* *Pseudoephedrine/Terfenadine B.I.D., Pseudoephedrine 120 mg B.I.D.*

Pseudoephedrine may cause ephedrine-like reactions such as tachycardia, palpitations, headache, dizziness, or nausea. Sympathomimetic drugs have also been associated with certain untoward reactions including fear, anxiety, tenseness, restlessness, tremor, weakness, pallor, respiratory difficulty, dysuria, insomnia, hallucinations, convulsions, CNS depression, arrhythmias, and cardiovascular collapse with hypotension.

In controlled clinical trials with Terfenadine, using the recommended daily dose of 60 mg b.i.d., the incidence of adverse events in patients receiving Terfendadine was similar to that reported in patients receiving placebo. These effects included.

Central Nervous System: Drowsiness, headache, fatigue, dizziness, nervousness, weakness, appetite increase;

◆ RATED THERAPEUTICALLY EQUIVALENT; ◇ THERAPEUTIC EQUIVALENCE UNCONFIRMED; ○ UNRATED

Gastrointestinal System: Abdominal distress, nausea, vomiting, change in bowel habits.

Eye, Ear, Nose and Throat: Dry mouth/nose/throat, cough, sore throat, epistaxis.

Skin: Eruption (including rash and urticaria) or itching.

Also reported spontaneously during the marketing of Terfenadine were: alopecia (hair loss or thinning), anaphylaxis, angioedema, bronchospasm, confusion, depression, galactorrhea, insomnia, menstrual disorders (including dysmenorrhea), musculoskeletal symptoms, nightmares, paresthesia, photosensitivity, rapid flare of psoriasis, seizures, sinus tachycardia, sweating, thrombocytopenia, tremor, urinary frequency, and visual disturbances.

Also in clinical trials, several instances of mild or, in one case, moderate transaminase elevations were seen in patients receiving Terfenadine. Mild elevations were also seen in placebo treated patients. Marketing experiences include isolated reports of jaundice, cholestatic hepatitis, and hepatitis. In most cases available information is incomplete.

OVERDOSAGE

Acute overdosage with Pseudoephedrine/Terfenadine tablets may produce clinical signs of CNS stimulation or depression and various cardiovascular effects, including cardiac collapse and death. Sympathomimetic amines should be used with great caution in the presence of Pseudoephedrine. Patients with signs of stimulation should be treated conservatively.

Adverse cardiac events including cardiac arrest, ventricular arrhythmias including torsades de pointes and QT prolongation have been reported at overdoses of 360 mg or more of Terfenadine and occur more frequently at doses in excess of 600 mg, and QTc prolongations of up to 30% have been observed at a dose of 300 mg b.i.d. Seizures and syncope have also been reported. USE OF DOSES IN EXCESS OF ONE TABLET B.I.D. IS NOT RECOMMENDED. (See *"Warning"* Box, *"Clinical Pharmacology"*, and *"Adverse Reactions"*.)

In overdose cases, where ventricular arrhythmias are associated with significant QTc prolongation, treatment with antiarrhythmics known to prolong QTc intervals is not recommended.

Therefore, in cases of overdosage, cardiac monitoring for at least 24 hours is recommended and for as long as QTc is prolonged, along with standard measures to remove any unabsorbed drug. Limited experience with the use of hemoperfusion (N = 1) or hemodialysis (N = 3) was not successful in completely removing the acid metabolite of Terfenadine from the blood.

Oral LD_{50} values for Terfenadine were greater than 5000 mg/kg in mature mice and rats. The oral LD_{50} was 438 mg/kg in newborn rats. The LD_{50} of Pseudoephedrine Hydrochloride alone in male and female rats was 1674 mg/kg, while the LD_{50} of Pseudoephedrine Hydrochloride administered with Terfenadine was 3017 mg/kg.

DOSAGE AND ADMINISTRATION

Adults and children 12 years and older: one tablet swallowed whole, morning and night.

USE OF DOSES IN EXCESS OF ONE TABLET B.I.D. IS NOT RECOMMENDED BECAUSE OF THE INCREASED POTENTIAL FOR QT INTERVAL PROLONGATION AND ADVERSE CARDIAC EVENTS. (See *"Warning"* Box.) USE OF PSEUDOEPHEDRINE/TERFENADINE IN PATIENTS WITH SIGNIFICANT HEPATIC DYSFUNCTION AND IN PATIENTS TAKING KETOCONAZOLE, ITRACONAZOLE, CLARITHROMYCIN, ERYTHROMYCIN, OR TROLEANDOMYCIN IS CONTRAINDICATED. (See *"Contraindications"*, *"Warnings"*, and *"Precautions: Drug Interactions"*.)

HOW SUPPLIED

TABLET, EXTENDED RELEASE: 120 MG-60 MG

BRAND/MANUFACTURER	NDC	SIZE	AWP
○ **BRAND**			
➤ SELDANE-D: Marion Merrell Dow	00068-0722-61	100s	$103.86
➤ SELDANE-D: Marion Merrell Dow	00068-0722-03	3000s	$3116.88

Psorcon *SEE* DIFLORASONE DIACETATE

Pulmozyme *SEE* DORNASE ALFA

Purinethol *SEE* MERCAPTOPURINE

P-V-Tussin *SEE* CHLORPHENIRAMINE MALEATE/HYDROCODONE BITARTRATE/PSEUDOEPHEDRINE HYDROCHLORIDE *AND* HYDROCODONE BITARTRATE WITH PSEUDOEPHEDRINE HYDROCHLORIDE

Pyrazinamide

DESCRIPTION

Pyrazinamide, the pyrazine analogue of nicotinamide, is an antituberculous agent. It is a white crystalline powder, stable at room temperature, and sparingly soluble in water. Pyrazinamide has the following molecular weight: 123.11. Each Pyrazinamide tablet for oral administration contains 500 mg of Pyrazinamide.

Following is its chemical structure:

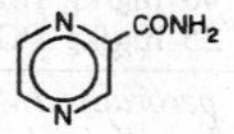

CLINICAL PHARMACOLOGY

Pyrazinamide is well absorbed from the GI tract and attains peak plasma concentrations within 2 hours. Plasma concentrations generally range from 30 to 50 mcg/mL with doses of 20 to 25 mg/kg. It is widely distributed in body tissues and fluids including the liver, lungs and cerebrospinal fluid (CSF). The CSF concentration is approximately equal to concurrent steady-state plasma concentrations in patients with inflamed meninges.[1] Pyrazinamide is approximately 10% bound to plasma proteins.[2]

The half-life (t1/2) of Pyrazinamide is 9 to 10 hours in patients with normal renal and hepatic function. The plasma half-life may be prolonged in patients with impaired renal or hepatic function. Pyrazinamide is hydrolyzed in the liver to its major active metabolite, pyrazinoic acid. Pyrazinoic acid is hydroxylated to the main excretory product, 5-hydroxypyrazinoic acid.[3]

Approximately 70% of an oral dose is excreted in urine, mainly by glomerular filtration within 24 hours.[3]

Pyrazinamide may be bacteriostatic or bactericidal against *Mycobacterium tuberculosis* depending on the concentration of the drug attained at the site of infection. The mechanism of action is unknown. *In vitro* and *in vivo* the drug is active only at a slightly acidic pH.

INDICATIONS AND USAGE

Pyrazinamide is indicated for the initial treatment of active tuberculosis in adults and children when combined with other antituberculous agents. (The current recommendation of the CDC for drug-susceptible disease is to use a six-month regimen for initial treatment of active tuberculosis, consisting of isoniazid, rifampin and pyrazinamide given for 2 months, followed by isoniazid and rifampin for 4 months.)*

(Patients with drug-resistant disease should be treated with regimens individualized to their situation. Pyrazinamide frequently will be an important component of such therapy.) (In patients with concomitant HIV infection, the physician should be aware of current recommendations of CDC. It is possible these patients may require a longer course of treatment.)

It is also indicated after treatment failure with other primary drugs in any form of active tuberculosis.

Pyrazinamide should only be used in conjunction with other effective antituberculous agents.

CONTRAINDICATIONS

Pyrazinamide is contraindicated in persons:
- with severe hepatic damage.
- who have shown hypersensitivity to it.
- with acute gout.

WARNINGS

Patients started on Pyrazinamide should have baseline serum uric acid and liver function determinations. Those patients with preexisting liver disease or those at increased risk for drug related hepatitis (e.g., alcohol abusers) should be followed closely.

Pyrazinamide should be discontinued and not be resumed if signs of hepatocellular damage or hyperuricemia accompanied by an acute gouty arthritis appear.

PRECAUTIONS

General: Pyrazinamide inhibits renal excretion of urates, frequently resulting in hyperuricemia which is usually asymptomatic. If hyperuricemia is accompanied by acute gouty arthritis, Pyrazinamide should be discontinued.

Pyrazinamide should be used with caution in patients with a history of diabetes mellitus, as management may be more difficult.

Primary resistance of *M. tuberculosis* to Pyrazinamide is uncommon. In cases with known or suspected drug resistance, *in vitro* susceptibility tests with recent cultures of *M. tuberculosis* against Pyrazinamide and the usual primary drugs should be performed. There are few reliable *in vitro* tests for Pyrazinamide resistance. A reference laboratory capable of performing these studies must be employed.

Information for Patients: Patients should be instructed to notify their physicians promptly if they experience any of the following: fever, loss of appetite, malaise, nausea and vomiting, darkened urine, yellowish discoloration of the skin and eyes, pain or swelling of the joints.

Compliance with the full course of therapy must be emphasized, and the importance of not missing any doses must be stressed.

* See recommendations of Center for Disease Control (CDC) and American Thoracic Society for complete regimen and dosage recommendations.[4]

➤ SHOWN IN PRODUCT IDENTIFICATION GUIDE

RECOMMENDED DRUGS FOR THE INITIAL TREATMENT OF TUBERCULOSIS IN CHILDREN AND ADULTS

Drug	Daily Dose*		Maximal Daily Dose in Children and adults	Twice Weekly Dose	
	Children	Adults		Children	Adults
Isoniazid	10 to 20 mg/kg PO or IM	5 mg/kg PO or IM	300 mg	20 to 40 mg/kg Max. 900 mg	15 mg/kg Max. 900 mg
Rifampin	10 to 20 mg/kg PO	10 mg/kg PO	600 mg	10 to 20 mg/kg Max. 600 mg	10 mg/kg Max. 600 mg
Pyrazinamide	15 to 30 mg/kg PO	15 to 30 mg/kg PO	2 g	50 to 70 mg/kg	50 to 70 mg/kg
Streptomycin	20 to 40 mg/kg IM	15 mg/kg**IM	1 g**	25 to 30 mg/kg IM	25 to 30 mg/kg IM
Ethambutol	15 to 25 mg/kg PO	15 to 25 mg/kg PO	2.5 g	50 mg/kg	50 mg/kg

Definition of abbreviations: PO = perorally; IM = intramuscularly.
* Doses based on weight should be adjusted as weight changes
** In persons older than 60 yrs of age the daily dose of streptomycin should be limited to 10 mg/kg with a maximal dose of 750 mg.

Laboratory Tests: Baseline liver function studies [especially ALT (SGPT), AST (SGOT) determinations] and uric acid levels should be determined prior to therapy. Appropriate laboratory testing should be performed at periodic intervals and if any clinical signs or symptoms occur during therapy.

Drug/Laboratory Test Interactions: Pyrazinamide has been reported to interfere with ACETEST® and KETOSTIX® urine tests to produce a pink-brown color.[5].

Carcinogenicity, Mutagenicity, Impairment of Fertility[6,7,8]: In lifetime bioassays in rats and mice, Pyrazinamide was administered in the diet at concentrations of up to 10,000 ppm. This resulted in estimated daily doses for the mouse of 2 g/kg, or 40 times the maximum human dose, and for the rat of 0.5 g/kg, or 10 times the maximum human dose. Pyrazinamide was not carcinogenic in rats or male mice and no conclusion was possible for female mice due to insufficient numbers of surviving control mice.

Pyrazinamide was not mutagenic in the Ames bacterial test, but induced chromosomal aberrations in human lymphocyte cell cultures.

Pregnancy: Teratogenic Effects—Pregnancy Category C: Animal reproduction studies have not been conducted with Pyrazinamide. It is also not known whether Pyrazinamide can cause fetal harm when administered to a pregnant woman or can affect reproduction capacity. Pyrazinamide should be given to a pregnant woman only if clearly needed.

Nursing Mothers: Pyrazinamide has been found in small amounts in breast milk. Therefore, it is advised that Pyrazinamide be used with caution in nursing mothers taking into account the risk-benefit of this therapy.[9]

Usage in Children: Pyrazinamide regimens employed in adults are probably equally effective in children.[4,10,11] Pyrazinamide appears to be well tolerated in children.

Geriatric Use[12]: Clinical studies of Pyrazinamide did not include sufficient numbers of patients aged 65 and over to determine whether they respond differently from younger patients. Other reported clinical experience has not identified differences in responses between the elderly and younger patients. In general, dose selection for an elderly patient should be cautious, usually starting at the low end of the dosing range, reflecting the greater frequency of decreased hepatic or renal function, and of concomitant disease or other drug therapy.

It does not appear that patients with impaired renal function require a reduction in dose. It may be prudent to select doses at the low end of the dosing range, however.[13]

ADVERSE REACTIONS
General: Fever porphyria and dysuria have rarely been reported. Gout (see "Precautions").

Gastrointestinal: The principal adverse effect is a hepatic reaction (see "Warnings"). Hepatotoxicity appears to be dose related, and may appear at any time during therapy. GI disturbances including nausea, vomiting and anorexia have also been reported.

Hematologic and Lymphatic: Thrombocytopenia and sideroblastic anemia with erythroid hyperplasia, vacuolation of erythrocytes and increased serum iron concentration have occurred rarely with this drug. Adverse effects on blood clotting mechanisms have also been rarely reported.

Other: Mild arthralgia and myalgia have been reported frequently. Hypersensitivity reactions including rashes, urticaria, and pruritus have been reported. Fever, acne, photosensitivity, porphyria, dysuria and interstital nephritis have been reported rarely.

OVERDOSAGE
Overdosage experience is limited. In one case report of overdose, abnormal liver function tests developed. These spontaneously reverted to normal when the drug was stopped. Clinical monitoring and supportive therapy should be employed. Pyrazinamide is dialyzable.[13]

DOSAGE AND ADMINISTRATION
Pyrazinamide should always be administered with other effective antituberculous drugs. It is administered for the initial 2 months of a 6-month or longer treatment regimen for drug-susceptible patients. Patients who are known or suspected to have drug-resistant disease should be treated with regimens individualized to their situation. Pyrazinamide frequently will be an important component of such therapy.

Patients with concomitant HIV infection may require longer courses of therapy. Physicians treating such patients should be alert to any revised recommendations from CDC for this group of patients.

Usual dose: Pyrazinamide is administered orally, 15 to 30 mg/kg once daily. Older regimens employed 3 to 4 divided doses daily, but most current recommendations are for once a day. Three grams per day should not be exceeded. The CDC recommendations do not exceed 2 g per day when given as a daily regimen (see table).

Alternatively, a twice weekly dosing regimen (50 to 70 mg/kg twice weekly based on lean body weight) has been developed to promote patient compliance with a regimen on an outpatient basis. In studies evaluating the twice weekly regimen, doses of Pyrazinamide in excess of 3 g twice weekly have been administered. This exceeds the recommended maximum 3 g/daily dose. However, an increased incidence of adverse reactions has not been reported.

The table is taken from the CDC-American Thoracic Society joint recommendations.[4] (See related table).

Store in a well-closed container at controlled room temperature 15°-30°C (59°-86°F).

REFERENCES
1. *Drug Information, American Hospital Formulary Service.* American Society of Hospital Pharmacists. Bethesda, Md. 1991. 2. *USPDI, Drug Information for the Health Care Professional.* United States Pharmacopeial Convention, Inc. Rockville, Md. 1991:1B:2226-2227. 3. Goodman-Gilman A, Rall TW, Nies As, Taylor P. *The Pharmacological Basis of Therapeutics*, ed 8. New York, Pergamon Press. 1990;1154. 4. Treatment of tuberculosis and tuberculosis infection in adults and children. *Am Rev Respir Dis.* 1986:134-363-368. 5. Reynolds JEF, Parfitt K, Parsons AV, Sweetman, SC. *Martindale The Extra Pharmacopoeia*, ed 29. London, The pharmaceutical Press. 1989;569-570. 6. Bioassay of pyrazinamide for possible carcinogenicity. National Cancer Institute Carcinogenesis Technical Report Series No. 48, 1978. 7. Zerger E, Anderson B, Haworth S, Lawlor T, Mortelmans K, Speck W. Salmonell mutagenicity tests: III. Results from the testing of 255 chemicals. *Environ Mutagen.* 1987;9(Suppl 9):1-109. 8. Roman IC, Georgian L. Cytogenetic effects of some antituberculosis drugs in vitro. *Mutation Research.* 1977;48:215-224. 9. Holdiness M. Antituberculosis drugs and breast-feeding. *Arch Intern Med.* 1984;144:1888. 10. Turcios N, Evans H. Preventing and managing turberculosis in children. *J Resp Dis.* 1989;10(6)(Jun):23. 11. Starke JR. Multidrug therapy for tuberculosis in children. *Pediatr Infec Dis J.* 1990;9:785-793. 12. Specific requirements on content and format of labeling for human prescription drugs; proposed addition of "geriatric use" subsection in the labeling. *Federal Register.* 1990;55(212) (Nov 1):46134-46137. 13. Stamathakis G, Montes C, Trouvin JH, et al. Pyrazinamide and pyrazinoic acid pharmacokinetics in patients with chronic renal failure. *Clinical Nephrology.* 1988;30:230-234.

HOW SUPPLIED
TABLETS: 500 MG

AVERAGE UNIT PRICE (AVAILABLE SIZES)		GENERIC A-RATED AVERAGE PRICE (GAAP)	
		100s	$100.95
GENERIC	$0.98	500s	$460.33

BRAND/MANUFACTURER	NDC	SIZE	AWP
◆ GENERICS			
Effcon	55806-0012-03	100s	$87.38
Lederle Std Prod	00005-5093-23	100s	$105.90
Effcon	55806-0012-21	100s ud	$93.62
UDL	51079-0691-20	100s ud	$116.88
Effcon	55806-0012-04	500s	$414.13
Lederle Std Prod	00005-5093-31	500s	$506.53

Pyridium *SEE* PHENAZOPYRIDINE HYDROCHLORIDE

Pyridostigmine Bromide

DESCRIPTION
Pyridostigmine Bromide is an active cholinesterase inhibitor. Chemically, Pyridostigmine Bromide is 3-hydroxy-1-methylpyridinium bromide dimethylcarbamate. Pyridostigmine Bromide is available in the following forms: syrup, tablets, slow-release tablets, and injection.

◆ RATED THERAPEUTICALLY EQUIVALENT; ◇ THERAPEUTIC EQUIVALENCE UNCONFIRMED; ○ UNRATED

Each ml of injection contains
Pyridostigmine Bromide ....5 mg

Each slow release tablet contains
Pyridostigmine Bromide ....180 mg

Each 5 ml syrup contains
Pyridostigmine Bromide ....60 mg

Each tablet contains
Pyridostigmine Bromide ....60 mg

Following is its chemical structure:

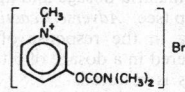

ACTIONS
Pyridostigmine Bromide inhibits the destruction of acetylcholine by cholinesterase and thereby permits freer transmission of nerve impulses across the neuromuscular junction. Pyridostigmine is an analog of neostigmine, but differs from it in certain clinically significant respects; for example, Pyridostigmine is characterized by a longer duration of action and fewer gastrointestinal side effects. Currently available data indicate that Pyridostigmine may have a significantly lower degree and incidence of bradycardia, salivation and gastrointestinal stimulation. Animal studies using the injectable form of Pyridostigmine and human studies using the oral preparation have indicated that Pyridostigmine has a longer duration of action than does neostigmine measured under similar circumstances.

INDICATION
Pyridostigmine Bromide is useful in the treatment of myasthenia gravis; the injectable form is also useful as a reversal agent or antagonist to nondepolarizing muscle relaxants such as curariform drugs and gallamine triethiodide.

UNLABELED USES
Pyridostigmine Bromide is used alone or as an adjunct in the treatment of chronic pain syndromes, including thalamic pain and causalgia, constipation, Lambert-Eaton syndrome, and motion sickness.

CONTRAINDICATIONS
Pyridostigmine Bromide is contraindicated in mechanical intestinal or urinary obstruction, and particular caution should be used in its administration to patients with bronchial asthma. Care should be observed in the use of atropine for counteracting side effects, as discussed below. Known hypersensitivity to anticholinesterase agents is a contraindication.

WARNINGS
Although failure of patients to show clinical improvement may reflect underdosage, it can also be indicative of overdosage. As is true of all cholinergic drugs, overdosage of Pyridostigmine Bromide may result in cholinergic crisis, a state characterized by increasing muscle weakness which, through involvement of the muscles of respiration, may lead to death. Myasthenic crisis due to an increase in the severity of the disease is also accompanied by extreme muscle weakness, and thus may be difficult to distinguish from cholinergic crisis on a symptomatic basis. Such differentiation is extremely important, since increases in doses of Pyridostigmine Bromide or other drugs of this class in the presence of cholinergic crisis or of a refractory or "insensitive" state could have grave consequences. Osserman and Genkins[1] indicate that the differential diagnosis of the two types of crisis may require the use of edrophonium chloride as well as clinical judgment. The treatment of the two conditions obviously differs radically. Whereas the presence of myasthenic crisis suggests the need for more intensive anticholinesterase therapy, the diagnosis of cholinergic crisis, according to Osserman and Genkins,[1] calls for the prompt *withdrawal* of all drugs of this type. The immediate use of atropine in cholinergic crisis is also recommended. A syringe containing 1 mg of atropine sulfate should be immediately available to be given in aliquots intravenously to counteract severe cholinergic reactions.

Atropine may also be used to abolish or obtund gastrointestinal side effects or other muscarinic reactions; but such use, by masking signs of overdosage, can lead to inadvertent induction of cholinergic crisis.

For detailed information on the management of patients with myasthenia gravis, the physician is referred to one of the excellent reviews such as those by Osserman and Genkins,[2] Grob[3] or Schwab.[4,5]

Pyridostigmine Bromide injectable should be used with particular caution in patients with bronchial asthma or cardiac dysrhythmias. Transient bradycardia may occur and be relieved by atropine sulfate. Atropine should also be used with caution in patients with cardiac dysrhythmias. When large doses of Pyridostigmine Bromide injectable are administered, as during reversal of muscle relaxants, the prior or simultaneous injection of atropine sulfate is advisable. Because of the possibility of hypersensitivity in an occasional patient, atropine and antishock medication should always be readily available.

When Pyridostigmine Bromide injectable is used as an antagonist to nondepolarizing muscle relaxants, adequate recovery of voluntary respiration and neuromuscular transmission must be obtained prior to discontinuation of respiratory assistance and there should be continuous patient observation.

Satisfactory recovery may be defined by a combination of clinical judgment, respiratory measurements and observation of the effects of peripheral nerve stimulation. If there is any doubt concerning the adequacy of recovery from the effects of the nondepolarizing muscle relaxant, artificial ventilation should be continued until all doubt has been removed.

Usage in Pregnancy: The safety of Pyridostigmine Bromide during pregnancy or lactation in humans has not been established. Therefore, use of Pyridostigmine Bromide in women who may become pregnant requires weighing the drug's potential benefits against its possible hazards to mother and child.

ADVERSE REACTIONS
The side effects of Pyridostigmine Bromide are most commonly related to overdosage and generally are of two varieties, muscarinic and nicotinic. Among those in the former group are nausea, vomiting, diarrhea, abdominal cramps, increased peristalsis, increased salivation, increased bronchial secretions, miosis and diaphoresis. Nicotinic side effects are comprised chiefly of muscle cramps, fasciculation and weakness. Muscarinic side effects can usually be counteracted by atropine, but for reasons shown in the preceding section the expedient is not without danger. As with any compound containing the Bromide radical, a skin rash may be seen in an occasional patient. Such reactions usually subside promptly upon discontinuance of the medication.

Thrombophlebitis has been reported subsequent to intravenous administration.

DOSAGE AND ADMINISTRATION
ORAL PYRIDOSTIGMINE BROMIDE
Dosage: The size and frequency of the dosage must be adjusted to the needs of the individual patient.

Syrup and Conventional Tablets: The average dose is ten 60-mg tablets or ten 5-ml teaspoonfuls daily, spaced to provide maximum relief when maximum strength is needed. In severe cases as many as 25 tablets or teaspoonfuls a day may be required, while in mild cases one to six tablets or teaspoonfuls a day may suffice.

Slow-release Tablets: One to three 180-mg tablets, once or twice daily, will usually be sufficient to control symptoms; however, the needs of certain individuals may vary markedly from this average. The interval between doses should be at least six hours. For optimum control, it may be necessary to use the more rapidly acting regular tablets or syrup in conjunction with slow-release therapy.

Note: For information on a diagnostic test for myasthenia gravis, and for the evaluation and stabilization of therapy, please see product literature on edrophonium chloride.

PYRIDOSTIGMINE BROMIDE INJECTABLE
For Myasthenia Gravis: To supplement oral dosage, pre- and postoperatively, during labor and postpartum, during myasthenic crisis, or whenever oral therapy is impractical, approximately 1/30th of the oral dose of Pyridostigmine Bromide may be given parenterally, either by intramuscular or *very slow* intravenous injection. *The patient must be closely observed for cholinergic reactions, particularly if the intravenous route is used.*

For details regarding the management of myasthenic patients who are to undergo major surgical procedures, see the article by Foldes.[6]

Neonates of myasthenic mothers may have transient difficulty in swallowing, sucking and breathing. Injectable Pyridostigmine Bromide may be indicated—by symptomatology and use of the edrophonium chloride test—until Pyridostigmine Bromide syrup can be taken. To date the world literature consists of less than 100 neonate patients.[7] Of these only 5 were treated with injectable Pyridostigmine, with the vast majority of the remaining neonates receiving neostigmine. Dosage requirements of Pyridostigmine Bromide injectable are minute, ranging from 0.05 mg to 0.15 mg/kg of body weight given intramuscularly. It is important to differentiate between cholinergic and myasthenic crises in neonates. (See *"Warnings".*)

Pyridostigmine Bromide given parenterally one hour before completion of second stage labor enables patients to have adequate strength during labor and provides protection to infants in the immediate postnatal state. For further information on the use of Pyridostigmine Bromide injectable in neonates of myasthenic mothers, see the article by Namba[7].

For Reversal of Nondepolarizing Muscle Relaxants: When Pyridostigmine Bromide injectable is given intravenously to reverse the action of muscle relaxant drugs, it is recommended that atropine sulfate (0.6 to 1.2 mg) also be given intravenously immediately prior to the Pyridostigmine Bromide. Side effects, notably excessive secretions and bradycardia, are thereby minimized. Usually 10 or 20 mg of Pyridostigmine Bromide will be sufficient for antagonism of the effects of the nondepolarizing muscle relaxants. Although full recovery may occur within 15 minutes in most patients, others may require a half hour or more. Satisfactory reversal can be evident by adequate voluntary respiration, respiratory measurements and use of a peripheral nerve stimulator device. It is recommended that the patient be well ventilated and a patent airway maintained until complete recovery of normal respiration is assured. Once satisfactory reversal has been attained, recurarization has not been reported. For additional information on the use of Pyridostigmine Bromide for antagonism of nondepolarizing muscle relaxants see the article by Katz[8] and McNall[9].

Failure of Pyridostigmine Bromide Injectable to provide prompt (within 30 minutes) reversal may occur, *e.g.*, in the presence of extreme debilitation, carcinomatosis, or with concomitant use of certain broad spectrum antibiotics or anesthetic agents, notably ether. Under these circumstances ventilation must be supported by artificial means until the patient has resumed control of his respiration.

REFERENCES

1. K. E. Osserman and G. Genkins, *J.A.M.A., 183*: 97, 1963. 2. K. E. Osserman and G. Genkins, *New York State J. Med., 61*: 2076, 1961. 3. D. Grob, *Arch. Intern. Med., 108*: 615, 1961. 4. R. S. Schwab, *New Eng. J. Med., 268*: 596,1963. 5. R. S. Schwab, *New Eng. J. Med., 268*: 717, 1963. 6. F. F. Foldes and P. McNall, *Anesthesiology, 23*: 837, 1962. 7. T. Namba *et al., Pediatrics, 45*: 488, 1970. 8. R. L. Katz, *Anesthesiology, 28*: 528, 1967. 9. P. McNall *et al., Anesthesia and Analgesia, 48*: 1026, 1969.

HOW SUPPLIED
INJECTION: 5 MG/ML

AVERAGE UNIT PRICE (AVAILABLE SIZES)

BRAND	$0.66			
BRAND/MANUFACTURER		NDC	SIZE	AWP
◆ BRAND				
REGONOL: Organon		00052-0460-02	2 ml 25s	$32.95
		00052-0460-05	5 ml 25s	$82.50

INJECTION: 10 MG

BRAND/MANUFACTURER	NDC	SIZE	AWP
◆ BRAND			
MESTINON: ICN	00187-3011-10	2 ml 10s	$50.40

SYRUP: 60 MG/5 ML

BRAND/MANUFACTURER	NDC	SIZE	AWP
○ BRAND			
MESTINON: ICN	00187-3012-20	480 ml	$32.10

TABLET, EXTENDED RELEASE: 180 MG

BRAND/MANUFACTURER	NDC	SIZE	AWP
○ BRAND			
MESTINON: ICN	00187-3013-50	100s	$82.32

TABLETS: 60 MG

BRAND/MANUFACTURER	NDC	SIZE	AWP
○ BRAND			
MESTINON: ICN	00187-3010-30	100s	$37.62
	00187-3010-40	500s	$185.58

Pyrimethamine

DESCRIPTION
Pyrimethamine is an antiparasitic available in tablet form for oral administration. Each scored tablet contains 25 mg Pyrimethamine.

Pyrimethamine is known chemically as 2,4-diamino-5-(*p*-chlorophenyl)-6-ethylpyrimidine.

Following is its chemical structure:

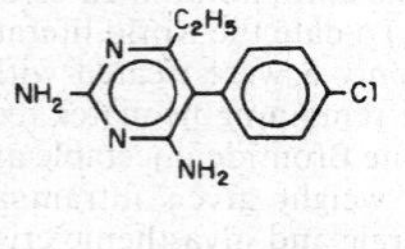

CLINICAL PHARMACOLOGY
Pyrimethamine is well absorbed, with peak levels occuring between 2 to 6 hours following administration. It is eliminated slowly and has a plasma half-life of approximately 96 hours. Pyrimthamine is 87% bound to human plasma proteins.

Microbiology: Pyrimethamine is a folic acid antagonist and the rationale for its therapeutic action is based on the differential requirement between host and parasite for nucleic acid precursors involved in growth. This activity is highly selective against plasmodia and *Toxoplasma gondii.*

Pyrimethamine possesses blood schizonticidal and some tissue schizonticidal activity against malaria parasites of humans. However, its blood schizonticidal activity may be slower than that of 4-aminoquinoline compounds. It does not destroy gametocytes, but arrests sporogony in the mosquito. The action of Pyrimethamine against *Toxoplasma gondii* is greatly enhanced when used in conjunction with sulfonamides. This was demonstrated by Eyles and Coleman[1] in the treatment of experimental toxoplasmosis in the mouse. Jacobs et al[2] demonstrated that combination of the two drugs effectively prevented the development of severe uveitis in most rabbits following the inoculation of the anterior chamber of the eye with toxoplasma.

INDICATIONS AND USAGE
Pyrimethamine is indicated for the chemoprophylaxis of malaria due to susceptible strains of plasmodia. It should not be used alone to treat an acute attack of malaria. Fast-acting schizonticides such as chloroquine or quinine are indicated and preferable for the treatment of acute attacks. However, conjoint use of Pyrimethamine will initiate *transmission control* and *suppressive cure* for susceptible strains of plasmodia.

Pyrimethamine is also indicated for the treatment of toxoplasmosis. For this purpose the drug should be used conjointly with a sulfonamide since synergism exists with this combination.

CONTRAINDICATIONS
Use of Pyrimethamine is contraindicated in patients with known hypersensitivity to Pyrimethamine. Use of the drug is also contraindicated in patients with documented megaloblastic anemia due to folate deficiency.

WARNINGS
The dosage of Pyrimethamine required for the treatment of toxoplasmosis is 10 to 20 times the recommended antimalaria dosage and approaches the toxic level. If signs of folate deficiency develop (see *"Adverse Reactions"*), reduce the dosage or discontinue the drug according to the response of the patient. Folinic acid (leucovorin) should be administered in a dosage of 5 to 15 mg daily (orally, IV or IM) until normal hematopoiesis is restored.

Pyrimethamine should be kept out of the reach of children as children and infants are extremely susceptible to adverse effects from an overdose. Deaths in children have been reported after accidental ingestion.

PRECAUTIONS
General: The recommended dosage for chemoprophylaxis of malaria should not be exceeded. A small "starting" dose for toxoplasmosis is recommended in patients with convulsive disorders to avoid the potential nervous system toxicity of Pyrimethamine. Pyrimethamine should be used with caution in patients with impaired renal or hepatic function or in patients with possible folate deficiency, such as individuals with malabsorption syndrome, alcoholism, or pregnancy, and those receiving therapy, such as phenytoin, affecting folate levels (see *"Pregnancy"* subsection).

Information for Patients: Patients should be warned that at the first appearance of a skin rash they should stop use of Pyrimethamine and seek medical attention immediately. Patients should also be warned that the appearance of sore throat, pallor, purpura, or glossitis may be early indications of serious disorders which require prophylactic treatment to be stopped, and medical treatment to be sought. Patients should be warned to keep Pyrimethamine out of the reach of children. Patients should be warned that if anorexia and vomiting occur, they may be minimized by taking the drug with meals.

Laboratory Tests: In patients receiving high dosage, as for the treatment of toxoplasmosis, semiweekly blood counts, including platelet counts, should be done.

Drug Interactions: Pyrimethamine may be used with sulfonamides, quinine, and other antimalarials, and with other antibiotics. However, the concomitant use of other antifolic drugs, such as sulfonamides or trimethoprim-sulfamethoxazole combinations, while the patient is receiving Pyrimethamine for antimalarial prophylaxis, may increase the risk of bone marrow suppression. If signs of folate deficiency develop, Pyrimethamine should be discontinued. Folinic acid (leucovorin) should be administered until normal hematopoiesis is restored (see *"Warnings"*). Mild hepatotoxicity has been reported in some patients when lorazepam and Pyrimethamine were administered concomitantly.

CARCINOGENESIS, MUTAGENESIS, IMPAIRMENT OF FERTILITY:
Carcinogenesis: Pyrimethamine has been reported to produce a significant increase in the number of lung tumors per mouse when given intraperitoneally at high doses (0.025 g/kg).[3] There have been two reports of cancer associated with Pyrimethamine administration: a 51-year-old female who developed chronic granulocytic leukemia after taking Pyrimethamine for two years for toxoplasmosis,[4] and a 56-year-old patient who developed reticulum cell sarcoma after 14 months of Pyrimethamine for toxoplasmosis.[5]

Mutagenesis: Pyrimethamine has been shown to be non-mutagenic in the following in vitro assays: the Ames point mutation assay, the Rec assay and the *E. coli* WP2 assay. It was positive in the L5178Y/TK +/- mouse lymphoma assay in the absence of exogenous metabolic activation.[6] Human blood lymphocytes cultured in vitro had structural chromosome aberrations induced by Pyrimethamine.

In vivo, chromosomes analyzed from the bone marrow of rats dosed with Pyrimethamine showed an increased number of structural and numerical aberrations.

Impairment of Fertility: The effects of Pyrimethamine on rat pregnancy seem to indicate that the fertility index of rats treated with Pyrimethamine is lowered only when the higher dosage is used, suggesting a possible toxic effect upon the whole organism and/or the conceptuses.[7]

Pregnancy: Teratogenic Effects: Pregnancy Category C. Pyrimethamine has been shown to be teratogenic in rats, hamsters, and Goettingen miniature pigs. There are no adequate and well-controlled studies in pregnant women. Pyrimethamine should be used during pregnancy only if the potential benefit justifies the potential risk to the fetus. Concurrent administration of folinic acid is strongly recommended when used for the treatment of toxoplasmosis during pregnancy. Thiersch[8] reported that when rats were given an oral dose of Pyrimethamine of 12.5 mg/kg from day 7 to 9 of the gestation period, there was 66.2% resorption and 32.8% of the live fetuses were stunted. When lower doses of 1 mg/kg and 0.5 mg/kg were given for 10 days, days 4 to 13 of gestation, there was 15% and 8.5% resorption, respectively, and 16.6% and 6.9% of the live fetuses were stunted. A

---

daily oral dose as low as 0.3 mg/kg given for days 7 to 16 of gestation still resulted in 2.7% of the fetuses being stunted.

Sullivan and Takacs[9] found that less than 10% of hamster fetuses died or were malformed following single doses of 20 mg to the mother, which on a mg/kg basis was eight to nine times greater than that given to rats.

Hayama and Kokue[10] reported on the administration of Pyrimethamine to pregnant female Goettingen miniature pigs. Sows given 0.9 mg/kg/day, during days 11 to 35 of pregnancy, i.e., the period of organogenesis in the pig, delivered, normal offspring. Sows administered a high dose 3.6 mg/kg/day during the same gestational period delivered offspring with a high incidence of malformations including cleft palate, club foot, and micrognathia.

Nursing Mother: Pyrimethamine is excreted in human milk. Milk samples obtained from lactating mothers after treatment with Pyrimethamine were found to have measurable concentrations of the drug, with peak concentration at 6 hours postadministration. It is estimated that after a single 75 mg dose of oral Pyrimethamine, approximately 3 to 4 mg of the drug would be passed on to the feeding child over a 48-hour period.

Because of the potential for serious adverse reactions in nursing infants from Pyrimethamine, a decision should be made whether to discontinue nursing or to discontinue the drug, taking into account the importance of the drug to the mother. (See *"Carcinogenesis, Mutagenesis, Impairment of Fertility"* and *"Pregnancy"* subsections.)

Pediatric Use: (See *"Dosage and Administration".*)

ADVERSE REACTIONS

Hypersensitivity reactions, occasionally severe, can occur at any dose, particularly when Pyrimethamine is administered concomitantly with a sulfonamide. With large doses of Pyrimethamine, anorexia and vomiting may occur. Vomiting may be minimized by giving the medication with meals; it usually disappears promptly upon reduction of dosage. Doses used in toxoplasmosis may produce megaloblastic anemia, leukopenia, thrombocytopenia, pancytopenia, atrophic glositis, hematuria, and disorders of cardiac rhythm. Hematologic effects, however, may also occur at low doses in certain individuals (see *"Precautions—General"*).

Insomnia, diarrhea, headache, light-headedness, dryness of the mouth or throat, fever, malaise, dermatitis, abnormal skin pigmentation, depression, seizures, pulmonary eosinophilia, and hyperphenyltalaninemia have been reported rarely.

OVERDOSAGE

Acute intoxication may follow the ingestion of an excessive amount of Pyrimethamine. Gastrointestinal and/or central nervous system signs may be present, including convulsions. The initial symptoms are usually gastrointestinal and may include abdominal pain, nausea, severe and repeated vomiting, possibly including hematemesis. Central nervous system toxicity may be manifest by initial excitability, generalized and prolonged convulsions which may be followed by respiratory depression, circulatory collapse and death within a few hours. Neurological symptoms appear rapidly (30 minutes to 2 hours after drug ingestion), suggesting that in gross over-dosage Pyrimethamine has a direct toxic effect on the central nervous system.

The fatal dose is variable, with the smallest reported fatal single dose being 250 mg to 300 mg. There are, however, reports of children who have recovered after taking 375 mg to 625 mg.

There is no specific antidote to acute Pyrimethamine poisoning. Gastric lavage is recommended and is effective if carried out very soon after drug ingestion. A parenteral barbiturate may be indicated to control convulsions. Folinic acid may also be given to counteract effects on the hematopoietic system (see *"Warnings"*).

DOSAGE AND ADMINISTRATION

For Chemoprophylaxis of Malaria: Adults and children over 10 years—25 mg (1 tablet) once weekly

　Children 4 through 10 years—12.5 mg (½ tablet) once weekly

　Infants and children under 4 years—6.25 mg (¼ tablet) once weekly

　Regimens planned to include *suppressive cure* should be extended through any characteristic periods of early recrudescence and late relapse for at least 10 weeks in each case.

For Treatment of Acute Attacks: Pyrimethamine is recommended in areas where only susceptible plasmodia exist. This drug is not recommended alone in the treatment of acute attacks of malaria in nonimmune persons. Fast-acting schizonticides such as chloroquine or quinine are indicated for treatment of acute attacks. However, conjoint Pyrimethamine dosage of 25 mg daily for 2 days will initiate *transmission control* and *suppressive cure.* Should circumstances arise wherein Pyrimethamine must be used alone in semi-immune persons, the adult dosage for an acute attack is 50 mg for 2 days; children 4 through 10 years old may be given 25 mg daily for 2 days. In any event, clinical cure should be followed by the once-weekly regimen described above.

For Toxoplasmosis: The dosage of Pyrimethamine for the treatment of toxoplasmosis must be carefully adjusted so as to provide maximum therapeutic effect and a minimum of side effects. At the high dosage required, there is a marked variation in the tolerance to the drug. Young patients may tolerate higher doses than older individuals.

The adult *starting* dose is 50 to 75 mg of the drug daily, together with 1 to 4 g daily of a sulfonamide of the sulfapyrimidine type, e.g., sulfadiazine. This dosage is ordinarily continued for 1 to 3 weeks, depending on the response of the patient and his tolerance of the therapy. The dosage may then be reduced to about one-

half that previously given for each drug and continued for an additional 4 to 5 weeks.

The pediatric dosage of Pyrimethamine is 1 mg/kg per day divided into 2 equal daily doses, after 2 to 4 days this dose may be reduced to one-half and continued for approximately one month. The usual pediatric sulfonamide dosage is used in conjunction with Pyrimethamine.

Store at 15° to 25°C (59° to 77°F) in a dry place and protect from light.

REFERENCES

1. Eyles DE, Coleman N. Synergistic effect of sulfadiazine and Pyrimethamine against experimental toxoplasmosis in the mouse. *Antibiot Chemother.* 1953;3:483-490. 2. Jacobs L, Melton ML, Kaufman HE. Treatment of experimental ocular toxoplasmosis, *Arch Ophthalmol.* 1964;71:111-118. 3. Bahna L. Pyrimethamine, *LARC Monogr Eval Carcinog Risk Chem.* 1977; 13:233-242. 4. Jim RTS, Elizaga FV. Development of chronic granulocytic leukemia in a patient treated with Pyrimethamine. *Hawaii Med J.* 1977;36:173-176. 5. Sadoff L. Antimalarial drugs and Burkitt's lymphoma. *Lancet.* 1973; 2:1262-1263. 6. Clive D, Johnson KO, Spector JKS, et al. Validation and characterization of the L5178Y/TK +/- mouse lymphoma mutagen assay system. *Mut Res.* 1979;59:61-108. 7. Andrade ATL, Guerra MO, Silva NOG, et al. Antifertility effects of Pyrimethamine. *Excerpta Med Int Cong Ser.* 1976;370:317-321. 8. Thiersch JB. Effects of certain 2,4-diaminopyrimidine antagonists of folic acid on pregnancy and rat fetus. *Proc Soc Exp Biol Med.* 1954;87:571-577. 9. Sullivan GE, Takacs E. Comparative teratogenicity of Pyrimethamine in rats and hamsters. *Teratology.* 1971;4:205-210. 10. Hayama T, Kokue E. Use of Goettingen miniature pigs for studying Pyrimethamine teratogenesis, *CRC Crit Rev Toxicol.* 1985;14:403-421.

HOW SUPPLIED
TABLETS: 25 MG

BRAND/MANUFACTURER	NDC	SIZE	AWP
○ BRAND DARAPRIM: Burr Wellcome	00081-0201-55	100s	$36.22

Pyrimethamine and Sulfadoxine

> **WARNING:**
> FATALITIES ASSOCIATED WITH THE ADMINISTRATION OF PYRIMETHAMINE/SULFADOXINE HAVE OCCURRED DUE TO SEVERE REACTIONS, INCLUDING STEVENS-JOHNSON SYNDROME AND TOXIC EPIDERMAL NECROLYSIS. PYRIMETHAMINE/SULFADOXINE PROPHYLAXIS SHOULD BE DISCONTINUED AT THE FIRST APPEARANCE OF SKIN RASH, IF A SIGNIFICANT REDUCTION IN THE COUNT OF ANY FORMED BLOOD ELEMENTS IS NOTED, OR UPON THE OCCURRENCE OF ACTIVE BACTERIAL OR FUNGAL INFECTIONS.

DESCRIPTION

Pyrimethamine/Sulfadoxine is an antimalarial agent, each tablet containing 500 mg N^1-(5,6-dimethoxy-4-pyrimidinyl) sulfanilamide (Sulfadoxine) and 25 mg 2,4-diamino-5-(p-chlorophenyl)-6-ethyl-pyrimidine (Pyrimethamine).

CLINICAL PHARMACOLOGY

Pyrimethamine/Sulfadoxine is an antimalarial agent which acts by reciprocal potentiation of its two components, achieved by a sequential blockade of two enzymes involved in the biosynthesis of folinic acid within the parasites. Pyrimethamine/Sulfadoxine is effective against certain strains of *Plasmodium falciparum* that are resistant to chloroquine.

Both the Sulfadoxine and Pyrimethamine of Pyrimethamine/Sulfadoxine are absorbed orally and are excreted mainly by the kidney. Following a single tablet administration, Sulfadoxine peak plasma concentrations of 51 to 76 mcg/ml are achieved in 2.5 to 6 hours and the Pyrimethamine peak plasma concentrations of 0.13 to 0.4 mcg/ml were achieved in 1.5 to 8 hours. The apparent half-life of elimination of Sulfadoxine ranged from 100 to 231 hours with a mean of 169 hours, whereas Pyrimethamine half-lives ranged from 54 to 148 hours with a mean of 111 hours. Both drugs appear in breast milk of nursing mothers.

INDICATIONS AND USAGE

Pyrimethamine/Sulfadoxine is indicated for the treatment of *P. falciparum* malaria for those patients in whom chloroquine resistance is suspected. Malaria prophylaxis with Pyrimethamine/Sulfadoxine is indicated for travelers to areas where chloroquine-resistant *P. falciparum* malaria is endemic. However, strains of *P. falciparum* may be encountered which have developed resistance to Pyrimethamine/Sulfadoxine.

CONTRAINDICATIONS

Prophylactic (repeated) use of Pyrimethamine/Sulfadoxine is contraindicated in patients with severe renal insufficiency, marked liver parenchymal damage or blood dyscrasias. Hypersensitivity to Pyrimethamine or sulfonamides. Patients with documented megaloblastic anemia due to folate deficiency. Infants less than two months of age. Pregnancy at term and during the nursing period because sulfonamides pass the placenta and are excreted in the milk and may cause kernicterus.

WARNINGS

> FATALITIES ASSOCIATED WITH THE ADMINISTRATION OF PYRIMETHA-
> MINE/SULFADOXINE HAVE OCCURRED DUE TO SEVERE REACTIONS,
> INCLUDING STEVENS-JOHNSON SYNDROME AND TOXIC EPIDERMAL
> NECROLYSIS. PYRIMETHAMINE/SULFADOXINE PROPHYLAXIS SHOULD
> BE DISCONTINUED AT THE FIRST APPEARANCE OF SKIN RASH, IF A
> SIGNIFICANT REDUCTION IN THE COUNT OF ANY FORMED BLOOD
> ELEMENTS IS NOTED, OR UPON THE OCCURRENCE OF ACTIVE BACTERI-
> AL OR FUNGAL INFECTIONS.

Fatalities associated with the administration of sulfonamides, although rare, have occurred due to severe reactions, including fulminant hepatic necrosis, agranulocytosis, aplastic anemia and other blood dyscrasias. Pyrimethamine/Sulfadoxine prophylaxis regimen has been reported to cause leukopenia during a treatment of two months or longer. This leukopenia is generally mild and reversible.

PRECAUTIONS

1. *General:* Pyrimethamine/Sulfadoxine should be given with caution to patients with impaired renal or hepatic function, to those with possible folate deficiency and to those with severe allergy or bronchial asthma. As with some sulfonamide drugs, in glucose-6-phosphate dehydrogenase-deficient individuals, hemolysis may occur. Urinalysis with microscopic examination and renal function tests should be performed during therapy of those patients who have impaired renal function.

2. *Information for the Patient:* Patients should be warned that at the first appearance of a skin rash, they should stop use of Pyrimethamine/Sulfadoxine and seek medical attention immediately. Adequate fluid intake must be maintained in order to prevent crystalluria and stone formation.

Patients should also be warned that the appearance of sore throat, fever, arthralgia, cough, shortness of breath, pallor, purpura, jaundice or glossitis may be early indications of serious disorders which require prophylactic treatment to be stopped and medical treatment to be sought.

Females should be cautioned against becoming pregnant and should not breast feed their infants during Pyrimethamine/Sulfadoxine therapy or prophylactic treatment.

Patients should be warned to keep Pyrimethamine/Sulfadoxine out of reach of children.

3. *Laboratory Tests:* Periodic blood counts and analysis of urine for crystalluria are desirable during prolonged prophylaxis.

4. *Drug Interactions:* There have been reports which may indicate an increase in incidence and severity of adverse reactions when chloroquine is used with Pyrimethamine/Sulfadoxine as compared to the use of Pyrimethamine/Sulfadoxine alone. Pyrimethamine/Sulfadoxine is compatible with quinine and with antibiotics. However, antifolic drugs such as sulfonamides or trimethoprim-sulfamethoxazole combinations should not be used while the patient is receiving Pyrimethamine/Sulfadoxine for antimalarial prophylaxis Pyrimethamine/Sulfadoxine has not been reported to interfere with antidiabetic agents.

If signs of folic acid deficiency develop Pyrimethamine/Sulfadoxine should be discontinued. Folinic acid (leucovorin) may be administered in doses of 5 mg to 15 mg intramuscularly daily, for 3 days or longer, for depressed platelet or white blood cell counts in patients with drug-induced folic acid deficiency when recovery is too slow.

5. *Carcinogenesis, Mutagenesis, Impairment of Fertility:* Pyrimethamine was not found carcinogenic in female mice or in male and female rats. The carcinogenic potential of Pyrimethamine in male mice could not be assessed from the study because of markedly reduced life-span. Pyrimethamine was found to be mutagenic in laboratory animals and also in human bone marrow following 3 or 4 consecutive daily doses totaling 200 mg to 300 mg. Pyrimethamine was not found mutagenic in the Ames test. Testicular changes have been observed in rats treated with 105 mg/kg/day of Pyrimethamine/Sulfadoxine and with 15 mg/kg/day of Pyrimethamine alone. Fertility of male rats and the ability of male or female rats to mate were not adversely affected at dosages of up to 210 mg/kg/day of Pyrimethamine/Sulfadoxine. The pregnancy rate of female rats was not affected following their treatment with 10.5 mg/kg/day, but was significantly reduced at dosages of 31.5 mg/kg/day or higher, a dosage approximately 30 times the weekly human prophylactic dose or higher.

6. *Pregnancy:* Teratogenic effects: Pregnancy Category C. Pyrimethamine/Sulfadoxine has been shown to be teratogenic in rats when given in weekly doses approximately 12 times the weekly human prophylactic dose. Teratology studies with Pyrimethamine plus Sulfadoxine (1:20) in rats showed the minimum oral teratogenic dose to be approximately 0.9 mg/kg Pyrimethamine plus 18 mg/kg Sulfadoxine. In rabbits, no teratogenic effects were noted at oral doses as high as 20 mg/kg Pyrimethamine plus 400 mg/kg Sulfadoxine.

There are no adequate and well-controlled studies in pregnant women. However, due to the teratogenic effect shown in animals and because Pyrimethamine plus Sulfadoxine may interfere with folic acid metabolism, Pyrimethamine/Sulfadoxine therapy should be used during pregnancy only if the potential benefit justifies the potential risk to the fetus. Women of childbearing potential who are traveling to areas where malaria is endemic should be warned against becoming pregnant.

Nonteratogenic effects: See *"Contraindications"* section.

7. *Nursing Mothers:* See *"Contraindication"* section.

8. *Pediatric Use:* Pyrimethamine/Sulfadoxine should not be given to infants less than two months of age because of inadequate development of the glucuronide-forming enzyme system.

ADVERSE REACTIONS

For completeness, all major reactions to Sulfonamides and to Pyrimethamine are included below, even though they may not have been reported with Pyrimethamine/Sulfadoxine. See *"Warnings"* and *"Precautions"* (*"Information for the Patient"*) sections.

Blood Dyscrasias: Agranulocytosis, aplastic anemia, megaloblastic anemia, thrombopenia, leukopenia, hemolytic anemia, purpura, hypoprothrombinemia, methemoglobinemia and eosinophilia.

Allergic Reactions: Erythema multiforme, Stevens-Johnson syndrome, generalized skin eruptions, toxic epidermal necrolysis, urticaria, serum sickness, pruritus, exfoliative dermatitis, anaphylactoid reactions, periorbital edema, conjunctival and scleral injection, photosensitization, arthralgia and allergic myocarditis.

Gastrointestinal Reactions: Glossitis, stomatitis, nausea, emesis, abdominal pains, hepatitis, hepatocellular necrosis, diarrhea and pancreatitis.

C.N.S. Reactions: Headache, peripheral neuritis, mental depression, convulsions, ataxia, hallucinations, tinnitus, vertigo, insomnia, apathy, fatigue, muscle weakness and nervousness.

Respiratory Reactions: Pulmonary infiltrates.

Miscellaneous Reactions: Drug fever, chills, and toxic nephrosis with oliguria and anuria. Periarteritis nodosa and L. E. phenomenon have occurred.

The sulfonamides bear certain chemical similarities to some goitrogens, diuretics (acetazolamide and the thiazides) and oral hypoglycemic agents. Diuresis and hypoglycemia have occurred rarely in patients receiving sulfonamides. Cross-sensitivity may exist with these agents. Rats appear to be especially susceptible to the goitrogenic effects of sulfonamides, and long-term administration has produced thyroid malignancies in the species.

OVERDOSAGE

Acute intoxication may be manifested by anorexia, vomiting and central nervous system stimulation (including convulsions), followed by megaloblastic anemia, leukopenia, thrombocytopenia, glossitis and crystalluria. In acute intoxication, emesis and gastric lavage followed by purges may be of benefit. The patient should be adequately hydrated to prevent renal damage. The renal and hematopoietic systems should be monitored for at least one month after an overdosage. If the patient is having convulsions, the use of a parenteral barbiturate is indicated. For depressed platelet or white blood cell counts, folinic acid (leucovorin) should be administered in a dosage of 5 mg to 15 mg intramuscularly daily for 3 days or longer.

DOSAGE AND ADMINISTRATION

(See *"Indications and Usage"* Section).

(A) TREATMENT OF ACUTE ATTACK OF MALARIA
A single dose of the following number of Pyrimethamine/Sulfadoxine Tablets is used in sequence with quinine or alone:

Adults	2 to 3 tablets
9 to 14 years	2 tablets
4 to 8 years	1 tablet
Under 4 years	½ tablet

(B) MALARIA PROPHYLAXIS
The first dose Pyrimethamine/Sulfadoxine should be taken one of two days before departure to an endemic area; administration should be continued during the stay and for four to six weeks after return.

	Once Weekly	Once Every Two Weeks
Adults	1 tablet	2 tablets
9 to 14 years	¾ tablet	1½ tablets
4 to 8 years	½ tablet	1 tablet
Under 4 years	¼ tablet	½ tablet

HOW SUPPLIED
TABLETS:

BRAND/MANUFACTURER	NDC	SIZE	AWP
BRAND			
FANSIDAR: Roche Labs	00004-0161-03	25s ud	$80.19

Quadrinal *SEE* EPHEDRINE HYDROCHLORIDE/ PHENOBARBITAL/POTASSIUM IODIDE/THEOPHYLLINE

Quarzan-T *SEE* CLIDINIUM BROMIDE

Quazepam

DESCRIPTION

Quazepam, a trifluoroethyl benzodiazepine hypnotic agent, having the chemical name 7-chloro-5-(o-fluorophenyl)-1,3-dihydro-(2,2, 2-trifluoroethyl)-2*H*-1,4-benzodiazepine-2-thione.

Quazepam has the empirical formula $C_{17}H_{11}ClF_4N_2S$, and a molecular weight of 386.8. It is a white crystalline compound, soluble in ethanol and insoluble in water.

Following is its chemical structure:

CLINICAL PHARMACOLOGY

Central nervous system agents of the 1,4-benzodiazepine class presumably exert their effects by binding to stereo-specific receptors at several sites within the central nervous system (CNS). Their exact mechanism of action is unknown. In a sleep laboratory study, Quazepam significantly decreased sleep latency and total wake time, and significantly increased total sleep time and percent sleep time, for one or more nights. Quazepam 15 mg was effective on the first night of administration. Sleep latency, total wake time and wake time after sleep onset were still decreased and percent sleep time was still increased for several nights after the drug was discontinued. Percent slow wave sleep was decreased, and REM sleep was essentially unchanged. No transient sleep disturbance, such as "rebound insomnia," was observed after withdrawal of the drug in sleep laboratory studies in 12 patients using 15 mg doses.

In outpatient studies, Quazepam improved all subjective measures of sleep including sleep induction time, duration of sleep, number of nocturnal awakening occurrence of early morning awakening, and sleep quality. Some effects were evident on the first night of administration of Quazepam (sleep induction time, number of nocturnal awakenings, and duration of sleep). Residual medication effects ("hangover") were minimal.

Quazepam is rapidly (absorption half-life of about 30 minutes) and well absorbed from the gastrointestinal tract. The peak plasma concentration of Quazepam is approximately 20 ng/ml after a 15 mg dose and is obtained at about 2 hours. Quazepam, the active parent compound, is extensively metabolized in the liver; two of the plasma metabolites are 2-oxoquazepam and N-desalkyl-2-oxoquazepam. All three compounds show pharmacological central nervous system activity in animals.

Following administration of ^{14}C-Quazepam, approximately 31% of the dose appears in the urine and 23% in the feces over a five-day period; only trace amounts of unchanged drug are present in the urine.

The mean elimination half-life of Quazepam and 2-oxoquazepam is 39 hours and that of N-desalkyl-2-oxoquazepam is 73 hours. Steady-state levels of Quazepam and 2-oxoquazepam are attained by the seventh daily dose and that of N-desalkyl-2-oxoquazepam by the thirteenth daily dose.

The pharmacokinetics of Quazepam and 2-oxoquazepam in geriatric subjects are comparable to those seen in young adults; as with desalkyl metabolites of other benzodiazepines, the elimination half-life of N-desalkyl-2-oxoquazepam in geriatric patients is about twice that of young adults.

The degree of plasma protein binding for Quazepam and its two major metabolites is greater than 95%. The absorption, distribution, metabolism, and excretion of benzodiazepines may be altered in various disease states including alcoholism, impaired hepatic function, and impaired renal function. The type and duration of hypnotic effects and the profile of unwanted effects during administration of benzodiazepine drugs may be influenced by the biologic half-life of administered drug and any active metabolites formed. When half-lives are long, drug or metabolites may accumulate during periods of nightly administration and be associated with impairments of cognitive and/or motor performance during waking hours; the possibility of interaction with other psychoactive drugs or alcohol will be enhanced. In contrast, if half-lives are short, drug and metabolites will be cleared before the next dose is ingested, and carry-over effects related to excessive sedation or CNS depression should be minimal or absent. However, during nightly use for an extended period, pharmacodynamic tolerance or adaptation to some effects of benzodiazepine hypnotics may develop. If the drug has a short half-life of elimination, it is possible that a relative deficiency of the drug or its active metabolites (i.e., in relationship to the receptor site) may occur at some point in the interval between each night's use. This sequence of events may account for two clinical findings reported to occur after several weeks of nightly use of rapidly eliminated benzodiazepine hypnotics, namely, increased wakefulness during the last third of the night, and the appearance of increased signs of daytime anxiety in selected patients.

Quazepam crosses the placental barrier of mice. Quazepam, 2-oxoquazepam and N-desalkyl-2-oxoquazepam are present in breast milk of lactating women, but the total amount found in the milk represents only about 0.1% of the administered dose.

INDICATIONS AND USAGE

Quazepam is indicated for the treatment of insomnia characterized by difficulty in falling asleep, frequent nocturnal awakenings, and/or early morning awakenings. The effectiveness of Quazepam has been established in placebo-controlled clinical studies of 5 nights duration in acute and chronic insomnia. The sustained effectiveness of Quazepam has been established in chronic insomnia in a sleep lab (polysomnographic) study of 28 nights duration.

Because insomnia is often transient and intermittent, the prolonged administration of Quazepam is generally not necessary or recommended. Since insomnia may be a symptom of several other disorders, the possibility that the complaint may be related to a condition for which there is a more specific treatment should be considered.

CONTRAINDICATIONS

Quazepam is contraindicated in patients with known hypersensitivity to this drug or other benzodiazepines, and in patients with established or suspected sleep apnea.

Usage in Pregnancy: Benzodiazepines may cause fetal damage when administered during pregnancy. An increased risk of congenital malformations associated with the use of diazepam and chlordiazepoxide during the first trimester of pregnancy has been suggested in several studies. Transplacental distribution has resulted in neonatal CNS depression following the ingestion of therapeutic doses of a benzodiazepine hypnotic during the last weeks of pregnancy.

Quazepam is contraindicated in pregnancy because the potential risks outweigh the possible advantages of their use during this period. If there is a likelihood of the patient becoming pregnant while receiving Quazepam, she should be warned of the potential risk to the fetus. Patients should be instructed to discontinue the drug prior to becoming pregnant. The possibility that a woman of childbearing potential may be pregnant at the time of institution of therapy should be considered. (See *"Pregnancy, Teratogenic Effects: Pregnancy Category X"*.)

WARNINGS

Patients receiving benzodiazepines should be cautioned about possible combined effects with alcohol and other CNS depressants. Also, caution patients that an additive effect may occur if alcoholic beverages are consumed during the day following the use of benzodiazepines for nighttime sedation. The potential for this interaction continues for several days following their discontinuance until serum levels of psychoactive metabolites have declined.

Patients should also be cautioned about engaging in hazardous occupations requiring complete mental alertness, such as operating machinery or driving a motor vehicle, after ingesting benzodiazepines, including potential impairment of the performance of such activities which may occur the day following ingestion.

Withdrawal symptoms of the type associated with sedatives/hypnotics (e.g., barbiturates, bromides, etc.) and alcohol have been reported after the discontinuation of benzodiazepines. While these symptoms have been more frequently reported after the discontinuation of excessive benzodiazepine doses, there have also been controlled studies demonstrating the occurrence of such symptoms after discontinuation of therapeutic doses of benzodiazepines, generally following prolonged use (but in some instances after periods as brief as six weeks). It is generally believed that the gradual reduction of dosage will diminish the occurrence of such symptoms (see *"Drug Abuse and Dependence"*).

PRECAUTIONS

General: Impaired motor and/or cognitive performance attributable to the accumulation of benzodiazepines and their active metabolites following several days of repeated use at their recommended doses is a concern in certain vulnerable patients (e.g., those especially sensitive to the effects of benzodiazepines or those with a reduced capacity to metabolize and eliminate them). Consequently, elderly or debilitated patients and those with impaired renal or hepatic function should be cautioned about the risk and advised to monitor themselves for signs of excessive sedation or impaired coordination.

The possibility of respiratory depression in patients with chronic pulmonary insufficiency should be considered.

When benzodiazepines are administered to depressed patients, there is a risk that the signs and symptoms of depression may be intensified. Consequently, appropriate precautions (e.g., limiting the total prescription size and increased monitoring for suicidal ideation) should be considered.

Information for Patients: It is suggested that physicians discuss the following information with patients. This information is intended to aid in the safe and effective use of this medication. It is not a disclosure of all possible adverse or intended effects.

1. Inform your physician about any alcohol consumption and medicine you are taking now, including drugs you may buy without a prescription. Alcohol should generally not be used during treatment with hypnotics.

2. Inform you physician if you are planning to become pregnant, if you are pregnant, or if you become pregnant while you are taking this medicine.

3. Inform your physician if you are nursing.

4. Until you experience how this medicine affects you, do not drive a car or operate potentially dangerous machinery, etc.

5. Benzodiazepines may cause daytime sedation, which may persist for several days following drug discontinuation.

6. Patients should be told not to increase the dose on their own and should inform their physician if they believe the drug "does not work anymore."

7. If benzodiazepines are taken on a prolonged and regular basis (even for periods as brief as six weeks), patients should be advised not to stop taking them

abruptly or to decrease the dose without consulting their physician, because withdrawal symptoms may occur.

Laboratory Tests: Laboratory tests are not ordinarily required in otherwise healthy patients when Quazepam is used as recommended.

Drug Interactions: The benzodiazepines, including Quazepam, produce additive CNS depressant effects when co-administered with psychotropic medications, anticonvulsants, antihistaminics, ethanol, and other drugs which produce CNS depression.

Carcinogenesis, Mutagenesis, Impairment of Fertility: Quazepam showed no evidence of carcinogenicity or other significant pathology in oral oncogenicity studies in mice and hamsters.

Quazepam was tested for mutagenicity using the L5178Y TK ± Mouse Lymphoma Mutagenesis Assay and Ames Test. The L5178Y TK ± Assay was equivocal and the Ames Test did not show mutagenic activity.

Reproduction studies in mice conducted with Quazepam at doses equal to 60 and 180 times the human dose of 15 mg, and with diazepam at 67 times the human dose, produced slight reductions in the pregnancy rate. Similar reduction in pregnancy rates have been reported in mice dosed with other benzodiazepines, and is believed to be related to the sedative effect of these drugs at high doses.

Pregnancy: Teratogenic Effects: Pregnancy Category X: (see "Contraindications, Usage in Pregnancy" section). Reproduction studies of Quazepam in mice at doses up to 400 times the human dose revealed no major drug-related malformations. Minor developmental variations that occurred were delayed ossification of the sternum, vertebrae, distal phalanges and supraoccipital bones, at doses of 66 and 400 times the human dose. Studies with diazepam at 200 times the human dose showed a similar or greater incidence than Quazepam. A reproduction study of Quazepam in New Zealand rabbits at doses up to 134 times the human dose demonstrated no effect on fetal morphology or development of offspring.

Nonteratogenic Effects: The child born of a mother who is taking benzodiazepines may be at some risk of withdrawal symptoms from the drug during the postnatal period. Neonatal flaccidity has been reported in children born of mothers who had been receiving benzodiazepines.

Labor and Delivery: Quazepam has no established use in labor or delivery.

Nursing Mothers: Quazepam and its metabolites are excreted in the milk of lactating women. Therefore, administration of Quazepam to nursing women is not recommended.

Pediatric Use: Safety and effectiveness in children below the age of 18 years have not been established.

ADVERSE REACTIONS

Adverse events most frequently encountered in patients treated with Quazepam are drowsiness and headache.

Accurate estimates of the incidence of adverse events associated with the use of any drug are difficult to obtain. Estimates are influenced by drug dose, detection technique, setting, physician judgments, etc. Consequently, the table below is presented solely to indicate the relative frequency of adverse events reported in representative controlled clinical studies conducted to evaluate the safety and efficacy of Quazepam. The figures cited cannot be used to predict precisely the incidence of such events in the course of usual medical practice. These figures, also, cannot be compared with those obtained from other clinical studies involving related drug products and placebo.

The figures cited below are estimates of untoward clinical event incidences of 1% or greater among subjects who participated in the relatively short duration placebo-controlled clinical trials of Quazepam.

Number of Patients	Quazepam* 267	Placebo 268
% of Patients Reporting		
Central Nervous System		
Daytime Drowsiness	12.0	3.3
Headache	4.5	2.2
Fatigue	1.9	0
Dizziness	1.5	< 1
Autonomic Nervous System		
Dry Mouth	1.5	< 1
Gastrointestinal System		
Dyspepsia	1.1	< 1

* *Quazepam 15 mg*

The following incidences of laboratory abnormalities occurred at a rate of 1% or greater in patients receiving Quazepam and the corresponding placebo group. None of these changes were considered to be of physiological significance.

	Quazepam		Placebo	
Number of Patients	234		244	
% of Patients Reporting	Low	High	Low	High
Hematology				
Hemoglobin	1.4	0	1.2	0
Hematocrit	1.5	0	1.7	0
Lymphocyte	1.3	1.6	1.2	1.9

	Quazepam		Placebo	
Number of Patients	234		244	
% of Patients Reporting	Low	High	Low	High
Eosinophil	*	1.5	*	1.3
SEG	1.1	*	1.6	*
Monocyte	*	1.1	*	*
Blood Chemistry				
Glucose	*	*	*	1.2
SGOT	*	1.3	*	1.1
Urinalysis				
Specific Gravity	*	*	*	1.1
WBC	0	2.6	0	3.0
RBC	0	*	0	1.1
Epithelial Cells	0	2.5	0	3.2
Crystals	0	*	0	1.0

* *These laboratory abnormalities occurred in less than 1% of patients. In addition, abnormalities in the following laboratory tests were observed in less than 1% of the patients evaluated: WBC count, platelet count, total protein, albumin, BUN, creatinine, total bilirubin, alkaline phosphatase and SGPT.*

The following additional events occurred among individuals receiving Quazepam at doses equivalent to or greater than those recommended during its clinical testing and development. There is no way to establish whether or not the administration of Quazepam caused these events.

Hypokinesia, ataxia, confusion, incoordination, hyperkinesia, speech disorder and tremor were reported.

Also depression, nervousness, agitation, amnesia, anorexia, anxiety, apathy, euphoria, impotence, decreased libido, paranoid reaction, nightmare, abnormal thinking, abnormal taste perception, abnormal vision, and cataract were reported.

Also reported were urinary incontinence, palpitations, nausea, constipation, diarrhea, abdominal pain, pruritus, rash, asthenia, and malaise.

The following list provides an overview of adverse experiences that have been reported and are considered to be reasonably related to the administration of benzodiazepines: incontinence, slurred speech, urinary retention, jaundice, dysarthria, dystonia, changes in libido, irritability, and menstrual irregularities.

As with all benzodiazepines, paradoxical reactions such as stimulation, agitation, increased muscle spasticity, sleep disturbances, hallucinations, and other adverse behavioral effects may occur in rare instances and in a random fashion. Should these occur, use of the drug should be discontinued. There have been reports of withdrawal signs and symptoms of the type associated with withdrawal from CNS depressant drugs following the rapid decrease or the abrupt discontinuation of benzodiazepines (see "Drug Abuse and Dependence" section).

DRUG ABUSE AND DEPENDENCE

Controlled Substance: Quazepam is a controlled substance under the Controlled Substance Act and has been assigned by the Drug Enforcement Administration to Schedule IV.

Abuse and Dependence: Withdrawal symptoms similar in character to those noted with barbiturates and alcohol (e.g., convulsions, tremor, abdominal and muscle cramps, vomiting and sweating) have occurred following abrupt discontinuance of benzodiazepines. The more severe withdrawal symptoms have usually been limited to those patients who received excessive doses over an extended period of time. Generally milder withdrawal symptoms (e.g., dysphoria and insomnia) have been reported following abrupt discontinuance of benzodiazepines taken continuously at therapeutic levels for several months. Consequently, after extended therapy, abrupt discontinuation should generally be avoided and a gradual dosage tapering schedule followed. Addiction-prone individuals (such as drug addicts or alcoholics) should be under careful surveillance when receiving Quazepam or other psychotropic agents because of the predisposition of such patients to habituation and dependence.

OVERDOSAGE

Manifestations of overdosage seen with other benzodiazepines include somnolence, confusion, and coma. In the event that an overdose occurs, the following is the recommended treatment. Respiration, pulse, and blood pressure should be monitored, as in all cases of drug overdosage. General supportive measures should be employed, along with immediate gastric lavage. Intravenous fluids should be administered and an adequate airway maintained. Hypotension may be treated with the use of norepinephrine bitartrate or metaraminol bitartrate. Dialysis is of limited value. Animal experiments suggest that forced diuresis or hemodialysis are probably of little value in treating overdosage. As with the management of intentional overdosing with any drug, it should be borne in mind that multiple agents may have been ingested.

The oral LD$_{50}$ in mice was greater than 5,000 mg/kg.

DOSAGE AND ADMINISTRATION

Adults: Initiate therapy at 15 mg until individual responses are determined. In some patients, the dose may then be reduced to 7.5 mg.

Elderly and debilitated patients: Because the elderly and debilitated may be more sensitive to benzodiazepines, attempts to reduce the nightly dosage after the first one or two nights of therapy are suggested.

Storage: Store between 2°-30°C (36°-86°F). Protect from excessive moisture.

HOW SUPPLIED
TABLETS (C-IV): 7.5 MG

BRAND/MANUFACTURER	NDC	SIZE	AWP
○ **BRAND**			
DORAL: Wallace	00037-9000-01	100s	$87.06
	00037-9000-02	100s ud	$87.06

TABLETS (C-IV): 15 MG

BRAND/MANUFACTURER	NDC	SIZE	AWP
○ **BRAND**			
DORAL: Wallace	00037-9002-01	100s	$95.14
	00037-9002-02	100s ud	$95.14

Quelicin Chloride *SEE* SUCCINYLCHOLINE CHLORIDE

Questran *SEE* CHOLESTYRAMINE

Quibron *SEE* GUAIFENESIN AND THEOPHYLLINE

Quibron T *SEE* THEOPHYLLINE

Quinaglute Dura-Tabs *SEE* QUINIDINE GLUCONATE

Quinamm *SEE* QUININE SULFATE

Quinapril Hydrochloride

> **USE IN PREGNANCY**
> WHEN USED IN PREGNANCY DURING THE SECOND AND THIRD TRIMESTERS, ACE INHIBITORS CAN CAUSE INJURY AND EVEN DEATH TO THE DEVELOPING FETUS. WHEN PREGNANCY IS DETECTED, QUINAPRIL HYDROCHLORIDE SHOULD BE DISCONTINUED AS SOON AS POSSIBLE. SEE *"WARNINGS, FETAL/NEONATAL MORBIDITY AND MORTALITY."*

DESCRIPTION
Quinapril Hydrochloride is the Hydrochloride salt of Quinapril, the ethyl ester of a nonsulfhydryl, angiotensin-converting enzyme (ACE) inhibitor, quinaprilat.

Quinapril Hydrochloride is chemically described as [3S[2[R*(R*)], 3R*]]-2-[2-[2-[[1-(ethoxycarbonyl)-3-phenylpropyl] amino]-1-oxopropyl]-1,2,3,4-tetrahydro-3-isoquinolinecarboxylic acid, monohydrochloride. Its empirical formula is $C_{25}H_{30}N_2O_5 \cdot HCl$.

Quinapril Hydrochloride is a white to off-white amorphous powder that is freely soluble in aqueous solvents.

Quinapril HCl tablets contain 5 mg, 10 mg, 20 mg, or 40 mg of Quinapril for oral administration.

Following is its chemical structure:

CLINICAL PHARMACOLOGY
Mechanism of Action: Quinapril is deesterified to the principal metabolite, quinaprilat, which is an inhibitor of ACE activity in human subjects and animals. ACE is a peptidyl dipeptidase that catalyzes the conversion of angiotensin I to the vasoconstrictor, angiotensin II. The effect of Quinapril in hypertension and in congestive heart failure (CHF) appears to result primarily from the inhibition of circulating and tissue ACE activity, thereby reducing angiotensin II formation. Quinapril inhibits the elevation in blood pressure caused by intravenously administered angiotensin I, but has no effect on the pressor response to angiotensin II, norepinephrine or epinephrine. Angiotensin II also stimulates the secretion of aldosterone from the adrenal cortex, thereby facilitating renal sodium and fluid reabsorption. Reduced aldosterone secretion by Quinapril may result in

a small increase in serum potassium. In controlled hypertension trials, treatment with Quinapril HCl alone resulted in mean increases in potassium of 0.07 mmol/L (see *"Precautions"*). Removal of angiotensin II negative feedback on renin secretion leads to increased plasma renin activity (PRA).

While the principal mechanism of antihypertensive effect is thought to be through the renin-angiotensin-aldosterone system, Quinapril exerts antihypertensive actions even in patients with low renin hypertension. Quinapril HCl was an effective antihypertensive in all races studied, although it was somewhat less effective in blacks (usually a predominantly low renin group) than in nonblacks. ACE is identical to kininase II, an enzyme that degrades bradykinin, a potent peptide vasodilator; whether increased levels of bradykinin play a role in the therapeutic effect of quinapril remains to be elucidated.

Pharmacokinetics and Metabolism: Following oral administration, peak plasma Quinapril concentrations are observed within one hour. Based on recovery of Quinapril and its metabolites in urine, the extent of absorption is at least 60%. The rate and extent of quinapril absorption are diminished moderately (approximately 25-30%) when quinapril tablets are administered during a high-fat meal. Following absorption, Quinapril is deesterified to its major active metabolite, quinaprilat (about 38% of oral dose), and to other minor inactive metabolites. Following multiple oral dosing of Quinapril, there is an effective accumulation half-life of quinaprilat of approximately 3 hours, and peak plasma quinaprilat concentrations are observed approximately 2 hours post-dose. Quinaprilat is eliminated primarily by renal excretion, up to 96% of an IV dose, and has an elimination half-life in plasma of approximately 2 hours and a prolonged terminal phase with a half-life of 25 hours. The pharmacokinetics of Quinapril and quinaprilat are linear over a single-dose range of 5-80 mg doses and 40-160 mg in multiple daily doses. Approximately 97% of either Quinapril or quinaprilat circulating in plasma is bound to proteins.

In patients with renal insufficiency, the elimination half-life of quinaprilat increases as creatinine clearance decreases. There is a linear correlation between plasma quinaprilat clearance and creatinine clearance. In patients with end-stage renal disease, chronic hemodialysis or continuous ambulatory peritoneal dialysis has little effect on the elimination of Quinapril and quinaprilat. Elimination of quinaprilat may be reduced in elderly patients ($\geq$ 65 years) and in those with heart failure; this reduction is attributable to decrease in renal function (see *"Dosage and Administration"*). Quinaprilat concentrations are reduced in patients with alcoholic cirrhosis due to impaired deesterification of Quinapril. Studies in rats indicate that Quinapril and its metabolites do not cross the blood-brain barrier.

PHARMACODYNAMICS AND CLINICAL EFFECTS
Hypertension: Single doses of 20 mg of Quinapril HCl provide over 80% inhibition of plasma ACE for 24 hours. Inhibition of the pressor response to angiotensin I is shorter-lived, with a 20 mg dose giving 75% inhibition for about 4 hours, 50% inhibition for about 8 hours, and 20% inhibition at 24 hours. With chronic dosing, however, there is substantial inhibition of angiotensin II levels at 24 hours by doses of 20-80 mg. Administration of 10 to 80 mg of Quinapril HCl to patients with mild to severe hypertension results in a reduction of sitting and standing blood pressure to about the same extent with minimal effect on heart rate. Symptomatic postural hypotension is infrequent although it can occur in patients who are salt- and/or volume-depleted (see *"Warnings"*). Antihypertensive activity commences within 1 hour with peak effects usually achieved by 2 to 4 hours after dosing. During chronic therapy, most of the blood pressure lowering effect of a given dose is obtained in 1-2 weeks. In multiple-dose studies, 10-80 mg per day in single or divided doses lowered systolic and diastolic blood pressure throughout the dosing interval, with a trough effect of about 5-11/3-7 mm Hg. The trough effect represents about 50% of the peak effect. While the dose-response relationship is relatively flat, doses of 40-80 mg were somewhat more effective at trough than 10-20 mg, and twice daily dosing tended to give a somewhat lower trough blood pressure than once daily dosing with the same total dose. The antihypertensive effect of Quinapril HCl continues during long-term therapy, with no evidence of loss of effectiveness.

Hemodynamic assessments in patients with hypertension indicate that blood pressure reduction produced by Quinapril is accompanied by a reduction in total peripheral resistance and renal vascular resistance with little or no change in heart rate, cardiac index, renal blood flow, glomerular filtration rate, or filtration fraction.

Use of Quinapril HCl with a thiazide diuretic gives a blood-pressure lowering effect greater than that seen with either agent alone.

In patients with hypertension, Quinapril HCl 10-40 mg was similar in effectiveness to captopril, enalapril, propranolol, and thiazide diuretics.

Therapeutic effects appear to be the same for elderly ($\geq$ 65 years of age) and younger adult patients given the same daily dosages, with no increase in adverse events in elderly patients.

Heart Failure: In baseline-controlled trials involving patients with congestive heart failure treated with digitalis and diuretics, parenteral quinaprilat, the active metabolite of Quinapril, reduced pulmonary capillary wedge pressure, and systemic vascular resistance and increased cardiac output/index. Similiar favorable hemodynamic effects were seen with oral Quinapril, and such effects appeared to be maintained during chronic oral Quinapril therapy. Quiniapril reduced renal hepatic vascular resistance and increased renal and hepatic blood flow with glomerular filtration rate remaining unchanged.

A significant dose response relationship for improvement in maximal exercise tolerance has been observed with Quinapril HCl therapy. Beneficial effects on the severity of heart failure as measured by New York Heart Association (NYHA) classification and Quality of Life and on symptoms of dyspnea, fatigue, and edema were evident after 6 months in a double blind, placebo controlled study. Favorable effects were maintained for up to two years of open label therapy. The effects of Quinapril on long-term mortality in heart failure have not been evaluated.

INDICATIONS AND USAGE

Hypertension: Quinapril HCl is indicated for the treatment of hypertension. It may be used alone or in combination with thiazide diuretics.

Heart Failure: Quinapril HCl is indicated in the management of heart failure as adjunctive therapy when added to conventional therapy including diuretics and/or digitalis.

In using Quinapril HCl, consideration should be given to the fact that another angiotensin converting enzyme inhibitor, captopril, has caused agranulocytosis, particularly in patients with renal impairment or collagen vascular disease. Available data are insufficient to show that Quinapril HCl does not have a similar risk (see *"Warnings"*).

CONTRAINDICATIONS

Quinapril HCl is contraindicated in patients who are hypersensitive to this product and in patients with a history of angioedema related to previous treatment with an ACE inhibitor.

WARNINGS

Angioedema: Angioedema of the face, extremities, lips, tongue, glottis, and larynx has been reported in patients treated with ACE inhibitors and has been seen in 0.1% of patients receiving Quinapril HCl. Angioedema associated with laryngeal edema can be fatal. If laryngeal stridor or angioedema of the face, tongue, or glottis occurs, treatment with Quinapril HCl should be discontinued immediately, the patient treated in accordance with accepted medical care, and carefully observed until the swelling disappears. In instances where swelling is confined to the face and lips, the condition generally resolves without treatment; antihistamines may be useful in relieving symptoms. **Where there is involvement of the tongue, glottis, or larynx likely to cause airway obstruction, emergency therapy including but not limited to, subcutaneous epinephrine solution 1:1000 (0.3 to 0.5 mL) should be promptly administered** (see *"Adverse Reactions"*).

Hypotension: Excessive hypotension is rare in patients with uncomplicated hypertension treated with Quinapril HCl alone. Patients with heart failure given Quinapril HCl commonly have some reduction in blood pressure, but discontinuation of therapy because of continuing symptomatic hypotension usually is not necessary when dosing instructions are followed. Caution should be observed when initiating therapy in patients with heart failure (see *"Dosage and Administration"*). In controlled studies, syncope was observed in 0.4% of patients (N = 3203); this incidence was similar to that observed for captopril (1%) and enalapril (0.8%).

Patients at risk of excessive hypotension, sometimes associated with oliguria and/or progressive azotemia, and rarely with acute renal failure and/or death, include patients with the following conditions or characteristics: heart failure, hyponatremia, high dose diuretic therapy, recent intensive diuresis or increase in diuretic dose, renal dialysis, or severe volume and/or salt depletion of any etiology. It may be advisable to eliminate the diuretic (except in patients with heart failure), reduce the diuretic dose or cautiously increase salt intake (except in patients with heart failure) before initiating therapy with Quinapril HCl in patients at risk for excessive hypotension who are able to tolerate such adjustments.

In patients at risk of excessive hypotension, therapy with Quinapril HCl should be started under close medical supervision. Such patients should be followed closely for the first two weeks of treatment and whenever the dose of Quinapril HCl and/or diuretic is increased. Similar considerations may apply to patients with ischemic heart or cerebrovascular disease in whom an excessive fall in blood pressure could result in a myocardial infarction or a cerebrovascular accident.

If excessive hypotension occurs, the patient should be placed in the supine position and, if necessary, receive an intravenous infusion of normal saline. A transient hypotensive response is not a contraindication to further doses of Quinapril HCl, which usually can be given without difficulty once the blood pressure has stabilized. If symptomatic hypotension develops, a dose reduction or discontinuation of Quinapril HCl or concomitant diuretic may be necessary.

Neutropenia/Agranulocytosis: Another ACE inhibitor, captopril, has been shown to cause agranulocytosis and bone marrow depression rarely in patients with uncomplicated hypertension, but more frequently in patients with renal impairment, especially if they also have a collagen vascular disease, such as systemic lupus erythematosus or scleroderma. Agranulocytosis did occur during Quinapril HCl treatment in one patient with a history of neutropenia during previous captopril therapy. Available data from clinical trials of Quinapril HCl are insufficient to show that, in patients without prior reactions to other ACE inhibitors Quinapril HCl does not cause agranulocytosis at similar rates. As with other ACE inhibitors, periodic monitoring of white blood cell counts in patients with collagen vascular disease and/or renal disease should be considered.

Fetal/Neonatal Morbidity and Mortality: ACE inhibitors can cause fetal and neonatal morbidity and death when administered to pregnant women. Several dozen cases have been reported in the world literature. When pregnancy is detected, ACE inhibitors should be discontinued as soon as possible.

The use of ACE inhibitors during the second and third trimesters of pregnancy has been associated with fetal and neonatal injury, including hypotension, neonatal skull hypoplasia, anuria, reversible or irreversible renal failure, and death. Oligohydramnios has also been reported, presumably resulting from decreased fetal renal function; oligohydramnios in this setting has been associated with fetal limb contractures, craniofacial deformation, and hypoplastic lung development. Prematurity, intrauterine growth retardation, and patent ductus arteriosus have also been reported, although it is not clear whether these occurrences were due to the ACE inhibitor exposure.

These adverse effects do not appear to have resulted from intrauterine ACE inhibitor exposure that has been limited to the first trimester. Mothers whose embryos and fetuses are exposed to ACE inhibitors only during the first trimester should be so informed. Nonetheless, when patients become pregnant, physicians should make every effort to discontinue the use of Quinapril HCl as soon as possible.

Rarely (probably less often than once in every thousand pregnancies), no alternative to ACE inhibitors will be found. In these rare cases, the mothers should be apprised of the potential hazards to their fetuses, and serial ultrasound examinations should be performed to assess the intraamniotic environment.

If oligohydramnios is observed Quinapril HCl should be discontinued unless it is considered life-saving for the mother. Contraction stress testing (CST), a non-stress test (NST), or biophysical profiling (BPP) may be appropriate, depending upon the week of pregnancy. Patients and physicians should be aware, however, that oligohydramnios may not appear until after the fetus has sustained irreversible injury.

Infants with histories of *in utero* exposure to ACE inhibitors should be closely observed for hypotension, oliguria, and hyperkalemia. If oliguria occurs, attention should be directed toward support of blood pressure and renal perfusion. Exchange transfusion or dialysis may be required as a means of reversing hypotension and/or substituting for disordered renal function. Removal of Quinapril HCl, which crosses the placenta, from the neonatal circulation is not significantly accelerated by these means.

No teratogenic effects of Quinapril HCl were seen in studies of pregnant rats and rabbits. On a mg/kg basis, the doses used were up to 180 times (in rats) and one time (in rabbits) the maximum recommended human dose.

PRECAUTIONS

GENERAL

Impaired Renal Function: As a consequence of inhibiting the renin-angiotensin-aldosterone system, changes in renal function may be anticipated in susceptible individuals. In patients with severe heart failure whose renal function may depend on the activity of the renin-angiotensin-aldosterone system, treatment with ACE inhibitors, including Quinapril HCl may be associated with oliguria and/or progressive azotemia and rarely acute renal failure and/or death.

In clinical studies in hypertensive patients with unilateral or bilateral renal artery stenosis, increases in blood urea nitrogen and serum creatinine have been observed in some patients following ACE inhibitor therapy. These increases were almost always reversible upon discontinuation of the ACE inhibitor and/or diuretic therapy. In such patients, renal function should be monitored during the first few weeks of therapy.

Some patients with hypertension or heart failure with no apparent preexisting renal vascular disease have developed increases in blood urea and serum creatinine, usually minor and transient, especially when Quinapril HCl has been given concomitantly with a diuretic. This is more likely to occur in patients with preexisting renal impairment. Dosage reduction and/or discontinuation of any diuretic and/or Quinapril HCl may be required.

Evaluation of patients with hypertension or heart failure should always include assessment of renal function (see "Dosage and Administration").

DOSAGE AND ADMINISTRATION

Hyperkalemia and Potassium-Sparing Diuretics: In clinical trials, hyperkalemia (serum potassium) ≥ 5.8 mmol/L) occurred in approximately 2% of patients receiving Quinapril HCl. In most cases, elevated serum potassium levels were isolated values which resolved despite continued therapy. Less than 0.1% of patients discontinued therapy due to hyperkalemia. Risk factors for the development of hyperkalemia include renal insufficiency, diabetes mellitus, and the concomitant use of potassium-sparing diuretics, potassium supplements, and/or potassium-containing salt substitutes, which should be used cautiously, if at all, with Quinapril HCl (see *"Precautions, Drug Interactions"*).

Cough: Cough has been reported with the use of ACE inhibitors. Characteristically, the cough is nonproductive, persistent, and resolves after discontinuation of therapy. ACE inhibitor-induced cough should be considered as part of the differential diagnosis of cough.

Surgery/Anesthesia: In patients undergoing major surgery or during anesthesia with agents that produce hypotension, Quinapril HCl will block angiotensin II formation secondary to compensatory renin release. If hypotension occurs and is considered to be due to this mechanism, it can be corrected by volume expansion.

INFORMATION FOR PATIENTS

Pregnancy: Female patients of childbearing age should be told about the consequences of second- and third-trimester exposure to ACE inhibitors, and they should also be told that these consequences do not appear to have resulted from intrauterine ACE-inhibitor exposure that has been limited to the first trimester. These patients should be asked to report pregnancies to their physicians as soon as possible.

Angioedema: Angioedema, including laryngeal edema, can occur with treatment with ACE inhibitors, especially following the first dose. Patients should be so advised and told to report immediately any signs or symptoms suggesting angioedema (swelling of face, extremities, eyes, lips, tongue, difficulty in swallowing or breathing) and to stop taking the drug until they have consulted with their physician (see "Warnings").

Symptomatic Hypotension: Patients should be cautioned that lightheadedness can occur, especially during the first few days of Quinapril HCl therapy, and that it should be reported to a physician. If actual syncope occurs, patients should be told to not take the drug until they have consulted with their physician (see "Warnings").

All patients should be cautioned that inadequate fluid intake or excessive perspiration, diarrhea, or vomiting can lead to an excessive fall in blood pressure because of reduction in fluid volume, with the same consequences of lightheadedness and possible syncope.

Patients planning to undergo any surgery and/or anesthesia should be told to inform their physician that they are taking an ACE inhibitor.

Hyperkalemia: Patients should be told not to use potassium supplements or salt substitutes containing potassium without consulting their physician (see "Precautions").

Neutropenia: Patients should be told to report promptly any indication of infection (eg, sore throat, fever) which could be a sign of neutropenia.

Note: As with many other drugs, certain advice to patients being treated with Quinapril HCl is warranted. This information is intended to aid in the safe and effective use of this medication. It is not a disclosure of all possible adverse or intended effects.

DRUG INTERACTIONS
Concomitant Diuretic Therapy: As with other ACE inhibitors, patients on diuretics, especially those on recently instituted diuretic therapy, may occasionally experience an excessive reduction of blood pressure after initiation of therapy with Quinapril HCl. The possiblity of hypotensive effects with Quinapril HCl may be minimized by either discontinuing the diuretic or cautiously increasing salt intake prior to initiation of treatment with Quinapril HCl. If it is not possible to discontinue the diuretic, the starting dose of Quinapril should be reduced (see "Dosage and Administration").

Agents Increasing Serum Potassium: Quinapril can attenuate potassium loss caused by thiazide diuretics and increase serum potassium when used alone. If concomitant therapy of Quinapril HCl with potassium-sparing diuretics (eg, spironolactone, triamterene, or amiloride), potassium supplements, or potassium-containing salt substitutes is indicated, they should be used with caution along with appropriate monitoring of serum potassium (see "Precautions").

Tetracycline and Other Drugs that Interact with Magnesium: Simultaneous administration of tetracycline with Quinapril HCl reduced the absorption of tetracycline by approximately 28% to 37% possibly due to the high magnesium content in Quinapril HCl tablets. This interaction should be considered if coprescribing Quinapril HCl and tetracycline or other drugs that interact with magnesium.

Lithium: Increased serum lithium levels and symptoms of lithium toxicity have been reported in patients receiving concomitant lithium and ACE inhibitor therapy. These drugs should be coadministered with caution and frequent monitoring of serum lithium levels is recommended. If a diuretic is also used, it may increase the risk of lithium toxicity.

Other Agents: Drug interaction studies of Quinapril HCl with other agents showed:

■ Multiple dose therapy with propranolol or cimetidine has no effect on the pharmacokinetics of single doses of Quinapril HCl.

■ The anticoagulant effect of a single dose of warfarin (measured by prothrombin time) was not significantly changed by Quinapril coadministration twice-daily.

■ Quinapril HCl treatment did not affect the pharmacokinetics of digoxin.

■ No pharmacokinetic interaction was observed when single doses of Quinapril HCl and hydrochlorothiazide were administered concomitantly.

CARCINOGENESIS, MUTAGENESIS, IMPAIRMENT OF FERTILITY
Quinapril hydrochloride was not carcinogenic in mice or rats when given in doses up to 75 or 100 mg/kg/day (50 to 60 times the maximum human daily dose, respectively, on an mg/kg basis and 3.8 to 10 times the maximum human daily dose when based on an mg/m^2 basis) for 104 weeks. Female rats given the highest dose level had an increased incidence of mesenteric lymph node hemangiomas and skin/subcutaneous lipomas. Neither Quinapril nor quinaprilat were mutagenic in the Ames bacterial assay with or without metabolic activation. Quinapril was also negative in the following genetic toxicology studies: *in vitro* mammalian cell point mutation, sister chromatid exchange in cultured mammalian cells, micronucleus test with mice, *in vitro* chromosome aberration with V79 cultured lung cells, and in an *in vitro* cytogetic study with rat bone marrow. There were no adverse effects on fertility or reproduction in rats at doses up to 100 mg/kg/day (60 and 10 times the maximum daily human dose when based on mg/kg and mg/m^2, respectively).

PREGNANCY
Pregnancy Categories C (first trimester) and D (second and third trimesters): See "Warnings", Fetal/Neonatal Morbidity and Mortality."

NURSING MOTHERS
It is not known if Quinapril or its metabolites are secreted in human milk. Quinapril is secreted to a limited extent, however, in milk of lactating rats (5% or less of the plasma drug concentration was found in rat milk). Because many drugs are secreted in human milk, caution should be exercised when Quinapril HCl is given to a nursing mother.

GERIATRIC USE
Elderly patients exhibited increased area under the plasma concentration time curve (AUC) and peak levels for quinaprilat compared to values observed in younger patients; this appeared to relate to decreased renal function rather than to age itself. In controlled and uncontrolled studies of Quinapril HCl where 918 (21%) patients were 65 years and older, no overall differences in effectiveness or safety were observed between older and younger patients. However, greater sensitivity of some older individual patients cannot be ruled out.

PEDIATRIC USE
The safety and effectiveness of Quinapril HCl in children have not been established.

ADVERSE REACTIONS
HYPERTENSION
Quinapril HCl has been evaluated for safety in 4960 subjects and patients. Of these, 3203 patients, including 655 elderly patients, participated in controlled clinical trials. Quinapril HCl has been evaluated for long-term safety in over 1400 patients treated for 1 year or more.

Adverse experiences were usually mild and transient.

In placebo-controlled trials, discontinuation of therapy because of adverse events was required in 4.7% of patients with hypertension.

Adverse experiences probably or possibly related to therapy or of unknown relationship to therapy occurring in 1% or more of the 1563 patients in placebo-controlled hypertension trials who were treated with Quinapril HCl are shown below.

ADVERSE EVENTS IN PLACEBO-CONTROLLED TRIALS

	Quinapril HCl (N = 1563) Incidence (Discontinuance)	Placebo (N = 579) Incidence (Discontinuance)
Headache	5.6 (0.7)	10.9 (0.7)
Dizziness	3.9 (0.8)	2.6 (0.2)
Fatigue	2.6 (0.3)	1.0
Coughing	2.0 (0.5)	0.0
Nausea and/or Vomiting	1.4 (0.3)	1.9 (0.2)
Abdominal Pain	1.0 (0.2)	0.7

Heart Failure: Quinapril HCl has been evaluated for safety in 1222 Quinapril HCl treated patients. Of these, 632 patients participated in controlled clinical trials. In placebo-controlled trials, discontinuation of therapy because of adverse events was required in 6.8% of patients with congestive heart failure.

Adverse experiences probably or possibly related or of unknown relationship to therapy occurring in 1% or more of the 585 patients in placebo-controlled congestive heart failure trials who were treated with Quinapril HCl are shown below.

	Quinapril HCl (N = 585) Incidence (Discontinuance)	Placebo (N = 295) Incidence (Discontinuance)
Dizziness	7.7 (0.7)	5.1 (1.0)
Coughing	4.3 (0.3)	1.4
Fatigue	2.6 (0.2)	1.4
Nausea and/or Vomiting	2.4 (0.2)	0.7
Chest Pain	2.4	1.0
Hypotension	2.9 (0.5)	1.0
Dyspnea	1.9 (0.2)	2.0
Diarrhea	1.7	1.0
Headache	1.7	1.0 (0.3)
Myalgia	1.5	2.0
Rash	1.4 (0.2)	1.0
Back Pain	1.2	0.3

See "Precautions, Cough."

Hypertension and/or Heart Failure: Clinical adverse experience probably, possibly, or definitely related, or of uncertain relationship, to therapy occurring in 0.5% to 1.0% (except as noted) of the patients with CHF or hypertension treated with Quinapril HCl with or without concomitant diuretic in controlled or uncontrolled trials (N = 4847) and less frequent, clinically significant events seen in clinical trials or post-marketing experience (the rarer events are in italics) include (listed by body system):

General: back pain, malaise, viral infections

Cardiovascular: palpitation, vasodilation, tachycardia, *heart failure, hyperkalemia, myocardial infarction, cerebrovascular accident, hypertensive crisis, angina pectoris, orthostatic hypotension, cardiac rhythm disturbances, cardiogenic shock*

Gastrointestinal: dry mouth or throat, constipation, *gastrointestinal hemorrhage, pancreatitis, abnormal liver function tests*

Nervous/Psychiatric: somnolence, vertigo, syncope, nervousness, depression

Integumentary: increased sweating, pruritus, *exfoliative dermatitis, photosensitivity reaction, dermatopolymyositis*

Urogenital: acute renal failure, worsening renal failure

Other: amblyopia, pharyngitis, *agranulocytosis, thrombocytopenia*

FETAL/NEONATAL MORBIDITY AND MORTALITY
See *"Warnings, Fetal/Neonatal Morbidity and Mortality."*

ANGIOEDEMA
Angioedema has been reported in patients receiving Quinapril HCl (0.1%). Angioedema associated with laryngeal edema may be fatal. If angioedema of the face, extremities, lips, tongue, glottis, and/or larynx occurs, treatment with Quinapril HCl should be discontinued and appropriate therapy instituted immediately. (See *"Warnings."*)

CLINICAL LABORATORY TEST FINDINGS
Hematology: (See *"Warnings"*).

Hyperkalemia: (See *"Precautions"*).

Creatinine and Blood Urea Nitrogen: Increases (> 1.25 times the upper limit of normal) in serum creatinine and blood urea nitrogen were observed in 2% and 2%, respectively, of all patients treated with Quinapril HCl alone. Increases are more likely to occur in patients receiving concomitant diuretic therapy than in those on Quinapril HCl alone. These increases often remit on continued therapy. In controlled studies of heart failure, increases in blood urea nitrogen and serum creatinine were observed in 11% and 8%, respectively, of patients treated with Quinapril HCl most often these patients were receiving diuretics with or without digitalis.

OVERDOSAGE
No data are available with respect to overdosage in humans. Doses of 1440 to 4280 mg/kg of Quinapril cause significant lethality in mice and rats

The most likely clinical manifestation would be symptoms attributable to severe hypotension.

Laboratory determinations of serum levels of Quinapril and its metabolites are not widely available, and such determinations have, in any event, no established role in the management of Quinapril overdose.

No data are available to suggest physiological maneuvers (eg. maneuvers to change pH of the urine) that might accelerate elimination of Quinapril and its metabolites.

Hemodialysis and peritoneal dialysis have little effect on the elimination of Quinapril and quinaprilat. Angiotensin II could presumably serve as a specific antagonist-antidote in the setting of Quinapril overdose, but angiotensin II is essentially unavailable outside of scattered research facilities. Because the hypotensive effect of Quinapril is achieved through vasodilation and effective hypovolemia, it is reasonable to treat Quinapril overdose by infusion of normal saline solution.

DOSAGE AND ADMINISTRATION
Hypertension: Monotherapy: The recommended initial dosage of Quinapril HCl in patients not on diuretics is 10 mg once daily. Dosage should be adjusted according to blood pressure response measured at peak (2-6 hours after dosing) and trough (predosing). Generally, dosage adjustments should be made at intervals of at least 2 weeks. Most patients have required dosages of 20, 40, or 80 mg/day, given as a single dose or in two equally divided doses. In some patients treated once daily, the antihypertensive effect may diminish toward the end of the dosing interval. In such patients an increase in dosage or twice daily administration may be warranted. In general, doses of 40-80 mg and divided doses give a somewhat greater effect at the end of the dosing interval.

Concomitant Diuretics: If blood pressure is not adequately controlled with Quinapril HCl monotherapy, a diuretic may be added. In patients who are currently being treated with a diuretic, symptomatic hypotension occasionally can occur following the initial dose of Quinapril HCl. To reduce the likelihood of hypotension, the diuretic should, if possible, be discontinued 2 to 3 days prior to beginning therapy with Quinapril HCl (see *"Warnings"*). Then, if blood pressure is not controlled with Quinapril HCl alone, diuretic therapy should be resumed.

If the diuretic cannot be discontinued, an initial dose of 5 mg Quinapril HCl should be used with careful medical supervision for several hours and until blood pressure has stabilized. The dosage should subsequently be titrated (as described above) to the optimal response (see *"Warnings," "Precautions"* and *"Drug Interactions"*).

Renal Impairment: Kinetic data indicate that the apparent elimination half-life of quinaprilat increases as creatinine clearance decreases. Recommended starting doses, based on clinical and pharmacokinetic data from patients with renal impairment, are as follows:

Creatinine Clearance	Maximum Recommend Initial Dose
> 60 mL/min	10 mg
30-60 mL/min	5 mg
10-30 mL/min	2.5 mg
< 10 mL/min	Insufficient data for dosage recommendation

Patients should subsequently have their dosage titrated (as described above) to the optimal response.

Elderly (≥ 65 years): The recommended initial dosage of Quinapril HCl in elderly patients is 10 mg given once daily followed by titration (as described above) to the optimal response.

Heart Failure: Quinapril HCl is indicated as adjunctive therapy when added to conventional therapy including diuretics and/or digitalis. The recommended starting dose is 5 mg twice daily. This dose may improve symptoms of heart failure, but increases in exercise duration have generally required higher doses. Therefore, if the initial dosage of Quinapril HCl is well tolerated, patients should then be titrated at weekly intervals until an effective dose, usually 20 to 40 mg daily given in two equally divided doses, is reached or undesirable hypotension, orthostatis, or azoteia (see *"Warnings"*) prohibit reaching this dose.

Following the initial dose of Quinapril HCl the patient should be observed under medical supervision for at least two hours for the presence of hypotension or orthostatis and, if present, until blood pressure stabilizes. The appearance of hypotension, orthostasis, or azoteia early in dose titration should not preclude further careful dose titration. Consideration should be given to reducing the dose of concomitant diuretics.

DOSE ADJUSTMENTS IN PATIENTS WITH HEART FAILURE AND RENAL IMPAIRMENT OR HYPONATREMIA
Pharmacokinetic data indicate that Quinapril elimination is dependent on level of renal function. In patients with heart failure and renal impairment, the recommended initial dose of Quinapril HCl is 5 mg in patients with a creatinine clearance above 30 mL/min and 2.5 mg in patients with a creatinine clearance of 10 to 30 mL/min. There is insufficient data for dosage recommendation in patients with a creatinine clearance less than 10 mL/min. (See *"Dosage and Administration, Heart Failure," "Warnings,"* and *"Precautions, Drug Interactions"*).

If the initial dose is well tolerated, Quinapril HCl may be administered the following day as a twice daily regimen. In the absence of excessive hypotension or significant deterioration of renal function, the dose may be increased at weekly intervals based on clinical and hemodynamic response.

Storage: Store at controlled room temperature 15°-30°C (59°-86°F). Dispense in well-closed containers as defined in the USP.

HOW SUPPLIED
TABLETS: 5 MG

BRAND/MANUFACTURER	NDC	SIZE	AWP
○ BRAND			
◆ ACCUPRIL: Parke-Davis	00071-0527-23	90s	$81.81

TABLETS: 10 MG

BRAND/MANUFACTURER	NDC	SIZE	AWP
○ BRAND			
◆ ACCUPRIL: Parke-Davis	00071-0530-23	90s	$81.81
	00071-0530-40	100s ud	$90.92

TABLETS: 20 MG

BRAND/MANUFACTURER	NDC	SIZE	AWP
○ BRAND			
◆ ACCUPRIL: Parke-Davis	00071-0532-23	90s	$81.81
	00071-0532-40	90s ud	$90.92

TABLETS: 40 MG

BRAND/MANUFACTURER	NDC	SIZE	AWP
○ BRAND			
◆ ACCUPRIL: Parke-Davis	00071-0535-23	90s	$81.81

Quinestrol

> ## WARNING
> *1. ESTROGENS HAVE BEEN REPORTED TO INCREASE THE RISK OF ENDOMETRIAL CARCINOMA.*
>
> THREE INDEPENDENT CASE CONTROL STUDIES HAVE SHOWN AN INCREASED RISK OF ENDOMETRIAL CANCER IN POSTMENOPAUSAL WOMEN EXPOSED TO EXOGENOUS ESTROGENS FOR PROLONGED PERIODS.[1-3] THIS RISK WAS INDEPENDENT OF THE OTHER KNOWN RISK FACTORS FOR ENDOMETRIAL CANCER. THESE STUDIES ARE FURTHER SUPPORTED BY THE FINDING THAT INCIDENCE RATES OF ENDOMETRIAL CANCER HAVE INCREASED SHARPLY SINCE 1969 IN EIGHT DIFFERENT AREAS OF THE UNITED STATES WITH POPULATION-BASED CANCER REPORTING SYSTEMS, AN INCREASE WHICH MAY BE RELATED TO THE RAPIDLY EXPANDING USE OF ESTROGENS DURING THE LAST DECADE.[4]
>
> THE THREE CASE CONTROL STUDIES REPORTED THAT THE RISK OF ENDOMETRIAL CANCER IN ESTROGEN USERS WAS ABOUT 4.5 TO 13.9

TIMES GREATER THAN IN NONUSERS. THE RISK APPEARS TO DEPEND ON BOTH DURATION OF TREATMENT[1] AND ON ESTROGEN DOSE.[3] IN VIEW OF THESE FINDINGS, WHEN ESTROGENS ARE USED FOR THE TREATMENT OF MENOPAUSAL SYMPTOMS, THE LOWEST DOSE THAT WILL CONTROL SYMPTOMS SHOULD BE UTILIZED AND MEDICATION SHOULD BE DISCONTINUED AS SOON AS POSSIBLE. WHEN PROLONGED TREATMENT IS MEDICALLY INDICATED, THE PATIENT SHOULD BE REASSESSED ON AT LEAST A SEMIANNUAL BASIS TO DETERMINE THE NEED FOR CONTINUED THERAPY. ALTHOUGH THE EVIDENCE MUST BE CONSIDERED PRELIMINARY, ONE STUDY SUGGESTS THAT CYCLIC ADMINISTRATION OF LOW DOSES OF ESTROGEN MAY CARRY LESS RISK THAN CONTINUOUS ADMINISTRATION.[3] THEREFORE, WHILE IT APPEARS PRUDENT TO UTILIZE SUCH A REGIMEN WITH OTHER ORALLY ADMINISTERED ESTROGENS, ESTROVIS MAY BE ADMINISTERED, FOLLOWING A SEVEN-DAY PRIMING SCHEDULE, ON A ONCE WEEKLY MAINTENANCE DOSAGE BEGINNING TWO WEEKS AFTER THE START OF TREATMENT.

CLOSE CLINICAL SURVEILLANCE OF ALL WOMEN TAKING ESTROGENS IS IMPORTANT. IN ALL CASES OF UNDIAGNOSED PERSISTENT OR RECURRING ABNORMAL VAGINAL BLEEDING, ADEQUATE DIAGNOSTIC MEASURES SHOULD BE UNDERTAKEN TO RULE OUT MALIGNANCY.

THERE IS NO EVIDENCE AT PRESENT THAT "NATURAL" ESTROGENS ARE MORE OR LESS HAZARDOUS THAN "SYNTHETIC" ESTROGENS AT EQUIESTROGENIC DOSES.

2. ESTROGENS SHOULD NOT BE USED DURING PREGNANCY.

THE USE OF FEMALE SEX HORMONES, BOTH ESTROGENS AND PROGESTOGENS, DURING EARLY PREGNANCY MAY SERIOUSLY DAMAGE THE OFFSPRING. IT HAS BEEN SHOWN THAT FEMALES EXPOSED *IN UTERO* TO DIETHYLSTILBESTROL, A NONSTEROIDAL ESTROGEN, HAVE AN INCREASED RISK OF DEVELOPING IN LATER LIFE A FORM OF VAGINAL OR CERVICAL CANCER THAT IS ORDINARILY EXTREMELY RARE.[5-6] THIS RISK HAS BEEN ESTIMATED AS NOT GREATER THAN 4 PER 1,000 EXPOSURES.[7] FURTHERMORE, A HIGH PERCENTAGE OF SUCH EXPOSED WOMEN (FROM 30 TO 90%) HAVE BEEN FOUND TO HAVE VAGINAL ADENOSIS,[8-12] EPITHELIAL CHANGES OF THE VAGINA AND CERVIX. ALTHOUGH THESE CHANGES ARE HISTOLOGICALLY BENIGN, IT IS NOT KNOWN WHETHER THEY ARE PRECURSORS OF MALIGNANCY. ALTHOUGH SIMILAR DATA ARE NOT AVAILABLE WITH THE USE OF OTHER ESTROGENS, IT CANNOT BE PRESUMED THEY WOULD NOT INDUCE SIMILAR CHANGES.

SEVERAL REPORTS SUGGEST AN ASSOCIATION BETWEEN INTRA-UTERINE EXPOSURE TO FEMALE SEX HORMONES AND CONGENITAL ANOMALIES, INCLUDING CONGENITAL HEART DEFECTS AND LIMB-REDUCTION DEFECTS.[13-16] ONE CASE CONTROL STUDY[16] ESTIMATED A 4.7-FOLD INCREASED RISK OF LIMB-REDUCTION DEFECTS IN INFANTS EXPOSED *IN UTERO* TO SEX HORMONES (ORAL CONTRACEPTIVES, HORMONE WITHDRAWAL TESTS FOR PREGNANCY, OR ATTEMPTED TREATMENT FOR THREATENED ABORTION). SOME OF THESE EXPOSURES WERE VERY SHORT AND INVOLVED ONLY A FEW DAYS OF TREATMENT. THE DATA SUGGEST THAT THE RISK OF LIMB-REDUCTION DEFECTS IN EXPOSED FETUSES IS SOMEWHAT LESS THAN 1 PER 1,000.

IN THE PAST, FEMALE SEX HORMONES HAVE BEEN USED DURING PREGNANCY IN AN ATTEMPT TO TREAT THREATENED OR HABITUAL ABORTION. THERE IS CONSIDERABLE EVIDENCE THAT ESTROGENS ARE INEFFECTIVE FOR THESE INDICATIONS, AND THERE IS NO EVIDENCE FROM WELL-CONTROLLED STUDIES THAT PROGESTOGENS ARE EFFECTIVE FOR THESE USES.

IF QUINESTROL IS USED DURING PREGNANCY, OR IF THE PATIENT BECOMES PREGNANT WHILE TAKING THIS DRUG, SHE SHOULD BE APPRISED OF THE POTENTIAL RISKS TO THE FETUS AND THE ADVISABILITY OF PREGNANCY CONTINUATION.

DESCRIPTION

Quinestrol is the 3-cyclopentylether of ethinyl estradiol. It is an estrogenic agent for oral administration. Each tablet contains 100 mcg quinestrol, USP. The chemical name is 3-cyclopentyloxy-17α-ethynylestra-1,3,5(10)-trien-17β-ol.

It is a white, essentially odorless powder, insoluble in water and soluble in alcohol, chloroform, and ether.

Following is its chemical structure:

CLINICAL PHARMACOLOGY

Quinestrol is an orally effective estrogen as judged by conventional assay procedures employing vagina and uterine end-points in mice, rats and rabbits.

The estrogenic effects of Quinestrol have been demonstrated in clinical studies by its effects on the endometrium, maturation of the vaginal epithelium, thinning of cervical mucus, suppression of pituitary gonadotropin, inhibition of ovulation, and prevention of postpartum breast discomfort.

INDICATIONS

Quinestrol is indicated in the treatment of:
1. Moderate to severe vasomotor symptoms associated with the menopause. (There is no evidence that estrogens are effective for nervous symptoms or depression which might occur during menopause, and they should not be used to treat these conditions.)
2. Atrophic vaginitis
3. Kraurosis vulvae
4. Female hypogonadism
5. Female castration
6. Primary ovarian failure

Quinestrol has not been shown to be effective for any purpose during pregnancy and its use may cause severe harm to the fetus (see Boxed "Warning").

UNLABELED USES
Quinestrol is used alone or as an adjunct in the prevention of cardiovascular disease.

CONTRAINDICATIONS

Estrogens should not be used in women (or men) with any of the following conditions:
1. Known or suspected cancer of the breast except in appropriately selected patients being treated for metastatic disease
2. Known or suspected estrogen-dependent neoplasia
3. Known or suspected pregnancy (See Boxed *"Warning"*)
4. Undiagnosed abnormal genital bleeding
5. Active thrombophlebitis or thromboembolic disorders
6. A past history of thrombophlebitis, thrombosis, or thromboembolic disorders associated with previous estrogen use (except when used in treatment of breast or prostatic malignancy)

WARNINGS

1. Induction of Malignant Neoplasms: Long-term continuous administration of natural and synthetic estrogens in certain animal species increases the frequency of carcinomas of the breast, cervix, vagina, and liver. There is now evidence that estrogens increase the risk of carcinoma of the endometrium in humans. (See Boxed *"Warning"*.)

At the present time, there is no satisfactory evidence that estrogens given to postmenopausal women increase the risk of cancer of the breast,[18] although a recent long-term follow up of a single physician's practice has raised this possibility.[18a] Because of the animal data, there is a need for caution in prescribing estrogens for women with a strong family history of breast cancer or who have breast nodules, fibrocystic disease, or abnormal mammograms.

2. Gallbladder Disease: A recent study has reported a 2- to 3-fold increase in the risk of surgically confirmed gallbladder disease in women receiving postmenopausal estrogens,[18] similar to the 2-fold increase previously noted in users of oral contraceptives.[19-24] In the case of oral contraceptives, the increased risk appeared after two years of use.[24]

3. Effects Similar to Those Caused by Estrogen-Progestogen Oral Contraceptives: There are several serious adverse effects of oral contraceptives, most of which have not, up to now, been documented as consequences of postmenopausal estrogen therapy. This may reflect the comparatively low doses of estrogen used in postmenopausal women. It would be expected that the larger doses of estrogen used to treat prostatic or breast cancer or postpartum breast engorgement are more likely to result in these adverse effects, and, in fact, it has been shown that there is an increased risk of thrombosis in men receiving estrogens for prostatic cancer and women for postpartum breast engorgement.[20-23]

a. Thromboembolic Disease: It is now well established that users of oral contraceptives have an increased risk of various thromboembolic and thrombotic vascular diseases, such as thrombophlebitis, pulmonary embolism, stroke, and myocardial infarction.[24-31] Cases of retinal thrombosis, mesenteric thrombosis, and optic neuritis have been reported in oral contraceptive users. There is evidence that the risk of several of these adverse reactions is related to the dose of the drug.[32,33] An increased risk of postsurgery thromboembolic complications has also been reported in users of oral contraceptives.[34,35] If feasible, estrogen should be discontinued at least 4 weeks before surgery of the type associated with an increased risk of thromboembolism, or during periods of prolonged immobilization.

While an increased rate of thromboembolic and thrombotic disease in postmenopausal users of estrogens has not been found,[18,36] this does not rule out the possibility that such an increase may be present or that subgroups of women who have underlying risk factors or who are receiving relatively large doses of estrogens may have increased risk. Therefore, estrogens should not be used in persons with active thrombophlebitis or thromboembolic disorders, and they should not be used (except in treatment of malignancy) in persons with a history of such disorders in association with estrogen use. They should be used with caution in patients with cerebral vascular or coronary artery disease and only for those in whom estrogens are clearly needed.

Large doses of estrogen (5 mg conjugated estrogens per day), comparable to those used to treat cancer of the prostate and breast, have been shown in a large prospective clinical trial in men[37] to increase the risk of nonfatal myocardial infarction, pulmonary embolism, and thrombophlebitis. When estrogen doses of this size are used, any of the thromboembolic and thrombotic adverse effects associated with oral contraceptive use should be considered a clear risk.

b. Hepatic Adenoma: Benign hepatic adenomas appear to be associated with the use of oral contraceptives.[38-40] Although benign, and rare, these may rupture and may cause death through intra-abdominal hemorrhage. Such lesions have not yet been reported in association with other estrogen or progestogen preparations but should be considered in estrogen users having abdominal pain and tenderness, abdominal mass, or hypovolemic shock. Hepatocellular carcinoma has also been reported in women taking estrogen-containing oral contraceptives.[39] The relationship of this malignancy to these drugs is not known at this time.

c. Elevated Blood Pressure: Increased blood pressure is not uncommon in women using oral contraceptives. There is now a report that this may, occur with use of estrogens in the menopause[11] and blood pressure should be monitored with estrogen use, especially if high doses are used.

d. Glucose Tolerance: A worsening of glucose tolerance has been observed in a significant percentage of patients on estrogen-containing oral contraceptives. For this reason, diabetic patients should be carefully observed while receiving estrogen.

4. Hypercalcemia: Administration of estrogens may lead to severe hypercalcemia in patients with breast cancer and bone metastases. If this occurs, the drug should be stopped and appropriate measures taken to reduce the serum calcium level.

PRECAUTIONS

A. GENERAL PRECAUTIONS

1. A complete medical and family history should be taken prior to the initiation of any estrogen therapy. The pretreatment and periodic physical examinations should include special reference to blood pressure, abdomen, and pelvic organs, and should include a Papanicolaou smear. As a general rule, estrogen should not be prescribed for longer than one year without another physical examination being performed.

2. Fluid retention—Because estrogens may cause some degree of fluid retention, conditions which might be influenced by this factor, such as epilepsy, migraine, and cardiac or renal dysfunction, require careful observation.

3. Certain patients may develop undesirable manifestations of excessive estrogenic stimulation, such as abnormal or excessive uterine bleeding, mastodynia, etc.

4. Oral contraceptives appear to be associated with an increased incidence of mental depression.[24] Although it is not clear whether this is due to the estrogenic or progestogenic component of the contraceptive, patients with a history of depression should be carefully observed.

5. Preexisting uterine leiomyomata may increase in size during estrogen use.

6. The pathologist should be advised of estrogen therapy when relevant specimens are submitted.

7. Patients with a past history of jaundice during pregnancy have an increased risk of recurrence of jaundice while receiving estrogen-containing oral contraceptive therapy. If jaundice develops in any patient receiving estrogen, the medication should be discontinued while the cause is investigated.

8. Estrogens may be poorly metabolized in patients with impaired liver function and they should be administered with caution in such patients.

9. Because estrogens influence the metabolism of calcium and phosphorus, they should be used with caution in patients with metabolic bone diseases that are associated with hypercalcemia or in patients with renal insufficiency.

10. Because of the effects of estrogens on epiphyseal closure, they should be used judiciously in young patients in whom bone growth is not complete.

11. Certain endocrine and liver function tests may be affected by estrogen-containing oral contraceptives. The following similar changes may be expected with larger doses of estrogen:

a. Increased sulfobromophthalein retention.

b. Increased prothrombin and factors VII, VIII, IX, and X; decreased antithrombin 3; increased norepinephrine-induced platelet aggregability.

c. Increased thyroid binding globulin (TBG) leading to increased circulating total thyroid hormone, as measured by PHI, T4 by column, or T4 by radioimmunoassay. Free T3 resin uptake is decreased, reflecting the elevated TBG; free T4 concentration is unaltered.

d. Impaired glucose tolerance.

e. Decreased pregnanediol excretion.

f. Reduced response to metyrapone test.

g. Reduced serum folate concentration.

h. Increased serum triglyceride and phospholipid concentration.

B. CONCOMITANT PROGESTIN USE

The lowest effective dose appropriate for the specific indication should be utilized. Studies of the addition of a progestin for seven or more days of a cycle of estrogen administration have reported a lowered incidence of endometrial hyperplasia. Morphological and biochemical studies of endometrium suggest that 10 to 13 days of progestin are needed to provide maximal maturation of the endometrium and to eliminate any hyperplastic changes. Whether this will provide protection from endometrial carcinoma has not been clearly established. There are possible additional risks which may be associated with the inclusion of progestin in estrogen replacement regimens. The potential risks include adverse effects on carbohydrate and lipid metabolism. The choice of progestin and dosage may be important in minimizing these adverse effects.

C. INFORMATION FOR THE PATIENTS
See text of *"Patient Package Insert".*

D. PREGNANCY
See *"Contraindications"* and Boxed *"Warning".*

E. NURSING MOTHERS
As a general principle, the administration of any drug to nursing mothers should be done only when clearly necessary because many drugs are excreted in human milk.

ADVERSE REACTIONS
(See *"Warnings"* regarding induction of neoplasia, adverse effects on the fetus, increased incidence of gallbladder disease, and adverse effects similar to those of oral contraceptives, including thromboembolism.) The following additional adverse reactions have been reported with estrogenic therapy, including oral contraceptives:

1. Genitourinary system:
Breakthrough bleeding, spotting, change in menstrual flow
Dysmenorrhea
Premenstrual-like syndrome
Amenorrhea during and after treatment
Increase in size of uterine fibromyomata
Vaginal candidiasis
Change in cervical eversion and in degree of cervical secretion
Cystitis-like syndrome

2. Breasts:
Tenderness, enlargement, secretion

3. Gastrointestinal:
Nausea, vomiting
Abdominal cramps, bloating
Cholestatic jaundice

4. Skin:
Chloasma or melasma which may persist when drug is discontinued
Erythema multiforme
Erythema nodosum
Hemorrhagic eruption
Loss of scalp hair
Hirsutism

5. Eyes:
Steepening of corneal curvature
Intolerance to contact lenses

6. CNS:
Headache, migraine, dizziness
Mental depression
Chorea

7. Miscellaneous:
Increase or decrease in weight
Reduced carbohydrate tolerance
Aggravation of porphyria
Edema
Changes in libido

ACUTE OVERDOSAGE
Numerous reports of ingestion of large doses of estrogen-containing oral contraceptives by young children indicate that serious ill effects do not occur. Overdosage of estrogen may cause nausea, and withdrawal bleeding may occur in females.

DOSAGE AND ADMINISTRATION
For treatment of moderate to severe vasomotor symptoms associated with the menopause, and for atrophic vaginitis, kraurosis vulvae, female hypogonadism, female castration, and primary ovarian failure.

One Quinestrol 100-mcg tablet once daily for seven days, followed by one 100-mcg tablet weekly as a maintenance schedule, commencing two weeks after inception of treatment. The dosage may be increased to 200 mcg weekly if the therapeutic response is not that which may be desirable or considered optimal.

The lowest maintenance dose that will control symptoms should be chosen and medication should be discontinued as promptly as possible.

Attempts to discontinue or taper medication should be made at three- to six-month intervals.

Treated patients with an intact uterus should be monitored closely for signs of endometrial cancer and appropriate diagnostic measures should be taken to rule out malignancy in the event of persistent or recurring abnormal vaginal bleeding.

Store between 15°-30°C (59°-86°F).

PHYSICIAN REFERENCES
1. Ziel, H.K. and W.D. Finkle, "Increased Risk of Endometrial Carcinoma Among Users of Conjugated Estrogens." *New England Journal of Medicine,* 293:1167-1170,

---

◆ RATED THERAPEUTICALLY EQUIVALENT; ◇ THERAPEUTIC EQUIVALENCE UNCONFIRMED; ○ UNRATED

1975. 2. Smith, D.C., R. Prentic, D.J. Thompson, and W.L. Hermann, "Association of Exogenous Estrogen and Endometrial Carcinoma." *New England Journal of Medicine*, 293:1164-1167, 1975. 3. Mack, T.M., M.C. Pike, B.E. Henderson, R.I. Pfeffer, V.R. Gerkins, M. Arthur, and S.E. Brown, "Estrogens and Endometrial Cancer in a Retirement Community." *New England Journal of Medicine*, 294:1262-1267, 1976. 4. Weiss, N.D., D.R. Szekely and D.F. Austin, "Increasing Incidence of Endometrial Cancer in the United States." *New England Journal of Medicine*, 294:1259-1262, 1976. 5. Herbst, A.L., H. Ulfelder and D.C. Poskanzer, "Adenocarcinoma of Vagina." *New England Journal of Medicine*, 284:878-881, 1971. 6. Greenwald, P., J. Barlow, P. Nasca, and W. Burnett, "Vaginal Cancer after Maternal Treatment with Synthetic Estrogens." *New England Journal of Medicine*, 285:390-392, 1971. 7. Lanier, A., K. Noller, D. Decker, L. Elveback, and L. Kurland, "Cancer and Stilbestrol, A Follow-Up of 1719 Persons Exposed to Estrogens in *Utero* and Born 1943-1959." *Mayo Clinic Proceedings*, 48:793-799, 1973. 8. Herbst, A., R. Kurman, and R. Scully, "Vaginal and Cervical Abnormalities After Exposure to Stilbestrol in Utero." *Obstetrics and Gynecology*, 40:287-298,1972. 9. Herbst, A., S. Robboy, G. Macdonald, and R. Scully, "The Effects of Local Progesterone on Stilbestrol-Associated Vaginal Adenosis." *American Journal of Obsterics and Gynecology*, 118:607-615, 1974. 10. Herbst, A., D. Poskanzer, S. Robboy, L. Friedlander, and R. Scully, "Prenatal Exposure to Stilbestrol, A Prospective Comparison of Exposed Female Offspring with Unexpected Controls." *New England Journal of Medicine*, 292:334-339, 1975. 11. Stafl. A., R. Mattingly, D. Foley, and W. Fetherston, "Clinical Diagnosis of Vaginal Adenosis." *Obstetrics and Gynecology*, 43:118-128, 1974. 12. Sherman, A.I., M. Goldrath, A. Berlin, V. Vakhariya, F. Banooni, W. Michaels, P. Goodman, S. Brown, "Cervical-Vaginal Adenosis After *In Utero* Exposure to Synthetic Estrogens," *Obstetrics and Gynecology*, 44:531-545, 1974. 13. Gal, I., B. Kirman, and J. Stern. "Hormone Pregnancy Tests and Congenital Malformation," *Nature*, 216:83, 1967. 14. Levy, E.P., A. Cohen, and F.C. Fraser, "Hormone Treatment During Pregnancy and Congenital Heart Defects," *Lancet*, 1:611, 1973. 15. Nora, J. and A. Nora, "Birth Defects and Oral Contraceptives," *Lancet*, 1:941-942, 1973. 16. Janerich, D.T., J.M. Piper, and D.M. Glebatis, "Oral Contraceptives and Congenital Limb-Reduction Defects," *New England Journal of Medicine*, 291:697-700, 1974. 17. "Estrogens for Oral or Parenteral Use," *Federal Register*, 40:8212, 1975. 18. Boston Collaborative Drug Surveillance Program "Surgically Confirmed Gallbladder Disease, Venous Thromboembolism and Breast Tumors in Relation to Post-Menopausal Estrogen Therapy," *New England Journal of Medicine*, 210:15-19, 1974. 18a. Hoover, R., L.A. Gray, Sr., P. Cole, and B. MacMahon, "Menopausal Estrogens and Breast Cancer." *New England Journal of Medicine*, 295:401-405, 1976. 19. Boston Collaborative Drug Surveillance Program, "Oral Contraceptives and Venous Thromboembolic Disease, Surgically Confirmed Gallbladder Disease, and Breast Tumors," *Lancet*, 1:1399-1404, 1973. 20. Daniel, D.G., H. Campbell, and A.C. Turnbull, "Puerperal Thromboembolism and Suppression of Lactation." *Lancet*, 2:287-289, 1967. 21. The Veterans Administration Cooperative Urological Research Group, "Carcinoma of the Prostate: Treatment Comparison," *Journal of Urology*, 98:516-522, 1967. 22. Ballar, J.C., "Thromboembolism and Oestrogen Therapy," *Lancet*, 2,560. 1967. 23. Blackard, C., R. Doe, G. Mellinger, and D. Byar, "Incidence of Cardiovascular Disease and Death in Patients Receiving Diethylstibestrol for Carcinoma of the Prostate," *Cancer*, 26:249-256, 1970. 24. Royal College of General Practitioners, "Oral Contraception and Thromboembolic Disease," *Journal of the Royal College of General Practitioners*, 13, 267-279, 1967. 25. Inman, W.H.W. and M.P. Vessey, "Investigation of Deaths from Pulmonary, Coronary, and Cerebral Thrombosis and Embolism in Women of Child-Bearing Age." *British Medical Journal*, 2:193-199, 1968. 26. Vessey, M.P. and R. Doll, "Investigation of Relation Between Use of Oral Contraceptives and Thromboembolic Disease, A Further Report," *British Medical Journal*, 2:651-657, 1969. 27. Sartwell, P.E., A.T. Masi, F.G. Arthes, G.R. Greene and H.E. Smith, "Thromboembolism and Oral Contraceptives: An Epidemiological Case Control Study." *American Journal of Epidemiology*, 90:365-380, 1969. 28. Collaborative Group for the Study of Stroke in Young Women, "Oral Contraception and Increased Risk of Cerebral Ischemia or Thrombosis," *New England Journal of Medicine*, 288:871-878, 1973. 29. Collaborative Group for the Study of Stroke in Young Women: "Oral Contraceptives and Stroke in Young Women: Associated Risk Factors," 231:718-722, 1975. *Journal of the American Medical Assoc.* 231:718-722, 1975. 30. Mann, J.I. and W.H.W. Inman, "Oral Contraceptives and Death from Myocardial Infarction," *British Medical Journal*, 2:245-248, 1975. 31. Mann, J.I., M.P. Vessey, M. Thorogood, and R. Doll, "Myocardial Infarction in Young Women with Special Reference to Oral Contraceptive Practice," *British Medical Journal*, 2:241-245, 1975. 32. Inman, W.H.W., M.P. Vessey, B. Westerholm, and A. Engelund. "Thromboembolic Disease and the Steroidal Content of Oral Contraceptives," *British Medical Journal*, 2:203-209, 1970. 33. Stolley, P.D., J.A. Tonascia, M.S. Tockman, P.E. Sartwell, A.H. Rutledge, and M.P. Jacobs, "Thrombosis with Low-Estrogen Oral Contraceptives," *American Journal of Epidemiology*, 102:197-208, 1975. 34. Vessey, M.P., R. Doll, A.S. Fairbairn, and G. Glober, "Post-Operative Thromboembolism and the use of the Oral Contraceptives," *British Medical Journal*, 3:123-126, 1970. 35. Greene, G.R. and P.E. Sartwell, "Oral Contraceptive Use in Patients with Thromboembolism Following Surgery, Trauma or Infection," *American Journal of Public Health*, 62:680-685, 1972. 36. Rosenberg, L., M.B. Armstrong and H. Jick "Myocardial Infarction and Estrogen Therapy in Post-menopausal Women," *New England Journal of Medicine*, 294:1256-1259, 1976. 37. Coronary Drug Project Research Group, "The Coronary Drug Project: Initial Findings Leading to Modifications of Its Research Protocol," *Journal of the American Medical Association*, 214:1303-1313, 1970. 38. Baum, J., F. Holtz, J.J. Bookstein, and E.W. Klein, "Possible Association between Benign Hepatomas and Oral Contraceptives," *Lancet*, 2:926-928, 1973. 39. Mays, E.T., W.M. Christopherson, M.M. Mahr, and H.C. Williams, "Hepatic Changes in Young Women Ingesting Contraceptive Steroids, Hepatic Hemorrhage and Primary Hepatic Tumors," *Journal of the American Medical Association*, 235:780-782, 1976. 40. Edmondson, H.A., B. Henderson, and B. Benton, "Liver Cell Adenomas Association with the Use of Oral Contraceptives," *New England Journal of Medicine*, 294:470-472, 1976. 41. Pfeffer, A.I. and S. Van Den Noore, "Estrogen use and Stroke Risk in Post-menopausal Women," *American Journal of Epidemiology*, 103:545-546, 1976.

HOW SUPPLIED

TABLETS: 100 MCG

BRAND/MANUFACTURER	NDC	SIZE	AWP
○ **BRAND**			
ESTROVIS: Parke-Davis	00071-0437-24	100s	$141.70

Quinethazone

DESCRIPTION

Quinethazone is a quinazoline derivative, in which a cyclic carbamyl group replaces the cyclic sulfamyl group present in the thiazide derivatives.

Quinethazone is 7-chloro-2-ethyl-1,2,3,4-tetrahydro-4-oxo-6-quinazolinesulfonamide.

Following is its chemical structure:

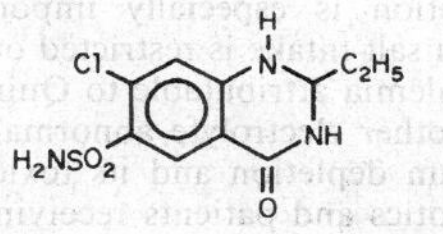

ACTIONS

Quinethazone produces urinary excretion of sodium and chloride in approximately equivalent amounts (saluresis), while potassium is excreted to a much lesser degree. The saluretic effect of Quinethazone is rapid and relatively prolonged, beginning within 2 hours after administration, reaching a peak at 6 hours, and lasting for 18 to 24 hours. While Quinethazone is chemically different, it is pharmacologically genetic to the benzothiadiazine group of drugs.

The dominant action of Quinethazone is to increase the renal excretion of sodium and chloride and an accompanying volume of water. This results from inhibition of the tubular mechanism of electrolyte reabsorption. The renal effect is virtually independent of alterations in acid-base balance. Quinethazone, like other drugs in this class, inhibits the proximal reabsorption of sodium and chloride. The excretion of potassium results from increased potassium secretion by the distal tubule where potassium is exchanged for sodium. Quinethazone may exert its antihypertensive effect by diuresis and sodium loss and/or on vascular function to reduce peripheral resistance.

INDICATIONS

Quinethazone, a nonmercurial oral diuretic agent, is indicated as adjunctive therapy in edema associated with congestive heart failure, hepatic cirrhosis and corticosteroid and estrogen therapy.

Quinethazone has also been found useful in edema due to various forms of renal dysfunction such as: nephrotic syndrome; acute glomerulonephritis; and chronic renal failure. Quinethazone is indicated in the management of hypertension either as the sole therapeutic agent or to enhance the effectiveness of other antihypertensive drugs in the more severe forms of hypertension.

Usage in Pregnancy: The routine use of diuretics in an otherwise healthy woman is inappropriate and exposes mother and fetus to unnecessary hazard. Diuretics do not prevent development of toxemia of pregnancy, and there is no satisfactory evidence that they are useful in the treatment of developed toxemia.

Edema during pregnancy may arise from pathological causes or from the physiologic and mechanical consequences of pregnancy. Diuretics are indicated in pregnancy when edema is due to pathologic causes, just as they are in the absence of pregnancy (however, see *"Warnings,"* below). Dependent edema in pregnancy, resulting from restriction of venous return by the expanded uterus, is properly treated through elevation of the lower extremities and use of support hose; use of diuretics to lower intravascular volume in this case is illogical and unnecessary. There is hypervolemia during normal pregnancy which is harmful to neither the fetus nor the mother (in the absence of cardiovascular disease), but which is associated with edema, including generalized edema, in the majority of pregnant women. If this edema produces discomfort, increased recumbency will often provide relief. In rare instances, this edema may cause extreme discomfort which is not relieved by rest. In these cases, a short course of diuretics may provide relief and may be appropriate.

CONTRAINDICATIONS

A. Anuria.

B. Hypersensitivity to this or other sulfonamide derived drugs.

WARNINGS

Diuretics should be used with caution in severe renal disease. In patients with renal disease, diuretics may precipitate azotemia. Cumulative effects of the drug may develop in patients with impaired renal function.

Diuretics should be used with caution in patients with impaired hepatic function or progressive liver disease, since minor alterations of fluid and electrolyte balance may precipitate hepatic coma.

Quinethazone may add to or potentiate the action of other antihypertensive drugs. Potentiation occurs with ganglionic or peripheral adrenergic blocking drugs.

Sensitivity reactions may occur in patients with a history of allergy or bronchial asthma.

The possibility of exacerbation or activation of systemic lupus erythematosus has been reported.

Usage in Pregnancy: Quinethazone crosses the placental barrier and appears in cord blood. The use of Quinethazone in pregnant women requires that the anticipated benefit be weighed against possible hazards to the fetus. These hazards include fetal or neonatal jaundice, thrombocytopenia, and possible other adverse reactions which have occurred in the adult.

➤ SHOWN IN PRODUCT IDENTIFICATION GUIDE

Nursing Mothers: Quinethazone appears in breast milk. If use of the drug is deemed essential, the patient should stop nursing.

PRECAUTIONS

(1) Quinethazone should be used with caution in patients with impaired hepatic function or progressive liver disease, since minor alterations of fluid and electrolyte balance may precipitate hepatic coma.

(2) Whereas electrolyte abnormalities are often present in such conditions as heart failure and cirrhosis as a result of underlying disease process, they may also be aggravated or may be produced independently by any potent diuretic affecting electrolyte excretion. Caution is especially important during prolonged or intensive therapy and when salt intake is restricted or during concomitant use of steroids or ACTH. Hypokalemia attributable to Quinethazone therapy has been mild and infrequent, and other electrolyte abnormalities have been rare.

The possibility of potassium depletion and its toxic sequelae must be kept in mind, particularly in cirrhotics and patients receiving digitalis. As a preventive measure the use of foods rich in potassium, such as orange juice, or supplements of potassium chloride may be desirable.

(3) In patients with impaired renal function, azotemia and/or excessive drug accumulation may develop.

(4) As with other potent diuretics, when Quinethazone is added to a regimen that includes ganglionic-blocking agents, the dosage of these latter preparations should be reduced to avoid a sudden drop in blood pressure. Reduction of dosage is also necessary when one or more of these antihypertensive agents is added to an established Quinethazone regimen.

(5) As with the thiazide diuretics, increases of serum uric acid may occur but precipitation of gout has been rare.

(6) A decreased glucose tolerance as evidenced by hyperglycemia and glycosuria thus aggravating or provoking diabetes mellitus has occurred.

(7) Quinethazone may decrease arterial responsiveness to norepinephrine and therefore should be withdrawn 48 hours before elective surgery. If emergency surgery is indicated, preanesthetic and anesthetic agents should be administered in reduced dosage. Quinethazone may also increase the responsiveness to tubocurarine. The antihypertensive effects of the drug may be enhanced in the postsympathectomy patient.

(8) Sensitivity reactions may be more likely to occur in patients with a history of allergy or bronchial asthma.

(9) The possibility of exacerbation or activation of systemic lupus erythematosus has been suggested for sulfonamide derived drugs.

ADVERSE REACTIONS

The following adverse reactions have been reported with the diuretic drugs, some of which may be expected to occur with Quinethazone:

A. Gastrointestinal System Reactions
1. anorexia
2. gastric irritation
3. nausea
4. vomiting
5. cramping
6. diarrhea
7. constipation
8. jaundice (intrahepatic cholestatic jaundice)
9. pancreatitis
10. hyperglycemia
11. glycosuria

B. Central Nervous System Reactions
1. dizziness
2. vertigo
3. paresthesias
4. headache
5. xanthopsia

C. Hematologic Reactions
1. leukopenia
2. thrombocytopenia
3. agranulocytosis
4. aplastic anemia

D. Dermatologic—Hypersensitivity Reactions
1. purpura
2. photosensitivity
3. rash
4. urticaria
5. necrotizing angiitis (vasculitis) (cutaneous vasculitis)

E. Cardiovascular Reactions
1. orthostatic hypotension may occur and may be potentiated by alcohol, barbiturates, or narcotics

F. Miscellaneous
1. muscle spasm
2. weakness
3. restlessness

Whenever adverse reactions are moderate or severe, thiazide dosage should be reduced or therapy withdrawn.

DOSAGE AND ADMINISTRATION

Average Adult Dosage: One or two 50 mg tablets, orally, once a day. Because of its relatively prolonged duration of activity, a single daily dose is generally sufficient. Occasionally, one tablet (50 mg) is administered twice a day. Infrequently, a total daily dose of three to four tablets (150 to 200 mg) may be necessary. The dosage employed depends upon the severity of the condition being treated and the responsiveness of the patient, and often must be adjusted at the beginning or during the course of therapy. When Quinethazone is used in combination with other antihypertensive agents, the dosage of each drug may often be reduced because of potentiation. (See under "Precautions" concerning the necessity for dosage adjustment when one or more of these drugs is added to an already established therapeutic regime.)

Store at controlled room temperature, 15°-30°C (59°-86°F).

HOW SUPPLIED

Current prices are unavailable. Check wholesaler for further information.

Quinidex Extentabs *SEE* QUINIDINE SULFATE

Quinidine Gluconate

DESCRIPTION

Each Quinidine Gluconate sustained-release tablet contains 324 mg Quinidine Gluconate (equivalent to 202 mg Quinidine base) in a tablet matrix specially designed for the sustained-release (8 to 12 hours) of the drug in the gastrointestinal tract. Quinidine Gluconate Sustained Release Tablets are to be administered orally.

Quinidine Gluconate is the Gluconate salt of Quinidine [6-methoxy-α-(5-vinyl-2-quinuclidinyl)-4-quinoline-methanol], a dextrorotatory isomer of quinine.

Quinidine Gluconate contains 62.3% of the anhydrous quinidine alkaloid, whereas quinidine sulfate contains 82.86%. In prescribing Quinidine Gluconate Sustained Release Tablets, this factor should be considered.

Therapeutic category: Type I antiarrhythmic.

Following is its chemical structure:

CLINICAL PHARMACOLOGY

The antiarrhythmic activity consists of the following basic actions:

1. In arrhythmias due to enhanced automaticity, Quinidine decreases the rate of rise of slow diastolic (Phase 4) depolarization, thereby depressing automaticity, particularly in ectopic foci.

2. In addition to the above, Quinidine slows depolarization, repolarization and amplitude of the action potential, thus increasing its duration leading to an increase in the refractoriness of atrial and ventricular tissue. Prolongation of the effective refractory period and an increase in conduction time may prevent the reentry phenomenon.

3. Quinidine exerts an indirect anticholinergic effect through blockade of vagal innervation. This anticholinergic effect may facilitate conduction in the atrioventricular junction.

Quinidine absorption from Quinidine Gluconate Sustained Release Tablets proceeds at a slower rate than the immediate-release products. In a single-dose pharmacokinetic study conducted in normal volunteers, the time of peak Quinidine serum concentration was 1.6 hours for Quinidine sulfate tablets and 3.6 hours for Quinidine Gluconate Sustained Release Tablets.

The apparent elimination half-life of Quinidine ranges from 4 to 10 hours in healthy persons with a usual mean value of 6 to 7 hours. The half-life may be prolonged in elderly persons. From 60% to 80% of the dose is metabolized by the liver. Renal excretion of the intact drug comprises the remainder of the total clearance. Quinidine is approximately 75% bound to serum proteins.

In the past, plasma levels of 1.5 to 5 µg/mL have been reported as therapeutic, based on nonspecific assay methodology that quantitates Quinidine metabolites as well as intact Quinidine. The therapeutic plasma level range using newer, more specific assays has not been definitively established; however, effective reduction of premature ventricular contractions has been reported with blood levels less than 1.0 µg/mL. In general, plasma Quinidine levels are lower using specific assays. Clinicians requesting serum Quinidine determinations should therefore also ask that the method of analysis be specified.

◆ RATED THERAPEUTICALLY EQUIVALENT; ◇ THERAPEUTIC EQUIVALENCE UNCONFIRMED; ○ UNRATED

Due to the wide individual variation in response to Quinidine therapy, the usefulness of serum Quinidine levels in the planning of optimal Quinidine therapy has not been clearly established. A serum Quinidine concentration within the reported therapeutic range may not necessarily be the optimal concentration for some patients. In the absence of toxicity, such patients may warrant an increase in dose to achieve the desired therapeutic effect. However, for those patients in whom a high blood level has been achieved without significant therapeutic response, increasing the dose to potentially toxic levels is not warranted and consideration should be given to combination or alternate therapy. In all cases, the physician should carefully consider the patient response and evidence of toxicity along with blood levels in determining optimal Quinidine therapy.

INDICATIONS AND USAGE
Quinidine Gluconate Sustained Release Tablets are indicated in the prevention and/or treatment of:

1. *Ventricular arrhythmias:* Premature ventricular contractions
Ventricular tachycardia (when not associated with complete heartblock)

2. *Junctional (nodal) arrhythmias:* AV junctional premature complexes
Paroxysmal junctional tachycardia

3. *Supraventricular (atrial) arrhythmias:* Premature atrial contractions
Paroxysmal atrial tachycardia
Atrial flutter
Atrial fibrillation (chronic and paroxysmal)

CONTRAINDICATIONS
1. Idiosyncrasy or hypersensitivity to Quinidine.
2. Complete AV block.
3. Complete bundle branch block or other severe intraventricular conduction defects, especially those exhibiting a marked grade of QRS widening.
4. Digitalis intoxication manifested by AV conduction disorders.
5. Myasthenia gravis.
6. Aberrant impulses and abnormal rhythms due to escape mechanisms.

WARNINGS
1. In the treatment of atrial flutter, reversion to sinus rhythm may be preceded by a progressive reduction in the degree of AV block to a 1:1 ratio resulting in an extremely rapid ventricular rate. This possible hazard may be reduced by digitalization prior to administration of Quinidine.
2. Recent reports indicate that plasma concentrations of digoxin increase and may even double when Quinidine is administered concurrently. Patients on concomitant therapy should be carefully monitored. Reduction of digoxin dosage may have to be considered.
3. Manifestations of Quinidine cardiotoxicity such as excessive prolongation of the QT interval, widening of the QRS complex and ventricular tachyarrhythmias mandate immediate discontinuation of the drug and/or close clinical and electrocardiographic monitoring.
4. In susceptible individuals, such as those with marginally compensated cardiovascular disease, Quinidine may produce clinically important depression of cardiac function such as hypotension, bradycardia, or heartblock. Quinidine therapy should be carefully monitored in such individuals.
5. Quinidine should be used with extreme caution in patients with incomplete AV block since complete block and asystole may be produced. Quinidine may cause abnormalities of cardiac rhythm in digitalized patients and therefore should be used with caution in the presence of digitalis intoxication.
6. Quinidine should be used with caution in patients exhibiting renal, cardiac or hepatic insufficiency because of potential accumulation of Quinidine in plasma leading to toxicity.
7. Patients taking Quinidine occasionally have syncopal episodes, usually resulting from ventricular tachycardia or fibrillation. This syndrome has not been shown to be related to dose or plasma levels. Syncopal episodes frequently terminate spontaneously or in response to treatment, but sometimes are fatal.
8. A few cases of hepatotoxicity, including granulomatous hepatitis, due to Quinidine hypersensitivity have been reported in patients taking Quinidine. Unexplained fever and/or elevation of hepatic enzymes, particularly in the early stages of therapy, warrant consideration of possible hepatotoxicity. Monitoring liver function during the first 4 to 8 weeks should be considered. Cessation of Quinidine in these cases usually results in the disappearance of toxicity.

PRECAUTIONS
General: The precautions to be observed include all those applicable to Quinidine. A preliminary test dose of a single tablet of Quinidine sulfate may be administered to determine if the patient has an idiosyncrasy to Quinidine. Hypersensitivity to Quinidine, although rare, should constantly be considered, especially during the first weeks of therapy.

Hospitalization for close clinical observation, electrocardiographic monitoring, and possible determination of plasma Quinidine levels is indicated when large doses are used, or with patients who present an increased risk.

Information for Patients: As with all solid oral dosage medications Quinidine Glucomate Sustained Release Tablets should be taken with an adequate amount of fluid, preferably in an upright position, to facilitate swallowing.

Drug Interactions:

Drug	Effect
Quinidine with anticholinergic drugs	Additive vagolytic effect
Quinidine with cholinergic drugs	Antagonism of cholinergic effects
Quinidine with carbonic anhydrase inhibitors, sodium bicarbonate, thiazide diuretics	Alkalinization of urine resulting in decreased excretion of quinidine
Quinidine with coumarin anticoagulants	Reduction of clotting factor concentrations
Quinidine with tubocurare, succinylcholine and decamethonium	Potentiation of neuromuscular blockade
Quinidine with phenothiazines and reserpine	Additive cardiac depressive effects
Quinidine with hepatic enzyme-inducing drugs (phenobarbital, phenytoin, rifampin)	Potential for reduction of Quinidine plasma levels
Quinidine with cimetidine	Potential for elevation of Quinidine plasma levels
Quinidine with digoxin	Increased plasma concentrations of digoxin (See "Warnings")

Carcinogenesis, Mutagenesis and Impairment of Fertility: Long-term studies in animals have not been performed to evaluate the carcinogenic potential of Quinidine. There is currently no evidence of Quinidine-induced mutagenesis or impairment of fertility.

Pregnancy: Teratogenic Effects: Pregnancy Category C. Animal reproduction studies have not been conducted with Quinidine. There are no adequate and well controlled studies in pregnant women. Quinidine Gluconate Sustained Release Tablets should be administered to a pregnant woman only if clearly indicated.

Nonteratogenic Effects: Like quinine, Quinidine has been reported to have oxytocic properties. The significance of this property in the clinical setting has not been established.

Nursing Mothers: Because of passage of the drug into breast milk, caution should be exercised when Quinidine Gluconate Sustained Release Tablets are administered to a nursing woman.

Pediatric Use: There are no adequate and well-controlled studies establishing the safety and effectiveness of Quinidine Gluconate Sustained Release Tablets in children.

ADVERSE REACTIONS
Symptoms of cinchonism, ringing in ears, headache, nausea, and/or disturbed vision may appear in sensitive patients after a single dose of the drug.

The most frequently encountered side effects to Quinidine are gastrointestinal in nature. These gastrointestinal effects include nausea, vomiting, abdominal pain, diarrhea, and rarely, esophagitis.

Less frequently encountered adverse reactions:

Cardiovascular: Widening of QRS complex, cardiac asystole, ventricular ectopic beats, idioventricular rhythms including ventricular tachycardia and fibrillation, paradoxical tachycardia, arterial embolism and hypotension.

Hematologic: Acute hemolytic anemia, hypoprothrombinemia, thrombocytopenia (purpura), agranulocytosis.

Central Nervous System: Headache, fever, vertigo, apprehension, excitement, confusion, delirium and syncope, disturbed hearing (tinnitus, decreased auditory acuity), disturbed vision (mydriasis, blurred vision, disturbed color perception, reduced vision field, photophobia, diplopia, night blindness, scotomata), optic neuritis.

Dermatologic: Rash, cutaneous flushing with intense pruritus, urticaria. Photosensitivity has also been reported.

Hypersensitivity Reactions: Angioedema, acute asthmatic episode, vascular collapse, respiratory arrest, hepatotoxicity including granulomatous hepatitis (See "Warnings").

Although rare, there have been reports of lupus erythematosus in patients taking Quinidine.

OVERDOSAGE
If ingestion of Quinidine is recent, gastric lavage, emesis and/or administration of activated charcoal may reduce absorption. Management of overdosage includes symptomatic treatment, ECG and blood pressure monitoring, cardiac pacing if indicated, and acidification of the urine. Artificial respiration and other supportive measures may be required. IV infusion of 1/6 molar sodium lactate reportedly reduces the cardiotoxic effects of Quinidine. Since marked CNS depression may occur even in the presence of convulsions, CNS depressants should not be administered. Hypotension may be treated, if necessary, with metaraminol or norepinephrine after adequate fluid volume replacement. Hemo-

dialysis has been reported to be effective in the treatment of Quinidine overdosage in adults and children, but is rarely warranted.

DOSAGE AND ADMINISTRATION

The dosage varies considerably depending upon the general condition and cardiovascular state of the patient. The quantity and frequency of administration of Quinidine Gluconate Sustained Release Tablets that will achieve the desired clinical results must be determined for each patient.

The ideal dosage is the minimum amount of total dose and frequency of daily administration that will prevent premature contractions, paroxysmal tachycardias and maintain normal sinus rhythm.

Prevention of premature atrial, nodal or ventricular contractions: 1 to 2 tablets every 8 or 12 hours.

Maintenance of normal sinus rhythm following conversion of paroxysmal tachycardias: 2 tablets every 12 hours or 1 1/2 to 2 tablets every 8 hours are usually required.

Although most patients may be maintained in normal rhythm on a dosage of 1 Quinidine Gluconate Sustained Release. Tablet every 8 or 12 hours, other patients may require larger doses or more frequent administration (ie every 6 hours) than the usually recommended schedule. Such increased dosage should be instituted only after careful clinical and laboratory evaluation of the patient, including monitoring of plasma Quinidine levels and, if possible, serial electrocardiograms.

Quinidine Gluconate Sustained Release Tablets are generally well tolerated. Gastrointestinal disturbances, if they occur, may be minimized by administering the drug with food.

It is frequently desirable to determine if a patient can tolerate maintenance Quinidine therapy prior to electrical conversion. Therefore, maintenance therapy may be initiated 2 to 3 days before electrical conversion is attempted.

Quinidine Gluconate Sustained Release Tablets are well suited for such a program and can be administered at a maintenance dose felt necessary for a given patient as indicated above.

Note: Dosage may be titrated by breaking the tablet in half. Do not crush or chew since sustained-release properties will be lost.

Store at controlled room temperature, between 15° and 30°C (59° and 86°F).

HOW SUPPLIED
TABLET, EXTENDED RELEASE: 324 MG

AVERAGE UNIT PRICE (AVAILABLE SIZES)		GENERIC A-RATED AVERAGE PRICE (GAAP)	
BRAND	$0.51	100s	$33.85
GENERIC	$0.30	250s	$64.73
HCFA FUL (100s ea)	$0.16	500s	$127.19

BRAND/MANUFACTURER	NDC	SIZE	AWP
◆ **BRAND**			
QUINAGLUTE DURA-TABS: Berlex Labs	50419-0101-10	100s	$52.20
	50419-0101-11	100s ud	$54.55
	50419-0101-25	250s	$126.75
	50419-0101-50	500s	$238.55
◆ **GENERICS**			
Rugby	00536-4434-01	100s	$24.68
Goldline	00182-1382-01	100s	$25.15
Geneva	00781-1804-01	100s	$27.35
QUIN-RELEASE: Major	00904-2202-60	100s	$27.50
Schein	00364-0604-01	100s	$27.75
Caremark	00339-5327-12	100s	$28.10
Qualitest	00603-5598-21	100s	$28.96
URL	00677-0675-01	100s	$29.00
Aligen	00405-4910-01	100s	$29.00
Mutual	53489-0141-01	100s	$29.00
Parmed	00349-7040-01	100s	$30.82
Moore,H.L.	00839-6473-06	100s	$34.63
Raway	00686-0027-20	100s ud	$29.00
Schein	00364-0604-90	100s ud	$37.95
Auro	55829-0461-10	100s ud	$41.48
Vangard	00615-1583-13	100s ud	$43.02
QUIN-RELEASE: Major	00904-2202-61	100s ud	$45.81
Geneva	00781-1804-13	100s ud	$45.81
UDL	51079-0027-20	100s ud	$45.99
Medirex	57480-0388-01	100s ud	$45.99
Rugby	00536-4434-02	250s	$57.38
Goldline	00182-1382-02	250s	$57.45
Schein	00364-0604-04	250s	$57.50
Aligen	00405-4910-04	250s	$57.94
QUIN-RELEASE: Major	00904-2202-70	250s	$61.85
Moore,H.L.	00839-6473-09	250s	$65.19
Geneva	00781-1804-25	250s	$70.95
URL	00677-0675-03	250s	$72.10
Mutual	53489-0141-03	250s	$72.10
Parmed	00349-7040-25	250s	$74.85
Rugby	00536-4434-05	500s	$109.35
Goldline	00182-1382-05	500s	$109.40
QUIN-RELEASE: Major	00904-2202-40	500s	$114.50
Schein	00364-0604-05	500s	$114.51
Moore,H.L.	00839-6473-12	500s	$132.96
Geneva	00781-1804-05	500s	$134.95
Qualitest	00603-5598-28	500s	$136.80
URL	00677-0675-05	500s	$137.50
Mutual	53489-0141-05	500s	$137.50

BRAND/MANUFACTURER	NDC	SIZE	AWP
Parmed	00349-7040-05	500s	$144.40
Parmed	00349-7040-10	1000s	$257.60

Quinidine Polygalacturonate

DESCRIPTION

Quinidine Polygalacturonate, an antiarrhythmic, is a polymer of Quinidine and Polygalacturonic acid which occurs as a creamy white, amorphous powder and is sparingly soluble in water, and freely soluble in hot 40% alcohol.

Chemically, Quinidine Polygalacturonate is $C_{20}H_{24}N_2O_2C_6H_{10}O_7 \cdot H_2O$.

Quinidine Polygalacturonate Tablets, for oral administration, contain 275 mg Quinidine Polygalacturonate equivalent in content to 200 mg (3 grains) of quinidine sulfate.

Following is its chemical structure:

ACTIONS

The Quinidine component slows conduction time, prolongs the refractory period, and depresses the excitability of heart muscle. Polygalacturonate slows ionization of the drug and protects the gastrointestinal tract by its demulcent effect.

INDICATIONS

Quinidine Polygalacturonate Tablets are indicated as maintenance therapy after spontaneous and electrical conversion of atrial tachycardia, flutter or fibrillation and in the treatment of:

■ Premature atrial and ventricular contractions.
■ Paroxysmal atrial tachycardia.
■ Paroxysmal A-V junctional rhythm.
■ Atrial flutter.
■ Paroxysmal atrial fibrillation.
■ Established atrial fibrillation when therapy is appropriate.
■ Paroxysmal ventricular tachycardia when not associated with complete heartblock.

CONTRAINDICATIONS

1. History of hypersensitivity to Quinidine manifested by thrombocytopenia, skin eruptions, febrile reactions, etc.
2. Complete A-V block.
3. Complete bundle branch block or other severe intraventricular conduction defects exhibiting marked QRS widening or bizarre complexes.
4. Myasthenia gravis.
5. Arrhythmias associated with digitalis toxicity.

WARNINGS

1. In the treatment of atrial fibrillation with rapid ventricular response, ventricular rate should be controlled with digitalis glycosides *prior* to administration of Quinidine.
2. In the treatment of atrial flutter with Quinidine, reversion to sinus rhythm may be preceded by progressive reduction in the degree of A-V block to a 1:1 ratio resulting in an extremely high ventricular rate. This potential hazard may be reduced by digitalization prior to administration of Quinidine.
Recent reports have described increased, potentially toxic, digoxin plasma levels when Quinidine is administered concurrently. When concurrent use is necessary, digoxin dosage should be reduced and plasma concentration should be monitored and patients observed closely for digitalis intoxication.
3. Quinidine cardiotoxicity may be manifested by increased P-R and Q-T intervals, 50% widening of QRS, and/or ventricular ectopic beats or tachycardia. Appearance of these toxic signs during Quinidine administration mandates immediate discontinuation of the drug and/or close clinical and electrocardiographic monitoring. Note: Quinidine effect is enhanced by potassium and reduced in the presence of hypokalemia.
4. Quinidine syncope may occur as a complication of long-term therapy. It is manifested by sudden loss of consciousness and by ventricular arrhythmias with bizarre QRS complexes. This syndrome does not appear to be related to dose or plasma levels, but occurs more often with prolonged Q-T intervals.
5. Because Quinidine antagonizes the effect of vagal excitation upon the atrium and the A-V node, the administration of parasympathomimetic drugs (choline esters) or the use of any other procedure to enhance vagal activity may fail to terminate paroxysmal supraventricular tachycardia in patients receiving Quinidine.
6. Quinidine should be used with extreme caution in:
a) The presence of incomplete A-V block, since a complete block and asystole may result.
b) Quinidine may cause unpredictable abnormalities of rhythm in digitalized hearts. Therefore, it should be used with caution in the presence of digitalis intoxication (see 2 above).
c) Partial bundle branch block.

◆ RATED THERAPEUTICALLY EQUIVALENT; ◇ THERAPEUTIC EQUIVALENCE UNCONFIRMED; ○ UNRATED

d) Severe congestive heart failure and hypotensive states due to the depressant effects of Quinidine on myocardial contractility and arterial pressure.
e) Poor renal function, especially renal tubular acidosis, because of the potential accumulation of Quinidine in plasma leading to toxic concentrations.

PRECAUTIONS

1. Test Dose: A preliminary test dose of a single tablet of quinidine *sulfate* should be administered prior to the initiation of treatment with Quinidine Polygalacturonate Tablets to determine whether the patient has an idiosyncrasy to the Quinidine molecule.

2. Hypersensitivity: During the first weeks of therapy, hypersensitivity to Quinidine, although rare, should be considered (e.g., angioedema, purpura., acute asthmatic episode, vascular collapse).

3. Long-Term Therapy: Periodic blood counts and liver and kidney function tests should be performed during long-term therapy, and the drug should be discontinued if blood dyscrasias or signs of hepatic or renal disorders occur.

4. Large Doses: ECG monitoring and determination of plasma Quinidine levels are recommended when doses greater than 2.5 g/day are administered.

5. Usage in Pregnancy: The use of Quinidine in pregnancy should be reserved only for those cases where the benefits outweigh the possible hazards to the patient and fetus.

6. Nursing Mothers: The drug should be used with extreme caution in nursing mothers because the drug is excreted in breast milk.

7. General: In patients exhibiting asthma, muscle weakness and infection with fever prior to Quinidine administration, hypersensitivity reactions to the drug may be masked.

DRUG INTERACTIONS

1. Caution should be used when Quinidine and its analogs are administered concurrently with coumarin anticoagulants. This combination may reduce prothrombin levels and cause bleeding.
2. Quinidine, a weak base, may have its half-life prolonged in patients who are concurrently taking drugs that can alkalize the urine, such as thiazide diuretics, sodium bicarbonate, and carbonic anhydrase inhibitors. Quinidine and drugs which alkalize the urine should be used together cautiously.
3. Quinidine exhibits a distinct anticholinergic activity in the myocardial tissues. An additive vagolytic effect may be seen when Quinidine and drugs having anticholinergic blocking activity are used together. Drugs having cholinergic activity may be antagonized by Quinidine.
4. Quinidine and other antiarrhythmic agents may produce additive cardiac depressant effects when administered together.
5. Quinidine interaction with cardiac glycosides (digoxin). See *"Warnings."*
6. Antacids may delay absorption of Quinidine but appear unlikely to cause incomplete absorption.
7. Phenobarbital and phenytoin may reduce plasma half life of Quinidine by 50%.
8. Quinidine may potentiate the neuromuscular blocking effect in ventilatory depression of patients receiving decamethonium, tubocarare or succinylcholine.

ADVERSE REACTIONS

Symptoms of cinchonism (ringing in the ears, headache, disturbed vision) may appear in sensitive patients after a single dose of the drug.

Gastrointestinal: The most common side effects encountered with Quinidine are referable to this system. Diarrhea frequently occurs, but it rarely necessitates withdrawal of the drug. Nausea, vomiting and abdominal pain also occur. Some of these effects may be minimized by administering the drug with meals.

Cardiovascular: Widening of QRS complex, cardiac asystole, ventricular ectopic beats, idioventricular rhythms including ventricular tachycardia and fibrillation; paradoxical tachycardia, arterial embolism, and hypotension.

Hematologic: Acute hemolytic anemia, hypoprothrombinemia, thrombocytopenic purpura, agranulocytosis.

CNS: Headache, fever, vertigo, apprehension, excitement, confusion, delirium, and syncope, disturbed hearing (tinnitus, decreased auditory acuity), disturbed vision (mydriasis, blurred vision, disturbed color perception, photophobia, diplopia, night blindness, scotomata), optic neuritis.

Dermatologic: Cutaneous flushing with intense pruritus.

Hypersensitivity Reactions: Angioedema, acute asthmatic episode, vascular collapse, respiratory arrest, hepatic dysfunction.

OVERDOSAGE

Cardiotoxic effects of Quinidine may be reversed in part by molar sodium lactate; the hypotension may be reversed by vasoconstrictors and by catecholamines (since vasodilation is partly due to alpha-adrenergic blockage).

DOSAGE AND ADMINISTRATION

Each tablet contains 275 mg Quinidine Polygalacturonate, equivalent to a 3-grain tablet of quinidine sulfate. Dosage must be adjusted to individual patient's needs, both for conversion and maintenance. An initial dose of 1 to 3 tablets may be used to terminate arrhythmia, and may be repeated in 3-4 hours. If normal sinus rhythm is not restored after 3 or 4 equal doses, the dose may be increased by 1/2 to 1 tablet (137.5 to 275 mg) and administered three to four times before any further dosage increase. For maintenance, one tablet may be used two or three times a day.

Store tablets at controlled room temperature 15° to 30°C (59°-86°F).

OVERDOSAGE

Cardiotoxic effects of Quinidine may be reversed in part by molar sodium lactate; the hypotension may be reversed by vasoconstrictors and by catecholamines (since vasodilation is partly due to alpha-adrenergic blockage).

HOW SUPPLIED
TABLETS:

BRAND/MANUFACTURER	NDC	SIZE	AWP
○ **BRAND**			
CARDIOQUIN: Purdue Frederick	00034-5470-80	100s	$96.35
	00034-5470-90	500s	$460.23

Quinidine Sulfate

DESCRIPTION

Quinidine Sulfate extended-release tablets are constructed to release one-third of their alkaloidal salt, Quinidine Sulfate (100 mg), on reaching the stomach, to begin absorption in the upper intestinal tract. The remaining two-thirds of the active drug (200 mg) is evenly distributed throughout a homogeneous core which slowly dissolves as it moves along the intestinal tract, releasing the Quinidine Sulfate for continuous absorption over an 8-12 hour period. Each Quinidine Sulfate tablet contains 300 mg of Quinidine Sulfate, the equivalent of 248.6 mg of the anhydrous Quinidine alkaloid.

Chemically, Quinidine Sulfate is cinchonan-9-ol,6'-methoxy-, (9s)-sulfate(2:1) (salt) dihydrate.

Following is its chemical structure:

ACTION

The action of Quinidine in preventing aberrant cardiac rhythms of atrial and ventricular origin resides in its ability to (a) depress excitability of cardiac muscle, (b) slow the rate of spontaneous rhythm, (c) decrease vagal tone, and (d) prolong conduction and effective refractory period.

INDICATIONS AND USAGE

Quinidine Sulfate is indicated for the treatment of:
- Premature atrial and ventricular contractions.
- Paroxysmal atrial tachycardia.
- Paroxysmal A-V junctional rhythm.
- Atrial flutter.
- Paroxysmal atrial fibrillation.
- Established atrial fibrillation when therapy is appropriate.
- Paroxysmal ventricular tachycardia when not associated with complete heartblock.
- Maintenance therapy after electrical conversion of atrial fibrillation and/or flutter.

CONTRAINDICATIONS

Intraventricular conduction defects. Complete A-V block. A-V conduction disorders caused by digitalis intoxication. Aberrant impulses and abnormal rhythms due to escape mechanisms. Idiosyncrasy or hypersensitivity to quinidine or related cinchona derivatives. Myasthenia gravis.

WARNINGS

In the treatment of atrial flutter, reversion to sinus rhythm may be preceded by a progressive reduction in the degree of A-V block to a 1:1 ratio, resulting in an extremely rapid ventricular rate. This possible hazard may be reduced by digitalization prior to administration of quinidine.

Reports in the literature indicate that serum concentrations of digoxin may increase and may even double when Quinidine is administered concurrently. Patients on concomitant therapy should be carefully monitored for digitalis toxicity. Reduction of digoxin dosage may have to be considered.

Manifestations of Quinidine cardiotoxicity such as excessive prolongation of the QT interval, widening of the QRS complex and ventricular tachyarrhythmias mandate immediate discontinuation of the drug and/or close clinical and electrocardiographic monitoring.

In susceptible individuals, such as those with marginally compensated cardiovascular disease, Quinidine may produce clinically important depression of cardiac function manifested by hypotension, bradycardia, or heartblock. Quinidine therapy should be carefully monitored in such individuals. Quinidine should be used with extreme caution in patients with incomplete AV block since complete AV block and asystole may be produced. Quinidine may cause abnormalities of cardiac rhythm in digitalized patients and therefore should be used with caution in the presence of digitalis intoxication. Quinidine should be used with caution in patients exhibiting renal, cardiac or hepatic insufficiency because of potential accumulation of Quinidine in serum, leading to toxicity.

➤ SHOWN IN PRODUCT IDENTIFICATION GUIDE

Patients taking Quinidine occasionally have syncopal episodes which usually result from ventricular tachycardia or fibrillation. This syndrome has not been shown to be related to dose or serum levels. Syncopal episodes frequently terminate spontaneously or in response to treatment, but sometimes are fatal.

Cases of hepatotoxicity, including granulomatous hepatitis, due to Quinidine hypersensitivity have been reported. Unexplained fever and/or elevation of hepatic enzymes, particularly in the early stages of therapy, warrant consideration of possible hepatotoxicity. Monitoring liver function during the first 4-8 weeks should be considered. Cessation of Quinidine in these cases usually results in the disappearance of toxicity.

PRECAUTIONS
GENERAL
All the precautions applying to regular Quinidine therapy apply to this product. Hypersensitivity or anaphylactoid reactions to Quinidine, although rare, should be considered, especially during the first weeks of therapy. Hospitalization for close clinical observation, electrocardiographic monitoring, and determination of serum quinidine levels are indicated when large doses of Quinidine are used or with patients who present an increased risk.

Information for Patients: As with all solid dosage medications, Quinidine Sulfate should be taken with an adequate amount of fluid, preferably with the patient in an upright position to facilitate swallowing. They should be swallowed whole in order to preserve the controlled-release mechanism.

Laboratory Tests: Periodic blood counts and liver and kidney function tests should be performed during long-term therapy; the drug should be discontinued if blood dyscrasias or evidence of hepatic or renal dysfunction occurs.

Drug Interactions:

Drug	Effect
Quinidine with anticholinergic drugs	Additive vagolytic effect
Quinidine with cholinergic drugs	Antagonism of cholinergic effects
Quinidine with carbonic anhydrase inhibitors, sodium bicarbonate, thiazide diuretics	Alkalinization of urine resulting in decreased excretion of Quinidine
Quinidine with coumarin anticoagulants	Reduction of clotting factor concentrations
Quinidine with tubocurare, succinylcholine, and decamethonium	Potentiation of neuromuscular blockade
Quinidine with phenothiazines and reserpine	Additive cardiac depressive effects
Quinidine with hepatic enzyme-inducing drugs (phenobarbital, phenytoin, rifampin)	Decreased plasma half-life of Quinidine
Quinidine with digoxin	Increased serum concentration of digoxin (See *"Warnings"*)
Quinidine with amiodarone	Increased serum concentration of Quinidine
Quinidine with cimetidine	Prolonged Quinidine half-life and an increase in serum Quinidine level
Quinidine with ranitidine	Premature ventricular contractions and/or bigeminy
Quinidine with verapamil	Increased Quinidine half-life and an increase in serum Quinidine level; potential hypotensive reactions
Quinidine with nifedipine	Decreased serum concentrations of Quinidine

Carcinogenesis: Studies in animals have not been performed to evaluate the carcinogenic potential of Quinidine.

Pregnancy, Teratogenic Effects: Pregnancy Category C. Animal reproduction studies have not been conducted with Quinidine. There are no adequate and well-controlled studies in pregnant women. Quinidine Sulfate should be administered to a pregnant woman only if clearly indicated.

Nonteratogenic Effects: Like quinine, Quinidine has been reported to have oxytocic properties. The significance of this property in the clinical setting has not been established.

Labor and Delivery: There is no known use for Quinidine Sulfate in labor and delivery. However, Quinidine has been reported to have oxytocic properties. The significance of this property in the clinical setting has not been established.

Nursing Mothers: Because of passage of the drug into breast milk, caution should be exercised when Quinidine Sulfate is administered to a nursing woman.

Pediatric Use: There are no adequate and well-controlled studies establishing the safety and effectiveness of Quinidine Sulfate in children.

ADVERSE REACTIONS
Symptoms of cinchonism, such as ringing in the ears, loss of hearing, dizziness, light-headedness, headache, nausea, and/or disturbed vision may appear in sensitive patients after a single dose of the drug. The most frequently encountered side effects to Quinidine are gastrointestinal.

Gastrointestinal: Nausea, vomiting, abdominal pain, diarrhea, anorexia, granulomatous hepatitis (which may be preceded by fever), esophagitis.

Cardiovascular: Ventricular extrasystoles occurring at a rate of one or more every 6 normal beats; widening of the QRS complex and prolonged QT interval; complete A-V block; ventricular tachycardia and fibrillation; ventricular flutter; torsade de pointes; arterial embolism; hypotension; syncope.

Central Nervous System: Headache, vertigo, apprehension, excitement, confusion, delirium, dementia, ataxia, depression.

Ophthalmologic and Otologic: Disturbed hearing (tinnitus, decreased auditory acuity), disturbed vision (mydriasis, blurred vision, disturbed color perception, photophobia, diplopia, night blindness, scotomata), optic neuritis, reduced visual field.

Dermatologic: Cutaneous flushing with intense pruritus, photosensitivity, urticaria, rash, eczema, exfoliative eruptions, psoriasis, abnormalities of pigmentation.

Hypersensitivity: Angioedema, acute asthmatic episode, vascular collapse, respiratory arrest, hepatotoxicity, granulomatous hepatitis (see *"Warnings"*), purpura, vasculitis.

Hematologic: Thrombocytopenia, thrombocytopenic purpura, agranulocytosis, acute hemolytic anemia, hypoprothrombinemia, leukocytosis, shift to left in WBC differential, neutropenia.

Immunologic: Systemic lupus erythematosus, lupus nephritis.

Miscellaneous: Fever, increase in serum skeletal muscle creatine phosphokinase, arthralgia, myalgia.

OVERDOSAGE
Symptoms: Overdosage of Quinidine can lead to accelerated idioventricular rhythm, morphologic appearance of QRS complexes, prolonged QT intervals, intermittent sinus capture beats, paroxysms of tachycardia, ventricular arrhythmias, hypotension, oliguria, respiratory depression, pulmonary edema, acidosis, seizures, and coma.

Treatment: Early treatment to empty the stomach using syrup of ipecac and/or gastric lavage is recommended. Since Quinidine Sulfate cannot be removed through a nasogastric tube, gastric lavage should be followed by saline cathartics. Administration of activated charcoal may reduce absorption. Other general supportive measures should be employed as indicated by patient response. In severe cases, circulation should be stabilized and measurements of pulmonary capillary wedge pressure should be performed to assure adequate left ventricular filling pressure. Electrolyte and blood gas abnormalities should be corrected. In Quinidine-induced vasodilation, catecholamines and other alpha-adrenergic agonists may be tried. Arrhythmias may be treated with lidocaine, pacing, and cardioversion. Administration of sodium lactate reportedly reduces the cardiotoxicity of Quinidine; however, sodium lactate is contraindicated in the presence of alkalosis as increased urinary pH can lead to an increase in the renal tubular absorption of Quinidine. Acidification of the urine may enhance the urinary excretion of Quinidine.

DOSAGE AND ADMINISTRATION
One or two Quinidine Sulfate tablets every 8 to 12 hours as may be required to achieve the desired therapeutic effect.

Store at controlled room temperature, between 15°C and 30°C (59°F and 86°F). Dispense in well-closed, light-resistant container.

HOW SUPPLIED
CAPSULE: 300 MG

BRAND/MANUFACTURER	NDC	SIZE	AWP
◆ **BRAND**			
CIN-QUIN: Solvay	00032-4020-01	100s	$37.38

TABLET, EXTENDED RELEASE: 300 MG

AVERAGE UNIT PRICE (AVAILABLE SIZES)			
GENERIC	$0.64		

BRAND/MANUFACTURER	NDC	SIZE	AWP
◆ **GENERICS**			
Copley	38245-0175-10	100s	$65.30
Copley	38245-0175-25	250s	$156.15

TABLET, EXTENDED RELEASE: 300 MG

BRAND/MANUFACTURER	NDC	SIZE	AWP
○ **BRAND**			
▶ QUINIDEX EXTENTABS: Robins Pharm	00031-6649-63	100s	$74.20
	00031-6649-64	100s ud	$75.81
	00031-6649-67	250s	$177.41

TABLETS: 200 MG

AVERAGE UNIT PRICE (AVAILABLE SIZES)		GENERIC A-RATED AVERAGE PRICE (GAAP)	
BRAND	$0.17	100s	$12.75
GENERIC	$0.11	1000s	$92.96
HCFA FUL (100s ea)	$0.09		

BRAND/MANUFACTURER	NDC	SIZE	AWP
◆ **BRAND**			
CIN-QUIN: Solvay	00032-4028-01	100s	$16.45

◆ RATED THERAPEUTICALLY EQUIVALENT; ◇ THERAPEUTIC EQUIVALENCE UNCONFIRMED; ○ UNRATED

BRAND/MANUFACTURER	NDC	SIZE	AWP
◆ **GENERICS**			
Eon	00185-4346-01	100s	$7.50
Major	00904-2201-60	100s	$9.25
Goldline	00182-0144-01	100s	$10.50
Halsey Pharm	00879-0358-01	100s	$10.50
Lederle Std Prod	00005-3558-23	100s	$11.00
Parmed	00349-2149-01	100s	$11.03
Moore,H.L.	00839-5063-06	100s	$11.27
Rugby	00536-4432-01	100s	$11.30
Schein	00364-0229-01	100s	$11.44
Geneva	00781-1900-01	100s	$11.50
URL	00677-0122-01	100s	$11.65
Mutual	53489-0461-01	100s	$11.65
Aligen	00405-4916-01	100s	$12.56
Purepac	00228-2356-10	100s	$12.56
Richlyn	00115-4380-01	100s	$15.41
UDL	51079-0031-20	100s ud	$12.50
Schein	00364-0229-90	100s ud	$12.98
Vangard	00615-0515-13	100s ud	$14.04
Raway	00686-0031-20	100s ud	$15.00
Roxane	00054-8733-25	100s ud	$17.76
Major	00904-2201-61	100s ud	$17.91
Medirex	57480-0359-01	100s ud	$21.25
Eon	00185-4346-10	1000s	$65.00
Major	00904-2201-80	1000s	$75.75
Schein	00364-0229-02	1000s	$82.29
Mason Dist	11845-0168-04	1000s	$83.93
Purepac	00228-2356-96	1000s	$84.67
Lederle Std Prod	00005-3558-34	1000s	$86.00
Goldline	00182-0144-10	1000s	$86.55
URL	00677-0122-10	1000s	$87.50
Geneva	00781-1900-10	1000s	$87.75
Qualitest	00603-5594-32	1000s	$88.80
Mutual	53489-0461-10	1000s	$89.85
Halsey Pharm	00879-0358-10	1000s	$89.95
Rugby	00536-4432-10	1000s	$91.25
Parmed	00349-2149-10	1000s	$94.10
Aligen	00405-4916-03	1000s	$96.56
Moore,H.L.	00839-5063-16	1000s	$98.96
Richlyn	00115-4380-03	1000s	$118.50
Roxane	00054-4736-31	1000s	$165.79

TABLETS: 300 MG

AVERAGE UNIT PRICE (AVAILABLE SIZES)		GENERIC A-RATED AVERAGE PRICE (GAAP)	
BRAND	$0.28	100s	$21.84
GENERIC	$0.21	1000s	$176.37
HCFA FUL (100s ea)	$0.15		

BRAND/MANUFACTURER	NDC	SIZE	AWP
◆ **BRAND**			
CIN-QUIN: Solvay	00032-4032-01	100s	$27.67
◆ **GENERICS**			
Eon	00185-1047-01	100s	$13.50
Geneva	00781-1902-01	100s	$16.89
Goldline	00182-1724-01	100s	$18.00
Moore,H.L.	00839-6605-06	100s	$18.62
Qualitest	00603-5595-21	100s	$18.70
Schein	00364-0582-01	100s	$19.95
URL	00677-1209-01	100s	$20.00
Mutual	53489-0460-01	100s	$20.00
Rugby	00536-4429-01	100s	$20.10
Major	00904-2203-60	100s	$20.15
Aligen	00405-4917-01	100s	$20.32
Parmed	00349-8278-01	100s	$21.56
QUINORA: Key	00085-0073-01	100s	$31.35
Roxane	00054-4735-25	100s	$32.22
Schein	00364-0582-90	100s ud	$21.50
Geneva	00781-1902-13	100s ud	$22.95
Goldline	00182-1724-89	100s ud	$23.20
Roxane	00054-8735-25	100s ud	$34.16
Eon	00185-1047-10	1000s	$125.00
Mutual	53489-0460-10	1000s	$155.00
Rugby	00536-4429-10	1000s	$166.65
Major	00904-2203-80	1000s	$167.05
Roxane	00054-4735-31	1000s	$268.13

Quinine Sulfate

DESCRIPTION

Quinine Sulfate is available as tablets for oral administration. Each tablet contains 260 mg Quinine Sulfate.

Quinine Sulfate occurs as a white, crystalline powder, which darkens on exposure to light. It is odorless and has a persistent, very bitter taste. It is slightly soluble in water, alcohol, chloroform, and ether.

Following is its chemical structure:

CLINICAL PHARMACOLOGY

Quinine, a cinchona alkaloid, acts on skeletal muscle by three mechanisms: it increases the refractory period by direct action on the muscle fiber, it decreases the excitability of the motor end-plate, an action similar to that of curare, and it affects the distribution of calcium within the muscle fiber. Quinine is readily absorbed when given orally. Absorption occurs mainly from the upper part of the small intestine, and is almost complete even in patients with marked diarrhea. The cinchona alkaloids in large measure are metabolically degraded in the body, especially in the liver; less than 5% of an administered dose is excreted unaltered in the urine. It is reported that there is no accumulation of the drugs in the body upon continued administration. The metabolic degradation products are excreted in the urine, where many of them have been identified as hydroxy derivatives, but small amounts also appear in the feces, gastric juice, bile, and saliva. Renal excretion of Quinine is twice as rapid when the urine is acidic as when it is alkaline, due to the greater tubular reabsorption of the alkaloidal base that occurs in an alkaline media. Excretion is also limited by the binding of a large fraction of cinchona alkaloids to plasma proteins.

Peak plasma concentrations of cinchona alkaloids occur within 1 to 3 hours after a single oral dose. The half-life is 4 to 5 hours. After chronic administration of total daily doses of 1 g of drug, the average plasma quinine concentration is approximately 7µg/ml. After termination of Quinine therapy, the plasma level falls rapidly and only a negligible concentration is detectable after 24 hours.

A large fraction (approximately 70%) of the plasma Quinine is bound to proteins. This explains in part why the concentration of the alkaloid in cerebrospinal fluid is only 2 to 5% of that in the plasma. However, it can traverse the placental membrane and readily reach fetal tissues.

Tinnitus and impairment of hearing rarely should occur at plasma Quinine concentrations of less than 10 µg/ml. While this level would not be anticipated from use of 1 or 2 tablets of Quinine Sulfate daily, an occasional patient may have some evidence of cinchonism on this dosage, such as tinnitus. (See "Warnings" section.)

INDICATIONS AND USAGE

For the prevention and treatment of nocturnal recumbency leg muscle cramps.

Chloroquine-resistant falciparum malaria: Oral Quinine Sulfate should be reserved for treating chloroquine-resistant strains of *P falciparum*. It should be given in conjunction with pyrimethamine, sulfonamide, clindamycin, or tetracycline.

UNLABELED USES

Quinine Sulfate is used as an adjunct with clindamycin in the treatment of babesia microti infections.

CONTRAINDICATIONS

Quinine Sulfate may cause fetal harm when administered to a pregnant woman. Congenital malformations in the human have been reported with the use of Quinine, primarily with large doses (up to 30 g) for attempted abortion. In about half of these reports, the malformation was deafness related to auditory nerve hypoplasia. Among the other abnormalities reported were limb anomalies, visceral defects, and visual changes. In animal tests, teratogenic effects were found in rabbits and guinea pigs and were absent in mice, rats, dogs, and monkeys. Quinine Sulfate is contraindicated in women who are or may become pregnant. If this drug is used during pregnancy, or if the patient becomes pregnant while taking this drug, the patient should be apprised of the potential hazard to the fetus.

Because of the Quinine content, Quinine Sulfate is contraindicated in patients with known Quinine hypersensitivity and in patients with glucose-6-phosphate dehydrogenase (G-6-PD) deficiency.

Since thrombocytopenic purpura may follow the administration of Quinine in highly sensitive patients, a history of this occurrence associated with previous Quinine ingestion contraindicates its further use. Recovery usually occurs following withdrawal of the medication and appropriate therapy. This drug should not be used in patients with tinnitus or optic neuritis or in patients with a history of blackwater fever.

WARNINGS

Repeated doses or overdosage of Quinine in some individuals may precipitate a cluster of symptoms referred to as cinchonism. Such symptoms, in the mildest form, include ringing in the ears, headache, nausea, and slightly disturbed vision; however, when medication is continued or after large single doses, symptoms also involve the gastrointestinal tract, the nervous and cardiovascular systems, and the skin.

Hemolysis (with the potential for hemolytic anemia) has been associated with a G-6-PD deficiency in patients taking Quinine. Quinine Sulfate should be stopped immediately if evidence of hemolysis appears.

If symptoms occur, drug should be discontinued and supportive measures instituted. In case of overdosage, see *"Overdosage"* section of prescribing information.

PRECAUTIONS
GENERAL
Quinine Sulfate should be discontinued if there is any evidence of hypersensitivity. (See *"Contraindications."*) Cutaneous flushing, pruritus, skin rashes, fever, gastric distress, dyspnea, ringing in the ears, and visual impairment are the usual expressions of hypersensitivity, particularly if only small doses of Quinine have been taken. Extreme flushing of the skin accompanied by intense, generalized pruritus is the most common form. Hemoglobinuria and asthma from Quinine are rare types of idiosyncrasy.

In patients with atrial fibrillation, the administration of Quinine requires the same precautions as those for quinidine. (See *"Drug Interactions."*)

DRUG INTERACTIONS
Increased plasma levels of digoxin have been demonstrated in individuals after concomitant Quinine administration. Increased plasma levels of digitoxin have been demonstrated in individuals after concomitant quinidine administration. It is therefore recommended that plasma levels of digoxin or digitoxin be determined periodically for those individuals taking either of these glycosides and Quinine Sulfate concomitantly.

Concurrent use of aluminum-containing antacids may delay or decrease absorption of Quinine.

Cinchona alkaloids, including Quinine, have the potential to depress the hepatic enzyme system that synthesizes the vitamin K-dependent factors. The resulting hypoprothrombinemic effect may enhance the action of warfarin and other oral anticoagulants.

The effects of neuromuscular blocking agents (particularly pancuronium, succinylcholine, and tubocurarine) may be potentiated with Quinine, and result in respiratory difficulties.

Urinary alkalizers (such as acetazolamide and sodium bicarbonate) may increase quinine blood levels with potential for toxicity.

DRUG/LABORATORY INTERACTIONS
Quinine may produce an elevated value for urinary 17-ketogenic steroids when the Zimmerman method is used.

CARCINOGENESIS, MUTAGENESIS, IMPAIRMENT OF FERTILITY
A study of Quinine Sulfate administered in drinking water (0.1%) to rats for periods up to 20 months showed no evidence of neoplastic changes.

Mutation studies of Quinine (dihydrochloride) in male and female mice gave negative results by the micronucleus test. Intraperitoneal injections (0.5 mM/kg) were given twice, 24 hours apart. Direct *Salmonella typhimurium* tests were negative: when mammalian liver homogenate was added, positive results were found.

Mutation studies of Quinine Hydrochloride, 100 mg/kg, p.o. in Chinese hamsters showed no genotoxic activity in the sister chromatid exchange (SCE) test, micronucleus test, or chromosome aberration test. In mice given Quinine Hydrochloride, 100 mg/kg, p.o., the micronucleus test and chromosome aberration test were negative; the SCE test exhibited an increase of SCEs/cell. Tests were repeated in two inbred strains of mice using 55, 75, and 110 mg/kg p.o. The effect was more pronounced in these mice and the increase in SCEs/cell demonstrated a linear dose relationship. One of the inbred strains had positive micronucleus test findings. The chromosome aberration test also revealed an increase of chromatid breaks. The Ames test system results were negative for point mutation.

No information relating to the effect of Quinine upon fertility in animal or in man has been found.

PREGNANCY
Category X. See *"Contraindications."*

NONTERATOGENIC EFFECTS
Because Quinine crosses the placenta in humans, the potential for fetal effects is present. Stillbirths in mothers taking Quinine have been reported in which no obvious cause for the fetal deaths was shown. Quinine in toxic amounts has been associated with abortion. Whether this action is always due to direct effect on the uterus is questionable.

NURSING MOTHERS
Caution should be exercised when Quinine Sulfate is given to nursing women because Quinine is excreted in breast milk (in small amounts).

ADVERSE REACTIONS
The following adverse reactions have been reported with Quinine Sulfate in therapeutic or excessive dosage. (Individual or multiple symptoms may represent cinchonism or hypersensitivity.)

Hematologic: acute hemolysis, disseminated intravascular coagulation, thrombocytopenic purpura, agranulocytosis, hypoprothrombinemia

CNS: visual disturbances, including blurred vision with scotomata, photophobia, diplopia, diminished visual fields, and disturbed color vision; tinnitus, deafness, and vertigo; headache, nausea, vomiting, fever, apprehension, restlessness, confusion, and syncope

Dermatologic/allergic: cutaneous rashes (urticarial, the most frequent type of allergic reaction, papular, or scarlatinal), pruritus, flushing of the skin, sweating, occasional edema of the face

Respiratory: asthmatic symptoms

Cardiovascular: anginal symptoms

Gastrointestinal: nausea and vomiting (may be CNS-related), epigastric pain, hepatitis

DRUG ABUSE AND DEPENDENCE
Tolerance, abuse, or dependence with Quinine Sulfate has not been reported.

OVERDOSAGE
The more common signs and symptoms of Quinine overdosage are tinnitus, dizziness, skin rash, and gastrointestinal disturbance (intestinal cramping). With higher doses, cardiovascular and CNS effects may occur, including headache, fever, vomiting, apprehension, confusion, and convulsions. Blindness and deafness, (with partial to total recovery, although persistent visual and/or auditory nerve damage have been reported) and hypoglycemia and hypokalemia may also occur. Other potential adverse effects are listed in the *"Adverse Reactions"* section.

Fatalities with Quinine have been reported from single oral doses of 2 to 8 grams; a single fatality reported with 1.5 grams may reflect an idiosyncratic effect.

TREATMENT
Gastrointestinal decontamination should be considered for the treatment of Quinine overdosage. Vital signs, electrocardiogram (ECG), blood glucose and serum electrolytes should be monitored. Supportive measures should be instituted as necessary. Caution should be used in administering antiarrhythmics since Quinine has Class I antiarrhythmic properties that can be potentiated by such agents. It is theoretically likely that mild hypokalemia may protect the heart from the toxic effects of Quinine, and so the correction of only severe hypokalemia is advisable.

Fluid and electrolyte balance should be maintained with intravenous fluids. Although acidification of the urine will promote renal excretion of Quinine, forced acid diuresis has had little impact on Quinine elimination by the kidney. In addition, peritoneal dialysis, hemodialysis, hemoperfusion, exchange transfusion and plasmapharesis have not been shown to effectively treat Quinine overdosage.

Stellate ganglion block has not been shown to effectively treat Quinine-induced blindness, and may result in complications.

DOSAGE AND ADMINISTRATION
1 tablet upon retiring. If needed, 2 tablets may be taken nightly—1 following the evening meal and 1 upon retiring. After several consecutive nights in which recumbency leg cramps do not occur, Quinine Sulfate may be discontinued in order to determine whether continued therapy is needed.

Store at room temperature, below 86°F (30°C).

HOW SUPPLIED
CAPSULE: 325 MG

AVERAGE UNIT PRICE (AVAILABLE SIZES)				
GENERIC	$0.19			
BRAND/MANUFACTURER		NDC	SIZE	AWP
◆ GENERICS				
Interpharm		53746-0251-01	100s	$20.00
Interpharm		53746-0251-05	500s	$91.00
Interpharm		53746-0251-10	1000s	$195.00

TABLETS: 260 MG

AVERAGE UNIT PRICE (AVAILABLE SIZES)		GENERIC A-RATED AVERAGE PRICE (GAAP)		
GENERIC	$0.13	100s		$15.72
BRAND/MANUFACTURER		NDC	SIZE	AWP
◆ GENERICS				
QUIN-260: Major		00904-0564-60	100s	$10.45
QUIN-260: Major		00904-0564-61	100s ud	$20.99
QUIN-260: Major		00904-0564-70	250s	$24.55
QUIN-260: Major		00904-0564-40	500s	$44.95

TABLETS: 260 MG

BRAND/MANUFACTURER	NDC	SIZE	AWP
○ BRAND			
QUINAMM: Marion Merrell Dow	00068-0547-15	100s	$63.00

R-Gene 10 *SEE* ARGININE HYDROCHLORIDE

Rabies Immune Globulin (Human)

DESCRIPTION
Rabies Immune Globulin (Human) is a sterile solution of antirabies immunoglobulin for intramuscular administration. This product is prepared from human

plasma. It is prepared by cold alcohol fractionation from the plasma of donors hyperimmunized with rabies vaccine.

CLINICAL PHARMACOLOGY

The usefulness of prophylactic rabies antibody in preventing rabies in man when administered immediately after exposure was dramatically demonstrated in a group of persons bitten by a rabid wolf in Iran.[1,2] Similarly, beneficial results were later reported from the U.S.S.R.[3] Studies coordinated by WHO helped determine the optimal conditions under which antirabies serum of equine origin and rabies vaccine can be used in man.[4-7] These studies showed that serum can interfere to a variable extent with the active immunity induced by the vaccine, but could be minimized by booster doses of vaccine after the end of the usual dosage series.

Preparation of Rabies Immune Globulin of human origin with adequate potency was reported by Cabasso et al.[8] In carefully controlled clinical studies, this globulin was used in conjunction with rabies vaccine of duck-embryo origin (DEV).[8,9] These studies determined that a human globulin dose of 20 IU/kg of rabies antibody, given simultaneously with the first DEV dose, resulted in amply detectable levels of passive rabies antibody 24 hours after injection in all recipients. The injections produced minimal, if any, interference with the subject's endogenous antibody response to DEV.

More recently, human diploid cell rabies vaccines (HDCV) prepared from tissue culture fluids containing rabies virus have received substantial clinical evaluation in Europe and the United States.[10-16] In a study in adult volunteers, the administration of Rabies Immune Globulin (Human) did not interfere with antibody formation induced by HDCV when given in a dose of 20 IU per kilogram body weight simultaneously with the first dose of vaccine.[15]

INDICATIONS AND USAGE

Rabies vaccine and Rabies Immune Globulin (Human) should be given to all persons suspected of exposure to rabies with one exception: persons who have been previously immunized with rabies vaccine and have a confirmed adequate rabies antibody titer should receive only vaccine. Rabies Immune Globulin (Human) should be administered as promptly as possible after exposure, but can be administered up to the eighth day after the first dose of vaccine is given.

Recommendations for use of passive and active immunization after exposure to an animal suspected of having rabies have been detailed by the U.S. Public Health Service Advisory Committee on Immunization Practices (ACIP).[17]

Every exposure to possible rabies infection must be individually evaluated. The following factors should be considered before specific antirabies treatment is initiated:

1. SPECIES OF BITING ANIMAL

Carnivorous wild animals (especially skunks, foxes, coyotes, raccoons, and bobcats) and bats are the animals most commonly infected with rabies and have caused most of the indigenous cases of human rabies in the United States since 1960.[18] Unless the animal is tested and shown not to be rabid, postexposure prophylaxis should be initiated upon bite or nonbite exposure to these animals (see item 3 below). If treatment has been initiated and subsequent testing in a competent laboratory shows the exposing animal is not rabid, treatment can be discontinued.

In the United States, the likelihood that a domestic dog or cat is infected with rabies varies from region to region; hence, the need for postexposure prophylaxis also varies. However, in most of Asia and all of Africa and Latin America, the dog remains the major source of human exposure; exposures to dogs in such countries represent a special threat. Travelers to those countries should be aware that > 50% of the rabies cases among humans in the United States result from exposure to dogs outside the United States.

Rodents (such as squirrels, hamsters, guinea pigs, gerbils, chipmunks, rats, and mice) and lagomorphs (including rabbits and hares) are rarely found to be infected with rabies and have not been known to cause human rabies in the United States. However, from 1971 through 1988, woodchucks accounted for 70% of the 179 cases of rabies among rodents reported to CDC.[19] In these cases, the state or local health department should be consulted before a decision is made to initiate postexposure antirabies prophylaxis.

2. CIRCUMSTANCES OF BITING INCIDENT

An unprovoked attack is more likely to mean that the animal is rabid. (Bites during attempts to feed or handle an apparently healthy animal may generally be regarded as provoked.)

3. TYPES OF EXPOSURE

Rabies is transmitted only when the virus is introduced into open cuts or wounds in skin or mucous membranes. If there has been no exposure (as described in this section), postexposure treatment is not necessary. Thus, the likelihood that rabies infection will result from exposure to a rabid animal varies with the nature and extent of the exposure. Two categories of exposure should be considered:

Bite: any penetration of the skin by teeth. Bites to the face and hands carry the highest risk, but the site of the bite should not influence the decision to begin treatment.[20]

Nonbite: scratches, abrasions, open wounds or mucous membranes contaminated with saliva or any potentially infectious material, such as brain tissue, from a rabid animal constitute nonbite exposures. If the material containing the virus is dry, the virus can be considered noninfectious. Casual contact, such as petting a rabid animal and contact with the blood, urine, or feces (e.g., guano) of a rabid animal, does not constitute an exposure and is not an indication for prophylaxis. Instances of airborne rabies have been reported rarely. Adherence to respiratory precautions will minimize the risk of airborne exposure.[21] The only documented cases of rabies from human-to-human transmission have occurred in patients who received corneas transplanted from persons who died of rabies undiagnosed at the time of death. Stringent guidelines for acceptance of donor corneas have reduced this risk.

Bite and nonbite exposures from humans with rabies theoretically could transmit rabies, although no cases of rabies acquired this way have been documented.

4. VACCINATION STATUS OF BITING ANIMAL

A properly immunized animal has only a minimal chance of developing rabies and transmitting the virus.

5. PRESENCE OF RABIES IN REGION

If adequate laboratory and field records indicate that there is no rabies infection in a domestic species within a given region, local health officials are justified in considering this in making recommendations on antirabies treatment following a bite by that particular species. Such officials should be consulted for current interpretations.

RABIES POSTEXPOSURE PROPHYLAXIS

The following recommendations are only a guide. In applying them, take into account the animal species involved, the circumstances of the bite or other exposure, the vaccination status of the animal, and presence of rabies in the region. Local or state public health officials should be consulted if questions arise about the need for rabies prophylaxis.

Local Treatment of Wounds: Immediate and thorough washing of all bite wounds and scratches with soap and water is perhaps the most effective measure for preventing rabies. In experimental animals, simple local wound cleansing has been shown to reduce markedly the likelihood of rabies.

Tetanus prophylaxis and measures to control bacterial infection should be given as indicated.

Active Immunization: Active immunization should be initiated as soon as possible after exposure. Many dosage schedules have been evaluated for the currently available rabies vaccines and their respective manufacturers' literature should be consulted.

Passive Immunization: A combination of active and passive immunization (vaccine and immune globulin) is considered the acceptable postexposure prophylaxis except for those persons who have been previously immunized with rabies vaccine and who have documented adequate rabies antibody titer. These individuals should receive vaccine only. For passive immunization, Rabies Immune Globulin (Human) is preferred over antirabies serum, equine.[16,17] It is recommended both for treatment of all bites by animals suspected of having rabies and for nonbite exposure inflicted by animals suspected of being rabid. Rabies Immune Globulin (Human) should be used in conjunction with rabies vaccine and can be administered through the seventh day after the first dose of vaccine is given. Beyond the seventh day, Rabies Immune Globulin (Human) is not indicated since an antibody response to cell culture vaccine is presumed to have occurred.

RABIES POSTEXPOSURE PROPHYLAXIS GUIDE[17]

Animal species	Condition of animal at time of attack	Treatment of exposure person [1]
Dog and cat	Healthy and available for 10 days of observation	None, unless animal develops rabies [2]
	Rabid or suspected rabid	RIGH [3] and HDCV
	Unknown (escaped)	Consult public health officials
Skunk, bat, fox, coyote raccoon, bobcat, and other carnivores; woodchuck	Regard as rabid unless geographic area is known to be free of rabies or proven negative by laboratory tests [4]	RIGH [3] and HDCV
Livestock, rodents, and lagomorphs (rabbits and hares)	Consider individually. Local and state public health officials should be consulted on questions about the need for rabies prophylaxis. In most geographical areas bites of squirrels, hamsters, guinea pigs, gerbils, chipmunks, rats, mice, other rodents, rabbits, and hares almost never call for antirabies prophylaxis.	

[1] ALL BITES AND WOUNDS SHOULD IMMEDIATELY BE THOROUGHLY CLEANSED WITH SOAP AND WATER. If antirabies treatment is indicated, both Rabies Immune Globulin (Human) [RIGH] and human diploid cell rabies vaccine (HDCV) should be given as soon as possible, REGARDLESS of the interval from exposure.
[2] During the usual holding period of 10 days, begin treatment with RIGH and vaccine (HDCV) at first sign of rabies in a dog or cat that has bitten someone. The symptomatic animal should be killed immediately and tested.
[3] If RIGH is not available, use antirabies serum, equine (ARS). Do not use more than the recommended dosage.

[4] The animal should be killed and tested as soon as possible. Holding for observation is not recommended. Discontinue vaccine if immunofluorescence test results of the animal are negative.

CONTRAINDICATONS
None known.

WARNINGS
Rabies Immune Globulin (Human) should be given with caution to patients with a history of prior systemic allergic reactions following the administration of human immunoglobulin preparations or in patients who are known to have had an allergic response to thimerosal.

The attending physician who wishes to administer Rabies Immune Globulin (Human) to persons with isolated immunoglobulin A (IgA) deficiency must weigh the benefits of immunization against the potential risks of hypersensitivity reactions. Such persons have increased potential for developing antibodies to IgA and could have anaphylactic reactions to subsequent administration of blood products that contain IgA.[22]

As with all preparations administered by the intramuscular route, bleeding complications may be encountered in patients with thrombocytopenia or other bleeding disorders.

PRECAUTIONS
GENERAL
Rabies Immune Globulin (Human) should not be administered intravenously because of the potential for serious reactions. Although systemic reactions to immunoglobulin preparations are rare, epinephrine should be available for treatment of acute anaphylactoid symptoms.

DRUG INTERACTIONS
Repeated doses of Rabies Immune Globulin (Human) should not be administered once vaccine treatment has been initiated as this could prevent the full expression of active immunity expected from the rabies vaccine. Other antibodies in the Rabies Immune Globulin (Human) preparation may interfere with the response to live vaccines such as measles, mumps, polio or rubella. Therefore, immunization with live vaccines should not be given within 3 months after Rabies Immune Globulin (Human) administration.

PREGNANCY CATEGORY C
Animal reproduction studies have not been conducted with Rabies Immune Globulin (Human). It is also not known whether Rabies Immune Globulin (Human) can cause fetal harm when administered to a pregnant woman or can affect reproduction capacity. Rabies Immune Globulin (Human) should be given to a pregnant woman only if clearly needed.

ADVERSE REACTIONS
Soreness at the site of injection and mild temperature elevations may be observed at times. Sensitization to repeated injections has occurred occasionally in immunoglobulin-deficient patients. Angioneurotic edema, skin rash, nephrotic syndrome, and anaphylactic shock have rarely been reported after intramuscular injection, so that a causal relationship between immunoglobulin and these reactions is not clear.

DOSAGE AND ADMINISTRATION
The recommended dose for Rabies Immune Globulin (Human) is 20 IU/kg (0.133 mL/kg) of body weight given preferably at the time of the first vaccine dose.[8,9] It may also be given through the seventh day after the first dose of vaccine is given. If anatomically feasible, up to one-half the dose of Rabies Immune Globulin (Human) should be thoroughly infiltrated in the area around the wound and the rest should be administered intramuscularly in the gluteal area. Because of risk of injury to the sciatic nerve, the central region of the gluteal area MUST be avoided: only the upper outer quadrant should be used.[23] Rabies Immune Globulin (Human) should never be administered in the same syringe or into the same anatomical site as vaccine.

Parenteral drug products should be inspected visually for particulate matter and discoloration prior to administration, whenever solution and container permit.

Rabies Immune Globulin (Human) should be stored under refrigeration (2°-8°C, 35°-46°F). Solution that has been frozen should not be used.

REFERENCES
1. Baltazard M, Bahmanyar M, Ghodssi M, et al: Essai pratique du sérum antirabique chez les mordus par loups enragéa. *Bull WHO* 13:747-72, 1955.   2. Habel K, Koprowski H: Laboratory data supporting the clinical trial of antirabies serum in persons bitten by a rabid wolf. *Bull WHO* 13:773-9, 1995.   3. Selimov M, Boltucij L, Semenova E, et al: [The use of antirabies gamma globulin in subjects severely bitten by rabid wolves or other animals.] *J Hyg Epidemiol Microbiol Immunol (Praha)* 3:168-80, 1959.   4. Atanasiu P, Bahmanyar M, Baltazard M, et al: Rabies neutralizing antibody response to different schedules of serum and vaccine inoculations in non-exposed persons: *Bull WHO* 14:593-611, 1956.   5. Atanasiu P, Bahmanyar M, Baltazard M, et al: Rabies neutralizing antibody response to different schedules of serum and vaccine inoculations in non-exposed persons: Part II. *Bull WHO* 17:911-32, 1957.   6. Atansiu P, Cannon DA, Dean DJ, et al: Rabies neutralizing antibody response to different schedules of serum and vaccine inoculations in non-exposed persons: Part 3. *Bull WHO* 25:103-14, 1961.   7. Atanasiu P, Dean DJ, Habel K, et al: Rabies neutralizing antibody response to different schedules of serum and vaccine inoculations in non-exposed persons: Part 4. *Bull WHO* 36:361-5, 1967.   8. Cabasso VJ, Loofbourow JC, Roby RE, et al: Rabies immune globulin of human origin: preparation and dosage determination in non-exposed volunteer subjects. *Bull WHO* 45:303-15, 1971.   9. Loofbourow JC, Cabasso VJ, Roby RE, et al: Rabies immune globulin (human): clinical trials and dose determination. *JAMA* 217(13): 1825-31, 1971.   10. Plotkin SA: New rabies vaccine halts disease — without severe reactions. *Mod Med* 45(20):45-8, 1977.   11. Plotkin SA, Wiktor TJ, Koprowski H, et al: Immunization schedules for the new human diploid cell vaccine against rabies. *Am J Epidemiol* 103(1):75-80, 1976.   12. Hafkin B, Hattwick MA, Smith JS, et al: A comparison of a WI-38 vaccine and duck embryo vaccine for preexposure rabies prophylaxis. *AM J Epidemiol* 107(5):439-43, 1978.   13. Kuwert EK, Marcus I, Höher PG; Neutralizing and complement-fixing antibody responses in pre- and post-exposure vaccinees to a rabies vaccine produced in human diploid cells. *J Biol Stand* 4(4):249-62, 1976.   14. Grandien M: Evaluation of tests for rabies antibody and analysis of serum responses after administration of three different types of rabies vaccines. *J Clin Microbiol* 5(3):263-7, 1977.   15. Kuwert EK, Marcus I, Werner J, et al: Postexpositionelle Schutzimpfung des Menschen gegen Tollwut mit einer neuentwickelten Gewebekulturvakzine (HDCS-Impfstoff). *Zentralbl Bakteriol [A]* 239(4):437-58, 1977.   16. Bahmanyar M, Fayaz A, Nour-Salehi S, et al: Successful protection of humans exposed to rabies infection: postexposure treatment with the new human diploid cell rabies vaccine and antirabies serum. *JAMA* 236(24):2751-4, 1976.   17. Recommendations of the Immunization Practices Advisory Committee (ACIP): Rabies prevention—United States, 1991. *MMWR* 40(RR-3):1-19, 1991.   18. Reid-Sanden FL, Dobbins JG, Smith JS, et al: Rabies surveillance in the United States during 1989. *J Am Vet Med Assoc* 197(12):1571-83, 1990.   19. Fishbein DB, Belotto AJ, Pacer Re et al: Rabies in rodents and lagomorphs in the United States, 1971-1984: increased cases in the woodchuck (*Marmota monax*) in mid-Atlantic states. *J Wildl Dis* 22(2):151-5, 1986.   20. Hattwick MAW: Human rabies. *Public Health Rev* 3(3):229-74, 1974.   21. Garner JS, Simmons BP: Guideline for isolation precautions in hospitals. *Infect Control* .   22. Fudenberg HH: Sensitization to immunoglobulins and hazards of gamma globulin therapy. In: Merler E (ed.): Immunoglobulins: biologic aspects and clinical uses. Washington, DC, Nat Acad Sci, 1970, pp 211-20.   23. Recommendations of the Immunization Practices Advisory Committee (ACIP): General recommendations on immunization. *MMWR* 38(13):205-14; 219-27, 1989.

HOW SUPPLIED
INJECTION:

BRAND/MANUFACTURER	NDC	SIZE	AWP
○ **BRAND**			
HYPERAB: Miles Biol	00192-0608-02	2 ml	$85.00
	00192-0608-10	10 ml	$335.00

INJECTION: 150 IU/ML

BRAND/MANUFACTURER	NDC	SIZE	AWP
○ **BRAND**			
IMOGAM RABIES: Connaught	49281-0180-20	2 ml	$124.75
	49281-0180-10	10 ml	$522.94

Rabies Vaccine

DESCRIPTION
Rabies Vaccine is a sterile, stable, freeze-dried suspension of rabies virus.

The virus is harvested from infected human diploid cells MRC 5 strain.

Rabies Vaccine is available for intramuscular (IM) and low-dose intradermal (ID) use.

The vaccine should be used immediately after reconstitution, and if not administered promptly, contents should be discarded.

CLINICAL PHARMACOLOGY
PRE-EXPOSURE IMMUNIZATION
High titer antibody responses of the Rabies Vaccine made in human diploid cells have been demonstrated in trials conducted in England[1], Germany[2, 3], France[4] and Belgium[5], Seroconversion was often obtained with only one dose. With two doses one month apart, 100% of the recipients developed specific antibody and the geometric mean titer of the group was approximately 10 international units. In the U.S., Rabies Vaccine resulted in geometric mean titers (GMT) of 12.9 I.U./ml at Day 49 and 5.1 I.U./ml at Day 90 when three doses were given intramuscularly during the course of one month. The range of antibody responses was 2.8 to 55.0 I.U./ml at Day 49 and 1.8 to 12.4 I.U. at Day 90.[6] The definition of a minimally accepted antibody titer varies among laboratories and is influenced by the type of test conducted. CDC currently specifies a 1:5 titer (complete inhibition) by the rapid fluorescent focus inhibition test (RFFIT) as acceptable. The World Health Organization (WHO) specifies a titer of 0.5 I.U.

POSTEXPOSURE IMMUNIZATION
Post-exposure efficacy of Rabies Vaccine was successfully proven during clinical experience in Iran[7] in conjunction with antirabies serum. Forty-five persons severely bitten by rabid dogs and wolves received Rabies Vaccine within hours of and up to 14 days after the bites. All individuals were fully protected against rabies.

There have been reports of possible vaccine failure when the vaccine has been administered in the gluteal area. Presumably subcutaneous fat in the gluteal area may interfere with the immunogenicity of human diploid cell rabies vaccine (HDCV)[26, 29]. For adults and children, Rabies Vaccine should be administered in the deltoid muscle. (See *"Dosage and Administration"*).

Studies in Europe[1, 2, 30-33] and in the United States[6, 34] to investigate the efficacy and safety of low dose intradermal vaccination schedules have shown that satisfactory levels of antibody were produced in all subjects with two or more inoculations.

Studies in the United States[6, 8, 34] using three doses of Rabies Vaccine demonstrated adequate rabies antibody titers in 100% of persons receiving intradermal injections. The geometric mean titer in these subjects 49 days after immunization was approximately 7.5 to 8.9 I.U. compared with 12.9 to 13.8 I.U. in controls receiving 1.0 ml of vaccine intramuscularly[6].

The definition of a minimally acceptable antibody titer varies both among laboratories and according to the purposes for which immunization is given. The Centers for Disease Control (CDC) currently specifies complete virus neutralization at a 1:5 serum dilution in the rapid fluorescent focus inhibition test (RFFIT) as an acceptable response to pre-exposure immunization. After studies of post-exposure immunization, the World Health Organization (WHO) specifies a titer of 0.5 I.U. as an acceptable response.

INDICATIONS AND USAGE

I. RATIONALE OF TREATMENT

Physicians must evaluate each possible rabies exposure. Local or state public health officials should be consulted if questions arise about the need for prophylaxis.[8]

In the United States and Canada, the following factors should be considered before antirabies treatment is initiated.

SPECIES OF BITING ANIMAL

Carnivorous wild animals (especially skunks, raccoons, foxes, coyotes, and bobcats) and bats are the animals most commonly infected with rabies and have caused most of the indigenous cases of human rabies in the United States since 1960. Unless an animal is tested and shown not to be rabid, post-exposure prophylaxis should be initiated upon bite or nonbite exposure to the animals. (See definition in "Type of Exposure" below.) If treatment has been initiated and subsequent testing in a competent laboratory shows the exposing animal is not rabid, treatment can be discontinued. 8

The likelihood that a domestic dog or cat is infected with rabies varies from region to region; hence the need for post-exposure prophylaxis also varies.[8]

Rodents (such as squirrels, hamsters, guinea pigs, gerbils, chipmunks, rats and mice) and lagomorphs (including rabbits and hares) are rarely found to be infected with rabies and have not been known to cause human rabies in the United States. In these cases, the state or local health department should be consulted before a decision is made to initiate post-exposure antirabies prophylaxis.[8]

CIRCUMSTANCES OF BITING INCIDENT

An UNPROVOKED attack is more likely than a provoked attack to indicate the animal is rabid. Bites inflicted on a person attempting to feed or handle an apparently healthy animal should generally be regarded as PROVOKED.

TYPE OF EXPOSURE

Rabies is transmitted by introducing the virus into open cuts or wounds in skin or via mucous membranes. The likelihood of rabies infection varies with the nature and extent of exposure. Two categories of exposure should be considered.

Bite: Any penetration of the skin by teeth.

Nonbite: Scratches, abrasions, open wounds, or mucous membranes contaminated with saliva or other potentially infectious material, such as brain tissue, from a rabid animal. Casual contact, such as petting a rabid animal (without a bite or nonbite exposure as described above), does not constitute an exposure and is not an indication for prophylaxis. There have been two instances of airborne rabies acquired in laboratories and two probable airborne rabies cases acquired in a bat-infested cave in Texas.[8, 9]

The only documented cases for rabies from human-to-human transmission occurred in four patients in the United States and overseas who received corneas transplanted from persons who died of rabies, undiagnosed at the time of death.[9, 10] Stringent guidelines for acceptance of donor corneas should reduce this risk. Bite and nonbite exposure from humans with rabies theoretically could transmit rabies, although no cases of rabies acquired this way have been documented. Each potential exposure to human rabies should be carefully evaluated to minimize unnecessary rabies prophylaxis.[8, 11]

II. PRE- AND POSTEXPOSURE TREATMENT OF RABIES

A. PRE-EXPOSURE—SEE TABLE 1

Pre-exposure immunization may be offered to persons in high risk groups, such as veterinarians, animal handlers, certain laboratory workers, and persons spending time (e.g. 1 month or more) in foreign countries where rabies is a constant threat. For persons traveling abroad into endemic areas, human diploid cell vaccine (HDCV) may be administered by the ID dose and route if the 3- dose series is completed 30 days or more before departure. If pre-exposure vaccination is performed for travelers at other times, a vaccine intended for intramuscular use should be used. Persons whose vocational or avocational pursuits bring them into contact with potentially rabid dogs, cats, foxes, skunks, bats, or other species at risk of having rabies should also be considered for pre-exposure prophylaxis.[8]

Vaccination is recommended for children living in or visiting countries where exposure to rabid animals is a constant threat. Worldwide statistics indicate children are more at risk than adults.

Pre-exposure prophylaxis is given for several reasons. First, it may provide protection to persons with inapparent exposure to rabies. Secondly, it may protect persons whose post-exposure therapy might be expected to be delayed. Finally, although it does not eliminate the need for additional therapy after a rabies exposure, it simplifies therapy by eliminating the need for globulin and decreasing the number of doses of vaccine needed. This is of particular importance for persons at high risk of being exposed in countries where the available rabies immunizing products may carry a higher risk of adverse reactions.

Pre-exposure immunization does not eliminate the need for prompt prophylaxis following an exposure. It only reduces the post-exposure treatment regimen.[8]

PRE-EXPOSURE RABIES TREATMENT GUIDE

1. Pre-exposure Immunization: Consists of the three doses of HDCV, 1.0 mL, intramuscularly (deltoid area), or 0.1 mL intradermally (deltoid area) one each on Days 0,7 and 21 or 28. Administration of routine booster doses of vaccine depends on exposure risk category as noted in Table 1. Pre-exposure immunization of immunosuppressed persons is not recommended.[8] (See related table).

B. POSTEXPOSURE—SEE TABLE 2

The essential components of rabies postexposure prophylaxis are local treatment of wounds and immunization, including administration, in most instances, of both globulin and vaccine (Table 2).[8,13]

1. Local Treatment of Wounds: Immediate and thorough washing of all bite wounds and scratches with soap and water is perhaps the most effective measure for preventing rabies. In experimental animals, simple local wound cleansing has been shown to reduce markedly the likelihood of rabies.[8,11]

Tetanus prophylaxis and measures to control bacterial infection should be given as indicated.

2. Specific Treatment: Postexposure antirabies immunization should always include administration of both antibody (preferably RIG) and vaccine, with one exception: persons who have been previously immunized with the recommended preexposure or postexposure regimens with HDCV or who have been immunized with other types of vaccines and have a history of documented adequate rabies antibody titer should receive only vaccine. The combination of globulin and vaccine is recommended for both bite exposures and nonbite exposures regardless of the interval between exposure and treatment.[14,15] The sooner treatment is begun after exposure, the better. However, there have been instances in which the decision to begin treatment was made as late as 6 months or longer after the exposure due to delay in recognition that an exposure had occurred.[8,13]

3. Treatment outside the United States: If postexposure is begun outside the United States with locally produced biologics, it may be desirable to provide additional treatment when the patient reaches the U.S. State health departments should be contacted for specific advice in such cases.[8]

POSTEXPOSURE TREATMENT GUIDE

The following recommendations are only a guide. In applying them, take into account the animal species involved, the circumstances of the bite or other exposure, the vaccination status of the animal, and presence of rabies in the region. Local or state public health officials should be consulted if questions arise about the need for rabies prophylaxis.[8]

Table 2[8]

Animal species	Condition of animal at time of attack	Treatment of exposed person*
Domestic Dog and cat	Healthy and available for 10 days of observation	None unless animal develops rabies†
	Rabid or suspected rabid	RIG § and HDCV
	Unknown (escaped)	Consult public health officials If treatment is indicated, give RIG§ and HDCV
Wild Skunk, bat, fox, coyote, raccoon, bobcat and other carnivores	Regard as rabid unless proven negative by laboratory test £	RIG § and HDCV
Other Livestock, rodents and lagomorphs (rabbits and hares)	Consider individually. Local and state public health officials should be consulted on questions about the need for rabies prophylaxis. Bites of squirrels, hamsters, guinea pigs, gerbils, chipmunks, rats, mice, other rodents, rabbits and hares, almost never call for antirabies prophylaxis.	

* *All bites and wounds should immediately be thoroughly cleansed with soap and water. If antirabies treatment is indicated, both rabies immune globulin (RIG) and human diploid cell rabies vaccine (HDCV) should be given as soon as possible regardless of the interval from exposure. Local reactions to vaccines are common and do not contraindicate continuing treatment. Discontinue vaccine if fluorescent antibody tests of the animal are negative.*

† *During the usual holding period of 10 days, begin treatment with RIG and HDCV at first sign of rabies in a dog or cat that has bitten someone. The symptomatic animal should be killed immediately and tested.*

§ *If RIG is not available, use antirabies serum, equine (ARS). Do not use more than the recommended dosage.*

£ *The animal should be killed and tested as soon as possible. Holding for observation is not recommended.*

CONTRAINDICATIONS

For postexposure treatment, there are no known specific contraindications to the use of Rabies Vaccine. In cases of pre-exposure immunization, there are no known specific contraindications other than situations such as developing febrile illness, etc.

WARNINGS

IM Rabies vaccine must not be used intradermally. In both pre-exposure and post exposure immunization, the full 1.0 ml dose should be given intramuscularly. ID Rabies Vaccine must not be used for post-exposure immunization. The full 0.1 ml dose should be given intradermally.

In the case of pre-exposure immunization, recently a significant increase has been noted in "immune complex-like" reactions in persons receiving booster doses of HDCV.[16,36] The illness characterized by onset 2-21 days post-booster, presents with a generalized urticaria and may also include arthralgia, arthritis, angioedema, nausea, vomiting, fever, and malaise. In no cases were the illness life-threatening. Preliminary data suggest this "immune complex-like" illness may occur in up to 6% of persons receiving booster vaccines and much less frequently in persons receiving primary immunization. Additional experience with this vaccine is needed to define more clearly the risk of these adverse reactions.[8,17]

There is preliminary evidence that beta propiolactone altered human albumin induces most of the allergic reactions.[8,37]

Two cases of neurologic illness resembling Guillain-Barre syndrome[18,19], a transient neuroparalytic illness, that resolved without sequelae in 12 weeks and a focal subacute central nervous system disorder temporally associated with HDCV, have been reported.[20]

All serious systemic neuroparalytic or anaphylactic reactions to a Rabies Vaccine should be immediately reported to the state health department or to the Division of Viral Diseases, Center for Infectious Diseases, CDC, (404) 329-3095 during working hours or (404) 329-2888 at other times.[8]

Persons who travel from the U.S. to developing countries and receive their pre-exposure vaccination abroad or within 30 days before leaving should be immunized by the intramuscular (IM) route (3 x 1.0 ml).

Persons previously vaccinated successfully against rabies and who come in contact with a rabid or potentially rabid animal, should have the wounds cleansed and receive a post-exposure dose of 1.0 ml of Rabies Vaccine intramuscularly, followed by a second 1.0 ml dose on Day 3. Intradermal immunization must not be used. Rabies immune globulin should NOT be given.

PRECAUTIONS

IN ADULTS AND CHILDREN THE VACCINE SHOULD BE INJECTED INTO THE DELTOID MUSCLE. IN INFANTS AND SMALL CHILDREN THE MID-LATERAL ASPECT OF THE THIGH MAY BE PREFERABLE.

GENERAL

When a person with a history of hypersensitivity must be given Rabies Vaccine, antihistamines may be given; epinephrine (1:1000) should be readily available to counteract anaphylactic reactions, and the person should be carefully observed after immunization.

While the concentration of antibiotics in each dose of vaccine is extremely small, persons with known hypersensitivity to any of these agents could manifest an allergic reaction. While the risk is small, it should be weighed in light of the potential risk of contracting rabies.

DRUG INTERACTIONS

Corticosteroids, other immunosuppressive agents, and immunosuppressive illnesses can interfere with the development of active immunity and predispose the patient to developing rabies. Immunosuppressive agents should not be administered during post-exposure therapy, unless essential for the treatment of other conditions. When rabies post-exposure prophylaxis is administered to persons receiving steroids or other immunosuppressive therapy, it is especially important

that serum be tested for rabies antibody to ensure that an adequate response has developed.[8]

Antimalarial drugs such as chloroquine have been associated with a reduction in the antibody response to Rabies Vaccine administered by the intradermal route. Although it is apparent that antimalarial agents are not the sole factor responsible for the reduced antibody response, it is recommended that persons on corticosteroids and other immunosuppressive drugs receive Rabies Vaccine (3 doses/1.0 ml each) by the intramuscular route until more definitive data is available.[38, 39, 40]

USAGE IN PREGNANCY

Pregnancy Category C. Animal reproduction studies have not been conducted with Rabies Vaccine. It is also not known whether the product can cause fetal harm when administered to a pregnant woman or can affect reproductive capacity. Rabies vaccine should be given to a pregnant woman only if clearly needed.

Because of the potential consequences of inadequately treated rabies exposure and limited data that indicate that fetal abnormalities have not been associated with rabies vaccination, pregnancy is not considered a contraindication to post-exposure prophylaxis.[8,21] If there is substantial risk of exposure to rabies, pre-exposure prophylaxis may also be indicated during pregnancy.[8]

PEDIATRIC USE

Both safety and efficacy in children have been established.

Although specific intradermal studies in children have not been conducted vaccine given to children intramuscularly (1.0 ml) has been shown to be safe. There are no known specific hazards expected from intradermal use of the vaccine in children.[41]

ADVERSE REACTIONS

Also See *"Warnings and Contraindications"* sections for additional statements.

Once initiated, rabies prophylaxis should not be interrupted or discontinued because of local or mild systemic adverse reactions to rabies vaccine. Usually such reactions can be successfully managed with anti-inflammatory and antipyretic agents (e.g. aspirin).

Reactions after vaccination with HDCV are less common than with previously available vaccines.[12,16,17,37] In a study using five doses of HDCV, administered intramuscularly local reactions such as pain, erythema, and swelling or itching at the injection site were reported in about 25% of recipients of HDCV, and mild systemic reactions such as headache, nausea, abdominal pain, muscle aches and dizziness were reported in about 20% of recipients.[8]

Serious systemic anaphylactic or neuroparalytic reactions occurring during the administration of rabies vaccines pose a dilemma for the attending physician. A patient's risk of developing rabies must be carefully considered before deciding to discontinue vaccination. Moreover, the use of corticosteroids to treat life-threatening neuroparalytic reactions carries the risk of inhibiting the development of active immunity to rabies. It is especially important in these cases that the serum of the patient be tested for rabies antibodies. Clinical experience with Rabies Vaccine has resulted in a low incidence of adverse reactions comparable to those following intramuscular vaccination when administered by the intradermal route except that a slight increase in transient local reactions has been observed following intradermal vaccination, especially when the vaccine is given in the forearm rather than in the lateral aspect of the upper arm. Local reactions consist of redness, itching, mild pain and minimal swelling at the site of injection. Generalized reactions are uncommon.[6] Mild local or systemic reactions can be treated with anti-inflammatory, antipyretic agents, e.g., aspirin and antihistamines. Systemic allergic or anaphylactic reactions following primary immunization have been reported to be less than 1%.[19] If an anaphylactic reaction should

---

Table 1[8]

CRITERIA FOR PRE-EXPOSURE IMMUNIZATION

Risk category	Nature of risk	Typical populations	Pre-exposure regimen
Continuous	Virus present continuously, often in high concentrations. Aerosol, mucous membrane, bite or nonbite exposure possible. Specific exposures may be unrecognized.	Rabies research lab workers*. Rabies biologics production workers.	Primary pre-exposure immunization course. Serology every 6 months. Booster immunization when antibody titer falls below acceptable level†.
Frequent	Exposure usually episodic, with source recognized, but exposure may also be unrecognized. Aerosol, mucous membrane, bite or nonbite exposure.	Rabies diagnostic lab workers*, spelunkers, veterinarians, and animal control and wildlife workers in rabies epizootic areas.	Primary pre-exposure immunization course. Booster immunization or serology every 2 years†.
Infrequent (greater than population-at-large)	Exposure nearly always episodic with source recognized. Mucous membrane, bite or nonbite exposure.	Veterinarians and animal control and wildlife workers in areas of low rabies endemicity. Certain travelers to foreign rabies epizootic areas. Veterinary students.	Primary pre-exposure immunization course. No routine booster immunization or serology.
Rare (population-at-large)	Exposure always episodic, mucous membrane, or bite with source recognized.	U.S. population-at-large, including individuals in rabies epizootic areas.	No pre-exposure immunization.

* *Judgment of relative risk and extra monitoring of immunization status of laboratory workers is the responsibility of the laboratory supervisor (see U.S. Department of Health and Human Service's Biosafety in Microbiological and Biomedical Laboratories, 1984).*

† *Pre-exposure booster immunization consists of one dose of HDCV, 1.0 ml/dose, IM or 0.1 ml ID (deltoid area). Acceptable antibody level is 1:5 titer (complete inhibition of infectious foci in RFFIT at 1:5 serum dilution). See Clinical Pharmacology. Boost if titer falls below 1:5.*

◆ RATED THERAPEUTICALLY EQUIVALENT; ◇ THERAPEUTIC EQUIVALENCE UNCONFIRMED; ○ UNRATED

occur, epinephrine is indicated. For "immune complex-like" reactions in persons receiving booster doses of HDCV see "Warnings".

Advice and assistance on the management of serious adverse reactions in persons receiving primary or booster rabies vaccines may be sought from the state health department or the CDC.[8]

DOSAGE AND ADMINISTRATION

Parenteral drug products should be inspected visually for particulate matter and discoloration prior to administration, whenever solution and container permit IM Rabies Vaccine: Reconstitute the freeze-dried vaccine in a single-dose vial with 1.0 ml of diluent. Gently swirl the contents until completely dissolved and withdraw the total amount of dissolved vaccine into the syringe by setting the vial in an upright position on the table.

The reconstituted vaccine should be used immediately.

After preparation of the injection site, immediately inject the vaccine intramuscularly. For adults and children, the vaccine should be injected into the deltoid muscle.[22-27, 29] In infants and small children, the mid- lateral aspect of the thigh may be preferable. Care should be taken to avoid injection into or near blood vessels and nerves. After aspiration, if blood or any suspicious discoloration appears in the syringe, do not inject but discard contents and repeat procedure using a new dose of vaccine, at a different site.

Note: The freeze-dried vaccine is creamy white to orange. After reconstitution it is pink to red.

A. PRE-EXPOSURE DOSAGE

1. Primary vaccination: In the United States, the Immunization Practices Advisory Committee (ACIP) recommends three injections of 1.0 ml each of IM Rabies Vaccine or 0.1 ml each of ID Rabies Vaccine one injection on Day 0 and one on Day 7 and one either on Day 21 or 28. The ACIP, in making this recommendation for ID Rabies Vaccines cites studies conducted in the United States and Europe in which more than 1500 persons received 0.1 ml of vaccine intradermally as the 2 or 3-dose pre-exposure vaccination. All subjects developed antibody as shown by the rapid fluorescent focus inhibition test (RFFIT). The ACIP suggests that routine serologic testing to confirm a satisfactory antibody response is not necessary.[28]

If the intradermal inoculation was not performed satisfactorily (vaccine injected subcutaneously) another dose should be given intradermally at a different site.

2. Booster dose: Persons working with live rabies virus in research laboratories and in vaccine production facilities should have rabies antibody titers checked every six months and boosters given as needed to maintain an adequate titer. (For definition of adequate titer, see *"Clinical Pharmacology"*) Only laboratory workers, such as those doing rabies diagnostic tests, spelunkers and veterinarians, animal control and wildlife officers in areas where rabies is epizootic should have boosters every 2 years or have their serum tested for rabies antibody every 2 years and, if the titer is inadequate, have a booster dose. Veterinarians and animal control and wildlife officers, if working in areas of low rabies endemicity, do not require routine booster doses of HDCV after completion of primary pre-exposure immunization (Table 1).[8]

Persons who have experienced "immune complex-like" hypersensitivity reactions should receive no further doses of HDCV unless they are exposed to rabies or they are truly likely to be inapparently and/or unavoidably exposed to rabies virus and have unsatisfactory antibody titers.

B. POSTEXPOSURE DOSAGE

The World Health Organization established a recommendation for six intramuscular doses of human diploid cell vaccine (HDCV) based on studies in Germany and Iran.[3,7] Used in this way, a total of 6 injections of a 1.0 ml dose of vaccine is given according to the following schedule: On Day 0, 3, 7, 14, 30 and 90. The first dose should be accompanied by rabies immune globulin (RIG) or antirabies serum (ARS). If possible, up to half the dose of RIG or ARS should be used to infiltrate the wound, and the rest administered intramuscularly, in a different site from the rabies vaccine, preferably in the gluteal region.

Studies conducted at the CDC in the United States have shown that a regimen of 1 dose of rabies immune globulin (RIG) and 5 doses of HDCV induced an excellent antibody response in all recipients. Of 511 persons bitten by proven rabid animals and so treated, none developed rabies.[8]

Based on these data, the ACIP recommends a 5-dose regimen for postexposure situations. Five 1.0 ml doses are given intramuscularly on Day 0, 3, 7, 14 and 28 in conjunction with RIG on Day 0.[8]

Because the antibody response following the recommended vaccination regimen with HDCV has been so satisfactory, routine post-vaccination serologic testing is not recommended. Serologic testing is indicated in unusual circumstances, as when the patient is known to be immunosuppressed. Contact state health department or CDC for recommendations.[8,28]

C. POSTEXPOSURE THERAPY OF PREVIOUSLY IMMUNIZED PERSONS

When an immunized person who was vaccinated by the recommended regimen with HDCV or who had previously demonstrated rabies antibody is exposed to rabies, that person should receive two IM doses (1.0 ml each) of HDCV, one immediately and one 3 days later. RIG should not be given in these cases. If the immune status of a previously vaccinated person who did not receive the recommended HDCV regimen is not known, full primary post-exposure antirabies treatment (RIG plus 5 doses of HDCV) may be necessary. In such cases, if

antibody can be demonstrated in a serum sample collected before vaccine is given, treatment can be discontinued after at least two doses of HDCV.[8]

STORAGE

The freeze-dried vaccine is stable if stored in the refrigerator between 2°C and 8°C (36°F to 46°F). Do not freeze.

REFERENCES

1. Aoki FY, Tyrell DAJ, Hill LE. Immunogenicity and acceptability of a human diploid cell culture rabies vaccine in volunteers. The Lancet, March 22, pp. 660-2 (1975). 2. Cox JH, Schneider LG. Prophylactic immunization of humans against rabies by intradermal inoculation of human diploid cell culture vaccine. J Clin Microbiol 3:96-101 (1976). 3. Kuwert EK, Marcus 1, Werner J, Iwand A, Thraenhart O. Some experiences with human diploid cell strain—(HDCS) rabies vaccine in pre- and post-exposure vaccinated humans. Developed Biol Standard 40:79-88 (1978). 4. Ajjan N, Soulebot J-P, Stellmann C, Biron G, Charbonnier C, Triau R, Merieux C, Resultats de la vaccination antirabique preventive par le vaccin inactiv' concentr' souche rabies PM/W138-1503-3M cultiv's sur cellules diplödes humaines. Develop Biol Standard 40:89-199 (1978). 5. Coty-Berger F. Vaccination antirabique preventive par du vaccin prepare sur cellules diploides humaines. Develop Biol Standard 40:101-4 (1978). 6. Bernard KW, Roberts MA, Summer J, Winkler WG, Mallonee J, Baer GM, Chaney R. Human diploid cell rabies vaccine JAMA 247:1138-42 (1982). 7. Bahmanyar M, Fayaz A, Nour-Salehi S, Mohammadi M, Koprowski H. Successful protection of humans exposed to rabies infection. JAMA 236: 2751-4 (1976). 8. CDC. Recommendations of the Immunization Practices Advisory Committee (ACIP). Rabies Prevention—United States, 1984, MMWR 33: 393-402, 407-8 (1984). 9. Anderson U, Nicholson KG, Tauxe RV, Winkler WG. Human rabies in the United States, 1960 to 1979, epidemiology, diagnosis and prevention. Ann Intern Med 100: 728-35 (1984). 10. WHO. Sixth report of the Expert Committee on Rabies. Geneva Switzerland: World Health Organization. (WHO technical report No. 523) (1973). 11. Baer GM, ed. The natural history of rabies. New York: Academic Press. (1975). 12. Greenberg M, Childress J. Vaccination against rabies with duck-embryo and Semple vaccines. JAMA 173:333-7 (1960). 13. Helmick CG. The epidemiology of human rabies post-exposure prophylaxis. JAMA 250: 1990-6 (1983). 14. Devriendt J, Staroukine M, Costy F, Vanderhaegen, J-J Fatal encephalitis apparently due to rabies. JAMA 248: 2304-6 (1982). 15. CDC. Human Rabies—Rwanda. MMWR 31: 135 (1982). 16. CDC. Systemic allergic reactions following immunization with human diploid cell rabies vaccine. MMWR 33:185-7 (1984). 17. Rubin RH, Hattwick MAW, Jones S, Gregg MB, Schwartz VD. Adverse reactions to duck embryo rabies vaccine. Ann Intern Med 78: 643-9 (1973). 18. Boe E, Nyland H. Guillain-Barre syndrome after vaccination with human diploid cell rabies vaccine. Scand J Infect Dis 12:231-2 (1980). 19. CDC. Adverse reactions to human diploid cell rabies vaccine. MMWR 29: 609-10 (1980). 20. Bernard KW, Smith PW, Kader FJ, Moran MJ. Neuroparalytic illness and human diploid cell rabies vaccine. JAMA 248: 3136-8 (1982). 21. Varner MW, McGuinness GA, Galask RP. Rabies vaccination in pregnancy. Am J of Obst and Gyn 143:717-18 (1982). 22. Cockshott WP, Thompson GT, Howlett U, Seely ET. Intramuscular or intralipomatous injections? N Eng J Med 307: 356-58 (1982). 23. CDC. General Recommendations on Immunization, ACIP, MMWR 32: 1-8, 13-17 (1983). 24. Committee on Immunization Council of Medical Societies, American College of Physicians. Guide for Adult Immunizations. (1985). 25. CDC. Rabies post-exposure prophylaxis with HDCV: Lower neutralizing antibody titers with Wyeth vaccine. MMWR 34: 90-92 (1985). 26. Shill M, Baynes Rd, Miller SD. Fatal rabies encephalitis despite appropriate post-exposure prophylaxis. N Engl J Med 316:1257-58 (1987). 27. Baer GM, Fishbein DB. Rabies post-exposure prophylaxis. N Engl J Med 316: 1270-72 (1987). 28. CDC. Recommendations of the Immunization Practices Advisory Committee (ACIP). Supplementary statement on rabies vaccine and serologic testing. MMWR 30: 535-6 (1981). 29. CDC. Human rabies despite treatment with Rabies Immune Globulin and Human Diploid Cell Rabies Vaccine—Thailand. MMWR 36: 759-765 (1987). 30. Turner GS, Aoki FY Nicholson KG, Tyrrell DA, Hill LE: Human diploid cell strain rabies vaccine: Rapid prophylactic immunization of volunteers with small doses. Lancet 1: 1379-81 (1976). 31. Nicholson KG, Turner GS, Aoki FY: Immunization with a human diploid cell strain of rabies virus vaccine: Two-year results, J Infect. Dis 137: 783-88 (1978). 32. Nicholson KG, Turner GS: Studies with human diploid cell strain rabies vaccine and human antirabies globulin in man. Dev. Biol. Stand. 40:115-20 (1978). 33. Ajjan N, Soulebot JP, Triau R, Biron G: Intradermal Immunization with rabies vaccine: Inactivated Wistar strain cultivated in human diploid cells. JAMA 244: 2528-31 (1980). 34. Dreesen DW, Brown WJ, Kemp DT, Brown J, Reid FL, Baer GM: Pre-exposure rabies prophylaxis: efficacy of a new packaging and delivery system for intradermal administration of human diploid cell vaccine Vaccine 2: 185-88 (1984). 36. Dreesen DW, Bernard KW, Parker RA, Deutsch AJ, Brown J: Immune complex-like disease in 23 persons following a booster dose of rabies human diploid cell vaccine. Vaccine 4: 45-49 (1986). 37. Baer H. Anderson HC, Bernard K, Quinnan G: Beta propiolactone treated human serum albumin (BPL HSA) an allergen for humans receiving rabies vaccine (Abstract). J Allergy and Clin Immunol 75: (No: 1 Part 2 suppl) (1985). 38. Taylor DN, Wasi C, Bernard K: Chloroquine prophylaxis associated with a poor antibody response to human diploid cell rabies vaccine. Lancet 1: 1408 (1984). 39. Pappaioanou M. Fishbein DB, Dreesen DW, Schwartz IK, Campbell GH, Sumner JW Patchen LC, Brown WJ: Antibody response to pre-exposure human diploid cell rabies vaccine given concurrently with chloroquine. N. Engl. J. Med. 314: 280-84 (1986). 40. Bernard KW, Fishbein DB, Miller KD, Parker RA, Waterman S, Sumner JW, Reid FL, Johnson BK, Rollins AJ, Oster CN, Schonberger LB, Baer GM, Winkler WG: Pre-exposure rabies immunization with human diploid cell vaccine. Decreased antibody responses in persons immunized in developing countries. Am. J. Trop. Med. Hyg. 34: 633-47 (1985). 41. Fridell E. Grandien M, Johansson R: Pre-exposure prophylaxis against rabies in children by human diploid cell vaccine. Lancet 1: 623 (1984). 42. CDC ACIP Recommendations: Supplementary statement on pre-exposure rabies prophylaxis by the intradermal route. MMWR 31: 279-85 (1982).

HOW SUPPLIED
INJECTION:

BRAND/MANUFACTURER	NDC	SIZE	AWP
○ GENERICS			
SK Beecham Pharm	00007-4840-01	1 ml	$119.45

POWDER FOR INJECTION:

BRAND/MANUFACTURER	NDC	SIZE	AWP
○ **BRAND**			
IMOVAX RABIES I.D.: Connaught	49281-0251-20	1s	$56.25
IMOVAX RABIES: Connaught	49281-0250-10	1s ud	$130.00

Rabies Vaccine Adsorbed

DESCRIPTION

Rabies Vaccine Adsorbed is a sterile, cell-culture derived rabies vaccine for pre- and post-exposure prophylaxis in humans. It is prepared with the CVS Kissling/MDPH strain of rabies virus. The virus is propagated in a diploid cell line derived from fetal rhesus lung cells (FRhL-2 cell line) in a serum-free, chemically defined, antibiotic-free medium. The virus harvest, which is clarified by centrifugation and filtration, is inactivated with betapropiolactone. After inactivation, the virus is adsorbed to aluminum phosphate.

The final vaccine is a suspension containing 2.5 international units or more of rabies antigen per 1.0 mL dose. It contains no more than 2.0 mg aluminum phosphate per mL and also contains 0.01% sodium ethylmercurithiosalicylate (thimerosal) as a preservative. The solution is a light pink color due to the presence of phenol red.

Rabies Vaccine Adsorbed is intended for intramuscular (LM) injection. CAUTION: THIS VACCINE IS NOT FOR USE BY THE INTRADERMAL (ID) ROUTE.

CLINICAL PHARMACOLOGY

The immune response to rabies vaccines can be ascertained by measuring antibody directed against rabies virus by means of the rapid fluorescent focus inhibition test (RFFIT). Serum antibody levels against rabies virus are usually expressed in terms of international units or serum titers. The definition of a minimally acceptable antibody titer in vaccinees varies among laboratories and is dependent on the type of test performed. The Centers for Disease Control considers complete virus neutralization at a 1:5 serum dilution by the RFFIT a minimally acceptable response to pre-exposure vaccination. The World Health Organization specifies that a minimum titer of 0.5 international units is an adequate response to vaccination.

In field trials of Rabies Vaccine Adsorbed, 99% or greater of 1,567 persons who had not been immunized previously against rabies responded with serum titers of 0.5 international units (a dilution titer of approximately 1:25) or greater by 2 weeks after the last of 3 IM injections of Rabies Vaccine Adsorbed given over a 3- or 4-week period. At 9 to 12 months post-immunization, 97% of 605 persons had antibody titers at or above a level of 0.1 international units (a 1:5 dilution of serum). In addition, 97% or more of 2,148 persons previously immunized with Duck Embryo Rabies Vaccine, Human Diploid Rabies Vaccine or Rabies Vaccine Adsorbed showed 4-fold increased antibody titers following a single booster injection of Rabies Vaccine Adsorbed.

In post-exposure field trials and clinical simulations of post-exposure prophylaxis, 5 doses of Rabies Vaccine Adsorbed, in conjunction with Rabies Immune Globulin, induced active antibody production in all previously unvaccinated persons between the seventh and fourteenth day following initiation of treatment. In post-exposure rabies prophylaxis, Rabies Immune Globulin is given concomitantly with the first injection of rabies vaccine to provide immediate passive immunoprophylaxis. If not given when vaccination was begun, Rabies Immune Globulin may be given up to 7 days after administration of the first dose of vaccine.

Rabies Vaccine Adsorbed has been used successfully to immunize both adults and children 6 years of age and older.

There have been reports of possible vaccine failures when human diploid cell rabies vaccine (HDCV) has been administered in the gluteal area. Subcutaneous fat in the gluteal area may interfere with the immunogenicity of HDCV.[1-3] It is not known if an adequate response would be obtained after gluteal administration of Rabies Vaccine Adsorbed. Therefore, adults and older children should receive this vaccine in the deltoid muscle. For younger children the anterolateral aspect of the thigh is also acceptable.

INDICATIONS AND USAGE

Rabies Vaccine Adsorbed is indicated for immunization against rabies in the following circumstances: *primary pre-exposure immunization* which is intended to induce immunity before exposure to the virus; *pre-exposure booster immunization* which is intended to augment or reinforce the level of immunity induced by previous immunization against rabies; or *post-exposure prophylaxis* which is given to persons who, in the judgment of the treating physician, may have been exposed to rabies virus. Each circumstance requires a different schedule of injections.

A. Primary Pre-Exposure Vaccination (see Table 1): Pre-exposure vaccination is given to persons who are at greater than usual risk of possible rabies exposure by reason of occupation or avocation. The list of such persons includes, but is not limited to, veterinarians and staff, certain laboratory workers, animal handlers and persons spending time (e.g., 1 month or more) in foreign countries where canine rabies is enzootic. Persons whose vocational or avocational pursuits bring them into contact with potentially rabid dogs, cats, foxes, skunks, raccoons, bats or other species at risk of having rabies should also be considered for pre-exposure prophylaxis.

Pre-exposure vaccination is given as a series of 3 individual injections of Rabies Vaccine Adsorbed with the second and third injections being given 7 and 21 or 28 days after the first injection, respectively. Pre-exposure vaccination does *not* eliminate the need for prompt post-exposure prophylaxis following an exposure; it only eliminates the need for Rabies Immune Globulin and reduces the number of injections of rabies vaccine needed for post-exposure prophylaxis. Criteria for pre-exposure vaccination are summarized in Table 1.

B. Pre-Exposure Booster Vaccination (see Table 1): Pre-exposure booster vaccination is given to persons who have received previous rabies vaccination and remain at increased risk of rabies exposure by reasons of occupation or avocation. Persons who work with live rabies virus in research laboratories or vaccine production facilities (continuous-risk category; see Table 1) should have a serum sample tested for rabies antibody every 6 months. Booster doses of vaccine should be given to maintain a serum titer corresponding to at least complete neutralization at a 1:5 serum dilution by the RFFIT. The frequent-risk category includes other laboratory workers, such as those doing rabies diagnostic testing, spelunkers, veterinarians and staff, animal-control and wildlife officers in areas where animal rabies is epizootic, and international travelers living or visiting (for > 30 days) in areas where canine rabies is endemic. Persons among this group should have a serum sample tested for rabies antibody every 2 years and, if the titer is less than complete neutralization at a 1:5 serum dilution by the RFFIT, should have a booster dose of vaccine. Alternatively, a booster can be administered in lieu of a titer determination. Veterinarians and animal-control and wildlife officers working in areas of low rabies enzooticity (infrequent-exposure group) do not require routine pre-exposure booster doses of Rabies Vaccine Adsorbed after completion of primary pre-exposure vaccination (Table 1).

A single booster injection of Rabies Vaccine Adsorbed has been shown to increase antibody titers in persons who have previously been immunized with Rabies Vaccine Adsorbed or Human Diploid Cell Rabies Vaccine. Persons who have been shown to have developed antibody responses to a previous series of injections of Duck Embryo Rabies Vaccine also respond to a single booster dose of Rabies Vaccine Adsorbed.

Table 1
PRE-EXPOSURE VACCINATION CRITERIA*

PRE-EXPOSURE VACCINATION. Primary pre-exposure vaccination consists of 3 doses of Rabies Vaccine Adsorbed, 1.0 mL, IM (i.e., deltoid area), 1 each on days 0, 7 and 21 or 28. Administration of routine booster doses of vaccine depends on exposure risk category as noted below.

Criteria for Pre-Exposure Vaccination			
Risk Category	Nature of Risk	Typical Populations	Pre-Exposure Regimen
Continuous	Virus present continuously, often in high concentrations. Aerosol, mucous membrane, bite or non-bite exposure possible. Exposure may go unrecognized.	Rabies research laboratory workers†; rabies biologics production workers.	Primary course. Serology every 6 months; booster vaccination when antibody level falls below acceptable level.‡
Frequent	Exposure usually episodic, with source recognized, but exposure may also be unrecognized. Aerosol, mucous membrane, bite or non-bite exposure.	Rabies diagnostic laboratory workers,† spelunkers, veterinarians and staff, and animal-control and wildlife workers in rabies enzootic areas; travelers visiting foreign areas of enzootic rabies for more than 30 days.	Primary course. Serologic testing or booster vaccination every 2 years.‡
Infrequent (greater than population at large)	Exposure nearly always episodic with source recognized. Mucous membrane, bite or non-bite exposure.	Veterinarians and animal-control and wildlife workers in areas of low rabies enzooticity. Veterinary students.	Primary course. No serologic testing or booster vaccination.
Rare (population at large)	Exposure always episodic. Mucous membrane or bite with source recognized.	U.S. population at large, including individuals in rabies enzootic areas.	No vaccination necessary.

*   References 4 and 5.

◆ RATED THERAPEUTICALLY EQUIVALENT; ◇ THERAPEUTIC EQUIVALENCE UNCONFIRMED; ○ UNRATED

† *Judgment of relative risk and extra monitoring of immunization status is the responsibility of the laboratory supervisor (see U.S. Department of Health and Human Services' Biosafety in Microbiological and Biomedical Laboratories, 1984).*
‡ *Pre-exposure booster vaccination consists of 1 dose of Rabies Vaccine Adsorbed, 1.0 mL dose intramuscular (deltoid muscle). Minimum acceptable antibody level is complete virus neutralization at a 1:5 serum dilution by RFFIT. Administer booster dose if titer falls below 1:5.*

Table 2
RABIES POST-EXPOSURE PROPHYLAXIS GUIDE*

Animal Type	Evaluation and Disposition of Animal	Post-Exposure Prophylaxis Recommendations
Dogs and cats	Healthy and available for 10 days' observation	Should not begin prophylaxis unless animal develops symptoms of rabies†
	Rabid or suspected rabid Unknown (escaped)	Immediate vaccination Consult public health officials
Skunks, raccoons, bats, foxes and most other carnivores; woodchucks	Regarded as rabid unless geographic area is known to be free of rabies or until animal proven negative by laboratory tests‡	Immediate vaccination
Livestock, rodents and lagomorphs (rabbits and hares)	Consider individually	Consult public health officials. Bites of squirrels, hamsters, guinea pigs, gerbils, chipmunks, rats, mice, other rodents, rabbits and hares almost never require antirabies treatment.

* *References 4 and 5.*
† *During the 10-day holding period, begin treatment with Rabies Vaccine Adsorbed with or without Rabies Immune Globulin (Human) at first sign of rabies in a dog or cat that has bitten someone (see "Post-Exposure Prophylaxis below"). The symptomatic animal should be killed immediately and tested.*
‡ *The animal should be killed and tested as soon as possible. Holding for observation is not recommended. Discontinue vaccine if immunofluorescence test results of the animal are negative.*

C. Postexposure Prophylaxis: Factors to be considered for appropriate post-exposure antirabies treatment are given in Table 2.[4,5] These include the species of animal with which the person has had contact, the circumstances of the biting incident and vaccination status of the exposing animal, the type of exposure and the previous rabies immunization history of the person exposed. Carnivorous wild animals (especially skunks, raccoons and foxes) and bats are the animals most commonly infected with rabies and the cause of most of the indigenous cases of human rabies in the United States since 1960. In contrast, with the exception of woodchucks, rodents (such as squirrels, hamsters, guinea pigs, gerbils, chipmunks, rats and mice) and lagomorphs (including rabbits and hares) are rarely found to be infected with rabies and have not been known to cause human rabies in the United States. The likelihood that a domestic dog or cat is infected with rabies varies from region to region and depends, in part, on the vaccination history of the animal. In addition, an unprovoked attack is more likely than a provoked attack to indicate that an animal is rabid. Moreover, rabies is transmitted by introducing the virus into open wounds or mucous membranes. Thus, the likelihood of rabies infection depends, in part, on whether the exposure occurred by penetrating the skin or by contamination of mucous membranes by saliva or other potentially infectious material. Physicians should evaluate each possible exposure to rabies and, if necessary, consult with their state or local public health officials regarding the need for rabies prophylaxis.

1. Local Treatment of Wounds: Immediate and thorough washing of all bite wounds and scratches with soap and water is perhaps the most effective measure for preventing rabies. In experimental animals, simple local wound cleaning has been shown to reduce markedly the likelihood of rabies. Tetanus prophylaxis and measures to control bacterial infection should be given as indicated.

2. Specific Treatment: RABIES VACCINE ADSORBED IS NOT INTENDED FOR USE IN PATIENTS KNOWN TO HAVE CLINICAL MANIFESTATION OF RABIES. The injection schedule for post-exposure prophylaxis depends on whether the patient has had or has not had previous vaccination against rabies. *For persons who have not previously been vaccinated against rabies*, the schedule consists of an initial injection IM of Rabies Immune Globulin (Human) (HRIG), 20 international units per kilogram body weight in total. If anatomically feasible, up to half the dose of HRIG should be thoroughly infiltrated around the wound(s) and the remainder should be administered IM in the gluteal region (for specific instructions for HRIG use, see the product package insert). The HRIG injection is followed by a series of 5 individual injections of Rabies Vaccine Adsorbed given IM on days 0, 3, 7, 14 and 28. The HRIG and Rabies Vaccine Adsorbed should be given at separate sites using separate syringes. Post-exposure rabies prophylaxis should begin the same day exposure occurred or as soon after exposure as possible. The combined use of HRIG and Rabies Vaccine Adsorbed is recommended for both bite and non-bite exposures, regardless of the interval between exposure and initiation of treatment. The sooner treatment is begun after exposure, the better. However, there have been instances in which the decision to begin treatment was made as late as 6 months or longer after exposure due to delay in recognition that an exposure had occurred. Post-exposure antirabies vaccine should always include administration of both passive antibody and vaccination with the exception of persons who have previously received complete vaccination regimens (pre-exposure or post-exposure) with a cell culture vaccine, or persons who have been vaccinated with other types of vaccines and have had documented rabies antibody titers. *Persons who have previously received rabies vaccination are given 2 IM doses of Rabies Vaccine Adsorbed: 1 on day 0 and another on day 3. They should not be given HRIG.*

3. Treatment Outside the United States: If post-exposure prophylaxis is begun outside the United States with locally produced biologics, it may be desirable to provide additional treatment when the patient reaches the United States. State health departments should be contacted for specific advice in each case.[4]

CONTRAINDICATIONS
Rabies Vaccine Adsorbed is contraindicated in persons who have had life-threatening allergic reactions to previous injections of this vaccine or to components of this vaccine, including thimerosal. No such reactions have been seen to date but are theoretically possible since less severe allergic reactions have been observed. Persons who have experienced nonlife-threatening allergic reactions to Rabies Vaccine Adsorbed may receive additional injections under appropriate medical supervision, if the indications for vaccination justify the risk and vaccines are not available to which the patient has not had a reaction.

WARNINGS
Pre-exposure immunization should be delayed in persons with an acute intercurrent illness.
Rabies Vaccine Adsorbed should be injected into the deltoid muscle unless the use of that muscle is contraindicated. As is the case in giving any adsorbed vaccine, care should be taken to avoid accidently depositing Rabies Vaccine Adsorbed in close approximation to a peripheral nerve or in adipose and subcutaneous tissue.

PRECAUTIONS
General: In adults and children, the vaccine should be injected into the deltoid muscle. In small children, the mid-lateral aspect of the thigh area may be preferable.
As with the injection of any biologic material that may induce an allergic reaction, epinephrine injection (1:1,000) should be available for immediate use should an anaphylactic reaction occur.
This vaccine should be given with caution to persons who are known to be sensitive to or allergic to monkey proteins. If a patient known to be allergic to monkey proteins has been exposed to a known rabid animal, and if no other rabies vaccine is available, then administration of Rabies Vaccine Adsorbed to the allergic patient should be done under the supervision of a physician qualified in the management of allergic reactions. Local or mild post-vaccination reactions are not a contraindication to continuing immunization.

Drug Interactions: Immunosuppressive agents, antimalarials and immunosuppressive diseases can interfere with development of active immunity after vaccination and may reduce the effectiveness of rabies vaccine. Immunosuppressive agents should not be given during post-exposure therapy unless essential for treatment of other conditions. When post-exposure prophylaxis is given to immunosuppressed persons, it is important that serum be tested for rabies antibody to ensure that an adequate response occurred.

Laboratory Tests: Routine testing for rabies antibody response to vaccination is not necessary. Experience from clinical trials documented that antibodies can be detected consistently in serum samples obtained approximately 2 weeks after the last injection. For immunosuppressed persons see Drug Interactions.

Pregnancy Category C: Animal reproduction studies have not been conducted with Rabies Vaccine Adsorbed. It is also not known whether Rabies Vaccine Adsorbed can cause fetal harm when administered to a pregnant woman or can affect reproductive capacity. Rabies Vaccine Adsorbed should be given to a pregnant woman only if clearly needed.

Pediatric Use: Rabies Vaccine Adsorbed has been administered to children as young as 6 years old without noticeable difference in effects from its administration to adults. All children from whom post-vaccination serum was obtained showed rabies antibody titers greater than 1:5. However, because of the limited experience with this vaccine in children, special precautions should be taken for unexpected adverse events.

ADVERSE REACTIONS
Once initiated, rabies prophylaxis should not be interrupted due to mild local or systemic reactions.

Local: Approximately 65% to 70% of persons given IM injections of Rabies Vaccine Adsorbed reported subjective mild, transient discomfort localized to the injection site. In a few, aching of the injected muscle and a mild local inflammatory reaction consisting of swelling, induration or erythema were present for 48 hours. These local complaints can usually be successfully treated with simple analgesics.

Systemic: Mild, transient constitutional reactions have been reported by 8% to 10% of Rabies Vaccine Adsorbed recipients. These consisted chiefly of headache, nausea, slight fever or fatigue. Also, serum-sickness-like reactions, some with arthralgia, suggestive of hypersensitivity to Rabies Vaccine Adsorbed, have been reported in less than 1% of vaccinees between 7 and 14 days after vaccination. These hypersensitivity reactions have occurred after booster vaccination, but have not been seen following primary immunization with Rabies Vaccine Adsorbed.

The occurrence of allergic reactions in patients receiving either Rabies Vaccine Adsorbed or Human Diploid Cell Rabies Vaccine raises special difficulties for the managing physician. The use of pre-exposure booster doses of Human Diploid Cell Rabies Vaccine has been limited by the observation of serum-sickness-like allergic reactions that occur in approximately 6% of individuals who receive boosters with that vaccine.[5] These reactions are thought to be due to small amounts of human serum albumin that have been rendered allergenic by betapropiolactone. Human serum albumin is not used in the medium used to grow the rabies virus for Rabies Vaccine Adsorbed and therefore is not present when betapropiolactone is added to inactivate the virus. Nevertheless, systemic allergic reactions have also occurred in some individuals following booster doses of Rabies Vaccine Adsorbed at a rate of less than 1%. However, it is not known whether patients who are allergic to Rabies Vaccine Adsorbed are also allergic to Human Diploid Cell Rabies Vaccine and vice versa. Thus, judgments must be made regarding whether or not to continue the vaccination schedule and whether or not to change the vaccines.

Other: Neurologic reactions such as those reported to be temporally associated with the administration of other viral vaccines, including Human Diploid Cell Rabies Vaccine, for example, allergic peripheral neuritis, encephalomyelitis or transverse myelitis, have not been reported in recipients of Rabies Vaccine Adsorbed.

If serious adverse reactions are noted, report them promptly to the manufacturer: Michigan Department of Public Health, 517-335-8050 during working hours or 517-335-9030 at other times. Reports may also be submitted directly to the FDA on form FDA-1639, single copies of which may be obtained from the Division of Epidemiology and Surveillance (HFN-730), 5600 Fishers Lane, Rockville, MD 20857.

DOSAGE AND ADMINISTRATION

Each vial of Rabies Vaccine Adsorbed contains a sufficient volume of vaccine to enable withdrawing a full dose of 1.0 mL. The vial should be shaken gently before withdrawing the vaccine to ensure complete suspension of the aluminum phosphate adjuvant. The vaccine should be given IM. THIS VACCINE IS NOT FOR USE BY THE ID ROUTE. Before injecting the vaccine, the syringe barrel should be retracted sufficiently to create a back-pressure to ascertain whether the needle is in the lumen of a blood vessel.

In adults and children, the site of the injection is the deltoid muscle. Administration into the buttock is not recommended since experience with other vaccines has shown that acceptable antibody titers may not be obtained.[3] In small children, who may have insufficient deltoid muscle mass, the anterolateral aspect of the thigh is an acceptable injection site.

Pre-Exposure Vaccination: Pre-exposure vaccination consists of three 1.0 mL IM injections of rabies vaccine, 1 each given at 0, 7 and 21 or 28 days. (Also see Table 1.)

Booster Vaccination: Booster vaccination consists of a single 1.0 mL IM injection of vaccine.

Post-Exposure Prophylaxis: Post-exposure prophylaxis for persons *not* previously vaccinated against rabies consists of an injection of HRIG, 20 international units per kilogram body weight, and five 1.0 mL injections of Rabies Vaccine Adsorbed, intramuscularly, 1 each to be given on days 0, 3, 7, 14 and 28. The amount of HRIG administered should not exceed the recommended amount. Post-exposure prophylaxis for persons who *have* been previously vaccinated against rabies consists of two 1.0 mL IM injections of Rabies Vaccine Adsorbed: 1 at day 0 and the second on day 3. HRIG should not be given. Persons should be considered to *have* been immunized previously if they received pre- or post-exposure prophylaxis with Rabies Vaccine Adsorbed or Human Diploid Cell Rabies Vaccine or have been documented to have had an adequate antibody response to Duck Embryo Rabies Vaccine. (Also see Table 2.)

Parenteral drug products should be inspected for particulate matter and discoloration prior to administration, whenever solution and container permit. This vaccine should have a light pink color due to the presence of phenol red in a neutral solution. Do not use vials that are discolored or contain particulate matter.

Storage: Rabies Vaccine Adsorbed should be stored at 2° to 8°C (35° to 46°F). Do not freeze; discard if product has been frozen.

REFERENCES

1. Shill, M., Baynes, R.D., and Miller, S.D.: Fatal Rabies Encephalitis Despite Appropriate Post-Exposure Prophylaxis. *N. Engl. J. Med.* 316:1257-1258, 1987. 2. Baer, G.M., and Fishbein, D.B.: Rabies Post-Exposure Prophylaxis. *N. Engl. J. Med.* 316:1270-1272, 1987. 3. Centers for Disease Control: Human Rabies Despite Treatment with Rabies Immune Globulin and Human Diploid Cell Rabies Vaccine—Thailand. *MMWR.* 36:(November 27) 757-760, 765, 1987. 4. Centers for Disease Control: Rabies Prevention—United States, 1991: Recommendations of the Immunization Practices Advisory Committee (ACIP). *MMWR.* 40 (No. RR-3): 1-19, 1991. 5. Centers for Disease Control: Rabies Vaccine Adsorbed: A New Rabies Vaccine for Use in Humans. *MMWR.* April 1988. 6. Corey, L., and Hattwick, M.A.W.: Treatment of Persons Exposed to Rabies. *JAMA.* 232:272-276, 1975. 7. Burgoyne, G.H., Kajiya, K.D., Brown, D.W., and Mitchell, J.R.: Rhesus Diploid Rabies Vaccine (Adsorbed): A New Rabies Vaccine Using FRhL-2 Cells. *J. Infect Dis.* 152:204-210, 1985. 8. Berlin, B.S., Mitchell, J.R., Burgoyne, G.H., et al.: Rhesus Diploid Rabies Vaccine (Adsorbed), A New Rabies Vaccine: Results of Initial Clinical Studies of Pre-Exposure Vaccination. *JAMA.* 247:1726-1728, 1982. 9. Berlin, B.S., Mitchell, J.R., Burgoyne, G.H., et al.: Rhesus Diploid Rabies Vaccine (Adsorbed), A New Rabies Vaccine II. Results of Clinical Studies Simulating Prophylactic Therapy for Rabies Exposure. *JAMA.* 249:2663-2665, 1983. 10. Bahmanyar, M., Fayaz, A., Nour-Salehi, S., et al.: Successful Protection of Humans Exposed to Rabies Infection. *JAMA.* 236:2751-2754, 1976.

HOW SUPPLIED
INJECTION:

BRAND/MANUFACTURER	NDC	SIZE	AWP
○ GENERICS			
SK Beecham Pharm	00007-4840-01	1 ml	$119.45

POWDER FOR INJECTION:

BRAND/MANUFACTURER	NDC	SIZE	AWP
○ BRAND			
IMOVAX RABIES I.D.: Connaught	49281-0251-20	1s	$56.25
IMOVAX RABIES: Connaught	49281-0250-10	1s ud	$130.00

Racemethionine

DESCRIPTION

Racemethionine is DL-2 amino-4 (methylthio)-butyric acid. A white, crystalline powder or platelets amino acid having a characteristic odor with the following chemical formula: CH_3 SCH_2 CH_2 CH (NH_2) COOH.

Composition:
CAPSULES - 200 mg Racemethionine
LIQUID - 75 mg Racemethionine per 5 mL.
Soluble in water, very slightly soluble in alcohol.

Following is its chemical structure:

$$CH_3SCH_2CH_2 - \overset{\overset{H}{|}}{\underset{\underset{NH_2}{|}}{C}} - COOH$$

ACTIONS AND INDICATIONS

An ammonia-free urine is produced by the acidifying effect of Racemethionine on the pH of urine. Racemethionine is indicated for the control of urine odor, dermatitis and ulcerations caused by ammoniacal urine in the incontinent adult patient. In infants, for the treatment of diaper rash caused by ammoniacal urine.

CONTRAINDICATIONS

Do not administer to patients with history of liver disease as large doses of Racemethionine may exaggerate the toxemia of the disease.

PRECAUTIONS

It has been pointed out by Goldstein[*] and in animal studies that excessive dosages of racemethionine added alone to the diet over extended periods may result in a weight gain below normal when protein intake is insufficient. Thus it is essential that adequate protein intake be maintained during therapy and that recommended dosage not be exceeded.

DOSAGE AND ADMINISTRATION

Capsules: Adults: One capsule three times daily with meals for odor control in incontinence. Where there is severe ulceration or eruption, one capsule four times a day. When the patient cannot take the capsule, the contents may be added to his food.

Infants and Children: Contents of one capsule added to the evening bottle of formula preferably while it is still warm or before sterilization or it may be given in juice or water. Liquid: Infants: 2 to 6 months; one teaspoonful (5 mL) three times per day for 3-5 days, 6 to 14 months; one teaspoonful (5 mL) four times per day for 3-5 days. In severe cases or when the infant is more than 1 year old, it may be necessary to double the dosage the first two days of treatment.

Note: Goldstein[**] reported no ill effects when prophylactic doses of 0.2 gm racemethionine were given daily to 50 infants continuously from an age of 2 months to age 6 months. However if there is no evidence of improvements after 10 days therapy, probable cause of rash is other than ammoniacal urine.

HOW SUPPLIED
CAPSULE:

BRAND/MANUFACTURER	NDC	SIZE	AWP
○ BRAND			
PEDAMETH: Forest Pharm	00456-0355-50	50s	$24.25
	00456-0355-02	500s	$198.29
PETAMETH: Forest Pharm	00456-1054-00	1000s	$127.74

* Goldstein, L. ARCHIVES OF PEDIATRICS, 17(285), 1953
** Goldstein, L.S., CLINICAL MEDICINE 59(455-458), 1952

◆ RATED THERAPEUTICALLY EQUIVALENT; ◇ THERAPEUTIC EQUIVALENCE UNCONFIRMED; ○ UNRATED

LIQUID:

BRAND/MANUFACTURER	NDC	SIZE	AWP
○ BRAND PEDAMETH: Forest Pharm	00456-1039-16	480 ml	$40.38

POWDER:

BRAND/MANUFACTURER	NDC	SIZE	AWP
○ GENERICS	17137-0361-04	125 gm	$7.00
	00395-1653-01	454 gm	$16.69

TABLETS: 0.5 GM

BRAND/MANUFACTURER	NDC	SIZE	AWP
○ GENERICS			
Lannett	00527-1155-01	100s	$2.50
Lannett	00527-1155-05	500s	$9.55
Lannett	00527-1155-10	1000s	$17.00

TABLETS: 500 MG

BRAND/MANUFACTURER	NDC	SIZE	AWP
○ GENERICS			
Interstate	00814-2641-30	1000s	$26.93

Ramipril

USE IN PREGNANCY

WHEN USED IN PREGNANCY DURING THE SECOND AND THIRD TRIMESTERS, ACE INHIBITORS CAN CAUSE INJURY AND EVEN DEATH TO THE DEVELOPING FETUS. WHEN PREGNANCY IS DETECTED, RAMIPRIL SHOULD BE DISCONTINUED AS SOON AS POSSIBLE. SEE "WARNINGS." FETAL/NEONATAL MORBIDITY AND MORTALITY.

DESCRIPTION

Ramipril is a 2-aza-bicyclo [3.3.0]-octane-3-carboxylic acid derivative. It is a white, crystalline substance soluble in polar organic solvents and buffered aqueous solutions. Ramipril melts between 105°C and 112°C.

The CAS Registry Number is 87333-19-5. Ramipril's chemical name is $(2S,3aS,6aS)$-1[(S)-N-](S)-1 -Carboxy-3-phenylpropyl] alanyl]octa-hydrocyclopenta[b]pyrrole-2 -carboxylic acid, 1-ethyl ester.

Its empiric formula is $C_{23}H_{32}N_2O_5$, and its molecular weight is 416.5.

Ramiprilat, the diacid metabolite of Ramipril, is a non-sulfhydryl angiotensin converting enzyme inhibitor. Ramipril is converted to ramiprilat by hepatic cleavage of the ester group.

Ramipril is supplied as hard shell capsules for oral administration containing 1.25 mg, 2.5 mg, 5 mg, and 10 mg of Ramipril.

Following is its chemical structure:

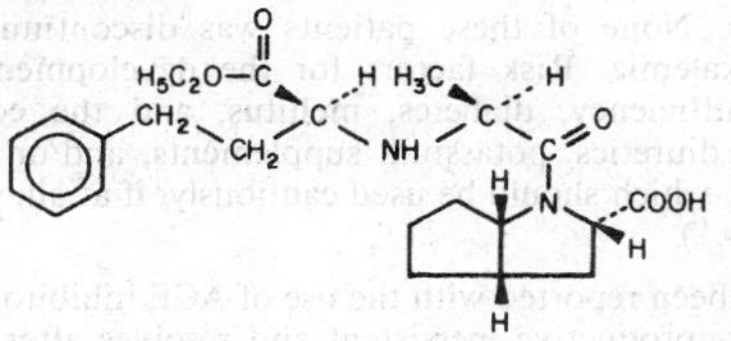

CLINICAL PHARMACOLOGY

MECHANISM OF ACTION

Ramipril and ramiprilat inhibit angiotensin-converting enzyme (ACE) in human subjects and animals. ACE is a peptidyl dipeptidase that catalyzes the conversion of angiotensin I to the vasoconstrictor substance, angiotensin II. Angiotensin II also stimulates aldosterone secretion by the adrenal cortex. Inhibition of ACE results in decreased plasma angiotensin II, which leads to decreased vasopressor activity and to decreased aldosterone secretion. The latter decrease may result in a small increase of serum potassium. In hypertensive patients with normal renal function treated with Ramipril alone for up to 56 weeks, approximately 4 percent of patients during the trial had an abnormally high serum potassium and an increase from baseline greater than 0.75 mEq/L, and none of the patients had an abnormally low potassium and a decrease from baseline greater than 0.75 mEq/L. In the same study, approximately 2% of patients treated with Ramipril and hydrochlorothiazide for up to 56 weeks had abnormally high potassium values and an increase from baseline of 0.75 mEq/L or greater, and approximately 2% had abnormally low values and decreases from baseline of 0.75 mEq/L or greater. (See "Precautions.") Removal of angiotensin II negative feedback on renin secretion leads to increased plasma renin activity.

ACE is identical to kininase, an enzyme that degrades bradykinin. Whether increased levels of bradykinin, a potent vasodepressor peptide, play a role in the therapeutic effects of Ramipril remains to be elucidated.

While the mechanism through which Ramipril lowers blood pressure is believed to be primarily suppression of the renin-angiotensin-aldosterone system, Ramipril has an antihypertensive effect even in patients with low-renin hypertension. Although Ramipril was antihypertensive in all races studied, black hypertensive patients (usually a low-renin hypertensive population) had a smaller average response to monotherapy than non-black patients.

PHARMACOKINETICS AND METABOLISM

Following oral administration of Ramipril, peak plasma concentrations of Ramipril are reached within one hour. The extent of absorption is at least 50-60% and is not significantly influenced by the presence of food in the GI tract, although the rate of absorption is reduced.

Cleavage of the ester group (primarily in the liver) converts Ramipril to its active diacid metabolite, ramiprilat. Peak plasma concentrations of ramiprilat are reached 2-4 hours after drug intake. The serum protein binding of Ramipril is about 73% and that of ramipralat about 56%; in vitro, these percentages are independent of concentration over the range of 0.01 to 10μg/ml.

Ramipril is almost completely metabolized to ramiprilat, which has about 6 times the ACE inhibitory activity of Ramipril, and to the diketopiperazine ester, the diketopiperazine acid, and the glucuronides of Ramipril and ramiprilat, all of which are inactive. After oral administration of Ramipril, about 60% of the parent drug and its metabolites are eliminated in the urine, and about 40% is found in the feces. Drug recovered in the feces may represent both biliary excretion of metabolites and/or unabsorbed drug, however the proportion of a dose eliminated by the bile has not been determined. Less than 2% of the administered dose is recovered in urine as unchanged Ramipril.

Blood concentrations of Ramipril and ramiprilat increase with increased dose, but are not strictly dose-proportional. The 24-hour AUC for ramiprilat, however, is dose-proportional over the 2.5-20 mg dose range. The absolute bioavailabilities of Ramipril and ramiprilat were 28% and 44%, respectively, when 5 mg of oral Ramipril was compared with the same dose of Ramipril given intravenously.

Plasma concentrations of ramiprilat decline in a triphasic manner (initial rapid decline, apparent elimination phase, terminal elimination phase). The initial rapid decline, which represents distribution of the drug into a large peripheral compartment and subsequent binding to both plasma and tissue ACE, has a half-life of 2-4 hours. Because of its potent binding to ACE and slow dissociation from the enzyme, ramiprilat shows two elimination phases. The apparent elimination phase corresponds to the clearance of free ramiprilat and has a half-life of 9-18 hours. The terminal elimination phase has a prolonged half-life (> 50 hours) and probably represents the binding/dissociation kinetics of the ramiprilat/ACE complex. It does not contribute to the accumulation of the drug. After multiple daily doses of Ramipril 5-10 mg, the half-life of ramiprilat concentrations within the therapeutic range was 13-17 hours.

After once-daily dosing, steady-state plasma concentrations of ramiprilat are reached by the fourth dose. Steady-state concentrations of ramiprilat are somewhat higher than those seen after the first dose of Ramipril, especially at low doses (2.5 mg), but the difference is clinically insignificant.

The urinary excretion of Ramipril, ramiprilat, and their metabolites is reduced in patients with impaired renal function. Compared to normal subjects, patients with creatinine clearance less than 40 ml/min/1.73m² had higher peak and trough ramiprilat levels and slightly longer times to peak concentrations. (See "Dosage and Administration.") In patients with impaired liver function, the metabolism of Ramipril to ramiprilat appears to be slowed, possibly because of diminished activity of hepatic esterases, and plasma Ramipril levels in these patients are increased about 3-fold. Peak concentrations of ramiprilat in these patients, however, are not different from those seen in subjects with normal hepatic function, and the effect of a given dose on plasma ACE activity does not vary with hepatic function.

PHARMACODYNAMICS

Single doses of Ramipril of 2.5-20 mg produce approximately 60-80% inhibition of ACE activity 4 hours after dosing with approximately 40-60% inhibition after 24 hours. Multiple oral doses of Ramipril of 2.0 mg or more cause plasma ACE activity to fall by more than 90% 4 hours after dosing, with over 80% inhibition of ACE activity remaining 24 hours after dosing. The more prolonged effect of even small multiple doses presumably reflects saturation of ACE binding sites by Ramiprilat and relatively slow release from those sites.

Administration of Ramipril to patients with mild to moderate hypertension results in a reduction of both supine and standing blood pressure to about the same extent with no compensatory tachycardia. Symptomatic postural hypotension is in infrequent, although it can occur in patients who are salt- and/or volume-depleted. (See "Warnings.") Use of Ramipril in combination with thiazide diuretics gives a blood pressure lowering effect greater than that seen with either agent alone.

In single-dose studies, doses of 5-20 mg of Ramipril lowered blood pressure within 1-2 hours, with peak reductions achieved 3-6 hours after dosing. The antihypertensive effect of a single dose persisted for 24 hours. In longer term (4-12 weeks) controlled studies, once-daily doses of 2.5-10 mg were similar in their effect, lowering supine or standing systolic and diastolic blood pressures 24 hours after dosing by about 6/4 mm Hg more than placebo. In comparisons of peak vs trough effect, the trough effect represented about 50-60% of the peak response. In a titration study comparing divided (bid) vs qd treatment, the divided regimen was superior, indicating that for some patients the antihypertensive effect with once-daily dosing is not adequately maintained. (See "Dosage and Administration.")

In most trials, the antihypertensive effect of Ramipril increased during the first several weeks of repeated measurements. The antihypertensive effect of Ramipril has been shown to continue during long-term therapy for at least 2 years. Abrupt withdrawal of Ramipril has not resulted in a rapid increase in blood pressure.

Ramipril has been compared with other ACE inhibitors, beta-blockers, and thiazide diuretics. It was approximately as effective as other ACE inhibitors and as atenolol. In both caucasians and blacks, hydrochlorothiazide (25 or 50 mg) was significantly more effective than Ramipril.

Except for thiazides, no formal interaction studies of Ramipril with other antihypertensive agents have been carried out. Limited experience in controlled and uncontrolled trials combining Ramipril with a calcium channel blocker, a loop diuretic, or triple therapy (beta-blocker, vasodilator, and a diuretic) indicate no unusual drug-drug interactions. Other ACE inhibitors have had less than additive effects with beta adrenergic blockers, presumably because both drugs lower blood pressure by inhibiting parts of the renin-angiotensin system.

Ramipril was less effective in blacks than in caucasians. The effectiveness of Ramipril was not influenced by age, sex, or weight.

In a baseline controlled study of 10 patients with mild essential hypertension, blood pressure reduction was accompanied by a 15% increase in renal blood flow. In healthy volunteers, glomerular filtration rate was unchanged.

INDICATIONS AND USAGE

Ramipril is indicated for the treatment of hypertension. It may be used alone or in combination with thiazide diuretics. In using Ramipril consideration should be given to the fact that another angiotensin converting enzyme inhibitor, captopril, has caused agranulocytosis, particularly in patients with renal impairment or collagen-vascular disease. Available data are insufficient to show that Ramipril does not have a similar risk. (See "Warnings.")

UNLABELED USES

Ramipril is used alone or as an adjunct in the treatment of congestive heart failure.

CONTRAINDICATIONS

Ramipril is contraindicated in patients who are hypersensitive to this product and in patients with history of angioedema related to previous treatment with an angiotensin converting enzyme inhibitor.

WARNINGS

ANGIOEDEMA

Angioedema of the face, extremities, lips, tongue, glottis, and larynx has been reported in patients treated with angiotensin converting enzyme inhibitors. Angioedema associated with laryngeal edema can be fatal. If laryngeal stridor or angioedema of the face, tongue, or glottis occurs, treatment with Ramipril should be discontinued and appropriate therapy instituted immediately. **Where there is involvement of the tongue, glottis, or larynx, likely to cause airway obstruction, appropriate therapy, e.g., subcutaneous epinephrine solution 1:1,000 (0.3 ml to 0.5 ml) should be promptly administered.** (See *"Adverse Reactions."*)

HYPOTENSION

Ramipril can cause symptomatic hypotension, after either the initial dose or a later dose when the dosage has been increased. Like other ACE inhibitors, Ramipril has been only rarely associated with hypotension is uncomplicated hypertensive patients. Symptomatic hypotension is most likely to occur in patients who have been volume- and/or salt-depleted as a result of prolonged diuretic therapy, dietary salt restriction, dialysis, diarrhea, or vomiting. Volume and/or salt depletion should be corrected before initiating therapy with Ramipril.

In patients with congestive heart failure, with or without associated renal insufficiency, ACE inhibitor therapy may cause excessive hypotension, which may be associated with oliguria or azotemia and, rarely with acute renal failure and death. In such patients, Ramipril therapy should be started under close medical supervision; they should be followed closely for the first 2 weeks of treatment and whenever the dose of Ramipril or diuretic is increased.

If hypotension occurs, the patient should be placed in a supine position and, if necessary, treated with intravenous infusion of physiological saline. Ramipril treatment usually can be continued following restoration of blood pressure and volume.

NEUTROPENIA/AGRANULOCYTOSIS

Another angiotensin converting enzyme inhibitor, captopril, has been shown to cause agranulocytosis and bone marrow depression, rarely in uncomplicated patients, but more frequently in patients with renal impairment, especially if they also have a collagen-vascular disease such as systemic lupus erythematosus or scleroderma. Available data from clinical trials of Ramipril are insufficient to show that Ramipril does not cause agranulocytosis at similar rates. Monitoring of white blood cell counts should be considered in patients with collagen-vascular disease, especially if the disease is associated with impaired renal function.

FETAL/NEONATAL MORBIDITY AND MORTALITY

ACE inhibitors can cause fetal and neonatal morbidity and mortality when administered to pregnant women. Over 100 cases have been reported in the world literature. When pregnancy is detected, ACE inhibitors should be discontinued as soon as possible.

The use of ACE inhibitors during the second and third trimesters of pregnancy has been associated with fetal and neonatal injury, including hypotension, neonatal skull hypoplasia, anuria, reversible or irreversible renal failure, and death. Oligohydramnios has also been reported, presumably resulting from decreased fetal renal function; oligohydramnios in this setting has been associated with fetal limb contractures, craniofacial deformations, and hypoplastic lung development. Prematurity, intrauterine growth retardation, and patent ductus

arteriosus have been reported, although it is not clear whether these occurrences were due to the ACE-inhibitor exposure.

These adverse effects do not appear to have resulted from intrauterine ACE-inhibitor exposure that has been limited to the first trimester. Mothers whose embryos and fetuses are exposed to ACE inhibitors only during the first trimester should be so informed. Nonetheless, when patients become pregnant, physicians should make every effort to discontinue the use of Ramipril as soon as possible.

Rarely (probably less often than once in every thousand pregnancies), no alternative to ACE inhibitors will be found. In these rare cases, the mothers should be apprised of the potential hazards to their fetuses, and serial ultrasound examinations should be performed to assess the intraamniotic environment.

If oligohydramnios is observed, Ramipril should be discontinued unless it is considered life-saving for the mother. Contraction stress testing (CST), a non-stress test (NST), or biophysical profiling (BPP) may be appropriate, depending upon the week of pregnancy. Patients and physicians should be aware, however, that oligohydramnios may not appear until after the fetus has sustained irreversible injury.

Infants with histories of *in utero* exposure to ACE inhibitors should be closely observed for hypotension, oliguria, and hypokalemia. If oliguria occurs, attention should be directed toward support of blood pressure and renal perfusion. Exchange transfusion or dialysis may be required as means of reversing hypotension and/or substituting for disordered renal function. Ramipril which crosses the placenta can be removed from the neonatal circulation by these means, but limited experience has not shown that such removal is central to the treatment of these infants.

No teratogenic effects of Ramipril were seen in studies of pregnant rats, rabbits, and cynomolgus monkeys. On a mg/kg basis, the doses used were up to 2500 times (in rats), 6.25 times (in rabbits), and 1250 times (in monkeys) the maximum recommended human dose.

PRECAUTIONS

GENERAL

Impaired Renal Function: As a consequence of inhibiting the renin-angiotensin-aldosterone system, changes in renal function may be anticipated in susceptible individuals. In patients with severe congestive heart failure whose renal function may depend on the activity of the renin-angiotensin-aldosterone system, treatment with angiotensin converting enzyme inhibitors, including Ramipril, may be associated with oliguria and/or progressive azotemia and (rarely) with acute renal failure and/or death.

In hypertensive patients with unilateral or bilateral renal artery stenosis, increases in blood urea nitrogen and serum creatinine may occur. Experience with another angiotensin converting enzyme inhibitor suggests that these increases are usually reversible upon discontinuation of Ramipril and/or diuretic therapy. In such patients renal function should be monitored during the first few weeks of therapy. Some hypertensive patients with no apparent pre-existing renal vascular disease have developed increases in blood urea nitrogen and serum creatinine, usually minor and transient, especially when Ramipril has been given concomitantly with a diuretic. This is more likely to occur in patients with pre-existing renal impairment. Dosage reduction of Ramipril and/or discontinuation of the diuretic may be required. *Evaluation of the hypertensive patient should always include assessment of renal function.* (See *"Dosage and Administration."*)

Hyperkalemia: In clinical trials, hyperkalemia (serum potassium greater than 5.7 m Eq/L) occurred in approximately 1% of hypertensive patients receiving Ramipril. In most cases, these were isolated values, which resolved despite continued therapy. None of these patients was discontinued from the trials because of hyperkalemia. Risk factors for the development of hyperkalemia include renal insufficiency, diabetes, mellitus, and the concomitant use of potassium-sparing diuretics, potassium supplements, and/or potassium-containing salt substitutes, which should be used cautiously, if at all, with Ramipril. (See *"Drug Interactions."*)

Cough: Cough has been reported with the use of ACE inhibitors. Characteristically, the cough is nonproductive, persistent and resolves after discontinuation of therapy. ACE inhibitor-induced cough should be considered as part of the diferential diagnosis of cough.

Impaired Liver Function: Since Ramipril is primarily metabolized by hepatic esterases to its active moiety, ramiprilat, patients with impaired liver function could develop markedly elevated plasma levels of Ramipril. No formal pharmacokinetic studies have been carried out in hypertensive patients with impaired liver function.

Surgery/Anesthesia: In patients undergoing surgery or during anesthesia with agents that produce hypotension, Ramipril may block angiotensin II formation that would otherwise occur secondary to compensatory renin release. Hypotension that occurs as a result of this mechanism can be corrected by volume expansion.

INFORMATION FOR PATIENTS

Pregnancy: Female patients of childbearing age should be told about the consequences of second- and third-trimester exposure to ACE inhibitors, and they should also be told that these consequences do not appear to have resulted from intrautrine ACE-inhibitor exposure that has been limited to the first trimester. These patients should be asked to report pregnancies to their physicians as soon as possible.

Angioedema: Angioedema, including laryngeal edema, can occur with treatment with ACE inhibitors, especially following the first dose. Patients should be so

---

◆ RATED THERAPEUTICALLY EQUIVALENT; ◇ THERAPEUTIC EQUIVALENCE UNCONFIRMED; ○ UNRATED

advised and told to report immediately any signs or symptoms suggesting angioedema (swelling of face, eyes, lips, or tongue, or difficulty in breathing) and to take no more drug until they have consulted with the prescribing physician.

Symptomatic Hypotension: Patients should be cautioned that lightheadedness can occur, especially during the first days of therapy, and it should be reported. Patients should be told that if syncope occurs, Ramipril should be discontinued until the physician has been consulted.

All patients should be cautioned that inadequate fluid intake or excessive perspiration, diarrhea, or vomiting can lead to an excessive fall in blood pressure, with the same consequences of lightheadedness and possible syncope.

Hyperkalemia: Patients should be told not to use salt substitutes containing potassium without consulting their physician.

Neutropenia: Patients should be told to promptly report any indication of infection (e.g., sore throat, fever), which could be a sign of neutropenia.

DRUG INTERACTIONS
With Diuretics: Patients on diuretics, especially those in whom diuretic therapy was recently instituted, may occasionally experience an excessive reduction of blood pressure after initiation of therapy with Ramipril. The possibility of hypotensive effects with Ramipril can be minimized by either discontinuing the diuretic or increasing the salt intake prior to initiation of treatment with Ramipril. If this is not possible, the starting dose should be reduced. (See *"Dosage and Administration."*)

With Potassium Supplements and Potassium-Sparing Diuretics: Ramipril can attenuate potassium loss caused by thiazide diuretics. Potassium-sparing diuretics (spironolactone, amiloride, triamterene, and others) or potassium supplements can increase the risk of hyperkalemia. Therefore, if concomitant use of such agents is indicated, they should be given with caution, and the patient's serum potassium should be monitored frequently.

With Lithium: Increased serum lithium levels and symptoms of lithium toxicity have been reported in patients receiving ACE inhibitors during therapy with lithium. These drugs should be coadministered with caution, and frequent monitoring of serum lithium levels is recommended. If a diuretic is also used, the risk of lithium toxicity may be increased.

Other: Neither Ramipril nor its metabolites have been found to interact with food, digoxin, or antacid.

CARCINOGENESIS, MUTAGENESIS, IMPAIRMENT OF FERTILITY
No evidence of a tumorigenic effect was found when ramipril was given by gavage to rats (up to 500 mg/kg/day for 24 months) or to mice (up to 1,000 mg/kg/day for 18 months). Dosages greatly in excess of those recommended for humans produced hypertrophy of the renal juxtaglomerular apparatus in mice, rats, dogs, and monkeys. No mutagenic activity was detected in the Ames test in bacteria, the micronucleus test in mice, unscheduled DNA synthesis in a human cell line, or a forward gene-mutation assay in a Chinese hamster ovary cell line. Several metabolites and degradation products of Ramipril were also negative in the Ames test. A study in rats with dosages as great as 500 mg/kg/day did not produce adverse effects on fertility.

PREGNANCY
Pregnancy Category C: (first trimester) and D (second and third trimesters). See *"Warnings: Fetal/neonatal morbidity and mortality."*

NURSING MOTHERS
Ingestion of a single 10 mg oral dose of Ramipril resulted in undetectable amounts of Ramipril and its metabolites in breast milk. However, because multiple doses may produce low milk concentrations that are not predictable from single doses. Ramipril should not be administered to nursing mothers.

GERIATRIC USE
Of the total number of patients who received Ramipril in US clinical studies of Ramipril 11.0% were 65 and over while 0.2% were 75 and over. No overall differences in effectiveness or safety were observed between these patients and younger patients, and other reported clinical experience has not identified differences in responses between the elderly and younger patients, but greater sensitivity of some older individuals cannot be ruled out.

One pharmacokinetic study conducted in hospitalized elderly patients indicated that peak ramiprilat levels and area under the plasma concentration time curve (AUC) for ramiprilat are higher in older patients.

PEDIATRIC USE
Safety and effectiveness in children have not been established.

ADVERSE REACTIONS
Ramipril has been evaluated for safety in over 4,000 patients with hypertension: of these, 1,230 patients were studied in US controlled trials, and 1,107 were studied in foreign controlled trials. Almost 700 of these patients were treated for at least one year. The overall incidence of reported adverse events was similar in Ramipril and placebo patients. The most frequent clinical side effects (possibly or probably related to study drug) reported by patients receiving Ramipril in US placebo-controlled trials were: headache (5.4%), "dizziness" (2.2%) and fatigue or asthenia (2.0%), but only the last was more common in Ramipril patients than in patients given placebo. Generally, the side effects were mild and transient, and there was no relation to total dosage within the range of 1.25 to 20 mg. Discontinuation of therapy because of a side effect was required in approximately

3% of US patients treated with Ramipril. The most common reasons for discontinuation were: cough (1.0%), "dizziness" (0.5%), and impotence (0.4%).

The side effects considered possibly or probably related to study drug that occurred in US placebo-controlled trials in more than 1% of patients treated with Ramipril are shown below.

PATIENTS IN US PLACEBO CONTROLLED STUDIES

	Ramipril (N = 651)		Placebo (N = 286)	
	n	%	n	%
Headache	35	5.4	17	5.9
"Dizziness"	14	2.2	9	3.1
Asthenia (Fatigue)	13	2.0	2	0.7
Nausea/ Vomiting	7	1.1	3	1.0

In placebo-controlled trials, there was also an excess of upper respiratory infection and flu syndrome in the Ramipril group. As these studies were carried out before the relationship of cough to ACE inhibitors was recognized, some of these events may represent Ramipril-induced cough. In a later 1-year study, increased cough was seen in almost 12% of Ramipril patients, with about 4% of these patients, requiring discontinuation of treatment. Other adverse experiences reported in controlled clinical trials (in less than 1% of Ramipril patients), or rarer events seen in postmarketing experience, include the following (In some, a causal relationship to drug use is uncertain.):

Cardiovascular: Symptomatic hypotension (reported in 0.5% of patients in US trials) (see *"Precautions"* and *"Warnings"*), syncope (not reported in US trials), angina pectoris, arrhythmia, chest pain, palpitations, myocardial infarction- and cerebrovascular events.

Renal: Some hypertensive patients with no apparent pre-existing renal disease have developed minor, usually transient, increases in blood urea nitrogen and serum creatinine when taking Ramipril, particularly when Ramipril was given concomitantly with a diuretic. (See *"Warnings."*)

Angioneurotic Edema: angioneurotic edema has been reported in 0.3% of patients in US clinical trials. (See *"Warnings"*).

Cough: A tickling, dry, persistent, nonproductive cough has been reported with the use of ACE inhibitors. Approximately 1% of patients treated with Ramipril have required discontinuation because of cough. The cough disappears shortly after discontinuation of treatment. (See *"Precautions, Cough"* subsection.)

Gastrointestinal: Abdominal pain (sometimes with enzyme changes suggesting pancreatitis), anorexia, constipation, diarrhea, dry mouth, dyspepsia, dysphagia, gastroenteritis, nausea, increased salivation, taste disturbance, and vomiting.

Dermatologic: Apparent hypersensitivity reactions (manifested by dermatitis, pruritis, or rash, with or without fever), photosensitivity, and purpura.

Neurologic and Psychiatric: Anxiety, amnesia, convulsions, depression, hearing loss, insomnia, nervousness, neuralgia, neuropathy, paresthesia, somnolence, tinnitus, tremor, vertigo, and vision disturbances.

FETAL/NEONATAL MORBIDITY AND MORTALITY
(See *"Warnings: Fetal/Neonatal Morbidity and Mortality."*)

Other: arthralgia, arthritis, dyspnea, edema, epistaxis, impotence, increased sweating, malaise, myalgia, and weight gain.

CLINICAL LABORATORY TEST FINDINGS
Creatinine and Blood Urea Nitrogen: Increases in creatinine levels occurred in 1.2% of patients receiving Ramipril alone, and in 1.5% of patients receiving Ramipril and a diuretic. Increases in blood urea nitrogen levels occurred in 0.5% of patients receiving Ramipril alone and in 3% of patients receiving Ramipril with a diuretic. None of these increases required discontinuation of treatment. Increases in these laboratory values are more likely to occur in patients with renal insufficiency or those pretreated with a diuretic and, based on experience with other ACE inhibitors, would be expected to be especially likely in patients with renal artery stenosis. (See *"Precautions"* and *"Warnings."*)

Since Ramipril decreases aldosterone secretion, elevation of serum potassium can occur. Potassium supplements and potassium-sparing diuretics should be given with caution, and the patient's serum potassium should be monitored frequently. (See *"Precautions"* and *"Warnings."*)

Hemoglobin and Hematocrit: Decreases in hemoglobin or hematocrit (a low value and a decrease of 5 g/dl or 5% respectively) were rare, occurring in 0.4% of patients receiving Ramipril alone and in 1.5% of patients receiving Ramipril plus a diuretic. No US patients discontinued treatment because of decreases in hemoglobin or hematocrit.

Other (causal relationships unknown): Clinically important changes in standard laboratory tests were rarely associated with Ramipril administration. Elevations of liver enzymes, serum bilirubin, uric acid, and blood glucose have been reported, as have scattered incidents of leukopenia, eosinophilia, and proteinuria. In US trials, less than 0.2% of patients discontinued treatment for laboratory abnormalities: all of these were cases of proteinuria or abnormal liver-function tests.

OVERDOSAGE

The oral LD_{50} of rats and mice is 10-11 g/kg. In dogs, oral doses as high as 1 g/kg induced only mild gastrointestinal distress. Human overdoses of Ramipril have not been reported, but the most common manifestation of human Ramipril overdosage is likely to be hypotension.

Laboratory determinations of serum levels of Ramipril and its metabolites are not widely available, and such determinations have, in any event, no established role in the management of Ramipril overdose.

No data are available to suggest physiological maneuvers (e.g., maneuvers to change the pH of the urine) that might accelerate elimination of Ramipril and its metabolites. Similarly, it is not known which, if any, of these substances can be usefully removed from the body by hemodialysis.

Angiotensin II could presumably serve as a specific antagonist-antidote in the setting of Ramipril overdose, but angiotensin II is essentially unavailable outside of scattered research facilities. Because the hypotensive effect of Ramipril is achieved through vasodilation and effective hypovolemia, it is reasonable to treat Ramipril overdose by infusion of normal saline solution.

DOSAGE AND ADMINISTRATION

The recommended initial dose for patients not receiving a diuretic is 2.5 mg once a day. Dosage should be adjusted according to the blood pressure response. The usual maintenance dosage range is 2.5 to 20 mg per day administered as a single dose or in two equally divided doses. In some patients treated once daily, the antihypertensive effect may diminish toward the end of the dosing interval. In such patients, an increase in dosage or twice daily administration should be considered. If blood pressure is not controlled with Ramipril alone, a diuretic can be added.

Concomitant administration of Ramipril with potassium supplements, potassium salt substitutes, or potassium-sparing diuretics can lead to increases of serum potassium. (See *"Precautions"*.)

In patients who are currently being treated with a diuretic, symptomatic hypotension occasionally can occur following the initial dose of Ramipril. To reduce the likelihood of hypotension, the diuretic should, if possible, be discontinued two to three days prior to beginning therapy with Ramipril (see *"Warnings"*). Then, if blood pressure is not controlled with Ramipril alone, diuretic therapy should be resumed.

If the diuretic cannot be discontinued, an initial dose of 1.25 mg Ramipril should be used to avoid excess hypotension.

DOSAGE ADJUSTMENT IN RENAL IMPAIRMENT

For patients with a creatinine clearance < 40 ml/min/1.73m² (serum creatinine > 2.5 mg/dl), the recommended initial dose is 1.25 mg Ramipril once daily. Dosage may be titrated upward until blood pressure is controlled or to a maximum total daily dose of 5 mg.

STORAGE

Dispense in well-closed container with safety closure. Store at controlled room temperature (59° to 86°F).

HOW SUPPLIED
CAPSULE: 1.25 MG

BRAND/MANUFACTURER	NDC	SIZE	AWP
○ **BRAND**			
► ALTACE: Hoechst	00039-0103-10	100s	$59.08
	00039-0103-11	100s ud	$59.08

CAPSULE: 2.5 MG

BRAND/MANUFACTURER	NDC	SIZE	AWP
○ **BRAND**			
► ALTACE: Hoechst	00039-0104-10	100s	$69.31
	00039-0104-11	100s ud	$69.31

CAPSULE: 5 MG

BRAND/MANUFACTURER	NDC	SIZE	AWP
○ **BRAND**			
► ALTACE: Hoechst	00039-0105-10	100s	$74.18
	00039-0105-11	100s ud	$74.18

CAPSULE: 10 MG

BRAND/MANUFACTURER	NDC	SIZE	AWP
○ **BRAND**			
► ALTACE: Hoechst	00039-0106-10	100s	$86.00

Ranitidine Hydrochloride

DESCRIPTION

The active ingredient in Ranitidine tablets, capsules, syrup, and injection is Ranitidine Hydrochloride (HCl), a histamine H_2-receptor antagonist. Chemically it is N[2-[[[5-[(dimethylamino)methyl]-2-furanyl] methyl]thio]ethyl]-N′-methyl-2-nitro-1,1-ethenediamine, HCl.

The empirical formula is $C_{13}H_{22}N_4O_3S\cdot HCl$, representing a molecular weight of 350.87.

Ranitidine HCl is a white to pale yellow, granular substance that is soluble in water. It has a slightly bitter taste and sulfurlike odor.

Ranitidine Injection is a clear, colorless to yellow, nonpyrogenic liquid. The yellow color of the liquid tends to intensify without adversely affecting potency. The pH of the injection solution is 6.7-7.3.

Each Ranitidine HCl 150 Tablet for oral administration contains 168 mg of Ranitidine HCl equivalent to 150 mg of Ranitidine.

Each Ranitidine HCl 300 Tablet for oral administration contains 336 mg of Ranitidine HCl equivalent to 300 mg of Ranitidine.

Ranitidine HCl 150 Capsules and Ranitidine HCl 300 Capsules for oral administration are soft gelatin capsules containing 168 mg of Ranitidine HCl equivalent to 150 mg of Ranitidine and 336 mg of Ranitidine HCl equivalent to 300 mg of Ranitidine, respectively.

Each 1 mL of Ranitidine HCl Syrup contains 16.8 mg of Ranitidine HCl equivalent to 15 mg of Ranitidine.

Sterile Injection for Intramuscular or Intravenous Administration: Each 1 mL of aqueous solution contains Ranitidine 25 mg (as the hydrochloride).

A pharmacy bulk package is a container of a sterile preparation for parenteral use that contains many single doses. The contents are intended for use in a pharmacy admixture program and are restricted to the preparation of admixtures for intravenous (IV) infusion.

Sterile, Premixed Solution for Intravenous Administration in Single-Dose, Flexible Plastic Containers: Each 50 mL contains Ranitidine HCl equivalent to 50 mg of Ranitidine. The osmolarity of this solution is 180 mOsm/L (approx.), and the pH is 6.7-7.3.

Following is its chemical structure:

$$(CH_3)_2NCH_2 \diagup\!\!\!\diagup O \diagdown\!\!\!\diagdown CH_2SCH_2CH_2NHCNHCH_3$$
$$\overset{CHNO_2}{\underset{\parallel}{}}$$

CLINICAL PHARMACOLOGY

Ranitidine HCl is a competitive, reversible inhibitor of the action of histamine at the histamine H_2-receptors, including receptors on the gastric cells. Ranitidine HCl does not lower serum Ca^{++} in hypercalcemic states. Ranitidine HCl is not an anticholinergic agent.

ANTISECRETORY ACTIVITY

1. Effects on Acid Secretion: Ranitidine HCl inhibits both daytime and nocturnal basal gastric acid secretion as well as gastric acid secretion stimulated by food, betazole, and pentagastrin, as shown in the following tables: (See related table).

It appears that basal-, nocturnal-, and betazole-stimulated secretions are most sensitive to inhibition by Oral Ranitidine HCl, responding almost completely to doses of 100 mg or less, while pentagastrin- and food-stimulated secretions are more difficult to suppress. (See related table).

In a group of 10 known hypersecretors, Ranitidine plasma levels of 71, 180, and 376 ng/mL inhibited basal acid secretion by 76%, 90%, and 99.5%, respectively.

It appears that basal- and betazole-stimulated secretions are most sensitive to inhibition by IV Ranitidine HCl, while pentagastrin-stimulated secretion is more difficult to suppress.

2. Effects on Other Gastrointestinal Secretions: Pepsin: Ranitidine HCl does not affect pepsin secretion. Total pepsin output is reduced in proportion to the decrease in volume of gastric juice.

Intrinsic Factor: Ranitidine HCl has no significant effect on pentagastrin-stimulated intrinsic factor secretion.

Serum Gastrin: Ranitidine HCl has little or no effect on fasting or postprandial serum gastrin.

OTHER PHARMACOLOGIC ACTIONS

a. Gastric bacterial flora—increase in nitrate-reducing organisms, significance not known.

b. Prolactin levels—no effect in recommended oral or intravenous (IV) dosage, but small, transient, dose-related increases in serum prolactin have been reported after IV bolus injections of 100 mg or more.

c. Other pituitary hormones—no effect on serum gonadotropins, TSH, or GH. Possible impairment of vasopressin release.

d. No change in cortisol, aldosterone, androgen, or estrogen levels.

e. No antiandrogenic action.

f. No effect on count, motility, or morphology of sperm.

Pharmacokinetics: Ranitidine HCl is 50% absorbed after oral administration, compared to an IV injection with mean peak levels of 440-545 ng/mL occurring at 2-3 hours after a 150-mg dose. The tablet and syrup formulations are bioequivalent, and the capsule and tablet are bioequivalent. The elimination half-life is 2.5-3 hours.

Absorption is not significantly impaired by the administration of food or antacids. Propantheline slightly delays and increases peak blood levels of Oral Ranitidine HCl, probably by delaying gastric emptying and transit time. In one study, simultaneous administration of high-potency antacid (150 mmol) in fasting subjects has been reported to decrease the absorption of Oral Ranitidine HCl.

◆ RATED THERAPEUTICALLY EQUIVALENT; ◇ THERAPEUTIC EQUIVALENCE UNCONFIRMED; ○ UNRATED

EFFECT OF ORAL RANITIDINE HCl ON GASTRIC ACID SECRETION

	Time After Dose, h	% Inhibition of Gastric Acid Output by Dose, mg			
		75-80	100	150	200
Basal	Up to 4		99	95	
Nocturnal	Up to 13	95	96	92	
Betazole	Up to 3		97	99	
Pentagastrin	Up to 5	58	72	72	80
Meal	Up to 3		73	79	95

EFFECT OF IV RANITIDINE HCL ON GASTRIC ACID SECRETION

	Time After Dose, h	% Inhibition of Gastric Acid Output by IV Dose, mg		
		20 mg	60 mg	100 mg
Betazole	Up to 2	93	99	99
Pentagastrin	Up to 3	47	66	77

Serum concentrations necessary to inhibit 50% of stimulated gastric acid secretion are estimated to be 36-94 ng/mL. Following a single oral dose of 150 mg, serum concentrations of Ranitidine HCl are in this range up to 12 hours. However, blood levels bear no consistent relationship to dose or degree of acid inhibition.

The principal route of excretion is the urine, with approximately 30% of the orally administered dose collected in the urine as unchanged drug in 24 hours. Renal clearance is about 410 mL per minute, indicating active tubular excretion. Four patients with clinically significant renal function impairment (creatinine clearance 25-35 mL per minute) administered 50 mg of Ranitidine IV had an average plasma half-life of 4.8 hours, a Ranitidine clearance of 29 mL per minute, and a volume of distribution of 1.76 L/g. In general, these parameters appear to be altered in proportion to creatinine clearance (see "Dosage and Administration").

Serum concentrations necessary to inhibit 50% of stimulated gastric acid secretion are estimated to be 36-94 ng/mL. Following single IV or intramuscular (IM) 50-mg doses, serum concentrations of Ranitidine HCl are in this range for 6-8 hours.

Following IV injection, approximately 70% of the dose is recovered in the urine as unchanged drug. Renal clearance averages 530 mL per minute, with a total clearance of 760 mL per minute. The volume of distribution is 1.4 L/kg, and the elimination half-life is 2-2.5 hours.

Ranitidine HCl is absorbed very rapidly after IM injection. Mean peak levels of 576 ng/mL occur within 15 minutes or less following a 50-mg IM dose. Absorption from IM sites is virtually complete, with a bioavailability of 90%-100% compared with IV administration.

In man, the N-oxide is the principal metabolite in the urine; however, this amounts to less than 4% of the dose. Other metabolites are the S-oxide (1%) and the desmethyl Ranitidine (1%). The remainder of the administered dose is found in the stool. Studies in patients with hepatic dysfunction (compensated cirrhosis) indicate that there are minor, but clinically insignificant, alterations in Ranitidine half-life, distribution, clearance, and bioavailability.

The volume of distribution is about 1.4 L/kg. Serum protein binding averages 15%.

CLINICAL TRIALS
Active Duodenal Ulcer: In a multicenter, double-blind, controlled, US study of endoscopically diagnosed duodenal ulcers, earlier healing was seen in the patients treated with oral Ranitidine HCl as shown in the following table: (See related table).

In these studies patients treated with Oral Ranitidine HCl reported a reduction in both daytime and nocturnal pain, and they also consumed less antacid than the placebo-treated patients.

	Mean Daily Doses of Antacid	
	Ulcer Healed	Ulcer Not Healed
Oral Ranitidine HCl	0.06	0.71
Oral Placebo	0.71	1.43

Foreign studies have shown that patients heal equally well with 150 mg b.i.d. and 300 mg h.s. (85% versus 84%, respectively) during a usual 4-week course of therapy. If patients require extended therapy of 8 weeks, the healing rate may be higher for 150 mg b.i.d. as compared to 300 mg h.s. (92% versus 87%, respectively).

Studies have been limited to short-term treatment of acute duodenal ulcer. Patients whose ulcers healed during therapy had recurrences of ulcers at the usual rates. There have been no systematic studies to evaluate whether continued treatment with Oral Ranitidine HCl alters recurrence rates.

Maintenance Therapy in Duodenal Ulcer: Oral Ranitidine HCl has been found to be effective as maintenance therapy for patients following healing of acute duodenal ulcers. In two independent, double-blind, multicenter, controlled trials, the number of duodenal ulcers observed was significantly less in patients treated with Oral Ranitidine HCl (150 mg h.s.) than in patients treated with placebo over a 12-month period.

DUODENAL ULCER PREVALENCE

Double-blind, Multicenter, Placebo-Controlled Trials

Multicenter Trial	Drug	Duodenal Ulcer Prevalence			No. of Patients
		0-4 Month	0-8 Months	0-12 Months	
USA	RAN	20%*	24%*	35%*	138
	PLC	44%	54%	59%	139
Foreign	RAN	12%*	21%*	28%*	174
	PLC	56%	64%	68%	165

% = Life table estimate.
* = p < 0.005 (Oral Ranitidine) versus comparator HCl.
RAN = Ranitidine.
PLC = placebo.

As with other H_2-antagonists, the factors responsible for the significant reduction in the prevalence of duodenal ulcers include prevention of recurrence of ulcers, more rapid healing of ulcers that may occur during maintenance therapy, or both.

Gastric Ulcer: In a multicenter, double-blind, controlled, US study of endoscopically diagnosed gastric ulcers, earlier healing was seen in the patients treated with Oral Ranitidine HCl as shown in the following table:

	Oral Ranitidine HCl*		Placebo*	
	Number Entered	Healed/ Evaluable	Number Entered	Healed/ Evaluable
Outpatients				
Week 2	92	16/83 (19%)	94	10/83 (12%)
Week 6		50/73 (68%)†		35/69 (51%)

* All patients were permitted p.r.n. antacids for relief of pain.
† p = 0.009.

In this multicenter trial, significantly more patients treated with oral Ranitidine HCl became pain-free during therapy.

Pathological Hypersecretory Conditions (such as Zollinger-Ellison syndrome): Ranitidine HCl inhibits gastric acid secretion and reduces occurrence of diarrhea, anorexia, and pain in patients with pathological hypersecretion associated with Zollinger-Ellison syndrome, systemic mastocytosis, and other pathological hy-

	Oral Ranitidine*		Oral Placebo*	
	Number Entered	Healed/ Evaluable	Number Entered	Healed/ Evaluable
Outpatients				
Week 2	195	69/182 (38%)†	188	31/164 (19%)
Week 4		137/187 (73%)†		76/168 (45%)

* All patients were permitted p.r.n. antacids for relief of pain.
† p < 0.0001.

► SHOWN IN PRODUCT IDENTIFICATION GUIDE

persecretory conditions (e.g., postoperative, "short-gut" syndrome, idiopathic). Use of Ranitidine HCl was followed by healing of ulcers in 8 of 19 (42%) patients who were intractable to previous therapy.

In a retrospective review of 52 Zollinger-Ellison patients given Ranitidine HCl as a continuous IV infusion for up to 15 days, no patients developed complications of acid-peptic disease such as bleeding or perforation. Acid output was controlled to less than or equal to 10 mEq per hour.

Gastroesophageal Reflux Disease (GERD): In two multicenter, double-blind, placebo-controlled, 6-week trials performed in the United States and Europe Ranitidine HCl 150 mg b.i.d. was more effective than placebo for the relief of heartburn and other symptoms associated with GERD. Ranitidine-treated patients consumed significantly less antacid than did placebo-treated patients.

The US trial indicated that Ranitidine HCl 150 mg b.i.d. significantly reduced the frequency of heartburn attacks and severity of heartburn pain within 1-2 weeks after starting therapy. The improvement was maintained throughout the 6-week trial period. Moreover, patient response rates demonstrated that the effect on heartburn extends through both the day and night time periods.

Erosive Esophagitis: In two multicenter, double-blind, randomized, placebo-controlled 12-week trials performed in the United States, Ranitidine HCl 150 mg q.i.d. was significantly more effective than placebo in healing endoscopically diagnosed erosive esophagitis and in relieving associated heartburn. The erosive esophagitis healing rates were as follows:

EROSIVE ESOPHAGITIS PATIENT HEALING RATES

	Healed/Evaluable	
	Placebo* n = 229	Ranitidine HCl 150 mg q.i.d n = 215
Week 4	43/198 (22%)	96/206 (47%)†
Week 8	63/176 (36%)	142/200 (71%)†
Week 12	92/159 (58%)	162/192 (84%)†

* *All patients were permitted p.r.n. antacids for relief of pain.*
† *p < 0.001 versus placebo.*

No additional benefit in healing of esophagitis or in relief of heartburn was seen with a Ranitidine dose of 300 mg q.i.d.

INDICATIONS AND USAGE
Oral Ranitidine HCl is indicated in:

1. Short-term treatment of active duodenal ulcer. Most patients heal within 4 weeks. Studies available to date have not assessed the safety of Ranitidine in uncomplicated duodenal ulcer for periods of more than 8 weeks.
2. Maintenance therapy for duodenal ulcer patients at reduced dosage after healing of acute ulcers. No placebo-controlled comparative studies have been carried out for periods of longer than 1 year.
3. The treatment of pathological hypersecretory conditions (e.g., Zollinger-Ellison syndrome and systemic mastocytosis).
4. Short-term treatment of active, benign gastric ulcer. Most patients heal within 6 weeks and the usefulness of further treatment has not been demonstrated. Studies available to date have not assessed the safety of Ranitidine in uncomplicated, benign gastric ulcer for periods of more than 6 weeks.
5. Treatment of GERD. Symptomatic relief commonly occurs within 1 or 2 weeks after starting therapy with Ranitidine HCl 150 mg b.i.d.
6. Treatment of endoscopically diagnosed erosive esophagitis. Healing of endoscopically diagnosed erosive esophagitis occurs at 4 weeks (47%), 8 weeks (71%), and 12 weeks (84%) of therapy with Ranitidine HCl 150 mg q.i.d. Symptomatic relief of heartburn commonly occurs within 24 hours of therapy initiation with Ranitidine HCl.

Concomitant antacids should be given as needed for pain relief to patients with active duodenal ulcer; active, benign gastric ulcer; hypersecretory states; GERD; and erosive esophagitis.

Ranitidine HCl Injection and Ranitidine HCl Injection Premixed are indicated in some hospitalized patients with pathological hypersecretory conditions or intractable duodenal ulcers, or as an alternative to the oral dosage form for short-term use in patients who are unable to take oral medication.

UNLABELED USES
Ranitidine is used alone or as an adjunct in the treatment of Mendelson's syndrome (for prophylaxis of aspiration pneumonitis), drug-induced gastritis, and acute upper gastrointestinal hemorrhage.

CONTRAINDICATIONS
Ranitidine HCl is contraindicated for patients known to have hypersensitivity to the drug or any of the ingredients.

PRECAUTIONS
GENERAL
1. Symptomatic response to Ranitidine HCl therapy does not preclude the presence of gastric malignancy.
2. Since Ranitidine HCl is excreted primarily by the kidney, dosage should be adjusted in patients with impaired renal function (see "Dosage and Administration"). Caution should be observed in patients with hepatic dysfunction since Ranitidine HCl is metabolized in the liver.

3. Rare reports suggest that Ranitidine HCl may precipitate acute porphyria attacks in patients with acute porphyria. Ranitidine HCl should therefore be avoided in patients with a history of acute porphyria.
4. In controlled studies in normal volunteers, elevations in SGPT have been observed when H₂-antagonists have been administered intravenously at greater than recommended dosages for 5 days or longer. Therefore, it seems prudent in patients receiving IV Ranitidine at dosages greater than or equal to 100 mg q.i.d. for periods of 5 days or longer to monitor SGPT daily (from day 5) for the remainder of IV therapy.
5. Bradycardia in association with rapid administration of Ranitidine HCl Injection has been reported rarely, usually in patients with factors predisposing to cardiac rhythm disturbances. Recommended rates of administration should not be exceeded (see "Dosage and Administration").

Laboratory Tests: False-positive tests for urine protein with Multistix® may occur during Ranitidine HCl therapy, and therefore testing with sulfosalicylic acid is recommended.

Drug Interactions: Although Ranitidine HCl has been reported to bind weakly to cytochrome P-450 *in vitro*, recommended doses of the drug do not inhibit the action of the cytochrome P-450-linked oxygenase enzymes in the liver. However, there have been isolated reports of drug interactions that suggest that Ranitidine HCl may affect the bioavailability of certain drugs by some mechanism as yet unidentified (e.g., a pH-dependent effect on absorption or a change in volume of distribution).

Increased or decreased prothrombin times have been reported during concurrent use of Ranitidine and warfarin. However, in human pharmacokinetic studies with dosages of Ranitidine up to 400 mg per day, no interaction occurred; Ranitidine had no effect on warfarin clearance or prothrombin time. The possibility of an interaction with warfarin at dosages of Ranitidine higher than 400 mg per day has not been investigated.

Carcinogenesis, Mutagenesis, Impairment of Fertility: There was no indication of tumorigenic or carcinogenic effects in life-span studies in mice and rats at dosages up to 2,000 mg/kg per day.

Ranitidine was not mutagenic in standard bacterial tests (*Salmonella, Escherichia coli*) for mutagenicity at concentrations up to the maximum recommended for these assays. In a dominant lethal assay, a single oral dose of 1,000 mg/kg to male rats was without effect on the outcome of two matings per week for the next 9 weeks.

Pregnancy: Teratogenic Effects: Pregnancy Category B: Reproduction studies have been performed in rats and rabbits at oral doses up to 160 times the human oral dose and have revealed no evidence of impaired fertility or harm to the fetus due to Ranitidine HCl. There are, however, no adequate and well-controlled studies in pregnant women. Because animal reproduction studies are not always predictive of human response, this drug should be used during pregnancy only if clearly needed.

Nursing Mothers: Ranitidine HCl is secreted in human milk. Caution should be exercised when Ranitidine HCl is administered to a nursing mother.

Pediatric Use: Safety and effectiveness in children have not been established.

Use in Elderly Patients: Ulcer healing rates in elderly patients (65-82 years of age) treated with oral Ranitidine HCl were no different from those in younger age-groups. The incidence rates for adverse events and laboratory abnormalities were also not different from those seen in other age-groups.

ADVERSE REACTIONS
The following have been reported as events in clinical trials or in the routine management of patients treated with oral Ranitidine HCl. The relationship to Ranitidine HCl therapy has been unclear in many cases. Headache, sometimes severe, seems to be related to Ranitidine HCl administration.

Central Nervous System: Rarely, malaise, dizziness, somnolence, insomnia, and vertigo. Rare cases of reversible mental confusion, agitation, depression, and hallucinations have been reported, predominantly in severely ill elderly patients. Rare cases of reversible blurred vision suggestive of a change in accommodation have been reported. Rare reports of reversible involuntary motor disturbances have been received.

Cardiovascular: As with other H₂-blockers, rare reports of arrhythmias such as tachycardia, bradycardia, asystole, atrioventricular block, and premature ventricular beats.

Gastrointestinal: Constipation, diarrhea, nausea/vomiting, abdominal discomfort/pain, and rare reports of pancreatitis.

Hepatic: In normal volunteers, SGPT values were increased to at least twice the pretreatment levels in 6 of 12 subjects receiving 100 mg q.i.d. IV for 7 days, and in 4 of 24 subjects receiving 50 mg q.i.d. IV for 5 days. There have been occasional reports of hepatitis, hepatocellular or hepatocanalicular or mixed, with or without jaundice. In such circumstances, Ranitidine should be immediately discontinued. These events are usually reversible, but in exceedingly rare circumstances death has occurred.

Musculoskeletal: Rare reports of arthralgias and myalgias.

Hematologic: Blood count changes (leukopenia, granulocytopenia, and thrombocytopenia) have occurred in a few patients. These were usually reversible. Rare cases of agranulocytosis, pancytopenia, sometimes with marrow hypoplasia, and aplastic anemia and exceedingly rare cases of acquired immune hemolytic anemia have been reported.

◆ RATED THERAPEUTICALLY EQUIVALENT; ◇ THERAPEUTIC EQUIVALENCE UNCONFIRMED; ○ UNRATED

Endocrine: Controlled studies in animals and man have shown no stimulation of any pituitary hormone by Ranitidine HCl and no antiandrogenic activity, and cimetidine-induced gynecomastia and impotence in hypersecretory patients have resolved when Ranitidine HCl has been substituted. However, occasional cases of gynecomastia, impotence, and loss of libido have been reported in male patients receiving Ranitidine HCl, but the incidence did not differ from that in the general population.

Integumentary: Rash, including rare cases suggestive of mild erythema multiforme, and, rarely, alopecia.

Other: Rare cases of hypersensitivity reactions (e.g., bronchospasm, fever, rash, eosinophilia), anaphylaxis, angioneurotic edema, and small increases in serum creatinine.

Transient pain at the site of IM injection has been reported. Transient local burning or itching has been reported with IV administration of Ranitidine HCl.

OVERDOSAGE

There has been limited experience with overdosage with oral Ranitidine and virtually no experience with overdosage with Ranitidine Injection. Reported acute ingestions of up to 18 g orally have been associated with transient adverse effects similar to those encountered in normal clinical experience (see *"Adverse Reactions"*). In addition, abnormalities of gait and hypotension have been reported.

When overdosage occurs, the usual measures to remove unabsorbed material from the gastrointestinal tract, clinical monitoring, and supportive therapy should be employed.

Studies in dogs receiving dosages of Ranitidine HCl in excess of 225 mg/kg per day have shown muscular tremors, vomiting, and rapid respiration. Single oral doses of 1,000 mg/kg in mice and rats were not lethal. Intravenous LD$_{50}$ values in mice and rats were 77 and 83 mg/kg, respectively.

DOSAGE AND ADMINISTRATION

Active Duodenal Ulcer: The current recommended adult oral dosage of Ranitidine HCl for duodenal ulcer is 150 mg or 10 mL (2 teaspoonfuls equivalent to 150 mg of Ranitidine) twice daily. An alternative dosage of 300 mg or 20 mL (4 teaspoonfuls equivalent to 300 mg of Ranitidine) once daily after the evening meal or at bedtime can be used for patients in whom dosing convenience is important. The advantages of one treatment regimen compared to the other in a particular patient population have yet to be demonstrated (see *"Clinical Trials: Active Duodenal Ulcer"*). Smaller doses have been shown to be equally effective in inhibiting gastric acid secretion in US studies, and several foreign trials have shown that 100 mg b.i.d. is as effective as the 150-mg dose.

Antacid should be given as needed for relief of pain (see *"Clinical Pharmacology: Pharmacokinetics"*).

Maintenance Therapy: The current recommended adult oral dosage is 150 or 10 mL (2 teaspoonfuls equivalent to 150 mg of Ranitidine) at bedtime.

Pathological Hypersecretory Conditions (such as Zollinger-Ellison syndrome): The current recommended adult oral dosage is 150 mg or 10 mL (2 teaspoonfuls equivalent to 150 mg of Ranitidine) twice a day. In some patients it may be necessary to administer Ranitidine HCl 150-mg doses more frequently. Dosages should be adjusted to individual patient needs, and should continue as long as clinically indicated. Dosages up to 6 g per day have been employed in patients with severe disease.

Benign Gastric Ulcer: The current recommended adult oral dosage is 150 mg or 10 mL (2 teaspoonfuls equivalent to 150 mg or Ranitidine) twice a day.

GERD: The current recommended adult oral dosage is 150 mg or 10 mL (2 teaspoonfuls equivalent to 150 mg of Ranitidine) twice a day.

Erosive Esophagitis: The current recommended adult oral dosage is 150 mg or 10 mL (2 teaspoonfuls equivalent to 150 mg of Ranitidine) four times a day.

Dosage Adjustment for Patients With Impaired Renal Function: On the basis of experience with a group of subjects with severely impaired renal function treated with Ranitidine HCl, the recommended dosage in patients with a creatinine clearance less than 50 mL per minute is 150 mg or 10 mL (2 teaspoonfuls equivalent to 150 mg of Ranitidine) every 24 hours. Should the patient's condition require, the frequency of dosing may be increased to every 12 hours or even further with caution. Hemodialysis reduces the level of circulating Ranitidine. Ideally, the dosing schedule should be adjusted so that the timing of a scheduled dose coincides with the end of hemodialysis.

Parenteral Administration: In some hospitalized patients with pathological hypersecretory conditions or intractable duodenal ulcers or in patients who are unable to take oral medication, Ranitidine HCl may be administered parenterally according to the following recommendations:

Intramuscular Injection: 50 mg (2 mL) every 6-8 hours. (No dilution necessary.)

Intermittent Intravenous Injection:

a. *Intermittent Bolus:* 50 mg (2 mL) every 6-8 hours. Dilute Ranitidine HCl Injection, 50 mg, in 0.9% sodium chloride injection or other compatible IV solution (see *"Stability"*) to a concentration no greater than 2.5 mg/mL (20 mL). Inject at a rate no greater than 4 mL per minute (5 minutes).

b. *Intermittent Infusion:* 50 mg (2 mL) every 6-8 hours. Dilute Ranitidine HCl Injection, 50 mg, in 5% dextrose injection or other compatible IV solution (see *"Stability"*) to a concentration no greater than 0.5 mg/mL (100 mL). Infuse at a rate no greater than 5-7 mL per minute (15-20 minutes).

Ranitidine HCl Injection Premixed solution, 50 mg, in 0.45% sodium chloride, 50 mL, requires no dilution and should be infused over 15-20 minutes.

In some patients it may be necessary to increase dosage. When this is necessary, the increases should be made by more frequent administration of the dose, but generally should not exceed 400 mg per day.

Continuous Intravenous Infusion: Add Ranitidine HCl Injection to 5% dextrose injection or other compatible IV solution (see *"Stability"*). Deliver at a rate of 6.25 mg per hour (e.g., 150 mg [6 mL] Ranitidine HCl Injection in 250 mL of 5% dextrose injection at 10.7 mL per hour).

For Zollinger-Ellison patients, dilute Ranitidine HCl Injection in 5% dextrose injection or other compatible IV solution (see *"Stability"*) to a concentration no greater than 2.5 mg/mL. Start the infusion at a rate of 1.0 mg/kg per hour. If after 4 hours either a measured gastric acid output is greater than 10 mEq per hour or the patient becomes symptomatic, the dose should be adjusted upward in 0.5-mg/kg per hour increments, and the acid output should be remeasured. Dosages up to 2.5 mg/kg per hour and infusion rates as high as 220 mg per hour have been used.

Ranitidine HCl Injection Premixed in Flexible Plastic Containers:

Instructions for Use: To Open: Tear outer wrap at notch and remove solution container. Check for minute leaks by squeezing container firmly. If leaks are found, discard unit as sterility may be impaired.

Preparation for Administration: Use aseptic technique.

1. Close flow control clamp of administration set.
2. Remove cover from outlet port at bottom of container.
3. Insert piercing pin of administration set into port with a twisting motion until the pin is firmly seated. *NOTE:* See full directions on administration set carton.
4. Suspend container from hanger.
5. Squeeze and release drip chamber to establish proper fluid level in chamber during infusion of Ranitidine HCl Injection Premixed.
6. Open flow control clamp to expel air from set. Close clamp.
7. Attach set to venipuncture device. If device is not indwelling, prime and make venipuncture.
8. Perform venipuncture.
9. Regulate rate of administration with flow control clamp.

Caution: Ranitidine HCl Injection Premixed in flexible plastic containers is to be administered by slow IV drip infusion only.

Additives should not be introduced into this solution: If used with a primary IV fluid system, the primary solution should be discontinued during Ranitidine HCl Injection Premixed infusion. Do not administer unless solution is clear and container is undamaged.

Warning: Do not use flexible plastic container in series connections.

Dosage Adjustment for Patients with Impaired Renal Function: The administration of Ranitidine as a continuous infusion has not been evaluated in patients with impaired renal function. On the basis of experience with a group of subjects with severely impaired renal function treated with Ranitidine HCl the recommended dosage in patients with a creatinine clearance less than 50 mL per minute is 50 mg every 18-24 hours. Should the patient's condition require, the frequency of dosing may be increased to every 12 hours or even further with caution. Hemodialysis reduces the level of circulating Ranitidine. Ideally, the dosing schedule should be adjusted so that the timing of a scheduled dose coincides with the end of hemodialysis.

Stability: Undiluted Ranitidine HCl Injection tends to exhibit a yellow color that may intensify over time without adversely affecting potency. Ranitidine HCl Injection is stable for 48 hours at room temperature when added to or diluted with most commonly used IV solutions, e.g., 0.9% sodium chloride injection, 5% dextrose injection, 10% dextrose injection, lactated ringer's injection, or 5% sodium bicarbonate injection.

Ranitidine HCl Injection Premixed in flexible plastic containers is sterile through the expiration date on the label when stored under recommended conditions.

Note: Parenteral drug products should be inspected visually for particulate matter and discoloration before administration whenever solution and container permit.

Directions for Dispensing: Pharmacy Bulk Package—Not for Direct Infusion: The pharmacy bulk package is for use in a pharmacy admixture service only under a laminar flow hood. The closure should be penetrated only once with a sterile transfer set or other sterile dispensing device, which allows measured distribution of the contents, and the contents dispensed in aliquots using aseptic technique. *Contents should be used as soon as possible following initial closure puncture, discard any un-used portion within 24 hours of first entry.* Following closure puncture, container should be maintained below 30°C (86°F) under a laminar flow hood until contents are dispensed.

Storage: Store injection between 4° and 30°C (39° and 86°F). Protect from light. Store the 40-mL pharmacy bulk vial in carton until time of use.

Store premixed injection between 2° and 25°C (36° and 77°F). Protect from light. Exposure of pharmaceutical products to heat should be minimized. Avoid excessive heat; however, brief exposure up to 40°C does not adversely affect the product. Protect from freezing.

Store tablets between 15° and 30°C (59° and 86°F) in a dry place. Protect from light. Replace cap securely after each opening.

Store capsules between 2° and 25°C (36° and 77°F) in a dry place. Protect from light. Replace cap securely after each opening.

Store syrup between 4° and 25°C (39° and 77°F). Dispense in tight, light-resistant containers as defined in the USP/NF.

HOW SUPPLIED
CAPSULE: 150 MG

BRAND/MANUFACTURER	NDC	SIZE	AWP
○ BRAND			
➤ ZANTAC 150 GELDOSE: Glaxo	00173-0428-00	60s	$95.66
	00173-0428-02	60s ud	$97.10

CAPSULE: 300 MG

BRAND/MANUFACTURER	NDC	SIZE	AWP
○ BRAND			
➤ ZANTAC 300 GELDOSE: Glaxo	00173-0429-00	30s	$86.27
	00173-0429-02	30s ud	$86.99

GRANULE FOR RECONSTITUTION: 150 MG

BRAND/MANUFACTURER	NDC	SIZE	AWP
○ BRAND			
ZANTAC 150 EFFERDOSE: Glaxo	00173-0451-00	30s	$47.83
	00173-0451-01	60s	$95.66

INJECTION: 25 MG/ML

BRAND/MANUFACTURER	NDC	SIZE	AWP
○ BRAND			
ZANTAC: Glaxo	00173-0363-01	6 ml	$9.26
	00173-0363-00	40 ml	$60.54
	00173-0362-38	2 ml 10s	$39.91

INJECTION: 50 MG/ML

BRAND/MANUFACTURER	NDC	SIZE	AWP
○ BRAND			
ZANTAC: Glaxo	00173-0441-00	50 ml 24s	$141.86

SYRUP: 150 MG/10 ML

BRAND/MANUFACTURER	NDC	SIZE	AWP
○ BRAND			
ZANTAC: Glaxo	00173-0383-54	480 ml	$186.74

TABLET, EFFERVESCENT: 150 MG

BRAND/MANUFACTURER	NDC	SIZE	AWP
○ BRAND			
➤ ZANTAC 150 EFFERDOSE: Glaxo	00173-0427-00	30s	$47.83
	00173-0427-02	60s	$95.66

TABLETS: 150 MG

BRAND/MANUFACTURER	NDC	SIZE	AWP
○ BRAND			
➤ ZANTAC: Glaxo	00173-0344-42	60s	$99.20
	00173-0344-09	100s	$165.35
	00173-0344-47	100s ud	$167.80
	00173-0344-16	180s	$297.61
	00173-0344-14	500s	$826.69
	00173-0344-12	1000s	$1653.18

TABLETS: 300 MG

BRAND/MANUFACTURER	NDC	SIZE	AWP
○ BRAND			
➤ ZANTAC 300: Glaxo	00173-0393-40	30s	$90.06
	00173-0393-47	100s ud	$302.51
ZANTAC: Glaxo	00173-0393-06	250s	$750.53

Rauzide SEE BENDROFLUMETHIAZIDE AND RAUWOLFIA SERPENTINA

Recombinate SEE ANTIHEMOPHILIC FACTOR

Recombivax HB SEE HEPATITIS B VACCINE, RECOMBINANT

Regitine SEE PHENTOLAMINE MESYLATE

Reglan SEE METOCLOPRAMIDE HYDROCHLORIDE

Regonol SEE PYRIDOSTIGMINE BROMIDE

Regroton SEE CHLORTHALIDONE WITH RESERPINE

Relafen SEE NABUMETONE

Renacidin SEE CITRIC ACID/GLUCONO-DELTA-LACTONE/ MAGNESIUM CARBONATE

RenAmin SEE AMINO ACIDS, INJECTABLE AND AMINO ACIDS/CALCIUM CHLORIDE/DEXTROSE/ELECTROLYTES

Renese R SEE POLYTHIAZIDE AND POLYTHIAZIDE AND RESERPINE

Reno-M SEE DIATRIZOATE MEGLUMINE

Renovue SEE IODAMIDE MEGLUMINE

Reserpine

DESCRIPTION
Reserpine USP, is an antihypertensive, available as 0.1-mg and 0.25-mg tablets for oral administration. Its chemical name is methyl 18β-hydroxy-11,17 α-dimethoxy-3β, 20α-yohimban-16β-carboxylate 3,4,5-trimethoxybenzoate (ester).

Reserpine USP, a pure crystalline alkaloid of rauwolfia, is a white or pale buff to slightly yellowish, odorless crystalline powder. It darkens slowly on exposure to light, but more rapidly when in solution. It is insoluble in water, freely soluble in acetic acid and in chloroform, slightly soluble in benzene, and very slightly soluble in alcohol and in ether. Its molecular weight is 608.69.

Following is its chemical structure:

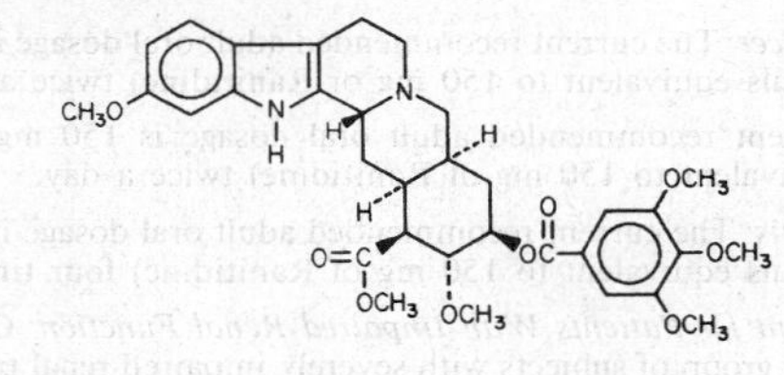

CLINICAL PHARMACOLOGY
Reserpine depletes stores of catecholamines and 5-hydroxytryptamine in many organs, including the brain and adrenal medulla. Most of its pharmacological effects have been attributed to this action. Depletion is slower and less complete in the adrenal medulla than in other tissues. The depression of sympathetic nerve function results in a decreased heart rate and a lowering of arterial blood pressure. The sedative and tranquilizing properties of Reserpine are thought to be related to depletion of catecholamines and 5-hydroxytryptamine from the brain.

Reserpine, like other rauwolfia compounds, is characterized by slow onset of action and sustained effects. Both cardiovascular and central nervous system effects may persist for a period of time following withdrawal of the drug.

Mean maximum plasma levels of 1.54 ng/mL were attained after a median of 3.5 hours in six normal subjects receiving a single oral dose of four 0.25-mg Reserpine tablets. Bioavailability was approximately 50% of that of a corresponding intravenous dose. Plasma levels of Reserpine after intravenous administration declined with a mean half-life of 33 hours. Reserpine is extensively bound (96%) to plasma proteins. No definitive studies on the human metabolism of Reserpine have been made.

INDICATIONS AND USAGE
Mild essential hypertension; also useful as adjunctive therapy with other antihypertensive agents in the more severe forms of hypertension; relief of symptoms in agitated psychotic states (e.g., schizophrenia), primarily in those

---

◆ RATED THERAPEUTICALLY EQUIVALENT; ◇ THERAPEUTIC EQUIVALENCE UNCONFIRMED; ○ UNRATED

individuals unable to tolerate phenothiazine derivatives or in those who also require antihypertensive medication.

UNLABELED USES
Reserpine is also used alone or as an adjunct in the treatment of cerebral vasospasm, refractory depression, hyperthyroidism, and tardive dyskinesia. It is also used to reduce the frequency and severity of migraine headache and in the treatment of Raynaud's disease.

CONTRAINDICATIONS
Known hypersensitivity, mental depression or history of mental depression (especially with suicidal tendencies), active peptic ulcer, ulcerative colitis, and patients receiving electroconvulsive therapy.

WARNINGS
Extreme caution should be exercised in treating patients with a history of mental depression. Reserpine may cause mental depression. Recognition of depression may be difficult because this condition may often be disguised by somatic complaints (Masked Depression). The drug should be discontinued at first signs of depression such as despondency, early morning insomnia, loss of appetite, impotence, or self-depreciation. Drug-induced depression may persist for several months after drug withdrawal and may be severe enough to result in suicide.

PRECAUTIONS
GENERAL
Since Reserpine increases gastrointestinal motility and secretion, it should be used cautiously in patients with a history of peptic ulcer, ulcerative colitis, or gallstones (biliary colic may be precipitated).

Caution should be exercised when treating hypertensive patients with renal insufficiency, since they adjust poorly to lowered blood pressure levels.

Preoperative withdrawal of Reserpine does not assure that circulatory instability will not occur. It is important that the anesthesiologist be aware of the patient's drug intake and consider this in the overall management, since hypotension has occurred in patients receiving rauwolfia preparations. Anticholinergic and/or adrenergic drugs (e.g., metaraminol, norepinephrine) have been employed to treat adverse vago-circulatory effects.

INFORMATION FOR PATIENTS
Patients should be informed of possible side effects and advised to take the medication regularly and continuously as directed.

DRUG INTERACTIONS
MAO inhibitors should be avoided or used with extreme caution.

Concurrent use of tricyclic antidepressants may decrease the antihypertensive effect of Reserpine.

Concurrent use of Reserpine and direct-or-indirect acting sympathomimetics should be closely monitored. The action of direct-acting amines (epinephrine, isoproterenol, phenylephrine, metaraminol) may be prolonged when given to patients taking Reserpine. The action of indirect-acting amines (ephedrine, tyramine, amphetamines) is inhibited.

Reserpine should be used cautiously with digitalis and quinidine, since cardiac arrhythmias have occurred with rauwolfia preparations.

Concomitant use of Reserpine with other antihypertensive agents necessitates careful titration of dosage with each agent.

CARCINOGENESIS, MUTAGENESIS, IMPAIRMENT OF FERTILITY
Animal Tumorigenicity: Rodent studies have shown that Reserpine is an animal tumorigen, causing an increased incidence of mammary fibroadenomas in female mice, malignant tumors of the seminal vesicles in male mice, and malignant adrenal medullary tumors in male rats. These findings arose in 2-year studies in which the drug was administered in the feed at concentrations of 5 to 10 ppm-about 100 to 300 times the usual human dose. The breast neoplasms are thought to be related to Reserpine's prolactin-elevating effect. Several other prolactin-elevating drugs have also been associated with an increased incidence of mammary neoplasia in rodents.

The extent to which these findings indicate a risk to humans is uncertain. Tissue culture experiments show that about one third of human breast tumors are prolactin-dependent *in vitro*, a factor of considerable importance if the use of the drug is contemplated in a patient with previously detected breast cancer. The possibility of an increased risk of breast cancer in Reserpine users has been studied extensively; however, no firm conclusion has emerged. Although a few epidemiologic studies have suggested a slightly increased risk (less than twofold in all studies except one) in women who have used Reserpine, other studies of generally similar design have not confirmed this. Epidemiologic studies conducted using other drugs (neuroleptic agents) that, like Reserpine, increase prolactin levels and therefore would be considered rodent mammary carcinogens have not shown an association between chronic administration of the drug and human mammary tumorigenesis. While long-term clinical observation has not suggested such an association, the available evidence is considered too limited to be conclusive at this time. An association of Reserpine intake with pheochromocytoma or tumors of the seminal vesicles has not been explored.

PREGNANCY CATEGORY C
Reserpine administered parenterally has been shown to be teratogenic in rats at doses up to 2 mg/kg and to have an embryocidal effect in guinea pigs given dosages of 0.5 mg daily.

There are no adequate and well-controlled studies of Reserpine in pregnant women. Reserpine should be used during pregnancy only if the potential benefit justifies the potential risk to the fetus.

Nonteratogenic Effects: Reserpine crosses the placental barrier, and increased respiratory tract secretions, nasal congestion, cyanosis, and anorexia may occur in neonates of Reserpine-treated mothers.

NURSING MOTHERS
Reserpine is excreted in maternal breast milk, and increased, respiratory tract secretions, nasal congestion, cyanosis, and anorexia may occur in breast-fed infants. Because of the potential for adverse reactions in nursing infants and the potential for tumorigenicity shown for Reserpine in animal studies, a decision should be made whether to discontinue nursing or to discontinue the drug, taking into account the importance of the drug to the mother.

PEDIATRIC USE
Safety and effectiveness in children have not been established by means of controlled clinical trials, although there is experience with the use of Reserpine in children. (See *"Dosage and Administration".*) Because of adverse effects such as emotional depression and lability, sedation, and stuffy nose, Reserpine is not usually recommended as a step-2 drug in the treatment of hypertension in children.

ADVERSE REACTIONS
The following adverse reactions have been observed with rauwolfia preparations, but there has not been enough systematic collection of data to support an estimate of their frequency. Consequently the reactions are categorized by organ system and are listed in decreasing order of severity and not frequency.

Digestive: Vomiting, diarrhea, nausea, anorexia, dryness of mouth, hypersecretion.

Cardiovascular: Arrhythmias (particularly when used concurrently with digitalis or quinidine), syncope, angina-like symptoms, bradycardia, edema.

Respiratory: Dyspnea, epistaxis, nasal congestion.

Neurologic: Rare parkinsonian syndrome and other extrapyramidal tract symptoms; dizziness; headache; paradoxical anxiety; depression; nervousness; nightmares; dull sensorium; drowsiness.

Musculoskeletal: Muscular aches.

Genitourinary: Pseudolactation, impotence, dysuria, gynecomastia, decreased libido, breast engorgement.

Metabolic: Weight gain.

Special Senses: Deafness, optic atrophy, glaucoma, uveitis, conjunctival injection.

Hypersensitive Reactions: Purpura, rash, pruritus.

OVERDOSAGE
ACUTE TOXICITY
No deaths due to acute poisoning with Reserpine have been reported.

Highest known doses survived; children, 1000 mg (age and sex not specified); young children, 200 mg (20-month-old boy).

Oral LD$_{50}$'s in animals (mg/kg): rat, 2993; mouse, 47 and 500.

SIGNS AND SYMPTOMS
The clinical picture of acute poisoning is characterized chiefly by signs and symptoms due to the reflex parasympathomimetic effect of Reserpine.

Impairment of consciousness may occur and may range from drowsiness to coma, depending upon the severity of overdosage. Flushing of the skin, conjunctival injection, and pupillary constriction are to be expected. Hypotension, hypothermia, central respiratory depression, and bradycardia may develop in cases of severe overdosage. Increased salivary and gastric secretion and diarrhea may also occur.

TREATMENT
There is no specific antidote.

Stomach contents should be evacuated, taking adequate precautions against aspiration and for protection of the airway. Activated charcoal slurry should be instilled.

The effects of Reserpine overdosage should be treated symptomatically. If hypotension is severe enough to require treatment with a vasopressor, one having a direct action upon vascular smooth muscle (e.g., phenylephrine, levarterenol, metaraminol) should be used. Since Reserpine is long-acting, the patient should be observed carefully for at least 72 hours, and treatment administered as required.

DOSAGE AND ADMINISTRATION
HYPERTENSION
In the average patient not receiving other antihypertensive agents, the usual initial dosage is 0.5 mg daily for 1 or 2 weeks. For maintenance, reduce to 0.1-0.25 mg daily. Higher dosages should be used cautiously, because occurrence of serious mental depression and other side effects may increase considerably.

PSYCHIATRIC DISORDERS
The usual initial dosage is 0.5 mg daily, but may range from 0.1 mg to 1.0 mg. Adjust dosage upward or downward according to the patient's response.

CHILDREN

Reserpine is not recommended for use in children (see *"Precautions, Pediatric Use"*). If it is to be used in treating a child, the usual recommended starting dose is 20 ug/kg daily. The maximum recommended dose is 0.25 mg (total) daily.

Storage

Store at controlled room temperature 15°-30°C (59°-86°F). Protect from moisture.

HOW SUPPLIED
TABLETS: 0.1 MG

BRAND/MANUFACTURER	NDC	SIZE	AWP
◇ GENERICS			
Eon	00185-0032-01	100s	$4.95
Geneva	00781-1086-10	1000s	$31.27
Eon	00185-0032-10	1000s	$39.95
Major	00904-2198-80	1000s	$40.45
Rugby	00536-4454-10	1000s	$44.42
Moore,H.L.	00839-1585-16	1000s	$52.64

TABLETS: 0.25 MG

BRAND/MANUFACTURER	NDC	SIZE	AWP
◇ GENERICS			
Eon	00185-0134-01	100s	$6.95
Richlyn	00115-4428-03	1000s	$14.10
Geneva	00781-1096-10	1000s	$49.84
Eon	00185-0134-10	1000s	$55.00
URL	00677-0126-10	1000s	$57.96
Moore,H.L.	00839-5128-16	1000s	$58.01
Major	00904-2199-80	1000s	$64.45
Rugby	00536-4458-10	1000s	$69.80

Reserpine and Trichlormethiazide

> **WARNING**
> THIS FIXED COMBINATION DRUG IS NOT INDICATED FOR INITIAL THERAPY OF HYPERTENSION. HYPERTENSION REQUIRES THERAPY TITRATED TO THE INDIVIDUAL PATIENT. IF THE FIXED COMBINATION REPRESENTS THE DOSAGE SO DETERMINED, ITS USE MAY BE MORE CONVENIENT IN PATIENT MANAGEMENT. THE TREATMENT OF HYPERTENSION IS NOT STATIC, BUT MUST BE REEVALUATED AS CONDITIONS IN EACH PATIENT WARRANT.

DESCRIPTION

Each tablet contains Reserpine 0.1 mg and Trichlormethiazide USP 2 mg or 4 mg.

Trichlormethiazide is an orally effective diuretic and antihypertensive of the thiazide class. Chemically, Trichlormethiazide is 2H-1,2,4-benzothiadiazine-7-sulfonamide, 6-chloro-3-(dichloromethyl)-3, 4-dihydro-,1,1-diazide. It differs from other thiazides by the inclusion of a dichloromethyl radical at the 3 position on the benzothiadiazine structure.

Reserpine is a pure crystalline alkaloid derived from the root of *Rauwolfia serpentina*. Chemically, Reserpine is methyl 18β-hydroxy-11, 17α-dimethoxy-3β, 20α-yohimban-16β-carboxylate 3,4,5-trimeth-oxybenzonate.

ACTION
TRICHLORMETHIAZIDE

The mechanism of action involves interference with the renal tubular mechanism of electrolyte reabsorption. At maximal therapeutic dosage, all thizides are approximately equal in their diuretic potency. The mechanism whereby thiazides function in the control of hypertension is unknown.

RESERPINE

Reserpine probably produces its antihypertensive effects through depletion of tissue stores of epinephrine and norepinephrine from peripheral sites. By contrast, its sedative and tranquilizing properties are thought to be related to depletion of 5-hydroxytryptamine from the brain.

Reserpine is characterized by slow onset of action and sustained effect. Both its cardiovascular and central nervous system effects may persist following withdrawal of the drug.

MEDICATIONS

Hypertension (See boxed *"Warning."*)

CONTRAINDICATIONS
TRICHLORMETHIAZIDE

Trichlormethiazide is contraindicated in patients with anuria and in patients known to be hypersensitive to this or other sulfonamide derivatives.

RESERPINE

Reserpine is contraindicated in patients with hypersensitivity to the drug, history of mental depression (especially with suicidal tendencies), active peptic ulcer, or ulcerative colitis.

WARNINGS

Trichlormethiazide: Use with caution in severe renal disease. In patients with renal disease, thiazides may precipitate azotemia. Cumulative effects of the drug may develop in patients with impaired renal function.

Thiazides should be used with caution in patients with impaired hepatic function or progressive liver disease, since minor alterations of fluid and electrolyte balance way precipitate hepatic coma.

Thiazides may add to or potentiate the action of other antihypertensive drugs. Potentiation occurs with ganglionic or peripheral adrenergic-blocking drugs.

Sensitivity reactions may occur in patients with a history of allergy or bronchial asthma. Exacerbation or activation of systemic lupus erythematosus has been reported.

Reserpine: Reserpine may cause mental depression. Recognition of depression may be difficult because this condition may often be disguised by somatic complaints (masked depression). The drug should be discontinued at the first signs of depression, such as despondency, early morning insomnia, loss of appetite, impotence, or self-deprecation. Drug-induced depression may persist for several months after drug withdrawal and may be severe enough to result in suicide.

Reserpine may induce peptic ulceration; discontinue use if peptic ulcer develops.

Electroshock therapy should not be given to patients taking Reserpine, since severe and even fatal reactions have been reported. The drug should be discontinued for two weeks before giving electroshock therapy.

Monoamine oxidase (MAO) inhibitors should be avoided or used with extreme caution.

USAGE IN PREGNANCY

Trichlormethiazide: Thiazides cross the placental barrier and appear in cord blood. The use of thiazides in pregnant women requires that the anticipated benefit be weighed against possible hazards to the fetus. These hazards include fetal or neonatal jaundice. thrombocytopenia, and possibly other adverse reactions which have occurred in the adult.

Reserpine: The safety of Reserpine for use during pregnancy has not been established; therefore, the drug should be used in pregnant patients or in woman of childbearing potential only when, in the judgment of the physician. It is essential to the welfare of the patient, increased respiratory secretions, nasal congestion, cyanosis, and anorexia may occur in infants born to Reserpine-treated mothers, since Reserpine crosses the placental barrier and appears in maternal breast milk.

NURSING MOTHERS

Reserpine and thiazides appear in breast milk. If use of Reserpine/Trichlormethiazide is deemed essential, the patient should stop nursing.

PRECAUTIONS

Certain brands of Reserpine 0.1 mg and Trichlormethiazide 2 mg tablets contain FD&C Yellow No. 5 (tartrazine), which may cause allergic-type reactions (including bronchial asthma) in certain susceptible individuals. Although the overall incidence of tartrazine sensitivity in the general population is low, it is frequently seen in patients who also have aspirin hypersensitivity.

TRICHLORMETHIAZIDE

Periodic determinations of serum electrolytes to detect possible electrolyte imbalance should be performed at appropriate intervals.

All patients receiving thiazide therapy should be observed for clinical signs of fluid or electrolyte imbalance; namely, hyponatremia, hypochloremic alkalosis, and hypokalemia. Serum and urine electrolyte determinations are particularly important when the patient is vomiting excessively or receiving parenteral fluids.

Medication, such as digitalis, may also influence serum electrolytes. Warning signs, irrespective of cause, are: dryness of the mouth, thirst, weakness, lethargy, drowsiness, restlessness, muscle pains or cramps, muscular fatigue, hypotension, oliguria, tachycardia, and gastrointestinal disturbances, such as nausea and vomiting.

Hypokalemia may develop with thiazides as with any other potent diuretic, especially with brisk diuresis, when severe cirrhosis is present, or during concomitant use of corticosteroids or ACTH.

Interference with adequate oral electrolyte intake will also contribute to hypokalemia. Digitalis therapy may exaggerate metabolic effects of hypokalemia, especially with reference to myocardial activity.

Any chloride deficit is generally mild and usually does not require specific treatment except under extraordinary circumstances (as in liver disease or renal disease). Dilutional hyponatremia may occur in adematous patients in hot weather; appropriate therapy is water restriction rather than administration of salt, except in rare instances when the hyponatremia is threatening. In actual salt depletion, appropriate replacement is the therapy of choice. Hyperuricemia may occur or frank gout may be precipitated in certain patients receiving thiazide therapy.

Insulin requirements in diabetic patients may be increased, decreased, or unchanged. Latent diabetes mellitus may become manifest during thiazide administration.

Thiazide drugs may increase the responsiveness to tubocurarine.

The antihypertensive effects of the drug may be enhanced in the postsympathectomy patient.

◆ RATED THERAPEUTICALLY EQUIVALENT; ◇ THERAPEUTIC EQUIVALENCE UNCONFIRMED; ○ UNRATED

Thiazides may decrease arterial responsiveness to norepinephrine. This diminution is not sufficient to preclude effectiveness of the pressor agent for therapeutic use.

If progressive renal impairment becomes evident, as indicated by a rising nonprotein nitrogen or blood area nitrogen, a careful reappraisal of therapy is necessary with consideration given to withholding or discontinuing diuretic therapy.

Thiazides may decrease serum PBI levels without signs of thyroid disturbance.

RESERPINE

Caution should be used in treating hypertensive patients with renal insufficiency.

Cardiac arrhythmias have occurred in patients receiving digitalis and quinidine with Reserpine.

Reserpine potentiates many anesthetic agents; hypotension and bradycardia have been noted during anesthesia. In addition, a relative sensitivity to norepinephrine or other pressor agents may exist due to the previous action of Reserpine; thus, usual amounts of the pressor agent may be excessive.

Use with caution in patients with a history of depression, peptic ulcer or other gastrointestinal disorders, and in hypertensive patients with functionally severe coronary artery disease.

Animal Tumorigenicity: Rodent studies have shown that Reserpine is an animal tumorigen, causing an increased incidence of mammary fibroadenomas in female mice, malignant tumors of the seminal vesicles in male mice, and malignant adrenal medullary tumors in male rats. These findings arose in 2 year studies in which the drug was administered in the feed at concentrations of 5 and 10 ppm (about 100 to 300 times the usual human dose). The breast neoplasms are thought to be related to Reserpine's prolactin-elevating effect. Several other prolactin-elevating drugs have also been associated with an increased incidence of mammary neoplasia in rodents.

The extent to which these findings indicate a risk to humans is uncertain. Tissue culture experiments show that about one-third of human breast tumors are prolactin-dependent *in vitro*, a factor of considerable importance if the use of the drug is contemplated in a patient with previously detected breast cancer. The possibility of an increased risk of breast cancer in Reserpine users has been studied extensively; however, no firm conclusion has emerged. Although a few epidemiologic studies have suggested a slightly increased risk (less than twofold in all studies except one) in women who have used Reserpine, other studies of generally similar design have not confirmed this. Epidemiologic studies conducted using other drugs (neuroleptic agents) like Reserpine that increase prolactin levels and, therefore, would be considered rodent mammary carcinogens, have not shown an association between chronic administration of the drug and human mammary tumorigenesis. While long-term clinical observation has not suggested such an association, the available evidence is considered too limited to be conclusive at this time. An association of Reserpine intake with pheochromocytoma or tumors of the seminal vesicles has not been explored.

ADVERSE REACTIONS

TRICHLORMETHIAZIDE

1. *Gastrointestinal:* anorexia, gastric irritation, nausea, diarrhea, constipation, jaundice (intrahepatic cholestatic jaundice), vomiting, cramping, pancreatitis.

2. *Central Nervous System:* dizziness, vertigo, paresthesia, headache, xanthopsia.

3. *Hematologic:* leukopenia, agranulocytosis, thrombocytopenia, aplastic anemia.

4. *Dermatologic-Hypersensitivity:* purpura, photosensitivity, rash, urticaria, necrotizing angiitis (vasculitis), cutaneous vasculitis.

5. *Cardiovascular:* orthostatic hypotension (possibly aggravated by alcohol, barbiturates, or narcotics).

6. *Other:* hyperglycemia, glycosuria, hyperuricemia, muscle spasm, weakness, restlessness.

RESERPINE

Gastric hypersecretion; vomiting; nervousness; paradoxical anxiety; CNS sensitization manifested by deafness, glaucoma, uveitis, and optic atrophy; purpura; nasal stuffiness; loose stools; reversible parkinsonism; muscular fatigue and weakness; and nightmares. Mental depression has been reported, particularly when Reserpine doses of over 1 mg daily are used. Other side effects of Reserpine reported include anorexia, nausea, dizziness, headaches, impotence, flushing of the skin, dryness of the mouth, biliary colic, blurred vision, muscular aches, and pruritus. Hypotension including the orthostatic variety may occur in some patients. Angina pectoris, arrhythmias, and congestive heart failure have also been reported but are uncommon.

After the onset of therapy with Reserpine, a turbulent phase of short duration may occur. Very rare additional adverse effects that have been observed in association with Reserpine therapy include epistaxis, skin eruptions, and edema due to sodium retention. Bradycardia may occur as an exaggerated response related to the pharmacodynamic effect of Reserpine.

DOSAGE

As determined by individual titration. (See boxed *"Warning."*)

In the stabilized hypertensive patient, administration may be continued on a once-daily basis administered in the morning. The maximum single effective dose of Reserpine/Trichlormethiazide is 8 mg (in some patients 4 mg). Doses in excess of 8 mg normally will not produce any increase in sodium and water excretion and in refractory patients may increase excretion of potassium.

Keep tightly closed. Store at room temperature, preferably below 86°F (30°C). Protect from excessive heat.

HOW SUPPLIED

TABLETS: 2 MG

BRAND/MANUFACTURER	NDC	SIZE	AWP
◇ **BRAND**			
METATENSIN #2: Marion Merrell Dow	00068-0064-01	100s	$57.18

TABLETS: 4 MG

BRAND/MANUFACTURER	NDC	SIZE	AWP
◇ **BRAND**			
METATENSIN #4: Marion Merrell Dow	00068-0065-01	100s	$85.50

Respbid *SEE* THEOPHYLLINE

Respiratory Vaccine, Mixed

DESCRIPTION

A polyvalent bacterial vaccine, Mixed Respiratory Vaccine is a sterile suspension of various strains of bacterial organisms and intended for subcutaneous injection.

Many of these strains were isolated in the preparation of autogenous vaccines for patients subject to respiratory infections. These organisms consist of two general classes of streptococci (a variety of viridans and non-hemolytic types). The staphylococci are a mixture of several aureus strains. Four types of pneumococci are included in this product. The other organisms contained in the vaccine are Neisseria (Branhamella) catarrhalis, Klebsiella pneumoniae (Friedlanders bacillus) and Haemophilus influenzae.

The organisms are grown in artificial media suited for rapid growth, washed with physiological salt solution, centrifuged, resuspended in salt solution and killed with phenol. The suspensions are standardized by direct microscopic count, mixed in required amounts and filled in rubber stoppered bottles. The filled bottles are tested for sterility and safety in the approved manner.

Active ingredients are as follows:

Staphylococcus aureus	1200 million
Streptococcus (viridans & non-hemolytic)	200 million
Streptococcus (Diplococcus) pneumoniae	150 million
Branhamella (Neisseria) catarrhalis	150 million
Klebsiella pneumoniae	150 million
Haemophilus influenzae	150 million
Total in each mL	2000 million

Mixed Respiratory Vaccine is available as a 20 ml multidose vial containing 2,000 million organisms per ml.

CLINICAL PHARMACOLOGY

The mechanism of action of Mixed Respiratory Vaccine is not known. In general, antigens injected into the skin are processed locally or in satellite lymph nodes by macrophages or lymphocytes. Subsequently, this may lead to production of blocking antibody to specific antigens or activation of suppressor cells or helper cells that alter the immunologic status of the patient.[1]

The antigens are apparently metabolized in the macrophages of the immune system. It is not known how much, if any, of the antigenic material in bacterial vaccines passes through the immune barriers to be excreted or detoxified by other organs.

INDICATIONS AND USAGE

BASED ON A REVIEW BY THE PANEL ON THE SAFETY, EFFECTIVENESS, AND LABELING OF BACTERIAL VACCINES AND BACTERIAL ANTIGENS THAT HAVE "NO U.S. STANDARD OF POTENCY" AND OTHER INFORMATION, THE FOOD AND DRUG ADMINISTRATION HAS DIRECTED THAT FURTHER INVESTIGATION BE CONDUCTED BEFORE THIS PRODUCT IS DETERMINED TO BE FULLY EFFECTIVE FOR THE LABELED INDICATIONS.

In recurrent and chronic infections of the respiratory tract and occasionally of the skin, the exact host-parasite relationships of the presumed offending organisms are so obscure that the factors that determine infection and resistance remain undefined. Thus many diseases such as rhinitis, infectious asthma, chronic sinusitis, nasal polyposis and chronic, serous otitis are of unknown etiology or obscure pathogenesis. Because bacterial or viral infection seems to play a prominent, though nebulous, role in these ill-defined disorders, and because these disorders may respond transiently or incompletely to appropriate antibiotic, surgical, antihistamine and antiflammatory treatment, bacterial vaccines have been used in the hopes of favorably altering the course of the chronic inflammatory process.

There are numerous uncontrolled, testimonial reports which indicate the benefits from the use of mixed respiratory vaccines for a variety of common chronic disorders, including those listed above.

A very few controlled studies have been made to evaluate the effectiveness of Mixed Respiratory Vaccine or to delineate the kinds of illness likely to respond to

Mixed Respiratory Vaccine administration. Infectious asthma, chronic bronchitis, rhino-bronchitis and secretory otitis were conditions treated, but exact criteria for these diagnoses were generally vague. Criteria for judging severity of symptoms were generally subjective, but the same criteria were applied to both treated and control patients.

A variety of vaccines were used for treatment. The closest to Mixed Respiratory Vaccine was a bacterial vaccine manufactured in France by Laboratories des Stallergenes. The genera and species were used in the same proportions as Mixed Respiratory Vaccine, but different strains were used.

To various degrees, these studies indicated that patients given bacterial vaccines did better over the period fo study and in some cases did less well later, after vaccines were discontinued.[2, 3, 4, 5, 6] Many of the reports on the effectiveness of Mixed Respiratory Vaccine have come from pediatric practices. The youngest patient reported is age 3.[3]

CONTRAINDICATIONS
Mixed Respiratory Vaccine should not be given to patients with known hypersensitivity to any component of the product. Occasionally a patient will develop excessively large, delayed local reactions after injections of Mixed Respiratory Vaccine and rarely vague malaise or myalgia. Subsequent doses should be drastically reduced or administration stopped. Patients with rheumatoid arthritis, lupus erythematosis or other connective tissue disease, should not be given bacterial vaccines because of the sensitizing role bacteria may play in these diseases and the damage that can occur from antigen-antibody complexes.

WARNINGS
Systemic reactions to Mixed Respiratory Vaccine are very rare because immediate hypersensitivity to bacterial products is rare. However, delayed hypersensitivity to bacterial products is common and, if severe, may limit the dose of Mixed Respiratory Vaccine that can comfortably be administered.

If delayed skin reactions are accompanied by any systemic symptoms, administration of Mixed Respiratory Vaccine should be stopped.

PRECAUTIONS
General: Always agitate the suspension to insure uniform distribution while withdrawing dose from vial.

Systemic reactions are rare. If any do occur, they should be treated like other allergenic reactions using epinephrine and antihistamines. In the event that a severe systemic or anaphylactic reaction occurs, apply a tourniquet above the site of the injection and inject 0.3 mL to 0.5 mL of 1:1000 Epinephrine HCl into the other arm. The dose may be repeated every 5 to 10 minutes, since a succession of small doses is more effective (and less dangerous) than a single large dose. Loosen the tourniquet at least every 10 minutes. A maximum of 0.1 mL of Epinephrine HCl 1:1000 also should be injected at the treatment injection site to delay absorption. If more than one injection had been given, distribute the 0.1 mL evenly among these sites.

The 1:1000 Epinephrine HCl dose for infants to 2 years is 0.05 to 0.1 mL; for children 2 to 6 years it is 0.15 mL; for children 6 to 12 years it is 0.2 mL.

After adequate Epinephrine has been given and in cases where symptoms of angioedema, urticaria, rhinitis, or conjunctivitis are not responding rapidly, intravenous or intramuscular antihistamines, given according to the manufacturer's directions, should be tried.

Reactions characterized by severe asthma or bronchospasm in the absence of shock and not responding to Epinephrine may be treated with intravenous aminophylline, again administered according to the manufacturer's directions.

Other measures which may be necessary are oxygen for cyanosis; endotrachial intubation or tracheotomy for laryngeal edema; resuscitation, difibrillation, intravenous sodium biocarbonate, and proper medication for cardiac arrest; mechanical airway use if the patient becomes unconscious; oral or intravenous corticosteroids if it is likely that the reactions may be prolonged. Hypotension should be monitored, and if necessary, vasopressors administered, along with adequate plasma volume replacement.

Rarely are all of the above measures necessary, the tourniquet and Epinephrine usually producing prompt responses. However, the physician should be prepared in advance for all contingencies, and promptness in beginning emergency treatment measures is of utmost importance.

Severe systemic reactions mandate a decrease of at least 50% in the next dose, followed by cautious increases. Repeated systemic reactions, even of a mild nature, are sufficient reason for the cessation of further attempts to reach the reaction-causing dose.

Drug Interactions: There are no known interactions with other drugs or allergens.

Carcinogenesis, Mutagenesis, Impairment of Fertility: No prospective, long-term studies are anticipated for carcinogenesis, mutagenesis, or impairment of fertility.

However, bacterial vaccines have been in use for 50 years, with no reports of carcinogenesis, mutagenesis, or impairment of fertility.

Pregnancy: Pregnancy Category C. Mixed Respiratory Vaccine. Animal reproduction studies have not been conducted with Mixed Respiratory Vaccine. It is also not known whether Mixed Respiratory Vaccine can cause fetal harm when administered to a pregnant woman or can affect reproduction capacity. Mixed Respiratory Vaccine should be given to a pregnant woman only if clearly needed. There have been no reports of untoward effects on the mother, the fetus or on the course of pregnancy or delivery.

Nursing Mothers: It is not known if bacterial products appear in the milk of nursing mothers after Mixed Respiratory Vaccine injections.

Pediatric Use: See "Indications and Usage".

ADVERSE REACTIONS
Immediate systemic reactions are rare. When suspicion has arisen, other antigens were given that were known to be associated with immediate hypersensitivity. Delayed, local reactions are frequent, but are no cause for alarm unless accompanied by some systemic manifestations such as fever, malaise or myalgia. No fatal adverse reactions have been reported.

DOSAGE AND ADMINISTRATION
Parenteral drug products should be inspected visually for particulate matter and discoloration prior to administration, whenever solution and container permit.

Mixed Respiratory Vaccine is a white suspension of bacterial cells. Always agitate the suspension to insure uniform distribution while withdrawing dose from vial. If discoloration occurs or particles are clumped and will not disperse, discard the material.

A variety of dose schedules have been advocated for this product. Most commonly, a schedule modeled after other hyposensitization schedules is used.

Mixed Respiratory Vaccine is supplied at a concentration of 2,000 million organisms per mL, of which an initial prophylactic dose of 0.05 mL, given subcutaneously, is recommended. Doses may be increased by 0.05 mL to 0.1 mL at 4 to 7 days intervals until a maximum dose of 0.5 mL to 1 mL has been reached. In acute conditions an initial dose of 0.02 mL should be given and increments of 0.02 mL to 0.05 mL administered at 3-to-5-day intervals. Patient sensitivity varies and for some, doses may be increased faster; for others, more slowly. Another dose should never be given until all local reaction resulting from the previous dose has disappeared.

Increasingly large delayed reactions may occur after administering maintenance doses for many months. Further administration of vaccine, even at smaller doses, may continue to increase the reaction. Stop vaccine immediately. A rest period of 2 to 6 months may allow the delayed hypersensitivity to subside, and injections may be resumed at a lower dose if still needed by the patient. Each patient is an individual problem, and therefore, only a general dose schedule can be outlined. Smaller increments in doses may be necessary for extremely sensitive patients.

When doses are being advanced, the time interval can be every three to four days with the lower concentrations. It may be necessary to increase the time interval to five or seven days when the more concentrated vaccine is given. Local reaction and generalized symptoms determine the terminal maintenance dose.

Generally, the maintenance dose of 0.5 mL of the 2,000 million per mL concentration should be given at weekly or alternate-week intervals. The hyposensitizing dose for children is the same as for adults. The maximum volume of antigen tolerated without undue pain and swelling may be less for the smaller individual so that the maximum dose administered to any patient should be individualized.

General reactions such as fatigue, drowsiness, etc., or a definite aggravation of allergic symptoms require a reduction in the size of the subsequent doses or the vaccine itself may also require further diluting.

Store at 2° to 8°C. Expiration date is shown on both the package and vial labels. Reorder when outdated.

REFERENCES
1. Kasuga, S. K. and C. M. Cordes, "The *In Vitro* Determination of Delayed-Type Hypersensitivity in Individuals Receiving Multiple Respiratory Vaccine MRV®." Unpublished communication. 2. Boutin, C., P. Cargino, J. P. Girbal and J. Levrand, "Study in Double-Blind of the Antibronchitis MRV Vaccine." Unpublished communication. 3. Mueller, H. L. and M. Lanz, "Hyposensitization with Bacterial Vaccine in Infectious Asthma," *The Journal of the American Medical Association*, 208 (2):1379-1383, 1969. 4. Johnstone, D. E., "Study of the Value of Bacterial Vaccines in the Treatment of Bronchial Asthma Associated with Respiratory Infections," *Pediatrics*, 24:427-433, 1959. 5. Fernandez, A. A., J. P. McGovern, "Secretory Otitis Media in Allergic Infants and Children," *Southern Medical Journal*, 58:581-586, 1965. 6. Barr, S. E., H. Brown, M. Fuchs, H. Orvis, A. Connor, F. J. Murray and A. Seltzer, "A Double-Blind Study of the Effects of Bacterial Vaccine on Infective Asthma," *Journal of Allergy*, 36:47-61, 1965.

HOW SUPPLIED
INJECTION: 2000 MILLION ORG/ML

BRAND/MANUFACTURER	NDC	SIZE	AWP
○ **BRAND**			
MRV: Miles Allergy	00118-9978-01	20 ml	$43.24

Restoril SEE TEMAZEPAM

Retin-A SEE TRETINOIN

Retrovir SEE ZIDOVUDINE

Rev-Eyes SEE DAPIPRAZOLE HYDROCHLORIDE

◆ RATED THERAPEUTICALLY EQUIVALENT; ◇ THERAPEUTIC EQUIVALENCE UNCONFIRMED; ○ UNRATED

Reversol *SEE* EDROPHONIUM CHLORIDE

Rheomacrodex *SEE* DEXTRAN 40

Rhinocort *SEE* BUDESONIDE

Rh$_o$(D) Immune Globulin

DESCRIPTION

Rh$_o$(D) Immune Globulin (Human) is a sterile solution of immune globulin containing antibodies to Rh$_o$(D) which is intended for intramuscular injection. This product has been prepared from large pools of human plasma. It contains 15%-18% protein. Rh$_o$(D) Immune Globulin is available in a full dose and a mini dose formulation. The potency of the full dose is equal to or greater than that of the U.S. Food and Drug Administration Reference Rh$_o$(D) Immune Globulin. Each single dose vial or syringe contains sufficient anti-Rh$_o$(D) (approximately 300 µg*) to effectively suppress the immunizing potential of 15 mL of Rh$_o$(D) positive packed red blood cells.[2-4]

One dose of Rh$_o$(D) Immune Globulin mini dose contains not less than one-sixth the quantity of Rh$_o$(D) antibody contained in one standard dose of Rh$_o$(D) Immune Globulin (Human), USP and it will suppress the immunizing potential of 2.5 mL of Rh$_o$(D) positive packed red blood cells or the equivalent of whole blood (5 mL). The quantity of Rh$_o$(D) antibody in Rh$_o$(D) Immune Globulin mini dose is not less than one-sixth of that contained in 1 mL of the U.S. Food and Drug Administration Reference Rh$_o$(D) Immune Globulin (Human).

CLINICAL PHARMACOLOGY

Rh$_o$(D) Immune Globulin is used to prevent isoimmunization in the Rh$_o$(D) negative individual exposed to Rh$_o$(D) positive blood as a result of a fetomaternal hemorrhage occurring during a delivery of an Rh$_o$(D) positive infant, abortion (either spontaneous or induced), or following amniocentesis or abdominal trauma. The risk of sensitization is higher in women undergoing induced abortions than in those aborting spontaneously.[5-7] Similarly, immunization resulting in the production of anti-Rh$_o$(D) following transfusion of Rh positive red cells to an Rh$_o$(D) negative recipient may be prevented by administering Rh$_o$(D) Immune Globulin (Human).[8,9]

Rh hemolytic disease of the newborn is the result of the active immunization of an Rh$_o$(D) negative mother by Rh$_o$(D) positive red cells entering the maternal circulation during a previous delivery, abortion, amniocentesis, abdominal trauma, or as a result of red cell transfusion.[7,11] Rh$_o$(D) Immune Globulin acts by suppressing the immune response of Rh$_o$(D) negative individuals to Rh$_o$(D) positive red blood cells. The mechanism of action of Rh$_o$(D) Immune Globulin is not fully understood.

The administration of Rh$_o$(D) Immune Globulin within 72 hours of a full-term delivery of an Rh$_o$(D) positive infant by an Rh$_o$(D) negative mother reduces the incidence of Rh isoimmunization from 12%-13% to 1%-2%.[12] The 1%-2% treatment failures are probably due to isoimmunization occurring during the latter part of pregnancy or following delivery.[13] Bowman and Pollock[14] have reported that the incidence of isoimmunization can be further reduced from approximately 1.6% to less than 0.1% by administering Rh$_o$(D) Immune Globulin in two doses, one antenatal at 28 weeks' gestation and another following delivery.

Rh$_o$(D) Immune Globulin mini dose is used to prevent the formation of anti-Rho(D) antibody in Rh$_o$(D) negative women who are exposed to the Rh$_o$(D) antigen at the time of spontaneous or induced abortion (up to 12 weeks' gestation).[7,15,16] Rh$_o$(D) Immune Globulin mini dose suppresses the stimulation of active immunity by Rh$_o$(D) positive fetal erythrocytes that may enter the maternal circulation at the time of termination of the pregnancy. The amount of anti-Rh$_o$(D) in Rh$_o$(D) Immune Globulin mini dose has been shown to effectively prevent maternal isosensitization to the Rh$_o$(D) antigens following spontaneous or induced abortion occurring up to the 12th week of gestation.[17-19] After the 12th week of gestation, a standard dose of Rh$_o$(D) Immune Globulin is indicated.

INDICATIONS AND USAGE

PREGNANCY AND OTHER OBSTETRIC CONDITIONS

Rh$_o$(D) Immune Globulin full dose is recommended for the prevention of Rh hemolytic disease of the newborn by its administration to the Rh$_o$(D) negative mother within 72 hours after birth of an Rh$_o$(D) positive infant,[20] providing the following criteria are met:

1. The mother must be Rh$_o$(D) negative, and must not already be sensitized to the Rh$_o$(D) factor.

---

* A full dose of Rh$_o$(D) Immune Globulin has traditionally been referred to as a "300 µg" dose and this usage is employed here for convenience in terminology. **It should not be constructed as the actual anti-D content.** Each full dose of Rh$_o$(D) Immune Globulin must contain at least as much anti-D as 1 mL of the U.S. Reference Rh$_o$(D) Immune Globulin. Studies performed at the FDA have shown that the U.S. Reference contains 820 international units (IU) of anti-D per mL. When the conversion factor determined for the International (WHO) Reference Preparation[1] is used, 820 IU per mL is equivalent to 164 µg per mL of anti-D.

---

2. Her child must be Rh$_o$(D) positive and should have a negative direct antiglobulin test (see "*Precautions*").

If Rh$_o$(D) Immune Globulin is administered antepartum, it is essential that the mother receive another dose of Rh$_o$(D) Immune Globulin after delivery of an Rh$_o$(D) positive infant.

If the father can be determined to be Rh$_o$(D) negative, Rh$_o$(D) Immune Globulin need not be given.

Rh$_o$(D) Immune Globulin should be administered within 72 hours to all nonimmunized Rh$_o$(D) negative women who have undergone spontaneous or induced abortion, following ruptured tubal pregnancy, amniocentesis, or abdominal trauma unless the blood group of the fetus or the father is known to be Rh$_o$(D) negative.[7,11] If the fetal blood group cannot be determined, one must assume that it is Rh$_o$(D) positive,[2] and Rh$_o$(D) Immune Globulin should be administered to the mother.

Rh$_o$(D) Immune Globulin mini dose is recommended to prevent the isoimmunization of Rh$_o$(D) negative women at the time of spontaneous or induced abortion of up to 12 weeks' gestation provided the following criteria are met:

1. The mother must be Rh$_o$(D) negative and must not already be sensitized to the Rh$_o$(D) antigen.

2. The father is not known to be Rh$_o$(D) negative.

3. Gestation is not more than 12 weeks at termination.

Note: Rh$_o$(D) Immune Globulin prophylaxis is not indicated if the fetus or father can be determined to be Rh negative. If the Rh status of the fetus is unknown, the fetus must be assumed to be Rh$_o$(D) positive, and Rh$_o$(D) Immune Globulin mini dose should be administered to the mother.

FOR ABORTIONS OR MISCARRIAGES OCCURRING AFTER 12 WEEKS' GESTATION, A STANDARD DOSE OF RH$_o$(D) IMMUNE GLOBULIN IS INDICATED.

Rh$_o$(D) Immune Globulin mini dose should be administered within 3 hours or as soon as possible after spontaneous passage or surgical removal of the products of conception. However, if Rh$_o$(D) Immune Globulin mini dose is not given within this time period, consideration should still be given to its administration since clinical studies in male volunteers have demonstrated the effectiveness of Rh$_o$(D) Immune Globulin in preventing isoimmunization as long as 72 hours after infusion of Rh$_o$(D) positive red cells.[21]

TRANSFUSION

Rh$_o$(D) Immune Globulin full dose may be used to prevent isoimmunization in Rh$_o$(D) negative individuals who have been transfused with Rh$_o$(D) positive red blood cells or blood components containing red blood cells.[8,22]

CONTRAINDICATIONS

None known.

WARNINGS

NEVER ADMINISTER RH$_o$(D) IMMUNE GLOBULIN INTRAVENOUSLY. INJECT ONLY INTRAMUSCULARLY. NEVER ADMINISTER TO THE NEONATE. ADMINISTER THE MINI DOSE ONLY TO WOMEN POST-ABORTION OR POST-MISCARRIAGE OF UP TO 12 WEEKS' GESTATION.

Rh$_o$(D) Immune Globulin should be given with caution to patients with a history of prior systemic allergic reactions following the administration of human immunoglobulin preparations or to patients who are known to have had an allergic response to thimerosal, an ingredient of some brands. The attending physician who wishes to administer Rh$_o$(D) Immune Globulin to persons with isolated immunoglobulin A (IgA) deficiency must weigh the benefits of immunization against the potential risks of hypersensitivity reactions. Such persons have increased potential for developing antibodies to IgA and could have anaphylactic reactions to subsequent administration of blood products that contain IgA.

As with all preparations administered by the intramuscular route, bleeding complications may be encountered in patients with thrombocytopenia or other bleeding disorders.

PRECAUTIONS

GENERAL

A large fetomaternal hemorrhage late in pregnancy or following delivery may cause a weak mixed field positive D^u test result. If there is any doubt about the mother's Rh type, she should be given Rh$_o$(D) Immune Globulin. A screening test to detect fetal red blood cells may be helpful in such cases.

If more than 15 mL of D-positive fetal red blood cells are present in the mother's circulation, more than a single dose of Rh$_o$(D) Immune Globulin is required. Failure to recognize this may result in the administration of an inadequate dose.

Although systemic reactions to human immunoglobulin preparations are rare, epinephrine should be available for treatment of acute anaphylactic reactions.

DRUG INTERACTIONS

Other antibodies in the Rh$_o$(D) Immune Globulin preparation may interfere with the response to live vaccines such as measles, mumps, polio or rubella. Therefore, immunization with live vaccines should not be given within 3 months after Rh$_o$(D) Immune Globulin administration.

DRUG/LABORATORY INTERACTIONS

Babies born of women given Rh$_o$(D) Immune Globulin antepartum may have a weakly positive direct antiglobulin test at birth.

Passively acquired anti-Rh$_o$(D) may be detected in maternal serum if antibody screening tests are performed subsequent to antepartum or postpartum administration of Rh$_o$(D) Immune Globulin.

➤ SHOWN IN PRODUCT IDENTIFICATION GUIDE

PREGNANCY CATEGORY C

Animal reproduction studies have not been conducted with $Rh_o(D)$ Immune Globulin. It is also not known whether $Rh_o(D)$ Immune Globulin can cause fetal harm when administered to a pregnant woman or can affect reproduction capacity. $Rh_o(D)$ Immune Globulin should be given to a pregnant woman only if clearly needed.

It should be again noted that $Rh_o(D)$ Immune Globulin mini dose is not indicated for use during pregnancy and it should be administered only post-abortion or post-miscarriage.

ADVERSE REACTIONS

Reactions to $Rh_o(D)$ Immune Globulin are infrequent in $Rh_o(D)$ negative individuals and consist primarily of slight soreness at the site of injection and slight temperature elevation. While sensitization to repeated injections of human immune globulin is extremely rare, it has occurred. Elevated bilirubin levels have been reported in some individuals receiving multiple doses of $Rh_o(D)$ Immune Globulin full dose following mismatched transfusions. This is believed to be due to a relatively rapid rate of foreign red cell destruction.

DOSAGE AND ADMINISTRATION

PREGNANCY AND OTHER OBSTETRIC CONDITIONS

1. For postpartum prophylaxis, administer one vial or syringe of $Rh_o(D)$ Immune Globulin full dose (300 µg*), preferably within 72 hours of delivery. Although a lesser degree of protection is afforded if Rh antibody is administered beyond the 72-hour period, $Rh_o(D)$ Immune Globulin full dose may still be given.[7,23] Full-term deliveries can vary in their dosage requirements depending on the magnitude of the fetomaternal hemorrhage. One 300 µg* vial or syringe of $Rh_o(D)$ Immune Globulin full dose provides sufficient antibody to prevent Rh sensitization if the volume of red blood cells that has entered the circulation is 15 mL or less.[2-4] In instances where a large (greater than 30 mL of whole blood or 15 mL red blood cells) fetomaternal hemorrhage is suspected, a fetal red cell count by an approved laboratory technique (e.g., modified Kleihauer-Betke acid elution stain technique) should be performed to determine the dosage of immune globulin required.[11,24] The red blood cell volume of the calculated fetomaternal hemorrhage is divided by 15 mL to obtain the number of vials or syringes of $Rh_o(D)$ Immune Globulin for administration.[3,11,22] If more than 15 mL of red cells is suspected or if the dose calculation results in a fraction, administer the next higher whole number of vials or syringes (e.g., if 1.4, give 2 vials or syringes).

2. For antenatal prophylaxis, one 300 µg* vial or syringe of $Rh_o(D)$ Immune Globulin full dose is administered at approximately 28 weeks' gestation. This **must** be followed by another 300 µg* dose, preferably within 72 hours following delivery, if the infant is Rh positive.

3. Following threatened abortion at any stage of gestation with continuation of pregnancy, it is recommended that 300 µg* of $Rh_o(D)$ Immune Globulin full dose be given. If more than 15 mL of red cells is suspected due to fetomaternal hemorrhage, the same dose modification in No. 1 above applies.

4. Following miscarriage, abortion, or termination of ectopic pregnancy at or beyond 13 weeks' gestation, it is recommended that 300 µg* of $Rh_o(D)$ Immune Globulin full dose be given. If more than 15 mL of red blood cells is suspected due to fetomaternal hemorrhage, the same dose modification in No. 1 above applies. If pregnancy is terminated prior to 13 weeks' gestation, a single dose of $Rh_o(D)$ Immune Globulin mini dose (approximately 50 µg*) may be used instead of $Rh_o(D)$ Immune Globulin full dose.

One syringe of $Rh_o(D)$ Immune Globulin mini dose provides sufficient antibody to prevent Rh sensitization to 2.5 mL $Rh_o(D)$ positive packed red cells or the equivalent (5 mL) of whole blood. This dose is sufficient to provide protection against maternal Rh sensitization for women undergoing spontaneous or induced abortion of up to 12 weeks' gestation.

$Rh_o(D)$ Immune Globulin mini dose should be administered within 3 hours or as soon as possible following spontaneous or induced abortion. If prompt administration is not possible, $Rh_o(D)$ Immune Globulin mini dose should be given within 72 hours following termination of the pregnancy.

5. Following amniocentesis at either 15 to 18 weeks' gestation or during the third trimester, or following abdominal trauma in the second or third trimester, it is recommended that 300 µg* of $Rh_o(D)$ Immune Globulin full dose be administered. If there is a fetomaternal hemorrhage in excess of 15 mL of red cells, the same dose modification in No. 1 applies.

If abdominal trauma, amniocentesis, or other adverse event requires the administration of $Rh_o(D)$ Immune Globulin full dose at 13 to 18 weeks' gestation, another 300 µg* dose should be given at 26 to 28 weeks. To maintain protection throughout pregnancy, the level of passively acquired anti-D(Rh_o) should not be allowed to fall below the level required to prevent an immune response to Rh positive red cells. The half-life of IgG is 23 to 26 days. In any case, a dose of $Rh_o(D)$ Immune Globulin full dose should be given within 72 hours after delivery if the baby is Rh positive. If delivery occurs within 3 weeks after the last dose, the postpartum dose may be withheld unless there is a fetomaternal hemorrhage in excess of 15 mL of red blood cells.[25] *(See footnote under *"Description".*)

TRANSFUSION

In the case of a transfusion of $Rh_o(D)$ positive red cells to an $Rh_o(D)$ negative recipient, the volume of Rh positive whole blood administered is multiplied by the hematocrit of the donor unit giving the volume of red blood cells transfused. The volume of red blood cells is divided by 15 mL which provides the number of vials or syringes of $Rh_o(D)$ Immune Globulin full dose to be administered.

If the dose calculated results in a fraction, the next higher whole number of vials or syringes should be administered (e.g., if 1.4, give 2 vials or 2 syringes).

$Rh_o(D)$ Immune Globulin full dose should be administered within 72 hours after an incompatible transfusion, but preferably as soon as possible.

INJECTION PROCEDURE

DO NOT INJECT INTRAVENOUSLY. DO NOT INJECT NEONATE. $Rh_o(D)$ Immune Globulin full or mini dose is administered **intramuscularly**, preferably in the anterolateral aspects of the upper thigh and the deltoid muscle of the upper arm. The gluteal region should not be used routinely as an injection site because of the risk of injury to the sciatic nerve. If the gluteal region is used, the central region MUST be avoided; only the upper, outer quadrant should be used.[26]

A. Single Vial or Syringe Dose

INJECT ENTIRE CONTENTS OF THE VIAL OR SYRINGE INTO THE INDIVIDUAL INTRAMUSCULARLY.

B. Multiple Vial or Syringe Dose

1. Calculate the number of vials or syringes of $Rh_o(D)$ Immune Globulin full dose to be given (See *"Dosage"* section above).

2. The total volume of $Rh_o(D)$ Immune Globulin full dose can be given in divided doses at different sites at one time or the total dose may be divided and injected at intervals, provided the total dosage is given within 72 hours of the fetomaternal hemorrhage or transfusion. USING STERILE TECHNIQUE, INJECT THE ENTIRE CONTENTS OF THE CALCULATED NUMBER OF VIALS OR SYRINGES INTRAMUSCULARLY INTO THE PATIENT.

Parenteral drug products should be inspected visually for particulate matter and discoloration prior to administration, whenever solution and container permit.

STORAGE

Store at 2°-8°C (35°-46°F). Do not freeze.

REFERENCES

1. Gunson HH, Bowell PJ, Kirkwood TBL. Collaborative study to recalibrate the International Reference Preparation of Anti-D Immunoglobulin. *J Clin Pathol* 33:249-53, 1980. 2. $Rh_o(D)$ immune globulin (human). *Med Lett Drugs Ther* 16(1):3-4, 1974. 3. Pollack W, Ascari WQ, Kochesky RJ, et al: Studies on Rh prophylaxis I. Relationship between doses of anti-Rh and size of antigenic stimulus. *Transfusion* 11 (6):333-9, 1971. 4. Unpublished data in files of Miles Inc., Cutter Biological. 5. Queenan JT, Shah S, Kubarych SF, *et al*: Role of induced abortion in rhesus immunisation. *Lancet* 1(7704): 815-7, 1971. 6. Goldman JA, Eckerling B; Prevention of Rh immunization after abortion with anti-D-immunoglobulin. *Obstet Gynecol* 40(3):366-70, 1972. 7. *The selective use of $Rh_o(D)$ Immune Globulin (Rh)G). ACOG Tech Bull* 61, 1981. 8. Pollack W, Asceri WQ, Crispen JF, et al: Studies on Rh prophylaxis. II. Rh immune prophylaxis after transfusion with Rh-positive blood. *Transfusion* 11 (6):340-4, 1971. 9. Keith LG, Houser GH: Anti-Rh immune globulin after a massive transfusion accident. *Transfusion* 11(3):176, 1971. 11. Current uses of Rh_o immune globulin and detection of antibodies. *ACOG Tech Bull* 35, 1976. 12. Pollack W: Rh hemolytic disease of the newborn; its cause and prevention. *Prog Clin Biol Res* 70:185-203, 1981. 13. Bowman JM, Chown B, Lewis M, et al: Rh isoimmunization during pregnancy: antenatal prophylaxis. *Can Med Assoc J* 118(6):623-7, 1978. 14. Bowman JM, Pollack JM: Antenatal prophylaxis of Rh isoimmunization: 28-weeks'-gestation service program. *Can Med Assoc J* 118(6):627-30, 1978. 15. Prevention of Rh sensitization. *WHO Tech Rep Ser* 468, 1971. 16. Recommendation of the Public Health Service Advisory Committee on Immunization Practices: Rh immune globulin. *MMWR* 21(15):126-7, 1972. 17. Stewart FH, Burnhill MS, Bozorgi N: Reduced dose of Rh immunoglobulin following first trimester pregnancy termination. *Obstet Gynecol* 51(3):318-22, 1978. 18. McMaster conference on prevention of Rh immunization, 28-30 September, 1977. *Vox Sang* 36(1):50-64, 1979. 19. Simonovits I: Efficiency of anti-D IgG prevention after induced abortion. *Vox Sang* 26(4):361-7, 1974. 20. Ascari WQ Allen AE, Baker WJ, et al: $Rh_o(D)$ immune globulin (human): evaluation in women at risk of Rh immunization. *JAMA* 205(1): 1-4, 1968. 21. Freda VJ, Gorman JG, Pollack W: Prevention of Rh-hemolytic disease with Rh-immune globulin. *Am J Obstet Gynecol* 128(4):456-60, 1977. 22. Prevention of Rh sensitization, *WHO Tech Rep Ser* 468:25, 1971. 23. Samson D, Mollison PL: Effect on primary Rh immunization of delayed administration of anti-Rh. *Immunology* 28:349-57, 1975. 24. Finn R, Harper DT, Stallings, SA, et al: Transplacental hemorrhage. *Transfusion* 3(2):114-24, 1963. 25. Garraty G (ed): Hemolytic disease of the newborn. Arlington, VA, American Association of Blood Banks, 1984, p 78. 26. Recommendations of the Immunization Practices Advisory Committee (ACIP): General recommendations on immunization. *MMWR* 38(13):205-14: 219-27, 1989.

J CODES

1 dose package IM—J2790

HOW SUPPLIED
INJECTION:

BRAND/MANUFACTURER	NDC	SIZE	AWP
○ **BRAND**			
MINI-GAMULIN RH: Armour	00053-7591-04	1 ml 6s	$86.80
GAMULIN RH: Armour	00053-7590-02	3 ml 6s	$351.68
MINI-GAMULIN RH: Armour	00053-7591-06	1 ml 10s	$168.00
GAMULIN RH: Armour	00053-7590-06	3 ml 10s	$546.14
MINI-GAMULIN RH: Armour	00053-7591-03	1 ml 25s	$370.00
GAMULIN RH: Armour	00053-7590-03	3 ml 25s	$1167.00

INJECTION: 50 U/GM

BRAND/MANUFACTURER	NDC	SIZE	AWP
○ **BRAND**			
HYPRHO-D MINI-DOSE: Miles Biol	00192-0621-05	0.17 ml 10s	$262.50

INJECTION: 50 MCG

BRAND/MANUFACTURER		NDC	SIZE	AWP
○ **BRAND**				
MICRHOGAM: Ortho Diagnostic		00562-8080-80	1 ea 5s	$140.00
		00562-8080-82	1 ea 25s	$650.00

INJECTION: 300 U/GM

BRAND/MANUFACTURER	NDC	SIZE	AWP
○ **BRAND**			
HYPRHO-D MINI-DOSE: Miles Biol	00192-0621-01	1 ml	$43.88
	00192-0621-10	1 ml 10s	$438.75
	00192-0621-22	1 ml 10s	$438.75

INJECTION: 300 MCG

BRAND/MANUFACTURER	NDC	SIZE	AWP
○ **BRAND**			
RHOGAM: Ortho Diagnostic	00562-8070-20	1 ea 25s	$1125.00
	00562-8070-90	1 ea 100s	$4265.00

RhoGAM SEE GLOBULIN, IMMUNE RHO₀(D) AND RHO(D)
IMMUNE GLOBULIN

Ribavirin

> **WARNINGS**
>
> USE OF AEROSOLIZED RIBAVIRIN IN PATIENTS REQUIRING MECHANICAL VENTILATOR ASSISTANCE SHOULD BE UNDERTAKEN ONLY BY PHYSICIANS AND SUPPORT STAFF FAMILIAR WITH THE SPECIFIC VENTILATOR BEING USED AND THIS MODE OF ADMINISTRATION OF THE DRUG. STRICT ATTENTION MUST BE PAID TO PROCEDURES THAT HAVE BEEN SHOWN TO MINIMIZE THE ACCUMULATION OF DRUG PRECIPITATE, WHICH CAN RESULT IN MECHANICAL VENTILATOR DYSFUNCTION AND ASSOCIATED INCREASED PULMONARY PRESSURES (SEE "WARNINGS").
>
> SUDDEN DETERIORATION OF RESPIRATORY FUNCTION HAS BEEN ASSOCIATED WITH INITIATION OF AEROSOLIZED RIBAVIRIN USE IN INFANTS. RESPIRATORY FUNCTION SHOULD BE CAREFULLY MONITORED DURING TREATMENT. IF INITIATION OF AEROSOLIZED RIBAVIRIN TREATMENT APPEARS TO PRODUCE SUDDEN DETERIORATION OF RESPIRATORY FUNCTION, TREATMENT SHOULD BE STOPPED AND REINSTITUTED ONLY WITH EXTREME CAUTION, CONTINUOUS MONITORING AND CONSIDERATION OF CONCOMITANT ADMINISTRATION OF BRONCHODILATORS (SEE "WARNINGS").
>
> RIBAVIRIN IS NOT INDICATED FOR USE IN ADULTS. PHYSICIANS AND PATIENTS SHOULD BE AWARE THAT RIBAVIRIN HAS BEEN SHOWN TO PRODUCE TESTICULAR LESIONS IN RODENTS AND TO BE TERATOGENIC IN ALL ANIMAL SPECIES IN WHICH ADEQUATE STUDIES HAVE BEEN CONDUCTED (RODENTS AND RABBITS); (SEE "CONTRAINDICATIONS").

DESCRIPTION
Ribavirin is a synthetic nucleoside with antiviral activity. Ribavirin for inhalation solution is a sterile, lyophilized powder to be reconstituted for aerosol administration. Each 100 ml glass vial contains 6 grams of Ribavirin, and when reconstituted to the recommended volume of 300 ml with sterile water for injection or sterile water for inhalation, will contain 20 mg of Ribavirin per ml, pH approximately 5.5. Aerosolization is to be carried out in a Small Particle Aerosol Generator (SPAG-2) nebulizer only.

Ribavirin is 1-beta-D-ribofuranosyl-1H-1,2,4-triazole-3-carboxa- mide.

Ribavirin is a stable, white, crystalline compound with a maximum solubility in water of 142 mg/ml at 25°C and with only a slight solubility in ethanol. The empirical formula is $C_8H_{12}N_4O_5$ and the molecular weight is 244.21.

Following is its chemical structure:

CLINICAL PHARMACOLOGY
MECHANISM OF ACTION
In cell cultures the inhibitory activity of Ribavirin for respiratory syncytial virus (RSV) is selective. The mechanism of action is unknown. Reversal of the *in vitro* antiviral activity by guanosine or xanthosine suggests Ribavirin may act as an analogue of these cellular metabolites.

MICROBIOLOGY
Ribavirin has demonstrated antiviral activity against RSV *in vitro*[1] and in experimentally infected cotton rats.[2] Several clinical isolates of RSV were evaluated for Ribavirin susceptibility by plaque reduction in tissue culture. Plaques were reduced 85-98% by 16 µg/ml; however, results may vary with the test system. The development of resistance has not been evaluated *in vitro* or in clinical trials.

In addition to the above, Ribavirin has been shown to have *in vitro* activity against influenza A and B viruses and herpes simplex virus, but the clinical significance of these data is unknown.

IMMUNOLOGIC EFFECTS
Neutralizing antibody responses to RSV were decreased in aerosolized Ribavirin treated infants compared to placebo treated infants.[3] One study also showed that RSV-specific IgE antibody in bronchial secretions was decreased in patients treated with aerosolized Ribavirin. In rats, Ribavirin administration resulted in lymphoid atrophy of the thymus, spleen, and lymph nodes. Humoral immunity was reduced in guinea pigs and ferrets. Cellular immunity was also mildly depressed in animal studies. The clinical significance of these observations is unknown.

PHARMACOKINETICS
Assay for Ribavirin in human materials is by a radioimmunoassay which detects Ribavirin and at least one metabolite.

Ribavirin, when administered by aerosol, is absorbed systemically. Four pediatric patients inhaling Ribavirin aerosol administered by face mask for 2.5 hours each day for 3 days had plasma concentrations ranging from 0.44 to 1.55 µM, with a mean concentration of 0.76 µM. The plasma half-life was reported to be 9.5 hours. Three pediatric patients inhaling aerosolized Ribavirin administered by face mask or mist tent for 20 hours each day for 5 days had plasma concentrations ranging from 1.5 to 14.3 µM, with a mean concentration of 6.8 µM.

The bioavailability of aerosolized Ribavirin is unknown and may depend on the mode of aerosol delivery. After aerosol treatment, peak plasma concentrations of Ribavirin are 85% to 98% less than the concentration that reduced RSV plaque formation in tissue culture. After aerosol treatment, respiratory tract secretions are likely to contain Ribavirin in concentrations many fold higher than those required to reduce plaque formation. However, RSV is an intracellular virus and it is unknown whether plasma concentrations or respiratory secretion concentrations of the drug better reflect intracellular concentrations in the respiratory tract. In man, rats, and rhesus monkeys, accumulation of Ribavirin and/or metabolites in the red blood cells has been noted, plateauing in red cells in man in about 4 days and gradually declining with an apparent half-life of 40 days (the half-life of erythrocytes). The extent of accumulation of Ribavirin following inhalation therapy is not well defined.

ANIMAL TOXICOLOGY
Ribavirin, when administered orally or as an aerosol, produced cardiac lesions in mice, rats, and monkeys, when given at doses of 30, 36 and 120 mg/kg or greater for 4 weeks or more (estimated human equivalent dose of 4.8, 12.3 and 111.4 mg/kg for a 5 kg child, or 2.5, 5.1 and 40 mg/kg for a 60 kg adult, based on body surface area adjustment). Aerosolized Ribavirin administered to developing ferrets at 60 mg/kg for 10 or 30 days resulted in inflammatory and possibly emphysematous changes in the lungs. Proliferative changes were seen in the lungs following exposure at 131 mg/kg for 30 days. The significance of these findings to human administration is unknown.

INDICATIONS AND USAGE
Ribavirin is indicated for the treatment of hospitalized infants and young children with severe lower respiratory tract infections due to respiratory syncytial virus. Treatment early in the course of severe lower respiratory tract infection may be necessary to achieve efficacy.

Only severe RSV lower respiratory tract infection should be treated with Ribavirin. The vast majority of infants and children with RSV infection have disease that is mild, self-limited, and does not require hospitalization or antiviral treatment. Many children with mild lower respiratory tract involvement will require shorter hospitalization than would be required for a full course of Ribavirin aerosol (3 to 7 days) and should not be treated with the drug. Thus the decision to treat with Ribavirin should be based on the severity of the RSV infection.

The presence of an underlying condition such as prematurity, immunosuppression or cardiopulmonary disease may increase the severity of clinical manifestations and complications of RSV infection.

Use of aerosolized Ribavirin in patients requiring mechanical ventilator assistance should be undertaken only by physicians and support staff familiar with this mode of administration and the specific ventilator being used (see "Warnings," and "Dosage and Administration").

DIAGNOSIS
RSV infection should be documented by a rapid diagnostic method such as demonstration of viral antigen in respiratory tract secretions by immunofluorescence[3,4] or ELISA[5] before or during the first 24 hours of treatment. Treatment may be initiated while awaiting rapid diagnostic test results. However, treatment should not be continued without documentation of RSV infection.

➤ SHOWN IN PRODUCT IDENTIFICATION GUIDE

Nonculture antigen detection techniques may have false positive or false negative results. Assessment of the clinical situation, the time of year and other parameters may warrant reevaluation of the laboratory diagnosis.

DESCRIPTION OF STUDIES

Non-Mechanically-Ventilated Infants: In two placebo controlled trials in infants hospitalized with RSV lower respiratory tract infection, aerosolized Ribavirin treatment had a therapeutic effect, as judged by the reduction in severity of clinical manifestations of disease by treatment day 3.[3,4] Treatment was most effective when instituted within the first 3 days of clinical illness. Virus titers in respiratory secretions were also significantly reduced with Ribavirin in one of these original studies.[4] Additional controlled studies conducted since these initial trials of aerosolized Ribavirin in the treatment of RSV infection have supported these data.

Mechanically-Ventilated Infants: A randomized, double-blind, placebo controlled evaluation of aerosolized Ribavirin at the recommended dose was conducted in 28 infants requiring mechanical ventilation for respiratory failure caused by documented RSV infection.[6] Mean age was 1.4 months (SD, 1.7 months). Seven patients had underlying diseases predisposing them to severe infection and 21 were previously normal. Aerosolized Ribavirin treatment significantly decreased the duration of mechanical ventilation required (4.9 vs. 9.9 days, $p = 0.01$) and duration of required supplemental oxygen (8.7 vs 13.5 says, $p = 0.01$). Intensive patient management and monitoring techniques were employed in this study. These included endotracheal tube suctioning every 1 to 2 hours; recording of proximal airway pressure, ventilatory rate, and F_1O_2 every hour; and arterial blood gas monitoring every 2 to 6 hours. To reduce the risk of Ribavirin precipitation and ventilator malfunction, heated wire tubing, two bacterial filters connected in series in the expiratory limb of the ventilator (with filter changes every 4 hours), and water column pressure release valves to monitor internal ventilator pressures were used in connecting ventilator circuits to the SPAG-2.

Employing these techniques, no technical difficulties with Ribavirin administration were encountered during the study. Adverse events consisted of bacterial pneumonia in one case, staphyloccus bacteremia in one case and two cases of post-extubation stridor. None were felt to be related to Ribavirin administration.

UNLABELED USES

Ribavirin is used alone or as an adjunct in the treatment of Hantaan virus infections, hemorrhagic fever, and AIDS-related complex. It is also used against herpes simplex infections, Lassa fever, influenza virus infections, viral hepatitis A and B, and measles.

CONTRAINDICATIONS

Ribavirin is contraindicated in individuals who have shown hypersensitivity to the drug or its components, and in women who are or may become pregnant during exposure to the drug. Ribavirin has demonstrated significant teratogenic and/or embryocidal potential in all animals species in which adequate studies have been conducted (rodents and rabbits). Therefore, although clinical studies have not been performed, it should be assumed that Ribavirin may cause fetal harm in humans. Studies in which the drug has been administered systemically demonstrate that Ribavirin is concentrated in the red blood cells and persists for the life of the erythrocyte.

WARNINGS

SUDDEN DETERIORATION OF RESPIRATORY FUNCTION HAS BEEN ASSOCIATED WITH INITIATION OF AEROSOLIZED RIBAVIRIN USE IN INFANTS. Respiratory function should be carefully monitored during treatment. If initiation of aerosolized Ribavirin treatment appears to produce sudden deterioration of respiratory function, treatment should be stopped and reinstituted only with extreme caution, continuous monitoring, and consideration of concomitant administration of bronchodilators.

USE WITH MECHANICAL VENTILATORS

USE OF AEROSOLIZED RIBAVIRIN IN PATIENTS REQUIRING MECHANICAL VENTILATOR ASSISTANCE SHOULD BE UNDERTAKEN ONLY BY PHYSICIANS AND SUPPORT STAFF FAMILIAR WITH THIS MODE OF ADMINISTRATION AND THE SPECIFIC VENTILATOR BEING USED. Strict attention must be paid to procedures that have been shown to minimize the accumulation of drug precipitate, which can result in mechanical ventilator dysfunction and associated increased pulmonary pressures. These procedures include the use of bacteria filters in series in the expiratory limb of the ventilator circuit with frequent changes (every 4 hours), water column pressure release valves to indicate elevated ventilator pressures, frequent monitoring of these devices and verification that Ribavirin crystals have not accumulated within the ventilator circuitry, and frequent suctioning and monitoring of the patient (see *"Clinical Studies"*).

Those administering aersolized Ribavirin in conjunction with mechanical ventilator use should be thoroughly familiar with detailed descriptions of these procedures as outlined in the SPAG-2 manual.

PRECAUTIONS

General: Patients with severe lower respiratory tract infection due to respiratory syncytial virus require optimum monitoring and attention to respiratory and fluid status (see SPAG-2 manual).

DRUG INTERACTIONS

Clinical studies of interactions of Ribavirin with other drugs commonly used to treat infants with RSV infections, such as digoxin, bronchodilators, other antiviral agents, antibiotics, or anti-metabolites have not been conducted. Interference by Ribavirin with laboratory tests has not been evaluated.

CARCINOGENESIS AND MUTAGENESIS

Ribavirin increased the incidence of cell transformations and mutations in mouse Balb/c 3T3 (fibroblasts) and L5178Y (lymphoma) cells at concentrations of 0.015 and 0.03-5.0 mg/ml, respectively (without metabolic activation.) Modest increases in mutation rates (3-4x) were observed at concentrations between 3.75-10.0 mg/ml in L5178Y cells *in vitro* with the addition of a metabolic activation fraction. In the mouse micronucleus assay, Ribavirin was clastogenic at intravenous doses of 20-200 mg/kg, (estimated human equivalent of 1.67-16.7 mg/kg, based on body surface area adjustment for a 60 kg adult). Ribavirin was not mutagenic in a dominant lethal assay in rats at intraperitoneal doses between 50-200 mg/kg when administered for 5 days (estimated human equivalent of 7.14-28.6 mg/kg, based on body surface area adjustment; see *"Pharmacokinetics"*).

In vivo carcinogenicity studies with Ribavirin are incomplete. However, results of a chronic feeding study with Ribavirin in rats, at doses of 16-100 mg/kg/day (estimated human equivalent of 2.3-14.3 mg/kg/day, based on body surface area adjustment for the adult), suggest that Ribavirin may induce benign mammary, pancreatic, pituitary and adrenal tumors. Preliminary results of 2 oral gavage oncogenicity studies in the mouse and rat (18-24 months; doses of 20-75 and 10-40 mg/kg/day, respectively [estimated human equivalent of 1.67 6.25 and 1.43 5.71 mg/kg/day, respectively, based on body surface area adjustment for the adult]) are inconclusive as to the carcinogenic potential of Ribavirin (see *"Pharmacokinetics"*). However, these studies have demonstrated a relationship between chronic Ribavirin exposure and increased incidences of vascular lesions (microscopic hemorrhages in mice) and retinal degeneration (in rats).

IMPAIRMENT OF FERTILITY

The fertility of Ribavirin-treated animals (male or female) has not been fully investigated. However, in the mouse, administration of Ribavirin at doses between 35-150 mg/kg/day (estimated human equivalent of 2.92-12.5 mg/kg/day, based on body surface area adjustment for the adult) resulted in significant seminiferous tubule atrophy, decreased sperm concentrations, and increased numbers of sperm with abnormal morphology. Partial recovery of sperm production was apparent 3-6 months following dose cessation. In several additional toxicology studies, Ribavirin has been shown to cause testicular lesions (tubular atrophy), in adult rats at oral dose levels as low as 16 mg/kg/day (estimated human equivalent of 2.29 mg/kg/day, based on body surface area adjustment; see *"Pharmacokinetics"*). Lower doses were not tested. The reproductive capacity of treated male animals has not been studied.

PREGNANCY: CATEGORY X

Ribavirin has demonstrated significant teratogenic and/or embryocidal potential in all animal species in which adequate studies have been conducted. Teratogenic effects were evident after single oral doses of 2.5 mg/kg or greater in the hamster, and after daily oral doses of 0.3 and 1.0 mg/kg in the rabbit and rat, respectively (estimated human equivalent doses of 0.12 and 0.14 mg/kg, based on body surface area adjustment for the adult). Malformation of the skull, palate, eye, jaw, limbs, skeleton, and gastrointestinal tract were noted. The incidence and severity of teratogenic effects increased with escalation of the drug dose. Survival of fetuses and offspring was reduced. Ribavirin caused embryolethality in the rabbit at daily oral dose levels as low as 1 mg/kg. No teratogenic effects were evident in the rabbit and rat administered daily oral doses of 0.1 and 0.3 mg/kg, respectively with estimated human equivalent doses of 0.01 and 0.04 mg/kg, based on body surface area adjustment (see *"Pharmacokinetics"*). These doses are considered to define the "No Observable Teratogenic Effects Level" (NOTEL) for Ribavirin in the rabbit and rat.

Following oral administration of Ribavirin in the pregnant rat (1.0 mg/kg) and rabbit (0.3 mg/kg), mean plasma levels of drug ranged from 0.10-0.20 μM [0.024-0.049 μg/ml] at 1 hour after dosing, to undetectable levels at 24 hours. At 1 hour following the administration of 0.3 or 0.1 mg/kg in the rat and rabbit (NOTEL), respectively, mean plasma levels of drug in both species were near or below the limit of detection (0.05 μM; see *"Pharmacokinetics"*).

Although clinical studies have not been performed, Ribavirin may cause fetal harm in humans. As noted previously, Ribavirin is concentrated in red blood cells and persists for the life of the cell. Thus the terminal half-life for the systemic elimination of Ribavirin is essentially that of the half-life of circulating erythrocytes. The minimum interval following exposure to Ribavirin before pregnancy may be safely initiated is unknown (see *"Contraindications," "Warnings,"* and *"Information for Health Care Personnel"*).

NURSING MOTHERS

Ribavirin has been shown to be toxic to lactating animals and their offspring. It is not known if Ribavirin is excreted in human milk.

INFORMATION FOR HEALTH CARE PERSONNEL

Health care workers directly providing care to patients receiving aerosolized Ribavirin should be aware that Ribavirin has been shown to be teratogenic in all animal species in which adequate studies have been conducted (rodents and rabbits). Although no reports of teratogenesis in offspring of mothers who were exposed to aerosolized Ribavirin during pregnancy have been confirmed, no controlled studies have been conducted in pregnant women. Studies of environmental exposure in treatment settings have shown that the drug can disperse into the immediate bedside area during routine patient care activities with highest ambient levels closest to the patient and extremely low levels outside of the immediate bedside area. Adverse reactions resulting from actual occupational

---

◆ RATED THERAPEUTICALLY EQUIVALENT; ◇ THERAPEUTIC EQUIVALENCE UNCONFIRMED; ○ UNRATED

exposure in adults are described below (see *"Adverse Events in Health Care Workers"*). Some studies have documented ambient drug concentrations at the bedside that could potentially lead to systemic exposures above those considered safe for exposure during pregnancy (1/1000 of the NOTEL dose in the most sensitive animal species).[7,8,9]

A 1992 study conducted by the National Institute of Occupational Safety and Health (NIOSH) demonstrated measurable urine levels of Ribavirin in health care workers exposed to aerosol in the course of direct patient care.[7] Levels were lowest in workers caring for infants receiving aerosolized Ribavirin with mechanical ventilation and highest in those caring for patients being administered the drug via an oxygen tent or hood. This study employed a more sensitive assay to evaluate Ribavirin levels in urine than was available for several previous studies of environmental exposure that failed to detect measurable Ribavirin levels in exposed workers. Creatinine adjusted urine levels in the NIOSH study ranged from less than 0.001 to 0.140 μM of Ribavirin per gram of creatinine in exposed workers. However, the relationship between urinary Ribavirin levels in exposed workers, plasma levels in animal studies, and the specific risk of teratogenesis in exposed pregnant women is unknown.

It is good practice to avoid unnecessary occupational exposure to chemicals wherever possible. Hospitals are encouraged to conduct training programs to minimize potential occupational exposure to Ribavirin. Health care workers who are pregnant should consider avoiding direct care of patients receiving aerosolized Ribavirin. If close patient contact cannot be avoided, precautions to limit exposure should be taken. These include administration of Ribavirin in negative pressure rooms; adequate room ventilation (at least six air exchanges per hour); the use of Ribavirin aerosol scavenging devices; turning off the SPAG-2 device for 5 to 10 minutes prior to prolonged patient contact, and wearing appropriately fitted respiratory masks. Surgical masks do not provide adequate filtration of Ribavirin particles. Further information is available from NIOSH's Hazard Evaluation and Technical Assistance Branch and additional recommendations have been published in an Aerosol Consensus Statement by the American Respiratory Care Foundation and the American Association for Respiratory Care.[10]

ADVERSE REACTIONS
The description of adverse reactions is based on events from clinical studies (approximately 200 patients) conducted prior to 1986, and the controlled trial of aerosolized Ribavirin conducted in 1989-1990. Additional data from spontaneous post-marketing reports of adverse events in individual patients have been available since 1986.

DEATHS
Deaths during or shortly after treatment with aerosolized Ribavirin have been reported in 20 cases of patients treated with Ribavirin; 12 of these patients were being treated for RSV infections). Several cases have been characterized as "possibly related" to Ribavirin by the treating physician; these were in infants who experienced worsening respiratory status related to bronchospasm while being treated with the drug. Several other cases have been attributed to mechanical ventilator malfunction in which Ribavirin precipitation within the ventilator apparatus led to excessively high pulmonary pressures and diminished oxygenation. In these cases the monitoring procedures described were not employed (see *"Description of Studies," "Warnings,"* and *"Dosage and Administration"*).

PULMONARY AND CARDIOVASCULAR
Pulmonary function significantly deteriorated during aerosolized Ribavirin treatment in six of six adults with chronic obstructive lung disease and in four of six asthmatic adults. Dyspnea and chest soreness were also reported in the latter group. Minor abnormalities in pulmonary function were also seen in healthy adult volunteers.

In the original study population of approximately 200 infants who received aerosolized Ribavirin several serious adverse events occurred in severely ill infants with life-threatening underlying diseases, many of whom required assisted ventilation. The role of Ribavirin in these events is indeterminate. Since the drug's approval in 1986, additional reports of similar serious, though non-fatal, events have been filed infrequently. Events associated with aerosolized Ribavirin use have included the following:

Pulmonary: Worsening of respiratory status, bronchospasm, pulmonary edema, hypoventilation, cyanosis, dyspnea, bacterial pneumonia, pneumothorax, apnea, atelectasis and ventilator dependence.

Cardiovascular: Cardiac arrest, hypotension, bradycardia and digitalis toxicity. Bigeminy, bradycardia and tachycardia have been described in patients with underlying congenital heart disease.

Some subjects requiring assisted ventilation experienced serious difficulties, due to inadequate ventilation and gas exchange. Precipitation of drug within the ventilation apparatus, including the endotracheal tube, has resulted in increased positive end expiratory pressure and increased positive inspiratory pressure. Accumulation of fluid in tubing ("rain out") has also been noted. Measures to avoid these complications should be followed carefully (see *"Dosage and Administration"*).

HEMATOLOGIC
Although anemia was not reported with use of aerosolized Ribavirin in controlled clinical trials, most infants treated with the aerosol have not been evaluated 1 to 2 weeks post-treatment when anemia is likely to occur. Anemia has been shown to occur frequently with experimental oral and intravenous Ribavirin in humans.

Also, cases of anemia (type unspecified), reticulocytosis and hemolytic anemia associated with aerosolized Ribavirin use have been reported through postmarketing reporting systems. All have been reversible with discontinuation of the drug.

Other: Rash and conjunctivitis have been associated with the use of aerosolized Ribavirin. These usually resolve within hours of discontinuing therapy. Seizures and asthenia associated with experimental intravenous Ribavirin therapy have also been reported.

Adverse Events in Health Care Workers: Studies of environmental exposure to aerosolized Ribavirin in health care workers administering care to patients receiving the drug have not detected adverse signs or symptoms related to exposure. However, 152 health care workers have reported experiencing adverse events through post-marketing surveillance. Nearly all were in individuals providing direct care to infants receiving aerosolized Ribavirin. Of 358 events from these 152 individual health care worker reports, the most common signs and symptoms were headache (51% of reports), conjunctivitis (32%), and rhinitis, nausea, rash, dizziness, pharyngitis, or lacrimation (10-20% each). Several cases of bronchospasm and/or chest pain were also reported, usually in individuals with known underlying reactive airway disease. Several case reports of damage to contact lenses after prolonged close exposure to aerosolized Ribavirin have also been reported. Most signs and symptoms reported as having occurred in exposed health care workers resolved within minutes to hours of discontinuing close exposure to aerosolized Ribavirin (also see *"Information for Health Care Personnel"*).

The symptoms of RSV in adults can include headache, conjunctivitis, sore throat and/or cough, fever, hoarseness, nasal congestion and wheezing, although RSV infections in adults are typically mild and transient. Such infections represent a potential hazard to uninfected hospital patients. It is unknown whether certain symptoms cited in reports from health care workers were due to exposure to the drug or infection with RSV. Hospitals should implement appropriate infection control procedures.

OVERDOSAGE
No overdosage with Ribavirin by aerosol administration has been reported in humans. The LD_{50} in mice is 2 gm orally and is associated with hypoactivity and gastrointestinal symptoms (estimated human equivalent dose of 0.17 gm/kg, based on body surface area conversion). The mean plasma half-life after administration of aerosolized Ribavirin for pediatric patients is 9.5 hours. Ribavirin is concentrated and persists in red blood cells for the life of the erythrocyte (see *"Pharmacokinetics"*).

DOSAGE AND ADMINISTRATION
BEFORE USE, READ THOROUGHLY THE VIRATEK SMALL PARTICLE AEROSOL GENERATOR (SPAG) MODEL SPAG-2 OPERATOR'S MANUAL FOR SMALL PARTICLE AEROSOL GENERATOR OPERATING INSTRUCTIONS AEROSOLIZED RIBAVIRIN SHOULD NOT BE ADMINISTERED WITH ANY OTHER AEROSOL GENERATING DEVICE.

The recommended treatment regimen is 20 mg/ml Ribavirin as the starting solution in the drug reservoir of the SPAG-2 unit, with continuous aerosol administration for 12-18 hours per day for 3 to 7 days. Using the recommended drug concentration of 20 mg/ml the average aerosol concentration for a 12 hour delivery period would be 190 micrograms/liter of air. Aerosolized Ribavirin should not be administered in a mixture for combined aerosolization or simultaneously with other aerosolized medications.

NON-MECHANICALLY VENTILATED INFANTS
Ribavirin should be delivered to an infant oxygen hood from the SPAG-2 aerosol generator. Administration by face mask or oxygen tent may be necessary if a hood cannot be employed (see SPAG-2 manual). However, the volume and condensation area are larger in a tent and this may alter delivery dynamics of the drug.

MECHANICALLY VENTILATED INFANTS
The recommended dose and administration schedule for infants who require mechanical ventilation is the same as for those who do not. Either a pressure or volume cycle ventilator may be used in conjunction with the SPAG-2. In either case, patients should have their endotracheal tubes suctioned every 1-2 hours, and their pulmonary pressures monitored frequently (every 2-4 hours). For both pressure and volume ventilators, heated wire connective tubing and bacteria filters in series in the expiratory limb of the system (which must be changed frequently, i.e., every 4 hours) must be used to minimize the risk of Ribavirin precipitation in the system and the subsequent risk of ventilator dysfunction. Water column pressure release valves should be used in the ventilator circuit for pressure cycled ventilators, and may be utilized with volume cycled ventilators (*see SPAG-2 Manual for Detailed Instructions*).

METHOD OF PREPARATION
Ribavirin is supplied as 6 grams of lyophilized powder per 100 ml vial for aerosol administration only. By sterile technique, solubilize drug with Sterile Water for Injection, USP, or Inhalation in the 100 ml vial. Transfer to the clean, sterilized 500 ml SPAG-2 reservoir and further dilute to a final volume of 300 ml with Sterile Water for Injection, USP, or Inhalation. The final concentration should be 20 mg/ml. **Important:** This water should NOT have had any antimicrobial agent or other substance added. The solution should be inspected visually for particulate matter and discoloration prior to administration. Solutions that have been placed in the SPAG-2 unit should be discarded at least every 24 hours and when the liquid level is low before adding newly reconstituted solution.

REFERENCES

1. Hruska JF, Bernstein JM, Douglas Jr., RG, and Hall CB. Effects of Virazole on respiratory syncytial virus in vitro. Antimicrob Agents Chemother 17:770-775, 1 1980. 2. Hruska JF, Morrow PE, Suffin SC, and Douglas Jr., RG. In vivo inhibition of respiratory syncytial virus by Virazole. Antimicrob Agents Chemother 21:125-130, 1982. 3. Taber LH, Knight V, Gilbert BE, McClung HW et al. Virazole aerosol treatment of bronchiolitis associated with respiratory tract infection in infants. Pediatrics 72:613-618, 1983. 4. Hall CB, McBride JT, Walsh EE, Bell DM et al. Aerosolized Virazole treatment of infants with respiratory syncytial viral infection. N Engl J Med 308:1443-7, 1983. 5. Hendry RM, McIntosh K, Fahnestock ML, and Pierik LT. Enzyme-linked immunosorbent assay for detection of respiratory syncytial virus infection. J Clin Microbiol 16:329-33, 1982. 6. Smith, David W., Frankel, Lorry R., Mather, Larry H., Tang, Allen T.S., Ariagno, Ronald L., Prober, Charles G. A Controlled Trial of Aerosolized Ribavirin in Infants Receiving Mechanical Ventilation for Severe Respiratory Syncytial Virus Infection. The New England Journal of Medicine 1991; 325:24-29. 7. Decker, John, Shultz, Ruth A., Health Hazard Evaluation Report: Florida Hospital, Orlando, Florida, Cincinnati OH: U.S. Department of Health and Human Services, Public Health Service, Centers for NIOSH Report No. HETA 91-104-2229.* 8. Barnes, D.J. and Doursew, M. Reference dose: Description and use in health risk assessments. Regul Tox. and Pharm. Vol. 8; p. 471-486, 1988. 9. Federal Register Vol. 53 No. 126 Thurs. June 30, 1988 p. 24834-24847. 10. American Association for Respirtory Care [1991*. Aerosol Consensus Statement-1991. Respiratory Care 36(9):916-921.

HOW SUPPLIED
POWDER FOR INJECTION:

BRAND/MANUFACTURER	NDC	SIZE	AWP
○ BRAND VIRAZOLE: ICN	53095-0007-14	4s	$5279.40

Ridaura *SEE* AURANOFIN

Rifabutin

DESCRIPTION

Rifabutin is an antimycobacterial agent. It is a semisynthetic ansamycin antibiotic derived from rifamycin S Rifabutin capsules for oral administration contain 150 mg of Ribabutin per capsule, along with the inactive ingredients microcrystalline cellulose, magnesium stearate, red iron oxide, silica gel, sodium lauryl sulfate, titanium dioxide, and edible white ink.

The chemical name for Rifabutin is 1',4-didehydro-1-deoxy-1,4-dihydro-5'-(2-methylpropyl)-1-oxorifam ycin XIV (Chemical Abstracts Service, 9th Collective Index) or (9S,12E,14S,15R,16S,17R, 18R,19R,20S, 21S,22E,24Z)-6,16, 18,20-tetrahydroxy-1'-isobutyl-14-methoxy-7,9,15,17,19,21, 25-heptamethyl-spiro [9,4-(epoxypentadeca[1,11,13]trienimino)-2H-furo [2',3':7,8] naphth [1,2-d] imidazole-2,4'-piperidine]-5,10,26-(3H,9H)-trione-16-acetate. Rifabutin has a molecular formula of $C_{46}H_{62}N_4O_{11}$, a molecular weight of 847.02.

Rifabutin is a red-violet powder soluble in chloroform and methanol, sparingly soluble in ethanol, and very slightly soluble in water (0.19 mg/mL). Its log P value (the base 10 logarithm of the partition coefficient between n-octanol and water) is 3.2 (n-octanol/water).

Following is its chemical structure:

CLINICAL PHARMACOLOGY
PHARMACOKINETICS

Following a single oral dose of 300 mg to nine healthy adult volunteers, Rifabutin was readily absorbed from the gastrointestinal tract with mean (± SD) peak plasma levels (C_{max}) of 375 (± 267) ng/mL (range: 141 to 1033 ng/mL) attained in 3.3 (± 0.9) hours (T_{max} range: 2 to 4 hours). Plasma concentrations post-C_{max} declined in an apparent biphasic manner. Kinetic dose-proportionality has been established over the 300 to 600 mg dose range in nine healthy adult volunteers (crossover design) and in 16 early symptomatic human immunodeficiency virus (HIV)-positive patients over a 300 to 900 mg dose range. Rifabutin was slowly eliminated from plasma in seven healthy adult volunteers, presumably because of *distribution-limited elimination*, with a mean terminal half-life of 45 (± 17) hours (range: 16 to 69 hours). Although the systemic levels of Rifabutin following multiple dosing decreased by 38%, its terminal half-life remained unchanged.

---

* Copies of the Report may be purchased from National Technical Information Service, 5285 Port Royal Road, Springfield, VA 22161; Ask for Publication PB 93119-345.

Rifabutin, due to its high lipophilicity, demonstrates a high propensity for distribution and intracellular tissue uptake. Estimates of apparent steady-state distribution volume (9.3 ± 1.5 L/kg) in five HIV-positive patients, following I.V. dosing, exceed total body water by approximately 15-fold. Substantially higher intracellular tissue levels than those seen in plasma have been observed in both rat and man. The lung to plasma concentration ratio, obtained at 12 hours, was found to be approximately 6.5 in four surgical patients administered an oral dose. Mean Rifabutin steady-state trough levels ($C_{p.min}^{ss}$; 24-hour post-dose) ranged from 50 to 65 ng/mL in HIV-positive patients and in healthy adult volunteers. About 85% of the drug is bound in a concentration-independent manner to plasma proteins over a concentration range of 0.05 to 1 μg/mL. Binding does not appear to be influenced by renal or hepatic dysfunction.

Mean systemic clearance (CL_s/F) in healthy adult volunteers following a single oral dose was 0.69 (± 0.32) L/hr/kg (range: 0.46 to 1.34 L/hr/kg). Renal and biliary clearance of unchanged drug each contribute approximately 5% to CL_s/F. About 30% of the dose is excreted in the feces. A mass-balance study in three healthy adult volunteers with ^{14}C-labeled drug has shown that 53% of the oral dose was excreted in the urine, primarily as metabolites. Of the five metabolites that have been identified, 25-O-desacetyl and 31-hydroxy are the most predominant, and show a plasma metabolite:parent area under the curve ratio of 0.10 and 0.07, respectively. The former has an activity equal to the parent drug and contributes up to 10% to the total antimicrobial activity.

Absolute bioavailability assessed in five HIV-positive patients, who received both oral and I.V. doses, averaged 20%. Total recovery of radioactivity in the urine indicates that at least 53% of the orally administered Rifabutin dose is absorbed from the G.I. tract. The bioavailability of Rifabutin from the capsule dosage form, relative to a solution, was 85% in 12 healthy adult volunteers. High-fat meals slow the rate without influencing the extent of absorption from the capsule dosage form. The overall pharmacokinetics of Rifabutin are modified only slightly by alterations in hepatic function or age. Rifabutin steady-state kinetics in early symptomatic HIV-positive patients are similar to healthy volunteers. Compared to healthy volunteers, steady-state kinetics of Rifabutin are more variable in elderly patients (> 70 years) and in symptomatic HIV-positive patients. Somewhat reduced drug distribution and faster elimination of rifabutin in patients with compromised renal function may result in decreased drug concentrations. The clinical implications of this are unknown.

No rifabutin disposition information is currently available in children or adolescents under 18 years of age.

MICROBIOLOGY

Mechanism of Action: Rifabutin inhibits DNA-dependent RNA polymerase in susceptible strains of *Escherichia coli* and *Bacillus subtilis* but not in mammalian cells. In resistant strains of *E. coli*, rifabutin, like rifampin, did not inhibit this enzyme. It is not known whether rifabutin inhibits DNA-dependent RNA polymerase in *Mycobacterium avium* or in *M. intracellulare* which comprise *M. avium* complex (MAC).

Susceptibility Testing: In vitro susceptibility testing methods and diagnostic products used for determining minimum inhibitory concentration (MIC) values against *M. avium* complex (MAC) organisms have not been standardized. Breakpoints to determine whether clinical isolates of MAC and other mycobacterial species are susceptible or resistant to rifabutin have not been established.

In Vitro Studies: Rifabutin has demonstrated *in vitro* activity against *M avium* complex (MAC) organisms isolated from both HIV-positive and HIV-negative people. While gene probe techniques may be used to identify these two organisms, many reported studies did not distinguish between these two species. The vast majority of isolates from MAC-infected, HIV-positive people are *M. avium*, whereas in HIV-negative people, about 40% of the MAC isolates are *M. intracellulare*.

Various *in vitro* methodologies employing broth or solid media, with and without polysorbate 80 (Tween 80), have been used to determine Rifabutin MIC values for mycobacterial species. In general, MIC values determined in broth are several fold lower than that observed with methods employing solid media. Utilization of Tween 80 in these assays has been shown to further lower MIC values. However, MIC values were substantially higher for egg based compared to agar based solid media.

Rifabutin activity against 211 MAC isolates from HIV-positive people was evaluated *in vitro* utilizing a radiometric broth and an agar dilution method. Results showed that 78% and 82% of these isolates had MIC99 values of ≤ 0.25 μg/mL and ≤ 1.0 μg/mL, respectively, when evaluated by these two methods. Rifabutin was also shown to be active against phagocytized, *M. avium* complex in a mouse macrophage cell culture model.

Rifabutin has *in vitro* activity against many strains of *Mycobacterium tuberculosis*. In one study, utilizing the radiometric broth method, each of 17 and 20 rifampin-naive clinical isolates tested from the United States and Taiwan, respectively, were shown to be susceptible to rifabutin concentrations of ≤ 0.125 μg/mL.

Cross-resistance between rifampin and Rifabutin is commonly observed with *M. tuberculosis and M. avium* complex isolates. Isolates of *M. tuberculosis* resistant to rifampin are likely to be resistant to Rifabutin. Rifampicin and Rifabutin MIC99 values against 523 isolates of *M. avium* complex were determined utilizing the agar dilution method (Ref. Heifets, Leonid B. and Iseman, Michael D. 1985. Determination of *in vitro* susceptibility of Mycobacteria to Ansamycin. Am. Rev. Respir. Dis. 132 (3):710-711. (See related table).

◆ RATED THERAPEUTICALLY EQUIVALENT; ◇ THERAPEUTIC EQUIVALENCE UNCONFIRMED; ○ UNRATED

INDICATIONS AND USAGE
Rifabutin is indicated for the prevention of disseminated *Mycobacterium avium* complex (MAC) disease in patients with advanced HIV infection.

CLINICAL STUDIES
Two randomized, double-blind clinical trials (study 023 and study 027) compared Rifabutin (300 mg/day to placebo in patients with CDC-defined AIDS and CD4 counts ≤ 200 cells/μL. These studies accrued patients from 2/90 through 2/92. Study 023 enrolled 590 patients, with a median CD4 cell count at study entry of 42 cells/μL (mean 61). Study 027 enrolled 556 patients, with a median CD4 cell count at study entry of 40 cells/μL (mean 58).

Endpoints included the following:

(1) MAC bacteremia, defined as at least one blood culture positive for *M. avium* complex bacteria.

(2) Clinically significant disseminated MAC disease, defined as MAC bacteremia accompanied by signs or symptoms of serious MAC infection, including one or more of the following: fever, night sweats, rigors, weight loss, worsening anemia, and/or elevations in alkaline phosphatase.

(3) Survival

MAC BACTEREMIA
Participants who received Rifabutin were one-third to one-half as likely to develop MAC bacteremia as were participants who received placebo. These results were statistically significant (study 023: p < 0.001; study 027: p = 0.002).

In study 023, the one-year cumulative incidence of MAC bacteremia, on an intent to treat basis, was 9% for patients randomized to Rifabutin and 22% for patients randomized to placebo. In study 027, these rates were 13% and 28% for Rifabutin treated and placebo-treated patients, respectively.

Most cases of MAC bacteremia (approximately 90% in these studies) occurred among participants whose CD4 count at study entry was ≤ 100 cells/μL. The median and mean CD4 counts at onset of MAC bacteremia were 13 cells/μL and 24 cells/μL, respectively. These studies did not investigate the optimal time to begin MAC prophylaxis.

CLINICALLY SIGNIFICANT DISSEMINATED MAC DISEASE
In association with the decreased incidence of bacteremia, patients on Rifabutin showed reductions in the signs and symptoms of disseminated MAC disease, including fever, night sweats, weight loss, fatigue, abdominal pain, anemia, and hepatic dysfunction.

SURVIVAL
The one year survival rates in study 023 were 77% for the Rifabutin group and 77% for the placebo group. In study 027, the one year survival rates were 77% for the Rifabutin group and 70% for the placebo group. These differences were not statistically significant.

UNLABELED USE
Rifabutin is used alone or as an adjunct in the treatment of pediatric mycobactderium intracellulare infection and mycobacterium tubercu- losis.

CONTRAINDICATIONS
Rifabutin is contraindicated in patients who have had clinically significant hypersensitivity to this drug, or to any other rifamycins.

WARNINGS
Rifabutin prophylaxis must not be administratered to patients with *active* tuberculosis. Tuberculosis in HIV-positive patients is common and may present with atypical or extrapulmonary findings. Patients are likely to have a nonreactive purified protein derivative (PPD) despite active disease. In addition to chest X-ray and sputum culture, the following studies may be useful in the diagnosis of tuberculosis in the HIV-positive patient: blood culture, urine culture, or biopsy of a suspicious lymph node.

Patients who develop complaints consistent with active tuberculosis while on Rifabutin prophylaxis should be evaluated immediately, so that those with active disease may be given an effective combination regimen of anti-tuberculosis medications. Administration of single-agent Rifabutin to patients with active tuberculosis is likely to lead to the development of tuberculosis that is resistant both to Rifabutin and to rifampin.

There is no evidence that Rifabutin is effective prophylaxis against *M. tuberculosis*. Patients requiring prophylaxis against both *M. tuberculosis* and *Mycobacterium avium* complex may be given isoniazid and Rifabutin concurrently.

PRECAUTIONS
Because Rifabutin may be associated with neutropenia, and more rarely thrombocytopenia, physicians should consider obtaining hematologic studies periodically in patients receiving Rifabutin prophylaxis.

INFORMATION FOR PATIENTS
Patients should be advised of the signs and symptoms of both MAC and tuberculosis, and should be instructed to consult their physicians if they develop new complaints consistent with either of these diseases. In addition, since Rifabutin may rarely be associated with myositis and uveitis, patients should be advised to notify their physicians if they develop signs or symptoms suggesting either of these disorders.

Urine, feces, saliva, sputum, perspiration, tears, and skin may be colored brown-orange with rifabutin and some of its metabolites. Soft contact lenses may be permanently stained. Patients to be treated with Rifabutin should be made aware of these possibilities.

DRUG INTERACTIONS
In 10 healthy adult volunteers and 8 HIV-positive patients, steady-state plasma levels of zidovudine (ZDV), an antiretroviral agent which is metabolized mainly through glucuronidation, were decreased after repeated Rifabutin dosing; the mean decrease in C_{max} and AUC was 48% and 32%, respectively. *In vitro* studies have demonstrated that Rifabutin does not affect the inhibition of HIV by ZDV.

Steady-state kinetics in 12 HIV-positive patients show that both the rate and extent of systemic availability of didanosine (ddI), was not altered after repeated dosing of Rifabutin.

Rifabutin has liver enzyme-inducing properties. The related drug rifampin is known to reduce the activity of a number of other drugs, including dapsone, narcotics (including methadone), anticoagulants, corticosteroids, cyclosporine, cardiac glycoside preparations, quinidine, oral contraceptives, oral hypoglycemic agents (sulfonylureas), and analgesics. Rifampin has also been reported to decrease the effects of concurrently administered ketoconazole, barbiturates, diazepam, verapamil, beta-adrenergic blockers, clofibrate, progestins, disopyramide, mexiletine, theophylline, chloramphenicol, and anticonvulsants. Because of the structural similarity of Rifabutin and rifampin, Rifabutin may be expected to have some effect on these drugs as well. However, unlike rifampin Rifabutin appears not to affect the acetylation of isoniazid. When Rifabutin was compared with rifampin in a study with 8 healthy normal volunteers, Rifabutin appeared to be a less potent enzyme inducer than rifampin. The significance of this finding for clinical drug interactions is not known. Dosage adjustment of drugs listed above may be necessary if they are given concurrently with Rifabutin. Patients using oral contraceptives should consider changing to nonhormonal methods of birth control.

CARCINOGENESIS, MUTAGENESIS, IMPAIRMENT OF FERTILITY
Long term carcinogenicity studies were conducted with Rifabutin in mice and in rats. Rifabutin was not carcinogenic in mice at doses up to 180 mg/kg/day, or approximately 36 times the recommended human daily dose. Rifabutin was not carcinogenic in the rat at doses up to 60 mg/kg/day, about 12 times the recommended human dose.

Rifabutin was not mutagenic in the bacterial mutation assay (Ames Test) using both Rifabutin-susceptible and resistant strains. Rifabutin was not mutagenic in *Schizosaccharomyces pombe P_1* and was not genotoxic in V-79 Chinese hamster cells, human lymphocytes *in vitro*, or mouse bone marrow cells *in vivo*.

Fertility was impaired in male rats given 160 mg/kg (32 times the recommended human daily dose).

PREGNANCY
Pregnancy Category B: Reproduction studies have been carried out in rats and rabbits given Rifabutin using dose levels up to 200 mg/kg (40 times the recommended human daily dose). No teratogenicity was observed in either species. In rats, given 200 mg/kg/day, there was a decrease in fetal viability. In rats, at 40 mg/kg/day (8 times the recommended human daily dose), Rifabutin caused an increase in fetal skeletal variants. In rabbits, at 80 mg/kg/day (16 times the recommended human daily dose), Rifabutin caused maternotoxicity and increase in fetal skeletal anomalies. There are no adequate and well-controlled studies in pregnant women. Because animal reproduction studies are not always predictive of human response, Rifabutin should be used in pregnant women only if the potential benefit justifies the potential risk to the fetus.

SUSCEPTIBILITY OF *M. AVIUM* COMPLEX STRAINS TO RIFAMPIN AND RIFABUTIN

Susceptibility to Rifampin (μg/mL)	Number of Strains	% of Strains Susceptible/Resistant to Different Concentrations of Rifabutin (μg/mL)			
		Susceptible to 0.5	Resistant to 0.5 only	Resistant to 1.0	Resistant to 2.0
Susceptible to 1.0	30	100.0	0.0	0.0	0.0
Resistant to 1.0 only	163	88.3	11.7	0.0	0.0
Resistant to 5.0	105	38.0	57.1	2.9	2.0
Resistant to 10.0	225	20.0	50.2	19.6	10.2
TOTAL	523	49.5	36.7	9.0	4.8

Rifabutin in vitro MIC$_{99}$ values of ≤ 0.5 μg/mL, determined by the agar dilution method, for M. kansasii, M. gordonae and M. marinum have been reported; however, the clinical significance of these results is unknown.

➤ SHOWN IN PRODUCT IDENTIFICATION GUIDE

NURSING MOTHERS

It is not known whether Rifabutin is excreted in human milk. Because many drugs are excreted in human milk and because of the potential for serious adverse reactions in nursing infants, a decision should be made whether to discontinue nursing or discontinue the drug, taking into account the importance of the drug to the mother.

PEDIATRIC USE

Safety and effectiveness of Rifabutin for prophylaxis of MAC in children have not been established. Limited safety data are available from treatment use in 22 HIV-positive children with MAC who received Rifabutin in combination with at least two other antimycobacterials for periods from 1 to 183 weeks. Mean doses (mg/kg) for these children were: 18.5 (range 15.0 to 25.0) for infants one year of age; 8.6 (range 4.4 to 18.8) for children 2 to 10 years of age; and 4.0 (range 2.8 to 5.4) for adolescents 14 to 16 years of age. There is no evidence that doses greater than 5 mg/kg daily are useful. Adverse experiences were similar to those observed in the adult population, and included leukopenia, neutropenia and rash. Doses of Rifabutin may be administered mixed with foods such as applesauce.

ADVERSE REACTIONS

Rifabutin was generally well tolerated in the controlled clinical trials. Discontinuation of therapy due to an adverse event was required in 16% of patients receiving Rifabutin compared to 8% of patients receiving placebo in these trials. Primary reasons for discontinuation of Rifabutin were rash (4% of treated patients), gastrointestinal intolerance (3%), and neutropenia (2%).

The following table enumerates adverse experiences that occurred at a frequency of 1% or greater, among the patients treated with Rifabutin in studies 023 and 027.

CLINICAL ADVERSE EXPERIENCES REPORTED IN ≥ 1% OF PATIENTS TREATED WITH RIFABUTIN

Adverse Event	Rifabutin (n = 566) %	Placebo (n = 580) %
Body as a Whole		
Abdominal Pain	4	3
Asthenia	1	1
Chest Pain	1	1
Fever	2	1
Headache	3	5
Pain	1	2
Digestive System		
Anorexia	2	2
Diarrhea	3	3
Dyspepsia	3	1
Eructation	3	1
Flatulence	2	1
Nausea	6	5
Nausea and Vomiting	3	1
Vomiting	1	1
Musculoskeletal System		
Myalgia	2	1
Nervous System		
Insomnia	1	1
Skin and Appendages		
Rash	11	8
Special Senses		
Taste Perversion	3	1
Urogenital System		
Discolored Urine	30	6

CLINICAL ADVERSE EVENTS REPORTED IN < 1% OF PATIENTS WHO RECEIVED RIFABUTIN

Considering data from the 023 and 027 pivotal trials, and from other clinical studies, Rifabutin appears to be a likely cause of the following adverse events which occurred in less than 1% of treated patients: flu-like syndrome, hepatitis, hemolysis, arthralgia, myositis, chest pressure or pain with dyspnea, and skin discoloration.

The following adverse events have occurred in more than one patient receiving Rifabutin, but an etiologic role has not been established; seizure, paresthesia, aphasia, confusion, and non-specific T wave changes on electrocardiogram. When Rifabutin was administered at doses from 1050 mg/day to 2400 mg/day, generalized arthralgia and uveitis were reported. These adverse experiences abated when Rifabutin was discontinued.

The following table enumerates the changes in laboratory values that were considered as laboratory abnormalities in studies 023 and 027.

PERCENTAGE OF PATIENTS WITH LABORATORY ABNORMALITIES

Laboratory Abnormalities	Rifabutin (n = 566) %	Placebo (n = 580) %
Chemistry:		
Increased Alkaline Phosphatase[1]	< 1	3
Increased SGOT[2]	7	12
Increased SGPT[2]	9	11

Hematology:

Laboratory Abnormalities	Rifabutin (n = 566) %	Placebo (n = 580) %
Anemia[3]	6	7
Eosinophilia	1	1
Leukopenia[4]	17	16
Neutropenia[5]	25	20
Thrombocytopenia[6]	5	4

INCLUDES GRADE 3 OR 4 TOXICITIES AS SPECIFIED:
[1] all values > 450 U/L
[2] all values > 150 U/L
[3] all hemoglobin values < 8.0 g/dL
[4] all WBC values < 1,500/mm^3
[5] all ANC values < 750/mm^3
[6] all platelet count values < 50,000/mm^3

The incidence of neutropenia in patients treated with Rifabutin was significantly greater than in patients treated with placebo (p = 0.03). Although thrombocytopenia was not significantly more common among Rifabutin treated patients in these trials, Rifabutin has been clearly linked to thrombocytopenia in rare cases. One patient in study 023 developed thrombotic thrombocytopenic purpura, which was attributed to Rifabutin.

ANIMAL TOXICOLOGY

Liver abnormalities, (increased bilirubin and liver weight), occurred in all species tested, in rats at doses 5 times, in monkeys at doses 8 times, and in mice at doses 6 times the recommended human daily dose. Testicular atrophy occurred in baboons at doses 4 times the recommended human dose, and in rats at doses 40 times the recommended human daily dose.

OVERDOSAGE

No information is available on accidental overdosage in humans.

TREATMENT

While there is no experience in the treatment of overdose with Rifabutin clinical experience with rifamycins suggest that gastric lavage to evacuate gastric contents (within a few hours of overdose), followed by instillation of an activated charcoal slurry into the stomach, may help absorb any remaining drug from the gastrointestinal tract.

Rifabutin is 85% protein bound and distributed extensively into tissues (Vss:8 to 9 L/kg). It is not primarily excreted via, the urinary route (less than 10% as unchanged drug); therefore, neither hemodialysis nor forced diuresis is expected to enhance the systemic elimination of unchanged Rifabutin from the body in a patient with Rifabutin overdose.

DOSAGE AND ADMINISTRATION

It is recommended that 300 mg of Rifabutin be administered once daily. For those patients with propensity to nausea, vomiting, or other gastrointestinal upset, administration of Rifabutin at doses of 150 mg twice daily taken with food may be useful.

Keep tightly closed and dispense in a tight container as defined in the USP. Store at controlled room temperature, 15° to 30°C (59° to 86°F).

HOW SUPPLIED
CAPSULE: 150 MG

BRAND/MANUFACTURER	NDC	SIZE	AWP
○ **BRAND**			
MYCOBUTIN: Pharmacia	00013-5301-17	100s	$356.25

Rifadin *SEE* RIFAMPIN

Rifamate *SEE* ISONIAZID AND RIFAMPIN

Rifampin

DESCRIPTION

Rifampin is available as capsules and injection.

Each capsule contains: Rifampin 150 or 300 mg.

Each vial contains: Rifampin 600 mg.

Rifampin is a semisynthetic antibiotic derivative of rifamycin B. The chemical name for Rifampin is 3-(4-methyl-1-piperazinyl-iminomethyl)-rifamycin SV.

Rifampin USP is a red-brown crystalline powder very slightly soluble in water, freely soluble in chloroform, and soluble in ethyl acetate and in methanol. Its molecular weight is 822.95.

◆ RATED THERAPEUTICALLY EQUIVALENT; ◇ THERAPEUTIC EQUIVALENCE UNCONFIRMED; ○ UNRATED

Following is its chemical structure:

CLINICAL PHARMACOLOGY

Human Pharmacology-Oral: Rifampin is readily absorbed from the gastrointestinal tract. Peak blood levels in normal adults vary widely from individual to individual. The peak level averages 7 μg/mL but may vary from 4 to 32 μg/mL. Absorption of Rifampin is reduced when the drug is ingested with food.

In normal subjects, the biological half-life of Rifampin in serum averages about 3 hours after a 600 mg oral dose, with increases up to 5.1 hours reported after a 900 mg dose. With repeated administration, the half-life decreases and reaches average values of approximately 2-3 hours. It does not differ in patients with renal failure at doses not exceeding 600 mg daily and, consequently, no dosage adjustment is required. Refer to *"Warnings"* for information regarding patients with hepatic insufficiency.

After absorption, Rifampin is rapidly eliminated in the bile, and an enterohepatic circulation ensues. During this process, Rifampin undergoes progressive deacetylation so that nearly all the drug in the bile is in this form in about 6 hours. This metabolite is microbiologically active. Intestinal reabsorption is reduced by deacetylation, and elimination is facilitated. Up to 30% of a dose is excreted in the urine, with about half of this being unchanged drug.

Rifampin is widely distributed throughout the body. It is present in effective concentrations in many organs and body fluids, including cerebrospinal fluid. Rifampin is about 80% protein bound. Most of the unbound fraction is not ionized and therefore diffuses freely into tissues.

Serum Levels in Children: In one recent study, children 6-58 months old were given Rifampin suspended in simple syrup or as dry powder mixed with applesauce at a dose of 10 mg/kg body weight. Peak serum levels of 10.7 and 11.5 μg/mL were obtained 1 hour after preprandial ingestion of the drug suspension and the applesauce mixture, respectively. The calculated $t_{1/2}$ for both preparations was 2.9 hrs. It should be noted that in other studies in children, at doses of 10 mg/kg body weight, mean peak serum levels of 3.5 μg/mL to 15 μg/mL have been reported.

Human Pharmacology—V: After intravenous administration of a 300 or 600 mg dose of Rifampin infused over 30 minutes to healthy male volunteers (n = 12), mean peak plasma concentrations were 9.0 and 17.5 μg/mL, respectively. The average plasma concentrations in these volunteers remained detectable for 8 and 12 hours, respectively (see table).

PLASMA CONCENTRATIONS (μg/mL)

Rifampin Dosage I.V.	30 min	1 hr	2 hr	4 hr	8 hr	12 hr
300 mg	8.9	4.9	4.0	2.5	< 2	< 2
600 mg	17.4	11.7	9.4	6.4	3.5	< 2

Plasma concentrations after the 600 mg dose, which were disproportionately higher (up to 30% greater than expected) than those found after the 300 mg dose, indicated that the elimination of larger doses was not as rapid.

After repeated once-a-day infusions (3 hr duration) of 600 mg in patients (n = 5) for 7 days, concentrations of intravenous Rifampin decreased from 5.8 μg/mL 8 hours after the infusion on day 1 to 2.6 μg/mL 8 hours after the infusion on day 7. The Rifampin dose is widely distributed throughout the body. It is present in effective concentrations in many organs and body fluids, including cerebrospinal fluid. Rifampin is about 80% protein bound. Most of the unbound fraction is not ionized and therefore diffuses freely into tissues.

Rifampin is rapidly eliminated in the bile and undergoes progressive enterohepatic circulation and deacetylation to the primary metabolite, 25-desacetyl-Rifampin. This metabolite is microbiologically active. Less than 30% of the dose is excreted as Rifampin or metabolites. Serum concentrations do not differ in patients with renal failure and, consequently, no dosage adjustment is required.

Serum Concentration of Rifampin in Children: In patients 0.25 to 12.8 years old (n = 12), the mean peak serum concentration of Rifampin at the end of a 30 minute infusion of approximately 300 mg/m² was 26 μg/mL. In these patients, peak concentrations 1 to 4 days after initiation of therapy ranged from 11.7 to 41.5 μg/mL; peak concentrations 5 to 14 days after initiation of therapy were 13.6 to 37.4 μg/mL. The serum half-life of Rifampin decreased significantly from 1.34 to 3.24 hours early in therapy to 1.17 to 3.19 hours 5 to 14 days after therapy was initiated.

Microbiology: Rifampin inhibits DNA-dependent RNA polymerase activity in susceptible cells. Specifically, it interacts with bacterial RNA polymerase but does not inhibit the mammalian enzyme. Rifampin is particularly active against rapidly growing extracellular organisms but has been demonstrated to have intracellular bactericidal activity against susceptible organisms as well.

Cross-resistance to Rifampin has been shown only with other rifamycins.

Rifampin has bactericidal activity against slow and intermittently growing *M. tuberculosis.* It also has significant activity against *Neisseria meningitidis* (see *"Indications and Usage"*).

In the treatment of both tuberculosis and the meningococcal carrier state (see *"Indications and Usage"*), the small number of resistant cells present within large populations of susceptible cells can rapidly become predominant. In addition, resistance to Rifampin has been determined to occur as single-step mutations of the DNA-dependent RNA polymerase. Since resistance can emerge rapidly, appropriate susceptibility tests should be performed in the event of persistent positive cultures.

Rifampin has been shown to have initial in vitro activity against the following organisms; however, clinical efficacy has not been established (see *"Indications and Usage"*): *Mycobacterium leprae, Haemophilus influenzae, Staphylococcus aureus,* and *Staphylococcus epidermidis.* Both penicillinase-producing and nonpenicillinase-producing strains, and β-lactam resistant staphylococci (Methicillin Resistant *S. aureus*/MRSA) are initially susceptible to Rifampin *in vitro.*

Susceptibility Testing: Use only diagnostic products and methods approved by the Food and Drug Administration for Rifampin susceptibility testing of *Mycobacterium tuberculosis* and *Neisseria meningitidis.* Consult the Food and Drug Administration-approved labeling of the diagnostic products for interpretation criteria and quality control parameters.

For the other organisms listed in the microbiology subsection of the labeling, *in vitro* susceptibility testing should be assessed by standardized methods developed by the National Committee for Clinical Laboratory Standards.

INDICATIONS AND USAGE

Tuberculosis: Rifampin is indicated in the treatment of all forms of tuberculosis. Rifampin must always be used in conjunction with at least one other antituberculosis drug. Frequently used regimens are Rifampin and isoniazid; Rifampin, isoniazid, and pyrazinamide; Rifampin, isoniazid, and ethambutol; and Rifampin and ethambutol.

Intravenous Rifampin is indicated for the initial treatment and retreatment of tuberculosis when the drug cannot be taken by mouth.

Meningococcal Carriers: Rifampin is indicated for the treatment of asymptomatic carriers of *N. meningitidis* to eliminate meningococci from the nasopharynx. *Rifampin is not indicated for the treatment of meningococcal infection because of the possibility of the rapid emergence of resistant organisms.* (See *"Warnings."*)

Rifampin should not be used indiscriminately, and therefore diagnostic laboratory procedures, including serotyping and susceptibility testing, should be performed for establishment of the carrier state and the correct treatment. So that the usefulness of Rifampin in the treatment of asymptomatic meningococcal carriers is preserved, the drug should be used only when the risk of meningococcal disease is high.

In the treatment of both tuberculosis and the meningococcal carrier state, the small number of resistant cells present within large populations of susceptible cells can rapidly become predominant. Since resistance can emerge rapidly, susceptibility tests should be performed in the event of persistent positive cultures.

UNLABELED USES
Rifampin is used alone or as an adjunct in the treatment of lepromatous leprosy (Hansen's disease), *Hemophilus influenzae* prophylaxis, gonorrhea, and Legionnaires' disease. It is also used as an adjunct in *Mycobacterium kansasii* infections, *Legionella micadei* infections and *Mycobacterium avium* infections in patients with acquired immunodeficiency syndrome (AIDS). Rifampin is also prescribed in patients with pruritus due to primary biliary corrhosis (PBC) and *Staphylococcus aureus* infections, including endocarditis caused by *S aureus* or *S epidermis.*

CONTRAINDICATIONS

Rifampin is contraindicated in patients with a history of hypersensitivity to any of the rifamycins. (See *"Warnings".*)

WARNINGS

Rifampin has been shown to produce liver dysfunction. Fatalities associated with jaundice have occurred in patients with liver disease and in patients taking Rifampin with other hepatotoxic agents. Patients with impaired liver function should only be given Rifampin in cases of necessity and then with caution and under strict medical supervision.

In these patients, careful monitoring of liver function, especially serum glutamic pyruvic transaminase (SGPT) and serum glutamic oxaloacetic transaminase (SGOT) should be carried out prior to therapy and then every two to four weeks during therapy. If signs of hepatocellular damage occur, Rifampin should be withdrawn.

In some cases, hyperbilirubinemia resulting from competition between Rifampin and bilirubin for excretory pathways of the liver at the cell level can occur in the early days of treatment. An isolated report showing a moderate rise in bilirubin and/or transaminase level is not in itself an indication for interrupting treatment; rather, the decision should be made after repeating the tests, noting trends in the levels, and considering them in conjunction with the patient's clinical condition.

Rifampin has enzyme-inducing properties, including induction of delta amino levulinic acid synthetase. Isolated reports have associated porphyria exacerbation with Rifampin administration.

The possibility of rapid emergence of resistant meningococci restricts the use of Rifampin to short-term treatment of the asymptomatic carrier state. Rifampin *is not to be used for the treatment of meningococcal disease.*

PRECAUTIONS

General: For the treatment of tuberculosis, Rifampin is usually administered on a daily basis. High doses of Rifampin (greater than 600 mg) given once or twice weekly have resulted in a high incidence of adverse reactions, including the "flu syndrome" (fever, chills and malaise), hematopoietic reactions (leukopenia, thrombocytopenia, or acute hemolytic anemia), cutaneous, gastrointestinal, and hepatic reactions, shortness of breath, shock and renal failure. Recent studies indicate that regimens using twice-weekly doses of Rifampin 600 mg plus isoniazid 15 mg/kg are much better tolerated.

Intermittent therapy may be used if the patient cannot or will not self-administer drugs on a daily basis. Patients on intermittent therapy should be closely monitored for compliance and cautioned against intentional or accidental interruption of prescribed therapy because of the increased risk of serious adverse reactions.

INTRAVENOUS RIFAMPIN.

For intravenous infusion only. Must not be administered by intramuscular or subcutaneous route: Avoid extravasation during injection; local irritation and inflammation due to extravascular infiltration of the infusion have been observed. If these occur, the infusion should be discontinued and restarted at another site.

Information for Patients: The patient should be told that this medication may cause the urine, feces, saliva, sputum, sweat, and tears to turn red-orange. Permanent discoloration of soft contact lenses may occur.

The patient should be advised that the reliability of oral contraceptives may be affected; consideration should be given to using alternative contraceptive measures.

Laboratory Tests: A complete blood count (CBC) should be obtained prior to instituting therapy and periodically throughout the course of therapy. Because of a possible transient rise in transaminase and bilirubin values, blood for baseline clinical chemistries should be obtained before Rifampin dosing.

Drug Interactions: Rifampin has liver enzyme-inducing properties and may reduce the activity of a number of drugs, including anticoagulants, corticosteroids, cyclosporine, cardiac glycoside preparations, quinidine, oral contraceptives, oral hypoglycemic agents (sulfonylureas), dapsone, narcotics, and analgesics. Rifampin also has been reported to diminish the effects of concurrently administered methadone, barbiturates, diazepam, verapamil, beta-adrenergic blockers, clofibrate, progestins, disopyramide, mexiletine, theophylline, chloramphenicol, and anticonvulsants. It may be necessary to adjust the dosages of these drugs if they are given concurrently with Rifampin.

Patients using oral contraceptives should be advised to change to nonhormonal methods of birth control during Rifampin therapy. Also, diabetes may become more difficult to control.

When Rifampin is taken with para-aminosalicylic acid (PAS), Rifampin levels in the serum may decrease. Therefore, the drugs should be taken at least 8 hours apart.

Probenecid has been reported to increase Rifampin blood levels. Halothane, when given concomitantly with Rifampin, has been reported to increase the hepatotoxicity of both drugs.

Ketoconazole, when given concomitantly with Rifampin, has been reported to diminish the serum concentrations of both drugs. Dosage should be adjusted if indicated by the patient's clinical condition. An interaction has also been reported with Rifampin-isoniazid and Vitamin D.

Drug/Laboratory Interactions: Therapeutic levels of Rifampin have been shown to inhibit standard microbiological assays for serum folate and Vitamin B_{12}. Thus, alternate assay methods should be considered. Transient abnormalities in liver function tests (e.g., elevation in serum bilirubin, abnormal bromsulphalein [BSP] excretion, alkaline phosphatase, and serum transaminases), and reduced biliary excretion of contrast media used for visualization of the gall-bladder have also been observed. Therefore, these tests should be performed before the morning dose of Rifampin.

Carcinogenesis, Mutagenesis, Impairment of Fertility: There are no known human data on long-term potential for carcinogenicity, mutagenicity, or impairment of fertility. A few cases of accelerated growth of lung carcinoma have been reported in man, but a causal relationship with the drug has not been established. An increase in the incidence of hepatomas in female mice (of a strain known to be particularly susceptible to the spontaneous development of hepatomas) was observed when Rifampin was administered in doses 2 to 10 times the average daily human dose for 60 weeks followed by an observation period of 46 weeks. No evidence of carcinogenity was found in male mice of the same strain, mice of a different strain, or rats, under similar experimental conditions.

Rifampin has been reported to possess immunosuppressive potential in rabbits, mice, rats, guinea pigs, human lymphocytes *in vitro,* and humans. Antitumor activity in vitro has also been shown with Rifampin.

There was no evidence of mutagenicity in bacteria, *Drosophila melanogaster,* or mice, nor did Rifampin induce chromosome aberrations in human lymphocytes treated *in vitro.* However, an increase in chromatid breaks was noted when whole-blood cell cultures were treated with Rifampin.

Pregnancy—Teratogenic Effects: Pregnancy—Category C: Rifampin has been shown to be teratogenic in rodents give oral doses of Rifampin 15 to 25 times the human dose. Although Rifampin has been reported to cross the placental barrier and appear in cord blood, the effect of Rifampin, alone or in combination with other antituberculosis drugs, on the human fetus is not known. Neonates of Rifampin-treated mothers should be carefully observed for any evidence of adverse effects. Isolated cases of fetal malformations have been reported; however, there are no adequate and well-controlled studies in pregnant women. Rifampin should be used during pregnancy only if the potential benefit justifies the potential risk to the fetus. Rifampin in oral doses of 150 to 250 mg/kg produced teratogenic effects in mice and rats. Malformations were primarily cleft palate in the mouse and spina bifida in the rat. The incidence of these anomalies was dose-dependent. When Rifampin was given to pregnant rabbits in doses up to 20 times the usual daily human dose, imperfect osteogenesis and embryotoxicity were reported.

When administered during the last few weeks of pregnancy, Rifampin can cause post-natal hemorrhages in the mother and infant for which treatment with vitamin K may be indicated.

Nursing Mothers: Because of the potential for tumorigenicity shown for Rifampin in animal studies, a decision should be made whether to discontinue nursing or discontinue the drug, taking into account the importance of the drug to the mother.

Pediatric Use: See *"Clinical Pharmacology—Serum Levels in Children";* see also *"Dosage and Administration".*

ADVERSE REACTIONS

Gastrointestinal: Heartburn, epigastric distress, anorexia, nausea, vomiting, jaundice, flatulence, cramps, and diarrhea have been noted in some patients. Although *C. difficile* has been shown in vitro to be sensitive to Rifampin, pseudomembranous colitis has been reported with the use of Rifampin (and other broad spectrum antibiotics). Therefore, it is important to consider this diagnosis in patients who develop diarrhea in association with antibiotic use. Rarely, hepatitis or a shock-like syndrome with hepatic involvement and abnormal liver function tests has been reported.

Hematologic: Thrombocytopenia has occurred primarily with high dose intermittent therapy, but has also been noted after resumption of interrupted treatment. It rarely occurs during well supervised daily therapy. This effect is reversible if the drug is discontinued as soon as purpura occurs. Cerebral hemorrhage and fatalities have been reported when Rifampin administration has been continued or resumed after the appearance of purpura.

Transient leukopenia, hemolytic anemia, and decreased hemoglobin have been observed.

Central Nervous System: Headache, fever, drowsiness, fatigue, ataxia, dizziness, inability to concentrate, mental confusion, behavioral changes, muscular weakness, pains in extremities, and generalized numbness have been observed. Rare reports of myopathy have also been observed.

Ocular: Visual disturbances have been observed.

Endocrine: Menstrual disturbances have been observed.

Renal: Elevations in BUN and serum uric acid have been reported. Rarely, hemolysis, hemoglobinuria, hematuria, interstitial nephritis, renal insufficiency, and acute renal failure have been noted. These are generally considered to be hypersensitivity reactions. They usually occur during intermittent therapy or when treatment is resumed following intentional or accidental interruption of a daily dosage regimen, and are reversible when Rifampin is discontinued and appropriate therapy instituted.

Dermatologic: Cutaneous reactions are mild and self-limiting and do not appear to be hypersensitivity reactions. Typically, they consist of flushing and itching with or without a rash. More serious cutaneous reactions which may be due to hypersensitivity occur but are uncommon.

Hypersensitivity Reactions: Occasionally, pruritus, urticaria, rash, pemphigoid reaction, eosinophilia, sore mouth, sore tongue, and conjunctivitis have been observed.

Miscellaneous: Edema of the face and extremities has been reported. Other reactions reported to have occurred with intermittent dosage regimens include "flu" syndrome (such as episodes of fever, chills, headache, dizziness, and bone pain), shortness of breath, wheezing, decrease in blood pressure, and shock. The "flu" syndrome may also appear if Rifampin is taken irregularly by the patient of if daily administration is resumed after a drug free interval.

OVERDOSAGE

Signs and Symptoms: Nausea, vomiting, and increasing lethargy will probably occur within a short time after ingestion; unconsciousness may occur when there is severe hepatic disease. Brownish-red or orange discoloration of the skin, urine, sweat, saliva, tears, and feces will occur, and its intensity is proportional to the amount ingested.

Liver enlargement, possibly with tenderness, may develop within a few hours after severe overdosage; jaundice may develop rapidly. Hepatic involvement may be more marked in patients with prior impairment of hepatic function. Other physical findings remain essentially normal.

Bilirubin levels may increase rapidly with severe overdosage; hepatic enzyme levels may be affected, especially with prior impairment of hepatic function. A direct effect upon the hematopoietic system, electrolyte levels, or acid-base balance is unlikely.

Acute Toxicity: In animal studies, the LD_{50} of Rifampin is approximately 885 mg/kg in the mouse, 1720 mg/kg in the rat, and 2120 mg/kg in the rabbit.

◆ RATED THERAPEUTICALLY EQUIVALENT; ◇ THERAPEUTIC EQUIVALENCE UNCONFIRMED; ○ UNRATED

Nonfatal overdoses with as high as 12 g of Rifampin have been reported. In one patient who swallowed 12 g of Rifampin, vomiting occurred four times within 1 hour of ingestion. Gastric lavage with 20 liters of water was initiated 5 hours after ingestion. Twelve hours after ingestion of Rifampin, a plasma concentration of 400 µg of Rifampin/mL was measured by microbiological assay. The plasma concentration fell to 64 µg/mL on the following day, and to 0.1 µg/mL on the third day. Urinary Rifampin concentration was 313 µg/mL approximately 30 hours after ingestion of the drug, 625 µg/mL after 36 hours, and 78 µg/mL after 40 hours. By the fourth day following the dose, only 0.1 µg/mL Rifampin was present in the urine. There was biochemical evidence of mild impairment of liver function. Liver function tests had returned to normal within 5 days, and the patient's recovery was described as uneventful.

One case of fatal overdose is known: a 26-year-old man died after self-administering 60 g of Rifampin.

Treatment: Since nausea and vomiting are likely to be present, gastric lavage is probably preferable to induction of emesis. Following evacuation of the gastric contents, the instillation of activated charcoal slurry into the stomach may help absorb any remaining drug from the gastrointestinal tract. Antiemetic medication may be required to control severe nausea and vomiting.

Active diuresis (with measured intake and output) will help promote excretion of the drug. Hemodialysis may be of value in some patients. In patients with previously adequate hepatic function, reversal of liver enlargement and of impaired hepatic excretory function probably will be noted within 72 hours, with a rapid return toward normal thereafter.

DOSAGE AND ADMINISTRATION
Rifampin can be administered by the oral route or by intravenous infusion (see *"Indications and Usage"*).

TUBERCULOSIS
Adults: 600 mg in a single daily administration, oral or intravenous.

Children: 10-20 mg/kg, not to exceed 600 mg/day, oral or intravenous.

It is recommended that oral Rifampin be administered once daily, either one hour before or two hours after a meal. In the treatment of tuberculosis, Rifampin should always be administered with at least one other antituberculosis drug. In general, therapy for tuberculosis should be continued for 6 to 9 months or until at least 6 months have elapsed from conversion of sputum to culture negativity. In patients who cannot be relied on for compliance, intermittent therapy with 600 mg/day two or three times/week under close supervision may be prescribed and substituted for the daily regimen after 1-2 months of an initial daily phase of therapy. The 9-Month Regimen ordinarily consists of Rifampin and isoniazid, usually supplemented during the initial phase by pyrazinamide, streptomycin, or ethambutol.

The 6-Month Regimen ordinarily consists of an initial 2-month phase of Rifampin, isoniazid and pyrazinamide, and, if clinically indicated, streptomycin or ethambutol, followed by 4 months of Rifampin and isoniazid.

Either of the above regimens is recommended as standard therapy.

The above recommendations apply to patients with drug-susceptible organisms. Patients with drug-resistant organisms may require longer treatment with other drug regimens.

MENINGOCOCCAL CARRIERS
Adults: For adults, it is recommended that 600 mg Rifampin be administered twice daily for two days.

Infants and Children: Children 1 month of age or older 10 mg/kg every 12 hours for two days.

Children under 1 month of age: 5 mg/kg every 12 hours for two days.

PREPARATION OF SOLUTION FOR INTRAVENOUS INFUSION.
Reconstitute the lyophilized powder by transferring 10 mL of sterile water for injection to a vial containing 600 mg of Rifampin for injection. Swirl vial gently to completely dissolve the antibiotic. The reconstituted solution contains 60 mg Rifampin per mL and is stable at room temperature for 24 hours. Immediately prior to administration, withdraw from the reconstituted solution a volume equivalent to the amount of Rifampin calculated to be administered and add to 500 mL of infusion medium. Mix well and infuse at a rate allowing for complete infusion in 3 hours. In some cases, the amount of Rifampin calculated to be administered may be added to 100 mL of infusion medium and infused in 30 minutes. The 500 mL and 100 mL infusion solutions should be prepared and used within a total 4-hour period. Precipitation of Rifampin from the infusion solution may occur beyond this time.

Caution: Dextrose 5% for injection is the recommended infusion medium. Sterile saline may be used when dextrose is contraindicated, but the stability of Rifampin is slightly reduced. Other infusion media are not recommended.

PREPARATION OF EXTEMPORANEOUS ORAL SUSPENSION
For pediatric and adult patients in whom capsule swallowing is difficult or where lower doses are needed, a liquid suspension may be prepared as follows.

Rifampin 1% w/v suspension (10 mg/mL) can be compounded using a syrup.

1. Empty contents of four Rifampin 300 mg capsules or eight Rifampin 150 mg capsules onto a piece of weighing paper.

2. If necessary, gently crush the capsule contents with a spatula to produce a fine powder.

3. Transfer Rifampin powder blend to a 4-ounce amber glass prescription bottle.

4. Rinse the paper and spatula with 20 mL of syrup and add the rinse to the bottle. Shake vigorously.

5. Add 100 mL of syrup to the bottle and shake vigorously. This compounding procedure results in a 1% w/v suspension containing 10 mg Rifampin/mL. Stability studies indicate that the suspension is stable when stored at room temperature (25 ± 3°C) or in a refrigerator (2-8°C) for four weeks. This extemporaneously prepared suspension must be shaken well prior to administration.

STORAGE
Capsules: Keep tightly closed. Store in a dry place. Avoid excessive heat.

Injection: Avoid excessive heat (temperatures above 40°C or 104°F). Protect from light.

REFERENCES
1. National Committee for Clinical Laboratory Standards, Approved Standard; Performance Standards for Antimicrobial Disk Susceptibility Tests (M7-A2), Second Edition; Approved Standard (1990). 2. National Committee for Clinical Laboratory Standards, Approved Standard: Methods for Dilution Antimicrobial Susceptibility Tests for Bacteria that Grow Aerobically (M2-A4), Fourth Edition; Approved Standard (1990).

HOW SUPPLIED
CAPSULE: 150 MG

BRAND/MANUFACTURER	NDC	SIZE	AWP
◆ BRAND			
RIFADIN: Marion Merrell Dow	00068-0510-30	30s	$44.70

CAPSULE: 300 MG

AVERAGE UNIT PRICE (AVAILABLE SIZES)			
BRAND	$1.97		

BRAND/MANUFACTURER	NDC	SIZE	AWP
◆ BRAND			
RIFADIN: Marion Merrell Dow	00068-0508-30	30s	$63.36
	00068-0508-60	60s	$126.66
RIMACTANE: Ciba Pharm	00083-0154-30	100s	$154.64
RIFADIN: Marion Merrell Dow	00068-0508-61	100s	$211.20

POWDER FOR INJECTION: 600 MG

BRAND/MANUFACTURER	NDC	SIZE	AWP
○ BRAND			
RIFADIN IV: Marion Merrell Dow	00068-0597-01	1s	$79.38

Rifater SEE ISONIAZID/PYRAZINAMIDE/RIFAMPIN

Rimactane SEE RIFAMPIN

Rimantadine Hydrochloride

DESCRIPTION
Rimantadine is a synthetic antiviral drug. Rimantadine is available as a 100 mg tablet and as a oral syrup containing 50 mg of Rimantadine per 5 mL.

Rimantadine Hydrochloride is a white to off-white crystalline powder which is freely soluble in water (50 mg/mL at 20°C). Chemically, Rimantadine Hydrochloride is alpha-methyltricyclo-(3.3.1.1/3.7)decane-1-methanamine hydrochloride, with an empirical formula of $C_{12}H_{21}N \cdot HCl$, and a molecular weight of 215.77.

Following is its chemical structure:

CLINICAL PHARMACOLOGY
Mechanism of Action: The mechanism of action of Rimantadine is not fully understood. Rimantadine appears to exert its inhibitory effect early in the viral replicative cycle, possibly inhibiting the uncoating of the virus. Genetic studies suggest that a virus protein specified by the virion M_2 gene plays an important role in the susceptibility of influenza A virus to inhibition by Rimantadine.

Microbiology: Rimantadine is inhibitory to the in vitro replication of influenza A virus isolates from each of the three antigenic subtypes, i.e., H1N1, H2N2 and H3N2, that have been isolated from man. Rimantadine has little or no activity against influenza B virus (Ref. 1,2). Rimantadine does not appear to interfere with the immunogenicity of inactivated influenza A vaccine.

A quantitative relationship between the *in vitro* susceptibility of influenza A virus to Rimantadine and clinical response to therapy has not been established.

Susceptibility test results, expressed as the concentration of the drug required to inhibit virus replication by 50% or more in a cell culture system, vary greatly (from 4 ng/mL to 20 μg/mL) depending upon the assay protocol used, size of the virus inoculum, isolates of the influenza A virus strains tested, and the cell types used (Ref. 2).

Rimantadine-resistant strains of influenza A virus have emerged among freshly isolated epidemic strains in closed settings where Rimantadine has been used. Resistant viruses have been shown to be transmissible and to cause typical influenza illness. (Ref. 3)

Pharmacokinetics: Although the pharmacokinetics profile of Rimantadine has been described, no pharmacodynamic data establishing a correlation between plasma concentration and its antiviral effect are available.

The tablet and syrup formulations of Rimantadine are equally absorbed after oral administration. The mean ±SD peak plasma concentration after a single 100 mg dose of Rimantadine was 74 ± 22 ng/mL (range: 45 to 138 ng/mL). The time to peak concentration was 6 ± 1 hours in healthy adults (age 20 to 44 years). The single dose elimination half-life in this population was 25.4 ± 6.5 hours (range: 13 to 65 hours). The single dose elimination half-life in a group of healthy 71 to 79 year-old subjects was 32 ± 16 hours (range: 20 to 65 hours).

After the administration of Rimantadine 100 mg twice daily to healthy volunteers (age 18 to 70 years) for 10 days, area under the curve (AUC) values were approximately 30% greater than predicted from a single dose. Plasma trough levels at steady state ranged between 118 and 468 ng/mL. In these patients no age-related differences in pharmacokinetics were detected. However, in a comparison of three groups of healthy older subjects) age 50-60, 61-70 and 71-79 years), the 71 to 79 year-old group had average AUC values, peak concentrations and elimination half-life values at steady state that were 20 to 30% higher than the other two groups. Steady-state concentrations in elderly nursing home patients (age 68 to 102 years) were 2- to 4-fold higher than those seen in healthy young and elderly adults.

The pharmacokinetic profile of Rimantadine in children has not been established. In a group (n=10) of children 4 to 8 years old who were given a single dose (6.6 mg/kg) of Rimantadine syrup, plasma concentrations of Rimantadine ranged from 446 to 988 ng/mL at 5 to 6 hours and from 170 to 424 ng/mL at 24 hours. In some children drug was detected in plasma 72 hours after the last dose.

Following oral administration, Rimantadine is extensively metabolized in the liver with less than 25% of the dose excreted in the urine as unchanged drug. Three hydroxylated metabolites have been found in plasma. These metabolites, an additional conjugated metabolite, and parent drug account for 74 ± 10% (n=4) of a single 200 mg dose of Rimantadine excreted in urine over 72 hours.

In a group (n=14) of patients with chronic liver disease, the majority of whom were stabilized cirrhotics, the pharmacokinetics of Rimantadine were not appreciably altered following a single 200 mg oral dose compared to 6 healthy subjects who were sex, age and weight matched to 6 of the patients with liver disease. After administration of a single 200 mg dose to patients (n=10) with severe hepatic dysfunction, AUC was approximately 3-fold larger, elimination half-life was approximately 2-fold longer and apparent clearance was about 50% lower when compared to historic data from healthy subjects.

Studies of the effects of renal insufficiency on the pharmacokinetics of Rimantadine have given inconsistent results. Following administration of a single 200 mg oral dose of Rimantadine to 8 patients with a creatinine clearance (CLcr) of 31-50 mL/min and 6 patients with a CLcr of 11-30 mL/min, the apparent clearance was 37% and 16% lower, respectively, and plasma metabolite concentrations were higher when compared to weight-, age-, and sex-matched healthy subjects (n=9, CLcr > 50 mL/min). After a single 200 mg oral dose of Rimantadine was given to 8 hemodialysis patients (CLcr 0-10 mL/min), there was a 1.6-fold increase in the elimination half-life and a 40% decrease in apparent clearance compared to age-matched healthy subjects. Hemodialysis did not contribute to the clearance of Rimantadine.

The *in vitro* human plasma protein binding of Rimantadine is about 40% over typical plasma concentrations. Albumin is the major binding protein.

INDICATIONS AND USAGE

Rimantadine is indicated for the prophylaxis and treatment of illness caused by various strains of influenza A virus in adults.

Rimantadine is indicated for prophylaxis against influenza A virus in children.

Prophylaxis: In controlled studies of children over the age of 1 year, healthy adults and elderly patients, Rimantadine has been shown to be safe and effective in preventing signs and symptoms of infection caused by various strains of influenza A virus. Early vaccination on an annual basis, as recommended by the Centers for Disease Control's Immunization Practices Advisory Committee, is the method of choice in the prophylaxis of influenza unless vaccination is contraindicated, not available or not feasible. Since Rimantadine does not completely prevent the host immune response to influenza A infection, individuals who take this drug may still develop immune responses to natural disease or vaccination and may be protected when later exposed to antigenically-related viruses. Following vaccination during an influenza outbreak. Rimantadine prophylaxis should be considered for the 2 to 4 week time period required to develop an antibody response. However, the safety and effectiveness of Rimantadine prophylaxis have not been demonstrated for longer than 6 weeks.

Treatment: Rimantadine therapy should be considered for adults who develop an influenza-like illness during known or suspected influenza A infection in the community. When administered within 48 hours after onset of signs and symptoms of infection caused by influenza A virus strains, Rimantadine has been shown to reduce the duration of fever and systemic symptoms.

CONTRAINDICATIONS

Rimantadine is contraindicated in patients with known hypersensitivity to drugs of the adamantane class, including Rimantadine and amantadine.

PRECAUTIONS

General: An increased incidence of seizures has been reported in patients with a history of epilepsy who received the related drug amantadine. In clinical trials of Rimantadine, the occurrence of seizure-like activity was observed in a small number of patients with a history of seizures who were not receiving anticonvulsant medication while taking Rimantadine. If seizures develop, Rimantadine should be discontinued.

The safety and pharmacokinetics of Rimantadine in renal and hepatic insufficiency have only been evaluated after single dose administration. In a single dose study of patients with anuric renal failure, the apparent clearance of Rimantadine was approximately 40% lower and the elimination half-life was 1.6-fold greater than that in healthy age-matched controls. In a study of 14 persons with chronic liver disease (mostly stabilized cirrhotics), no alterations in the pharmacokinetics were observed after the administration of a single dose of Rimantadine. However, the apparent clearance of Rimantadine following a single dose to 10 patients with severe liver dysfunction was 50% lower than reported for healthy subjects. Because of the potential for accumulation of Rimantadine and its metabolites in plasma, caution should be exercised when patients with renal or hepatic insufficiency are treated with Rimantadine.

Transmission of Rimantadine-resistant virus should be considered when treating patients whose contacts are at high risk for influenza A illness. Influenza A virus strains resistant to Rimantadine can emerge during treatment and such resistant strains have been shown to be transmissible and to cause typical influenza illness [Ref.3]. Although the frequency, rapidity, and clinical significance of the emergence of drug-resistant virus are not yet established, several small studies have demonstrated that 10% to 30% of patients with initially sensitive virus, upon treatment with Rimantadine, shed Rimantadine-resistant virus. [Ref.3,4,5,6]

Clinical response to Rimantadine, although slower in those patients who subsequently shed resistant virus, was not significantly different from those who did not shed resistant virus. [Ref.3] No data is available in humans that addresses the activity or effectiveness of Rimantadine therapy in subjects infected with resistant virus.

Drug Interactions: Cimetidine: The effects of chronic cimetidine use on the metabolism of Rimantadine are not known. When a single 100 mg dose of Rimantadine was administered one hour after the initiation of cimetidine (300 mg four times a day), the apparent total Rimantadine clearance of this single dose in normal healthy adults was reduced by 18% (compared to the apparent total Rimantadine clearance in the same subjects in the absence of cimetidine).

Acetaminophen: Rimantadine 100 mg, was given twice daily for 13 days to 12 healthy volunteers. On day 11, acetaminophen (650 mg four times daily) was started and continued for 8 days. The pharmacokinetics of Rimantadine were assessed on days 11 and 13. Co-administration with acetaminophen reduced the peak concentration and AUC values for Rimantadine by approximately 11%.

Aspirin: Rimantadine, 100 mg, was given twice daily for 13 days to 12 healthy volunteers. On day 11, aspirin (650 mg, four times daily) was started and continued for 8 days. The pharmacokinetics of Rimantadine were assessed on days 11 and 13. Peak plasma concentrations and AUC of Rimantadine were reduced approximately 10% in the presence of aspirin.

Carcinogenesis, Mutagenesis, and Impairment of Fertility: Carcinogenesis: Carcinogenicity studies in animals have not been performed.

Mutagenesis: No mutagenic effects were seen when Rimantadine was evaluated in several standard assays for mutagenicity.

Impairment of Fertility: A reproduction study in male and female rats did not show detectable impairment of fertility at dosages up to 60 mg/kg/day (3 times the maximum human dose based on body surface area comparisons).

Pregnancy Teratogenic Effects: Pregnancy Category (C). There are no adequate and well-controlled studies in pregnant women. Rimantadine is reported to cross the placenta in mice. Rimantadine has been shown to be embryotoxic in rats when given at a dose of 200 mg/kg/day (11 times the recommended human dose based on body surface are comparisons). At this dose the embryotoxic effect consisted of increased fetal resorption in rats; this dose also produced a variety of maternal effects including ataxia, tremors, convulsions and significantly reduced weight gain. No embryotoxicity was observed when rabbits were given doses up to 50 mg/kg/day (5 times the recommended human dose based on body surface area comparisons). However, there was evidence of a developmental abnormality in the form of a change in the ratio of fetuses with 12 or 13 ribs. This ratio is normally about 50:50 in a litter but was 80:20 after Rimantadine treatment.

Nonteratogenic Effects: Rimantadine was administered to pregnant rats in a peri- and postnatal reproduction toxicity study at doses of 30, 60 and 120 mg/kg/day (1.7, 3.4 and 6.8 times the recommended human dose based on body surface area comparisons). Maternal toxicity during gestation was noted at the two higher doses of Rimantadine, and at the highest dose, 120 mg/kg/day, there was an increase in pup mortality during the first 2 to 4 days postpartum. Decreased fertility of the F1 generation was also noted for the two higher doses.

For these reasons, Rimantandine should be used during pregnancy only if the potential benefit justifies the risk to the fetus.

Nursing Mothers: Rimantadine should not be administered to nursing mothers because of the adverse effects noted in offspring of rats treated with Rimantadine during the nursing period. Rimantadine is concentrated in rat milk in a dose-related manner: 2 to 3 hours following administration of Rimantadine, rat breast milk levels were approximately twice those observed in the serum.

Pediatric Use: In children, Rimantadine is recommended for the prophylaxis of influenza A. The safety and effectiveness of Rimantadine in the treatment of symptomatic influenza infection in children have not been established. Prophylaxis studies with Rimantadine have not been performed in children below the age of 1 year.

ADVERSE REACTIONS

In 1,027 patients treated with Rimantadine in controlled clinical trials at the recommended dose of 200 mg daily, the most frequently reported adverse events involved the gastrointestinal and nervous systems.

Incidence > 1%: Adverse events reported most frequently (1-3%) at the recommended dose in controlled clinical trials are shown in the table below.

	Rimantadine (n = 1027)	Control (n = 986)
Nervous System		
Insomnia	2.1%	0.9%
Dizziness	1.9%	1.1%
Headache	1.4%	1.3%
Nervousness	1.3%	0.6%
Fatigue	1.0%	0.9%
Gastrointestinal System		
Nausea	2.8%	1.6%
Vomiting	1.7%	0.6%
Anorexia	1.6%	0.8%
Dry mouth	1.5%	0.6%
Abdominal Pain	1.4%	0.8%
Body as a Whole		
Asthenia	1.4%	0.5%

Less frequent adverse events (0.3 to 1%) at the recommended dose in controlled clinical trials were:

Gastrointestinal System: diarrhea, dyspepsia;

Nervous System: Impairment of concentration, ataxia, somnolence, agitation, depression;

Skin and Appendages: rash;

Hearing and Vestibular: tinnitus;

Respiratory: dyspnea.

Additional adverse events (less than 0.3%) reported at recommended doses in controlled clinical trials were.

Nervous System: gait abnormality, euphoria, hyperkinesia, tremor, hallucination, confusion, convulsions;

Respiratory: bronchospasm, cough;

Cardiovascular: pallor, palpitation, hypertension, cerebrovascular disorder, cardiac failure, pedal edema, heart block, tachycardia, syncope;

Reproduction: non-puerperal lactation;

Special Senses: taste loss/change, parosmia.

Rates of adverse events, particularly those involving the gastrointestinal and nervous systems, increased significantly in controlled studies using higher than recommended doses of Rimantadine. In most cases, symptoms resolved rapidly with discontinuation of treatment. In addition to the adverse events reported above, the following were also reported at higher than recommended doses: increased lacrimation, increased micturition frequency, fever, rigors, agitation, constipation, diaphoresis, dysphagia, stomatitis, hypesthesia and eye pain.

Adverse Reactions in Trials of Rimantadine and Amantadine: In a six-week prophylaxis study of 436 healthy adults comparing Rimantadine with amantadine and placebo, the following adverse reactions were reported with an incidence > 1%.

	Rimantadine 200 mg/day (n = 145)	Placebo (n = 143)	Amantadine 200 mg/day (n = 148)
Nervous System			
Insomnia	3.4%	0.7%	7.0%
Nervousness	2.1%	0.7%	2.8%
Impaired			
Concentration	2.1%	1.4%	2.1%
Dizziness	0.7%	0.0%	2.1%
Depression	0.7%	0.7%	3.5%
Total % of subjects with adverse reactions	6.9%	4.1%	14.7%
Total % of subjects withdrawn due to adverse reactions	6.9%	3.4%	14.0%

Usage in the Elderly: In general, the incidence of adverse events in controlled clinical trials in the elderly was higher in both the Rimantadine and placebo-treated groups compared to younger adults and children. Most of these patients had other chronic illnesses. In a placebo-controlled study of 83 nursing home patients with influenza, 10.6% of those treated with Rimantadine compared with 8.3% in the placebo group experienced events related to the central nervous system. The profile of these events was similar to that for the most frequent adverse events reported in other controlled trials (see list above).

Pooled data from controlled studies of prophylaxis and treatment of influenza with Rimantadine in persons over 65 years of age showed an increase in adverse clinical events associated with the recommended dose of Rimantadine (100 mg twice a day) compared to controls as follows: central and peripheral nervous systems, 12.5% for Rimantadine versus 8.7% for control patients; gastrointestinal system, 17.0% for Rimantadine versus 11.3% for controls.

OVERDOSAGE

As with any overdose, supportive therapy should be administered as indicated. Overdoses of a related drug, amantadine, have been reported with adverse reactions consisting of agitation, hallucinations, cardiac arrhythmia and death. The administration of intravenous physostigmine (a cholinergic agent) at doses of 1 to 2 mg in adults (Ref. 7) and 0.5 mg in children (Ref. 8) repeated as needed as long as the dose did not exceed 2 mg/hour has been reported anecdotally to be beneficial in patients with central nervous system effects from overdoses of amantadine.

DOSAGE AND ADMINISTRATION

For Prophylaxis in Adults and Children:

Adults: The recommended adult dose of Rimantadine is 100 mg twice a day. In patients with severe hepatic dysfunction, renal failure (CrCl ≤ 10 mL/min.) and elderly nursing home patients, a dose reduction to 100 mg daily is recommended. There are currently no data available regarding the safety of Rimantadine during multiple dosing in subjects with renal or hepatic impairment. Because of the potential for accumulation of Rimantadine metabolites during multiple dosing, patients with any degree of renal insufficiency should be monitored for adverse effects, with dosage adjustments being made as necessary.

Children: In children less than 10 years of age, Rimantadine should be administered once a day, at a dose of 5 mg/kg but not exceeding 150 mg. For children 10 years of age or older, use the adult dose.

For Treatment in Adults: The recommended adult dose of Rimantadine is 100 mg twice a day. In patients with severe hepatic dysfunction, renal failure (CrCl ≤ 10 mL/min) and elderly nursing home patients, a dose reduction to 100 mg daily is recommended. There are currently no data available regarding the safety of Rimantadine during multiple dosing in subjects with renal or hepatic impairment. Because of the potential for accumulation of Rimantadine metabolites during multiple dosing, patients with any degree of renal insufficiency should be monitored for adverse effects, with dosage adjustments being made as necessary. Rimantadine therapy should be initiated as soon as possible, preferably within 48 hours after onset of signs and symptoms of influenza A infection. Therapy should be continued for approximately seven days from the initial onset of symptoms.

Storage: Tablets and syrup should be stored at 15° - 30°C (59° - 86°F).

REFERENCES
1. Belshe, R.B., Burk, B., Newman, F., Cerruti, R.L. and Sim, I.S. (1989) J. Infect. Dis. 159, 430-435. 2. Sim, I.S., Cerruti, R.L. and Connell, E.V., (1989) J. Resp. Dis. (Suppl.), S46-S51. 3. Hayden, F.G., Belshe, R.B., Clover, R.D. et al (1989) N. Engl. J. Med. 321 (25), 1696-1702. 4. Hall, C.B., Dolin, R., Gala, C.L., et al (1987) Pediatrics 80, 275-282. 5. Thompson, J., Fleet, W., Lawrence, E. et al (1987) J. Med. Vir. 21, 249-255. 6. Belshe, R.B., Smith, M.H., Hall, C.B., et al (1988) J. Virol. 62, 1508-1512. 7. Casey, D.F.N. Engl. J. Med. 1978:298:516., 8. Berkowitz, C.D.J. Pediatrics 1979:95:144.

HOW SUPPLIED
SYRUP: 50 MG/5 ML

BRAND/MANUFACTURER	NDC	SIZE	AWP
○ **BRAND**			
FLUMADINE: Forest Pharm	00456-0527-08	240 ml	$25.80

TABLETS: 100 MG

BRAND/MANUFACTURER	NDC	SIZE	AWP
○ **BRAND**			
► FLUMADINE: Forest Pharm	00456-0521-01	100s	$127.57

Rimso-50 *SEE* DIMETHYL SULFOXIDE

Ringer's, Injectable

DESCRIPTION

This product is a sterile, nonpyrogenic solution of electrolytes without dextrose in water for injection intended for intravenous administration as a fluid and nutrient and/or electrolyte replenisher. It contains no bacteriostat, antimicrobial agent or added buffer (except for pH adjustment).

Each 100 ml of Ringer's Injection, USP contains sodium chloride 860 mg, potassium chloride 30 mg and calcium chloride, dihydrate 33 mg. A liter provides sodium (Na^+) 147.5 mEq, potassium (K^+) 4 mEq, calcium (Ca^{++}) 4.5 mEq and chloride (Cl^-) 156 mEq. The electrolyte content is isotonic (309 mOsm/liter; calc.) in relation to the extracellular fluid (approx. 280 mOsm/liter). The pH of the solution is 5.8 (approx.).

Calcium Chloride, USP is chemically designated $CaCl_2 \cdot 2H_2O$, white fragments or granules freely soluble in water.

Potassium Chloride, USP is chemically designated KCl, a white granular powder freely soluble in water.

Sodium Chloride, USP is chemically designated NaCl, a white crystalline compound freely soluble in water.

Water for Injection, USP is chemically designated H_2O.

CLINICAL PHARMACOLOGY

When administered intravenously, these solutions provide variable sources of water, electrolytes and carbohydrate calories.

Solutions containing carbohydrate in the form of dextrose restore blood glucose levels and provide calories.

Calcium chloride in water dissociates to provide calcium (Ca^{++}) and chloride (Cl^-) ions. They are normal constituents of the body fluids and are dependent on various physiologic mechanisms for maintenance of balance between intake and output. Approximately 80% of body calcium is excreted in the feces as insoluble salts; urinary excretion accounts for the remaining 20%.

Potassium chloride in water dissociates to provide potassium (K^+) and chloride (Cl^-) ions. Potassium is found in low concentration in plasma and extracellular fluids (3.5 to 5.0 mEq/liter in a healthy adult). It is the chief cation of body cells (160 mEq/liter of intracellular water). Potassium plays an important role in electrolyte balance. Normally about 80 to 90% of the potassium intake is excreted in the urine; the remainder in the stools and to a small extent, in the perspiration. The kidney does not conserve potassium well so that during fasting or in patients on a potassium-free diet, potassium loss from the body continues resulting in potassium depletion.

Sodium chloride in water dissociates to provide sodium (Na^+) and chloride (Cl^-) ions. Sodium (Na^+) is the principal cation of the extracellular fluid and plays a large part in the therapy of fluid and electrolyte disturbances. Chloride (Cl^-) has an integral role in buffering action when oxygen and carbon dioxide exchange occurs in the red blood cells. The distribution and excretion of sodium (Na^+) and chloride (Cl^-) are largely under the control of the kidney which maintains a balance between intake and output.

Water is an essential constituent of all body tissues and accounts for approximately 70% of total body weight. Average normal adult daily requirement ranges from two to three liters (1.0 to 1.5 liters each for insensible water loss by perspiration and urine production).

Water balance is maintained by various regulatory mechanisms. Water distribution depends primarily on the concentration of electrolytes in the body compartments and sodium (Na^+) plays a major role in maintaining physiologic equilibrium.

INDICATIONS AND USAGE

These solutions are indicated for parenteral replacement of extracellular losses of fluid and electrolytes, plus minimal calories, as required by the clinical condition of the patient.

CONTRAINDICATIONS

Do not administer unless the solution is clear and seal is intact. Discard unused portion.

WARNINGS

Solutions containing calcium ions should not be administered simultaneously through the same administration set as blood because of the likelihood of coagulation.

Solutions which contain potassium should be used with great care, if at all, in patients with hyperkalemia, severe renal failure and in conditions in which potassium retention is present.

Solutions containing sodium ions should be used with great care, if at all, in patients with congestive heart failure, severe renal insufficiency and in clinical states in which there exists edema with sodium retention.

In patients with diminished renal function, administration of solutions containing sodium or potassium ions may result in sodium or potassium retention.

The intravenous administration of these solutions can cause fluid and/or solute overloading resulting in dilution of serum electrolyte concentrations, overhydration, congested states or pulmonary edema. The risk of dilutional states is inversely proportional to the electrolyte concentrations of administered parenteral solutions.

The risk of solute overload causing congested states with peripheral and pulmonary edema is directly proportional to the electrolyte concentrations of such solutions.

Additives may be incompatible. Consult with pharmacist if available. When introducing additives, use aseptic technique, mix thoroughly and do not store.

PRECAUTIONS

Clinical evaluation and periodic laboratory determinations are necessary to monitor changes in fluid balance, electrolyte concentrations and acid-base balance during prolonged parenteral therapy or whenever the condition of the patient warrants such evaluation.

Caution must be exercised in the administration of parenteral fluids, especially those containing sodium ions, to patients receiving corticosteroids or corticotropin.

Potassium containing solutions should be used with caution in the presence of cardiac disease, particularly in digitalized patients or in the presence of renal disease.

Solutions containing lactate ions should be used with caution as excess administration may result in metabolic alkalosis.

Pregnancy Category C. Animal reproduction studies have not been conducted with Ringer's Injection, USP, Dextrose and Ringer's Injection, Lactated Ringer's Injection, USP or Dextrose and Lactated Ringer's Injection. It is also not known whether these injections can cause fetal harm when administered to a pregnant woman or can affect reproduction capacity. These injections should be given to a pregnant woman only if clearly needed.

ADVERSE REACTIONS

Reactions which may occur because of the solution or the technique of administration include febrile response, infection at the site of injection, venous thrombosis or phlebitis extending from the site of injection, extravasation and hypervolemia.

If an adverse reaction does occur, discontinue the infusion, evaluate the patient, institute appropriate therapeutic countermeasures and save the remainder of the fluid for examination if deemed necessary.

OVERDOSAGE

In the event of overhydration or solute overload, re-evaluate the patient and institute appropriate corrective measures. See *"Warnings"* and *"Precautions"*.

DOSAGE AND ADMINISTRATION

The dose is dependent upon the age, weight and clinical condition of the patient.

Parenteral drug products should be inspected visually for particulate matter and discoloration prior to administration, whenever solution and container permit. See *"Contraindications"*.

Protect from freezing and extreme heat.

HOW SUPPLIED
INJECTION:

AVERAGE UNIT PRICE (AVAILABLE SIZES)		GENERIC A-RATED AVERAGE PRICE (GAAP)	
GENERIC	$0.02	1000 ml 12s	$149.76
		500 ml 24s	$262.56

BRAND/MANUFACTURER	NDC	SIZE	AWP
◆ GENERICS			
McGaw	00264-1380-10	500 ml	$11.04
Baxter	00338-0105-04	1000 ml 12s	$148.32
Abbott Hosp	00074-7982-09	1000 ml 12s	$151.19
Baxter	00338-0105-03	500 ml 24s	$260.06
Abbott Hosp	00074-7982-24	500 ml 24s	$265.05

Ringer's Solution, Irrigation

DESCRIPTION

These products are sterile nonpyrogenic solutions of electrolytes in water for injection intended only for sterile irrigation, washing and rinsing purposes.

Each 100 mL of Ringer's Solution for Irrigation, USP contains: Sodium chloride 860 mg; potassium chloride 30 mg; calcium chloride dihydrate 33 mg. The pH is 5.7 (5.0 - 7.5). The solution is isotonic (309 mOsmol/liter, calc.) and has the following electrolyte content (mEq/liter): Na^+ 147.5; K^+ 4; Ca^{++} 4.5; Cl^- 156.

The solution contains no bacteriostat, antimicrobial agent or added buffer and is intended only for use as single-dose or short procedure irrigation. When smaller volumes are required the unused portion should be discarded. Ringer's Solution for Irrigation, USP may be classified as a sterile irrigant, wash, rinse and pharmaceutical vehicle.

Calcium Chloride, USP is chemically designated calcium chloride dihydrate ($CaCl_2 \cdot 2H_2O$), white fragments or granules freely soluble in water.

Potassium Chloride, USP is chemically designated KCl, a white granular powder freely soluble in water.

Sodium Chloride, USP is chemically designated NaCl, a white crystalline powder freely soluble in water.

Water for Injection, USP is chemically designated H_2O.

The semi-rigid container is fabricated from a specially formulated polyolefin. It is a copolymer of ethylene and propylene. The safety of the plastic has been confirmed by tests in animals according to USP biological standards for plastic containers. The container requires no vapor barrier to maintain the proper drug concentration.

◆ RATED THERAPEUTICALLY EQUIVALENT; ◇ THERAPEUTIC EQUIVALENCE UNCONFIRMED; ○ UNRATED

CLINICAL PHARMACOLOGY

Ringer's Solution for Irrigation, USP, exerts a mechanical cleansing action for sterile irrigation of body cavities, tissues or wounds, indwelling urethral catheters and surgical drainage tubes, and for washing, rinsing or soaking surgical dressings, instruments and laboratory specimens. It also serves as a vehicle for drugs used for irrigation or other pharmaceutical preparations.

Ringer's Solution for Irrigation, USP, provides an isotonic irrigation with the same ionic constituents as Ringer's Injection, USP, a modification of Ringer's solution (also called Ringer's mixture) originally used only as a topical physiologic salt solution.

Ringer's Solution for Irrigation, USP, is considered generally compatible with living tissues and organs.

Calcium Chloride in water dissociates to provide calcium (Ca^{++}) and chloride (Cl^-) ions. They are normal constituents of the body fluids and are dependent on various physiologic mechanisms for maintenance of balance between intake and output. Approximately 80% of body calcium is excreted in the feces as insoluble salts; urinary excretion accounts for the remaining 20%.

Potassium chloride in water dissociates to provide potassium (K^+) and chloride (Cl^-) ions. Potassium is the chief cation of body cells (160 mEq/liter of intracellular water). It is found in low concentration in plasma and extracellular fluids (3.5 to 5.0 mEq/liter in a healthy adult). Potassium plays an important role in electrolyte balance.

Normally about 80 to 90% of the potassium intake is excreted in the urine; the remainder in the stools and to a small extent, in the perspiration. The kidney does not conserve potassium well so that during fasting or in patients on a potassium free diet, potassium loss from the body continues resulting in potassium depletion.

Sodium chloride in water dissociates to provide sodium (Na^+) and chloride (Cl^-) ions. Sodium (Na^+) is the principal cation of the extracellular fluid and plays a large part in the therapy of fluid and electrolyte disturbances. Chloride (Cl^-) has an integral role in buffering action when oxygen and carbon dioxide exchange occurs in the red blood cells. The distribution and excretion of sodium (Na^+) and chloride (Cl^-) are largely under the control of the kidney which maintains a balance between intake and output.

Water is an essential constituent of all body tissues and accounts for approximately 70% of total body weight. Average normal adult daily requirement ranges from two to three liters (1.0 to 1.5 liters each for insensible water loss by perspiration and urine production).

Water balance is maintained by various regulatory mechanisms. Water distribution depends primarily on the concentration of electrolytes in the body compartments and sodium (Na^+) plays a major role in maintaining physiologic equilibrium.

INDICATIONS AND USAGE

Ringer's Solution for Irrigation, USP is indicated for all general irrigation, washing and rinsing purposes which permit use of a sterile, nonpyrogenic electrolyte solution.

CONTRAINDICATIONS

Not for injection by usual parenteral routes.

An electrolyte solution should not be used for irrigation during electrosurgical procedures.

WARNINGS

FOR IRRIGATION ONLY. NOT FOR INJECTION.

Irrigating fluids have been demonstrated to enter the systemic circulation in relatively large volumes; thus this irrigation must be regarded as a systemic drug. Absorption of large amounts can cause fluid and/or solute overloading resulting in dilution of serum electrolyte concentrations, overhydration, congested states or pulmonary edema.

The risk of dilutional states is inversely proportional to the electrolyte concentrations of administered parenteral solutions. The risk of solute overload causing congested states with peripheral and pulmonary edema is directly proportional to the electrolyte concentrations of such solutions.

Do not heat over 66° C (150° F).

PRECAUTIONS

Do not use for irrigation that may result in absorption into the blood.

Caution should be observed when the solution is used for continuous irrigation or allowed to "dwell" inside body cavities because of possible absorption into the blood stream and the production of circulatory overload.

Aseptic technique is essential with the use of sterile solutions for irrigation of body cavities, wounds and urethral catheters or for wetting dressings that come in contact with body tissues.

When used as a "pour" irrigation, no part of the contents should be allowed to contact the surface below the outer protected thread area of the semi-rigid wide mouth container. When used for irrigation via irrigation equipment, the administration set should be attached promptly. Unused portions should be discarded and a fresh container of appropriate size used for the start-up of each cycle or repeat procedure. For repeated irrigations of urethral catheters, a separate container should be used for each patient.

Do not administer unless solution is clear, seal is intact and container is undamaged. Discard unused portion.

Pregnancy Category C. Animal reproduction studies have not been conducted with Ringer's Solution for Irrigation. It is also not known whether it can cause fetal harm when administered to a pregnant woman or can affect reproduction capacity. It should be given to a pregnant woman only if clearly needed.

ADVERSE REACTIONS

Possible adverse effects arising from the irrigation of body cavities, tissues, or indwelling catheters and tubes are usually avoidable when proper procedures are followed. Displaced catheters or drainage tubes can lead to irrigation or infiltration of unintended structures or cavities. Excessive volume or pressure during irrigation of closed cavities may cause undue distention or disruption of tissues. Accidental contamination from careless technique may transmit infection.

Should any adverse reaction occur, discontinue the irrigant, evaluate the patient, institute appropriate therapeutic countermeasures and save the remainder of the fluid for examination if deemed necessary.

OVERDOSAGE

In the event of overhydration or solute overload, re-evaluate the patient and institute appropriate corrective measures. See *"Warnings", "Precautions"* and *"Adverse Reactions".*

DOSAGE AND ADMINISTRATION

The dose is dependent upon the capacity or surface area of the structure to be irrigated and the nature of the procedure. When used as a vehicle for other drugs, the manufacturer's recommendations should be followed.

Parenteral drug products should be inspected visually for particulate matter and discoloration prior to administration, whenever solution container permits. See *"Precautions".*

DRUG INTERACTIONS

Additives may be incompatible. Consult with pharmacist, if available. When introducing additives, use aseptic technique, mix thoroughly and do not store.

STORAGE

Exposure of pharmaceutical products to heat should be minimized. Avoid excessive heat. Protect from freezing. It is recommended that the product be stored at room temperature (25° C); however, brief exposure up to 40° C does not adversely affect the product.

HOW SUPPLIED
SOLUTION:

AVERAGE UNIT PRICE (AVAILABLE SIZES)		GENERIC A-RATED AVERAGE PRICE (GAAP)		
GENERIC	$0.02	1000 ml 12s		$240.93
BRAND/MANUFACTURER		NDC	SIZE	AWP
◆ GENERICS				
McGaw		00264-2202-00	1000 ml	$15.22
McGaw		00264-2203-00	1000 ml	$15.31
McGaw		00264-2203-50	2000 ml	$25.55
McGaw		00264-2202-50	2000 ml	$25.80
McGaw		00264-2203-70	4000 ml	$32.92
Baxter		00338-0104-04	1000 ml 12s	$238.61
Abbott Hosp		00074-6140-09	1000 ml 12s	$243.25

Risperdal *SEE* RISPERIDONE

Risperidone

DESCRIPTION

Risperidone is an antipsychotic agent belonging to a new chemical class, the benzisoxazole derivatives. The chemical designation is 3-[2-[4-(6-fluoro-1,2-benzisoxazol-3-yl)-1-piperidinyl]ethyl]-6, 7, 8, 9-tetrahydro-2-methyl-4*H*-pyrido[1,2-a]pyrimidin-4-one. Its molecular formula is $C_{28}H_{27}FN_4O_2$ and its molecular weight is 410.49.

Risperidone is a white to slightly beige powder. It is practically insoluble in water, freely soluble in methylene chloride, and soluble in methanol and 0.1 *N* HCl.

Risperidone for oral use is available in tablets of 1 mg, 2 mg, 3 mg, and 4 mg.

Following is its chemical structure:

CLINICAL PHARMACOLOGY
PHARMACODYNAMICS

The mechanism of action of Risperidone, as with other antipsychotic drugs, is unknown. However, it has been proposed that this drug's antipsychotic activity is mediated through a combination of dopamine type 2 (D_2) and serotonin type 2 ($5HT_2$) antagonism. Antagonism at receptors other than D_2 and $5HT_2$ may explain some of the other effects of Risperidone.

Risperidone is a selective monoaminergic antagonist with high affinity (Ki of 0.12 to 7.3 nM) for the serotonin type 2 ($5HT_2$), dopamine type 2 (D_2), α_1 and α_2 adrenergic, and H_1 histaminergic receptors. Risperidone antagonizes other receptors, but with lower potency. Risperidone has low to moderate affinity (Ki of

47 to 253 nM) for the serotonin $5HT_{1C}$, $5HT_{1D}$, and $5HT_{1A}$ receptors, weak affinity (Ki of 620 to 800 nM) for the dopamine D_1 and haloperidol-sensitive sigma site, and no affinity (when tested at concentration $> 10^{-5}$ M) for cholinergic muscarinic or β_1 and β_2 adrenergic receptors.

PHARMACOKINETICS

Risperidone is well absorbed, as illustrated by a mass balance study involving a single 1 mg oral dose of ^{14}C-Risperidone as a solution in three healthy male volunteers. Total recovery of radioactivity at one week was 85%, including 70% in the urine and 15% in the feces.

Risperidone is extensively metabolized in the liver by cytochrome $P_{450}IID_6$ to a major active metabolite, 9-hydroxyrisperidone, which is the predominant circulating specie, and appears approximately equi-effective with Risperidone with respect to receptor binding activity and some effects in animals. (A second minor pathway is N-dealkylation). Consequently, the clinical effect of the drug likely results from the combined concentrations of Risperidone plus 9-hydroxyrisperidone. Plasma concentrations of Risperidone, 9-hydroxyrisperidone, and Risperidone plus 9-hydroxyrisperidone are dose proportional over the dosing range of 1 to 16 mg daily (0.5 to mg BID). The relative oral bioavailability of Risperidone from a tablet was 94% (CV = 10%) when compared to a solution. Food does not affect either the rate or extent of absorption of Risperidone. Thus, Risperidone can be given with or without meals. The absolute oral bioavailability of Risperidone was 70% (CV = 25%).

The enzyme catalyzing hydroxylation of Risperidone to 9-hydroxyrisperidone is cytochrome $P_{450}IID_6$, also called debrisoquin hydroxylase, the enzyme responsible for metabolism of many neuroleptics, antidepressants, antiarrhythmics, and other drugs. Cytochrome $P_{450}IID_6$ is subject to genetic polymorphism (about 6-8% of caucasians, and a very low percent of Asians have little or no activity and are "poor metabolizers") and to inhibition by a variety of substrates and some non-substrates, notably quinidine. Extensive metabolizers convert Risperidone rapidly into 9-hydroxyrisperidone, while poor metabolizers convert it much more slowly. Extensive metabolizers, therefore, have lower Risperidone and higher 9-hydroxyrisperidone concentrations than poor metabolizers. Following oral administration of solution or tablet, mean peak plasma concentrations occurred at about 1 hour. Peak 9-hydroxyrisperidone occurred at about 3 hours in extensive metabolizers, and 17 hours in poor metabolizers. The apparent half-life of Risperidone was three hours (CV = 30%) in extensive metabolizers and 20 hours (CV = 40%) in poor metabolizers. The apparent half-life of 9-hydroxyrisperidone was about 21 hours (CV = 20%) in extensive metabolizers and 30 hours (CV = 25%) in poor metabolizers. Steady-state concentrations of Risperidone are reached in 1 day in extensive metabolizers and would be expected to reach steady state in about 5 days in poor metabolizers. Steady-state concentrations of 9-hydroxyrisperidone are reached in 5-6 days (measured in extensive metabolizers). Because Risperidone and 9-hydroxyrisperidone are approximately equi-effective, the sum of their concentrations is pertinent. The pharmacokinetics of the sum of Risperidone and 9-hydroxyrisperidone, after single and multiple doses, were similar in extensive and poor metabolizers, with an overall mean elimination half-life of about 20 hours. In analyses comparing adverse reaction rates in extensive and poor metabolizers in controlled and open studies, no important differences were seen.

Risperidone could be subject to two kinds of drug-drug interactions. First, inhibitors of cytochrome $P_{450}IID_6$ could interfere with conversion of Risperidone to 9-hydroxyrisperidone. This in fact occurs with quinidine, giving essentially all recipients a Risperidone pharmacokinetic profile typical of poor metabolizers. The favorable and adverse effects of Risperidone in patients receiving quinidine have not been evaluated, but observations in a modest number (n is approximately equal to 70) of poor metabolizers given Risperidone do not suggest important differences between poor and extensive metabolizers. It would also be possible for Risperidone to interfere with metabolism of other drugs metabolized by cytochrome $P_{450}IID_6$. Relatively weak binding of Risperidone to the enzyme suggests this is unlikely (see "Precautions" and "Drug Interactions").

The plasma protein binding of Risperidone was about 90% over the *in vitro* concentration range of 0.5 to 200 ng/mL and increased with increasing concentrations of α_1-acid glycoprotein. The plasma binding of 9-hydroxyrisperidone was 77%. Neither the parent nor the metabolite displaced each other from the plasma binding sites. High therapeutic concentrations of sulfamethazine (100 µg/mL), warfarin (10 µg/mL) and carbamazepine (10 µg/mL) caused only a slight increase in the free fraction of Risperidone at 10 ng/mL and 9-hydroxyrisperidone at 50 ng/mL, changes of unknown clinical significance.

SPECIAL POPULATIONS

Renal Impairment: In patients with moderate to severe renal disease, clearance of the sum of Risperidone and its active metabolite decreased by 60% compared to young healthy subjects. Risperidone doses should be reduced in patients with renal disease (see "Precautions" and "Dosage and Administration").

Hepatic Impairment: While the pharmacokinetics of Risperidone in subjects with liver disease were comparable to those in young healthy subjects, the mean free fraction of Risperidone in plasma was increased by about 35% because of the diminished concentration of both albumin and α_1-acid glycoprotein. Risperidone doses should be reduced in patients with liver disease (see "Precautions" and "Dosage and Administration").

Elderly: In healthy elderly subjects renal clearance of both Risperidone and 9-hydroxyrisperidone was decreased, and elimination half-lives were prolonged compared to young healthy subjects. Dosing should be modified accordingly in the elderly patients (see "Dosage and Administration").

Race and Gender Effects: No specific pharmacokinetic study was conducted to investigate race and gender effects, but a population pharmacokinetic analysis did not identify important differences in the disposition of Risperidone due to gender (whether corrected for body weight or not) or race.

CLINICAL TRIALS

The efficacy of Risperidone in the management of the manifestations of psychotic disorders was established in three short-term (6- to 8-week) controlled trials of psychotic inpatients who met DSM III-R criteria for schizophrenia.

Several instruments were used for assessing psychiatric signs and symptoms in these studies, among them the Brief Psychiatric Rating Scale (BPRS), a multi-item inventory of general psychopathology traditionally used to evaluate the effects of drug treatment in psychosis. The BPRS psychosis cluster (conceptual disorganization, hallucinatory behavior, suspiciousness, and unusual thought content) is considered a particularly useful subset for assessing actively psychotic schizophrenic patients. A second traditional assessment, the Clinical Global Impression (CGI), reflects the impression of a skilled observer, fully familiar with the manifestation of schizophrenia, about the overall clinical state of the patient. In addition, two more recently developed, but less well evaluated scales, were employed; these included the Positive and Negative Symptoms Scale (PANSS) and the Scale for Assessing Negative Symptoms (SANS).

The results of the trials follow:

(1) In a 6-week, placebo-controlled trial (n = 160) involving titration of Risperidone in doses up to 10 mg/day (BID schedule), Risperidone was generally superior to placebo on the BPRS total score, on the BPRS psychosis cluster, and marginally superior to placebo on the SANS.

(2) In an 8-week, placebo-controlled trial (n = 513) involving 4 fixed doses of Risperidone (2, 6, 10, and 16 mg/day, on a BID schedule), all 4 Risperidone groups were generally superior to placebo on the BPRS total score, BPRS psychosis cluster, and CGI severity score; the 3 highest Risperidone dose groups were generally superior to placebo on the PANSS negative subscale. The most consistently positive responses on all measures were seen for the 6 mg dose group, and there was no suggestion of increased benefit from larger doses.

(3) In an 8-week, dose comparison trial (n = 1356) involving 5 fixed doses of Risperidone (1,4,8,12, and 16 mg/day, on a BID schedule), the four highest Risperidone, dose groups were generally superior to the 1 mg Risperidone dose group on BPRS total score, BPRS psychosis cluster, and CGI severity score. None of the dose groups were superior to the 1 mg group on the PANSS negative subscale. The most consistently positive responses were seen for the 4 mg dose group.

INDICATIONS AND USAGE

Risperidone is indicated for the management of the manifestations of psychotic disorders.

The antipsychotic efficacy of Risperidone was established in short-term (6 to 8 weeks) controlled trials of schizophrenic inpatients (see "Clinical Pharmacology").

The effectiveness of Risperidone in long-term use, that is, more than 6 to 8 weeks, has not been systematically evaluated in controlled trials. Therefore, the physician who elects to use Risperidone for extended periods should periodically re-evaluate the long-term usefulness of the drug for the individual patient. (See "Dosage and Administration".)

UNLABELED USES

Risperidone is used as an adjunct for treatment of behavioral problems in patients with mental deficiency.

CONTRAINDICATIONS

Risperidone is contraindicated in patients with a known hypersensitivity to the product.

WARNINGS

NEUROLEPTIC MALIGNANT SYNDROME (NMS)

A potentially fatal symptom complex sometimes referred to as Neuroleptic Malignant Syndrome (NMS) has been reported in association with antipsychotic drugs. Clinical manifestations of NMS are hyperpyrexia, muscle rigidity, altered mental status and evidence of autonomic instability (irregular pulse or blood pressure, tachycardia, diaphoresis and cardiac dysrhythmia). Additional signs may include elevated creatine phosphokinase, myoglobinuria (rhabdomyolysis), and acute renal failure.

The diagnostic evaluation of patients with this syndrome is complicated. In arriving at a diagnosis, it is important to identify cases where the clinical presentation includes both serious medical illness (e.g., pneumonia, systemic infection, etc.) and untreated or inadequately treated extrapyramidal signs and symptoms (EPS). Other important considerations in the differential diagnosis include central anticholinergic toxicity, heat stroke, drug fever, and primary central nervous system pathology.

The management of NMS should include: 1) immediate discontinuation of antipsychotic drugs and other drugs not essential to concurrent therapy; 2) intensive symptomatic treatment and medical monitoring; and 3) treatment of any concomitant serious medical problems for which specific treatments are available. There is no general agreement about specific pharmacological treatment regimens for uncomplicated NMS.

If a patient requires antipsychotic drug treatment after recovery from NMS, the potential reintroduction of drug therapy should be carefully considered. The patient should be carefully monitored, since recurrences of NMS have been reported.

◆ RATED THERAPEUTICALLY EQUIVALENT; ◇ THERAPEUTIC EQUIVALENCE UNCONFIRMED; ○ UNRATED

TARDIVE DYSKINESIA

A syndrome of potentially irreversible, involuntary, dyskinetic movements may develop in patients treated with antipsychotic drugs. Although the prevalence of the syndrome appears to be highest among the elderly, especially elderly women, it is impossible to rely upon prevalence estimates to predict, at the inception of antipsychotic treatment, which patients are likely to develop the syndrome. Whether antipsychotic drug products differ in their potential to cause tardive dyskinesia is unknown.

The risk of developing tardive dyskinesia and the likelihood that it will become irreversible are believed to increase as the duration of treatment and the total cumulative dose of antipsychotic drugs administered to the patient increase. However, the syndrome can develop, although much less commonly, after relatively brief treatment periods at low doses.

There is no known treatment for established cases of tardive dyskinesia, although the syndrome may remit, partially or completely, if antipsychotic treatment is withdrawn. Antipsychotic treatment, itself, however, may suppress (or partially suppress) the signs and symptoms of the syndrome and thereby may possibly mask the underlying process. The effect that symptomatic suppression has upon the long-term course of the syndrome is unknown.

Given these considerations, Risperidone should be prescribed in a manner that is most likely to minimize the occurrence of tardive dyskinesia. Chronic antipsychotic treatment should generally be reserved for patients who suffer from a chronic illness that (1) is known to respond to antipsychotic drugs, and (2) for whom alternative, equally effective, but potentially less harmful treatments are not available or appropriate. In patients who do require chronic treatment, the smallest dose and the shortest duration of treatment producing a satisfactory clinical response should be sought. The need for continued treatment should be reassessed periodically.

If signs and symptoms of tardive dyskinesia appear in a patient on Risperidone, drug discontinuation should be considered. However, some patients may require treatment with Risperidone despite the presence of the syndrome.

Potential for Proarrhythmic Effects: Risperidone and/or 9-hydroxyrisperidone appears to lengthen the QT interval in some patients, although there is no average increase in treated patients, even at 12-16 mg/day, well above the recommended dose. Other drugs that prolong the QT interval have been associated with the occurrence of torsades de pointes, a life-threatening arrhythmia. Bradycardia, electrolyte imbalance, concomitant use with other drugs that prolong QT, or the presence of congenital prolongation in QT can increase the risk for occurrence of this arrhythmia.

PRECAUTIONS
GENERAL

Orthostatic Hypotension: Risperidone may induce orthostatic hypotension associated with dizziness, tachycardia, and in some patients, syncope, especially during the initial dose-titration period, probably reflecting its alpha-adrenergic antagonistic properties. Syncope was reported in 0.2% (6/2607) of Risperidone treated patients in phase 2-3 studies. The risk of orthostatic hypotension and syncope may be minimized by limiting the initial dose to 1 mg BID in normal adults and 0.5 mg BID in the elderly and patients with renal or hepatic impairment (see *"Dosage and Administration"*). A dose reduction should be considered if hypotension occurs. Risperidone should be used with particular caution in patients with known cardiovascular disease (history of myocardial infarction or ischemia, heart failure, or conduction abnormalities), cerebrovascular disease, and conditions which would predispose patients to hypotension (dehydration, hypovolemia, and treatment with antihypertensive medications).

Seizures: During premarketing testing, seizures occurred in 0.3% (9/2607) of Risperidone treated patients, two in association with hyponatremia. Risperidone should be used cautiously in patients with a history of seizures.

Hyperprolactinemia: As with other drugs that antagonize dopamine D_2 receptors, Risperidone elevates prolactin levels and the elevation persists during chronic administration. Tissue culture experiments indicate that approximately one-third of human breast cancers are prolactin dependent in vitro, a factor of potential importance if the prescription of these drugs is contemplated in a patient with previously detected breast cancer. Although disturbances such as galactorrhea, amenorrhea, gynecomastia, and impotence have been reported with prolactin-elevating compounds, the clinical significance of elevated serum prolactin levels is unknown for most patients. As is common with compounds which increase prolactin release, an increase in pituitary gland, mammary gland, and pancreatic islet cell hyperplasia and/or neoplasia was observed in the Risperidone carcinogenicity studies conducted in mice and rats (see *"Carcinogenesis"*). However, neither clinical studies nor epidemiologic studies conducted to date have shown an association between chronic administration of this class of drugs and tumorigenesis in humans; the available evidence is considered too limited to be conclusive at this time.

Potential for Cognitive and Motor Impairment: Somnolence was a commonly reported adverse event associated with Risperidone treatment, especially when ascertained by direct questioning of patients. This adverse event is dose related, and in a study utilizing a checklist to detect adverse events, 41% of the high dose patients (Risperidone 16 mg/day) reported somnolence compared to 16% of placebo patients. Direct questioning is more sensitive for detecting adverse events than spontaneous reporting, by which 8% of Risperidone 16 mg/day patients and 1% of placebo patients reported somnolence as an adverse event. Since Risperidone has the potential to impair judgment, thinking, or motor skills, patients should be cautioned about operating hazardous machinery, including automobiles, until they are reasonably certain that Risperidone therapy does not affect them adversely.

Priapism: A single case of priapism was reported in a 50-year-old patient receiving Risperidone in a large, open premarketing experience (approximately 1300 patients). This event occurred after 11 months of treatment with Risperidone alone, and required surgical intervention. While the relationship of this event to Risperidone use cannot be established on the basis of a single case, other drugs with alpha-adrenergic blocking effects have been reported to induce priapism, and it is possible that Risperidone may share this capacity.

Thrombotic Thrombocytopenic Purpura (TTP): A single case of TTP was reported in a 28 year-old female patient receiving Risperidone in a large, open premarketing experience (approximately 1300 patients). She experienced jaundice, fever, and bruising, but eventually recovered after receiving plasmapheresis. The relationship to Risperidone therapy is unknown.

Antiemetic Effect: Risperidone has an antiemetic effect in animals; this effect may also occur in humans, and may mask signs and symptoms of overdosage with certain drugs or of conditions such as intestinal obstruction, Reye's syndrome, and brain tumor.

Body Temperature Regulation: Although not reported with Risperidone, disruption of body temperature regulation has been attributed to other antipsychotic agents. Caution is advised when prescribing for patients who will be exposed to extreme heat.

Suicide: The possibility of a suicide attempt is inherent in schizophrenia, and close supervision of high risk patients should accompany drug therapy. Prescriptions for Risperidone should be written for the smallest quantity of tablets consistent with good patient management, in order to reduce the risk of overdose.

Use in Patients with Concomitant Illness: Clinical experience with Risperidone in patients with certain concomitant systemic illnesses is limited. Caution is advisable in using Risperidone in patients with diseases or conditions that could affect metabolism or hemodynamic responses.

Risperidone has not been evaluated or used to any appreciable extent in patients with a recent history of myocardial infarction or unstable heart disease. Patients with these diagnoses were excluded from clinical studies during the product's premarket testing. The electrocardiograms of approximately 380 patients who received Risperidone and 120 patients who received placebo in two double-blind, placebo-controlled trials were evaluated and the date revealed one finding of potential concern, i.e., 8 patients taking Risperidone whose baseline QTc interval was less than 450 msec were observed to have QTc intervals greater than 450 msec during treatment; no such prolongations were seen in the smaller placebo group. There were 3 such episodes in the approximately 125 patients who received haloperidol. Because of the risks of orthostatic hypotension and QT prolongation, caution should be observed in cardiac patients (see *"Warnings"* and *"Precautions"*).

Increased plasma concentrations of Risperidone and 9-hydroxyrisperidone occur in patients with severe renal impairment (creatinine clearance < 30 mL/min/1.73 m^2), and an increase in the free fraction of the Risperidone is seen in patients with severe hepatic impairment. A lower starting dose should be used in such patients (see *"Dosage and Administration"*).

Information for Patients: Physicians are advised to discuss the following issues with patients for whom they prescribe Risperidone.

Orthostatic Hypotension: Patients should be advised of the risk of orthostatic hypotension, especially during the period of initial dose titration.

Interference With Cognitive and Motor Performance: Since Risperidone has the potential to impair judgment, thinking, or motor skills, patients should be cautioned about operating hazardous machinery, including automobiles, until they are reasonably certain that Risperidone therapy does not affect them adversely.

Pregnancy: Patients should be advised to notify their physician if they become pregnant or intend to become pregnant during therapy.

Nursing: Patients should be advised not to breast feed an infant if they are taking Risperidone.

Concomitant Medication: Patients should be advised to inform their physicians if they are taking, or plan to take, any prescription or over-the-counter drugs, since there is a potential for interaction.

Alcohol: Patients should be advised to avoid alcohol while taking Risperidone.

LABORATORY TESTS
No specific laboratory tests are recommended.

DRUG INTERACTIONS
The interactions of Risperidone and other drugs have not been systematically evaluated. Given the primary CNS effects of Risperidone, caution should be used when Risperidone is taken in combination with other centrally acting drugs and alcohol.

Because of its potential for inducing hypotension, Risperidone may enhance the effects of certain antihypertensive agents.

Risperidone may antagonize the effects of levodopa and dopamine agonists. Chronic administration of carbamazepine with Risperidone may increase the clearance of Risperidone.

Chronic administration of clozapine with Risperidone may decrease the clearance of Risperidone.

Drugs that Inhibit Cytochrome $P_{450}IID_6$ and Other P_{450} Isozymes: Risperidone is metabolized to 9-hydroxyrisperidone by cytochrome $P_{450}IID_6$, an enzyme that is polymorphic in the population and that can be inhibited by a variety of psychotropic and other drugs (see *"Clinical Pharmacology"*). Drug interactions that reduce the metabolism of Risperidone to 9-hydroxyrisperidone would increase the plasma concentrations of Risperidone and lower the concentrations of 9-hydroxyrisperidone. Analysis of clinical studies involving a modest number of poor metabolizers (n is approximately equal to 70) does not suggest that poor and extensive metabolizers have different rates of adverse effects. No comparison of effectiveness in the two groups has been made.

In vitro studies showed that drugs metabolized by other P_{450} isozymes, including 1A1, 1A2, IIC9, MP, and IIIA4, are only weak inhibitors of Risperidone metabolism.

Drugs Metabolized by Cytochrome $P_{450}IID_6$: In vitro studies indicate that Risperidone is a relatively weak inhibitor of cytochrome $P_{450}IID_6$. Therefore, Risperidone is not expected to substantially inhibit the clearance of drugs that are metabolized by this enzymatic pathway. However, clinical data to confirm this expectation are not available.

CARCINOGENESIS, MUTAGENESIS, IMPAIRMENT OF FERTILITY
Carcinogenesis: Carcinogenicity studies were conducted in Swiss albino mice and Wistar rats. Risperidone was administered in the diet at doses of 0.63, 2.5, and 10 mg/kg for 18 months to mice and for 25 months to rats. These doses are equivalent to 2.4, 9.4 and 37.5 times the maximum human dose (16 mg/day) on a mg/kg basis or 0.2, 0.75 and 3 times the maximum human dose (mice) or 0.4, 1.5, and 6 times the maximum human dose (rats) on a mg/m^2 basis. A maximum tolerated dose was not achieved in male mice. There were statistically significant increases in pituitary gland adenomas, endocrine pancreas adenomas and mammary gland adenocarcinomas. The following table summarizes the multiples of the human dose on a mg/m^2 (mg/kg) basis at which these tumors occurred.

Tumor Type	Species	Sex	Multiple of Maximum Human Dose in mg/m^2 (mg/kg)	
			Lowest Effect Level	Highest No Effect
Pituitary adenomas	mouse	female	0.75 (9.4)	0.2 (2.4)
Endocrine pancreas adenomas	rat	male	1.5 (9.4)	0.4 (2.4)
Mammary gland adeno-carcinomas	mouse	female	0.2 (2.4)	none
	rat	female	0.4 (2.4)	none
	rat	male	6 (37.5)	1.5 (9.4)
Mammary gland neoplasms Total	rat	male	1.5 (9.4)	0.4 (2.4)

Antipsychotic drugs have been shown to chronically elevate prolactin levels in rodents. Serum prolactin levels were not measured during the Risperidone carcinogenicity studies; however, measurements during subchronic toxicity studies showed that Risperidone elevated serum prolactin levels 5 to 6 fold in mice and rats at the same doses used in the carcinogenicity studies. An increase in mammary, pituitary, and endocrine pancreas neoplasms has been found in rodents after chronic administration of other antipsychotic drugs and is considered to be prolactin mediated. The relevance for human risk of the findings of prolactin-mediated endocrine tumors in rodents in unknown (see *"Hyperprolactinemia"* under *"Precautions, General"*).

Mutagenesis: No evidence of mutagenic potential for Risperidone was found in the Ames reverse mutation test, mouse lymphoma assay, *in vitro* rat hepatocyte DNA-repair assay, *in vivo* micronucleus test in mice, the sex-linked recessive lethal test in Drosophila, or the chromosomal aberration test in human lymphocytes or Chinese hamster cells.

Impairment of Fertility: Risperidone (0.16 to 5 mg/kg) was shown to impair mating, but not fertility, in Wistar rats in three reproductive studies (two Segment I and a multigenerational study) at doses 0.1 to 3 times the maximum recommended human dose on a mg/m^2 basis. The effect appeared to be in females since impaired mating behavior was not noted in the Segment I study in which males only were treated. In a subchronic study in Beagle dogs in which Risperidone was administered at doses of 0.31 to 5 mg/kg, sperm motility and concentration were decreased at doses 0.6 to 10 times the human dose on a mg/m^2 basis. Dose-related decreases were also noted in serum testosterone at the same doses. Serum testosterone and sperm parameters partially recovered but remained decreased after treatment was discontinued. No no-effect doses were noted in either rat or dog.

PREGNANCY
Pregnancy Category C: The teratogenic potential of Risperidone was studied in three Segment II studies in Sprague-Dawley and Wistar rats and in one Segment II study in New Zealand rabbits. The incidence of malformations was not increased compared to control in offspring of rats or rabbits given 0.4 to 6 times the human dose on a mg/m^2 basis. In three reproductive studies in rats (two Segment III and a multigenerational study), there was an increased in pup deaths during the first 4 days of lactation at doses 0.1 to 3 times the human dose on a mg/m^2 basis. It is not known whether these deaths were due to a direct effect on the fetuses or pups or to effects on the dams. There was no no-effect dose for increased rat pup mortality. In one Segment III study, there was an increase in stillborn rat pups at a dose 1.5 times higher than the human dose on a mg/m^2 basis.

Placental transfer of Risperidone occurs in rat pups. There are no adequate and well-controlled studies in pregnant women. However, there was one report of a case of agenesis of the corpus callosum in an infant exposed to Risperidone in utero. The causal relationship to Risperidone therapy is unknown.

Risperidone should be used during pregnancy only if the potential benefit justifies the potential risk to the fetus.

LABOR AND DELIVERY
The effect of Risperidone on labor and delivery in humans is unknown.

NURSING MOTHERS
It is not known whether or not Risperidone is excreted in human milk. In animal studies, Risperidone and 9-hydroxyrisperidone were excreted in breast milk. Therefore, women receiving Risperidone should not breastfeed.

PEDIATRIC USE
Safety and effectiveness in children have not been established.

GERIATRIC USE
Clinical studies of Risperidone did not include sufficient numbers of patients aged 65 and over to determine whether they respond differently from younger patients. In general, a lower starting dose is recommended for an elderly patient, reflecting a decreased pharmacokinetic clearance in the elderly, as well as a greater frequency of decreased hepatic, renal, or cardiac function, and a greater tendency to postural hypotension (see *"Clinical Pharmacology"* and *"Dosage and Administration"*).

ADVERSE REACTIONS
ASSOCIATED WITH DISCONTINUATION OF TREATMENT
Approximately 9% percent (244/2607) of Risperidone-treated patients in phase 2-3 studies discontinued treatment due to an adverse event, compared with about 7% on placebo and 10% on active control drugs. The more common events ($\geq$ 0.3%) associated with discontinuation and considered to be possibly or probably drug-related included:

Adverse Event	Risperidone	Placebo
Extrapyramidal symptoms	2.1%	0%
Dizziness	0.7%	0%
Hyperkinesia	0.6%	0%
Somnolence	0.5%	0%
Nausea	0.3%	0%

Suicide attempt was associated with discontinuation in 1.2% of Risperidone treated patients compared to 0.6% of placebo patients, but, given the almost 40-fold greater exposure time in Risperidone compared to placebo patients, it is unlikely that suicide attempt is a Risperidone related adverse event (see *"Precautions"*). Discontinuation for extrapyramidal symptoms was 0% in placebo patients but 3.8% in active-control patients in the phase 2-3 trials.

INCIDENCE IN CONTROLLED TRIALS
Commonly Observed Adverse Events in Controlled Clinical Trials: In two 6- to 8-week placebo-controlled trials, spontaneously-reported, treatment-emergent adverse events with an incidence of 5% or greater in at least one of the Risperidone groups and at least twice that of placebo were: anxiety, somnolence, extrapyramidal symptoms, dizziness, constipation, nausea, dyspepsia, rhinitis, rash, and tachycardia.

Adverse events were also elicited in one of these two trials (i.e., in the fixed-dose trial comparing Risperidone at doses of 2, 6, 10, and 16 mg/day with placebo) utilizing a checklist for detecting adverse events, a method that is more sensitive than spontaneous reporting. By this method, the following additional common and drug-related adverse events were present at least 5% and twice the rate of placebo: increased dream activity, increased duration of sleep, accommodation disturbances, reduced salivation, micturition disturbances, diarrhea, weight gain, menorrhagia, diminished sexual desire, erectile dysfunction, ejaculatory dysfunction, and orgastic dysfunction.

Adverse Events Occurring at an Incidence of 1% or More Among Risperidone Treated Patients: The table that follows enumerates adverse events that occurred at an incidence of 1% or more, and were at least as frequent among Risperidone treated patients treated at doses of $\leq$ 10 mg/day than among placebo-treated patients in the pooled results of two 6- to 8-week controlled trials. Patients received Risperidone doses of 2, 6, 10, or 16 mg/day in the dose comparison trial, or up to a maximum dose of 10 mg/day in the titration study. This table shows the percentage of patients in each dose group ($\leq$ 10 mg/day or 16 mg/day) who spontaneously reported at least one episode of an event at some time during their treatment. Patients given doses of 2, 6, or 10 mg did not differ materially in these rates. Reported adverse events were classified using the World Health Organization preferred terms.

The prescriber should be aware that these figures cannot be used to predict the incidence of side effects in the course of usual medical practice where patient

---

characteristics and other factors differ from those which prevailed in this clinical trial. Similarly, the cited frequencies cannot be compared with figures obtained from other clinical investigations involving different treatments, uses and investigators. The cited figures, however, do provide the prescribing physician with some basis for estimating the relative contribution of drug and nondrug factors to the side effect incidence rate in the population studied.

Table 1
TREATMENT-EMERGENT ADVERSE EXPERIENCE INCIDENCE IN 6- TO 8-WEEK CONTROLLED CLINICAL TRIALS[1]

Body System /Preferred Term	Risperidone ≤ 10 mg/day (N = 324)	Risperidone 16 mg/day (N = 77)	Placebo (N = 142)
Psychiatric Disorders			
Insomnia	26%	23%	19%
Agitation	22%	26%	20%
Anxiety	12%	20%	9%
Somnolence	3%	8%	1%
Aggressive reaction	1%	3%	1%
Nervous System			
Extrapyramidal symptoms [2]	17%	34%	16%
Headache	14%	12%	12%
Dizziness	4%	7%	1%
Gastrointestinal System			
Constipation	7%	13%	3%
Nausea	6%	4%	3%
Dyspepsia	5%	10%	4%
Vomiting	5%	7%	4%
Abdominal pain	4%	1%	0%
Saliva increased	2%	0%	1%
Toothache	2%	0%	0%
Respiratory System			
Rhinitis	10%	8%	4%
Coughing	3%	3%	1%
Sinusitis	2%	1%	1%
Pharyngitis	2%	3%	0%
Dyspnea	1%	0%	0%
Body as a Whole			
Back pain	2%	0%	1%
Chest pain	2%	3%	1%
Fever	2%	3%	0%
Dermatological			
Rash	2%	5%	1%
Dry skin	2%	4%	0%
Seborrhea	1%	0%	0%
Infections			
Upper respiratory	3%	3%	1%
Visual			
Abnormal vision	2%	1%	1%
Musculo-Skeletal			
Arthralgia	2%	3%	0%
Cardiovascular			
Tachycardia	3%	5%	0%

[1] Events reported by at least 1% of patients with Risperidone < 10 mg/day are included, and are rounded to the nearest %. Comparative rates for Risperidone 16 mg/day and placebo are provided as well. Events for which the Risperidone incidence (in both dose groups) was equal to or less than placebo are not listed in the table, but included the following: nervousness, injury, and fungal infection.

[2] Includes tremor, dystonia, hypokinesia, hypertonia, hyperkinesia, oculogyric crisis, ataxia, abnormal gait, involuntary muscle contractions, hyporeflexia, and extrapyramidal disorders. Although the incidence of "extrapyramidal symptoms" does not appear to differ for the '≤ 10 mg/ day' group and placebo, the data for individual dose groups in fixed dose trials do suggest a dose/response relationship (see "Dose Dependency of Adverse Events").

DOSE DEPENDENCY OF ADVERSE EVENTS:
Extrapyramidal Symptoms: Data from two fixed dose trials provided evidence of dose-relatedness for extrapyramidal symptoms associated with Risperidone treatment.

Two methods were used to measure extrapyramidal symptoms (EPS) in an 8-week trial comparing four fixed doses of Risperidone (2, 6, 10, and 16 mg/day), including (1) a parkinsonism score (mean change from baseline) from the Extrapyramidal Symptom Rating Scale and (2) incidence of spontaneous complaints of EPS:

Dose Groups	Placebo	Ris 2	Ris 6	Ris 10	Ris 16
Parkinsonism	1.2	0.9	1.8	2.4	2.6
EPS Incidence	13%	13%	16%	20%	31%

Similar methods were used to measure extrapyramidal symptoms (EPS) in an 8-week trial comparing five fixed doses of Risperidone (1, 4, 8, 12, and 16 mg/day):

Dose Groups	Ris 1	Ris 4	Ris 8	Ris 12	Ris 16
Parkinsonism	0.6	1.7	2.4	2.9	4.1
EPS Incidence	7%	12%	18%	18%	21%

Other Adverse Events: Adverse event data elicited by a checklist for side effects from a large study comparing 5 fixed doses of Risperidone (1, 4, 8, 12, and 16 mg/ day) were explored for dose-relatedness of adverse events. A Cochran-Armitage Test for trend in these data revealed a positive trend ($\rho < 0.05$) for the following adverse events: sleepiness, increased duration of sleep, accommodation disturbances, orthostatic dizziness, palpitations, weight gain, erectile dysfunction, ejaculatory dysfunction, orgastic dysfunction, asthenia/lassitude/increased fatigability, and increased pigmentation.

Vital Sign Changes: Risperidone is associated with orthostatic hypotension and tachycardia (see *"Precautions"*).

Weight Changes: The proportions of Risperidone and placebo-treated patients meeting a weight gain criterion of ≥ 7% of body weight were compared in a pool of 6- to 8-week placebo-controlled trials, revealing a statistically significantly greater incidence of weight gain for Risperidone (18%) compared to placebo (9%).

Laboratory Changes: A between group comparison for 6- to 8-week placebo-controlled trials revealed no statistically significant Risperidone/placebo differences in the proportions of patients experiencing potentially important changes in routine serum chemistry, hematology, or urinalysis parameters. Similarly, there were no Risperidone placebo differences in the incidence of discontinuations for changes in serum chemistry, hematology, or urinalysis. However, Risperidone administration was associated with increases in serum prolactin (see *"Precautions"*).

ECG Changes: The electrocardiograms of approximately 380 patients who received Risperidone and 120 patients who received placebo in two double-blind, placebo-controlled trials were evaluated and revealed one finding of potential concern; i.e., 8 patients taking Risperidone whose baseline QTc interval was less than 450 msec were observed to have QTc intervals greater than 450 msec during treatment (see *"Warnings"*). Changes of this type were not seen among about 120 placebo patients, but were seen in patients receiving haloperidol (3/126).

OTHER EVENTS OBSERVED DURING THE PRE-MARKETING EVALUATION OF RISPERIDONE
During its premarketing assessment, multiple doses of Risperidone were administered to 2607 patients in phase 2 and 3 studies. The conditions and duration of exposure to Risperidone varied greatly, and included (in overlapping categories) open and double-blind studies, uncontrolled and controlled studies, inpatient and outpatient studies, fixed-dose and titration studies, and short-term or longer-term exposure. In most studies, untoward events associated with this exposure were obtained by spontaneous report and recorded by clinical investigators using terminology of their own choosing. Consequently, it is not possible to provide a meaningful estimate of the proportion of individuals experiencing adverse events without first grouping similar types of untoward events into a smaller number of standardized event categories. In two large studies, adverse events were also elicited utilizing the UKU (direct questioning) side effect rating scale, and these events were not further categorized using standard terminology *Note:* These events are marked with an asterisk in the listings that follow).

In the listings that follow, spontaneously reported adverse events were classified using World Health Organization (WHO) preferred terms. The frequencies presented, therefore, represent the proportion of the 2607 patients exposed to multiple doses of Risperidone who experienced an event of the type cited on at least one occasion while receiving Risperidone. All reported events are included except those already listed in Table 1, those events for which a drug cause was remote, and those event terms which were so general as to be uninformative. It is important to emphasize that, although the events reported occurred during treatment with Risperidone, they were not necessarily caused by it.

Events are further categorized by body system and listed in order of decreasing frequency according to the following definitions: frequent adverse events are those occurring in at least 1/100 patients (only those not already listed in the tabulated results from placebo controlled trials appear in this listing); infrequent adverse events are those occurring in 1/100 to 1/1000 patients; rare events are those occurring in fewer than 1/1000 patients.

Psychiatric Disorders: Frequent: increased dream actvity*, diminished sexual desire*, nervousness. *Infrequent:* impaired concentration, depression, apathy, catatonic reaction, euphoria, increased libido, amnesia. *Rare:* emotional lability, nightmares, delirium, withdrawal syndrome, yawning.

Central and Peripheral Nervous System Disorders: Frequent: increased sleep duration*. *Infrequent:* dysarthria, vertigo, stupor, paraesthesia, confusion. *Rare:* aphasia, cholinergic syndrome, hyposthesia, tongue paralysis, leg cramps, torticollis, hypotonia, coma, migraine, hyperreflexia, choreoathetosis.

Gastro-intestinal Disorders: Frequent: anorexia, reduced salivation*. *Infrequent:* flatulence, diarrhea, increased appetite, stomatitis, melena, dysphagia, hemorrhoids, gastritis. *Rare:* fecal incontinence, eructation, gastroesophageal reflux,

* Incidence based on elicited reports.

➤ SHOWN IN PRODUCT IDENTIFICATION GUIDE

gastroenteritis, esophagitis, tongue discoloration, cholelithiasis, tongue edema, diverticulitis, gingivitis, discolored feces, GI hemorrhage, hematemesis.

Body as a Whole/General Disorders: Frequent: fatigue. *Infrequent:* edema, rigors, malaise, influenza-like symptoms. *Rare:* pallor, enlarged abdomen, allergic reaction, ascites, sarcoidosis, flushing.

Respiratory System Disorders: Infrequent: hyperventilation, bronchospasm, pneumonia, stridor. *Rare:* asthma, increased sputum, aspiration.

Skin and Appendage Disorders: Frequent: increased pigmentation*, photosensitivity*. *Infrequent:* increased sweating, acne, decreased sweating, alopecia, hyperkeratosis, pruritus, skin exfoliation. *Rare:* bullous eruption, skin ulceration, aggravated psoriasis, furunculosis, verruca, dermatitis lichenoid, hypertrichosis, genital pruritus, urticaria.

Cardiovascular Disorders: Infrequent: palpitation, hypertension, hypotension, AV block, myocardial infarction. *Rare:* ventricular tachycardia, angina pectoris, premature atrial contractions, T wave inversions, ventricular extrasystoles, ST depression, myocarditis.

Vision Disorders: Infrequent: abnormal accommodation, xerophthalmia. *Rare:* diplopia, eye pain, blepharitis, photopsia, photophobia, abnormal lacrimation.

Metabolic and Nutritional Disorders: Infrequent: hyponatremia, weight increase, creatine phosphokinase increase, thirst, weight decrease, diabetes mellitus. *Rare:* decreased serum iron, cachexia, dehydration, hypokalemia, hypoproteinemia, hyperphosphatemia, hypertriglyceridemia, hyperuricemia, hypoglycemia.

Urinary System Disorders: Frequent: polyuria/polydipsia*. *Infrequent:* urinary incontinence, hematuria, dysuria. *Rare:* urinary retention, cystitis, renal insufficiency.

Musculo-skeletal System Disorders: Infrequent: myalgia. *Rare:* arthrosis, synostosis, bursitis, arthritis, skeletal pain.

Reproductive Disorders, Female: Frequent: menorrhagia*, orgastic dysfunction*, dry vagina*. *Infrequent:* nonpuerperal lactation, amenorrhea, female breast pain, leukorrhea, mastitis, dysmenorrhea, female perineal pain, intermenstrual bleeding, vaginal hemorrhage.

Liver and Biliary System Disorders: Infrequent: increased SGOT, increased SGPT. *Rare:* hepatic failure, cholestatic hepatitis, cholecystitis, cholelithiasis, hepatitis, hepatocellular damage.

Platelet, Bleeding and Clotting Disorders: Infrequent: epistaxis, purpura. *Rare:* hemorrhage, superficial phlebitis, thrombophlebitis, thrombocytopenia.

Hearing and Vestibular Disorders: Rare: tinnitus, hyperacusis, decreased hearing.

Red Blood Cell Disorders: Infrequent: anemia, hypochromic anemia. *Rare:* normocytic anemia.

Reproductive Disorders, Male: Frequent: erectile dysfunction*. *Infrequent:* ejaculation failure.

White Cell and Resistance Disorders: Rare: leukocytosis, lymphadenopathy, leucopenia, Pelger-Huet anomaly.

Endocrine Disorders: Rare: gynecomastia, male breast pain, antidiuretic hormone disorder.

Special Senses: Rare: bitter taste.

DRUG ABUSE AND DEPENDENCE
Controlled Substance Class: Risperidone is not a controlled substance.

Physical and Psychologic Dependence: Risperidone has not been systematically studied in animals or humans for its potential for abuse, tolerance or physical dependence. While the clinical trials did not reveal any tendency for any drug-seeking behavior, these observations were not systematic and it is not possible to predict on the basis of this limited experience the extent to which a CNS-active drug will be misused, diverted and/or abused once marketed. Consequently, patients should be evaluated carefully for a history of drug abuse, and such patients should be observed closely for signs of Risperidone misuse or abuse (e.g., development of tolerance, increases in dose, drug-seeking behavior).

OVERDOSAGE
Human Experience: Experience with Risperidone in acute overdosage was limited in the premarketing database (8 reports), with estimated doses ranging from 20 to 300 mg and no fatalities. In general, reported signs and symptoms were those resulting from an exaggeration of the drug's known pharmacological effects, i.e., drowsiness and sedation, tachycardia and hypotension, and extrapyramidal symptoms. One case, involving an estimated overdose of 240 mg, was associated with hyponatremia, hypokalemia, prolonged QT, and widened QRS. Another case, involving an estimated overdose of 36 mg, was associated with a seizure.

Management of Overdosage: In case of acute overdosage, establish and maintain an airway and ensure adequate oxygenation and ventilation. Gastric lavage (after intubation, if patient is unconscious) and administration of activated charcoal together with a laxative should be considered. The possibility of obtundation, seizures or dystonic reaction of the head and neck following overdose may create a risk of aspiration with induced emesis. Cardiovascular monitoring should commence immediately and should include continuous electrocardiographic monitoring to detect possible arrhythmias. If antiarrhythmic therapy is administered, disopyramide, procainamide and quinidine carry a theoretical hazard of QT-prolonging effects that might be additive to those of Risperidone. Similarly, it

is reasonable to expect that the alpha-blocking properties of bretylium might be additive to those of Risperidone, resulting in problematic hypotension.

There is no specific antidote to Risperidone. Therefore appropriate supportive measures should be instituted. The possibility of multiple drug involvement should be considered. Hypotension and circulatory collapse should be treated with appropriate measures such as intravenous fluids and/or sympathomimetic agents (epinephrine and dopamine should not be used, since beta stimulation may worsen hypotension in the setting of Risperidone-induced alpha blockade). In cases of severe extrapyramidal symptoms, anticholinergic medication should be administered. Close medical supervision and monitoring should continue until the patient recovers.

DOSAGE AND ADMINISTRATION
Usual Initial Dose: Risperidone should be administered on a BID schedule, generally beginning with 1 mg BID initially, with increases in increments of 1 mg BID on the second and third day, as tolerated, to a target dose of 3 mg BID by the third day. Further dosage adjustments, if indicated, should generally occur at intervals of not less than 1 week, since steady state for the active metabolite would not be achieved for approximately 1 week in the typical patient. When dosage adjustments are necessary, small dose increments/decrements of 1 mg BID are recommended.

Antipsychotic efficacy was demonstrated in a dose range of 4 to 16 mg/day in the clinical trials supporting effectiveness of Risperidone, however, maximal effect was generally seen in a range of 4 to 6 mg/day. Doses above 6 mg/day were not demonstrated to be more efficacious than lower doses, were associated with more extrapyramidal symptoms and other adverse effects, and are not generally recommended. The safety of doses above 16 mg/day has not been evaluated in clinical trials.

Dosage in Special Populations: The recommended initial dose is 0.5 mg BID in patients who are elderly or debilitated, patients with severe renal or hepatic impairment, and patients either predisposed to hypotension or for whom hypotension would pose a risk. Dosage increases in these patients should be in increments of 0.5 mg BID. Dosage increases above 1.5 mg BID should generally occur at intervals of not less than 1 week. Elderly or debilitated patients, and patients with renal impairment, may have less ability to eliminate Risperidone than normal adults. Patients with impaired hepatic function may have increases in the free fraction of the Risperidone, possibly resulting in an enhanced effect (see "Clinical Pharmacology"). Patients with a predisposition to hypotensive reactions or for whom such reactions would pose a particular risk likewise need to be titrated cautiously and carefully monitored (see "Precautions").

Maintenance Therapy: While there is no body of evidence available to answer the question of how long the patient treated with Risperidone should remain on it, the effectiveness of maintenance treatment is well established for many other antipsychotic drugs. It is recommended that responding patients be continued on Risperidone, but at the lowest dose needed to maintain remission. Patients should be periodically reassessed to determine the need for maintenance treatment.

Reinitiation of Treatment in Patients Previously Discontinued: Although there are no data to specifically address reinitiation of treatment, it is recommended that when restarting patients who have had an interval off Risperidone, the initial 3-day dose titration schedule should be followed.

Switching from Other Antipsychotics: Although there are no data to specifically address switching from other antipsychotics to Risperidone, immediate discontinuation of the previous antipsychotic treatment upon initiation of Risperidone therapy is recommended when medically appropriate. In all cases, the period of overlapping antipsychotic administration should be minimized. When switching patients from depot antipsychotics, initiate Risperidone therapy in place of the next scheduled injection. The need for continuing existing EPS medications should be reevaluated periodically.

Storage and Handling: Risperidone should be stored at room temperature (59°-86°F/15°-30°C). Risperidone should be protected from light and moisture.

HOW SUPPLIED
TABLETS: 1 MG

BRAND/MANUFACTURER	NDC	SIZE	AWP
○ BRAND			
▶ RISPERDAL: Janssen	50458-0300-06	60s	$113.76
	50458-0300-01	100s ud	$189.60

TABLETS: 2 MG

BRAND/MANUFACTURER	NDC	SIZE	AWP
○ BRAND			
▶ RISPERDAL: Janssen	50458-0320-06	60s	$189.36
	50458-0320-01	100s ud	$315.60

TABLETS: 3 MG

BRAND/MANUFACTURER	NDC	SIZE	AWP
○ BRAND			
▶ RISPERDAL: Janssen	50458-0330-06	60s	$236.88
	50458-0330-01	100s ud	$394.80

◆ RATED THERAPEUTICALLY EQUIVALENT; ◇ THERAPEUTIC EQUIVALENCE UNCONFIRMED; ○ UNRATED

TABLETS: 4 MG

BRAND/MANUFACTURER

	NDC	SIZE	AWP
○ **BRAND**			
▶ RISPERDAL: Janssen	50458-0350-06	60s	$315.36
	50458-0350-01	100s ud	$525.60

Ritalin *SEE* METHYLPHENIDATE HYDROCHLORIDE

Ritodrine Hydrochloride

DESCRIPTION

Ritodrine Hydrochloride, which contains a betamimetic (beta sympathomimetic amine), is available in two dosage forms. Ritodrine Hydrochloride for parenteral (intravenous) use is a clear, colorless, sterile, aqueous solution; each milliliter contains either 10 mg or 15 mg of Ritodrine Hydrochloride.

FOR INTRAVENOUS USE ONLY. MUST BE DILUTED BEFORE USE. FOR DOSAGE AND ADMINISTRATION INSTRUCTIONS, SEE PRODUCT INFORMATION BELOW. DO NOT USE IF INJECTION IS DISCOLORED OR CONTAINS A PRECIPITATE.

Each Ritodrine Hydrochloride tablet contains 10 mg of Ritodrine Hydrochloride.

Ritodrine Hydrochloride is a white, odorless crystalline powder, freely soluble in water, with a melting point between 196° and 205°C. The chemical name of Ritodrine Hydrochloride is erythro-p-hydroxy-α-[1[p-hydroxyphenethyl)-amino]ethyl] benzyl alcohol Hydrochloride.

Following is its chemical structure:

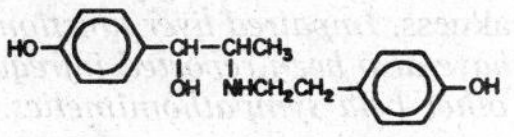

CLINICAL PHARMACOLOGY

Ritodrine Hydrochloride is a beta-receptor agonist, which has been shown by *in vitro* and *in vivo* pharmacologic studies in animals to exert a preferential effect on the β_2 adrenergic receptors such as those in the uterine smooth muscle. Stimulation of the β_2 receptors inhibits contractility of the uterine smooth muscle.

In humans, intravenous infusions of 0.05 to 0.30 mg/min. or single oral doses of 10 to 20 mg decreased the intensity and frequency of uterine contractions. These effects were antagonized by beta-blocking compounds. Intravenous administration induced an immediate dose-related elevation of heart rate with maximum mean increases between 19 and 40 beats per minute. Widening of the pulse pressure was also observed; the average increase in systolic blood pressure was 4.0 mm Hg, and the average decrease in diastolic pressure was 12.3 mm Hg With oral intake, the increase in heart rate was mild and delayed.

During intravenous infusion in humans, transient elevations of blood glucose, insulin, and free fatty acids have been observed. Decreased serum potassium has also been found, but effects on other electrolytes have not been reported.

Serum kinetics in humans (nonpregnant females) of an intravenous infusion of 60 minutes duration were determined by measuring serum Ritodrine levels by a radioimmunoassay technique. The distribution half-life was found to be 6 to 9 minutes, and the effective half-life 1.7 to 2.6 hours. In a study of serum kinetics after oral ingestion (male subjects), the decline of serum drug levels could be described in terms of a two-phase decay with an initial half-life of 1.3 hours and a final half-life of 12 hours. With either route of administration, 90% of the excretion was completed within 24 hours after the dose.

Comparison of Ritodrine serum levels after intravenous administration with those after oral dosage indicates the oral bioavailability is about 30%. Intravenous infusion at a rate of 0.15 mg./min. for 1 hour yielded maximum serum levels ranging between 32 and 52 ng./mL in a group of 6 non-pregnant female volunteers; maximum serum levels following single and repeated (4 × 10 mg/24 hr.) 10 mg. oral doses ranged between 5 and 15 ng/mL and were obtained within 30 to 60 minutes after ingestion.

Placental transfer was confirmed by measurement of drug concentrations in cord blood showing that Ritodrine and its conjugates reach the fetal circulation.

INDICATIONS AND USAGE

Ritodrine Hydrochloride is indicated for the management of preterm labor in suitable patients.

Administered intravenously, the drug will decrease uterine activity and thus prolong gestation in the majority of such patients. After intravenous Ritodrine Hydrochloride has arrested the acute episode, oral administration may help to avert relapse. Additional acute episodes may be treated by repeating the intravenous infusion. The incidence of neonatal mortality and respiratory distress syndrome increases when the normal gestation period is shortened.

Since successful inhibition of labor is more likely with early treatment, therapy with Ritodrine Hydrochloride should be instituted as soon as the diagnosis of preterm labor is established and contraindications ruled out in pregnancies of 20 or more weeks' gestation. The efficacy and safety of Ritodrine Hydrochloride in advanced labor, that is, when cervical dilatation is more than 4 cm or effacement is more than 80%, have not been established.

CONTRAINDICATIONS

Ritodrine Hydrochloride is contraindicated before the 20th week of pregnancy.

Ritodrine Hydrochloride is also contraindicated in those conditions of the mother or fetus in which continuation of pregnancy is hazardous specific contraindications include:
1. Antepartum hemorrhage which demands immediate delivery
2. Eclampsia and severe preeclampsia
3. Intrauterine fetal death
4. Chorioamnionitis
5. Maternal cardiac disease
6. Pulmonary hypertension
7. Maternal hyperthyroidism
8. Uncontrolled maternal diabetes mellitus (See *"Precautions"*.)
9. Pre-existing maternal medical conditions that would be seriously affected by the known pharmacologic properties of a betamimetic drug; such as: hypovolemia, cardiac arrhythmias associated with tachycardia or digitalis intoxication, uncontrolled hypertension, pheochromocytoma, bronchial asthma already treated by betamimetics and/or steroids
10. Known hypersensitivity to any component of the product.

WARNINGS

MATERNAL PULMONARY EDEMA HAS BEEN REPORTED IN PATIENTS TREATED WITH RITODRINE HYDROCHLORIDE SOMETIMES AFTER DELIVERY. IT HAS OCCURRED MORE OFTEN WHEN PATIENTS WERE TREATED CONCOMITANTLY WITH CORTICOSTEROIDS. MATERNAL DEATH FROM THIS CONDITION HAS BEEN REPORTED WITH OR WITHOUT CORTICOSTEROIDS GIVEN CONCOMITANTLY WITH DRUGS OF THIS CLASS.

PATIENTS SO TREATED MUST BE CLOSELY MONITORED IN THE HOSPITAL. THE PATIENT'S STATE OF HYDRATION SHOULD BE CAREFULLY MONITORED: FLUID OVERLOAD MUST BE AVOIDED. (SEE *"DOSAGE AND ADMINISTRATION"*.) INTRAVENOUS FLUID LOADING MAY BE AGGRAVATED BY THE USE OF BETAMIMETICS WITH OR WITHOUT CORTICOSTEROIDS AND MAY TURN INTO MANIFEST CIRCULATORY OVERLOADING WITH SUBSEQUENT PULMONARY EDEMA. IF PULMONARY EDEMA DEVELOPS DURING ADMINISTRATION, THE DRUG SHOULD BE DISCONTINUED. EDEMA SHOULD BE MANAGED BY CONVENTIONAL MEANS.

Intravenous administration of Ritodrine Hydrochloride should be supervised by persons having knowledge of the pharmacology of the drug and who are qualified to identify and manage complications of drug administration and pregnancy. Beta-adrenergic drugs increase cardiac output, and even in a normal healthy heart this added myocardial oxygen demand can sometimes lead to myocardial ischemia. Complications may include: myocardial necrosis, which may result in death; arrhythmias, including premature atrial and ventricular contractions, ventricular tachycardia, and bundle branch block; anginal pain, with or without ECG changes. *Because cardiovascular responses are common and more pronounced during intravenous administration of Ritodrine Hydrochloride cardiovascular effects, including maternal pulse rate and blood pressure and fetal heart rate, should be closely monitored. Care should be exercised for maternal signs and symptoms of pulmonary edema. A persistent high tachycardia (over 140 beats per minute) may be one of the signs of impending pulmonary edema with drugs of this class. Occult cardiac disease may be unmasked with the use of Ritodrine Hydrochloride. If the patient complains of chest pain or tightness of chest, the drug should be temporarily discontinued and an ECG should be done as soon as possible.* The drug should not be administered to patients with mild to moderate preeclampsia, hypertension, or diabetes unless the attending physician considers that the benefits clearly outweigh the risks.

Ritodrine Hydrochloride Injection contains sodium metabisulfite, a sulfite that may cause serious allergic-type reactions including anaphylactic symptoms and life-threatening or less severe asthmatic episodes in certain susceptible people. The overall prevalence of sulfite sensitivity in the general population is unknown and probably low. Sulfite sensitivity is seen more frequently in asthmatic than in nonasthmatic people.

PRECAUTIONS

When Ritodrine Hydrochloride is used for the management of preterm labor in a patient with premature rupture of the membranes, the benefits of delaying delivery should be balanced against the potential risks of development of chorioamnionitis.

Among low birth weight infants, approximately 9% may be growth retarded for gestational age. Therefore, Intra-Uterine Growth Retardation (IUGR) should be considered in the differential diagnosis of preterm labor; this is especially important when the gestational age is in doubt. The decision to continue or reinitiate the administration of Ritodrine Hydrochloride will depend on an assessment of fetal maturity. In addition to clinical parameters, other studies, such as sonography or amniocentesis, may be helpful in establishing the state of fetal maturity if it is in doubt.

BASELINE EKG
This should be done to rule out occult maternal heart disease.

LABORATORY TESTS
Because intravenous administration of Ritodrine Hydrochloride has been shown to elevate plasma insulin and glucose and to decrease plasma potassium

concentrations, monitoring of glucose and electrolyte levels is recommended during protracted infusions. Decrease of plasma potassium concentrations is usually transient, returning to normal within 24 hours. Special attention should be paid to biochemical variables when treating diabetic patients or those receiving potassium-depleting diuretics.

Serial hemograms may be helpful as an index of state of hydration.

DRUG INTERACTIONS
Corticosteroids used concomitantly may lead to pulmonary edema. (See *"Warnings".*)

Cardiovascular effects of Ritodrine Hydrochloride injection (especially cardiac arrhythmia or hypotension) may be potentiated by concomitant use of the following drugs.

1. magnesium sulfate
2. diazoxide
3. meperidine
4. potent general anesthetic agents

Systemic hypertension may be exaggerated in the presence of parasympatholytic agents such as atropine.

The effects of other sympathomimetic amines may be potentiated when concurrently administered and these effects may be additive. A sufficient time interval should elapse prior to administration of another sympathomimetic drug. With either oral or intravenous administration, 90% of the excretion of Ritodrine Hydrochloride is completed within 24 hours after the dose.

(See *"Clinical Pharmacology".*)

Beta-adrenergic blocking drugs inhibit the action of Ritodrine Hydrochloride; coadministration of these drugs should, therefore, be avoided.

With anesthetics used in surgery, the possibility that hypotensive effects may be potentiated should be considered.

MIGRAINE HEADACHE
Transient cerebral ischemia associated with beta sympathomimetic therapy has been reported in two patients with migraine headache.

CARCINOGENESIS, MUTAGENESIS, IMPAIRMENT OF FERTILITY
In rats given oral doses of 1, 10 and 150 mg/kg/day of Ritodrine Hydrochloride for 82 weeks, benign and malignant tumors were found in the various dosage groups. Since there were no important differences between untreated controls and treated groups and no dose-related trends, it was concluded that there was no evidence of tumorigenicity. The incidence (2-4%) of tumors of the type found in this study is not unusual in this species.

Reproduction studies in rats and rabbits have revealed no evidence of impaired fertility due to Ritodrine Hydrochloride.

PREGNANCY
Teratogenic Effects: (Pregnancy Category B): Reproduction studies were performed in rats and rabbits. The doses employed intravenously were +1/9 (1 mg/kg), ⅓ (3 mg/kg), and 1 (9 mg/kg) times the maximum human daily intravenous dose (but given to the animals as a bolus rather than by infusion). The oral doses, 10 and 100 mg/kg represented 5 and 50 times the maximum human daily oral maintenance dose. The results of these studies have revealed no evidence of impaired fertility or harm to the fetus due to Ritodrine Hydrochloride.

No adverse fetal effects were encountered when single intravenous doses of 1, 3, and 9 mg/kg/day or oral doses of 10 and 100 mg/kg/day were given to rats and rabbits on Days 6 through 15 and 6 through 18 of gestation, respectively. Intravenous doses of 1 and 8 mg/kg/day or oral doses of 10 and 100 mg/kg/day administered to the mother from Day 15 of pregnancy to Day 21 postpartum did not affect perinatal or postnatal development in rats. A slight increase in fetal weight in the rat was observed. Oral administration to both sexes did not impair fertility or reproductive performance. Lethal doses to pregnant rats did not cause immediate fetal demise. There are no adequate and well-controlled studies of Ritodrine Hydrochloride effects in pregnant women before 20 weeks' gestation; *therefore, this drug should not be used before the 20th week of pregnancy.* Studies of Ritodrine Hydrochloride administered to pregnant women from the 20th week of gestation have not shown increased risk of fetal abnormalities. Follow-up of selected variables in a small number of children for up to 2 years has not revealed harmful effects on growth, developmental or functional maturation. Nonetheless, although clinical studies did not demonstrate a risk of permanent adverse fetal effects from Ritodrine Hydrochloride the possibility cannot be excluded; therefore Ritodrine Hydrochloride should be used only when clearly indicated.

Some studies indicate that infants born before 36 weeks' gestation make up less than 10% of all births but account for as many as 75% of perinatal deaths and one-half of all neurologically handicapped infants. There are data available indicating that infants born at any time prior to full term may manifest a higher incidence of neurologic or other handicaps than occurs in the total population of infants born at or after full term. In delaying or preventing preterm labor, the use of Ritodrine Hydrochloride should result in an overall increase in neonatal survival. Handicapped infants who might not have otherwise survived may survive.

ADVERSE REACTIONS
The unwanted effects of Ritodrine Hydrochloride are related to its betamimetic activity and usually are controlled by suitable dosage adjustment.

EFFECTS ASSOCIATED WITH INTRAVENOUS ADMINISTRATION
Usual Effects (80-100% of Patients): Intravenous infusion of Ritodrine Hydrochloride leads almost invariably to dose-related alterations in maternal and fetal heart rates and in maternal blood pressure. During clinical studies in which the maximum infusion rate was limited to 0.35 mg/min (one patient received 0.40 mg/min), the maximum maternal and fetal heart rates averaged, respectively, 130 (range 60 to 180) and 164 (range 130 to 200) beats per minute. The maximum maternal systolic blood pressures averaged 128 mm Hg (range 96 to 162 mm Hg), an average increase of 12 mm Hg from pretreatment levels. The minimum maternal diastolic blood pressures averaged 48 mm Hg (range 0 to 76 mm Hg), an average decrease of 23 mm Hg from pretreatment levels. While the more severe effects were usually managed effectively by dosage adjustments, in less than 1% of patients, persistent maternal tachycardia or decreased diastolic blood pressure required withdrawal of the drug. A persistent high tachycardia (over 140 beats per minute) may be one of the signs of impending pulmonary edema. (See *"Warnings".*)

Ritodrine Hydrochloride infusion is associated with transient elevation of blood glucose and insulin, which decreases toward normal values after 48 to 72 hours despite continued infusion. Elevation of free fatty acids and cAMP has been reported. Reduction of potassium levels should be expected; other biochemical effects have not been reported.

Frequent Effects (10-50% of Patients): Intravenous Ritodrine Hydrochloride in about one-third of the patients, was associated with palpitation. Tremor, nausea, vomiting, headache, or erythema was observed in 10 to 15% of patients.

Occasional Effects (5-10% of Patients): Nervousness, jitteriness, restlessness, emotional upset, or anxiety was reported in 5 to 6% of patients and malaise in similar numbers.

Infrequent Effects (1-3% of Patients): Cardiac symptoms including chest pain or tightness (rarely associated with abnormalities of ECG) and arrhythmia were reported in 1 to 2% of patients. (See *"Warnings".*)

Other infrequently reported maternal effects included: anaphylactic shock, rash, heart murmur, epigastric distress, ileus, bloating, constipation, diarrhea, dyspnea, hyperventilation, hemolytic icterus, glycosuria, lactic acidosis, sweating, chills, drowsiness, and weakness. *Impaired liver function (i.e., increased transaminase levels and hepatitis) have also been reported infrequently (less than 1%) with the use of Ritodrine and other beta sympathomimetics.*

NEONATAL EFFECTS
Infrequently reported neonatal symptoms include hypoglycemia and ileus. In addition, hypocalcemia and hypotension have been reported in neonates whose mothers were treated with other betamimetic agents.

EFFECTS ASSOCIATED WITH ORAL ADMINISTRATION
Frequent Effects (< 50% of Patients): Oral Ritodrine in clinical studies was often associated with small increases in maternal heart rate, but little or no effect upon either maternal systolic or diastolic blood pressure or upon fetal heart rate was found.

Oral Ritodrine in 10 to 15% of patients was associated with palpitation or tremor. Nausea and jitteriness were less frequent (5 to 8%), while rash was observed in some patients (3 to 4%), and arrhythmia was infrequent (about 1%). *Impaired liver function (i.e., increased transaminase levels and hepatitis) have also been reported infrequently (less than 1%) with the use of Ritodrine and other beta sympathomimetics.*

OVERDOSAGE
The symptoms of overdosage are those of excessive beta-adrenergic stimulation including exaggeration of the known pharmacologic effects, the most prominent being tachycardia (maternal and fetal), palpitation, cardiac arrhythmia, hypotension, dyspnea, nervousness, tremor, nausea, and vomiting. If an excess of Ritodrine tablets is ingested, gastric lavage or induction of emesis should be carried out followed by administration of activated charcoal. When symptoms of overdose occur as a result of intravenous administration, Ritodrine should be discontinued; an appropriate beta-blocking agent may be used as an antidote. Ritodrine Hydrochloride is dialyzable.

Acute intravenous toxicity was studied in rats and rabbits and acute oral toxicity in mice, rats, guinea pigs, and dogs. The LD50 values in the most sensitive of the species used were 64 mg/kg intravenously in the nonpregnant rabbit and 540 mg/kg orally in the nonpregnant mouse. The intravenous LD50 value in the pregnant rat was 85 mg/kg The amount of drug required to produce symptoms of overdose in humans is individually variable. No reports of human mortality due to overdose have been received.

DOSAGE AND ADMINISTRATION
In the management of preterm labor, the initial intravenous treatment should usually be followed by oral administration. The optimum dose of Ritodrine Hydrochloride is determined by a clinical balance of uterine response and unwanted effects.

INTRAVENOUS THERAPY
Do not use intravenous Ritodrine Hydrochloride if the solution is discolored or contains any precipitate or particulate matter. Ritodrine Hydrochloride injection should be used promptly after preparation, but in no case after 48 hours of preparation.

Method of Administration: To minimize the risks of hypotension, the patient should be maintained in the left lateral position throughout infusion and careful attention given to her state of hydration, but fluid overload must be avoided. For appropriate control and dose titration, a controlled infusion device is recommended to adjust the rate of flow in drops/minute. An IV microdrip chamber (60 drops/mL) can provide a convenient range of infusion rates within the recommended dose range for Ritodrine Hydrochloride.

Recommended Dilution: 150 mg Ritodrine Hydrochloride in 500 mL fluid yielding a final concentration of 0.3 mg/mL*. Ritodrine for intravenous infusion should be diluted with 5% w/v dextrose solution. Because of the increased probability of pulmonary edema, saline diluents such as:

—0.9% w/v sodium chloride solution,

—compound sodium chloride solution (Ringer's solution)

—and Hartmann's solution, should be reserved for cases where dextrose solution is medically undesirable e.g. diabetes mellitus.

Intravenous therapy should be started as soon as possible after diagnosis. The usual initial dose is 0.1 mg/minute (0.33 mL/min, 20 drops/min using a microdrip chamber at the recommended dilution), to be gradually increased according to the results by 0.05 mg/minute (0.17 mL/min., 10 drops/min. using a microdrip chamber at the recommended dilution) every 10 minutes until the desired result is attained. The effective dosage usually lies between 0.15 and 0.35 mg/minute (0.50 to 1.17 mL/min, 30-70 drops/min using a microdrip chamber at the recommended dilution). Frequent monitoring of maternal uterine contractions, heart rate, and blood pressure, and of fetal heart rate is required, with dosage individually titrated according to response. If other drugs need to be given intravenously, the use of "piggyback" or other site of intravenous administration permits the continued independent control of the rate of infusion of the Ritodrine Hydrochloride.

The infusion should generally be continued for at least 12 hours after uterine contractions cease. With the recommended dilution, the maximum volume of fluid that might be administered after 12 hours at the highest dose (0.35 mg/min) will be approximately 840 mL.

The amount of IV fluids administered and the rate of administration should be monitored to avoid circulatory fluid overload (over-hydration). (See "Precautions, Laboratory Tests".)

ORAL MAINTENANCE

One tablet (10 mg) may be given approximately 30 minutes before the termination of intravenous therapy. The usual dosage schedule for the first 24 hours of oral administration is 1 tablet (10 mg) every two hours. Thereafter, the usual maintenance is 1 or 2 tablets (10 to 20 mg) every four to six hours, the dose depending on uterine activity and unwanted effects. The total daily dose of oral Ritodrine should not exceed 120 mg. The treatment may be continued as long as the physician considers it desirable to prolong pregnancy.

Recurrence of unwanted preterm labor may be treated with repeated infusion of Ritodrine Hydrochloride.

STORAGE

Both the tablet and intravenous dosage forms should be stored at room temperature, preferably below 86°F, (30°C). Protect from excessive heat.

HOW SUPPLIED
INJECTION: 10 MG/ML

AVERAGE UNIT PRICE (AVAILABLE SIZES)

BRAND			$17.40

BRAND/MANUFACTURER	NDC	SIZE	AWP
◆ BRAND			
YUTOPAR: Astra	00186-0569-13	5 ml 10s	$844.51
	00186-0599-03	5 ml 10s	$895.18
◆ GENERICS			
Abbott Hosp	00074-3193-01	5 ml 10s	$340.34

INJECTION: 15 MG/ML

BRAND/MANUFACTURER	NDC	SIZE	AWP
◆ BRAND			
YUTOPAR: Astra	00186-0597-12	10 ml	$220.23
◆ GENERICS			
Abbott Hosp	00074-3195-01	10 ml	$122.53

INJECTION: 150 MG

BRAND/MANUFACTURER	NDC	SIZE	AWP
◆ BRAND			
YUTOPAR: Astra	00186-0644-01	10 ml 10s	$216.05

TABLETS: 10 MG

BRAND/MANUFACTURER	NDC	SIZE	AWP
○ BRAND			
YUTOPAR: Astra	00186-0595-60	60s	$143.59
	00186-0595-78	100s ud	$256.18

Robaxin *SEE* METHOCARBAMOL

Robaxisal *SEE* ASPIRIN AND METHOCARBAMOL

* In those cases where fluid restriction is medically desirable, a more concentrated solution may be prepared.

Robinul *SEE* GLYCOPYRROLATE

Robitussin-AC *SEE* CODEINE PHOSPHATE WITH GUAIFENESIN

Robitussin-DAC *SEE* CODEINE PHOSPHATE/ GUAIFENESIN/PSEUDOEPHEDRINE HYDROCHLORIDE

Rocaltrol *SEE* CALCITRIOL

Rocephin *SEE* CEFTRIAXONE SODIUM

Rocuronium Bromide

This drug should be administered by adequately-trained individuals familiar with its actions, characteristics, and hazards.

DESCRIPTION
Rocuronium Bromide Injection is a non-depolarizing neuromuscular blocking agent with a rapid to intermediate onset depending on dose and intermediate duration. Rocuronium Bromide is chemically designated as 1[17β-(acetyloxy)-3α-hydroxy-2β-(4-morpho-linyl)-5α-androstan -16β-yl]-1-(2-propenyl)pyrrolidinium bromide.

The chemical formula is $C_{32}H_{53}BrN_2O_4$ with a molecular weight of 609.70. The partition coefficient of Rocuronium Bromide in n-octanol/water is 0.5 at 20°C.

Rocuronium Bromide Injection is supplied as a sterile, nonpyrogenic, isotonic solution for intravenous injection only. Each mL contains 10 mg Rocuronium Bromide and 2 mg soldium acetate. The aqueous solution is adjusted to isotonicity with sodium chloride and to a pH to 4 with acetic acid and/or sodium hydroxide.

Following is its chemical structure:

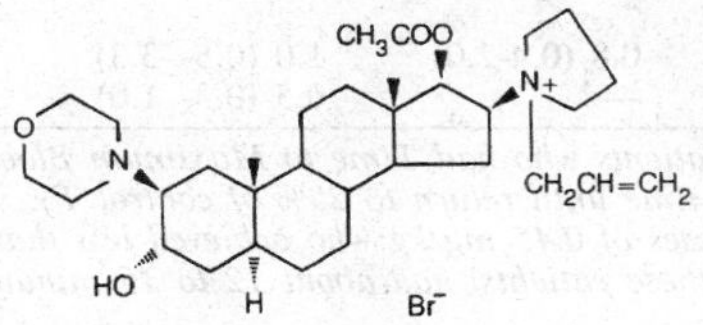

CLINICAL PHARMACOLOGY
Rocuronium Bromide Injection is a non-depolarizing neuromuscular blocking agent with a rapid to intermediate onset depending on dose and intermediate duration. It acts by competing for cholinergic receptors at the motor end-plate. This action is antagonized by acetylcholinesterase inhibitors, such as neostigmine and edrophonium.

Pharmacodynamics: The ED_{95}(dose required to produce 95% suppression of the first [T_1] mechanomyographic [MMG] response of the adductor pollicis muscle [thumb] to indirect supramaximal train-of-four stimulation of the ulnar nerve) during opioid/nitrous oxide/oxygen anesthesia is approximately 0.3 mg/kg. Patient variability around the ED_{95} dose suggests that 50% of patients will exhibit T_1 depressional of 91-97%.

Table 1 presents intubating conditions in patients with intubation initiated at 60 to 70 seconds.

Table 1
INTUBATING CONDITIONS IN PATIENTS WITH INTUBATION INITIATED AT 60 TO 70 SECONDS.
PERCENT, MEDIAN (RANGE)

Rocuronium Bromide Dose (mg/kg) Administered over 5 sec	Percent of patients with excellent or good intubating conditions	Time to completion of intubation (min)
Adults* 18-64 yr		
0.45 (n = 43)	86%	1.6 (1.0-7.0)
0.6 (n = 51)	96%	1.6 (1.0-3.2)
Pediatric 3 mo-1 yr		
0.6 (n = 18)	100%	1.0 (1.0-1.5)

➤ SHOWN IN PRODUCT IDENTIFICATION GUIDE

Rocuronium Bromide Dose (mg/kg) Administered over 5 sec	Percent of patients with excellent or good intubating conditions	Time to completion of intubation (min)
Pediatric 1-12 yr		
0.6 (n = 12)	100%	1.0 (0.5-2.3)

* *Excludes patients undergoing cesarean section*
Excellent intubating conditions = jaw relaxed, vocal cords apart and immobile, no diaphragmatic movement.
Good intubating conditions = same as excellent but with some diaphragmatic movement.

Table 2 presents the time to onset and clinical duration for the initial dose of Rocuronium Bromide under opioid/nitrous oxide/oxygen anesthesia in adults and geriatric patients, and under halothane anesthesia in children.

Table 2
TIME TO ONSET AND CLINICAL DURATION FOLLOWING INITIAL (INTUBATING) DOSE DURING OPIOID/NITROUS OXIDE/OXYGEN ANESTHESIA (ADULTS) AND HALOTHANE ANESTHESIA (CHILDREN), MEDIAN (RANGE)

Rocuronium Bromide Dose (mg/kg) Administered over 5 sec	Time to ≥ 80% Block (min)	Time to Maximum Block (min)	Clinical Duration (min)
Adults 18-64 yr			
0.45 (n = 50)	1.3 (0.8-6.2)	3.0 (1.3- 8.2)	22 (12-31)
0.6 (n = 142)	1.0 (0.4-6.0)	1.8 (0.6-13.0)	31 (15-85)
0.9 (n = 20)	1.1 (0.3-3.8)	1.4 (0.8- 6.2)	58 (27-111)
1.2 (n = 18)	0.7 (0.4-1.7)	1.0 (0.6- 4.7)	67 (38-160)
Geriatric ≥ 65 yr			
0.6 (n = 31)	2.3 (1.0-8.3)	3.7 (1.3-11.3)	46 (22-73)
0.9 (n = 5)	2.0 (1.0-3.0)	2.5 (1.2- 5.0)	62 (49-75)
1.2 (n = 7)	1.0 (0.8-3.5)	1.3 (1.2- 4.7)	94 (64-138)
Pediatric 3 mo-1 yr			
0.6 (n = 17)	—	0.8 (0.3- 3.0)	41 (24-68)
0.8 (n = 9)	—	0.7 (0.5- 0.8)	40 (27-70)
Pediatric 1-12 yr			
0.6 (n = 27)	0.8 (0.4-2.0)	1.0 (0.5- 3.3)	26 (17-39)
0.8 (n = 18)	—	0.5 (0.3- 1.0)	30 (17-56)

n - the number of patients who had Time to Maximum Block recorded.
Clinical duration = time until return to 25% of control T_1.
Patients receiving doses of 0.45 mg/kg who achieved less than 90% block (16% of these patients) had about 12 to 15 minutes to 25% recovery.

The time to ≥ 80% block and clinical duration as a function of dose are presented in Figures 1 and 2.

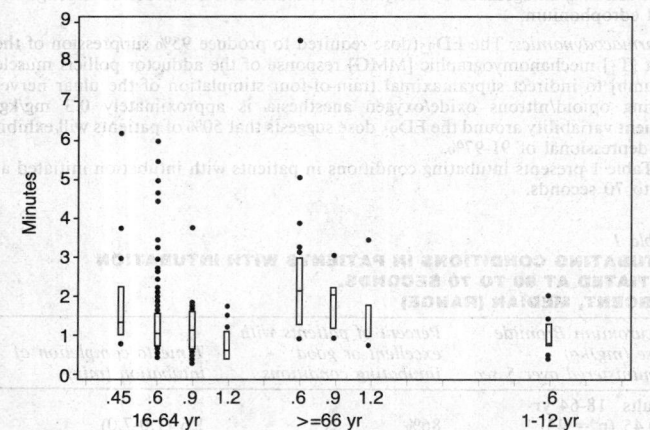

Figure 1. Time to ≥ 80% Block vs. Initial Dose of Rocuronium Bromide By Age Group (Median, 25th and 75th percentile, and individual values).

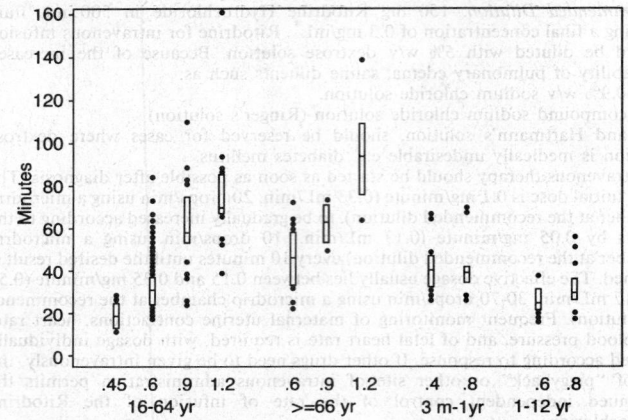

Figure 2. Duration of Clinical Effect vs. Initial Dose of Rocuronium Bromide By Age Group (Median, 25th and 75th percentile, and individual values).

The clinical durations for the first maintenance doses, in patients receiving five or more maintenance doses are represented in Figure 3 (see also *"Maintenance Dosing"* subsection of *"Dosage And Administration"*).

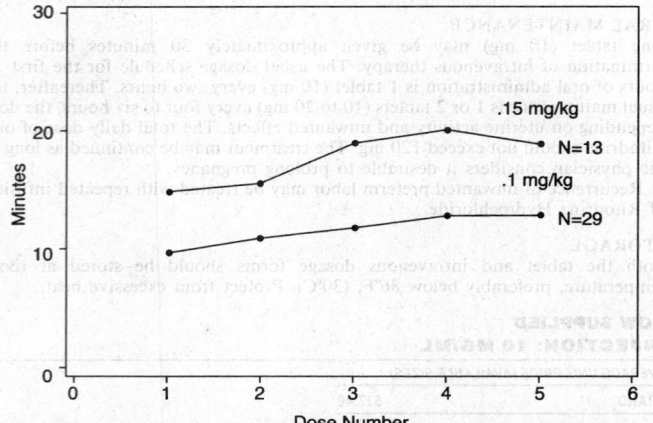

Figure 3. Duration of Clinical Effect vs. Number of Rocuronium Bromide Maintenance Doses, by Dose.

Once spontaneous recovery has reached 25% of control T_1, the neuromuscular block produced by Rocuronium Bromide is readily reversed with anticholinesterase agents, e.g., edrophonium or neostigmine.

The median spontaneous recovery from 25 to 75% T_1 was 13 minutes in adult patients. When neuromuscular block was reversed in 36 adults at a T_1 of 22-27%, recovery to a T_1 of 89 (50-132)% and T_4/T_1 of 69 (38-92)% was achieved within 5 minutes. Only five of 320 adults reversed received an additional dose of reversal agent. The median (range) dose of neostigmine was 0.04 (0.01 to 0.09) mg/kg and the median (range) dose of edrophonium was 0.5 (0.3 to 1.0) mg/kg.

In geriatric patients (n = 51) reversed with neostigmine, the median T_4/T_1 increased from 40 to 88% in 5 minutes.

Children (n = 27) who received 0.5 mg/kg edrophonium had increases in the median T_4/T_1 from 37% at reversal to 93% after 2 minutes. Children (n = 58) who received 1 mg/kg edrophonium had increases in the median T_4/T_1 from 72% at reversal to 100% after 2 minutes. Infants (n = 10) who were reversed with 0.03 mg/kg neostigmine recovered from 25 to 75% T_1 within 4 minutes.

There were no reports of less than satisfactory clinical recovery of neuromuscular function.

The neuromuscular blocking action of Rocuronium Bromide may be enhanced in the presence of potent inhalation anesthetics (see *"Inhalation Anesthetics"* subsection of *"Precautions"*). Hemodynamics: There were no dose-related effects on the incidence of changes from baseline (≥ 30%) in mean arterial blood pressure (MAP) or heart rate associated with Rocuronium Bromide Injection administration over the dose range of 0.12 to 1.2 mg/kg (4 x ED_{95}) within 5 minutes after Rocuronium Bromide administration and prior to intubation. Increases or decreases in MAP were observed in 2-5% of geriatric and other adult patients, and in about 1% of pediatric patients. Heart rate changes (≥ 30%) occurred in 0-2% of geriatric and other adult patients. Tachycardia (≥ 30%) occurred in 12 of 127 children. Most of the children developing tachycardia were from a single study where the patients were anesthetized with halothane and who did not receive atropine for induction (see *"Pediatric"* subsection of *"Clinical Trials"*). In U.S. studies, laryngoscopy and tracheal intubation following Rocuronium Bromide administration were accompanied by transient tachycardia (≥ 30% increases) in about one-third of adult patients under opioid/ nitrous oxide/oxygen anesthesia. Animal studies have indicated that the ratio of uromuscular block following Rocuronium Bromide administration is less than vecuronium but greater than pancuronium. The tachycardia observed in some patients may result from this vagal blocking activity.

Histamine Release: In studies of histamine release, clinically significant concentrations of plasma histamine occurred in 1 of 88 patients. Clinical signs of histamine release (flushing, rash, or bronchospasm) associated with the administration of Rocuronium Bromide Injection were assessed in clinical trials and reported in 9 of 1137 (0.8%) patients.

Pharmocokinetics: In an effort to maximize the information gathered in the in vivo pharmacokinetic studies, the data from the studies was used to develop population estimates of the parameters for the subpopulations represented (e.g., geriatric, pediatric, renal, and hepatic insufficiency). These population based estimates and a measure of the estimate variability are contained in the following section.

Following IV administration of Rocuronium Bromide Injection, plasma levels of Rocuronium follow a three compartment open model. The rapid distribution half-life is 1-2 minutes and the slower distribution half-life is 14-18 minutes. Rocuronium is approximately 30% bound to human plasma proteins. In geriatric and other adult surgical patients undergoing either opioid/nitrous oxide/oxygen or inhalational anesthesia the observed pharmacokinetic profile was essentially unchanged.

Table 3
PHARMACOKINETIC IN ADULTS (N = 22; AGES 27-58 YR) AND GERIATRIC (N = 20; ≥ 65 YR) DURING OPIOID/NITROUS OXIDE/OXYGEN ANESTHESIA (MEAN ± SD)

PK Parameters	Adults (Ages 27-58 yr)	Geriatrics (≥ 65 yr)
Clearance (L/kg/hr)	0.25 ± 0.08	0.21 ± 0.06
Volume of Distribution at Steady State (L/kg)	0.25 ± 0.04	0.22 ± 0.03
$T_{1/2}$ β Elimination (hr)	1.4 ± 0.4	1.5 ± 0.4

In general, studies with normal adult subjects did not reveal any differences in the pharmacokinetics of Rocuronium due to gender. Studies of distribution, metabolism, and excretion in cats and dogs indicate that Rocuronium is eliminated primarily by the liver. The Rocuronium analog 17-desacetyl-Rocuronium, a metabolite, has been rarely observed in the plasma or urine of humans administered single doses of 0.5-1 mg/kg with or without a subsequent infusion (for up to 12 hr) of Rocuronium. In the cat, 17-desacetyl-Rocuronium has approximately one-twentieth the neuromuscular blocking potency of Rocuronium. The effects of renal failure and hepatic disease on the pharmacokinetics and pharmacodynamics of Rocuronium in humans are consistent with these findings.

In general, patients undergoing cadaver kidney transplant have a small reduction in clearance which is offset pharmacokinetically by a corresponding increase in volume, such that the net effect is an unchanged plasma half-life. Patients with demonstrated liver cirrhosis have a marked increase in their volume of distribution resulting in a plasma half-life approximately twice that of patients with normal hepatic function. Table 4 shows the pharmacokinetic parameters in subjects with either impaired renal or hepatic function.

Table 4
PHARMACOKINETIC PARAMETERS IN ADULTS WITH NORMAL RENAL AND HEPATIC FUNCTION (N = 10, AGES 23-65). RENAL TRANSPLANT PATIENTS (N = 10, AGES 21-45) AND HEPATIC DYSFUNCTION PATIENTS (N = 9, AGES 31-67) DURING ISOFLURANE ANESTHESIA (MEAN ± SD)

PK Parameters	Normal Renal and Hepatic Function	Renal Transplant Patients	Hepatic Dysfunction Patients
Clearance (L/kg/hr)	0.16 ± 0.05*	0.13 ± 0.04	0.13 ± 0.06
Volume of Distribution at Steady State (L/kg)	0.26 ± 0.03	0.34 ± 0.11	0.53 ± 0.14
$T_{1/2}$ β Elimination (hr)	2.4 ± 0.8*	2.4 ± 1.1	4.3 ± 2.6

* Differences in the calculated $T_{1/2}$ β and Cl between this study and the study in young adults vs. geriatrics (≥ 65 years) is related to the different sample populations and anesthetic techniques.

The net result of these findings is that subjects with renal failure have clinical durations that are similar to but somewhat more variable than the duration that one would expect in subjects with normal renal function. Hepatically-impaired patients, due to the large increase in volume, may demonstrate clinical durations approaching 1.5 times that of subjects with normal hepatic function. In both populations the clinician should individualize the dose to the needs of the patient (see *"Individualization of Dosage"*).

Tissue redistribution accounts for most (about 80%) of the initial amount of Rocuronium administered. As tissue compartments fill with continued dosing (4-8 hours), less drug is redistributed away from the site of action and, for an infusion-only dose, the rate to maintain neuromuscular blockade falls to about 20% of the initial infusion rate. The use of a loading dose and a smaller infusion rate reduces the need for adjustment of dose.

Special Population—Pediatrics: The clinical duration of effects of Rocuronium Bromide Injection did not vary with age in patients 4 months to 8 years of age. The terminal half-life and other pharmacokinetic parameters of Rocuronium in these children are presented in Table 5.

Table 5
PHARMACOKINETIC PARAMETERS OF ROCURONIUM IN PEDIATRIC PATIENTS (AGES 3- < 12 MO, N = 6; 1- < 3 YR, N = 5; 3- < 8 YR, N = 7) DURING HALOTHANE ANESTHESIA (MEAN ± SD)

PK Parameters	Patient Age Range 3- < 12 mo	1- < 3 yr	3- < 8 yr
Clearance (L/kg/hr)	0.35 ± 0.08	0.32 ± 0.07	0.44 ± 0.16
Volume of Distribution of Steady State (L/kg)	0.30 ± 0.04	0.26 ± 0.06	0.21 ± 0.03
$T_{1/2}$ β Elimination (hr)	1.3 ± 0.5	1.1 ± 0.7	0.8 ± 0.3

CLINICAL TRIALS
In U.S. clinical trials a total of 1,137 patients received Rocuronium Bromide Injection including 176 pediatric, 140 geriatric, 55 obstetric, and 766 other adults. Most patients (90%) were ASA physical status I or II, about 9% were ASA III, and 10 patients (undergoing coronary artery bypass grafting or valvular surgery) were ASA IV. In European clinical trials, a total of 1,394 patients received Rocuronium Bromide including 52 pediatric, 128 geriatric (≥ 65 years) and 1,214 other adults.

Adult Patients: Intubation using doses of Rocuronium Bromide Injection 0.6 to 0.85 mg/kg was evaluated in 203 adults in 11 clinical trials. Excellent to good intubating conditions were generally achieved within 2 minutes and the maximum block occurred within 3 minutes in most patients. Doses within this range provide clinical relaxation for a median (range) time of 33 (14-85) minutes under opioid/nitrous oxide/oxygen anesthesia. Larger doses (0.9 and 1.2 mg/kg) were evaluated in two trials with 19 and 16 patients under opioid/nitrous oxide/oxygen anesthesia and provided 58 (27-111) and 67 (38-160) minutes of clinical relaxation, respectively.

Cardiovascular Disease: In one clinical trial, 10 patients with clinically significant cardiovascular disease undergoing coronary artery bypass graft received an initial dose of 0.6 mg/kg Rocuronium Bromide Injection. Neuromuscular block was maintained during surgery with bolus maintenance doses of 0.3 mg/kg. Following induction, continuous 0.008 mg/kg/min infusion of Rocuronium Bromide produced relaxation sufficient to support mechanical ventilation for 6 to 12 hours in the surgical intensive care unit (SICU) while the patients were recovering from surgery. Hypertension and tachycardia were reported in some patients but these occurrences were less frequent in patients receiving beta or calcium channel blocking drugs. In 7 of these 10 patients Rocuronium Bromide was associated with transient increases (≥ 30%) in pulmonary vascular resistance. In another clinical trial of 17 patients undergoing abdominal aortic surgery, transient increases (≥ 30%) in pulmonary vascular resistance were observed in 4 of 17 patients receiving Rocuronium Bromide 0.6 or 0.9 mg/kg.

Rapid Sequence Intubation: Intubating conditions were assessed in 230 patients in six clinical trials where anesthesia was induced with either thiopental (3 to 6 mg/kg) or propofol (1.5 to 2.5 mg/kg) in combination with either fentanyl (2 to 5 mcg/kg) or alfentanil (1 mg). Most of the patients also received a premedication such as midazolam or temazepam. Most patients had intubation attempted within 60 to 90 seconds of administration of Rocuronium Bromide Injection 0.6 mg/kg or succinylcholine 1 to 1.5 mg/kg. Excellent or good intubating conditions were achieved in 119/120 (99% [95% confidence interval 95-99.9%]) patients receiving Rocuronium Bromide and in 108/110 (98% [94-99.8%]) patients receiving succinylcholine. The duration of action of Rocuronium Bromide 0.6 mg/kg is longer than succinylcholine and at this dose is approximately equivalent to the duration of other intermediate acting neuromuscular blocking drugs.

Geriatric Patients: Rocuronium Bromide Injection was evaluated in 55 geriatric patients (ages 65-80 years) in six clinical trials. Doses of 0.6 mg/kg provided excellent to good intubating conditions in a median (range) time of 2.3 (1-8) minutes. Recovery times from 25% to 75% after these doses were not prolonged in geriatric patients compared to other adult patients.

Pediatric Patients: Rocuronium Bromide Injection 0.6 or 0.8 mg/kg was evaluated for intubation in 75 pediatric patients (n = 28; age 3-12 months, n = 47; age 1-12 years) in three trials using halothane (1-5%) nitrous oxide (60-70%) in oxygen. Of the children anesthetized with halothane who did not receive atropine for induction, about 80% experienced a transient increase (≥ 30%) in heart rate after intubation. One of the 19 infants anesthetized with halothane and fentanyl who received atropine for induction experienced this magnitude of change.

Obese Patients: Rocuronium Bromide Injection was dosed according to actual body weight (ABW) in most clinical trials. The administration of Rocuronium Bromide in the 47 of 330 (14%) patients who were at least 30% or more above their ideal body weight (IBW) was not associated with clinically significant differences in the onset, duration, recovery, or reversal of Rocuronium Bromide-induced neuromuscular block.

In one clinical trial in obese patients, Rocuronium Bromide 0.6 mg/kg was dosed according to ABW (n = 12) or IBW (n = 11). Obese patients dosed according to IBW had a longer time to maximum block, a shorter clinical duration of 25 (14-29) minutes, and did not achieve intubating conditions comparable to those dosed based on ABW. These results support the recommendation that obese patients be dosed based on actual body weight.

Obstetric Patients: Rocuronium Bromide Injection 0.6 mg/kg was administered with thiopental, 3-4 mg/kg (n = 13) or 4-6 mg/kg (n = 42), for rapid sequence induction of anesthesia for cesarean section. No neonate had APGAR scores < 7 at 5 minutes. The umbilical venous plasma concentrations were 18% of maternal concentrations at delivery. Intubating conditions were poor or inadequate in 5 of 13 women receiving 3-4 mg/kg thiopental when intubation was attempted 60 seconds after drug injection. Therefore, Rocuronium Bromide is not recommended for rapid sequence induction in cesarean section patients.

INDIVIDUALIZATION OF DOSAGE

Doses of Rocuronium Bromide Injection should be individualized and a peripheral nerve stimulator should be used to measure neuromuscular function during Rocuronium Bromide administration in order to monitor drug effect, determine the need for additional doses, and confirm recovery from neuromuscular block.

Based on the known actions of Rocuronium Bromide, the following factors should be considered when administering Rocuronium Bromide.

Renal or Hepatic Impairment: No differences from patients with normal hepatic and kidney function were observed for onset time at a dose of 0.6 mg/kg Rocuronium Bromide Injection. When compared to patients with normal renal and hepatic function, the mean clinical duration is similar in patients with end-stage renal disease undergoing renal transplant, and is about 1.5 times longer in patients with hepatic disease. Patients with renal failure may have a greater variation in duration of effect (see *"Pharmacokinetics"* subsection of *"Clinical Pharmacology"* and *"Renal Failure"* and *"Hepatic Disease"* subsections of *"Precautions"*).

Reduced Plasma Cholinesterase Activity: No differences from patients with normal plasma cholinesterase activity is expected since Rocuronium metabolism does not depend on plasma cholinesterase.

Drugs or Conditions Causing Potentiation of or Resistance to Neuromuscular Block: The neuromuscular blocking action of Rocuronium Bromide Injection is potentiated by isoflurane and enflurane anesthesia. Potentiation is minimal when administration of the recommended dose of Rocuronium Bromide occurs prior to the administration of these potent inhalation agents. The median clinical duration of a dose of 0.57-0.85 mg/kg was 34, 38, and 42 minutes under opioid/nitrous oxide/oxygen, enflurane and isoflurane maintenance anesthesia, respectively. During 1-2 hr of infusion, the infusion rate of Rocuronium Bromide required to maintain about 95% block was decreased by as much as 40% under enflurane and isoflurane anesthesia (see *"Inhalation Anesthetics"* subsection of *"Precautions"*).

When Rocuronium Bromide is administered to patients chronically receiving anticonvulsant agents such as carbamazepine or phenytoin, shorter durations of neuromuscular block may occur and infusion rates may be higher due to the development of resistance to nondepolarizing muscle relaxants (see *"Anticonvulsants"* subsection of *"Precautions"*).

Pulmonary Hypertension: Rocuronium Bromide Injection may be associated with increased pulmonary vascular resistance, so caution is appropriate in patients with pulmonary hypertension or valvular heart disease (see *"Clinical Trials"* subsection of *"Clinical Pharmacology"*).

Obesity: In obese patients, the initial dose of Rocuronium Bromide Injection 0.6 mg/kg should be based upon the patient's actual body weight (see *"Obese Patients"* subsection of *"Clinical Trials"*).

Based on the known actions of other nondepolarizing neuromuscular blocking agents the following additional factors should be considered when administering Rocuronium Bromide:

Drugs or Conditions Causing Potentiation of or Resistance to Neuromuscular Block: Resistance to nondepolarizing agents, consistent with up-regulation of skeletal muscle acetylcholine receptors, is associated with burns, disuse atrophy, denervation, and direct muscle trauma. Receptor up-regulation may also contribute to the resistance to non-depolarizing muscle relaxants which sometimes develops in patients with cerebral palsy, patients chronically receiving anticonvulsant agents such as carbamazepine or phenytoin or with chronic exposure to nondepolarizing agents (see *"Precautions"*).

Other nondepolarizing neuromuscular blocking agents have been found to exhibit profound neuromuscular blocking effects in cachectic or debilitated patients, patients with neuromuscular diseases, and patients with carcinomatosis. In these or other patients in whom potentiation of neuromuscular block or difficulty with reversal may be anticipated, a decrease from the recommended initial dose should be considered.

Certain antibiotics, magnesium salts, lithium, local anesthetics, procainamide, and quinidine have been shown to increase the duration of neuromuscular block and decrease infusion requirements of other neuromuscular blocking agents. In patients in whom potentiation of neuromuscular block may be anticipated, a decrease from the recommended initial dose should be considered (see *"Antibiotics"* and *"Other"* subsections of *"Precautions"*).

Severe acid-base and/or electrolyte abnormalities may potentiate or cause resistance to the neuromuscular blocking action of Rocuronium Bromide

Injection (see *"Other"* subsection of *"Precautions"*). No data are available in such patients and no dosing recommendations can be made.

Burns: Patients with burns are known to develop resistance to nondepolarizing neuromuscular blocking agents, probably due to up-regulation of postsynaptic skeletal muscle cholinergic receptors (see *"Individualization of Dosage"*).

INDICATIONS AND USAGE

Rocuronium Bromide Injection is a non-depolarizing neuromuscular blocking agent with a rapid to intermediate onset depending on dose and intermediate duration and is indicated for inpatients and outpatients as an adjunct to general anesthesia to facilitate both rapid sequence and routine tracheal intubation, and to provide skeletal muscle relaxation during surgery or mechanical ventilation.

CONTRAINDICATIONS

Rocuronium Bromide Injection is contraindicated in patients known to have hypersensitivity to Rocuronium Bromide.

WARNINGS

ROCURONIUM BROMIDE INJECTION SHOULD BE ADMINISTERED IN CAREFULLY ADJUSTED DOSAGES BY OR UNDER THE SUPERVISION OF EXPERIENCED CLINICIANS WHO ARE FAMILIAR WITH THE DRUG'S ACTIONS AND THE POSSIBLE COMPLICATIONS OF ITS USE. THE DRUG SHOULD NOT BE ADMINISTERED UNLESS FACILITIES FOR INTUBATION, ARTIFICIAL RESPIRATION, OXYGEN THERAPY, AND AN ANTAGONIST ARE IMMEDIATELY AVAILABLE. IT IS RECOMMENDED THAT CLINICIANS ADMINISTERING NEUROMUSCULAR BLOCKING AGENTS SUCH AS ROCURONIUM BROMIDE EMPLOY A PERIPHERAL NERVE STIMULATOR TO MONITOR DRUG RESPONSE, NEED FOR ADDITIONAL RELAXANT, AND ADEQUACY OF SPONTANEOUS RECOVERY OR ANTAGONISM.

ROCURONIUM BROMIDE HAS NO KNOWN EFFECT ON CONSCIOUSNESS, PAIN THRESHOLD, OR CEREBRATION. THEREFORE, ITS ADMINISTRATION MUST BE ACCOMPANIED BY ADEQUATE ANESTHESIA OR SEDATION.

In patients with myasthenia gravis or myasthenia gravis or myasthenic (Eaton-Lambert) syndrome, small doses of nondepolarizing neuromuscular blocking agents may have profound effects. In such patients, a peripheral nerve stimulator and use of a small test dose may be of value in monitoring the response to administration of muscle relaxants.

Rocuronium Bromide, which has an acid pH, should not be mixed with alkaline solutions (e.g., barbiturate solutions) in the same syringe or administered simultaneously during intravenous infusion through the same needle.

PRECAUTIONS

Long-term Use in I.C.U.: Rocuronium Bromide Injection has not been studied for long-term use in the I.C.U. As with other nondepolarizing neuromuscular blocking drugs, apparent tolerance to Rocuronium Bromide may develop rarely during chronic administration in the I.C.U. While the mechanism for development of this resistance is not known, receptor up-regulation may be a contributing factor. It is STRONGLY RECOMMENDED THAT NEUROMUSCULAR TRANSMISSION BE MONITORED CONTINUOUSLY DURING ADMINISTRATION AND RECOVERY WITH THE HELP OF A NERVE STIMULATOR. ADDITIONAL DOSES OF ROCURONIUM BROMIDE OR ANY OTHER NEUROMUSCULAR BLOCKING AGENT SHOULD NOT BE GIVEN UNTIL THERE IS A DEFINITE RESPONSE (ONE TWITCH OF THE TRAIN-OF-FOUR) TO NERVE STIMULATION. Prolonged paralysis and/or skeletal muscle weakness may be noted during initial attempts to wean from the ventilator patients who have chronically received neuromuscular blocking drugs in the I.C.U. Therefore, Rocuronium Bromide should only be used in this setting if, in the opinion of the prescribing physician, the specific advantages of the drug outweigh the risk.

Labor and Delivery: The use of Rocuronium Bromide Injection in cesarean section has been studied in a limited number of patients. Rocuronium Bromide is not recommended for rapid sequence induction in cesarean section patients (see *"Clinical Trials"* subsection of *"Clinical Pharmacology"*).

Hepatic Disease: Since Rocuronium Bromide Injection is primarily excreted by the liver it should be used with caution in patients with clinically significant heaptic disease. Rocuronium Bromide 0.6 mg/kg has been studied in a limited number of patients (n = 9) with clinically significant hepatic disease under steady-state isoflurane anesthesia. After Rocuronium Bromide 0.6 mg/kg, the median (range) clinical duration of 60 (35-166) minutes was moderately prolonged compared to 42 minutes in patients with normal hepatic function. The median recovery time of 53 minutes was also prolonged in patients with cirrhosis compared to 20 minutes in patients with normal hepatic function. Four of eight patients with cirrhosis, who received Rocuronium Bromide 0.6 mg/kg under opioid/nitrous oxide/oxygen anesthesia, did not achieve complete block. These findings are consistent with the increase in volume of distribution at steady state observed in patients with significant hepatic disease (see Pharmacokinetics subsection of *"Clinical Pharmacology"*). If used for rapid sequence induction in patients with ascites, an increased initial dosage may be necessary to assure complete block. Duration will be prolonged in these cases. The use of doses higher than 0.6 mg/kg has not been studied.

Renal Failure: Due to the limited role of the kidney in the excretion of Rocuronium Bromide Injection, usual dosing guidelines should be adequate. Rocuronium Bromide 0.6 mg/kg has been evaluated in three single center trials (n = 30, ages 19-61 years) in patients undergoing renal transplant surgery, or shunt

---

procedures in preparation for dialysis. After Rocuronium Bromide 0.6 mg/kg, the time to maximum block was about 1-2 minutes and was not different from patients without renal dysfunction. The mean ± SD clinical duration of 54 ± 22 minutes was not considered prolonged compared to 46 ± 12 minutes in normal patients: however, there was substantial variation (range, 22-90 minutes). The spontaneous recovery rate from 25 to 75% of control in renal dysfunction patients of 27 ± 11 minutes was similar to 28 ± 20 minutes in normal patients (see "Pharmacokinetics" subsection of "Clinical Pharmacology").

Malignant Hyperthermia (MH): Malignant hyperthermia has not been reported with the administration of Rocuronium Bromide Injection. Because Rocuronium Bromide is always used with other agents, and the occurrence of malignant hyperthermia during anesthesia is possible even in the absence of known triggering agents, clinicians should be familiar with early signs, confirmatory diagnosis and treatment of malignant hyperthermia prior to the start of any anesthetic. In an animal study in MH-susceptible swine, the administration of Rocuronium Bromide did not appear to trigger malignant hyperthermia.

Altered Circulation Time: Conditions associated with slower circulation time, e.g., cardiovascular disease or advanced age, may be associated with a delay in onset time. Because higher doses of Rocuronium Bromide Injection produce a longer duration of action, the initial dosage should usually not be increased in these patients to reduce onset time; instead, when feasible, more time should be allowed for the drug to achieve onset of effect.

Drug Interactions: The use of Rocuronium Bromide Injection before succinylcholine, for the purpose of attenuating some of the side effects of succinylcholine, has not been studied.

If Rocuronium Bromide is administered following administration of succinylcholine, it should not be given until recovery from succinylcholine has been observed. The median duration of action of Rocuronium Bromide 0.6 mg/kg administered after a 1 mg/kg dose of succinylcholine when T_1 returned to 75% of control was 36 minutes (range 14-57, n = 12) vs. 28 minutes (17-51, n = 12) without succinylcholine.

There are no controlled studies documenting the use of Rocuronium Bromide before or after other nondepolarizing muscle relaxants. Interactions have been observed when other non-depolarizing muscle relaxants have been administered in succession.

Inhalation Anesthetics: Use of inhalation anesthetics has been shown to enhance the activity of other neuromuscular blocking agents, enflurane > isoflurane > halothane.

Isoflurane and enflurane may also prolong the duration of action of initial and maintenance doses of Rocuronium Bromide Injection and decrease the average infusion requirement of Rocuronium Bromide by 40% compared to opioid/nitrous oxide/oxygen anesthesia. No definite interaction between Rocuronium Bromide and halothane has been demonstrated. In one study, use of enflurane in 10 patients resulted in a 20% increase in mean clinical duration of the initial intubating dose, and a 37% increase in the duration of subsequent maintenance doses, when compared in the same study to 10 patients under opioid/nitrous oxide/oxygen anesthesia. The clinical duration of initial doses of Rocuronium Bromide of 0.57-0.85 mg/kg under enflurane or isoflurane anesthesia, as used clinically, was increased by 11% and 23%, respectively. The duration of maintenance doses was affected to a greater extent, increasing by 30 to 50% under either enflurane or isoflurane anesthesia. Potentiation by these agents is also observed with respect to the infusion rates of Rocuronium Bromide required to maintain approximately 95% neuromuscular block. Under isoflurane and enflurane anesthesia, the infusion rates are decreased by approximately 40% compared to opioid/nitrous oxide/oxygen anesthesia. The median spontaneous recovery time (from 25 to 75% of control T_1) is not affected by halothane, but is prolonged by enflurane (15% longer) and isoflurane (62% longer). Reversal-induced recovery of Rocuronium Bromide neuromuscular block is minimally affected by anesthetic technique.

Intravenous Anesthetics: The use of propofol for induction and maintenance of anesthesia does not alter the clinical duration or recovery characteristics following recommended doses of Rocuronium Bromide Injection.

Anticonvulsants: In 2 of 4 patients receiving chronic anticonvulsant therapy apparent resistance to the effects of Rocuronium Bromide Injection was observed in the form of diminished magnitude of neuromuscular block, or shortened clinical duration. As with other nondepolarizing neuromuscular blocking drugs, if Rocuronium Bromide is administered to patients chronically receiving anticonvulsant agents such as carbamazepine or phenytoin, shorter durations of neuromuscular block may occur and infusion rates may be higher due to the development of resistance to nondepolarizing muscle relaxants. While the mechanism for development of this resistance is not known, receptor up-regulation may be a contributing factor (see "Individualization of Dosage").

Antibiotics: Drugs which may enhance the neuromuscular blocking action of nondepolarizing agents such as Rocuronium Bromide Injection include certain antibiotics (e.g., aminoglycosides; vancomycin; tetracyclines; bacitracin; polymyxins; colistin; and sodium colistimethate). If these antibiotics are used in conjunction with Rocuronium Bromide, prolongation of neuromuscular block should be considered a possibility.

Other: Experience concerning injection of quinidine during recovery from use of other muscle relaxants suggests that recurrent paralysis may occur. This possibility must also be considered for Rocuronium Bromide Injection.

Rocuronium Bromide-induced neuromuscular blockade was modified by alkalosis and acidosis in experimental pigs. Both respiratory and metabolic

acidosis prolonged the recovery time. The potency of Rocuronium Bromide was significantly enhanced in metabolic acidosis and alkalosis, but was reduced in respiratory alkalosis. In addition, experience with other drugs has suggested that acute (e.g., diarrhea) or chronic (e.g., adrenocortical insufficiency) electrolyte imbalance may alter neuromuscular blockade. Since electrolyte imbalance and acid-base imbalance are usually mixed, either enhancement or inhibition may occur. Magnesium salts, administered for the management of toxemia of pregnancy, may enhance neuromuscular blockade.

A local tolerance study in rabbits demonstrated that Rocuronium Bromide was well tolerated following intravenous, intra-arterial and perivenous administration with only a slight irritation of surrounding tissues observed after perivenous administration. In humans, if extravasation occurs it may be associated with signs or symptoms of local irritation: the injection or infusion should be terminated immediately and restarted in another vein (see "Dosage and Administration").

Drug/Laboratory Test Interactions: None known.

Carcinogenesis, Mutagenesis, Impairment of Fertility: Studies in animals have not been performed to evaluate carcinogenic potential or impairment of fertility. Mutagenicity studies (Ames test, analysis of chromosomal aberrations in mammalian cells, and micronucleus test) conducted with Rocuronium Bromide Injection did not suggest mutagenic potential.

Pregnancy Category B: A teratogenicity study has been conducted in rats using intravenously administered doses of Rocuronium Bromide Injection approximating the clinical dose in humans (0.3 mg/kg). No teratogenic effects were observed in this study. There are no adequate and well-controlled studies in pregnant women. Rocuronium Bromide should be used during pregnancy only if the potential benefit justifies the potential risk to the fetus.

Pediatric Use: The use of Rocuronium Bromide Injection in children less than 3 months of age has not been studied. see "Pharmacodynamics" subsection of "Clinical Pharmacology" and "Use in Pediatrics" subsection of "Dosage and Administration" for clinical experience and recommendations for use in infants and children 3 months to 14 years of age.

ADVERSE REACTIONS

Clinical studies in the U.S. (n = 1,137) and Europe (n = 1,394) totaled 2,531 patients. Prolonged neuromuscular block is associated with neuromuscular blockers as a class. Prolonged neuromuscular block (166 minutes) occurred after 0.6 mg/kg Rocuronium Bromide Injection in an obese, 67-year-old female with hepatic dysfunction who had received gentamicin before surgery. The patients exposed in the U.S. clinical studies provide the basis for calculation of adverse reaction rates. The following adverse experiences were reported in patients administered Rocuronium Bromide (all events judged by investigators during the clinical trials to have a possible causal relationship):

Adverse experiences in greater than 1% patients: None adverse experiences in less than 1% of patients: probably related or relationship unknown):

Cardiovascular:	arrhythmia, abnormal electrocardiogram, tachycardia
Digestive:	nausea, vomiting
Respiratory:	asthma (bronchospasm, wheezing, or rhonchi), hiccup
Skin and Appendages:	rash, injection site edema, pruritus

In the European studies, the most commonly reported adverse experiences were transient hypotension (2%) and hypertension (2%); it is in greater frequency than the U.S. studies (0.1% and 0.1%). Changes in heart rate and blood pressure were defined differently from the U.S. studies in which changes in cardiovascular parameters were not considered as adverse events unless judged by the investigator as unexpected, clinically significant, or thought to be histamine-related.

OVERDOSAGE

No cases of significant accidental or intentional overdose with Rocuronium Bromide Injection have been reported. Overdosage with neuromuscular blocking agents may result in neuromuscular block beyond the time needed for surgery and anesthesia. The primary treatment is maintenance of a patent airway and controlled ventilation until recovery of normal neuromuscular function is assured. Once evidence of recovery from neuromuscular block is observed, further recovery may be facilitated by administration of an anticholinesterase agent (e.g., neostigmine, edrophonium) in conjunction with an appropriate anticholinergic agent (see "Antagonism of Neuromuscular Blockade").

ANTAGONISM OF NEUROMUSCULAR BLOCKADE

Antagonists (such as Neostigmine) should not be Administered Prior to the Demonstration of some Spontaneous Recovery from neuromuscular Blockade. The use of a nerve Stimulator to Document Recovery and Antagonism of Neuromuscular Blockade is Recommended.

Patients should be evaluated for adequate clinical evidence of antagonism, e.g., 5 sec head lift, adequate phonation, ventilation, and upper airway maintenance. Ventilation must be supported until no longer required.

Antagonism may be delayed in the presence of debilitation, carcinomatosis, and concomitant use of certain broad spectrum antibiotics, or anesthetic agents and other drugs which enhance neuromuscular blockade or separately cause respiratory depression. Under such circumstances, the management is the same as that of prolonged neuromuscular blockade.

DOSAGE AND ADMINISTRATION

ROCURONIUM BROMIDE INJECTION IS FOR INTRAVENOUS USE ONLY. THIS DRUG SHOULD BE ADMINISTERED BY OR UNDER THE SUPERVISION OF EXPERIENCED CLINICIANS FAMILIAR WITH THE USE OF NEUROMUSCULAR BLOCKING AGENTS. INDIVIDUALIZATION OF DOSAGE SHOULD BE CONSIDERED IN EACH CASE (see *"Individualization of Dosage"* subsection of *"Clinical Pharmacology"*).

The dosage information which follows is derived from studies based upon units of drug per unit of body weight. It is expressed in this section in units of mg/kg to assist the clinician in calculating individual patient dosage requirements relative to the product as supplied for clinical use. It is intended to serve as an initial guide to clinicians familiar with other neuromuscular blocking agents to acquire experience with Rocuronium Bromide. The monitoring of twitch response is recommended to evaluate recovery from Rocuronium Bromide and decrease the hazards of overdosage if additional doses are administered (see *"Pharmacodynamics"* subsection of *"Clinical Pharmacology"* and *"Maintenance Dosing"* subsection).

It is recommended that clinicians administering neuromuscular blocking agents such as Rocuronium Bromide employ a peripheral nerve stimulator to monitor drug response, determine the need for additional relaxant and adequacy of spontaneous recovery or antagonism.

Rapid Sequence Intubation: In appropriately premedicated and adequately anesthetized patients, Rocuronium Bromide Injection 0.6-1.2 mg/kg will provide excellent or good intubating conditions in most patients in less than 2 minutes (see *"Clinical Trials"* subsection of *"Clinical Pharmacology"*).

Dose for Tracheal Intubation: The recommended initial dose regardless of anesthetic technique is 0.6 mg/kg. Neuromuscular block sufficient for intubation ($\geq$ 80% block) is attained in a median (range) time of 1 (0.4-6) minute(s) and most patients have intubation completed within 2 minutes. Maximum blockade is achieved in most patients in less than 3 minutes. This dose may be expected to provide 31 (15-85) minutes of clinical relaxation under opioid/nitrous oxide oxygen anesthesia. Under halothane, isoflurane, and enflurane anesthesia, some extension of the period of clinical relaxation should be expected (see *"Inhalation Anesthetics"* subsection of *"Precautions"*).

A lower dose of Rocuronium Bromide Injection (0.45 mg/kg) may be used. Neuromuscular block sufficient for intubation ($\geq$ 80% block) is attained in a median (range) time of 1.3 (0.8-6.2) minute(s) and most patients have intubation completed within 2 minutes. Maximum blockade is achieved in most patients in less than 4 minutes. This dose may be expected to provide 22 (12-31) minutes of clinical relaxation under opioid/nitrous oxide/oxygen anesthesia. Patients receiving this low dose of 0.45 mg/kg who achieve less than 90% block (about 16% of these patients) may have a more rapid time to 25% recovery, 12-15 minutes.

Should there be reason for the selection of a larger bolus dose in individual patients, initial doses of 0.9 or 1.2 mg/kg can be administered during surgery under opioid/nitrous oxide/oxygen anesthesia without adverse effects to the cardiovascular system. These doses will provide $\geq$ 80% block in most patients in less than 2 minutes, with maximum blockade occurring in most patients in less than 3 minutes. Doses of 0.9 and 1.2 mg/kg may be expected to provide 58 (27-111) and 67 (38-160) minutes, respectively, of clinical relaxation under opioid/nitrous oxide/oxygen anesthesia.

Maintenance Dosing: Maintenance doses of 0.1, 0.15, and 0.2 mg/kg Rocuronium Bromide Injection, administered at 25% recovery of control T_1 (defined as 3 twiches of train-of-four), provide a median (range of 12 (2-31), 17 (6-50) and 24 (7-69) minutes of clinical duration under opioid/nitrous oxide/oxygen anesthesia (see *"Pharmacodynamics"* subsection of *"Clinical Pharmacology"*). In all cases, dosing should be guided based on the clinical duration following initial dose or prior maintenance dose and not administered until recovery of neuromuscular function is evident. A clinically insignificant cumulation of effect with repetitive maintenance dosing has been observed (see *"Pharmacodynamics"* subsection of *"Clinical Pharmacology"*).

Use by Continuous Infusion: Infusion at an initial rate of 0.01 to 0.012 mg/kg/min of Rocuronium Bromide Injection should be initiated only after early evidence of spontaneous recovery from an intubating dose. Due to rapid redistribution (see *"Pharmacokinetics"* subsection of *"Clinical Pharmacology"*) and the associated rapid spontaneous recovery, initiation of the infusion after substantial return of neuromuscular function (more than 10% of control T_1), may necessitate additional bolus doses to maintain adequate block for surgery.

Upon reaching the desired level of neuromuscular block, the infusion of Rocuronium Bromide must be individualized for each patient. The rate of administration should be adjusted according to the patient's twitch response as monitored with the use of a peripheral nerve stimulator. In clinical trials, infusion rates have ranged from 0.004 to 0.016 mg/kg/min. Inhalation anesthetics, particularly enflurane and isoflurane may enhance the neuromuscular blocking action of nondepolarizing muscle relaxants. In the presence of steady-state concentrations of enflurane or isoflurane, it may be necessary to reduce the rate of infusion by 30 to 50%, at 45-60 minutes after the intubating dose.

Spontaneous recovery and reversal of neuromuscular blockade following discontinuation of Rocuronium Bromide infusion may be expected to proceed at rates comparable to that following comparable total doses administered by repetitive bolus injections (see *"Pharmacodynamics"* subsection of *"Clinical Pharmacology"*).

Infusion solutions of Rocuronium Bromide can be prepared by mixing Rocuronium Bromide with an appropriate infusion solution such as 5% glucose in water or Lactated Ringers (see *"Compatibility"*). Unused portions of infusion solutions should be discarded.

Use in Pediatrics: Initial doses of 0.6 mg/kg in children under halothane anesthesia produce excellent to good intubating conditions within 1 minute. The median (range) time to maximum block was 1 (0.5-3.3) minute(s). This dose will provide a median (range) time of clinical relaxation of 41 (24-68) minutes in 3 months-1 year pediatric patients and 27 (17-41) minutes in 1-12-year-old children. Maintenance doses of 0.075-0.125 mg/kg, administered upon return of T_1 to 25% of control, provide clinical relaxation for 7-10 minutes.

Spontaneous recovery proceeds at approximately the same rate in pediatric patients (3 months-1 year) as in adults, but is more rapid in pediatric patients (1-12 years) than adults (see Tables 2 and 4 in *"Pharmacodynamics"* subsection of *"Clinical Pharmacology"*). A continuous infusion of Rocuronium Bromide Injection, initiated at a rate of 0.012 mg/kg/min upon return of T_1 to 10% of control (one twitch present in the train-of-four), may also be used to maintain neuromuscular blockade in children. The infusion of Rocuronium Bromide must be individualized for each patient. The rate of administration should be adjusted according to the patient's twitch response as monitored with the use of a peripheral nerve stimulator. Spontaneous recovery and reversal of neuromuscular blockade following discontinuation of Rocuronium Bromide infusion may be expected to proceed at rates comparable to that following similar total exposure to single bolus doses (see *"Pharmacodynamics"* subsection of *"Clinical Pharmacology"*).

Use in Obese Patients: An analysis across all U.S.- controlled clinical studies indicates that the pharmacodynamics of Rocuronium Bromide. Injection are not different between obese and non-obese patients when dosed based upon their actual body weight.

Use in Geriatrics: Geriatric patients ($\geq$ 65 year) exhibited a slightly prolonged median (range) clinical duration of 46 (22-73). 62 (49-75), and 94 (64-138) minutes under opioid/nitrous oxide/oxygen anesthesia following doses of 0.6, 0.9 and 1.2 mg/kg, respectively. Maintenance doses of 0.1 and 0.15 mg/kg Rocuronium Bromide Injection, administered at 25% recovery of T_1, provide approximately 13 and 33 minutes of clinical duration under opioid/nitrous oxide/oxygen anesthesia. The median (range) rate of spontaneous recovery of T_1, from 25 to 75% in geriatric patients, is 17 (7-56) minutes which is not different from that in other adults (see *"Pharmacokinetics"* and *"Pharmacodynamics"* subsections of *"Clinical Pharmacology"*).

Compatibility: Rocuronium Bromide Injection is compatible in solution with:
0.9% NaCl solution   Sterile water for injection
5% glucose in water   Lactate Ringers
5% glucose in saline

Use within 24 hours of mixing with the above solutions. Parenteral drug products should be inspected visually for particulate matter and clarity prior to administration whenever solution and container permit. Do not use solution if particulate matter is present.

Safety and Handling: There is no specific work exposure limit for Rocuronium Bromide Injection. In case of eye contact, flush with water for at least 10 minutes.

Storage: Rocuronium Bromide Injection should be stored under refrigeration, 2 to 8°C (36 to 46°F). DO NOT FREEZE. Upon removal from refrigeration to room temperature storage conditions (25°C/77°F), use Rocuronium Bromide Injection within 30 days.

HOW SUPPLIED
INJECTION: 10 MG/ML

BRAND/MANUFACTURER	NDC	SIZE	AWP
○ BRAND			
ZEMURON: Organon	00052-0450-15	5 ml	$149.17

Roferon-A *SEE* INTERFERON ALFA-2A

Rogaine *SEE* MINOXIDIL, TOPICAL

Romazicon *SEE* FLUMAZENIL

Rondec *SEE* CARBINOXAMINE MALEATE WITH PSEUDOEPHEDRINE HYDROCHLORIDE

Rondec DM *SEE* CARBINOXAMINE MALEATE/DEXTROMETHORPHAN HYDROBROMIDE/PSEUDOEPHEDRINE HYDROCHLORIDE

◆ RATED THERAPEUTICALLY EQUIVALENT; ◇ THERAPEUTIC EQUIVALENCE UNCONFIRMED; ○ UNRATED

Rowasa *SEE MESALAMINE*

Roxicodone *SEE OXYCODONE HYDROCHLORIDE*

Rubella and Mumps Vaccine

DESCRIPTION

Rubella and Mumps Vaccine is a live virus vaccine for immunization against rubella (German measles) and mumps.

Rubella and Mumps Vaccine is a sterile lyophilized preparation of the Wistar RA 27/3 strain of live attenuated rubella virus grown in human diploid cell (WI-38) culture; and the Jeryl Lynn (B level) strain of mumps virus grown in cell cultures of chick embryo. The vaccine viruses are the same as those used in the manufacture of (Rubella Virus Vaccine Live, and (Mumps Virus Vaccine Live. The two viruses are mixed before being lyophilized. The reconstituted vaccine is for subcutaneous administration. When reconstituted as directed, the dose for injection is 0.5 mL and contains not less than the equivalent of 1,000 TCID$_{50}$ of the U.S. Reference Rubella Virus and 20,000 TCID$_{50}$ of the U.S. Reference Mumps Virus. Each dose contains approximately 25 mcg of neomycin. The product contains no preservative.

CLINICAL PHARMACOLOGY

Clinical studies of 73 double seronegative children 12 months to 2 years of age demonstrated that Rubella and Mumps Vaccine is highly immunogenic and generally well tolerated. In these studies, a single injection of the vaccine induced rubella hemagglutination-inhibition (HI) antibodies in 100 percent, and mumps neutralizing antibodies in 97 percent of the susceptible children.

The RA 27/3 rubella strain in Rubella and Mumps Vaccine elicits higher immediate post-vaccination HI, complement-fixing and neutralizing antibody levels than other strains of rubella vaccine and has been shown to induce a broader profile of circulating antibodies including anti-theta and anti-iota precipitating antibodies. The RA 27/3 rubella strain immunologically simulates natural infection more closely than other rubella vaccine viruses. The increased levels and broader profile of antibodies produced by RA 27/3 strain rubella virus vaccine appear to correlate with greater resistance to subclinical reinfection with the wild virus, and provide greater confidence for lasting immunity.

Vaccine induced antibody levels following administration of Rubella and Mumps Vaccine have been shown to persist for at least two years without substantial decline. Antibody levels after immunization with Rubella and Mumps Vaccine containing the HPV-77 strain of rubella, have persisted for 10.5 years without substantial decline. If the present pattern continues, it will provide a basis for the expectation that immunity following vaccination will be permanent. However, continued surveillance will be required to demonstrate this point.

INDICATIONS AND USAGE

Rubella and Mumps Vaccine is indicated for simultaneous immunization against rubella and mumps in persons 12 months of age or older. A booster is not needed.

The vaccine is not recommended for infants younger than 12 months because they may retain maternal rubella and mumps neutralizing antibodies which may interfere with the immune response.

Previously unimmunized children of susceptible pregnant women should receive live attenuated rubella vaccine, because an immunized child will be less likely to acquire natural rubella and introduce the virus into the household.

Individuals planning travel outside the United States, if not immune, can acquire measles, mumps or rubella and import these diseases to the United States. Therefore, prior to international travel, individuals known to be susceptible to one or more of these diseases can receive either a single antigen vaccine (measles, mumps, or rubella), or a combined antigen vaccine as appropriate. However, Measles, Mumps, and Rubella Virus Vaccine is preferred for persons likely to be susceptible to mumps and rubella; and if a single-antigen measles vaccine is not readily available, travelers should receive Measles, Mumps, and Rubella Virus Vaccine regardless of their immune status to mumps or rubella.

NONPREGNANT ADOLESCENT AND ADULT FEMALES

Immunizations of susceptible non-pregnant adolescent and adult females of childbearing age with live attenuated rubella virus vaccine is indicated if certain precautions are observed (see below and *"Precautions"*). Vaccinating susceptible postpubertal females confers individual protection against subsequently acquiring rubella infection during pregnancy, which in turn prevents infection of the fetus and consequent congenital rubella injury.

Women of childbearing age should be advised not to become pregnant for three months after vaccination and should be informed of the reasons for this precaution.*

---

* *NOTE:* The Immunization Practices Advisory Committee (ACIP) has recommended "In view of the importance of protecting this age group against rubella, reasonable precautions in a rubella immunization program include asking females if they are pregnant, excluding those who say they are, and explaining the theoretical risks to the others."

It is recommended that rubella susceptibility be determined by serologic testing prior to immunization.** If immune, as evidenced by a specific rubella antibody titer of 1:8 or greater (hemagglutination-inhibition test), vaccination is unnecessary. Congenital malformations do occur in up to seven percent of all live births. Their chance appearance after vaccination could lead to misinterpretation of the cause, particularly if the prior rubella-immune status of vaccinees is unknown.

Postpubertal females should be informed of the frequent occurrence of generally self-limited arthralgia and/or arthritis beginning 2 to 4 weeks after vaccination (see *"Adverse Reactions"*).

POSTPARTUM WOMEN

It has been found convenient in many instances to vaccinate rubella-susceptible women in the immediate postpartum period. (See *"Nursing Mothers"*.)

Revaccination: Children vaccinated when younger than 12 months of age should be revaccinated. Based on available evidence, there is no reason to routinely revaccinate persons who were vaccinated originally when 12 months of age or older. However, persons should be revaccinated if there is evidence to suggest that initial immunization was ineffective.

USE WITH OTHER VACCINES

Routine administration of DTP (diphtheria, tetanus, pertussis) and/or OPV (oral poliovirus vaccine) concomitantly with measles, mumps and rubella vaccines is not recommended because there are insufficient data relating to the simultaneous administration of these antigens. However, the American Academy of Pediatrics has noted that in some circumstances, particularly when the patient may not return, some practitioners prefer to administer all these antigens on a single day. If done, separate sites and syringes should be used for DTP and Rubella and Mumps Vaccine.

Rubella and Mumps Vaccine should not be given less than one month before or after administration of other virus vaccines.

CONTRAINDICATIONS

Do not give Rubella and Mumps Vaccine to pregnant females; the possible effects of the vaccine on fetal development are unknown at this time. If vaccination of postpubertal females is undertaken, pregnancy should be avoided for three months following vaccination. (See *"Precautions, Pregnancy"*.)

Anaphylactic or anaphylactoid reactions to neomycin (each dose of reconstituted vaccine contains approximately 25 mcg of neomycin).

History of anaphylactic or anaphylactoid reactions to eggs (see *"Hypersensitivity to Eggs" below*).

Any febrile respiratory illness or other active febrile infection.

Active untreated tuberculosis.

Patients receiving immunosuppressive therapy. This contraindication does not apply to patients who are receiving corticosteroids as replacement therapy, e.g., for Addison's disease.

Individuals with blood dyscrasias, leukemia, lymphomas of any type, or other malignant neoplasms affecting the bone marrow or lymphatic systems.

Primary and acquired immunodeficiency states, including patients who are immunosuppressed in association with AIDS or other clinical manifestations of infection with human immunodeficiency viruses; cellular immune deficiencies; and hypogammaglobulinemic and dysgammaglobulinemic states.

Individuals with a family history of congenital or hereditary immunodeficiency, until the immune competence of the potential vaccine recipient is demonstrated.

HYPERSENSITIVITY TO EGGS

Live mumps vaccine is produced in chick embryo cell culture. Persons with a history of anaphylactic, anaphylactoid, or other immediate reactions (e.g., hives, swelling of the mouth and throat, difficulty breathing, hypotension, or shock) subsequent to egg ingestion should not be vaccinated. Evidence indicates that persons are not at increased risk if they have egg allergies that are not anaphylactic or anaphylactoid in nature. Such persons may be vaccinated in the usual manner. There is no evidence to indicate that persons with allergies to chickens or feathers are at increased risk of reaction to the vaccine.

PRECAUTIONS

GENERAL

Adequate treatment provisions including epinephrine, should be available for immediate use should an anaphylactic or anaphylactoid reaction occur.

Children and young adults who are known to be infected with human immunodeficiency viruses but without overt clinical manifestations of immunosuppression may be vaccinated; however, the vaccinees should be monitored closely for vaccine-preventable diseases because immunization may be less effective than for uninfected persons.

Vaccination should be deferred for at least 3 months following blood or plasma transfusions, or administration of human immune serum globulin.

Excretion of small amounts of the live attenuated rubella virus from the nose and throat has occurred in the majority of susceptible individuals 7-28 days after

---

** *NOTE:* The Immunization Practices Advisory Committee (ACIP) has stated "When practical, and when reliable laboratory services are available, potential vaccinees of childbearing age can have serologic tests to determine susceptibility to rubella. However, routinely performing serologic tests for all females of childbearing age to determine susceptibility so that vaccine is given only to proven susceptibles is expensive and has been ineffective in some areas. Accordingly, the ACIP believes that rubella vaccination of a woman who is not known to be pregnant and has no history of vaccination is justifiable without serologic testing."

vaccination. There is no confirmed evidence to indicate that such virus is transmitted to susceptible persons who are in contact with the vaccinated individuals. Consequently, transmission through close personal contact, while accepted as a theoretical possibility, is not regarded as a significant risk. However, transmission of the rubella vaccine virus to infants via breast milk has been documented (see *"Nursing Mothers"*).

There are no reports of transmission of live attenuated mumps virus from vaccines to susceptible contacts.

It has been reported that live attenuated rubella and mumps virus vaccines given individually may result in a temporary depression of tuberculin skin sensitivity. Therefore, if a tuberculin test is to be done, it should be administered either before or simultaneously with Rubella and Mumps Vaccine.

As for any vaccine, vaccination with Rubella and Mumps Vaccine may not result in seroconversion in 100% of susceptible persons given the vaccine.

PREGNANCY
PREGNANCY CATEGORY C
Animal reproduction studies have not been conducted with Rubella and Mumps Vaccine. It is also not known whether Rubella and Mumps Vaccine can cause fetal harm when administered to a pregnant woman or can affect reproduction capacity. Therefore, the vaccine should not be administered to pregnant females; furthermore, pregnancy should be avoided for three months following vaccination (see *"Contraindications"*).

In counseling women who are inadvertently vaccinated when pregnant or who become pregnant within 3 months of vaccination, the physician should be aware of the following: (1) In a 10 year survey involving over 700 pregnant women who received rubella vaccine within 3 months before or after conception, (of whom 189 received the Wistar RA 27/3 strain) none of the newborns had abnormalities compatible with congenital rubella syndrome; and (2) although mumps virus is capable of infecting the placenta and fetus, there is no good evidence that it causes congenital malformations in humans. Mumps vaccine virus also has been shown to infect the placenta, but the virus has not been isolated from the fetal tissues from susceptible women who were vaccinated and underwent elective abortions.

NURSING MOTHERS
It is not known whether mumps vaccine virus is secreted in human milk. Recent studies have shown that lactating post-partum women immunized with live attenuated rubella vaccine may secrete the virus in breast milk and transmit it to breast-fed infants. In the infants with serological evidence of rubella infection, none exhibited severe disease; however, one exhibited mild clinical illness typical of acquired rubella. Caution should be exercised when Rubella and Mumps Vaccine is administered to a nursing woman.

ADVERSE REACTIONS
Burning and/or stinging of short duration at the injection site have been reported.

The adverse clinical reactions associated with the use of Rubella and Mumps Vaccine are those expected to follow administration of the monovalent vaccines given separately. These may include malaise, sore throat, cough, rhinitis, headache, dizziness, fever, rash, nausea, vomiting or diarrhea; mild local reactions such as erythema, induration, tenderness and regional lymphadenopathy; parotitis, orchitis, nerve deafness, thrombocytopenia and purpura; allergic reactions such as wheal and flare at the injection site or urticaria; polyneuritis; and arthralgia and/or arthritis (usually transient and rarely chronic).

Anaphylaxis and anaphylactoid reactions have been reported.

Vasculitis has been reported rarely.

Moderate fever [101-102.9°F (38.3-39.4°C)] occurs occasionally, and high fever [above 103°F (39.4°C)] occurs less commonly. On rare occasions, children developing fever may exhibit febrile convulsions. Syncope, particularly at the time of mass vaccination, has been reported. Rash occurs infrequently and is usually minimal, but rarely may be generalized. Erythema multiforme has also been reported rarely. Forms of optic neuritis, including retrobulbar neuritis and papillitis may infrequently follow viral infections, and have been reported to occur 1 to 3 weeks following inoculation with some live virus vaccines.

Isolated reports of polyneuropathy including Guillain-Barre syndrome have been reported after immunization with rubella-containing vaccines.

Clinical experience with live attenuated rubella and mumps virus vaccines given individually indicates that encephalitis and other nervous system reactions have occurred very rarely. These might occur also with Rubella and Mumps Vaccine.

Arthralgia and/or arthritis (usually transient and rarely chronic), and polyneuritis are features of natural rubella and vary in frequency and severity with age and sex, being greatest in adult females and least in prepubertal children. This type of involvement as well as myalgia and paresthesia have also been reported following administration of Rubella Virus Vaccine Live.

Chronic arthritis has been associated with natural rubella infection and has been related to persistent virus and/or viral antigen isolated from body tissues. Only rarely have vaccine recipients developed chronic joint symptoms.

Following vaccination in children, reactions in joints are uncommon and generally of brief duration. In women, incidence rates for arthritis and arthralgia are generally higher than those seen in children (children: 0-3%; women: 12-20%), and the reactions tend to be more marked and of longer duration. Symptoms may persist for a matter of months or on rare occasions for years. In adolescent girls, the reactions appear to be intermediate in incidence between those seen in children and in adult women. Even in older women (35-45 years), these reactions are generally well tolerated and rarely interfere with normal activities.

DOSAGE AND ADMINISTRATION
FOR SUBCUTANEOUS ADMINISTRATION
Do not inject intravenously: The dosage of vaccine is the same for all persons. Inject the total volume (about 0.5 mL) of reconstituted vaccine subcutaneously, preferably into the outer aspect of upper arm. *Do not give immune globulin (IG) concurrently with* Rubella and Mumps Vaccine. During shipment, to insure that there is no loss of potency, the vaccine must be maintained at a temperature of 10°C (50°F) or less.

Before reconstitution, store Rubella and Mumps Vaccine at 2-8°C (36-46°F). *Protect from light.*

Caution: A sterile syringe free of preservatives, antiseptics, and detergents should be used for each injection of the vaccine because these substances may inactivate the live virus vaccine. A 25 gauge, ⅝″ needle is recommended.

To reconstitute, use only the diluent supplied, since it is free of preservatives or other antiviral substances which might inactivate the vaccine. First withdraw the entire volume of diluent into the syringe to be used for reconstitution. Inject all the diluent in the syringe into the vial of lyophilized vaccine, and agitate to mix thoroughly. Withdraw the entire contents into a syringe and inject the total volume of restored vaccine subcutaneously.

It is important to use a separate sterile syringe and needle for each individual patient to prevent transmission of hepatitis B virus and other infectious agents from one person to another.

It is recommended that the vaccine be used as soon as possible after reconstitution. Protect the vaccine from light at all times, since such exposure may inactivate the virus. Store reconstituted vaccine in the vaccine vial in a dark place at 2-8°C (36-46°F) and discard if not used within eight hours.

Each dose of Rubella and Mumps Vaccine contains not less than the equivalent of 1,000 $TCID_{50}$ of the U.S. Reference Rubella Virus and 20,000 $TCID_{50}$ of the U.S. Reference Mumps Virus.

Parenteral drug products should be inspected visually for particulate matter and discoloration prior to administration. Rubella and Mumps Vaccine, when reconstituted, is clear yellow.

HOW SUPPLIED
INJECTION:

BRAND/MANUFACTURER	NDC	SIZE	AWP
○ BRAND			
BIAVAX II: Merck	00006-4746-00	1 ml	$22.46
	00006-4669-00	1 ml 10s	$197.75

Rubella Virus Vaccine

DESCRIPTION
Rubella Virus Vaccine Live is a live virus vaccine for immunization against rubella (German measles).

Rubella Virus Vaccine is a sterile lyophilized preparation of the Wistar Institute RA 27/3 strain of live attenuated rubella virus. The virus was adapted to and propagated in human diploid cell (WI-38) culture.

The reconstituted vaccine is for subcutaneous administration. When reconstituted as directed, the dose for injection is 0.5 mL and contains not less than the equivalent of 1,000 $TCID_{50}$ (tissue culture infectious doses) of the U.S. Reference Rubella Virus. Each dose also contains approximately 25 mcg of neomycin.

CLINICAL PHARMACOLOGY
Rubella Virus Vaccine produces a modified, non-communicable rubella infection in susceptible persons.

Extensive clinical trials of rubella virus vaccines, prepared using RA 27/3 strain rubella virus, have been carried out in more than 28,000 human subjects (approximately 11,000 with Rubella Virus Vaccine in the U.S.A. and more than 20 additional countries. A single injection of the vaccine has been shown to induce rubella hemagglutination-inhibiting (HI) antibodies in 97% or more of susceptible persons. The RA 27/3 rubella strain elicits higher immediate post-vaccination HI, complement-fixing and neutralizing antibody levels than other strains of rubella vaccine and has been shown to induce a broader profile of circulating antibodies including anti-theta and anti-iota precipitating antibodies. The RA 27/3 rubella strain immunologically simulates natural infection more closely than other rubella vaccine viruses. The increased levels and broader profile of antibodies produced by RA 27/3 strain rubella virus vaccine appear to correlate with greater resistance to subclinical reinfection with the wild virus, and provide greater confidence for lasting immunity.

Vaccine-induced antibody levels have been shown to persist for at least 10 years without substantial decline. If the present pattern continues, it will provide a basis for the expectation that immunity following vaccination will be permanent. However, continued surveillance will be required to demonstrate this point.

INDICATIONS AND USAGE[†]
1. Children Between 12 Months of Age and Puberty: Rubella Virus Vaccine is indicated for immunization against Rubella (German measles) in persons from 12 months of age to puberty. A booster is not needed. It is not recommended for

---

† Based in part on the recommendation for rubella vaccine use of the Immunization Practices Advisory Committee (ACIP), Morbidity and Mortality Weekly Report: *33* (22); 301-310, 315-318, June 8, 1984.

infants younger than 12 months because they may retain maternal rubella neutralizing antibodies that may interfere with the immune response. Children in kindergarten and the first grades of elementary school deserve priority for vaccination because often they are epidemiologically the major source of virus dissemination in the community. A history of rubella illness is usually not reliable enough to exclude children from immunization.

Previously unimmunized children of susceptible pregnant women should receive live attenuated Rubella Vaccine, because an immunized child will be less likely to acquire natural rubella and introduce the virus into the household.

2. Adolescent and Adult Males: Vaccination of adolescent or adult males may be a useful procedure in preventing or controlling outbreaks of rubella in circumscribed population groups (e.g., military bases and schools).

3. Non-Pregnant Adolescent and Adult Females: Immunization of susceptible non-pregnant adolescent and adult females of childbearing age with live attenuated Rubella Virus Vaccine is indicated if certain precautions are observed (see *below* and *"Precautions"*). Vaccinating susceptible postpubertal females confers individual protection against subsequently acquiring rubella infection during pregnancy, which in turn prevents infection of the fetus and consequent congenital rubella injury.

Women of childbearing age should be advised not to become pregnant for three months after vaccination and should be informed of the reason for this precaution.*

It is recommended that rubella susceptibility be determined by serologic testing prior to immunization.** If immune, as evidenced by a specific Rubella antibody titer of 1:8 or greater (hemagglutination-inhibition test), vaccination is unnecessary. Congenital malformations do occur in up to seven percent of all live births. Their chance appearance after vaccination could lead to misinterpretation of the cause, particularly if the prior rubella-immune status of vaccinees is unknown.

Postpubertal females should be informed of the frequent occurrence of generally self-limited arthralgia and/or arthritis beginning 2 to 4 weeks after vaccination (see *"Adverse Reactions"*).

4. Postpartum Women: It has been found convenient in many instances to vaccinate rubella-susceptible women in the immediate postpartum period (see *"Nursing Mothers"*).

5. International Travelers: Individuals planning travel outside the United States, if not immune, can acquire measles, mumps or rubella and import these diseases to the United States. Therefore, prior to International travel, individuals known to be susceptible to one or more of these diseases can receive either a single antigen vaccine (measles, mumps or rubella), or a combined antigen vaccine as appropriate. However, Measles, Mumps, and Rubella Virus Vaccine Live, is preferred for persons likely to be susceptible to mumps and rubella; and if single-antigen measles vaccine is not readily available, travelers should receive Measles, Mumps, and Rubella Virus Vaccine Live regardless of their immune status to mumps or rubella.

Revaccination: Children vaccinated when younger than 12 months of age should be revaccinated. Based on available evidence, there is no reason to routinely revaccinate persons who were vaccinated originally when 12 months of age or older. However, persons should be revaccinated if there is evidence to suggest that initial immunization was ineffective.

USE WITH OTHER VACCINES

Routine administration of DTP (diphtheria, tetanus, pertussis) and/or OPV (oral poliovirus vaccines concomitantly with Measles, Mumps and Rubella Vaccines is not recommended because there are insufficient data relating to the simultaneous administration of these antigens. However, the American Academy of Pediatrics has noted that in some circumstances, particularly when the patient may not return, some practitioners prefer to administer all these antigens on a single day. If done, separate sites and syringes should be used for DTP and Rubella Virus Vaccine.

Rubella Virus Vaccine should not be given less than one month before or after administration of other virus vaccines.

CONTRAINDICATIONS

Do not give Rubella Virus Vaccine to pregnant females; the possible effects of the vaccine on fetal development are unknown at this time. If vaccination of postpubertal females is undertaken, pregnancy should be avoided for three months following vaccination. (See *"Precautions, Pregnancy"*.)

Anaphylactic or anaphylactoid reactions to neomycin (each dose of reconstituted vaccine contains approximately 25 mcg of neomycin).

Any febrile respiratory illness or other active febrile infection.

Active untreated tuberculosis.

---

* *Note:* The Immunization Practices Advisory Committee (ACIP) has recommended "In view of the importance of protecting this age group against rubella, reasonable precautions in a rubella immunization program include asking females if they are pregnant, excluding those who say they are, and explaining the theoretical risks to the others."

** *Note:* The Immunization Practices Advisory Committee (ACIP) has stated. "When practical, and when reliable laboratory services are available, potential vaccinees of childbearing age can have serologic tests to determine susceptibility to rubella. However, routinely performing serologic tests for all females of childbearing age to determine susceptibility so that vaccine is given only to proven susceptibles is expensive and has been ineffective in some areas. Accordingly, the ACIP believes that rubella vaccination of a women who is not known to be pregnant and has no history of vaccination is justifiable without serologic testing."

Patients receiving immunosuppressive therapy. This contraindication does not apply to patients who are receiving corticosteroids as replacement therapy, e.g., for Addison's disease.

Individuals with blood dyscrasias, leukemia, lymphomas of any type, or other malignant neoplasms affecting the bone marrow or lymphatic systems.

Primary and acquired immunodeficiency states, including patients who are immunosuppressed in association with AIDS or other clinical manifestations of infection with human immunodeficiency viruses; cellular immune deficiencies; and hypogammaglobulinemic and dysgammaglobulinemic states.

Individuals with a family history of congenital or hereditary immunodeficiency, until the immune competence of the potential vaccine recipient is demonstrated.

PRECAUTIONS

GENERAL

Adequate treatment provisions including epinephrine, should be available for immediate use should an anaphylactic or anaphylactoid reaction occur.

Excretion of small amounts of the live attenuated rubella virus from the nose or throat has occurred in the majority of susceptible individuals 7-28 days after vaccination. There is no confirmed evidence to indicate that such virus is transmitted to susceptible persons who are in contact with the vaccinated individuals. Consequently, transmission through close personal contact, while accepted as a theoretical possibility, is not regarded as a significant risk. However, transmission of the vaccine virus to infants via breast milk has been documented (see *"Nursing Mothers"*).

There is no evidence that live Rubella Virus Vaccine given after exposure to natural Rubella Virus will prevent illness. There is, however, no contraindication to vaccinating children already exposed to natural rubella.

Children and young adults who are known to be infected with human immunodeficiency viruses but without overt clinical manifestations of immunosuppression may be vaccinated; however, the vaccinees should be monitored closely for vaccine-preventable diseases because immunization may be less effective than for uninfected persons.

Vaccination should be deferred for at least three months following blood or plasma transfusions, or administration of human immune serum globulin. However, susceptible postpartum patients who received blood products may receive Rubella Virus Vaccine prior to discharge provided that a repeat HI titer is drawn 6-8 weeks after vaccination to insure seroconversion. Similarly, although studies with other live Rubella Virus Vaccines suggest that Rubella Virus Vaccine may be given in the immediate postpartum period to those non-immune women who have received anti-Rho (D) globulin (human) without interfering with vaccine effectiveness, a follow-up post vaccination HI titer should also be determined.

It has been reported that attenuated Rubella Virus Vaccine, live, may result in a temporary depression of tuberculin skin sensitivity. Therefore, if a tuberculin test is to be done, it should be administered either before or simultaneously with Rubella Virus Vaccine.

As for any vaccine, vaccination with Rubella Virus Vaccine may not result in seroconversion in 100% of susceptible persons given the vaccine.

PREGNANCY

Pregnancy Category C: Animal reproduction studies have not been conducted with Rubella Virus Vaccine. It is also not known whether Rubella Virus Vaccine can cause fetal harm when administered to a pregnant woman or can affect reproduction capacity. There is evidence suggesting transmission of Rubella Vaccine viruses to products of conception. Therefore, Rubella Vaccine should not be administered to pregnant females (see *"Contraindications"*).

In counseling women who are inadvertently vaccinated when pregnant or who become pregnant within 3 months of vaccination, the physician should be aware of the following: In a 10 year survey involving over 700 pregnant women who received Rubella Vaccine within 3 months before or after conception. (of whom 189 received the Wistar RA 27/3 strain) none of the newborns had abnormalities compatible with congenital Rubella syndrome.

Nursing Mothers: Recent studies have shown that lactating postpartum women immunized with live attenuated Rubella Vaccine may secrete the virus in breast milk and transmit it to breast-fed infants. In the infants with serological evidence of Rubella infection, none exhibited severe disease; however, one exhibited mild clinical illness typical of acquired Rubella. Caution should be exercised when Rubella Virus Vaccine is administered to a nursing woman.

ADVERSE REACTIONS

Burning and/or stinging of short duration at the injection site have been reported.

Symptoms of the same kind as those seen following natural Rubella may occur after vaccination. These include mild regional lymphadenopathy, urticaria, rash, malaise, sore throat, fever, headache, dizziness, nausea, vomiting, diarrhea polyneuritis, and arthralgia and/or arthritis (usually transient and rarely chronic). Local pain, wheal and flare, induration, and erythema may occur at the site of injection. Reactions are usually mild and transient. Erythema multiforme has also been reported rarely.

Cough and rhinitis have also been reported.

Vasculitis has been reported rarely.

Anaphylaxis and anaphylactoid reactions have been reported.

Moderate fever [101-102.9°F (38.3-39.4°C)] occurs occasionally, and high fever [over 103°F (39.4°C)] occurs less commonly.

Syncope, particularly at the time of mass vaccination, has been reported.

Chronic arthritis has been associated with natural rubella infection and has been related to persistent virus and/or viral antigen isolated from body tissues. Only rarely have vaccine recipients developed chronic joint symptoms.

Following vaccination in children, reactions in joints are uncommon and generally of brief duration. In women, incidence rates for arthritis and arthralgia are generally higher than those seen in children (children: 0-3%; women: 12-20%) and the reactions tend to be more marked and of longer duration. Symptoms may persist for a matter of months or on rare occasions for years. In adolescent girls, the reactions appear to be intermediate in incidence between those seen in children and in adult women. Even in older women (35-45 years), these reactions are generally well tolerated and rarely interfere with normal activities. Myalgia and paresthesia have been reported rarely after administration of Rubella Virus Vaccine.

Forms of optic neuritis, including retrobulbar neuritis and papillitis may infrequently follow viral infections, and have been reported to occur 1 to 3 weeks following inoculation with some live virus vaccines.

Isolated reports of polyneuropathy including Guillain-Barré syndrome have been reported after immunization with rubella-containing vaccines.

Clinical experience with live rubella vaccines thus far indicates that encephalitis and other nervous system reactions have occurred very rarely in subjects who were given the vaccines, but a cause and effect relationship has not been established.

Thrombocytopenia with or without purpura has been reported.

DOSAGE AND ADMINISTRATION
FOR SUBCUTANEOUS ADMINISTRATION
Do not inject intravenously: The dosage of vaccine is the same for all persons. Inject the total volume of the single dose vial (about 0.5 mL) or 0.5 mL of the multiple dose vial of reconstituted vaccine subcutaneously, preferably into the outer aspect of upper arm. *Do not give immune globulin (IG) concurrently with* Rubella Virus Vaccine. To insure that there is no loss of potency during shipment, the vaccine must be maintained at a temperature of 10°C (50°F) or less.

Before reconstitution, store Rubella Virus Vaccine at 2-8°C (36-46°F). *Protect from light.*

Caution: A sterile syringe free of preservatives, antiseptics, and detergents should be used for each injection and/or reconstitution of the vaccine because these substances may inactivate the live virus vaccine. A 25 gauge, ⅝" needle is recommended.

To reconstitute, use only the diluent supplied, since it is free of preservatives or other antiviral substances which might inactivate the vaccine.

Single Dose Vial: First withdraw the entire volume of diluent into the syringe to be used for reconstitution. Inject all the diluent in the syringe into the vial of lyophilized vaccine, and agitate to mix thoroughly. Withdraw the entire contents into a syringe and inject the total volume of restored vaccine subcutaneously.

It is important to use a separate sterile syringe and needle for each individual patient to prevent transmission of hepatitis B and other infectious agents from one person to another.

10 Dose Vial (available only to government agencies/institutions): Withdraw the entire contents (7 mL) of the diluent vial into the sterile syringe to be used for reconstitution, and introduce into the 10 dose vial of lyophilized vaccine. Agitate to ensure thorough mixing. The outer labeling suggests "For Jet Injector or Syringe Use". Use with separate sterile syringes is permitted for containers of 10 doses or less. The vaccine and diluent do not contain preservatives; therefore, the user must recognize the potential contamination hazards and exercise special precautions to protect the sterility and potency of the product. The use of aseptic techniques and proper storage prior to and after restoration of the vaccine and subsequent withdrawal of the individual doses is essential. Use 0.5 mL of the reconstituted vaccine for subcutaneous injection.

It is important to use a separate sterile syringe and needle for each individual patient to prevent transmission of hepatitis B and other infectious agents from one person to another.

50 Dose Vial (available only to government agencies/institutions): Withdraw the entire contents (30 mL) of diluent vial into the sterile syringe to be used for reconstitution and introduce into the 50 dose vial of lyophilized vaccine. Agitate to ensure thorough mixing. With full aseptic precautions, attach the vial to the sterilized multidose jet injector apparatus. Use 0.5 mL of the reconstituted vaccine for subcutaneous injection.

Each dose contains not less than the equivalent of 1,000 $TCID_{50}$ of the U.S. Reference Rubella Virus.

Parenteral drug products should be inspected visually for particulate matter and discoloration prior to administration. Rubella Virus Vaccine, when reconstituted, is clear yellow.

STORAGE
It is recommended that the vaccine be used as soon as possible after reconstitution. Protect vaccine from light at all times, since such exposure may inactivate the virus. Store reconstituted vaccine in the vaccine vial in a dark place at 2-8°C (36-46°F) and discard if not used within 8 hours.

HOW SUPPLIED
INJECTION:

BRAND/MANUFACTURER	NDC	SIZE	AWP
○ BRAND			
MERUVAX II: Merck	00006-4747-00	1 ml	$13.38
	00006-4673-00	1 ml 10s	$113.00

Rubex SEE DOXORUBICIN HYDROCHLORIDE

Ryna-CX SEE CODEINE PHOSPHATE/GUAIFENESIN/ PSEUDOEPHEDRINE HYDROCHLORIDE

Rynatan SEE CHLORPHENIRAMINE TANNATE/ PHENYLEPHRINE TANNATE/PYRILAMINE TANNATE

Rynatuss SEE CARBETAPENTANE/CHLORPHENIRAMINE/ EPHEDRINE/PHENYLEPHRINE

Salagen SEE PILOCARPINE HYDROCHLORIDE, ORAL

Salflex SEE SALSALATE

Salmeterol Xinafoate

DESCRIPTION
Salmeterol Xinafoate Inhalation Aerosol contains Salmeterol Xinafoate as the racemic form of the 1-hydroxy-2-naphthoic acid salt of salmeterol. The active component of the formulation is salmeterol base, a highly selective beta$_2$-adrenergic bronchodilator. The chemical name of Salmeterol Xinafoate is 4-hydroxy-alpha-^{1}-[[[6-(4-phenyl-butoxy) hexyl] amino]methyl]-1,3-benzenedimethanol, 1-hydroxy-2-naphtha- lenecarboxylate.

The molecular weight of Salmeterol Xinafoate is 603.8, and the empirical formula is $C_{25}H_{37}NO_4.C_{11}H_8O_3$. Salmeterol Xinafoate is a white to off-white powder. It is freely soluble in methanol; slightly soluble in ethanol, chloroform, and isopropanol; and sparingly soluble in water.

Salmeterol Xinafoate Inhalation Aerosol is a pressurized, metered-dose aerosol unit for oral inhalation. It contains a microcrystalline suspension of Salmeterol Xinafoate in a mixture of two chlorofluorocarbon propellants (trichlorofluoromethane and dichlorodifluoromethane) with lecithin. 36.25 mcg of Salmeterol Xinafoate is equivalent to 25 mcg of salmeterol base. Each actuation delivers 25 mcg of Salmeterol base (as Salmeterol Xinafoate) from the valve and 21 mcg of Salmeterol base (as Salmeterol Xinafoate) from the actuator.

Following is its chemical structure:

CLINICAL PHARMACOLOGY
Mechanism of Action: Salmeterol is a long-acting beta-adrenergic agonist. *In vitro* studies and *in vivo* pharmacologic studies demonstrate that Salmeterol is selective for beta$_2$-adrenoceptors compared with isoproterenol, which has approximately equal agonist activity on beta$_1$- and beta$_2$-adrenoceptors. *In vitro* studies show Salmeterol to be at least 50 times more selective for beta$_2$-adrenoceptors than albuterol. Although beta$_2$-adrenoceptors are the predominant adrenergic receptors in bronchial smooth muscle and beta$_1$-adrenoceptors are the predominant receptors in the heart, there are also beta$_2$-adrenoceptors in the human heart comprising 10% to 50% of the total beta-adrenoceptors. The precise function of these is not yet established, but they raise the possibility that even highly selective beta$_2$-agonists may have cardiac effects.

◆ RATED THERAPEUTICALLY EQUIVALENT; ◇ THERAPEUTIC EQUIVALENCE UNCONFIRMED; ○ UNRATED

The pharmacologic effects of beta₂-adrenoceptor agonist drugs, including Salmeterol, are at least in part attributable to stimulation of intracellular adenyl cyclase, the enzyme that catalyzes the conversion of adenosine triphosphate (ATP) to cyclic-3',5'-adenosine monophosphate (cyclic AMP). Increased cyclic AMP levels cause relaxation of bronchial smooth muscle and inhibition of release of mediators of immediate hypersensitivity from cells, especially from mast cells.

In vitro tests show that Salmeterol is a potent and long-lasting inhibitor of the release of mast cell mediators, such as histamine, leukotrienes, and prostaglandin D₂, from human lung. Salmeterol inhibits histamine-induced plasma protein extravasation and inhibits platelet activating factor-induced eosinophil accumulation in the lungs of guinea pigs when administered by the inhaled route. In humans, Salmeterol inhibits both the early- and late-phase responses to inhaled allergens, the latter persisting for over 30 hours after a single dose when the bronchodilator effect is no longer evident. Single doses of Salmeterol also attenuate allergen-induced bronchial hyper-responsiveness.

Pharmacokinetics: Salmeterol acts locally in the lung; plasma levels therefore do not predict therapeutic effect. Because of the low therapeutic dose, systemic levels of Salmeterol are low or undetectable after inhalation of recommended doses (42 mcg twice daily). Following chronic administration of an inhaled dose of 42 mcg twice daily, Salmeterol was detected in plasma within 5 to 10 minutes in six asthmatic patients; plasma concentrations were very low, with peak concentrations of 150 pg/mL and no accumulation with repeated doses. Larger inhaled doses gave approximately proportionally increased blood levels. In these patients, a second peak concentration of 115 pg/mL occurred at about 45 minutes, probably due to absorption of the swallowed portion of the dose (most of the dose delivered by a metered-dose inhaler is swallowed). Oral administration of 1 mg of radiolabeled Salmeterol (as Salmeterol Xinafoate) to two healthy subjects gave peak plasma Salmeterol concentrations of about 650 pg/mL at about 45 minutes; the terminal elimination half-life was about 5.5 hours (one volunteer only).

Salmeterol Xinafoate, as ionic salt, dissociates in solution so that the Salmeterol and 1-hydroxy-2-naphthoic acid Xinafoate moieties are absorbed, distributed, metabolized, and excreted independently. Salmeterol base is extensively metabolized by hydroxylation, with subsequent elimination predominantly in the feces. In the two subjects discussed above, approximately 25% and 60% of orally administered radioactivity was eliminated in urine and feces, respectively, over a period of 7 days. No significant amount of unchanged salmeterol base was detected in either urine or feces.

Salmeterol is 94% to 98% bound to human plasma proteins *in vitro* over the concentration range of 8 to 7,722 ng of base per milliliter, much higher concentrations than those achieved following therapeutic doses of Salmeterol.

The Xinafoate moiety has no apparent pharmacologic activity, is highly protein bound (>99%), and has a long elimination half-life of 11 days.

The pharmacokinetics of Salmeterol base have not been studied in elderly patients nor in patients with hepatic or renal impairment. Since Salmeterol is predominantly cleared by hepatic metabolism, liver function impairment may lead to accumulation of Salmeterol in plasma. Therefore, patients with hepatic disease should be closely monitored.

Pharmacodynamics and Clinical Trials: Inhaled Salmeterol meterol, like other beta-adrenergic agonist drugs, can in some patients produce cardiovascular effects (see "Precautions"). The cardiovascular effects (heart rate, blood pressure) associated with Salmeterol administration occur with similar frequency, and are of similar type and severity, as those noted following albuterol administration.

The effects of rising inhaled doses of Salmeterol and standard inhaled doses of albuterol were studied in volunteers and in patients with asthma. Salmeterol doses up to 84 mcg resulted in heart rate increases of 3 to 16 beats/minute, about the same as albuterol (4 to 10 beats/minute). In two double-blind studies, patients receiving either Salmeterol (n = 81) or albuterol (n = 80) underwent continuous electrocardiographic monitoring during four 24-hour periods; no clinically significant dysrhythmias were noted.

Beta-agonists and methylxanthines administered concurrently in laboratory animals (minipigs, rodents, and dogs) cause cardiac arrhythmias and sudden death (with histologic evidence of myocardial necrosis). Whether these findings are relevant to humans is not known.

In placebo- and albuterol-controlled, single-dose clinical trials with Salmeterol Xinafoate Inhalation Aerosol, the time to onset of effective bronchodilation (> 15% improvement in forced expiratory volume in 1 second [FEV₁]) was 10 to 20 minutes after a 42-mcg dose. Maximum improvement in FEV₁ generally occurred within 180 minutes, and clinically significant improvement continued for 12 hours in most patients.

In two large, randomized, double-blind studies, Salmeterol Xinafoate Inhalation Aerosol was compared with albuterol and placebo in patients with mild-to-moderate asthma, including both patients who did and who did not receive concomitant inhaled corticosteroids. The efficacy of Salmeterol Xinafoate Inhalation Aerosol was demonstrated over the 12-week period with no change in effectiveness over this period of time. There were no gender-related differences in safety and efficacy. No development of tachyphylaxis to the bronchodilator effect has been noted in these studies. FEV₁ measurements (percent of predicted) from these two 12-weeks trials are shown below for both the first and last treatment days.

FEV₁ as Percent of Predicted, From Two Large 12-Week Clinical Trials

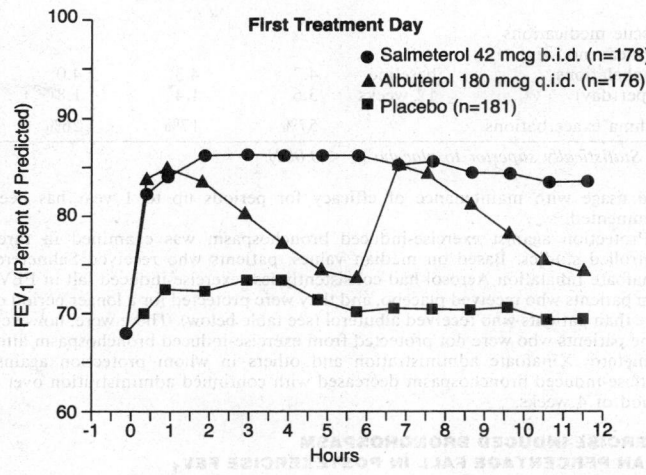

First Treatment Day
- Salmeterol 42 mcg b.i.d. (n=178)
- Albuterol 180 mcg q.i.d. (n=176)
- Placebo (n=181)

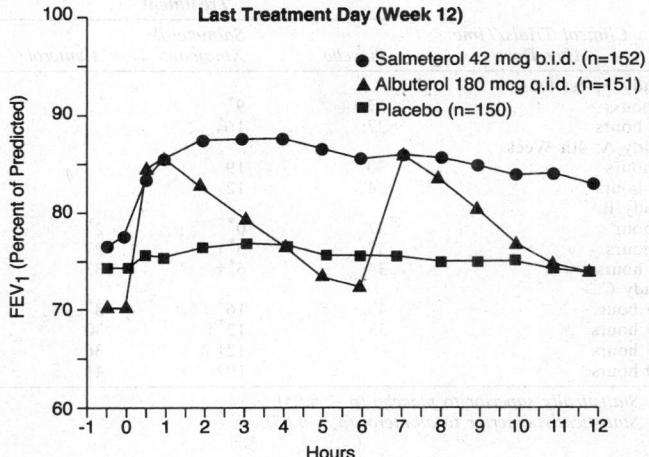

Last Treatment Day (Week 12)
- Salmeterol 42 mcg b.i.d. (n=152)
- Albuterol 180 mcg q.i.d. (n=151)
- Placebo (n=150)

During daily treatment with Salmeterol Xinafoate Inhalation Aerosol for 12 weeks in patients with asthma, the following treatment effects were seen:

TWO LARGE 12-WEEK CLINICAL TRIALS: EFFICACY PARAMETERS
MULTICENTER STUDY 1

Parameter	Time	Placebo	Salmeterol Xinafoate	Albuterol
Mean AM PEFR (L/min)	baseline	410	420	404
	12 weeks	409	443*	395
Mean % days with no symptoms	baseline	12	15	15
	12 weeks	17	35*	27
Mean % nights with no awakenings	baseline	71	77	70
	12 weeks	79	89†	75
Rescue medications (mean no. of inhalations per day)	baseline	3.9	3.8	4.0
	12 weeks	2.9	1.2‡	1.9
Asthma exacerbations		53%	16%	31%

* Statistically superior to placebo (p = 0.002).
† Statistically superior to placebo (p = 0.008).
‡ Statistically superior to placebo (p < 0.001).

MULTICENTER STUDY 2

Parameter	Time	Placebo	Salmeterol Xinafoate	Albuterol
Mean AM PEFR (L/min)	baseline	409	406	390
	12 weeks	412	451*	388
Mean % days with no symptoms	baseline	11	8	14
	12 weeks	17	36*	21
Mean % nights with no awakenings	baseline	64	59	62
	12 weeks	70	85*	74

Parameter	Time	Placebo	Salmeterol Xinafoate	Albuterol
Rescue medications (mean no. of inhalations per day)	baseline	4.7	4.3	4.0
	12 weeks	3.6	1.4*	1.8
Asthma exacerbations		57%	17%	26%

* *Statistically superior to placebo (p < 0.001).*

Safe usage with maintenance of efficacy for periods up to 1 year has been documented.

Protection against exercise-induced bronchospasm was examined in three controlled studies. Based on median values, patients who received Salmeterol Xinafoate Inhalation Aerosol had consistently less exercise-induced fall in FEV_1 than patients who received placebo, and they were protected for a longer period of time than patients who received albuterol (see table below). There were, however, some patients who were not protected from exercise-induced bronchospasm after Salmeterol Xinafoate administration and others in whom protection against exercise-induced bronchospasm decreased with continued administration over a period of 4 weeks.

EXERCISE-INDUCED BRONCHOSPASM
MEAN PERCENTAGE FALL IN POSTEXERCISE FEV_1

Clinical Trials/Time After Dose	Treatment		
	Placebo	Salmeterol Xinafoate	Albuterol
Study A: 1st Dose			
6 hours	37	9*	
12 hours	27	16*	
Study A: 4th Week			
6 hours	30	19	
12 hours	24	12	
Study B:			
1 hour	37	0*	2*
6 hours	37	5*†	27
12 hours	34	6*†	33
Study C:			
0.5 hour	43	16*	8*
2.5 hours	33	12*†	30
4.5 hours	-	12†	36
6.0 hours	-	19†	41

* *Statistically superior to placebo (p ≤ 0.05).*
† *Statistically superior to albuterol (p ≤ 0.05).*

INDICATIONS AND USAGE
Salmeterol Xinafoate Inhalation Aerosol is indicated for long-term, twice-daily (morning and evening) administration in the maintenance treatment of asthma and in the prevention of bronchospasm in patients 12 years of age and older with reversible obstructive airway disease, including patients with symptoms of nocturnal asthma, who require regular treatment with inhaled, short-acting beta$_2$-agonists. It should not be used in patients whose asthma can be managed by occasional use of short-acting, inhaled beta$_2$-agonists.

Salmeterol Xinafoate Inhalation Aerosol may be used with or without concurrent inhaled or systemic corticosteroid therapy.

Salmeterol Xinafoate Inhalation Aerosol is also indicated for prevention of exercise-induced bronchospasm in patients 12 years of age and older.

CONTRAINDICATIONS
Salmeterol Xinafoate Inhalation Aerosol is contraindicated in patients with a history of hypersensitivity to any of the components.

WARNINGS
1. Not for Use to Treat Acute Symptoms: Watch for Increased Need for Short-Acting Beta$_2$-Agonists: Salmeterol Xinafoate Inhalation Aerosol should not be used to relieve acute asthma symptoms. If the patient's short-acting, inhaled beta$_2$-agonist becomes less effective, e.g., the patient needs more inhalations than usual, medical evaluation must be obtained immediately and increasing use of Salmeterol Xinafoate Inhalation Aerosol in this situation is inappropriate. Salmeterol Xinafoate Inhalation Aerosol should not be used more frequently than twice daily (morning and evening) at the recommended dose. When prescribing Salmeterol Xinafoate Inhalation Aerosol, patients must be provided with a short-acting, inhaled beta$_2$-agonist (e.g., albuterol) for treatment of symptoms that occur despite regular twice-daily (morning and evening) use of Salmeterol Xinafoate.

Asthma may deteriorate acutely over a period of hours or chronically over several days. In this setting, increased use of inhaled, short-acting beta$_2$-agonists is a marker of destabilization of asthma and requires re-evaluation of the patient and consideration of alternative treatment regimens, especially inhaled or systemic corticosteroids. If the patient uses four or more inhalations per day of a short-acting beta$_2$-agonist on a regular basis, or if more than one canister (200 inhalations per canister) is used in an 8-week period, then the patient should see the physician for re-evaluation of treatment.

2. Use With Short-Acting Beta$_2$-Agonists: When patients begin treatment with Salmeterol Xinafoate Inhalation Aerosol, those who have been taking short-acting, inhaled beta$_2$-agonists on a regular daily basis should be advised to discontinue their regular daily-dosing regimen and should be clearly instructed to use short-acting, inhaled beta$_2$-agonists only for symptomatic relief if they develop asthma symptoms while taking Salmeterol Xinafoate Inhalation Aerosol (see *"Precautions: Drug Interactions"*).

3. Salmeterol Xinafoate Inhalation Aerosol is Not a Substitute for Oral or Inhaled Corticosteroids: Patients must be warned not to stop or reduce corticosteroid therapy without medical advice, even if they feel better when they are being treated with Salmeterol Xinafoate.

4. Do Not Exceed Recommended Dose: As with other beta-adrenergic aerosols, Salmeterol Xinafoate Inhalation Aerosol should not be used in excess. Fatalities have been reported in association with excessive use of inhaled sympathomimetic drugs. Large doses of inhaled or oral salmeterol (12 to 20 times the recommended dose) have been associated with clinically significant prolongation of the QT_c interval, which has the potential for producing ventricular arrhythmias.

5. Paradoxical Bronchospasm: As with other inhaled asthma medications, paradoxical bronchospasm (which can be life-threatening) has been reported following the use of Salmeterol Xinafoate Inhalation Aerosol. If it occurs, treatment with Salmeterol Xinafoate Inhalation Aerosol should be discontinued immediately and alternative therapy instituted.

6. Immediate Hypersensitivity Reactions: Immediate hypersensitivity reactions may occur after administration of Salmeterol Xinafoate Inhalation Aerosol, as demonstrated by rare cases of urticaria, rash, and bronchospasm.

PRECAUTIONS
GENERAL
1. Use with Space or Other Devices: The safety and effectiveness of Salmeterol Xinafoate Inhalation Aerosol when used with a spacer or other devices have not been adequately studied.

2. Cardiovascular and Other Effects: No effect on the cardiovascular system is usually seen after the administration of inhaled Salmeterol in recommended doses, but the cardiovascular and central nervous system effects seen with all sympathomimetic drugs (e.g., increased blood pressure, heart rate, excitement) can occur after use of Salmeterol Xinafoate Inhalation Aerosol and may require discontinuation of the drug. Salmeterol, like all sympathomimetic amines, should be used with caution in patients with cardiovascular disorders, especially coronary insufficiency, cardiac arrhythmias, and hypertension; in patients with convulsive disorders or thyrotoxicosis; and in patients who are unusually responsive to sympathomimetic amines.

As has been described with other beta-adrenergic agonist bronchodilators, clinically significant changes in systolic and/or diastolic blood pressure, pulse rate, and electrocardiograms have been seen infrequently in individual patients in controlled clinical studies with Salmeterol.

3. Metabolic Effects: Doses of the related beta$_2$-adrenoceptor agonist albuterol, when administered intravenously, have been reported to aggravate pre-existing diabetes mellitus and ketoacidosis. No effects on glucose have been seen with Salmeterol Xinafoate Inhalation Aerosol at recommended doses.

Administration of beta$_2$-adrenoceptor agonists may cause a decrease in serum potassium, possibly through intracellular shunting, which has the potential to increase the likelihood of arrythmias. The decrease is usually transient, not requiring supplementation.

Clinically significant changes in blood glucose and/or serum potassium were seen rarely during clinical studies with long-term administration of Salmeterol Xinafoate Inhalation Aerosol at recommended doses.

INFORMATION FOR PATIENTS
See illustrated Patient's Instructions for Use. **SHAKE WELL BEFORE USING.** Patients should be given the following information:

1. Not for Use to Treat Acute Symptoms: Salmeterol Xinafoate Inhalation Aerosol is not meant to relieve acute asthmatic symptoms. Acute symptoms should be treated with an inhaled, short-acting bronchodilator that has been prescribed by a physician for symptom relief.

2. Do Not Exceed Recommended Dose: The bronchodilator action of Salmeterol Xinafoate usually lasts for at least 12 hours. Therefore it should not be used more often than every 12 hours.

3. Use With Other Medications: While using Salmeterol Xinafoate Inhalation Aerosol, other inhaled medicines should be taken only as directed by the physician.

4. Use with Short-Acting, Inhaled Beta-Agonists: While using Salmeterol Xinafoate Inhalation Aerosol, medical attention should be sought immediately if the short-acting bronchodilator treatment becomes less effective for symptom relief, if more inhalations than usual are needed, or if more than the maximum number of inhalations of short-acting bronchodilator treatment prescribed for a 24-hour period are needed. If the patient uses four or more inhalations per day of a short-acting beta$_2$-agonist on a regular basis, or if more than one canister (200 inhalations per canister) is used in an 8-week period, then the patient should see the physician for re-evaluation of treatment.

Patients should be cautioned regarding potential adverse cardiovascular effects, such as palpitations or chest pain, related to the use of additional beta$_2$-agonist.

◆ RATED THERAPEUTICALLY EQUIVALENT; ◇ THERAPEUTIC EQUIVALENCE UNCONFIRMED; ○ UNRATED

5. *Use of Systemic or Inhaled Steroids:* Salmeterol Xinafoate Inhalation Aerosol does not replace oral or inhaled corticosteroids; the dosage of these medicines should not be changed and they should not be stopped without consulting the physician, even if the patient feels better.

6. *Use for Exercise-Induced Bronchospasm:* When using Salmeterol Xinafoate Inhalation Aerosol to prevent exercise-induced bronchospasm, the dose should be administered at least 30 to 60 minutes before exercise.

DRUG INTERACTIONS
Short-Acting Beta-Agonists: In the two 3-month, repetitive-dose clinical trials (n = 184), the mean daily need for additional beta2-agonists use was 1 to 1 ½ inhalations per day, but some patients used more. Eight percent of patients used at least eight inhalations per day at least on one occasion. Six percent used 9 to 12 inhalations at least once. There were 15 patients (8%) who averaged over four inhalations per day. Four of these used an average of 8 to 11 inhalations per day. In these 15 patients there was no observed increase in frequency of cardiovascular adverse events. The safety of concomitant use of more than eight inhalations per day of short-acting beta2-agonists with Salmeterol Xinafoate Inhalation Aerosol has not been established. In 15 patients who experienced worsening of asthma while receiving Salmeterol Xinafoate Inhalation Aerosol, nebulized albuterol (one dose in most) led to improvement in FEV_1 and no increase in occurrence of cardiovascular adverse events.

Monoamine Oxidase Inhibitors and Tricyclic Antidepressants: Salmeterol should be administered with extreme caution to patients being treated with monoamine oxidase inhibitors or tricyclic antidepressants because the action of Salmeterol on the vascular system may be potentiated by these agents.

Corticosteroids and Cromoglycate: In clinical trials, inhaled corticosteroids and/or inhaled cromolyn sodium did not alter the safety profile of Salmeterol Xinafoate Inhalation Aerosol when administered concurrently.

Methylxanthines: The concurrent use of intravenously or orally administered methylxanthines (e.g., aminophylline, theophylline) by patients receiving Salmeterol Xinafoate Inhalation Aerosol has not been completely evaluated. In one clinical trial, 87 patients receiving Salmeterol Xinafoate Inhalation Aerosol 42 mcg twice daily concurrently with a theophylline product had adverse event rates similar to those in 71 patients receiving Salmeterol Xinafoate Inhalation Aerosol without theophylline. Resting heart rates were slightly higher in the patients on theophylline but were little affected by Salmeterol Xinafoate Inhalation Aerosol therapy.

CARCINOGENESIS, MUTAGENESIS, IMPAIRMENT OF FERTILITY
In an 18-month oral carcinogenicity study in CD-mice, Salmeterol Xinafoate caused a dose-related increase in the incidence of smooth muscle hyperplasia, cystic glandular hyperplasia, and leiomyomas of the uterus and a dose-related increase in the incidence of cysts in the ovaries. A higher incidence of leiomyosarcomas was not statistically significant; tumor findings were observed at oral doses of 1.4 and 10 mg/kg, which gave 9 and 63 times, respectively, the human exposure based on rodent: human AUC comparisons. Salmeterol caused a dose-dependent increase in the incidence of mesovarian leiomyomas and ovarian cysts in Sprague Dawley rats in a 24-month inhalation/oral carcinogenicity study. Tumors were observed in rats receiving doses of 0.68 and 2.58 mg/kg per day (about 55 and 215 times the recommended clinical dose [mg/m²]). These findings in rodents are similar to those reported previously for other beta-adrenergic agonist drugs. The relevance of these findings to human use is unknown.

No significant effects occurred in mice at 0.2 mg/kg (1.3 times the recommended clinical dose based on comparisons of the AUCs) and in rats at 0.21 mg/kg (15 times the recommended clinical dose on a mg/m² basis).

Salmeterol Xinafoate produced no detectable or reproducible increases in microbial and mammalian gene mutation *in vitro.* No blastogenic activity occurred *in vitro* in human lymphocytes or *in vivo* in a rat micronucleus test. No effects on fertility were identified in male and female rats treated orally with Salmeterol Xinafoate at doses up to 2 mg/kg orally (about 160 times the recommended clinical dose on a mg/m² basis).

PREGNANCY
Teratogenic Effects: Pregnancy Category C: No significant effects of maternal exposure to oral Salmeterol Xinafoate occurred in the rat at doses up to the equivalent of about 160 times the recommended clinical dose on a mg/m² basis. Dutch rabbit fetuses exposed to Salmeterol Xinafoate *in utero* exhibited effects characteristically resulting from beta-adrenoceptor stimulation; these included precocious eyelid openings, cleft palate, sternebral fusion, limb and paw flexures, and delayed ossification of the frontal cranial bones. No significant effects occurred at 0.6 mg/kg given orally (12 times the recommended clinical dose based on comparison of the AUCs).

New Zealand White rabbits were less sensitive since only delayed ossification of the frontal bones was seen at 10 mg/kg given orally (approximately 1,600 times the recommended clinical dose on a mg/m² basis). Extensive use of other beta-agonists has provided no evidence that these class effects in animals are relevant to use in humans. There are no adequate and well-controlled studies with Salmeterol Xinafoate Inhalation Aerosol in pregnant women. Salmeterol Xinafoate Inhalation Aerosol should be used during pregnancy only if the potential benefit justifies the potential risk to the fetus.

USE IN LABOR AND DELIVERY
There are no well-controlled human studies that have investigated effects of Salmeterol on preterm labor or labor at term. Because of the potential for beta-agonist interference with uterine contractility, use of Salmeterol Xinafoate Inhalation Aerosol during labor should be restricted to those patients in whom the benefits clearly outweigh the risks.

NURSING MOTHERS
Plasma levels of Salmeterol after inhaled therapeutic doses are very low (85 to 200 pg/mL) in humans. In lactating rats dosed with radiolabeled Salmeterol, levels of radioactivity were similar in plasma and milk. In rats, concentrations of Salmeterol in plasma and milk were similar. The Xinafoate moiety is also transferred to milk in rats at concentrations of about half the corresponding level in plasma. However, since there is no experience with use of Salmeterol Xinafoate Inhalation Aerosol by nursing mothers, a decision should be made whether to discontinue nursing or to discontinue the drug, taking into account the importance of the drug to the mother. Caution should be exercised when Salmeterol Xinafoate is administered to a nursing women.

PEDIATRIC USE
The safety and effectiveness of Salmeterol Xinafoate Inhalation Aerosol in children younger than 12 years of age have not been established.

GERIATRIC USE
Of the total number of patients who received Salmeterol Xinafoate Inhalation Aerosol in all clinical studies, 241 were 65 years and older. Geriatric patients (65 years and older) with reversible obstructive airway disease were evaluated in four well-controlled studies of 3 weeks' to 3 months' duration. Two placebo-controlled, crossover studies evaluated twice-daily dosing with Salmeterol for 21 to 28 days in 45 patients. An additional 75 geriatric patients were treated with Salmeterol for 3 months in two large parallel-group, multicenter studies. These 120 patients experienced increases in AM and PM peak expiratory flow rate and decreases in diurnal variation in peak expiratory flow rate similar to responses seen in the total populations of the two latter studies. The adverse event type and frequency in geriatric patients were not different from those of the total populations studied.

No apparent differences in the efficacy and safety of Salmeterol Xinafoate Inhalation Aerosol were observed when geriatric patients were compared with younger patients in clinical trials. As with other beta2-agonists, however, special caution should be observed when using Salmeterol Xinafoate Inhalation Aerosol in elderly patients who have concomitant cardiovascular disease that could be adversely affected by this class of drug. Based on available data, no adjustment of Salmeterol dosage in geriatric patients is warranted.

ADVERSE REACTIONS
Adverse reactions to Salmeterol are similar in nature to reactions to other selective beta2-adrenoceptor agonists, i.e., tachycardia; palpitations; immediate hypersensitivity reactions, including urticaria, rash, bronchospasm (see *"Warnings"*); headache; tremor; nervousness; and paradoxical bronchospasm (see *"Warnings"*).

Two multicenter, 12-week, controlled studies have evaluated twice-daily doses of Salmeterol Xinafoate Inhalation Aerosol in patients 12 years of age and older with asthma. The following table reports the incidence of adverse events in these two studies.

ADVERSE EXPERIENCE INCIDENCE IN TWO LARGE 12-WEEK CLINICAL TRIALS*

	Percent of Patients		
Adverse Event Type	Placebo n = 187	Salmeterol Xinafoate 42 mcg b.i.d. n = 184	Albuterol 180 mcg q.i.d. n = 185
Ear, nose, and throat			
Upper respiratory tract infection	13	14	16*
Nasopharyngitis	12	14	11
Disease of nasal cavity/sinus	4	6	1
Sinus headache	2	4	< 1
Gastrointestinal			
Stomachache	0	4	0
Neurological			
Headache	23	28	27
Tremor	2	4	3
Respiratory			
Cough	6	7	3
Lower respiratory infection	2	4	2

* *The only adverse experience classified as serious was one case of upper respiratory tract infection in a patient treated with albuterol.*

The table above includes all events (whether considered drug related or nondrug related by the investigator) that occurred at a rate of over 3% in the Salmeterol Xinafoate Inhalation Aerosol treatment group and were more common in the Salmeterol Xinafoate Inhalation Aerosol group than in the placebo group.

Pharyngitis, allergic rhinitis, dizziness/giddiness, and influenza occurred at 3% or more but were equally common on placebo. Other events occurring in the Salmeterol Xinafoate Inhalation Aerosol treatment group at a frequency of 1% to 3% were as follows:

Cardiovascular: Tachycardia, palpitations.

Ear, Nose, and Throat: Rhinitis, laryngitis.

Gastrointestinal: Nausea, viral gastroenteritis, nausea and vomiting, diarrhea, abdominal pain.

Hypersensitivity: Urticaria.

Mouth and Teeth: Dental pain.

Musculoskeletal: Pain in joint, back pain, muscle cramp/contraction, myalgia/myositis, muscular soreness.

Neurological: Nervousness, malaise/fatigue.

Respiratory: Tracheitis/bronchitis.

Skin: Rash/skin eruption.

Urogenital: Dysmenorrhea.

In small dose-response studies, tremor, nervousness, and palpitations appeared to be dose related.

OVERDOSAGE

Overdosage with Salmeterol may be expected to result in exaggeration of the pharmacologic adverse effects associated with beta-adrenoceptor agonists, including tachycardia and/or arrhythmia, tremor, headache, and muscle cramps. Overdosage with Salmeterol can lead to clinically significant prolongation of the QT_c interval, which can produce ventricular arrhythmias. Other signs of overdosage may include hypokalemia and hyperglycemia.

In these cases, therapy with Salmeterol Xinafoate Inhalation Aerosol and all beta-adrenergic-stimulant drugs should be stopped, supportive therapy provided, and judicious use of a beta-adrenergic blocking agent should be considered, bearing in mind the possibility that such agents can produce bronchospasm. Cardiac monitoring is recommended in cases of overdosage.

As with all sympathomimetic pressurized aerosol medications, cardiac arrest and even death may be associated with abuse of Salmeterol Xinafoate Inhalation Aerosol.

Rats and dogs survived the maximum practicable inhalation doses of Salmeterol of 2.9 and 0.7 mg/kg, respectively. The maximum nonlethal oral doses in mice and rats were approximately 150 mg/kg and > 1,000 mg/kg, respectively. Dialysis is not appropriate treatment for overdosage of Salmeterol Xinafoate Inhalation Aerosol.

DOSAGE AND ADMINISTRATION

Salmeterol Xinafoate Inhalation Aerosol should be administered by the orally inhaled route only (see *"Patient's Instructions for Use"*). For maintenance of bronchodilatation and prevention of symptoms of asthma, including the symptoms of nocturnal asthma, the usual dosage for adults and children 12 years of age and older is two inhalations (42 mcg) twice daily (morning and evening, approximately 12 hours apart). Adverse effects are more likely to occur with higher doses of Salmeterol, and more frequent administration or administration of a larger number of inhalations is not recommended.

To gain full therapeutic benefit, Salmeterol Xinafoate Inhalation Aerosol should be administered twice daily (morning and evening) in the treatment of reversible airway obstruction.

If a previously effective dosage regimen fails to provide the usual response, medical advice should be sought immediately as this is often a sign of destabilization of asthma. Under these circumstances, the therapeutic regimen should be re-evaluated and additional therapeutic options, such as inhaled or systemic corticosteroids, should be considered. If symptoms arise in the period between doses, a short-acting, inhaled beta₂-agonist should be taken for immediate relief.

Prevention of Exercise-Induced Brochospasm: Two inhalations at least 30 to 60 minutes before exercise have been shown to protect against exercise-induced bronchospasm in many patients for up to 12 hours. *Additional doses of Salmeterol Xinafoate Inhalation Aerosol should not be used for 12 hours after the administration of this drug. Patients who are receiving Salmeterol Xinafoate Inhalation Aerosol twice daily (morning and evening) should not use additional Salmeterol Xinafoate Inhalation Aerosol for prevention of exercise-induced bronchospasm. If this dose is not effective, other appropriate therapy for exercise-induced bronchospasm should be considered.*

Geriatric Use: In studies where geriatric patients (65 years of age or older, see *"Precautions"*) have been treated with Salmeterol Xinafoate Inhalation Aerosol, efficacy and safety of 42 mcg given twice daily (morning and evening) did not differ from that in younger patients. Consequently, no dosage adjustment is recommended.

Storage: Avoid spraying in eyes. Contents under pressure. Do not puncture or incinerate. Do not store at temperatures above 120°F. Keep out of reach of children. As with most inhaled medications in aerosol canisters, the therapeutic effect of this medication may decrease when the canister is cold; for best results, the canister should be at room temperature before use. Shake well before using.

Note: The indented statement below is required by the Federal government's Clean Air Act for all products containing or manufactured with chlorofluorocarbons (CFCs).

WARNING: Contains trichlorofluoromethane and dichlorodifluoromethane, substances which harm public health and environment by destroying ozone in the upper atmosphere.

HOW SUPPLIED
AEROSOL SOLID INGREDIENTS: 21 MCG/INH

BRAND/MANUFACTURER	NDC	SIZE	AWP
○ **BRAND**			
SEREVENT: Allen & Hanburys	00173-0467-00	6.5 gm	$29.94
	00173-0465-00	13 gm	$46.30

AEROSOL SOLID W/ADAPTER: 21 MCG/INH

BRAND/MANUFACTURER	NDC	SIZE	AWP
○ **BRAND**			
SEREVENT: Allen & Hanburys	00173-0464-00	13 gm	$47.95

Salsalate

DESCRIPTION
Salsalate is a nonsteroidal anti-inflammatory agent for oral administration. Chemically, Salsalate (salicylsalicylic acid or 2-hydroxy-benzoic acid, 2-carboxyphenyl ester) is a dimer of salicylic acid. Empirical formula: $C_{14}H_{10}O_5$; molecular weight: 258.2. The ingredient in this product is of the following classes: nonsteroidal anti-inflammatory agent and analgesic.

Each Salsalate tablet contains 500 mg or 750 mg. Certain brands of Salsalate are available as 500 mg capsules also.

Following is its chemical structure:

CLINICAL PHARMACOLOGY
Salsalate is insoluble in acid gastric fluids (< 0.1 mg/ml at pH 1.0), but readily soluble in the small intestine where it is partially hydrolyzed to two molecules of salicylic acid. A significant portion of the parent compound is absorbed unchanged and undergoes rapid esterase hydrolysis in the body; its half-life is about one hour. About 13% is excreted through the kidneys as a glucuronide conjugate of the parent compound, less than 1% as unchanged Salsalate, and the remainder as salicylic acid and its metabolites. Thus, the amount of salicylic acid available from Salsalate is about 15% less than from aspirin, when the two drugs are administered on a salicylic acid molar equivalent basis (3.6 g Salsalate/5 g aspirin). Salicylic acid biotransformation is saturated at anti-inflammatory doses of Salsalate. Such capacity-limited biotransformation results in an increase in the half-life of salicylic acid from 3.5 to 16 or more hours. Thus, dosing with Salsalate twice a day will satisfactorily maintain blood levels within the desired therapeutic range (10 to 30 mg/100 ml) throughout the 12-hour intervals. Therapeutic blood levels continue for up to 16 hours after the last dose. Salsalate produces more sustained serum salicylate levels than does acetylsalicylic acid. The reasons for this probably relate to the slower rate of hydrolysis of Salsalate than acetylsalicylic acid. The parent compound does not show capacity-limited biotransformation, nor does it accumulate in the plasma on multiple dosing. Food slows the absorption of all salicylates including Salsalate.

The mode of anti-inflammatory action of Salsalate and other nonsteroidal anti-inflammatory drugs is not fully defined. Although salicylic acid (the primary metabolite of Salsalate is a weak inhibitor of prostaglandin synthesis *in vitro* Salsalate appears to selectively inhibit prostaglandin synthesis *in vivo*,[1] providing anti-inflammatory activity equivalent to aspirin[2] and indomethacin.[3] Unlike aspirin, Salsalate does not inhibit platelet aggregation.[4]

The usefulness of salicylic acid, the active *in vivo* product of Salsalate, in the treatment of arthritic disorders has been established.[5,6] In contrast to aspirin, Salsalate causes no greater fecal gastrointestinal blood loss than placebo.[7]

INDICATIONS AND USAGE
Salsalate is indicated for the temporary relief of the signs and symptoms of rheumatoid arthritis, osteoarthritis, and related rheumatic disorders.

CONTRAINDICATIONS
Salsalate is contraindicated in patients hypersensitive to Salsalate.

WARNINGS
Reye's Syndrome may develop in individuals who have chicken pox, influenza, or flu symptoms. Some studies suggest possible association between the development of Reye's Syndrome and the use of medicines containing salicylate or aspirin. Salsalate contains a salicylate and therefore is not recommended for use in patients with chicken pox, influenza, or flu symptoms.

PRECAUTIONS
General Precautions: Great care should be exercised when Salsalate is prescribed in the presence of chronic renal insufficiency or peptic ulcer disease. Protein binding of salicylic acid can be influenced by nutritional status, competitive binding of other drugs, and fluctuations in serum proteins caused by disease (rheumatoid arthritis, etc.).

Although cross reactivity, including bronchospasm, has been reported occasionally with non-acetylated salicylates, including Salsalate, in aspirin-sensitive patients,[8,9] Salsalate is less likely than aspirin to induce asthma in such patients.[10]

Information for Patients: Patients on long-term treatment should be warned not to take other salicylates so as to avoid potentially toxic concentrations. They should also be warned that if symptoms of overdosage, such as tinnitus, vertigo, headache, confusion, drowsiness, sweating, hyperventilation, vomiting or diarrhea appear, the drug should be stopped and physician notified.

Laboratory Tests: Plasma salicylic acid concentrations should be periodically monitored during long-term treatment with Salsalate to aid maintenance of therapeutically effective levels: 10 to 30 mg/100 ml. Toxic manifestations are not usually seen until plasma concentrations exceed 30 mg/100 ml (see *"Overdosage"*). Urinary pH should also be regularly monitored: sudden acidification, as from pH 6.5 to 5.5, can double the plasma level, resulting in toxicity.

An increase in urinary pH will increase renal clearance and urinary excretion of salicylic acid, thus lowering plasma levels.

Drug Interactions: Salicylates antagonize the uricosuric action of drugs used to treat gout. ASPIRIN AND OTHER SALICYLATE DRUGS WILL BE ADDITIVE TO SALSALATE AND MAY INCREASE PLASMA CONCENTRATIONS OF SALICYLIC ACID TO TOXIC LEVELS. Drugs and foods that raise urine pH will increase renal clearance and urinary excretion of salicylic acid, thus lowering plasma levels; acidifying drugs or foods will decrease urinary excretion and increase plasma levels. Salicylates given concomitantly with anticoagulant drugs may competitively displace anticoagulant drugs from plasma protein binding sites and thereby predispose to systemic bleeding. Salicylates may enhance the hypoglycemic effect of oral antidiabetic drugs of the sulfonylurea class. Salicylate competes with a number of drugs for protein binding sites, notably penicillin, thiopental, throxine, triiodothyronine, phenytoin, sulfinpyrazone, naproxen, warfarin, methotrexate, and possibly corticosteroids.

Drug/Laboratory Test Interactions: Salicylate competes with thyroid hormone for binding to plasma proteins, which may be reflected in a depressed plasma T_4 value in some patients; thyroid function and basal metabolism are unaffected.

Carcinogenesis: No long-term animal studies have been performed with Salsalate to evaluate its carcinogenic potential; however, several such studies using aspirin and other salicylates have failed to demonstrate any association of these agents with cancerous cell changes.

Use in Pregnancy: Pregnancy Category C: Salsalate and salicyclic acid have been shown to be teratogenic and embryocidal in rats when given in doses 4 to 5 times the usual human dose. These effects were not observed at doses twice as great as the usual human dose. There are no adequate and well-controlled studies in pregnant women. Salsalate should be used during pregnancy only if the potential benefit justifies the potential risk to the fetus.

Labor and Delivery: There exist no adequate and well-controlled studies in pregnant women. Although adverse effects on mother or infant have not been reported with Salsalate use during labor, caution is advised when anti-inflammatory dosage is involved. However, other salicylates have been associated with prolonged gestation and labor, maternal and neonatal bleeding sequelae, potentiation of narcotic and barbiturate effects (respiratory or cardiac arrest in the mother), delivery problems and stillbirth.

Nursing Mothers: It is not known whether Salsalate per se is excreted in human milk; salicylic acid, the primary metabolite of Salsalate, has been shown to appear in human milk in concentrations approximating the maternal blood level. Thus, the infant of a mother on Salsalate therapy might ingest in mother's milk 30 to 80% as much salicylate per kg body weight as the mother is taking. Accordingly, caution should be exercised when Salsalate is administered to a nursing woman.

Pediatric Use: Safety and effectiveness of Salsalate use in children have not been established. (See *"Warnings"* section.)

ADVERSE REACTIONS

In two well-controlled clinical trials (n = 280 patients), the following reversible adverse experiences characteristic of salicylates were most commonly reported with Salsalate, listed in descending order of frequency: tinnitus, nausea, hearing impairment, rash, and vertigo. These common symptoms of salicylates, i.e., tinnitus or reversible hearing impairment, are often used as a guide to therapy.

Although cause-and-effect relationships have not been established, spontaneous reports over a ten-year period have included the following additional medically significant adverse experiences: abdominal pain, abnormal hepatic function, anaphylactic shock, angioedema, bronchospasm, decreased creatinine clearance, diarrhea, G.I. bleeding, hepatitis, hypotension, nephritis and urticaria.

DRUG ABUSE AND DEPENDENCE

Drug abuse and dependence have not been reported with Salsalate.

OVERDOSAGE

IN ALL CASES OF SUSPECTED OVERDOSE, IMMEDIATELY CALL YOUR REGIONAL POISON CENTER AND/OR SEEK PROFESSIONAL ASSISTANCE.

Death has followed ingestion of 10 to 30 g of salicylates in adults, but much larger amounts have been ingested without fatal outcome.

Symptoms: The usual symptoms of salicylism—tinnitus, vertigo, headache, confusion, drowsiness, sweating, hyperventilation, vomiting and diarrhea—will occur. More severe intoxication will lead to disruption of electrolyte balance and blood pH, and hyperthermia and dehydration.

Treatment: Further absorption of Salsalate from the G.I. tract should be prevented by emesis (syrup of ipecac) and, if necessary, by gastric lavage.

Fluid and electrolyte imbalance should be corrected by the administration of appropriate I.V. therapy. Adequate renal function should be maintained. Hemodialysis or peritoneal dialysis may be required in extreme cases.

DOSAGE AND ADMINISTRATION

Adults: The usual dosage is 3000 mg daily, given in divided doses as follows: 1) two doses of two 750 mg tablets; 2) four doses of one 750 mg tablet; 3) two doses of three 500 mg tablets/capsules; or 4) three doses of two 500 mg tablets/capsules. Some patients, e.g., the elderly, may require a lower dosage to achieve therapeutic blood concentrations and to avoid the more common side affects such as auditory.

Dosage should be adjusted according to the severity of the disease and the response of the patient.

Alleviation of symptoms is gradual, and full benefit may not be evident for 3 to 4 days, when plasma salicylate levels have achieved steady state. There is no evidence for development of tissue tolerance (tachyphylaxis), but salicylate therapy may induce increased activity of metabolizing liver enzymes, causing a greater rate of salicyluric acid production and excretion, with a resultant increase in dosage requirement for maintenance of therapeutic serum salicylate levels.

Children: Dosage recommendations and indications for Salsalate use in children have not been established.

Store at controlled room temperature 15°–30°C (59°–86°F). Dispense in a tight, light-resistant container as defined in the USP.

REFERENCES

1. Morris HG, et al. Effects of salsalate (non-acetylated salicylate) and aspirin on serum prostaglandins in humans. Thera Drug Mon 1985;7:435-438. 2. April PA, et al. Does the acetyl group of aspirin contribute to the antiinflammatory efficacy of salicylic acid in the treatment of rheumatoid arthritis? Sem Arth & Rheum 1990;19:(4)2:20-28 3. Deodhar SD, et al. A short term comparative trial of salsalate and indomethacin in rheumatoid arthritis. Curr Med Res Opin 1977;5:185-188. 4. Estes D, Kaplan K. Lack of platelet effect with the aspirin analog, salsalate. Arth & Rheum 1980;23:1303-1307. 5. Dick C, et al. Effect of anti-inflammatory drug therapy on clearance of ^{133}Xe from knee joints of patients with rheumatoid arthritis. Br Med J 1969;3:278-280. 6. Dick WC, et al. Indices of inflammatory activity. Ann of Rheum Dis 1970;29:643-648. 7. Cohen A. Fecal blood loss and plasma salicylate study of salicylsalicylic acid and aspirin. J. Clin Pharmacol 1979;19:242-247. 8. Chudwin DS, et al. Sensitivity to non-acetylated salicylates in a patient with asthma, nasal polyps, and rheumatoid arthritis. Ann of Allergy 1986;57:133-134. 9. Spector SL, et al. Aspirin and concomitant idiosyncrasies in adult asthmatic patients. J Allergy Clin Immunol 1979;64;500-506. 10. Stevenson DD, et al. Salsalate cross sensitivity in aspirin-sensitive asthmatics. J Allergy Clin Immunol 1990;86:749-758.

HOW SUPPLIED

CAPSULE: 500 MG

BRAND/MANUFACTURER	NDC	SIZE	AWP
BRAND			
DISALCID: 3M Pharm	00089-0148-10	100s	$42.12
GENERICS			
Geneva	00781-1108-01	100s	$10.28
Geneva	00781-1108-05	500s	$42.05

CAPSULE: 750 MG

BRAND/MANUFACTURER	NDC	SIZE	AWP
GENERICS			
Geneva	00781-1109-01	100s	$13.52
Geneva	00781-1109-05	500s	$61.24

TABLETS:

BRAND/MANUFACTURER	NDC	SIZE	AWP
GENERICS			
MARTHRITIC: Marnel	00682-0810-01	100s	$22.40

TABLETS: 500 MG

BRAND/MANUFACTURER	NDC	SIZE	AWP
BRAND			
SALFLEX: Carnrick	00086-0071-10	100s	$21.95
DISALCID: 3M Pharm	00089-0149-10	100s	$40.38
	00089-0149-50	500s	$191.46
GENERICS			
Southwood	58016-0219-10	10s	$4.21
Allscrips	54569-2544-01	20s	$3.04
Southwood	58016-0219-20	20s	$6.77
Southwood	58016-0219-28	28s	$8.85
Allscrips	54569-2544-00	30s	$4.57
Southwood	58016-0219-30	30s	$9.28
Allscrips	54569-2544-02	60s	$9.13
Copley	38245-0143-10	100s	$7.62
Mutual	53489-0465-01	100s	$11.75
Schein	00364-0832-01	100s	$11.88
Qualitest	00603-5754-21	100s	$11.90
URL	00677-1024-01	100s	$11.99
Goldline	00182-1802-01	100s	$12.00
Major	00904-1253-60	100s	$12.10
Major	00904-1250-60	100s	$12.10
Martec	52555-0247-01	100s	$12.16
AMIGESIC: Amide	52152-0019-02	100s	$12.95
Rugby	00536-4522-01	100s	$13.20

▶ **SHOWN IN PRODUCT IDENTIFICATION GUIDE**

BRAND/MANUFACTURER	NDC	SIZE	AWP
Moore,H.L.	00839-7167-06	100s	$14.16
Eon	00185-0761-01	100s	$16.95
Eon	00185-0856-01	100s	$16.95
Rosemont	00832-1037-00	100s	$17.65
SALSITAB: Upsher-Smith	00245-0153-11	100s	$17.65
Duramed	51285-0296-02	100s	$20.77
Invamed	52189-0243-24	100s	$20.77
Aligen	00405-4934-01	100s	$21.25
Sidmak	50111-0390-01	100s	$21.25
R.I.D.	54807-0140-01	100s	$30.18
Barre	00472-0132-10	100s	$33.37
Goldline	00182-1802-89	100s ud	$11.00
Auro	55829-0469-10	100s ud	$16.89
SALSITAB: Upsher-Smith	00245-0153-01	100s ud	$19.21
Major	00904-1250-61	100s ud	$22.01
Medirex	57480-0411-01	100s ud	$23.00
Copley	38245-0143-50	500s	$34.62
Major	00904-1253-40	500s	$37.45
Major	00904-1250-40	500s	$37.45
Mutual	53489-0465-05	500s	$42.00
Martec	52555-0247-05	500s	$49.21
Parmed	00349-8481-05	500s	$50.69
Moore,H.L.	00839-7167-12	500s	$53.04
Rosemont	00832-1037-50	500s	$55.00
Eon	00185-0761-05	500s	$79.95
Eon	00185-0856-05	500s	$79.95
SALSITAB: Upsher-Smith	00245-0153-15	500s	$83.64
Duramed	51285-0296-04	500s	$98.66
Invamed	52189-0243-29	500s	$98.66
Aligen	00405-4934-02	500s	$99.50
Sidmak	50111-0390-02	500s	$99.50
Barre	00472-0132-50	500s	$158.44

TABLETS: 750 MG

BRAND/MANUFACTURER	NDC	SIZE	AWP
○ **BRAND**			
SALFLEX: Carnrick	00086-0072-10	100s	$28.65
MONO-GESIC: Central	00131-2164-37	100s	$28.80
DISALCID: 3M Pharm	00089-0151-10	100s	$51.66
SALFLEX: Carnrick	00086-0072-50	500s	$115.00
MONO-GESIC: Central	00131-2164-41	500s	$138.95
DISALCID: 3M Pharm	00089-0151-50	500s	$244.86
○ **GENERICS**			
Southwood	58016-0221-10	10s	$4.47
Allscrips	54569-1712-05	12s	$2.34
Southwood	58016-0221-20	20s	$7.74
Allscrips	54569-1712-01	28s	$5.45
Cheshire	55175-0088-08	28s	$7.18
Allscrips	54569-1712-04	30s	$5.84
Cheshire	55175-0088-00	30s	$7.70
Allscrips	54569-1712-00	40s	$7.79
Cheshire	55175-0088-04	40s	$8.21
Southwood	58016-0221-40	40s	$9.46
Southwood	58016-0221-60	60s	$10.98
Allscrips	54569-1712-03	60s	$11.68
Copley	38245-0144-10	100s	$9.15
Major	00904-1254-60	100s	$13.50
Major	00904-1251-60	100s	$13.50
Parmed	00349-8482-01	100s	$13.77
Qualitest	00603-5755-21	100s	$14.40
Schein	00364-0833-01	100s	$14.85
URL	00677-1025-01	100s	$14.95
Mutual	53489-0466-01	100s	$14.95
Goldline	00182-1803-01	100s	$15.00
Southwood	58016-0221-00	100s	$15.56
Rosemont	00832-1038-00	100s	$15.75
Martec	52555-0248-01	100s	$16.16
AMIGESIC: Amide	52152-0020-02	100s	$16.95
Moore,H.L.	00839-7168-06	100s	$17.75
Allscrips	54569-1712-02	100s	$19.47
ANAFLEX 750: Blansett	51674-0013-01	100s	$22.25
Eon	00185-0762-01	100s	$22.50
Eon	00185-0857-01	100s	$22.50
SALSITAB: Upsher-Smith	00245-0154-11	100s	$25.08
Duramed	51285-0297-02	100s	$26.56
Invamed	52189-0244-24	100s	$26.56
Aligen	00405-4935-01	100s	$28.00
Sidmak	50111-0391-01	100s	$28.00
R.I.D.	54807-0141-01	100s	$42.43
Barre	00472-0133-10	100s	$42.71
Goldline	00182-1803-89	100s ud	$15.00
Auro	55829-0470-10	100s ud	$23.22
Major	00904-1251-61	100s ud	$26.86
SALSITAB: Upsher-Smith	00245-0154-01	100s ud	$26.98
Medirex	57480-0412-01	100s ud	$27.00
Copley	38245-0144-50	500s	$42.31
Goldline	00182-1803-05	500s	$46.50
Major	00904-1254-40	500s	$58.45

Saluron *SEE* HYDROFLUMETHIAZIDE

Salutensin *SEE* HYDROFLUMETHIAZIDE WITH RESERPINE

Sandimmune *SEE* CYCLOSPORINE

Sandoglobulin *SEE* GLOBULIN, IMMUNE

Sandostatin *SEE* OCTREOTIDE ACETATE

Sanorex *SEE* MAZINDOL

Sansert *SEE* METHYSERGIDE MALEATE

Santyl *SEE* COLLAGENASE

Sargramostim

DESCRIPTION

Sargramostim is a recombinant human granulocyte-macrophage colony stimulating factor (rhu GM-CSF) produced by recombinant DNA technology in a yeast (*S. cerevisiae*) expression system. GM-CSF is a hematopoietic growth factor which stimulates proliferation and differentiation of hematopoietic progenitor cells. Sargramostim is a glycoprotein of 127 amino acids characterized by 3 primary molecular species having molecular masses of 19,500, 16,800, and 15,500 daltons. The amino acid sequence of Sargramostim differs from the natural human GM-CSF by a substitution of leucine at position 23, and the carbohydrate moiety may be different from the native protein. Sargramostim has been selected as the proper name for yeast-derived rhu GM-CSF. Sargramostim is formulated as a sterile, white, preservative-free, lyophilized powder and is intended for IV infusion following reconstitution with 1 ml Sterile Water for Injection USP. Each single-use vial of Sargramostim contains either 250 mcg or 500 mcg Sargramostim; 40 mg Mannitol, USP; 10 mg Sucrose, NF; and 1.2 mg Tromethamine, USP. The pH of the reconstituted, isotonic solution is 7.4 + 0.3. The specific activity of Sargramostim is approximately 5×10^7 colony forming units per mg in a normal human bone marrow colony formation assay.

Following is its chemical structure:

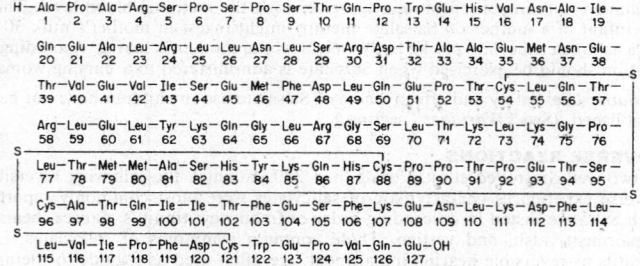

CLINICAL PHARMACOLOGY

GENERAL

Granulocyte-macrophage colony stimulating factor belongs to a group of growth factors termed colony stimulating factors which support survival, clonal expansion, and differentiation of hematopoietic progenitor cells. GM-CSF induces partially committed progenitor cells to divide and differentiate in the granulocyte-macrophage pathways.

GM-CSF is also capable of activating mature granulocytes and macrophages. GM-CSF is a multilineage factor and, in addition to dose-dependent effects on the myelomonocytic lineage, can promote the proliferation of megakaryocytic and erythroid progenitors.[1] However, other factors are required to induce complete maturation in these two lineages.

The various cellular responses (i.e., division, maturation, activation) are induced through GM-CSF binding to specific receptors expressed on the cell surface of target cells.[2]

IN VITRO STUDIES OF SARGRAMOSTIM IN HUMAN CELLS

The biological activity of GM-CSF is species-specific. Consequently, *in vitro* studies have been performed on human cells to characterize the pharmacological activity of Sargramostim. *In vitro* exposure of human bone marrow cells to

Sargramostim at concentrations ranging from 1-100 ng/ml results in the proliferation of hematopoietic progenitors and in the formation of pure granulocyte, pure macrophage, and mixed granulocyte-macrophage colonies.[3] Chemotactic, antifungal, and antiparasitic[4] activities of granulocytes and monocyte are increased by exposure to Sargramostim in vitro. Sargramostim increases the cytotoxicity of monocytes toward certain neutrophils to inhibit the growth of tumor cells.

IN VIVO PRIMATE STUDIES OF SARGRAMOSTIM
Pharmacology/toxicology studies of Sargramostim were performed in cynomolgus monkeys. An acute toxicity study revealed an absence of treatment-related toxicity following a single IV bolus injection at a dose of 300 mcg/kg. Two subacute studies were performed using IV injection (maximum dose 200 mcg/kg/day × 14 days) and subcutaneous injection (maximum dose 200 mcg/kg/day × 28 days). No major visceral organ toxicity was documented. Notable histopathology findings included increased cellularity in hematologic organs, heart, and lung tissues. A dose-dependent increase in leukocyte count occurred during the dosing period which consisted primarily of segmented neutrophils; increases in monocytes, basophils, eosinophils, and lymphocytes were also noted. Leukocyte counts decreased to pretreatment values over a 1-2 week recovery period.

PHARMACOKINETICS
Pharmacokinetic profiles have been analyzed in patients with various neoplastic diseases following intravenous administration of Sargramostim. In 2 patients receiving 250 mcg/m^2 of Sargramostim by 2 hour IV infusion, serum concentration ranged from 22,000 pg/ml to 23,000 pg/ml at the termination of the infusion. The pharmacokinetic profile, calculated on samples from 5 patients receiving 500-750 mcg/m^2 of Sargramostim by 2 hour IV infusion, revealed a rapid initial decline in GM-CSF serum concentration ($t_{1/2\alpha} \sim$ 12 to 17 minutes) followed by a slower decrease ($t_{1/2\beta} \sim$ 2 hours). In four patients treated with Sargramostim by subcutaneous injection (125 mcg/m^2 every 12 hours), Sargramostim was detected in the serum within 5 minutes after administration (range 55-450 pg/ml). Peak levels were observed 2 hours after injection (range 350-3,900 pg/ml), and Sargramostim remained at detectable levels 6 hours following injection (range 150-2,700 pg/ml).[5]

ANTIBODY FORMATION
Serum samples collected before and after Sargramostim treatment from 165 patients with a variety of underlying diseases have been examined for the presence of antibodies. Neutralizing antibodies were detected in 5 of 165 patients (3.0%) after receiving Sargramostim by continuous IV infusion (3 patients) or subcutaneous injection (2 patients) for 28 to 84 days in multiple courses. All 5 patients had impaired hematopoiesis before the administration of Sargramostim and consequently the effect of the development of anti-GM-CSF antibodies on normal hematopoiesis could not be assessed. Drug-induced neutropenia, neutralization of endogenous GM-CSF activity, and diminution of the therapeutic effect of Sargramostim secondary to formation of neutralizing antibody remain a theoretical possibility. A systematic screening program to evaluate antibody formation is ongoing for patients enrolled in clinical trials.

INDICATIONS AND USAGE
USE IN MYELOID RECONSTITUTION AFTER AUTOLOGOUS BONE MARROW TRANSPLANTATION
Sargramostim is indicated for acceleration of myeloid recovery in patients with nonHodgkin's lymphoma (NHL), acute lymphoblastic leukemia (ALL), and Hodgkin's disease undergoing autologous bone marrow transplantation (BMT). After autologous BMT in patients with NHL, ALL, or Hodgkin's disease Sargramostim has been found to be safe and effective in accelerating myeloid engraftment, decreasing median duration of antibiotic administration, reducing the median duration of infectious episodes and shortening the median duration of hospitalization. Hematologic response to Sargramostim can be detected by complete blood count (CBC) with differential performed twice per week.

Insufficient data are presently available to support the efficacy of Sargramostim in accelerating myeloid recovery following peripheral blood stem cell transplantation.

USE IN BONE MARROW TRANSPLANTATION FAILURE OR ENGRAFTMENT DELAY
Sargramostim is indicated in patients who have undergone allogeneic or autologous bone marrow transplantation (BMT) in whom engraftment is delayed or has failed. Sargramostim has been found to be safe and effective in prolonging survival of patients who are experiencing graft failure or engraftment delay, in the presence or absence of infection, following autologous or allogeneic BMT. Survival benefit may be relatively greater in those patients who demonstrate one or more of the following characteristics: autologous BMT failure or engraftment delay, no previous total body irradiation, malignancy other than leukemia or a multiple organ failure (MOF) score ≤ 2 (see "Clinical Experience"). Hematologic response to Sargramostim can be detected by complete blood count (CBC) with differential performed twice per week.

CLINICAL EXPERIENCE
Effects on Myeloid Reconstitution after Autologous Bone Marrow Transplantation.[6] Following a dose-ranging Phase I/II trial in patients undergoing autologous BMT for lymphoid malignancies,[7,8] three single-center, randomized, placebo-controlled and double-blinded studies were conducted to evaluate the safety and efficacy of Sargramostim or promoting hematopoietic reconstitution following autologous BMT. A total of 128 patients (65 Sargramostim, 63 placebo) were enrolled in these 3 studies. The majority of the patients had lymphoid malignancy

(87 NHL, 17 ALL), 23 patients had Hodgkin's disease, and 1 patient had acute myeloblastic leukemia (AML). In 72 patients with NHL or ALL, the bone marrow harvest was purged prior to storage with one of several monoclonal antibodies. No chemical agent was used for in vitro treatment of the bone marrow. Preparative regimens in the 3 studies included cyclophosphamide (total dose 120-150 mg/kg) and total body irradiation (total dose 1,200-1,575 rads). Other regimens used in patients with Hodgkin's disease and NHL without radiotherapy consisted of 3 or more of the following in combination (expressed as total dose): cytosine arabinoside (400 mg/m^2) and carmustine (300 mg/m^2), cyclophosphamide (140-150 mg/kg), hydroxyurea (4.5 gm/m^2), and etoposide (375-450 mg/m^2).

Compared to placebo, administration of Sargramostim in 2 studies (n = 44 and 47) significantly improved the following hematologic and clinical endpoints: time to neutrophil engraftment, duration of hospitalization, and infection experience or antibacterial usage. In the third study (n = 37) there was a positive trend toward earlier myeloid engraftment in favor of Sargramostim. This latter study differed from the other 2 in having enrolled a large number of patients with Hodgkin's disease who had also received extensive radiation and chemotherapy prior to harvest of autologous bone marrow. A subgroup analysis of the data from all three studies revealed that the median time to engraftment for patients with Hodgkin's disease, regardless of treatment, was 6 days longer when compared to patients with NHL and ALL, but that the overall beneficial Sargramostim treatment effect was the same. In the following combined analysis of the 3 studies, these 2 subgroups (NHL and ALL vs. Hodgkin's disease) are presented separately.

Patients with Lymphoid Malignancy (Non-Hodgkin's Lymphoma and Acute Lymphoblastic Leukemia): Myeloid engraftment (absolute neutrophil count [ANC] ≥ 500 cells/mm^3) in 54 patients receiving Sargramostim was observed 6 days earlier than in 50 patients treated with placebo (see table below). Accelerated myeloid engraftment was associated with significant clinical benefits. The median duration of hospitalization was 6 days shorter for the Sargramostim group than for the placebo group. Median duration of infectious episodes (defined as fever and neutropenia; or 2 positive cultures of the same organism; or fever > 38°C and 1 positive blood culture; or clinical evidence of infection) was 3 days less in the group treated with Sargramostim. The median duration of antibacterial administration in the post-transplantation period was 4 days shorter for the patients treated with Sargramostim than for placebo-treated patients. The study was unable to detect a significant difference between the treatment groups in rate of disease relapse 24 months post-transplantation. As a group, leukemic subjects receiving Sargramostim derived less benefit than NHL subjects. However, both the leukemic and NHL groups receiving Sargramostim engrafted earlier than controls. (See related table).

Patients with Hodgkin's Disease: If patients with Hodgkin's disease are analyzed separately, a trend toward earlier myeloid engraftment was noted. Sargramostim treated patients engrafted earlier (by 5 days) than the placebo-treated subjects (p = 0.189, Wilcoxon) but the number of patients was small (n = 22); 1 patient (#23) from one site was noncontrolled and was excluded from the analysis. Studies are in progress to confirm statistically the trend toward earlier engraftment of Sargramostim in patients with Hodgkin's disease.

EFFECTS IN BONE MARROW TRANSPLANTATION FAILURE OR ENGRAFTMENT DELAY
A historically-controlled study was conducted in patients experiencing graft failure following allogeneic or autologous BMT to determine whether Sargramostim improved survival after BMT failure.

Three categories of patients were eligible for this study:
1) patients displaying a delay in engraftment (ANC ≤ 100 cells/mm^3 by day 28 post-transplantation);
2) patients displaying a delay in engraftment (ANC ≤ 100 cells/mm^3 by day 21 post-transplantation) and who had evidence of an active infection; and
3) patients who lost their marrow graft after a transient engraftment (manifested by an average of ANC ≥ 500 cells/mm^3 for at least one week followed by loss of engraftment with ANC > 500 cells/mm^3 for at least one week beyond day 21 post-transplantation).

A total of 140 eligible patients from 35 institutions treated with Sargramostim were evaluated in comparison to 103 historical control patients from a single institution. One hundred sixty-three patients had lymphoid or myeloid leukemia, 24 patients had nonHodgkin's lymphoma, 19 patients had Hodgkin's disease and 37 patients had other diseases, such as aplastic anemia, myelodysplasia or non-hematologic malignancy. The majority of patients (223 out of 243) had received prior chemotherapy with or without radiotherapy and/or immunotherapy prior to preparation for transplantation.

One hundred day survival was improved in favor of the patients treated with Sargramostim after graft failure following either autologous or allogeneic BMT. In addition, the median survival was improved by greater than 2-fold. The median survival of patients treated with Sargramostim after autologous failure was 474 days versus 161 days for the historical patients. Similarly, after allogeneic failure, the median survival was 97 days with Sargramostim treatment and 35 days for the historical controls. Improvement in survival was better in patients with fewer impaired organs. (See related table).

The MOF score is a simple clinical and laboratory assessment of 7 major organ systems: cardiovascular, respiratory, gastrointestinal, hematologic, renal, hepatic and neurologic.[9] Assessment of the MOF score is recommended as an additional method of determining the need to initiate treatment with Sargramostim in patients with graft failure or delay in engraftment following autologous or allogeneic BMT.

Factors that Contribute to Survival: The probability of survival was relatively greater for patients with any one of the following characteristics: autologous BMT failure or delay in engraftment, exclusion of total body irradiation from the preparative regimen, a non-leukemic malignancy or MOF score ≤ 2 (0, 1 or 2 dysfunctional organ systems). Leukemic subjects derived less benefit than other subjects.

UNLABELED USES
Sargramostim is used alone or as an adjunct in the treatment of chemotherapy-induced myelosuppression.

CONTRAINDICATIONS
Sargramostim is contraindicated in patients with:
1) excessive leukemic myeloid blasts in the bone marrow or peripheral blood ($\geq 10\%$).
2) known hypersensitivity to GM-CSF, yeast-derived products, or any component of the product.

WARNINGS
FLUID RETENTION
Peripheral edema, capillary leak syndrome, pleural and/or pericardial effusion have been reported in patients after Sargramostim administration. In 156 patients enrolled in placebo-controlled studies using Sargramostim at a dose of 250 mcg/m^2/day by 2 hour IV infusion, the reported incidences of fluid retention (Sargramostim vs. placebo) were as follows: peripheral edema, 11% vs. 7%; pleural effusion, 1% vs. 0%; and pericardial effusion, 4% vs. 1%. Capillary leak syndrome was not observed in this limited number of studies; based on other uncontrolled studies and post-marketing reports, the incidence is estimated to be less than 1%. In patients with preexisting pleural and pericardial effusions, administration of Sargramostim may aggravate fluid retention; however, fluid retention associated with or worsened by Sargramostim has been reversible after interruption or dose reduction of Sargramostim with or without diuretic therapy. Sargramostim should be used with caution in patients with preexisting fluid retention, pulmonary infiltrates, or congestive heart failure.

RESPIRATORY SYMPTOMS
Sequestration of granulocytes in the pulmonary circulation has been documented following Sargramostim infusion,[10] and dyspnea has been reported occasionally in patients treated with Sargramostim. Special attention should be given to respiratory symptoms during or immediately following Sargramostim infusion, especially in patients with preexisting lung disease. In patients displaying dyspnea during Sargramostim administration, the rate of infusion should be reduced by half. If respiratory symptoms worsen despite infusion rate reduction, the infusion should be discontinued. Subsequent IV infusions may be administered following the standard dose schedule with careful monitoring. Sargramostim should be administered with caution in patients with hypoxia.

CARDIOVASCULAR SYMPTOMS
Occasional transient supraventricular arrhythmia has been reported in uncontrolled studies during Sargramostim administration, particularly in patients with a previous history of cardiac arrhythmia. However, these arrhythmias have been reversible after discontinuation of Sargramostim. Sargramostim should be used with caution in patients with preexisting cardiac disease.

RENAL AND HEPATIC DYSFUNCTION
In some patients with preexisting renal or hepatic dysfunction enrolled in uncontrolled clinical trials, administration of Sargramostim has induced elevation of serum creatinine or bilirubin and hepatic enzymes. Dose reduction or interruption of Sargramostim administration has resulted in a decrease in pretreatment values. However, in controlled clinical trials the incidences of renal and hepatic dysfunction were comparable between Sargramostim (250 mcg/m^2/day by 2 hour IV infusion) and placebo-treated patients. Monitoring of renal and hepatic function in patients displaying renal or hepatic dysfunction prior to initiation of treatment is recommended at least biweekly during Sargramostim administration.

PRECAUTIONS
GENERAL
Parenteral administration of recombinant proteins should be attended by appropriate precautions in case an allergic or untoward reaction occurs. Transient rashes and local injection site reactions have occasionally been observed concomitantly with Sargramostim treatment. Serious allergic or anaphylactic reactions have been reported rarely. If any serious allergic or anaphylactic reaction occurs, Sargramostim therapy should immediately be discontinued and appropriate therapy initiated (see *"Warnings"*).

Rarely, hypotension with flushing and syncope has been reported following the first administration of Sargramostim. These signs have resolved with symptomatic treatment and have not recurred with subsequent doses in the same cycle of treatment.

Stimulation of marrow precursors with Sargramostim may result in a rapid rise in white blood cell (WBC) count. If the ANC exceeds 20,000 cells/mm^3 or if the platelet count exceeds 500,000/mm^3, Sargramostim administration should be interrupted or the dose reduced by half. The decision to reduce the dose or interrupt treatment should be based on the clinical condition of the patient. Excessive blood counts have returned to normal or baseline levels within 3 to 7 days following cessation of Sargramostim therapy. Twice weekly monitoring of CBC with differential (including examination for the presence of blast cells) should be performed to preclude development of excessive counts.

GROWTH FACTOR POTENTIAL
Sargramostim is a growth factor that primarily stimulates normal myeloid precursors. However, the possibility that Sargramostim can act as a growth factor for any tumor type, particularly myeloid malignancies, cannot be excluded. Because of the possibility of tumor growth potentiation, precaution should be exercised when using this drug in any malignancy with myeloid characteristics.

Sargramostim has been administered to patients with AML and myelodysplastic syndromes (MDS) in uncontrolled studies without evidence of increased relapse rates.[11,12,13] Controlled studies have not been performed in patients with AML or MDS. Sargramostim may be administered to those patients with AML or MDS who experience graft failure or delay in engraftment after bone marrow ablation and transplantation.

Progression of the underlying neoplastic disease (NHL, ALL, or Hodgkin's disease) was not observed during Sargramostim administration in clinical trials; however, should disease progression be detected during Sargramostim treatment, Sargramostim therapy should be discontinued. In controlled studies, the 24 month relapse rate was comparable in patients treated with Sargramostim or placebo.

USE IN PATIENTS RECEIVING PURGED BONE MARROW
Sargramostim is effective in accelerating myeloid recovery in patients receiving bone marrow purged by anti-B lymphocyte monoclonal antibodies. Data obtained from uncontrolled studies suggest that if *in vitro* marrow purging with chemical agents causes a significant decrease in the number of responsive hematopoietic progenitors, the patient may not respond to Sargramostim. When the bone marrow purging process preserves a sufficient number of progenitors ($> 1.2 \times 10^4$/kg), a beneficial effect of Sargramostim on myeloid engraftment has been reported.[14]

AUTOLOGOUS BMT: COMBINED ANALYSIS FROM PLACEBO-CONTROLLED CLINICAL TRIALS OF RESPONSES IN PATIENTS WITH NHL AND ALL

	ANC $\geq 500/mm^3$	ANC $\geq 1000/mm^3$	Median Values (days)		
			Duration of Hospitalization	Duration of Infection	Duration of Antibacterial Therapy
Sargramostim (n = 54)	18 *#	24 *#	25 *	1 *	21 *
Placebo (n = 50)	4	32	31	4	25

* $p < 0.05$ Wilcoxon or CMH ridit chi-square
\# $p < 0.05$ Log rank
Note: The single AML patient was not included.

MEDIAN SURVIVAL BY MULTIPLE ORGAN FAILURE (MOF) CATEGORY

	Median Survival (Days)		
	MOF ≤ 2 Organs	MOF > 2 Organs	MOF (Composite of Both Groups)
Autologous BMT			
Sargramostim	474 (n = 58)	78.5 (n = 10)	474 (n = 68)
Historical	165 (n = 14)	39 (n = 3)	161 (n = 17)
Allogeneic BMT			
Sargramostim	174 (n = 50)	27 (n = 22)	97 (n = 72)
Historical	52.5 (n = 60)	15.5 (n = 26)	35 (n = 86)

◆ RATED THERAPEUTICALLY EQUIVALENT; ◇ THERAPEUTIC EQUIVALENCE UNCONFIRMED; ○ UNRATED

USE IN PATIENTS PREVIOUSLY EXPOSED TO INTENSIVE CHEMOTHERAPY/RADIOTHERAPY

In patients who before autologous BMT, have received extensive radiotherapy to hematopoietic sites for the treatment of primary disease in the abdomen or chest, or have been exposed to multiple myelotoxic agents (alkylating agents, anthracycline antibiotics, and antimetabolites), the effect of Sargramostim on myeloid reconstitution may be limited.

PATIENT MONITORING

Sargramostim can induce variable increases in WBC and/or platelet counts. In order to avoid potential complications of excessive leukocytosis (WBC > 50,000 cells/mm³; ANC > 20,000 cells/mm³), a CBC is recommended twice per week during Sargramostim therapy. Monitoring of renal and hepatic function in patients displaying renal or hepatic dysfunction prior to initiation of treatment is recommended at least bi-weekly during Sargramostim administration. Body weight and hydration status should be carefully monitored during Sargramostim administration.

DRUG INTERACTION

Interactions between Sargramostim and other drugs have not been fully evaluated. Drugs which may potentiate the myeloproliferative effects of Sargramostim, such as lithium and corticosteroids, should be used with caution.

CONCOMITANT USE WITH CHEMOTHERAPY AND RADIOTHERAPY

The safety and efficacy of Sargramostim given simultaneously with cytotoxic chemotherapy or radiotherapy have not been established. Because of potential sensitivity of rapidly dividing hematopoietic progenitor cells to cytotoxic chemotherapeutic or radiologic therapies, Sargramostim should not be administered within 24 hours preceding or following chemotherapy, or within 12 hours preceding or following radiotherapy.

CARCINOGENESIS, MUTAGENESIS, IMPAIRMENT OF FERTILITY

Animal studies have not been conducted with Sargramostim to evaluate the carinogenic potential or the effect on fertility.

PREGNANCY (CATEGORY C)

Animal reproduction studies have not been conducted with Sargramostim. It is not known whether Sargramostim can cause fetal harm when administered to a pregnant woman or can affect reproductive capability. Sargramostim should be given to a pregnant woman only if clearly needed.

NURSING MOTHERS

It is not known whether Sargramostim is excreted in human milk. Because many drugs are excreted in human milk, Sargramostim should be administered to a nursing woman only if clearly needed.

PEDIATRIC USE

Safety and effectiveness in children have not been established; however, available safety data indicate that Sargramostim does not exhibit any greater toxicity in children than adults. A total of 113 pediatric subjects between the ages of 4 months and 18 years have been treated with Sargramostim in clinical trials at doses ranging from 60-1,000 mcg/m²/day intravenously and 4-1,500 mcg/m²/day subcutaneously. In 53 pediatric patients enrolled in controlled studies at a dose of 250 mcg/m²/day by 2 hour IV infusion, the type and frequency of adverse events were comparable to those reported for the adult population.

ADVERSE REACTIONS

Sargramostim is generally well tolerated. In 3 placebo-controlled studies enrolling a total of 156 patients after autologous BMT or peripheral stem cell transplantation, events reported in at least 10% of patients in Sargramostim or placebo groups were:

PERCENT OF PATIENTS REPORTING EVENTS

Events by Body System	Sargramostim (n = 79)	Placebo (n = 77)
Body, General		
Fever	95	96
Mucous membrane disorder	75	78
Asthenia	66	51
Malaise	57	51
Sepsis	11	14
Digestive System		
Nausea	90	96
Diarrhea	89	82
Vomiting	85	90
Anorexia	54	58
GI disorder	37	47
GI hemorrhage	27	33
Stomatitis	24	29
Liver damage	13	14
Skin and Appendages		
Alopecia	73	74
Rash	44	38
Metabolic/Nutritional Disorder		
Edema	34	35

Events by Body System	Sargramostim (n = 79)	Placebo (n = 77)
Peripheral edema	11	7
Respiratory System		
Dyspnea	28	31
Lung disorder	20	23
Hemic and Lymphatic System		
Blood dyscrasis	25	27
Cardiovascular System		
Hemorrhage	23	30
Urogenital System		
Urinary tract disorder	14	13
Kidney function abnormal	8	10
Nervous System		
CNS disorder	11	16

The frequency and type of adverse events were similar between Sargramostim and placebo control groups. Diarrhea, asthenia, rash, and malaise were the only events observed for 5% more subjects in the Sargramostim group than in the placebo group.

No significant differences were observed between Sargramostim and placebo-treated patients in the type or frequency of laboratory abnormalities, including renal and hepatic parameters. In some patients with preexisting renal or hepatic dysfunction enrolled in uncontrolled clinical trials, administration of Sargramostim has induced elevation of serum creatinine or bilirubin and hepatic enzymes (see "Warnings"). In addition, there was no significant difference in relapse rate and 24 month survival between the Sargramostim and placebo-treated patients.

Adverse events observed for the patients treated with Sargramostim in the historically controlled BMT failure study were similar to those reported in the placebo-controlled studies. In addition, headache (26%), pericardial effusion (25%), arthralgia (21%) and myalgia (18%) were also reported in patients treated with Sargramostim in the graft failure study.

In uncontrolled Phase I/II studies with Sargramostim in 215 patients, the most frequent adverse events were fever, asthenia, headache, bone pain, chills, and myalgia. These systemic events were generally mild or moderate and were usually prevented or reversed by the administration of analgesics and antipyretics such as acetaminophen. In these uncontrolled trials, other infrequent events reported were dyspnea, peripheral edema, and rash.

In patients with preexisting peripheral edema, capillary leak syndrome, pleural and/or pericardial effusion, administration of Sargramostim may aggravate fluid retention (see "Warnings"). Body weight and hydration status should be carefully monitored during Sargramostim administration.

Adverse events observed in pediatric patients in controlled studies were comparable to those observed in adult patients.

OVERDOSAGE

The maximum amount of Sargramostim that can be safely administered in single or multiple doses has not been determined. Doses up to 100 mcg/kg/day (4,000 mcg/m²/day or 16 times the recommended dose) were administered to 4 patients in a Phase I uncontrolled clinical study by continuous IV infusion for 7 to 18 days. Increases in WBC up to 200,000 cells/mm³ were observed. Adverse events reported were: dyspnea, malaise, nausea, fever, rash, sinus tachycardia, headache, and chills. All these events were reversible after discontinuation of Sargramostime.

In case of overdosage, Sargramostim therapy should be discontinued and the patient carefully monitored for WBC increase and respiratory symptoms.

DOSAGE AND ADMINISTRATION

MYELOID RECONSTITUTION AFTER AUTOLOGOUS BONE MARROW TRANSPLANTATION

The recommended dose is 250 mcg/m²/day for 21 days as a 2 hour IV infusion beginning 2 to 4 hours after the autologous bone marrow infusion, and not less than 24 hours after the last dose of chemotherapy and 12 hours after the last dose of radiotherapy. If a severe adverse reaction occurs, the dose can be reduced or temporarily discontinued until the reaction abates. If blast cells appear or disease progression occurs, the treatment should be discontinued.

In order to avoid potential complications of excessive leukocytosis (WBC > 50,000 cells/mm³; ANC > 20,000 cells/mm³), a CBC with differential is recommended twice per week during Sargramostim therapy. Sargramostim treatment should be interrupted or the dose reduced by half if the ANC exceeds 20,000 cells/mm³.

BONE MARROW TRANSPLANTATION FAILURE OR ENGRAFTMENT DELAY

The recommended dose is 250 mcg/m²/day for 14 days as a 2 hour IV infusion. The dose can be repeated after 7 days off therapy if engraftment has not occurred. If engraftment still has not occurred, a third course of 500 mcg/m²/day for 14 days may be tried after another 7 days off therapy. If there is still no improvement, it is unlikely that further dose escalation will be beneficial. If a severe adverse reaction occurs, the dose can be reduced or temporarily discontinued until the reaction abates. If blast cells appear or disease progression occurs, the treatment should be discontinued.

2478 / PRODUCT INFORMATION

In order to avoid potential complications of excessive leukocytosis (WBC > 50,000 cells/mm^3, ANC > 20,000 cells/mm^3) a CBC with differential is recommended twice per week during Sargramostim therapy. Sargramostim treatment should be interrupted or the dose reduced by half if the ANC exceeds 20,000 cells/mm^3.

PREPARATION OF SARGRAMOSTIM

1. Sargramostim is a sterile, white, preservative-free, lyophilized powder suitable for IV infusion upon reconstitution. Sargramostim (250 mcg or 500 mcg vials) should be reconstituted aseptically with 1.0 ml Sterile Water for Injection, USP (without preservative). The reconstituted Sargramostim solutions are clear, colorless, isotonic with a pH of 7.4 ± 0.3, and contain 250 or 500 mcg/ml of Sargramostim. The single-use vial should not be re-entered or reused. Do not save any unused portion for later administration.

2. During reconstitution the Sterile Water for Injection, USP should be directed at the side of the vial and the contents gently swirled to avoid foaming during dissolution. Avoid excessive or vigorous agitation; do not shake.

3. Dilution for IV infusion should be performed in 0.9% Sodium Chloride Injection, USP. If the final concentration of Sargramostim is below 10 mcg/ml, Albumin (Human) at a final concentration of 0.1% should be added to the saline prior to addition of Sargramostim to prevent adsorption to the components of the drug delivery system. To obtain a final concentration of 0.1% Albumin (Human), add 1 mg Albumin (Human) per 1 ml 0.9% Sodium Chloride Injection, USP (e.g. use 1 ml 5% Albumin [Human] in 50 ml 0.9% Sodium Chloride Injection, USP).

4. An in-line membrane filler should not be used for intravenous infusion of Sargramostim.

5. Sargramostim contains no antibacterial preservative and therefore should be administered as soon as possible, and within 6 hours following reconstitution and/or dilution for IV infusion. Store Sargramostim solutions under refrigeration at 2-8°C (36-46°F): do not freeze. Sargramostim vials are intended for single use only; discard any unused solution after 6 hours.

6. In the absence of compatibility and stability information, no other medication should be added to infusion solutions containing Sargramostim. Use only 0.9% Sodium Chloride Injection, USP to prepare IV infusion solutions.

7. Aseptic technique should be employed in the preparation of all Sargramostim solutions. To assure correct concentration following reconstitution, care should be exercised to eliminate any air bubbles from the needle hub of the syringe used to prepare the diluent. Parenteral drug products should be inspected visually for particulate matter and discoloration prior to administration whenever solution and container permit.

STORAGE

The sterile powder, the reconstituted solution, and the diluted solution for injection should be refrigerated at 2-8°C (36-46°F). Do not freeze or shake. Do not use beyond the expiration date printed on the vial.

REFERENCES

1. Metcalf D. The molecular biology and functions of the granulocyte-macrophage colony-stimulating factors. Blood 1986; 67(2):257-267. 2. Park LS, Friend D, Gillis S, Urdal DL. Characterization of the cell surface receptor for human granulocyte/macrophage colony stimulating factor. J. Exp Med 1986: 164:251-262. 3. Grabstein KH, Urdal DL, Tushinski RJ, et al. Induction of macrophage tumoricidal activity by granulocyte-macrophage colony-stimulating factors. Science 1986; 232:506-508. 4. Reed SG, Nathan CF, Pihl DL, et al. Recombinant granulocyte/macrophage colony-stimulating factor activates macrophages to inhibit Trypanosoma cruzi and release hydrogen peroxide. J Exp Med 1987: 166:1734-1746. 5. Shadduck RK, Washeed A, Evans C, et al. Serum and urinary levels of recombinant human granulocyte-macrophage colony stimulating factor. Assessment after intravenous infusion and subcutaneous injection. Exp Hem 1990: 18:601. 6. Nemunaitis J, Rabinowe SN, Singer JW, et al. Recombinant human granulocyte-macrophage colony-stimulating factor after autologous bone marrow transplantation for lymphoid malignancy: Pooled results of a randomized, double-blind, placebo controlled trial. NEJM 1991: 324(25):1773-1778. 7. Nemunaitis J, Singer JW, Buckner CD, et al. Use of recombinant human granulocyte-macrophage colony stimulating factor in autologous bone marrow transplantation for lymphoid malignancies. Blood 1988; 72(2):834-836. 8. Nemunaitis J, Singer JW, Buckner CD, et al. Long-term follow-up of patients who received recombinant human granulocyte-macrophage colony stimulating factor after autologous bone marrow transplantation for lymphoid malignancy. BMT 1991; 7:49-52. 9. Goris RJA, Boekhorst TPA, Nuytinck JKS, et al Multiple organ failure: Generalized auto-destructive inflammation? Arch Surg 1985; 120:1109-1115. 10. Hermann F, Schulz G, Lindemann A, et al. Yeast-expressed granulocyte-macrophage colony-stimulating factor in cancer patients. A phase Ib clinical study. In Behring Institute Research Communications. Colony Stimulating Factors-CSF. International Symposium, Garmisch-Partenkirchen, West Germany. 1988; 83:107-118. 11. Estey EH, Dixon D, Kantarjian H, et al. Treatment of poor-prognosis, newly diagnosed acute myeloid leukemia with Ara-C and recombinant human granulocyte-macrophage colony-stimulating factor. Blood 1990; 75(9): 1766-1769. 12. Vadhan-Raj S, Keating M. LeMaistre A, et al. Effects of recombinant human granulocyte-macrophage colony-stimulating factor in patients with myelodysplastic syndromes. NEJM 1987: 317:1545-1552. 13. Buchner T, Hiddemann W, Koenigsmann M, et al. Recombinant human granulocyte-macrophage colony stimulating factor after chemotherapy in patients with acute myeloid leukemia at higher age or after relapse. Blood 1991: 78(5):1190-1197. 14. Blazar BR, Kersey JH, McGlave PB, et al, In vivo administration of recombinant human granulocyte/macrophage colony-stimulating factor in acute lymphoblastic leukemia patients receiving purged autografts. Blood 1989: 73(3):849-857.

J CODES
250 mcg IV—J2820

HOW SUPPLIED
POWDER FOR INJECTION: 250 MCG

BRAND/MANUFACTURER	NDC	SIZE	AWP
○ BRAND LEUKINE: Immunex	58406-0002-01	1s	$106.00

POWDER FOR INJECTION: 500 MCG

BRAND/MANUFACTURER	NDC	SIZE	AWP
○ BRAND LEUKINE: Immunex	58406-0001-01	1s	$200.00

Sclavo Test-PPD SEE TUBERCULIN

Scopolamine

DESCRIPTION

Scopolamine is available as an injection and in a transdermal delivery system. Scopolamine hydrobromide injection is a sterile solution of Scopolamine ($C_{17}H_{21}NO_4$•HBr·3H_2O) in water for injection. Scopolamine hydrobromide injection is intended for intramuscular intravenous and subcutaneous use. Its pH is 3.5-6.5.

The Scopolamine transdermal delivery system is designed for continuous release of Scopolamine following application to an area of intact skin on the head, behind the ear. Clinical evaluation has demonstrated that the system provides effective antiemetic and antinauseant actions when tested against motion-sickness stimuli in adults.

Release Rate Concept: The Scopolamine transdermal system is programmed to deliver 0.5 mg of Scopolamine at an approximately constant rate to the systemic circulation over the 3-day lifetime of the system. An initial priming dose of Scopolamine, saturates the skin binding sites and rapidly brings the plasma concentration of Scopolamine to the required steady-state level. A continuous controlled release of Scopolamine maintains the plasma level constant.

Each ml of solution for injection contains:
Scopolamine Hydrobromide ....0.3, 0.4, or 1 mg

The transdermal system contains:
Scopolamine ....1.5 mg

Following is its chemical structure:

CLINICAL PHARMACOLOGY

Scopolamine, a belladonna alkaloid, is one of the major antimuscarinic agents that inhibit the action of acetylcholine (ACh) on autonomic effectors innervated by postganglionic cholinergic nerves as well as on smooth muscles that lack cholinergic innervation. It exerts little effect on the actions of ACh at nicotinic receptor sites such as autonomic ganglia. The major action of this antimuscarinic agent is a surmountable antagonism to ACh and other muscarinic agents.

As compared with atropine, Scopolamine differs only quantitatively in antimuscarinic actions. Scopolamine has a stronger action on the iris, ciliary body and certain secretory glands such as salivary, bronchial and sweat. Scopolamine, in therapeutic doses, normally causes drowsiness, euphoria, amnesia, fatigue and dreamless sleep with a reduction in rapid-eye-movement sleep. However, the same doses occasionally cause excitement, restlessness, hallucinations, or delirium, especially in the presence of severe pain. Scopolamine depresses the EEG arousal response to photostimulation. It is more potent than atropine on the antitremor activity (parkinsonism) in animals induced by surgical lesions. Scopolamine is effective in preventing motion sickness by acting on the maculae of the utricle and saccule.

Scopolamine, although less potent than atropine, has been used frequently in preanesthetic medication for the purpose of inhibiting the secretions of the nose, mouth, pharynx and bronchi and reduces the occurrence of laryngospasm during general anesthesia. Scopolamine is less potent in the decrease of cardiac rate, but not in the changes of blood pressure or cardiac output. Like other antimuscarinic agents, Scopolamine has been used widely in the treatment of peptic ulcers and as an antispasmodic agent for G.I. disorders. This is due to the fact that Scopolamine reduces salivary secretion, the gastric secretion (both the volume and acid content), and also it inhibits the motor activity of the stomach, duodenum, jejunum, ileum and colon, characterized by a decrease in tone, amplitude and frequency of peristaltic contractions.

The ability of Scopolamine to prevent motion-induced nausea is believed to be associated with inhibition of vestibular input to the CNS, which results in inhibition of the vomiting reflex. In addition, Scopolamine may have a direct action on the vomiting center within the reticular formation of the brain stem.

◆ RATED THERAPEUTICALLY EQUIVALENT; ◇ THERAPEUTIC EQUIVALENCE UNCONFIRMED; ○ UNRATED

Applied to the postauricular skin, Scopolamine transdermal system provides for a gradual release of Scopolamine.

INDICATIONS AND USAGE

Scopolamine HBr injection is indicated as a sedative and tranquilizing depressant to the central nervous system. In its peripheral actions, Scopolamine differs from atropine in that it is a stronger blocking agent for the iris, ciliary body and salivary, bronchial and sweat glands but is weaker in its action on the heart (in which it is incapable of exerting actions in tolerated doses), the intestinal tract and bronchial musculature.

In addition to the usual uses for antimuscarinic drugs, Scopolamine is employed for its central depressant actions as a sedative. Frequently it is given as a preanesthetic medicament for both its sedative-tranquilizing and antisecretory actions. It is an effective antiemetic. It is used in maniacal states, in delirium tremens and in obstetrics. As a mydriatic and cycloplegic, it has a somewhat shorter duration (3 to 7 days) and intraocular pressure is affected less markedly than with atropine.

Scopolamine transdermal system is indicated for prevention of nausea and vomiting associated with motion sickness in adults. It should be applied only to skin in the postauricular area.

Clinical Results: Scopolamine transdermal system provides antiemetic protection within several hours following application behind the ear. In 195 adult subjects of different racial origins who participated in clinical efficacy studies at sea or in a controlled motion environment, there was a 75% reduction in the incidence of motion-induced nausea and vomiting, Scopolamine transdermal system provided significantly greater protection than that obtained with oral dimenhydrinate.

UNLABELED USES

Scopolamine is used alone or as an adjunct in the treatment of sialorrhea, duodenal ulcer, and postoperative vomiting.

CONTRAINDICATIONS

Scopolamine HBr is contraindicated in patients with narrow-angle glaucoma, since administration of the drug could raise the intraocular pressure to dangerous levels. However, this will not happen for side-angle glaucoma patients. Repeated administration of Scopolamine to a patient with chronic lung disease is considered to be potentially hazardous. Patients hypersensitive to belladonna or to barbiturates may be hypersensitive to Scopolamine hydrobromide.

Scopolamine transdermal system should not be used in patients with known hypersensitivity to Scopolamine or any of the components of the adhesive matrix making up the therapeutic system, or in patients with glaucoma.

WARNINGS

Addiction does not occur, although vomiting, malaise, sweating and salivation have been reported in patients with parkinsonism upon sudden withdrawal of large doses of Scopolamine. Scopolamine is one of the most important drugs of the belladonna group from the standpoint of poisoning; infants and young children are especially susceptible to the belladonna alkaloids. Scopolamine is usually stated to be more toxic than atropine. Idiosyncrasy is more common with Scopolamine than with atropine and ordinary therapeutic doses sometimes cause alarming reactions.

Scopolamine transdermal system should not be used in children and should be used with special caution in the elderly. See *"Precautions"*.

Since drowsiness, disorientation, and confusion may occur with the use of Stcopolamine, patients should be warned of the possibility and cautioned against engaging in activities that require mental alertness, such as driving a motor vehicle or operating dangerous machinery.

Potentially alarming idiosyncratic reactions may occur with ordinary therapeutic doses of Scopolamine.

PRECAUTIONS

GENERAL

If there is mydriasis and photophobia, dark glasses should be worn. Appropriate dosage precautions must be taken with infants, children, persons with mongolism, brain damage, spasticity, or light irides. Elevated intraocular pressure, urinary difficulty and retention and constipation are more probable in elderly persons. Men with prostatic hypertrophy should especially be monitored for urinary function. Because of the tachycardic effects of the drugs, care must be exercised when tachycardia, other tachyarrhythmias, coronary heart disease, congestive heart disease or hyperthyroidism preexist. Persons with hypertension may experience both exaggerated orthostatic hypotension and tachycardia. Similarly, autonomic neuropathy requires caution. Persons with a history of allergies or bronchial asthma will show a higher than normal incidence of hypersensitivity reactions.

Scopolamine should be used with caution in patients with pyloric obstruction, or urinary bladder neck obstruction. Caution should be exercised when administering an antiemetic or antimuscarinic drug to patients suspected of having intestinal obstruction.

Scopolamine transdermal system should be used with special caution in the elderly or in individuals with impaired metabolic, liver, or kidney functions, because of the increased likelihood of CNS effects.

INFORMATION FOR PATIENTS

Since Scopolamine can cause temporary dilation of the pupils and blurred vision if it comes in contact with the eyes, patients should be strongly advised to wash their hands thoroughly with soap and water immediately after handling the system.

Patients should be advised to remove the system immediately and contact a physician in the unlikely event that they experience symptoms of acute narrow-angle glaucoma (pain in and reddening of the eyes accompanied by dilated pupils). Patients should be warned against driving a motor vehicle or operating dangerous machinery.

LABORATORY TESTS

Barbiturates may increase bromosulfonphthalein (BSP) levels; administration is not recommended during the 24 hours preceding the test.

DRUG INTERACTIONS

Other drugs, such as phenothiazines, tricyclic antidepressants, certain antihistamines, meperidine, etc., which have weak antimuscarinic activity, may considerably intensify the effects of antimuscarinic drugs. Aluminum- and magnesium trisilicate-containing antacids have been shown to decrease the absorption of some antimuscarinic drugs and may possibly do so with all of them.

Scopolamine should be used with care in patients taking drugs, including alcohol, capable of causing CNS effects. Special attention should be given to drugs having anticholinergic properties, e.g., belladonna alkaloids, antihistamines (including meclizine), and antidepressants.

CARCINOGENESIS, MUTAGENESIS, IMPAIRMENT OF FERTILITY

No long-term studies in animals have been performed to evaluate carcinogenic potential. Fertility studies were performed in female rats and revealed no evidence of impaired fertility or harm to the fetus due to Scopolamine HBr administered by daily subcutaneous injection. In the highest-dose group (plasma level approximately 500 times the level achieved in humans using a transdermal system), reduced maternal body weights were observed.

PREGNANCY CATEGORY C

Teratogenic studies were performed in pregnant rats and rabbits with Scopolamine HBr administered by daily intravenous injection. No adverse effects were recorded in the rats. In the rabbits, the highest dose (plasma level approximately 100 times the level achieved in humans using a transdermal system) of drug administered had a marginal embryotoxic effect.

Scopolamine HBr can pass the placental barrier; the threat to the fetus *in utero* is unknown, but use during pregnancy may cause respiratory depression in the neonate and may contribute to neonatal hemorrhage due to reduction in vitamin K-dependent clotting factors in the neonate.

Scopolamine should be used during pregnancy only if the potential benefit justifies the potential risk to the fetus.

NURSING MOTHERS

Problems in humans have not been documented; however, risk-benefit must be considered since barbiturates and belladonna alkaloids are excreted in breast milk.

It is not known whether Scopolamine is excreted in human milk. Because many drugs are excreted in human milk, caution should be exercised when transdermal Scopolamine system is administered to a nursing woman.

PEDIATRIC USE

Children are particularly susceptible to the side effects of belladonna alkaloids. Scopolamine transdermal system should not be used in children because it is not known whether this system will release an amount of Scopolamine that could produce serious adverse effects in children.

ADVERSE REACTIONS

With nearly all antimuscarinic drugs, dry mouth is the first and dry skin is the second most common side effect. Thirst and difficulty in swallowing occur when the mouth and esophagus become sufficiently dry; chronic dry mouth also fosters dental caries. Suppression of sweating causes reflexive flushing and heat intolerance and can result in heat exhaustion or heat stroke in a hot environment; it also contributes to the hyperthermia seen in intoxication. Mydriasis frequently occurs, especially with Scopolamine; photophobia and blurring of vision are consequences of mydriasis. Cycloplegia (which exacerbates blurred vision) occurs approximately concomitantly with mydriasis, but usually higher doses are required. In susceptible persons, especially the elderly, cycloplegia may contribute to an elevation of intraocular pressure. Difficulty in urination and urinary retention may occur. Tachycardia is a common side effect. Constipation, even bowel stasis, may occur.

In the larger therapeutic doses, Scopolamine may cause dizziness, restlessness, tremors, fatigue and locomotor difficulties.

The following additional adverse reactions have been reported during the use of Scopolamine transdermal system: drowsiness, disorientation; memory disturbances; dizziness; restlessness; hallucinations; confusion; rashes and erythema; acute narrow-angle glaucoma; and dry, itchy, or red eyes.

Drug Withdrawal: Symptoms including dizziness, nausea, vomiting, headache and disturbances of equilibrium have been reported in a few patients following discontinuation of the use of the Scopolamine transdermal system. These symptoms have occurred most often in patients who have used the systems for more than three days.

OVERDOSAGE

Serious systemic intoxication can occur even from topical ophthalmologic application, especially in children, since both local absorption and nasolacrimal drainage into the gut can deliver considerable amounts to the circulation. In serious intoxication, hyperpyrexia, flushing, nausea, vomiting, drowsiness, disorientation, memory disturbances, dizziness, restlessness, confusion, stupor, hallucinations, leukocytosis, nonallergenic rashes, circulatory or respiratory collapse, even death, in addition to all aforenamed effects, may occur. Children, especially infants and children with mongolism, spastic paralysis or brain damage, are more sensitive than adults to the toxic effects.

If marked excitement is present and more specific treatment is not available, diazepam is most suitable for sedation and for control of convulsions. Large doses should be avoided because the central depressant action may coincide with the depression occurring late in belladonna poisoning. Phenothiazines should not be used because their antimuscuranic action is likely to intensify toxicity and may plunge the patient into coma. Artificial respiration with oxygen may be necessary. Ice bags and alcohol sponges help to reduce fever, especially in children.

Should any symptoms occur, the Scopolamine transdermal system should be immediately removed. Appropriate parasympathomimetic therapy should be initiated if these symptoms are severe.

DOSAGE AND ADMINISTRATION
SCOPOLAMINE HBR INJECTION
Adult: For obstetric amnesia or preoperative sedation, 0.32 to 0.65 mg (320 to 650 µg).

For sedation or tranquilization, 0.6 mg (600 µg) 3 or 4 times a day.

Subcutaneous, as an antiemetic, 0.6 to 1 mg.

Pediatric: Age 6 mo. to 3 yr., 0.1 to 0.15 mg (100 to 150 µg). Age 3 to 6 yr., 0.2 to 0.3 mg (200 to 300 µg).

Subcutaneous, as antiemetic, 0.006 mg (6 µg) per kg.

DOSAGE EQUIVALENTS

1 mg (1000 µg)/mL		
1 mg	(1000 µg)	1 mL
0.8 mg	(800 µg)	0.8 mL
0.6 mg	(600 µg)	0.6 mL
0.5 mg	(500 µg)	0.5 mL
0.4 mg	(400 µg)	0.4 mL
0.3 mg	(300 µg)	0.3 mL
0.2 mg	(200 µg)	0.2 mL
0.1 mg	(100 µg)	0.1 mL
0.4 mg (400 µg)/mL		
0.4 mg	(400 µg)	1 mL
0.3 mg	(300 µg)	0.75 mL
0.25 mg	(250 µg)	0.63 mL
0.2 mg	(200 µg)	0.50 mL
0.15 mg	(150 µg)	0.38 mL
0.3 mg (300 µg)/mL		
0.3 mg	(300 µg)	1 mL
0.25 mg	(250 µg)	0.83 mL
0.2 mg	(200 µg)	0.66 mL
0.15 mg	(150 µg)	0.5 mL

Belladonna alkaloids provide a therapeutic effect in about 1 or 2 hours with a duration of about 4 hours.

Geriatric and debilitated patients may respond to the usual doses with excitement, agitation, drowsiness or confusion; lower doses may be required in such patients.

Close supervision is recommended for infants, blondes, mongoloids and children with spastic paralysis or brain damage, since an increased responsiveness to belladonna alkaloids has been reported in these patients and dosage adjustments are often required.

Administration of belladonna alkaloids and barbiturates 30 to 60 minutes before meals is recommended to maximize absorption and, when issued for reducing stomach acid formation, to allow its effect to coincide better with antacid administration following the meal.

Parenteral drug products should be inspected visually for particulate matter prior to administration, whenever solution and container permit.

SCOPOLAMINE TRANSDERMAL DELIVERY SYSTEM
Initiation of Therapy: One Scopolamine transdermal system (programmed to deliver 0.5 mg of Scopolamine over 3 days) should be applied to the hairless area behind one ear at least 4 hours before the antiemetic effect is required. Only one should be worn at any time.

Handling: After the system is applied on dry skin behind the ear, the hands should be washed thoroughly with soap and water and dried. Upon removal of the system, it should be discarded, and the hands and application site washed thoroughly with soap and water and dried, to prevent any traces of Scopolamine from coming into direct contact with the eyes.

Continuation of Therapy: Should the system become displaced, it should be discarded, and a fresh one placed on the hairless area behind the other ear. If therapy is required for longer than 3 days, the first system should be discarded, and a fresh one placed on the hairless area behind the other ear.

STORAGE
Protect from light.

Use only if solution is clear and seal intact.

The system should be stored between 59° - 86°F (15° - 30°C).

HOW SUPPLIED

SCOPOLAMINE
FILM, EXTENDED RELEASE: 1.5 MG

BRAND/MANUFACTURER	NDC	SIZE	AWP
○ BRAND			
TRANSDERM-SCOP: Ciba Pharm	00083-4345-04	12s	$44.95

SCOPOLAMINE HYDROBROMIDE
INJECTION: 0.4 MG/ML

BRAND/MANUFACTURER	NDC	SIZE	AWP
◆ GENERICS			
Fujisawa	00469-0268-25	1 ml	$1.76

INJECTION: 1 MG/ML

BRAND/MANUFACTURER	NDC	SIZE	AWP
◆ GENERICS			
Fujisawa	00469-0270-25	1 ml	$1.76

Scopolamine Hydrobromide, Ophthalmic

DESCRIPTION
Scopolamine Hydrobromide is an anticholinergic prepared as a sterile topical ophthalmic solution.

Established name: Scopolamine Hydrobromide

Chemical name: Benzeneacetic acid, α-(hydroxy-methyl)-, 9-methyl-3-oxa-9-aza-tricyclo[3.3.1.0^{2,4}]non-7-yl ester, hydrobromide, trihydrate, [7(S)-(1α,2β,4β,5α,7β)-].

Each mL contains: Active: Scopolamine Hydrobromide 0.25%.

Following is its chemical structure:

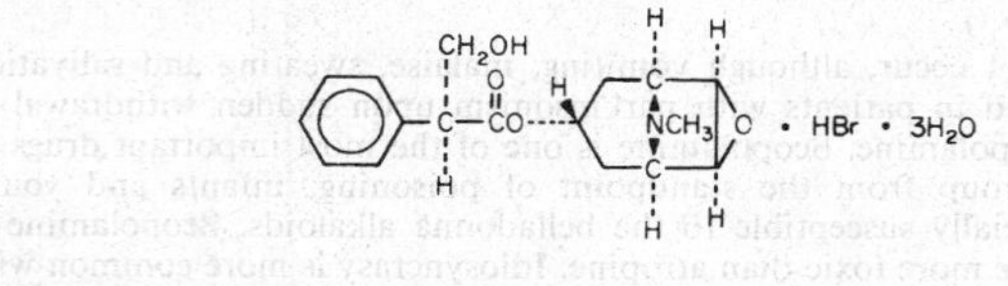

CLINICAL PHARMACOLOGY
This anticholinergic preparation blocks the responses of the sphincter muscle of the iris and the accommodative muscle of the ciliary body to cholinergic stimulation, producing pupillary dilation (mydriasis) and paralysis of accommodation (cycloplegia).

INDICATIONS AND USAGE
For mydriasis and cycloplegia in diagnostic procedures. For some pre- and postoperative states when a mydriatic and cycloplegic is needed in the treatment of iridocyclitis.

CONTRAINDICATIONS
Contraindicated in persons with primary glaucoma or a tendency toward glaucoma, e.g., narrow anterior chamber angle; and in those showing hypersensitivity to any component of this preparation.

WARNINGS
Do not touch dropper tip to any surface, as this may contaminate the solution. For topical use only—not for injection. In infants and small children, use with extreme caution.

PRECAUTIONS
To avoid excessive absorption, the lacrimal sac should be compressed by digital pressure for two to three minutes after instillation. To avoid inducing angle closure glaucoma, an estimation of the depth of the angle of the anterior chamber should be made.

Patient Warning: Patient should be advised not to drive or engage in other hazardous activities when drowsy or while pupils are dilated. Patient may experience sensitivity to light and should protect eyes in bright illumination during dilation. Parents should be warned not to get this preparation in their child's mouth and to wash their own hands and the child's hands following administration.

ADVERSE REACTIONS
Prolonged use may produce local irritation, characterized by follicular conjunctivitis, vascular congestion, edema, exudate, and an eczematoid dermatitis. Somnolence, dryness of the mouth, or visual hallucinations may occur.

◆ RATED THERAPEUTICALLY EQUIVALENT; ◇ THERAPEUTIC EQUIVALENCE UNCONFIRMED; ○ UNRATED

DOSAGE AND ADMINISTRATION

For refraction, administer one or two drops topically in the eye(s) one hour before refracting. For uveitis, administer one or two drops topically in the eye(s) up to four times daily.

Store at 46° to 80°F. Protect from light.

HOW SUPPLIED
DROP: 0.25%

BRAND/MANUFACTURER	NDC	SIZE	AWP
○ **BRAND**			
ISOPTO HYOSCINE: Alcon Ophthalmic	00998-0331-05	5 ml	$10.94
	00998-0331-15	15 ml	$15.13

Sebizon *SEE* SULFACETAMIDE SODIUM, TOPICAL

Secobarbital Sodium

DESCRIPTION
WARNING: MAY BE HABIT-FORMING

The barbiturates are nonselective central nervous system (CNS) depressants that are primarily used as sedative-hypnotics. In subhypnotic doses, they are also used as anticonvulsants. The barbiturates and their sodium salts are subject to control under the Federal Controlled Substances Act.

Secobarbital Sodium is a barbituric acid derivative and occurs as a white, odorless, bitter powder that is very soluble in water, soluble in alcohol, and practically insoluble in ether. Chemically, the drug is sodium 5-ally-5-(1-methyl-butyl)barbiturate, with the empirical formula $C_{12}H_{17}N_2NaO_3$. Its molecular weight is 260.27.

Each Capsule contains 100 mg (0.38 mmol) of Secobarbital Sodium.

Following is its chemical structure:

CLINICAL PHARMACOLOGY
Barbiturates are capable of producing all levels of CNS mood alteration, from excitation to mild sedation, hypnosis, and deep coma. Overdosage can produce death. In high enough therapeutic doses, barbiturates induce anesthesia. Barbiturates depress the sensory cortex, decrease motor activity, alter cerebellar function, and produce drowsiness, sedation, and hypnosis.

Barbiturate-induced sleep differs from physiologic sleep. Sleep laboratory studies have demonstrated that barbiturates reduce the amount of time spent in the rapid eye movement (REM) phase, or dreaming stage of sleep. Also, Stages III and IV sleep are decreased. Following abrupt cessation of regularly used barbiturates, patients may experience markedly increased dreaming, nightmares, and/or insomnia. Therefore, withdrawal of a single therapeutic dose over 5 or 6 days has been recommended to lessen the REM rebound and disturbed sleep that contribute to drug withdrawal syndrome (for example, decreasing the dose from 3 to 2 doses a day for 1 week).

In studies, Secobarbital Sodium and pentobarbital sodium have been found to lose most of their effectiveness for both inducing and maintaining sleep by the end of 2 weeks of continued drug administration, even with the use of multiple doses. As with Secobarbital Sodium and pentobarbital sodium, other barbiturates (including amobarbital) might be expected to lose their effectiveness for inducing and maintaining sleep after about 2 weeks. The short-, intermediate-, and to a lesser degree, long-acting barbiturates have been widely prescribed for treating insomnia. Although the clinical literature abounds with claims that the short-acting barbiturates are superior for producing sleep whereas the intermediate-acting compounds are more effective in maintaining sleep, controlled studies have failed to demonstrate these differential effects. Therefore, as sleep medications, the barbiturates are of limited value beyond short-term use.

Barbiturates have little analgesic action at subanesthetic doses. Rather, in subanesthetic doses, these drugs may increase the reaction to painful stimuli. All barbiturates exhibit anticonvulsant activity in anesthetic doses. However, of the drugs in this class, only phenobarbital, mephobarbital, and metharbital are effective as oral anticonvulsants in subhypnotic doses.

Barbiturates are respiratory depressants, and the degree of depression is dependent on the dose. With hypnotic doses, respiratory depression is similar to that which occurs during physiologic sleep accompanied by a slight decrease in blood pressure and heart rate.

Studies in laboratory animals have shown that barbiturates cause reduction in the tone and contractility of the uterus, ureters, and urinary bladder. However, concentrations of the drugs required to produce this effect in humans are not reached with sedative-hypnotic doses.

Barbiturates do not impair normal hepatic function, but have been shown to induce liver microsomal enzymes, thus increasing and/or altering the metabolism of barbiturates and other drugs (see *"Drug Interactions"* under *"Precautions"*).

Pharmacokinetics: Barbiturates are absorbed in varying degrees following oral or parenteral administration. The salts are more rapidly absorbed than are the acids. The rate of absorption is increased if the sodium salt is ingested as a dilute solution or taken on an empty stomach.

Duration of action, which is related to the rate at which the barbiturates are redistributed throughout the body, varies among persons and in the same person from time to time. Secobarbital Sodium is classified as a short-acting barbiturate when taken orally. Its onset of action is 10 to 15 minutes and its duration of action ranges from 3 to 4 hours.

Barbiturates are weak acids that are absorbed and rapidly distributed to all tissues and fluids, with high concentrations in the brain, liver, and kidneys. Lipid solubility of the barbiturates is the dominant factor in their distribution within the body. The more lipid soluble the barbiturate, the more rapidly it penetrates all tissues of the body. Barbiturates are bound to plasma and tissue proteins to a varying degree, with the degree of binding increasing directly as a function of lipid solubility.

Phenobarbital has the lowest lipid solubility, lowest plasma binding, lowest brain protein binding, the longest delay in onset of activity, and the longest duration of action. At the opposite extreme is secobarbital, which has the highest lipid solubility, highest plasma protein binding, highest brain protein binding, the shortest delay in onset of activity, and the shortest duration of action. The plasma half-life for secobarbital sodium in adults ranges between 15 to 40 hours, with a mean of 28 hours. No data are available for children and newborns.

Barbiturates are metabolized primarily by the hepatic microsomal enzyme system, and the metabolic products are excreted in the urine and, less commonly, in the feces. The excretion of unmetabolized barbiturate is 1 feature that distinguishes the long-acting category from those belonging to other categories, which are almost entirely metabolized. The inactive metabolites of the barbiturates are excreted as conjugates of glucuronic acid.

INDICATIONS AND USAGE
A. Hypnotic, for the short-term treatment of insomnia, since it appears to lose its effectiveness for sleep induction and sleep maintenance after 2 weeks (see *"Clinical Pharmacology"*).

B. Preanesthetic

CONTRAINDICATIONS
Secobarbital Sodium is contraindicated in patients who are hypersensitive to barbiturates. It is also contraindicated in patients with a history of manifest or latent porphyria, marked impairment of liver function, or respiratory disease in which dyspnea or obstruction is evident.

WARNINGS
1. Habit-Forming: Secobarbital Sodium may be habit-forming. Tolerance and psychological and physical dependence may occur with continued use (see *"Drug Abuse and Dependence"* and *"Pharmacokinetics"* under *"Clinical Pharmacology"*). Patients who have psychological dependence on barbiturates may increase the dosage or decrease the dosage interval without consulting a physician and subsequently may develop a physical dependence on barbiturates. To minimize the possibility of overdosage or development of dependence, the prescribing and dispensing of sedative-hypnotic barbiturates should be limited to the amount required for the interval until the next appointment. The abrupt cessation after prolonged use in a person who is dependent on the drug may result in withdrawal symptoms, including delirium, convulsions, and possibly death. Barbiturates should be withdrawn gradually from any patient known to be taking excessive doses over long periods of time (see *"Drug Abuse and Dependence"*).

2. Acute or Chronic Pain: Caution should be exercised when barbiturates are administered to patients with acute or chronic pain, because paradoxical excitement could be induced or important symptoms could be masked.

3. Usage in Pregnancy: Barbiturates can cause fetal harm when administered to a pregnant woman, Retrospective, case-controlled studies have suggested that there may be a connection between the maternal consumption of barbiturates and a higher than expected incidence of fetal abnormalities. Barbiturates readily cross the placental barrier and are distributed throughout fetal tissues; the highest concentrations are found in the placenta, fetal liver, and brain. Fetal blood levels approach maternal blood levels following parenteral administration.

Withdrawal symptoms occur in infants born to women who receive barbiturates throughout the last trimester of pregnancy (see *"Drug Abuse and Dependence"*). If Secobarbital Sodium is used during pregnancy or if the patient becomes pregnant while taking this drug, the patient should be apprised of the potential hazard to the fetus.

4. Synergistic Effects: The concomitant use of alcohol or other CNS depressants may produce additive CNS-depressant effects.

PRECAUTIONS
General: Barbiturates may be habit-forming. Tolerance and psychological and physical dependence may occur with continuing use (see *"Drug Abuse and Dependence"*). *Barbiturates should be administered with caution, if at all, to patients who are mentally depressed, have suicidal tendencies, or have a history of drug abuse.*

Elderly or debilitated patients may react to barbiturates with marked excitement, depression, or confusion. In some persons, especially children, barbiturates repeatedly produce excitement rather than depression.

In patients with hepatic damage, barbiturates should be administered with caution and initially in reduced doses. Barbiturates should not be administered to patients showing the premonitory signs of hepatic coma.

Information for Patients: The following information should be given to patients receiving Secobarbital Sodium:

1. The use of Secobarbital Sodium carries with it an associated risk of psychological and/or physical dependence. The patient should be warned against increasing the dose of the drug without consulting a physician.

2. Secobarbital Sodium may impair the mental and/or physical abilities required for the performance of potentially hazardous tasks, such as driving a car or operating machinery. The patient should be cautioned accordingly.

3. Alcohol should not be consumed while taking Secobarbital Sodium. The concurrent use of Secobarbital Sodium with other CNS depressants (eg, alcohol, narcotics, tranquilizers, and antihistamines) may result in additional CNS-depressant effects.

Laboratory Tests: Prolonged therapy with barbiturates should be accompanied by periodic laboratory evaluation of organic systems, including hematopoietic, renal, and hepatic systems (see *"General"* under *"Precautions* and *"Adverse Reactions"*).

Drug Interactions: Most reports of clinically significant drug interactions occurring with the barbiturates have involved phenobarbital. However, the application of these data to other barbiturates appears valid and warrants serial blood level determinations of the relevant drugs when there are multiple therapies.

1. Anticoagulants: Phenobarbital lowers the plasma levels of dicumarol and causes a decrease in anticoagulant activity as measured by the prothrombin time. Barbiturates can induce hepatic microsomal enzymes, resulting in increased metabolism and decreased anticoagulant response of oral anticoagulants (eg, warfarin, acenocoumarol, dicumarol, and phenprocoumon). Patients stabilized on anticoagulant therapy may require dosage adjustments if barbiturates are added to or withdrawn from their dosage regimen.

2. Corticosteroids: Barbiturates appear to enhance the metabolism of exogenous corticosteroids, probably through the induction of hepatic microsomal enzymes. Patients stabilized on corticosteroid therapy may require dosage adjustments if barbiturates are added to or withdrawn from their dosage regimen.

3. Griseofulvin: Phenobarbital appears to interfere with the absorption of orally administered griseofulvin, thus decreasing its blood level. The effect of the resultant decreased blood levels of griseofulvin on therapeutic response has not been established. However, it would be preferable to avoid concomitant administration of these drugs.

4. Doxycycline: Phenobarbital has been shown to shorten the half-life of doxycycline for as long as 2 weeks after barbiturate therapy is discontinued.

This mechanism is probably through the induction of hepatic microsomal enzymes that metabolize the antibiotic. If barbiturates and doxycycline are administered concurrently, the clinical response to doxycycline should be monitored closely.

5. Phenytoin, Sodium Valproate, Valproic Acid: The effect of barbiturates on the metabolism of phenytoin appears to be variable. Some investigators report an accelerating effect, whereas others report no effect. Because the effect of barbiturates on the metabolism of phenytoin is not predictable, phenytoin and barbiturate blood levels should be monitored more frequently if these drugs are given concurrently. Sodium valproate and valproic acid increase Secobarbital Sodium serum levels; therefore, Secobarbital Sodium blood levels should be monitored closely and appropriate dosage adjustment made as clinically indicated.

6. CNS Depressants: The concomitant use of other CNS depressants, including other sedatives or hypnotics, antihistamines, tranquilizers, or alcohol, may produce additive depressant effects.

7. Monoamine Oxidase Inhibitors (MAOIs): MAOIs prolong the effects of barbiturates, probably because metabolism of the barbiturate is inhibited.

8. Estradiol, Estrone, Progesterone, and Other Steroidal Hormones: Pretreatment with or concurrent administration of phenobarbital may decrease the effect of estradiol by increasing its metabolism. There have been reports of patients treated with antiepileptic drugs (eg, phenobarbital) who become pregnant while taking oral contraceptives. An alternate contraceptive method might be suggested to women taking barbiturates.

Carcinogenesis:

1. Animal Data: Phenobarbital sodium is carcinogenic in mice and rats after lifetime administration. In mice, it produced benign and malignant liver cell tumors. In rats, benign liver cell tumors were observed very late in life.

2. Human Data: In a 29-year epidemiologic study of 9,136 patients who were treated on an anticonvulsant protocol that included phenobarbital, results indicated a higher than normal incidence of hepatic carcinoma. Previously, some of these patients had been treated with thorotrast, a drug that is known to produce hepatic carcinomas. Thus, this study did not provide sufficient evidence that phenobarbital sodium is carcinogenic in humans.

A retrospective study of 84 children with brain tumors matched to 73 normal controls and 78 cancer controls (malignant disease other than brain tumors) suggested an association between exposure to barbiturates prenatally and an increased incidence of brain tumors.

Usage in Pregnancy:

1. Teratogenic Effects Pregnancy Category D: See *"Usage in Pregnancy"* under *"Warnings".*

2. Nonteratogenic Effects: Reports of infants suffering from long-term barbiturate exposure in utero included the acute withdrawal syndrome of seizures and hyperirritability from birth to a delayed onset of up to 14 days (see *"Drug Abuse and Dependence"*).

Labor and Delivery: Hypnotic doses of barbiturates do not appear to impair uterine activity significantly during labor. Full anesthetic doses of barbiturates decrease the force and frequency of uterine contractions. Administration of sedative-hypnotic barbiturates to the mother during labor may result in respiratory depression in the newborn. Premature infants are particularly susceptible to the depressant effects of barbiturates. If barbiturates are used during labor and delivery, resuscitation equipment should be available.

Data are not available to evaluate the effect of barbiturates when forceps delivery or other intervention is necessary or to determine the effect of barbiturates on the later growth, development, and functional maturity of the child.

Nursing Mothers: Caution should be exercised when Secobarbital Sodium is administered to a nursing woman, because small amounts of barbiturates are excreted in the milk.

ADVERSE REACTIONS

The following adverse reactions and their incidences were compiled from surveillance of thousands of hospitalized patients who received barbiturates. Because such patients may be less aware of some of the milder adverse effects of barbiturates, the incidence of these reactions may be somewhat higher in fully ambulatory patients.

MORE THAN 1 IN 100 PATIENTS
The most common adverse reaction estimated to occur at a rate of 1 to 3 patients per 100 is the following:

Nervous System: Somnolence

LESS THAN 1 IN 100 PATIENTS
Adverse reactions estimated to occur at a rate of less than 1 in 100 patients are listed below, grouped by organ system and by decreasing order of occurrence.

Nervous System: Agitation, confusion, hyperkinesia, ataxia, CNS depression, nightmares, nervousness, psychiatric disturbance, hallucinations, insomnia, anxiety, dizziness, abnormality in thinking.

Respiratory System: Hypoventilation, apnea

Cardiovascular System: Bradycardia, hypotension, syncope

Digestive System: Nausea, vomiting, constipation

Other Reported Reactions: Headache, injection site reactions, hypersensitivity reactions (angioedema, skin rashes, exfoliative dermatitis), fever, liver damage, megaloblastic anemia following chronic phenobarbital use.

DRUG ABUSE AND DEPENDENCE

Controlled Substance: Secobarbital Sodium is a Schedule II drug.

Dependence: Barbiturates may be habit-forming; tolerance, psychological dependence, and physical dependence may occur, especially following prolonged use of high doses of barbiturates. Daily administration in excess of 400 mg of Secobarbital Sodium for approximately 90 days is likely to produce some degree of physical dependence. A dosage of 600 to 800 mg for at least 35 days is sufficient to produce withdrawal seizures. The average daily dose for the barbiturate addict is usually about 1.5 g. As tolerance to barbiturates develops, the amount needed to maintain the same level of intoxication increases; tolerance to a fatal dosage, however, does not increase more than twofold. As this occurs, the margin between intoxicating dosage and fatal dosage becomes smaller. Symptoms of acute intoxication with barbiturates include unsteady gait, slurred speech, and sustained nystagmus. Mental signs of chronic intoxication include confusion, poor judgment, irritability, insomnia, and somatic complaints.

Symptoms of barbiturate dependence are similar to those of chronic alcoholism. If an individual appears to be intoxicated with alcohol to a degree that is radically disproportionate to the amount of alcohol in his or her blood, the use of barbiturates should be suspected. The lethal dose of a barbiturate is far less if alcohol is also ingested.

The symptoms of barbiturate withdrawal can be severe and may cause death. Minor withdrawal symptoms may appear 8 to 12 hours after the last dose of a barbiturate. These symptoms usually appear in the following order: anxiety, muscle twitching, tremor of hands and fingers, progressive weakness, dizziness, distortion in visual perception, nausea, vomiting, insomnia, and orthostatic hypotension. Major withdrawal symptoms (convulsions and delirium) may occur within 16 hours and last up to 5 days after abrupt cessation of barbiturates. Intensity of withdrawal symptoms gradually declines over a period of approximately 15 days. Individuals susceptible to barbiturate abuse and dependence include alcoholics and opiate abusers, as well as other sedative-hypnotic and amphetamine abusers.

Drug dependence on barbiturates arises from repeated administration on a continuous basis, generally in amounts exceeding therapeutic dose levels. The characteristics of drug dependence on barbiturates include the following: (a) a strong desire or need to continue taking the drug; (b) a tendency to increase the dose; (c) a psychic dependence on the effects of the drug related to subjective and individual appreciation of those effects; and (d) a physical dependence on the effects of the drug, requiring its presence for maintenance of homeostasis and resulting in a definite, characteristic, and self-limited abstinence syndrome when the drug is withdrawn.

Treatment of barbiturate dependence consists of cautious and gradual withdrawal of the drug. Barbiturate-dependent patients can be withdrawn by using a

---

number of withdrawal regimens. In all cases, withdrawal takes an extended period. One method involves substituting a 30-mg dose of phenobarbital for each 100- to 200-mg dose of barbiturate that the patient has been taking. The total daily amount of phenobarbital is then administered in 3 or 4 divided doses, not to exceed 600 mg daily. Should signs of withdrawal occur on the first day of treatment, a loading dose of 100 to 200 mg of phenobarbital may be administered IM in addition to the oral dose. After stabilization on phenobarbital, the total daily dose is decreased by 30 mg a day as long as withdrawal is proceeding smoothly. A modification of this regimen involves initiating treatment at the patient's regular dosage level and decreasing the daily dosage by 10% as tolerated by the patient.

Infants that are physically dependent on barbiturates may be given phenobarbital, 3 to 10 mg/kg/day. After withdrawal symptoms (hyperactivity, disturbed sleep, tremors, and hyperreflexia) are relieved, the dosage of phenobarbital should be gradually decreased and completely withdrawn over a 2-week period.

OVERDOSAGE

The toxic dose of barbiturates varies considerably. In general, an oral dose of 1 g of most barbiturates produces serious poisoning in an adult. Death commonly occurs after 2 to 10 g of ingested barbiturate. The sedated, therapeutic blood levels of Secobarbital range between 0.5 to 5 μg/mL; the usual lethal blood level ranges from 15 to 40 μg/mL. Barbiturate intoxication may be confused with alcoholism, bromide intoxication, and various neurologic disorders. Potential tolerance must be considered when evaluating significance of dose and plasma concentration.

Signs and Symptoms: Symptoms of oral overdose may occur within 15 minutes and begin with central nervous system depression, underventilation, hypotension, and hypothermia, which may progress to pulmonary edema and death. Hemorrhagic blisters may develop, especially at pressure points.

In extreme overdose, all electrical activity in the brain may cease, in which case a "flat" EEG normally equated with clinical death cannot be accepted as indicative of brain death. This effect is fully reversible unless hypoxic damage occurs. Consideration should be given to the possibility of barbiturate intoxication even in situations that appear to involve trauma.

Complications such as pneumonia, pulmonary edema, cardiac arrhythmias, congestive heart failure, and renal failure may occur. Uremia may increase CNS sensitivity to barbiturates if renal function is impaired. Differential diagnosis should include hypoglycemia, head trauma, cerebrovascular accidents, convulsive states, and diabetic coma.

Treatment: To obtain up-to-date information about the treatment of overdose, a good resource is your certified Regional Poison Control Center. Telephone numbers of certified poison control centers are listed in the *Physicians' Desk Reference (PDR).* In managing overdosage, consider the possibility of multiple drug overdoses, interaction among drugs, and unusual drug kinetics in your patient.

Protect the patient's airway and support ventilation and perfusion. Meticulously monitor and maintain, within acceptable limits, the patient's vital signs, blood gases, serum electrolytes, etc. Absorption of drugs from the gastrointestinal tract may be decreased by giving activated charcoal, which, in many cases, is more effective than emesis or lavage; consider charcoal instead of or in addition to gastric emptying. Repeated doses of charcoal over time may hasten elimination of some drugs that have been absorbed. Safeguard the patient's airway when employing gastric emptying or charcoal.

Diuresis and peritoneal dialysis are of little value; hemodialysis and hemoperfusion enhance drug clearance and should be considered in serious poisoning. If the patient has chronically abused sedatives, withdrawal reactions may be manifest following acute overdose.

DOSAGE AND ADMINISTRATION

Dosages of barbiturates must be individualized with full knowledge of their particular characteristics. Factors of consideration are the patient's age, weight, and condition.

Adults: As a hypnotic, 100 mg at bedtime. Preoperatively, 200 to 300 mg 1 to 2 hours before surgery.

Children: Preoperatively, 2 to 6 mg/kg, with a maximum dosage of 100 mg.

Special Patient Population: Dosage should be reduced in the elderly or debilitated because these patients may be more sensitive to barbiturates. Dosage should be reduced for patients with impaired renal function or hepatic disease.

Storage: Store at controlled room temperature, 15° to 30°C (59° to 86°F). Dispense in a tight container.

J CODES
Up to 250 mg IM,IV—J2860

HOW SUPPLIED
CAPSULE (C-II): 100 MG

AVERAGE UNIT PRICE (AVAILABLE SIZES)

BRAND		$0.22	
BRAND/MANUFACTURER	NDC	SIZE	AWP
◆ BRAND			
SECONAL SODIUM: Lilly	00002-0640-02	100s	$20.08
	00002-0640-33	100s ud	$24.46

Seconal Sodium *SEE* SECOBARBITAL SODIUM

Secran Prenatal *SEE* VITAMINS, PRENATAL

Secretin

DESCRIPTION
Secretin is a gastrointestinal peptide hormone that was first extracted from porcine duodenum by Jorpes & Mutt (1961). The heptacosa-peptide was subsequently sequenced and synthesized by Mutt, Bodansky and their co-workers at the Karolinska Institute. Secretin is a highly purified naturally occurring porcine hormone with a potency of not less than 3000 clinical units (CU) per mg peptide. Secretin is chemically defined as follows:

Molecular Weight 3055.5
Empirical Formula: $C_{130}H_{220}N_{44}O_{41}$
Structural Formula: H-His-Ser-Asp-Gly-Thr-Phe-Thr-Ser-Glu-Leu-Ser-Arg-Leu-Arg-Asp-Ser -Ala-Arg-Leu- Gln-Arg-Leu-Leu-Gln-Gly-Leu-Val-NH$_2$

Secretin contains 75 CU of lyophilized, sterile purified Secretin per vial. When reconstituted in 7.5 ml of Sodium Chloride Injection USP, each mL of solution contains 10 CU secretin for intravenous use. The pH of the reconstituted solution has a range of 2.5-5.0

Following is its chemical structure:

1							9
His-Ser-Asp-Gly-Thr-Phe-Thr-Ser-Glu-							

10							18
Leu-Ser-Arg-Leu-Arg-Asp-Ser-Ala-Arg-							

19							27
Leu-Gln-Arg-Leu-Leu-Gln-Gly-Leu-Val							

CLINICAL PHARMACOLOGY
The primary action of Secretin is to increase the volume and bicarbonate content of secreted pancreatic juices. The standard unit of activity used for Secretin is the clinical unit defined by Jorgs L Mutt in 1966. In a study of 6 healthy subjects the t(1/2) for Secretin approximated 4 minutes with a clearance rate of 540 mL/min (Kolts and McGuigan, 1977). Normal ranges for pancreatic secretory response to intravenous secretin in patients with defined pancreatic diseases have been shown to vary. The variation is related to the Secretin product used as well as inter-investigator differences in operative technique. However, it has been demonstrated that properly performed tests with Secretin will identify pancreatic disease (Gutierrez and Baron, 1972, Lagerloef et al., 1967).

The pancreatic secretory responses to Secretin in normal subjects and patients with well-documented pancreatitis are shown in Table 1 (Gutierrez and Baron, 1972).

Table 1

	Normal male subjects (10)[a]	Chronic Pancreatitis (5)
Volume secreted (ml/kg/ hr	3.6±0.8[b]	1.1±0.6
HCO$_3$ content (mEq/l)	114±20	71±33
HCO$_3$ output (mEq/kg/ hr)	0.436±0.141	0.105±0.093

[a]*number of subjects.*
[b] $x \pm S.D.$

The values obtained for Table 1 are derived from a single study by investigators skilled in performing the Secretin test and are to be taken only as guidelines. These results should not be generalized to results of Secretin testing conducted in other laboratories. However, a volume response of less than 2.0 mL/kg/hr, bicarbonate concentration of less than 90 mEq/liter and bicarbonate concentration of less than 0.2 mEq/Kg/hr are consistent with impaired pancreatic function. A physician or institution planning to perform Secretin testing for diagnosis of pancreatic disease should begin by assessing enough normal subjects ($\geq$ 5) to develop proficiency in proper technique and to generate normal response ranges for the three commonly assessed parameters of pancreatic exocrine response to Secretin.

Proper technique for carrying out the Secretin test of pancreatic function is described in *"Dosage and Administration"*.

Secretin administered intravenously stimulates gastrin release in patients with gastrinoma (Zollinger-Ellison syndrome), whereas no or only small changes in serum gastrin concentrations occur in normal subjects. Secretin may produce a small decrease in serum gastrin levels in patients with duodenal ulcer disease. This gastrin response is the basis for the use of Secretin as a provocative test in the evaluation of patients in whom gastrinoma is a diagnostic consideration. Accepted technique for carrying out the Secretin provocation test is detailed in *"Dosage and Administration"*.

➤ SHOWN IN PRODUCT IDENTIFICATION GUIDE

INDICATIONS AND USAGE
Secretin is indicated for:
(1) Diagnosis of pancreatic exocrine disease.
(2) As an adjunct in obtaining desquamated pancreatic cells for cytopathologic examination.
(3) Diagnosis of gastrinoma (Zollinger-Ellison syndrome).

CONTRAINDICATIONS
Patients suffering from actue pancreatitis should not receive Secretin until the attack has subsided.

WARNING
Because of a potential allergic reaction to Secretin, patients should receive an initial intravenous test dose of 0.1-1.0 CU. If no allergic reaction is noted after one minute the recommended dose may be injected slowly over 1 minute. A test dose is especially important in patients with a history of atopic allergy and/or asthma. Appropriate measures for the treatment of acute hypersensitivity reactions should be immediately available.

PRECAUTIONS
General: Patients who have undergone vagotomy, or are receiving anticholinergics at the time of Secretin testing, or who have inflammatory bowel disease may be hyporesponsive to Secretin stimulation. This response does not indicate pancreatic disease. A greater than normal volume response to Secretin stimulation, which can mask coexisting pancreatic disease, is occasionally encountered in patients with alcoholic or other liver disease.

Drug/Laboratory Test Interaction: The concomitant use of anticholinergic agents may make patients hyporesponsive (false positive).

Carcinogenesis, Mutagenesis, Impairment of Fertility: Long term studies in animals have not been performed to evaluate the carcinogenic, mutagenic potential or possible impairment of fertility effects of Secretin.

Pregnancy Category C: Animal reproduction studies have not been conducted with Secretin. It is also not known whether Secretin can cause fetal harm when administered to a pregnant woman or can affect reproductive capacity. Secretin should be given to a pregnant woman for diagnosis of gastrinoma (Zollinger-Ellison syndrome) only if clearly needed. Insofar as fluoroscopic guidance is usually necessary to position the double-lumen tube used in the pancreatic function test, this test should be postponed until after delivery.

Nursing Mothers: It is not known whether Secretin is excreted in human milk. Because many drugs are excreted in human milk, caution is advised when Secretin is administered to a nursing woman. Further, normal values for pancreatic secretory response to Secretin and for serum gastrin response have not been established for nursing women.

Pediatric Use: Safety and effectiveness in children have not been established.

ADVERSE REACTIONS
No adverse reactions to Secretin have been reported.

DOSAGE AND ADMINISTRATION
Secretin should be prepared immediately prior to use. The contents of a vial are dissolved in 7.5 mL of Sodium Chloride Injection USP, to yield a concentration of 10 CU per ml. Avoid vigorous shaking. Discard any unused portion after reconstitution.
The reconstituted drug product should be inspected visually prior to administration. If particulate matter or discoloration are seen, the product should be discarded.

DOSAGE
PANCREATIC FUNCTION TESTING AND PROCEDURE FOR OBTAINING DESQUAMATED PANCREATIC CELLS FOR CYTOPATHOLOGY: 1 CU per kg body weight by slow intravenous injection over 1 minute.

Diagnosis of Gastrinoma: (Zollinger-Ellison syndrome): 2 CU per kg body weight by slow intravenous injection over 1 minute.

ADMINISTRATION
1. Pancreatic Function Testing: A Dreiling type, radioopaque, double-lumen tube is passed through the mouth following a 12-15 hour fast. The proximal lumen of the tube is placed in the gastric antrum and the distal lumen just beyond the pailla of Vater with the aid of fluoroscopic guidance. The positioning of the tube must be confirmed and the tube secured prior to Secretin testing. A negative pressure of 25-40 mm Hg is applied to both lumens and maintained throughout the test. Interruption of suction at 1 minute intervals improves the reliability of fluid collections. When uncontaminated duodenal contents are obtained -i.e., when these secretions are clear, although possibly bile stained, and have a pH of $\geq$ 6.0 - a baseline sample of duodenal fluids is collected for 2 consecutive 10 minute periods. Subsequent to the baseline collections, Secretin at a dose of 1 CU/kg of body weight is injected intravenously in approximately 1 minute. Duodenal fluid is then collected for 60 minutes after Secretin administration. The aspirate is fractioned into four collection periods, the first two at 10 minute intervals, and the last two at 20 minute intervals. The duodenal lumen of the tube is cleared with an injection of air after collection of each fraction. Wide variations in volume of the aspirate will be indicative of incomplete aspiration or contamination. Each fraction of duodenal fluid is to be chilled and subsequently analyzed for volume and bicarbonate concentration.

2. Procedure for Obtaining Desquamated Pancreatic cells for cytopathology: A duodenal aspirate obtained as under Pancreatic Function Testing is submitted for cytopathological examination.

3. Secretin Testing For Gastrinoma (Zollinger-Ellison syndrome). The patient should have fasted for at least 12 hours prior to beginning the test. Prior to injection of Secretin two blood samples are drawn for determination of fasting serum gastrin levels (baseline values). Subsequently, 2 CU of Secretin per kg of body weight are administered intravenously over 1 minute: post-injection blood samples are collected after 1,2,5,10 and 30 minutes for determination of serum gastrin concentrations.
Gastrinoma is strongly indicated in patients with elevated fasting serum gastrin concentrations in the 120-500 pg/ml range (determined by RIA using an antibody to gastrin similar to that prepared by Rehfeld) and in patients who show an increase in serum gastrin concentration of more than 110 pg per ml over basal level.
The unreconstituted product should be stored at -20°C (freezer). However, the biological activity of Secretin will not be significantly decreased by storage at temperatures up to 25°C for up to 3 weeks.

REFERENCES
1. Jorpes, E., and Mutt, V. On the biological activity and amino acid composition of Secretin. *Acta Chem Scand* 15 (1961) 1790-1791. 2. Jorpes, E., and Mutt V. On the biological assay of Secretin. The reference standard. *Acta Physiol Scand* 66 (1966) 316-325. 3. Kolts, B.E. and Mc Guigan, J.E. Radioimmunoassay Measurement of Secretin Half-Life in Man. *Gastroenterol.* 72 (1977) 55-60. 4. Lagerlof, H.O. et al. A Secretin test with high doses of Secretin and correction for incomplete recovery of duodenal juice. *Gastroenterol* 52 (1967) 67-77. 5. Gutierrez, L.V., and Baron, J.H. A comparison of Boots and GIH Secretin as stimuli of pancreatic Secretin in human subjects with or without chronic pancreatitis. *Gut* 13 (1972) 721-725.

HOW SUPPLIED
POWDER FOR INJECTION: 75 CU/VIAL

BRAND/MANUFACTURER	NDC	SIZE	AWP
○ BRAND			
SECRETIN-FERRING: Ferring	55566-1075-01	1s	$131.64

Secretin-Ferring *SEE* SECRETIN

Sectral *SEE* ACEBUTOLOL HYDROCHLORIDE

Seldane *SEE* TERFENADINE

Seldane-D *SEE* PSEUDOEPHEDRINE HYDROCHLORIDE
AND TERFENADINE

Selegiline Hydrochloride

DESCRIPTION
Selegiline Hydrochloride is a levorotatory acetylenic derivative of phenethylamine. It is commonly referred to in the clinical and pharmacological literature as l-deprenyl.

The chemical name is: (R)-(-)-N,2-dimethyl-N-2-propynyl-phenethylamine hydrochloride. It is a white to near white crystalline power, freely soluble in water, chloroform, and methanol, and has a molecular weight of 223.75.

Following is its chemical structure:

CLINICAL PHARMACOLOGY
The mechanisms accounting for Selegiline's beneficial adjunctive action in the treatment of Parkinson's disease are not fully understood. Inhibition of monoamine oxidase, type B, activity is generally considered to be of primary importance; in addition, there is evidence that Selegiline may act through other mechanisms to increase dopaminergic activity.
Selegiline is best known as an irreversible inhibitor of monoamine oxidase (MAO), an intracellular enzyme associated with the outer membrane of mitochondria. Selegiline inhibits MAO by acting as a "sucide" substrate for the enzyme; that is, it is converted by MAO to an active moiety which combines irreversibly with the active site and/or the enzyme's essential FAD cofactor. Because Selegiline has greater affinity for type B than for Type A active sites, it can serve as a selective inhibitor of MAO type B if it is administered at the recommended dose.

MAOs are widely distributed throughout the body; their concentration is especially high in liver, kidney, stomach, intestinal wall, and brain. MAOs are currently subclassified into two types, A and B, which differ in their substrate specificity and tissue distribution. In humans, intestinal MAO is predominantly type A, while most of that in brain is type B.

In CNS neurons, MAO plays an important role in the catabolism of catecholamines (dopamine, norepinephrine and epinephrine) and serotonin. MAOs are also important in the catabolism of various exogenous amines found in a variety of foods and drugs. MAO in the GI tract and liver (primarily type A), for example, is thought to provide vital protection from exogenous amines (e.g., tyramine) that have the capacity, if absorbed intact, to cause a "hypertensive crisis," the so-called "cheese reaction." (If large amounts of certain exogenous amines gain access to the systemic circulation—e.g., from fermented cheese, red wine, herring, over-the-counter cough/cold medications, etc.—they are taken up by adrenergic neurons and displace norepinephrine from storage sites within membrane bound vesicles. Subsequent release of the displace norepinephrine causes the rise in systemic blood pressure, etc.)

In theory, therefore, because MAO A of the gut is not inhibited, patients treated with selegiline at a dose of 10 mg a day can take medications containing pharmacologically active amines and consume tyramine-containing foods without risk of uncontrolled hypertension. To date, clinical experience appears to confirm this prediction; cheese reactions have not been reported in Selegiline treated patients. The pathophysiology of the 'cheese reaction' is complicated and, in addition to its ability to inhibit MAO B selectively, Selegiline's apparent freedom from this reaction has been attributed to an ability to prevent tyramine and other indirect acting sympathomimetics from displacing norepinephrine from adrenergic neurons.

However, until the pathophysiology of the cheese reaction is more completely understood, it seems prudent to assume that Selegiline can only be used safely without dietary restrictions at doses where it presumably selectively inhibits MAO B (e.g., 10 mg/day). **In short, attention to the dose dependent nature of Selegiline's selectivity is critical if it is to be used without elaborate restrictions being placed on diet and concomitant drug use.** (See *"Warnings"* and *"Precautions"*).

It is important to be aware that Selegiline may have pharmacologic effects unrelated to MAO B inhibition. As noted above, there is some evidence that it may increase dopaminergic activity by other mechanisms, including interfering with dopamine re-uptake at the synapse. Effects resulting from Selegiline administration may also be mediated through its metabolites. Two of its three principal metabolites, amphetamine and methamphetamine, have pharmacological actions of their own; they interfere with neuronal uptake and enhance release of several neurotransmitters (e.g., norepinephrine, dopamine, serotonin). However, the extent to which these metabolites contribute to the effects of Selegiline are unknown.

RATIONALE FOR THE USE OF A SELECTIVE MONOAMINE OXIDASE TYPE B INHIBITOR IN PARKINSON'S DISEASE

Many of the prominent symptoms of Parkinson's disease are due to a deficiency of striatal dopamine that is the consequence of a progressive degeneration and loss of a population of dopaminergic neurons which originate in the substantia nigra of the midbrain and project to the basal ganglia or striatum. Early in the course of Parkinson's, the deficit in the capacity of these neurons to synthesize dopamine can be overcome by administration of exogenous levodopa, usually given in combination with a peripheral decarboxylase inhibitor (carbidopa).

With the passage of time, due to the progression of the disease and/or the effect of sustained treatment, the efficacy and quality of the therapeutic response to levodopa diminishes. Thus, after several years of levodopa treatment, the response, for a given dose of levodopa, is shorter, has less predictable onset and offset (i.e., there is "wearing off"), and is often accompanied by side effects (e.g., dyskinesia, akinesias, on-off phenomena, freezing, etc.)

This deteriorating response is currently interpreted as a manifestation of the inability of the ever decreasing population of intact nigrostriatal neurons to synthesize and release adequate amounts of dopamine.

MAO B inhibition may be useful in this setting because, by blocking the catabolism of dopamine, it would increase the net amount of dopamine available (i.e., it would increase the pool of dopamine). Whether or not this mechanism or an alternative one actually accounts for the observed beneficial effects of adjunctive Selegiline is unknown.

Selegiline's benefit in Parkinson's disease has only been documented as an adjunct to levodopa/carbidopa. Whether or not it might be effective as a sole treatment is unknown, but past attempts to treat Parkinson's disease with nonselective MAOI monothotherapy are reported to have been unsuccessful. It is important to note that attempts to treat Parkinsonian patients with combinations of levodopa and currently marketed nonselective MAO inhibitors were abandoned because of multiple side effects including hypertension, increase in involuntary movement and toxic delirium.

PHARMACOKINETIC INFORMATION (ABSORPTION, DISTRIBUTION, METABOLISM AND ELIMINATION—ADME)

Only preliminary information about the details of the pharmacokinetics of Selegiline and its metabolites is available. Data obtained in a study of 12 healthy subjects that was intended to examine the effects of Selegiline on the ADME of an oral hypoglycemic agent, however, provides some information. Following the oral administration of a single dose of 10 mg of Selegiline Hydrochloride to these subjects, serum levels of intact Selegiline were below the limit of detection (less than 10 ng/ml). Three metabolites, N-desmethyldeprenyl, the major metabolite (mean half-life 2.0 hours), amphetamine (mean half-life 17.7 hours), and

methamphetamine (mean half-life 20.5 hours), were found in serum and urine. Over a period of 48 hours, 45% of the dose administered appeared in the urine as these 3 metabolites. In an extension of this study intended to examine the effects of steady state conditions, the same subjects were given a 10 mg dose of Selegiline Hydrochloride for seven consecutive days. Under these conditions, the mean trough serum levels for amphetamine were 3.5 ng/ml and 8.0 ng/ml for methamphetamine; trough levels of N-desmethyldeprenyl were below the levels of detection.

The rate of MAO B regeneration following discontinuation of treatment has not been quantitated. It is this rate, dependent upon de novo protein synthesis, which seems likely to determine how fast normal MAO B activity can be restored.

INDICATIONS AND USAGE

Selegiline Hydrochloride is indicated as an adjunct in the management of Parkinsonian patients being treated with levodopa/carbidopa who exhibit deterioration in the quality of their response to this therapy. There is no evidence from controlled studies that Selegiline has any beneficial effect in the absence of concurrent levodopa therapy.

Evidence supporting this claim was obtained in randomized controlled clinical investigations that compared the effects of added Selegiline or placebo in patients receiving levodopa/carbidopa. Selegiline was significantly superior to placebo on all three principal outcome measures employed; change from baseline in daily levodopa/carbidopa dose, the amount of 'off' time, and patient self-rating of treatment success. Beneficial effects were also observed on other measures of treatment success (e.g., measures of reduced end of dose akinesia, decreased tremor and sialorrhea, improved speech and dressing ability and improved overall disability as assessed by walking and comparison to previous state).

UNLABELED USES

Selegiline is used alone or as an adjunct in the treatment of dementia of the Alzheimer's type and in endogenous depression.

CONTRAINDICATIONS

Selegiline Hydrochloride is contraindicated in patients with a known hypersensitivity to this drug.

Selegiline Hydrochloride is contraindicated for use with meperidine. This contraindication is often extended to other opioids (see *"Drug Interactions"*).

WARNINGS

Selegiline should not be used at daily doses exceeding those recommended (10 mg/day) because of the risks associated with non-selective inhibition of MAO. (See *"Clinical Pharmacology"*.)

The selectivity of Selegiline for MAO B may not be absolute even at the recommended daily dose of 10 mg a day and selectivity is further diminished with increasing daily doses. The precise dose at which Selegiline becomes a nonselective inhibitor of all MAO is unknown, but may be in the range of 30 to 40 mg a day.

Definitive clinical data on the concomitant use of Selegiline Hydrochloride and fluoxetine hydrochloride (PROZAC) is not available. Death has been reported to occur following the initiation of therapy with nonselective MAOIs (NARDIL, PARNATE) shortly after discontinuation of fluoxetine. To date, this reaction has not been reported with Selegiline Hydrochloride; however, since the mechanism of this reaction is not fully understood it seems prudent, in general, to avoid this combination. Because of the long half-lives of fluoxetine and its active metabolite, at least five weeks (approximately 5 half-lives) should elapse between discontinuation of fluoxetine and initiation of MAOI therapy. Based on experience with the combined use of MAOIs and tricyclic antidepressants, at least 14 days should elapse between discontinuation of an MAOI and initiation of treatment with fluoxetine.

PRECAUTIONS

GENERAL

Some patients given Selegiline may experience an exacerbation of levodopa associated side effects, presumably due to the increased amounts of dopamine reacting with supersensitive postsynaptic receptors. These effects may often be mitigated by reducing the dose of levodopa/carbidopa by approximately 10 to 30%.

The decision to prescribe Selegiline should take into consideration that the MAO system of enzymes is complex and incompletely understood and there is only a limited amount of carefully documented clinical experience with Selegiline. Consequently, the full spectrum of possible responses to Selegiline may not have been observed in premarketing evaluation of the drug. It is advisable, therefore, to observe patients closely for atypical responses.

INFORMATION FOR PATIENTS

Patients should be advised of the possible need to reduce levodopa dosage after the initiation of Selegiline Hydrochloride therapy. Patients (or their families if the patient is incompetent) should be advised not to exceed the daily recommended dose of 10 mg. The risk of using higher daily doses of Selegiline should be explained, and a brief description of the 'cheese reaction' provided. While hypertensive reactions with Selegiline have not been reported, documented experience is limited. Consequently, it may be useful to inform patients (or their families) about the signs and symptoms associated with MAOI induced hypertensive reactions. In particular, patients should be urged to report, immediately, any severe headache or other atypical or unusual symptoms not previously experienced.

LABORATORY TESTS

No specific laboratory tests are deemed essential for the management of patients on Selegiline Hydrochloride. Periodic routine evaluation of all patients, however, is appropriate.

DRUG INTERACTIONS

The occurrence of stupor, muscular rigidity, severe agitation, and elevated temperature has been reported in a man receiving Selegiline and meperidine, as well as other medications. Symptoms resolved over days when the combination was discontinued. This case is typical of the interaction of meperidine and MAOIs. Other serious reactions (including severe agitation, hallucinations, and death) have been reported in patients receiving this combination. While it cannot be said definitively that all of these reactions were caused by this combination, they are all compatible with this well recognized interaction. No other interactions attributed to the combined use of Selegiline and other drugs have been reported. However, because the database of documented clinical experience is limited, the level of reassurance provided by this lack of adverse reporting is uncertain. (See *"Warning and Precautions".*)

CARCINOGENESIS, MUTAGENESIS, AND IMPAIRMENT OF FERTILITY

Studies have not been performed to date to evaluate the carcinogenic potential of Selegiline Hydrochloride.

PREGNANCY

Pregnancy Category C: Insufficient animal reproduction studies have been done with Selegiline to conclude that Selegiline poses no teratogenic risk. However, one rat study carried out at doses as much as 180 fold the recommended human dose revealed no evidence of a teratogenic effect. It is not known whether Selegiline can cause fetal harm when administered to a pregnant woman or can affect reproduction capacity. Selegiline should be given to a pregnant woman only if clearly needed.

NURSING MOTHERS

It is not known whether Selegiline Hydrochloride is excreted in human milk. Because many drugs are excreted in human milk, consideration should be given to discontinuing the use of all but absolutely essential drug treatments in nursing women.

PEDIATRIC USE

The effects of Selegiline Hydrochloride in children have not been evaluated.

ADVERSE REACTIONS

INTRODUCTION

The number of patients who received Selegiline in prospectively monitored premarketing studies is limited. While other sources of information about the use of Selegiline are available (e.g., literature reports, foreign postmarketing reports, etc.) they do not provide the kind of information necessary to estimate the incidence of adverse events. Thus, overall incidence figures for adverse reactions associated with the use of Selegiline cannot be provided. Many of the adverse reactions seen have been also reported as symptoms of dopamine excess.

Moreover, the importance and severity of various reactions reported often cannot be ascertained. One index of relative importance, however, is whether or not a reaction caused treatment discontinuation. In prospective pre-marketing studies, the following events led, in decreasing order of frequency, to discontinuation of treatment with Selegiline: nausea, hallucinations, confusion, depression, loss of balance, insomnia, orthostatic hypotension, increased akinetic involuntary movements, agitation, arrhythmia, bradykinesia, chorea, delusions, hypertension, new or increased angina pectoris and syncope. Events reported only once as a cause of discontinuation are ankle edema, anxiety, burning lips/mouth, constipation, drowsiness/lethargy, dystonia, excess perspiration, increased freezing, gastrointestinal bleeding, hair loss, increased tremor, nervousness, weakness and weight loss.

Experience with Selegiline Hydrochloride obtained in parallel, placebo controlled, randomized studies provides only a limited basis for estimates of adverse reaction rates. The following reactions that occurred with greater frequency among the 49 patients assigned to Selegiline as compared to the 50 patients assigned to placebo in the only parallel, placebo controlled trial performed in patients with Parkinson's disease are shown in the following table. None of these adverse reactions led to a discontinuation of treatment.

INCIDENCE OF TREATMENT-EMERGENT ADVERSE EXPERIENCES IN THE PLACEBO-CONTROLLED CLINICAL TRIAL

Adverse Event	Number of Patients Reporting Events	
	Selegiline Hydrochloride N = 49	Placebo N = 50
Nausea	10	3
Dizziness/Light-headed/Fainting	7	1
Abdominal Pain	4	2
Confusion	3	0
Hallucinations	3	1
Dry mouth	3	1
Vivid Dreams	2	0
Dyskinesias	2	5

Adverse Event	Number of Patients Reporting Events	
	Selegiline Hydrochloride N = 49	Placebo N = 50
Headache	2	1

The following events were reported once in either or both groups:

Ache, generalized	1	0
Anxiety/Tension	1	1
Anemia	0	1
Diarrhea	1	0
Hair Loss	0	1
Insomnia	1	0
Lethargy	1	0
Leg pain	1	0
Low back pain	1	0
Malaise	0	1
Palpitations	1	0
Urinary Retention	1	0
Weight Loss	1	0

In all prospectively monitored clinical investigations, enrolling approximately 920 patients, the following adverse events, classified by body system, were reported.

CENTRAL NERVOUS SYSTEM

Motor/Coordination/Extrapyramidal: increased tremor, chorea, loss of balance, restlessness, blepharospasm, increased bradykinesia, facial grimace, falling down, heavy leg, muscle twitch*, myoclonic jerks*, stiff neck, tardive dyskinesia, dystonic symptoms, dyskinesia, involuntary movements, freezing, festination, increased apraxia, muscle cramps.

Mental Status/Behavioral/Psychiatric: hallucinations, dizziness, confusion, anxiety, depression, drowsiness, behavior/mood change, dreams*/nightmares, tiredness, delusions, disorientation, lightheadedness, impaired memory*, increased energy*, transient high*, hollow feeling, lethargy/malaise, apathy, overstimulation, vertigo, personality change, sleep disturbance, restlessness, weakness, transient irritability.

Pain/Altered Sensation: headache, back pain, leg pain, tinnitus, migraine, supraorbital pain, throat burning, generalized ache, chills, numbness of toes/fingers, taste disturbance.

AUTONOMIC NERVOUS SYSTEM

dry mouth, blurred vision, sexual dysfunction.

CARDIOVASCULAR

orthostatic hypotension, hypertension, arrhythmia, palpitations, new or increased angina pectoris, hypotension, tachycardia, peripheral edema, sinus bradycardia, syncope.

GASTROINTESTINAL

nausea/vomiting, constipation, weight loss, anorexia, poor appetite, dysphagia, diarrhea, heartburn, rectal bleeding, bruxism*, gastrointestinal bleeding (exacerbation of preexisting ulcer disease).

GENITOURINARY/GYNECOLOGIC/ENDOCRINE

slow urination, transient anorgasmia*, nocturia, prostatic hypertrophy, urinary hesitancy, urinary retention, decreased penile sensation*, urinary frequency.

SKIN AND APPENDAGES

increased sweating, diaphoresis, facial hair, hair loss, hematoma, rash, photosensitivity.

MISCELLANEOUS

asthma, diplopia, shortness of breath, speech affected.

POSTMARKETING REPORTS

The following experiences were described in spontaneous postmarketing reports. These reports do not provide sufficient information to establish a clear causal relationship with the use of Selegiline Hydrochloride.

CNS: Seizure in dialyzed chronic renal failure patient on concomitant medications.

OVERDOSAGE

SELEGILINE

No specific information is available about clinically significant overdoses with Selegiline Hydrochloride. However, experience gained during Selegiline's development reveals that some individuals exposed to doses of 600 mg d,l-Selegiline suffered severe hypotension and psychomotor agitation.

Since the selective inhibition of MAO B by Selegiline Hydrochloride is achieved only at doses in the range recommended for the treatment of Parkinson's disease (e.g., 10 mg/day), overdoses are likely to cause significant inhibition of both MAO A and MAO B. Consequently, the signs and symptoms of overdose may resemble those observed with marketed non-selective MAO inhibitors [e.g., tranylcypromine, isocarboxazide, and phenelzine].

* indicates events reported only at doses greater than 10 mg/day.

◆ RATED THERAPEUTICALLY EQUIVALENT; ◇ THERAPEUTIC EQUIVALENCE UNCONFIRMED; ○ UNRATED

OVERDOSE WITH NONSELECTIVE MAO INHIBITION

Note: This section is provided for reference; it does not describe events that have actually been observed with Selegiline in overdose.

Characteristically, signs and symptoms of non selective MAOI overdose may not appear immediately. Delays of up to 12 hours between ingestion of drug and the appearance of signs may occur. Importantly, the peak intensity of the syndrome may not be reached for upwards of a day following the overdose. Death has been reported following overdosage. Therefore, immediate hospitalization, with continuous patient observation and monitoring for a period of at least two days following the ingestion of such drugs in overdose, is strongly recommended.

The clinical picture of MAOI overdose varies considerably; its severity may be a function of the amount of drug consumed. The central nervous and cardiovascular systems are prominently involved.

Signs and symptoms of overdosage may include, alone or in combination, any of the following: drowsiness, dizziness, faintness, irritability, hyperactivity, agitation, severe headache, hallucinations, trismus, opisthotonus, convulsions, and coma; rapid and irregular pulse, hypertension, hypotension and vascular collapse; precordial pain, respiratory depression and failure, hyperpyrexia, diaphoresis, and cool, clammy skin.

TREATMENT SUGGESTIONS FOR OVERDOSE

Note: **Because there is no recorded experience with Selegiline overdose, the following suggestions are offered based upon the assumption that Selegiline overdose may be modeled by non-selective MAOI poisoning. In any case, up-to-date information about the treatment of overdose can often be obtained from a certified Regional Poison Control Center. Telephone numbers of certified Poison Control Centers are listed in the *Physicians' Desk Reference (PDR)*.**

Treatment of overdose with nonselective MAOIs is symptomatic and supportive. Induction of emesis or gastric lavage with instillation of charcoal slurry may be helpful in early poisoning, provided the airway has been protected against aspiration. Signs and symptoms of central nervous system stimulation, including convulsions, should be treated with diazepam, given slowly intravenously. Phenothiazine derivatives and central nervous system stimulants should be avoided. Hypotension and vascular collapse should be treated with intravenous fluids and, if necessary, blood pressure titration with an intravenous infusion of a dilute pressor agent. It should be noted that adrenergic agents may produce a markedly increased pressor response.

Respiration should be supported by appropriate measures, including management of the airway, use of supplemental oxygen, and mechanical ventilatory assistance, as required.

Body temperature should be monitored closely. Intensive management of hyperpyrexia may be required. Maintenance of fluid and electrolyte balance is essential.

DOSAGE AND ADMINISTRATION

Selegiline Hydrochloride is intended for administration to Parkinsonian patients receiving levodopa/carbidopa therapy who demonstrate a deteriorating response to this treatment. The recommended regimen for the administration of Selegiline Hydrochloride is 10 mg per day administered as divided doses of 5 mg each taken at breakfast and lunch. There is no evidence that additional benefit will be obtained from the administration of higher doses. Moreover, higher doses should ordinarily be avoided because of the increased risk of side effects.

After two to three days of Selegiline treatment, an attempt may be made to reduce the dose of levodopa/carbidopa. A reduction of 10 to 30% was achieved with the typical participant in the domestic placebo controlled trials who was assigned to Selegiline treatment. Further reductions of levodopa/carbidopa may be possible during continued Selegiline therapy.

Store at controlled room temperature, 59° to 86°F (15° to 30°C).

HOW SUPPLIED
TABLETS: 5 MG

BRAND/MANUFACTURER	NDC	SIZE	AWP
○ **BRAND**			
▶ ELDEPRYL: Somerset	39506-0011-25	60s	$128.19

Selenious Acid

DESCRIPTION

Selenious Acid is a sterile, nonpyrogenic solution for use as an additive to solutions for total parenteral nutrition (TPN).

Each mL contains:

Ingredients	Single-Dose Preparation (10 mL)	Multiple-Dose Preparation (30 mL)
Selenium (as Selenious Acid)	40 mcg	40 mcg
Benzyl Alchol	-	0.9%
Water for Injection	q.s.	q.s.

Nitric acid may have been added for pH adjustment (1.8-2.4).

CLINICAL PHARMACOLOGY

Selenium is part of glutathione peroxidase which protects cell components from oxidative damage due to peroxides produced in cellular metabolism. Prolonged TPN support in humans has resulted in selenium deficiency symptoms which include muscle pain and tenderness. The symptoms have been reported to respond to supplementation of TPN solutions with selenium. Pediatric conditions, Keshan disease and Kwashiorkor have been associated with low dietary intake of selenium. The conditions are endemic to geographical areas with low selenium soil content. Dietary supplementation with selenium salts has been reported to reduce the incidence of the conditions among affected children.

Normal blood levels of selenium in different human populations have been found to vary and depend on the selenium content of the food consumed. Results of surveys carried out in some countries are tabulated below: (See related table).

Plasma selenium levels of 0.3 and 0.9 mcg/100 mL have been reported to produce deficiency symptoms in humans.

Selenium is eliminated primarily in urine. However, significant endogenous losses through feces also occur. The rate of excretion and the relative importance of two routes varies with the chemical form of selenium used in supplementation. Ancillary routes of elimination are lungs and skin.

INDICATIONS AND USAGE

Selenious Acid is indicated for use as a supplement to intravenous solutions given for TPN. Administration of Selenious Acid in TPN solutions helps to maintain plasma selenium levels and to prevent depletion of endogenous stores and subsequent deficiency symptoms.

CONTRAINDICATIONS

Selenious Acid should not be given undiluted by direct injection into a peripheral vein because of the potential for infusion phlebitis.

WARNINGS

Selenium can be toxic if given in excessive amounts. Supplementation of TPN solution with selenium should be immediately discontinued if toxicity symptoms are observed. Frequent determination of plasma selenium levels during TPN support and close medical supervision are recommended.

Selenious Acid is a hypotonic solution and should be administered in admixtures only.

PRECAUTIONS

As selenium is eliminated in urine and feces, selenium supplements may be adjusted, reduced or omitted in renal dysfunction and/or gastrointestinal malfunction. In patients receiving blood transfusion, contribution from such transfusions should also be considered. Frequent selenium plasma level determinations are suggested as a guideline.

In animals, selenium has been reported to enhance the action of vitamin E and decrease the toxicity of mercury, cadmium and arsenic.

PREGNANCY CATEGORY C

Selenium at high dosage levels (15 to 30 mcg/egg) has been reported to have adverse embryological effects among chickens. There are, however, no adequate and well-controlled studies in pregnant women. Selenious Acid should be used during pregnancy only if potential benefit justifies the potential risk to the fetus.

Presence of selenium in placenta and umbilical cord blood has been reported in humans.

ADVERSE REACTIONS

The amount of selenium present in Selenious Acid is small. Symptoms of toxicity from selenium are unlikely to occur at the recommended dosage level.

OVERDOSAGE

Chronic toxicity in humans resulting from exposure to selenium in industrial environments, intake of foods grown in seleniferous soils, use of selenium-contaminated water and application of cosmetics containing selenium has been reported in literature. Toxicity symptoms include hair loss, weakened nails, dermatitis, dental defects, gastrointestinal disorders, nervousness, mental depression, metallic taste, vomiting and garlic odor of breath and sweat. Acute poisoning due to ingestion of large amounts of selenium compounds has resulted in death with histopathological changes including fulminating peripheral vascular collapse, internal vascular congestion, diffusely hemorrhagic, congested and edematous lungs, brick-red color gastric mucosa. The death was preceded by coma.

No effective antidote to selenium poisoning in humans is known. Animal studies have shown casein and linseed oil in feeds, reduced glutathione, arsenic, magnesium sulfate and bromobenzene to afford limited protection.

DOSAGE AND ADMINISTRATION

Selenious Acid provides 40 mcg selenium/mL. For metabolically stable adults receiving TPN, the suggested additive dosage level is 20 to 40 mcg selenium/day. For pediatric patients, the suggested additive dosage level is 3 mcg/kg/day.

In adults, selenium deficiency states resulting from long-term TPN support, selenium as selenomethionine or Selenious Acid, administered intravenously at 100 mcg/day for a period of 24 and 31 days, respectively, has been reported to reverse deficiency symptoms without toxicity.

Aseptic addition of Selenious Acid to the TPN solution under a laminar flow hood is recommended. Selenium is physically compatible with the electrolytes and other trace elements usually present in amino acid/dextrose solution used for TPN. Frequent monitoring of plasma selenium levels is suggested as a guideline for subsequent administration. The normal whole blood range for selenium is approximately 10 to 37 mcg/100 mL.

Parenteral drug products should be inspected visually for discoloration and particulate matter prior to administration, whenever solution and container permit.

Country	Number of Samples	Whole Blood	*Selenium (mcg/100 mL)[a]* Blood Cells	Plasma/Serum
Canada	254 Adults	(37.9 ± 7.8)	(23.6 ± 6)	(14.4 ± 2.9)
England	8[b]	26-37 (32)	—	—
Guatemala & Southern USA	10 Adults 9 Children[c]	19-28 (22) (23 ± 5)	(36 ± 12)	(15 ± 5)
New Zealand[d]	113 Adults	(5.4 ± 0.1)	(6.6 ± 0.3)	(4.3 ± 0.1)
Thailand	3 Adults	14.4-20.2	17.8-35.8	8.1-12.5
	9 Children[e]	(12 ± 3.6)	(19.5 ± 8.2)	(8.3 ± 2.2)
USA	210 Adults	15.7-25.6 (20.6)		

[a] Mean values with or without standard deviation in parentheses, all other ranges.
[b] Age Group unknown.
[c] Three children recovered from Kwashiorkor, the other six under treatment for other diseases.
[d] Low selenium-content soil area.
[e] Well-nourished children, three recovered from Kwashiorkor and the other six under treatment for other diseases.
[f] Mean values from seven subjects.

Store at controlled room temperature 15°-30°C (59°-86°F). Do not permit to freeze.

HOW SUPPLIED
INJECTION: 40 MCG/ML

AVERAGE UNIT PRICE (AVAILABLE SIZES)			
BRAND	$0.93		

BRAND/MANUFACTURER	NDC	SIZE	AWP
◆ BRAND			
SELEPEN: Fujisawa	00469-8820-30	10 ml	$8.65
	00469-5400-50	30 ml	$29.93

Selenium Sulfide

DESCRIPTION
A liquid antiseborrheic, antifungal preparation for topical application. Contains: Selenium Sulfide 2½% w/v in aqueous suspension; also contains: bentonite, lauric diethanolamide, ethylene glycol monostearate, titanium dioxide, amphoteric-2, sodium lauryl sulfate, sodium phosphate (monobasic), glyceryl monoricinoleate, citric acid, captan and perfume.

CLINICAL PHARMACOLOGY
Selenium Sulfide appears to have a cytostatic effect on cells of the epidermis and follicular epithelium, reducing corneocyte production.

INDICATIONS AND USAGE
Treatment of tinea versicolor, seborrheic dermatitis of scalp and treatment of dandruff.

CONTRAINDICATIONS
Not to be used by patients allergic to ingredients.

PRECAUTIONS
General: Not to be used when inflammation or exudation is present as increased absorption may occur.

Information for Patients: See "Warnings and Precautions" section under "Application Instructions".

Carcinogenesis: Dermal application of 25% and 50% solutions of 2.5% Selenium Sulfide lotion on mice over an 88 week period, indicated no carcinogenic effects.

Pregnancy: WHEN USED FOR THE TREATMENT OF TINEA VERSICOLOR, SELENIUM SULFIDE IS CLASSIFIED AS PREGNANCY CATEGORY C. Animal reproduction studies have not been conducted with Selenium Sulfide. It is also not known whether Selenium Sulfide can cause fetal harm when applied to body surfaces of a pregnant woman or an can affect reproduction capacity. Under ordinary circumstances Selenium Sulfide should not be used for the treatment of tinea versicolor in pregnant women.

Pediatric Use: Safety and effectiveness in infants have not been established.

ADVERSE REACTIONS
In decreasing order of severity; skin irritation; occasional reports of increase in normal hair loss; discoloration of hair (can be avoided or minimized by thorough rinsing of hair after treatment). As with other shampoos, oiliness or dryness of hair and scalp may occur.

OVERDOSAGE
Accidental Oral Ingestion: No documented reports of serious toxicity in humans resulting from acute ingestion of Selenium Sulfide, however, acute toxicity studies in animals suggest that ingestion of large amounts could result in potential human toxicity. Evacuation of the stomach contents should be considered in cases of acute oral ingestion.

DOSAGE AND ADMINISTRATION
See application instructions.

Treatment of tinea versicolor: Apply to affected areas and lather with a small amount of water. Allow product to remain on skin for 10 minutes, then rinse thoroughly. Repeat procedure once a day for 7 days.

Treatment of seborrheic dermatitis and dandruff: Usually two applications each week for two weeks will afford control. After this, may be used at less frequent intervals —weekly, every two weeks, or every 3 or 4 weeks in some cases. Should not be applied more frequently than required to maintain control.

APPLICATION INSTRUCTIONS: KEEP TIGHTLY CAPPED.
Shake well before using. Product may damage jewelry; remove jewelry before use.
For treatment of tinea versicolor:

1. Apply to affected areas and lather with a small amount of water.
2. Allow to remain on skin for 10 minutes.
3. Rinse body thoroughly.
4. Repeat this procedure once a day for 7 days.

For treatment of dandruff and seborrheic dermatitis of the scalp:

1. Massage about 1 or 2 teaspoonfuls of shampoo into wet scalp.
2. Allow to remain on scalp for 2 to 3 minutes.
3. Rinse scalp thoroughly.
4. Repeat application and rinse thoroughly.
5. After treatment, wash hands well.
6. Repeat treatments as directed by physician.

WARNINGS AND PRECAUTIONS
For External Use Only. Do not use on broken skin or inflamed areas. If allergic reactions occur, discontinue use. Avoid getting shampoo in eyes or in contact with genital area and skin folds as it may cause irritation and burning. These areas should be thoroughly rinsed after application. Keep this and all other medicines out of reach of children.
Store Below 86°F (30°C).

HOW SUPPLIED
LOTION: 2.5%

AVERAGE UNIT PRICE (AVAILABLE SIZES)		GENERIC A-RATED AVERAGE PRICE (GAAP)	
BRAND	$0.10	120 ml	$3.33
GENERIC	$0.04	120 ml	$3.05
HCFA FUL (120 ml)	$0.02		

BRAND/MANUFACTURER	NDC	SIZE	AWP
◆ BRAND			
SELSUN: Ross Pharm	00074-2660-04	120 ml	$11.99
◆ GENERICS			
GLO-SEL: Syosset	47854-0605-22	60 ml	$11.00
Thames	49158-0112-34	120 ml	$2.10
Barre	00472-1533-04	120 ml	$3.05
Schein	00364-7169-77	120 ml	$3.10
URL	00677-0552-41	120 ml	$3.20
Major	00904-1533-20	120 ml	$3.20
Major	00904-1533-00	120 ml	$3.30
Rugby	00536-1980-97	120 ml	$3.45
Qualitest	00603-1674-54	120 ml	$3.55

SHAMPOO: 2.5%

AVERAGE UNIT PRICE (AVAILABLE SIZES)		GENERIC A-RATED AVERAGE PRICE (GAAP)	
BRAND	$0.11	120 ml	$3.48
GENERIC	$0.03		

BRAND/MANUFACTURER	NDC	SIZE	AWP
◆ BRAND			
EXSEL: Allergan Herbert	00023-0817-99	120 ml	$12.86
◆ GENERICS			
Clay-Park	45802-0040-64	120 ml	$2.80
Goldline	00182-6088-37	120 ml	$3.00
Moore,H.L.	00839-5435-65	120 ml	$3.98
Geneva	00781-7100-04	120 ml	$4.13

◆ RATED THERAPEUTICALLY EQUIVALENT; ◇ THERAPEUTIC EQUIVALENCE UNCONFIRMED; ○ UNRATED

Selepen SEE SELENIOUS ACID

Selsun SEE SELENIUM SULFIDE

Semprex-D SEE ACRIVASTINE AND PSEUDOEPHEDRINE HYDROCHLORIDE

Sensorcaine SEE BUPIVACAINE, BUPIVACAINE WITH EPINEPHRINE, AND BUPIVACAINE SPINAL IN DEXTROSE

Septisol SEE HEXACHLOROPHENE

Septra SEE SULFAMETHOXAZOLE AND TRIMETHOPRIM

Ser-Ap-Es SEE HYDRALAZINE HYDROCHLORIDE/ HYDROCHLOROTHIAZIDE/RESERPINE

Serax SEE OXAZEPAM

Serentil SEE MESORIDAZINE BESYLATE

Serevent SEE SALMETEROL XINAFOATE

Sermorelin Acetate

DESCRIPTION

Sermorelin Acetate is a sterile, nonpyrogenic lyophilized preparation containing 50 mcg, 5 mg mannitol, 0.66 mg monobasic sodium phosphate, and 0.04 mg dibasic sodium phosphate. Sermorelin Acetate is an acetate salt of a synthetic, 29-amino acid polypeptide that is the amino-terminal segment of the naturally occurring human growth hormone-releasing hormone (GHRH or GRH) consisting of 44 amino acid residues.

The free base of Sermorelin has the empirical formula $C_{14}H_{246}N_{44}O_{42}S_1$ and a molecular weight of 3.358 daltons. Sermorelin Acetate appears to be equivalent to GRH (1-44) in its ability to stimulate growth hormone secretion in humans. It has also been called GRH (1-29) and GHRH (1-29).

Following is its chemical structure:

H—Tyr—Ala—Asp—Ala—Ile—Phe—Thr—Asn—Ser—Tyr—Arg—Lys—Val—
1   2   3   4   5   6   7   8   9   10   11   12   13

Leu—Gly—Gln—Leu—Ser—Ala—Arg—Lys—Leu—Leu—Gln—Asp—Ile—
14   15   16   17   18   19   20   21   22   23   24   25   26

Met—Ser—Arg—NH$_2$ • $xC_2H_4O_2$ • yH_2O
27   28   29

CLINICAL PHARMACOLOGY

Sermorelin Acetate increases plasma growth hormone (GH) concentrations by direct stimulation of the pituitary gland to release GH.

Because baseline GH levels are generally very low (< 4 ng/mL), provocative tests may be useful in determining the functional GH-secreting capability of the pituitary somatotroph. Adults and children with normal responses to standard provocative tests of GH secretion were used to define the range of normal plasma GH-level responses to Sermorelin Acetate. It was found that the absolute peak GH level following Sermorelin Acetate infusion and the time elapsed from infusion to that peak are appropriate measures to evaluate the response to GH infusion. Doses of Sermorelin Acetate used in children and adults in these studies ranged from 0.3 to 6.06 mcg/kg with a majority of patients receiving 1 mcg/kg. Based on these studies and published reports, 1 mcg/kg was chosen as the recommended dose for diagnostic purposes.

A total of 71 Sermorelin Acetate Injection tests were performed on 47 boys and 24 girls who showed normal responses to standard, indirect provocative tests such

as clonidine, L-dopa, and arginine. The GH peak plasma response to Sermorelin Acetate was 28 ± 15 ng/mL (average ± S.D.) and the time to this peak was 30 ± 27 minutes (average ± S.D.).

Of all children who had GH responses of > 7 ng/mL to standard provocative tests, 96% also had responses to Sermorelin Acetate of > 7 ng/mL. In 77 patients who failed to respond to standard provocative tests, mean GH peak responses to Sermorelin Acetate were significantly lower compared to the mean GH peak response of normal control children. However, 53% of the children who failed to respond to standard tests had a GH response to Sermorelin Acetate of more than 7 ng/mL, suggesting that clinical GH deficiency is frequently not due to somatotroph failure.

The following figure shows the time course of average plasma GH-level responses to Sermorelin Acetate injection in normal children and those with subnormal responses to standard provocative tests, i.e. growth hormone-deficient (GHD) children.

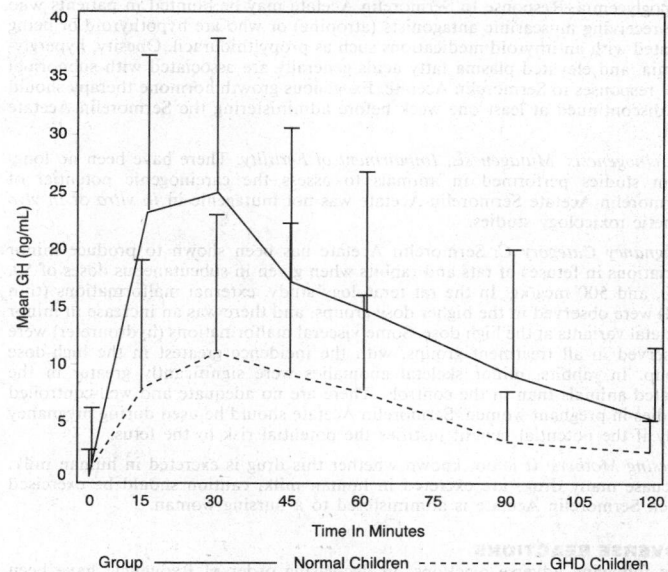

Mean (& SD) of GH Response to Sermorelin Acetate in Normal and GHD Children

Group ——— Normal Children - - - - - GHD Children

In 14 published reports that utilized different forms of GRH including GRH (1-44), GRH (1-40), and formulations of GRH (1-29) other than Sermorelin Acetate, 167 normal young adults of both sexes, 19 to 40 years old, were tested with approximately 1 mcg/kg GRH peptide. The data derived from pooling these results are similar to the results obtained from 14 normal male adults, 19 to 30 years old tested with Sermorelin Acetate:

ADULT VOLUNTEERS

Source	N	Age Range	Range of Mean Peak GH (ng/mL)	Mean Peak GH (ng/mL)
14 Studies	167	19-40	10-41	22
Sermoreline Acetate	14	19-30	—	24

In adults, time to peak GH response to Sermorelin Acetate was 35 ± 29 minutes (average ± S.D.).

Preliminary studies have demonstrated a decline in GH responsiveness to GRH with age in persons over 40 years old, but the normal range of GH response to Sermorelin Acetate in older adults has not been established.

INDICATIONS AND USAGE

Sermorelin Acetate as a single intravenous injection is indicated for evaluating the ability of the somatotroph of the pituitary gland to secrete growth hormone (GH). A normal plasma GH response to Sermorelin Acetate demonstrates that the somatotroph is intact. However, a normal response does not exclude GH deficiency because this deficiency is frequently the result of hypothalamic dysfunction in the presence of an intact somatotroph. The Sermorelin Acetate stimulation test is most easily interpreted when there is a subnormal response to conventional provocative testing and a normal response to Sermoreline Acetate.

Such findings suggest that hypothalamic dysfunction is the cause for the growth hormone deficiency. When both conventional and Sermorelin Acetate testing result in subnormal GH responses, the site of dysfunction cannot be determined with certainty because some patients with GH deficiency due to hypothalamic dysfunction require repeated Sermorelin Acetate administration before demonstrating a normal response.

The Sermorelin Acetate test has not been found useful in the diagnosis of acromegaly.

➤ SHOWN IN PRODUCT IDENTIFICATION GUIDE

CONTRAINDICATIONS

Sermorelin Acetate is contraindicated in patients hypersensitive to Sermorelin Acetate or any of the excipients.

WARNINGS

Although hypersensitivity reactions have been observed with other polypeptide hormones, to date no such reactions have been reported following the administration of a single dose of Sermorelin Acetate. Antibody formation has been reported in humans after chronic subcutaneous administration of large doses of Sermorelin Acetate (see "Adverse Reactions" sections).

PRECAUTIONS

Drug Interactions: The Sermorelin Acetate test should not be conducted in the presence of drugs that directly affect the pituitary secretion of somatotropin. These include preparations that contain or release somatostatin, insulin, glucocorticoids, or cyclooxygenase inhibitors such as aspirin or indomethacin. Somatotropin levels may be transiently elevated by clonidine, levodopa, and insulin-induced hypoglycemia. Response to Sermorelin Acetate may be blunted in patients who are receiving muscarinic antagonists (atropine) or who are hypothyroid or being treated with antithyroid medications such as propylthiouracil. Obesity, hyperglycemia, and elevated plasma fatty acids generally are associated with subnormal GH responses to Sermorelin Acetate. Exogenous growth hormone therapy should be discontinued at least one week before administering the Sermorelin Acetate test.

Carcinogenesis, Mutagenesis, Impairment of Fertility: There have been no long-term studies performed in animals to assess the carcinogenic potential of Sermorelin Acetate Sermorelin Acetate was not mutagenic in *in vitro* or *in vivo* genetic toxicology studies.

Pregnancy Category C: Sermorelin Acetate has been shown to produce minor variations in fetuses of rats and rabbits when given in subcutaneous doses of 50, 150, and 500 mcg/kg. In the rat teratology study, external malformations (thin tail) were observed in the higher dose groups, and there was an increase in minor skeletal variants at the high dose. Some visceral malformations (hydroureter) were observed in all treatment groups, with the incidence greatest in the high-dose group. In rabbits, minor skeletal anomalies were significantly greater in the treated animals than in the controls. There are no adequate and well-controlled studies in pregnant women. Sermorelin Acetate should be used during pregnancy only if the potential benefit justifies the potential risk to the fetus.

Nursing Mothers: It is not known whether this drug is excreted in human milk. Becuase many drugs are excreted in human milk, caution should be exercised when Sermorelin Acetate is administered to a nursing woman.

ADVERSE REACTIONS

The following adverse reactions, in decreasing order of frequency, have been reported following Sermorelin Acetate administration:

  Transient warmth and/or flushing of the face
  Injection site pain
  Redness and/or swelling at injection site
  Nausea
  Headache
  Vomiting
  Strange taste in the mouth
  Paleness
  Tightness in the chest

Approximately one in four patients given repeated doses of one or more of the three forms of GRH (1-29, 1-40, and 1-44) has developed antibodies to GRH. The clinical significance of these antibodies is unknown. One patient who developed antibodies to GRH (1-44) also experienced an allergic reaction described as severe redness, swelling, and urticaria at the injection sites. No long-lasting effects from this reaction were reported. No symptomatic allergic reactions to GRH (1-29) have been reported.

OVERDOSAGE

Changes of heart rate and blood pressure have been reported with the various GRH peptides in intravenous doses exceeding 10 mcg/kg. Cardiovascular collapse is a conceivable, but as of yet, unreported, complication of overdosage with GRH (1-29).

DOSAGE AND ADMINISTRATION

Sermorelin Acetate dosage should be individualized for each patient according to his/her weight. It is recommended that Sermorelin Acetate be administered in a single intravenous dose of 1.0 mcg/kg body weight in the morning following an overnight fast.

DIRECTIONS

Children (or subjects less than 50 kg):

1) Reconstitute the contents of one 50 mcg ampule of Sermorelin Acetate with a minimum of 0.5 mL of the accompanying sterile diluent.
2) Venous blood samples for growth hormone determinations should be drawn 15 minutes before and immediately prior to Sermorelin Acetate administration.
3) Administer a bolus of 1 mcg/kg body weight Sermorelin Acetate intravenously followed by a 3 mL normal saline flush.
4) Draw venous blood samples for growth hormone determinations at 15, 30, 45, and 60 minutes after Sermorelin Acetate administration

Adults (or subjects over 50 kg):

1) Determine the number of ampules needed, based on a dose of 1 mcg/kg body weight.
2) Reconstitute the contents of each ampule with a minimum of 0.5 mL of the accompanying sterile diluent.
3) Follow steps 2-4 above.

Parenteral drug products should be inspected visually for particulate matter and discoloration prior to administration, whenever solution and container permit. The drug should be discarded if not dissolved or if the reconstituted solution is cloudy or discolored.

The lyophilized product must be stored refrigerated (2° - 8°C/36° - 46°F). Use immediately after reconstitution. Discard unused material.

HOW SUPPLIED
POWDER FOR INJECTION: 50 MCG

BRAND/MANUFACTURER	NDC	SIZE	AWP
○ BRAND GEREF: Serono	44087-4050-01	1s	$40.00

Seromycin *SEE* CYCLOSERINE

Serophene *SEE* CLOMIPHENE CITRATE

Sertraline Hydrochloride

DESCRIPTION

Sertraline Hydrochloride is an antidepressant for oral administration. It is chemically unrelated to tricylic, tetracyclic, or other available antidepressant agents. It has a molecular weight of 342.7. Sertraline Hydrochloride has the following chemical name: (1S-cis)-4-(3,4-dichlorophenyl)-1,2,3,4-tetrahydro-N-methyl-1-nap hthalenamine hydrochloride. Sertraline Hydrochloride is a white crystalline powder that is slightly soluble in water and isopropyl alcohol, and sparingly soluble in ethanol.

Following is its chemical structure:

CLINICAL PHARMACOLOGY
PHARMACODYNAMICS

The mechanism of action of Sertraline Hydrochloride is presumed to be linked to its inhibition of CNS neuronal uptake of serotonin (5HT). Studies at clinically relevant doses in man have demonstrated that Sertraline Hydrochloride blocks the uptake of serotonin into human platelets. *In vitro* studies in animals also suggest that Sertraline Hydrochloride is a potent and selective inhibitor of neuronal serotonin reuptake and has only very weak effects on norepinephrine and dopamine neuronal reuptake. *In vitro* studies have shown that Sertraline Hydrochloride has no significant affinity for adrenergic (alpha$_1$, alpha$_2$, beta), cholinergic, GABA, dopaminergic, histaminergic, serotonergic (5HT$_{1A}$, 5HT$_{1B}$, 5HT$_2$), or benzodiazepine receptors; antagonism of such receptors has been hypothesized to be associated with various anticholinergic, sedative, and cardiovascular effects for other psychotropic drugs. The chronic administration of Sertraline Hydrochloride was found in animals to downregulate brain norepinephrine receptors, as has been observed with other clinically effective antidepressants. Sertraline Hydrochloride does not inhibit monoamine oxidase.

PHARMACOKINETICS

Systemic Bioavailability: In man, following oral once-daily dosing over the range of 50 to 200 mg for 14 days, mean peak plasma concentrations (Cmax) of Sertraline Hydrochloride occurred between 4.5 to 8.4 hours postdosing. The average terminal elimination half-life of plasma sertraline is about 26 hours. Based on this pharmacokinetic parameter, steady-state sertraline plasma levels should be achieved after approximately one week of once-daily dosing. Linear dose-proportional pharmacokinetics were demonstrated in a single dose study in which the Cmax and area under the plasma concentration time curve (AUC) of Sertraline Hydrochloride were proportional to dose over a range of 50 to 200 mg. Consistent with the terminal elimination half-life, there is an approximately two-fold accumulation, compared to a single dose, of Sertraline Hydrochloride with repeated dosing over a 50 to 200 mg dose range. The single-dose bioavailability of Sertraline Hydrochloride tablets is approximately equal to an equivalent dose of solution.

The effects of food on the bioavailability of Sertraline Hydrochloride were studied in subjects administered a single-dose with and without food. AUC was slightly increased when drug was administered with food but the Cmax was 25% greater, while the time to reach peak plasma concentration decreased from 8 hours post-dosing to 5.5 hours.

Metabolism: Sertraline Hydrochloride undergoes extensive first pass metabolism. The principal initial pathway of metabolism for Sertraline Hydrochloride is N-demethylation. N-desmethylsertraline has a plasma terminal elimination half-life of 62 to 104 hours. Both *in vitro* biochemical and *in vivo* pharmacological testing have shown N-desmethylsertraline to be substantially less active than Sertraline Hydrochloride. Both Sertraline Hydrochloride and N-desmethyl-sertraline undergo oxidative deamination and subsequent reduction, hydroxylation, and glucuronide conjugation. In a study of radiolabeled Sertraline Hydrochloride, involving two healthy male subjects, sertraline accounted for less than 5% of the plasma radioactivity. About 40-45% of the administered radioactivity was recovered in urine in 9 days. Unchanged Sertraline Hydrochloride was not detectable in the urine. For the same period, about 40-45% of the administered radioactivity was accounted for in feces, including 12-14% unchanged Sertraline Hydrochloride. Desmethylsertraline exhibits time-related, dose dependent increases in AUC (0-24 hour), Cmax and Cmin, with about a 5-9 fold increase in these pharmacokinetic parameters between day 1 and day 14.

Protein Binding: In vitro protein binding studies performed with radiolabeled ^{3}H-sertraline showed that Sertraline Hydrochloride is highly bound to serum proteins (98%) in the range of 20 to 500 ng/mL. However, at up to 300 and 200 ng/mL concentrations, respectively. Sertraline Hydrochloride and N-desmethylsertraline did not alter the plasma protein binding of two other highly protein bound drugs, viz., warfarin and propranolol (see *"Precautions"*).

Age: Sertraline Hydrochloride plasma clearance in a group of 16 (8 male, 8 female) elderly patients treated for 14 days at dose of 100 mg/day was approximately 40% lower than in a similarly studied group of younger (25 to 32 y.c.) individuals. Steady state, therefore, should be achieved after 2 to 3 weeks in older patients. The same study showed a decreased clearance of desmethylsertraline in older males, but not in older females.

Liver Disease: As might be predicted from its primary site of metabolism, liver impairment can affect the elimination or Sertraline Hydrochloride. The elimination half-life of Sertraline Hydrochloride was prolonged in a single dose study of patients with mild, stable cirrhosis, with a mean of 52 hours compared to 22 hours seen in subjects without liver disease. This suggests that the use of Sertraline Hydrochloride in patients with liver disease must be approached with caution. If Sertraline Hydrochloride is administered to patients with liver disease a lower or less frequent dose should be used (see *"Precautions"* and *"Dosage and Administration"*).

Renal Disease: The pharmacokinetics of Sertraline Hydrochloride in patients with significant renal dysfunction have not been determined.

INDICATIONS AND USAGE

Sertraline Hydrochloride is indicated for the treatment of depression. The efficacy of Sertraline Hydrochloride in the treatment of a major depressive episode was established in six to eight week controlled trials of outpatients whose diagnoses corresponded most closely to the DSM-III category of major depressive disorder.

A major depressive episode implies a prominent and relatively persistent depressed or dysphoric mood that usually interferes with daily functioning (nearly every day for at least 2 weeks); it should include at least 4 of the following 8 symptoms: change in appetite, change in sleep, psychomotor agitation or retardation, loss of interest in usual activities or decrease in sexual drive, increased fatigue, feelings of guilt or worthlessness, slowed thinking or impaired concentration, and a suicide attempt or suicidal ideation.

The antidepressant action of Sertraline Hydrochloride in hospitalized depressed patients has not been adequately studied.

A study of depressed outpatients who had responded to Sertraline Hydrochloride during an initial eight-week open treatment phase and were then randomized to continuation on Sertraline Hydrochloride or placebo demonstrated a significantly lower relapse rate over the next eight weeks for patients taking Sertraline Hydrochloride compared to those on placebo. However, the effectiveness of Sertraline Hydrochloride in long-term use, that is, for more than 16 weeks, has not been systematically evaluated in controlled trials. Therefore, the physician who elects to use Sertraline Hydrochloride for extended periods should periodically reevaluate the long-term usefulness of the drug for the individual patient.

UNLABELED USES

Sertraline Hydrochloride is used alone or as an adjunct in the treatment of obsessive compulsive disorder and obesity.

CONTRAINDICATIONS

None known.

WARNINGS

Cases of serious reactions have been reported in patients receiving Sertraline Hydrochloride in combination with a monoamine oxidase inhibitor (MAOI). The symptoms have included mental status changes such as memory changes, confusion and irritability, chills, pyrexia and muscle rigidity. In patients receiving another serotonin reuptake inhibitor drug in combination with a monoamine oxidase inhibitor (MAOI), there have been reports of serious, sometimes fatal, reactions including hyperthermia, rigidity, myoclonus, autonomic instability with possible rapid fluctuations of vital signs, mental status changes that include extreme agitation progressing to delirium and coma. These reactions have also been reported in patients who have recently discontinued that drug and have been started on an MAOI. Some cases presented with features resembling neuroleptic malignant syndrome. Therefore, it is recommended that Sertraline Hydrochloride not be used in combination with an MAOI, or within 14 days of discontinuing treatment with an MAOI. Similarly, at least 14 days should be allowed after stopping Sertraline Hydrochloride before starting an MAOI.

PRECAUTIONS

GENERAL

Activation of Mania/Hypomania: During premarketing testing, hypomania or mania occurred in approximately 0.4% of Sertraline Hydrochloride treated patients. Activation of mania/hypomania has also been reported in a small proportion of patients with Major Affective Disorder treated with other marketed antidepressants.

Weight Loss: Significant weight loss may be an undesirable result of treatment with Sertraline Hydrochloride for some patients, but on average, patients in controlled trials had minimal, 1 to 2 pound weight loss versus smaller changes on placebo. Only rarely have Sertraline Hydrochloride patients been discontinued for weight loss.

Seizure: Sertraline Hydrochloride has not been evaluated in patients with a seizure disorder. These patients were excluded from clinical studies during the product's premarket testing. Accordingly, like other antidepressants, Sertraline Hydrochloride should be introduced with care in epileptic patients.

Suicide: The possibility of a suicide attempt is inherent in depression and may persist until significant remission occurs. Close supervision of high-risk patients should accompany initial drug therapy. Prescriptions for Sertraline Hydrochloride should be written for the smallest quantity of tablets consistent with good patient management, in order to reduce the risk of overdose.

Weak Uricosuric Effect: Sertraline Hydrochloride is associated with a mean decrease in serum uric acid of approximately 7%. The clinical significance of this weak uricosuric effect is unknown, and there have been no reports of acute renal failure with Sertraline Hydrochloride.

Use in Patients with Concomitant Illness: Clinical experience with Sertraline Hydrochloride in patients with certain concomitant systemic illness is limited. Caution is advisable in using Sertraline Hydrochloride in patients with diseases or conditions that could affect metabolism or hemodynamic responses.

Sertraline Hydrochloride has not been evaluated or used to any appreciable extent in patients with a recent history of myocardial infarction or unstable heart disease. Patients with these diagnoses were excluded from clinical studies during the product's premarket testing. However, the electrocardiograms of 774 patients who received Sertraline Hydrochloride in double-blind trials were evaluated and the data indicate that Sertraline Hydrochloride is not associated with the development of significant ECG abnormalities. Sertraline Hydrochloride is extensively metabolized by the liver. In subjects with mild, stable cirrhosis of the liver, the clearance of sertraline was decreased, thus increasing the elimination half-life. A lower or less frequent dose should be used in patients with cirrhosis.

Since Sertraline Hydrochloride is extensively metabolized, excretion of unchanged drug in urine is a minor route of elimination. However, until the pharmacokinetics of Sertraline Hydrochloride have been studied in patients with renal impairment and until adequate numbers of patients with severe renal impairment have been evaluated during chronic treatment with Sertraline Hydrochloride, it should be used with caution in such patients.

Interference with Cognitive and Motor Performance: In controlled studies, Sertraline Hydrochloride did not cause sedation and did not interfere with psychomotor performance.

Hyponatremia: Several cases of hyponatremia have been reported. The hyponatremia appeared to be reversible when Sertraline Hydrochloride was discontinued. The majority of these occurrences have been in elderly individuals, some in patients taking diuretics or who were otherwise volume depleted.

Platelet Function: There have been rare reports of altered platelet function and/or abnormal results from laboratory studies in patients taking Sertraline Hydrochloride. While there have been reports of abnormal bleeding or purpura in several patients taking Sertraline Hydrochloride, it is unclear whether Sertraline Hydrochloride had a causative role.

INFORMATION FOR PATIENTS

Physicians are advised to discuss the following issues with patients for whom they prescribe Sertraline Hydrochloride:

Patients should be told that although Sertraline Hydrochloride has not been shown to impair the ability of normal subjects to perform tasks requiring complex motor and mental skills in laboratory experiments, drugs that act upon the central nervous system may affect some individuals adversely.

Patients should be told that although Sertraline Hydrochloride has not been shown in experiments with normal subjects to increase the mental and motor skill impairments caused by alcohol, the concomitant use of Sertraline Hydrochloride and alcohol in depressed patients is not advised.

Patients should be told that while no adverse intreaction of Sertraline Hydrochloride with over-the-counter (OTC) drug products is known to occur, the potential for interaction exists. Thus, the use of any OTC product should be initiated cautiously according to the directions of use given for the OTC product. Patients should be advised to notify their physician if they become pregnant or intend to become pregnant during therapy.

Patients should be advised to notify their physician if they are breast feeding an infant.

LABORATORY TESTS

None.

DRUG INTERACTIONS

Potential Effects of Coadministration of Drugs Highly Bound to Plasma Proteins: Because Sertraline Hydrochloride is tightly bound to plasma protein, the administration of Sertraline Hydrochloride to a patient taking another drug which is tightly bound to protein, (e.g., warfarin, digitoxin) may cause a shift in plasma concentrations potentially resulting in an adverse effect. Conversely, adverse effects may result from displacement of protein bound Sertraline Hydrochloride by other tightly bound drugs.

In a study comparing prothrombin time AUC (0-120 hr) following dosing with warfarin (0.75 mg/kg) before and after 21 days of dosing with either Sertraline Hydrochloride (50-200 mg/day) or placebo, there was a mean increase in prothrombin time of 8% relative to baseline for Sertraline Hydrochloride compared to a 1% decrease for placebo (p < 0.02). The normalization of prothrombin time for the Sertraline Hydrochloride group was delayed compared to the placebo group. The clinical significance of this change is unknown. Accordingly, prothrombin time should be carefully monitored when Sertraline Hydrochloride therapy is initiated or stopped.

Cimetidine: In a study assessing disposition of Sertraline Hydrochloride (100mg) on the second of 8 days of cimetidine administration (800mg daily), there were increases in Sertraline Hydrochloride mean AUC (50%), Cmax (24%) and half-life (26%) compared to the placebo group. The clinical significance of these changes is unknown.

CNS Active Drugs: In a study comparing the disposition of intravenously administered diazepam before and after 21 days of dosing with either Sertraline Hydrochloride (50 to 200 mg/day escalating dose) or placebo, there was a 32% decrease relative to baseline in diazepam clearance for the Sertraline Hydrochloride group compared to a 19% decrease relative to baseline for the placebo group (p < 0.03). There was a 23% increase in Tmax for desmethyldiazepam in the Sertraline Hydrochloride group compared to a 20% decrease in the placebo group (p < 0.03). The clinical significance of these changes is unknown.

In a placebo-controlled trial in normal volunteers, the administration of two doses of Sertraline Hydrochloride did not significantly alter steady-state lithium levels or the renal clearance of lithium.

Nonetheless, at this time, it is recommended that plasma lithium levels be monitored following initiation of Sertraline Hydrochloride therapy with appropriate adjustments to the lithium dose. The risk of using Sertraline Hydrochloride in combination with other CNS active drugs has not been systematically evaluated. Consequently, caution is advised if the concomitant administration of Sertraline Hydrochloride and such drugs is required.

There is limited controlled experience regarding the optimal timing of switching from other antidepressants to Sertraline Hydrochloride: Care and prudent medical judgment should be exercised when switching, particularly from long-acting agents. The duration of an appropriate washout period which should intervene before switching from one selective serotonin reuptake inhibitor (SSRI) to another has not been established.

Hypoglycemic Drugs: In a placebo-controlled trial in normal volunteers, administration of Sertraline Hydrochloride for 22 days (including 200 mg/day for the final 13 days) caused a statistically significant 16% decrease from baseline in the clearance of tolbutamide following an intravenous 1000 mg dose. Sertraline Hydrochloride administration did not noticeably change either the plasma protein binding or the apparent volume of distribution of tolbutamide, suggesting that the decreased clearance was due to a change in the metabolism of the drug. The clinical significance of this decrease in tolbutamide clearance is unknown.

Atenolol: Sertraline Hydrochloride (100 mg) when administered to 10 healthy male subjects had no effect on the beta-adrenergic blocking ability of atenolol.

Digoxin: In a placebo-controlled trial in normal volunteers, administration of Sertraline Hydrochloride for 17 days (including 200 mg/day for the last 10 days) did not change mean serum digoxin levels or digoxin renal clearance.

Microsomal Enzyme Induction: Preclinical studies have shown Sertraline Hydrochloride to induce hepatic microsomal enzymes, in clinical studies, Sertraline Hydrochloride was shown to induce hepatic enzymes minimally as determined by a small (5%) but statistically significant decrease in antipyrine half-life following administration of 200 mg/day for 21 days. This small change in antipyrine half-life reflects a clinically insignificant change in hepatic metabolism.

Electroconvulsive Therapy: There are no clinical studies establishing the risks or benefits of the combined use of electroconvulsive therapy (ECT) and Sertraline Hydrochloride.

Alcohol: Although Sertraline Hydrochloride did not potentiate the cognitive and psychomotor effects of alcohol in experiments with normal subjects, the concomitant use of Sertraline Hydrochloride and alcohol in depressed patients is not recommended.

CARCINOGENESIS, MUTAGENESIS, IMPAIRMENT OF FERTILITY

Lifetime carcinogenicity studies were carried out in CD-1 mice and Long-Evans rats at doses up to 40 mg/kg in mice (10 times, on a mg/kg basis, and the same, on a mg/m² basis, as the maximum recommended human dose) and at doses up to 40 mg/kg in rats (10 times, on a mg/kg basis, and 2 times, on a mg/m² basis, the maximum recommended human dose). There was a dose-related increase in the incidence of liver adenomas in male mice receiving sertraline at 10-40 mg/kg. No increase was seen in female mice or in rats of either sex receiving the same treatments, nor was there an increase in hepatocellular carcinomas. Liver adenomas have a variable rate of spontaneous occurrence in the CD-1 mouse and are of unknown significance to humans. There was an increase in follicular

adenomas of the thyroid in female rats receiving Sertraline Hydrochloride at 40 mg/kg; this was not accompanied by thyroid hyperplasia. While there was an increase in uterine adenocarcinomas in rats receiving Sertraline Hydrochloride at 10-40 mg/kg compared to placebo controls, this effect was not clearly drug related.

Sertraline Hydrochloride had no genotoxic effects, with or without metabolic activation, based on the following assays: bacterial mutation assay; mouse lymphoma mutation assay; and tests for cytogenetic aberrations *in vitro* in mouse bone marrow and *in vitro* in human lymphocytes.

A decrease in fertility was seen in one of two rat studies at a dose of 80 mg/kg (20 times the maximum human dose on a mg/kg basis and 4 times on a mg/m² basis).

PREGNANCY-PREGNANCY CATEGORY B

Teratogenic Effects: Reproduction studies have been performed in rats and rabbits at doses up to approximately 20 times and 10 times the maximum daily human mg/kg dose (4 to 4.5 times the mg/m² dose), respectively.

There was no evidence of teratogenicity at any dose level. At doses approximately 2.5-10 times the maximum daily human mg/kg dose, Sertraline Hydrochloride was associated with delayed ossification in fetuses, probably secondary to effects on the dams.

There are no adequate and well-controlled studies in pregnant women. Because animal reproduction studies are not always predictive of human response, this drug should be used during pregnancy only if clearly needed.

Non-teratogenic Effects: There was also decreased neonatal survival following maternal administration of Sertraline Hydrochloride at doses as low as approximately 5 times the maximum human mg/kg dose. The decrease in pup survival was shown to be most probably due to *in utero* exposure to Sertraline Hydrochloride. The clinical significance of these effects is unknown.

Labor and Delivery: The effect of Sertraline Hydrochloride on labor and delivery in humans is unknown.

Nursing Mothers: It is not known whether, and if so in what amount, Sertraline Hydrochloride or its metabolites are excreted in human milk. Because many drugs are excreted in human milk, caution should be exercised when Sertraline Hydrochloride is administered to a nursing woman.

Pediatric Use: Safety and effectiveness in children have not been established.

Geriatric Use: Several hundred elderly patients have participated in clinical studies with Sertraline Hydrochloride. The pattern of adverse reactions in the elderly was similar to that in younger patients.

ADVERSE REACTIONS

Commonly Observed: The most commonly observed adverse events associated with the use of Sertraline Hydrochloride and not seen at an equivalent incidence among placebo-treated patients were: gastrointestinal complaints, including nausea, diarrhea/loose stools and dyspepsia; tremor; dizziness; insomnia; somnolence; increased sweating; dry mouth; and male sexual dysfunction (primarily ejaculatory delay).

Associated with Discontinuation of Treatment: Fifteen percent of 2710 subjects who received Sertraline Hydrochloride in premarketing multiple dose clinical trials discontinued treatment due to an adverse event. The more common events (reported by at least 1% of subjects) associated with discontinuation included agitation, insomnia, male sexual dysfunction (primarily ejaculatory delay), somnolence, dizziness, headache, tremor, anorexia, diarrhea/loose stools, nausea, and fatigue.

Incidence in Controlled Clinical Trials: The table that follows enumerates adverse events that occurred at a frequency of 1% or more among Sertraline Hydrochloride patients who participated in controlled trials comparing titrated Sertraline Hydrochloride with placebo. Most patients received doses of 50 to 200 mg per day. The prescriber should be aware that these figures cannot be used to predict the incidence of side effects in the course of usual medical practice where patient characteristics and other factors differ from those which prevailed in the clinical trials. Similarly, the cited frequencies cannot be compared with figures obtained from other clinical investigations involving different treatments, uses, and investigators. The cited figures, however, do provide the prescribing physician with some basis for estimating the relative contribution of drug and non-drug factors to the side effect incidence rate in the population studied.

TREATMENT-EMERGENT ADVERSE EXPERIENCE INCIDENCE IN PLACEBO-CONTROLLED CLINICAL TRIALS*

Adverse Experience	(Percent of Patients Reporting)	
	Sertraline Hydrochloride (N = 861)	Placebo (N = 853)
Autonomic Nervous System Disorders		
Mouth Dry	16.3	9.3
Sweating Increased	8.4	2.9
Cardiovascular		
Palpitations	3.5	1.6
Chest Pain	1.0	1.6
Centr. & Periph. Nerv. System Disorders		
Headache	20.3	19.0
Dizziness	11.7	6.7
Tremor	10.7	2.7
Paresthesia	2.0	1.8

Adverse Experience	(Percent of Patients Reporting)	
	Sertraline Hydrochloride (N = 861)	Placebo (N = 853)
Hypoesthesia	1.7	0.6
Twitching	1.4	0.1
Hypertonia	1.3	0.4
Disorders of Skin and Appendages		
Rash	2.1	1.5
Gastrointestinal Disorders		
Nausea	26.1	11.8
Diarrhea/Loose Stools	17.7	9.3
Constipation	8.4	6.3
Dyspepsia	6.0	2.8
Vomiting	3.8	1.8
Flatulence	3.3	2.5
Anorexia	2.8	1.6
Abdominal Pain	2.4	2.2
Appetite Increased	1.3	0.9
General		
Fatigue	10.6	8.1
Hot Flushes	2.2	0.5
Fever	1.6	0.6
Back Pain	1.5	0.9
Metabolic and Nutritional Disorders		
Thirst	1.4	0.9
Musculoskeletal System Disorders		
Myalgia	1.7	1.5
Psychiatric Disorders		
Insomnia	16.4	8.8
Sexual Dysfunction-Male (1)	15.5	2.2
Somnolence	13.4	5.9
Agitation	5.6	4.0
Nervousness	3.4	1.9
Anxiety	2.6	1.3
Yawning	1.9	0.2
Sexual Dysfunction-Female (2)	1.7	0.2
Concentration Impaired	1.3	0.5
Reproductive		
Menstrual Disorder (2)	1.0	0.5
Respiratory System Disorders		
Rhinitis	2.0	1.5
Pharyngitis	1.2	0.9
Special Senses		
Vision Abnormal	4.2	2.1
Tinnitus	1.4	1.1
Taste Perversion	1.2	0.7
Urinary System Disorders		
Micturition Frequency	2.0	1.2
Micturition Disorder	1.4	0.5

* *Events reported by at least 1% of patients treated with Sertraline Hydrochloride are included.*

(1) *—Primarily ejaculatory delay; % based on male patients only; 271 Sertraline Hydrochloride and 271 placebo patients.*

(2) *—% based on female patients only; 590 Sertraline Hydrochloride and 582 placebo patients.*

Other Events Observed During the Premarketing Evaluation of Sertraline Hydrochloride: During its premarketing assessment, multiple doses of Sertraline Hydrochloride were administered to approximately 2700 subjects. The conditions and duration of exposure to Sertraline Hydrochloride varied greatly, and included (in overlapping categories) clinical pharmacology studies, open and double-blind studies, uncontrolled and controlled studies, inpatient and outpatient studies, fixed-dose and titration studies, and studies for indications other than depression. Untoward events associated with this exposure were recorded by clinical investigators using terminology of their own choosing. Consequently, it is not possible to provide a meaningful estimate of the proportion of individuals experiencing adverse events without first grouping similar types of untoward events into a smaller number of standardized event categories.

In the tabulations that follow, a World Health Organization dictionary of terminology has been used to classify reported adverse events. The frequencies presented, therefore, represent the proportion of the approximately 2700 individuals exposed to multiple doses of Sertraline Hydrochloride who experienced an event of the type cited on at least one occasion while receiving Sertraline Hydrochloride. All events are included except those already listed in the previous table and those reported in terms so general as to be uninformative. It is important to emphasize that although the events reported occurred during treatment with Sertraline Hydrochloride, they were not necessarily caused by it. Events are further categorized by body system and listed in order of decreasing frequency according to the following definitions: frequent adverse events are those occurring on one or more occasions in at least 1/100 patients (only those not already listed in the tabulated results from placebo controlled trials appear in this listing); infrequent adverse events are those occurring in 1/100 to 1/1000 patients; rare events are those occurring in fewer than 1/1000 patients. Events of major clinical importance are also described in the *"Precautions"* section.

Autonomic Nervous System Disorders: Infrequent: flushing, mydriasis, increased saliva, cold clammy skin; *Rare:* pallor.

Cardiovascular: Infrequent: postural dizziness, hypertension, hypotension, postural hypotension, edema, dependent edema, periorbital edema, peripheral edema, peripheral ischemia, syncope, tachycardia; *Rare:* precordial chest pain, substernal chest pain, aggravated hypertension, myocardial infarction, varicose veins.

Central and Peripheral Nervous System Disorders: Frequent: confusion; *Infrequent:* ataxia, abnormal coordination, abnormal gait, hyperesthesia, hyperkinesia, hypokinesia, migraine, nystagmus, vertigo; *Rare:* local anesthesia, coma, convulsions, dyskinesia, dysphonia, hyporeflexia, hypotonia, ptosis.

Disorders of Skin and Appendages: Infrequent: acne, alopecia, pruritus, erythematous rash, maculopapular rash, dry skin; *Rare:* bullous eruption, dermatitis, erythema multiforme, abnormal hair texture, hypertrichosis, photosensitivity reaction, follicular rash, skin discoloration, abnormal skin odor, urticaria.

Endocrine Disorders: Rare: exophthalmos, gynecomastia.

Gastrointestinal Disorders: Infrequent: dysphagia, eructation; *Rare:* diverticulitis, fecal incontinence, gastritis, gastroenteritis, glossitis, gum hyperplasia, hemorrhoids, hiccup, melena, hemorrhagic peptic ulcer, proctitis, stomatitis, ulcerative stomatitis, tenesmus, tongue edema, tongue ulceration.

General: Frequent: asthenia; *Infrequent:* malaise, generalized edema, rigors, weight decrease, weight increase; *Rare:* enlarged abdomen, halitosis, otitis media, aphthous stomatitis.

Hematopoietic and Lymphatic: Infrequent: lymphadenopathy, purpura; *Rare:* anemia, anterior chamber eye hemorrhage.

Metabolic and Nutritional Disorders: Rare: dehydration, hypercholesterolemia, hypoglycemia.

Musculoskeletal System Disorders: Infrequent: arthralgia, arthrosis, dystonia, muscle cramps, muscle weakness; *Rare:* hernia.

Psychiatric Disorders: Infrequent: abnormal dreams, aggressive reaction, amnesia, apathy, delusion, depersonalization, depression, aggravated depression, emotional lability, euphoria, hallucination, neurosis, paranoid reaction, suicide ideation and attempt, teeth-grinding, abnormal thinking; *Rare:* hysteria, somnambulism, withdrawal syndrome.

Reproductive: Infrequent: dysmenorrhea (2), intermenstrual bleeding (2); *Rare:* amenorrhea (2), balanoposthitis (1), breast enlargement (2), female breast pain (2), leukorrhea (2), menorrhagia (2), atrophic vaginitis (2). (1)—% based on male subjects only; 1005. (2)—% based on female subjects only; 1705.

Respiratory System Disorders: Infrequent: bronchospasm, coughing, dyspnea, epistaxis; *Rare:* bradypnea, hyperventilation, sinusitis, stridor.

Special Senses: Infrequent: abnormal accommodation, conjunctivitis, diplopia, earache, eye pain, xerophthalmia; *Rare:* abnormal lacrimation, photophobia, visual field defect.

Urinary System Disorders: Infrequent: dysuria, face edema, nocturia, polyuria, urinary incontinence; *Rare:* oliguria, renal pain, urinary retention.

Laboratory Tests: In man, asymptomatic elevations in serum transaminases (SGOT [or AST] and SGPT [or ALT]) have been reported infrequently (approximately 0.8%) in association with Sertraline Hydrochloride administration. These hepatic enzyme elevations usually occurred within the first 1 to 9 weeks of drug treatment and promptly diminished upon drug discontinuation. Sertraline Hydrochloride therapy was associated with small mean increases in total cholesterol (approximately 3%) and triglycerides (approximately 5%), and a small mean decrease in serum uric acid (approximately 7%) of no apparent clinical importance.

DRUG ABUSE AND DEPENDENCE
Controlled Substance Class: Sertraline Hydrochloride is not a controlled substance.

Physical and Psychological Dependence: Sertraline Hydrochloride has not been systematically studied, in animals or humans, for its potential for abuse, tolerance, or physical dependence. However, the premarketing clinical experience with Sertraline Hydrochloride did not reveal any tendency for a withdrawal syndrome or any drug-seeking behavior. As with any CNS active drug, physicians should carefully evaluate patients for history of drug abuse and follow such patients closely, observing them for signs of Sertraline Hydrochloride misuse or abuse (e.g., development of tolerance, incrementation of dose, drug-seeking behavior).

OVERDOSAGE
Human Experience: As of November, 1992, there were 79 reports of non-fatal acute overdoses involving Sertraline Hydrochloride, of which 28 were overdoses of Sertraline Hydrochloride alone and the remainder involved a combination of other drugs and/or alcohol in addition to Sertraline Hydrochloride. In those cases of overdose involving only Sertraline Hydrochloride, the reported doses ranged from 500mg to 600mg. In a subset of 18 of these patients in whom Sertraline Hydrochloride blood levels were determined, plasma concentrations ranged from < 5ng/mL to 554ng/mL. Symptoms of overdose with Sertraline Hydrochloride alone included somnolence, nausea, vomiting, tachycardia, ECG changes, anxiety and dilated pupils. Treatment was primarily supportive and included monitoring and use of activated charcoal, gastric lavage or cathartics and hydration. Although there were no reports of death when Sertraline Hydrochloride was taken alone,

there were 4 deaths involving overdoses of Sertraline Hydrochloride in combination with other drugs and/or alcohol. Therefore, any overdosage should be treated aggressively.

Management of Overdoses: Establish and maintain an airway, insure adequate oxygenation and ventilation. Activated charcoal, which may be used with sorbitol, may be as or more effective than emesis or lavage, and should be considered in treating overdose.

Cardiac and vital signs monitoring is recommended along with general symptomatic and supportive measures.

There are no specific antidotes for Sertraline Hydrochloride.

Due to the large volume of distribution of Sertraline Hydrochloride, forced diuresis, dialysis, hemoperfusion, and exchange transfusion are unlikely to be of benefit.

In managing overdosage, consider the possibility of multiple drug involvement. The physician should consider contacting a poison control center on the treatment of any overdose.

DOSE AND ADMINISTRATION

Initial Treatment: Sertraline Hydrochloride, treatment should be initiated with a dose of 50 mg once daily. While a relationship between dose and antidepressant effect has not been established, patients were dosed in a range of 50-200 mg/day in the clinical trials demonstrating the anti-depressant effectiveness of Sertraline Hydrochloride. Consequently, patients not responding to a 50 mg dose may benefit from dose increases up to a maximum of 200 mg/day. Given the 24-hour elimination half-life of Sertraline Hydrochloride, dose changes should not occur at intervals of less than 1 week.

Sertraline Hydrochloride should be administered once daily, either in the morning or evening.

As indicated under *"Precautions,"* a lower or less frequent dosage should be used in patients with hepatic impairment. In addition, particular care should be used in patients with renal impairment.

Maintenance/Continuation/Extended Treatment: There is evidence to suggest that depressed patients responding during an initial 8-week treatment phase will continue to benefit during an additional 8 weeks of treatment. While there are insufficient data regarding any benefits from treatment beyond 16 weeks, it is generally agreed among expert psychopharmacologists that acute episodes of depression require several months or longer of sustained pharmacological therapy. Whether the dose of antidepressant needed to induce remission is identical to the dose needed to maintain and/or sustain euthymia is unknown.

Storage: Store at controlled room temperature, 59° F to 86° F (15° to 30° C).

HOW SUPPLIED
TABLETS: 50 MG

BRAND/MANUFACTURER	NDC	SIZE	AWP
○ BRAND			
▶ ZOLOFT: Roerig,J.B.	00049-4900-66	100s	$194.41
	00049-4900-41	100s ud	$194.41

TABLETS: 100 MG

BRAND/MANUFACTURER	NDC	SIZE	AWP
○ BRAND			
▶ ZOLOFT: Roerig,J.B.	00049-4910-66	100s	$200.04
	00049-4910-41	100s ud	$200.04

Shellcap *SEE* BROMPHENIRAMINE MALEATE AND PSEUDOEPHEDRINE HYDROCHLORIDE

Silvadene *SEE* SILVER SULFADIAZINE

Silver Nitrate

DESCRIPTION
Silver Nitrate is available as a solution, an ophthalmic solution, and an ointment.
Silver Nitrate ophthalmic solution is an ophthalmic anti-infective.

Each fl. oz. of solution contains:	
Silver Nitrate	.3, 7.5, or 15 gm

The ophthalmic solution contains:	
Silver Nitrate	1%

Each fl. oz. of ointment contains:	
Silver Nitrate	.3 gm

CLINICAL PHARMACOLOGY
Silver Nitrate in weak solutions is used as a germicide and astringent to mucous membranes. The germicidal action is due to precipitation of bacterial proteins by liberated silver ions.

Mechanism of Action of Silver: "The attachment of silver to a reactive group of a protein sharply decreases the solubility of the protein, and the conformation of the protein may also be altered; that is, denaturation may occur. Precipitation of the protein generally results. When the concentration of silver is low, precipitation is confined to proteins in the interstices, and an astringent action is said to have occurred. When the concentration is high, membrane and intracellular structures are damaged, and there is a caustic or corrosive effect. Because silver ions attach so readily to the various active groups of proteins, the silver ions are captured before they diffuse far into the tissues. Precipitation of silver as silver chloride also limits the extent of movement of the ions. Thus, the local effects of silver are self-limiting, and the spread of damage occurs only when the dose of silver overwhelms the capacity of the tissues to fix the ion at the site of application. The antiseptic effects of silver probably also derive in part from the reactions with bacterial and viral proteins."

From: *The Pharmacological Basis of Therapeutics* — 3rd edition by Goodman and Gilman.

Also: *Remington's Pharmaceutical Sciences* — 14th edition—pg. 406.

INDICATIONS AND USAGE
Silver Nitrate is used in medical practice to provide antiseptic, astringent, germicidal, local (epithelial) stimulant or caustic action externally.[1,5] It can be used for local treatment of infected aphthous ulcers,[2] for treatment of indolent wounds, to destroy exuberant granulations, to freshen the edges of ulcers, fissures, to touch the basis of vesicular bullous or aphthous lesions, and to provide styptic action.[1,2]

Silver Nitrate in a 10% solution is also indicated in the treatment of Impetigo Vulgarie (when the bases of lesions present considerable oozing upon removal of crust).[3]

In podiatry, the product is used to treat neurovascular helomas, to cauterize and destroy small nerve endings and blood vessels. It forms a protective covering after the removal of corns and callouses. It is also one of the cauterant chemotherapeutic methods employed in the treatment of plantar warts.[7] It is used in the chemo-surgical destruction of plantar warts, granulation tissue, papillomatous growths. It is used as an escharotic agent for the treatment of granuloma pyogenicum.[8] It is considered a strong caustic and escharotic.

In the treatment of pruritus, the moist and macerated perianal and intergluteal dermatitis is best treated with desiccating agents such as Silver Nitrate solution (painted on daily by a physician in concentrations up to 10% or higher.[4]

Silver Nitrate ophthalmic solution is indicated for the prevention of gonorrheal ophthalmia neonatorum.

Silver Nitrate has not been effective for prevention of neonatal chlamydial conjunctivitis.[9]

CONTRAINDICATIONS
Do not apply to wounds, cuts or broken skin. There are no known contraindications to use of the ophthalmic solution.

WARNINGS
Prolonged or frequent use may result in permanent discoloration of the skin. However, topical silver for localized application to suppress granulation tissue apparently does not develop argyria.[6]

A 1% ophthalmic solution is considered optimal; however, it must be used with caution, since cauterization of the cornea and blindness may result, especially with repeated applications.

When ingested, Silver Nitrate is highly toxic to the gastrointestinal tract and central nervous system. Swallowing can cause severe gastroenteritis that may end fatally. Sodium chloride may be used by gastric lavage to remove the chemical.

Silver Nitrate is caustic and irritating to the skin and mucous membranes.

PRECAUTIONS
General: Solutions of Silver Nitrate must be handled carefully, since they tend to stain skin and utensils. Silver Nitrate stains may be removed from linen by applications of iodine tincture followed by sodium thiosulfate solution.

Preserve in tight, light-resistant containers. Keep lids tightly closed.

ADVERSE REACTIONS
Discontinue use if redness or irritation occurs.

A mild chemical conjunctivitis should result from a properly performed Credé prophylaxis using Silver Nitrate ophthalmic solution. With the 1% solution of Silver Nitrate, chemical conjunctivitis occurs in 20% or less of cases.

OVERDOSAGE
In case of accidental ingestion, give a tablespoonful of salt in a glass of warm water and repeat until vomit fluid is clear. Have patient lie down and keep warm. Give milk or whites of eggs beaten with water. If accidently splashed in or touched on the eye, wash copiously with water and see a physician.

When a solution of 2% or higher Silver Nitrate concentration is used in the eye, conjunctivitis may be produced. The eye should be irrigated with an isotonic solution of sodium chloride after solutions of Silver Nitrate stronger than 1% are instilled.

DOSAGE AND ADMINISTRATION
Apply a cotton applicator dipped in solution on the affected area or lesion two or three times weekly for two or three weeks as needed.

Apply in an apertured pad on affected area or lesion for approximately 5 days as needed.

Ophthalmic Solution: Immediately after the child is born, the eyelids should be cleaned with sterile absorbent cotton or gauze and sterile water. A separate

---

◆ RATED THERAPEUTICALLY EQUIVALENT; ◇ THERAPEUTIC EQUIVALENCE UNCONFIRMED; ○ UNRATED

pledget should be used for each eye, and the lids, without being opened, should be washed from the nose outward until free of all blood, mucus, or meconium.

Next, the lids should be separated, and 2 drops of 1% Silver Nitrate solution should be dropped into the eye. The lids should be separated and elevated away from the eyeball so that a lake of Silver Nitrate may lie for a half minute or longer between them, coming in contact with every portion of the conjunctival sac.

The American Academy of Pediatrics has endorsed a statement from the Committee on Ophthalmia Neonatorum of the National Society for the Prevention of Blindness, which does not recommend irrigation of the eyes following instillation of the Silver Nitrate.

Storage: The ophthalmic solution should be kept at controlled room temperature, 59° to 86°F (15° to 30°C). Do not freeze. It should not be used when cold. Protect from light.

REFERENCES

1. Stewart C. Harvey, in "Pharmacological Basis of Principles of Therapeutics", eds. Goodman and Gilman, chp. 50. 2. Sultzberger, M.B. and Wolf, Jack, "Dermatology, Essentials of Diagnosis and Treatment", chp. 1 pg. 73, Yearbook Publishers, Chicago, Ill. 1952. 3. ibid., pg. 282. 4. ibid., pg. 455. 5. S.M. Pack & George Klein, "Therapy of Dermatological Disorders", Lea & Febinger, Philadelphia, Pa. 1951, pg. 338. 6. Herman Beerman & Bernard A. Kirshbaum, chp. 7 "Drug Eruptions (Dermatitis Medicamentosa) pg. 381, "Dermatology" eds. Moschella-Pillsbury-Hurley, W.B. Saunders, publishers, Philadelphia, Pa. 1975. 7. Joseph W. Burnett & William A. Cnitcher, in "Dermatology" chp. 12, "Viral and Rickettsial infections", eds. Moschella-Pillsbury-Hurley, W.B. Saunders, publishers, Philadelphia, Pa. 1975. 8. "Dermatology" eds. Pillsbury, Shelley & Kligman, W.B. Saunders, Publishers, Philadelphia, Pa. 1956. chp. 48 "Tumors of the Skin." 9. Schachter J. et al: Prospective study of chlamydial infection in neonates. *Lancet* 1979;2:377.

HOW SUPPLIED
DROP: 1%

BRAND/MANUFACTURER	NDC	SIZE	AWP
○ GENERICS			
Lilly	00002-1608-02	1 ml 100s	$136.16

DROP: 10%

BRAND/MANUFACTURER	NDC	SIZE	AWP
○ GENERICS			
Gordon	10481-1051-01	30 ml	$17.50

DROP: 25%

BRAND/MANUFACTURER	NDC	SIZE	AWP
○ GENERICS			
Gordon	10481-1052-01	30 ml	$28.75

DROP: 50%

BRAND/MANUFACTURER	NDC	SIZE	AWP
○ GENERICS			
Gordon	10481-1053-01	30 ml	$42.50

GRANULAR:

BRAND/MANUFACTURER	NDC	SIZE	AWP
○ GENERICS			
	00574-0653-25	25 gm	$22.28
	00574-0653-01	100 gm	$78.64

OINTMENT: 10%

BRAND/MANUFACTURER	NDC	SIZE	AWP
○ GENERICS			
Gordon	10481-3011-01	30 gm	$27.50

SWAB:

BRAND/MANUFACTURER	NDC	SIZE	AWP
○ GENERICS			
Raway	00686-1590-10	100s dozdoz	$117.00

Silver Sulfadiazine

DESCRIPTION
Silver Sulfadiazine Cream, 1%, is a topical antibacterial preparation which has as its active antimicrobial ingredient Silver Sulfadiazine. The active moiety is contained within an opaque, white, water-miscible cream base.

Each 1000 grams of Silver Sulfadiazine Cream contains 10 grams of Silver Sulfadiazine.

Silver Sulfadiazine has an empirical formula of $C_{10}H_9AgN_4O_2S$ and molecular weight of 357.14.

Following is its chemical structure:

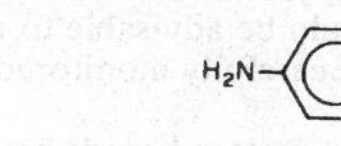

CLINICAL PHARMACOLOGY
Silver Sulfadiazine has broad antimicrobial activity. It is bactericidal for many gram-negative and gram-positive bacteria as well as being effective against yeast. Results from *in vitro* testing are listed below.

Sufficient data have been obtained to demonstrate that Silver Sulfadiazine will inhibit bacteria that are resistant to other antimicrobial agents and that the compound is superior to Sulfadiazine.

Studies utilizing radioactive micronized Silver Sulfadiazine, electron microscopy, and biochemical techniques have revealed that the mechanism of action of Silver Sulfadiazine on bacteria differs from silver nitrate and sodium Sulfadiazine. Silver Sulfadiazine acts only on the cell wall to produce its bactericidal effect.

RESULTS OF IN VITRO TESTING WITH CONCENTRATIONS OF SILVER SULFADIAZINE

Genus & Species	Number of Sensitive Strains/ Total Number of Strains Tested	
	50 μg/mL	100 μg/mL
Pseudomonas aeruginosa	130/130	130/130
Pseudomonas maltophilia	7/7	7/7
Enterobacter species	48/50	50/50
Enterobacter cloacae	24/24	24/24
Klebsiella species	53/54	54/54
Escherichia coli	63/63	63/63
Serratia species	27/28	28/28
Providencia mirabilis	53/53	53/53
Morganella morganii	10/10	10/10
Proteus rettgeri	2/2	2/2
Proteus vulgaris	2/2	2/2
Providencia species	1/1	1/1
Citrobacter species	10/10	10/10
Acinetobacter calcoaceticus	10/11	11/11
Staphylococcus aureus	100/101	101/101
Staphylococcus epidermidis	51/51	51/51
β-Hemolytic Streptococcus	4/4	4/4
Enterococcus species	52/53	53/53
Corynebacterium diphtheriae	2/2	2/2
Clostridium perfringens	0/2	2/2
Candida albicans	43/50	50/50

Silver Sulfadiazine is not a carbonic anhydrase inhibitor and may be useful in situations where such agents are contraindicated.

INDICATIONS AND USAGE
Silver Sulfadiazine Cream is a topical antimicrobial drug indicated as an adjunct for the prevention and treatment of wound sepsis in patients with second and third degree burns.

CONTRAINDICATIONS
Silver Sulfadiazine Cream is contraindicated in patients who are hypersensitive to Silver Sulfadiazine or any of the other ingredients in the preparation.

Because sulfonamide therapy is known to increase the possibility of kernicterus, Silver Sulfadiazine Cream should not be used on pregnant women approaching or at term, on premature infants, or on newborn infants during the first 2 months of life.

WARNINGS
There is potential cross-sensitivity between Silver Sulfadiazine and other sulfonamides. If allergic reactions attributable to treatment with Silver Sulfadiazine occur, continuation of therapy must be weighed against the potential hazards of the particular allergic reaction.

Fungal proliferation in and below the eschar may occur. However, the incidence of clinically reported fungal superinfection is low.

The use of Silver Sulfadiazine Cream in some cases of glucose-6-phosphate dehydrogenase-deficient individuals may be hazardous, as hemolysis may occur.

PRECAUTION
General: If hepatic and renal functions become impaired and elimination of drug decreases, accumulation may occur and discontinuation of Silver Sulfadiazine Cream should be weighed against the therapeutic benefit being achieved.

In considering the use of topical proteolytic enzymes in conjunction with Silver Sulfadiazine Cream, the possibility should be noted that silver may inactivate such enzymes.

► SHOWN IN PRODUCT IDENTIFICATION GUIDE

Laboratory Tests: In the treatment of burn wounds involving extensive areas of the body, the serum sulfa concentrations may approach adult therapeutic levels (8 to 12 mg%). Therefore, in these patients it would be advisable to monitor serum sulfa concentrations. Renal function should be carefully monitored and the urine should be checked for sulfa crystals.

Absorption of the propylene glycol vehicle in certain brands has been reported to affect serum osmolality, which may affect the interpretation of laboratory tests.

Carcinogenesis, Mutagenesis, Impairment of Fertility: Long-term term dermal toxicity studies of 24 months duration in rats and 18 months in mice with concentrations of Silver Sulfadiazine three to ten times the concentration in Silver Sulfadiazine Cream revealed no evidence of carcinogenicity.

Pregnancy: Pregnancy category B. A reproductive study has been performed in rabbits at doses up to three to ten times the concentration of Silver Sulfadiazine in Silver Sulfadiazine Cream and has revealed no evidence of harm to the fetus due to Silver Sulfadiazine. There are, however, no adequate and well-controlled studies in pregnant women. Because animal reproduction studies are not always predictive of human response, this drug should be used during pregnancy only if clearly justified, especially in pregnant women approaching or at term (see *"Contraindications"*).

Nursing Mothers: It is not known whether Silver Sulfadiazine Cream is excreted in human milk. However, sulfonamides are known to be excreted in human milk, and all sulfonamide derivatives are known to increase the possibility of kernicterus. Because of the possibility for serious adverse reactions in nursing infants from sulfonamides, a decision should be made whether to discontinue nursing or to discontinue the drug, taking into account the importance of the drug to the mother.

Pediatric Use: Safety and effectiveness in children have not been established (see *"Contraindications"*).

ADVERSE REACTIONS

Several cases of transient leukopenia have been reported in patients receiving Silver Sulfadiazine therapy. Leukopenia associated with Silver Sulfadiazine administration is primarily characterized by decreased neutrophil count. Maximal white blood cell depression occurs within two to four days of initiation of therapy. Rebound to normal leukocyte levels follows onset within two to three days. Recovery is not influenced by continuation of Silver Sulfadiazine therapy. The incidence of leukopenia in various reports averages about 20%. A higher incidence has been seen in patients treated concurrently with cimetidine.

Other infrequently occurring events include skin necrosis, erythema multiforme, skin discoloration, burning sensation, rashes, and interstitial nephritis.

Reduction in bacterial growth after application of topical antibacterial agents has been reported to permit spontaneous healing of deep partial-thickness burns by preventing conversion of the partial thickness to full thickness by sepsis. However, reduction in bacterial colonization has caused delayed separation, in some cases necessitating escharotomy in order to prevent contracture.

Absorption of Silver Sulfadiazine varies depending upon the percent of body surface area and the extent of the tissue damage. Although few have been reported, it is possible that any adverse reaction associated with sulfonamides may occur. Some of the reactions which have been associated with sulfonamides are as follows: blood dyscrasias, including agranulocytosis, aplastic anemia, thrombocytopenia, leukopenia and hemolytic anemia; dermatologic and allergic reactions, including Stevens-Johnson syndrome and exfoliative dermatitis; gastrointestinal reactions; hepatitis and hepatocellular necrosis; CNS reactions; and toxic nephrosis.

DOSAGE AND ADMINISTRATION

FOR TOPICAL USE ONLY - NOT FOR OPHTHALMIC USE.

Prompt institution of appropriate regimens for care of the burned patient is of prime importance and includes the control of shock and pain. The burn wounds are then cleansed and debrided and Silver Sulfadiazine Cream is applied under sterile conditions. The burn areas should be covered with Silver Sulfadiazine Cream at all times. The cream should be applied once to twice daily to a thickness of approximately 1/16 inch. Whenever necessary, the cream should be reapplied to any areas from which it has been removed by patient activity. Administration may be accomplished in minimal time because dressings are not required. However, if individual patient requirements make dressings necessary, they may be used.

Reapply immediately after hydrotherapy.

Treatment with Silver Sulfadiazine Cream should be continued until satisfactory healing has occurred or until the burn site is ready for grafting. The drug should not be withdrawn from the therapeutic regimen while there remains the possibility of infection except if a significant adverse reaction occurs.

Store at controlled room temperature 15°-30°C (59°-86°F).

HOW SUPPLIED
CREAM:

AVERAGE UNIT PRICE (AVAILABLE SIZES)

BRAND	$0.06

BRAND/MANUFACTURER	NDC	SIZE	AWP
◆ BRAND			
SSD AF: Boots Pharm	00048-2110-70	400 gm	$24.75
	00048-2110-73	1000 gm	$48.10

CREAM: 1%

AVERAGE UNIT PRICE (AVAILABLE SIZES)		GENERIC A-RATED AVERAGE PRICE (GAAP)	
BRAND	$0.12	50 gm	$5.42
GENERIC	$0.10	85 gm	$10.13
HCFA FUL (50 gm)	$0.12	400 gm	$23.44
HCFA FUL (400 gm)	$0.07	1000 gm	$48.26
HCFA FUL (1000 gm)	$0.06		

BRAND/MANUFACTURER	NDC	SIZE	AWP
◆ BRAND			
SILVADENE: Marion Merrell Dow	00088-1050-20	20 gm	$4.00
SSD AF: Boots Pharm	00048-2110-71	50 gm	$5.85
SILVADENE: Marion Merrell Dow	00088-1050-50	50 gm	$6.50
	00088-1050-85	85 gm	$11.63
	00088-1050-72	400 gm	$27.69
	00088-1050-58	1000 gm	$54.00
◆ GENERICS			
THERMAZENE: Sherwood	08880-9505-02	20 gm	$3.80
Boots Pharm	00048-2100-77	25 gm	$3.40
Par	49884-0521-46	30 gm	$4.75
Rugby	00536-6415-80	50 gm	$4.90
Qualitest	00603-7840-84	50 gm	$4.94
Boots Pharm	00048-2100-71	50 gm	$4.95
Boots Labs	00524-0500-71	50 gm	$5.05
Boots Pharm	00048-2100-78	50 gm	$5.30
Goldline	00182-5055-67	50 gm	$5.63
Moore,H.L.	00839-7644-81	50 gm	$5.74
THERMAZENE: Sherwood	08880-9505-05	50 gm	$6.15
Par	49884-0521-36	50 gm	$6.15
Boots Pharm	00048-2100-79	85 gm	$9.25
THERMAZENE: Sherwood	08880-9505-85	85 gm	$11.00
Boots Pharm	00048-2100-70	400 gm	$21.00
Boots Labs	00524-0500-70	400 gm	$21.10
Rugby	00536-6415-37	400 gm	$23.09
THERMAZENE: Sherwood	08880-9505-40	400 gm	$26.00
Par	49884-0521-40	400 gm	$26.00
Boots Labs	00524-0500-73	1000 gm	$43.32
Boots Pharm	00048-2100-73	1000 gm	$47.70
THERMAZENE: Sherwood	08880-9505-10	1000 gm	$51.00
Par	49884-0521-39	1000 gm	$51.00

Simvastatin

DESCRIPTION

Simvastatin is a cholesterol lowering agent that is derived synthetically from a fermentation product of *Aspergillus terreus.* After oral ingestion, Simvastatin, which is an inactive lactone, is hydrolyzed to the corresponding β-hydroxyacid form. This is an inhibitor of 3-hydroxy-3-methyl-glutaryl-coenzyme A (HMG-CoA) reductase. This enzyme catalyzes the conversion of HMG-CoA to mevalonate, which is an early and rate-limiting step in the biosynthesis of cholesterol.

Simvastatin is butanoic acid, 2,2-dimethyl-, 1,2,3,7,8,8a-hexahydro-3,7-dimethyl-8-[2-(tetrahydro-4-hydroxy- 6-oxo-2 *H*-pyran-2-yl) ethyl]-1-napthalenyl ester, [1*S*-[1α,3α,7β, 8β(2*S**, 4*S**),-8aβ]]. The empirical formula of Simvastatin is $C_{25}H_{38}O_5$ and its molecular weight is 418.57.

Simvastatin is a white to off-white, nonhygroscopic, crystalline powder that is practically insoluble in water, and freely soluble in chloroform, methanol and ethanol.

Following is its chemical structure:

CLINICAL PHARMACOLOGY

The involvement of low-density lipoprotein (LDL) cholesterol in atherogenesis has been well-documented in clinical and pathological studies, as well as in many animal experiments. Epidemiological studies have established that high LDL (low-density lipoprotein) cholesterol and low HDL (high-density lipoprotein) cholesterol are both risk factors for coronary heart disease. The Lipid Research Clinics Coronary Primary Prevention Trial (LRC-CPPT), coordinated by the National Institutes of Health (NIH), studied men aged 35-59 with total cholesterol levels of 265 mg/dL (6.8 mmol/L) or greater, LDL cholesterol values 175 mg/dL (4.5 mmol/L) or greater, and triglyceride levels not more than 300 mg/dL (3.4 mmol/L). This seven-year, double-blind, placebo-controlled study demonstrated that lowering LDL cholesterol with diet and cholestyramine decreased the combined rate of coronary heart disease death plus non-fatal myocardial infarction. Simvastatin has been shown to reduce both normal and elevated LDL cholesterol concentrations. The effect of Simvastatin-induced changes in lipoprotein levels, including reduction of serum cholesterol, on cardiovascular morbidity or mortality has not been established.

LDL is formed from very-low-density lipoprotein (VLDL) and is catabolized predominantly by the high affinity LDL receptor. The mechanism of the LDL-

---

◆ RATED THERAPEUTICALLY EQUIVALENT; ◇ THERAPEUTIC EQUIVALENCE UNCONFIRMED; ○ UNRATED

lowering effect of Simvastatin may involve both reduction of VLDL cholesterol concentration, and induction of the LDL receptor, leading to reduced production and/or increased catabolism of LDL cholesterol. Apolipoprotein B also falls substantially during treatment with Simvastatin. Since each LDL particle contains one molecule of apolipoprotein B, and since little apolipoprotein B is found in other lipoproteins, this strongly suggests that Simvastatin does not merely cause cholesterol to be lost from LDL, but also reduces the concentration of circulating LDL particles. In addition, Simvastatin modestly reduces VLDL cholesterol and plasma triglycerides and can produce increases of variable magnitude in HDL cholesterol. The effects of Simvastatin on Lp(a), fibrinogen, and certain other independent biochemical risk markers for coronary heart disease are unknown.

Simvastatin is a specific inhibitor of HMG-CoA reductase, the enzyme that catalyzes the conversion of HMG-CoA to mevalonate. The conversion of HMG-CoA to mevalonate is an early step in the biosynthetic pathway for cholesterol.

PHARMACOKINETICS

Simvastatin is a lactone that is readily hydrolyzed in vivo to the corresponding β-hydroxyacid, a potent inhibitor of HMG-CoA reductase. Inhibition of HMG-CoA reductase is the basis for an assay in pharmacokinetic studies of the β-hydroxyacid metabolites (active inhibitors) and, following base hydrolysis, active plus latent inhibitors (total inhibitors) in plasma following administration of Simvastatin.

Following an oral dose of ^{14}C-labeled Simvastatin in man, 13% of the dose was excreted in urine and 60% in feces. The latter represents absorbed drug equivalents excreted in bile, as well as any unabsorbed drug. Plasma concentrations of total radioactivity (Simvastatin plus ^{14}C-metabolites) peaked at 4 hours and declined rapidly to about 10% of peak by 12 hours postdose. Absorption of Simvastatin, estimated relative to an intravenous reference dose, in each of two animal species tested, averaged about 85% of an oral dose. In animal studies, after oral dosing, Simvastatin achieved substantially higher concentrations in the liver than in nontarget tissues. Simvastatin undergoes extensive first-pass extraction in the liver, its primary site of action, with subsequent excretion of drug equivalents in the bile. As a consequence of extensive hepatic extraction of Simvastatin (estimated to be > 60% in man), the availability of drug to the general circulation is low. In a single-dose study in nine healthy subjects, it was estimated that less than 5% of an oral dose of Simvastatin reaches the general circulation as active inhibitors. Following administration of Simvastatin tablets, the coefficient of variation, based on between-subject variability, was approximately 48% for the area under the concentration-time curve (AUC) for total inhibitory activity in the general circulation. Both Simvastatin and its β-hydroxyacid metabolite are highly bound (approximately 95%) to human plasma proteins. Animals studies have not been performed to determine whether Simvastatin crosses the blood-brain and placental barriers. However, when radiolabeled Simvastatin was administered to rats, Simvastatin-derived radioactivity crossed the blood-brain barrier.

The major active metabolites of Simvastatin present in human plasma are the β-hydroxyacid of Simvastatin and its 6'-hydroxy, 6'-hydroxy methyl, and 6'-exomethylene derivatives. Peak plasma concentrations of both active and total inhibitors were attained within 1.3 to 2.4 hours postdose. While the recommended therapeutic dose range is 5 to 40 mg/day, there was no substantial deviation from linearity of AUC of inhibitors in the general circulation with an increase in dose to as high as 120 mg. Relative to the fasting state, the plasma profile of inhibitors was not affected when Simvastatin was administered immediately before an A.H.A. recommended low-fat meal.

Kinetic studies with another reductase inhibitor, having a similar principal route of elimination, have suggested that for a given dose level higher systemic exposure may be achieved in patients with severe renal insufficiency (as measured by creatinine clearance).

CLINICAL STUDIES

Simvastatin has been shown to be highly effective in reducing total and LDL cholesterol in heterozygous familial and nonfamilial forms of hypercholesterolemia and in mixed hyperlipidemia. A marked response was seen within 2 weeks, and the maximum therapeutic response occurred within 4-6 weeks. The response was maintained during chronic therapy.

In a multicenter, double-blind, placebo-controlled, dose-response study in patients with familial or non-familial hypercholesterolemia, Simvastatin given as a single-dose in the evening (the recommended dosing) was similarly effective as when given on a twice-daily basis. Simvastatin consistently and significantly decreased total plasma cholesterol (TOTAL-C), LDL cholesterol (LDL-C), total cholesterol/HDL cholesterol (TOTAL-C/HDL-C) ratio, and LDL cholesterol/HDL cholesterol (LDL-C/HDL-C) ratio. Simvastatin also modestly decreased triglycerides (TRIG) and produced increases of variable magnitude in HDL cholesterol (HDL-C).

The results of a dose response study in patients with primary hypercholesterolemia are presented in Table 1. (See related table).

Simvastatin was compared to cholestyramine, probucol, or gemfibrozil, respectively, in double-blind parallel studies involving 1102 patients. All studies were performed in patients who were at moderate to high risk of coronary events based on serum cholesterol levels. At all dosage levels tested, Simvastatin produced a significantly greater reduction of total plasma cholesterol, LDL cholesterol, VLDL cholesterol, triglycerides, and total cholesterol/HDL cholesterol ratio when compared to cholestyramine or probucol. The increase in HDL seen with Simvastatin was not significantly greater than the increase seen with cholestyramine but was significantly different from the decrease seen with probucol (see Tables 2 and 3). (See related tables).

In a study designed to evaluate the possible effects of Simvastatin on reproductive hormones and sperm characteristics in men with familial hypercholesterolemia, there was a small decrease in the mean percentage of vital sperm and a small increase in the mean percentage of abnormal forms, with these changes achieving statistical significance at week 14. However, there was no effect on numbers or concentration of motile sperm. Simvastatin had no effect on basal reproductive hormone levels (prolactin, luteinizing hormone, follicle-stimulating hormone, and plasma testosterone). Provocative testing (HCG stimulation) was not done. Treatment with another HMG-CoA reductase inhibitor resulted in a statistically significant decrease in plasma testosterone response to HCG.

In a study to evaluate the effect of Simvastatin on adrenocortical function in patients with Type II hypercholesterolemia, Simvastatin had no effect on basal adrenocortical function as assessed by determination of morning plasma cortisol levels, urine free cortisol, and urinary excretion of 17-hydroxy steroids. Simvastatin also had no effect on adrenocortical reserve as evaluated by the plasma cortisol response to ACTH stimulation and insulin-induced hypoglycemia.

INDICATIONS AND USAGE

Therapy with lipid-altering agents should be a component of multiple risk factor intervention in those individuals at significantly increased risk for atherosclerotic vascular disease due to hypercholesterolemia. Simvastatin is indicated as an adjunct to diet for the reduction of elevated total and LDL cholesterol levels in patients with primary hypercholesterolemia (Types IIa and IIb[1]), when the response to a diet restricted in saturated fat and cholesterol and other nonpharmacological measures alone has been inadequate.

Prior to initiating therapy with Simvastatin, secondary causes for hypercholesterolemia (e.g., poorly controlled diabetes mellitus, hypothyroidism, nephrotic syndrome, dysproteinemias, obstructive liver disease, other drug therapy, alcoholism) should be excluded, and a lipid profile performed to measure TOTAL-C, HDL-C, and triglycerides (TG). For patients with TG less than 400 mg/dL (< 4.5 mmol/L), LDL-C can be estimated using the following equation:

LDL-C = Total cholesterol — [0.20 × (triglycerides) — HDL-C]

For TG levels > 400 mg/dL (> 4.5 mmol/L), this equation is less accurate and LDL-C concentrations should be determined by ultracentrifugation. In many hypertriglyceridemic patients, LDL-C may be low or normal despite elevated TOTAL-C. In such cases, Simvastatin is not indicated.

Lipid determinations should be performed at intervals of no less than four weeks and dosage adjusted according to the patient's response to therapy.

The National Cholesterol Education Program (NCEP) Treatment Guidelines are summarized below:

Definite Atherosclerotic Disease*	Two or More Other Risk Factors**	LDL-Cholesterol mg/dL (mmol/L)	
		Initiation Level	Goal
NO	NO	≥ 190 (≥ 4.9)	< 160 (< 4.1)
NO	YES	≥ 160 (≥ 4.1)	< 130 (< 3.4)
YES	YES or NO	≥ 130 (≥ 3.4)	≤ 100 (≤ 2.6)

* Coronary heart disease or peripheral vascular disease (including symptomatic carotid artery disease).

** Other risk factors for coronary heart disease (CHD) include: age (males: ≥ 45 years; females: ≥ 55 years or premature menopause without estrogen replacement therapy); family history of premature CHD; current cigarette smoking; hypertension; confirmed HDL-C < 35 mg/dL (< 0.91 mmol/L); and diabetes mellitus. Subtract one risk factor if HDL-C is ≥ 60 mg/dL (≥ 1.6 mmol/L).

Table 1
DOSE RESPONSE IN PATIENTS WITH PRIMARY HYPERCHOLESTEROLEMIA (MEAN PERCENT CHANGE FROM BASELINE AFTER 8 WEEKS)

Treatment	N	Total-C	LDL-C	HDL-C	LDL-C/HDL-C	Total-C/HDL-C	TRIG
Placebo	28	−3	−4	+2	−4	−3	+7
Simvastatin							
5 mg q.p.m.	28	−17	−24	+7	−27	−22	−10
10 mg q.p.m.	27	−24	−33	+9	−37	−29	−10
20 mg q.p.m.	26	−25	−33	+11	−36	−30	−19
40 mg q.p.m.	29	−28	−40	+12	−46	−36	−19

Since the goal of treatment is to lower LDL-C, the NCEP recommends that LDL-C levels be used to initiate and assess treatment response. Only if LDL-C levels are not available, should the TOTAL-C be used to monitor therapy.

Although Simvastatin may be useful to reduce elevated LDL cholesterol levels in patients with combined hypercholesterolemia and hypertriglyceridemia where hypercholesterolemia is the major abnormality (Type IIb hyperlipoproteinemia), it has not been studied in conditions where the major abnormality is elevation of chylomicrons, VLDL or IDL (i.e., hyperlipoproteinemia types I, III, IV, or V, see table below).

The effect of Simvastatin-induced changes in lipoprotein levels, including reduction of serum cholesterol, on cardiovascular morbidity or mortality has not been established.

CLASSIFICATION OF HYPERLIPOPROTEINEMIAS

Type	Lipoproteins elevated	Lipid Elevations major	minor
I (rare)	chylomicrons	TG	→ C
IIa	LDL	C	—
IIb	LDL, VLDL	C	TG
III (rare)	IDL	C/TG	—
IV	VLDL	TG	→ C
V (rare)	chylomicrons, VLDL	TG	→ C

C = cholesterol, TG = triglycerides, LDL = low-density lipoprotein, VLDL = very-low-density lipoprotein, IDL = intermediate-density lipoprotein.

† For adult diabetics, a modification of these guidelines is recommended — see: American Diabetes Association Consensus Statement: Role of cardiovascular risk factors in prevention and treatment of macrovascular disease in diabetes, Diabetes Care 12(8): 573-79, 1989.

CONTRAINDICATIONS

Hypersensitivity to any component of this medication. Active liver disease or unexplained persistent elevations of serum transaminases (see "Warnings").

Pregnancy and lactation: Atherosclerosis is a chronic process and the discontinuation of lipid-lowering drugs during pregnancy should have little impact on the outcome of long-term therapy of primary hypercholesterolemia. Moreover, cholesterol and other products of the cholesterol biosynthesis pathway are essential components for fetal development, including synthesis of steroids and cell membranes. Because of the ability of inhibitors of HMG-CoA reductase such as Simvastatin to decrease the synthesis of cholesterol and possibly other products of the cholesterol biosynthesis pathway, Simvastatin may cause fetal harm when administered to a pregnant woman. Therefore, Simvastatin is contraindicated during pregnancy and in nursing mothers. Simvastatin should be administered to women of childbearing age only when such patients are highly unlikely to conceive. If the patient becomes pregnant while taking this drug, Simvastatin should be discontinued and the patient should be apprised of the potential hazard to the fetus.

WARNINGS

LIVER DYSFUNCTION

Persistent increases (to more than 3 times the upper limit of normal) in serum transaminases have occurred in 1% of patients who received Simvastatin in clinical trials. When drug treatment was interrupted or discontinued in these patients, the transaminase levels usually fell slowly to pretreatment levels. The increases were not associated with jaundice or other clinical signs or symptoms. There was no evidence of hypersensitivity.

It is recommended that liver function tests be performed during therapy with Simvastatin. Serum transaminase levels, including ALT (SGPT), should be monitored before treatment begins, every six weeks for the first three months, every eight weeks during the remainder of the first year, and periodically thereafter (e.g., at approximately 6 month intervals). Special attention should be paid to patients who develop elevated serum transaminase levels, and in these patients, measurements should be repeated promptly and then performed more frequently. If the transaminase levels show evidence of progression, particularly if they rise to three times the upper limit of normal and are persistent, the drug should be discontinued. Liver biopsy should be considered if elevations persist beyond discontinuation of drug.

The drug should be used with caution in patients who consume substantial quantities of alcohol and/or have a past history of liver disease. Active liver diseases or unexplained transaminase elevations are contraindications to the use of Simvastatin.

As with other lipid-lowering agents, moderate (less than three times the upper limit of normal) elevations of serum transaminases have been reported following therapy with Simvastatin. These changes appeared soon after initiation of therapy with Simvastatin, were often transient, were not accompanied by any symptoms and did not require interruption of treatment.

SKELETAL MUSCLE

Rare cases of rhabdomyolysis with acute renal failure secondary to myoglobinuria have been associated with Simvastatin therapy. Rhabdomyolysis has also been associated with other HMG-CoA reductase inhibitors when they were administered alone or concomitantly with 1) immunosuppressive therapy, including cyclosporine in cardiac transplant patients; 2) gemfibrozil or lipid-lowering doses (≥ 1 g/day) of nicotinic acid in non-transplant patients, or 3) erythromycin in seriously ill patients. Some of the patients who had rhabdomyolysis in association with the reductase inhibitors had preexisting renal insufficiency, usually as a consequence of long-standing diabetes. In most subjects who have had an unsatisfactory lipid response to either Simvastatin or gemfibrozil alone, the possible benefits of combined therapy with these drugs are not considered to outweigh the risk of severe myopathy, rhabdomyolysis, and acute renal failure. While it is not known whether this interaction occurs with fibrates other than gemfibrozil, myopathy and rhabdomyolysis have occasionally been associated with the use of other fibrates alone, including clofibrate. Therefore, the combined use of Simvastatin with other fibrates should generally be avoided. Physicians contemplating combined therapy with Simvastatin and lipid-lowering doses of nicotinic acid, or with immunosuppressive drugs should carefully weigh the potential benefits and risks and should carefully monitor patients for any signs and symptoms of muscle pain, tenderness, or weakness, particularly during the initial months of therapy and during any periods of upward dosage titration of either drug. Periodic creatine phosphokinase (CPK) determinations may be considered in such situations, but there is no assurance that such monitoring will prevent the occurrence of severe myopathy.

Because of an apparent relationship between increased plasma levels of active metabolites derived from other HMG-CoA reductase inhibitors and myopathy, in patients taking cyclosporine, the daily dosage should not exceed 10 mg/day (see "Dosage and Administration").

Simvastatin therapy should be temporarily withheld or discontinued in any patient with an acute, serious condition suggestive of a myopathy or having a risk factor predisposing to the development of renal failure secondary to rhabdomyolysis, (e.g., severe acute infection, hypotension, major surgery, trauma, severe metabolic, endocrine and electrolyte disorders, and uncontrolled seizures.)

Myopathy should be considered in any patient with diffuse myalgias, muscle tenderness or weakness, and/or marked elevation of CPK. Patients should be advised to report promptly unexplained muscle pain, tenderness or weakness, particularly if accompanied by malaise or fever. Simvastatin therapy should be

Table 2
SIMVASTATIN VS. CHOLESTYRAMINE (PERCENT CHANGE FROM BASELINE AFTER 12 WEEKS)

Treatment	N	Total-C (mean)	LDL-C (mean)	HDL-C (mean)	LDL-C/ HDL-C (mean)	Total-C/HDL-C (mean)	VLDL-C (median)	TRIG (mean)
Simvastatin								
20 mg q.p.m.	84	−27	−32	+10	−36	−31	−8	−13
40 mg q.p.m.	82	−33	−41	+10	−45	−38	−28	−21
Cholestyramine								
4-24 g/day*	85	−15	−21	+8	−25	−19	+7	+15

* maximum tolerated dose (mean dose taken, 18 g/day)

Table 3
SIMVASTATIN VS. PROBUCOL (PERCENT CHANGE FROM BASELINE AFTER 12 WEEKS)

Treatment	N	TOTAL-C (mean)	LDL-C (mean)	HDL-C (mean)	LDL-C/ HDL-C (mean)	Total-C/HDL-C (mean)	VLDL-C (median)	TRIG (mean)
Simvastatin								
20 mg q.p.m.	82	−27	−34	+10	−39	−34	−18	−17
40 mg q.p.m.	80	−30	−40	+13	−45	−37	−14	−19
Probucol								
500 mg b.i.d.	81	−13	−8	−27	+31	+25	+11	−0.4

◆ RATED THERAPEUTICALLY EQUIVALENT; ◇ THERAPEUTIC EQUIVALENCE UNCONFIRMED; ○ UNRATED

discontinued if markedly elevated CPK levels occur or myopathy is diagnosed or suspected.

PRECAUTIONS
GENERAL
Before instituting therapy with Simvastatin, an attempt should be made to control hypercholesterolemia with appropriate diet, exercise, and weight reduction in obese patients, and to treat other underlying medical problems (see *"Indications and Usage"*).

Simvastatin may cause elevation of creatine phosphokinase and transaminase levels (see *"Warnings"* and *"Adverse Reactions"*). This should be considered in the differential diagnosis of chest pain in a patient on therapy with Simvastatin.

HOMOZYGOUS FAMILIAL HYPERCHOLESTEROLEMIA
Simvastatin is less effective in patients with the rare homozygous familial hypercholesterolemia, possibly because these patients have few functional LDL receptors.

INFORMATION FOR PATIENTS
Patients should be advised to report promptly unexplained muscle pain, tenderness, or weakness, particularly if accompanied by malaise or fever.

DRUG INTERACTIONS
Immunosuppressive Drugs: Gemfibrozil, Niacin (Nicotinic Acid), Erythromycin: See *"Warnings: Skeletal Muscle"*.

Antipyrine: Because Simvastatin had no effect on the pharmocokinetics of antipyrine, interactions with other drugs metabolized via the same cytochrome isozymes are not expected.

Propranolol: In healthy male volunteers there was a significant decrease in mean C_{max}, but no change in AUC, for Simvastatin total and active inhibitors with concomitant administration of single doses of Simvastatin and propranolol. The clinical relevance of this finding is unclear. The pharmacokinetics of the enantiomers of propranolol were not affected.

Digoxin: Concomitant administration of a single dose of digoxin in healthy male volunteers receiving Simvastatin resulted in a slight elevation (less than 0.3 ng/mL) in digoxin concentrations in plasma (as measured by a radioimmunoassay) compared to concomitant administration of placebo and digoxin. Patients taking digoxin should be monitored appropriately when Simvastatin is initiated.

Warfarin: Simvastatin therapy appeared to enhance slightly the anticoagulant effect of warfarin (mean changes in prothrombin time less than two seconds) in normal volunteers maintained in a state of low therapeutic anticoagulation. With other reductase inhibitors, clinically evident bleeding and/or increased prothrombin time has been reported in a few patients taking coumarin anticoagulants concomitantly. In such patients, prothrombin time should be determined before starting Simvastatin and frequently enough during early therapy to insure that no significant alteration of prothrombin time occurs. Once a stable prothrombin time has been documented, prothrombin times can be monitored at the intervals usually recommended for patients on coumarin anticoagulants. If the dose of Simvastatin is changed, the same procedure should be repeated. Simvastatin therapy has not been associated with bleeding or with changes in prothrombin time in patients not taking anticoagulants.

Other Concomitant Therapy: Although specific interaction studies were not performed, in clinical studies, Simvastatin was used concomitantly with angiotensin-converting enzyme (ACE) inhibitors, beta blockers, calcium-channel blockers, diuretics and nonsteroidal anti-inflammatory drugs (NSAIDs) without evidence of clinically significant adverse interactions. The effect of cholestyramine on the absorption and kinetics of Simvastatin has not been determined.

ENDOCRINE FUNCTION
HMG-CoA reductase inhibitors interfere with cholesterol synthesis and as such might theoretically blunt adrenal and/or gonadal steroid production. However, clinical studies have shown that Simvastatin does not reduce basal plasma cortisol concentration or impair adrenal reserve and does not reduce basal plasma testosterone concentration (see *"Clinical Pharmacology, Clinical Studies"*). Another HMG-CoA reductase inhibitor has been shown to reduce the plasma testosterone response to HCG: the effect of Simvastatin on HCG-stimulated testosterone secretion has not been studied.

Results of clinical trials with drugs in this class have been inconsistent with regard to drug effects on basal and reserve steroid levels. The effects of HMG-CoA reductase inhibitors on male fertility have not been studied in adequate numbers of male patients. The effects, if any, on the pituitary-gonadal axis in premenopausal women are unknown. Patients treated with Simvastatin who develop clinical evidence of endocrine dysfunction should be evaluated appropriately. Caution should also be exercised if an HMG-CoA reductase inhibitor or other agent used to lower cholesterol levels is administered to patients also receiving other drugs (e.g., ketoconazole, spironolactone, cimetidine) that may decrease the levels or activity of endogenous steroid hormones.

CNS TOXICITY
Optic nerve degeneration was seen in clinically normal dogs treated with Simvastatin for 14 weeks at 180 mg/kg/day, a dose that produced mean plasma drug levels about 44 times higher than the mean drug level in humans taking 40 mg/day.

CNS vascular lesions, characterized by perivascular hemorrhage and edema, mononuclear cell infiltration of perivascular spaces, perivascular fibrin deposits and necrosis of small vessels were seen in dogs treated with Simvastatin at a dose of 360 mg/kg/day, a dose that produced plasma drug levels that were about 50 times higher than the mean drug levels in humans taking 40 mg/day. Similar CNS vascular lesions have been observed with several other drugs of this class. A chemically similar drug in this class also produced optic nerve degeneration (Wallerian degeneration of retinogeniculate fibers) in clinically normal dogs in a dose-dependent fashion starting at 60 mg/kg/day, a dose that produced mean plasma drug levels about 30 times higher than the mean drug level in humans taking the highest recommended dose (as measured by total enzyme inhibitory activity). This same drug also produced vestibulocochlear Wallerian-like degeneration and retinal ganglion cell chromatolysis in dogs treated for 14 weeks at 180 mg/kg/day, a dose that resulted in a mean plasma drug level similar to that seen with the 60 mg/kg/day dose.

CARCINOGENESIS, MUTAGENESIS, IMPAIRMENT OF FERTILITY
In a 72-week carcinogenicity study, mice were administered daily doses of Simvastatin of 25, 100, and 400 mg/kg body weight, which resulted in mean plasma drug levels approximately 3, 15, and 33 times higher than the mean human plasma drug concentration (as total inhibitory activity) after a 40 mg oral dose. Liver carcinomas were significantly increased in high-dose females and mid- and high-dose males with a maximum incidence of 90 percent in males. The incidence of adenomas of the liver was significantly increased in mid- and high-dose females. Drug treatment also significantly increased the incidence of lung adenomas in mid- and high-dose males and females. Adenomas of the Harderian gland (a gland of the eye of rodents) were significantly higher in high-dose mice than in controls. No evidence of a tumorigenic effect was observed at 25 mg/kg/day. Although mice were given up to 500 times the human dose (HD) on a mg/kg/body weight basis, blood levels of HMG-CoA reductase inhibitory activity were only 3-33 times higher in mice than in humans given 40 mg of Simvastatin.

In a separate 92-week carcinogenicity study in mice at doses up to 25 mg/kg/day, no evidence of a tumorigenic effect was observed. Although mice were given up to 31 times the human dose on a mg/kg basis, plasma drug levels were only 2-4 times higher than humans given 40 mg Simvastatin as measured by AUC.

In a two-year study in rats, there was a statistically significant increase in the incidence of thyroid follicular adenomas in female rats exposed to approximately 45 times higher levels of Simvastatin than humans given 40 mg Simvastatin (as measured by AUC). Preliminary results from a second two-year rat study indicate an increase in the incidence of thyroid and liver tumors in male and female rats at doses that produce exposure levels ≥ 29 times (based on AUC) that achieved in humans at a dosage of 40 mg/day. Liver tumors are found in rodents with all the chemically similar drugs of this class. No increased incidence of tumors was observed at doses that produce exposure levels 15 times (based on AUC) those seen in man.

No evidence of mutagenicity was observed in a microbial mutagen test using mutant strains of *Salmonella typhimurium* with or without rat or mouse liver metabolic activation. In addition, no evidence of damage to genetic material was noted in an *in vitro* alkaline elution assay using rat hepatocytes, a V-79 mammalian cell forward mutation study, an *in vitro* chromosome aberration study in CHO cells, or in *in vivo* chromosomal aberration assay in mouse bone marrow.

There was decreased fertility in male rats treated with Simvastatin for 34 weeks at 25 mg/kg body weight (15 times the maximum human exposure level, based on AUC, in patients receiving 40 mg/day); however, this effect was not observed during a subsequent fertility study in which Simvastatin was administered at this same dose level to male rats for 11 weeks (the entire cycle of spermatogenesis including epididymal maturation). No microscopic changes were observed in the testes of rats from either study. At 180 mg/kg/day, (which produces exposure levels 44 times higher than those in humans taking 40 mg/day), seminiferous tubule degeneration (necrosis and loss of spermatogenic epithelium) was observed. In dogs, there was drug-related testicular atrophy, decreased spermatogenesis, spermatocytic degeneration and giant cell formation at 10 mg/kg/day (approximately 7 times the human exposure level, based on AUC, at 40 mg/day). The clinical significance of these findings is unclear.

PREGNANCY
Pregnancy Category X: See *"Contraindications"*.

Safety in pregnant women has not been established. Simvastatin was not teratogenic in rats at doses of 25 mg/kg/day or in rabbits at doses up to 10 mg/kg daily. These doses resulted in 6 times (rat) or 4 times (rabbit) the human exposure based on mg/m^2 surface area. However, in studies with another structurally-related HMG-CoA reductase inhibitor, skeletal malformations were observed in rats and mice. Rare reports of congenital anomalies have been received following intrauterine exposure to HMG-CoA reductase inhibitors. There has been one report of severe congenital bony deformity, tracheo-esophageal fistula, and anal atresia (VATER association) in a baby born to a woman who took another HMG-CoA reductase inhibitor with dextroamphetamine sulfate during the first trimester of pregnancy. Simvastatin should be administered to women of childbearing potential only when such patients are highly unlikely to conceive and have been informed of the potential hazards. If the woman becomes pregnant while taking Simvastatin, it should be discontinued and the patient advised again as to the potential hazards to the fetus.

NURSING MOTHERS
It is not known whether Simvastatin is excreted in human milk. Because a small amount of another drug in this class is excreted in human milk and because of the potential for serious adverse reactions in nursing infants, women taking Simvastatin should not nurse their infants (see *"Contraindications"*).

➤ SHOWN IN PRODUCT IDENTIFICATION GUIDE

PEDIATRIC USE
Safety and effectiveness in children and adolescents have not been established. Because children and adolescents are not likely to benefit from cholesterol lowering for at least a decade and because experience with this drug is limited (no studies in subjects below the age of 20 years), treatment of children or adolescents with Simvastatin is not recommended at this time.

ADVERSE REACTIONS
In the controlled clinical studies and their open extensions (2423 patients with mean duration of follow-up of approximately 18 months), 1.4% of patients were discontinued due to adverse experiences attributable to Simvastatin. Adverse reactions have usually been mild and transient. Simvastatin has been evaluated for serious adverse reactions in more than 21,000 patients and is generally well-tolerated.

CLINICAL ADVERSE EXPERIENCES
Adverse experiences occurring at an incidence of 1 percent or greater in patients treated with Simvastatin, regardless of causality, in controlled clinical studies are shown in the table below:

	Simvastatin (N = 1583) %	Placebo (N = 157) %	Cholestyramine (N = 179) %	Probucol (N = 81) %
Body as a Whole				
Abdominal pain	3.2	3.2	8.9	2.5
Asthenia	1.6	2.5	1.1	1.2
Gastrointestinal				
Constipation	2.3	1.3	29.1	1.2
Diarrhea	1.9	2.5	7.8	3.7
Dyspepsia	1.1	—	4.5	3.7
Flatulence	1.9	1.3	14.5	6.2
Nausea	1.3	1.9	10.1	2.5
Nervous System/ Psychiatric				
Headache	3.5	5.1	4.5	3.7
Respiratory				
Upper respiratory infection	2.1	1.9	3.4	6.2

The following effects have been reported with drugs in this class. Not all effects listed below have necessarily been associated with Simvastatin therapy.

Skeletal: myopathy, rhabdomyolysis, arthralgias.

Neurological: dysfunction of certain cranial nerves (including alteration of taste, impairment of extra-ocular movement, facial paresis), tremor, vertigo, memory loss, paresthesia, peripheral neuropathy, peripheral nerve palsy, anxiety, insomnia, depression.

Hypersensitivity Reactions: An apparent hypersensitivity syndrome has been reported rarely which has included one or more of the following features: anaphylaxis, angioedema, lupus erythematous-like syndrome, polymyalgia rheumatica, vasculitis, purpura, thrombocytopenia, leukopenia, hemolytic anemia, positive ANA, ESR increase, eosinophilia, arthritis, arthralgia, urticaria, asthenia, photosensitivity, fever, chills, flushing, malaise, dyspnea, toxic epidermal necrolysis, erythema multiforme, including Stevens-Johnson syndrome.

Gastrointestinal: pancreatitis, hepatitis, including chronic active hepatitis, cholestatic jaundice, fatty change in liver, and, rarely, cirrhosis, fulminant hepatic necrosis, and hepatoma: anorexia, vomiting.

Skin: alopecia, pruritus. A variety of skin changes (e.g., nodules, discoloration, dryness of skin/mucous membranes, changes to hair/nails) has been reported.

Reproductive: gynecomastia, loss of libido, erectile dysfunction.

Eye: progression of cataracts (lens opacities), ophthalmoplegia.

Laboratory Abnormalities: elevated transaminases, alkaline phosphatase, and bilirubin; thyroid function abnormalities.

LABORATORY TESTS
Marked persistent increases of serum transaminases have been noted (see *"Warnings, Liver Dysfunction"*). About 5% of patients had elevations of creatine phosphokinase (CPK) levels of 3 or more times the normal value on one or more occasions. This was attributable to the noncardiac fraction of occasions. This was attributable to the noncardiac fraction of CPK. Muscle pain or dysfunction usually was not reported (see *"Warnings, Skeletal Muscle"*).

CONCOMITANT THERAPY
In controlled clinical studies in which Simvastatin was administered concomitantly with cholestyramine, no adverse reactions peculiar to this concomitant treatment were observed. The adverse reactions that occurred were limited to those reported previously with Simvastatin or cholestyramine. The combined use of Simvastatin with fibrates should generally be avoided (see *"Warnings, Skeletal Muscle"*).

OVERDOSAGE
Significant lethality was observed in mice after a single oral dose of 9 g/m². No evidence of lethality was observed in rats or dogs treated with doses of 30 and 100 g/m², respectively. No specific diagnostic signs were observed in rodents. At these doses the only signs seen in dogs were emesis and mucoid stools.

A few cases of overdosage with Simvastatin have been reported; no patients had any specific symptoms, and all patients recovered without sequelae. The maximum dose taken was 450 mg. Until further experience is obtained, no specific treatment of overdosage with Simvastatin can be recommended. The dializability of Simvastatin and its metabolites in man is not known at present.

DOSAGE AND ADMINISTRATION
The patient should be placed on a standard cholesterol-lowering diet before receiving Simvastatin and should continue on this diet during treatment with Simvastatin (see NCEP Treatment Guidelines for details on dietary therapy).

The recommended starting dose is 5-10 mg once a day in the evening. The recommended dosing range is 5-40 mg/day as a single dose in the evening; the maximum recommended dose is 40 mg/day. Doses should be individualized according to baseline LDL-C levels, the recommended goal of therapy (see NCEP Guidelines) and the patient's response. A starting dose of 5 mg/day should be considered for patients with LDL-C (on diet) of ≤ 190 mg/dL (4.9 mmol/L) and for the elderly. Patients with LDL-C levels > 190 mg/dL (4.9 mmol/L) should be started on 10 mg/day. Adjustments of dosage should be made at intervals of 4 weeks or more.

In the elderly, maximum reductions in LDL cholesterol may be achieved with daily doses of 20 mg or less.

Cholesterol levels should be monitored periodically and consideration should be given to reducing the dosage of Simvastatin if cholesterol falls below the targeted range.

CONCOMITANT THERAPY
Simvastatin is effective alone or when used concomitantly with bile-acid sequestrants. Use of Simvastatin with fibrate-type drugs such as gemfibrozil or clofibrate should generally be avoided (see *"Warnings, Skeletal Muscle"*).

In patients taking immunosuppressive drugs concomitantly with Simvastatin (see *"Warnings, Skeletal Muscle"*), therapy should begin with 5 mg of Simvastatin and should not exceed 10 mg/day.

DOSAGE IN PATIENTS WITH RENAL INSUFFICIENCY
Because Simvastatin does not undergo significant renal excretion, modification of dosage should not be necessary in patients with mild to moderate renal insufficiency. However, caution should be exercised when Simvastatin is administered to patients with severe renal insufficiency; such patients should be started at 5 mg/day and be closely monitored (see *"Clinical Pharmacology, Pharmacokinetics"*).

STORAGE
Store between 5-30°C (41-86°F).

HOW SUPPLIED
TABLETS: 5 MG

BRAND/MANUFACTURER	NDC	SIZE	AWP
○ BRAND			
▶ ZOCOR: Merck	00006-0726-61	60s	$102.34
	00006-0726-54	90s	$153.51
	00006-0726-28	100s ud	$170.58

TABLETS: 10 MG

BRAND/MANUFACTURER	NDC	SIZE	AWP
○ BRAND			
▶ ZOCOR: Merck	00006-0735-61	60s	$108.03
	00006-0735-54	90s	$162.05
	00006-0735-28	100s ud	$180.06
	00006-0735-82	1000s	$1800.50
	00006-0735-87	10000s	$18005.00

TABLETS: 20 MG

BRAND/MANUFACTURER	NDC	SIZE	AWP
○ BRAND			
▶ ZOCOR: Merck	00006-0740-61	60s	$195.76
	00006-0740-82	1000s	$3262.78
	00006-0740-87	10000s	$32627.83

TABLETS: 40 MG

BRAND/MANUFACTURER	NDC	SIZE	AWP
○ BRAND			
▶ ZOCOR: Merck	00006-0749-61	60s	$206.25

Sincalide

DESCRIPTION
Sincalide is a cholecystopancreatic-gastrointestinal hormone peptide for parenteral administration. The agent is a synthetically-prepared C-terminal octapeptide of cholecystokinin. Each vial of Sincalide provides a sterile nonpyrogenic lyophilized white powder consisting of 5 mcg Sincalide. Sincalide is designated chemically as L-aspartyl-L-tyrosyl-L-methionylglycyl-L-tryptophyl-L-methionyl-L- aspartylphenyl-L-alaninamide hydrogen sulfate (ester).

The empirical formula is $C_{49}H_{62}N_{10}O_{16}S_3$ and the molecular weight is 1143.27.

Following is its chemical structure:

$$\text{Asp - Tyr - Met - Gly - Trp - Met - Asp - Phe} - NH_2$$

with an SO_3H group on Tyr (position 2), and positions numbered 1 2 3 4 5 6 7 8.

CLINICAL PHARMACOLOGY

When injected intravenously, Sincalide produces a substantial reduction in gallbladder size by causing this organ to contract. The evacuation of bile that results is similar to that which occurs physiologically in response to endogenous cholecystokinin. The intravenous (bolus) administration of Sincalide causes a prompt contraction of the gallbladder that becomes maximal in 5 to 15 minutes, as compared with the stimulus of a fatty meal which causes a progressive contraction that becomes maximal after approximately 40 minutes. Generally, a 40 percent reduction in radiographic area of the gallbladder is considered satisfactory contraction, although some patients will show area reduction of 60 to 70 percent.

Like cholecystokinin, Sincalide stimulates pancreatic secretion; concurrent administration with secretin increases both the volume of pancreatic secretion and the output of bicarbonate and protein (enzymes) by the gland. This combined effect of secretin and Sincalide permits the assessment of specific pancreatic function through measurement and analysis of the duodenal aspirate. The parameters usually determined are: volume of the secretion; bicarbonate concentration; and amylase content (which parallels the content of trypsin and total protein).

Both cholecystokinin and Sincalide stimulate intestinal motility, and may cause pyloric contraction which retards gastric emptying.

INDICATIONS AND USAGE

Sincalide may be used: (1) to stimulate gallbladder contraction, as may be assessed by contrast agent cholecystography or ultrasonography, or to obtain by duodenal aspiration a sample of concentrated bile for analysis of cholesterol, bile salts, phospholipids, and crystals; (2) to stimulate pancreatic secretion (especially in conjunction with secretin) prior to obtaining a duodenal aspirate for analysis of enzyme activity, composition, and cytology; (3) to accelerate the transit of a barium meal through the small bowel, thereby decreasing the time and extent of radiation associated with fluoroscopy and x-ray examination of the intestinal tract.

CONTRAINDICATIONS

Sincalide is contraindicated in patients hypersensitive to it and in patients with intestinal obstruction.

WARNINGS

Because of Sincalide's effect on smooth muscle, pregnant patients should be advised that spontaneous abortion or premature induction of labor may occur (see "Pregnancy Category B").

PRECAUTIONS

GENERAL

The possibility exists that stimulation of gallbladder contraction in patients with small gallbladder stones could lead to the evacuation of the stones from the gallbladder, resulting in their lodging in the cystic duct or in the common bile duct. The risk of such an event is considered to be minimal because Sincalide, when given as directed, does not ordinarily cause complete contraction of the gallbladder.

CARCINOGENESIS, MUTAGENESIS, IMPAIRMENT OF FERTILITY

Long-term studies in animals have not been performed to evaluate carcinogenic or mutagenic potential, or possible impairment of fertility in males or females.

TERATOGENIC EFFECTS *PREGNANCY CATEGORY B*:

Reproduction studies in rats in which Sincalide was administered subcutaneously at doses up to 12.5 times the maximum recommended human dose revealed no evidence of harm to the fetus due to Sincalide. There are, however, no adequate and well-controlled studies in pregnant women. Because animal reproduction studies are not always predictive of human response, this drug should be used during pregnancy only if clearly needed (see "Warnings").

LABOR AND DELIVERY

Sincalide should not be administered to pregnant women near term because of its effect on smooth muscle; the possibility of inducing labor prematurely exists. The effects of Sincalide on labor, delivery and lactation in animals has not been determined (see "Warnings").

NURSING MOTHERS

It is not known whether this drug is excreted in human milk. Because many drugs are excreted in human milk, caution should be exercised when Sincalide is administered to a nursing woman.

PEDIATRIC USE

Safety and effectiveness in children have not been established.

ADVERSE REACTIONS

Reactions to Sincalide are generally mild and of short duration. The most frequent adverse reactions were abdominal discomfort or pain, and nausea; rapid intravenous injection of 0.04 mcg Sincalide per kg expectably causes transient abdominal cramping. These phenomena are usually manifestations of the physiologic action of the drug, including delayed gastric emptying and increased intestinal motility. These reactions occurred in approximately 20 percent of patients; they are not to be construed as necessarily indicating an abnormality of the biliary tract unless there is other clinical or radiologic evidence of disease.

The incidence of other adverse reactions, including vomiting, flushing, sweating, rash, hypotension, hypertension, shortness of breath, urge to defecate, headache, diarrhea, sneezing, and numbness was less than 1 percent; dizziness was reported in approximately 2 percent of patients. These manifestations are usually lessened by slower injection rate.

OVERDOSAGE

Although no overdosage reports have been received, gastrointestinal symptoms (abdominal cramps, nausea, vomiting and diarrhea) would be expected. Hypotension with dizziness or fainting might also occur. Overdosage symptoms should be treated symptomatically and should be of short duration. Starting with single bolus i.v. injection comparable to the human dose of 0.4 mg/kg, Sincalide caused hypotension and bradycardia in dogs. Higher doses injected once or repeatedly in dogs caused syncope and ECG changes in addition. These effects were attributed to Sincalide-induced vagal stimulation in that all were prevented by pretreatment with atropine or bilateral vagotomy.

DOSAGE AND ADMINISTRATION

RECONSTITUTION

To reconstitute, aseptically add 5 mL of sterile water for injection USP to the vial; any additional dilution should be made with sodium chloride injection USP, 0.9%.

Parenteral drug products should be inspected visually for particulate matter and discoloration prior to administration, whenever solution and container permit.

For prompt contraction of the gallbladder, a dose of 0.02 mcg Sincalide per kg (1.4 mcg/70 kg) is injected intravenously over a 30- to 60-second interval; if satisfactory contraction of the gallbladder does not occur in 15 minutes, a second dose, 0.04 mcg Sincalide per kg, may be administered. To reduce the intestinal side effects (see "Adverse Reactions"), an intravenous infusion may be prepared at a dose of 0.12 mcg/kg in 100 mL of Sodium Chloride Injection USP and given at a rate of 2 mL per minute; alternatively, an intramuscular dose of 0.1 mcg/kg may be given. When Sincalide is used in cholecystography, roentgenograms are usually taken at five-minute intervals after the injection. For visualization of the cystic duct, it may be necessary to take roentgenograms at one-minute intervals during the first five minutes after the injection.

For the secretin-Sincalide test of pancreatic function, the patient receives a dose of 0.25 units secretin per kg by intravenous infusion over a 60-minute period. Thirty minutes after the initiation of the secretin infusion, a separate IV infusion of Sincalide at a total dose of 0.02 mcg per kg is administered over a 30-minute interval. For example, the total dose for a 70 kg patient is 1.4 mcg of Sincalide; therefore, dilute 1.4 mL of reconstituted Sincalide solution to 30 mL with sodium chloride injection USP and administer at a rate of 1 mL per minute.

To accelerate the transit time of a barium meal through the small bowel, administer Sincalide after the barium meal is beyond the proximal jejunum. (Sincalide, like cholecystokinin, may cause pyloric contraction.) The recommended dose is 0.04 mcg Sincalide per kg (2.8 mcg/70 kg) injected intravenously over a 30- to 60-second interval; if satisfactory transit of the barium meal has not occurred in 30 minutes, a second dose of 0.04 mcg Sincalide per kg may be administered. For reduction of side effects, a 30-minute IV infusion of Sincalide [0.12 mcg per kg (8.4 mcg/70 kg) diluted to approximately 100 mL with sodium chloride injection USP] may be administered.

STORAGE

Store at room temperature, 15°-30° C (59°-86° F), prior to reconstitution. After reconstitution, the solution may be kept at room temperature; it should be used within 24 hours of reconstitution, after which time any unused portion should be discarded.

HOW SUPPLIED
POWDER FOR INJECTION: 5 MCG

BRAND/MANUFACTURER	NDC	SIZE	AWP
○ **BRAND**			
KINEVAC: Bracco Diag	00003-0556-15	10s	$274.34

Sinemet *SEE* CARBIDOPA AND LEVODOPA

Sinequan *SEE* DOXEPIN HYDROCHLORIDE

Sinografin *SEE* DIATRIZOATE MEGLUMINE AND
IODIPAMIDE MEGLUMINE

➤ SHOWN IN PRODUCT IDENTIFICATION GUIDE

Skelaxin *SEE* METAXALONE

Skin Test Antigens, Multiple

DESCRIPTION

Skin Test Antigens, Multiple, for Cellular Hypersensitivity is a disposable, plastic applicator consisting of eight sterile test heads preloaded with the following seven delayed hypersensitivity skin test antigens and glycerin negative control for percutaneous administration: Tetanus Toxoid Antigen, Diphtheria Toxoid Antigen, Streptococcus Antigen, Old Tuberculin, Candida Antigen Trichophyton Antigen, and Proteus Antigen. Skin Test Antigens, Multiple provides a quick, convenient and uniform procedure for delayed cutaneous hypersensitivity testing.

The eight test heads of the Skin Test Antigens, Multiple applicator are numbered 1 through 8 and are preloaded with the following test substances:

TEST HEAD NO. 1 - TETANUS TOXOID ANTIGEN
Tetanus Toxoid Antigen is a sterile solution containing tetanus toxoid prepared from the culture filtrate of *Clostridium tetani* inactivated and detoxified with formaldehyde. Residual formaldehyde does not exceed 0.02%. The potency of each lot is determined by a comparison of responses obtained by the intradermal injection of the lot and a reference Tetanus Toxoid into sensitized guinea pigs. Each ml of Tetanus Toxoid Antigen is biologically equivalent to 550,000 Merieux Tetanus Units.

TEST HEAD NO. 2 - DIPHTHERIA TOXOID ANTIGEN
Diphtheria Toxoid Antigen is a sterile, solution containing diphtheria toxoid prepared from the culture filtrate of *Corynebacterium diphtheriae*, inactivated and detoxified with formaldehyde. Residual formaldehyde does not exceed 0.02%. The potency of each lot is determined by a comparison of responses obtained by the intradermal injection of the lot and a reference Diphtheria Toxoid into sensitized guinea pigs.

Each ml of Diphtheria Toxoid Antigen is biologically equivalent to 1,100,000 Merieux Diphtheria Units.

TEST HEAD NO. 3 - STREPTOCOCCUS ANTIGEN
Streptococcus Antigen is a sterile solution containing culture filtrate of Streptococcus (Group C) inactivated with phenol. Residual phenol does not exceed 0.5%. The potency of each lot is determined by a comparison of responses obtained by the intradermal injection of the lot and a reference Streptococcus preparation into sensitized guinea pigs. Each ml of Streptococcus Antigen is biologically equivalent to 2,000 Merieux Streptococcus Units.

TEST HEAD NO. 4 - TUBERCULIN, OLD
Tuberculin, Old is a sterile, glycerinated solution containing culture filtrates of *Mycobacterium tuberculosis*(C, D and PN) and *Mycobacterium bovis* (Vallee). The potency of each lot is standardized by a comparison of responses obtained by the intradermal injection of the lot and the U.S. Standard Tuberculin, Old into sensitized guinea pigs. Each ml of Tuberculin, Old is biologically equivalent to 300,000 U.S. Tuberculin Units (TU).

TEST HEAD NO. 5 - GLYCERIN NEGATIVE CONTROL
Glycerin Negative Control is a 70% sterile glycerin solution identical to the glycerin solution that serves as a vehicle for the skin test antigens.

TEST HEAD NO. 6 - CANDIDA ANTIGEN
Candida Antigen is a sterile, solution containing culture filtrate of *Candida albicans* inactivated with phenol. Residual phenol does not exceed 0.5%. The potency of each lot is determined by a comparison of responses obtained by the intradermal injection of the lot and a reference Candida preparation into sensitized guinea pigs. Each ml of Candida Antigen in is biologically equivalent to 2,000 Merieux Candida Units.

TEST HEAD NO 7 - TRICHOPHYTON ANTIGEN
Trichophyton Antigen is a sterile solution containing culture filtrate of *Trichophyton mentagrophytes* inactivated by the addition of phenol. Residual phenol does not exceed 0.5%. The potency of each lot is determined by a comparison responses obtained by the intradermal injection of the lot and a reference Trcichophyton preparation into sensitized guinea pigs. Each ml of Trichophyton Antigen is biologically equivalent to 150 Merieux Trichophyton Units.

TEST HEAD NO. 8 - PROTEUS ANTIGEN
Proteus Antigen is a sterile solution containing culture filtrate of *Proteus Mirabilis* inactivated by the addition of phenol. Residual phenol does not exceed 0.5%. The potency of each lot is determined by a comparison of responses obtained by the intradermal injection of the lot and reference Proteus preparation into sensitized guinea pigs. Each ml of Proteus Antigen in glycerin is biologically equivalent to 150 Merieux Proteus Units.

CLINICAL PHARMACOLOGY
The delayed cutaneous responses associated with the ubiquitous antigens in the Skin Test Antigens, Multiple, battery appear to be typical cellular hypersensitivity reactions. A relatively small amount of soluble antigen is introduced into the epidermis and superficial dermal tissue by puncture. Circulating T-cells (lymphocytes), sensitized to the antigen from prior contact, react with the antigens in the skin and induce a specific immune response which includes mitosis (blastogene-

sis) and the release of many soluble mediators (lymphokines). Some lymphokines initiate inflammation (vasculitis and edema) that is manifest after several hours.[2] The intensity of the overall dermal inflammation reaches its peak 24 to 72 hours after antigen application and is resolved within days or weeks.

Delayed hypersensitivity skin testing may be useful in evaluating individuals suspected of having primary or acquired immune deficiency disorders in which cell-mediated immunity is decreased or absent.[3]

An assessment of cellular hypersensitivity reactions has been shown to be useful in many conditions with other products. Protein calorie malnutrition is often complicated by the increasing frequency and severity of infection.[4] Malnutrition of moderate-severe degree (weight for height less than 70% of standard) is almost invariably associated with impaired immune response. Delayed hypersensitivity is one of the immunocompetence response criteria in moderate to severe protein calorie malnutrition.[5] Even marginal malnutrition may be associated with alterations in immunocompetence. Delayed hypersensitivity tests again have been shown to be a comparative immunocompetence parameter. Marginal malnutrition has been shown to have a predictive value for morbidity and mortality.[6] The presence of minerals, other trace elements and certain vitamin deficiencies such as ascorbic acid has been associated with decreased delayed hypersensitivity response. Other factors such as diabetes mellitus, uremia, and certain acquired immune deficiency disorders can depress delayed hypersensitivity.[8] Skin testing at periodic intervals may be useful to determine if a state of immunodepression persists or if delayed hypersensitivity skin test responsiveness returns to normal limits. Delayed hypersensitivity testing has been used to assess nutritional and immunocompetence criteria in the pre-or post-surgical evaluations to detect high risk groups[9] and adopt improved nutritional support and therapeutic programs.[10]

INDICATIONS AND USAGE
For detection of anergy (nonresponsiveness to antigens) by means of delayed hypersensitivity skin testing.

Cutaneous anergy may indicate functional impairment of or abnormalities in, the cellular immune system. Delayed cellular hypersensitivity is a valuable measure of immune response because it involves a complex series of immunologic, cellular, mediator-associated, and vascular effects.

Numerous investigators have shown a positive correlation between defective cell-mediated immunity, as indicated by anergy to multiple skin test antigens, and disseminated cancer.[10-14]. The occurrence of anergy may be correlated to some extent with advanced stage disease.[11] The demonstration of anergy can be a negative prognostic factor in certain malignant diseases since diminished cutaneous reactivity has been associated with poor prognosis.[12] In general, patients capable of displaying normal delayed hypersensitivity skin test reactions to standard skin test antigens may have a better prognosis, whereas those who remain anergic or who exhibit significantly impaired reactivity, tend to have a poor response to therapy,[13] an increased incidence of recurrences and a shortened survival.[10]

The table below summarizes data obtained from studies with the Skin Test Antigens, Multiple antigens in France, in a normal population and in cancer patients. The table illustrates differences in skin test responses between the sexes and between healthy persons compared to those with cancer. Clinical studies conducted in the United States using similar products manufactured by Pasteur Merieux Serums et Vaccins S.A. show comparable results to those obtained in France.

SKIN TEST ANTIGENS, MULTIPLE RESULTS WITH SEVEN ANTIGENS*

	Normal Volunteers		Localized Cancer		Disseminated Cancer	
	Male	*Female*	*Male*	*Female*	*Male*	*Female*
Total Subjects Tested	315	299	393	296	229	164
Percent Anergic	1.2	4.3	14.8	24.7	22.3	33.5
Geometric Mean Scores (mm)	18.3	12.2	12.1	9.6	9.8	7.5
Mean No. Antigens Positive	4.5	3.5	3.3	2.8	2.8	2.3

* *Induration - 2 mm at 48 hours is considered a positive reaction.*

Delayed hypersensitivity skin testing is not an absolute determinant of immune system dysfunction, and any such interpretation must be avoided. Delayed cutaneous hypersensitivity may be diminished or absent when there is *in vitro* evidence that T-lymphocyte function remains intact, and when antibody-associated immunity and phagocytic function appear normal.

Until data are avaible for infants and children (to age 16), skin testing with Skin Test Antigens, Multiple is recommended only for subjects 17 years of age or greater.

CONTRAINDICATIONS
Do not apply at sites involving acneiform, infected or inflamed skin. Although severe systemic reactions are rare to diphtheria and tetanus, antigens, persons known to have a history of systemic reactions should be tested with Skin Test Antigens, Multiple only after the test heads containing these antigens have been removed.

◆ RATED THERAPEUTICALLY EQUIVALENT; ◇ THERAPEUTIC EQUIVALENCE UNCONFIRMED; ○ UNRATED

WARNINGS

Epinephrine should be available in case of severe reactions.

PRECAUTIONS

General: Discard the Skin Test Antigens, Multiple applicator after use. DO NOT REUSE.

The sterility of Skin Test Antigens, Multiple is guaranteed only when the seals on the individual test heads are intact. Do not attempt to resterilize the applicator as this may result in transmission of hepatitis and/or other infections.

If periodic testing is done more frequently than every two months, then the test sites should be rotated so that retesting is not conducted at the same site sooner than two months.

Reactivity to delayed hypersensitivity skin test antigens may decrease or disappear temporarily as a result of febrile illness; measles and other viral infections; live virus vaccination including measles, mumps, rubella, and poliomyelitis vaccines.

Individuals may acquire skin testing sensitivity resulting from either immunization or infection.

Epinephrine should be available in case of severe reactions.

Information for Patients: Patients should be informed of the types of test site reactions that may be expected.

Drug/Drug Interactions: It is possible to observe loss of reactivity in patients undergoing treatment with drugs or procedures that suppress immunity, such as: corticosteroids chemotherapeutic agents, antilymphocyte globulin and irradiation.[8]

Drug/Laboratory Test Interactions: The effect of repeated skin testing on specific antibody levels is not yet known, consequently those doing *in vitro* testing must be cognizant of the fact that repeated skin testing may alter antibody levels.

Pregnancy Category C: Animal reproduction studies have not been conducted with Skin Test Antigens, Multiple. It is also not known whether Skin Test Antigens, Multiple can cause fetal harm when administered to a pregnant woman or can affect reproduction capacity. Skin Test Antigens, Multiple should be given to a pregnant woman only if clearly needed. Pregnancy may result in a decreased level of sensitivity to the test antigens.

Pediatric Use: The safety and effectiveness of Skin Test Antigens, Multiple in children below the age of 17 have not been established.

ADVERSE REACTIONS

Vesiculation, ulceration or necrosis may occur in highly sensitive subjects at the test site. Pain or pruritis at the test site may be relieved by topical glucocorticoids or ice pack.

Systemic reactions may occur in those persons sensitive to allergenic media components.

DOSAGE AND ADMINISTRATION

Carefully follow each step of instructions below.

A. PREPARATION OF THE SITE AND SKIN TEST ANTIGENS, MULTIPLE

1. Remove Skin Test Antigens, Multiple from refrigeration approximately one hour before use.

2. Select only tests sites that permit sufficient surface area and subcutaneous tissue to allow adequate penetration of all points on all eight test heads. Preferred sites are the volar surfaces of the arms and the back. Skin of the posterior thighs may be used if necessary. If several tests are planned, alternating forearms is desirable.

Avoid hairy areas when possible because interpretation of reactions will be more difficult.

3. Cleanse test site with alcohol and allow to dry completely before testing. Ether or acetone may also be used.

4. Tear off the foil strip covering the test heads.

5. Tap the device on a hard surface, foil side up, to release antigen from top of cap.

6. Remove the protective plastic cap on each preloaded test head by twisting cap clockwise and counterclockwise. Carefully, lift cap away from points.

B. APPLICATION OF SKIN TEST ANTIGENS, MULTIPLE

1. Point "T-bar" end of Skin Test Antigens, Multiple toward a censtant reference point such as the elbow or head of the subject being tested to eliminate later identification problems with antigens or the control. The antigens and control are numbered clockwise, beginning top right through 8 on the round plastic platform supporting each test head.

2. Keep the skin at test site taut.

3. Press loaded unit into the skin with sufficient pressure to puncture the skin and allow adequate penetration of all points. Maintain firm contact for at least five seconds. Drug application the device should be "rocked" back and forth and side to side **without removing any of the test heads from the skin sites**. Bleeding rarely occurs with proper pressure.

4. If adequate pressure is applied it will be possible to observe:

a. The puncture marks of the nine tines on each of the eight test heads.

b. An imprint of the circular platform surrounding each test head.

c. Residual antigen and glycerin at each of the eight sites.

If any of the above 3 criteria are not fully followed, the test results may not be reliable.

5. Identify the area of tests sites by drawing one line above test sites No. 8 and No. 1, and another below test sites No. 5 and No. 4.

The lines should be drawn about one-quarter inch from the puncture patterns and made with an indelible marker so that they will remain clearly visible on the skin for at least 48 hours. (See "Skin Test Antigens, Multiple Results".)

6. Allow residual antigens and glycerin to remain on the skin surface for at least three minutes, then gently dab with a gauze and so as not to cross-contaminate test sites with antigen.

7. Discard Skin Test Antigens, Multiple applicator after use.

C. READING AND RECORDING SKIN TEST ANTIGENS, MULTIPLE RESULTS

1. Reading should be done in good light. Read the test sites at both 24 and 48 hours, if possible. The largest reaction recorded from the two readings at each test site should be used. If two readings are not possible, a single 48 hours reading is recommended. The time for maximal reactivity to the various antigens may vary in different people. This may depend on the presence of antibodies.

2. A positive reaction from any of the seven delayed hypersensitivity skin test antigens is **induration of 2 mm or greater** providing there is no induration at the negative control site. Fewer than 2% of healthy volunteers tested during clinical studies exhibited detectable induration from the glycerin negative control solution. Should induration occur at the negative control site, then indurated reactions from individual antigens must exceed the size of induration from the negative control solution by 2 mm or greater to be considered positive. Erythema without induration is of no significance. **The size of the induration reactions with Skin Test Antigens, Multiple may be smaller than those obtained with other intradermal procedures.**

3. Determine the size of an indurated area at each test site by inspection, palpation with gentle finger stroking, and measurements across two diameters at right angles. Record the average diameter of induration $\frac{a+b}{2}$

D. SCORING

Periodic testing with Skin Test Antigens, Multiple can be conducted to determine if a state of anergy persists, or if skin test reactivity return. A two-part scoring system has been developed for the test battery that consists of the number of positive antigens and the total induration resulting from all positive antigen test sites. Whenever positive skin test reactions occur, the scoring system can be used to assist in determining the degree of skin test reactivity and whether there is a trend over a period of time toward greater or lesser skin test responsiveness.

The scoring system can be illustrated by this hypothetical example: Three of the seven delayed hypersensitivity skin test antigens administered simultaneously produce indurated reactions measuring 3 mm, 2 mm and 5 mm respectively.

The resulting score in this hypothetical case is 3/10 mm.

The number 3 represents the number of antigens positive, while 10 mm represents the sum total of induration from all three positive test sites. If a patient is anergic the score is 0/0 mm signifying no reaction to any antigen and no resulting induration.

Occasionally, a small and diffused reaction (2 mm-3 mm) may be present at one time of testing and not at another. The disappearance or recurrence of such a reaction is probably not significant, providing positive reaction sizes to other antigens remain relatively constant. However, the disappearance or substantial reduction in size of a larger, well-defined reaction may be significant, even though the total score is not appreciably affected.

STORAGE

Store at 2 °C to 8 °C (35 ° to 46°F).

REFERENCES

1. Kniken, W.T., Anderson, C.T. and Roumiantzeff, M. The MULTITEST® System: A standarized approach to evaluation of delayed hypersensitivity and cell mediated immunity. *Annals Allergy* 43: 73-79 (1979). 2. Turk, J.L. Delayed Hypersensitivity. Research Monographs in Immunology. Vol 1, pp 97-109, Elsevier/North Holland. Biomedical Press. New York (1980). 3. Turk, J.L. Delayed Hypersensitivity. Research Monographs in Immunology, Vol 1, pp 111-157. Elsevier/North Holland. Biomedical Press. New York (1980). 4. Law, D. K., Dudrick, S.J. and Abdou, N.I. Immunocompetence of patients with protein-calorie malnutrition: The effects of nutritional repletion. *Ann. Intern. Med.*79: 545-550 (1973). 5. Bristrain, B.R. et al. Cellular immunity in adult marasmus. *Arch. Intern. Med.*137: 1408-1411 (1977) 7. Hoffman-Goetz, L. and Blackburn, G.L. Relationship of nutrition to immunology and cancer, pp 73-92 *Nutrition and Cancer: Etiology ad Treatment,*edited by Newell, G.R. and Ellison, N.M. Raven Press, N.Y. (1981). 8. Spitler, L.E. Delayed hypersensitivity skin testing, in *Manual of Clinical Immunology* pp 53-63, editors, Rose, N.R. and Friedman, H., A.S.M., Wash, D.C. (1976). 9. Meakins, J.L. et al. Delayed hypersensitivity: Indicator of acquired failure of host defenses in sepsis and trauma. *Ann. Surg.*1986: 241-250 (1977). 10. Johnson, W.C. et al. Role of delayed hypersensitivity in predicting postoperative morbidity and mortality. *Amen. J. Surgery* 137: 536-541 (1979). 11. Lamb, D., Pilney, F. Kelly, W.D. and Good, R.A. A comparative study of the incidence of energy in patients with carcinoma, leukemia, Hodgkin's disease and other lymphomas. *J. Immunology* 89: 555-558 (1962). 12. Eilber, F.R. and Morton, D.L. Impaired immunologic reactivity and recurrence following cancer surgery. *Cancer* 25: 362-367 (1970). 12. Hersh, E.M. et al. Chematherapy, immunocompetence, immunosuppression and prognosis in acute leukemia. *N. Engl. J. Med.*285: 1211-1216 (1971). 14. Fass, L. Herberman, R.B. and Ziegler, J. Delayed cutaneous hpersensitivity reactions to autologous extracts of Burkitt-lymphoma cells, *N. Engl. J. Med.*282:776-780 (1970).

HOW SUPPLIED
TEST:

BRAND/MANUFACTURER	NDC	SIZE	AWP
○ **BRAND**			
MULTITEST CMI: Connaught	49281-0780-80	1s	$41.00

► SHOWN IN PRODUCT IDENTIFICATION GUIDE

Slo-bid Gyrocaps *SEE* THEOPHYLLINE

Slo-Phyllin *SEE* THEOPHYLLINE

Slo-Phyllin GG *SEE* GUAIFENESIN AND THEOPHYLLINE

Slow-K *SEE* POTASSIUM CHLORIDE, ORAL

Sodium Benzoate and Sodium Phenylacetate

For oral use only. **Not for parenteral use.** Concentrated solution. Must be diluted to appropriate strength prior to administration. (See *"Dosage and Administration".*)

DESCRIPTION
10% Sodium Benzoate/10% Sodium Phenylacetate Oral Solution is a concentrated solution to be diluted and used as an oral adjunctive therapy in patients with urea cycle enzymopathies (UCE). Sodium Benzoate/Sodium Phenylacetate is an aqueous solution.

Each 100 mL contains:

Sodium Benzoate NF	10 g
Sodium Phenylacetate	10 g
Calculated Osmolarity:	Approx. 2620 mOsm/L

Electrolyte (mEq/100 mL): (Sodium 130)

10% Sodium Benzoate/10% Sodium Phenylacetate is supplied in multiple-unit amber glass bottles containing 100 mL, with child-resistant tamper-evident bottle caps. The bottle should not be used initially if the breakaway ring is separated.

CLINICAL PHARMACOLOGY
Sodium Benzoate and Sodium Phenylacetate are metabolically active compounds which decrease elevated blood ammonia concentrations in patients with inborn errors of ureagenesis. The mechanisms for this action are conjugation reactions involving acylation of amino acids. In primates, benzoate conjugates with glycine to form hippurate, and phenylacetate conjugates with glutamine to form phenylacetylglutamine. One mole of hippurate contains one mole of nitrogen, and one mole of phenylacetylglutamine contains two moles of nitrogen. Diversion of nitrogen to these conjugation products results in decreased ammonia formation.

The syntheses of hippurate and phenylacetylglutamine occur via two-step pathways requiring adenosine triphosphate and coenzyme A to form the acyl-coenzyme A intermediates and subsequent amino acid-specific transacylation of glycine and glutamine, respectively.

Studies have shown that Benzoate and Phenylacetate activate these conjugation pathways which then substitute for or supplement the defective ureagenic pathway in patients with urea cycle enzymopathies, and thereby help prevent the accumulation of ammonia. Sodium Benzoate and Sodium Phenylacetate have been used successfully as adjunctive therapy in UCE patients with deficiencies of the following urea cycle enzymes: carbamylphosphate synthetase, ornithine transcarbamylase, and argininosuccinate synthetase. The therapeutic regimens, which also included dietary manipulation and amino acid supplementation, were effective in the long term management of UCE patients. The survival rate in patients with complete enzyme deficiencies was approximately 80% with this combined regimen in what was previously an almost universally fatal disease within the first year of life. The survival rate for each complete enzyme deficiency studied was: carbamylphosphate synthetase - 75%, ornithine transcarbamylase (males) - 59%, argininosuccinate synthetase - 96%. Survival in heterozygous females with partial ornithine transcarbamylase deficiency was 95%, and for patients with other partial deficiencies, 86%. Results of clinical studies indicated that early diagnosis and treatment are important in minimizing developmental disabilities. Reversal of preexisting neurologic impairment is not likely to occur with treatment and neurologic deterioration may continue in some patients.

Pharmacokinetic studies have not been conducted in the primary patient population (neonates, infants, and children). Preliminary pharmacokinetic data were obtained from only three normal adult subjects and the overall disposition of Sodium Benzoate, Sodium Phenylacetate and their metabolites has not been fully characterized. These preliminary pharmacokinetic studies suggest that peak blood levels of Benzoate or Phenylacetate occur within one hour after a single oral dose of Sodium Benzoate or Sodium Phenylacetate, respectively. A majority of the administered compound (approximately 80-100%) was excreted by the kidney within 24 hours as the respective conjugation product, hippurate or phenylacetylglutamine.

The major sites for metabolism of Benzoate and Phenylacetate are the liver and kidney.

INDICATIONS AND USAGE
10% Sodium Benzoate and 10% Sodium Phenylacetate Oral Solution is indicated as adjunctive therapy for the prevention and treatment of hyperammonemia in the chronic management of patients with urea cycle enzymopathies involving partial or complete deficiencies of carbamylphosphate synthetase, ornithine transcarbamylase, or argininosuccinate synthetase.

CONTRAINDICATIONS
There are no known contraindications.

WARNINGS
There have been reports of a possible link between parenteral solutions preserved with benzyl alcohol and morbidity and mortality in low birthweight infants. Use of preserved parenteral solutions was associated with high blood and urine levels of benzyl alcohol and its metabolites, benzoate and hippurate. It is theorized that the immature liver may not be capable of adequately metabolizing these compounds. Therefore, 10% Sodium Benzoate/10% Sodium Phenylacetate should not be administered to low birthweight infants unless, in the opinion of the physician, the benefits outweigh the risks.

Solutions containing sodium ions should be used with great care, if at all, in patients with congestive heart failure, severe renal insufficiency, and in clinical states in which there is sodium retention with edema.

In patients with diminished renal function, administration of solutions containing sodium ions may result in sodium retention.

PRECAUTIONS
GENERAL
For oral use only. **Not for parenteral use.**

The bottle should not be used initially if the breakaway ring is separated.

10% Sodium Benzoate/10% Sodium Phenylacetate is a concentrated solution and should be diluted before use (see *"Dosage and Administration"*).

10% Sodium Benzoate/10% Sodium Phenylacetate is not intended as sole therapy for UCE patients. It should be combined as adjunctive therapy with dietary management (low protein diet) and amino acid supplementation for optimal results.

Caution should be exercised when administering 10% Sodium Benzoate/10% Sodium Phenylacetate to patients with neonatal hyperbilirubinemia since *in vitro* experiments suggest that benzoate competes for bilirubin binding sites on albumin.

The benefits of 10% Sodium Benzoate/10% Sodium Phenylacetate in treating neonatal hyperammonemic coma have not been established. The treatment of choice in neonatal hyperammonemic coma is hemodialysis. Peritoneal dialysis may be helpful if hemodialysis is not available.

Care should be exercised when administering solutions containing sodium to patients with renal or cardiovascular insufficiency, with or without congestive heart failure, particularly if they are postoperative.

10% Sodium Benzoate/10% Sodium Phenylacetate should not be administered to patients with known hypersensitivities to Sodium Benzoate or Sodium Phenylacetate. No such cases of hypersensitivities have been reported.

DRUG INTERACTIONS
Some antibiotics such as penicillin may compete with conjugated products of 10% Sodium Benzoate/10% Sodium Phenylacetate for active secretion by renal tubules which may affect the overall disposition of 10% Sodium Benzoate/10% Sodium Phenylacetate.

Probenecid is known to inhibit the renal transport of many organic compounds including amino hippuric acid and may affect renal excretion of the conjugation products of 10% Sodium Benzoate/10% Sodium Phenylacetate.

There have been reports that valproic acid can induce hyperammonemia. The proposed mechanism is direct inhibition of carbamylphosphate synthetase or interference with the synthesis of its activator, N-acetylglutamate. Therefore, administration of valproic acid to UCE patients may exacerbate their condition and be antagonistic to the efficacy of 10% Sodium Benzoate/10% Sodium Phenylacetate.

CARCINOGENESIS, MUTAGENESIS. IMPAIRMENT OF FERTILITY
Sodium Benzoate has been extensively tested as a food preservative and results indicate it is not mutagenic or carcinogenic and has not been found to impair fertility. Carcinogenicity, mutagenicity and fertility studies of Sodium Phenylacetate have not been conducted.

USAGE IN PREGNANCY
Pregnancy Category C. Animal reproduction studies have not been conducted with 10% Sodium Benzoate/10% Sodium Phenylacetate. It is also not known whether 10% Sodium Benzoate/10% Sodium Phenylacetate can cause fetal harm when administered to a pregnant woman or can affect reproduction capacity. 10% Sodium Benzoate/10% Sodium Phenylacetate should be given to a pregnant woman only if clearly needed.

NURSING MOTHERS
It is not known whether this drug is excreted in human milk. Because many drugs are excreted in human milk, caution should be exercised when 10% Sodium Benzoate/10% Sodium Phenylacetate is administered to a nursing woman.

PEDIATRIC USE
See *"Dosage and Administration"*.

◆ RATED THERAPEUTICALLY EQUIVALENT; ◇ THERAPEUTIC EQUIVALENCE UNCONFIRMED; ○ UNRATED

ADVERSE REACTIONS

Nausea and vomiting have occurred in patients treated with Sodium Benzoate and Sodium Phenylacetate, usually during intravenous administration of these compounds.

Due to structural similarities between benzoate and salicylates, 10% Sodium Benzoate and 10% Sodium Phenylacetate Oral Solution may have the potential to cause side effects associated with salicylates such as exacerbation of peptic ulcers, mild hyperventilation, and mild respiratory alkalosis.

In view of the Sodium content of this product, the possibility of hypernatremia should be considered. Hypernatremia may be associated with edema and exacerbation of congestive heart failure due to retention of water, resulting in an expanded extracellular fluid volume.

If an adverse reaction does occur, discontinue administration, evaluate the patient, and institute appropriate therapeutic countermeasures.

OVERDOSAGE

Four adverse experiences have been reported involving overdoses of Sodium Phenylacetate and/or Sodium Benzoate in UCE patients. One patient who was inadvertently given a ten-fold overdose of Sodium Benzoate and Sodium Phenylacetate by intravenous infusion died after experiencing severe metabolic acidosis and circulatory collapse. A patient who received a three-fold overdose of intravenous Sodium Benzoate and Sodium Phenylacetate experienced lethargy and vomiting which resolved after the drugs were discontinued. Two patients became irritable and vomited after receiving three-fold overdoses of oral Sodium Benzoate. Both patients recovered without treatment within 24 hours after the drug was discontinued.

In the event of an overdose of 10% Sodium Benzoate/10% Sodium Phenylacetate, discontinue the drug and institute supportive measures for metabolic acidosis and circulatory collapse. Hemodialysis or peritoneal dialysis may be beneficial.

DOSAGE AND ADMINISTRATION

For oral use only. Must be diluted before use.

The usual total daily dose for adjunctive therapy of UCE patients is 2.5 mL/kg/day (250 mg Sodium Benzoate and 250 mg Sodium Phenylacetate) in three to six equally divided doses. The total daily dose should not exceed 100 mL (10 g each of Sodium Benzoate and Sodium Phenylacetate).

Each dose of the drug should be diluted in four to eight ounces of infant formula or milk and administered with meals. If other beverages are used, particularly acidic beverages, precipitation of the drug may occur depending on pH and the final concentration. Therefore, the mixture should be inspected for compatibility before administration.

10% Sodium Benzoate/10% Sodium Phenylacetate is a concentrated solution and care should be taken in calculating the dose to avoid the possibility of overdosage.

10% Sodium Benzoate/10% Sodium Phenylacetate is not intended as sole therapy for UCE patients. It should be combined as adjunctive therapy with dietary management (low protein diet) and amino acid supplementation for optimal results.

Because Sodium Phenylacetate has a lingering odor, care should be taken in mixing and administering the drug to minimize contact with skin and clothing.

Store at room temperature. Avoid excessive heat.

HOW SUPPLIED
SOLUTION: 10%-10%

BRAND/MANUFACTURER	NDC	SIZE	AWP
○ BRAND			
UCEPHAN: McGaw	00264-6910-37	100 ml 6s	$71.06

Sodium Bicarbonate

DESCRIPTION

Sodium Bicarbonate Injection, USP is a sterile, nonpyrogenic, hypertonic solution of sodium bicarbonate ($NaHCO_3$) in water for injection for administration by the intravenous route as an electrolyte replenisher and systemic alkalizer.

Solutions are offered in concentrations of 4.2%, 5.0%, 7.5% and 8.4%.

Solutions containing no bacteriostat, antimicrobial agent or added buffer are intended only for use as a single-dose injection. When smaller doses are required, the unused portion should be discarded with the entire unit.

Sodium Bicarbonate, 84 mg is equal to one milliequivalent each of Na^+ and HCO_3^-. Sodium Bicarbonate, USP is chemically designated $NaHCO_3$, a white crystalline powder soluble in water.

Water for Injection, USP is chemically designated H_2O.

CLINICAL PHARMACOLOGY

Intravenous Sodium Bicarbonate therapy increases plasma Bicarbonate, buffers excess hydrogen ion concentration, raises blood pH and reverses the clinical manifestations of acidosis.

Sodium Bicarbonate in water dissociates to provide Sodium (Na^+) and Bicarbonate (HCO_3^-) ions. Sodium (Na^+) is the principal cation of the extracellular fluid and plays a large part in the therapy of fluid and electrolyte disturbances. Bicarbonate (HCO_3^-) is a normal constituent of body fluids and the normal plasma level ranges from 24 to 31 mEq/liter. Plasma concentration is regulated by the kidney through acidification of the urine when there is a deficit

or by alkalinization of the urine when there is an excess. Bicarbonate anion is considered "labile" since at a proper concentration of hydrogen ion (H^+) it may be converted to carbonic acid (H_2CO_3) and thence to its volatile form, carbon dioxide (CO_2) excreted by the lung. Normally a ratio of 1:20 (carbonic acid: Bicarbonate) is present in the extracellular fluid. In a healthy adult with normal kidney function, practically all the glomerular filtered Bicarbonate ion is reabsorbed; less than 1% is excreted in the urine.

INDICATIONS AND USAGE

Sodium Bicarbonate Injection, USP is indicated in the treatment of metabolic acidosis which may occur in severe renal disease, uncontrolled diabetes, circulatory insufficiency due to shock or severe dehydration, extracorporeal circulation of blood, cardiac arrest and severe primary lactic acidosis. Sodium bicarbonate is further indicated in the treatment of certain drug intoxications, including barbiturates (where dissociation of the barbiturate-protein complex is desired), in poisoning by salicylates or methyl alcohol and in hemolytic reactions requiring alkalinization of the urine to diminish nephrotoxicity of blood pigments. Sodium Bicarbonate also is indicated in severe diarrhea which is often accompanied by a significant loss of Bicarbonate.

Treatment of metabolic acidosis should, if possible, be superimposed on measures designed to control the basic cause of the acidosis — e.g., insulin in uncomplicated diabetes, blood volume restoration in shock. But since an appreciable time interval may elapse before all of the ancillary effects are brought about, bicarbonate therapy is indicated to minimize risks inherent to the acidosis itself.

Vigorous Bicarbonate therapy is required in any form of metabolic acidosis where a rapid increase in plasma total CO_2 content is crucial — e.g., cardiac arrest, circulatory insufficiency due to shock or severe dehydration, and in severe primary lactic acidosis or severe diabetic acidosis.

UNLABELED USES

Sodium Bicarbonate is used alone or as an adjunct in the treatment of Lesch-Nyhan syndrome, to correct metabolic acidosis in Lowe's syndrome, and in rhabdomyolysis. Sodium Bicarbonate vaginal solution is also used to enhance sperm penetration in endocervical mucus.

CONTRAINDICATIONS

Sodium Bicarbonate Injection, USP is contraindicated in patients who are losing chloride by vomiting or from continuous gastrointestinal suction, and in patients receiving diuretics known to produce a hypochloremic alkalosis.

WARNINGS

Solutions containing sodium ions should be used with great care, if at all, in patients with congestive heart failure, severe renal insufficiency and in clinical states in which there exists edema with sodium retention.

In patients with diminished renal function, administration of solutions containing Sodium ions may result in Sodium retention.

The intravenous administration of these solutions can cause fluid and/or solute overloading resulting in dilution of serum electrolyte concentrations, overhydration, congested states or pulmonary edema.

Extravascular infiltration should be avoided, see "Adverse Reactions."

PRECAUTIONS

The potentially large loads of sodium given with Bicarbonate require that caution be exercised in the use of Sodium Bicarbonate in patients with congestive heart failure or other edematous or Sodium-retaining states, as well as in patients with oliguria or anuria.

Caution must be exercised in the administration of parenteral fluids, especially those containing Sodium ions, to patients receiving corticosteroids or corticotropin.

Potassium depletion may predispose to metabolic alkalosis and coexistent hypocalcemia may be associated with carpopedal spasm as the plasma pH rises. These dangers can be minimized if such electrolyte imbalances are appropriately treated prior to or concomitantly with Bicarbonate infusion.

Rapid injection (10 mL/min) of hypertonic Sodium Bicarbonate Injection, USP, solutions into neonates and children under two years of age may produce hypernatremia, a decrease in cerebrospinal fluid pressure and possible intracranial hemorrhage. The rate of administration in such patients should therefore be limited to no more than 8 mEq/kg/day. A 4.2% solution may be preferred for such slow administration. In emergencies such as cardiac arrest, the risk of rapid infusion must be weighed against the potential for fatality due to acidosis.

DRUG INTERACTIONS

Additives may be incompatible; norepinephrine and dobutamine are incompatible with Sodium Bicarbonate solution.

The addition of Sodium Bicarbonate to parenteral solutions containing calcium should be avoided, except where compatibility has been previously established. Precipitation or haze may result from Sodium Bicarbonate-Calcium admixtures. *Note:* Do not use the injection if it contains precipitate.

Additives may be incompatible. Consult with pharmacist, if available. When introducing additives, use aseptic technique, mix thoroughly and do not store.

LABORATORY TESTS

The aim of all Bicarbonate therapy is to produce a substantial correction of the low total CO_2 content and blood pH, but the risks of overdosage and alkalosis should be avoided. Hence, repeated fractional doses and periodic monitoring by appropriate laboratory tests are recommended to minimize the possibility of overdosage.

Pregnancy Category C: Animal reproduction studies have not been conducted with Sodium Bicarbonate. It is also not known whether Sodium Bicarbonate can cause fetal harm when administered to a pregnant woman or can affect reproduction capacity. Sodium Bicarbonate should be given to a pregnant woman only if clearly needed.

ADVERSE REACTIONS

Overly agressive therapy wtih Sodium Bicarbonate Injection, USP can result in metabolic alkalosis (associated with muscular twitchings, irritability and tetany) and hypernatremia.

Inadvertent extravasation of intravenously administered hypertonic solutions of Sodium Bicarbonate have been reported to cause chemical cellulitis because of their alkalinity, with tissue necrosis, ulceration or sloughing at the site of infiltration. Prompt elevation of the part, warmth and local injection of lidocaine or hyaluronidase are recommended to prevent sloughing of extravasated I.V. infusions.

OVERDOSAGE

Should alkalosis result, the Bicarbonate should be stopped and the patient managed according to the degree of alkalosis present. 0.9% sodium chloride injection intravenous may be given; potassium chloride also may be indicated if there is hypokalemia. Severe alkalosis may be accompanied by hyperirritability or tetany and these symptoms may be controlled by calcium gluconate. An acidifying agent such as ammonium chloride may also be indicated in severe alkalosis. See *"Warnings"* and *"Precautions."*

DOSAGE AND ADMINISTRATION

Sodium Bicarbonate Injection, USP is administered by the intravenous route.

In cardiac arrest: a rapid intravenous dose of one to two 50 mL vials (44.6 to 100 mEq) may be given initially and continued at a rate of 50 mL (44.6 to 50 mEq) every 5 to 10 minutes if necessary (as indicated by arterial pH and blood gas monitoring) to reverse the acidosis. Caution should be observed in emergencies where very rapid infusion of large quantities of Bicarbonate is indicated. Bicarbonate solutions are hypertonic and may produce an undesirable rise in plasma sodium concentration in the process of correcting the metabolic acidosis. In cardiac arrest, however, the risks from acidosis exceed those of hypernatremia.

In infants: (up to two years of age), the 4.2% solution is recommended for intravenous administration at a dose not to exceed 8 mEq/kg/day. Slow administration rates and the 4.2% solution are recommended in neonates, to guard against the possibility of producing hypernatremia, decreasing cerebrospinal fluid pressure and inducing intracranial hemorrhage.

In less urgent forms of metabolic acidosis: Sodium Bicarbonate Injection USP may be added to other intravenous fluids. The amount of Bicarbonate to be given to older children and adults over a four-to-eight-hour period is approximately 2 to 5 mEq/kg of body weight – depending upon the severity of the acidosis as judged by the lowering of total CO_2 content, blood pH and clinical condition of the patient. In metabolic acidosis associated with shock, therapy should be monitored by measuring blood gases, plasma osmolarity, arterial blood lactate, hemodynamics and cardiac rhythm. Bicarbonate therapy should always be planned in a stepwise fashion since the degree of response from a given dose is not precisely predictable. Initially an infusion of 2 to 5 mEq/kg body weight over a period of 4 to 8 hours will produce a measurable improvement in the abnormal acid-base status of the blood. The next step of therapy is dependent upon the clinical response of the patient. If severe symptoms have abated, then the frequency of administration and the size of the dose may be reduced.

In general, it is unwise to attempt full correction of a low total CO_2 content during the first 24 hours of therapy, since this may be accompanied by an unrecognized alkalosis because of a delay in the readjustment of ventilation to normal. Owing to this lag, the achievement of total CO_2 content of about 20 mEq/liter at the end of the first day of therapy will usually be associated with a normal blood pH. Further modification of the acidosis to completely normal values usually occurs in the presence of normal kidney function when and if the cause of the acidosis can be controlled. Values for total CO_2 which are brought to normal or above normal within the first day of therapy are very likely to be associated with grossly alkaline values for blood pH, with ensuing undesired side effects.

Parenteral drug products should be inspected visually for particulate matter and discoloration prior to administration, whenever solution and container permit. See *"Precautions."*

Do not use unless solution is clear and the container or seal is intact. Discard unused portion.

Store at controlled room temperature, 15° to 30°C (59° to 86°F).

HOW SUPPLIED
INJECTION: 4%

BRAND/MANUFACTURER	NDC	SIZE	AWP
◆ **BRAND**			
NEUT: Abbott Hosp	00074-6609-02	5 ml 25s	$134.19

INJECTION: 4.2%

AVERAGE UNIT PRICE (AVAILABLE SIZES)		GENERIC A-RATED AVERAGE PRICE (GAAP)	
GENERIC	$1.17	10 ml 10s	$131.10

BRAND/MANUFACTURER	NDC	SIZE	AWP
◆ **GENERICS**			
Fujisawa	00469-0026-25	5 ml	$3.33
Abbott Hosp	00074-5534-01	10 ml 10s	$124.69
Abbott Hosp	00074-5534-23	10 ml 10s	$137.51
Abbott Hosp	00074-5534-33	10 ml 25s	$343.78

INJECTION: 4.2%

BRAND/MANUFACTURER	NDC	SIZE	AWP
○ **GENERICS**			
Astra	00186-0645-01	5 ml 10s	$39.40
Astra	00186-0646-01	10 ml 10s	$82.63
Intl Med Sys	00548-1031-00	10 ml 25s	$223.13

INJECTION: 5%

BRAND/MANUFACTURER	NDC	SIZE	AWP
○ **GENERICS**			
McGaw	00264-1498-10	500 ml	$38.81
Baxter	00338-0374-03	500 ml 12s	$470.74
Abbott Hosp	00074-1594-03	500 ml 12s	$479.80

INJECTION: 7.5%

AVERAGE UNIT PRICE (AVAILABLE SIZES)		GENERIC A-RATED AVERAGE PRICE (GAAP)	
GENERIC	$0.26	50 ml 10s	$183.17
		50 ml 25s	$326.71

BRAND/MANUFACTURER	NDC	SIZE	AWP
◆ **GENERICS**			
Fujisawa	00469-8400-60	50 ml	$2.89
Abbott Hosp	00074-4916-01	50 ml 10s	$176.70
Abbott Hosp	00074-4916-23	50 ml 10s	$189.64
Abbott Hosp	00074-4103-03	50 ml 25s	$179.31
Abbott Hosp	00074-4916-33	50 ml 25s	$474.11

For additional alternatives, turn to the section beginning on page 2859.

Sodium Chloride, Inhalation

INDICATIONS

For use in respiratory therapy. Contents of these vials are for use in apparatus for intermittent positive pressure-breathing (IPPB) and for tracheal lavage.

WARNING

Not for injection or in preparations to be used for injection.

DOSAGE AND ADMINISTRATION

To verify container integrity squeeze plastic container before use. Twist cap completely off plastic container, invert, squeeze prescribed volume in nebulizer cup of IPPB apparatus.

Can also be used for tracheal lavage.
Internal contents sterile.
External surface of vial not sterile.
Discard any unused portion of the contents of the single dose vial as well as any unused solution remaining in the nebulizer cup.
Store at controlled room temperature, 15°-30°C (59°-86°F).

HOW SUPPLIED
SOLUTION: 0.45%

BRAND/MANUFACTURER	NDC	SIZE	AWP
○ **GENERICS**			
Astra	00186-4101-01	3 ml 100s	$19.88
Astra	00186-4101-03	5 ml 100s	$19.88

SOLUTION: 0.9%

BRAND/MANUFACTURER	NDC	SIZE	AWP
○ **GENERICS**			
Southwood	58016-0603-01	3 ml	$5.27
Astra	00186-4100-01	3 ml 100s	$19.88
Wyeth-Ayerst	00008-0490-01	3 ml 100s	$22.10
Roxane	00054-8809-25	3 ml 100s	$31.82
Astra	00186-4100-03	5 ml 100s	$19.88
Wyeth-Ayerst	00008-0490-02	5 ml 100s	$22.10
Roxane	00054-8810-25	5 ml 100s	$31.82
Allscrips	54569-3078-00	5 ml 100s ud	$31.82

SOLUTION: 3%

BRAND/MANUFACTURER	NDC	SIZE	AWP
○ **GENERICS**			
Dey	49502-0640-15	15 ml 50s	$51.00

SOLUTION: 10%

BRAND/MANUFACTURER	NDC	SIZE	AWP
○ **GENERICS**			
Dey	49502-0641-15	15 ml 50s	$51.00

Sodium Chloride, Injectable

DESCRIPTION

Sodium Chloride Injection, USP, solutions are sterile and nonpyrogenic. They are parenteral solutions containing various concentrations of Sodium Chloride in water for injection intended for intravenous administration.

◆ RATED THERAPEUTICALLY EQUIVALENT; ◇ THERAPEUTIC EQUIVALENCE UNCONFIRMED; ○ UNRATED

See table for summary of content and characteristics of these solutions.

The solutions contain no bacteriostat, antimicrobial agent or added buffer and each is intended only as a single-dose injection. When smaller doses are required the unused portion should be discarded.

The solutions are parenteral fluid and electrolyte replenishers.

Sodium Chloride, USP, is chemically designated NaCl, a white crystalline powder freely soluble in water.

Water for Injection, USP, is chemically designated H_2O.

CLINICAL PHARMACOLOGY
When administered intravenously, these solutions provide a source of water and electrolytes.

Solutions which provide combinations of hypotonic or isotonic concentrations of Sodium Chloride are suitable for parenteral maintenance or replacement of water and electrolyte requirements.

Isotonic concentrations of Sodium Chloride are suitable for parenteral replacement of Chloride losses that exceed or equal the Sodium loss. Hypotonic concentrations of Sodium Chloride are suited for parenteral maintenance of water requirements when only small quantities of salt are desired. A hypertonic concentration of Sodium Chloride may be used to repair severe salt depletion syndrome.

Sodium Chloride in water dissociates to provide Sodium (Na^+) and Chloride (Cl^-) ions. Sodium (Na^+) is the principal cation of the extracellular fluid and plays a large part in the therapy of fluid and electrolyte disturbances. Chloride (Cl^-) has an integral role in buffering action when oxygen and carbon dioxide exchange occurs in the red blood cells. The distribution and excretion of Sodium (Na^+) and Chloride (Cl^-) are largely under the control of the kidney which maintains a balance between intake and output.

Water is an essential constituent of all body tissues and accounts for approximately 70% of total body weight. Average normal adult daily requirements range from two to three liters (1.0 to 1.5 liters each for insensible water loss by perspiration and urine production).

Water balance is maintained by various regulatory mechanisms. Water distribution depends primarily on the concentration of electrolytes in the body compartments and Sodium (Na^+) plays a major role in maintaining physiologic equilibrium.

INDICATIONS AND USAGE
Intravenous solutions containing Sodium Chloride are indicated for parenteral replenishment of fluid and Sodium Chloride as required by the clinical condition of the patient.

CONTRAINDICATIONS
None known.

WARNINGS
Solutions containing Sodium ions should be used with great care, if at all, in patients with congestive heart failure, severe renal insufficiency and in clinical states in which there exists edema with Sodium retention.

Excessive administration of potassium-free solutions may result in significant hypokalemia.

In patients with diminished renal function, administration of solutions containing Sodium ions may result in Sodium retention.

The intravenous administration of these solutions can cause fluid and/or solute overloading resulting in dilution of serum electrolyte concentrations, overhydration, congested states or pulmonary edema.

The risk of dilutional states is inversely proportional to the electrolyte concentrations of administered parenteral solutions. The risk of solute overload causing congested states with peripheral and pulmonary edema is directly proportional to the electrolyte concentrations of such solutions.

PRECAUTIONS
Clinical evaluation and periodic laboratory determinations are necessary to monitor changes in fluid balance, electrolyte concentrations and acid-base balance during prolonged parenteral therapy or whenever the condition of the patient warrants such evaluation.

Caution must be exercised in the administration of parenteral fluids, especially those containing Sodium ions to patients receiving corticosteroids or corticotropin.

Do not administer unless solution is clear and container is undamaged. Discard unused portion.

Pregnancy Category C: Animal reproduction studies have not been conducted with Sodium Chloride. It is also not known whether Sodium Chloride can cause fetal harm when administered to a pregnant woman or can affect reproduction capacity. Sodium Chloride should be given to a pregnant woman only if clearly needed.

ADVERSE REACTIONS
Reactions which may occur because of the solution or the technique of administration include febrile response, infection at the site of injection, venous thrombosis or phlebitis extending from the site of injection, extravasation and hypervolemia.

If an adverse reaction does occur, discontinue the infusion, evaluate the patient, institute appropriate therapeutic countermeasures and save the remainder of the fluid for examination if deemed necessary.

OVERDOSAGE
In the event of overhydration or solute overload, re-evaluate the patient and institute appropriate corrective measures. (See *"Warnings"*, *"Precautions"*, and *"Adverse Reactions".)*

DOSAGE AND ADMINISTRATION
The dose is dependent upon the age, weight and clinical condition of the patient.

DRUG INTERACTIONS
Additives may be incompatible. Consult with pharmacist, if available. When introducing additives, use aseptic technique, mix thoroughly and do not store.

Parenteral drug products should be inspected visually for particulate matter and discoloration prior to administration, whenever solution and container permit (see *"Precautions"*).

INSTRUCTIONS FOR USE
To Open: Tear outer wrap at notch and remove solution container. If supplemental medication is desired, follow directions below before preparing for administration. Some opacity of the plastic due to moisture absorption during the sterilization process may be observed. This is normal and does not affect the solution quality or safety. The opacity will diminish gradually.

To Add Medication:
1. Prepare additive port.
2. Using aseptic technique and an additive delivery needle of appropriate length, puncture resealable additive port at target area, inner diaphragm and inject. Withdrawal needle after injecting medication.
3. The additive port may be protected by covering with an additive cap.
4. Mix container contents thoroughly.

Preparation for Administration
(Use Aseptic Technique)
1. Close flow control clamp of administration set.
2. Remove cover from outlet port at bottom of container.
3. Insert piercing pin of administration set into port with a twisting motion until the set is firmly seated. *Note:* See full directions on administration set carton.
4. Suspend container from hanger.
5. Squeeze and release drip chamber to establish proper fluid level in chamber.
6. Open flow control clamp and clear air from set. Close clamp.
7. Attach set to venipuncture device. If device is not indwelling, prime and make venipuncture.
8. Regulate rate of administration with flow control clamp.

WARNING: Do not use flexible container in series connections.

STORAGE
Exposure of pharmaceutical products to heat should be minimized. Avoid excessive heat. Protect from freezing. It is recommended that the product be stored at room temperature (25° C); however, brief exposure to 40° C does not adversely affect the product.

J CODES
250 cc IV—J7050
1,000 cc IV—J7030
IV—J2912

HOW SUPPLIED
INJECTION: 0.45%

AVERAGE UNIT PRICE (AVAILABLE SIZES)		GENERIC A-RATED AVERAGE PRICE (GAAP)	
GENERIC	$0.02	500 ml	$9.77
		1000 ml	$10.75
		1000 ml 12s	$131.85
		500 ml 24s	$234.34

BRAND/MANUFACTURER	NDC	SIZE	AWP
◆ GENERICS			
McGaw	00264-1402-10	500 ml	$9.64
McGaw	00264-7802-10	500 ml	$9.89
McGaw	00264-7802-00	1000 ml	$10.69
McGaw	00264-1402-00	1000 ml	$10.80
Baxter	00338-0043-04	1000 ml 12s	$130.61
Abbott Hosp	00074-7985-09	1000 ml 12s	$133.10
Abbott Hosp	00074-7985-02	250 ml 24s	$236.55
Baxter	00338-0043-03	500 ml 24s	$232.13
Abbott Hosp	00074-7985-03	500 ml 24s	$236.55

➤ SHOWN IN PRODUCT IDENTIFICATION GUIDE

INJECTION: 0.9%

AVERAGE UNIT PRICE (AVAILABLE SIZES)		GENERIC A-RATED AVERAGE PRICE (GAAP)	
GENERIC	$0.14	3 ml	$2.26
		10 ml	$1.20
		30 ml	$1.32
		100 ml	$7.43
		500 ml	$10.10
		1000 ml	$10.23
		250 ml 12s	$97.95
		1000 ml 12s	$105.13
		250 ml 24s	$261.14
		500 ml 24s	$220.73
		10 ml 25s	$36.91
		20 ml 25s	$42.01
		50 ml 25s	$79.71
		25 ml 48s	$634.25
		50 ml 80s	$974.25
		100 ml 80s	$974.25
		50 ml 96s	$928.51
		100 ml 96s	$928.51

BRAND/MANUFACTURER	NDC	SIZE	AWP
◆ GENERICS			
Fujisawa	00469-5186-15	2 ml	$1.40
Fujisawa	00469-2005-86	3 ml	$2.17
Fujisawa	00469-2005-88	3 ml	$2.35
Fujisawa	00469-0248-15	10 ml	$1.08
Fujisawa	00469-2059-10	10 ml	$1.08
Fujisawa	00469-1186-15	10 ml	$1.44
Fujisawa	00469-4186-15	20 ml	$1.76
McGaw	00264-1800-36	25 ml	$14.65
Fujisawa	00469-2059-30	30 ml	$1.32
Fujisawa	00469-2248-15	30 ml	$1.32
Fujisawa	00469-0186-25	100 ml	$3.10
McGaw	00264-1800-31	100 ml	$9.60
McGaw	00264-1800-32	100 ml	$9.60
McGaw	00264-1400-23	150 ml	$9.36
McGaw	00264-7800-20	250 ml	$9.12
McGaw	00264-7800-10	500 ml	$9.90
McGaw	00264-1400-10	500 ml	$10.30
McGaw	00264-1400-00	1000 ml	$9.77
McGaw	00264-7800-00	1000 ml	$10.69
Abbott Hosp	00074-4888-99	100 ml 5s	$17.22
Abbott Hosp	00074-1584-01	50 ml 12s	$189.95
Abbott Hosp	00074-1584-11	100 ml 12s	$189.95
Abbott Hosp	00074-1583-01	150 ml 12s	$118.28
Baxter	00338-0045-02	250 ml 12s	$59.52
Baxter	00338-0044-02	250 ml 12s	$116.06
Abbott Hosp	00074-1583-02	250 ml 12s	$118.28
Baxter	00338-0046-04	1000 ml 12s	$76.32
Baxter	00338-0049-04	1000 ml 12s	$118.37
Abbott Hosp	00074-7983-09	1000 ml 12s	$120.70
Abbott Hosp	00074-7983-02	250 ml 24s	$222.87
Abbott Hosp	00074-7983-53	250 ml 24s	$222.87
Baxter	00338-0048-02	250 ml 24s	$277.34
Abbott Hosp	00074-7101-02	250 ml 24s	$321.48
Baxter	00338-0049-03	500 ml 24s	$218.59
Abbott Hosp	00074-7983-03	500 ml 24s	$222.87
Abbott Hosp	00074-1966-04	10 ml 25s	$34.73
Abbott Hosp	00074-4888-25	10 ml 25s	$37.70
Abbott Hosp	00074-7067-10	10 ml 25s	$38.30
Abbott Hosp	00074-1966-05	20 ml 25s	$40.08
Abbott Hosp	00074-4888-20	20 ml 25s	$43.94
Abbott Hosp	00074-1966-07	30 ml 25s	$44.23
Abbott Hosp	00074-4888-50	50 ml 25s	$65.61
Abbott Hosp	00074-1493-01	50 ml 25s	$93.81
Abbott Hosp	00074-1492-01	100 ml 25s	$97.67
Abbott Hosp	00074-7983-61	150 ml 32s	$297.16
Baxter	00338-0049-01	150 ml 36s	$327.89
Baxter	00338-0049-02	250 ml 36s	$327.89
Baxter	00338-0049-10	25 ml 48s	$542.88
Abbott Hosp	00074-7984-20	25 ml 48s	$725.61
Abbott Hosp	00074-7101-13	50 ml 48s	$531.24
Abbott Hosp	00074-7101-23	100 ml 48s	$531.24
Abbott Hosp	00074-7984-36	50 ml 80s	$788.50
Baxter	00338-0553-11	50 ml 80s	$1160.00
Abbott Hosp	00074-7984-37	100 ml 80s	$788.50
Baxter	00338-0553-18	100 ml 80s	$1160.00
Baxter	00338-0049-11	50 ml 96s	$928.51
Baxter	00338-0049-31	50 ml 96s	$928.51
Baxter	00338-0049-41	50 ml 96s	$928.51
Baxter	00338-0049-18	100 ml 96s	$928.51
Baxter	00338-0049-38	100 ml 96s	$928.51
Baxter	00338-0049-48	100 ml 96s	$928.51
Baxter	00338-0045-61	30 ml 100s	$85.00

INJECTION: 0.9%

BRAND/MANUFACTURER	NDC	SIZE	AWP
◇ GENERICS			
Insource	58441-1101-03	30 ml	$1.87

INJECTION: 2.5%

BRAND/MANUFACTURER	NDC	SIZE	AWP
◆ GENERICS			
Abbott Hosp	00074-4219-02	250 ml 12s	$298.11

INJECTION: 3%

BRAND/MANUFACTURER	NDC	SIZE	AWP
◆ GENERICS			
Baxter	00338-0054-03	500 ml 24s	$258.52

INJECTION: 5%

AVERAGE UNIT PRICE (AVAILABLE SIZES)	
GENERIC	$0.02

BRAND/MANUFACTURER	NDC	SIZE	AWP
◆ GENERICS			
Abbott Hosp	00074-1586-03	500 ml 12s	$145.35
Baxter	00338-0056-03	500 ml 24s	$285.12

INJECTION: 14.6%

AVERAGE UNIT PRICE (AVAILABLE SIZES)	
GENERIC	$0.09

BRAND/MANUFACTURER	NDC	SIZE	AWP
◆ GENERICS			
Fujisawa	00469-1390-40	20 ml	$2.26
Fujisawa	00469-1390-60	40 ml	$2.67

INJECTION: 23.4%

AVERAGE UNIT PRICE (AVAILABLE SIZES)	
GENERIC	$0.75

BRAND/MANUFACTURER	NDC	SIZE	AWP
◆ GENERICS			
Fujisawa	00469-1187-25	30 ml	$2.39
Fujisawa	00469-8801-00	100 ml	$9.30
Fujisawa	00469-8802-00	200 ml	$17.10
Abbott Hosp	00074-1130-02	250 ml 12s	$93.77
Abbott Hosp	00074-1141-01	50 ml 25s	$120.53
Abbott Hosp	00074-1141-02	100 ml 25s	$152.59

Sodium Fluoride

DESCRIPTION

Sodium Fluoride is available as liquid drops, gel, and tablets, for use as a dental caries preventive.

Each ml of liquid drops contains:
Sodium Fluoride ....1.1 mg, providing 0.5 mg Fluoride ion or
4.97 mg, providing 2.25 mg Fluoride ion (0.125 mg Fluoride)

The gel contains:
Sodium Fluoride 1.1%

Each tablet contains:
Sodium Fluoride ....2.2 mg, providing 1 mg Fluoride
1.1 mg, providing 0.5 mg Fluoride
0.55 mg, providing 0.25 mg Fluoride

CLINICAL PHARMACOLOGY

Sodium Fluoride acts systemically (before tooth eruption) and topically (posteruption) by increasing tooth resistance to acid dissolution, by promoting remineralization, inhibiting the cariogenic microbial process and by enhancing penetration of the Fluoride ion into tooth enamel.

INDICATIONS AND USAGE

It has been established that ingestion of fluoridated drinking water (1 ppm F) during the period of tooth development results in a significant decrease in the incidence of dental caries.[1] Sodium Fluoride drops and Sodium Fluoride tablets were developed to provide systemic Fluoride for use as a supplement in infants and children from birth to age 3 and older, living in areas where the drinking water Fluoride level does not exceed 0.7 ppm.

It is well established that 1.1% Sodium Fluoride is safe and extraordinarily effective as a caries preventive when applied frequently with mouthpiece applicators.[14] Sodium Fluoride gel in a squeeze tube is a particularly convenient dosage form which permits the application of a thin ribbon of gel onto a toothbrush as well as a mouthpiece tray.

CONTRAINDICATIONS

Do not use in areas where the drinking water exceeds 0.7 ppm F.

Some Sodium Fluoride tablets are contraindicated when the F-content of drinking water is 0.3 ppm or more and should not be administered to children under age 3.

◆ RATED THERAPEUTICALLY EQUIVALENT; ◇ THERAPEUTIC EQUIVALENCE UNCONFIRMED; ○ UNRATED

There are no contraindications to use of the gel. It may be used in areas where drinking water is fluoridated or not, because topical Fluoride cannot produce fluorosis.

WARNINGS
See "Contraindications" above. As in the case of all medications. keep out of reach of children. Some brands and/or formulations contain FD&C Yellow #6.

Use of the gel in children under age 6 requires special supervision to prevent repeated swallowing of gel which could cause dental fluorosis.

PRECAUTIONS
See "Overdosage" section below. Incompatibility of Fluoride with dairy foods has been reported due to formation of calcium fluoride which is poorly absorbed. Not for use in the eyes.

ADVERSE REACTIONS
Allergic rash and other idiosyncrasies have been rarely reported.

OVERDOSAGE
Prolonged daily ingestion of excessive Fluoride will result in varying degrees of dental fluorosis. (The total amount of Sodium Fluoride in the drops and tablets (25 mg F) conforms with recommendations of the American Dental Association for the maximum to be dispensed at one time for safety purposes.) Accidental ingestion of a usual treatment dose of the gel (1-2 mg F) is not harmful.

DOSAGE[2] AND ADMINISTRATION
DROPS

F-Content of Drinking Water	Daily Dosage		
	Birth to Age 2	Age 2-3	Age 3-12
< 0.3 ppm	2 drops or ½ dropper	4 drops or 1 dropper	8 drops or 2 droppers
0.3-0.7 ppm	One-half above dosage.		
> 0.7 ppm	Fluoride supplements contraindicated.		

Sodium Fluoride drops may be administered orally undiluted or mixed with fluids.

TABLETS

F-Content of Drinking Water	Daily Dosage (F ion)		
	Birth to Age 2	Age 2-3	Age 3-12
< 0.3 ppm	0.25 mg	0.5 mg	1.0 mg
0.3-0.7 ppm	One-half above dosages.		
> 0.7 ppm	Fluoride supplements contraindicated.		

One tablet daily, to be dissolved in the mouth or chewed before swallowing, preferably at bedtime after brushing teeth.

GEL
1. After brushing with toothpaste, rinse as usual. Adults and children 6 years of age or older, apply a thin ribbon of gel to the teeth with a toothbrush or mouthtrays for at least one minute, preferably at bedtime.

2. After use, adults expectorate gel. For best results, do not eat, drink, or rinse for 30 minutes. Children expectorate gel after use and rinse mouth thoroughly.

REFERENCES
1. Accepted Dental Therapeutics. Ed.40.American Dental Association, Chicago, 1984, p. 399-402. 2. Ibid. p. 401. American Academy of Pediatrics. Pediatrics 63:150-152, 1979. 3. Accepted Dental Therapeutics. Ed. 40, ADA. Chicago, p. 405-407, 1984. 4. Englander HR, Keyes PH and Gestwicki M: JADA 75:638-644, 1967. 5. Englander HR et al: JADA 78:783-787, 1969. 6. Englander HR et al: JADA 82:354-358, 1971.

HOW SUPPLIED
CHEW TABLET: 0.25 MG

BRAND/MANUFACTURER	NDC	SIZE	AWP
○ **BRAND**			
LURIDE: Colgate Oral	00126-0186-21	120s	$5.83

CHEW TABLET: 0.5 MG

BRAND/MANUFACTURER	NDC	SIZE	AWP
○ **BRAND**			
LURIDE: Colgate Oral	00126-0014-21	120s	$5.83
	00126-0014-81	1200s	$31.19
○ **GENERICS**			
Southwood	58016-0900-50	50s	$2.89
Southwood	58016-0900-00	100s	$4.23
NAFRINSE: Orachem	10733-0765-04	120s dozdoz	$19.80

BRAND/MANUFACTURER	NDC	SIZE	AWP
Copley	38245-0123-20	1000s	$7.15
Qualitest	00603-3622-32	1000s	$7.55
FLUORITAB: Fluoritab	00288-0006-04	1000s	$8.65
Major	00904-1125-80	1000s	$8.65
Perry Med	11763-0713-04	1000s	$8.83
Moore,H.L.	00839-6578-16	1000s	$8.84
FLUORITAB: Fluoritab	00288-0006-02	5000s	$32.00

CHEW TABLET: 1 MG

AVERAGE UNIT PRICE (AVAILABLE SIZES)		GENERIC A-RATED AVERAGE PRICE (GAAP)	
GENERIC	$0.01	100s	$1.82
		5000s	$32.00

BRAND/MANUFACTURER	NDC	SIZE	AWP
◆ **GENERICS**			
FLUORITAB: Fluoritab	00288-0001-01	100s	$1.82
FLUORITAB: Fluoritab	00288-0003-01	100s	$1.82
FLUORITAB: Fluoritab	00288-0003-04	1000s	$8.65
FLUORITAB: Fluoritab	00288-0001-02	5000s	$32.00
FLUORITAB: Fluoritab	00288-0003-02	5000s	$32.00

CHEW TABLET: 1 MG

BRAND/MANUFACTURER	NDC	SIZE	AWP
○ **BRAND**			
LURIDE: Colgate Oral	00126-0006-21	120s	$7.11
	00126-0143-21	120s	$7.11
LURIDE SF: Colgate Oral	00126-0007-21	120s	$7.11
KARIDIUM: Lorvic	00273-0101-01	180s	$5.50
	00273-0101-02	1000s	$19.95
LURIDE: Colgate Oral	00126-0006-10	1000s	$31.19
	00126-0143-10	1000s	$31.19
○ **GENERICS**			
Richlyn	00115-4631-01	100s	$0.99
FLUORABON: Perry Med	11763-0525-01	100s	$1.93
FLUORABON: Perry Med	11763-0526-01	100s	$1.93
FLUORABON: Perry Med	11763-0532-01	100s	$1.93
Southwood	58016-0978-00	100s	$4.84
NAFRINSE: Orachem	10733-0567-05	120s dozdoz	$19.80
Veratex	17022-4501-06	1000s	$4.95
Geneva	00781-1816-10	1000s	$6.73
Pharmacist's Choice	54979-0455-10	1000s	$7.10
Copley	38245-0131-20	1000s	$7.15
Rugby	00536-4547-10	1000s	$7.19
Rugby	00536-4548-10	1000s	$7.19
Qualitest	00603-3623-32	1000s	$7.55
Richlyn	00115-4631-03	1000s	$7.65
URL	00677-0132-10	1000s	$7.85
Perry Med	11763-0317-04	1000s	$8.83
Perry Med	11763-0318-04	1000s	$8.83
Moore,H.L.	00839-5035-16	1000s	$8.84
Schein	00364-0254-02	1000s	$8.91
Major	00904-1126-80	1000s	$10.15

DROP: 0.125 MG/DRP

BRAND/MANUFACTURER	NDC	SIZE	AWP
○ **BRAND**			
KARIDIUM: Lorvic	00273-0102-01	30 ml	$3.30
LURIDE: Colgate Oral	00126-0002-62	50 ml	$8.70
KARIDIUM: Lorvic	00273-0102-02	60 ml	$5.50
○ **GENERICS**			
Copley	38245-0600-11	30 ml	$2.80
Moore,H.L.	00839-7315-63	30 ml	$3.38
Liquipharm	54198-0105-30	30 ml	$3.50
Hi-Tech	50383-0629-30	30 ml	$3.60
Major	00904-1127-30	30 ml	$4.25
Qualitest	00603-1244-45	30 ml	$4.40
Tri-Med	55654-0014-02	30 ml	$5.00
Aligen	00405-3720-53	30 ml	$5.25
Rugby	00536-1981-75	30 ml	$5.76
Allscrips	54569-2959-00	30 ml	$5.76
Goldline	00182-6133-66	30 ml	$6.75
Southwood	58016-9077-01	30 ml	$7.70

DROP: 0.5 MG/ML

BRAND/MANUFACTURER	NDC	SIZE	AWP
○ **BRAND**			
PEDIAFLOR: Ross Pharm	00074-0101-50	50 ml	$12.38

► SHOWN IN PRODUCT IDENTIFICATION GUIDE

GEL: 1.1%

BRAND/MANUFACTURER	NDC	SIZE	AWP
○ **BRAND**			
PREVIDENT: Colgate Oral	00126-0088-02	60 gm	$7.29
PREVIDENT: Colgate Oral	00126-0089-02	60 gm	$7.29
	00126-0288-02	60 gm	$7.29
	00126-0289-02	60 gm	$7.29
	00126-0290-02	60 gm	$7.29
THERA-FLUR: Colgate Oral	00126-0048-54	24 ml	$5.31
THERA-FLUR-N: Colgate Oral	00126-0196-54	24 ml	$5.31
○ **GENERICS**			
KARIGEL-N: Lorvic	00273-0131-01	24 gm	$1.67
KARIGEL: Lorvic	00273-0103-01	30 gm	$1.67
KARIGEL: Lorvic	00273-0103-02	120 gm	$3.97
KARIGEL: Lorvic	00273-0103-03	240 gm	$6.63
KARIGEL-N: Lorvic	00273-0131-04	125 ml	$3.97

SOLUTION: 0.2%

BRAND/MANUFACTURER	NDC	SIZE	AWP
○ **BRAND**			
PREVIDENT DENTAL RINSE: Colgate Oral	00126-0179-99	250 ml	$5.73
FLUORINSE: Oral B Lab	00041-0350-07	480 ml	$7.49
	00041-0351-07	480 ml	$7.49

SOLUTION: 1 MG/5 ML

BRAND/MANUFACTURER	NDC	SIZE	AWP
○ **BRAND**			
PHOS-FLUR: Colgate Oral	00126-0129-99	250 ml	$5.20
	00126-0126-46	500 ml	$8.74
	00126-0129-46	500 ml	$8.74
	00126-0452-46	500 ml	$8.74
	00126-0453-46	500 ml	$8.74
	00126-0454-46	500 ml	$8.74
○ **GENERICS**			
Copley	38245-0616-07	500 ml	$6.00
Liquipharm	54198-0108-16	500 ml	$6.40
Liquipharm	54198-0109-16	500 ml	$6.40
Liquipharm	54198-0110-16	500 ml	$6.40
Liquipharm	54198-0111-16	500 ml	$6.40
LIQUIFLUR: Moore,H.L.	00839-7484-79	500 ml	$6.74

Sodium Fluoride/Vitamin A/ Vitamin C/Vitamin D

DESCRIPTION

One dropperful (1.0 mL) provides:

Fluoride ....0.25 mg

Vitamins			% U.S. RDA*	% U.S. RDA**
Vitamin A	1500	I.U.	100	60
Vitamin D	400	I.U.	100	100
Vitamin C	35	mg	100	87

Active Ingredients: Ascorbic acid, Vitamin A palmitate, Sodium Fluoride and ergocalciferol.
* % U.S. Recommended Daily Allowance for infants.
** % U.S. Recommended Daily Allowance for children under 4 years of age.

INDICATIONS AND USAGE

As an aid in the prevention of dental caries in infants and children, and in the prophylaxis of Vitamin A, D and C deficiencies.

CONTRAINDICATIONS

Should be used only where the Fluoride content of the drinking water supply is known to be 0.7 parts per million or less.

PRECAUTIONS

The recommended dosage should not be exceeded since chronic overdosage of Fluoride may result in mottling of tooth enamel and osseous changes.

OVERDOSAGE

In children, acute ingestion of 10 to 20 mg of Sodium Fluoride may cause excessive salivation and gastrointestinal disturbances; 500 mg may be fatal. Oral and/or intravenous fluids containing calcium may be indicated.

DOSAGE AND ADMINISTRATION

One dropperful daily, or as directed by physician or dentist.
  Store below 77°F (25°C).

HOW SUPPLIED

CHEW TABLET: 1 MG

BRAND/MANUFACTURER	NDC	SIZE	AWP
○ **BRAND**			
TRI VITA: Amide	52152-0002-02	100s	$5.95
TRI-VI-FLOR: Mead Johnson Nutr	00087-0477-01	100s	$13.54
○ **GENERICS**			
FLOR-DAC TRI-VITAMIN: Perry Med	11763-0530-01	100s	$2.99
Copley	38245-0176-10	100s	$4.00
Moore,H.L.	00839-7188-06	100s	$5.20
TRI-A-VITE W/FLUORIDE: Major	00904-7810-60	100s	$5.40
Rugby	00536-4737-01	100s	$5.45
Southwood	58016-0966-00	100s	$5.64
Schein	00364-0846-01	100s	$5.70
Qualitest	00603-6300-21	100s	$5.94
Goldline	00182-4539-01	100s	$6.15
R.I.D.	54807-0852-01	100s	$12.55
Copley	38245-0176-20	1000s	$39.00
Moore,H.L.	00839-7188-16	1000s	$46.40

For additional alternatives, turn to the section beginning on page 2859.

Sodium Fluoride and Vitamins, Multi

DESCRIPTION

CHEWABLE TABLETS

		Percentage of U.S. Recommended Daily Allowance	
		Children Age 2-3 Years	*Adults & Children Age 4 Years or More*
Each tablet supplies:			
Vitamin A	2500 IU	100	50
Vitamin D	400 IU	100	100
Vitamin E	15 IU	150	50
Vitamin C	60 mg	150	100
Folic acid	0.3 mg	150	75
Thiamine	1.05 mg	150	70
Riboflavin	1.2 mg	150	70
Niacin	13.5 mg	150	68
Vitamin B_6	1.05 mg	150	53
Vitamin B_{12}	4.5 µg	150	75

Sodium Fluoride/Vitamin, Multi Chewable Tablets come in 3 different strengths of Fluoride: 0.25 mg, 0.5 mg and 1 mg.

DROPS

		Percentage of U.S. Recommended Daily Allowance	
		Infants	*Children Under Age 4 Years*
Each 1.0 ml supplies:			
Vitamin A	1500 IU	100	60
Vitamin D	400 IU	100	100
Vitamin E	5 IU	100	60
Vitamin C	35 mg	100	88
Thiamine	0.5 mg	100	71
Riboflavin	0.6 mg	100	75
Niacin	8 mg	100	89
Vitamin B_6	0.4 mg	100	57
Vitamin B_{12}	2 µg	100	67

◆ RATED THERAPEUTICALLY EQUIVALENT; ◇ THERAPEUTIC EQUIVALENCE UNCONFIRMED; ○ UNRATED

Sodium Fluoride/Vitamins, Multi Drops are in two different strengths: Fluoride 0.25 g/ml, Fluoride 0.5 g/ml.

Active Ingredient for Caries Prophylaxis: Fluoride as Sodium Fluoride.

CLINICAL PHARMACOLOGY

It is well established that fluoridation of the water supply (1 ppm fluoride) during the period of tooth development leads to a significant decrease in the incidence of dental caries.

Sodium Fluoride/Vitamin Multi tablets provide Sodium Fluoride and ten essential vitamins in a chewable tablet. Because the tablets are chewable, they provide a topical as well as systemic source of Fluoride.

Hydroxyapatite is the principal crystal for all calcified tissue in the human body. The fluoride ion reacts with the hydroxyapatite in the tooth as it is formed to produce the more caries-resistant crystal, fluorapatite. The reaction may be expressed by the equation:[4]

$$Ca_{10}(PO_4)_6(OH)_2 + 2F^- \rightarrow Ca_{10}(PO_4)_6F_2 + 2OH^-$$
$$\text{(Hydroxyapatite)} \qquad \text{(Fluorapatite)}$$

Three stages of Fluoride deposition in tooth enamel can be distinguished.
1. Small amounts (reflecting the low levels of Fluoride in tissue fluids) are incorporated into the enamel crystals while they are being formed.
2. After enamel has been laid down, Fluoride deposition continues in the surface enamel. Diffusion of Fluoride from the surface inward is apparently restricted.
3. After eruption, the surface enamel acquires Fluoride from water, food, supplementary Fluoride and smaller amounts from saliva.

INDICATIONS AND USAGE

Supplementation of the diet with ten essential vitamins.
Supplementation of the diet with fluoride for caries prophylaxis.
Sodium Fluoride/Vitamin, Multi chewable tablets provide Fluoride in tablet form for children 2-3 years of age where the drinking water has a Fluoride content of less than 0.3 ppm, and for children 3 years of age and above where the drinking water contains 0.3 through 0.7 ppm of Fluoride.

Sodium Fluoride/Vitamin, Multi 0.25 mg drops were developed to provide Fluoride in drop form for infants and young children from birth to 2 years of age in areas where the drinking water contains less than 0.3 ppm of Fluoride and for children ages 2-3 years in areas where the drinking water contains 0.3 through 0.7 ppm of Fluoride. Each 1.0 mL supplies Sodium Fluoride (0.25 mg Fluoride) plus nine essential vitamins.

Sodium Fluoride/Vitamin Multi 0.5 mg (multivitamin and Fluoride supplement) drops provide Fluoride in drop form for children ages 2-3 years in areas where the drinking water contains less than 0.3 ppm fluoride; and for children 3 years of age and older in areas where the drinking water contains 0.3 through 0.7 ppm of Fluoride. Each 1.0 mL provides Sodium Fluoride (0.5 mg Fluoride) plus nine essential vitamins.

Sodium Fluoride/Vitamin, Multi chewable tablets supply significant amounts of vitamins A, D, E, C, thiamine, riboflavin, niacin, pyridodine, cyanocobalamin and folic acid to supplement the diet, and to help assure that nutritional deficiencies of these vitamins will not develop. Thus, in a single easy-to-use preparation, children obtain ten essential vitamins and the important mineral, Fluoride.

Sodium Fluoride/Vitamin, Multi drops supply significant amounts of vitamins A, D, E, C thiamine, riboflavin, niacin, pyridoxine, and cyanocobalamin to supplement the diet, and to help assure that nutritional deficiencies of these vitamins will not develop Thus, in a single easy-to-use preparation, infants and children obtain nine essential vitamins and Fluoride.

The American Academy of Pediatrics recommends that children up to age 16 years, in areas where drinking water contains less than optimal levels of Fluoride, receive daily Fluoride supplementation.

Children using Sodium Fluoride/Vitamin, Multi chewable tablets regularly should receive semi-annual dental examinations. The regular brushing of teeth and attention to good oral hygiene practices are also essential.

A comprehensive 5½ year series of studies of the effectiveness of vitamin-fluoride products in caries protection has been published.[6-7] Children in this continuing study lived in an area where the water supply contained only 0.05 ppm Flouride. The subjects were divided into two groups, one which used only nonfluoridated vitamin products and the other vitamin-Fluoride products.

The three-year interim report showed 63% fewer carious surfaces in primary teeth and 43% fewer carious surfaces in permanent teeth of the children taking vitamin-fluoride products.[1]

After four years the studies continued to support the effectiveness of vitamin-fluoride products, showing a reduction in carious surfaces of 68% in primary teeth and 46% in permanent teeth.[2]

Results at the end of 5½ years further confirmed the previous findings and indicated that significant reductions in dental caries are apparent with the continued use of vitamin-Fluoride products.[6]

WARNING

As in the case of all medications, keep out of the reach of children.

PRECAUTIONS

The suggested dose should not be exceeded, since dental fluorosis may result from continued ingestion of large amounts of Fluoride.

Before prescribing Sodium Fluoride/Vitamin Multi chewable tablets or drops:
1. determine the Fluoride content of the drinking water.
2. make sure the child is not receiving significant amounts of Fluoride from other medications.
3. periodically check to make sure that the child does not develop significant dental fluorosis.

The Council on Dental Therapeutics of the American Dental Association recommends that no more than 264 mg of Sodium Fluoride should be dispensed at one time.[6]

Sodium Fluoride/Vitamin Multi drops should be dispersed in the original plastic container, since contact with glass leads to instability and precipitation. (The amount of Sodium Fluoride in the 50-mL size is well below the maximum to be dispensed at one time according to recommendations of the American Dental Association.)

ADVERSE REACTIONS

Allergic rash and other idiosyncrasies have been rarely reported.

DOSAGE AND ADMINISTRATION

One tablet daily or as prescribed. 1.0 mL daily or as prescribed. May be dropped directly into mouth with a dropper or mixed with cereal, fruit juice or other food. *Use full dosage.*

REFERENCES

1. Hennon DK, Stookey GK, Muhler JC. The clinical anticariogenic effectiveness of supplementary fluoride-vitamin preparations—Results at the end of three years. J Denistry for Children, January 1966:33:3-12. 2. Hennon DK, Stookey GK, Muhler JC. The clinical anticariogenic effectiveness of supplementary fluoride-vitamin preparation—Results at the end of four years. J. Dentistry for Children, November 1967:34:439-449. 3. Hennon DK, Stookey GK, Muhler JC: The clinical anticariogenic effectiveness of supplementary fluoride-vitamin preparations—Results at the end of five and a half years. Pher and Ther in Dent 1970:1:1. 4. Brudevold F., McCann HG. Fluoride and caries control—Mechanism of action. In: Nizel AE, ed, The Science of Nutrition and Its Application in Clinical Dentistry. Philadelphia: WB Saunders Co: 1966:331-347. 5. American Academy of Pediatrics Committee on Nutrition: Fluoride supplementation. Pediatrics. 1988:77:768. 6. Council on Dental Therapeutics. Am Dental Assoc. Accepted Dental Therapeutics. 1977, 37th ed, p 294.

HOW SUPPLIED
CHEW TABLET: 0.25 MG

BRAND/MANUFACTURER	NDC	SIZE	AWP
○ **BRAND**			
▶ POLY-VI-FLOR: Mead Johnson Nutr	00087-0487-41	100s	$14.99

CHEW TABLET: 0.5 MG

BRAND/MANUFACTURER	NDC	SIZE	AWP
○ **BRAND**			
▶ POLY-VI-FLOR: Mead Johnson Nutr	00087-0468-41	100s	$14.99
○ **GENERICS**			
Allscrips	54569-3372-00	60s	$2.49
UNI MULTI FLUOR: URL	00677-1080-01	100s	$3.30
Copley	38245-0158-10	100s	$3.40
Moore,H.L.	00839-6589-06	100s	$3.44
Geneva	00781-1994-01	100s	$3.46
Qualitest	00603-4711-21	100s	$3.51
Schein	00364-1157-01	100s	$3.65
Amide	52152-0031-02	100s	$3.95
Allscrips	54569-3372-01	100s	$4.15
MULTI-VITE-FLOR: Parmed	00349-2044-01	100s	$4.40
POLYTABS-F: Major	00904-2683-60	100s	$4.65
Goldline	00182-1819-01	100s	$4.95
Balan,J.J.	00304-0810-01	100s	$4.98
Rugby	00536-4312-01	100s	$5.46
FLORVITE: Everett	00642-0081-10	100s	$11.15
Amide	52152-0031-05	1000s	$29.95
Balan,J.J.	00304-0810-00	1000s	$31.98
Copley	38245-0158-20	1000s	$33.00
Qualitest	00603-4711-32	1000s	$33.70
Rugby	00536-4312-10	1000s	$41.07
POLYTABS-F: Major	00904-2683-80	1000s	$41.95

For additional alternatives, turn to the section beginning on page 2859.

Sodium Hyaluronate

DESCRIPTION

Sodium Hyaluronate Viscoelastic Solution is a sterile, nonpyrogenic, viscoelastic preparation of a highly purified, noninflammatory, fraction of Sodium Hyaluronate. Sodium Hyaluronate contains 30 mg/mL of Sodium Hyaluronate, dissolved in a physiological balanced salt solution (pH 7.0 to 7.5). This polymer is made up of repeating disaccharide units of N-acetylglucosamine and sodium glucuronate linked by glycosidic bonds.

Sodium Hyaluronate is a physiological substance that is widely distributed in the extra-cellular matrix of connective tissues in both animals and man. For example, it is present in the vitreous and aqueous humor of the eye, the synovial fluid, the skin and the umbilical cord. Sodium Hyaluronates prepared from various human and animal tissues are not chemically different from each other.

Sodium Hyaluronate has been developed as an ophthalmic surgical aid for use in anterior segment surgery.

INDICATIONS

Sodium Hyaluronate is indicated for use as a surgical aid in the following ophthalmic surgical procedures:

- Cataract surgery with an intraocular lens
- Cataract surgery without an intraocular lens
- Secondary intraocular lens implantation
- Corneal transplant surgery
- Glaucoma filtration surgery

Sodium Hyaluronate aids in filling space left by the loss of ocular fluid or tissues during or after these surgical procedures and reduces endothelial cell damage during these procedures by acting as a protective layer, reducing endothelial trauma from instruments or intraocular lens touch.

CONTRAINDICATIONS

There are no known contraindications for the use of Sodium Hyaluronate other than contraindications for the specific surgical procedure.

APPLICATIONS

1. Cataract Surgery and IOL Implantation: The required amount of Sodium Hyaluronate is slowly infused through a needle or cannula into the anterior chamber. The protective effect of Sodium Hyaluronate as an aid is optimized when the injection is performed prior to cataract extraction and insertion of the IOL and may be performed prior to both intra- and extra-capsular cataract procedures. Sodium Hyaluronate may also be used to coat surgical instruments and the IOL prior to insertion. Additional Sodium Hyaluronate may be injected during surgery to replace any that is lost during manipulation (see *"Precautions"*).

2. Corneal Transplant Surgery: The corneal button is removed and the anterior chamber filled with Sodium Hyaluronate until it is level with the surface of the cornea. The donor graft is then placed on top of the Sodium Hyaluronate and sutured into place. Additional Sodium Hyaluronate can be used as required to aid in the surgical procedure (see *"Precautions"*).

3. Glaucoma Filtration Surgery: Sodium Hyaluronate is injected through a corneal paracentesis to restore and maintain the anterior chamber volume during the performance of the trabeculectomy. Additional Sodium Hyaluronate can be used as required to aid in the surgical procedure (see *"Precautions"*).

PRECAUTIONS

Those precautions normally considered during ophthalmic surgical procedure are recommended. There have been reports of significantly increased intraocular pressure following the use of Sodium Hyaluronate as an ophthalmic surgical aid. For this reason, the following precautions should be considered:

- The intraocular pressure of postoperative patients should be carefully monitored.
- An excess quantity of Sodium Hyaluronate should not be used.
- Sodium Hyaluronate should be removed from the anterior chamber at the end of surgery by irrigation or aspiration.
- If the postoperative intraocular pressure increases above expected values, correcting therapy should be administered.

Denaturation and particulate formation in viscoelastics with the repeated use of a reusable cannula has been reported in some studies. A single use cannula such as the one provided in this package should be used when instilling Sodium Hyaluronate into the eye.

Because Sodium Hyaluronate is a highly purified fraction extracted from avian tissues and may contain minute amounts of protein, the physician should be aware of potential risks of the type that can occur with the injection of biological material.

ADVERSE REACTIONS

The following adverse reactions have been reported following the use of Sodium Hyaluronate: increased intraocular pressure, secondary glaucoma, postoperative inflammatory reactions.

DOSAGE AND ADMINISTRATION

For Intraocular Use:

Store at room temperature: 15 - 30°C (59 - 86°F).

Protect from freezing.

Protect from light.

REFERENCES

1. Bourne, W., Liesegang, T., Walter, R., Illstrup, D: "The effect of sodium hyaluronate on endothelial cell damage during extracapsular cataract extraction and posterior chamber lens implantation," *Am. J. Ophthalmol,* 98:759-762, 1984. 2. Genstler, D., Keates, R.: "Am-Visc in extracapsular cataract extraction, *J. Am. Intraocul. Implant Soc.,* 9:317-320, 1983. 3. Miller, D., Stegmann, R.: "Use of Na-hyaluronate in anterior segment eye surgery," *Am. Intra-Ocular Implant Soc. J.,* 6:13-15, 1980. 4. Richter, W.: "Non-immunogenicity of purified hyaluronic acid preparations tested by passive

cutaneous anaphylaxis," *Int. Arch. All,* 47:211-217, 1974. 5. Richter, W., Ryde, M., Zetterstron, O.: "Non-immunogenicity of a purified sodium hyaluronate preparation in man," *Int. Arch Appl Immun,* 59:45-48, 1979. 6. Swann, D.A.: "Studies on Hyaluronic Acid. 1. The preparation and properties of rooster comb hyaluronic acid." *Blochim, Blophys. Acta,* 156:17-30, 1968.

HOW SUPPLIED
INJECTION:

BRAND/MANUFACTURER	NDC	SIZE	AWP
○ **BRAND**			
HEALON: Pharmacia	00016-0314-40	0.4 ml	$81.25
	00016-0310-55	0.55 ml	$118.75
HEALON YELLOW: Pharmacia	00016-0315-55	0.55 ml	$130.63
HEALON: Pharmacia	00016-0310-85	0.85 ml	$156.25
HEALON YELLOW: Pharmacia	00016-0315-85	0.85 ml	$171.88

INJECTION: 30 MG/ML

BRAND/MANUFACTURER	NDC	SIZE	AWP
○ **BRAND**			
VITRAX: Allergan Optical	00023-6663-05	0.5 ml	$120.00
	00023-6663-65	0.65 ml	$120.00

Sodium Iodide

DESCRIPTION

Sodium Iodide Injection is a sterile, nonpyrogenic solution for use as an additive to solutions for total parenteral nutrition.

Each mL contains:

Sodium Iodide (equivalent to 100 mcg Iodide) ....118 mcg

Following is its chemical structure:

$$Na-I$$

CLINICAL PHARMACOLOGY

Iodine is an integral part of thyroid hormones, triiodothyronine (T_3) and thyroxine (T_4). The hormones regulate basal metabolism. The thyroid function is modulated by hypothalmic-pituitary axis through thyroid-releasing hormone and thyroid-stimulating hormone by negative feed back of thyroxine levels in plasma. The essentiality of iodine in humans and animals is well established. Persistent iodine deficiency results in histological changes in thyroid gland and impaired thyroid function, which may culminate in goiter. Iodine deficiency in early stage in life has been reported to produce cretinism. Published reports on pharmacokinetics of iodine in humans and animals show that absorption of iodine from the gastrointestinal tract is rapid and complete.

Skin and lungs can also absorb iodine. Iodine is utilized as Iodide or iodated organic complexes. On administration Iodide equilibrates in extracellular fluids and although all body cells contain Iodide, it is specifically concentrated by thyroid gland, which, in humans, is estimated to contain 7 to 8 mg total iodine.

Other important organs to take up Iodide are salivary glands and gastric mucosa, and to a lesser extent, choroid plexus, skin, hair, mammary glands and placenta. Iodine in saliva and gastric mucosal secretions is reabsorbed and recycled. The circulating iodine is hormonal thyroxine of which 30 to 70 mcg is protein bound and 0.5 mcg is free thyroxine. The normal plasma inorganic Iodide levels are estimated between 0.5 and 1.5 mcg/100 mL. The major route of excretion is via kidneys. Some excretion of conjugated thyroid hormones takes place via bile.

INDICATIONS AND USAGE

Sodium Iodide Injection is indicated for use as a supplement to intravenous solutions given for total parenteral nutrition (TPN). Administration of Sodium Iodide Injection in TPN solutions helps to prevent depletion of endogenous stores and subsequent deficiency symptoms.

UNLABELED USES

Sodium Iodide is used as an adjunct in the treatment of severe thyrotoxicosis crisis (thyroid storm).

CONTRAINDICATIONS

Sodium Iodide Injection is contraindicated for patients with known hypersensitivity to iodine. Sodium Iodide Injection should not be given undiluted by direct injection into a peripheral vein because of potential for infusion phlebitis.

WARNINGS

Sensitization to Iodides and deaths due to anaphylactic shock following Iodide administration have been reported. The physician must evaluate the patient for hypersensitivity before initiating TPN supplementation with Sodium Iodide Injection.

Sodium Iodide Injection is a hypotonic solution and should be administered in admixtures only.

PRECAUTIONS

As iodine is eliminated in urine, iodine supplements in TPN solutions may be adjusted, reduced or omitted in patients with renal dysfunction.

◆ RATED THERAPEUTICALLY EQUIVALENT; ◇ THERAPEUTIC EQUIVALENCE UNCONFIRMED; ○ UNRATED

Iodine is constituent of several medications and diagnostic compounds, and is reported to be bioavailable from them. If the patients are using such compounds, consideration to their contribution should be given.

Iodine is readily absorbed through skin, lungs and mucous membrane. Consideration should be given to environmental, topical skin disinfection and wound treatment practices with surgical swabs and solutions containing iodine and povidone iodine. Air in the coastal areas is known to contain more iodine than inland areas.

ADVERSE REACTIONS
The amount of iodine present in Sodium Iodide Injection is small. In normal patients (see "Warnings"), symptoms of toxicity from iodine are unlikely to occur at the recommended dosage levels.

Hypersensitivity to Iodides may result in angioneurotic edema, cutaneous and mucosal hemorrhages, fever, arthralgia, lymph-node enlargement and eosinophilia. If patient develops a reaction, TPN supplementation with Sodium Iodide Injection should be immediately withdrawn and appropriate measures taken.

OVERDOSAGE
The symptoms of chronic Iodide poisoning in humans include metallic taste, soreness of the mouth, increased salivation, coryza, sneezing, swelling of the eyelids, severe headache, pulmonary edema, tenderness of salivary glands, acneform skin lesions and skin eruptions.

Abundant fluids and salt intake helps in elimination of Iodides.

DOSAGE AND ADMINISTRATION
Sodium Iodide Injection provides 100 mcg iodine per mL. For the metabolically stable adults receiving TPN, the suggested dosage level is 1 to 2 mcg iodine/kg/day (normal adults 75-150 mcg daily). For pregnant and lactating mothers and growing children, the suggested additive level is 2 to 3 mcg iodine/kg/day. Aseptic addition of Sodium Iodide Injection to TPN solutions under a laminar flow hood is recommended. Iodine is physically compatible with electrolytes and other trace elements usually present in amino-acid/dextrose solutions used for TPN.

Periodic monitoring for thyroid function is suggested as a guideline for adjusting dosage level.

Parenteral drug products should be inspected visually for particulate matter and discoloration prior to administration, whenever solution and container permit.

Store below 30°C (86°F). Do not permit to freeze.

HOW SUPPLIED
INJECTION: 118 MCG/ML

BRAND/MANUFACTURER	NDC	SIZE	AWP
◆ BRAND IODOPEN: Fujisawa	00469-1900-30	10 ml	$9.15

Sodium Lactate

DESCRIPTION
Sodium Lactate Injection is a fluid and electrolyte replenisher and a systemic alkalizer.

Sodium Lactate Injection, USP 50 mEq (5 mEq/mL), is a sterile, nonpyrogenic, concentrated solution of Sodium Lactate in water for injection. The solution is administered after dilution by the intravenous route. **It should not be administered undiluted.** Each 10 mL vial contains Sodium Lactate, anhydrous 5.6 g (50 mEq each of Na^+ and lactate anion). The solution contains no bacteriostat, antimicrobial agent or added buffer. Contains hydrochloric acid for pH adjustment. The osmolar concentration is 10 mOsm/mL (calc.). Sodium Lactate Injection, USP, 1/6 Molar is a sterile, nonpyrogenic, approximately isotonic solution of Sodium Lactate in water for injection for administration by the intravenous route.

The solution represents a one-sixth molar (0.167 M) concentration of Sodium Lactate, a racemic compound prepared by a synthetic route. Each 100 mL contains Sodium Lactate, anhydrous, 1.87 g and provides 167 mEq/liter of sodium (Na^+), 167 mEq/liter of lactate ($C_3H_5O_3$) and 55 calories/liter. The total osmolar concentration is 334 mOsmol/liter (calc.) which is slightly hypertonic in relation to the extracellular fluid (280 mOsmol/liter).

The solution contains no bacteriostat, antimicrobial agents or (except for pH adjustment) and is intended only as a single-dose injection. When smaller doses are required the unused portion should be discarded.

In a 1/6 molar solution or when diluted with water for injection to make a 1/6 molar solution, the pH of sodium lactate injection is 6.0 to 7.3.

Sodium Lactate, USP is chemically designated CH₃CH(OH)COONa, a 60% aqueous solution miscible in water.

Each single dose unit contains:

Sodium Lactate 50 meg (4 mEq/ml)	10 ml
Sodium Lactate 1/6 Molar	500 ml
Sodium Lactate 1/6 Molar	1000 ml

or

Each single dose vial of Sodium Lactate Injection 50 mEq contains:

Sodium Lactate	10 ml

Each single dose flexible plastic container of Sodium Lactate Injection 1/6 molar contains:

Sodium Lactate	500 ml or 1000 ml

CLINICAL PHARMACOLOGY
Lactate anion ($CH_3CH(OH)COO^-$) serves the import purpose of providing "raw material" for subsequent regneration of bicarbonate (HCO_3^-) and thus acts as a source (alternate) of bicarbonate when normal production and utilization of lactic acid is not impaired as a result of disordered lactate metabolism. Lactate anion is usually present in extracellular fluid at a level of less than 1 mEq/liter, but may attain a level of 10 mEq/liter during exercise. It is seldom measured as such as thus is one of the "unmeasured anions" ("anion gap") in determinations of the ionic composition of plasma.

Since metabolic conversion of lactate to bicarbonate is dependent on the integrity of cellular oxidative processes, lactate may be inadeauate or ineffective as a source of bicarbonate in patients suffering from acidosis associated with shock or other disorders involving reduced perfusion of body tissues. When oxidative activity is intact, one to two hours time is required for conversion of lactate to bicarbonate.

The lactate anion is in equilibrium with pyruvate and has an alkalizing effect resulting from simultaneous removal by the liver of lactate and hydrogen ions. In the liver, lactate is metabolized to glycogen which is ultimately converted to carbon dioxide and water by oxidative metabolism.

The sodium (Na^+) ion combines with bicarbonate ion produced from carbon dioxide of the body and thus retains bicarbonate to combat metabolic acidosis (bicarbonate deficiency). The normal plasma level of lactate ranges from 0.9 to 1.9 mEq/liter.

Sodium is the principal cation of extracellular fluid. It comprises more than 90% of total cations at its normal plasma concentration of approximately 140 mEq/liter. The sodium ion exerts a primary role in controlling total body water and its distribution.

INDICATIONS AND USAGE
Sodium Lactate Injection, USP 50 mEq (5 mEq/mL) (after dilution) and 1/6 molar are primarily indicated as a source of bicarbonate for prevention or control of mild to moderate metabolic acidosis in patients with restricted oral intake whose oxidative processes are not seriously impaired. It is not intended nor effective for correcting severe acidotic states which require immediate restoration of plasma bicarbonate levels. Sodium lactate has no advantage over sodium bicarbonate and may be detrimental in the management of lactic acidosis.

UNLABELED USES
Sodium Lactate is used alone or as an adjunct in the treatment of hypovolemia, urolithiasis, and panic disorder with or without agoraphobia.

CONTRAINDICATIONS
Sodium Lactate Injection is contraindicated in patients suffering from hypernatremia or fluid retention.

It should not be used in conditions in which lactate levels are increased (e.g., shock, congestive heart failure, respiratory alkalosis) or in which utilization of lactate is diminished (e.g., anoxia, beriberi).

NOT FOR USE IN THE TREATMENT OF LACTIC ACIDOSIS.

WARNINGS
Solutions containing sodium ions should be used with great care, if at all, in patients with congestive heart failure, severe renal insufficiency and in clinical states in which there exists edema with sodium retention.

In patients with diminished renal function, administration of solutions containing sodium ions may result in sodium retention.

The intravenous administration of this solution (after appropriate dilution when necessary) can cause fluid and/or solute overloading resulting in dilution of other serum electrolyte concentrations, overhydration, congested states or pulmonary edema. The risk of dilutional states is inversely proportional to the electrolyte concentrations of administration parenteral solutions.

The risk of solute overload causing congested states with peripheral and pulmonary edema is directly proportional to the electrolyte concentrations of such solutions.

Excessive administration of potassium-free solutions may result in significant hypokalemia.

PRECAUTIONS
Clinical evaluation and periodic laboratory determinations are necessary to monitor changes in fluid balance, electrolyte concentrations and acid-base balance during prolonged parenteral therapy or whenever the condition of the patient warrants such evaluation.

Sodium Lactate Injection, USP 50 mEq must be suitably diluted before infusion to avoid a sudden increase in the level of sodium or lactate. Too rapid administration and overdosage should be avoided.

The potentially large loads of sodium given with lactate require that caution be exercised in patients with congestive heart failure or other edematous or sodium-retaining states, as well as in patients with oliguria or anuria.

Solutions containing lactate ions should be used with caution as excess administration may result in metabolic alkalosis.

Do not administer unless solution is clear and seal is intact or container is undamaged. Discard unused portion.

Pregnancy Category C: Animal reproduction studies have not been conducted with Sodium Lactate. It is also not known whether Sodium Lactate can cause fetal harm when administered to a pregnant woman or can affect reproduction capacity. Sodium Lactate should be given to a pregnant woman only if clearly needed.

Additives may be incompatible. Consult with pharmacist, if available. When introducing additives, use aseptic technique, mix thoroughly and do not store.

Caution must be exercised in the administration of parenteral fluids, especially those containing sodium ions, to patients receiving corticosteroids or corticotropin.

ADVERSE REACTIONS

Reactions which may occur because of the solution or the technique of administration include febrile response, infection at the site of injection, venous thrombosis or phlebitis extending from the site of injection, extravasation and hypovolemia.

Adverse effects of Sodium Lactate are essentially limited to overdosage of either sodium or lactate ions. See "Warnings" and "Precautions".

If an adverse reaction does occur, discontinue the infusion, evaluate the patient, institute appropriate therapeutic countermeasures and save the remainder of the fluid for examination, if deemed necessary.

OVERDOSAGE

In the event of overhydration or overdosage, discontinue infusion containing Sodium Lactate immediately and institute corrective therapy as indicated to reduce elevated serum sodium levels and restore acid-base balance if necessary. See "Warnings" and "Precautions", and "Adverse Reactions".

DOSAGE AND ADMINISTRATION

The dose is dependent upon the age, weight and clinical condition of the patient.

Sodium Lactate Injection, USP 50 mEq (5 mEq/mL) is administered intravenously only after addition to a larger volume of fluid. The amount of sodium ion and lactate ion to be added to larger volume intravenous fluids should be determined in accordance with the electrolyte requirements of each individual patient.

All or part of the content(s) of one (50 mEq in 10 mL) or more vial containers may be added to other intravenous solutions to provide any desired number of milliequivalents of lactate anion (with the same number of milliequivalents of Na$^+$). The contents of one container (50 mEq in 10 mL) added to 290 mL of a nonelectrolyte solution or of sterile water for injection will provide 300 mL of an approximately isotonic (1/6 molar) concentration of sodium lactate (1.9%), containing 167 mEq/liter each of Na$^+$ and lactate anion.

Parenteral drug products should be inspected visually for particulate matter and discoloration prior to administration. See "Precautions".

Store Sodium Lactate Injection 50 mEq at controlled room temperature 15° to 30°C (59° to 86°F). Store Sodium Lactate Injection 1/6 molar at room temperature (25°C). Avoid excessive heat. Protect from freezing.

HOW SUPPLIED
INJECTION:

AVERAGE UNIT PRICE (AVAILABLE SIZES)			
GENERIC		$0.02	

BRAND/MANUFACTURER	NDC	SIZE	AWP
◆ **GENERICS**			
McGaw	00264-7810-00	1000 ml	$17.78
Baxter	00338-0129-04	1000 ml 12s	$215.71
Baxter	00338-0129-03	500 ml 24s	$341.28

INJECTION: 5 MEQ/ML

BRAND/MANUFACTURER	NDC	SIZE	AWP
◆ **GENERICS**			
Fujisawa	00469-3750-30	10 ml	$2.99

INJECTION: 50 MEQ

BRAND/MANUFACTURER	NDC	SIZE	AWP
◆ **GENERICS**			
Abbott Hosp	00074-6664-02	10 ml 25s	$119.64

INJECTION: 167 MEQ/1,000 ML

AVERAGE UNIT PRICE (AVAILABLE SIZES)			
GENERIC		$0.02	

BRAND/MANUFACTURER	NDC	SIZE	AWP
◆ **GENERICS**			
Abbott Hosp	00074-7987-09	1000 ml 12s	$219.88
Abbott Hosp	00074-7987-03	500 ml 24s	$347.99

Sodium Nitroprusside

AFTER RECONSTITUTION WITH APPROPRIATE DILUENT, STERILE SODIUM NITROPRUSSIDE, USP IS NOT SUITABLE FOR DIRECT INJECTION. THE RECONSTITUTED SOLUTION MUST BE FURTHER DILUTED IN STERILE 5% DEXTROSE INJECTION BEFORE INFUSION.

STERILE SODIUM NITROPRUSSIDE, USP CAN CAUSE PRECIPITOUS DECREASES IN BLOOD PRESSURE (SEE "DOSAGE AND ADMINISTRATION"). IN PATIENTS NOT PROPERLY MONITORED, THESE DECREASES CAN LEAD TO IRREVERSIBLE ISCHEMIC INJURIES OR DEATH. SODIUM NITROPRUSSIDE SHOULD BE USED ONLY WHEN AVAILABLE EQUIPMENT AND PERSONNEL ALLOW BLOOD PRESSURE TO BE CONTINUOUSLY MONITORED.

EXCEPT WHEN USED BRIEFLY OR AT LOW (< 2 μG/KG/MIN) INFUSION RATES, SODIUM NITROPRUSSIDE GIVES RISE TO IMPORTANT QUANTITIES OF CYANIDE ION, WHICH CAN REACH TOXIC, POTENTIALLY LETHAL LEVELS (SEE "WARNINGS"). THE USUAL DOSE RATE IS 0.5 - 10 μG/KG/MIN, BUT INFUSION AT THE MAXIMUM DOSE RATE SHOULD NEVER LAST MORE THAN 10 MINUTES. IF BLOOD PRESSURE HAS NOT BEEN ADEQUATELY CONTROLLED AFTER 10 MINUTES OF INFUSION AT THE MAXIMUM RATE, ADMINISTRATION OF SODIUM NITROPRUSSIDE SHOULD BE TERMINATED IMMEDIATELY.

ALTHOUGH ACID-BASE BALANCE AND VENOUS OXYGEN CONCENTRATION SHOULD BE MONITORED AND MAY INDICATE CYANIDE TOXICITY, THESE LABORATORY TESTS PROVIDE IMPERFECT GUIDANCE.

THIS PACKAGE INSERT SHOULD BE THOROUGHLY REVIEWED BEFORE ADMINISTRATION OF STERILE SODIUM NITROPRUSSIDE, USP.

DESCRIPTION

Sodium Nitroprusside is disodium pentacyanonitrosylferrate(2-)dihydrate, an inorganic hypotensive agent. Its molecular formula is $Na_2[Fe(CN)_5NO] \cdot 2H_2O$ and molecular weight is 297.95.

Dry Sodium Nitroprusside is a reddish-brown powder, soluble in water. In an aqueous solution infused intravenously, Sodium Nitroprusside is a rapid-acting vasodilator, active on both arteries and veins.

Sodium Nitroprusside solution is rapidly degraded by trace contaminants, often with resulting color changes. (See "Dosage and Administration".) The solution is also sensitive to certain wavelengths of light, and it must be protected from light in clinical use.

Each 5 mL *Single Use* vial contains the equivalent of 50 mg of Sodium Nitroprusside dihydrate.

Following is its chemical structure:

CH₂OH
H-C-OH
O
=O
NaO   OH

CLINICAL PHARMACOLOGY

The principal pharmacological action of Sodium Nitroprusside is relaxation of vascular smooth muscle and consequent dilatation of peripheral arteries and veins. Other smooth muscle (e.g., uterus, duodenum) is not affected. Sodium Nitroprusside is more active on veins than on arteries, but this selectivity is much less marked than that of nitroglycerin. Dilatation of the veins promotes peripheral pooling of blood and decreases venous return to the heart, thereby reducing left ventricular end-diastolic pressure and pulmonary capillary wedge pressure (preload). Arteriolar relaxation reduces systemic vascular resistance, systolic arterial pressure and mean arterial pressure (afterload). Dilatation of the coronary arteries also occurs.

In association with the decrease in blood pressure, Sodium Nitroprusside administered intravenously to hypertensive and normotensive patients produces slight increases in heart rate and a variable effect on cardiac output. In hypertensive patients, moderate doses induce renal vasodilation roughly proportional to the decrease in systemic blood pressure, so there is no appreciable change in renal blood flow or glomerular filtration rate.

In normotensive subjects, acute reduction of mean arterial pressure to 60 - 75 mm Hg by infusion of Sodium Nitroprusside caused a significant increase in renin activity. In the same study, ten renovascular-hypertensive patients given Sodium Nitroprusside had significant increases in renin release from the involved kidney at mean arterial pressures of 90 - 137 mm Hg.

The hypotensive effect of Sodium Nitroprusside is seen within a minute or two after the start of an adequate infusion, and it dissipates almost as rapidly after an infusion is discontinued. The effect is augmented by ganglionic blocking agents and inhaled anesthetics.

PHARMACOKINETICS AND METABOLISM

Infused Sodium Nitroprusside is rapidly distributed to a volume that is approximately coextensive with the extracellular space. The drug is cleared from this volume by intraerythrocytic reaction with hemoglobin (Hgb), and Sodium Nitroprusside's resulting circulatory half-life is about 2 minutes.

The products of the Nitroprusside/hemoglobin reaction are cyanmethemoglobin (cyanmetHgb) and cyanide ion (CN$^-$). Safe use of Sodium Nitroprusside injection must be guided by knowledge of the further metabolism of these products.

As shown in the diagram below, the essential features of Nitroprusside metabolism are:

■ one molecule of Sodium Nitroprusside is metabolized by combination with hemoglobin to produce one molecule of cyanmethemoglobin and four CN^- ions;
■ methemoglobin, obtained from hemoglobin, can sequester cyanide as cyanmethemoglobin;
■ thiosulfate reacts with cyanide to produce thiocyanate;
■ thiocyanate is eliminated in the urine;
■ cyanide not otherwise removed binds to cytochromes; and
■ cyanide is much more toxic than methemoglobin or thiocyanate.

Metabolism of Sodium Nitroprusside

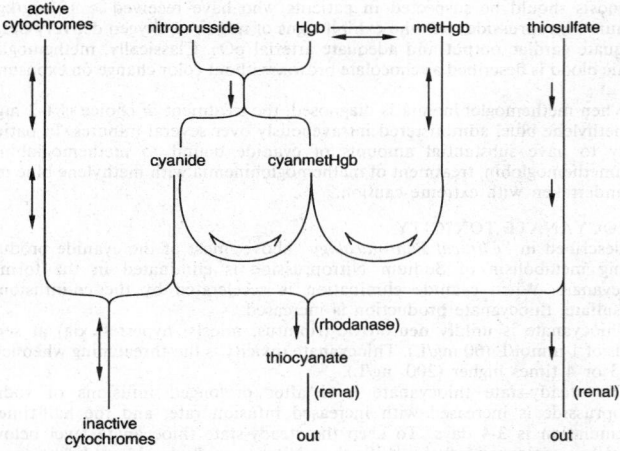

Cyanide ion is normally found in serum; it is derived from dietary substrates and from tobacco smoke. Cyanide binds avidly (but reversibly) to ferric ion (Fe^{+++}), most body stores of which are found in erythrocyte methemoglobin (metHgb) and in mitochondrial cytochromes. When CN^- is infused or generated within the bloodstream, essentially all of it is bound to methemoglobin until intraerythrocytic methemoglobin has been saturated.

When the Fe^{++} of cytochromes is bound to cyanide, the cytochromes are unable to participate in oxidative metabolism. In this situation, cells may be able to provide for their energy needs by utilizing anaerobic pathways, but they thereby generate an increasing body burden of lactic acid. Other cells may be unable to utilize these alternate pathways and they may die hypoxic deaths.

CN^- levels in packed erythrocytes are typically less than 1 µmol/L (less than 25 µg/L); levels are roughly doubled in heavy smokers.

At healthy steady state, most people have less than 1% of their hemoglobin in the form of methemoglobin. Nitroprusside metabolism can lead to methemoglobin formation (a) through dissociation of cyanmethemoglobin formed in the original reaction of Sodium Nitroprusside with Hgb and (b) by direct oxidation of Hgb by the released nitroso group. Relatively large quantities of Sodium Nitroprusside, however, are required to produce significant methemoglobinemia.

At physiologic methemoglobin levels, the CN^- binding capacity of packed red cells is a little less than 200 µmol/L (5 mg/L). Cytochrome toxicity is seen at levels only slightly higher, and death has been reported at levels from 300 to 3000 µmol/L (8-80 mg/L). Put another way, a patient with a normal red cell mass (35 mL/kg) and normal methemoglobin levels can buffer about 175 µg/kg of CN^-, corresponding to a little less than 500 µg/kg of infused Sodium Nitroprusside. Some cyanide is eliminated from the body as expired hydrogen cyanide, but most is enzymatically converted to thiocyanate (SCN^-) by thiosulfate-cyanide sulfur transferase (rhodanese, EC 2.8.1.1), a mitochondrial enzyme. The enzyme is normally present in great excess, so the reaction is rate-limited by the availability of sulfur donors, especially thiosulfate, cystine and cysteine.

Thiosulfate is a normal constituent of serum, produced from cysteine by way of β-mercaptopyruvate. Physiological levels of thiosulfate are typically about 0.1 mmol/L (11 mg/L), but they are approximately twice this level in children and in adults who are not eating. Infused thiosulfate is cleared from the body (primarily by the kidneys) with a half-life of about 20 minutes. When thiosulfate is being supplied only by normal physiologic mechanisms, conversion of CN^- to SCN^- generally proceeds at about 1 µg/kg/min. This rate of CN^- clearance corresponds to steady-state processing of a Sodium Nitroprusside infusion of slightly more than 2 µg/kg/min. CN^- begins to accumulate when Sodium Nitroprusside infusions exceed this rate.

Thiocyanate (SCN^-) is also a normal physiological constituent of serum, with normal levels typically in the range of 50-250 µmol/L (3-15 mg/L). Clearance of SCN^- is primarily renal, with half-life of about 3 days. In renal failure, the half-life can be doubled or tripled.

Clinical Trials: Baseline-controlled clinical trials have uniformly shown that Sodium Nitroprusside has a prompt hypotensive effect, at least initially, in all populations. With increasing rates of infusion, Sodium Nitroprusside has been able to lower blood pressure without an observed limit of effect.

Clinical trials have also shown that the hypotensive effect of Sodium Nitroprusside is associated with reduced blood loss in a variety of major surgical procedures.

In patients with acute congestive heart failure and increased peripheral vascular resistance, administration of Sodium Nitroprusside causes reductions in peripheral resistance, increases in cardiac output and reductions in left ventricular filling pressure.

Many trials have verified the clinical significance of the metabolic pathways described above. In patients receiving unopposed infusions of Sodium Nitroprusside, cyanide and thiocyanate levels have increased with increasing rates of Sodium Nitroprusside infusion. Mild to moderate metabolic acidosis has usually accompanied higher cyanide levels, but peak base deficits have lagged behind the peak cyanide levels by an hour or more.

Progressive tachyphylaxis to the hypotensive effects of Sodium Nitroprusside has been reported in several trials and numerous case reports. This tachyphylaxis has frequently been attributed to concomitant cyanide toxicity, but the only evidence adduced for this assertion has been the observation that in patients treated with Sodium Nitroprusside and found to be resistant to its hypotensive effects, cyanide levels are often found to be elevated. In the only reported *comparisons* of cyanide levels in resistant and nonresistant patients, cyanide levels did *not* correlate with tachyphylaxis. The mechanism of tachyphylaxis to Sodium Nitroprusside remains unknown.

INDICATIONS AND USAGE

Sodium Nitroprusside is indicated for the immediate reduction of blood pressure of patients in hypertensive crises. Concomitant longer-acting antihypertensive medication should be administered so that the duration of treatment with Sodium Nitroprusside can be minimized.

Sodium Nitroprusside is also indicated for producing controlled hypotension in order to reduce bleeding during surgery. Sodium Nitroprusside is also indicated for the treatment of acute congestive heart failure.

UNLABELED USES
Sodium Nitroprusside is used alone or as an adjunct in the treatment of pulmonary hypertension and acute myocardial infarction.

CONTRAINDICATIONS

Sodium Nitroprusside should not be used in the treatment of compensatory hypertension, where the primary hemodynamic lesion is aortic coarctation or arteriovenous shunting.

Sodium Nitroprusside should not be used to produce hypotension during surgery in patients with known inadequate cerebral circulation, or in moribund patients (A.S.A. Class 5E) coming to emergency surgery.

Patients with congenital (Leber's) optic atrophy or with tobacco amblyopia have unusually high cyanide/thiocyanate ratios. These rare conditions are probably associated with defective or absent rhodanese, and Sodium Nitroprusside should be avoided in these patients.

Sodium Nitroprusside should not be used for the treatment of acute congestive heart failure associated with reduced peripheral vascular resistance such as high-output heart failure that may be seen in endotoxic sepsis.

WARNINGS

(See also the boxed *"Warning"* at the beginning of this prescribing information.)

The principal hazards of Nitroprusside administration are excessive hypotension and excessive accumulation of cyanide (see also *"Overdosage"* and *"Dosage and Administration"*).

EXCESSIVE HYPOTENSION
Small transient excesses in the infusion rate of Sodium Nitroprusside can result in excessive hypotension, sometimes to levels so low as to compromise the perfusion of vital organs. These hemodynamic changes may lead to a variety of associated symptoms (see *"Adverse Reactions"*). Nitroprusside-induced hypotension will be self-limited within 1-10 minutes after discontinuation of the Nitroprusside infusion; during these few minutes, it may be helpful to put the patient into a head-down (Trendelenburg) position to maximize venous return. If hypotension persists more than a few minutes after discontinuation of the infusion of Sterile Sodium Nitroprusside, USP, then Nitroprusside is not the cause and the true cause must be sought.

CYANIDE TOXICITY
As described in *"Clinical Pharmacology"* above, Sodium Nitroprusside infusions at rates above 2 µg/kg/min generate cyanide ion (CN^-) faster than the body can normally dispose of it. (When sodium thiosulfate is given, as described under *"Dosage and Administration"*, the body's capacity for CN^- elimination is greatly increased.) Methemoglobin normally present in the body can buffer a certain amount of CN^-, but the capacity of this system is exhausted by the CN^- produced from about 500 µg/kg of Sodium Nitroprusside. This amount of Sodium Nitroprusside is administered in less than an hour when the drug is administered at 10 µg/kg/min (the maximum recommended rate). Thereafter, the toxic effects of CN^- may be rapid, serious and even lethal.

The true rates of clinically important cyanide toxicity cannot be assessed from spontaneous reports or published data. Most patients reported to have experienced such toxicity have received relatively prolonged infusions, and the only patients whose deaths have been unequivocally attributed to Nitroprusside-induced cyanide toxicity have been patients who had received Nitroprusside infusions at rates (30-120 µg/kg/min) much greater than those now recommended.

Elevated cyanide levels, metabolic acidosis and marked clinical deterioration, however, have occasionally been reported in patients who received infusions at recommended rates for only a few hours and even, in one case, for only 35 minutes. In some of these cases, infusion of sodium thiosulfate caused dramatic clinical improvement, supporting the diagnosis of cyanide toxicity.

Cyanide toxicity may manifest itself as venous hyperoxemia with bright red venous blood, as cells become unable to extract the oxygen delivered to them; metabolic (lactic) acidosis; air hunger; confusion and death. Cyanide toxicity due to causes other than Nitroprusside has been associated with angina pectoris and myocardial infarction; ataxia, seizures and stroke; and other diffuse ischemic damage.

Hypertensive patients, and patients concomitantly receiving other antihypertensive medications, may be more sensitive to the effects of Sodium Nitroprusside than normal subjects.

PRECAUTIONS

GENERAL
Like other vasodilators, Sodium Nitroprusside can cause increases in intracranial pressure. In patients whose intracranial pressure is already elevated, Sodium Nitroprusside should be used only with extreme caution.

HEPATIC
Use caution when administering Nitroprusside to patients with hepatic insufficiency.

USE IN ANESTHESIA
When Sodium Nitroprusside (or any other vasodilator) is used for controlled hypotension during anesthesia, the patient's capacity to compensate for anemia and hypovolemia may be diminished. If possible, pre-existing anemia and hypovolemia should be corrected prior to administration of Sterile Sodium Nitroprusside, USP.

Hypotensive anesthetic techniques may also cause abnormalities of the pulmonary ventilation/perfusion ratio. Patients intolerant of these abnormalities may require a higher fraction of inspired oxygen.

Extreme caution should be exercised in patients who are especially poor surgical risks (A.S.A. Class 4 and 4E).

LABORATORY TESTS
The cyanide-level assay is technically difficult, and cyanide levels in body fluids other than packed red blood cells are difficult to interpret. Cyanide toxicity will lead to lactic acidosis and venous hyperoxemia, but these findings may not be present until an hour or more after the cyanide capacity of the body's red-cell mass has been exhausted.

DRUG INTERACTIONS
The hypotensive effect of Sodium Nitroprusside is augmented by that of most other hypotensive drugs, including ganglionic blocking agents, negative inotropic agents and inhaled anesthetics.

CARCINOGENESIS, MUTAGENESIS, IMPAIRMENT OF FERTILITY
Animal studies assessing Sodium Nitroprusside's carcinogenicity and mutagenicity have not been conducted. Similarly, Sodium Nitroprusside has not been tested for effects on fertility.

PREGNANCY
Teratogenic Effects: Pregnancy Category C: There are no adequate, well-controlled studies of Sterile Sodium Nitroprusside, USP in either laboratory animals or pregnant women. It is not known whether Nitroprusside can cause fetal harm when administered to a pregnant woman or can affect reproductive capacity. Sterile Sodium Nitroprusside, USP should be given to a pregnant woman only if clearly needed.

Nonteratogenic Effects: In three studies in pregnant ewes, Nitroprusside was shown to cross the placental barrier. Fetal cyanide levels were shown to be dose-related to maternal levels of Nitroprusside. The metabolic transformation of sodium Nitroprusside given to pregnant ewes led to fatal levels of cyanide in the fetuses. The infusion of 25 µg/kg/min of Sodium Nitroprusside for one hour in pregnant ewes resulted in the death of all fetuses. Pregnant ewes infused with 1 µg/kg/min of Sodium Nitroprusside for one hour delivered normal lambs.

According to one investigator, a pregnant woman at 24 weeks gestation was given Sodium Nitroprusside to control gestational hypertension secondary to mitral valve disease. Sodium Nitroprusside was infused at 3.9 mcg/kg/min for a total of 3.5 mg/kg over 15 hours prior to delivery of a 478 gram stillborn infant without any obvious anomalies. Cyanide levels in the fetal liver were less than 10 mcg/mL. Toxic levels have been reported to be more than 30-40 mcg/mL. The mother demonstrated no cyanide toxicity.

The effects of administering Sodium Thiosulfate in pregnancy, either by itself or as a co-infusion with Sodium Nitroprusside, are completely unknown.

NURSING MOTHERS
It is not known whether Sodium Nitroprusside and its metabolites are excreted in human milk. Because many drugs are excreted in human milk and because of the potential for serious adverse reactions in nursing infants from Sodium Nitroprusside, a decision should be made whether to discontinue nursing or to discontinue the drug, taking into account the importance of the drug to the mother.

PEDIATRIC USE
See *"Dosage and Administration"*.

ADVERSE REACTIONS
The most important adverse reactions to Sodium Nitroprusside are the avoidable ones of excessive hypotension and cyanide toxicity, described under *"Warnings"*. The adverse reactions described in this section develop less rapidly and, as it happens, less commonly.

METHEMOGLOBINEMIA
As described in *"Clinical Pharmacology"* above, Sodium Nitroprusside infusions can cause sequestration of hemoglobin as methemoglobin. The back-conversion process is normally rapid, and clinically significant methemoglobinemia (>10%) is seen only rarely in patients receiving Sterile Sodium Nitroprusside, USP. Even patients congenitally incapable of back-converting methemoglobin should demonstrate 10% methemoglobinemia only after they have received about 10 mg/kg of Sodium Nitroprusside, and a patient receiving Sodium Nitroprusside at the maximum recommended rate (10 µg/kg/min) would take over 16 hours to reach this total accumulated dose.

Methemoglobin levels can be measured by most clinical laboratories. The diagnosis should be suspected in patients who have received > 10 mg/kg of Sodium Nitroprusside and who exhibit signs of impaired oxygen delivery despite adequate cardiac output and adequate arterial pO_2. Classically, methemoglobinemic blood is described as chocolate brown, without color change on exposure to air.

When methemoglobinemia is diagnosed, the treatment of choice is 1-2 mg/kg of methylene blue, administered intravenously over several minutes. In patients likely to have substantial amounts of cyanide bound to methemoglobin as cyanmethemoglobin, treatment of methemoglobinemia with methylene blue must be undertaken with extreme caution.

THIOCYANATE TOXICITY
As described in *"Clinical Pharmacology"* above, most of the cyanide produced during metabolism of Sodium Nitroprusside is eliminated in the form of thiocyanate. When cyanide elimination is accelerated by the co-infusion of thiosulfate, thiocyanate production is increased.

Thiocyanate is mildly neurotoxic (tinnitus, miosis, hyperreflexia) at serum levels of 1 mmol/L (60 mg/L). Thiocyanate toxicity is life-threatening when levels are 3 or 4 times higher (200 mg/L).

The steady-state thiocyanate level after prolonged infusions of sodium nitroprusside is increased with increased infusion rate, and the half-time of accumulation is 3-4 days. To keep the steady-state thiocyanate level below 1 mmol/L, a prolonged infusion of Sodium Nitroprusside should not be more rapid than 3 µ/kg/min; in anuric patients, the corresponding limits is just 1 µg/kg/min. When prolonged infusions are more rapid than these, thiocyanate levels should be measured daily. Physiologic maneuvers (e.g., those that alter the pH of the urine) are not known to increase the elimination of thiocyanate. Thiocyanate clearance rates during dialysis, on the other hand, can approach the blood flow rate of the dialyzer.

Thiocyanate interferes with iodine uptake by the thyroid.

Abdominal pain, apprehension, diaphoresis, "dizziness", headache, muscle twitching, nausea, palpitations, restlessness, retching and retrosternal discomfort have been noted when the blood pressure was too rapidly reduced. These symptoms quickly disappeared when the infusion was slowed or discontinued, and they did not reappear with a continued (or resumed) slower infusion.

Other adverse reactions reported are—

Cardiovascular: Bradycardia, electrocardiographic changes, tachycardia.

Dermatologic: Rash.

Endocrine: Hypothyroidism.

Gastrointestinal: Ileus.

Hematologic: Decreased platelet aggregation.

Neurologic: Increased intracranial pressure.

Miscellaneous: Flushing, venous streaking, irritation of the infusion site.

OVERDOSAGE
Overdosage of Nitroprusside can be manifested as excessive hypotension or cyanide toxicity (see *"Warnings"*) or as thiocyanate toxicity (see *"Adverse Reactions"*).

The acute intravenous mean lethal doses (LD_{50}) of Nitroprusside in rabbits, dogs, mice and rats are 2.8, 5.0, 8.4 and 11.2 mg/kg, respectively.

TREATMENT OF CYANIDE TOXICITY
Cyanide levels can be measured by many laboratories, and blood-gas studies that can detect venous hyperoxemia or acidosis are widely available. **Acidosis may not appear until more than an hour after the appearance of dangerous cyanide levels, and laboratory tests should not be awaited. Reasonable suspicion of cyanide toxicity is adequate grounds for initiation of treatment.**

Treatment of cyanide toxicity consists of:

■ discontinuing the administration of Sodium Nitroprusside;
■ providing a buffer for cyanide by using sodium nitrite to convert as much hemoglobin into methemoglobin as the patient can safely tolerate; and then
■ infusing sodium thiosulfate in sufficient quantity to convert the cyanide into thiocyanate.

The necessary medications for this treatment are contained in commercially available Cyanide Antidote Kits. Alternatively, discrete stocks of medications can be used.

◆ RATED THERAPEUTICALLY EQUIVALENT; ◇ THERAPEUTIC EQUIVALENCE UNCONFIRMED; ○ UNRATED

Hemodialysis is ineffective in removal of cyanide, but it will eliminate most thiocyanate.

Cyanide Antidote Kits contain both amyl nitrite and sodium nitrite for induction of methemoglobinemia. The amyl nitrite is supplied in the form of inhalant ampuls, for administration in environments where intravenous administration of sodium nitrite may be delayed. In a patient who already has a patent intravenous line, use of amyl nitrite confers no benefit that is not provided by infusion of sodium nitrite.

Sodium nitrite is available in a 3% solution, and 4-6 mg/kg (about 0.2 mL/kg) should be injected over 2-4 minutes. This dose can be expected to convert about 10% of the patient's hemoglobin into methemoglobin; this level of methemoglobinemia is not associated with any important hazard of its own. The nitrite infusion may cause transient vasodilatation and hypotension, and this hypotension must, if it occurs, be routinely managed.

Immediately after infusion of the sodium nitrite, sodium thiosulfate should be infused. This agent is available in 10% and 25% solutions, and the recommended dose is 150-200 mg/kg; a typical adult dose is 50 mL of the 25% solution. Thiosulfate treatment of an acutely cyanide-toxic patient will raise thiocyanate levels, but not to a dangerous degree.

The nitrite/thiosulfate regimen may be repeated, at half the original doses, after two hours.

DOSAGE AND ADMINISTRATION
The contents of a 50 mg Sterile Sodium Nitroprusside, USP *Single Use* vial should be dissolved in 2 to 3 mL of 5% dextrose injection, USP. **NO OTHER DILUENT SHOULD BE USED.**

DILUTION TO PROPER STRENGTH FOR INFUSION
Depending on the desired concentration, the initially reconstituted solution containing 50 mg of Sterile Sodium Nitroprusside, USP must be further diluted in 250-1000 mL of sterile 5% dextrose injection. The diluted solution should be protected from light, using aluminum foil or other opaque material. It is not necessary to cover the infusion drip chamber or the tubing.

VERIFICATION OF THE CHEMICAL INTEGRITY OF THE PRODUCT
Sodium nitroprusside solution can be inactivated by reactions with trace contaminants. The products of these reactions are often blue, green or red, much brighter than the faint brownish color of unreacted Sterile Sodium Nitroprusside, USP. Discolored solutions, or solutions in which particulate matter is visible, should not be used. If properly protected from light, the freshly reconstituted and diluted solution is stable for 24 hours.

No other drugs should be administered in the same solution with Sodium Nitroprusside.

AVOIDANCE OF EXCESSIVE HYPOTENSION
While the average effective rate in adults and children is about 3 μg/kg/min, some patients will become dangerously hypotensive when they receive Sterile Sodium Nitroprusside, USP at this rate. Infusion of Sodium Nitroprusside should therefore be started at a very low rate (0.3 μg/kg/min), with upward titration every few minutes until the desired effect is achieved or the maximum recommended infusion rate (10 μg/kg/min) has been reached.

Because Sodium Nitroprusside's hypotensive effect is very rapid in onset and in dissipation, small variations in infusion rate can lead to wide, undesirable variations in blood pressure. **Sodium Nitroprusside should not be infused through ordinary IV apparatus, regulated only by gravity and mechanical clamps. Only an infusion pump, preferably a volumetric pump, should be used.**

Because Sodium Nitroprusside can induce essentially ulimited blood pressure reduction, **the blood pressure of a patient receiving this drug must be continuously monitored,** using either a continually reinflated sphygmomanometer or (preferably) an intra-arterial pressure sensor. Special caution should be used in elderly patients, since they may be more sensitive to the hypotensive effects of the drug.

When Sodium Nitroprusside is used in the treatment of acute congestive heart failure, titration of the infusion rate must be guided by the results of invasive hemodynamic monitoring with simultaneous monitoring of urine output. Sodium Nitroprusside can be titrated by increasing the infusion rate until:

■ measured cardiac output is no longer increasing.
■ systemic blood pressure cannot be further reduced without compromising the perfusion of vital organs, or
■ the maximum recommended infusion rate has been reached

whichever comes earliest. Specific hemodynamic goals must be tailored to the clinical situation, but improvements in cardiac output and left ventricular filling pressure must not be purchased at the price of undue hypotension and consequent hypoperfusion.

The table below shows the infusion rates corresponding to the recommended initial and maximal doses (0.3 μg/kg/min and 10 μg/kg/min, respectively) for both adults and children of various weights. Some of the listed infusion rates are so slow or so rapid as to be impractical, and these practicalities must be considered when the concentration to be used is selected. Note that when the concentration used in a given patient is changed the tubing is still filled with a solution at the previous concentration.

AVOIDANCE OF CYANIDE TOXICITY
As described in *"Clinical Pharmacology"* above, when more than 500 μg/kg of Sodium Nitroprusside is administered faster than 2 μg/kg/min, cyanide is generated faster than the unaided patient can eliminate it. Administration of sodium thiosulfate has been shown to increase the rate of cyanide processing, reducing the hazard of cyanide toxicity. Although toxic reactions to sodium thiosulfate have not been reported, the co-infusion regimen has not been

extensively studied, and it cannot be recommended without reservation. In one study, sodium thiosulfate appeared to potentiate the hypotensive effects of Sodium Nitroprusside.

Co-infusions of sodium thiosulfate have been administered at rates of 5 - 10 times that of Sodium Nitroprusside. Care must be taken to avoid the indiscriminate use of prolonged or high doses of Sodium Nitroprusside with Sodium thiosulfate as this may result in thiocyanate toxicity and hypovolemia. Incautious administration of Sodium Nitroprusside must still be avoided, and all of the precautions concerning Sodium Nitroprusside administration must still be observed.

INFUSION RATES (mL/HOUR) TO ACHIEVE INITIAL (0.3 μg/kg/min) AND MAXIMAL (10 μg/kg/min) DOSING OF STERILE SODIUM NITROPRUSSIDE, USP

Volume Sodium Nitroprusside Concentration		250 mL 50 mg 200 μg/mL		500 mL 50 mg 100 μg/mL		1000 mL 50 mg 50 μg/mL
pt weight						
kg	*lbs*	*init*	*max*	*init*	*max*	*init*	*max*
10	22	1	30	2	60	4	120
20	44	2	60	4	120	7	240
30	66	3	90	5	180	11	360
40	88	4	120	7	240	14	480
50	110	5	150	9	300	18	600
60	132	5	180	11	360	22	720
70	154	6	210	13	420	25	840
80	176	7	240	14	480	29	960
90	198	8	270	16	540	32	1080
100	220	9	300	18	600	36	1200

CONSIDERATION OF METHEMOGLOBINEMIA AND THIOCYANATE TOXICITY
Rare patients receiving more than 10 mg/kg of Sodium Nitroprusside will develop methemoglobinemia; other patients, especially those with impaired renal function, will predictably develop thiocyanate toxicity after prolonged, rapid infusions. In accordance with the descriptions in *"Adverse Reactions"* above, patients with suggestive findings should be tested for these toxicities.

Parenteral drug products should be inspected visually for particulate matter and discoloration prior to administration whenever solution and container permit. (See above.)

STORAGE
Store freeze-dried product, reconstituted solution and prepared intravenous infusion at controlled room temperature 15°-30° C (59°-86° F). Keep freeze-dried vial enclosed in box until ready to use. Sodium Nitroprusside solutions are extremely sensitive to light. Protect reconstituted solution and intravenous infusion from light. Promptly wrap intravenous infusion with aluminum foil supplied in package or with other opaque material to protect from light.

THE RECONSTITUTED SOLUTION AND INTRAVENOUS INFUSION SHOULD BE DISCARDED AFTER 24 HOURS.

HOW SUPPLIED
POWDER FOR INJECTION: 50 MG

AVERAGE UNIT PRICE (AVAILABLE SIZES)

BRAND	$9.08	*GENERIC A-RATED AVERAGE PRICE (GAAP)*		
GENERIC	$5.75	1s		$5.75

BRAND/MANUFACTURER		*NDC*	*SIZE*	*AWP*
◆ **BRAND**				
NITROPRESS: Abbott Hosp		00074-3024-01	1s	$7.75
		00074-3034-44	1s	$8.19
NITROPRESS ADVANTAGE KIT: Abbott Hosp		00074-3250-01	10s	$113.05
◆ **GENERICS**				
Gensia		00703-1802-01	1s	$5.25
Elkins-Sinn		00641-0125-21	1s	$6.25

Sodium Phosphate

DESCRIPTION
Sodium Phosphates Injection, USP, 3 mM P/mL (millimoles/mL), is a sterile, nonpyrogenic, *concentrated solution* containing a mixture of monobasic Sodium Phosphate and dibasic Sodium Phosphate in water for injection.

The solution is administered after dilution by the intravenous route as an electrolyte replenisher. *It must not be administered undiluted.*

Each mL contains 276 mg of monobasic Sodium Phosphate, monohydrate and 142 mg of dibasic Sodium Phosphate, anhydrous (equivalent to 268 mg of dibasic Sodium Phosphate, heptahydrate).

One mM of phosphorus weighs 31 mg, and the product provides 93 mg (approximately 3 mM) of phosphorus/mL plus 92 mg (4 mEq) of sodium/mL. Note: 1 mM P = 1 mM PO_4. The pH is 5.5 (5.0 to 6.0). The osmolar concentration is 12 mOsmol/mL (calc).

The solution is intended as an alternative to potassium phosphate to provide phosphorus for addition to large volume infusion fluids for intravenous use.

It is provided as a 15 mL partial fill single-dose vial; when lesser amounts are required, the unused portion should be discarded with the entire unit.

Monobasic Sodium Phosphate, USP (monohydrate) is chemically designated $NaH_2PO_4 \cdot H_2O$, white, odorless crystals or granules freely soluble in water.

Dibasic Sodium Phosphate, USP (anhydrous) is chemically designated Na_2HPO_4, colorless or white granular salt freely soluble in water.

CLINICAL PHARMACOLOGY

Phosphorus in the form of organic and inorganic phosphate has a variety of important biochemical functions in the body and is involved in many significant metabolic and enzyme reactions in almost all organs and tissues. It exerts a modifying influence on the steady state of calcium levels, a buffering effect on acid-base equilibrium and a primary role in the renal excretion of hydrogen ion.

Phosphorus is present in plasma and other extracellular fluid, in cell membranes and intracellular fluid, as well as in collagen and bone tissues. Phosphorus in the extracellular fluid is primarily in inorganic form and plasma levels may vary somewhat with age. The ratio of disodium phosphate and monosodium phosphate in the extracellular fluid is 4 to 1 (80% to 20%) at the normal pH of 7.4. This buffer ratio varies with the pH, but owing to its relatively low concentration, it contributes little to the buffering capacity of the extracellular fluid.

Phosphorus, present in large amounts in erythrocytes and other tissue cells, plays a significant intracellular role in the synthesis of high energy organic phosphates. It has been shown to be essential to maintain red cell glucose utilization, lactate production, and the concentration of both erythrocyte adenosine triphosphate (ATP) and 2,3 diphosphoglycerate (DPG), and must be deemed as important to other tissue cells. Hypophosphatemia should be avoided during periods of total parenteral nutrition, or other lengthy periods of intravenous infusions. It has been suggested that patients receiving total parenteral nutrition receive 12 to 15 mM phosphorus per 250 g of dextrose. Serum phosphorus levels should be regularly monitored and appropriate amounts of phosphorus should be added to the infusions to maintain normal serum phosphorus levels. Intravenous infusion of inorganic phosphorus may be accompanied by a decrease in the serum level and urinary excretion of calcium. The normal level of serum phosphorus is 3.0 to 4.5 mg/100 mL in adults; 4.0 to 7.0 mg/100 mL in children.

Intravenously infused phosphorus not taken up by the tissues is excreted almost entirely in the urine. Plasma phosphorus is believed to be filterable by the renal glomeruli, and the major portion of filtered phosphorus (greater than 80%) is actively reabsorbed by the tubules. Many modifying influences tend to alter the amount excreted in the urine.

Sodium is the principal cation of extracellular fluid. It comprises more than 90% of the total cations at its normal plasma concentration of approximately 142 mEq/liter. While the sodium ion can diffuse across cell membranes, intracellular sodium is maintained at a much lower concentration than extracellular sodium through the expenditure of energy by the cell (so called "sodium cation pump"). Loss of intracellular potassium ion is usually accompanied by an increase in intracellular sodium ion.

When serum sodium concentration is low, the secretion of antidiuretic hormone (ADH) by the pituitary is inhibited, thereby preventing water reabsorption by the distal renal tubules. On the other hand, adrenal secretion of aldosterone increases renal tubular reabsorption of sodium in an effort to re-establish normal serum sodium concentration.

INDICATIONS AND USAGE

Sodium Phosphates Injection, USP, 3 mM P/mL is indicated as a source of phosphorus, for addition to large volume intravenous fluids, to prevent or correct hypophosphatemia in patients with restricted or no oral intake. It is also useful as an additive for preparing specific parenteral fluid formulas when the needs of the patient cannot be met by standard electrolyte or nutrient solutions.

The concomitant amount of sodium (Na+ 4 mEq/mL) must be calculated into total electrolyte dose of such prepared solutions.

CONTRAINDICATIONS

Sodium Phosphate is contraindicated in diseases where high phosphorus or low calcium levels may be encountered, and in patients with hypernatremia.

WARNINGS

Sodium Phosphates Injection, USP, 3 mM P/mL must be diluted and thoroughly mixed before use.

To avoid phosphorus intoxication, infuse solutions containing Sodium Phosphate slowly. Infusing high concentrations of phosphorus may result in a reduction of serum calcium and symptoms of hypocalcemic tetany. Calcium levels should be monitored.

Solutions containing sodium ion should be used with great care, if at all, in patients with congestive heart failure, severe renal insufficiency and in clinical states in which there exists edema with sodium retention.

In patients with diminished renal function, administration of solutions containing sodium ions may result in sodium retention.

PRECAUTIONS

Do not administer unless solution is clear and seal is intact. Discard unused portion.

Phosphorus replacement therapy with Sodium Phosphate should be guided primarily by the serum phosphorus level and the limits imposed by the accompanying sodium (Na+) ion.

Use with caution in patients with renal impairment, cirrhosis, cardiac failure and other edematous or sodium-retaining states.

Caution must be exercised in the administration of parenteral fluids, especially those containing sodium ion, to patients receiving corticosteroids or corticotropin.

Pregnancy Category C. Animal reproduction studies have not been conducted with Sodium Phosphate. It is also not known whether Sodium Phosphate can cause fetal harm when administered to a pregnant woman or can affect reproduction capacity. Sodium Phosphate should be given to a pregnant woman only if clearly needed.

ADVERSE REACTIONS

Adverse reactions involve the possibility of phosphorus intoxication. Phosphorus intoxication results in a reduction of serum calcium and the symptoms are those of hypocalcemic tetany. See *"Warnings"*.

OVERDOSAGE

In the event of overdosage, discontinue infusions containing Sodium Phosphate immediately and institute corrective therapy to restore depressed serum calcium and to reduce elevated serum sodium levels. See *"Warnings," "Precautions"* and *"Adverse Reactions."*

DOSAGE AND ADMINISTRATION

Sodium Phosphates Injection, USP, 3 mM P/mL is administered intravenously *only after dilution and thorough mixing in a larger volume of fluid.* The dose and rate of administration are dependent upon the individual needs of the patient. Serum Sodium, phosphorus and calcium levels should be monitored as a guide to dosage.

Using aseptic technique, all or part of the contents of one or more vials may be added to other intravenous fluids to provide any desired number of millimoles (mM) of phosphorus.

In patients on total parenteral nutrition, approximately 12 to 15 mM of phosphorus (equivalent to 372 to 465 mg elemental phosphorus) per liter bottle of TPN solution containing 250 g dextrose is usually adequate to maintain normal serum phosphorus, though larger amounts may be required in hypermetabolic states. The amount of sodium and phosphorus which accompanies the addition of Sodium Phosphate also should be kept in mind, and if necessary, serum sodium levels should be monitored.

The suggested dose of phosphorus for infants receiving TPN is 1.5 to 2 mM P/kg/day.

Parenteral drug products should be inspected visually for particulate matter and discoloration prior to administration, whenever solution and container permit. See *"Precautions"*.

Store at controlled room temperature, 15° to 30° C (59° to 86° F).

HOW SUPPLIED
INJECTION: 3 MM/ML

BRAND/MANUFACTURER	NDC	SIZE	AWP
○ **GENERICS**			
Fujisawa	00469-1170-25	10 ml	$1.32
Fujisawa	00469-2170-25	15 ml	$2.63
Fujisawa	00469-1180-60	50 ml	$9.08
Amer Regent	00517-3405-25	5 ml 25s	$20.94
Amer Regent	00517-3415-25	15 ml 25s	$32.19
Abbott Hosp	00074-7391-72	15 ml 25s	$120.83
Amer Regent	00517-3450-25	50 ml 25s	$85.94
Abbott Hosp	00074-3295-51	50 ml 25s	$244.03
Raway	00686-3405-25	10 ml 100s	$170.00
Raway	00686-3415-25	30 ml 100s	$185.00

Sodium Polystyrene Sulfonate

DESCRIPTION

Sodium Polystyrene Sulfonate Suspension USP can be administered orally or in an enema; the suspension contains per 60 mL:

Sodium Polystyrene Sulfonate USP .... 15 g

The drug is also available as a light brown to brown, finely ground, powdered form of Sodium Polystyrene Sulfonate, a cation-exchange resin.

Sodium Polystyrene Sulfonate is a benzene, diethenyl-, polymer with ethenylbenzene, sulfonated, sodium salt.

The Sodium content of the suspension is 1500 mg (65 mEq) per 60 mL; of the powder approximately 100 mg (4.1 mEq) per gram. It is a brown, slightly viscous suspension. The suspension and powder have an *in-vitro* exchange capacity of approximately 3.1 mEq (*in-vivo* approximately 1 mEq) of potassium per 4 mL (1 gram) of suspension or 1 gram of powder.

CLINICAL PHARMACOLOGY

As the resin passes along the intestine or is retained in the colon after administration by enema, the Sodium ions are partially released and are replaced by potassium ions. For the most part, this action occurs in the large intestine, which excretes potassium ions to a greater degree than does the small intestine. The efficiency of this process is limited and unpredictably variable. It commonly approximates the order of 33%, but the range is so large that definite indices of electrolyte balance must be clearly monitored. Metabolic data are unavailable.

INDICATIONS AND USAGE

Sodium Polystyrene Sulfonate is indicated for the treatment of hyperkalemia.

UNLABELED USES
Sodium Polystyrene Sulfonate is used as an adjunct in the treatment of lithium intoxication.

CONTRAINDICATIONS
Sodium Polystyrene Sulfonate is contraindicated in patients with hypokalema or those patients who are hypersensitive to it.

WARNINGS

ALTERNATIVE THERAPY IN SEVERE HYPERKALEMIA
Since the effective lowering of serum potassium with Sodium Polystyrene Sulfonate may take hours to days, treatment with this drug alone may be insufficient to rapidly correct severe hyperkalemia associated with states of rapid tissue breakdown (e.g., burns and renal failure) or hyperkalemia so marked as to constitute a medical emergency. Therefore, other definitive measures, including dialysis, should always be considered and may be imperative.

HYPOKALEMIA
Serious potassium deficiency can occur from Sodium Polystyrene Sulfonate therapy. The effect must be carefully controlled by frequent serum potassium determinations within each 24 hour period. Since intracellular potassium deficiency is not always reflected by serum potassium levels, the level at which treatment with Sodium Polystyrene Sulfonate should be discontinued must be determined individually for each patient. Important aids in making this determination are the patient's clinical condition and electrocardiogram. Early clinical signs of severe hypokalemia include a pattern of irritable confusion and delayed thought processes. Electocardiographically, severe hypokalemia is often associated with a lengthened Q-T interval, widening, flattening, or inversion of the T wave, and prominent U waves. Also, cardiac arrhythmias may occur, such as premature atrial, nodal, and ventricular contractions, and supraventricular and ventricular tachycardias. The toxic effects of digitalis are likely to be exaggerated. Marked hypokalemia can also be manifested by severe muscle weakness, at times extending into frank paralysis.

ELECTROLYTE DISTURBANCES
Like all cation-exchange resins, Sodium Polystyrene Sulfonate is not totally selective (for potassium) in its actions, and small amounts of other cations such as magnesium and calcium can also be lost during treatment. Accordingly, patients receiving Sodium Polystyrene Sulfonate should be monitored for all applicable electrolyte disturbances.

SYSTEMIC ALKALYSIS
Systemic alkalosis has been reported after cation-exchange resins were administered orally in combination with nonabsorbable cation-donating antacids and laxatives such as magnesium hydroxide and aluminum carbonate. Magnesium hydroxide should not be administered with Sodium Polystyrene Sulfonate. One case of grand mal seizure has been reported in a patient with chronic hypocalcemia of renal failure who was given Sodium Polystyrene Sulfonate with magnesium hydroxide as a laxative. (See *"Precautions, Drug Interactions"*.)

PRECAUTIONS
Caution is advised when Sodium Polystyrene Sulfonate is administered to patients who cannot tolerate even a small increase in Sodium loads (i.e., severe congestive heart failure, severe hypertension, or marked edema). In such instances compensatory restriction of sodium intake from other sources may be indicated.

If constipation occurs, patients should be treated with sorbitol (from 10 to 20 mL of 70% syrup every 2 hours or as needed to produce 1 to 2 watery stools daily) a measure which also reduces any tendency to fecal impaction.

DRUG INTERACTIONS
Antacids: The simultaneous oral administration of Sodium Polystyrene Sulfonate with nonabsorbable cation-donating antacids and laxatives may reduce the resin's potassium exchange capability.

Systemic alkalosis has been reported after cation-exchange resins were administered orally in combination with nonabsorbable cation-donating antacids and laxatives such as magnesium hydroxide and aluminum carbonate. Magnesium hydroxide should not be administered with Sodium Polystyrene Sulfonate. One case of grand mal seizure has been reported in a patient with chronic hypocalcemia of renal failure who was given Sodium Polystyrene Sulfonate with magnesium hydroxide as a laxative. Intestinal obstruction due to concretions of aluminum hydroxide when used in combination with Sodium Polystyrene Sulfonate has been reported.

Digitalis: The toxic effects of digitalis on the heart, especially various ventricular arrhythmias and A-V nodal dissociation, are likely to be exaggerated by hypokalemia, even in the face of serum digoxin concentrations in the "normal range". (See *"Warnings."*)

Carcinogenesis, Mutagenesis, Impairment of Fertility: Studies have not been performed.

Pregnancy Category C: Animal reproduction studies have not been conducted with Sodium Polystyrene Sulfonate. It is also not known whether Sodium Polystyrene Sulfonate can cause fetal harm when administered to a pregnant woman or can affect reproduction capacity. Sodium Polystyrene Sulfonate should be given to a pregnant woman only if clearly needed.

Nursing Mothers: It is not known whether this drug is excreted in human milk. Because many drugs are excreted in human milk, caution should be exercised when Sodium Polystyrene Sulfonate is administered to a nursing woman.

ADVERSE REACTIONS
Sodium Polystyrene Sulfonate may cause some degree of gastric irritation. Anorexia, nausea, vomiting, and constipation may occur especially if high doses are given. Also, hypokalemia, hypocalcemia, and significant sodium retention may occur. Occasionally diarrhea develops. Large doses in elderly individuals may cause fecal impaction (see *"Precautions"*). This effect may be obviated through usage of the resin in enemas as described under *"Dosage and Administration."* Rare instances of colonic necrosis have been reported. Intestinal obstruction due to concretions of aluminum hydroxide, when used in combination with Sodium Polystyrene Sulfonate, has been reported.

DOSAGE AND ADMINISTRATION
Suspension of this drug should be freshly prepared and not stored beyond 24 hours. If making a suspension from the powder, it should be freshly prepared and not stored beyond 24 hours.

ORAL ADMINISTRATION
The average daily adult dose is 15 g (60 mL) to 60 g (240 mL). This is best provided by administering 15 g (60 mL or approximately 4 *level* teaspoons) of Sodium Polystyrene Sulfonate suspension one to four times daily. Each 60 mL of Sodium Polystyrene Sulfonate suspension contains 1500 mg (65 mEq) of Sodium. One gram of Sodium Polystyrene Sulfonate powder contains 4.1 mEq of Sodium; one level teaspoon contains approximately 3.5 g of Sodium Polystyrene Sulfonate and 15 mEq of sodium. (A heaping teaspoon may contain as much as 10 g to 12 g of Sodium Polystyrene Sulfonate.) Since the *in-vivo* efficiency of Sodium-potassium exchange resins is approximately 33%, about one-third of the resin's actual Sodium content is being delivered to the body.

In smaller children and infants, lower doses should be employed by using as a guide a rate of 1 mEq of potassium per gram of resin as the basis for calculation.

Each dose of the powder should be given as a suspension in a small quantity of water or, for greater palatability, in syrup. The amount of fluid usually ranges from 20 mL to 100 mL, depending on the dose, or may be simply determined by allowing 3 mL to 4 mL per gram of resin. Sorbitol may be administered in order to combat constipation.

The suspension or powder may be introduced into the stomach through a plastic tube and, if desired, mixed with a diet appropriate for a patient in renal failure.

RECTAL ADMINISTRATION
The suspension may also be given, although with less effective results, as a retention enema for adults of 30 g (120 mL) to 50 g (200 mL) every six hours. Each dose is administered as a warm emulsion (at body temperature) in 100 mL of aqueous vehicle, such as sorbitol. The emulsion should be agitated gently during administration. The enema should be retained as long as possible and followed by a cleansing enema.

After an initial cleansing enema, a soft, large size (French 28) rubber tube is inserted into the rectum for a distance of 20 cm, with the tip well into the sigmoid color, and taped in place. The suspension, or powder suspended in the appropriate amount of aqueous vehicle, is introduced at body temperature by gravity. The powder particles are kept in suspension by stirring. The suspension is flushed with 50 or 100 mL of fluid, following which the tube is clamped and left in place. If back leakage occurs, the hips are elevated on pillows or a knee-chest position is taken temporarily. A somewhat thicker suspension may be used, but care should be taken that no paste is formed, because the latter has a greatly reduced exchange surface and will be particularly ineffective if deposited in the rectal ampulla. The suspension is kept in the sigmoid colon for several hours, if possible. Then the colon is irrigated with a nonsodium-containing solution at body temperature in order to remove the resin. Two quarts of flushing solution may be necessary. The returns are drained constantly through a Y tube connection. Particular attention should be paid to this cleansing enema when sorbitol has been used.

The intensity and duration of therapy depend upon the severity and resistance of hyperkalemia.

Note: Sodium Polystyrene Sulfonate suspension should not be heated for to do say may alter the exchange properties of the resin.

SHAKE WELL BEFORE USING

STORAGE
Dispense in a tight container as defined in the USP/NF. Store at controlled room temperature 15°-30°C (59°-86°F).

HOW SUPPLIED
POWDER FOR RECONSTITUTION:

BRAND/MANUFACTURER	NDC	SIZE	AWP
◆ **BRAND**			
KAYEXALATE: Sanofi Winthrop	00024-1075-01	480 gm	$159.79
◆ **GENERICS**			
Carolina	46287-0012-16	480 gm	$48.75

➤ SHOWN IN PRODUCT IDENTIFICATION GUIDE

SUSPENSION: 15 GM/60 ML

AVERAGE UNIT PRICE (AVAILABLE SIZES)			
GENERIC	$0.10		

AVERAGE UNIT PRICE (AVAILABLE SIZES)		GENERIC A-RATED AVERAGE PRICE (GAAP)	
GENERIC	$0.16	60 ml 10s	$69.43

BRAND/MANUFACTURER	NDC	SIZE	AWP
◆ GENERICS			
Roxane	00054-8815-01	120 ml	$19.67
Carolina	46287-0006-01	480 ml	$29.70
Roxane	00054-3805-63	500 ml	$47.86
Carolina	46287-0006-04	120 ml 6s	$66.60
Carolina	46287-0006-60	60 ml 10s ud	$52.36
Roxane	00054-8816-11	60 ml 10s ud	$86.49

SUSPENSION: 50 GM/200 ML

BRAND/MANUFACTURER	NDC	SIZE	AWP
◆ GENERICS			
Roxane	00054-8817-55	200 ml	$29.50

Sodium Sulamyd *SEE* SULFACETAMIDE SODIUM, OPHTHALMIC

Sodium Tetradecyl Sulfate

DESCRIPTION

Sodium Tetradecyl Sulfate is an anionic surfactant which occurs as a white, waxy solid. The chemical name of Sodium Tetradecyl Sulfate is 7-Ethyl-2-methyl-4-hendecanol sulfate sodium salt. Its molecular formula is $C_{14}H_{29}NaSO_4$ and its molecular weight is 316.44.

Sodium Tetradecyl Sulfate Injection is a sterile nonpyrogenic solution for intravenous use as a sclerosing agent. Each mL contains Sodium Tetradecyl Sulfate 10 mg or 30 mg, benzyl alcohol 0.02 mL and dibasic sodium phosphate, anhydrous 0.72 mg in Water for Injection. pH 7.9; monobasic sodium phosphate and/or sodium hydroxide added, if needed, for pH adjustment.

CLINICAL PHARMACOLOGY

Sodium Tetradecyl Sulfate Injection is a mild sclerosing agent. Intravenous injection causes intima inflammation and thrombus formation. This usually occludes the injected vein. Subsequent formation of fibrous tissue results in partial or complete vein obliteration.

INDICATIONS AND USAGE

Indicated in the treatment of small uncomplicated varicose veins of the lower extremities that show simple dilation with competent valves. The benefit-to-risk ratio should be considered in selected patients who are great surgical risks due to conditions such as old age.

CONTRAINDICATIONS

Contraindicated in previous hypersensitivity reactions to the drug; in acute superficial thrombophlebitis; significant valvular or deep vein incompetence; huge superficial veins with wide open communications to deeper veins; phlebitis migrans; acute cellulitis; allergic conditions; acute infections; varicosities caused by abdominal and pelvic tumors unless the tumor has been removed; bedridden patients; such uncontrolled systemic diseases as diabetes, toxic hyperthyroidism, tuberculosis, asthma, neoplasm, sepsis, blood dyscrasias and acute respiratory or skin diseases.

WARNINGS

Since severe adverse local effects, including tissue necrosis, may occur following extravasation, Sodium Tetradecyl Sulfate Injection should be administered only by a physician familiar with proper injection technique. Extreme care in needle placement and using the minimal effective volume at each injection site are, therefore, important. Allergic reactions have been reported. Therefore, as a precaution against anaphylactoid shock, it is recommended that 0.5 mL of Sodium Tetradecyl Sulfate be injected into a varicosity, followed by observation of the patient for several hours before administration of a second or larger dose. The possibility of an anaphylactoid reaction should be kept in mind, and the physician should be prepared to treat it appropriately. In extreme emergencies, 0.25 mL of 1:1000 Epinephrine Injection (0.25 mg) intravenously should be used and side reactions controlled with antihistamines.

PRECAUTIONS

GENERAL

Venous sclerotherapy should not be undertaken if tests, such as the Trendelenberg and Perthes, and angiography show significant valvular or deep venous incompetence. The physician should bear in mind the fact that injection necrosis is likely to result from extravascular injection of sclerosing agents.

Extreme caution must be exercised in the presence of underlying arterial disease such as marked peripheral arteriosclerosis or thromboangiitis obliterans (Buerger's Disease).

The drug should only be administered by physicians who are familiar with an acceptable injection technique. Because of the danger of thrombosis extension into the deep venous system, thorough preinjection evaluation for valvular competency should be carried out and slow injections with a small amount (not over 2 mL) of the preparation should be injected into the varicosity. In particular, deep venous patency must be determined by angiography and/or the Perthes test before sclerotherapy is undertaken.

Embolism may occur as much as four weeks after injection of Sodium Tetradecyl Sulfate.

The incidence of recurrence is low if the patient wears elastic stockings.

DRUG INTERACTIONS

No well-controlled studies have been performed on patients taking antiovulatory agents. The physician must use judgment and evaluate any patient taking antiovulatory drugs prior to initiating treatment with Sodium Tetradecyl Sulfate Injection. (See *"Adverse Reactions".*) Heparin should not be included in the same syringe as Sodium Tetradecyl Sulfate since the two are incompatible.

CARCINOGENESIS, MUTAGENESIS, IMPAIRMENT OF FERTILITY

When tested in the L5178YTK-/- mouse lymphoma assay, Sodium Tetradecyl Sulfate did not induce a dose-related increase in the frequency of thymidine kinase-deficient mutants and, therefore, was judged to be nonmutagenic in this system. However, no long-term animal carcinogenicity studies with Sodium Tetradecyl Sulfate have been performed.

PREGNANCY

Teratogenic Effects: Pregnancy Category C. Adequate reproduction studies have not been performed in animals to determine whether this drug affects fertility in males or females, has teratogenic potential, or has other adverse effects on the fetus. There are no well-controlled studies in pregnant women, but investigational and marketing experience does not include any positive evidence of adverse effects on the fetus. Although there is no clearly defined risk, such experience cannot exclude the possibility of infrequent or subtle damage to the human fetus.

NURSING MOTHERS

It is not known whether this drug is excreted in human milk. Because many drugs are excreted in human milk, caution should be exercised when Sodium Tetradecyl Sulfate Injection is administered to a nursing woman.

ADVERSE REACTIONS

Local reactions consisting of pain, urticaria or ulceration may occur at the site of injection. A permanent discoloration, usually small and hardly noticeable but which may be objectionable from a cosmetic viewpoint, may remain along the path of the sclerosed vein segment. Sloughing and necrosis of tissue may occur following extravasation of the drug. Systemic reactions, except for allergic ones, have been slight. These include headache, nausea and vomiting. Allergic reactions such as hives, asthma, hayfever and anaphylactoid shock have been reported. (See *"Warnings".*)

One death has been reported in a patient who received Sodium Tetradecyl Sulfate Injection and who had been receiving an antiovulatory agent.

Another death (fatal pulmonary embolism) has been reported in a 36-year-old female treated with Sodium Tetradecyl *acetate* and who was not taking oral contraceptives.

DOSAGE AND ADMINISTRATION

For intravenous use only. Do not use if precipitated or discolored. The strength of solution required depends on the size and degree of varicosity. In general, the 1% solution will be found most useful with the 3% solution preferred for larger varicosities. The dosage should be kept small, using 0.5 to 2 mL (preferably 1 mL maximum) for each injection, and the maximum single treatment should not exceed 10 mL.

Parenteral drug products should be inspected visually for particulate matter and discoloration prior to administration, whenever solution and container permit.

Store at controlled room temperature 15°-30°C (59°-86° F).

ANIMAL TOXICOLOGY

The intravenous LD_{50} of Sodium Tetradecyl Sulfate in mice was reported to be 90 ± 5 mg/kg.

In the rat, the acute intravenous LD_{50} of Sodium Tetradecyl Sulfate was estimated to be between 72 mg/kg and 108 mg/kg.

Purified Sodium Tetradecyl Sulfate was found to have an LD_{50} of 2 g/kg when administered orally by stomach tube as a 25% aqueous solution to rats. In rats given 0.15 g/kg in drinking water for 30 days, no appreciable toxicity was seen although some growth inhibition was discernible.

HOW SUPPLIED
INJECTION: 1%

BRAND/MANUFACTURER	NDC	SIZE	AWP
◆ GENERICS			
SOTRADECOL: Elkins-Sinn	00641-1514-34	2 ml 5s	$57.86

◆ RATED THERAPEUTICALLY EQUIVALENT; ◇ THERAPEUTIC EQUIVALENCE UNCONFIRMED; ○ UNRATED

INJECTION: 3%

BRAND/MANUFACTURER	NDC	SIZE	AWP
◆ GENERICS			
SOTRADECOL: Elkins-Sinn	00641-1516-34	2 ml 5s	$68.58

Sodium Thiosalicylate

DESCRIPTION
Sodium Thiosalicylate Injection (an analgesic, antipyretic agent) is a sterile solution manufactured from Thiosalicylic Acid with the aid of Sodium Bicarbonate (30 mL vial) for intramuscular administration. Each mL contains 50 mg Sodium Thiosalicylate in Water for Injection.

Following is its chemical structure:

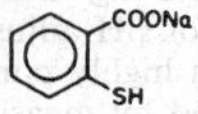

CLINICAL PHARMACOLOGY
In common with the various salicylate compounds, Thiosalicylate exerts analgesic and antipyretic effects. In antipyretic drugs, the ability to lower temperature is most readily seen in febrile patients, while normal temperatures do not show much change, action being primarily upon hypothalamic nuclei. The selective central depressant action of salicylates produces analgesia without any apparent cortical effects.

Given intramuscularly, Thiosalicylate is readily absorbed and appreciable amounts detected in the blood within 1 1/2 hours. Salicylates are rapidly distributed through the body tissues. Sodium bicarbonate tends to lower plasma salicylate levels while ammonium chloride tends to elevate the level. Metabolic changes appear to be made in the kidney and while approximately 50 percent of the salicylate is excreted in 24 hours, some traces are found in urine for periods up to 48 hours.

INDICATIONS AND USAGE
Palliative relief of muscular pains, acute gout, arthritis, rheumatic fever, and muscular skeletal disturbances.

CONTRAINDICATIONS
Hemophilia, bleeding ulcers, and hemorrhagic states are absolute contraindications. Hypersensitivity to salicylates is not an absolute contraindication, but a sensitivity test with 0.05 or 0.1 mL of Sodium Thiosalicylate Injection should be made before continuing therapy.

Note: This product contains benzyl alcohol. Benzyl alcohol has been associated with a fatal "Gasping Syndrome" in premature infants and infants of low birth weight.

Contraindicated in those persons who have shown hypersensitivity to any component of this preparation.

WARNING
Salicylates have been reported to be associated with the development of Reye's Syndrome in children and teenagers with chicken pox, influenze and influenze-like infections. Since Sodium Thiosalicylate is structurally and pharmacologically related to the salicylates and appears to share the toxic potentials of the salicylates, Sodium Thiosalicylate Injection is not recommended for use in children and teenagers with chicken pox, influenze and influenze-like infections.

PRECAUTIONS
Febrile children suffering dehydration appear quite prone to salicylate intoxication. Exercise caution with patients suffering oral diseases.

Pregnancy And Lactation: Safe use of Sodium Thiosalicylate during pregnancy or lactation has not been established.

ADVERSE REACTIONS
Large continued doses of salicylate may produce dizziness, tinnitus, headache, lassitude, profuse sweating, thirst, mental confusion, tremor, delirium and coma, as well as skin eruptions. Disturbances of acid-base and electrolytic balances have also been observed. Hemorrhagic disturbances from prolonged larger doses of salicylates are not uncommon. Prescribe sodium bicarbonate per os concurrent with Thiosalicylate. Long-term usage indicates administration of vitamin K.

DOSAGE AND ADMINISTRATION
It is advisable to administer this product intramuscularly in order to obviate the usual problems associated with intravenous administration.

The usual adult dosage for the symptomatic treatment of muscular pain and musculoskeletal disorders is 50-100 mg once daily or once every other day.

In the symptomatic treatment of rheumatic fever, the usual adult IM dosage is 100-150 mg every 4-8 hours for 3 days, followed by 100 mg twice daily until the patient is asymptomatic.

In the symptomatic treatment of acute gout, the usual adult IM dosage is 100 mg every 3-4 hours for two days, followed by 100 mg once daily until the patient is asymptomatic.

Parenteral drug products should be inspected visually for particulate matter and discoloration prior to administration, whenever the solution and container permit.

A slight precipitate may form due to oxidation. If the precipitate does not redissolve when the container is shaken well, the injection should not be used.

HOW SUPPLIED
INJECTION:

BRAND/MANUFACTURER	NDC	SIZE	AWP
○ GENERICS			
REXOLATE: Hyrex	00314-0762-30	30 ml	$29.50

INJECTION: 50 MG/ML

BRAND/MANUFACTURER	NDC	SIZE	AWP
○ GENERICS			
TUSAL: Roberts/Hauck	59441-0617-30	30 ml	$9.44
Hyrex	00314-5720-30	30 ml	$14.00
Clint	55553-0009-30	30 ml	$29.50

Sodium Thiosulfate

DESCRIPTION
Sodium Thiosulfate is a preservative free, sterile solution for slow intravenous injection only. It is available as a 10% (100 mg/mL) solution and as a 25% (250 mg/mL) solution. Each mL contains: Sodium Thiosulfate Pentahydrate 100 mg or 250 mg. Sodium Thiosulfate is designated as $Na_2S_2O_3$. The pentahydrate form, $(NA_2S_2O_2 \cdot 5H_2O$; molecular weight 248.17) occurs as odorless granules or crystals that are soluble in water and insoluble in alcohol.

CLINICAL PHARMACOLOGY
Sodium Thiosulfate is used as an antidote for cyanide poisoning. The primary mechanism of cyanide detoxification involves the conversion of cyanide to the thiocyanate ion, which is relatively nontoxic. This reaction involves the enzyme rhodanese (thiosulfate: cyanide sulfurtransferase) which is found in many body tissues, but with the major activity in the liver. The body has the capability to detoxify cyanide; however, the rhodanese enzyme system is slow to respond to large amounts of cyanide. The rhodanese enzyme reaction can be accelerated by supplying an exogenous source of sulfur. This is commonly accomplished by administering Sodium Thiosulfate. Sodium Thiosulfate may be used alone or in combination with nitrite compounds such as amyl nitrite or sodium nitrite.

Following intravenous injection, Sodium Thiosulfate is distributed throughout the extracellular fluid and is excreted unchanged in the urine. The biological half life is reported to be 0.65 hours.

INDICATIONS AND USAGE
Sodium Thiosulfate is indicated for the treatment of cyanide poisoning.

CONTRAINDICATIONS
None known.

WARNINGS
None known.

PRECAUTIONS
Sodium Thiosulfate is essentially nontoxic. However, studies conducted in dogs, with a constant infusion of Sodium Thiosulfate, showed hypovolemia which was considered to be due to an osmotic diuretic effect of Sodium Thiosulfate.

Pregnancy: Teratogenic Effects - Pregnancy Category C: Animal reproduction studies have not been conducted with Sodium Thiosulfate. It is also not known whether Sodium Thiosulfate can cause fetal harm when administered to a pregnant woman or can affect reproduction capacity. Sodium Thiosulfate should be given to a pregnant woman only if clearly needed.

ADVERSE REACTIONS
None known.

DRUG ABUSE AND DEPENDENCE
None known.

DOSAGE AND ADMINISTRATION
Death from cyanide poisoning occurs rapidly. Delays in administering the antidote should be avoided.

Slow Intravenous Use Only: The dose of Sodium Thiosulfate whether used alone or in combination with other cyanide antidotes is 12.5 grams given intravenously over approximately 10 minutes. The dosage for children is 7 grams per square meter of body surface area, with a maximum dose of 12.5 grams.

Patients should be closely monitored for 24 to 48 hours for symptoms of cyanide poisoning to reappear. In the event symptoms return, Sodium Thiosulfate administration should be repeated at one half the original dose.

Parenteral drug products should be inspected visually for particulate matter and discoloration prior to administration, whenever solution and container permit.

Storage: Store at controlled room temperature 15°-30°C (59°-86°F).

► SHOWN IN PRODUCT IDENTIFICATION GUIDE

2522 / PRODUCT INFORMATION

HOW SUPPLIED
GRANULAR:

BRAND/MANUFACTURER	NDC	SIZE	AWP
○ GENERICS			
	00395-2745-01	454 gm	$5.05
	17137-0533-01	500 gm	$6.30

INJECTION: 1 GM

BRAND/MANUFACTURER	NDC	SIZE	AWP
○ GENERICS			
Pasadena	00418-1854-10	10 ml 25s	$170.50

INJECTION: 10%

BRAND/MANUFACTURER	NDC	SIZE	AWP
○ GENERICS			
Amer Regent	00517-1019-05	10 ml 5s	$37.50
CMC-Cons	00223-8570-10	10 ml 5s	$55.50

INJECTION: 12.5 GM

BRAND/MANUFACTURER	NDC	SIZE	AWP
○ GENERICS			
Pasadena	00418-1861-50	50 ml	$19.28

INJECTION: 25%

BRAND/MANUFACTURER	NDC	SIZE	AWP
○ GENERICS			
Amer Regent	00517-5019-01	50 ml	$22.50
CMC-Cons	00223-8573-50	50 ml	$45.00
Raway	00686-5019-01	50 ml 5s	$180.00

INJECTION: 100 MG/ML

BRAND/MANUFACTURER	NDC	SIZE	AWP
○ GENERICS			
Raway	00686-1019-05	10 ml 20s	$240.00

LOTION:

BRAND/MANUFACTURER	NDC	SIZE	AWP
○ BRAND			
TINASTAT: Vita Elixir	00181-0676-00	120 ml	$6.00

Solaquin Forte SEE HYDROQUINONE

Solatene SEE BETA CAROTENE

Solfoton SEE PHENOBARBITAL

Solganal SEE AUROTHIOGLUCOSE

Solu-Cortef SEE HYDROCORTISONE, SYSTEMIC

Solu-Medrol SEE METHYLPREDNISOLONE

Soma SEE CARISOPRODOL, ASPIRIN/CARISOPRODOL/CODEINE PHOSPHATE AND ASPIRIN AND CARISOPRODOL

Somatrem

DESCRIPTION

Somatrem is a polypeptide hormone which is of recombinant DNA origin. Somatrem has 192 amino acid residues and a molecular weight of about 22,000 daltons. The product contains the identical sequence of 191 amino acids constituting pituitary-derived human growth hormone plus an additional amino acid, methionine, on the N-terminus of the molecule. Somatrem growth hormone is synthesized in a special laboratory strain of *E. coli* bacteria which has been modified by the addition of the gene for human growth hormone production.

Somatrem growth hormone, a sterile, white, lyophilized powder, is intended for intramuscular or subcutaneous administration after reconstitution with Bacteriostatic Water for Injection, USP (benzyl alcohol preserved).

The quantitative composition of the lyophilized drug per vial is:

5 mg (approximately 13 IU) Vial:
Somatrem 5.0 mg (approximately 13 IU)
Mannitol 40.0 mg
Sodium phosphates 1.7 mg
(Monobasic sodium phosphate 0.1 mg and dibasic sodium phosphate 1.6 mg)

10 mg (approximately 26 IU) Vial:
Somatrem 10.0 mg (approximately 26 IU)
Mannitol 80.0 mg
Sodium phosphates 3.4 mg
(Monobasic sodium phosphate 0.2 mg and dibasic sodium phosphate 3.2 mg)
Phosphoric acid may be used for pH adjustment.
Somatrem growth hormone is a highly purified preperation.
Biological potency is determined by measuring the increase in body weight induced in hypophysectomized rats.

Following is its chemical structure:

```
H-Met-Phe-Pro-Thr-Ile - Pro-Leu-Ser-Arg-Leu-Phe-Asp-Asn-Ala-Met-Leu-
   1   2   3   4   5    6   7   8   9  10  11  12  13  14  15
Arg-Ala-His-Arg-Leu-His-Gln-Leu-Ala-Phe-Asp-Thr-Tyr-Gln-Glu-Phe-
 16  17  18  19  20  21  22  23  24  25  26  27  28  29  30  31
Glu-Glu-Ala-Tyr-Ile-Pro-Lys-Glu-Gln-Lys-Tyr-Ser-Phe-Leu-Gln-Asn-
 32  33  34  35  36  37  38  39  40  41  42  43  44  45  46  47
Pro-Gln-Thr-Ser-Leu-Cys-Phe-Ser-Glu-Ser-Ile-Pro-Thr-Pro-Ser-Asn-
 48  49  50  51  52  53  54  55  56  57  58  59  60  61  62  63
Arg-Glu-Glu-Thr-Gln-Gln-Lys-Ser-Asn-Leu-Glu-Leu-Leu-Arg-Ile-Ser-
 64  65  66  67  68  69  70  71  72  73  74  75  76  77  78  79
Leu-Leu-Leu-Ile-Gln-Ser-Trp-Leu-Glu-Pro-Val-Gln-Phe-Leu-Arg-Ser-
 80  81  82  83  84  85  86  87  88  89  90  91  92  93  94  95
Val-Phe-Ala-Asn-Ser-Leu-Val-Tyr-Gly-Ala-Ser-Asp-Ser-Asn-Val-Tyr-
 96  97  98  99 100 101 102 103 104 105 106 107 108 109 110 111
Asp-Leu-Leu-Lys-Asp-Leu-Glu-Glu-Gly-Ile-Gln-Thr-Leu-Met-Gly-Arg-
112 113 114 115 116 117 118 119 120 121 122 123 124 125 126 127
Leu-Glu-Asp-Gly-Ser-Pro-Arg-Thr-Gly-Gln-Ile-Phe-Lys-Gln-Thr-Tyr-
128 129 130 131 132 133 134 135 136 137 138 139 140 141 142 143
Ser-Lys-Phe-Asp-Thr-Asn-Ser-His-Asn-Asp-Asp-Ala-Leu-Leu-Lys-Asn-
144 145 146 147 148 149 150 151 152 153 154 155 156 157 158 159
Tyr-Gly-Leu-Leu-Tyr-Cys-Phe-Arg-Lys-Asp-Met-Asp-Lys-Val-Glu-Thr-
160 161 162 163 164 165 166 167 168 169 170 171 172 173 174 175
Phe-Leu-Arg-Ile-Val-Gln-Cys-Arg-Ser-Val-Glu-Gly-Ser-Cys-Gly-Phe-OH
176 177 178 179 180 181 182 183 184 185 186 187 188 189 190 191
```

CLINICAL PHARMACOLOGY

Linear Growth: The primary and most intensively studied action of Somatrem for injection is the stimulation of linear growth. This effect is demonstrated in patients lacking adequate endogenous growth hormone production.

In vitro, preclinical, and clinical testing has demonstrated that Somatrem growth hormone is therapeutically equivalent to somatropin (human growth hormone, pituitary origin). Short-term clinical studies in normal adults show equivalent pharmacokinetics. Treatment of growth hormone deficient children with Somatrem growth hormone results in an increase in growth rate and somatomedin-C levels similar to that seen with somatropin therapy.

Other actions that have been demonstrated for Somatrem and/or somatropin include:

A. Tissue Growth: 1) Skeletal Growth: Somatrem stimulates skeletal growth in patients with growth hormone deficiency. The measurable increase in body length after administration of somatropin results from its effect on the epiphyseal growth plates of long bones. Studies *in vitro* have shown that the incorporation of sulfate into proteoglycans is not due to a direct effect of somatropin, but rather is accomplished by a mediator called somatomedin-C. Somatomedin-C is low in the serum of growth hormone deficient children but increases during treatment with Somatrem. 2) Cell Growth: It has been shown that the total number of skeletal muscle cells is markedly decreased in short-stature children lacking endogenous growth hormone compared with normal children. Treatment with somatropin results in an increase in both the number and the size of muscle cells. 3) Organ Growth: Somatropin influences the size of internal organs, and it also increases red cell mass.

B. Protein Metabolism: Linear growth is facilitated in part by increased cellular protein synthesis. This is reflected by nitrogen retention as demonstrated by a decline in urinary nitrogen excretion and blood urea nitrogen following the initiation of somatropin therapy. Treatment with Somatrem results in a similar decline in blood urea nitrogen.

C. Carbohydrate Metabolism: Both somatropin and Somatrem have been found to influence carbohydrate metabolism. It is recognized that children with hypopituitarism sometimes experience fasting hypoglycemia. In normal healthy subjects, large doses of Somatrem growth hormone may impair glucose tolerance. Administration of either somatropin or Somatrem to normal adults resulted in an increase in serum insulin levels. Although the precise mechanism by which somatropin and Somatrem induce insulin resistance is presently not known, it is attributed to a decrease in insulin sensitivity. An increase in serum glucose levels is observed during treatment with somatropin.

D. Lipid Metabolism: In growth hormone deficient subjects, long-term administration of somatropin often results in a general reduction in body fat stores. Acute administration of somatropin to humans results in lipid mobilization. Nonesterified fatty acids increase in plasma within two hours of somatropin administration.

◆ RATED THERAPEUTICALLY EQUIVALENT; ◇ THERAPEUTIC EQUIVALENCE UNCONFIRMED; ○ UNRATED

E. Mineral Metabolism: The retention of total body potassium and phosphorus, which is induced by somatropin administration, is thought to be due to cell growth. Sodium retention also occurs.

Serum levels of inorganic phosphate increase in patients with growth hormone deficiency after somatropin or Somatrem therapy due to metabolic activity associated with bone growth as well as increased tubular reabsorption of phosphate by the kidney. Serum calcium is not significantly altered in patients treated with either somatropin or Somatrem.

Although calcium excretion in the urine is increased, there is a simultaneous increase in calcium absorption from the intestine.

F. Connective Tissue Metabolism: Somatropin stimulates the synthesis of chondroitin sulfate and collagen as well as the urinary excretion of hydroxyproline.

INDICATIONS AND USAGE

Somatrem is indicated only for the long-term treatment of children who have growth failure due to a lack of adequate endogenous growth hormone secretion. Other etiologies of short stature should be excluded.

UNLABELED USES
Somatrem is used alone or as an adjunct in the treatment of growth hormone deficiency in adults and growth retardation in Down syndrome. It is also used to treat Turner's syndrome.

CONTRAINDICATIONS

Somatrem should not be used in subjects with closed epiphyses.

Somatrem growth hormone should not be used in patients with active neoplasia. Intracranial lesions must be inactive and antitumor therapy complete prior to instituting therapy. Somatrem growth hormone should be discontinued if there is evidence of recurrent tumor growth.

Somatrem growth hormone, when reconstituted with Bacteriostic Water for Injection, USP (benzyl alcohol preserved) should not be used in patients with a known sensitivity to benzyl alcohol.

WARNINGS

Benzyl alcohol as a preservative in Bacteriostatic Water for Injection has been associated with toxicity in newborns. When administering Somatrem to newborns, reconstitute with Sterile Water for Injection, USP. USE ONLY ONE DOSE PER VIAL AND DISCARD THE UNUSED PORTION.

PRECAUTIONS

General: Somatrem should be used only by physicians experienced in the diagnosis or management of patients with pituitary growth hormone deficiency. Patients with growth hormone deficiency secondary to an intracranial lesion should be examined frequently for progression or recurrence of the underlying disease process. Because Somatrem may induce a state of insulin resistance, patients should be observed for evidence of glucose intolerance.

Hypothyroidism may develop during Somatrem treatment. Untreated hypothyroidism prevents optimal response to Somatrem growth hormone. Therefore, patients should have periodic thyroid function tests and should be treated with thyroid hormone when indicated.

Leukemia has been reported in a small number of growth hormone deficient patients, treated with growth hormone. On the basis of current evidence, experts cannot conclude that growth hormone therapy is responsible for these occurrences. If there is any risk to an individual patient, it is minimal.

Slipped capital femoral epiphysis may occur more frequently in patients with endocrine disorders. Physicians and parents should be alert to the development of a limp or complaints of hip or knee pain in Somatrem-treated patients.

As for any protein, a systemic allergic reaction may occur.

See *"Warnings"* for use of Bacteriostatic Water for Injection, USP (benzyl alcohol preserved) in newborns.

Drug Interactions: Concomitant glucocorticoid therapy may inhibit the growth promoting effect of Somatrem growth hormone. Patients with coexisting ACTH deficiency should have their glucocorticoid replacement dose carefully adjusted to avoid an inhibitory effect on growth.

Carcinogenesis, Mutagenesis, Impairment of Fertility: Carcinogenicity, mutagenicity and reproduction studies have not been conducted with Somatrem growth hormone.

Pregnancy: Pregnancy (Category C). Animal reproduction studies have not been conducted with Somatrem growth hormone. It is also not known whether Somatrem growth hormone can cause fetal harm when administered to a pregnant woman or can affect reproduction capacity. Somatrem growth hormone should be given to a pregnant woman only if clearly needed.

Nursing Mothers: It is not known whether this drug is excreted in human milk. Because many drugs are excreted in human milk, caution should be exercised when Somatrem growth hormone is administered to a nursing woman.

ADVERSE REACTIONS

A. Somatrem.

Approximately 30 percent of all Somatrem-treated patients developed persistent antibodies to growth hormone.

In patients who had been previously treated with pituitary-derived growth hormone, one of twenty-two subjects developed persistent antibodies to growth hormone in response to Somatrem therapy.

In children not previously treated with any exogenous growth hormone approximately 40 percent developed persistent antibodies to growth hormone.

In general, the growth hormone antibodies are not neutralizing and do not interfere with the growth response to Somatrem growth hormone. One of eighty-four subjects treated with Somatrem growth hormone for 6 to 36 months developed antibodies associated with high binding capacities and failed to respond to treatment with Somatrem growth hormone.

In addition to an evaluation of compliance with treatment program and thyroid status, testing for antibodies to human growth hormone should be carried out in any patient who fails to respond to therapy.

Additional short-term immunologic and renal function studies were carried out in group of patients after approximately two years of treatment to detect other potential adverse effects of antibodies to growth hormone. The antibody was determined to be of the IgG class; no antibodies to growth hormone of the IgE class were detected. Testing included immune complex determination, measurement of total hemolytic complement and specific complement components, and immunochemical analyses. No adverse effects of growth hormone antibody formation were observed.

These findings are supported by a toxicity study conducted in a primate model in which a similar antibody response to growth hormone was observed. Somatrem, administered to monkeys by intramuscular injection at doses of 125 and 625 µg/kg TIW, was compared to pituitary-human growth hormone at the same doses and with placebo over a period of 90 days. Most monkeys treated with high-dose Somatrem growth hormone developed persistent antibodies at week four. There were no biologically significant drug related changes in standard laboratory variables. Histopathologic examination of the kidney and other selected organs (pituitary, lungs, liver and pancreas) showed no treatment related toxicity. There was no evidence of immune complexes or immune complex toxicity when the kidney was also examined for the presence of immune complexes and possible toxic effects of immune complexes by immunohistochemistry and electron microscopy.

B. Bacteriostatic Water for Injection. USP (benzyl alcohol preserved)

Toxicity in newborns has been associated with benzyl alcohol as a preservative (see *"Warnings"*).

OVERDOSAGE

The recommended dosage of up to 0.1 mg (0.26 IU) per kg body weight three times per week should not be exceeded due to the potential risk of side effects.

DOSAGE AND ADMINISTRATION

The Somatrem dosage must be individualized for each patient. A dosage and schedule of up to 0.1 mg/kg (0.26 IU/kg) body weight administered three times per week (TIW) by intramuscular or subcutaneous injection is recommended.

After the dose has been determined, reconstitute as follows: each 5 mg vial with 1-5 mL of Bacteriostatic Water for Injection, USP (benzyl alcohol preserved); or each 10 mg vial with 1-10 mL of Bacteriostatic Water for Injection, USP (benzyl alcohol preserved) only. For use in newborns see *"Warnings"*. The pH of Somatrem after reconstitution is approximately 7.8.

To prepare the Somatrem solution, inject the Bacteriostatic Water for Injection, USP (benzyl alcohol preserved) into the vial of Somatrem growth hormone, aiming the stream of liquid against the glass wall. Then swirl the product vial with a **GENTLE** rotary motion until the contents are completely dissolved. **DO NOT SHAKE.** Because Somatrem growth hormone is a protein, shaking can result in a cloudy solution. Immediately after reconstitution, the Somatrem solution should be clear. Occasionally, after refrigeration, you may notice that small colorless particles of protein are present in the Somatrem solution. This is not unusual for proteins like Somatrem growth hormone. If the solution is cloudy immediately after reconstitution or refrigeration, the contents **MUST NOT** be injected. Before and after injections the septum of the vial should be wiped with an antiseptic solution to prevent contamination of the contents after repeated needle insertions. It is recommended that Somatrem growth hormone be administered using sterile, disposable syringes and needles. The syringes should be of small enough volume that the prescribed dose can be drawn from the vial with reasonable accuracy.

STORAGE
Somatrem, before and after reconstitution with Bacteriostatic Water for Injection, USP (benzyl alcohol preserved), must be stored at 2°-8°C/36°-46°F (refrigerator).

Reconstituted vials should be used within 14 days after reconstitution.

Avoid freezing the reconstituted vial of Somatrem growth hormone and the Bacteriostatic Water for Injection, USP (benzyl alcohol preserved).

Expiration dates are stated on the labels.

HOW SUPPLIED
POWDER FOR INJECTION: 5 MG

BRAND/MANUFACTURER	NDC	SIZE	AWP
○ **BRAND** PROTROPIN: Genentech	50242-0015-02	2s	$420.00

POWDER FOR INJECTION: 10 MG

BRAND/MANUFACTURER	NDC	SIZE	AWP
○ **BRAND** PROTROPIN: Genentech	50242-0016-20	2s	$840.00

► SHOWN IN PRODUCT IDENTIFICATION GUIDE

Somatropin

DESCRIPTION

Somatropin for injection is a human growth hormone (hGH) produced by recombinant DNA technology. Somatropin has 191 amino acid residues and a molecular weight of 22,125 daltons. The amino acid sequence of the product is identical to that of pituitary-derived human growth hormone. The protein is synthesized by the addition of the gene for human growth hormone.

Somatropin is a highly purified preparation. Biological potency is determined by measuring the increase in body weight induced in hypophysectomized rats.

Somatropin is a sterile, white, lyophilized powder intended for subcutaneous administration after reconstitution; some brands may also be administered intramuscularly.

Each 5 mg vial contains 5 mg (approximately 13 IU or 225 picomoles) Somatropin.

Each 10 mg vial contains 10 mg (approximately 26 IU) Somatropin.

Following is its chemical structure:

```
H—Phe—Pro—Thr—Ile—Pro—Leu—Ser—Arg—Leu—Phe—Asp—Asn—Ala—Met—Leu—Arg—Ala—His—Arg—
    1    2    3    4    5    6    7    8    9   10   11   12   13   14   15   16   17   18   19

Leu—His—Gln—Leu—Ala—Phe—Asp—Thr—Tyr—Gln—Glu—Phe—Glu—Glu—Ala—Tyr—Ile—Pro—Lys—Glu—
 20   21   22   23   24   25   26   27   28   29   30   31   32   33   34   35   36   37   38   39

Gln—Lys—Tyr—Ser—Phe—Leu—Gln—Asn—Pro—Gln—Thr—Ser—Leu—Cys—Phe—Ser—Glu—Ser—Ile—Pro—
 40   41   42   43   44   45   46   47   48   49   50   51   52   53   54   55   56   57   58   59

Thr—Pro—Ser—Asn—Arg—Glu—Glu—Thr—Gln—Gln—Lys—Ser—Asn—Leu—Glu—Leu—Leu—Arg—Ile—Ser—
 60   61   62   63   64   65   66   67   68   69   70   71   72   73   74   75   76   77   78   79

Leu—Leu—Leu—Ile—Gln—Ser—Trp—Leu—Glu—Pro—Val—Gln—Phe—Leu—Arg—Ser—Val—Phe—Ala—
 80   81   82   83   84   85   86   87   88   89   90   91   92   93   94   95   96   97   98

Asn—Ser—Leu—Val—Tyr—Gly—Ala—Ser—Asn—Ser—Asp—Val—Tyr—Asp—Leu—Leu—Lys—Asp—Leu—Glu—
 99  100  101  102  103  104  105  106  107  108  109  110  111  112  113  114  115  116  117  118

Glu—Gly—Ile—Gln—Thr—Leu—Met—Gly—Arg—Leu—Glu—Asp—Gly—Ser—Pro—Arg—Thr—Gly—Gln—Ile—
119  120  121  122  123  124  125  126  127  128  129  130  131  132  133  134  135  136  137  138

Phe—Lys—Gln—Thr—Tyr—Ser—Lys—Phe—Asp—Thr—Asn—Ser—His—Asn—Asp—Asp—Ala—Leu—Leu—Lys—
139  140  141  142  143  144  145  146  147  148  149  150  151  152  153  154  155  156  157  158

Asn—Tyr—Gly—Leu—Leu—Tyr—Cys—Phe—Arg—Lys—Asp—Met—Asp—Lys—Val—Glu—Thr—Phe—Leu—
159  160  161  162  163  164  165  166  167  168  169  170  171  172  173  174  175  176  177

Arg—Ile—Val—Gln—Cys—Arg—Ser—Val—Glu—Gly—Ser—Cys—Gly—Phe—OH
178  179  180  181  182  183  184  185  186  187  188  189  190  191
```

CLINICAL PHARMACOLOGY

GENERAL

In vitro, preclinical, and clinical testing have demonstrated that Somatropin is therapeutically equivalent to pituitary-derived human growth hormone and achieves equivalent pharmacokinetic profiles in normal adults. Treatment of children who lack adequate endogenous growth hormone secretion with Somatropin resulted in an increase in growth rate and an increase in insulin-like growth factor-I/Somatomedin-C levels similar to that seen with pituitary-derived human growth hormone.

Actions that have been demonstrated for Somatropin somatrem and/or pituitary-derived human growth hormone include:

A. Tissue Growth: 1) Skeletal Growth: Somatropin stimulates skeletal growth in children with growth failure due to a lack of adequate secretion of endogenous growth hormone or secondary to chronic renal insufficiency. The measurable increase in body length after administration of either Somatropin or human growth hormone of pituitary origin is accomplished at the epiphyseal plates at the ends of a growing bone. Growth and metabolism of epiphyseal plate cells are directly stimulated by growth hormone and one of its mediators, insulin-like growth factor-I. Serum levels of insulin-like growth factor-I are low in children and adolescents who are growth hormone deficient, but increase during treatment with Somatropin. New bone is formed at the epiphyses in response to growth hormone. This results in linear growth until these growth plates fuse at the end of puberty. Elevations in mean serum alkaline phosphatase concentrations are also seen. 2) Cell Growth: It has been shown that there are fewer skeletal muscle cells in short-statured children who lack endogenous growth hormone as compared with normal children. Treatment with pituitary-derived human growth hormone results in an increase in both the number and the size of skeletal muscle cells. 3) Organ Growth: Growth hormone of human pituitary origin influences the size of internal organs, including kidneys, and increases red cell mass. Treatment of hypophysectomized or genetic dwarf rats with Somatropin results in organ growth that is proportional to the overall body growth. In normal rats subjected to nephrectomy-induced uremia, Somatropin promoted skeletal and body growth.

B. Protein Metabolism: Linear growth is facilitated in part by growth hormone-stimulated protein synthesis. This is reflected by nitrogen retention as demonstrated by a decline in urinary nitrogen excretion and blood urea nitrogen during therapy with human growth hormone of pituitary origin. Treatment with Somatropin results in a similar decrease in serum urea nitrogen.

C. Carbohydrate Metabolism: Growth hormone is a modulator of carbohydrate metabolism. For example, children with inadequate secretion of growth hormone or hypopituitarism, sometimes experience fasting hypoglycemia that is improved by treatment with Somatropin. Somatropin therapy may decrease glucose tolerance. Administration of Somatropin to normal adults, patients with chronic renal insufficiency, and patients who lack adequate secretion of endogenous growth hormone resulted in increases in mean serum fasting and postprandial insulin levels. However, glucose and hemoglobin A_{1C} levels remained in the normal range.

D. Lipid Metabolism: Acute administration of pituitary-derived human growth hormone to growth-hormone-deficient patients results in lipid mobilization. Nonesterified fatty acids increase in plasma within two hours of pituitary-derived human growth hormone administration. In growth hormone deficient patients, long-term growth hormone administration often decreases body fat. Mean cholesterol levels decreased in patients treated with Somatropin.

E. Mineral Metabolism: The retention of total body potassium in response to pituitary-derived growth hormone administration apparently results from cellular growth. Serum levels of inorganic phosphorus may increase slightly in patients with inadequate secretion of endogenous growth hormone or chronic renal insufficiency after growth hormone or Somatropin therapy due to metabolic activity associated with bone growth as well as increased tubular reabsorption of phosphate by the kidney. Serum calcium is not significantly altered in these patients. Sodium retention also occurs. (See "Precautions: Laboratory Tests.")

F. Connective Tissue Metabolism: Growth hormone stimulates the synthesis of chondroitin sulfate and collagen as well as the urinary excretion of hydroxyproline.

PHARMACOKINETICS

The pharmacokinetics of Somatropin have been investigated in healthy men after the subcutaneous administration of 0.1 mg/kg of body weight. A mean peak concentration (C_{max}) of 56.1 ng/mL occurred at a mean time of 7.5 hrs. The extent of absorption of Somatropin, assessed by area under the concentration versus time curve (AUC), was 626 ng•hr/mL and closely compares with that of somatrem (590 ng•hr/mL). The AUC of Somatropin is similar regardless of injection site.

Growth hormone localizes to highly perfused organs, most notably liver and kidney. In the kidney, growth hormone is filtered by the glomerulus, reabsorbed in the proximal tubule, and is broken down within renal cells into amino acids which return to the circulation.

In both normal and growth hormone deficient adults and children, the intramuscular and subcutaneous pharmacokinetic profiles of Somatropin are similar regardless of type of growth hormone or dosing regimen used. The subcutaneous pharmacokinetic profile of Somatropin is comparable to estimates in the published literature. A small number of dose-ranging studies suggest that clearance and AUC of Somatropin is proportional to dose in the therapeutic dose range. Consistent with the role of the liver and kidney as major elimination organs for exogenously administered human growth hormone, there is a reduction in growth hormone clearance in patients with severe liver or kidney dysfunction.

EFFECTS OF SOMATROPIN GROWTH FAILURE DUE TO CHRONIC RENAL INSUFFICIENCY (CRI)

Two multicenter, randomized, controlled clinical trials were conducted to determine whether treatment with Somatropin prior to renal transplantation in children with chronic renal insufficiency could improve their growth rates and height deficits. One study was a double-blinded, placebo-controlled trial and the other was an open-label, randomized trial. The dose of Somatropin in both controlled studies was 0.05 mg/kg/day (0.35 mg/kg/wk) administered daily by subcutaneous injection. Combining the data from those patients completing two years in the two controlled studies results in 62 children treated with Somatropin and 28 children in the control groups (either placebo-treated or untreated). The mean first year growth rate was 10.8 cm/yr for Somatropin treated patients, compared with a mean growth rate of 6.5 cm/yr for placebo/untreated controls (p < 0.00005). The mean second year growth rate was 7.8 cm/yr for the Somatropin-treated group, compared with 5.5 cm/yr for controls (p < 0.00005). There was a significant increase in mean height standard deviation score in the Somatropin group (- 2.9 at baseline to - 1.5 at Month 24, n = 62) but no significant change in the controls (- 2.8 at baseline - 2.9 at Month 24, n = 28). The mean third year growth rate of 7.6 cm/yr in the Somatropin treated patients (n = 27) suggests that Somatropin stimulates growth beyond two years. However, there are no control data for the third year because control patients crossed over to growth hormone treatment after two years of participation. The gains in height were accompanied by appropriate advancement of skeletal age. These data demonstrate that Somatropin therapy improves growth rate and corrects the acquired height deficit associated with chronic renal insufficiency. *Currently there are insufficient data regarding the benefit of treatment beyond three years. Although predicted final height was improved during Somatropin therapy, the effect of Somatropin on final adult height remains to be determined.*

POST-TRANSPLANT GROWTH

The North American Pediatric Renal Transplant Cooperative Study (NAPRTCS) has reported data for growth post-transplant in children who did not receive growth hormone. The average change in height SD score during the initial two years post-transplant was 0.18 (n = 300, J Ped 1993; 122;397-402).

Controlled studies of growth hormone treatment for the short stature associated with CRI were not designed to compare the growth of treated or untreated patients after they received renal transplants. However, growth data are available from a small number of patients who have been followed for at least 11 months. Of the 7 control patients, 4 increased their height SD score and 3 had either no significant change or a decrease in height SD score. The 13 patients treated with Somatropin prior to transplant had either no significant change or an increase in height SD score after transplantation, indicating that the individual gains achieved with growth hormone therapy prior to transplant were maintained after transplantation. The differences in the height deficit narrowed between the treated and untreated groups in the post-transplant period.

INDICATIONS AND USAGE

Somatropin is indicated for the long-term treatment of children who have growth failure due to a lack of endogenous growth hormone secretion.

Some brands of Somatropin are also indicated for the treatment of children who have growth failure associated with chronic renal insufficiency up to the time of renal transplantation. Somatropin therapy should be used in conjunction with optimal management of chronic renal insufficiency.

UNLABELED USES

Somatropin is used alone or as an adjunct in the treatment of growth hormone deficiency in adults, in prepubertal children with chronic renal failure and severe growth retardation, and osteoporosis. It is also used in Hand-Schuller-Christian disease, kwashiorkor, in conjunction with menotropins to induce ovulation, short stature children who do not have documented deficiency of growth hormone, Turner's syndrome, and in massive gastrointestinal hemorrhage induced by stress ulcers.

CONTRAINDICATIONS

Somatropin should not be used in subjects with closed epiphyses.

Somatropin should not be used in patients with active neoplasia. Intracranial lesions must be inactive and antitumor therapy complete prior to the institution of therapy. Growth hormone therapy should be discontinued if evidence of neoplasia develops.

Somatropin should not be used in patients with a known sensitivity to any components of the diluent used for reconstitution.

WARNINGS

Some diluents contain benzyl alcohol as a preservative, which has been associated with toxicity in newborns. When administering Somatropin to newborns, or sensitivity to the diluent should occur, the vials may be reconstituted with Sterile Water for Injection, USP. When Somatropin is reconstituted in this manner, (1) use only 1 reconstituted dose per vial, (2) refrigerate the solution (36° to 46°F [2° to 8°C]) if it is not used immediately after reconstitution, (3) use the reconstituted dose within 24 hours, and (4) discard the unused portion.

PRECAUTIONS

General: Therapy with Somatropin should be prescribed and directed by physicians experienced in the diagnosis and management of patients with chronic renal insufficiency or growth hormone deficiency. No studies have been performed of Somatropin therapy in children who have received renal transplants. Currently, treatment of patients with functioning renal allografts is not indicated. Because Somatropin may induce a state of insulin resistance, patients should be monitored for evidence of glucose intolerance.

Patients with growth hormone deficiency secondary to an intra- cranial lesion taking Somatropin should be examined frequently for progression or recurrence of the lesion.

Patients with growth failure secondary to chronic renal insufficiency should be examined periodically for evidence of progression of renal osteodystrophy. Slipped capital femoral epiphysis or avascular necrosis of the femoral head may be seen in children with advanced renal osteodystrophy, and it is uncertain whether these problems are affected by growth hormone therapy. X-rays of the hip should be obtained prior to initiating therapy. Physicians and parents should be alert to the development of a limp or complaints of hip or knee pain in patients treated with Somatropin.

Slipped capital femoral epiphysis may occur more frequently in patients with endocrine disorders, including growth hormone deficiency, or in patients undergoing rapid growth.

Intracranial hypertension (IH) with papilledema, visual changes, headache, nausea and/or vomiting has been reported in a small number of patients treated with growth hormone products. Symptoms usually occurred within the first eight (8) weeks of the initiation of growth hormone therapy. In all reported cases, IH-associated signs and symptoms resolved after termination of therapy or a reduction of the growth hormone dose. Funduscopic examination of patients is recommended at the initiation and periodically during the course of growth hormone therapy.

As for any protein, local or systemic allergic reactions may occur. Parents/Patient should be informed that such reactions are possible and that prompt medical attention should be sought if allergic reactions occur.

Laboratory Tests: Serum levels of inorganic phosphorus, alkaline phosphatase, and parathyroid hormone (PTH) may increase with Somatropin therapy. Changes in thyroid hormone laboratory measurements may develop during Somatropin treatment in children who lack adequate endogenous growth hormone secretion. Untreated hypothyroidism prevents optimal response to Somatropin. Therefore, patients should have periodic thyroid function tests and should be treated with thyroid hormone when indicated.

Drug Interaction: The use of Somatropin in patients with chronic renal insufficiency receiving glucocorticoid therapy has not been evaluated. Concomitant glucocorticoid therapy may inhibit the growth promoting effect of Somatropin. Patients with coexisting ACTH deficiency should have their glucocorticoid replacement dose carefully adjusted to avoid an inhibitory effect on growth.

There was no evidence in the controlled studies of Somatropin's interaction with drugs commonly used in chronic renal insufficiency patients. However, formal drug interaction studies have not been conducted.

Carcinogenesis, Mutagenesis, Impairment of Fertility: Long-term animal studies for carcinogenicity and impairment of fertility with this human growth hormone Somatropin have not been performed. There has been no evidence to date of Somatropin-induced mutagenicity.

Pregnancy: Pregnancy (Category C): Animal reproduction studies have not been conducted with Somatropin. It is also not known whether Somatropin can cause fetal harm when administered to a pregnant woman or can affect reproduction capacity. Somatropin should be given to a pregnant woman only if clearly needed.

Nursing Mothers: There have been no studies conducted with Somatropin in nursing mothers. It is not known whether Somatropin is excreted in human milk. Because many drugs are excreted in human milk, caution should be exercised when Somatropin is administered to a nursing mother.

Information for Patients: Patients being treated with growth hormone and/or their parents should be informed of the potential benefits and risks associated with treatment. If home use is determined to be desirable by the physician, instructions on appropriate use should be given.

If home use is prescribed, a puncture resistant container for the disposal of used syringes and needles should be recommended to the patient. Patients and/or parents should be thoroughly instructed in the importance of proper disposal and cautioned against any reuse of needles and syringes.

ADVERSE REACTIONS

Approximately 2% of 481 naive and previously treated clinical trial patients treated with Somatropin, have developed antibodies to growth hormone, as demonstrated by a binding capacity determination threshold ≥ 0.02 µg/mL. Nevertheless, even these patients experienced increases in linear growth and other salutary effects of Somatropin and did not experience any unusual adverse events. In some cases when binding capacity exceeds 2 mg/L, growth attenuation has been observed. In clinical studies of patients that were treated with Somatropin for the first time, 0/107 growth hormone inadequate (GHI) patients and 0/125 CRI patients screened for antibody production developed antibodies with binding capacities ≥ 2 mg/L at six months. Although growth-limiting antibodies have been observed with other growth hormone preparations (including products of pituitary origin), antibodies in patients treated with Somatropin have not limited growth. The long-term implications of antibody development are uncertain at this time.

Of the 232 naive and previously treated clinical trial patients receiving Somatropin for 6 months or more, 4.7% had serum binding of radiolabeled growth hormone in excess of twice the binding observed in control sera when the serum samples were assayed at a tenfold dilution. Among these patients were 160 naive patients, of whom 6.9% had positive serum binding.

Additional short-term immunologic and renal function studies were carried out in a group of patients with chronic renal insufficiency after approximately one year of treatment to detect other potential adverse effects of antibodies to growth hormone. Testing included measurements of C1q, C3, C4, rheumatoid factor, creatinine, creatinine clearance and BUN. No adverse effects of growth hormone antibodies were noted.

In addition to an evaluation of compliance with the prescribed treatment program and thyroid status, testing for antibodies to human growth hormone should be carried out in any patient who fails to respond to therapy.

In studies in children treated with Somatropin, injection site pain was reported infrequently.

In clinical studies in which high doses of Somatropin were administered to healthy adult volunteers, the following events have occurred infrequently: headache, localized muscle pain, weakness, mild hyperglycemia, and glucosuria. A mild and transient edema, which appeared in 2.5% of patients, was observed early during the course of treatment.

Leukemia has been reported in a small number of growth hormone deficient patients treated with growth hormone. It is uncertain whether this increased risk is related to the pathology of growth hormone deficiency itself, growth hormone therapy, or other associated treatments such as radiation therapy for intracranial tumors. On the basis of current evidence, experts cannot conclude that growth hormone therapy is responsible for these occurrences. There have been no reports of leukemia in growth hormone-treated CRI patients. The risk to GHI and CRI patients, if any, remains to be established.

OVERDOSAGE

The recommended dosage for GHI is 0.30 mg/kg (approximately 0.78 IU/kg) of body weight weekly to up to 0.06 mg/kg (0.16 IU/kg) of body weight 3 times per week. The recommended dosage for CRI is 0.35 mg/kg (approximately 0.91 IU/kg) of body weight weekly. Acute overdosage could lead initially to hypoglycemia and subsequently to hyperglycemia. Long-term overdosage could result in signs and symptoms of gigantism and/or acromegaly consistent with the known effects of excess human growth hormone.

DOSAGE AND ADMINISTRATION

GROWTH HORMONE INADEQUACY (GHI)

Depending on the brand, a weekly dosage of 0.30 mg/kg (approximately 0.78 IU/kg) of body weight administered by daily subcutaneous injection or up to 0.6 mg/kg (0.16 IU/kg) of body weight administered 3 times per week by subcutaneous or intramuscular injection is recommended.

The Somatropin dosage and administration schedule for GHI should be individualized for each patient. Therapy should not be continued if final height is achieved or epiphyseal fusion occurs. Patients who fail to respond adequately while on Somatropin therapy should be evaluated to determine the cause of unresponsiveness.

CHRONIC RENAL INSUFFICIENCY (CRI)

For brands with this indication, a weekly dosage of 0.35 mg/kg (approximately 0.91 IU/kg) of body weight administered by daily subcutaneous injection is recommended.

The duration of Somatropin therapy for CRI should be individualized for each patient.

Somatropin therapy may be continued up to the time of renal transplantation. Therapy should not be continued if final height is achieved or epiphyseal fusion occurs. Patients who fail to respond adequately while on Somatropin therapy should be evaluated to determine the cause of unresponsiveness. In order to optimize therapy for patients who require dialysis, the following guidelines for injection schedule are recommended:

1. Hemodialysis patients should receive their injection at night just prior to going to sleep or at least 3-4 hours after their hemodialysis to prevent hematoma formation due to the heparin.

2. Chronic Cycling Peritoneal Dialysis (CCPD) patients should receive their injection in the morning after they have completed dialysis.

3. Chronic Ambulatory Peritoneal Dialysis (CAPD) patients should receive their injection in the evening at the time of the overnight exchange.

After the dose has been determined, reconstitute as follows: each 5 mg vial should be reconstituted with 1-5 mL of diluent; or each 10 mg vial should be reconstituted with 1-10 mL of diluent. For use in newborns see *"Warnings"*.

To prepare the Somatropin solution, inject the diluent into the Somatropin vial, aiming the stream of liquid against the glass wall. Then swirl the product vial with a *Gentle* rotary motion until the contents are completely dissolved. *Do Not Shake*. Because Somatropin is a protein, shaking can result in a cloudy solution. The Somatropin solution should be clear immediately after reconstitution. Occasionally, after refrigeration, you may notice that small colorless particles of protein are present in the Somatropin solution. This is not unusual for solutions containing proteins. If the solution is cloudy immediately after reconstitution or refrigeration, the contents **MUST NOT** be injected. Some brands should not contain particulate matter; check product labeling.

Before needle insertion, wipe the septum of both the Somatropin and diluent vials with rubbing alcohol or an antiseptic solution to prevent contamination of the contents by microorganisms that may be introduced by repeated needle insertions. It is recommended that Somatropin be administered using sterile, disposable syringes and needles. The syringes should be of small enough volume that the prescribed dose can be drawn from the vial with reasonable accuracy.

STABILITY AND STORAGE

Before Reconstitution: Somatropin and any diluent other than Sterile Water for Injection, must be stored at 2-8°C/36-46°F (under refrigeration). **Avoid freezing.** Expiration dates are stated on the labels.

After Reconstitution: Vial contents are stable for up to 14 days when reconstituted and stored at 2-8°C/36-46°F (under refrigeration). **Avoid freezing.**

HOW SUPPLIED
POWDER FOR INJECTION: 5 MG

BRAND/MANUFACTURER	NDC	SIZE	AWP
○ **BRAND**			
NUTROPIN: Genentech	50242-0072-02	2s	$420.00
HUMATROPE: Lilly	00002-7335-16	6s ud	$1260.05

POWDER FOR INJECTION: 10 MG

BRAND/MANUFACTURER	NDC	SIZE	AWP
○ **BRAND**			
NUTROPIN: Genentech	50242-0018-20	2s	$840.00

Sorbitol

DESCRIPTION

3% Sorbitol Urologic Irrigating Solution is a sterile, nonpyrogenic, nonhemolytic, electrically nonconductive solution in a single dose plastic container for use as a urologic irrigating solution. Each liter contains 30 g Sorbitol in Water for Injection. pH 5.0 (4.5 to 6.5). Osmolarity 165 mOsmol/L (calc.).

Sorbitol is a reduced form of dextrose and is designated chemically as D-Glucitol.

The Uromatic® plastic container is fabricated from a specially formulated polyvinyl chloride (PL 146® plastic). The amount of water that can permeate from inside the container into the overwrap is insufficient to affect the solution significantly. Solutions in contact with the plastic container can leach out certain at its chemical components in very small amounts within the expiration period, e.g., di-2-ethylhexyl phthalate (DEHP), up to 5 parts per million; however, the safety of the plastic has been confirmed in tests in animals according to USP biological tests for plastic containers as well as by tissue culture toxicity studies.

CLINICAL PHARMACOLOGY

3% Sorbitol Urologic Irrigating Solution is useful as an irrigating fluid for the urinary bladder because the sorbitol solution is nonhemolytic, electrically nonconductive, and provides a high degree of visibility for urologic procedures requiring endoscopy. During transurethral surgical procedures, the solution acts as a lavage for removing blood and tissue fragments. It is also useful as an irrigating fluid to maintain the patency of an indwelling catheter in the immediate postoperative period. If absorbed either intravascularly or extravascularly during transurethral resections, the Sorbitol will be either metabolized to carbon dioxide and water or excreted by a normally functioning kidney.

INDICATIONS AND USAGE

3% Sorbitol Urologic Irrigating Solution is indicated for use as a urologic irrigating fluid with endoscopic instruments during transurethral procedures requiring distension, irrigation, and lavage of the urinary bladder. It may be used for lavage of an indwelling catheter to maintain patency.

UNLABELED USES

Sorbitol is used alone or as an adjunct in the treatment of hepatic encephalopathy.

CONTRAINDICATIONS

Anuria.

WARNINGS

Not for injection.

Solutions for urologic irrigation must be used with caution in patients with severe cardiopulmonary or renal dysfunction.

Irrigating fluids used during transurethral prostatectomy have been demonstrated to enter the systemic circulation in relatively large volumes; thus Sorbitol irrigating solution must be regarded as a systemic drug. Absorption of large amounts of fluids containing Sorbitol may significantly alter cardiopulmonary and renal dynamics.

Hyperglycemia from metabolism of absorbed Sorbitol may occur in patients with diabetes mellitus.

The contents of an opened container should be used promptly to minimize the possibility of bacterial growth of pyrogen formation. Discard the unused portion of irrigating solution since no antimicrobial agent has been added.

PRECAUTIONS

The cardiovascular status, especially of the patient with cardiac disease, should be carefully observed before and during transurethral resection of the prostate when using 3% Sorbitol Urologic Irrigating Solution. Because the quantity of fluid absorbed into the systemic circulation by opened prostatic veins may produce significant expansion of the intravascular fluid and lead to fulminating congestive heart failure.

Shift of sodium free intracellular fluid into the extracellular compartment. Following systemic absorption may lower serum concentration and aggravate preexisting hyponatremia.

Excessive loss of water and electrolytes may lead to serious imbalances. With continuous administration of solution, loss of water may occur in excess of electrolytes, producing hypernatremia.

Sustained diuresis that results from transurethral irrigation with sorbitol irrigating solutions may obscure and intensity inadequate hydration or hypovolemia.

PREGNANCY TERATOGENIC EFFECTS

Pregnancy Category C. Animal reproduction studies have not been conducted with 3% Sorbitol Urologic Irrigating Solution. It is not known whether 3% Sorbitol Urologic Irrigating Solution can cause fetal harm when administered to a pregnant woman or can affect reproductive capacity. 3% Sorbitol Urologic Irrigating Solution should be given to a pregnant woman only if clearly needed.

Do not administer unless the solution is clear and the seal is intact.

ADVERSE REACTIONS

The literature reports occasional adverse reactions for intravenous Sorbitol infusions. These include disturbances such as acidosis, electrolyte loss, marked diuresis, urinary retention, edema, dryness of mouth and thirst, and dehydration; cardiovascular/pulmonary disorders such as pulmonary congestion, hypotension, tachycardia, angina-like pains, and other general reactions such as blurred vision, convulsions, nausea, vomiting, diarrhea, rhinitis, chills, vertigo, and backache. Allergic reactions reported to occur from Sorbitol include urticaria.

Should adverse reactions occur, discontinue the irrigant and reevaluate the clinical status of the patient.

DOSAGE AND ADMINISTRATION

The volume of solution needed will vary with the nature and duration of the urologic procedure.

If desired, warm in overwrap to near body temperature in a water bath or oven heated to not more than 45°C.

Parenteral drug products should be inspected visually for particulate matter and discoloration prior to administration whenever solution and container permit.

DIRECTIONS FOR USE

Tear overwrap down side at slit and remove solution container. Some opacity of the plastic due to moisture absorption during the sterilization process may be observed. This is normal and does not affect the solution quality or safety. The opacity will diminish gradually. Check for minute leaks by squeezing bag firmly. If leaks are found, discard solution as sterility may be impaired.

USE ASEPTIC TECHNIQUE

1. Suspend container using hanger hole.
2. Remove plastic protector from outlet port (red tip).
3. Attach irrigation set. Refer to complete directions accompanying set.

◆ RATED THERAPEUTICALLY EQUIVALENT; ◇ THERAPEUTIC EQUIVALENCE UNCONFIRMED; ○ UNRATED

Exposure of pharmaceutical products to heat should be minimized. Avoid excessive heat. It is recommended the product be stored at room temperature (25°C): brief exposure up to 40°C does not adversely affect the product.

HOW SUPPLIED
SOLUTION: 3%

AVERAGE UNIT PRICE (AVAILABLE SIZES)

GENERIC	$0.007

BRAND/MANUFACTURER	NDC	SIZE	AWP
◆ GENERICS			
Baxter	00338-0295-49	5000 ml 2s	$65.75
Baxter	00338-0295-47	3000 ml 4s	$81.36

Sorbitrate SEE ISOSORBIDE DINITRATE

Sotalol Hydrochloride

DESCRIPTION
Sotalol Hydrochloride is an antiarrhythmic drug with Class II (beta-adrenoreceptor blocking) and Class III (cardiac action potential duration prolongation) properties. Sotalol Hydrochloride is a white, crystalline solid with a molecular weight of 308.8. It is hydrophilic, soluble in water, propylene glycol and ethanol, but is only slightly soluble in chloroform. Chemically, Sotalol Hydrochloride is d,l-N-[4-[1-hydroxy-2-[(1-methylethyl)amino]ethyl]pheny/l]methane-sulfonamide monohydrochloride. The molecular formula is $C_{12}H_{20}N_2O_3S \cdot HCl$

Following is its chemical structure:

$$CH_3SO_2NH - \bigcirc - \overset{OH}{\underset{|}{C}}HCH_2NHCH(CH_3)_2 \cdot HCl$$

CLINICAL PHARMACOLOGY
Mechanism of Action: Sotalol Hydrochloride has both beta-adrenoreceptor blocking (Vaughan Williams Class II) and cardiac action potential duration prolongation (Vaughan Williams Class III) antiarrhythmic properties. Sotalol Hydrochloride is a racemic mixture of d- and l-isomers. Both isomers have similar Class III antiarrhythmic effects, while the l-isomer is responsible for virtually all of the beta-blocking activity. The beta-blocking effect of Sotalol Hydrochloride is non-cardioselective, half maximal at about 80 mg/day and maximal at doses between 320 and 640 mg/day. Sotalol Hydrochloride does not have partial agonist or membrane stabilizing activity. Although significant beta-blockade occurs at oral doses as low as 25 mg, Class III effects are seen only at daily doses of 160 mg and above.

Electrophysiology: Sotalol Hydrochloride prolongs the plateau phase of the cardiac action potential in the isolated myocyte, as well as in isolated tissue preparations of ventricular or atrial muscle (Class III activity). In intact animals it slows heart rate, decreases AV nodal conduction and increases the refractory periods of atrial and ventricular muscle and conduction tissue.

In man, the Class II (beta-blockade) electrophysiological effects of Sotalol Hydrochloride are manifested by increased sinus cycle length (slowed heart rate), decreased AV nodal conduction and increased AV nodal refractoriness. The Class III electrophysiological effects in man include prolongation of the atrial and ventricular monophasic action potentials, and effective refractory period prolongation of atrial muscle, ventricular muscle, and atrio-ventricular accessory pathways (where present) in both the anterograde and retrograde directions. With oral doses of 160 to 640 mg/day, the surface ECG shows dose-related mean increases of 40-100 msec in QT and 10-40 msec in QT_c. (See *"Warnings"* for description of relationship between QT_c and torsade de pointes type arrhythmias.) No significant alteration in QRS interval is observed.

In a small study (n = 25) of patients with implanted defibrillators treated concurrently with Sotalol Hydrochloride, the average defibrillatory threshold was 6 joules (range 2-15 joules) compared to a mean of 16 joules for a non-randomized comparative group primarily receiving amiodarone.

Hemodynamics: In a study of systemic hemodynamic function measured invasively in 12 patients with a mean LV ejection fraction of 37% and ventricular tachycardia (9 sustained and 3 non-sustained), a median dose of 160 mg twice daily of Sotalol Hydrochloride produced a 28% reduction in heart rate and a 24% decrease in cardiac index at 2 hours post dosing at steady-state. Concurrently, systemic vascular resistance and stroke volume showed non-significant increases of 25% and 8%, respectively. Pulmonary capillary wedge pressure increased significantly from 6.4 mmHg to 11.8 mmHg in the 11 patients who completed the study. One patient was discontinued because of worsening congestive heart failure. Mean arterial pressure, mean pulmonary artery pressure and stroke work index did not significantly change. Exercise and isoproterenol induced tachycardia are antagonized by Sotalol Hydrochloride, and total peripheral resistance increases by a small amount.

In hypertensive patients, Sotalol Hydrochloride produces significant reductions in both systolic and diastolic blood pressures. Although Sotalol Hydrochloride is usually well-tolerated hemodynamically, caution should be exercised in patients with marginal cardiac compensation as deterioration in cardiac performance may occur. (See *"Warnings: Congestive Heart Failure"*.)

Clinical Actions: Sotalol Hydrochloride has been studied in life-threatening and less severe arrhythmias. In patients with frequent premature ventricular complexes (VPC), Sotalol Hydrochloride was significantly superior to placebo in reducing VPCs paired VPCs and nonsustained ventricular tachycardia (NSVT); the response was dose-related through 640 mg/day with 80-85% of patients having at least a 75% reduction of VPCs. Sotalol Hydrochloride was also superior, at the doses evaluated, to propranolol (40-80 mg TID) and similar to quinidine (200-400 mg QID) in reducing VPCs. In patients with life-threatening arrhythmias [sustained ventricular tachycardia/fibrillation (VT/VF)]. Sotalol Hydrochloride was studied acutely [by suppression of programmed electrical stimulation (PES) induced VT and by suppression of Holter monitor evidence of sustained VT] and, in acute responders, chronically.

In a double-blind, randomized comparison of Sotalol Hydrochloride and procainamide given intravenously (total of 2 mg/kg Sotalol Hydrochloride vs. 19 mg/kg of procainamide over 90 minutes), Sotalol Hydrochloride suppressed PES induction in 30% of patients vs. 20% of procainamide (p = 0.2).

In a randomized clinical trial [Electrophysiologic Study Versus Electrocardiographic Monitoring (ESVEM) Trial] comparing choice of antiarrhythmic therapy by PES suppression vs. Holter monitor selection (in each case followed by treadmill exercise testing) in patients with a history of sustained VT/VF who were also inducible by PES, the effectiveness acutely and chronically of Sotalol Hydrochloride was compared with 6 other drugs (procainamide, quinidine, mexiletine, propafenone, imipramine and pirmenol). Overall response, limited to first randomized drug, was 39% for Sotalol Hydrochloride and 30% for the pooled other drugs. Acute response rate for first drug randomized using suppression of PES induction was 36% for Sotalol Hydrochloride vs. a mean of 13% for the other drugs. Using the Holter monitoring endpoint (complete suppression of sustained VT, 90% suppression of NSVT, 80% suppression of VPC pairs, and at least 70% suppression of VPCs), Sotalol Hydrochloride yielded 41% response vs. 45% for the other drugs combined. Among responders placed on long-term therapy identified acutely as effective (by either PES or Holter), Sotalol Hydrochloride, when compared to the pool of other drugs, had the lowest two-year mortality (13% vs. 22%), the lowest two-year VT recurrence rate (30% vs. 60%), and the lowest withdrawal rate (38% vs. about 75-80%). The most commonly used doses of Sotalol Hydrochloride in this trial were 320-480 mg/day (66% of patients), with 16% receiving 240 mg/day or less and 18% receiving 640 mg or more.

It cannot be determined, however, in the absence of a controlled comparison of Sotalol Hydrochloride vs. no pharmacologic treatment (e.g., in patients with implanted defibrillators) whether Sotalol Hydrochloride response causes improved survival or identifies a population with a good prognosis.

In a large double-blind, placebo controlled secondary prevention (post-infarction) trial (n = 1,456), Sotalol Hydrochloride was given as a non-titrated initial dose of 320 mg once daily. Sotalol Hydrochloride did not produce a significant increase in survival (7.3% mortality on Sotalol Hydrochloride vs 8.9% on placebo, p = 0.3), but overall did not suggest an adverse effect on survival. There was, however, a suggestion of an early (i.e., first 10 days) excess mortality (3% on Sotalol Hydrochloride vs. 2% on placebo). In a second small trial (n = 17 randomized to Sotalol) where Sotalol Hydrochloride was administered at high doses (e.g., 320 mg twice daily) to high-risk post-infarction patients (ejection fraction < 40% and either > 10 VPC/hr or VT on Holter), there were 4 fatalities and 3 serious hemodynamic/electrical adverse events within two weeks of initiating Sotalol Hydrochloride.

Pharmacokinetics: In healthy subjects, the oral bioavailability of Sotalol Hydrochloride is 90-100%. After oral administration, peak plasma concentrations are reached in 2.5 to 4 hours, and steady-state plasma concentrations are attained within 2-3 days (i.e. after 5-6 doses when administered twice daily). Over the dosage range 160-640 mg/day Sotalol Hydrochloride displays dose proportionality with respect to plasma concentrations. Distribution occurs to a central (plasma) and to a peripheral compartment with a mean elimination half-life of 12 hours. Dosing every 12 hours results in trough plasma concentrations which are approximately one-half of those at peak.

Sotalol Hydrochloride does not bind to plasma proteins and is not metabolized. Sotalol Hydrochloride shows very little intersubject variability in plasma levels. The pharmacokinetics of the d and l enantiomers of Sotalol are essentially identical. Sotalol Hydrochloride crosses the blood brain barrier poorly. Excretion is predominantly via the kidney in the unchanged form, and therefore lower doses are necessary in conditions of renal impairment (see *"Dosage And Administration"*). Age per se does not significantly alter the pharmacokinetics of Sotalol Hydrochloride, but impaired renal function in geriatric patients can increase the terminal elimination half-life, resulting in increased drug accumulation. The absorption of Sotalol Hydrochloride was reduced by approximately 20% compared to fasting when it was administered with a standard meal. Since Sotalol Hydrochloride is not subject to first-pass metabolism, patients with hepatic impairment show no alteration in clearance of Sotalol Hydrochloride.

INDICATIONS AND USAGE
Oral Sotalol Hydrochloride is indicated for the treatment of documented ventricular arrhythmias, such as sustained ventricular tachycardia, that in the judgment of the physician are life-threatening. Because of the proarrhythmic effects of Sotalol Hydrochloride (see *"Warnings"*), including a 1.5 to 2% rate of torsade de pointes or new VT/VF in patients with either NSVT or supraventricular arrhythmias, its use in patients with less severe arrhythmias, even if the

patients are symptomatic, is generally not recommended. Treatment of patients with asymptomatic ventricular premature contractions should be avoided.

Initiation of Sotalol Hydrochloride treatment or increasing doses, as with other antiarrhythmic agents used to treat life-threatening arrhythmias, should be carried out in the hospital. The response to treatment should then be evaluated by a suitable method (e.g., PES or Holter monitoring) prior to continuing the patient on chronic therapy. Various approaches have been used to determine the response to antiarrhythmic therapy, including Sotalol Hydrochloride.

In the ESVEM Trial, response by Holter monitoring was tentatively defined as 100% suppression of ventricular tachycardia, 90% suppression of non-sustained VT, 80% suppression of paired VPCs, and 75% suppression of total VPCs in patients who had at least 10 VPCs/hour at baseline; this tentative response was confirmed if VT lasting 5 or more beats was not observed during treadmill exercise testing using a standard Bruce protocol. The PES protocol utilized a maximum of three extrastimuli at three pacing cycle lengths and two right ventricular pacing sites. Response by PES was defined as prevention of induction of the following: 1) monomorphic VT lasting over 15 seconds; 2) non-sustained polymorphic VT containing more than 15 beats of monomorphic VT in patients with a history of monomorphic VT; 3) polymorphic VT or VF greater than 15 beats in patients with VF or a history of aborted sudden death without monomorphic VT; and 4) two episodes of polymorphic VT or VF of greater than 15 beats in a patient presenting with monomorphic VT. Sustained VT or NSVT producing hypotension during the final treadmill test was considered a drug failure.

In a multicenter open-label long-term study of Sotalol Hydrochloride in patients with life-threatening ventricular arrhythmias which had proven refractory to other antiarrhythmic medications, response by Holter monitoring was defined as in ESVEM. Response by PES was defined as non-inducibility of sustained VT by at least double extrastimuli delivered at a pacing cycle length of 400 msec. Overall survival and arrhythmia recurrence rates in this study were similar to those seen in ESVEM, although there was no comparative group to allow a definitive assessment of outcome.

Antiarrhythmic drugs have not been shown to enhance survival in patients with ventricular arrhythmias.

UNLABELED USES
Sotalol Hydrochloride is used alone or as an adjunct in the treatment of angina pectoris and essential hypertension.

CONTRAINDICATIONS

Sotalol Hydrochloride, is contraindicated in patients with bronchial asthma, sinus bradycardia, second and third degree AV block, unless a functioning pacemaker is present, congenital or acquired long QT syndromes, cardiogenic shock, uncontrolled congestive heart failure, and previous evidence of hypersensitivity to Sotalol Hydrochloride.

WARNINGS

Mortality: **The National Heart Lung and Blood Institute conducted the Cardiac Arrhythmia Suppression Trial (CAST), a long-term, multicenter, randomized, double-blind study in patients with asymptomatic nonlife-threatening ventricular ectopy who had a myocardial infarction more than six days but less than two years previously. An excess of mortality rate or nonfatal cardiac arrest rate was seen in patients treated with encainide or flecainide (56/730) compared with that seen in patients assigned to matched placebo-treated groups (22/725), and a similar excess has been seen with moricizine. The average duration of treatment with encainide or flecainide in this study was ten months.**

The applicability of these results to other populations (e.g., those without recent myocardial infarction) and to other than Class I antiarrhythmic agents is uncertain. Sotalol Hydrochloride is devoid of Class I effects, and in a large (n = 1,456) controlled trial in patients with a recent myocardial infarction, who did not necessarily have ventricular arrhythmias, Sotalol Hydrochloride did not produce increased mortality at doses up to 320 mg/day (see "Clinical Actions"). On the other hand, in the large post-infarction study using a non-titrated initial dose of 320 mg once daily and in a second small randomized trial in high-risk post-infarction patients treated with high doses (320 mg BID), there have been suggestions of an excess of early sudden deaths.

Proarrhythmia: Like other antiarrhythmic agents Sotalol Hydrochloride can provoke new or worsened ventricular arrhythmias in some patients, including sustained ventricular tachycardia or ventricular fibrillation, with potentially fatal consequences. Because of its effect on cardiac repolarization (QT_c interval prolongation), torsade de pointes, a polymorphic ventricular tachycardia with prolongation of the QT interval and a shifting electrical axis is the most common form of proarrhythmia associated with Sotalol Hydrochloride, occurring in about 4% of high risk (history of sustained VT/VF) patients. The risk of torsade de pointes progressively increases with prolongation of the QT interval, and is worsened also by reduction in heart rate and reduction in serum potassium (see "Electrolyte Disturbances").

Because of the variable temporal recurrence of arrhythmias, it is not always possible to distinguish between a new or aggravated arrhythmic event and the patient's underlying rhythm disorder. (Note, however, that torsade de pointes is usually a drug-induced arrhythmia in people with an initially normal QT_c.) Thus, the incidence of drug-related events cannot be precisely determined, so that the occurrence rates provided must be considered approximations. Note also that drug-induced arrhythmias may often not be identified, particularly if they occur long after starting the drug, due to less frequent monitoring. It is clear from the NIH-sponsored CAST (see "Warnings: Mortality") that some antiarrhythmic drugs can cause increased sudden death mortality, presumably due to new

arrhythmias or asystole, that do not appear early in treatment but that represent a sustained increased risk.

Overall in clinical trials with Sotalol Hydrochloride, 4.3% of 3257 patients experienced a new or worsened ventricular arrhythmia. Of this 4.3%, there was a new or worsened sustained ventricular tachycardia in approximately 1% of patients and torsade de pointes in 2.4%. Additionally, in approximately 1% of patients, deaths were considered possibly drug-related; such cases, although difficult to evaluate, may have been associated with proarrhythmic events. **In patients with a history of sustained ventricular tachycardia, the incidence of torsade de pointes was 4% and worsened VT in about 1%; in patients with other, less serious, ventricular arrhythmias and supraventricular arrhythmias, the incidence of torsade de pointes was 1% and 1.4%, respectively.**

Torsade de pointes arrhythmias were dose related, as is the prolongation of QT (QT_c) interval, as shown in the table below.

PERCENT INCIDENCE OF TORSADE DE POINTES AND MEAN QT_c INTERVAL BY DOSE FOR PATIENTS WITH SUSTAINED VT/VF

Daily Dose (mg)	Incidence of Torsade de pointes	Mean QT_c* (msec)
80	0 (69)	463 (17)
160	0.5 (832)	467 (181)
320	1.6 (835)	473 (344)
480	4.4 (459)	483 (234)
640	3.7 (324)	490 (185)
> 640	5.8 (103)	512 (62)

( ) Number of patients assessed
* *highest on-therapy value*

In addition to dose and presence of sustained VT, other risk factors for torsade de pointes were gender (females had a higher incidence), excessive prolongation of the QT_c interval (see table below) and history of cardiomegaly or congestive heart failure. Patients with sustained ventricular tachycardia and a history of congestive heart failure appear to have the highest risk for serious proarrhythmia (7%). Of the patients experiencing torsade de pointes, approximately two-thirds spontaneously reverted to their baseline rhythm. The others were either converted electrically (D/C cardioversion or overdrive pacing) or treated with other drugs (see "Overdosage"). It is not possible to determine whether some sudden deaths represented episodes of torsade de pointes, but in some instances sudden death did follow a documented episode of torsade de pointes. Although Sotalol Hydrochloride therapy was discontinued in most patients experiencing torsade de pointes, 17% were continued on a lower dose. Nonetheless, Sotalol Hydrochloride should be used with particular caution if the QT_c is greater than 500 msec on-therapy and serious consideration should be given to reducing the dose or discontinuing therapy when the QT_c exceeds 550 msec. Due to the multiple risk-factors associated with torsade de pointes, however, caution should be exercised regardless of the QT_c interval. The table below relates the incidence of torsade de pointes to on-therapy QT_c and change in QT_c from baseline. It should be noted, however, that the highest on-therapy QT_c was in many cases the one obtained at the time of the torsade de pointes event, so that the table overstates the predictive value of a high QT_c. (See related table).

Proarrhythmic events must be anticipated not only on initiating therapy, but with every upward dose adjustment. Proarrhythmic events most often occur within 7 days of initiating therapy or of an increase in dose; 75% of serious proarrhythmia (torsade de pointes and worsened VT) occurred within 7 days of initiating Sotalol Hydrochloride therapy, while 60% of such events occurred within 3 days of initiation or a dosage change. Initiating therapy at 80 mg BID with gradual upward dose titration and appropriate evaluations for efficacy (e.g., PES or Holter) and safety (e.g., QT interval, heart rate and electrolytes) prior to dose escalation, should reduce the risk of proarrhythmia. Avoiding excessive accumulation of Sotalol Hydrochloride in patients with diminished renal function, by appropriate dose reduction, should also reduce the risk of proarrhythmia (see "Dosage and Administration").

Congestive Heart Failure: Sympathetic stimulation is necessary in supporting circulatory function in congestive heart failure, and beta-blockade carries the potential hazard of further depressing myocardial contractility and precipitating more severe failure. In patients who have congestive heart failure controlled by digitalis and/or diuretics, Sotalol Hydrochloride should be administered cautiously. Both digitalis and Sotalol Hydrochloride slow AV conduction. As with all beta-blockers, caution is advised when initiating therapy in patients with any evidence of left ventricular dysfunction. In premarketing studies, new or worsened congestive heart failure (CHF) occurred in 3.3% (n = 3257) of patients and led to discontinuation in approximately 1% of patients receiving Sotalol Hydrochloride. The incidence was higher in patients presenting with sustained ventricular tachycardia/fibrillation (4.6%, n = 1363), or a prior history of heart failure (7.3%, n = 696). Based on a life-table analysis, the one-year incidence of new or worsened CHF was 3% in patients without a prior history and 10% in patients with a prior history of CHF. NYHA Classification was also closely associated to the incidence of new or worsened heart failure while receiving Sotalol Hydrochloride (1.8% in 1395 Class I patients, 4.9% in 1254 Class II patients and 6.1% in 278 Class III or IV patients).

Electrolyte Disturbances: Sotalol Hydrochloride should not be used in patients with hypokalemia or hypomagnesemia prior to correction of imbalance, as these conditions can exaggerate the degree of QT prolongation, and increase the potential for torsade de pointes. Special attention should be given to electrolyte and acid-base balance in patients experiencing severe or prolonged diarrhea or patients receiving concomitant diuretic drugs.

Conduction Disturbances: Excessive prolongation of the QT interval (> 550 msec) can promote serious arrhythmias and should be avoided (see *"Proarrhythmias"* above). Sinus bradycardia (heart rate less than 50 bpm) occurred in 13% of patients receiving Sotalol Hydrochloride in clinical trials, and led to discontinuation in about 3% of patients. Bradycardia itself increases the risk of torsade de pointes. Sinus pause, sinus arrest and sinus node dysfunction occur in less than 1% of patients. The incidence of 2nd- or 3rd-degree AV block is approximately 1%.

Recent Acute MI: Sotalol Hydrochloride can be used safely and effectively in the long-term treatment of life-threatening ventricular arrhythmias following a myocardial infarction. However, experience in the use of Sotalol Hydrochloride to treat cardiac arrhythmias in the early phase of recovery from acute MI is limited and at least at high initial doses is not reassuring. (See *"Warnings: Mortality".*) In the first 2 weeks post-MI caution is advised and careful dose titration is especially important, particularly in patients with markedly impaired ventricular function.

The following warnings are related to the beta-blocking activity of Sotalol Hydrochloride.

Abrupt Withdrawal: Hypersensitivity to catecholamines has been observed in patients withdrawn from beta-blocker therapy. Occasional cases of exacerbation of angina pectoris, arrhythmias and, in some cases, myocardial infarction have been reported after abrupt discontinuation of beta-blocker therapy. Therefore, it is prudent when discontinuing chronically administered Sotalol Hydrochloride, particularly in patients with ischemic heart disease, to carefully monitor the patient and consider the temporary use of an alternate beta-blocker if appropriate. If possible, the dosage of Sotalol Hydrochloride should be gradually reduced over a period of one to two weeks. If angina or acute coronary insufficiency develops, appropriate therapy should be instituted promptly. Patients should be warned against interruption or discontinuation of therapy without the physician's advice. Because coronary artery disease is common and may be unrecognized in patients receiving Sotalol Hydrochloride, abrupt discontinuation in patients with arrhythmias may unmask latent coronary insufficiency.

Nonallergic Bronchospasm: (e.g., chronic bronchitis and emphysema): **PATIENTS WITH BRONCHOSPASTIC DISEASES SHOULD IN GENERAL NOT RECEIVE BETA-BLOCKERS.** It is prudent, if Sotalol Hydrochloride is to be administered, to use the smallest effective dose, so that inhibition of bronchodilation produced by endogenous or exogenous catecholamine stimulation of beta$_2$ receptors may be minimized.

Anaphylaxis: While taking beta-blockers, patients with a history of anaphylactic reaction to a variety of allergens may have a more severe reaction on repeated challenge, either accidental, diagnostic or therapeutic. Such patients may be unresponsive to the usual doses of epinephrine used to treat the allergic reaction.

Anesthesia: The management of patients undergoing major surgery who are being treated with beta-blockers is controversial. Protracted severe hypotension and difficulty in restoring and maintaining normal cardiac rhythm after anesthesia have been reported in patients receiving beta-blockers.

Diabetes: In patients with diabetes (especially labile diabetes) or with a history of episodes of spontaneous hypoglycemia, Sotalol Hydrochloride should be given with caution since beta-blockade may mask some important premonitory signs of acute hypoglycemia; e.g., tachycardia.

Sick Sinus Syndrome: Sotalol Hydrochloride should be used only with extreme caution in patients with sick sinus syndrome associated with symptomatic arrhythmias, because it may cause sinus bradycardia, sinus pauses or sinus arrest.

Thyrotoxicosis: Beta-blockade may mask certain clinical signs (e.g., tachycardia) of hyperthyroidism. Patients suspected of developing thyrotoxicosis should be managed carefully to avoid abrupt withdrawal of beta-blockade which might be followed by an exacerbation of symptoms of hyperthyroidism, including thyroid storm.

PRECAUTIONS

Renal Impairment: Sotalol Hydrochloride is mainly eliminated via the kidneys through glomerular filtration and to a small degree by tubular secretion. There is a direct relationship between renal function, as measured by serum creatinine or creatinine clearance, and the elimination rate of Sotalol Hydrochloride. Guidance for dosing in conditions of renal impairment can be found under *"Dosage and Administration".*

DRUG INTERACTIONS

Antiarrhythmics: Class Ia antiarrhythmic drugs, such as disopyramide, quinidine and procainamide and other Class III drugs (e.g., amiodarone) are not recommended as concomitant therapy with Sotalol Hydrochloride because of their potential to prolong refractoriness (see *"Warnings"*). There is only limited experience with the concomitant use of Class Ib or Ic antiarrhythmics. Additive Class II effects would also be anticipated with the use of other beta-blocking agents concomitantly with Sotalol Hydrochloride.

Digoxin: Single and multiple doses of Sotalol Hydrochloride do not substantially affect serum digoxin levels. Proarrhythmic events were more common in Sotalol Hydrochloride treated patients also receiving digoxin; it is not clear whether this represents an interaction or is related to the presence of CHF, a known risk factor for proarrhythmia, in the patients receiving digoxin.

Calcium Blocking Drugs: Sotalol Hydrochloride should be administered with caution in conjunction with calcium blocking drugs because of possible additive effects on atrioventricular conduction or ventricular function. Additionally, concomitant use of these drugs may have additive effects on blood pressure, possibly leading to hypotension.

Catecholamine-depleting Agents: Concomitant use of catecholamine-depleting drugs, such as reserpine and guanethidine, with a beta-blocker may produce an excessive reduction of resting sympathetic nervous tone. Patients treated with Sotalol Hydrochloride plus a catecholamine depletor should therefore be closely monitored for evidence of hypotension and or marked bradycardia which may produce syncope.

Insulin and Oral Antidiabetics: Hyperglycemia may occur, and the dosage of insulin or antidiabetic drugs may require adjustment. Symptoms of hypoglycemia may be masked.

Beta-2-receptor Stimulants: Beta-agonists such as salbutamol, terbutaline and isoprenaline may have to be administered in increased dosages when used concomitantly with Sotalol Hydrochloride.

Clonidine: Beta-blocking drugs may potentiate the rebound hypertension sometimes observed after discontinuation of clonidine; therefore, caution is advised when discontinuing clonidine in patients receiving Sotalol Hydrochloride.

Other: No pharmacokinetic interactions were observed with hydrochlorothiazide or warfarin.

Drugs Prolonging the QT Interval: Sotalol Hydrochloride should be administered with caution in conjunction with other drugs known to prolong the QT interval such as Class I antiarrhythmic agents, phenothiazines, tricyclic antidepressants, terfenadine and astemizole (see *"Warnings"*).

Carcinogenesis, Mutagenicity, Impairment of Fertility: No evidence of carcinogenic potential was observed in rats during a 24-month study at 137-275 mg/kg/day (approximately 30 times the maximum recommended human oral dose (MRHD) as mg/kg or 5 times the MRHD as mg/m^2) or in mice, during a 24-month study at 4141-7122 mg/kg/day (approximately 450-750 times the MRHD as mg/kg or 36-63 time the MRHD as mg/m^2).

Sotalol Hydrochloride has not been evaluated in any specific assay of mutagenicity or clastogenicity.

No significant reduction in fertility occurred in rats at oral doses of 1000 mg/kg/day (approximately 100 times the MRHD as mg/kg or 9 times the MRHD as mg/m^2) prior to mating, except for a small reduction in the number of offspring per litter.

Pregnancy Category B: Reproduction studies in rats and rabbits during organogenesis at 100 and 22 times the MRHD as mg/kg (9 and 7 times the MRHD as mg/m^2), respectively, did not reveal any teratogenic potential associated with Sotalol Hydrochloride. In rabbits, a high dose of Sotalol Hydrochloride (160 mg/kg/day) at 16 times the MRHD as mg/kg (6 times the MRHD as mg/m$_2$) produced a slight increase in fetal death likely due to maternal toxicity. Eight times the maximum dose (80 mg/kg/day or 3 times the MRHD as mg/m$_2$) did not result in an increased incidence of fetal deaths. In rats, 1000 mg/kg/day Sotalol Hydrochloride, 100 times the MRHD (18 times the MRHD as mg/m$_2$), increased the number of early resorptions, while at 14 times the maximum dose (2.5 times the MRHD as mg/m$_2$), no increase in early resorptions was noted. However, animal reproduction studies are not always predictive of human response.

Although there are no adequate and well-controlled studies in pregnant women, Sotalol Hydrochloride has been shown to cross the placenta, and is found in

RELATIONSHIP BETWEEN QT$_c$ INTERVAL PROLONGATION AND TORSADE DE POINTES

On-Therapy QT$_c$ Interval (msec)	Incidence of Torsade de pointes	Change in QT$_c$ Interval From Baseline (msec)	Incidence of Torsade de pointes
less than 500	1.3% (1787)	less than 65	1.6% (1516)
500-525	3.4% (236)	65-80	3.2% (158)
525-550	5.6% (125)	80-100	4.1% (146)
> 550	10.8% (157)	100-130	5.2% (115)
		> 130	7.1% (99)

( ) Number of patients assessed

➤ SHOWN IN PRODUCT IDENTIFICATION GUIDE

INCIDENCE (%) OF ADVERSE EVENTS AND DISCONTINUATIONS

Body System	Daily Dose 160mg (n = 832)	240mg (n = 263)	320mg (n = 835)	480mg (n = 459)	640mg (n = 324)	% Patients Any Dose* (n = 1292)	Discontinued (n = 1292)
Body as a whole							
infection	1	2	2	2	3	4	< 1
fever	1	2	3	2		4	< 1
localized pain	1	2	2	2		3	< 1
Cardiovascular							
dyspnea	5	8	11	15	15	21	2
bradycardia	8	8	9	7	5	16	< 1
chest pain	4	3	10	10	6	16	< 1
palpitation	3	2	8	9	12	14	< 1
edema	2	2	5	3	5	8	1
ECG abnormal	4	2	4	2	7	6	1
hypotension	3	4	3	2	5	6	1
proarrhythmia	< 1	< 1	2	4	5	3	1
syncope	1	1	3	2	2	4	1
heart failure	3	2	3	2	2	5	1
presyncope	3	2	3	4	5		
peripheral vascular disorder	1	2	1	1	2	3	< 1
cardiovascular disorder	1	< 1	2	2	2	3	< 1
vasodilation	1	< 1	1	2	2	4	< 1
AICD Discharge	< 1	2	2	2	2	3	< 1
hypertension	< 1	1	1	1	2	2	< 1
Nervous							
fatigue	5	8	12	12	13	20	2
dizziness	7	6	11	11	14	20	2
asthenia	4	5	7	8	10	13	1
light-headed	4	3	6	6	7	12	< 1
headache	3	4	6	5	4	8	< 1
sleep problem	1	1	5	4	6	8	< 1
perspiration	1	2	3	4	6	6	< 1
altered consciousness	2	3	1	2	3	4	< 1
depression	1	2	2	2	3	4	< 1
paresthesia	1	1	2	3	4	4	< 1
anxiety	2	2	2	3	4	4	< 1
mood change	< 1	< 1	1	3		3	< 1
appetite disorder	1	2	1	1	3	3	< 1
stroke	< 1	< 1	1	1		2	< 1
Digestive							
nausea/vomiting	5	4	4	6	6	10	1
diarrhea	2	3	3	3	5	5	< 1
dyspepsia	2	2	3	3	2	6	< 1
abdominal pain	< 1	< 1	2	2	3	3	< 1
colon problem	2	1	1	< 1	2	2	< 1
flatulence	1	< 1	1	1		2	< 1
Respiratory							
pulmonary problem	3	4	5	3	6	8	< 1
upper respiratory tract problem	1	1	3	4	5	5	< 1
asthma	1	1	1	1	1	2	< 1
Urogenital							
genitourinary disorder	1	0	1	1	2	3	< 1
sexual dysfunction	< 1	1	1	1		3	< 1
Metabolic							
abnormal lab value	1	1	2	2	2	4	< 1
weight change	1	1	1	< 1	2	2	< 1
Musculoskeletal							
extremity pain	2	2	4	5	3	7	< 1
back pain	1	< 1	2	2	2	3	< 1
Skin and Appendages							
rash	2	3	2	3	4	5	< 1
Hematologic							
bleeding	1	< 1	1	< 1	2	2	< 1
Special Senses							
visual problem	1	1	2	4	5	5	< 1

* *Because patients are counted at each dose level tested, the Any Dose column cannot be determined by adding across the doses.*

◆ RATED THERAPEUTICALLY EQUIVALENT; ◇ THERAPEUTIC EQUIVALENCE UNCONFIRMED; ○ UNRATED

amniotic fluid. There has been a report of subnormal birth weight with Sotalol Hydrochloride. Therefore, Sotalol Hydrochloride should be used during pregnancy only if the potential benefit outweighs the potential risk.

Nursing Mothers: Sotalol Hydrochloride is excreted in the milk of laboratory animals and has been reported to be present in human milk. Because of the potential for adverse reactions in nursing infants from Sotalol Hydrochloride, a decision should be made whether to discontinue nursing or to discontinue the drug, taking into account the importance of the drug to the mother.

Pediatric Use: The safety and effectiveness of Sotalol Hydrochloride in children have not been established.

ADVERSE REACTIONS
During premarketing trials, 3186 patients with cardiac arrhythmias (1363 with sustained ventricular tachycardia) received oral Sotalol Hydrochloride, of whom 2451 received the drug for at least two-weeks. The most important adverse effects are torsade de pointes and other serious new ventricular arrhythmias (see *"Warnings"*), occurring at rates of almost 4% and 1%, respectively, in the VT/VF population. Overall, discontinuation because of unacceptable side-effects was necessary in 17% of all patients in clinical trials, and in 13% of patients treated for at least two-weeks. The most common adverse reactions leading to discontinuation of Sotalol Hydrochloride are as follows: fatigue 4%, bradycardia (less than 50 bpm) 3%, dyspnea 3%, proarrhythmia 3%, asthenia 2%, and dizziness 2%.

Occasional reports of elevated serum liver enzymes have occurred with Sotalol Hydrochloride therapy but no cause and effect relationship has been established. One case of peripheral neuropathy which resolved on discontinuation of Sotalol Hydrochloride and recurred when the patient was rechallenged with the drug was reported in an early dose tolerance study. Elevated blood glucose levels and increased insulin requirements can occur in diabetic patients.

The following table lists as a function of dosage the most common (incidence of 2% or greater) adverse events, regardless of relationship to therapy and the percent of patients discontinued due to the event, as collected from clinical trials involving 1292 patients with sustained VT/VF. (See related table).

Potential Adverse Effects: Foreign marketing experience with Sotalol Hydrochloride shows an adverse experience profile similar to that described above from clinical trials. Voluntary reports since introduction include rare reports (less than one report per 10,000 patients) of: emotional lability, slightly clouded sensorium, incoordination, vertigo, paralysis, thrombocytopenia, eosinophilia, leukopenia, photosensitivity reaction, fever, pulmonary edema, hyperlipidemia, myalgia, pruritis, alopecia.

The oculomucocutaneous syndrome associated with the beta-blocker practolol has not been associated with Sotalol Hydrochloride during investigational use and foreign marketing experience.

OVERDOSAGE
Intentional or accidental overdosage with Sotalol Hydrochloride has rarely resulted in death.

Symptoms and Treatment of Overdosage: The most common signs to be expected are bradycardia, congestive heart failure, hypotension, bronchospasm and hypoglycemia. In cases of massive intentional overdosage (2-16 grams) of Sotalol Hydrochloride the following clinical findings were seen: hypotension, bradycardia, prolongation of QT interval, torsade de pointes, ventricular tachycardia, and premature ventricular complexes. If overdosage occurs, therapy with Sotalol Hydrochloride should be discontinued and the patient observed closely. Because of the lack of protein binding, hemodialysis is useful for reducing Sotalol Hydrochloride plasma concentrations. Patients should be carefully observed until QT intervals are normalized. In addition, if required, the following therapeutic measures are suggested:

Bradycardia: Atropine, another anticholinergic drug, a beta-adrenergic agonist or transvenous cardiac pacing.

Heart Block: (second and third degree) transvenous cardiac pacemaker.

Hypotension: (depending on associated factors) epinephrine rather than isoproterenol or norepinephrine may be useful.

Bronchospasm: Aminophylline or aerosol beta-2-receptor stimulant.

Torsade de pointes: DC cardioversion, transvenous cardiac pacing, epinephrine, magnesium sulfate.

DOSAGE AND ADMINISTRATION
As with other antiarrhythmic agents, Sotalol Hydrochloride should be initiated and doses increased in a hospital with facilities for cardiac rhythm monitoring and assessment (see *"Indications and Usage"*). Sotalol Hydrochloride should be administered only after appropriate clinical assessment (see *"Indications And Usage"*), and the dosage of Sotalol Hydrochloride must be individualized for each patient on the basis of therapeutic response and tolerance. Proarrhythmic events can occur not only at initiation of therapy, but also with each upward dosage adjustment.

Dosage of Sotalol Hydrochloride should be adjusted gradually, allowing 2-3 days between dosing increments in order to attain steady-state plasma concentrations, and to allow monitoring of QT intervals. Graded dose adjustment will help prevent the usage of doses which are higher than necessary to control the arrhythmia. The recommended initial dose is 80 mg twice daily. This dose may be increased, if necessary, after appropriate evaluation to 240 or 320 mg/day. In most patients, a therapeutic response is obtained at a total daily dose of 160 to 320 mg/day, given in two or three divided doses. Some patients with life-

threatening refractory ventricular arrhythmias may require doses as high as 480-640 mg/day; however, these doses should only be prescribed when the potential benefit outweighs the increased risk of adverse events, in particular proarrhythmia. Because of the long terminal elimination half-life of Sotalol Hydrochloride, dosing on more than a BID regimen is usually not necessary.

Because Sotalol Hydrochloride is excreted predominantly in urine and its terminal elimination half-life is prolonged in conditions of renal impairment, the dosing interval of Sotalol Hydrochloride should be modified (when creatinine clearance is lower than 60 mL/min) according to the following table.

Creatinine Clearance mL/min	Dosing Interval (hours)
> 60	12
30-60	24
10-30	36-48
< 10	Dose should be individualized

Since the terminal elimination half-life of Sotalol Hydrochloride is increased in patients with renal impairment, a longer duration of dosing is required to reach steady-state. Dose escalations in renal impairment should be done after administration of at least 5-6 doses at appropriate intervals (see table above).

Transfer to Sotalol Hydrochloride: Before starting Sotalol Hydrochloride, previous antiarrhythmic therapy should generally be withdrawn under careful monitoring for a minimum of 2-3 plasma half-lives if the patient's clinical condition permits (see *"Drug Interactions"*). Treatment has been initiated in some patients receiving I.V. lidocaine without ill effect. After discontinuation of amiodarone, Sotalol Hydrochloride should not be initiated until the QT interval is normalized (see *"Warnings"*).

Storage: Store at controlled room temperature, between 15° to 30°C (59° to 86°F).

HOW SUPPLIED
TABLETS: 80 MG

BRAND/MANUFACTURER	NDC	SIZE	AWP
BRAND			
▶ BETAPACE: Berlex Labs	50419-0105-10	100s	$153.65
	50419-0105-11	100s ud	$156.35

TABLETS: 160 MG

BRAND/MANUFACTURER	NDC	SIZE	AWP
BRAND			
▶ BETAPACE: Berlex Labs	50419-0106-10	100s	$256.15
	50419-0106-11	100s ud	$258.85

TABLETS: 240 MG

BRAND/MANUFACTURER	NDC	SIZE	AWP
BRAND			
▶ BETAPACE: Berlex Labs	50419-0107-10	100s	$333.05
	50419-0107-11	100s ud	$335.75

Sparine SEE PROMAZINE HYDROCHLORIDE

Spectazole SEE ECONAZOLE NITRATE

Spectinomycin Hydrochloride

DESCRIPTION
Spectinomycin Hydrochloride Sterile Powder is an aminocyclitol antibiotic produced by a species of soil microorganism designated as *Streptomyces spectabilis*. Sterile Spectinomycin Hydrochloride is the pentahydrated dihydrochloride salt of Spectinomycin.

Spectinomycin Hydrochloride is isolated as a white to pale buff crystalline dihydrochloride pentahydrate powder, molecular weight 495, and is stable in the dry state for 36 months.

Following is its chemical structure:

CLINICAL PHARMACOLOGY

Spectinomycin Hydrochloride is an inhibitor of protein synthesis in the bacterial cell; the site of action is the 30S ribosomal subunit.

In vitro studies have shown Spectinomycin Hydrochloride to be active against most strains of *Neisseria gonorrhoeae* (minimum inhibitory concentration < 7.5 to 20 mcg/ml).

Definitive *in vitro* studies have shown no cross-resistance of *N. gonorrhoeae* between Spectinomycin Hydrochloride and penicillin. The antibiotic is not significantly bound to plasma protein.

INDICATIONS AND USAGE

Spectinomycin Hydrochloride Sterile Powder is indicated in the treatment of acute gonorrheal urethritis and proctitis in the male and acute gonorrheal cervicitis and proctitis in the female when due to susceptible strains of *Neisseria gonorrhoeae*. Men and women with known recent exposure to gonorrhea should be treated as those known to have gonorrhea.

The *in vitro* susceptibility of *Neisseria gonorrhoeae* to Spectinomycin Hydrochloride can be tested by agar dilution methods. Spectinomycin Hydrochloride Susceptibility Powder is available for this purpose, and its package insert should be consulted for details.

CONTRAINDICATIONS

The use of Spectinomycin Hydrochloride Sterile Powder is contraindicated in patients previously found hypersensitive to it.

WARNINGS

Spectinomycin Hydrochloride is not effective in the treatment of syphilis. Antibiotics used in high doses for short periods of time to treat gonorrhea may mask or delay the symptoms of incubating syphilis. Since the treatment of syphilis demands prolonged therapy with any effective antibiotic, patients being treated for gonorrhea should be closely observed clinically. All patients with gonorrhea should have a serologic test for syphilis at the time of diagnosis. Patients treated with Spectinomycin Hydrochloride should have a follow-up serologic test for syphilis after three months.

Usage in pregnancy: Safety for use in pregnancy has not been established.

Usage in infants and children: Safety for use in infants and children has not been established.

The diluent provided with this product contains benzyl alcohol which has been associated with a fatal gasping syndrome in infants.

PRECAUTIONS

The usual precautions should be observed with atopic individuals.

The clinical effectiveness of Spectinomycin Hydrochloride Sterile Powder should be monitored to detect evidence of development of resistance by *Neisseria gonorrhoeae*.

ADVERSE REACTIONS

The following reactions were observed during the single dose clinical trials: soreness at the injection site, urticaria, dizziness, nausea, chills, fever and insomnia.

During multiple dose subchronic tolerance studies in normal human volunteers, the following were noted: a decrease in hemoglobin, hematocrit and creatinine clearance; elevation of alkaline phosphatase, BUN and SGPT. In single and multiple dose studies in normal volunteers, a reduction in urine output was noted. Extensive renal function studies demonstrated no consistent changes indicative of renal toxicity. Although no clearly defined case of anaphylaxis has been reported with Spectinomycin Hydrochloride Sterile Powder, the possibility of such reactions should be considered particularly when using antibiotics.

A few cases of anaphylaxis or anaphylactoid reactions have been reported. If serious allergic reactions occur, the usual agents (epinephrine, corticosteroids, and/or antihistamines) should be available for emergency use. In cases of severe anaphylaxis, airway support and oxygen may also be required.

DOSAGE AND ADMINISTRATION

PREPARATION OF DRUG FOR INTRAMUSCULAR INJECTION
Spectinomycin Hydrochloride Sterile Powder, 2 grams: reconstitute with 3.2 ml of the accompanying diluent.[*]

Spectinomycin Hydrochloride Sterile Powder, 4 grams: reconstitute with 6.2 ml of the accompanying diluent.[*]

Shake vials vigorously immediately after adding diluent and before withdrawing dose. It is recommended that disposable syringes and needles be used to avoid contamination with penicillin residue, especially when treating patients known to be highly sensitive to penicillin. **Use of 20 gauge needle is recommended.**

DOSAGE
Intramuscular injections should be made deep into the upper outer quadrant of the gluteal muscle.

Adults (Men and Women): **Inject 5 ml intramuscularly** for a 2 gram dose. This is also the recommended dose for patients being treated after failure of previous antibiotic therapy.

In geographic areas where antibiotic resistance is known to be prevalent, initial treatment with 4 grams (10 ml) intramuscularly is preferred. The 10 ml injection may be divided between two gluteal injection sites.

---

[*] Bacteriostatic Water for Injection with Benzyl Alcohol 0.945% w/v added as preservative.

STORAGE CONDITIONS

Store unreconstituted product at controlled room temperature 15°-30°C (59°-86°F). Store prepared suspension at controlled room temperature 15°-30°C (59°-86°F) and use within 24 hours.

HUMAN PHARMACOLOGY

Spectinomycin Hydrochloride Sterile Powder is rapidly absorbed after intramuscular injection. A single, two gram injection produces peak serum concentrations averaging about 100 mcg/ml at one hour; a single, four gram injection produces peak serum concentrations averaging 160 mcg/ml at two hours. Average serum concentrations of 15 mcg/ml for the two gram dose and 31 mcg/ml for the four gram dose were present eight hours after dosing.

J CODES

Up to 2 g IM—J3320

HOW SUPPLIED

POWDER FOR INJECTION: 2 GM

BRAND/MANUFACTURER	NDC	SIZE	AWP
○ **BRAND**			
TROBICIN: Upjohn	00009-0566-01	1s	$16.13

Spectrobid *SEE* BACAMPICILLIN HYDROCHLORIDE

Spinal-22 Whitacre W/Lidocaine
SEE **LIDOCAINE HYDROCHLORIDE, LOCAL ANESTHESIA**

Spironolactone

> **WARNING**
> SPIRONOLACTONE HAS BEEN SHOWN TO BE A TUMORIGEN IN CHRONIC TOXICITY STUDIES IN RATS (SEE *"WARNINGS"*). SPIRONOLACTONE SHOULD BE USED ONLY IN THOSE CONDITIONS DESCRIBED UNDER *INDICATIONS AND USAGE*. UNNECESSARY USE OF THIS DRUG SHOULD BE AVOIDED.

DESCRIPTION

Spironolactone oral tablets contain 25 mg, 50 mg, or 100 mg of the aldosterone antagonist Spironolactone, 17-hydroxy-7α-mercapto-3-oxo-17α-pregn-4-ene-21-carboxylic acid γ-lactone acetate.

Spironolactone is practically insoluble in water, soluble in alcohol, and freely soluble in benzene and in chloroform.

Following is its chemical structure:

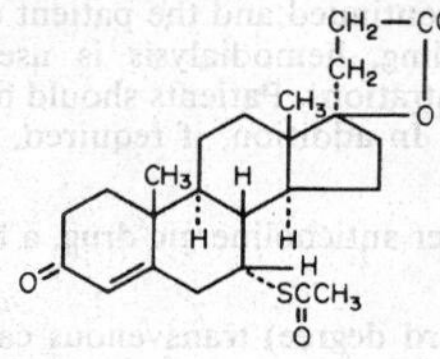

CLINICAL PHARMACOLOGY

Mechanism of Action: Spironolactone is a specific pharmacologic antagonist of aldosterone, acting primarily through competitive binding of receptors at the aldosterone-dependent sodium-potassium exchange site in the distal convoluted renal tubule. Spironolactone causes increased amounts of sodium and water to be excreted while potassium is retained. Spironolactone acts both as a diuretic and as an antihypertensive drug by this mechanism. It may be given alone or with other diuretic agents which act more proximally in the renal tubule.

Aldosterone Antagonist Activity: Increased levels of the mineralocorticoid, aldosterone, are present in primary and secondary hyperaldosteronism. Edematous states in which secondary aldosteronism is usually involved include congestive heart failure, hepatic cirrhosis, and the nephrotic syndrome. By competing with aldosterone for receptor sites, Spironolactone provides effective therapy for the edema and ascites in those conditions. Spironolactone counteracts secondary aldosteronism induced by the volume depletion and associated sodium loss caused by active diuretic therapy.

Spironolactone is effective in lowering the systolic and diastolic blood pressure in patients with primary hyperaldosteronism. It is also effective in most cases of essential hypertension, despite the fact that aldosterone secretion may be within normal limits in benign essential hypertension.

Through its action in antagonizing the effect of aldosterone, Spironolactone inhibits the exchange of sodium for potassium in the distal renal tubule and helps

---

to prevent potassium loss. Spironolactone has not been demonstrated to elevate serum uric acid, to precipitate gout, or to alter carbohydrate metabolism.

Pharmacokinetics: Spironolactone is rapidly and extensively metabolized. Sulfur-containing products are the predominant metabolites and are thought to be primarily responsible, together with spironolactone, for the therapeutic effects of the drug. The following pharmacokinetic data were obtained from 12 healthy volunteers following the administration of 100 mg of spironolactone daily for 15 days. On the 15th day, Spironolactone was given immediately after a low-fat breakfast and blood was drawn thereafter.

	Accumulation Factor: AUC (0-24 hr, day 15)/ AUC (0-24 hr, day 1)	Mean Peak Serum Concentration	Mean (SD) Post-Steady State Half-life
7-α-(thiomethyl) spirolactone (TMS)	1.25	391 ng/mL at 3.2 hr	13.8 hr (6.4) (terminal)
6-β-hydroxy-7-α-(thiomethyl) spirolactone (HTMS)	1.50	125 ng/mL at 5.1 hr	15.0 hr (4.0) (terminal)
Canrenone (C)	1.41	181 ng/mL at 4.3 hr	16.5 hr (6.3) (terminal)
Spironolactone	1.30	80 ng/mL at 2.6 hr	Approximately 1.4 hr (0.5) (β-half-life)

The pharmacological activity of Spironolactone metabolites in man is not known. However, in the adrenalectomized rat the antimineralocorticoid activities of the metabolites C, TMS, and HTMS, relative to Spironolactone, were 1.10, 1.28, and 0.32, respectively. Relative to Spironolactone, their binding affinites to the aldosterone receptors in rat kidney slices were 0.19, 0.86, and 0.06, respectively.

In humans the potencies of TMS and 7-α-thiospirolactone in reversing the effects of the synthetic mineralocorticoid, fludrocortisone, on urinary electrolyte composition were 0.33 and 0.26, respectively, relative to Spironolactone. However, since the serum concentrations of these steroids were not determined, their incomplete absorption and/or first-pass metabolism could not be ruled out as a reason for their reduced *in vivo* activities.

Both Spironolactone and canrenone are more than 90% bound to plasma proteins. The metabolites are excreted primarily in the urine and secondarily in bile.

The effect of food on Spironolactone absorption (two 100-mg Spironolactone tablets) was assessed in a single dose study of 9 healthy, drug free volunteers. Food increased the bioavailability of unmetabolized Spironolactone by almost 100%. The clinical importance of this finding is not known.

INDICATIONS AND USAGE
Spironolactone is indicated in the management of:

Primary Hyperaldosteronism: for:

Establishing the diagnosis of primary hyperaldosteronism by therapeutic trial.
Short-term preoperative treatment of patients with primary hyperaldosteronism.
Long-term maintenance therapy for patients with discrete aldosterone-producing adrenal adenomas who are judged to be poor operative risks or who decline surgery.
Long-term maintenance therapy for patients with bilateral micro- or macronodular adrenal hyperplasia (idiopathic hyperaldosteronism).

Edematous Conditions: for patients with:

Congestive Heart Failure: For the management of edema and sodium retention when the patient is only partially responsive to, or is intolerant of, other therapeutic measures. Spironolactone is also indicated for patients with congestive heart failure taking digitalis when other therapies are considered inappropriate.

Cirrhosis of the Liver Accompanied by Edema and/or Ascites: Aldosterone levels may be exceptionally high in this condition. Spironolactone is indicated for maintenance therapy together with bed rest and the restriction of fluid and sodium.

The Nephrotic Syndrome: For nephrotic patients when treatment of the underlying disease, restriction of fluid and sodium intake, and the use of other diuretics do not provide an adequate response.

Essential Hypertension: Usually in combination with other drugs, Spironolactone is indicated for patients who cannot be treated adequately with other agents or for whom other agents are considered inappropriate.

Hypokalemia: For the treatment of patients with hypokalemia when other measures are considered inappropriate or inadequate. Spironolactone is also indicated for the prophylaxis of hypokalemia in patients taking digitalis when other measures are considered inadequate or inappropriate.

Usage in Pregnancy: The routine use of diuretics in an otherwise healthy woman is inappropriate and exposes mother and fetus to unnecessary hazard. Diuretics do not prevent development of toxemia of pregnancy, and there is no satisfactory evidence that they are useful in the treatment of developing toxemia.

Edema during pregnancy may arise from pathologic causes or from the physiologic and mechanical consequences of pregnancy.

Spironolactone is indicated in pregnancy when edema is due to pathologic causes just as it is in the absence of pregnancy (however, see *"Warnings"* section). Dependent edema in pregnancy, resulting from restriction of venous return by the expanded uterus, is properly treated through elevation of the lower extremities and use of support hose; use of diuretics to lower intravascular volume in this case is unsupported and unnecessary. There is hypervolemia during normal pregnancy which is not harmful to either the fetus or the mother (in the absence of cardiovascular disease), but which is associated with edema, including generalized edema, in the majority of pregnant women. If this edema produces discomfort, increased recumbency will often provide relief. In rare instances, this edema may cause extreme discomfort which is not relieved by rest. In these cases, a short course of diuretics may provide relief and may be appropriate.

UNLABELED USES
Spironolactone is used alone or as an adjunct in the treatment of hirsutism in women with polycystic ovary syndrome, in the management of premenstrual syndrome, and in familial male precocious puberty. It is also used to minimize the occurrence of acute mountain sickness, in infants with bronchopulmonary dysplasia, and in the treatment of acne vulgaris.

CONTRAINDICATIONS
Spironolactone is contraindicated for patients with anuria, acute renal insufficiency, significant impairment of renal excretory function, or hyperkalemia.

WARNINGS
Potassium supplementation, either in the form of medication or as a diet rich in potassium, should not ordinarily be given in association with Spironolactone therapy. Excessive potassium intake may cause hyperkalemia in patients receiving Spironolactone (see *"Precautions"* section). Spironolactone should not be administered concurrently with other potassium-sparing diuretics. Spironolactone, when used with ACE inhibitors, even in the presence of a diuretic, has been associated with severe hyperkalemia. Extreme caution should be exercised when Spironolactone is given concomitantly with ACE inhibitors (see *"Precautions: Drug Interactions"*).

Spironolactone has been shown to be a tumorigen in chronic toxicity studies performed in rats, with its proliferative effects manifested on endocrine organs and the liver. In one study using 25, 75, and 250 times the usual daily human dose (2 mg/kg) there was a statistically significant dose-related increase in benign adenomas of the thyroid and testes. In female rats there was a statistically significant increase in malignant mammary tumors at the mid-dose only. In male rats there was a dose-related increase in proliferative changes in the liver. At the highest dosage level (500 mg/kg) the range of effects included hepatocytomegaly, hyperplastic nodules, and hepatocellular carcinoma; the last was not statistically significant at a value of p = 0.05. A dose-related (above 20 mg/kg/day) incidence of myelocytic leukemia was observed in rats fed daily doses of potassium canrenoate for a period of one year. In long-term (two-year) oral carcinogenicity studies of potassium canrenoate in the rat, myelocytic leukemia and hepatic, thyroid, testicular, and mammary tumors were observed. Potassium canrenoate did not produce a mutagenic effect in tests using bacteria or yeast. It did produce a positive mutagenic effect in several *in vitro* tests in mammalian cells following metabolic activation. In an *in vivo* mammalian system potassium canrenoate was not mutagenic. Canrenone and canrenoic acid are the major metabolites of potassium canrenoate. Spironolactone is also metabolized to canrenone. An increased incidence of leukemia was not observed in chronic rat toxicity studies conducted with Spironolactone at doses up to 500 mg/kg/day.

PRECAUTIONS
General: Because of the diuretic action of Spironolactone, patients should be carefully evaluated for possible disturbances of fluid and electrolyte balance. Hyperkalemia may occur in patients with impaired renal function or excessive potassium intake and can cause cardiac irregularities, which may be fatal. Consequently, no potassium supplement should ordinarily be given with Spironolactone. Hyperkalemia can be treated promptly by the rapid intravenous administration of glucose (20% to 50%) and regular insulin, using 0.25 to 0.5 units of insulin per gram of glucose. This is a temporary measure to be repeated as required. Spironolactone use should be discontinued and potassium intake (including dietary potassium) restricted.

Reversible hyperchloremic metabolic acidosis, usually in association with hyperkalemia, has been reported to occur in some patients with decompensated hepatic cirrhosis, even in the presence of normal renal function.

Hyponatremia, manifested by dryness of the mouth, thirst, lethargy, and drowsiness, and confirmed by a low serum sodium level, may be caused or aggravated, especially when Spironolactone is administered in combination with other diuretics.

Gynecomastia may develop in association with the use of Spironolactone; physicians should be alert to its possible onset. The development of gynecomastia appears to be related to both dosage level and duration of therapy and is normally reversible when Spironolactone is discontinued. In rare instances some breast enlargement may persist when Spironolactone is discontinued.

Spironolactone therapy may cause a transient elevation of BUN, especially in patients with preexisting renal impairment. Spironolactone may cause mild acidosis.

A determination of serum electrolytes to detect possible electrolyte imbalance should be performed at periodic intervals.

Drug Interactions: When used in combination with other diuretics or antihypertensive agents, Spironolactone potentiates their effects. Therefore, the dosage of such drugs, particularly the ganglionic blocking agents, should be reduced by at least 50% when Spironolactone is added to the regimen.

Concomitant administration of potassium-sparing diuretics with ACE inhibitors or indomethacin has been associated with severe hyperkalemia.

Spironolactone reduces the vascular responsiveness to norepinephrine. Therefore, caution should be exercised in the management of patients subjected to regional or general anesthesia while they are being treated with Spironolactone. Spironolactone has been shown to increase the half-life of digoxin. This may result in increased serum digoxin levels and subsequent digitalis toxicity. It may be necessary to reduce the maintenance and digitalization doses when Spironolactone is administered, and the patient should be carefully monitored to avoid over- or underdigitalization.

Drug/Laboratory Test Interactions: Several reports of possible interference with digoxin radioimmunoassays by Spironolactone or its metabolites, have appeared in the literature. Neither the extent nor the potential clinical significance of its interference (which may be assay-specific) has been fully established.

Usage in Pregnancy: Spironolactone or its metabolites may cross the placental barrier. Therefore, the use of Spironolactone in pregnant women requires that the anticipated benefit be weighed against possible hazard to the fetus.

Nursing Mothers: Canrenone, a metabolite of Spironolactone, appears in breast milk. If use of the drug is deemed essential, an alternative method of infant feeding should be instituted.

ADVERSE REACTIONS

Gynecomastia is observed not infrequently. A few cases of agranulocytosis have been reported in patients taking Spironolactone. Other adverse reactions that have been reported in association with Spironolactone are: gastrointestinal symptoms including cramping and diarrhea, drowsiness, lethargy, headache, maculopapular or erythematous cutaneous eruptions, urticaria, mental confusion, drug fever, ataxia, inability to achieve or maintain erection, irregular menses or amenorrhea, postmenopausal bleeding, hirsutism, deepening of the voice, gastric bleeding, ulceration, gastritis, and vomiting. Carcinoma of the breast has been reported in patients taking Spironolactone, but a cause and effect relationship has not been established.

Adverse reactions are usually reversible upon discontinuation of the drug.

DOSAGE AND ADMINISTRATION

Primary Hyperaldosteronism: Spironolactone may be employed as an initial diagnostic measure to provide presumptive evidence of primary hyperaldosteronism while patients are on normal diets.

Long Test: Spironolactone is administered at a daily dosage of 400 mg for three to four weeks. Correction of hypokalemia and of hypertension provides presumptive evidence for the diagnosis of primary hyperaldosteronism.

Short Test: Spironolactone is administered at a daily dosage of 400 mg for four days. If serum potassium increases during Spironolactone administration but drops when Spironolactone is discontinued, a presumptive diagnosis of primary hyperaldosteronism should be considered.

After the diagnosis of hyperaldosteronism has been established by more definitive testing procedures, Spironolactone may be administered in doses of 100 to 400 mg daily in preparation for surgery. For patients who are considered unsuitable for surgery, Spironolactone may be employed for long-term maintenance therapy at the lowest effective dosage determined for the individual patient.

Edema in Adults (congestive heart failure, hepatic cirrhosis, or nephrotic syndrome). An initial daily dosage of 100 mg of Spironolactone administered in either single or divided doses is recommended, but may range from 25 to 200 mg daily. When given as the sole agent for diuresis, Spironolactone should be continued for at least five days at the initial dosage level, after which it may be adjusted to the optimal therapeutic or maintenance level administered in either single or divided daily doses. If, after five days, an adequate diuretic response to Spironolactone has not occurred, a second diuretic which acts more proximally in the renal tubule may be added to the regimen. Because of the additive effect of Spironolactone when administered concurrently with such diuretics, an enhanced diuresis usually begins on the first day of combined treatment; combined therapy is indicated when more rapid diuresis is desired. The dosage of Spironolactone should remain unchanged when other diuretic therapy is added.

Edema in Children: The initial daily dosage should provide approximately 1.5 mg of Spironolactone per pound of body weight (3.3 mg/kg) administered in either single or divided doses.

Essential Hypertension: For adults, an initial daily dosage of 50 to 100 mg of Spironolactone administered in either single or divided doses is recommended. Spironolactone may also be given with diuretics which act more proximally in the renal tubule or with other antihypertensive agents. Treatment with Spironolactone should be continued for at least two weeks, since the maximum response may not occur before this time. Subsequently, dosage should be adjusted according to the response of the patient.

Hypokalemia: Spironolactone in a dosage ranging from 25 mg to 100 mg daily is useful in treating a diuretic-induced hypokalemia, when oral potassium supplements or other potassium-sparing regimens are considered inappropriate.

Storage: Store below 86°F (30°C).

HOW SUPPLIED
TABLETS: 25 MG

AVERAGE UNIT PRICE (AVAILABLE SIZES)		GENERIC A-RATED AVERAGE PRICE (GAAP)	
BRAND	$0.35	100s	$9.48
GENERIC	$0.08	500s	$31.77
HCFA FUL (100s ea)	$0.05	1000s	$60.41

BRAND/MANUFACTURER	NDC	SIZE	AWP
◆ BRAND			
➤ ALDACTONE: Searle	00025-1001-31	100s	$37.22
	00025-1001-51	500s	$176.64
	00025-1001-55	2500s	$830.72
◆ GENERICS			
Major	00904-0343-60	100s	$5.80
Rugby	00536-4575-01	100s	$6.90
Qualitest	00603-5766-21	100s	$6.90
Mylan	00378-2146-01	100s	$6.95
Caremark	00339-5355-12	100s	$7.12
Mutual	53489-0143-01	100s	$7.25
Goldline	00182-1157-01	100s	$7.25
Geneva	00781-1599-01	100s	$7.46
Aligen	00405-4940-01	100s	$7.57
URL	00677-0625-01	100s	$7.71
Moore, H.L.	00839-6330-06	100s	$7.76
Parmed	00349-2305-01	100s	$7.95
Purepac	00228-2388-10	100s	$9.18
U.S. Trading	56126-0304-11	100s ud	$5.13
Raway	00686-0103-20	100s ud	$7.95
Major	00904-0343-61	100s ud	$10.72
Vangard	00615-1535-13	100s ud	$16.12
Auro	55829-0471-10	100s ud	$16.64
UDL	51079-0103-20	100s ud	$17.28
Geneva	00781-1599-13	100s ud	$20.00
Major	00904-0343-70	250s	$12.90
Major	00904-0343-40	500s	$21.40
Mylan	00378-2146-05	500s	$26.52
Qualitest	00603-5766-28	500s	$30.76
Rugby	00536-4575-05	500s	$31.20
Mutual	53489-0143-05	500s	$34.85
Purepac	00228-2388-50	500s	$45.90
Major	00904-0343-80	1000s	$42.75
Moore, H.L.	00839-6330-16	1000s	$46.31
Geneva	00781-1599-10	1000s	$57.69
URL	00677-0625-10	1000s	$58.80
Mutual	53489-0143-10	1000s	$58.80
Goldline	00182-1157-10	1000s	$58.80
Aligen	00405-4940-03	1000s	$61.89
Rugby	00536-4575-10	1000s	$62.30
Parmed	00349-2305-10	1000s	$64.95
Purepac	00228-2388-96	1000s	$91.80

TABLETS: 50 MG

BRAND/MANUFACTURER	NDC	SIZE	AWP
○ BRAND			
➤ ALDACTONE: Searle	00025-1041-31	100s	$65.35
	00025-1041-34	100s ud	$68.45

TABLETS: 100 MG

BRAND/MANUFACTURER	NDC	SIZE	AWP
○ BRAND			
➤ ALDACTONE: Searle	00025-1031-31	100s	$109.56
	00025-1031-34	100s ud	$114.87

Sporanox *SEE* ITRACONAZOLE

SSD AF *SEE* SILVER SULFADIAZINE

Stadol *SEE* BUTORPHANOL TARTRATE

Stannous Fluoride

DESCRIPTION
A stable, water-free gel containing 0.4% Stannous Fluoride for use as a dental caries preventive. This is a Fluoride treatment gel, not a toothpaste. Read directions carefully before using.

◆ RATED THERAPEUTICALLY EQUIVALENT; ◇ THERAPEUTIC EQUIVALENCE UNCONFIRMED; ○ UNRATED

CLINICAL PHARMACOLOGY

Frequent topical application to the teeth with preparations having a relatively high fluoride content increases tooth resistance to acid dissolution, promotes remineralization, and inhibits the canogenic microbial process.

INDICATIONS AND USAGE

It is well established that a 0.4% Stannous Fluoride gel is a convenient way to apply fluoride to the surfaces of teeth to aid in the prevention of decalcification and dental caries. This is accomplished by increasing the resistance of tooth surfaces to acid dissolution.

CONTRAINDICATIONS

None (may be used whether drinking water is fluoridated or not, since topical fluoride cannot produce fluorosis.)

WARNINGS

As with all medication, keep out of reach of children. Children under 12 years of age should be supervised in the use of this product. Use in children under 6 years of age requires special supervision to prevent swallowing of gel which could cause dental fluorosis in developing teeth. Consult a dentist or physician.

PRECAUTIONS

DO NOT SWALLOW.

ADVERSE REACTION

Allergic reactions or other idiosyncrasies are rarely reported.

OVERDOSAGE

Accidental ingestion of a usual treatment dose (1-2 mg F) is not harmful.

DOSAGE AND ADMINISTRATION

Adults and children 6 years and older: For maximum benefits Stannous Fluoride should be applied daily or more often if your dentist recommends additional therapy. Following regular brushing and flossing, shake excess water from your toothbrush and liberally cover bristle surface with Stannous Fluoride. Brush onto all tooth surfaces for one minute, then vigorously swish for one minute, then spit out. DO NOT SWALLOW gel. Children under 12 years of age should be supervised in the use of the gel.

Children under 6 years of age: Consult a dentist or physician.

HOW SUPPLIED
GEL:

BRAND/MANUFACTURER	NDC	SIZE	AWP
○ **BRAND**			
PERFECT CHOICE: Challenge	50467-0110-04	129 gm	$8.15
	50467-0811-04	129 gm	$8.15
	50467-0812-04	129 gm	$8.15
	50467-0813-04	129 gm	$8.15
	50467-0814-04	129 gm	$8.15
	50467-0815-04	129 gm	$8.15
	50467-0816-04	129 gm	$8.15
	50467-0817-04	129 gm	$8.15

GEL: 0.4%

BRAND/MANUFACTURER	NDC	SIZE	AWP
○ **BRAND**			
STOP: Oral B Lab	00041-0710-34	120 gm	$6.02
	00041-0711-34	120 gm	$6.02
	00041-0712-34	120 gm	$6.02
GEL-KAM: Colgate Oral	00126-2328-93	129 gm	$7.81
	00126-2342-93	129 gm	$7.81
	00126-2350-93	129 gm	$7.81
	00126-2351-93	129 gm	$7.81
	00126-2352-93	129 gm	$7.81
	00126-2361-93	129 gm	$7.81
GEL-KAM DENTAL THERAPY PAK: Colgate Oral	00126-2328-98	105 gm 2s	$12.08
	00126-2342-98	105 gm 2s	$12.08
	00126-2350-98	105 gm 2s	$12.08
	00126-2351-98	105 gm 2s	$12.08
	00126-2352-98	105 gm 2s	$12.08
	00126-2361-98	105 gm 2s	$12.08

GEL: 0.63%

BRAND/MANUFACTURER	NDC	SIZE	AWP
○ **GENERICS**			
PERIO MED: Omnii Intl	00217-3315-35	300 gm	$6.00
PERIO MED: Omnii Intl	00217-3316-35	300 gm	$6.00
OMNI PERIO-MED: Dunhall	00217-3310-35	300 gm	$6.00

LIQUID:

BRAND/MANUFACTURER	NDC	SIZE	AWP
○ **GENERICS**			
OMNII-MED: Dunhall	00217-3010-30	210 ml	$5.00
OMNII-MED: Dunhall	00217-3020-30	210 ml	$5.00
OMNII-MED: Dunhall	00217-3030-30	210 ml	$5.00
OMNII-MED: Dunhall	00217-3040-30	210 ml	$5.00
OMNII-MED: Dunhall	00217-3050-30	210 ml	$5.00
OMNII-MED: Dunhall	00217-3060-30	210 ml	$5.00

LIQUID: 0.63%

BRAND/MANUFACTURER	NDC	SIZE	AWP
○ **GENERICS**			
STANIMAX PERIO RINSE: SDI Labs	58640-4010-01	300 ml 12s	$91.00

SOLUTION: 0.63%

BRAND/MANUFACTURER	NDC	SIZE	AWP
○ **BRAND**			
GEL-KAM: Colgate Oral	00126-2310-02	300 ml	$14.27
	00126-2312-02	300 ml	$14.27

Stanozolol

DESCRIPTION

Stanozolol is an anabolic steroid, a synthetic derivative of testosterone. Each tablet contains 2 mg of Stanozolol. It is designated chemically as 17-methyl-2'*H*-5α-androst-2-eno[3,2-*c*]pyrazol-17β-ol.

Following is its chemical structure:

CLINICAL PHARMACOLOGY

Anabolic steroids are synthetic derivatives of testosterone. Certain clinical effects and adverse reactions demonstrate the androgenic properties of this class of drugs. Complete dissociation of anabolic and androgenic effects has not been achieved. The actions of anabolic steroids are therefore similar to those of male sex hormones with the possibility of causing serious disturbances of growth and sexual development if given to young children. They suppress the gonadotropic functions of the pituitary and may exert a direct effect upon the testes.

Stanozolol has been found to increase low-density lipoproteins and decrease high-density lipoproteins. These changes are not associated with any increase in total cholesterol or triglyceride levels and revert to normal on discontinuation of treatment.

Hereditary angioedema (HAE) is an autosomal dominant disorder caused by a deficient or nonfunctional C1 esterase inhibitor (C1 INH) and clinically characterized by episodes of swelling of the face, extremities, genitalia, bowel wall, and upper respiratory tract.

In small scale clinical studies, Stanozolol was effective in controlling the frequency and severity of attacks of angioedema and in increasing serum levels of C1 INH and C4. Stanozolol is not effective in stopping HAE attacks while they are under way. The effect of Stanozolol on increasing serum levels of C1 INH and C4 may be related to an increase in protein anabolism.

INDICATIONS AND USAGE

Hereditary Angioedema: Stanozolol is indicated prophylactically to decrease the frequency and severity of attacks of angioedema.

UNLABELED USES

Stanozolol is used alone or as an adjunct in the treatment of liposilerosis, postmenopausal osteoporosis, rheumatoid arthritis, and postoperative deep venous thrombosis. It is also used in patients with hemophilia A and in patients with familid antithrombin III deficiency.

CONTRAINDICATIONS

The use of Stanozolol is contraindicated in the following:

1. Male patients with carcinoma of the breast, or with known or suspected carcinoma of the prostate.
2. Carcinoma of the breast in females with hypercalcemia; androgenic anabolic steroids may stimulate osteolytic resorption of bone.
3. Nephrosis or the nephrotic phase of nephritis.
4. Stanozolol can cause fetal harm when administered to a pregnant woman.

Stanozolol is contraindicated in women who are or may become pregnant. If this drug is used during pregnancy, or if the patient becomes pregnant while taking this drug, the patient should be apprised of the potential hazard to the fetus.

WARNINGS

PELIOSIS HEPATIS, A CONDITION IN WHICH LIVER AND SOMETIMES SPLENIC TISSUE IS REPLACED WITH BLOOD-FILLED CYSTS, HAS BEEN REPORTED IN PATIENTS RECEIVING ANDROGENIC ANABOLIC STEROID THERAPY. THESE CYSTS ARE SOMETIMES PRESENT WITH MINIMAL HEPATIC DYSFUNCTION, BUT AT OTHER TIMES THEY HAVE BEEN ASSOCIATED WITH LIVER FAILURE. THEY ARE OFTEN NOT RECOGNIZED UNTIL LIFE-THREATENING LIVER FAILURE OR INTRA-ABDOMINAL HEMORRHAGE DEVELOPS. WITHDRAWAL OF DRUG USUALLY RESULTS IN COMPLETE DISAPPEARANCE OF LESIONS.

➤ SHOWN IN PRODUCT IDENTIFICATION GUIDE

LIVER CELL TUMORS ARE ALSO REPORTED. MOST OFTEN THESE TUMORS ARE BENIGN AND ANDROGEN-DEPENDENT, BUT FATAL MALIGNANT TUMORS HAVE BEEN REPORTED. WITHDRAWAL OF DRUG OFTEN RESULTS IN REGRESSION OR CESSATION OF PROGRESSION OF THE TUMOR. HOWEVER, HEPATIC TUMORS ASSOCIATED WITH ANDROGENS OR ANABOLIC STEROIDS ARE MUCH MORE VASCULAR THAN OTHER HEPATIC TUMORS AND MAY BE SILENT UNTIL LIFE-THREATENING INTRA-ABDOMINAL HEMORRHAGE DEVELOPS.

BLOOD LIPID CHANGES THAT ARE KNOWN TO BE ASSOCIATED WITH INCREASED RISK OF ATHEROSCLEROSIS ARE SEEN IN PATIENTS TREATED WITH ANDROGENS AND ANABOLIC STEROIDS. THESE CHANGES INCLUDE DECREASED HIGH-DENSITY LIPOPROTEIN AND SOMETIMES INCREASED LOW-DENSITY LIPOPROTEIN. THE CHANGES MAY BE VERY MARKED AND COULD HAVE A SERIOUS IMPACT ON THE RISK OF ATHEROSCLEROSIS AND CORONARY ARTERY DISEASE.

Cholestatic hepatitis and jaundice occur with 17-alpha-alkylated androgens at relatively low doses. If cholestatic hepatitis with jaundice appears, the anabolic steroid should be discontinued. If liver function tests become abnormal, the patient should be monitored closely and the etiology determined. Generally, the anabolic steroid should be discontinued although in cases of mild abnormalities, the physician may elect to follow the patient carefully at a reduced drug dosage.

In patients with breast cancer, anabolic steroid therapy may cause hypercalcemia by stimulating osteolysis. In this case, the drug should be discontinued.

Edema with or without congestive heart failure may be a serious complication in patients with preexisting cardiac, renal, or hepatic disease. Concomitant administration of adrenal cortical steroids or ACTH may add to the edema.

Geriatric male patients treated with androgenic anabolic steroids may be at an increased risk for the development of prostatic hypertrophy and prostatic carcinoma.

In children, anabolic steroid treatment may accelerate bone maturation without producing compensatory gain in linear growth. This adverse effect may result in compromised adult stature. The younger the child, the greater the risk of compromising final mature height. The effect on bone maturation should be monitored by assessing bone age of the wrist and hand every six months.

Anabolic steroids have not been shown to enhance athletic ability.

PRECAUTIONS
GENERAL
Anabolic steroids may cause suppression of clotting factors II, V, VII, and X, and an increase in prothrombin time.

Women should be observed for signs of virilization (deepening of the voice, hirsutism, acne, and clitoromegaly). To prevent irreversible change, drug therapy must be discontinued, or the dosage significantly reduced when mild virilism is first detected. Such virilization is usual following androgenic anabolic steroid use at high doses. Some virilizing changes in women are irreversible even after prompt discontinuance of therapy and are not prevented by concomitant use of estrogens. Menstrual irregularities may also occur.

The insulin or oral hypoglycemic dosage may need adjustment in diabetic patients who receive anabolic steroids.

INFORMATION FOR THE PATIENT
The physician should instruct patients to report any of the following side effects of androgens:

Adult or Adolescent Males: Too frequent or persistent erections of the penis, appearance or aggravation of acne.

Women: Hoarseness, acne, changes in menstrual periods, or more hair on the face.

All Patients: Any nausea, vomiting, changes in skin color, or ankle swelling.

Laboratory Tests: Women with disseminated breast carcinoma should have frequent determination of urine and serum calcium levels during the course of androgenic anabolic steroid therapy (see "Warnings").

Because of the hepatotoxicity associated with the use of 17-alpha-alkylated androgens, liver function tests should be obtained periodically.

Periodic (every 6 months) x-ray examinations of bone age should be made during treatment of prepubertal patients to determine the rate of bone maturation and the effects of androgenic anabolic steroid therapy on the epiphyseal centers.

In common with other anabolic steroids, Stanozolol, has been reported to lower the level of high-density lipoproteins and raise the level of low-density lipoproteins. These changes usually revert to normal on discontinuation of treatment. Increased low-density lipoproteins and decreased high-density lipoproteins are considered cardiovascular risk factors. Serum lipids and high-density lipoprotein cholesterol should be determined periodically.

Hemoglobin and hematocrit should be checked periodically for polycythemia in patients who are receiving high doses of anabolic steroids.

Drug Interaction: Anabolic steroids may increase sensitivity to anticoagulants; therefore, dosage of an anticoagulant may have to be decreased in order to maintain the prothrombin time at the desired therapeutic level.

Drug/Laboratory Test Interferences: Therapy with androgenic anabolic steroids may decrease levels of thyroxine-binding globulin resulting in decreased total T_4 serum levels and increase resin uptake of T_3 and T_4. Free thyroid hormone levels remain unchanged and there is no clinical evidence of thyroid dysfunction.

Carcinogenesis, Mutagenesis, Impairment of Fertility:

Animal data: Testosterone has been tested by subcutaneous injection and implantation in mice and rats. The implant induced cervical-uterine tumors in mice, which metastasized in some cases. There is suggestive evidence that injection of testosterone into some strains of female mice increases their susceptibility to hepatoma. Testosterone is also known to increase the number of tumors and decrease the degree of differentiation of chemically-induced carcinomas of the liver in rats.

Human Data: There are rare reports of hepatocellular carcinoma in patients receiving long-term therapy with androgens in high doses. Withdrawal of the drugs did not lead to regression of the tumors in all cases.

Geriatric patients treated with androgens may be at an increased risk of developing prostatic hypertrophy and prostatic carcinoma although conclusive evidence to support this concept is lacking.

This compound has not been tested for mutagenic potential. However, as noted above, cacinogenic effects have been attributed to treatment with androgenic hormones. The potential carcinogenic effects likely occur through a hormonal mechanism rather than by a direct chemical interaction mechanism.

Impairment of fertility was not tested directly in animal species. However, as noted below under "Adverse Reactions", oligospermia in males and amenorrhea in females are potential adverse effects of treatment with Stanozolol. Therefore, impairment of fertility is a possible outcome of treatment with Stanozolol.

Pregnancy Category X: See "Contraindications" section.

Nursing Mothers: It is not known whether anabolic steroids are excreted in human milk. Many drugs are excreted in human milk and because of the potential for adverse reactions in nursing infants from Stanozolol, a decision should be made whether to discontinue nursing or discontinue the drug, taking into account the importance of the drug to the mother.

Pediatric Use: Anabolic agents may accelerate epiphyseal maturation more rapidly than linear growth in children, and the effect may continue for 6 months after the drug has been stopped. Therefore, therapy should be monitored by x-ray studies at 6 month intervals in order to avoid the risk of compromising the adult height. The safety and efficacy of Stanozolol in children with hereditary angioedema have not been established.

ADVERSE REACTIONS
Hepatic: Cholestatic jaundice with, rarely, hepatic necrosis and death. Hepatocellular neoplasms and peliosis hepatis have been reported in association with long-term androgenic-anabolic steroid therapy (see "Warnings"). Reversible changes in liver function tests also occur including increased bromsulphalein (BSP) retention and increases in serum bilirubin, glutamic oxaloacetic transaminase (SGOT), and alkaline phosphatase.

Genitourinary System: In men. Prepubertal: Phallic enlargement and increased frequency of erections.

Postpubertal: Inhibition of testicular function, testicular atrophy and oligospermia, impotence, chronic priapism, epididymitis and bladder irritability.

In women: Clitoral enlargement, menstrual irregularities.

In both sexes: Increased or decreased libido.

CNS: Habituation, excitation, insomnia, depression.

Gastrointestinal: Nausea, vomiting, diarrhea.

Hematologic: Bleeding in patients on concomitant anticoagulant therapy.

Breast: Gynecomastia.

Larynx: Deepening of the voice in women.

Hair: Hirsutism and male pattern baldness in women.

Skin: Acne (especially in women and prepubertal boys).

Skeletal: Premature closure of epiphyses in children (see "Precautions, Pediatric Use").

Fluid and Electrolytes: Edema, retention of serum electrolytes (sodium, chloride, potassium, phosphate, calcium).

Metabolic/Endocrine: Decreased glucose tolerance (see "Precautions"), increased serum levels of low-density lipoproteins and decreased levels of high-density lipoproteins (see "Precautions, Laboratory Tests"), increased creatine and creatinine excretion, increased serum levels of creatinine phosphokinase (CPK).

Some virilizing changes in women are irreversible even after prompt discontinuance of therapy and are not prevented by concomitant use of estrogens (see "Precautions").

DRUG ABUSE AND DEPENDENCE
Stanozolol is classified by the Anabolic Steroids Control Act as a schedule III controlled substance.

DOSAGE AND ADMINISTRATION
The use of anabolic steroids may be associated with serious adverse reactions, many of which are dose related; therefore, patients should be placed on the lowest possible effective dose.

Hereditary Angioedema: The dosage requirements for continuous treatment of hereditary angioedema with Stanozolol should be individualized on the basis of the clinical response of the patient. It is recommended that the patient be started on 2 mg, three times a day. After a favorable initial response is obtained in terms of prevention of episodes of edematous attacks, the proper continuing dosage should be determined by decreasing the dosage at intervals of one to three months to a maintenance dosage of 2 mg a day. Some patients may be successfully managed on a 2 mg alternate day schedule. During the dose adjusting phase, close monitoring of the patient's response is indicated, particularly if the patient has a history of airway involvement.

The prophylactic dose of Stanozolol to be used prior to dental extraction or other traumatic or stressful situations has not been established and may be substantially larger.

Attacks of hereditary angioedema are generally infrequent in childhood and the risks from Stanozolol administration are substantially increased. Therefore, long-term prophylactic therapy with this drug is generally not recommended in children, and should only be undertaken with due consideration of the benefits and risks involved (see "Precautions, Pediatric Use").

HOW SUPPLIED
TABLETS (C-III): 2 MG

BRAND/MANUFACTURER	NDC	SIZE	AWP
○ **BRAND**			
WINSTROL: Sanofi Winthrop	00024-2253-04	100s	$63.95

Staphage Lysate (SPL)

DESCRIPTION
Staphage Lysate is a bacteriologically sterile staphylococcal vaccine containing components of *S. aureus*, bacteriophage, and some culture medium ingredients (sodium chloride and ultrafiltered beef heart infusion broth).

Staphage Lysate is prepared by lysing parent cultures of *S. aureus*, Serologic Types I & III,[1] with a poly-valent staphylococcus bacteriophage.[2] Bacteriologic sterility is achieved by ultrafiltration. Neither heat nor preservative is used in its preparation.

Staphage Lysate is standardized on the basis of bacterial cell content before phage lysis. Each milliliter contains: 120-180 million colony-forming units of *S. aureus* and 100-1000 million staphylococcus bacteriophage plaque-forming units.

Staphage Lysate is administered by several routes, according to the directions of the physician. These include subcutaneous injection, intranasal aerosol inhalation or nasal drop instillation, oral administration, topical application or irrigation, and combinations of these routes.

CLINICAL PHARMACOLOGY
In experimental conditions, *S. aureus* or its cellular components may induce cell-mediated immunity.[3,4]

In uncontrolled studies in humans, favorable results have been reported using Staphage Lysate for a variety of staphylococcal disease,[5-9] as well as for Herpes virus and aphthous ulcers (essentially treatment failures with other therapeutic modalities).[10]

In vitro, Staphage Lysate has been shown to stimulate lymphoproliferative responses in both T- and B-cell subpopulations present in peripheral and cord blood of normal human subjects.[11-13]

These findings appear to support the interpretation that Staphage Lysate in staphylococcal-hypersensitive subjects acts as an immunopotentiator of nonspecific cell-mediated immunity.

Pharmacokinetic data in humans are unavailable.

ANIMAL PHARMACOLOGY
An increased capability of macrophages to inactive staphylococci has been demonstrated in laboratory animals[4,14-16] following Staphage Lysate treatment.

It further has been demonstrated that laboratory animals hypersensitized to staphylococcus and elicited specifically with Staphage Lysate are protected nonspecifically against challenge with vaccinia virus,[17] influenza virus,[18] virulent field strains of *E. coli*,[19,20] and *K. pneumoniae*.[21]

In laboratory animals, Staphage Lysate has been shown to act as an immunomodulator.[22]

INDICATIONS AND USAGE

BASED ON A REVIEW BY THE PANEL ON BACTERIAL VACCINES AND BACTERIAL ANTIGENS WITH NO U.S. STANDARD OF POTENCY AND OTHER INFORMATION, THE FOOD AND DRUG ADMINISTRATION HAS DIRECTED THAT FURTHER INVESTIGATION BE CONDUCTED BEFORE THIS PRODUCT IS DETERMINED FULLY EFFECTIVE FOR THE LABELED INDICATION(S).

Staphage Lysate is indicated in the treatment of either staphylococcal infections or polymicrobial infections with a staphylococcal component.

Caution should be exercised when administering Staphage Lysate intranasally to patients with known allergies (see "Intranasal Aerosol Inhalation" under "Dosage and Administration").

Although Staphage Lysate has been used in infants and children, its safety and effectiveness in these patient groups have not been established.

The use of Staphage Lysate has not been shown to adversely affect other treatment modalities.

CONTRAINDICATIONS
During an acute asthmatic episode, Staphage Lysate should not be used intranasally.

WARNINGS
In common with all antigens employed to stimulate the production of antibodies that are protective in the event of subsequent disease, Staphage Lysate presents the remote potential of host sensitization to staphylococcal or bovine protein. Anaphylaxis has never been observed in the more than 10 million doses administered, but the physician must bear this possibility in mind and be prepared to deal with such an emergency by having at hand appropriate resuscitation equipment and medications.

Caution should be observed when administering Staphage Lysate intranasally to patients with known allergies (see "Intranasal Aerosol Inhalation" under "Dosage and Administration").

PRECAUTIONS

STAPHAGE LYSATE DOES NOT CONTAIN A PRESERVATIVE; THEREFORE, IT MUST BE HANDLED ASEPTICALLY.
STAPHAGE LYSATE MUST NOT BE USED IF IT BECOMES CLOUDY OR TURBID. (THIS WOULD INDICATE CONTAMINATION.)
STAPHAGE LYSATE MUST BE STORED IN THE REFRIGERATOR (2-8°C). DO NOT FREEZE.

General: A separate, sterile tuberculin syringe and needle should be used for each patient to prevent transmission of homologous serum hepatitis and other disease entities from one patient to another.

Staphage Lysate in the 1-ml ampule should be used for subcutaneous injection and intranasal aerosol inhalation. When a parenteral dose of Staphage Lysate is withdrawn from the 1-ml ampule, the remainder must either be used immediately (by intranasal, oral, or topical administration depending on the condition being treated) or discarded.

Staphage Lysate in the 10-ml vial should be used only for intranasal (aerosol or drop instillation), oral, or topical administration; it should not be used for subcutaneous injection.

When using the 10-ml vial, the rubber cap should be wiped carefully and completely with an appropriate antiseptic before introducing the needle to withdraw the solution.

Caution should be exercised when administering Staphage Lysate intranasally to patients with known allergies (see "Intranasal Aerosol Inhalation" under "Dosage and Administration").

In common with all antigens employed to stimulate the production of antibodies that are protective in the event of subsequent disease, Staphage Lysate presents the remote potential of host sensitization to staphylococcal or bovine protein. Anaphylaxis has never been observed in the more than 10 million doses administered, but the physician must bear this possibility in mind and be prepared to deal with such an emergency by having at hand appropriate resuscitation equipment and medications.

Information for Patients: The physician may wish to inform the patient that Staphage Lysate may cause vaccine-type or site-of-injection reactions (see under "Adverse Reactions") and, if excessive, these reactions may be lessened by dose reduction at the discretion of the physician.

Pregnancy: Pregnancy Category B. Reproduction studies[23-26] have been performed in rats and rabbits at doses up to 250 times the human dose and have revealed no evidence of impaired fertility or harm to the fetus due to Staphage Lysate. There are, however, no adequate and well-controlled studies in pregnant women. Because animal reproduction studies are not always predictive of human response, Staphage Lysate should be used during pregnancy only if clearly indicated.

Nursing Mothers: It is not known whether Staphage Lysate is excreted in human milk. Because many drugs are excreted in human milk, caution should be exercised when Staphage Lysate is administered to a nursing woman.

Pediatric Use: Safety and effectiveness in children have not been established.

ADVERSE REACTIONS
Staphage Lysate may cause general vaccine-type reactions (i.e., malaise, fever, or chills). If excessive, these reactions may be lessened by dose reduction at the discretion of the physician.

Reactions at the site of injection (i.e., redness, itching, and/or swelling) may occur in 2 to 3 hours and may last up to 3 days, steadily decreasing. These reactions indicate a normal response to Staphage Lysate and, if excessive, may be lessened by dose reduction at the discretion of the physician.

Caution should be exercised when administering Staphage Lysate intranasally to patients with known allergies (see "Intranasal Aerosol Inhalation" under "Dosage and Administration").

DOSAGE AND ADMINISTRATION
Staphage Lysate is administered by several routes, according to the directions of the physician. These include subcutaneous injection, intranasal aerosol inhalation or nasal drop instillation, oral administration, topical application or irrigation, and combinations of these routes. The severity of the infection and the response of the patient should be the guiding factors in determining the proper dosage regimen.

Parenteral drug products should be inspected visually for particulate matter and discoloration prior to administration, whenever solution and container permit.

It is highly recommended that all new patients first be skin-tested with 0.025 to 0.05 ml intracutaneously to assess their relative sensitivity to Staphage Lysate. Based on relative sensitivity to the skin test, the initial dose of Staphage Lysate is small, followed by incremental increases at prescribed intervals (according to urgency and tolerance), to a maximum dose. This dose is continued until improvement is certain, then the interval may be lengthened gradually to the longest interval that maintains adequate clinical control.

The limit of tolerance is the maximum quantity of Staphage Lysate that can be given to a patient without producing signs of a general vaccine-type reaction (i.e., malaise, fever, or chills).

For chronic, recurrent, refractory, or deep-seated infections, it may be necessary to increase cautiously the frequency and/or the dose to achieve the desired therapeutic response.

Children usually should receive about ½ the adult dose. Infants are best treated with nasal drop instillation, sprays, or topical application.

Subcutaneous Injection: Staphage Lysate is administered in the deltoid region. Following the initial injection, subsequent injections are given in alternate arms, avoiding a previous site.

If an undue amount of local redness, itching, and/or swelling ensues, await a partial subsidence of the reactions, proceed with ½ the previous dose, and make incremental increases at longer intervals.

Following a subcutaneous injection, the unused contents of the 1-ml ampule may be given orally, topically, or intranasally to reinforce the subcutaneous dose.

Acute Infections: The initial dose varies from 0.05 to 0.2 ml, followed by incremental increases (according to urgency and tolerance) of 0.1 to 0.2 ml at 1- to 2-day intervals, to a maximum dose of up to 0.5 ml. This dose is continued until improvement is certain, then the interval may be lengthened gradually to the longest interval that maintains adequate clinical control.

Subacute and Chronic Infections: The initial dose varies from 0.05 to 0.1 ml, followed by incremental increases (according to urgency and tolerance) of 0.1 to 0.2 ml at 2- to 4-day intervals, to a maximum dose of 0.2 to 0.5 ml. This dose is continued until improvement is certain, then the interval may be lengthened gradually to the longest interval that maintains adequate clinical control.

Intranasal Aerosol Inhalation: Staphage Lysate is rapidly absorbed through the anterior nares, the main reservoir of pathogenic staphylococci. The nose often contains the identical strain isolated from infections in other parts of the body.

The importance of intranasal aerosol inhalation is stressed because of the high-absorptive characteristics of the nasal mucosa.

When using this route, some patients may experience transient general vaccine-type reactions (i.e., malaise, fever, or chills). If excessive, these reactions may be lessened by dose reduction at the discretion of the physician.

Intranasal aerosol inhalation allows direct access to the sinuses, throat, and bronchi; when this route is combined with subcutaneous injection, better clinical results may be obtained.

A nebulizer with nasal tips is used, attached by rubber tubing having a hand-controlled air valve to an air supply (e.g., a DeVilbiss Air Compressor, 561 Series). The nebulizer should be cleaned after each use according to the manufacturer's directions.

A measured dose of Staphage Lysate is placed in the nebulizer, adding sufficient sterile preservative-free water or isotonic saline to a total volume of 1.0 ml for efficient atomization. Nebulization is achieved by closing the air valve during inspiration, holding the breath a few seconds, and exhaling through the mouth, avoiding hyperventilation.

Patients without Allergies: The usual initial dose is 0.1 ml, followed by incremental increases (according to urgency and tolerance) of up to 0.2 ml at 1- to 3-day intervals, to a maximum dose of 0.5 to 1.0 ml. This dose is continued until improvement is certain, then the interval may be lengthened gradually to the longest interval that maintains adequate clinical control.

Patients With Known Allergies: Caution should be exercised when administering Staphage Lysate by this route to patients with allergies such as bronchial asthma, pulmonary fibrosis, emphysema, bronchiectasis, hay fever, and multiple allergies.

It is highly recommended that these patients first be skin-tested with 0.025 to 0.05 ml intracutaneously to assess their relative sensitivity to Staphage Lysate.

Based on relative sensitivity to the skin test, the initial dose varies from 0.05 to 0.1 ml, followed by incremental increases (according to urgency and tolerance) of 0.05 to 0.1 ml at weekly intervals, to a maximum dose of 0.25 to 0.5 ml. This dose is continued until improvement is certain, then the interval may be lengthened gradually to the longest interval that maintains adequate clinical control.

These doses can be increased cautiously at shorter intervals if the patient tolerates Staphage Lysate well.

For faster immunologic response, Staphage Lysate may be given concomitantly by subcutaneous injection or orally without aftereffects.

Nasal Drop Instillation: If intranasal aerosol inhalation equipment is not available, the physician may administer Staphage Lysate by nasal drop instillation, particularly to patients with upper respiratory symptoms. Staphage Lysate may be given by this route either alone or concomitantly with other routes of administration.

Before using Staphage Lysate by nasal drop instillation, review all information under "Intranasal Aerosol Inhalation."

When using this route, withdraw the appropriate dose (see under "Intranasal Aerosol Inhalation") with a sterile tuberculin syringe and needle, remove the needle, and use the syringe as a dropper. The dose should be divided equally between each nostril and should remain in contact with the nasal mucosa for a minimum of 2 minutes to achieve adequate absorption.

Oral Administration: The specific therapy of staphylococcal enterocolitis should include an oral dose of 1 to 2 ml, in water, 1 to 3 times a day as long as necessary to maintain adequate clinical control.

For systemic action, Staphage Lysate by subcutaneous injection or intranasally will reinforce the oral dose.

Topical Application: Concomitantly with other routes of administration, Staphage Lysate in the form of sprays, drops, packs, or irrigations may be used to treat accessible lesions of the skin and mucous membranes, including eye and ear infections, burns, sinus tracts, and ulcers. The usual dose varies from 0.25 to 2 ml, as often as indicated to maintain adequate clinical control.

Storage: Staphage Lysate must be stored in the refrigerator (2-8°C). Do not freeze.

REFERENCES
1. Oeding P: Serologic typing of staphylococci. *Acta Pathol Microbiol (Scandinav)* 33:312-324, 1953.   2. Smith PB, Mudd S: The Gratia polyvalent staphylococcal bacteriophage. *Proc Soc Exp Biol Med* 134(1): 225-229, 1970.   3. Shayegani M: Failure of immune sera to enhance significantly phagocytosis of *Staphylococcus aureus*: Nonspecific adsorption of phagocytosis-promoting factors. *Infec Immun* 2: 742-749, 1970.   4. Mudd S: Resistance against *Staphylococcus aureus. JAMA* 218(11): 1671-1673, 1971.   5. Baker AG: The treatment of chronic bronchial asthma. *Am Pract Dig Treat* 9(4): 591-598,1958.   6. Baker AG: Staphylococcal bacteriophage lysate. Topical and parenteral use in allergic patients. *Pa Med J* 66: 25-28, 1963.   7. Salmon GG Jr, Symonds M: Staphage Lysate therapy in chronic staphylococcal infections. *J Med Soc NJ* 60: 188-193, 1963.   Kress DW, *et al.*: A preliminary report on the use of Staphage Lysate for treatment of hidradenitis suppurativa. *Ann Plastic Surg* 6(5): 393-395, 1981.   9. Vymola F. *et al.*: Staphylococcal osteomyelitis. *Ann NY Acad Sci* 236: 508-514, 1974.   10. Mudd S, Baker AG: Nonspecific cell-mediated immunity in the treatment of recurrent Herpes-virus and aphthous ulcers. In Hasagawa T, ed: *Proceedings of the First Intersectional Congress of IAMS* (Science Council of Japan) 4: 459-470, 1975.   11. Dean JH, *et al.*: *In vitro* human reactivity to staphylococcal phage lysate. *J Immunol* 115(4): 1060-1064, 1975.   12. Dean JH, *et al.*: Functional activities of rosette separated human peripheral blood leukocytes. *J Immunol* 115(5): 1449-1445, 1975.   13. Padarathsingh ML, Dean JH: Development of potency assay for evaluating staphylococcal phage lysate. Unpublished institutional report, 1979.   14. Lenhart N, Mudd S: The staphylococcidal capability of rabbit macrophages. *Bacteriol Proc*: M276, 1971.   15. Shayegani M, De Courcy SJ Jr, Mudd S. Cell-mediated immunity in mice infected with *S. aureus* and elicited with specific bacterial antigens. *J Reticuloendothel Soc* 14: 44-51, 1973.   16. Mudd S, Shayegani M: Delayed-type hypersensitivity to *S. aureus* and its uses. *Ann NY Acad Sci* 236: 244-251, 1974.   17. Allen EG, Mudd S: Protection of mice against vaccinia virus by bacterial infection and sustained stimulation with specific baterial antigens. *Infec Immun* 7(1): 62-67, 1973.   18. Shayegani M, Lief FS, Mudd S: Specific and nonspecific cell-mediated resistance to influenza virus in mice. *Infec Immun* 9(6): 991-998, 1974.   19. Shayegani M, Parsons LM: Nonspecific resistance to *Escherichia* coli in mice. *Infec Immun* 12(4): 779-784, 1975.   20. Shayegani M, Parsons LM, Maupin PS: Correlation of staphylococci-induced delayed-type hypersensitivity and nonspecific resistance during their development, long-term duration and adoptive transfer. *J Reticuloendothel Soc* 28(3): 265-274, 1980.   21. Esber HJ, De Courcy SJ Jr, Bogdon AE: Specific and nonspecific immune resistance enhancing activity of Staphage Lysate. *J Immunopharmacol* 3(1): 79-92, 1981.   22. Aoki T, *et al.*: Staphage Lysate and lentinan as immunomodulators and/or immunopotentiators in clinical and experimental systems. In Hersh EM, *et al.*, eds, *Augmenting Agents in Cancer Therapy* (Raven, New York): 101-112, 1981.   23. Hirayama H, *et al.*: Acute toxicity test and subacute subcutaneous toxicity test of staphylococcal phage lysate (SPL) in rabbits. *Pharmacometrics (Japan)* 20(3): 455-471, 1980.   24. Hirayama H, *et al.*: Chronic subcutaneous toxicity test of staphylococcal phage lysate (SPL) in rabbits. *Pharmacometrics (Japan)* 20(3): 473-485, 1980.   25. Hirayama H, *et al.*: Reproductive evaluation of staphylococcal phage lysate (SPL). 1. Fertility study in rats. *Pharmacometrics (Japan)* 20(3): 487-499, 1980. 2. Embryotoxic and teratogenic study in rats and rabbits. *Ibid.* 20(4): 575-594, 1980. 3. Peri- and postnatal study in rats. *Ibid.* 20(4): 595-608, 1980.   26. Hirayama H, *et al.*: Long-term subcutaneous toxicity test on staphylococcal phage lysate (SPL) as a bacterial antigen, and its effects on the ultrastructure of mononuclear phagocyte system in rabbits. *Pharmacometrics (Japan)* 20(4): 609-637, 1980.

HOW SUPPLIED
INJECTION:

BRAND/MANUFACTURER	NDC	SIZE	AWP
○ **BRAND**			
STAPHAGE LYSATE (SPL): Delmont	48532-0299-01	10 ml	$30.50
	48532-0299-02	1 ml 10s	$32.50

Staphcillin *SEE* METHICILLIN SODIUM

Stavudine

WARNING

STAVUDINE CAPSULES IS INDICATED FOR THE TREATMENT OF ADULTS WITH ADVANCED HIV INFECTION WHO ARE INTOLERANT OF APPROVED THERAPIES WITH PROVEN CLINICAL BENEFIT OR WHO HAVE EXPERIENCED SIGNIFICANT CLINICAL OR IMMUNOLOGIC DETERIORATION WHILE RECEIVING THESE THERAPIES OR FOR WHOM

SUCH THERAPIES ARE CONTRAINDICATED. THIS INDICATION IS BASED ON ANALYSES OF SURROGATE END-POINT RESPONSES. AT PRESENT, THERE ARE NO RESULTS FROM CONTROLLED TRIALS EVALUATING THE EFFECT OF STAVUDINE THERAPY ON THE CLINICAL PROGRESSION OF HIV INFECTION, SUCH AS THE INCIDENCE OF OPPORTUNISTIC INFECTIONS OR SURVIVAL. BECAUSE THERAPY WITH ZIDOVUDINE HAS BEEN SHOWN TO PROLONG SURVIVAL IN PATIENTS WITH ADVANCED HIV DISEASE, ZIDOVUDINE SHOULD BE CONSIDERED INITIAL THERAPY FOR THE TREATMENT OF HIV INFECTION.

THE MAJOR CLINICAL TOXICITY OF STAVUDINE IS PERIPHERAL NEUROPATHY. THIS OCCURRED IN 15 TO 21 PERCENT OF PATIENTS IN THE CONTROLLED TRIALS.

PATIENTS RECEIVING STAVUDINE OR ANY OTHER ANTIRETROVIRAL THERAPY MAY CONTINUE TO DEVELOP OPPORTUNISTIC INFECTIONS AND OTHER COMPLICATIONS OF HIV INFECTION, AND THEREFORE SHOULD REMAIN UNDER CLOSE CLINICAL OBSERVATION BY PHYSICIANS EXPERIENCED IN THE TREATMENT OF PATIENTS WITH HIV-ASSOCIATED DISEASES.

DESCRIPTION

Stavudine (formerly called d4T) is a synthetic thymidine nucleoside analogue, active against the Human Immunodeficiency Virus (HIV). *Each capsule contains*: Stavudine 15, 20, 30, or 40 mg.

The chemical name for Stavudine is 2',3'-didehydro-3'-deoxy-thymidine.

Stavudine is a white to off-white crystalline solid with the molecular formula $C_{10}H_{12}N_2O_4$ and a molecular weight of 224.2. The solubility of Stavudine at 23°C is approximately 83 mg/mL in water and 30 mg/mL in propylene glycol. The n-octanol/water partition coefficient of Stavudine at 23°C is 0.144.

Following is its chemical structure:

CLINICAL PHARMACOLOGY

MECHANISM OF ACTION

Stavudine, a nucleoside analogue of thymidine, inhibits the replication of HIV in human cells *in vitro*. Stavudine is phosphorylated by cellular kinases to Stavudine triphosphate which exerts antiviral activity. Stavudine triphosphate has an intracellular half-life of 3.5 hours in CEM and peripheral blood mononuclear cells. Stavudine triphosphate inhibits HIV replication by two known mechanisms: 1) it inhibits HIV reverse transcriptase by competing with the natural substrate deoxythymidine triphosphate ($K_1 = 0.0083$ to 0.032 μM); and 2) it inhibits viral DNA synthesis by causing DNA chain termination because Stavudine lacks the 3'-hydroxyl group necessary for DNA elongation. In addition to the inhibitory effect on HIV reverse transcriptase, Stavudine triphosphate inhibits cellular DNA polymerase beta and gamma, and markedly reduces the synthesis of mitochondrial DNA.

MICROBIOLOGY

Antiviral activity in vitro: The relationship between *in vitro* susceptibility of HIV to Stavudine and the inhibition of HIV replication in humans or clinical response to therapy has not been established. *In vitro* sensitivity test results vary greatly depending upon the time between virus infection and Stavudine treatment, size of virus inoculum, the cell type employed, and the particular assay method used. Results of several studies on the *in vitro* antiviral activity of Stavudine against HIV-1 conducted in a number of cell types, and on the *in vitro* cytotoxicity of Stavudine are summarized in Table 1.

Table 1

Cell Type	ED^a_{50} (μg/mL)*	CC^b_{50} (μg/mL)*
T-cell (MT-4, ATH8, CEM)	0.002-0.92	0.27-25
PBMCs[c]	0.002-0.009	16
Monocyte/macrophage	0.0132-0.112	> 2.25

* *1μg/mL = 4.46 μM*

(a) *ED_{50} = The concentration required to inhibit viral replication by 50% (measured by either inhibition of HIV-1 induced cytopathic effect, supernatant reverse transcriptase activity or p24 antigen production).*

(b) *CC_{50} = The concentration required to inhibit cell viability or growth by 50% (determined by trypan blue exclusion method or incorporation of ^{3}H-thymidine in DNA).*

(c) *PBMCs = Peripheral blood mononuclear cells.*

DRUG RESISTANCE

Preclinical studies: In vitro selection studies have yieled HIV-1 (strains HXB2 and IIIb) with reduced (7 to 30-fold) sensitivity to Stavudine.

Clinical studies: The development of resistance to Stavudine was studied using HIV-1 isolates obtained from 13 patients treated with Stavudine for 18 to 22 months. Ten of the 13 patients had been treated with zidovudine before Stavudine treatment and 3 patients were reported to be zidovudine-naive. Eleven pairs of these pre- and post-therapy HIV-1 clinical isolates were evaluated for *in vitro* sensitivity to Stavudine, zidovudine, and didanosine. Drug sensitivity testing indicated that 3 of the 11 post-treatment isolates displayed 4 to 12-fold decreases in their sensitivity to Stavudine. Five of the 11 Stavudine post-treatment isolates became resistant (9 to 176-fold) to zidovudine. In addition, 3 of the 11 Stavudine post-treatment isolates were resistant to didanosine. A Stavudine-resistant HIV-1 isolate from one patient was cross-resistant to both zidovudine and didanosine. Of the other two isolates, one was cross-resistant to zidovudine, and the other to didanosine.

Genotypic analysis of 13 pairs of pre- and post-treatment clinical isolates identified multiple mutations in the reverse transcriptase gene. Mutations which confer resistance to zidovudine were observed in 7 of the 13 isolates from patients after Stavudine treatment, and correlated with the observed zidovudine-resistant phenotype. However, no genetic basis for the observed changes in Stavudine and didanosine sensitivity was identified. The relationship between Stavudine treatment and the appearance of zidovudine and didanosine resistance remains unexplained.

DRUG COMBINATION STUDIES

In vitro studies were used to assess the antiviral activity of Stavudine with zidovudine at different molar ratios by the extent of inhibition of HIV-1 induced cytopathic effects in CEM-SS cells. At a molar ratio of 20 (Stavudine to zidovudine), an antagonistic antiviral effect was detected, while at molar ratios of 100 and 500, an additive antiviral effect was apparent. Similarly, the combination of Stavudine with didanosine (molar ratios of Stavudine to didanosine of 0.05, 0.10, 0.16 and 0.5) showed an additive antiviral effect.

PHARMACOKINETICS

The pharmacokinetics of Stavudine have been evaluated in 142 HIV-infected patients following administration of oral doses ranging from 0.03 to 4 mg/kg administered as single doses and as multiple doses every 6, 8, or 12 hours. Stavudine pharmacokinetics have also been evaluated in 44 HIV-infected patients after single intravenous doses ranging from 0.0625 to 1 mg/kg administered as 1-hour infusions.

ABSORPTION AND BIOAVAILABILITY

Following oral administration to HIV-infected patients, Stavudine was rapidly absorbed with a mean ± SD absolute bioavailability of 86.4 ± 18.2% (n = 25). Peak plasma concentrations (C_{max}) increased in a dose-related manner for doses (n = 4 to 10 per dose level) ranging from 0.03 to 4 mg/kg and occurred ≤ 1 hour after dosing. Area under the plasma concentration-time curve (AUC) increased in proportion to dose after both single and multiple doses. There was no significant accumulation of Stavudine with repeated administration every 6, 8, or 12 hours.

When Stavudine (70 mg) was administered to 16 asymptomatic HIV-infected patients under fasting conditions, 1 hour before a standardized high-fat meal (773 Kcal, 53% fat), or immediately after the meal, systemic exposure (AUC) was similar. Mean ± SD C_{max} of Stavudine was reduced from 1.44 ± 0.49 μg/mL in the fasting state to 0.75 ± 16 μg/mL after the meal, and the median time to reach C_{max} was prolonged from 0.6 to 1.5 hours.

DISTRIBUTION

Following 1-hour intravenous infusions (n = 44) of Stavudine doses ranging from 0.0625 to 1 mg/kg, mean ± SD volume of distribution was 58 ± 21 L, suggesting that Stavudine distributes into extravascular spaces. Mean ± SD apparent volume of distribution following administration of single oral doses (n = 71) ranging from 0.03 to 4 mg/kg was 66 ± 22 L. Volume of distribution was independent of doses and did not correlate with body weight.

In three patients who received oral Stavudine doses of 1.3, 3, or 4 mg/kg, Stavudine was measured in cerebrospinal fluid samples at concentrations of 0.08, 0.20, and 0.48 μg/mL at 0.5, 1.75, and 5 hours post-dose, respectively. Stavudine concentrations from simultaneously collected plasma samples were not available.

Binding of Stavudine to serum proteins was negligible over the concentration range of 0.01-11.4 μg/mL. Stavudine distributes equally between red blood cells and plasma.

METABOLISM

After incubation of [^{14}C]-Stavudine for 6 hours with human liver slices, 87% of radioactivity was accounted for by parent drug, 2% was metabolized to thymine, and 7% was associated with unidentified polar compounds. The metabolic fate of Stavudine has not been elucidated in humans.

ELIMINATION

Plasma clearance and terminal elimination half-life were independent of dose over an intravenous dosing range of 0.0625 to 1 mg/kg and an oral dosing range of 0.03 to 4 mg/kg. Following 1-hour infusions (n = 44), plasma concentrations of Stavudine declined in a biphasic manner with a mean ± SD terminal elimination half-life of 1.15 ± 0.35 hours. After single oral doses (n = 115), the mean ± SD terminal elimination half-life was 1.44 ± 0.30 hours. Mean ± SD total body clearance, after intravenous infusion was 594 ± 164 mL/min (8.3 ± 2.3 mL/min/kg), and was independent of dose and body weight. Following single-dose oral administration (n = 113), mean ± SD apparent oral clearance was independent of dose having a value of 559 ± 168 mL/min (8.03 ± 2.54 mL/min/kg). Renal elimination accounted for about 40% of the overall clearance regardless of the

Table 3
INCIDENCE OF PERIPHERAL NEUROPATHY*

			Phase 1 Trials			
Stavudine Dose (mg/kg/day)	0.5	1.0	2.0	4.0	8.0	12.0
N	21	26	17	20	12	11
Peripheral Neuropathy	6 (29%)	5 (19%)	9 (53%)	14 (70%)	8 (67%)	7 (64%)

		Controlled Trials		
	Study AI455-019		*Parallel Track Program*	
	Stavudine (40 mg BID)	zidovudine (200 mg TID)	Stavudine (40 mg BID)	Stavudine (20 mg BID)
N	172	185	4623	4603
Peripheral Neuropathy	25 (15%)	11 (6%)	959 (21%)	713 (15%)

* requiring dose modification, and regardless of grade leading to modification

route of administration. The mean renal clearance was about twice the average endogenous creatinine clearance, indicating active tubular secretion in addition to glomerular filtration. Mean ± SD (n = 88) cumulative urinary excretion of unchanged drug over 6 to 24 hours after administration of an oral dose was 39 ± 23% of the dose.

SPECIAL POPULATIONS
Pediatric: Stavudine pharmacokinetics have been evaluated in 19 HIV-infected pediatric patients after single intravenous doses ranging from 0.125 to 2 mg/kg administered as 1-hour infusions. The pharmacokinetics of Stavudine have been evaluated in 10 children (age 8 months to 4.5 years) who received Stavudine oral solution and 8 children (age 6 to 15 years) who received Stavudine capsules at oral doses ranging from 0.125 to 2 mg/kg administered every 12 hours.

Absorption: Stavudine was rapidly absorbed following oral administration to HIV-infected children with a mean ± SD absolute bioavailability of 78.5 ± 35% and 69.2 ± 23% for capsule and solution formulations, respectively. First-dose and multiple-dose (after 12 weeks of treatment) pharmacokinetic profiles were similar, indicating no accumulation of Stavudine.

Distribution: Following intravenous infusions (n = 19) of Stavudine at doses ranging from 0.125 to 2 mg/kg, the mean ± SD volume of distribution was 13.2 ± 8.95 L (0.68 ± 0.29 L/kg), suggesting that Stavudine distributes into extravascular spaces. After 12 weeks of treatment, the concentration of Stavudine in cerebrospinal fluid samples collected from seven patients ranged from 0.01 to 0.12 µg/mL at times ranging from 2 to 3 hours post-dose (doses ranging from 0.125 to 1 mg/kg). The cerebrospinal fluid concentrations corresponded to 16% to 97% (mean, 55%; n = 6) of the concentration in simultaneous plasma samples.

Elimination: Plasma concentrations of Stavudine declined with a mean ± SD terminal elimination half-life of 1.09 ± 0.28 hours following the end of a 1-hour infusion (n = 19). After a single oral dose (n = 18), the mean ± SD terminal half-life was 0.91 ± 0.24 hours. The mean ± SD total body clearance after intravenous infusion was 181.13 ± 98.36 mL/min (9.64 ± 3.10 mL/min/kg). The mean ± SD apparent oral clearance after administration of solution (n = 10, age < 6 years)

and capsule (n = 8, age > 6 years) formulations was 16.45 ± 4.28 and 11.01 ± 2.94 mL/min/kg, respectively.

Renal insufficiency: Preliminary data from 14 non-HIV-infected subjects with reduced renal function and 5 subjects with normal renal function indicated that the apparent oral clearance (CL/F) of Stavudine decreased as creatinine clearance (CL_{cr}) decreased (see Table 2). The terminal elimination half-life ($t_{1/2}$) was prolonged up to 8 hours. C_{max} and T_{max} were not significantly affected by reduced renal function. Based on these preliminary observations, it is recommended that Stavudine Capsules dosage be modified in patients with reduced creatinine clearance (see *"Dosage and Administration"*).

Table 2
MEAN ± SD PHARMACOKINETIC PARAMETER VALUES SINGLE 40-MG ORAL DOSE OF STAVUDINE

	Creatinine Clearance		
	> 50 mL/min (n = 10)	26-50 mL/min (n = 5)	9-25 mL/min (n = 4)
CL_{cr}(mL/min)	104 ± 28	41 ± 5	15 ± 6
CL/F (mL/min)	335 ± 57	191 ± 39	106 ± 12
CL_R(mL/min)*	167 ± 65	73 ± 18	16 ± 3
$t_{1/2}$ (h)	1.7 ± 0.4	3.5 ± 2.5	4.8 ± 0.8

* CL_R = renal clearance

Geriatric: Stavudine pharmacokinetics have not been specifically investigated in patients > 65 years of age.

Gender: Stavudine pharmacokinetics have not been studied as a function of gender.

Race: Pharmacokinetic differences due to race have not been evaluated.

Hepatic Insufficiency: Stavudine pharmacokinetics in patients with hepatic insufficiency have not been investigated.

Table 5
CONTROLLED CLINICAL TRIALS: INCIDENCE OF ADULT LABORATORY ABNORMALITIES[a]

			%	
	Study AI455-019		*Parallel Track Program*	
Lab Tests (units)	Stavudine (40 mg BID) (n = 172)	Zidovudine (200 mg TID) (n = 185)	Stavudine (40 mg BID) (n = 4623)	Stavudine (20 mg BID) (n = 4603)
AST (SGOT) (> 5.0 × ULN[b])	8	13	5	5
ALT (SGPT) (> 5.0 × ULN)	12	13	10	9
Alkaline Phosphatase (> 5.0 × ULN)	1	0	4	4
Bilirubin (> 2.5 × ULN)	1	3	N/A[c]	N/A[c]
Anemia (< 8.0 g/dL)	0	2	3	3
Leukopenia (WBC < 1000/mm³)	0	1	1	1
Neutropenia (neutrophils < 750/mm³)	3	8	11	12
Thrombocytopenia (platelets < 50,000/mm³)	1	2	4	4
Amylase (> 1.4 × ULN)	9	8	N/A[c]	N/A[c]

a data presented for patients for whom laboratory evaluations were performed.
b ULN = upper limit of normal.
c collection of this data was not required per protocol.

◆ RATED THERAPEUTICALLY EQUIVALENT; ◊ THERAPEUTIC EQUIVALENCE UNCONFIRMED; ○ UNRATED

INDICATIONS AND USAGE

Stavudine Capsules is indicated for the treatment of adults with advanced HIV infection who are intolerant of approved therapies with proven clinical benefit or who have experienced significant clinical or immunologic deterioration while receiving these therapies or for whom such therapies are contraindicated.

This indication is based on analyses of surrogate endpoint responses. At present, there are no results from controlled trials evaluating the effect of Stavudine therapy on the clinical progression of HIV infection, such as the incidence of opportunistic infections or survival.

Because therapy with zidovudine has been shown to prolong survival in patients with advanced HIV disease, zidovudine should be considered initial therapy for the treatment of HIV infection.

CLINICAL STUDIES

STUDY AI455-019

This was a Phase 3, multi-center, randomized, double-blind trial of Stavudine vs. continued zidovudine in HIV-infected adults who had received at least 24 weeks of prior zidovudine treatment. Stavudine was administered in dosages of 40 mg BID for patients weighing $\geq$ 60 kg, and 30 mg BID for those weighing < 60 kg. The zidovudine dosage was 200 mg TID. An interim analysis included data from 359 patients with a median baseline CD4 cell count of 250 cells/mm^3 (range: 10 to 735 cells/mm^3), and a median duration of prior zidovudine treatment of 85 weeks (range: 24 to 246 weeks). At 12 weeks, the mean change from baseline in CD4 cell counts was + 22 cells/mm^3 (range: - 185 to + 375 cells/mm^3) in patients taking Stavudine. At 12 weeks, the mean change in CD4 cell counts from baseline among patients who were continued on zidovudine was - 22 cells/mm^3 (range: - 215 to + 430 cells/mm^3).

STAVUDINE PARALLEL TRACK PROGRAM (STUDY AI455-900)

This program provided access to Stavudine for HIV-infected patients with CD4 cell counts < 300/mm^3 who had failed, were intolerant of, or had contraindications to therapy with zidovudine and didanosine. The program was a randomized, double-blind, comparative trial of Stavudine, 20 or 40 mg twice daily for patients weighing < 60 kg (15 or 30 mg twice daily for patients weighing 40 to 60 kg, and 10 or 20 mg twice daily for patients weighing < 40 kg).

The Parallel Track Program began patient enrollment and randomization in October 1992. An interim analysis was conducted on 10,438 patients randomized through December 1993. Prior to randomization, over 99% of patients had received zidovudine for a median of 91 weeks, and 98% of patients had received didanosine for a median of 22 weeks. Ninety-five percent of the patients were male, and 85% were white. The median CD4 cell count at entry was 41 cells/mm^3 (range: 0 to 426). For the 9,226 patients who had received Stavudine at the time the interim analysis, the median duration of drug treatment was 18 weeks (range: < 1 to 60 weeks).

In an intent-to-treat analysis of randomized subjects, the 40-week survival rates were similar for the two dose groups (79% for each group).

CONTRAINDICATIONS

Stavudine is contraindicated in patients with clinically significant hypersensitivity to Stavudine or to any of the components contained in the formulation.

WARNINGS

The major clinical toxicity of Stavudine is peripheral neuropathy. This occurred in 15% to 21% of patients in the controlled trials.

Patients should be monitored for the development of neuropathy that is usually characterized by numbness, tingling, or pain in the feet or hands. Stavudine-related peripheral neuropathy may resolve if therapy is withdrawn promptly. In some cases, symptoms may worsen temporarily following discontinuation of therapy. If symptoms resolve completely, resumption of treatment may be considered at a reduced dose (see *"Dosage and Administration"*).

Patients with a history of peripheral neuropathy are at increased risk for the development of neuropathy. If Stavudine must be administered in this clinical setting, careful monitoring is essential.

The effect of pre-existing hepatic dysfunction on Stavudine pharmacokinetics is unknown. Therefore, no recommendation for dose adjustments can be made.

Pancreatitis was reported in 1% of patients enrolled in controlled clinical trials and was associated with 14 deaths, five of which were attributed to drug toxicity.

PRECAUTIONS

INFORMATION FOR PATIENTS

Patients should be informed that Stavudine is not a cure for HIV infection, and that they may continue to acquire illnesses associated with AIDS or ARC, including opportunistic infections. Stavudine has not been shown to reduce the incidence or frequency of such illnesses, and patients should be advised to remain under the care of a physician when using Stavudine.

Patients should be informed that the most common toxicity of Stavudine is peripheral neuropathy. Symptoms of peripheral neuropathy include tingling, burning, pain, or numbness in the hands or feet. Patients should be counseled that this toxicity occurs with greater frequency in patients with a history of peripheral neuropathy. They should be advised that these symptoms should be reported to their physicians and that dose changes may be necessary. They should also be cautioned about the use of other medications that may exacerbate peripheral neuropathy.

Patients should be told that the long-term effects of Stavudine are unknown at this time. They should be advised that Stavudine therapy has not been shown to reduce the risk of transmission of HIV to others through sexual contact or blood contamination.

LABORATORY TESTS

Mild to moderate increases in AST (SGOT) and ALT (SGPT) occurred commonly in clinical trials, and tended to resolve following interruption of therapy (see *"Dosage and Administration"*).

CARCINOGENESIS, MUTAGENESIS, IMPAIRMENT OF FERTILITY

Long-term carcinogenicity studies of Stavudine in animals have not been completed. Stavudine was not mutagenic in the Ames, *E. coli* reverse mutation, or the CHO/HGPRT mammalian cell forward gene mutation assays, with and without metabolic activation. Stavudine produced positive results in the *in vitro* human lymphocyte clastogenesis and mouse fibroblast assays, and in the *in vivo* mouse micronucleus test. In the *in vitro* assays, Stavudine elevated the frequency of chromosome aberrations in human lymphocytes (concentrations of 25 to 250 μg/mL, without metabolic activation) and increased the frequency of transformed foci in mouse fibroblast cells (concentrations of 25 to 2500 μg/mL, with and without metabolic activation). In the *in vivo* micronucleus assay, Stavudine was clastogenic in bone marrow cells following oral Stavudine administration to mice at dosages of 600 to 2000 mg/kg/day for 3 days.

No evidence of impaired fertility was seen in rats with exposures (based on C$_{max}$) up to 216 times that observed following a clinical dosage of 1 mg/kg/day.

PREGNANCY

Pregnancy "Category C". Reproduction studies have been performed in rats and rabbits with exposures (based on C$_{max}$) up to 399 and 183 times, respectively, of that seen at a clinical dosage of 1 mg/kg/day and have revealed no evidence of teratogenicity. The incidence in fetuses of a common skeletal variation, unossified or incomplete ossification of sternebra, was increased in rats at 399 times human exposure, while no effect was observed at 216 times human exposure. A slight post-implantation loss was noted at 216 times the human exposure with no effect noted at approximately 135 times the human exposure. An increase in early rat neonatal mortality (birth to 4 days of age) occurred at 399 times the human exposure, while survival of neonates was unaffected at approximately 135 times the human exposure. A study in rats showed that Stavudine is transferred to the fetus through the placenta. The concentration in fetal tissue was approximately one-half the concentration in maternal plasma. There are no adequate and well-controlled studies in pregnant women. Because animal reproduction studies are not always predictive of human response, Stavudine should be used during pregnancy only if clearly needed.

NURSING MOTHERS

Studies in which lactating rats were administered a single dose (5 or 100 mg/kg) of Stavudine demonstrated that Stavudine is readily excreted into breast milk. It is not known whether Stavudine is excreted in human milk. Because many drugs are excreted in human milk, and because of the potential for adverse reactions from Stavudine in nursing infants, mothers should be instructed to discontinue nursing if they are receiving Stavudine Capsules.

PEDIATRIC USE

Safety and effectiveness of Stavudine for treatment of HIV infection in children have not been established. Limited data are available from 37 children aged 5 months to 15 years who received Stavudine in doses ranging from 0.125 to 4.0 mg/kg/day for a median duration of 37 weeks (range 8 to 75 weeks). Serious adverse events that have been observed include AST (SGOT) and ALT (SGPT) elevations and one case of neuropathy. (See *"Clinical Pharmacology"*).

ADVERSE REACTIONS

The major clinical toxicity of Stavudine is peripheral neuropathy (see *"Warnings"*). This toxicity is dose related (see Table 3). Modest elevation of hepatic transaminases was commonly observed in controlled trials.

Adverse events that occurred in $\geq$ 1% of adult patients receiving Stavudine in the Phase 3 controlled comparative trial (Study AI455-019) and in the Parallel Track Program (study AI455-900) are provided in Table 4. (See related tables).

Laboratory abnormalities reported in the Phase 3 controlled comparative trial (Study AI455-019) and the Parallel Track Program (Study AI455-900) are shown in Table 5. (See related table).

OVERDOSAGE

Experience with adults treated with 12 to 24 times the recommended daily dosage revealed no acute toxicity. Complications of chronic overdosage include peripheral neuropathy and hepatic toxicity. It is not known whether Stavudine is eliminated by peritoneal dialysis or hemodialysis.

DOSAGE AND ADMINISTRATION

Adults: The interval between oral doses should be 12 hours. C$_{max}$ was decreased by approximately 45% when Stavudine was administered with food; however, the systemic availability (AUC) was unchanged (see *"Clinical Pharmacology"*). Thus, it appears that Stavudine may be taken without regard to meals. The recommended starting dose based on body weight is as follows:

40 mg twice daily for patients $\geq$ 60 kg.
30 mg twice daily for patients < 60 kg.

Dosage Adjustment: Patients should be monitored for the development of peripheral neuropathy, which is usually characterized by numbness, tingling, or pain in the feet or hands. If these symptoms develop on treatment, Stavudine therapy should be interupted. Symptoms may resolve if therapy is withdrawn promptly. In some cases, symptoms may worsen temporarily following discontinuation of therapy. If symptoms resolve completely, resumption of treatment may be considered using the following dosage schedule:

20 mg twice daily for patients $\geq$ 60 kg.
15 mg twice daily for patients < 60 kg.

Table 4

CLINICAL ADVERSE EVENTS: INCIDENCE > 1% FOR STAVUDINE IN THE PHASE 3 CONTROLLED COMPARATIVE TRIAL (STUDY AI455-019)[1] AND IN THE PARALLEL TRACK PROGRAM (STUDY AI455-900)

			%	
Adverse Events	*Study AI455-019*		*Parallel Track Program*	
	Stavudine (40 mg BID) (n = 172)	*Zidovudine (200 mg TID) (n = 185)*	*Stavudine (40 mg BID) (n = 4623)*	*Stavudine (20 mg BID) (n = 4603)*
Body as a Whole				
Headache	55	52	3	3
Chills/Fever	38	49	5	6
Asthenia	28	36	2	2
Abdominal Pain	26	27	4	5
Back Pain	20	17	*	*
Pain	18	21	3	2
Malaise	17	17	*	*
Allergic Reaction	9	7	*	*
Flu Syndrome	9	6	*	*
Pelvic Pain	2	2	*	*
Neoplasms	2	1	*	*
Death	*	0	5	5
Cardiovascular				
Chest Pain	8	11	*	*
Vasodilation	3	1	*	*
Hypertension	2	3	*	*
Peripheral Vascular Disorder	2	*	*	*
Syncope	1	1	*	*
Digestive				
Diarrhea	50	47	4	5
Nausea and Vomiting	35	46	6	6
Anorexia	10	21	*	*
Dyspepsia	9	15	*	*
Constipation	7	4	*	*
Ulcerative Stomatitis	3	6	*	*
Aphthous Stomatitis	1	2	*	*
Pancreatitis	1	*	1	1
Hemic/Lymphatic				
Lymphadenopathy	5	4	*	*
Metabolic/Nutritional				
Weight Loss	10	11	*	*
Musculoskeletal				
Myalgia	35	36	2	1
Arthralgia	19	19	*	*
Nervous				
Other peripheral neurologic symptoms[2]	40	36	5	6
Insomnia	26	34	1	1
Anxiety	22	17	*	*
Neuropathy (requiring dose modification)[3]	15	6	21	15
Depression	14	21	*	*
Nervousness	10	11	*	*
Dizziness	9	8	*	*
Confusion	3	2	*	*
Migraine	3	2	*	0
Somnolence	2	1	*	*
Tremor	2	0	*	*
Neuralgia	1	0	*	*
Dementia	0	2	1	2
Respiratory				
Dyspnea	13	10	*	1
Pneumonia	3	1	4	5
Asthma	2	1	*	*
Skin and Appendages				
Rash	33	32	3	3
Sweating	19	18	*	*
Pruritus	12	11	*	1
Maculopapular Rash	6	6	*	*
Skin Benign Neoplasm	4	5	*	*
Urticaria	3	3	*	*
Exfoliative Dermatitis	1	*	0	*
Special Senses				
Conjunctivitis	5	2	*	*
Abnormal Vision	3	8	*	*
Urogenital				
Dysuria	3	1	*	*
Genital Pain	2	1	0	0
Dysmenorrhea	2	0	0	0
Vaginitis	2	0	0	0
Urinary Frequency	1	2	*	*
Hematuria	1	*	*	*
Impotence	1	*	*	*
Neoplasm Urogenital	1	*	0	0

* *This event occurred in fewer than 1% of patients.*
1 *Includes all clinical complaints.*
2 *Peripheral neurologic symptoms not requiring dose modification.*
3 *Neuropathy regardless of grade leading to dose modification.*

◆ **RATED THERAPEUTICALLY EQUIVALENT;** ◇ **THERAPEUTIC EQUIVALENCE UNCONFIRMED;** ○ **UNRATED**

Clinically significant elevations of hepatic transaminases should be managed in the same fashion.

Stavudine Capsules may be administered to adult patients with impaired renal function. The following schedule is recommended:

Table 6

Creatinine Clearance (mL/min)	Recommended Stavudine Dose by Patient Weight	
	≥ 60 kg	< 60 kg
> 50	40 mg every 12 hours	30 mg every 12 hours
26-50	20 mg every 12 hours	15 mg every 12 hours
10-25	20 mg every 24 hours	15 mg every 24 hours

There are insufficient data to recommend a dose for patients with creatinine clearance < 10 mL/min or for patients undergoing dialysis.

Storage: Stavudine Capsules should be stored in tightly closed containers at controlled room temperature, 59° to 86°F (15° to 30°C).

HOW SUPPLIED
CAPSULE: 15 MG

BRAND/MANUFACTURER	NDC	SIZE	AWP
○ **BRAND**			
➤ ZERIT: Bristol-Myer Onc/Hiv	00003-1964-01	60s	$200.01

CAPSULE: 20 MG

BRAND/MANUFACTURER	NDC	SIZE	AWP
○ **BRAND**			
➤ ZERIT: Bristol-Myer Onc/Hiv	00003-1965-01	60s	$208.00

CAPSULE: 30 MG

BRAND/MANUFACTURER	NDC	SIZE	AWP
○ **BRAND**			
➤ ZERIT: Bristol-Myer Onc/Hiv	00003-1966-01	60s	$217.00

CAPSULE: 40 MG

BRAND/MANUFACTURER	NDC	SIZE	AWP
○ **BRAND**			
➤ ZERIT: Bristol-Myer Onc/Hiv	00003-1967-01	60s	$225.00

Stelazine SEE TRIFLUOPERAZINE HYDROCHLORIDE

S-T Forte SEE GUAIFENESIN/HYDROCODONE BITARTRATE/ PHENIRAMINE MALEATE/PHENYLEPHRINE HYDROCHLORIDE/ PHENYLPROPANOLAMINE HYDROCHLORIDE

Stilphostrol SEE DIETHYLSTILBESTROL

Stimate SEE DESMOPRESSIN ACETATE

Stop SEE STANNOUS FLUORIDE

Streptase SEE STREPTOKINASE

Streptokinase

DESCRIPTION

Streptokinase is a sterile, purified preparation of a bacterial protein elaborated by group C β-hemolytic streptococci. It is supplied as a lyophilized white powder containing 25 mg cross-linked gelatin polypeptides, 25 mg sodium L-glutamate, sodium hydroxide to adjust pH, and 100 mg albumin (human) per vial as stabilizers. The preparation contains no preservatives and is intended for intravenous and intracoronary administration.

CLINICAL PHARMACOLOGY

Streptokinase acts with plasminogen to produce an "activator complex" that converts plasminogen to the proteolytic enzyme plasmin. The $t_{1/2}$ of the activator complex is about 23 minutes; the complex is inactivated, in part, by antistreptococcal antibodies. The mechanism by which Streptokinase is eliminated is unknown; no metabolites of Streptokinase have been identified. Plasmin degrades fibrin clots as well as fibrinogen and other plasma proteins. Plasmin is inactivated by circulating inhibitors, such as α-2-plasmin inhibitor or α-2-macroglobulin. These inhibitors are rapidly consumed at high doses of Streptokinase.

Intravenous infusion of Streptokinase is followed by increased fibrinolytic activity, which decreases plasma fibrinogen levels for 24 to 36 hours. The decrease in plasma fibrinogen is associated with decreases in plasma and blood viscosity and red blood cell aggregation. The hyperfibrinolytic effect disappears within a few hours after discontinuation, but a prolonged thrombin time may persist for up to 24 hours due to the decrease in plasma levels of fibrinogen and an increase in the amount of circulating fibrinogen degradation products (FDP). Depending upon the dosage and duration of infusion of Streptokinase, the thrombin time will decrease less than two times the normal control value within 4 hours, and return to normal by 24 hours.

Intravenous administration has been shown to reduce blood pressure and total peripheral resistance with a corresponding reduction in cardiac afterload. These expected responses were not studied with the intracoronary administration of Streptokinase. The quantitative benefit has not been evaluated.

Variable amounts of circulating antistreptokinase antibody are present in individuals as a result of recent streptococcal infection. The recommended dosage schedule usually obviates the need for antibody titration.

Two large randomized, placebo-controlled studies conducted with a 60 minute intravenous infusion of 1,500.000 IU of Streptokinase for the treatment of acute myocardial infarction within 6 hours of the onset of symptoms have reported reductions in acute mortality from 20-25%.(1,2)

In the GISSI study, the reduction in mortality was time dependent; there was a 47% reduction in mortality among patients treated within one hour of the onset of chest pain, a 23% reduction among patients treated within three hours, and a 17% reduction among patients treated between three and six hours. There was also a reduction in mortality in patients treated between six and twelve hours from the onset of symptoms, but the reduction was not statistically significant.

One of eight smaller studies using a similar dosing schedule showed statistically significant reduction in mortality. When all of these studies were pooled, the overall decrease in mortality was approximately 23%. Results from pooling several studies using different dosages with long term infusion corroborate these observations.

In addition, studies measuring left ventricular ejection fraction (LVEF) at discharge showed the mean LVEFs were approximately 3-6 percentage points higher in the Streptokinase group when compared to the control group. This difference was statistically significant in some of the studies.(3,4) Furthermore, some studies reported greater improvement in LVEF among patients treated within three hours than in patients treated later. Fewer Streptokinase treated patients had very low ejection fractions associated with congestive heart failure, and the number of patients with clinical symptoms of CHF was reduced.

The rate of reocclusion of the infarct-related vessel has been reported to be approximately 20%. The rate of reocclusion depends on dosage, additional anticoagulant therapy and residual stenosis. When the reinfarctions were evaluated in studies involving 8,800 Streptokinase treated patients, the overall rate was 3.8% (range 2-15%). In over 8,500 control patients, the rate of reinfarction was 2.4%.

Streptokinase administered by the intracoronary route has resulted in thrombolysis usually within one hour, and ensuing reperfusion results in limitation of infarct size, improvement of cardiac function, and reduction of mortality.(5,6) LVEF was increased in patients treated with Streptokinase when compared to patients treated with conventional therapy. When the initial LVEF was low, the Streptokinase-treated patients showed greater improvement than did the controls. Spontaneous reperfusion is known to occur and has been observed with angiography at various time points after infarction. Data from one study show that 73% of the Streptokinase-treated patients and 47% of the placebo-allocated patients reperfused during hospitalization.

Studies with thrombolytic therapy for pulmonary embolism show no significant difference in lung perfusion scan between the thrombolysis group and the heparin group at one year follow-up. However, measurements of pulmonary capillary blood volumes and diffusing capacities at two weeks and one year after therapy indicate that a more complete resolution of thrombotic obstruction and normalization of pulmonary physiology was achieved with thrombolytic therapy, thus preventing the long term sequelae of pulmonary hypertension and pulmonary failure.(7)

The long term benefit of Streptokinase therapy for deep vein thrombosis (DVT) has been evaluated venographically.(8) The combined results of five randomized studies show no residual thrombotic material in 60-75% of patients treated with Streptokinase versus only 10% of those treated with heparin. Thrombolytic therapy also preserves venous valve function in a majority of cases, thus avoiding the pathologic venous changes that produce the clinical post-phlebitic syndrome which occurs in 90% of the DVT patients treated with heparin.

There is a time-related decrease in effectiveness when Streptokinase is used in the management of peripheral arterial thromboembolism. When administered three to ten days after onset of obstruction, rates of clearance of 50-75% were reported.

INDICATIONS AND USAGE
ACUTE EVOLVING TRANSMURAL MYOCARDIAL INFARCTION
Streptokinase is indicated for use in the management of acute myocardial infarction (AMI) in adults, for the lysis of intracoronary thrombi, for the improvement of ventricular function, for the reduction of the incidence of congestive heart failure associated with AMI, and for the reduction of mortality when administered by either the intravenous or intracoronary route. Earlier administration of Streptokinase is correlated with greater clinical benefit. (See "Clinical Pharmacology" section.)

PULMONARY EMBOLISM
Streptokinase is indicated for the lysis of objectively diagnosed (angiography or lung scan) pulmonary emboli, involving obstruction of blood flow to a lobe or multiple segments, with or without unstable hemodynamics.

DEEP VEIN THROMBOSIS
Streptokinase is indicated for the lysis of objectively diagnosed (preferably ascending venography), acute, extensive thrombi of the deep veins such as those involving the popliteal and more proximal vessels.

ARTERIAL THROMBOSIS OR EMBOLISM
Streptokinase is indicated for the lysis of acute arterial thrombi and emboli. Streptokinase is not indicated for arterial emboli originating from the left side of the heart due to the risk of new embolic phenomena such as cerebral embolism.

OCCLUSION OF ARTERIOVENOUS CANNULAE
Streptokinase is indicated as an alternative to surgical revision for clearing totally or partially occluded arteriovenous cannulae when acceptable flow cannot be achieved.

UNLABELED USES
Streptokinase is used alone or as an adjunct in the treatment of retinal vein thrombosis.

CONTRAINDICATIONS
Because thrombolytic therapy increases the risk of bleeding Streptokinase is contraindicated in the following situations:

- active internal bleeding
- recent (within 2 months) cerebrovascular accident, intracranial or intraspinal surgery (see "Warnings")
- Intracranial neoplasm
- severe uncontrolled hypertension

Streptokinase should not be administered to patients having experienced severe allergic reaction to the product.

WARNINGS
BLEEDING
Streptokinase will cause lysis of hemostatic fibrin deposits such as those occuring at sites of needle punctures, and bleeding may occur from such sites. In order to minimize the risk of bleeding during treatment with Streptokinase, venipunctures and physical handling of the patient should be performed carefully and as infrequently as possible, and intramuscular injections must be avoided.

Should arterial puncture be necessary during intravenous therapy, upper extremity vessels are preferable. Pressure should be applied for at least 30 minutes, a pressure dressing applied, and the puncture site checked frequently for evidence of bleeding.

In the following conditions, the risks of therapy may be increased and should be weighed against the anticipated benefits.

- Recent (within 10 days) major surgery, obstetrical delivery, organ biopsy, previous puncture of noncompressible vessels.
- Recent (within 10 days) serious gastrointestinal bleeding
- Recent (within 10 days) trauma including cardiopulmonary resuscitation
- Hypertension: systolic BP $\leq$ 180 mm Hg and/or diastolic BP $\leq$ 110 mm Hg
- High likelihood of left heart thrombus, e.g., mitral stenosis with artrial fibrillation
- Subacute bacterial endocarditis
- Hemostatic defects including those secondary to severe hepatic or renal disease
- Pregnancy
- Age $\leq$ 75 years
- Cerebrovascular disease
- Diabetic hemorrhagic retinopathy
- Septic thrombophlebitis or occluded AV cannula at seriously infected site
- Any other condition in which bleeding constitutes a significant hazard or would be particularly difficult to manage because of its location.

Should serious spontaneous bleeding (not controllable by local pressure) occur, the infusion of Streptokinase should be terminated immediately and treatment instituted as described under (see "Adverse Reactions").

ARRHYTHMIAS
Rapid lysis of coronary thrombi has been shown to cause reperfusion atrial or ventricular dysrhythmias requiring immediate treatment. Careful monitoring for arrhythmia is recommended during and immediately following administration of Streptokinase for acute myocardial infarction.

HYPOTENSION
Hypotension, sometimes severe, not secondary to bleeding or anaphylaxis has been observed during intravenous Streptokinase infusion in 1% to 10% of patients. Patients should be monitored closely and, should symptomatic or alarming hypotension occur, appropriate treatment should be administered. This treatment may include a decrease in the intravenous Streptokinase infusion rate. Smaller hypotensive effects are common and have not required treatment.

OTHER
Noncardiogenic pulmonary edema has been reported rarely in patients treated with Streptokinase. The risk of this appears greatest in patients who have large myocardial infarctions and are undergoing thrombolytic therapy by the intracoronary route.

Rarely, polyneuropathy has been temporally related to the use of Streptokinase.

Should pulmonary embolism or recurrent pulmonary embolism occur during Streptokinase therapy, the originally planned course of treatment should be completed in an attempt to lyse the embolus. While pulmonary embolism may occasionally occur during Streptokinase treatment, the incidence is no greater than when patients are treated with heparin alone.

PRECAUTIONS
GENERAL
Because of the increased likelihood of resistance, due to Antistreptokinase antibody, Streptokinase may not be effective if administered between five days and twelve months of prior Streptokinase or Anistreplase administration or streptococcal infections, such as streptoccal pharyngitis, acute rheumatic fever, or acute glomerulonephritis secondary to a streptococcal infection.

LABORATORY TESTS
Intravenous or Intracoronary Infusion for Myocardial Infarction: Intravenous administration of Streptokinase will cause marked decreases in plasminogen and fibrinogen and increases in thrombin time (TT), activated partial thromboplastin time (APTT), and prothrombin time (PT). These changes may also occur in some patients with intracoronary administration of Streptokinase.

Intravenous Infusion for Other Indications: Before commencing thrombolytic therapy, it is desirable to obtain an activated partial thromboplastin time (APTT), a prothrombin time (PT), a thrombin time (TT), fibrinogen levels, and a hematocrit and platelet count. If heparin has been given, it should be discontinued and the TT or APTT should be less than twice the normal control value before thrombolytic therapy is started.

During the infusion, decreases in plasminogen and fibrinogen levels and an increase in the level of FDP (the latter two causing a prolongation in the clotting times of coagulation tests) will generally confirm the existence of a lytic state. Therefore, lytic therapy can be confirmed by performing the TT, APTT, PT, or fibrinogen levels approximately 4 hours after initiation of therapy.

If heparin is to be (re)instituted following the Streptokinase infusion, the TT or APTT should be less than twice the normal control value (see manufacturer's prescribing information for proper use of heparin).

DRUG INTERACTIONS
The interaction of Streptokinase with other drugs has not been well studied.

Use of Anticoagulants and Antiplatelet Agents: Streptokinase alone or in combination with antiplatelet agents and anticoagulants, may cause bleeding complications. Therefore, careful monitoring is advised.

Anticoagulation After Treatment for Myocardial Infarction: Administration of anticoagulant and/or antiplatelet drugs following administration of Streptokinase appears to increase the risk of bleeding (see "Adverse Reactions"). These agents have been used in an attempt to prevent reocclusion of the target vessel. Use of anticoagulants following administration of Streptokinase has not yet been shown to be of unequivocal clinical benefit. Therefore, the use of anticoagulant regimens should be individualized.

Anticoagulation After IV Treatment for Other Indications: Continuous intravenous infusion of heparin, without a loading dose, has been recommended following termination of Streptokinase infusion for treatment of pulmonary embolism or deep vein thrombosis to prevent rethrombosis. The effect of Streptokinase on thrombin time (TT) and activated partial thromboplastin time (APTT) will usually diminish with 3 to 4 hours after Streptokinase therapy, and heparin therapy without a loading dose can be initiated when the TT or the APTT is less than twice the normal control value.

PREGNANCY
Pregnancy Category C: Animal reproduction studies have not been conducted with Streptokinase. It is also not known whether Streptokinase can cause fetal harm when administered to a pregnant woman or can affect reproduction capacity. Streptokinase should be given to a pregnant woman only if clearly needed.

PEDIATRIC USE
Safety and effectiveness in children have not been established.

ADVERSE REACTIONS
The following adverse reactions have been associated with intravenous therapy and may also occur with intracoronary artery infusion:

♦ RATED THERAPEUTICALLY EQUIVALENT; ◇ THERAPEUTIC EQUIVALENCE UNCONFIRMED; ○ UNRATED

BLEEDING

The incidence of bleeding (major or minor) varied widely from study to study depending on dosage, patient population and concomitant therapy.

Minor bleeding can be anticipated mainly at invaded or disturbed sites. If such bleeding occurs, local measures should be taken to control the bleeding.

Severe internal bleeding involving gastrointestinal, genitourinary, retroperitoneal, or intracerebral sites has occurred and has resulted in fatalites. In three studies in which anticoagulation was optional following intravenous administration of Streptokinase for acute myocardial infarction, the incidence of major bleeding ranged from 0.3%-6.2%. In 21 studies in which anticoagulation was compulsory, the incidence of major bleeding ranged from 0-16%. The overall incidence of major bleeding with high-dose intravenous infusion was 1.2%.

Major bleed rates are difficult to determine for other dosages and patient populations because of the different dosing and intervals of infusions. The rates reported appear to be within the ranges reported for intravenous administration in acute myocardial infarction.

Should uncontrollable bleeding occur, Streptokinase infusion should be terminated immediately. Slowing the rate of administration of Streptokinase will not help correct bleeding and may make it worse. If necessary, bleeding can be reversed and blood loss effectively managed with appropriate replacement therapy. Although the use of aminocaproic acid in humans as an antidote for streptokinase has not been documented, it may be considered in an emergency situation.

ALLERGIC REACTIONS

Anaphylactic and anaphylactoid reactions have been observed rarely in patients treated intravenously with Streptokinase. These ranged in severity from minor breathing difficulty to bronchospasm, periorbital swelling or angioneurotic edema. Other milder allergic effects such as urticaria, itching, flushing, nausea, headache and musculoskeletal pain have also been observed, as have delayed hypersensitivity reactions such as vasculitis and interstitial nephritis. Anaphylactic shock was reported in one study with an incidence rate of 0.1%.

Mild or moderate allergic reactions may be managed with concomitant antihistamine and/or corticosteroid therapy. Severe allergic reactions require immediate discontinuation of Streptokinase with adrenergic, antihistamine, and/or corticosteroid agents administered intravenously as required.

FEVER

Although Streptokinase is nonpyrogenic in standard animal tests, recent reports in the literature have noted an incidence of fever ranging from 0 to 21% in patients treated intravenously with Streptokinase. Symptomatic treatment is usually sufficient to alleviate discomfort.

DOSAGE AND ADMINISTRATION

ACUTE EVOLVING TRANSMURAL MYOCARDIAL INFARCTION

Administer Streptokinase as soon as possible after onset of symptoms: The greatest benefit in mortality reduction was observed when Streptokinase was administered within one hour; statistically significant benefits were observed up to six hours and some benefit was observed up to 12 hours without statistical significance. (See *"Clinical Pharmacology".*)

Route	Total Dose	Dosage/Duration
Intravenous infusion	1,500,000 IU	1,500,000 IU within 60 min.
Intracoronary infusion	140,000 IU	2,000 IU by bolus followed by 2,000 IU/min. for 60 min.

PULMONARY EMBOLISM, DEEP VEIN THROMBOSIS, ARTERIAL THROMBOSIS OR EMBOLISM

Streptokinase treatment should be instituted as soon as possible after onset of the thrombotic event, preferably within 7 days. Any delay in instituting lytic therapy to evaluate the effect of heparin therapy decreases the potential for optimal efficacy. Since human exposure to streptococci is common, antibodies to Streptokinase are prevalent. Thus, a loading dose of Streptokinase sufficient to neutralize these antibodies is required. A dose of 250,000 IU of Streptokinase infused into a peripheral vein over 30 minutes has been found appropriate in over 90% of patients. Furthermore, if the thrombin time or any other parameter of lysis after 4 hours of therapy is not significantly different from the normal control level, discontinue Streptokinase because excessive resistance is present.

Indication	Loading Dose	IV Infusion Dosage/Duration
Pulmonary Embolism	250,000 IU/30 min.	100,000 IU/hr. for 24 hr. (72 hrs. if concurrent DVT is suspected).
Deep Vein Thrombosis	250,000 IU/30 min.	100,000 IU/hr. for 72 hr./
Arterial Thrombosis or Embolism	250,000 IU/30 min.	100,000 IU/hr. for 24-72 hr./

ARTERIOVENOUS CANNULAE OCCLUSION

Before using Streptokinase an attempt should be made to clear the cannula by careful syringe technique, using heparinized saline solution. If adequate flow is not reestablished, Streptokinase may be employed. Allow the effect of any pretreatment anticoagulants to diminish. Instill 250,000 IU Streptokinase in 2 mL of solution into each occluded limb of the cannula slowly. Clamp off cannula limb(s) for 2 hours. Observe the patient closely for possible adverse effects. After treatment, aspirate contents of infused cannula limb(s), flush with saline, reconnect cannula.

RECONSTITUTION AND DILUTION

The protein nature and lyophilized form of Streptokinase require careful reconstitution and dilution. Slight flocculation (described as thin translucent fibers) of reconstituted Streptokinase occurred occasionally during clinical trials but did not interfere with the safe use of the solution. The following reconstitution and dilution procedures are recommended:

1. Slowly add 5 mL Sodium Chloride Injection, USP or Dextrose (5%) Injection, USP to the Streptokinase vial, directing the diluent at the side of the vacuum-packed vial rather than into the drug powder.

2. Roll and tilt the vial gently to reconstitute. *Avoid shaking.* (Shaking may cause foaming.)

3. Withdraw the entire reconstituted contents of the vial; slowly and carefully dilute further to a total volume as recommended in Table 1. Avoid shaking and agitation on dilution. (If necessary, total volume may be increased to a maximum of 500 mL in glass or 50 mL in plastic containers, and the infusion pump rate in Table 1 should be adjusted accordingly.) To facilitate setting the infusion pump rate, a total volume of 45 mL, or a multiple thereof, is recommended.

4. When diluting the 1,500,000 IU infusion bottle (50 mL), slowly add 5 mL Sodium Chloride Injection, USP, or Dextrose (5%) Injection, USP, directing it at the side of the bottle rather than into the drug powder. Roll and tilt the bottle gently to reconstitute. Avoid shaking as it may cause foaming. Add an additional 40 mL of diluent to the bottle, avoiding shaking and agitation (total volume = 45 mL). Administer by infusion pump at the rate indicated in Table 1.

5. Parenteral drug products should be inspected visually for particulate matter and discoloration prior to administration. (The albumin (human) may impart a slightly yellow color to the solution.)

6. The reconstituted solution can be filtered through a 0.8 μm or larger pore size filter.

7. Because Streptokinase contains no preservatives, it should be reconstituted immediately before use. The solution may be used for direct intravenous administration within eight hours following reconstitution if stored at 2-8°C (36-46° F)

8. Do add other medication to the container of Streptokinase. (See related table).

FOR USE IN ARTERIOVENOUS CANNULAE

Slowly reconstitute the contents of 250,000 IU Streptokinase vacuum-packed vial with 2 mL Sodium Chloride Injection, USP or Dextrose (5%) Injection, USP.

STORAGE:

Store unopened vials at controlled room temperature 15°-30° C or (59°-86° F). Unused reconstituted drug should be discarded.

REFERENCES

1. GISSI: Effectiveness of intravenous thrombolytic treatment in acute myocardial infarction. Lancet I: 397-402, 1986. 2. ISIS Steering Committee: Intravenous streptokinase given within 0-4 hours of onset of myocardial infarction reduced mortality in ISIS-2. Lancet I: 502, 1987. 3. White, H., Norris, R., Brown, M., et al: Effect of intravenous streptokinase on left ventricular function and early survival after acute myocardial infarction. N Engl J Med 317: 850-5, 1987. 4. The I.S.A.M. Study Group: A prospective trial of intravenous streptokinase in acute myocardial infarction (I.S.A.M.). N Engl J Med 314: 1465-1471, 1986. 5. Anderson, J., Marshall, H., Bray, B., et al: A randomized trial of intracoronary streptokinase in the treatment of acute myocardial infarction. N Engl J Med 308: 1312-18, 1983. 6. Kennedy, J., Ritchie, J., Davis, K., Fritz, J.: Western Washington randomized trial of intracoronary streptokinase in acute myocardial infarction. N Engl J Med 309: 1477-82, 1983. 7. Sharma, G., Burleson, V., Sasahara, A.: Effect of thrombolytic therapy on pulmonary-capillary blood volume in patients with pulmonary embolism. N Engl J Med 303: 842-5, 1980. 8. Arneson, H., Heilo, A., Jakobsen, E., et al: A prospective study of streptokinase and heparin in the treatment of venous thrombosis. Acta Med Scand 203: 457-463, 1978.

J CODES
IV—J2995

HOW SUPPLIED
POWDER FOR INJECTION: 1.5 MILLION U

BRAND/MANUFACTURER	NDC	SIZE	AWP
○ **BRAND**			
STREPTASE: Astra	00186-1773-01	1s	$473.84

POWDER FOR INJECTION: 1.5 MILLION IU

BRAND/MANUFACTURER	NDC	SIZE	AWP
○ **BRAND**			
STREPTASE: Astra	00186-1774-01	1s	$478.56
KABIKINASE: Pharmacia	00016-0111-75	10s	$4120.00

Table 1
SUGGESTED DILUTIONS AND INFUSION RATES

Dosage	Vial Size (IU)	Total Solution Volume	Infusion Rate
I. Acute Myocardial Infarction			
A. Intravenous Infusion	1,500,000	45 mL	Infuse 45 mL within 60 minutes
B. Intracoronary Infusion	250,000	125 mL	
1. 20,000 IU bolus			1. Loading dose of 10 mL
2. 2,000 IU/minute for 60 minutes			2. Then 60 mL/hour
II. Pulmonary Embolism, Deep Vein Thrombosis, Arterial Thrombosis or Ebolism			
A. Intravenous Infusion			
1. 250,000 IU loading dose over 30 minutes	1,500,000	90 mL	1. Infuse 30 mL/hour for 30 minutes
2. 100,000 IU/hour maintenance dose			2. Infuse 6 mL/hour
B. Same	1,500,000 infusion bottle	45 mL	1. 15 mL/hour for 30 minutes
			2. Infuse 3 mL/hour

POWDER FOR INJECTION: 250,000 IU

BRAND/MANUFACTURER	NDC	SIZE	AWP
○ **BRAND**			
STREPTASE: Astra	00186-1770-01	1s	$107.34
KABIKINASE: Pharmacia	00016-0110-59	10s	$772.50

POWDER FOR INJECTION: 600,000 IU

BRAND/MANUFACTURER	NDC	SIZE	AWP
○ **BRAND**			
KABIKINASE: Pharmacia	00016-0110-67	10s	$1600.00

POWDER FOR INJECTION: 750,000 IU

BRAND/MANUFACTURER	NDC	SIZE	AWP
○ **BRAND**			
STREPTASE: Astra	00186-1771-01	1s	$236.91
KABIKINASE: Pharmacia	00016-0119-35	10s	$2188.75

Streptomycin Sulfate

WARNING

THE RISK OF SEVERE NEUROTOXIC REACTIONS IS SHARPLY INCREASED IN PATIENTS WITH IMPAIRED RENAL FUNCTION OR PRE-RENAL AZOTEMIA. THESE INCLUDE DISTURBANCES OF VESTIBULAR AND COCHLEAR FUNCTION. OPTIC NERVE DYSFUNCTION, PERIPHERAL NEURITIS, ARACHNOIDITIS, AND ENCEPHALOPATHY MAY ALSO OCCUR. THE INCIDENCE OF CLINICALLY DETECTABLE, IRREVERSIBLE VESTIBULAR DAMAGE IS PARTICULARLY HIGH IN PATIENTS TREATED WITH STREPTOMYCIN.

RENAL FUNCTION SHOULD BE MONITORED CAREFULLY; PATIENTS WITH RENAL IMPAIRMENT AND/OR NITROGEN RETENTION SHOULD RECEIVE REDUCED DOSAGES. THE PEAK SERUM CONCENTRATION IN INDIVIDUALS WITH KIDNEY DAMAGE SHOULD NOT EXCEED 20 TO 25 MCG/ML.

THE CONCURRENT OR SEQUENTIAL USE OF OTHER NEUROTOXIC AND/OR NEPHROTOXIC DRUGS WITH STREPTOMYCIN SULFATE, INCLUDING NEOMYCIN, KANAMYCIN, GENTAMICIN, CEPHALORIDINE, PAROMOMYCIN, VIOMYCIN, POLYMYXIN B. COLISTIN, TOBRAMYCIN AND CYCLOSPORINE SHOULD BE AVOIDED.

THE NEUROTOXICITY OF STREPTOMYCIN CAN RESULT IN RESPIRATORY PARALYSIS FROM NEUROMUSCULAR BLOCKAGE, ESPECIALLY WHEN THE DRUG IS GIVEN SOON AFTER THE USE OF ANESTHESIA OR OF MUSCLE RELAXANTS.

THE ADMINISTRATION OF STREPTOMYCIN IN PARENTERAL FORM SHOULD BE RESERVED FOR PATIENTS WHERE ADEQUATE LABORATORY AND AUDIOMETRIC TESTING FACILITIES ARE AVAILABLE DURING THERAPY.

DESCRIPTION

Streptomycin is a water-soluble aminoglycoside derived from *Streptomyces griseus*. It is marketed as the sulfate salt of streptomycin. The chemical name of streptomycin sulfate is D-Streptamine, O-2-deoxy-2-(methylamino)-α-L-glucopyranosyl-(1,2)-O-5-deoxy-3-C-formyl-α-L-lyxofuranosyl-(1-4-)N,N',bis(aminoiminomethyl)-, sulfate (2:3)(salt). The empirical formula for Streptomycin Sulfate is $(C_{21}H_{39}H_7O_{12})_2 \cdot 3H_2SO_4$ and the molecular weight is 1457.38. Streptomycin Sulfate Injection, 1 g/2.5 mL (400 mg/mL), is supplied as a sterile, nonpyrogenic solution for intramuscular use.

Each mL contains: Streptomycin Sulfate equivalent to 400 mg of Streptomycin. Certain brands of Streptomycin contain sodium metabisulfite. (See *"Warnings"*.)

Following is its chemical structure:

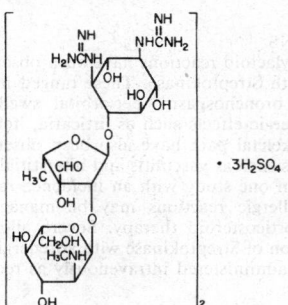

CLINICAL PHARMACOLOGY

Following intramuscular injection of 1 g of Streptomycin, as the Sulfate, a peak serum level of 25 to 50 mcg/mL is reached within 1 hour, diminishing slowly to about 50 percent after 5 to 6 hours.

Appreciable concentrations are found in all organ tissues except the brain. Significant amounts have been found in pleural fluid and tuberculous cavities. Streptomycin passes through the placenta with serum levels in the cord blood similar to maternal levels. Small amounts are excreted in milk, saliva, and sweat.

Streptomycin is excreted by glomerular filtration. In patients with normal kidney function, between 29% and 89% of a single 600 mg dose is excreted in the urine within 24 hours. Any reduction of glomerular function results in decreased excretion of the drug and concurrent rise in serum and tissue levels.

Microbiology: Streptomycin Sulfate is a bacterial antibiotic. It acts by interfering with normal protein synthesis.

Streptomycin has been shown to be active against most strains of the following organisms both *in vitro* and in clinical infection (see *"Indications and Usage"*):

Brucella (brucellosis)
Calymmatobacterium granulomatis (donovanosis, granuloma inguinale),
Escherichia coli, Proteus spp., Aerobacter aerogenes, Klebsiella pneumoniae, and *Enterococcus faecalis* in urinary tract infections.
Francisella tularensis,
Haemophilus ducreyi (chancroid),
Haemophilus influenzae (in respiratory, endocardial, and meningeal infections—concomitantly with another antibacterial agent).
Klebsiella pneumoniae pneumonia (concomitantly with another antibacterial agent).
Mycobacterium tuberculosis,
Pasteurella pestis
Streptococcus viridans, *Enterococcus faecalis* (in endocardial infections—concomitantly with penicillin).

SUSCEPTIBILITY TESTS

Diffusion Techniques: Quantitative methods that require measurement of zone diameters give the most precise estimate of the susceptibility of bacteria to antimicrobial agents. One such standard procedure[1] which has been recommended for use with disks to test susceptibilty of organisms to Streptomycin uses the 10 mcg Streptomycin disk. Interpretation involves the correlation of the diameter obtained in the disk test with the minimum inhibitory concentration (MIC) for Streptomycin.

Reports from the laboratory giving results of the standard single disk susceptibility test with a 10 mcg Streptomycin disk should be interpreted according to the following criteria:

Zone Diameter (mm)	Interpretation
≥ 15	(S) Susceptible

◆ RATED THERAPEUTICALLY EQUIVALENT; ◇ THERAPEUTIC EQUIVALENCE UNCONFIRMED; ○ UNRATED

Zone Diameter (mm)	Interpretation
11-12	(I) Intermediate
≤ 10	(R) Resistant

A report of "Susceptible" indicates that the pathogen is likely to respond to monotherapy with Streptomycin. A report of "Intermediate" indicates that the result be considered equivocal, and, if the organism is not fully susceptible to alternative clinically feasible drugs, the test should be repeated. This category provides a buffer zone which prevents small uncontrolled technical factors from causing major discrepancies in interpretations. A report of "Resistant" indicates that achievable drug concentrations are unlikely to be inhibitory and other therapy should be selected.

Standardized procedures require the use of laboratory control organisms. The 10 mcg Streptomycin disk should give the following zone diameter:

Organism	Zone diameter (mm)
E. coli ATCC 25922	12-20
S. aureus ATCC 25923	14-22

METHODS SECTION:
Two standardized in vitro susceptibility methods are available for testing Streptomycin against Mycobacterium tuberculosis organisms. The agar proportion method (CDC or NCCLS M24-P) utilizes middlebrook 7H10 medium impregnated with Streptomycin at two final concentrations, 2.0 and 10.0 mcg/mL. MIC$_{90}$ values are calculated by comparing the quantity of organisms growing in the medium containing drug to the control cultures. Mycobacterial growth in the presence of drug $\geq 1\%$ of the control indicates resistance.

The radiometric broth method employs the BACTEC 460 machine to compare the growth index from untreated control cultures grown in the presence of 6.0 mcg/mL of Streptomycin. Strict adherence to the manufacturer's instructions for sample processing and data interpretation is required for this assay.

Susceptibility test results obtained by these two different methods cannot be compared unless equivalent drug concentrations are evaluated.

The clinical relevance of in vitro susceptibility test results for mycobacterial species other than M. tuberculosis using either the BACTEC or the proportion method has not been determined.

INDICATIONS AND USAGE

Streptomycin is indicated for the treatment of individuals with moderate to severe infections caused by susceptible strains of microorganisms in the specific conditions listed below:

1. Mycobacterium tuberculosis: The Advisory Council for the Elimination of Tuberculosis, the American Thoracic Society, and the Center for Disease Control recommend that either Streptomycin or ethambutol be added as a fourth drug in a regimen containing isoniazid (INH), rifampin and pyrazinamide for initial treatment of tuberculosis unless the likelihood of INH or rifampin resistance is very low. The need for a fourth drug should be reassessed when the results of susceptibility testing are known. In the past when the national rate of primary drug resistance to isoniazid was known to be less than 4% and was either stable or declining, therapy with two and three drug regimens was considered adequate. If community rates of INH resistance are currently less than 4%, an initial treatment regimen with less than four drugs may be considered.

Streptomycin is also indicated for therapy of tuberculosis when one or more of the above drugs is contraindicated because of toxicity or intolerance. The management of tuberculosis has become more complex as a consequence of increasing rates of drug resistance and concomitant HIV infection. Additional consultation from experts in the treatment of tuberculosis may be desirable in those settings.

2. Nontuberculosis infections: The use of Streptomycin should be limited to the treatment of infections caused by bacteria which have been shown to be susceptible to the antibacterial effects of Streptomycin and which are not amenable to therapy with less potentially toxic agents.

a. Pasteurella pestis (plague),
b. Francisella tularensis (tularemia),
c. Brucella,
d. Calymmatobacterium granulomatis (donovanosis, granuloma inguinale),
e. H. ducreyi (chancroid),
f. H. influenzae (in respiratory, endocardial, and meningeal infections—concomitantly with another antibacterial agent),
g. K. pneumoniae pneumonia (concomitantly with another antibacterial agent),
h. E. coli, Proteus, A. aerogenes, K. pneumoniae, and Enterococcus faecalis in urinary tract infections,
i. Streptococcus viridans, Enterococcus faecalis (in endocardial infections—concomitantly with penicillin),
j. Gram-negative bacillary bacteremia (concomitantly with another antibacterial agent).

UNLABELED USES
Streptomycin Sulfate is also used alone or as an adjunct in the treatment of Whipple's disease, certain infections in AIDS patients, Haverphill fever, and Ménière's disease.

CONTRAINDICATIONS

A history of clinically significant hypersensitivity to Streptomycin is a contraindication to its use. Clinically significant hypersensitivity to other aminoglycosides

may contraindicate the use of Streptomycin because of the known cross-sensitivity of patients to drugs in this class.

WARNINGS

Ototoxicity: Both vestibular and auditory dysfunction can follow the administration of Streptomycin. The degree of impairment is directly proportional to the dose and duration of Streptomycin administration, to the age of the patient, to the level of renal function and to the amount of underlying existing auditory dysfunction. The ototoxic effects of the aminoglycosides, including Streptomycin, are potentiated by the co-administration of ethacrynic acid, mannitol, furosemide and possibly other diuretics.

The vestibulotoxic potential of Streptomycin exceeds that of its capacity for cochlear toxicity. Vestibular damage is heralded by headache, nausea, vomiting and disequilibrium. Early cochlear injury is demonstrated by the loss of high frequency hearing. Appropriate monitoring and early discontinuation of the drug may permit recovery prior to irreversible damage to the sensorineural cells.

Sulfites: Streptomycin contains sodium metabisulfite, a sulfite that may cause allergic type reactions including anaphylactic symptoms and life-threatening or less severe asthmatic episodes in certain susceptible people. The over-all prevalence of sulfite sensitivity in the general population is unknown and probably low. Sulfite sensitivity is seen more frequently in asthmatic than in non-asthmatic people.

Pregnancy: Streptomycin can cause fetal harm when administered to a pregnant woman. Because Streptomycin readily crosses the placental barrier, caution in use of the drug is important to prevent ototoxicity in the fetus. If this drug is used during pregnancy, or if the patient becomes pregnant while taking this drug, the patient should be apprised of the potential hazard to the fetus.

PRECAUTIONS

General: Baseline and periodic caloric stimulation tests and audiometric tests are advisable with extended Streptomycin therapy. Tinnitus, roaring noises, or a sense of fullness in the ears indicates need for audiometric examination or termination of Streptomycin therapy or both.

Care should be taken by individuals handling Streptomycin for injection to avoid skin sensitivity reactions. As with all intramuscular preparations, Streptomycin Sulfate Injection should be injected well within the body of a relatively large muscle and care should be taken to minimize the possibility of damage to peripheral nerves. (See "Dosage and Administration").

Extreme caution must be exercised in selecting a dosage regimen in the presence of pre-existing renal insufficiency. In severely uremic patients a single dose may produce high blood levels for several days and the cumulative effect may produce ototoxic sequelae. When Streptomycin must be given for prolonged periods of time alkalinization of the urine may minimize or prevent renal irritation.

A syndrome of apparent central nervous system depression, characterized by stupor and flaccidity, occasionally coma and deep respiratory depression, has been reported in very young infants in whom Streptomycin dosage had exceeded the recommended limits. Thus, infants should not receive Streptomycin in excess of the recommended dosage.

In the treatment of venereal infections such as granuloma inguinale, and chancroid, if concomitant syphilis is suspected, suitable laboratory procedures such as a dark field examination should be performed before the start of treatment, and monthly serologic tests should be done for at least four months.

As with other antibiotics, use of this drug may result in overgrowth of nonsusceptible organisms, including fungi. If superinfection occurs, appropriate therapy should be instituted.

Drug Interactions: The ototoxic effects of the aminoglycosides, including Streptomycin, are potentiated by the co-administration of ethacrynic acid, furonsemide, mannitol and possibly other diuretics.

Pregnancy: Category D: See "Warnings" section.

Nursing Mothers: Because of the potential for serious adverse reactions in nursing infants from Streptomycin, a decision should be made whether to discontinue nursing or to discontinue the drug, taking into account the importance of the drug to the mother.

Pediatric Use: See "Dosage and Administration".

ADVERSE REACTIONS

The following reactions are common: vestibular ototoxicity (nausea, vomiting, and vertigo); paresthesia of face; rash; fever; urticaria; angioneurotic edema; and eosinophilia.

The following reactions are less frequent: cochlear ototoxicity (deafness); exfoliative dermatitis; anaphylaxis; azotemia; leucopenia; thrombocytopenia; pancytopenia; hemolytic anemia; muscular weakness; and amblyopia.

Vestibular dysfunction resulting from the parenteral administration of Streptomycin is cumulatively related to the total daily dose. When 1.8 to 2 g/day are given, symptoms are likely to develop in the large percentage of patients—especially in the elderly or patients with impaired renal function—within four weeks. Therefore, it is recommended that caloric and audiometric tests be done prior to, during, and following intensive therapy with Streptomycin in order to facilitate detection of any vestibular dysfunction and/or impairment of hearing which may occur.

Vestibular symptoms generally appear early and usually are reversible with early detection and cessation of Streptomycin administration. Two to three months after stopping the drug, gross vestibular symptoms usually disappear, except for the relative inability to walk in total darkness or on very rough terrain.

Although Streptomycin is the least nephrotoxic of the aminoglycosides, nephrotoxicity does occur rarely.

Clinical judgment as to termination of therapy must be exercised when side effects occur.

DOSAGE AND ADMINISTRATION

INTRAMUSCULAR ROUTE ONLY

Adults: The preferred site is the upper outer quadrant of the buttock. (i.e., gluteus maximus), or the mid-lateral thigh.

Children: It is recommended that intramuscular injections be given preferably in the mid-lateral muscles of the thigh. In infants and small children the periphery of the upper outer quadrant of the gluteal region should be used only when necessary, such as in burn patients, in order to minimize the possibility of damage to the sciatic nerve.

The deltoid area should be used only if well developed such as in certain adults and older children, and then only with caution to avoid radial nerve injury. Intramuscular injections should not be made into the lower and mid-third of the upper arm. As with all intramuscular injections, aspiration is necessary to help avoid inadvertent injection into a blood vessel.

Injection sites should be alternated. As higher doses or more prolonged therapy with Streptomycin may be indicated for more severe or fulminating infections (endocarditis, meningitis, etc.), the physician should always take adequate measures to be immediately aware of any toxic signs or symptoms occurring in the patient as a result of Streptomycin therapy.

1. Tuberculosis: The standard regimen for the treatment of drug susceptible tuberculosis has been two months of INH, rifampin and pyrazinamide followed by four months of INH and rifampin (patients with concomitant infection with tuberculosis and HIV may require treatment for a longer period). When Streptomycin is added to this regimen because of suspected or proven drug resistance (see *"Indications and Usage"* section), the recommended dosing for Streptomycin is as follows:

	Daily	Twice Weekly	Thrice Weekly
Children	20-40 mg/kg Max 1 g	25-30 mg/kg Max 1.5 g	25-30 mg/kg Max 1.5 g
Adults	15 mg/kg Max 1 g	25-30 mg/kg Max 1.5 g	25-30 mg/kg Max 1.5 g

Streptomycin is usually administered daily as a single intramuscular injection. A total dose of not more than 120 g over the course of therapy should be given unless there are no other therapeutic options. In patients older than 60 years of age the drug should be used at a reduced dosage due to the risk of increased toxicity. (See boxed *"Warning"*).

Therapy with Streptomycin may be terminated when toxic symptoms have appeared, when impending toxicity is feared, when organisms become resistant, or when full treatment effect has been obtained. The total period of drug treatment of tuberculosis is a minimum of 1 year; however, indications for terminating therapy with Streptomycin may occur at any time as noted above.

2. Tularemia: One to 2 g daily in divided doses for 7 to 14 days until the patient is afebrile for 5 to 7 days.

3. Plague: Two grams of Streptomycin daily in two divided doses should be administered intramuscularly. A minimum of 10 days of therapy is recommended.

4. Bacterial Endocarditis:

a. Streptococcal endocarditis: In penicillin-sensitive alpha and non-hemolytic streptococcal endocarditis (penicillin MIC ≤ 0.1 mcg/mL), Streptomycin may be used for 2-week treatment concomitantly with penicillin. The Streptomycin regimen is 1 g b.i.d. for the first week, and 500 mg b.i.d. for the second week. If the patient is over 60 years of age, the dosage should be 500 mg b.i.d. for the entire 2-week period.

b. Enterococcal Endocarditis: Streptomycin in doses of 1 g b.i.d. for 2 weeks and 500 mg b.i.d. for an additional 4 weeks is given in combination with penicillin. Ototoxicity may require termination of the Streptomycin prior to completion of the 6-week course of treatment.

5. Concomitant use with other agents: For concomitant use with other agents to which the infecting organism is also sensitive: Streptomycin is considered a second-line agent for the treatment of gram-negative bacillary bacteremia, meningitis, and pneumonia; brucellosis; granuloma inguinale; chancroid, and urinary tract infection.

For adults: 1 to 2 grams in divided doses every six to twelve hours for moderate to severe infections. Doses should generally not exceed 2 grams per day.

For children: 20 to 40 mg/kg/day (8 to 20 mg/lb/day) in divided doses every 6 to 12 hours. (Particular care should be taken to avoid excessive dosage in children.)

Parenteral drug products should be inspected visually for particulate matter and discoloration prior to administration, whenever solution and container permit.

Storage: Store under refrigeration at 36° to 46°F (2° to 8°C).

REFERENCES

1. National Committee for Clinical Laboratory Standards. Performance Standards for Antimicrobial Disk Susceptibility Tests—Fourth Edition. Approved Standard NCCLS Document M2-A4. Vol. 10, No. 7, NCCLS, Villanova, PA 1990.

J CODES
Up to 1 g IM—J3000

HOW SUPPLIED
POWDER FOR INJECTION: 1 GM

BRAND/MANUFACTURER	NDC	SIZE	AWP
○ GENERICS			
Allscrips	54569-2373-00	1s	$8.35

Streptozocin

> **WARNING**
>
> STREPTOZOCIN STERILE POWDER SHOULD BE ADMINISTERED UNDER THE SUPERVISION OF A PHYSICIAN EXPERIENCED IN THE USE OF CANCER CHEMOTHERAPEUTIC AGENTS.
>
> A PATIENT NEED NOT BE HOSPITALIZED BUT SHOULD HAVE ACCESS TO A FACILITY WITH LABORATORY AND SUPPORTIVE RESOURCES SUFFICIENT TO MONITOR DRUG TOLERANCE AND TO PROTECT AND MAINTAIN A PATIENT COMPROMISED BY DRUG TOXICITY. RENAL TOXICITY IS DOSE-RELATED AND CUMULATIVE AND MAY BE SEVERE OR FATAL. OTHER MAJOR TOXICITIES ARE NAUSEA AND VOMITING WHICH MAY BE SEVERE AND AT TIMES TREATMENT-LIMITING. IN ADDITION, LIVER DYSFUNCTION, DIARRHEA, AND HEMATOLOGICAL CHANGES HAVE BEEN OBSERVED IN SOME PATIENTS. STREPTOZOCIN IS MUTAGENIC. WHEN ADMINISTERED PARENTERALLY, IT HAS BEEN FOUND TO BE TUMORIGENIC OR CARCINOGENIC IN SOME RODENTS.
>
> THE PHYSICIAN MUST JUDGE THE POSSIBLE BENEFIT TO HIS PATIENT AGAINST THE KNOWN TOXIC EFFECTS OF THIS DRUG IN CONSIDERING THE ADVISABILITY OF THERAPY WITH STREPTOZOCIN. HE SHOULD BE FAMILIAR WITH THE FOLLOWING TEXT BEFORE MAKING HIS JUDGMENT AND BEGINNING TREATMENT.

DESCRIPTION
Each vial of Streptozocin Sterile Powder contains 1 g of the active ingredient Streptozocin 2 - deoxy - 2 - [[(methylnitrosoamino)carbonyl]amino]- α(and β) - D - glucopyranose and 220 mg citric acid anhydrous. Streptozocin is available as a sterile, pale yellow, freeze-dried preparation for intravenous administration. The pH was adjusted with sodium hydroxide. When reconstituted as directed, the pH of the solution will be between 3.5 and 4.5. Streptozocin is a synthetic antineoplastic agent that is chemically related to other nitrosoureas used in cancer chemotherapy. Streptozocin is an ivory-colored crystalline powder with a molecular weight of 265.2. It is very soluble in water or physiological saline and is soluble in alcohol.

Following is its chemical structure:

CLINICAL PHARMACOLOGY
Streptozocin inhibits DNA synthesis in bacterial and mammalian cells. In bacterial cells, a specific interaction with cytosine moieties leads to degradation of DNA. The biochemical mechanism leading to mammalian cell death has not been definitely established; Streptozocin inhibits cell proliferation at a considerably lower level than that needed to inhibit precursor incorporation into DNA or to inhibit several of the enzymes involved in DNA synthesis. Although Streptozocin inhibits the progression of cells into mitosis, no specific phase of the cell cycle is particularly sensitive to its lethal effects.

Streptozocin is active in the L1210 leukemic mouse over a fairly wide range of parenteral dosage schedules. In experiments in many animal species, Streptozocin induced a diabetes that resembles human hyperglycemic nonketotic diabetes mellitus. This phenomenon, which has been extensively studied, appears to be mediated through a lowering of beta cell nicotinamide adenine dinucleotide (NAD) and consequent histopathologic alteration of pancreatic islet beta cells.

The metabolism and the chemical dissociation of Streptozocin that occurs under physiologic conditions has not been extensively studied. When administered intravenously to a variety of experimental animals, Streptozocin disappears from the blood very rapidly. In all species tested, it was found to concentrate in the liver and kidney. As much as 20% of the drug (or metabolites containing an N-nitrosourea group) is metabolized and/or excreted by the kidney. Metabolic products have not yet been identified.

INDICATIONS AND USAGE

Streptozocin Sterile Powder is indicated in the treatment of metastatic islet cell carcinoma of the pancreas. Responses have been obtained with both functional and nonfunctional carcinomas. Because of its inherent renal toxicity, therapy with this drug should be limited to patients with symptomatic or progressive metastatic disease.

UNLABELED USES

Streptozocin is used alone or as an adjunct in the treatment of colon carcinoma and Hodgkin's Disease.

WARNINGS

RENAL TOXICITY

Many patients treated with Streptozocin Sterile Powder have experienced renal toxicity, as evidenced by azotemia, anuria hypophosphatemia, glycosuria and renal tubular acidosis.

Such toxicity is dose-related and cumulative and may be severe or fatal. Renal function must be monitored before and after each course of therapy. Serial urinalysis, blood urea nitrogen, plasma creatinine, serum electrolytes and creatinine clearance should be obtained prior to, at least weekly during, and for four weeks after drug administration. Serial urinalysis is particularly important for the early detection of proteinuria and should be quantitated with a 24 hour collection when proteinuria is detected. Mild proteinuria is one of the first signs of renal toxicity and may herald further deterioration of renal function. Reduction of the dose of Streptozocin or discontinuation of treatment is suggested in the presence of significant renal toxicity.

Use of Streptozocin in patients with preexisting renal disease requires a judgment by the physician of potential benefits as opposed to the known risk of serious renal damage.

This drug should not be used in combination with or concomitantly with other potential nephrotoxins.

When exposed dermally, some rats developed benign tumors at the site of application of Streptozocin. Consequently, Streptozocin may pose a carcinogenic hazard following topical exposure if not properly handled (see *"Dosage and Administration"*).

See additional warnings at the beginning of this monograph.

PRECAUTIONS

Laboratory Tests: Patients who are treated with Streptozocin Sterile Powder must be monitored closely, particularly for evidence of renal, hepatic, and hematopoietic toxicity. Renal function tests are described in the *"Warnings"* section. Patients should also be monitored closely for evidence of hematopoietic and hepatic toxicities. Complete blood counts and liver function tests should be done at least weekly. Dosage adjustments or discontinuance of the drug may be indicated, depending upon the degree of toxicity noted.

Mutagenesis, Carcinogenesis, Impairment of Fertility: Streptozocin is mutagenic in bacteria, plants, and mammalian cells. When administered parenterally, it has been shown to induce renal tumors in rats and to induce liver tumors and other tumors in hamsters. Stomach and pancreatic tumors were observed in rats treated orally with Streptozocin. Streptozocin has also been shown to be carcinogenic in mice.

Streptozocin adversely affected fertility when administered to male and female rats.

Pregnancy Category C: Reproduction studies revealed that Streptozocin is teratogenic in the rat and has abortifacient effects in rabbits. When administered intravenously to pregnant monkeys, it appears rapidly in the fetal circulation. There are no studies in pregnant women. Streptozocin should be used during pregnancy only if the potential benefit justifies the potential risk to the fetus.

Nursing Mothers: It is not known whether Streptozocin is excreted in human milk. Because many drugs are excreted in human milk and because of the potential for serious adverse reactions in nursing infants, nursing should be discontinued in patients receiving Streptozocin.

ADVERSE REACTIONS

Renal: See *"Warnings"*.

Gastrointestinal: Most patients treated with Streptozocin Sterile Powder have experienced severe nausea and vomiting, occasionally requiring discontinuation of drug therapy. Some patients experienced diarrhea. A number of patients have experienced hepatic toxicity, as characterized by elevated liver enzyme (SGOT and LDH) levels and hypoalbuminemia.

Hematological: Hematological toxicity has been rare, most often involving mild decreases in hematocrit values. However, *fatal hematological toxicity with substantial reductions in leukocyte and platelet count* has been observed.

Metabolic: Mild to moderate abnormalities of glucose tolerance have been noted in some patients treated with Streptozocin. These have generally been reversible, but insulin shock with hypoglycemia has been observed.

Genitourinary: Two cases of nephrogenic diabetes insipidus following therapy with Streptozocin have been reported. One had spontaneous recovery and the second responded to indomethacin.

OVERDOSAGE

No specific antidote for Streptozocin is known.

DOSAGE AND ADMINISTRATION

Streptozocin Sterile Powder should be administered intravenously. It is not active orally. Although it has been administered intra-arterially, this is not recommended pending further evaluation of the possibility that adverse renal effects may be evoked more rapidly by this route of administration. Two different dosage schedules have been employed successfully with Streptozocin.

Daily Schedule: The recommended dose for daily intravenous administration is 500 mg/m^2 of body surface area for five consecutive days every six weeks until maximum benefit or until treatment-limiting toxicity is observed. Dose escalation on this schedule is not recommended.

Weekly Schedule: The recommended initial dose for weekly intravenous administration is 1000 mg/m^2 of body surface area at weekly intervals for the first two courses (weeks). In subsequent courses, drug doses may be escalated in patients who have not achieved a therapeutic response and who have not experienced significant toxicity with the previous course of treatment. However A SINGLE DOSE OF 1500 MG/M^2 BODY SURFACE AREA SHOULD NOT BE EXCEEDED as a greater dose may cause azotemia. When administered on this schedule, the median time to onset of response is about 17 days and the median time to maximum response is about 35 days. The median *total* dose to onset of response is about 2000 mg/m^2 body surface area and the median *total* dose to maximum response is about 4000 mg/m^2 body surface area. The ideal duration of maintenance therapy with Streptozocin has not yet been clearly established for either of the above schedules.

For patients with functional tumors, serial monitoring of fasting insulin levels allows a determination of biochemical response to therapy. For patients with either functional or nonfunctional tumors, response to therapy can be determined by measurable reductions of tumor size (reduction of organomegaly, masses, or lymph nodes).

Reconstitute Streptozocin with 9.5 ml of Dextrose Injection USP, or 0.9% Sodium Chloride Injection USP. The resulting pale-gold solution will contain 100 mg of Streptozocin and 22 mg of citric acid per ml. Where more dilute infusion solutions are desirable, further dilution in the above vehicles is recommended. The total storage time for Streptozocin after it has been placed in solution should not exceed 12 hours. This product contains no preservatives and is not intended as a multiple-dose vial.

Caution in the handling and preparation of the powder and solution should be exercised, and the use of gloves is recommended. If Streptozocin Sterile Powder or a solution prepared from Streptozocin contacts the skin or mucosae, immediately wash the affected area with soap and water.

Procedures for proper handling and disposal of anticancer drugs should be considered. Several guidelines on this subject have been published.[4-9] There is no general agreement that all of the procedures recommended in the guidelines are necessary or appropriate.

Unopened vials of Streptozocin should be stored at refrigeration temperatures (2-8° C) and protected from light (preferably stored in carton).

REFERENCES

1. Broder LE and Carter SK: *Ann Int Med, 79*:101-118, 1972.   2. Schein PS, O'Connell MJ, Blom J, Hubbard S. Magrath IT, Bergevin P, Wiernik PH, Ziegler TL, and DeVita VT: *Cancer, 34*:993-1000, 1974.   3. Moertel CG, *et al: Cancer Chemother Rep, 55*:303-307, 1972.   4. Recommendations for the Safe Handling of Parenteral Antineoplastic Drugs, NIH Publication No. 83-2621. For sale by the Superintendent of Documents, US Government Printing Office, Washington, DC 20402.   5. AMA Council Report. Guidelines for Handling Parenteral Antineoplastics. JAMA, March 15, 1985.   6. National Study Commission on Cytotoxic Exposure-Recommendations for Handling Cytotoxic Agents. Available from Louis P. Jeffrey, ScD, Director of Pharmacy Services, Rhode Island Hospital, 593 Eddy Street, Providence, Rhode Island 02902.   7. Clinical Oncological Society of Australia: Guidelines and recommendations for safe handling of antineoplastic agents. *Med J Australia* 1:426-428, 1983.   8. Jones RB, et al, Safe handling of chemotherapeutic agents: A report from the Mount Sinai Medical Center CA-A Cancer Journal for Clinicians Sept/Oct., 1983, pp. 258-263.   9. American Society of Hospital Pharmacists Technical assistance bulletin on handling cytotoxic drugs in hospitals. *AmJ Hosp Pharm* 42:131-137, 1985.

J CODES

1 gm IV—J9320

HOW SUPPLIED
POWDER FOR INJECTION: 1 GM

BRAND/MANUFACTURER	NDC	SIZE	AWP
○ BRAND ZANOSAR: Upjohn	00009-0844-01	1s	$59.01

Strontium-89 Chloride

DESCRIPTION

Strontium-89 Chloride is a sterile, nonpyrogenic, aqueous solution of Strontium-89 Chloride for intravenous administration. The solution contains no preservative.

Each milliliter contains:

Strontium Chloride	10.9 - 22.6 mg
Water for Injection	q.s. to 1 mL

► SHOWN IN PRODUCT IDENTIFICATION GUIDE

The radioactive concentration is 37 MBq/mL, 1 mCi/mL, and the specific activity is 2.96-6.17 MBq/mg, 80-167 μCi/mg at calibration. The pH of the solution is 4 - 7.5.

Strontium-89 Chloride is supplied in a 10 mL vial containing 148 MBq, 4 mCi. The vial is shipped in a transportation shield with approximately 3 mm lead wall thickness, package insert, and two therapeutic agent warning labels.

PHYSICAL CHARACTERISTICS
Strontium-89 decays by beta emission with a physical half-life of 50.5 days. The maximum beta energy is 1.463 MeV (100%). The maximum range of β- from Strontium-89 in tissue is approximately 8 mm.

Radioactive decay factors to be applied to the stated value for radioactive concentration at calibration, when calculating injection volumes at the time of administration, are given in Table 1.

Table 1:
DECAY OF STRONTIUM-89

Day*	Factor	Day*	Factor
-24	1.39	+6	0.92
-22	1.35	+8	0.90
-20	1.32	+10	0.87
-18	1.28	+12	0.85
-16	1.25	+14	0.83
-14	1.21	+16	0.80
-12	1.18	+18	0.78
-10	1.15	+20	0.76
-8	1.12	+22	0.74
-6	1.09	+24	0.72
-4	1.06	+26	0.70
-2	1.03	+28	0.68
0=calibration	1.00		

* *Days before (−) or after (+) the calibration date stated on the vial.*

Following is its chemical structure:

$$^{89}SrCl_2$$

CLINICAL PHARMACOLOGY
Following intravenous injection, soluble strontium compounds behave like their calcium analogs, clearing rapidly from the blood and selectively localizing in bone mineral. Uptake of Strontium by bone occurs preferentially in sites of active osteogenesis; thus primary bone tumors and areas of metastatic involvement (blastic lesions) can accumulate significantly greater concentrations of Strontium than surrounding normal bone.

Strontium-89 Chloride is retained in metastatic bone lesions much longer than in normal bone, where turnover is about 14 days. In patients with extensive skeletal metastases, well over half of the injected dose is retained in the bones.

Excretion pathways are two-thirds urinary and one-third fecal in patients with bone metastases. Urinary excretion is higher in people without bone lesions. Urinary excretion is greatest in the first two days following injection.

Strontium-89 is a pure beta emitter and Strontium-89 Chloride selectively irradiates sites of primary and metastatic bone involvement with minimal irradiation of soft tissues distant from the bone lesions. (The maximum range in tissue is 8 mm; maximum energy is 1.463 MeV.) Mean absorbed radiation doses are listed under the *"Radiation Dosimetry"* section.

Clinical trials have examined relief of pain in cancer patients who have received therapy for bone metastases (external radiation to indexed sites) but in whom persistent pain recurred. In a multicenter Canadian placebo-controlled trial of 126 patients, pain relief occurred in more patients treated with a single injection of Strontium-89 Chloride than in patients treated with an injection of placebo. Results are given in the following tables.

Table 2 compares the percentage and number of patients treated with Strontium-89 Chloride or placebo who had reduced pain and no increase in analgesic or radiotherapy re-treatment.

Table 2:
COMPARISON OF THE EFFECTS OF STRONTIUM-89 AND PLACEBO, AS ADJUNCT TO RADIOTHERAPY, ON TREATMENT OUTCOME OVER TIME.

	Months Post treatment					
	1	*2*	*3*	*4*	*5*	*6*
Strontium-89 Chloride	71.4%	78.9%	60.6%	59.3%	36.4%	63.6%
	(n=42)	(n=38)	(n=33)	(n=27)	(n=22)	(n=22)
Placebo	61.4%	57.1%	55.9%	25.0%	31.8%	35.0%
	(n=44)	(n=35)	(n=34)	(n=24)	(n=22)	(n=20)

At each visit, treatment success, defined as a reduction in a patient's pain score without any increase in analgesic intake and without any supplementary radiotherapy at the index site, was more frequent among patients assigned to Strontium-89 Chloride than to placebo.

Table 3 compares the number and percentage of patients treated with Strontium-89 Chloride or placebo as an adjunct to radiotherapy who were pain free without analgesic at the intervals shown. (See related table).

The number of patients classified at each visit as treatment successes who were pain free at the index site and required no analgesics was consistently higher in the Strontium-89 Chloride group.

New pain sites were less frequent in patients treated with Strontium-89 Chloride.

In another clinical trial, pain relief was greater in a group of patients treated with Strontium-89 Chloride compared with a group treated with non-radioactive Strontium-88.

INDICATIONS AND USAGE
Strontium-89 Chloride Injection is indicated for the relief of bone pain in patients with painful skeletal metastases.

The presence of bone metastases should be confirmed prior to therapy.

CONTRAINDICATIONS
None known.

WARNINGS
Use of Strontium-89 Chloride in patients with evidence of seriously compromised bone marrow from previous therapy or disease infiltration is not recommended unless the potential benefit of the treatment outweighs its risks. Bone marrow toxicity is to be expected following the administration of Strontium-89 Chloride, particularly white blood cells and platelets. The extent of toxicity is variable. It is recommended that the patient's peripheral blood cell counts be monitored at least once every other week. Typically, platelets will be depressed by about 30% compared to pre-administration levels. The nadir of platelet depression in most patients is found between 12 and 16 weeks following administration of Strontium-89 Chloride. White blood cells are usually depressed to a varying extent compared to pre-administration levels. Thereafter, recovery occurs slowly, typically reaching pre-administration levels six months after treatment unless the patient's disease or additional therapy intervenes.

In considering repeat administration of Strontium-89 Chloride, the patient's hematologic response to the initial dose, current platelet level and other evidence of marrow depletion should be carefully evaluated.

Verification of dose and patient identification is necessary prior to administration because Strontium-89 Chloride delivers a relatively high dose of radioactivity.

Strontium-89 Chloride may cause fetal harm when administered to a pregnant woman. There are no adequate and well-controlled studies in pregnant women. If this drug is used during pregnancy, or if the patient becomes pregnant while receiving this drug, the patient should be apprised of the potential hazard to the fetus. Women of childbearing potential should be advised to avoid becoming pregnant.

PRECAUTIONS
Strontium-89 Chloride is not indicated for use in patients with cancer not involving bone. Strontium-89 Chloride should be used with caution in patients with platelet counts below 60,000 and white cell counts below 2,400.

Radiopharmaceuticals should only be used by physicians who are qualified by training and experience in the safe use and handling of radionuclides and whose experience and training have been approved by the appropriate government agency authorized to license the use of radionuclides.

Strontium-89 Chloride, like other radioactive drugs, must be handled with care and appropriate safety measures taken to minimize radiation to clinical personnel.

In view of the delayed onset of pain relief, typically 7 to 20 days postinjection, administration of Strontium-89 Chloride to patients with very short life expectancy is not recommended.

A calcium-like flushing sensation has been observed in patients following a rapid (less than 30 second injection) administration.

Special precautions, such as urinary catheterization, should be taken following administration to patients who are incontinent to minimize the risk of radioactive contamination of clothing, bed linen and the patient's environment.

CARCINOGENESIS, MUTAGENESIS, IMPAIRMENT OF FERTILITY
Data from a repetitive dose animal study suggests that Strontium 89 Chloride is a potential carcinogen. Thirty-three of 40 rats injected with Strontium-89 Chloride in ten consecutive monthly doses of either 250 or 350 μCi/kg developed malignant bone tumors after a latency period of approximately 9 months. No neoplasia was observed in the control animals. Treatment with Strontium-89 Chloride should be restricted to patients with well documented metastatic bone disease.

Adequate studies with Strontium-89 Chloride have not been performed to evaluate mutagenic potential or effects on fertility.

PREGNANCY
Teratogenic effects.
Pregnancy Category D. See *"Warnings"* section.

NURSING MOTHERS
Because Strontium acts as a calcium analog, secretion of Strontium-89 Chloride into human milk is likely. It is recommended that nursing be discontinued by mothers about to receive intravenous Strontium-89 Chloride. It is not known whether this drug is excreted in human milk.

PEDIATRIC USE
Safety and effectiveness in children below the age of 18 years have not been established.

◆ RATED THERAPEUTICALLY EQUIVALENT; ◇ THERAPEUTIC EQUIVALENCE UNCONFIRMED; ○ UNRATED

Table 3:
COMPARISON OF THE EFFECTS OF STRONTIUM-89 AND PLACEBO, AS ADJUNCT TO RADIOTHERAPY, ON REDUCTION OF PAIN SCORE AND ANALGESIC SCORE TO ZERO.

	Months Post treatment						
	1	2	3	4	5	6	9
Strontium-89 Chloride	6 14.3% (n=42)	5 13.2% (n=38)	5 15.2% (n=33)	3 11.1% (n=27)	4 18.2% (n=22)	4 18.2% (n=22)	2 18.2% (n=11)
Placebo	3 6.8% (n=44)	3 8.6% (n=35)	2 5.9% (n=34)	0 (n=24)	1 4.5% (n=22)	1 5% (n=20)	0 (n=17)

ADVERSE REACTIONS
A single case of fatal septicemia following leukopenia was reported during clinical trials. Most severe reactions of marrow toxicity can be managed by conventional means.

A small number of patients have reported a transient increase in bone pain at 36 to 72 hours after injection. This is usually mild and self-limiting, and controllable with analgesics. A single patient reported chills and fever 12 hours after injection without long-term sequelae.

DOSAGE AND ADMINISTRATION
The recommended dose of Strontium-89 Chloride is 148 MBq, 4 mCi, administered by slow intravenous injection (1-2 minutes). Alternatively, a dose of 1.5 - 2.2 MBq/kg, 40-60 μCi/kg body weight may be used.

Repeated administrations of Strontium-89 Chloride should be based on an individual patient's response to therapy, current symptoms, and hematologic status, and are generally not recommended at intervals of less than 90 days.

The patient dose should be measured by a suitable radioactivity calibration system immediately prior to administration.

RADIATION DOSIMETRY
The estimated radiation dose that would be delivered over time by the intravenous injection of 37 MBq, 1 mCi of Strontium-89 to a normal healthy adult is given in Table 4. Data are taken from the ICRP publication "Radiation Dose to Patients from Radiopharmaceuticals", ICRP #53, Vol. 18, No. 1-4, Page 171, Pergamon Press, 1988.

Table 4:
STRONTIUM-89 DOSIMETRY

Organ	mGy/MBq	rad/mCi
Bone Surface	17.0	63.0
Red Bone Marrow	11.0	40.7
Lower Bowel Wall	4.7	17.4
Bladder Wall	1.3	4.8
Testes	0.8	2.9
Ovaries	0.8	2.9
Uterine Wall	0.8	2.9
Kidneys	0.8	2.9

When blastic osseous metastases are present, significantly enhanced localization of the radiopharmaceutical will occur with correspondingly higher doses to the metastases compared with normal bones and other organs.

The radiation dose hazard in handling Strontium-89 Chloride injection during dose dispensing and administration is similar to that from phosphorus-32. The beta emission has a range in water of about 8 mm (max.) and in glass of about 3 mm, but the bremsstrahlung radiation may augment the contact dose.

Measured values of the dose on the surface of the unshielded vial are about 65 mR/minute/mCi.

It is recommended that the vial be kept inside its transportation shield whenever possible.

The vial and its contents should be stored inside its transportation container at room temperature (15-25 °C, 59-77 °F).

The calibration date (for radioactivity content) and expiration date are quoted on the vial label. The expiration date will be 28 days after calibration. Stability studies have shown no change in any of the product characteristics monitored during routine product quality control over the period from manufacture to expiration.

This radiopharmaceutical is licensed by the Illinois Department of Nuclear Safety for distribution to persons licensed pursuant to 32 Illinois Adm. Code 330.260 (a) and Part 335 Subpart F.335.5010 or under equivalent licenses of the USNRC or an Agreement State.

HOW SUPPLIED
INJECTION: 10.9-22.6 MG/ML

BRAND/MANUFACTURER	NDC	SIZE	AWP
○ **BRAND**			
METASTRON: Medi-Physics	17156-0524-01	10 ml ud	$1924.00

Stuartnatal Plus SEE VITAMINS, PRENATAL

Sublimaze SEE FENTANYL

Succimer

DESCRIPTION
Succimer is an orally active, heavy metal chelating agent. The chemical name for Succimer is meso 2, 3-dimercaptosuccinic acid (DMSA). Its empirical formula is $C_4H_6O_4S_2$ and molecular weight is 182.2.

Succimer is a white crystalline powder with an unpleasant, characteristic mercaptan odor and taste.

Each Succimer capsule for oral administration contains beads coated with 100 mg of Succimer.

Following is its chemical structure:

```
        COOH
        |
    H—C—SH
        |
    H—C—SH
        |
        COOH
```

CLINICAL PHARMACOLOGY
Succimer is a lead chelator; it forms water soluble chelates and, consequently, increases the urinary excretion of lead.

Preclinical Toxicology: In an ongoing six month chronic oral toxicity study in dogs, thrombocytopenia was observed in animals receiving Succimer at 80 or 140 mg/kg/day after three months of dosing. Preliminary gross pathology findings in the affected dogs included ecchymoses in a number of organs. No depressed platelet counts were observed in dogs receiving Succimer at 10 mg/kg/day for three months. Platelets were not enumerated in previous oral toxicity studies up to 28 days. In those studies, daily doses of Succimer up to 200 mg/kg/day did not produce any significant overt toxicity in rats and dogs. However, six and twenty-eight day oral toxicity studies in dogs have shown that doses of 300 mg/kg/day or higher were toxic and lethal to some dogs. Kidney and gastrointestinal tract were the major target organs for Succimer toxicity.

Toxicity was manifested by anorexia, emesis, mucoid and/or bloody diarrhea, increased blood urea nitrogen concentration, increased SGPT, SGOT and alkaline phosphatase levels, renal tubular necrosis, purulent nephritis and severe gastrointestinal bleeding and ulceration. Deaths were due to renal failure.

Pharmacokinetics: In a study performed in healthy adult volunteers, after a single dose of ^{14}C-Succimer at 16,32, or 48 mg/kg, absorption was rapid but variable with peak blood radioactivity levels between one and two hours. On average, 49% of the radiolabeled dose was excreted: 39% in the feces, 9% in the urine and 1% as carbon dioxide from the lungs. Since fecal excretion probably represented non-absorbed drug, most of the absorbed drug was excreted by the kidneys. The apparent elimination half-life of the radio-labeled material in the blood was about two days.

In other studies of healthy adult volunteers receiving a single oral dose of 10 mg/kg, the chemical analysis of Succimer and its metabolites in the urine showed that Succimer was rapidly and extensively metabolized. Approximately 25% of the administered dose was excreted in the urine with the peak blood level and urinary excretion occurring between two and four hours. Of the total amount of drug eliminated in the urine, approximately 90% was eliminated in altered form as mixed Succimer-cysteine disulfides; the remaining 10% was eliminated unchanged. The majority of mixed disulfides consisted of Succimer in disulfide linkages with two molecules of L-cysteine, the remaining disulfides contained one L-cysteine per Succimer molecule.

Pharmacodynamics: Dose ranging studies were performed in 18 men with blood lead levels of 44-96 μg/dL. Three groups of 6 patients received either 10.0, 6.7 or 3.3 mg/kg Succimer orally every 8 hours for 5 days. After five days the mean blood levels of the three groups decreased 72.5%, 58.3% and 35.5% respectively. The mean urinary lead excretions in the initial 24 hours were 28.6, 18.6 and 12.3 times the pretreatment 24 hour urinary lead excretion. As the chelatable pool was reduced during therapy, urinary lead output decreased. A mean of 19 mg of lead was excreted during a five-day course of 30 mg/kg/day Succimer. Clinical symptoms, such as headache and colic, and biochemical indices of lead toxicity also improved. Decrease in urinary excretion of d-aminolevulinic acid (ALA) and coproporphyrin paralleled the improvement in erythrocyte d-aminolevulinic acid dehydratase (ALA-D). Three control patients with lead poisoning of similar severity received CaNa$_2$EDTA intravenously at a dose of 50 mg/kg/day for five days. The mean blood lead level decreased 47.4% and the mean urinary lead excretion was 21 mg in the control patients.

Effect on Essential Minerals: In the above studies Succimer had no significant effect on the urinary elimination of iron, calcium or magnesium. Zinc excretion doubled during treatment. The effect of Succimer on the excretion of essential minerals was small compared to that of CaNa$_2$EDTA, which can induce more than a ten-fold increase in urinary excretion of zinc and doubling of copper and iron excretion.

Efficacy: A dose ranging study was performed in 15 children aged 2 to 7 years with blood lead levels of 30-49 μg/dL and positive CaNa$_2$EDTA lead mobilization tests. Each group of five patients received 350, 233 or 116 mg/m^2 Succimer every 8 hours for 5 days. These doses corresponded to 10, 6.7 and 3.3 mg/kg. Six control patients received 1000 mg/m^2/day CaNa$_2$EDTA intravenously for 5 days. Following therapy, the mean blood lead levels decreased 78, 63 and 42% respectively in the three groups treated with Succimer. The response of the 350 mg/m^2 every 8 hours (10 mg/kg q 8 hr) group was significantly better than that of the other Succimer treated groups as well as that of the control group, whose mean blood lead level fell 48%. No adverse reactions or changes in essential mineral excretion were reported in the Succimer treated groups. In the CaNa$_2$EDTA treated group, the cumulative amount of urinary lead excreted was slightly but significantly greater than in the Succimer group. After CaNa$_2$EDTA, the urinary excretion of copper, zinc, iron and calcium were significantly increased.

As with other chelators, both adults and children experienced a rebound in blood lead levels after discontinuation of Succimer. In these studies, after treatment with a dose of 350 mg/m^2 (10 mg/kg) every 8 hours for five days, the mean lead level rebounded and plateaued at 60-85% of pretreatment levels two weeks after therapy. The rebound plateau was somewhat higher with lower doses of Succimer and with intravenous CaNa$_2$EDTA.

In an attempt to control rebound of blood lead levels, 19 children, ages 1-7 years, with blood lead levels of 42-67 μg/dL, were treated with 350 mg/m^2 Succimer every 8 hours for five days and then divided into three groups. One group was followed for two weeks with no further therapy, the second group was treated for two weeks with 350 mg/m^2 daily, and the third with 350 mg/m^2 every 12 hours. After the initial 5 days of therapy, the mean blood lead level in all subjects declined 61%. While the untreated group and the group treated with 350 mg/m^2 daily experienced rebound during the ensuing two weeks, the group who received the 350 mg/m^2 every 12 hours experienced no such rebound during the treatment period and less rebound following cessation of therapy.

In another study, ten children, ages 21 to 72 months, with blood lead levels of 30-57 μg/dL were treated with Succimer 350 mg/m^2 every eight hours for five days followed by an additional 19-22 days of therapy at a dose of 350 mg/m^2 every 12 hours. The mean blood lead levels decreased and remained stable at under 15 μg/dL during the extended dosing period.

In addition to the controlled studies, approximately 250 patients with lead poisoning have been treated with Succimer either orally or parenterally in open U.S. and foreign studies with similar results reported. Succimer has been used for the treatment of lead poisoning in one patient with sickle cell anemia and in five patients with glucose-6-phosphodehydrogenase (G6PD) deficiency without adverse reactions.

Lead Encephalopathy: Three adults with lead encephalopathy have been reported in the literature to have improved with Succimer therapy. However, data are not available regarding the use of Succimer for the treatment of this rare and sometimes fatal complication of lead poisoning in children.

Other Heavy Metal Poisoning: No controlled clinical studies have been conducted with Succimer in poisoning with other heavy metals. A limited number of patients have received Succimer for mercury or arsenic poisoning. These patients showed increased urinary excretion of the heavy metal and varying degrees of symptomatic improvement.

INDICATIONS AND USAGE
Succimer is indicated for the treatment of lead poisoning in children with blood lead levels above 45 μg/dL. Succimer is not indicated for prophylaxis of lead poisoning in a lead-containing environment; the use of Succimer should always be accompanied by identification and removal of the source of the lead exposure.

CONTRAINDICATIONS
Succimer should not be administered to patients with a history of allergy to the drug.

WARNINGS
Keep out of reach of children. Succimer is not a substitute for effective abatement of lead exposure.

Mild to moderate neutropenia has been observed in some patients receiving Succimer. While a causal relationship to Succimer has not been definitely established, neutropenia has been reported with other drugs in the same chemical class. A complete blood count with <u>white blood cell differential</u> and <u>direct platelet counts</u> should be obtained prior to and weekly during treatment with Succimer. Therapy should either be withheld or discontinued if the absolute neutrophil count (ANC) is below 1200/μL and the patient followed closely to document recovery of the ANC to above 1500/μL or to the patient's baseline neutrophil count. There is limited experience with reexposure in patients who have developed neutropenia. Therefore, such patients should be rechallenged only if the benefit of Succimer therapy clearly outweighs the potential risk of another episode of neutropenia and then only with careful patient monitoring.

Patients treated with Succimer should be instructed to promptly report any signs of infection. If infection is suspected, the above laboratory tests should be conducted immediately.

PRECAUTIONS
The extent of clinical experience with Succimer is limited. Therefore, patients should be carefully observed during treatment.

General: Elevated blood lead levels and associated symptoms may return rapidly after discontinuation of Succimer because of redistribution of lead from bone stores to soft tissues and blood. After therapy, patients should be monitored for rebound of blood lead levels, by measuring blood lead levels at least once weekly until stable. However, the severity of lead intoxication (as measured by the initial blood lead level and the rate and degree of rebound of blood lead) should be used as a guide for more frequent blood lead monitoring. All patients undergoing treatment should be adequately hydrated. Caution should be exercised in using Succimer therapy in patients with compromised renal function. Limited data suggests that Succimer is dialyzable, but that the lead chelates are not.

Transient mild elevations of serum transaminases have been observed in 6-10% of patients during the course of Succimer therapy. Serum transaminases should be monitored before the start of therapy and at least weekly during therapy. Patients with a history of liver disease should be monitored closely. No data are available regarding the metabolism of Succimer in patients with liver disease.

Clinical experience with repeated courses is limited. The safety of uninterrupted dosing longer than three weeks has not been established and it is not recommended.

The possibility of allergic or other mucocutaneous reactions to the drug must be borne in mind on readministration (as well as during initial courses). Patients requiring repeated courses of Succimer should be monitored during each treatment course. One patient experienced recurrent mucocutaneous vesicular eruptions of increasing severity affecting the oral mucosa, the external urethral meatus and the perianal area on the third, fourth and fifth courses of the drug. The reaction resolved between courses and upon discontinuation of therapy.

Information for Patients: Patients should be instructed to maintain adequate fluid intake. If rash occurs, patients should consult their physician. Patients should be instructed to promptly report any indication of infection, which may be a sign of neutropenia (see "*Warning*" and "*Adverse Reactions*").

In young children unable to swallow capsules, the contents of the capsule can be administered in a small amount of food (see "*Dosage and Administration*").

Drug Interaction: Succimer is not known to interact with other drugs including iron supplements; interactions have not been systematically studied. Concomitant administration of Succimer with other chelation therapy, such as CaNa$_2$EDTA is not recommended.

Drug/Laboratory Tests Interaction: Succimer may interfere with serum and urinary laboratory tests. *In vitro* studies have shown Succimer to cause false positive results for ketones in urine using nitroprusside reagents and falsely decreased measurements of serum uric acid and CPK.

Carcinogenesis, Mutagenesis and Impairment of Fertility: Succimer has not been tested for carcinogenic potential in long-term animal studies. Succimer has not been tested in animals for its effect on fertility and reproductive performance in males and females. It was not mutagenic in the Ames bacterial assay and in the mammalian cell forward gene mutation assay.

Pregnancy: Teratogenic Effects — Pregnancy Category C. Succimer has been shown to be teratogenic and fetoxic in pregnant mice when given subcutaneously in a dose range of 410 to 1640 mg/kg/day during the period of organogenesis. There are no adequate and well controlled studies in pregnant women. Succimer should be used during pregnancy only if the potential benefit justifies the potential risk to the fetus.

Nursing Mothers: It is not known whether this drug is excreted in human milk. Because many drugs and heavy metals are excreted in human milk, nursing mothers requiring Succimer therapy should be discouraged from nursing their infants.

Pediatric Use: Refer to the "*Indications*" and "*Dosage and Administration*" sections. There is no therapeutic experience with Succimer in children under one year of age.

ADVERSE REACTIONS
Clinical experience with Succimer has been limited. Consequently, the full spectrum and incidence of adverse reactions including the possibility of hypersensitivity or idiosyncratic reactions have not been determined. The most common events attributable to Succimer, i.e., gastrointestinal symptoms or increases in serum transaminases, have been observed in about 10% of patients (see "*Precautions*"). Rashes, some necessitating discontinuation of therapy, have been reported in about 4% of patients. If rash occurs, other causes (e.g. measles) should be considered before ascribing the reaction to Succimer. Rechallenge with Succimer may be considered if lead levels are high enough to warrant retreatment. One allergic mucocutaneous reaction has been reported on repeated administration of the drug (see "*Precautions*"). Mild to moderate neutropenia has been observed in some patients receiving Succimer (see "*Warnings*"). Table 1 presents

adverse events reported with the administration of Succimer for the treatment of lead and other heavy metal intoxication.

Table 1
INCIDENCE OF ADVERSE EVENTS IN DOMESTIC STUDIES REGARDLESS OF ATTRIBUTION OR SUCCIMER DOSAGE

	Children (191)		*Adults (134)*	
	%	(n)	%	(n)
DIGESTIVE:	12.0	23	20.9	28
Nausea, vomiting, diarrhea, appetite loss, hemorrhoidal symptoms, loose stools, metallic taste in mouth.				
BODY AS A WHOLE:	5.2	10	15.7	21
Back pain, abdominal cramps, stomach pains, head pain, rib pain, chills, flank pain, fever, flu-like symptoms, heavy head/tired, head cold, headache, moniliasis.				
METABOLIC:	4.2	8	10.4	14
Elevated SGPT, SGOT, alkaline phosphatase, elevated serum cholesterol.				
NERVOUS:	1.0	2	12.7	17
Drowsiness, dizziness, sensorimotor neuropathy, sleepiness, paresthesia.				
SKIN AND APPENDAGES:	2.6	5	11.2	15
Papular rash, herpetic rash, rash, mucocutaneous eruptions, pruritus.				
SPECIAL SENSES:	1.0	2	3.7	5
Cloudy film in eye, ears plugged, otitis media, eyes watery.				
RESPIRATORY:	3.7	7	0.7	1
Throat sore, rhinorrhea, nasal congestion, cough.				
UROGENITAL:	0.0		3.7	5
Decreased urination, voiding difficulty, proteinuria increased.				
CARDIOVASCULAR:	0.0		1.8	2
Arrhythmia				
HEME/LYMPHATIC:	0.5*	1	1.5*	2
Mild to moderate neutropenia				
Increased platelet count, intermittent eosinophilia.				
MUSCULOSKELETAL:	0.0		3.0	4
Kneecap pain, leg pains.				

* *Does not include neutropenia — see "Warnings"*

OVERDOSAGES
Doses of 2300 mg/kg in the rat and 2400 mg/kg in the mouse produced ataxia, convulsions, labored respiration and frequently death. No case of overdosage has been reported in humans. Limited data indicate that Succimer is dialyzable. In case of acute overdosage, induction of vomiting or gastric lavage followed by administration of an activated charcoal slurry and appropriate supportive therapy are recommended.

DOSAGE AND ADMINISTRATION
Start dosage at 10 mg/kg or 350 mg/m^2 every eight hours for five days. Initiation of therapy at higher doses is not recommended. (See Table 2 for dosing chart and number of capsules.) Reduce frequency of administration to 10 mg/kg or 350 mg/m^2 every 12 hours (two-thirds of initial daily dosage) for an additional two weeks of therapy. A course of treatment lasts 19 days. Repeated courses may be necessary if indicated by weekly monitoring of blood lead concentration. A minimum of two weeks between courses is recommended unless blood lead levels indicate the need for more prompt treatment.

Table 2
SUCCIMER PEDIATRIC DOSING CHART

Lbs	KG	Dose (MG)*	Number of Capsules*
18-35	8-15	100	1
36-55	16-23	200	2
56-75	24-34	300	3
76-100	35-44	400	4
> 100	> 45	500	5

* *To be administered every 8 hours for 5 days, followed by dosing every 12 hours for 14 days.*

In young children who cannot swallow capsules, Succimer can be administered by separating the capsule and sprinkling the medicated beads on a small amount of soft food or putting them in a spoon and following with fruit drink. Identification of the source of lead in the child's environment and its abatement are critical to a successful therapy outcome. Chelation therapy is not a substitute for preventing further exposure to lead and should not be used to permit continued exposure to lead.

Patients who have received CaNa$_2$EDTA with or without BAL may use Succimer for subsequent treatment after an interval of four weeks. Data on the concomitant use of Succimer with CaNa$_2$EDTA with or without BAL are not available, and such use is not recommended.

Store between 15°C and 25°C and avoid excessive heat.

HOW SUPPLIED
CAPSULE: 100 MG

BRAND/MANUFACTURER	NDC	SIZE	AWP
○ **BRAND**			
CHEMET: McNeil Cons	00045-0134-10	100s	$318.00

Succinylcholine Chloride

THIS DRUG SHOULD BE USED ONLY BY INDIVIDUALS FAMILIAR WITH ITS ACTIONS, CHARACTERISTICS AND HAZARDS.

DESCRIPTION
Sucanylcholine Chloride is an ultra short-acting depolarizing-type, skeletal muscle relaxant for intravenous administration.

Succinylcholine Chloride is a white, odorless, slightly bitter powder and very soluble in water. The drug is unstable in alkaline solutions but relatively stable in acid solutions, depending upon the concentration of the solution and the storage temperature. Solutions of Succinylcholine Chloride should be stored under refrigeration to preserve potency. Injection is a sterile non-pyrogenic solution for intravenous injection, containing 20 mg Succinylcholine Chloride in each mL and made isotonic with sodium chloride. The pH is adjusted to 3.5 with hydrochloric acid. Methylparaben (0.1%) is added as a preservative. Succinylcholine Chloride sterile powder is packed in a vial, containing either 500 mg or 1000 mg of Succinylcholine. The chemical name for Succinylcholine Chloride is 2,2'-[(1,4-dioxo-1,4-butanediyl)bis(oxy)] bis[*N,N,N*- trimethylethanaminium] dichloride.

Following is its chemical structure:

$$\begin{array}{c} COOCH_2CH_2N^+(CH_3)_3 \\ (CH_2)_2 \\ COOCH_2CH_2N^+(CH_3)_3 \end{array} \; 2Cl^-$$

CLINICAL PHARMACOLOGY
Succinylcholine is a depolarizing skeletal muscle relaxant. As does acetylcholine, it combines with the cholinergic receptors of the motor end plate to produce depolarization. This depolarization may be observed as fasciculations. Subsequent neuromuscular transmission is inhibited so long as adequate concentration of Succinylcholine remains at the receptor site. Onset of flaccid paralysis is rapid (less than one minute after intravenous administration), and with single administration lasts approximately 4 to 6 minutes.

Succinylcholine is rapidly hydrolyzed by plasma cholinesterase to succinylmonocholine (which possesses clinically insignificant depolarizing muscle relaxant properties) and then more slowly to succinic acid and choline (see *"Precautions"*). About 10% of the drug is excreted unchanged in the urine. The paralysis following administration of Succinylcholine is progressive, with differing sensitivities of different muscles. This initially involves consecutively the levator muscles of the face, muscles of the glottis and finally the intercostals and the diaphragm and all other skeletal muscles. Succinylcholine has no direct action on the uterus or other smooth muscle structures. Because it is highly ionized and has low fat solubility, it does not readily cross the placenta. Tachyphylaxis occurs with repeated administration (see *"Precautions"*).

Depending on the dose and duration of Succinylcholine administration, the characteristic depolarizing neuromuscular block (Phase 1 block) may change to a block with characteristics superficially resembling a nondepolarizing block (Phase II block). This may be associated with prolonged respiratory muscle paralysis or weakness in patients who manifest the transition to Phase II block. When this diagnosis is confirmed by peripheral nerve stimulation, it may sometimes be reversed with anticholinesterase drugs such as neostigmine (see *"Precautions"*).

Anticholinesterase drugs may not always be effective. If given before Succinylcholine is metabolized by cholinesterase, anticholinesterase drugs may prolong rather than shorten paralysis. Succinylcholine has no direct effect on the myocardium. Succinylcholine stimulates both autonomic ganglia and muscarinic receptors which may cause changes in cardiac rhythm, including cardiac arrest. Changes in rhythm including cardiac arrest may also result from vagal stimulation, which may occur during surgical procedures or from hyperkalemia. These effects are enhanced by halogenated anesthetics.

Succinylcholine causes an increase in intraocular pressure immediately after its injection and during the fasiculation phase, and slight increases which may persist after onset of complete paralysis. Succinylcholine may cause slight increases in intracranial pressure immediately after its injection and during the fasciculation phase (See *"Precautions"*).

As with other neuromuscular blocking agents, the potential for releasing histamine is present following Succinylcholine administration. Signs and symptoms of histamine mediated release such as flushing, hypotension and bronchoconstriction are, however, uncommon in normal clinical usage.

Succinylcholine has no effect on consciousness, pain threshold or cerebration. It should be used only with adequate anesthesia. (See *"Warnings"*).

INDICATIONS AND USAGE
Succinylcholine Chloride is indicated as an adjunct to general anesthesia, to facilitate tracheal intubation, and to provide skeletal muscle relaxation during surgery or mechanical ventilation.

CONTRAINDICATIONS
Succinylcholine is contraindicated in persons with personal or familial history of malignant hyperthermia, skeletal muscle myopathies, and known hypersensitivity to the drug. It is also contraindicated in patients after the acute phase of injury following major burns, multiple trauma, extensive denervation of skeletal muscle, or upper motor neuron injury, because Succinylcholine administered to such

➤ SHOWN IN PRODUCT IDENTIFICATION GUIDE

individuals may result in severe hyperkalemia which may result in cardiac arrest (see *"Warnings"*). The risk of hyperkalemia in these patients increases over time and usually peaks at 7 to 10 days after the injury. The precise time of onset and the duration of the risk period are not known.

Except when used for emergency tracheal intubation or in instances where immediate securing of the airway is necessary, Succinylcholine is contraindicated in children and adolescent patients. Acute rhabdomyolysis with hyplerkalemia can occur when used in these individuals with a skeletal muscle myopathy (diagnosed or undiagnosed) such as Duchenne's muscular dystrophy (see *"Pediatric Use"* subsection of *"Precautions"*).

WARNINGS

SUCCINYLCHOLINE SHOULD BE USED ONLY BY THOSE SKILLED IN THE MANAGEMENT OF ARTIFICIAL RESPIRATION AND ONLY WHEN FACILITIES ARE INSTANTLY AVAILABLE FOR TRACHEAL INTUBATION AND FOR PROVIDING ADEQUATE VENTILATION OF THE PATIENT, INCLUDING THE ADMINISTRATION OF OXYGEN UNDER POSITIVE PRESSURE AND THE ELIMINATION OF CARBON DIOXIDE. THE CLINICIAN MUST BE PREPARED TO ASSIST OR CONTROL RESPIRATION.

TO AVOID DISTRESS TO THE PATIENT, SUCCINYLCHOLINE SHOULD NOT BE ADMINISTERED BEFORE UNCONSCIOUSNESS HAS BEEN INDUCED IN EMERGENCY SITUATIONS. HOWEVER, IT MAY BE NECESSARY TO ADMINISTER SUCCINYLCHOLINE BEFORE UNCONSCIOUSNESS IS INDUCED.

SUCCINYLCHOLINE IS METABOLIZED BY PLASMA CHOLINESTERASE AND SHOULD BE USED WITH CAUTION, IF AT ALL, IN PATIENTS KNOWN TO BE OR SUSPECTED OF BEING HOMOZYGOUS FOR THE ATYPICAL PLASMA CHOLINESTERASE GENE.

Hyperkalemia: Succinylcholine should be administered with **GREAT CAUTION** to patients suffering from electrolyte abnormalities and those who may have massive digitalis toxicity, because in these circumstances Succinylcholine may induce serious cardiac arrhythmias or cardiac arrest due to hyperkalemia.

GREAT CAUTION should be observed if Succinylcholine is administered to patients during the acute phase of injury following major burns, multiple trauma, extensive denervation of skeletal muscle, or upper motor neuron injury (see *"Contraindications"*). The risk of hyperkalemia in these patients increases over time and usually peaks at 7 to 10 days after the injury. The risk is dependent on the extent and location of the injury. The precise time of onset and the duration of the risk period are undetermined. Patients with chronic abdominal infection, subarachnoid hemorrhage, or conditions causing degeneration of central and peripheral nervous systems should receive Succinylcholine with **GREAT CAUTION** because of the potential for developing severe hyperkalemia.

Malignant Hyperthermia: Succinylcholine administration has been associated with acute onset of malignant hyperthermia, a potentially fatal hypermetabolic state of skeletal muscle. The risk of developing malignant hyperthermia following Succinylcholine administration increases with the concomitant administration of volatile anesthetics. Malignant hyperthermia frequently presents as intractable spasm of the jaw muscles (masseter spasm) which may progress to generalized rigidity, increased oxygen demand, tachycardia, tachypnea and profound hyperpyrexia. Successful outcome depends on recognition of early signs, such as jaw muscle spasm, acidosis, or generalized ridigity to initial administration of Succinylcholine for tracheal intubation, or failure of tachycardia to respond to deepening anesthesia. Skin mottling, rising temperature and coagulopathies may occur later in the course of the hypermetabolic process. Recognition of the syndrome is a signal for discontinuance of anesthesia, attention to increased oxygen consumption, correction of acidosis, support of circulation, assurance of adequate urinary output and institution of measures to control rising temperature. Intravenous dantrolene sodium is recommended as an adjunct to supportive measures in the management of this problem. Consult literature references and the dantrolene prescribing information for additional information about the management of malignant hyperthermic crisis. Continuous monitoring of temperature and expired CO_2 is recommended as an aid to early recognition of malignant hyperthermia.

Other: In both adults and children the incidence of bradycardia, which may progress to asystole, is higher following a second dose of Succinylcholine. The incidence and severity of bradycardia is higher in children than adults. Pretreatment with anticholinergic agents (e.g., atropine) may reduce the occurrence of bradyarrhythmias.

Succinylcholine causes an increase in intraocular pressure. It should not be used in instances in which an increase in intraocular pressure is undesirable (e.g., narrow angle glaucoma, penetrating eye injury) unless the potential benefit of its use outweighs the potential risk.

Succinylcholine is acidic (pH = 3.5) and should not be mixed with alkaline solutions having a pH greater than 8.5 (e.g., barbiturate solutions).

PRECAUTIONS

General: When Succinylcholine is given over a prolonged period of time, the characteristic depolarization block of the myoneural junction (Phase I block) may change to a block with characteristics superficially resembling a non-depolarizing block (Phase II block). Prolonged muscle paralysis or weakness may be observed in patients manifesting this transition to Phase II block. The transition from Phase I to Phase II block has been reported in 7 of 7 patients studied under halothane anesthesia after an accumulated dose of 2 to 4 mg/kg Succinylcholine (administered in repeated, divided doses). The onset of Phase II block coincided

with the onset of tachyphlaxis and prolongation of spontaneous recovery. In another study, using balanced anesthesia (N_2O/O_2/narcotic-thiopental) and Succinylcholine infusion, the transition was less abrupt, with great individual variability in the dose of Succinylcholine required to produce Phase II block. Of 32 patients studied, 24 developed Phase II block. Tachyphylaxis was not associated with the transition to Phase II block, and 50% of the patients who developed Phase II block experienced prolonged recovery.

When Phase II block is suspected in cases of prolonged neuromuscular blockade, positive diagnosis should be made by peripheral nerve stimulation, prior to administration of any anticholinesterase drug. Reversal of Phase II block is a medical decision which must be made upon the basis of the individual clinical pharmacology and the experience and judgment of the physician. The presence of Phase II block is indicated by fade of responses to successive stimuli (preferably "train of four"). The use of an anticholinesterase drug to reverse Phase II block should be accompanied by appropriate doses of an anticholinergic drug to prevent disturbances of cardiac rhythm. After adequate reversal of Phase II block with an anticholinesterase agent, the patient should be continually observed for at least 1 hour for signs of return of muscle relaxation. Reversal should not be attempted unless: (1) a peripheral nerve stimulator is used to determine the presence of Phase II block (since anticholinesterase agents will potentiate Succinylcholine-induced Phase I block), and (2) spontaneous recovery of muscle twitch has been observed for at least 20 minutes and has reached a plateau with further recovery proceeding slowly; this delay is to ensure complete hydrolysis of Succinylcholine by plasma cholinesterase prior to administration of the anticholinesterase agent. Should the type of block be misdiagnosed, depolarization of the type initially induced by Succinylcholine (i.e., Phase I block) will be prolonged by an anticholinesterase agent.

Succinylcholine should be employed with caution in patients with fractures or muscle spasm because the initial muscle fasciculations may cause additional trauma.

Succinylcholine may cause a transient increase in intracranial pressure; however, adequate anesthetic induction prior to administration of Succinylcholine will minimize this effect.

Succinylcholine may increase intragastric pressure, which could result in regurgitation and possible aspiration of stomach contents.

Neuromuscular blockade may be prolonged in patients with bypokalemia or hypocalemia.

Reduced Plasma Cholinesterace Activity: Succinylcholine should be used carefully in patients with reduced plasma cholinesterase (pseudocholinesterase) activity. The likelihood of prolonged neuromuscular block following administration of Succinylcholine must be considered in such patients (see *"Dosage and Administration"*).

Plasma cholinesterase activity may be diminished in the presence of genetic abnormalities of plasma cholinesterase (e.g., patients heterozygous or homozygous for atypical plasma cholinesterase gene), pregnancy, severe liver or kidney disease, malignant tumors, infections, burns, anemia, decompensated heart disease, peptic ulcer, or myxedema. Plasma cholinesterase activity may also be diminished by chronic administration of oral contraceptives, glucocorticoids, or certain monoamine oxidase inhibitors and by irreversible inhibitors of plasma cholinesterase (e.g., organophosphate insecticides, echothiophate, and certain antineoplastic drugs).

Patients homozygous for atypical plasma cholinesterase gene (1 in 2500 patients) are extremely sensitive to the neuromuscular blocking effect of Succinylcholine. In these patients, a 5 to 10 mg test dose of Succinylcholine may be administered to evaluate sensitivity to Succinylcholine, or neuromuscular blockade may be produced by the cautious administration of a 1 mg/mL solution of Succinylcholine by slow intravenous infusion. Apnea or prolonged muscle paralysis should be treated with controlled respiration.

Drug Interactions: Drugs which may enhance the neuromuscular blocking action of Succinylcholine include: promazine, oxytocin, aprotinin, certain non-penicillin antibiotics, quinidine, +1b-adrenergic blockers, procainamide, lidocaine, trimethaphan, lithium carbonate, magnesium salts, quinine, chloroquine, diethylether, isoflurane, desflurane, metoclopramide and terbutaline. The neuromuscular blocking effect of Succinylcholine may be enhanced by drugs that reduce plasma cholinesterase activity (e.g., chronically administered oral contraceptives, glucocorticoids, or certain monoamine oxidase inhibitors) or by drugs that irreversibly inhibit plasma cholinesterase (see *"Precautions"*).

If other neuromuscular blocking agents are to be used during the same procedure, the possibility of a synergistic or antagonistic effect should be considered.

Carcinogenesis, Mutagenesis, Impairment of Fertility: There have been no long-term studies performed in animals to evaluate carcinogenic potential.

Pregnancy: Teratogenic Effects: Pregnancy Category C. Animal reproduction studies have not been conducted with Succinylcholine Chloride. It is also not known whether Succinylcholine can cause fetal harm when administered to a pregnant woman or can affect reproduction capacity. Succinylcholine should be given to a pregnant woman only if clearly needed.

Nonteratogenic Effects: Plasma cholinesterase levels are decreased by approximately 24% during pregnancy and for several days postpartum. Therefore, a higher proportion of patients may be expected to show increased sensitivity (prolonged apnea) to Succinylcholine when pregnant than when nonpregnant.

Labor and Delivery: Succinylcholine is commonly used to provide muscle relaxation during delivery by caesarean section. While small amounts of Succinylcholine are known to cross the placental barrier, under normal conditions the quantity of drug that enters fetal circulation after a single dose of 1 mg/kg to the mother should not endanger the fetus. However, since the amount of drug that crosses the placental barrier is dependent on the concentration gradient between the maternal and fetal circulations, residual neuromuscular blockade (apnea and flaccidity) may occur in the newborn after repeated high doses to, or in the presence of atypical plasma cholinesterase in the mother.

Nursing Mothers: It is not known whether Succinylcholine is excreted in human milk. Because many drugs are excreted in human milk, caution should be exercised following Succinylcholine administration to a nursing woman.

Pediatric Use: There are rare reports of ventricular dysrhythmias and cardiac arrest secondary to acute rhabdomyolysis with hyperkalemia in apparently healthy children and adolescents who receive Succinylcholine (see *"Contraindications"*). Several of these individuals were subsequently found to be suffering from a myopathy such as Duchenne's muscular dystrophy whose clinical signs were not obvious. When a healthy appearing child or adolescent suddenly develops cardiac arrest soon after administration of Succinylcholine immediate treatment of hyperkalemia should be considered, including hyperventilation, bicarbonate, calcium, glucose and insulin. Treatment for acute rhabdomyolysis, including a single intravenous dose of dantrolene, should also be considered.

As in adults, the incidence of bradycardia in children is higher following the second dose of Succinylcholine. The incidence and severity of bradycardia is higher in children than adults. Pretreatment with anticholinergic agents, e.g., atropine, may reduce the occurrence of bradyarrhythmias.

ADVERSE REACTIONS
Adverse reactions to Succinylcholine consist primarily of an extension of its pharmacological actions. Succinylcholine causes profound muscle relaxation resulting in respiratory depression to the point of apnea; this effect may be prolonged. Hypersensitivity reactions, including anaphylaxis, may occur in rare instances. The following additional adverse reactions have been reported; cardiac arrest, malignant hyperthermia, arrhythmias, bradycardia, tachycardia, hypertension, hypotension, hyperkalemia, prolonged respiratory depression or apnea, increased intraocular pressure, muscle fasciculation, jaw rigidity, postoperative muscle pain, rhabdomyolysis with possible myoglobinuric acute renal failure, excessive salivation, and rash.

OVERDOSAGE
Overdosage with Succinylcholine may result in neuromuscular block beyond the time needed for surgery and anesthesia. This may be manifested by skeletal muscle weakness, decreased respiratory reserve, low tidal volume, or apnea. The primary treatment is maintenance of a patent airway and respiratory support until recovery of normal respiration is assured. Depending on the dose and duration of Succinylcholine administration, the characteristic depolarizing neuromuscular block (Phase I) may change to a block with characteristics superficially resembling a nondepolarizing block (Phase II) (see *"Precautions"*).

DOSAGE AND ADMINISTRATION
The dosage of Succinylcholine should be individualized and should always be determined by the clinician after careful assessment of the patient (see *"Warnings"*).

Parenteral drug products should be inspected visually for particulate matter and discoloration prior to administration whenever solution and container permit. Solutions which are not clear and colorless should not be used.

ADULTS
For Short Surgical Procedures: The average dose required to produce neuromuscular blockade and to facilitate tracheal intubation is 0.6 mg/kg Succinylcholine Chloride Injection given intravenously. The optimum dose will vary among individuals and may be from 0.3 to 1.1 mg/kg for adults. Following administration of doses in this range, neuromuscular blockade develops in about 1 minutes; maximum blockade may persist for about 2 minutes, after which recovery takes place within 4 to 6 minutes. However, very large doses may result in more prolonged blockade. A 5 to 10 mg test dose may be used to determine the sensitivity of the patient and the individual recovery time.

For Long Surgical Procedures: The dose of Succinylcholine administered by infusion depends upon the duration of the surgical procedure and the need for muscle relaxation. The average rate for an adult ranges between 2.5 and 4.3 mg per minute.

Solutions containing from 1 to 2 mg per mL Succinylcholine have commonly been used for continuous infusion. The more dilute solution (1 mg per mL) is probably preferable from the standpoint of ease of control of the rate of administration of the drug and, hence, of relaxation. This intravenous solution containing 1 mg per mL may be administered at a rate of 0.5 mg (0.5 mL) to 10 mg (10 mL) per minute to obtain the required amount of relaxation. The amount required per minute will depend upon the individual response as well as the degree of relaxation required. Avoid overburdening the circulation with a large volume of fluid. It is recommended that neuromuscular function be carefully monitored with a peripheral nerve stimulator when using Succinylcholine by infusion in order to avoid overdose, detect development of Phase II block, follow its rate of recovery, and assess the effects of reversing agents (see *"Precautions"*).

Intermittent intravenous injections of Succinylcholine may also be used to provide muscle relaxation for long procedures. An intravenous injection of 0.3 to 1.1 mg/kg may be given initially, followed, at appropriate intervals, by further injections of 0.04 to 0.07 mg/kg to maintain the degree of relaxation required.

Pediatric Use: For emergency tracheal intubation or in instances where immediate securing of the airway is necessary, the intravenous dose of Succinylcholine is 2 mg/kg for infants and small children: for older children and adolescents the dose is 1 mg/kg (see *"Contraindications"* and *"Pediatric Use"* subsection of *"Precautions"*).

Rarely, IV bolus administration of Succinylcholine in infants and children may result in malignant ventricular arrythmias and cardiac arrest secondary to acute rhabdomyolysis with hyperkalemia. In such situations, an underlying myopathy should be suspected.

Intravenous bolus administration of Succinylcholine in infants or children may result in profound bradycardia or, rarely, asystole. As in adults, the incidence of bradycardia in children is higher following a second dose of Succinylcholine. The occurrence of bradyarrhythmias may be reduced by pretreatment with atropine (see *"Pediatric Use"* subsection of *"Precautions"*).

Intramuscular Use: If necessary, Succinylcholine may be given intramuscularly to infants, older children or adults when a suitable vein is inaccessible. A dose of up to 3 to 4 mg/kg may be given, but not more than 150 mg total dose should be administered by this route. The onset of effect of Succinylcholine given intramuscularly is usually observed in about 2 to 3 minutes.

Compatibility and Admixtures: Succinylcholine is acidic (pH 3.5) and should not be mixed with alkaline solutions having a pH greater than 8.5 (e.g., barbiturate solutions). Admixture containing 1 to 2 mg/mL may be prepared by adding 1 g Succinylcholine to 1000 or 500 mL sterile solution, such as 5% Dextrose Injection USP or 0.9% Sodium Chloride Injection USP. Admixtures of Succinylcholine must be used within 24 hours after preparation. Aseptic techniques should be used to prepare the diluted product. Admixtures of Succinylcholine should be prepared for single patient use only. The unused portion of diluted Succinylcholine should be discarded.

Storage: Store in refrigerator at 2° to 8°C (36° to 46°F). The multi-dose vials are stable for up to 14 days at room temperature without significant loss of potency.

J CODES
Up to 20 mg IV,IM—J0330

HOW SUPPLIED
INJECTION: 20 MG/ML
AVERAGE UNIT PRICE (AVAILABLE SIZES)

BRAND	$0.79

BRAND/MANUFACTURER	NDC	SIZE	AWP
◆ **BRAND**			
SUCOSTRIN: Apothecon	00003-0719-15	10 ml	$3.98
QUELICIN CHLORIDE: Abbott Hosp	00074-8065-01	5 ml 10s	$103.08
ANECTINE: Burr Wellcome	00081-0071-95	10 ml 12s	$41.22
QUELICIN CHLORIDE: Abbott Hosp	00074-6629-02	10 ml 25s	$89.66
◆ **GENERICS**			
Organon	00052-0445-10	10 ml 25s	$19.75

INJECTION: 50 MG/ML
BRAND/MANUFACTURER	NDC	SIZE	AWP
◆ **BRAND**			
QUELICIN CHLORIDE: Abbott Hosp	00074-6642-02	10 ml 25s	$128.55

INJECTION: 100 MG/ML
BRAND/MANUFACTURER	NDC	SIZE	AWP
◆ **BRAND**			
QUELICIN CHLORIDE: Abbott Hosp	00074-6970-10	10 ml 25s	$198.31

POWDER FOR INJECTION: 500 MG
BRAND/MANUFACTURER	NDC	SIZE	AWP
◆ **BRAND**			
ANECTINE FLO-PACK: Burr Wellcome	00081-0085-15	12s	$101.20

POWDER FOR INJECTION: 1000 MG
BRAND/MANUFACTURER	NDC	SIZE	AWP
◆ **BRAND**			
ANECTINE FLO-PACK: Burr Wellcome	00081-0086-15	12s	$165.22

Sucostrin *SEE* SUCCINYLCHOLINE CHLORIDE

Sucralfate

DESCRIPTION
Sucralfate is an α-D-glucopyranoside, β-D-fructofuranosyl-, octakis-(hydrogen sulfate), aluminum complex. Its molecular formula is $R = SO_3[Al_2(OH)_5.(H_2O)_2]$.

Tablets for oral administration contain 1 gm of Sucralfate. The suspension contains 1 gm per 10 ml.

Therapeutic category: antiulcer.

➤ SHOWN IN PRODUCT IDENTIFICATION GUIDE

Following is its chemical structure:

$(R \text{ is } SO_3[Al_2(OH)_x(H_2O)_y])$

CLINICAL PHARMACOLOGY

Sucralfate is only minimally absorbed from the gastrointestinal tract. The small amounts of the sulfated disaccharide that are absorbed are excreted primarily in the urine.

Although the mechanism of Sucralfate's ability to accelerate healing of duodenal ulcers remains to be fully defined, it is known that it exerts its effect through a local, rather than systemic, action. The following observations also appear pertinent:

1. Studies in human subjects and with animal models of ulcer disease have shown that Sucralfate forms an ulcer-adherent complex with proteinaceous exudate at the ulcer site.
2. *In vitro*, a Sucralfate-albumin film provides a barrier to diffusion of hydrogen ions.
3. In human subjects, Sucralfate given in doses recommended for ulcer therapy inhibits pepsin activity in gastric juice by 32%.
4. *In vitro* Sucralfate absorbs bile salts.

These observations suggest that Sucralfate's antiulcer activity is the result of formation of an ulcer-adherent complex that covers the ulcer site and protects it against further attack by acid, pepsin, and bile salts. There are approximately 14-16 mEq of acid-neutralizing capacity per 1-gm dose of Sucralfate.

CLINICAL TRIALS

ACUTE DUODENAL ULCER

Over 600 patients have participated in well-controlled clinical trials worldwide. Multicenter trials conducted in the United States, both of them placebo-controlled studies with endoscopic evaluation at 2 and 4 weeks, showed:

Study 1 Treatment Groups	Ulcer Healing/No. Patients	
	2 wk	4 wk (Overall)
Sucralfate	37/105 (35.2%)	82/109 (75.2%)
Placebo	26/106 (24.5%)	68/107 (63.6%)

Study 2 Treatment Groups	Ulcer Healing/No. Patients	
	2 wk	4 wk (Overall)
Sucralfate	8/24 (33%)	22/24 (92%)
Placebo	4/31 (13%)	18/31 (58%)

The Sucralfate-placebo differences were statistically significant in both studies at 4 weeks but not at 2 weeks. The poorer result in the first study may have occurred because Sucralfate was given 2 hours after meals and at bedtime rather than 1 hour before meals and at bedtime, the regimen used in international studies and in the second United States study. In addition, in the first study liquid antacid was utilized as needed, whereas in the second study antacid tablets were used.

In a multicenter, double-blind, placebo-controlled study of Sucralfate Suspension, a dosage regimen of 1 g (10 mL) four times daily was demonstrated to be superior to placebo in ulcer healing.

RESULTS FROM CLINICAL TRIALS HEALING RATES FOR ACUTE DUODENAL ULCER

Treatment	N	Week 2 Healing Rates	Week 4 Healing Rates	Week 8 Healing Rates
Sucralfate Suspension	145	23(16%)*	66(46%)†	95(66%)‡
Placebo	147	10(7%)	39(27%)	58(39%)

* P = 0.016
† P = 0.001
‡ P = 0.0001

Equivalence of Sucralfate Suspension to Sucralfate tablets has not been demonstrated.

MAINTENANCE THERAPY AFTER HEALING OF DUODENAL ULCER

Two double-blind randomized placebo-controlled U.S. multicenter trials have demonstrated that Sucralfate tablets (1 gm bid) are effective as maintenance therapy following healing of duodenal ulcers.

In one study, endoscopies were performed monthly for 4 months. Of the 254 patients who enrolled, 239 were analyzed in the intention-to-treat life table analysis presented below.

DUODENAL ULCER RECURRENCE RATE (%)

Drug	N	Months of Therapy			
		1	2	3	4
Sucralfate	122	20*	30*	38**	4**
Placebo	117	33	46	55	63

* p < 0.05, ** p < 0.01
Prn antacids were not permitted in this study.

In the other study, scheduled endoscopies were performed at 6 and 12 months, but for cause endoscopies were permitted as symptoms dictated. Median symptom scores between the Sucralfate and placebo groups were not significantly different. A life table intention-to-treat analysis for the 94 patients enrolled in the trial had the following results:

DUODENAL ULCER RECURRENCE RATE (%)

Drug	N	6 months	12 months
Sucralfate	48	19*	27*
Placebo	46	54	65

* p < 0.002
Prn antacids were permitted in this study.

Data from placebo-controlled studies longer than 1 year are not available.

INDICATIONS AND USAGE

Sucralfate tablets and suspension are indicated in:
- Short-term treatment (up to 8 weeks) of active duodenal ulcer. Antacids may be prescribed as needed for relief of pain. While healing with Sucralfate may occur during the first week or two, treatment should be continued for 4 to 8 weeks unless healing has been demonstrated by x-ray or endoscopic examination.

Sucralfate tablets are also indicated in:
- Maintenance therapy for duodenal ulcer patients at reduced dosage after healing of acute ulcers.

UNLABELED USES

Sucralfate is used alone or as an adjunct in treatment and maintenance therapy for gastric ulcer, hemorrhagic gastritis, reflux esophagitis, and radiation-induced diarrhea. It is also used in the treatment of hyperphosphatemia, stomatitis, and decubitus ulcers, and has been used to prevent stress ulcers.

CONTRAINDICATIONS

There are no known contraindications to the use of Sucralfate.

PRECAUTIONS

Duodenal ulcer is a chronic recurrent disease. While short-term treatment with Sucralfate can result in complete healing of the ulcer, a successful course of treatment with Sucralfate should not be expected to alter the posthealing frequency or severity of duodenal ulceration.

SPECIAL POPULATIONS: CHRONIC RENAL FAILURE AND DIALYSIS PATIENTS:

When Sucralfate is administered orally, small amounts of aluminum are absorbed from the gastrointestinal tract. Concomitant use of Sucralfate with other products that contain aluminum, such as aluminum-containing antacids, may increase the total body burden of aluminum. Patients with normal renal function receiving the recommended doses of Sucralfate and aluminum-containing products adequately excrete aluminum in the urine. Patients with chronic renal failure or those receiving dialysis have impaired excretion of absorbed aluminum. In addition, aluminum does not cross dialysis membranes because it is bound to albumin and transferrin plasma proteins. Aluminum accumulation and toxicity (aluminum osteodystrophy, osteomalacia, encephalopathy) have been described in patients with renal impairment. Sucralfate should be used with caution in patients with chronic renal failure.

DRUG INTERACTIONS

Some studies have shown that simultaneous Sucralfate administration in healthy volunteers reduced the extent of absorption (bioavailability) of single doses of the following drugs: cimetidine, ciprofloxacin, digoxin, ketoconazole, norfloxacin, phenytoin, ranitidine, tetracycline, and theophylline. Subtherapeutic prothrombin times with concomitant warfarin and Sucralfate therapy have been reported in spontaneous and published case reports. However, two clinical studies have demonstrated no change in either serum warfarin concentration or prothrombin time with the addition of Sucralfate to chronic warfarin therapy.

The mechanism of these interactions appears to be nonsystemic in nature, presumably resulting from Sucralfate binding to the concomitant agent in the gastrointestinal tract. In all cases studied to date (cimetidine, ciprofloxacin, digoxin, ranitidine, and warfarin), dosing the concomitant medication 2 hours before Sucralfate eliminated the interaction. Because of the potential of Sucralfate to alter the absorption of some drugs, Sucralfate should be administered separately from other drugs when alterations in bioavailability are felt to be critical. In these cases, patients should be monitored appropriately.

CARCINOGENESIS, MUTAGENESIS, IMPAIRMENT OF FERTILITY

Chronic oral toxicity studies of 24 months' duration were conducted in mice and rats at doses up to 1 gm/kg (12 times the human dose). There was no evidence of drug-related tumorigenicity. A reproduction study in rats at doses up to 38 times the human dose did not reveal any indication of fertility impairment. Mutagenicity studies were not conducted.

PREGNANCY
Teratogenic effects. Pregnancy Category B: Teratogenicity studies have been performed in mice, rats, and rabbits at doses up to 50 times the human dose and have revealed no evidence of harm to the fetus due to Sucralfate. There are, however, no adequate and well-controlled studies in pregnant women. Because animal reproduction studies are not always predictive of human response, this drug should be used during pregnancy only if clearly needed.

NURSING MOTHERS
It is not known whether this drug is excreted in human milk. Because many drugs are excreted in human milk, caution should be exercised when Sucralfate is administered to a nursing woman.

PEDIATRIC USE
Safety and effectiveness in children have not been established.

ADVERSE REACTIONS
Adverse reactions to Sucralfate tablets in clinical trials were minor and only rarely led to discontinuation of the drug. In studies involving over 2700 patients treated with Sucralfate tablets, adverse effects were reported in 129 (4.7%).

Constipation was the most frequent complaint (2%). Other adverse effects reported in less than 0.5% of the patients are listed below by body system:

Gastrointestinal: diarrhea, nausea, vomiting, gastric discomfort, indigestion, flatulence, dry mouth

Dermatological: pruritus, rash

Nervous System: dizziness, insomnia, sleepiness, vertigo

Other: back pain, headache

Postmarketing reports with Sucralfate tablets of hypersensitivity reactions, including urticaria (hives), angioedema, respiratory difficulty, and rhinitis have been received. Similar reactions were reported with Sucralfate suspension. In addition, laryngospasm and facial swelling have been reported with Sucralfate suspension. However, a causal relationship has not been established.

OVERDOSAGE
There is no experience in humans with overdosage. Acute oral toxicity studies in animals, however, using doses up to 12 gm/kg body weight, could not find a lethal dose. Risks associated with overdosage should, therefore, be minimal.

DOSAGE AND ADMINISTRATION
Active Duodenal Ulcer: The recommended adult oral dosage for duodenal ulcer is 1 g (1 tablet or 10 mL/2 teaspoonful) four times a day on an empty stomach.

Antacids may be prescribed as needed for relief of pain but should not be taken within one-half hour before or after Sucralfate.

While healing with Sucralfate may occur during the first week or two, treatment should be continued for 4 to 8 weeks unless healing has been demonstrated by x-ray or endoscopic examination.

Maintenance Therapy: The recommended adult oral dosage is 1 g twice a day.
Shake The Suspension Well Before Using.

Storage: Store Sucralfate Suspension at controlled room temperature, 59-86°F (15-30°C).
Avoid freezing.

HOW SUPPLIED
SUSPENSION: 1 GM/10 ML

BRAND/MANUFACTURER	NDC	SIZE	AWP
○ BRAND			
CARAFATE: Marion Merrell Dow	00088-1700-15	420 ml	$29.01
	00088-1700-22	420 ml 2s	$58.02

TABLETS: 1 GM

BRAND/MANUFACTURER	NDC	SIZE	AWP
○ BRAND			
➤ CARAFATE: Marion Merrell Dow	00088-1712-47	100s	$73.69
	00088-1712-49	100s ud	$84.00
	00088-1712-53	120s	$88.38
	00088-1712-55	500s	$350.63
	00088-1712-73	6000s	$4208.88

Sufenta *SEE* SUFENTANIL CITRATE

Sufentanil Citrate

DESCRIPTION
Sufentanil Citrate is a potent opioid analgesic chemically designated as N-[-4-(methyoxymethyl)-1-[2-(2-thienyl)ethyl]-4-piperidinyl]-N-phenylpropanamide 2-hydroxy-1,2,3-propanetricarboxylate (1:1) with a molecular weight of 578.68.

Sufentanil Citrate is a sterile, preservative free, aqueous solution containing 50 µg per ml of Sufentanil base for intravenous and epidural injection. The solution has a pH range of 3.5-6.0.

Following is its chemical structure:

CLINICAL PHARMACOLOGY
PHARMACOLOGY
Sufentanil Citrate is an opioid analgesic. When used in balanced general anesthesia, Sufentanil Citrate has been reported to be as much as 10 times as potent as fentanyl. When administered intravenously as a primary anesthetic agent with 100% oxygen, Sufentanil Citrate is approximately 5 to 7 times as potent as fentanyl. Assays of histamine in patients administered Sufentanil Citrate have shown no elevation in plasma histamine levels and no indication of histamine release. (See dosage chart for more complete information on the intravenous use of Sufentanil Citrate.)

PHARMACODYNAMICS
Intravenous Use: At intravenous doses of up to 8 µg/kg, Sufentanil Citrate is an analgesic component of general anesthesia: at intravenous doses ≥ 8 µg/kg, Sufentanil Citrate produces a deep level of anesthesia. Sufentanil Citrate produces a dose related attenuation of catecholamine release, particularly norepinephrine.

At intravenous dosages of ≥ 8 µg/kg, Sufentanil Citrate produces hypnosis and anesthesia without the use of additional anesthetic agents. A deep level of anesthesia is maintained at these dosages, as demonstrated by EEG patterns. Dosages of up to 25 µg/kg attenuate the sympathetic response to surgical stress. The catecholamine response, particularly norepinephrine, is further attenuated at doses of Sufentanil Citrate of 25-30 µg/kg, with hemodynamic stability and preservation of favorable myocardial oxygen balance.

Sufentanil Citrate has an immediate onset of action, with relatively limited accumulation. Rapid elimination from tissue storage sites allows for relatively more rapid recovery as compared with equipotent dosages of fentanyl. At dosages of 1-2 µg/kg, recovery times are comparable to those observed with fentanyl; at dosages of > 2-6 µg/kg, recovery times are comparable to enflurane, isoflurane and fentanyl. Within the anesthetic dosage range of 8-30 µg/kg of Sufentanil Citrate, recovery times are more rapid compared to equipotent fentanyl dosages.

The vagolytic effects of pancuronium may produce a dose dependent elevation in heart rate during Sufentanil Citrate-oxygen anesthesia. The use of moderate doses of pancuronium or of a less vagolytic neuromuscular blocking agent may be used to maintain a stable lower heart rate and blood pressure during Sufentanil Citrate-oxygen anesthesia. The vagolytic effects of pancuronium may be reduced in patients administered nitrous oxide with Sufentanil Citrate.

Preliminary data suggest that in patients administered high doses of Sufentanil Citrate, initial dosage requirements for neuromuscular blocking agents are generally lower as compared to patients given fentanyl or halothane, and comparable to patients given enflurane.

Bradycardia is infrequently seen in patients administered Sufentanil Citrate-oxygen anesthesia. The use of nitrous oxide with high doses of Sufentanil Citrate may decrease mean arterial pressure, heart rate and cardiac output.

Sufentanil Citrate at 20 µg/kg has been shown to provide more adequate reduction in intracranial volume than equivalent doses of fentanyl, based upon requirements for furosemide and anesthesia supplementation in one study of patients undergoing craniotomy. During carotid endarterectomy, Sufentanil Citrate-nitrous oxide/oxygen produced reductions in cerebral blood flow comparable to those of enflurane-nitrous oxide/oxygen. During cardiovascular surgery, Sufentanil Citrate-oxygen produced EEG patterns similar to fentanyl-oxygen; these EEG changes were judged to be compatible with adequate general anesthesia.

The intraoperative use of Sufentanil Citrate at anesthetic dosages maintains cardiac output, with a slight reduction in systemic vascular resistance during the initial postoperative period. The incidence of postoperative hypertension, need for vasoactive agents and requirements for postoperative analgesics are generally reduced in patients administered moderate or high doses of Sufentanil Citrate as compared to patients given inhalation agents.

Skeletal muscle rigidity is related to the dose and speed of administration of Sufentanil Citrate. This muscular rigidity may occur unless preventative measures are taken (see *"Warnings"*).

Decreased respiratory drive and increased airway resistance occur with Sufentanil Citrate. The duration and degree of respiratory depression are dose related when Sufentanil Citrate is used at sub-anesthetic dosages. At high doses, a pronounced decrease in pulmonary exchange and apnea may be produced.

Epidural Use in Labor and Delivery: Onset of analgesic effect occurs within approximately 10 minutes of administration of epidural doses of Sufentanil Citrate and bupivacaine. Duration of analgesia following a single epidural injection of 10-15 µg Sufentanil Citrate and bupivacaine 0.125% averaged 1.7 hours.

During labor and vaginal delivery, the addition of 10-15 µg Sufentanil Citrate to 10 mL 0.125% bupivacaine provides an increase in the duration of analgesia compared to bupivacaine without an opioid. Analgesia from 15 µg Sufentanil Citrate plus 10 mL 0.125% bupivacaine is comparable to analgesia from 10 mL of

0.25% bupivacaine alone. Apgar scores of neonates following epidural administration of both drugs to women in labor were comparable to neonates whose mothers received bupivacaine without an opioid epidurally.

PHARMACOKINETICS

Intravenous Use: The pharmacokinetics of intravenous Sufentanil Citrate can be described as a three-compartment model, with a distribution time of 1.4 minutes, redistribution of 17.1 minutes and an elimination half-life of 164 minutes. The liver and small intestine are the major sites of biotransformation. Approximately 80% of the administered dose is excreted within 24 hours and only 2% of the dose is eliminated as unchanged drug. Plasma protein binding of Sufentanil Citrate, related to the alpha$_1$ acid glycoprotein concentration, was approximately 93% in healthy males, 91% in mothers and 79% in neonates.

Epidural Use in Labor and Delivery: After epidural administration of incremental doses totaling 5-40 µg Sufentanil Citrate during labor and delivery, maternal and neonatal Sufentanil Citrate plasma concentrations were at or near the 0.05-0.1 ng/mL limit of detection, and were slightly higher in mothers than in their infants.

CLINICAL STUDIES

Epidural Use in Labor and Delivery: Epidural Sufentanil Citrate was tested in 340 patients in two (one single-center and one multicenter) double-blind, parallel studies. Doses ranged from 10 to 15 µg Sufentanil Citrate and were delivered in a 10 mL volume of 0.125% bupivacaine with and without epinephrine 1:200,000. In all cases Sufentanil Citrate was administered following a dose of local anesthetic to test proper catheter placement. Since epidural opioids and local anesthetics potentiate each other, these results may not reflect the dose or efficacy of epidural Sufentanil Citrate by itself.

Individual doses of 10-15 µg Sufentanil Citrate plus bupivacaine 0.125% with epinephrine provided analgesia during the first stage of labor with a duration of 1-2 hours. Onset was rapid (within 10 minutes). Subsequent doses (equal dose) tended to have shorter duration. Analgesia was profound (complete pain relief) in 80% to 100% of patients and a 25% incidence of pruritus was observed. The duration of initial doses of Sufentanil Citrate plus bupivacaine with epinephrine is approximately 95 minutes, and of subsequent doses, 70 minutes.

There are insufficient data to critically evaluate neonatal neuromuscular and adaptive capacity following recommended doses of maternally administered epidural Sufentanil Citrate with bupivacaine. However, if larger than recommended doses are used for combined local and systemic analgesia, e.g. after administration of a single dose of 50 µg epidural Sufentanil Citrate during delivery, then impaired neonatal adaption to sound and light can be detected for 1 to 4 hours, and if a dose of 80 µg is used, impaired neuromuscular coordination can be detected for more than 4 hours.

INDICATIONS AND USAGE

Sufentanil Citrate is indicated for intravenous administration: as an analgesic adjunct in the maintenance of balanced general anesthesia in patients who are intubated and ventilated, as a primary anesthetic agent for the induction and maintenance of anesthesia with 100% oxygen in patients undergoing major surgical procedures, in patients who are intubated and ventilated, such as cardiovascular surgery or neurosurgical procedures in the sitting position, to provide favorable myocardial and cerebral oxygen balance or when extended postoperative ventilation is anticipated.

Sufentanil Citrate is indicated for epidural administration as an analgesic combined with low dose bupivacaine, usually 12.5 mg per administration, during labor and vaginal delivery.

See *"Dosage and Administration"* section for more complete information on the use of Sufentanil Citrate.

CONTRAINDICATIONS

Sufentanil Citrate is contraindicated in patients with known hypersensitivity to the drug.

WARNINGS

SUFENTANIL CITRATE SHOULD BE ADMINISTERED ONLY BY PERSONS SPECIFICALLY TRAINED IN THE USE OF INTRAVENOUS AND EPIDURAL ANESTHETICS AND MANAGEMENT OF THE RESPIRATORY EFFECTS OF POTENT OPIOIDS.

AN OPIOID ANTAGONIST, RESUSCITATIVE AND INTUBATION EQUIPMENT AND OXYGEN SHOULD BE READILY AVAILABLE.

PRIOR TO CATHETER INSERTION, THE PHYSICIAN SHOULD BE FAMILIAR WITH PATIENT CONDITIONS (SUCH AS INFECTION AT THE INJECTION SITE, BLEEDING DIATHESIS, ANTICOAGULANT THERAPY, ETC.) WHICH CALL FOR SPECIAL EVALUATION OF THE BENEFIT VERSUS RISK POTENTIAL.

Intravenous Use: Intravenous administration or unintentional intravascular injection during epidural administration of Sufentanil Citrate may cause skeletal muscle rigidity, particularly of the truncal muscles. The incidence and severity of muscle rigidity is dose related. Administration of Sufentanil Citrate may produce muscular rigidity with a more rapid onset of action than that seen with fentanyl. Sufentanil Citrate may produce muscular rigidity that involves the skeletal muscles of the neck and extremities. As with fentanyl, muscular rigidity has been reported to occur or recur infrequently in the extended postoperative period. The incidence of muscular rigidity associated with intravenous Sufentanil Citrate can be reduced by: 1) administration of up to ¼ of the full paralyzing dose of a non-depolarizing neuromuscular blocking agent just prior to administration of Sufentanil Citrate at dosages of up to 8 µg/kg, 2) administration of a full paralyzing dose of a neuromuscular blocking agent following loss of consciousness

when Sufentanil Citrate is used in anesthetic dosages (above 8 µg/kg) titrated by slow intravenous infusion, or, 3) simultaneous administration of Sufentanil Citrate and a full paralyzing dose of a neuromuscular blocking agent when Sufentanil Citrate is used in rapidly administered anesthetic dosages (above 8 µg/kg).

The neuromuscular blocking agents used should be compatible with the patient's cardiovascular status. Adequate facilities should be available for postoperative monitoring and ventilation of patients administered Sufentanil Citrate. It is essential that these facilities be fully equipped to handle all degrees of respiratory depression.

PRECAUTIONS

General: The initial dose of Sufentanil Citrate should be appropriately reduced in elderly and debilitated patients. The effect of the initial dose should be considered in determining supplemental doses.

Vital signs should be monitored routinely.

Nitrous oxide may produce cardiovascular depression when given with high doses of Sufentanil Citrate (see *"Clinical Pharmacology"*).

Bradycardia has been reported infrequently with Sutentanil Citrate-oxygen anesthesia and has been responsive to atropine.

Respiratory depression caused by opioid analgesics can be reversed by opioid antagonists such as naloxone. Because the duration of respiratory depression produced by Sufentanil Citrate may last longer than the duration of the opioid antagonist action, appropriate surveillance should be maintained. As with all potent opioids, profound analgesia is accompanied by respiratory depression and diminished sensitivity to CO_2 stimulation which may persist into or recur in the postoperative period. Respiratory depression may be enhanced when Sufentanil Citrate is administered in combination with volatile inhalational agents and/or other central nervous system depressants such as barbiturates, tranquilizers, and other opioids. Appropriate postoperative monitoring should be employed to ensure that adequate spontaneous breathing is established and maintained prior to discharging the patient from the recovery area. Respiration should be closely monitored following each administration of an epidural injection of Sufentanil Citrate.

Proper placement of the needle or catheter in the epidural space should be verified before Sufentanil Citrate is injected to assure that unintentional intravascular or intrathecal administration does not occur. Unintentional intravascular injection of Sufentanil Citrate could result in a potentially serious overdose, including acute truncal muscular rigidity and apnea. Unintentional intrathecal injection of the full Sufentanil Citrate/bupivacaine epidural doses and volume could produce effects of high spinal anesthesia including prolonged paralysis and delayed recovery. If analgesia is inadequate, the placement and integrity of the catheter should be verified prior to the administration of any additional epidural medications. Sufentanil Citrate should be administered epidurally by slow injection.

Neuromuscular Blocking Agents: The hemodynamic effects and degree of skeletal muscle relaxation required should be considered in the selection of a neuromuscular blocking agent. High doses of pancuronium may produce increases in heart rate during Sufentanil Citrate-oxygen anesthesia; this effect may be more pronounced in the presence of calcium channel and/or beta blockers. Muscle relaxants with no clinically significant effect on heart rate (at recommended doses) would not counteract the vagotonic effect of Sufentanil Citrate, therefore a lower heart rate would be expected. Rare reports of bradycardia associated with the concomitant use of succinylcholine and Sufentanil Citrate have been reported.

Interaction with Calcium Channel and Beta Blockers: The incidence and degree of bradycardia and hypotension during induction with Sufentanil Citrate may be greater in patients on chronic calcium channel and beta blocker therapy. (See *"Neuromuscular Blocking Agents"*.)

Interaction with Other Central Nervous System Depressants: Both the magnitude and duration of central nervous system and cardiovascular effects may be enhanced when Sufentanil Citrate is administered to patients receiving barbiturates, tranquilizers, other opioids, general anesthetics or other CNS depressants. In such cases of combined treatment, the dose of Sufentanil Citrate and/or these agents should be reduced.

The use of benzodiazepines with Sufentanil Citrate during induction may result in a decrease in mean arterial pressure and systemic vascular resistance.

Head Injuries: Sufentanil Citrate may obscure the clinical course of patients with head injuries.

Impaired Respiration: Sufentanil Citrate should be used with caution in patients with pulmonary disease, decreased respiratory reserve or potentially compromised respiration. In such patients, opioids may additionally decrease respiratory drive and increase airway resistance. During anesthesia, this can be managed by assisted or controlled respiration.

Impaired Hepatic or Renal Function: In patients with liver or kidney dysfunction, Sufentanil Citrate should be administered with caution due to the importance of these organs in the metabolism and excretion of Sufentanil Citrate.

Carcinogenesis, Mutagenesis and Impairment of Fertility: No long-term animal studies of Sufentanil Citrate have been performed to evaluate carcinogenic potential. The micronucleus test in female rats revealed that single intravenous doses of Sufentanil Citrate as high as 80 µg/kg (approximately 2.5 times the upper human dose) produced no structural chromosome mutations. The Ames *Salmonella typhimurium* metabolic activating test also revealed no mutagenic activity. See *"Animal Toxicology"* for reproduction studies in rats and rabbits.

◆ RATED THERAPEUTICALLY EQUIVALENT; ◇ THERAPEUTIC EQUIVALENCE UNCONFIRMED; ○ UNRATED

Pregnancy Category C: Sufentanil Citrate has been shown to have an embryocidal effect in rats and rabbits when given in doses 2.5 times the upper human dose for a period of 10 days to over 30 days. These effects were most probably due to maternal toxicity (decreased food consumption with increased mortality) following prolonged administration of the drug. No evidence of teratogenic effects have been observed after administration of Sufentanil Citrate in rats or rabbits.

Labor and Delivery: The use of epidurally administered Sufentanil Citrate in combination with bupivacaine 0.125% with or without epinephrine is indicated for labor and delivery. (See *"Indications and Usage"* and *"Dosage and Administration"* sections.) Sufentanil Citrate is not recommended for intravenous use or for use of larger epidural doses during labor and delivery because of potential risks to the newborn infant after delivery. In clinical trials, one case of severe fetal bradycardia associated with maternal administration of Sufentanil Citrate 15 μg plus bupivacaine 0.125% (10 mL total volume).

Nursing Mothers: It is not known whether Sufentanil Citrate is excreted in human milk. Because fentanyl analogs are excreted in human milk, caution should be exercised when Sufentanil Citrate is administered to a nursing woman.

Pediatric Use: The safety and efficacy of intravenous Sufentanil Citrate in children under two years of age undergoing cardiovascular surgery has been documented in a limited number of cases.

Animal Toxicology: The intravenous LD$_{50}$ of Sufentanil Citrate is 16.8 to 18.0 mg/kg in mice, 11.8 to 13.0 mg/kg in guinea pigs and 10.1 to 19.5 mg/kg in dogs. Reproduction studies performed in rats and rabbits given doses of up to 2.5 times the upper human dose for a period of 10 to over 30 days revealed high maternal mortality rates due to decreased food consumption and anoxia, which preclude any meaningful interpretation of the results. Epidural and intrathecal injections of Sufentanil Citrate in dogs and epidural injections in rats were not associated with neurotoxicity.

ADVERSE REACTIONS

The most common adverse reactions of opioids are respiratory depression and skeletal muscle rigidity, particularly of the truncal muscles. Sufentanil Citrate may produce muscular rigidity that involves the skeletal muscles of the neck and extremities. See *"Clinical Pharmacology," "Warnings"* and *"Precautions"* on the management of respiratory depression and skeletal muscle rigidity.

Urinary retention has been associated with the use of epidural opioids but was not reported in the clinical trials of epidurally administered Sufentanil Citrate due to the use of indwelling catheters. The incidence of urinary retention in patients without urinary catheters receiving epidural Sufentanil Citrate is unknown; return of normal bladder activity may be delayed. The following adverse reaction information is derived from controlled clinical trials in 320 patients who received intravenous Sufentanil Citrate during surgical anesthesia and in 340 patients who received epidural Sufentanil Citrate plus bupivacaine 0.125% for analgesia during labor and is presented below. Based on the observed frequency, none of the reactions occurring with an incidence less than 1% were observed during clinical trials of epidural Sufentanil Citrate used during labor and delivery (N = 340).

In general cardiovascular and musculoskeletal adverse experiences were not observed in clinical trials of epidural Sufentanil Citrate. Hypotension was observed 7 times more frequently in intravenous trials than in epidural trials. The incidence of central nervous system, dermatological and gastrointestinal adverse experiences was approximately 4 to 25 times higher in studies of epidural use in labor and delivery.

PROBABLY CAUSALLY RELATED: INCIDENCE GREATER THAN 1%— DERIVED FROM CLINICAL TRIALS
(See preceding paragraph).
    Cardiovascular: bradycardia,* hypertension,* hypotension.*
    Musculoskeletal: chest wall rigidity.*
    Central Nervous System: somnolence.*
    Dermatological: pruritus (25%).
    Gastrointestinal: nausea,* vomiting.*

PROBABLY CAUSALLY RELATED: INCIDENCE LESS THAN 1%— DERIVED FROM CLINICAL TRIALS
(Adverse events reported in post-marketing surveillance, not seen in clinical trials, are *italicized*.)

Cardiovascular: arrhythmia,** tachycardia.**

Central Nervous System: chills.**

Dermatological: erythema.**

Musculoskeletal: skeletal muscle rigidity of neck and extremities.

Respiratory: apnea,** bronchospasm,** postoperative respiratory depression.**

*Miscellaneous: intraoperative muscle movement.***

DRUG ABUSE AND DEPENDENCE

Sufentanil Citrate is a Schedule II controlled drug substance that can produce drug dependence of the morphine type and therefore has the potential for being abused.

* Incidence 3% to 9%
** 0.3% to 1%

OVERDOSAGE

Overdosage is manifested by an extension of the pharmacological actions of Sufentanil Citrate (see *"Clinical Pharmacology"*) as with other potent opioid analgesics. The most serious and significant effect of overdose for both intravenous and epidural administration of Sufentanil Citrate is respiratory depression. Intravenous administration of an opioid antagonist such as naloxone should be employed as a specific antidote to manage respiratory depression. The duration of respiratory depression following overdosage with Sufentanil Citrate may be longer than the duration of action of the opioid antagonist. Administration of an opioid antagonist should not preclude more immediate countermeasures. In the event of overdosage, oxygen should be administered and ventilation assisted or controlled as indicated for hypoventilation or apnea. A patent airway must be maintained, and a nasopharyngeal airway or endotracheal tube may be indicated. If depressed respiration is associated with muscular rigidity, a neuromuscular blocking agent may be required to facilitate assisted or controlled respiration. Intravenous fluids and vasopressors for the treatment of hypotension and other supportive measures may be employed.

DOSAGE AND ADMINISTRATION

The dosage of Sufentanil Citrate should be individualized in each case according to body weight, physical status, underlying pathological condition, use of other drugs, and type of surgical procedure and anesthesia. In obese patients (more than 20% above ideal total body weight), the dosage of Sufentanil Citrate should be determined on the basis of lean body weight. Dosage should be reduced in elderly and debilitated patients (see *"Precautions"*).

Vital signs should be monitored routinely.

Parenteral drug products should be inspected visually for particulate matter and discoloration prior to administration, whenever solution and container permit.

Intravenous Use: Sufentanil Citrate may be administered intravenously by slow injection or infusion 1) in doses of up to 8 μg/kg as an analgesic adjunct to general anesthesia, and 2) in doses ≥ 8 μg/kg as a primary anesthetic agent for induction and maintenance of anesthesia (see Dosage Range Chart). If benzodiazepines, barbiturates, inhalation agents, other opioids or other central nervous system depressants are used concomitantly, the dose of Sufentanil Citrate and/or these agents should be reduced (see *"Precautions"*). In all cases dosage should be titrated to individual patient response.

Usage in Children: For induction and maintenance of anesthesia in children less than 12 years of age undergoing cardiovascular surgery, an anesthetic dose of 10-25 μg/kg administered with 100% oxygen is generally recommended. Supplemental dosages of up to 25-50 μg are recommended for maintenance, based on response to initial dose and as determined by changes in vital signs indicating surgical stress or lightening of anesthesia.

Premedication: The selection of preanesthetic medications should be based upon the needs of the individual patient.

Neuromuscular Blocking Agents: The neuromuscular blocking agent selected should be compatible with the patient's condition, taking into account the hemodynamic effects of a particular muscle relaxant and the degree of skeletal muscle relaxation required (see *"Clinical Pharmacology," "Warnings"* and *"Precautions"*).

ADULT DOSAGE RANGE CHART FOR INTRAVENOUS USE

Analgesic Component to General Anesthesia • Total Dosage Requirements of 1 μg/kg/hr or Less are Recommended	
Total Dosage	Maintenance Dosage
Analgesic Dosages	
INCREMENTAL OR INFUSION: 1-2 μg/kg (expected duration of anesthesia 1-2 hours). Approximately 75% or more of total Sufentanil Citrate dosage may be administered prior to intubation by either slow injection or infusion titrated to individual patient response. Dosages in this range are generally administered with nitrous oxide/oxygen in patients undergoing general surgery in which endotracheal intubation and mechanical ventilation are required.	**INCREMENTAL:** 10-25 μg (0.2-0.5 mL) may be administered in increments as needed when movement and/or changes in vital signs indicate surgical stress or lightening of analgesia. Supplemental dosages should be individualized and adjusted to remaining operative time anticipated. **INFUSION:** Sufentanil Citrate may be administered as an intermittent or continuous infusion as needed in response to signs of lightening of analgesia. In absence of signs of lightening of analgesia, infusion rates should always be adjusted downward until there is some response to surgical stimulation. Maintenance infusion rates should be adjusted

Analgesic Component to General Anesthesia
• *Total Dosage Requirements of 1 µg/kg/hr or Less are Recommended*

Total Dosage	Maintenance Dosage

Analgesic Dosages

INCREMENTAL OR INFUSION:

2-8 µg/kg (expected duration of anesthesia 2-8 hours). Approximately 75% or less of the total calculated Sufentanil Citrate dosage may be administered by slow injection or infusion prior to intubation, titrated to individual patient response. Dosages in this range are generally administered with nitrous oxide/oxygen in patients undergoing more complicated major surgical procedures in which endotracheal intubation and mechanical ventilation are required. At dosages in this range, Sufentanil Citrate has been shown to provide some attenuation of sympathetic reflex activity in response to surgical stimuli, provide hemodynamic stability, and provide relatively rapid recovery.

based upon the induction dose of Sufentanil Citrate so that the total dose does not exceed 1 µg/kg/hr of expected surgical time. Dosage should be individualized and adjusted to remaining operative time time anticipated.

INCREMENTAL:

10-50 µg (0.2-1 mL) may be administered in increments as needed when movement and/or changes in vital signs indicate surgical stress or lightening of analgesia. Supplemental dosages should be individualized and adjusted to the remaining operative time anticipated.

INFUSION:

Sufentanil Citrate may be administered as an intermittent or continuous infusion as needed in response to signs of lightening of analgesia. In the absence of signs of lightening of analgesia, infusion rates should always be adjusted downward until there is some response to surgical stimulation. Maintenance infusion rates should be adjusted based upon the induction dose of Sufentanil Citrate so that the total dose does not exceed 1 µg/kg/hr of expected surgical time. Dosage should be individualized and adjusted to remaining operative time anticipated.

Anesthetic Dosages

INCREMENTAL OR INFUSION:

8-30 µg/kg (anesthetic doses). At this anesthetic dosage range Sufentanil Citrate is generally administered as a slow injection, as an infusion, or as an injection followed by an infusion. Sufentanil Citrate with 100% oxygen and a muscle relaxant has been found to produce sleep at dosages ≥ 8 µg/kg and to maintain a deep level of anesthesia without the use of additional anesthetic agents. The addition of N₂O to these dosages will reduce systolic blood pressure. At dosages in this range of up to 25 µg/kg, catecholamine release is attenuated. Dosages of 25-30 µg/kg have been shown to block sympathetic response including catecholamine release. High doses are indicated in patients undergoing major surgical procedures, in which endotracheal intubation and mechanical ventilation are required, such as cardiovascular surgery and neurosurgery in the sitting position

INCREMENTAL:

Depending on the initial dose, maintenance doses of 0.5-10 µg/kg may be administered by slow injection in anticipation of surgical stress such as incision, sternotomy or cardiopulmonary bypass.

Anesthetic Dosages

with maintenance of favorable myocardial and cerebral oxygen balance. Postoperative observation is essential and postoperative mechanical ventilation may be required at the higher dosage range due to extended postoperative respiratory depression. Dosage should be titrated to individual patient response.

INFUSION:

Sufentanil Citrate may be administered by continuous or intermittent infusion as needed in response to signs of lightening of anesthesia. In the absence of lightening of anesthesia, infusion rates should always be adjusted downward until there is some response to surgical stimulation. The maintenance infusion rate for Sufentanil Citrate should be based upon the induction dose so that the total dose for the procedure does not exceed 30 µg/kg.

In patients administered high doses of Sufentanil Citrate, it is essential that qualified personnel and adequate facilities are available for the management of postoperative respiratory depression.

Also see *"Warnings"* and *"Precautions"* sections.

For purposes of administering small volumes of Sufentanil Citrate accurately, the use of a tuberculin syringe or equivalent is recommended.

EPIDURAL USE IN LABOR AND DELIVERY

Proper placement of the needle or catheter in the epidural space should be verified before Sufentanil Citrate is injected to assure that unintentional intravascular or intrathecal administration does not occur. Unintentional intravascular injection of Sufentanil Citrate could result in a potentially serious overdose, including acute truncal muscular rigidity and apnea. Unintentional intrathecal injection of the full Sufentanil Citrate, bupivacaine epidural doses and volume could produce effects of high spinal anesthesia including prolonged paralysis and delayed recovery. If analgesia is inadequate, the placement and integrity of the catheter should be verified prior to the administration of any additional epidural medications. Sufentanil Citrate should be administered by slow injection. Respiration should be closely monitored following each administration of an epidural injection of Sufentanil Citrate.

Dosage for Labor and Delivery: The recommended dosage is Sufentanil Citrate 10-15 µg administered with 10 mL bupivacaine 0.125% with or without epinephrine. Sufentanil Citrate and bupivacaine should be mixed together before administration. Doses can be repeated twice (for a total of three doses) at not less than one-hour intervals until delivery.

Protect from light. Store at room temperature 15°-30°C (59°-86°F).

HOW SUPPLIED
INJECTION (C-II):

BRAND/MANUFACTURER	NDC	SIZE	AWP
○ **BRAND**			
SUFENTA: Janssen	50458-0050-01	1 ml 10s	$129.83
	50458-0050-02	2 ml 10s	$230.27
	50458-0050-05	5 ml 10s	$478.51

Sulconazole Nitrate

DESCRIPTION

Sulconazole Nitrate Cream, 1.0% is a broad-spectrum antifungal agent intended for topical application. Sulconazole Nitrate, the active ingredient in Sulconazole Nitrate Cream, is an imidazole derivative with in vitro antifungal and antiyeast activity. Its chemical name is (±)-1-[2.4-dichloro-β-[(p-chlorobenzyl)-thio]-phen-ethyl] imidazole mononitrate. Sulconazole Nitrate is a white to off-white crystalline powder with a molecular weight of 460.77. It is freely soluble in pyridine: slightly soluble in ethanol, acetone, and chloroform; and very slightly soluble in water. It has a melting point of about 130°C.

Sulconazole Nitrate Cream contains Sulconazole Nitrate 10 mg/g in an emollient cream base consisting of propylene glycol, stearyl alcohol, isopropyl myristate, cetyl alcohol, polysorbate 60, sorbitan monostearate, glyceryl stearate and PEG-100 stearate, ascorbyl palmitate, and purified water, with sodium hydroxide and/or nitric acid added to adjust the pH.

♦ RATED THERAPEUTICALLY EQUIVALENT; ◇ THERAPEUTIC EQUIVALENCE UNCONFIRMED; ○ UNRATED

Following is its chemical structure:

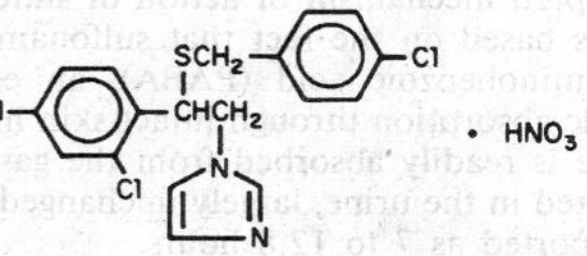

CLINICAL PHARMACOLOGY

Sulconazole Nitrate is an imidazole derivative with broad-spectrum antifungal activity that inhibits the growth in vitro of the common pathogenic dermatophytes including *Trichophyton rubrum, Trichophyton mentagraphytes, Epidermophyton floccosum* and *Microsporum canis*. It also inhibits (*in vitro*) the organism responsible for tinea versicolor, *Malossezia furfur*. Sulconazole Nitrate has been shown to be active *in vivo* against the following microorganisms, although clinical efficacy has not been established: *Candida albicans* and certain gram positive bacteria.

A modified Draize test showed no allergic contact dermatitis and a phototoxicity study showed no phototoxic or photoallergic reaction to Sulconazole Nitrate Cream. Maximization tests with Sulconazole Nitrate Cream showed no evidence of contact sensitization or irritation.

INDICATIONS AND USAGE

Sulconazole Nitrate Cream, 1.0% is an antifungal agent indicated for the treatment of tinea pedis (athlete's foot), tinea cruris, and tinea corporis caused by *Trichophyton rubrum, Trichophyton mentagrophytes, Epidermophyton floccosum, and Microsporum canis*,* and for the treatment of tinea versicolor.

UNLABELED USES
Sulconazole Nitrate is used alone or as an adjunct in the treatment of cutaneous candidiasis.

CONTRAINDICATIONS

Sulconazole Nitrate Cream, 1.0% is contraindicated in patients who have a history of hypersensitivity to any of its ingredients.

PRECAUTIONS

General: Sulconazole Nitrate Cream, 1.0% is for external use only. Avoid contact with the eyes. If irritation develops, the cream should be discontinued and appropriate therapy instituted.

Information for Patients: Patients should be told to use Sulconazole Nitrate Cream as directed by the physician, to use it externally only, and to avoid contact with the eyes.

Carcinogenesis, Mutagenesis, Impairment of Fertility: Long-term animal studies to determine carcinogenic potential have not been performed. *In vitro* studies have shown no mutagenic activity.

Pregnancy (Category C): There are no adequate and well controlled studies in pregnant women. Sulconazole Nitrate should be used during pregnancy only if clearly needed. Sulconazole Nitrate has been shown to be embryotoxic in rats when given in doses of 125 times the adult human dose (in mg/kg). The drug was not teratogenic in rats or rabbits at oral doses of 50 mg/kg/day.

Sulconazole Nitrate given orally to rats at a dose 125 times the human dose resulted in prolonged gestation and dystocia. Several females died during the prenatal period, most likely due to labor complications.

Nursing Mothers: It is not known whether Salconazole Nitrate is excreted in human milk. Caution should be exercised when Sulconazole Nitrate is administered to a nursing woman.

Pediatric Use: Safety and effectiveness in children have not been established.

ADVERSE REACTIONS

There were no systemic effects and only infrequent cutaneous adverse reactions in 1185 patients treated with Sulconazole Nitrate Cream in controlled clinical trials. Approximately 3% of these patients reported itching, 3% burning or stinging, and 1% redness. These complaints did not usually interfere with treatment.

CLINICAL STUDIES

In a vehicle-controlled study for the treatment of tinea pedis (moccasin type) due to *T. rubrum*, after 4-6 weeks of treatment 69% of patients on the active drug and 19% of patients on the drug vehicle had become KOH and culture negative. In addition, 68% of patients on the active drug and 20% of patients on the drug vehicle showed a good or excellent clinical response.

DOSAGE AND ADMINISTRATION

A small amount of cream should be gently massaged into the affected and surrounding skin areas once or twice daily, except in tinea pedis, where administration should be twice daily.

Early relief of symptoms is experienced by the majority of patients and clinical improvement may be seen fairly soon after treatment is begun; however, tinea corporis/cruris and tinea versicolor should be treated for 3 weeks and tinea pedis for 4 weeks to reduce the possibility of recurrence.

---

* Efficacy for this organism in the organ system was studied in fewer than ten infections

If significant clinical improvement is not seen after 4 to 6 weeks of treatment, an alternate diagnosis should be considered.

Avoid excessive heat, above 40°C (104°F).

HOW SUPPLIED
CREAM: 1%

BRAND/MANUFACTURER	NDC	SIZE	AWP
○ **BRAND**			
EXELDERM: Westwood-Squibb	00072-8200-15	15 gm	$9.34
	00072-8200-30	30 gm	$16.42
	00072-8200-60	60 gm	$27.20

SOLUTION: 1%

BRAND/MANUFACTURER	NDC	SIZE	AWP
○ **BRAND**			
EXELDERM: Westwood-Squibb	00072-8400-30	30 ml	$20.10

Sulf-10 SEE SULFACETAMIDE SODIUM, OPHTHALMIC

Sulfabenzamide/Sulfacetamide/Sulfathiazole

DESCRIPTION

Sulfabenzamide/Sulfacetamide/Sulfathiazole Cream contains Sulfathiazole (Benzenesulfonamide, 4-amino-N-2-thiazolyl-N[1]-2-thiazolysulfanilamide) 3.42%, Sulfacetamide (Acetamide,N-[(4-aminophenyl) sulfonyl]-N-Sulfanilylacetamide) 2.86%, and Sulfabenzamide (Benzamide,N-[(4-aminophenyl) sulfonyl]-N-Sulfanilylbenzamide) 3.7% compounded with cetyl alcohol 2%, cholesterol, diethylaminoethyl stearamide, glyceryl monostearate, lanolin, lecithin, methylparaben, peanut oil, phosphoric acid, propylene glycol, propylparaben, purified water, stearic acid and urea.

Each Sulfabenzamide/Sulfacetamide/Sulfathiazole Tablet contains Sulfathiazole (Benzene-Sulfonamide,4-amino-N-2-thiazolyl-N[1]-2-thiazolyls ulfanilamide) 172.5 mg, Sulfacetamide (Acetamide,N-[(4-aminophenyl) sulfonyl]-N-Sulfanilylacetamide) 143.75 mg and sulfabenzamide (Benzamide,N-[(4-aminophenyl)sulfonyl]-N-Sulfanilybenzamide) 184.0 mg, compounded with guar gum, lactose, magnesium stearate, starch and urea. Sulfabenzamide/Sulfacetamide/Sulfathiazole Cream and Sulfabenzamide/Sulfacetamide/Sulfathiazole Tablets are topical antibacterial preparations available for intravaginal administration.

CLINICAL PHARMACOLOGY

The mode of action of Sulfabenzamide/Sulfacetamide/Sulfathiazole is not completely known. Sulfabenzamide/Sulfacetamide/Sulfathiazole Cream and Sulfabenzamide/Sulfacetamide/Sulfathiazole Tablets are topical antibacterial preparations used intravaginally against *Haemophilus (Gardnerella) vaginalis* bacteria. Indirect effects, such as lowering the vaginal pH, may be equally important mechanisms.

INDICATIONS AND USAGE

Sulfabenzamide/Sulfacetamide/Sulfathiazole Cream and Sulfabenzamide/Sulfacetamide/Sulfathiazole Tablets are indicated for the treatment of vaginitis caused by *Haemophilus (Gardnerella) vaginalis* bacteria.

The diagnosis of a *Haemophilus (Gardnerella) vaginalis* vaginitis should be firmly established before initiation of treatment with Sulfabenzamide/Sulfacetamide/Sulfathiazole.

CONTRAINDICATIONS

Sulfabenzamide/Sulfacetamide/Sulfathiazole is contraindicated in the following circumstances: kidney disease; hypersensitivity to sulfonamides; in pregnancy at term and during the nursing period because sulfonamides cross the placenta, are excreted in breast milk and may cause Kernicterus.

WARNINGS

Deaths associated with the administration of sulfonamides have been reported from hypersensitivity reactions, agranulocytosis, aplastic anemia and other blood dyscrasias. The presence of clinical signs such as sore throat, fever, palor, purpura or jaundice may be early indications of serious blood disorders.

PRECAUTIONS

Because sulfonamides may be absorbed from the vaginal mucosa, the usual precautions for oral sulfonamides apply. Patients should be observed for skin rash or evidence of systemic toxicity, and if these develop, the medications should be discontinued.

Laboratory Tests: Standard office diagnostic procedures for vaginitis are usually sufficient to establish the diagnosis of *Haemophilus (Gardnerella) vaginalis* and to rule out a trichomonal or monilial infection. These include noting a fish-like odor upon addition of 10% KOH to vaginal discharge and microscopic identification of "clue cells" in a wet mount preparation. If cultures are obtained, care must be taken to use appropriate media and methods for *Haemophilus (Gardnerella) vaginalis*.

Carcinogenesis, Mutagenesis, Impairment of Fertility: The sulfonamides bear certain chemical similarities to some goitrogens. Rats appear to be especially susceptible to the goitrogenic effects of sulfonamides, and long-term administration has produced thyroid malignancies in this species.

PREGNANCY

Teratogenic Effects: Pregnancy Category C. The safe use of sulfonamides in pregnancy has not been established. The teratogenicity potential of most sulfonamides has not been thoroughly investigated in either animals or humans. However, a significant increase in the incidence of cleft palate and other bony abnormalities of offspring has been observed when certain sulfonamides of the short, intermediate and long-acting types were given to pregnant rats and mice at high oral doses (7 to 25 times the human therapeutic dose).

Nursing Mothers: Because of the potential for serious adverse reactions in nursing infants from Sulfabenzamide/Sulfacetamide/Sulfathiazole, a decision should be made whether to discontinue nursing or to discontinue the drug, taking into account the importance of the drug to the mother. (See *"Contraindications"*.)

Pediatric Use: Safety and effectiveness in children have not been established.

ADVERSE REACTIONS

There has been one reported case of Agranulocytosis in a patient receiving Sulfabenzamide/Sulfacetamide/Sulfathiazole Cream. The most frequent adverse reactions to Sulfabenzamide/Sulfacetamide/Sulfathiazole are localized irritation and/or allergy including rare reports of Stevens Johnson syndrome which may be fatal.

DOSAGE AND ADMINISTRATION

Sulfabenzamide/Sulfacetamide/Sulfathiazole Cream: One full applicator intravaginally twice daily for four to six days. This course of therapy may be repeated if necessary; the dosage may be reduced one-half to one-quarter.

Sulfabenzamide/Sulfacetamide/Sulfathiazole Vaginal Tablets: One tablet intravaginally before retiring and again in the morning for ten days. This course may be repeated, if necessary.

HOW SUPPLIED
CREAM:

AVERAGE UNIT PRICE (AVAILABLE SIZES)		GENERIC A-RATED AVERAGE PRICE (GAAP)	
BRAND	$0.35	78 gm	$9.88
GENERIC	$0.08	82.5 gm	$4.97

BRAND/MANUFACTURER	NDC	SIZE	AWP
◆ BRAND			
SULTRIN TRIPLE SULFA: Ortho Pharm	00062-5440-77	78 gm	$27.36
◆ GENERICS			
Moore,H.L.	00839-6329-46	78 gm	$3.63
NMC	23317-0700-78	78 gm	$4.94
TRYSUL: Savage	00281-3790-47	78 gm	$21.07
GYNE SULF: G&W	00713-0214-33	82.5 gm	$4.20
Clay-Park	45802-0156-45	82.5 gm	$4.21
Qualitest	00603-7880-86	82.5 gm	$4.75
URL	00677-0754-48	82.5 gm	$5.33
Rugby	00536-5280-69	82.5 gm	$5.37
Fougera	00168-0018-33	82.5 gm	$5.37
Goldline	00182-1215-75	82.5 gm	$5.55
Schein	00364-7284-37	82.5 gm	$6.70
V.V.S.: EconoMed	38130-0049-03	82.5 gm	$8.98
Geneva	00781-7020-33	90 gm	$4.22
Parmed	00349-9025-09	90 gm	$7.68

TABLETS:

AVERAGE UNIT PRICE (AVAILABLE SIZES)	
GENERIC	$0.10

BRAND/MANUFACTURER	NDC	SIZE	AWP
◆ GENERICS			
Richlyn	00115-4711-01	100s	$10.90
Richlyn	00115-4711-03	1000s	$83.85

TABLETS:

BRAND/MANUFACTURER	NDC	SIZE	AWP
○ BRAND			
SULTRIN TRIPLE SULFA: Ortho Pharm	00062-5441-64	20s	$29.76

Sulfacet-R *SEE SULFACETAMIDE SODIUM AND SULFUR*

Sulfacetamide Sodium and Sulfur

DESCRIPTION

Each mL of Sulfacetamide Sodium/Sulfur Acne Lotion (sulfacetamide sodium 10% and sulfur 5%), as dispensed, contains 100 mg of Sodium Sulfacetamide and 50 mg of sulfur.

Sodium Sulfacetamide is a sulfonamide with antibacterial activity while sulfur acts as a keratolytic agent. Chemically Sodium Sulfacetamide is N′-[(4-aminophenyl)sulfonyl]-acetamide, monosodium salt, monohydrate.

CLINICAL PHARMACOLOGY

The most widely accepted mechanism of action of sulfonamides is the Woods-Fildes theory which is based on the fact that sulfonamides act as competitive antagonists to para-aminobenzoic acid (PABA), an essential component for bacterial growth. While absorption through intact skin has not been determined, Sodium Sulfacetamide is readily absorbed from the gastrointestinal tract when taken orally and excreted in the urine, largely unchanged. The biological half-life has variously been reported as 7 to 12.8 hours.

The exact mode of action of sulfur in the treatment of acne is unknown, but it has been reported that it inhibits the growth of *p. acnes* and the formation of free fatty acids.

INDICATIONS

Sulfacetamide Sodium/Sulfur is indicated in the topical control of acne vulgaris, acne rosacea and seborrheic dermatitis.

CONTRAINDICATIONS

Sulfacetamide Sodium/Sulfur Acne Lotion is contraindicated for use by patients having known hypersensitivity to sulfonamides, sulfur, or any other component of this preparation. Sulfacetamide Sodium/Sulfur Acne Lotion is not to be used by patients with kidney disease.

WARNINGS

Although rare, sensitivity to Sodium Sulfacetamide may occur. Therefore, caution and careful supervision should be observed when prescribing this drug for patients who may be prone to hypersensitivity to topical sulfonamides. Systemic toxic reactions such as agranulocytosis, acute hemolytic anemia, purpura hemorrhagica, drug fever, jaundice and contact dermatitis indicate hypersensitivity to sulfonamides. Particular caution should be employed if areas of denuded or abraded skin are involved. Contains sodium bisulfite, a sulfite that may cause allergic-type reactions including anaphylactic symptoms and life-threatening or less severe asthmatic episodes in certain susceptible people. The overall prevalence of sulfite sensitivity in the general population is unknown and probably low. Sulfite sensitivity is seen more frequently in asthmatic than in nonasthmatic people.

PRECAUTIONS

General: if irritation develops, use of the product should be discontinued and appropriate therapy instituted. For external use only. Keep away from eyes. Patients should be carefully observed for possible local irritation or sensitization during long-term therapy. The object of this therapy is to achieve desquamation without irritation, but Sodium Sulfacetamide and sulfur can cause reddening and scaling of epidermis. These side effects are not unusual in the treatment of acne vulgaris, but patients should be cautioned about the possibility. Keep out of the reach of children.

Carcinogenesis, Mutagenesis and Impairment of Fertility: Long-term studies in animals have not been performed to evaluate carcinogenic potential.

Pregnancy: Pregnancy Category C. Animal reproduction studies have not been conducted with Sulfacetamide Sodium/Sulfur Acne Lotion. It is also not known whether Sulfacetamide Sodium/Sulfur Acne Lotion can cause fetal harm when administered to a pregnant woman or can affect reproduction capacity Sulfacetamide Sodium/Sulfur Acne Lotion should be given to a pregnant woman only if clearly needed.

Nursing Mothers: It is not known whether Sodium Sulfacetamide is excreted in the human milk following topical use of Sulfacetamide Sodium/Sulfur Acne Lotion. However, small amounts of orally administered sulfonamides have been reported to be eliminated in human milk. In view of this and because many drugs are excreted in human milk, caution should be exercised when Sulfacetamide Sodium/Sulfur Acne Lotion is administered to a nursing woman.

Pediatric Use: Safety and effectiveness in children under the age of 12 have not been established.

ADVERSE REACTIONS

Although rare, Sodium Sulfacetamide may cause local irritation.

DOSAGE AND ADMINISTRATION

Shake well before using. Apply a thin film to affected areas with light massaging to blend in each application 1 to 3 times daily.

HOW SUPPLIED
LOTION: 10%-5%

BRAND/MANUFACTURER	NDC	SIZE	AWP
○ BRAND			
SULFACET-R: Dermik	00066-0028-25	25 ml	$20.44
NOVACET: Genderm	52761-0530-30	30 ml	$20.46
○ GENERICS			
Glades	59366-2762-03	25 gm	$17.34
Glades	59366-2762-05	30 gm	$17.34

Sulfacetamide Sodium, Ophthalmic

DESCRIPTION

Sulfacetamide Sodium Ophthalmic Solution and Ointment 10% are topical anti-infective agents for ophthalmic use.

◆ RATED THERAPEUTICALLY EQUIVALENT; ◇ THERAPEUTIC EQUIVALENCE UNCONFIRMED; ○ UNRATED

CHEMICAL NAME
N-Sulfanilylacetamide monosodium salt monohydrate.

Sulfacetamide Sodium-10 solution contains:

Sulfacetamide Sodium 10%

with: polyvinyl alcohol 1.4%; benzalkonium chloride (0.005%); sodium thiosulfate; sodium phosphate dibasic; sodium phosphate monobasic; edetate disodium; polysorbate 80; hydrochloric acid and/or sodium hydroxide to adjust the pH; and purified water.

Sulfacetamide Sodium-10 ointment contains:

Sulfacetamide Sodium 10%

with: phenylmercuric acetate (0.0008%), white petrolatum, mineral oil, and petrolatum (and) lanolin alcohol.

Following is its chemical structure:

$$H_2N-\langle\text{ring}\rangle-SO_2NCOCH_3 \cdot H_2O$$
$$\overset{Na}{|}$$

CLINICAL PHARMACOLOGY
Sulfonamides exert a bacteriostatic effect against a wide range of gram-positive and gram-negative organisms by restricting, through competition with para-aminobenzoic acid, the synthesis of folic acid which bacteria require for growth.

INDICATIONS AND USAGE
Sulfacetamide Sodium Ophthalmic is indicated for the treatment of conjunctivitis, corneal ulcer and other superficial ocular infections caused by susceptible microorganisms, and as adjunctive treatment in systemic sulfonamide therapy of trachoma.

CONTRAINDICATIONS
Sulfacetamide Sodium Ophthalmic is contraindicated in individuals who have a hypersensitivity to sulfonamide preparations or to any of the ingredients of the preparation.

WARNINGS
Sulfacetamide Sodium solution is **FOR TOPICAL EYE USE ONLY—NOT FOR INJECTION.** As with all sulfonamide preparations, severe sensitivity reactions, e.g., Stevens-Johnson syndrome, fever, skin rash, GI disturbances and bone marrow depression have been identified in individuals with no prior history of sulfonamide hypersensitivity. A significant percentage of staphylococcal isolates are completely resistant to sulfa drugs.

PRECAUTIONS
Sulfacetamide preparations are incompatible with silver preparations. Nonsusceptible organisms, including fungi, may proliferate with the use of this preparation. Sulfonamides are inactivated by the aminobenzoic acid present in purulent exudates. Sensitization may occur when a sulfonamide is readministered irrespective of the route of administration, and cross-sensitivity between different sulfonamides may occur. If signs of sensitivity or other untoward reactions occur, discontinue use of the preparation.

Ophthalmic ointments may retard corneal healing.

Do not touch dropper tip to any surface since this may contaminate the contents.

ADVERSE REACTIONS
Sulfacetamide Sodium Ophthalmic may cause local irritation, stinging and burning. While the irritation may be transient, occasionally, use of the medication has to be discontinued.

Although sensitivity reactions to Sulfacetamide Sodium are rare, an isolated incident of Stevens-Johnson syndrome was reported in a patient who had experienced a previous bullous drug reaction to an orally administered sulfonamide, and a single instance of local hypersensitivity was reported which progressed to a fatal syndrome resembling systemic lupus erythematosus. The development of secondary infection has occurred after the use of antimicrobials.

DOSAGE AND ADMINISTRATION
Sulfacetamide Sodium Ophthalmic 10% solution: One to two drops into the lower conjunctival sac every 2 or 3 hours during the day, less often at night.

Sulfacetamide Sodium Ophthalmic 10% ointment: Apply a small amount of ointment in the conjunctival sac 4 times daily and at bedtime.

Storage: Store ointment away from heat. Store solution between 8°-25°C (46°-77°F). Protect from light. Do not use if solution is discolored (dark brown).

HOW SUPPLIED
DROP: 10%

AVERAGE UNIT PRICE (AVAILABLE SIZES)		GENERIC A-RATED AVERAGE PRICE (GAAP)	
BRAND	$1.67	2 ml	$2.50
GENERIC	$0.42	5 ml	$2.62
		15 ml	$3.38

BRAND/MANUFACTURER	NDC	SIZE	AWP
◆ BRAND			
BLEPH-10: Allergan Optical	11980-0011-03	2.5 ml	$4.08
	11980-0011-05	5 ml	$12.24
SULF-10: Iolab	00058-0732-15	15 ml	$9.24
SODIUM SULAMYD: Schering	00085-0946-06	15 ml	$17.08
BLEPH-10: Allergan Optical	11980-0011-15	15 ml	$17.13
SULF-10: Iolab	00058-0786-12	1 ml 12s	$24.96
SODIUM SULAMYD: Schering	00085-0946-03	5 ml 25s	$332.50
◆ GENERICS			
OCUSULF-10: Optopics	52238-0650-02	2 ml	$2.25
AK-SULF: Akorn	17478-0221-20	2 ml	$2.44
SULFAC: Ocusoft	54799-0782-02	2 ml	$2.80
OCUSULF-10: Optopics	52238-0650-05	5 ml	$2.60
AK-SULF: Akorn	17478-0221-10	5 ml	$2.63
Qualitest	00603-7280-41	15 ml	$2.50
Bausch&Lomb Pharm	24208-0670-04	15 ml	$2.75
Moore,H.L.	00839-5523-31	15 ml	$2.82
Martec	52555-0993-01	15 ml	$2.85
AK-SULF: Akorn	17478-0221-12	15 ml	$2.94
OCUSULF-10: Optopics	52238-0650-15	15 ml	$2.95
Geneva	00781-7120-85	15 ml	$2.97
URL	00677-0917-30	15 ml	$3.25
Rugby	00536-3502-72	15 ml	$3.29
Major	00904-2728-35	15 ml	$3.30
Fougera	00168-0220-15	15 ml	$3.37
Goldline	00182-0671-64	15 ml	$3.45
Parmed	00349-8472-85	15 ml	$3.49
Schein	00364-7136-72	15 ml	$3.50
Aligen	00405-6135-15	15 ml	$3.50
Steris	00402-0782-15	15 ml	$3.50
SULFAC: Ocusoft	54799-0782-15	15 ml	$7.05
Bausch&Lomb Pharm	24208-0670-59	2 ml 12s	$27.00

DROP: 15%

AVERAGE UNIT PRICE (AVAILABLE SIZES)	
BRAND	$1.76
GENERIC	$0.87

BRAND/MANUFACTURER	NDC	SIZE	AWP
◆ BRAND			
ISOPTO CETAMIDE: Alcon Ophthalmic	00998-0522-05	5 ml	$12.25
	00998-0522-15	15 ml	$16.13
◆ GENERICS			
Bausch&Lomb Pharm	24208-0665-04	15 ml	$2.48
Alcon Surg	00065-0731-12	2 ml 12s	$37.80

DROP: 30%

AVERAGE UNIT PRICE (AVAILABLE SIZES)		GENERIC A-RATED AVERAGE PRICE (GAAP)	
BRAND	$1.21	15 ml	$6.09
GENERIC	$0.41		

BRAND/MANUFACTURER	NDC	SIZE	AWP
◆ BRAND			
SODIUM SULAMYD: Schering	00085-0717-06	15 ml	$18.12
◆ GENERICS			
Aligen	00405-6137-15	15 ml	$5.26
SULFAIR FORTE: Bausch&Lomb Pharm	24208-0695-64	15 ml	$5.90
Schein	00364-7137-72	15 ml	$6.00
Steris	00402-0783-15	15 ml	$6.00
Qualitest	00603-7281-41	15 ml	$6.30
Rugby	00536-3520-72	15 ml	$7.10

OINTMENT: 10%

AVERAGE UNIT PRICE (AVAILABLE SIZES)		GENERIC A-RATED AVERAGE PRICE (GAAP)	
BRAND	$3.78	3.5 gm	$2.79
GENERIC	$0.80		
HCFA FUL (3.5 gm)	$0.81		

BRAND/MANUFACTURER	NDC	SIZE	AWP
◆ BRAND			
BLEPH-10: Allergan Optical	00023-0311-04	3.5 gm	$12.18
CETAMIDE: Alcon Ophthalmic	00065-0526-35	3.5 gm	$13.50
SODIUM SULAMYD: Schering	00085-0066-03	3.5 gm	$13.98
◆ GENERICS			
AK-SULF: Akorn	17478-0227-35	3.5 gm	$2.69
Moore,H.L.	00839-5501-43	3.5 gm	$2.70
Bausch&Lomb Pharm	24208-0771-35	3.5 gm	$2.70
Fougera	00168-0079-38	3.5 gm	$3.08

► SHOWN IN PRODUCT IDENTIFICATION GUIDE

Sulfacetamide Sodium, Topical

DESCRIPTION

Sulfacetamide Sodium lotion contains in each gram 100 mg Sulfacetamide Sodium, USP. This bland lotion, containing surface active agents which allow the medication to come into intimate contact with the skin, is greaseless and disappears when rubbed into the skin or scalp. The hair can be combed and arranged as usual after application. The Lotion rinses easily from the scalp with water.

Sulfacetamide Sodium is $C_8H_9N_2NaO_3S \cdot H_2O$ with a molecular weight of 254.24. Chemically it is Acetamide, N-[(4-aminophenyl) sulfonyl]-, monosodium salt, monohydrate.

Sulfacetamide Sodium is an odorless, white, crystalline powder with a bitter taste. It is freely soluble in water, sparingly soluble in alcohol, while practically insoluble in benzene, in chloroform, and in either.

Following is its chemical structure:

$$H_2N-\!\!\bigcirc\!\!-SO_2NCOCH_3 \cdot H_2O$$

CLINICAL PHARMACOLOGY

Sulfacetamide Sodium exerts a bacteriostatic effect against sulfonamide-sensitive gram-positive and gram-negative microorganisms commonly isolated from secondary cutaneous pyogenic infections. It acts by restricting the synthesis of folic acid required by bacteria for growth, by its competition with para-aminobenzoic acid. There are no clinical data available on the degree and rate of systemic absorption of Sulfacetamide Sodium lotion when applied to the skin or scalp. However, significant absorption of Sulfacetamide Sodium through the skin has been reported.

The following *in vitro* data are available but their clinical significance is unknown. Organisms which show susceptibility to Sulfacetamide Sodium are: *Streptococci, Staphylocci, E. coli, Klebsiella pneumoniae, Pseudomonas pyocyanea, Salmonella* species, *Proteus vulgaris, Nocardia,* and *Actinomyces.*

INDICATIONS AND USAGE

Sulfacetamide Sodium Lotion is intended for topical application in the following scaling dermatoses: seborrheic dermatitis and seborrhea sicca (dandruff). It is also indicated for the treatment of secondary bacterial infections of the skin due to organisms susceptible to sulfonamides.

UNLABELED USES

Sodium Sulfacetamide is used alone or as anadjunct in the treatment of Acne vulgaris.

CONTRAINDICATIONS

Sulfacetamide Sodium lotion is contraindicated in persons with known or suspected hypersensitivity to sulfonamides or to any of the ingredients of the preparation.

WARNINGS

Sulfonamides are known to cause Stevens-Johnson syndrome in hypersensitive individuals. Stevens-Johnson syndrome has also been reported following the use of Sulfacetamide Sodium topically. Cases of drug-induced systemic lupus erythematosus from topical sulfacetamide have also been reported. In one of these cases there was a fatal outcome.

PRECAUTIONS

General: Nonsusceptible organisms, including fungi, may proliferate with the use of this preparation. Hypersensitivity reactions may recur when a sulfonamide is re-administered, irrespective of the route of administration, and cross hypersensitivity between different sulfonamides may occur. If Sulfacetamide Sodium Lotion produces signs of hypersensitivity or other untoward reactions, discontinue use of the preparation. Systemic absorption of topical sulfonamides is greater following application to large, infected, abraded, denuded or severely burned areas. Under these circumstances, potentially any of the adverse effects produced by the systemic administration of these agents could occur and appropriate observations and laboratory determinations should be performed.

Information for Patients: Patients should discontinue Sulfacetamide Sodium lotion if the condition becomes worse, or if a rash develops in the area being treated or elsewhere. Sulfacetamide Sodium Lotion should also be discontinued promptly and the physician notified if any arthritis, fever, or sores in the month develop.

Drug Interactions: Sulfacetamide Sodium lotion is incompatible with silver preparations.

Carcinogenesis, Mutagenesis, and Impairment of Fertility: Long-term animal studies for carcinogenic potential have not been performed on Sulfacetamide Sodium Lotion to date. Studies on reproduction and fertility have also not been performed. One author detected chromosomal non-dysjunction in the yeast, *Saccharomyces cerevisiae,* following application of Sulfacetamide Sodium. The significance of this finding to the topical use of Sulfacetamide Sodium in the human is unknown.

Pregnancy Category C: Animal reproduction studies have not been conducted with Sulfacetamide Sodium lotion. It is also not known whether Sulfacetamide Sodium lotion can cause fetal harm when administered to a pregnant woman or can affect reproduction capacity. Sulfacetamide Sodium Lotion should be used by a pregnant woman only if clearly needed.

Nursing Mothers: It is not known whether this drug is excreted in human milk. Because many drugs are excreted in human milk, caution should be exercised when Sulfacetamide Sodium Lotion is administered to a nursing woman.

Pediatric Use: Safety and effectiveness in children below the age of 12 years have not been established.

ADVERSE REACTIONS

Reports of irritation and hypersensitivity to Sulfacetamide Sodium are uncommon. The following adverse reactions, reported after administration of sterile ophthalmic Sulfacetamide Sodium, are noteworthy: instances of Stevens-Johnson syndrome and instances of local hypersensitivity which progressed to a syndrome resembling systemic lupus erythematosus; in one case a fatal outcome has been reported. (See *"Warnings".*)

OVERDOSAGE

The oral LD_{50} of Sulfacetamide in mice is 16.5 g/kg. In the event of overdosage, emergency treatment should be started immediately.

Manifestations: Overdosage may cause nausea and vomiting. Large doses may cause hematuria, crystalluria and renal shutdown due to precipitation of sulfa crystals in the renal tubules and urinary tract.

Treatment: The patient should be induced to vomit, even if emesis has occurred spontaneously. Pharmacologic vomiting by the administration of ipecac syrup is a preferred method. However, vomiting should not be induced in patients with impaired consciousness. The action of ipecac is facilitated by physical activity and by the administration of eight to twelve fluid ounces of water. If emesis does not occur within fifteen minutes, the dose of ipecac should be repeated. Precautions against aspiration must be taken, especially in infants and children. Following emesis, any drug remaining in the stomach may be adsorbed by activated charcoal administered as a slurry with water. If vomiting is unsuccessful or contraindicated, gastric lavage should be performed. Isotonic and one-half isotonic saline are the lavage solutions of choice. Saline cathartics, such as milk of magnesia, draw water into the bowel by osmosis and therefore may be valuable for their action in rapid dilution of bowel content. After emergency treatment the patient should continue to be medically monitored.

Observe kidney function for up to one week and have the patient ingest copious amounts of fluid during this period. Mannitol infusions may be helpful at the first sign of oliguria. Alkalinization of the urine by ingestion of bicarbonate is very helpful in preventing crystallization of sulfa drug in the kidney.

DOSAGE AND ADMINISTRATION

Seborrheic Dermatitis Including Seborrhea Sicca: In mild cases involving the scalp and adjacent skin areas, including noninflammatory types with scaling (dandruff), the Lotion should be applied at bedtime and allowed to remain overnight. Its application should be preceded by a shampoo if the hair and scalp are oily or greasy or if there is considerable debris. In severe cases with crusting, heavy scaling, and inflammation involving the scalp or the scalp and other skin, the Lotion should be applied twice daily. Initially, the hair and scalp should be cleansed with a nonirritating shampoo. To insure intimate contact of the medication with the affected skin, cleaning should be repeated as frequently as necessary thereafter.

The plastic tube is convenient for applying Sulfacetamide Sodium lotion, especially for patients with thick hair. The hair should be parted a section at a time and a small quantity of Lotion squeezed on the scalp from the inverted tube. The scalp should be completely moistened and the Lotion gently rubbed in with the finger tips. The hair should be brushed thoroughly for 2 to 3 minutes. The following morning the hair and scalp may be washed, if desired. The hair should be washed at least once a week. (Rinsing with plain water or thorough brushing will remove any excess medication.) The application of the Lotion at bedtime as described should be repeated 8 to 10 times. As the eruption subsides, the interval between applications may be lengthened. Applications once or twice weekly or every other week may prevent recurrence. Should the eruption recur after stopping therapy, the application of Sulfacetamide Sodium Lotion should be reinitiated as at the beginning of treatment.

Secondary Cutaneous Bacterial Infections: The Lotion should be applied to affected areas 2 to 4 times daily until the infection has cleared.

Occasionally, a slight yellowish discoloration may occur when an excessive amount of the Lotion is used and comes in contact with white fabrics. This discoloration, however, presents no problem, as it is readily removed by ordinary laundering without bleaches.

Note: Store between 2° and 30°C (36° and 86°F). The Lotion may tend to darken slightly on prolonged standing. Slight discoloration does not impair the efficacy or safety of the product.

◆ RATED THERAPEUTICALLY EQUIVALENT; ◇ THERAPEUTIC EQUIVALENCE UNCONFIRMED; ○ UNRATED

HOW SUPPLIED
LOTION: 10%

BRAND/MANUFACTURER

	NDC	SIZE	AWP
○ **BRAND** SEBIZON: Schering	00085-0600-05	85 ml	$17.17

Sulfadiazine

DESCRIPTION
Sulfadiazine is an oral sulfonamide anti-bacterial agent. Each tablet, for oral administration, contains 500 mg Sulfadiazine.

Sulfadiazine occurs as a white or slightly yellow powder. It is odorless, or nearly so, and slowly darkens on exposure to light. It is practically insoluble in water and slightly soluble in alcohol. The chemical name of Sulfadiazine is N^1-2-pyrimidinyl sulfanilamide. The molecular formula is $C_{10}H_{10}N_4O_2S$. It has a molecular weight of 250.27.

Most sulfonamides slowly darken on exposure to light.

Following is its chemical structure:

CLINICAL PHARMACOLOGY
The systemic sulfonamides are bacteriostatic agents having a similar spectrum of activity. Sulfonamides competitively inhibit bacterial synthesis of folic acid (pteroylglutamic acid) from aminobenzoic acid. Resistant strains are capable of utilizing folic acid precursors or preformed folic acid.

Sulfonamides exist in the blood in 3 forms — free, conjugated (acetylated and possibly others), and protein bound. The free form is considered to be the therapeutically active one.

Sulfadiazine given orally is readily absorbed from the gastrointestinal tract. After a single 2 g oral dose, a peak of 6.04 mg/100 mL is reached in 4 hours; of this, 4.65 mg/100 mL is free drug.

When a dose of 100 mg/kg of body weight is given initially and followed by 50 mg/kg every 6 hours, blood levels of free Sulfadiazine are about 7 mg/100 mL. Protein binding is 38 to 48%.

Sulfadiazine diffuses into the cerebrospinal fluid; free drug reaches 32 to 65% of blood levels and total drug 40 to 60%.

Sulfadiazine is excreted largely in the urine, where concentrations are 10 to 25 times greater than serum levels. Approximately 10% of a single oral dose is excreted in the first 6 hours, 50% within 24 hours, and 60 to 85% in 48 to 72 hours. Of the amount excreted in the urine, 15% to 40% is in the acetyl form.

INDICATIONS AND USAGE
Sulfadiazine tablets are indicated in the following conditions:
Chancroid
Trachoma
Inclusion conjunctivitis
Nocardiosis
Urinary tract infections (primarily pyelonephritis, pyelitis, and cystitis) in the absence of obstructive uropathy or foreign bodies, when these infections are caused by susceptible strains of the following organisms: *Escherichia coli*, *Klebsiella* species, *Enterobacter* species, *Staphylococcus aureus*, *Proteus mirabilis*, and *P. vulgaris*. Sulfadiazine should be used for urinary tract infections only after use of more soluble sulfonamides has been unsuccessful. Toxoplasmosis, as adjunctive therapy with pyrimethamine.
Malaria due to chloroquine-resistant strains of *Plasmodium falciparum*, when used as adjunctive therapy.
Prophylaxis of meningococcal meningitis when sulfonamide-sensitive group A strains are known to prevail in family groups or larger closed populations (the prophylactic usefulness of sulfonamides when group B or C infections are prevalent is not proved and may be harmful in closed population groups.)
Meningococcal meningitis, when the organism has been demonstrated to be susceptible.
Acute otitis media due to *Haemophilus influenzae*, when used concomitantly with adequate doses of penicillin.
Prophylaxis against recurrences of rheumatic fever, as an alternative to penicillin.
H. influenzae meningitis, as adjunctive therapy with parental streptomycin.

Important Notes: In vitro sulfonamide susceptibility tests are not always reliable. The test must be carefully coordinated with bacteriologic and clinical response. When the patient is already taking sulfonamides, follow-up cultures should have aminobenzoic acid added to the culture media.

Currently, the increasing frequency of resistant organisms limits the usefulness of antibacterial agents, including the sulfonamides, especially in the treatment of recurrent and complicated urinary tract infections.

Wide variation in blood levels may result with identical doses. Blood levels should be measured in patients receiving sulfonamides for serious infections. Free sulfonamide blood levels of 5 to 15 mg per 100 mL may be considered therapeutically effective for most infections, and blood levels of 12 to 15 mg per 100 mL may be considered optimal for serious infections. Twenty mg per 100 mL

should be the maximum total sulfonamide level, since adverse reactions occur more frequently above this level.

CONTRAINDICATIONS
Sulfadiazine is contraindicated in the following circumstances: Hypersensitivity to sulfonamides.

In infants less than 2 months of age (except as adjunctive therapy with pyrimethamine in the treatment of congenital toxoplasmosis).

In pregnancy at term and during the nursing period, because sulfonamides cross the placenta and are excreted in breast milk and may cause kernicterus.

WARNINGS
The sulfonamides should *not* be used for the *treatment* of group A beta-hemolytic streptococcal infections. In an established infection, they will not eradicate the streptococcus and, therefore, will not prevent sequelae such as rheumatic fever and glomerulonephritis.

Deaths associated with the administration of sulfonamides have been reported from hypersensitivity reactions, agranulocytosis, aplastic anemia, and other blood dyscrasias.

The presence of such clinical signs as sore throat, fever, pallor, purpura, or jaundice may be early indications of serious blood disorders.

The frequency of renal complications is considerably lower in patients receiving the more soluble sulfonamides.

PRECAUTIONS
General: Sulfonamides should be given with caution to patients with impaired renal or hepatic function and to those with severe allergy or bronchial asthma.

Hemolysis may occur in individuals deficient in glucose-6-phosphate dehydrogenase. This reaction is dose related.

Adequate fluid intake must be maintained in order to prevent crystalluria and stone formation.

Information for Patients: Patients should be instructed to drink an eight ounce glass of water with each dose of medication and at frequent intervals throughout the day. Caution patients to report promptly the onset of sore throat, fever, pallor, purpura, or jaundice when taking this drug, since these may be early indications of serious blood disorders.

Laboratory Tests: Complete blood counts and urinalyses with careful microscopic examinations should be done frequently in patients receiving sulfonamides.

Drug Interactions: Administration of a sulfonamide may increase the effect of oral anticoagulants and methotrexate, probably by displacement of these drugs from binding sites on plasma albumin. Potentiation of the action of sulfonylurea hypoglycemic agents, thiazide diuretics, and uricosuric agents may also be noted. This may also be due to displacement of the drugs from albumin, or a pharmacodynamic mechanism may play a role. Conversely, agents such as indomethacin, probenecid, and salicylates may displace sulfonamides from plasma albumin and increase the concentrations of free drug in plasma.

Carcinogenesis, Mutagenesis, Impairment of Fertility: The sulfonamides bear certain chemical similarities to some goitrogens. Rats appear to be especially susceptible to the goitrogenic effects of sulfonamides, and long-term administration has produced thyroid malignancies in rats.

Pregnancy: Teratogenic Effects: Pregnancy Category C: The safe use of sulfonamides in pregnancy has not been established. The teratogenic potential of most sulfonamides has not been thoroughly investigated in either animals or humans. However, a significant increase in the incidence of cleft palate and other bony abnormalities in offspring has been observed when certain sulfonamides of the short, intermediate, and long acting types were given to pregnant rats and mice in high oral doses (7 to 25 times the human therapeutic dose).

Nursing Mothers: Sulfadiazine is contraindicated for use in nursing mothers because the sulfonamides cross the placenta, are excreted in breast milk and may cause kernicterus.

Because of the potential for serious adverse reactions in nursing infants from Sulfadiazine, a decision should be made whether to discontinue nursing or to discontinue the drug, taking into account the importance of the drug to the mother. See *"Contraindications"*.

Pediatric Use: Sulfadiazine is contraindicated in infants less than 2 months of age (except as adjunctive therapy with pyrimethamine in the treatment of congenital toxoplasmosis). See *"Contraindications"* and *"Dosage and Administration"*.

ADVERSE REACTIONS
Blood Dyscrasias: Agranulocytosis, aplastic anemia, thrombocytopenia, leukopenia, hemolytic anemia, purpura, hypoprothrombinemia, and methemoglobinemia.

Allergic Reactions: Erythema multiforme (Stevens-Johnson syndrome), generalized skin eruptions, epidermal necrolysis, urticaria, serum sickness, pruritus, exfoliative dermatitis, anaphylactoid reactions, periorbital edema, conjunctival and scleral injection, photosensitization, arthralgia, allergic myocarditis, drug fever, and chills.

Gastrointestinal Reactions: Nausea, emesis, abdominal pains, hepatitis, diarrhea, anorexia, pancreatitis, and stomatitis.

C.N.S. Reactions: Headache, peripheral neuritis, mental depression, convulsions, ataxia, hallucinations, tinnitus, vertigo, and insomnia.

Renal: Crystalluria, stone formation, toxic nephrosis with oliguria and anuria; periarteritis nodosa and lupus erythematosus phenomenon have been noted.

► SHOWN IN PRODUCT IDENTIFICATION GUIDE

Miscellaneous Reactions: The sulfonamides bear certain chemical similarities to some goitrogens, diuretics (acetazolamide and the thiazides), and oral hypoglycemic agents. Goiter production, diuresis, and hypoglycemia have occurred rarely in patients receiving sulfonamides. Cross-sensitivity may exist with these agents.

DOSAGE AND ADMINISTRATION

Systemic sulfonamides are Contraindicated in infants under 2 months of age except as adjunctive therapy with pyrimethamine in the treatment of congenital toxoplasmosis.

Usage Dosage for Infants over 2 Months of Age and Children: Initially, one-half the 24-hour dose. Maintenance, 150 mg/kg or 4 g/m^2, divided into 4 to 6 doses, every 24 hours, with a maximum of 6 g every 24 hours. Rheumatic fever prophylaxis, under 30 kg (66 pounds), 500 mg every 24 hours; over 30 kg (66 pounds), 1 g every 24 hours.

Usual Adult Dosage: Initially, 2 to 4 g. Maintenance, 2 to 4 g, divided into 3 to 6 doses, every 24 hours.

Storage: Store at controlled room temperature 15°-30°C (59°-86°F).

Dispense in a tight, light-resistant container as defined in the USP.

HOW SUPPLIED
TABLETS: 500 MG

AVERAGE UNIT PRICE (AVAILABLE SIZES)		GENERIC A-RATED AVERAGE PRICE (GAAP)	
GENERIC	$0.41	100s	$42.38
		1000s	$358.48

BRAND/MANUFACTURER	NDC	SIZE	AWP
◆ GENERICS			
Goldline	00182-1996-01	100s	$37.45
Eon	00185-0757-01	100s	$37.50
Aligen	00405-4955-01	100s	$39.47
Rugby	00536-5656-01	100s	$47.75
Major	00904-7870-60	100s	$49.75
Goldline	00182-1996-10	1000s	$358.45
Eon	00185-0757-10	1000s	$358.50

Sulfamethizole

DESCRIPTION
Sulfamethizole is an antibacterial sulfonamide available in tablet form for oral administration.

Chemical name: N'-(5-methyl-1,3,4-thiadiazol-2-yl) sulfanilamide.

Sulfamethizole is a 5-membered heterocyclic sulfanilamide, occurring as a white or light buff-colored crystalline powder. Solubility in water is dependent upon the pH (1 g/5 mL at pH 7.5; 1 g/4000 mL at pH 6.5). It is soluble in alcohol, and practically insoluble in benzene.

Following is its chemical structure:

CLINICAL PHARMACOLOGY
MECHANISM OF SULFONAMIDE BACTERIOSTATIC ACTION
The primary mechanism of bacteriostatic action by Sulfamethizole is the same as that of most sulfonamides. By competing with the precursor para-aminobenzoic acid, sulfonamides inhibit bacterial synthesis of folic (pteroylglutamic) acid which is required for bacterial growth. Resistant strains are capable of utilizing folic acid precursors or performed folic acid.

ANTIBACTERIAL SPECTRUM
The antibacterial spectrum of all sulfonamides is similar. *In vitro* sensitivity of bacteria to sulfonamides does not always reflect *in vivo* sensitivity. Therefore, efficacy must be carefully evaluated with bacteriologic and clinical responses in the individual patient. (See *"Warnings"*.)

FACTORS DETERMINING EFFICACY
Efficacy of antimicrobial therapy is dependent upon a number of factors including the *in vivo* sensitivity of the involved organisms, the concentration of the drug required for bacteriostasis, and the achievable concentration of the sulfonamide at the desired site of action.

Because of the very rapid renal clearance of Sulfamethizole, the blood levels attained are low, and accumulation of the drug in tissues outside the urinary tract is very limited. Therefore, Sulfamethizole is not appropriate for treatment of systemic infections such as nocardiosis or for local lesions outside the urinary tract such as chancroid and trachoma. However, its low degree of acetylation and its rapid renal clearance permit high concentrations of active Sulfamethizole to occur in the urinary tract, making it especially applicable for the treatment of infections of this tract. In addition, the possibility of crystalluria is minimized because of the high solubility of the drug in urine.

Approximately 95% of a given dose of Sulfamethizole is not metabolized; less than 5% is acetylated. As a consequence, almost all of a given dose of Sulfamethizole is present in its active form in the body.

Approximately 80% of an administered dose is recoverable within eight hours; approximately 98% is cleared within 15 to 24 hours. Sulfamethizole is cleared by the kidney at a rate only 10 to 20% lower than that for creatinine.

BLOOD CONCENTRATIONS
Following a single 2 g dose of Sulfamethizole, peak total drug levels in whole blood are in the range of 6 mg %, the levels fall to about 50% in four hours, and are negligible at eight hours. Approximately the same concentrations are found in children following a single dose of 100 mg/kg.

URINE CONCENTRATIONS
The following average values of free drug in mg/mL were found after a single 4 g dose of Sulfamethizole:

0 to 2 hours	—	7.01
2 to 4 "	—	10.97
4 to 6 "	—	5.93
6 to 10 "	—	1.09
10 to 24 "	—	0.31

Following a single 2 g dose, the following average concentrations of total drug in mg/mL of urine were found:

0 to 4 hours	—	5.15
4 to 8 "	—	1.8
8 to 12 "	—	0.4
16 to 24 "	—	0.1

Following a single 1 g dose of Sulfamethizole, the average concentration of total drug during the first 3.5 hours was 2.9 mg/mL.

SOLUBILITY IN URINE
Sulfamethizole is highly soluble in urine. The solubilities of free and acetylated drug in buffered urine at 37° C at various pH's, in mg/mL, are given below:

pH	free	acetylated
4.5	108	33
5.3	220	.....
5.6	480	278
6.0	729	310
6.5	5,650	380
7.0	8,250	1,500
7.5	54,000	.....

INDICATIONS AND USAGE
Sulfamethizole is indicated in the treatment of urinary tract infections (primarily pyelonephritis, pyelitis, and cystitis) in the absence of obstructive uropathy or foreign bodies, when these infections are caused by susceptible strains of the following organisms: *Escherichia coli, Klebsiella-Enterobacter, Staphylococcus aureus, Proteus mirabilis,* and *Proteus vulgaris.*

Important Note. In vitro sulfonamide sensitivity tests are not always reliable. The test must be carefully coordinated with bacteriologic and clinical reponse. When the patient is already taking sulfonamides, follow-up cultures should have aminobenzoic acid added to the culture media. Currently, the increasing frequency of resistant organisms is a limitation of the usefulness of antibacterial agents, including the sulfonamides, especially in the treatment of recurrent and complicated urinary tract infections.

Wide variation in blood levels may result with identical doses. Blood levels should be measured in patients receiving sulfonamides for serious infections. Free sulfonamide blood levels of 5-15 mg per 100 mL may be considered therapeutically effective for most infections, with blood levels of 12-15 mg per 100 mL optimal for serious infections; 20 mg per 100 mL should be the maximum total sulfonamide level, as adverse reactions occur more frequently above this level.

CONTRAINDICATIONS
Sulfonamides should not be used in patients hypersensitive to sulfa drugs. They should not be used in infants less than two months of age, in pregnancy at term, and during the nursing period because sulfonamides cross the placenta and are excreted in breast milk and may cause kernicterus.

WARNINGS
Deaths associated with the administration of sulfonamides have been reported from hypersensitivity reactions, agranulocytosis, aplastic anemia, and other blood dyscrasias. The occurrence of sore throat, fever, pallor, purpura, or jaundice during sulfonamide administration may be an early indication of serious blood dyscrasias.

PRECAUTIONS
GENERAL
The usual precautions used in sulfonamide therapy should be observed, including the maintenance of an adequate fluid intake. Sulfonamides should be used with caution in patients with impairment of hepatic or renal function, severe allergy or bronchial asthma, and in patients with glucose-6-phosphate dehydrogenase deficiency since sulfas may cause hemolysis in this latter group.

◆ RATED THERAPEUTICALLY EQUIVALENT; ◇ THERAPEUTIC EQUIVALENCE UNCONFIRMED; ○ UNRATED

INFORMATION FOR THE PATIENT

Adequate fluid intake should be maintained while taking Sulfamethizole. Patients should drink a full 8 oz. glass of water with each dose of Sulfamethizole and drink additional fluids at frequent intervals throughout the day. Patients should immediately report any adverse side effects to their physician.

LABORATORY TESTS

Frequent blood counts and renal function tests should be carried out during sulfonamide treatment, especially during prolonged administration. Microscopic urinalyses should be done once a week when a patient is treated for longer than two weeks. Urine cultures should be made to confirm eradication of bacteriuria.

DRUG INTERACTIONS

The most important interactions between the sulfonamides and other drugs involve those with oral anticoagulants, the sulfonylurea hypoglycemic agents, and the hydantoin anticonvulsants. In each case, sulfonamides can potentiate the effects of the other drug. Dosage adjustments may have to be made when these drugs are given concomitantly. Cross sensitivity may exist with these agents. PABA and certain local anesthetics such as procaine that are esters of PABA, antagonize the effects of sulfonamides and therefore decrease their effectiveness.

An insoluble precipitate may form in acidic urine when Sulfamethizole is used concomitantly with methenamine mandelate.

Tolbutamide, diphenylhydantoin, phenytoin, and warfarin may have prolonged half-lives when administered with Sulfamethizole.

CARCINOGENESIS, MUTAGENESIS, IMPAIRMENT OF FERTILITY

Rats appear to be especially susceptible to the goitrogenic effects of sulfonamides, and long-term administration has produced thyroid malignancies in the species.

No long-term fertility or mutagenicity studies have been conducted in animals or humans.

Pregnancy: Teratogenic Effects. Pregnancy Category C:

USAGE IN PREGNANCY

The safe use of sulfonamides in pregnancy has not been established. The teratogenicity potential of most sulfonamides has not been thoroughly investigated in either animals or humans. However, a significant increase in the incidence of cleft palate and other bony abnormalities of offspring has been observed when certain sulfonamides of the short-, intermediate-, and long-acting types were given to pregnant rats and mice at high oral doses (7 to 25 times the human dose). Sulfamethizole should be used during pregnancy only if the potential benefit justifies the potential risk to the fetus.

NURSING MOTHERS

Sulfamethizole is contraindicated in pregnant women and nursing mothers. Sulfonamides cross the placenta and are excreted in breast milk to a significant degree. Because of the potential for serious adverse reactions in nursing infants from sulfonamides, a decision should be made whether to discontinue nursing or to discontinue the drug, taking into account the importance of the drug to the mother. See *"Contraindications"*.

PEDIATRIC USE

Sulfamethizole is not indicated for use in infants less than two months old. See *"Contraindications"* and *"Dosage and Administration"*.

ADVERSE REACTIONS

BLOOD DYSCRASIAS

Agranulocytosis, aplastic anemia, thrombocytopenia, leukopenia, hemolytic anemia, purpura, hypoprothrombinemia, and methemoglo- binemia.

ALLERGIC REACTIONS

Drug fever, erythema multiforme (Stevens-Johnson syndrome), generalized skin eruptions, epidermal necrolysis, urticaria, serum sickness, pruritus, exfoliative dermatitis, anaphylactoid reactions, periorbital edema, conjunctival and scleral injection, photosensitization, arthralgia, and allergic myocarditis.

GASTROINTESTINAL REACTIONS

Nausea, emesis, abdominal pains, hepatitis, diarrhea, anorexia, pancreatitis, and stomatitis.

CNS REACTIONS

Headache, peripheral neuritis, mental depression, convulsions, ataxia, hallucinations, tinnitus, vertigo, and insomnia.

RENAL

Crystalluria, toxic nephrosis with oliguria and anuria.

MISCELLANEOUS REACTIONS

Chills, periarteritis nodosum, and LE phenomenon.

The sulfonamides bear certain chemical similarities to some goitrogens, diuretics (acetazolamide and the thiazides), and oral hypoglycemic agents. Goiter production, diuresis, and hypoglycemia have occurred rarely in patients receiving sulfonamides. Cross-sensitivity may exist with these agents. (See *"Precautions—Carcinogenesis, Mutagenesis, Impairment of Fertility"*.)

OVERDOSAGE

The maximum tolerated single dose of sulfa drug has not been established. Sulfamethoxazole has been given in single doses up to 2000 mg. The acute signs and symptoms associated with sulfonamide overdose include anorexia, nausea, colicky abdominal pain, vertigo, headache, drowsiness and unconsciousness.

Pyrexia, hematuria and crystalluria have been reported. Blood dyscrasias and jaundice are late manifestations of overdosing.

General treatment of overdose for sulfonamides includes induction of emesis and gastric lavage. Urine output should be maintained by either oral or I.V. fluid administration in patients with normal renal function. Renal function with appropriate blood chemistries including electrolytes should be monitored closely in the acute period. Hematologic parameters should be followed over the next 10 days to two weeks after the overdose ingestion. Methemoglobinuria can be acutely reversed with intravenous 1% methylene blue. Sulfamethizole is only minimally dialyzable by hemodialysis and is not dialyzable by peritoneal dialysis. Other supportive measures should be instituted appropriate to signs and symptoms.

DOSAGE AND ADMINISTRATION

USUAL DOSAGE

Adults: 500 mg to 1 g, three or four times daily.

Children and Infants (over 2 months of age): 30 to 45 mg/kg/24 hours, divided into 4 doses.

Storage: Store at room temperature (approximately 25° C)

HOW SUPPLIED
TABLETS: 500 MG

BRAND/MANUFACTURER	NDC	SIZE	AWP
◆ **BRAND**			
THIOSULFIL FORTE: Wyeth-Ayerst	00046-0786-81	100s	$53.88

Sulfamethoxazole

DESCRIPTION

Sulfamethoxazole is an intermediate-dosage antibacterial sulfonamide available in tablets and suspension. Each tablet contains 0.5 g sulfamethoxazole. Each teaspoonful (5 mL) of the suspension contains 0.5 g Sulfamethoxazole.

Sulfamethoxazole is N^1-(5-methyl-3-isoxazolyl) sulfanilamide. It is an almost white, odorless, tasteless compound with a molecular weight of 253.28.

Following is its chemical structure:

$$H_2N - \bigcirc - SO_2NH - \underset{O}{\overset{N}{\diagup}} CH_3$$

CLINICAL PHARMACOLOGY

Sulfamethoxazole is rapidly absorbed following oral administration. It exists in the blood as unbound, protein-bound, metabolized and conjugated forms. The metabolism of Sulfamethoxazole occurs predominately by N_4-acetylation, although the glucuronide conjugate has been identified. The free form is considered to be the therapeutically active form. Approximately 70% of Sulfamethoxazole is bound to plasma proteins; of the unbound portion, 80% to 90% is in the nonacetylated form.

Following a single 1-gram oral dose in 12 volunteer male subjects, the mean peak plasma concentration of 38 mcg/mL of intact Sulfamethoxazole was achieved by 2 hours. The mean half-life of Sulfamethoxazole is approximately 10 hours. However, patients with severely impaired renal function, as shown by a creatinine clearance of less than 30 mL/minute, exhibit an increase of the half-life of Sulfamethoxazole, requiring dosage regimen adjustment.

Sulfamethoxazole is excreted primarily by the kidneys chiefly through glomerular filtration but also through tubular secretion. Urine concentrations of Sulfamethoxazole are considerably higher than are the concentrations in blood. Eighty percent to 100 percent of the dose is excreted in the urine as total Sulfamethoxazole, of which 30% is intact drug with the remaining as the N_4-acetylated metabolite.

Sulfamethoxazole diffuses into cerebrospinal fluid, with peak concentrations occurring at 8 hours and reaching approximately 14% of simultaneous plasma concentrations. The drug has also been shown to distribute to aqueous humor, vaginal fluid and middle ear fluid; it also passes the placental barrier and is excreted in breast milk.

Microbiology: The systemic sulfonamides are bacteriostatic agents and the spectrum of activity is similar for all. Sulfonamides inhibit bacterial synthesis of dihydrofolic acid by competing with *para*-aminobenzoic acid (PABA). Resistant strains are capable of utilizing folic acid precursors or preformed folic acid.

INDICATIONS AND USAGE

Acute, recurrent or chronic urinary tract infections (primarily pyelonephritis, pyelitis and cystitis) due to susceptible organisms (usually *E. coli, Klebsiella-Enterbacter*, staphylococcus, *Proteus mirabilis* and, less frequently, *Proteus vulgaris*) in the absence of obstructive uropathy or foreign bodies.

Meningococcal meningitis prophylaxis when sulfonamide-sensitive group A strains are known to prevail in family groups or larger closed populations. (The prophylactic usefulness of sulfonamides when group B or C infections are prevalent has not been proven and in closed population groups may be harmful.)

Acute otitis media due to *Haemophilus influenzae* when used concomitantly with adequate doses of penicillin.

Trachoma, Inclusion conjunctivitis, Nocardiosis, Chancroid. Toxoplasmosis as adjunctive therapy with pyrimethamine. Malaria due to chloroquine-resistant strains of *Plasmodium falciparum*, when used as adjunctive therapy.

Important note: In vitro sulfonamide susceptibility tests are not always reliable. The test must be carefully coordinated with bacteriologic and clinical response. When the patient is already taking sulfonamides, follow-up cultures should have aminobenzoic acid added to the culture media. Currently, the increasing frequency of resistant organisms is a limitation of the usefulness of antibacterial agents including the sulfonamides, especially in the treatment of chronic and recurrent urinary tract infections.

Wide variation in blood concentrations may result with identical doses. Blood concentrations should be measured in patients receiving sulfonamides for serious infections. Free sulfonamide blood concentrations of 5 to 15 mg/100 mL may be considered therapeutically effective for most infections, with blood concentrations of 12 to 15 mg/100 mL optimal for serious infections; 20 mg/100 mL should be the maximum total sulfonamide concentration, since adverse reactions occur more frequently above this concentration.

CONTRAINDICATIONS

Hypersensitivity to sulfonamides. Infants less than 2 months of age (except in the treatment of congenital toxoplasmosis as adjunctive therapy with pyrimethamine). Pregnancy at term and during the nursing period because sulfonamides pass the placenta and are excreted in the milk and may cause kernicterus.

WARNINGS

The sulfonamides should not be used for the treatment of group A beta-hemolytic streptococcal infections. In an established infection, they will not eradicate the streptococcus, and therefore will not prevent sequelae such as rheumatic fever and glomerulonephritis.

Deaths associated with the administration of sulfonamides have been reported from hypersensitivity reactions, hepatocellular necrosis, agranulocytosis, aplastic anemia and other blood dyscrasias.

The presence of clinical signs such as sore throat, fever, arthralgia, cough, shortness of breath, pallor, purpura or jaundice may be early indications of serious reactions, including serious blood disorders.

PRECAUTIONS

General: Sulfonamides should be given with caution to patients with impaired renal or hepatic function and to those with severe allergy or bronchial asthma. In glucose-6-phosphate dehydrogenase-deficient individuals, hemolysis may occur. This reaction is frequently dose-related.

Information for Patients: Patients should be instructed to maintain an adequate fluid intake in order to prevent crystalluria and stone formation.

Laboratory Tests: Complete blood counts should be done frequently in patients receiving sulfonamides. If a significant reduction in the count of any formed blood element is noted, Sulfamethoxazole should be discontinued. Urinalyses with careful microscopic examination and renal function tests should be performed during therapy, particularly for those patients with impaired renal function.

Drug Interactions: In elderly patients concurrently receiving certain diuretics, primarily thiazides, an increased incidence of thrombopenia with purpura has been reported.

It has been reported that Sulfamethoxazole may prolong the prothrombin time in patients who are receiving the anticoagulant warfarin. This interaction should be kept in mind when Sulfamethoxazole is given to patients already on anticoagulant therapy, and the coagulation time should be reassessed.

Sulfamethoxazole may inhibit the hepatic metabolism of phenytoin. At a 1.6 Gm dose Sulfamethoxazole produced a slight but significant increase in the half-life of phenytoin but did not produce a corresponding decrease in the metabolic clearance rate. When administering these drugs concurrently, one should be alert for possible excessive phenytoin effect.

Sulfonamides can also displace methotrexate from plasma protein-binding sites, thus increasing free methotrexate concentrations.

The presence of Sulfamethoxazole may interfere with the Jaffe alkaline picrate reaction assay for creatinine, resulting in overestimations of about 10% in the range of normal values.

Carcinogenesis, Mutagenesis, Impairment of Fertility: Carcinogenesis: Sulfamethoxazole has not been adequately tested in animals to permit an evaluation of its carcinogenic potential. Mutagenesis: Bacterial mutagenic studies have not been performed with Sulfamethoxazole. No chromosomal damage was observed in human leukocytes cultured *in vitro* with Sulfamethoxazole; the concentrations used exceeded blood levels of Sulfamethoxazole following therapy with Sulfamethoxazole. Impairment of fertility: No adverse effects on fertility or general reproductive performance were observed in rats given Sulfamethoxazole in oral dosages as high as 350 mg/kg/day.

Pregnancy: Teratogenic Effects: Pregnancy Category C. In rats, oral doses of 533 mg/kg of Sulfamethoxazole produced teratologic effects manifested mainly as cleft palates. The highest dose which did not cause cleft palates in rats was 512 mg/kg of Sulfamethoxazole. In rabbits, 150 to 350 mg/kg/day increased maternal mortality but had no deleterious effects on fetal development.

There are no adequate and well-controlled studies of Sulfamethoxazole in pregnant women. Sulfamethoxazole should be used during pregnancy only if the potential benefit justifies the potential risk to the fetus.

Nonteratogenic effects: see *"Contraindications"* section.

Nursing mothers: See "Contraindications" section.

Pediatric Use: Sulfamethoxazole is not recommended in infants under 2 months of age, except in the treatment of congenital toxoplasmosis as adjunctive therapy

with pyrimethamine. (See *"Contraindications"* section.) At the present time there are insufficient clinical data on prolonged or recurrent therapy in chronic renal diseases of children under 6 years of age.

ADVERSE REACTIONS

Included in the listing that follows are adverse reactions that have not been reported with this specific drug; however, the pharmacologic similarities among the sulfonamides require that each of the reactions be considered with Sulfamethoxazole administration.

Hematologic: Agranulocytosis, aplastic anemia, thrombocytopenia, leukopenia, hemolytic anemia, purpura, hypoprothrombinemia, methemoglobinemia, neutropenia, eosinophilia.

Allergic Reactions: Anaphylaxis, allergic myocarditis, serum sickness, conjunctival and scleral injection, generalized allergic reactions. In addition, periarteritis nodosa and systemic lupus erythematosus have been reported.

Dermatologic: Stevens-Johnson syndrome, epidermal necrolysis, erythema multiforme, exfoliative dermatitis, photosensitivity, pruritus, urticaria, rash, generalized skin eruptions.

Gastrointestinal: Hepatitis, hepatocellular necrosis, pseudomembranous enterocolitis, pancreatitis, stomatitis, glossitis, nausea, emesis, abdominal pain, diarrhea, anorexia.

Genitourinary: Creatinine elevation, toxic nephrosis with oliguria and anuria. The frequency of renal complications is considerably lower in patients receiving the more soluble sulfonamides.

Neurologic: Convulsions, peripheral neuritis, ataxia, vertigo, tinnitus, headache.

Psychiatric: Hallucinations, depression, apathy.

Endocrine: The sulfonamides bear certain chemical similarities to some goitrogens, diuretics (acetazolamide and the thiazides) and oral hypoglycemic agents. Cross-sensitivity may exist with these agents. Diuresis and hypoglycemia have occurred rarely in patients receiving sulfonamides.

Musculoskeletal: Arthralgia, myalgia.

Respiratory: Pulmonary infiltrates.

Miscellaneous: Edema (including periorbital), pyrexia, chills, weakness, fatigue, insomnia.

OVERDOSAGE

Acute: The amount of a single dose of Sulfamethoxazole that is either associated with symptoms of overdosage or is likely to be life-threatening has not been reported. Signs and symptoms of overdosage reported with sulfonamides include anorexia, colic, nausea, vomiting, dizziness, headache, drowsiness and unconsciousness. Pyrexia, hematuria and crystalluria may be noted. Blood dyscrasias and jaundice are potential late manifestations of overdosage.

General principles of treatment include the institution of gastric lavage or emesis; forcing oral fluids; and the administration of intravenous fluids if urine output is low and renal function is normal. The patient should be monitored with blood counts and appropriate blood chemistries, including electrolytes. If a significant blood dyscrasia or jaundice occurs, specific therapy should be instituted for these complications. Peritoneal dialysis is not effective and hemodialysis is only moderately effective in eliminating sulfamethoxazole.

Chronic: Use of Sulfamethoxazole at high doses and/or for extended periods of time may cause bone marrow depression manifested as thrombocytopenia, leukopenia and/or megaloblastic anemia. If signs of bone marrow depression occur, the patient should be given leucovorin 3 to 6 mg intramuscularly daily for three days, or as required to restore normal hematopoiesis.

Animal Toxicity: The oral LD_{50} of Sulfamethoxazole is 2300 mg/kg in mice, 3000 mg/kg in rats and > 2000 mg/kg in rabbits.

DOSAGE AND ADMINISTRATION

Systemic sulfonamides are contraindicated in infants under 2 months of age, except in the treatment of congenital toxoplasmosis as adjunctive therapy with pyrimethamine. The usual dosage schedules are as follows:

Children:

Infants (2 Months or Older) and Children	Initial Dose (50-60 mg/kg)	Dose Morning and Evening Daily Thereafter (25-30 mg/kg)
20 lbs	1 tablet or 1 teasp. (0.5 g)	½ tablet or ½ teasp. (0.25 g)
40 lbs	2 tablets or 2 teasp. (1 g)	1 tablet or 1 teasp. (0.5 g)
60 lbs	3 tablets or 3 teasp. (1.5 g)	1 ½ tablets or 1 ½ teasp. (0.75 g)
80 lbs	4 tablets or 4 teasp. (2 g)	2 tablets or 2 teasp. (1 g)

The maximum dose for children should not exceed 75 mg/kg/24 hours.

Adults

Mild to Moderate Infections	4 tablets or 4 teasp. (2 g)	2 tablets or 2 teasp. (1 g)

Note: One teaspoonful equals 5 mL.

Adults

Severe Infections: 4 tablets or 4 teaspoonfuls (2 Gm) initially, followed by 2 tablets or 2 teaspoonfuls (1 Gm) three times daily thereafter.

Patients with impaired renal function (creatinine clearance below 20 to 30 mL/min) require decreased dosage adjustment.

HOW SUPPLIED
TABLETS: 500 MG

AVERAGE UNIT PRICE (AVAILABLE SIZES)			
BRAND			$0.51

BRAND/MANUFACTURER	NDC	SIZE	AWP
◆ BRAND			
▶ GANTANOL: Roche Labs	00004-0010-01	100s	$49.80
	00004-0010-49	100s ud	$51.86

TABLETS: 0.5 GM

AVERAGE UNIT PRICE (AVAILABLE SIZES)		GENERIC A-RATED AVERAGE PRICE (GAAP)	
GENERIC	$0.10	100s	$9.81

BRAND/MANUFACTURER	NDC	SIZE	AWP
◆ GENERICS			
GAMAZOLE: Major	00904-1150-60	100s	$8.31
UROBAK: Shionogi	45809-0711-11	100s	$11.30

Sulfamethoxazole and Trimethoprim

DESCRIPTION
Sulfamethoxazole/Trimethoprim is a synthetic antibacterial combination product. Each Sulfamethoxazole/Timethoprim Tablet contains 80 mg Trimethoprim and 400 mg Sulfamethoxazole.

Each Sulfamethoxazole Trimethoprim DS (double strength) Tablet contains 160 mg Trimethoprim and 800 mg Sulfamethoxazole.

Each teaspoonful (5 mL) of Sulfamethoxazole Trimethoprim Suspension contains 40 mg Trimethoprim and 200 mg Sulfamethoxazole. Both tablet and suspension forms are for oral administration.

Sulfamethoxazole/Trimethoprim I.V. infusion is a sterile solution for intravenous infusion only. Each mL contains 16 mg Trimethoprim and 80 mg Sulfamethoxazole.

Trimethoprim is 2,4-diamino-5-(3,4,5-trimethoxybenzyl)pyrimidine. It is a white to light yellow, odorless, bitter compound with a molecular weight of 290.3, and the molecular formula $C_{14}H_{18}N_4O_3$.

Sulfamethoxazole is N^1-(5-methyl-3-isoxazolyl) sulfanilamide. It is an almost white, odorless, tasteless compound with a molecular weight of 253.28, and the molecular formula $C_{10}H_{11}N_3O_3S$.

CLINICAL PHARMACOLOGY
Sulfamethoxazole/Trimethoprim is rapidly absorbed following oral administration. Both Sulfamethoxazole and Trimethoprim exist in the blood as unbound, protein-bound and metabolized forms: Sulfamethoxazole also exists as the conjugated form. The metabolism of Sulfamethoxazole occurs predominantely by N_4-acetylation, although the glucuronide conjugate has been identified. The principal metabolites of Trimethoprim are the 1- and 3-oxides and the 3'- and 4'-hydroxy derivatives. The free forms of Sulfamethoxazole and Trimethoprim are considered to be the therapeutically active forms. Approximately 44% of Trimethoprim and 70% of Sulfamethoxazole are bound to plasma proteins. The presence of 10 mg percent Sulfamethoxazole in plasma decreases the protein binding of Trimethoprim by an insignificant degree; Trimethoprim does not influence the protein binding of Sulfamethoxazole.

Peak blood levels for the individual components occur 1 to 4 hours after oral administration. The mean serum half-lives of Sulfamethoxazole and Trimethoprim are 10 and 8 to 10 hours, respectively. However, patients with severely impaired renal function exhibit an increase in the half-lives of both components, requiring dosage regimen adjustment (see *"Dosage And Administration"* section). Detectable amounts of Trimethoprim and Sulfamethoxazole are present in the blood 24 hours after drug administration. During administration of 160 mg Trimethoprim and 800 mg Sulfamethoxazole b.i.d. the mean steady state plasma concentration of Trimethoprim was 1.72 µg/mL. The steady state minimal plasma levels of free and total Sulfamethoxazole were 57.4 µg/mL and 68.0 µg/mL, respectively. These steady state levels were achieved after three days of drug administration.[1]

Following a one-hour intravenous infusion of a single dose of 160 mg Trimethoprim and 800 mg Sulfamethoxazole to 11 patients whose weight ranged from 105 lbs. to 165 lbs. (mean, 143 lbs.), the mean peak plasma concentrations of Trimethoprim and Sulfamethoxazole were 3.4 ± 0.3 µg/mL and 46.3 ± 2.7 µg/mL, respectively. Following repeated intravenous administration of the same dose at eight-hour intervals, the mean plasma concentrations just prior to and immediately after each infusion at steady state were 5.6 ± 0.6 µg/mL and 8.8 ± 0.9 µg/mL for Trimethoprim and 70.6 ± 7.3 µg/mL and 105.6 ± 10.9 µg/mL for Sulfamethoxazole. The mean plasma half-life was 11.3 ± 0.7 hours for Trimethoprim and 12.8 ± 1.8 hours for Sulfamethoxazole. All of these 11 patients had normal renal function and their ages ranged from 17 to 78 years (median, 60 years).[6]

Pharmacokinetic studies in children and adults suggest an age-dependent half-life of Trimethoprim as indicated in the following table.[7]

Age (years)	No. of Patients	Mean Trimethoprim Half-life (hours)
< 1	2	7.67
1-10	9	5.49
10-20	5	8.19
20-63	6	12.82

Excretion of Sulfamethoxazole and Trimethoprim is primarily by the kidneys through both glomerular filtration and tubular secretion. Urine concentrations of both Sulfamethoxazole and Trimethoprim are considerably higher than are the concentrations in the blood. The average percentage of the dose recovered in urine from 0 to 72 hours after a single oral dose is 84.5% for total sulfonamide and 66.8% for free Trimethoprim. Thirty percent of the total sulfonamide is excreted as free Sulfamethoxazole, with the remaining as N_4-acetylated metabolite.[2] The percent of dose excreted in urine over a 12-hour period following the intravenous administration of the first dose of 240 mg of Trimethoprim and 1200 mg of Sulfamethoxazole on day 1 ranged from 17% to 42.4% as free Trimethoprim; 7% to 12.7% as free Sulfamethoxazole; and 36.7% to 56% as total (free plus the N_4-acetylated metabolite) Sulfamethoxazole. When administered together, neither Sulfamethoxazole nor Trimethoprim affects the urinary excretion pattern of the other.

Both Trimethoprim and Sulfamethoxazole distribute to sputum, vaginal fluid, and middle ear fluid; Trimethoprim also distributes to bronchial secretion and both pass the placental barrier and are excreted in human milk.

Microbiology: Sulfamethoxazole inhibits bacterial synthesis of dihydrofolic acid by competing with *para*-aminobenzoic acid (PABA). Trimethoprim blocks the production of tetrahydrofolic acid from dihydrofolic acid by binding to and reversibly inhibiting the required enzyme, dihydrofolate reductase. Thus, Sulfamethoxazole/Trimethoprim blocks two consecutive steps in the biosynthesis of nucleic acids and proteins essential to many bacteria.

In vitro studies have shown that bacterial resistance develops more slowly with Sulfomethoxazole/Trimethoprim than with either Trimethoprim or Sulfamethoxazole alone.

In vitro serial dilution tests have shown that the spectrum of antibacterial activity of Sulfomethoxazole/Trimethoprim includes the common urinary tract pathogens with the exception of *Pseudomonas aeruginosa*. The following organisms are usually susceptible: *Escherichia coli*, *Klebsiella* species, *Enterobacter* species, *Morganella morganii*, *Proteus mirabilis* and indole-positive *Proteus* species including *Proteus vulgaris*.

The usual spectrum of antimicrobial activity of Sulfamethazole/Trimethoprim includes bacterial pathogens isolated from middle ear exudate and from bronchial secretions (*Haemophilus influenzae*, including ampicillin-resistant strains, and *Streptococcus pneumoniae*), and enterotoxigenic strains of *Escherichia coli* (ETEC) causing bacterial gastroenteritis. *Shigella flexneri* and *Shigella sonnei* are also usually susceptible. It should be noted, however, that there are little clinical data on the use of Sulfamethoxazole/Trimethoprim I.V. Infusion in serious systemic infections due to *Haemophilus influenzae* and *Streptococcus pneumoniae*. (See related table.)

Susceptibility Testing: The recommended quantitative disc susceptibility method may be used for estimating the susceptibility of bacteria to Sulfamethoxazole/Trimethoprim.[3,4] With this procedure, a report from the laboratory of "Susceptible to Trimethoprim and Sulfamethoxazole" indicates that the infection is likely to respond to therapy with Sulfamethoxazole/Trimethoprim. If the infection is confined to the urine, a report of "Intermediate susceptibility to Trimethoprim and Sulfamethoxazole" also indicates that the infection is likely to respond. A report of "Resistant to Trimethoprim and Sulfamethoxazole" indicates that the infection is unlikely to respond to therapy with Sulfamethoxazole/Trimethoprim.

INDICATIONS AND USAGE
Urinary Tract Infections (Oral and Parenteral): For the treatment of urinary tract infections due to susceptible strains of the following organisms: *Escherichia coli*, *Klebsiella* species, *Enterbacter* species, *Morganella morganii*, *Proteus mirabilis*, and *Proteus vulgaris*. It is recommended that initial episodes of uncomplicated urinary tract infections be treated with a single effective antibacterial agent rather than the combination.

Sulfamethoxazole/Trimethoprim I.V. Infusion is indicated when oral administration of Sulfamethoxazole/Trimethoprim is not feasible and when the organism is not susceptible to single agent antibacterials effective in the urinary tract.

Acute Otitis Media (Oral): For the treatment of acute otitis media in children due to susceptible strains of *Streptococcus pneumoniae* or *Haemophilus influenzae* when in the judgment of the physician Sulfamethoxazole/Trimethoprim offers some advantage over the use of other antimicrobial agents. To date, there are limited data on the safety of repeated use of Sulfamethoxazole/Trimethoprim in children under two years of age Sulfamethoxazole/Triemthoprim is not indicated for prophylactic or prolonged administration in otitis media at any age.

Acute Exacerbations of Chronic Bronchitis in Adults (Oral): For the treatment of acute exacerbations of chronic bronchitis due to susceptible strains of *Streptococ-*

cus pneumoniae or Haemophilus influenzae when in the judgment of the physician, Sulfamethoxazole/Trimethoprim offers some advantage over the use of a single antimicrobial agent.

Travelers' Diarrhea in Adults (Oral): For the treatment of travelers' diarrhea due to susceptible strains of enterotoxigenic E. coli.

Shigellosis (Oral and Parenteral): For the treatment of enteritis caused by susceptible strains of Shigella flexneri and Shigella sonnei when antibacterial therapy is indicated.

Pneumocystis Carinii Pneumonia (Oral and parenteral): For the treatment of documented pneumocystis carinii pneumonia.

The oral forms are also indicated for prophylaxis against Pneumocystis carinii pneumonia in individuals who are immunosuppressed and considered to be at an increased risk of developing Pneumocystis carinii pneumonia.

Although appropriate culture and susceptibility studies should be performed, therapy may be started while awaiting the results of these studies.

CONTRAINDICATIONS
Sulfamethoxazole/Trimethoprim is contraindicated in patients with a known hypersensitivity to Trimethoprim or sulfonamides, and in patients with documented megaloblastic anemia due to folate deficiency. Sulfamethoxazole/Trimethoprim is also contraindicated in pregnant patients at term and in nursing mothers, because sulfonamides pass the placenta and are excreted in the milk and may cause kernicterus. Sulfamethoxazole/Trimethoprim is contraindicated in infants less than two months of age.

WARNINGS
FATALITIES ASSOCIATED WITH THE ADMINISTRATION OF SULFONAMIDES, ALTHOUGH RARE, HAVE OCCURRED DUE TO SEVERE REACTIONS, INCLUDING STEVENS-JOHNSON SYNDROME, TOXIC EPIDERMAL NECROLYSIS, FULMINANT HEPATIC NECROSIS, AGRANULOCYTOSIS, APLASTIC ANEMIA, OTHER BLOOD DYSCRASIAS AND HYPERSENSITIVITY OF THE RESPIRATORY TRACT.

SEPTRA SHOULD BE DISCONTINUED AT THE FIRST APPEARANCE OF SKIN RASH OR ANY SIGN OF ADVERSE REACTION. Clinical signs, such as rash, sore throat, fever, arthralgia, cough, shortness of breath, pallor, purpura, or jaundice may be early indications of serious reactions. Cough, shortness of breath, and/or pulmonary infiltrates may be indicators of pulmonary hypersensitivity to sulfonamides. In rare instances a skin rash may be followed by more severe reactions, such as Stevens-Johnson syndrome, toxic epidermal necrolysis, hepatic necrosis, or serious blood disorder. Complete blood counts should be done frequently in patients receiving sulfonamides.

Sulfamethoxazole/Trimethoprim Should Not Be Used in the Treatment of Streptococcal Pharyngitis: Clinical studies have documented that patients with group A β-hemolytic streptococcal tonsillopharyngitis have a greater incidence of bacteriologic failure when treated with Sulfamethoxazole/Trimethoprim than do those patients treated with penicillin, as evidenced by failure to eradicate this organism from the tonsillopharyngeal area.

Some brands contain sodium metabisulfite, a sulfite that may cause allergic-type reactions including anaphylactic symptoms and life-threatening or less severe asthmatic episodes in certain susceptible people. The overall prevalence of sulfite sensitivity in the general population is unknown and probably low. Sulfite sensitivity is seen more frequently in asthmatic than in nonasthmatic people.

Some brands contain benzyl alcohol. In newborn infants, benzyl alcohol has been associated with an increased incidence of neurological and other complications which are sometimes fatal.

PRECAUTIONS
General: Sulfamethoxazole/Trimethoprim should be given with caution to patients with impaired renal or hepatic function, to those with possible folate deficiency (e.g., the elderly, chronic alcoholics, patients receiving anticonvulsant therapy, patients with malabsorption syndrome, and patients in malnutrition states), and to those with severe allergy or bronchial asthma. In glucose-6-phosphate dehydrogenase-deficient individuals, hemolysis may occur. This

reaction is frequently dose-related. (See "Clinical Pharmacology" and "Dosage and Administration").

Local irritation and inflammation due to extravascular infiltration of the infusion has been observed with Sulfamethoxazole/Trimethoprim I.V. Infusion. If these occur the infusion should be discontinued and restarted at another site.

Use In the Elderly: There may be an increased risk of severe adverse reactions in elderly patients, particularly when complicating conditions exist, e.g., impaired kidney and/or liver function, or concomitant use of other drugs. Severe skin reactions or generalized bone marrow suppression (see "Warnings" and "Adverse Reactions" sections), or a specific decrease in platelets (with or without purpura) are the most frequently reported severe adverse reactions in elderly patients. In those concurrently receiving certain diuretics, primarily thiazides, an increased incidence of thrombocytopenia with purpura has been reported. Appropriate dosage adjustments should be made for patients with impaired kidney function (see "Dosage and Administration" section).

Use in the Treatment of and Prophylaxis (Oral) for Pneumocystis carinii *Pneumonia in Patients with Acquired Immunodeficiency Syndrome (AIDS):* The incidence of side effects, particularly rash, fever, leukopenia, elevated aminotransferase (transaminase) values, hypokalemia, and hyponatremia in AIDS patients who are being treated with Sulfamethoxazole/Trimethoprim for *Pneumocystis carinii* pneumonia has been reported to be greatly increased compared with the incidence normally associated with the use of Sulfamethoxazole/Trimethoprim in non-AIDS patients. Adverse effects are generally less severe in patients receiving Sulfamethoxazole/Trimethoprim for prophylaxis. A history of mild intolerance to Sulfamethoxazole/Trimethoprim in AIDS patients does not appear to predict intolerance of subsequent secondary prophylaxis. However, if a patient develops skin rash or any sign of adverse reaction, therapy with Sulfamethoxazole/Trimethoprim should be re-evaluated (see "Warnings").

Information for Patients: Patients should be instructed to maintain an adequate fluid intake in order to prevent crystalluria and stone formation.

Laboratory Tests: Appropriate culture and susceptibility studies should be performed before and throughout treatment. Complete blood counts should be done frequently in patients receiving Sulfamethoxazole/Trimethoprim; if a significant reduction in the count of any formed blood element is noted, Sulfamethoxazole/Trimethoprim should be discontinued. Urinalysis with careful microscopic examination and renal function tests should be performed during therapy, particularly for those patients with impaired renal function.

Drug Interactions: In elderly patients concurrently receiving certain diuretics, primarily thiazides, an increased incidence of thrombocytopenia with purpura has been reported. It has been reported that Sulfamethoxazole/Trimethoprim may prolong the prothrombin time in patients who are receiving the anticoagulant warfarin. This interaction should be kept in mind when Sulfamethoxazole/Trimethoprim is given to patients already on anticoagulant therapy, and the coagulation time should be reassessed.

Sulfamethoxazole/Trimethoprim may inhibit the hepatic metabolism of phenytoin. Sulfamethoxazole/Trimethoprim given at a common clinical dosage, increased the phenytoin half-life by 39% and decreased the phenytoin metabolic clearance rate by 27%. When administering these drugs concurrently, one should be alert for possible excessive phenytoin effect.

Sulfonamides can also displace methotrexate from plasma protein binding sites, thus increasing free methotrexate concentrations.

Drug/Laboratory Test Interactions: Sulfamethoxazole/Trimethoprim, specifically the Trimethoprim component, can interfere with a serum methotrexate assay as determined by the competitive binding protein technique (CBPA) when a bacterial dihydrofolate reductase is used as the binding protein. No interference occurs, however, if methotrexate is measured by a radioimmunoassay (RIA).

The presence of Trimethoprim and Sulfamethoxazole may also interfere with the Jaff alkaline picrate reaction assay for creatinine resulting in over-estimations of about 10% in the range of normal values.

Carcinogenesis: Long-term studies in animals to evaluate carcinogenic potential have not been conducted with Sulfamethoxazole/Trimethoprim.

REPRESENTATIVE MINIMUM INHIBITORY CONCENTRATION VALUES FOR ORGANISMS SUSCEPTIBLE TO SEPTRA (MIC.µg/mL)

Bacteria	TMP Alone	SMX Alone	TMP/SMX (1:19) TMP	SMX
Escherichia coli	0.05-1.5	1.0-245	0.05-0.5	0.95-9.5
Escherichia coli (enterotoxigenic strains)	0.015-0.15	0.285-> 950	0.005-0.15	0.095-2.85
Proteus species (indole positive)	0.5-5.0	7.35-300	0.05-1.5	0.95-28.5
Morganella morganii	0.5-5.0	7.35-300	0.05-1.5	0.95-28.5
Proteus mirabilis	0.5-1.5	7.35-30	0.05-0.15	0.95-2.85
Klebsiella species	0.15-5.0	2.45-245	0.05-1.5	0.95-28.5
Enterobacter species	0.15-5.0	2.45-245	0.05-1.5	0.95-28.5
Haemophilus Influezae	0.15-1.5	2.85-95	0.015-0.15	0.285-2.85
Streptococcus pneumoniae	0.15-1.5	7.35-24.5	0.05-0.15	0.95-2.85
Shigella flexneri†	< 0.01-0.04	< 0.16-> 320	< 0.002-0.03	0.04-0.625
Shigella sonei†	0.02-0.08	0.625-> 320	0.004-0.06	0.08-1.25

TMP = Trimethoprim SMX = Sulfamethoxazole
† Rudoy RC, Nelson JD, Haltalin KC, Antimicrobial Agents and Chemotherapy. 1974; 5:439-443.

◆ RATED THERAPEUTICALLY EQUIVALENT; ◇ THERAPEUTIC EQUIVALENCE UNCONFIRMED; ○ UNRATED

Mutagenesis: Bacterial mutagenic studies have not been performed with Sulfamethoxazole and Trimethoprim in combination. Trimethoprim was demonstrated to be non-mutagenic in the Ames assay. In studies at two laboratories no chromosomal damage was detected in cultured Chinese hamster ovary cells at concentrations approximately 500 times human plasma levels; at concentrations approximately 1000 times human plasma levels in these same cells a low level of chromosomal damage was induced at one of the laboratories. No chromosomal abnormalities were observed in cultured human leukocytes at concentrations of Trimethoprim up to 20 times human steady state plasma levels. No chromosomal effects were detected in peripheral lymphocytes of human subjects receiving 320 mg of Trimethoprim in combination with up to 1600 mg of Sulfamethoxazole per day for as long as 112 weeks.

Impairment of Fertility: No adverse effects on fertility or general reproductive performance were observed in rats given oral dosages as high as 70 mg/kg/day Trimethoprim plus 350 mg/kg/day Sulfamethoxazole. Sulfamethoxazole/Trimethoprim I.V. infusion has not been studied in animals for evidence of impairment of fertility.

Pregnancy: Teratogenic Effects: Pregnancy Category C. In rats, oral doses of 533 mg/kg Sulfamethoxazole or 200 mg/kg Trimethoprim produced teratological effects manifested mainly as cleft palates. The highest dose which did not cause cleft palates in rats was 512 mg/kg Sulfamethoxazole or 192 mg/kg Trimethoprim when administered separately. In two studies in rats, no teratology was observed when 512 mg/kg of Sulfamethoxazole was used in combination with 128 mg/kg of Trimethoprim. In one study, however, cleft palates were observed in one litter out of 9 when 355 mg/kg of Sulfamethoxazole was used in combination with 88 mg/kg of Trimethoprim.

In some rabbit studies, an overall increase in fetal loss (dead and resorbed and malformed conceptuses) was associated with doses of Trimethoprim 6 times the human therapeutic dose.

While there are no large, well-controlled studies on the use of Trimethoprim and Sulfamethoxazole in pregnant women, Brumfitt and Pursell,[5] in a retrospective study, reported the outcome of 186 pregnancies during which the mother received either placebo or oral Trimethoprim and Sulfamethoxazole. The incidence of congenital abnormalities was 4.5% (3 of 66) in those who received placebo and 3.3% (4 of 120) in those receiving Trimethoprim and Sulfamethoxazole. There were no abnormalities in the 10 children whose mothers received the drug during the first trimester. In a separate survey, Brumfitt and Pursell also found no congenital abnormalities in 35 children whose mothers had received oral Trimethoprim and Sulfamethoxazole at the time of conception or shortly thereafter.

Because Trimethoprim and Sulfamethoxazole may interfere with folic acid metabolism, Sulfamethoxazole/Trimethoprim should be used during pregnancy only if the potential benefit justifies the potential risk to the fetus.

Nonteratogenic Effects: see *"Contraindications"* sections.

Nursing Mothers: see *"Contraindications"* sections.

Pediatric use: Sulfomethoxazole/Trimethoprim is not recommended for infants younger than two months of age (see *"Indications And Usage"* and *"Contraindications"* sections).

ADVERSE REACTIONS

The most common adverse effects are gastrointestinal disturbances (nausea, vomiting, anorexia) and allergic skin reactions (such as rash and urticaria). **FATALITIES ASSOCIATED WITH THE ADMINISTRATION OF SULFONAMIDES, ALTHOUGH RARE, HAVE OCCURRED DUE TO SEVERE REACTIONS, INCLUDING STEVENS-JOHNSON SYNDROME, TOXIC EPIDERMAL NECROLYSIS, FULMINANT HEPATIC NECROSIS, AGRANULOCYTOSIS, APLASTIC ANEMIA, OTHER BLOOD DYSCRASIA AND HYPERSENSITIVITY OF THE RESPIRATORY TRACT** (see *"Warnings Sections"*). Local reaction, pain, and slight irritation on I.V. administration are infrequent. Thrombophlebitis has rarely been observed.

Hematologic: Agranulocytosis, aplastic anemia, thrombocytopenia, leukopenia, neutropenia, hemolytic anemia, megaloblastic anemia, hypoprothrombinemia, methemoglobinemia, eosinophilia.

Allergic: Stevens-Johnson syndrome, toxic epidermal necrolysis, anaphylaxis, allergic myocarditis, erythema multiforme, exfoliative dermatitis, angioedema, drug fever, chills, Henoch-Schoenlein purpura, serum sickness-like syndrome, generalized allergic reactions, generalized skin eruptions, photosensitivity, conjunctival and scleral injection, pruritus, urticaria and rash. In addition, periarteritis nodosa, and systemic lupus erythematosus have been reported.

Gastrointestinal: Hepatitis including cholesterol jaundice and hepatic necrosis, evaluation of serum transaminase and bilirubin, pseudomembranous enterocolitis, pancreatitis, stomatitis, glossitis, nausea, emesis, abdominal pain, diarrhea, anorexia.

Genitourinary: Renal failure, interstitial nephritis, BUN and serum creatinine elevation, toxic nephrosis with oliguria and anuria, and crystalluria.

Metabolic: Hyperkalemia, hyponatremia (see *"Precautions: Use in the Treatment and Prophylaxis (Oral) of Pneumocystis carinii Pneumonia in Patients with Acquired Immunodeficiency Syndrome"*).

Neurologic: Aseptic meningitis, convulsions, peripheral neuritis, ataxia, vertigo, tinnitus, headache.

Psychiatric: Hallucinations, depression, apathy, nervousness.

Endocrine: The sulfonamides bear certain chemical similarities to some goitrogens, diuretics (acetazolamide and the thiazides), and oral hypoglycemic agents. Cross-sensitivity may exist with these agents. Diuresis and hypoglycemia have occurred rarely in patients receiving sulfonamides.

Musculoskeletal: Arthralgia and myalgia.

Respiratory System: Pulmonary infiltrates, cough, shortness of breath.

Miscellaneous: Weakness, fatigue, insomnia.

OVERDOSAGE

Acute: The amount of a single dose of Sulfomethazole/Trimethoprim that is either associated with symptoms of overdosage or is likely to be life-threatening has not been reported. Since there has been no extensive experience in humans with single doses of Sulfamethoxazole Trimethoprim I.V. Infusion in excess of 25 mL (400 mg Trimethoprim and 2000 mg Sulfamethoxazole), the maximum tolerated dose in humans is unknown. Signs and symptoms of overdosage reported with sulfonamides include anorexia, colic, nausea, vomiting, dizziness, headache, drowsiness and unconsciousness. Pyrexia, hematuria, and crystalluria may be noted. Blood dyscrasias and jaundice are potential late manifestations of overdosage. Signs of acute overdosage with trimethoprim include nausea, vomiting, dizziness, headache, mental depression, confusion, and bone marrow depression. General principles of treatment include the institution of gastric lavage or emesis: forcing oral fluids: and the administration of intravenous fluids if urine output is low and renal function is normal. Acidification of the urine will increase renal elimination of Trimethoprim. The patient should be monitored with blood counts and appropriate blood chemistries, including electrolytes. If a significant blood dyscrasia or jaundice occurs, specific therapy should be instituted for these complications. Peritoneal dialysis is not effective and hemodialysis is only moderately effective in eliminating Trimethoprim and Sulfamethoxazole.

Chronic: Use of Sulfamethoxazole/Trimethoprim at high doses and/or for extended periods of time may cause bone marrow depression manifested as thrombocytopenia, leukopenia and/or megaloblastic anemia. If signs of bone marrow depression occur, the patient should be given leucovorin; 5 to 15 mg leucovorin daily has been recommended by some investigators.

Animal Toxicity: The LD_{50} of Sulfamethoxazole/Trimethoprim I.V. Infusion in mice is 700 mg/kg or 7.3 mL/kg; in rats and rabbits the LD_{50} is > 500 mg/kg or > 5.2 mL/kg. The vehicle produced the same LD_{50} in each of these species as the active drug.

The signs and symptoms noted in mice, rats and rabbits with Sulfamethoxazole/Trimethoprim I.V. Infusion or its vehicle at the high I.V. doses used in acute toxicity studies included ataxia, decreased motor activity, loss of righting reflex, tremors or convulsions, and/or respiratory depression.

DOSAGE AND ADMINISTRATION

ORAL SULFAMETHOXAZOLE/TRIMETHOPRIM:
Not recommended for use in infants less than two months of age.

URINARY TRACT INFECTIONS AND SHIGELLOSIS IN ADULTS AND CHILDREN AND ACUTE OTITIS MEDIA IN CHILDREN
Adults: The usual adult dosage in the treatment of urinary tract infections is one Sulfamethoxazole/Trimethoprim DS (double strength) tablet, two Sulfamethoxazole/Trimethoprim tablets or four teaspoonfuls (20 mL) Sulfamethoxazole/Trimethoprim Suspension every 12 hours for 10 to 14 days. An identical daily dosage is used for 5 days in the treatment of shigellosis.

Children: The recommended dose for children with urinary tract infections or acute otitis media is 8 mg/kg Trimethoprim and 40 mg/kg Sulfamethoxazole per 24 hours, given in two divided doses every 12 hours for 10 days. An identical daily dosage is used for 5 days in the treatment of shigellosis. The following table is a guideline for the attainment of this dosage:

Children: Two months of age or older:

| Weight | | | Dose-every 12 hours | |
lb	kg		Teaspoonfuls	Tablets
22	10		1 (5 mL)	
44	20		2 (10 mL)	1
66	30		3 (15 mL)	1 ½
88	40		4 (20 mL)	2 (or 1 DS Tablet)

For Patients with Impaired Renal Function: When renal function is impaired, a reduced dosage should be employed using the following table:

Creatinine Clearance (mL/min)	Recommended Dosage Regimen
Above 30	Use Standard Regimen
15-30	½ the Usual Regimen
Below 15	Use Not Recommended

ACUTE EXACERBATIONS OF CHRONIC BRONCHITIS IN ADULTS
The usual adult dosage in the treatment of acute exacerbations of chronic bronchitis is one Sulfamethoxazole/Trimethoprim DS (double strength) tablet,

two Sulfamethoxazole/Trimethoprim tablets or four teaspoonfuls (20 mL) Sulfamethoxazole/Trimethoprim Suspension every 12 hours for 14 days.

TRAVELERS' DIARRHEA IN ADULTS

For the treatment of travelers' diarrhea, the usual adult dosage is one Sulfamethoxazole/Trimethoprim DS (double strength) tablet, two Sulfamethoxazole/Trimethoprim tablets or four teaspoonfuls (20 mL) of Sulfamethoxazole/Trimethoprim Suspension every 12 hours for 5 days.

PNEUMOCYSTIS CARINII PNEUMONIA

Treatment: Adults and Children: The recommended dosage for treatment of patients with documented *Pneumocystis carinii* pneumonia is 15 to 20 mg/kg Trimethoprim and 75 to 100 mg/kg Sulfamethoxazole per 24 hours given in equally divided doses every 6 hours for 14 to 21 days. The following table is a guideline for the upper limit of this dosage:

Weight		Dose-every 6 hours	
lb	kg	Teaspoonfuls	Tablets
18	8	1 (5 mL)	
35	16	2 (10 mL)	1
53	24	3 (15 mL)	1 ½
70	32	4 (20 mL)	2 (or 1 DS Tablet)
88	40	5 (25 mL)	2 ½
106	48	6 (30 mL)	3 (or 1 ½ DS Tablets)
141	64	8 (40 mL)	4 (or 2 DS Tablets)
176	80	10 (50 mL)	5 (or 2 ½ DS Tablets)

For the lower limit dose (15 mg/kg Trimethoprim and 75 mg/kg Sulfamethoxazole per 24 hours) administer 75% of the dose in the above table.

PROPHYLAXIS

Adults: The recommended dosage for prophylaxis in adults is one Sulfamethoxazole/Trimethoprim DS (double strength) tablet daily.

Children: For children, the recommended dose is 150 mg/m² day Trimethoprim with 750 mg/m²/day Sulfamethoxazole given orally in equally divided doses twice a day, on 3 consecutive days per week. The total daily dose: should not exceed 320 mg Trimethoprim and 1600 mg Sulfamethoxazole. The following table is a guideline for the attainment of this dosage in children:

	Dose—every 12 hours	
Body Surface Area (m²)	Teaspoonfuls	Tablets
0.26	1/2 (2.5 mL)	
0.53	1 (5 mL)	1/2
1.06	2 (10 mL)	1

SULFAMETHOXAZOLE/TRIMETHOPRIM I.V. INFUSION

Contraindicated in infants less than two months of age. *Caution—Sulfmethoxazole/Trimethoprim I.V. infusion must be diluted in 5% Dextrose in Water solution prior to administration. Do not mix Sulfamethoxazole/Trimethoprim I.V. infusion with other drugs or solutions. Rapid infusion or bolus injection must be avoided.*

CHILDREN AND ADULTS

Pneumocystis Carinii Pneumonia: Total daily dose is 15 to 20 mg/kg (based on the Trimethoprim component) given in three to four equally divided doses every 6 to 8 hours for up to 14 days. One investigator noted that a total daily dose of 10 to 15 mg/kg was sufficient in 10 adult patients with normal renal function.[9]

Severe Urinary Tract Infections and Shigellosis: Total daily dose is 8 to 10 mg/kg (based on the Trimethoprim component) given in two to four equally divided doses every 6, 8 or 12 hours for up to 14 days for severe urinary tract infections and 5 days for shigellosis. The maximum recommended daily dose is 60 mL per day.

METHOD OF PREPARATION

Sulfamethoxazole/Trimethoprim I.V. infusion must be diluted. *Each 5 mL should be added to 125 mL of 5% Dextrose in water. Each 10 mL vial should be added to 250 mL of 5% Dextrose in Water and used within six (6) hours.* After diluting with 5% dextrose in water the solution should not be refrigerated and should be used within 6 hours, or the specified time. If a dilution of 5 mL per 100 mL of 5% Dextrose in Water is desired, it should be used within 4 hours. If upon visual inspection there is cloudiness or evidence of crystallization after mixing, the solution should be discarded and a fresh solution prepared.

Multiple Dose Vial: After initial entry into the vial, the remaining contents must be used within 48 hours.

The following infusion systems have been tested and found satisfactory: unit-dose glass containers; unit-dose polyvinyl chloride and polyolefin containers. No other systems have been tested and therefore no others can be recommended.

Dilution: Each 5 mL of Sulfamethoxazole/Trimethoprim I.V. infusion should be added to 125 mL of 5% Dextrose in Water.

Note: In those instances where fluid restriction is desirable, each 5 mL may be added to 75 mL of 5% Dextrose in Water. Under these circumstances the solution should be mixed just prior to use and should be administered within two (2) hours. If upon visual inspection there is cloudiness or evidence of crystallization after mixing, the solution should be discarded and a fresh solution prepared.

Do not mix Sulfamethoxazole/Trimethoprim I.V. infusion-5% Dextrose in Water with drugs or solutions in the same container.

ADMINISTRATION

The solution should be given by intravenous infusions over a period of 60 to 90 minutes. Rapid infusion or bolus injections must be avoided. Sulfamethoxazole/Trimethoprim I.V. Infusion should not be given intramuscularly.

INSTRUCTIONS FOR USE - VIALS

To Open Diluent Container: Peel overwrap from the corner and remove container. Some opacity of the plastic due to moisture absorption during the sterilization process may be observed. This is normal and does not affect the solution quality or safety. The opacity will diminish gradually.

To Assemble Vial and Flexible Diluent Container: (Use Aseptic Technique):
  1. Remove the protective covers from the top of the vial and the vial port on the diluent container as follows:
    a. To remove the breakaway vial cap, swing the pull ring over the top of the vial and pull down far enough to start the opening, then pull straight up to remove the cap. *Note:* Once the breakaway cap has been removed, do not access vial with syringe.
    b. To remove the vial port cover, grasp the tab on the pull ring, pull up to break the three tie strings, then pull back to remove the cover.
  2. Screw the vial into the vial port until it will go no further. *The vial must be screwed in tightly to assure a seal.* This occurs approximately ½ turn (180°) after the first audible click. The clicking sound does not assure a seal; the vial must be turned as far as it will go. *Note:* Once vial is seated, do not attempt to remove.
  3. Recheck the vial to assure that it is tight by trying to turn it further in the direction of assembly.
  4. Label appropriately.

To Prepare Admixture:
  1. Squeeze the bottom of the diluent container gently to inflate the portion of the container surrounding the end of the drug vial.
  2. With the other hand, push the drug vial down into the container telescoping the walls of the container. Grasp the inner cap of the vial through the walls of the container.
  3. Pull the inner cap from the drug vial. Verify that the rubber stopper has been pulled out, allowing the drug and diluent to mix.
  Mix contents thoroughly and use within the specified time.

Preparation for Administration: (Use Aseptic Technique):
  1. Confirm the activation and admixture of vial contents.
  2. Check for leaks by squeezing container firmly. If leaks are found, discard unit as sterility may be impaired.
  3. Close flow control clamp of administration set.
  4. Remove cover from outlet port at bottom of container.
  5. Insert piercing pin of administration set into port with a twisting motion until the pin is firmly seated. *Note:* See full directions on administration set carton.
  6. Lift the free end of the hanger loop on the bottom of the vial, breaking the two tie strings. Bend the loop outward to lock it in the upright position, then suspend container from hanger.
  7. Squeeze and release drip chamber to establish proper fluid level in chamber.
  8. Open flow control clamp and clear air from set. Close clamp.
  9. Attach set to venipuncture device. If device is not indwelling, prime and make venipuncture.
  10. Regulate rate of administration with flow control clamp.

Warning: Do not use flexible container in series connections.

STORAGE

Tablets should be stored at 15° to 25°C (59°-77°F) in a dry place and protected from light.

Suspension should be stored at 15° to 25°C (59°-77°F) and protected from light.

REFERENCES

1. Kremers P, Duvivier J, Heusghem C. Pharmacokinetic studies of co-trimoxazole in man after single and repeated doses. *J Clin Pharmacol.* 1974; 14:112-117. 2. Kaplan SA, Weinfeld RE, Abruzzo CW, McFaden K, Jack ML, Weissman L. Pharmacokinetic profile of trimethoprim-sulfamethoxazole in man. *J Infect Dis.* November 1973; 128(suppl):S547-S555. 3. Antibiotic susceptibility discs: certification procedure. Fed Reg. 37:20527-20529, 1972. 4. Bauer AW, Kirby WMM, Sherris JC, Turck M. Antibiotic susceptibility testing by standardized single disk method. *Am J Clin Pathol.* 1966; 45:493-496. 5. Brumfitt W, Pursell R. Trimethoprim-sulfamethoxazole in the treatment of bacteriuria in women. *J Infect Dis.* November 1973; 128(suppl):S657-S663. 6. Grose WE, Bodey GP, Loo TL. Clinical pharmacology of intravenously administered trimethoprim-sulfamethoxazole. *Antimicrob Agents Chemother.* 1979:15:447-451. 7. Siber GR, Gorham C, Durbin W, Lesko L, Levin MJ, Pharmacology of intravenous trimethoprim-sulfamethoxazole in children and adults. In: Nelson JD, Grassi C, eds. *Current Chemotherapy of Infectious Disease.* Washington, DC: American Society for Microbiology; 1980:1:691-692. 8. National Committee for Clinical Laboratory Standards, Performance standards for antimicrobial disk susceptibility tests. 2nd ed. Villanova, PA, 1979. 9. Winston DJ, Lau WK, Gale RP, Young LS. Trimethoprim-sulfamethoxazole for the treatment of *Pneumocystis carinii* pneumonia. *Ann Intern Med.* 1980:92:762-769.

HOW SUPPLIED
INJECTION: 80 MG/ML-16 MG/ML

AVERAGE UNIT PRICE (AVAILABLE SIZES)		GENERIC A-RATED AVERAGE PRICE (GAAP)	
BRAND	$0.96	5 ml 10s	$50.51
GENERIC	$0.94	10 ml 10s	$94.46

BRAND/MANUFACTURER	NDC	SIZE	AWP
◆ BRAND			
BACTRIM I.V.: Roche Labs	00004-1958-01	30 ml	$42.51
SEPTRA I.V.: Burr Wellcome	00081-0856-44	5 ml 10s	$36.19
	00081-0856-95	10 ml 10s	$70.92
	00081-0856-47	10 ml 10s	$72.40
BACTRIM I.V.: Roche Labs	00004-1955-01	10 ml 10s	$152.48
SEPTRA I.V.: Burr Wellcome	00081-0856-01	20 ml 10s	$131.70
◆ GENERICS			
Elkins-Sinn	00641-2766-41	30 ml	$35.35
Gensia	00703-9526-01	30 ml	$15.15
Gensia	00703-9503-03	5 ml 10s	$27.88
Elkins-Sinn	00641-1532-33	5 ml 10s	$58.89
Elkins-Sinn	00641-2764-43	5 ml 10s	$64.75
Gensia	00703-9514-03	10 ml 10s	$62.00
Elkins-Sinn	00641-2765-43	10 ml 10s	$126.91

SUSPENSION: 200 MG-40 MG/5 ML

AVERAGE UNIT PRICE (AVAILABLE SIZES)		GENERIC A-RATED AVERAGE PRICE (GAAP)	
BRAND	$0.09	100 ml	$3.86
GENERIC	$0.03	480 ml	$11.33
HCFA FUL (100 ml)	$0.06	20 ml 50s	$55.42
HCFA FUL (480 ml)	$0.01		

BRAND/MANUFACTURER	NDC	SIZE	AWP
◆ BRAND			
SEPTRA: Burr Wellcome	00081-0854-96	480 ml	$40.81
	00081-0855-96	480 ml	$40.81
BACTRIM PEDIATRIC: Roche Labs	00004-1033-28	480 ml	$42.33
SEPTRA: Burr Wellcome	00081-0855-03	100 ml 6s	$51.74
	00081-0855-01	150 ml 6s	$77.64
	00081-0855-02	200 ml 6s	$103.50
◆ GENERICS			
Biocraft	00332-6100-32	100 ml	$3.76
SULFATRIM PEDIATRIC: Barre	00472-1285-33	100 ml	$3.95
Apothecon	00003-1201-10	473 ml	$11.27
SULFATRIM: Mason Dist	11845-0442-13	480 ml	$9.68
Raway	00686-6100-38	480 ml	$9.75
Schein	00364-2076-16	480 ml	$10.00
Geneva	00781-6062-16	480 ml	$10.30
Geneva	00781-6063-16	480 ml	$10.30
SULFATRIM: Mason Dist	11845-0443-13	480 ml	$10.42
Schein	00364-2077-16	480 ml	$10.73
Rugby	00536-1715-85	480 ml	$10.77
Major	00904-0406-16	480 ml	$10.80
Warner Chilcott	00047-2903-23	480 ml	$10.98
SULFATRIM SUSPENSION: URL	00677-0840-33	480 ml	$11.50
SULFATRIM PEDIATRIC: Qualitest	00603-1687-58	480 ml	$11.58
Rugby	00536-1725-85	480 ml	$11.62
SULFATRIM PEDIATRIC: Barre	00472-1285-16	480 ml	$11.65
Goldline	00182-1558-40	480 ml	$11.65
URL	00677-0841-33	480 ml	$11.70
Moore,H.L.	00839-6718-69	480 ml	$11.73
Moore,H.L.	00839-7709-69	480 ml	$11.73
Moore,H.L.	00839-6699-69	480 ml	$11.73
Major	00904-0405-16	480 ml	$11.95
Biocraft	00332-6100-38	480 ml	$12.04
Aligen	00405-3675-16	480 ml	$12.04
SULFATRIM: Qualitest	00603-1688-58	480 ml	$12.16
COTRIM PEDIATRIC: Lemmon	00093-0190-16	480 ml	$12.25
Lemmon	00093-0562-16	480 ml	$12.25
SULFATRIM: Barre	00472-1284-16	480 ml	$12.30
Goldline	00182-1559-40	480 ml	$12.30
UDL	51079-0638-20	20 ml 50s ud	$45.84
Raway	00686-0638-10	20 ml 50s ud	$65.00

TABLET: 400 MG-80 MG

AVERAGE UNIT PRICE (AVAILABLE SIZES)		GENERIC A-RATED AVERAGE PRICE (GAAP)	
BRAND	$0.71	100s	$18.93
GENERIC	$0.18	500s	$80.79
HCFA FUL (100s ea)	$0.07		

BRAND/MANUFACTURER	NDC	SIZE	AWP
◆ BRAND			
▶ SEPTRA: Burr Wellcome	00081-0852-55	100s	$70.00
▶ BACTRIM: Roche Labs	00004-0050-01	100s	$72.59
◆ GENERICS			
Raway	00686-2130-09	100s	$8.75
Roxane	00054-4800-25	100s	$12.14
Geneva	00781-1062-01	100s	$12.46
UROPLUS: Shionogi	45809-0910-11	100s	$12.69
Qualitest	00603-5778-21	100s	$12.70
Rugby	00536-4692-01	100s	$12.72

BRAND/MANUFACTURER	NDC	SIZE	AWP
Interpharm	53746-0271-01	100s	$12.85
Schein	00364-2068-01	100s	$13.81
Major	00904-2726-01	100s	$13.85
Martec	52555-0341-01	100s	$15.57
Moore,H.L.	00839-6487-06	100s	$16.88
URL	00677-0783-01	100s	$18.50
COTRIM: Lemmon	00093-0188-01	100s	$18.50
Lemmon	00093-0088-01	100s	$18.50
▶ Mutual	53489-0145-01	100s	$18.50
Biocraft	00332-2130-09	100s	$23.24
Goldline	00182-1478-01	100s	$23.24
Apothecon	00003-0138-50	100s	$23.42
Sidmak	50111-0341-01	100s	$24.00
Aligen	00405-4928-01	100s	$24.00
Parmed	00349-2364-01	100s	$25.00
U.S. Trading	56126-0139-11	100s ud	$7.92
Vangard	00615-0171-13	100s ud	$14.80
Raway	00686-0171-13	100s ud	$15.50
Roxane	00054-8800-25	100s ud	$16.70
Geneva	00781-1062-13	100s ud	$28.00
Medirex	57480-0436-01	100s ud	$28.00
Schein	00364-2068-90	100s ud	$37.95
Goldline	00182-8843-89	100s ud	$38.65
UROPLUS: Shionogi	45809-0910-12	500s	$55.94
Rugby	00536-4692-05	500s	$58.40
Major	00904-2726-40	500s	$58.40
Interpharm	53746-0271-05	500s	$60.00
Schein	00364-2068-05	500s	$63.51
URL	00677-0783-05	500s	$67.50
▶ Mutual	53489-0145-05	500s	$67.50
Parmed	00349-2364-05	500s	$71.64
COTRIM: Lemmon	00093-0188-05	500s	$83.50
Lemmon	00093-0088-05	500s	$83.50
Biocraft	00332-2130-13	500s	$104.59
Sidmak	50111-0341-02	500s	$106.00
Aligen	00405-4928-02	500s	$106.00
Lederle Std Prod	00005-3117-31	500s	$112.58
Apothecon	00003-0138-60	500s	$112.72

For additional alternatives, turn to the section beginning on page 2859.

For additional alternatives, turn to the section beginning on page 2859.

Sulfamylon Acetate *SEE* MAFENIDE ACETATE

Sulfanilamide

DESCRIPTION
Sulfanilamide is a preparation for vaginal administration for the treatment of *Candida albicans* infections and available in the following forms:

SULFANILAMIDE CREAM

Each tube contains:

Sulfanilamide 15.0%

SULFANILAMIDE SUPPOSITORIES

Each suppository contains:

Sulfanilamide .... 1.05 g

Sulfanilamide is an anti-infective agent. It is *p*-aminobenzene- sulfonamide.

Sulfanilamide occurs as a white odorless crystalline powder with a slightly bitter taste and sweet aftertaste. It is slightly soluble in water, alcohol, acetone, glycerin, propylene glycol, hydrochloric acid, and solutions of potassium and sodium hydroxide. It is practically insoluble in chloroform, ether, benzene, and petroleum ether.

Following is its chemical structure:

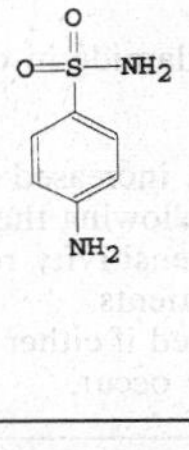

CLINICAL PHARMACOLOGY

Sulfanilamide has been a useful ingredient of vaginal formulations for about four decades. It blocks certain metabolic processes essential for the growth of susceptible bacteria. In Sulfanilamide, the Sulfanilamide is in a specifically compounded base buffered to the pH (about 4.3) of the normal vagina to encourage the presence of the normally occurring Döderlein's bacilli of the vagina.

The use of Sulfanilamide for the treatment of vulvovaginitis caused by *Candida albicans* is supported by three clinical investigations. The three studies show Sulfanilamide to be significantly more effective ($p \leq 0.01$) than placebo as follows:

In Study I, the ratio of effectiveness was 71% for the Sulfanilamide versus 49% for placebo with 30 days of treatment;
In Study II, the percentages were 48% and 24%, respectively, with 15 days of treatment;
In Study III, the percentages were 66% versus 33%, respectively, with 30 days of treatment.

INDICATIONS AND USAGE

For the treatment of vulvovaginitis caused by *Candida albicans*. (See *"Clinical Pharmacology"*.)

CONTRAINDICATIONS

Sulfanilamide should not be used in patients known to be sensitive to this product or to the sulfonamides.

PRECAUTIONS

GENERAL

Because sulfonamides are absorbed from the vaginal mucosa, the usual precautions for oral sulfonamides apply. Patients should be observed for skin rash or evidence of systemic toxicity, and if these develop, the medications should be discontinued.

Deaths associated with administration of oral sulfonamides have reportedly occurred from hypersensitivity reactions, agranulocytosis, aplastic anemia, and other blood dyscrasias. Goiter production, diuresis, and hypoglycemia have reportedly occurred rarely in patients receiving oral sulfonamides. Cross-sensitivity may exist with these agents. Rats appear to be especially susceptible to the goitrogenic effects of sulfonamides, and long-term administration has reportedly produced thyroid malignancies in this species.

Vaginal applicators or inserters should be used with caution after the seventh month of pregnancy.

INFORMATION FOR PATIENTS

The doctor should advise the patient that in the event unusual local itching and burning occur, or other unusual symptoms develop, medication should be discontinued and not re-started without further consultation.

DRUG INTERACTIONS

Drug interactions have not been documented with Sulfanilamide.

CARCINOGENESIS, MUTAGENESIS, IMPAIRMENT OF FERTILITY

No data are available on long-term potential of Sulfanilamide for carcinogenicity, mutagenicity, or impairment of fertility in animals or humans.

PREGNANCY TERATOGENIC EFFECTS

Pregnancy Category C: Animal reproductive studies have been conducted with sulfonamides, including Sulfanilamide (see below). It is not known whether Sulfanilamide can cause fetal harm when administered to a pregnant woman or can affect reproductive capacity. Sulfanilamide should be given to a pregnant woman only if clearly needed.

Sulfonamides, including Sulfanilamide, readily pass through the placenta and reach fetal circulation. The concentration in the fetus is from 50-90% of that in the maternal blood and if high enough, can cause toxic effects. The safe use of sulfonamides, including Sulfanilamide, in pregnancy has not been established. The teratogenic potential of most sulfonamides has not been thoroughly investigated in either animals or humans. However, a significant increase in the incidence of cleft palate and other bony abnormalities of offspring has been observed when certain sulfonamides of the short, intermediate, and long-acting types (including Sulfanilamide) were given to pregnant rats and mice at high oral doses (seven to 25 times the human therapeutic oral dose).

NURSING MOTHERS

Sulfanilamide should be avoided in nursing mothers because absorbed sulfonamides will appear in maternal milk, and have caused kernicterus in the newborn. Because of the potential for serious adverse reactions in nursing infants from sulfonamides, a decision should be made whether to discontinue nursing or to discontinue the drug.

PEDIATRIC USE

Safety and effectiveness of Sulfanilamide in children have not been established.

ADVERSE REACTIONS

Local sensitivity reactions such as increased discomfort or a burning sensation have occasionally been reported following the use of topical sulfonamides. With the use of Sulfanilamide Cream, sensitivity reactions (only local) were reported for 0.2% of the investigational patients.

Treatment should be discontinued if either local or systemic manifestations of sulfonamide toxicity or sensitivity occur.

DRUG ABUSE AND DEPENDENCE

Tolerance, abuse, or dependence with Sulfanilamide have not been reported.

OVERDOSAGE

There have been no reports of accidental overdosage with Sulfanilamide.
The acute oral LD_{50} of Sulfanilamide is 3700-4200 mg/kg in mice.
The minimum human lethal dose of Sulfanilamide has not been established.
It is not known if Sulfanilamide is dialyzable.

DOSAGE AND ADMINISTRATION

One applicatorful (about 6 g) or one suppository intravaginally once or twice daily. Improvements in symptoms should occur within a few days, but treatment should be continued for a period of 30 days.

Douching with a suitable solution before insertion may be recommended for hygienic purposes.

Sulfanilamide Cream and Suppositories: Store room temperature, below 86°F. Protect from cold and moisture.

HOW SUPPLIED
CREAM: 15%

BRAND/MANUFACTURER	NDC	SIZE	AWP
◆ BRAND			
AVC: Marion Merrell Dow	00068-0099-04	120 gm	$28.92

SUPPOSITORY:

BRAND/MANUFACTURER	NDC	SIZE	AWP
◆ BRAND			
AVC: Marion Merrell Dow	00068-0098-16	16s	$31.50

Sulfasalazine

DESCRIPTION

Sulfasalazine 500 mg enteric-coated tablets for oral administration are film coated with cellulose acetate phthalate to prevent disintegration of the tablet in the stomach and thus reduce possible irritation of the gastric mucosa.

Sulfasalazine tablets, 500 mg, for oral administration are also available.

Therapeutic Classification: Anti-inflammatory agent.

Chemical Designation: 5-([p-(2-Pyridylsulfamoyl) phenyl] azo) salicylic acid.

Following is its chemical structure:

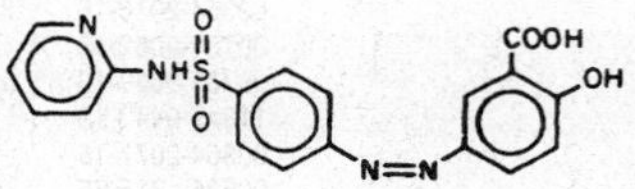

CLINICAL PHARMACOLOGY

After oral administration, Sulfasalazine is partially absorbed and extensively metabolized as described below.

About one-third of a given dose of Sulfasalazine (SS) is absorbed from the small intestine. The remaining two-thirds pass to the colon where the compound is split (presumably by intestinal bacteria) into its components, 5-aminosalicylic acid (5-ASA) and sulfapyridine (SP). Most of the SP thus liberated is absorbed whereas only about one-third of the 5-ASA is absorbed, the remainder being excreted in the feces. The distribution metabolism and excretion of SS and its two components are as follows:

SULFASALAZINE (ENTERIC-COATED TABLETS)

Sulfasalazine (SS): Detectable serum concentrations of SS have been found in healthy subjects within 90 minutes after the ingestion of a single 2 g dose of Sulfasalazine EN-tabs. Maximum concentrations of SS occur between 3 and 12 hours, with the mean peak concentration (6 mcg/ml) occurring at 6 hours. Small amounts of SS are excreted unchanged in the urine.

Sulfapyridine (SP): Following absorption and distribution, SP is acetylated and hydroxylated in the liver, and then conjugated with glucuronic acid. After ingestion of a single 2 g dose of Sulfasalazine by healthy subjects, peak concentrations of SP and its various metabolities appear in the serum between 12 and 24 hours, with the peak concentration (13 mcg/mL) occurring at 12 and lasting until 24 hours. The total recovery of SS and its SP metabolites from the urine of healthy subjects 3 days after the administration of a single 2 g dose of Sulfasalazine averaged 81%.

5-Aminosalicylic Acid (5-ASA): The serum concentration of 5-ASA in patients with ulcerative colitis was found to range from 0 to 4 mcg/mL, and to exist mainly in the form of acetyl-5-ASA. The urinary recovery of this compound was mostly in the acetylated form.

SULFASALAZINE TABLETS

Sulfasalazine Detectable serum concentrations of SS have been found in healthy subjects within 90 minutes after the ingestion of a single 2 g dose of Sulfasalazine Tablets. Maximum concentrations of SS occur between 1.5 and 6 hours, with the mean peak concentration (14 mcg/ml) occurring at 3 hours. Small amounts of SS are excreted unchanged in the urine.

Sulfapyridine (SP): Following absorption and distribution, SP is acetylated and hydroxylated in the liver, and then conjugated with glucuronic acid. After ingestion of a single 2 g dose of Sulfasalazine Tablets by healthy subjects, SP and its various metabolites appear in the serum within 3 to 6 hours. Maximum concentrations of total SP occur between 6 and 24 hours, with the mean peak concentration (21 mcg/ml) occurring at 12 hours. The total recovery of SS and its SP metabolites from the urine of healthy subjects 3 days after the administration of a single 2 g dose of Sulfasalazine Tablets averaged 91%.

5-Aminosalicylic Acid (5-ASA): The serum concentration of 5-ASA in patients with ulcerative colitis was found to range from 0 to 4 mcg/ml, and to exist mainly in the form of acetyl-5-ASA. The urinary recovery of this compound was mostly in the acetylated form.

Mean serum concentrations of total SP, i.e. SP and its metabolites, tend to be significantly greater in patients with a slow acetylator phenotype than in those with a fast acetylator phenotype. Total serum sulfapyridine concentrations greater than 50 mcg/ml appear to be associated with an increased incidence of adverse reactions.

The mode of action of Sulfasalazine is still under investigation. It may be related to the immunosuppressant properties that have been observed in animal and *in vitro* models, to its affinity for connective tissue, and/or to the relatively high concentration it reaches in serous fluids, the liver and intestinal walls, as demonstrated in autoradiographic studies in animals. Sulfasalazine has also been described as a highly efficient vehicle for carrying its principal metabolites, SP and 5-ASA, to the colon, where a local action for both of them has been postulated. Recent clinical studies utilizing rectal administration of SS, SP, and 5-ASA have indicated that the major therapeutic action may reside in the 5-ASA moiety.

INDICATIONS AND USAGE
Sulfasalazine is indicated:

a. in the treatment of mild to moderate ulcerative colitis, and as adjunctive therapy in severe ulcerative colitis.
b. for the prolongation of the remission period between acute attacks of ulcerative colitis.

Sulfasalazine enteric-coated tablets are particularly indicated in patients who cannot take the regular Sulfasalazine tablet because of gastrointestinal intolerance, and in whom there is evidence that this intolerance is not primarily due to high blood levels of sulfapyridine and its metabolites, e.g. patients experiencing nausea, vomiting, etc., when taking the first few doses of the drug or patients in whom a reduction in dosage does not alleviate the gastrointestinal side effects.

UNLABELED USES
Sulfasalazine is used alone or as an adjunct in the treatment of ankylosing spondylitis, Crohn's disease, and juvenile arthritis. It is also used in the treatment of psoriasis and rheumatoid arthritis.

CONTRAINDICATIONS
Hypersensitivity to Sulfasalazine, its metabolites, sulfonamides or salicylates. In infants under 2 years of age. Intestinal and urinary obstruction. Patients with porphyria should not receive sulfonamides as these drugs have been reported to precipitate an acute attack.

WARNINGS
Only after critical appraisal should Sulfasalazine be used in patients with hepatic or renal damage or blood dyscrasias. Deaths associated with the administration of Sulfasalazine have been reported from hypersensitivity reactions, agranulocytosis, aplastic anemia, other blood dyscrasias, renal and liver damage, irreversible neuromuscular and CNS changes, and fibrosing alveolitis. The presence of clinical signs such as sore throat, fever, pallor, purpura, or jaundice may be indications of serious blood disorders. Complete blood counts as well as urinalysis with careful microscopic examination should be done frequently in patients receiving Sulfasalazine. Oligospermia and infertility have been observed in men treated with Sulfasalazine. Withdrawal of the drug appears to reverse these effects.

PRECAUTIONS
General: Sulfasalazine should be given with caution to patients with severe allergy or bronchial asthma. Adequate fluid intake must be maintained in order to prevent crystalluria and stone formation. Patients with glucose-6-phosphate dehydrogenase deficiency should be observed closely for signs of hemolytic anemia. This reaction is frequently dose related. If toxic or hypersensitivity reactions occur, the drug should be discontinued immediately.

Isolated instances have been reported when Sulfasalazine enteric-coated tablets have passed undisintegrated. This may be due to a lack of intestinal esterases in these patients. If this is observed, the administration of Sulfasalazine should be discontinued immediately.

Information for Patients: Patients should be informed of the possibility of adverse reactions and of the need for careful medical supervision. They should also be made aware that ulcerative colitis rarely remits completely, and that the risk of relapse can be substantially reduced by continued administration of Sulfasalazine (at a maintenance dosage). Patients should be instructed to take Sulfasalazine in evenly divided doses preferably after meals. Additionally, patients should be advised that Sulfasalazine may produce an orange-yellow discoloration of the urine or skin.

Laboratory Tests: The progress of the disease during treatment can be evaluated by clinical criteria, including the presence of fever, weight changes, degree and frequency of diarrhea and bleeding as well as by sigmoidoscopy and the evaluation of biopsy samples. The determination of serum sulfapyridine levels may be useful since concentrations greater than 50 mcg/ml appear to be associated with an increased incidence of adverse reactions. Complete blood counts, as well as a urinalysis with careful microscopic examination should be done frequently in patients receiving Sulfasalazine.

Drug Interactions: Reduced absorption of folic acid and digoxin have been reported when administered concomitantly with Sulfasalazine.

Drug/Laboratory Test Interactions: The presence of Sulfasalazine or its metabolites in body fluids has not been reported to interfere with laboratory test procedures.

Carcinogenesis, Mutagenesis, Impairment of Fertility: There have been no long-term studies of the carcinogenic or mutagenic potential of Sulfasalazine. Impairment of male fertility was observed in reproductive studies performed in rats and rabbits at doses up to six times the human dose. Oligospermia and infertility have been described in men treated with Sulfasalazine. Withdrawal of the drug appears to reverse these effects (see *"Warnings"*).

PREGNANCY
Teratogenic Effects: Pregnancy Category B: Reproduction studies have been performed in rats and rabbits at doses up to 6 times the human dose and have revealed no evidence of impaired female fertility or harm to the fetus due to Sulfasalazine.

There are, however, no adequate and well-controlled studies in pregnant women. Because animal reproduction studies are not always predictive of human response, this drug should be used during pregnancy only if clearly needed. A national survey evaluated the outcome of pregnancies associated with inflammatory bowel disease (IBD). In a group of 186 women treated with Sulfasalazine alone or Sulfasalazine and concomitant steroid therapy, the incidence of fetal morbidity and mortality was comparable to that for 245 untreated IBD pregnancies as well as with population data from the National Center for Health Statistics.[1] Another study of 1,445 pregnancies associated with exposure to sulfonamides in which Sulfasalazine was included indicated that this group of drugs appeared to be devoid of any association with fetal malformation.[2] A review of the medical literature covering 1,155 pregnancies which occurred in women having ulcerative colitis suggested that the outcome was similar to what was expected in the general population[3].

No clinical studies have been performed which indicate the effect of Sulfasalazine on the later growth development and functional maturation of children whose mothers received the drug during pregnancy.

Nonteratogenic Effects: Sulfasalazine and sulfapyridine pass the placental barrier. Although sulfapyridine has been shown to have a poor bilirubin displacing capacity, the potential for kernicterus in newborns should be kept in mind. A case of agranulocytosis has been reported in an infant whose mother was taking both Sulfasalazine and prednisone throughout pregnancy.

Nursing Mothers: Caution should be exercised when Sulfasalazine is administered to a nursing woman. Sulfonamides are excreted in the milk. In the newborn, they compete with bilirubin for binding sites on the plasma proteins and may thus cause kernicterus. Insignificant amounts of uncleaved sulfasalazine have been found in milk, whereas the sulfapyridine levels in milk are about 30-60 per cent of those in the serum. Sulfapyridine has been shown to have a poor bilirubin displacing capacity.

Pediatric Use: Safety and effectiveness in children below the age of two years have not been established.

ADVERSE REACTIONS
The most common adverse reactions associated with Sulfasalazine are anorexia, headache, nausea, vomiting, gastric distress and apparently reversible oligospermia. These occur in about one-third of the patients. Less frequent adverse reactions are skin rash, pruritus, urticaria, fever, Heinz body anemia, hemolytic anemia and cyanosis which may occur at a frequency of one in every thirty patients or less. Experience suggests that with a daily dosage of 4 g or more, or total serum sulfapyridine levels above 50 mcg/ml, the incidence of adverse reactions tends to increase.

Although the listing which follows includes a few adverse reactions which have not been reported with this specific drug, the pharmacological similarities among the sulfonamides require that each of these reactions be considered when Sulfasalazine is administered.

Other adverse reactions which occur rarely, in approximately 1 in 1000 patients or less are:

Blood Dyscrasias: aplastic anemia, agranulocytosis, leukopenia, megaloblastic (macrocytic) anemia, purpura, thrombocytopenia, hypoprothrombinemia and methemoglobinemia, and congenital neutropenia.

Hypersensitivity Reactions: erythema multiforme (Stevens Johnson syndrome), exfoliative dermatitis, epidermal necrolysis (Lyell's syndrome) with corneal damage, anaphylaxis, serum sickness syndrome, pneumonitis with or without eosinophilia, vasculitis, fibrosing alveolitis, pleuritis, pericarditis with or without tamponade, allergic myocarditis, polyarteritis nodosa, L.E. syndrome, hepatitis and hepatic necrosis with or without immune complexes, parapsoriasis varioliformis acuta (Mucha Haberman syndrome), rhabdomyolysis, photosensitization, arthralgia, periorbital edema, conjuctival and scleral injection and alopecia.

Gastrointestinal Reactions: hepatitis, pancreatitis, bloody diarrhea, impaired folic acid absorption, impaired digoxin absorption, stomatitis, diarrhea and abdominal pains.

CNS Reactions: transverse myelitis, convulsions, meningitis, transient lesions of the posterior spinal column, cauda equina syndrome, Guillain-Barre syndrome, peripheral neuropathy, mental depression, vertigo, hearing loss, insomnia, ataxia, hallucinations, tinnitus and drowsiness.

Renal Reactions: toxic nephrosis with oliguria and anuria, nephritis, nephrotic syndrome, hematuria, crystalluria and proteinuria.

Other Reactions: urine discoloration and skin discoloration. The sulfonamides bear certain chemical similarities to some goitrogens, diuretics, (acetazolamide and the thiazides), and oral hypoglycemic agents. Goiter production, diuresis, and hypoglycemia have occurred rarely in patients receiving sulfonamides. Cross-sensitivity may exist with these agents. Rats appear to be especially susceptible to the goitrogenic effects of sulfonamides and long-term administration has produced thyroid malignancies in this species.

DRUG ABUSE AND DEPENDENCE
None reported.

OVERDOSAGE
There is evidence that the incidence and severity of toxicity are directly related to the total serum sulfapyridine concentration. Symptoms of overdosage may include nausea, vomiting, gastric distress and abdominal pains. In more advanced cases, CNS symptoms such as drowsiness, convulsions, etc. may be observed. Serum sulfapyridine concentrations may be used to monitor the progress of recovery from overdosage.

Experience suggests that with a daily dosage of 4 g or more or total serum sulfapyridine levels above 50 mcg/ml the incidence of adverse reactions tends to increase. There are no documented reports of deaths due to ingestion of large single doses of Sulfasalazine.

It has not been possible to determine the oral LD_{50} in laboratory animals such as mice, since the highest daily oral dose which can be given (12 g/kg) is not lethal. Doses of Sulfasalazine of 16 g per day have been given to patients without mortality.

Instructions for Overdosage: Gastric lavage or emesis plus catharsis as indicated. Alkalinize urine. If kidney function is normal, force fluids. If anuria is present, restrict fluids and salt, and treat appropriately. Catheterization of the ureters may be indicated for complete renal blockage by crystals. The low molecular weight of Sulfasalazine and its metabolites may facilitate their removal by dialysis. For agranulocytosis, discontinue the drug immediately, hospitalize the patient and institute appropriate therapy.

For hypersensitivity reactions, discontinue treatment immediately. Such reactions may be controlled with antihistamines and, if necessary, systemic corticosteroids.

When in the physician's opinion, reinstitution of Sulfasalazine is warranted, regimens modeled upon desensitization procedures may be attempted approximately two weeks after Sulfasalazine has been discontinued and symptoms have disappeared (see *"Dosage and Administration"*).

DOSAGE AND ADMINISTRATION
Dosage should be adjusted to each individual's response and tolerance. The drug should be given in evenly divided doses over each 24-hour period; intervals between nighttime doses should not exceed 8 hours, with administration after meals recommended when feasible. Experience suggests that with daily dosages of 4 g or more, the incidence of adverse reactions tends to increase; hence, patients receiving these dosages should be instructed about and carefully observed for the appearance of adverse effects.

Various desensitization-like regimens have been reported to be effective in 34 of 53 patients,[4] 7 of 8 patients[5] and 19 of 20 patients.[6] Upon reinstituting Sulfasalazine such regimens comprise a total daily dose of 50 to 250 mg which, every 4 to 7 days thereafter, is doubled until the desired therapeutic level is achieved. If the symptoms of sensitivity recur, Sulfasalazine should be discontinued. Desensitization should not be attempted in patients who have a history of agranulocytosis or who have experienced an anaphylactoid reaction while on a previous course of Sulfasalazine therapy.

USUAL DOSAGE OF SULFASALAZINE TABLETS AND SULFASALAZINE (ENTERIC-COATED TABLETS)
Initial Therapy:
ADULTS: 3-4 g daily in evenly divided doses. In some cases it is advisable to initiate therapy with a small dosage, e.g. 1-2 g daily, to lessen adverse gastrointestinal effects. If daily doses exceeding 4 g are required to achieve desired effects, the increased risk of toxicity should be kept in mind.
CHILDREN TWO YEARS OF AGE AND OLDER: 40-60 mg per kg body weight in each 24-hour period, divided into 3-6 doses.

Maintenance Therapy:
ADULTS: 2 g daily.
CHILDREN TWO YEARS OF AGE AND OLDER: 30 mg per kg body weight in each 24-hour period, divided into 4 doses.
Response to therapy and adjustment of dosage should be determined by periodic examination. It is often necessary to continue medication, even when clinical symptoms, including diarrhea, have been controlled. When endoscopic examination confirms satisfactory improvement, dosage is reduced to a maintenance level. If symptoms of gastric intolerance (anorexia, nausea, vomiting, etc.)

occur after the first few doses of Sulfasalazine they are probably due to mucosal irritation and may be alleviated by distributing the total daily dose more evenly over the day or by giving Sulfasalazine enteric-coated tablets. If diarrhea recurs, dosage should be increased to previous effective levels. If such symptoms occur after the first few days of treatment with Sulfasalazine they are probably due to increased serum levels of total sulfapyridine, and may be alleviated by halving the dose and subsequently increasing it gradually over several days. If symptoms continue, the drug should be stopped for 5-7 days, then reinstituted at a lower daily dose.

Storage: Store at room temperature, 15-30°C (59-86°F).

REFERENCES
1. Mogadam M, et al: Pregnancy in inflammatory bowel disease: Effect of sulfasalazine and corticosteroids on fetal outcome *Gastroenterol* 80:72-76, 1981.   2. Kaufman D W (ed): *Birth Defects and Drugs in Pregnancy.* Littleton, MA, Publishing Sciences Group, Inc. 1977, pp 296-313.   3. Jarnerot G: Fertility, sterility and pregnancy in chronic inflammatory bowel disease. *Scand J Gastroenterol* 17:1-4, 1982.   4. Korelitz BI, et al: *Gastroenterol* 82:1104, 1982.   5. Holdsworth C G: *Brit Med J* 282:110, 1981.   6. Taffet S L, Das K M: *Amer J Med* 73:520-524, 1982.

HOW SUPPLIED
ENTERIC COATED TABLETS: 500 MG

AVERAGE UNIT PRICE (AVAILABLE SIZES)	
BRAND	$0.23

BRAND/MANUFACTURER		NDC	SIZE	AWP
◆ BRAND				
AZULFIDINE ENTABS: Pharmacia		00016-0102-01	100s	$23.63
		00016-0102-05	500s	$111.63

TABLETS: 500 MG

AVERAGE UNIT PRICE (AVAILABLE SIZES)		GENERIC A-RATED AVERAGE PRICE (GAAP)	
BRAND	$0.20	100s	$13.77
GENERIC	$0.13	500s	$63.29
HCFA FUL (100s ea)	$0.12		

BRAND/MANUFACTURER	NDC	SIZE	AWP
◆ BRAND			
▶ AZULFIDINE: Pharmacia	00016-0101-01	100s	$19.69
	00016-0101-11	100s ud	$22.06
	00016-0101-05	500s	$86.81
◆ GENERICS			
Mason Dist	11845-0121-01	100s	$11.25
Moore,H.L.	00839-6098-06	100s	$12.68
URL	00677-0483-01	100s	$13.50
Major	00904-1152-60	100s	$13.50
Mutual	53489-0147-01	100s	$13.50
Qualitest	00603-5802-21	100s	$13.88
Rugby	00536-4617-01	100s	$14.39
Goldline	00182-1016-01	100s	$14.40
Aligen	00405-4956-01	100s	$15.55
U.S. Trading	56126-0306-11	100s ud	$10.74
Major	00904-1152-61	100s ud	$11.90
Raway	00686-0044-20	100s ud	$19.95
Major	00904-1152-70	250s	$23.90
Mason Dist	11845-0121-03	500s	$52.87
Moore,H.L.	00839-6098-12	500s	$57.23
Major	00904-1152-40	500s	$60.95
URL	00677-0483-05	500s	$62.00
Mutual	53489-0147-05	500s	$62.00
Schein	00364-0444-05	500s	$63.85
Qualitest	00603-5802-28	500s	$63.95
Rugby	00536-4617-05	500s	$68.33
Aligen	00405-4956-02	500s	$70.42
Goldline	00182-1016-05	500s	$71.25
Rugby	00536-4617-10	1000s	$129.00

Sulfinpyrazone

DESCRIPTION
Sulfinpyrazone is a uricosuric agent available as 100 mg tablets and 200 mg capsules for oral administration. Its chemical name is 1,2-diphenyl-4-[2-(phenyl-sulfinyl)ethyl]-3,5-pyrazolidinedione.

Sulfinpyrazone is a white to off-white powder practically insoluble in water and in solvent hexane, soluble in alcohol and in acetone, and sparingly soluble in dilute alkali. Its molecular weight is 404.48.

Following is its chemical structure:

CLINICAL PHARMACOLOGY

Its pharmacologic activity is the potentiation of the urinary excretion of uric acid. It is useful for reducing the blood urate levels in patients with chronic tophaceous gout and acute intermittent gout, and for promoting the resorption of tophi.

INDICATIONS

Sulfinpyrazone is indicated for the treatment of:

1. Chronic gouty arthritis
2. Intermittent gouty arthritis.

UNLABELED USES

Sulfinpyrazone is used alone or as an adjunct in the treatment of cerebral ischemia and coronary artery disease.

CONTRAINDICATIONS

Patients with an active peptic ulcer or symptoms of gastrointestinal inflammation or ulceration should not receive the drug.

The drug is contraindicated in patients with a history or the presence of:

1. Hypersensitivity to phenylbutazone or other pyrazoles
2. Blood dyscrasias

WARNINGS

Studies on the teratogenicity of pyrazole compounds in animals have yielded inconclusive results. Up to the present time, however, there have been no reported cases of human congenital malformation proved to be due to the use of the drug.

It is suggested that Sulfinpyrazone be used with caution in pregnant women, weighing the potential risks against the possible benefits.

PRECAUTIONS

As with all pyrazole compounds, patients receiving Sulfinpyrazone should be kept under close medical supervision and periodic blood counts are recommended. It may be administered with care to patients with a history of healed peptic ulcer.

Recent reports have indicated that Sulfinpyrazone potentiates the action of certain sulfonamides, such as sulfadiazine and sulfisoxazole. In addition, other pyrazole compounds (phenylbutazone) have been observed to potentiate the hypoglycemic sulfonylurea agents, as well as insulin. In view of these observations, it is suggested that Sulfinpyrazone be used with caution in conjunction with sulfa drugs, the sulfonylurea hypoglycemic agents and insulin.

Because Sulfinpyrazone is a potent uricosuric agent, it may precipitate urolithiasis and renal colic, especially in the initial stages of therapy. For this reason, an adequate fluid intake and alkalinization of the urine are recommended. In cases with significant renal impairment, periodic assessment of renal function is indicated. Occasional cases of renal failure have been reported; but a cause-and-effect relationship has not always been clearly established.

Salicylates antagonize the uricosuric action of Sulfinpyrazone and for this reason their concomitant use is contraindicated in gouty arthritis.

Sulfinpyrazone may accentuate the action of coumarin-type anticoagulants and further depress prothrombin activity when these medications are employed simultaneously.

NOTE

Sulfinpyrazone has minimal anti-inflammatory effect and is not intended for the relief of an acute attack of gout.

In the initial stages of therapy, because of the marked ability of Sulfinpyrazone to mobilize urates, acute attacks of gouty arthritis may be precipitated.

ADVERSE REACTIONS

The most frequently reported adverse reactions with Sulfinpyrazone have been upper gastrointestinal disturbances. In these patients it is advisable to administer the drug with food, milk, or antacids. Despite this precaution, Sulfinpyrazone may aggravate or reactivate peptic ulcer.

Rash has been reported. In most instances, this reaction did not necessitate discontinuation of therapy. In general Sulfinpyrazone has not been observed to affect electrolyte balance.

Blood dyscrasias (anemia, leukopenia, agranulocytosis, thrombocytopenia and aplastic anemia) have rarely been reported. There has also been a published report associating Sulfinpyrazone administered concomitantly with other drugs including colchicine, with leukemia following long-term treatment of patients with gout. However, the circumstances involved in the two cases reported are such that a cause-and-effect relationship to Sulfinpyrazone has not been clearly established.

OVERDOSAGE

Symptoms: Nausea, vomiting, diarrhea, epigastric pain, ataxia, labored respiration, convulsions, coma. Possible symptoms, seen after overdosage with other pyrazolone derivatives: anemia, jaundice, ulceration.

Treatment: No specific antidote. Induce emesis; gastric lavage; supportive treatment (intravenous glucose infusions, analeptics).

DOSAGE AND ADMINISTRATION

Initial: 200-400 mg daily in two divided doses, with meals or milk, gradually increasing when necessary to full maintenance dosage in one week.

Maintenance: 400 mg daily, given in two divided doses, as above. This dosage may be increased to 800 mg daily, if necessary, and may sometimes be reduced to as low as 200 mg daily after the blood urate level has been controlled. Treatment should be continued without interruption even in the presence of acute exacerbations, which can be concomitantly treated with phenylbutazone or colchicine. Patients previously controlled with other uricosuric therapy may be transferred to Sulfinpyrazone at full maintenance dosage.

Do not store above 86°F (30°C).

Dispense in tight container (USP).

HOW SUPPLIED

CAPSULE: 200 MG

AVERAGE UNIT PRICE (AVAILABLE SIZES)		GENERIC A-RATED AVERAGE PRICE (GAAP)	
BRAND	$0.53	100s	$31.60
GENERIC	$0.29	500s	$120.82
HCFA FUL (100s ea)	$0.19		

BRAND/MANUFACTURER	NDC	SIZE	AWP
◆ BRAND			
ANTURANE: Ciba Pharm	00083-0168-30	100s	$52.69
◆ GENERICS			
Moore,H.L.	00839-6638-06	100s	$25.77
Rugby	00536-4616-01	100s	$26.06
Major	00904-1187-60	100s	$27.80
Barr	00555-0272-02	100s	$28.48
Goldline	00182-1544-01	100s	$28.50
Schein	00364-0652-01	100s	$38.71
Zenith	00172-2969-60	100s	$38.75
Aligen	00405-4962-01	100s	$38.75
Moore,H.L.	00839-7891-12	500s	$86.87
Moore,H.L.	00839-6638-12	500s	$86.92
Barr	00555-0272-04	500s	$121.99
Zenith	00172-2969-70	500s	$187.50

TABLETS: 100 MG

AVERAGE UNIT PRICE (AVAILABLE SIZES)		GENERIC A-RATED AVERAGE PRICE (GAAP)	
BRAND	$0.33	100s	$14.13
GENERIC	$0.14		
HCFA FUL (100s ea)	$0.13		

BRAND/MANUFACTURER	NDC	SIZE	AWP
◆ BRAND			
ANTURANE: Ciba Pharm	00083-0041-30	100s	$32.73
◆ GENERICS			
Moore,H.L.	00839-6604-06	100s	$12.14
Barr	00555-0271-02	100s	$13.22
Aligen	00405-4961-01	100s	$14.65
Goldline	00182-1426-01	100s	$14.65
Major	00904-1186-60	100s	$14.80
Rugby	00536-4615-01	100s	$15.31

Sulfisoxazole Diolamine, Ophthalmic

DESCRIPTION

Sulfisoxazole Diolamine Ophthalmic Solution is an antibacterial sulfonamide preparation specifically intended for topical ophthalmic use. The solution is a sterile, isotonic preparation containing 4% (40 mg/mL) Sulfisoxazole in the form of the Dolamine salt, and phenylmercuric nitrate 1:100,000 as a preservative. The solution has a physiologic pH, and does not cause significant stinging or burning on application.

Chemically, Sulfisoxazole Diolamine is N^1-(3,4-dimethyl-5-isoxazolyl) sulfanilamide compound with 2,2'-iminodiethanol (1:1). It is a white to off-white, odorless, crystalline powder that is freely soluble in water and soluble in alcohol. Sulfisoxazole Diolamine has a molecular weight of 372.44.

Following is its chemical structure:

$$NH_2 - \phenyl - SO_2NH - \isoxazole(CH_3)(CH_3)$$

CLINICAL PHARMACOLOGY

Sulfonamides do not appear to be appreciably absorbed from mucous membranes.

Microbiology: Sulfonamides exert a bacteriostatic effect against a wide range of gram-positive and gram-negative microorganisms. Sulfonamides inhibit bacterial synthesis of dihydrofolic acid by competing with *para*-aminobenzoic acid (PABA). Resistant strains are capable of utilizing folic acid precursors or preformed folic acid. Currently, the increasing frequency of resistant organisms is a limitation of the usefulness of antibacterial agents, including the sulfonamides.

INDICATIONS

For the treatment of conjunctivitis, corneal ulcers and other superficial ocular infections due to susceptible microorganisms, and as an adjunct in systemic sulfonamide therapy of trachoma.

CONTRAINDICATIONS

Hypersensitivity to sulfonamides or to other ingredients in the formulation. Infants less than 2 months of age. Pregnancy at term and during the nursing period because sulfonamides pass the placenta and are excreted in the milk and may cause kernicterus.

PRECAUTIONS

General: Nonsusceptible organisms, including fungi, may proliferate with the use of this preparation. Sulfonamides are inactivated by the *para*-aminobenzoic acid present in purulent exudates. Should undesirable reactions occur, discontinue Sulfisoxazole Diolamine immediately.

Information for Patients: Patients using Sulfisoxazole Diolamine Ophthalmic Solution should be instructed not to touch the dropper tip to any surface, since contamination of the solution may result.

Drug Interactions: Sulfisoxazole Diolamine Ophthalmic Solution is incompatible with preparations containing silver. *In vitro* antagonism with Sulfisoxazole Diolamine and gentamicin sulfate Sulfisoxazole Diolamine has been reported.

Carcinogenesis, Mutagenesis, Impairment of Fertility Carcinogensis: Carcinogenic studies have not been performed with ophthalmic preparations of Sulfisoxazole Diolamine. Sulfisozole Diolamine was not carcinogenic in either sex when administered by gavage for 103 weeks at dosages up to 2000 mg/kg/day in mice or 400 mg/kg/day in rats.

Mutagenesis: Bacterial mutagenic studies have not been performed with Sulfisoxazole Diolamine. However, Sulfisoxazole Diolamine was not observed to be mutagenic in *E. coli* Sd-4-73 when tested in the absence of a metabolic activating system.

Impairment of Fertility: Fertility studies have not been performed with ophthalmic preparations of Sulfisoxazole. No effects on mating behavior, conception rate or fertility index (percent pregnant) were observed in a reproduction study in rats given oral dosages of 800 mg/kg/day Sulfisoxazole Diolamine.

Pregnancy: Teratogenic Effects: Pregnancy Category C. Teratogenic studies of ophthalmic preparations of Sulfisoxazole have not been performed in laboratory animals. Sulfisoxazole was not teratogenic in either rats or rabbits at oral dosages of 800 mg/kg/day. However, in another teratogenicity study, cleft palates developed in both rats and mice after oral administration of 1000 mg/kg/day Sulfisoxazole; skeletal defects were also observed in rats. This dose is 9 to 18 times the usual adult dosage for oral Sulfisoxazole Diolamine.

There are no adequate and well-controlled studies of Sulfisoxazole Diolamine in pregnant women. Sulfisoxazole Diolamine Ophthalmic Solution should be used during pregnancy only if the potential benefit justifies the potential risk to the fetus.

Nursing Mothers: (See "Contraindications" section.)

Pediatric Use: Sulfisoxazole Diolamine Ophthalmic Solution is not recommended for use in infants younger than 2 months of age.

ADVERSE REACTIONS

Topical application of the sulfonamides may produce sensitization and preclude later systemic use of these drugs. In addition, patients who have been sensitized by systemic sulfonamide administration may exhibit hypersensitivity reactions following topical application of the drugs.

Ophthalmic: Ocular irritation, chemosis, itching. Included in the listing that follows are adverse reactions that have not been reported with this dosage form but have been reported for the systemically absorbed sulfonamides.

Hematologic: Agranulocytosis, aplastic anemia, thrombocytopenia, leukopenia, hemolytic anemia, purpura, hypoprothrombinemia and methemoglobinemia.

Allergic Reactions: Erythema multiforme (Stevens-Johnson syndrome), generalized skin eruptions, epidermal necrolysis, urticaria, serum sickness, pruritus, exfoliative dermatitis, anaphylactoid reactions, periorbital edema, conjunctival and scleral injection, photosensitization, arthralgia and allergic myocarditis.

Gastrointestinal Reactions: Nausea, emesis, abdominal pains, hepatitis, hepatocellular necrosis, diarrhea, anorexia, pancreatitis and stomatitis.

C.N.S. Reactions: Headache, peripheral neuritis, mental depression, convulsions, ataxia, hallucinations, tinnitus, vertigo and insomnia.

Miscellaneous Reactions: Drug fever, chills, and toxic nephrosis with oliguria and anuria. Periarteritis, nodosa and L.E. phenomenon have occurred.

Endocrine: The sulfonamides bear certain chemical similarities to some goitrogen, diuretics (acetazolamide and the thiazides) and oral hypoglycemic agents. Goiter production, diuresis and hypoglycemia have occurred rarely in patients receiving sulfonamides. Cross sensitivity may exist with these agents.

DOSAGE AND ADMINISTRATION

Solution: Instill 2 or 3 drops in the eye 3 or more times daily. Care should be taken not to touch dropper tip to any surface, since contamination of the solution may result.

Solution is stable at room temperature and does not require refrigeration.

HOW SUPPLIED
DROP: 4%

BRAND/MANUFACTURER	NDC	SIZE	AWP
○ BRAND			
GANTRISIN OPHTHALMIC: Roche Labs	00004-1702-39	15 ml	$9.44

Sulfisoxazole, Oral

DESCRIPTION

Sulfisoxazole is an antibacterial sulfonamide available in tablets, pediatric suspension and syrup for oral administration. Each tablet contains 0.5 gm Sulfisoxazole with corn starch, gelatin, lactose and magnesium stearate. Each teaspoonful (5 mL) of the pediatric suspension contains the equivalent of approximately 0.5 gm Sulfisoxazole in the form of acetyl Sulfisoxazole in a vehicle containing 0.3% alcohol, carboxymethylcellulose (sodium), citric acid, methylcellulose, parabens (methyl and propyl), partial invert sugar, sodium citrate, sorbitan monolaurate, sucrose, flavors and water. Each teaspoonful (5 mL) of the syrup contains the equivalent of approximately 0.5 gm Sulfisoxazole in the form of acetyl Sulfisoxazole in a vehicle containing 0.9% alcohol, benzoic acid, carrageenan, citric acid, cocoa, sodium citrate, sorbitan monolaurate, sucrose, flavors and water.

Sulfisoxazole is N^1-(3,4-dimethyl-5-isoxazoly)sulfanilamide. It is a white to slightly yellowish, odorless, slightly bitter, crystalline powder that is soluble in alcohol and very slightly soluble in water. Sulfisoxazole has a molecular weight of 267.30.

Acetyl Sulfisoxazole, the tasteless form of Sulfisoxazole, is N^1 acetyl Sulfisoxazole and must be distinguished from N^4 acetyl Sulfisoxazole, which is a metabolite of Sulfisoxazole. Acetyl Sulfisoxazole is a white or slightly yellow, crystalline powder that is slightly soluble in alcohol and practically insoluble in water. Acetyl Sulfisoxazole has a molecular weight of 309.34.

Following is its chemical structure:

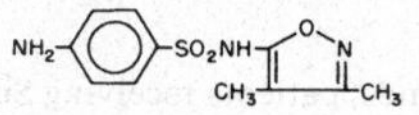

CLINICAL PHARMACOLOGY

Following oral administration, Sulfisoxazole is rapidly and completely absorbed; the small intestine is the major site of absorption, but some of the drug is absorbed from the stomach. Sulfonamides are present in the blood as free, conjugated (acetylated and possibly other forms) and protein-bound forms. The amount present as "free" drug is considered to be the therapeutically active form. Approximately 85% of a dose of Sulfisoxazole is bound to plasma proteins, primarily to albumin; 65% to 72% of the unbound portion is in the nonacetylated form.

Maximum plasma concentrations of intact Sulfisoxazole following a single 2-gm oral dose of Sulfisoxazole to healthy adult volunteers ranged from 127 to 211 mcg/mL (mean, 169 mcg/mL) and the time of peak plasma concentration ranged from 1 to 4 hours (mean, 2.5 hours). The elimination half-life of Sulfisoxazole ranged from 4.6 to 7.8 hours after oral administration. The elimination of Sulfisoxazole has been shown to be slower in elderly subjects (63 to 75 years) with diminished renal function (creatinine clearance, 37 to 68 mL/min).[1] After multiple-dose oral administration of 500 mg q.id. to healthy volunteers, the average steady-state plasma concentrations of intact Sulfisoxazole ranged from 49.9 to 88.8 mcg/mL (mean, 63.4 mcg/mL).[2]

Wide variation in blood levels may result following identical doses of a sulfonamide. Blood levels should be measured in patients receiving sulfonamides at the higher recommended doses or being treated for serious infections. Free sulfonamide blood levels of 50 to 150 mcg/mL may be considered therapeutically effective for most infections, with blood levels of 120 to 150 mcg/mL being optimal for serious infections. The maximum sulfonamide level should not exceed 200 mcg/mL, since adverse reactions occur more frequently above this concentration.

N^1-acetyl Sulfisoxazole is metabolized to Sulfisoxazole by digestive enzymes in the gastrointestinal tract and is absorbed as Sulfisoxazole. This enzymatic splitting is presumed to be responsible for slower absorption and lower peak blood concentrations than are attained following administration of an equal oral dose of Sulfisoxazole. With continued administration of acetyl Sulfisoxazole, blood concentrations approximate those of Sulfisoxazole. Following a single 4-gm dose of acetyl Sulfisoxazole to healthy volunteers, maximum plasma concentrations of Sulfisoxazole ranged from 122 to 282 mcg/mL (mean, 181 mcg/mL) for the pediatric suspension and from 101 to 202 mcg/mL (mean, 144 mcg/mL) for the syrup, and occurred between 2 and 6 hours postadministration. The half-lives of elimination from plasma ranged from 5.4 to 7.4 and from 5.9 to 8.5 hours, respectively.

Sulfisoxazole and its acetylated metabolites are excreted primarily by the kidneys through glomerular filtration. Concentrations of Sulfisoxazole are considerably higher in the urine than the blood. The mean urinary excretion recovery following oral administration of Sulfisoxazole is 97% within 48 hours, of which 52% is intact drug, with the remaining as the N^4-acetylated metabolite. Following administration of Acetyl Sulfisoxazole syrup or suspension, approximately 58% is excreted in the urine as total drug within 72 hours.

Sulfisoxazole is distributed only in extracellular body fluid. It is excreted in human milk. It readily crosses the placental barrier and enters into fetal circulation and also crosses the blood-brain barrier. In healthy subjects, cerebrospinal fluid concentrations of Sulfisoxazole vary; in patients with meningitis, however, concentrations of free drug in cerebrospinal fluid as high as 94 mcg/mL have been reported.

Microbiology: The sulfonamides are bacteriostatic agents and the spectrum of activity is similar for all. Sulfonamides inhibit bacterial synthesis of dihydrofolic

---

◆ RATED THERAPEUTICALLY EQUIVALENT; ◇ THERAPEUTIC EQUIVALENCE UNCONFIRMED; ○ UNRATED

acid by preventing the condensation of the pteridine with aminobenzoic acid through competitive inhibition of the enzyme dihydropteroate synthetase. Resistant strains have altered dihydropteroate synthetase with reduced affinity for sulfonamides or produce increased quantities of aminobenzoic acid.

Susceptibility Tests: Diffusion Techniques: Quantitative methods that require measurement of zone diameters give the most precise estimate of the susceptibility of bacteria to antimicrobial agents. One such standard procedure[3] which has been recommended for use with disks to test susceptibility of organisms to Sulfisoxazole uses the 250- or 300-mcg Sulfisoxazole disk. Interpretation involves the correlation of the diameter obtained in the disk test with the minimum inhibitory concentration (MIC) to Sulfisoxazole.

Reports from the laboratory giving results of the standard single-disk susceptibility test with a 250- or 300-mcg Sulfisoxazole disk should be interpreted according to the following criteria:

Zone Diameter (mm)	Interpretation
≥ 17	Susceptible
13-16	Moderately susceptible
≤ 12	Resistant

A report of "susceptible" indicates that the pathogen is likely to be inhibited by generally achievable blood levels. A report of "moderately susceptible" suggests that the organism would be susceptible if high dosage is used or if the infection is confined to tissues and fluids in which high antimicrobial levels are attained. A report of "resistant" indicates that achievable concentrations are unlikely to be inhibitory, and other therapy should be selected.

Standardized procedures require the use of laboratory control organisms. The 250- or 300-mcg Sulfisoxazole disk should give the following zone diameters:

Organism	Zone Diameter (mm)
E. coli ATCC 25922	18-26 mm
S. aureus ATCC 25923	24-34 mm

Dilution Techniques: Use a standardized dilution method[4] (broth, agar, microdilution) or equivalent with Sulfisoxazole powder. The MIC values obtained should be interpreted according to the following criteria:

MIC (mcg/mL)	Interpretation
≤ 256	Susceptible
≥ 512	Resistant

As with standard diffusion techniques, dilution methods require the use of laboratory control organisms. Dilutions of standard Sulfisoxazole powder should provide the following MIC values:

Organism	MIC (mcg/mL)
S. aureus ATCC 29213	32-128
E. faecalis ATCC 29212	32-128
E. coli ATCC 25922	8-32

INDICATIONS AND USAGE

Acute, recurrent or chronic urinary tract infections (primarily pyelonephritis, pyelitis and cystitis) due to susceptible organisms (usually *Escherichia coli, Klebsiella-Enterobacter,* staphylococcus, *Proteus mirabilis* and, less frequently, *Proteus vulgaris*) in the absence of obstructive uropathy or foreign bodies.

Meningococcal meningitis where the organism has been demonstrated to be susceptible. *Haemophilus influenzae* meningitis as adjunctive therapy with parenteral streptomycin.

Meningococcal meningitis prophylaxis when sulfonamide-sensitive group A strains are known to prevail in family groups or larger closed populations. (The prophylactic usefulness of sulfonamides when group B or C infections are prevalent has not been proven and in closed population groups may be harmful.)

Acute otitis media due to *Haemophilus influenzae* when used concomitantly with adequate doses of penicillin or erythromycin (see appropriate labeling for prescribing information). Trachoma. Inclusion conjunctivitis. Nocardiosis. Chancroid. Toxoplasmosis as adjunctive therapy with pyrimethamine. Malaria due to chloroquine-resistant strains of *Plasmodium falciparum,* when used as adjunctive therapy.

Currently, the increasing frequency of resistant organisms is a limitation of the usefulness of antibacterial agents including the sulfonamides, especially in the treatment of chronic and recurrent urinary tract infections.

Important Note: In vitro sulfonamide susceptibility tests are not always reliable. The test must be carefully coordinated with bacteriologic and clinical response. When the patient is already taking sulfonamides, follow-up cultures should have aminobenzoic acid added to the culture media.

UNLABELED USES

Sulfisoxazole oral is used alone or as an adjunct in the treatment of lymphogranuloma venereum.

CONTRAINDICATIONS

Sulfisoxazole is contraindicated in the following patient populations: patients with a known hypersensitivity to sulfonamides; children younger than 2 months (except in the treatment of congenital toxoplasmosis as adjunctive therapy with pyrimethamine); pregnant women *at term*; and mothers nursing infants less than 2 months of age.

Use in pregnant women at term, in children less than 2 months of age and in mothers nursing infants less than 2 months of age is contraindicated because sulfonamides may promote kernicterus in the newborn by displacing bilirubin from plasma proteins.

WARNINGS

FATALITIES ASSOCIATED WITH THE ADMINISTRATION OF SULFONAMIDES, ALTHOUGH RARE, HAVE OCCURRED DUE TO SEVERE REACTIONS, INCLUDING STEVENS-JOHNSON SYNDROME, TOXIC EPIDERMAL NECROLYSIS, FULMINANT HEPATIC NECROSIS, AGRANULOCYTOSIS, APLASTIC ANEMIA AND OTHER BLOOD DYSCRASIAS.

SULFONAMIDES, INCLUDING SULFISOXAZOLE, SHOULD BE DISCONTINUED AT THE FIRST APPEARANCE OF SKIN RASH OR ANY SIGN OF AN ADVERSE REACTION. In rare instances, a skin rash may be followed by more severe reactions such as Stevens-Johnson syndrome, toxic epidermal necrolysis, hepatic necrosis and serious blood disorders. (See *"Precautions"*).

Clinical signs such as rash, sore throat, fever, arthralgia, pallor, purpura or jaundice may be early indications of serious reactions.

Cough, shortness of breath and pulmonary infiltrates are hypersensitivity reactions of the respiratory tract that have been reported in association with sulfonamide treatment. The sulfonamides should not be used for the treatment of group A beta-hemolytic streptococcal infections. In an established infection, they will not eradicate the streptococcus and, therefore, will not prevent sequelae such as rheumatic fever.

Pseudomembranous colitis has been reported with nearly all antibacterial agents, including Sulfisoxazole, and may range in severity from mild to life-threatening. Therefore, it is important to consider this diagnosis in patients who present with diarrhea subsequent to the administration of antibacterial agents.

Treatment with antibacterial agents alters the normal flora of the colon and may permit overgrowth of clostridia. Studies indicate that toxin produced by *Clostridium difficile* is one primary cause of "antibiotic-associated colitis."

After the diagnosis of pseudomembranous colitis has been established, therapeutic measures should be initiated. Mild cases of pseudomembranous colitis usually respond to drug discontinuation alone. In moderate to severe cases, consideration should be given to management with fluids and electrolytes, protein supplementation, and treatment with an antibacterial drug clinically effective against *C. difficile* colitis.

PRECAUTIONS

General: Sulfonamides should be given with caution to patients with impaired renal or hepatic function and to those with severe allergy or bronchial asthma. In glucose-6-phosphate dehydrogenase-deficient individuals, hemolysis may occur; this reaction is frequently dose-related.

The frequency of resistant organisms limits the usefulness of antibacterial agents, including the sulfonamides, as sole therapy in the treatment of urinary tract infections. Since sulfonamides are bacteriostatic and not bactericidal, a complete course of therapy is needed to prevent immediate regrowth and the development of resistant uropathogens.

Information for Patients: Patients should maintain an adequate fluid intake to prevent crystalluria and stone formation.

Laboratory Tests: Complete blood counts should be done frequently in patients receiving sulfonamides. If a significant reduction in the count of any formed blood element is noted, sulfonamide therapy should be discontinued. Urinalyses with careful microscopic examination and renal function tests should be performed during therapy, particularly for those patients with impaired renal function. Blood levels should be measured in patients receiving a sulfonamide for serious infections. (See *"Indications and Usage"*)

Drug Interactions: It has been reported that Sulfisoxazole may prolong the prothrombin time in patients who are receiving anticoagulants, including warfarin. This interaction should be kept in mind when Sulfisoxazole is given to patients already on anticoagulant therapy, and prothrombin time or other suitable coagulation test should be monitored.

It has been proposed that Sulfisoxazole competes with thiopental for plasma protein binding. In one study involving 48 patients, intravenous Sulfisoxazole resulted in a decrease in the amount of thiopental required for anesthesia and in a shortening of the awakening time. It is not known whether chronic oral doses of Sulfisoxazole would have a similar effect. Until more is known about this interaction, physicians should be aware that patients receiving Sulfisoxazole might require less thiopental for anesthesia.

Sulfonamides can displace methotrexate from plasma protein-binding sites, thus increasing free methotrexate concentrations. Studies in man have shown Sulfisoxazole infusions to decrease plasma protein-bound methotrexate by one-fourth.

Sulfisoxazole can also potentiate the blood sugar lowering activity of sulfonylureas, as well as cause hypoglycemia by itself.

Carcinogenesis, Mutagenesis, Impairment of Fertility: Carcinogenesis: Sulfisoxazole was not carcinogenic to mice in either sex when administered by gavage for 103 weeks at dosages up to approximately 18 times the highest recommended human daily dose or to rats at 4 times the highest recommended human daily dose. Rats appear to be especially susceptible to the goitrogenic effects of sulfonamides and long-term administration of sulfonamides has resulted in thyroid malignancies in this species.

Mutagenesis: There are no studies available that adequately evaluate the mutagenic potential of Sulfisoxazole. Ames mutagenic assays have not been performed with Sulfisoxazole. However, Sulfisoxazole was not observed to be mutagenic in *E. coli* Sd-4-73 when tested in the absence of a metabolic activating system.

Impairment of Fertility: Sulfisoxazole has not undergone adequate trials relating to impairment of fertility. In a reproduction study in rats given 7 times the highest recommended human dose per day of Sulfisoxazole, no effects were observed regarding mating behavior, conception rate or fertility index (percent pregnant).

Pregnancy: Teratogenic Effects: Pregnancy Category C. At dosages 7 times the highest recommended human daily dose, Sulfisoxazole was not teratogenic in either rats or rabbits. However, in two other teratogenicity studies, cleft palates developed in both rats and mice, and skeletal defects were also observed in rats after administration of 9 times the highest recommended human daily dose of Sulfisoxazole.

There are no adequate and well-controlled studies of Sulfisoxazole in pregnant women. It is not known whether Sulfisoxazole can cause fetal harm when administered to a pregnant woman prior to term or can affect reproduction capacity. Sulfisoxazole should be used during pregnancy only if the potential benefit justifies the potential risk to the fetus.

Nonteratogenic Effects: Kernicterus may occur in the newborn as a result of treatment of a pregnant woman *at term* with sulfonamides. (See *"Contraindications"*.)

Nursing Mothers: Sulfisoxazole is excreted in human milk. Because of the potential for the development of kernicterus in neonates due to the displacement of bilirubin from plasma proteins by Sulfisoxazole, a decision should be made whether to discontinue nursing or discontinue the drug taking into account the importance of the drug to the mother. (See *"Contraindications"*.)

Pediatric Use: Sulfisoxazole is not recommended for use in infants younger than 2 months of age except in the treatment of congenital toxoplasmosis as adjunctive therapy with pyrimethamine. (See *"Contraindications"*.)

ADVERSE REACTIONS
The listing that follows includes adverse reactions both that have been reported with Sulfisoxazole and some which have not been reported with this specific drug: however, the pharmacologic similarities among the sulfonamides require that each of the reactions be considered with the administration of any of the Sulfisoxazole dosage forms.

Allergic/Dermatologic: Anaphylaxis, erythema multiforme (Stevens-Johnson syndrome), toxic epidermal necrolysis, exfoliative dermatitis, angioedema, arteritis and vasculitis, allergic myocarditis, serum sickness, rash, urticaria, pruritus, photosensitivity, and conjunctival and scleral injection, generalized allergic reactions and generalized skin eruptions. In addition, periarteritis nodosa and systemic lupus erythematosus have been reported. (See *"Warnings"*.)

Cardiovascular: Tachycardia, palpitations, syncope, cyanosis.

Endocrine: The sulfonamides bear certain chemical similarities to some goitrogens, diuretics (acetazolamide and thiazides) and oral hypoglycemia agents. Cross-sensitivity may exist with these agents. Development of goiter, diuresis and hypoglycemia have occurred rarely in patients receiving sulfonamides.

Gastrointestinal: Hepatitis, hepatocellular necrosis, jaundice, pseudomembranous colitis, nausea, emesis, anorexia, abdominal pain, diarrhea, gastrointestinal hemorrhage, melena, flatulence, glossitis, stomatitis, salivary gland enlargement, pancreatitis.

Onset of pseudomembranous colitis symptoms may occur during or after treatment with Sulfisoxazole. (See *"Warnings"*.)

Sulfisoxazole has been reported to cause increased elevations of liver-associated enzymes in patients with hepatitis.

Genitourinary: Crystalluria, hematuria, BUN and creatinine elevations, nephritis and toxic nephrosis with oliguria and anuria. Acute renal failure and urinary retention have also been reported. The frequency of renal complications, commonly associated with some sulfonamides, is lower in patients receiving the more soluble sulfonamides such as Sulfisoxazole.

Hematologic: Leukopenia, agranulocytosis, aplastic anemia, thrombocytopenia, purpura, hemolyticanemia, anemia, eosinophilia, clotting disorders including hypoprothombinemia, and hypofibrinogenemia, sulfhemoglobinemia, methemoglobinemia.

Musculoskeletal: Arthralgia, myalgia.

Neurologic: Headache, dizziness, peripheral neuritis, paresthesia, convulsions, tinnitus, vertigo, ataxia, intracranial hypertension.

Psychiatric: Psychosis, hallucination, disorientation, depression, anxiety, apathy.

Respiratory: Cough, shortness of breath, pulmonary infiltrates. (See *"Warnings"*.)

Vascular: Angioedema, arteritis, vasculitis.

Miscellaneous: Edema (including periorbital), pyrexia, drowsiness, weakness, fatigue, lassitude, rigors, flushing, hearing loss, insomnia, pneumonitis, chills.

OVERDOSAGE
The amount of a single dose of Sulfisoxazole that is associated with symptoms of overdosage or is likely to be life-threatening has not been reported. Signs and symptoms of overdosage reported with sulfonamides include anorexia, colic, nausea, vomiting, dizziness, headache, drowsiness and unconsciousness. Pyrexia, hematuria and crystalluria may be noted. Blood dyscrasias and jaundice are potential late manifestations of overdosage.

General principles of treatment include the immediate discontinuation of the drug; institution of gastric lavage or emesis; forcing oral fluids; and the administration of intravenous fluids if urine output is low and renal function is normal. The patient should be monitored with blood counts and appropriate blood chemistries, including electrolytes. If the patient becomes cyanotic, the possibility of methemoglobinemia should be considered and, if present, the condition should be treated appropriately with intravenous 1% methylene blue. If a significant blood dyscrasia or jaundice occurs, specific therapy should be instituted for these complications.

Peritoneal dialysis is not effective and hemodialysis is only moderately effective in eliminating sulfonamides.

DOSAGE AND ADMINISTRATION
Systemic sulfonamides are contraindicated in infants under 2 months of age, except in the treatment of congenital toxoplasmosis as adjunctive therapy with pyrimethamine.

Usual Dose for Infants over 2 Months of Age and Children: Initial dose: One half of the 24-hour dose. Maintenance dose: 150 mg/kg/24 hours or 4 gm/M^2/24 hours—dose to be divided into 4 to 6 doses/24 hours. The maximum dose should not exceed 6 gm/24 hours.

Usual Adult Dose: Initial dose: 2 to 4 gm. Maintenance dose: 4 to 8 gm/24 hours, divided in 4 to 6 doses/24 hours.

REFERENCES
1. Boisvert A, Barbeau G, Belanger PM: Pharmacokinetics of sulfisoxazole in young and elderly subjects. *Gerontology*, 1984: 30: 125-131. 2. Oie S, Gambertoglio JG, Fleckenstein L: Comparison of the disposition of total and unbound sulfisoxazole after single and multiple dosing. *J Pharmacokinet Biopharm*. 1982; 10: 157-172. 3. National Committee for Clinical Laboratory Standards. *Performance Standards for Antimicrobial Disk Susceptibility Tests*. 4th ed. Villanova, PA: April 1990. Approved Standard NCCLS Document M2-A4. Vol. 10, No. 7 NCCLS. 4. National Committee for Clinical Laboratory Standards. *Methods for Dilution Antimicrobial Susceptibility Tests for Bacteria that Grow Aerobically*. 2nd ed. Villanova, PA; April 1990. Approved Standard NCCLS Document M7-A2, Vol. 10, No. 8 NCCLS.

HOW SUPPLIED
SUSPENSION: 500 MG/5 ML

BRAND/MANUFACTURER	NDC	SIZE	AWP
◆ BRAND			
GANTRISIN PEDIATRIC: Roche Labs	00004-1003-30	120 ml	$11.40

SUSPENSION: 500 MG/5 ML

BRAND/MANUFACTURER	NDC	SIZE	AWP
◇ BRAND			
GANTRISIN PEDIATRIC: Roche Labs	00004-1003-28	480 ml	$39.57

TABLETS: 500 MG

AVERAGE UNIT PRICE (AVAILABLE SIZES)		GENERIC A-RATED AVERAGE PRICE (GAAP)	
BRAND	$0.23	100s	$12.27
GENERIC	$0.11	1000s	$90.27
HCFA FUL (100s ea)	$0.09		

BRAND/MANUFACTURER	NDC	SIZE	AWP
◆ BRAND			
▶ GANTRISIN: Roche Labs	00004-0009-01	100s	$22.48
	00004-0009-49	100s ud	$24.48
	00004-0009-14	500s	$111.35
◆ GENERICS			
Zenith	00172-2218-60	100s	$10.45
Aligen	00405-4971-01	100s	$11.00
Moore,H.L.	00839-1649-06	100s	$11.19
Schein	00364-0265-01	100s	$11.70
URL	00677-0143-01	100s	$12.25
Martec	52555-0323-01	100s	$12.25
Richlyn	00115-4747-01	100s	$12.87
Goldline	00182-0497-01	100s	$12.90
Geneva	00781-1015-01	100s	$12.98
Major	00904-2218-60	100s	$13.45
Rugby	00536-4618-01	100s	$13.97
Parmed	00349-2220-10	1000s	$59.51
Major	00904-2218-80	1000s	$81.40
Zenith	00172-2218-80	1000s	$84.50
Richlyn	00115-4747-03	1000s	$99.00
Rugby	00536-4618-10	1000s	$126.92

Sulfoxyl *SEE* BENZOYL PEROXIDE WITH SULFUR

◆ RATED THERAPEUTICALLY EQUIVALENT; ◇ THERAPEUTIC EQUIVALENCE UNCONFIRMED; ○ UNRATED

Sulindac

DESCRIPTION

Sulindac is a nonsteroidal, anti-inflammatory indene derivative designated chemically as (Z)-5-fluoro-2-methyl-1-[[p-(methylsulfinyl) phenyl]methylene]-1H-indene-3-acetic acid. It is not a salicylate, pyrazolone or propionic acid derivative. Its empirical formula is $C_{20}H_{17}FO_3S$, with a molecular weight of 356.42. Sulindac, a yellow crystalline compound, is a weak organic acid practically insoluble in water below pH 4.5, but very soluble as the sodium salt or in buffers of pH 6 or higher.

Following absorption, Sulindac undergoes two major biotransformations—reversible reduction to the sulfide metabolite, and irreversible oxidation to the sulfone metabolite. Available evidence indicates that the biological activity resides with the sulfide metabolite.

Following is its chemical structure:

CLINICAL PHARMACOLOGY

Sulindac is a nonsteroidal anti-inflammatory drug, also possessing analgesic and antipyretic activities. Its mode of action, like that of other nonsteroidal, anti-inflammatory agents, is not known; however, its therapeutic action is not due to pituitary-adrenal stimulation. Inhibition of prostaglandin synthesis by the sulfide metabolite may be involved in the anti-inflammatory action of Sulindac.

Sulindac is approximately 90% absorbed in man after oral administration. The peak plasma concentrations of the biologically active sulfide metabolite are achieved in about two hours when Sulindac is administered in the fasting state, and in about three to four hours when Sulindac is administered with food. The mean half-life of Sulindac is 7.8 hours while the mean half-life of the sulfide metabolite is 16.4 hours. Sustained plasma levels of the sulfide metabolite are consistent with a prolonged anti-inflammatory action which is the rationale for a twice per day dosage schedule.

Sulindac and its sulfone metabolite undergo extensive enterohepatic circulation relative to the sulfide metabolite in animals. Studies in man have also demonstrated that recirculation of the parent drug, Sulindac, and its sulfone metabolite, is more extensive than that of the active sulfide metabolite. The active sulfide metabolite accounts for less than six percent of the total intestinal exposure to Sulindac and its metabolites.

The primary route of excretion in man is via the urine as both Sulindac and its sulfone metabolite (free and glucuronide conjugates). Approximately 50% of the administered dose is excreted in the urine, with the conjugated sulfone metabolite accounting for the major portion. Less than 1% of the administered dose of Sulindac appears in the urine as the sulfide metabolite. Approximately 25% is found in the feces, primarily as the sulfone and sulfide metabolites.

The bioavailability of Sulindac, as assessed by urinary excretion, was not changed by concomitant administration of an antacid containing magnesium hydroxide 200 mg and aluminum hydroxide 225 mg per 5 mL.

Because Sulindac is excreted in the urine primarily as biologically inactive forms, it may possibly affect renal function to a lesser extent than other nonsteroidal anti-inflammatory drugs, however, renal adverse experiences have been reported with Sulindac (see "Adverse Reactions"). In a study of patients with chronic glomerular disease treated with therapeutic doses of Sulindac, no effect was demonstrated on renal blood flow, glomerular filtration rate, or urinary excretion of prostaglandin E_2 and the primary metabolite of prostacyclin, 6-keto-$PGF_1\alpha$. However, in other studies in healthy volunteers and patients with liver disease, Sulindac was found to blunt the renal responses to intravenous furosemide, i.e., the diuresis, natriuresis, increments in plasma renin activity and urinary excretion of prostaglandins. These observations may represent a differentiation of the effects of Sulindac on renal functions based on differences in pathogenesis of the renal prostaglandin dependence associated with differing dose-response relationships of different NSAIDs to the various renal functions influenced by prostaglandins. These observations need further clarification and in the interim, Sulindac should be used with caution in patients whose renal function may be impaired (see "Precautions").

In healthy men, the average fecal blood loss, measured over a two-week period during administration of 400 mg per day of Sulindac, was similar to that for placebo, and was statistically significantly less than that resulting from 4800 mg per day of aspirin.

In controlled clinical studies Sulindac was evaluated in the following five conditions:

1. OSTEOARTHRITIS

In patients with osteoarthritis of the hip and knee, the anti-inflammatory and analgesic activity of Sulindac was demonstrated by clinical measurements that included: assessments by both patient and investigator of overall response; decrease in disease activity as assessed by both patient and investigator; improvement in ARA Functional Class; relief of night pain; improvement in overall evaluation of pain, including pain on weight bearing and pain on active and passive motion; improvement in joint mobility, range of motion, and functional activities; decreased swelling and tenderness; and decreased duration of stiffness following prolonged inactivity.

In clinical studies in which dosages were adjusted according to patient needs, Sulindac 200 to 400 mg daily was shown to be comparable in effectiveness to aspirin 2400 to 4800 mg daily. Sulindac was generally well tolerated, and patients on it had a lower overall incidence of total adverse effects, of milder gastrointestinal reactions, and of tinnitus than did patients on aspirin. (See "Adverse Reactions".)

2. RHEUMATOID ARTHRITIS

In patients with rheumatoid arthritis, the anti-inflammatory and analgesic activity of Sulindac was demonstrated by clinical measurements that included: assessments by both patient and investigator of overall response; decrease in disease activity as assessed by both patient and investigator; reduction in overall joint pain; reduction in duration and severity of morning stiffness; reduction in day and night pain; decrease in time required to walk 50 feet; decrease in general pain as measured on a visual analog scale improvement in the Ritchie articular index; decrease in proximal interphalangeal joint size; improvement in ARA Functional Class; increase in grip strength; reduction in painful joint count and score; reduction in swollen joint count and score; and increased flexion and extension of the wrist.

In clinical studies in which dosages were adjusted according to patient needs, Sulindac 300 to 400 mg daily was shown to be comparable in effectiveness to aspirin 3600 to 4800 mg daily. Sulindac was generally well tolerated, and patients on it had a lower overall incidence of total adverse effects of milder gastrointestinal reactions, and of tinnitus than did patients on aspirin. (See "Adverse Reactions".)

In patients with rheumatoid arthritis, Sulindac may be used in combination with gold salts at usual dosage levels. In clinical studies, Sulindac added to the regimen of gold salts usually resulted in additional symptomatic relief but did not alter the course of the underlying disease.

3. ANKYLOSING SPONDYLITIS

In patients with ankylosing spondylitis, the anti-inflammatory and analgesic activity of Sulindac was demonstrated by clinical measurements that included: assessments by both patient and investigator of overall response; decrease in disease activity as assessed by both patient and investigator; improvement in ARA Functional Class; improvement in patient and investigator evaluation of spinal pain tenderness and/or spasm: reduction in the duration of morning stiffness; increase in the time to onset of fatigue; relief of night pain; increase in chest expansion; and increase in spinal mobility evaluated by fingers-to-floor distance, occiput to wall distance, the Schober Test, and the Wright Modification of the Schober Test. In a clinical study in which dosages were adjusted according to patient need, Sulindac 200 to 400 mg daily was as effective as indomethacin 75 to 150 mg daily. In a second study, Sulindac 300 to 400 mg daily was comparable in effectiveness to phenylbutazone 400 to 600 mg daily. Sulindac was better tolerated than phenylbutazone. (See "Adverse Reactions".)

4. ACUTE PAINFUL SHOULDER (ACUTE SUBACROMIAL BURSITIS/ SUPRASPINATUS TENDINITIS)

In patients with acute painful shoulder (acute subacromial bursitis/supraspinatus tendinitis), the anti-inflammatory and analgesic activity of Sulindac was demonstrated by clinical measurements that included: assessments by both patient and investigator of overall response; relief of night pain, spontaneous pain, and pain on active motion; decrease in local tenderness; and improvement in range of motion measured by abduction, and internal and external rotation. In clinical studies in acute painful shoulder, Sulindac 300 to 400 mg daily and oxyphenbutazone 400 to 600 mg daily were shown to be equally effective and well tolerated.

5. ACUTE GOUTY ARTHRITIS

In patients with acute gouty arthritis, the anti-inflammatory and analgesic activity of Sulindac was demonstrated by clinical measurements that included: assessments by both the patient and investigator of overall response; relief of weight-bearing pain; relief of pain at rest and on active and passive motion; decrease in tenderness; reduction in warmth and swelling; increase in range of motion; and improvement in ability to function. In clinical studies, Sulindac at 400 mg daily and phenylbutazone at 600 mg daily were shown to be equally effective. In these short-term studies in which reduction of dosage was permitted according to response, both drugs were equally well tolerated.

INDICATIONS AND USAGE

Sulindac is indicated for acute or long-term use in the relief of signs and symptoms of the following:

1. Osteoarthritis
2. Rheumatoid arthritis*
3. Ankylosing spondylitis
4. Acute painful shoulder (Acute subacromial bursitis/ supraspinatus tendinitis)
5. Acute gouty arthritis

---

* The safety and effectiveness of Sulindac have not been established in rheumatoid arthritis patients who are designated in the American Rheumatism Association classification as Functional Class IV (incapacitated, largely or wholly bedridden, or confined to wheelchair; little or no self-care).

► SHOWN IN PRODUCT IDENTIFICATION GUIDE

UNLABELED USES

Sulindac is used alone or as an adjunct in the treatment of colon polyposis, including Gardner's syndrome or familial polyposis coli. It is also used in the treatment of adult respiratory distress syndrome, diabetic neuropathy, fever, and juvenile rheumatoid arthritis.

CONTRAINDICATIONS

Sulindac should not be used in:

Patients who are hypersensitive to this product.

Patients in whom acute asthmatic attacks, urticaria, or rhinitis are precipitated by aspirin or other nonsteroidal anti-inflammatory agents.

WARNINGS

GASTROINTESTINAL EFFECTS

Peptic ulceration and gastrointestinal bleeding have been reported in patients receiving Sulindac. Fatalities have occurred. Gastrointestinal bleeding is associated with higher morbidity and mortality in patients acutely ill with other conditions, the elderly and patients with hemorrhagic disorders. In patients with active gastrointestinal bleeding or an active peptic ulcer, an appropriate ulcer regimen should be instituted, and the physician must weigh the benefits of therapy with Sulindac against possible hazards, and carefully monitor the patient's progress. When Sulindac is given to patients with a history of either upper or lower gastrointestinal tract disease, it should be given under close supervision and only after consulting the *"Adverse Reactions"* section.

RISK OF GI ULCERATIONS, BLEEDING AND PERFORATION WITH NSAID THERAPY

Serious gastrointestinal toxicity such as bleeding, ulceration, and perforation, can occur at any time, with or without warning symptoms, in patients treated chronically with NSAID therapy. Although minor upper gastrointestinal problems, such as dyspepsia, are common, usually developing early in therapy, physicians should remain alert for ulceration and bleeding in patients treated chronically with NSAIDs even in the absence of previous GI tract symptoms. In patients observed in clinical trials of several months to two years duration, symptomatic upper GI ulcers, gross bleeding or perforation appear to occur in approximately 1% of patients treated for 3-6 months, and in about 2-4% of patients treated for one year. Physicians should inform patients about the signs and/or symptoms of serious GI toxicity and what steps to take if they occur.

Studies to date have not identified any subset of patients not at risk of developing peptic ulceration and bleeding. Except for a prior history of serious GI events and other risk factors known to be associated with peptic ulcer disease, such as alcoholism, smoking, etc., no risk factors (e.g., age, sex) have been associated with increased risk. Elderly or debilitated patients seem to tolerate ulceration or bleeding less well than other individuals and most spontaneous reports of fatal GI events are in this population. Studies to date are inconclusive concerning the relative risk of various NSAIDs in causing such reactions. High doses of any NSAID probably carry a greater risk of these reactions, although controlled clinical trials showing this do not exist in most cases. In considering the use of relatively large doses (within the recommended dosage range), sufficient benefit should be anticipated to offset the potential increased risk of GI toxicity.

HYPERSENSITIVITY

Rarely, fever and other evidence of hypersensitivity (see *"Adverse Reactions"*) including abnormalities in one or more liver function tests and severe skin reactions have occurred during therapy with Sulindac. Fatalities have occurred in these patients. Hepatitis, jaundice, or both, with or without fever, may occur usually within the first one to three months of therapy. Determinations of liver function should be considered whenever a patient on therapy with Sulindac develops unexplained fever, rash or other dermatologic reactions or constitutional symptoms. If unexplained fever or other evidence of hypersensitivity occurs, therapy with Sulindac should be discontinued. The elevated temperature and abnormalities in liver function caused by Sulindac characteristically have reverted to normal after discontinuation of therapy. Administration of Sulindac should not be reinstituted in such patients.

HEPATIC EFFECTS

In addition to hypersensitivity reactions involving the liver, in some patients the findings are consistent with those of cholestatic hepatitis. As with other nonsteroidal anti-inflammatory drugs, borderline elevations of one or more liver tests without any other signs and symptoms may occur in up to 15% of patients. These abnormalities may progress, may remain essentially unchanged, or may be transient with continued therapy. The SGPT (ALT) test is probably the most sensitive indicator of liver dysfunction. Meaningful (3 times the upper limit of normal) elevations of SGPT or SGOT (AST) occurred in controlled clinical trials in less than 1% of patients. A patient with symptoms and/or signs suggesting liver dysfunction, or in whom an abnormal liver test has occurred, should be evaluated for evidence of the development of more severe hepatic reaction while on therapy with Sulindac. Although such reactions as described above are rare, if abnormal liver tests persist or worsen, if clinical signs and symptoms consistent with liver disease develop, or if systemic manifestations occur (e.g. eosinophilia, rash, etc.), Sulindac should be discontinued.

In clinical trials with Sulindac the use of doses of 600 mg/day has been associated with an increased incidence of mild liver test abnormalities (see *"Dosage and Administration"* for maximum dosage recommendation).

PRECAUTIONS

GENERAL

Non-steroidal anti-inflammatory drugs, including Sulindac may mask the usual signs and symptoms of infection. Therefore, the physician must be continually on the alert for this and should use the drug with extra care in the presence of existing infection.

Although Sulindac has less effect on platelet function and bleeding time than aspirin, it is an inhibitor of platelet function; therefore, patients who may be adversely affected should be carefully observed when Sulindac is administered.

Pancreatitis has been reported in patients receiving Sulindac (see *"Adverse Reactions"*). Should pancreatitis be suspected the drug should be discontinued and not restarted, supportive medical therapy instituted, and the patient monitored closely with appropriate laboratory studies (e.g., serum and urine amylase, amylase/creatinine clearance ratio, electrolytes, serum calcium, glucose, lipase, etc.). A search for other causes of pancreatitis as well as those conditions which mimic pancreatitis should be conducted.

Because of reports of adverse eye findings with nonsteroidal anti-inflammatory agents, it is recommended that patients who develop eye complaints during treatment with Sulindac have ophthalmologic studies.

In patients with poor liver function, delayed, elevated and prolonged circulating levels of the sulfide and sulfone metabolites may occur. Such patients should be monitored closely; a reduction of daily dosage may be required.

Edema has been observed in some patients taking Sulindac. Therefore, as with other non-steroidal anti-inflammatory drugs, Sulindac should be used with caution in patients with compromised cardiac function, hypertension, or other conditions predisposing to fluid retention.

Sulindac may allow a reduction in dosage or the elimination of chronic corticosteroid therapy in some patients with rheumatoid arthritis. However, it is generally necessary to reduce corticosteroids gradually over several months in order to avoid an exacerbation of disease or signs and symptoms of adrenal insufficiency. Abrupt withdrawal of chronic corticosteroid treatment is generally not recommended even when patients have had a serious complication of chronic corticosteroid therapy.

RENAL EFFECTS

As with other nonsteroidal anti-inflammatory drugs, long term administration of Sulindac to animals has resulted in renal papillary necrosis and other abnormal renal pathology. In humans, there have been reports of acute interstitial nephritis with hematuria, proteinuria, and occasionally nephrotic syndrome.

A second form of renal toxicity has been seen in patients with prerenal and renal conditions leading to a reduction in renal blood flow or blood volume, where the renal prostaglandins have a supportive role in the maintenance of renal perfusion. In these patients administration of an NSAID may cause a dose dependent reduction in prostaglandin formation and may precipitate overt renal decompensation. Sulindac may affect renal function less than other NSAIDs in patients with chronic glomerular renal disease (see *"Clinical Pharmacology"*). Until these observations are better understood and clarified, however, and because renal adverse experiences have been reported with Sulindac (see *"Adverse Reactions"*), caution should be exercised when administering the drug to patients with conditions associated with increased risk of the effects of nonsteroidal anti-inflammatory drugs on renal function, such as those with renal or hepatic dysfunction, diabetes mellitus, advanced age, extracellular volume depletion from any cause, congestive heart failure, septicemia, pyelonephritis, or concomitant use of any nephrotoxic drug. Discontinuation of NSAID therapy is typically followed by recovery to the pretreatment state.

Since Sulindac is eliminated primarily by the kidneys, patients with significantly impaired renal function should be closely monitored; a lower daily dosage should be anticipated to avoid excessive drug accumulation.

Sulindac metabolites have been reported rarely as the major or a minor component in renal stones in association with other calculus components. Sulindac should be used with caution in patients with a history of renal lithiasis and they should be kept well hydrated while receiving Sulindac.

INFORMATION FOR PATIENTS

Sulindac, like other drugs of its class, is not free of side effects. The side effects of these drugs can cause discomfort and, rarely, there are more serious side effects such as gastrointestinal bleeding, which may result in hospitalization and even fatal outcomes.

NSAIDs (Nonsteroidal Anti-inflammatory Drugs) are often essential agents in the management of arthritis, but they also may be commonly employed for conditions which are less serious.

Physicians may wish to discuss with their patients the potential risks (see *"Warnings," "Precautions"* and *"Adverse Reactions"*) and likely benefits of NSAID treatment, particularly when the drugs are used for less serious conditions where treatment without NSAIDs may represent an acceptable alternative to both the patient and physician.

LABORATORY TESTS

Because serious GI tract ulceration and bleeding can occur without warning symptoms, physicians should follow chronically treated patients for the signs and symptoms of ulceration and bleeding and should inform them of the importance of this follow-up (see *"Warnings, Risk of GI Ulcerations, Bleeding and Perforation with NSAID Therapy"*).

USE IN PREGNANCY

Sulindac is not recommended for use in pregnant women, since safety for use has not been established, and because of the known effect of drugs of this class on the

---

human fetus (closure of the ductus arteriosus, platelet dysfunction with resultant bleeding, renal dysfunction or failure with oligohydramnios, gastrointestinal bleeding or perforation, and myocardial degenerative changes) during the third trimester of pregnancy. In reproduction studies in the rat, a decrease in average fetal weight and an increase in numbers of dead pups were observed on the first day of the postpartum period at dosage levels of 20 and 40 mg/kg/day (2 ½ and 5 times the usual maximum daily dose in humans), although there was no adverse effect on the survival and growth during the remainder of the postpartum period Sulindac prolongs the duration of gestation in rats, as do other compounds of this class which also may cause dystocia and delayed parturition in pregnant animals. Visceral and skeletal malformations observed in low incidence among rabbits in some teratology studies did not occur at the same dosage levels in repeat studies, nor at a higher dosage level in the same species.

NURSING MOTHERS
Nursing should not be undertaken while a patient is on Sulindac. It is not known whether Sulindac is secreted in human milk; however, it is secreted in the milk of lactating rats.

USE IN CHILDREN
Safety and effectiveness in children have not been established.

DRUG INTERACTIONS
DMSO should not be used with Sulindac. Concomitant administration has been reported to reduce the plasma levels of the active sulfide metabolite and potentially reduce efficacy. In addition, this combination has been reported to cause peripheral neuropathy.

Although Sulindac and its sulfide metabolite are highly bound to protein, studies, in which Sulindac was given at a dose of 400 mg daily, have shown no clinically significant interaction with oral anticoagulants or oral hypoglycemic agents. However, patients should be monitored carefully until it is certain that no change in the anticoagulant or hypoglycemic dosage is required. Special attention should be paid to patients taking higher doses than those recommended and to patients with renal impairment or other metabolic defects that might increase Sulindac blood levels.

The concomitant administration of aspirin with Sulindac significantly depressed the plasma levels of the active sulfide metabolite. A double-blind study compared the safety and efficacy of Sulindac 300 or 400 mg daily given alone or with aspirin 2.4 g/day for the treatment of osteoarthritis. The addition of aspirin did not alter the types of clinical or laboratory adverse experiences for Sulindac; however, the combination showed an increase in the incidence of gastrointestinal adverse experiences. Since the addition of aspirin did not have a favorable effect on the therapeutic response to Sulindac, the combination is not recommended.

Caution should be used if Sulindac is administered concomitantly with methotrexate. Nonsteroidal anti-inflammatory drugs have been reported to decrease the tubular secretion of methotrexate and to potentiate its toxicity.

Administration of nonsteroidal anti-inflammatory drugs concomitantly with cyclosporine has been associated with an increase in cyclosporine-induced toxicity, possibly due to decreased synthesis of renal prostacyclin. NSAIDs should be used with caution in patients taking cyclosporine, and renal function should be carefully monitored.

The concomitant administration of Sulindac and diflunisal in normal volunteers resulted in lowering of the plasma levels of the active Sulindac sulfide metabolite by approximately one-third.

Probenecid given concomitantly with Sulindac had only a slight effect on plasma sulfide levels, while plasma levels of Sulindac and sulfone were increased. Sulindac was shown to produce a modest reduction in the uricosuric action of probenecid, which probably is not significant under most circumstances.

Neither propoxyphene hydrochloride nor acetaminophen had any effect on the plasma levels of Sulindac or its sulfide metabolite.

ADVERSE REACTIONS
The following adverse reactions were reported in clinical trials or have been reported since the drug was marketed. The probability exists of a causal relationship between Sulindac and these adverse reactions. The adverse reactions which have been observed in clinical trials encompass observations in 1,865 patients, including 232 observed for at least 48 weeks.

INCIDENCE GREATER THAN 1%
Gastrointestinal: The most frequent types of adverse reactions occurring with Sulindac are gastrointestinal; these include gastrointestinal pain (10%), dyspepsia*, nausea* with or without vomiting, diarrhea*, constipation*, flatulence, anorexia and gastrointestinal cramps.

Dermatologic: Rash*, pruritus.

Central Nervous System: Dizziness*, headache*, nervousness.

Special Senses: Tinnitus.

Miscellaneous: Edema (see "Precautions").

INCIDENCE LESS THAN 1 IN 100
Gastrointestinal: Gastritis, gastroenteritis or colitis. Peptic ulcer and gastrointestinal bleeding have been reported. GI perforation has been reported rarely.

Liver function abnormalities; jaundice, sometimes with fever; cholestasis; hepatitis; hepatic failure.

* Incidence between 3% and 9%. Those reactions occurring in 1 to 3% of patients are not marked with an asterisk.

There have been rare reports of Sulindac metabolites in common bile duct "sludge" and in biliary calculi in patients with symptoms of cholecystitis who underwent a cholecystectomy.
Pancreatitis (see "Precautions").
Ageusia; glossitis.

Dermatologic: Stomatitis, sore or dry mucous membranes, alopecia, photosensitivity.
Erythema multiforme, toxic epidermal necrolysis, Stevens-Johnson syndrome, and exfoliative dermatitis have been reported.

Cardiovascular: Congestive heart failure, especially in patients with marginal cardiac function; palpitation; hypertension.

Hematologic: Thrombocytopenia; ecchymosis; purpura; leukopenia; agranulocytosis; neutropenia; bone marrow depression, including aplastic anemia; hemolytic anemia; increased prothrombin time in patients on oral anticoagulants (see "Precautions").

Genitourinary: Urine discoloration, dysuria; vaginal bleeding; hematuria; proteinuria; crystalluria; renal impairment, including renal failure; interstitial nephritis; nephrotic syndrome.
Renal calculi containing Sulindac metabolites have been observed rarely.

Metabolic: Hyperkalemia.

Musculoskeletal: Muscle weakness.

Psychiatric: Depression: psychic disturbances including acute psychosis.

Nervous System: Vertigo; insomnia; somnolence; paresthesia; convulsions; syncope; aseptic meningitis.

Special Senses: Blurred vision; visual disturbances; decreased hearing; metallic or bitter taste.

Respiratory: Epistaxis.

Hypersensitivity Reactions:
Anaphylaxis; angioneurotic edema: bronchial spasm; dyspnea.
Hypersensitivity vasculitis.
A potentially fatal apparent hypersensitivity syndrome has been reported. This syndrome may include constitutional symptoms (fever, chills, diaphoresis, flushing), cutaneous findings (rash or other dermatologic reactions—see above), conjunctivitis, involvement of major organs (changes in liver function including hepatic failure, jaundice, pancreatitis, pneumonitis with or without pleural effusion, leukopenia, leukocytosis, eosinophilia, disseminated intravascular coagulation, anemia, renal impairment, including renal failure), and other less specific findings (adenitis, arthralgia, arthritis, myalgia, fatigue, malaise, hypotension, chest pain, tachycardia).

CAUSAL RELATIONSHIP UNKNOWN
A rare occurrence of fulminant necrotizing fasciitis, particularly in association with Group A beta-hemolytic streptococcus, has been described in persons treated with non-steroidal anti-inflammatory agents, sometimes with fatal outcome (see "Precautions, General").

Other reactions have been reported in clinical trials or since the drug was marketed, but occurred under circumstances where a causal relationship could not be established. However, in these rarely reported events, that possibility cannot be excluded. Therefore, these observations are listed to serve as alerting information to physicians.

Cardiovascular: Arrhythmia.

Metabolic: Hyperglycemia.

Nervous System: Neuritis.

Special Senses: Disturbances of the retina and its vasculature.

Miscellaneous: Gynecomastia.

MANAGEMENT OF OVERDOSAGE
Cases of overdosage have been reported and rarely, deaths have occurred. The following signs and symptoms may be observed following overdosage: stupor, coma, diminished urine output and hypotension.

In the event of overdosage, the stomach should be emptied by inducing vomiting or by gastric lavage, and the patient carefully observed and given symptomatic and supportive treatment.

Animal studies show that absorption is decreased by the prompt administration of activated charcoal and excretion is enhanced by alkalinization of the urine.

DOSAGE AND ADMINISTRATION
Sulindac should be administered orally twice a day with food. The maximum dosage is 400 mg per day. Dosages above 400 mg per day are not recommended.

In osteoarthritis, rheumatoid arthritis, and ankylosing spondylitis, the recommended starting dosage is 150 mg twice a day. The dosage may be lowered or raised depending on the response.

A prompt response (within one week) can be expected in about one-half of patients with osteoarthritis, ankylosing spondylitis, and rheumatoid arthritis. Others may require longer to respond.

In acute painful shoulder (acute subacromial bursitis/supraspinatus tendinitis) and acute gouty arthritis, the recommended dosage is 200 mg twice a day. After a satisfactory response has been achieved, the dosage may be reduced according to the response. In acute painful shoulder, therapy for 7-14 days is usually adequate. In acute gouty arthritis, therapy for 7 days is usually adequate.

HOW SUPPLIED
TABLETS: 150 MG

AVERAGE UNIT PRICE (AVAILABLE SIZES)		GENERIC A-RATED AVERAGE PRICE (GAAP)	
BRAND	$0.95	100s	$77.72
GENERIC	$0.76	500s	$357.37
HCFA FUL (100s ea)	$0.29	1000s	$665.66

BRAND/MANUFACTURER	NDC	SIZE	AWP
◆ BRAND			
➤ CLINORIL: Merck	00006-0941-68	100s	$93.25
	00006-0941-28	100s ud	$97.34
	00006-0941-54	720s	$672.43
◆ GENERICS			
Schein	00364-2441-06	60s	$47.75
Warner Chilcott	00047-0773-24	100s	$71.14
Schein	00364-2441-01	100s	$71.50
Qualitest	00603-5872-21	100s	$71.50
Lederle Std Prod	00005-3550-43	100s	$74.71
Moore,H.L.	00839-7621-06	100s	$75.53
Major	00904-3378-60	100s	$77.50
Goldline	00182-1705-01	100s	$77.50
Mason Dist	11845-0415-01	100s	$77.66
➤ West Point	59591-0170-68	100s	$78.35
Mylan	00378-0427-01	100s	$78.95
URL	00677-1173-01	100s	$79.90
Aligen	00405-4973-01	100s	$79.90
Mutual	53489-0478-01	100s	$79.90
Geneva	00781-1811-01	100s	$80.20
Rugby	00536-5645-01	100s	$81.75
Du Pont Multi	00056-0220-70	100s	$81.81
Parmed	00349-8887-01	100s	$84.25
Raway	00686-0666-20	100s ud	$60.00
Major	00904-3378-61	100s ud	$68.48
Schein	00364-2441-90	100s ud	$74.65
Vangard	00615-3528-13	100s ud	$78.88
Goldline	00182-1705-89	100s ud	$80.00
Geneva	00781-1811-13	100s ud	$83.71
UDL	51079-0666-20	100s ud	$87.60
Medirex	57480-0399-01	100s ud	$87.60
Moore,H.L.	00839-7621-12	500s	$302.39
Schein	00364-2441-05	500s	$321.80
Mason Dist	11845-0415-03	500s	$343.43
Major	00904-3378-40	500s	$344.65
Goldline	00182-1705-05	500s	$346.50
➤ West Point	59591-0170-74	500s	$359.90
Rugby	00536-5645-05	500s	$361.50
URL	00677-1173-05	500s	$364.70
Mutual	53489-0478-05	500s	$364.70
Geneva	00781-1811-05	500s	$372.93
Du Pont Multi	00056-0220-85	500s	$388.60
Parmed	00349-8887-05	500s	$417.30
Sandocare	58345-0829-65	640s	$544.00
Warner Chilcott	00047-0773-32	1000s	$640.22
Lederle Std Prod	00005-3550-34	1000s	$691.09

TABLETS: 200 MG

AVERAGE UNIT PRICE (AVAILABLE SIZES)		GENERIC A-RATED AVERAGE PRICE (GAAP)	
BRAND	$1.16	100s	$94.66
GENERIC	$0.92	500s	$432.01
HCFA FUL (100s ea)	$0.36	1000s	$828.37

BRAND/MANUFACTURER	NDC	SIZE	AWP
◆ BRAND			
➤ CLINORIL: Merck	00006-0942-68	100s	$114.60
	00006-0942-28	100s ud	$118.65
	00006-0942-54	720s	$826.11
	00006-0942-78	1200s	$1376.25
◆ GENERICS			
Warner Chilcott	00047-0774-24	100s	$86.34
➤ Schein	00364-2442-01	100s	$87.90
Qualitest	00603-5873-21	100s	$87.90
Lederle Std Prod	00005-3551-43	100s	$89.91
Moore,H.L.	00839-7622-06	100s	$93.49
URL	00677-1174-01	100s	$95.00
Aligen	00405-4974-01	100s	$95.00
Mutual	53489-0479-01	100s	$95.00
Goldline	00182-1706-01	100s	$95.00
Goldline	00182-1721-01	100s	$95.00
Mason Dist	11845-0416-01	100s	$95.33
➤ West Point	59591-0154-68	100s	$95.75
Major	00904-3379-60	100s	$96.50
Mylan	00378-0531-01	100s	$96.95
Geneva	00781-1812-01	100s	$99.70
Rugby	00536-5646-01	100s	$100.35
Du Pont Multi	00056-0221-70	100s	$106.15
Raway	00686-0667-20	100s ud	$65.00
Major	00904-3379-61	100s ud	$83.47
➤ Schein	00364-2442-90	100s ud	$91.00
Vangard	00615-3529-13	100s ud	$99.05
Goldline	00182-1706-89	100s ud	$99.95
Geneva	00781-1812-13	100s ud	$103.23
Medirex	57480-0400-01	100s ud	$106.75

BRAND/MANUFACTURER	NDC	SIZE	AWP
UDL	51079-0667-20	100s ud	$106.78
Moore,H.L.	00839-7622-12	500s	$371.24
➤ Schein	00364-2442-05	500s	$395.50
Major	00904-3379-40	500s	$418.00
Mason Dist	11845-0416-03	500s	$421.80
Goldline	00182-1706-05	500s	$423.00
➤ West Point	59591-0154-74	500s	$430.87
URL	00677-1174-05	500s	$440.10
Mutual	53489-0479-05	500s	$440.10
Rugby	00536-5646-05	500s	$443.70
Geneva	00781-1812-05	500s	$463.61
Du Pont Multi	00056-0221-85	500s	$504.21
Sandocare	58345-0830-65	640s	$645.00
Goldline	00182-1721-10	1000s	$790.00
Lederle Std Prod	00005-3551-34	1000s	$831.70
Warner Chilcott	00047-0774-32	1000s	$863.40

Sultrin Triple Sulfa *SEE SULFABENZAMIDE/* SULFACETAMIDE/SULFATHIAZOLE

Sumatriptan Succinate

DESCRIPTION

Sumatriptan Succinate injection is a selective 5-hydroxytryptamine$_1$ receptor subtype agonist. Sumatriptan (as the Succinate), is chemically designated as 3-[2-(dimethylamino)ethyl]-N-methyl -1H-indole -5- methanesulfonamide butane-1,4-dioate(1:1). The empirical formula is $C_{14}H_{21}N_3O_2S \cdot C_4H_6O_4$, representing a molecular weight of 413.5.

Sumatriptan Succinate is a white to off-white powder that is readily soluble in water and in saline.

Sumatriptan Succinate is a clear, colorless to pale yellow, sterile, nonpyrogenic solution for subcutaneous injection. Each 0.5 mL of solution contains 6 mg of Sumatriptan (base) as the Succinate salt. The pH range of the solution is approximately 4.2 to 5.3. The osmolality of the injection is 291 mOsmol.

Following is its chemical structure:

CLINICAL PHARMACOLOGY

Mechanism of Action: Sumatriptan has been demonstrated to be a selective agonist for a vascular 5-hydroxytryptamine$_1$ receptor subtype (probably a member of the 5-HT$_{1D}$ family) with no significant affinity (as measured using standard radioligand binding assays) or pharmacological activity at 5-HT$_2$, 5-HT$_3$ receptor subtypes or at alpha$_1$-, alpha$_2$-, or beta-adrenergic; dopamine$_1$; dopamine$_2$; muscarinic; or benzodiazepine receptors.

The vascular 5-HT$_1$ receptor subtype to which Sumatriptan binds selectively, and through which it presumably exerts its antimigrainous effect, has been shown to be present on cranial arteries in both dog and primate, on the human basilar artery, and in the vasculature of the isolated dura mater of humans. In these tissues, Sumatriptan activates this receptor to cause vasoconstriction, an action in humans correlating with the relief of migraine. In the anesthetized dog, Sumatriptan selectively reduces the carotid arterial blood flow with little or no effect on arterial blood pressure or total peripheral resistance. In the cat, Sumatriptan selectively constricts the carotid arteriovenous anastomoses while having little effect on blood flow or resistance in cerebral or extracerebral tissues.

Pharmacokinetics: Pharmacokinetic parameters following a 6-mg subcutaneous injection into the deltoid area of the arm in nine males (*mean age, 33 years; mean weight, 77 kg*) were systemic clearance; 1,194 ± 149 mL per minute (*mean ± S.D.*), distribution half-life: 15 ± 2 minutes, terminal half-life: 115 ± 19 minutes, and volume of distribution central compartment: 50 ± 8 liters. Of this dose, 22 ± 4% was excreted in the urine as unchanged Sumatriptan and 38 ± 7% as the indole acetic acid metabolite.

After a single 6-mg subcutaneous manual injection into the deltoid area of the arm in 18 healthy males (*age, 24 ± 6 years; weight, 70 kg*), the maximum serum concentration (C_{max}) was (*mean ± standard deviation*) 74 ± 15 ng/mL and the time to peak concentration (T_{max}) was 12 minutes after injection (*range, 5 to 20 minutes*). In this study, the same dose injected subcutaneously in the thigh gave a C_{max} of 61 ± 15 ng/mL by manual injection versus 52 ± 15 ng/mL by autoinjector techniques. The T_{max} or amount absorbed were not significantly altered by either the site or technique of injection.

The bioavailability of Sumatriptan via subcutaneous site injection to 18 healthy male subjects was 97 ± 16% of that obtained following intravenous injection. Protein binding, determined by equilibrium dialysis over the concentration range of 10-1,000 ng/mL, is low, approximately 14% to 21%. The effect of Sumatriptan on the protein binding of other drugs has not been evaluated.

◆ RATED THERAPEUTICALLY EQUIVALENT; ◇ THERAPEUTIC EQUIVALENCE UNCONFIRMED; ○ UNRATED

The pharmacokinetics of Sumatriptan in the elderly (*mean age, 72 years; two males and four females*) and in patients with migraine (*mean age, 38 years; 25 males and 155 females*) were similar to that in healthy male subjects (*mean age, 30 years*). The systemic clearance and C_{max} of Sumatriptan were similar in black ($n = 34$) and Caucasian ($n = 38$) healthy male subjects.

In vitro studies with human microsomes suggest that Sumatriptan is metabolized by monoamine oxidase (MAO), predominantly the A isoenzyme. In a study of 42 healthy females, pretreatment with MAO-A inhibitor resulted in a marked increase in Sumatriptan area under the curve, a marked increase in half-life, and a marked decrease in CL_p/F. No significant effect was seen with a MAO-B inhibitor.

The effect of hepatic and renal impairment on the pharmacokinetics of Sumatriptan has not been evaluated.

PHARMACODYNAMICS
TYPICAL PHYSIOLOGIC RESPONSES
A. CARDIOVASCULAR
Blood Pressure: Transient increases in systolic and diastolic blood pressure may be observed after 6 mg of Sumatriptan Succinate injection. In a placebo-controlled study of 12 hypertensive migraineurs with documented diastolic blood pressure of ≥ 95 mmHg on two occasions during a migraine-free period, administration of 6 mg of Sumatriptan subcutaneously caused transient (usually less than 1 hour) elevations of blood pressure. Mean peak systolic and diastolic blood pressures were both 6 mmHg above baseline; peak increases were usually within 30 minutes of injection. The greatest observation of increased blood pressure was in one individual with increases of 33 mmHg systolic and 17 mmHg diastolic postdose; this greatest response was maintained less than 20 minutes, occurred during the first half-hour after injection, and was without any other clinically significant effect.

In two placebo-controlled trials of 6 mg of Sumatriptan Succinate during migraine attacks ($n = 547$ treated with Sumatriptan Succinate; $n = 370$, placebo), there were no differences between treatment groups for the number of patients who experienced clinically significant increases in blood pressure (defined prospectively as 20 mmHg above baseline and ≥ 180 mmHg for systolic blood pressure, or 15 mmHg above baseline and ≥ 105 mmHg diastolic blood pressure). These studies did not exclude patients with a history of hypertension ($n = 25$ for placebo and $n = 66$ for Sumatriptan Succinate hypertension subgroups). Withdrawal of antihypertensive medications (if any) was not a requirement in these studies; some patients were taking beta-adrenergic receptor blocking drugs ($n = 12$), calcium channel blocking drugs ($n = 3$), diuretics ($n = 4$), or enalapril ($n = 1$). Mean blood pressures for these hypertension subgroups were 138/89 for placebo and 132/86 for Sumatriptan Succinate pretreatment. Neither placebo nor Sumatriptan Succinate was associated with changes in mean blood pressure in these hypertension subgroups. One patient in the placebo subgroup experienced a clinically significant (see definition above) elevation of diastolic blood pressure, and one patient treated with Sumatriptan Succinate experienced a clinically significant elevation in systolic blood pressure (see definition above); both these observations were transient and not accompanied by rises in systolic and diastolic blood pressure, respectively.

In controlled studies of 2,306 migraine patients receiving 4 to 8 mg of Sumatriptan Succinate, clinically significant increases or decreases (increases as defined above, decreases prospectively defined as 20 mmHg below baseline and ≤ 90 mmHg systolic or 15 mmHg below baseline and ≤ 50 mmHg diastolic) were present in $\leq 1\%$ of patients. Identical results were observed in placebo-treated patients.

Peripheral (small) Arteries: In healthy volunteers ($n = 18$), weighted mean toe-arm systolic blood pressure gradients were used to study the possible effects of Sumatriptan on peripheral (small vessel) arterial reactivity. After 8 mg of Sumatriptan, the mean toe-arm pressure gradient fell by 6.6 mmHg systolic during the first 2 hours postdose. The maximum decrease in systolic toe-arm gradient occurred at 1 hour postdose, and returned to baseline values (a mean decrease of 8.3 mmHg) by 4 hours. Clinically insignificant changes in ordinary systolic blood pressure, similar to those described in the preceding paragraphs, were also observed in this study. These changes in toe-arm systolic gradient are interpreted as being slight and not indicating a clinically significant risk of peripheral vasospasm in healthy volunteers.

Heart Rate: The transient increases in blood pressure observed in the clinical trials described above were not accompanied by any clinically significant changes in heart rate. This was also true for the hypertensive subgroups in the two pivotal trials. Overall, there was observed a mean decrease of 4 bpm associated with Sumatriptan Succinate in the two large pivotal studies; while not of clinical significance, it is possible that this was associated with relief of migraine.

B. OTHER PHYSIOLOGIC EFFECTS
Respiratory Rate: Respiratory rate was monitored in many of the studies described in this section. There is no evidence for an effect of Sumatriptan on respiratory rate, and neither is there any theoretical reason to expect such an effect.

Clinical Studies: In US controlled clinical trials enrolling more than 1,000 patients during migraine attacks who were experiencing moderate or severe pain and one or more of the symptoms enumerated in Table 2 below, onset of relief began as early as 10 minutes following a 6-mg dose of Sumatriptan Succinate. Smaller doses of Sumatriptan may also prove effective, although the proportion of patients obtaining adequate relief is decreased and the latency to that relief is greater.

In one well-controlled study where placebo ($n = 62$) was compared to six different doses of Sumatriptan Succinate ($n = 30$ each group) in a single-attack, parallel-group design, the dose response relationship was found to be as shown in the following Table 1.

Table 1
DOSE RESPONSE RELATIONSHIP FOR EFFICACY

Sumatriptan Succinate Dose (mg)	% Patients With Relief† at 10 Minutes	% Patients With Relief† at 30 Minutes	% Patients With Relief† at 1 Hour	% Patients With Relief† at 2 Hours	Adverse Events Incidence (%)
placebo	5	15	24	21	55
1	10	40	43	40	63
2	7	23	57	43	63
3	17	47	57	60	77
4	13	37	50	57	80
6	10	63	73	70	83
8	23	57	80	83	93

† *Relief is defined as the reduction of moderate or severe pain to no or mild pain after dosing without use of rescue medication.*

In two US well-controlled clinical trials in 1,104 migraine patients with moderate and severe migraine pain, the onset of relief was rapid (less than 10 minutes). Headache relief, as evidenced by a reduction in pain from severe or moderately severe to mild or no headache, was achieved in 70% of the patients within 1 hour of a single 6-mg subcutaneous dose of Sumatriptan Succinate. Headache relief was achieved in approximately 82% of patients within 2 hours, and 65% of all patients were pain free within 2 hours.

The following table shows the 1- and 2-hour efficacy results.

Table 2
EFFICACY DATA FROM US PHASE III TRIALS

One-Hour Data	Study 1 Placebo ($n = 190$)	Study 1 Sumatriptan Succinate 6 mg ($n = 384$)	Study 2 Placebo ($n = 180$)	Study 2 Sumatriptan Succinate 6 mg ($n = 350$)
Patients with pain relief (grade 0/1)	18%	70%*	26%	70%*
Patients with no pain	5%*	48%*	13%	49%*
Patients without nausea	48%	73%*	50%	73%*
Patients without photophobia	23%	56%*	25%	58%*
Patients with little or no clinical disability§	34%	76%*	34%	76%*

Two-Hour Data	Study 1 Placebo†	Study 1 Sumatriptan Succinate 6 mg‡	Study 2 Placebo†	Study 2 Sumatriptan Succinate 6 mg‡
Patients with pain relief (grade 0/1)	31%	81%	39%	82%*
Patients with no pain	11%	63%*	19%	65%*
Patients without nausea	56%	82%*	63%	81%*
Patients without photophobia	31%	72%*	35%	71%*
Patients with little or no clinical disability§	42%	85%*	49%	84%*

* *$p < 0.05$ versus placebo.*
† *Includes patients that may have received an additional placebo injection 1 hour after the initial injection.*
‡ *Includes patients that may have received an additional 6 mg of Sumatriptan Succinate 1 hour after the initial injection.*
§ *A successful outcome in terms of clinical disability was defined prospectively as able to work mildly impaired or able to work and function normally.*

Sumatriptan Succinate also relieved photophobia, phonophobia (sound sensitivity), nausea, and vomiting associated with migraine attacks. Similar efficacy was seen when patients self-administered Sumatriptan Succinate using an autoinjector. The efficacy of Sumatriptan Succinate is unaffected by whether or not migraine is associated with aura, duration of attack, gender of the patient, or concomitant use of common migraine prophylactic drugs (e.g., beta-blockers).

INDICATIONS AND USAGE
Sumatriptan Succinate is indicated for the acute treatment of migraine attacks with or without aura.

Sumatriptan Succinate is not for use in the management of hemiplegic or basilar migraine (see *"Warnings"*).

Safety and effectiveness have also not been established for cluster headache, which is present in an older, predominantly male population.

UNLABELED USES

Sumatriptan is used alone or as an adjunct in the treatment of cluster headache.

CONTRAINDICATIONS

Sumatriptan Succinate should not be given intravenously because of its potential to cause coronary vasospasm. For similar reasons, Sumatriptan Succinate should not be given subcutaneously to patients with ischemic heart disease (angina pectoris, history of myocardial infarction, or documented silent ischemia) or to patients with Prinzmetal's s angina. Also, patients with symptoms or signs consistent with ischemic heart disease should not receive Sumatriptan Succinate. Because Sumatriptan Succinate can give rise to increases in blood pressure (usually small), it should not be given to patients with uncontrolled hypertension.

Sumatriptan Succinate should not be used concomitantly with ergotamine containing preparations.

Sumatriptan Succinate is contraindicated in patients with hypersensitivity to Sumatriptan.

WARNINGS

Sumatriptan Succinate should only be used where a clear diagnosis of migraine has been established.

Sumatriptan Succinate should not be administered to patients with basilar or hemiplegic migraine.

There is a potential for MAO inhibitors to alter Sumatriptan pharmacokinetics (increased systemic exposure). In patients receiving MAO inhibitors, decreased doses of Sumatriptan should be considered (see *"Clinical Pharmacology"*).

Hypersensitivity (anaphylaxis/anaphylactoid) reactions have occurred on rare occasions in patients receiving Sumatriptan. Such reactions can be life threatening or fatal. In general, hypersensitivity reactions to drugs are more likely to occur in individuals with a history of sensitivity to multiple allergens.

Cardiac Events/Coronary Constriction: Serious coronary events, including some that have been fatal, following Sumatriptan injection have occurred but are extremely rare. Although it is not clear how many of these can be attributed to Sumatriptan, because of its potential to cause coronary vasospam, Sumatriptan injection should not be given to patients in whom unrecognized coronary artery disease (CAD) is likely without a prior evaluation for underlying cardiovascular disease. Such patients include postmenopausal women, males over 40, and patients with risk factors for CAD such as hypertension, hypercholesterolemia, obesity, diabetes, smokers, and strong family history. Following a satisfactory cardiovascular assessment, it is strongly recommended that the first dose of Sumatriptan Succinate be administered in the physician's office for these patients. If symptoms consistent with angina occur, electrocardiographic (ECG) evaluation should be carried out to look for ischemic changes.

Sumatriptan may cause coronary vasospasm in patients with a history of coronary artery disease, who are known to be more susceptible than others to coronary artery vasospasm, and, rarely, in patients without prior history suggestive coronary artery disease. There were eight patients among the more than 1,900 who participated in controlled trials who sustained clinical events during or shortly after receiving subcutaneous Sumatriptan that may have reflected coronary vasospasm. Six of these eight patients had ECG changes consistent with transient ischemia, but without symptoms or signs. Of the eight patients, four had some findings suggestive or coronary artery disease prior to treatment. None of these adverse events was associated with a serious clinical outcome.

There have been rare reports from countries in which Sumatriptan Succinate has been marketed of serious and/or life-threatening arrhythmias, including atrial fibrillation, ventricular fibrillation, ventricular tachycardia; myocardial infarction; and marked ischemic ST elevations associated with Sumatriptan Succinate. In addition, there have been rare, but more frequent, reports of chest and arm discomfort thought to represent angina pectoris.

Drug-Associated Fatalities: In extensive worldwide postmarketing experience, deaths have been reported following the use of Sumatriptan. In most cases, these have occurred well after Sumatriptan use (i.e., 3 or more hours postinjection) and probably reflect underlying disease and spontaneous events.

There have, however, been several fatalities that occurred within a few hours after Sumatriptan's use. The specific contribution of sumatriptan to most of these deaths cannot be determined, but in one case, a 41-year-old woman with a 6-day history of unilateral headache, uncertain history of cardiovascular disease with known risk factors (positive family history, postmenopausal woman, and smoking) and a history of asthma and codeine allergy, experienced nausea, vomiting, a sense of warmth, chest pressure, and sweating within 7 minutes of dosing. This was followed by hypotension at about one-half hour, and ventricular tachycardia/ventricular fibrillation leading to death. In most other cases, death was attributed to myocardial infarctions occurring hours after drug administration.

Deaths attributed to strokes, cerebral hemorrhage, and other cerebrovascular events have also been reported in patients treated with Sumatriptan. In many cases, it appears possible that the cerebrovascular events were primary, Sumatriptan having been administered in the incorrect belief that the symptoms experienced were migrainous in origin when they were not. Accordingly, it is important to advise patients not to administer Sumatriptan if a headache being experienced were migrainous in origin when they were not. Accordingly, it is important to advise patients not to administer Sumatriptan if a headache being experienced is atypical.

Use in Women of Childbearing Potential: (see *"Precautions"*).

PRECAUTIONS

General: Chest, jaw, or neck tightness is relatively common after Sumatriptan Succinate but has only rarely been associated with ischemic ECG changes.

Sumatriptan Succinate may cause mild, transient elevation of blood pressure and peripheral vascular resistance (see *"Clinical Pharmacology"*).

Sumatriptan Succinate should also be administered with caution to patients with diseases that may alter the absorption, metabolism, or excretion of drugs, such as impaired hepatic or renal function.

There have been rare reports of seizure following administration of Sumatriptan.

As with other acute migraine therapies, before treating headaches in patients diagnosed as migraineurs and in migraineurs who present with atypical symptoms, care should be taken to exclude other potentially serious neurological conditions. There have been rare reports where patients received Sumatriptan for severe headaches that were subsequently shown to have been secondary to an evolving neurological lesion (cerebrovascular accident, subarachnoid hemorrhage). For a given attack, if a patient does not respond to the first dose, the diagnosis of migraine should be reconsidered before administration of a second dose. In this regard, it should be noted that migraineurs may be at increased risk of certain cerebrovascular events (e.g., cerebrovascular accident, transient ischemic attack).

Although written instructions are supplied with the autoinjector, patients who are advised to self-administer Sumatriptan Succinate in medically unsupervised situations should receive instruction on the proper use of the product from the physician or other suitably qualified health care professional prior to doing so for the first time.

Information for Patients: See patient information supplied with the product.

Laboratory Tests: No specific laboratory tests are recommended for monitoring patients prior to and/or after treatment with Sumatriptan Succinate.

Drug Interactions: There is no evidence that concomitant use of migraine prophylactic medications has any effect on the efficacy or unwanted effects of Sumatriptan Succinate. In two Phase III trials in the US, a retrospective analysis of 282 patients who had been using prophylactic drugs (verapamil n = 63, amitriptyline n = 57, propranolol n = 94, for 45 other drugs n = 123) were compared to those who had not used prophylaxis (n = 452). There were no differences in relief rates at 60 minutes postdose for Sumatriptan Succinate whether or not prophylactic medications were used. There were also no differences in overall adverse event rates between the two groups.

Ergot-containing drugs have been reported to cause prolonged vasospasm reactions. Because there is a theoretical basis that these effects *may* be additive, use of ergotamine and Sumatriptan within 24 hours of each other should be avoided (see *"Contraindications"*).

There is a potential for MAO inhibitors to alter sumatriptan pharmacokinetics (increased systemic exposure). Sumatriptan should be administered with caution to patients receiving MAO inhibitors.

Drug/Laboratory Test Interactions: Sumatriptan Succinate is not known to interfere with commonly employed clinical laboratory tests.

Carcinogenesis, Mutagenesis, Impairment of Fertility: In a 104-week lifetime study in rats given Sumatriptan by oral gavage, serum concentrations achieved were dose related, ranging at the low dose from approximately twice the peak concentration of the drug after the recommended human subcutaneous dose of 6 mg to more than 100 times this concentration at the high dose. There was no evidence of an increase in tumors considered to be related to Sumatriptan administration.

In a 78-week study in which mice received Sumatriptan continuously in drinking water, there was no evidence for an increase in tumors considered to be related to Sumatriptan administration. That study, however, did not use the maximum tolerated dose and therefore did not fully explore the carcinogenic potential of Sumatriptan Succinate in the mouse.

A segment I rat fertility study by the subcutaneous route has shown no evidence of impaired fertility.

Pregnancy: Pregnancy Category C: Sumatriptan has been shown to be embryolethal in rabbits when given in daily doses producing plasma levels 3-fold higher than those attained following a 6-mg subcutaneous injection (i.e., recommended dose) to humans. There is no evidence that establishes that Sumatriptan is a human teratogen; however, there are no adequate and well-controlled studies in pregnant women. Sumatriptan Succinate should be used during pregnancy only if the potential benefit justifies the potential risk to the fetus.

In assessing this information, the following additional findings should be considered.

Embryolethality: When given intravenously to pregnant rabbits daily throughout the period of organogenesis, Sumatriptan caused embryolethality at doses at or close to those producing maternal toxicity. The mechanism of the embryolethality is not known. At these doses, peak concentrations of drug in plasma were more than 3-fold higher than the range observed in humans after the recommended subcutaneous dose of 6 mg.

The intravenous administration of Sumatriptan to pregnant rats throughout organogenesis at doses producing plasma concentrations more than 50 times those seen after the recommended Subcutaneous human dose did not cause embryolethality. In a study of pregnant rats given subcutaneous Sumatriptan daily prior to and throughout pregnancy, there was no evidence of increased embryo/fetal lethality.

Teratogenicity: Term fetuses from Dutch Stride rabbits treated during organogenesis with oral Sumatriptan exhibited an increased incidence of cervicothoracic

---

◆ RATED THERAPEUTICALLY EQUIVALENT; ◇ THERAPEUTIC EQUIVALENCE UNCONFIRMED; ○ UNRATED

vascular defects and minor skeletal abnormalities. The functional significance of these abnormalities is not known.

In a study in rats dosed daily with subcutaneous Sumatriptan prior to and throughout pregnancy, there was no evidence of teratogenicity.

Studies in rats and rabbits evaluating the teratogenic potential of Sumatriptan administered subcutaneously only during organogenesis (standard Segment II studies) have not been performed.

Nursing Mothers: Sumatriptan is excreted in breast milk in animals. No data exist in humans. Therefore, caution should be exercised when considering the administration of Sumatriptan Succinate to a nursing woman.

Pediatric Use: Safety and effectiveness of Sumatriptan Succinate in children have not been established.

Use in the Elderly: The safety and effectiveness of Sumatriptan Succinate in individuals over age 65 have not been systematically evaluated. However, the pharmacokinetic disposition of Sumatriptan Succinate in the elderly is similar to that seen in younger adults. No unusual adverse, age-related phenomena have been identified in patients over the age of 60 who participated in clinical trials with Sumatriptan Succinate.

ADVERSE REACTIONS

(See also *"Precautions"*.) Sumatriptan may cause coronary vasospasm in patients with a history of coronary artery disease, known to be susceptible to coronary artery vasospasm, and, very rarely, without prior history suggestive of coronary artery disease. There have been rare reports from countries in which Sumatriptan Succinate has been marketed of serious and/or life-threatening arrhythmias, including atrial fibrillation, ventricular fibrillation, ventricular tachycardia; myocardial infarction; and marked ischemic ST elevations associated with Sumatriptan Succinate (see *"Warnings"*). More often, there has been chest discomfort that appeared to represent angina pectoris.

Other untoward clinical events associated with the use of subcutaneous Sumatriptan Succinate are: pain or redness at the injection site, atypical sensations (such as sensations of warmth, cold, tingling or paresthesia, pressure, burning, numbness, tightness, all of which may be localized or generalized), flushing, chest symptoms (pressure, pain, or tightness), fatigue, dizziness, and drowsiness. All these untoward effects are usually transient, although they may be severe in some patients. Transient rises in blood pressure soon after treatment have been recorded.

Among patients in clinical trials of subcutaneous Sumatriptan Succinate (n = 6,218), up to 3.5% of patients withdrew for reasons related to adverse events.

Incidence in Controlled Clinical Trials: The following Table 3 lists adverse events that occurred in two large US, Phase III, placebo-controlled clinical trials following either a single dose of Sumatriptan Succinate or placebo. Only events that occurred at a frequency of 1% or more in Sumatriptan Succinate treatment groups and were at least as frequent as in the placebo group are included in Table 3.

Table 3
TREATMENT-EMERGENT ADVERSE EXPERIENCE INCIDENCE IN TWO LARGE PLACEBO-CONTROLLED CLINICAL TRIALS: EVENTS REPORTED BY AT LEAST 1% OF SUMATRIPTAN SUCCINATE PATIENTS

	Percent of Patients Reporting	
Adverse Event Type	Sumatriptan Succinate 6 mg SC n = 547	Placebo n = 370
Atypical sensations	42.0	9.2
Tingling	13.5	3.0
Warm/hot sensation	10.8	3.5
Burning sensation	7.5	0.3
Feeling of heaviness	7.3	1.1
Pressure sensation	7.1	1.6
Feeling of tightness	5.1	0.3
Numbness	4.6	2.2
Feeling strange	2.2	0.3
Tight feeling in head	2.2	0.3
Cold sensation	1.1	0.5
Cardiovascular		
Flushing	6.6	2.4
Chest discomfort	4.5	1.4
Tightness in chest	2.7	0.5
Pressure in chest	1.8	0.3
Ear, nose, and throat		
Throat discomfort	3.3	0.5
Discomfort; nasal cavity/sinuses	2.2	0.3
Eye		
Vision alterations	1.1	0.0
Gastrointestinal		
Abdominal discomfort	1.3	0.8
Dysphagia	1.1	0.8
Injection site reaction	58.7	23.8
Miscellaneous		
Jaw discomfort	1.8	0.0

	Percent of Patients Reporting	
Adverse Event Type	Sumatriptan Succinate 6 mg SC n = 547	Placebo n = 370
Mouth and teeth		
Discomfort of mouth/tongue	4.9	4.6
Musculoskeletal		
Weakness	4.9	0.3
Neck pain/stiffness	4.8	0.5
Myalgia	1.8	0.5
Muscle cramp(s)	1.1	0.0
Neurological		
Dizziness/vertigo	11.9	4.3
Drowsiness/sedation	2.7	2.2
Headache	2.2	0.3
Anxiety	1.1	0.5
Malaise/fatigue	1.1	0.8
Skin		
Sweating	1.6	1.1

The sum of the percentages cited are greater than 100% because patients may experience more than one type of adverse event. Only events that occurred at a frequency of 1% or more in Sumatriptan Succinate treatment groups and were at least as frequent as in the placebo groups are included.

Other Events Observed in Association With the Administration of Sumatriptan Succinate: In the paragraphs that follow, the frequencies of less commonly reported adverse clinical events are presented. Because the reports cite events observed in open and uncontrolled studies, the role of Sumatriptan Succinate in their causation cannot be reliably determined. Furthermore, variability associated with reporting requirements, the terminology used to describe adverse events, etc., limit the value of the quantitative frequency estimates provided.

Event frequencies are calculated as the number of patients reporting an event divided by the total number of patients (n = 6,218) exposed to subcutaneous Sumatriptan Succinate. Given their imprecision, frequencies for specific adverse event occurrences are defined as follows: "infrequent" indicates a frequency estimated as falling between 1/1,000 and 1/100; "rare," a frequency less than 1/1,000.

Cardiovascular: Infrequent were hypertension, hypotension, bradycardia, tachycardia, palpitations, pulsating sensations, various transient ECG changes (nonspecific ST or T wave changes, prolongation of PR or QTc intervals, sinus arrhythmia, nonsustained ventricular premature beats, isolated junctional ectopic beats, atrial ectopic beats, delayed activation of the right ventricle), and syncope. Rare were pallor, arrhythmia, abnormal pulse, vasodilatation, and Raynaud's syndrome.

Endocrine and Metabolic: Infrequent was thirst. Rare were polydipsia and dehydration.

Eye: Infrequent was irritation of the eye.

Gastrointestinal: Infrequent were gastroesophageal reflux, diarrhea, and disturbances of liver function tests. Rare were peptic ulcer, retching, flatulence/eructation, and gallstones.

Musculoskeletal: Infrequent were various joint disturbances (pain, stiffness, swelling, ache). Rare were muscle stiffness, need to flex calf muscles, backache, muscle tiredness, and swelling of the extremities.

Neurological: Infrequent were mental confusion, euphoria, agitation, relaxation, chills, sensation of lightness, tremor, shivering, disturbances of taste, prickling sensations, paresthesia, stinging sensations, headaches, facial pain, photophobia, and lacrimation. Rare were transient hemiplegia, hysteria, globus hystericus, intoxication, depression, myoclonia, monoplegia/diplegia, sleep disturbance, difficulties in concentration, disturbances of smell, hyperesthesia, dysesthesia, simultaneous hot and cold sensations, tickling sensations, dysarthria, yawning, reduced appetite, hunger, and dystonia.

Respiratory: Infrequent was dyspnea. Rare were influenza, diseases of the lower respiratory tract, and hiccoughs.

Dermatological: Infrequent were erythema, pruritus, and skin rashes and eruptions. Rare was skin tenderness.

Urogenital: Rare were dysuria, frequency, dysmenorrhea, and renal calculus.

Miscellaneous: Infrequent were miscellaneous laboratory abnormalities, including minor disturbances in liver function tests, "serotonin agonist effect," and hypersensitivity to various agents. Rare was fever.

Postmarketing Experience: Episodes of Prinzmetal's angina, myocardial infarction, acute renal failure, seizure, cerebrovascular accident, dysphasia, subarachnoid hemorrhage, arrhythmias (atrial fibrillation, ventricular fibrillation, and ventricular tachycardia, photosensitivity, and exacerbation of sunfurn; for many of these reports, frequency and causality for Sumatriptan have not been established.) The following hypersensitivity reactions have been reported: rash, urticaria, pruritus, erythema, and shortness of breath. In addition, severe anaphylaxis/anaphylactoid reactions have been reported (see *"Warnings"*).

DRUG ABUSE AND DEPENDENCE

The abuse potential of Sumatriptan Succinate cannot be fully delineated in advance of extensive marketing experience. One clinical study enrolling 12 patients with a history of substance abuse failed to induce subjective behavior and/or physiologic response ordinarily associated with drugs that have an established potential for abuse.

OVERDOSAGE

Patients (n = 269) have received single injections of 8 to 12 mg without significant adverse effects. Volunteers (n = 47) have received single subcutaneous doses of up to 16 mg without serious adverse events.

No gross overdoses in clinical practice have been reported. Coronary vasospasm was observed after intravenous administration of Sumatriptan Succinate (see "Contraindications"). Overdoses would be expected from animal data (dogs at 0.1 g/kg, rats at 2 g/kg) to possibly cause convulsions, tremor, inactivity, erythema of the extremities, reduced respiratory rate, cyanosis, ataxia, mydriasis, injection site reactions (desquamation, hair loss, and scab formation), and paralysis. The half-life of elimination of Sumatriptan is about 2 hours (see "Clinical Pharmacology"), and therefore monitoring of patients after overdose with Sumatriptan Succinate should continue while symptoms or signs persist, and for at least 10 hours.

It is unknown what effect hemodialysis or peritoneal dialysis has on the serum concentrations of sumatriptan.

DOSAGE AND ADMINISTRATION

The maximum single recommended adult dose of Sumatriptan Succinate is 6 mg injected subcutaneously. Controlled clinical trials have failed to show that clear benefit is associated with the administration of a second 6-mg dose in patients who have failed to respond to a first injection.

The maximum recommended dose that may be given in 24 hours is two 6-mg injections separated by at least one hour. Although the recommended dose is 6 mg, if side effects are dose limiting, then lower doses may be used (see "Clinical Pharmacology"). In patients receiving MAO inhibitors, decreased doses of Sumatriptan should be considered (see "Clinical Pharmacology"). In patients receiving doses lower than 6 mg, only the single-dose vial dosage form should be used. An autoinjection device is available for use with 6-mg prefilled syringes to facilitate self-administration in patients in whom this dose is deemed necessary.

Parenteral drug products should be inspected visually for particulate matter and discoloration before administration whenever solution and container permit.

Storage: Store Injection between 2° and 30°C (36° and 86°F). Protect from light.

HOW SUPPLIED
INJECTION: 6 MG/0.5 ML

BRAND/MANUFACTURER	NDC	SIZE	AWP
○ **BRAND**			
IMITREX: Cerenex	00173-0449-02	0.5 ml 5s	$164.88

KIT: 6 MG/0.5 ML

BRAND/MANUFACTURER	NDC	SIZE	AWP
○ **BRAND**			
IMITREX: Cerenex	00173-0449-01	1s	$66.95
	00173-0449-03	1s	$70.68

Supprelin *SEE* HISTRELIN ACETATE

Suprane *SEE* DESFLURANE

Suprax *SEE* CEFIXIME

Suprofen

DESCRIPTION

Suprofen 1% ophthalmic solution is a topical nonsteroidal anti-inflammatory product for ophthalmic use. Suprofen chemically is α-methyl-4-(2-thienyl-carbonyl) benzeneacetic acid, with an empirical formula of $C_{14}H_{12}O_3S$, and a molecular weight of 260.3.

Following is its chemical structure:

CLINICAL PHARMACOLOGY

Suprofen is one of a series of phenylalkanoic acids that have shown analgesic, antipyretic, and anti-inflammatory activity in animal inflammatory diseases. Its mechanism of action is believed to be through inhibition of the cyclo-oxygenase enzyme that is essential in the biosynthesis of prostaglandins.

Prostaglandins have been shown in many animal models to be mediators of certain kinds of intraocular inflammation. In studies performed on animal eyes, prostaglandins have been shown to produce disruption of the blood-aqueous humor barrier, vasodilatation, increased vascular permeability, leukocytosis, and increased intraocular pressure. Prostaglandins appear to play a role in the miotic response produced during ocular surgery by constricting the iris sphincter independently of cholinergic mechanisms. In clinical studies, Suprofen has been shown to inhibit the miosis induced during the course of cataract surgery. Suprofen could possibly interfere with the miotic effect of intraoperatively administered acetylcholine chloride.

Results from clinical studies indicate that Suprofen ophthalmic solution has no significant effect on intraocular pressure.

There are no data available on the systemic absorption of ocularly applied Suprofen. The oral dose of Suprofen is 200 mg every four to six hours. If Suprofen 1% ophthalmic solution is applied as two drops (1 mg Suprofen) to one eye five times on the day prior to surgery and three times on the day of surgery, the total applied dose over the two days would be about 25 times less than a single 200 mg oral dose.

INDICATIONS AND USAGE

Suprofen ophthalmic solution is indicated for inhibition of intraoperative miosis.

CONTRAINDICATIONS

Suprofen is contraindicated in epithelial herpes simplex keratitis (dendritic keratitis) and in individuals hypersensitive to any component of the medication.

WARNINGS

The potential exists for cross sensitivity to acetylsalicylic acid and other nonsteroidal anti-inflammatory drugs. Therefore, caution should be used when treating individuals who have previously exhibited sensitivities to these drugs.

With nonsteroidal anti-inflammatory drugs, the potential exists for increased bleeding time due to interference with thrombocyte aggregation. There have been reports that ocularly applied nonsteroidal anti-inflammatory drugs may cause increased bleeding tendency of ocular tissues in conjunction with ocular surgery.

PRECAUTIONS

General: Use of oral Suprofen has been associated with a syndrome of acute flank pain and generally reversible renal insufficiency, which may present as acute uric acid nephropathy. This syndrome occurs in approximately 1 in 3500 patients and has been reported with as few as one to two doses of a 200 mg capsule. If Suprofen 1% ophthalmic solution is applied as two drops (1 mg Suprofen) to one eye five times on the day prior to surgery and three times on the day of surgery, the total applied dose over the two days would be about 25 times less than a single 200 mg oral dose. Do not touch dropper tip to any surface, as this may contaminate the solution.

Ocular: Patients with histories of herpes simplex keratitis should be monitored closely. Suprofen is contraindicated in patients with active herpes simplex keratitis.

The possibility of increased ocular bleeding during surgery associated with nonsteroidal anti-inflammatory drugs should be considered.

CARCINOGENESIS, MUTAGENESIS, IMPAIRMENT OF FERTILITY

In an 18-month study in mice, an increased incidence of benign hepatomas occurred in females at a dose of 40 mg/kg/day. Male mice, treated at doses of 2, 5, 10 and 40 mg/kg/day, also had an increased incidence of hepatomas when compared to control animals. No evidence of carcinogenicity was found in long term studies in doses as high as 40 mg/kg/day in the rat and mouse. Based on a battery of mutagenicity tests (Ames, micronucleus, and dominant lethal) Suprofen does not appear to have mutagenic potential. Reproductive studies in rats at a dose of up to 40 mg/kg/day revealed no impairment of fertility and only slight reductions of fertility at doses of 80 mg/kg/day. However, testicular atrophy/hypoplasia was observed in a six-month dog study (at 80 mg/kg/day) and a 12-month rat study (at 40 mg/kg/day).

PREGNANCY CATEGORY C

Reproductive studies have been performed in rabbits at doses up to 200 mg/kg/day and in rats at doses up to 80 mg/kg/day. In rats, doses of 40 mg/kg/day and above, and in rabbits, doses of 80 mg/kg/day and above, resulted in an increased incidence of fetal resorption associated with maternal toxicity. There was an increase in stillbirths and a decrease in postnatal survival in pregnant rats treated with Suprofen at 2.5 mg/kg/day and above. An increased incidence of delayed parturition occurred in rats. As there are no adequate and well-controlled studies in pregnant women, this drug should be used during pregnancy only if the potential benefit justifies the potential risk to the fetus. Because of the known effect of nonsteroidal anti-inflammatory drugs on the fetal cardiovascular system (closure of ductus arteriosus), use during late pregnancy should be avoided.

NURSING MOTHERS

Suprofen is excreted in human milk after a single oral dose. Based on measurements of plasma and milk levels in women taking oral Suprofen, the milk concentration is about 1% of the plasma level. Because systemic absorption may occur from topical ocular administration, a decision should be considered to discontinue nursing while receiving Suprofen, since the safety of Suprofen in human neonates has not been established.

PEDIATRIC USE
Safety and effectiveness in children have not been established.

DRUG INTERACTIONS
Clinical studies with acetylcholine chloride revealed no interference, and there is no known pharmacological basis for such an interaction. However, with other topical nonsteroidal anti-inflammatory products, there have been reports that acetylcholine chloride and carbachol have been ineffective when used in patients treated with these agents.

Interaction of Suprofen with other topical ophthalmic medications has not been fully investigated.

ADVERSE REACTIONS
Ocular: The most frequent adverse reactions reported are burning and stinging of short duration. Instances of discomfort, itching and redness have been reported. Other reactions occurring in less than 0.5% of patients include allergy, iritis, pain, chemosis, photophobia, irritation, and punctate epithelial staining.

SYSTEMIC
Systemic reactions related to therapy were not reported in the clinical studies. It is known that some systemic absorption does occur with ocularly applied drugs, and that nonsteroidal anti-inflammatory drugs have been shown to increase bleeding time by interference with thrombocyte aggregation. It is recommended that Suprofen be used with caution in patients with bleeding tendencies and those taking anticoagulants.

OVERDOSAGE
Overdosage will not ordinarily cause acute problems. If accidently ingested, drink fluids to dilute.

DOSAGE AND ADMINISTRATION
On the day of surgery, instill two drops into the conjunctival sac at three, two and one hour prior to surgery. Two drops may be instilled into the conjunctival sac every four hours, while awake, the day preceding surgery.

HOW SUPPLIED
DROP: 1%

BRAND/MANUFACTURER	NDC	SIZE	AWP
○ **BRAND**			
PROFENAL: Alcon Surg	00065-0348-25	2.5 ml 12s	$87.95

Surmontil *SEE* TRIMIPRAMINE MALEATE

Survanta Intratracheal *SEE* BERACTANT

Sutilains

DESCRIPTION
Sutilains Ointment, USP is a sterile topical preparation containing proteolytic enzymes, elaborated by *Bacillus subtilis*, in a hydrophobic ointment base consisting of 95% mineral oil and 5% polyethylene. One gram of ointment contains approximately 82,000 USP Casein Units of proteolytic activity.

One USP Casein Unit of proteolytic activity is contained in the amount of Sutilains which, when incubated with 35 mg of denatured casein at 37°C, produces in one minute a hydrolysate whose absorbance at 275 nm is equal to that of a tyrosine solution containing 1.5 micrograms of USP Tyrosine Reference Standard per mL.

CLINICAL PHARMACOLOGY
Sutilains Ointment selectively digests necrotic soft tissue by proteolytic action, thus facilitating the removal of necrotic tissue and purulent exudates that impair formation of granulation tissue and delay wound healing.

At body temperatures these proteolytic enzymes have optimal activity in the pH range from 6.0 to 6.8.

INDICATIONS AND USAGE
For wound debridement: Sutilains Ointment is indicated as an adjunct to established methods of wound care for biochemical debridement of:

Second and third degree burns,
Decubitus ulcers,
Incisional, traumatic, and pyogenic wounds,
Ulcers secondary to peripheral vascular disease.

CONTRAINDICATIONS
Application of Sutilains Ointment is contraindicated in:

Wounds communicating with major body cavities,
Wounds containing exposed major nerves or nervous tissue, and
Fungating neoplastic ulcers.

WARNING
Do not permit Sutilains Ointment to come into contact with the eyes. In the case of inadvertent contact, the eyes should be immediately rinsed with copious amounts of preferably sterile water.

PRECAUTIONS
A moist environment is essential for optimal activity of the enzyme. *In vitro*, several detergents and antiseptics (benzalkonium chloride, hexachlorophene, iodine, and nitrofurazone) may render the substrate indifferent to the action of the enzyme. Compounds such as thimerosal, containing metallic ions, interfere directly with enzyme activity to a slight degree, whereas neomycin, sulfamylon, streptomycin, and penicillin do not affect enzyme activity. If used concurrently with adjunctive topical therapy for 24-48 hours and no dissolution of slough occurs, then further therapy is not likely to be effective.

In cases of existent or threatening invasive infection, appropriate systemic antibiotic therapy should be instituted.

Although studies in humans have shown that there may be antibody response to absorbed enzyme material, there have been no reports of systemic allergic reaction to Sutilains Ointment.

Pregnancy: Pregnancy category B: Studies in rabbits at doses up to two times the maximum human dose revealed no evidence of impaired fertility or fetal harm. There are, however, no adequate and well controlled studies in women. Because animal reproductive studies are not always predicative of human response, this drug should be used during pregnancy only if no adequate alternatives are available.

Pediatric Use: Safety and effectiveness in children have not been established.

ADVERSE REACTIONS
Adverse reactions consist of mild, transient pain, paresthesias, bleeding and transient dermatitis. Pain usually can be controlled by administration of mild analgesics. Side effects severe enough to warrant discontinuation of therapy have occurred occasionally.

If bleeding or dermatitis occurs as a result of the application of (Sutilains Ointment, USP) therapy should be discontinued. No systemic toxicity has been observed as a result of the topical application of Sutilains Ointment.

DOSAGE AND ADMINISTRATION
FOR TOPICAL USE ONLY—NOT FOR OPHTHALMIC USE
ADHERENCE TO THE FOLLOWING IS SUGGESTED FOR OPTIMIZING THERAPEUTIC AFFECT:

1. Thoroughly cleanse and irrigate wound with sodium chloride solution or tap water. Wounds **MUST** be cleansed of antiseptics (e.g., hexachlorophene, benzalkonium chloride, nitrofurazone) or heavy-metal antibacterials (e.g., silver nitrate, thimerosal) which may alter substrate characteristics or denature the enzyme.

2. Thoroughly moisten wound area by tubbing, showering, or wet soaks (e.g., sodium chloride solution or tap water).

3. Apply approximately ⅛ inch (3mm) thick layer extending to ¼ to ½ inch (6mm to 12mm) beyond the area to be debrided, assuring intimate contact with necrotic tissue.

4. Apply a dressing that provides and maintains a moist environment.

5. Repeat entire procedure 3 to 4 times per day for best results.

Refrigerate at 2° to 8°C (36°-46°F).

HOW SUPPLIED
OINTMENT:

BRAND/MANUFACTURER	NDC	SIZE	AWP
○ **BRAND**			
TRAVASE: Boots Pharm	00048-1500-52	14.2 gm	$38.85

Symmetrel *SEE* AMANTADINE HYDROCHLORIDE

Syn-Rx *SEE* GUAIFENESIN AND PSEUDOEPHEDRINE HYDROCHLORIDE

Synalar *SEE* FLUOCINOLONE ACETONIDE

Synalgos-DC *SEE* ASPIRIN/CAFFEINE/DIHYDROCODEINE BITARTRATE

Synarel *SEE* NAFARELIN ACETATE

Synemol *SEE* FLUOCINOLONE ACETONIDE

► SHOWN IN PRODUCT IDENTIFICATION GUIDE

Synthroid *SEE* LEVOTHYROXINE SODIUM

Syntocinon *SEE* OXYTOCIN

Syprine *SEE* TRIENTINE HYDROCHLORIDE

T-Diet *SEE* PHENTERMINE

T-Phyl *SEE* THEOPHYLLINE

Tac 3 *SEE* TRIAMCINOLONE ACETONIDE, INJECTABLE

Tacaryl *SEE* METHDILAZINE HYDROCHLORIDE

Tace *SEE* CHLOROTRIANISENE

Tacrine Hydrochloride

DESCRIPTION

Tacrine Hydrochloride is a reversible cholinesterase inhibitor, known chemically as 1,2,3,4-tetrahydro-9-acridinamine monohydrochloride monohydrate. Tacrine Hydrochloride is commonly referred to in the clinical and pharmacological literature as THA. It has an empirical formula of $C_{13}H_{14}N_2 \cdot HCl \cdot H_2O$ and a molecular weight of 252.74.

Tacrine Hydrochloride is a white solid and is freely soluble in distilled water, 0.1N hydrochloric acid, acetate buffer (pH 4.0), phosphate buffer (pH 7.0 to 7.4), methanol, dimethylsulfoxide (DMSO), ethanol, and propylene glycol. The compound is sparingly soluble in linoleic acid and PEG 400.

Each 10-, 20-, 30-, and 40-mg Tacrine Hydrochloride capsule for oral administration contains 12.75, 25.50, 38.25, and 51.00 mg of Tacrine Hydrochloride, respectively.

Following is its chemical structure:

CLINICAL PHARMACOLOGY

Although widespread degeneration of multiple CNS neuronal systems eventually occurs, early pathological changes in Alzheimer's Disease involve, in a relatively selective manner, cholinergic neuronal pathways that project from the basal forebrain to the cerebral cortex and hippocampus. The resulting deficiency of cortical acetylcholine is believed to account for some of the clinical manifestations of mild to moderate dementia. Tacrine, an orally bioavailable, centrally active, reversible cholinesterase inhibitor, presumably acts by elevating acetylcholine concentrations in the cerebral cortex by slowing the degeneration of acetylcholine released by still intact cholinergic neurons. If this theoretical mechanism of action is correct, Tacrine's effects may lessen as the disease process advances and fewer cholinergic neurons remain functionally intact. There is no evidence that Tacrine alters the course of the underlying dementing process.

CLINICAL TRIAL DATA

The conclusion that Tacrine HCl is an effective treatment for Alzheimer's Disease derives from two adequate and well controlled clinical investigations that evaluated Tacrine's effects in patients with probable Alzheimer's disease of mild to moderate severity (NINCDS criteria, Mini-Mental State Examination (MMSE) of Folstein, Folstein and McHugh scores of 10 to 26).

In each study, outcomes during treatment with Tacrine and placebo were assessed on two primary measures: (1) the cognitive subscale of the Alzheimer's Disease Assessment Scale (ADAS cog) of Rosen, Mohs, and Davis and (2) a clinician's rated clinical global impression of change.

STUDY ENDPOINTS

The ADAS cog is a multi-item test battery administered by a psychometrician that examines aspects of memory, attention, praxis, reason, and language. The worst possible score is 70. Elderly, normal adults may score as low as 0 or 1 unit, but individuals judged not to be demented can score higher. The mean score of patients entering each study was approximately 28 units (range 7 to 62). The ADAS cog score is reported to deteriorate at a rate of about 6 to 10 units per year for untreated patients at this stage of dementia.

The clinician's global assessments used in the two studies relied on a clinician's judgment about the overall clinical change observed in patients over the course of the study. Although the conditions for obtaining the clinical assessment differed in each study, the global assessment was rated on a 7-point scale in both studies. A rating of four (4) represents no change; lower ratings indicate improvement from baseline and higher ratings deterioration.

TWELVE-WEEK STUDY

In one study of 12 weeks duration, patients were randomized to sequences that provided a comparison between placebo, 20, 40, and 80 mg/day by study's end. Statistically significant drug-placebo differences were detected on both primary outcome measures for the group titrated to 80 mg/day. Estimates of the size of the treatment effect varied between 2 and 4 ADAS cog units. The imprecision in these estimates reflects the fact that different analyses, conducted in attempts to account for the effects of the failure of a substantial fraction of the patients randomized to complete the full 12 weeks of the study, yielded different results.

The placebo-80 mg/day comparison also achieved statistical significance on the clinician's global impression of change (CGIC) with a 0.3 to 0.4 unit mean difference. The following diagram illustrates the percentages of patients falling into each global category at trial's end for the patients given placebo or 80 mg/day.

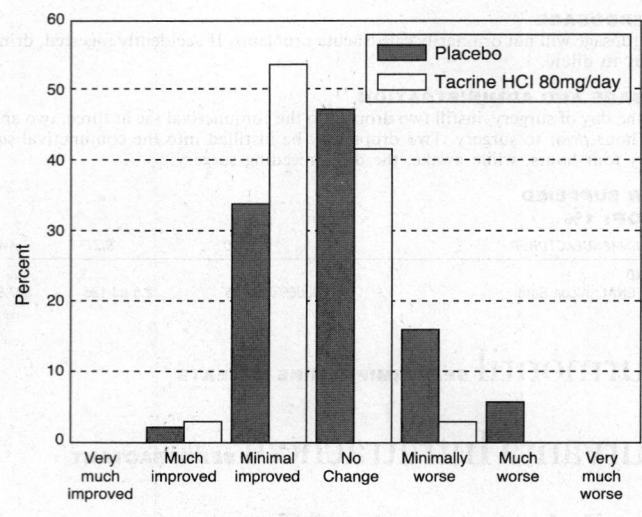

FIGURE 1. Percent of Patients in Each of the Seven Outcome Categories on the Clinician-Rated CGIC for Patients Completing 12 Weeks of Treatment (83% of patients randomized to placebo completed 12 weeks of treatment and are represented above; 56% of those randomized to the 80 mg day Tacrine HCl sequence completed 12 weeks).

THIRTY-WEEK STUDY

The second study was 30 weeks long. Six hundred sixty-three patients were randomized to 4 treatment sequences (placebo and 3 drug groups) that called for the daily dose of Tacrine to be increased at 6-week intervals, starting with a 40-mg/day dose. By study's end, a comparison between placebo, 80, 120, and 160 mg/day was possible. Patients in the 160 mg group received this dose for the final 12 weeks; the 120 mg group received that dose for 18 weeks.

The study showed statistically significant drug-placebo differences for the 80 and 120 mg/day groups at 18 weeks and for the 120 and 160 mg/day groups at 30 weeks on both a performance-based test of cognitive function (the ADAS cog) and a clinician's assessment of global change (Clinician Interview Based Impression: CIBI). Because many patients failed to complete 30 weeks on treatment, analyses that used each patient's last on-study value or retrieved patients' (see below) 30-week value, even if they were no longer in the study ("intent-to-treat" analysis) were also carried out. All analyses confirmed the effectiveness of Tarcine, although the estimated mean treatment effect was different in each analysis.

Effects on ADAS Cog: The results for the ADAS cog are shown in Figure 2 for the subset of patients actually completing the full 30 weeks of the study. They show that individual patients, whether assigned to Tacrine or to placebo, had a wide range of responses. This variability in response is illustrated in the display that follows (Figure 2).

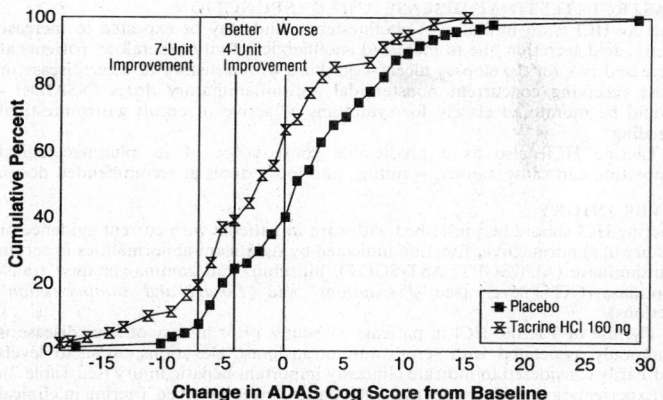

FIGURE 2. Cumulative Percent of Patients Completing 30 Weeks of Treatment Who Attained a Change in ADAS Cog Score From Baseline at Least as Large as the Value on the X Axis. The display is based on scores obtained from a subset of patients (ie, 64% of the 184 randomized to placebo and 27% of the 239 randomized to the 160 mg/day treatment group).

Figure 2 presents the cumulative percentage (Y axis) of patients assigned to placebo or 160 mg/day who actually completed 30 weeks on treatment and who attained a change in ADAS cog score from baseline at least as large as the ADAS cog change score value given on the X axis. A negative change from baseline represents improvement; a positive change deterioration. Thus, in a display of this type, the curve for an effective treatment is shifted to the left of the curve for placebo. The frequency in each group of any response, e.g., an improvement of 7 ADAS cog units, can be found by plotting the change on the X axis, then reading upward along the Y axis. The variability of response is apparent from the fact that the distribution of responses under both treatment conditions range from large negative to large positive values. Nonetheless, the mean drug-placebo ADAS cog difference for the 30-week 160 mg/day completer patients is 4.8 units, a statistically significant difference.

Effects on CIBI: The results on the CIBI are shown in Figure 3.

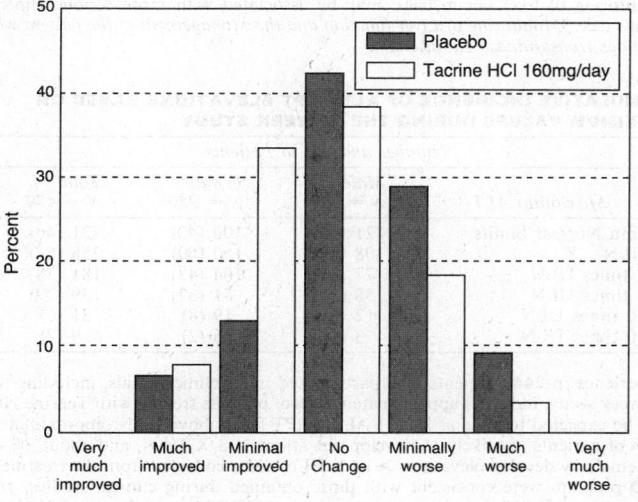

CIBI Rating at Week 30

FIGURE 3. Percent of Patients in Each of the Seven Outcome Categories of the CIBI Among Those Completing 30 Weeks. The display is based on scores obtained from the same subset of patients as Figure 2.

Figure 3 is a histogram of the frequency distribution of CIBI scores attained by patients assigned to placebo or the 160 mg/day Tacrine dose group who actually completed the full 30 weeks of the study. The mean Tacrine-placebo difference for this group of patients on the CIBI was 0.5 units and was statistically significant.

Expected Responses in Newly Treated Patients: Although the results described clearly document Tacrine effectiveness, they are based on only a fraction of the patients initially randomized to Tacrine, those who could tolerate Tacrine and remain on treatment uninterrupted for the full 30 weeks. In considering the expected outcome in a group of patients newly started on Tacrine, account must be taken both of the likelihood of staying on therapy and the responses in patients who do so.

Table 1 provides 3 estimates of the proportion of patients assigned to treatment with Tacrine at 160 mg a day or with placebo who attained a particular measure of improvement (i.e., a 7 point improvement from baseline in ADAS cog score). The criterion has been chosen entirely for illustrative purposes.

Table 1

PROPORTION OF PATIENTS ATTAINING ≥ 7 UNIT IMPROVEMENT ON THE ADAS COF AT THE WEEK 30 ASSESSMENT

Treatment Group N Randomized	I N (%) of Those Randomized	II N (%) of Those Completing Week 30	III N (%) of Those With Week 30 Assessments
Placebo (N = 184)	10/184 (5.4)	10/117 (8.5)	11/143[1] (7.7)
160 mg/day (N = 239)	13/239 (5.4)	13/64 (20.3)	25/172[2] (14.5)

[1] *13 of the 143 were receiving Tacrine when evaluated.*
[2] *41 of the 172 were not receiving Tacrine when evaluated.*

The first column of the table is based on all patients participating in the study. The proportion provides an estimate of the likelihood that a patient entering the study will (1) still be on his or her assigned treatment at week 30 **and** (2) will improve 7 or more ADAS cognitive points over his or her baseline score. The estimate of response derived in this manner is conservative because the rules under which the 30-week study was conducted required the withdrawal of patients with relatively low (> 3 × ULN), asymptomatic, transaminase elevations. In actual clinical practice under the conditions of treatment recommended in the Dosage and Administration Section, a larger fraction of these patients would be able to remain on Tacrine and the proportion of those improving 7 or more points on Tacrine would be expected, therefore, to be increased (the third column illustrates this).

The second column of the table presents the proportion of 7 unit responders based on the number of patients who (1) were able to complete the full 30 weeks of the study and (2) attained an ADAS cognitive score at week 30 that was 7 or more points better than their baseline score. This analysis provides an optimistic estimate of Tacrine's effects because it reflects experience gained only with the minority of patients who were able to remain on treatment to the study's end. The comparison between the proportions of placebo and 160 mg patients attaining a 7 or more point improvement is complicated further by the fact that a larger proportion of Tacrine assigned patients withdrew prematurely.

The third column of the table presents the proportion of patients who had evaluations made at 30 weeks and had a 7-point or greater response. The analysis includes data from patients still on their assigned treatment at week 30 as well as patients who withdrew from the study prior to that time, but were retrieved for a week 30 evaluation. Because patients who withdrew prior to week 30 were permitted to receive Tacrine under "open label" conditions, retrieved patients included in this analysis could be receiving either no treatment or treatment with Tacrine. In this analysis, patients are considered under the treatment to which they were randomized, regardless of the treatment they were actually receiving at week 30. Thus, some placebo patients could have received Tacrine and some Tacrine patients could have been receiving no Tacrine. Like the analysis based on percent randomized (column I), this analysis, therefore, tends to provide a conservative view of the expected effects of Tacrine treatment.

Effects of Tacrine HCl Over Time: Figure 4 shows for each dose group the time course of change from baseline in ADAS cog scores for patients completing 30 weeks of treatment. There appears to be a persistent difference between groups, but all groups, after initial improvement, deteriorate with time.

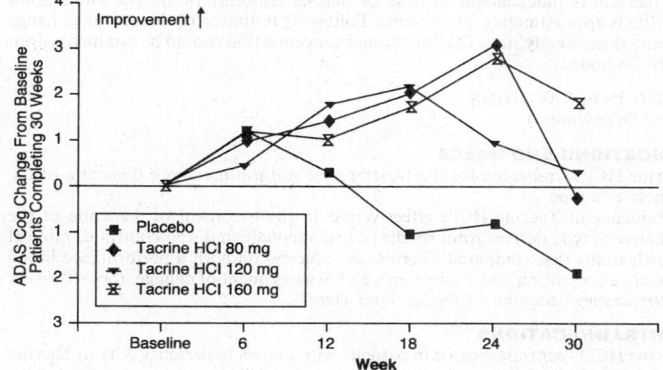

FIGURE 4. ADAS Cog Change From Baseline Over Time for the Subset of Patients Completing 30 Weeks of Treatment. In all Tacrine treatment groups dosing was initiated at 40 mg/day and increased in increments of 40 mg every 6 weeks until the target dose was achieved.

Patient age, gender, and other baseline patient characteristics were not found to predict clinical outcome.

CLINICAL PHARMACOKINETICS (ABSORPTION, DISTRIBUTION, METABOLISM, AND ELIMINATION)
Absorption: Tacrine HCl is rapidly absorbed after oral administration; maximal plasma concentrations occur within 1 to 2 hours. The rate and extent of Tacrine absorption following administration of Tacrine capsules and solution are virtually

indistinguishable. Absolute bioavailability of Tacrine is approximately 17 (SD ± 13) %. Food reduces Tacrine bioavailability by approximately 30-40%; however, there is no food effect if Tacrine is administered at least an hour before meals. The effect of achlorhydria on the absorption of Tacrine is unknown.

Distribution: Mean volume of distribution of Tacrine is approximately 349 (SD ± 193) L. Tacrine is about 55% bound to plasma proteins. The extent and degree of Tacrine's distribution within various body compartments has not been systematically studied. However, 336 hours after the administration of a single radiolabeled dose, approximately 25% of the radiolabel was not recovered in a mass balance study, suggesting the possibility that Tacrine and/or one or more of its metabolites may be retained.

Metabolism: Tacrine is extensively metabolized by the cytochrome P450 system to multiple metabolites, not all of which have been identified. The vast majority of radiolabeled species present in the plasma following a single dose of ^{14}C radiolabeled Tacrine are unidentified (ie, only 5% of radioactivity in plasma has been identified [Tacrine and 3-hydroxylated metabolites; 1-, 2-, and 4-hydroxytacrine]).

Studies utilizing human liver preparations demonstrated that cytochrome P450 IA2 is the principal isozyme involved in Tacrine metabolism. These findings are consistent with the observation that Tacrine and/or one of its metabolites inhibits the metabolism of theophylline in humans (see *"Precautions: Drug-Drug Interactions: theophylline"*). Results from a study utilizing quinidine to inhibit cytochrome P450 IID6 indicate that Tacrine is not metabolized extensively by this enzyme system.

Following aromatic ring hydroxylation, Tacrine's metabolites undergo glucuronidation. Whether Tacrine and/or its metabolites undergo biliary excretion or entero-hepatic circulation is unknown.

Special Populations: Age: Based on pooled pharmacokinetic studies (n = 192), there is no clinically relevant influence of age (50 to 84 years) on Tacrine clearance.

Gender: Average Tacrine plasma concentrations are approximately 50% higher in females than in males. This is not explained by differences in body surface area or elimination half-life. The difference is probably due to higher systemic availability after oral dosing and may reflect the known lower activity of cytochrome P450 IA2 in women.

Race: The effect of race on Tacrine clearance has not been studied.

Smoking: Mean plasma Tacrine concentrations in current smokers are approximately one third the concentrations in nonsmokers. Cigarette smoking is known to induce cytochrome P450 IA2.

Renal disease: Renal disease does not appear to affect the clearance of Tacrine.

Liver disease: Although studies in patients with liver disease have not been done, it is likely that functional hepatic impairment will reduce the clearance of Tacrine and its metabolites.

Presystemic Clearance/Elimination/Excretion: Tacrine undergoes presystemic clearance (ie, first pass metabolism). The extent of this first pass metabolism depends upon the dose of Tacrine administered. Because the enzyme system involved can be saturated at relatively low doses, a larger fraction of a high dose of Tacrine will escape first pass elimination than of a smaller dose. Thus, when a 40 mg daily dose is increased by 40 mg, the average plasma concentration will be increased by approximately 6 ng/mL. However, when a daily dose of 80 or 120 mg is increased by 40 mg, the increment in average plasma concentration is approximately 10 ng/mL.

Elimination of Tacrine from the plasma, however, is not dose dependent (ie, the half-life is independent of dose or plasma concentration). The elimination half-life is approximately 2 to 4 hours. Following initiation of therapy or a change in daily dose, steady state Tacrine plasma concentration should be attained within 24 to 36 hours.

DRUG INTERACTIONS
(See *"Precautions"*).

INDICATIONS AND USAGE
Tacrine HCl is indicated for the treatment of mild to moderate dementia of the Alzheimer's type.

Evidence of Tacrine HCl's effectiveness in the treatment of dementia of the Alzheimer's type derives from results of two adequate and well-controlled clinical investigations that compared Tacrine and placebo on both a performance based measure of cognition and a clinician's global assessment of change. (See *"Clinical Pharmacology"* section: *"Clinical Trial Data"*).

CONTRAINDICATIONS
Tacrine HCl is contraindicated in patients with known hypersensitivity to Tacrine or acridine derivatives.

Tacrine HCl is contraindicated in patients previously treated with Tacrine HCl who developed treatment-associated jaundice confirmed by elevated total bilirubin greater than 3.0 mg/dL.

WARNINGS
ANESTHESIA
Tacrine HCl, as a cholinesterase inhibitor, is likely to exaggerate succinylcholine-type muscle relaxation during anesthesia.

CARDIOVASCULAR CONDITIONS
Because of its cholinomimetic action, Tacrine HCl may have vagotonic effects on the heart rate (eg, bradycardia). This action may be particularly important to patients with a "sick sinus syndrome," etc.

GASTROINTESTINAL DISEASE AND DYSFUNCTION
Tacrine HCl is an inhibitor of cholinesterase and may be expected to increase gastric acid secretion due to increased cholinergic activity. Therefore, patients at increased risk for developing ulcers - eg, those with a history of ulcer disease or those receiving concurrent nonsteroidal anti-inflammatory drugs (NSAIDs) - should be monitored closely for symptoms of active or occult gastrointestinal bleeding.

Tacrine HCl, also as a predictable consequence of its pharmacological properties, can cause nausea, vomiting, and loose stools at recommended doses.

LIVER INJURY
Tacrine HCl should be prescribed with care in patients with current evidence or history of abnormal liver function indicated by significant abnormalities in serum transaminase (ALT/SGPT; AST/SGOT), bilirubin, and gamma-glutamyl transpeptidase (GGT) levels (see *"Precautions"* and *"Dosage and Administration"* sections).

The use of Tacrine HCl in patients without a prior history of liver disease is commonly associated with serum aminotransferase elevations, some to levels ordinarily considered to indicate clinically important hepatic injury (see Table 2).

Experience gained in more than 8000 patients who received Tacrine in clinical studies and the treatment IND program indicates that if Tacrine is promptly withdrawn following detection of these elevations, clinically evident signs and symptoms of liver injury are rare.

Long-term follow up of patients who experience transaminase elevations, however, is limited and it is impossible, therefore, to exclude, with certainty, the possibility of chronic sequelae.

CLINICAL EXPERIENCE IN CONTROLLED TRIALS AND TREATMENT IND
Experience with Tacrine in controlled trials and in a large, less closely monitored experience (a treatment IND) is summarized below:

Clinically Evident Liver Toxicity: One of more than 8000 patients exposed to Tacrine in clinical studies and the treatment IND program had documented elevated billirubin (5.3 x Upper Limit of Normal, ULN) and jaundice with transaminase levels (AST/SGOT) nearly 20 x ULN.

Blood Chemistry Signs of Liver Injury: Experience from the 30-week clinical study (described earlier) provides a representative estimate of the frequency of ALT/SGPT elevations expected for patients who receive Tacrine HCl according to the conditions of use recommended in labeling (Table 2). A dosing regimen employing a more rapid escalation of the daily dose of Tacrine, or less frequent monitoring of liver chemistries, may be associated with more serious clinical events (see *"Monitoring of Liver function and the Management of the patient who develops transaminase elevations"*).

Table 2
CUMULATIVE INCIDENCE OF ALT/SGPT ELEVATIONS BASED ON MAXIMUM VALUES DURING THE 30-WEEK STUDY

Maximum ALT	Number and (%) of Patients		
	Males N = 229	Females N = 250	Total N = 479
Within Normal Limits	121 (53)	100 (40)	221 (46)
> ULN	108 (47)	150 (60)	258 (54)
> 2 times ULN	77 (34)	104 (42)	181 (38)
> 3 times ULN	58 (25)	81 (32)	139 (29)
> 10 times ULN	12 (5)	19 (8)	31 (6)
> 20 times ULN	3 (1)	6 (2)	9 (2)

Experience in 2446 patients who participated in all clinical trials, including the 30-week study, indicates approximately 50% of patients treated with Tacrine HCl can be expected to have at least 1 ALT/SGPT level above ULN; approximately 25% of patients are likely to develop elevations > 3 X ULN, and about 7% of patients may develop elevations > 10 X ULN. Data collected from the treatment IND program were consistent with those obtained during clinical studies, and showed 3% of 5665 patients experiencing an ALT/SGPT elevation > 10 X ULN.

In clinical trials where transaminases were monitored weekly, the median time to onset of the first ALT/SGPT elevation above ULN was approximately 6 weeks, with maximum ALT/SGPT occurring 1 week later, even in instances when Tacrine HCL treatment was stopped. Under the conditions of forced slow upwards dose titration (increases of 40 mg a day every 6 weeks) employed in clinical studies, 95% of transaminase elevations > 3 X ULN occurred within the first 18 weeks of Tacrine HCl therapy, and 99% of the 10-fold elevations occurred by the 12th week and on not more than 80 mg; note, however, that for most patients ALT was monitored weekly and Tacrine HCl was stopped when liver enzymes exceeded 3 X ULN. With less frequent monitoring or the less stringent discontinuation criteria recommended below (see *"Dosage and Administration"*), it is possible that marked elevations might be more common. It must also be appreciated that experience with prolonged exposure to the high dose (160 mg/day) is limited. In all cases, transaminase levels returned to within normal limits upon discontinuation of Tacrine HCl treatment or following dosage reduction, usually within 4 to 6 weeks.

This relatively benign experience may be the consequence of careful laboratory monitoring that facilitated the discontinuation of patients early on after the onset of their transaminase elevations. Consequently, frequent monitoring of serum transaminase levels is recommended (see *"Dosage and Administration"*, *"Warn-*

ings: Liver Injury: Monitoring of Liver Function and the Management of the Patient Who Develops Transaminase Elevations" and *"Precautions: Laboratory Tests"*).

Liver biopsy Experience: Liver biopsy results in 7 patients who received Tacrine (1 in a Parke-Davis sponsored study and 6 in studies reported in the literature) revealed hepatocellular necrosis in 6 patients, and granulomatous changes in the seventh. In all cases, liver function tests returned to normal with no evidence of persisting hepatic dysfunction.

Experience with the Rechallenge of Patients with Transaminase Elevations following recovery: Two hundred and twelve patients among the 866 patients assigned to Tacrine in the 12 and 30 week studies were withdrawn because they developed transaminase elevations > 3 X ULN. One hundred and forty-five of these patients were subsequently rechallenged. During their initial exposure to Tacrine, 20 of these 145 had experienced initial elevations > 10 times ULN, while the remainder had experienced elevations between 3 and 10 X ULN.

Upon rechallenge with an initial dose of 40 mg/day, only 48 (33%) of the 145 patients developed transaminase elevations greater than 3 X ULN. Of these patients, 44 had elevations that were between 3 and 10 X ULN and 4 had elevations that were > 10 X ULN.

The mean time to onset of elevations occurred earlier on rechallenge than on initial exposure (22 versus 48 days). Of the 145 patients rechallenged, 127 (88%) were able to continue Tacrine HCl treatment, and 91 of these 127 patients titrated to doses higher than those associated with the initial transaminase elevation.

Predictors of the Risk of Transaminase Elevations: The incidence of transaminase elevations is higher among females. There are no other known predictors of the risk of hepatocellular injury.

MONITORING OF LIVER FUNCTION AND THE MANAGEMENT OF THE PATIENT WHO DEVELOPS TRANSAMINASE ELEVATIONS.
(See also *"Dosage and Administration"* and *"Precautions: Laboratory Tests."*)

Blood Chemistries: Serum transaminase levels (specifically ALT/SGPT) should be monitored weekly for at least the first 18 weeks following initiation of Tacrine HCl treatment, after which monitoring may be decreased to every 3 months. Weekly monitoring should be resumed for a minimum of 6 weeks on each occasion that the dose of Tacrine HCl is increased. Continued weekly monitoring (beyond 18 weeks) may be indicated in patients with modest elevations (greater than twice the upper limit of normal).

A full monitoring sequence should be repeated in the event that a patient suspends treatment with Tacrine for more than 4 weeks.

It transaminase elevations occur, the dose of Tacrine should be modified according to the table shown below in *"Dosage and Administration"*.

Rechallenge: Patients with clinical jaundice confirmed by a significant elevation in total bilirubin (> 3 mg/dL) should permanently discontinue Tacrine HCl and not be rechallenged. Patients who are required to discontinue Tacrine HCl treatment because of transaminase elevations may be rechallenged once transaminase levels return to within normal limits. (See *"Dosage and Administration"*.)

Rechallenge of patients with transaminase elevations less than 10 X ULN has not resulted in serious liver injury. However, because experience in the rechallenge of patients who had elevations greater than 10 X ULN is limited, the risks associated with the rechallenge of these patients are not well characterized. Careful, frequent (weekly) monitoring of serum ALT should be undertaken when rechallenging such patients.

If rechallenged, patients should be given an initial dose of 40 mg/day (10 mg QID) and transaminase levels monitored weekly. If, after 6 weeks on 40 mg/day, the patient is tolerating the dosage with no unacceptable elevations in transaminases, recommended dose-titration and transaminase monitoring may be resumed.

Liver Biopsy: Liver biopsy is not indicated in cases of uncomplicated transaminase elevation.

GENITOURINARY
Cholinomimetics may cause bladder outflow obstruction.

NEUROLOGICAL CONDITIONS
Seizures: Cholinomimetics are believed to have some potential to cause generalized convulsions; seizure activity may, however, also be a manifestation of Alzheimer's disease.

Sudden Worsening of the Degree of Cognitive Impairment: Worsening of cognitive function has been reported following abrupt discontinuation of Tacrine HCl or after a large reduction in total daily dose (80 mg/day or more).

PULMONARY CONDITIONS
Because of its cholinomimetic action, Tacrine HCl should be prescribed with care to patients with a history of asthma.

PRECAUTIONS
GENERAL
LIVER INJURY
See *"Warnings"*.

HEMATOLOGY
An absolute neutrophil count (ANC) less than 500/μL occurred in 4 patients who received Tacrine HCl during the course of clinical trials. Three of the 4 patients had concurrent medical conditions commonly associated with a low ANC; 2 of these patients remained on Tacrine HCl. The fourth patient, who had a history of

hypersensitivity (penicillin allergy), withdrew from the study as a result of a rash and also developed an ANC ≥ 500/μL, which returned to normal; this patient was not rechallenged and, therefore, the role played by Tacrine HCl in this reaction is unknown.

Six patients had an absolute neutrophil count ≤ 1500/μL, associated with an elevation of ALT/SGPT.

The total clinical experience in more than 8000 patients does not indicate a clear association between Tacrine HCl treatment and serious white blood cell abnormalities.

INFORMATION FOR PATIENTS AND CAREGIVERS
Patients and caregivers should be advised that the effect of Tacrine HCl therapy is thought to depend upon its administration at regular intervals, as directed.

The caregiver should be advised about the possibility of adverse effects. Two types should be distinguished: (1) those occurring in close temporal association with the initiation of treatment or an increase in dose (eg, nausea, vomiting, loose stools, diarrhea, etc) and (2) those with a delayed onset (eg, rash, jaundice, changes in the color of stool—black, very dark or light [ie, acholic]).

Patients and caregivers should be encouraged to inform the physician about the emergence of new events or any increase in the severity of existing adverse clinical events.

Caregivers should be advised that abrupt discontinuation of Tacrine HCl or a large reduction in total daily dose (80 mg/day or more) may cause a decline in cognitive function and behavioral disturbances. Unsupervised increases in the dose of Tacrine also have serious consequences. Consequently, changes in dose should not be undertaken in the absence of direct instruction of a physician.

LABORATORY TESTS
(See *"Warnings: Liver Injury"* and *"Dosage and Administration"*.)

Serum transaminase levels (specifically ALT/SGPT) should be monitored in patients given Tacrine HCl (see *"Warnings: Liver Injury"*).

DRUG-DRUG INTERACTIONS
Possible metabolic basis for interactions: Tacrine is primarily eliminated by hepatic metabolism via cytochrome P450 drug metabolizing enzymes. Drug-drug interactions may occur when Tacrine HCl is given concurrently with agents such as theophylline that undergo extensive metabolism via cytochrome P450 IA2. **Theophylline.** Coadministration of Tacrine HCl with theophylline increased theophylline elimination half-life and average plasma theophylline concentrations by approximately 2-fold. Therefore, monitoring of plasma theophylline concentrations and appropriate reduction of theophylline dose are recommended in patients receiving Tacrine HCl and theophylline concurrently. The effect of theophylline on Tacrine HCl pharmacokinetics has not been assessed.

Cimetidine: Cimetidine increased the Cmax and AUC of Tacrine by approximately 54% and 64%, respectively.

Anticholinergics: Because of its mechanism of action. Tacrine HCl has the potential to interfere with the activity of anticholinergic medications.

Cholinomimetics and Cholinesterase Inhibitors: A synergistic effect is expected when Tacrine HCl is given concurrently with succinylcholine (see *"Warnings"*), cholinesterase inhibitors, or cholinergic agonists such as bethanechol.

Other Interactions: Rate and extent of Tacrine absorption were not influenced by the coadministration of an antacid containing magnesium and aluminum. Tacrine had no major effect on digoxin or diazepam pharmacokinetics or the anticoagulant activity of warfarin.

CARCINOGENESIS, MUTAGENESIS, IMPAIRMENT OF FERTILITY
Tacrine was mutagenic to bacteria in the Ames test. Unscheduled DNA synthesis was induced in rat and mouse hepatocytes *in vitro*. Results of cytogenetic (chromosomal aberration) studies were equivocal. Tacrine was not mutagenic in an *in vitro* mammalian mutation test. Overall, the results of these tests, along with the fact that Tacrine belongs to a chemical class (acridines) containing some members which are animal carcinogens, suggest that Tacrine may be carcinogenic.

Studies of the effects of Tacrine on fertility have not been performed.

PREGNANCY
Category C: Animal reproduction studies have not been conducted with Tacrine. It is also not known whether Tacrine HCl can cause fetal harm when administered to a pregnant woman or can affect reproductive capacity.

NURSING MOTHERS
It is not known whether this drug is excreted in human milk.

PEDIATRIC USE
There are no adequate and well-controlled trials to document the safety and efficacy of Tacrine in any dementing illness occurring in children.

ADVERSE REACTIONS
COMMON ADVERSE EVENTS LEADING TO DISCONTINUATION
In clinical trials, approximately 17% of the 2706 patients who received Tacrine HCl and 5% of the 1886 patients who received placebo withdrew permanently because of adverse events. It should be noted that some of the placebo-treated patients were exposed to Tacrine HCl prior to receiving placebo due to the variety of study designs used, including crossover studies. Transaminase elevations were the most common reason for withdrawals during Tacrine HCl treatment (8% of all Tacrine HCl-treated patients, or 212 of 456 patients withdrawn). The controlled clinical trial protocols required that any patient with an ALT/SGPT elevation > 3 X ULN be withdrawn, because of concern about potential hepatotoxicity. Apart

from withdrawals due to transaminase elevations, 244 patients (9%) withdrew for adverse events while receiving Tacrine HCl.

Other adverse events that most frequently led to the withdrawal of Tacrine-treated patients in clinical trials were nausea and/or vomiting (1.5%), agitation (0.9%), rash (0.7%), anorexia (0.7%), and confusion (0.5%). These adverse events also most frequently led to the withdrawal of placebo-treated patients, although at lower frequencies (0.1% to 0.2%).

MOST FREQUENT ADVERSE CLINICAL EVENTS SEEN IN ASSOCIATION WITH THE USE OF TACRINE
The events identified here are those that occurred at an absolute incidence of at least 5% of patients treated with Tacrine HCl, and at a rate at least 2-fold higher in patients treated with Tacrine HCl than placebo.

The most common adverse events associated with the use of Tacrine HCl were elevated transaminases, nausea and/or vomiting, diarrhea, dyspepsia, myalgia, anorexia, and ataxia. Of these events, nausea and/or vomiting, diarrhea, dyspepsia, and anorexia appeared to be dose-dependent.

ADVERSE EVENTS REPORTED IN CONTROLLED TRIALS
The events cited in the tables below reflect experience gained under closely monitored conditions of clinical trials with a highly selected patient population. In actual clinical practice or in other clinical trials, these frequency estimates may not apply, as the conditions of use, reporting behavior, and the kinds of patients treated may differ.

Table 3 lists treatment-emergent signs and symptoms that occurred in at least 2% of patients with Alzheimer's disease in placebo-controlled trials and who received the recommended regimen for dose introduction and titration of Tacrine HCl (see *"Dosage and Administration"*).

Table 3
ADVERSE EVENTS OCCURRING IN AT LEAST 2% OF PATIENTS RECEIVING TACRINE HCl USING THE RECOMMENDED REGIMEN FOR DOSE INTRODUCTION AND TITRATION IN CONTROLLED CLINICAL TRIALS

[Number (%) of Patients]

Body System/Adverse Events	Tacrine N = 634	Placebo N = 342
Laboratory Deviations		
Elevated Transaminase	184(29)	5 (2)
Body As a Whole		
Headache	67(11)	52(15)
Fatigue	26 (4)	9 (3)
Chest Pain	24 (4)	18 (5)
Weight Decrease	21 (3)	4 (1)
Back Pain	15 (2)	14 (4)
Asthenia	15 (2)	7 (2)
Digestive System		
Nausea and/or Vomiting	178(28)	29 (9)
Diarrhea	99(16)	18 (5)
Dyspepsia	57 (9)	22 (6)
Anorexia	54 (9)	11 (3)
Abdominal Pain	48 (8)	24 (7)
Flatulence	22 (4)	5 (2)
Constipation	24 (4)	8 (2)
Hemic and Lymphatic System		
Purpura	15 (2)	8 (2)
Musculoskeletal System		
Myalgia	54 (9)	18 (5)
Nervous System		
Dizziness	73(12)	39(11)
Confusion	42 (7)	24 (7)
Ataxia	36 (6)	12 (4)
Insomnia	37 (6)	18 (5)
Somnolence	22 (4)	11 (3)
Tremor	14 (2)	2 (< 1)
Psychobiologic Function		
Agitation	43 (7)	30 (9)
Depression	22 (4)	14 (4)
Thinking Abnormal	17 (3)	14 (4)
Anxiety	16 (3)	7 (2)
Hallucination	15 (2)	12 (4)
Hostility	15 (2)	5 (2)
Respiratory System		
Rhinitis	51 (8)	22 (6)
Upper Respiratory Infection	18 (3)	11 (3)
Coughing	17 (3)	18 (5)
Skin and Appendages		
Rash	46 (7)	18 (5)
Facial Flushing, Skin Flushing	16 (3)	3 (< 1)
Urogenital System		
Urination Frequency	21 (3)	12 (4)
Urinary Tract Infection	21 (3)	20 (6)
Urinary Incontinence	16 (3)	9 (3)

a   ALT or AST value of approximately 3 X ULN or greater or that resulted in a change in patient management.

b   Includes COSTART terms: rash, rash-erythematous, rash-maculopapular, urticaria, petechial rash, rash-vesiculobullous, and pruritus.

OTHER ADVERSE EVENTS OBSERVED DURING ALL CLINICAL TRIALS
Tacrine HCl has been administered to 2706 individuals during clinical trials. A total of 1471 patients were treated for at least 3 months, 1137 for at least 6 months, and 773 for at least 1 year. Any untoward reactions that occurred during these trials were recorded as adverse events by the clinical investigators using terminology of their own choosing. To provide a meaningful estimate of the proportion of individuals having similar types of events, the events were grouped into a smaller number of standardized categories using a modified COSTART dictionary. These categories are used in the listing below. The frequencies represent the proportion of the 2706 individuals exposed to Tacrine HCl who experienced that event while receiving Tacrine HCl. All adverse events are included except those already listed on the previous table and those COSTART terms too general to be informative. Events are further classified by body system categories and listed using the following definitions: frequent adverse events are defined as those occurring in at least 1/100 patients; infrequent adverse events are those occurring in 1/100 to 1/1000 patients; and rare adverse events are those occurring in less than 1/1000 patients. These adverse events are not necessarily related to Tacrine HCl treatment. Only rare adverse events deemed to be potentially important are included.

Body As a Whole: Frequent: Chill, fever, malaise, peripheral edema. *Infrequent:* Face edema, dehydration, weight increase, cachexia, edema (generalized), lipoma. *Rare:* Heat exhaustion, sepsis, cholingeric crisis, death.

Cardiovascular System: Frequent: Hypotension, hypertension: *Infrequent:* Heart failure, myocardial infarction, angina pectoris, cerebrovascular accident, transient ischemic attack, phlebitis, venous insufficiency, abdominal aortic aneurysm, atrial fibrillation or flutter, palpitation, tachycardia, bradycardia, pulmonary embolus, migraine, hypercholesterolemia. *Rare:* Heart arrest, premature atrial contractions, A-V block, bundle branch block.

Digestive System: Infrequent: Glossitis, gingivitis, mouth or throat dry, stomatitis, increased salivation, dysphagia, esophagitis, gastritis, gastroenteritis, GI hemorrhage, stomach ulcer, hiatal hernia, hemorrhoids, stools bloody, diverticulitis, fecal impaction, fecal incontinence, hemorrhage (rectum), cholelithiasis, cholecystitis, increased appetite. *Rare:* Duodenal ulcer, bowel obstruction.

Endocrine System: Infrequent: Diabetes. *Rare:* Hyperthyroid, hypothyroid.

Hemic and Lymphatic: Infrequent: Anemia, lymphadenopathy. *Rare:* Leukopenia, thrombocytopenia, hemolysis, pancytopenia.

Musculoskeletal: Frequent: Fracture, arthralgia, arthritis, hypertonia. *Infrequent:* Osteoporosis, tendinitis, bursitis, gout. *Rare:* Myopathy.

Nervous System: Frequent: Convulsions, vertigo, syncope, hyperkinesia, paresthesia. *Infrequent:* Dreaming abnormal, dysarthria, aphasia, amnesia, wandering, twitching, hypesthesia, delirium, paralysis, bradykinesia, movement disorder, cogwheel rigidity, paresis, neuritis, hemiplegia, Parkinson's disease, neuropathy, extrapyramidal syndrome, reflexes decreased/absent. *Rare:* Tardive dyskinesia, dysesthesia, dystonia, encephalitis, coma, apraxia, oculogyric crisis, akathisia, oral facial dyskinesia, Bell's palsy.

Psychobiologic Function: Frequent: Nervousness. *Infrequent:* Apathy, increased libido, paranoia, neurosis. *Rare:* Suicidal, psychosis, hysteria.

Respiratory System: Frequent: Pharyngitis, sinusitis, bronchitis, pneumonia, dyspnea. *Infrequent:* Epistaxis, chest congestion, asthma, hyperventilation, lower respiratory infection. *Rare:* Hemoptysis, lung edema, lung cancer, acute epiglottitis.

Skin and Appendages: Frequent: Sweating increased. *Infrequent:* Acne, alopecia, dermatitis, eczema, skin dry, herpes zoster, psoriasis, cellulitis, cyst, furunculosis, herpes simplex, hyperkeratosis, basal cell carcinoma, skin cancer. *Rare:* Desquamation, seborrhea, squamous cell carcinoma, ulcer (skin), skin necrosis, melanoma.

Urogenital System: Infrequent: Hematuria, renal stone, kidney infection, glycosuria, dysuria, polyuria, nocturia, pyuria, cystitis, urinary retention, urination urgency, vaginal hemorrhage, pruritus (genital), breast pain, impotence, prostate cancer. *Rare:* Bladder tumor, renal tumor, renal failure, urinary obstruction, breast cancer, epididymitis, carcinoma (ovary).

Special Senses: Frequent: Conjunctivitis. *Infrequent:* Cataract, eyes dry, eye pain, visual field defect, diplopia, amblyopia, glaucoma, hordeolum, deafness, earache, tinnitus, inner ear infection, otitis media, unusual taste. *Rare:* Vision loss, ptosis, blepharitis, labyrinthitis, inner ear disturbance.

OVERDOSAGE
As in any case of overdose, general supportive measures should be utilized. Overdosage with cholinesterase inhibitors can cause a cholinergic crisis characterized by severe nausea/vomiting, salivation, sweating, bradycardia, hypotension, collapse, and convulsions. Increasing muscle weakness is a possibility and may result in death if respiratory muscles are involved.

Tertiary anticholinergics such as atropine may be used as an antidote for Tacrine HCl overdosage Intravenous atropine sulfate titrated to effect is recommended: initial dose of 1.0 to 2.0 mg IV with subsequent doses based upon clinical response. Atypical increases in blood pressure and heart rate have been reported with other cholinomimetics when coadministered with quaternary anticholinergics such as glycopyrrolate.

It is not known whether Tacrine HCl or its metabolites can be eliminated by dialysis (hemodialysis, peritoneal dialysis, or hemofiltration).

The estimated median lethal dose of Tacrine HCl following a single oral dose in rats is 40 mg/kg, or approximately 12 times the maximum recommended human dose of 160 mg/day. Dose-related signs of cholinergic stimulation were observed in animals and included vomiting, diarrhea, salivation, lacrimation, ataxia, convulsions, tremor, and stereotypic head and body movements.

DOSAGE AND ADMINISTRATION
The recommendations for dose titration are based on experience from clinical trials. The rate of dose escalation may be slowed if a patient is intolerant to the titration schedule recommended below. It is not advisable, however, to accelerate the dose incrementation plan.

Following initiation of therapy, or any dosage increase, patients should be observed carefully for adverse effects. Tacrine HCl should be taken between meals whenever possible; however, if minor GI upset occurs, Tacrine HCl may be taken with meals to improve tolerability. Taking Tacrine HCl with meals can be expected to reduce plasma levels approximately 30% to 40%.

INITIATION OF TREATMENT
The initial dose of Tacrine HCl is 40 mg/day (10 mg QID). This dose should be maintained for a minimum of 6 weeks with weekly monitoring of transaminase levels. It is important that the dose not be increased during this period because of the potential for delayed onset of transaminase elevations.

DOSE TITRATION
Following 6 weeks of treatment at 40 mg/day, the dose of Tacrine HCl should then be increased to 80 mg/day (20 mg QID), providing there are no significant transaminase elevations and the patient is tolerating treatment. Patients should be titrated to higher doses (120 and 160 mg/day, in divided doses on a QID schedule) at 6-week intervals on the basis of tolerance.

DOSE ADJUSTMENT
Serum transaminase levels (specifically ALT/SGPT) should be monitored weekly for at least the first 18 weeks following initiation of Tacrine HCl treatment, after which monitoring may be decreased to every 3 months. Weekly monitoring should be resumed for at least an additional interval of 6 weeks on each occasion that the dose of Tacrine is increased. Continued weekly monitoring (beyond 18 weeks) may be indicated in patients with modest elevations (greater than twice the upper limit of normal).

A full monitoring and dose titration sequence must be repeated in the event that a patient suspends treatment with Tacrine for more than 4 weeks.

If transaminase elevations occur, the dose of Tacrine HCl should be modified according to the table below:

Table 4
RECOMMENDED DOSE REGIMEN MODIFICATION IN RESPONSE TO TRANSAMINASE ELEVATIONS

Transaminase Level	Treatment Regimen
≤ 3 × ULN	Continue treatment according to recommended titration.
> 3 to ≤ 5 × ULN	Reduce the daily dose of Tacrine HCl by 40 mg/day. Resume dose-titration when transaminases return to within normal limits.
> 5 × ULN	Stop Tacrine HCl treatment. Monitor transaminase levels until within normal limits. See Rechallange section below.
	Experience is limited with patients with ALT > 10 X ULN. The risk of rechallenge must be considered against demonstrated clinical benefit.
	Patients with clinical jaundice confirmed by a significant elevation in total bilirubin (> 3 mg/dL) should permanently discontinue Tacrine HCl and not be rechallenged.

RECHALLENGE
Patients who are required to discontinue Tacrine HCl treatment because of transaminase elevations may be rechallenged once transaminase levels return to within normal limits.

Rechallenge of patients exposed to transaminase elevations less than 10 X ULN has not resulted in serious liver injury. However, because experience in the rechallenge of patients who had elevations greater than 10 X ULN is limited, the risks associated with the rechallenge of these patients are not well characterized. Careful, frequent (weekly) monitoring of serum ALT should be undertaken when rechallenging such patients.

If rechallenged, patients should be given an initial dose of 40 mg/day (10 mg QID) and transaminase levels monitored weekly. If, after 6 weeks on 40 mg/day, the patient is tolerating the dosage with no unacceptable elevations in transaminases, recommended dose-titration and transaminase monitoring may be resumed.

STORAGE
Store at controlled room temperature, 15°C to 30°C (59°F to 86°F), away from moisture.

HOW SUPPLIED
CAPSULE: 10 MG

BRAND/MANUFACTURER	NDC	SIZE	AWP
○ **BRAND**			
COGNEX: Parke-Davis	00071-0096-40	100s ud	$119.69
	00071-0096-25	120s	$114.74

CAPSULE: 20 MG

BRAND/MANUFACTURER	NDC	SIZE	AWP
○ **BRAND**			
COGNEX: Parke-Davis	00071-0097-40	100s ud	$119.69
	00071-0097-25	120s	$114.74

CAPSULE: 30 MG

BRAND/MANUFACTURER	NDC	SIZE	AWP
○ **BRAND**			
➤ COGNEX: Parke-Davis	00071-0095-40	100s ud	$119.69
	00071-0095-25	120s	$114.74

CAPSULE: 40 MG

BRAND/MANUFACTURER	NDC	SIZE	AWP
○ **BRAND**			
➤ COGNEX: Parke-Davis	00071-0098-40	100s ud	$119.69
	00071-0098-25	120s	$114.74

Tacrolimus

> **WARNING**
> INCREASED SUSCEPTIBILITY TO INFECTION AND THE POSSIBLE DEVELOPMENT OF LYMPHOMA MAY RESULT FROM IMMUNOSUPPRESSION. ONLY PHYSICIANS EXPERIENCED IN IMMUNOSUPPRESSIVE THERAPY AND MANAGEMENT OF ORGAN TRANSPLANT PATIENTS SHOULD PRESCRIBE TACROLIMUS. PATIENTS RECEIVING THE DRUG SHOULD BE MANAGED IN FACILITIES EQUIPPED AND STAFFED WITH ADEQUATE LABORATORY AND SUPPORTIVE MEDICAL RESOURCES. THE PHYSICIAN RESPONSIBLE FOR MAINTENANCE THERAPY SHOULD HAVE COMPLETE INFORMATION REQUISITE FOR THE FOLLOW-UP OF THE PATIENT.

DESCRIPTION
Tacrolimus is available for oral administration as capsules and as a sterile solution for administration by intravenous infusion only.

Each capsule contains: Tacrolimus (anhydrous) 1 or 5 mg (equivalent)
Each ml of solution contains: Tacrolimus (anhydrous) 5 mg (equivalent)

Tacrolimus injection must be diluted with 0.9% Sodium Chloride Injection or 5% Dextrose Injection before use.

Tacrolimus, previously known as FK506, is a macrolide immunosuppressant produced by *Streptomyces tsukubaensis*. Chemically, tacrolimus is designated as [3 S-[3R*[E(1S*,3S*,4S*)],-4S*, 5R*,8S*,9E, 12R*, 14R*,15S*,16R*,18S*,19S*,26a-R*]]-5, 6, 8, 11, 12, 13, 14, 15, 16, 17, 18, 19, 24, 25, 26, 26a-hexadecahydro-5,19-dihydroxy-3-[2-(4- hydroxy-3-methoxycyclohex-yl)- 1-methylethenyl]-14, 16-dimethoxy 4,10,12,18-teramethyl-8-(2-propenyl)-15,19-epoxy-3H-pyrido [2,1-c][1,4] oxaazacyclotricosine-1, 7, 20, 21 (4H,23H)-tetrone, monohydrate.

Tacrolimus has an empirical formula of $C_{44}H_{69}NO_{12} \cdot H_2O$ and a formula weight of 822.05. Tacrolimus appears as white crystals or crystalline powder. It is practically insoluble in water, freely soluble in ethanol, and very soluble in methanol and chloroform.

Following is its chemical structure:

CLINICAL PHARMACOLOGY

MECHANISM OF ACTION

Tacrolimus prolongs the survival of the host and transplanted graft in animal transplant models of liver, kidney, heart, bone marrow, small bowel and pancreas, lung and trachea, skin, cornea, and limb.

In animals, Tacrolimus has been demonstrated to suppress some humoral immunity and, to a greater extent, cell-mediated reactions such as allograft rejection, delayed type hypersensitivity, collagen-induced arthritis, experimental allergic encephalomyelitis, and graft versus host disease.

Tacrolimus inhibits T-lymphocyte activation, although the exact mechanism of action is not known. Experimental evidence suggests that Tacrolimus binds to an intracellular protein, FKBP-12. A complex of Tacrolimus-FKBP-12, calcium, calmodulin, and calcineurin is then formed and the phosphatase activity of calcineurin inhibited. This effect may prevent the generation of nuclear factor of activated T-cells (NF-AT), a nuclear component thought to initiate gene transcription for the formation of lymphokines (interleukin-2, gamma interferon). The net result is the inhibition of T-lymphocyte activation (i.e., immunosuppression).

PHARMACOKINETICS

Absorption of Tacrolimus from the gastrointestinal tract after oral administration is variable. The absorption half-life of Tacrolimus in 16 liver transplant patients averaged 5.7 hours (standard deviation 4.6 hours). Peak concentrations (Cmax) in blood and plasma were achieved at approximately 1.5-3.5 hours. Mean (standard deviation) pharmacokinetic parameters of Tacrolimus in whole blood after oral administration were: (See related table).

The disposition of Tacrolimus from whole blood was biphasic with a terminal elimination half-life of 11.7 ($\pm$ 3.9) hours in liver transplant patients and 21.2 ($\pm$ 8.5) hours in healthy volunteers. The volume of distribution and total body clearance for Tacrolimus following intravenous administration were:

Population	Number of Subjects	Dose (mg/kg/12h)	Vd (l/kg)	Cl (L/h/kg)
Health Volunteers	27	0.01	0.88 (0.31)	0.042 (0.016)
Liver Transplant Patients	17	0.05	0.85 (0.3)	0.053 (0.017)
Mean (SD)	Vd Volume of distribution Cl Total body clearance			

Pharmacokinetic data indicate that whole blood rather than plasma may serve as the more appropriate medium to describe the pharmacokinetic characteristics of Tacrolimus. The results of a single-dose bioequivalence study conducted in 27 healthy volunteers indicated that the absolute bioavailability of the 5-mg capsule was 14.4% and that of five 1-mg capsules was 17.4%. This study failed to establish the bioequivalence of these two formulations.

The effect of food was studied in 11 liver transplant patients. Tacrolimus was administered in the fasting state or 15 minutes after a breakfast of measured fat content (34% of 400 total calories). The results indicate that the presence of food reduces the absorption of Tacrolimus (decrease in AUC and Cmax, and increase in Tmax). The relative oral bioavailability (whole blood) was reduced by 27.0 ($\pm$ 18.2%) when compared to administration in the fasting state.

The protein-binding of Tacrolimus reported in two studies was 75% and 99% over a range of concentrations of 0.1-100 ng/mL. Tacrolimus is bound to proteins, mainly albumins and alpha-1-acid glycoprotein, and is highly bound to erythrocytes. The distribution of Tacrolimus between whole blood and plasma depends on several factors such as hematocrit, temperature of separation of plasma, drug concentration, and plasma protein concentration. In a U.S. study, the ratio of whole blood concentration to plasma concentration ranged from 12 to 67 (mean 35).

Tacrolimus trough concentrations from 10 to 60 ng/mL measured at 10-12 hours post-dose (Cmin) correlated well with the area under the plasma or whole blood concentration-time curve (AUC). In 28 liver transplant patients, the correlation coefficient was 0.94.

Pharmacokinetic studies in pediatric patients have not been conducted. However, trough concentrations obtained from 30 children (less than 12 years old) showed that children need higher doses than adults to achieve similar Tacrolimus trough concentrations, suggesting that the pharmacokinetic characteristics of Tacrolimus are different in children as compared to adults. (See "Dosage and Administration").

Tacrolimus is extensively metabolized by the mixed-function oxidase system, primarily the cytochrome P-450 enzyme system (P-450 IIIA). In man, less than 1% of the dose administered is excreted unchanged in the urine. The major metabolic pathway has not been determined. Demethylation and hydroxylation were identified as the primary mechanisms of biotransformation in vitro. The major metabolite identified in incubations with human liver microsomes is 13-demethyl Tacrolimus. Ten possible metabolites have been identified in human plasma. Two metabolites, a demethylated and a double-demethylated Tacrolimus, were shown to retain 10% and 7%, respectively, of the inhibitory effect of Tacrolimus on T-lymphocyte activation.

CLINICAL STUDIES

The safety and efficacy of Tacrolimus-based immunosuppression following orthotopic liver transplantation were assessed in two prospective, randomized, non-blinded multicenter studies. The active control groups were treated with a cyclosporine-based immunosuppressive regimen. Both studies used concomitant adrenal corticosteroids as part of the immunosuppressive regimens. These studies were designed to evaluate whether the two regimens were therapeutically equivalent, with patient and graft survival at 12 months following transplantation as the primary endpoints. The Tacrolimus-based immunosuppressive regimen was found to be equivalent to the cyclosporine-based immunosuppressive regimens. In one trial, 529 patients were enrolled at 12 clinical sites in the United States; prior to surgery, 263 were randomized to the Tacrolimus-based immunosuppressive regimen and 266 to a cyclosporine-based immunosuppressive regimen (CBIR). In 10 of the 12 sites, the same CBIR protocol was used, while 2 sites used different control protocols. This trial excluded patients with renal dysfunction, fulminant hepatic failure with Stage IV encephalopathy, and cancers; pediatric patients ($\leq$ 12 years old) were allowed.

In the second trial, 545 patients were enrolled at 8 clinical sites in Europe; prior to surgery, 270 were randomized to the Tacrolimus-based immunosuppressive regimen and 275 to a CBIR. In this study, each center used its local standard CBIR protocol in the active-control arm. This trial excluded pediatric patients, but did allow enrollment of subjects with renal dysfunction, fulminant hepatic failure in Stage IV encephalopathy, and cancers other than primary hepatic with metastases.

One-year patient survival and graft survival in the Tacrolimus-based treatment groups were equivalent to those in the CBIR treatment groups in both studies. The overall one-year patient survival (CBIR and Tacrolimus-based treatment groups combined) was 88% in the U.S. study and 78% in the European study. The overall one-year graft survival (CBIR and Tacrolimus-based treatment groups combined) was 81% in the U.S. study and 73% in the European study. In both studies, the median time to convert from IV to oral Tacrolimus dosing was 2 days.

Information on secondary outcomes (incidence of acute rejection, use of OKT3 for steroid-resistant rejection, and incidence of refractory rejection) was also collected. Because of the nature of the study designs, comparisons of differences between the study arms for these secondary endpoints could not be reliably assessed.

INDICATIONS AND USAGE

Tacrolimus is indicated for the prophylaxis of organ rejection in patients receiving allogeneic liver transplants. It is recommended that Tacrolimus be used concomitantly with adrenal corticosteroids. Because of the risk of anaphylaxis, Tacrolimus injection should be reserved for patients unable to take Tacrolimus capsules orally.

CONTRAINDICATIONS

Tacrolimus is contraindicated in patients with a hypersensitivity to or to any other component of the product.

WARNINGS

(See boxed "Warning")

Tacrolimus can cause neurotoxicity, and nephrotoxicity particularly when used in high doses. Nephrotoxicity has been noted in 40% and 33% of liver

Population	No. of Subjs/Study	Dose mg/kg/12h	Cmax ng/mL	Tmax hours	AUC ng/ml.h	F%
Healthy Volunteers	27	0.07 (1×5mg)	28.6 (8.6)	1.4 (0.62)	271 (122)	14.4 (6.0)
		0.07 (5×1 mg)	36.2 (13.8)	1.3 (0.43)	329 (174)	17.4 (7.0)
Liver Transplant Patients	17	0.15	68.5 (30.0)	2.3 (1.5)	519 (179)	21.8 (6.3)
	11 Effect of Food	0.15 (Food)	27.1 (14.7)	3.2 (1.3)	223 (125)	-
		0.15 (Fasting)	52.4 (17.0)	1.5 (1.2)	290 (117)	-
Mean (SD)	Cmax maximum concentration AUC area under the conc-time curve			Tmax time to maximum concentration F absolute bioavailability		

◆ RATED THERAPEUTICALLY EQUIVALENT; ◇ THERAPEUTIC EQUIVALENCE UNCONFIRMED; ○ UNRATED

transplantation patients receiving Tacrolimus in the U.S. and European randomized trials, respectively (see *"Adverse Reactions"*). More overt nephrotoxicity is seen early after transplantation, characterized by increasing serum creatinine and a decrease in urine output. Patients with impaired renal function should be monitored closely, and the dosage of Tacrolimus may need to be reduced. In patients with persistent elevations of serum creatinine who are unresponsive to dosage adjustments, consideration should be given to changing to another immunosuppressive therapy. Care should be taken in using Tacrolimus and other nephrotoxic drugs. **In particular, to avoid excess nephrotoxicity, Tacrolimus should not be used simultaneously with cyclosporine. Tacrolimus for cyclosporine should be discontinued at least 24 hours prior to initiating the other. In the presence of elevated Tacrolimus or cyclosporine concentrations, dosing with the other drug usually should be further delayed.**

Mild to severe hyperkalemia has been noted in 44% and 10% of liver transplant recipients treated with Tacrolimus in the U.S. and European randomized trials and may require treatment (see *"Adverse Reactions"*). **Serum potassium levels should be monitored and potassium-sparing diuretics should be used during Tacrolimus therapy** (see *"Precautions"*).

Neurotoxicity, including tremor, headache, and other changes in motor function, mental status, and sensory function were reported in approximately 55% of liver transplant recipients in the two randomized studies (see *"Adverse Reactions"*). Tremor and headache have been associated with high whole-blood concentrations of Tacrolimus and may respond to dosage adjustment. Seizures have occurred in adult and pediatric patients receiving Tacrolimus (see *"Adverse Reactions"*). Coma and delirium also have been associated with high plasma concentrations of Tacrolimus. As in patients receiving other immunosuppressants, patients receiving Tacrolimus are at increased risk of developing lymphomas and other malignancies, particularly of the skin. The risk appears to be related to the intensity and duration of immunosuppression rather than to the use of any specific agent. A lymphoproliferative disorder (LPD) related to Epstein-Barr Virus (EBV) infection has been reported in immunosuppressed organ transplant recipients. The risk of LPD appears greatest in young children who are at risk for primary EBV infection while immunosuppressed or who are switched to Tacrolimus following long-term immunosuppression therapy. Because of the danger of oversuppression of the immune system, which can increase susceptibility to infection, Tacrolimus should not be administered with other immunosuppressive agents except adrenal corticosteroids. The efficacy and safety of the use of Tacrolimus in combination with other immunosuppressive agents has not been determined. A few patients receiving Tacrolimus injection have experienced anaphylactic reactions. Although the exact cause of these reactions is not known, drugs with castor oil derivatives in the formulation have been associated with anaphylaxis in a small percentage of patients; some brands of Tacrolimus contain castor oil. Because of this potential risk of anaphylaxis, Tacrolimus injection should be reserved for patients who are unable to take Tacrolimus capsules.

Patients receiving Tacrolimus injection should be under continuous observation for at least the first 30 minutes following the start of the infusion and at frequent intervals thereafter. If signs or symptoms of anaphylaxis occur, the infusion should be stopped. An aqueous solution of epinephrine 1:1000 should be available at the bedside as well as a source of oxygen.

PRECAUTIONS
GENERAL
Hypertension is a common adverse effect of Tacrolimus therapy (see *"Adverse Reactions"*). Mild or moderate hypertension is more frequently reported than severe hypertension. Antihypertensive therapy may be required; the control of blood pressure can be accomplished with any of the common antihypertensive agents. Since Tacrolimus can cause hyperkalemia, potassium-sparing diuretics should be avoided. While calcium-channel blocking agents can be effective in treating Tacrolimus-associated hypertension, care should be taken since interference with Tacrolimus metabolism may require a dosage reduction (see *"Drug Interactions"*).

Hyperglycemia was associated with the use of Tacrolimus in 47% and 29% of liver transplant recipients in the U.S. and European randomized studies, respectively, and may require treatment (see *"Adverse Reactions"*).

RENALLY AND HEPATICALLY IMPAIRED PATIENTS
For patients with renal insufficiency some evidence suggests that lower doses should be used (see *"Dosage and Administration"*).

The use of Tacrolimus in liver transplant recipients experiencing post-transplant hepatic impairment may be associated with increased risk of developing renal insufficiency related to high whole-blood levels of Tacrolimus. These patients should be monitored closely and dosage adjustments should be considered. Some evidence suggests that lower doses should be used in these patients (see *"Dosage and Administration"*).

INFORMATION FOR PATIENTS
Patients should be informed of the need for repeated appropriate laboratory tests while they are receiving Tacrolimus. They should be given complete dosage instructions, advised of the potential risks during pregnancy, and informed of the increased risk of neoplasia.

LABORATORY TESTS
Serum creatinine and potassium should be assessed regularly. Routine monitoring of metabolic and hematologic systems should be performed as clinically warranted.

DRUG INTERACTIONS
Drug interaction studies with Tacrolimus have not been conducted. Due to the potential for additive or synergistic impairment of renal function, care should be taken when administering Tacrolimus with drugs that may be associated with renal dysfunction. These include, but are not limited to, aminoglycosides, amphotericin B, and cisplatin. Initial clinical experience with the co-administration of Tacrolimus and cyclosporine resulted in additive/synergistic nephrotoxicity. Patients switched from cyclosporine to Tacrolimus should receive the first Tacrolimus dose no sooner than 24 hours after the last cyclosporine dose. Dosing may be further delayed in the presence of elevated cyclosporine levels.

DRUGS THAT MAY ALTER TACROLIMUS CONCENTRATIONS
Since Tacrolimus is metabolized mainly by the cytochrome P-450 IIIA enzyme systems, substances known to inhibit these enzymes may decrease the metabolism of Tacrolimus with resultant increases in whole blood or plasma levels. Drugs known to induce these enzyme systems may result in an increased metabolism of Tacrolimus and decreased whole blood or plasma levels. Monitoring of blood levels and appropriate dosage adjustments are essential when such drugs are used concomitantly.

DRUGS THAT MAY INCREASE TACROLIMUS BLOOD LEVELS

Calcium Channel Blockers	Antifungal Agents	Other Drugs
diltiazem	clotrimazole	bromocriptine
nicardipine	fluconazole	cimetidine
verapamil	itraconazole	clarithromycin
	ketoconazole	cyclosporine
		danazol
		erythromycin
		methylprednisolone
		metoclopramide

DRUGS THAT MAY DECREASE TACROLIMUS BLOOD LEVELS

Anticonvulsants	Antibiotics
carbamazepine	rifabutin
phenobarbital	rifampin
phenytoin	

OTHER DRUG INTERACTIONS
Immunosuppressants may affect vaccination. Therefore, during treatment with Tacrolimus, vaccination may be less effective. The use of live vaccines should be avoided; live vaccines may include, but are not limited to measles, mumps, rubella, oral polio, BCG, yellow fever, and TY 21a typhoid.[1]

CARCINOGENESIS, MUTAGENESIS AND IMPAIRMENT OF FERTILITY
An increased incidence of malignancy is a recognized complication of immunosuppression in recipients of organ transplants. The most common forms of neoplasms are non-Hodgkin's lymphomas and carcinomas of the skin. As with other immunosuppressive therapies, the risk of malignancies in Tacrolimus recipients may be higher than in the normal, healthy population. Lymphoproliferative disorders associated with Epstein-Barr Virus infection have been seen. It has been reported that reduction or discontinuance of immunosuppression may cause the lesions to regress.

No evidence of genotoxicity was seen in bacterial (Salmonella and E. coli) or mammalian (Chinese hamster lung-derived cells) *in vitro* assays of mutagenicity, the *in vitro* CHO/HGPRT assay of mutagenicity, or *in vivo* clastogenicity assays performed in mice; Tacrolimus did not cause unscheduled DNA synthesis in rodent hepatocytes.

Although studies are ongoing, no adequate studies to evaluate the carcinogenic potential of Tacrolimus have been completed.

No impairment of fertility was demonstrated in studies of male and female rats. Tacrolimus, given orally in 1.0 mg/kg (0.5 × the recommended clinical dose based on body surface area corrections) to male and female rats, prior to and during mating, as well as to dams during gestation and lactation, was associated with embryolethality and with adverse effects on female reproduction. Effects on female reproductive function (parturition) and embryolethal effects were indicated by a higher rate of pre-implantation loss and increased numbers of undelivered and nonviable pups. When given at 3.2 mg/kg (1.5 × the recommended clinical dose based on body surface area correction), Tacrolimus was associated with maternal and paternal toxicity as well as reproductive toxicity including marked adverse effects on estrus cycles, parturition, pup viability, and pup malformations.

PREGNANCY: CATEGORY C
In reproduction studies in rats and rabbits, adverse effects on the fetus were observed mainly at dose levels that were toxic to dams. Tacrolimus at oral doses of 0.32 and 1.0 mg/kg during organogenesis in rabbits was associated with maternal toxicity as well as an increase in incidence of abortions; these doses are equivalent to 0.33× and 1.0× (based on body surface area corrections) the recommended clinical dose (0.3 mg/kg). At the higher dose only, an increased incidence of malformations and developmental variations was also seen. Tacrolimus, at oral doses of 3.2 mg/kg during organogenesis in rats, was associated with maternal toxicity and caused an increase in late resorptions, decreased numbers of live births, and decreased pup weight and viability. Tacrolimus, given orally at 1.0 and 3.2 mg/kg (equivalent to 0.5× and 1.5× the recommended clinical dose based on body surface area corrections) to pregnant rats after organogenesis and during

lactation, was associated with reduced pup weights. No reduction in male or female fertility was evident.

There are no adequate and well-controlled studies in pregnant women. Tacrolimus is transferred across the placenta. The use of Tacrolimus during pregnancy has been associated with neonatal hyperkalemia and renal dysfunction. Tacrolimus should be used during pregnancy only if the potential benefit to the mother justifies potential risk to the fetus.

NURSING MOTHERS
Since Tacrolimus is excreted in human milk, nursing should be avoided.

PEDIATRIC PATIENTS
Successful liver transplants have been performed in pediatric patients (age less than 12 years) using Tacrolimus. One of the two randomized active-controlled trials of Tacrolimus in primary liver transplantation included 51 pediatric patients. Thirty patients were randomized to Tacrolimus-based and 21 to cyclosporine-based therapies. Additionally, 22 pediatric patients were studied in an uncontrolled trial of Tacrolimus in living related donor liver transplantation. Pediatric patients generally required higher doses to maintain blood trough levels of Tacrolimus similar to adult patients (see *"Dosage and Administration"*).

ADVERSE REACTIONS
The principal adverse reactions of Tacrolimus are tremor, headache, diarrhea, hypertension, nausea, and renal dysfunction. These occur with oral and intravenous administration of Tacrolimus and may respond to a reduction in dosing. Diarrhea was sometimes associated with other gastrointestinal complaints such as nausea and vomiting.

Hyperkalemia, hypomagnesemia and hyperuricemia have occurred in patients receiving Tacrolimus therapy. Hyperglycemia has been noted in many patients; some may require insulin therapy.

The incidence of adverse events was determined in two randomized comparative liver transplant trials among 512 patients receiving Tacrolimus and steroids and 511 patients receiving a cyclosporine-based regimen (CBIR). The proportion of patients reporting more than one adverse event was 99.8% in the Tacrolimus group and 99.6% in the CBIR group. Precautions must be taken when comparing the incidence of adverse events in the U.S. study to that in the European study. Only adverse events occurring up to 12-months post-transplant in the U.S. study and up to 6-months in the European study are presented. The two studies also included different patient populations and patients were treated with immunosuppressive regimens of differing intensities. Adverse events reported in > 15% in Tacrolimus patients (combined study results) are presented below for the two controlled trials in liver transplantation: (See related table).

The following adverse events, not mentioned above, were reported with greater than 3% incidence in Tacrolimus-treated patients.

Nervous System: (see *"Warnings"*) abnormal dreams, agitation, anxiety, confusion, convulsion, depression, dizziness, emotional lability, hallucinations, hypertonia, incoordination, myoclonus nervousness, neuropathy, psychosis, somnolence, thinking abnormal.

Special Senses: abnormal vision, amblyopia, tinnitus.

Gastrointestinal: cholangitis, cholestatic jaundice, dyspepsia, dysphasia, flatulence, gastrointestinal hemorrhage, GGT increase, GI performance, hepatitis, ileus, increased appetite, jaundice, liver damage, oral moniliasis.

Cardiovascular: chest pain, abnormal ECG, hemorrhage, hypotension, tachycardia.

Urogenital: (see *"Warnings"*) hematuria, kidney failure.

Metabolic Nutritional: acidosis, alkaline phosphatase increased, alkalosis, bilirubinemia, healing abnormal, hyperlipemia, hyperphosphatemia, hyperuricemia, hypocalcemia, hypophosphatemia, hyponatremia, hypoproteinemia, AST (SGOT) increased, ALT (SGPT) increased.

Endocrine: (see *"Precautions"*) diabetes mellitus.

Hemic/Lymphatic: Coagulation disorder, ecchymosis hypochromic anemia, leukopenia, prothrombin decreased.

Miscellaneous: abdomen enlarged, abscess, chills, hernia, peritonitis, photosensitivity reaction.

Musculoskeletal: arthralgia, generalized spasm, leg cramps, myalgia, myasthenia, osteoporosis.

Respiratory: asthma, bronchitis, cough increased, lung disorder, pulmonary edema, pharyngitis, pneumonia, respiratory disorder, rhinitis, sinusitis, voice alteration.

Skin: alopecia, herpes simplex, hirsutism, skin disorder, sweating.

OVERDOSAGE
There is minimal experience with overdosage. In patients who have received inadvertent overdosage of Tacrolimus no adverse reactions different from those reported in patients receiving therapeutic doses have been described. General supportive measures and systemic treatment should be followed in all cases of overdosage. Based on the poor aqueous solubility and extensive erythrocyte and plasma protein binding, it is anticipated that Tacrolimus is not dialyzable to any significant extent.

In acute oral and intravenous toxicity studies, mortalities were seen at and above the following doses: in adult rats, 52× the recommended human oral dose; in immature rats, 16× the recommended oral dose; and in adult rats, 16× the recommended human intravenous dose (all based on body surface area corrections).

DOSAGE AND ADMINISTRATION
TACROLIMUS INJECTION
For Intravenous Infusion Only

Note: Anaphylactic reactions have occurred with injectables containing castor oil derivatives. See *"Warnings"* section.

In patients unable to take oral Tacrolimus capsules, therapy may be initiated with Tacrolimus injection. The initial dose of Tacrolimus should be administered no sooner than 6 hours after transplantation. The recommended starting dose of Tacrolimus injection is 0.05-0.10 mg/kg/day as a continuous intravenous infusion. Adult patients receive doses at the lower end of the dosing range. Concomitant adrenal corticosteroid therapy is recommended early post-transplantation. Continuous intravenous infusion of Tacrolimus injection should be continued only until the patient can tolerate oral administration of Tacrolimus capsules.

PREPARATION FOR ADMINISTRATION/STABILITY
Tacrolimus injection must be diluted with 0.9% Sodium Chloride Injection or 5% Dextrose Injection to a concentration between 0.004 mg/mL and 0.02 mg/mL prior to use. Diluted infusion solution should be stored in glass or polyethylene containers and should be discarded after 24 hours. The diluted infusion solution should not be stored in a PVC container due to decreased stability and the potential for extraction of phthalates. Parenteral drug products should be inspected visually for particulate matter and discoloration prior to administration, whenever solution and container permit.

TACROLIMUS CAPSULES
It is recommended that patients be converted from intravenous to oral Tacrolimus capsules as soon as oral therapy can be tolerated. This usually occurs within 2-3 days. The first dose of oral therapy should be given 8-12 hours after discontinuing the IV infusion. The recommended starting oral dose of Tacrolimus capsules is 0.15-0.30 mg/kg/day administered in two divided daily doses every 12 hours. The initial dose of Tacrolimus should be administered no sooner than 6 hours after transplantation. Adult patients should receive doses at the lower end of the dosing range.

Dosing should be titrated based on clinical assessments of rejection and tolerability. Lower Tacrolimus dosages may be sufficient as maintenance therapy. Adjunct therapy with adrenal corticosteroids is recommended early post transplant.

PEDIATRIC PATIENTS
Pediatric patients without pre-existing renal or hepatic dysfunction have required and tolerated higher doses than adults to achieve similar blood concentrations. Therefore, it is recommended that therapy be initiated in pediatric patients at the high end of the recommended adult intravenous and oral dosing ranges (0.1 mg/kg/day intravenous and 0.3 mg/kg/day oral). Dose adjustments may be required.

PATIENTS WITH HEPATIC OR RENAL DYSFUNCTION
Due to the potential for nephrotoxicity, patients with renal or hepatic impairment should receive doses at the lowest value of the recommended intravenous and oral dosing ranges. Further reductions in dose below these ranges may be required. Tacrolimus therapy usually should be delayed up to 48 hours or longer in patients with post-operative oliguria.

CONVERSION FROM ONE IMMUNOSUPPRESSIVE REGIMEN TO ANOTHER
Tacrolimus should not be used simultaneously with cyclosporine. Tacrolimus or cyclosporine should be discontinued at least 24 hours before initiating the other. In the presence of elevated Tacrolimus or cyclosporine concentrations, dosing with the other drug usually should be further delayed.

BLOOD CONCENTRATION MONITORING
Most study centers have found Tacrolimus blood-concentration monitoring helpful in patient management. While no fixed relationship has been established, such blood monitoring may assist in the clinical evaluation of rejection and toxicity, dose adjustments, and the assessment of compliance. Various assays have been used to measure blood concentrations of Tacrolimus. Comparison of the concentrations in published literature to patient concentrations using current assays must be made with detailed knowledge of the assay methods employed.

Data from the U.S. clinical trail show that Tacrolimus whole blood concentrations, as measured by ELISA, were most variable during the first week post-transplantation. After this early period, the median trough blood concentrations, measured at intervals from the second week to one year posttransplantation, ranged from 9.8 ng/mL to 19.4 ng/mL.

STORE AND DISPENSE
Store capsules at controlled room temperature, 15°C-30°C (59°F-86°F). Store solution for intravenous infusion between 5°C and 25°C (41°F and 77°F).

REFERENCE
1. CDC: Recommendations of the Advisory Committee on Immunization Practices: Use of vaccines and immune globulins in persons with altered immunocompetence. MMWR 1993;42(RR-4): 1-18.

	U.S. Study (%)		European Study (%)	
	Tacrolimus (N = 250)	CBIR (N = 250)	Tacrolimus (N = 262)	CBIR (N = 261)
Nervous System				
Headache (See "Warnings")	64	60	31	20
Tremor (See "Warnings")	56	46	44	30
Insomnia	64	68	29	21
Paresthesia	40	30	15	13
Gastrointestinal				
Diarrhea	72	47	32	23
Nausea	46	37	30	22
Constipation	24	27	19	20
LFT Abnormal	36	30	5	2
Anorexia	34	24	6	4
Vomiting	27	15	12	9
Cardiovascular				
Hypertension (See "Precautions")	47	56	31	35
Urogenital				
Kidney Function Abnormal (See "Warnings")	40	27	33	18
Creatinine Increased (See "Warnings")	39	25	19	16
BUN Increased (See "Warnings")	30	22	8	7
Urinary Tract Infection	16	18	19	18
Oliguria	18	15	16	8
Metabolic and Nutritional				
Hyperkalemia (See "Warnings")	45	26	10	7
Hypokalemia	29	34	11	14
Hyperglycemia (See "Precautions")	47	38	29	16
Hypomagnesemia	48	45	15	8
Hemic and Lymphatic				
Anemia	47	38	4	1
Leukocytosis	32	26	8	7
Thrombocytopenia	24	20	10	14
Miscellaneous				
Abdominal Pain	59	54	26	20
Pain	63	57	19	14
Fever	48	56	15	18
Asthenia	52	48	7	4
Back Pain	30	29	13	14
Ascites	27	22	5	6
Peripheral Edema	26	26	10	11
Respiratory System				
Pleural Effusion	30	32	32	29
Atelectasis	28	30	5	4
Dyspnea	29	23	3	2
Skin and Appendages				
Pruritus	36	20	11	5
Rash	24	19	8	3

HOW SUPPLIED
CAPSULE: 1 MG

BRAND/MANUFACTURER	NDC	SIZE	AWP
○ BRAND PROGRAF: Fujisawa	00469-0617-71	100s	$218.40

CAPSULE: 5 MG

BRAND/MANUFACTURER	NDC	SIZE	AWP
○ BRAND PROGRAF: Fujisawa	00469-0657-71	100s	$1092.00

INJECTION: 5 MG/ML

BRAND/MANUFACTURER	NDC	SIZE	AWP
○ BRAND PROGRAF: Fujisawa	00469-3016-01	1 ml 10s	$2220.00

Tagamet SEE CIMETIDINE

Talacen SEE ACETAMINOPHEN AND PENTAZOCINE HYDROCHLORIDE

Talwin SEE ASPIRIN AND PENTAZOCINE HYDROCHLORIDE

Talwin Lactate SEE PENTAZOCINE LACTATE

Talwin Nx SEE NALOXONE HYDROCHLORIDE AND PENTAZOCINE HYDROCHLORIDE

Tambocor SEE FLECAINIDE ACETATE

Tamoxifen Citrate

DESCRIPTION
Tamoxifen Citrate tablets for oral administration contain 15.2 mg of tamoxifen citrate, which is equivalent to 10 mg of tamoxifen. It is a nonsteroidal antiestrogen. Chemically, Tamoxifen Citrate is the trans-isomer of a triphenylethylene derivative. The chemical name is (Z)2-[4-(1,2-diphenyl-1-butenyl) phenoxy]-N, N-dimethylethanamine 2-hydroxy-1,2,3-propanetricarboxylate (1:1).

Tamoxifen Citrate has a molecular weight of 563.62, the pKa' is 8.85, the equilibrium solubility in water at 37°C is 0.5 mg/mL and in 0.02 N HCl at 37°C, it is 0.2 mg/mL.

Tamoxifen Citrate is intended only for oral administration; the tablets should be protected from heat and light.

Following is its chemical structure:

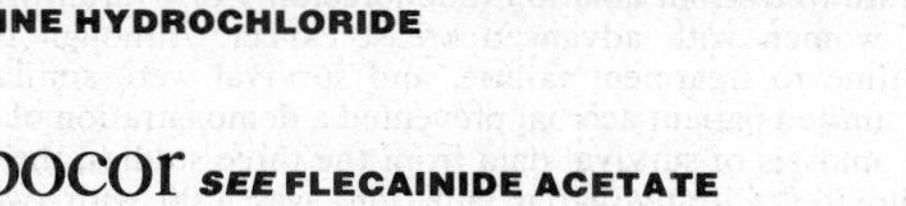

CLINICAL PHARMACOLOGY
Tamoxifen Citrate is a nonsteroidal agent which has demonstrated potent antiestrogenic properties in animal test systems. The antiestrogenic effects may be

➤ SHOWN IN PRODUCT IDENTIFICATION GUIDE

related to its ability to compete with estrogen for binding sites in target tissues such as breast. Tamoxifen inhibits the induction of rat mammary carcinoma induced by dimethylbenzanthracene (DMBA) and causes the regression of already established DMBA-induced tumors. In this rat model, Tamoxifen appears to exert its antitumor effects by binding the estrogen receptors.

In cytosols derived from human breast adenocarcinomas, Tamoxifen competes with estradiol for estrogen receptor protein. Preliminary pharmacokinetics in women using radiolabeled Tamoxifen has shown that most of the radioactivity is slowly excreted in the feces, with only small amounts appearing in the urine. The drug is excreted mainly as conjugates, with unchanged drug and hydroxylated metabolites accounting for 30% of the total.

Blood levels of total radioactivity following single oral doses of approximately 0.3 mg/kg reached peak values of 0.06-0.14 µg/mL at 4-7 hours after dosing, with only 20%-30% of the drug present as Tamoxifen. There was an initial half-life of 7-14 hours with secondary peaks four or more days later. The prolongation of blood levels and fecal excretion is believed to be due to enterohepatic circulation.

Two studies (Hubay and NSABP B-09) demonstrated an improved disease-free survival following radical or modified radical mastectomy in postmenopausal women or women 50 years of age or older with surgically curable breast cancer with positive axillary nodes when Tamoxifen Citrate was added to adjuvant cytotoxic chemotherapy. In the Hubay study, Tamoxifen Citrate was added to "low-dose" CMF (cyclophosphamide, methotrexate and fluorouracil). In the NSABP B-09 study, Tamoxifen Citrate was added to melphalan [L-phenylalanine mustard (P)] and fluorouracil (F).

Tumor hormone receptors may help predict which patients will benefit from the adjuvant theapy, but not all breast cancer adjuvant Tamoxifen Citrate studies have shown a clear relationship between hormone receptor status and treatment effect. In the Hubay study, patients with a positive (more than 3 fmol) estrogen receptor were more likely to benefit. In the NSABP B-09 study in women age 50-59 years, only women with both estrogen and progesterone receptor levels 10 fmol or greater clearly benefited, while there was a nonstatistically significant trend toward adverse effect in women with both estrogen and progesterone receptor levels less than 10 fmol. In women age 60-70 years, there was a trend toward a beneficial effect of Tamoxifen Citrate without any clear relationship to estrogen or progestrone receptor status.

Three prospective studies (ECOG-1178, Toronto, NATO) using Tamoxifen Citrate adjuvantly as a single agent demonstrated an improved disease-free survival following total mastectomy and axillary dissection for postmenopasal women with positive axillary nodes compared to placebo/no treatment controls. The NATO study also demonstrated an overall survival benefit.

One prospective, double-blind, randomized study (NSABP-14) demonstrated a significant improvement in disease-free survival for Tamoxifen Citrate compared to placebo when used adjuvantly following total mastectomy and axillary dissection or segmental resection, axillary dissection, and breast radiation in women with axillary node-negative breast cancer whose tumors were estrogen receptor positive (≥ 10 fmol/mg cytosol protein). The benefit was apparent in both women under age 50 and those aged 50 years or more. One additional randomized study (NATO) demonstrated improved disease-free survival for Tamoxifen Citrate compared to no adjuvant therapy following total mastectomy and axillary dissection in postmenopausal women with axillary node-negative breast cancer. In this study, the benefits of Tamoxifen Citrate appeared to be independent of estrogen receptor status.

Three prospective, randomized studies (Ingle, Pritchard, Buchanan) compared Tamoxifen Citrate to ovarian ablation (oophorectomy or ovarian irradiation) in premenopausal women with advanced breast cancer. Although the objective response rate, time to treatment failure, and survival were similar with both treatments, the limited patient accrual prevented a demonstration of equivalence. In an overview analysis of survival data from the three studies, the hazard ratio for death (Tamoxifen Citrate/ovarian ablation) was 1.00 with two-sided 95% confidence intervals of 0.73 to 1.37. Elevated serum and plasma estrogens have been observed in premenopausal women receiving Tamoxifen Citrate. However, the data from the randomized studies do not suggest an adverse effect. A limited number of premenopausal patients with disease progression during Tamoxifen Citrate therapy responded to subsequent ovarian ablation.

Published results from 122 patients (119 evaluable) and case reports in 16 patients (13 evaluable) treated with Tamoxifen Citrate have shown that Tamoxifen Citrate is effective for the pallative treatment of male breast cancer. Sixty-six of these 132 evaluable patients responded to Tamoxifen Citrate which constitutes a 50% objective response rate.

INDICATIONS AND USAGE

Adjuvant Therapy: Tamoxifen Citrate is effective in delaying recurrence following total mastectomy and axillary dissection or segmental mastectomy, axillary dissection, and breast irradiation in women with axillary node-negative breast cancer. Data are insufficient to predict which women are most likely to benefit and to determine if Tamoxifen Citrate provides any benefit in women with tumors less than 1 cm. Tamoxifen Citrate is effective in delaying recurrence following total mastectomy and axillary dissection in postmenopausal women with breast cancer ($T_{1\text{-}3}$, N_1, M_0). In some Tamoxifen Citrate adjuvant studies, most of the benefit to date has been in the subgroup with 4 or more positive axillary nodes.

The estrogen and progesterone receptor values may help to predict whether adjuvant Tamoxifen Citrate therapy is likely to be beneficial.

Therapy for Advanced Disease: Tamoxifen Citrate is effective in the treatment of metastatic breast cancer in women and men. In premenopausal women with metastatic breast cancer, Tamoxifen Citrate is an alternative to oophorectomy or ovarian irradiation. Available evidence indicates that patients whose tumors are estrogen receptor positive are more likely to benefit from Tamoxifen Citrate therapy.

UNLABELED USES

Tamoxifen Citrate is used alone or as an adjunct in treatment to induce ovulation in women with anovulatory infertility, to improve normal sperm motility and sperm density in normogonadotrophic oligospermia, and to treat patients with small cell lung cancer. It is also used in the treatment of mastalgia or breast pain, biopsy–proven ductal adenocarcinoma of the pancreas, and idiopathic gynecomastia. Tamoxifen is also prescribed in hyperlipidemia and renal cell carcinoma, and is used in prophylaxis of osteoporosis in postmenopausal women.

CONTRAINDICATIONS

Tamoxifen Citrate is contraindicated in patients with known hypersensitivity to the drug.

WARNINGS

Visual disturbance including corneal changes, cataracts and retinopathy have been reported in patients receiving Tamoxifen Citrate.

As with other additive hormonal therapy (estrogens and androgens), hypercalcemia has been reported in some breast cancer patients with bone metastases within a few weeks of starting treatment with Tamoxifen Citrate. If hypercalcemia does occur, appropriate measures should be taken and, if severe, Tamoxifen Citrate should be discontinued.

An increased incidence of endometrial changes including hyperplasia, polyps, and endometrial cancer has been reported in association with Tamoxifen Citrate treatment. The incidence and pattern of this increase suggest that the underlying mechanism is related to the estrogenic properties of Tamoxifen Citrate. Any patients receiving Tamoxifen Citrate who report abnormal vaginal bleeding should be promptly evaluated.

In a large randomized trial in Sweden of adjuvant Tamoxifen Citrate 10 mg/day for 2-5 years, an increased incidence of endometrial cancer was noted. Thirteen of 931 Tamoxifen Citrate treated patients versus 2 of 915 controls developed cancer of the body of the uterus [RR = 6.4 (1.4 - 28), $P < 0.01$]. After approximately 7 years of follow-up in the ongoing NSABP B-14 trial, 9 of the 1,439 women randomized to receive Tamoxifen Citrate developed Stage I endometrial cancer. Two of the 1,440 women randomized to receive placebo, who subsequently had recurrent breast cancer and were treated with Tamoxifen Citrate, also developed Stage 1 endometrial cancer. Patients receiving Tamoxifen Citrate should have routine gynecological care and report any abnormal vaginal bleeding to their physician.

In the same Swedish trial, the incidence of second primary breast tumors was reduced in the Tamoxifen arm ($P < 0.05$). In the NSABP, B-14 trial in which patients were randomized to Tamoxifen Citrate 20 mg/day for 5 years versus placebo, the incidence of second primary breast cancers is also reduced. Tamoxifen Citrate has been associated with changes in liver enzyme levels, and on rare occasions, a spectrum of more severe liver abnormalities including fatty liver, cholestasis, hepatitis and hepatic necrosis. A few of these serious cases included fatalities. In most reported cases the relationship to Tamoxifen Citrate is uncertain. However, some positive rechallenges and dechallenges have been reported.

Pregnancy Category D: Tamoxifen Citrate may cause fetal harm when administered to a pregnant woman. Individuals should not become pregnant while taking Tamoxifen Citrate and should use barrier or nonhormonal contraceptive measures. Effects on reproductive functions are expected from the antiestrogenic properties of the drug. In reproductive studies in rats at dose levels equal to or below the human dose, nonteratogenic developmental skeletal changes were seen and were found to be reversible. In addition, in fertility studies in rats and in teratology studies in rabbits using doses at or below those used in humans, a lower incidence of embryo implantation and a higher incidence of fetal death or retarded in utero growth were observed, with slower learning behavior in some rat pups. The impairment of learning behavior did not achieve statistical significance in one study, and, in another study where significance was reported, this was by comparing dosed animals with controls of another study. Several pregnant marmosets were dosed during organogenesis or in the last half of pregnancy. No deformations were seen, and although the dose was high enough to terminate pregnancy in some animals, those that did maintain pregnancy showed no evidence of teratogenic malformations. There are no adequate and well-controlled studies in pregnant women. There have been reports of spontaneous abortions, birth defects, fetal deaths, and vaginal bleeding. If this drug is used during pregnancy or the patient becomes pregnant while taking this drug, the patient should be apprised of the potential hazard to the fetus.

PRECAUTIONS

General: Tamoxifen Citrate should be used cautiously in patients with existing leukopenia or thrombocytopenia. Observations of leukopenia and thrombocytopenia occasionally have been reported. Decreases in platelet counts, usually to 50,000-100,000/mm^3, infrequently lower, have been occasionally reported in patients taking Tamoxifen Citrate for breast cancer. In patients with significant thrombocytopenia, rare hemorrhagic episodes have occurred but it is uncertain if these episodes are due to Tamoxifen Citrate therapy.

Information for Patients: Women taking Tamoxifen Citrate should be instructed to report abnormal vaginal bleeding which should be promptly investigated.

Laboratory Tests: Periodic complete blood counts, including platelet counts, may be appropriate.

Drug Interactions: When Tamoxifen Citrate is used in combination with coumarin-type anticoagulants, a significant increase in anticoagulant effect may occur. Where such coadministration, exists, careful monitoring of the patient's prothrombin time is recommended.

One patient receiving Tamoxifen Citrate with concomitant phenobarbital exhibited a steady state serum level of Tamoxifen lower than that observed for other patients (ie, 26 ng/mL vs. mean value of 122 ng/mL). However, the clinical significance of this finding is not known.

Concomitant bromocriptine therapy has been shown to elevate serum tamoxifen and N-desmethyltamoxifen.

Drug/Laboratory Testing Interactions: During postmarketing surveillance, T_4 elevations were reported for a few postmenopausal patients which may be explained by increases in thyroid-binding globulin. These elevations were not accompanied by clinical hyperthyroidism.

Variations in the karyopyknotic index on vaginal smears and various degrees of estrogen effect on Pap smears have been infrequently seen in postmenopausal patients given Tamoxifen Citrate.

In the postmarketing experience with Tamoxifen Citrate, infrequent cases of hyperlipidemias have been reported. Periodic monitoring of plasma triglycerides and cholesterol may be indicated in patients with pre-existing hyperlipidemias.

Carcinogenesis: A conventional carcinogenesis study in rats, (doses of 5, 20, and 35 mg/kg/day for up to 2 years) revealed hepatocellular carcinoma at all doses, and the incidence of these tumors was significantly greater among rats given 20 or 35 mg/kg/day (69%) than those given 5 mg/kg/day (14%). The incidence of these tumors in rats given 5 mg/kg/day (29.5 mg/m^2) was significantly greater than in controls.

In addition, preliminary data from 2 independent reports of 6-month studies in rats reveal liver tumors which in one study are classified as malignant.

Endocrine changes in immature and mature mice were investigated in a 13-month study. Granulosa cell ovarian tumors and interstitial cell testicular tumors were found in mice receiving Tamoxifen Citrate, but not in the controls.

Mutagenesis: No genotoxic potential has been found in a battery of *in vivo* and *in vitro* tests with pro- and eukaryotic test systems with drug metabolizing systems present.

Impairment of Fertility: Fertility in female rats was decreased following administration of 0.04 mg/kg for two weeks prior to mating through day 7 of pregnancy. There was a decreased number of implantations, and all fetuses were found dead.

Following administration to rats of 0.16 mg/kg from days 7-17 of pregnancy, there were increased numbers of fetal deaths. Administration of 0.125 mg/kg to rabbits during days 6-18 of pregnancy resulted in abortion or premature delivery. Fetal deaths occurred at higher doses. There were no teratogenic changes in either rat or rabbit segment II studies. Several pregnant marmosets were dosed with 10 mg/kg/day either during organogenesis or in the last half of pregnancy. No deformations were seen, and although the dose was high enough to terminate pregnancy in some animals, those that did maintain pregnancy showed no evidence of teratogenic malformations. Rats given 0.16 mg/kg from day 17 of pregnancy to 1 day before weaning demonstrated increased numbers of dead pups at parturition. It was reported that some rat pups showed slower learning behavior, but this did not achieve statistical significance in one study, and in another study where significance was reported, this was obtained by comparing dosed animals with controls of another study.

The recommended daily human dose of 20-40 mg corresponds to 0.4-0.8 mg/kg for an average 50 kg woman.

Pregnancy Category D: See "Warnings".

Nursing Mothers: It is not known whether this drug is excreted in human milk. Because many drugs are excreted in human milk and because of the potential for serious adverse reactions in nursing infants from Tamoxifen Citrate, a decision should be made whether to discontinue nursing or to discontinue the drug, taking into account the importance of the drug to the mother.

ADVERSE REACTIONS

Adverse reactions to Tamoxifen Citrate are relatively mild and rarely severe enough to require discontinuation of treatment. If adverse reactions are severe, it is sometimes possible to control them by a simple reduction of dosage without loss of control of the disease.

In patients treated with Tamoxifen Citrate for metastatic breast cancer, the most frequent adverse reactions to Tamoxifen Citrate are hot flashes and nausea and/or vomiting. These may occur in up to one-fourth of patients.

Less frequently reported adverse reactions are vaginal bleeding, vaginal discharge, menstrual irregularities and skin rash. Usually these have not been of sufficient severity to require dosage reduction or discontinuation of treatment. Increased bone and tumor pain and, also, local disease flare have occurred, which are sometimes associated with a good tumor response. Patients with increased bone pain may require additional analgesics. Patients with soft tissue disease may have sudden increases in the size of preexisting lesions, sometimes associated with marked erythema within and surrounding the lesions and/or the development of new lesions. When they occur, the bone pain or disease flare are seen shortly after starting Tamoxifen Citrate and generally subside rapidly.

Other adverse reactions which are seen infrequently are hypercalcemia, peripheral edema, distaste for food, pruritus vulvae, depression, dizziness, light-headedness, headache, and hair thinning and/or partial hair loss.

There have been infrequent reports of thromboembolic events occurring during Tamoxifen Citrate therapy. Since for cancer patients in general an increased incidence of thromboembolic events is known to occur, a causal relationship to

Tamoxifen Citrate remains conjectural. An increased incidence has been reported when cytotoxic agents are combined with Tamoxifen Citrate.

Tamoxifen Citrate has been associated with changes in liver enzyme levels, and on rare occasions, a spectrum of more severe liver abnormalities including fatty liver, cholestatis, hepatitis and hepatic necrosis. A few of these serious cases included fatalities. In most reported cases the relationship to Tamoxifen Citrate is uncertain. However, some positive rechallenges and dechallenges have been reported.

Ovarian cysts have been observed in a small number of pre-menopausal menopausal patients with advanced breast cancer who have been treated with Tamoxifen Citrate.

Continued clinical studies have resulted in further information which better indicates the incidence of adverse reactions with Tamoxifen Citrate as compared to placebo.

In the ongoing NSABP study B-14, women with axillary node-negative breast cancer were randomized to 5 years of Tamoxifen Citrate or placebo following primary surgery. The reported adverse effects are tabulated below (mean follow-up of 29 months). The incidence of hot flashes (57% v 41%), vaginal discharge (24% v 12%), and irregular menses (19% v 15%) were higher with Tamoxifen Citrate compared with placebo. The incidence of all other adverse effects were similar in the two treatment groups with the exception of thromboembolic events (phlebitis), which although rare, were more common with Tamoxifen Citrate than with placebo.

NSABP B-14 STUDY

	No. of Women (%)			
Adverse Effect	Tamoxifen Citrate (n = 1376)		Placebo (n = 1396)	
Hot Flashes	787	(57)	566	(41)
Fluid Retention	339	(25)	326	(23)
Vaginal discharge	330	(24)	160	(12)
Irregular menses	264	(19)	203	(15)
Nausea	255	(19)	235	(17)
Skin rash	180	(13)	150	(11)
Diarrhea	106	(8)	129	(9)
Vomiting	25	(2)	16	(1)
Phlebitis	15	(1)	2	(< 1)
Thrombocytopenia*	10	(1)	4	(< 1)
Leukopenia**	7	(1)	10	(1)

* *Defined as a platelet count of < 100,000/mm^3*
** *Defined as a white blood cell count of < 3000/mm^3*

In the Eastern Cooperative Oncology Group (ECOG) adjuvant breast cancer trial, Tamoxifen Citrate or placebo was administered for 2 years to women following mastectomy. When compared to placebo, Tamoxifen Citrate showed a significantly higher incidence of hot flashes (19% versus 8% for placebo). The incidence of all other adverse reactions was similar in the 2 treatment groups with the exception of thrombocytopenia where the incidence for Tamoxifen Citrate was 10% versus 3% for placebo, an observation of borderline statistical significance.

The other adverse reactions reported equally in the ECOG study for Tamoxifen Citrate and placebo include abnormal renal function tests, fatigue, dyspnea, anorexia, cough, and abdominal cramps. A relationship of these reactions to the administration of Tamoxifen Citrate has not been demonstrated since the frequency was not significantly different from that reported in placebo treated women.

In other adjuvant studies, Toronto and Tamoxifen Citrate Adjuvant Trial Organization (NATO), women received either Tamoxifen Citrate or no therapy. In the Toronto study, hot flashes and nausea and/or vomiting were observed in 29% and 19% of patients, respectively, for Tamoxifen Citrate versus 0% and 0% in the untreated group. In the NATO trial, hot flashes, nausea and/or vomiting and vaginal bleeding were reported in 2.8%, 2.1%, and 2.0% of women, respectively, for Tamoxifen Citrate versus 0.2% for each in the untreated group. The following table summarizes the incidence of adverse reactions reported at a frequency of 2% or greater from clinical trials (Ingle, Pritchard, Buchanan) which compared Tamoxifen Citrate therapy to ovarian ablation in premenopausal patients with metastatic breast cancer.

	Tamoxifen Citrate All Effects Number of Women (%)		Ovarian Ablation All Effects Number of Women (%)	
Adverse Reactions*	n = 104		n = 100	
Flush	34	(32.7)	46	(46)
Amenorrhea	17	(16.3)	69	(69)
Altered Menses	13	(12.5)	5	(5)
Oligomenorrhea	9	(8.7)	1	(1)
Bone Pain	6	(5.7)	6	(6)
Menstrual Disorder	6	(5.7)	4	(4)
Nausea	5	(4.8)	4	(4)
Cough/Coughing	4	(3.8)	1	(1)
Edema	4	(3.8)	1	(1)
Fatigue	4	(3.8)	1	(1)
Musculoskeletal Pain	3	(2.8)	0	(0)
Pain	3	(2.8)	4	(4)
Ovarian Cyst(s)	3	(2.8)	2	(2)

Adverse Reactions*	Tamoxifen Citrate All Effects Number of Women (%) n = 104		Ovarian Ablation All Effects Number of Women (%) n = 100	
Depression	2	(1.9)	2	(2)
Abdominal Cramps	1	(1)	2	(2)
Anorexia	1	(1)	2	(2)

* *Some women had more than one adverse reaction.*

Tamoxifen Citrate is well tolerated in males with breast cancer. Reports from the literature and case reports suggest that the safety profile of Tamoxifen Citrate in males is similar to that seen in women. Loss of libido and impotence had resulted in male patients stopping therapy when treated with Tamoxifen. Also, in oligospermic males treated with Tamoxifen, LH, FSH, testosterone and estrogen levels were elevated. No significant changes were reported.

OVERDOSAGE
Signs observed at the highest doses following studies to determine LD_{50} in animals were respiratory difficulties and convulsions.

Acute overdosage in humans has not been reported. In a study of advanced metastic cancer patients which specifically determined the maximum tolerated dose of Tamoxifen Citrate in evaluating the use of very high doses to reverse multidrug resistance, acute neurotoxicity manifested by tremor, hyperreflexia, unsteady gait and dizziness were noted. These symptoms occurred within 3-5 days of beginning Tamoxifen Citrate and cleared within 2-5 days after stopping therapy. No permanent neurologic toxicity was noted. One patient experienced a seizure several days after Tamoxifen Citrate was discontinued and neurotoxic symptoms had resolved. The causal relationship of the seizure to Tamoxifen Citrate therapy is unknown. Doses given in these patients were all greater than 400 mg/m² loading dose followed by maintenance doses of 150 mg/m² of Tamoxifen Citrate given twice a day.

In the same study, prolongation of the QT interval on the electrocardiogram was noted when patients were given doses higher than 250 mg/m² loading dose, followed by maintenance doses of 80 mg/m² of Tamoxifen Citrate given twice a day. For a woman with a body surface area of 1.5 m² the minimal loading dose and maintenance doses given at which neurological symptoms and QT changes occurred were at least 6 fold higher in respect to the maximum recommended dose. No specific treatment for overdosage is known; treatment must be symptomatic.

DOSAGE AND ADMINISTRATION
In women and men with metastatic breast cancer, one or two 10 mg tablets are administered twice a day (morning and evening). In three single agent adjuvant studies in women, one 10 mg Tamoxifen Citrate tablet was administered two (ECOG and NATO) or three (Toronto) times a day for two years (See "Clinical Pharmacology"). In B-14, the ongoing NSABP adjuvant study in women, one 10 mg Tamoxifen Citrate tablet is being given twice a day for five years. The optimal duration of adjuvant therapy is not known.

Protect tablets from heat and light.

HOW SUPPLIED
TABLETS: 10 MG

BRAND/MANUFACTURER	NDC	SIZE	AWP
○ **BRAND**			
▶ NOLVADEX: Zeneca	00310-0600-60	60s	$86.14
	00310-0600-25	250s	$358.86
○ **GENERICS**			
Barr	00555-0446-09	60s	$81.74
Barr	00555-0446-03	250s	$340.58

Tanafed SEE CHLORPHENIRAMINE TANNATE WITH PSEUDOEPHEDRINE TANNATE

Tao SEE TROLEANDOMYCIN

Tapazole SEE METHIMAZOLE

Tavist SEE CLEMASTINE FUMARATE

Taxol SEE PACLITAXEL

Tazicef SEE CEFTAZIDIME

Tazidime SEE CEFTAZIDIME

Teebacin SEE AMINOSALICYLIC ACID

Tegison SEE ETRETINATE

Tegopen SEE CLOXACILLIN SODIUM

Tegretol SEE CARBAMAZEPINE

Telepaque SEE IOPANOIC ACID

Temaril SEE TRIMEPRAZINE TARTRATE

Temazepam

DESCRIPTION
Temazepam is a benzodiazepine hypnotic agent. The chemical name is 7-chloro-1,3-dihydro-3-hydroxy-1-methyl-5-phenyl-2H-1, 4-benzodiazepin-2-one. The molecular formula is $C_{16}H_{13}ClN_2O_2$. The molecular weight is 300.74.

Temazepam is a white, crystalline substance, very slightly soluble in water and sparingly soluble in alcohol, USP.

Temazepam capsules, 7.5 mg, 15 mg, and 30 mg, are for oral administration.

Following is its chemical structure:

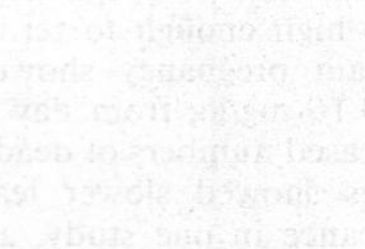

CLINICAL PHARMACOLOGY
PHARMACOKINETICS
In a single and multiple dose absorption, distribution, metabolism, and excretion (ADME) study, using ³H labeled drug, Temazepam was well absorbed and found to have minimal (8%) first pass metabolism. There were no active metabolites formed and the only significant metabolite present in blood was the O-conjugate. The unchanged drug was 96% bound to plasma proteins. The blood level decline of the parent drug was biphasic with the short half-life ranging from 0.4-0.6 hours and the terminal half-life from 3.5-18.4 hours (mean 8.8 hours), depending on the study population and method of determination. Metabolites were formed with a half-life of 10 hours and excreted with a half-life of approximately 2 hours. Thus, formation of the major metabolite is the rate limiting step in the biodisposition of Temazepam. There is no accumulation of metabolites. A dose-proportional relationship has been established for the area under the plasma concentration/time curve over the 15-30 mg dose range.

Temazepam was completely metabolized through conjugation prior to excretion; 80%-90% of the dose appeared in the urine. The major metabolite was the O-conjugate of Temazepam (90%), the O-conjugate of N-desmethyl Temazepam was a minor metabolite (7%).

BIOAVAILABILITY, INDUCTION, AND PLASMA LEVELS
Following ingestion of a 30 mg Temazepam capsule, measurable plasma concentrations were achieved 10-20 minutes after dosing with peak plasma levels ranging from 666-982 ng/mL (mean 865 ng/mL) occurring approximately 1.2-1.6 hours (mean 1.5 hours) after dosing.

In a 7 day study, in which subjects were given a 30 mg Temazepam capsule 1 hour before retiring, steady-state (as measured by the attainment of maximal trough concentrations) was achieved by the third dose. Mean plasma levels of Temazepam (for days 2-7) were 260 ± 210 ng/mL at 9 hours and 75 ± 80 ng/mL at 24 hours after dosing. A slight trend toward declining 24 hour plasma levels was seen after day 4 in the study, however, the 24 hour plasma levels were quite variable.

At a dose of 30 mg once-a-day for 8 weeks, no evidence of enzyme induction was found in man.

◆ RATED THERAPEUTICALLY EQUIVALENT; ◇ THERAPEUTIC EQUIVALENCE UNCONFIRMED; ○ UNRATED

ELIMINATION RATE OF BENZODIAZEPINE HYPNOTICS AND PROFILE OF COMMON UNTOWARD EFFECTS

The type and duration of hypnotic effects and the profile of unwanted effects during administration of benzodiazepine hypnotics may be influenced by the biologic half-life of the administered drug and for some hypnotics, the half-life of any active metabolites formed. Benzodiazepine hypnotics have a spectrum of half-lives from short (< 4 hours) to long (> 20 hours). When half-lives are long, drug (and for some drugs their active metabolites) may accumulate during periods of nightly administration and be associated with impairments of cognitive and/or motor performance during waking hours; the possibility of interaction with other psychoactive drugs or alcohol will be enhanced. In contrast, if half-lives are shorter, drug (and, where appropriate, its active metabolites) will be cleared before the next dose is ingested, and carry-over effects related to excessive sedation or CNS depression should be minimal or absent. However, during nightly use for an extended period, pharmacodynamic tolerance or adaptation to some effects of benzodiazepine hypnotics may develop. If the drug has a short elimination half-life, it is possible that a relative deficiency of the drug, or, if appropriate, its active metabolites (i.e., in relationship to the receptor site) may occur at some point in the interval between each night's use. This sequence of events may account for 2 clinical findings reported to occur after several weeks of nightly use of rapidly eliminated benzodiazepine hypnotics, namely, increased wakefulness during the last third of the night, and the appearance of increased signs of daytime anxiety.

CONTROLLED TRIALS SUPPORTING EFFICACY

Temazepam improved sleep parameters in clinical studies. Residual medication effects ("hangover") were essentially absent. Early morning awakening, a particular problem in the geriatric patient, was significantly reduced. Patients with chronic insomnia were evaluated in 2 week, placebo controlled sleep laboratory studies with Temazepam at doses of 7.5 mg, 15 mg, and 30 mg, given 30 minutes prior to bedtime. There was a linear dose-response improvement in total sleep time and sleep latency, with significant drug-placebo differences at 2 weeks occurring only for total sleep time at the 2 higher doses, and for sleep latency only at the highest dose.

In these sleep laboratory studies, REM sleep was essentially unchanged and slow wave sleep was decreased. No measurable effects on daytime alertness or performance occurred following Temazepam treatment or during the withdrawal period, even though a transient sleep disturbance in some sleep parameters was observed following withdrawal of the higher doses. There was no evidence of tolerance development in the sleep laboratory parameters when patients were given Temazepam nightly for at least 2 weeks.

In addition, normal subjects with transient insomnia associated with first night adaptation to the sleep laboratory were evaluated in 24 hour, placebo controlled sleep laboratory studies with Temazepam at doses of 7.5 mg, 15 mg, and 30 mg, given 30 minutes prior to bedtime. There was a linear dose-response improvement in total sleep time, sleep latency and number of awakenings, with significant drug-placebo differences occurring for sleep latency at all doses, for total sleep time at the 2 higher doses and for number of awakenings only at the 30 mg dose.

INDICATIONS AND USAGE

Temazepam is indicated for the short-term treatment of insomnia (generally 7-10 days). For patients in whom the drug is used for more than 2-3 weeks, periodic reevaluation is recommended to determine whether there is a continuing need. (See *"Warnings"*.)

For patients with short-term insomnia, instructions in the prescription should indicate that Temazepam should be used for short periods of time (7-10 days).

Temazepam should not be prescribed in quantities exceeding a 1-month supply.

Insomnia is characterized by complaints of difficulty in falling asleep, frequent nocturnal awakenings, and/or early morning awakenings. Both sleep laboratory and outpatient studies provide support for the effectiveness of Temazepam administered 30 minutes before bedtime in decreasing sleep latency and improving sleep maintenance in patients with chronic insomnia. In addition, sleep laboratory studies have confirmed similar effects in normal subjects with transient insomnia (see *"Clinical Pharmacology"*).

UNLABELED USES

Temazepam is used alone or as an adjunct in the treatment of anxiety disorders.

CONTRAINDICATIONS

Benzodiazepines may cause fetal damage when administered during pregnancy. An increased risk of congenital malformations associated with the use of diazepam and chlordiazepoxide during the first trimester of pregnancy has been suggested in several studies. Transplacental distribution has resulted in neonatal CNS depression following the ingestion of therapeutic doses of a benzodiazepine hypnotic during the last weeks of pregnancy.

Reproduction studies in animals with Temazepam were performed in rats and rabbits. In a perinatal-postnatal study in rats, oral doses of 60 mg/kg/day resulted in increasing nursling mortality. Teratology studies in rats demonstrated increased fetal resorptions at doses of 30 and 120 mg/kg in one study and increased occurrence of rudimentary ribs, which are considered skeletal variants, in a second study at doses of 240 mg/kg or higher. In rabbits, occasional abnormalities such as exencephaly and fusion or asymmetry of ribs were reported without dose relationship.

Although these abnormalities were not found in the concurrent control group, they have been reported to occur randomly in historical controls. At doses of 40 mg/kg or higher, there was an increased incidence of the 13th rib variant when compared to the incidence in concurrent and historical controls.

Temazepam is contraindicated in pregnant women. If there is a likelihood of the patient becoming pregnant while receiving Temazepam, she should be warned of the potential risk to the fetus. Patients should be instructed to discontinue the drug prior to becoming pregnant. The possibility that a woman of childbearing potential may be pregnant at the time of institution of therapy should be considered.

WARNINGS

Sleep disturbance may be the presenting manifestation of an underlying physical and/or psychiatric disorder. Consequently, a decision to initiate symptomatic treatment of insomnia should only be made after the patient has been carefully evaluated.

The failure of insomnia to remit after 7-10 days of treatment may indicate the presence of a primary psychiatric and/or medical illness.

Worsening of insomnia may be the consequence of an unrecognized psychiatric or physical disorder as may the emergence of new abnormalities of thinking or behavior. Such abnormalities have also been reported to occur in association with the use of drugs with central nervous system depressant activity, including those of the benzodiazepine class. Some of these changes may be characterized by decreased inhibition, e.g., aggressiveness and extroversion that seem out of character, similar to that seen with alcohol. Other kinds of behavioral changes can also occur, for example, bizarre behavior, agitation, hallucinations, depersonalization, and, in primarily depressed patients, the worsening of depression, including suicidal thinking. In controlled clinical trials involving 1076 patients on Temazepam and 783 patients on placebo, reports of hallucinations, agitation, and overstimulation occurred at rates less than 1 in 100 patients. Hallucinations were reported in 2 Temazepam patients and 1 placebo patient; agitation was reported in 1 Temazepam patient; 2 Temazepam patients reported overstimulation. There were no reports of worsening of depression or suicidal ideation, aggressiveness, extroversion, bizarre behavior or depersonalization in these controlled clinical trials.

It can rarely be determined with certainty whether a particular instance of the abnormal behaviors listed above is drug induced, spontaneous in origin, or a result of an underlying psychiatric or physical disorder. Nonetheless, the emergence of any new behavioral sign or symptom of concern requires careful and immediate evaluation.

Because some of the worrisome adverse effects of benzodiazepines, including Temazepam appear to be dose related (see *"Precautions"* and *"Dosage and Administration"*), it is important to use the lowest possible effective dose. Elderly patients are especially at risk.

Patients receiving Temazepam should be cautioned about possible combined effects with alcohol and other CNS depressants.

Withdrawal symptoms (of the barbiturate type) have occurred after the abrupt discontinuation of benzodiazepines (see *"Drug Abuse and Dependence"*).

PRECAUTIONS

GENERAL

Since the risk of the development of oversedation, dizziness, confusion, and/or ataxia increases substantially with larger doses of benzodiazepines in elderly and debilitated patients, 7.5 mg of Temazepam is recommended as the initial dosage for such patients.

Temazepam should be administered with caution in severely depressed patients or those in whom there is any evidence of latent depression; it should be recognized that suicidal tendencies may be present and protective measures may be necessary.

The usual precautions should be observed in patients with impaired renal or hepatic function and in patients with chronic pulmonary insufficiency.

If Temazepam is to be combined with other drugs having known hypnotic properties or CNS-depressant effects, consideration should be given to potential additive effects.

The possibility of a synergistic effect exists with the co-administration of Temazepam and diphenhydramine. One case of stillbirth at term has been reported 8 hours after a pregnant patient received Temazepam and diphenhydramine. A cause and effect relationship has not yet been determined. (See *"Contraindications."*)

INFORMATION FOR PATIENTS

The text of a patient package insert is printed at the end of this insert. To assure safe and effective use of Temazepam the information and instructions provided in this patient package insert should be discussed with patients.

LABORATORY TESTS

The usual precautions should be observed in patients with impaired renal or hepatic function and in patients with chronic pulmonary insufficiency. Abnormal liver function tests as well as blood dyscrasias have been reported with benzodiazepines.

DRUG INTERACTIONS

The pharmacokinetic profile of Temazepam does not appear to be altered by orally administered cimetidine dosed according to labeling.

CARCINOGENESIS, MUTAGENESIS, IMPAIRMENT OF FERTILITY

Carcinogenicity studies were conducted in rats at dietary Temazepam doses up to 160 mg/kg/day for 24 months and in mice at dietary dose of 160 mg/kg/day for 18 months. No evidence of carcinogenicity was observed although hyperplastic liver nodules were observed in female mice exposed to the highest dose. The clinical significance of this finding is not known.

Fertility in male and female rats was not adversely affected by Temazepam. No mutagenicity tests have been done with Temazepam.

PREGNANCY
Pregnancy Category X (see "Contraindications").

NURSING MOTHERS
It is not known whether this drug is excreted in human milk. Because many drugs are excreted in human milk, caution should be exercised when Temazepam is administered to a nursing woman.

PEDIATRIC USE
Safety and effectiveness in children below the age of 18 years have not been established.

ADVERSE REACTIONS
During controlled clinical studies in which 1076 patients received Temazepam at bedtime, the drug was well tolerated. Side effects were usually mild and transient. Adverse reactions occurring in 1% or more of patients are presented in the following table:

	Temzepam % incidence (n = 1076)	Placebo % incidence (n = 783)
Drowsiness	9.1	5.6
Headache	8.5	9.1
Fatigue	4.8	4.7
Nervousness	4.6	8.2
Lethargy	4.5	3.4
Dizziness	4.5	3.3
Nausea	3.1	3.8
Hangover	2.5	1.1
Anxiety	2.0	1.5
Depression	1.7	1.8
Dry Mouth	1.7	2.2
Diarrhea	1.7	1.1
Abdominal Discomfort	1.5	1.9
Euphoria	1.5	0.4
Weakness	1.4	0.9
Confusion	1.3	0.5
Blurred Vision	1.3	1.3
Nightmares	1.2	1.7
Vertigo	1.2	0.8

The following adverse events have been reported less frequently (0.5-0.9%):

Central Nervous System: anorexia, ataxia, equilibrium loss, tremor, increased dreaming

Cardiovascular: dyspnea, palpitations

Gastrointestinal: vomiting

Musculoskeletal: backache

Special Senses: hyperhidrosis, burning eyes

Amnesia, hallucinations, horizontal nystagmus, and paradoxical reactions including restlessness, overstimulation and agitation were rare (less than 0.5%).

DRUG ABUSE AND DEPENDENCE
CONTROLLED SUBSTANCE
Temazepam is a controlled substance in Schedule IV.

ABUSE AND DEPENDENCE
Withdrawal symptoms, similar in character to those noted with barbiturates and alcohol (convulsions, tremor, abdominal, and muscle cramps, vomiting, and sweating), have occurred following abrupt discontinuance of benzodiazepines. The more severe withdrawal symptoms have usually been limited to those patients who received excessive doses over an extended period of time. Generally milder withdrawal symptoms (e.g., dysphoria and insomnia) have been reported following abrupt discontinuance of benzodiazepines taken continuously at therapeutic levels for several months. Consequently, after extended therapy at doses higher than 15 mg, abrupt discontinuation should generally be avoided and a gradual dosage tapering schedule followed. As with any hypnotic, caution must be exercised in administering Temazepam to individuals known to be addiction-prone or to those whose history suggests they may increase the dosage on their own initiative. It is desirable to limit repeated prescriptions without adequate medical supervision.

OVERDOSAGE
Manifestations of acute overdosage of Temazepam can be expected to reflect the CNS effects of the drug and include somnolence, confusion, and coma, with reduced or absent reflexes, respiratory depression, and hypotension. If the patient is conscious, vomiting should be induced mechanically or with emetics. Gastric lavage should be employed utilizing concurrently a cuffed endotracheal tube if the patient is unconscious to prevent aspiration and pulmonary complications. Maintenance of adequate pulmonary ventilation is essential. The use of pressor agents intravenously may be necessary to combat hypotension. Fluids should be administered intravenously to encourage diuresis. The value of dialysis has not been determined. If excitation occurs, barbiturates should not be used. It should be borne in mind that multiple agents may have been ingested.

The oral LD_{50} was 1963 mg/kg in mice, 1833 mg/kg in rats, and > 2400 mg/kg in rabbits.

DOSAGE AND ADMINISTRATION
While the recommended usual adult dose is 15 mg before retiring, 7.5 mg may be sufficient for some patients, and others may need 30 mg. In transient insomnia, a 7.5 mg dose may be sufficient to improve sleep latency. In elderly or debilitated patients, it is recommended that therapy be initiated with 7.5 mg until individual responses are determined.

Store in a tight, light-resistant container, below 86°F (30°C).

PATIENT INFORMATION
INTRODUCTION
Your doctor has prescribed Temazepam to help you sleep. The following information is intended to guide you in the safe use of this medicine. It is not meant to take the place of your doctor's instructions. If you have any questions about Temazepam capsules be sure to ask your doctor or pharmacist.

Temazepam is used to treat different types of sleep problems, such as:
- trouble falling asleep
- waking up too early in the morning
- waking up often during the night

Some people may have more than one of these problems.

Temazepam belongs to a group of medicines known as the "benzodiazepines." There are many different benzodiazepine medicines used to help people sleep better. Sleep problems are usually temporary, requiring treatment for only a short time, usually 7-10 days. However, if your sleep problems continue, consult your doctor. He/she will determine whether other measures are needed to overcome your sleep problems. Some people have chronic sleep problems that may require more prolonged use of sleep medicine. However, you should not use these medicines for long periods without talking with your doctor about the risks and benefits of prolonged use.

SIDE EFFECTS
Common side effects: All medicines have side effects. The most common side effects of benzodiazepine sleeping medicines include:
- drowsiness
- dizziness
- light-headedness
- difficulty with coordination

You may find that these medicines make you sleepy during the day. How drowsy you feel depends upon how your body reacts to the medicine, which benzodiazepine sleeping medicine you are taking, and how large a dose your doctor has prescribed. Day-time drowsiness is best avoided by taking the lowest dose possible that will still help you to sleep at night. Your doctor will work with you to find the dose of Temazepam that is best for you.

To manage these side effects while you are taking this medicine:
- Use extreme care while doing anything that requires complete alertness, such as driving a car, operating machinery, or piloting an aircraft. As with any medicines used to help people sleep better, you should be very careful when you first start taking Temazepam until you know how the medicine will affect you.
- NEVER drink alcohol while you are being treated with Temazepam or any benzodiazepine medicine. Alcohol can increase the side effects of Temazepam or any other benzodiazepine medicine.
- Do not take any other medicines without asking your doctor first. This includes medicines you can buy without a prescription. Some medicines can cause drowsiness and are best avoided while taking Temazepam.

Always take the exact dose of Temazepam prescribed by your doctor. Never change your dose without talking to your doctor first.

SPECIAL CONCERNS
There are some special problems that may occur while taking benzodiazepine sleeping medicines.

Memory problems: Benzodiazepine sleeping medicines may cause a special type of memory loss or "amnesia". When this occurs, a person may not remember what has happened for several hours after taking the medicine. This is usually not a problem since most people fall asleep after taking the medicine.

Memory loss can be a problem, however, when sleeping medicines are taken while traveling, such as during an airplane flight and the person wakes up before the effect of the medicine is gone. This has been called "traveler's amnesia". Memory problems were noticed in fewer than 1 in 100 patients taking Temazepam in clinical trials. Memory problems can be avoided if you take Temazepam only when you are able to get a full night's sleep (7-8 hours) before you need to be active again. Be sure to talk to your doctor if you think you are having memory problems.

Tolerance: When benzodiazepine sleeping medicines are used every night for more than a few weeks, they may lose their effectiveness to help you sleep. This is known as "tolerance".

If tolerance to the medicine develops, other effects may occur depending upon which benzodiazepine sleeping medicine you are taking. Tolerance to benzodiazepine sleeping medicines that are shorter-acting may cause you to:
- wake up during the last third of the night
- become anxious or nervous while you are awake

These effects are less common with Temazepam because it is intermediate-acting.

Dependence: All the benzodiazepine sleeping medicines can cause dependence, especially when these medicines are used regularly for longer than a few weeks or at high doses. Some people develop a need to continue taking their medicines. This is known as dependence or "addiction."

When people develop dependence, they may have difficulty stopping the benzodiazepine sleeping medicine. If the medicine is suddenly stopped, the body is not able to function normally and unpleasant symptoms may occur (see *"Withdrawal"*). They may find they have to keep taking the medicine either at the prescribed dose or at increasing doses just to avoid withdrawal symptoms.

All people taking benzodiazepine sleeping medicines have some risk of becoming dependent on the medicine. However, people who have been dependent on alcohol or other drugs in the past may have a higher chance of becoming addicted to benzodiazepine medicines. This possibility must be considered before using these medicines for more than a few weeks. If you have been addicted to alcohol or drugs in the past, it is important to tell your doctor before starting Temazepam or any benzodiazepine sleeping medicine.

Withdrawal: Withdrawal symptoms may occur when a benzodiazepine sleeping medicine is stopped suddenly after being used daily for a long time. But these symptoms can occur even if the medicine has been used for only a week or two.

In mild cases, withdrawal symptoms may include unpleasant feelings. In more severe cases, abdominal and muscle cramps, vomiting, sweating, shakiness, and rarely, seizures may occur. These more severe withdrawal symptoms are very uncommon.

Another problem that may occur when benzodiazepine sleeping medicines are stopped is known as "rebound insomnia". This means that a person may have more trouble sleeping the first few nights after the medicine is stopped than before starting the medicine. If you should experience rebound insomnia, do not get discouraged. This problem usually goes away on its own after 1 or 2 nights.

If you have been taking Temazepam or any other benzodiazepine sleeping medicine for more than 1 or 2 weeks, do not stop taking it on your own. Your doctor may give you special directions on how to gradually decrease your dose before stopping the medicine. Always follow your doctor's directions.

Changes in behavior and thinking: Some people using benzodiazepine sleeping medicines have experienced unusual changes in their thinking and/or behavior, including; more outgoing or aggressive behavior than normal; loss of personal identity; confusion; strange behavior; agitation; hallucinations; worsening of depression; and suicidal thoughts.

How often these effects occur depends on several factors, such as a person's general health or the use of other medicines. Clinical studies with Temazepam revealed that unusual behavior changes occurred in less than 1 in 100 patients.

It is also important to realize that it is rarely clear whether these behavior changes are caused by the medicine, an illness, or occur on their own. In fact, sleep problems that do not improve may be due to illnesses that were present before the medicine was used. If you or your family notice any changes in your behavior, or if you have any unusual or disturbing thoughts, call your doctor immediately.

Pregnancy: Certain benzodiazepines have been linked to birth defects when taken by a pregnant woman in the early months of pregnancy. These medicines can also cause sedation of the unborn baby when used during the last weeks of pregnancy. Temazepam should not be taken at any time during pregnancy. Be sure to tell your doctor if you are pregnant, if you are planning to become pregnant, or if you become pregnant while taking Temazepam.

SAFE USE OF BENZODIAZEPINE SLEEPING MEDICINES
To ensure the safe and effective use of Temazepam or any other benzodiazepine sleeping medicine, you should observe the following cautions:

1. Temazepam is a prescription medicine and should be used ONLY as directed by your doctor. Follow your doctor's instructions about how to take, when to take, and how long to take Temazepam.

2. Never use Temazepam or any other benzodiazepine sleeping medicine for longer than 1 or 2 weeks without first asking your doctor.

3. If you notice any unusual or disturbing thoughts or behavior during treatment with Temazepam or any other benzodiazepine sleeping medicine, contact your doctor.

4. Tell your doctor about any medicines you may be taking, including medicines you may buy without a prescription. You should also tell your doctor if you drink alcohol. DO NOT use alcohol while taking Temazepam or any other benzodiazepine sleeping medicine.

5. Do not take Temazepam or any other benzodiazepine sleeping medicine unless you are able to get a full night's sleep before you must be active again. For example, Temazepam or any other benzodiazepine sleeping medicine should not be taken on an overnight airplane flight of less than 7-8 hours since "traveler's amnesia" may occur.

6. Do not increase the prescribed dose of Temazepam or any other benzodiazepine sleeping medicine unless instructed by your doctor.

7. Use extreme care while doing anything that requires complete alertness, such as driving a car, operating machinery, or piloting an aircraft when you first start taking Temazepam or any other benzodiazepine sleeping medicine until you know whether the medicine will still have some carryover effect in you the next day.

8. Be aware that you may have more sleeping problems (rebound insomnia) the first night or two after stopping Temazepam. Temazepam or any other benzodiazepine sleeping medicine.

9. Be sure to tell your doctor if you are pregnant, if you are planning to become pregnant, or if you become pregnant while taking Temazepam. Temazepam or any other benzodiazepine sleeping medicine should not be taken at any time during pregnancy.

10. As with all prescription medicines, never share Temazepam or any other benzodiazepine sleeping medicine with anyone else. Always store Temazepam or any other benzodiazepine sleeping medicine in the original container out of reach of children.

HOW SUPPLIED
CAPSULE (C-IV): 7.5 MG

AVERAGE UNIT PRICE (AVAILABLE SIZES)		GENERIC A-RATED AVERAGE PRICE (GAAP)	
GENERIC	$0.47	100s	$47.33

BRAND/MANUFACTURER	NDC	SIZE	AWP
◆ **GENERICS**			
Creighton	50752-0271-05	100s	$46.67
Creighton	50752-0271-06	100s ud	$47.99

CAPSULE (C-IV): 7.5 MG

BRAND/MANUFACTURER	NDC	SIZE	AWP
○ **BRAND**			
➤ RESTORIL: Sandoz Pharm	00078-0140-05	100s	$54.90
	00078-0140-06	100s	$56.46
➤ RESTORIL: Sandocare	00078-0140-65	640s	$360.72

CAPSULE (C-IV): 15 MG

AVERAGE UNIT PRICE (AVAILABLE SIZES)		GENERIC A-RATED AVERAGE PRICE (GAAP)	
BRAND	$0.63	100s	$25.08
GENERIC	$0.23	500s	$103.54
HCFA FUL (100s ea)	$0.05		

BRAND/MANUFACTURER	NDC	SIZE	AWP
◆ **BRAND**			
➤ RESTORIL: Sandoz Pharm	00078-0098-13	25s ud	$17.40
	00078-0098-05	100s	$61.38
	00078-0098-06	100s ud	$62.94
	00078-0098-08	500s	$287.76
➤ RESTORIL: Sandocare	00078-0098-65	640s ud	$402.00
◆ **GENERICS**			
Warner Chilcott	00047-0977-24	100s	$15.16
Qualitest	00603-5895-21	100s	$17.35
Rugby	00536-4628-01	100s	$17.37
Major	00904-2810-60	100s	$17.40
Schein	00364-0815-01	100s	$17.50
Goldline	00182-1822-01	100s	$17.95
➤ Geneva	00781-2201-01	100s	$19.95
Purepac	00228-2076-10	100s	$20.72
Parmed	00349-8927-01	100s	$21.35
UDL	51079-0418-21	100s	$21.80
URL	00677-1069-01	100s	$23.33
Mylan	00378-4010-01	100s	$23.38
Par	49884-0240-01	100s	$23.75
Moore,H.L.	00839-7164-06	100s	$23.75
Martec	52555-0242-01	100s	$24.20
Aligen	00405-0185-01	100s	$25.04
Creighton	50752-0272-05	100s	$52.17
UDL	51079-0418-20	100s ud	$21.80
Goldline	00182-1822-89	100s ud	$26.90
Vangard	00615-0470-13	100s ud	$27.31
Vangard	00615-0470-47	100s ud	$27.31
Auro	55829-0875-10	100s ud	$28.68
Major	00904-2810-61	100s ud	$29.40
➤ Geneva	00781-2201-13	100s ud	$29.95
Creighton	50752-0272-06	100s ud	$53.50
Schein	00364-0815-05	500s	$69.50
Major	00904-2810-40	500s	$72.00
Warner Chilcott	00047-0977-30	500s	$72.65
Qualitest	00603-5895-28	500s	$73.40
Rugby	00536-4628-05	500s	$73.63
Goldline	00182-1822-05	500s	$77.95
Geneva	00781-2201-05	500s	$85.00
Purepac	00228-2076-50	500s	$99.98
Aligen	00405-0185-02	500s	$105.24
Parmed	00349-8927-05	500s	$106.47
Mylan	00378-4010-05	500s	$111.26
Moore,H.L.	00839-7164-12	500s	$114.20
Par	49884-0240-05	500s	$115.00
Mason Dist	11845-0344-03	500s	$115.00
Moore,H.L.	00839-7899-12	500s	$120.76
Creighton	50752-0272-08	500s	$244.60

➤ SHOWN IN PRODUCT IDENTIFICATION GUIDE

CAPSULE (C-IV): 30 MG

AVERAGE UNIT PRICE (AVAILABLE SIZES)		GENERIC A-RATED AVERAGE PRICE (GAAP)	
BRAND	$0.71	100s	$28.57
GENERIC	$0.27	500s	$119.24
HCFA FUL (100s ea)	$0.06		

BRAND/MANUFACTURER	NDC	SIZE	AWP
◆ **BRAND**			
➤ RESTORIL: Sandoz Pharm	00078-0099-13	25s ud	$19.20
	00078-0099-05	100s	$68.64
	00078-0099-06	100s ud	$70.14
	00078-0099-08	500s	$333.18
➤ RESTORIL: Sandocare	00078-0099-65	640s ud	$449.94
◆ **GENERICS**			
Warner Chilcott	00047-0978-24	100s	$17.75
Schein	00364-0816-01	100s	$19.75
Goldline	00182-1823-01	100s	$20.95
Qualitest	00603-5896-21	100s	$21.10
Rugby	00536-4629-01	100s	$21.13
Major	00904-2811-60	100s	$21.25
➤ Geneva	00781-2202-01	100s	$22.50
Purepac	00228-2077-10	100s	$23.74
UDL	51079-0419-21	100s	$24.13
Parmed	00349-8488-01	100s	$25.60
Aligen	00405-0186-01	100s	$25.80
URL	00677-1070-01	100s	$26.45
➤ Mylan	00378-5050-01	100s	$26.50
Par	49884-0241-01	100s	$27.50
Moore,H.L.	00839-7165-06	100s	$27.66
Martec	52555-0243-01	100s	$28.05
Moore,H.L.	00839-7900-06	100s	$28.88
Creighton	50752-0273-05	100s	$58.34
UDL	51079-0419-20	100s ud	$24.13
Goldline	00182-1823-89	100s ud	$30.50
Vangard	00615-0471-13	100s ud	$30.89
Vangard	00615-0471-47	100s ud	$30.89
Auro	55829-0876-10	100s ud	$31.84
Major	00904-2811-61	100s ud	$32.76
➤ Geneva	00781-2202-13	100s ud	$35.00
Creighton	50752-0273-06	100s ud	$59.62
Qualitest	00603-5896-28	500s	$84.25
Rugby	00536-4629-05	500s	$84.31
Major	00904-2811-40	500s	$84.35
Warner Chilcott	00047-0978-30	500s	$86.60
Schein	00364-0816-05	500s	$88.50
Goldline	00182-1823-05	500s	$89.95
➤ Geneva	00781-2202-05	500s	$97.50
Purepac	00228-2077-50	500s	$115.27
Aligen	00405-0186-02	500s	$121.33
Parmed	00349-8488-05	500s	$124.50
➤ Mylan	00378-5050-05	500s	$126.50
Par	49884-0241-05	500s	$128.50
Mason Dist	11845-0345-03	500s	$128.50
Moore,H.L.	00839-7165-12	500s	$129.05
Moore,H.L.	00839-7900-12	500s	$135.53
Creighton	50752-0273-08	500s	$283.20

Temovate *SEE* CLOBETASOL PROPIONATE

Ten-K *SEE* POTASSIUM CHLORIDE, ORAL

Tenex *SEE* GUANFACINE HYDROCHLORIDE

Teniposide

WARNING

TENIPOSIDE FOR INJECTION CONCENTRATE IS A CYTOTOXIC DRUG, WHICH SHOULD BE ADMINISTERED UNDER THE SUPERVISION OF A QUALIFIED PHYSICIAN EXPERIENCED IN THE USE OF CANCER CHEMOTHERAPEUTIC AGENTS. APPROPRIATE MANAGEMENT OF THERAPY AND COMPLICATIONS IS POSSIBLE ONLY WHEN ADEQUATE TREATMENT FACILITIES ARE READILY AVAILABLE.

SEVERE MYELOSUPPRESSION WITH RESULTING INFECTION OR BLEEDING MAY OCCUR. HYPERSENSITIVITY REACTIONS, INCLUDING ANAPHYLAXIS-LIKE SYMPTOMS, MAY OCCUR WITH INITIAL DOSING OR AT REPEATED EXPOSURE TO TENIPOSIDE. EPINEPHRINE, WITH OR WITHOUT CORTICOSTEROIDS AND ANTIHISTAMINES, HAS BEEN EMPLOYED TO ALLEVIATE HYPERSENSITIVITY REACTION SYMPTOMS.

DESCRIPTION

Teniposide for Injection Concentrate (also commonly known as VM-26), is supplied as a sterile nonpyrogenic solution in a nonaqueous medium intended for dilution with a suitable parenteral vehicle prior to intravenous infusion. Teniposide is available in 50 mg (5 mL) ampules. Each mL contains 10 mg Teniposide, 30 mg benzyl alcohol, 60 mg N,N-dimethylacetamide, 500 mg polyoxyethylated castor oil and 42.7 percent (V/V) dehydrated alcohol. The pH of the clear solution is adjusted to approximately 5 with maleic acid.

Teniposide is a semisynthetic derivative of podophyllotoxin. The chemical name for Teniposide is 4'-demethylepipodophyllotoxin 9-[4,6-0-(R)-2-thenyli-dene-β-D-glucopyranoside]. Teniposide differs from etoposide, another podophyllotoxin derivative, by the substitution of a thenylidene group on the glucopyranoside ring.

Teniposide is a white to off-white crystalline powder with the empirical formula $C_{32}H_{32}O_{13}S$ and a molecular weight of 656.66. It is a lipophilic compound with a partition coefficient value (octanol/water) of approximately 100. Teniposide is insoluble in water and ether. It is slightly soluble in methanol and very soluble in acetone and dimethylformamide.

Following is its chemical structure:

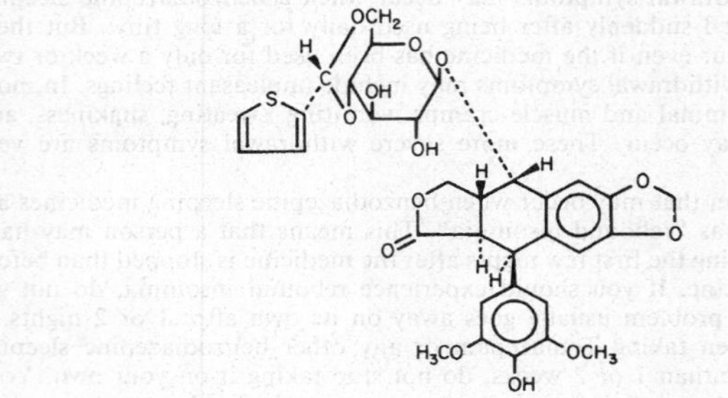

CLINICAL PHARMACOLOGY

Teniposide is a phase-specific cytotoxic drug, acting in the late S or early G_2 phase of the cell cycle, thus preventing cells from entering mitosis.

Teniposide causes dose-dependent single- and double-stranded breaks in DNA and DNA: protein cross-links. The mechanism of action appears to be related to the inhibition of type II topoisomerase activity since Teniposide does not intercalate into DNA or bind strongly to DNA. The cytotoxic effects of Teniposide are related to the relative number of double-stranded DNA breaks produced in cells, which are a reflection of the stabilization of a topoisomerase II-DNA intermediate.

Teniposide has a broad spectrum of *in vivo* antitumor activity against murine tumors, including hematologic malignancies and various solid tumors. Notably, Teniposide is active against sublines of certain murine leukemias with acquired resistance to cisplatin, doxorubicin, amsacrine, daunorubicin, mitoxantrone or vincristine.

Plasma drug levels declined biexponentially following intravenous infusion (155 mg/m² over 1 to 2.5 hours) of Teniposide given to eight children (4-11 years old) with newly diagnosed acute lymphoblastic leukemia (ALL). The observed average pharmacokinetic parameters and associated coefficients of variation ($CV^6/_9$) based on a two-compartment model analysis of the data are as follows:

Parameter	Mean	CV%
Total body clearance (mL/min/m²)	10.3	25
Volume at steady-state (L/m²)	3.1	30
Terminal half-life (hours)	5.0	44
Volume of central compartment (L/m²)	1.5	36
Rate constant central to peripheral (1/hours)	0.47	62
Rate constant, peripheral to central (1/hours)	0.42	37

There appears to be some association between an increase in serum alkaline phosphatase or gamma glutamyl-transpeptidase and a decrease in plasma clearance of Teniposide. Therefore, caution should be exercised if Teniposide is to be administered to patients with hepatic dysfunction.

In adults, at doses of 100 to 333 mg/m²/day, plasma levels increased linearly with dose. Drug accumulation in adult patients did not occur after daily administration of Teniposide for 3 days. In pediatric patients, maximum plasma concentrations (Cmax) after infusions of 137 to 203 mg/m² over a period of one to two hours exceeded 40 μg/mL; by 20 to 24 hours after infusion plasma levels were generally < 2μg/mL.

Renal clearance of parent Teniposide accounts for about 10 percent of total body clearance. In adults, after intravenous administration of 10 mg/kg or 67 mg/m² of tritium-labeled Teniposide, 44 percent of the radiolabel was recovered in urine (parent drug and metabolites) within 120 hours after dosing. From 4 to 12 percent of a dose is excreted in urine as parent drug. Fecal excretion of radioactivity within 72 hours after dosing accounted for 0 to 10 percent of the dose.

◆ RATED THERAPEUTICALLY EQUIVALENT; ◇ THERAPEUTIC EQUIVALENCE UNCONFIRMED; ○ UNRATED

Mean steady-state volumes of distribution range from 8 to 44 L/m^2 for adults and 3 to 11 L/m^2 for children. The blood-brain barrier appears to limit diffusion of Teniposide into the brain, although in a study in patients with brain tumors, CSF levels of Teniposide were higher than CSF levels reported in other studies of patients who did not have brain tumors.

Teniposide is highly protein bound. *In vitro* plasma protein binding of Teniposide is > 99 percent. The high affinity of Teniposide for plasma proteins may be an important factor in limiting distribution of drug within the body. Steady state volume of distribution of the drug increases with a decrease in plasma albumin levels. Therefore, careful monitoring of children with hypoalbuminemia is indicated during therapy. Levels of Teniposide in saliva, CSF and malignant ascites fluid are low relative to simultaneously measured plasma levels.

The pharmacokinetic characteristics of Teniposide differ from those of etoposide, another podophyllotoxin. Teniposide is more extensively bound to plasma proteins, and its cellular uptake is greater. Teniposide also has a lower systemic clearance, a longer elimination half-life, and is excreted in the urine as parent drug to a lesser extent than etoposide. In a study at St. Jude Children's Research Hospital (SJCRH), 9 children with acute lymphocytic leukemia (ALL) failing induction therapy with a cytarabine-containing regimen, were treated with Teniposide plus cytarabine. Three of these patients were induced into complete remission with durations of remission of 30 weeks, 59 weeks, and 13 years. In another study at SJCRH, 16 children with ALL refractory to vincristine/prednisone-containing regimens were treated with Teniposide plus vincristine and predinisone. Three of these patients were induced into complete remission with durations of remission of 5, 5, 37, and 73 weeks. In these two studies patients served as their owen control based on the premise that long term complete remissions could not be achieved by re-treatment with drugs to which they had previously failed to respond.

INDICATIONS AND USAGE

Teniposide in combination with other approved anticancer agents, is indicated for induction therapy in patients with refractory childhood acute lymphoblastic leukemia.

UNLABELED USES
Teniposide is used as an adjunct in the treatment of multiple myeloma.

CONTRAIDICATIONS

Teniposide is generally contraindicated in patients who have demonstrated a previous hypersensitivity to Teniposide and/or polyoxyethylated castor oil.

WARNINGS

Teniposide is a potent drug and should be used only by physicians experienced in the administration of cancer chemotherapeutic drugs. Blood counts as well as renal and hepatic function tests should be carefully monitored prior to and during therapy.

Patients being treated with Teniposide should be observed frequently for myelosuppression both during and after therapy. Dose-limiting bone marrow suppression is the most significant toxicity associated with Teniposide therapy. Therefore, the following studies should be obtained at the start of therapy and prior to each subsequent dose of Teniposide: hemoglobin, white blood cell count and differential and platelet count. If necessary, repeat bone marrow examination should be performed prior to the decision to continue therapy in the setting of severe myelosuppression.

Physicians should be aware of the possible occurrence of a hypersensitivity reaction variably manifested by chills, fever, urticaria, tachycardia, bronchospasm, dyspnea, hypertension or hypotension and facial flushing. This reaction may occur with the first dose of Teniposide and may be life threatening if not treated promptly with antihistamines, corticosteroids, epinephrine, intravenous fluids and other supportive measures as clinically indicated. The exact cause of these reactions is unknown. They may be due to the polyoxyethylated castor oil component of the vehicle or to Teniposide itself[1]. Patients who have experienced prior hypersensitivity reactions to Teniposide are at risk for recurrence of symptoms and should only be retreated with Teniposide if the antileukemic benefit already demonstrated clearly outweighs the risk of a probable hypersensitivity reaction for that patient. When a decision is made to re-treat a patient with Teniposide in spite of an earlier hypersensitivity reaction, the patient should be pretreated with corticosteroids and antihistamines and receive careful clinical observation during and after Teniposide infusion. In the clinical experience with Teniposide at SJCRH and the National Cancer Institute (NCI), re-treatment of patients with prior hypersensitivity reactions has been accomplished using measures described above. To date, there is no evidence to suggest cross-sensitization between Teniposide and VePesid.

One episode of sudden death, attributed to probable arrhythmia and intractable hypotension has been reported in an elderly patient receiving Teniposide combination therapy for a nonleukemic malignancy. (See "Adverse Reactions" section.) Patients receiving Teniposide treatment should be under continuous observation for at least the first 60 minutes following the start of the infusion and at frequent intervals thereafter. If symptoms or signs of anaphylaxis occur, the infusion should be stopped immediately, followed by the administration of epinephrine, corticosteroids, antihistamines, pressor agents, or volume expanders at the discretion of the physician. An aqueous solution of epinephrine 1:1000 and a source of oxygen should be available at the bedside.

For parenteral administration, Teniposide should be given only by slow intravenous infusion (lasting at least 30- to 60-minutes) since hypotension has been reported as a possible side effect of rapid intravenous injection, perhaps due to a direct effect of Polyoxyethylated Castor oil[2,3]. If clinically significant hypotension develops, the Teniposide infusion should be discontinued. The blood pressure usually normalizes within hours in response to cessation of the infusion and administration of fluids or other supportive therapy as appropriate. If the infusion is restarted, a slower administration rate should be used and the patient should be carefully monitored.

Acute central nervous system depression and hypotension have been observed in patients receiving investigational infusions of high-dose Teniposide who were pretreated with antiemetic drugs. The depressant effects of the antiemetic agents and the alcohol content of the Teniposide formulation may place patients receiving higher than recommended doses of Teniposide at risk for central nervous system depression.

Pregnancy: Pregnancy "Category D." Teniposide may cause fetal harm when administered to a pregnant woman. Teniposide has been shown to be teratogenic and embryotoxic in laboratory animals. In pregnant rats intravenous administration of Teniposide 0. 1-3 mg/kg (0.6-18 mg/m^2), every second day from day 6 to day 16 post coitum caused dose-related embryotoxicity and teratogenicity. Major anomalies included spinal and rib defects, deformed extremities, anophthalmia and celosomia.

There are no adequate and well-controlled studies in pregnant women. If Teniposide is used during pregnancy, or if the patient becomes pregnant while receiving this drug, the patient should be apprised of the potential hazard to the fetus. Women of childbearing potential should be advised to avoid becoming pregnant during therapy with Teniposide.

PRECAUTIONS

General: In all instances where the use of Teniposide is considered for chemotherapy, the physician must evaluate the need and usefulness of the drug against the risk of adverse reactions. Most such adverse reactions are reversible if detected early. If severe reactions occur, the drug should be reduced in dosage or discontinued and appropriate corrective measures should be taken according to the clinical judgment of the physician. Reinstitution of Teniposide therapy should be carried out with caution, and with adequate consideration of the further need for the drug and alertness as to possible recurrence of toxicity.

Teniposide must be administered as an intravenous infusion. Care should be taken to ensure that the intravenous catheter or needle is in the proper position and functional prior to infusion. Improper administration of Teniposide may result in extravasation causing local tissue necrosis and/or thrombophlebitis. In some instances, occlusion of central venous access devices has occurred during 24-hour infusion of Teniposide at a concentration of 0.1 to 0.2 mg/mL. Frequent observation during these infusions is necessary to minimize this risk[4,5].

Laboratory Tests: Periodic complete blood counts and assessments of renal and hepatic function should be done during the course of Teniposide treatment. They should be performed prior to therapy and at clinically appropriate intervals during and after therapy. There should be at least one determination of hematologic status prior to therapy with Teniposide.

Drug Interactions: In a study in which 34 different drugs were tested, therapeutically relevant concentrations of tolbutamide, sodium salicylate and sulfamethizole displaced protein-bound Teniposide in fresh human serum to a small but significant extent. Because of the extremely high binding of Teniposide to plasma proteins, these small decreases in binding could cause substantial increases in free drug levels in plasma which could result in potentiation of drug toxicity. Therefore, caution should be used in administering Teniposide to patients receiving these other agents. There was no change in the plasma kinetics of Teniposide when coadministered with methotrexate. However, the plasma clearance of methotrexate was slightly increased. An increase in intracellular levels of methotrexate was observed *in vitro* in the presence of Teniposide.

Carcinogenesis, Mutagenesis, Impairment of Fertility: Children at SJCRH with ALL in remission who received maintenance therapy with Teniposide weekly or twice weekly doses (plus other chemotherapeutic agents), had a relative risk of developing secondary acute nonlymphocytic leukemia (ANLL) approximately 12 times that of patients treated according to other less intensive schedules[6].

A short course of Teniposide for remission-induction and/or consolidation therapy was not associated with an increased risk of secondary ANLL, but the number of patients assessed was small. The potential benefit from Teniposide must be weighed on a case by case basis against the potential risk of the induction of a secondary leukemia. The carcinogenicity of teniposide has not been studied in laboratory animals. Compounds with similar mechanisms of action and mutagenicity profiles have been reported to be carcinogenic and teniposide should be considered a potential carcinogen in humans. Teniposide has been shown to be mutagenic in various bacterial and mammalian genetic toxicity tests. These include positive mutagenic effects in the Ames/Salmonella and *B. subtilis* bacterial mutagenicity assays. Teniposide caused gene mutations in both Chinese hamster ovary cells and mouse lymphoma cells and DNA damage as measured by alkaline elution in human lung carcinoma derived cell lines. In addition, Teniposide induced aberrations in chromosome structure in primary cultures of human lymphocytes *in vitro* and in L5178y/TK + /-mouse lymphoma cells *in vitro*. Chromosome aberrations were observed *in vivo* in the embryonic tissue of pregnant. Swiss albino mice treated with Teniposide. Teniposide also caused a dose-related increase in sister chromatid exchanges in Chinese hamster ovary cells and it has been shown to be embryotoxic and teratogenic in rats receiving Teniposide during organogenesis. Treatment of pregnant rats IV with doses between 1.0 and 3.0 mg/kg/day on alternate days from day 6 to 16 post coitum caused retardation of embryonic development, prenatal mortality and fetal abnormalities.

Pregnancy: Pregnancy "Category D." (See *"Warnings"* section.)

Nursing Mothers: It is not known whether this drug is excreted in human milk. Because many drugs are excreted in human milk and because of the potential for serious adverse reactions in nursing infants, a decision should be made whether to discontinue nursing or to discontinue the drug, taking into account the importance of Teniposide therapy to the mother.

Patients with Down's Syndrome: Patients with both Down's Syndrome and leukemia may be especially sensitive to myelosuppressive chemotherapy, therefore, initial dosing with Teniposide should be reduced in these patients. It is suggested that the first course of Teniposide should be given at half the usual dose. Subsequent courses may be administered at higher dosages depending on the degree of myelosuppression and mucositis encountered in earlier courses in an individual patient.

ADVERSE REACTIONS

The table below presents the incidences of adverse reactions derived from an analysis of data contained within literature reports of 7 studies involving 303 pediatric patients in which Teniposide was administered by injection as a single agent in a variety of doses and schedules for a variety of hematologic malignancies and solid tumors. The total number of patients evaluable for a given event was not 303 since the individual studies did not address the occurrence of each event listed. Five of these 7 studies assessed Teniposide activity in hematologic malignancies, such as leukemia. Thus, many of these patients had abnormal hematologic status at start of therapy with Teniposide and were expected to develop significant myelo-suppression as an endpoint of treatment.

SINGLE-AGENT TENIPOSIDE SUMMARY OF TOXICITY FOR ALL EVALUABLE PEDIATRIC PATIENTS

Toxicity	Incidence in Evaluable Patients (%)
Hematologic toxicity	
Myelosuppression, nonspecified	75
Leukopenia (< 3,000 WBC/ μL)	89
Neutropenia (< 2,000 ANC/μL)	95
Thrombocytopenia (< 100,000 plt/μL)	85
Anemia	88
Non-Hematologic Toxicity	
Mucositis	76
Diarrhea	33
Nausea/vomiting	29
Infection	12
Alopecia	9
Bleeding	5
Hypersensitivity reactions	5
Rash	3
Fever	3
Hypotension/Cardiovascular	2
Neurotoxicity	< 1
Hepatic dysfunction	< 1
Renal dysfunction	< 1
Metabolic abnormalities	< 1

Hematologic Toxicity: Teniposide when used with other chemotherapeutic agents for the treatment of ALL, results in severe myelosuppression. Early onset of profound myelosuppression with delayed recovery can be expected when using the doses and schedules of Teniposide necessary for treatment of refractory ALL, since bone marrow hypoplasia is a desired endpoint of therapy. The occurrence of acute non-lymphocytic leukemia (ANLL), with or without a preleukemic phase, has been reported in patients treated with Teniposide in combination with other antineoplastic agents. See *"Precautions"* subsection *"Carcinogenesis, Mutagenesis, Impairment of Fertility".*

Gastrointestinal Toxicity: Nausea and vomiting are the most common gastrointestinal toxicities, having occurred in 29 percent of evaluable pediatric patients. The severity of this nausea and vomiting is generally mild to moderate.

Hypotension: Transient hypotension following rapid intravenous administration has been reported in 2 percent of evaluable pediatric patients. One episode of sudden death, attributed to probable arrhythmia and intractable hypotension, has been reported in an elderly patient receiving Teniposide combination therapy for a non-leukemic malignancy. No other cardiac toxicity or electrocardiographic changes have been documented. No delayed hypotension has been noted.

Allergic Reactions: Hypersentivity reactions characterized by chills, fever, tachycardia, flushing, bronchospasm, dyspnea, and blood pressure changes (hypertension or hypotension) have been reported to occur in approximately 5 percent of evaluable pediatric patients receiving intravenous Teniposide. The incidence of hypersensitivity reactions to Teniposide appears to be increased in patients with brain tumors, and in patients with neuroblastoma[1].

Central Nervous System: Acute central nervous system depression and hypotension have been observed in patients receiving investigational infusions of high-dose Teniposide who were pretreated with antiemetic drugs. The depressant effects of the antiemetic agents and the alcohol content of the Teniposide formulation may place patients receiving higher than recommended doses of Teniposide at risk for central nervous system depression.

Alopecia: Alopecia, sometimes progressing to total baldness, was observed in 9 percent of evaluable pediatric patients who received Teniposide as single agent therapy. It was usually reversible.

OVERDOSE

There is no known antidote for Teniposide overdosage. The anticipated complications of overdosage are secondary to bone marrow suppression. Treatment should consist of supportive care including blood products and antibotics as indicated.

DOSAGE AND ADMINISTRATION

Note: Contact of undiluted Teniposide for injection concentrate with plastic equipment or devices used to prepare solutions for infusion may result in softening or cracking and possible drug product leakage. This effect has *not* been reported with *diluted solutions* of Teniposide.

In order to prevent extraction of the plasticizer DEHP[di(2-ethylhexyl)phtalate], solutions of Teniposide for injection concentrate should be prepared in non-DEHP containing LVP containers such as glass or polyolefin plastic bags or containers.

Teniposide solutions should be administered with non-DEHP containing IV administration sets.

In one study, childhood ALL patients failing induction therapy with a cytarabine-containing regimen were treated with the combination of Teniposide 165 mg/m^2 and cytarabine 300 mg/m^2 intravenously, twice weekly for 8-9 doses. In another study, patients with childhood ALL refractory to vincristine/prednisone-containing regimens were treated with the combination of Teniposide 250 mg/m^2 and vincristine 1.5 mg/m^2 intravenously, weekly for 4-8 weeks and prednisone 40 mg/m^2 orally × 28 days.

Adequate data in patients with hepatic insufficiency and/or renal insufficiency are lacking, but dose adjustments may be necessary for patients with significant renal or hepatic impairment.

Preparation and Administration Precautions: Teniposide is a cytotoxic anticancer drug and, as with other potentially toxic compounds, caution should be exercised in handling and preparing the solution of Teniposide. Skin reactions associated with accidental exposure to Teniposide may occur. The use of gloves is recommended. If Teniposide solution contacts the skin, immediately wash the skin thoroughly with soap and water. If Teniposide contacts mucous membranes, the membranes should be flushed thoroughly with water.

Preparation for Intravenous Administration: Teniposide must be diluted with either 5 percent Dextrose Injection, USP or 0.9 percent Sodium Chloride Injection, USP, to give final Teniposide concentrations of 0.1 mg/mL, 0.2 mg/mL, 0.4 mg/mL or 1.0 mg/mL. Solutions prepared in 5 percent Dextrose Injection, USP or 0.9 percent Sodium Chloride Injection, USP at Teniposide concentrations of 0.1 mg/mL, 0.2 mg/mL or 0.4 mg/mL are stable at room temperature for up to 24 hours after preparation. Teniposide solutions prepared at a final Teniposide concentration of 1.0 mg/mL should be administered within 4 hours of preparation to reduce the potential for precipitation. *Refrigeration of Teniposide solutions is not recommended.* Stability and use times are identical in glass and plastic parenteral solution containers.

Although solutions are chemically stable under the conditions indicated, precipitation of Teniposide may occur at the recommended concentrations, especially if the diluted solution is subjected to more agitation than is recommended to prepare the drug solution for parenteral administration[7]. In addition, storage time prior to administration should be minimized and care should be taken to avoid contact of the diluted solution with other drugs or fluids. Parenteral drug products should be inspected visually for particulate matter and discoloration prior to administration whenever solution and container permit. *Precipitation has been reported during 24-hour infusions of Teniposide diluted to Teniposide concentrations of 0.1 to 0.2 mg/mL, resulting in occlusion of central venous access catheters in several patients[4,5]. Heparin solution can cause precipitation of Teniposide, therefore, the administration apparatus should be flushed thoroughly with 5 percent Dextrose Injection or 0.9 percent Sodium Chloride Injection, USP before and after administration of Teniposide[5].*

Hypotension has been reported following rapid intravenous administration; it is recommended that the Teniposide solution be administered over at least a 30 to 60-minute period. *Teniposide should not be given by rapid intravenous injection.* In a 24-hour study under simulated conditions of actual use of the product relative to dilution strength, diluent and administration rates, dilutions at 0.1 to 1.0 mg/mL were chemically stable for at least 24 hours. Data collected for the presence of the extractable DEHP [di(2-ethylhexyl)phtalate] from PVC containers show that levels increased with time and concentration of the solutions. The data appeared similar for 0.9 percent Sodium Chloride Injection, USP, and 5 percent Dextrose Injection, USP. Consequently, the use of PVC containers is not recommended.

Similarly, the use of non-DEHP IV administration sets is recommended. Lipid administration sets or low DEHP containing nitroglycerin sets will keep patients' exposure to DEHP at low levels and are suitable for use. The diluted solutions are chemically and physically compatible with the recommended IV administration sets and LVP containers for up to 24 hours at ambient room temperature and lighting conditions. *Because of the potential for precipitation, compatibility with other drugs, infusion materials or IV pumps cannot be assured.*

Stability: Unopened ampules of Teniposide Injection Concentrate are stable until the date indicated on the package when stored under refrigeration (2°—8°C) in the original package. Freezing does not adversely affect the product.

Storage: Store the unopened ampules under refrigeration (2°—8°C). Retain in original package to protect from light.

Handling and Disposal: Procedures for proper handling and disposal of anticancer drugs should be considered. Several guidelines on this subject have been published[6-14]. There is no general agreement that all of the procedures recommended in the guidelines are necessary or appropriate.

REFERENCES
1. O'Dwyer PJ, King SA, Fortner CL and Leyland-Jones B: Hypersensitivity reactions to teniposide (VM-26): an analysis. *J Clin Oncol.* 1986: 4(8):1262-1269. 2. Lorenz W, Perlmann H-J, Schmall A, et al: Histamine release in dogs by Cremophor® EL and its derivatives. *Agents and Actions.* 1977; 7(1):63-67. 3. Lassus M, Scott D, and Leyland-Jones B: Allergic reactions associated with cremophor containing antineoplastics. *Proc Am Soc Clin Oncol* 1985; 4:268 (Abstract C-1042). 4. Strong D, Morris L: Precipitation of teniposide during infusion. *Am J Hosp Pharm* Mar 1990: Letter, 47:512,518. 5. Bogardus J, Kaplan M, Carpenter J: Precipitation of Teniposide During Infusion. *Am J Hosp Pharm*; Mar 1990: Letter, 47:518-519. 6. Pul C-H, et al: Acute Myeloid Leukemia in Children Treated with Epipodophyllotoxins for Acute Lymphoblastic Leukemia. *N Engl J Med.* 1991: 325:1682-1687. 7. Deardoff D, Schmidt C: Mixing additives in plastic LVPs. *Am J Hosp Phar.* Dec 1980: Letter, 37:1610, 1613. 8. Recommendations for the Safe Handling of Parenteral Antineoplastic Drugs. NIH Publication No. 83-2621. For sale by the Superintendent of Documents, US Government Printing office, Washington, DC 20402. 9. AMA Council Report. Guidelines for handling parenteral antineoplastics. *JAMA* 1985; 253 (11); 1590-1592. 10. National Study Commission on Cytotoxic Exposure—Recommendations for Handling Cytotoxic Agents. Available from Louis P. Jeffrey, Chairman, ScD, National Study Commission on Cytotoxic Exposure. Massachusetts College of Pharmacy and Allied Health Sciences, 179 Longwood Avenue, Boston, Massachusetts, 02115. 11. Clinical Oncological Society of Australia. Guidlines and Recommendations for Safe Handling of Antineoplastic Agents. *Med J Australia* 1983; 1:426-428. 12. Jones RB, et al: Safe handling of chemotherapeutic agents: a report from the Mount Sinai Medical Center. *CA-A Cancer Journal for Clinicians* 1983; Sept./Oct. 258-263. 13. American Society of Hospital Pharmacists Technical Assistance Bulletin on Handling Cytotoxic Drugs in Hospitals. *Am J Hosp Pharm* 1990: 47:1033-1049. 14. OSHA Work-Practice Guidelines for Personnel Dealing With Cytotoxic (Antineoplastic) drugs. *Am J Hosp Pharm* 1986: 43:1193-1204.

HOW SUPPLIED
INJECTION: 50 MG/5 ML

BRAND/MANUFACTURER	NDC	SIZE	AWP
○ **BRAND**			
VUMON: Bristol-Myer Onc/Hiv	00015-3075-19	5 ml	$150.39
	00015-3075-97	5 ml 10s	$1503.90

Tenoretic *SEE* ATENOLOL WITH CHLORTHALIDONE

Tenormin *SEE* ATENOLOL

Tensilon *SEE* EDROPHONIUM CHLORIDE

Tenuate *SEE* DIETHYLPROPION HYDROCHLORIDE

Terazol *SEE* TERCONAZOLE

Terazosin Hydrochloride

DESCRIPTION
Terazosin Hydrochloride an alpha-l-selective adrenoceptor blocking agent, is a quinazoline derivative represented by the following chemical name and structural formula:
(RS)-Piperazine, 1-(4-amino-6,7-dimethoxy-2-quinazolinyl)-4-[(tetra-hydro- 2-furanyl)carbonyl]-, monohydrochloride, dihydrate.

Terazosin Hydrochloride is a white, crystalline substance, freely soluble in water and isotonic saline and has a molecular weight of 459.93. Terazosin Hydrochloride tablets for oral ingestion are supplied in four dosage strengths containing Terazosin Hydrochloride equivalent to 1 mg, 2 mg, 5 mg, or 10 mg of Terazosin.

Following is its chemical structure:

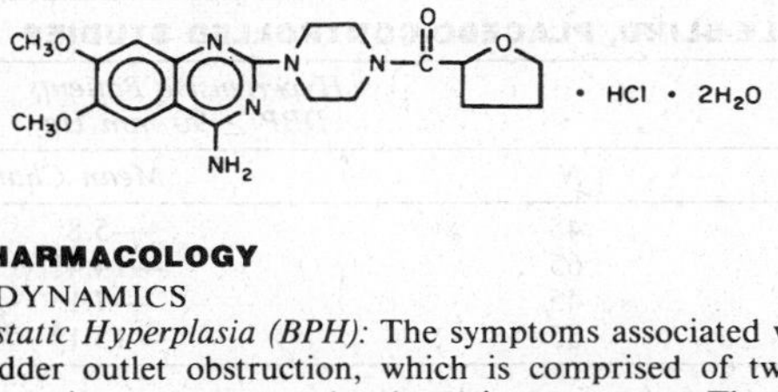

CLINICAL PHARMACOLOGY
PHARMACODYNAMICS
A. Benign Prostatic Hyperplasia (BPH): The symptoms associated with BPH are related to bladder outlet obstruction, which is comprised of two underlying components: a static component and a dynamic component. The static compo-

nent is a consequence of an increase in prostate size. Over time, the prostate will continue to enlarge. However, clinical studies have demonstrated that the size of the prostate does not correlate with the severity of BPH symptoms or the degree of urinary obstruction.[1]. The dynamic component is a function of an increase in smooth muscle tone in the prostate and bladder neck, leading to constriction of the bladder outlet. Smooth muscle tone is mediated by sympathetic nervous stimulation of alpha-1 adrenoceptors, which are abundant in the prostate, prostatic capsule and bladder neck. The reduction in symptoms and improvement in urine flow rates following administration of Terazosin is related to relaxation of smooth muscle produced by blockade of alpha-1 adrenoceptors in the bladder neck and prostate. Because there are relatively few alpha-1 adrenoceptors in the bladder body, Terazosin is able to reduce the bladder outlet obstruction without affecting bladder contractility.

Terazosin has been extensively studied in 1222 men with symptomatic BPH. In three placebo-controlled studies, symptom evaluation and uroflowmetric measurements were performed approximately 24 hours following dosing. Symptoms were systematically quantified using the Boyarsky Index. The questionnaire evaluated both obstructive (hesitancy, intermittency, terminal dribbling, impairment of size and force of stream, sensation of incomplete bladder emptying) and irritative (nocturia, daytime frequency, urgency, dysuria) symptoms by rating each of the 9 symptoms from 0-3, for a total score of 27 points. Results from these studies indicated that Terazosin statistically significantly improved symptoms and peak urine flow rates over placebo as follows: (See related table).

In all three studies, both symptoms scores and peak urine flow rates showed statistically significant improvement from baseline in patients treated with Terazosin Hydrochloride from week 2 (or the first clinic visit) and throughout the study duration.

Analysis of the effect of Terazosin Hydrochloride on individual urinary symptoms demonstrated that compared to placebo, Terazosin Hydrochloride significantly improved the symptoms of hesitancy, intermittency, impairment in size and force of urinary stream, sensation of incomplete emptying, terminal dribbling, daytime frequency and nocturia.

Global assessments of overall urinary function and symptoms were also performed by investigators who were blinded to patient treatment assignment. In studies 1 and 3, patients treated with Terazosin Hydrochloride had a significantly (p ≤ 0.001) greater overall improvement compared to placebo treated patients. In a short term study (Study 1) patients were randomized to either 2, 5 or 10 mg of Terazosin Hydrochloride or placebo. Patients randomized to the 10 mg group achieved a statistically significant response in both symptoms and peak flow rate compared to placebo.

In a long-term, open-label, non-placebo controlled clinical trial, 181 men were followed for 2 years and 58 of these men were followed for 30 months. The effect Terazosin Hydrochloride on urinary symptom scores and peak flow rates was maintained throughout the study duration.

In this long-term trial, both symptom scores and peak urinary flow rates showed statistically significant improvement suggesting a relaxation of smooth muscle cells.

Although blockade of alpha-1 adrenoceptors also lowers blood pressure in hypertensive patients with increased peripheral vascular resistance, Terazosin treatment of normotensive men with BPH did not result in a clinically significant blood pressure lowering effect: (See related table).

B. Hypertension: In animals, Terazosin causes a decrease in blood pressure by decreasing total peripheral vascular resistance. The vasodilatory hypotensive action of Terazosin appears to be produced mainly by blockade of alpha-1 adrenoceptors. Terazosin decreases blood pressure gradually within 15 minutes following oral administration.

Patients in clinical trials of Terazosin were administered once daily (the great majority) and twice daily regimens with total doses usually in the range of 5-20 mg/day, and had mild (about 77%, diastolic pressure 95-105 mmHg) or moderate (23%, diastolic pressure 105-115 mmHg) hypertension. Because Terazosin, like all alpha antagonists, can cause unusually large falls in blood pressure after the first dose or first few doses, the initial dose was 1 mg in virtually all trials, with subsequent titration to a specified fixed dose or titration to some specified blood pressure end point (usually a supine diastolic pressure of 90 mmHg).

Blood pressure responses were measured at the end of the dosing interval (usually 24 hours) and effects were shown to persist throughout the interval, with the usual supine responses 5-10 mmHg systolic and 3.5-8 mmHg diastolic greater than placebo. The responses in the standing position tended to be somewhat larger, by 1-3 mmHg, although this was not true in all studies. The magnitude of the blood pressure responses was similar to prazosin and less than hydrochlorothiazide (in a single study of hypertensive patients). In measurements 24 hours after dosing, heart rate was unchanged.

Limited measurements of peak response (2-3 hours after dosing) during chronic Terazosin administration indicate that it is greater than about twice the trough (24 hour) response, suggesting some attenuation of response at 24 hours, presumably due to a fall in blood Terazosin concentrations at the end of the dose interval. This explanation is not established with certainty, however, and is not consistent with the similarity of blood pressure response to once daily and twice daily dosing and with the absence of an observed dose-response relationship over a range of 5-20 mg, i.e., if blood concentrations had fallen to the point of providing less than full effect at 24 hours, a shorter dosing interval or larger dose should have led to increased response.

Further dose response and dose duration studies are being carried out. Blood pressure should be measured at the end of the dose interval; if response is not satisfactory, patients may be tried on a larger dose or twice daily dosing regimen. The latter should also be considered if possibly blood pressure-related side effects, such as dizziness, palpitations, or orthostatic complaints, are seen within a few hours after dosing. The greater blood pressure effect associated with peak plasma concentrations (first few hours after dosing) appears somewhat more position-dependent (greater in the erect position) than the effect of Terazosin at 24 hours and in the erect position there is also a 6-10 beat per minute increase in heart rate in the first few hours after dosing. During the first 3 hours after dosing 12.5% of patients had a systolic pressure fall of 30 mmHg or more from supine to standing, or standing systolic pressure below 90 mmHg with a fall of at least 20 mmHg, compared to 4% of a placebo group.

There was a tendency for patients to gain weight during Terazosin therapy. In placebo-controlled monotherapy trials, male and female patients receiving Terazosin gained a mean of 1.7 and 2.2 pounds respectively, compared to losses of 0.2 and 1.2 pounds respectively in the placebo group. Both differences were statistically significant.

During controlled clinical trials, patients receiving Terazosin monotherapy had a small but statistically significant decrease (a 3% fall) compared to placebo in total cholesterol and the combined low-density and very-low-density lipoprotein fractions. No significant changes were observed in high-density lipoprotein fraction and triglycerides compared to placebo.

Analysis of clinical laboratory data following administration of Terazosin suggested the possibility of hemodilution based on decreases in hematocrit, hemoglobin, white blood cells, total protein and albumin. Decreases in hematocrit and total protein have been observed with alpha-blockade and are attributed to hemodilution.

PHARMACOKINETICS
Relative to solution, Terazosin Hydrochloride administered as tablets is essentially completely absorbed in man. Food had little or no effect on the extent of absorption but food delayed the time to peak concentration by about 1 hour. Terazosin has been shown to undergo minimal hepatic first-pass metabolism and nearly all of the circulating dose is in the form of parent drug. The plasma levels peak about one hour after dosing, and then decline with a half-life of approximately 12 hours. In a study that evaluated the effect of age on Terazosin pharmacokinetics, the mean plasma half-lives were 14.0 and 11.4 hours for the age group $\geq$ 70 years and the age group of 20-39 years, respectively. After oral administration the plasma clearance was decreased by 31.7% in patients 70 years of age or older compared to that in patients 20-39 years of age.

The drug is highly bound to plasma proteins and binding is constant over the clinically observed concentration range. Approximately 10% of an orally administered dose is excreted as parent drug in the urine and approximately 20% is excreted in the feces. The remainder is eliminated as metabolites. Impaired renal function had no significant effect on the elimination of Terazosin, and dosage adjustment of Terazosin to compensate for the drug removal during hemodialysis (approximately 10%) does not appear to be necessary. Overall, approximately 40% of the administered dose is excreted in the urine and approximately 60% in the feces. The disposition of the compound in animals is qualitatively similar to that in man.

INDICATIONS AND USAGE
Terazosin Hydrochloride is indicated for the treatment of symptomatic benign prostatic hyperplasia (BPH). There is a rapid response, with approximately 70% of patients experiencing an increase in urinary flow and improvement in symptoms of BPH when treated with Terazosin Hydrochloride. The long-term effects of Terazosin Hydrochloride on the incidence of surgery, acute urinary obstruction or other complications of BPH are yet to be determined.

Terazosin Hydrochloride tablets are also indicated for the treatment of hypertension. Terazosin Hydrochloride tablets can be used alone or in combination with other antihypertensive agents such as diuretics or beta-adrenergic blocking agents.

UNLABELED USES
Terazosin is used alone or as an adjunct in the treatment of congestive heart failure and hyperlipidemia.

CONTRAINDICATIONS
Terazosin Hydrochloride tablets are contraindicated in patients known to be hypersensitive to Terazosin Hydrochloride.

WARNINGS
Syncope and "First-Dose" Effect: **Terazosin Hydrochloride tablets, like other alpha-adrenergic blocking agents, can cause marked lowering of blood pressure, especially postural hypotension, and syncope in association with the first dose or first few days of therapy. A similar effect can be anticipated if therapy is interrupted for several days and then restarted. Syncope has also been reported with other alpha-adrenergic blocking agents in association with rapid dosage increases or the introduction of another antihypertensive drug. Syncope is believed to be due to an excessive postural hypotensive effect, although occasionally the syncopal episode has been preceded by a bout of severe supraventricular tachycardia with heart rates of 120-160 beats per minute. Additionally, the possibility of the contribution of hemodilution to the symptoms of postural hypotension should be considered.**

To decrease the likelihood of syncope or excessive hypotension, treatment should always be initiated with a 1 mg dose of Terazosin Hydrochloride tablets, given at bedtime. The 2 mg, 5 mg and 10 mg tablets are not indicated as initial therapy. Dosage should then be increased slowly, according to recommendations in the *"Dosage and Administration"* section and additional antihypertensive agents should be added with caution. The patient should be cautioned to avoid situations, such as driving or hazardous tasks, where injury could result should syncope occur during initiation of therapy.

In early investigational studies, where increasing single doses up to 7.5 mg were given at 3 day intervals, tolerance to the first dose phenomenon did not necessarily develop and the "first-dose" effect could be observed at all doses. Syncopal episodes occurred in 3 of the 14 subjects given Terazosin Hydrochloride tablets at doses of 2.5, 5 and 7.5 mg, which are higher than the recommended initial dose; in addition, severe orthostatic hypotension (blood pressure falling to 50/0 mmHg) was seen in two others and dizziness, tachycardia, and lightheadedness occurred in most subjects. These adverse effects all occurred within 90 minutes of dosing.

	N	Symptom Score (Range 0-27)		N	Peak Flow Rate (mL/sec)	
		Mean Baseline	Mean Change (%)		Mean Baseline	Mean Change (%)
Study 1 (10 mg)[a]						
Titration to fixed dose (12 wks)						
Placebo	55	9.7	—2.3(24)	54	10.1	+1.0 (10)
Terazosin	54	10.1	—4.5(45)*	52	8.8	+3.0 (34)*
Study 2 (2, 5, 10, 20 mg)[b]						
Titration to response (24 wks)						
Placebo	89	12.5	—3.8 (30)	88	8.8	+1.4 (16)
Terazosin	85	12.2	—5.3 (43)*	84	8.4	+2.9 (35)*
Study 3 (1, 2, 5, 10 mg)[c]						
Titration to response (24 wks)						
Placebo	74	10.4	—1.1 (11)	74	8.8	+1.2 (14)
Terazosin	73	10.9	—4.6 (42)*	73	8.6	+2.6 (30)*

a Highest dose 10 mg shown.
b 23% of patients on 10 mg, 41% of patients on 20 mg.
c 67% of patients on 10 mg.
* Significantly ($p \leq 0.05$) more improvement than placebo.

MEAN CHANGES IN BLOOD PRESSURE FROM BASELINE TO FINAL VISIT IN ALL DOUBLE-BLIND, PLACEBO-CONTROLLED STUDIES

		Normotensive Patients DBP < 90 mm Hg		Hypertensive Patients DBP ≥ 90 mm Hg	
	Group	N	Mean Change	N	Mean Change
SBP	Placebo	293	—0.1	45	—5.8
(mm Hg)	Terazosin	519	—3.3*	65	—14.4*
DBP	Placebo	293	+ 0.4	45	—7.1
(mm Hg)	Terazosin	519	—2.2*	65	—15.1*

* $p \geq 0.05$ vs. placebo

◆ RATED THERAPEUTICALLY EQUIVALENT; ◇ THERAPEUTIC EQUIVALENCE UNCONFIRMED; ○ UNRATED

In three placebo-controlled BPH studies 1, 2, and 3 (see *"Clinical Pharmacology"*), the incidence of postural hypotension in the Terazosin treated patients was 5.1%, 5.2%, and 3.7% respectively.

In multiple dose clinical trials involving nearly 2000 hypertensive patients treated with Terazosin Hydrochloride tablets, syncope was reported in about 1% of patients. Syncope was not necessarily associated only with the first dose.

If syncope occurs, the patient should be placed in a recumbent position and treated supportively as necessary. There is evidence that the orthostatic effect of Terazosin Hydrochloride tablets is greater, even in chronic use, shortly after dosing. The risk of the events is greatest during the initial seven days of treatment, but continues at all time intervals.

PRECAUTIONS
GENERAL
Prostatic Cancer: Carcinoma of the prostate and BPH cause many of the same symptoms. These two diseases frequently co-exist. Therefore, patients thought to have BPH should be examined prior to starting Terazosin Hydrochloride therapy to rule out the presence of carcinoma of the prostate.

Orthostatic Hypotension: While syncope is the most severe orthostatic effect of Terazosin Hydrochloride tablets (see *"Warnings"*), other symptoms of lowered blood pressure, such as dizziness, lightheadedness and palpitations, were more common and occurred in some 28% of patients in clinical trials of hypertension. In BPH clinical trials, 21% of the patients experienced one or more of the following: dizziness, hypotension, postural hypotension, syncope, and vertigo. Patients with occupations in which such events represent potential problems should be treated with particular caution.

Information for Patients (see Patient Package Insert): Patients should be made aware of the possibility of syncopal and orthostatic symptoms, especially at the initiation of therapy, and to avoid driving or hazardous tasks for 12 hours after the first dose, after a dosage increase and after interruption of therapy when treatment is resumed. They should be cautioned to avoid situations where injury could result should syncope occur during initiation of Terazosin Hydrochloride therapy. They should also be advised of the need to sit or lie down when symptoms of lowered blood pressure occur, although these symptoms are not always orthostatic, and to be careful when rising from a sitting or lying position. If dizziness, lightheadedness, or palpitations are bothersome they should be reported to the physician, so that dose adjustment can be considered.

Patients should also be told that drowsiness or somnolence can occur with Terazosin Hydrochloride tablets, requiring caution in people who must drive or operate heavy machinery.

Laboratory Tests: Small but statistically significant decreases in hematocrit, hemoglobin, white blood cells, total protein and albumin were observed in controlled clinical trials. These laboratory findings suggested the possibility of hemodilution. Treatment with Terazosin Hydrochloride for up to 24 months had no significant effect on prostate specific antigen (PSA) levels.

Drug Interactions: In controlled trials, Terazosin Hydrochloride tablets have been added to diuretics, and several beta-adrenergic blockers; no unexpected interactions were observed. Terazosin Hydrochloride tablets have also been used in patients on a variety of concomitant therapies; while these were not formal interaction studies, no interactions were observed. Terazosin Hydrochloride tablets have been used concomitantly in at least 50 patients on the following drugs or drug classes: 1) analgesic/anti-inflammatory (e.g., acetaminophen, aspirin, codeine, ibuprofen, indomethacin); 2) antibiotics (e.g., erythromycin, trimethoprim and sulfamethoxazole); 3) anticholinergic/sympathomimetics (e.g., phenylephrine hydrochloride, phenylpropanolamine hydrochloride, pseudoephedrine hydrochloride); 4) antigout (e.g., allopurinol); 5) antihistamines (e.g., chlorpheniramine); 6) cardiovascular agents (e.g., atenolol, hydrochlorothiazide, methyclothiazide, propranolol); 7) corticosteroids; 8) gastro-intestinal agents (e.g., antacids); 9) hypoglycemics; 10) sedatives and tranquilizers (e.g., diazepam).

Use with Other Drugs: In a study (n = 24) where Terazosin Hydrochloride and verapamil were administered concomitantly, Terazosin's mean AUC_{0-24} increased 11% after the first verapamil dose and after 3 weeks of verapamil treatment it increased by 24% with associated increases in C_{max} (25%) and C_{min} (32%) means. Terazosin mean T_{max} decreased from 1.3 hours to 0.8 hours after 3 weeks of verapamil treatment. Statistically significant differences were not found in the verapamil level with and without Terazosin. In a study (n = 6) where Terazosin and captopril were administered concomitantly, plasma disposition of captopril was not influenced by concomitant administration of Terazosin and Terazosin maximum plasma concentrations increased linearly with dose at steady-state after administration of Terazosin plus captopril (see *"Dosage and Administration"*).

Carcinogenesis, Mutagenesis, Impairment of Fertility: Terazosin Hydrochloride was devoid of mutagenic potential when evaluated *in vivo* and *in vitro* (the Ames test, *in vivo* cytogenetics, the dominant lethal test in mice, *in vivo* Chinese hamster chromosome aberration test and V79 forward mutation assay). Terazosin Hydrochloride, administered in the feed to rats at doses of 8, 40, and 250 mg/kg/day for two years, was associated with a statistically significant increase in benign adrenal medullary tumors of male rats exposed to the 250 mg/kg dose. This dose is 695 times the maximum recommended human dose of 20 mg/55kg patient. Female rats were unaffected. Terazosin Hydrochloride was not oncogenic in mice when administered in feed for 2 years at a maximum tolerated dose of 32 mg/kg/day. The absence of mutagenicity in a battery of tests, of tumorigenicity of any cell type in the mouse carcinogenicity assay, of increased total tumor incidence in either species, and of proliferative adrenal lesions in female rats, suggests a male rat species-specific event. Numerous other diverse pharmaceutical and chemical compounds have also been associated with benign adrenal medullary tumors in male rats without supporting evidence for carcinogenicity in man.

The effect of Terazosin Hydrochloride on fertility was assessed in a standard fertility/reproductive performance study in which male and female rats were administered oral doses of 8, 30 and 120 mg/kg/day. Four of 20 male rats given 30 mg/kg and five of 19 male rats given 120 mg/kg failed to sire a litter. Testicular weights and morphology were unaffected by treatment. Vaginal smears at 30 and 120 mg/kg/day, however, appeared to contain less sperm than smears from control matings and good correlation was reported between sperm count and subsequent pregnancy.

Oral administration of Terazosin Hydrochloride for one or two years elicited a statistically significant increase in the incidence of testicular atrophy in rats exposed to 40 and 250 mg/kg/day, but not in rats exposed to 8 mg/kg/day (> 20 times the maximum recommended human dose). Testicular atrophy was also observed in dogs dosed with 300 mg/kg/day (> 800 times the maximum recommended human dose) for three months but not after one year when dosed with 20 mg/kg/day. This lesion has also been seen with prazosin, another (marketed) selective-alpha-1 blocking agent.

Pregnancy: Teratogenic effects: Pregnancy Category C. Terazosin Hydrochloride was not teratogenic in either rats or rabbits when administered at oral doses up to 1330 and 165 times, respectively, the maximum recommended human dose. Fetal resorptions occurred in rats dosed with 480 mg/kg/day, approximately 1330 times the maximum recommended human dose. Increased fetal resorptions, decreased fetal weight and an increased number of supernumerary ribs were observed in offspring of rabbits dosed with 165 times the maximum recommended human dose. These findings (in both species) were most likely secondary to maternal toxicity. There are no adequate and well-controlled studies in pregnant women and the safety of Terazosin in pregnancy has not been established. Terazosin Hydrochloride is not recommended during pregnancy unless the potential benefit justifies the potential risk to the mother and fetus. Nonteratogenic effects: In a peri- and post-natal development study in rats, significantly more pups died in the group dosed with 120 mg/kg/day (> 300 times the maximum recommended human dose) than in the control group during the three-week postpartum period.

Nursing Mothers: It is not known whether Terazosin is excreted in breast milk. Because many drugs are excreted in breast milk, caution should be exercised when Terazosin Hydrochloride tablets are administered to a nursing woman.

Pediatric Use: Safety and effectiveness in children have not been determined.

ADVERSE REACTIONS
BENIGN PROSTATIC HYPERPLASIA
The incidence of treatment-emergent adverse events has been ascertained from clinical trials conducted worldwide. All adverse events reported during these trials were recorded as adverse reactions. The incidence rates presented below are based on combined data from six placebo-controlled trials involving once-a-day administration of Terazosin at doses ranging from 1 to 20 mg. Table 1 summarizes those adverse events reported for patients in these trials when the incidence rate in the Terazosin group was at least 1% and was greater than that for the placebo group, or where the reaction is of clinical interest. Asthenia, postural hypotension, dizziness, somnolence, nasal congestion/rhinitis, and impotence were the only events that were significantly (p ≤ 0.05) more common in patients receiving Terazosin than in patients receiving placebo. The incidence of urinary tract infection was significantly lower in the patients receiving Terazosin than in patients receiving placebo. An analysis of the incidence rate of hypotensive adverse events (see *"Precautions"*) adjusted for the length of drug treatment has shown that the risk of the events is greatest during the initial seven days of treatment, but continues at all time intervals.

Table 1
ADVERSE REACTIONS DURING PLACEBO-CONTROLLED TRIALS BENIGN PROSTATIC HYPERPLASIA

Body System	Terazosin (N = 636)	Placebo (N = 360)
Body as a Whole		
† Asthenia	7.4%*	3.3%
Flu Syndrome	2.4%	1.7%
Headache	4.9%	5.8%
Cardiovascular System		
Hypotension	0.6%	0.6%
Palpitations	0.9%	1.1%
Postural Hypotension	3.9%	0.8%
Syncope	0.6%	0.0%
Digestive System		
Nausea	1.7%	1.1%
Metabolic And Nutritional Disorders		
Peripheral Edema	0.9%	0.3%
Weight Gain	0.5%	0.0%
Nervous System		
Dizziness	9.1%*	4.2%
Somnolence	3.6%*	1.9%
Vertigo	1.4%	0.3%
Respiratory System		
Dyspnea	1.7%	0.8%

Body System	Terazosin (N = 636)	Placebo (N = 360)
Nasal Congestion/Rhinitis	1.9%*	0.0%
Special Senses		
Blurred Vision/Amblyopia	1.3%	0.6%
Urogenital System		
Impotence	1.6%*	0.6%
Urinary Tract Infection	1.3%	3.9%*

† Includes weakness, tiredness, lassitude and fatigue.
* ≤ 0.05 comparison between groups.

Additional adverse events have been reported, but these are, in general, not distinguishable from symptoms that might have occurred in the absence of exposure to Terazosin. The safety profile of patients treated in the long-term open-label study was similar to that observed in the controlled studies. The adverse events were usually transient and mild or moderate in intensity, but sometimes were serious enough to interrupt treatment. In the placebo-controlled clinical trials, the rates of premature termination due to adverse events were not statistically different between the placebo and Terazosin groups. The adverse events that were bothersome, as judged by their being reported as reasons for discontinuation of therapy by at least 0.5% of the Terazosin group and being reported more often than in the placebo group, are shown in Table 2.

Table 2
DISCONTINUATION DURING PLACEBO-CONTROLLED TRIALS BENIGN PROSTATIC HYPERPLASIA

Body System	Terazosin (N = 636)	Placebo (N = 360)
Body as a Whole		
Fever	0.5%	0.0%
Headache	1.1%	0.8%
Cardiovascular System		
Postural Hypotension	0.5%	0.0%
Syncope	0.5%	0.0%
Digestive System		
Nausea	0.5%	0.3%
Nervous System		
Dizziness	2.0%	1.1%
Vertigo	0.5%	0.0%
Respiratory System		
Dyspnea	0.5%	0.3%
Special Senses		
Blurred Vision/Amblyopia	0.6%	0.0%
Urogenital System		
Urinary Tract Infection	0.5%	0.3%

HYPERTENSION
The prevalence of adverse reactions has been ascertained from clinical trials conducted primarily in the United States. All adverse experiences (events) reported during these trials were recorded as adverse reactions. The prevalence rates presented below are based on combined data from fourteen placebo-controlled trials involving once-a-day administration of Terazosin, as monotherapy or in combination with other antihypertensive agents, at doses ranging from 1 to 40mg. Table 3 summarizes those adverse experiences reported for patients in these trials where the prevalence rate in the Terazosin group was at least 5%, where the prevalence rate for the Terazosin group was at least 2% and was greater than the prevalence rate for the placebo group, or where the reaction is of particular interest. Asthenia, blurred vision, dizziness, nasal congestion, nausea, peripheral edema, palpitations and somnolence were the only symptoms that were significantly (p < 0.05) more common in patients receiving Terazosin than in patients receiving placebo. Similar adverse reaction rates were observed in placebo-controlled monotherapy trials.

Table 3
ADVERSE REACTIONS DURING PLACEBO-CONTROLLED TRIALS HYPERTENSION

Body System	Terazosin (N = 859)	Placebo (N = 506)
Body as a Whole		
† Asthenia	11.3%*	4.3%
Back Pain	2.4%	1.2%
Headache	16.2%	15.8%
Cardiovascular System		
Palpitations	4.3%*	1.2%
Postural Hypotension	1.3%	0.4%
Tachycardia	1.9%	1.2%
Digestive System		
Nausea	4.4%*	1.4%

Body System	Terazosin (N = 859)	Placebo (N = 506)
Metabolic and Nutritional Disorders		
Edema	0.9%	0.6%
Peripheral Edema	5.5%*	2.4%
Weight Gain	0.5%	0.2%
Musculoskeletal System		
Pain-Extremities	3.5%	3.0%
Nervous System		
Depression	0.3%	0.2%
Dizziness	19.3%*	7.5%
Libido Decreased	0.6%	0.2%
Nervousness	2.3%	1.8%
Paresthesia	2.9%	1.4%
Somnolence	5.4%*	2.6%
Respiratory System		
Dyspnea	3.1%	2.4%
Nasal Congestion	5.9%*	3.4%
Sinusitis	2.6%	1.4%
Special Senses		
Blurred Vision	1.6%*	0.0%
Urogenital System		
Impotence	1.2%	1.4%

† Includes weakness, tiredness, lassitude and fatigue.
* Statistically significant at p = 0.05 level.

Additional adverse reactions have been reported, but these are, in general, not distinguishable from symptoms that might have occurred in the absence of exposure to Terazosin. The following additional adverse reactions were reported by at least 1% of 1987 patients who received Terazosin in controlled or open, short- or long-term clinical trials or have been reported during marketing experience:

Body as a Whole: chest pain, facial edema, fever, abdominal pain, neck pain, shoulder pain;

Cardiovascular System: arrhythmia, vasodilation;

Digestive System: constipation, diarrhea, dry mouth, dyspepsia, flatulence, vomiting;

Metabolic/Nutritional Disorders: gout;

Musculoskeletal System: arthralgia, arthritis, joint disorder, myalgia;

Nervous System: anxiety, insomnia;

Respiratory System: bronchitis, cold symptoms, epistaxis, flu symptoms, increased cough, pharyngitis, rhinitis;

Skin and Appendages: pruritus, rash, sweating;

Special Senses: abnormal vision, conjunctivitis, tinnitus;

Urogenital System: urinary frequency, urinary incontinence primarily reported in postmenopausal women, urinary tract infection. Postmarketing experience indicates that in rare instances patients may develop allergic reactions, including anaphylaxis, following administration of Terazosin tablets.

The adverse reactions were usually mild or moderate in intensity but sometimes were serious enough to interrupt treatment. The adverse reactions that were most bothersome, as judged by their being reported as reasons for discontinuation of therapy by at least 0.5% of the Terazosin group and being reported more often than in the placebo group, are shown in Table 4.

Table 4
DISCONTINUATIONS DURING PLACEBO-CONTROLLED TRIALS HYPERTENSION

Body System	Terazosin (N = 859)	Placebo (N = 506)
Body as a Whole		
Asthenia	1.6%	0.0%
Headache	1.3%	1.0%
Cardiovascular System		
Palpitations	1.4%	0.2%
Postural Hypotension	0.5%*	0.0%
Syncope	0.5%	0.2%
Tachycardia	0.5%	0.2%
Digestive System		
Nausea	0.8%	0.0%
Metabolic and Nutritional Disorders		
Peripheral Edema	0.6%	0.0%
Nervous System		
Dizziness	3.1%	0.4%
Paresthesia	0.8%	0.2%
Somnolence	0.6%	0.2%

Body System	Terazosin (N = 859)	Placebo (N = 506)
Respiratory System		
Dyspnea	0.9%	0.6%
Nasal Congestion	0.6%	0.0%
Special Senses		
Blurred Vision	0.6%	0.0%

OVERDOSAGE

Should overdosage of Terazosin Hydrochloride lead to hypotension, support of the cardiovascular system is of first importance. Restoration of blood pressure and normalization of heart rate may be accomplished by keeping the patient in the supine position. If this measure is inadequate, shock should first be treated with volume expanders. If necessary, vasopressors should then be used and renal function should be monitored and supported as needed. Laboratory data indicate that Terazosin Hydrochloride is highly protein bound; therefore, dialysis may not be of benefit.

DOSAGE AND ADMINISTRATION

If Terazosin Hydrochloride administration is discontinued for several days, therapy should be reinstituted using the initial dosing regimen.

BENIGN PROSTATIC HYPERPLASIA
Initial Dose: 1 mg at bedtime is the starting dose for all patients, and this dose should not be exceeded as an initial dose. Patients should be closely followed during initial administration in order to minimize the risk of severe hypotensive response.

Subsequent Doses: The dose should be increased in a stepwise fashion to 2 mg, 5mg, or 10 mg once daily to achieve the desired improvement of symptoms and/or flow rates. Doses of 10 mg once daily are generally required for the clinical response. Therefore, treatment with 10 mg for a minimum of 4-6 weeks may be required to assess whether a beneficial response has been achieved. Some patients may not achieve a clinical response despite appropriate titration. Although some additional patients responded at a 20 mg daily dose, there was an insufficient number of patients studied to draw definitive conclusions about this dose. There are insufficient data to support the use of higher doses for those patients who show inadequate or no response to 20 mg daily.

Use with Other Drugs: Caution should be observed when Terazosin Hydrochloride tablets are administered concomitantly with other antihypertensive agents, especially the calcium channel blocker verapamil, to avoid the possibility of developing significant hypotension. When using Terazosin Hydrochloride tablets and other antihypertensive agents concomitantly, dosage reduction and retitration of either agent may be necessary (see *"Precautions"*).

Hypertension: The dose of Terazosin Hydrochloride and the dose interval (12 or 24 hours) should be adjusted according to the patient's individual blood pressure response. The following is a guide to its administration.

Initial Dose: 1 mg at bedtime is the starting dose for all patients, and this dose should not be exceeded. This initial dosing regimen should be strictly observed to minimize the potential for severe hypotensive effects.

Subsequent Doses: The dose may be slowly increased to achieve the desired blood pressure response. The usual recommended dose range is 1 mg to 5 mg administered once a day; however, some patients may benefit from doses as high as 20 mg per day. Doses over 20 mg do not appear to provide further blood pressure effect and doses over 40 mg have not been studied. Blood pressure should be monitored at the end of the dosing interval to be sure control is maintained throughout the interval. It may also be helpful to measure blood pressure 2-3 hours after dosing to see if the maximum and minimum responses are similar, and to evaluate symptoms such as dizziness or palpitations which can result from excessive hypotensive response. If response is substantially diminished at 24 hours an increased dose or use of a twice daily regimen can be considered. **If Terazosin administration is discontinued for several days or longer, therapy should be reinstituted using the initial dosing regimen.** In clinical trials, except for the initial dose, the dose was given in the morning.

Use With Other Drugs: (see above).

Storage: Store tablets below 86°F (30°C).

REFERENCE
1. Lepor H. Role of alpha-adrenergic blockers in the treatment of benign prostatic hypertrophy. *Prostate* 1990; 3:75-84.

HOW SUPPLIED
TABLETS: 1 MG

BRAND/MANUFACTURER	NDC	SIZE	AWP
○ **BRAND**			
► HYTRIN: Abbott Pharm	00074-3322-13	100s	$122.23
	00074-3322-11	100s ud	$130.54
	00074-3322-53	500s	$611.15

TABLETS: 2 MG

BRAND/MANUFACTURER	NDC	SIZE	AWP
○ **BRAND**			
► HYTRIN: Abbott Pharm	00074-3323-13	100s	$122.23
	00074-3323-11	100s ud	$130.54
	00074-3323-53	500s	$611.15

TABLETS: 5 MG

BRAND/MANUFACTURER	NDC	SIZE	AWP
○ **BRAND**			
► HYTRIN: Abbott Pharm	00074-3324-13	100s	$122.23
	00074-3324-11	100s ud	$130.54
	00074-3324-53	500s	$611.15

TABLETS: 10 MG

BRAND/MANUFACTURER	NDC	SIZE	AWP
○ **BRAND**			
► HYTRIN: Abbott Pharm	00074-3325-13	100s	$122.23
	00074-3325-11	100s ud	$130.54
	00074-3325-53	500s	$566.14

Terbinafine Hydrochloride

DESCRIPTION
Terbinafine Hydrochloride Cream, 1%, contains the synthetic antifungal compound, Terbinafine Hydrochloride. It is intended for topical dermatologic use only.

Chemically, Terbinafine Hydrochloride is (E)-*N*-(6,6-dimethyl-2-hepten-4-ynyl)-*N*-methyl-1-naphthalenemethanamine hydrochloride. The compound has the empirical formula $C_{21}H_{26}ClN$, and a molecular weight of 327.90.

Terbinafine Hydrochloride is a white to off-white fine crystalline powder. It is freely soluble in methanol and methylene chloride, soluble in ethanol, and slightly soluble in water. Each gram of Terbinafine Hydrochloride Cream, 1%, contains 10 mg of Terbinafine Hydrochloride in a white cream base of benzyl alcohol NF, cetyl alcohol NF, cetyl palmitate, isopropyl myristate NF, polysorbate 60 NF, purified water USP, sodium hydroxide NF, sorbitan monostearate NF, and stearyl alcohol NF.

Following is its chemical structure:

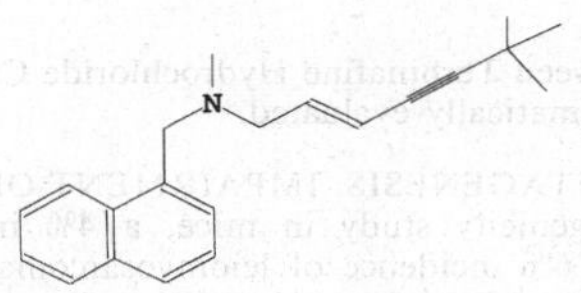

CLINICAL PHARMACOLOGY
PHARMACOKINETICS
Following a single application of 100 μL of Terbinafine Hydrochloride Cream, 1% (containing 1 mg of [14C-terbinafine) to a 30 cm² area of the ventral forearm of 6 healthy subjects, the recovery of radioactivity in urine and feces averaged 3.5% of the administered dose.

In a study of 16 healthy subjects, 8 of whose skin was artificially compromised by stripping the stratum corneum to the viable layer, single and multiple applications (average 0.1 mg/cm² B.I.D. for 5 days) of Terbinafine as Terbinafine Hydrochloride Cream, 1% were made to various sites. In this study, systemic absorption was highly variable. The maximum measured plasma concentration of terbinafine was 11.4 ng/mL, and the maximum measured plasma concentration of the de-methylated metabolite was 11.0 ng/mL. In many patients there were no detectable plasma levels of either parent compound or metabolite. Urinary excretion accounted for up to 9% of the topically applied dose; the majority excreted less than 4%. No measurement of fecal drug content was performed.

In a study of 10 patients with tinea cruris, once daily application of Terbinafine Hydrochloride Cream, 1% for 7 days resulted in plasma concentrations of terbinafine of 0-11 ng/mL on day 7. Plasma concentrations of the metabolites of Terbinafine ranged from 11-80 ng/mL in these patients.

Approximately 75% of cutaneously absorbed Terbinafine is eliminated in the urine predominantly as metabolites.

MICROBIOLOGY
Terbinafine Hydrochloride is a synthetic allylamine derivative. Terbinafine Hydrochloride exerts its antifungal effect by inhibiting squalene epoxidase, a key enzyme in sterol biosynthesis in fungi. This action results in a deficiency in ergosterol and a corresponding accumulation of squalene within the fungal cell and causes fungal cell death.

Terbinafine has been shown to be active against most strains of the following organisms both *in vitro* and in clinical infections at indicated body sites (see *"Indications and Usage"*):
Epidermophyton floccósum

Trichophyton mentagrophytes
Trichophyton rubrum

The following *in vitro* data are available: *however, their clinical significance is unknown.* Terbinafine exhibits satisfactory *in vitro* MIC's against most strains of the following organisms; however, the safety and efficacy of Terbinafine in treating clinical infections due to these organisms have not been established in adequate and well-controlled clinical trials.

Microsporum canis
Microsporum gypseum
Microsporum nanum
Trichophyton verrucosum

INDICATIONS AND USAGE
Terbinafine Hydrochloride Cream, 1% is indicated for the topical treatment of the following dermatologic infections: interdigital tinea pedis (athlete's foot), tinea cruris (jock itch), or tinea corporis (ringworm) due to *Epidermophyton floccosum, Trichophyton mentagrophytes, or Trichophyton rubrum* (see *"Dosage And Administration"*). Diagnosis of the disease should be confirmed either by direct microscopic examination of scrapings from infected tissue mounted in a solution of potassium hydroxide or by culture.

CONTRAINDICATIONS
Terbinafine Hydrochloride Cream, 1% is contraindicated in individuals who have known or suspected hypersensitivity to Terbinafine or any other of its components.

WARNINGS
Terbinafine Hydrochloride Cream, 1% is not for ophthalmic, oral, or intravaginal use.

PRECAUTIONS
GENERAL
If irritation or sensitivity develops with the use Terbinafine Hydrochloride Cream, 1%, treatment should be discontinued and appropriate therapy instituted.

INFORMATION FOR PATIENTS
The patient should be told to:
1. Use Terbinafine Hydrochloride Cream, 1% as directed by the physician and avoid contact with the eyes, nose, mouth, or other mucous membranes.
2. Use the medication for the treatment time recommended by the physician.
3. Inform the physician if the area of application shows signs of increased irritation or possible sensitization (redness, itching, burning, blistering, swelling, or oozing).
4. Avoid the use of occlusive dressings unless otherwise directed by the physician.

DRUG INTERACTIONS
Potential interactions between Terbinafine Hydrochloride Cream, 1% and other drugs have not been systematically evaluated.

CARCINOGENESIS, MUTAGENESIS, IMPAIRMENT OF FERTILITY
In a 2-year oral carcinogenicity study in mice, a 4% incidence of splenic hemangiosarcomas and a 6% incidence of leiomyosarcoma-like tumors of the seminal vesicles were observed in males at the highest dose level, 156 mg/kg/day (equivalent to at least 390 times the maximum potential exposure at the recommended human topical dose*). In a carcinogenicity study in rats at the highest dose level, 69 mg/kg/day (equivalent to at least 173 times the maximum potential exposure at the recommended human topical dose*), a 6% incidence of both liver tumors and skin lipomas were observed in males. In rats, the formation of liver tumors was associated with peroxisomal proliferation.

A battery of *in vitro* and *in vivo* genotoxicity tests, including Ames assay, mutagenicity evaluation in Chinese hamster ovarian cells, chromosome aberration test, sister chromatid exchanges, and mouse micronucleus test revealed no evidence for a mutagenic or clastogenic potential for the drug.

Reproductive studies in rats administered up to 300 mg/kg/day orally (equivalent to at least 750 times the maximum potential exposure at the recommended human topical dose*) did not reveal any adverse effects on fertility or other reproductive parameters. Intravaginal mucosal application of Terbinafine Hydrochloride at 150 mg/day in pregnant rabbits did not increase the incidence of abortions or premature deliveries or affect fetal parameters.

PREGNANCY
Pregnancy Category B: Oral doses of Terbinafine Hydrochloride, up to 300 mg/kg/day (equivalent to at least 750 times the maximum potential exposure at the recommended human topical dose*), during organogenesis in rats and rabbits were not teratogenic. Similarly, a subcutaneous study in rats at doses up to 100 mg/kg day (equivalent to at least 250 times the maximum potential exposure at the recommended human topical dose*) and a percutaneous study in rabbits, including doses up to 150 mg/kg/day (equivalent to at least 350 times the maximum potential exposure at the recommended human topical dose* did not reveal any teratogenic potential.

---

* The above comparisons between oral animal doses and maximum potential exposure at the recommended human topical doses are based upon the application to human skin of 0.1 mg of terbinafine/cm², the assumption of average human cutaneous exposure of 100 cm² [assuming the use of 1 gram of Terbinafine Hydrochloride Cream, 1% per dose] and the *theoretical* worst case scenario of 100% human cutaneous absorption. At present, comparative animal and human systemic exposure pharmacokinetic data are not available.

There are, however, no adequate and well-controlled studies in pregnant women. Because animal reproduction studies are not always predictive of human response, this drug should be used only if clearly indicated during pregnancy.

NURSING MOTHERS
After a single *oral* dose of 500 mg of Terbinafine Hydrochloride to 2 volunteers, the total dose of Terbinafine Hydrochloride secreted in human milk during the 72-hour post-dosing period was 0.65 mg in one person and 0.15 mg in the other. The total excretion of Terbinafine in human milk was 0.13% and 0.03% of the administered dose, respectively. The concentrations of the 1 metabolite measured in the human milk of these 2 volunteers were below the detection limit of the assay used (150 ng/mL of milk).

Because of the small amount of data on human neonatal exposure, a decision should be made whether to discontinue nursing or to discontinue the drug, taking into account the importance of the drug to the mother, as well as the findings of tumors in male mice and rats following *oral* administration of Terbinafine Hydrochloride and the lack of data on carcinogenicity in neonatal animals.

Nursing mothers should avoid application of Terbinafine Hydrochloride Cream, 1% to the breast.

PEDIATRIC USE
Safety and efficacy in children or infants below the age of 12 years have not been established.

ADVERSE REACTIONS
CLINICAL TRIALS
In clinical trials, 6 (0.2%) of 2265 patients treated with Terbinafine Hydrochloride Cream, 1% discontinued therapy due to adverse events and 52 (2.3%) reported adverse reactions thought to be possibly, probably, or definitely related to drug therapy. These reactions included irritation (1%), burning (0.8%), itching (0.2%), and dryness (0.2%).

OVERDOSAGE
Overdosage of Terbinafine Hydrochloride in humans has not been reported to date. Acute overdosage with topical application of Terbinafine Hydrochloride is unlikely due to the limited absorption of topically applied drug and would not be expected to lead to a life threatening situation.

Overdosage in rats and mice by the oral and intravenous routes of drug administration has produced sedation, drowsiness, ataxia, dyspnea, exophthalmus, and piloerection. The majority of deaths in animals occurred following oral administration of doses exceeding 3 grams/kilogram or following 200 mg/kg administered intravenously. In rabbits, overdosage produced erythema, edema, and scale formation following topical administration of doses in excess of 1.5 grams/kilogram.

When Terbinafine Hydrochloride Cream, 1% was administered as a single *oral* dose at 10 and 25 mL/kg (100 and 250 mg/kg, respectively) to rats and mice, no deaths or other drug-related toxicities were observed.

DOSAGE AND ADMINISTRATION
In the treatment of interdigital tinea pedis (athlete's foot), Terbinafine Hydrochloride Cream, 1% should be applied to cover the affected and immediately surrounding areas twice daily *until clinical signs and symptoms are significantly improved.* In many patients this occurs by day 7 of drug therapy. The duration of drug therapy should be for a minimum of 1 week and should not exceed 4 weeks. (See *"Clinical Studies"* and following *Note.*)

In the treatment of tinea cruris (jock itch) or tinea corporis (ringworm), Terbinafine Hydrochloride Cream, 1%, should be applied to cover the affected and immediately surrounding areas once or twice daily *until clinical signs and symptoms are significantly improved.* In many patients this occurs by day 7 of drug therapy. The duration of drug therapy should be for a minimum of 1 week and should note exceed 4 weeks. (See *"Clinical Studies"* and following *Note.*)

NOTE:
Many patients treated with shorter durations of therapy (1-2 weeks) continue to improve during the 2-4 weeks after drug therapy has been completed. As a consequence, patients should not be considered therapeutic failures until they have been observed for a period of 2-4 weeks off therapy. (See *"Clinical Studies".*)

If successful outcome is not achieved during the post-treatment observation period, the diagnosis should be reviewed.

CLINICAL STUDIES
In the following data presentations, the term "successful outcome" refers to those patients evaluated at a specific time point, who had both negative mycological results (culture and KOH preparation) and a *total* clinical score of less than 2. The clinical score is the sum of the scores of each sign and symptom graded on a scale from 0-absent to 3-severe. Mean clinical scores at entry ranged from 8-11 in the pivotal clinical trials. All studies included, at a minimum, clinical evaluation of erythema, desquamation, and pruritus.

A. TINEA PEDIS
In 3 studies of Terbinafine Hydrochloride Cream, 1% used B.I.D. in the treatment of tinea pedis, 2 (combined in the table below) were vehicle-controlled (placebo) evaluations of 1 week treatment duration. The third study (see following table) was of 4 weeks therapy compared to another active drug. (See related table).

SUCCESSFUL OUTCOMES

	1 Week Therapy			4 Weeks Therapy		
Therapy	At 1 wk. (end of Rx)	At 4 wks (3 wk f/up)	At 6 wks (5 wk f/up)	At 4 wks (end of Rx)	At 6 wks (2 wk f/up)	
Terbinafine Hydrochloride	14% (11/79)	51% (40/78)	65% (51/78)	71% (94/133)	73% (97/132)	
Vehicle	6% (5/79)	13% (10/75)	12% (8/69)			
Active Control	ND	ND	ND	63% (84/133)	59% (79/134)	

B. TINEA CORPORIS/CRURIS

Two studies (combined below) compared Terbinafine Hydrochloride Cream, 1% to vehicle (placebo), applied once daily for 1 week in the treatment of tinea corporis/cruris.

In the following table, sites of infection are separated into 2 groups: (1) tinea corporis and (2) tinea cruris. Patients with mixed tinea corporis/cruris are included in both groups.

SUCCESSFUL OUTCOMES AFTER 1 WEEK OF THERAPY

Disease	Drug	At 1 wk (end of Rx)	At 4 wks (3 wk f/up)
Corporis	Terbinafine Hydrochloride	21% (7/33)	83% (25/30)
	Vehicle	0% (0/31)	31% (4/13)
Cruris	Terbinafine Hydrochloride	43% (21/49)	92% (45/49)
	Vehicle	9% (5/58)	25% (7/28)

HOW SUPPLIED
CREAM: 1%

BRAND/MANUFACTURER	NDC	SIZE	AWP
○ **BRAND** LAMISIL: Sandoz Pharm	00078-0170-40	15 gm	$22.68
	00078-0170-46	30 gm	$40.80

Terbutaline Sulfate

DESCRIPTION

Terbutaline Sulfate USP, (±)α[(tert-butylamino) methyl]-3,5-dihydroxybenzyl-clcohol sulfate (2:1) (salt) is a beta-adrenergic agonist bronchodilator. The formula is $(C_{12}H_{19}NO_3)_2 \cdot M_2$ SO_4.

Terbutaline Sulfate is a bronchodilator available as tablets for oral administration, a subcutaneous injection, and an aerosol for oval inhalation.

Each tablet contains:
Terbutaline Sulfate ....2.5 mg or 5 mg
(2.05 or 4.1 mg of the free base)

Each ml of aerosol suspension contains:
Terbutaline Sulfate ....01 gm
(Each actuation delivers 0.20 mg from the mouthpiece)

Each ml of solution for injection contains:
Terbutaline Sulfate ....1 mg
(0.82 mg free base)

Terbutaline Sulfate USP is a white to gray-white crystalline powder. It is odorless or has a faint odor or acetic acid. It is soluble in water and in 0.1N hydrochloric acid, slightly soluble in methanol, and insoluble in chloroform. Its molecular weight is 548.65.

Following is its chemical structure:

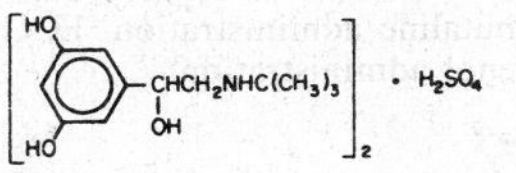

CLINICAL PHARMACOLOGY

Terbutaline Sulfate is a β-adrenergic-receptor agonist that has been shown by *in vitro* and *in vivo* studies in animals to exert a preferential effect on beta$_2$-adrenergic receptors. While it is recognized that beta$_2$-adrenergic receptors are the predominant receptors in bronchial smooth muscle, recent data indicate that there is a population of beta$_2$-receptors in the human heart existing in a concentration between 10-50%. The precise function of these, however, is not yet established (see "Precautions"). Controlled clinical studies in patients who were administered Terbutaline Sulfate subcutaneous injection or oral inhalation have not revealed a preferential beta$_2$-adrenergic effect. Controlled clinical studies in patients who were administered the drug orally have revealed proportionally greater changes in pulmonary function parameters than in heart rate or blood pressure. While this *suggests* a relative preference for the β$_2$ receptor in man, the usual cardiovascular effects commonly associated with sympathomimetic agents were also observed with Terbutaline Sulfate.

The pharmacologic effects of beta-adrenergic agonists, including Terbutaline Sulfate are at least in part attributable to stimulation through beta-adrenergic receptors of intracellular adenyl cyclase, the enzyme which catalyzes the conversion of adenosine triphosphate (ATP) to cyclic 3'5'-adenosine monophosphate (cAMP). Increased cAMP levels are associated with relaxation of bronchial smooth muscle and inhibition of release of mediators of immediate hypersensitivity from cells, especially from mast cells.

Terbutaline Sulfate has been shown in controlled clinical studies to relieve bronchospasm associated with chronic obstructive pulmonary disease such as asthma, chronic bronchitis, and emphysema. This action was manifested by a clinically significant improvement in pulmonary function as demonstrated by an increase in FEV$_1$ of 15% or more in some patients.

Following administration of Terbutaline Sulfate, a measurable change in flow rate is usually observed in 30 minutes, and a clinically significant improvement in pulmonary function occurs at 60-120 minutes. The maximum effect usually occurs within 120-180 minutes. Terbutaline Sulfate tablets also produce a clinically significant decrease in airway and pulmonary resistance which persists for at least four hours or longer. Significant bronchodilator action, as measured by various pulmonary function determinations (airway resistance, FEF$_{25-75\%}$, or PEFR), has been demonstrated in some studies for periods up to eight hours. Clinical studies were conducted in which the effectiveness of Terbutaline Sulfate tablets was evaluated in comparison with ephedrine over periods up to three months. Both drugs continued to produce significant improvement in pulmonary function throughout this period of treatment.

Following administration of 0.25 mg by subcutaneous injection, a measurable change in flow rate is usually observed within five minutes, and a clinically significant increase in FEV$_1$ occurs by 15 minutes following the injection. The maximum effect usually occurs within 30-60 minutes and clinically significant bronchodilator activity has been observed to persist for 90 minutes to four hours in most patients. The duration of clinically significant improvement is comparable to that found with equimilligram doses of epinephrine.

Subcutaneously administered Terbutaline Sulfate subcutaneous injection shows peak plasma concentrations 15-30 minutes after injection (0.5 mg dose, mean peak plasma level 7.6 μg/L). Approximately one-third is metabolized (inactive), the majority of the dose being excreted in urine unchanged. A half-life of 3-4 hours has been reported. Terbutaline Sulfate by inhaler also produced clinically significant increases in peak expiratory flow rate and instantaneous flow rates at 75, 50, and 25% of vital capacity. There were also clinically significant reductions in functional residual capacity, residual volume, and airway resistance in some patients. In controlled clinical trials the onset of improvement in pulmonary function was within 5 to 30 minutes. These studies also showed that maximum improvement in pulmonary function occurred at 120 minutes following two inhalations of Terbutaline Sulfate inhalation aerosol and that clinically significant improvement (i.e., 15% increase in FEV$_1$/predicted FEV$_1$) generally continued for 3 to 4 hours in most patients. In some studies there was a significant decrease in improvement of pulmonary function noted with continued administration of Terbutaline Sulfate aerosol. Continued effectiveness of Terbutaline Sulfate inhalation aerosol was demonstrated over a 14-week period in some patients in these clinical trials. Some patients with asthma, in single-dose studies only, have shown a therapeutic response that was still apparent at 6 hours.

Terbutaline crosses the placenta. After single dose IV administration of Terbutaline to 22 women in late pregnancy who were delivered by elective Caesarean section due to clinical reasons, umbilical blood levels of Terbutaline were found to range from 11 to 48% of the maternal blood levels.

Recent studies in laboratory animals (minipigs, rodents, and dogs), recorded the occurrence of cardiac arrhythmias and sudden death (with histologic evidence of myocardial necrosis) when beta agonists and methylxanthines were administered concurrently. The significance of these findings when applied to humans is currently unknown.

INDICATIONS AND USAGE

Terbutaline Sulfate is indicated as a bronchodilator for the relief of bronchospasm in patients with reversible obstructive airway disease. Such as asthma, brochitis, and emphysema.

UNLABELED USES
Terbutaline Sulfate is used alone or as an adjunct in the treatment of achalasia, congestive heart failure, cough, cystic fibrosis, and primary dysmenorrhea.

Terbutaline Sulfate is also used in the treatment of hyaline membrane disease, intrauterine fetal distress, status asthmatious, urticaria, prevention of preterm labor, and in the treatment of intraoperative penile erection.

CONTRAINDICATIONS

Terbutaline Sulfate is contraindicated in patients with a history of hypersensitivity to any of its components or to sympathomimetic amines.

WARNINGS

As with other adrenergic aerosols, the potential for paradoxical bronchospasm (which can be life-threatening) should be kept in mind. If it occurs, the preparation should be discontinued immediately and alternative therapy instituted.

Fatalities have been reported in association with excessive use of inhaled sympathomimetic drugs. The exact cause of death is unknown. As with other beta-adrenergic aerosols, Terbutaline Sulfate inhalers should not be used in excess.

Controlled clinical studies and other clinical experience have shown that Terbutaline Sulfate, like other beta-adrenergic agonists, can produce a significant cardiovascular effect in some patients, as measured by pulse rate, blood pressure, symptoms, and/or ECG changes.

There have been rare reports of seizures in patients receiving Terbutaline; seizures did not recur in these patients after the drug was discontinued.

The contents of Terbutaline Sulfate aerosol inhalers are under pressure. Do not puncture the container. Do not use or store it near heat or open flame. Exposure to temperatures above 120°F may cause bursting. Never throw the container into a fire or incinerator. Keep it out of children's reach.

PRECAUTIONS

GENERAL

Terbutaline Sulfate is a sympathomimetic amine and, as such, should be used with caution in patients with cardiovascular disorders, including arrhythmias, coronary insufficiency and hypertension, in patients with hyperthyroidism or diabetes mellitus, or history of seizures, and in patients who are unusually responsive to sympathomimetic amines.

Age related differences in the hemodynamic response to β-adrenergic receptor stimulation have been reported.

Patients susceptible to hypokalemia should be monitored because transient early falls in serum potassium levels have been reported with β agonists.

Immediate hypersensitivity reactions and exacerbation of bronchospasm have been reported after Terbutaline administration.

Large doses of intravenous Terbutaline Sulfate have been reported to aggravate preexisting diabetes and ketoacidosis. Terbutaline Sulfate should not be used for tocolysis.

The concomitant use of Terbutaline Sulfate with other sympathomimetic agents is not recommended, since their combined effect on the cardiovascular system may be deleterious to the patient. However, this does not preclude the use of an aerosol bronchodilator of the adrenergic stimulant type for the relief of an acute bronchospasm in patients receiving chronic oral Terbutaline Sulfate therapy.

Use of the subcutaneous injection for preparation of other dosage forms, e.g., IV infusion, is not appropriate. Sterility, stability, and accurate dosing cannot be assured if the solution for injection is not used in accordance with information in *"Dosage and Administration"*.

INFORMATION FOR PATIENTS

The action of Terbutaline Sulfate aerosol inhalation may last up to 6 hours and, therefore, it should not be used more frequently than recommended.

Patients should not increase the number or frequency of doses without consulting the physician. If symptoms get worse, patients should consult their physician promptly. While taking Terbutaline Sulfate aerosol inhalation, patients should not take other inhaled medicines that have not been prescribed by the physician.

DRUG INTERACTIONS

Other sympathomimetic bronchodilators or epinephrine should not be used concomitantly with Terbutaline Sulfate. Terbutaline Sulfate should be administered with caution to patients being treated with monoamine oxidase inhibitors or tricyclic antidepressants, since the action of Terbutaline Sulfate on the vascular system may be potentiated.

Beta-receptor-blocking agents and Terbutaline Sulfate inhibit the effect of each other. β-adrenergic receptor blocking agents not only block the pulmonary effect of Terbutaline but may produce severe asthmatic attacks in asthmatic patients. Therefore, patients requiring treatment for both bronchospastic disease and hypertension should be treated with medication other than β-adrenergic blocking agents for hypertension.

CARCINOGENESIS, MUTAGENESIS, IMPAIRMENT OF FERTILITY

A 2-year oral carcinogenesis bioassay of Terbutaline Sulfate (50, 500, 1000, and 2000 mg/kg, corresponding to 1042, 10,417, 20,833, and 41,667 times the recommended daily adult inhaled dose or 5,000, 50,000, 100,000, and 200,000 times the recommended adult subcutaneous dose) in Sprague-Dawley rats revealed drug-related changes in the female genital system. Female rats showed dose-related increases in leiomyomas of the mesovarium: 3 (5%) at 50 mg/kg, 17 (28%) at 500 mg/kg, 21 (35%) at 1000 mg/kg, and 23 (38%) at 2000 mg/kg, which were significant at the three highest levels. None occurred in female controls. The incidence of ovarian cysts was significantly elevated at all dose levels except 2000

mg/kg, and hyperplasia of the mesovarium was increased significantly at 500 and 2000 mg/kg.

A 21-month oral (feeding) study of Terbutaline Sulfate (5, 50, and 200 mg/kg, corresponding to 104, 1042, and 4167 times the recommended daily adult inhaled dose or 500, 5,000, and 20,000 times the recommended daily adult subcutaneous dose) in the mouse revealed no evidence of carcinogenicity.

Studies of Terbutaline Sulfate have not been conducted to determine mutagenic potential.

A Segment 1 oral reproduction study of Terbutaline Sulfate (up to 50 mg/kg corresponding to 1042 times the maximum clinical dose or 5,000 times the human subcutaneous dose) in the rat revealed no adverse effects on fertility.

PREGNANCY CATEGORY B

Reproduction studies have been performed in mice (up to 1.1 mg/kg subcutaneously, corresponding to 110 times the human subcutaneous dose) and in rats and rabbits at doses up to 1042 times the human aerosol dose or 5,000 times the subcutaneous dose and have revealed no evidence of impaired fertility or harm to the fetus due to Terbutaline Sulfate. There are, however, no adequate and well-controlled studies in pregnant women. Because animal reproduction studies are not always predictive of human response, this drug should be used during pregnancy only if clearly needed.

USAGE IN LABOR AND DELIVERY

Terbutaline Sulfate is not indicated and should not be used for the management of preterm labor. It has been reported that high doses of Terbutaline Sulfate administered intravenously inhibit uterine contractions.

Serious adverse reactions have been reported following administration of Terbutaline Sulfate to women in labor. In the mother, these include increased heart rate, transient hyperglycemia, hypokalemia, cardiac arrhythmias, pulmonary edema, and myocardial ischemia. Increased fetal heart rate and neonatal hypoglycemia may occur as a result of maternal administration. Maternal death has been reported with Terbutaline Sulfate and other drugs of this class.

NURSING MOTHERS

Terbutaline is excreted in breast milk.

Caution should be exercised when Terbutaline Sulfate is administered to a nursing woman.

PEDIATRIC USE

Safety and effectiveness in children below the age of 12 years have not been established.

ADVERSE REACTIONS

The adverse reactions of Terbutaline Sulfate are similar to those of other sympathomimetic agents. Commonly observed side effects include nervousness and tremor. These occur more frequently at subcutaneous doses in excess of 0.25 mg. Other reported reactions include headache, increased heart rate, palpitations, dizziness, drowsiness, nausea, vomiting, sweating, and muscle cramps. These reactions are generally transient in nature and usually do not require treatment. The frequency of these side effects appears to diminish with continued therapy. In general, all the side effects observed are characteristic of those commonly seen with sympathomimetic amines.

There have been rare reports of elevations in liver enzymes and of hypersensitivity vasculitis. A 14-week double-blind study compared Terbutaline Sulfate and isoproterenol aerosols in 259 asthmatic patients. The results of this study showed that the incidence of cardiovascular effects was as follows: palpitations, none with Terbutaline and fewer than 5 per 100 with isoproterenol; tachycardia, about 3 per 100 with Terbutaline and about 2 per 100 with isoproterenol; and increased blood pressure, fewer than 1 per 100 with Terbutaline and about 2 per 100 with isoproterenol; and increased blood pressure, fewer than 1 per 100 with Terbutaline and about 2 per 100 with isoproterenol. In the same study, both drugs caused headache and nausea or digestive disorder in fewer than 10 patients per 100, tremor or nervousness in fewer than 5 patients per 100, and drowsiness in fewer than 5 patients per 100. About 4% of patients receiving Terbutaline and about 1% of patients receiving isoproterenol had dysrhythmias. In addition, Terbutaline Sulfate, like other sympathomimetic agents, can cause adverse reactions such as angina, dyspnea and wheezing, vomiting, vertigo, central stimulation, insomnia, unusual taste, and drying or irritation of the oropharynx. Significantly more patients experienced dyspnea or wheezing, or both, after Terbutaline than after isoproterenol administration. ECG changes such as sinus pause, atrial premature beats, AV block, ventricular premature beats, ST-T-wave depression, T-wave inversion, sinus bradycardia, and atrial escape beat with aberrant conduction were described after Terbutaline administration. ECG changes were similar in frequency after isoproterenol administration.

OVERDOSAGE

Overdosage experience is limited. Excessive beta-adrenergic-receptor stimulation may augment the signs and symptoms listed under *"Adverse Reactions"* and may be accompanied by other adrenergic effects. In the case of Terbutaline overdosage, the patient should be treated symptomatically for the sympathomimetic overdosage with careful consideration given to the appropriateness of any chosen therapy and to the possible effect on the patient's underlying disease state.

Signs and symptoms of overdosage may include the following—

Cardiovascular: tachycardia of varying degrees, transient arrhythmias, and extrasystoles. A significant drop in blood pressure may occur due to peripheral vasodilation.

◆ RATED THERAPEUTICALLY EQUIVALENT; ◇ THERAPEUTIC EQUIVALENCE UNCONFIRMED; ○ UNRATED

Neuromuscular: tremors of varying degrees, nervousness, drowsiness, muscle cramps, headache, and sweating.

Gastrointestinal: nausea and vomiting.

Endocrine: varying degrees of hyperglycemia and rise in insulin levels which could be followed by rebound hypoglycemia. Hypokalemia in the early stages may occur. The duration of these signs and symptoms will be dependent on the degree of overdosage.

Studies in mice, rats, rabbits, and dogs have established the LD_{50} of Terbutaline to be 1-9 g/kg orally and 0.3-1.6 g/kg subcutaneously.

It is not known whether Terbutaline is dialyzable.

Treat the alert patient who has taken excessive oral medication by emptying the stomach by means of induced emesis, followed by gastric lavage. In the unconscious patient, secure the airway with a cuffed endotracheal tube before beginning lavage (do not induce emesis). Instillation of activated charcoal slurry may help reduce absorption of Terbutaline Sulfate. Maintain adequate respiratory exchange. Provide cardiac and respiratory support as needed. Continue observation until symptom-free.

DOSAGE AND ADMINISTRATION
INHALATION AEROSOL TABLETS
The usual oral dose of Terbutaline Sulfate tablets for adults is 5 mg administered at approximately six-hour intervals, three times daily, during the hours the patient is usually awake. If side effects are particularly disturbing, the dose may be reduced to 2.5 mg three times daily, and still provide a clinically significant improvement in pulmonary function. A dose of 2.5 mg, three times daily, also is recommended for children in the 12- to 15-year group Terbutaline Sulfate tablets are not recommended at present for use in children below the age of 12 years. In adults, a total dose of 15 mg should not be exceeded in a 24-hour period. In children, a total dose of 7.5 mg should not be exceeded in a 24-hour period.

SUBCUTANEOUS INJECTION
Parenteral drug products should be inspected visually for particulate matter and discoloration prior to administration, whenever solution and container permit.

The usual subcutaneous dose of Terbutaline Sulfate is 0.25 mg (0.25 ml) injected into the lateral deltoid area. If significant clinical improvement does not occur by 15-30 minutes, a second dose of 0.25 mg may be administered. A total dose of 0.5 mg should not be exceeded within a four-hour period. If a patient fails to respond to a second 0.25 mg (0.25 ml) dose within 15-30 minutes, other therapeutic measures should be considered.

The usual dosage for adults and children 12 years and older is two inhalations separated by a 60-second interval, repeated every 4 to 6 hours. Dosing should not be repeated more often than every 4 to 6 hours. The use of Terbutaline Sulfate inhalation aerosol can be continued as medically indicated to control recurring bouts of bronchospasm. During this time most patients gain optimal benefit from regular use of the inhaler. Safe usage for periods extending over several years has been documented.

If a previously effective dosage regimen fails to provide the usual relief, medical advice should be sought immediately, as this is often a sign of seriously worsening asthma, which would require reassessment of therapy.

Store all forms of Terbutaline Sulfate between 59°-86°F(15°-30°C).

Solutions of Terbutaline Sulfate are sensitive to excessive heat and light. The solution for injection should, therefore, be stored in the original carton to provide protection from light until dispensed. Solutions should not be used if discolored.

WARNING
Certain brands of Terbutaline Sulfate inhalers may contain CFC-11, CFC-12, and CFC-114, substances which harm public health and environment by destroying ozone in the upper atmosphere.

J CODES
Up to 1 mg SC,IV—J3105

HOW SUPPLIED
AEROSOL SOLID INGREDIENTS: 0.2 MG/INH

BRAND/MANUFACTURER	NDC	SIZE	AWP
◆ **BRAND**			
BRETHAIRE: Geigy	00028-5557-87	7.5 gm	$17.64

AEROSOL SOLID W/ADAPTER: 0.2 MG/INH

BRAND/MANUFACTURER	NDC	SIZE	AWP
◆ **BRAND**			
BRETHAIRE: Geigy	00028-5557-88	7.5 gm	$19.95

INJECTION: 1 MG/ML

AVERAGE UNIT PRICE (AVAILABLE SIZES)			
BRAND	$1.61		

BRAND/MANUFACTURER	NDC	SIZE	AWP
◆ **BRAND**			
BRETHINE: Geigy	00028-7507-23	1 ml 10s	$17.87
	00028-7507-01	1 ml 100s	$142.33
◆ **GENERICS**			
BRICANYL: Marion Merrell Dow	00068-0702-20	1 ml 10s	$26.16

TABLETS: 2.5 MG

BRAND/MANUFACTURER	NDC	SIZE	AWP
◇ **BRAND**			
▶ BRETHINE: Geigy	00028-0072-01	100s	$24.41
	00028-0072-61	100s ud	$26.85
	00028-0072-10	1000s	$230.65
	00028-0072-65	1200s	$294.41
◇ **GENERICS**			
▶ BRICANYL: Marion Merrell Dow	00068-0725-61	100s	$28.68

TABLETS: 5 MG

BRAND/MANUFACTURER	NDC	SIZE	AWP
◇ **BRAND**			
▶ BRETHINE: Geigy	00028-0105-01	100s	$35.15
	00028-0105-61	100s ud	$37.62
	00028-0105-10	1000s	$332.53
	00028-0105-65	1200s	$423.66
◇ **GENERICS**			
▶ BRICANYL: Marion Merrell Dow	00068-0750-61	100s	$41.16

Terconazole

DESCRIPTION
Terconazole Vaginal Suppositories are white to off-white suppositories for intravaginal administration containing 80 mg of the antifungal agent Terconazole, cis-1-[4-[[2-(2,4-dichlorophenyl)-2-(1H-1,2,4-triazol-1- ylmethyl) -1,3-dioxolan-4-yl]methoxy]phenyl]-4-(1-methylethyl)piperazine, in triglycerides derived from coconut and/or palm kernel oil (a base of hydrogenated vegetable oils) and butylated hydroxyanisole.

Terconazole, a triazole derivative, is a white to almost white powder with a molecular weight of 532.47. It is insoluble in water; sparingly soluble in ethanol; and soluble in butanol.

Following is its chemical structure:

$$(CH_3)_2CH-N \quad N-\langle\text{phenyl}\rangle-OCH_2 \quad O \quad CH_2 \quad Cl$$

CLINICAL PHARMACOLOGY
Microbiology: Terconazole exhibits fungicidal activity in *vitro* against *Candida albicans.* The MIC values for Terconazole against most species of lactic acid bacteria typically found in the human vagina were $\geq$ 128 mcg/ml, therefore, these beneficial bacteria are not affected by drug treatment. The exact pharmacologic mode of action of Terconazole is uncertain; however, it may exert its antifungal activity by the disruption of normal fungal cell membrane permeability. No resistance to Terconazole has developed during successive passages of *C. albicans.*

Human Pharmacology: Following intravaginal administration of Terconazole in humans, absorption ranged from 5-8% in three hysterectomized subjects and 12-16% in two non-hysterectomized subjects with tubal ligations. Following oral (30 mg) administration of ^{14}C-labelled Terconazole, the half-life of elimination from the blood for the parent Terconazole was 6 9 hours (range 4 0-11.3). Terconazole is extensively metabolized; the plasma AUC for Terconazole compared to the AUC for total radioactivity was 0.6%. Total radioactivity was eliminated from the blood with a half-life of 52.2 hours (range 44-60). Excretion of radioactivity was both by renal (32-56%) and fecal (47-52%) routes.

Photosensitivity reactions were observed in some normal volunteers following repeated dermal application of Terconazole 2.0% and 0.8% creams under conditions of filtered artificial ultraviolet light.

Photosensitivity reactions have not been observed in U.S. and foreign clinical trials in patients who were treated vaginally with Terconazole suppositories or cream.

INDICATIONS AND USAGE
Terconazole Vaginal Suppositories are indicated for the local treatment of vulvovaginal candidiasis (moniliasis). As Terconazole Vaginal Suppositories are effective only for vulvovaginitis caused by the genus *Candida,* the diagnosis should be confirmed by KOH smears and/or cultures.

CONTRAINDICATIONS
Patients known to be hypersensitive to Terconazole or to any components of the suppository.

WARNINGS
None.

PRECAUTIONS
General: Discontinue use and do not retreat with Terconazole if sensitization, irritation, fever, chills or flu-like symptoms are reported during use. The base contained in the suppository formulation may interact with certain rubber latex products, such as those used in vaginal contraceptive diaphragms, therefore

concurrent use is not recommended. If there is lack of response to Terconazole Vaginal Suppositories, appropriate microbiological studies (standard KOH smear and/or cultures) should be repeated to confirm the diagnosis and rule out other pathogens.

Drug Interactions: The therapeutic effect of Terconazole Vaginal Suppositories is not affected by oral contraceptive usage.

CARCINOGENESIS, MUTAGENESIS, IMPAIRMENT OF FERTILITY
Carcinogenesis: Studies to determine the carcinogenic potential of Terconazole have not been performed.

Mutagenicity: Terconazole was not mutagenic when tested *in vitro* for induction of microbial point mutations (Ames test), or for inducing cellular transformation, or *in vivo* for chromosome breaks (micronucleus test) or dominant lethal mutations in mouse germ cells.

Impairment of Fertility: No impairment of fertility occurred when female rats were administered Terconazole orally up to 40 mg/kg/day.

Pregnancy: Pregnancy Category C.

There was no evidence of teratogenicity when Terconazole was administered orally up to 40 mg/kg/day (25 x the recommended intravaginal human dose) in rats, or 20 mg/kg/day in rabbits, or subcutaneously in rats up to 20 mg/kg/day. Dosages at or below 10 mg/kg/day produced no embryotoxicity; however, there was a delay in fetal ossification at 10 mg/kg/day in rats. There was some evidence of embryotoxicity in rabbits and rats at 20-40 mg/kg. In rats this was reflected as a decrease in little size and number of viable young and reduced fetal weight. There was also delay in ossification and an increased incidence of skeletal variants.

The no-effect oral dose of 10 mg/kg/day resulted in a mean peak plasma level of Terconazole in pregnant rats of 0.176 mcg/ml which exceeds by 44 times the mean peak plasma level (0.004 mcg/ml) seen in normal subjects after intravaginal administration of Terconazole. This assessment does not account for possible exposure of the fetus through direct transfer of Terconazole from the irritated vagina to the fetus by diffusion across amniotic membranes.

Since Terconazole is absorbed from the human vagina, it should not be used in the first trimester of pregnancy unless the physician considers it essential to the welfare of the patient.

Nursing Mothers: It is not known whether Terconazole is excreted in human milk. Animal studies have shown that rat off-spring exposed via the milk of treated (40 mg/kg/orally) dams showed decreased survival during the first few post-partum days. Because many drugs are excreted in human milk, and because of the potential for adverse reaction in nursing infants from Terconazole, a decision should be made whether to discontinue nursing or to discontinue the drug, taking into account the importance of the drug to the mother.

Pediatric Use: Safety and efficacy in children have not been established.

ADVERSE REACTIONS
During controlled clinical studies conducted in the United States. 284 patients with vulvovaginal candidiasis were treated with Terconazole 80 mg vaginal suppositories. Based on comparative analyses with placebo (295 patients) the adverse experiences considered adverse reactions most likely related to Terconazole 80 mg vaginal suppositories were headache (30.3% vs 20.7% with placebo) and pain of the female genitalia (4.2% vs 0.7% with placebo). Adverse reactions that were reported but were not statistically significantly different from placebo were burning (15.2% vs 11.2% with placebo) and body pain (3.9% vs 1.7% with placebo). Fever (2.8% vs 1.4% with placebo) and chills (1.8% vs 0.7% with placebo) have also been reported. The therapy-related dropout rate was 3.5% and the placebo therapy-related dropout rate was 2.7%. The adverse drug experience on Terconazole most frequently causing discontinuation was burning (2.5% vs 1.4% with placebo) and pruritus (1.8% vs 1.4% with placebo).

DOSAGE AND ADMINISTRATION
One Terconazole Vaginal Suppository (80 mg Terconazole) is administered intravaginally once daily at bedtime for three consecutive days. Before prescribing another course of therapy, the diagnosis should be reconfirmed by smears and/or cultures and other pathogens commonly associated with vulvovaginitis ruled out. The therapeutic effect of Terconazole Vaginal Suppositories is not affected by menstruation.

Store at controlled room temperature (59°F-86°F or 15°C-30°C).

HOW SUPPLIED
CREAM: 0.4%

BRAND/MANUFACTURER	NDC	SIZE	AWP
○ **BRAND**			
TERAZOL 7: Ortho Pharm	00062-5350-01	45 gm	$22.26

CREAM: 0.8%

BRAND/MANUFACTURER	NDC	SIZE	AWP
○ **BRAND**			
TERAZOL 3: Ortho Pharm	00062-5356-01	20 gm	$22.26

SUPPOSITORY: 80 MG

BRAND/MANUFACTURER	NDC	SIZE	AWP
○ **BRAND**			
TERAZOL 3: Ortho Pharm	00062-5351-01	3s	$22.26

Terfenadine

WARNING BOX
QT INTERVAL PROLONGATION/VENTRICULAR ARRHYTHMIA
RARE CASES OF SERIOUS CARDIOVASCULAR ADVERSE EVENTS, INCLUDING DEATH, CARDIAC ARREST, TORSADES DE POINTES, AND OTHER VENTRICULAR ARRHYTHMIAS, HAVE BEEN OBSERVED IN THE FOLLOWING CLINICAL SETTINGS, FREQUENTLY IN ASSOCIATION WITH INCREASED TERFENADINE LEVELS WHICH LEAD TO ELECTROCARDIOGRAPHIC QT PROLONGATION:
1. CONCOMITANT ADMINISTRATION OF KETOCONAZOLE OR ITRACONAZOLE
2. OVERDOSE, INCLUDING SINGLE DOSES AS LOW AS 360 MG
3. CONCOMITANT ADMINISTRATION OF CLARITHROMYCIN, ERYTHROMYCIN, OR TROLEANDOMYCIN
4. SIGNIFICANT HEPATIC DYSFUNCTION
TERFENADINE IS CONTRAINDICATED IN PATIENTS TAKING KETOCONAZOLE, ITRACONAZOLE, ERYTHROMYCIN, CLARITHROMYCIN, OR TROLEANDOMYCIN, AND IN PATIENTS WITH SIGNIFICANT HEPATIC DYSFUNCTION.
DO NOT EXCEED RECOMMENDED DOSE.
IN SOME CASES, SEVERE ARRHYTHMIAS HAVE BEEN PRECEDED BY EPISODES OF SYNCOPE. SYNCOPE IN PATIENTS RECEIVING TERFENADINE SHOULD LEAD TO DISCONTINUATION OF TREATMENT AND FULL EVALUATION OF POTENTIAL ARRHYTHMIAS.
(SEE *"CONTRAINDICATIONS", "WARNINGS," "CLINICAL PHARMACOLOGY,"* AND *"PRECAUTIONS: DRUG INTERACTIONS."*)

DESCRIPTION
Terfenadine is available as tablets for oral administration. Each tablet contains 60 mg Terfenadine. Terfenadine is a histamine H_1-receptor antagonist with the chemical name α-[4-(1,1-Dimethylethyl) phenyl]-4-(hydroxy-diphenylmethyl)- 1-piperidinebutanol (±). The molecular weight is 471.68. The molecular formula is $C_{32}H_{41}NO_2$.

Terfenadine occurs as a white to off-white crystalline powder. It is freely soluble in chloroform, soluble in ethanol, and very slightly soluble in water.

Following is its chemical structure:

CLINICAL PHARMACOLOGY
Terfenadine is chemically distinct from other antihistamines.

Histamine skin wheal studies have shown that Terfenadine in single and repeated doses of 60 mg in 64 subjects has an antihistaminic effect beginning at 1-2 hours, reaching its maximum at 3-4 hours, and lasting in excess of 12 hours. The correlation between response on skin wheal testing and clinical efficacy is unclear. The four best controlled and largest clinical trials each lasted 7 days and involved about 1,000 total patients in comparisons of Terfenadine (60 mg b.i.d.) with an active drug (chlorpheniramine, 4 mg t.i.d.; dexchlorpheniramine, 2 mg t.i.d.; or clemastine 1 mg b.i.d.). About 50-70% of Terfenadine or other antihistamine recipients had moderate to complete relief of symptoms, compared with 30-50% of placebo recipients. The frequency of drowsiness with Terfenadine was similar to the frequency with placebo and less than with other antihistamines. None of these studies showed a difference between Terfenadine and other antihistamines in the frequency of anticholinergic effects. In studies which include 52 subjects in whom EEG assessments were made, no depressant effects have been observed.

Animal studies have demonstrated that Terfenadine is a histamine H_1-receptor antagonist. In these animal studies, no sedative or anticholinergic effects were observed at effective antihistaminic doses. Radioactive disposition and autoradiographic studies in rats and radioligand binding studies with guinea pig brain H_1-receptors indicate that, at effective antihistamine doses, neither Terfenadine nor its metabolites penetrate the blood brain barrier well.

On the basis of a mass balance study using ^{14}C labeled Terfenadine the oral absorption of Terfenadine was estimated to be at least 70%. Terfenadine itself undergoes extensive (99%) first pass metabolism to two primary metabolites, an active acid metabolite and an inactive dealkylated metabolite. Therefore, systemic availability of Terfenadine is low under normal conditions, and parent Terfenadine is not normally detectable in plasma at levels > 10 ng/mL. Although in rare cases there was measurable plasma Terfenadine in apparently normal individuals without identifiable risk factors, the implications of this finding with respect to the variability of Terfenadine metabolism in the normal population cannot be assessed without further study. Further studies of Terfenadine

---

metabolism in the general population are pending. From information gained in the ^{14}C study it appears that approximately forty percent of the total dose is eliminated renally (40% as acid metabolite, 30% dealkyl metabolite, and 30% minor unidentified metabolites). Sixty percent of the dose is eliminated in the feces (50% as the acid metabolite, 2% unchanged Terfenadine, and the remainder as minor unidentified metabolites). Studies investigating the effect of hepatic and renal insufficiency or the metabolism and excretion of Terfenadine are incomplete. Preliminary information indicates that in cases of hepatic impairment, significant concentrations of unchanged Terfenadine can be detected with the rate of acid metabolite formation being decreased. A single-dose study in patients with hepatic impairment revealed increased parent terfenadine and impaired metabolism, suggesting that additional drug accumulation may occur after repetitive dosing in such patients. Terfenadine is contraindicated for use in patients with significant hepatic dysfunction. (See "Contraindications" and "Warnings".) In subjects with normal hepatic function, unchanged terfenadine plasma concentrations have not been detected. **Elevated levels of parent Terfenadine, whether due to significant hepatic dysfunction, concomitant medications, or overdose, have been associated with QT interval prolongation and serious cardiac adverse events.** (See "Contraindications" and "Warnings".) In controlled clinical trials in otherwise normal patients with rhinitis, small increases in QTc interval were observed at doses of 60 mg b.i.d. In studies at 300 mg b.i.d. a mean increase in QTc of 10% (range –4% to +30%) (mean increase of 46 msec) was observed.

Data have been reported demonstrating that compared to young subjects, elderly subjects experience a 25% reduction in clearance of the acid metabolite after single-dose oral administration of 120 mg. Further studies are necessary to fully characterize pharmacokinetics in the elderly.

In vitro studies demonstrate that Terfenadine is extensively (97%) bound to human serum protein while the acid metabolite is approximately 70% bound to human serum protein. Based on data gathered from *in vitro* models of antihistaminic activity, the acid metabolite of Terfenadine has approximately 30% of the H_1 blocking activity of Terfenadine. The relative contribution of Terfenadine and the acid metabolite to the pharmacodynamic effects have not been clearly defined. Since unchanged Terfenadine is usually not detected in plasma, and active acid metabolite concentrations are relatively high, the acid metabolite may be the entity responsible for the majority of efficacy after oral administration of Terfenadine.

In a study involving the administration of a single 60 mg Terfenadine tablet to 24 subjects, mean peak plasma levels of the acid metabolite were 263 ng/mL (range 133-423 ng/mL) and occurred approximately 2.5 hours after dosing. Plasma concentrations of unchanged Terfenadine were not detected. The elimination profile of the acid metabolite was biphasic in nature with an initial mean plasma half-life of 3.5 hours followed by a mean plasma half-life of 6 hours. Ninety percent of the plasma level time curve was associated with these half-lives. Although the elimination profile is somewhat complex, the effective pharmacokinetic half-life can be estimated at approximately 8.5 hours. However, receptor binding and pharmacologic effects, both therapeutic and adverse, may persist well beyond that time.

INDICATIONS AND USAGE
Terfenadine is indicated for the relief of symptoms associated with seasonal allergic rhinitis such as sneezing, rhinorrhea, pruritus, and lacrimation.

Clinical studies conducted to date have not demonstrated effectiveness of terfenadine in the common cold.

UNLABELED USES
Terfenadine is used alone or as an adjunct in the treatment of asthma, exercise-induced asthma, and chronic idiopathic urticaria.

CONTRAINDICATIONS
CONCOMITANT ADMINISTRATION OF TERFENADINE WITH KETOCONAZOLE OR ITRACONAZOLE IS CONTRAINDICATED. TERFENADINE IS ALSO CONTRAINDICATED IN PATIENTS WITH DISEASE STATES OR OTHER CONCOMITANT MEDICATIONS KNOWN TO IMPAIR ITS METABOLISM, INCLUDING SIGNIFICANT HEPATIC DYSFUNCTION, AND CONCURRENT USE OF CLARITHROMYCIN, ERYTHROMYCIN, OR TROLEANDOMYCIN. QT PROLONGATION HAS BEEN DEMONSTRATED IN SOME PATIENTS TAKING TERFENADINE IN THESE SETTINGS, AND RARE CASES OF SERIOUS CARDIOVASCULAR EVENTS, INCLUDING DEATH, CARDIAC ARREST, AND TORSADES DE POINTES, HAVE BEEN REPORTED IN THESE PATIENT POPULATIONS. (See "Warnings" and "Precautions: Drug Interactions.")

Terfenadine is contraindicated in patients with a known hypersensitivity to Terfenadine or any of its ingredients.

WARNINGS
Terfenadine undergoes extensive metabolism in the liver by a specific cytochrome P450 isoenzyme. This metabolic pathway may be impaired in patients with hepatic dysfunction (alcoholic cirrhosis, hepatitis) or who are taking drugs such as ketoconazole, itraconazole, or clarithromycin, erythromycin, or troleandomycin (macrolide antibiotics), or other potent inhibitors of this isoenzyme. Interference with this metabolism can lead to elevated Terfenadine plasma levels associated with QT prolongation and increased risk of ventricular tachyarrhythmias (such as torsades de pointes, ventricular tachycardia, and ventricular fibrillation) at the recommended dose. Terfenadine is contraindicated for use by patients with these conditions (see "Warning" box, "Contraindications", and "Precautions: Drug Interactions").

Other patients who may be at risk for these adverse cardiovascular events include patients who may experience new or increased QT prolongation while receiving certain drugs or having conditions which lead to QT prolongation. These include patients taking certain antiarrhythmics, bepridil, certain psychotropics, probucol, or astemizole; patients with electrolyte abnormalities such as hypokalemia or hypomagnesemia, or taking diuretics with potential for inducing electrolyte abnormalities; and patients with congenital QT syndrome. Terfenadine is not recommended for use by patients with these conditions.

The relationship of underlying cardiac disease to the development of ventricular tachyarrhythmias while on Terfenadine therapy is unclear; nonetheless, Terfenadine should also be used with caution in these patients.

PRECAUTIONS
INFORMATION FOR PATIENTS
Patients taking Terfenadine should receive the following information and instructions. Antihistamines are prescribed to reduce allergic symptoms. Patients should be advised to take Terfenadine only as needed and *Not To Exceed The Prescribed Dose*. Patients should be questioned about use of any other prescription or over-the-counter medication, and should be cautioned regarding the potential for life-threatening arrhythmias with concurrent use of ketoconazole, itraconazole, clarithromycin, erythromycin, or troleandomycin. Patients should be advised to consult the physician before concurrent use of other medications with Terfenadine. Patients should be questioned about pregnancy or lactation before starting Terfenadine therapy, since the drug should be used in pregnancy or lactation only if the potential benefit justifies the potential risk to fetus or baby. Patients should also be instructed to store this medication in a tightly closed container in a cool, dry place, away from heat or direct sunlight, and away from children.

DRUG INTERACTIONS
Ketoconazole: Spontaneous adverse reaction reports of patients taking concomitant ketoconazole with recommended doses of terfenadine demonstrate QT interval prolongation and rare serious cardiac events, e.g. death, cardiac arrest, and ventricular arrhythmia including torsades de pointes. Pharmacokinetic data indicate that ketoconazole markedly inhibits the metabolism of Terfenadine, resulting in elevated plasma terfenadine levels. Presence of unchanged Terfenadine is associated with statistically significant prolongation of the QT and QTc intervals. **Concomitant administration of ketoconazole and Terfenadine is contraindicated** (see "Contraindications," "Warnings," and "Adverse Reactions").

Itraconazole: Torsades de pointes and elevated parent Terfenadine levels have been reported during concomitant use of Terfenadine and itraconazole in clinical trials of itraconazole and from foreign post-marketing sources. One death has also been reported from foreign post-marketing sources. **Concomitant administration of Itraconazole and Terfenadine is contraindicated** (see "Contraindications," "Warnings" and "Adverse Reactions").

Due to the clinical similarity of other azole-type antifungal agents (including fluconazole, metronidazole, and miconazole) to ketoconazole and itraconazole, concomitant use of these products with Terfenadine is not recommended pending full examination of potential interactions.

Macrolides: Clinical drug interaction studies indicate that erythromycin and clarithromycin can exert an effect on Terfenadine metabolism by a mechanism which may be similar to that of ketoconazole, but to lesser extent. Although erythromycin measurably decreases the clearance of the Terfenadine acid metabolite, its influence on Terfenadine plasma levels is still under investigation. A few spontaneous accounts of QT interval prolongation with ventricular arrhythmia including torsades de pointes have been reported in patients receiving erythromycin or troleandomycin. **Concomitant administration of Terfenadine with clarithromycin, erythromycin, or troleandomycin is contraindicated** (see "Contraindications," "Warnings" and "Adverse Reactions"). Pending full characterization of potential interactions, concomitant administration of terfenadine with other macrolide antibiotics, including azithromycin, is not recommended. Studies to evaluate the potential interaction of terfenadine with azithromycin are in progress.

CARCINOGENESIS, MUTAGENESIS, IMPAIRMENT OF FERTILITY
Oral doses of Terfenadine, corresponding to 63 times the recommended human daily dose, in mice for 18 months or in rats for 24 months, revealed no evidence of tumorigenicity. Microbial and micronucleus test assays with Terfendine have revealed no evidence of mutagenesis.

Reproduction and fertility studies in rats showed no effects on male or female fertility at oral doses of up to 21 times the human daily dose. At 63 times the human daily dose there was a small but significant reduction in implants and at 125 times the human daily dose reduced implants and increased post-implantation losses were observed, which were judged to be secondary to maternal toxicity.

PREGNANCY CATEGORY C
There was no evidence of animal teratogenicity. Reproduction studies have been performed in rats at doses 63 times and 125 times the human daily dose and have revealed decreased pup weight gain and survival when Terfenadine was administered throughout pregnancy and lactation. There are no adequate and well-controlled studies in pregnant women. Terfenadine should be used during pregnancy only if the potential benefit justifies the potential risk to the fetus.

NONTERATOGENIC EFFECTS
Terfenadine is not recommended for nursing women. The drug has caused decreased pup weight gain and survival in rats given doses 63 times and 125 times

ADVERSE EVENTS REPORTED IN CLINICAL TRIALS

	Percent Patients Reporting				
	Controlled Studies*			All Clinical Studies**	
Adverse Event	Terfenadine n = 781	Placebo n = 665	Control n = 626***	Terfenadine n = 2462	Placebo n = 1478
Central Nervous System					
Drowsiness	9.0	8.1	18.1	8.5	8.2
Headache	6.3	7.4	3.8	15.8	11.2
Fatigue	2.9	0.9	5.8	4.5	3.0
Dizziness	1.4	1.1	1.0	1.5	1.2
Nervousness	0.9	0.2	0.6	1.7	1.0
Weakness	0.9	0.6	0.2	0.6	0.5
Appetite Increase	0.6	0.0		0.5	0.0
Gastrointestinal System					
Gastrointestinal Distress (Abdominal distress, Nausea, Vomiting, Change in Bowel habits)	4.6	3.0	2.7	7.6	5.4
Eye, Ear, Nose, and Throat					
Dry Mouth/Nose/Throat	2.3	1.8	3.5	4.8	3.1
Cough	0.9	0.2	0.5	2.5	1.7
Sore Throat	0.5	0.3	0.5	3.2	1.6
Epistaxis	0.0	0.8	0.2	0.7	0.4
Skin					
Eruption (including rash and urticaria) or itching	1.0	1.7	1.4	1.6	2.0

* Duration of treatment in "Controlled Studies" was usually 7-14 DAYS.
** Duration of treatment in "All Clinical Studies" was up to 6 months.
*** Controlled Drugs: Chlorpheniramine (291 patients), d-Chlorpheniramine (189 patients), Clemastine (146 patients)

the human daily dose throughout pregnancy and lactation. Effects on pups exposed to Terfenadine only during lactation are not known, and there are no adequate and well-controlled studies in women during lactation.

PEDIATRIC USE
Safety and effectiveness of Terfenadine in children below the age of 12 years have not been established.

ADVERSE REACTIONS
CORDIOVASCULAR ADVERSE EVENTS
Rare reports of severe cardiovascular adverse effects have been received which include ventricular tachyarrhythmias (torsades de pointes, ventricular tachycardia, ventricular fibrillation, and cardiac arrest), hypotension, palpitations, syncope and dizziness. Rare reports of deaths resulting from ventricular tachyarrhythmias have been received (see "Contraindications," "Warnings", and "Precautions: Drug Interactions"). Hypotension, palpitations, syncope, and dizziness could reflect undetected ventricular arrhythmia. In some patients, death, cardiac arrest, or Torsades de Pointes have been preceded by episodes of syncope. (See "Warning" box.) Rare reports of serious cardiovascular adverse events have been received, some involving QT prolongation and torsades de pointes, in apparently normal individuals without identifiable risk factors, there is not conclusive evidence of a causal relationship of these events with Terfenadine. Although in rare cases there was measurable plasma Terfenadine, the implications of this finding with respect to the variability of terfenadine metabolism in the normal population cannot be assessed without further study. In controlled clinical trials in otherwise normal patients with rhinitis, small increases in QTc interval were observed at doses of 60 mg b.i.d. In studies at 300 mg b.i.d. a mean increase in QTc of 10% (range –4% to + 30%) (mean increase of 46 msec) was observed.

GENERAL ADVERSE EVENTS
Experience from clinical studies, including both controlled and uncontrolled studies involving more than 2,400 patients who received Terfenadine, provides information on adverse experience incidence for periods of a few days up to six months. The usual dose in these studies was 60 mg twice daily, but in a small number of patients, the dose was as low as 20 mg twice a day, or as high as 600 mg daily.

In controlled clinical studies using the recommended dose of 60 mg b.i.d., the incidence of reported adverse effects in patients receiving Terfenadine was similar to that reported in patients receiving placebo. (See table below.) (See related table).

In addition to the more frequent side effects reported in clinical trials (see table), adverse effects have been reported at a lower incidence in clinical trials and/or spontaneously during marketing of Terfenadine that warrant listing as possibly associated with drug administration. These include: alopecia (hair loss or thinning), anaphylaxis, angioedema, bronchospasm, confusion, depression, galactorrhea, insomnia, menstrual disorders (including dysmenorrhea), musculoskeletal symptoms, nightmares, paresthesia, photosensitivity, rapid flare of psoriasis, seizures, sinus tachycardia, sweating, thrombocytopenia, tremor, urinary frequency, and visual disturbances.

In clinical trials, several instances of mild, or in one case, moderate transaminase elevations were seen in patients receiving Terfenadine: Mild elevations were also seen in placebo treated patients. Marketing experiences

include isolated reports of jaundice, cholestatic hepatitis, and hepatitis. In most cases available information is incomplete.

OVERDOSAGE
Signs and symptoms of overdosate may be absent or mild (e.g. headache, nausea, confusion); but adverse cardiac events including cardiac arrest, ventricular arrhythmias including torsades de pointes and QT prolongation have been reported at overdoses of 360 mg or more and occur more frequently at doses in excess of 600 mg, and QTc prolongations of up to 30% have been observed at a dose of 300 mg b.i.d. Seizures and syncope have also been reported. Use of doses in excess of 60 mg b.i.d. is not recomemnded. (See "Warning" box, "Clinical Pharmacology", and "Adverse Reactions".)

In overdose cases, where ventricular arrhythmias are associated with significant QTc prolongation, treatment with antiarrhythmics known to prolong QTc intervals is not recommended.

Therefore, in cases of overdosage, cardiac monitoring for at least 24 hours is recommended and for as long as QTc is prolonged, along with standard measures to remove any unabsorbed drug. Limited experience with the use of hemoperfusion (N = 1) or hemodialysis (N = 3) was not successful in completely removing the acid metabolite of terfenadine from the blood.

Treatment of the signs and symptoms of overdosage should be symptomatic and supportive after the acute stage. Oral LD$_{50}$ values for Terfenadine were greater than 5000 mg/kg in mature mice and rats. The oral LD$_{50}$ was 438 mg/kg in newborn rats.

DOSAGE AND ADMINISTRATION
One tablet (60 mg) twice daily for adults and children 12 years and older.

USE OF DOSES IN EXCESS OF 60 MG B.I.D. IS NOT RECOMMENDED BECAUSE OF THE INCREASED POTENTIAL FOR QT INTERVAL PROLONGATION AND ADVERSE CARDIAC EVENTS. (See "Warning" box.) USE OF TERFENADINE IN PATIENTS WITH SIGNIFICANT HEPATIC DYSFUNCTION AND IN PATIENTS TAKING KETOCONAZOLE, ITRACONAZOLE, CLARITHROMYCIN, ERYTHROMYCIN, OR TROLEANDOMYCIN IS CONTRAINDICATED. (See "Contraindications," "Warnings", and "Precautions: Drug Interactions".)

Store tablets at controlled room temperature, 59-86°F (15°-30°C). Protect from exposure to temperatures above 104°F (40°C) and moisture.

HOW SUPPLIED
TABLETS: 60 MG

BRAND/MANUFACTURER	NDC	SIZE	AWP
○ **BRAND**			
► SELDANE: Marion Merrell Dow	00068-0723-30	30s	$36.78
	00068-0723-61	100s	$92.16
	00068-0723-65	500s	$460.74
	00068-0723-06	6000s	$5528.88

Teriparatide Acetate

DESCRIPTION
Teriparatide Acetate for Injection, Synthetic contains Teriparatide Acetate (hPTH 1-34), a synthetic polypeptide hormone consisting of the 1-34 fragment of

human parathyroid hormone, the biologically active N-terminal region of the 84 amino acid native hormone.

The structure of Teriparatide Acetate is represented by the following amino acid sequence:

H₂N-Ser-Val-Ser-Glu-Ile-Gln-Leu-Met-His-Asn-Leu-Gly-Lys-His-Leu-Asn- Ser-Met-Glu-Arg-Val-Glu-Trp-Leu-Arg-Lys-Lys-Leu-Gln-Asp- Val-His-Asn-Phe- OH XCH₃COOH, X= 6-9.

Teriparatide Acetate is a sterile, lyophilized powder providing 200 units hPTH activity per vial.

Following is its chemical structure:

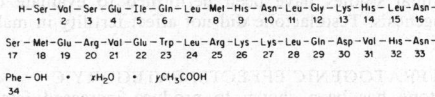

CLINICAL PHARMACOLOGY
Parathyroid hormone is secreted by the four parathyroid glands found on or embedded in the two lateral lobes of the thyroid gland. hPTH 1-34 acts on bone to mobilize calcium and on the kidney to reduce calcium clearance, increase phosphate excretion, stimulate the release of cyclic AMP in the urine, and stimulate the conversion of 25-hydroxyvitamin D₃ (25-OH-D₃) to the active form 1, 25-dihydroxyvitamin D₃[1,25(OH)₂D₃].

The initial effect of Teriparatide Acetate on bone is to promote an increased rate of release of calcium from bone mineral into blood. The action may be mediated by an effect on osteocytes or osteoclasts.

The kidney effects, which may be due to a direct action of the hormone on its receptors, include a reduction of calcium clearance and an inhibition of tubular phosphate reabsorption as well as an increased excretion of sodium and potassium. Parathyroid hormone stimulates the conversion of 25-OH-D to 1, 25 (OH)₂D by the kidney.

Intestinal transport of calcium is increased by the PTH indirectly by increasing renal, 1, 25 (OH)₂D production.

The primary mode of action is the stimulation of adenylate cyclase in the involved organ.

INDICATIONS AND USAGE
Teriparatide Acetate for Injection, Synthetic is indicated as a diagnostic agent to assist in establishing the diagnosis in patients presenting with clinical and laboratory evidence of hypocalcemia due to either hypoparathyroidism or pseudohypoparathyroidism. The test will distinguish between hypoparathyroidism and pseudohypoparathyroidism, but not between these conditions and normal. The discriminant power of Teriparatide Acetate effect on urinary cAMP is much greater than that of the effect on urinary phosphate.

CONTRAINDICATIONS
Known hypersensitivity to Teriparatide Acetate or to any components of the preparation.

WARNINGS
Allergic Reactions: Because Teriparatide Acetate is a peptide, the possibility of a systemic allergic reaction cannot be overlooked. The usual provisions should be made for the emergency treatment of such a reaction should it occur.

PRECAUTIONS
1. General: The administration of Teriparatide Acetate could lead to hypercalcemia. Teriparatide Acetate is not intended for recurrent or chronic use.

2. Carcinogenesis, Mutagenesis, Impairment of Fertility: No studies have been performed to evaluate the carcinogenic or mutagenic potential of Teriparatide Acetate or its effect on fertility.

3. Pregnancy/Teratogenic Effects: Pregnancy-Category C: Animal reproduction studies have not been conducted with Teriparatide Acetate. It is also not known whether Teriparatide Acetate can cause fetal harm when administered to a pregnant woman or can affect reproduction capacity. Teriparatide Acetate should be given to a pregnant woman only if clearly needed.

4. Nursing Mother: It is not known to what degree Teriparatide Acetate is excreted in human milk, but the peptide would not be expected to be absorbed in an active form from the infant's gastrointestinal tract. However, caution should be exercised when Teriparatide Acetate is administered to a nursing woman.

5. Pediatric Use: There is limited data on safety in children. The use of Teriparatide Acetate in children 3 years of age and older was uneventful and the response to the drug followed expected patterns.

ADVERSE REACTIONS
CARDIOVASCULAR
A hypertensive crisis occurred in one patient 8 hours after a study. This patient had had previous hypertensive episodes not related to Teriparatide Acetate injection.

METABOLIC/NUTRITIONAL
Hypocalcemia was not reversed in one patient, and a hypocalcemic convulsion occurred 4 ½ hours following injection; this was corrected by calcium administration.

GASTROINTESTINAL
Nausea, abdominal cramps, urge to defecate, and diarrhea was reported. The incidence of each of these adverse reactions was less than 2%.

OTHER
Tingling of the extremities, metallic taste, and pain at the injection site have been reported during or shortly following the infusion. The incidence of each of these adverse reactions was less than 2%.

OVERDOSAGE
Teriparatide Acetate given repeatedly in doses in excess of 500 units may produce hypercalcemia. In those who are borderline hypercalcemic (10.5 mg/dL), a dose of 200 units could produce mild hypercalcemia for a brief period. If hypercalcemia develops, the drug should be discontinued and steps should be taken to ensure adequate hydration.

DOSAGE AND ADMINISTRATION
Diagnostic Use in Patients with Hypocalcemia: The recommended dose for adults is 200 units of Teriparatide Acetate. Reconstitute by adding the 10 mL diluent to the 10 mL Teriparatide Acetate vial. The 10 mL of solution is infused intravenously over a 10-minute period. In children 3 years of age or older, the recommended dose is 3 units per kg of body weight, up to a maximum of 200 units. Reconstituted solution should be used within 4 hours. Discard any unused portion.

Parenteral drug products should be inspected visually for particulate matter and discoloration prior to administration, whenever solution and container permit.

Modified Ellsworth Howard Test: Test subjects should be in a fasting state when starting the test period. An active urine output should be initiated and maintained by the ingestion of 200 mL of water per hour for 2 hours prior to study and continuing through the study. A baseline urine collection should be made in the 60-minute period preceding the Teriparatide Acetate infusion. Following the hPTH (1-34) infusions (time 0), urine should be collected as separate collections in the 0-30 minutes, 30-60 minute and 60-120 minute postinfusion time periods. Confidence in the test will be influenced by adequate hydration and urine flow and complete collection of urine specimens.

INTERPRETATION OF TEST
The measurement of urinary cAMP and phosphate must be corrected for creatinine excretion.

In the clinical trials, patients with hypoparathyroidism showed a tenfold or greater increase over baseline of urinary cAMP at the 0-30 minute postinfusion period, and 92 percent of these patients showed a threefold or greater urinary phosphate excretion in the 0-60 minute collection.

Patients with end-organ resistance pseudohypoparathyroidism showed a blunted response of less than sixfold increase of urinary cAMP excretion over baseline in the 0-30 minute period, and 88 percent showed a less than threefold increase in urinary phosphate excretion in the 0-60 minute collection period.

Although this test does not discriminate between normal and abnormal in most cases, it does discriminate between hypoparathyroidism and pseudohypoparathyroidism. The change in the urinary cAMP excretion in the 0-30 minute period is the most sensitive indicator for separation of hypoparathyroidisms.

Storage: Store vials at controlled room temperature, 15°-30°C (59°-86°F).

HOW SUPPLIED
POWDER FOR INJECTION:

BRAND/MANUFACTURER	NDC	SIZE	AWP
BRAND PARATHAR: RPR	00075-2050-53	1s	$69.67

Terra-Cortril *SEE* HYDROCORTISONE ACETATE WITH OXYTETRACYCLINE HYDROCHLORIDE

Terramycin *SEE* LIDOCAINE HYDROCHLORIDE AND OXYTETRACYCLINE, OXYTETRACYCLINE HYDROCHLORIDE *AND* OXYTETRACYCLINE HYDROCHLORIDE WITH POLYMYXIN B SULFATE

Teslac *SEE* TESTOLACTONE

Tessalon Perles *SEE* BENZONATATE

Testoderm *SEE* TESTOSTERONE, TRANSDERMAL

➤ SHOWN IN PRODUCT IDENTIFICATION GUIDE

Testolactone

This product does NOT meet USP requirements. Testolactone exceeds USP Organic Volatile Impurities (OVI) Limit for Methylene Chloride. The USP limit for Methylene Chloride is 100 ppm. Testolactone normally contains 1,000 ppm.

DESCRIPTION

Testolactone Tablets are available for oral administration as tablets providing 50 mg Testolactone per tablet. Testolactone is a synthetic antineoplastic agent that is structurally distinct from the androgen steroid nucleus in possessing a six-membered lactone ring in place of the usual five-membered carbocyclic D-ring. Testolactone is chemically designated as 13-hydroxy-3-oxo-13,17-secoandrosta-1,4-dien-17-oic acid -lactone.

Testolactone is a white, odorless, crystalline solid, soluble in ethanol and slightly soluble in water. Its molecular formula is $C_{19}H_{24}O_3$ and its molecular weight in 300.40. CAS number for Testolactone is 968-93-4.

Following is its chemical structure:

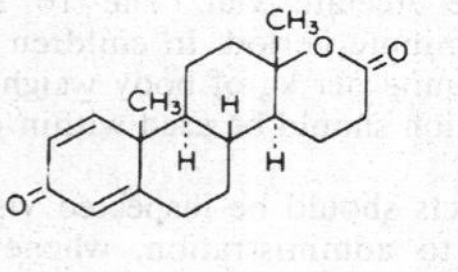

CLINICAL PHARMACOLOGY

Although the precise mechanism by which Testolactone produces its clinical antineoplastic effects has not been established, its principal action is reported to be inhibition of steroid aromatase activity and consequent reduction in estrone synthesis from adrenal androstenedione, the major source of estrogen in postmenopausal women. Based on *in vitro* studies, the aromatase inhibition may be noncompetitive and irreversible. This phenomenon may account for the persistence of Testolactone's effect on estrogen synthesis after drug withdrawal.

Despite some similarity to testosterone, Testolactone has no *in vivo* androgenic effect. No other hormonal effects have been reported in clinical studies in patients receiving Testolactone. In one study, Testolactone administered orally (1000 mg/day) was reported to increase renal tubular reabsorption of calcium but to have no effect on serum calcium concentration. The mechanism of the hypocalciuric effect is unknown. No clinical effects in humans of Testolactone on adrenal function have been reported; however, one study noted an increase in urinary excretion of 17-ketosteroids in most of the patients treated with 150 mg/day orally.

Testolactone is well absorbed from the gastrointestinal tract. It is metabolized to several derivatives in the liver, all of which preserve the lactone D-ring. These metabolites, as well as some unmetabolized drug, are excreted in the urine. Additional pharmacokinetic data in humans are unavailable.

For information concerning carcinogensis, mutagenesis, pregnancy, and lactation, see the corresponding *"Precautions"* sections.

In animals, parenteral but not oral Testolactone reduced cortisone acetate induced hepatic glycogen deposits. In animal tests conducted to detect any hormonal activity for Testolactone, some evidence of antiandrogenic and antiglucocorticoid activity was seen; increased growth rate in the newborn was suggested. However there was no clear manifestation of androgenic, estrogenic or antiestrogenic, progestational or antiprogestational, gonadotropin-like or antigonadotropic effects. Testolactone did not demonstrate anti-inflammatory, mineralocorticoid-like, or glucocorticoid-like properties.

INDICATIONS AND USAGE

Testolactone Tablets are recommended as adjunctive therapy in the palliative treatment of advanced or disseminated breast cancer in postmenopausal women when hormonal therapy is indicated. Testolactone may also be used in women who were diagnosed as having had disseminated breast carcinoma noma when premenopausal, in whom ovarian function has been subsequently terminated.

Testolactone Tablets were found to be effective in approximately 15% of patients with advanced or disseminated mammary cancer evaluated according to the following criteria: 1) those with a measurable decrease in size of all demonstrable tumor masses; 2) those in whom more than 50% of non-osseous lesions decreased in size although all bone lesions remained static; and 3) those in whom more than 50% of total lesions improved while the remainder were static.

CONTRAINDICATIONS

Testolactone is contraindicated in the treatment of breast cancer in men and in patients with a history of hypersensitivity to the drug.

PRECAUTIONS

INFORMATION FOR PATIENTS

The physician should be consulted regarding missed doses. Notify the physician if adverse reactions occur or become more pronounced.

LABORATORY TESTS

Plasma calcium levels should be routinely determined in any patient receiving therapy for mammary cancer, particularly during periods of active remission of bony metastases. If hypercalcemia occurs, appropriate measures should be instituted.

DRUG INTERACTIONS

When administered concurrently Testolactone may increase the effects of oral anticoagulants; monitor and adjust anticoagulant dosage accordingly.

DRUG/LABORATORY TEST INTERACTIONS

Physiologic effects of Testolactone may result in decreased estradiol concentrations with radioimmunoassays for estradiol, increased plasma calcium concentrations (see *"Precautions, Laboratory Tests"*), and increased 24-hour urinary excretion of creatine and 17-ketosteroids.

CARCINOGENESIS, MUTAGENESIS, IMPAIRMENT OF FERTILITY

No long-term animal studies have been performed to evaluate carcinogenic potential or mutagenesis. Testolactone did not affect fertility in male or female rats.

PREGNANCY: TERATOGENIC EFFECTS, CATEGORY C

In rats, Testolactone has been shown to produce increased fetal mortality, increased abnormal fetal development, and increased mortality in growing pups when given at doses 5 to 15 times the recommended human dose. In rabbits, no teratologic effects were observed at doses 2.5 to 7.5 times the recommended human dose. There are no adequate and well controlled studies in pregnant women. Testolactone is intended for use only in postmenopausal women and should not be used during pregnancy.

NURSING MOTHERS

It is not known whether this drug is excreted in human milk. Because many drugs are excreted in human milk, a decision should be made whether or not to discontinue nursing.

PEDIATRIC USE

Safety and effectiveness in children have not been established.

ADVERSE REACTIONS

Certain signs and symptoms have been reported in association with the use of this drug but, in these instances, it is often impossible to determine the relationship of the underlying disease and drug administration to the reported reaction. Such reactions include maculopapular erythema, increase in blood pressure, paresthesia, aches and edema of the extremities, glossitis, anorexia and nausea and vomiting. Alopecia alone and with associated nail growth disturbance have been reported rarely; these side effects subsided without interruption of treatment.

DRUG ABUSE AND DEPENDENCE

Testolactone is classified as a controlled substance under the Anabolic Steroids Control Act of 1990 and has been assigned to Schedule III.

OVERDOSAGE

There have been no reports of acute overdosage with Testolactone Tablets.

DOSAGE AND ADMINISTRATION

The recommended oral dose is 250 mg qid.

In order to evaluate the response, therapy with Testolactone should be continued for a minimum of three months unless there is active progression of the disease.

STORAGE

Store at room temperature; avoid excessive heat.

HOW SUPPLIED

TABLETS (C-III): 50 MG

BRAND/MANUFACTURER	NDC	SIZE	AWP
○ **BRAND**			
TESLAC: Bristol-Myer Onc/Hiv	00003-0690-50	100s	$124.11

Testosterone, Injectable

DESCRIPTION

Testosterone propionate injection is a sterile oleaginous solution of Testosterone propionate for intramuscular use. Testosterone propionate is the propionic acid ester of testosterone-delta-4-androstene-17-beta-ol-3-one. Testosterone is 17-beta-hydroxy-4-androsten-3-one, a white or off white crystal or crystalline powder. It is practically insoluble in water but is freely soluble in dehydrated alcohol and chloroform. It is soluble in dioxane and vegetable oils.

Empirical formula: $C_{22}H_{32}O_3$. Molecular weight: 344.49.

Chemical name: 17β-(1-oxopropoxy)androst-4-en-3-one.

Testosterone cypionate injection is a sterile solution of Testosterone cypionate for intramuscular use. Testosterone cypionate ($C_{27}H_{40}O_3$) MW 412.59 is a white or creamy white, crystalline powder, is odorless or has a slight odor. 17β-(3-cyclopentyl-1-oxopropoxy) androst-4-en-3-one.

It is insoluble in water, freely soluble in alcohol and ether and soluble in vegetable oil.

Testosterone enanthate injection is a clear, colorless to pale yellow sterile oleaginous solution of Testosterone enanthate for intramuscular use. Testosterone enanthate ($C_{26}H_{40}O_3$) MW 400.60, is a white or creamy white, crystalline powder. It is odorless or has a faint odor characteristic of heptanoic acid.

It is insoluble in water, very soluble in ether and soluble in vegetable oils.

Androgens are derivatives of cyclopentano-perhydrophenanthrene. Endogenous androgens are C-19 steroids with a side chain at C-17, and with two angular methyl groups. Testosterone is the primary endogenous androgen. In their active form, all drugs in the class have a 17-beta-hydroxy group. Esterification of the 17-beta-hydroxy group produces compounds (testosterone enanthate and testosterone propionate) which have a longer duration of action and are hydrolyzed in vivo to free Testosterone. Fluoxymesterone and methyltestosterone are synthetic derivatives of Testosterone.

Each mL injection contains: Testosterone 25, 50, or 100 mg or Testosterone Propionate 25, 50 or 100 mg or Testosterone Cypionate 100 or 200 mg or Testosterone Enanthate 100 or 200 mg.

The androgens are steroids that develop and maintain primary and secondary male sex characteristics.

Following is its chemical structure:

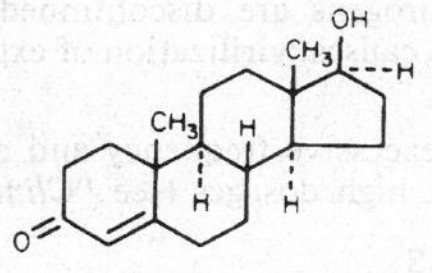

CLINICAL PHARMACOLOGY

Actions: Testosterone is an active androgen for intramuscular injection. It possesses the properties attributable to the testicular hormone.

Endogenous androgens are responsible for the normal growth and development of the male sex organs and for maintenance of secondary sex characteristics. These effects include the growth and maturation of prostate, seminal vesicles, penis, and scrotum, the development of male hair distribution, such, as beard, pubic, chest and axillary hair, laryngeal enlargement, vocal cord thickening, alterations in body musculature, and fat distribution. Drugs in this class also cause retention of nitrogen, sodium, potassium, phosphorus, and decreased urinary excretion of calcium. Androgens have been reported to increase protein anabolism and decrease protein catabolism. Nitrogen balance is improved only when there is sufficient intake of calories and protein. Androgens are responsible for the growth spurt of adolescence and for the eventual termination of linear growth which is brought about by fusion of the epiphyseal growth centers. In children, exogenous androgens accelerate linear growth rates, but may cause a disproportionate advancement in bone maturation. Use over long periods may result in fusion of the epiphyseal growth centers and termination of the growth process.

Androgens have been reported to stimulate the production of red blood cells by enhancing the production of erythropoietic stimulating factor.

During exogenous administration of androgens, endogenous Testosterone release is inhibited through feedback inhibition of pituitary luteinizing hormone (LH). At large doses of exogenous androgens, spermatogenesis may also be suppressed through feedback inhibition of pituitary follicle stimulating hormone (FSH).

There is a lack of substantial evidence that androgens are effective in fractures, surgery, convalescence, and functional uterine bleeding.

Testosterone cypionate is intended for androgen therapy, particularly when prolonged action is desirable. Following a single intramuscular injection, the androgenic effect is sustained over a period of about 4 weeks. This continuous flow of hormone is thought to resemble closely the endogenous production of testosterone.

Testosterone cypionate is primarily used for its protein anabolic effect and its catabolic inhibiting effect on tissue. Nitrogen balance is improved with anabolic agents but only when there is sufficient intake of calories and protein. Whether this positive nitrogen balance is of primary benefit in the utilization of protein-building dietary substances has not been established.

Pharmacokinetics: Testosterone esters are less polar than free testosterone. Testosterone esters in oil injected intramuscularly are absorbed slowly from the lipid phase; thus, Testosterone cypionate and enanthate can be given at intervals of two to four weeks. Suspensions of Testosterone or its esters in aqueous media may cause local irritation and the rate of absorption is not always uniform.

Testosterone in plasma is 98 percent bound to a specific Testosterone-estradiol binding globulin and about 2 percent is free. Generally, the amount of this sex-hormone binding globulin in the plasma will determine the distribution of Testosterone between free and bound forms, and the free Testosterone concentration will determine its half-life.

About 90 percent of a dose of Testosterone is excreted in the urine as glucuronic and sulfuric acid conjugates of Testosterone and its metabolites; about 6 percent of a dose is excreted in the feces, mostly in the unconjugated form. Inactivation of Testosterone occurs primarily in the liver. Testosterone is metabolized to various 17-keto steroids through two different pathways. There are considerable variations of the half-life of Testosterone as reported in the literature, ranging from 10 to 100 minutes.

In many tissues the activity of Testosterone appears to depend on reduction to dihydrotestosterone, which binds to cytosol receptor proteins. The steroid-receptor complex is transported to the nucleus where it initiates transcription events and cellular changes related to androgen action.

Suspensions of Testosterone or its esters in aqueous media may cause local irritation and the rate of absorption is not always uniform.

INDICATIONS AND USAGE

1. *Males:* Androgens are indicated for replacement therapy in conditions associated with a deficiency or absence of endogenous Testosterone.

a. Primary hypogonadism (congenital or acquired) — testicular failure due to cryptorchidism, bilateral torsion, orchitis, vanishing testis syndrome, or orchidectomy.

b. Hypogonadotropic hypogonadism (congenital or acquired) — idiopathic gonadotropin of or LHRH deficiency, or pituitary-hypothalamic injury from tumors, trauma, or radiation. (Appropriate adrenal cortical and thyroid hormone replacement therapy are still necessary, however, and are actually of primary importance.)

If the above conditions occur prior to puberty, androgen replacement therapy will be needed during the adolescent years for development of secondary sexual characteristics. Prolonged androgen treatment will be required to maintain sexual characteristics in these and other males who develop Testosterone deficiency after puberty.

c. Androgens may be used to stimulate puberty in carefully selected males with clearly delayed puberty. These patients usually have a familial pattern of delayed puberty that is not secondary to a pathological disorder; puberty is expected to occur spontaneously at a relatively late date. Brief treatment with conservative doses may occasionally be justified in these patients if they do not respond to psychological support. The potential adverse effect on bone maturation should be discussed with the patient and parents prior to androgen administration. An x-ray of the hand and wrist to determine bone age should be obtained every 6 months to assess the effect of treatment on the epiphyseal centers (see *"Warnings").*

2. *Females:* Androgens may be used secondarily in women with advancing inoperable metastatic (skeletal) mammary cancer who are 1 to 5 years postmenopausal. Primary goals of therapy in these women include ablation of the ovaries. Other methods of counteracting estrogen activity are adrenalectomy, hypophysectomy and/or antiestrogen therapy. This treatment has also been used in premenopausal women with breast cancer who have benefited from oophorectomy and are considered to have a hormone-responsive tumor. Judgment concerning androgen therapy should be made by an oncologist with expertise in this field.

Androgens (methyltestosterone, fluoxymesterone, and testosterone propionate) have been used for the management of postpartum breast pain and engorgement.

UNLABELED USES

Testosterone propionate is used alone or as an adjunct in the treatment of vulvar dystrophies, atrophic vaginitis (when used topically), and cluster headaches. It is also used in lichen sclerosis, sexual dysfunction in alcoholic, cirrhotic men, and anemia associated with chronic renal failure. The topical Testosterone therapy in prepuberty patients with micropenis is used to increase penis size, and as a male contraceptive to induce azoospermia.

CONTRAINDICATIONS

Androgens are contraindicated in men with carcinomas of the breast or with known or suspected carcinomas of the prostate, and in women who are or may become pregnant. When administered to pregnant women, androgens cause virilization of the external genitalia of the female fetus. This virilization includes clitoromegaly, abnormal vaginal development, and fusion of genital folds to form a scrotal-like structure. The degree of masculinization is related to the amount of drug given and the age of the fetus, and is most likely to occur in the female fetus when the drugs are given in the first trimester. If the patient becomes pregnant while taking these drugs, she should be apprised of the potential hazard to the fetus.

Androgens are also contraindicated in patients with nephrosis or the nephrotic phase of nephritis.

Hypersensitivity to any of the components of the product.

WARNINGS

This drug is not to be administered intravenously. Do not give Testosterone to elderly, asthenic males who may react adversely to overstimulation by androgens. Do not administer this product to patients who are sensitive/allergic to mercury compounds.

In patients with breast cancer, androgen therapy may cause hypercalcemia by stimulating osteolysis. In patients with cancer, hypercalcemia may indicate progression of bony metastasis. If hypercalcemia occurs, the drugs should be discontinued and appropriate measures instituted.

Prolonged use of high doses of androgens has been associated with the development of peliosis hepatis and hepatic neoplasms including hepatocellular carcinoma (See *"Precautions — Carcinogenesis")* Peliosis hepatis can be a life-threatening or fatal complication.

Cholestatic hepatitis and jaundice occur with 17-alpha-alkylandrogens at a relatively low dose. If cholestatic hepatitis with jaundice appears or if liver function tests become abnormal, the androgen should be discontinued and the etiology should be determined. Drug-induced jaundice is reversible when the medication is discontinued.

Geriatric patients treated with androgens may be at an increased risk for the development of prostatic hypertrophy and prostatic carcinoma.

Edema with or without congestive heart failure may be a serious complication in patients with preexisting cardiac, renal, or hepatic disease. In addition to discontinuation of the drug, diuretic therapy may be required. If the administration of Testosterone enanthate is restarted, a lower dose should be used.

Gynecomastia frequently develops and occasionally persists in patients being treated for hypogonadism.

Androgen therapy should be used cautiously in healthy males with delayed puberty. The effect on bone maturation should be monitored by assessing bone age of the wrist and hand every six months. In children, androgen treatment may accelerate bone maturation without producing compensatory gain in linear growth. This adverse effect may result in compromised adult stature. The younger the child the greater the risk of compromising final mature height.

This drug has not been shown to be safe and effective for the enhancement of athletic performance. Because of the potential risk of serious adverse health effects, this drug should not be used for such purpose.

PRECAUTIONS

General: Women should be observed for signs of virilization (deepening of the voice, hirsutism, acne, clitoromegaly and menstrual irregularities). Discontinuation of drug therapy at the time of evidence of mild virilism is necessary to prevent irreversible virilization. Such virilization is usual following androgen use at high doses and is not prevented by concomitant use of estrogens. A decision may be made by the patient and the physician that some virilization will be tolerated during treatment for breast carcinoma.

Because androgens may alter serum cholesterol concentration, caution should be used when administering these drugs to patients with a history of myocardial infarction or coronary artery disease. Serial determinations of serum cholesterol should be made and therapy adjusted accordingly. A causal relationship between myocardial infarction and hypercholesterolemia has not been established.

INFORMATION FOR THE PATIENT

The physician should instruct patients to report any of the following side effects of androgens:

Adults or Adolescents Males: Too-frequent or persistent erections of the penis.

Women: Hoarseness, acne, changes in menstrual periods, or more hair on the face.

All Patients: Any nausea, vomiting, changes in skin color or ankle swelling.

Any male adolescent patient receiving androgens for delayed puberty should have bone development checked every six months.

LABORATORY TESTS

1. Women with disseminated breast carcinoma should have frequent determination of urine and serum calcium levels during the course of androgen therapy. (See *"Warnings"*).

2. Because of the hepatotoxicity associated with the use of 17-alpha-alkylated androgens, liver function tests should be obtained periodically.

3. Periodic (every 6 months) x-ray examinations of bone age should be made during treatment of prepubertal males to determine the rate of bone maturation and the effects of androgen therapy on the epiphyseal centers.

4. Hemoglobin and hematocrit should be checked periodically for polycythemia in patients who are receiving high doses of androgens.

DRUG INTERACTIONS

Anticoagulants: C-17 substituted derivatives of testosterone, such as methandrostenolone, have been reported to decrease the anticoagulant requirements of patients receiving oral anticoagulants.

Patients receiving oral anticoagulant therapy require close monitoring, especially when androgens are started or stopped.

2. Oxyphenbutazone: Concurrent administration of oxyphenbutazone and androgens may result in elevated serum levels of oxyphenbutazone.

3. Insulin: In diabetic patients the metabolic effects of androgens may decrease blood glucose and insulin requirements.

4 ACTH and corticosteroids: Enhanced tendency towards edema. Use caution when giving these drugs together, especially in patients with hepatic or cardiac disease.

DRUG/LABORATORY TEST INTERFERENCES

Androgens may decrease levels of thyroxine-binding globulin, resulting in decreased total T^4 serum levels and increased resin uptake of T^3 and T^4. Free thyroid hormone levels remain unchanged, however, and there is no clinical evidence of thyroid dysfunction.

Carcinogenesis: Animal Data: Testosterone has been tested by subcutaneous injection and implantation in mice and rats. The implant induced cervical-uterine tumors in mice, which metastasized in some cases. There is suggestive evidence that injection of testosterone into some strains of female mice increases their susceptibility to hepatoma. Testosterone is also known to increase the number of tumors and decrease the degree of differentiation of chemically induced carcinomas of the liver in rats.

Human Data: There are rare reports of hepatocellular carcinoma in patients receiving long-term therapy with androgens in high doses. Withdrawal of the drugs did not lead to regression of the tumors in all cases.

Geriatric patients treated with androgens may be at an increased risk for the development of prostatic hypertrophy and prostatic carcinoma.

PREGNANCY

Teratogenic Effects: Pregnancy Category X (see *"Contraindications"*).

NURSING MOTHERS

It is not known whether androgens are excreted in human milk. Because many drugs are excreted in human milk and because of the potential for serious adverse reactions in nursing infants from androgens, a decision should be made whether to discontinue nursing or to discontinue the drug, taking into account the importance of the drug to the mother.

PEDIATRIC USE

Androgen therapy should be used very cautiously in children and only by specialists who are aware of the adverse effects on bone maturation. Skeletal maturation must be monitored every six months by an x-ray of hand and wrist (See *"Indications and Usage"* and *"Warnings"*).

ADVERSE REACTIONS

Injections can result in local irritation, redness, and pain.

ENDOCRINE AND UROGENITAL

Female: The most common side effects of androgen therapy are amenorrhea and other menstrual irregularities, inhibition of gonadotropin secretion, and virilization, including deepening of the voice and clitoral enlargement. The latter usually is not reversible after androgens are discontinued. When administered to a pregnant woman androgens causes, virilization of external genitalia of the female fetus.

Male: Gynecomastia, and excessive frequency and duration of penile erections. Oligospermia may occur at high dosages (see *"Clinical Pharmacology"*).

SKIN AND APPENDAGES

Hirsutism, male pattern baldness, and acne.

FLUID AND ELECTROLYTE DISTURBANCES

Retention of sodium, chloride, water, potassium, calcium and inorganic phosphates.

GASTROINTESTINAL

Nausea, cholestatic jaundice, alterations in liver function tests, rarely hepatocellular neoplasms and peliosis hepatis (See *"Warnings"*).

HEMATOLOGIC

Suppression of clotting factors II, V, VII, and X. Bleeding in patients on concomitant anticoagulant therapy, and polycythemia.

NERVOUS SYSTEM

Increased or decreased libido, headache, anxiety depression, and generalized paresthesia.

METABOLIC

Increased serum cholesterol.

MISCELLANEOUS

Inflammation and pain at the site of intramuscular injection or subcutaneous implantation of Testosterone containing pellets, stomatitis with buccal preparations, and rarely anaphylactoid reactions.

DRUG ABUSE AND DEPENDENCE

Testosterone Enanthate Injection is classified as a Schedule III controlled substance under the Anabolic Steroids Control Act of 1990.

OVERDOSAGE

There have been no reports of acute overdosage with the androgens.

DOSAGE AND ADMINISTRATION

Androgens are administered as oral or buccal tablets, intramuscular injections, or subcutaneous pellets.

Androgens should not be given intravenously. Intramuscular injections should be given deep in the gluteal muscle. Shake well prior to withdrawal. Care should be taken to inject the preparation deeply into the gluteal muscle following the usual precautions for intramuscular administration. In general, total doses above 400 mg of Testosterone cypionate or enanthate per month are not required because of the prolonged action of the preparation. Injections more frequently than every two weeks are rarely indicated *"Note"*: Use of a wet needle or wet syringe may cause the solution to become cloudy; however, this does not affect the potency of the material.

The suggested dosage for androgens varies depending on the age, sex, and diagnosis of the individual patient. Dosage is adjusted according to the patient's response and the appearance of adverse reactions.

ANDROGEN REPLACEMENT

Testosterone propionate: 25-50 mg 2 to 3 times/week.

Testosterone cypionate: 50-400 mg every 2 to 4 weeks.

Testosterone enanthate: 50-400 mg every 2 to 4 weeks.

Testosterone: 25-50 mg 2 to 3 times/week.

Various dosage regimens have been used to induce pubertal changes in hypogonadal males, some experts have advocated lower dosages initially, gradually increasing the dose as puberty progresses, with or without a decrease to maintenance levels.

Other experts emphasize that higher dosages are needed to induce pubertal changes and lower dosages can be used for maintenance after puberty. The chronological and skeletal ages must be taken into consideration, both in determining the initial dose and in adjusting the dose. X-ray should be taken at appropriate intervals to determine the amount of bone maturation and skeletal development (See *"Indications and Usage"*, and *"Warnings"*).

DELAYED PUBERTY

Testosterone propionate: lower ranges for 4 to 6 months.

Testosterone cypionate: lower ranges for 4 to 6 months.

◆ RATED THERAPEUTICALLY EQUIVALENT; ◇ THERAPEUTIC EQUIVALENCE UNCONFIRMED; ○ UNRATED

Testosterone enanthate: 50-200 mg every 2 to 4 weeks for 4 to 6 months.

Testosterone: lower ranges for 4 to 6 months.

Women with metastatic breast carcinoma must be followed closely because androgen therapy occasionally appears to accelerate the disease. Thus many experts prefer to use the shorter-acting androgen preparations rather than those with prolonged activity for treating breast carcinoma, particularly during the early stages of androgen therapy.

PALLIATION OF MAMMARY CANCER
Testosterone propionate: 50-100 mg 3 times/week.

Testosterone cypionate: 200-400 mg every 2 to 4 weeks.

Testosterone enanthate: 200-400 mg every 2 to 4 weeks.

Testosterone: 50-100 mg 3 times/week.

POSTPARTUM BREAST ENGORGEMENT
Testosterone propionate: 25 to 50 mg for 3 to 4 days, starting at the time of delivery.

Parenteral drug products should be inspected visually for particulate matter and discoloration prior to administration whenever the solution and container permit.

STORAGE
Store at room temperature 15° - 30° C (59° - 86° F). Do not freeze. PROTECT FROM LIGHT.

Storage at low temperature may produce crystal formation. If present, dissolve by warming to 85° F and shaking vial.

J CODES
Up to 100 mg IM—J3150
Up to 50 mg IM—J3140
Up to 200 mg IM—J3130
Up to 100 mg IM—J3120
1 cc, 50 mg IM—J1090
1 cc, 200 mg IM—J1080
Up to 100 mg IM—J1070

HOW SUPPLIED

TESTOSTERONE
INJECTION (C-III): 100 MG/ML

AVERAGE UNIT PRICE (AVAILABLE SIZES)		GENERIC A-RATED AVERAGE PRICE (GAAP)	
GENERIC	$1.20	10 ml	$13.35

BRAND/MANUFACTURER		NDC	SIZE	AWP
◆ GENERICS				
Geneva		00781-3093-70	10 ml	$10.95
Rugby		00536-9500-70	10 ml	$15.75
Rugby		00536-9500-75	30 ml	$28.20

TESTOSTERONE CYPIONATE
INJECTION (C-III): 100 MG/ML

AVERAGE UNIT PRICE (AVAILABLE SIZES)		GENERIC A-RATED AVERAGE PRICE (GAAP)	
BRAND	$3.20	10 ml	$11.62
GENERIC	$1.16		

BRAND/MANUFACTURER	NDC	SIZE	AWP
◆ BRAND			
DEPO-TESTOSTERONE: Upjohn	00009-0347-02	10 ml	$32.01
◆ GENERICS			
Schein	00364-6609-54	10 ml	$8.02
Steris	00402-0255-10	10 ml	$8.02
Geneva	00781-3096-70	10 ml	$11.80
DEPOTEST: Hyrex	00314-0815-70	10 ml	$12.80
Goldline	00182-0712-63	10 ml	$13.35
Rugby	00536-9480-70	10 ml	$15.75

INJECTION (C-III): 200 MG/ML

AVERAGE UNIT PRICE (AVAILABLE SIZES)		GENERIC A-RATED AVERAGE PRICE (GAAP)	
BRAND	$8.12	10 ml	$17.61
GENERIC	$1.76		

BRAND/MANUFACTURER	NDC	SIZE	AWP
◆ BRAND			
DEPO-TESTOSTERONE: Upjohn	00009-0417-01	1 ml	$10.49
	00009-0417-02	10 ml	$57.44
◆ GENERICS			
Schein	00364-6610-54	10 ml	$8.70
Steris	00402-0256-10	10 ml	$8.70
URL	00677-0980-21	10 ml	$13.50
DEPOTEST: Hyrex	00314-0835-70	10 ml	$17.80
Goldline	00182-0713-63	10 ml	$19.50
Geneva	00781-3097-70	10 ml	$19.99
Rugby	00536-9490-70	10 ml	$26.25
VIRILON IM: Star	00076-0301-10	10 ml	$26.40

TESTOSTERONE ENANTHATE
INJECTION (C-III): 100 MG/ML

AVERAGE UNIT PRICE (AVAILABLE SIZES)		GENERIC A-RATED AVERAGE PRICE (GAAP)	
GENERIC	$0.77	10 ml	$7.74

BRAND/MANUFACTURER	NDC	SIZE	AWP
◆ GENERICS			
Schein	00364-6616-54	10 ml	$4.58
EVERONE: Hyrex	00314-0650-70	10 ml	$10.90

INJECTION (C-III): 200 MG/ML

AVERAGE UNIT PRICE (AVAILABLE SIZES)		GENERIC A-RATED AVERAGE PRICE (GAAP)	
BRAND	$14.96	10 ml	$13.31
GENERIC	$1.33		

BRAND/MANUFACTURER	NDC	SIZE	AWP
◆ BRAND			
DELATESTRYL: BTG Pharm Corp	54396-0328-16	1 ml	$18.69
	54396-0328-40	5 ml	$56.19
◆ GENERICS			
Schein	00364-6617-54	10 ml	$8.40
Steris	00402-0356-10	10 ml	$8.40
URL	00677-0313-21	10 ml	$13.05
Geneva	00781-3105-70	10 ml	$16.55
ANDROPOSITORY 200: Rugby	00536-1670-70	10 ml	$16.58
EVERONE: Hyrex	00314-0652-70	10 ml	$16.90

TESTOSTERONE PROPIONATE
INJECTION (C-III): 100 MG/ML

AVERAGE UNIT PRICE (AVAILABLE SIZES)		GENERIC A-RATED AVERAGE PRICE (GAAP)	
GENERIC	$1.18	10 ml	$13.03

BRAND/MANUFACTURER	NDC	SIZE	AWP
◆ GENERICS			
Schein	00364-6686-54	10 ml	$8.49
Steris	00402-0383-10	10 ml	$8.49
URL	00677-0309-21	10 ml	$10.80
Major	00904-0868-10	10 ml	$13.35
Goldline	00182-1197-63	10 ml	$15.75
Geneva	00781-3102-70	10 ml	$15.97
Rugby	00536-8900-70	10 ml	$18.38
Major	00904-0868-30	30 ml	$9.84

Testosterone, Transdermal

DESCRIPTION
The Testosterone Transdermal system is designed to release controlled amounts of the primary circulating endogenous androgen continuously upon application to scrotal skin.

Two sizes are available to provide nominal in vivo transdermal delivery of 4 or 6 mg Testosterone for one day (patients vary in their ability to absorb Testosterone, see *"Clinical Studies"*); they have a contact surface area of 40 or 60 cm^2 and contain 10 or 15 mg Testosterone USP, respectively. The composition of the two sizes per unit area is identical. Testosterone USP is a white or creamy-white crystalline powder or crystals chemically described as 17-beta hydroxyand-rost-4-en-3-one. Its empirical formula is $C_{19}H_{28}O_2$ and molecular weight is 288.43.

The Testosterone Transdermal system comprises two layers. Proceeding from the outer surface to the film in contact with the skin, these layers are a soft flexible backing of polyethylene terephthalate and a Testosterone-containing film of ethylenevinyl acetate copolymer that contacts the skin surface and modulates the availability of the steroid. A protective liner of fluorocarbon diacrylate or silicone-coated polyester covers the drug film and must be removed before the system can be used.

The active component of the system is Testosterone. The remaining components of the system are pharmacologically inactive.

Following is its chemical structure:

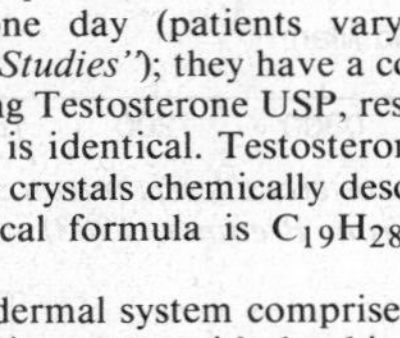

CLINICAL PHARMACOLOGY
The Testosterone Transdermal system releases the primary endogenous androgenic hormone. Endogenous androgens, including Testosterone and dihydrotestosterone (DHT), are responsible for the normal growth and development of the male sex organs and for maintenance of secondary sex characteristics. These effects include the growth and maturation of prostate, seminal vesicles, penis, and scrotum; the development of male hair distribution, such as facial, pubic, chest,

and axillary hair; laryngeal enlargement, vocal chord thickening, alterations in body musculature, and fat distribution. DHT is necessary for the normal development of secondary sex characteristics.

Drugs in this class also cause retention of nitrogen, sodium, potassium, phosphorus, and decreased urinary excretion of calcium. Androgens have been reported to increase protein anabolism and decrease protein catabolism. Nitrogen balance is improved only when there is sufficient intake of calories and protein.

Androgen are responsible for the growth spurt of adolescence and for the eventual termination of linear growth brought about by fusion of the epiphyseal growth centers. In children, exogenous androgens accelerate linear growth rates but may cause a disproportionate advancement in bone maturation. Use over long periods may result in fusion of the epiphyseal growth centers and termination of the growth process. Androgens have been reported to stimulate the production of red blood cells by enhancing the production of erythropoietin.

During exogenous administration of androgens, endogenous Testosterone release may be inhibited through feedback inhibition of pituitary luteinizing hormone (LH). At large doses of exogenous androgens, spermatogenesis may also be suppressed through feedback inhibition of pituitary follicle-stimulating hormone (FSH).

There is a lack of substantial evidence that androgens are effective in fractures, surgery, or convalescence.

PHARMACOKINETICS

Endogenous total Testosterone serum concentrations in normal males follow a diurnal pattern. Young men and old men have slightly different patterns (Figure A). Daily application of a Testosterone Transdermal system approximates the natural endogenous pattern of serum Testosterone of normal males. Following placement of a Testosterone Transdermal system on scrotal skin, the serum Testosterone concentration rises to a maximum at 2 to 4 hours and returns toward baseline within approximately 2 hours after system removal. Serum levels reach a plateau at 3 to 4 weeks. Hypogonadal men using Testosterone Transdermal therapy have trough serum Testosterone concentrations that are about 15% of peak levels. The Testosterone levels achieved with Testosterone Transdermal therapy generally are within the range for normal men (see also "Clinical Studies"). The typical pattern achieved with nominal Testosterone delivery of 6 mg/daily from Testosterone Transdermal systems is shown in Figure B. Scrotal skin is at least five times more permeable to Testosterone than other skin sites. The Testosterone Transdermal system will not produce adequate serum Testosterone concentration if it is applied to nongenital skin.

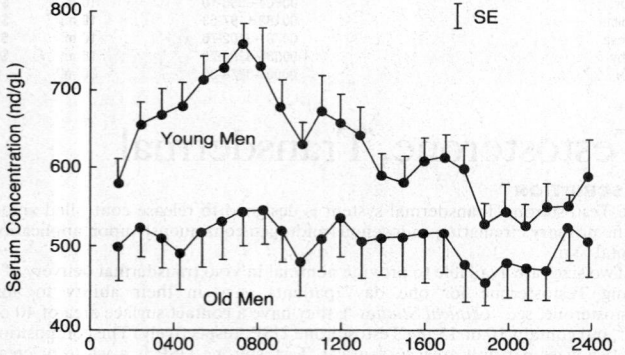

Figure A. Hourly serum Testosterone levels (mean ± SE) in normal young (n = 17) and old (n = 12) men. (From Bremner, 1983)

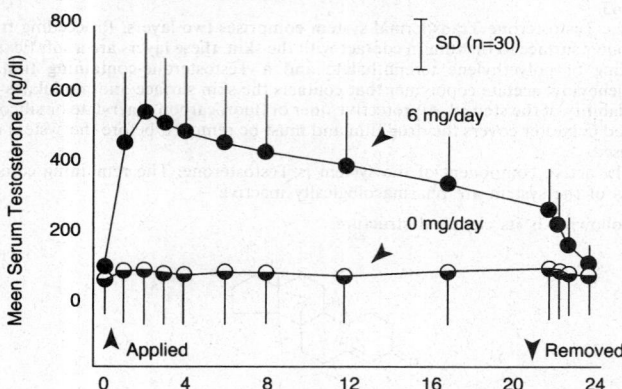

Figure B. Serum concentration of Testosterone (mean ± SD) while wearing a Testosterone Transdermal system or placebo (n=30). Systems were applied at 0 hours and removed at 22 hours.

There is considerable variation in the half-life of Testosterone as reported in the literature, ranging from 10 to 100 minutes.

Circulating Testosterone is chiefly bound in the serum to sex hormone-binding globulin (SHBG) and albumin. The albumin-bound fraction of Testosterone easily

dissociates from albumin and is presumed to be bioactive. The portion of Testosterone bound to SHBG is not considered biologically active. The amount of SHBG in the serum and the total Testosterone level will determine the distribution of bioactive and nonbioactive androgen. SHBG-binding capacity is high in prepubertal children, declines during puberty and adulthood and increases again during the later decades of life.

Testosterone is a substrate for conversion to an active metabolite dihydrotestosterone (DHT).

About 90 percent of a dose of Testosterone given intramuscularly is excreted in the urine as glucuronic and sulfuric acid conjugates of Testosterone and its metabolites; about 6 percent of a dose is excreted in the feces, mostly in the unconjugated form. Inactivation of Testosterone occurs primarily in the liver. Testosterone is metabolized to various 17-keto steroids through two different pathways, and the major active metabolites are estradiol and dihydrotestosterone (DHT). Normal concentrations of estradiol in men are 0.8 to 3.5 ng/dL. DHT concentrations in normal male serum are 30 to 85 ng/dL. DHT binds with greater affinity to SHBG than does Testosterone. In reproductive tissues, DHT is further metabolized to 3-alpha and 3-beta androstanediol.

In many tissues the activity of Testosterone appears to depend on reduction to dihydrotestosterone, which binds to cytosol receptor proteins. The steroid-receptor complex is transported to the nucleus where it initiates transcription and cellular changes related to androgen action.

CLINICAL STUDIES

After at least 3 weeks of Testosterone Transdermal therapy when steady state is obtained, 30 hypogonadal men treated with 6 mg/d systems for 22 hours daily achieved mean maximum serum Testosterone concentrations of 593 ng/dL at 2 to 4 hours post-application. Sixty percent of the patients achieved individual maximal Testosterone concentrations >500 ng/dL. The mean 24-hour steady-state AUC (area under the curve) value was 9132 ng/dL. The mean DHT serum concentrations ranged from 134 to 162 ng/dL. Normal levels of Testosterone have been maintained in patients who have worn the systems for up to six years. DHT levels also remain stable. The increase in serum Testosterone concentration is proportional to the size of the system.

The variability of total Testosterone concentrations among patients receiving Testosterone Transdermal treatment had a coefficient of variation from 35% to 49%. The coefficient of variation of total Testosterone concentrations within individual patients was 30% to 41%. This variability is comparable to the values reported in the literature for both normal and hypogonadal men.

In two 12-week clinical studies in 72 hypogonadal men, Testosterone Transdermal therapy produced positive effects on mood and sexual behavior. By 5 weeks, 45 patients not previously treated with Testosterone Transdermal systems showed statistically significant increases in sexual activity. Compared to baseline, mean sexual events per week increased for sexual intercourse (0.3 to 0.8), orgasm (0.4 to 1.2), waking erections (1.0 to 3.5), and spontaneous erections (0.4 to 2.8).

Changes in nonfasting serum lipid concentrations were observed during Testosterone Transdermal therapy. By three months total cholesterol and high-density lipoprotein cholesterol decreased an average of 8% and 13%, respectively. High-density lipoprotein cholesterol remained stable thereafter. Total cholesterol continued to decrease through two years. At the end of two years, the total cholesterol/high-density lipoprotein cholesterol ratio was not different from pretreatment values.

Composite results of all studies show elevated dihydrotestosterone concentrations and a change in the ratio of Testosterone to dihydrotestosterone (T/DHT) during treatment. The range in this ratio was 0.7-12.5, as compared with a ratio of 3.6-15.2 in normal untreated men. The long-term effects of the change in this ratio are not known.

Estradiol levels increased to the normal range with treatment. Sporadic elevations of estradiol above the normal range for men were observed in 3 of 72 patients and these were not associated with feminizing side effects.

INDICATIONS AND USAGE

The Testosterone Transdermal system is indicated for replacement therapy in males for conditions associated with a deficiency or absence of endogenous Testosterone.

1. Primary hypogonadism (congenital or acquired)—testicular failure due to cryptorchidism, bilateral torsion, orchitis, vanishing testis syndrome, orchidectomy, Klinefelter's syndrome, chemotherapy, or toxic damage from alcohol or heavy metals. These men usually have low serum Testosterone levels and gonadotropins (FSH, LH) above the normal range.

2. Hypogonadotropic hypogonadism (congenital or acquired)—idiopathic gonadotropin or LHRH deficiency or pituitary-hypothalamic injury from tumors, trauma, or radiation. These men have low Testosterone serum levels but have gonadotropins in the normal or low range.

Testosterone Transdermal therapy has not been evaluated clinically in males under 18 years of age.

CONTRAINDICATIONS

Androgens are contraindicated in men with carcinoma of the breast or known or suspected carcinoma of the prostate.

Testosterone Transdermal therapy has not been evaluated in women and must not be used in women. Testosterone may cause fetal harm.

Testosterone Transdermal systems should not be used in patients with known hypersensitivity to any components of the system.

◆ RATED THERAPEUTICALLY EQUIVALENT; ◇ THERAPEUTIC EQUIVALENCE UNCONFIRMED; ○ UNRATED

WARNINGS

Prolonged use of high doses of orally active 17-alpha-alkyl androgens (eg, methyltestosterone) has been associated with serious hepatic adverse effects (peliosis hepatitis, hepatic neoplasms, cholestatic hepatitis, and jaundice). Long-term therapy with Testosterone enanthate, which elevates blood levels for prolonged periods, has produced multiple hepatic adenomas. Testosterone is not known to produce these adverse effects.

Geriatric patients treated with androgens may be at an increased risk for the development of prostatic hypertrophy and prostatic carcinoma (see *"Precautions: Carcinogenesis, Mutagenesis, Impairment of Fertility"*).

Edema with or without congestive heart failure may be a serious complication in patients with preexisting cardiac, renal, or hepatic disease. In addition to discontinuation of the drug, diuretic therapy may be required.

Gynecomastia frequently develops and occasionally persists in patients being treated for hypogonadism.

PRECAUTIONS
INFORMATION FOR THE PATIENT
A booklet containing instructions for use of the Testosterone Transdermal system is available.

The physician should instruct patients to report any of the following side effects of androgens:

■ Too frequent or presistent erections of the penis.
■ Any nausea, vomiting, changes in skin color or ankle swelling.

Virilization of female partners has been reported with use of a topical Testosterone solution. Percutaneous creams leave as much as 90 mg residual Testosterone on the skin. Results from one study indicated that the potential for transfer of Testosterone to a sexual partner from a Testosterone Transdermal system is 6 μg/d, 1/45th the daily endogenous Testosterone production by the female body. Changes in body hair distribution or significant increase in acne of the female partner should be brought to the attention of a physician.

LABORATORY TESTS
1. Hemoglobin and hematocrit levels should be checked periodically (to detect polycythemia) in patients on long-term androgen therapy.
2. Liver function, prostatic acid phosphatase, prostatic specific antigen, cholesterol, and high-density lipoproteins should be checked periodically.

DRUG INTERACTIONS
1. Anticoagulants, C-17 substituted derivatives of Testosterone, such as methandrostenolone, have been reported to decrease the anticoagulant requirements of patients receiving oral anticoagulants. Patients receiving oral anticoagulant therapy require close monitoring, especially when androgens are started or stopped.
2. Oxyphenbutazone. Concurrent administration of oxyphenbutazone and androgens may result in elevated serum levels of oxyphenbutazone.
3. Insulin. In diabetic patients the metabolic effects of androgens may decrease blood glucose and, therefore, insulin requirements.

DRUG/LABORATORY TEST INTERACTIONS
Androgens may decrease levels of thyroxin-binding globulin, resulting in decreased total T_4 serum levels and increased resin uptake of T_3 and T_4. Free thyroid hormone levels remain unchanged, however, and there is no clinical evidence of thyroid dysfunction.

CARCINOGENESIS, MUTAGENESIS, IMPAIRMENT OF FERTILITY
Animal Data: Testosterone has been tested by subcutaneous injection and implantation in mice and rats. In mice, the implant induced cervical-uterine tumors, which metastasized in some cases. There is suggestive evidence that injection of Testosterone into some strains of female mice increases their susceptibility to hepatoma. Testosterone is also known to increase the number of tumors and decrease the degree of differentiation of chemically induced carcinomas of the liver in rats.

Human Data: There are rare reports of hepatocellular carcinoma in patients receiving long-term therapy with androgens in high doses. Withdrawal of the drugs did not lead to regression of the tumors in all cases.

Geriatric Use: Geriatric patients treated with androgens may be at an increased risk for the development of prostatic hypertrophy and prostatic carcinoma.

PREGNANCY CATEGORY X
(See *"Contraindications"*.)

Teratogenic Effects: Testosterone Transdermal therapy must not be used in women.

Nursing Mothers: Testosterone Transdermal therapy must not be used in women.

Pediatric Use: Testosterone Transdermal therapy has not been evaluated clinically in males under 18 years of age.

ADVERSE REACTIONS
ADVERSE REACTIONS WITH THE TESTOSTERONE TRANSDERMAL SYSTEM
In clinical studies of 104 patients treated with the Testosterone Transdermal system the most common adverse effects reported were local effects. In US clinical trials, most of the 72 patients filling out a daily questionnaire reported scrotal itching, discomfort, or irritation at some time during therapy. Of all the daily questionnaire responses, 7% reported itching, 4% discomfort, and 2% irritation. All topical reactions decreased with duration of use.

The following adverse effects were reported in association with Testosterone Transdermal therapy in 104 patients using the product for up to three years; a causal relationship to Testosterone Transdermal treatment was not always determined. These effects are listed in decreasing order of occurrence with the number of patients reporting the effect in parentheses: Gynecomastia (5), acne (4), prostatitis/urinary tract infection (4), breast tenderness (3), stroke (2), memory loss (1), pupillary dilation (1), abnormal liver enzymes (1), scrotal cellulitis (1), deep vein phlebitis (1), benign prostatic hypertrophy (1), rectal mucosal lesion over prostate (1), hematuria/bladder cancer (1), papilloma on scrotum (1), and congestive heart failure (1). See *"Clinical Pharmacology, Clinical Studies"* subsection, regarding effects on serum lipids.

ADVERSE REACTIONS WITH INJECTION OR ORAL ANDROGEN THERAPY
Skin and Appendages: Hirsutism, male pattern of baldness, seborrhea, and acne.

Endocrine and Urogenital: Gynecomastia and excessive frequency and duration of penile erections. Oligospermia may occur at high dosages (see *"Clinical Pharmacology"*).

Fluid and Electrolyte Disturbances: Retention of sodium, chloride, water, potassium, calcium, and inorganic phosphates.

Gastrointestinal: Nausea, cholestatic jaundice, alterations in liver function tests. Rare instances of hepatocellular neoplasms and peliosis hepatitis have occurred (see *"Warnings"*).

Hematologic: Suppression of clotting factors II, V, VII, and X, bleeding in patients on concomitant anticoagulant therapy, and polycythemia.

Nervous System: Increased or decreased libido, headache, anxiety, depression, and generalized paresthesia.

Metabolic: Increased serum cholesterol.

Miscellaneous: Rarely, anaphylactoid reactions.

DRUG ABUSE AND DEPENDENCE
Testosterone Transdermal system is a Schedule III controlled substance under the Anabolic Steroids Control Act.

With oral administration, it is not possible to achieve clinically significant serum Testosterone concentrations in the target organs using the Testosterone in the Testosterone, Transdermal system due to extensive first-pass metabolism. The half-life of an IM injection of Testosterone is about 10 minutes.

Because scrotal skin is at least five times more permeable to Testosterone than other skin sites, the Testosterone Transdermal system will not produce adequate serum Testosterone concentrations if it is applied to nongenital skin.

OVERDOSAGE
There is one report of acute overdosage with Testosterone enanthate: Testosterone levels of up to 11,400 ng/dL were implicated in a cerebrovascular accident.

DOSAGE AND ADMINISTRATION
Patients should start therapy with a 6 mg/d system applied daily; if scrotal area is inadequate, a 4 mg/d system should be used. The Testosterone, Transdermal system should be placed on clean, dry, scrotal skin. Scrotal hair should be dry-shaved for optimal skin contact. Chemical depilatories should not be used (see *"Patient Information"*). The Testosterone Transdermal system should be worn 22-24 hours.

After 3-4 weeks of daily system use, blood should be drawn 2-4 hours after system application for determination of serum total Testosterone. Because of variability in analytical values among diagnostic laboratories, this laboratory work and later analyses for assessing the effect of the Testosterone Transdermal therapy should be performed at the same laboratory.

If patients have not achieved desired results by the end of 6-8 weeks of therapy with the Testosterone, Transdermal system, another form of Testosterone replacement therapy should be considered.

Testosterone Transdermal system is a Schedule III controlled substance under the Anabolic Steroids Control Act.

Store at room temperature, 15-30°C.

REFERENCE
Bremner WJ, Vitiello MV, Prinz PN. *Loss of Circadian Rhythmicity in Blood Testosterone Levels with Aging in Normal Men.* J Clin Endocrin Metab (1983) 56 (6): 1278-1281.

HOW SUPPLIED
FILM, EXTENDED RELEASE (C-III): 4 MG

BRAND/MANUFACTURER	NDC	SIZE	AWP
BRAND			
TESTODERM: Alza	17314-4608-03	30s	$67.68

FILM, EXTENDED RELEASE (C-III): 6 MG

BRAND/MANUFACTURER	NDC	SIZE	AWP
BRAND			
TESTODERM: Alza	17314-4609-03	30s	$67.68

➤ SHOWN IN PRODUCT IDENTIFICATION GUIDE

Tetanus Immune Globulin

DESCRIPTION

Tetanus Immune Globulin (Human), USP is a sterile solution of tetanus hyperimmune immunoglobulin, primarily immunoglobulin G (IgG), containing 15%-18% protein, of which not less than 90% is gamma globulin. This product has been prepared from large pools of plasma obtained from individuals immunized with tetanus toxoid. Tetanus Immune Globulin is stabilized with 0.21-0.32 M glycine and contains the mercurial preservative sodium ethylmercurithiosalicylate (thimerosal), 80-120 μg per mL as measured by mercury assay. The pH is adjusted to 6.4-7.2 with sodium carbonate or acetic acid as required. The product is standardized against the U.S. Standard Antitoxin and the U.S. Control Tetanus Toxin and contains not less than 250 tetanus antitoxin units per container. Tetanus Immune Globulin must be administered intramuscularly.

CLINICAL PHARMACOLOGY

Tetanus Immune Globulin supplies passive immunity to those individuals who have low or no immunity to the toxin produced by the tetanus organism, *Clostridium tetani*. The antibodies act to neutralize the free form of the powerful exotoxin produced by this bacterium. Historically, such passive protection was provided by antitoxin derived from equine or bovine serum; however, the foreign protein in these heterologous products often produced severe allergic manifestations, even in individuals who demonstrated negative skin and/or conjunctival tests prior to administration. Estimates of the frequency of these foreign protein reactions following antitoxin of equine origin varied from 5%-30%.[1-4]

Several studies suggest the value of human tetanus anti-toxin in the treatment of active tetanus.[5,6] In 1961 and 1962, Nation et al,[5] using Tetanus Immune Globulin treated 20 patients with tetanus using single doses of 3,000 to 6,000 antitoxin units in combination with other accepted clinical and nursing procedures. Six patients, all over 45 years of age, died of causes other than tetanus. The authors felt that the mortality rate (30%) compared favorably with their previous experience using equine antitoxin in larger doses and that the results were much better than the 60% national death rate for tetanus reported from 1951 to 1954.[7] Blake et al, however, found in a data analysis of 545 cases of tetanus reported to the Centers for Disease Control from 1965 to 1971 that survival was no better with 8,000 units of human Tetanus Immune Globulin (TIG) than with 500 units; however, an optimal dose could not be determined.

Passive immunization with Tetanus Immune Globulin may be undertaken concomitantly with active immunization using tetanus toxoid in those persons who must receive an immediate injection of tetanus antitoxin and in whom it is desirable to begin the process of active immunization. Based on the work of Rubbo,[9] McComb and Dwyer,[10] and Levine at al,[11] the physician may thus supply immediate passive protection against tetanus, and at the same time begin formation of active immunization in the injured individual which upon completion of a *full toxoid series* will preclude future need for antitoxin. Peak blood levels of IgG are obtained approximately 2 days after intramuscular injection. The half-life of IgG in the circulation of individuals with normal IgG levels is approximately 23 days.[12]

INDICATIONS AND USAGE

Tetanus Immune Globulin (Human), USP—is indicated for prophylaxis against tetanus following injury in patients whose immunization is incomplete or uncertain (see below). It is also indicated, although evidence of effectiveness is limited, in the regimen of treatment of active cases of tetanus.[5,6,13]

The following table is a summary guide to tetanus prophylaxis in wound management:

GUIDE TO TETANUS PROPHYLAXIS IN WOUND MANAGEMENT[14]

History of Tetanus Immunization (Doses)	Clean, Minor Wounds		All Other Wounds	
	Td*	TIG§	Td	TIG
Uncertain or less than 3	Yes	No	Yes	Yes
3 or more†	No‡	No	No£	No

* *Adult type tetanus and diphtheria toxoids. If the patient is less than 7 years old, DT or DTP is given (see "Dosage and Administration").*
§ *Tetanus Immune Globulin (Human)*
† *If only three doses of fluid tetanus toxoid have been received, a fourth dose of toxoid, preferably an adsorbed toxoid, should be given.*
‡ *Yes if more than 10 years since the last dose.*
£ *Yes if more than 5 years since the last dose.*

CONTRAINDICATIONS

None known.

WARNINGS

Tetanus Immune Globulin should be given with caution to patients with a history of prior systemic allergic reactions following the administration of human immunoglobulin preparations, or in patients who are known to have had an allergic response to thimerosal.

In patients who have severe thrombocytopenia or any coagulation disorder that would contraindicate intramuscular injections, Tetanus Immune Globulin should be given only if the expected benefits outweigh the risks.

PRECAUTIONS

GENERAL

Tetanus Immune Globulin should not be given intravenously. Intravenous injection of immunoglobulin intended for intramuscular use can, on occasion, cause a precipitous fall in blood pressure, and a picture not unlike anaphylaxis. Injections should only be made *intramuscularly* and care should be taken to draw back on the plunger of the syringe before injection in order to be certain that the needle is not in a blood vessel. Intramuscular injections are preferably administered in the anterolateral aspects of the upper thigh and the deltoid muscle of the upper arm. The gluteal region should not be used routinely as an injection site because of the risk of injury to the sciatic nerve. If the gluteal region is used, the central region MUST be avoided; only the upper, outer quadrant should be used.[15]

Skin tests should not be done. The intradermal injection of concentrated IgG solutions often causes a localized area of inflammation which can be misinterpreted as a positive allergic reaction. In actuality, this does not represent an allergy: rather, it is localized tissue irritation. Misinterpretation of the results of such tests can lead the physician to withhold needed human antitoxin from a patient who is not actually allergic to this material. True allergic responses to human IgG given in the prescribed intramuscular manner are rare.

Although systemic reactions to human immunoglobulin preparations are rare, epinephrine should be available for treatment of acute anaphylactic reactions.

DRUG INTERACTIONS

Antibodies in immunoglobulin preparations may interfere with the response to live viral vaccines such as measles, mumps, polio, and rubella. Therefore, use of such vaccines should be deferred until approximately 3 months after Tetanus Immune Globulin (Human), USP—administration.

No interactions with other products are known.

PREGNANCY CATEGORY C

Animal reproduction studies have not been conducted with Tetanus Immune Globulin. It is also not known whether Tetanus Immune Globulin can cause fetal harm when administered to a pregnant woman or can affect reproduction capacity. Tetanus Immune Globulin should be given to a pregnant woman only if clearly needed.

ADVERSE REACTIONS

Slight soreness at the site of injection and slight temperature elevation may be noted at times. Sensitization to repeated injections of human immunoglobulin is extremely rare.

In the course of routine injections of large numbers of persons with immunoglobulin there have been a few isolated occurrences of angioneurotic edema, nephrotic syndrome, and anaphylactic shock after injection.

OVERDOSAGE

Although no data are available, clinical experience with other immunoglobulin preparations suggests that the only manifestations would be pain and tenderness at the injection site.

DOSAGE AND ADMINISTRATION

ROUTINE PROPHYLACTIC DOSAGE SCHEDULE

Adults and children 7 years and older: Tetanus Immune Globulin 250 units should be given by deep intramuscular injection (see *"Precautions"*). At the same time, but in a different extremity and with a separate syringe, Tetanus and Diphtheria Toxoids Adsorbed (For Adult Use) (Td) should be administered according to the manufacturer's package insert.

Children less than 7 years old: In small children the routine prophylactic dose of Tetanus Immune Globulin may be calculated by the body weight (4.0 units/kg). However, it may be advisable to administer the entire contents of the vial or syringe of Tetanus Immune Globulin (250 units) regardless of the child's size, since theoretically the same amount of toxin will be produced in the child's body by the infecting tetanus organism as it will in an adult's body. At the same time but in a different extremity and with a different syringe, diphtheria and tetanus toxoids and pertussis vaccine adsorbed (DTP) or diphtheria and tetanus toxoids adsorbed (for pediatric use)(DT), if pertussis vaccine is contraindicated, should be administered per the manufacturer's package insert.

Note: The single injection of tetanus toxoid only initiates the series for producing active immunity in the recipient. The physician must impress upon the patient the need for further toxoid injections in 1 month and 1 year. Without such, the active immunization series is incomplete.

Current recommendations for wound management of patients definitely known to have completed a full tetanus toxoid series indicate tetanus toxoid booster only if more than 5 to 10 years have elapsed since the last dose of toxoid.[14] The prophylactic dosage schedule for these patients and for those with incomplete or uncertain immunity is shown on the table in *"Indications and Usage"*.

Since tetanus is actually a local infection, proper initial wound care is of paramount importance. The use of antitoxin is adjunctive to this procedure. However, in approximately 10% of the recent tetanus cases, no wound or other breach in skin or mucous membrane could be implicated.[16]

TREATMENT OF ACTIVE CASES OF TETANUS

Standard therapy for the treatment of active tetanus including the use of Tetanus Immune Globulin must be implemented immediately. The dosage should be adjusted according to the severity of the infection.[5,6]

◆ RATED THERAPEUTICALLY EQUIVALENT; ◇ THERAPEUTIC EQUIVALENCE UNCONFIRMED; ○ UNRATED

Parenteral drug products should be inspected visually for particulate matter and discoloration prior to administration, whenever solution and container permit. They should not be used if particulate matter and/or discoloration are present.

STORAGE
Store at 2°-8°C (35°-46°F). Solution that has been frozen should not be used.

LIMITED WARRANTY
A number of factors beyond the manufacturer's control could reduce the efficacy of this product or even result in an ill effect following its use. These include improper storage and handling of the product after it leaves the manufacturer's hands, diagnosis, dosage, method of administration, and biological differences in individual patients. Because of these factors it is important that this product be stored properly and that the directions be followed carefully during use.

REFERENCES
1. Moynihan NH: Tetanus prophylaxis and serum sensitivity tests. *Br Med J* 1:260-4, 1956. 2. Scheibel I: The uses and results of active tetanus immunization. *Bull WHO* 13:381-94, 1955. 3. Edsall G: Specific prophylaxis of tetanus. *JAMA* 171(4):417-27, 1959. 4. Bardenwerper HW: Serum neuritis from tetanus antitoxin. *JAMA* 179(10):763-6, 1962. 5. Nation NS, Pierce NF, Adler SJ, et al: Tetanus: the use of human hyperimmune globulin in treatment. *Calif Med* 98(6):305-6, 1963. 6. Ellis M: Human antitetanus serum in the treatment of tetanus. *Br Med J* 1(5338):1123-6, 1963. 7. Axnick NW, Alexander ER: Tetanus in the United States: A review of the problem. *Am J Public Health* 47(12):1493-1501, 1957. 8. Blake PA, Feldman RA, Buchanan TM, et al: Serologic therapy of tetanus in the United States, 1965-1971. *JAMA* 235(1):42-4, 1976. 9. Rubbo SD: New approaches to tetanus prophylaxis. *Lancet* 2(7461):449-53, 1966. 10. McComb JA, Dwyer RC: Passive-active immunization with tetanus immune globulin (human). *N Engl J Med* 268(16):857-62, 1963. 11. Levine L., McComb JA, Dwyer RC, et al: Active-passive tetanus immunization; choice of toxoid, dose of tetanus immune globulin and timing of injections. *N Engl J Med* 274(4):186-90, 1966. 12. Waldmann TA, Strober W, Blaese RM: Variations in the metabolism of immunoglobulins measured by turnover rates. In Merler E (ed.): Immunoglobulins; biologic aspects and clinical uses. Washington, DC, Nat Acad Sci, 1970, p 33-51. 13. McCracken GH Jr., Dowell DL, Marshall FN: Double-blind trial of equine antitoxin and human immune globulin in tetanus neonatorum. *Lancet* 1(7710):1146-9, 1971. 14. American Academy of Pediatrics, Committee on Infectious Diseases: Report ed. 20. Evanston, 1986, p. 355-9. 15. Recommendations of the Immunization Practices Advisory Committee (ACIP): General recommendations on immunization. *MMWR* 38(13): 205-14; 219-27, 1989. 16. Tetanus-Rates by year, United States, 1955-1984. Annual Summary 1984. *MMWR* 33 (54):61, 1986.

J CODES
Up to 250 units IM—J1670

HOW SUPPLIED
INJECTION: 250 U

BRAND/MANUFACTURER	NDC	SIZE	AWP
○ BRAND			
HYPER-TET: Miles Biol	00192-0614-01	1 ml	$23.44
	00192-0614-70	1 ml 10s	$234.38

Tetanus Toxoid Adsorbed

DESCRIPTION
Tetanus Toxoid Adsorbed is a sterile preparation of refined Tetanus toxoid for intramuscular use only. After shaking, the product is a homogeneous white suspension.

The Tetanus toxin is produced according to the method of Mueller and Miller[1] and is detoxified by use of formaldehyde. The Toxoid is refined by the Pillemer alcohol fractionation method[2] and is diluted with a solution containing sodium phosphate dibasic, sodium phosphate monobasic, glycine sodium chloride and thimerosal (mercury derivative) in a final concentration of 1:10,000 as a preservative and aluminum phosphate as adjuvant. The aluminum content does not exceed 0.80 mg per 0.5 mL dose.

Each 0.5 mL dose is formulated to contain 5 Lf units of Tetanus Toxoid.

CLINICAL PHARMACOLOGY
Tetanus is an intoxication manifested primarily by neuromuscular dysfunction, caused by a potent exotoxin elaborated by *Clostridium tetani*. The incidence of tetanus in the U.S. has dropped dramatically with the routine use of Tetanus Toxoid, remaining relatively constant over the last decade at about 90 cases reported annually[3]. Spores of *C tetani* are ubiquitous, and there is essentially no natural immunity to tetanus toxin. Thus, universal primary immunization with Tetanus Toxoid, and subsequent maintenance of adequate antitoxin levels by means of timed boosters, is necessary to protect all age groups[3]. Tetanus Toxoid is a highly effective antigen, and a completed primary series generally induces protective levels of serum antitoxin that persist for at least 10 years[3].

INDICATIONS AND USAGE
Tetanus Toxoid Adsorbed is indicated for active immunization against tetanus in adults and children 2 months of age or older.

Immunization of persons 7 years of age or older may be accomplished by the use of Tetanus and Diphtheria Toxoids Adsorbed, for Adult Use (Td), Tetanus Toxoid Adsorbed, or Tetanus Toxoid Fluid. The Immunization Practices Advisory Committee (ACIP) of the U.S. Public Health Service recommends the use of the combined Toxoids vaccine rather than single component vaccines for both primary and booster injections, including active Tetanus immunization in wound management[3]. Individuals for whom the use of a vaccine containing diphtheria toxoid is contraindicated should receive a single-component Tetanus Toxoid-containing vaccine. Immunization of infants and children 2 months of age up to the seventh birthday is usually accomplished by the use of Diphtheria and Tetanus Toxoids and Pertussis Vaccine Adsorbed (DTP) or Diphtheria and Tetanus Toxoids Adsorbed, for pediatric use (DT). Tetanus Toxoid Adsorbed may be used for immunizing infants and children for whom the use of a vaccine containing diphtheria toxoid and pertussis antigen is contraindicated.

Comparative tests have shown that the adsorbed toxoids are superior to the fluid toxoids in antibody titers produced and in the durability of protection achieved. The promptness of antibody response to booster doses of either fluid or adsorbed toxoid is not sufficiently different to be of clinical importance. When Tetanus immune globulin (TIG) is to be administered at the same visit as Tetanus Toxoid, the Adsorbed Toxoid should be used.[3,4]

Persons Recovering from Tetanus: Tetanus infection may not confer immunity; therefore, initiation or completion of active immunization is indicated at the time of recovery from this infection.[3]

Neonatal Tetanus Prevention: There is no evidence that Tetanus Toxoid is teratogenic. A previously unimmunized pregnant woman who may deliver her child under nonhygienic circumstances and/or surroundings should receive two properly spaced doses of a Tetanus Toxoid-containing preparation before delivery, preferably during the last two trimesters. Incompletely immunized pregnant women should complete the three-dose series. Those immunized more than 10 years previously should have a booster dose.[3] (See also pregnancy information under *"Precautions".*)

CONTRAINDICATIONS
HYPERSENSITIVITY TO ANY COMPONENT OF THE VACCINE INCLUDING THIMEROSAL, A MERCURY DERIVATIVE, IS A CONTRAINDICATION.

THE OCCURRENCE OF ANY TYPE OF NEUROLOGICAL SYMPTOMS OR SIGNS FOLLOWING ADMINISTRATION OF THIS PRODUCT IS A CONTRAINDICATION TO FURTHER USE.

IMMUNIZATION SHOULD BE DEFERRED DURING THE COURSE OF ANY FEBRILE ILLNESS OR ACUTE INFECTION. A MINOR AFEBRILE ILLNESS SUCH AS A MILD UPPER RESPIRATORY INFECTION IS NOT USUALLY REASON TO DEFER IMMUNIZATION.[3]

The clinical judgment of the attending physician should prevail at all times.

Routine immunization should be deferred during an outbreak of poliomyelitis, providing the patient has not sustained an injury that increases the risk of tetanus.

WARNINGS
THE OCCURRENCE OF A NEUROLOGICAL OR SEVERE HYPERSENSITIVITY REACTION FOLLOWING A PREVIOUS DOSE IS A CONTRAINDICATION TO FURTHER USE OF THIS PRODUCT.[3]

THE ADMINISTRATION OF BOOSTER DOSES MORE FREQUENTLY THAN RECOMMENDED (see *"Dosage and Administration"*) MAY BE ASSOCIATED WITH INCREASED INCIDENCE AND SEVERITY OF REACTIONS.[3]

Persons who experience Arthus-type hypersensitivity reactions or temperature greater than 39.4°C (103°F) after a previous dose of Tetanus Toxoid usually have very high serum tetanus antitoxin levels and should not be given even emergency doses of Tetanus Toxoid more frequently than every 10 years, even if they have a wound that is neither clean nor minor.[3]

If a contraindication to using Tetanus Toxoid exists in a person who has not completed a primary immunizing course of Tetanus Toxoid, and other than a clean, minor wound is sustained, only passive immunization should be given using human Tetanus Immune Globulin (TIG).[3]

Tetanus Toxoid Adsorbed should not be given to individuals with thrombocytopenia or any coagulation disorder that would contraindicate intramuscular injection, unless the potential benefit clearly outweighs the risk of administration.

Patients with impaired immune responsiveness, whether due to the use of immunosuppressive therapy (including irradiation, corticosteroids, antimetabolites, alkylating agents, and cytotoxic agents), a genetic defect, human immunodeficiency virus (HIV) infection, or other causes, may have a reduced antibody response to active immunization procedures.[3,5] Deferral of administration of vaccine may be considered in individuals receiving immunosuppressive therapy.[3,4]

Special care should be taken to prevent injection into a blood vessel.

PRECAUTIONS
GENERAL
1. PRIOR TO ADMINISTRATION OF ANY DOSE OF VACCINE THE PARENT, GUARDIAN, OR ADULT PATIENT SHOULD BE ASKED ABOUT THE RECENT HEALTH STATUS AND IMMUNIZATION HISTORY OF THE PATIENT TO BE IMMUNIZED IN ORDER TO DETERMINE THE EXISTENCE OF ANY CONTRAINDICATIONS TO IMMUNIZATION (SEE *"CONTRAINDICATIONS," "WARNINGS"*).

2. WHEN THE PATIENT RETURNS FOR THE NEXT DOSE IN A SERIES, THE PARENT, GUARDIAN, OR ADULT PATIENT SHOULD BE QUESTIONED CONCERNING OCCURRENCE OF ANY SYMPTOM AND/OR SIGN OF AN ADVERSE REACTION AFTER THE PREVIOUS DOSE (SEE *"CONTRAINDICATIONS," "ADVERSE REACTIONS"*).

3. BEFORE THE INJECTION OF ANY BIOLOGICAL, THE PHYSICIAN SHOULD TAKE ALL PRECAUTIONS KNOWN FOR PREVENTION OF ALLERGIC OR ANY OTHER SIDE REACTIONS. This should include: a

review of the patient's history regarding possible sensitivity; the ready availability of epinephrine 1:1,000 and other appropriate agents used for control of immediate allergic reactions; and a knowledge of the recent literature pertaining to use of the biological concerned, including the nature of side effects and adverse reactions that may follow its use.

4. A separate sterile syringe and needle or a sterile disposable unit should be used for each individual patient to prevent transmission of hepatitis or other infectious agents from one person to another.

5. *Shake vigorously before withdrawing each dose to resuspend the contents of the vial.*

6. NATIONAL CHILDHOOD VACCINE INJURY ACT OF 1986 (AS AMENDED IN 1987)

This Act requires that the manufacturer and lot number of the vaccine administered be recorded by the health care provider in the vaccine recipient's permanent record, along with the date of administration of the vaccine and the name, address and title of the person administering the vaccine.

The Act further requires the health care provider to report to a health department or to the FDA the occurrence following immunization of any event set forth in the Vaccine Injury Table including: anaphylaxis or anaphylactic shock within 24 hours, encephalopathy or encephalitis within 7 days, residual seizure disorder, any acute complication or sequelae (including death) of above events, or any event that would contraindicate further doses of vaccine, according to this package insert.[6]

Information for the Patient: PRIOR TO ADMINISTRATION OF THIS VACCINE, HEALTH CARE PERSONNEL SHOULD INFORM THE PARENT, GUARDIAN, OR ADULT PATIENT OF THE BENEFITS AND RISKS OF VACCINATION AGAINST TETANUS.

Use in Pregnancy: Pregnancy Category C: Animal reproductive studies have not been conducted with this product. There is no evidence that Tetanus Toxoid is teratogenic. An appropriate Tetanus Toxoid-containing preparation (usually Td) should be given to inadequately immunized women because it affords protection against neonatal tetanus.[7] Waiting until the second trimester is a reasonable precaution to minimize any theoretical concern.[4] Maintenance of adequate immunization by routine boosters in nonpregnant women of child-bearing age (see *"Dosage and Administration"*) can obviate the need to vaccinate women during pregnancy.

ADVERSE REACTIONS

Local reactions, such as erythema, induration, and tenderness, are common after the administration of Tetanus Toxoid.[8-10] Such local reactions are usually self-limiting and require no therapy. Nodule,[11] sterile abscess formation, or subcutaneous atrophy may occur at the site of injection. Systemic reactions, such as fever, chills, myalgia, and headaches also may occur.[8-10]

Arthus-type hypersensitivity reactions, or high fever, may occur in persons who have very high serum antitoxin antibodies due to overly frequent injections of Toxoid.[3] (See *"Warnings"*.)

NEUROLOGICAL COMPLICATIONS,[12] SUCH AS CONVULSIONS,[13] ENCEPHALOPATHY,[13,14] AND VARIOUS MONO- AND POLYNEUROPATHIES,[14-20] INCLUDING GUILLAIN-BARRÉ SYNDROME,[21,22] HAVE BEEN REPORTED FOLLOWING ADMINISTRATION OF PREPARATIONS CONTAINING TETANUS ANTIGEN.

URTICARIA, ERYTHEMA MULTIFORME OR OTHER RASH, ARTHRALGIAS[13] AND, MORE RARELY, A SEVERE ANAPHYLACTIC REACTION (IE, URTICARIA WITH SWELLING OF THE MOUTH, DIFFICULTY BREATHING, HYPOTENSION, OR SHOCK) HAVE BEEN REPORTED FOLLOWING ADMINISTRATION OF PREPARATIONS CONTAINING TETANUS ANTIGEN.

DOSAGE AND ADMINISTRATION

For Intramuscular Use Only: Shake vigorously before withdrawing each dose to resuspend the contents of the vial or syringe.

Parenteral drug products should be inspected visually for particulate matter and discoloration prior to administration. (See *"Description"*.)

Preferred injection sites for intramuscular injection include the anterolateral aspect of the upper thigh and the deltoid area of the upper arm. Care should be taken to avoid major peripheral nerve trunks.

Before injection, the skin at the injection site should be cleansed and prepared with a suitable germicide.

After insertion of the needle, aspirate to help avoid inadvertent injection into a blood vessel.

The primary immunizing course for unimmunized individuals 1 year of age or older consists of *two* doses of 0.5 mL each, 4 to 8 weeks apart, followed by a *third* (reinforcing) dose of 0.5 mL, 6 to 12 months after the second dose. The reinforcing dose is an integral part of the primary immunizing course. If, after beginning combined immunization against diphtheria, tetanus, and pertussis, further doses of vaccine containing pertussis and diphtheria antigens become contraindicated, Tetanus Toxoid Adsorbed may be substituted for each of the remaining doses.

When immunization with Tetanus Toxoid Adsorbed is begun in the first year of life, the primary series consists of *three* doses of 0.5 mL each, 4 to 8 weeks apart, followed by a *fourth* (reinforcing) dose of 0.5 mL, 6 to 12 months after the third dose.

Interruption of the recommended schedule with a delay between doses does not interfere with the final immunity achieved with Tetanus Toxoid Adsorbed. There is no need to start the series over again, regardless of the length of time elapsed between doses.[3]

Booster Doses: A single injection of 0.5 mL of Tetanus Toxoid Adsorbed is given 10 years after completion of primary immunization and every 10 years thereafter. If a dose is given sooner as part of wound management, the next booster is not needed for 10 years thereafter. MORE FREQUENT BOOSTER DOSES ARE NOT INDICATED AND MAY BE ASSOCIATED WITH INCREASED INCIDENCE AND SEVERITY OF REACTIONS.[3]

Tetanus Prophylaxis in Wound Management: The need for active immunization with a Tetanus Toxoid-containing preparation, with or without passive immunization with human Tetanus Immune Globulin (TIG) depends on both the condition of the wound and the patient's immunization history. Tetanus has rarely occurred among persons with a documented primary series of Toxoid injections. A thorough attempt must be made to determine whether a patient has completed primary immunization.[3]

Individuals who have completed primary immunization against tetanus, and who sustain wounds which are minor and uncontaminated, should receive a booster dose of the appropriate Tetanus Toxoid-containing preparation (see *"Indications and Usage"*) only if they have not received Tetanus Toxoid within the preceding 10 years. For other wounds, a booster is appropriate if the patient has not received Tetanus Toxoid within the preceding 5 years. Antitoxin antibodies develop rapidly in persons who have previously received at least two doses of Tetanus Toxoid.[3]

Individuals who have not completed primary immunization against tetanus, or whose immunization history is unknown or uncertain, should be immunized with the appropriate Tetanus Toxoid-containing product (see *"Indications and Usage"*). Completion of primary immunization thereafter should be ensured. In addition, if these individuals have sustained a tetanus-prone wound, the use of human Tetanus immune globulin (TIG) is recommended. A separate syringe and site of administration should be used. When TIG is to be administered at the same visit as Tetanus Toxoid, an adsorbed Tetanus Toxoid-containing preparation should be used.[3]

SUMMARY GUIDE TO TETANUS PROPHYLAXIS IN ROUTINE WOUND MANAGEMENT[3]*

History of Tetanus Toxoid (doses)	Clean, minor wounds		All other wounds†	
	Td‡	TIG	Td‡	TIG
Unknown or < three	Yes	No	Yes	Yes
≥ three§	No"	No	No£	No

* *Important details are in the text.*
† *Such as, but not limited to, wounds contaminated with dirt, feces, soil, saliva, etc; puncture wounds; avulsions; and wounds resulting from missiles, crushing, burns and frostbite.*
‡ *For children under 7 years old DTP (DT, if pertussis vaccine is contraindicated) is preferred to Tetanus Toxoid alone. For persons 7 years and older, Td is preferred to Tetanus Toxoid alone.*
§ *If only three doses of fluid Toxoid have been received, a fourth dose of Toxoid, preferably an Adsorbed Toxoid, should be given.*
" *Yes, if more than 10 years since last dose.*
£ *Yes, if more than 5 years since last dose. (More frequent boosters are not needed and can accentuate side effects.)*

In order to enhance diphtheria protection in the population, the ACIP recommends Tetanus and diphtheria Toxoid For Adult Use as the preferred preparation for active Tetanus immunization in wound management of patients 7 years of age or older.[3]

Storage: DO NOT FREEZE. STORE REFRIGERATED, AWAY FROM FREEZER COMPARTMENT, AT 2°C to 8°C (36°F to 46°F).

REFERENCES
1. Mueller JH, Miller PA: Factors influencing the production of tetanal toxin. *J Immunol* 1947;56:143-147. 2. Pillemer L, Grossberg DB, Wittler RG: The immunochemistry of toxins and toxoids. II. The preparation and immunological evaluation of purified tetanal toxoid. *J Immunol* 1946;54:213-224. 3. Recommendation of the Immunization Practices Advisory Committee (ACIP): Diphtheria, Tetanus and pertussis: Guidelines for vaccine prophylaxis and other preventive measures. *MMWR* 1985;34:405-426. 4. Committee on Immunization, Council of Medical Societies, American College of Physicians: Guide for Adult Immunization, 1st Edition 1985; Philadelphia, PA. 5. Recommendation of the ACIP: Immunization of children infected with Human T-Lymphotrophic Virus Type III/Lymphadenopathy associated virus. *MMWR* 1986;35(38):595-606. 6. National Childhood Vaccine Injury Act: Requirements for permanent vaccination records and for reporting of selected events after vaccination. *MMWR* 1988;37(13):197-200. 7. Recommendations of the ACIP: General recommendations on immunization. *MMWR* 1983;32(1):1-17. 8. Macko MB, Powell CE: Comparison of the morbidity of Tetanus Toxoid boosters with Tetanus-diphtheria Toxoid boosters. *Ann Energy Med* 1985;14:(1):33-35. 9. Deacon SP, et al: A comparative clinical study of Adsorbed Tetanus vaccine and adult-type Tetanus-diphtheria vaccine. *J Hyg (Cambridge)* 1982;89:513-519. 10. Jacobs RL, et al: Adverse reactions to Tetanus Toxoid. *JAMA* 1982;247:(1):40-42. 11. Fawcett HA, Smith N: Injection-site granuloma due to aluminum. *Arch Dermatol* 1984;120:1318-1322. 12. Rutledge SL, Snead OC: Neurologic complications of immunizations. *J Pediatr* 1986;109:917-924. 13. Adverse Events Following Immunization. *MMWR* 1985;34(3):43-47. 14. Schlenska GK: Unusual neurological complications following Tetanus Toxoid administration. *J Neurol* 1977;215:299-302. 15. Blumstein GI, Kreithen H: Peripheral neuropathy following Tetanus Toxoid administration. *JAMA*

1966;198:1030-1031. 16. Reinstein L, Pargament JM, Goodman JS: Peripheral neuropathy after multiple Tetanus Toxoid injections. *Arch Phys Med Rehabil* 1982;63:332-334. 17. Tsairis P, Duck PJ, Mulder DW: Natural history of brachial plexus neuropathy. *Arch Neurol* 1972;27:109-117. 18. Quast U, Hennessen W, Widmark RM: Mono- and polyneuritis after Tetanus vaccination. *Devel Bio Stand* 1979;43:25-32. 19. Holliday PL, Bauer RB: Polyradiculoneuritis secondary to immunization with Tetanus and diphtheria Toxoids. *Arch Neurol* 1983;40:56-57. 20. Fenichel GM: Neurological complications of Tetanus Toxoid. *Arch Neurol* 1983;40:390. 21. Pollard JD, Selby G: Relapsing neuropathy due to Tetanus Toxoid. *J Neurol Sci* 1978;37:113-125. 22. Newton N, Janati A: Guillain-Barré syndrome after vaccination with purified Tetanus Toxoid. *S Med J* 1987;80:1053-1054.

J CODES

Up to 1 ml IM,SC—J3180

HOW SUPPLIED
INJECTION:

BRAND/MANUFACTURER	NDC	SIZE	AWP
○ **GENERICS**			
Sclavo	42021-0110-23	5 ml	$7.00
Berna	58337-1301-01	5 ml	$9.50
Wyeth-Ayerst	00008-0339-03	5 ml	$11.18
Connaught	49281-0800-83	5 ml	$13.13
Lederle Labs	00005-1938-31	5 ml	$13.85
Wyeth-Ayerst	00008-0340-02	7.5 ml	$11.18
Connaught	49281-0812-84	7.5 ml	$13.50
Berna	58337-1301-02	0.5 ml 10s	$22.20
Allscrips	54569-2540-00	0.5 ml 10s	$29.95
Lederle Labs	00005-1938-47	0.5 ml 10s ud	$29.80

INJECTION: 10 Lf U/0.5 ML

BRAND/MANUFACTURER	NDC	SIZE	AWP
○ **GENERICS**			
Sclavo	42021-0110-19	1 ml	$2.04
Wyeth-Ayerst	00008-0339-01	1 ml 10s	$20.33
Wyeth-Ayerst	00008-0340-01	1 ml 10s	$20.33

Tetracaine Hydrochloride, Injectable

DESCRIPTION

Tetracaine Hydrochloride is 2-(Dimethylamino)ethyl *p*-(butylamino) benzoate monohydrochloride. It is a white crystalline, odorless powder that is readily soluble in water, physiologic saline solution, and dextrose solution.

Tetracaine Hydrochloride is a local anesthetic of the ester-linkage type, related to procaine.

Tetracaine Hydrochloride is supplied in two forms for prolonged spinal anesthesia: instantly soluble particles and 1% Solution. A sterile, instantly soluble form consisting of a network of extremely fine, highly purified particles, resembling snow.

1% Solution: A sterile, isotonic, isobaric solution, each 1 mL containing 10 mg Tetracaine Hydrochloride, 6.7 mg.

Following is its chemical structure:

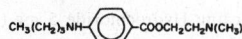

$CH_3(CH_2)_3NH$—⬡—$COOCH_2CH_2N(CH_3)_2$

CLINICAL PHARMACOLOGY

Parenteral administration of Tetracaine Hydrochloride, Injectable stabilizes the neuronal membrane and prevents initiation and transmission of nerve impulses thereby effecting local anesthesia. The onset of action is rapid, and the duration prolonged (up to two or three hours or longer of surgical anesthesia).

Tetracaine Hydrochloride, Injectable is detoxified by plasma esterases to aminobenzoic acid and diethylaminoethanol.

INDICATIONS AND USAGE

Tetracaine Hydrochloride, Injectable is indicated for the production of spinal anesthesia for procedures requiring two to three hours.

CONTRAINDICATIONS

Spinal anesthesia with Tetracaine Hydrochloride, Injectable is contraindicated in patients with known hypersensitivity to tetracaine hydrochloride or to drugs of a similar chemical configuration (ester-type local anesthetics), or aminobenzoic acid or its derivatives; and in patients for whom spinal anesthesia as a technique is contraindicated.

The decision as to whether or not spinal anesthesia should be used for an individual patient should be made by the physician after weighing the advantages with the risks and possible complications. Contraindications to spinal anesthesia as a technique can be found in standard reference texts, and usually include generalized septicemia, infection at the site of injection, certain diseases of the cerebrospinal system, uncontrolled hypotension, etc.

WARNINGS

RESUSCITATIVE EQUIPMENT AND DRUGS SHOULD BE IMMEDIATELY AVAILABLE WHENEVER ANY LOCAL ANESTHETIC DRUG IS USED.

Large doses of local anesthetics should not be used in patients with heartblock.

Reactions resulting in fatality have occurred on rare occasions with the use of local anesthetics, even in the absence of a history of hypersensitivity.

Contains acetone sodium bisulfite, a sulfite that may cause allergic-type reactions including anaphylactic symptoms and life-threatening or less severe asthmatic episodes in certain susceptible people. The overall prevalence of sulfite sensitivity in the general population is unknown and probably low. Sulfite sensitivity is seen more frequently in asthmatic than in nonasthmatic people.

PRECAUTIONS

The safety and effectiveness of any spinal anesthetic depend upon proper dosage, correct technique, adequate precautions, and readiness for emergencies. The lowest dosage that results in effective anesthesia should be used to avoid high plasma levels and serious systemic side effects. Tolerance varies with the status of the patient; debilitated, elderly patients or acutely ill patients should be given reduced doses commensurate with their weight, age, and physical status. Reduced doses are also indicated for obstetric patients and those with increased intra-abdominal pressure.

Caution should be used in administering Tetracaine Hydrochloride, Injectable to patients with abnormal or reduced levels of plasma esterases.

Blood pressure should be frequently monitored during spinal anesthesia and hypotension immediately corrected.

Spinal anesthetics should be used with caution in patients with severe disturbances of cardiac rhythm, shock, or heartblock.

Drug Interactions: Tetracaine Hydrochloride, Injectable should not be used if the patient is being treated with a sulfonamide because aminobenzoic acid inhibits the action of sulfonamides.

Carcinogenesis, Mutagenesis, Impairment of Fertility: Long-term animal studies to evaluate carcinogenic potential and reproduction studies in animals have not been performed. There is no evidence from human data that Tetracaine Hydrochloride, Injectable may be carcinogenic or that it impairs fertility.

Pregnancy Category C: Animal reproduction studies have not been conducted with Tetracaine Hydrochloride, Injectable. It is not known whether Tetracaine Hydrochloride, Injectable can cause fetal harm when administered to a pregnant woman or can affect reproduction capacity. Tetracaine Hydrochloride, Injectable should be given to a pregnant woman only if clearly needed and the potential benefits outweigh the risk.

Labor and Delivery: Vasopressor agents administered for the treatment of hypotension resulting from spinal anesthesia may result in severe persistent hypertension and/or rupture of cerebral blood vessels if oxytocic drugs have also been administered; therefore, vasopressors should be used with extreme caution in the presence of oxytocic drugs.

Tetracaine Hydrochloride, Injectable has a recognized use during labor and delivery; the effect of the drug on duration of labor, incidence of forceps delivery, status of the newborn, and later growth and development of the child have not been studied.

Nursing Mothers: It is not known whether Tetracaine Hydrochloride, Injectable is excreted in human milk, however, it is rapidly metabolized following absorption into the plasma. Because many drugs are excreted in human milk, caution should be exercised when Tetracaine Hydrochloride, Injectable brand of tetracaine hydrochloride, is administered to a nursing woman.

Pediatric Use: Safety and effectiveness of Tetracaine Hydrochloride, Injectable in children have not been established.

ADVERSE REACTIONS

Systemic adverse reactions to Tetracaine Hydrochloride, Injectable are characteristic of those associated with other local anesthetics and can involve the central nervous system and the cardiovascular system. Systemic reactions usually result from high plasma levels due to excessive dosage, rapid absorption, or inadvertent intravascular injection.

A small number of reactions to Tetracaine Hydrochloride, Injectable may result from hypersensitivity, idiosyncrasy, or diminished tolerance to normal dosage.

Central Nervous System: effects are characterized by excitation or depression. The first manifestation may be nervousness, dizziness, blurred vision, or tremors, followed by drowsiness, convulsions, unconsciousness and possibly respiratory and cardiac arrest. Since excitement may be transient or absent, the first manifestation may be drowsiness, sometimes merging into unconsciousness and respiratory and cardiac arrest. Other central nervous system effects may be nausea, vomiting, chills, constriction of the pupils, or tinnitus.

Cardiovascular: system reactions include depression of the myocardium, blood pressure changes (usually hypotension), and cardiac arrest.

Allergic: reactions, which may be due to hypersensitivity, idiosyncrasy, or diminished tolerance, are characterized by cutaneous lesions (eg, urticaria), edema, and other manifestations of allergy. Detection of sensitivity by skin testing is of limited value. Severe allergic reactions including anaphylaxis have occurred rarely and are not usually dose-related.

SUGGESTED DOSAGE FOR SPINAL ANESTHESIA

Extent of anesthesia	Using Tetracaine Hydrochloride instantly soluble particles		Using 1% Solution		
	Dose of Tetracaine Hydrochloride instantly soluble particles (mg)	Volume of spinal fluid (mL)	Dose of solution (mL)	Volume of spinal fluid (mL)	Site of injection (lumbar interspace)
Perineum	5*	1	0.5 (= 5 mg)*	0.5	4th
Perineum and lower extremities	10	2	1 (= 10 mg)	1	3d or 4th
Up to costal margin	15 to 20†	3	1.5 to 2 (= 15 mg to 20 mg)†	1.5 to 2	2d, 3d, or 4th

* For vaginal delivery (saddle block), from 2 mg to 5 mg in dextrose.

† Doses exceeding 15 mg are rarely required and should be used only in exceptional cases. Inject solution at rate of about 1 mL per 5 seconds.

Reactions Associated with Spinal Anesthesia Techniques:

Central Nervous System: post-spinal headache, meningismus, arachnoiditis, palsies, or spinal nerve paralysis.

Cardiovascular: hypotension due to vasomotor paralysis and pooling of the blood in the venous bed.

Respiratory: respiratory impairment or paralysis due to the level of anesthesia extending to the upper thoracic and cervical segments.

Gastrointestinal: nausea and vomiting.

Treatment of Reactions: Toxic effects of local anesthetics require symptomatic treatment; there is no specific cure. **The most important measure is oxygenation of the patient by maintaining an airway and supporting ventilation.** Supportive treatment of the cardiovascular system includes intravenous fluids and, when appropriate, vasopressors (preferably those that stimulate the myocardium). Convulsions are usually controlled with adequate oxygenation alone but intravenous administration in small increments of a barbiturate (preferably an ultrashort-acting barbiturate such as thiopental and thiamylal) or diazepam can be utilized. Intravenous barbiturates or anticonvulsant agents should only be administered by those familiar with their use and only if ventilation and oxygenation have first been assured. In spinal anesthesia, sympathetic blockade also occurs as a pharmacological action, resulting in peripheral vasodilation and often hypotension. The extent of the hypotension will usually depend on the number of dermatomes blocked. The blood pressure should therefore be monitored in the early phases of anesthesia. If hypotension occurs, it is readily controlled by vasoconstrictors administered either by the intramuscular or the intravenous route, the dosage of which would depend on the severity of the hypotension and the response to treatment.

DOSAGE AND ADMINISTRATION

As with all anesthetics, the dosage varies and depends upon the area to be anesthetized, the number of neuronal segments to be blocked, individual tolerance, and the technique of anesthesia. The lowest dosage needed to provide effective anesthesia should be administered. For specific techniques and procedures, refer to standard textbooks. (See related table).

The extent and degree of spinal anesthesia depend upon dosage, specific gravity of the anesthetic solution, volume of solution used, force of the injection, level of puncture, position of the patient during and immediately after injection, etc.

When spinal fluid is added to either the Tetracaine Hydrochloride, instantly soluble particles or solution, some turbidity results, the degree depending on the pH of the spinal fluid, the temperature of the solution during mixing, as well as the amount of drug and diluent employed. This cloudiness is due to the release of the *base* from the hydrochloride. Liberation of base (which is completed within the spinal canal) is held to be essential for satisfactory results with any spinal anesthetic.

The specific gravity of spinal fluid at 25°C/25°C varies under normal conditions from 1.0063 to 1.0075. A solution of the instantly soluble form Tetracaine Hydrochloride, instantly soluble particles in spinal fluid has only a slightly greater specific gravity. The 1% concentration in saline solution has a specific gravity of 1.0060 to 1.0074 at 25°C/25°C.

A hyperbaric solution may be prepared by mixing equal volumes of the 1% Solution and Dextrose Solution 10% (which is available in ampuls of 3 mL).

If the Tetracaine Hydrochloride, instantly soluble particles form is preferred, it is first dissolved in Dextrose Solution 10% in a ratio of 1 mL dextrose to 10 mg of the anesthetic. Further dilution is made with an equal volume of spinal fluid. The resulting solution now contains 5% dextrose with 5 mg of anesthetic agent per milliliter.

A hypobaric solution may be prepared by dissolving the Tetracaine Hydrochloride, instantly soluble particles in Sterile Water for Injection, USP (1 mg per milliliter). The specific gravity of this solution is essentially the same as that of water, 1.000 at 25°C/25°C.

Examine ampuls carefully before use. Do not use solution if crystals, cloudiness, or discoloration is observed.

These formulations of tetracaine hydrochloride do not contain preservatives; therefore, unused portions should be discarded and the reconstituted Tetracaine Hydrochloride, instantly soluble particles should be used immediately.

STERILIZATION OF AMPULS

The drug in intact ampuls is sterile. The preferred method of destroying bacteria on the exterior of ampuls before opening is heat sterilization (autoclaving). Immersion in antiseptic solution is not recommended.

Autoclave at 15-pound pressure, at 121°C (250°F), for 15 minutes. The Tetracaine Hydrochloride, instantly soluble particles form may also be autoclaved in the same way but may lose its snowlike appearance and tend to adhere to the sides of the ampul. This may slightly decrease the rate at which the drug dissolves but does not interfere with its anesthetic potency.

Autoclaving increases likelihood of crystal formation. Unused autoclaved ampuls should be discarded. Under no circumstance should unused ampuls which have been autoclaved be returned to stock.

Protect ampuls from light and store solution under refrigeration.

HOW SUPPLIED
INJECTION:

BRAND/MANUFACTURER	NDC	SIZE	AWP
○ **BRAND** PONTOCAINE HCL/DEXTROSE 6%: Sanofi Winthrop	00024-1594-02	2 ml 10s	$50.08
	00024-1595-02	5 ml 10s	$63.96

INJECTION: 1%

BRAND/MANUFACTURER	NDC	SIZE	AWP
○ **BRAND** PONTOCAINE HCL: Sanofi Winthrop	00024-1574-25	2 ml 25s	$128.59

POWDER FOR INJECTION: 20 MG

BRAND/MANUFACTURER	NDC	SIZE	AWP
○ **BRAND** PONTOCAINE HCL: Sanofi Winthrop	00024-1577-06	100s	$1039.46

Tetracaine Hydrochloride, Ophthalmic

DESCRIPTION

Tetracaine Hydrochloride is a sterile aqueous topical anesthetic ophthalmic solution. The molecular weight is 300.83 and molecular formula is $C_{15}H_{24}N_2O_2 \cdot HCl$.

Benzoic acid,4-[butylamino]-,2-[dimethylamino]ethyl ester, monohydrochloride.

Each mL contains: Tetracaine Hydrochloride 5 mg (0.5%).

Following is its chemical structure:

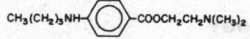

$$CH_3(CH_2)_3NH \text{—} \bigcirc \text{—} COOCH_2CH_2N(CH_3)_2$$

CLINICAL PHARMACOLOGY

Topical anesthetics stabilize the neuronal membrane and prevent the initiation and transmission nerve impulses, thereby effecting local anesthesia. The onset of anesthesia usually begins within 30 seconds and lasts a relatively short period of time.

INDICATIONS AND USAGE

For procedures in which a rapid and short-acting topical ophthalmic anesthetic is indicated such as in tonometry, gonioscopy, removal of corneal foreign bodies, conjunctival scraping for diagnostic purposes, suture removal from the cornea, other short corneal and conjunctival procedures.

CONTRAINDICATIONS

Should not be used by the patient without physician supervision, or in those persons showing hypersensitivity to any component of this preparation. This product should never be prescribed for the patient's own use.

WARNINGS

Prolonged use results in diminished duration of anesthesia and retarded healing. This may cause the drug to be used more frequently creating a 'vicious circle.' Subsequent corneal infection and/or corneal opacification with accompanying permanent visual loss or corneal perforation may occur.

PRECAUTIONS
FOR TOPICAL USE ONLY—NOT FOR INJECTION.

To prevent contaminating the dropper tip and solution, care should be taken not to touch the eyelids or surrounding area with the dropper tip. Patient should be advised not to touch or rub the eye(s) until the effect of the anesthetic has worn off.

Information to the Patient:

After instillation of this product, the surface of the eye is insensitive and can be scratched without feeling it. Do not rub eye. Do not instill this product repeatedly because severe eye damage may occur.

Note: DO NOT USE IF SOLUTION CONTAINS CRYSTALS, OR IS CLOUDY OR DISCOLORED.

ADVERSE REACTIONS
Transient symptoms (signs) such as stinging, burning and conjunctival redness may occur. A rare, severe, immediate allergic cornea reaction has been reported, characterized by acute diffuse epithelial keratitis with filament formation and/or sloughing of large areas of necrotic epithelium, diffuse stromal edema, descemetitis and iritis.

DOSAGE AND ADMINISTRATION
For tonometry and other procedures of short duration, instill one or two drops just prior to evaluation. For minor surgical procedures such as foreign body or suture removal, administer one to two drops every five to ten minutes for one to three instillations. For prolonged anesthesia as in cataract extraction, instill one or two drops in the eye(s) every five to ten minutes for three to five doses.

Store between 15°-30° (59°-86°F). Keep tightly closed.

Keep out of reach of children.

HOW SUPPLIED
DROP: 0.5%

BRAND/MANUFACTURER	NDC	SIZE	AWP
◆ GENERICS			
Rugby	00536-5002-72	15 ml	$2.31

DROP: 0.5%

BRAND/MANUFACTURER	NDC	SIZE	AWP
○ BRAND			
PONTOCAINE HCL: Sanofi Winthrop	00024-1583-01	15 ml	$16.28
	00024-1584-01	60 ml	$31.21

DROP: 2%

BRAND/MANUFACTURER	NDC	SIZE	AWP
○ BRAND			
PONTOCAINE HCL: Sanofi Winthrop	00024-1585-01	30 ml	$21.39
	00024-1585-02	120 ml	$61.66

OINTMENT: 0.5%

BRAND/MANUFACTURER	NDC	SIZE	AWP
○ BRAND			
PONTOCAINE HCL: Sanofi Winthrop	00024-1586-01	3.75 gm	$11.79

Tetracycline Hydrochloride, Ophthalmic

DESCRIPTION
Tetracycline Hydrochloride, Ophthalmic is available as a suspension and an ointment. Tetracycline Hydrochloride Ophthalmic suspension, USP, Sterile contains 10 mg of Tetracycline Hydrochloride per mL; Tetracycline Hydrochloride Ophthalmic Ointment contains 10 mg of Tetracycline Hydochloride per gm.

Chemically, Tetracycline Hydrochloride, Ophthalmic is: [4S-(4α,4aα,5aα,6β,12aα)]-4-(dimethylamino)-1,4, 4a, 5, 5a, 6, 11, 12a-octahydro-3, 6, 10, 12, 12a-pentahydroxy-6-methyl-1,11-dioxo-2-naphthacenecarboxamide monohydrochloride.

Following is its chemical structure:

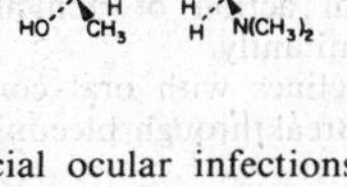

INDICATIONS
For the treatment of superficial ocular infections susceptible to Tetracycline Hydrochloride, Ophthalmic.

For prophylaxis of ophthalmia neonatorum due to *Neisseria gonorrhoeae or Chlamydia trachomatis.* The Centers for Disease Control (USPHS) and the Committee on Drugs, the Committee on Fetus and Newborn, and the Committee on Infectious Diseases of the American Academy of Pediatrics recommend 1 percent silver nitrate solution in single-dose ampoules or single-use tubes of an ophthalmic ointment containing 0.5 percent erythromycin or 1 percent tetracycline as "effective and acceptable regimens for prophylaxis of gonococcal ophthalmia neonatorum."[1] (For infants born to mothers with clinically apparent gonorrhea, intravenous or intramuscular injections of aqueous crystalline penicillin G should be given: a single dose of 50,000 units for term infants or 20,000 units for infants of low birth weight. Topical prophylaxis alone is inadequate for these infants.[1])

The following organisms have demonstrated susceptibility to Tetracycline Hydrochloride, Ophthalmic:

Staphylococcus aureus
Streptococci including *Streptococcus pneumoniae*
Escherichia coli
Neisseria species
Chlamydia trachomatis

When treating trachoma, a concomitant oral Tetracycline is helpful.

Other organisms, not known to cause superficial eye infections, but with demonstrated susceptibility to Tetracycline Hydrochloride, Ophthalmic, have been omitted from the above list.

Tetracycline Hydrochloride, Ophthalmic, does not provide adequate coverage against:

Haemophilus influenzae
Klebsiella/Enterobacter species
Pseudomonas aeruginosa
Serratia marcescens

CONTRAINDICATIONS
This product is contraindicated in persons who have shown hypersensitivity to any of the tetracyclines.

PRECAUTIONS
The use of antibiotics occasionally may result in overgrowth of nonsusceptible organisms. Constant observation of the patient is essential. If new infections appear during therapy, appropriate measures should be taken.

ADVERSE REACTIONS
Dermatitis and allied symptomatology have been reported.

If adverse reaction or idiosyncrasy occurs, discontinue medication and institute appropriate therapy.

DOSAGE AND ADMINISTRATION
Suspension: For most susceptible bacterial infections shake well, then gently squeeze the plastic dropper bottle to instill 2 drops in the affected eye, or if necessary, in both eyes, 2 or 4 times daily, or more frequently, depending upon the severity of the infection. Very severe infections may require days of treatment, whereas other cases may be cured by instillation with much less frequency for 48 hours.

In acute and chronic trachoma, instill 2 drops in each eye 2 to 4 times daily. This treatment should be continued for 1 to 2 months, except that certain individual or complicated cases may require a longer duration. A concomitant oral tetracycline is helpful.

For unit dose administration and convenience, a dispenser may be used. Immediately prior to use, simultaneously roll, invert and squeeze dispenser between thumb and fingers. Repeat several times to mix contents well. Use aseptic technique to cut the tip of the dispenser, thereby maintaining sterility. Discard first two drops before instilling drops in eye(s). Instill two drops in eye(s), then discard dispenser.

Ointment: Apply directly to the affected area every 2 hours or more often, as the severity of the infection and the degree of response indicate. Severe or stubborn ocular infections may require treatment for many days, and may also require oral therapy. Mild infections may respond within 48 hours.

Storage: Store at controlled room temperature, 15°-30°C (59°-86°F).

REFERENCE:
1 American Academy of Pediatrics. Prophylaxis and treatment of neonatal gonococcal infections. *Pediatrics.* 1980; 65:1047.

HOW SUPPLIED
DROP: 1%

BRAND/MANUFACTURER	NDC	SIZE	AWP
○ BRAND			
ACHROMYCIN: Storz/Lederle	00005-3505-18	4 ml	$20.89

OINTMENT: 1%

BRAND/MANUFACTURER	NDC	SIZE	AWP
○ BRAND			
ACHROMYCIN: Storz/Lederle	00005-3501-51	3.75 gm	$13.14

Tetracycline Hydrochloride, Oral

DESCRIPTION
Tetracycline Hydrochloride, Oral is an antibiotic isolated from *Streptomyces aureofaciens.* Chemically it is the monohydrochloride of [4S-(4α,4aα,5aα,6β,12aα,)] -4- (Dimethylamino)- 1,4,4a,5a,6,11,12a-octa- hydro-3, 6, 10, 12, 12a-pentahydroxy-6-methyl-1,11-dioxo-2-naphtha- cenecarboxamide.

Following is its chemical structure:

CLINICAL PHARMACOLOGY
The Tetracyclines are primarily bacteriostatic and are thought to exert their antimicrobial effect by the inhibition of protein synthesis. Tetracyclines are active against a wide range of gram-negative and gram-positive organisms.

The drugs in the Tetracycline class have closely similar antimicrobial spectra, and cross-resistance among them is common. Microorganisms may be considered susceptible if the MIC (minimum inhibitory concentration) is not more than 4 mcg/mL and intermediate if the MIC is 4 to 12.5 mcg/mL. Susceptibility plate testing: A Tetracycline disc may be used to determine microbial susceptibility to drugs in the Tetracycline class. If the Kirby-Bauer method of disc susceptibility testing is used, a 30 mcg Tetracycline Hydrochloride disc should give a zone of at least 19 mm when tested against a Tetracycline-susceptible bacterial strain.

Tetracyclines are readily absorbed and are bound to plasma proteins in varying degrees. They are concentrated by the liver in the bile and excreted in the urine and feces at high concentrations and in a biologically active form.

INDICATIONS
Tetracycline Hydrochloride is indicated in infections caused by the following microorganisms.
Rickettsiae: (Rocky Mountain spotted fever, typhus fever, and the typhus group, Q fever, rickettsialpox, tick fevers).
Mycoplasma pneumoniae (PPLO Eaton agent).
Agents of psittacosis and ornithosis.
Agents of lymphogranuloma venereum and granuloma inguinale.
The spirochetal agent of relapsing fever (*Borrelia recurrentis*).
The following gram-negative microorganisms:
Haemophilus ducreyi (chancroid).
Yersinia pestis and *Francisella tulcrenisis*, formerly *Pasteurella restis* and *Pasteurella tularensis*,
Bartonella bacilliformis,
Bacteroides species,
Vibrio comma and *Vibrio fetus*,
Brucella species (in conjunction with streptomycin).

Because many strains of the following groups of microorganisms have been shown to be resistant to Tetracyclines, culture and susceptibility testing are recommended.
Tetracycline Hydrochloride is indicated for treatment of infections caused by the following gram-negative microorganisms, when bacteriologic testing indicates appropriate susceptibility to the drug.
Escherichia coli,
Enterobacter aerogenes (formerly *Aerobacter aerogenes*),
Shigella species,
Mima species and *Herellea* species,
Haemophilus influenzae (respiratory infections),
Klebsiella species (respiratory and urinary infections).

Tetracycline Hydrochloride is indicated for treatment of infections caused by the following gram-positive microorganisms when bacteriologic testing indicates appropriate susceptibility to the drug:
Streptococcus species:
Up to 44% of strains of *Streptococcus pyogenes* and 74% of *Streptococcus faecalis* have been found to be resistant to tetracycline drugs. Therefore, tetracyclines should not be used for streptococcal disease unless the organism has been demonstrated to be sensitive.

For upper respiratory infections due to Group A beta-hemolytic streptococci, penicillin is the usual drug of choice, including prophylaxis of rheumatic fever.
Streptococcus pneumoniae,
Staphylococcus aureus, skin and soft tissue infections.

Tetracyclines are not the drug of choice in the treatment of any type of staphylococcal infection.
When penicillin is contraindicated, tetracyclines are alternative drugs in the treatment of infections due to:
Neisseria gonorrhoeae,
Treponema pallidum and *Treponema pertenue* (syphilis and yaws),
Listeria monocytogenes,
Clostridium species,
Bacillus anthracis,
Fusobacterium fusiforme (Vincent's infection),
Actinomyces species.

In acute intestinal amebiasis, the Tetracyclines may be a useful adjunct to amebicides.
In severe acne, the Tetracyclines may be useful adjunctive therapy.
Tetracycline Hydrochloride is indicated in the treatment of trachoma, although the infectious agent is not always eliminated, as judged by immunofluorescence.
Inclusion conjunctivitis may be treated with oral Tetracyclines or with a combination of oral and topical agents.

Tetracycline Hydrochloride is indicated for the treatment of uncomplicated urethral, endocervical or rectal infections in adults caused by *Chlamydia trachomatis*.[1]

UNLABELED USES
Tetracycline HCl is used alone or as an adjunct in the treatment of *Borrelia burgdorferi* infections (Lyme disease), bullous pemphigoid, epididymitis, and malaria (*Plasmodium falciparum* malaria). It is also prescribed in the treatment of nongonococcal urethritis (gonorrhoea occurring simultaneously with *Chlamydia trachomatis* infection), chronic blepharitis, including meibomian keratoconjunctivitis, Reiter's syndrome, and Whipple's disease. Tetracycline is also prescribed in the treatment of periodontitis, including juvenile periodontitis.

CONTRAINDICATIONS
This drug is contraindicated in persons who have shown hypersensitivity to any of the Tetracyclines.

WARNINGS
THE USE OF DRUGS OF THE TETRACYCLINE CLASS DURING TOOTH DEVELOPMENT (LAST HALF OF PREGNANCY, INFANCY AND CHILDHOOD TO THE AGE OF 8 YEARS) MAY CAUSE PERMANENT DISCOLORATION OF THE TEETH (YELLOW-GRAY-BROWN).

This adverse reaction is more common during long-term use of the drugs but has been observed following repeated short-term courses. Enamel hypoplasia has also been reported. TETRACYCLINE DRUGS, THEREFORE, SHOULD NOT BE USED IN THIS AGE GROUP UNLESS OTHER DRUGS ARE NOT LIKELY TO BE EFFECTIVE OR ARE CONTRAINDICATED.

If renal impairment exists, even usual oral or parenteral doses may lead to excessive systemic accumulation of the drug and possible liver toxicity. Under such conditions, lower than usual total doses are indicated and, if therapy is prolonged, serum level determinations of the drug may be advisable.

Photosensitivity manifested by an exaggerated sunburn reaction has been observed in some individuals taking Tetracyclines. Patients apt to be exposed to direct sunlight or ultraviolet light should be advised that this reaction can occur with Tetracycline drugs, and treatment should be discontinued at the first evidence of skin erythema.

The antianabolic action of the Tetracyclines may cause an increase in BUN. While this is not a problem in those with normal renal function, in patients with significantly impaired function, higher serum levels of Tetracycline may lead to azotemia, hyperphosphatemia, and acidosis.

Usage in Pregnancy: (See above "Warnings" about use during tooth development.) Results of animal studies indicate that Tetracyclines cross the placenta, are found in fetal tissues and can have toxic effects on the developing fetus (often related to retardation of skeletal development). Evidence of embryotoxicity has also been noted in animals treated early in pregnancy.

Usage in Newborns, Infants, and Children: (See above "Warnings" about use during tooth development.)
All Tetracyclines form a stable calcium complex in any bone-forming tissue. A decrease in the fibula growth rate has been observed in prematures given oral Tetracycline in doses of 25 mg/kg every 6 hours. This reaction was shown to be reversible when the drug was discontinued.

Tetracyclines are present in the milk of lactating women who are taking a drug in this class.

PRECAUTIONS
General: Pseudotumor cerebri (benign intracranial hypertension) in adults has been associated with the use of Tetracyclines. The usual clinical manifestations are headache and blurred vision. Bulging fontanels have been associated with the use of Tetracyclines in infants. While both of these conditions and related symptoms usually resolve soon after discontinuation of the Tetracycline, the possibility for permanent sequelae exists.

As with other antibiotic preparations, use of this drug may result in overgrowth of nonsusceptible organisms, including fungi. If superinfection occurs, the antibiotic should be discontinued and appropriate therapy should be instituted.

In venereal diseases when coexistent syphilis is suspected, darkfield examination should be done before treatment is started and the blood serology repeated monthly for at least 4 months.

In long-term therapy, periodic laboratory evaluation of organ systems, including hematopoietic, renal and hepatic studies should be performed.

All infections due to Group A beta-hemolytic streptococci should be treated for at least 10 days.

Drug Interactions: Because Tetracyclines have been shown to depress plasma prothrombin activity, patients who are on anticoagulant therapy may require downward adjustment of their anticoagulant dosage.

Since bacteriostatic drugs, such as the Tetracycline class of antibiotics, may interfere with the bactericidal action of penicillins, it is not advisable to administer these drugs concomitantly.

Concurrent use of Tetracyclines with oral contraceptives may render oral contraceptives less effective. Breakthrough bleeding has been reported.

ADVERSE REACTIONS
Gastrointestinal: Anorexia, nausea, vomiting, diarrhea, glossitis, dysphagia, enterocolitis, pancreatitis, and inflammatory lesions (with monilial overgrowth) in the anogenital region, increases in liver enzymes, and hepatic toxicity have been reported rarely. Rare instances of esophagitis and esophageal ulcerations have been reported in patients taking the Tetracycline-class antibiotics in capsule

and tablet form. Most of these patients took the medication immediately before going to bed (see *"Dosage and Administration"*).

Skin: Maculopapular and erythematous rashes. Exfoliative dermatitis has been reported but is uncommon. Photosensitivity is discussed above. (See *"Warnings"*.)

Renal toxicity: Rise in BUN has been reported and is apparently dose related. (See *"Warnings"*.)

Hypersensitivity reactions: Urticaria, angioneurotic edema, anaphylaxis, anaphylactoid purpura, pericarditis and exacerbation of systemic lupus erythematosus.

Blood: Hemolytic anemia, thrombocytopenia, neutropenia and eosinophilia have been reported.

CNS: Pseudotumor cerebri (benign intracranial hypertension) in adults and bulging fontanels in infants. (See *"Precautions—General"*.) Dizziness, tinnitus, and visual disturbances have been reported. Myasthenic syndrome has been reported rarely.

Other: When given over prolonged periods, tetracyclines have been reported to produce brown-black microscopic discoloration of thyroid glands. No abnormalities of thyroid function studies are known to occur.

DOSAGE AND ADMINISTRATION
Therapy should be continued for at least 24 to 48 hours after symptoms and fever have subsided.

Concomitant Therapy: Antacids containing aluminum, calcium, or magnesium impair absorption and should not be given to patients taking Oral Tetracycline.

Foods and some dairy products also interfere with absorption. Oral forms of Tetracycline should be given 1 hour before or 2 hours after meals.

In patients with renal impairment: (See *"Warnings"*.) Total dosage should be decreased by reduction of recommended individual doses and/or by extending time intervals between doses.

In the treatment of streptococcal infections, a therapeutic dose of Tetracycline should be administered for at least 10 days.

Adults: Usual daily dose, 1 to 2 grams divided in two or four equal doses, depending on the severity of the infection.

For children above 8 years of age: Usual daily dose, 10 to 20 mg (25 to 50 mg/kg) per pound of body weight divided in two or four equal doses.

For treatment of brucellosis, 500 mg Tetracycline four times daily for 3 weeks should be accompanied by streptomycin, 1 gram intramuscularly twice daily the first week and once daily the second week.

For treatment of syphilis, a total of 30 to 40 grams in equally divided doses over a period of 10 to 15 days should be given. Close follow-up, including laboratory tests, is recommended. Gonorrhea patients sensitive to penicillin may be treated with Tetracycline, administered as an initial oral dose of 1.5 grams followed by 0.5 gram every 6 hours for 4 days to a total dosage of 9 grams.

Uncomplicated urethral, endocervical, or rectal infection in adults caused by *Chlamydia trachomatis*: 500 mg, by mouth, 4 times a day for at least 7 days.[1]

Storage: Store at controlled room temperature, 15°-30°C (59°-86°F).

REFERENCE
1. CDC Sexually Transmitted Diseases Treatment Guidelines 1982.

HOW SUPPLIED
CAPSULE: 100 MG

BRAND/MANUFACTURER	NDC	SIZE	AWP
◆ GENERICS			
Richlyn	00115-1399-03	1000s	$31.20

CAPSULE: 250 MG

AVERAGE UNIT PRICE (AVAILABLE SIZES)		GENERIC A-RATED AVERAGE PRICE (GAAP)	
BRAND	$0.05	100s	$5.70
GENERIC	$0.05	1000s	$41.45
HCFA FUL (100s ea)	$0.03		

BRAND/MANUFACTURER	NDC	SIZE	AWP
◆ BRAND			
➤ ACHROMYCIN V: Lederle Std Prod	00005-4880-23	100s	$3.83
PANMYCIN: Upjohn	00009-0782-01	100s	$5.23
➤ ACHROMYCIN V: Lederle Std Prod	00005-4880-61	480s	$33.20
	00005-4880-34	1000s	$31.49
PANMYCIN: Upjohn	00009-0782-03	1000s	$45.69
➤ ACHROMYCIN V: Lederle Std Prod	00005-4880-65	1200s	$45.90
◆ GENERICS			
Med-Derm	45565-0040-01	100s	$3.95
Warner Chilcott	00047-0407-24	100s	$4.51
ROBITET 250: Robins Pharm	00031-8417-63	100s	$4.88
Purepac	00228-2404-10	100s	$5.14
➤ SUMYCIN: Apothecon	00003-0655-40	100s	$5.39
➤ SUMYCIN: Apothecon	00003-0655-46	100s	$5.39
Halsey Pharm	00879-0158-01	100s	$5.60
Rugby	00536-1820-01	100s	$5.62
URL	00677-0376-01	100s	$5.75
Major	00904-2416-60	100s	$5.75
Qualitest	00603-5919-21	100s	$5.75
Zenith	00172-2416-60	100s	$5.80

BRAND/MANUFACTURER	NDC	SIZE	AWP
Richlyn	00115-1400-01	100s	$5.83
URL	00677-0144-01	100s	$5.85
Richlyn	00115-1405-01	100s	$5.87
Moore,H.L.	00839-1656-06	100s	$5.87
Goldline	00182-0112-01	100s	$6.00
Schein	00364-2026-01	100s	$6.25
Aligen	00405-4981-01	100s	$6.31
U.S. Trading	56126-0362-11	100s ud	$4.79
Auro	55829-0696-10	100s ud	$6.11
Vangard	00615-0151-13	100s ud	$6.28
Goldline	00182-0112-89	100s ud	$6.30
Schein	00364-2026-90	100s ud	$7.75
Med-Derm	45565-0040-03	1000s	$25.00
Warner Chilcott	00047-0407-32	1000s	$31.93
Geneva	00781-2529-10	1000s	$37.88
Purepac	00228-2404-96	1000s	$38.76
Mason Dist	11845-0138-04	1000s	$39.82
Barr	00555-0011-05	1000s	$40.15
➤ Mylan	00378-0101-10	1000s	$40.62
Halsey Pharm	00879-0158-10	1000s	$41.00
Parmed	00349-8930-10	1000s	$41.03
Rugby	00536-1820-10	1000s	$41.92
Major	00904-2416-80	1000s	$41.95
Moore,H.L.	00839-1656-16	1000s	$42.11
ROBITET 250: Robins Pharm	00031-8417-74	1000s	$42.55
Qualitest	00603-5919-32	1000s	$42.88
Schein	00364-2026-02	1000s	$42.95
Richlyn	00115-1400-03	1000s	$44.85
Goldline	00182-0112-10	1000s	$45.00
Richlyn	00115-1405-03	1000s	$45.15
Zenith	00172-2416-80	1000s	$45.80
Aligen	00405-4981-03	1000s	$45.80
Parmed	00349-2426-10	1000s	$45.95
➤ SUMYCIN: Apothecon	00003-0655-60	1000s	$48.89

CAPSULE: 500 MG

AVERAGE UNIT PRICE (AVAILABLE SIZES)		GENERIC A-RATED AVERAGE PRICE (GAAP)	
BRAND	$0.06	100s	$10.04
GENERIC	$0.09	500s	$42.05
HCFA FUL (100s ea)	$0.05	1000s	$76.85

BRAND/MANUFACTURER	NDC	SIZE	AWP
◆ BRAND			
➤ ACHROMYCIN V: Lederle Std Prod	00005-4875-23	100s	$6.40
	00005-4875-34	1000s	$57.14
◆ GENERICS			
Allscrips	54569-2501-06	56s	$4.98
Warner Chilcott	00047-0697-24	100s	$7.41
ROBITET 500: Robins Pharm	00031-8427-63	100s	$7.93
Purepac	00228-2406-10	100s	$8.42
Schein	00364-2029-01	100s	$8.50
Moore,H.L.	00839-5075-06	100s	$8.63
Mylan	00378-0102-01	100s	$8.88
URL	00677-0377-01	100s	$8.89
Geneva	00781-2466-01	100s	$8.90
Goldline	00182-0679-01	100s	$8.90
Qualitest	00603-5920-21	100s	$8.90
Rugby	00536-1870-01	100s	$8.93
Major	00904-2407-60	100s	$8.95
Halsey Pharm	00879-0159-01	100s	$9.45
Barr	00555-0010-02	100s	$10.15
Aligen	00405-4976-01	100s	$10.20
Zenith	00172-2407-60	100s	$10.30
➤ SUMYCIN: Apothecon	00003-0763-40	100s	$10.48
Richlyn	00115-1402-01	100s	$11.39
U.S. Trading	56126-0363-11	100s ud	$7.40
Raway	00686-0162-13	100s ud	$10.50
Auro	55829-0697-10	100s ud	$11.04
Vangard	00615-0162-13	100s ud	$11.48
Schein	00364-2029-90	100s ud	$16.75
Goldline	00182-0679-89	100s ud	$18.55
ROBITET 500: Robins Pharm	00031-8427-70	500s	$36.15
Mylan	00378-0102-05	500s	$41.54
Purepac	00228-2406-50	500s	$42.24
➤ SUMYCIN: Apothecon	00003-0763-50	500s	$48.26
Barr	00555-0010-05	1000s	$70.76
Purepac	00228-2406-96	1000s	$70.77
Moore,H.L.	00839-5075-16	1000s	$73.51
Mason Dist	11845-0139-04	1000s	$73.74
Schein	00364-2029-02	1000s	$75.00
Goldline	00182-0679-10	1000s	$75.00
Geneva	00781-2466-10	1000s	$75.20
Qualitest	00603-5920-32	1000s	$75.25
Aligen	00405-4976-03	1000s	$75.55
Rugby	00536-1870-10	1000s	$77.62
Major	00904-2407-80	1000s	$77.75
Halsey Pharm	00879-0159-10	1000s	$78.80
Richlyn	00115-1402-03	1000s	$87.60
Zenith	00172-2407-80	1000s	$89.30

HOW SUPPLIED
SYRUP: 125 MG/5 ML

BRAND/MANUFACTURER	NDC	SIZE	AWP
◆ GENERICS			
SUMYCIN: Apothecon	00003-0815-50	473 ml	$9.88

TABLETS: 250 MG

AVERAGE UNIT PRICE (AVAILABLE SIZES)			
GENERIC	$0.05		

BRAND/MANUFACTURER	NDC	SIZE	AWP
◆ GENERICS			
SUMYCIN: Apothecon	00003-0663-45	100s	$5.39
SUMYCIN: Apothecon	00003-0663-75	1000s	$48.89

TABLETS: 500 MG

AVERAGE UNIT PRICE (AVAILABLE SIZES)			
GENERIC	$0.10		

BRAND/MANUFACTURER	NDC	SIZE	AWP
◆ GENERICS			
SUMYCIN: Apothecon	00003-0603-43	100s	$10.48
SUMYCIN: Apothecon	00003-0603-50	500s	$48.26

Tetracycline Hydrochloride, Topical

DESCRIPTION
Tetracycline Hydrochloride, Topical is a topical antibiotic preparation containing 2.2 mg of Tetracyline Hydrochloride per ml as the active ingredient, as well as 4-epitetracycline Hydrochloride and sodium bisulfite in an aqueous base of 40% ethanol, citric acid and n-decyl methyl sulfoxide. Tetracycline is 4-(dimethylamino)-1,4,4a,5,5a,6,11,12a-octahydro-3,6,10,12,12a pentahydroxy-6-methyl-1,11-dioxo-2-naphthacenecarboxamide.

Following is its chemical structure:

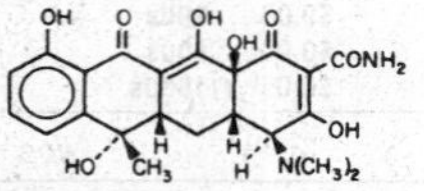

CLINICAL PHARMACOLOGY
Tetracycline Hydrochloride, Topical delivers Tetracycline to the pilosebaceous apparatus and the adjacent tissues. Tetracycline Hydrochloride, Topical on the face and neck twice daily delivered to the skin an average dose of 2.9 mg of Tetracycline Hydrochloride per day. Patients who used the medication twice daily on other acne-involved areas in addition to the face and neck applied an average dose of 4.8 mg of Tetracycline Hydrochloride per day. Tetracycline Hydrochloride, Topical has been formulated such that the recrystallization properties of the tetracyclines on the skin greatly reduce or eliminate the yellow color often associated with topical Tetracycline.

INDICATIONS AND USAGE
Tetracycline Hydrochloride, Topical is indicated in the treatment of acne vulgaris.

CONTRAINDICATIONS
Tetracycline Hydrochloride, Topical is contraindicated in persons who have shown hypersensitivity to any of its ingredients or to any of the other tetracyclines.

WARNINGS
Contains sodium bisulfite, a sulfite that may cause allergic type reactions including anaphylactic symptoms and life threatening or less severe asthmatic episodes in certain susceptible people. The overall prevalence of sulfite sensitivity in the general population is unknown and probably low. Sulfite sensitivity is seen more frequently in asthmatic than in nonasthmatic people.

PRECAUTIONS
General: This drug is for external use only and care should be taken to keep it out of the eyes, nose, and mouth.
Carcinogenesis, Mutagenesis, and Impairment of Fertility: A two year dermal study in mice has been performed with Tetracycline Hydrochloride, Topical and indicates there is no carcinogenic potential with this drug.
Pregnancy: Pregnancy Category B. Reproduction studies have been performed in rats and rabbits at doses of up to 246 times the human dose (assuming the human dose to be 1.3 ml/40kg/day) and have revealed no evidence of impaired fertility or harm to the fetus from Tetracycline Hydrochloride, Topical. There are, however, no adequate and well-controlled studies in pregnant women. Because animal reproduction studies are not always predictive of human response, this drug should be used during pregnancy only if clearly needed.
Nursing Mothers: It is not known whether tetracycline or any other component of Tetracycline Hydrochloride, Topical administered in this topical form is excreted in human milk. Because many drugs are excreted in human milk, caution should be exercised when Tetracycline Hydrochloride, Topical is administered to a nursing woman.

Pediatric Use: Safety and effectiveness in children below the age of eleven have not been established.

ADVERSE REACTIONS
Among the 838 patients treated with Tetracycline Hydrochloride, Topical under normal usage conditions during clinical evaluation, there was one instance of severe dermatitis requiring systemic steroid therapy. About one-third of patients are likely to experience a stinging or burning sensation upon application of Tetracycline Hydrochloride, Topical. The sensation ordinarily lasts no more than a few minutes, and does not occur at every application. There has been no indication that patients experience sufficient discomfort to reduce the frequency of use or to discontinue use of the product. The kinds of side effects often associated with oral or parenteral administration of tetracycline (e.g., various gastrointestinal complaints, vaginitis, hematologic abnormalities, manifestations of systemic hypersensitivity reactions, and dental and skeletal disorders) have not been observed with Tetracycline Hydrochloride, Topical. Because of the topical form of administration, it is highly unlikely that such side effects will occur from its use.

DOSAGE AND ADMINISTRATION
It is recommended that Tetracycline Hydrochloride, Topical be applied generously twice daily to the entire affected area (not just to individual lesions) until the skin is thoroughly wet. Instructions to the patient for proper application are provided on the Tetracycline Hydrochloride, Topical bottle label. Patients may continue their normal use of cosmetics. Concomitant use with benzoyl peroxide or oral tetracycline has been reported without observed problems.
Tetracycline Hydrochloride, Topical should be kept at controlled room temperature 59°F-86°F (15°C-30°C) or below.

HOW SUPPLIED
SOLUTION: 2.2 MG/ML

BRAND/MANUFACTURER	NDC	SIZE	AWP
○ BRAND			
TOPICYCLINE: Roberts Pharm	54092-0315-70	70 ml	$46.79

Tetrahydrozoline Hydrochloride

DESCRIPTION
Tetrahydrozoline Hydrochloride, 2-(1,2,3,4-Tetrahydro-1-naphthyl)-2-imidazoline monohydrochloride, is a nasal decongestant.
Tetrahydrozoline Hydrochloride nasal solution is available for topical nasal application as 0.1% nasal solution to be used as drops or spray and as 0.05% pediatric nasal drops.

Following is its chemical structure:

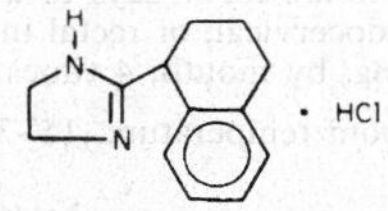

CLINICAL PHARMACOLOGY
Tetrahydrozoline HCl nasal solution, a sympathomimetic amine, possesses vasoconstrictor and decongestant actions when applied to the nasal mucosa, resulting in vasoconstriction of the smaller arterioles of the nasal passages. Information on the absorption, distribution and elimination of the drug is not available.

INDICATIONS AND USAGE
Tetrahydrozoline HCl nasal solution is indicated for decongestion of nasal and nasopharyngeal mucosa.

CONTRAINDICATIONS
Tetrahydrozoline HCl nasal solution is contraindicated for patients who have shown previous hypersensitivity to its components. The 0.1% solution is contraindicated in children under six years of age. Tetrahydrozoline HCl nasal solution is not to be used for infants under two years of age. Tetrahydrozoline HCl pediatric nasal drops solution should be used for children between the ages of 2 and 6 years (see *"Dosage and Administration"*). Tetrahydrozoline HCl nasal solution should not be used by patients under treatment with monoamine oxidase (MAO) inhibitors.

WARNINGS
Overdosage in children may produce profound sedation. This may be accompanied by profuse sweating, hypotension or even shock (see *"Overdosage"*).

GENERAL
Avoid doses greater or more frequent than those recommended below. Excessive dosage in children may, on rare occasions, cause severe drowsiness. Profuse sweating may accompany this effect. Overdosage may also cause marked hypotension or even shock. Use cautiously in patients with cardiovascular disease (e.g., coronary artery disease, hypertension), and metabolic-endocrine diseases (e.g., hyperthyroidism, diabetes).

INFORMATION FOR PATIENTS
Patients should be advised to follow the prescribed dosage regimen. The spray should be administered with the head held upright. To spray, squeeze bottle quickly and firmly and sniff briskly. Instillation of the nose drops can be most conveniently accomplished with the patient in the lateral head-low position.

◆ RATED THERAPEUTICALLY EQUIVALENT; ◇ THERAPEUTIC EQUIVALENCE UNCONFIRMED; ○ UNRATED

DRUG INTERACTIONS

Drug	Effect
Monoamine oxidase (MAO) inhibitors	Hypertension

PREGNANCY

Pregnancy Category C. Animal reproduction studies have not been conducted with Tetrahydrozoline HCl. It is also not known whether Tetrahydrozoline HCl nasal solution can cause fetal harm when administered to a pregnant woman or can affect reproduction capacity. Tetrahydrozoline HCl nasal solution should be given to a pregnant woman only if clearly needed.

NURSING MOTHERS

It is not known whether this drug is secreted in human milk. Because many drugs are secreted in human milk, caution should be exercised when Tetrahydrozoline HCl nasal solution is administered to a nursing woman.

ADVERSE REACTIONS

Local application of Tetrahydrozoline HCl nasal solution can be associated with burning, stinging, sneezing, or dryness of the mucosa. Occasionally, systemic sympathomimetic effects can occur, including headaches, drowsiness, weakness, tremors, light-headedness, insomnia, and palpitations. Rebound congestion can also occur, and is characterized by chronic swelling of the nasal mucosa resulting in chronic redness, swelling and rhinitis. If adverse reactions occur, discontinue use.

OVERDOSAGE

The administration or ingestion of overdoses of Tetrahydrozoline HCl nasal solution may result in oversedation in young children. Overdoses have caused hypertension, bradycardia, drowsiness and rebound hypotension in adults; a shock-like syndrome with hypotension and bradycardia may also occur. In either case, the treatment of overdosage is usually that of watchful expectancy and general supportive measures. The patient should be kept warm, fluid balance should be maintained orally, if possible, and parenterally, if necessary.

If the respiratory rate drops to 10 or below, the patient should be given oxygen, and respiration assisted. Blood pressure should be watched carefully to prevent a hypotensive crisis.

There is no known antidote for Tetrahydrozoline HCl nasal solution. The use of stimulants is contraindicated. To date, there have been no reports of fatalities resulting from overdosages of Tetrahydrozoline HCl nasal solution and while the symptoms resulting from Tetrahydrozoline HCl nasal solution overdosage may be alarming, they are self-limiting and the patient recovers with no sequelae.

DOSAGE AND ADMINISTRATION

ADULTS AND CHILDREN 6 YEARS AND OVER
Tetrahydrozoline HCl 0.1% Nasal Solution: It is recommended that 2 to 4 drops of Tetrahydrozoline HCl 0.1% nasal solution be instilled in each nostril as needed, never more often than every three hours. Less frequent administration is usually sufficient since relief is maintained for four hours or longer in most cases, and often for as long as eight hours. Bedtime instillation usually assures sleep undisturbed by the need for remediation before morning, or by insomnia from central stimulation.

Tetrahydrozoline HCl 0.1% Nasal Spray: It is recommended to squeeze quickly and firmly three or four times Tetrahydrozoline HCl 0.1% nasal spray in each nostril as needed, never more often than every three hours. Less frequent administration is usually sufficient since relief is maintained for four hours or longer in most cases, and often for as long as eight hours. Bedtime instillation usually assures sleep undisturbed by the need for remediation before morning, or by insomnia from central stimulation.

CHILDREN 2 TO 6 YEARS OF AGE
Tetrahydrozoline HCl 0.05% Pediatric Nasal Drops

Note: Do *not* use Tetrahydrozoline HCl 0.1% nasal solution or Tetrahydrozoline HCl 0.1% nasal spray.

It is recommended that 2 to 3 drops of Tetrahydrozoline HCl 0.05% pediatric nasal drops be instilled in each nostril as needed, and never more often than every three hours. Relief usually lasts for several hours, so that instillations are usually needed only every four to six hours. Instillation of nose drops can be most conveniently accomplished with the patient in the lateral head-low position.

Storage: Store below 86° F (30°C).

HOW SUPPLIED

DROP: 0.05%

BRAND/MANUFACTURER	NDC	SIZE	AWP
○ **BRAND**			
TYZINE PEDIATRIC NASAL: Kenwood	00482-4770-15	15 ml	$7.80

SOLUTION: 0.1%

BRAND/MANUFACTURER	NDC	SIZE	AWP
○ **BRAND**			
TYZINE NASAL: Kenwood	00482-4760-30	30 ml	$9.92

SPRAY: 0.1%

BRAND/MANUFACTURER	NDC	SIZE	AWP
○ **BRAND**			
TYZINE NASAL: Kenwood	00482-4760-15	15 ml	$8.14

Tetramune *SEE* DIPHTHERIA/HAEMOPHILUS B/ PERTUSSIS/TETANUS VACCINE

Texacort *SEE* HYDROCORTISONE, TOPICAL

Thalitone *SEE* CHLORTHALIDONE

Tham *SEE* TROMETHAMINE

Theo-24 *SEE* THEOPHYLLINE

Theo-Dur *SEE* THEOPHYLLINE

Theo-Sav *SEE* THEOPHYLLINE

Theobid *SEE* THEOPHYLLINE

Theolair *SEE* THEOPHYLLINE

Theophylline

DESCRIPTION

Theophylline is a bronchodilator structurally classified as a xanthine derivative. It is available as extended-release tablets and capsules, sustained-action capsules, immediate-release capsules, elixir, and solution for injection.

Each extended-release tablet contains:	
Theophylline (anhydrous)	100, 200, 300, and 450 mg
Each extended-release capsule contains:	
Theophylline (anhydrous)	100, 200, 300, or 400 mg
Each sustained-action capsule contains:	
Theophylline (anhydrous)	50, 75, 125, or 200 mg
Each immediate-release capsule contains:	
Theophylline (anhydrous)	100 or 200 mg
Each 15 ml (tablespoonful) of elixir contains:	
Theophylline (anhydrous)	80 mg
Each 100 ml of solution for injection contains:	
Theophylline (anhydrous)	40, 80, 160, 200, 320, or 400 mg

The chemical formula of Theophylline is 1H-Purine-2, 6-dione, 3, 7-dihydro-1, 3-dimethyl. Its molecular weight is 180.17.

Anhydrous Theophylline is a white odorless, crystalline powder having a bitter taste.

Following is its chemical structure:

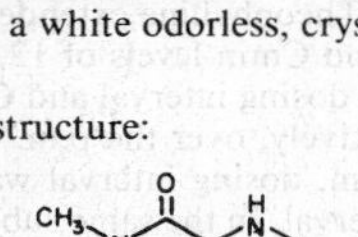

CLINICAL PHARMACOLOGY

Theophylline directly relaxes the smooth muscle of the bronchial airways and pulmonary blood vessels, thus acting mainly as a bronchodilator and smooth muscle relaxant. It has also been demonstrated that aminophylline has a potent effect on diaphragmatic contractility in normal persons and may then be capable of reducing fatigability and thereby improve contractility in patients with chronic

➤ SHOWN IN PRODUCT IDENTIFICATION GUIDE

obstructive airways disease. The exact mode of action remains unsettled. The drug also possesses other actions typical of the xanthine derivatives: coronary vasodilation, diuresis, and cardiac, cerebral, and skeletal muscle stimulation. Although Theophylline does cause inhibition of phosphodiesterase with a resultant increase in intracellular cyclic AMP, which could mediate smooth muscle relaxation, other agents similarly inhibit the enzyme, producing a rise of cyclic AMP but are unassociated with any demonstrable bronchodilation. Other mechanisms proposed include an effect on translocation of intracellular calcium; prostaglandin antagonism; stimulation of catecholamines endogenously; inhibition of cyclic guanosine monophosphate metabolism and adenosine receptor antagonism. None of these mechanisms has been proved, however. At concentrations higher than those attained *in vivo,* Theophylline also inhibits the release of histamine by mast cells.

In vitro, Theophylline has been shown to act synergistically with beta agonists which increase intracellular cyclic AMP through the stimulation of adenyl cyclase, and there are now available data which demonstrate an additive effect *in vitro* with combined use.

Pharmacokinetics: The half-life of Theophylline is influenced by a number of known variables. It may be prolonged in chronic alcoholics, particularly those with liver disease (cirrhosis or alcoholic disease) or in patients with chronic obstructive pulmonary disease, impaired renal function, cor pulmonale or other causes of heart failure and in patients taking certain other drugs (see *"Precautions, Drug Interactions").*

Older adults (over age 55) and patients with chronic obstructive pulmonary disease, with or without cor pulmonale, also may have much slower clearance rates. For such patients, the Theophylline half-life may exceed 24 hours.

Newborns have extremely slow clearance rates compared to older infants and children (i.e. those over 6 months to 1 year of age), and may also have a Theophylline half-life of over 24 hours. Not until 3 to 6 months of age do these rates approach those seen in older children. Older children have rapid clearance rates while most non-smoking adults have clearance rates between these two extremes. In premature neonates the decreased clearance is related to metabolic pathways that have yet to be established.

High fever for prolonged periods may also reduce the rate of theophylline elimination.

THEOPHYLLINE ELIMINATION CHARACTERISTICS

Theophylline

Clearance Rates (mean ± S.D.)	Half-Life Average (mean ± S.D.)
Children (over 6 months of age)	
1.45 ± 0.58 mL/kg/min	3.7 ± 1.1 hrs
Adult nonsmokers uncomplicated asthma	
0.65 ± 0.19 mL/kg/min	8.7 ± 2.2 hrs

The half-life of Theophylline in smokers (1 to 2 packs/day) averages 4-5 hours, much shorter than the half-life in nonsmokers which averages 7-9 hours. The increase in Theophylline clearance caused by smoking is probably the result of induction of drug-metabolizing enzymes that do not readily normalize after cessation of smoking. It appears that between 3 months and 2 years may be necessary for normalization of the effect of smoking on Theophylline pharmacokinetics.

Extended-Release Tablets: Theophylline extended-release tablets at 8 mg/kg body weight (300-700 mg/dose) produced mean peak Theophylline plasma levels of 7.5 ± 1.9 mcg/mL at 9.2 ± 1.9 hours following administration. In multiple dose, steady-state, 3 and 5 day studies with 12 normal subjects, Theophylline extended-release tablets administered at 8 mg/kg (300-600 mg/dose) twice daily, achieved an average peak-trough difference of 4 mcg/mL. The Cmax and Cmin were 13.9 ± 6.9 and 9.9 ± 6.0, respectively. The mean % fluctuation ± S.D. of the plasma concentration at steady state [% fluctuation = 100 (Cmax-Cmin)/Cmin] was 54.2 ± 45.7%. These pharmacokinetic parameters were measured under fasting conditions.

In a multiple dose (300-500 mg BID) steady-state, 5 day study involving 14 normal, nonfasting subjects with Theophylline half-lives between 5.8 and 12.3 hours (mean 8.0 ± 1.8 hours). Theophylline extended-release tablets, dosed twice daily, produced mean Cmax and Cmin levels of 12.2 ± 2.0 and 10.2 ± 1.6 mcg/mL, respectively, over the a.m. dosing interval and Cmax and Cmin of 11.6 ± 1.6 and 8.7 ± 1.8 mcg/mL, respectively, over the p.m. dosing interval. The mean % fluctuation ± S.D. over the a.m. dosing interval was 30.4 ± 12.9% and 33.7 ± 13.1% over the p.m. dosing interval. In the same subjects, Theophylline extended-release tablets given once daily, in the morning, in doses ranging from 600-1000 mg (same daily dose as for BID, above) produced a mean Cmax and Cmin of 14.4 ± 2.2 and 5.5 ± 2.0, respectively and a mean % fluctuation ± S.D. of 195.8 ± 106.0%. Average peak-through differences over 24 hours were 8.9 ± 1.3 and 3.7 ± 1.2 mcg/mL when Theophylline extended-release tablets was given once or twice daily, respectively. In both the twice daily and once daily dosing regimens, Theophylline extended-release tablets exhibited complete bioavailability when compared to an immediate release product.

In a single-dose bioavailability study in eleven subjects, 1000 mg of Theophylline extended-release tablets was administered under fasting conditions and immediately following a high fat content (62 g) breakfast of approximately 1100 kcal. The rate and extent of absorption of Theophylline from Theophylline extended-release tablets administered in fasting and fed conditions were similar.

Extended-Release Capsules: In a 6-day multiple-dose study involving 18 subjects (with Theophylline clearance rates between 0.57 and 1.02 ml/kg/min) who had fasted overnight and 3 hours after morning dosing, Theophylline extended-release capsules given once daily in a dose of 1500 mg produced serum Theophylline levels that ranged between 5.7 mcg/ml and 22 mcg/ml. The mean minimum and maximum values were 11.6 mcg/ml and 18.1 mcg/ml, respectively, with an average peak-trough difference of 6.5 mcg/ml. The mean percent fluctuation [(Cmax-Cmin/Cmin) x 100] equals 80%. A 24-hour single-dose study demonstrated an approximately proportional increase in serum levels as the dose was increased from 600 to 1500 mg.

Taking Theophylline extended-release capsules with a high-fat-content meal may result in a significant increase in the peak serum level and in the extent of absorption of Theophylline as compared to administration in the fasted state (see *"Precautions: Drug/Food Interactions").*

Following the single-dose administration (8 mg/kg) of Theophylline extended-release capsules to 20 normal subjects who had fasted overnight and 2 hours after morning dosing, peak serum Theophylline concentrations of 4.8 ± 1.5 (SD) mcg/ml were obtained at 13.3 ± 4.7 (SD) hours. The amount of the dose absorbed was approximately 13% at 3 hours, 31% at 6 hours, 55% at 12 hours, 70% at 16 hours, and 88% at 24 hours. The extent of Theophylline bioavailability from Theophylline extended-release capsules for 24 hour dosing was comparable to the most widely used 12-hour extended-release product when both products were administered every 12 hours.

In two separate single-dose studies utilizing different subjects, the following bioavailability variables were observed. Theophylline sustained-action capsule administered in a 500-mg dose sprinkled on applesauce to 6 healthy adults produced mean peak Theophylline serum levels of 9.03 ± 2.59 mcg/mL at 8.67 ± 1.03 hours following administration. Administration of two lots of Theophylline sustained-action capsules as intact capsules in a 600-mg dose to 6 healthy adults produced mean peak Theophylline serum levels of 9.08 ± 1.30 mcg/mL and 7.60 ± 0.95 mcg/mL at 8.33 ± 1.50 and 8.67 ± 3.01 hours after administration respectively. In these studies, Theophylline sustained-action capsules exhibited complete bioavailability when compared with an immediate-release product. In both of these studies, the subjects fasted for 10 hours prior to dosing and for 4 hours after dosing.

In a multiple-dose, two-way, crossover study with 18 healthy, normal adults, the bioavailability from Theophylline sustained-action capsules administered as intact capsules was evaluated using Theophylline extended-release tablets as the reference product. Fifteen subjects received 400 mg at 7:00 AM and 7:00 PM while 3 subjects received 200 mg because of low Theophylline clearance. All meals and snacks were provided to the subjects during the course of this study, with breakfast at 9:00 AM, lunch at 12:30 PM, a snack at 3:00 PM, and dinner at 9:00 PM. Theophylline sustained-action capsules produced mean Cmax and Cmin Theophylline serum levels of 10.4 ± 2.6 and 6.9 ± 1.8 mcg/mL as compared with a Cmax and Cmin of 10.5 ± 2.8 and 7.5 ± 2.7 mcg/mL for Theophylline extended-release tablets. The mean percent fluctuation normalized to Css was 38.8 ± 8.5% for the capsules and 33.4 ± 9.7% for the tablets [% fluctuation =100(Cmax-Cmin)/Css, where Css = AUC$_{0-12}$/dosing interval]. The mean percent fluctuation when normalized to Cmin was 51.9 ± 15.4% for the capsules and 43.9 ± 17.4% for the tablets [% fluctuation = 100 (Cmax-Cmin/Cmin]. The average peak through differences over 12 hours for the capsules and the tablets were 3.5 ± 1.2 and 3.0 ± 0.7 mcg/mL, respectively. The AUC for the capsules was 108.4 ± 26.0 while that for the tablets was 112.1 ± 32.5 mcg-hr/mL. In a separate study, Theophylline, extended-release, showed complete bioavailability when compared to an immediate-release product. This would suggest that bioavailability from Theophylline sustained-action capsules was complete and not statistically different from that of the Theophylline extended-release tablets.

INDICATIONS AND USAGE

For relief and/or prevention of symptoms from asthma and reversible broncho-spasm associated with chronic bronchitis and emphysema.

UNLABELED USES

Theophylline is used alone or as an adjunct in the treatment of Cheyne-Stokes respiration, cystic fibrosis, essential tremor, and severe headache. It is also used to improve exercise-induced myocardial ischemia in patients with stable angina pectoris, in bronchchopulmonary dysplasia, and cerebral vasospasm.

CONTRAINDICATIONS

This product is contraindicated in individuals who have shown hypersensitivity to its components. It is also contraindicated in patients with active peptic ulcer disease, and in individuals with underlying seizure disorders (unless receiving appropriate anticonvulsant medication).

Intravenous solutions containing dextrose may be contraindicated in patients with known allergy to corn or corn products.

WARNINGS

Serum levels above 20 mcg/ml are rarely found after appropriate administration of recommended doses. However, in individuals in whom Theophylline plasma clearance is reduced *for any reason,* even conventional doses may result in increased serum levels and potential toxicity. Reduced Theophylline clearance has been documented in the following readily identifiable groups: 1) patients with impaired liver function, 2) patients over 55 years of age, particularly males and those with chronic lung disease; 3) those with cardiac failure from any cause; 4) patients with sustained high fever; 5) neonates and infants under 1 year of age; 6) those patients taking certain drugs (see *"Precautions, Drug Interactions"*), or 7) patients with lowered body plasma clearance (due to transient cardiac decompensation). Frequently, such patients have markedly prolonged Theophylline serum levels following discontinuation of the drug.

Reduction of dosage and laboratory monitoring is especially appropriate in the above individuals.

Morphine, curare, and stilbamidine should be used with caution in patients with airflow obstruction because they stimulate histamine release and may also suppress respiration leading to respiratory failure. Alternate drugs should be chosen whenever possible.

Serious side effects such as ventricular arrhythmias, convulsions or even death may appear as the first sign of toxicity without any previous warning. Less serious signs of Theophylline toxicity (i.e. nausea and restlessness) may occur frequently when initiating therapy, but are usually transient; when signs are persistent during maintenance therapy, they are often associated with serum concentrations above 20 mcg/mL. Stated differently: *serious toxicity is not reliably proceded by less severe side effects.* Serum concentration measurements may contribute significant information towards predicting potential life-threatening toxicity.

Many patients who require Theophylline may exhibit tachycardia due to their underlying disease process so that the cause/effect relationship to elevated serum Theophylline concentrations may not be appreciated. Theophylline products may cause or worsen arrhythmias and any pre-existing arrhythmias, and any significant change in rate and/or rhythm warrants monitoring and further investigation.

Status asthmaticus is a medical emergency. Optimal therapy frequently requires additional medication including corticosteroids when the patient is not rapidly responsive to bronchodilators.

Halothane anesthesia in the presence of Theophylline may produce sinus tachycardia or ventricular arrhythmias. Studies in laboratory animals (minipigs, rodents, and dogs) recorded the occurrence of cardiac arrhythmias and sudden death (with histologic evidence of myocardial necrosis) when beta-agonists and methylxanthines were administered concurrently. The significance of these findings when applied to humans is currently unknown.

Solutions containing dextrose without electrolytes should not be administered simultaneously with blood through the same infusion set because of the possibility of agglomeration of erythrocytes.

The intravenous administration of these solutions may cause fluid overloading resulting in dilution of serum electrolyte concentrations, overhydration, congested states or pulmonary edema.

Because dosages of these drugs are titrated to response (see *"Dosage and Administration"*), *no additives should be made to Theophylline solution for injection.*

PRECAUTIONS

THEOPHYLLINE EXTENDED-RELEASE TABLETS OR SUSTAINED-ACTION CAPSULES SHOULD NOT BE CHEWED OR CRUSHED.

General: On the average Theophylline half-life is shorter in cigarette and marijuana smokers than in non-smokers, but smokers can have half-lives as long as non-smokers. Theophylline should not be administered concurrently with other xanthine medications. Use with caution in patients with hypoxemia, hypertension severe cardiac disease, hyperthyroidism, acute myocardial injury, cor pulmonale, congestive heart failure, liver disease, in the elderly (especially males), and in neonates. In particular, great caution should be used in giving Theophylline to patients with congestive heart failure. Frequently such patients have markedly prolonged Theophylline serum levels with Theophylline persisting in serum for long periods following discontinuation of the drug or those with a history of peptic ulcer. Theophylline may occasionally act as a local irritant to the G.I. tract although gastrointestinal symptoms are more commonly centrally mediated and associated with serum drug concentrations over 20 mcg/mL.

Clinical evaluation and periodic laboratory determinations are necessary to monitor changes in fluid balance, electrolyte concentrations, and acid-base balance during prolonged intravenous therapy or whenever the condition of the patient warrants such evaluation.

If intravenous administration is controlled by a pumping device, care must be taken to discontinue pumping action before the container runs dry or air embolism may result.

It is recommended that intravenous administration apparatus be replaced at least once every 24 hours.

Use only if solution is clear and container and seals are intact.

Information for Patients: This information is intended to aid in the safe and effective use of this medication. It is not a disclosure of all possible adverse or intended effects.

Patients who require a relatively high dose of Theophylline (ie, a dose equal to or greater than 900 mg of 13 mg/kg, whichever is less) should be informed of important considerations relating to time of drug administration and meal content (see *"Precautions: Drug/Food Interactions"* and *"Dosage and Administration"*).

The physician should reinforce the importance of taking only the prescribed dose and time interval between doses. Theophylline extended-release tablets and capsules should not be chewed or crushed. When dosing Theophylline extended-release tablets on a once daily (q24h) basis, tablets should be taken whole and not split. As with any controlled-release Theophylline product, the patient should alert the physician if symptoms occur repeatedly, especially near the end of the dosing interval.

When prescribing administration by the sprinkle method, details of the proper technique should be explained to the patient (see *"Dosage and Administration, Sprinkling Contents on Food"*). Patients should be informed of the need to take this drug in the fasting state, and that drug administration should be 1 hour before or 2 hours after meals (see *"Precautions, Drug-Food Interactions,"* and *"Dosage and Administration"*).

Laboratory Tests: Serum Theophylline levels should be monitored periodically to assure achievement of optimal levels for safety and efficacy and as a method of predicting toxicity. For such measurements, the serum sample should be obtained at the time of peak concentration, 3 to 6 hours when medication is taken every 8 hours, 4 to 8 hours when medication is taken every 12 hours, or 8 hours when taken once daily, or 12 hours after administration of a morning dose of extended-release capsules for 24-hour dosing. It is important that the patient has not missed or taken additional doses during the previous 48 hours or 72 hours for extended-release capsules for 24-hour dosing, and that dosing intervals were reasonably equally spaced. DOSAGE ADJUSTMENT BASED ON SERUM THEOPHYLLINE MEASUREMENTS WHEN THESE INSTRUCTIONS HAVE NOT BEEN FOLLOWED MAY RESULT IN RECOMMENDATIONS THAT PRESENT RISK OF TOXICITY TO THE PATIENT.

Drug Interactions: Toxic synergism with ephedrine has been documented and may occur with some other sympathomimetic bronchodilators. Halothane anesthesia in the presence of Theophylline may produce sinus tachycardia or ventricular arrhythmias. In addition, the following drug interactions have been demonstrated:

Theophylline with:	
Allopurinol (high dose)	Increased serum Theophylline levels
Cimetidine	Increased serum Theophylline levels
Ciprofloxacin	Increased serum Theophylline levels
Clindamycin	Increased serum Theophylline levels
Erythromycin, Troleandomycin	Increased serum Theophylline levels
Lithium carbonate	Increased renal excretion of lithium
Oral contraceptives	Increased serum Theophylline levels
Phenytoin	Decreased Theophylline and phenytoin serum levels
Propranolol	Increased serum Theophylline levels or antagonism of propranolol effect
Rifampin	Decreased serum Theophylline levels
Carbamazepine	Decreased serum Theophylline levels
Phenobarbital	Decreased serum Theophylline levels

Drug-Food Interactions: Theophylline extended-release tablets and Theophylline sustained-action capsules *100 mg* have not been adequately studied to determine whether their bioavailability is altered when given with food. Available data suggest that drug administration at the time of food ingestion may influence the absorption characteristics of Theophylline controlled-release products resulting in serum values different from those found after administration in the fasting state. Data indicate that administration of sustained-action capsules at the time of food ingestion will result in significantly lower peak-serum concentrations and reduced extent of absorption (bioavailability). The influence of the type and amount of food as well as the time interval between drug and food on performance of the drug is under study.

A drug-food effect, if any, would likely have its greatest clinical significance when high Theophylline serum levels are being maintained and/or when large single doses (greater than 13 mg/kg or 900 mg) of a controlled-release Theophylline product are given.

The rate and extent of absorption of Theophylline from Theophylline 200 mg, 300 mg, and 450 mg extended-release tablets are similar when administered fasting or immediately after a high fat content breakfast such as 8 oz. whole milk, egg/cheese/bacon on muffin, 1 blueberry muffin with margarine, and 1 serving of hash brown potatoes (about 1100 kcal, including approximately 62 g of fat). (See *"Clinical Pharmacology, Pharmacokinetics"*.) Taking Theophylline extended-release capsules 24-hour less than one hour before a high-fat-content meal, such as 8 oz whole milk, 2 fried eggs, 2 bacon strips, 2 oz hashed brown potatoes, and 2 slices of buttered toast (about 985 calories, including approximately 71 g of fat) may result in a significant increase in peak serum level and in the extent of absorption of Theophylline as compared to administration in the fasted state. In some cases (especially with doses of 900 mg or more taken less than one hour before a high-fat-content meal) serum Theophylline levels may exceed the 20 mcg/ml level, above which Theophylline toxicity is more likely to occur.

Drug-Laboratory Test Interactions: Currently available analytical methods, including high pressure liquid chromatography and immunoassay techniques, for measuring serum Theoophylline levels are specific. Metabolites and other drugs generally do not affect the results. Other new analytic methods are also now in use. The physician should be aware of the laboratory method used and whether other drugs will interfere with the assay for Theophylline.

When plasma levels of Theophylline are measured by spectrophotometric methods, the ingestion of coffee, tea, cola beverages, chocolate and acetaminophen may contribute to falsely high values.

Carcinogenesis, Mutagenesis, and Impairment of Fertility: Long-term carcinogenicity studies have not been performed with Theophylline. Theophylline has been shown to be mutagenic in *Escherichia coli* and other lower organisms *(Euglena gracilis* and *Ophiostoma multiannulatum).*

Chromosome-breaking activity was detected in human cell cultures at concentrations of Theophylline up to 50 times the therapeutic serum concentration in humans. Theophylline was not mutagenic in the dominant lethal assay in male mice given Theophylline intraperitoneally in doses up to 30 times the maximum daily human oral dose.

Studies to determine the effects on fertility have not been performed with Theophylline.

Pregnancy: Category C. Limited animal studies have shown teratogenic activity of Theophylline in mice and rats. There are no adequate and well-controlled studies in pregnant women. Theophylline should be used during pregnancy only if the potential benefit justifies the potential risk to the fetus.

Nursing Mothers: Theophylline is distributed into breast milk and may cause irritability or other signs of toxicity in nursing infants. Because of the potential for serious adverse reactions in nursing infants from Theophylline, a decision should be made whether to discontinue nursing or to discontinue the drug, taking into account the importance of the drug to the mother.

Pediatric Use: Safety and effectiveness of Theophylline extended-release tablets administered:

1. Every 24 hours in children under 12 years of age, have not been established.
2. Every 12 hours in children under 6 years of age, have not been established.
Safety and efficacy of Theophylline sustained-action capsules in children under 6 years of age have not been established.

Sufficient numbers of infants under the age of 1 year have not been studied in clinical trials to support use of intravenous Theophylline in this age group; however there is evidence recorded that the use of dosage recommendations for older infants and young children (16 mg/kg/24 hours) may result in the development of toxic serum levels. Such findings very probably reflect differences in the metabolic handling of the drug related to absent or undeveloped enzyme systems. Consequently, the use of the drug in this age group should carefully consider the associated benefits and risks. If used, the maintenance dose must be conservative and in accord with the following guidelines.

Initial Maintenance Dosage (of Theophylline anhydrous intravenous): Premature Infants:

Up to 24 days postnatal age -1 mg/kg q 12 h
Beyond 24 days postnatal age - 1.5 mg/kg q 12 h
Infants 6 to 52 weeks:
$[(0.2 \times \text{age in weeks}) + 51 \times \text{kg body wt} = 24 \text{ hour dose in mg}$
Up to 26 weeks, divide into q 8 h dosing intervals
From 26 to 52 weeks, divide into q 6 h dosing intervals

Final dosage should be guided by serum concentration after a steady state (no further accumulation of drug) has been achieved.

ADVERSE REACTIONS

The following adverse actions have been observed, but there has not been enough systematic collection of data to support an estimate of their frequency. The most consistent adverse reactions are usually due to overdosage:

1. *Gastrointestinal:* nausea, vomiting, epigastric pain, hematemesis, diarrhea.

2. *Central Nervous System:* headaches, irritability, restlessness, insomnia, reflex hyperexcitability, muscle twitching, clonic and tonic generalized convulsions.

3. *Cardiovascular:* palpitation, tachycardia, extrasystole, flushing, hypotension, circulatory failure, ventricular arrhythmia.

4. *Respiratory:* tachypnea.

5. *Renal:* potentiation of diuresis, albuminuria, increased excretion of renal tubular and red blood cells.

6. *Others:* alopecia, hyperglycemia inappropriate ADH syndrome, rash.

Reactions which may occur because of the intravenous solution or the technique of administration include febrile response, infection at the site of injection, venous thrombosis or phlebitis extending from the site of injection, extravasation and hypervolemia.

MANAGEMENT OF ADVERSE REACTIONS TO INTRAVENOUS THEOPHYLLINE

1. In the of severe reaction, discontinue the use of the drug.
2. Institute emergency resuscitative procedures and administer the emergency drug necessary to manage the severe reaction (see *"Overdosage"*).
3. Save the remainder of the fluid for examination if deemed necessary.

OVERDOSAGE

Management: It is suggested that the management principles (consistent with the clinical status of the patient when first seen) outlined below be instituted and that simultaneous contact with a Regional Poison Control Center be established. In this way both updated information and individualization regarding the required therapy may be provided.
1. When potential oral overdose is established and seizure has not occurred:

a) If patient is alert and seen within the early hours after ingestion, induction of emesis may be of value. Gastric lavage has been demonstrated to be of no value in influencing outcome in patients who present more than 1 hour after ingestion.
b) Administer a cathartic. Sorbitol solution is reported to be of value.
c) Administer repeated doses of activated charcoal and monitor theophylline serum levels.
d) Prophylactic administration of phenobarbital has been shown to elevate the seizure threshold in laboratory animals, and administration of this drug can be considered.

2. If patient presents with a seizure:

a) Establish an airway.
b) Administer oxygen.
c) Treat the seizure with intravenous diazepam, 0.1 to 0.3 mg/kg up to 10 mg. If seizures cannot be controlled, the use of general anesthesia should be considered.
d) Monitor vital signs, maintain blood pressure and provide adequate hydration.

3. If post-seizure coma is present:
a) Maintain airway and oxygenation.
b) If result of oral medication, follow above recommendations to prevent absorption of the drug, but intubation and lavage will have to be performed instead of inducing emesis, and the cathartic and charcoal will need to be introduced via a large bore gastric lavage tube.
c) Continue to provide full supportive care and adequate hydration until the drug is metabolized. In general drug metabolism is sufficiently rapid so as not to warrant dialysis. If repeated oral activated charcoal is ineffective (as noted by stable or rising serum levels) charcoal hemoperfusion may be indicated.

DOSAGE AND ADMINISTRATION

Theophylline extended-release tablets. The rate and extent of absorption of Theophylline from Theophylline extended-release tablets 200, 300 and 450 mg when administered fasting or immediately after a high fat content breakfast are similar (see *"Clinical Pharmacology, Pharmacokinetics"*).

Theopylline extended-release tablets have not been adequately studied for their bioavailability when administered with food (see *"Precautions, Drug-Food Interactions"*).

Patients who require a relatively high dose of Theophylline (ie, a dose equal to or greater than 900 mg or 13 mg/kg, whichever is less) should not take Theophylline extended-release capsules 24-hour less than 1 hour before a high-fat-content meal since this may result in a significant increase in peak serum level and in the extent of absorption of Theophylline as compared to administration in the fasted state (see *"Precautions, Drugs–Food Interactions"*).

There are data to indicate that administration of Theophylline sustained-action capsules at the time of food ingestion will result in significantly lower peak-serum concentrations and reduced extent of absorption (bioavailability).

Therefore, the patient should be instructed to take this medication at least one hour before or two hours after a meal (see *"Precautions, Drug-Food Interactions"*).

Effective use of Theophylline (i.e., the concentration of drug in the serum associated with optimal benefit and minimal risk of toxicity) is considered to occur when the Theophylline concentration is maintained from 10 to 20 mcg/ml. The early studies from which these levels were derived were carried out in patients immediately or shortly after recovery from acute exacerbations of their disease (some hospitalized with status asthmaticus).

Although the 20 mcg/mL remains appropriate as a critical value (above which toxicity is more likely to occur) for safety purposes, additional data are now available which indicate that the serum Theophylline concentrations required to produce maximum physiologic benefit may, in fact, fluctuate with the degree of bronchospasm present and with the rate of elimination and are variable. Therefore, the physician should individualize the range appropriate to the patient's requirements, based on both symptomatic response and improvement in pulmonary function. It should be stressed that serum Theophylline concentrations maintained at the upper level of the 10 to 20 mcg/mL range may be associated with potential toxicity when factors known to reduce Theophylline clearance are operative (see *"Warnings"*).

If it is not possible to obtain serum level determinations, restriction of the daily dose (in otherwise healthy adults) to not greater than 13 mg/kg/day, to a maximum of 900 mg of Theophylline will result in relatively few patients exceeding serum levels of 20 mcg/ml and the resultant greater risk of toxicity.

Caution should be exercised for younger children who cannot complain of minor side effects. Older adults, particularly those with cor pulmonale, congestive heart failure, and/or liver disease may have unusually low dosage requirements and thus may have unusually low dosage requirements and thus may experience toxicity at the maximal dosage recommended below. It is important that no patient be maintained on any dosage that is not tolerated. In instructing patients to increase dosage according to the schedule above, they should be instructed not to take a subsequent dose if apparent side effects occur and to resume therapy at a lower dose once adverse effects have disappeared.

Theophylline does not distribute into fatty tissue. Dosage should be calculated on the basis of lean (ideal) body weight where mg/kg doses are presented.

Frequency of Dosing: When immediate release products with rapid absorption are used, dosing to maintain serum levels generally requires administration every 6 hours. This is particularly true in children, but dosing intervals up to 8 hours may be satisfactory in adults since they eliminate the drug at a slower rate. Some children, and adults requiring higher than average doses (those having rapid rates of clearance, e.g. half-lives of under 6 hours) may benefit and be more effectively controlled during chronic therapy when given products with extended-release characteristics since these provide longer dosing intervals and/or less fluctuation in serum concentration between dosing.

Extended-release Theophylline products are intended for patients with relatively continuous or recurring symptoms who have a need to maintain therapeutic serum levels of Theophylline. They are not intended for patients experiencing an acute episodes of bronchospasm (associated with asthma, chronic bronchitis, or emphysema). Such patients require rapid relief of symptoms and should be treated with an immediate-release or intravenous Theophylline preparation (or other bronchodilators) and not with extended-release products.

Patients who metabolize Theophylline at a normal or slow rate are reasonable candidates for once-daily dosing with Theophylline extended release capsules 24-hour. Patients who metabolize Theophylline rapidly (eg, the young, smokers, and some nonsmoking adults) and who have symptoms repeatedly at the end of a dosing interval, will require either increased doses given once a day or prefereably, are likely to be better controlled by a schedule of twice-daily dosing. Those patients who require increased daily doses are more likely to experience relatively wide peak-trough differences and may be candidates for twice-a-day dosing with Theophylline extended-release capsules 24-hour.

Patients should be instructed to take this medication each morning at approximately the same time and not to exceed the prescribed dose.

Recent studies suggest that dosing of extended-release Theophylline products at night (after the evening meal) results in serum concentrations of Theophylline which are not identical to those recorded during waking hours and may be characterized by early trough and delayed peak levels. This appears to occur whether the drug is given as an immediate-release, extended-release, or intravenous product. To avoid this phenomenon when two doses per day are prescribed, it is recommended that the second dose be given 10 to 12 hours after the morning dose and before the evening meal.

Food and posture, along with changes associated with circadian rhythm, may influence the rate of absorption and/or clearance rates of Theophylline from extended-release dosage forms administered at night. The exact relationship of these and other factors to nighttime serum concentrations and the clinical significance of such findings require additional study. Therefore, it is not recommended that Theophylline extended-release capsule 24 hours (when used as a once-a-day product) be administered at night.

Since there is a wide variation from patient to patient in the total dose of Theophylline required to attain the desired level in the serum, it is essential that the dose be titrated and that serum levels be monitored before and after transfer to any sustained-release product.

When serum levels are not measured, the initial dosage should be restricted to the amount recommended below (see *"Initiation of Therapy"*.)

Dosage guidelines are approximations only and the wide range of Theophylline clearance between individuals (particularly those with concomitant disease) makes indiscriminate usage hazardous.

DOSAGE GUIDELINES
Warning: Do not attempt to maintain any dose that is not tolerated.

It is recommended that dosing be considered in two stages: initiation of therapy with Theophylline extended-release tablets and titration, adjustment, and chronic maintenance.

Initiation of Therapy:

It is recommended that the appropriate dosage be established using an immediate-release preparation. Slow clinical titration is generally preferred to help assure acceptance and safety of the medication, and to allow the patient to develop tolerance to the transient caffeine-like side effects. Then, if the total 24 hour dose can be given by use of the available strengths of this product, the patient can usually be switched to Theophylline extended-release tablets giving one-half of the daily dose at 12 hour intervals. However, certain patients, such as the young smokers and some non-smoking adults are likely to metabolize Theophylline rapidly and require dosing at 8 hour intervals. Such patients can generally be identified as having trough serum concentrations lower than desired or repeatedly exhibiting symptoms near the end of a dosing interval.

Alternatively, therapy can be initiated with Theophylline extended-release tablets since it is available in dosage forms/strengths which permit titration and adjustment in dosage as outlined in the following dosing guidelines. It is recommended that for children under 25 kg, proper dosage be established with a liquid preparation to permit titration in small increments.

The Average Initial Adult and Children's (over 25 kg) *Dose is one* Theophylline extended-release tablet 200 mg q12h.

Titration and Adjustment and Chronic Maintenance: If the desired response is not achieved with the above *Average Initial Dose* recommendations, there are no adverse reactions and the serum Theophylline level cannot be measured, dosage adjustment should proceed by increasing the dose in approximately 25% increments at three day intervals. Following each adjustment, the clinical response should be assessed. If the clinical response is satisfactory, then that dosage level should be maintained. Dosage increases may be made in this manner up to the following.

MAXIMUM DOSE WITHOUT MEASUREMENT OF SERUM CONCENTRATION

	Dose Per Interval
Children (25-35 kg)	250 mg q12h
Adults and Children (35-70 kg)	300 mg q12h
Adults (over 70 kg)	450 mg q12h

It is important that no patient be maintained on any dosage that is not tolerated. In instructing patients to increase dosage according to the schedule above, they should be instructed not to take a subsequent dose if apparent side effects occur and to resume therapy at a lower dose once adverse effects have disappeared.

If an increased dose is not tolerated because of headaches or stomach upset (nausea, vomiting, diarrhea, etc.), decrease dose to previous tolerated level. Do not exceed the above recommended doses unless serum Theophylline levels can be measured.

If serum Theophylline levels can be measured and the concentration is between 10 and 20 mcg/ml, maintain dose if tolerated. *Check serum concentration at approximately 8 hours after a dose when none have been missed or added for at least 3 days. Recheck serum Theophylline concentration at 6 to 12 month intervals.* This interval may need to be more frequent in some individuals. Take the following action if the measured serum Theophylline concentration is too high.

20 to 25 mcg/ml—Decrease dose by about 10% and serum Theophylline levels should be rechecked after 3 days.[*]

25 to 30 mcg/ml—Skip next dose and decrease subsequent doses by 25% and serum Theophylline levels should be rechecked after 3 days.

Over 30 mcg/ml—Skip next 2 doses and decrease subsequent doses by 50% and serum Theophylline levels should be rechecked after 3 days.

Take the following action if the measured serum Theophylline concentration is too low.

7.5 to 10 mcg/ml—Increase dose by 25%[**]

5 to 7.5 mcg/ml—Increase dose by 25%.

Recheck Serum Theophylline for Guidance in Further Dosage Adjustment.

DOSAGE ADJUSTMENT BASED ON SERUM THEOPHYLLINE CONCENTRATION MEASUREMNTS WHEN THESE INSTRUCTIONS HAVE NOT BEEN FOLLOWED MAY RESULT IN RECOMMENDATIONS THAT PRESENT RISK OF TOXICITY TO THE PATIENT.

Once-Daily Dosing: The slow absorption rate of this preparation may allow once-daily administration in adult non-smokers with appropriate total body clearance and other patients with low dosage requirements. Once-daily dosing should be considered only after the patient has been gradually and satisfactorily titrated to therapeutic levels with q12h dosing. Once-daily dosing should be based on twice the q12h dose and should be initiated at the end of the last q12h dosing interval. The trough concentration (Cmin) obtained following conversion to once-daily dosing may be lower (especially in high clearance patients) and the peak concentration (Cmax) may be higher (especially in low clearance patients) than that obtained with q12h dosing. If symptoms recur, or signs of toxicity appear during the once-daily dosing interval, dosing on the q12h basis should be reinstituted.

It is essential that serum Theophylline concentrations be monitored before and after transfer to once-daily dosing.

Food and posture, along with changes associated with circadian rhythm, may influence the rate of absorption and/or clearance rates of Theophylline from controlled-release dosage forms administered at night. The exact relationship of these and other factors to nighttime serum concentrations and the clinical significance of such findings require additional study. Therefore, it is not recommended that Theophylline extended-release tablets, when used as a once-a-day product, be administered at night. Theophylline extended-release tablets, when used as a once-a-day product, must be taken whole and not broken.

Theophylline extended-release capsules 24-hour: because a high-fat-content meal may significantly increase the peak level and extent of absorption of Theophylline from Theophylline extended-release capsules 24-hour, patients receiving large single doses (ie, equal to or greater than 900 mg or 13 mg/kg, whichever is less) should be instructed to avoid eating a high-fat-content morning meal or to take their medication at least 1 hour before eating. If the physician cannot be assured that the patient will follow the regimen, then the patient should be placed on a twice-daily dosing regimen.

For patients receiving lower once-daily single doses (less than 900 mg), very high peak levels are less likely to occur when Theophylline extended-release capsules 24-hour is taken with food. With close monitoring, patients less certain to observe the fasting requirements could be treated with once-daily dosing.

It is recommended that dosing be considered in three stages: (I) initiation of therapy with Theophylline extended-release capsules 24-hour, (II) titration and adjustment, and (III) chronic maintenance.

I. INITIATION OF THERAPY WITH THEOPHYLLINE EXTENDED-RELEASE CAPSULES 24-HOUR

A. *Transfer of patients* already on established daily doses of Theophylline (whether stabilized on immediate- or extended-release products) can be accomplished by administering the total daily dosage as a single dose given in the morning (eg, 300 mg of an immediate-release product given t.i.d. should be given as 900 mg of Theophylline extended-release capsules 24-hour). The initial transfer should not be made at doses exceeding 900 mg/day or 13 mg/kg/day, whichever is less. Subsequent dose titration should be done on the basis of serum levels and with appropriate attention to the time of drug administration and meal content as noted above.

It must be recognized that the peak and trough serum Theophylline levels produced by once-daily dosing may vary (usually wider peak-trough differences) from those produced by the previous product and/or dosage regimen.

B. *For initiation of therapy with Theophylline extended-release capsules 24-hour* in patients who are not currently taking a Theophylline product, the total daily dose, administered in the morning, must be established in accordance with the following guidelines:

Body Weight	Daily Dose
Children 35 kg and above	400 mg
Adults	400 mg

* Finer adjustments in dosage may be needed for some patients.
** Dividing the daily dosage into 3 doses administered at 8 hour intervals may be indicated if symptoms occur repeatedly at the end of a dosing interval.

► SHOWN IN PRODUCT IDENTIFICATION GUIDE

If appropriate serum Theophylline concentrations or adequate improvement in pulmonary function is not obtained after 3 days, the instructions in Part II (below) should be followed.

II. TITRATION AND ADJUSTMENT OF DOSE

This phase of adjustment should be implemented either by the use of serum concentration measurements or by empiric principles when serum level determinations are not available.

A. If serum levels can be measured: After 3 days' therapy with Theophylline extended-release capsules 24-hour, serum levels should be determined for peak concentration (sample obtained 12 hours after the morning dose) and trough concentration (24 hours after the morning dose). It is important that the patient has not missed or added any dose during the 72-hour period and that dosing intervals have been reasonably consistent. Dose adjustment based on measurements when these instructions have not been followed may result in toxicity.

Based on the results of the peak-trough values obtained, three possibilities exist:

1. The values of serum Theophylline concentration fall within the desired range. If this result is obtained, the dosage should be maintained if it is tolerated.

2. If the serum Theophylline concentration is too high, the dosage should be reduced as follows:

a. If the values are between 20 and 25 mcg/ml, the daily dose may be reduced by about 10% and serum Theophylline levels should be rechecked after 3 days.

b. If the values are between 25 and 30 mcg/ml, the next dose should be skipped and the daily dose reduced by about 25%. The serum concentration should be rechecked after 3 days.

c. If the values are over 30 mcg/ml, the next dose should be skipped and the daily dose reduced by 50%. The serum concentration should be rechecked after 3 days.

3. If the serum Theophylline concentration is too low, the dosage should be increased at 3-day intervals by 100 mg or 200 mg (but not greater than 25% of the current dose), depending upon the desired goal. The serum concentration may be rechecked at appropriate intervals, but at least at the end of this adjustment period.

B. If serum levels cannot be measured:

1. If the clinical response is satisfactory then the total daily dose should be maintained.

2. If the response is unsatisfactory (due to persistence of symptoms or minimal improvement in measured function) after 3 days, then the dose may be increased by 100-mg increments. Reevaluation should be undertaken every 3 days.

3. If the response is still unsatisfactory and there are no adverse reactions, the dose may be cautiously adjusted upward in increments of 100 mg/day at 3- to 5-day intervals up to 900 mg (or 13 mg/kg/day, whichever is less).

4. If a response is accompanied by adverse reactions, then the next dose should be withheld or reduced by 25% depending on the severity of the reactions.

III. CHRONIC MAINTENANCE

After the dose is established, Theophylline serum concentrations usually remain stable. However, as noted elsewhere (see "Warnings" and "Precautions"), certain exogenous and endogenous factors alter Theophylline elimination (including concomitant disease and drug interactions) which require drug monitoring and adjustments in total daily dose requirements while such factors are operative.

If the patient's condition is otherwise clinically stable and none of the recognized factors that alter elimination is present, measurement of serum levels need be repeated only every 6 to 12 months.

THEOPHYLLINE SUSTAINED-ACTION CAPSULES

Sprinkling Contents on Food: Theophylline sustained-action capsule may be administered by carefully opening the capsule and sprinkling the contents on a spoonful of soft food such as applesauce or pudding. The soft food should be swallowed immediately without chewing and followed with a glass of cool water or juice to ensure complete swallowing of the drug. It is recommended that the food used should not be hot and should be soft enough to be swallowed without chewing. Any drug/food mixture should be used immediately and not stored for future use. The small amount of food (one spoonful) used to administer the dose will not alter the bioavailability of Theophylline sustained-action capsules; however, the dosing should be at least 1 hour before or 2 hours after a meal. SUBDIVIDING THE CONTENTS OF A CAPSULE IS NOT RECOMMENDED.

Dosage Guidelines: Because administration of Theophylline sustained-action capsules at the time of food ingestion has been shown to result in significantly lower peak-serum concentrations and reduced extent of absorption (bioavailability), patients should be instructed to take this medication at least 1 hour before or 2 hours after a meal (see "Precautions, Drug-Food Interactions").

Taking Theophylline sustained-action capsules at 12-hour intervals under the above restrictive recommendations in regard to food ingestion may be difficult for the patient to follow. Under such circumstances, consideration should be given to prescribing this drug every 8 hours (giving one-third of the 24-hour dosage requirement with each dose), if this regimen would more easily permit dosing under fasting conditions.

I. ACUTE SYMPTOMS

Note: Status asthmaticus should be considered a medical emergency and is defined as that degree of bronchospasm which is not rapidly responsive to usual doses of conventional bronchodilators. Optimal therapy for such patients frequently require both *additional medication*, parenterally administered and *close monitoring*, preferably in an intensive care setting.

II. CHRONIC THERAPY

A. Initiating Therapy with an Immediate-Release Product: It is recommended that the appropriate dosage be established using an immediate-release preparation. Children weighing less than 25 kg should have their daily dosage requirements established with a liquid preparation to permit small dosage increments. Slow clinical titration is generally preferred to help assure acceptance and safety of the medication, and to allow the patient to develop tolerance to transient caffeine-like side effects. Then, if the total 24-hour dose can be given by use of the sustained-release product, the patient can usually be switched to Theophylline sustained-action capsules, giving one-half of the daily dose at 12-hour intervals. Patients who metabolize Theophylline rapidly such as the young, smokers, and some nonsmoking adults, are the most likely candidates for dosing at 8-hour intervals. Such patients can generally be identified as having trough-serum concentrations lower than desired or repeatedly exhibiting symptoms near the end of a dosing interval.

B. Initiating Therapy with Theophylline sustained-action capsules: Alternatively, therapy can be initiated with Theophylline sustained-action capsules since it is available in dosage strengths which permit titration and adjustments of dosage in adults and older children:

Initial Dose: 16 mg/kg/24 hours or 400 mg/24 hours (whichever is less) of anhydrous Theophylline in 2 divided doses, 12-hour intervals.

Increasing Dose: The above dosage may be increased in approximately 25% increments at 3-day intervals so long as the drug is tolerated; until clinical response is satisfactory or the maximum dose as indicated in Section III (below) is reached. The serum concentration may be checked at these intervals, but at a minimum, should be checked at the end of this adjustment period.

III. MAINTENANCE DOSE OF THEOPHYLLINE WHERE THE SERUM CONCENTRATION IS NOT MEASURED

WARNING: DO NOT ATTEMPT TO MAINTAIN ANY DOSE THAT IS NOT TOLERATED.

Not to exceed the following:			Dose per 12 hours
Age	6-9 years	24 mg/kg/day	12.0 mg/kg
Age	9-12 years	20 mg/kg/day	10.0 mg/kg
Age	12-16 years	18 mg/kg/day	9.0 mg/kg
Age	Over 16 years	13 mg/kg/day or 900 mg (WHICHEVER IS LESS)	6.5 mg/kg

IV. MEASUREMENT OF SERUM THEOPHYLLINE CONCENTRATIONS DURING CHRONIC THERAPY

If the above maximum doses are to be maintained or exceeded, serum Theophylline measurement is recommended. The serum sample should be obtained at the time of peak absorption: 1 to 2 hours after administration for immediate-release products and 5 to 10 hours after dosing for Theophylline sustained-action capsules. It is important that the patient will have missed no doses during the previous 48 hours and that the dosing intervals will have been reasonably typical with no added doses during that period of time. *Dosage adjustment based on serum Theophylline concentration measurements when these instructions have not been followed may result in recommendations that present risk of toxicity to the patient.*

V. FINAL ADJUSTMENT OF DOSAGE (SEE TABLE 1)

Table 1

DOSAGE ADJUSTMENT AFTER SERUM THEOPHYLLINE MEASUREMENT

If serum Theophylline is:		Directions:
Within Normal Limits	10 to 20 mcg/mL	Maintain dosage if tolerated. Recheck serum Theophylline concentration at 6- to 12-month intervals*
Too High	20 to 25 mcg/mL	Decrease doses by about 10%. Serum Theophylline concentration should be checked until within normal limits. Recheck at 6 to 12 months.
	25 to 30 mcg/mL	Skip next dose and decrease subsequent doses by about 25%. Serum Theophylline concentrations should be checked until within normal limits. Recheck at 6 to 12 months.

◆ RATED THERAPEUTICALLY EQUIVALENT; ◇ THERAPEUTIC EQUIVALENCE UNCONFIRMED; ○ UNRATED

If serum Theophylline is:		Directions:
	over 30 mcg/mL	Skip next 2 doses and decrease subsequent doses by 50%. Serum Theophylline concentrations should be checked until within normal limits. Recheck at 6 to 12 months.
Too low	7.5 to 10 mcg/mL	Increase dose by about 25%.** Serum Theophylline concentrations should be checked for guidance in further dosage adjustment. Recheck serum Theophylline concentration at 6- to 12-month intervals.*
	5 to 7.5 mcg/mL	Increase dose by about 25% to the nearest dose increment and recheck serum Theophylline for guidance in further dosage adjustment (another increase will probably be needed, but this provides a safety check).

* *Finer adjustments in dosage may be needed for some patients.*
** *The total daily dose may need to be administered at more frequent intervals if asthma symptoms occur repeatedly at the end of a dosing interval.*

When given intravenously or when rapidly absorbed products such as Theophylline are used, dosing to maintain around-the-clock blood levels generally requires administration every 6 hours to obtain the greatest efficacy for clinical use in children; dosing intervals up to 8 hours may be satisfactory for adults because they eliminate Theophylline more slowly. Children, and adults requiring higher than average doses, may benefit from products with slower absorption which may allow longer dosing intervals and/or less fluctuation in serum concentration over a dosing interval during chronic therapy.

Due to the marked variation in Theophylline metabolism in infants under 6 months of age, intravenous Theophylline is not recommended for infants under 6 months of age.

Both the loading and maintenance dosage of Theophylline may be given intravenously via either intermittent or continuous infusion. With either, the rate should not exceed 25 mg per minute; and the total amount should be selected according to the following schedule.

THEOPHYLLINE DOSAGE SCHEDULE
(see "Pediatric Use")

1. Patients not currently receiving Theophylline products:

Group	Loading Dose	Dose for 1st 12 Hours	Maintenance Dose Beyond 12 Hours
Children 6 months to 9 yrs	5 mg/kg	4 mg/kg q 4 hrs × 3 doses or 0.95 mg/kg/h	4 mg/kg q 6 hrs or 0.79 mg/kg/h
Children, 9-16 yrs, and young adult smokers	5 mg/kg	3 mg/kg q 4 hrs × 3 doses or 0.79 mg/kg/h	3 mg/kg q 6 hrs or 0.63 mg/kg/h
Otherwise healthy nonsmoking adults	5 mg/kg	3 mg/kg q 6 hrs × 2 doses or 0.56 mg/kg/h	3 mg/kg q 8 hrs or 0.4 mg/kg/h
Older patients and patients with cor pulmonale	5 mg/kg	2 mg/kg q 6 hrs × 2 doses or 0.4 mg/kg/h	2 mg/kg q 8 hrs or 0.24 mg/kg/h
Patients with congestive heart failure, liver disease	5 mg/kg	1.5 mg/kg q 6 hrs × 2 doses or 0.3 mg/kg/h	1-2 mg/kg q 12 hrs or 0.08- 0.16 mg/kg/h

2. *Patients currently receiving Theophylline products:* Determine, where possible, the time, amount, route of administration, and form of the patient's last dose. (1 mg of Theophylline anhydrous is equivalent to approximately 1.25 mg of aminophylline dihydrate.)

The loading dose for Theophylline will be based on the principle that each 0.5 mg/kg of Theophylline administered as a loading dose will result in a 1 mcg/mL increase in serum Theophylline concentration. Ideally, then, the loading dose should be deferred if a serum Theophylline concentration can be rapidly obtained. If this is not possible, the clinician must exercise judgment in selecting a dose that has a potential for benefit with minimum additional risk. When there is sufficient respiratory distress to warrant a small risk, 2.5 mg/kg of intravenous Theophylline is likely to increase the serum concentration when administered as a loading dose in rapidly absorbed form by approximately 5 mcg/mL. If the patient is not already experiencing Theophylline toxicity, the risk of dangerous adverse effects from this dose is low.

After this modified loading dose, the maintenance dosage recommendations in this group of patients are the same as those described above.

Comments: It is recommended that serum Theophylline concentrations be monitored in order to obtain optimal therapeutic theophylline dosage. However, it is not always possible or practical to obtain a serum theophylline level. Therefore, patients should be closely monitored for signs of toxicity. The present data suggest that the above dosage recommendations will achieve therapeutic serum concentrations with minimal risk of toxicity for most patients. However, some risk of toxic serum concentrations is still present.

Adverse reactions to Theophylline often occur when serum Theophylline levels exceed 20 mcg/mL.

Oral therapy should be substituted for intravenous Theophylline as soon as adequate improvement is achieved.

When an intravenous solution containing Theophylline is given piggyback, the intravenous system already in place should be turned off while the Theophylline is infused if there is a potential problem with solution incompatibility in the administration set.

The following may be incompatible when mixed with Theophylline in intravenous fluids:

anileridine HCl, ascorbic acid, chlorpromazine, codeine phosphate, cortico-tropin, dimenhydrinate, epinephrine HCl, erythromycin gluceptate, hydralazine HCl, hydroxyzine HCl, insulin, levorphanol tartrate, meperidine HCl, methadone HCl, methicillin sodium, morphine sulfate, norepinephrine bitartrate, oxytetracycline HCl, papaverine HCl, penicillin G potassium, phenobarbital sodium, phenytoin sodium, procaine HCl, prochlorperazine maleate, promazine HCl, promethazine HCl, tetracycline HCl, vancomycin HCl, vitamin B complex with C.

Parenteral drug products should be inspected visually for particulate matter and discoloration prior to administration, whenever solution and container permit.

STORAGE CONDITIONS
Keep tightly closed. Store at controlled room temperature 15-30°C (59-86°F).

Exposure of pharmaceutical products to heat should be minimized. Avoid excessive heat. Protect from freezing. It is recommended that solution for injection be stored at room temperature (25°C); however, brief exposure up to 40°C does not adversely affect the product.

J CODES
Up to 2 ml—J2810

HOW SUPPLIED
CAPSULE: 100 MG

BRAND/MANUFACTURER	NDC	SIZE	AWP
◆ BRAND			
ELIXOPHYLLIN: Forest Pharm	00456-0642-01	100s	$47.10
◆ GENERICS			
U.S. Trading	56126-0436-11	100s ud	$10.50

CAPSULE: 100 MG

BRAND/MANUFACTURER	NDC	SIZE	AWP
◇ BRAND			
BRONKODYL: Sanofi Winthrop	00024-1036-10	100s	$39.02

CAPSULE: 200 MG

AVERAGE UNIT PRICE (AVAILABLE SIZES)

BRAND	$0.62		

BRAND/MANUFACTURER	NDC	SIZE	AWP
◆ BRAND			
ELIXOPHYLLIN: Forest Pharm	00456-0643-01	100s	$62.59
	00456-0643-02	500s	$304.34
◆ GENERICS			
U.S. Trading	56126-0437-11	100s ud	$16.37

CAPSULE: 200 MG

BRAND/MANUFACTURER	NDC	SIZE	AWP
◇ BRAND			
BRONKODYL: Sanofi Winthrop	00024-1037-10	100s	$51.93

CAPSULE: 300 MG

BRAND/MANUFACTURER	NDC	SIZE	AWP
◆ GENERICS			
U.S. Trading	56126-0438-11	100s ud	$20.82

CAPSULE, EXTENDED RELEASE: 50 MG

BRAND/MANUFACTURER	NDC	SIZE	AWP
◇ BRAND			
➤ THEO-DUR SPRINKLE: Key	00085-0928-01	100s	$15.83
➤ SLO-BID GYROCAPS: RPR	00075-0057-00	100s	$19.31
	00075-0057-62	100s ud	$20.07

➤ SHOWN IN PRODUCT IDENTIFICATION GUIDE

CAPSULE, EXTENDED RELEASE: 65 MG

BRAND/MANUFACTURER	NDC	SIZE	AWP
◇ GENERICS			
AEROLATE III: Fleming	00256-0150-01	100s	$17.00

CAPSULE, EXTENDED RELEASE: 75 MG

BRAND/MANUFACTURER	NDC	SIZE	AWP
◇ BRAND			
➤ THEO-DUR SPRINKLE: Key	00085-0875-01	100s	$18.04
➤ SLO-BID GYROCAPS: RPR	00075-1075-00	100s	$21.31
	00075-1075-62	100s ud	$22.59

CAPSULE, EXTENDED RELEASE: 100 MG

AVERAGE UNIT PRICE (AVAILABLE SIZES)		GENERIC A-RATED AVERAGE PRICE (GAAP)	
BRAND	$0.24	100s	$20.13
GENERIC	$0.20		

BRAND/MANUFACTURER	NDC	SIZE	AWP
◆ BRAND			
➤ SLO-BID GYROCAPS: RPR	00075-0100-00	100s	$23.28
	00075-0100-62	100s ud	$24.79
	00075-0100-99	1000s	$229.38
◆ GENERICS			
Inwood	00258-3637-01	100s	$19.61
Warner Chilcott	00047-0196-24	100s	$19.62
Lemmon	00093-0934-01	100s	$19.65
Thrift Drug Svcs	59198-0252-01	100s	$19.65
Arcola	00070-2340-00	100s	$19.76
Major	00904-7846-60	100s	$20.55
Qualitest	00603-5949-21	100s	$20.57
Goldline	00182-1311-01	100s	$20.59
Schein	00364-2585-01	100s	$20.59
Moore,H.L.	00839-7885-06	100s	$20.73

CAPSULE, EXTENDED RELEASE: 100 MG

BRAND/MANUFACTURER	NDC	SIZE	AWP
◇ BRAND			
THEO-24: Whitby	50474-0100-01	100s	$22.03
	50474-0100-60	100s ud	$33.05

CAPSULE, EXTENDED RELEASE: 125 MG

AVERAGE UNIT PRICE (AVAILABLE SIZES)		GENERIC A-RATED AVERAGE PRICE (GAAP)	
BRAND	$0.30	100s	$25.13
GENERIC	$0.25		

BRAND/MANUFACTURER	NDC	SIZE	AWP
◆ BRAND			
➤ SLO-BID GYROCAPS: RPR	00075-1125-00	100s	$29.17
	00075-1125-62	100s ud	$29.92
◆ GENERICS			
Warner Chilcott	00047-0197-24	100s	$24.50
Inwood	00258-3638-01	100s	$24.55
Lemmon	00093-0936-01	100s	$24.60
Thrift Drug Svcs	59198-0253-01	100s	$24.60
Arcola	00070-2341-00	100s	$24.77
Major	00904-7847-60	100s	$25.75
Qualitest	00603-5950-21	100s	$25.78
Goldline	00182-1312-01	100s	$25.79
Schein	00364-2586-01	100s	$25.79

CAPSULE, EXTENDED RELEASE: 125 MG

BRAND/MANUFACTURER	NDC	SIZE	AWP
◇ BRAND			
➤ THEO-DUR SPRINKLE: Key	00085-0381-01	100s	$20.56
➤ SLO-PHYLLIN 125: RPR	00075-1355-00	100s	$34.86
THEOVENT: Schering	00085-0402-01	100s	$36.17

CAPSULE, EXTENDED RELEASE: 130 MG

BRAND/MANUFACTURER	NDC	SIZE	AWP
◇ GENERICS			
➤ THEOCLEAR L.A.-130: Central	00131-4247-37	100s	$16.00
AEROLATE JR: Fleming	00256-0114-01	100s	$18.25

CAPSULE, EXTENDED RELEASE: 200 MG

AVERAGE UNIT PRICE (AVAILABLE SIZES)		GENERIC A-RATED AVERAGE PRICE (GAAP)	
BRAND	$0.34	100s	$29.94
GENERIC	$0.30		

BRAND/MANUFACTURER	NDC	SIZE	AWP
◆ BRAND			
➤ SLO-BID GYROCAPS: RPR	00075-0200-00	100s	$34.71
	00075-0200-62	100s ud	$32.88
	00075-0200-99	1000s	$341.07
◆ GENERICS			
Warner Chilcott	00047-0198-24	100s	$29.20
Inwood	00258-3634-01	100s	$29.23
Lemmon	00093-0938-01	100s	$29.25
Thrift Drug Svcs	59198-0254-01	100s	$29.25
Rugby	00536-5633-01	100s	$29.47
Arcola	00070-2342-00	100s	$29.48
Qualitest	00603-5951-21	100s	$30.60
Goldline	00182-1313-01	100s	$30.69
Major	00904-7848-60	100s	$30.70
Schein	00364-2587-01	100s	$30.70
Aligen	00405-4984-01	100s	$30.77

CAPSULE, EXTENDED RELEASE: 200 MG

BRAND/MANUFACTURER	NDC	SIZE	AWP
◇ BRAND			
➤ THEO-DUR SPRINKLE: Key	00085-0620-01	100s	$23.45
THEO-24: Whitby	50474-0200-01	100s	$32.85
	50474-0200-60	100s ud	$41.02
	50474-0200-50	500s	$157.62

For additional alternatives, turn to the section beginning on page 2859.

Theovent SEE THEOPHYLLINE

Thera-Flur SEE SODIUM FLUORIDE

Theracys SEE BCG

Theragran Hematinic SEE FERROUS FUMARATE/FOLIC ACID/MINERALS/VITAMINS, MULTI

Thiabendazole

DESCRIPTION

Thiabendazole is an anthelmintic provided as 500 mg chewable tablets, and as a suspension, containing 500 mg Thiabendazole per 5 mL. The suspension also contains sorbic acid 0.1% added as a preservative.

Thiabendazole is a white to off-white odorless powder with a molecular weight of 201.26, which is practically insoluble in water but readily soluble in dilute acid and alkali. Its chemical name is 2-(4-thiazolyl)-1H-benzimidazole. The empirical formula is $C_{10}H_7N_3S$.

Following is its chemical structure:

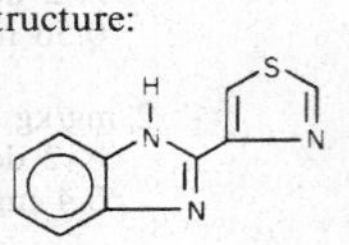

CLINICAL PHARMACOLOGY

In man, Thiabendazole is rapidly absorbed and peak plasma concentration is reached within 1 to 2 hours after the oral administration of a suspension. It is metabolized almost completely to the 5-hydroxy form which appears in the urine as glucuronide or sulfate conjugates. In 48 hours, about 5% of the administered dose is recovered from the feces and about 90% from the urine. Most is excreted in the first 24 hours.

MECHANISM OF ACTION

The precise mode of action of Thiabendazole on the parasite is unknown, but it may inhibit the helminth-specific enzyme fumarate reductase.

Thiabendazole is vermicidal and/or vermifugal against *Ascaris lumbricoides* ("common roundworm"), *Strongloides stercorglis* (threadworm). *Necator americanus*, and *Ancylostoma duodenale* (hookworm), *Trichuris trichiura* (whip-worm), *Ancylostoma braziliense* (dog and cat hookworm), *Toxocara canis* and *Toxocara cati* (ascarids), and *Enterobius vermicularis* (pinworm).

Its effect on larvae of *Trichinella spiralis* that have migrated to muscle is questionable.

◆ RATED THERAPEUTICALLY EQUIVALENT; ◇ THERAPEUTIC EQUIVALENCE UNCONFIRMED; ○ UNRATED

Thiabendazole also suppresses egg and/or larval production and may inhibit the subsequent development of those eggs or larvae which are passed in the feces.

INDICATIONS AND USAGE

Thiabendazole is indicated for the treatment of:

Strongyloidiasis (threadworm)

Cutaneous larva migrans (creeping eruption)

Visceral larva migrans

Trichinosis: Relief of symptoms and fever and a reduction of eosinophilia have followed the use of Thiabendazole during the invasion stage of the disease.

Although not indicated as primary therapy, when enterobiasis (pinworm) occurs with any of the conditions listed above, additional therapy is not required for most patients. Thiabendazole should be used only in the following infestations when more specific therapy is not available or cannot be used or when further therapy with a second agent is desirable: Uncinariasis (hookworm: *Necator americanus* and *Ancylostoma duodenale*); Trichuriasis (whipworm); Ascariasis (large roundworm).

CONTRAINDICATION

Hypersensitivity to this product.

WARNINGS

If hypersensitivity reactions occur, the drug should be discontinued immediately and not be resumed. Erythema multiforme has been associated with Thiabendazole therapy; in severe cases (Stevens-Johnson syndrome), fatalities have occurred.

Because CNS side effects may occur quite frequently, activities requiring mental alertness should be avoided.

PRECAUTIONS

GENERAL

Thiabendazole is not suitable for the treatment of mixed infections with ascaris because it may cause these worms to migrate.

Ideally, supportive therapy is indicated for anemic, dehydrated or malnourished patients prior to initiation of the anthelmintic therapy.

In the presence of hepatic or renal dysfunction, patients should be carefully monitored.

Thiabendazole should be used only in patients in whom susceptible worm infestation has been diagnosed and should not be used prophylactically.

INFORMATION FOR PATIENTS

Because CNS side effects may occur quite frequently, activities requiring mental alertness should be avoided.

LABORATORY TESTS

Rarely, a transient rise in cephalin flocculation and SGOT has occurred in patients receiving Thiabendazole.

DRUG INTERACTIONS

Thiabendazole may compete with other drugs, such as theophylline, for sites of metabolism in the liver, thus elevating the serum levels of such compounds to potentially toxic levels. Therefore, when concomitant use of Thiabendazole and xanthine derivatives is anticipated, it may be necessary to monitor blood levels and/or reduce the dosage of such compounds. Such concomitant use should be administered under careful medical supervision.

CARCINOGENESIS, MUTAGENESIS, IMPAIRMENT OF FERTILITY

Thiabendazole has been used in numerous short- and long-term studies in animals at doses up to 15 times the usual human dose and was without carcinogenic effects. It did not adversely affect fertility in the mouse at 2½ times the usual human dose or in the rat at a dose equivalent to the usual human dose. Thiabendazole had no mutagenic activity in the *in vitro* microbial mutagen test, the micronucleus test and the host mediated assay *in vivo*.

PREGNANCY

Pregnancy Category C: Reproduction and teratogenic studies done in the rabbit at a dose up to 15 times the usual human dose, in the rat at a dose equivalent to the human dose, and in the mouse at a dose up to 2 ½ times the usual human dose, revealed no evidence of harm to the fetus. In an additional study in the mouse, no defects were observed when Thiabendazole was given in an aqueous suspension, at a dose 10 times the usual human dose; however, cleft palate and axial skeletal defects were observed when Thiabendazole was suspended in olive oil and given at the same dose. There are no adequate and well controlled studies in pregnant women. Thiabendazole should be used during pregnancy only if the potential benefit justifies the potential risk to the fetus.

NURSING MOTHERS

It is not known whether this drug is excreted in human milk. Because of the potential for serious adverse reactions in nursing infants from Thiabendazole, a decision should be made whether to discontinue nursing or to discontinue the drug, taking into account the importance of the drug to the mother.

PEDIATRIC USE

The safety and effectiveness of Thiabendazole for the treatment of Strongyloidiasis, Ascariasis, Uncinariasis, Trichuriasis and Trichinosis in children weighing less than 30 lbs has been limited.

ADVERSE REACTIONS

Gastrointestinal: anorexia, nausea, vomiting, diarrhea, epigastric distress, jaundice, cholestasis and parenchymal liver damage.

Central Nervous System: dizziness, weariness, drowsiness, giddiness, headache, numbness, hyperiritability, convulsions, collapse, psychic disturbances.

Special Senses: tinnitus, abnormal sensation in eyes, xanthopsia, blurring of vision, drying of mucous membranes (mouth, eyes, etc.)

Cardiovascular: hypotension.

Metabolic: hyperglycemia.

Hematologic: transient leukopenia.

Genitourinary: hematuria, enuresis, malodor of the urine, crystalluria.

Hypersensitivity: pruritus, fever, facial flush, chills, conjunctival injection, angioedema, anaphylaxis, skin rashes (including perianal), erythema multiforme (including Stevens-Johnson syndrome), and lymphadenopathy.

Miscellaneous: appearance of live Ascaris in the mouth and nose.

OVERDOSAGE

Overdosage may be associated with transient disturbances of vision and psychic alterations.

There is no specific antidote in the event of overdosage. Therefore, symptomatic and supportive measures should be employed. Emesis should be induced or gastric lavage performed carefully.

The oral LD_{20} of Thiabendazole is 3.6 g/kg, 3.1 g/kg and 3.8 g/kg in the mouse, rat, and rabbit respectively.

DOSAGE AND ADMINISTRATION

The recommended maximum daily dose of Thiabendazole is 3 grams: Thiabendazole should be given after meals if possible. Thiabendazole tablets should be chewed before swallowing. Dietary restriction, complementary medications and cleansing enemas are not needed.

The usual dosage schedule for all conditions is two doses per day. The dosage is determined by the patient's weight. A weight-dose chart follows:

THERAPEUTIC REGIMENS

Indication	Regimen	Comments
*Strongyloidiasis	2 doses per day for 2 successive days.	A single dose of 20 mg/lb or 50 mg/kg may be employed as an alternative schedule, but a higher incidence of side effects should be expected.
Cutaneous Larva Migrans (Creeping Eruption)	2 doses per day for 2 successive days.	If active lesions are still present 2 days after completion of therapy, a second course is recommended.
Visceral Larva Migrans	2 doses per day for 7 successive days.	Safety and efficacy data on the seven-day treatment course are limited.
*Trichinosis	2 doses per day for 2-4 successive days according to the response of the patient.	The optimal dosage for the treatment of trichinosis has not been established.
Other Indications		
*Intestinal roundworms (including Ascariasis, Uncinariasis and Trichuriasis)	2 doses per day for 2 successive days.	A single dose of 20 mg/lb or 50 mg/kg may be employed as an alternative schedule, but a higher incidence of side effects should be expected.

* *Clinical experience with Thiabendazole for treatment of each of these conditions in children weighing less than 30 lbs has been limited.*

► SHOWN IN PRODUCT IDENTIFICATION GUIDE

Weight	Each Dose	
	g	mL
30 lb	0.25 (½ tablet)	2.5 (½ teaspoon)
50 lb	0.5 (1 tablet)	5.0 (1 teaspoon)
75 lb	0.75 (1½ tablets)	7.5 (1½ teaspoons)
100 lb	1.0 (2 tables)	10.0 (2 teaspoons)
125 lb	1.25 (2½ tablets)	12.5 (2½ teaspoons)
150 lb & over	1.5 (3 tablets)	15.0 (3 teaspoons)

The regimen for each indication follows: (See related table).

HOW SUPPLIED
CHEW TABLET: 500 MG

BRAND/MANUFACTURER	NDC	SIZE	AWP
○ BRAND MINTEZOL: Merck	00006-0907-36	36s	$35.14

SUSPENSION: 500 MG/5 ML

BRAND/MANUFACTURER	NDC	SIZE	AWP
○ BRAND MINTEZOL: Merck	00006-3331-60	120 ml	$20.41

Thioguanine

CAUTION: Thioguanine is a potent drug. It should not be used unless a diagnosis of acute nonlymphocytic leukemia has been adequately established and the responsible physician is knowledgeable in assessing response to chemotherapy.

DESCRIPTION
Thioguanine is one of a large series of purine analogues which interfere with nucleic acid biosynthesis, and has been found active against selected human neoplastic diseases.[1]

Thioguanine, known chemically as 2-amino-1,7-dihydro-6H-purine-6-thione, is an analogue of the nucleic acid constituent guanine, and is closely related structurally and functionally to mercaptopurine.

Thiogunine is available in tablets for oral administration.

Following is its chemical structure:

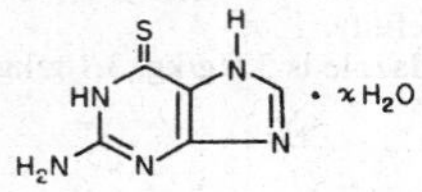

CLINICAL PHARMACOLOGY
Clinical studies have shown that the absorption of an oral dose of Thioguanine in man is incomplete and variable, averaging approximately 30% of the administered dose (range: 1%-46%).[2,3] Following oral administration of ^{35}S-6-Thioguanine, total plasma radioactivity reached a maximum at eight hours and declined slowly thereafter. Parent drug represented only a very small fraction of the total plasma radioactivity at any time, being virtually undetectable throughout the period of measurements.

The oral administration of radiolabeled Thioguanine revealed only trace quantities of parent drug in the urine. However, a methylated metabolite, 2-amino-6-methyl-thiopurine (MTG), appeared very early, rose to a maximum six to eight hours after drug administration, and was still being excreted after 12 to 22 hours. Radiolabeled sulfate appeared somewhat later than MTG but was the principal metabolite after eight hours. Thiouric acid and some unidentified products were found in the urine in small amounts.[3] Intravenous administration of ^{35}S-6-Thioguanine disclosed a median plasma half-disappearance time of 80 minutes (range: 25 to 240 minutes) when the compound was given in single doses of 65 to 300 mg/m². Although initial plasma levels of Thioguanine did correlate with the dose level, there was no correlation between the plasma half-disappearance time and the dose.[2]

Thioguanine is incorporated into the DNA and the RNA of human bone marrow cells. Studies with intravenous ^{35}S-6-Thioguanine have shown that the amount of Thioguanine incorporated into nucleic acids is more than 100 times higher after five daily doses than after a single dose. With the 5-dose schedule, from one-half to virtually all of the guanine in the residual DNA was replaced by Thioguanine.[2] Tissue distribution studies of ^{35}S-6-Thioguanine in mice showed only traces of radioactivity in brain after oral administration. No measurements have been made of Thioguanine concentrations in human cerebrospinal fluid, but observations on tissue distribution in animals, together with the lack of CNS penetration by the closely related compound, mercaptopurine, suggest that Thioguanine does not reach therapeutic concentrations in the CSF.

Monitoring of plasma levels of Thioguanine during therapy is of questionable value.[3] There is technical difficulty in determining plasma concentrations, which are seldom greater than 1 to 2 µg/mL after a therapeutic oral dose. More significantly, Thioguanine enters rapidly into the anabolic and catabolic pathways for purines, and the active intracellular metabolites have appreciably longer half-lives than the parent drug. The biochemical effects of a single dose of Thioguanine are evident long after the parent drug has disappeared from plasma. Because of this rapid metabolism of Thioguanine to active intracellular derivatives, hemodialysis would not be expected to appreciably reduce toxicity of the drug. Thioguanine competes with hypoxanthine and guanine for the enzyme hypoxanthine-guanine phosphoribosyltransferase (HGPRTase) and is itself converted to 6-thioguanylic acid (TGMP). This nucleotide reaches high intracellular concentrations at therapeutic doses. TGMP interferes at several points with the synthesis of guanine nucleotides. It inhibits de novo purine biosynthesis by pseudo-feedback inhibition of glutamine-5-phosphoribosylpyrophosphate amidotransferase—the first enzyme unique to the de novo pathway for purine ribonucleotide synthesis. TGMP also inhibits the conversion of inosinic acid (IMP) to xanthylic acid (XMP) by competition for the enzyme IMP dehydrogenase. At one time TGMP was felt to be a significant inhibitor of ATP:GMP phosphotransferase (guanylate kinase),[4] but recent results have shown this not to be so.[5]

Thioguanylic acid is further converted to the di- and tri-phosphates, thioguanosine diphosphate (TGDP) and thioguanosine triphosphate (TGTP) (as well as their 2'-deoxyribosyl analogues) by the same enzymes which metabolize guanine nucleotides.[6] Thioguanine nucleotides are incorporated into both the RNA and the DNA by phosphodiester linkages[2] and it has been argued that incorporation of such fraudulent bases contributes to the cytotoxicity of Thioguanine.

Thus, Thioguanine has multiple metabolic effects and at present it is not possible to designate one major site of action. Its tumor inhibitory properties may be due to one or more of its effects on (a) feedback inhibition of de novo purine synthesis; (b) inhibition of purine nucleotide interconversions; or (c) incorporation into the DNA and the RNA. The net consequence of its actions is a sequential blockade of the synthesis and utilization of the purine nucleotides.[4,6,7]

The catabolism of Thioguanine and its metabolites is complex and shows significant differences between man and the mouse.[2,3] In both humans and mice, after oral administration of ^{35}S-6-Thioguanine, urine contains virtually no detectable intact Thioguanine. While deamination and subsequent oxidation to thiouric acid occurs only to a small extent in man, it is the main pathway in mice. The product of deamination by guanase, 6-thioxanthine, is inactive, having negligible antitumor activity. This pathway of Thioguanine inactivation is not dependent on the action of xanthine oxidase and an inhibitor of that enzyme (such as allopurinol), will not block the detoxification of Thioguanine even though the inactive 6-thioxanthine is normally further oxidized by xanthine oxidase to thiouric acid before it is eliminated. In man, methylation of Thioguanine is much more extensive than in the mouse. The product of methylation, 2-amino-6-methyl-thiopurine, is also substantially less active and less toxic than Thioguanine and its formation is likewise unaffected by the presence of allopurinol. Appreciable amounts of inorganic sulfate are also found in both murine and human urine, presumably arising from further metabolism of the methylated derivatives.

In some animal tumors, resistance to the effect of Thioguanine correlates with the loss of HGPRTase activity and the resulting inability to convert Thioguanine to thioguanylic acid. However, other resistance mechanisms, such as increased catabolism of TGMP by a nonspecific phosphatase, may be operative. Although not invariable, it is usual to find cross-resistance between Thioguanine and its close analogue, mercaptopurine.

INDICATIONS AND USAGE
a) Acute Nonlymphocytic Leukemias: Thiogunine is indicated for remission induction, remission consolidation, and maintenance therapy of acute nonlymphocytic leukemias.[8,9] The response to this agent depends upon the age of the patient (younger patients faring better than older), and whether Thioguanine is used in previously treated or previously untreated patients. Reliance upon Thioguanine alone is seldom justified for initial remission induction of acute nonlymphocytic leukemias because combination chemotherapy including Thioguanine results in more frequent remission induction and longer duration of remission than Thioguanine alone.

b) Other Neoplasms: Thioguanine is not effective in chronic lymphocytic leukemia, Hodgkin's lymphoma, multiple myeloma, or solid tumors. Although Thioguanine is one of several agents with activity in the treatment of the chronic phase of chronic myelogenous leukemia, more objective responses are observed with busulfan, and therefore busulfan is usually regarded as the preferred drug.

CONTRAINDICATIONS
Thioguanine should not be used in patients whose disease has demonstrated prior resistance to this drug. In animals and man, there is usually complete cross-resistance between mercaptopurine and Thioguanine.

WARNINGS
SINCE DRUGS USED IN CANCER CHEMOTHERAPY ARE POTENTIALLY HAZARDOUS, IT IS RECOMMENDED THAT ONLY PHYSICIANS EXPERIENCED WITH THE RISKS OF THIOGUANINE AND KNOWLEDGEABLE IN THE NATURAL HISTORY OF ACUTE NONLYMPHOCYTIC LEUKEMIAS ADMINISTER THIS DRUG.

The most consistent, dose-related toxicity is bone marrow suppression. This may be manifested by anemia, leukopenia, thrombocytopenia, or any combination of these. Any one of these findings may also reflect progression of the underlying disease. Since Thioguanine may have a delayed effect, it is important to withdraw the medication temporarily at the first sign of an abnormally large fall in any of the formed elements of the blood.

It is recommended that evaluation of the hemoglobin concentration or hematocrit, total white blood cell count and differential count, and quantitative platelet count be obtained frequently while the patient is on Thioguanine therapy. In cases where the cause of fluctuations in the formed elements in the peripheral blood is obscure, bone marrow examination may be useful for the evaluation of marrow status. The decision to increase, decrease, continue, or discontinue a given dosage of Thioguanine must be based not only on the absolute hematologic values, but also upon the rapidity with which changes are occurring. In many instances, particularly during the induction phase of acute leukemia, complete blood counts will need to be done more frequently in order to evaluate the effect of the therapy. The dosage of Thioguanine may need to be reduced when this agent is combined with other drugs whose primary toxicity is myelosuppression.

Myelosuppression is often unavoidable during the induction phase of adult acute nonlymphocytic leukemias if remission induction is to be successful. Whether or not this demands modification or cessation of dosage depends both upon the response of the underlying disease and a careful consideration of supportive facilities (granulocyte and platelet transfusions) which may be available. Life-threatening infections and bleeding have been observed as consequences of Thioguanine-induced granulocytopenia and thrombocytopenia. The effect of Thioguanine on the immunocompetence of patients is unknown.

Pregnancy: Pregnancy Category D: Drugs such as Thioguanine are potential mutagens and teratogens. Thioguanine may cause fetal harm when administered to a pregnant woman. Thioguanine has been shown to be teratogenic in rats when given in doses five (5) times the human dose. When given to the rat on the 4th and 5th days of gestation, 13% of surviving placentas did not contain fetuses, and 19% of offspring were malformed or stunted. The malformations noted included generalized edema, cranial defects, and general skeletal hypoplasia, hydrocephalus, ventral hernia, situs inversus, and incomplete development of the limbs.[10] There are no adequate and well-controlled studies in pregnant women. If this drug is used during pregnancy, or if the patient becomes pregnant while taking the drug, the patient should be apprised of the potential hazard to the fetus. Women of childbearing potential should be advised to avoid becoming pregnant.

PRECAUTIONS
General: Although the primary toxicity of Thioguanine is myelosuppression, other toxicities have occasionally been observed, particularly when Thioguanine is used in combination with other cancer chemotherapeutic agents.

A few cases of jaundice have been reported in patients with leukemia receiving Thioguanine. Among these were two adult male patients and four children with acute myelogenous leukemia and an adult male with acute lymphocytic leukemia who developed veno-occlusive hepatic disease while receiving chemotherapy for their leukemia.[11,12] Six patients had received cytarabine prior to treatment with Thioguanine, and some were receiving other chemotherapy in addition to Thioguanine when they became symptomatic. While veno-occlusive hepatic disease has not been reported in patients treated with Thioguanine alone, it is recommended that Thioguanine be withheld if there is evidence of toxic hepatitis or biliary stasis, and that appropriate clinical and laboratory investigations be initiated to establish the etiology of the hepatic dysfunction. Deterioration in liver function studies during Thioguanine therapy should prompt discontinuation of treatment and a search for an explanation of the hepatotoxicity.

Information for Patients: Patients should be informed that the major toxicities of Thioguanine are related to myelosuppression, hepatotoxicity, and gastrointestinal toxicity. Patients should never be allowed to take the drug without medical supervision and should be advised to consult their physician if they experience fever, sore throat, jaundice, nausea, vomiting, signs of local infection, bleeding from any site, or symptoms suggestive of anemia. Women of childbearing potential should be advised to avoid becoming pregnant.

Laboratory Tests: It is advisable to monitor liver function tests (serum transaminases, alkaline phosphatase, bilirubin) at weekly intervals when first beginning therapy and at monthly intervals therafter. It may be advisable to perform liver function tests more frequently in patients with known pre-existing liver disease or in patients who are receiving Thioguanine and other hepatotoxic drugs. Patients should be instructed to discontinue Thioguanine immediately if clinical jaundice is detected (see *"Warnings"* section).

Drug Interactions: There is usually complete cross-resistance between mercaptopurine and Thioguanine.

In one study, 12 of approximately 330 patients receiving continuous busulfan and Thioguanine therapy for treatment of chronic myelogenous leukemia were found to have esophageal varices associated with abnormal liver function tests.[13] Subsequent liver biopsies were performed in four of these patients, all of which showed evidence of nodular regenerative hyperplasia. Duration of combination therapy prior to the appearance of esophageal varices ranged from 6 to 45 months. With the present analysis of the data, no cases of hepatotoxicity have appeared in the busulfan alone arm of the study. Long-term continuous therapy with Thioguanine and busulfan should be used with caution.

Carcinogenesis, Mutagenesis, Impairment of Fertility: In view of its action on cellular DNA, Thioguanine is potentially mutagenic and carcinogenic, and consideration should be given to the theoretical risk of carcinogenesis when Thioguanine is administered (see *"Warnings"* section).

Pregnancy: Teratogenic Effects: Pregnancy Category D. See *"Warnings"* section.

Nursing Mothers: It is not known whether this drug is excreted in human milk. Because of the potential for tumorigenicity shown for Thioguanine, a decision should be made whether to discontinue nursing or to discontinue the drug, taking into account the importance of the drug to the mother.

ADVERSE REACTIONS
The most frequent adverse reaction to Thioguanine is myelosuppression. The induction of complete remission of acute myelogenous leukemia usually requires combination chemotherapy in dosages which produce marrow hypoplasia.[14] Since consolidation and maintenance of remission are also effected by multiple drug regimens whose component agents cause myelosuppression, pancytopenia is observed in nearly all patients. Dosages and schedules must be adjusted to prevent life-threatening cytopenias whenever these adverse reactions are observed.

Hyperuricemia frequently occurs in patients receiving Thioguanine as a consequence of rapid cell lysis accompanying the antineoplastic effect. Adverse effects can be minimized by increased hydration, urine alkalinization, and the prophylactic administration of a xanthine oxidase inhibitor such as Allopurinol. Unlike mercaptopurine and azathioprine, Thioguanine may be continued in the usual dosage when allopurinol is used conjointly to inhibit uric acid formation.

Less frequent adverse reactions include nausea, vomiting, anorexia, and stomatitis. Intestinal necrosis and perforation have been reported in patients who received multiple drug chemotherapy including Thioguanine.

Hepatic Effects: Liver enzyme and other liver function studies are occasionally abnormal. If jaundice, hepatomegaly, or anorexia with tenderness in the right hypochondrium occurs, Thioguanine should be withheld until the exact etiology can be determined. There have been reports of veno-occlusive liver disease occurring in patients who received combination chemotherapy including Thioguanine.[11,12] Esophageal varices have been reported in patients receiving continuous busulfan and Thioguanine therapy for treatment of chronic myelogenous leukemia (see *"Precautions: Drug Interactions"* section).

OVERDOSAGE
Signs and symptoms of overdosage may be immediate, such as nausea, vomiting, malaise, hypertension, and diaphoresis; or delayed, such as myelosuppression and azotemia.[15] It is not known whether Thioguanine is dialyzable. Hemodialysis is thought to be of marginal use due to the rapid intracellular incorporation of Thioguanine into active metabolites with long persistence. The oral LD_{50} of Thioguanine was determined to be 823 mg/kg $\pm$ 50.73 mg/kg and 740 mg/kg $\pm$ 45.24 mg/kg for male and female rats respectively.[16] Symptoms of overdosage may occur after a single dose of as little as 2.0 to 3.0 mg/kg Thioguanine. As much as 35 mg/kg has been given in a single oral dose with reversible myelosuppression observed. There is no known pharmacologic antagonist of Thioguanine. The drug should be discontinued immediately if unintended toxicity occurs during treatment. Severe hematologic toxicity may require supportive therapy with platelet transfusions for bleeding, and granulocyte transfusions and antibiotics if sepsis is documented. If a patient is seen immediately following an accidental overdosage of the drug, it may be useful to induce emesis.

DOSAGE AND ADMINISTRATION
Thioguanine is administered orally. The dosage which will be tolerated and effective varies according to the stage and type of neoplastic process being treated. Because the usual therapies for adult and childhood acute nonlymphocytic leukemias involve the use of Thioguanine with other agents in combination, physicians responsible for administering these therapies should be experienced in the use of cancer chemotherapy and in the chosen protocol.

Ninety-six (59%) of one hundred sixty-three children with previously untreated acute nonlymphocytic leukemia obtained complete remission with a multiple drug protocol including Thioguanine, prednisone, cytarabine, cyclophosphamide, and vincristine. Remission was maintained with daily Thioguanine, four-day pulses of cytarabine and cyclophosphamide, and a single dose of vincristine every 28 days. The median duration of remission was 11.5 months.[8]

Fifty-three percent of previously untreated adults with acute nonlymphocytic leukemias attained remission following use of the combination of Thioguanine and cytarabine according to a protocol developed at The Memorial Sloan-Kettering Cancer Center. A median duration of remission of 8.8 months was achieved with the multiple drug maintenance regimen which included Thioguanine.[9]

On those occasions when single agent chemotherapy with Thioguanine may be appropriate, the usual initial dosage for children and adults is approximately 2 mg/kg of body weight per day. If, after four weeks on this dosage, there is no clinical improvement and no leukocyte or platelet depression, the dosage may be cautiously increased to 3 mg/kg per day. The total daily dose may be given at one time.

The dosage of Thioguanine used does not depend on whether or not the patient is receiving allopurinol; **this is in contradistinction to the dosage reduction which is mandatory when mercaptopurine or azathioprine is given simultaneously with allopurinol.**

Procedures for proper handling and disposal of anticancer drugs should be considered. Several guidelines on this subject have been published.[17-23]

There is no general agreement that all of the procedures recommended in the guidelines are necessary or appropriate.

Store at 15° to 25°C (59° to 77°F) in a dry place.

REFERENCES
1. Hitchings GH, Elion GB. The chemistry and biochemistry of purine analogs. *Ann NY Acad Sci.* 1954;60:195-199. 2. LePage GA, Whitecar JP Jr. Pharmacology of 6-thioguanine in man. *Cancer Res.* 1971;31:1627-1631. 3. Elion GB. Biochemistry and pharmacology of purine analogues. *Fed Proc.* 1967; 26:898-904. 4. Miech RP, Parks RE

Jr, Anderson JH Jr, Sartorelli AC. An hypothesis on the mechanism of action of 6-thioguanine. *Biochem Pharmacol.* 1967; 16:2222-2227. 5. Miller RL, Adamczyk DL, Spector T, Agarwal KC, Miech RP, Panks RE Jr. Reassessment of the interactions of guanylate kinase and 6-thioguanine 5'-phosphate. *Biochem Pharmacol.* 1977;26:1573-1576. 6. Paterson ARP, Tidd DN. 6-Thiopurines. In: Sartorelli AC, Johns DG, eds. *Antineoplastic and Immunosuppressive Agents,* Part II. Berlin: Springer Verlag; 1975:384-403. 7. Nelson JA, Carpenter JW, Rose LM, Adamson DJ. Mechanisms of action of 6-thioguanine, 6-mercaptopurine, and 8-azaguanine. *Cancer Res.* 1975;35:2872-2878. 8. Chard RL Jr, Finklestein JZ, Sonley MJ, et al. Increased survival in childhood acute nonlymphocytic leukemia after treatment with prednisone, cytosine arabinoside, 6-thioguanine, cyclophosphamide, and oncovin (PATCO) combination therapy. *Med Ped Oncol.* 1978;4:263-273. 9. Mertelsmann R, Drapkin RL, Gee TS, et al. Treatment of acute nonlymphocytic leukemia in adults: response to 2,2-anhydro-1-B-D-arabinofuranosyl-5-fluorocytosine and thioguanine on the L-12 protocol. *Cancer.* 1981;48:2136-2142. 10. Thiersch JB: Effect of 2-6 diaminopurine (2-6DP): 6 chlorpurine (CIP) and thioguanine (ThG) on rat litter *in utero. Proc Soc Exp Biol Med.* 1957;94:40-43. 11. Griner PF, Elbadawi A, Packman CH. Veno-occlusive disease of the liver after chemotherapy of acute leukemia: report of two cases. *Ann Intern Med.* 1976; 85:578-582. 12. Gill RA, Onstad GR, Cardamone JM, Maneval DC, Sumner HW. Hepatic veno-occlusive disease caused by 6-thioguanine. *Ann Intern Med.* 1982;96:58-60. 13. Key NS, Kelly PMA, Emerson PM, Chapman RWG, Allan NC, McGee JO'D. Oesophageal varices associated with busulfan-thioguanine combination therapy for chronic myeloid leukaemia. *Lancet.* 1987;2:1050-1052. 14. Clarkson BD, Dowling MD, Gee TS, Cunningham IB, Burchenal JH. Treatment of acute leukemia in adults. *Cancer.* 1975;36:775-795. 15. Presant CA, Denes AE, Klein L, Garrett S, Metter GE. Phase I and preliminary phase II observations of high-dose intermittent 6-thioguanine. *Cancer Treat Rep.* 1980;64:1109-1113. 16. Unpublished data on file with Burroughs Wellcome Co. 17. Recommendations for the safe handling of parenteral antineoplastic drugs. Washington, DC: Division of Safety, National Institutes of Health; 1983. US Dept. of Health and Human Services, Public Health Service publication NIH 83-2621. 18. AMA Council on Scientific Affairs. Guidelines for handling parenteral antineoplastics. *JAMA.* 1985;253: 1590-1591. 19. National Study Commission on Cytotoxic Exposure. Recommendations for handling cytotoxic agents. 1984. Available from Louis P. Jeffrey, ScD, Director of Pharmacy Services, Rhode Island Hospital, 593 Eddy Street, Providence, RI 02902. 20. Clinical Oncological Society of Australia. Guidelines and recommendations for safe handling of antineoplastic agents. *Med J Australia.* 1983;1:426-428. 21. Jones RB, Frank R, Mass T. Safe handling of chemotherapeutic agents: A report from the Mount Sinai Medical Center. *CA—A Cancer J for Clin.* 1983;33:258-263. 22. American Society of Hospital Pharmacists. ASHP technical assistance bulletin on handling cytotoxic and hazardous drugs. *Am J Hosp Pharm.* 1990;47:1033-1049. 23. Yodaiken RE, Bennett D. OSHA work-practice guidelines for personnel dealing with cytotoxic (antineoplastic) drugs. *Am. J Hosp Pharm.* 1986;43:1193-1204.

HOW SUPPLIED

TABLETS: 40 MG

BRAND/MANUFACTURER	NDC	SIZE	AWP
○ BRAND			
THIOGUANINE: Burr Wellcome	00081-0880-25	25s	$70.00

Thioguanine *SEE* THIOGUANINE

Thiola *SEE* TIOPRONIN

Thiopental Sodium

DESCRIPTION

Each Kit Contains:

Thipental Sodium	1 g
Thiopental Sodium	2.5 g
Thiopental Sodium	5 g

Each Ready-to-Mix Syringe Contains:

Thiopental Sodium	250 mg
Thipental Sodium	400 mg
Thipental Sodium	500 mg

Each Vial Contains:

Thiopental Sodium	500 mg
Thiopental Sodium	1 g

Thiopental Sodium for Injection, USP is a thiobarbiturate, the sulfur analogue of sodium pentobarbital.

The drug is prepared as a sterile powder and after reconstitution with an appropriate diluent is administered by the intravenous route.

Thiopental Sodium is chemically designated Sodium 5-ethyl-5-(1-methylbutyl)-2-thiobarbiturate.

The drug is a yellowish, hygroscopic powder, stabilized with anhydrous sodium carbonate as a buffer (60 mg/g of Thiopental Sodium).

Following is its chemical structure:

CLINICAL PHARMACOLOGY

Thiopental Sodium is an ultrashort-acting depressant of the central nervous system which induces hypnosis and anesthesia, but not analgesia. It produces hypnosis within 30 to 40 seconds of intravenous injection. Recovery after a small dose is rapid, with some somnolence and retrograde amnesia. Repeated intravenous doses lead to prolonged anesthesia because fatty tissues act as a reservoir; they accumulate Thiopental Sodium in concentrations 6 to 12 times greater than the plasma concentration, and then release the drug slowly to cause prolonged anesthesia.

The half-life of the elimination phase after a single intravenous dose is three to eight hours.

The distribution and fate of Thiopental Sodium (as with other barbiturates) is influenced chiefly by its lipid solubility (partition coefficient), protein binding and extent of ionization. Thiopental Sodium has a partition coefficient of 580.

Approximately 80% of the drug in the blood is bound to plasma protein. Thiopental Sodium is largely degraded in the liver and to a smaller extent in other tissues, especially the kidney and brain. It has a pK_a of 7.4.

Concentration in spinal fluid is slightly less than in the plasma.

Biotransformation products of Thiopental are pharmacologically inactive and mostly excreted in the urine.

INDICATIONS AND USAGE

Thiopental Sodium is indicated (1) as the sole anesthetic agent for brief (15 minute) procedures, (2) for induction of anesthesia prior to administration of other anesthetic agents, (3) to supplement regional anesthesia, (4) to provide hypnosis during balanced anesthesia with other agents for analgesia or muscle relaxation, (5) for the control of convulsive states during or following inhalation anesthesia, local anesthesia, or other causes, (6) in neurosurgical patients with increased intracranial pressure, if adequate ventilation is provided, and (7) for narcoanalysis and narcosynthesis in psychiatric disorders.

UNLABELED USES

Thiopental Sodium is used alone or as an adjunct in the treatment of phantom limb pain and status epilepticus refractory to other therapies.

CONTRAINDICATIONS

ABSOLUTE CONTRAINDICATIONS

(1) Absence of suitable veins for intravenous administration, (2) hypersensitivity (allergy) to barbiturates and (3) variegate porphyria (South African) or acute intermittent porphyria.

RELATIVE CONTRAINDICATIONS

(1) Severe cardiovascular disease, (2) hypotension or shock, (3) conditions in which the hypnotic effect may be prolonged or potentiated—excessive premedication, Addison's disease, hepatic or renal dysfunction, myxedema, increased blood urea, severe anemia, asthma, myasthenia gravis, and (4) status asthmaticus.

WARNINGS

KEEP RESUSCITATIVE AND ENDOTRACHEAL INTUBATION EQUIPMENT AND OXYGEN READILY AVAILABLE. MAINTAIN PATENCY OF THE AIRWAY AT ALL TIMES.

This drug should be administered only by persons qualified in the use of intravenous anesthetics.

Avoid extravasation or intra-arterial injection.

WARNING: MAY BE HABIT FORMING.

PRECAUTIONS

Observe aseptic precautions at all times in preparation and handling of Thiopental Sodium solutions.

If used in conditions involving relative contraindications, reduce dosage and administer slowly.

Care should be taken in administering the drug to patients with advanced cardiac disease, increased intracranial pressure, ophthalmoplegia plus, asthma, myasthenia gravis and endocrine insufficiency (pituitary, thyroid, adrenal, pancreas).

Drug Interactions: The following drug interactions have been reported with Thiopental.

Drug	Effect
Probenecid	Prolonged action of Thiopental
Diazoxide	Hypotension
Zimelidine	Thiopental antagonism
Opioid analgesics	Decreased antinociceptive action
Aminophylline	Thiopental antagonism
Midazolam	Synergism

Pregnancy Category C: Animal reproduction studies have not been conducted with Thiopental Sodium. It is also not known whether Thiopental Sodium can cause fetal harm when administered to a pregnant woman or can affect reproduction capacity. Thiopental Sodium should be given to a pregnant woman only if clearly needed.

Nursing Mothers: Thiopental Sodium readily crosses the placental barrier and small amounts may appear in the milk of nursing mothers following administration of large doses.

◆ RATED THERAPEUTICALLY EQUIVALENT; ◇ THERAPEUTIC EQUIVALENCE UNCONFIRMED; ○ UNRATED

ADVERSE REACTIONS

Adverse reactions include respiratory depression, myocardial depression, cardiac arrhythmias, prolonged somnolence and recovery, sneezing, coughing, bronchospasm, laryngospasm and shivering. Anaphylactic and anaphylactoid reactions to Thiopental Sodium have been reported. Symptoms, e.g., urticaria, bronchospasm, vasodilation and edema should be managed by conventional means.

Rarely, immune hemolytic anemia with renal failure and radial nerve palsy have been reported.

DRUG ABUSE AND DEPENDENCE

WARNING: MAY BE HABIT FORMING.

Thiopental Sodium is classified as a Schedule III controlled substance.

OVERDOSAGE

Overdosage may occur from too rapid or repeated injections. Too rapid injection may be followed by an alarming fall in blood pressure even to shock levels. Apnea, occasional laryngospasm, coughing and other respiratory difficulties with excessive or too rapid injections may occur. In the event of suspected or apparent overdosage, the drug should be discontinued, a patent airway established (intubate if necessary) or maintained, and oxygen should be administered, with assisted ventilation if necessary. The lethal dose of barbiturates varies and cannot be stated with certainty. Lethal blood levels may be as low as 1 mg/100 mL for short-acting barbiturates; less if other depressant drugs or alcohol are also present.

MANAGEMENT OF OVERDOSAGE

It is generally agreed that respiratory depression or arrest due to unusual sensitivity to Thiopental Sodium or overdosage is easily managed if there is no concomitant respiratory obstruction. If the airway is patent, any method of ventilating the lungs (that prevents hypoxia) should be successful in maintaining other vital functions. Since depression of respiratory activity is one of the characteristic actions of the drug, it is important to observe respiration closely.

Should laryngeal spasm occur, it may be relieved by one of the usual methods, such as the use of a relaxant drug or positive pressure oxygen. Endotracheal intubation may be indicated in difficult cases.

DOSAGE AND ADMINISTRATION

Thiopental Sodium is administered by the intravenous route only. Individual response to the drug is so varied that there can be no fixed dosage. The drug should be titrated against patient requirements as governed by age, sex and body weight. Younger patients require relatively larger doses than middle-aged and elderly persons; the latter metabolize the drug more slowly. Pre-puberty requirements are the same for both sexes, but adult females require less than adult males. Dose is usually proportional to body weight and obese patients require a larger dose than relatively lean persons of the same weight.

PREMEDICATION

Premedication usually consists of atropine or scopolamine to suppress vagal reflexes and inhibit secretions. In addition, a barbiturate or an opiate is often given. Sodium pentobarbital injection is suggested because it provides a preliminary indication of how the patient will react to barbiturate anesthesia. Ideally, the peak effect of these medications should be reached shortly before the time of induction.

TEST DOSE

It is advisable to inject a small "test" dose of 25 to 75 mg (1 to 3 mL of a 2.5% solution) of Thiopental Sodium to assess tolerance or unusual sensitivity to Thiopental Sodium, and pausing to observe patient reaction for at least 60 seconds. If unexpectedly deep anesthesia develops or if respiratory depression occurs, consider these possibilities: (1) the patient may be unusually sensitive to Thiopental Sodium, (2) the solution may be more concentrated than had been assumed, or (3) the patient may have received too much premedication.

USE IN ANESTHESIA

Moderately slow induction can usually be accomplished in the "average" adult by injection of 50 to 75 mg (2 to 3 mL of a 2.5% solution) at intervals of 20 to 40 seconds, depending on the reaction of the patient. Once anesthesia is established, additional injections of 25 to 50 mg can be given whenever the patient moves.

Slow injection is recommended to minimize respiratory depression and the possibility of overdosage. The smallest dose consistent with attaining the surgical objective is the desired goal. Momentary apnea following each injection is typical, and progressive decrease in the amplitude of respiration appears with increasing dosage. Pulse remains normal or increases slightly and returns to normal. Blood pressure usually falls slightly but returns toward normal. Muscles usually relax about 30 seconds after unconsciousness is attained, but this may be masked if a skeletal muscle relaxant is used. The tone of jaw muscles is a fairly reliable index. The pupils may dilate but later contract; sensitivity to light is not usually lost until a level of anesthesia deep enough to permit surgery is attained. Nystagmus and divergent strabismus are characteristic during early stages, but at the level of surgical anesthesia, the eyes are central and fixed. Corneal and conjunctival reflexes disappear during surgical anesthesia.

When Thiopental Sodium is used for induction in balanced anesthesia with a skeletal muscle relaxant and an inhalation agent, the total dose of Thiopental Sodium can be estimated and then injected in two to four fractional doses. With this technique, brief periods of apnea may occur which may require assisted or controlled pulmonary ventilation. Aas an initial dose, 210 to 280 mg (3 to 4 mg/kg) of Thiopental Sodium is usually required for rapid induction in the average adult (70 kg).

When Thiopental Sodium is used as the sole anesthetic agent, the desired level of anesthesia can be maintained by injection of small repeated doses as needed or by using a continuous intravenous drip in a 0.2% or 0.4% concentration. (Sterile water should not be used as the diluent in these concentrations, since hemolysis will occur.) With continuous drip, the depth of anesthesia is controlled by adjusting the rate of infusion.

USE IN CONVULSIVE STATES

For the control of convulsive states following anesthesia (inhalation or local) or other causes, 75 to 125 mg (3 to 5 mL of a 2.5% solution) should be given as soon as possible after the convulsion begins. Convulsions following the use of a local anesthetic may require 125 to 250 mg of Thiopental Sodium given over a ten minute period. If the convulsion is caused by a local anesthetic, the required dose of Thiopental Sodium will depend upon the amount of local anesthetic given and its convulsant properties.

USE IN NEUROSURGICAL PATIENTS WITH INCREASED INTRACRANIAL PRESSURE

In neurosurgical patients, intermittent bolus injections of 1.5 to 3.5 mg/kg of body weight may be given to reduce intraoperative elevations of intracranial pressure, if adequate ventilation is provided.

USE IN PSYCHIATRIC DISORDERS

For narcoanalysis and narcosynthesis in psychiatric disorders, premedication with an anticholinergic agent may precede administration of Thiopental Sodium. After a test dose, is injected at a slow rate of 100 mg/min (4 mL/min of a 2.5% solution) with the patient counting backwards from 100. Shortly after counting becomes confused but before actual sleep is produced, the injection is discontinued. Allow the patient to return to a semidrowsy state where conversation is coherent. Alternatively, Thiopental Sodium may be administered by rapid I.V. drip using a 0.2% concentration in 5% dextrose and water. At this concentration, the rate of administration should not exceed 50 mL/min.

MANAGEMENT OF SOME COMPLICATIONS

Respiratory depression (hypoventilation, apnea), which may result from either unusual responsiveness to Thiopental Sodium or overdosage, is managed as stated above. Thiopental Sodium should be considered to have the same potential for producing respiratory depression as an inhalation agent, and patency of the airway must be protected at all times.

Laryngospasm may occur with light Thiopental Sodium narcosis at intubation, or in the absence of intubation if foreign matter or secretions in the respiratory tract create irritation. Laryngeal and bronchial vagal reflexes can be suppressed, and secretions minimized by giving atropine or scopolamine premedication and a barbiturate or opiate. Use of a skeletal muscle relaxant or positive pressure oxygen will usually relieve laryngospasm. Tracheostomy may be indicated in difficult cases.

Myocardial depression, proportional to the amount of drug in direct contact with the heart, can occur and may cause hypotension, particularly in patients with an unhealthy myocardium. Arrhythmias may appear if PCO_2 is elevated, but they are uncommon with adequate ventilation. Management of myocardial depression is the same as for overdosage. Thiopental Sodium does not sensitize the heart to epinephrine or other sympathomimetic amines.

Extravascular infiltration should be avoided. Care should be taken to insure that the needle is within the lumen of the vein before injection of Thiopental Sodium. Extravascular injection may cause chemical irritation of the tissues varying from slight tenderness to venopasm, extensive necrosis and sloughing. This is due primarily to the high alkaline pH (10 to 11) of clinical concentrations of the drug. If extravasation occurs, the local irritant effects can be reduced by injection of 1% procaine locally to relieve pain and enhance vasodilatation. Local application of heat also may help to increase local circulation and removal of the infiltrate.

Intra-arterial injection can occur inadvertently, especially if an aberrant superficial artery is present at the medial aspect of the antecubital fossa. The area selected for intravenous injection of the drug should be palpated for detection of an underlying pulsating vessel. Accidental intra-arterial injection can cause arteriospasm and severe pain along the course of the artery with blanching of the arm and fingers. Appropriate corrective measures should be instituted promptly to avoid possible development of gangrene. Any patient complaint of pain warrants stopping the injection. Methods suggested for dealing with this complication vary with the severity of symptoms. The following have been suggested:

1. Dilute the injected Thiopental Sodium by removing the tourniquet and any restrictive garments.
2. Leave the needle in place, if possible.
3. Inject the artery with a dilute solution of papaverine, 40 to 80 mg, or 10 mL of 1% procaine, to inhibit smooth muscle spasm.
4. If necessary, perform sympathetic block of the brachial plexus and/or stellate ganglion to relieve pain and assist in opening collateral circulation. Papaverine can be injected into the subclavian artery, if desired.
5. Unless otherwise contraindicated, institute immediate heparinization to prevent thrombus formation.
6. Consider local infiltration of an alpha-adrenergic blocking agent such as phentolamine into the vasospastic area.
7. Provide additional symptomatic treatment as required.

Shivering after Thiopental Sodium anesthesia, manifested by twitching face muscles and occasional progression to tremors of the arms, head, shoulder and body, is a thermal reaction due to increased sensitivity to cold. Shivering appears if the room environment is cold and if a large ventilatory heat loss has been sustained with balanced inhalation anesthesia employing nitrous oxide. Treatment consists of warming the patient with blankets, maintaining room temperature near 22° C (72° F), and administration of chlorpromazine or methylphenidate.

PREPARATION OF SOLUTIONS

Thiopental Sodium is supplied as a yellowish, hygroscopic powder in a variety of different containers. Solutions should be prepared aseptically with one of the three following diluents: Sterile Water for Injection, USP, 0.9% Sodium Chloride Injection, USP or 5% Dextrose Injection, USP. Clinical concentrations used for intermittent intravenous administration vary between 2.0% and 5.0%. A 2.0% or 2.5% solution is most commonly used. A 3.4% concentration in sterile water for injection is isotonic; concentrations less than 2.0% in this diluent are not used because they cause hemolysis. For continuous intravenous drip administration, concentrations of 0.2% or 0.4% are used. Solutions may be prepared by adding Thiopental Sodium to 5% Dextrose Injection, USP, 0.9% Sodium Chloride Injection, USP or Normosol®-R pH 7.4.

Since Thiopental Sodium contains no added bacteriostatic agent, extreme care in preparation and handling should be exercised at all times to prevent the introduction of microbial contaminants. Solutions should be freshly prepared and used promptly; when reconstituted for administration to several patients, unused portions should be discarded after 24 hours. Sterilization by heating should not be attempted.

Warning: The 2.5 g and larger sizes contain adequate medication for several patients.

COMPATIBILITY

Any solution of Thiopental Sodium with a visible precipitate should not be administered. The stability of Thiopental Sodium solutions depends upon several factors, including the diluent, temperature of storage and the amount of carbon dioxide from room air that gains access to the solution. Any factor or condition which tends to lower pH (increase acidity) of Thiopental Sodium solutions will increase the likelihood of precipitation of Thiopental acid. Such factors include the use of diluents which are too acidic and the absorption of carbon dioxide which can combine with water to form carbonic acid.

Solutions of succinylcholine, tubocurarine or other drugs which have an acid pH should not be mixed with Thiopental Sodium solutions. The most stable solutions are those reconstituted in water or isotonic saline, kept under refrigeration and tightly stoppered. The presence or absence of a visible precipitate offers a practical guide to the physical compatibility of prepared solutions of Thiopental Sodium.

CALCULATIONS FOR VARIOUS CONCENTRATIONS

Concentration Desired		Amounts to Use	
Percent	mg/mL	Thiopental Sodium g	Diluent mL
0.2	2	1	500
0.4	4	1	250
		2	500
2.0	20	5	250
		10	500
2.5	25	1	40
		5	200
5	50	1	20
		5	100

Reconstituted solutions of Thiopental Sodium should be inspected visually for particulate matter and discoloration, whenever solution and container permit.

READY-TO-MIX SYRINGE

USE ASEPTIC TECHNIQUE

Do not assemble until ready to use.

1. Remove caps from diluent barrel and injector.

2. Insert diluent barrel into injector. Rotate diluent barrel clockwise (approximately three turns) until barrel is securely attached to injector.

3. Remove protective luer adapter covers from both injector/barrel assembly and Thiopental Sodium drug vial. With drug vial on flat surface, attach luer adapter of injector/barrel assembly to luer connector of Thiopental Sodium drug vial.

4. Firmly press luer connection together until connector of drug vial is depressed into neck of drug vial.

5. With drug vial still on flat surface, slowly push down on injector until diluent is transferred into drug vial. Shake syringe assembly, if necessary, to aid Thiopental Sodium reconstitution.

6. To transfer reconstitution solution back into syringe assembly, invert syringe assembly, with injector fully depressed, so that drug vial is on top. Release pressure on injector to allow solution to fill syringe barrel.

7. To remove empty drug vial, grasp neck of drug vial and exert twisting motion to separate connection from syringe. Adhere additive label. Replace luer cover on syringe until ready for use.

DILUENTS IN THIOPENTAL SODIUM KITS

READY-TO-MIX SYRINGES AND VIALS

(For preparing solutions of Thiopental Sodium for Injection, USP)

DESCRIPTION

The following diluents in various container, syringe and vial sizes are provided in Thiopental Sodium Kits, Thiopental Sodium Ready-to-Mix Syringes and Vials for preparing solutions of Thiopental Sodium for clinical use:

Sterile Water for Injection, USP is a sterile, nonpyrogenic preparation of water for injection which contains no bacteriostat, antimicrobial agents or added buffers. The pH is 5.7 (5.0 to 7.0).

Sterile Water for Injection, USP is a pharmaceutic aid (solvent) for intravenous administration only after addition of a solute.

Water is chemically designated H_2O.

0.9% Sodium Chloride Injection, USP is a sterile, nonpyrogenic, isotonic solution of sodium chloride and water for injection. Each mL contains sodium chloride 9 mg (308 mOsmol/liter calc). It contains no bacteriostat, antimicrobial agents or added buffers except for pH adjustment. May contain hydrochloric acid and/or sodium hydroxide for pH adjustment. pH is 5.7 (4.5 to 7.0).

0.9% Sodium Chloride Injection, USP is an isotonic vehicle for intravenous administration of another solute.

Sodium chloride is chemically designated NaCl, a white crystalline compound freely soluble in water.

The semi-rigid vial is fabricated from a specially formulated polyolefin. It is a copolymer of ethylene and propylene. The safety of the plastic has been confirmed by tests in animals according to USP biological standards for plastic containers. The container requires no vapor barrier to maintain the proper labeled volume.

CLINICAL PHARMACOLOGY

Sterile Water for Injection, USP serves only as a pharmaceutic aid for diluting or dissolving drugs prior to administration.

Water is an essential constituent of all body tissues and accounts for approximately 70% of total body weight. Average normal adult daily requirement ranges from two to three liters (1.0 to 1.5 liters each for insensible water loss by perspiration and urine excretion).

Water balance is maintained by various regulatory mechanisms. Water distribution depends primarily on the concentration of dissociated electrolytes in the body comparments and sodium (Na+) plays a major role in maintaining a physiologic equilibrium between fluid intake and output.

0.9% Sodium Chloride Injection, USP serves only as an isotonic vehicle for drugs prior to administration.

Sodium chloride in water is an electrolyte solution of sodium (Na+) and chloride (Cl⁻) ions. These ions are normal constituents of the body fluids (principally extracellular) and are essential for maintaining electrolyte balance.

The distribution and excretion of sodium (Na+) and chloride (Cl⁻) are largely under the control of the kidney which maintains a balance between intake and output of these ions.

The small volumes of fluid and amounts of sodium chloride provided by 0.9% Sodium Chloride Injection in Ready-to-Mix Syringes are unlikely to produce a significant effect on fluid or electrolyte balance.

INDICATIONS AND USAGE

These products are indicated only for preparing Thiopental Sodium solutions for clinical use.

CONTRAINDICATIONS

Do not use unless the diluent is clear and the bottle or vial seal or syringe package is undamaged.

Diluents in Thiopental Sodium Kits, Ready-to-Mix Syringes or Vials should not be used for fluid or sodium chloride replacement.

WARNINGS

Intravenous administration of Sterile Water for Injection, USP without a solute may result in hemolysis.

Use aseptic technique for preparing Thiopental Sodium solutions when using Thiopental Sodium Kits, Syringes or Vials and during withdrawal from reconstituted single or multiple-use containers.

Administer only clear reconstituted solutions.

Use within 24 hours after reconstitution. Discard unused portions.

PRECAUTIONS

Do not use unless solution is clear and container is undamaged.

Inspect reconstituted (mixed) solutions of Thiopental Sodium for clarity and freedom from precipitation or discoloration prior to administration. Use reconstituted solution only if it is clear, free from precipitate and not discolored.

Use Transfer Label in each Thiopental Sodium Kit and affix to container of reconstituted solution to show concentration and time of preparation.

Pregnancy Category C: Animal reproduction studies have not been conducted with sterile water for injection or sodium chloride injection. It is also not known whether sterile water or sodium chloride injection containing additives can cause fetal harm when administered to a pregnant woman or can affect reproduction capacity. Sterile water for injection or sodium chloride injection with additives should be given to a pregnant woman only if clearly needed.

ADVERSE REACTIONS

Reactions which may occur because of the diluents, technique of preparation or mixing, or administration of reconstituted solutions of Thiopental Sodium

---

include febrile response or infection at the site of injection, venous thrombosis or phlebitis extending from the site of injection and extravasation.

If an adverse reaction does occur, discontinue the injection, evaluate the patient, institute appropriate therapeutic countermeasures and save the remainder of unused solution (or the used container or syringe) for examination if deemed necessary.

DRUG ABUSE AND DEPENDENCE
None known.

OVERDOSAGE
Used as diluents for preparing solutions of Thiopental Sodium the small volumes of administered fluid (from Sterile Water for Injection in bottles and vials) and amounts of sodium chloride (from 0.9% Sodium Chloride Injection in Ready-to-Mix Syringes) are unlikely to pose a threat of fluid or sodium chloride overload.

DOSAGE AND ADMINISTRATION
Thiopental Sodium solutions should be administered only by intravenous injection and by individuals experienced in the conduct of intravenous anesthesia.

The volume and choice of diluent for preparing Thiopental Sodium solutions for clinical use depends on the concentration and vehicle desired. Thiopental Sodium Kits provide only Sterile Water for Injection as the diluent for individual or multi-patient use; Thiopental Sodium Ready-to-Mix Syringes provide only 0.9% Sodium Chloride Injection, USP as the diluent for individual patient use; vials provide only Sterile Water for Injection, USP as the diluent for individual patient use.

Parenteral drug products should be inspected visually for particulate matter and discoloration prior to administration, whenever solution and container permit. See *"Precautions"*.

Table (See related table).

STORAGE
Store at controlled room temperature, 15° to 30°C (59° to 86°F). Keep reconstituted solution in a cool place.

J CODES
IV—J2520

HOW SUPPLIED
INJECTION (C-III): 1 GM

BRAND/MANUFACTURER	NDC	SIZE	AWP
○ BRAND			
PENTOTHAL: Abbott Hosp	00074-6435-01	1 ml 25s	$397.22

POWDER FOR INJECTION (C-III): 2.5 MG

BRAND/MANUFACTURER	NDC	SIZE	AWP
○ GENERICS			
Gensia	00703-2540-01	1s	$23.13

POWDER FOR INJECTION (C-III): 250 MG

BRAND/MANUFACTURER	NDC	SIZE	AWP
○ BRAND			
PENTOTHAL: Abbott Hosp	00074-6418-01	25s	$213.16
	00074-6241-03	25s	$217.61
	00074-3351-01	25s	$234.83

POWDER FOR INJECTION (C-III): 400 MG

BRAND/MANUFACTURER	NDC	SIZE	AWP
○ BRAND			
PENTOTHAL: Abbott Hosp	00074-6419-01	25s	$264.22
	00074-6246-03	25s	$268.67
	00074-3352-01	25s	$285.89

POWDER FOR INJECTION (C-III): 500 MG

BRAND/MANUFACTURER	NDC	SIZE	AWP
○ BRAND			
PENTOTHAL: Abbott Hosp	00074-3329-01	25s	$230.08
	00074-6420-01	25s	$295.39
	00074-6243-01	25s	$302.81
	00074-3353-01	25s	$319.73
○ GENERICS			
Gensia	00703-2580-01	1s	$8.44

POWDER FOR INJECTION (C-III): 1 GM

BRAND/MANUFACTURER	NDC	SIZE	AWP
○ GENERICS			
Gensia	00703-2530-01	1s	$17.75

POWDER FOR INJECTION (C-III): 1 GM (2.5%)

BRAND/MANUFACTURER	NDC	SIZE	AWP
○ BRAND			
PENTOTHAL: Abbott Hosp	00074-6244-01	25s	$396.33

POWDER FOR INJECTION (C-III): 2.5 GM (2%)

BRAND/MANUFACTURER	NDC	SIZE	AWP
○ BRAND			
PENTOTHAL: Abbott Hosp	00074-6259-01	25s	$878.16

POWDER FOR INJECTION (C-III): 2.5 GM (2.5%)

BRAND/MANUFACTURER	NDC	SIZE	AWP
○ BRAND			
PENTOTHAL: Abbott Hosp	00074-6260-01	25s	$854.70

POWDER FOR INJECTION (C-III): 5 GM

BRAND/MANUFACTURER	NDC	SIZE	AWP
○ GENERICS			
Gensia	00703-2550-01	1s	$34.75

POWDER FOR INJECTION (C-III): 5 GM (2%)

BRAND/MANUFACTURER	NDC	SIZE	AWP
○ BRAND			
PENTOTHAL: Abbott Hosp	00074-6108-01	25s	$1356.13

POWDER FOR INJECTION (C-III): 5 GM (2.5%)

BRAND/MANUFACTURER	NDC	SIZE	AWP
○ BRAND			
PENTOTHAL: Abbott Hosp	00074-6504-01	25s	$1343.36

THIOPENTAL SODIUM AND DILUENT IN KITS AND READY-TO-MIX SYRINGES

	Thiopental Sodium	Thiopental Sodium Container	Diluent (mL)*	Diluent Container	Theoretical Reconstituted Conc.
Kit	2.5 g	Squeeze Bottle	W (125)	PF Bottle	2% (20 mg/mL)
Kit	5 g	Squeeze Bottle	W (250)	PF Bottle	2% (20 mg/mL)
Kit	1 g	Squeeze Bottle	W (40)	PF Bottle	2.5% (25 mg/mL)
Kit	2.5 g	Squeeze Bottle	W (100)	PF Bottle	2.5% (25 mg/mL)
Kit	5 g	Squeeze Bottle	W (200)	Bottle	2.5% (25 mg/mL)
Kit	1 g	Vial	W (50)	Plastic Vial	2% (20 mg/mL)
Kit	500 mg	Vial	W (20)	Plastic Vial	2.5% (25 mg/mL)
Ready-to-Mix-Syringe	400 mg	Syringe	S (20)	Syringe	2% (20 mg/mL)
Ready-to-Mix Syringe	250 mg	Syringe	S (10)	Syringe	2.5% (25 mg/mL)
Ready-to-Mix Syringe	500 mg	Syringe	S (20)	Syringe	2.5% (25 mg/mL)
Ready-to-Mix Syringe	250 mg	Syringe	S (10)	Plastic Vial	2.5% (25 mg/mL)
Ready-to-Mix Syringe	400 mg	Syringe	S (20)	Plastic Vial	2% (20 mg/mL)
Ready-to-Mix Syringe	500 mg	Syringe	S (20)	Plastic Vial	2.5% (25 mg/mL)
Ready-to-Mix Syringe	250 mg	Syringe	W (10)	Plastic Vial	2.5% (25 mg/mL)
Ready-to-Mix Syringe	400 mg	Syringe	W (20)	Plastic Vial	2% (20 mg/mL)
Ready-to-Mix Syringe	500 mg	Syringe	W (20)	Plastic Vial	2.5% (25 mg/mL)

PF — Denotes partial-fill
W — Denotes Sterile Water for Injection, USP
S — Denotes 0.9% Sodium Chloride Injection, USP

SUSPENSION (C-III): 2 GM

BRAND/MANUFACTURER	NDC	SIZE	AWP
○ **BRAND**			
PENTOTHAL: Abbott Hosp	00074-7236-04	1 ml	$34.26

Thioridazine Hydrochloride

DESCRIPTION
Thioridazine Hydrochloride is 2-methylmercapto-10-[2-(N-methyl-2-piperidyl) ethyl] phenothiazine.

The presence of a thiomethyl radical (S-CH$_3$) in position 2, conventionally occupied by a halogen, is unique and could account for the greater toleration obtained with recommended doses of Thioridazine Hydrochloride as well as a greater specificity of psychotherapeutic action.

Thioridazine Hydrochloride is available in 10 mg, 15 mg, 25 mg, 50 mg, 100 mg, 150 mg, and 200 mg Tablets.

Following is its chemical structure:

CLINICAL PHARMACOLOGY
Thioridazine Hydrochloride is effective in reducing excitement, hypermotility, abnormal initiative, affective tension, and agitation through its inhibitory effect on psychomotor functions. Successful modification of such symptoms is the prerequisite for, and often the beginning of, the process of recovery in patients exhibiting mental and emotional disturbances.

Thioridazine Hydrochloride's basic pharmacological activity is similar to that of other phenothiazines, but certain specific qualities have come to light which support the observation that the clinical spectrum of this drug shows significant differences from those of the other agents of this class. Minimal antiemetic activity and minimal extrapyramidal stimulation, notably pseudoparkinsonism, are distinctive features of this drug.

INDICATIONS
For the management of manifestations of psychotic disorders.

For the short-term treatment of moderate to marked depression with variable degrees of anxiety in adult patients and for the treatment of multiple symptoms such as agitation, anxiety, depressed mood, tension, sleep disturbances, and fears in geriatric patients.

For the treatment of severe behavioral problems in children marked by combativeness and/or explosive hyperexcitable behavior (out of proportion to immediate provocations), and in the short-term treatment of hyperactive children who show excessive motor activity with accompanying conduct disorders consisting of some or all of the following symptoms: impulsivity, difficulty sustaining attention, aggressivity, mood lability, and poor frustration tolerances.

UNLABELED USES
Thioridazine is used alone or as an adjunct in the treatment of sexual disorders, including inhibition of nocturnal emissions and to control premature ejaculation. It is also used for the symptomatic relief of acute alcohol withdrawal.

CONTRAINDICATIONS
In common with other phenothiazines, Thioridazine Hydrochloride is contraindicated in severe central nervous system depression or comatose states from any cause. It should also be noted that hypertensive or hypotensive heart disease of extreme degree is a contraindication of phenothiazine administration.

WARNINGS
TARDIVE DYSKINESIA
Tardive dyskinesia, a syndrome consisting of potentially irreversible, involuntary, dyskinetic movements may develop in patients treated with neuroleptic (antipsychotic) drugs. Although the prevalence of the syndrome appears to be highest among the elderly, especially elderly women, it is impossible to rely upon prevalence estimates to predict, at the inception of neuroleptic treatment, which patients are likely to develop the syndrome. Whether neuroleptic drug products differ in their potential to cause tardive dyskinesia is unknown.

Both the risk of developing the syndrome and the likelihood that it will become irreversible are believed to increase as the duration of treatment and the total cumulative dose of neuroleptic drugs administered to the patient increase. However, the syndrome can develop, although much less commonly, after relatively brief treatment periods at low doses. There is no known treatment for established cases of tardive dyskinesia, although the syndrome may remit, partially or completely, if neuroleptic treatment is withdrawn. Neuroleptic treatment itself, however, may suppress (or partially suppress) the signs and symptoms of the syndrome and thereby may possibly mask the underlying disease process. The effect that symptomatic suppression has upon the long-term course of the syndrome is unknown.

Given these considerations, neuroleptics should be prescribed in a manner that is most likely to minimize the occurrence of tardive dyskinesia. Chronic neuroleptic treatment should generally be reserved for patients who suffer from a chronic illness that, 1) is known to respond to neuroleptic drugs, and, 2) for whom alternative, equally effective, but potentially less harmful treatments are *not* available or appropriate. In patients who do require chronic treatment, the smallest dose and the shortest duration of treatment producing a satisfactory clinical response should be sought. The need for continued treatment should be reassessed periodically.

If signs and symptoms of tardive dyskinesia appear in a patient on neuroleptics, drug discontinuation should be considered. However, some patients may require treatment despite the presence of the syndrome.

(For further information about the description of tardive dyskinesia and its clinical detection, please refer to the sections on "Information for Patients" and "Adverse Reactions".)

It has been suggested in regard to phenothiazines in general, that people who have demonstrated a hypersensitivity reaction (e.g. blood dyscrasias, jaundice) to one may be more prone to demonstrate a reaction to others. Attention should be paid to the fact that phenothiazines are capable of potentiating central nervous system depressants (e.g. anesthetics, opiates, alcohol, etc.) as well as atropine and phosphorus insecticides. Physicians should carefully consider benefit versus risk when treating less severe disorders.

Reproductive studies in animals and clinical experience to date have failed to show a teratogenic effect with Thioridazine Hydrochloride. However, in view of the desirability of keeping the administration of all drugs to a minimum during pregnancy, Thioridazine Hydrochloride should be given only when the benefits derived from treatment exceed the possible risks to mother and fetus.

NEUROLEPTIC MALIGNANT SYNDROME (NMS)
A potentially fatal symptom complex sometimes referred to as Neuroleptic Malignant Syndrome (NMS) has been reported in association with antipsychotic drugs. Clinical manifestations of NMS are hyperpyrexia, muscle rigidity, altered mental status, and evidence of autonomic instability (irregular pulse or blood pressure, tachycardia, diaphoresis, and cardiac dysrhythmias).

The diagnostic evaluation of patients with this syndrome is complicated. In arriving at a diagnosis, it is important to identify cases where the clinical presentation includes both serious medical illness (e.g. pneumonia, systemic infection, etc.) and untreated or inadequately treated extrapyramidal signs and symptoms (EPS). Other important considerations in the differential diagnosis include central anticholinergic toxicity, heat stroke, drug fever, and primary central nervous system (CNS) pathology.

The management of NMS should include, 1) immediate discontinuation of antipsychotic drugs and other drugs not essential to concurrent therapy, 2) intensive symptomatic treatment and medical monitoring, and 3) treatment of any concomitant serious medical problems for which specific treatments are available. There is no general agreement about specific pharmacological treatment regimens for uncomplicated NMS.

If a patient requires antipsychotic drug treatment after recovery from NMS, the potential reintroduction of drug therapy should be carefully considered. The patient should be carefully monitored, since recurrences of NMS have been reported.

PRECAUTIONS
Leukopenia and/or agranulocytosis and convulsive seizures have been reported but are infrequent. Thioridazine Hydrochloride has been shown to be helpful in the treatment of behavioral disorders in epileptic patients, but anticonvulsant medication should also be maintained. Pigmentary retinopathy, which has been observed primarily in patients taking larger than recommended doses, is characterized by diminution of visual acuity, brownish coloring of vision, and impairment of night vision; examination of the fundus discloses deposits of pigment. The possibility of this complication may be reduced by remaining within the recommended limits of dosage.

Where patients are participating in activities requiring complete mental alertness (e.g. driving) it is advisable to administer the phenothiazines cautiously and to increase the dosage gradually. Female patients appear to have a greater tendency to orthostatic hypotension than male patients. The administration of epinephrine should be avoided in the treatment of drug-induced hypotension in view of the fact that phenothiazines may induce a reversed epinephrine effect on occasion. Should a vasoconstrictor be required, the most suitable are levarterenol and phenylephrine.

Neuroleptic drugs elevate prolactin levels; the elevation persists during chronic administration. Tissue culture experiments indicate that approximately one-third of human breast cancers are prolactin dependent *in vitro,* a factor of potential importance if the prescription of these drugs is contemplated in a patient with a previously detected breast cancer. Although disturbances such as galactorrhea, amenorrhea, gynecomastia, and impotence have been reported, the clinical significance of elevated serum prolactin levels is unknown for most patients. An increase in mammary neoplasms has been found in rodents after chronic administration of neuroleptic drugs. Neither clinical studies nor epidemiologic studies conducted to date, however, have shown an association between chronic administration of these drugs and mammary tumorigenesis; the available evidence is considered too limited to be conclusive at this time.

Concurrent administration of propranolol (100-800 mg daily) has been reported to produce increases in plasma levels of thioridazine (approximately 50%-400%) and its metabolites (approximately 80%-300%).

Pindolol: Concurrent administration of pindolol and Thioridazine have resulted in moderate, dose-related increases in the serum levels of Thioridazine and two of its metabolites, as well as higher than expected serum pindolol levels.

◆ RATED THERAPEUTICALLY EQUIVALENT; ◇ THERAPEUTIC EQUIVALENCE UNCONFIRMED; ○ UNRATED

It is recommended that a daily dose in excess of 300 mg be reserved for use only in severe neuropsychiatric conditions.

Information for Patients: Given the likelihood that some patients exposed chronically to neuroleptics will develop tardive dyskinesia, it is advised that all patients in whom chronic use is contemplated be given, if possible, full information about this risk. The decision to inform patients and/or their guardians must obviously take into account the clinical circumstances and the competency of the patient to understand the information provided.

ADVERSE REACTIONS

In the recommended dosage ranges with Thioridazine Hydrochloride, most side effects are mild and transient.

Central Nervous System: Drowsiness may be encountered on occasion, especially where large doses are given early in treatment. Generally, this effect tends to subside with continued therapy or a reduction in dosage. Pseudoparkinsonism and other extrapyramidal symptoms may occur but are infrequent. Nocturnal confusion, hyperactivity, lethargy, psychotic reactions, restlessness, and headache have been reported but are extremely rare.

Autonomic Nervous System: Dryness of mouth, blurred vision, constipation, nausea, vomiting, diarrhea, nasal stuffiness, and pallor have been seen.

Endocrine System: Galactorrhea, breast engorgement, amenorrhea, inhibition of ejaculation, and peripheral edema have been described.

Skin: Dermatitis and skin eruptions of the urticarial type have been observed infrequently. Photosensitivity is extremely rare.

Cardiovascular System: ECG changes have been reported. (see *"Phenothiazine Derivatives: Cardiovascular Effects"*).

Other: Rare cases described as parotid swelling have been reported following administration of Thioridazine Hydrochloride.

POST INTRODUCTION REPORTS

These are voluntary reports of adverse events temporally associated with Thioridazine Hydrochloride that were received since marketing, and there may be no causal relationship between Thioridazine Hydrochloride use and these events; priapism.

PHENOTHIAZINE DERIVATIVES

It should be noted that efficacy, indications, and untoward effects have varied with the different phenothiazines. It has been reported that old age lowers the tolerance for phenothiazines. The most common neurological side effects in these patients are parkinsonism and akathisia. There appears to be an increased risk of agranulocytosis and leukopenia in the geriatric population. The physician should be aware that the following have occurred with one or more phenothiazines and should be considered whenever one of these drugs is used:

Autonomic Reactions: Miosis, obstipation, anorexia, paralytic ileus.

Cutaneous Reactions: Erythema, exfoliative dermatitis, contact dermatitis.

Blood Dyscrasias: Agranulocytosis, leukopenia, eosinophilia, thrombocytopenia, anemia, aplastic anemia, pancytopenia.

Allergic Reactions: Fever, laryngeal edema, angioneurotic edema, asthma.

Hepatotoxicity: Jaundice, biliary stasis.

Cardiovascular Effects: Changes in the terminal portion of the electrocardiogram, including prolongation of the Q-T interval, lowering and inversion of the T-wave, and appearance of a wave tentatively identified as a bifid T or a U wave have been observed in some patients receiving the phenothiazine tranquilizers, including Thioridazine Hydrochloride. To date, these appear to be due to altered repolarization and not related to myocardial damage. They appear to be reversible.

While there is no evidence at present that these changes are in any way precursors of any significant disturbance of cardiac rhythm, it should be noted that several sudden and unexpected deaths apparently due to cardiac arrest have occurred in patients previously showing characteristic electrocardiographic changes while taking the drug. The use of periodic electrocardiograms has been proposed but would appear to be of questionable value as a predictive device. Hypotension, rarely resulting in cardiac arrest.

Extrapyramidal Symptoms: Akathisia, agitation, motor restlessness, dystonic reactions, trismus, torticollis, opisthotonus, oculogyric crises, tremor, muscular rigidity, akinesia.

Tardive Dyskinesia: Chronic use of neuroleptics may be associated with the development of tardive dyskinesia. The salient features of this syndrome are described in the *"Warnings"* section and subsequently.

The syndrome is characterized by involuntary choreoathetoid movements which variously involve the tongue, face, mouth, lips or jaw (e.g. protrusion of the tongue, puffing of cheeks, puckering of the mouth, chewing movements), trunk, and extremities. The severity of the syndrome and the degree of impairment produced vary widely.

The syndrome may become clinically recognizable either during treatment, upon dosage reduction, or upon withdrawal of treatment. Movements may decrease in intensity and may disappear altogether if further treatment with neuroleptics is withheld. It is generally believed that reversibility is more likely after short rather than long-term neuroleptic exposure. Consequently, early detection of tardive dyskinesia is important. To increase the likelihood of detecting the syndrome at the earliest possible time, the dosage of neuroleptic

drug should be reduced periodically (if clinically possible) and the patient observed for signs of the disorder. This maneuver is critical, for neuroleptic drugs may mask the signs of the syndrome.

Neuroleptic Malignant Syndrome (NMS): Chronic use of neuroleptics may be associated with the development of Neuroleptic Malignant Syndrome. The salient features of this syndrome are described in the *"Warnings"* section and subsequently. Clinical manifestations of NMS are hyperpyrexia, muscle rigidity, altered mental status, and evidence of autonomic instability (irregular pulse or blood pressure, tachycardia, diaphoresis, and cardiac dysrhythmias).

Endocrine Disturbances: Menstrual irregularities, altered libido, gynecomastia, lactation, weight gain, edema. False positive pregnancy tests have been reported.

Urinary Disturbances: Retention, incontinence.

Others: Hyperpyrexia. Behavioral effects suggestive of a paradoxical reaction have been reported. These include excitement, bizarre dreams, aggravation of psychoses, and toxic confusional states. More recently, a peculiar skin-eye syndrome has been recognized as a side effect following long-term treatment with phenothiazines. This reaction is marked by progressive pigmentation of areas of the skin or conjunctiva and/or accompanied by discoloration of the exposed sclera and cornea. Opacities of the anterior lens and cornea described as irregular or stellate in shape have also been reported. Systemic lupus erythematosus-like syndrome.

DOSAGE

Dosage must be individualized according to the degree of mental and emotional disturbance. In all cases, the smallest effective dosage should be determined for each patient.

ADULTS

Psychotic Manifestations: The usual starting dose is 50-100 mg three times a day, with a gradual increment to a maximum of 800 mg daily if necessary. Once effective control of symptoms has been achieved, the dosage may be reduced gradually to determine the minimum maintenance dose. The total daily dosage ranges from 200-800 mg, divided into two to four doses.

For the short-term treatment of moderate to marked depression with variable degrees of anxiety in adult patients and for the treatment of multiple symptoms such as agitation, anxiety, depressed mood, tension, sleep disturbances, and fears in geriatric patients: The usual starting dose is 25 mg three times a day. Dosage ranges from 10 mg two to four times a day in milder cases to 50 mg three or four times a day for more severely disturbed patients. The total daily dosage range is from 20 mg to a maximum of 200 mg.

CHILDREN

Thioridazine Hydrochloride is not intended for children under 2 years of age. For children aged 2-12 the dosage of Thioridazine Hydrochloride ranges from 0.5 mg to a maximum of 3.0 mg/kg/day. For children with moderate disorders, 10 mg two or three times a day is the usual starting dose. For hospitalized, severely disturbed, or psychotic children, 25 mg two or three times daily is the usual starting dose. Dosage may be increased gradually until optimum therapeutic effect is obtained or the maximum has been reached.

STORAGE

Tablets: Below 86°F (30°C); tight container.

Concentrate: Below 86°F (30°C): tight, amber glass bottle.

The concentrate may be diluted with distilled water, acidified tap water, or suitable juices. Each dose should be so diluted just prior to administration — preparation and storage of bulk dilutions is not recommended.

Oral Suspension: Below 77°F (25°C); tight, amber glass bottle.

HOW SUPPLIED
CONCENTRATE: 30 MG/ML

AVERAGE UNIT PRICE (AVAILABLE SIZES)		GENERIC A-RATED AVERAGE PRICE (GAAP)	
BRAND	$0.26	120 ml	$15.79
GENERIC	$0.13	120 ml	$13.00
HCFA FUL (120 ml)	$0.11		

BRAND/MANUFACTURER	NDC	SIZE	AWP
◆ **BRAND**			
MELLARIL: Sandoz Pharm	00078-0001-31	120 ml	$30.78
◆ **GENERICS**			
Copley	38245-0608-14	120 ml	$11.23
Moore,H.L.	00839-7056-65	120 ml	$13.76
Roxane	00054-3860-50	120 ml	$14.76
Qualitest	00603-1756-54	120 ml	$15.24
Geneva	00781-6150-04	120 ml	$15.85
Schein	00364-2119-77	120 ml	$16.75
Rugby	00536-2200-97	120 ml	$17.33

➤ SHOWN IN PRODUCT IDENTIFICATION GUIDE

CONCENTRATE: 100 MG/ML

AVERAGE UNIT PRICE (AVAILABLE SIZES)		GENERIC A-RATED AVERAGE PRICE (GAAP)	
BRAND	$0.67	120 ml	$39.35
GENERIC	$0.29		
HCFA FUL (120 ml)	$0.45		

BRAND/MANUFACTURER	NDC	SIZE	AWP
◆ BRAND			
MELLARIL: Sandoz Pharm	00078-0009-31	120 ml	$80.40
◆ GENERICS			
Copley	38245-0609-14	120 ml	$25.77
Roxane	00054-3861-50	120 ml	$35.64
Barre	00472-1451-94	120 ml	$43.05

SUSPENSION: 25 MG/5 ML

BRAND/MANUFACTURER	NDC	SIZE	AWP
◆ BRAND			
MELLARIL-S: Sandoz Pharm	00078-0068-33	480 ml	$48.42

SUSPENSION: 100 MG/5 ML

BRAND/MANUFACTURER	NDC	SIZE	AWP
◆ BRAND			
MELLARIL-S: Sandoz Pharm	00078-0069-33	480 ml	$99.60

TABLET: 10 MG

AVERAGE UNIT PRICE (AVAILABLE SIZES)		GENERIC A-RATED AVERAGE PRICE (GAAP)	
BRAND	$0.29	100s	$12.36
GENERIC	$0.11	1000s	$79.90
HCFA FUL (100s ea)	$0.04		

BRAND/MANUFACTURER	NDC	SIZE	AWP
◆ BRAND			
➤ MELLARIL: Sandoz Pharm	00078-0002-05	100s	$28.50
	00078-0002-06	100s ud	$30.60
	00078-0002-09	1000s	$274.20
◆ GENERICS			
Medirex	57480-0362-06	30s	$5.81
Goldline	00182-1578-01	100s	$5.25
Aligen	00405-4993-01	100s	$5.56
Qualitest	00603-5992-21	100s	$5.90
Rugby	00536-4641-01	100s	$6.68
Parmed	00349-8268-01	100s	$6.96
Major	00904-1614-60	100s	$8.20
Moore,H.L.	00839-6703-06	100s	$8.49
Mutual	53489-0148-01	100s	$8.70
URL	00677-0823-01	100s	$8.90
Geneva	00781-1604-01	100s	$8.95
Schein	00364-2317-01	100s	$9.00
Mylan	00378-0612-01	100s	$9.01
Creighton	50752-0264-05	100s	$22.85
Raway	00686-0565-20	100s ud	$8.75
Vangard	00615-2504-13	100s ud	$17.00
U.S. Trading	56126-0096-11	100s ud	$17.36
UDL	51079-0565-20	100s ud	$17.89
Geneva	00781-1604-13	100s ud	$18.50
Creighton	50752-0264-06	100s ud	$24.53
Medirex	57480-0362-01	100s ud	$28.80
Parmed	00349-8268-10	1000s	$52.95
Rugby	00536-4641-10	1000s	$54.50
Major	00904-1614-80	1000s	$54.50
Goldline	00182-1578-10	1000s	$54.55
Moore,H.L.	00839-6703-16	1000s	$72.23
URL	00677-0823-10	1000s	$72.90
Aligen	00405-4993-03	1000s	$72.90
Mutual	53489-0148-10	1000s	$72.90
Schein	00364-2317-02	1000s	$76.66
Mylan	00378-0612-10	1000s	$76.75
Geneva	00781-1604-10	1000s	$77.87
Creighton	50752-0264-09	1000s	$220.07

TABLET: 15 MG

AVERAGE UNIT PRICE (AVAILABLE SIZES)		GENERIC A-RATED AVERAGE PRICE (GAAP)	
BRAND	$0.34	100s	$15.36
GENERIC	$0.14		
HCFA FUL (100s ea)	$0.05		

BRAND/MANUFACTURER	NDC	SIZE	AWP
◆ BRAND			
➤ MELLARIL: Sandoz Pharm	00078-0008-05	100s	$33.60
◆ GENERICS			
Schein	00364-0669-01	100s	$10.00
Geneva	00781-1614-01	100s	$12.95
Aligen	00405-4994-01	100s	$15.80
Creighton	50752-0265-05	100s	$26.93
U.S. Trading	56126-0097-11	100s ud	$4.97
Geneva	00781-1614-13	100s ud	$21.50
Major	00904-1801-80	1000s	$57.75

TABLET: 25 MG

AVERAGE UNIT PRICE (AVAILABLE SIZES)		GENERIC A-RATED AVERAGE PRICE (GAAP)	
BRAND	$0.40	100s	$17.00
GENERIC	$0.15	1000s	$111.20
HCFA FUL (100s ea)	$0.05		

BRAND/MANUFACTURER	NDC	SIZE	AWP
◆ BRAND			
➤ MELLARIL: Sandoz Pharm	00078-0003-05	100s	$40.08
	00078-0003-06	100s ud	$42.54
	00078-0003-09	1000s	$385.50
◆ GENERICS			
Medirex	57480-0363-06	30s	$7.76
Qualitest	00603-5993-21	100s	$8.91
Rugby	00536-4642-01	100s	$8.95
Goldline	00182-1579-01	100s	$9.00
Schein	00364-0662-01	100s	$10.75
Major	00904-1616-60	100s	$11.60
URL	00677-0824-01	100s	$13.50
Aligen	00405-4995-01	100s	$13.50
Geneva	00781-1624-01	100s	$13.50
Mutual	53489-0149-01	100s	$13.50
Moore,H.L.	00839-6704-06	100s	$13.57
➤ Mylan	00378-0614-01	100s	$13.65
Parmed	00349-8269-01	100s	$13.75
Creighton	50752-0266-05	100s	$32.13
U.S. Trading	56126-0098-11	100s ud	$5.54
Raway	00686-0566-20	100s ud	$11.35
Major	00904-1795-61	100s ud	$16.91
Major	00904-1802-61	100s ud	$16.91
Vangard	00615-2506-13	100s ud	$23.33
Geneva	00781-1624-13	100s ud	$24.00
UDL	51079-0566-20	100s ud	$25.34
Creighton	50752-0266-06	100s ud	$34.12
Medirex	57480-0363-01	100s ud	$40.10
Goldline	00182-1579-10	1000s	$63.75
Major	00904-1616-80	1000s	$82.50
Qualitest	00603-5993-32	1000s	$86.51
Rugby	00536-4642-10	1000s	$87.90
Schein	00364-0662-02	1000s	$87.90
Parmed	00349-8269-10	1000s	$93.73
URL	00677-0824-10	1000s	$105.25
Aligen	00405-4995-03	1000s	$105.25
Mutual	53489-0149-10	1000s	$105.25
Geneva	00781-1624-10	1000s	$105.45
Moore,H.L.	00839-6704-16	1000s	$105.71
➤ Mylan	00378-0614-10	1000s	$106.95
Creighton	50752-0266-09	1000s	$309.42

For additional alternatives, turn to the section beginning on page 2859.

Thiosulfil Forte *SEE* SULFAMETHIZOLE

Thiotepa

THIOTEPA is a polyfunctional alkylating agent used in the chemotherapy of certain neoplastic diseases.

DESCRIPTION

Thiotepa is an ethylenimine-type compound, 1,1',1''-phosphinothioylidynetris-aziridine available in powder form in vials which contain a sterile mixture of 15 mg Thiotepa. Thiotepa has also been known as TESPA and TSPA and is not the same as TEPA. Thiotepa is stable in alkaline medium and unstable in acid medium. When reconstituted with Sterile Water for Injection, the resulting solution has a pH of approximately 7.6.

Following is its chemical structure:

ACTION

Thiotepa is a cytotoxic agent of the polyfunctional alkylating type (more than one reactive ethylenimine group) related chemically and pharmacologically to nitrogen mustard. Its radiomimetic action is believed to occur through the release of ethylenimine radicals which, like irradiation, disrupt the bonds of DNA. One of the principal bond disruptions is initiated by alkylation of guanine at the N-7 position, which severs the linkage between the purine base and the sugar and liberates alkylated guanines.

On the basis of tissue concentration studies, it is reported that Thiotepa has no differential affinity for neoplasms. Most of the drug appears to be excreted unchanged in the urine.

◆ RATED THERAPEUTICALLY EQUIVALENT; ◇ THERAPEUTIC EQUIVALENCE UNCONFIRMED; ○ UNRATED

INDICATIONS

Thiotepa has been tried with varying results in the palliation of a wide variety of neoplastic diseases. However, the most consistent results have been seen in the following tumors:

1. Adenocarcinoma of the breast.
2. Adenocarcinoma of the ovary.
3. For controlling intracavitary effusions secondary to diffuse or localized neoplastic diseases of various serosal cavities.

For the treatment of superficial papillary carcinoma of the urinary bladder.

While now largely superseded by other treatments, Thiotepa has been effective against other lymphomas, such as lymphosarcoma and Hodgkin's disease.

UNLABELED USES

Thiotepa is also used alone or as an adjunct in the treatment of Hodgkin's disease and pterygium.

CONTRAINDICATIONS

Therapy is probably contraindicated in cases of existing hepatic, renal, or bone marrow damage. However, if the need outweighs the risk in such patients, Thiotepa may be used in low dosage, and accompanied by hepatic, renal, and hemopoietic function tests.

Thiotepa is contraindicated in patients with a known hypersensitivity (allergy) to this preparation.

WARNINGS

The administration of Thiotepa to pregnant women is not recommended except in cases where the benefit to be gained outweights the risk of teratogenicity involved.

Thiotepa is highly toxic to the hematopoietic system. A rapidly falling white blood cell or platelet count indicates the necessity for discontinuing or reducing the dosage of Thiotepa. Weekly blood and platelet counts are recommended during therapy and for at least 3 weeks after therapy has been discontinued.

Thiotepa is a polyfunctional alkylating agent, capable of cross-linking the DNA within a cell and changing its nature. The replication of the cell is, therefore, altered, and Thiotepa may be described as mutagenic. An in vitro study has shown that it causes chromosomal aberrations of the chromatid type and that the frequency of induced aberrations increases with the age of the subject.

Like all alkylating agents, Thiotepa is carcinogenic. Carcinogenicity is shown most clearly in mouse studies, but there is strong circumstantial evidence of carcinogenicity in man.

PRECAUTIONS

The serious complication of excessive Thiotepa therapy, or sensitivity to the effects of Thiotepa, is bone marrow depression. If proper precautions are not observed, Thiotepa may cause leukopenia, thrombocytopenia, and anemia. Death from septicemia and hemorrhage has occured as a direct result of hematopoietic depression by Thiotepa.

It is not advisable to combine, simultaneously or sequentially, cancer chemotherapeutic agents or a cancer chemotherapeutic agent and a therapeutic modality having the same mechanism of action. Therefore, Thiotepa combined with other alkylating agents such as nitrogen mustard or cyclophosphamide or Thiotepa combined with irradiation would serve to intensify toxicity rather than to enhance therapeutic response. If these agents must follow each other, it is important that recovery from the first agent, as indicated by white blood cell count, be complete before therapy with the second agent is instituted.

The most reliable guide to Thiotepa toxicity is the white blood cell count. If this falls to 3000 or less, the dose should be discontinued. Another good index of Thiotepa toxicity is the platelet count; if this falls to 150,000, therapy should be discontinued. Red blood cell count is a less accurate indicator of Thiotepa toxicity.

Other drugs which are known to produce bone marrow depression should be avoided.

There is no known antidote for overdosage with Thiotepa. Transfusions of whole blood or platelets or leukocytes have proved beneficial to the patient in combating hematopoietic toxicity.

ADVERSE REACTIONS

Apart from its effect on the blood-forming elements, Thiotepa may cause other adverse reactions. These include pain at the site of injection, nausea, vomiting, anorexia, dizziness, headache, amenorrhea, and interference with spermatogenesis.

Febrile reaction and weeping from a subcutaneous lesion may occur as the result of breakdown of tumor tissue.

Allergic reactions are rare, but hives and skin rash have been noted occasionally. One case of alopecia has been reported. In addition, a patient who has received Thiotepa and other anticancer agents experienced prolonged apnea after succinylcholine was administered prior to surgery. It was theorized that this was caused by decrease of pseudocholinesterase activity caused by the anticancer drugs.

There have been rare reports of chemical cystitis or hemorrhagic cystitis following intravesical, but not parenteral administration of Thiotepa.

DOSAGE

Parenteral routes of administration are most reliable since absorption of Thiotepa from the gastrointestinal tract is variable.

Since Thiotepa is nonvesicant, intravenous doses may be given directly and rapidly without need for slow drip or large volumes of diluent. Some physicians prefer to give Thiotepa directly into the tumor mass. This may be effected transrectally, transvaginally, or intracerebrally. The technique is discussed in the appropriate section which follows. For the control of malignant effusions, Thiotepa is instilled directly into the cavity involved.

Dosage must be carefully individualized. A slow response to Thiotepa may be deceptive and may occasion unwarranted frequency of administration with subsequent signs of toxicity. After maximum benefit is obtained by initial therapy, it is necessary to continue patient on maintenance therapy (1-to 4-week intervals). In order to continue optimal effect, maintenance doses should be no more frequent than weekly in order to preserve correlation between dose and blood counts.

Initial and Maintenance Doses: Initially the higher dose in the given range is commonly administered. The maintenance dose should be adjusted weekly on the basis of pre-treatment control blood counts and subsequent blood counts.

Intravenous Administration: Thiotepa may be given by rapid intravenous administration in doses of 0.3 to 0.4 mg/kg. Doses should be given at 1- to 4-week intervals.

For conversion of mg/kg of body weight to mg/M^2 of body surface or the reverse, a ratio of 1:30 is given as a guideline. The conversion factor varies between 1:20 and 1:40 depending on age and body build.

Intratumor Administration: Thiotepa in initial doses of 0.6 to 0.8 mg/kg may be injected directly into a tumor by means of a 22-gauge needle. A small amount of local anesthetic is injected first; then the syringe is removed and the Thiotepa solution is injected through the same needle. The drug is diluted in Sterile Water for Injection, 10 mg per 1 mL. Maintenance doses at 1- to 4-week intervals range from 0.07 mg/kg to 0.8 mg/kg depending on the condition of the patient.

Intracavitary Administration: The dosage recommended is 0.6 to 0.8 mg/kg. Administration is usually effected through the same tubing which is used to remove the fluid from the cavity involved.

Intravesical Administration: Patients with papillary carcinoma of the bladder are dehydrated for 8 to 12 hours prior to treatment. Then 60 mg of Thiotepa in 30 to 60 mL of Sterile Water for Injection is instilled into the bladder by catheter. For maximum effect, the solution should be retained for 2 hours. If the patient finds it impossible to retain 60 mL for 2 hours, the dose may be given in a volume of 30 mL. If desired, the patient may be positioned every 15 minutes for maximum area contact. The usual course of treatment is once a week for 4 weeks. The course may be repeated if necessary, but second and third courses must be given with caution since bone marrow depression may be increased. Deaths have occurred after intravesical administration, caused by bone marrow depression from systemically absorbed drug.

Preparation of Solution: The powder should be reconstituted preferably in Sterile Water for Injection. The amount of diluent most often used is 1.5 mL resulting in a drug concentration of 5 mg in each 0.5 mL of solution. Larger volumes are usually employed for intracavitary use, intravenous drip, or perfusion therapy. The 1.5 mL reconstituted preparation may be added to larger volumes of other diluents: Sodium Chloride Injection USP, Dextrose Injection USP, Dextrose and Sodium Chloride Injection USP, Ringer's Injection USP, or Lactated Ringer's Injection USP. Reconstituted solutions should be clear to slightly opaque but solutions that are grossly opaque or precipitated should not be used.

Since the original powder form contains 15 mg Thiotepa, 80 mg NaCl, and 50 mg NaHCO$_3$, reconstitution and further dilution of the powder with Sterile Water for Injection to a concentration of approximately 1 mg/mL produces an isotonic solution. Reconstitution and further dilution with other diluents may result in hypertonic solutions, which may cause mild to moderate discomfort on injection.

For local use into single or multiple sites, Thiotepa may be mixed with procaine HCl 2%, epinephrine HCl 1:1000, or both.

Procedures for proper handling and disposal of anti-cancer drugs should be considered. Several guidelines on this subject have been published.[1-6] There is no general agreement that all of the procedures recommended in the guidelines are necessary or appropriate.

Whether in its original powder form or in reconstituted solution, Thiotepa must be stored in the refrigerator at 2°-8° C (36°-46° F). Reconstituted solutions may be kept for 5 days in a refrigerator without substantial loss of potency.

REFERENCES

1. Recommendations for the Safe Handling of Parenteral Antineoplastic Drugs. NIH Publication No. 83-2621. For sale by the Superintendent of Documents, U.S. Government Printing Office, Washington, D.C. 20402. 2. AMA Council Report. Guidelines for Handling Parenteral Antineoplastics. JAMA, March 15, 1985. 3. National Study Commission on Cytotoxic Exposure—Recommendations for Handling Cytotoxic Agents. Available from Louis P. Jeffrey, ScD, Director of Pharmacy Services, Rhode Island Hospital, 593 Eddy Street, Providence, Rhode Island 02902. 4. Clinical Oncological Society of Australia: Guidelines and recommendations for safe handling of antineoplastic agents. Med J Australia. 1983; 1:426-428. 5. Jones, RB, et al. Safe handling of chemotherapeutic agents: A report from the Mount Sinai Medical Center. CA—A Cancer Journal for Clinicians Sept/Oct 1983; 258-263. 6. American Society of Hospital Pharmacists technical assistance bulletin on handling cytotoxic drugs in hospitals. Am J Hosp Pharm. 1985; 42:131-137.

HOW SUPPLIED
POWDER FOR INJECTION: 15 MG

BRAND/MANUFACTURER	NDC	SIZE	AWP
○ BRAND			
THIOTEPA: Immunex	00005-4650-91	1s	$62.88

➤ SHOWN IN PRODUCT IDENTIFICATION GUIDE

Thiotepa *SEE* THIOTEPA

Thiothixene

DESCRIPTION

Thiothixene is a Thioxanthene derivative. Specifically, Thiothixene is the *cis* isomer of N,N-dimethyl-9-[3-(4-methyl-1-piperazinyl)-propylidene]thioxa nthene-2-sulfonamide.

The thioxanthenes differ from the phenothiazines by the replacement of nitrogen in the central ring with a carbon-linked side chain fixed in space in a rigid structural configuration. An N,N-dimethyl sulfonamide functional group is bonded to the thioxanthene nucleus.

ACTIONS

Thiothixene is a psychotropic agent of the thioxanthene series. Thiothixene possesses certain chemical and pharmacological similarities to the piperazine phenothiazines and differences from the aliphatic group of phenothiazines. Thiothixene's mode of action has not been clearly established.

INDICATIONS

Thiothixene is effective in the management of manifestations of psychotic disorders. Thiothixene has not been evaluated in the management of behavioral complications in patients with mental retardation.

UNLABELED USES

Thiothixene is used alone or as an adjunct in the treatment of depression and senile psychosis.

CONTRAINDICATIONS

Thiothixene is contraindicated in patients with circulatory collapse, comatose states, central nervous system depression due to any cause, and blood dyscrasias. Thiothixene is contraindicated in individuals who have shown hypersensitivity to the drug. It is not known whether there is a cross sensitivity between the thioxanthenes and the phenothiazine derivatives, but this possibility should be considered.

WARNINGS

Tardive Dyskinesia: Tardive dyskinesia, a syndrome consisting of potentially irreversible, involuntary, dyskinetic movements may develop in patients treated with neuroleptic (antipsychotic) drugs. Although the prevalence of the syndrome appears to be highest among the elderly, especially elderly women, it is impossible to rely upon prevalence estimates to predict, at the inception of neuroleptic treatment, which patients are likely to develop the syndrome. Whether neuroleptic drug products differ in their potential to cause tardive dyskinesia is unknown.

Both the risk of developing the syndrome and the likelihood that it will become irreversible are believed to increase as the duration of treatment and the total cumulative dose of neuroleptic drugs administered to the patient increase. However, the syndrome can develop, although much less commonly, after relatively brief treatment periods at low doses. There is no known treatment for established cases of tardive dyskinesia, although the syndrome may remit, partially or completely, if neuroleptic treatment is withdrawn. Neuroleptic treatment, itself, however, may suppress (or partially suppress) the signs and symptoms of the syndrome and thereby may possibly mask the underlying disease process. The effect that symptomatic suppression has upon the long-term course of the syndrome is unknown.

Given these considerations, neuroleptics should be prescribed in a manner that is most likely to minimize the occurrence of tardive dyskinesia. Chronic neuroleptic treatment should generally be reserved for patients who suffer from a chronic illness that, 1) is known to respond to neuroleptic drugs, and, 2) for whom alternative, equally effective, but potentially less harmful treatments are *not* available or appropriate. In patients who do require chronic treatment, the smallest dose and the shortest duration of treatment producing a satisfactory clinical response should be sought. The need for continued treatment should be reassessed periodically.

If signs and symptoms of tardive dyskinesia appear in a patient on neuroleptics, drug discontinuation should be considered. However, some patients may require treatment despite the presence of the syndrome.

(For further information about the description of tardive dyskinesia and its clinical detection, please refer to "Information for Patients" in the "Precautions" section, and to the "Adverse Reactions" section.)

Neuroleptic Malignant Syndrome (NMS): A potentially fatal symptom complex sometimes referred to as Neuroleptic Malignant Syndrome (NMS) has been reported in association with antipsychotic drugs. Clinical manifestations of NMS are hyperpyrexia, muscle rigidity, altered mental status and evidence of autonomic instability (irregular pulse or blood pressure, tachycardia, diaphoresis, and cardiac dysrhythmias).

The diagnostic evaluation of patients with this syndrome is complicated. In arriving at a diagnosis, it is important to identify cases where the clinical presentation includes both serious medical illness (e.g., pneumonia, systemic infection, etc.) and untreated or inadequately treated extrapyramidal signs and symptoms (EPS). Other important considerations in the differential diagnosis include central anticholinergic toxicity, heat stroke, drug fever and primary central nervous system (CNS) pathology.

The management of NMS should include 1) immediate discontinuation of antipsychotic drugs and other drugs not essential to concurrent therapy, 2) intensive symptomatic treatment and medical monitoring, and 3) treatment of any concomitant serious medical problems for which specific treatments are available. There is no general agreement about specific pharmacological treatment regimens for uncomplicated NMS.

If a patient requires antipsychotic drug treatment after recovery from NMS, the potential reintroduction of drug therapy should be carefully considered. The patient should be carefully monitored, since recurrences of NMS have been reported.

Usage in Pregnancy: Safe use of Thiothixene during pregnancy has not been established. Therefore, this drug should be given to pregnant patients only when, in the judgment of the physician, the expected benefits from treatment exceed the possible risks to mother and fetus. Animal reproductive studies and clinical experience to date have not demonstrated any teratogenic effects.

In the animal reproduction studies with Thiothixene, there was some decrease in conception rate and litter size, and an increase in resorption rate in rats and rabbits, changes which have been similarly reported with other psychotropic agents. After repeated oral administration of Thiothixene to rats (5 to 15 mg/kg/day), rabbits (3 to 50 mg/kg/day), and monkeys (1 to 3 mg/kg/day) before and during gestation, no teratogenic effects were seen. (See "Precautions".)

Usage in Children: The use of Thiothixene in children under 12 years of age is not recommended because safety and efficacy in the pediatric age group have not been established.

As is true with many CNS drugs, Thiothixene may impair the mental and/or physical abilities required for the performance of potentially hazardous tasks such as driving a car or operating machinery, especially during the first few days of therapy. Therefore, the patient should be cautioned accordingly.

As in the case of other CNS-acting drugs, patients receiving Thiothixene should be cautioned about the possible additive effects (which may include hypotension) with CNS depressants and with alcohol.

PRECAUTIONS

General: An antiemetic effect was observed in animal studies with Thiothixene since this effect may also occur in man, it is possible that Thiothixene may mask signs of overdosage of toxic drugs and may obscure conditions such as intestinal obstruction and brain tumor.

In consideration of the known capability of Thiothixene and certain other psychotropic drugs to precipitate convulsions, extreme caution should be used in patients with a history of convulsive disorders, or those in a state of alcohol withdrawal since it may lower the convulsive threshold. Although Thiothixene potentiates the actions of the barbiturates, the dosage of the anticonvulsant therapy should not be reduced when Thiothixene is administered concurrently.

Caution as well as careful adjustment of the dosage is indicated when Thiothixene is used in conjunction with other CNS depressants other than anticonvulsant drugs.

Though exhibiting rather weak anticholinergic properties, Thiothixene should be used with caution in patients who are known or suspected to have glaucoma, or who might be exposed to extreme heat, or who are receiving atropine or related drugs.

Use with caution in patients with cardiovascular disease. Also, careful observation should be made for pigmentary retinopathy, and lenticular pigmentation (fine lenticular pigmentation has been noted in a small number of patients treated with Thiothixene for prolonged periods). Blood dyscrasias (agranulocytosis, pancytopenia, thrombocytopenic purpura), and liver damage (jaundice, biliary stasis), have been reported with related drugs.

Undue exposure to sunlight should be avoided. Photosensitive reactions have been reported in patients on Thiothixene. As with all intramuscular preparations, Thiothixene Intramuscular should be injected well within the body of a relatively large muscle. The preferred sites are the upper outer quadrant of the buttock (i.e., gluteus maximus) and the mid-lateral thigh.

The deltoid area should be used only if well developed such as in certain adults and older children, and then only with caution to avoid radial nerve injury. Intramuscular injections should not be made into the lower and mid-thirds of the upper arm. As with all intramuscular injections, aspiration is necessary to help avoid inadvertent injection into a blood vessel.

Neuroleptic drugs elevate prolactin levels; the elevation persists during chronic administration. Tissue culture experiments indicate that approximately one-third of human breast cancers are prolactin dependent *in vitro*, a factor of potential importance if the prescription of these drugs is contemplated in a patient with a previously detected breast cancer. Although disturbances such as galactorrhea, amenorrhea, gynecomastia, and impotence have been reported, the clinical significance of elevated serum prolactin levels is unknown for most patients. An increase in mammary neoplasms has been found in rodents after chronic administration of neuroleptic drugs. Neither clinical studies nor epidemiologic studies conducted to date, however, have shown an association between chronic administration of these drugs and mammary tumorigenesis; the available evidence is considered too limited to be conclusive at this time.

Information for Patients: Given the likelihood that some patients exposed chronically to neuroleptics will develop tardive dyskinesia, it is advised that all patients in whom chronic use is contemplated be given, if possible, full information about this risk. The decision to inform patients and/or their guardians must obviously take into account the clinical circumstances and the competency of the patient to understand the information provided.

◆ RATED THERAPEUTICALLY EQUIVALENT; ◇ THERAPEUTIC EQUIVALENCE UNCONFIRMED; ○ UNRATED

ADVERSE REACTIONS

Note: Not all of the following adverse reactions have been reported with Thiothixene. However, since Thiothixene has certain chemical and pharmacologic similarities to the phenothiazines, all of the known side effects and toxicity associated with phenothiazine therapy should be borne in mind when Thiothixene is used.

Cardiovascular Effects: Tachycardia, hypotension, lightheadedness, and syncope. In the event hypotension occurs, epinephrine should not be used as a pressor agent since a paradoxical further lowering of blood pressure may result. Nonspecific EKG changes have been observed in some patients receiving Thiothixene. These changes are usually reversible and frequently disappear on continued Thiothixene therapy. The incidence of these changes is lower than that observed with some phenothiazines.

The clinical significance of these changes is not known.

CNS Effects: Drowsiness, usually mild, may occur although it usually subsides with continuation of Thiothixene therapy. The incidence of sedation appears similar to that of the piperazine group of phenothiazines, but less than that of certain aliphatic phenothiazines. Restlessness, agitation and insomnia have been noted with Thiothixene Seizures and paradoxical exacerbation of psychotic symptoms have occurred with Thiothixene infrequently.

Hyperreflexia has been reported in infants delivered from mothers having received structurally related drugs.

In addition, phenothiazine derivatives have been associated with cerebral edema and cerebrospinal fluid abnormalities. Extrapyramidal symptoms, such as pseudo-parkinsonism, akathisia, and dystonia have been reported. Management of these extrapyramidal symptoms depends upon the type and severity. Rapid relief of acute symptoms may require the use of an injectable antiparkinson agent. More slowly emerging symptoms may be managed by reducing the dosage of Thiothixene and/or administering an oral antiparkinson agent.

Persistent Tardive Dyskinesia: As with all antipsychotic agents tardive dyskinesia may appear in some patients on long term therapy or may occur after drug therapy has been discontinued. The syndrome is characterized by rhythmical involuntary movements of the tongue, face, mouth or jaw (e.g., protrusion of tongue, puffing of cheeks, puckering of mouth, chewing movements). Sometimes these may be accompanied by involuntary movements of extremities.

Since early detection of tardive dyskinesia is important, patients should be monitored on an ongoing basis. It has been reported that fine vermicular movement of the tongue may be an early sign of the syndrome. If this or any other presentation of the syndrome is observed, the clinician should consider possible discontinuation of neuroleptic medication. (See *"Warnings"* section.)

Hepatic Effects: Elevations of serum transaminase and alkaline phosphatase, usually transient, have been infrequently observed in some patients. No clinically confirmed cases of jaundice attributable to Thiothixene have been reported.

Hematologic Effects: As is true with certain other psychotropic drugs, leukopenia and leucocytosis, which are usually transient, can occur occasionally with Thiothixene. Other antipsychotic drugs have been associated with agranulocytosis, eosinophilia, hemolytic anemia, thrombocytopenia and pancytopenia.

Allergic Reactions: Rash, pruritus, urticaria, photosensitivity, and rare cases of anaphylaxis have been reported with Thiothixene. Undue exposure to sunlight should be avoided. Although not experienced with Thiothixene exfoliative dermatitis and contact dermatitis (in nursing personnel), have been reported with certain phenothiazines.

Endocrine Disorders: Lactation, moderate breast enlargement and amenorrhea have occurred in a small percentage of females receiving Thiothixene. If persistent, this may necessitate a reduction in dosage or the discontinuation of therapy. Phenothiazines have been associated with false positive pregnancy tests, gynecomastia, hypoglycemia, hyperglycemia, and glycosuria.

Autonomic Effects: Dry mouth, blurred vision, nasal congestion, constipation, increased sweating, increased salivation, and impotence have occurred infrequently with Thiothixene therapy. Phenothiazines have been associated with miosis, mydriasis, and adynamic ileus.

Other Adverse Reactions: Hyperpyrexia, anorexia, nausea, vomiting, diarrhea, increase in appetite and weight, weakness or fatigue, polydipsia and peripheral edema.

Although not reported with Thiothixene, evidence indicates there is a relationship between phenothiazine therapy and the occurrence of a systemic lupus erythematosus-like syndrome.

Neuroleptic Malignant Syndrome (NMS): Please refer to the text regarding NMS in the *"Warnings"* section.

Note: Sudden deaths have occasionally been reported in patients who have received certain phenothiazine derivatives. In some cases the cause of death was apparently cardiac arrest or asphyxia due to failure of the cough reflex. In others, the cause could not be determined nor could it be established that death was due to phenothiazine administration.

OVERDOSAGE

Manifestations include muscular twitching, drowsiness, and dizziness. Symptoms of gross overdosage may include CNS depression, rigidity, weakness, torticollis, tremor, salivation, dysphagia, hypotension, disturbances of gait, or coma.

Treatment: Essentially symptomatic and supportive. Early gastric lavage (oral overdose) is helpful. Keep patient under careful observation and maintain an open airway, since involvement of the extrapyramidal system may produce dysphagia and respiratory difficulty in severe overdosage. If hypotension occurs, the standard measures for managing circulatory shock should be used (I.V. fluids and/or vasoconstrictors).

If a vasoconstrictor is needed, levarterenol and phenylephrine re the most suitable drugs. Other pressor agents, including epinephrine, are not recommended, since phenothiazine derivatives may reverse the usual pressor elevating action of these agents and cause further lowering of blood pressure.

If CNS depression is marked, symptomatic treatment is indicated. Extrapyramidal symptoms may be treated with antiparkinson drugs.

There are no data on the use of peritoneal or hemodialysis, but they are known to be of little value in phenothiazine intoxication.

DOSAGE AND ADMINISTRATION

PREPARATION

Thiothixene Intramuscular Solution is ready for use as supplied.

Thiothixene Intramuscular For Injection must be reconstituted with 2.2 ml of Sterile Water for Injection.

FOR INTRAMUSCULAR USE ONLY

Dosage of Thiothixene should be individually adjusted depending on the chronicity and severity of the condition. In general, small doses should be used initially and gradually increased to the optimal effective level, based on patient response.

Usage in children under 12 years of age is not recommended. Where more rapid control and treatment of acute behavior is desirable, the intramuscular form of Thiothixene may be indicated. It is also of benefit where the very nature of the patient's symptomatology, whether acute or chronic, renders oral administration impractical or even impossible.

For treatment of acute symptomatology or in patients unable or unwilling to take oral medication, the usual dose is 4 mg of Thiothixene Intramuscular administered 2 to 4 times daily. Dosage may be increased or decreased depending on response. Most patients are controlled on a total daily dosage of 16 to 20 mg. The maximum recommended dosage is 30 mg/day. An oral form should supplant the injectable form as soon as possible. It may be necessary to adjust the dosage when changing from the intramuscular to oral dosage forms.

CAPSULES AND CONCENTRATE

Dosage of Thiothixene should be individually adjusted depending on the chronicity and severity of the condition. In general, small doses should be used initially and gradually increased to the optimal effective level, based on patient response.

Some patients have been successfully maintained on once-a-day Thiothixene therapy.

The use of Thiothixene in children under 12 years of age is not recommended because safe conditions for its use have not been established.

In milder conditions, an initial dose of 2 mg three times daily. If indicated, a subsequent increase to 15 mg/day total daily dose is often effective.

In more severe conditions, an initial dose of 5 mg twice daily. The usual optimal dose is 20 to 30 mg daily. If indicated, an increase to 60 mg/day total daily dose is often effective. Exceeding a total daily dose of 60 mg rarely increases the beneficial response.

The reconstituted solution of Thiothixene Intramuscular For Injection may be stored for 48 hours at room temperature before discarding.

J CODES

Up to 4 mg IM—J2330

HOW SUPPLIED

THIOTHIXENE

CAPSULE: 1 MG

AVERAGE UNIT PRICE (AVAILABLE SIZES)		GENERIC A-RATED AVERAGE PRICE (GAAP)		
BRAND	$0.38	100s		$19.90
GENERIC	$0.20			
HCFA FUL (100s ea)	$0.10			

BRAND/MANUFACTURER	NDC	SIZE	AWP
◆ BRAND			
➤ NAVANE: Roerig	00049-5710-66	100s	$38.03
◆ GENERICS			
Rugby	00536-4951-01	100s	$15.75
Qualitest	00603-6018-21	100s	$15.77
Aligen	00405-5004-01	100s	$16.20
Major	00904-2890-60	100s	$17.50
Major	00904-2955-60	100s	$17.50
Schein	00364-2166-01	100s	$17.55
Geneva	00781-2226-01	100s	$17.60
Mylan	00378-1001-01	100s	$20.95
Moore,H.L.	00839-7288-06	100s	$21.06
U.S. Trading	56106-0378-11	100s ud	$12.23
UDL	51079-0586-20	100s ud	$28.80
Vangard	00615-1302-13	100s ud	$28.80
Geneva	00781-2226-13	100s ud	$28.95

➤ SHOWN IN PRODUCT IDENTIFICATION GUIDE

CAPSULE: 2 MG

AVERAGE UNIT PRICE (AVAILABLE SIZES)		GENERIC A-RATED AVERAGE PRICE (GAAP)	
BRAND	$0.48	100s	$27.23
GENERIC	$0.25	500s	$86.42
HCFA FUL (100s ea)	$0.13	1000s	$218.78

BRAND/MANUFACTURER	NDC	SIZE	AWP
◆ BRAND			
➤ NAVANE: Roerig	00049-5720-66	100s	$51.28
	00049-5720-82	1000s	$456.14
◆ GENERICS			
Qualitest	00603-6019-21	100s	$20.89
Rugby	00536-4952-01	100s	$21.00
Goldline	00182-1836-01	100s	$24.75
Geneva	00781-2227-01	100s	$24.80
Major	00904-2891-60	100s	$24.85
Aligen	00405-5005-01	100s	$25.38
Schein	00364-2167-01	100s	$26.80
Parmed	00349-8664-01	100s	$27.16
Mylan	00378-2002-01	100s	$27.25
Moore,H.L.	00839-7289-06	100s	$27.54
U.S. Trading	56126-0379-11	100s ud	$15.02
Vangard	00615-1303-13	100s ud	$38.05
UDL	51079-0587-20	100s ud	$38.81
Geneva	00781-2227-13	100s ud	$38.85
Major	00904-2891-40	500s	$79.75
Major	00904-2956-40	500s	$79.75
Rugby	00536-4952-05	500s	$99.75
Schein	00364-2167-02	1000s	$192.85
Parmed	00349-8664-10	1000s	$223.79
Mylan	00378-2002-10	1000s	$239.71

CAPSULE: 5 MG

AVERAGE UNIT PRICE (AVAILABLE SIZES)		GENERIC A-RATED AVERAGE PRICE (GAAP)	
BRAND	$0.76	100s	$41.88
GENERIC	$0.38	500s	$124.86
HCFA FUL (100s ea)	$0.18	1000s	$313.74

BRAND/MANUFACTURER	NDC	SIZE	AWP
◆ BRAND			
➤ NAVANE: Roerig	00049-5730-66	100s	$80.18
	00049-5730-82	1000s	$712.70
◆ GENERICS			
Rugby	00536-4516-01	100s	$35.25
Major	00904-2892-60	100s	$36.80
Major	00904-2957-60	100s	$36.80
Qualitest	00603-6020-21	100s	$37.11
Aligen	00405-5006-01	100s	$38.25
Goldline	00182-1837-01	100s	$38.25
Geneva	00781-2228-01	100s	$38.26
Schein	00364-2168-01	100s	$41.05
Mylan	00378-3005-01	100s	$41.50
Moore,H.L.	00839-7290-06	100s	$42.46
Parmed	00349-8665-01	100s	$42.71
U.S. Trading	56126-0380-11	100s ud	$18.77
Vangard	00615-1304-13	100s ud	$59.50
UDL	51079-0588-20	100s ud	$60.76
Geneva	00781-2228-13	100s ud	$60.80
Rugby	00536-4516-05	500s	$124.68
Major	00904-2892-40	500s	$124.95
Major	00904-2957-40	500s	$124.95
Schein	00364-2168-02	1000s	$219.25
Parmed	00349-8665-10	1000s	$358.78
Mylan	00378-3005-10	1000s	$363.20

CAPSULE: 10 MG

AVERAGE UNIT PRICE (AVAILABLE SIZES)		GENERIC A-RATED AVERAGE PRICE (GAAP)	
BRAND	$1.04	100s	$55.48
GENERIC	$0.52	500s	$191.20
HCFA FUL (100s ea)	$0.27	1000s	$469.56

BRAND/MANUFACTURER	NDC	SIZE	AWP
◆ BRAND			
➤ NAVANE: Roerig	00049-5740-66	100s	$110.49
	00049-5740-82	1000s	$983.47
◆ GENERICS			
Rugby	00536-4954-01	100s	$45.75
Major	00904-2893-60	100s	$47.15
Major	00904-2958-60	100s	$47.15
Qualitest	00603-6021-21	100s	$52.70
URL	00677-1152-01	100s	$53.50
Geneva	00781-2229-01	100s	$53.60

BRAND/MANUFACTURER	NDC	SIZE	AWP
Aligen	00405-5007-01	100s	$55.80
Schein	00364-2169-01	100s	$56.05
Parmed	00349-8666-01	100s	$58.44
Mylan	00378-5010-01	100s	$59.25
Moore,H.L.	00839-7291-06	100s	$59.93
U.S. Trading	56126-0381-11	100s ud	$27.17
Vangard	00615-0347-13	100s ud	$52.46
UDL	51079-0589-20	100s ud	$80.08
Geneva	00781-2229-13	100s ud	$80.10
Major	00904-2893-40	500s	$178.15
Major	00904-2958-40	500s	$178.15
Rugby	00536-4954-05	500s	$217.31
Schein	00364-2169-02	1000s	$378.25
Parmed	00349-8666-10	1000s	$499.60
Mylan	00378-5010-10	1000s	$530.83

CAPSULE: 20 MG

AVERAGE UNIT PRICE (AVAILABLE SIZES)	
BRAND	$1.55

BRAND/MANUFACTURER	NDC	SIZE	AWP
◆ BRAND			
➤ NAVANE: Roerig	00049-5770-66	100s	$155.04
	00049-5770-41	100s ud	$170.46
➤ NAVANE: Roerig	00049-5770-73	500s	$692.81
◆ GENERICS			
U.S. Trading	56126-0416-11	100s ud	$5.07

For additional alternatives, turn to the section beginning on page 2859.

Thorazine *SEE* CHLORPROMAZINE

Thrombate III *SEE* ANTITHROMBIN III (HUMAN)

Thrombin

DESCRIPTION

Thrombin is a protein substance produced through a conversion reaction in which prothrombin of bovine origin is activated by tissue thromboplastin in the presence of calcium chloride. It is supplied as a sterile powder that has been freeze-dried in the final container.

CLINICAL PHARMACOLOGY

Thrombin requires no intermediate physiological agent for its action. It clots the fibrinogen of the blood directly. **Failure to clot blood occurs in the rare case where the primary clotting defect is the absence of fibrinogen itself.** The speed with which Thrombin clots blood is dependent upon its concentration. For example, 5000 units of Thrombin dissolved in 5 ml of saline diluent is capable of clotting an equal volume of blood in less than a second, or 1000 ml in less than a minute.

INDICATIONS AND USAGE

Thrombin is indicated as an aid in hemostasis wherever oozing blood from capillaries and small venules is accessible.

In various types of surgery, solutions of Thrombin may be used in conjunction with absorbable gelatin sponge for hemostasis.

CONTRAINDICATIONS

Thrombin is contraindicated in persons known to be sensitive to any of its components and/or to material of bovine origin.

WARNING

Because of its action in the clotting mechanism, Thrombin must not be injected or otherwise allowed to enter large blood vessels. Extensive intravascular clotting and even death may result. Thrombin is an antigenic substance and has caused sensitivity and allergic reactions when injected into animals.

PRECAUTIONS

General: Consult the absorbable gelatin sponge product labeling for complete information for use prior to utilizing the Thrombin-saturated sponge procedure.

Pregnancy — Teratogenic effects: Pregnancy Category C. Animal reproduction studies have not been conducted with Thrombin. It is also not known whether Thrombin can cause fetal harm when administered to a pregnant woman or can

◆ RATED THERAPEUTICALLY EQUIVALENT; ◇ THERAPEUTIC EQUIVALENCE UNCONFIRMED; ○ UNRATED

affect reproduction capacity. Thrombin, should be given to a pregnant woman only if clearly indicated.

Pediatric Use: Safety and effectiveness in children have not been established.

ADVERSE REACTIONS
Allergic reactions may be encountered in persons known to be sensitive to bovine materials.

DOSAGE AND ADMINISTRATION
General: Solutions of Thrombin may be prepared in sterile distilled water or isotonic saline. The intended use determines the strength of the solution to prepare. For general use in plastic surgery, dental extractions, skin grafting, neurosurgery, etc., solutions containing approximately 100 units per mL are frequently used. For this, an appropriate dilution of Thrombin should be prepared to yield a concentration of 100 units per mL. Where bleeding is profuse, as from cut surfaces of liver and spleen, concentrations as high as 1000 to 2000 units per mL may be required. For this, 5000 unit dissolved in 5 mL or 2.5 mL, respectively, of diluent is appropriate. Intermediate strengths to suit the needs of the case may be prepared by selecting the proper strength and dissolving the powder in an appropriate volume of diluent. In many situations, it may be advantageous to use Thrombin in dry form on oozing surfaces.

Caution: Solutions should be used immediately upon reconstitution. If necessary, refrigerate the solution and use within 3 hours of reconstitution.

The following techniques are suggested for the topical application of Thrombin.

1. The recipient surface should be sponged (not wiped) free of blood before Thrombin is applied.

2. A spray may be used or the surface may be flooded using a sterile syringe and small gauge needle. The most effective hemostasis results when the Thrombin mixes freely with the blood as soon as it reaches the surface.

3. In instances where Thrombin in dry form is needed, the dried Thrombin is broken up into a powder by means of a sterile glass rod or other suitable sterile instrument.

4. Sponging of treated surfaces should be avoided in order that the clot remain securely in place.

Thrombin may be used in conjunction with absorbable gelatin sponge as follows:

1. Prepare Thrombin solution of the desired strength.

2. Immerse sponge strips of the desired size in the Thrombin solution. Knead the sponge strips vigorously with moistened gloved fingers to remove trapped air, thereby facilitating saturation of the sponge.

3. Apply saturated sponge to bleeding area. Hold in place for 10 to 15 seconds with a pledget of cotton or a small gauze sponge.

Storage: Store at room temperature 15° to 30°C (59° to 86°F).

HOW SUPPLIED
KIT: 10,000 U

BRAND/MANUFACTURER	NDC	SIZE	AWP
○ BRAND			
THROMBOSTAT: Parke-Davis	00071-4176-37	1s	$42.54
THROMBINAR: Jones Medical	00053-7104-02	1s	$44.25

KIT: 20,000 U

BRAND/MANUFACTURER	NDC	SIZE	AWP
○ BRAND			
THROMBOSTAT: Parke-Davis	00071-4180-36	1s	$71.26
THROMBINAR: Jones Medical	00053-7105-02	1s	$74.10

KIT: 5000 U

BRAND/MANUFACTURER	NDC	SIZE	AWP
○ BRAND			
THROMBINAR: Jones Medical	00053-7102-02	1s	$24.00

POWDER FOR RECONSTITUTION: 10,000 U

BRAND/MANUFACTURER	NDC	SIZE	AWP
○ BRAND			
THROMBOSTAT: Parke-Davis	00071-4176-35	1s	$34.15
	00071-4176-36	1s	$39.71
THROMBINAR: Jones Medical	00053-7104-03	1s	$40.60
THROMBOGEN: J&J Medical	00137-0019-12	10 ml 10s	$323.91
	00137-0019-14	10 ml 10s	$351.38

POWDER FOR RECONSTITUTION: 20,000 U

BRAND/MANUFACTURER	NDC	SIZE	AWP
○ BRAND			
THROMBOSTAT: Parke-Davis	00071-4180-35	1s	$65.63
THROMBINAR: Jones Medical	00053-7105-03	1s	$73.10
THROMBOGEN: J&J Medical	00137-0019-13	20 ml 10s	$657.12
	00137-0019-15	20 ml 10s	$713.14

POWDER FOR RECONSTITUTION: 50,000 U

BRAND/MANUFACTURER	NDC	SIZE	AWP
○ BRAND			
THROMBINAR: Jones Medical	00053-7106-01	1s	$135.60

POWDER FOR RECONSTITUTION: 1000 U

BRAND/MANUFACTURER	NDC	SIZE	AWP
○ BRAND			
THROMBINAR: Jones Medical	00053-7100-01	1s	$6.55
THROMBOGEN: J&J Medical	00137-0019-10	1 ml 10s	$52.46

POWDER FOR RECONSTITUTION: 5000 U

BRAND/MANUFACTURER	NDC	SIZE	AWP
○ BRAND			
THROMBOSTAT: Parke-Davis	00071-4173-35	1s	$18.56
THROMBINAR: Jones Medical	00053-7102-01	1s	$21.20
THROMBOSTAT: Parke-Davis	00071-4173-36	1s	$21.59
THROMBOGEN: J&J Medical	00137-0019-11	5 ml 10s	$176.07

Thrombinar *SEE* THROMBIN

Thrombogen *SEE* THROMBIN

Thrombostat *SEE* THROMBIN

Thyrel TRH *SEE* PROTIRELIN

Thyroid

DESCRIPTION
Thyroid tablets for oral use are natural preparations derived from porcine thyroid glands. (T_3 liothyronine is approximately four times as potent as T_4 levothyroxine on a microgram for microgram basis.) They provide 38 mcg levothyroxine (T_4) and 9 mcg liothyronine (T_3) per grain of Thyroid.

Pork Thyroid "liquid" capsules are prepared by special process from cleaned, fresh pork thyroid glands, deprived of connective tissue, defatted and suspended in soy bean oil and encapsulated in gelatin for greater oral absorption. The active hormones (T_4 and T_3) are available in their natural state in a ratio of approximately 2.5:1, as in humans, to insure therapeutic availability. Capsules are standardized by USP method for iodine content and also biologically to insure 100% metabolic potency.

CLINICAL PHARMACOLOGY
The steps in the synthesis of the thyroid hormones are controlled by thyrotropin (Thyroid Stimulating Hormone, TSH) secreted by the anterior pituitary. This hormone's secretion is in turn controlled by a feedback mechanism effected by the thyroid hormones themselves and by thyrotropin releasing hormone (TRH), a tripeptide of hypothalamic origin. Endogenous thyroid hormone secretion is suppressed when exogenous thyroid hormones are administered to euthyroid individuals in excess of the normal gland's secretion.

The mechanisms by which thyroid hormones exert their physiologic action are not well understood. These hormones enhance oxygen consumption by most tissues of the body, increase the basal metabolic rate, and the metabolism of carbohydrates, lipids, and proteins. Thus, they exert a profound influence on every organ system in the body and are of particular importance in the development of the central nervous system. Thyroid is replacement therapy for diminished or absent thyroid function. Effect develops slowly and is fully reached in 10-14 days per grain increase in most instances.

The normal thyroid gland contains approximately 200 mcg of levothyroxine (T_4) per gram of gland, and 15 mcg of liothyronine (T_3) per gram. The ratio of these two hormones in the circulation does not represent the ratio in the thyroid gland, since about 80 percent of peripheral liothyronine (T_3) comes from monodeiodination of levothyroxine (T_4). Peripheral monodeiodination of levothyroxine (T_4) at the 5 position (inner ring) also results in the formation of reverse liothyronine (T_3), which is calorigenically inactive.

Liothyronine (T_3) levels are low in the fetus and newborn, in old age, in chronic caloric deprivation, hepatic cirrhosis, renal failure, surgical stress, and chronic illnesses representing what has been called the "T_3 thyronine syndrome."

Pharmacokinetics: Animal studies have shown that levothyroxine (T_4) is only partially absorbed from the gastrointestinal tract. The degree of absorption is dependent on the vehicle used for its administration and by the character of the intestinal contents, the intestinal flora, including plasma protein, and soluble dietary factors, all of which bind thyroid and thereby make it unavailable for diffusion. Only 41 percent is absorbed when given in a gelatin capsule as opposed to a 74 percent absorption when given with an albumin carrier.

► SHOWN IN PRODUCT IDENTIFICATION GUIDE

Depending on other factors, absorption has varied from 48 to 79 percent of the administered dose. Fasting increases absorption. Malabsorption syndromes, as well as dietary factors, (children's soybean formula, concomitant use of anionic exchange resins such (as cholestyramine) cause excessive fecal loss. Liothyronine (T_3) is almost totally absorbed, 95 percent in 4 hours. The hormones contained in the natural preparations are absorbed in a manner similar to the synthetic hormones.

More than 99 percent of circulating hormones are bound to serum proteins, including thyroid-binding globulin (TBg), thyroid-binding prealbumin (TBPA), and albumin (TBa), whose capacities and affinities vary for the hormones. The higher affinity of levothyroxine (T_4) for both TBg and TBPA as compared to liothyronine (T_3) partially explains the higher serum levels and longer half-life of the former hormone. Both protein-bound hormones exist in reverse equilibrium with minute amounts of free hormone, the latter accounting for the metabolic activity.

Deiodination of levothyroxine (T_4) occurs at a number of sites, including liver, kidney, and other tissues. The conjugated hormone, in the form of glucuronide or sulfate, is found in the bile and gut where it may complete an enterohepatic circulation. Eighty-five percent of levothyroxine (T_4) metabolized daily is deiodinated.

INDICATIONS AND USAGE
Thyroid tablets are indicated:

1. As replacement or supplemental therapy in patients with hypothyroidism of any etiology, except transient hypothyroidism during the recovery phase of subacute thyroiditis. This category includes cretinism, myxedema, and ordinary hypothyroidism in patients of any age (children, adults, the elderly), or state (including pregnancy); primary hypothyroidism resulting from functional deficiency, primary atrophy, partial or total absence of thyroid gland, or the effects of surgery, radiation, or drugs, with or without the presence of goiter; and secondary (pituitary), or tertiary (hypothalamic) hypothyroidism (See *"Warnings"*).

2. As pituitary TSH suppressants, in the treatment or prevention of various types of euthyroid goiters, including thyroid nodules, subacute or chronic lymphocytic thyroiditis (Hashimoto's), multinodular goiter, and in the management of thyroid cancer.

3. As diagnostic agents in suppression tests to differentiate suspected mild hyperthyroidism or thyroid gland autonomy.

CONTRAINDICATIONS
Thyroid hormone preparations are generally contraindicated in patients with diagnosed but as yet uncorrected adrenal cortical insufficiency, untreated thyrotoxicosis, angina pectoris, myocardial infarction, hypertension unless complicated by hypothyroidism, and apparent hypersensitivity to any of their active or extraneous constituents. There is no well-documented evidence from the literature, however, of true allergic or idiosyncratic reactions to thyroid hormone.

WARNINGS

DRUGS WITH THYROID HORMONE ACTIVITY, ALONE OR TOGETHER WITH OTHER THERAPEUTIC AGENTS, HAVE BEEN USED FOR THE TREATMENT OF OBESITY. IN EUTHYROID PATIENTS, DOSES WITHIN THE RANGE OF DAILY HORMONAL REQUIREMENTS ARE INEFFECTIVE FOR WEIGHT REDUCTION. LARGER DOSES MAY PRODUCE SERIOUS OR EVEN LIFE-THREATENING MANIFESTATIONS OF TOXICITY, PARTICULARLY WHEN GIVEN IN ASSOCIATION WITH SYMPATHOMIMETIC AMINES SUCH AS THOSE USED FOR THEIR ANORECTIC EFFECTS.

The use of thyroid hormones in the therapy of obesity, alone or combined with other drugs, is unjustified and has been shown to be ineffective. Neither is their use justified for the treatment of male or female infertility unless this condition is accompanied by hypothyroidism.

PRECAUTIONS
General: Thyroid hormones should be used with great caution in a number of circumstances where the integrity of the cardiovascular system, particularly the coronary arteries, is suspected. These include patients with angina pectoris or the elderly, in whom there is a greater likelihood of occult cardiac disease. In these patients therapy should be initiated with low doses, i.e., 15-30 mg Thyroid. When, in such patients, a euthyroid state can only be reached at the expense of an aggravation of the cardiovascular disease, thyroid hormone dosage should be reduced.

Thyroid hormone therapy in patients with concomitant diabetes mellitus or diabetes insipidus or adrenal cortical insufficiency aggravates the intensity of their symptoms. Appropriate adjustments of the various therapeutic measures directed at these concomitant endocrine diseases are required. The therapy of myxedema coma requires simultaneous administration of glucocorticoids (see *"Dosage and Administration"*).

Hypothyroidism decreases and hyperthyroidism increases the sensitivity to oral anticoagulants. Prothrombin time should be closely monitored in thyroid-treated patients on oral anticoagulants and dosage of the latter agents adjusted on the basis of frequent prothrombin time determinations. In infants, excessive doses of thyroid hormone preparations may produce craniosynostosis.

Information for the Patient: Patients on thyroid hormone preparations and parents of children on thyroid therapy should be informed that:

1. Replacement therapy is to be taken essentially for life, with the exception of cases of transient hypothyroidism, usually associated with thyroiditis, and in those patients receiving a therapeutic trial of the drug.

2. They should immediately report during the course of therapy any signs or symptoms of thyroid hormone toxicity, e.g., chest pain, increased pulse rate, palpitations, excessive sweating, heat intolerance, nervousness, or any other unusual event.

3. In case of concomitant diabetes mellitus, the daily dosage of antidiabetic medication may need readjustment as thyroid hormone replacement is achieved. If thyroid medication is stopped, a downward readjustment of the dosage of insulin or oral hypoglycemic agent may be necessary to avoid hypoglycemia. At all times, close monitoring of urinary glucose levels is mandatory in such patients.

4. In case of concomitant oral anticoagulant therapy, the prothrombin time should be measured frequently to determine if the dosage of oral anticoagulants is to be readjusted.

5. Partial loss of hair may be experienced by children in the first few months of thyroid therapy, but this is usually a transient phenomenon and later recovery is usually the rule.

Laboratory Tests: Treatment of patients with thyroid hormones requires the periodic assessment of thyroid status by means of appropriate laboratory tests besides the full clinical evaluation. The TSH suppression test can be used to test the effectiveness of any thyroid preparation bearing in mind the relative insensitivity of the infant pituitary to the negative feedback effect of thyroid hormones. Serum T_4 levels can be used to test the effectiveness of all thyroid medications except T_3. When the total serum T_4 is low but TSH is normal, a test specific to assess unbound (free) T_4 levels is warranted. Specific measurements of T_4 and T_3 by competitive protein binding or radioimmunoassay are not influenced by blood levels of organic or inorganic iodine.

Drug Interactions: Oral Anticoagulants: Thyroid hormones appear to increase catabolism of vitamin K-dependent clotting factors. If oral anticoagulants are also being given, compensatory increases in clotting factor synthesis are impaired. Patients stabilized on oral anticoagulants who are found to require thyroid replacement therapy should be watched very closely when thyroid is started. If a patient is truly hypothyroid, it is likely that a reduction in anticoagulant dosage will be required. No special precautions appear to be necessary when oral anticoagulant therapy is begun in a patient already stabilized on maintenance thyroid replacement therapy.

Insulin or Oral Hypoglycemics: Initiating thyroid replacement therapy may cause increases in insulin or oral hypoglycemic requirements. The effects seen are poorly understood and depend upon a variety of factors such as dose and type of thyroid preparations and endocrine status of the patient. Patients receiving insulin or oral hypoglycemics should be closely watched during initiation of thyroid replacement therapy.

Cholestyramine or Colestipol: Cholestyramine or colestipol binds both levothyroxine (T_4) and liothyronine (T_3) in the intestine, thus impairing absorption of these thyroid hormones. *In vitro* studies indicate that the binding is not easily removed. Therefore, four to five hours should elapse between administration of cholestyramine or colestipol and thyroid hormones.

Estrogen, Oral Contraceptives: Estrogens tend to increase serum thyroxine-binding globulin (TBg). In a patient with a nonfunctioning thyroid gland who is receiving thyroid replacement therapy, free levothyroxine (T_4) may be decreased when estrogens are started thus increasing thyroid requirements. However, if the patient's thyroid gland has sufficient function, the decreased free levothyroxine (T_4) will result in a compensatory increase in levothyroxine (T_4) output by the thyroid. Therefore, patients without a functioning thyroid gland who are on thyroid replacement therapy may need to increase their thyroid dose if estrogens or estrogen-containing oral contraceptives are given.

Drug/Laboratory Test Interactions: The following drugs or moieties are known to interfere with laboratory tests performed in patients on thyroid hormone therapy: androgens, corticosteroids, estrogens, oral contraceptives containing estrogens, iodine-containing preparations, and the numerous preparations containing salicylates.

1. Changes in TBg concentration should be taken into consideration in the interpretation of levothyroxine (T_4) and liothyronine (T_3) values. In such cases, the unbound (free) hormone should be measured. Pregnancy, estrogens, and estrogen-containing oral contraceptives increase TBg concentrations. TBg may also be increased during infectious hepatitis. Decreases in TBg concentrations are observed in nephrosis, acromegaly, and after androgen or corticosteroid therapy. Familial hyper- or hypothyroxine-binding-globulinemias have been described. The incidence of TBg deficiency approximates 1 in 9,000. The binding of levothyroxine by TBPA is inhibited by salicylates.

2. Medicinal or dietary iodine interferes with all *in vivo* tests of radio-iodine uptake, producing low uptakes which may not be relative of a true decrease in hormone synthesis.

3. The persistence of clinical and laboratory evidence of hypothyroidism in spite of adequate dosage replacement indicates either poor patient compliance, poor absorption, excessive fecal loss, or inactivity of the preparation. Intracellular resistance to thyroid hormone is quite rare.

Carcinogenesis, Mutagenesis, and Impairment of Fertility: A reportedly apparent association between prolonged thyroid therapy and breast cancer has not been confirmed and patients on thyroid for established indications should not discontinue therapy. No confirmatory long-term studies in animals have been performed to evaluate carcinogenic potential, mutagenicity, or impairment of fertility in either males or females.

Pregnancy-Category A: Thyroid hormones do not readily cross the placental barrier. The clinical experience to date does not indicate any adverse effect on fetuses when thyroid hormones are administered to pregnant women. On the basis of current knowledge, thyroid replacement therapy to hypothyroid women should not be discontinued during pregnancy.

Nursing Mothers: Minimal amounts of thyroid hormones are excreted in human milk. Thyroid is not associated with serious adverse reactions and does not have a known tumorigenic potential. However, caution should be exercised when thyroid is administered to a nursing woman.

Pediatric Use: Pregnant mothers provide little or no thyroid hormone to the fetus. The incidence of congenital hypothyroidism is relatively high (1:4,000) and the hypothyroid fetus would not derive any benefit from the small amounts of hormone crossing the placental barrier. Routine determinations or serum T_4 and/or TSH is strongly advised in neonates in view of the deleterious effects of thyroid deficiency on growth and development.

Treatment should be initiated immediately upon diagnosis, and maintained for life, unless transient hypothyroidism is suspected; in which case, therapy may be interrupted for 2 to 8 weeks after the age of 3 years to reassess the condition. Cessation of therapy is justified in patients who have maintained a normal TSH during those 2 to 8 weeks.

ADVERSE REACTIONS

Adverse reactions other than those indicative of hyperthyroidism because of therapeutic overdosage, either initially or during the maintenance period, are rare (see *"Overdosage"*).

OVERDOSAGE

Signs and Symptoms: Excessive doses of thyroid result in a hypermetabolic state resembling in every respect the condition of endogenous origin. The condition may be self-induced.

Overdosage may cause tachycardia, angina pectoris, diarrhea, nervousness, sweating, headache and increased pulse action. In most cases, reduction of dosage overcomes side effects.

Treatment of Overdosage: Dosage should be reduced or therapy temporarily discontinued if signs and symptoms of overdosage appear.

Treatment may be reinstituted at a lower dosage. In normal individuals, normal hypothalamic-pituitary-thyroid axis function is restored in 6 to 8 weeks after thyroid suppression.

Treatment of acute massive thyroid hormone overdosage is aimed at reducing gastrointestinal absorption of the drugs and counteracting central and peripheral effects, mainly those of increased sympathetic activity. Vomiting may be induced initially if further gastrointestinal absorption can reasonably be prevented and barring contraindications such as coma, convulsions, or loss of the gagging reflex. Treatment is symptomatic and supportive. Oxygen may be administered and ventilation maintained. Cardiac glycosides may be indicated if congestive heart failure develops. Measures to control fever, hypoglycemia, or fluid loss should be instituted if needed. Antiadrenergic agents, particularly propranolol, have been used advantageously in the treatment of increased sympathetic activity. Propranolol may be administered intravenously at a dosage of 1 to 3 mg, over a 10-minute period or orally, 80 to 160 mg/day, initially, especially when no contraindications exist for its use.

Other adjunctive measures may include administration of cholestyramine to interfere with thyroxine absorption, and glucocorticoids to inhibit conversion of T_4 to T_3.

DOSAGE AND ADMINISTRATION

The dosage of thyroid hormones is determined by the indication and must in every case be individualized according to patient response and laboratory findings.

Thyroid hormones are given orally. In acute, emergency conditions, injectable levothyroxine sodium (T_4) may be given intravenously when oral administration is not feasible or desirable, as in the treatment of myxedema coma, or during total parenteral nutrition. Intramuscular administration is not advisable because of reported poor absorption.

Hypothyroidism: Therapy is usually instituted using low doses, with increments which depend on the cardiovascular status of the patient. The usual starting dose is 30 mg Thyroid, with increments of 15 mg every 2 to 3 weeks. A lower starting dosage, 15 mg/day, is recommended in patients with long-standing myxedema, particularly if cardiovascular impairment is suspected, in which case extreme caution is recommended. The appearance of angina is an indication for a reduction in dosage. Most patients require 60 to 120 mg/day. Failure to respond to doses of 180 mg suggests lack of compliance or malabsorption. Maintenance dosages 60 to 120 mg/day usually result in normal serum T_4 and T_3 levels. Adequate therapy usually results in normal TSH and T_4 levels after 2 to 3 weeks of therapy.

Readjustment of thyroid hormone dosage should be made within the first four weeks of therapy, after proper clinical and laboratory evaluations, including serum levels of T_4, bound and free, and TSH.

Liothyronine (T_3) may be used in preference to levothyroxine (T_4) during radio-isotope scanning procedures, since induction of hypothyroidism in those cases is more abrupt and can be of shorter duration. It may also be preferred when impairment of peripheral conversion of levothyroxine (T_4) and liothyronine (T_3) is suspected.

Myxedema Coma: Myxedema coma is usually precipitated in the hypothyroid patient of long-standing by intercurrent illness or drugs such as sedatives and anesthetics and should be considered a medical emergency. Therapy should be directed at the correction of electrolyte disturbances and possible infection besides the administration of thyroid hormones. Corticosteroids should be administered routinely. Levothyroxine (T_4) and liothyronine (T_3) may be administered via a nasogastric tube but the preferred route of administration of both hormones is intravenous. Levothyroxine sodium (T_4) is given at a starting dose of 400 mcg (100 mcg/mL) given rapidly, and is usually well tolerated, even in the elderly. This initial dose is followed by daily supplements of 100 to 200 mcg given IV. Normal T_4 levels are achieved in 24 hours followed in 3 days by threefold elevation of T_3. Oral therapy with thyroid hormone would be resumed as soon as the clinical situation has been stabilized and the patient is able to take oral medication.

Thyroid Cancer: Exogenous thyroid hormone may produce regression of metastases from follicular and papillary carcinoma of the thyroid and is used as ancillary therapy of these conditions with radioactive iodine. TSH should be suppressed to low or undetectable levels. Therefore, larger amounts of thyroid hormone than those used for replacement therapy are required. Medullary carcinoma of the thyroid is usually unresponsive to this therapy.

Thyroid Suppression Therapy: Administration of thyroid hormone in doses higher than those produced physiologically by the gland results in suppression of the production of endogenous hormone. This is the basis for the thyroid suppression test and is used as an aid in the diagnosis of patients with signs of mild hyperthyroidism in whom base line laboratory tests appear normal, or to demonstrate thyroid gland autonomy in patients with Grave's ophthalmopathy. ^{131}I uptake is determined before and after the administration of the exogenous hormone. A 50 percent or greater suppression of uptake indicates a normal thyroid-pituitary axis and thus rules out thyroid gland autonomy.

For adults, the usual suppressive dose of levothyroxine (T_4) is 1.56 mg/kg of body weight per day given for 7 to 10 days. These doses usually yield normal serum T_4 and T_3 levels and lack of response to TSH.

Thyroid hormones should be administered cautiously to patients in whom there is strong suspicion of thyroid gland autonomy. In view of the fact that the exogenous hormone effects will be additive to the endogenous source.

Pediatric Dosage: Pediatric dosage should follow the recommendations summarized in Table 1. In infants with congenital hypothyroidism, therapy with full doses should be instituted as soon as the diagnosis has been made.

RECOMMENDED PEDIATRIC DOSAGE FOR CONGENITAL HYPOTHYROIDISM

Age	Dose per day	Daily dose per kg of body weight
0-6 mos	15-30 mg	4.8-6 mg
6-12 mos	30-45 mg	3.6-4.8 mg
1-5 yrs	45-60 mg	3-3.6 mg
6-12 yrs	60-90 mg	2.4-3 mg
Over 12 yrs	Over 90 mg	1.2-1.8 mg

Note: T_3 liothyronine is approximately four times as potent as T_4 levothyroxine on a microgram for microgram basis.

STORAGE
Tablets should be stored at controlled room temperature, 59°–86°F (15°-30°C), in capped bottles or unbroken plastic strip packing.

HOW SUPPLIED
TABLET: 15 MG

BRAND/MANUFACTURER	NDC	SIZE	AWP
○ **BRAND**			
▶ ARMOUR THYROID: Forest Pharm	00456-0457-01	100s	$7.50

TABLET: 30 MG

BRAND/MANUFACTURER	NDC	SIZE	AWP
○ **BRAND**			
▶ ARMOUR THYROID: Forest Pharm	00456-0458-01	100s	$8.77
	00456-0458-63	100s ud	$15.42
	00456-0458-00	1000s	$70.14
○ **GENERICS**			
Major	00904-7865-60	100s	$4.50
Norton,HN	50732-0685-01	100s	$7.50
Time-Cap	49483-0021-01	100s	$7.60
Moore,H.L.	00839-7931-06	100s	$8.36
Jones Medical	52604-0686-01	100s	$10.50
Jones Medical	52604-0626-01	100s	$10.85
Veratex	17022-8622-06	1000s	$7.50
Rugby	00536-4694-10	1000s	$9.13
URL	00677-0150-10	1000s	$11.65
Qualitest	00603-6045-32	1000s	$12.35
Major	00904-7865-80	1000s	$13.45
Jones Medical	52604-0776-02	1000s	$15.10

▶ SHOWN IN PRODUCT IDENTIFICATION GUIDE

BRAND/MANUFACTURER	NDC	SIZE	AWP
Truxton	00463-6199-10	1000s	$16.80
WESTHROID: Jones-Western	52604-7070-02	1000s	$18.08
Norton,HN	50732-0685-10	1000s	$34.51
Time-Cap	49483-0021-10	1000s	$34.70
Moore,H.L.	00839-7931-16	1000s	$38.14
Jones Medical	52604-0686-02	1000s	$93.70
WESTHROID: Jones-Western	52604-7070-08	1008s	$18.84

For additional alternatives, turn to the section beginning on page 2859.

Thyrolar SEE LIOTRIX

Thyrotropin

DESCRIPTION
Thyrotropin is a highly purified and lyophilized thyrotropic or thyroid stimulating hormone (TSH) isolated from bovine anterior pituitary. The potency of Thyrotropin is designated in terms of international Thyrotropin units and is free of significant amounts of adreno-corticotropic, gonadotropic, somatotropic and posterior pituitary hormones. It is soluble throughout a wide pH range and is stable at room temperature when kept in the dry state. It dissolves readily in physiologic saline and will retain its potency when in solution for at least two weeks if refrigerated.

It is a sterile preparation for intramuscular or subcutaneous use only. It is a glyco-protein with a molecular weight in the range of 28,000 - 30,000.

CLINICAL PHARMACOLOGY
The action of Thyrotropin produces increased uptake of iodine by the thyroid, increased formation of thyroid hormone, increased release of thyroid hormone, and cellular hyperplasia of the thyroid on prolonged stimulation.

After injection, the effect on the thyroid in normal individuals is evident within 8 hours reaching a maximum in 24-48 hours.

INDICATIONS AND USAGE
Thyrotropin is indicated for use as a diagnostic agent. It is used to differentiate thyroid failure from pituitary failure and to establish a diagnosis of decreased thyroid reserve.

CONTRAINDICATIONS
1. Hypersensitivity to Thyrotropin
2. Coronary thrombosis
3. Untreated Addison's disease

WARNINGS
Anaphylactic reactions have been reported on repeated administration.

PRECAUTIONS
General: Since Thyrotropin can stimulate thyroid secretion, caution must be observed when using in patients with cardiac disease who are unable to tolerate additional stress.

Drug Interactions: Thyrotropin can be used with PBI or I^{131} uptake determinations.

Pregnancy Category C: Animal reproduction studies have not been conducted with Thyrotropin. It is also not known whether Thyrotropin can cause fetal harm when administered to a pregnant woman or can affect reproduction capacity. Thyrotropin should be given to a pregnant woman only if clearly needed.

Nursing Mothers: It is not known whether this drug is excreted in human milk. Because many drugs are excreted in human milk, caution should be exercised when Thyrotropin is administered to a nursing woman.

Pediatric Use: Safety and effectiveness in children have not been established.

ADVERSE REACTIONS
Nausea, vomiting, headache, and urticaria are the most commonly seen reactions. Also seen and probably related to a sensitivity type reaction is transitory hypotension and tachycardia. Anaphylactic reactions with patient collapse have been reported.

Thyroid gland swelling has been reported particularly with larger doses (> 10μ).

DRUG ABUSE AND DEPENDENCE
Drug abuse and dependence have not been reported.

OVERDOSAGE
Symptoms: Headache, irritability, nervousness, sweating, tachycardia, increased bowel mobility, menstrual irregularities. Angina pectoris or congestive heart failure may be induced or aggravated. Shock may also develop. Excessive doses may result in symptoms resembling thyroid storm. Chronic excessive dosage will produce the signs and symptoms of hyperthyroidism.

Treatment: In shock, supportive measures and treatment of unrecognized adrenal insufficiency should be considered. Thyrotropin is discontinued.

DOSAGE AND ADMINISTRATION
Thyrotropin is injected intramuscularly or subcutaneously in a dose of 10 IU for 1 to 3 days followed by a radioiodine uptake study 24 hours after the last injection. In thyroid failure, no response will be seen; in pituitary failure, a substantial response should be seen.

Parenteral drug products should be inspected visually for particulate matter and discoloration prior to administration whenever solution and container permit.

Thyrotropin should be stored at controlled room temperature, 15°-30°C (59°-86°F). After reconstitution store between 2°-8°C (36°-46°F), for not longer than two weeks.

J CODES
Up to 10 IU IM, SC—J3240

HOW SUPPLIED
POWDER FOR INJECTION: 10 IU

BRAND/MANUFACTURER	NDC	SIZE	AWP
○ BRAND			
THYTROPAR: RPR	00075-3610-01	1s	$193.98

Thytropar SEE THYROTROPIN

Ticar SEE TICARCILLIN DISODIUM

Ticarcillin Disodium

DESCRIPTION
Ticarcillin Disodium is a semisynthetic injectable penicillin derived from the penicillin nucleus, 6-aminopenicillanic acid. Chemically, it is N-(2-Carboxy-3,3-dimethyl-7-oxo-4-thia-1-azabicyclo [3.2.0]hept-6-yl)-3-thiophenemaloamic acid disodium salt.

It is supplied as a white to pale yellow powder for reconstitution. The reconstituted solution is clear, colorless or pale yellow, having a pH of 6.0 to 8.0. Ticarcillin is very soluble in water; its solubility is greater than 600 mg/mL.

Following is its chemical structure:

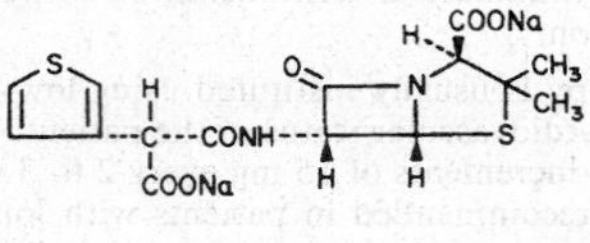

ACTIONS
PHARMACOLOGY
Ticarcillin is not absorbed orally; therefore, it must be given intravenously or intramuscularly. Following intramuscular administration, peak serum concentrations occur within ½ to 1 hour. Somewhat higher and more prolonged serum levels can be achieved with the concurrent administration of probenecid.

The minimum inhibitory concentrations (MICs) for many strains of *Pseudomonas* are relatively high by usual standards; serum levels of 60 mcg/mL or greater are required. However, the low degree of toxicity of Ticarcillin permits the use of doses large enough to achieve inhibitory levels for these strains in serum or tissues. Other susceptible organisms usually require serum levels in the 10 to 25 mcg/mL range. (See related table).

As with other pencillins, Ticarcillin is eliminated by glomerular filtration and tubular secretion. It is not highly bound to serum protein (approximately 45%) and is excreted unchanged in high concentrations in the urine. After the administration of a 1 to 2 gram IM dose, a urine concentration of 2000 to 4000

---

mcg/mL may be obtained in patients with normal renal function. The serum half-life of Ticarcillin in normal individuals is approximately 70 minutes.

An inverse relationship exists between serum half-life and creatinine clearance, but the dosage of Ticarcillin Disodium need only be adjusted in cases of severe renal impairment (see *"Dosage And Administration"*). The administered Ticarcillin Disodium may be removed from patients undergoing dialysis; the actual amount removed depends on the duration and type of dialysis.

Ticarcillin can be detected in tissues and interstitial fluid following parental administration. Penetration into the cerebrospinal fluid, bile and pleural fluid has been demonstrated.

MICROBIOLOGY

Ticarcillin is bactericidal and demonstrates substaintial *in vitro* activity against both gram-positive and gram-negative organisms. Many strains of the following organisms were found to be susceptible to Ticarcillin *in vitro*:

Pseudomonas aeruginosa (and other species)
Escherichia coli
Proteus mirabilis
Morganella morganii (formerly Proteus morganii)
Providencia rettgeri (formerly Proteus rettgeri)
Proteus vulgaris
Enterobacter species
Haemophilus influenzae
Neisseria species
Salmonella species
Staphylococcus aureus (non-penicillinase producing)
Staphylococcus epidermidis
Beta-hemolytic streptococci (Group A)
Streptococcus faecalis (Entercoccus)
Streptococcus pneumoniae
Anaerobic bacteria, including:
Bacteroides species including *B. fragilis*
Fusobacterium species
Veillonella species
Clostridium species
Eubacterium species
Peptococcus species
Peptostreptococcus species

In vitro synergism between Ticarcillin and gentamicin sulfate, tobramycin sulfate or amikacin sulfate against certain strains of *Pseudomonas aeruginosa* has been demonstrated.

Some strains of such microorganisms as *Mima-Herellea (Acinetobacter)*, *Citrobacter* and *Serratia* have shown susceptibility.

Ticarcillin is not stable in the presence of penicillinase.

Some strains of *Pseudomonas* have developed resistance fairly rapidly.

DISK SUSCEPTIBILITY TESTS
Susceptibility Tests: Ticarcillin disks or powders should be used for testing susceptibility to Ticarcillin. However, organisms reportedly susceptible to carbenicillin are susceptible to Ticarcillin.

Diffusion Techniques: For the disk diffusion method of susceptibility testing a 75 mcg Ticarcillin disk should be used. The method for the this test is the one outlined in NCCLS publication M2-A3[*] with the following interpretative criteria:

Culture	Susceptible	Intermediate	Resistant
P. aeruginosa and *Enterobacteriaceae*	≥ 15 mm	12 to 14 mm	≤ 11 mm
The MIC correlates are:	Resistant > 128 mcg/mL		
	Susceptible ≤ 64 mcg/mL		

Dilution Techniques: Dilution techniques for determining the MIC (minimum inhibitory concentration) are published by NCCLS for the broth and agar dilution procedures. The MIC data should be interpreted in light of the concentrations present in serum, tissue and body fluids. Organisms with MIC ≤ 64 are considered susceptible when they are in tissue but organisms with MIC ≤ 128 would be susceptible in urine where the Ticarcillin Disodium concentrations are

[*] Performance Standards for Antimicrobial Disc Susceptibility Tests, National Committee for Clinical Laboratory Standards, Vol. 4, No. 16, pp. 369-402, 1984.

much greater. At present, only dilution methods can be recommended for testing antibiotic susceptibility of obligate anaerobes.

Susceptibility testing methods require the use of control organisms. The 75 mcg Ticarcillin; disk should give zone diameters between 22 and 28 mm for *P. aeruginosa* ATCC 27853 and 24 and 30 mm for *E. coli* ATCC 25922. Reference strains are available for dilution testing of Ticarcillin; 95% of the MICs should fall within the following MIC ranges and the majority of MICs should be at values close to the center of the pertinent range (reference NCCLS publication M7-A[†]).

S. aureus ATCC 29213, 2.0 to 8.0 mcg/mL; *S. faecalis* ATCC 29212, 16 to 64 mcg/mL; *E. coli* ATCC 25922, 2.0 to 8.0 mcg/mL; *P. aeruginosa* ATCC 27853, 8.0 to 32 mcg/mL.

INDICATIONS
Ticarcillin Disodium is indicated for the treatment of the following infections:
    Bacterial septicemia‡
    Skin and soft-tissue infections‡
    Acute and chronic respiratory tract infections‡§
Genitourinary tract infections (complicated and uncomplicated) due to susceptible strains of *Pseudomonas aeruginosa, Proteus* species (both indole-positive and indole-negative), *Escherichia coli, Enterobacter* and *Streptococcus faecalis* (enterococcus).

Ticarcillin is also indicated in the treatment of the following infections due to susceptible anaerobic bacteria:
1. Bacterial septicemia.
2. Lower respiratory tract infections such as empyema, anaerobic pneumonitis and lung abscess.
3. Intra-abdominal infections such as peritonitis and intra-abdominal abscess (typically resulting from anaerobic organisms resident in the normal gastrointestinal tract).
4. Infections of the female pelvis and genital tract, such as endometritis, pelvic inflammatory disease, pelvic abscess and salpingitis.
5. Skin and soft-tissue infections.

Although Ticarcillin is primarily indicated in gram-negative infections, its *in vitro* activity against gram-positive organisms should be considered in treating infections caused by both gram-negative and gram-positive organisms (see Microbiology).

Based on the *in vitro* synergism between Ticarcillin, and gentamicin sulfate, tobramycin sulfate or amikacin sulfate against certain strains of *Pseudomonas aeruginosa*, combined therapy has been successful, using full therapeutic dosages. (For additional prescribing information, see the gentamicin sulfate, tobramycin sulfate and amikacin sulfate package inserts.)

Note: Culturing and susceptibility testing should be performed initially and during treatment to monitor the effectiveness of therapy and the susceptibility of the bacteria.

CONTRAINDICATIONS
A history of allergic reaction to any of the pencicllins is a contraindication.

WARNINGS
Serious and occasionally fatal hypersensitivity (anaphylactoid) reactions have been reported in patients receiving penicillin. These reactions are more likely to occur in persons with a history of sensitivity to multiple allergens.

There are reports of patients with a history of penicillin hypersensitivity reactions who experience severe hypersensitivity reactions when treated with a cephalosporin. Before therapy with a penicillin, carefully inquiry should be made about previous hypersensitivity reactions to penicillins, cephalosporins and other allergens. If a reaction occurs, the drug should be discontinued unless, in the opinion of the physician, the condition being treated is life-threatening and amenable only to Ticarcillin therapy. **Serious anaphylactoid reactions require immediate emergency treatment with epinephrine. Oxygen, intravenous steroids and airway management, including intubation, should also be administered as indicated.**

Some patients receiving high doses of Ticarcillin may develop hemorrhagic manifestations associated with abnormalities of coagulation tests, such as bleeding time and platelet aggregation. On withdrawal of the drug, the bleeding

† Methods for Dilution Antimicrobial Susceptibility Tests for Bacteria That Grow Aerobically, Vol. 5, No. 22, pp. 579-618, 1985.
‡ Caused by susceptible strains of *Pseudomonas aeruginosa, Proteus* species (both indole-positive and indole-negative) and *Escherichia coli*.
§ Though clinical improvement has been shown, bacteriological cures cannot be expected in patients with chronic respiratory disease or cystic fibrosis.

TICARCILLIN SERUM LEVELS

Dosage	Route	1/4 hr.	1/2 hr.	1 hr.	2hr.	3 hr.	4 hr.	6 hr.
				mcg/mL				
Adults:								
500 mg	I.M.	-	7.7	8.6	6.0	4.0	-	2.9
1 gram	I.M.	-	31.0	18.7	15.7	9.7	-	3.4
2 grams	I.M.	-	63.6	39.7	32.3	18.9	-	3.4
3 grams	I.V. -	190.0	140.0	107.0	52.2	31.3	13.8	4.2
5 grams	I.V.	327.0	28.0	175.0	106.0	63.0	28.5	9.6
3 grams + I.V. gram probenecid	Oral	223.0	166.0	123.0	78.0	54.0	35.4	17.1

		½ hr.	1 hr.	1 ½ hr.	2 hr.	4 hr.	8 hr.	
Neonates:								
50 mg/kg	I.M.	64.0	70.7	63.7	60.1	33.2	11.6	

should cease and coagulation abnormalities revert to normal. Other causes of abnormal bleeding should also be considered. Patients with renal impairment, in whom excretion of Ticarcillin is delayed, should be observed for bleeding manifestations. Such patients should be dosed strictly according to recommendations (see *"Dosage and Administration"*). If bleeding manifestations appear, Ticarcillin treatment should be discontinued and appropriate therapy instituted.

Pseudomembraneous colitis has been reported with nearly all antibacterial agents, including Ticarcillin Disodium and has ranged in severity from mild to life-threatening. Therefore, it is important to consider this diagnosis in patients who present with diarrhea subsequent to the administration of antibacterial agents.

Treatment with antibacterial agents alters the normal flora of the colon and may permit overgrowth of clostridia. Studies indicate that a toxin produced by *Clostridium difficile* is one primary cause of "antibiotic-associated colitis."

Mild cases of pseudomembranous colitis usually respond to drug discontinuation alone. In moderate to severe cases, consideration should be given to management with fluids and electrolytes, protein supplementation and treatment with an antibacterial drug effective against *C. difficile*.

PRECAUTIONS

Although *Ticarcillin Disodium* exhibits the characteristic low toxicity of the penicillins, as with any other potent agent, it is advisable to check periodically for organ system dysfunction (including renal, hepatic and hematopoietic) during prolonged treatment. If overgrowth of resistant organisms occurs, the appropriate therapy should be initiated.

Since the theoretical sodium content is 5.2 mEq (120 mg) per gram of Ticarcillin and the actual vial content can be as high as 6.5 mEq/gram, electrolyte and cardiac status should be monitored carefully.

In a few patients receiving intravenous Ticarcillin, hypokalemia has been reported. Serum potassium should be measured periodically, and, if necessary, corrective therapy should be implemented.

As with any penicillin, the possibility of an allergic response, including anaphylaxis, exists, particularly in hypersensitive patients.

USAGE DURING PREGNANCY

Reproduction studies have been performed in mice and rats and have revealed no evidence of impaired fertility or harm to the fetus due to Ticarcillin. There are no well-controlled studies in pregnant women, but investigational experience does not include any positive evidence of adverse effects on the fetus. Although there is no clearly defined risk, such experience cannot exclude the possibility of infrequent or subtle damage to the fetus. Ticarcillin should be used in pregnant women only when clearly needed.

ADVERSE REACTIONS

The following adverse reactions may occur:

Hypersensitivity Reactions: Skin rashes, pruritus, urticaria, drug fever.

Gastrointestinal Disturbances: Nausea and vomiting, pseudomembranous colitis. Onset of pseudomembranous colitis symptoms may occur during or after antibiotic treatment. (See *"Warnings"*).

Hemic and Lymphatic Systems: As with other penicillins, anemia, thrombocytopenia, leukopenia, neutropenia and eosinophilia.

Abnormalities of Blood, Hepatic and Renal Laboratory Studies: As with other semisynthetic penicillins, SGOT and SGPT elevations have been reported. To date, clinical manifestations of hepatic or renal disorders have not been observed which could be ascribed solely to Ticarcillin.

CNS: Patients, especially those with impaired renal function, may experience convulsions or neuromuscular excitability when very high doses of the drug are administered.

Other: Local reactions such as pain (rarely accompanied by induration) at the site of the injection have been reported. Vein irritation and phlebitis can occur, particularly when undiluted solution is directly injected into the vein.

DOSAGE AND ADMINISTRATION

Clinical experience indicates that in serious urinary tract and systemic infections, intravenous therapy in the higher doses should be used. Intramuscular injections should not exceed 2 grams per injection. (See related table).

CHILDREN UNDER 40 KG (88 LBS)

The daily dose for children should not exceed the adult dosage.

Bacterial septicemia Respiratory tract infections Skin and soft-tissue infections Intra-abdominal infections Infections of the female pelvis and genital tract	200 to 300 mg/kg/day by I.V. infusion in divided doses every 4 or 6 hours.
Urinary tract infections Complicated:	150 to 200 mg/kg/day by I.V. infusion in divided doses every 4 or 6 hours.
Uncomplicated:	50 to 100 mg/kg/day I.M. or direct I.V. in divided doses every 6 or 8 hours.
Infections complicated by renal insufficiency:	Clinical data are insufficient to recommended an optimum dose.

Children weighing more than 40 kg (88 lbs) should receive adult dosages.

NEONATES

In the neonate, for severe infections (sepsis) due to susceptible strains of Pseudomonas, Proteus and E. coli, the following Ticarcillin Disodium dosages may be given I.M. or by 10 to 20 minute I.V. infusion:

Infants under 2000 grams body weight:	Infants over 2000 grams body weight:
Aged 0 to 7 days 75 mg/kg/12 hours (150 mg/kg/day)	Aged 0 to 7 days 75 mg/kg/8 hours (225 mg/kg/day)
Aged over 7 days 75 mg/kg/8 hours (225 mg/kg/day)	Aged over 7 days 100 mg/kg/8 hours (300 mg/kg/day)

This dosage schedule is intended to produce peak serum concentrations of 125 to 150 mcg/mL 1 hour after a dose of Ticarcillin; and trough concentrations of 25 to 50 mcg/mL immediately before the next dose.

Note: Gentamicin, tobramycin or amikacin may be used concurrently with Ticarcillin Disodium for initial therapy until results of culture and susceptibility studies are known.

Seriously ill patients should receive the higher doses. Ticarcillin Disodium has proved to be useful in infections in which protective mechanisms are impaired, such as in acute leukemia and during therapy with immunosuppressive or oncolytic drugs.

DIRECTIONS FOR USE

1 gram, 3 gram and 6 gram Standard Vials

Intramuscular Use: (concentration of approximately 385 mg/mL): For initial reconstitution use Sterile Water for Injection, USP, Sodium Chloride Injection, USP, or 1% Lidocaine Hydrochloride solution‡ (without epinephrine).

Each gram of Ticarcillin Disodium should be reconstituted with 2 mL of Sterile Water for Injection, USP, Sodium Chloride Injection, USP, or 1% Lidocaine Hydrochloride solution‡ (without epinephrine) and **used promptly.** Each 2.6 mL of the resulting solution will then contain 1 gram of Ticarcillin Disodium.

Only the 1 gram vial should be used for intramuscular administration: As with all intramuscular preparations, (Ticarcillin Disodium) should be injected well within the body of a relatively large muscle using usual techniques and precautions.

Intravenous Administration: (concentration of approximately 200 mg/mL): For initial reconstitution use Sodium Chloride Injection, USP, Dextrose Injection 5% or Lactated Ringer's Injection.

Reconstitute each gram of Ticarcillin Disodium with 4 mL of the appropriate diluent. After the addition of 4 mL of diluent per gram of Ticarcillin Disodium, each 1.0 mL of the resulting solution will have an approximate concentration of 200 mg. Once dissolved, further dilute if desired.

Direct Intravenous Injection: In order to avoid vein irritation, administer solution as slowly as possible.

Intravenous Infusion: Administer by continuous or intermittent intravenous drip. Intermittent infusion should be administered over a 30 minute to 2-hour period in equally divided doses.

3 gram Piggyback Bottle Intravenous Infusion: (concentrations of approximately 29 mg/mL to 100 mg/mL): The 3 gram bottle should be reconstituted with a minimum of 30 mL of the desired intravenous solution listed below.

Amount of Diluent	Concentration of Solution
100 mL	1 gram/34 mL (~ 29 mg/mL)
60 mL	1 gram/20 mL (50 mg/mL)
30 mL	1 gram/10 mL (100 mg/mL)

In order to avoid vein irritation, the solution should be administered as slowly as possible. A dilution of approximately 50 mg/mL or more will further reduce the incidence of vein irritation.

Intravenous Infusion: Stability studies in the intravenous solutions listed below indicate that Ticarcillin Disodium will provide sufficient activity at room temperature 21° to 24°C (70° to 75°F) within the stated time periods at concentrations between 10 mg/mL and 50 mg/mL — see *Stability Period* section below.

After reconstitution and prior to administration Ticarcillin Disodium as with other parenteral drugs should be inspected visually for particulate matter and discoloration.

STABILITY PERIOD

Intravenous Solution (concentration of 10 mg/mL to 100 mg/mL)	Room Temperature 21° to 24°C (70° to 75°F)	Refrigeration 4°C (40°F)
Sodium Chloride Injection, USP	72 hours	14 days
Dextrose Injection 5%	72 hours	14 days
Lactated Ringer's Injection	48 hours	14 days

‡ For full product information, refer to manufacturer's package insert for Lidocaine Hydrochloride.

◆ RATED THERAPEUTICALLY EQUIVALENT; ◇ THERAPEUTIC EQUIVALENCE UNCONFIRMED; ○ UNRATED

ADULTS

Bacterial septicemia Respiratory tract infections Skin and soft-tissue infections Intra-abdominal infections Infections of the female pelvis and genital tract	200 to 300 mg/kg/day by I.V. infusion in divided doses every 4 or 6 hours. (The usual dose is 3 grams given every 4 hours [18 grams/day] or 4 grams given every 6 hours [16 grams/day] depending on weight and the severity of the infection.)

Urinary tract infections Complicated:	150 to 200 mg/kg/day by I.V. infusion in divided doses every 4 or 6 hours. (Usual recommended dosage for average [70 kg] adults: 3 grams q.i.d.)
Uncomplicated:	1 gram I.M. or direct I.V. every 6 hours.

Infections complicated by renal insufficiency*: Initial loading dose of 3 grams I.V. followed by I.V. doses, based on creatinine clearance and type of dialysis, as indicated below:

Creatinine clearance mL/min.:		
over 60	3 grams every 4 hours	To calculate creatinine clearance† from a serum creatinine value use the following formula:
30 to 60	2 grams every 4 hours	
10 to 30	2 grams every 8 hours	
less than 10	2 grams every 12 hours	$C_{cr}= \dfrac{(140-Age)(wt.\ in\ Kg)}{72 \times S_{cr}(mg/100\ mL)}$
less than 10	(or 1 gram I.M. every 6 hours)	This is the calculated creatinine clearance
with hepatic dysfunction	2 grams every 24 hours	for adult males; for females it is 15% less.
patients on peritoneal	(or 1 gram I.M. every 12 hours)	†Cockcroft, D.W., et al: Prediction of
dialysis	3 grams every 12 hours	Creatinine Clearance from Serum
patients on hemodialysis	2 grams every 12 hours	Creatinine. *Nephron* 16:31–41, 1976.
	supplemented with 3 grams after each dialysis	

* The half-life of Ticarcillin in patients with renal failure is approximately 13 hours.

Refrigerated solutions stored longer than 72 hours should *not* be used for multidose purposes.

After reconstitution and dilution to a concentration of 10 mg/mL to 100 mg/mL, this solution can be frozen — 18°C (0°F) and stored for up to 30 days. The thawed solution must be used within 24 hours.

Unused solutions should be discarded after the time periods mentioned above.

It is recommended that Ticarcillin Disodium and gentamicin sulfate, tobramycin sulfate or amikacin sulfate *not* be mixed together in the same I.V. solution due to the gradual inactivation of gentamicin sulfate tobramycin sulfate or amikacin sulfate under these circumstances. The therapeutic effect of Ticarcillin Disodium and these aminoglycoside drugs remains unimpaired when administered separately.

Storage: Store dry powder at room temperature or below.

HOW SUPPLIED
POWDER FOR INJECTION: 1 GM

BRAND/MANUFACTURER	NDC	SIZE	AWP
○ BRAND			
TICAR: Abbott Pharm	00029-6550-22	1s	$3.10

POWDER FOR INJECTION: 3 GM

BRAND/MANUFACTURER	NDC	SIZE	AWP
○ BRAND			
TICAR: Abbott Pharm	00029-6552-26	1s	$9.30
	00029-6552-40	1s	$9.60
	00029-6552-21	1s	$9.95

POWDER FOR INJECTION: 6 GM

BRAND/MANUFACTURER	NDC	SIZE	AWP
○ BRAND			
TICAR: Abbott Pharm	00029-6555-26	1s	$17.50

POWDER FOR INJECTION: 20 GM

BRAND/MANUFACTURER	NDC	SIZE	AWP
○ BRAND			
TICAR: Abbott Pharm	00029-6558-21	1s	$57.15

POWDER FOR INJECTION: 30 GM

BRAND/MANUFACTURER	NDC	SIZE	AWP
○ BRAND			
TICAR: Abbott Pharm	00029-6559-21	1s	$83.95

Tice BCG Vaccine *SEE BCG*

Ticlopidine Hydrochloride

DESCRIPTION
Ticlopidine Hydrochloride is a platelet aggregation inhibitor. Chemically it is 5-[(2-chlorophenyl)methyl]-4,5,6,7-tetrahydrothieno[3,2-c] pyridine hydrochloride.

Ticlopidine Hydrochloride is a white crystalline solid. It is freely soluble in water and self buffers to a pH of 3.6. It also dissolves freely in methanol, is sparingly soluble in methylene chloride and ethanol, slightly soluble in acetone, and insoluble in a buffer solution of pH 6.3. It has a molecular weight of 300.25.

Ticlopidine Hydrochloride tablets for oral administration are provided as white, oval, film coated, blue imprinted tablets containing 250 mg of Ticlopidine Hydrochloride.

Following is its chemical structure:

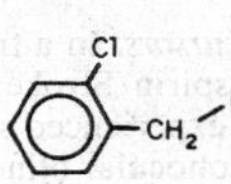

CLINICAL PHARMACOLOGY
MECHANISM OF ACTION
When taken orally Ticlopidine HCl causes a time and dose-dependent inhibition of both platelet aggregation and release of platelet granule constituents, as well as a prolongation of bleeding time. The intact drug has no significant *in vitro* activity at the concentrations attained *in vivo*, and, although analysis of urine and plasma indicates at least twenty metabolites, no metabolite which accounts for the activity of Ticlopidine HCl has been isolated.

Ticlopidine HCl, after oral ingestion, interferes with platelet membrane function by inhibiting ADP-induced platelet-fibrinogen binding and subsequent platelet-platelet interactions. The effect on platelet function is irreversible for the life of the platelet, as shown both by persistent inhibition of fibrinogen binding after washing platelets ex vivo and by inhibition of platelet aggregation after resuspension of platelets in buffered medium.

PHARMACOKINETICS AND METABOLISM
After oral administration of a single 250 mg dose, Ticlopidine HCl is rapidly absorbed, with peak plasma levels occurring at approximately 2 hours after dosing, and is extensively metabolized. Absorption is greater than 80%. Administration after meals results in a 20% increase in the AUC of Ticlopidine HCl.

Ticlopidine HCl displays non-linear pharmacokinetics and clearance decreases markedly on repeated dosing. In older volunteers the apparent half-life of Ticlopidine HCl after a single 250 mg dose is about 12.6 hours, with repeat dosing at 250 mg BID, the terminal elimination half-life rises to 4-5 days and steady state levels of Ticlopidine HCl in plasma are obtained after approximately 14-21 days.

Ticlopidine HCl binds reversibly (98%) to plasma proteins, mainly to serum albumin and lipoproteins. The binding to albumin and lipoproteins is nonsaturable over a wide concentration range. Ticlopidine HCl also binds to alpha-1 acid glycoprotein. At concentrations attained with the recommended dose, only 15% or less Ticlopidine HCl in plasma is bound to this protein.

Ticlopidine HCl is metabolized extensively by the liver; only trace amounts of intact drug are detected in the urine. Following an oral dose of radioactive Ticlopidine HCl administered in solution, 60% of the radioactivity is recovered in the urine and 23% in the feces. Approximately, ⅓ of the dose excreted in the feces is intact Ticlopidine HCl, possibly excreted in the bile. Ticlopidine HCl is a minor component in plasma (5%) after a single dose, but at steady state is the major component (15%). Approximately 40-50% of the radioactive metabolites circulating in plasma are covalently bound to plasma proteins, probably by acylation.

Clearance of Ticlopidine HCl decreases with age. Steady state trough values in elderly patients (mean age 70 years) are about twice those in young volunteer populations.

Hepatically Impaired Patients: The effect of decreased hepatic function on the pharmacokinetics of Ticlopidine HCl was studied in 17 patients with advanced cirrhosis. The average plasma concentration of Ticlopidine HCl in these subjects was slightly higher than that seen in older subjects in a separate trial. (See "Contraindications")

Renally Impaired Patients: Patients with mildly (Ccr 50-80 ml/min) or moderately (Ccr 20-50 ml/min) impaired renal function were compared to normal subjects (Ccr 80-150 ml/min) in a study of the pharmacokinetic and platelet pharmacodynamic effects of Ticlopidine HCl (250 mg BID) for 11 days. Concentrations of unchanged Ticlopidine HCl were measured after a single 250 mg dose and after the final 250 mg dose on Day 11. AUC values of Ticlopidine HCl increased by 28 and 60% in mild and moderately impaired patients respectively and plasma clearance decreased by 37 and 52% respectively, but there were no statistically significant differences in ADP-induced platelet aggregation. In this small study (26 patients) bleeding times showed significant prolongation only in the moderately impaired patients.

PHARMACODYNAMICS
In healthy volunteers over the age of 50 substantial inhibition (over 50%) of ADP-induced platelet aggregation is detected within 4 days after administration of Ticlopidine HCl 250 mg BID and maximum platelet aggregation inhibition (60-70%) is achieved after 8 to 11 days. Lower doses cause less, and more delayed, platelet aggregation inhibition, while doses above 250 mg BID give little additional effect on platelet aggregation, but an increased rate of adverse effects. The dose of 250 mg BID is the only dose that has been evaluated in controlled clinical trials.

After discontinuation of Ticlopidine HCl, bleeding time and other platelet function tests return to normal within two weeks in the majority of patients.

At the recommended therapeutic dose (250 mg BID) Ticlopidine HCl has no known significant pharmacological actions in man other than inhibition of platelet function and prolongation of the bleeding time.

CLINICAL TRIALS
The effect of Ticlopidine HCl on the risk of stroke and cardiovascular events was studied in two multi-center randomized double-blind trials.

1. Study in patients experiencing stroke precursors: In a trial comparing Tichlopidine HCl and aspirin (The Ticlopidine Aspirin Stroke Study or TASS), 3069 patients (1987 men, 1082 women) who had experienced such stroke precursors as transient ischemic attack (TIA), transient monocular blindness (amaurosis fugax), reversible ischemic neurological deficit, or minor stroke were randomized to Ticlopidine HCl 250 mg BID or aspirin 650 mg BID. The study was designed to follow patients for at least 2 and up to 5 years.

Over the duration of the study Ticlopidine HCl significantly reduced the risk of fatal and nonfatal stroke by 24% (p = .011) from 18.1 to 13.8 per 100 patients followed for five years, compared to aspirin. During the first year, when the risk of stroke is greatest, the reduction in risk of stroke (fatal and nonfatal) compared to aspirin was 48%, the reduction was similar in men and women.

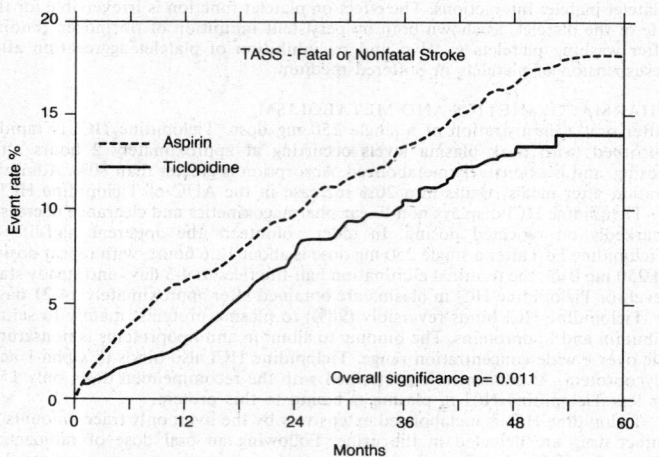

2. Study in patients who had a completed atherothrombotic stroke: In a trial comparing Ticlopidine HCl with placebo (The Canadian American Ticlopidine Study, or CATS) 1073 patients who had experienced a previous atherothrombotic stroke were treated with Ticlopidine HCl 250 mg BID or placebo for up to 3 years.

Ticlopidine HCl significantly reduced the overall risk of stroke by 24% (p = .017) from 24.6 to 18.6 per 100 patients followed for three years, compared to placebo. During the first year the reduction in risk of fatal and nonfatal stroke over placebo was 33%.

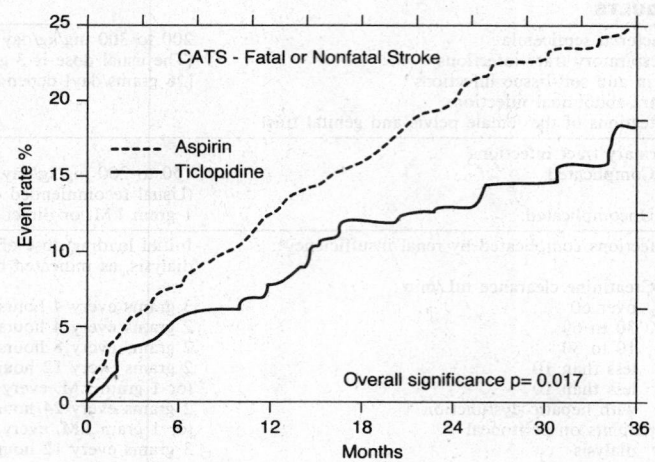

INDICATIONS AND USAGE
Ticlopidine HCl is indicated to reduce the risk of thrombotic stroke (fatal or nonfatal) in patients who have experienced stroke precursors, and in patients who have had a completed thrombotic stroke.

Because Ticlopidine HCl is associated with a risk of neutropenia/agranulocytosis, which may be life-threatening (see "Warnings"), Ticlopidine HCl should be reserved for patients who are intolerant to aspirin therapy where indicated to prevent stroke.

UNLABELED USES
Ticlopidine Hydrochloride is used alone or as an adjunct in the treatment of diabetic micrangiopathy, including diabetic nephropathy and diabetic retinopathy. It is also used to reduce infarct size after myocardial infarction, transient ischemic attacks, and in rheumatoid arthritis.

CONTRAINDICATIONS
The use of Ticlopidine HCl is contraindicated in the following conditions:
- Hypersensitivity to the drug.
- Presence of hematopoietic disorders such as neutropenia and thrombocytopenia.
- Presence of a hemostatic disorder or active pathological bleeding (such as bleeding peptic ulcer or intracranial bleeding).
- Patients with severe liver impairment.

WARNINGS

NEUTROPENIA

NEUTROPENIA DEFINED IN THESE STUDIES AS AN ANC < 1200 NEUTROPHILIS/MM^3 OCCURRED IN 50 OF 2,048 (2.4%) STROKE PATIENTS WHO RECEIVED TICLOPIDINE HCL IN CLINICAL TRIALS.

SEVERE NEUTROPENIA (< 450 NEUTROPHILS/MM^3): SEVERE NEUTROPENIA AND/OR AGRANULOCYTOSIS OCCURRED IN 17 OF THE 2,048 (0.8%) PATIENTS WHO RECEIVED TICLOPIDINE HCL. WHEN THE DRUG WAS DISCONTINUED IN THESE PATIENTS, THE NEUTROPHIL COUNTS RETURNED TO NORMAL (> 1200 NEUTROPHILS/MM^3) WITHIN 1-3 WEEKS.

MILD TO MODERATE NEUTROPENIA (451-1200 NEUTROPHILS/MM^3): MILD TO MODERATE NEUTROPENIA OCCURRED IN 33 OF THE 2,048 (1.6%) PATIENTS WHO RECEIVED TICLOPIDINE HCL. ELEVEN OF THE PATIENTS DISCONTINUED TREATMENT AND RECOVERED WITHIN A FEW DAYS. IN THE REMAINING 22 PATIENTS, THE NEUTROPENIA WAS TRANSIENT AND DID NOT REQUIRE DISCONTINUATION OF THERAPY.

THE ONSET OF SEVERE NEUTROPENIA OCCURRED 3 WEEKS TO 3 MONTHS AFTER THE START OF THERAPY WITH TICLOPIDINE HCL WITH NO DOCUMENTED CASES OF SEVERE NEUTROPENIA BEYOND THAT TIME IN THE LARGE CONTROLLED TRIALS. THE BONE MARROW TYPICALLY SHOWED A REDUCTION IN MYELOID PRECURSORS.

IT IS THEREFORE ESSENTIAL THAT CBCS AND WHITE CELL DIFFERENTIALS BE PERFORMED EVERY TWO WEEKS STARTING AT BASELINE BEFORE TREATMENT IS INITIATED TO THE END OF THE THIRD MONTH OF THERAPY WITH TICLOPIDINE HCL, BUT MORE FREQUENT MONITORING IS NECESSARY FOR PATIENTS WHOSE ABSOLUTE NEUTROPHIL COUNTS HAVE BEEN CONSISTENTLY DECLINING OR ARE 30% LESS THAN THE BASELINE COUNT. BECAUSE OF THE LONG PLASMA HALF-LIFE OF TICLOPIDINE HCL, IT IS RECOMMENDED THAT ANY PATIENT WHO DISCONTINUES TICLOPIDINE HCL FOR ANY REASON WITHIN THE FIRST 90 DAYS CONTINUE TO HAVE CBC MONITORING AND WHITE CELL DIFFERENTIAL FOR AT LEAST ANOTHER TWO WEEKS AFTER DISCONTINUATION OF THERAPY.

NEUTROPENIA (AN ABSOLUTE NEUTROPHIL COUNT (ANC) OF LESS THAN 1200 NEUTROPHILS/MM^3) IS CALCULATED AS FOLLOWS: ANC = WBC × % NEUTROPHILS. IF CLINICAL EVALUATION AND REPEAT LABORATORY TESTING CONFIRM THE PRESENCE OF NEUTROPENIA (> 1200/MM^3), THE DRUG SHOULD BE DISCONTINUED.

IN CLINICAL TRIALS, WHEN THERAPY WAS DISCONTINUED IMMEDIATELY UPON DETECTION OF NEUTROPENIA, THE NEUTROPHIL COUNTS RETURNED TO NORMAL WITHIN 1-3 WEEKS.

AFTER THE FIRST THREE MONTHS OF THERAPY, CBCS NEED BE OBTAINED ONLY FOR PATIENTS WITH SIGNS OR SYMPTOMS SUGGESTIVE OF INFECTION.

Thrombocytopenia: Rarely, thrombocytopenia may occur in isolation or together with neutropenia.

If clinical evaluation and repeat laboratory testing confirm the presence of thrombocytopenia (< 80,000 cells/mm^3), the drug should be discontinued.

Cholesterol Elevation: Ticlopidine HCl therapy causes increased serum cholesterol and triglycerides. Serum total cholesterol levels are increased 8-10% within one month of therapy and persist at that level. The ratios of the lipoprotein subfractions are unchanged.

Other Hematological Effects: Rare cases of pancytopenia and thrombotic thrombocytopenic purpura, some of which have been fatal, have been reported in Post-Marketing Surveillance.

Anticoagulant Drugs: The tolerance and safety of coadministration of Ticlopidine HCl with heparin, oral anticoagulants, or fibrinolytic agents has not been established. If a patient is switched from an anticoagulant or fibrinolytic drug to Ticlopidine HCl the former drug should be discontinued prior to Ticlopidine HCl administration.

PRECAUTIONS
GENERAL
Ticlopidine HCl should be used with caution in patients who may be at risk of increased bleeding from trauma, surgery, or pathological conditions. If it is desired to eliminate the antiplatelet effects of Ticlopidine HCl prior to elective surgery, the drug should be discontinued 10-14 days prior to surgery. Several controlled clinical studies have found increased surgical blood loss in patients undergoing surgery during treatment with Ticlopidine. In TASS and CATS it was recommended that patients have Ticlopidine discontinued prior to elective surgery. Several hundred patients underwent surgery during the trials, and no excessive surgical bleeding was reported. Prolonged bleeding time is normalized within two hours after administration of 20 mg methylprednisolone i.v. Platelet transfusions may also be used to reverse the effect of Ticlopidine HCl on bleeding.

GI BLEEDING
Ticlopidine HCl prolongs template bleeding time. The drug should be used with caution in patients who have lesions with a propensity to bleed (such as ulcers). Drugs that might induce such lesions should be used with caution in patients on Ticlopidine HCl. (See *"Contraindications"*).

USE IN HEPATICALLY IMPAIRED PATIENTS
Because of limited experience in patients with severe hepatic disease, who may have bleeding diatheses, the use of Ticlopidine HCl is not recommended in this population. (See *"Clinical Pharmacology"* and *"Contraindications"*).

USE IN RENALLY IMPAIRED PATIENTS
There is limited experience in patients with renal impairment. In controlled clinical trials, no unexpected problems have been encountered in patients having mild renal impairment and there is no experience with dosage adjustment in patients with greater degrees of renal impairment. Nevertheless, for renally impaired patients it may be necessary to reduce the dosage of Ticlopidine or discontinue it altogether, if hemorrhagic or hematopoietic problems are encountered. (See *"Clinical Pharmacology"*).

INFORMATION FOR THE PATIENT (SEE PPI)
Patients should be told that a decrease in the number of white blood cells (neutropenia) can occur with Ticlopidine HCl, especially during the first three months of treatment, and that if neutropenia is severe, it could result in an increased risk of infection. They should be told it is critically important to obtain the scheduled blood tests to detect neutropenia. Patients should also be reminded to contact their physicians if they experience any indication of infection such as fever, chills, and sore throat, all of which may be consequences of neutropenia.

All patients should be told that it may take them longer than usual to stop bleeding when they take Ticlopidine HCl and that they should report any unusual bleeding to their physician. Patients should tell physicians and dentists that they are taking Ticlopidine HCl before any surgery is scheduled and before any new drug is prescribed.

Patients should be told to report promptly side effects of Ticlopidine HCl such as severe or persistent diarrhea, skin rashes, or subcutaneous bleeding, or any signs of cholestasis, such as yellow skin or sclera, dark urine or light colored stools.

Patients should be told to take Ticlopidine HCl with food or just after eating in order to minimize gastrointestinal discomfort.

LABORATORY TESTS
Liver Function: Ticlopidine HCl therapy has been associated with elevations of alkaline phosphatase and transaminases which generally occurred within 1-4 months of therapy initiation. In controlled clinical trials, the incidence of elevated alkaline phosphatase (greater than 2 times upper limit of normal) was 7.6% in Ticlopidine HCl patients, 6.0% in placebo patients and 2.5% in aspirin patients. The incidence of elevated AST (SGOT) (greater than 2 times upper limit of normal) was 3.1% in ticlopidine patients, 4.0% in placebo patients and 2.1% in aspirin patients. No progressive increases were observed in closely monitored clinical trials (e.g. no transaminase greater than 10 times the upper limit of normal was seen), but most patients with these abnormalities had therapy discontinued. Occasionally patients had developed minor elevations in bilirubin.

Based on post-marketing and clinical trials experiences, liver function testing should be considered whenever liver dysfunction is suspected, particularly during the first four months of treatment.

DRUG INTERACTIONS
Therapeutic doses of Ticlopidine HCl caused a 30% increase in the plasma half-life of antipyrine and may cause analogous effect on similarly metabolized drugs. Therefore the dose of drugs metabolized by hepatic microsomal enzymes with low therapeutic ratios, or being given to patients with hepatic impairment, may require adjustment to maintain optimal therapeutic blood levels when starting or stopping concomitant therapy with Ticlopidine HCl. Studies of specific drug interactions yielded the following results:

Aspirin: Aspirin did not modify the Ticlopidine-mediated inhibition of ADP-induced platelet aggregation, but Ticlopidine HCl potentiated the effect of aspirin on collagen-induced platelet aggregation. The safety of this combination has not been established and concomitant use of aspirin and Ticlopidine HCl is not recommended (See *"Precautions—GI Bleeding"*).

Antacids: Administration of Ticlopidine HCl after antacids resulted in an 18% decrease in plasma levels of Ticlopidine HCl.

Cimetidine: Chronic administration of cimetidine reduced the clearance of a single dose of Ticlopidine HCl by 50%.

Digoxin: Co-administration of Ticlopidine HCl with digoxin resulted in a slight decrease (approximately 15%) in digoxin plasma levels. Little or no change in therapeutic efficacy of digoxin would be expected.

Theophylline: In normal volunteers, concomitant administration of Ticlopidine HCl resulted in a significant increase in the theophylline elimination half-life from 8.6 to 12.2 hr and a comparable reduction in total plasma clearance of theophylline.

Phenobarbital: In six normal volunteers, the inhibitory effects of Ticlopidine HCl on platelet aggregation were not altered by chronic administration of phenobarbital.

Phenytoin: In vitro studies demonstrated that Ticlopidine HCl does not alter the plasma protein binding of phenytoin. However, the protein binding interactions of Ticlopidine HCl and its metabolites have not been studies in vivo. Several cases of elevated phenytoin plasma levels with associated somnolence and lethargy have been reported following coadministration with Ticlopidine HCl. Caution should be exercised in coadministering this drug with Ticlopidine HCl and it may be useful to remeasure phenytoin blood concentrations.

Propranolol: In vitro studies demonstrated that Ticlopidine HCl does not alter the plasma protein binding of propranolol. However, the protein binding interactions of Ticlopidine HCl and its metabolites have not been studies in vivo. Caution should be exercised in coadministering this drug with Ticlopidine HCl.

Other Concomitant Therapy: Although specific interaction studies were not performed, in clinical studies, Ticlopidine HCl was used concomitantly with beta blockers, calcium channel blockers, diuretics, and nonsteroidal anti-inflammatory drugs without evidence of clinically significant adverse interactions. (See *"Precautions"*.)

Food Interaction: The oral bioavailability of Ticlopidine HCl is increased by 20% when taken after a meal. Administration of Ticlopidine HCl with food is recommended to maximize gastrointestinal tolerance. In controlled trials, Ticlopidine HCl was taken with meals.

CARCINOGENESIS, MUTAGENESIS, IMPAIRMENT OF FERTILITY
In a two-year oral carcinogenicity study in rats Ticlopidine HCl at daily doses of up to 100 mg/kg (610 mg/m^2) was not tumorigenic. For a 70 kg person (1.73m^2 body surface area), the dose represents 14 times the recommended clinical dose on a mg/kg basis and 2 times the clinical dose on body surface area basis. In a 78 week oral carcinogenicity study in mice Ticlopidine HCl at daily doses up to 275 mg/kg (1180 mg/m^2) was not tumorigenic. The dose represents 40 times the recommended clinical dose on a mg/kg basis and 4 times the clinical dose on body surface area basis.

Ticlopidine HCl was not mutagenic in in vitro Ames test, rat hepatocyte DNA-repair assay, and Chinese hamster fibroblast chromosomal aberration test and in vivo mouse spermatozoid morphology test, Chinese hamster micronucleus test and Chinese hamster bone marrow cell sister chromatid exchange test. Ticlopidine HCl was found to have no effect on fertility of male and female rats at oral doses up to 400 mg/kg/day.

PREGNANCY: TERATOGENIC EFFECTS
Pregnancy Category B. Teratology studies have been conducted in mice (doses up to 200 mg/kg/day), rats (doses up to 400 mg/kg/day) and rabbits (doses up to 200 mg/kg/day). Doses of 400 mg/kg in rats, 200 mg/kg/day in mice, and 100 mg/kg in rabbits produced maternal toxicity as well as fetal toxicity, but there was no evidence of a teratogenic potential of Ticlopidine. There are, however, no

adequate and well-controlled studies in pregnant women. Because animal reproduction studies are not always predictive of a human response, this drug should be used during pregnancy only if clearly needed.

NURSING MOTHERS
Studies in rats have shown Ticlopidine HCl is excreted in the milk. It is not known whether this drug is excreted in human milk. Because many drugs are excreted in human milk and because of the potential for serious adverse reactions in nursing infants from Ticlopidine HCl, a decision should be made whether to discontinue nursing or to discontinue the drug, taking into account the importance of the drug to the mother.

PEDIATRIC USE
Safety and efficacy in patients under the age of 18 have not been established.

GERIATRIC USE
Clearance of Ticlopidine HCl is somewhat lower in elderly patients and trough levels are increased. The major clinical trials with Ticlopidine HCl were conducted in an elderly population with an average age of 64 years. Of the total number of patients in the therapeutic trials, 45% of patients were over 65 years old and 12% were over 75 years old. No overall differences in effectiveness or safety were observed between these patients and younger patients, and other reported clinical experience has not identified differences in responses between the elderly and younger patients, but greater sensitivity of some older individuals cannot be ruled out.

ADVERSE REACTIONS
Adverse reactions were relatively frequent, with over 50% of patients reporting at least one. Most (30 to 40%) involved the gastrointestinal tract. Most adverse effects are mild, but 21% of patients discontinued therapy because of an adverse event, principally diarrhea, rash, nausea, vomiting, G.I. pain, and neutropenia. Most adverse effects occur early in the course of treatment, but a new onset of adverse effects can occur after several months.

The incidence rates of adverse events listed in the following table were derived from multicenter, controlled clinical trials described above comparing Ticlopidine HCl, placebo, and aspirin over study periods of up to 5.8 years. Adverse events considered by the investigator to be probably drug-related that occurred in at least one percent of patients treated with Ticlopidine HCl are shown in the following table:

PERCENT OF PATIENTS WITH ADVERSE EVENTS IN CONTROLLED STUDIES

Event	Ticlopidine HCl (n = 2048) Incidence	Aspirin (n = 1527) Incidence	Placebo (n = 536) Incidence
Any Event	60.0 (20.9)	53.2 (14.5)	34.3 (6.1)
Diarrhea	12.5 (6.3)	5.2 (1.8)	4.5 (1.7)
Nausea	7.0 (2.6)	6.2 (1.9)	1.7 (0.9)
Dyspepsia	7.0 (1.1)	9.0 (2.0)	0.9 (0.2)
Rash	5.1 (3.4)	1.5 (0.8)	0.6 (0.9)
GI Pain	3.7 (1.9)	5.6 (2.7)	1.3 (0.4)
Neutropenia	2.4 (1.3)	0.8 (0.1)	1.1 (0.4)
Purpura	2.2 (0.2)	1.6 (0.1)	0.0 (0.0)
Vomiting	1.9 (1.4)	1.4 (0.9)	0.9 (0.4)
Flatulence	1.5 (0.1)	1.4 (0.3)	0.0 (0.0)
Pruritus	1.3 (0.8)	0.3 (0.1)	0.0 (0.0)
Dizziness	1.1 (0.4)	0.5 (0.4)	0.0 (0.0)
Anorexia	1.0 (0.4)	0.5 (0.3)	0.0 (0.0)
Abnormal Liver Function test	1.0 (0.7)	0.3 (0.3)	0.0 (0.0)

Incidence of discontinuation, regardless of relationship therapy, is shown in parentheses

NEUTROPENIA/THROMBOCYTOPENIA
See "Warnings".

GASTROINTESTINAL
Ticlopidine HCl therapy has been associated with a variety of gastrointestinal complaints including diarrhea and nausea. The majority of cases are mild, but about 13% of patients discontinued therapy because of these. They usually occur within 3 months of initiation of therapy and typically are resolved within 1-2 weeks without discontinuation of therapy. If the effect is severe or persistent, therapy should be discontinued.

HEMORRHAGIC
Ticlopidine HCl has been associated with a number of bleeding complications such as ecchymosis, epistaxis, hematuria, conjunctival hemorrhage, gastrointestinal bleeding and perioperative bleeding.

Intracerebral bleeding was rare in clinical trials with Ticlopidine HCl with an incidence no greater than that seen with comparator agents. (Ticlopidine 0.5%, aspirin 0.6%, placebo 0.75%.)

RASH
Ticlopidine HCl has been associated with a maculopapular or urticarial rash (often with pruritus). Rash usually occurs within 3 months of initiation of therapy, with a mean onset time of 11 days. If drug is discontinued, recovery occurs within several days. Many rashes do not recur on drug rechallenge. There have been rare reports of severe rashes.

LESS FREQUENT ADVERSE REACTIONS (PROBABLY RELATED)
Clinical adverse experiences occurring in 0.5 to 1.0 percent of patients in the controlled trials include:

Digestive System: GI fullness.

Skin and Appendages: urticaria.

Nervous System: headache.

Body as a Whole: asthenia, pain.

Hemostatic System: epistaxis.

Special Senses: tinnitus.

In addition, rarer, relatively serious events have also been reported, mainly from foreign post marketing experience: Pancytopenia, hemolytic anemia with reticulocytosis, allergic pneumonitis, systemic lupus (positive ANA), peripheral neuropathy, vasculitis, serum sickness, arthropathy, hepatitis, cholestatic jaundice, nephrotic syndrome, myositis, hyponatremia, immune thrombocytopenia and thrombocytopenic thrombotic purpura (TTP).

OVERDOSAGE
One case of deliberate overdosage with Ticlopidine HCl has been reported by foreign postmarketing surveillance program. A 38 year old male took a single 6000 mg dose of Ticlopidine HCl (equivalent to 24 standard 250 mg tablets). The only abnormalities reported were increased bleeding time and increased SGPT. No special therapy was instituted and the patient recovered without sequelae.

Single oral doses of Ticlopidine at 1600 mg/kg and 500 mg/kg were lethal to rats and mice, respectively. Symptoms of acute toxicity were GI hemorrhage, convulsions, hypothermia, dyspnea, loss of equilibrium and abnormal gait.

DOSAGE AND ADMINISTRATION
The recommended dose of Ticlopidine HCl is 250 mg BID taken with food. Other doses have not been studied in controlled trials for these indications.

STORAGE
Store at 15—30°C (59—86°F).

HOW SUPPLIED
TABLETS: 250 MG

BRAND/MANUFACTURER	NDC	SIZE	AWP
○ BRAND			
► TICLID: Syntex	00033-0431-38	30s	$40.94
	00033-0431-53	100s	$136.49

Tigan SEE TRIMETHOBENZAMIDE HYDROCHLORIDE

Tilade SEE NEDOCROMIL SODIUM

Timentin SEE CLAVULANATE POTASSIUM WITH
TICARCILLIN DISODIUM

Timolide 10-25 SEE HYDROCHLOROTHIAZIDE AND
TIMOLOL MALEATE

Timolol Maleate, Ophthalmic

DESCRIPTION
Timolol Maleate is a nonselective beta-adrenergic receptor blocking agent. Its chemical name is (-)-1-(*tert*-butyl-amino)-3-[(4-morpholino-1,2,5-thiadiazol-3-yl)oxy]-2-propanol maleate (1:1) (salt). Timolol Maleate possesses an asymmetric carbon atom in its structure and is provided as the levo-isomer. The nominal optical rotation of Timolol Maleate is: $[\alpha]_{405\,nm}^{25}$ in 0.1 N HCl (C = 5%) = - 12.2°.

Its molecular formula is $C_{13}H_{24}N_4O_3S \cdot C_4H_4O_4$.

Timolol Maleate has a molecular weight of 432.49. It is a white odorless, crystalline powder which is soluble in water, methanol, and alcohol. Timolol Maleate, Ophthalmic, is available as a sterile ophthalmic gel and a sterile ophthalmic solution in 0.25% and 0.5% strengths. Each mL of Timolol Maleate 0.25% contains 2.5 mg of Timolol (3.4 mg of Timolol Maleate). Each mL of Timolol Maleate 0.05% contains 5.0 mg of Timolol (6.8 mg of Timolol Maleate).

Following is its chemical structure:

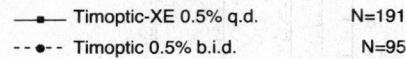

CLINICAL PHARMACOLOGY

MECHANISM OF ACTION

Timolol Maleate is a beta$_1$ and beta$_2$ (nonselective) adrenergic receptor blocking agent that does not have significant intrinsic sympathomimetic, direct myocardial depressant, or local anesthetic (membrane-stabilizing) activity.

Timolol Maleate, Ophthalmic, when applied topically in the eye, has the action of reducing elevated, as well as normal, intraocular pressure, whether or not accompanied by glaucoma. Elevated intraocular pressure is a major risk factor in the pathogenesis of glaucomatous visual field loss. The higher the level of intraocular pressure, the greater the likelihood of glaucomatous visual field loss and optic nerve damage.

The onset of reduction in intraocular pressure following administration of Timolol Maleate can usually be detected within one-half hour after a single dose. The maximum effect usually occurs in one to two hours and significant lowering of intraocular pressure can be maintained for periods as long as 24 hours with a single dose. Repeated observations over a period of one year indicate that the intraocular pressure-lowering effect of Timolol Maleate is well maintained.

The precise mechanism of the ocular hypotensive action of Timolol Maleate is not clearly established at this time. Tonography and fluorophotometry studies of Timolol Maleate in man suggest that its predominant action may be related to reduced aqueous formation. However, in some studies, a slight increase in outflow facility was also observed.

Unlike miotics, Timolol Maleate reduces intraocular pressure with little or no effect on accommodation or pupil size. Thus, changes in visual acuity due to increased accommodation are uncommon, and dim or blurred vision and night blindness produced by miotics are not evident. In addition, in patients with cataracts the inability to see around lenticular opacities when the pupil is constricted is avoided.

Beta-adrenergic receptor blockade reduces cardiac output in both healthy subjects and patients with heart disease. In patients with severe impairment of myocardial function beta-adrenergic receptor blockade may inhibit the stimulatory effect of the sympathetic nervous system necessary to maintain adequate cardiac function.

Beta-adrenergic receptor blockade in the bronchi and bronchioles results in increased airway resistance from unopposed parasympathetic activity. Such an effect in patients with asthma or other bronchospastic conditions is potentially dangerous.

PHARMACOKINETICS

In a study of plasma drug concentration in six subjects, the systemic exposure to Timolol was determined following once daily administration of Timolol Maleate gel forming solution 0.5% in the morning.

The mean peak plasma concentration following this morning dose was 0.28 ng/mL.

CLINICAL STUDIES

In the clinical studies which are reported below, ocular pressure reductions to less than 22 mmHg were used as a reasonable reference point to allow comparisons between treatments. Reduction of ocular pressure to just below 22 mmHG may not be optimal for all patients; therapy should be individualized.

In controlled multiclinic studies in patients with untreated intraocular pressures of 22 mmHg or greater, Timolol Maleate 0.25 percent or 0.5 percent administered twice a day produced a greater reduction in intraocular pressure than 1, 2, 3, or 4 percent pilocarpine solution administered four times a day or 0.5, 1, or 2 percent epinephrine hydrochloride solution administered twice a day.

In the multiclinic studies comparing Timolol Maleate with pilocarpine, 61 percent of patients treated with Timolol Maleate had intraocular pressure reduced to less than 22 mmHg compared to 32 percent of patients treated with pilocarpine. For patients completing these studies, the mean reduction in pressure at the end of the study from pretreatment was 30.7 percent for patients treated with Timolol Maleate and 21.7 percent for patients treated with pilocarpine.

In the multiclinic studies comparing Timolol Maleate with epinephrine, 69 percent of patients treated with Timolol Maleate had intraocular pressure reduced to less than 22 mmHg compared to 42 percent of patients treated with epinephrine. For patients completing these studies, the mean reduction in pressure at the end of the study from pretreatment was 33.2 percent for patients treated with Timolol Maleate and 28.1 percent for patients treated with epinephrine.

In these studies, Timolol Maleate was generally well tolerated and produced fewer and less severe side effects than either pilocarpine or epinephrine. A slight reduction of resting heart rate in some patients receiving Timolol Maleate (mean reduction 2.9 beats/minute standard deviation 10.2) was observed.

Timolol Maleate has also been used in patients with glaucoma wearing conventional (PMMA) hard contact lenses, and has generally been well tolerated. Timolol Maleate has not been studied in patients wearing lenses made with materials other than PMMA (see *"Precautions, Information for Patients"*).

In controlled, double-masked, multicenter clinical studies comparing Timolol Maleate gel-forming solution to Timolol Maleate, Ophthalmic, solution, Timolol Maleate gel administered once a day was shown to be equally effective in lowering intraocular pressure as the equivalent concentration of Timolol Maleate gel administered twice a day. The effect of timolol in lowering intraocular pressure was evident for 24 hours with a single dose of Timolol Maleate. Repeated observations over a period of six months indicate that the intraocular pressure-lowering effect of Timolol Maleate gel-forming solution was consistent. The results from the largest U.S. and international clinical trials comparing Timolol Maleate gel-forming solution 0.5% to Timolol Maleate, Ophthmalic, solution 0.5% are shown in Figure 1.

US STUDY

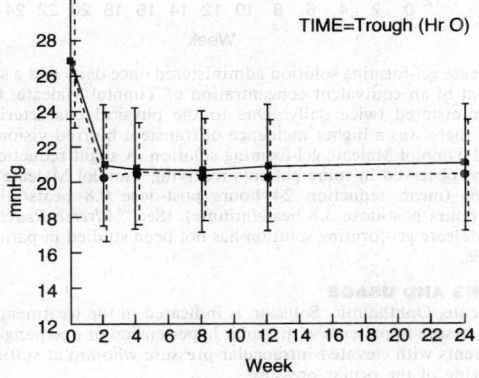

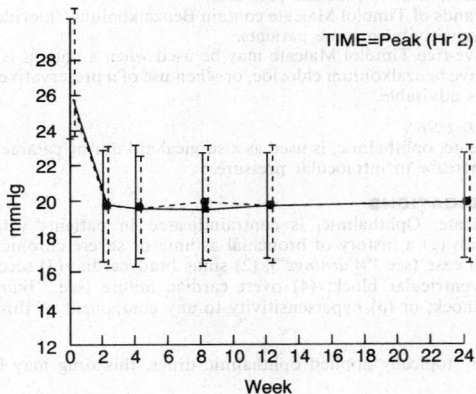

International Study

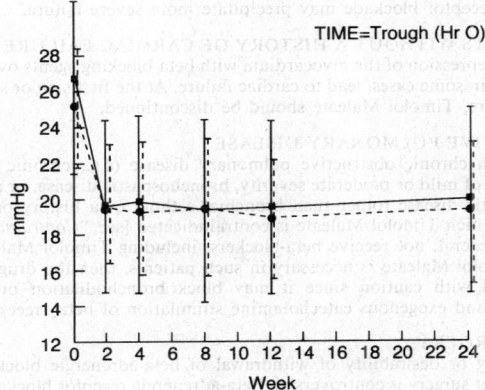

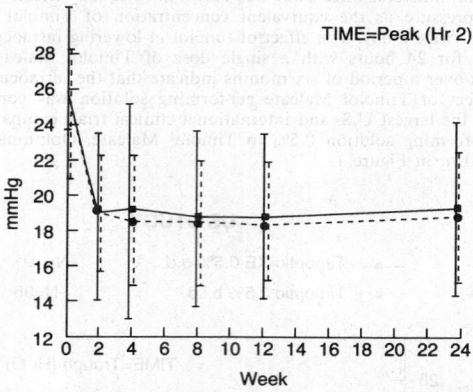

TIME=Peak (Hr 2)

Timolol Maleate gel-forming solution administered once daily had a safety profile similar to that of an equivalent concentration of Timolol Maleate, Ophthmalic, solution administered twice daily. Due to the physical characteristics of the formulation, there was a higher incidence of transient blurred vision in patients administered Timolol Maleate gel-forming solution. A slight reduction in resting heart rate was observed in some patients receiving Timolol Maleate gel-forming solution 0.5% (mean reduction 24 hours post-dose 0.8 beats/minute, mean reduction 2 hours post-dose 3.8 beats/minute). (See "Adverse Reactions").

Timolol Maleate gel-forming solution has not been studied in patients wearing contact lenses.

INDICATIONS AND USAGE

Timolol Maleate, Ophthalmic, Solution is indicated in the treatment of elevated intraocular pressure in patients with ocular hypertension or open-angle glaucoma.

Other patients with elevated intraocular pressure who are at sufficient risk to require lowering of the ocular pressure.

Clinical trials have also shown that in patients who respond inadequately to multiple antiglaucoma drug therapy the addition of Timolol Maleate may produce a further reduction of intraocular pressure.

Certain brands of Timolol Maleate contain Benzalkonium Chloride which may cause some sensitivity in some patients.

Preservative-free Timolol Maleate may be used when a patient is sensitive to the preservative benzalkonium chloride, or when use of a preservative-free topical medication is advisable.

UNLABELED USES

Timolol Maleate, ophthalmic, is used as a surgical aid during cataract extraction, to prevent increase in intraocular pressure.

CONTRAINDICATIONS

Timolol Maleate, Ophthalmic, is contraindicated in patients with bronchial asthma or with (1) a history of bronchial asthma or severe chronic obstructive pulmonary disease (see "Warnings"); (2) sinus bradycardia; (3) second or third degree atrioventricular block; (4) overt cardiac failure (see "Warnings"); (5) cardiogenic shock; or (6) hypersensitivity to any component of this product.

WARNINGS

As with many topically applied ophthalmic drugs, this drug may be absorbed systemically.

The same adverse reactions found with systemic administration of beta-adrenergic blocking agents may occur with topical ophthalmic administration. For example, severe respiratory reactions and cardiac reactions, including death due to bronchospasm in patients with asthma, and rarely death in association with cardiac failure, have been reported following systemic or ophthalmic administration of Timolol Maleate. (See "Contraindications".)

CARDIAC FAILURE

Sympathetic stimulation may be essential for support of the circulation in individuals with diminished myocardial contractility, and its inhibition by beta-adrenergic receptor blockade may precipitate more severe failure.

IN PATIENTS WITHOUT A HISTORY OF CARDIAC FAILURE

Continued depression of the myocardium with beta-blocking agents over a period of time can, in some cases, lead to cardiac failure. At the first sign or symptom of cardiac failure, Timolol Maleate should be discontinued.

OBSTRUCTIVE PULMONARY DISEASE

Patients with chronic obstructive pulmonary disease (e.g., chronic bronchitis, emphysema) of mild or moderate severity, bronchospastic disease, or a history of bronchospastic disease (other than bronchial asthma or a history of bronchial asthma, in which Timolol Maleate is contraindicated [see "Contraindications"]) should, in general, not receive beta-blockers, including Timolol Maleate. However, if Timolol Maleate is necessary in such patients, then the drug should be administered with caution since it may block bronchodilation produced by endogenous and exogenous catecholamine stimulation of $beta_2$ receptors.

MAJOR SURGERY

The necessity or desirability of withdrawal of beta-adrenergic blocking agents prior to major surgery is controversial. Beta-adrenergic receptor blockade impairs the ability of the heart to respond to beta-adrenergically mediated reflex stimuli. This may augment the risk of general anesthesia in surgical procedures. Some patients receiving beta-adrenergic receptor blocking agents have experienced protracted, severe hypotension during anesthesia. Difficulty in restarting and maintaining the heartbeat has also been reported. For these reasons, in patients undergoing elective surgery, some authorities recommend gradual withdrawal of beta-adrenergic receptor blocking agents.

If necessary during surgery, the effects of beta-adrenergic blocking agents may be reversed by sufficient doses of such adrenergic agonists as isoproterenol, dopamine, dobutamine, or levarterenol.

DIABETES MELLITUS

Beta-adrenergic blocking agents should be administered with caution in patients subject to spontaneous hypoglycemia or to diabetic patients (especially those with labile diabetes) who are receiving insulin or oral hypoglycemic agents. Beta-adrenergic receptor blocking agents may mask the signs and symptoms of acute hypoglycemia.

THYROTOXICOSIS

Beta-adrenergic blocking agents may mask certain clinical signs (e.g., tachycardia) of hyperthyroidism. Patients suspected of developing thyrotoxicosis should be managed carefully to avoid abrupt withdrawal of beta-adrenergic blocking agents that might precipitate a thyroid storm.

PRECAUTIONS

GENERAL

Because of potential effects of beta-adrenergic blocking agents on blood pressure and pulse, these agents should be used with caution in patients with cerebrovascular insufficiency. If signs or symptoms suggesting reduced cerebral blood flow develop following initiation of therapy with Timolol Maleate alternative therapy should be considered. There have been reports of bacterial keratitis associated with the use of multiple dose containers of topical ophthalmic products. These containers had been inadvertently contaminated by patients who, in most cases, had a concurrent corneal disease or a disruption of the ocular epithelial surface. (See "Precautions, Information for Patients".)

Angle-closure Glaucoma: In patients with angle-closure glaucoma, the immediate objective of treatment is to reopen the angle. This may require constricting the pupil with a miotic. Timolol Maleate has little or no effect on the pupil. Timolol Maleate gel-forming solution should not be used alone in the treatment of angle-closure glaucoma. When Timolol Maleate is used to reduce elevated intraocular pressure in angle-closure glaucoma, it should be used with a miotic and not alone.

As with the use of other antiglaucoma drugs, diminished responsiveness to Timolol Maleate after prolonged therapy has been reported in some patients. However, in one long-term study in which 96 patients have been followed for at least 3 years, no significant difference in mean intraocular pressure has been observed after initial stabilization.

Anaphylaxis: While taking beta-blockers, patients with a history of atopy or a history of severe anaphylactic reactions to a variety of allergens may be more reactive to repeated accidental, diagnostic, or therapeutic challenge with such allergens. Such patients may be unresponsive to the usual doses of epinephrine used to treat anaphylactic reactions.

Muscle Weakness: Beta-adrenergic blockade has been reported to potentiate muscle weakness consistent with certain myasthenic symptoms (e.g., diplopia, ptosis, and generalized weakness). Timolol has been reported rarely to increase muscle weakness in some patients with myasthenia gravis or myasthenic symptoms.

INFORMATION FOR PATIENTS

Patients should be instructed to avoid allowing the tip of the dispensing container to contact the eye or surrounding structures.

Since sterility cannot be maintained after the individual unit is opened, if the product comes in individual units, patients should be instructed to use the product immediately after opening, and to discard the individual unit and any remaining contents immediately after use. Patients should also be instructed that ocular solutions, if handled improperly, can become contaminated by common bacteria known to cause ocular infections. Serious damage to the eye and subsequent loss of vision may result from using contaminated solutions. (See "Precautions, General").

Patients should also be advised that if they develop an intercurrent ocular condition (e.g., trauma, ocular surgery, or infection), they should immediately seek their physician's advice concerning the continued use of the present multidose container.

Patients should be instructed to invert the closed container and shake once before each use. It is not necessary to shake the container more than once.

Patients requiring concomitant topical ophthalmic medications should be instructed to administer these at least 10 minutes before instilling certain brands of Timolol Maleate contain benzalkonium chloride, which may be absorbed by soft contact lenses. Patients wearing soft contact lenses should be instructed to wait at least 15 minutes after instilling Timolol Maleate before they insert their lenses.

Patients with bronchial asthma, a history of bronchial asthma, severe chronic obstructive pulmonary disease, sinus bradycardia, second or third degree atrioventricular block, or cardiac failure should be advised not to take this product. (See "Contraindications").

DRUG INTERACTIONS
Beta-adrenergic blocking agents: Patients who are receiving a beta-adrenergic blocking agent orally and Timolol Maleate should be observed for potential additive effects of beta-blockade, both systemic and on intraocular pressure. Patients should not usually receive two topical ophthalmic beta-adrenergic blocking agents concurrently.

Calcium Antagonists: Caution should be used in the coadministration of beta-adrenergic blocking agents, such as Timolol Maleate and oral or intravenous calcium antagonists because of possible atrioventricular conduction disturbances, left ventricular failure, or hypotension. In patients with impaired cardiac function, coadministration should be avoided.

Catecholamine-depleting Drugs: Close observation of the patient is recommended when a beta blocker is administered to patients receiving catecholamine-depleting drugs such as reserpine, because of possible additive effects and the production of hypotension and/or marked bradycardia, which may result in vertigo, syncope, or postural hypotension.

Digitalis and Calcium Antagonists: The concomitant use of beta-adrenergic blocking agents with digitalis and calcium antagonists may have additive effects in prolonging atrioventricular conduction time.

Epinephrine: (See *"Precautions, General, Anaphylaxis"*.)

ANIMAL STUDIES
No adverse ocular effects were observed in rabbits and dogs administered Timolol Maleate topically in studies lasting one and two years respectively.

Although Timolol Maleate used alone has little or no effect on pupil size, mydrasis resulting from concomitant therapy with Timolol Maleate and epinephrine has been reported occasionally.

CARCINOGENESIS, MUTAGENESIS, IMPAIRMENT OF FERTILITY
In a two-year oral study of Timolol Maleate administered orally to rats, there was a statistically significant increase in the incidence of adrenal pheochromocytomas in male rats administered 300 mg/kg/day 250 times the maximum recommended daily human oral dose of 60 mg, based on a patient weight of 50 kg; (approximately 42,000 times the systemic exposure following the maximum recommended human man ophthalmic dose). Similar differences were not observed in rats administered oral doses equivalent to approximately 20 or 80 times the maximum recommended daily human oral dose or 14,000 times the maximum recommended human ophthalmic dose.

In a lifetime oral study in mice, there were statistically significant increases in the incidence of benign and malignant pulmonary tumors, benign uterine polyps, and mammary adenocarcinomas in female mice at 500 mg/kg/day (approximately 400 times the maximum daily human oral dose or 71,000 times the systemic exposure following the maximum recommended human ophthalmic dose), but not at 5 or 50 mg/kg/day (approximately 700 or 7,000, respectively, times the systemic exposure following the maximum recommended human ophthalmic dose). In a subsequent study in female mice, in which post-mortem examinations were limited to the uterus and the lungs, a statistically significant increase in the incidence of pulmonary tumors was again observed at 500 mg/kg/day.

The increased occurrence of mammary adenocarcinomas was associated with elevations in serum prolactin, which occurred in female mice administered oral Timolol at 500 mg/kg, but not at oral doses of 5 or 50 mg/kg/day. An increased incidence of mammary adenocarcinomas in rodents has been associated with administration of several other therapeutic agents that elevate serum prolactin, but no correlation between serum prolactin levels and mammary tumors has been established in humans. Furthermore, in adult human female subjects who received oral dosages of up to 60 mg of Timolol Maleate (the maximum recommended human oral dosage), there were no clinically meaningful changes in serum prolactin.

Timolol Maleate was devoid of mutagenic potential when tested *in vivo* (mouse) in the micronucleus test and cytogenetic assay (doses up to 800 mg/kg) and *in vitro* in a neoplastic cell transformation assay (up to 100 µg/mL). In Ames tests, the highest concentrations of Timolol employed, 5,000 or 10,000 µg/plate, were associated with statistically significant elevations of revertants observed with tester strain TA100 (in seven replicate assays), but not in the remaining three strains. In the assays with tester strain TA100, no consistent dose response relationship was observed, and the ratio of test to control revertants did not reach 2. A ratio of 2 is usually considered the criterion for a positive Ames test. Reproduction and fertility studies in rats demonstrated no adverse effect on male or female fertility at doses up to 125 times the maximum recommended daily human oral dose or 21,000 times the systemic exposure following the maximum recommended human ophthalmic dose.

PREGNANCY—TERATOGENIC EFFECTS
Pregnancy Category: Teratogenicity studies with Timolol in mice and rabbits at oral doses up to 50 mg/kg/day (approximately 40 times the maximum recommended daily human dose or 7,000 times the systemic exposure following the maximum recommended human ophthalmic dose) demonstrated no evidence of fetal malformations. Although delayed fetal ossification was observed at this dose in rats, there were no adverse effects on postnatal development of offspring. Doses of 1000 mg/kg/day (approximately 830 times the maximum recommended daily human oral dose or 142,000 times the systemic exposure following the maximum recommended human ophthalmic dose) were maternotoxic in mice and resulted in an increased number of fetal resorptions. Increased fetal resorptions were also seen in rabbits at doses of approximately 40 times the maximum recommended daily human oral dose or 14,000 times the systemic exposure following the

maximum recommended human ophthalmic dose, in this case without apparent maternotoxicity.

There are no adequate and well-controlled studies in pregnant women. Timolol Maleate should be used during pregnancy only if the potential benefit justifies the potential risk to the fetus.

NURSING MOTHERS
Timolol Maleate has been detected in human milk following oral and ophthalmic drug administration. Because of the potential for serious adverse reactions in nursing infants from Timolol, a decision should be made whether to discontinue nursing or to discontinue the drug, taking into account the importance of the drug to the mother.

PEDIATRIC USE
Safety and effectiveness in children have not been established.

GERIATRIC USE
Of the total number of patients in clinical studies of Timolol Maleate 46% were 65 years of age and over, while 14% were 75 years of age and over. No overall differences in effectiveness or safety were observed between these patients and younger patients, but greater sensitivity of some older individuals to the product cannot be ruled out.

ADVERSE REACTIONS
In clinical trials, transient blurred vision upon instillation of the drop was reported in approximately one in three patients (lasting from 30 seconds to 5 minutes). Less than 1% of patients discontinued from the studies due to blurred vision. The frequency of patients reporting burning and stinging upon instillation was comparable between Timolol Maleate Gel Forming Solution and Timolol Maleate Ophthmalic Solution (approximately one in eight patients).

Adverse experiences reported in 1-5% of patients were:

Ocular: Pain, conjunctivitis, discharge (e.g., crusting), foreign body sensation, itching and tearing;

Systemic: Headache, dizziness, and upper respiratory infections.

The following additional adverse experiences have been reported with the ocular administration of Timolol Maleate formulations:

Body as a Whole: Asthenia, chest pain, fatigue.

Cardiovascular: Bradycardia, arrhythmia, hypotension, hypertension, syncope, heart block, cerebral vascular accident, cerebral ischemia, cardiac failure, worsening of angina pectoris, palpitation, cardiac arrest, pulmonary edema.

Digestive: Nausea, diarrhea, dyspepsia, anorexia, dry mouth.

Immunologic: Systemic lupus erythematosus

Nervous System/Psychiatric: Depression, dizziness, increase in signs and symptoms of myasthenia gravis, paresthesia, behavioral changes including confusion, hallucinations, anxiety, disorientation, nervousness, somnolence and other psychic disturbances.

Skin: Hypersensitivity, including localized and generalized rash; urticaria; alopecia.

Respiratory: Bronchospasm (predominantly in patients with preexisting bronchospastic disease), respiratory failure, dyspnea, nasal congestion, cough.

Endocrine: Masked symptoms of hypoglycemia in insulin-dependent diabetics (see *"Warnings"*).

Special Senses: Signs and symptoms of ocular irritation, including conjunctivitis, blepharitis, keratitis, blepharoptosis, decreased corneal sensitivity, aphakic cystoid macular edema, and visual disturbances including refractive changes (due to withdrawal of miotic therapy in some cases), diplopia, and ptosis.

Urogenital: Retroperitoneal fibrosis, impotence.

The following additional adverse effects have been reported in clinical experience with ORAL Timolol Maleate or other ORAL beta-blocking agents and may be considered potential effects of ophthalmic Timolol Maleate.

Allergic: Erythematous rash, fever combined with aching and sore throat, laryngospasm with respiratory distress.

Body as a Whole: Extremity pain, decreased exercise tolerance, weight loss.

Cardiovascular: Edema, worsening of arterial insufficiency, Raynaud's phenomenon, vasodilatation.

Digestive: Gastrointestinal pain, hepatomegaly, vomiting, mesenteric arterial thrombosis, ischemic colitis.

Hematologic: Nonthrombocytopenic purpura, thrombocytopenic purpura, agranulocytosis.

Endocrine: Hyperglycemia, hypoglycemia.

Skin: Pruritus skin irritation, increased pigmentation, sweating, cold hands and feet.

Musculoskeletal: Arthralgia, claudication.

Nervous System/Psychiatric: Vertigo, local weakness, decreased libido, nightmares, insomnia, diminished concentration, reversible mental depression progressing to catatonia, an acute reversible syndrome characterized by disorientation for time and place, short term memory loss, emotional lability, slightly clouded sensorium, and decreased performance on neuropsychometrics.

Respiratory: Rales, bronchial obstruction.

Special Senses: Tinnitus, dry eyes.

Urogenital: Urination difficulties, Peyronie's disease.

Causal Relationship Unknown: The following adverse effects have been reported, and a causal relationship to therapy with Timolol Maleate, Ophthalmic, has not been established.

Cardiovascular: Hypertension, pulmonary edema, worsening of angina pectoris.

Digestive: Dyspepsia, anorexia, dry mouth.

Nervous System/Psychiatric: Behavioral changes including confusion, hallucinations, anxiety, disorientation; nervousness, somnolence, and other psychic disturbances.

Special Senses: Aphakic cystoid macular edema.

Urogenital: Retroperitoneal fibrosis, impotence.

There have been reports of a syndrome comprising psoriasiform skin rash, conjunctivitis sicca, otitis and sclerosing serositis attributed to the beta- adrenergic receptor blocking agent, practolol. This syndrome has not been reported with Timolol Maleate.

OVERDOSAGE

There have been reports of inadvertent overdosage with Timolol Maleate, Ophthalmic solution resulting in systemic effects such as dizziness, headache, shortness of breath, bradycardia, bronchospasm, and cardiac arrest.

Overdosage has been reported with Timolol Maleate tablets. A 30 year old female ingested 650 mg of Timolol Maleate tablets, maximum recommended oral daily dose is 60 mg) and experienced second and third degree heart block. She recovered without treatment but approximately two months later developed irregular heartbeat, hypertension, dizziness, tinnitus, faintness, increased pulse rate, and borderline first degree heart block.

Significant lethality (oral LD_{50}) was observed in female rats and female mice after a single oral dose of 900 and 1190 mg/kg (5310 and 3570 mg/m^2) of Timolol, respectively.

An *in vitro* hemodialysis study, using ^{14}C Timolol added to human plasma or whole blood showed that Timolol was readily dialyzed from these fluids; however, a study of patients with renal failure showed that Timolol did not dialyze readily.

The most common signs and symptoms to be expected with overdosage with administration of a systemic beta-adrenergic receptor blocking agent are symptomatic bradycardia, hypotension, bronchospasm, and acute cardiac failure.

The following therapeutic measures should be considered:

(1) Gastric lavage: If ingested.

(2) Symptomatic bradycardia: Use atropine sulfate intravenously in a dosage of 0.25 mg to 2 mg to induce vagal blockade. If bradycardia persists, intravenous isoproterenol hydrochloride should be administered cautiously. In refractory cases the use of a transvenous cardiac pacemaker may be considered.

(3) Hypotension: Use sympathomimetic pressor drug therapy, such as dopamine, dobutamine or levarterenol. In refractory cases the use of glucagon hydrochloride has been reported to be useful.

(4) Bronchospasm: Use isoproterenol hydrochloride. Additional therapy with aminophylline may be considered.

(5) Acute cardiac failure: Conventional therapy with digitalis, diuretics, and oxygen should be instituted immediately. In refractory cases the use of intravenous aminophylline is suggested. This may be followed if necessary by glucagon hydrochloride which has been reported to be useful.

(6) Heart block (second or third degree): Use isoproterenol hydrochloride or a transvenous cardiac pacemaker.

DOSAGE AND ADMINISTRATION

Patients should be instructed to invert the closed container and shake once before each use. It is not necessary to shake the container more than once. Other topically applied ophthalmic medications should be administered at least 10 minutes before Timolol Maleate. (See "Precautions, Information for Patients".)

The usual starting dose is one drop of 0.25 percent Timolol Maleate, regular and preservative-free, in the affected eye(s) twice a day. If the clinical response is not adequate, the dosage may be changed to one drop of 0.5 percent solution in the affected eye(s) twice a day. The dose is one drop of Timolol Maleate Gel Forming Solution (either 0.25% or 0.5%) in the affected eye(s) once a day.

Because in some patients the pressure-lowering response to Timolol Maleate Ophthmalic Solution may require a few weeks to stabilize, evaluation should include a determination of intraocular pressure after approximately 4 weeks of treatment with Timolol Maleate Ophthalmic Solution.

Dosages higher than one drop of 0.5% Timolol Maleate Ophthmalic Solution once a day have not been studied. If the patient's intraocular pressure is still not at a satisfactory level on this regimen, concomitant therapy can be considered.

When patients have been switched from therapy with Timolol Maleate Ophthmalic Solution administered twice daily to Timolol Maleate Gel Forming Solution administered once daily, the ocular hypotensive effect has remained consistent.

Since in some patients the pressure-lowering response to Timolol Maleate may require a few weeks to stabilize, evaluation should include a determination of intraocular pressure after approximately 4 weeks of treatment with Timolol Maleate. if the intraocular pressure is maintained at satisfactory levels, the dosage schedule of Timolol Maleate may be changed to one drop once a day in the

affected eye(s). Because of diurnal variations in intraocular pressure, satisfactory response to the once-a-day dose is best determined by measuring the intraocular pressure at different times during the day.

Dosages above one drop of 0.5 percent Timolol Maleate twice a day generally have not been shown to produce further reduction in intraocular pressure. If the patient's intraocular pressure is still not at a satisfactory level on this regimen, concomitant therapy with pilocarpine and other miotics, and/or epinephrine, and/or systemically administered carbonic anhydrase inhibitors, such as acetazolamide, can be instituted. (For patients using preservative-free Timolol Maleate, taking into consideration that the preparation(s) used concomitantly may contain one or more preservatives).

When a patient is transferred from another topical ophthalmic beta-adrenergic blocking agent, that agent should be discontinued after proper dosing on one day and treatment with Timolol Maleate started on the following day with 1 drop of 0.25 percent Timolol Maleate in the affected eye(s) twice a day. The dose may be increased to one drop of 0.5 percent Timolol Maleate twice a day if the clinical response is not adequate.

When a patient is transferred from a single antiglaucoma agent, other than a topical ophthalmic beta-adrenergic blocking agent, continue the agent already being used and add one drop of 0.25 percent Timolol Maleate in the affected eye(s) twice a day. On the following day, discontinue the previously used antiglaucoma agent completely and continue with Timolol Maleate. If a higher dosage of Timolol Maleate is required, substitute one drop of 0.5 percent solution in the affected eye(s) twice a day.

When a patient is transferred from several concomitantly administered antiglaucoma agents, individualization is required. If any of the agents is an ophthalmic beta-adrenergic blocker, it should be discontinued before starting Timolol Maleate. Additional adjustments should involve one agent at a time and usually should be made at intervals of not less than one week. A recommended approach is to continue the agents being used and to add one drop of 0.25 percent Timolol Maleate in the affected eye(s) twice a day. On the following day, discontinue one of the other antiglaucoma agents. The remaining antiglaucoma agents may be decreased or discontinued according to the patient's response to treatment. If a higher dosage of Timolol Maleate is required, substitute one drop of 0.5 percent solution in the affected eye(s) twice a day. The physician may be able to discontinue some or all of the other antiglaucoma agents.

Preservative-free Timolol Maleate is a sterile solution that does not contain a preservative. The solution from one individual unit is to be used immediately after opening for administration to one or both eyes. Since sterility cannot be guaranteed after the individual unit is opened, the remaining contents should be discarded immediately after administration.

Storage: Store Timolol Maleate, Ophthalmic, solution at room temperature. Store gel-forming solution between 15° and 25°C (59° and 77°F). **AVOID FREEZING.** Protect from light.

HOW SUPPLIED
DROP: 0.25%

BRAND/MANUFACTURER	NDC	SIZE	AWP
○ **BRAND**			
TIMOPTIC OCUMETER: Merck	00006-3366-32	2.5 ml	$7.34
TIMOPTIC-XE: Merck	00006-3557-32	2.5 ml	$11.83
TIMOPTIC OCUMETER: Merck	00006-3366-03	5 ml	$14.36
TIMOPTIC-XE: Merck	00006-3557-03	5 ml	$20.86
TIMOPTIC OCUMETER: Merck	00006-3366-10	10 ml	$27.74
	00006-3366-12	15 ml	$41.50
TIMOPTIC-XE: Merck	00006-3557-91	2.5 ml 3s	$35.10
TIMOPTIC OCUDOSE: Merck	00006-3542-60	0.45 ml 60s ud	$83.55

DROP: 0.5%

BRAND/MANUFACTURER	NDC	SIZE	AWP
○ **BRAND**			
TIMOPTIC OCUMETER: Merck	00006-3367-32	2.5 ml	$8.74
TIMOPTIC-XE: Merck	00006-3558-32	2.5 ml	$13.98
TIMOPTIC OCUMETER: Merck	00006-3367-03	5 ml	$16.99
TIMOPTIC-XE: Merck	00006-3558-03	5 ml	$24.78
TIMOPTIC OCUMETER: Merck	00006-3367-10	10 ml	$32.95
	00006-3367-12	15 ml	$49.30
TIMOPTIC-XE: Merck	00006-3558-91	2.5 ml 3s	$41.70
TIMOPTIC OCUDOSE: Merck	00006-3543-60	0.45 ml 60s ud	$100.59

Timolol Maleate, Oral

DESCRIPTION

Timolol Maleate, Oral is a nonselective beta-adrenergic receptor blocking agent. The chemical name for Timolol Meleate is (S)-1-[(1,1-dimethylethyl)amino] -3-[[4-(4-morpholinyl)-1,2,5-thiadiazol-3-yl]oxy]-2-propanol (Z)-2-butenedioate (1:1) salt. It possesses an asymmetric carbon atom in its structure and is provided as the levo isomer. Its empirical formula is $C_{13}H_{24}N_4O_3S.C_4H_4O_4$. Timolol Maleate has a molecular weight of 432.49. It is a white, odorless, crystalline powder which is soluble in water, methanol, and alcohol.

Timolol Maleate, Oral is supplied as tablets in three strengths containing 5 mg, 10 mg or 20 mg Timolol Maleate for oral administration.

Following is its chemical structure:

CLINICAL PHARMACOLOGY

Timolol Maleate, Oral is a beta$_1$ and beta$_2$ (nonselective) adrenergic receptor blocking agent that does not have significant intrinsic sympathomimetic, direct myocardial depressant, or local anesthetic activity.

PHARMACODYNAMICS

Clinical pharmacology studies have confirmed the beta-adrenergic blocking activity as shown by (1) changes in resting heart rate and response of heart rate to changes in posture; (2) inhibition of isoproterenol-induced tachycardia; (3) alteration of the response to the Valsalva maneuver and amyl nitrite administration; and (4) reduction of heart rate and blood pressure changes on exercise.

Timolol Maleate, Oral decreases the positive chronotropic, positive inotropic, bronchodilator, and vasodilator responses caused by beta-adrenergic receptor agonists. The magnitude of this decreased response is proportional to the existing sympathetic tone and the concentration of Timolol Maleate at receptor sites.

In normal volunteers, the reduction in heart rate response to a standard exercise was dose dependent over the test range of 0.5 to 20 mg, with a peak reduction at 2 hours of approximately 30% at higher doses.

Beta-adrenergic receptor blockade reduces cardiac output in both healthy subjects and patients with heart disease. In patients with severe impairment of myocardial function beta-adrenergic receptor blockade may inhibit the stimulatory effect of the sympathetic nervous system necessary to maintain adequate cardiac function.

Beta-adrenergic receptor blockade in the bronchi and bronchioles results in increased airway resistance from unopposed parasympathetic activity. Such an effect in patients with asthma or other bronchospastic conditions is potentially dangerous.

Clinical studies indicate that Timolol Maleate at a dosage of 20-60 mg/day reduces blood pressure without causing postural hypotension in most patients with essential hypertension. Administration of Timolol Maleate to patients with hypertension results initially in a decrease in cardiac output, little immediate change in blood pressure, and an increase in calculated peripheral resistance. With continued administration of Timolol Maleate blood pressure decreases within a few days, cardiac output usually remains reduced, and peripheral resistance falls toward pretreatment levels. Plasma volume may decrease or remain unchanged during therapy with Timolol Maleate. In the majority of patients with hypertension, Timolol Maleate also decreases plasma renin activity. Dosage adjustment to achieve optimal antihypertensive effect may require a few weeks. When therapy with Timolol Maleate is discontinued, the blood pressure tends to return to pretreatment levels gradually. In most patients the antihypertensive activity of Timolol Maleate is maintained with long-term therapy and is well tolerated.

The mechanism of the antihypertensive effects of beta-adrenergic receptor blocking agents is not established at this time. Possible mechanisms of action include reduction in cardiac output, reduction in plasma renin activity, and a central nervous system sympatholytic action.

A Norwegian multicenter, double-blind study compared the effects of Timolol Maleate with placebo in 1,884 patients who had survived the acute phase of a myocardial infarction. Patients with systolic blood pressure below 100 mm Hg, sick sinus syndrome and contraindications to beta blockers, uncontrolled heart failure, second or third degree AV block and bradycardia ($<$ 50 beats per minute), were excluded from the multi-center trial. Therapy with Timolol Maleate, begun 7 to 28 days following infarction, was shown to reduce overall mortality; this was primarily attributable to a reduction in cardiovascular mortality. Timolol Maleate significantly reduced the incidence of sudden deaths (deaths occurring without symptoms or within 24 hours of the onset of symptoms), including those occurring within one hour, and particularly instantaneous deaths (those occurring without preceding symptoms). The protective effect of Timolol Maleate was consistent regardless of age, sex or site of infarction. The effect was clearest in patients with a first infarction who were considered at a high risk of dying, defined as those with one or more of the following characteristics during the acute phase: transient left ventricular failure, cardiomegaly, newly appearing atrial fibrillation or flutter, systolic hypotension, or SGOT (ASAT) levels greater than four times the upper limit of normal. Therapy with Timolol Maleate also reduced the incidence of non-fatal reinfarction. The mechanism of the protective effect of Timolol Maleate is unknown.

Timolol Maleate was studied for the prophylactic treatment of migraine headache in placebo-controlled clinical trials involving 400 patients, mostly women between the ages of 18 and 66 years. Common migraine was the most frequent diagnosis. All patients had at least two headaches per month at baseline. Approximately 50 percent of patients who received Timolol Maleate had a reduction in the frequency of migraine headache of at least 50 percent, compared to a similar decrease in frequency in 30 percent of patients receiving placebo. The most common cardiovascular adverse effect was bradycardia (5%).

PHARMACOKINETICS AND METABOLISM

Timolol Maleate is rapidly and nearly completely absorbed (about 90%) following oral ingestion. Detectable plasma levels of timolol occur within one-half hour and peak plasma levels occur in about one to two hours. The drug half-life in plasma is approximately 4 hours and this is essentially unchanged in patients with moderate renal insufficiency. Timolol is partially metabolized by the liver and timolol and its metabolites are excreted by the kidney. Timolol is not extensively bound to plasma proteins; i.e., $<$ 10% by equilibrium dialysis and approximately 60% by ultrafiltration. An in vitro hemodialysis study, using ^{14}C Timolol added to human plasma or whole blood, showed that Timolol was readily dialyzed from these fluids; however, a study of patients with renal failure showed that Timolol did not dialyze readily. Plasma levels following oral administration are about half those following intravenous administration, indicating approximately 50% first pass metabolism. The level of beta sympathetic activity varies widely among individuals, and no simple correlation exists between the dose or plasma level of Timolol Maleate and its therapeutic activity. Therefore, objective clinical measurements such as reduction of heart rate and/or blood pressure should be used as guides in determining the optimal dosage for each patient.

INDICATIONS AND USAGE

HYPERTENSION

Timolol Maleate is indicated for the treatment of hypertension. It may be used alone or in combination with other antihypertensive agents, especially thiazide-type diuretics.

MYOCARDIAL INFARCTION

Timolol Maleate is indicated in patients who have survived the acute phase of a myocardial infarction, and are clinically stable, to reduce cardiovascular mortality and the risk of reinfarction.

MIGRAINE

Timolol Maleate is indicated for the prophylaxis of migraine headache.

UNLABLED USES

Timolol Maleate is used alone or as an adjunct in the treatment of angina pectoris, situational anxiety, and atrial fibrillation. Timolol Maleate is also used in the treatment of essential tremor and hyperthyroidism, and is prescribed to inhibit tachycardia due to air travel phobia and to reduce intraocular pressure before cataract extraction.

CONTRAINDICATIONS

Timolol Maleate is contraindicated in patients with bronchial asthma or with a history of bronchial asthma, or severe chronic obstructive pulmonary disease (see "Warnings"); sinus bradycardia; second and third degree atrioventricular block; overt cardiac failure (see "Warnings"); cardiogenic shock; hypersensitivity to this product.

WARNINGS

CARDIAC FAILURE

Sympathetic stimulation may be essential for support of the circulation in individuals with diminished myocardial contractility, and its inhibition by beta-adrenergic receptor blockade may precipitate more severe failure. Although beta blockers should be avoided in overt congestive heart failure, they can be used, if necessary, with caution in patients with a history of failure who are well-compensated, usually with digitalis and diuretics. Both digitalis and Timolol Maleate slow AV conduction. If cardiac failure persists, therapy with Timolol Maleate should be withdrawn.

In Patients Without a History of Cardiac Failure continued depression of the myocardium with beta-blocking agents over a period of time can, in some cases, lead to cardiac failure. At the first sign or symptom of cardiac failure patients receiving Timolol Maleate should be digitalized and/or be given a diuretic, and the response observed closely. If cardiac failure continues, despite adequate digitalization and diuretic therapy, Timolol Maleate should be withdrawn.

EXACERBATION OF ISCHEMIC HEART DISEASE FOLLOWING ABRUPT WITHDRAWAL: HYPERSENSITIVITY TO CATECHOLAMINES HAS BEEN OBSERVED IN PATIENTS WITHDRAWN FROM BETA BLOCKER THERAPY; EXACERBATION OF ANGINA AND, IN SOME CASES, MYOCARDIAL INFARCTION HAVE OCCURRED AFTER *ABRUPT* DISCONTINUATION OF SUCH THERAPY. WHEN DISCONTINUING CHRONICALLY ADMINISTERED TIMOLOL MALEATE, PARTICULARLY IN PATIENTS WITH ISCHEMIC HEART DISEASE, THE DOSAGE SHOULD BE GRADUALLY REDUCED OVER A PERIOD OF ONE TO TWO WEEKS AND THE PATIENT SHOULD BE CAREFULLY MONITORED. IF ANGINA MARKEDLY WORSENS OR ACUTE CORONARY INSUFFICIENCY DEVELOPS, TIMOLOL MALEATE ADMINISTRATION SHOULD BE REINSTITUTED PROMPTLY, AT LEAST TEMPORARILY, AND OTHER MEASURES APPROPRIATE FOR THE MANAGEMENT OF UNSTABLE ANGINA SHOULD BE TAKEN. PATIENTS SHOULD BE WARNED AGAINST INTERRUPTION OR DISCONTINUATION OF THERAPY WITHOUT THE PHYSICIAN'S ADVICE. BECAUSE CORONARY ARTERY DISEASE IS COMMON AND MAY BE UNRECOGNIZED, IT MAY BE PRUDENT NOT TO DISCONTINUE TIMOLOL MALEATE THERAPY ABRUPTLY EVEN IN PATIENTS TREATED ONLY FOR HYPERTENSION.

OBSTRUCTIVE PULMONARY DISEASE
PATIENTS WITH CHRONIC OBSTRUCTIVE PULMONARY DISEASE (e.g., CHRONIC BRONCHITIS, EMPHYSEMA) OF MILD OR MODERATE SEVERITY, BRONCHOSPASTIC DISEASE OR A HISTORY OF BRONCHOS-

PASTIC DISEASE (OTHER THAN BRONCHIAL ASTHMA OR A HISTORY OF BRONCHIAL ASTHMA, IN WHICH TIMOLOL MALEATE IS CONTRAINDICATED, (see *"CONTRAINDICATIONS"*), SHOULD IN GENERAL NOT RECEIVE BETA BLOCKERS, INCLUDING TIMOLOL MALEATE. However, if Timolol Maleate is necessary in such patients, then the drug should be administered with caution since it may block bronchodilation produced by endogenous and exogenous catecholamine stimulation of beta$_2$ receptors.

MAJOR SURGERY
The necessity or desirability of withdrawal of beta-blocking therapy prior to major surgery is controversial. Beta-adrenergic receptor blockade impairs the ability of the heart to respond to beta-adrenergically mediated reflex stimuli. This may augment the risk of general anesthesia in surgical procedures. Some patients receiving beta-adrenergic receptor blocking agents have been subject to protracted severe hypotension during anesthesia. Difficulty in restarting and maintaining the heartbeat has also been reported. For these reasons, in patients undergoing elective surgery, some authorities recommend gradual withdrawal of beta-adrenergic receptor blocking agents.

If necessary during surgery, the effects of beta-adrenergic blocking agents may be reversed by sufficient doses of such agonists as isoproterenol, dopamine, dobutamine or levarterenol (see *"Overdosage"*).

DIABETES MELLITUS
Timolol Maleate should be administered with caution in patients subject to spontaneous hypoglycemia or to diabetic patients (especially those with labile diabetes) who are receiving insulin or oral hypoglycemic agents. Beta-adrenergic receptor blocking agents may mask the signs and symptoms of acute hypoglycemia.

THYROTOXICOSIS
Beta-adrenergic blockade may mask certain clinical signs (e.g., tachycardia) of hyperthyroidism. Patients suspected of developing thyrotoxicosis should be managed carefully to avoid abrupt withdrawal of beta blockade which might precipitate a thyroid storm.

PRECAUTIONS
GENERAL
Impaired Hepatic or Renal Function: Since Timolol Maleate is partially metabolized in the liver and excreted mainly by the kidneys, dosage reductions may be necessary when hepatic and/or renal insufficiency is present.

Dosing in the Presence of Marked Renal Failure: Although the pharmacokinetics of Timolol Maleate are not greatly altered by renal impairment, marked hypotensive responses have been seen in patients with marked renal impairment undergoing dialysis after 20 mg doses. Dosing in such patients should therefore be especially cautious.

Muscle Weakness: Beta-adrenergic blockade has been reported to potentiate muscle weakness consistent with certain myasthenic symptoms (e.g., diplopia, ptosis, and generalized weakness). Timolol has been reported rarely to increase muscle weakness in some patients with myasthenia gravis or myasthenic symptoms.

Cerebrovascular Insufficiency: Because of potential effects of beta-adrenergic blocking agents relative to blood pressure and pulse, these agents should be used with caution in patients with cerebrovascular insufficiency. If signs or symptoms suggesting reduced cerebral blood flow are observed, consideration should be given to discontinuing these agents.

DRUG INTERACTIONS
Close observation of the patient is recommended when Timolol Maleate is administered to patients receiving catecholamine-depleting drugs such as reserpine, because of possible additive effects and the production of hypotension and/or marked bradycardia, which may produce vertigo, syncope, or postural hypotension.

Blunting of the antihypertensive effect of beta-adrenoceptor blocking agents by nonsteroidal anti-inflammatory drugs has been reported. When using these agents concomitantly, patients should be observed carefully to confirm that the desired therapeutic effect has been obtained.

Literature reports suggest that oral calcium antagonists may be used in combination with beta-adrenergic blocking agents when heart function is normal, but should be avoided in patients with impaired cardiac function. Hypotension, AV conduction disturbances, and left ventricular failure have been reported in some patients receiving beta-adrenergic blocking agents when an oral calcium antagonist was added to the treatment regimen. Hypotension was more likely to occur if the calcium antagonist were a dihydropyridine derivative, e.g. nifedipine, while left ventricular failure and AV conduction disturbances were more likely to occur with either verapamil or diltiazem.

Intravenous calcium antagonists should be used with caution in patients receiving beta-adrenergic blocking agents. The concomitant use of beta-adrenergic blocking agents with digitalis and either diltiazem or verapamil may have additive effects in prolonging AV conduction time.

Risk from Anaphylactic Reaction: While taking beta-blockers, patients with a history of atopy or a history of severe anaphylactic reaction to a variety of allergens may be more reactive to repeated accidental, diagnostic, or therapeutic challenge with such allergens. Such patients may be unresponsive to the usual doses of epinephrine used to treat anaphylactic reactions.

CARCINOGENESIS, MUTAGENESIS, IMPAIRMENT OF FERTILITY
In a two-year study of Timolol Maleate in rats, there was a statistically significant increase in the incidence of adrenal pheochromocytomas in male rats administered 300 mg/kg/day (250 times* the maximum recommended human dose). Similar differences were not observed in rats administered doses equivalent to approximately 20 or 80 times* the maximum recommended human dose.

In a lifetime study in mice, there were statistically significant increases in the incidence of benign and malignant pulmonary tumors, benign uterine polyps and mammary adenocarcinoma in female mice at 500 mg/kg/day (approximately 400 times* the maximum recommended human dose), but not at 5 or 50 mg/kg/day. In a subsequent study in female mice, in which postmortem examinations were limited to uterus and lungs, a statistically significant increase in the incidence of pulmonary tumors was again observed at 500 mg/kg/day.

The increased occurrence of mammary adenocarcinoma was associated with elevations in serum prolactin that occurred in female mice administered timolol at 500 mg/kg/day, but not at doses of 5 or 50 mg/kg/day. An increased incidence of mammary adenocarcinomas in rodents has been associated with administration of several other therapeutic agents which elevate serum prolactin, but no correlation between serum prolactin levels and mammary tumors has been established in man. Furthermore, in adult human female subjects who received oral dosages of up to 60 mg of Timolol Maleate, the maximum recommended human oral dosage, there were no clinically meaningful changes in serum prolactin.

Timolol Maleate was devoid of mutagenic potential when evaluated *in vivo* (mouse) in the micronucleus test and cytogenetic assay (doses up to 800 mg/kg) and *in vitro* in a neoplastic cell transformation assay (up to 100 μg/mL). In Ames tests the highest concentrations of Timolol employed, 5000 or 10,000 μg/plate, were associated with statistically significant elevations of revertants observed with tester strain TA100 (in seven replicate assays), but not in the remaining three strains. In the assays with tester strain TA100, no consistent dose response relationship was observed, nor did the ratio of test to control revertants reach 2. A ratio of 2 is usually considered the criterion for a positive Ames test.

Reproduction and fertility studies in rats showed no adverse effect on male or female fertility at doses up to 125 times* the maximum recommended human dose.

PREGNANCY
Pregnancy Category C: Teratogenicity studies with Timolol in mice, rats and rabbits at doses up to 50 mg/kg/day (approximately 40 times the maximum recommended daily human dose) showed no evidence of fetal malformations. Although delayed fetal ossification was observed at this dose in rats, there were no adverse effects on postnatal development of offspring. Doses of 1000 mg/kg/day (approximately 830 times the maximum recommended daily human dose) were maternotoxic in mice and resulted in an increased number of fetal resorptions. Increased fetal resorptions were also seen in rabbits at doses of approximately 40 times the maximum recommended daily human dose, in this case without apparent maternotoxicity. There are no adequate and well-controlled studies in pregnant women Timolol Maleate should be used during pregnancy only if the potential benefit justifies the potential risk to the fetus.

NURSING MOTHERS
Timolol Maleate has been detected in human milk. Because of the potential for serious adverse reactions from Timolol in nursing infants, a decision should be made whether to discontinue nursing or to discontinue the drug, taking into account the importance of the drug to the mother.

PEDIATRIC USE
Safety and effectiveness in children have not been established.

ADVERSE REACTIONS
Timolol Maleate is usually well tolerated in properly selected patients. Most adverse effects have been mild and transient. In a multicenter (12-week) clinical trial comparing Timolol Maleate and placebo in hypertensive patients, the following adverse reactions were reported spontaneously and considered to be causally related to Timolol Maleate:

	Timolol Maleate (n = 176) %	Placebo (n = 168) %
Body as a Whole		
fatigue/tiredness	3.4	0.6
headache	1.7	1.8
chest pain	0.6	0
asthenia	0.6	0
Cardiovascular		
bradycardia	9.1	0
arrhythmia	1.1	0.6
syncope	0.6	0
edema	0.6	1.2
Digestive		
dyspepsia	0.6	0.6
nausea	0.6	0
Skin		
pruritus	1.1	0

* Based on patient weight of 50 kg

◆ RATED THERAPEUTICALLY EQUIVALENT; ◇ THERAPEUTIC EQUIVALENCE UNCONFIRMED; ○ UNRATED

Nervous System		
dizziness	2.3	1.2
vertigo	0.6	0
paresthesia	0.6	0
Psychiatric		
decreased		
libido	0.6	0
Respiratory		
dyspnea	1.7	0.6
bronchial		
spasm	0.6	0
rales	0.6	0
Special Senses		
eye irritation	1.1	0.6
tinnitus	0.6	0

These data are representative of the incidence of adverse effects that may be observed in properly selected patients treated with Timolol Maleate, i.e., excluding patients with bronchospastic disease, congestive heart failure or other contraindications to beta blocker therapy.

In patients with migraine the incidence of bradycardia was 5 percent.

In a coronary artery disease population studied in the Norwegian multi-center trial (see "Clinical Pharmacology"), the frequency of the principal adverse reactions and the frequency with which these resulted in discontinuation of therapy in the Timolol and placebo groups were:

Timolol Maleate	Adverse Reaction†		Withdrawal‡	
	Timolol (n = 945) %	Placebo (n = 939) %	Timolol (n = 945) %	Placebo (n = 939) %
Asthenia or Fatigue	5	1	< 1	< 1
Heart Rate < 40 beats/ minute	5	< 1	4	< 1
Cardiac Failure— Nonfatal	8	7	3	2
Hypotension	3	2	3	1
Pulmonary Edema— Nonfatal	2	< 1	< 1	< 1
Claudication	3	3	1	< 1
AV Block 2nd or 3rd degree	< 1	< 1	< 1	< 1
Sinoatrial Block	< 1	< 1	< 1	< 1
Cold Hands and Feet	8	< 1	< 1	0
Nausea or Digestive Disorders	8	6	1	< 1
Dizziness	6	4	1	0
Bronchial Obstruction	2	< 1	1	< 1

† When an adverse reaction recurred in a patient, it is listed only once.
‡ Only principal reason for withdrawal in each patient is listed.
These adverse reactions can also occur in patients treated for hypertension.

The following additional adverse effects have been reported in clinical experience with the drug.

Body as a Whole: extremity pain, decreased exercise tolerance, weight loss, fever;

Cardiovascular: cardiac arrest, cardiac failure, cerebrovascular accident, worsening of angina pectoris, worsening of arterial insufficiency, Raynaud's phenomenon, palpitations, vasodilatation.

Digestive: gastrointestinal pain, hepatomegaly, vomiting, diarrhea, dyspepsia.

Hematologic: nonthrombocytopenic purpura.

Endocrine: hyperglycemia, hypoglycemia.

Skin: rash, skin irritation, increased pigmentation, sweating, alopecia.

Musculoskeletal: arthralgia;

Nervous System: local weakness, increase in signs and symptoms of myasthenia gravis.

Psychiatric: depression, nightmares, somnolence, insomnia, nervousness, diminished concentration, hallucinations.

Respiratory: cough.

Special Senses: visual disturbances, diplopia, ptosis, dry eyes.

Urogenital: impotence, urination difficulties.

There have been reports of retroperitoneal fibrosis in patients receiving Timolol Maleate and in patients receiving other beta-adrenergic blocking agents. A causal relationship between this condition and therapy with beta-adrenergic blocking agents has not been established.

Potential Adverse Effects: In addition, a variety of adverse effects not observed in clinical trials with Timolol Maleate, but reported with other beta-adrenergic blocking agents, should be considered potential adverse effects of Timolol Maleate.

Nervous System: Reversible mental depression progressing to catatonia; an acute reversible syndrome characterized by disorientation for time and place, short-term memory loss, emotional lability, slightly clouded sensorium, and decreased performance on neuropsychometrics.

Cardiovascular: Intensification of AV block (see "Contraindications").

Digestive: Mesenteric arterial thrombosis, ischemic colitis.

Hematologic: Agranulocytosis, thrombocytopenic purpura.

Allergic: Erythematous rash, fever combined with aching and sore throat, laryngospasm with respiratory distress.

Miscellaneous: Peyronie's disease.

There have been reports of a syndrome comprising psoriasiform skin rash, conjunctivitis sicca, otitis, and sclerosing serositis attributed to the beta-adrenergic receptor blocking agent, practolol. This syndrome has not been reported with Timolol Maleate.

Clinical Laboratory Test Findings: Clinically important changes in standard laboratory parameters were rarely associated with the administration of Timolol Maleate. Slight increases in blood urea nitrogen, serum potassium, uric acid, and triglycerides, and slight decreases in hemoglobin, hematocrit and HDL cholesterol occurred, but were not progressive or associated with clinical manifestations. Increases in liver function tests have been reported.

OVERDOSAGE

Overdosage has been reported with Timolol Maleate tablets. A 30-year-old female ingested 650 mg of Timolol Maleate (maximum recommended daily dose—60 mg) and experienced second and third degree heart block. She recovered without treatment but approximately two months later developed irregular heart beat, hypertension, dizziness, tinnitus, faintness, increased pulse rate and borderline first degree heart block.

The oral LD_{50} of the drug is 1190 and 900 mg/kg in female mice and female rats, respectively.

An *in vitro* hemodialysis study, using ^{14}C Timolol added to human plasma or whole blood, showed that Timolol was readily dialyzed from these fluids; however, a study of patients with renal failure showed that Timolol did not dialyze readily.

The most common signs and symptoms to be expected with overdosage with a beta-adrenergic receptor blocking agent are symptomatic bradycardia, hypotension, bronchospasm, and acute cardiac failure. Therapy with Timolol Maleate should be discontinued and the patient observed closely. The following additional therapeutic measures should be considered:

(1) *Gastric lavage*
(2) *Symptomatic bradycardia*: Use atropine sulfate intravenously in a dosage of 0.25 mg to 2 mg to induce vagal blockade. If bradycardia persists, intravenous isoproterenol hydrochloride should be administered cautiously. In refractory cases the use of a transvenous cardiac pacemaker may be considered.
(3) *Hypotension*: Use sympathomimetic pressor drug therapy, such as dopamine, dobutamine or levarterenol. In refractory cases the use of glucagon hydrochloride has been reported to be useful.
(4) *Bronchospasm*: Use isoproterenol hydrochloride. Additional therapy with aminophylline may be considered.
(5) *Acute cardiac failure*: Conventional therapy with digitalis, diuretics, and oxygen should be instituted immediately. In refractory cases the use of intravenous aminophylline is suggested. This may be followed if necessary by glucagon hydrochloride which has been reported to be useful.
(6) *Heart block (second or third degree)*: Use isoproterenol hydrochloride or a transvenous cardiac pacemaker.

DOSAGE AND ADMINISTRATION

HYPERTENSION

The usual initial dosage of Timolol Maleate is 10 mg twice a day, whether used alone or added to diuretic therapy. Dosage may be increased or decreased depending on heart rate and blood pressure response. The usual total maintenance dosage is 20-40 mg per day. Increases in dosage to a maximum of 60 mg per day divided into two doses may be necessary. There should be an interval of at least seven days between increases in dosages.

Timolol Maleate may be used with a thiazide diuretic or with other antihypertensive agents. Patients should be observed carefully during initiation of such concomitant therapy.

MYOCARDIAL INFARCTION

The recommended dosage for long-term prophylactic use in patients who have survived the acute phase of a myocardial infarction is 10 mg given twice daily (see "Clinical Pharmacology").

MIGRAINE

The usual initial dosage of Timolol Maleate is 10 mg twice a day. During maintenance therapy the 20 mg daily dosage may be administered as a single dose. Total daily dosage may be increased to a maximum of 30 mg, given in divided doses, or decreased to 10 mg once per day, depending on clinical response and tolerability. If a satisfactory response is not obtained after 6-8 weeks use of the maximum daily dosage, therapy with Timolol Maleate should be discontinued.

STORAGE

Store in a well-closed container, protected from light.

HOW SUPPLIED
TABLETS: 5 MG

AVERAGE UNIT PRICE (AVAILABLE SIZES)		GENERIC A-RATED AVERAGE PRICE (GAAP)	
BRAND	$0.41		
GENERIC	$0.27		
HCFA FUL (100s ea)	$0.18	100s	$26.51

BRAND/MANUFACTURER	NDC	SIZE	AWP
◆ BRAND			
➤ BLOCADREN: Merck	00006-0059-68	100s	$41.41
◆ GENERICS			
Moore,H.L.	00839-7584-06	100s	$23.80
Qualitest	00603-6071-21	100s	$25.95
Schein	00364-2357-01	100s	$26.50
➤ Geneva	00781-1126-01	100s	$27.10
Mylan	00378-0055-01	100s	$27.15
Novopharm	55953-0916-40	100s	$28.56

TABLETS: 10 MG

AVERAGE UNIT PRICE (AVAILABLE SIZES)		GENERIC A-RATED AVERAGE PRICE (GAAP)	
BRAND	$0.53	100s	$33.55
GENERIC	$0.34		
HCFA FUL (100s ea)	$0.28		

BRAND/MANUFACTURER	NDC	SIZE	AWP
◆ BRAND			
➤ BLOCADREN: Merck	00006-0136-68	100s	$51.21
	00006-0136-28	100s ud	$55.49
◆ GENERICS			
Rugby	00536-4696-01	100s	$30.48
Qualitest	00603-6072-21	100s	$31.80
Schein	00364-2358-01	100s	$33.00
Aligen	00405-5020-01	100s	$33.70
➤ Geneva	00781-1127-01	100s	$34.20
Mylan	00378-0221-01	100s	$34.25
Novopharm	55953-0972-40	100s	$35.25
Moore,H.L.	00839-7936-06	100s	$35.71

TABLETS: 20 MG

AVERAGE UNIT PRICE (AVAILABLE SIZES)		GENERIC A-RATED AVERAGE PRICE (GAAP)	
BRAND	$0.95	100s	$64.69
GENERIC	$0.65		
HCFA FUL (100s ea)	$0.53		

BRAND/MANUFACTURER	NDC	SIZE	AWP
◆ BRAND			
➤ BLOCADREN: Merck	00006-0437-68	100s	$94.46
◆ GENERICS			
Schein	00364-2359-01	100s	$60.50
Geneva	00781-1128-01	100s	$64.89
Mylan	00378-0715-01	100s	$64.95
Novopharm	55953-0984-40	100s	$65.09
Moore,H.L.	00839-7937-06	100s	$68.03

Timoptic *SEE* TIMOLOL MALEATE, OPHTHALMIC

Tinastat *SEE* SODIUM THIOSULFATE

Tioconazole

DESCRIPTION
Tioconazole, 1-[2-[(2-chloro-3-thienyl)methoxy]-2(2,4- dichlorophenyl)ethyl]-1H-imidazole, is a topical antifungal agent. Its chemical formula is $C_{16}H_{13}Cl_3N_2OS$ with a molecular weight of 387.7.

Tioconazole vaginal ointment contains 6.5% of Tioconazole.

Each applicator-full of Tioconazole provides approximately 4.6 grams of ointment containing 300 mg of Tioconazole.

Following is its chemical structure:

CLINICAL PHARMACOLOGY
Tioconazole is a broad-spectrum antifungal agent that inhibits the growth of human pathogenic yeasts. Tioconazole exhibits fungicidal activity *in vitro* against *Candida albicans*, other species of the genus *Candida*, and against *Torulopsis glabrata*.

Pharmacokinetics: Systemic absorption of Tioconazole after a single intravaginal application of Tioconazole in nonpregnant patients is negligible.

INDICATIONS AND USAGE
Tioconazole is indicated for the local treatment of vulvovaginal candidiasis (moniliasis). As Tioconazole has been shown to be effective only for candidal vulvovaginitis, the diagnosis should be confirmed by KOH smears and/or cultures. Other pathogens commonly associated with vulvovaginitis should be ruled out by appropriate methods.

Studies have shown that women taking oral contraceptives have a cure rate similar to those not taking such agents when treated with Tioconazole.

Safety and effectiveness in pregnant and diabetic patients have not been established (see *"Precautions"*).

UNLABELED USES
Tioconazole is used alone or as an adjunct in the treatment of vaginal trichomoniasis, trichophyton mentagrophytes, including pityriasis versicolor; dermatomycosis, and onychomycosis.

CONTRAINDICATIONS
Tioconazole is contraindicated in individuals who have been shown to be sensitive to imidazole antifungal agents or to other components of the ointment.

PRECAUTIONS
General: Tioconazole is intended for intravaginal administration only. Applicators should be opened just prior to administration to prevent contamination. Administration of Tioconazole just prior to bedtime may be preferred. The Tioconazole ointment base may interact with rubber or latex products such as condoms or vaginal contraceptive diaphragms; therefore, use of such products within 72 hours following treatment is not recommended.

If clinical symptoms persist, appropriate microbiological tests should be repeated to rule out other pathogens and to confirm the diagnosis.

Information for Patients: The Tioconazole ointment base may interact with rubber or latex products such as condoms or vaginal contraceptive diaphragms; therefore, use of such products within 72 hours following treatment is not recommended.

Carcinogenesis: No long-term studies in animals have been performed to evaluate the carcinogenic potential of Tioconazole.

Mutagenesis: Tioconazole did not demonstrate mutagenic activity at the levels examined in tests at either the chromosomal or subchromosomal level.

Impairment of Fertility: No impairment of fertility was seen in male rats administered Tioconazole hydrochloride in oral doses up to 150 mg/kg/day. However, there was evidence of preimplantation loss in female rats at oral dose levels above 35 mg/kg/day.

Pregnancy—Pregnancy Category C: Tioconazole hydrochloride had no adverse effects on fetal viability or growth when administered orally to pregnant rats at doses of 55, 110, and 165 mg/kg/day during the period of organogenesis. A drug-related increase in the incidence of dilated ureters, hydroureters, and hydronephrosis observed in the fetuses of this study was transient and no longer evident in pups raised to 21 days of age. These effects did not occur following intravaginal administration of approximately 10 mg/kg/day in a 2% cream. There was no evidence of major structural anomalies. No embryotoxic or teratogenic effects were observed in rabbits receiving oral dose levels as high as 165 mg/kg/day or daily intravaginal application of approximately 2-3 mg/kg in a 2% Tioconazole cream during organogenesis. Tioconazole hydrochloride, like other azole antimycotic agents, causes dystocia in rats when treatment is extended through parturition. Associated effects in rats include prolongation of pregnancy, *in utero* deaths, and impaired pup survival. The "no-effect" level for this phenomenon is 20 mg/kg/day orally and approximately 9 mg/kg/day intravaginally. No effect on parturition occurred in rabbits at 50 mg/kg/day orally.

There are no adequate and well-controlled studies in pregnant women. Tioconazole should be used during pregnancy only if the potential benefit justifies the potential risk to the fetus.

Nursing Mothers: It is not known whether this drug is excreted in human milk. Because many drugs are excreted in human milk, nursing should be temporarily discontinued while Tioconazole is administered.

Pediatric Use: Safety and effectiveness in children have not been established.

ADVERSE REACTIONS
The incidence of adverse reactions to Tioconazole is based on clinical trials involving 1000 patients. Burning and itching were the most frequent side effects occurring in approximately 6% and 5% of the patients, respectively. In most instances these did not interfere with the course of therapy. There were occasional reports (less than 1%) of other side effects including irritation, discharge, vulvar edema and swelling, vaginal pain, dysuria, nocturia, dyspareunia, dryness of vaginal secretions, desquamation, and burning sensation.

DOSAGE AND ADMINISTRATION
Tioconazole has been found to be effective as a single-dose treatment for vulvovaginal candidiasis. Using the prefilled applicator, insert one applicator-full

---

intravaginally. Administration of Tioconazole just prior to bedtime may be preferred.

WARNING
Manufactured with 1,1,1-trichloroethane, a substance which harms public health and environment by destroying ozone in the upper atmosphere.

Store at controlled room temperature, 15°-30°C (59°-86°F).

HOW SUPPLIED
OINTMENT: 6.5%

BRAND/MANUFACTURER	NDC	SIZE	AWP
○ BRAND			
VAGISTAT-1: Mead Johnson Labs	00087-0657-40	4.6 gm	$24.20

Tiopronin

DESCRIPTION
Tiopranin is a reducing and complexing thiol compound. Tiopronin is N-(2-Mercaptopropionyl) glycine.

Tiopronin has the empirical formula $C_5H_9NO_3S$ and a molecular weight of 163.20. In this drug product Tiopranin exists as a dl racemic mixture.

Tiopronin is a white crystalline powder which is freely soluble in water.

Tiopronin tablets are sugar coated tablets, each containing 100 mg. of Tiopronin, and are taken orally.

Following is its chemical structure:

$$H_3C-CH-CO-NH-CH_2-COOH$$
$$| $$
$$SH$$

CLINICAL PHARMACOLOGY
Tiopronin is an active reducing agent which undergoes thiol-disulfide exchange with cystine to form a mixed disulfide of Thiola-cysteine.

$$2R\text{-}SH + R'\text{-}S\text{-}S\text{-}R' \quad 2R\text{-}S\text{-}S\text{-}R' + 2H^+$$

Thiola Cystine $\rightleftharpoons$ Thiola-cysteine

From this reaction, a water-soluble mixed disulfide is formed and the amount of sparingly soluble cystine is reduced. When Tiopronin is given orally, up to 48% of dose appears in urine during the first 4 hours and up to 78% by 72 hours. Thus, in patients with cystinuria, sufficient amount of Tiopronin or its active metabolites could appear in urine to react with cystine, lowering cystine excretion.

The decrement in urinary cystine produced by Tiopronin is generally proportional to the dose. A reduction in urinary cystine of 250-350 mg/day at a Tiopronin dosage of 1 g/day, and a decline of approximately 500 mg/day at a dosage of 2 g/day, might be expected. Tiopronin causes a sustained reduction in cystine excretion without apparent loss of effectiveness. Tiopronin has a rapid onset and offset of action, showing a fall in cystine excretion on the first day of administration and a rise on the first day of drug withdrawal.

INDICATIONS AND USAGE
Tiopronin is indicated for the prevention of cystine (kidney) stone formation in patients with severe homozygous cystinuria with urinary cystine greater than 500 mg/day, who are resistant to treatment with conservative measures of high fluid intake, alkali and diet modification, or who have adverse reactions to d-penicillamine.

Cystine stones typically occur in approximately 10,000 persons in the United States who are homozygous for cystinuria. These persons excrete abnormal amounts of cystine in urine of over 250 mg/g creatinine, as well as excessive amounts of other dibasic amino acids (lysine, arginine and ornithine). In addition, they show varying intestinal transport defects for these same amino acids. The stone formation is the result of poor aqueous solubility of cystine.

Since there are no known inhibitors of the crystallization of cystine, the stone formation is determined primarily by the urinary supersaturation of cystine. Thus, cystine stones could theoretically form whenever urinary cystine concentration exceeds the solubility limit. Cystine solubility in urine is pH-dependent, and ranges from 170-300 mg/liter at pH 5, 190-400 mg/liter at pH 7 and 220-500 mg/liter at pH 7.5.

The goal of therapy is to reduce urinary cystine concentration below its solubility limit. It may be accomplished by dietary means aimed at reducing cystine synthesis and by a high fluid intake in order to increase urine volume and thereby lower cystine concentration.

Unfortunately, the above conservative measures alone may be ineffective in controlling cystine stone formation in some homozygous patients with severe cystinuria (urinary cystine exceeding 500 mg/day). In such patients, d-penicillamine has been used as an additional therapy. Like Tiopronin, d-penicillamine undergoes thiol-disulfide exchange with cystine, thereby lowering the amount of sparingly soluble cystine in urine.

However, d-penicillamine treatment is frequently accompanied by adverse reactions, such as dermatologic complications, hypersensitivity reactions, hematologic abnormalities and renal disturbances. Tiopronin may have a particular therapeutic role in such patients.

UNLABELED USES
Tiopronin is used alone or as an adjunct in the treatment of senile cataracts, chronic active hepatitis, and rheumatoid arthritis.

CONTRAINDICATIONS
The use of Tiopronin during pregnancy is contraindicated, except in those with severe cystinuria where the anticipated benefit of inhibited stone formation clearly outweighs possible hazards of treatment (See "Precautions").

Tiopronin should not be begun again in patients with a prior history of developing agranulocytosis, aplastic anemia or thrombocytopenia on this medication.

Mothers maintained on Tiopronin treatment should not nurse their infants.

WARNINGS
Despite apparent lower toxicity of Tiopronin, Tipronin may potentially cause all the serious adverse reactions reported for d-penicillamine. Thus, although no death has been reported to result directly from Tiopronin treatment, a fatal outcome from Tiopronin is possible, as has been reported with d-penicillamine therapy from such complications as aplastic anemia, agranulocytosis, thrombocytopenia, Goodpasture's syndrome or myasthenia gravis.

Leukopenia of the granulocytic series may develop without eosinophilia. Thrombocytopenia may be immunologic in origin or occur on an idiosyncratic basis. The reduction in peripheral blood white count to less than 3500/cubic mm or in platelet count to below 100,000 cubic mm mandates cessation of therapy. Patients should be instructed to report promptly the occurrence of any symptom or sign of these hematological abnormalities, such as fever, sore throat, chills, bleeding or easy bruisability.

Proteinuria, sometimes sufficiently severe to cause nephrotic syndrome, may develop from membranous glomerulopathy. A close observation of affected patients is mandatory.

The following complications, though rare, have been reported during d-penicillamine therapy and could occur during Tiopronin treatment. When there are abnormal urinary findings associated with hemoptysis and pulmonary infiltrates suggestive of Goodpasture's syndrome, Tiopronin treatment should be stopped. Appearance of myasthenic syndrome or myasthenia gravis requires cessation of treatment. When pemphigus-type reactions develop, Tiopronin therapy should be stopped. Steroid treatment may be necessary.

PRECAUTIONS
Patients should be advised of the potential development of complications and to report promptly the occurrence of any symptom or sign of them.

To help monitor potential complications, the following tests are recommended; peripheral blood counts, direct platelet count, hemoglobin; serum albumin, liver function tests; 24-hour urinary protein and routine urinalysis at 3-6 month intervals during treatment. In order to assess effect on stone disease, urinary cystine analysis should be monitored frequently during the first 6 months when the optimum dose schedule is being determined, and at 6-month intervals thereafter. Abdominal roentgenogram (KUB) is advised on a yearly basis to monitor the size and appearance/disappearance of stone(s).

CARCINOGENESIS, MUTAGENESIS, IMPAIRMENT OF FERTILITY:
Longterm carcinogenicity studies in animals have not been performed. High doses of Tiopronin in experimental animals have been shown to interfere with maintenance of pregnancy and viability of the fetus.

USE IN PREGNANCY
Pregnancy category C. D-penicillamine has been shown to cause skeletal defects and cleft palates in the fetus when given to pregnant rats at 10 times the dose recommended for human use. A similar teratogenicity might be expected for Tiopronin although no such findings could be related to the drug in studies in mice and rats at doses up to 10 times the highest recommended human dose.

There are no adequate and well-controlled studies in pregnant women. Tiopronin should be used during pregnancy only if the potential benefit justifies potential risk to the fetus.

NURSING MOTHERS
Because Tiopronin may be excreted in milk, and because of the potential serious adverse reactions of nursing infants from Tiopronin mothers taking Tiopronin should not nurse their infants.

PEDIATRIC USE
Safety and effectiveness below the age of 9 have not been established.

ADVERSE REACTIONS
Some patients may develop drug fever, usually during the first month of therapy. Tiopronin treatment should be discontinued until the fever subsides. It may be reinstated at a small dose, with a gradual increase in dosage until the desired level is achieved.

A generalized rash (erythematous, maculopapular or morbilliform) accompanied by pruritis may develop during the first few months of treatment. It may be controlled by antihistamine therapy, typically recedes when Tiopronin treatment is discontinued, and seldom recurs when Tiopronin treatment is restarted at a lower dosage. Less commonly, rash may appear late in the course of treatment (of more than 6 months). Located usually in the trunk, the late rash is associated with intense pruritis, recedes slowly after discontinuing treatment, and usually recurs upon resumption of treatment.

A drug reaction simulating lupus erythematous, manifested by fever, arthralgia and lymphadenopathy may develop. It may be associated with a positive antinuclear antibody test, but not necessarily with nephropathy. It may require discontinuance of Tiopronin treatment.

A reduction in taste perception may develop. It is believed to be the result of chelation of trace metals by Tiopronin. Hypogeusia is often self-limiting.

► SHOWN IN PRODUCT IDENTIFICATION GUIDE

Unlike during d-pencillamine therapy, vitamin B$_6$ deficiency is uncommonly associated with Tiopronin treatment.

Some patients may complain of wrinkling and friability of skin. This complication usually occurs after long-term treatment, and is believed to result from the effect of Tiopronin on collagen.

A multiclinic trial involving 66 cystinuric patients in the United States indicated that Tiopronin is associated with fewer or less severe adverse reactions than d-pencillamine. Among those who had to stop taking d-penicillamine due to toxicity, 64.7% could take Tiopronin. In those without prior history of d-penicillamine treatment, only 5.9% developed reactions of sufficient severity to require Tiopronin withdrawal. A review of available literature support the findings from this trial.

Despite this apparent reduced toxicity to Tiopronin relative to d-penicillamine, Tiopronin treatment may potentially be associated with all the adverse reactions reported with d-pencillamine. They include:

Gastrointestinal side-effects (nausea, emesis, diarrhea or soft-stools, anorexia, abdominal pain, bloating or flatus) in about 1 in 6 patients;

Impairment in taste and smell in about 1 in 25 patients;

Dermatologic complications (pharyngitis, oral ulcers, rash, ecchymosis, prurites, uritcaria, warts, skin wrinkling, pemphigus, elastosis perforans serpiginosa) in about 1 in 6 patients;

Hypersensitivity reactions (laryngeal edema, dyspnea, respiratory distress, fever, chills, arthralgia, weakness, fatigue, myalgia, adenopathy) in about 1 in 25 patients;

Hematologic abnormalities (increased bleeding, anemia, leukopenia, thrombocytopenia, eosinophilia) in about 1 in 25 patients;

Renal complications (proteinuria, nephrotic syndrome, hematuria) in about 1 in 20 patients;

Pulmonary manifestations (bronchiolitis, hemoptysis, pulmonary infiltrates, dyspnea) in about 1 in 50 patients;

Neurologic complications (myasthenic syndrome) in about 1 in 50 patients.

These reactions are more likely to develop during Tiopronin therapy among patients who had previously shown toxicity to d-penicillamine.

In patients who had previously manifested adverse reactions to d-penicillamine, adverse reactions to Tiopronin are more likely to occur than in patients who took Tiopronin for the first time. A close supervision with a careful monitoring of potential side effects is mandatory during Tiopronin treatment. Patients should be told to report promptly any symptoms suggesting toxicity. The treatment with Tiopronin should be stopped if severe toxicity develops.

DOSAGE AND ADMINISTRATION

It is recommended that a conservative treatment program should be attempted first. At least 3 liters of fluid (10-10 oz glassfuls) should be provided, including two glasses with each meal and at bedtime. The patients should be expected to awake at night to urinate; they should drink two more glasses of fluids before returning to bed. Additional fluids should be consumed if there is excessive sweating or intestinal fluid loss. A minimum urine output of 2 liters/day on a consistent basis should be sought. A modest amount of alkali should be provided in order to maintain urinary pH at a high normal range (6.5-7.0). Potassium alkali are advantageous over sodium alkali, because they do not cause hypercalciuria and are less likely to cause the complication of calcium stones.

Excessive alkali therapy is not advisable. When urinary pH increases above 7.0 with alkali therapy, the complication of calcium phosphate nephrolithiasis may ensue because of the enhanced urinary supersaturation of hydroxyapatite in an alkaline environment.

In patients who continue to form cystine stones on the above conservative program, Tiopronin may be added to the treatment program. Tiopronin may also be substituted for d-penicillamine in patients who have developed toxicity to the latter drug. In both situations, the conservative treatment program should be continued.

The dose of Tiopronin should not be arbitrary but should be based on that amount required to reduce urinary cystine concentration to below its solubility limit (generally < 250 mg/liter). The extent of the decline in cystine excretion is generally dependent on the Tiopronin dosage.

Tiopronin may be begun at a dosage of 800 mg/day in adult patients with cystine stones. In a multiclinic trial, average dose of Tiopronin was about 1000 mg/day. However, some patients required a smaller dose. In children, initial dosage may be based on 15 mg/kg/day. Urinary cystine should be measured at 1 month after Tiopronin treatment, and every 3 months thereafter. Tiopronin dosage should be readjusted depending on the urinary cystine value. Whenever possible, Tiopronin should be given in divided doses 3 times/day at least one hour before or 2 hours after meals.

In patients who had shown severe toxicity to d-penicillamine, Tiopronin might be begun at a lower dosage.

Store in a dry place at controlled room temperature, 15°C-30°C (59°F-86°F).

HOW SUPPLIED
TABLETS: 100 MG

BRAND/MANUFACTURER	NDC	SIZE	AWP
○ **BRAND**			
THIOLA: Mission	00178-0900-01	100s	$65.00

Tobradex *SEE* DEXAMETHASONE AND TOBRAMYCIN

Tobramycin, Ophthalmic

DESCRIPTION

Tobramycin 0.3% is a sterile topical ophthalmic antibiotic formulation prepared specifically for topical therapy of external ophthalmic infections. This product is supplied in solution and ointment forms.

Each mL of Tobramycin, Ophthalmic solution contains: Active: Tobramycin 0.3% (3 mg). Preservative: Benzalkonium Chloride 0.01%.

Each gram of Tobramycin, Ophthalmic ointment contains: Active: Tobramycin 0.3% (3 mg). Preservative: Chlorobutanol 0.5%.

Chemical name: 0-{3-amino-3-deoxy-α-D-gluco-pyranosyl-(1→4)}-0-{2,6-di-amino-2,3,6-trideoxy-α-D-ribohexo-pyranosyl-(1→6)}-2-deoxystreptamine.

Tobramycin is a water-soluble aminoglycoside antibiotic active against a wide variety of gram-negative and gram-positive ophthalmic pathogens.

Following is its chemical structure:

CLINICAL PHARMACOLOGY

In Vitro Data: *In vitro* studies have demonstrated Tobramycin, Ophthalmic (Tobramycin) is active against susceptible strains of the following microorganisms:

Staphylococci, including *S. aureus* and *S. epidermidis* (coagulase-positive and coagulase-negative), including penicillin-resistant strains.

Streptococci, including some of the Group A-betahemolytic species, some nonhemolytic species, and some *Streptococcus pneumoniae*.

Pseudomonas aeruginosa, Escherichia coli, Klebsiella pneumoniae, Enterobacter aerogenes, Proteus mirabilis, Morganella morganii, most *Proteus vulgaris* strains, *Haemophilus influenzae* and *H. aegyptius, Moraxella lacunata*, and *Acinetobacter calcoaceticus* and some *Neisseria* species. Bacterial susceptibility studies demonstrate that in some cases, microorganisms resistant to gentamicin retain susceptibility to Tobramycin.

INDICATIONS AND USAGE

Tobramycin is a topical antibiotic indicated in the treatment of external infections of the eye and its adnexa caused by susceptible bacteria. Appropriate monitoring of bacterial response to topical antibiotic therapy should accompany the use of Tobramycin.

Clinical studies have shown Tobramycin to be safe and effective for use in children.

CONTRAINDICATIONS

Tobramycin Ophthalmic Solution and Ointment are contraindicated in patients with known hypersensitivity to any of their components.

WARNINGS

NOT FOR INJECTION INTO THE EYE. Do not touch tube or dropper tip to any surface, as this may contaminate the contents. Sensitivity to topically applied aminoglycosides may occur in some patients. If a sensitivity reaction to Tobramycin occurs, discontinue use.

PRECAUTIONS

As with other antibiotic preparations, prolonged use may result in overgrowth of nonsusceptible organisms, including fungi. If superinfection occurs, appropriate therapy should be initiated. Ophthalmic ointments may retard corneal wound healing.

Pregnancy Category B: Reproduction studies in three types of animals at doses up to thirty-three times the normal human systemic dose have revealed no evidence of impaired fertility or harm to the fetus due to Tobramycin. There are, however, no adequate and well-controlled studies in pregnant women. Because animal studies are not always predictive of human response, this drug should be used during pregnancy only if clearly needed.

Nursing Mothers: Because of the potential for adverse reactions in nursing infants from Tobramycin a decision should be made whether to discontinue nursing the infant or discontinue the drug, taking into account the importance of the drug to the mother.

ADVERSE REACTIONS

The most frequent adverse reactions to Tobramycin Ophthalmic Solution and Ointment are hypersensitivity and localized ocular toxicity, including lid itching and swelling, and conjunctival erythema. These reactions occur in less than three of 100 patients treated with Tobramycin. Similar reactions may occur with the topical use of other aminoglycoside antibiotics. Other adverse reactions have not been reported from Tobramycin therapy; however, if topical ocular Tobramycin is administered concomitantly with systemic aminoglycoside antibiotics, care should be taken to monitor the total serum concentration.

In clinical trials, Tobramycin Ophthalmic Ointment produced significantly fewer adverse reactions (3.7%) than did Garamycin Ophthalmic Ointment (10.6%).

OVERDOSAGE

Clinically apparent signs and symptoms of an overdose of Tobramycin Ophthalmic Solution or Ointment (punctate keratitis, erythema, increased lacrimation, edema and lid itching) may be similar to adverse reaction effects seen in some patients.

DOSAGE AND ADMINISTRATION

Solution: In mild to moderate disease, instill one or two drops into the affected eye(s) every four hours. In severe infections, instill two drops into the eye(s) hourly until improvement, following which treatment should be reduced prior to discontinuation.

Ointment: In mild to moderate disease, apply a half-inch ribbon into the affected eye(s) two or three times per day. In severe infections, instill a half-inch ribbon into the affected eye(s) every three to four hours until improvement, following which treatment should be reduced prior to discontinuation.

HOW TO APPLY TOBRAMYCIN OINTMENT
1. Tilt your head back.
2. Place a finger on your cheek just under your eye and gently pull down until a "V" pocket is formed between your eyeball and your lower lid.
3. Place a small amount (about 1/2 inch) of Tobramycin in the "V" pocket. Do not let the tip of the tube touch your eye.
4. Look downward before closing your eye.
Tobramycin Ointment may be used in conjunction with Tobramycin Solution.

Store at 8°-27°C (46°-80°F).

J CODES
Up to 80 mg IM,IV—J3260

HOW SUPPLIED
DROP: 0.3%

AVERAGE UNIT PRICE (AVAILABLE SIZES)		GENERIC A-RATED AVERAGE PRICE (GAAP)		
GENERIC	$2.75	5 ml		$13.56

BRAND/MANUFACTURER	NDC	SIZE	AWP
◆ GENERICS			
AKTOB: Akorn	17478-0290-10	5 ml	$11.88
Bausch&Lomb Pharm	24208-0290-05	5 ml	$12.72
Moore,H.L.	00839-7610-85	5 ml	$13.16
Aligen	00405-6145-05	5 ml	$13.38
Qualitest	00603-7345-37	5 ml	$13.44
URL	00677-1535-20	5 ml	$14.82
Major	00904-2970-05	5 ml	$14.95
Rugby	00536-2980-65	5 ml	$15.52

DROP: 0.3%

BRAND/MANUFACTURER	NDC	SIZE	AWP
○ BRAND			
TOBREX: Alcon Ophthalmic	00998-0643-05	5 ml	$18.13

OINTMENT: 0.3%

BRAND/MANUFACTURER	NDC	SIZE	AWP
○ BRAND			
TOBREX: Alcon Ophthalmic	00065-0644-35	3.5 gm	$18.13

Tobramycin Sulfate, Injectable

WARNINGS

PATIENTS TREATED WITH TOBRAMYCIN SULFATE AND OTHER AMINOGLYCOSIDES SHOULD BE UNDER CLOSE CLINICAL OBSERVATION, BECAUSE THESE DRUGS HAVE AN INHERENT POTENTIAL FOR CAUSING OTOTOXICITY AND NEPHROTOXICITY.

NEUROTOXICITY, MANIFESTED AS BOTH AUDITORY AND VESTIBULAR OTOTOXICITY, CAN OCCUR. THE AUDITORY CHANGES ARE IRREVERSIBLE, ARE USUALLY BILATERAL, AND MAY BE PARTIAL OR TOTAL. EIGHTH-NERVE IMPAIRMENT AND NEPHROTOXICITY MAY DEVELOP, PRIMARILY IN PATIENTS HAVING PREEXISTING RENAL DAMAGE AND IN THOSE WITH NORMAL RENAL FUNCTION TO WHOM AMINOGLYCOSIDES ARE ADMINISTERED FOR LONGER PERIODS OR IN HIGHER DOSES THAN THOSE RECOMMENDED. OTHER MANIFESTATIONS OF NEUROTOXICITY MAY INCLUDE NUMBNESS, SKIN TINGLING, MUSCLE TWITCHING, AND CONVULSIONS. THE RISK OF AMINOGLYCOSIDE-INDUCED HEARING LOSS INCREASES WITH THE DEGREE OF EXPOSURE TO EITHER HIGH PEAK OR HIGH TROUGH SERUM

CONCENTRATIONS. PATIENTS WHO DEVELOP COCHLEAR DAMAGE MAY NOT HAVE SYMPTOMS DURING THERAPY TO WARN THEM OF EIGHTH-NERVE TOXICITY, AND PARTIAL OR TOTAL IRREVERSIBLE BILATERAL DEAFNESS MAY CONTINUE TO DEVELOP AFTER THE DRUG HAS BEEN DISCONTINUED.

RARELY, NEPHROTOXICITY MAY NOT BECOME APPARENT UNTIL THE FIRST FEW DAYS AFTER CESSATION OF THERAPY. AMINOGLYCOSIDE-INDUCED NEPHROTOXICITY USUALLY IS REVERSIBLE. RENAL AND EIGHTH-NERVE FUNCTION SHOULD BE CLOSELY MONITORED IN PATIENTS WITH KNOWN OR SUSPECTED RENAL IMPAIRMENT AND ALSO IN THOSE WHOSE RENAL FUNCTION IS INITIALLY NORMAL BUT WHO DEVELOP SIGNS OF RENAL DYSFUNCTION DURING THERAPY. PEAK AND TROUGH SERUM CONCENTRATIONS OF AMINOGLYCOSIDES SHOULD BE MONITORED PERIODICALLY DURING THERAPY TO ASSURE ADEQUATE LEVELS AND TO AVOID POTENTIALLY TOXIC LEVELS. PROLONGED SERUM CONCENTRATIONS ABOVE 12 µG/ML SHOULD BE AVOIDED. RISING TROUGH LEVELS (ABOVE 2 µG/ML) MAY INDICATE TISSUE ACCUMULATION. SUCH ACCUMULATION, EXCESSIVE PEAK CONCENTRATIONS, ADVANCED AGE, AND CUMULATIVE DOSE MAY CONTRIBUTE TO OTOTOXICITY AND NEPHROTOXICITY (SEE PRECAUTIONS). URINE SHOULD BE EXAMINED FOR DECREASED SPECIFIC GRAVITY AND INCREASED EXCRETION OF PROTEIN, CELLS, AND CASTS. BLOOD UREA NITROGEN, SERUM CREATININE, AND CREATININE CLEARANCE SHOULD BE MEASURED PERIODICALLY. WHEN FEASIBLE, IT IS RECOMMENDED THAT SERIAL AUDIOGRAMS BE OBTAINED IN PATIENTS OLD ENOUGH TO BE TESTED, PARTICULARLY HIGH-RISK PATIENTS. EVIDENCE OF IMPAIRMENT OF RENAL, VESTIBULAR, OR AUDITORY FUNCTION REQUIRES DISCONTINUATION OF THE DRUG OR DOSAGE ADJUSTMENT.

TOBRAMYCIN SULFATE SHOULD BE USED WITH CAUTION IN PREMATURE AND NEONATAL INFANTS BECAUSE OF THEIR RENAL IMMATURITY AND THE RESULTING PROLONGATION OF SERUM HALF-LIFE OF THE DRUG. CONCURRENT AND SEQUENTIAL USE OF OTHER NEUROTOXIC AND/OR NEPHROTOXIC ANTIBIOTICS, PARTICULARLY OTHER AMINOGLYCOSIDES (EG, AMIKACIN, STREPTOMYCIN, NEOMYCIN, KANAMYCIN, GENTAMICIN, AND PAROMOMYCIN), CEPHALORIDINE, VIOMYCIN, POLYMYXIN B, COLISTIN, CISPLATIN, AND VANCOMYCIN, SHOULD BE AVOIDED. OTHER FACTORS THAT MAY INCREASE PATIENT RISK ARE ADVANCED AGE AND DEHYDRATION. AMINOGLYCOSIDES SHOULD NOT BE GIVEN CONCURRENTLY WITH POTENT DIURETICS, SUCH AS ETHACRYNIC ACID AND FUROSEMIDE. SOME DIURETICS THEMSELVES CAUSE OTOTOXICITY, AND INTRAVENOUSLY ADMINISTERED DIURETICS ENHANCE AMINOGLYCOSIDE TOXICITY BY ALTERING ANTIBIOTIC CONCENTRATIONS IN SERUM AND TISSUE.

AMINOGLYCOSIDES CAN CAUSE FETAL HARM WHEN ADMINISTERED TO A PREGNANT WOMAN (SEE "PRECAUTIONS").

DESCRIPTION

Tobramycin Sulfate, a water-soluble antibiotic of the aminoglycoside group, is derived from the actinomycete *Streptomyces tenebrarius*. Tobramycin Sulfate is a clear and colorless sterile aqueous solution for parenteral administration.

Tobramycin Sulfate is O-3-amino-3-deoxy-α-D-glucopyranosyl-1 → 4)-O-[2,6-diamino-2,3,6-trideoxy-α-D-ribo-hexopyranosyl-(1 → 6)]-2-deoxy-L-streptamine, sulfate (2:5)(salt) and has the chemical formula $(C_{18}H_{37}N_5O_9)_2.5H_2SO_4$. The molecular weight is 1,425.39.

Following is its chemical structure:

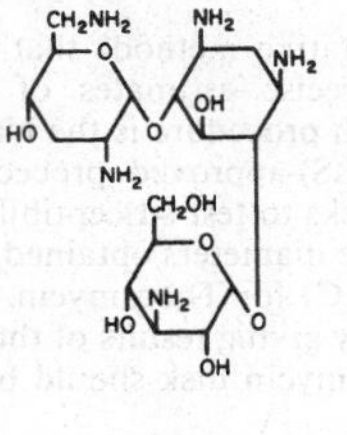

CLINICAL PHARMACOLOGY

Tobramycin is rapidly absorbed following intramuscular administration. Peak serum concentrations of tobramycin occur between 30 and 90 minutes after intramuscular administration. Following an intramuscular dose of 1 mg/kg of body weight, maximum serum concentrations reach about 4 µg/mL, and measurable levels persist for as long as 8 hours. Therapeutic serum levels are generally considered to range from 4 to 6 µg/mL. When Tobramycin Sulfate is administered by intravenous infusion over a 1-hour period, the serum concentrations are similar to those obtained by intramuscular administration. Tobramycin Sulfate is poorly absorbed from the gastrointestinal tract.

In patients with normal renal function, except neonates, Tobramycin Sulfate administered every 8 hours does not accumulate in the serum. However, in those patients with reduced renal function and in neonates, the serum concentration of the antibiotic is usually higher and can be measured for longer periods of time than in normal adults. Dosage for such patients must, therefore, be adjusted accordingly (see "Dosage and Administration").

Following parenteral administration, little, if any, metabolic transformation occurs, and Tobramycin is eliminated almost exclusively by glomerular filtration. Renal clearance is similar to that of endogenous creatinine. Ultrafiltration studies demonstrate that practically no serum protein binding occurs. In patients with normal renal function, up to 84% of the dose is recoverable from the urine in 8 hours and up to 93% in 24 hours.

Peak urine concentrations ranging from 75 to 100 µg/mL have been observed following the intramuscular injection of a single dose of 1 mg/kg. After several days of treatment, the amount of Tobramycin excreted in the urine approaches the daily dose administered. When renal function is impaired, excretion of Tobramycin Sulfate is slowed, and accumulation of the drug may cause toxic blood levels.

The serum half-life in normal individuals is 2 hours. An inverse relationship exists between serum half-life and creatinine clearance, and the dosage schedule should be adjusted according to the degree of renal impairment (see "Dosage and Administration"). In patients undergoing dialysis, 25% to 70% of the administered dose may be removed, depending on the duration and type of dialysis.

Tobramycin can be detected in tissues and body fluids after parenteral administration. Concentrations in bile and stools ordinarily have been low, which suggests minimum biliary excretion. Tobramycin has appeared in low concentration in the cerebrospinal fluid following parenteral administration, and concentrations are dependent on dose, rate of penetration, and degree of meningeal inflammation. It has also been found in sputum, peritoneal fluid, synovial fluid, and abscess fluids, and it crosses the placental membranes. Concentrations in the renal cortex are several times higher than the usual serum levels.

Probenecid does not affect the renal tubular transport of Tobramycin.

Tobramycin acts by inhibiting synthesis of protein in bacterial cells. In vitro tests demonstrate that Tobramycin is bactericidal.

Tobramycin has been shown to be active against most strains of the following organisms both in vitro and in clinical infections (see "Indications and Usage"):

GRAM-POSITIVE AEROBES
Staphylococcus aureus

GRAM-NEGATIVE AEROBES
Citrobacter species
  Enterobacter species
  Escherichia coli
  Klebsiella species
  Morganella morganii
  Pseudomonas aeruginosa
  Proteus mirabilis
  Proteus vulgaris
  Providencia species
  Serratia species

Aminoglycosides have a low order of activity against most gram-positive organisms, including *Streptococcus pyogenes, Streptococcus pneumoniae,*and enterococci.

Although most strains of enterococci demonstrate in vitro resistance, some strains in this group are susceptible. In vitro studies have shown that an aminoglycoside combined with an antibiotic that interferes with cell-wall synthesis affects some enterococcal strains synergistically. The combination of penicillin G and Tobramycin results in a synergistic bactericidal effect in vitro against certain strains of *Enterococcus faecalis*. However, this combination is not synergistic against other closely related organisms, eg, *Enterococcus faecium*. Speciation of enterococci alone cannot be used to predict susceptibility. Susceptibility testing and tests for antibiotic synergism are emphasized.

Cross resistance between aminoglycosides may occur.

SUSCEPTIBILITY TESTS
Diffusion Techniques: Quantitative methods that require measurement of zone diameters give the most precise estimates of susceptibility of bacteria to antimicrobial agents. One such procedure is the National Committee for Clinical Laboratory Standards (NCCLS)-approved procedure.[1] This method has been recommended for use with disks to test susceptibility to Tobramycin. Interpretation involves correlation of the diameters obtained in the disk test with minimum inhibitory concentrations (MIC) for Tobramycin.

Reports from the laboratory giving results of the standard single-disk susceptibility test with a 10-µg Tobramycin disk should be interpreted according to the following criteria:

Zone Diameter (mm)	Interpretation
≥ 15	(S) Susceptible
13-14	(I) Intermediate
≤ 12	(R) Resistant

A report of "Susceptible" indicates that the pathogen is likely to be inhibited by generally achievable blood levels. A report of "Intermediate" suggests that the organism would be susceptible if high dosage is used or if the infection is confined to tissues and fluids in which high antimicrobial levels are obtained. A report of "Resistant" indicates that achievable concentrations are unlikely to be inhibitory and other therapy should be selected.

Standardized procedures require the use of laboratory control organisms. The 10-µg Tobramycin disk should give the following zone diameters:

Organism	Zone Diameter (mm)
E. coli ATCC 25922	18-26
P. aeruginosa ATCC 27853	19-25
S. aureus ATCC 25923	19-29

Dilution Techniques: Broth and agar dilution methods, such as those recommended by the NCCLS,[2] may be used to determine MICs of Tobramycin. MIC test results should be interpreted according to the following criteria:

MIC (µg/mL)	Interpretation
≤ 4	(S) Susceptible
8	(I) Intermediate
≥ 16	(R) Resistant

As with standard diffusion methods, dilution procedures require the use of laboratory control organisms. Standard Tobramycin powder should give the following MIC values:

Organism	MIC Range (µg/mL)
E. faecalis ATCC 29212	8.0-32.0
E. coli ATCC 25922	0.25-1
P. aeruginosa ATCC 27853	0.12-2
S. aureus ATCC 29213	0.12-1

INDICATIONS AND USAGE
Tobramycin Sulfate is indicated for the treatment of serious bacterial infections caused by susceptible strains of the designated microorganisms in the diseases listed below:

Septicemia in the neonate, child, and adult caused by *P. aeruginosa, E. coli,* and *Klebsiella* sp

Lower respiratory tract infections caused by *P. aeruginosa, Klebsiella* sp, *Enterobacter* sp, *Serratia* sp, *E. coli*, and *S. aureus* (penicillinase- and nonpenicillinase-producing strains)

Serious central-nervous-system infections (meningitis) caused by susceptible organisms

Intra-abdominal infections, including peritonitis, caused by *E. coli, Klebsiella* sp, and *Enterobacter* sp

Skin, bone, and skin structure infections caused by *P. aeruginosa, Proteus* sp, *E. coli, Klebsiella* sp, *Enterobacter* sp, and *S. aureus*

Complicated and recurrent urinary tract infections caused by *P. aeruginosa, Proteus* sp (indole-positive and indole-negative), *E. coli, Klebsiella* sp, *Enterobacter* sp, *Serratia* sp, *S. aureus, Providencia* sp, and *Citrobacter* sp

Aminoglycosides, including Tobramycin Sulfate, are not indicated in uncomplicated initial episodes of urinary tract infections unless the causative organisms are not susceptible to antibiotics having less potential toxicity. Tobramycin Sulfate may be considered in serious staphylococcal infections when penicillin or other potentially less toxic drugs are contraindicated and when bacterial susceptibility testing and clinical judgment indicate its use.

Bacterial cultures should be obtained prior to and during treatment to isolate and identify etiologic organisms and to test their susceptibility to Tobramycin. If susceptibility tests show that the causative organisms are resistant to Tobramycin, other appropriate therapy should be instituted. In patients in whom a serious life-threatening gram-negative infection is suspected, including those in whom concurrent therapy with a penicillin or cephalosporin and an aminoglycoside may be indicated, treatment with Tobramycin Sulfate may be initiated before the results of susceptibility studies are obtained. The decision to continue therapy with Tobramycin Sulfate should be based on the results of susceptibility studies, the severity of the infection, and the important additional concepts discussed in the "Warnings" box above.

UNLABELED USES
Tobramycin is used as an adjunct in the treatment of pulmonary infections in patients with cystic fibrosis.

CONTRAINDICATIONS
A hypersensitivity to any aminoglycoside is a contraindication to the use of Tobramycin. A history of hypersensitivity or serious toxic reactions to aminoglycosides may also contraindicate the use of any other aminoglycoside because of the known cross-sensitivity of patients to drugs in this class.

WARNINGS
See "Warnings" box above.

Tobramycin Sulfate contains sodium bisulfite, a sulfite that may cause allergic-type reactions, including anaphylactic symptoms and life-threatening or less severe asthmatic episodes, in certain susceptible people. The overall prevalence of sulfite sensitivity in the general population is unknown and probably low. Sulfite sensitivity is seen more frequently in asthmatic than in nonasthmatic people.

PRECAUTIONS

Serum and urine specimens for examination should be collected during therapy, as recommended in the *"Warnings"* box. Serum calcium, magnesium, and sodium should be monitored.

Peak and trough serum levels should be measured periodically during therapy. Prolonged concentrations above 12 µg/mL should be avoided. Rising trough levels (above 2 µg/mL) may indicate tissue accumulation. Such accumulation, advanced age, and cumulative dosage may contribute to ototoxicity and nephrotoxicity. It is particularly important to monitor serum levels closely in patients with known renal impairment.

A useful guideline would be to perform serum level assays after 2 or 3 doses, so that the dosage could be adjusted if necessary, and at 3- to 4-day intervals during therapy. In the event of changing renal function, more frequent serum levels should be obtained and the dosage or dosage interval adjusted according to the guidelines provided in the *"Dosage and Administration"* section.

In order to measure the peak level, a serum sample should be drawn about 30 minutes following intravenous infusion or 1 hour after an intramuscular injection. Trough levels are measured by obtaining serum samples at 8 hours or just prior to the next dose of Tobramycin Sulfate. These suggested time intervals are intended only as guidelines and may vary according to institutional practices. It is important, however, that there be consistency within the individual patient program unless computerized pharmacokinetic dosing programs are available in the institution. These serum-level assays may be especially useful for monitoring the treatment of severely ill patients with changing renal function or of those infected with less susceptible organisms or those receiving maximum dosage.

Neuromuscular blockade and respiratory paralysis have been reported in cats receiving very high doses of Tobramycin (40 mg/kg). The possibility of prolonged or secondary apnea should be considered if Tobramycin is administered to anesthetized patients who are also receiving neuromuscular blocking agents, such as succinylcholine, tubocurarine, or decamethonium, or to patients receiving massive transfusions of citrated blood. If neuromuscular blockade occurs, it may be reversed by the administration of calcium salts.

Cross-allergenicity among aminoglycosides has been demonstrated.

In patients with extensive burns, altered pharmacokinetics may result in reduced serum concentrations of aminoglycosides. In such patients treated with Tobramycin Sulfate, measurement of serum concentration is especially recommended as a basis for determination of appropriate dosage.

Elderly patients may have reduced renal function that may not be evident in the results of routine screening tests, such as BUN or serum creatinine. A creatinine clearance determination may be more useful. Monitoring of renal function during treatment with aminoglycosides is particularly important in such patients.

An increased incidence of nephrotoxicity has been reported following concomitant administration of aminoglycoside antibiotics and cephalosporins.

Aminoglycosides should be used with caution in patients with muscular disorders, such as myasthenia gravis or parkinsonism, since these drugs may aggravate muscle weakness because of their potential curare-like effect on neuromuscular function.

Aminoglycosides may be absorbed in significant quantities from body surfaces after local irrigation or application and may cause neurotoxicity and nephrotoxicity.

Although not indicated for intraocular and/or subconjunctival use, there have been reports of macular necrosis following this type of injection of aminoglycosides, including tobramycin.

See *"Warnings"* box regarding concurrent use of potent diuretics and concurrent and sequential use of other neurotoxic or nephrotoxic drugs.

The inactivation of Tobramycin and other aminoglycosides by β-lactam-type antibiotics (penicillins or cephalosporins) has been demonstrated in vitro and in patients with severe renal impairment. Such inactivation has not been found in patients with normal renal function who have been given the drugs by separate routes of administration.

Therapy with Tobramycin may result in overgrowth of non-susceptible organisms. If overgrowth of nonsusceptible organisms occurs, appropriate therapy should be initiated.

Pregnancy Category D: Aminoglycosides can cause fetal harm when administered to a pregnant women. Aminoglycoside antibiotics cross the placenta, and there have been several reports of total irreversible bilateral congenital deafness in children whose mothers received streptomycin during pregnancy. Serious side effects to mother, fetus, or newborn have not been reported in the treatment of pregnant women with other aminoglycosides. If Tobramycin is used during pregnancy or if the patient becomes pregnant while taking Tobramycin, she should be apprised of the potential hazard to the fetus.

Usage in Children: See *"Indications and Usage"* and *"Dosage and Administration"*.

ADVERSE REACTIONS

Neurotoxicity: Adverse effects on both the vestibular and auditory branches of the eight nerve have been noted, especially in patients receiving high doses or prolonged therapy, in those given previous courses of therapy with an ototoxin, and in cases of dehydration. Symptoms include dizziness, vertigo, tinnitus, roaring in the ears, and hearing loss. Hearing loss is usually irreversible and is manifested initially by diminution of high-tone acuity. Tobramycin and gentamicin sulfates closely parallel each other in regard to ototoxic potential.

Nephrotoxicity: Renal function changes, as shown by rising BUN, NPN, and serum creatinine and by oliguria, cylindruria, and increased proteinuria, have been reported, especially in patients with a history of renal impairment who are treated for longer periods or with higher doses than those recommended. Adverse renal effects can occur in patients with initially normal renal function.

Clinical studies and studies in experimental animals have been conducted to compare the nephrotoxic potential of Tobramycin and gentamicin. In some of the clinical studies and in the animal studies, Tobramycin caused nephrotoxicity significantly less frequently than gentamicin. In some other clinical studies, no significant difference in the incidence of nephrotoxicity between Tobramycin and gentamicin was found.

Other reported adverse reactions possibly related to Tobramycin include anemia, granulocytopenia, and thrombocytopenia; and fever, rash, itching, urticaria, nausea, vomiting, diarrhea, headache, lethargy, pain at the injection site, mental confusion, and disorientation. Laboratory abnormalities possibly related to Nebcin include increased serum transaminases (AST [SGOT], ALT [SGPT]); increased serum LDH and bilirubin; decreased serum calcium, magnesium, sodium, and potassium; and leukopenia, leukocytosis, and eosinophilia.

OVERDOSAGE

Signs and Symptoms: The severity of the signs and symptoms following a Tobramycin overdose are dependent on the dose administered, the patient's renal function, state of hydration, and age and whether or not other medications with similar toxicities are being administered concurrently. Toxicity may occur in patients treated more than 10 days, in adults given more than 5 mg/kg/day, in children given more than 7.5 mg/kg/day, or in patients with reduced renal function where dose has not been appropriately adjusted.

Nephrotoxicity following the parenteral administration of an aminoglycoside is most closely related to the area under the curve of the serum concentration versus time graph. Nephrotoxicity is more likely if trough blood concentrations fail to fall below 2 µg/mL and is also proportional to the average blood concentration. Patients who are elderly, have abnormal renal function, are receiving other nephrotoxic drugs, or are volume depleted are at greater risk for developing acute tubular necrosis. Auditory and vestibular toxicities have been associated with aminoglycoside overdose. These toxicities occur in patients treated longer than 10 days, in patients with abnormal renal function, in dehydrated patients, or in patients receiving medications with additive auditory toxicities. These patients may not have signs or symptoms or may experience dizziness, tinnitus, vertigo, and a loss of high-tone acuity as ototoxicity progresses. Ototoxicity signs and symptoms may not begin to occur until long after the drug has been discontinued.

Neuromuscular blockade or respiratory paralysis may occur following administration of aminoglycosides. Neuromuscular blockade, respiratory failure, and prolonged respiratory paralysis may occur more commonly in patients with myasthenia gravis or Parkinson's disease. Prolonged respiratory paralysis may also occur in patients receiving decamethonium, tubocurarine, or succinylcholine. If neuromuscular blockade occurs, it may be reversed by the administration of calcium salts but mechanical assistance may be necessary.

If Tobramycin were ingested, toxicity would be less likely because aminoglycosides are poorly absorbed from an intact gastrointestinal tract.

Treatment: In all cases of suspected overdosage, call your regional poison control center to obtain the most up-to-date information about the treatment of overdose. This recommendation is made because, in general, information regarding the treatment of overdose may change more rapidly than the package insert. In managing overdosage, consider the possibility of multiple drug overdoses, interaction among drugs, and unusual drug kinetics in your patient.

The initial intervention in a Tobramycin overdose is to establish an airway and ensure oxygenation and ventilation. Resuscitative measures should be initiated promptly if respiratory paralysis occurs.

Patients who have received an overdose of Tobramycin and who have normal renal function should be adequately hydrated to maintain a urine output of 3 to 5 mL/kg/hr. Fluid balance, creatinine clearance, and Tobramycin plasma levels should be carefully monitored until the serum Tobramycin level falls below 2 µg/mL.

Patients in whom the elimination half-life is greater than 2 hours or whose renal function is abnormal may require more aggressive therapy. In such patients, hemodialysis may be beneficial.

DOSAGE AND ADMINISTRATION

Tobramycin Sulfate may be given intramuscularly or intravenously. ADD-Vantage vials are not for intramuscular administration. Recommended dosages are the same for both routes. The patient's pretreatment body weight should be obtained for calculation of correct dosage. It is desirable to measure both peak and trough serum concentrations (see *"Warnings"* and *"Precautions"*).

Administration for Patients with Normal Renal Function—Adults with Serious Infections: 3 mg/kg/day in 3 equal doses every 8 hours (see Table 1).

Adults With Life-Threatening Infections: Up to 5 mg/kg/day may be administered in 3 or 4 equal doses (see Table 1). The dosage should be reduced to 3 mg/kg/day as soon as clinically indicated. To prevent increased toxicity due to excessive blood levels, dosage should not exceed 5 mg/kg/day unless serum levels are monitored (see *"Warnings"* box and *"Precautions"*). (See related table).

Children: 6 to 7.5 mg/kg/day in 3 or 4 equally divided doses (2 to 2.5 mg/kg every 8 hours or 1.5 to 1.89 mg/kg every 6 hours).

Premature or Full-Term Neonates 1 Week of Age or Less: Up to 4 mg/kg/day may be administererd in 2 equal doses every 12 hours.

It is desirable to limit treatment to a short term. The usual duration of treatment is 7 to 10 days. A longer course of therapy may be necessary in difficult and complicated infections. In such cases, monitoring of renal, auditory, and vestibular functions is advised, because neurotoxicity is more likely to occur when treatment is extended longer than 10 days.

Administration for Patients With Impaired Penal Function: Whenever possible, serum tobramycin concentrations should be monitored during therapy.

Following a loading dose of 1 mg/kg, subsequent dosage in these patients must be adjusted, either with reduced doses administered at 8-hour intervals or with normal doses given at prolonged intervals. Both of these methods are suggested as guides to be used when serum levels of Tobramycin cannot be measured directly. They are based on either the creatinine clearance level or the serum creatinine level of the patient because these values correlate with the half-life of Tobramycin. The dosage schedule derived from either method should be used in conjunction with careful clinical and laboratory observations of the patient and should be modified as necessary. Neither method should be used when dialysis is being performed.

Reduced Dosage at 8-hour Intervals: When the creatinine clearance rate is 70 mL or less per minute or when the serum creatinine value is known, the amount of the reduced dose can be determined by multiplying the normal dose from Table 1 by the percent of normal dose from the accompanying nomogram.

REDUCED DOSAGE NOMOGRAM*
Creatinine Clearance (mL/min/1.73 m²)

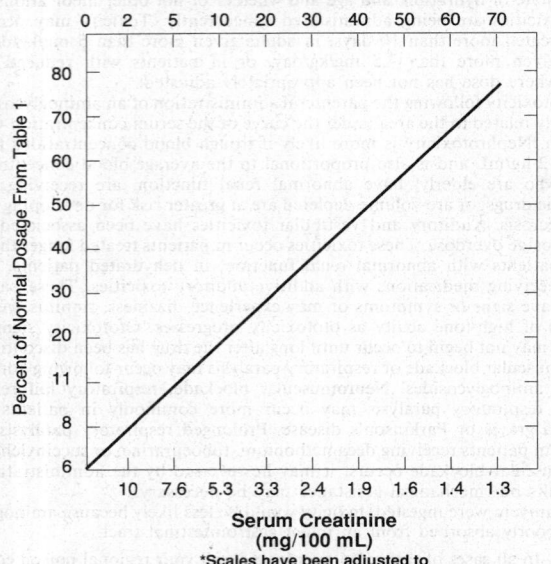

Scales have been adjusted to facilitate dosage calculations.

An alternate rough guide for determining reduced dosage at 8-hour intervals (for patients whose steady-state serum creatinine values are known) is to divide the normally recommended dose by the patient's serum creatinine.

Normal Dosage at Prolonged Intervals: If the creatinine clearance rate is not available and the patient's condition is stable, a dosage frequency *in hours* for the dosage given in Table 1 can be determined by multiplying the patient's serum creatinine by 6.

Dosage in Obese Patients: The appropriate dose may be calculated by using the patient's estimated lean body weight plus 40% of the excess as the basic weight on which to figure mg/kg.

Intramuscular Administration: Tobramycin Sulfate may be administered by withdrawing the appropriate dose directly from a vial or by using a prefilled Hyporet®. ADD-Vantage vials are not for intramuscular administration.

Intravenous Administration: For intravenous administration, the usual volume of diluent (0.9% Sodium Chloride Injection or 5% Dextrose Injection) is 50 to 100 mL for adult doses. For children, the volume of diluent should be proportionately less than that for adults. The diluted solution usually should be infused over a period of 20 to 60 minutes. Infusion periods of less than 20 minutes are not recommended, because peak serum levels may exceed 12 μg/mL (see "Warnings box").

Use of ADD Vantage Nebcin Vials: ADD-Vantage Nebcin vials are not intended for multiple use and should not be used with a syringe in the conventional way. These products are intended for use only with Abbott ADD-Vantage diluent containers and in those instances in which the physician's order specified 60-mg or 80-mg doses. Use within 24 hours after activation.

Tobramycin Sulfate Injection, USP should not be physically premixed with other drugs but should be administered separately according to the recommended dose and route.

Prior to administration, parenteral drug products should be inspected visually for particulate matter and discoloration whenever solution and container permit.

Storage: Store at controlled room temperature, 59° to 86°F (15° to 30°C).

REFERENCES
1 National Committee for Clinical Laboratory Standards, Performance standards for antimicrobial disk susceptibility tests—4th ed. Approved Standard NCCLS Document M2-A4, Vol 10, No 7, NCCLS, Villanova, PA 1990. 2. National Committee for Clinical Laboratory Standards, Methods for dilution antimicrobial susceptibility tests for bacteria that grow aerobically—2nd ed. Approved Standard NCCLS Document M7-A2, Vol 10, No 8, NCCLS, Villanova, PA, 1990.

J CODES
Up to 80 mg IM,IV—J3260

HOW SUPPLIED
INJECTION: 10 MG/ML

AVERAGE UNIT PRICE (AVAILABLE SIZES)				
BRAND	$1.83	GENERIC A-RATED AVERAGE PRICE (GAAP)		
GENERIC	$1.73	2 ml 25s		$100.62
BRAND/MANUFACTURER		NDC	SIZE	AWP
◆ BRAND				
NEBCIN PEDIATRIC: Lilly		00002-0501-01	2 ml	$3.65

Table 1
DOSAGE SCHEDULE GUIDE FOR TOBRAMYCIN SULFATE IN ADULTS WITH NORMAL RENAL FUNCTION

(Dosage at 8-Hour Intervals)

For Patient Weighing		Usual Dose for Serious Infections 1 mg/kg q8h (Total, 3 mg/kg/day)		Maximum Dose for Life Threatening Infections (Reduce as soon as possible) 1.66 mg/kg q8h (Total, 5 mg/kg/day)	
kg	lb	mg/dose q8h	mL/dose* q8h	mg/dose q8h	mL/dose* q8h
120	264	120 mg	3 mL	200 mg	5 mL
115	253	115 mg	2.9 mL	191 mg	4.75 mL
110	242	110 mg	2.75 mL	183 mg	4.5 mL
105	231	105 mg	2.6 mL	175 mg	4.4 mL
100	220	100 mg	2.5 mL	166 mg	4.2 mL
95	209	95 mg	2.4 mL	158 mg	4 mL
90	198	90 mg	2.25 mL	150 mg	3.75 mL
85	187	85 mg	2.1 mL	141 mg	3.5 mL
80	176	80 mg	2 mL	133 mg	3.3 mL
75	165	75 mg	1.9 mL	125 mg	3.1 mL
70	154	70 mg	1.75 mL	116 mg	2.9 mL
65	143	65 mg	1.6 mL	108 mg	2.7 mL
60	132	60 mg	1.5 mL	100 mg	2.5 mL
55	121	55 mg	1.4 mL	91 mg	2.25 mL
50	110	50 mg	1.25 mL	83 mg	2.1 mL
45	99	45 mg	1.1 mL	75 mg	1.9 mL
40	88	40 mg	1 mL	66 mg	1.6 mL

* *Applicable to all product forms except Tobramycin Sulfate, Pediatric, Injection.*

◆ RATED THERAPEUTICALLY EQUIVALENT; ◇ THERAPEUTIC EQUIVALENCE UNCONFIRMED; ○ UNRATED

BRAND/MANUFACTURER	NDC	SIZE	AWP
◆ GENERICS			
Apothecon	00003-2724-10	2 ml 25s	$82.20
Abbott Hosp	00074-3577-01	2 ml 25s	$119.05
Abbott Hosp	00074-3254-03	6 ml 25s	$233.94
Abbott Hosp	00074-3255-03	8 ml 25s	$262.73

INJECTION: 40 MG/ML

AVERAGE UNIT PRICE (AVAILABLE SIZES)		GENERIC A-RATED AVERAGE PRICE (GAAP)	
BRAND	$3.64	30 ml	$81.93
GENERIC	$4.66	2 ml 10s	$70.57
		2 ml 25s	$245.59

BRAND/MANUFACTURER	NDC	SIZE	AWP
◆ BRAND			
NEBCIN: Lilly	00002-1499-01	2 ml	$7.28
	00002-7090-16	30 ml 6s	$655.59
	00002-1499-25	2 ml 25s	$182.11
◆ GENERICS			
Apothecon	00003-2725-30	30 ml	$70.97
Geneva	00781-3775-90	30 ml	$92.88
Gensia	00703-9416-01	30 ml	$205.74
Lederle Std Prod	00205-3027-45	1.5 ml 10s	$65.63
Lederle Std Prod	00205-3027-04	2 ml 10s	$67.44
Lederle Std Prod	00205-3027-46	2 ml 10s	$73.69
Lederle Std Prod	00205-3027-08	30 ml 10s	$1011.50
Abbott Hosp	00074-3582-01	1 ml 25s	$228.30
Apothecon	00003-2725-10	2 ml 25s	$131.10
Abbott Hosp	00074-3578-01	2 ml 25s	$236.31
Abbott Hosp	00074-3583-01	2 ml 25s	$256.20
Gensia	00703-9402-04	2 ml 25s	$358.75

INJECTION: 40 MG/ML

BRAND/MANUFACTURER	NDC	SIZE	AWP
○ BRAND			
NEBCIN: Lilly	00002-0509-24	1.5 ml 24s	$169.06
	00002-0503-24	2 ml 24s	$189.22

INJECTION: 60 MG

BRAND/MANUFACTURER	NDC	SIZE	AWP
◆ GENERICS			
Abbott Hosp	00074-3469-13	50 ml 24s	$322.62

INJECTION: 80 MG/ML

BRAND/MANUFACTURER	NDC	SIZE	AWP
◆ GENERICS			
Geneva	00781-3772-72	2 ml 25s	$170.53

INJECTION: 80 MG

BRAND/MANUFACTURER	NDC	SIZE	AWP
◆ GENERICS			
Abbott Hosp	00074-3470-23	100 ml 24s	$338.01

POWDER FOR INJECTION: 40 MG/ML

BRAND/MANUFACTURER	NDC	SIZE	AWP
◆ GENERICS			
Abbott Hosp	00074-3590-02	1s	$236.31

POWDER FOR INJECTION: 60 MG

BRAND/MANUFACTURER	NDC	SIZE	AWP
◆ BRAND			
NEBCIN: Lilly	00002-7293-25	25s	$173.11

POWDER FOR INJECTION: 80 MG

BRAND/MANUFACTURER	NDC	SIZE	AWP
◆ BRAND			
NEBCIN: Lilly	00002-7294-25	25s	$194.11

POWDER FOR INJECTION: 1.2 GM

BRAND/MANUFACTURER	NDC	SIZE	AWP
◆ BRAND			
NEBCIN: Lilly	00002-7040-16	6s	$655.59

Tobrex *SEE* TOBRAMYCIN

Tocainide Hydrochloride

WARNINGS

BLOOD DYSCRASIAS: AGRANULOCYTOSIS, BONE MARROW DEPRESSION, LEUKOPENIA, NEUTROPENIA, APLASTIC/HYPOPLASTIC ANEMIA, THROMBOCYTOPENIA AND SEQUELAE SUCH AS SEPTICEMIA AND SEPTIC SHOCK HAVE BEEN REPORTED IN PATIENTS RECEIVING TOCAINIDE HYDROCHLORIDE (TOCAINIDE HCL). MOST OF THESE PATIENTS RECEIVED TOCAINIDE HCL WITHIN THE RECOMMENDED DOSAGE RANGE.

FATALITIES HAVE OCCURRED (WITH APPROXIMATELY 25 PERCENT MORTALITY IN REPORTED AGRANULOCYTOSIS CASES). SINCE MOST OF THESE EVENTS HAVE BEEN NOTED DURING THE FIRST 12 WEEKS OF THERAPY, IT IS RECOMMENDED THAT COMPLETE BLOOD COUNTS, INCLUDING WHITE CELL, DIFFERENTIAL AND PLATELET COUNTS BE PERFORMED, OPTIMALLY, AT WEEKLY INTERVALS FOR THE FIRST THREE MONTHS OF THERAPY; AND FREQUENTLY THEREAFTER. COMPLETE BLOOD COUNTS SHOULD BE PERFORMED PROMPTLY IF THE PATIENT DEVELOPS ANY SIGNS OF INFECTION (SUCH AS FEVER, CHILLS, SORE THROAT, OR STOMATITIS), BRUISING, OR BLEEDING. IF ANY OF THESE HEMATOLOGIC DISORDERS IS IDENTIFIED, TOCAINIDE HCL SHOULD BE DISCONTINUED AND APPROPRIATE TREATMENT SHOULD BE INSTITUTED IF NECESSARY. BLOOD COUNTS USUALLY RETURN TO NORMAL WITHIN ONE MONTH OF DISCONTINUATION. CAUTION SHOULD BE USED IN PATIENTS WITH PRE-EXISTING MARROW FAILURE OR CYTOPENIA OF ANY TYPE. (SEE *"ADVERSE REACTIONS"*.)

PULMONARY FIBROSIS: PULMONARY FIBROSIS, INTERSTITIAL PNEUMONITIS, FIBROSING ALVEOLITIS, PULMONARY EDEMA, AND PNEUMONIA HAVE BEEN REPORTED IN PATIENTS RECEIVING TOCAINIDE HCL. MANY OF THESE EVENTS OCCURRED IN PATIENTS WHO WERE SERIOUSLY ILL. FATALITIES HAVE BEEN REPORTED. THE EXPERIENCES ARE USUALLY CHARACTERIZED BY BILATERAL INFILTRATES ON X-RAY AND ARE FREQUENTLY ASSOCIATED WITH DYSPNEA AND COUGH. FEVER MAY OR MAY NOT BE PRESENT. PATIENTS SHOULD BE INSTRUCTED TO PROMPTLY REPORT THE DEVELOPMENT OF ANY PULMONARY SYMPTOMS SUCH AS EXERTIONAL DYSPNEA, COUGH OR WHEEZING. CHEST X-RAYS ARE ADVISABLE AT THAT TIME. IF THESE PULMONARY DISORDERS DEVELOP, TOCAINIDE HCL SHOULD BE DISCONTINUED. (SEE *"ADVERSE REACTIONS"*.)

DESCRIPTION

Tocainide Hydrochloride is a primary amine analog of lidocaine with antiarrhythmic properties useful in the treatment of ventricular arrhythmias. The chemical name for Tocainide Hydrochloride is 2-amino-*N*-(2,6-dimethylphenyl) propanamide hydrochloride. Its empirical formula is $C_{11}H_{16}N_2O.HCl$, with a molecular weight of 228.72.

Tocainide Hydrochloride is a white crystalline powder with a bitter taste and is freely soluble in water. It is supplied as 400 mg and 600 mg tablets for oral administration. Each tablet contains the following inactive ingredients: hydroxypropyl methylcellulose, iron oxide, magnesium stearate, methylcellulose, polyethylene glycol, and titanium dioxide.

Following is its chemical structure:

$$CH_3CHCONH- \underset{NH_2}{} $$

CLINICAL PHARMACOLOGY

ACTION

Tocainide, like lidocaine, produces dose dependent decreases in sodium and potassium conductance, thereby decreasing the excitability of myocardial cells. In experimental animal models, the dose-related depression of sodium current is more pronounced in ischemic tissue than in normal tissue.

ELECTROPHYSIOLOGY

Tocainide is a Class I antiarrhythmic compound with electrophysiologic properties in man similar to those of lidocaine, but dissimilar from quinidine, procainamide, and disopyramide.

In studies of isolated dog Purkinje fibers, Tocainide in concentrations of 1-50 mcg/mL had no significant effect on resting membrane potential, but reduced the amplitude and rate of depolarization (dv/dt) of the action potential. Tocainide decreased the effective refractory period (ERP) to a lesser extent than the action potential duration (APD) resulting in an increase in the ERP/APD ratio.

In patients with cardiac disease Tocainide HCl produced no clinically significant changes in sinus nodal function, effective refractory periods, or intracardiac conduction times when studied under electrophysiologic testing procedures.

Tocainide, like lidocaine, characteristically does not prolong ventricular depolarization (QRS duration) or repolarization (QT intervals) as measured by electrocardiography. Theoretically, therefore, Tocainide HCl may be useful in the treatment of ventricular arrhythmias associated with a prolonged QT interval.

Patients who respond to lidocaine also respond to Tocainide HCl in a majority of cases. Failure to respond to lidocaine usually predicts failure to respond to Tocainide HCl, but there are exceptions to this.

In a controlled comparison with quinidine, 600 mg b.i.d. of Tocainide HCl produced a mean reduction of 42 percent in PVC count, compared to a 54 percent reduction by quinidine 300 mg every 6 hours. Among all patients entered into the study, about one-fifth of Tocainide recipients and one-third of quinidine recipients had 75 percent or greater reductions in PVC count or had elimination of ventricular tachycardia.

PHARMACOKINETICS
Following oral administration of Tocainide, peak plasma concentrations occur within 0.5 to 2 hours. The average plasma half-life in patients is approximately 15 hours. Although the effective plasma concentration may vary from patient to patient, the usual therapeutic plasma range (as defined by 50-80 percent PVC suppression) is 4-10 mcg/mL (18-45 micromole/L), expressed as Tocainide Hydrochloride. Tocainide is approximately 10 percent bound to plasma protein.

In contrast to lidocaine, Tocainide undergoes negligible first pass hepatic degradation. Following oral administration, the bioavailability of Tocainide HCl approaches 100 percent. The extent of its bioavailability is unaffected by food. Tocainide has no cardioactive metabolites. Approximately 40 percent of the administered dose of Tocainide is excreted unchanged in the urine. Acidification of the urine has not been shown to significantly alter Tocainide excretion in the urine, but alkalinization of the urine results in a significant decrease in the percent of Tocainide excreted unchanged in the urine. Animal data indicate that Tocainide crosses the blood-brain barrier; however, it has less lipid solubility than lidocaine.

HEMODYNAMICS
Cardiac catheterization studies in man utilizing intravenous Tocainide infusions (0.5-0.75 mg/kg/min over 15 min) have shown that Tocainide usually produces a small degree of depression of parameters of left ventricular function, such as left ventricular dP/dt, and left ventricular end diastolic pressure. There were usually no changes in cardiac output or clinical evidence of increasing congestive heart failure in the well-compensated patients studied. Small but statistically significant increases in aortic and pulmonary arterial pressures have been consistently observed and are probably related to small increases in vascular resistance. When used concomitantly with a beta-blocking drug, Tocainide further reduced cardiac index and left ventricular dP/dt and further increased pulmonary wedge pressure.

No clinically significant changes in heart rate, blood pressure, or signs of myocardial depression were observed in a study of 72 post-myocardial infarction patients receiving long-term therapy with oral Tocainide HCl at usual doses (400 mg q8h). When Tocainide was administered orally at a dose of 120 mg/kg to anesthetized dogs (14 times the initial maximum dose recommended for humans), a negative inotropic effect was observed: the rate of change of left ventricular pressure decreased by up to 29 percent of control at 3 hours after administration. This effect was not observed at lower doses (60 mg/kg). Tocainide has been used safely in patients with acute myocardial infarction and various degrees of congestive heart failure. It has, however, a small negative inotropic effect and can increase peripheral resistance slightly. It therefore should be used cautiously in patients with known heart failure, particularly if a beta blocker is given as well. (See "Precautions".)

INDICATIONS AND USAGE
Tocainide HCl is indicated for the treatment of documented ventricular arrhythmias, such as sustained ventricular tachycardia, that, in the judgment of the physician, are life-threatening. Because of the proarrhythmic effects of Tocainide HCl, as well as its potential for other serious adverse effects (See "Warnings"), its use to treat lesser arrhythmias is not recommended. Treatment of patients with asymptomatic ventricular premature contractions should be avoided.

Initiation of treatment with Tocainide HCl, as with other antiarrhythmic agents used to treat life-threatening arrhythmias, should be carried out in the hospital. It is essential that each patient given Tocainide HCl be evaluated electrocardiographically and clinically prior to, and during, therapy with Tocainide HCl to determine whether the response to Tocainide HCl supports continued treatment.

Antiarrhythmic drugs have not been shown to enhance survival in patients with ventricular arrhythmias.

CONTRAINDICATIONS
Patients who are hypersensitive to this product or to local anesthetics of the amide type.

Patients with second or third degree atrioventricular block in the absence of an artificial ventricular pacemaker.

WARNINGS
Mortality: In the National Heart, Lung and Blood Institute's Cardiac Arrhythmia Suppression Trial (CAST), a long-term, multi-centered, randomized, double-blind study in patients with asymptomatic non-life-threatening ventricular arrhythmias who had had myocardial infarctions more than six days but less than two years previously, an excessive mortality or non-fatal

cardiac arrest rate was seen in patients treated with encainide or flecainide (56/730) compared with that seen in patients assigned to matched placebo-treated groups (22/725). The average duration of treatment with encainide or flecainide in this study was ten months.

The applicability of these results to other populations (e.g., those without recent myocardial infarctions) or to other antiarrhythmic drugs is uncertain, but at present it is prudent to consider any antiarrhythmic agent to have a significant risk in patients with structural heart disease.

Acceleration of Ventricular Rate: Acceleration of ventricular rate occurs infrequently when antiarrhythmics are administered to patients with atrial flutter or fibrillation (see "Adverse Reactions").

PRECAUTIONS
GENERAL
In patients with known heart failure or minimal cardiac reserve, Tocainide HCl should be used with caution because of the potential for aggravating the degree of heart failure.

Caution should be used in the institution or continuation of antiarrhythmic therapy in the presence of signs of increasing depression of cardiac conductivity.

In patients with severe liver or kidney disease, the rate of drug elimination may be significantly decreased (see "Dosage and Administration").

Since antiarrhythmic drugs may be ineffective in patients with hypokalemia, the possibility of a potassium deficit should be explored and, if present, the deficit should be corrected.

Like all other oral antiarrhythmics, Tocainide HCl has been reported to increase arrhythmias in some patients (see "Adverse Reactions").

INFORMATION FOR PATIENTS
Patients should be instructed to promptly report the development of bruising or bleeding; any signs of infections such as fever, chills, sore throat, or soreness and ulcers in the mouth; or any pulmonary symptoms, such as exertional dyspnea, cough, or wheezing; rash.

LABORATORY TESTS
As with other antiarrhythmics, abnormal liver function tests, particularly in the early stages of therapy, have been reported. Periodic monitoring of liver function should be considered. Hepatitis and jaundice have been reported in some patients.

DRUG INTERACTIONS
Tocainide and lidocaine are pharmacodynamically similar. The concomitant use of these two agents may cause an increased incidence of adverse reactions, including central nervous system adverse reactions such as seizure.

Specific interaction studies with cimetidine, digoxin, metoprolol and warfarin have been conducted; no clinically significant interaction was seen with cimetidine, digoxin or warfarin, but Tocainide and metoprolol had additive effects on wedge pressure and cardiac index. Tocainide HCl has also been used in open studies with digitalis, beta-blocking agents, other antiarrhythmic agents, anticoagulants, and diuretics, without evidence of clinically significant interactions. Nevertheless, caution should be exercised in the use of multiple drug therapy.

Tocainide HCl is equally effective in digitalized and non-digitalized patients. In 17 patients with refractory ventricular arrhythmias on concomitant therapy, serum digoxin levels (1.1 ± 0.4 ng/mL) remained in the expected normal range (0.5-2.5 ng/mL) during Tocainide administration.

CARCINOGENESIS, MUTAGENESIS, IMPAIRMENT OF FERTILITY
The carcinogenic potential of Tocainide was studied in mice using oral doses up to 300 mg/kg/day (about 6 times the maximum recommended human dose) for up to 94 weeks in males and 102 weeks in females and in rats at doses up to 200 mg/kg/day for 24 months. Tocainide did not affect the type or incidence of neoplasia in the two studies.

Tocainide did not show any mutagenic potential when evaluated *in vivo* in the micronucleus test using mice at oral doses up to 187.5 mg/kg/day (about 7 times the usual human dose). Also, no mutagenic activity was seen *in vitro* in the Ames microbial mutagen test or in the mouse lymphoma forward mutation assay.

Reproduction and fertility studies in rats showed no adverse effects on male or female fertility at oral doses up to 200 mg/kg/day (about 8 times the usual human dose).

PREGNANCY
Pregnancy Category C. In a teratogenicity study in rabbits, Tocainide was administered orally at doses of 25, 50, and 100 mg/kg/day (about 1 to 4 times the usual human dose). No evidence of a drug-related teratogenic effect was noted; however, these doses were maternotoxic and produced a dose-related increase in abortions and stillbirths. In a teratogenicity study in rats, an oral dose of 300 mg/kg/day (about 12 times the usual human dose) showed no evidence of treatment-related fetal malformations, but maternotoxicity and an increase in fetal resorptions were noted. An oral dose of 30 mg/kg/day (about twice the usual human dose) did not produce any adverse effects.

In reproduction studies in rats at maternotoxic oral doses of 200 and 300 mg/kg/day (about 8 and 12 times the usual human dose, respectively), dystocia, and delayed parturition occurred which was accompanied by an increase in stillbirths and decreased survival in offspring during the first week postpartum. Growth and viability of surviving offspring were not affected for the remainder of the lactation period.

There are no adequate and well-controlled studies in pregnant women. Tocainide HCl should be used during pregnancy only if the potential benefit justifies the potential risk to the fetus.

NURSING MOTHERS

It is not known whether Tocainide is secreted in human milk. Because many drugs are secreted in human milk and because of the potential for serious adverse reactions in nursing infants from Tocainide HCl, a decision should be made whether to discontinue nursing or to discontinue the drug, taking into account the importance of the drug to the mother.

PEDIATRIC USE

Safety and effectiveness in children have not been established.

ADVERSE REACTIONS

Tocainide HCl commonly produces minor, transient, nervous system and gastrointestinal adverse reactions, but is otherwise generally well tolerated. Tocainide HCl has been evaluated in both short-term (n = 1,358) and long-term (n = 262) controlled studies as well as a compassionate use program. Dosages were lower in most of the controlled studies (1200 mg/day) and higher in the compassionate use program (1800 mg and more). In long-term (2-6 months) controlled studies, the most frequent adverse reactions were dizziness/vertigo (15.3 percent), nausea (14.5 percent), paresthesia (9.2 percent), and tremor (8.4 percent). These reactions were generally mild, transient, dose-related and reversible with a reduction in dosage, by taking the drug with food, or by therapy discontinuation. Tremor, when present, may be useful as a clinical indicator that the maximum dose is being approached. Adverse reactions leading to therapy discontinuation occurred in 21 percent of patients in long-term controlled trials and were usually related to the nervous system or digestive system.

Adverse reactions occurring in greater than one percent of patients from the short-term and long-term controlled studies appear in the following table:

	Percent of Patients Controlled Studies	
	Short-term (n = 1,358)	Long-term (n = 262)
Body as a Whole		
Tiredness/ drowsiness/ fatigue/ lethargy/ lassitude/ sleepiness	1.6	0.8
Hot/cold feelings	0.5	1.5
Cardiovascular		
Hypotension	3.4	2.7
Bradycardia	1.8	0.4
Palpitations	1.8	0.4
Chest pain	1.6	0.4
Conduction disorders	1.5	0.0
Left ventricular failure	1.4	0.0
Digestive		
Nausea	15.2	14.5
Vomiting	8.3	4.6
Anorexia	1.2	1.9
Diarrhea/ loose stools	0.0	3.8
Nervous System/Psychiatric		
Dizziness/vertigo	8.0	15.3
Paresthesia	3.5	9.2
Tremor	2.9	8.4
Confusion/ disorientation/ hallucinations	2.1	2.7
Headache	2.1	4.6
Nervousness	1.5	0.4
Altered mood/ awareness	1.5	3.4
Incoordination/ unsteadiness/ walking disturbances	1.2	0.0
Anxiety	1.1	1.5
Ataxia	0.2	3.0
Skin		
Diaphoresis	5.1	2.3
Rash/skin lesion	0.4	8.4
Special Senses		
Blurred vision/ visual disturbances	1.3	1.5
Tinnitus/ hearing loss	0.4	1.5
Nystagmus	0.0	1.1

An additional group of about 2,000 patients has been treated in a program allowing for the use of Tocainide HCl under compassionate use circumstances.

These patients were seriously ill with the large majority on multiple drug therapy, and comparatively high doses of Tocainide HCl were used. Fifty-four percent of the patients continued in the program for one year or longer, and 12 percent were treated for longer than three years, with the longest duration of therapy being nine years. Adverse reactions leading to therapy discontinuation occurred in 12 percent of patients (usually central nervous system effects or rash). A tabulation of adverse reactions occurring in one percent or more of patients follows:

	Percent of Patients Compassionate Use (n = 1,927)
Cardiovascular	
Increased ventricular arrhythmias/PVCs	10.9
CHF/progression of CHF	4.0
Tachycardia	3.2
Hypotension	1.8
Conduction disorders	1.3
Bradycardia	1.0
Digestive	
Nausea	24.6
Anorexia	11.3
Vomiting	9.0
Diarrhea/loose stools	6.8
Musculoskeletal	
Arthritis/arthralgia	4.7
Myalgia	1.7
Nervous System/Psychiatric	
Dizziness/vertigo	25.3
Tremor	21.6
Nervousness	11.5
Confusion/disorientation/ hallucinations	11.2
Altered mood/awareness	11.0
Ataxia	10.8
Paresthesia	9.2
Skin	
Rash/skin lesion	12.2
Diaphoresis	8.3
Lupus	1.6
Special Senses	
Blurred vision/ vision disturbances	10.0
Nystagmus	1.1

Adverse reactions occurring in less than one percent of patients in either the controlled studies or the compassionate use program or since the drug was marketed are as follows:

Body as a Whole: Septicemia; septic shock; syncope; vasovagal episodes; edema; fever; chills; cinchonism; asthenia; malaise.

Cardiovascular: Ventricular fibrillation; extension of acute myocardial infarction; cardiogenic shock; pulmonary embolism; angina; AV block; hypertension; claudication; increased QRS duration; pleurisy/pericarditis; prolonged QT interval; right bundle branch block; cardiomegaly; sinus arrest; vasculitis; orthostatic hypotension; cold extremities.

Digestive: Hepatitis, jaundice (see "Precautions"), abnormal liver function tests; pancreatitis; abdominal pain/discomfort; constipation; dysphagia; gastrointestinal symptoms (including dyspepsia); stomatitis; dry mouth; thirst.

Hematologic: Agranulocytosis; bone marrow depression; aplastic/hypoplastic anemia; hemolytic anemia; anemia; leukopenia; neutropenia; thrombocytopenia; eosinophilia.

Metabolic and Immune: Hypersensitivity Reaction (including some of the following symptoms or signs: rash, fever, joint pains, abnormal liver function tests, eosinophilia); increased ANA.

Musculoskeletal: Muscle cramps; muscle twitching/spasm; neck pain; pain radiating from neck; pressure on shoulder.

Nervous System/Psychiatric: Coma; convulsions/seizures; myasthenia gravis; depression; psychosis; psychic disturbances; agitation; decreased mental acuity; dysarthria; impaired memory; increased stuttering/slurred speech; insomnia/ sleeping disturbances; local anesthesia; dream abnormalities.

Respiratory: Respiratory arrest; pulmonary edema; pulmonary fibrosis; fibrosing alveolitis; pneumonia; interstitial pneumonitis; dyspnea; hiccough; yawning.

Skin: Stevens-Johnson syndrome; exfoliative dermatitis; erythema multiforme; urticaria; alopecia; pruritus; pallor/flushed face.

Special Senses: Diplopia; earache; taste perversion/smell perversion.

Urogenital: Urinary retention; polyuria/increased diuresis.

Agranulocytosis, bone marrow depression, leukopenia, neutropenia, aplastic/ hypoplastic anemia, and thrombocytopenia have been reported (0.18 percent) in patients receiving Tocainide HCl in controlled trials and the compassionate use program. Most of these events have been noted during the firat 12 weeks of therapy. (See Box "Warnings").

Pulmonary fibrosis, interstitial pneumonitis, fibrosing alveolitis, pulmonary edema, and pneumonia, possibly drug related, have been reported in patients receiving Tocainide HCl. The incidence of pulmonary fibrosis (including interstitial pneumonitis and fibrosing alveolitis) was 0.11 percent in controlled trials and the compassionate use program. These events usually occurred in seriously ill patients. Symptoms of these pulmonary disorders and/or x-ray changes usually occurred following 3-18 weeks of therapy. Fatalities have been reported. (See Box "Warnings".)

A number of disorders, in which a causal relationship with Tocainide HCl has not been established, have been reported in seriously ill patients. These include: renal failure, renal dysfunction, myocardial infarction, cerebrovascular accidents and transient ischemic attacks. These disorders may be related to the patients underlying condition.

DRUG ABUSE AND DEPENDENCE

Drug withdrawal after chronic treatment has not shown any indication of psychological or physical dependence.

OVERDOSAGE

The initial and most important signs and symptoms of overdosage would be expected to be related to the central nervous system. Other adverse reactions, such as gastrointestinal disturbances, may follow. (see "Adverse Reactions").

Should convulsions or cardiopulmonary depression or arrest develop, the patency of the airway and adequacy of ventilation must be assured immediately. Should convulsions persist despite ventilatory therapy with oxygen, small increments of anticonvulsive agents may be given intravenously. Examples of such agents include a benzodiazepine (e.g., diazepam), an ultra-short-acting barbiturate (e.g., thiopental or thiamylal), or a short-acting barbiturate (e.g., pentobarbital or secobarbital).

The oral LD_{50} of Tocainide was calculated to be about 800 mg/kg in mice, 1000 mg/kg in rats, and 230 mg/kg in guinea pigs; deaths were usually preceded by convulsions.

Studies in normal individuals to date indicate that Tocainide has a hemodialysis clearance approximately equivalent to its renal clearance.

DOSAGE AND ADMINISTRATION

The dosage of Tocainide HCl must be individualized on the basis of antiarrhythmic response and tolerance, both of which are dose related Clinical and electrocardiographic evaluation (including Holter monitoring if necessary for evaluation) are needed to determine whether the desired antiarrhythmic response has been obtained and to guide titration and dose adjustment. Adverse effects appearing shortly after dosing, for example, suggest a need for dividing the dose further with a shorter dose-interval. Loss of arrhythmia control prior to the next dose suggests use of a shorter dose interval and/or a dose increase. Absence of a clear response suggests reconsideration of therapy.

The recommended initial dosage is 400 mg every 8 hours. The usual adult dosage is between 1200 and 1800 mg/day in a three dose daily divided regimen. Doses beyond 2400 mg per day have been administered infrequently. Patients who tolerate the t.i.d. regimen may be tried on a twice daily regimen with careful monitoring.

Some patients, particularly those with renal or hepatic impairment, may be adequately treated with less than 1200 mg/day.

Store below 40°C (104°F), preferably between 15 and 30°C (59 and 85°F). Store in a well-closed container.

HOW SUPPLIED
TABLETS: 400 MG

BRAND/MANUFACTURER	NDC	SIZE	AWP
○ BRAND			
▶ TONOCARD: Merck	00006-0707-68	100s	$83.78
	00006-0707-28	100s ud	$88.49

TABLETS: 600 MG

BRAND/MANUFACTURER	NDC	SIZE	AWP
○ BRAND			
▶ TONOCARD: Merck	00006-0709-68	100s	$106.78
	00006-0709-28	100s ud	$111.51

Tofranil SEE IMIPRAMINE

Tolazamide

DESCRIPTION

Tolazamide Tablets contain Tolazamide, an oral blood glucose lowering drug of the sulfonylurea class. Tolazamide is a white or creamy-white powder with a melting point of 165° to 173° C. The solubility to Tolazamide at pH 6.0 (mean urinary pH) is 27.8 mg per 100 mL.

The chemical names for Tolazamide are (1) Benzenesulfonamide, N-[[(hexahydro-1H -azepin-1-yl)amino]-carbonyl]-4-methyl-; (2) 1-(Hexahydro-1H-azepin-1-yl)-3-(p-tolylsulfonyl)-urea and its molecular weight is 311.40.

Tolazamide Tablets for oral administration are available as scored, white tablets containing 100 mg, 250 mg or 500 mg Tolazamide.

Following is its chemical structure:

$$CH_3 - \bigcirc - SO_2NHCONH - N$$

CLINICAL PHARMACOLOGY
ACTIONS

Tolazamide appears to lower the blood glucose acutely by stimulating the release of insulin from the pancreas, an effect dependent upon functioning beta cells in the pancreatic islets. The mechanism by which Tolazamide lowers blood glucose during long-term administration has not been clearly established. With chronic administration in type II diabetic patients, the blood glucose lowering effect persists despite a gradual decline in the insulin secretory response to the drug. Extrapancreatic effects may be involved in the mechanism of action of oral sulfonylurea hypoglycemic drugs.

Some patients who are initially responsive to oral hypoglycemic drugs, including (Tolazamide), may become unresponsive or poorly responsive over time. Alternatively, Tolazamide may be effective in some patients who have become unresponsive to one or more sulfonylurea drugs.

In addition to its blood glucose lowering actions, Tolazamide produces a mild diuresis by enhancement of renal free water clearance.

PHARMACOKINETICS

Tolazamide is rapidly and well absorbed from the gastrointestinal tract. Peak serum concentrations occur at three to four hours following a single oral dose of the drug. The average biological half-life of the drug is seven hours. The drug does not continue to accumulate in the blood after the first four to six doses are administered. A steady or equilibrium state is reached during which the peak and nadir values do not change from day to day after the fourth to sixth doses.

Tolazamide is metabolized to five major metabolites ranging in hypoglycemic activity from 0-70%. They are excreted principally in the urine. Following a single oral dose of tritiated Tolazamide, 85% of the dose was excreted in the urine and 7% in the feces over a five-day period. Most of the urinary excretion of the drug occurred within the first 24 hours postadministration.

When nomal fasting nondiabetic subjects are given a single 500 mg dose of Tolazamide orally, a hypoglycemic effect can be noted within 20 minutes after ingestion with a peak hypoglycemic effect occurring in two to four hours. Following a single oral dose of 500 mg Tolazamide, a statistically significant hypoglycemic effect was demonstrated in fasted nondiabetic subjects 20 hours after administration. With fasting diabetic patients, the peak hypoglycemic effect occurs at four to six hours. The duration of maximal hypoglycemic effect in fed diabetic patients is about ten hours, with the onset occurring at four to six hours and with the blood glucose levels beginning to rise at 14 to 16 hours. Single dose potency of Tolazamide in normal subjects has been shown to be 6.7 times that of tolbutamide on a milligram basis. Clinical experience in diabetic patients has demonstrated Tolazamide to be approximately five times more potent than tolbutamide on a milligram basis, and approximately equivalent in milligram potency to chlorpropamide.

INDICATIONS AND USAGE

Tolazamide is indicated as an adjunct to diet to lower the blood glucose in patients with noninsulin dependent diabetes mellitus (Type II) whose hyperglycemia cannot be satisfactorily controlled by diet alone.

In initiating treatment for noninsulin-dependent diabetes, diet should be emphasized as the primary form of treatment. Caloric restriction and weight loss are essential in the obese diabetic patient. Proper dietary management alone may be effective in controlling the blood glucose and symptoms of hyperglycemia. The importance of regular physical activity should also be stressed and cardiovascular risk factors should be identified and corrective measures taken where possible.

If this treatment program fails to reduce symptoms and/or blood glucose, the use of an oral sulfonylurea or insulin should be considered. Use of Tolazamide must be viewed by both the physician and patient as a treatment in addition to diet and not as a substitute for diet or as a convenient mechanism for avoiding dietary restraint. Furthermore, loss of blood glucose control on diet alone may be transient thus requiring only short-term administration of Tolazamide. During maintenance programs, Tolazamide should be discontinued if satisfactory lowering of blood glucose is no longer achieved. Judgments should be based on regular clinical and laboratory evaluations.

In considering the use of Tolazamide in asymptomatic patients, it should be recognized that controlling the blood glucose in noninsulin-dependent diabetes has not been definitely established to be effective in preventing the long-term cardiovascular or neural complications of diabetes.

CONTRAINDICATIONS

Tolazamide are contraindicated in patients with: 1) known hypersensitivity or allergy to Tolazamide; 2) diabetic ketoacidosis, with or without coma. This condition should be treated with insulin; 3) Type I diabetes, as sole therapy.

SPECIAL WARNING ON INCREASED RISK OF CARDIOVASCULAR MORALITY

The administration of oral hypoglycemic drugs has been reported to be associated with increased cardiovascular mortality as compared to treatment with diet alone or diet plus insulin. This warning is based on the study conducted by the University Group Diabetes Program (UGDP), a long-term prospective clinical trial designed to evaluate the effectiveness of glucose-lowering drugs in preventing or delaying vascular complications in patients with noninsulin-

---

◆ RATED THERAPEUTICALLY EQUIVALENT; ◇ THERAPEUTIC EQUIVALENCE UNCONFIRMED; ○ UNRATED

dependent diabetes. The study involved 823 patients who were randomly assigned to one of four treatment groups (*DIABETES*, 19 (supp. 2):747-830, 1970.)

UGDP reported that patients treated for five to eight years with diet plus a fixed dose of tolbutamide (1.5 grams per day) had a rate of cardiovascular mortality approximately 2 1/2 times that of patients with diet alone. A significant increase in total mortality was not observed, but the use of tolbutamide was discontinued based on the increase on cardiovascular mortality, thus limiting the opportunity for the study to show an increase in overall mortality. Despite controversy regarding the interpretation of these results, the findings of the UGDP study provide an adequate basis for this warning. The patient should be informed of the potential risks and advantages of Tolazamide and of alternative modes of therapy.

Although only one drug in the sulfonylurea class (tolbutamide) was included in this study, it is prudent from a safety standpoint to consider that this warning may also apply to other oral hypoglycemic drugs in this class, in view of their close similarities in mode of action and chemical structure.

PRECAUTIONS

GENERAL

Hypoglycemia: All sulfonylurea drugs are capable of producing severe hypoglycemia. Proper patient selection and dosage and instructions are important to avoid hypoglycemic episodes. Renal or hepatic insufficiency may cause elevated blood levels of Tolazamide and the latter may also diminish gluconeogenic capacity, both of which increase the risk of serious hypoglycemic reactions. Elderly, debilitated, or malnourished patients and those with adrenal or pituitary insufficiency are particularly susceptible to the hypoglycemic action of glucose lowering drugs. Hypoglycemia may be difficult to recognize in the elderly and in people who are taking beta-adrenergic blocking drugs. Hypoglycemia is more likely to occur when caloric intake is deficient, after severe or prolonged exercise, when alcohol is ingested, or when more than one glucose-lowering drug is used.

Loss of Control of Blood Glucose: When a patient stabilized on any diabetic regimen is exposed to stress such as fever, trauma, infection, or surgery, loss of control of blood glucose may occur. At such times it may be necessary to discontinue Tolazamide and administer insulin.

The effectiveness of any hypoglycemic drug, including Tolazamide, in lowering blood glucose to a desired level decreases in many patients over a period of time, which may be due to progression of the severity of the diabetes or to diminished responsiveness to the drug. This phenomenon is known as secondary failure to distinguish it from primary failure in which the drug is ineffective in an individual patient when first given. Adequate adjustment of dose and adherence to diet should be assessed before classifying a patient as a secondary failure.

INFORMATION FOR PATIENTS

Patients should be informed of the potential risks and advantages of Tolazamide and of alternative modes of therapy. They should also be informed about the importance of adherence to dietary instructions, of a regular exercise program, and of regular testing of urine and/or blood glucose.

The risks of hypoglycemia, its symptoms and treatment, and conditions that predispose to its development should be explained to patients and responsible family members. Primary and secondary failure should also be explained.

LABORATORY TESTS

Blood and urine glucose should be monitored periodically. Measurement of glycosylated hemoglobin may be useful in some patients.

DRUG INTERACTIONS

The hypoglycemia action of sulfonylureas may be potentiated by certain drugs including nonsteroidal anti-inflammatory agents and other drugs that are highly protein bound, salicylates, sulfonamides, chloramphenicol, probenecid, coumarins, monoamine oxidase inhibitors, and beta-adrenergic blocking agents. When such drugs are administered to a patient receiving Tolazamide, the patient should be closely observed for hypoglycemia. When such drugs are withdrawn from a patient receiving Tolazamide, the patient should be observed closely for loss of control.

Certain drugs tend to produce hyperglycemia and may lead to loss of control. These drugs include the thiazides and other diuretics, corticosteroids, phenothiazines, thyroid products, estrogens, oral contraceptives, phenytoin, nicotinic acid, sympathomimetics, calcium channel blocking drugs, and isoniazid. When such drugs are administered to a patient receiving Tolazamide the patient should be closely observed for loss of control. When such drugs are withdrawn from a patient receiving Tolazamide the patient should be observed closely for hypoglycemia.

A potential interaction between oral miconazole and oral hypoglycemic agents leading to severe hypoglycemia has been reported. Whether this interaction also occurs with the intravenous, topical or vaginal preparations of miconazole is not known.

CARCINOGENICITY

In a bioassay for carcinogenicity, rats and mice of both sexes were treated with Tolazamide for 103 weeks at low and high doses. No evidence of carcinogenicity was found.

PREGNANCY

Teratogenic Effects: Pregnancy Category C. Tolazamide, administered to pregnant rats at ten times the human dose, decreased litter size but did not produce teratogenic effects in the offspring. In rats treated at a daily dose of 14 mg/kg no reproductive aberrations or drug related fetal anomalies were noted. At an elevated dose of 100 mg/kg per day there was a reduction in the number of pups born and an increased perinatal mortality. There are, however, no adequate and well-controlled studies in pregnant women. Because animal reproduction studies are not always predictive of human response, Tolazamide is not recommended for the treatment of the pregnant diabetic patient. Serious consideration should also be given to the possible hazards of the use of Tolazamide in women of child bearing age and in those who might become pregnant while using the drug.

Because recent information suggests that abnormal blood glucose levels during pregnancy are associated with a higher incidence of congenital abnormalities, many experts recommend that insulin be used during pregnancy to maintain blood glucose levels as close to normal as possible.

Nonteratogenic Effects: Prolonged severe hypoglycemia (four to ten days) has been reported in neonates born to mothers who were receiving a sulfonylurea drug at the time of delivery. This has been reported more frequently with the use of agents with prolonged half-lives. If Tolazamide is used during pregnancy, it should be discontinued at least two weeks before the expected delivery date.

NURSING MOTHERS

Although it is not known whether Tolazamide is excreted in human milk, some sulfonylurea drugs are known to be excreted in human milk. Because the potential for hypoglycemia in nursing infants may exist, a decision should be made whether to discontinue nursing or to discontinue the drug, taking into account the importance of the drug to the mother. If the drug is discontinued and if diet alone is inadequate for controlling blood glucose, insulin therapy should be considered.

PEDIATRIC USE

Safety and effectiveness in children have not been established.

ADVERSE REACTIONS

Tolazamide has generally been well tolerated. In clinical studies in which more than 1,784 diabetic patients were specifically evaluated for incidence of side effects, only 2.1% were discontinued from therapy because of side effects.

Hypoglycemia: See "Precautions" and "Overdosage" sections.

Gastrointestinal Reactions: Cholestatic jaundice may occur rarely; Tolazamide Tablets should be discontinued if this occurs. Gastrointestinal disturbances, eg, nausea, epigastric fullness, and heartburn, are the most common reactions and occurred in 1% of patients treated during clinical trials. They tend to be dose-related and may disappear when dosage is reduced.

Dermatologic Reactions: Allergic skin reactions, eg, pruritus, erythema, urticaria, and morbilliform or maculopapular eruptions, occurred in 0.4% of patients treated during clinical trials. These may be transient and may disappear despite continued use of Tolazamide; if skin reactions persist, the drug should be discontinued.

Porphyria cutanea tarda and photosensitivity reactions have been reported with sulfonylureas.

Hematologic Reactions: Leukopenia, agranulocytosis, thrombocytopenia, hemolytic anemia, aplastic anemia, and pancytopenia have been reported with sulfonylureas.

Metabolic Reactions: Hepatic porphyria and disulfiram-like reactions have been reported with sulfonylureas; however, disulfiram-like reactions with Tolazamide have been reported very rarely.

Cases of hyponatremia have been reported with Tolazamide and all other sulfonylureas, most often in patients who are on other medications or have medical conditions known to cause hyponatremia or increase release of antidiuretic hormone. The syndrome of inappropriate antidiuretic hormone (SIADH) secretion has been reported with certain other sylfonylureas, and it has been suggested that these sulfonylureas may augment the peripheral (antidiuretic) action of ADH and/or increase release of ADH.

Miscellaneous: Weakness, fatigue, dizziness, vertigo, malaise and headache were reported infrequently in patients treated during clinical trials. The relationship to therapy with Tolazamide is difficult to assess.

OVERDOSAGE

Overdosage of sulfonylureas, including Tolazamide, can produce hypoglycemia.

Mild hypoglycemic symptoms without loss of consciousness or neurologic findings should be treated aggressively with oral glucose and adjustment in drug dosage and/or meal patterns. Close monitoring should continue until the physician is assured the patient is out of danger. Severe hypoglycemic reactions with coma, seizure, or other neurological impairment occur infrequently, but constitute medical emergencies requiring immediate hospitalization. If hypoglycemic coma is suspected or diagnosed, the patient should be given a rapid intravenous injection of concentrated (50%) glucose solution. This should be followed by a continuous infusion of a more dilute (10%) glucose solution at a rate which will maintain the blood glucose at a level above 100 mg/dl. Patients should be closely monitored for a minimum of 24 to 48 hours since hypoglycemia may recur after apparent clinical recovery.

DOSAGE AND ADMINISTRATION

There is no fixed dosage regimen for the management of diabetes mellitus with Tolazamide or any other hypoglycemic agent. In addition to the usual monitoring of urinary glucose, the patient's blood glucose must also be monitored periodically to determine the minimum effective dose for the patient; to detect primary failure, ie, inadequate lowering of blood glucose at the maximum recommended dose of medication; and to detect secondary failure, ie, loss of adequate blood glucose response after an initial period of effectiveness. Glycosylated hemoglobin levels may also be of value in monitoring the patient's response to therapy.

➤ SHOWN IN PRODUCT IDENTIFICATION GUIDE

Short-term administration of Tolazamide may be sufficient during periods of transient loss of control in patients usually controlled well on diet.

USUAL STARTING DOSE
The usual starting dose of Tolazamide Tablets for the mild to moderately severe Type II diabetic patient is 100-250 mg daily administered with breakfast or the first main meal. Generally, if the fasting blood glucose is less than 200 mg/dl, the starting dose is 100 mg/day as a single daily dose. If the fasting blood glucose value is greater than 200 mg/dl, the starting dose is 250 mg/day as a single dose. If the patient is malnourished, underweight, elderly, or not eating properly, the initial therapy should be 100 mg once a day. Failure to follow an appropriate dosage regimen may precipitate hypoglycemia. Patients who do not adhere to their prescribed dietary regimen are more prone to exhibit unsatisfactory response to drug therapy.

TRANSFER FROM OTHER HYPOGLYCEMIC THERAPY
Patients Receiving Other Oral Antidiabetic Therapy: Transfer of patients from other oral antidiabetes regimens to Tolazamide should be done conservatively. When transferring patients from oral hypoglycemic agents other than chlorpropamide to Tolazamide no transition period or initial or priming dose is necessary. When transferring from chlorpropamide, particular care should be exercised to avoid hypoglycemia.

Tolbutamide: If receiving less than 1 gm/day, begin at 100 mg of Tolazamide per day. If receiving 1 gm or more per day, initiate at 250 mg of Tolazamide per day as a single dose.

Chlorpropamide: 250 mg of chlorpropamide may be considered to provide approximately the same degree of blood glucose control as 250 mg of Tolazamide. The patient should be observed carefully for hypoglycemia during the transition period from chlorpropamide to Tolazamide (one to two weeks) due to the prolonged retention of chlorpropamide in the body and the possibility of a subsequent overlapping drug effect.

Acetohexamide: 100 mg of Tolazamide may be considered to provide approximately the same degree of blood glucose control as 250 mg of acetohexamide.

Patients Receiving Insulin: Some Type II diabetic patients who have been treated only with insulin may respond satisfactorily to therapy with Tolazamide. If the patient's previous insulin dosage has been less than 20 units, substitution of 100 mg of Tolazamide per day as a single daily dose may be tried. If the previous insulin dosage was less than 40 units, but more than 20 units, the patient should be placed directly on 250 mg of Tolazamide per day as a single dose. If the previous insulin dosage was greater than 40 units, the insulin dosage should be decreased by 50% and 250 mg of Tolazamide per day started. The dosage of Tolazamide should be adjusted weekly (or more often in the group previously requiring more than 40 units of insulin). During this conversion period when both insulin and Tolazamide are being used, hypoglycemia may rarely occur. During insulin withdrawal, patients should test their urine for glucose and acetone at least three times daily and report results to their physician. The appearance of persistent acetonuria with glycosuria indicates that the patient is a Type I diabetic who requires insulin therapy.

MAXIMUM DOSE
Daily doses of greater than 1000 mg are not recommended. Patients will generally have no further response to doses larger than this.

USUAL MAINTENANCE DOSE
The usual maintenance dose is in the range of 100-1000 mg/day with the average maintenance dose being 250-500 mg/day. Following initiation of therapy, dosage adjustment is made in increments of 100 mg to 250 mg at weekly intervals based on the patient's blood glucose response.

DOSAGE INTERVAL
Once a day therapy is usually satisfactory. Doses up to 500 mg/day should be given as a single dose in the morning. 500 mg once daily is as effective as 250 mg twice daily. When a dose of more than 500 mg/day is required, the dose may be divided and given twice daily.

In elderly patients, debilitated or malnourished patients, and patients with impaired renal or hepatic function, the initial and maintenance dosing should be conservative to avoid hypoglycemic reactions (see *"Precautions"* section).

Store at controlled room temperature 15-30° C (59-86° F).

HOW SUPPLIED
TABLETS: 100 MG

AVERAGE UNIT PRICE (AVAILABLE SIZES)		GENERIC A-RATED AVERAGE PRICE (GAAP)	
BRAND	$0.26	100s	$13.41
GENERIC	$0.13		
HCFA FUL (100s ea)	$0.06		

BRAND/MANUFACTURER	NDC	SIZE	AWP
◆ BRAND			
▶ TOLINASE: Upjohn	00009-0070-02	100s	$25.78
◆ GENERICS			
Schein	00364-0721-01	100s	$10.40
Goldline	00182-1677-01	100s	$10.50
Qualitest	00603-6096-21	100s	$10.50
Rugby	00536-4738-01	100s	$10.60
Zenith	00172-2978-60	100s	$10.65
Major	00904-0234-60	100s	$10.80

BRAND/MANUFACTURER	NDC	SIZE	AWP
Mutual	53489-0151-01	100s	$11.00
Martec	52555-0291-01	100s	$11.20
Aligen	00405-5024-01	100s	$11.24
URL	00677-0953-01	100s	$12.44
Moore,H.L.	00839-7014-06	100s	$12.49
Geneva	00781-1922-01	100s	$12.70
U.S. Trading	56126-0122-11	100s ud	$7.88
Major	00904-0234-61	100s ud	$17.15
Auro	55829-0510-10	100s ud	$18.53
Schein	00364-0721-90	100s ud	$19.89
Geneva	00781-1922-13	100s ud	$20.00
UDL	51079-0291-20	100s ud	$23.39
Rugby	00536-4738-02	250s	$25.90

TABLETS: 250 MG

AVERAGE UNIT PRICE (AVAILABLE SIZES)		GENERIC A-RATED AVERAGE PRICE (GAAP)	
BRAND	$0.55	100s	$26.22
GENERIC	$0.23	200s	$39.83
HCFA FUL (100s ea)	$0.09	500s	$90.46
		1000s	$188.93

BRAND/MANUFACTURER	NDC	SIZE	AWP
◆ BRAND			
▶ TOLINASE: Upjohn	00009-0114-05	100s	$54.43
	00009-0114-06	100s ud	$58.13
	00009-0114-04	200s	$107.38
	00009-0114-02	1000s	$524.24
◆ GENERICS			
Rugby	00536-4739-01	100s	$21.50
Schein	00364-0720-01	100s	$21.50
Qualitest	00603-6097-21	100s	$21.51
Zenith	00172-2979-60	100s	$21.80
Mylan	00378-0217-01	100s	$21.92
Moore,H.L.	00839-6755-06	100s	$22.26
URL	00677-0954-01	100s	$22.50
Mutual	53489-0152-01	100s	$22.50
Martec	52555-0292-01	100s	$22.90
Aligen	00405-5025-01	100s	$25.15
Interpharm	53746-0286-01	100s	$26.00
Geneva	00781-1932-01	100s	$26.50
U.S. Trading	56126-0103-11	100s ud	$19.07
Raway	00686-0292-20	100s ud	$20.00
Goldline	00182-1645-89	100s ud	$29.95
Geneva	00781-1932-13	100s ud	$32.00
Auro	55829-0511-10	100s ud	$33.45
Schein	00364-0720-90	100s ud	$33.50
Major	00904-0235-61	100s ud	$34.36
UDL	51079-0292-20	100s ud	$46.06
Goldline	00182-1645-04	200s	$34.50
Major	00904-0235-25	200s	$35.90
Qualitest	00603-6097-23	200s	$36.40
URL	00677-0954-04	200s	$40.75
Mutual	53489-0152-04	200s	$40.75
Zenith	00172-2979-61	200s	$42.00
Interpharm	53746-0286-02	200s	$48.50
Rugby	00536-4739-02	250s	$51.40
Major	00904-0235-40	500s	$66.30
Zenith	00172-2979-70	500s	$94.50
Rugby	00536-4739-03	500s	$99.80
Schein	00364-0720-05	500s	$101.25
Schein	00364-0720-02	1000s	$175.00
Goldline	00182-1645-10	1000s	$175.00
Zenith	00172-2979-80	1000s	$179.55
URL	00677-0954-10	1000s	$179.60
Moore,H.L.	00839-6755-16	1000s	$179.62
Martec	52555-0292-10	1000s	$188.90
Qualitest	00603-6097-32	1000s	$189.56
Mutual	53489-0152-10	1000s	$191.00
Aligen	00405-5025-03	1000s	$201.05
Interpharm	53746-0286-10	1000s	$230.00

TABLETS: 500 MG

AVERAGE UNIT PRICE (AVAILABLE SIZES)		GENERIC A-RATED AVERAGE PRICE (GAAP)	
BRAND	$1.04	100s	$48.17
GENERIC	$0.45	500s	$167.51
HCFA FUL (100s ea)	$0.18		

BRAND/MANUFACTURER	NDC	SIZE	AWP
◆ BRAND			
▶ TOLINASE: Upjohn	00009-0477-06	100s	$104.43
◆ GENERICS			
Aligen	00405-5026-01	100s	$31.45
Zenith	00172-2980-60	100s	$32.10
Mylan	00378-0551-01	100s	$38.20
Rugby	00536-4744-01	100s	$40.40
Qualitest	00603-6098-21	100s	$40.43
Major	00904-0236-60	100s	$40.45
Martec	52555-0293-01	100s	$40.45
Goldline	00182-1679-01	100s	$40.45
Schein	00364-0722-01	100s	$43.25

◆ RATED THERAPEUTICALLY EQUIVALENT; ◇ THERAPEUTIC EQUIVALENCE UNCONFIRMED; ○ UNRATED

BRAND/MANUFACTURER	NDC	SIZE	AWP
Moore,H.L.	00839-7016-06	100s	$43.34
URL	00677-0955-01	100s	$45.00
Mutual	53489-0153-01	100s	$45.00
Interpharm	53746-0287-01	100s	$48.50
Geneva	00781-1942-01	100s	$49.95
Raway	00686-0293-20	100s ud	$30.00
Geneva	00781-1942-13	100s ud	$66.66
Major	00904-0236-61	100s ud	$67.15
Schein	00364-0722-90	100s ud	$67.30
Auro	55829-0512-10	100s ud	$69.67
UDL	51079-0293-20	100s ud	$83.57
Rugby	00536-4744-02	250s	$97.50
Major	00904-0236-40	500s	$111.65
Zenith	00172-2980-70	500s	$152.80
Qualitest	00603-6098-28	500s	$153.12
Mutual	53489-0153-05	500s	$190.00
Interpharm	53746-0287-05	500s	$230.00

Tolazoline Hydrochloride

DESCRIPTION
Tolazoline Hydrochloride USP is a peripheral vasodilator available in ampuls for intravenous administration. Each milliliter of sterile, aqueous solution contains Tolazoline Hydrochloride USP, 25 mg; tartaric acid ACS, 6.5 mg; and hydrous sodium citrate USP, 6.5 mg. Tolazoline Hydrochloride is 4,5-dihydro-2-(phenyl-methyl)-1*H*-imidazole monohydrochloride.

Tolazoline Hydrochloride USP is a white to off-white crystalline powder. Its solutions are slightly acid to litmus. It is freely soluble in water and in alcohol. Its molecular weight is 196.68.

Following is its chemical structure:

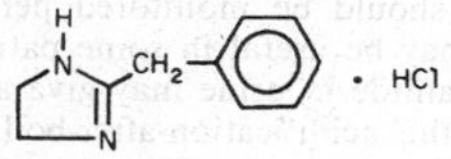

CLINICAL PHARMACOLOGY
Tolazoline Hydrochloride is a direct peripheral vasodilator with moderate competitive alpha-adrenergic blocking activity. It decreases peripheral resistance and increases venous capacitance. It has the following additional actions: (1) sympathomimetic, including cardiac stimulation; (2) parasympathomimetic, including gastrointestinal tract stimulation that is blocked by atropine; and (3) histamine-like, including stimulation of gastric secretion and peripheral vasodilatation. Tolazoline Hydrochloride given intravenously produces vasodilation, primarily due to a direct effect on vascular smooth muscle, and cardiac stimulation; the blood pressure response depends on the relative contributions of the two effects. Tolazoline Hydrochloride usually reduces pulmonary arterial pressure and vascular resistance. In neonates the half-life of Tolazoline Hydrochloride ranges from 3 to 10 hours.

INDICATIONS AND USAGE
Tolazoline Hydrochloride is indicated for the treatment of persistent pulmonary hypertension of the newborn ('persistent fetal circulation') when systemic arterial oxygenation cannot be satisfactorily maintained by usual supportive care (supplemental oxygen and/or mechanical ventilation).

Tolazoline Hydrochloride should be used in a highly supervised setting, where vital signs, oxygenation, acid-base status, fluid, and electrolytes can be monitored and maintained.

CONTRAINDICATIONS
Tolazoline Hydrochloride is contraindicated in patients with hypersensitivity to Tolazoline.

WARNINGS
Tolazoline Hydrochloride stimulates gastric secretion and may activate stress ulcers. Through this mechanism, it can produce significant hypochloremic alkalosis. Pretreatment of infants with antacids may prevent gastrointestinal bleeding.

Patients should be observed closely for signs of systemic hypotension, and supportive therapy should be instituted if needed.

In patients with mitral stenosis, parenterally administered Tolazoline Hydrochloride may produce a rise or fall in pulmonary artery pressure and total pulmonary resistance; therefore, it must be used with caution in patients with known or suspected mitral stenosis.

PRECAUTIONS
General: The effects of Tolazoline Hydrochloride on pulmonary vessels may be pH dependent. Acidosis may decrease the effect of Tolazoline Hydrochloride.

Carcinogenesis, Mutagenesis, Impairment of Fertility: Long-term carcinogenicity studies in animals have not been performed with Tolazoline Hydrochloride.

Pregnancy Category C: Animal reproduction studies have not been conducted with Tolazoline Hydrochloride. It is also not known whether Tolazoline Hydrochloride can cause fetal harm when administered to a pregnant woman or can affect reproduction capacity. Tolazoline Hydrochloride should be given to a pregnant woman only if clearly needed.

Nursing Mothers: It is not known whether this drug is excreted in human milk. Because many drugs are excreted in human milk, caution should be exercised when Tolazoline Hydrochloride is administered to a nursing woman.

ADVERSE REACTIONS
The following adverse reactions have been observed, but there are insufficient data to support an estimate of their frequency:

Cardiovascular: Hypotension, tachycardia, cardiac arrhythmias, hypertension, pulmonary hemorrhage.

Digestive and Hepatic: Gastrointestinal hemorrhage, nausea, vomiting, diarrhea, hepatitis.

Skin: Flushing, increased pilomotor activity with tingling or chilliness, rash.

Hematologic: Thrombocytopenia, leukopenia.

Renal: Edema, oliguria, hematuria.

OVERDOSAGE
ACUTE TOXICITY
Oral LD$_{50}$'s (mg/kg): mice, 400; rats, 1200.

SIGNS AND SYMPTOMS
Signs and symptoms of overdosage may include increased pilomotor activity, peripheral vasodilatation, skin flushing, and, in rare instances, hypotension and shock.

TREATMENT
In treating hypotension, it is most important to place the patient's head low and administer intravenous fluids. Epinephrine should not be used, since large doses of Tolazoline Hydrochloride may cause "epinephrine reversal" (further reduction in blood pressure, followed by an exaggerated rebound).

DOSAGE AND ADMINISTRATION
An initial dose of 1 to 2 mg/kg, via scalp vein, followed by an infusion of 1 to 2 mg/kg per hour have usually resulted in significant increases in arterial oxygen. There is very little experience with infusions lasting beyond 36 to 48 hours. Response, if it occurs, can be expected within 30 minutes after the initial dose.

Note: Parenteral drug products should be inspected visually for particulate matter and discoloration prior to administration, whenever solution and container permit.

Store between 15° and 30° C (59°-86° F). Protect from light.

J CODES
Up to 25 mg IV—J2670

HOW SUPPLIED
INJECTION: 25 MG/ML

BRAND/MANUFACTURER	NDC	SIZE	AWP
○ BRAND			
PRISCOLINE HYDROCHLORIDE: Ciba Pharm	00083-6733-04	4 ml 4s	$46.05

Tolbutamide

DESCRIPTION
Tolbutamide is an oral blood glucose lowering drug of the sulfonylurea category. It is a pure white crystalline compound practically insoluble in water but forming water-soluble salts with alkalies. The chemical names for Tolbutamide are (1) Benzenesulfonamide, N-[(butylamino) carbonyl]-4-methyl; (2) 1-Butyl-3-(ptolyl-sulfonyl)urea and its molecular weight is 270.35.

Each Tolbutamide Tablet for oral administration contains 500 mg Tolbutamide.

Following is its chemical structure:

$$CH_3 - \bigcirc - SO_2 - NHCONH(CH_2)_3CH_3$$

CLINICAL PHARMACOLOGY
ACTIONS
Tolbutamide appears to lower blood glucose acutely by stimulating the release of insulin from the pancreas, an effect dependent upon functioning beta cells in the pancreatic islets. The mechanism by which Tolbutamide lowers blood glucose during long-term administration has not been clearly established. With chronic administration in Type II diabetic patients, the blood glucose lowering effect persists despite a gradual decline in the insulin secretory response to the drug. Extrapancreatic effects may be involved in the mechanism of action of oral sulfonylurea hypoglycemic drugs.

Some patients who are initially responsive to oral hypoglycemic drugs, including Tolbutamide may become unresponsive or poorly responsive over time. Alternatively, Tolbutamide may be effective in some patients who have become unresponsive to one or more other sulfonylurea drugs.

PHARMACOKINETICS
When administered orally, Tolbutamide is readily absorbed from the gastrointestinal tract. Absorption is not impaired and glucose lowering and insulin releasing effects are not altered if the drug is taken with food. Detectable levels are present

➤ SHOWN IN PRODUCT IDENTIFICATION GUIDE

in the plasma within twenty minutes after oral ingestion of a 500 mg Tolbutamide Tablet, with peak levels occurring at three to four hours and only small amounts detectable at 24 hours. The half-life of Tolbutamide is 4.5 to 6.5 hours. As Tolbutamide has no pamino group, it cannot be acetylated, which is one of the common modes of metabolic degradation for the antibacterial sulfonamides. However, the presence of the p-methyl group renders Tolbutamide susceptible to oxidation, and this appears to be the principal manner of its metabolic degradation in man. The p-methyl group is oxidized to form a carboxyl group, converting tolbutamide into the totally inactive metabolite 1-butyl-3-p-carboxyphenylsulfonylurea, which can be recovered in the urine within 24 hours in amounts accounting for up to 75% of the administered dose.

The major Tolbutamide metabolite has been found to have no hypoglycemic or other action when administered orally and IV to both normal and diabetic subjects. This Tolbutamide metabolite is highly soluble over the critical acid range of urinary pH values, and its solubility increases with increase in pH. Because of the marked solubility of the Tolbutamide metabolite, crystalluria does not occur. A second metabolite, 1-butyl-3-(p-hydroxymethyl) phenyl sulfonylurea also occurs to a limited extent. It is an inactive metabolite.

The administration of 3 grams of Tolbutamide to either nondiabetic or Tolbutamide-responsive diabetic subjects will, in both instances, occasion a gradual lowering of blood glucose. Increasing the dose to 6 grams does not usually cause a response which is significantly different from that produced by the 3 gram dose. Following the administration of a 3 gram dose of Tolbutamide solution, nondiabetic fasting adults exhibit a 30% or greater reduction in blood glucose within one hour, following which the blood glucose gradually returns to the fasting level over six to twelve hours. Following the administration of a 3 gram dose of Tolbutamide solution, Tolbutamide responsive diabetic patients show a gradually progressive blood glucose lowering effect, the maximal response being reached between five to eight hours after ingestion of a single 3 gram dose. The blood glucose then rises gradually and by the 24th hour has usually returned to pretest levels. The magnitude of the reduction, when expressed in terms of percent of the protest blood glucose, tends to be similar to the response seen in the nondiabetic subject.

INDICATIONS AND USAGE

Tolbutamide Tablets are indicated as an adjunct to diet to lower the blood glucose in patients with noninsulin-dependent diabetes mellitus (type II) whose hyperglycemia cannot be satisfactorily controlled by diet alone. In initiating treatment for noninsulin-dependent diabetes, diet should be emphasized as the primary form of treatment. Caloric restriction and weight loss are essential in the obese diabetic patient. Proper dietary management alone may be effective in controlling the blood glucose and symptoms of hyperglycemia. The importance of regular physical activity should also be stressed and cardiovascular risk factors should be identified and corrective measures taken where possible.

If this treatment program fails to reduce symptoms and/or blood glucose, the use of an oral sulfonylurea or insulin should be considered. Use of Tolbutamide must be viewed by both the physician and patient as a treatment in addition to diet, and not as a substitute for diet or as a convenient mechanism for avoiding dietary restraint. Furthermore, loss of blood glucose control on diet alone may be transient, thus requiring only short-term administration of Tolbutamide.

During maintenance programs, Tolbutamide should be discontinued if satisfactory lowering of blood glucose is no longer achieved. Judgments should be based on regular clinical and laboratory evaluations.

In considering the use of Tolbutamide in asymptomatic patients, it should be recognized that controlling the blood glucose in noninsulin-dependent diabetes has not been definitely established to be effective in preventing the long-term cardiovascular or neural complications of diabetes.

CONTRAINDICATIONS

Tolbutamide Tablets are contraindicated in patients with: 1) known hypersensitivity or allergy to Tolbutamide; 2) diabetic ketoacidosis, with or without coma; this condition should be treated with insulin. 3) Type I diabetes, as sole therapy.

Special Warning on Increased Risk of Cardiovascular Mortality:

The administration of oral hypoglycemic drugs has been reported to be associated with increased cardiovascular mortality as compared to treatment with diet alone or diet plus insulin. This warning is based on the study conducted by the University Group Diabetes Program (UGDP), a long-term prospective clinical trial designed to evaluate the effectiveness of glucose-lowering drugs in preventing or delaying vascular complications in patients with noninsulin-dependent diabetes. The study involved 823 patients who were randomly assigned to one of four treatment groups (Diabetes, 19 (supp. 2): 747-830, 1970.)

UGDP reported that patients treated for five to eight years with diet plus a fixed dose of Tolbutamide (1.5 grams per day) had a rate of cardiovascular mortality approximately 2 ½ times that of patients treated with diet alone. A significant increase in total mortality was not observed, but the use of Tolbutamide was discontinued based on the increase in cardiovascular mortality, thus limiting the opportunity for the study to show an increase in overall mortality. Despite controversy regarding the interpretation of these results, the findings of the UGDP study provide an adequate basis for this warning. The patient should be informed of the potential risks and advantages of Tolbutamide Tablets and of alternative modes of therapy.

Although only one drug in the sulfonylurea class (Tolbutamide) was included in this study, it is prudent from a safety standpoint to consider that this warning may also apply to other oral hypoglycemic drugs in this class, in view of their close similarities in mode of action and chemical structure.

PRECAUTIONS

GENERAL

Hypoglycemia: All sulfonylurea drugs are capable of producing severe hypoglycemia. Proper patient selection and dosage and instructions are important to avoid hypoglycemic episodes. Renal or hepatic insufficiency may cause elevated blood levels of Tolbutamide and the latter may also diminish gluconeogenic capacity, both of which increase the risk of serious hypoglycemic reactions. Elderly, debilitated or malnourished patients and those with adrenal or pituitary insufficiency are particularly susceptible to the hypoglycemic action of glucose lowering drugs. Hypoglycemia may be difficult to recognize in the elderly and people who are taking beta-adrenergic blocking drugs. Hypoglycemia is more likely to occur when caloric intake is deficient, after severe or prolonged exercise, when alcohol is ingested, or when more than one glucose lowering drug is used.

Loss of Control of Blood Glucose: When a patient stabilized on any diabetic regimen is exposed to stress such as fever, trauma, infection, or surgery, loss of blood glucose control may occur. At such times it may be necessary to discontinue Tolbutamide and administer insulin.

The effectiveness of any hypoglycemic drug, including Tolbutamide in lowering blood glucose to a desired level decreases in patients over a period of time, which may be due to progression of the severity of the diabetes or to diminished responsiveness to the drug. This phenomenon is known as secondary drug failure to distinguish it from primary failure in which the drug is ineffective in an individual patient when first given. Adequate adjustment of dose and adherence to diet should be assessed before classifying a patient as a secondary failure.

INFORMATION FOR PATIENTS

Patients should be informed of the potential risks and advantages of Tolbutamide Tablets and of alternative modes of therapy. They should also be informed about the importance of adherence to dietary instructions, of a regular exercise program, and of regular testing of urine and/or blood glucose.

The risks of hypoglycemia, its symptoms and treatment, and conditions that predispose to its development should be explained to patients and responsible family members. Primary and secondary failure should also be explained.

LABORATORY TESTS

Blood and urine glucose should be monitored periodically. Measurement of glycosylated hemoglobin may be useful in some patients.

A metabolite of Tolbutamide in urine may give a false positive reaction for albumin if measured by the acidification-after-boiling test, which causes the metabolite to precipitate. There is no interference with the sulfosalicylic acid test.

DRUG INTERACTIONS

The hypoglycemic action of sulfonylureas may be potentiated by certain drugs including nonsteroidal anti-inflammatory agents and other drugs that are highly protein bound, salicylates, sulfonamides, chloramphenicol, probenecid, coumarins, monoamine oxidase inhibitors, and beta adrenergic blocking agents. When such drugs are administered to a patient receiving Tolbutamide the patient should be closely observed for hypoglycemia. When such drugs are withdrawn from a patient receiving Tolbutamide, the patient should be observed closely for loss of control.

Certain drugs tend to produce hyperglycemia and may lead to loss of control. These drugs include the thiazides and other diuretics, corticosteroids, phenothiazines, thyroid products, estrogens, oral contraceptives, phenytoin, nicotinic acid, sympathomimetics, calcium channel blocking drugs and isoniazid. When such drugs are administered to a patient receiving Tolbutamide the patient should be closely observed for loss of control of blood glucose. When such drugs are withdrawn from a patient receiving Tolbutamide, the patient should be observed closely for hypoglycemia.

A potential interaction between oral miconazole and oral hypoglycemic agents leading to severe hypoglycemia has been reported. Whether this interaction also occurs with the intravenous, topical or vaginal preparations of miconazole is not known.

CARCINOGENESIS AND MUTAGENICITY

Bioassay for carcinogenicity was performed in both sexes of rats and mice following ingestion of Tolbutamide for 78 weeks. No evidence of carcinogenicity was found.

Tolbutamide has also been demonstrated to be nonmutagenic in the Ames salmonella/mammalian microsome mutagenicity test.

PREGNANCY

Teratogenic Effects: Pregnancy Category C. Tolbutamide has been shown to be teratogenic in rats given in doses 25 to 100 times the human dose. In some studies, pregnant rats given high doses of Tolbutamide have shown increased mortality in offspring and ocular and bony abnormalities. Repeat studies in other species (rabbits) have not demonstrated a teratogenic effect. There are no adequate and well controlled studies in pregnant women. Tolbutamide is not recommended for the treatment of pregnant diabetic patients. Serious consideration should also be given to the possible hazards of the use of Tolbutamide in women of child-bearing age and in those who might become pregnant while using the drug.

Because recent information suggests that abnormal blood glucose levels during pregnancy are associated with a higher incidence of congenital abnormalities, many experts recommend that insulin be used during pregnancy to maintain blood glucose levels as close to normal as possible.

Nonteratogenic Effects: Prolonged severe hypoglycemia (four to ten days) has been reported in neonates born to mothers who were receiving a sulfonylurea drug at the time of delivery. This has been reported more frequently with the use of agents with prolonged half lives. If Tolbutamide is used during pregnancy, it should be discontinued at least two weeks before the expected delivery date.

NURSING MOTHERS

Although it is not known whether Tolbutamide is excreted in human milk, some sulfonylurea drugs are known to be excreted in human milk. Because the potential for hypoglycemia in nursing infants may exist, a decision should be made whether to discontinue nursing or to discontinue the drug, taking into account the importance of the drug to the mother. If the drug is discontinued and if diet alone is inadequate for controlling blood glucose, insulin therapy should be considered.

PEDIATRIC USE

Safety and effectiveness in children have not been established.

ADVERSE REACTIONS

Hypoglycemia: See *"Precautions"* and *"Overdosage"* sections.

Gastrointestinal Reactions: Cholestatic jaundice may occur rarely; Tolbutamide Tablets should be discontinued if this occurs. Gastrointestinal disturbances, eg, nausea, epigastric fullness, and heartburn, are the most common reactions and occurred in 1.4% of patients treated during clinical trials. They tend to be dose-related and may disappear when dosage is reduced.

Dermatologic Reactions: Allergic skin reactions, eg, pruritus, erythema, urticaria, and morbilliform or maculopapular eruptions, occurred in 1.1% of patients treated during clinical trials. These may be transient and may disappear despite continued use of Tolbutamide if skin reactions persist, the drug should be discontinued.

Porphyria cutanea tarda and photosensitivity reactions have been reported with sulfonylureas.

Hematologic Reactions: Leukopenia, agranulocytosis, thrombocytopenia, hemolytic anemia, aplastic anemia, and pancytopenia have been reported with sulfonylureas.

Metabolic Reactions: Hepatic porphria and disulfiram-like reactions have been reported with sulfonylureas.

Endocrine Reactions: Cases of hyponatremia and the syndrome of inappropriate antidiuretic hormone (SIADH) secretion have been reported with this and other sulfonylureas.

Miscellaneous Reactions: Headache and taste alterations have occasionally been reported with Tolbutamide administration.

OVERDOSAGE

Overdosage of sulfonylureas, including Tolbutamide Tablets, can produce symptoms of hypoglycemia.

Mild hypoglycemic symptoms without loss of consciousness or neurologic findings should be treated aggressively with oral glucose and adjustments in drug dosage and/or meal patterns. Close monitoring should continue until the physician is assured the patient is out of danger. Severe hypoglycemic reactions with coma, seizure, or other neurological impairment occur infrequently but constitute medical emergencies requiring immediate hospitalization. If hypoglycemic coma is suspected or diagnosed, the patient should be given a rapid intravenous injection of concentrated (50%) dextrose injection. This should be followed by a continuous infusion of a more dilute (10%) dextrose injection at a rate which will maintain the blood glucose level above 100 mg/dl. Patients should be closely monitored for a minimum of 24 to 48 hours, since hypoglycemia may recur after apparent clinical recovery.

DOSAGE AND ADMINISTRATION

There is no fixed dosage regimen for the management of diabetes mellitus with Tolbutamide Tablets or any other hypoglycemic agent. In addition to the usual monitoring of urinary glucose, the patient's blood glucose must also be monitored periodically to determine the minimum effective dose for the patient; to detect primary failure, ie, inadequate lowering of blood glucose at the maximum recommended dose of medication; and to detect secondary failure, ie, loss of adequate blood-glucose-lowering response after an initial period of effectiveness. Glycosylated hemoglobin levels may also be of value in monitoring the patient's response to therapy.

Short-term administration of Tolbutamide may be sufficient during periods of transient loss of control in patients usually controlled well on diet.

USUAL STARTING DOSE

The usual starting dose is 1 to 2 grams daily. This may be increased or decreased depending on individual patient response. Failure to follow an appropriate dosage regimen may precipitate hypoglycemia. Patients who do not adhere to their prescribed dietary regimens are more prone to exhibit unsatisfactory response to drug therapy.

TRANSFER FROM OTHER HYPOGLYCEMIC THERAPY

Patients Receiving Other Oral Antidiabetic Therapy: Transfer of patients from other oral antidiabetes regimens to Tolbutamide should be done conservatively. When transferring patients from oral hypoglycemic agents other than chlorpropamide to Tolbutamide no transition period and no initial or priming doses are necessary. When transferring patients from chlorpropamide, however, particular care should be exercised during the first two weeks because of the prolonged retention of chlorpropamide in the body and the possibility that subsequent overlapping drug effects might provoke hypoglycemia.

Patients Receiving Insulin: Patients requiring 20 units or less of insulin daily may be placed directly on Tolbutamide and insulin abruptly discontinued. Patients whose insulin requirement is between 20 and 40 units daily may be started on therapy with Tolbutamide with a concurrent 30 to 50% reduction in insulin dose,

with further daily reduction of the insulin when response to Tolbutamide is observed. In patients requiring more than 40 units of insulin daily, therapy with Tolbutamide may be initiated in conjunction with a 20% reduction in insulin dose the first day, with further careful reduction of insulin as response is observed. Occasionally, conversion to Tolbutamide in the hospital may be advisable in candidates who require more than 40 units of insulin daily. During this conversion period when both insulin and Tolbutamide are being used, hypoglycemia may rarely occur. During insulin withdrawal, patients should test their urine for glucose and acetone at least three times daily and report results to their physician. The appearance of persistent acetonuria with glycosuria indicates that the patient is a Type 1 diabetic patient who requires insulin therapy.

MAXIMUM DOSE

Daily doses of greater than 3 grams are not recommended.

USUAL MAINTENANCE DOSE

The maintenance dose is in the range of 0.25-3 grams daily. Maintenance doses above 2 grams are seldom required.

DOSAGE INTERVAL

The total daily dose may be taken either in the morning or in divided doses through the day. While either schedule is usually effective, the divided dose system is preferred by some clinicians from the standpoint of digestive tolerance.

In elderly, debilitated or malnourished patients and patients with impaired renal or hepatic function, the initial and maintenance dosing should be conservative to avoid hypoglycemic reactions (see *"Precautions"* section).

STORAGE

Store at controlled room temperature 15° to 30°C (59° to 86°F). Dispense in well-closed container with child-resistant closure.

HOW SUPPLIED
TABLETS: 500 MG

AVERAGE UNIT PRICE (AVAILABLE SIZES)		GENERIC A-RATED AVERAGE PRICE (GAAP)	
BRAND	$0.26	100s	$8.68
GENERIC	$0.07	500s	$25.19
HCFA FUL (100s ea)	$0.04	1000s	$63.08

BRAND/MANUFACTURER	NDC	SIZE	AWP
◆ BRAND			
➤ ORINASE: Upjohn	00009-0100-11	100s	$26.00
	00009-0100-02	200s	$51.41
	00009-0100-03	500s	$128.35
	00009-0100-05	1000s	$253.65
◆ GENERICS			
Goldline	00182-1084-01	100s	$5.55
Qualitest	00603-6121-21	100s	$5.80
Rugby	00536-4668-01	100s	$6.08
Major	00904-0223-60	100s	$6.30
Mylan	00378-0215-01	100s	$6.50
Zenith	00172-2245-60	100s	$6.65
URL	00677-0592-01	100s	$7.90
Moore,H.L.	00839-6253-06	100s	$7.95
Schein	00364-0477-01	100s	$11.06
Aligen	00405-5031-01	100s	$11.06
Raway	00686-0596-20	100s ud	$8.50
Major	00904-0223-61	100s ud	$9.77
Auro	55829-0515-10	100s ud	$10.39
Vangard	00615-1514-13	100s ud	$11.65
Goldline	00182-1084-89	100s ud	$11.70
UDL	51079-0560-20	100s ud	$12.00
Moore,H.L.	00839-6253-12	500s	$22.67
Mylan	00378-0215-05	500s	$23.55
Goldline	00182-1084-05	500s	$24.00
Major	00904-0223-40	500s	$25.30
URL	00677-0592-05	500s	$25.90
Zenith	00172-2245-70	500s	$26.50
Rugby	00536-4668-05	500s	$28.43
Moore,H.L.	00839-6253-16	1000s	$46.78
Zenith	00172-2245-80	1000s	$51.90
URL	00677-0592-10	1000s	$55.09
Rugby	00536-4668-10	1000s	$55.14
Major	00904-0223-80	1000s	$55.95
Aligen	00405-5031-03	1000s	$81.96
Schein	00364-0477-02	1000s	$94.76

Tolbutamide Sodium

DESCRIPTION

Tolbutamide Sodium sterile powder contains Tolbutamide Sodium which is a white to off-white, practically odorless, crystalline powder, having a slightly bitter taste. It is freely soluble in water, soluble in alcohol and in chloroform, very slightly soluble in ether.

Each vial contains the equivalent of 1.0 g of free Tolbutamide, present as 1.081 g of the Sodium salt of 1-Butyl-3-(p-tolylsulfonyl) urea. The 81 mg of Sodium present should not interdict the diagnostic use of this preparation in patients maintained on salt-poor regimens. The diluent consists of 20 ml of sterile water for injection.

The chemical name for Tolbutamide Sodium is 1-Butyl-3-(p-tolylsulfonyl) urea monosodium salt $C_{12}H_{17}N_2NaO_3S$.

Following is its chemical structure:

$$CH_3 - \text{(benzene ring)} - SO_2NCONH(CH_2)_2CH_3, \ Na$$

CLINICAL PHARMACOLOGY
The prompt decrease in blood glucose in normal individuals is associated with a prompt increase in serum insulin levels, as determined by immunoassay, which rise from a fasting mean value of 19 µU per ml to a peak mean value of approximately 40 µU per ml (range 27 to 89) 20 minutes after injection. In patients with functioning islet cell adenoma, Tolbutamide Sodium has a marked and prolonged blood glucose lowering effect associated with an excessive, prompt rise in serum insulin (118 to 1,055 µU/ml), resulting in a marked and prolonged blood glucose effect (Figure 1).

INDICATIONS AND USAGE
Tolbutamide Sodium sterile powder is indicated for use as an aid in the diagnosis of pancreatic islet cell adenoma.

The difficulties of differential diagnosis of spontaneous hypoglycemia have made clear the need for more definitive diagnostic procedures in order to avoid subtotal pancreatic resection in patients in whom surgery is not indicated. Fully 80% of cases of spontaneous hypoglycemia result from one of three causes: functional hyperinsulinism, organic hyperinsulinism, and hepatogenic hypoglycemia. Functional hyperinsulinism is by far the most common form of the disorder, accounting for 70% of all cases. This form of hyperinsulinism is believed to be basically a psychosomatic disorder associated with an imbalance of autonomic nervous system influences on blood glucose control. The management of such patients is dietary, as is that of patients with hepatogenic hypoglycemia. These must be distinguished from organic hyperinsulinism due to pancreatic islet cell adenoma which requires surgery.

Figure 1

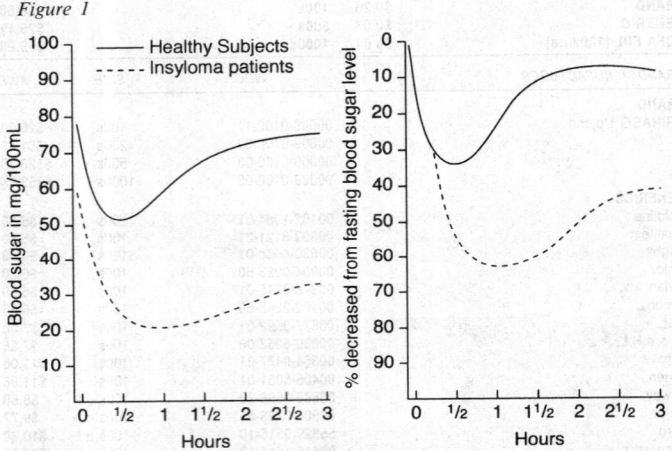

Effect of intravenous injection of Tolbutamide Sodium on blood glucose in healthy subjects and insulinoma patients.

Patients with functioning insulinomas exhibit hypoglycemic responses to intravenously administered Tolbutamide Sodium which are sufficiently distinctive to make this drug a valuable adjunct in the diagnosis of functioning insulinomas.

It will be noted from Figure 1 that the administration of 1.0 g of Tolbutamide Sodium to healthy subjects results in a rapid fall in blood glucose levels for 30 to 45 minutes, followed by a secondary rise of the blood glucose concentration into the normal range in the ensuing 90 to 180 minutes. The initial hypoglycemia results from the rapid release of insulin from the pancreatic beta cells, while the secondary rise is due to activation of counter-regulatory factors. In contrast, patients with insulinomas were found to exhibit Tolbutamide induced blood glucose decreases of greater magnitude than healthy persons. Of greater significance than the magnitude of blood glucose fall in these patients is the persistence of the hypoglycemia for three hours after the administration of Tolbutamide Sodium. It is this phenomenon of persistent Tolbutamide induced hypoglycemia for three hours rather than degree of blood glucose decrease which is of importance in the diagnosis of pancreatic islet cell adenomas. False positive responses have been observed in a few patients with liver disease, alcohol hypoglycemia, idiopatric hypoglycemia of infancy, severe under nutrition, azotemia, sarcoma, and other extrapancreatic insulin producing tumors.

CONTRAINDICATIONS
Because of the lack of data to establish ideal dosage and the inability to interpret results, use of Tolbutamide Sodium sterile powder is not recommended in children.

The test should not be performed on persons who have previously shown allergy to Tolbutamide or related sulfonylureas.

WARNINGS
Severe and prolonged hypoglycemia following oral administration of Tolbutamide has been reported in patients suffering from severe liver disease and severe renal disease.

Severe hypoglycemic symptoms may develop during the test, particularly in patients with fasting blood glucose levels in the hypoglycemic range. If they occur, the test should be terminated immediately by intravenously injecting 12.5 to 25 g of glucose in a 25 to 50% solution.

PRECAUTIONS
General: Although the hypoglycemic symptoms produced by this test dose are usually not severe, certain nondiabetics may develop moderate to severe symptoms. To avoid this occurrence, the diagnostic test should be terminated by the oral administration of carbohydrate immediately after the 30-minute blood sample has been withdrawn.

It is essential that only a true glucose procedure (Somogyl-Nelson, Modified Folin-Wu, AutoAnalyzer,® or glucose oxidase) be used to determine blood glucose in order to eliminate highly variable amounts of nonglucose reducing substances as a major source of error.

As with all intravenous injections, epinephrine and other resuscitative drugs should be at hand to administer in the event of anaphylaxis.

Because hypoglycemia of considerable magnitude can occur in certain nondiabetics, it would be wise to routinely terminate each test immediately upon withdrawal of the 30-minute blood sample by the oral administration of carbohydrate, especially in the testing of persons with atherosclerosis.

Drug Interactions: Certain drugs may potentiate the hypoglycemic action of Tolbutamide. These include dicumarol, phenyramidol, salicylates, sulfonamides, oxyphenbutazone, phenylbutazone, probenecid, monoamine oxidase inhibitors, beta-adrenergic blocking agents, and chloramphenicol. There is a danger of both increased and/or prolonged hypoglycemia if these drugs are used together.

Concomitant ingestion of salicylates, sulfonamides, oxyphenbutazone, phenylbutazone, probenecid, monoamine oxidase inhibitors may interfere with results of a Tolbutamide tolerance test.

Response to Tolbutamide is diminished in patients on therapy with beta-adrenergic blocking agents.

Drug-Laboratory Test Interactions: On very rare occasions, urine containing the Tolbutamide metabolite may give a false positive reaction for albumin by the usual test (acidification after boiling) since this procedure causes the metabolite to precipitate as flocculent particles. This problem may be circumvented by the use of bromphenol reagent stripe.

Carcinogenesis, Mutagenesis, Impairment of Fertility: Bioassay for carcinogenicity was performed in both sexes of rats and mice following Tolbutamide ingestion for 78 weeks. No evidence of carcinogenicity was found.

Tolbutamide has also been demonstrated to be nonmutagenic in the Ames salmonella/mammalian microsome mutagenicity test.

Pregnancy: Teratogenic Effects. Pregnancy Category C: Tolbutamide Sodium has been shown to be teratogenic in rats given doses 25 to 100 times the human dose. In some studies, pregnant rats given high doses of Tolbutamide have shown increased mortality in offspring and ocular and bony abnormalities. Repeat studies in other species (rabbits) have not demonstrated a teratogenic effect. There are no adequate and well controlled studies in pregnant women. Tolbutamide Sodium sterile powder is not recommended for the treatment of pregnant diabetic patients. Serious consideration should also be given to the possible hazards of the use of Tolbutamide Sodium in women of childbearing age and potential who might become pregnant while using the drug.

Nonteratogenic Effects: Prolonged severe hypoglycemia (four to ten days) has been reported in neonates born to mothers who were receiving a sulfonylurea drug at the time for delivery. This has been reported more frequently with the use of agents with prolonged half lives. Use of the drug in pregnant patients is not recommended.

Nursing Mothers: Tolbutamide is excreted in small amounts in the breast milk of nursing mothers. Because of the potential for serious adverse reactions in nursing infants, a decision should be made whether to discontinue nursing or to discontinue the drug, taking into account the importance of the drug to the mother.

Pediatric Use: Safety and effectiveness in children have not been established.

ADVERSE REACTIONS
Rarely a patient may experience a mild pain in the shoulder or slight burning sensation along the course of an arm vein during the intravenous injection. Such pain which lasts no more than 2 to 3 minutes, is attributed to venospasm and may be obviated by administering the test solution over a period of no less than two, preferably, three minutes. Thrombophlebitis with thrombosis of the injected vein has been found to occur in a small percentage of patients (0.8 to 2.4%). This is usually painless, detectable only by careful palpation and may not appear for one or two weeks after injection. No sequelae have been noted. The vein gradually shrinks or recanalizes.

OVERDOSAGE
Overdosage of sulfonylureas, including Tolbutamide Sodium sterile powder, will produce symptoms of hypoglycemia. The symptoms produced may be mild, consisting only of sweating, trembling, weakness, fatigue, nervousness, hunger, or nausea. They may be more severe, including lethargy, confusion, stupor, loss of

---

◆ RATED THERAPEUTICALLY EQUIVALENT; ◇ THERAPEUTIC EQUIVALENCE UNCONFIRMED; ○ UNRATED

consciousness, or coma. Seizures may occur with marked hypoglycemia. In these cases, laboratory evaluation will reveal a low blood glucose level.

Mild symptoms of hypoglycemia without loss of consciousness should be treated aggressively with oral glucose and appropriate adjustment in drug dosage and meal patterns. Monitoring should continue until such time as the patient is out of danger. Severe hypoglycemic reactions with coma, seizure, or other neurological impairment are rare, but constitute medical emergencies and require immediate hospitalization. If hypoglycemic coma is suspected or diagnosed, the patient should be given a rapid intravenous injection of concentrated (50%) dextrose solution. This can be repeated as needed. This should be followed by a continuous infusion of a more dilute (10%) dextrose solution at a rate which will maintain the blood glucose level above 100 mg/dl. Patients should be closely monitored in the hospital for a minimum of 24 to 48 hours, since hypoglycemia may recur after apparent clinical recovery.

Overdosage with sulfonylurea drugs has not been reported to be responsive to either peritoneal dialysis or hemodialysis. The experience, however, is quite limited.

The oral LD_{50} of Tolbutamide in the rat was greater than 2344 mg/kg.

The dose of medication which may cause hypoglycemia in humans is variable. In some individuals, usual therapeutic doses have been known to cause symptomatic hypoglycemia.

DOSAGE AND ADMINISTRATION

FAJANS TEST

1. The patient should receive a high carbohydrate diet of from 150 to 300 g daily for at least three days prior to the test.

2. On morning of test, after an overnight fast, withdraw a fasting blood specimen.

3. Inject entire volume (20 ml) of Tolbutamide Sodium solution intravenously at a constant rate over a two to three minute period.

4. Withdraw blood specimens at the following intervals (in minutes) after the midpoint of the injection: 20, 30, 45, 60, 90, 120, 150, and 180. Of greater significance than the magnitude of blood glucose fall in these patients is the persistence of the hypoglycemia for three hours after the administration of Tolbutamide Sodium. The determination of serum insulin levels before, and at 10, 20, and 30 minutes after the intravenous administration of the drug as described below, provides a specific and safer test for insulinoma. It also permits the performance of the test in the presence of moderate fasting hypoglycemia, since interpretation is not based on the decline of the blood glucose.

5. Blood glucose determinations are made by the true glucose procedures.

The procedure is terminated with a feeding of readily assimilable carbohydrate or breakfast.

Interpretation of Results—Healthy Subjects: A decrease to a blood glucose of 38 to 79% of the fasting level may be expected. At 90 to 120 minutes a level of from 78 to 100% of initial level may be seen. Similar responses are to be found in patients with functional hyperinsulinism.

Insulinoma Patients: Minimum blood glucose levels of 17 to 50% of fasting values are seen. In the 90 to 180 minute interval, levels are in the range of 40 to 64%. Some patients with liver disease may show the same type of blood glucose response as do patients with insulinomas. Therefore, appropriate laboratory and clinical tests must be employed to distinguish between these two conditions.

Use with Serum Insulin Determination in Insulinoma Patients: If a method of assay for serum insulin is available, the test for insulinoma may be made shorter and more specific. Using an immunoassay, serum insulin levels rose to peak values of 160 to 300µU per ml in five subjects with proven insulinoma (normal range 27 to 89). In four of the subjects the peak was attained in 20 to 30 minutes, the first determination being performed at 60 minutes in the fifth subject. Excessive increases in plasma insulin of five patients with insulinomas (range 118 to 1,055, mean 486µU/ml) were also found by immunoassay.

The serum insulin response returned to normal after the removal of the insulinoma in two other patients.

Accordingly, the determination of serum insulin levels before, and at 10, 20, and 30 minutes after the intravenous administration of the drug described above, provides a specific and safer test for insulinoma, and permits the performance of the test in the presence of moderate fasting hypoglycemia, since interpretation is not based on the decline of the blood glucose. The test may be terminated after the 30-minute specimen by the feeding of carbohydrate as described above.

PREPARATION OF TOLBUTAMIDE SODIUM SOLUTION

1. Remove the protective metal cap from the vial and sterilize the top of the rubber stopper with a suitable germicide.

2. Break off the neck of the glass ampoule.

3. Using a 20 ml syringe, withdraw all the diluent and inject it into the vial containing Tolbutamide Sodium sterile powder.

4. Shake thoroughly until solution is complete.

Parenteral drug products should be inspected visually for particulate matter and discoloration prior to administration, whenever solution and container permit.

Storage Conditions: Store unreconstituted product at controlled room temperature, 15°-30°C (59°-86°F). Use immediately after reconstitution (within one hour) but only if solution is complete and clear.

BRAND/MANUFACTURER	NDC	SIZE	AWP
○ **BRAND**			
ORINASE DIAGNOSTIC: Upjohn	00009-0741-02	1s	$54.88

Tolectin SEE TOLMETIN SODIUM

Tolinase SEE TOLAZAMIDE

Tolmetin Sodium

DESCRIPTION

Tolmetin Sodium tablets for oral administration contain Tolmetin Sodium as the dihydrate in an amount equivalent to 200 mg of Tolmetin (scored for 100 mg).

Tolmetin Sodium capsules for oral administration contain Tolmetin Sodium as the dihydrate in an amount equivalent to 400 mg of Tolmetin.

Tolmetin Sodium tablets for oral administration contain Tolmetin Sodium as the dihydrate in an amount equivalent to 600 mg of Tolmetin.

The pKa of Tolmetin is 3.5 and Tolmetin Sodium is freely soluble in water.

Tolmetin Sodium is a nonsteroidal anti-inflammatory agent.

The structural formula is: Sodium 1-methyl-5-(4-methylbenzoyl)-1*H*-pyrrole-2-acetate dihydrate.

Following is its chemical structure:

CLINICAL PHARMACOLOGY

Studies in animals have shown Tolmetin Sodium to possess anti-inflammatory, analgesic and antipyretic activity. In the rat Tolmetin Sodium prevents the development of experimentally induced polyarthritis and also decreases established inflammation.

The mode of action of Tolmetin Sodium is not known. However, studies in laboratory animals and man have demonstrated that the anti-inflammatory action of Tolmetin Sodium is *not* due to pituitary-adrenal stimulation. Tolmetin Sodium inhibits prostaglandin synthetase *in vitro* and lowers the plasma level of prostaglandin E in man. This reduction in prostaglandin synthesis may be responsible for the anti-inflammatory action. Tolmetin Sodium does not appear to alter the course of the underlying disease in man.

In patients with rheumatoid arthritis and in normal volunteers, Tolmetin Sodium is rapidly and almost completely absorbed with peak plasma levels being reached within 30-60 minutes after an oral therapeutic dose. In controlled studies, the time to reach peak Tolmetin plasma concentration is approximately 20 minutes longer following administration of a 600 mg tablet, compared to an equivalent dose given as 200 mg tablets. The clinical meaningfulness of this finding, if any, is unknown. Tolmetin displays a biphasic elimination from the plasma consisting of a rapid phase with a half-life of one to 2 hours followed by a slower phase with a half-life of about 5 hours. Peak plasma levels of approximately 40 µg/mL are obtained with a 400 mg oral dose. Essentially all of the administered dose is recovered in the urine in 24 hours either as an inactive oxidative metabolite or as conjugates of Tolmetin. An 18-day multiple dose study demonstrated no accumulation of Tolmetin when compared with a single dose.

In two fecal blood loss studies of 4 to 6 days duration involving 15 subjects each, Tolmetin Sodium did not induce an increase in blood loss over that observed during a 4-day drug-free control period. In the same studies, aspirin produced a greater blood loss than occurred during the drug-free control period, and a greater blood loss than occurred during the Tolmetin Sodium treatment period. In one of the two studies, indomethacin produced a greater fecal blood loss than occurred during the drug free control period; in the second study, indomethacin did not induce a significant increase in blood loss.

Tolmetin Sodium is effective in treating both the acute flares and in the long term management of the symptoms of rheumatoid arthritis, osteoarthritis and juvenile rheumatoid arthritis.

In patients with either rheumatoid arthritis or osteoarthritis Tolmetin Sodium is as effective as aspirin and indomethacin in controlling disease activity, but the frequency of the milder gastrointestinal adverse effects and tinnitus was less than in aspirin-treated patients, and the incidence of central nervous system adverse effects was less than in indomethacin-treated patients.

In patients with juvenile rheumatoid arthritis, Tolmetin Sodium is as effective as aspirin in controlling disease activity, with a similar incidence of adverse reactions. Mean SGOT values, initially elevated in patients on previous aspirin therapy, remained elevated in the aspirin group and decreased in the Tolmetin Sodium group.

Tolmetin Sodium has produced additional therapeutic benefit when added to a regimen of gold salts and, to a lesser extent, with corticosteroids. Tolmetin Sodium should not be used in conjunction with salicylates since greater benefit from the combination is not likely, but the potential for adverse reactions is increased.

INDICATIONS AND USAGE

Tolmetin Sodium is indicated for the relief of signs and symptoms of rheumatoid arthritis and osteoarthritis. Tolmetin Sodium is indicated in the treatment of acute flares and the long-term management of the chronic disease.

Tolmetin Sodium is also indicated for treatment of juvenile rheumatoid arthritis. The safety and effectiveness of Tolmetin Sodium have not been established in children under 2 years of age (see *"Precautions—Pediatric Use"* and *"Dosage and Administration"*).

CONTRAINDICATIONS

Anaphylactoid reactions have been reported with Tolmetin Sodium as with other nonsteroidal anti-inflammatory drugs. Because of the possibility of cross-sensitivity to other nonsteroidal anti-inflammatory drugs, particularly zomepirac sodium, anaphylactoid reactions may be more likely to occur in patients who have exhibited allergic reactions to these compounds. For this reason, Tolmetin Sodium should not be given to patients in whom aspirin and other nonsteroidal anti-inflammatory drugs induce symptoms of asthma, rhinitis, urticaria and other symptoms of allergic or anaphylactoid reactions. Patients experiencing anaphylactoid reactions on Tolmetin Sodium should be treated with conventional therapy, such as epinephrine, antihistamines and/or steroids.

WARNINGS

RISK OF GI ULCERATION, BLEEDING AND PERFORATION WITH NSAID THERAPY

Serious gastrointestinal toxicity such as bleeding, ulceration, and perforation, can occur at any time, with or without symptoms, in patients treated chronically with NSAID (Nonsteroidal Anti-Inflammatory Drug) therapy. Although minor upper gastrointestinal problems, such as dyspepsia, are common, usually developing early in therapy, physicians should remain alert for ulceration and bleeding in patients treated chronically with NSAID's even in the absence of previous GI tract symptoms. In patients observed in clinical trials of several months to two years duration, symptomatic upper GI ulcers, gross bleeding or perforation appear to occur in approximately 1% of patients treated for 3-6 months, and in about 2-4% of patients treated for one year. Physicians should inform patients about the signs and/or symptoms of serious GI toxicity and what steps to take if they occur.

Studies to date have not identified any subset of patients not at risk of developing peptic ulceration and bleeding. Except for a prior history of serious GI events and other risk factors known to be associated with peptic ulcer disease, such as alcoholism, smoking, etc., no risk factor (e.g., age, sex) have been associated with increased risk. Elderly or debilitated patients seem to tolerate ulceration or bleeding less well than other individuals and most spontaneous reports of fatal GI events are in this population. Studies to date are inconclusive concerning the relative risk of various NSAID's in causing such reactions. High doses of any NSAID probably carry a greater risk of these reactions, although controlled clinical trials showing this do not exist in most cases. In considering the use of relatively large doses (within the recommended dosage range), sufficient benefit should be anticipated to offset the potential increased risk of GI toxicity.

PRECAUTIONS

GENERAL

Because of ocular changes observed in animals and reports of adverse eye findings with nonsteroidal anti-inflammatory agents, it is recommended that patients who develop visual disturbances during treatment with Tolmetin Sodium have ophthalmologic evaluations.

As with other nonsteroidal anti-inflammatory drugs, longterm administration of Tolmetin to animals has resulted in renal papillary necrosis and other abnormal renal pathology. In humans, there have been reports of acute interstitial nephritis with hematuria, proteinuria, and occasionally nephrotic syndrome.

A second form of renal toxicity has been seen in patients with prerenal conditions leading to a reduction in renal blood flow or blood volume, where the renal prostaglandins have a supportive role in the maintenance of renal perfusion. In these patients administration of an NSAID may cause a dose dependent reduction in prostaglandin formation and may precipitate overt renal decompensation. Patients at greatest risk of this reaction are those with heart failure, liver dysfunction, those taking diuretics, and the elderly. Discontinuation of NSAID therapy is typically followed by recovery to the pretreatment state.

Since Tolmetin Sodium and its metabolites are eliminated primarily by the kidneys, patients with impaired renal function should be closely monitored, and it should be anticipated that they will require lower doses.

Tolmetin Sodium prolongs bleeding time. Patients who may be adversely affected by prolongation of bleeding time should be carefully observed when Tolmetin Sodium is administered.

In patients receiving concomitant Tolmetin Sodium steroid therapy, any reduction in steroid dosage should be gradual to avoid the possible complications of sudden steroid withdrawal.

Peripheral edema has been reported in some patients receiving Tolmetin Sodium therapy. Therefore, as with other nonsteroidal anti-inflammatory drugs, Tolmetin Sodium should be used with caution in patients with compromised cardiac function, hypertension, or other conditions predisposing to fluid retention.

The antipyretic and anti-inflammatory activities of the drug may reduce fever and inflammation, thus diminishing their utility as diagnostic signs in detecting complications of presumed noninfectious, non-inflammatory painful conditions. As with other nonsteroidal anti-inflammatory drugs, borderline elevations of one

or more liver tests may occur in up to 15% of patients. These abnormalities may progress, may remain essentially unchanged, or may be transient with continued therapy. The SGPT (ALT) test is probably the most sensitive indicator of liver dysfunction. Meaningful (3 times the upper limit of normal) elevations of SGPT or SGOT (AST) occurred in controlled clinical trials in less than 1% of patients. A patient with symptoms and/or signs suggesting liver dysfunction, or in whom an abnormal liver test has occurred, should be evaluated for evidence of the development of more severe hepatic reaction while on therapy with Tolmetin Sodium. Severe hepatic reactions, including jaundice and fatal hepatitis, have been reported with Tolmetin Sodium as with other nonsteroidal anti-inflammatory drugs. Although such reactions are rare, if abnormal liver tests persist or worsen, if clinical signs and symptoms consistent with liver disease develop, or if systemic manifestations occur (e.g. eosinophilia, rash, etc.), Tolmetin Sodium should be discontinued.

CARCINOGENESIS, MUTAGENESIS, IMPAIRMENT OF FERTILITY

Tolmetin Sodium did not possess any carcinogenic liability in the following long-term studies: a 24-month study in rats at doses as high as 75 mg/kg/day, and an 18-month study in mice at doses as high as 50 mg/kg/day.

No mutagenic potential of Tolmetin Sodium was found in the Ames Salmonella-Microsomal Activation Test.

Reproductive studies revealed no impairment of fertility in animals. Effects on parturition have been shown, however, as with other prostaglandin inhibitors. This information is detailed in the *"Pregnancy"* section below.

PREGNANCY

Pregnancy Category C. Reproduction studies in rats and rabbits at doses up to 50 mg/kg (1.5 times the maximum clinical dose based on a body weight of 60 kg) revealed no evidence of teratogenesis or impaired fertility due to Tolmetin Sodium. However, Tolmetin Sodium is an inhibitor of prostaglandin synthetase. Drugs in this class have known effects on the fetal cardiovascular system which may cause constriction of the ductus arteriosus *in utero* during the third trimester of pregnancy, which may result in persistent pulmonary hypertension of the newborn.

There are no adequate and well-controlled studies in pregnant women. Tolmetin Sodium should be used during pregnancy only if the potential benefit justifies the potential risk to the fetus.

NONTERATOGENIC EFFECTS

Prostaglandin inhibitors have also been shown to increase the incidence of dystocia and delayed parturition in animals.

NURSING MOTHERS

Tolmetin Sodium has been shown to be secreted in human milk. Because of the possible adverse effects of prostaglandin inhibiting drugs on neonates, use in nursing mothers should be avoided.

PEDIATRIC USE

The safety and effectiveness of Tolmetin Sodium in children under 2 years of age have not been established.

DRUG INTERACTIONS

The *in vitro* binding of warfarin to human plasma proteins is unaffected by Tolmetin, and Tolmetin does not alter the prothrombin time of normal volunteers. However, increased prothrombin time and bleeding have been reported in patients on concomitant Tolmetin Sodium and warfarin therapy. Therefore, caution should be exercised when administering Tolmetin Sodium to patients on anticoagulants.

In adult diabetic patients under treatment with either sulfonylureas or insulin there is no change in the clinical effects of either Tolmetin Sodium or the hypoglycemic agents.

Caution should be used if Tolmetin Sodium is administered concomitantly with methotrexate. Tolmetin Sodium and other nonsteroidal anti-inflammatory drugs have been reported to reduce the tubular secretion of methotrexate in an animal model, possibly enhancing the toxicity of methotrexate.

LABORATORY TESTS

Because serious GI tract ulceration and bleeding can occur without warning symptoms, physicians should follow chronically treated patients for the signs and symptoms of ulceration and bleeding and should inform them of the importance of this follow-up (see *"Warnings—Risk of GI Ulceration, Bleeding and Perforation with NSAID Therapy"*).

DRUG/LABORATORY TEST INTERACTION

The metabolites of Tolmetin Sodium in urine have been found to give positive tests for proteinuria using tests which rely on acid precipitation as their endpoint (e.g., sulfosalicylic acid). No interference is seen in the tests for proteinuria using dye-impregnated commercially available reagent strips (e.g., Albustix®, Uristix®, etc.).

DRUG-FOOD INTERACTION

In a controlled single dose study, administration of Tolmetin Sodium with milk had no effect on peak plasma Tolmetin concentrations, but decreased total Tolmetin bioavailability by 16%. When Tolmetin Sodium was taken immediately after a meal, peak plasma Tolmetin concentrations were reduced by 50% while total bioavailability was again decreased by 16%.

INFORMATION FOR PATIENTS

Tolmetin Sodium, like other drugs of its class, is not free of side effects. The side effects of these drugs can cause discomfort and, rarely, there are more serious side effects, such as gastrointestinal bleeding, which may result in hospitalization and even fatal outcomes.

NSAID's (Nonsteroidal Anti-Inflammatory Drugs) are often essential agents in the management of arthritis, but they also may be commonly employed for conditions which are less serious.

Physicians may wish to discuss with their patients the potential risks (see "Warnings", "Precautions" and "Adverse Reactions" sections) and likely benefits of NSAID treatment, particularly when the drugs are used for less serious conditions where treatment without NSAID's may represent an acceptable alternative to both the patient and physician.

ADVERSE REACTIONS

The adverse reactions which have been observed in clinical trials encompass observations in about 4370 patients treated with Tolmetin Sodium, over 800 of whom have undergone at least one year of therapy. These adverse reactions, reported below by body system, are among those typical of nonsteroidal anti-inflammatory drugs and, as expected, gastrointestinal complaints were most frequent. In clinical trials with Tolmetin Sodium about 10% of patients dropped out because of adverse reactions, mostly gastrointestinal in nature.

INCIDENCE GREATER THAN 1%

The following adverse reactions which occurred more frequently than 1 in 100 were reported in controlled clinical trials.

Gastrointestinal: Nausea (11%),* dyspepsia,* gastrointestinal distress,* abdominal pain,* diarrhea,* flatulence,* vomiting,* constipation, gastritis, and peptic ulcer. Forty percent of the ulcer patients had a prior history of peptic ulcer disease and/or were receiving concomitant anti-inflammatory drugs including corticosteroids, which are known to produce peptic ulceration.

Body as a Whole: Headache,* asthenia,* chest pain

Cardiovascular: Elevated blood pressure,* edema*

Central Nervous System: Dizziness,* drowsiness, depression

Metabolic/Nutritional: Weight gain,* weight loss*

Dermatologic: Skin irritation

Special Senses: Tinnitus, visual disturbance

Hematologic: Small and transient decreases in hemoglobin and hematocrit not associated with gastrointestinal bleeding have occurred. These are similar to changes reported with other nonsteroidal anti-inflammatory drugs.

Urogenital: Elevated BUN, urinary tract infection

INCIDENCE LESS THAN 1%
(Causal Relationship Probable)

The following adverse reactions were reported less frequently than 1 in 100 in controlled clinical trials or were reported since marketing. The probability exists that there is a causal relationship between Tolmetin Sodium and these adverse reactions.

Gastrointestinal: Gastrointestinal bleeding with or without evidence of peptic ulcer, perforation, glossitis, stomatitis, hepatitis, liver function abnormalities

Body as a Whole: Anaphylactoid reactions, fever, lymphadenopathy, serum sickness

Hematologic: Hemolytic anemia, thrombocytopenia, granulocytopenia, agranulocytosis

Cardiovascular: Congestive heart failure in patients with marginal cardiac function

Dermatologic: Urticaria, purpura, erythema multiforme, toxic epidermal necrolysis

Urogenital: Hematuria, proteinuria, dysuria, renal failure

INCIDENCE LESS THAN 1%
(Causal Relationship Unknown)

Other adverse reactions were reported less frequently than 1 in 100 in controlled clinical trials or were reported since marketing, but a causal relationship between Tolmetin Sodium and the reaction could not be determined. These rarely reported reactions are being listed as alerting information for the physician since the possibility of a causal relationship cannot be excluded.

Body as Whole: Epistaxis

Special Senses: Optic neuropathy, retinal and macular changes.

MANAGEMENT OF OVERDOSAGE

In the event of overdosage, the stomach should be emptied by inducing vomiting or by gastric lavage followed by the administration of activated charcoal.

DOSAGE AND ADMINISTRATION

In adults with rheumatoid arthritis or osteoarthritis, the recommended starting dose is 400 mg three times daily (1200 mg daily), preferably including a dose on arising and a dose at bedtime. To achieve optimal therapeutic effect the dose

should be adjusted according to the patient's response after one to two weeks. Control is usually achieved at doses of 600-1800 mg daily in divided doses (generally t.i.d.). Doses larger than 1800 mg/kg have not been studied and are not recommended.

The recommended starting dose for children (2 years and older) is 20 mg/kg/day in divided doses (t.i.d. or q.i.d.). When control has been achieved, the usual dose ranges from 15 to 30 mg/kg/day. Doses higher than 30 mg/kg/day have not been studied and, therefore, are not recommended.

A therapeutic response to Tolmetin Sodium can be expected in a few days to a week. Progressive improvement can be anticipated during succeeding weeks of therapy. If gastrointestinal symptoms occur, Tolmetin Sodium can be administered with antacids other than sodium bicarbonate. Tolmetin Sodium bioavailability and pharmacokinetics are not significantly affected by acute or chronic administration of magnesium and aluminum hydroxides; however, bioavailability is affected by food or milk (see "Precautions—Drug-Food Interaction").

Store at controlled room temperature, (15°-30°C, 59°-86°F).

Protect from light.

HOW SUPPLIED
CAPSULE: 400 MG

AVERAGE UNIT PRICE (AVAILABLE SIZES)		GENERIC A-RATED AVERAGE PRICE (GAAP)	
BRAND	$0.97	30s	$24.78
GENERIC	$0.77	100s	$78.44
HCFA FUL (100s ea)	$0.40	500s	$369.38
		1000s	$648.60

BRAND/MANUFACTURER	NDC	SIZE	AWP
◆ BRAND			
➤ TOLECTIN DS: McNeil Pharm	00045-0414-60	100s	$96.88
	00045-0414-10	100s ud	$101.26
	00045-0414-70	500s	$468.12
◆ GENERICS			
Allscrips	54569-3730-00	30s	$22.86
Medirex	57480-0360-06	30s	$26.70
Norton,HN	50732-0900-01	100s	$68.95
Goldline	00182-1931-01	100s	$69.50
Mutual	53489-0507-01	100s	$72.87
Schein	00364-2507-01	100s	$74.00
Geneva	00781-2182-01	100s	$74.50
Rugby	00536-5509-01	100s	$75.50
Duramed	51285-0847-02	100s	$75.50
Purepac	00228-2520-10	100s	$77.61
Major	00904-7653-60	100s	$78.45
Parmed	00349-8963-01	100s	$79.90
URL	00677-1424-01	100s	$79.95
Aligen	00405-5035-01	100s	$80.00
Qualitest	00603-6130-21	100s	$80.00
Novopharm	55953-0815-40	100s	$80.00
Moore,H.L.	00839-7671-06	100s	$80.99
Mylan	00378-5200-01	100s	$81.25
Vangard	00615-0351-13	100s ud	$79.40
Novopharm	55953-0815-01	100s ud	$82.00
Medirex	57480-0360-01	100s ud	$89.00
Goldline	00182-1931-89	100s ud	$89.50
Goldline	00182-1931-05	500s	$337.50
Mutual	53489-0507-05	500s	$353.49
Duramed	51285-0847-04	500s	$358.65
Rugby	00536-5509-05	500s	$365.50
URL	00677-1424-05	500s	$373.50
Purepac	00228-2520-50	500s	$373.58
Aligen	00405-5035-02	500s	$380.00
Novopharm	55953-0815-70	500s	$380.00
Major	00904-7653-40	500s	$383.45
Moore,H.L.	00839-7671-12	500s	$388.13
Major	00904-7653-80	1000s	$575.20
Novopharm	55953-0815-80	1000s	$722.00

TABLETS: 200 MG

AVERAGE UNIT PRICE (AVAILABLE SIZES)		GENERIC A-RATED AVERAGE PRICE (GAAP)	
BRAND	$0.61	100s	$49.58
GENERIC	$0.50		

BRAND/MANUFACTURER	NDC	SIZE	AWP
◆ BRAND			
➤ TOLECTIN: McNeil Pharm	00045-0412-60	100s	$61.07
◆ GENERICS			
Mutual	53489-0506-01	100s	$46.09
Duramed	51285-0846-02	100s	$49.75
URL	00677-1425-01	100s	$51.00
Moore,H.L.	00839-7729-06	100s	$51.49

TABLETS: 600 MG

AVERAGE UNIT PRICE (AVAILABLE SIZES)		GENERIC A-RATED AVERAGE PRICE (GAAP)	
BRAND	$1.16	100s	$95.94
GENERIC	$0.95	500s	$453.76

BRAND/MANUFACTURER	NDC	SIZE	AWP
◆ BRAND			
➤ TOLECTIN 600: McNeil Pharm	00045-0416-60	100s	$117.56
	00045-0416-70	500s	$568.13

* Reactions occurring in 3% to 9% of patients treated with Tolmetin Sodium. Reactions occurring in fewer than 3% of the patients are unmarked.

➤ SHOWN IN PRODUCT IDENTIFICATION GUIDE

BRAND/MANUFACTURER	NDC	SIZE	AWP
◆ **GENERICS**			
Aligen	00405-5034-01	100s	$85.92
Mason Dist	11845-0486-01	100s	$88.53
Schein	00364-2523-01	100s	$89.75
URL	00677-1447-01	100s	$89.89
Purepac	00228-2480-10	100s	$94.30
Geneva	00781-1428-01	100s	$94.90
Goldline	00182-1932-01	100s	$95.00
Novopharm	55953-0817-40	100s	$95.00
Moore,H.L.	00839-7690-06	100s	$95.03
Qualitest	00603-6131-21	100s	$95.06
Rugby	00536-4681-01	100s	$95.19
Major	00904-7694-60	100s	$95.25
Duramed	51285-0848-02	100s	$96.50
Parmed	00349-8964-01	100s	$99.00
Mylan	00378-0313-01	100s	$105.75
Goldline	00182-1932-89	100s ud	$120.00
Aligen	00405-5034-02	500s	$412.41
Moore,H.L.	00839-7690-12	500s	$451.37
Purepac	00228-2480-50	500s	$497.51

Tonocard SEE TOCAINIDE HYDROCHLORIDE

Topicort SEE DESOXIMETASONE

Topicycline SEE TETRACYCLINE HYDROCHLORIDE, TOPICAL

Toprol XL SEE METOPROLOL

Toradol SEE KETOROLAC TROMETHAMINE, SYSTEMIC

Torecan SEE TRIETHYLPERAZINE MALEATE

Tornalate SEE BITOLTEROL MESYLATE

Torsemide

DESCRIPTION
Torsemide is a diuretic of the pyridine-sulfonyl-urea class. Its chemical name is 1-isopropyl-3-[(4-*m*-toluidino-3-pyridyl)sulfonyl]urea.

Its empirical formula is $C_{16}H_{20}N_4O_3S$, its pKa is 7.1, and its molecular weight is 348.43.

Torsemide is a white to off-white crystalline powder. The tablets for oral administration also contain lactose NF, crospovidone NF, povidone USP, microcrystalline cellulose NF, and magnesium stearate NF. Torsemide ampuls for intravenous injection contain a sterile solution of Torsemide (10 mg/mL), polyethylene glycol-400 NF, tromethamine USP, and sodium hydroxide NF (as needed to adjust pH) in water for injection USP.

Following is its chemical structure:

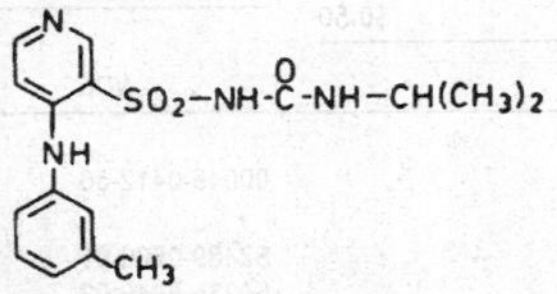

CLINICAL PHARMACOLOGY
Mechanism of Action: Micropuncture studies in animals have shown that Torsemide acts from within the lumen of the thick ascending portion of the loop of Henle, where it inhibits the Na+/K+/2Cl−-carrier system. Clinical pharmacology studies have confirmed this site of action in humans, and effects in other segments of the nephron have not been demonstrated. Diuretic activity thus correlates better with the rate of drug excretion in the urine than with the concentration in the blood.

Torsemide increases the urinary excretion of sodium, chloride, and water, but it does not significantly alter glomerular filtration rate, renal plasma flow, or acid-base balance.

Pharmacokinetics and Metabolism: The *bioavailability* of Torsemide Tablets is approximately 80%, with little intersubject variation; the 90% confidence interval is 75% to 89%. The drug is absorbed with little first-pass metabolism, and the serum concentration reaches its peak (C_{max}) within one hour after oral administration. C_{max} and area under the serum concentration-time curve (AUC) after oral administration are proportional to dose over the range of 2.5 to 200 mg. Simultaneous food intake delays the time to C_{max} by about 30 minutes, but overall bioavailability (AUC) and diuretic activity are unchanged. Absorption is essentially unaffected by renal or hepatic dysfunction.

The *volume of distribution* of Torsemide is 12 to 15 liters in normal adults or in patients with mild to moderate renal failure or congestive heart failure. In patients with hepatic cirrhosis, the volume of distribution is approximately doubled.

In normal subjects the *elimination half-life* of Torsemide is approximately 3.5 hours. Torsemide is cleared from the circulation by both hepatic metabolism (approximately 80% of total clearance) and excretion into the urine (approximately 20% of total clearance in patients with normal renal function). The major metabolite in humans is the carboxylic acid derivative, which is biologically inactive. Two of the lesser metabolites possess some diuretic activity, but for practical purposes metabolism terminates the action of the drug.

Because Torsemide is extensively bound to plasma protein (> 99%), very little enters tubular urine via glomerular filtration. Most renal clearance of Torsemide occurs via active secretion of the drug by the proximal tubules into tubular urine.

In patients with decompensated congestive heart failure, hepatic and renal clearance are both reduced, probably because of hepatic congestion and decreased renal plasma flow, respectively. The total clearance of Torsemide is approximately 50% of that seen in healthy volunteers, and the plasma half-life and AUC are correspondingly increased. Because of reduced renal clearance, a smaller fraction of any given dose is delivered to the intraluminal site of action, so at any given dose there is less natriuresis in patients with congestive heart failure than in normal subjects.

In patients with renal failure, renal clearance of Torsemide is markedly decreased but total plasma clearance is not significantly altered. A smaller fraction of the administered dose is delivered to the intraluminal site of action, and the natriuretic action of any given dose of diuretic is reduced. A diuretic response in renal failure may still be achieved if patients are given higher doses. The total plasma clearance and elimination half-life of Torsemide remain normal under the conditions of impaired renal function because metabolic elimination by the liver remains intact.

In patients with hepatic cirrhosis, the volume of distribution, plasma half-life, and renal clearance are all increased, but total clearance is unchanged.

The pharmacokinetic profile of Torsemide in healthy elderly subjects is similar to that in young subjects except for a decrease in renal clearance related to the decline in renal function that commonly occurs with aging. However, total plasma clearance and elimination half-life remain unchanged.

Clinical Effects: The diuretic effects of Torsemide begin within 10 minutes of intravenous dosing and peak within the first hour. With oral dosing, the onset of diuresis occurs within one hour and the peak effect occurs during the first or second hour. Independent of the route of administration, diuresis lasts about six to eight hours. In healthy subjects given single doses, the dose-response relationship for sodium excretion is linear over the dose range of 2.5 to 20 mg. The increase in potassium excretion is negligible after a single dose of up to 10 mg and only slight (5 to 15 mEq) after a single dose of 20 mg.

Torsemide has been studied in controlled trials in patients with New York Heart Association Class II to Class IV *congestive heart failure.* Patients who received 10 to 20 mg of daily Torsemide in these studies achieved significantly greater reductions in weight and edema than did patients who received placebo.

In single-dose studies in patients with *nonanuric renal failure,* high doses of Torsemide (20 to 200 mg) caused marked increases in water and sodium excretion. In patients with nonanuric renal failure severe enough to require hemodialysis, chronic treatment with up to 200 mg of daily Torsemide has not been shown to change steady-state fluid retention. Chronic use of any diuretic in renal disease has not been studied in adequate and well-controlled trials. When patients in a study of acute renal failure received total daily doses of 520 to 1200 mg of Torsemide, 26% experienced seizures; seizures were also seen in similar patients who received comparably high doses of furosemide, but not in similar patients who received placebo.

When given with aldosterone antagonists. Torsemide also caused increases in sodium and fluid excretion in patients with edema or ascites due to *hepatic cirrhosis.* Urinary sodium excretion rate relative to the urinary excretion rate of Torsemide is less in cirrhotic patients than in healthy subjects (possibly because of the hyperaldosteronism and resultant sodium retention that are characteristic of portal hypertension and ascites). However, because of the increased renal clearance of Torsemide in patients with hepatic cirrhosis, these factors tend to balance each other, and the result is an overall natriuretic response that is similar to that seen in healthy subjects. Chronic use of any diuretic in hepatic disease has not been studied in adequate and well-controlled trials.

In patients with *essential hypertension,* Torsemide has been shown in controlled studies to lower blood pressure when administered once a day at doses of 5 to 10 mg. The antihypertensive effect is near maximal after four to six weeks of treatment, but it may continue to increase for up to 12 weeks. Systolic and diastolic supine and standing blood pressures are all reduced. There is no significant orthostatic effect, and there is only a minimal peak-trough difference in blood-pressure reduction.

The antihypertensive effects of Torsemide are, like those of other diuretics, on the average greater in black patients (a low-renin population) than in nonblack patients. When Torsemide is first administered, daily urinary sodium excretion increases for at least a week. With chronic administration, however, daily sodium loss comes into balance with dietary sodium intake. If the administration of Torsemide is suddenly stopped, blood pressure returns to pretreatment levels over several days, without overshoot.

Torsemide has been administered together with β-adrenergic blocking agents, ACE inhibitors, and calcium-channel blockers. Adverse drug interactions have not been observed, and special dosage adjustment has not been necessary.

INDICATIONS AND USE

Torsemide is indicated for the treatment of edema associated with congestive heart failure, renal disease, or hepatic disease. Chronic use of any diuretic in renal or hepatic disease has not been studied in adequate and well-controlled trials.

Torsemide Intravenous Injection is indicated when a rapid onset of diuresis is desired or when oral administration is impractical.

Torsemide is indicated for the treatment of hypertension alone or in combination with other antihypertensive agents.

CONTRAINDICATIONS

Torsemide is contraindicated in patients with known hypersensitivity to Torsemide or to sulfonylureas.

Torsemide is contraindicated in patients who are anuric.

WARNINGS

Hepatic Disease with Cirrhosis and Ascites: Torsemide should be used with caution in patients with hepatic disease with cirrhosis and ascites, since sudden alterations of fluid and electrolyte balance may precipiatate hepatic coma. In these patients, diuresis with Torsemide (or any other diuretic) is best initiated in the hospital. To prevent hypokalemia and metabolic alkalosis, an aldosterone antagonist or potassium-sparing drug should be used concomitantly with Torsemide.

Ototoxicity: Tinnitus and hearing loss (usually reversible) have been observed after rapid intravenous injection of other loop diuretics and have also been observed after oral Torsemide. It is not certain that these events were attributable to Torsemide. Ototoxicity has also been seen in animal studies when very high plasma levels of Torsemide were induced. Administered intravenously, Torsemide should be injected slowly over two minutes, and single doses should not exceed 200 mg.

Volume and Electrolyte Depletion: Patients receiving diuretics should be observed for clinical evidence of electrolyte imbalance, hypovolemia, or prerenal azotemia. Symptoms of these disturbances may include one or more of the following: dryness of the mouth, thirst, weakness, lethargy, drowsiness, restlessness, muscle pains or cramps, muscular fatigue, hypotension, oliguria, tachycardia, nausea, and vomiting. Excessive diuresis may cause dehydration, blood-volume reduction, and possibly thrombosis and embolism, especially in elderly patients. In patients who develop fluid and electrolyte imbalances, hypovolemia, or prerenal azotemia, the observed laboratory changes may include hyper- or hyponatremia, hyper- or hypochloremia, hyper- or hypokalemia, acid-base abnormalities, and increased blood urea nitrogen. If any of these occur Torsemide should be discontinued until the situation is corrected, Torsemide may be restarted at a lower dose.

In controlled studies in the United States, Torsemide was administered to hypertensive patients at doses of 5 mg or 10 mg daily. After six weeks at these doses, the mean decrease in serum potassium was approximately 0.1 mEq/L. The percentage of patients who had a serum potassium level below 3.5 mEq/L at any time during the studies was essentially the same in patients who received Torsemide (1.5%) as in those who received placebo (3%). In patients followed for one year, there was no further change in mean serum potassium levels. In patients with congestive heart failure, hepatic cirrhosis, or renal disease treated with Torsemide at doses higher than those studied in U.S. antihypertensive trials, hypokalemia was observed with greater frequency, in a dose-related manner.

In patients with cardiovascular disease, especially those receiving digitalis glycosides, diuretic-induced hypokalemia may be a risk factor for the development of arrhythmias. The risk of hypokalemia is greatest in patients with cirrhosis of the liver, in patients experiencing a brisk diuresis, in patients who are receiving inadequate oral intake of electrolytes, and in patients receiving concomitant therapy with corticosteroids or ACTH.

Periodic monitoring of serum potassium and other electrolytes is advised in patients treated with Torsemide.

PRECAUTIONS

LABORATORY VALUES

Potassium: See statement in *"Warnings"*.

Calcium: Single doses of Torsemide increased the urinary excretion of calcium by normal subjects, but serum calcium levels were slightly increased in four-to six-week hypertension trials. In a long-term study of patients with congestive heart failure, the average one-year change in serum calcium was a decrease of 0.10 mg/dL (0.02 mmol/L). Among 426 patients treated with Torsemide for an average of 11 months, hypocalcemia was not reported as an adverse event.

Magnesium: Single doses of Torsemide caused healthy volunteers to increase their urinary excretion of magnesium, but serum magnesium levels were slightly increased in four- to six-week hypertension trials. In long-term hypertension studies, the average one year change in serum magnesium was an increase of 0.03 mg/dL (0.01 mmol/L). Among 426 patients treated with Torsemide for an average of 11 months, one case of hypomagnesemia [1.3 mg/dL (0.53 mmol/L)] was reported as an adverse event.

In a long-term clinical study of Torsemide in patients with congestive heart failure, the estimated annual change in serum magnesium was an increase of 0.2 mg/dL (0.08 mmol/L), but these data are confounded by the fact that many of these patients received magnesium supplements. In a four-week study in which magnesium supplementation was not given, the rate of occurrence of serum magnesium levels below 1.7 mg/dL (0.70 mmol/L) was 6% and 9% in the groups receiving 5 mg and 10 mg of Torsemide respectively.

Blood Urea Nitrogen (BUN), Creatinine, and Uric Acid: Torsemide produces small dose-related increases in each of these laboratory values. In hypertensive patients who received 10 mg of Torsemide daily for six weeks, the mean increase in blood urea nitrogen was 1.8 mg/dL (0.6 mmol/L), the mean increase in serum creatinine was 0.05 mg/dL (4 μmol/L), and the mean increase in serum uric acid was 1.2 mg/dL (70 μmol/L). Little further change occurred with long-term treatment, and all changes reversed when treatment was discontinued.

Symptomatic gout has been reported in patients receiving Torsemide, but its incidence has been similar to that seen in patients receiving placebo.

Glucose: Hypertensive patients who received 10 mg of daily Torsemide experienced a mean increase in serum glucose concentration of 5.5 mg/dL (0.3 mmol/L) after six weeks of therapy, with a further increase of 1.8 mg/dL (0.1 mmol/L) during the subsequent year. In long-term studies in diabetics, mean fasting glucose values were not significantly changed from baseline. Cases of hyperglycemia have been reported but are uncommon.

Serum Lipids: In the controlled short-term hypertension studies in the United States, daily doses of 5, 10, and 20 mg of Torsemide were associated with increases in total plasma cholesterol of 4, 4, and 8 mg/dL (0.10 to 0.20 mmol/L), respectively. The changes subsided during chronic therapy.

In the same short-term hypertension studies, daily doses of 5, 10, and 20 mg of Torsemide were associated with mean increases in plasma triglycerides of 16, 13, and 71 mg/dL (0.15 to 0.80 mmol/L), respectively.

In long-term studies of 5 to 20 mg Torsemide daily, no clinically significant differences from baseline lipid values were observed after one year of therapy.

Other: In long-term studies in hypertensive patients, Torsemide has been associated with small mean decreases in hemoglobin, hematocrit, and erythrocyte count and small mean increases in white blood cell count, platelet count, and serum alkaline phosphatase. Although statistically significant, all of these changes were medically inconsequential. No significant trends have been observed in any liver enzyme tests other than alkaline phosphatase.

DRUG INTERACTIONS

In patients with essential hypertension, Torsemide has been administered together with β-blockers, ACE inhibitors, and calcium-channel blockers. In patients with congestive heart failure, Torsemide has been administered together with digitalis glycosides, ACE inhibitors, and organic nitrates. None of these combined uses was associated with new or unexpected adverse events.

Torsemide does not affect the protein binding of *glyburide* or of *warfarin*, the anticoagulant effect of *phenprocoumon* (a related coumarin derivative), or the pharmacokinetics of *digoxin* or *carvedilol* (a vasodilator/β-blocker). In healthy subjects, coadministration of Torsemide was associated with significant reduction in the renal clearance of *spironolactone*, with corresponding increases in the AUC. However, clinical experience indicates that dosage adjustment of either agent is not required.

Because Torsemide and salicylates compete for secretion by renal tubules, patients receiving high doses of *salicylates* may experience salicylate toxicity when Torsemide is concomitantly administered. Also, although possible interactions between Torsemide and *nonsteroidal anti-inflammatory agents (including aspirin)* have not been studied, coadministration of these agents with another loop diuretic (furosemide) has occasionally been associated with renal dysfunction.

The natriuretic effect of Torsemide (like that of many other diuretics) is partially inhibited by the concomitant administration of *indomethacin*. This effect has been demonstrated for Torsemide under conditions of dietary sodium restriction (50 mEq/day) but not in the presence of normal sodium intake (150 mEq/day).

The pharmacokinetic profile and diuretic activity of Torsemide are not altered by *cimetidine* or *spironolactone*. Coadministration of *digoxin* is reported to increase the area under the curve for Torsemide by 50%, but dose adjustment of Torsemide is not necessary. Concomitant use of Torsemide and cholestyramine has not been studied in humans but, in a study in animals, coadministration of cholestyramine decreased the absorption of orally administered Torsemide. If Torsemide and cholestyramine are used concomitantly, simultaneous administration is not recommended.

Coadministration of *probenecid* reduces secretion of Torsemide into the proximal tubule and thereby decreases the diuretic activity of Torsemide.

Other diuretics are known to reduce the renal clearance of *lithium*, inducing a high risk of lithium toxicity, so coadministration of lithium and diuretics should be undertaken with great caution, if at all. Coadministration of lithium and Torsemide has not been studied.

Other diuretics have been reported to increase the ototoxic potential of *aminoglycoside antibiotics* and of *ethacrynic acid*, especially in the presence of impaired renal function. These potential interactions with Torsemide have not been studied.

CARCINOGENESIS, MUTAGENESIS, IMPAIRMENT OF FERTILITY

No overall increase in tumor incidence was found when Torsemide was given to rats and mice throughout their lives at doses up to 9 mg/kg/day (rats) and 32 mg/kg/day (mice). On a body-weight basis, these doses are 27 to 96 times a human

➤ SHOWN IN PRODUCT IDENTIFICATION GUIDE

dose of 20 mg; on a body-surface-area basis, they are 5 to 8 times this dose. In the rat study, the high-dose female group demonstrated renal tubular injury, interstitial inflammation, and a statistically significant increase in renal adenomas and carcinomas. The tumor incidence in this group was, however, not much higher than the incidence sometimes seen in historical controls. Similar signs of chronic non-neoplastic renal injury have been reported in high-dose animal studies of other diuretics such as furosemide and hydrochlorothiazide.

No mutagenic activity was detected in any of a variety of in vivo and in vitro tests of Torsemide and its major human metabolite. The tests included the Ames test in bacteria (with and without metabolic activation), tests for chromosome aberrations and sister-chromatid exchanges in human lymphocytes, tests for various nuclear anomalies in cells found in hamster and murine bone marrow, tests for unscheduled DNA synthesis in mice and rats, and others. In doses up to 25 mg/kg/day (75 times a human dose of 20 mg on a body-weight basis; 13 times this dose on a body-surface-area basis) Torsemide had no adverse effect on the reproductive performance of male or female rats.

PREGNANCY
Pregnancy Category B. There was no fetotoxicity or teratogenicity in rats treated with up to 5 mg/kg/day of Torsemide (on a mg/kg basis, this is 15 times a human dose of 20 mg/day; on a mg/m^2 basis, the animal dose is 10 times the human dose), or in rabbits treated with 1.6 mg/kg/day (on a mg/kg basis, 5 times the human dose of 20 mg/day; on a mg/m^2 basis, 1.7 times this dose). Fetal and maternal toxicity (decrease in average body weight, increase in fetal resorption, and delayed fetal ossification) occurred in rabbits and rats given doses 4 (rabbits) and 5 (rats) times larger. Adequate and well-controlled studies have not been carried out in pregnant women. Because animal reproduction studies are not always predictive of human response, this drug should be used during pregnancy only if clearly needed.

LABOR AND DELIVERY
The effect of Torsemide on labor and delivery is unknown.

NURSING MOTHERS
It is not known whether Torsemide is excreted in human milk. Because many drugs are excreted in human milk, caution should be exercised when Torsemide is administered to a nursing woman.

GERIATRIC USE
Of the total number of patients who received Torsemide in U.S. clinical studies, 24% were 65 or older while about 4% were 75 or older. No specific age-related differences in effectiveness or safety were observed between younger patients and elderly patients.

PEDIATRIC USE
Safety and effectiveness in children have not been established.

Administration of another loop diuretic to severely premature infants with edema due to patent ductus arteriosus and hyaline membrane disease has occasionally been associated with renal calcifications, sometimes barely visible on x-ray but sometimes in staghorn form, filling the renal pelves. Some of these calculi have been dissolved, and hypercalciuria has been reported to have decreased, when chlorothiazide has been coadministered along with the loop diuretic. In other premature neonates with hyaline membrane disease, another loop diuretic has been reported to increase the risk of persistent patent ductus arteriosus, possibly through a prostaglandin-E-mediated process. The use of Torsemide in such patients has not been studied.

ADVERSE REACTIONS
At the time of approval, Torsemide had been evaluated for safety in approximately 4000 subjects: over 800 of these subjects received Torsemide for at least six months, and over 380 were treated for more than one year. Among these subjects were 564 who received Torsemide during U.S.-based trials in which 274 other subjects received placebo.

The reported side effects of Torsemide were generally transient, and there was no relationship between side effects and age, sex, race, or duration of therapy. Discontinuation of therapy due to side effects occurred in 3.5% of U.S. patients treated with Torsemide and in 4.4% of patients treated with placebo. In studies conducted in the United States and Europe, discontinuation rates due to side effects were 3.0% (38/1250) with Torsemide and 3.4% (13/380) with furosemide in patients with congestive heart failure, 2.0% (8/409) with Torsemide and 4.8% (11/230) with furosemide in patients with renal insufficiency, and 7.6% (13/170) with Torsemide and 0% (0/33) with furosemide in patients with cirrhosis.

The most common reasons for discontinuation of therapy with Torsemide were (in descending order of frequency) dizziness, headache, nausea, weakness, vomiting, hyperglycemia, excessive urination, hyperuricemia, hypokalemia, excessive thirst, hypovolemia, impotence, esophageal hemorrhage, and dyspepsia. Dropout rates for these adverse events ranged from 0.1% to 0.5%.

The side effects considered possibly or probably related to study drug that occurred in U.S. placebo-controlled trials in more than 1% of patients treated with Torsemide are shown in the table below.

REACTIONS POSSIBLY OR PROBABLY DRUG-RELATED
U.S. PLACEBO-CONTROLLED STUDIES
INCIDENCE (PERCENTAGES OF PATIENTS)

	Torsemide (N = 564)	placebo (N = 274)
Headache	7.3	9.1
Excessive urination	6.7	2.2
Dizziness	3.2	4.0
Rhinitis	2.8	2.2
Asthenia	2.0	1.5
Diarrhea	2.0	1.1
ECG abnormality	2.0	0.4
Cough increase	2.0	1.5
Constipation	1.8	0.7
Nausea	1.8	0.4
Arthralgia	1.8	0.7
Dyspepsia	1.6	0.7
Sore throat	1.6	0.7
Myalgia	1.6	1.5
Chest pain	1.2	0.4
Insomnia	1.2	1.8
Edema	1.1	1.1
Nervousness	1.1	0.4

The daily doses of Torsemide used in these trials ranged from 1.25 to 20 mg, with most patients receiving 5 to 10 mg; the duration of treatment ranged from one to 52 days, with a median of 41 days. Of the side effects listed in the table, only "excessive urination" occurred significantly more frequently in patients treated with Torsemide than in patients treated with placebo. In the placebo-controlled hypertension studies whose design allowed side-effect rates to be attributed to dose, excessive urination was reported by 1% of patients receiving placebo, 4% of those treated with 5 mg of daily Torsemide, and 15% of those treated with 10 mg. The complaint of excessive urination was generally not reported as an adverse event among patients who received Torsemide for cardiac, renal, or hepatic failure.

Serious adverse events reported in the clinical studies for which a drug relationship could not be excluded were atrial fibrillation, chest pain, diarrhea, digitalis intoxication, gastrointestinal hemorrhage, hyperglycemia, hyperuricemia, hypokalemia, hypotension, hypovolemia, shunt thrombosis, rash, rectal bleeding, syncope, and ventricular tachycardia. Angioedema has been reported in a patient exposed to Torsemide who was later found to be allergic to sulfa drugs.

Of the adverse reactions during placebo-controlled trials listed without taking into account assessment of relatedness to drug therapy, arthritis and various other nonspecific musculoskeletal problems were more frequently reported in association with Torsemide than with placebo, even though gout was somewhat more frequently associated with placebo. These reactions did not increase in frequency or severity with the dose of Torsemide. One patient in the group treated with Torsemide withdrew due to myalgia, and one in the placebo group withdrew due to gout.

Hypokalemia: See statement in *"Warnings"*.

OVERDOSE
There is no human experience with overdoses of Torsemide, but the signs and symptoms of overdosage can be anticipated to be those of excessive pharmacologic effect: dehydration, hypovolemia, hypotension, hyponatremia, hypokalemia, hypochloremic alkalosis, and hemoconcentration. Treatment of overdosage should consist of fluid and electrolyte replacement.

Laboratory determinations of serum levels of Torsemide and its metabolites are not widely available.

No data are available to suggest physiological maneuvers (e.g., maneuvers to change the pH of the urine) that might accelerate elimination of Torsemide and its metabolites. Torsemide is not dialyzable, so hemodialysis will not accelerate elimination.

DOSAGE AND ADMINISTRATION
General: Torsemide Tablets may be given at any time in relation to a meal, as convenient. Special dosage adjustment in the elderly is not necessary.

Because of the high bioavailability of Torsemide, oral and intravenous doses are therapeutically equivalent, so patients may be switched to and from the intravenous form with no change in dose. Torsemide Intravenous Injection should be administered slowly over a period of two minutes.

Before administration, the solution of Torsemide should be visually inspected for discoloration and particulate matter. If either is found, the ampul should not be used.

Congestive Heart Failure: The usual initial dose is 10 mg or 20 mg of once-daily oral or intravenous Torsemide. If the diuretic response is inadequate, the dose should be titrated upward by approximately doubling until the desired diuretic response is obtained. Single doses higher than 200 mg have not been adequately studied.

Chronic Renal Failure: The usual initial dose of Torsemide is 20 mg of once-daily oral or intravenous Torsemide. If the diuretic response is inadequate, the dose should be titrated upward by approximately doubling until the desired diuretic response is obtained. Single doses higher than 200 mg have not been adequately studied.

Chronic use of any diuretic in renal disease has not been studied in adequate and well-controlled trials.

Hepatic Cirrhosis: The usual initial dose is 5 mg or 10 mg of once-daily oral or intravenous Torsemide, administered together with an aldosterone antagonist or a potassium-sparing diuretic. If the diuretic reponse is inadequate, the dose should be titrated upward by approximately doubling until the desired diuretic response is obtained. Single doses higher than 40 mg have not been adequately studied.

Chronic use of any diuretic in hepatic disease has not been studied in adequate and well-controlled trials.

Hypertension: The usual initial dose is 5 mg once daily. If the 5 mg dose does not provide adequate reduction in blood pressure within four to six weeks, the dose may be increased to 10 mg once daily. If the response to 10 mg is insufficient, an additional antihypertensive agent should be added to the treatment regimen.

Storage: Store all dosage forms at controlled room temperature, 15-30°C (59-86°F). Do not freeze.

HOW SUPPLIED
INJECTION: 10 MG/ML

BRAND/MANUFACTURER	NDC	SIZE	AWP
○ **BRAND**			
DEMADEX I.V.: Boehr Mann Pharm	53169-0108-80	2 ml 10s	$35.75
	53169-0108-81	5 ml 10s	$50.50

TABLETS: 5 MG

BRAND/MANUFACTURER	NDC	SIZE	AWP
○ **BRAND**			
► DEMADEX: Boehr Mann Pharm	53169-0102-01	100s	$43.75
	53169-0102-60	100s ud	$45.00

TABLETS: 10 MG

BRAND/MANUFACTURER	NDC	SIZE	AWP
○ **BRAND**			
► DEMADEX: Boehr Mann Pharm	53169-0103-01	100s	$47.50
	53169-0103-60	100s ud	$48.75

TABLETS: 20 MG

BRAND/MANUFACTURER	NDC	SIZE	AWP
○ **BRAND**			
► DEMADEX: Boehr Mann Pharm	53169-0104-01	100s	$51.25
	53169-0104-60	100s ud	$52.50

TABLETS: 100 MG

BRAND/MANUFACTURER	NDC	SIZE	AWP
○ **BRAND**			
► DEMADEX: Boehr Mann Pharm	53169-0105-01	100s	$216.25
	53169-0105-60	100s ud	$222.50

Touro SEE GUAIFENESIN AND GUAIFENESIN AND PSEUDOEPHEDRINE HYDROCHLORIDE

TPN Electrolytes SEE DEXTROSE AND ELECTROLYTES AND ELECTROLYTES, INJECTABLE

Trac Tabs 2x SEE ATROPINE SULFATE/BENZOIC ACID/ HYOSCYAMINE/METHENAMINE/METHYLENE BLUE/ PHENYLSALICYLATE

Tracelyte SEE DEXTROSE AND ELECTROLYTES AND ELECTROLYTES, INJECTABLE

Tracrium SEE ATRACURIUM BESYLATE

Trancopal SEE CHLORMEZANONE

Trandate SEE LABETALOL HYDROCHLORIDE

Tranexamic Acid

DESCRIPTION
Each tablet contains 500 mg of Tranexamic Acid.

Each ml of the sterile solution for intravenous injection contains 100 mg Tranexamic Acid and Water for Injection to 1 mL.

FORMULATION
Chemical Name: trans-4-(aminomethyl)cyclohexanecarboxylic acid.

Its empirical formula is $C_8H_{15}NO_2$ and molecular weight is 157.2.

Tranexamic Acid is a white crystalline powder. The aqueous solution for injection has a pH of 6.5-7.5.

Following is its chemical structure:

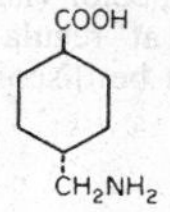

CLINICAL PHARMACOLOGY
Tranexamic Acid is a competitive inhibitor of plasminogen activation, and at much higher concentrations, a noncompetitive inhibitor of plasmin, i.e., actions similar to aminocaproic acid. Tranexamic Acid is about 10 times more potent *in vitro* than aminocaproic acid.

Tranexamic Acid binds more strongly than aminocaproic acid to both the strong and weak receptor sites of the plasminogen molecule in a ratio corresponding to the difference in potency between the compounds.

Tranexamic Acid in a concentration of 1 mg per mL does not aggregate platelets *in vitro*. Tranexamic Acid in concentrations up to 10 mg per mL blood has no influence on the platelet count, the coagulation time or various coagulation factors in whole blood or citrated blood from normal subjects. On the other hand, Tranexamic Acid in concentrations of 10 mg and 1 mg per mL blood prolongs the thrombin time.

The plasma protein binding of Tranexamic Acid is about 3 per cent at therapeutic plasma levels and seems to be fully accounted for by its binding to plasminogen. Tranexamic Acid does not bind to serum albumin.

Absorption of Tranexamic Acid after oral administration in humans represents approximately 30-50% of the ingested dose and bioavailability is not affected by food intake.

After an intravenous dose of 1 g, the plasma concentration time curve shows a triexponential decay with a half-life of about 2 hours for the terminal elimination phase. The initial volume of distribution is about 9-12 liters. Urinary excretion is the main route of elimination via glomerular filtration. Overall renal clearance is equal to overall plasma clearance (110-116 mL/min) and more than 95% of the dose is excreted in the urine as the unchanged drug. Excretion of Tranexamic Acid is about 90% at 24 hours after intravenous administration of 10 mg per kg body weight. After oral administration of 10-15 mg per kg body weight, the cumulative urinary excretion at 24 hours is 39% and at 48 hours, 41% of the ingested dose or 78% and 82% of the absorbed material. Only a small fraction of the drug is metabolized. After oral administration, 1% of the dicarboxylic acid and 0.5% of the acetylated compound are excreted.

The plasma peak level after 1 g orally is 8 mg per L and after 2 g, 15 mg per L, both obtained three hours after dosing. An antifibrinolytic concentration of Tranexamic Acid remains in different tissues for about 17 hours, and in the serum, up to seven or eight hours.

Tranexamic Acid passes through the placenta. The concentration in cord blood after an intravenous injection of 10 mg per kg to pregnant women is about 30 mg per L, as high as in the maternal blood. Tranexamic Acid diffuses rapidly into joint fluid and the synovial membrane. In the joint fluid the same concentration is obtained in the serum. The biological half-life of Tranexamic Acid in the joint fluid is about three hours.

The concentration of Tranexamic Acid in a number of other tissues is lower than in blood. In breast milk the concentration is about one hundredth of the serum peak concentration. Tranexamic Acid concentration in cerebrospinal fluid is about one tenth of that of the plasma. The drug passes into the aqueous humor, the concentration being about one tenth of the plasma concentration.

Tranexamic Acid has been detected in semen where it inhibits fibrinolytic activity but does not influence sperm migration.

INDICATIONS AND USAGE
Tranexamic Acid is indicated in patients with hemophilia for short term use (two to eight days) to reduce or prevent hemorrhage and reduce the need for replacement therapy during and following tooth extraction.

CONTRAINDICATIONS
Tranexamic Acid is contraindicated:
1. In patients with acquired defective color vision, since this prohibits measuring one endpoint that should be followed as a measure of toxicity (see *"Warnings"*).
2. In patients with subarachnoid hemorrhage. Anecdotal experience indicates that cerebral edema and cerebral infarction may be caused by Tranexamic Acid in such patients.

WARNINGS
Focal areas in retinal degeneration have developed in cats, dogs and rats following oral or intravenous Tranexamic Acid at doses between 250 to 1600 mg/kg/day (6 to 40 times the recommended usual human dose) from 6 days to 1 year. The incidence of such lesions has varied from 25% to 100% of animals treated and was dose-related. At lower doses some lesions have appeared to be reversible.

Limited data in cats and rabbits showed retinal changes in some animals with doses as low as 126 mg/kg/day (only about 3 times the recommended human dose) administered for several days to two weeks.

No retinal changes have been reported or noted in eye examinations in patients treated with Tranexamic Acid for weeks to months in clinical trials.

However, visual abnormalities, often poorly characterized, represent the most frequently reported postmarketing adverse reaction in Sweden. For patients who are to be treated continually for longer than several days, an ophthalmological examination, including visual acuity, color vision, eye-ground and visual fields, is advised, before commencing and at regular intervals during the course of treatment. Tranexamic Acid should be discontinued if changes in examination results are found.

PRECAUTIONS

General: The dose of Tranexamic Acid should be reduced in patients with renal insufficiency because of the risk of accumulation. See *"Dosage and Administration"*.

Carcinogenesis, mutagenesis, impairment of fertility: An increased incidence of leukemia in male mice receiving Tranexamic Acid in food at the concentration of 4.8% (equivalent to doses as high as 5 g/kg/day) may have been related to treatment. Female mice were not included in this experiment.

Hyperplasia of the biliary tract and cholangioma and adenocarcinoma of the intrahepatic biliary system have been reported in one strain of rats after dietary administration of doses exceeding the maximum tolerated dose for 22 months. Hyperplastic, but not neoplastic, lesions were reported at lower doses. Subsequent long term dietary administration studies in a different strain of rat, each with an exposure level equal to the maximum level employed in the earlier experiment, have failed to show such hyperplastic/neoplastic changes in the liver. No mutagenic activity has been demonstrated in several *in vitro* and *in vivo* test systems.

Pregnancy (Category B): Reproduction studies performed in mice, rats, and rabbits have not revealed any evidence of impaired fertility or adverse effects on the fetus due to Tranexamic Acid.

There are no adequate and well-controlled studies in pregnant women. However, Tranexamic Acid is known to pass the placenta and appears in cord blood at concentrations approximately equal to maternal concentration. Because animal reproduction studies are not always predictive of human response, this drug should be used during pregnancy only if clearly needed.

Labor and Delivery: See above under Pregnancy.

Nursing Mothers: Tranexamic Acid is present in the mother's milk at a concentration of about a hundredth of the corresponding serum levels. Caution should be exercised when Tranexamic Acid is administered to a nursing woman.

Pediatric Use: The drug has had limited use in children, principally in connection with tooth extraction. The limited data suggest that dosing instructions for adults can be used for children needing Tranexamic Acid therapy.

ADVERSE REACTIONS

Gastrointestinal disturbances (nausea, vomiting, diarrhea) may occur but disappear when the dosage is reduced. Giddiness and hypotension have been reported occasionally. Hypotension has been observed when intravenous injection is too rapid. To avoid this response, the solution should not be injected more rapidly than 1 mL per minute. This adverse reaction has not been reported with oral administration.

OVERDOSAGE

There is no known case of overdosage of Tranexamic Acid. Symptoms of overdosage may be nausea, vomiting, orthostatic symptoms and/or hypotension.

DOSAGE AND ADMINISTRATION

For dental extraction in patients with hemophilia: Immediately before surgery, substitution therapy is given together with Tranexamic Acid, 10 mg per kg body weight IV. After surgery, 25 mg per kg body weight are given orally three to four times daily for two to eight days.

Alternatively Tranexamic Acid can be administered entirely orally, 25 mg per kg body weight 3 to 4 times a day beginning one day prior to surgery.

Parenteral therapy, 10 mg per kg body weight 3 to 4 times daily can be used for patients unable to take oral medication. *Note*: For patients with moderate to severe impaired renal function, the following dosages are recommended:

TRANEXAMIC ACID DOSAGE

Serum Creatinine (µmol/L)	IV Dose	Tablets
120-250 (1.36-2.83 mg/dL)	10 mg/kg BID	15 mg/kg BID
250-500 (2.83-5.66 mg/dL)	10 mg/kg daily	15 mg/kg daily
> 500 (> 5.66 mg/dL)	10 mg/kg every 48 hours or 5 mg/kg every 24 hours	15 mg/kg every 48 hours or 7.5 mg/kg every 24 hours

For intravenous infusion Tranexamic Acid Injection may be mixed with most solutions for infusion such as electrolyte solutions, carbohydrate solutions, amino acid solutions and Dextran solutions. The mixture should be prepared the same day the solution is to be used. Heparin may be added to Tranexamic Acid Injection. Tranexamic Acid Injection should NOT be mixed with blood. The drug is a synthetic amino acid, and should NOT be mixed with solutions containing penicillin.

Store Tranexamic Acid tablets and injection at room temperature 15—30°C (59—86°F).

HOW SUPPLIED
INJECTION: 100 MG/ML

BRAND/MANUFACTURER	NDC	SIZE	AWP
○ BRAND CYKLOKAPRON: Pharmacia	00016-1114-08	10 ml 10s	$162.25

TABLETS: 500 MG

BRAND/MANUFACTURER	NDC	SIZE	AWP
○ BRAND CYKLOKAPRON: Pharmacia	00016-0114-00	100s	$315.00

Transderm-Nitro *SEE* NITROGLYCERIN

Transderm-Scōp *SEE* SCOPOLAMINE

Tranxene *SEE* CLORAZEPATE DIPOTASSIUM

Tranylcypromine Sulfate

Before prescribing, the physician should be familiar with the entire contents of this prescribing information.

DESCRIPTION

Chemically, Tranylcypromine Sulfate is (±)-*trans*-2-phenyl-cyclopropylamine sulfate (2:1).

Each coated tablet contains Tranylcypromine Sulfate equivalent to 10 mg of Tranylcypromine.

Following is its chemical structure:

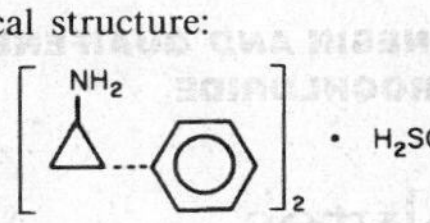

$$\left[\begin{array}{c} NH_2 \\ \triangle \cdots \bigcirc \end{array} \right]_2 \cdot H_2SO_4$$

CLINICAL PHARMACOLOGY

Tranylcypromine is a non hydrazine monoamine oxidase inhibitor with a rapid onset of activity. It increases the concentration of epinephrine, norepinephrine, and serotonin in storage sites throughout the nervous system, and in theory, this increased concentration of monoamines in the brain stem is the basis for its antidepressant activity. When Tranylcypromine is withdrawn, monoamine oxidase activity is recovered in 3 to 5 days, although the drug is excreted in 24 hours.

INDICATIONS

For the treatment of Major Depressive Episode without Melancholia.

Tranylcypromine Sulfate should be used in adult patients who can be closely supervised. It should rarely be the first antidepressant drug given. Rather, the drug is suited for patients who have failed to respond to the drugs more commonly administered for depression.

The effectiveness of Tranylcypromine Sulfate has been established in adult outpatients, most of whom had a depressive illness which would correspond to a diagnosis of Major Depressive Episode Without Melancholia. As described in the American Psychiatric Association's Diagnostic and Statistical Manual, third edition (DSM III), Major Depressive Episode implies a prominent and relatively persistent (nearly every day for at least two weeks) depressed or dysphoric mood that usually interferes with daily functioning and includes at least four of the following eight symptoms: change in appetite, change in sleep, psychomotor agitation or retardation, loss of interest in usual activities or decrease in sexual drive, increased fatigability, feelings of guilt or worthlessness, slowed thinking or impaired concentration, and suicidal ideation or attempts. The effectiveness of Tranylcypromine Sulfate in patients who meet the criteria for Major Depressive Episode with Melancholia (endogenous features) has not been established.

UNLABELED USES

Tranylcypromine Sulfate is used alone or as an adjunct in the treatment of bulimia, obsessive compulsive disorder, and manifestations of psychotic disorders. Tranylcypromine Sulfate is also used as an adjunct in the treatment of multiple sclerosis.

SUMMARY OF CONTRAINDICATIONS

Tranylcypromine Sulfate should not be administered in combination with any of the following: MAO inhibitors or dibenzazepine derivatives; sympathomimetics (including amphetamines); some central nervous system depressants (including narcotics and alcohol); antihypertensive, diuretic, antihistaminic, sedative or anesthetic drugs; bupropion HCl; buspirone HCl; dextromethorphan; cheese or other foods with a high tyramine content; or excessive quantities of caffeine.

Tranylcypromine Sulfate should not be administered to any patient with a confirmed or suspected cerebrovascular defect or to any patient with cardiovascular disease, hypertension or history of headache.

(For complete discussion of *"Contraindications"* and *"Warnings"* see below.)

CONTRAINDICATIONS

Tranylcypromine Sulfate is contraindicated:

1. In patients with cerebrovascular defects or cardiovascular disorders.

Tranylcypromine Sulfate should not be administered to any patient with a confirmed or suspected cerebrovascular defect or to any patient with cardiovascular disease or hypertension.

2. In the presence of pheochromocytoma: Tranylcypromine Sulfate should not be used in the presence of pheochromocytoma since such tumors secrete pressor substances.

3. In combination with MAO inhibitors or with dibenzaze-pine-related entities: Tranylcypromine Sulfate should not be administered together or in rapid succession with other MAO inhibitors or with dibenzazepine-related entities. Hypertensive crises or severe convulsive seizures may occur in patients receiving such combinations.

In patients being transferred to Tranylcypromine Sulfate from another MAO inhibitor or from a dibenzazepine-related entity, allow a medication-free interval of at least a week, then initiate *Tranylcypromine Sulfate* using half the normal starting dosage for at least the first week of therapy. Similarly, at least a week should elapse between the discontinuance of Tranylcypromine Sulfate and the administration of another MAO inhibitor or a dibenzazepine-related entity, or the readministration of Tranylcypromine Sulfate.

The following list includes some other MAO inhibitors, dibenzazepine-related entities and tricyclic antidepressants.

Other MAO Inhibitors
Furazolidone
Isocarboxazid
Pargyline HCl
Pargyline HCl and methyclothiazide
Phenelzine sulfate
Procarbazine HCl

Dibenzazepine-Related and Other Tricyclics
Amitriptyline HCl
Perphenazine and amitriptyline HCl
Clomipramine hydrochloride
Desipramine HCl
Imipramine HCl
Nortriptyline HCl
Protriptyline HCl
Doxepin HCl
Carbamazepine
Cyclobenzaprine HCl
Amoxapine
Maprotiline HCl
Trimipramine maleate

4. In combination with bupropion: The concurrent administration of a MAO inhibitor and bupropion hydrochloride is contraindicated. At least 14 days should elapse between discontinuation of a MAO inhibitor and initiation of treatment with bupropion hydrochloride.

5. In combination with selective serotonin reuptake inhibitors (SSRIs): As a general rule Tranylcypromine Sulfate should not be administered in combination with any SSRI. There have been reports of serious, sometimes fatal, reactions (including hyperthermia, rigidity, myoclonus, autonomic instability with possible rapid fluctuations of vital signs, and mental status changes that include extreme agitation progressing to delirium and coma) in patients receiving fluoxetine in combination with a monoamine oxidase inhibitor (MAOI), and in patients who have recently discontinued fluoxetine and are then started on a MAOI. Some cases presented with features resembling neuroleptic malignant syndrome. Therefore, fluoxetine and other SSRIs should not be used in combination with a MAOI, or within 14 days or discontinuing therapy with a MAOI. Since fluoxetine and its major metabolite have very long elimination half-lives, at least 5 weeks should be allowed after stopping fluoxetine before starting a MAOI.

At least 2 weeks should be allowed after stopping sertraline or paroxetine before starting a MAOI.

6. In combination with buspirone: Tranylcypromine Sulfate should not be used in combination with buspirone HCl since several cases of elevated blood pressure have been reported in patients taking MAO inhibitors who were then given buspirone HCl. At least 10 days should elapse between the discontinuation of Tranylcypromine Sulfate and the institution of buspirone HCl.

7. In combination with sympathomimetics: Tranylcypromine Sulfate should not be administered in combination with sympathomimetics, including amphetamines, and over-the-counter drugs such as cold, hay fever or weight-reducing preparations that contain vasoconstrictors.

During Tranylcypromine Sulfate therapy, it appears that certain patients are particularly vulnerable to the effects of sympathomimetics when the activity of certain enzymes is inhibited. Use of sympathomimetics and compounds such as guanethidine, methyldopa, reserpine, dopamine, levodopa and tryptophan with Tranylcypromine Sulfate may precipitate hypertension, headache and related symptoms. In addition, use with tryptophan may precipitate disorientation, memory impairment and other neurologic and behavioral signs.

8. In combination with meperidine: Do not use meperidine concomitantly with MAO inhibitors or within 2 or 3 weeks following MAOI therapy. Serious reactions have been precipitated with concomitant use, including coma, severe hypertension or hypotension, severe respiratory depression, convulsions, malignant hyperpyrexia, excitation, peripheral vascular collapse and death. It is thought that these reactions may be mediated by accumulation of 5-HT (serotonin) consequent to MAO inhibition.

9. In combination with dextromethorphan: The combination of MAO inhibitors and dextromethorphan has been reported to cause brief episodes of psychosis or bizarre behavior.

10. In combination with cheese or other foods with a high tyramine content: Hypertensive crises have sometimes occurred during Tranylcypromine Sulfate therapy after ingestion of foods with a high tyramine content. In general, the patient should avoid protein foods in which aging or protein breakdown is used to increase flavor. In particular, patient should be instructed not to take foods such as cheese (particularly strong or aged varieties), sour cream, Chianti wine, sherry, beer (including nonalcoholic beer), liqueurs, pickled herring, anchovies, caviar, liver, canned figs, raisins, bananas or avocados (particularly if overripe), chocolate, soy sauce, sauerkraut, the pods of broad beans (fava beans), yeast extracts, yogurt, meat extracts or meat prepared with tenderizers.

11. In patients undergoing elective surgery: Patients taking Tranylcypromine Sulfate should not undergo elective surgery requiring general anesthesia. Also, they should not be given cocaine or local anesthesia containing sympathomimetic vasoconstrictors. The possible combined hypotensive effects of Tranylcypromine Sulfate and spinal anesthesia should be kept in mind. Tranylcypromine Sulfate should be discontinued at least 10 days prior to elective surgery.

ADDITIONAL CONTRAINDICATIONS

In general, the physician should bear in mind the possibility of a lowered margin of safety when Tranylcypromine Sulfate is administered in combination with potent drugs.

1. Tranylcypromine Sulfate should not be used in combination with some central nervous system depressants such as narcotics and alcohol, or with hypotensive agents. A marked potentiating effect on these classes of drugs has been reported.

2. Antiparkinsonism drugs should be used with caution in patients receiving Tranylcypromine Sulfate since severe reactions have been reported.

3. Tranylcypromine Sulfate should not be used in patients with a history of liver disease or in those with abnormal liver function tests.

4. Excessive use of caffeine in any form should be avoided in patients receiving Tranylcypromine Sulfate.

WARNING TO PHYSICIANS

Tranylcypromine Sulfate is a potent agent with the capability of producing serious side effects. Tranylcypromine Sulfate is not recommended in those depressive reactions where other antidepressant drugs may be effective. **It should be reserved for patients who can be closely supervised and who have not responded satisfactorily to the drugs more commonly administered for depression.**

Before prescribing, the physician should be completely familiar with the full material on dosage, side effects, and contraindications on these pages, with the principles of MAO inhibitor therapy and the side effects of this class of drugs. Also, the physician should be familiar with the symptomatology of mental depressions and alternate methods of treatment to aid in the careful selection of patients for Tranylcypromine Sulfate therapy. In depressed patients, the possibility of suicide should always be considered and adequate precautions taken.

Pregnancy Warning: Use of any drug in pregnancy, during lactation, or in women of childbearing age requires that the potential benefits of the drug be weighed against its possible hazards to mother and child.

Animal reproductive studies show that Tranylcypromine Sulfate passes through the placental barrier into the fetus of the rat, and into the milk of the lactating dog. The absence of a harmful action of Tranylcypromine Sulfate on fertility or on postnatal development by either prenatal treatment or from the milk of treated animals has not been demonstrated. Tranylcypromine is excreted in human milk.

WARNING TO THE PATIENT

Patients should be instructed to report promptly the occurrence of headache or other unusual symptoms, i.e., palpitation and/or tachycardia, a sense of constriction in the throat or chest, sweating, dizziness, neck stiffness, nausea, or vomiting.

Patients should be warned against eating the foods listed in Section 9 under *"Contraindications"* while on Tranylcypromine Sulfate therapy. Also, they should be told not to drink alcoholic beverages. The patient should also be warned about the possibility of hypotension and faintness, as well as drowsiness sufficient to impair performance of potentially hazardous tasks such as driving a car or operating machinery.

Patients should also be cautioned not to take concomitant medications, whether prescription or over-the-counter drugs such as cold, hay fever or weight-reducing preparations, without the advice of a physician. They should be advised not to consume excessive amounts of caffeine in any form. Likewise, they should inform other physicians, and their dentist, about their use of Tranylcypromine Sulfate.

WARNINGS

Hypertensive Crises: **The most important reaction associated with Tranylcypromine Sulfate is the occurrence of hypertensive crises which have sometimes been fatal.**

These crises are characterized by some or all of the following symptoms: occipital headache which may radiate frontally, palpitation, neck stiffness or soreness, nausea or vomiting, sweating (sometimes with fever and sometimes with cold, clammy skin) and photophobia. Either tachycardia or bradycardia may be present, and associated constricting chest pain and dilated pupils may occur. **Intracranial bleeding, sometimes fatal in outcome, has been reported in association with the paradoxical increase in blood pressure.**

In all patients taking Tranylcypromine Sulfate blood pressure should be followed closely to detect evidence of any pressor response. It is emphasized that full reliance should not be placed on blood pressure readings, but that the patient should also be observed frequently.

Therapy should be discontinued immediately upon the occurrence of palpitation or frequent headaches during Tranylcypromine Sulfate therapy. These signs may be prodromal of a hypertensive crisis.

IMPORTANT RECOMMENDED TREATMENT IN HYPERTENSIVE CRISES

If a hypertensive crisis occurs, Tranylcypromine Sulfate should be discontinued and therapy to lower blood pressure should be instituted immediately. Headache tends to abate as blood pressure is lowered. On the basis of present evidence, phentolamine is recommended. (The dosage reported for phentolamine is 5 mg I.V.) Care should be taken to administer this drug slowly in order to avoid producing an excessive hypotensive effect. Fever should be managed by means of external cooling. Other symptomatic and supportive measures may be desirable in particular cases. Do not use parenteral reserpine.

PRECAUTIONS

HYPOTENSION

Hypotension has been observed during Tranylcypromine Sulfate therapy. Symptoms of postural hypotension are seen most commonly but not exclusively in patients with pre-existent hypertension; blood pressure usually returns rapidly to pretreatment levels upon discontinuation of the drug. At doses above 30 mg daily, postural hypotension is a major side effect and may result in syncope. Dosage increases should be made more gradually in patients showing a tendency toward hypotension at the beginning of therapy.

Postural hypotension may be relieved by having the patient lie down until blood pressure returns to normal.

Also, when Tranylcypromine Sulfate is combined with those phenothiazine derivatives or other compounds known to cause hypotension, the possibility of additive hypotensive effects should be considered.

OTHER PRECAUTIONS

There have been reports of drug dependency in patients using doses of Tranylcypromine significantly in excess of the therapeutic range. Some of these patients had a history of previous substance abuse. The following withdrawal symptoms have been reported: restlessness, anxiety, depression, confusion, hallucinations, headache, weakness and diarrhea. Drugs which lower the seizure threshold, including MAO inhibitors, should not be used with Disulfiran. As with other MAO inhibitors, Tranylcypromine Sulfate should be discontinued at least 48 hours before myelography (withdrawal should be gradual) and should not be resumed for at least 24 hours postprocedure.

In depressed patients, the possibility of suicide should always be considered and adequate precautions taken. Exclusive reliance on drug therapy to prevent suicidal attempts is unwarranted, as there may be a delay in the onset of therapeutic effect or an increase in anxiety and agitation. Also, some patients fail to respond to drug therapy or may respond only temporarily.

MAO inhibitors may have the capacity to suppress anginal pain that would otherwise serve as a warning of myocardial ischemia. The usual precautions should be observed in patients with impaired renal function since there is a possibility of cumulative effects in such patients.

Older patients may suffer more morbidity than younger patients during and following an episode of hypertension or malignant hyperthermia. Older patients have less compensatory reserve to cope with any serious adverse reaction. Therefore, Tranylcypromine Sulfate should be used with caution in the elderly population.

Although excretion of Tranylcypromine Sulfate is rapid, inhibition of MAO may persis up to 10 days following discontinuation.

Because the influence of Tranylcypromine Sulfate on the convulsive threshold is variable in animal experiments, suitable precautions should be taken if epileptic patients are treated.

Some MAO inhibitors have contributed to hypoglycemic episodes in diabetic patients receiving insulin or oral hypoglycemic agents. Therefore, Tranylcypromine Sulfate should be used with caution in diabetics using these drugs.

Tranylcypromine Sulfate may aggravate coexisting symptoms in depression, such as anxiety and agitation.

Use Tranylcypromine Sulfate with caution in hyperthyroid patients because of their increased sensitivity to pressor amines.

Tranylcypromine Sulfate should be administered with caution in patients receiving disulfiran. In a single study, rats given high intraperitoneal doses of *d* or *l* isomers of Tranylcypromine Sulfate plus disulfiram experienced severe toxicity including convulsions and death. Additional studies in rats given high oral doses of racemic Tranylcypromine Sulfate and disulfiram produced no adverse interaction.

ADVERSE REACTIONS

Overstimulation which may include increased anxiety, agitation and manic symptoms is usually evidence of excessive therapeutic action. Dosage should be reduced, or a phenothiazine tranquilizer should be administered concomitantly.

Patients may experience restlessness or insomnia; may notice some weakness, drowsiness, episodes of dizziness, or dry mouth; or may report nausea, diarrhea, abdominal pain, or constipation. Most of these effects can be relieved by lowering the dosage or by giving suitable concomitant medication. Tachycardia, significant anorexia, edema, palpitation, blurred vision, chills, and impotence have each been reported.

Headaches without blood pressure elevation have occurred. Rare instances of hepatitis and skin rash have been reported. Impaired water excretion compatible with the syndrome of inappropriate secretion of antidiuretic hormone (SIADH) has been reported.

Tinnitus, muscle spasm, tremors, myoclonic jerks, numbness, paresthesia, urinary retention and retarded ejaculation have been reported.

Hematologic disorders including anemia, leukopenia, agranulocytosis, and thrombocytopenia have been reported.

POST INTRODUCTION REPORTS

The following are spontaneously reported adverse events temporally associated with Tranylcypromine Sulfate therapy. No clear relationship between Tranylcypromine Sulfate and these events has been established. Localized scleroderma, flare-up of cystic acne, ataxia, confusion, disorientation, memory loss, urinary frequency, urinary incontinence, urticaria, fissuring in corner of mouth, akinesia.

OVERDOSAGE

Symptoms: The characteristic symptoms that may be caused by overdosage are usually those described on the preceding pages.

However, an intensification of these symptoms and sometimes severe additional manifestations may be seen, depending on the degree of overdosage and on individual susceptibility. Some patients exhibit insomnia, restlessness and anxiety, progressing in severe cases to agitation, mental confusion and incoherence. Hypotension, dizziness, weakness and drowsiness may occur, progressing in severe cases to extreme dizziness and shock. A few patients have displayed hypertension with severe headache and other symptoms. Rare instances have been reported in which hypertension was accompanied by twitching or myoclonic fibrillation of skeletal muscles with hyperpyrexia, sometimes progressing to generalized rigidity and coma.

Treatment: Gastric lavage is helpful if performed early. Treatment should normally consist of general supportive measures, close observation of vital signs and steps to counteract specific symptoms as they occur, since MAO inhibition may persist. The management of hypertensive crises is described under *"Warnings"* in the *"Hypertensive Crises"* section.

External cooling is recommended if hyperpyrexia occurs. Barbiturates have been reported to help relieve myoclonic reactions, but frequency of administration should be controlled carefully because Tranylcypromine Sulfate may prolong barbiturate activity. When hypotension requires treatment, the standard measures for managing circulatory shock should be initiated. If pressor agents are used, the rate of infusion should be regulated by careful observation of the patient because an exaggerated pressor response sometimes occurs in the presence of MAO inhibition. Remember that the toxic effect of Tranylcypromine Sulfate may be delayed or prolonged following the last dose of the drug. Therefore, the patient should be closely observed for at least a week. It is not known if Tranylcypromine is dialyzable.

DOSAGE AND ADMINISTRATION

Dosage should be adjusted to the requirements of the individual patient. Improvement should be seen within 48 hours to three weeks after starting therapy.

The usual effective dosage is 30 mg per day, usually given in divided doses. If there are no signs of improvement after a reasonable period (up to two weeks), then the dosage may be increased in 10 mg per day increments at intervals of one to three weeks; the dosage range may be extended to a maximum of 60 mg per day from the usual 30 mg per day.

Store at controlled room temperature (15° to 30°C; 59° to 86°F).

HOW SUPPLIED
TABLETS: 10 MG

BRAND/MANUFACTURER	NDC	SIZE	AWP
○ **BRAND**			
PARNATE: SK Beecham Pharm	00007-4471-20	100s	$43.60

Trasylol *SEE* APROTININ

Travase *SEE* SUTILAINS

◆ RATED THERAPEUTICALLY EQUIVALENT; ◇ THERAPEUTIC EQUIVALENCE UNCONFIRMED; ○ UNRATED

Travasol *SEE* AMINO ACIDS WITH ELECTROLYTES, INJECTABLE, AMINO ACIDS, INJECTABLE *AND* AMINO ACIDS/ CALCIUM CHLORIDE/DEXTROSE/ELECTROLYTES

Trazodone Hydrochloride

DESCRIPTION

Trazodone Hydrochloride is an antidepressant chemically unrelated to tricyclic, tetracyclic, or other known antidepressant agents. It is a triazolopyridine derivative designated as 2-[3-[4-(3-chlorophenyl)-1-piperazinyl] propyl]-1,2,4-triazolo[4, 3-a]pyridin-3(2*H*)-one hydrochloride. Trazodone Hydrochloride is a white odorless crystalline powder which is freely soluble in water. Its molecular weight is 408.3. The empirical formula is $C_{19}H_{22}CIN_5O \cdot HCl$

Trazodone Hydrochloride is supplied for oral administration in 50 mg, 100 mg, 150 mg and 300 mg tablets.

Following is its chemical structure:

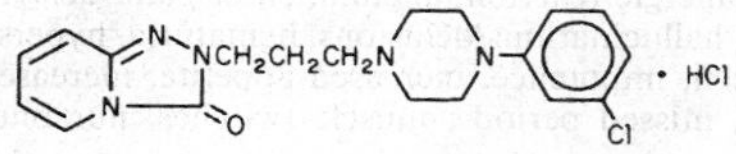

CLINICAL PHARMACOLOGY

The mechanism of Trazodone Hydrochloride's antidepressant action in man is not fully understood. In animals, Trazodone Hydrochloride selectively inhibits serotonin uptake by brain synaptosomes and potentiates the behavioral changes induced by the serotonin precursor, 5-hydroxytryptophan. Cardiac conduction effects of Trazodone Hydrochloride in the anesthetized dog are qualitatively disimilar and quantitatively less pronounced than those seen with tricyclic antidepressants. Trazodone Hydrochloride is not a monoamine oxidase inhibitor and, unlike amphetamine-type drugs, does not stimulate the central nervous system.

In man, Trazodone Hydrochloride is well absorbed after oral administration without selective localization in any tissue. When Trazodone Hydrochloride is taken shortly after ingestion of food, there may be an increase in the amount of drug absorbed, a decrease in maximum concentration, and a lengthening in the time to maximum concentration. Peak plasma levels occur approximately 1 hour after dosing when Trazodone Hydrochloride is taken on an empty stomach or 2 hours after dosing when taken with food. Elimination of Trazodone Hydrochloride is biphasic, consisting of an initial phase (half-life 3-6 hours) followed by a slower phase (half-life 5-9 hours), and is unaffected by the presence or absence of food. Since the clearance of Trazodone Hydrochloride from the body is sufficiently variable, in some patients Trazodone Hydrochloride may accumulate in the plasma.

For those patients who responded to Trazodone Hydrochloride one-third of the inpatients and one-half of the outpatients had a significant therapeutic response by the end of the first week of treatment. Three-fourths of all responders demonstrated a significant therapeutic effect by the end of the second week. One-fourth of responders required 2-4 weeks for a significant therapeutic response.

INDICATIONS AND USAGE

Trazodone Hydrochloride is indicated for the treatment of depression. The efficacy of Trazodone Hydrochloride has been demonstrated in both inpatient and outpatient settings and for depressed patients with and without prominent anxiety. The depressive illness of patients studied corresponds to the Major Depressive Episode criteria of the American Psychiatric Association's Diagnostic and Statistical Manual, III[1].

Major Depressive Episode implies a prominent and relatively persistent (nearly every day for at least 2 weeks) depressed or dysphoric mood that usually interferes with daily functioning, and includes at least four of the following eight symptoms: change in appetite, change in sleep, psychomotor agitation or retardation, loss of interest in usual activities or decrease in sexual drive, increased fatigability, feelings of guilt or worthlessness, slowed thinking or impaired concentration, and suicidal ideation or attempts.

UNLABELED USES

Trazodone Hydrochloride is used alone or as an adjunct in the treatment of bulimia, diabetic neuropathy, kleptomania, and in the prophylaxis of migraine headache. It is also used in reducing anxiety, panic symptoms and phobic symptoms in patients with panic disorder or agoraphobia with panic attacks and in the treatment of acute alcohol withdrawal syndrome.

CONTRAINDICATIONS

Trazodone Hydrochloride is contraindicated in patients hypersensitive to Trazodone Hydrochloride.

WARNINGS

TRAZODONE HAS BEEN ASSOCIATED WITH THE OCCURRENCE OF PRIAPISM. IN APPROXIMATELY ⅓ OF THE CASES REPORTED, SURGICAL INTERVENTION WAS REQUIRED AND, IN A PORTION OF THESE CASES, PERMANENT IMPAIRMENT OF ERECTILE FUNCTION OR IMPOTENCE RESULTED. MALE PATIENTS WITH PROLONGED OR INAPPROPRIATE ERECTIONS SHOULD IMMEDIATELY DISCONTINUE THE DRUG AND CONSULT THEIR PHYSICIAN.

If an erection should persist, promptly contact Bristol-Myers Squibb USPG Medical Services Department (800)321-1335.

The detumescence of priapism and drug-induced penile erections by the intracavernosal injection of alpha-adrenergic stimulants such as epinephrine and metaraminol has been reported.[2-7] For one case of priapism (of some 12-24 hours' duration) in a Trazodone Hydrochloride-treated patient in whom the intracavernosal injection of epinephrine was accomplished, prompt detumescence occurred with return of normal erectile activity.

This procedure should be performed under the supervision of a urologist or a physician familiar with the procedure and should not be initiated without urologic consultation if the priapism has persisted for more than 24 hours.

Trazodone Hydrochloride is not recommended for use during the initial recovery phase of myocardial infarction.

Caution should be used when administering Trazodone Hydrochloride to patients with cardiac disease, and such patients should be closely monitored, since antidepressant drugs (including Trazodone Hydrochloride have been associated with the occurrence of cardiac arrhythmias. Recent clinical studies in patients with pre-existing cardiac disease indicate that Trazodone Hydrochloride may be arrhythmogenic in some patients in that population. Arrhythmias identified include isolated PVCs, ventricular couplets, and in two patients short episodes (3-4 beats) of ventricular tachycardia.

PRECAUTIONS

General: The possibility of suicide in seriously depressed patients is inherent in the illness and may persist until significant remission occurs. Therefore, prescriptions should be written for the smallest number of tablets consistent with good patient management.

Hypotension, including orthostatic hypotension and syncope, has been reported to occur in patients receiving Trazodone Hydrochloride. Concomitant administration of antihypertensive therapy with Trazodone Hydrochloride may require a reduction in the dose of the antihypertensive drug.

Little is known about the interaction between Trazodone Hydrochloride and general anesthetics; therefore, prior to elective surgery, Trazodone Hydrochloride should be discontinued for as long as clinically feasible.

As with all antidepressants, the use of Trazodone Hydrochloride should be based on the consideration of the physician that the expected benefits of therapy outweigh potential risk factors.

Information for Patients: Because priapism has been reported to occur in patients receiving Trazodone Hydrochloride, patients with prolonged or inappropriate penile erection should immediately discontinue the drug and consult with the physician (see *"Warnings"*).

Antidepressants may impair the mental and/or physical ability required for the performance of potentially hazardous tasks, such as operating an automobile or machinery; the patient should be cautioned accordingly.

Trazodone Hydrochloride may enhance the response to alcohol, barbiturates, and other CNS depressants.

Trazodone Hydrochloride should be given shortly after a meal or light snack. Within any individual patient, total drug absorption may be up to 20% higher when the drug is taken with food rather than on an empty stomach. The risk of dizziness/light-headedness may increase under fasting conditions.

Laboratory Tests: Occasional low white blood cell and neutrophil counts have been noted in patients receiving Trazodone Hydrochloride. These were not considered clinically significant and did not necessitate discontinuation of the drug; however, the drug should be discontinued in any patient whose white blood cell count or absolute neutrophil count falls below normal levels. White blood cell and differential counts are recommended for patients who develop fever and sore throat (or other signs of infection) during therapy.

Drug Interactions: Increased serum digoxin or phenytoin levels have been reported to occur in patients receiving Trazodone Hydrochloride concurrently with either of those two drugs.

It is not known whether interactions will occur between monoamine oxidase (MAO) inhibitors and Trazodone Hydrochloride. Due to the absence of clinical experience, if MAO inhibitors are discontinued shortly before or are to be given concomitantly with Trazodone Hydrochloride, therapy should be initiated cautiously with gradual increase in dosage until optimum response is achieved.

Therapeutic Interactions: Concurrent administration with electroshock therapy should be avoided because of the absence of experience in this area.

There have been reports of increased and decreased prothrombin time occurring in Coumadinized patients who take Trazodone Hydrochloride.

Carcinogenesis, Mutagenesis, Impairment of Fertility: No drug- or dose-related occurrence of carcinogenesis was evident in rats receiving Trazodone Hydrochloride in daily oral doses up to 300 mg/kg for 18 months.

Pregnancy Category C: Trazodone Hydrochloride has been shown to cause increased fetal resorption and other adverse effects on the fetus in two studies using the rat when given at dose levels approximately 30-50 times the proposed maximum human dose. There was also an increase in congenital anomalies in one of three rabbit studies at approximately 15-50 times the maximum human dose. There are no adequate and well-controlled studies in pregnant women. Trazodone Hydrochloride should be used during pregnancy only if the potential benefit justifies the potential risk to the fetus.

Nursing Mothers: Trazodone Hydrochloride and/or its metabolites have been found in the milk of lactating rats, suggesting that the drug may be secreted in

➤ SHOWN IN PRODUCT IDENTIFICATION GUIDE

human milk. Caution should be exercised when Trazodone Hydrochloride is administered to a nursing woman.

Pediatric Use: Safety and effectiveness in children below the age of 18 have not been established.

ADVERSE REACTIONS
Because the frequency of adverse drug effects is affected by diverse factors (eg, drug dose, method of detection, physician judgment, disease under treatment, etc.), a single meaningful estimate of adverse event incidence is difficult to obtain. This problem is illustrated by the variation in adverse event incidence observed and reported from the inpatients and outpatients treated with Trazodone Hydrochloride. It is impossible to determine precisely what accounts for the differences observed.

Clinical Trial Reports: The table below is presented solely to indicate the relative frequency of adverse events reported in representative controlled clinical studies conducted to evaluate the safety and efficacy of Trazodone Hydrochloride.

The figures cited cannot be used to predict precisely the incidence of untoward events in the course of usual medical practice where patient characteristics and other factors often differ from those which prevailed in the clinical trials. These incidence figures, also, cannot be compared with those obtained from other clinical studies involving related drug products and placebo, as each group of drug trials is conducted under a different set of conditions.

| | Treatment-Emergent Symptom Incidence | | | |
| | Inpts. | | Outpts. | |
	T	P	T	P
Number of Patients	142	95	157	158
% of Patients Reporting				
Allergic				
Skin Condition/ Edema	2.8	1.1	7.0	1.3
Autonomic				
Blurred Vision	6.3	4.2	14.7	3.8
Constipation	7.0	4.2	7.6	5.7
Dry Mouth	14.8	8.4	33.8	20.3
Cardiovascular				
Hypertension	2.1	1.1	1.3	*
Hypotension	7.0	1.1	3.8	0.0
Shortness of Breath	*	1.1	1.3	0.0
Syncope	2.8	2.1	4.5	1.3
Tachycardia/ Palpitations	0.0	0.0	7.0	7.0
CNS				
Anger/Hostility	3.5	6.3	1.3	2.5
Confusion	4.9	0.0	5.7	7.6
Decreased Concentration	2.8	2.1	1.3	0.0
Disorientation	2.1	0.0	*	0.0
Dizziness/Light- headedness	19.7	5.3	28.0	15.2
Drowsiness	23.9	6.3	40.8	19.6
Excitement	1.4	1.1	5.1	5.7
Fatigue	11.3	4.2	5.7	2.5
Headache	9.9	5.3	19.8	15.8
Insomnia	9.9	10.5	6.4	12.0
Impaired Memory	1.4	0.0	*	*
Nervousness	14.8	10.5	6.4	8.2
Gastrointestinal				
Abdominal/Gastric Disorder	3.5	4.2	5.7	4.4
Bad Taste in Mouth	1.4	0.0	0.0	0.0
Diarrhea	0.0	1.1	4.5	1.9
Nausea/Vomiting	9.9	1.1	12.7	9.5
Musculoskeletal				
Musculoskeletal Aches/Pains	5.6	3.2	5.1	2.5
Neurological				
Incoordination	4.9	0.0	1.9	0.0
Paresthesia	1.4	0.0	0.0	*
Tremors	2.8	1.1	5.1	3.8
Sexual Function				
Decreased Libido	*	1.1	1.3	*
Other				
Decreased Appetite	3.5	5.3	0.0	*
Eyes Red/Tired/ Itching	2.8	0.0	0.0	0.0
Head Full-Heavy	2.8	0.0	0.0	0.0
Malaise	2.8	0.0	0.0	0.0
Nasal/Sinus Congestion	2.8	0.0	5.7	3.2

| | Treatment-Emergent Symptom Incidence | | | |
| | Inpts. | | Outpts. | |
	T	P	T	P
Nightmares/Vivid Dreams	*	1.1	5.1	5.7
Sweating/ Clamminess	1.4	1.1	*	*
Tinnitus	1.4	0.0	0.0	*
Weight Gain	1.4	0.0	4.5	1.9
Weight Loss	*	3.2	5.7	2.5

T = Trazodone Hydrochloride P = Placebo
*Incidence less than 1%

Occasional sinus bradycardia has occurred in long-term studies.

In addition to the relatively common (ie, greater than 1%) untoward events enumerated above, the following adverse events have been reported to occur in association with the use of Trazodone Hydrochloride in the controlled clinical studies: akathisia, allergic reaction, anemia, chest pain, delayed urine flow, early menses, flatulence, hallucinations/delusions, hematuria, hypersalivation, hypomania, impaired speech, impotence, increased appetite, increased libido, increased urinary frequency, missed periods; muscle twitches, numbness, and retrograde ejaculation.

Postintroduction Reports: Although the following adverse reactions have been reported in Trazodone Hydrochloride users, the causal association has neither been confirmed nor refuted.

Voluntary reports received since market introduction include the following: agitation, alopecia, apnea, ataxia, breast enlargement or engorgement, diplopia, edema, extrapyramidal symptoms, grand mal seizures, hallucinations, hemolytic anemia, hyperbilirubinemia, leukonychia, jaundice, lactation, liver enzyme alterations, methemoglobinemia, nausea/vomiting (most frequently), paresthesia, priapism (see *"Warnings"* and *"Precautions, Information for Patients"*); some patients have required surgical intervention), pruritus, psychosis, rash, stupor, inappropriate ADH syndrome, tardive dyskinesia, unexplained death, urinary incontinence, urinary retention, urticaria, vasodilation, vertigo, and weakness.

Cardiovascular system effects which have been reported include the following: conduction block, orthostatic hypotension and syncope, palpitations, bradycardia, atrial fibrillation, myocardial infarction, cardiac arrest, arrhythmia, and ventricular ectopic activity, including ventricular tachycardia (see *"Warnings"*).

OVERDOSE
Animal Oral LD$_{50}$: The oral LD$_{50}$ of the drug is 610 mg/kg in mice, 486 mg/kg in rats, and 560 mg/kg in rabbits.

Signs and Symptoms: Death from overdose has occurred in patients ingesting Trazodone Hydrochloride and other drugs concurrently (namely, alcohol; alcohol + chloral hydrate + diazepam; amobarbital; chlordiazepoxide; or meprobamate).

The most severe reactions reported to have occurred with overdose of Trazodone Hydrochloride alone have been priapism, respiratory arrest, seizures, and EKG changes. The reactions reported most frequently have been drowsiness and vomiting. Overdosage may cause an increase in incidence or severity of any of the reported adverse reactions (see *"Adverse Reactions"*).

Treatment: There is no specific antidote for Trazodone Hydrochloride. Treatment should be symptomatic and supportive in the case of hypotension or excessive sedation. Any patient suspected of having taken an overdose should have the stomach emptied by gastric lavage. Forced diuresis may be useful in facilitating elimination of the drug.

DOSAGE AND ADMINISTRATION
The dosage should be initiated at a low level and increased gradually, noting the clinical response and any evidence of intolerance. Occurrence of drowsiness may require the administration of a major portion of the daily dose at bedtime or a reduction of dosage. Trazodone Hydrochloride should be taken shortly after a meal or light snack. Symptomatic relief may be seen during the first week, with optimal antidepressant effects typically evident within 2 weeks. Twenty-five percent of those who respond to Trazodone Hydrochloride require more than 2 weeks (up to 4 weeks) of drug administration.

Usual Adult Dosage: An initial dose of 150 mg/day in divided doses is suggested. The dose may be increased by 50 mg/day every 3 to 4 days. The maximum dose for outpatients usually should not exceed 400 mg/day in divided doses. Inpatients (ie, more severely depressed patients) may be given up to but not in excess of 600 mg/day in divided doses.

Maintenance: Dosage during prolonged maintenance therapy should be kept at the lowest effective level. Once an adequate response has been achieved, dosage may be gradually reduced, with subsequent adjustment depending on therapeutic response.

Although there has been no systematic evaluation of the efficacy of Trazodone Hydrochloride beyond 6 weeks, it is generally recommended that a course of antidepressant drug treatment should be continued for several months.

Storage:
Store at room temperature. Protect from temperatures above 140°F (40°C). Dispense in tight, light-resistant container (USP).

◆ RATED THERAPEUTICALLY EQUIVALENT; ◇ THERAPEUTIC EQUIVALENCE UNCONFIRMED; ○ UNRATED

REFERENCES
1. Williams JBW, Ed: Diagnostic and Statistical Manual of Mental Disorders-III, American Psychiatric Association, May 1980. 2. Brindley GS: New treatment for priapism, *Lancet* July 28, 1984; ii:220. 3. Goldstein I, et al: Pharmacologic detumescence: The alternative to surgical shunting, *J Urology* April 1986; 135(4:PEII):308A. 4. Brindley GS: Pilot experiments on the actions of drugs injected into the human corpus cavernosum penis, *Br J Pharmacol* 1986; 87:495-500. 5. Padma-Nathan H, et al: Treatment of prolonged or priapistic erections following intracavernosal papaverine therapy, *Semin Urol* 1986; 4(4):236-238. 6. Lue TF, et al: Priapism: A refined approach to diagnosis and treatment, *J Urology* 1986; 136:104-110. 7. Fabre LF, Feighner JP: Long-term therapy for depression with trazodone, *J Clin Psychiatry* 1983; 44(1):17-21.

HOW SUPPLIED
TABLET: 50 MG

AVERAGE UNIT PRICE (AVAILABLE SIZES)		GENERIC A-RATED AVERAGE PRICE (GAAP)	
BRAND	$1.21	100s	$29.25
GENERIC	$0.27	500s	$120.34
HCFA FUL (100s ea)	$0.08	1000s	$236.74

BRAND/MANUFACTURER	NDC	SIZE	AWP
◆ BRAND			
➤ DESYREL: Apothecon	00087-0775-41	100s	$123.18
	00087-0775-42	100s ud	$131.27
	00087-0775-43	1000s	$1070.40
◆ GENERICS			
Medirex	57480-0369-06	30s	$13.50
Rugby	00536-4715-01	100s	$17.70
Barr	00555-0489-02	100s	$23.28
Warner Chilcott	00047-0577-24	100s	$23.29
Qualitest	00603-6144-21	100s	$24.07
Major	00904-3990-60	100s	$25.20
➤ Schein	00364-2109-01	100s	$25.75
Sidmak	50111-0433-01	100s	$26.00
Martec	52555-0260-01	100s	$26.80
Lemmon	00093-0637-01	100s	$28.41
Geneva	00781-1807-01	100s	$28.45
Aligen	00405-5036-01	100s	$28.60
URL	00677-1133-01	100s	$28.65
Mutual	53489-0510-01	100s	$28.65
Goldline	00182-1259-01	100s	$28.65
Purepac	00228-2439-10	100s	$28.72
Du Pont Multi	00056-0261-70	100s	$29.00
Moore,H.L.	00839-7251-06	100s	$30.71
Parmed	00349-8906-01	100s	$41.73
U.S. Trading	56126-0368-11	100s ud	$11.72
Raway	00686-0472-20	100s ud	$24.00
Geneva	00781-1807-13	100s ud	$30.32
Vangard	00615-2578-13	100s ud	$36.00
Major	00904-3990-61	100s ud	$36.40
UDL	51079-0427-20	100s ud	$42.42
Medirex	57480-0369-01	100s ud	$42.95
Goldline	00182-1259-89	100s ud	$43.00
Rugby	00536-4715-02	250s	$34.80
Major	00904-3990-40	500s	$63.80
Rugby	00536-4715-05	500s	$65.40
Qualitest	00603-6144-28	500s	$99.30
Barr	00555-0489-04	500s	$105.56
Sidmak	50111-0433-02	500s	$128.00
Goldline	00182-1259-05	500s	$128.00
Martec	52555-0260-05	500s	$131.85
Geneva	00781-1807-05	500s	$135.14
Parmed	00349-8906-05	500s	$143.38
Purepac	00228-2439-50	500s	$143.60
URL	00677-1133-05	500s	$150.00
Mutual	53489-0510-05	500s	$150.00
➤ Schein	00364-2109-02	1000s	$137.75
Sidmak	50111-0433-03	1000s	$221.65
Goldline	00182-1259-10	1000s	$221.65
Martec	52555-0260-10	1000s	$226.00
Geneva	00781-1807-10	1000s	$247.22
Mutual	53489-0510-10	1000s	$260.00
Aligen	00405-5036-03	1000s	$262.20
Lemmon	00093-0637-10	1000s	$269.90
Moore,H.L.	00839-7251-16	1000s	$284.30

TABLET: 100 MG

AVERAGE UNIT PRICE (AVAILABLE SIZES)		GENERIC A-RATED AVERAGE PRICE (GAAP)	
BRAND	$2.11	100s	$49.45
GENERIC	$0.44	250s	$98.33
HCFA FUL (100s ea)	$0.13	500s	$168.60
		1000s	$330.12

BRAND/MANUFACTURER	NDC	SIZE	AWP
◆ BRAND			
➤ DESYREL: Apothecon	00087-0776-41	100s	$215.27
	00087-0776-42	100s ud	$229.21
	00087-0776-43	1000s	$1870.58
◆ GENERICS			
Medirex	57480-0370-06	30s	$22.70
Barr	00555-0490-02	100s	$36.75
Warner Chilcott	00047-0578-24	100s	$36.90

BRAND/MANUFACTURER	NDC	SIZE	AWP
Rugby	00536-4688-01	100s	$38.69
Major	00904-3991-60	100s	$39.75
Sidmak	50111-0434-01	100s	$41.00
Qualitest	00603-6145-21	100s	$41.00
Moore,H.L.	00839-7252-06	100s	$41.78
Martec	52555-0261-01	100s	$42.25
Goldline	00182-1260-01	100s	$42.50
Schein	00364-2110-01	100s	$44.50
Lemmon	00093-0638-01	100s	$46.43
URL	00677-1134-01	100s	$47.45
Mutual	53489-0511-01	100s	$47.45
Geneva	00781-1808-01	100s	$47.56
Du Pont Multi	00056-0262-70	100s	$48.00
Purepac	00228-2441-10	100s	$48.66
Aligen	00405-5037-01	100s	$48.82
Parmed	00349-8907-01	100s	$70.18
U.S. Trading	56126-0369-11	100s ud	$23.90
Raway	00686-0428-20	100s ud	$30.00
Geneva	00781-1808-13	100s ud	$62.10
Vangard	00615-2579-13	100s ud	$63.42
Major	00904-3991-61	100s ud	$63.55
UDL	51079-0428-20	100s ud	$73.59
Medirex	57480-0370-01	100s ud	$74.25
Goldline	00182-1260-89	100s ud	$74.40
Rugby	00536-4688-02	250s	$80.51
Parmed	00349-8907-25	250s	$116.15
Major	00904-3991-40	500s	$97.05
Rugby	00536-4688-05	500s	$119.40
Qualitest	00603-6145-28	500s	$165.12
Barr	00555-0490-04	500s	$174.56
URL	00677-1134-05	500s	$180.00
Mutual	53489-0511-05	500s	$180.00
Sidmak	50111-0434-02	500s	$187.00
Goldline	00182-1260-05	500s	$187.00
Martec	52555-0261-05	500s	$190.70
Moore,H.L.	00839-7252-12	500s	$205.13
Schein	00364-2110-02	1000s	$227.50
Mutual	53489-0511-10	1000s	$300.00
Sidmak	50111-0434-03	1000s	$341.00
Goldline	00182-1260-10	1000s	$341.00
Lemmon	00093-0638-10	1000s	$441.08

For additional alternatives, turn to the section beginning on page 2859.

Trecator-SC *SEE* ETHIONAMIDE

Trental *SEE* PENTOXIFYLLINE

Tretinoin

DESCRIPTION
Tretinoin Gel, Cream and Liquid, containing Tretinoin are used for the topical treatment of acne vulgaris. Tretinoin Gel contains Tretinoin (retinoic acid, vitamin A acid) in either of two strengths. 0.025% or 0.01% by weight, in a gel. Tretinoin Cream contains Tretinoin in either of three strengths, 0.1%, 0.05%, or 0.025% by weight. Tretinoin Liquid contains Tretinoin 0.05% by weight. Chemically, Tretinoin is *all-trans*-retinoic acid.

Following is its chemical structure:

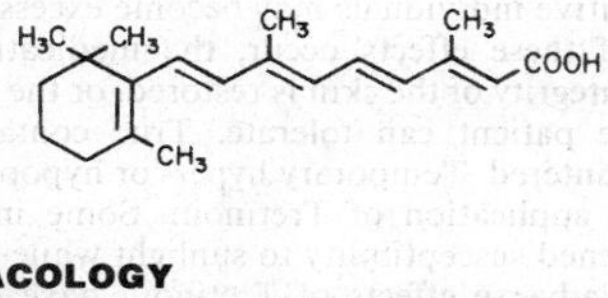

CLINICAL PHARMACOLOGY
Although the exact mode of action of Tretinoin is unknown, current evidence suggests that topical Tretinoin decreases cohesiveness of follicular epithelial cells with decreased microcomedo formation. Additionally, Tretinoin stimulates mitotic activity and increased turnover of follicular epithelial cells causing extrusion of the comedones.

➤ SHOWN IN PRODUCT IDENTIFICATION GUIDE

INDICATIONS AND USAGE

Tretinoin is indicated for topical application in the treatment of acne vulgaris. The safety and efficacy of the long-term use of this product in the treatment of other disorders have not been established.

UNLABELED USES

Tretinoin is used alone or as an adjunct in the treatment of photoaging, including hyperpigmented macules (liver spots) and premature wrinkles; drug-induced photosensitivity, and psoriasis. It is also used in epidermal wound healing, xerophthalmia, black hairy tongue caused by systemic antibiotic therapy, and keloids (hypertrophic scars). Tretinoin is also prescribed in the treatment of hyperkeratotic skin disease including keratinizing dermatoses, lamellar ichthyosis, ichthyosis vulgaris, and ichthyosiform erythroderma; oral lichen planus, and melasma.

CONTRAINDICATIONS

Use of the product should be discontinued if hypersensitivity to any of the ingredients is noted.

PRECAUTIONS

General: If a reaction suggesting sensitivity or chemical irritation occurs, use of the medication should be discontinued. Exposure to sunlight, including sunlamps, should be minimized during the use of Tretinoin, and patients with sunburn should be advised not to use the product until fully recovered because of heightened susceptibility to sunlight as a result of the use of Tretinoin. Patients who may be required to have considerable sun exposure due to occupation and those with inherent sensitivity to the sun should exercise particular caution. Use of sunscreen products and protective clothing over treated areas is recommended when exposure cannot be avoided. Weather extremes, such as wind or cold, also may be irritating to patients under treatment with Tretinoin.

Tretinoin acne treatment should be kept away from the eyes, the mouth, angles of the nose, and mucous membranes. Topical use may induce severe local erythema and peeling at the site of application. If the degree of local irritation warrants, patients should be directed to use the medication less frequently, discontinue use temporarily, or discontinue use altogether. Tretinoin has been reported to cause severe irritation on eczematous skin and should be used with utmost caution in patients with this condition.

Drug Interactions: Concomitant topical medication, medicated or abrasive soaps and cleansers, soaps and cosmetics that have a strong drying effect, and products with high concentrations of alcohol, astringents, spices or lime should be used with caution because of possible interaction with Tretinoin. Particular caution should be exercised in using preparations containing sulfur, resorcinol, or salicylic acid with Tretinoin. It also is advisable to "rest" a patient's skin until the effects of such preparations subside before use of Tretinoin is begun.

Carcinogenesis: Long-term animal studies to determine the carcinogenic potential of Tretinoin have not been performed. Studies in hairless albino mice suggest that Tretinoin may accelerate the tumorigenic potential of weakly carcinogenic light from a solar simulator. In other studies, when lightly pigmented hairless mice treated with Tretinoin were exposed to carcinogenic doses of UVB light, the incidence and rate of development of skin tumors was reduced. Due to significantly different experimental conditions, no strict comparison of these disparate data is possible. Although the significance of these studies to man is not clear, patients should avoid or minimize exposure to sun.

Pregnancy: Teratogenic effects. Pregnancy Category C. *Oral* Tretinoin has been shown to be teratogenic in rats when given in doses 1000 times the topical human dose. Oral Tretinoin has been shown to be fetotoxic in rats when given in doses 500 times the topical human dose. *Topical* Tretinoin has not been shown to be teratogenic in rats and rabbits when given in doses of 100 and 320 times the topical human dose, respectively (assuming a 50 kg adult applies 250 mg of 0.1% cream topically). However, at these topical doses, delayed ossification of a number of bones occurred in both species. These changes may be considered variants of normal development and are usually corrected after weaning. There are no adequate and well-controlled studies in pregnant women. Tretinoin should be used during pregnancy only if the potential benefit justifies the potential risk to the fetus.

Nursing mothers: It is not known whether this drug is excreted in human milk. Because many drugs are excreted in human milk, caution should be exercised when Tretinoin is administered to a nursing woman.

GELS ARE FLAMMABLE. *Note:* Keep away from heat and flame. Keep tube tightly closed.

ADVERSE REACTIONS

The skin of certain sensitive individuals may become excessively red, edematous, blistered, or crusted. If these effects occur, the medication should either be discontinued until the integrity of the skin is restored, or the medication should be adjusted to a level the patient can tolerate. True contact allergy to topical Tretinoin is rarely encountered. Temporary hyper- or hypopigmentation has been reported with repeated application of Tretinoin. Some individuals have been reported to have heightened susceptibility to sunlight while under treatment with Tretinoin. To date, all adverse effects of Tretinoin have been reversible upon discontinuance of therapy (see *"Dosage and Administration"* section).

OVERDOSAGE

If medication is applied excessively, no more rapid or better results will be obtained and marked redness, peeling, or discomfort may occur. Oral ingestion of the drug may lead to the same side effects as those associated with excessive oral intake of Vitamin A.

DOSAGE AND ADMINISTRATION

Tretinoin Gel, Cream or Liquid should be applied once a day, before retiring, to the skin where acne lesions appear, using enough to cover the entire affected area lightly. Liquid: The liquid may be applied using a fingertip, gauze pad or cotton swab. If gauze or cotton is employed, care should be taken not to oversaturate it to the extent that the liquid would run into areas where treatment is not intended. Gel: Excessive application results in 'pilling' of the gel, which minimizes the likelihood of overapplication by the patient.

Application may cause a transitory feeling of warmth or slight stinging. In cases where it has been necessary to temporarily discontinue therapy or to reduce the frequency of application, therapy may be resumed or frequency of application increased when the patients become able to tolerate the treatment.

Alterations of vehicle, drug concentration, or dose frequency should be closely monitored by careful observation of the clinical therapeutic response and skin tolerance.

During the early weeks of therapy, an *apparent* exacerbation of inflammatory lesions may occur. This is due to the action of the medication on deep, previously unseen lesions and should not be considered a reason to discontinue therapy.

Therapeutic results should be noticed after two to three weeks but more than six weeks of therapy may be required before definite beneficial effects are seen.

Once the acne lesions have responded satisfactorily, it may be possible to maintain the improvement with less frequent applications, or other dosage forms.

Patients treated with Tretinoin acne treatment may use cosmetics, but the areas to be treated should be cleansed thoroughly before the medication is applied. (See *"Precautions"*).

Storage: Tretinoin Liquid, 0.05%, and Tretinoin Gel, 0.025% and 0.01%: Store below 86°F.

Tretinoin Cream, 0.1%, 0.05%, and 0.025%: store below 80°F.

HOW SUPPLIED
CREAM: 0.025%

BRAND/MANUFACTURER	NDC	SIZE	AWP
○ **BRAND**			
RETIN-A: Ortho Pharm	00062-0165-01	20 gm	$24.90
	00062-0165-02	45 gm	$47.28

CREAM: 0.05%

BRAND/MANUFACTURER	NDC	SIZE	AWP
○ **BRAND**			
RETIN-A: Ortho Pharm	00062-0175-12	20 gm	$25.80
	00062-0175-13	45 gm	$48.60

CREAM: 0.1%

BRAND/MANUFACTURER	NDC	SIZE	AWP
○ **BRAND**			
RETIN-A: Ortho Pharm	00062-0275-23	20 gm	$30.12
	00062-0275-01	45 gm	$56.70

GEL: 0.01%

BRAND/MANUFACTURER	NDC	SIZE	AWP
○ **BRAND**			
RETIN-A: Ortho Pharm	00062-0575-44	15 gm	$20.10
	00062-0575-46	45 gm	$47.58

GEL: 0.025%

BRAND/MANUFACTURER	NDC	SIZE	AWP
○ **BRAND**			
RETIN-A: Ortho Pharm	00062-0475-42	15 gm	$20.28
	00062-0475-45	45 gm	$47.94

LIQUID: 0.05%

BRAND/MANUFACTURER	NDC	SIZE	AWP
○ **BRAND**			
RETIN-A: Ortho Pharm	00062-0075-07	28 ml	$39.66

Trexan *SEE* NALTREXONE HYDROCHLORIDE

TriVita *SEE* SODIUM FLUORIDE/VITAMIN A/VITAMIN C/VITAMIN D

Tri-Immunol *SEE* DIPHTHERIA/PERTUSSIS/TETANUS

◆ RATED THERAPEUTICALLY EQUIVALENT; ◇ THERAPEUTIC EQUIVALENCE UNCONFIRMED; ○ UNRATED

Tri-Levlen *SEE* ETHINYL ESTRADIOL WITH LEVONORGESTREL

Tri-Norinyl *SEE* ETHINYL ESTRADIOL AND NORETHINDRONE

Tri-Vi-Flor *SEE* SODIUM FLUORIDE/VITAMIN A/VITAMIN C/ VITAMIN D

Tri-Vi-Flor with Iron *SEE* FERROUS SULFATE/ SODIUM FLUORIDE/VITAMINS, MULTI

Triamcinolone

DESCRIPTION
Triamcinolone is a synthetic adrenocorticosteroid and has the chemical name 9-Fluoro-11β, 16α, 17, 21-tetrahydroxypregna- 1, 4-diene-3, 20-dione.

Each tablet contains:
Triamcinolone ....1, 2, 4, or 8 mg

Following is its chemical structure:

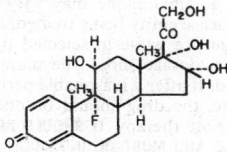

ACTION
Triamcinolone is primarily glucocorticoid in action and has potent anti-inflammatory, hormonal and metabolic effects common to cortisone-like drugs. It is essentially devoid of mineralocorticoid activity when administered in therapeutic doses, causing little or no sodium retention, with potassium excretion minimal or absent. The body's immune responses to diverse stimuli are also modified by its action.

INDICATIONS
1. Endocrine Disorders:
Primary or secondary adrenocortical insufficiency (hydrocortisone or cortisone is the first choice; synthetic analogs may be used in conjunction with mineralocorticoids where applicable; in infancy mineralocorticoid supplementation is of particular importance).
Congenital adrenal hyperplasia.
Nonsuppurative thyroiditis.
Hypercalcemia associated with cancer.

2. Rheumatic Disorders:
As adjunctive therapy for short-term administration (to tide the patient over an acute episode or exacerbation) in:
Psoriatic arthritis.
Rheumatoid arthritis, including juvenile rheumatoid arthritis (selected cases may require low-dose maintenance therapy).
Ankylosing spondylitis.
Acute and subacute bursitis.
Acute nonspecific tenosynovitis.
Acute gouty arthritis.
Posttraumatic osteoarthritis.
Synovitis of osteoarthritis.
Epicondylitis.

3. Collagen Diseases:
During an exacerbation or as maintenance therapy in selected cases of -
Systemic lupus erythematosus.
Acute rheumatic carditis.

4. Dermatologic Diseases:
Pemphigus.
Bullous dermatitis herpetiformis.
Severe erythema multiforme (Stevens-Johnson syndrome).
Exfoliative dermatitis.
Mycosis fungoides.
Severe psoriasis.
Severe seborrheic dermatitis.

5. Allergic States:
Control of severe or incapacitating allergic conditions intractable to adequate trials of conventional treatment:
Seasonal or perennial allergic rhinitis.
Bronchial asthma.
Contact dermatitis.
Atopic dermatitis.
Serum sickness.
Drug hypersensitivity reactions.

6. Ophthalmic Diseases:
Severe acute and chronic allergic and inflammatory processes involving the eye and its adnexa such as -
Allergic conjunctivitis.
Keratitis.
Allergic corneal marginal ulcers.
Herpes zoster ophthalmicus.
Iritis and iridocyclitis.
Chorioretinitis.
Anterior segment inflammation.
Diffuse posterior uveitis and choroiditis.
Optic neuritis.
Sympathetic ophthalmia.

7. Respiratory Diseases:
Symptomatic sarcoidosis.
Loeffler's syndrome not manageable by other means.
Berylliosis.
Fulminating or disseminated pulmonary tuberculosis when used concurrently with appropriate antituberculous chemotherapy.
Aspiration pneumonitis.

8. Hematologic Disorders:
Idiopathic thrombocytopenic purpura in adults.
Secondary thrombocytopenia in adults.
Acquired (autoimmune) hemolytic anemia.
Erythroblastopenia (RBC anemia).
Congenital (erythroid) hypoplastic anemia.

9. Neoplastic Diseases:
For palliative management of:
Leukemias and lymphomas in adults.
Acute leukemia of childhood.

10. Edematous States:
To induce a diuresis or remission of proteinuria in the nephrotic syndrome, without uremia, of the idiopathic type or that due to lupus erythematosus.

11. Gastrointestinal Diseases:
To tide the patient over a critical period of the disease in:
Ulcerative colitis.
Regional enteritis.

12. Nervous System:
Acute exacerbations of multiple sclerosis.

13. Miscellaneous:
Tuberculous meningitis with subarachnoid block or impending block when used concurrently with appropriate antituberculous chemotherapy.
Trichinosis with neurologic or myocardial involvement.

CONTRAINDICATIONS
Systemic fungal infections.
Sensitivity to the drug or any of its components.

WARNINGS
In patients on corticosteroid therapy subjected to unusual stress, increased dosage of rapidly acting corticosteroids before, during, and after the stressful situation is indicated.

Corticosteroids may mask some signs of infection, and new infections may appear during their use. There may be decreased resistance and inability to localize infection when corticosteroids are used.

Prolonged use of corticosteroids may produce posterior subcapsular cataracts, glaucoma with possible damage to the optic nerves, and may enhance the establishment of secondary ocular infections due to fungi or viruses.

Usage in Pregnancy: Since adequate human reproduction studies have not been done with corticosteroids, the use of these drugs in pregnancy, nursing mothers or women of childbearing potential requires that the possible benefits of the drug be weighed against the potential hazards to the mother and embryo or fetus. Infants born of mothers who have received substantial doses of corticosteroids during pregnancy should be carefully observed for signs of hypoadrenalism.

Average and large doses of hydrocortisone or cortisone can cause elevation of blood pressure, salt and water retention, and increased excretion of potassium. These effects are less likely to occur with Triamcinolone except when used in large doses. Dietary salt restriction and potassium supplementation may be necessary. All corticosteroids increase calcium excretion.

While on corticosteroid therapy patients should not be vaccinated against smallpox. Other immunization procedures should not be undertaken in patients who are on corticosteroids, especially on high doses, because of possible hazards of neurological complications and lack of antibody response.

The use of Triamcinolone in active tuberculosis should be restricted to those cases of fulminating or disseminated tuberculosis in which the corticosteroid is used for the management of the disease in conjunction with appropriate antituberculous regimen.

If corticosteroids are indicated in patients with latent tuberculosis or tuberculin reactivity, close observation is necessary as reactivation of the disease may occur. During prolonged corticosteroid therapy, these patients should receive chemoprophylaxis.

Persons who are on drugs which suppress the immune system are more susceptible to infections than healthy individuals. Chickenpox and measles, for example, can have a more serious or even fatal course in nonimmune children or adults on corticosteroids. In such children or adults who have not had these diseases, particular care should be taken to avoid exposure. How the dose, route and duration of corticosteroid administration affects the risk of developing a disseminated infection is not known. The contribution of the underlying disease and/or prior corticosteroid treatment to the risk is also not known. If exposed to chickenpox, prophylaxis with varicella zoster immune globulin (VZIG) may be indicated. If exposed to measles, prophylaxis with pooled intramuscular immunoglobulin (IG) may be indicated. (See the respective package inserts for complete VZIG and IG prescribing information.) If chickenpox develops, treatment with antiviral agents may be considered.

PRECAUTIONS

Drug-induced secondary adrenocortical insufficiency may be minimized by gradual reduction of dosage. This type of relative insufficiency may persist for months after discontinuation of therapy; therefore, in any situation of stress occurring during that period, hormone therapy should be reinstituted. Since mineralocorticoid secretion may be impaired, salt and/or a mineralocorticoid should be administered concurrently.

There is an enhanced effect of corticosteroids on patients with hypothyroidism and in those with cirrhosis.

Corticosteroids should be used cautiously in patients with ocular herpes simplex because of possible corneal perforation.

The lowest possible dose of corticosteroids should be used to control the condition under treatment, and when reduction in dosage is possible, the reduction should be gradual.

Psychic derangements may appear when corticosteroids are used, ranging from euphoria, insomnia, mood swings, personality changes, and severe depression to frank psychotic manifestations. Also, existing emotional instability or psychotic tendencies may be aggravated by corticosteroids.

Aspirin should be used cautiously in conjunction with corticosteroids in hypoprothrombinemia.

Steroids should be used with caution in nonspecific ulcerative colitis if there is a probability of impending perforation, abscess or other pyogenic infection, diverticulitis, fresh intestinal anastomoses, active or latent peptic ulcer, renal insufficiency, hypertension, osteoporosis, and myasthenia gravis.

Growth and development of infants and children on prolonged corticosteroid therapy should be carefully observed.

Although controlled clinical trials have shown corticosteroids to be effective in speeding the resolution of acute exacerbations of multiple sclerosis they do not show that they affect the ultimate outcome or natural history of the disease. The studies do show that relatively high doses of corticosteroids are necessary to demonstrate a significant effect. (See "Dosage and Administration".)

Since complications of treatment with glucocorticoid are dependent on the size of the dose and the duration of treatment of risk/benefit decision must be made in each individual case as to dose and duration of treatment and as to whether daily or intermittent therapy should be used.

INFORMATION FOR PATIENTS

Persons who are on immunosuppressant doses of corticosteroids should be warned to avoid exposure to chickenpox or measles and should also be advised that if they are exposed, medical advice should be sought without delay.

ADVERSE REACTIONS

Fluid and electrolyte disturbances:
Sodium retention.
Fluid retention.
Congestive heart failure in susceptible patients.
Potassium loss.
Hypokalemic alkalosis.
Hypertension.

Musculoskeletal:
Muscle weakness.
Steroid myopathy.
Loss of muscle mass.
Osteoporosis.
Vertebral compression fractures.
Aseptic necrosis of femoral and humeral heads.
Pathologic fracture of long bones.

Gastrointestinal:
Peptic ulcer with possible subsequent perforation and hemorrhage.
Pancreatitis.
Abdominal distention.
Ulcerative esophagitis.

Dermatologic:
Impaired wound healing.
Thin fragile skin.
Petechiae and ecchymoses.

Facial erythema.
Increased sweating.
May suppress reactions to skin tests.

Neurological:
Convulsions.
Increased intracranial pressure with papilledema (pseudotumor cerebri) usually after treatment.
Vertigo.
Headache.

Endocrine:
Menstrual irregularities.
Development of cushingoid state.
Suppression of growth in children.
Secondary adrenocortical and pituitary unresponsiveness, particu- larly in times of stress, as in trauma, surgery or illness.
Decreased carbohydrate tolerance.
Manifestations of latent diabetes mellitus.
Increased requirements for insulin or oral hypoglycemic agents in diabetics.

Ophthalmic:
Posterior subcapsular cataracts.
Increased intraocular pressure.
Glaucoma.
Exophthalmos.

Metabolic:
Negative nitrogen balance due to protein catabolism.

Hypersensitivity Reactions:
Anaphylactoid reactions have been reported rarely with products of this class.

DOSAGE AND ADMINISTRATION

GENERAL PRINCIPLES

1. The initial dosage of Triamcinolone may vary from 4 to 48 mg per day depending on the specific disease entity being treated. In situations of less severity lower doses will generally suffice while in selected patients higher initial doses may be required. The initial dosage should be maintained or adjusted until a satisfactory response is noted. If after a reasonable period of time there is a lack of satisfactory clinical response, the drug should be discontinued and the patient transferred to other appropriate therapy. **IT SHOULD BE EMPHASIZED THAT DOSAGE REQUIREMENTS ARE VARIABLE AND MUST BE INDIVIDUALIZED ON THE BASIS OF THE DISEASE UNDER TREATMENT AND THE RESPONSE OF THE PATIENT.** After a favorable response is noted, the proper maintenance dosage should be determined by decreasing the initial drug dosage in small increments at appropriate time intervals until the lowest dosage is reached which will maintain an adequate clinical response. It should be kept in mind that constant monitoring is needed in regard to drug dosage. Included in the situations which may make dosage adjustments necessary are changes in clinical status secondary to remissions or exacerbations in the disease process, the patient's individual drug responsiveness, and the effect of patient exposure to stressful situations not directly related to the disease entity under treatment; in this latter situation it may be necessary to increase the dosage of Triamcinolone for a period of time consistent with the patient's condition. If after long-term therapy the drug is to be stopped, it is recommended that it be withdrawn gradually rather than abruptly.

2. Dosage should be individualized according to the severity of the disease and the response of the patient. For infants and children, the recommended dosage should be governed by the same considerations rather than by strict adherence to the ratio indicated by age or body weight.

3. Hormone therapy is an adjunct to, and not a replacement for, conventional therapy.

4. The severity, prognosis and expected duration of the disease and the reaction of the patient to medication are primary factors in determining dosage.

5. If a period of spontaneous remission occurs in a chronic condition, treatment should be discontinued.

6. Blood pressure, body weight, routine laboratory studies, including 2-hour postprandial blood glucose and serum potassium, and a chest X-ray should be obtained at regular intervals during prolonged therapy. Upper GI X-rays are desirable in patients with known or suspected peptic ulcer disease.

7. Suppression of autogenous pituitary function, a common effect of exogenous corticosteroids administration, may be reduced, modified or minimized by revision of dose schedules. The time of maximum corticoid effect is from midnight to 8 AM and minimal during the intervening hours. Use of a single daily dose at or about 8 AM will be effective in most conditions, will lower corticoid overload and will cause the least interference with the diurnal system of endogenous secretion and hypothalamo-pituitary-adrenal function; alternate-day dosage in some conditions in certain severe disorders requiring long-term and/or high dose maintenance levels have proven both clinically effective and less likely to produce adverse reactions.

The maximum daily morning dose not associated with lasting adrenocorticoid suppression is 8 mg.

8. *Alternate-Day Therapy:* After the conventional dose has been established, some patients may be maintained on alternate-day therapy. It has been shown that the activity of the adrenal cortex varies throughout the day, being greatest from about midnight to 8:00 AM. Exogenous corticoid suppresses this activity least when given at the time of maximum activity. A 48 hour interval appears to be necessary since shorter intervals are accompanied by adrenal suppression similar to that of conventional daily divided doses. Therefore, with the alternate-day dose plan, a

---

◆ RATED THERAPEUTICALLY EQUIVALENT; ◇ THERAPEUTIC EQUIVALENCE UNCONFIRMED; ○ UNRATED

	Anti-Inflammatory Relative Potency		Frequently Used Tablet Strength (mg)		Tablet X Potency Equivalent Value
Hydrocortisone	1	X	20	=	20
Prednisolone	4	X	5	=	20
Triamcinolone	5	X	4	=	20
Dexamethasone	25	X	0.75	=	18.75

total 48-hour requirement is given every other day at 8:00 AM. As with other regimens, the minimum effective dose level should be sought.

SPECIFIC DOSAGE RECOMMENDATIONS

1. Endocrine Disorders: Wide variation in dosage requirements for the endocrine disorders such as *congenital adrenal hyperplasia, non-suppurative thyroiditis,* and *hypercalcemia* associated with *cancer* precludes specific recommendation except for *adrenocortical insufficiency* where the dose is usually 4-12 mg daily in addition to mineralocorticoid therapy.

2. Rheumatic Disorders: Rheumatoid arthritis; acute gouty arthritis; ankylosing spondylitis; and *selected cases of psoriatic arthritis;* in *acute* and *subacute bursitis;* and in *acute nonspecific tenosynovitis.* The initial suppressive dose of Triamcinolone in these conditions ranges from 8 to 16 mg per day, although the occasional patient may require higher doses.

Patients may show an early or a delayed effect, characterized by a reduction in the inflammatory reaction and in joint swelling, together with alleviation of pain and stiffness, resulting in an increased range of motion of the affected joints or tissues. Maintenance doses are adjusted to keep symptoms at a level tolerable to the patient. Rapid reduction of the steroid or its abrupt discontinuance may result in recurrence or even exacerbation of signs and symptoms. Short-term administration is desirable as a rule. Triamcinolone is ordinarily administered as a single morning dose, daily or on alternate days, depending on the need of the patient. Occasional patients may secure more effective relief on divided daily doses, either 2 to 4 times daily.

3. Collagen Diseases: Systemic Lupus Erythematosus: The initial dose is usually 20 to 32 mg daily continued until the desired response is obtained, when reduced maintenance levels are sought. Patients with more severe symptoms may require higher initial doses, 48 mg or more daily, and higher maintenance doses. Although some patients with systemic lupus erythematosus appear to have spontaneous remissions or to tolerate the disorder in its milder forms for prolonged periods of time, adjustment of dosage scheduling to reduce adverse suppression of the pituitary-adrenal axis may be useful.

Acute Rheumatic Carditis: In severely ill patients with carditis, pericardial effusion and/or congestive heart failure, corticosteroid therapy is effective in the control of the acute and severe inflammatory changes and may be lifesaving. Initial doses of Triamcinolone may be from 20 to 60 mg daily, and clinical response is usually rapid and the drug can then be reduced. Maintenance therapy should be continued for at least 6 to 8 weeks and is seldom required beyond a period of 3 months. Corticosteroid therapy does not preclude conventional treatment, including antibiotics and salicylization.

4. Dermatological Disorders: Pemphigus; bullous dermatitis herpetiformis; severe erythema multiforme (Stevens-Johnson syndrome); *exfoliative dermatitis;* and *mycosis fungoides.* The initial dose is 8 to 16 mg daily. In these conditions, as well as in certain allergic dermatoses, *alternate-day* administration has been found effective and apparently less likely to produce adverse side effects.

Severe psoriasis: Triamcinolone may produce reduction or remission of the disabling skin manifestations following initial doses of 8 to 16 mg daily. The period of maintenance is dependent on the clinical response. Corticosteroid reduction or discontinuation of therapy should be attempted with caution since relapse may occur and may appear in a more aggravated form, the so-called "rebound phenomenon."

5. Allergic States: Triamcinolone is administered in doses of 8 to 12 mg daily in acute seasonal or perennial *allergic rhinitis.* Intractable cases may require high initial and maintenance doses. In *bronchial asthma,* 8 to 16 mg daily are usually effective. The usual therapeutic measures for control of bronchial asthma should be carried out in addition to Triamcinolone therapy. In both allergic rhinitis and bronchial asthma, therapy is directed at alleviation of acute distress and chronic long-term use of corticosteroids is neither desirable nor often essential. Some patients may be maintained on alternate-day therapy. In such conditions as *contact dermatitis* and *atopic dermatitis,* topical therapy may be supplemented with short courses of Triamcinolone by mouth in doses of 8 to 16 mg daily. In severely ill patients with *serum sickness,* epinephrine may be the drug of choice for immediate therapy, often supplemented by antihistamines.

Triamcinolone is frequently useful as adjunctive treatment in such cases, with the dosage determined by the severity of the disorder, the speed with which therapeutic response is desired and the response of the patient to initial therapy.

6. Ophthalmological Diseases: Allergic conjunctivitis; keratitis; iridocyclitis; chorioretinitis; anterior segment inflammation; diffuse posterior uveitis and *choroiditis; optic neuritis* and *sympathetic ophthalmia.* Initial doses range from 12 to 40 mg daily depending on the severity of the condition, the nature and degree of involvement of ocular structure, but response is usually rapid and therapy of short-term duration.

7. Respiratory Diseases: Symptomatic sarcoidosis; Loeffler's syndrome; berylliosis; and in certain cases of *fulminating* or *disseminated pulmonary tuberculosis* when concurrently accompanied by appropriate antituberculous chemotherapy. Initial doses are usually in the range of 16 to 48 mg daily.

8. Hematologic Disorders: Idiopathic and *secondary thrombocytopenia* in *adults,* acquired *(autoimmune) hemolytic anemia; erythroblastopenia (RBC anemia); congenital (erythroid) hypoplastic anemia.* Triamcinolone is used to produce a remission of symptoms and may, in some instances, produce an apparent regression of abnormal cellular blood elements to normal states, temporary or permanent. The recommended dose varies between 16 and 60 mg daily, with reduction after adequate clinical response.

9. Neoplastic Diseases: Acute leukemia in childhood: The usual dose of Triamcinolone is 1 mg per kilogram of body weight daily, although as much as 2 mg per kilogram may be necessary. Initial response is usually seen within 6 to 21 days and therapy continued from 4 to 6 weeks.

Acute leukemia and lymphoma in adults: The usual dose of Triamcinolone is 16 to 40 mg daily, although it may be necessary to give as much as 100 mg daily in leukemia. Triamcinolone therapy in these neoplasias is only palliative and not curative. Other therapeutic and supportive measures must be used when appropriate.

10. Edematous States: Nephrotic Syndrome: Triamcinolone may be used to induce a diuresis or remission of proteinuria in the nephrotic syndrome, without uremia, of the idiopathic type or that due to lupus erythematosus. The average dose is 16 to 20 mg (up to 48 mg) daily until diuresis occurs. The diuresis may be massive and usually occurs by the 14th day, but occasionally may be delayed. After diuresis begins it is advisable to continue treatment until maximal or complete chemical and clinical remission occurs, at which time the dosage should be reduced gradually and then discontinued. In less severe cases maintenance dosages of as little as 4 mg daily may be adequate. Alternatively and when maintenance therapy may be prolonged, Triamcinolone may be administered on alternate-day dose schedules.

11. Miscellaneous: Tuberculous Meningitis: Triamcinolone may be useful when accompanied by appropriate antituberculous therapy when there is subarachnoid block or impending block. The average dosage is 32 to 48 mg daily in either single or divided doses. (See related table).

STORAGE
Store at controlled room temperature, 15°-30°C (59°-86°F).

HOW SUPPLIED
TABLETS: 1 MG

BRAND/MANUFACTURER	NDC	SIZE	AWP
◇ BRAND			
ARISTOCORT: Fujisawa	57317-0602-50	50s	$17.23

TABLETS: 2 MG

BRAND/MANUFACTURER	NDC	SIZE	AWP
◇ BRAND			
ARISTOCORT: Fujisawa	57317-0601-10	100s	$72.52

TABLETS: 4 MG

BRAND/MANUFACTURER	NDC	SIZE	AWP
◇ BRAND			
ARISTOPAK: Fujisawa	57317-0600-16	16s	$20.05
ARISTOCORT: Fujisawa	57317-0600-30	30s	$41.44
	57317-0600-10	100s	$131.23
◇ GENERICS			
Qualitest	00603-6170-14	16s	$9.72
Major	00904-0884-44	16s	$10.45
Horizon Pharm Inc	60904-0454-35	16s	$13.50
Major	00904-0884-60	100s	$7.90
Schein	00364-0352-01	100s	$7.95
Aligen	00405-5042-01	100s	$8.07
Richlyn	00115-4840-01	100s	$10.45
Richlyn	00115-4840-02	500s	$27.00
Richlyn	00115-4840-03	1000s	$80.40

TABLETS: 8 MG

BRAND/MANUFACTURER	NDC	SIZE	AWP
◇ BRAND			
ARISTOCORT: Fujisawa	57317-0603-50	50s	$107.57

Triamcinolone Acetonide, Inhalation

DESCRIPTION
Triamcinolone Acetonide, Inhalation, is a glucocorticosteroid with a molecular weight of 434.5 and with the chemical designation 9-Fluoro-11β, 16α, 17, 21-

tetrahydroxypregna-1, 4-diene-3, 20-dione cyclic 16, 17-acetal with acetone. ($C_{24}H_{31}FO_6$).

It is available as an oral and a nasal inhaler.

Triamcinolone Acetonide oral and nasal inhalers are metered-dose aerosol units containing a microcrystalline suspension of Triamcinolone Acetonide in propellant. Each canister of oral inhaler contains 60 mg Triamcinolone Acetonide; each canister of nasal inhaler contains 15 mg. Each actuation of the oral inhaler releases approximately 200 mcg Triamcinolone Acetonide, of which approximately 100 mcg are delivered from the unit (in-vitro testing). There are at least 240 actuations in one Triamcinolone Acetonide aerosol canister. After 240 actuations, the amount delivered per actuation may not be consistent and the unit should be discarded. Each actuation of the nasal inhaler releases approximately 55 mcg Triamcinolone Acetonide from the nasal actuator to the patient (estimated from in vitro testing). There are at least 100 actuations in one Triamcinolone Acetonide nasal inhaler canister. After 100 actuations, the amount delivered per actuation may not be consistent and the unit should be discarded.

Following is its chemical structure:

CLINICAL PHARMACOLOGY

The precise mechanism of the action of the inhaled drug is unknown. However, use of the inhaler makes it possible to provide effective local steroid activity with minimal systemic effect.

Triamcinolone Acetonide is a more potent derivative of Triamcinolone. Although Triamcinolone itself is approximately one to two times as potent as prednisone in animal models of inflammation, Triamcinolone Acetonide is approximately 8 times more potent than prednisone.

Although the precise mechanism of glucocorticoid antiallergic action is unknown, glucocorticoids are very effective. However, when allergic symptoms are very severe, local treatment with recommended doses (microgram) of any available aerosolized corticoid are not as effective as treatment with larger doses (milligram) of oral or parenteral formulations.

Corticoids do not have an immediate effect on allergic signs and symptoms. Treatment effects may be observed as early as 12 hours after onset of treatment and, generally, it takes 3-4 days to reach maximum benefit. Similarly when corticoids are prematurely discontinued symptoms may not recur for several days.

Pharmacokinetic studies with radiolabeled Triamcinolone Acetonide have been carried out by the oral route and intravenous route in several species. The pharmacokinetic behavior of the Triamcinolone Acetonide was similar in all species within each route of administration. The major portion of the dose was eliminated in the feces irrespective of route of administration with only one species (rabbit) showing significant urinary excretion of radioactivity.

The results of studies in which Triamcinolone Acetonide was administered as an aerosol showed rapid disappearance of radioactivity from the lungs comparable to that observed following oral administration with peak blood levels occurring in one to two hours. Virtually no radioactivity was present in the lung and trachea 24 hours after dosing.

Based upon intravenous dosing of Triamcinolone Acetonide phosphate ester, the half-life of Triamcinolone Acetonide was reported to be 88 minutes. The volume of distribution (Vd) reported was 99.5 L (SD ± 27.5) and clearance was 45.2 L/hour (SD ± 9.1) for Triamcinolone Acetonide. The plasma half-life of corticoids does not correlate well with the biologic half-life.

When administered intranasally to man at 440 mcg/day dose, the peak plasma concentration was < 1ng/mL and occurred on average at 3.4 hours (range 0.5-8.0 hours) post dosing. The apparent half-life was 4.0 hours (range 1.0-7.0 hours); however, this value probably reflects lingering absorption. Intranasal doses below 440 mcg/day gave sparse data and did not allow for the calculation of meaningful pharmacokinetic parameters.

Three metabolites of Triamcinolone Acetonide have been identified. They are 6β-hydroxytriamcinolone acetonide, 21-carboxytriamcinolone acetonide and 21-carboxy-6β-hydroxytriamcinolone acetonide. All three metabolites are expected to be substantially less active than the parent compound due to (a) the dependence of anti-inflammatory activity on the presence of a 21-hydroxyl group, (b) the decreased activity observed upon 6-hydroxylation, and (c) the markedly increased water solubility favoring rapid elimination. There appeared to be some quantitative differences in the metabolites among species. No differences were detected in metabolic pattern as a function of route of administration.

CLINICAL TRIALS

Nasal Inhaler: In double-blind, parallel, placebo-controlled clinical trials of seasonal and perennial allergic rhinitis, in fixed total daily doses of 110, 220 and 440 mcg per day, the responses to aerosolized Triamcinolone Acetonide demonstrated a statistically significant improvement over placebo. In open label trials where the doses were sometimes adjusted according to patient's signs and symptoms, the daily doses and regimens varied. The most commonly used dose was 110 mcg per day.

In attempting to determine if systemic absorption played a role in the response to Triamcinolone Acetonide nasal inhalation a clinical study comparing intranasal and depot intramuscular Triamcinolone Acetonide was conducted. The doses used were based on bioavailability studies of each formulation. The final doses of Triamcinolone Acetonide nasal inhalation 440 mcg once a day and Triamcinolone Acetonide suspension, 4 mg intramuscularly once a week, were chosen to deliver comparable total amounts of weekly Triamcinolone Acetonide. However, the weekly injection yielded sustained plasma levels throughout the dosing interval while the daily Triamcinolone Acetonide nasal inhalation resulted in daily peak and trough concentrations, the mean of which was 3.5 times below the plasma levels obtained with the Triamcinolone intramuscular injections. Both topical Triamcinolone Acetonide nasal inhalation, and intramuscular Triamcinolone Acetonide suspension were clinically effective. In addition, in some studies there was evidence of improvement of eye symptoms. This suggests that Triamcinolone Acetonide nasal inhalation, at least to some degree, is acting by a systemic mechanism.

In order to evaluate the effects of systemic absorption on the hypothalamic-pituitary-adrenal (HPA) axis, Triamcinolone Acetonide nasal inhalation in doses of 440 mcg once a day was compared to placebo and 42 days of a single morning dose of prednisone 10 mg. Adrenal response to a six-hour cosyntropin stimulation test suggests that intranasal Triamcinolone Acetonide 440 mcg/day for six weeks did not measurably affect adrenal activity. Conversely, oral prednisone at 10 mg/day significantly reduced the response to ACTH.

INDIVIDUALIZATION OF DOSAGE

Individual patients will experience a variable time to onset and degree of symptom relief when using Triamcinolone Acetonide nasal inhalation. It is recommended that dosing be started at 220 mcg once a day and the effect be assessed in four-seven days. Some relief can be expected in approximately two-thirds of patients within that time. If greater effect is desired an increase of dose to 440 mcg once a day can be tried. If adequate relief has not been obtained by the third week of Triamcinolone Acetonide nasal inhalation treatment, consideration to alternate forms of treatment should be given.

A dose-response between 110 mcg/day (one spray/nostril/day) and 440 mcg/day (four sprays/nostril/day) is not clearly discernible. In general, in the clinical trials the highest dose tended to provide relief sooner. This suggests an alternative approach to starting therapy with Triamcinolone Acetonide nasal inhalation, e.g., starting treatment with 440 mcg (four sprays/nostril/day) and then, depending on the patient's response, decreasing the dose by one spray per day every four to seven days.

Although Triamcinolone Acetonide nasal inhalation may be used at 220 mcg/day or 440 mcg/day divided into two or four times a day, the degree of relief does not seem to be significantly different compared to once-a-day dosing. As with other nasal corticoids, the vehicle used to deliver the corticoid may cause symptoms that are difficult to distinguish from the patient's rhinitis symptoms. Thus, depending upon the balance between these vehicle side effects and the benefits of treatment, in determining the optimal dose for the relief of symptoms, individual patients may need to have a trial of high and low doses.

After symptoms have been brought under control, reducing the daily dose to 110 mcg has been shown to be effective in control of symptoms in approximately one half of patients being treated long term for allergic rhinitis. It is always desirable to titrate an individual patient to the minimum effective dose to reduce the possibility of side effects (see *"Precautions"*, *"Warnings"*, *"Information for Patients"* and *"Adverse Reactions"* sections).

INDICATIONS

Triamcinolone Acetonide oral inhaler is indicated only for patients who require chronic treatment with corticosteroids for the control of the symptoms of bronchial asthma. Such patients would include those already receiving systemic corticosteroids and selected patients who are inadequately controlled on a non-steroid regimen and in whom steroid therapy has been withheld because of concern over potential adverse effects.

Triamcinolone Acetonide oral inhaler is *not* indicated:

1. For relief of asthma which can be controlled by bronchodilators and other non-steroid medications.
2. In patients who require systemic corticosteroid treatment infrequently.
3. In the treatment of non-asthmatic bronchitis.

Triamcinolone Acetonide nasal inhaler is indicated for the nasal treatment of seasonal and perennial allergic rhinitis symptoms.

CONTRAINDICATIONS

Triamcinolone Acetonide oral inhaler is contraindicated in the primary treatment of status asthmaticus or other acute episodes of asthma where intensive measures are required.

Hypersensitivity to any of the ingredients of either the oral or the nasal inhaler contraindicates its use.

WARNINGS

PARTICULAR CARE IS NEEDED IN PATIENTS WHO ARE TRANSFERRED FROM SYSTEMICALLY ACTIVE CORTICOSTEROIDS TO TRIAMCINOLONE ACETONIDE ORAL INHALER BECAUSE DEATHS DUE TO ADRENAL INSUFFICIENCY HAVE OCCURRED IN ASTHMATIC PATIENTS DURING AND AFTER TRANSFER FROM SYSTEMIC CORTICOSTEROIDS TO

AEROSOLIZED STEROIDS IN RECOMMENDED DOSES. AFTER WITHDRAWAL FROM SYSTEMIC CORTICOSTEROIDS, A NUMBER OF MONTHS IS USUALLY REQUIRED FOR RECOVERY OF HYPOTHALAMIC-PITUITARY-ADRENAL (HPA) FUNCTION. FOR SOME PATIENTS WHO HAVE RECEIVED LARGE DOSES OF ORAL STEROIDS FOR LONG PERIODS OF TIME BEFORE THERAPY WITH TRIAMCINOLONE ACETONIDE ORAL INHALER IS INITIATED, RECOVERY MAY BE DELAYED FOR ONE YEAR OR LONGER. DURING THIS PERIOD OF HPA SUPPRESSION, PATIENTS MAY EXHIBIT SIGNS AND SYMPTOMS OF ADRENAL INSUFFICIENCY WHEN EXPOSED TO TRAUMA, SURGERY OR INFECTIONS, PARTICULARLY GASTROENTERITIS OR OTHER CONDITIONS WITH ACUTE ELECTROLYTE LOSS. THE REPLACEMENT OF A SYSTEMIC CORTICOSTEROID WITH A TOPICAL CORTICOID CAN BE ACCOMPANIED BY SIGNS OF ADRENAL INSUFFICIENCY AND, IN ADDITION, SOME PATIENTS MAY EXPERIENCE SYMPTOMS OF WITHDRAWAL, *E.G.*, JOINT AND/OR MUSCULAR PAIN, LASSITUDE AND DEPRESSION. PATIENTS PREVIOUSLY TREATED FOR PROLONGED PERIODS WITH SYSTEMIC CORTICOSTEROIDS AND TRANSFERRED TO TOPICAL CORTICOIDS SHOULD BE CAREFULLY MONITORED FOR ACUTE ADRENAL INSUFFICIENCY IN RESPONSE TO STRESS. IN THOSE PATIENTS WHO HAVE ASTHMA OR OTHER CLINICAL CONDITIONS REQUIRING LONG-TERM SYSTEMIC CORTICOSTEROID TREATMENT, TOO RAPID A DECREASE IN SYSTEMIC CORTICOSTEROIDS MAY CAUSE A SEVERE EXACERBATION OF THEIR SYMPTOMS. ALTHOUGH TRIAMCINOLONE ACETONIDE ORAL INHALER MAY PROVIDE CONTROL OF ASTHMATIC SYMPTOMS DURING THESE EPISODES, IN RECOMMENDED DOSES IT SUPPLIES ONLY NORMAL PHYSIOLOGICAL AMOUNTS OF CORTICOSTEROID SYSTEMICALLY AND DOES NOT PROVIDE THE INCREASED SYSTEMIC STEROID WHICH IS NECESSARY FOR COPING WITH THESE EMERGENCIES.

DURING PERIODS OF STRESS OR A SEVERE ASTHMATIC ATTACK, PATIENTS WHO HAVE BEEN RECENTLY WITHDRAWN FROM SYSTEMIC CORTICOSTEROIDS SHOULD BE INSTRUCTED TO RESUME SYSTEMIC STEROIDS (IN LARGE DOSES) IMMEDIATELY AND TO CONTACT THEIR PHYSICIAN FOR FURTHER INSTRUCTION. THESE PATIENTS SHOULD ALSO BE INSTRUCTED TO CARRY A WARNING CARD INDICATING THAT THEY MAY NEED SUPPLEMENTARY SYSTEMIC STEROIDS DURING PERIODS OF STRESS OR A SEVERE ASTHMA ATTACK.

Localized infections with *Candida albicans* have occurred infrequently in the mouth and pharynx with Triamcinolone Acetonide oral inhaler. These areas should be examined by the treating physician at each patient visit. The percentage of positive mouth and throat cultures for *Candida albicans* did not change during a year of continuous therapy. The incidence of clinically apparent infection is low (2.5%). These infections may disappear spontaneously or may require treatment with appropriate antifungal therapy or discontinuance of treatment with Triamcinolone Acetonide oral inhaler.

In clinical studies with Triamcinolone Acetonide administered intranasally, the development of localized infections of the nose and pharynx with *Candida albicans* has rarely occurred. When such an infection develops it may require treatment with appropriate local therapy and discontinuance of treatment with Triamcinolone Acetonide nasal inhaler.

Children who are on immunosuppressant drugs are more susceptible to infections than healthy children. Chickenpox and measles, for example, can have a more serious or even fatal course in children on immunosuppressant doses of corticosteroids. In such children, or in adults who have not had these diseases, particular care should be taken to avoid exposure. If exposed, therapy with varicella zoster immune globulin (VZIG) or pooled intravenous immunoglobulin (IVIG), as appropriate, may be indicated. If chickenpox develops, treatment with antiviral agents may be considered.

Triamcinolone Acetonide oral inhaler is not to be regarded as a bronchodilator and is not indicated for rapid relief of bronchospasm. Patients should be instructed to contact their physician immediately when episodes of asthma which are not responsive to bronchodilators occur during the course of treatment with Triamcinolone Acetonide oral inhaler. During such episodes, patients may require therapy with systemic corticosteroids.

There is no evidence that control of asthma can be achieved by the administration of Triamcinolone Acetonide oral inhaler in amounts greater than the recommended doses, which appear to be the therapeutic equivalent of approximately 10 mg/day of oral prednisone.

The use of Triamcinolone Acetonide oral inhaler with alternate-day systemic prednisone could increase the likelihood of HPA suppression compared to a therapeutic dose of either one alone. Therefore Triamcinolone Acetonide oral or nasal inhaler should be used with caution in patients already receiving alternate-day prednisone treatment for any disease.

Transfer of patients from systemic steroid therapy to Triamcinolone Acetonide oral inhaler may unmask allergic conditions previously suppressed by the systemic steroid therapy, e.g., rhinitis, conjunctivitis, and eczema.

PRECAUTIONS
During withdrawal from oral steroids, some patients may experience symptoms of systemically active steroid withdrawal, e.g., joint and/or muscular pain, lassitude

and depression, despite maintenance or even improvement of respiratory function (see "*Dosage and Administration*" for details). Although steroid withdrawal effects are usually transient and not severe, severe and even fatal exacerbation of asthma can occur if the previous daily oral corticosteroid requirement had significantly exceeded 10 mg/day of prednisone or equivalent.

In responsive patients, inhaled corticosteroids will often permit control of asthmatic symptoms with less suppression of HPA function than therapeutically equivalent oral doses of prednisone. Since Triamcinolone Acetonide is absorbed into the circulation and can be systemically active, the beneficial effects of Triamcinolone Acetonide oral inhaler in minimizing or preventing HPA dysfunction may be expected only when recommended dosages are not exceeded.

Suppression of HPA function has been reported in volunteers who received 4000 mcg daily of Triamcinolone Acetonide. In addition, suppression of HPA function has been reported in some patients who have received recommended doses for as little as 6-12 weeks. Since the response of HPA function to inhaled corticosteroids is highly individualized, the physician should consider this information when treating patients.

Because of the possibility of systemic absorption of inhaled corticosteroids, patients treated with these drugs should be observed carefully for any evidence of systemic corticosteroid effects including suppression of growth in children. Particular care should be taken in observing patients post-operatively or during periods of stress for evidence of a decrease in adrenal function.

The long-term effects of Triamcinolone Acetonide inhaler in human subjects are not completely known, although patients have received Triamcinolone Acetonide oral inhaler on a continuous basis for periods of two years or longer. While there has been no clinical evidence of adverse experiences, the local effects of the agent on developmental or immunologic processes in the mouth, pharynx, trachea and lung are also unknown.

Triamcinolone Acetonide Oral Inhaler should be used with caution, if at all, in patients with active or quiescent tuberculous infections of the respiratory tract or in patients with untreated fungal, bacterial, or systemic viral infections or ocular herpes simplex. The potential effects of long-term administration of Triamcinolone Acetonide Oral Inhaler on lung or other tissues are unknown. However, pulmonary infiltrates with eosinophilia have occurred in patients receiving other inhaled corticosteroids.

When used at excessive doses, systemic corticosteroid effects such as hypercorticism and adrenal suppression may appear. If such changes occur, Triamcinolone Acetonide oral or nasal inhaler should be discontinued slowly, consistent with accepted procedures for discontinuing oral steroid therapy.

Triamcinolone Acetonide administered intranasally has been shown to be absorbed into the systemic circulation in humans. Patients with active rhinitis showed absorption similar to that found in normal volunteers. Triamcinolone Acetonide at 440 mcg/day for 42 days did not measurably affect adrenal response to a six hour cosyntropin test. In the same study prednisone 10 mg/day significantly reduced adrenal response to ACTH over the same period (see "*Clinical Trials*" section).

Triamcinolone Acetonide nasal inhaler should be used with caution, if at all, in patients with active or quiescent tuberculous infections of the respiratory tract or in patients with untreated fungal, bacterial, or systemic viral infections or ocular herpes simplex.

Because of the inhibitory effect of corticosteroids on wound healing in patients who have experienced recent nasal septal ulcers, nasal surgery or trauma, a corticosteroid should be used with caution until healing has occurred. As with other nasally inhaled corticosteroids, nasal septal perforations have been reported in rare instances.

Information for Patients: Patients who are on immunosuppressant doses of corticosteroids should be warned to avoid exposure to chickenpox or measles and, if exposed, to obtain medical advice.

Patients should use Triamcinolone Acetonide nasal inhaler at regular intervals since its effectiveness depends on its regular use. A decrease in symptoms may occur as soon as 12 hours after starting steroid therapy and generally can be expected to occur within a few days of initiating therapy in allergic rhinitis. The patient should take the medication as directed and should not exceed the prescribed dosage. The patient should contact the physician if symptoms do not improve after three weeks, or if the condition worsens. Nasal irritation and/or burning or stinging after use of the spray occur only rarely with this product. The patient should contact the physician if they occur.

Because that dispensed per puff may not be consistent, it is important to shake the canister well. Also, the canister should be discarded after 100 actuations.

Carcinogenesis, Mutagenesis: Animal studies of Triamcinolone Acetonide to tests its carcinogenic potential are underway.

Impairment of Fertility: Male and female rats which were administered oral Triamcinolone Acetonide at doses as high as 15 mcg/kg/day (110 mcg/m^2/day, as calculated on a surface area basis) exhibited no evidence of impaired fertility. The maximum human dose, for comparison, is 22.9 mcg/kg/day (889 mcg/m^2/day). However, a few female rats which received maternally toxic doses of 8 or 15 mcg/kg/day (60 mcg/m^2/day or 110 mcg/m^2/day, respectively, as calculated on a surface area basis) exhibited dystocia and prolonged delivery. Developmental toxicity, which included increases in fetal resorptions and stillbirths and decreases in pup body weight and survival, also occurred at the maternally toxic doses (2.5-15.0 mcg/kg/day or 20-110 mcg/m^2/day, as calculated on a surface area basis). Reproductive performance of female rats and effects on fetuses and offspring were comparable between groups that received placebo and non-toxic or marginally toxic doses (0.5 and 1.0 mcg/kg/day or 3.8 mcg/m^2/day and 7.0 mcg/m^2/day).

Pregnancy: Pregnancy Category C. Like other corticoids, Triamcinolone Acetonide has been shown to be teratogenic in rats and rabbits. Teratogenic effects, which occurred in both species at 0.02, 0.04 and 0.08 mg/kg/day (approximately 135, 270 and 540 mcg/m^2/day in the rat and 320, 640 and 1280 mcg/m^2/day in the rabbit, as calculated on a surface area basis), included a low incidence of cleft palate and/or internal hydrocephaly and axial skeletal defects. Teratogenic effects, including CNS and cranial malformations, have also been observed in non-human primates at 0.5 mg/kg/day (approximately 6.7 mg/m^2/day). The doses of 0.02, 0.04, 0.08, and 0.5 mg/kg/day used in these toxicology studies are approximately 12.8, 25.5, 51, and 318.7 times the minimum recommended dose of 110 mcg of Triamcinolone Acetonide nasal inhaler per day and 3.2, 6.4, 12.7, and 80 times the maximum recommended dose of 440 mcg of Triamcinolone Acetonide nasal inhaler per day based on a patient body weight of 70 kg. Administration of aerosol by inhalation to pregnant rats and rabbits produced embryotoxic and fetotoxic effects which were comparable to those produced by administration by other routes. There are no adequate and well-controlled studies in pregnant women. Triamcinolone Acetonide should be used during pregnancy only if the potential benefit justifies the potential risk to the fetus.

Experience with oral corticoids since their introduction in pharmacologic as opposed to physiologic doses suggests that rodents are more prone to teratogenic effects from corticoids than humans. In addition, because there is a natural increase in glucocorticoid production during pregnancy, most women will require a lower exogenous steroid dose and many will not need corticoid treatment during pregnancy.

Nonteratogenic Effects: Hypoadrenalism may occur in infants born of mothers receiving corticosteroids during pregnancy. Such infants should be carefully observed.

Nursing Mothers: It is not known whether Triamcinolone Acetonide is excreted in human milk. Because other corticosteroids are excreted in human milk, caution should be exercised when Triamcinolone Acetonide oral or nasal inhalation is administered to nursing women.

Pediatric Use: Safety and effectiveness of Triamcinolone Acetonide oral inhalation have not been established in children below the age of 6. Safety and effectiveness of Triamcinolone Acetonide nasal inhalation have not been established in children below the age of 12. Oral corticoids have been shown to cause growth suppression in children and teenagers, particularly with higher doses over extended periods. If a child or teenager on any corticoid appears to have growth suppression, the possibility that they are particularly sensitive to this effect of steroids should be considered.

ADVERSE REACTIONS
ORAL INHALATION
A few cases of oral candidiasis have been reported (see *"Warnings"*). In addition, some patients receiving Triamcinolone Acetonide oral inhaler have experienced hoarseness, dry throat, irritated throat and dry mouth. Increased wheezing and cough have been reported infrequently as has facial edema. These adverse effects have generally been mild and transient.

NASAL INHALATION
In controlled and uncontrolled studies, 1257 patients received treatment with intranasal Triamcinolone Acetonide. Adverse reactions are based on the 567 patients who received a product similar to Triamcinolone Acetonide nasal inhaler. These patients were treated for an average of 48 days (range 1 to 117 days). The 145 patients enrolled in uncontrolled studies received treatment from 1 to 820 days (average 332 days). The most prevalent adverse experience was headache, being reported by approximately 18% of the patients who received Triamcinolone Acetonide nasal inhaler. Nasal irritation was reported by 2.8% of the patients receiving Triamcinolone Acetonide nasal inhaler. Other nasopharyngeal side effects were reported by fewer than 5% of the patients who received Triamcinolone Acetonide nasal inhaler and included: dry mucous membranes, naso-sinus congestion, throat discomfort, sneezing, and epistaxis. The complaints do not usually interfere with treatment and in the controlled and uncontrolled studies approximately 1% of patients have discontinued because of these nasal adverse effects.

In the event of accidental overdose, an increased potential for these adverse experiences may be expected, but systemic adverse experiences are unlikely (see *"Overdosage"* section).

OVERDOSAGE
Acute overdosage with the nasal inhaler is unlikely. The acute topical application of the entire 15 mg of the canister would most likely cause nasal irritation and headache. One would be unlikely to see acute systemic adverse effects if the nasal application of 15 mg of Triamcinolone Acetonide were administered all at once.

DOSAGE AND ADMINISTRATION
ORAL INHALATION
All patients should be instructed that the Triamcinolone Acetonide oral inhaler must be used on a regular daily basis rather than *prn*. Reliable dosage delivery cannot be assured after 240 actuations and patients should be cautioned against longer use of individual canisters.

Good oral hygiene including rinsing of the mouth after inhalation is recommended.

Adults: The usual dosage is two inhalations (approximately 200 mcg) given three to four times a day. The maximal daily intake should not exceed 16 inhalations (1600 mcg) in adults. Higher initial doses (12-16 inhalations per day) may be

advisable in patients with more severe asthma, the dosage then being adjusted downward according to the response of the patient. In some patients maintenance can be accomplished when the total daily dose is given on a twice a day schedule.

Children 6 to 12 Years of Age: The usual dosage is one or two inhalations (100 to 200 mcg) given three to four times a day according to the response of the patient. The maximum daily intake should not exceed 12 inhalations (1200 mcg) in children 6 to 12 years of age. Insufficient clinical data exist with respect to the administration of Triamcinolone Acetonide Oral Inhaler in children below the age of 6. The long-term effects of inhaled steroids on growth are still under evaluation.

Patients receiving bronchodilators by inhalation should be advised to use the bronchodilator before Triamcinolone Acetonide oral inhaler in order to enhance penetration of Triamcinolone Acetonide into the bronchial tree. After use of an aerosol bronchodilator, several minutes should elapse before use of the Triamcinolone Acetonide oral inhaler to reduce the potential toxicity from the inhaled fluorocarbon propellants in the two aerosols.

Different considerations must be given to the following groups of patients in order to obtain the full therapeutic benefit of Triamcinolone Acetonide oral inhaler.

Patients Not Receiving Systemic Steroids: The use of Triamcinolone Acetonide oral inhaler is straightforward in patients who are inadequately controlled with non-steroid medications but in whom systemic steroid therapy has been withheld because of concern over potential adverse reactions. In patients who respond to Triamcinolone Acetonide, an improvement in pulmonary function is usually apparent within one to two weeks after the start of Triamcinolone Acetonide oral inhaler.

Patients Receiving Systemic Steroids: In those patients dependent on systemic steroids, transfer to Triamcinolone Acetonide oral inhaler and subsequent management may be more difficult because recovery from impaired adrenal function is usually slow. Such suppression has been known to last for up to 12 months or longer. Clinical studies, however, have demonstrated that Triamcinolone Acetonide oral inhaler may be effective in the management of these asthmatic patients and may permit replacement or significant reduction in the dosage of systemic corticosteroids.

The patient's asthma should be reasonably stable before treatment with Triamcinolone Acetonide oral inhaler is started. Initially, the inhaler should be used concurrently with the patient's usual maintenance dose of systemic steroid. After approximately one week, gradual withdrawal of the systemic steroid is started by reducing the dose. The next reduction is made after an interval of one of two weeks, depending on the response of the patient. Generally, these decrements should not exceed 2.5 mg of prednisone or its equivalent. A slow rate of withdrawal cannot be overemphasized. During withdrawal, some patients may experience symptoms of systemically active steroid withdrawal, e.g., joint and/or muscular pain, lassitude and depression, despite maintenance or even improvement of respiratory function. Such patients should be encouraged to continue with the inhaler but should be watched carefully for objective signs of adrenal insufficiency, such as hypotension and weight loss. If evidence of adrenal insufficiency occurs, the systemic steroid dose should be boosted temporarily and thereafter further withdrawal should continue more slowly. No clinical studies have been conducted evaluating Triamcinolone Acetonide with alternate day prednisone regimens. However, based on the results of such a study with another inhaled corticosteroid, inhaled corticosteroids generally are not recommended for chronic use with alternate day prednisone regimens (see *"Warnings"*).

During periods of stress or a severe asthma attack, transfer patients will require supplementary treatment with systemic steroids. Exacerbations of asthma which occur during the course of treatment with Triamcinolone Acetonide oral inhaler should be treated with a short course of systemic steroid which is gradually tapered as these symptoms subside. There is no evidence that control of asthma can be achieved by administration of Triamcinolone Acetonide oral inhaler in amounts greater than the recommended doses.

NASAL INHALATION
A decrease in symptoms may occur as soon as 12 hours after starting steroid therapy and generally can be expected to occur within a few days of initiating therapy in allergic rhinitis.

If improvement is not evident after 2-3 weeks, the patient should be re-evaluated. (See *"Individualization of Dosage"* section.)

Adults and Children 12 Years of Age and Older: The recommended starting dose of Triamcinolone Acetonide nasal inhaler is 220 mcg per day given as two sprays (approximately 55 mcg/spray) in each nostril once a day. If needed, the dose may be increased to 440 mcg per day (approximately 55 mcg/spray) either as once a day dosage or divided up to four times a day, *i.e.*, twice a day (two sprays/nostril), or four times a day (one spray/nostril). After the desired effect is obtained, some patients may be maintained on a dose of as little as one spray (approximately 55 mcg) in each nostril once a day (total daily dose 110 mcg per day).

WARNING
Some brands contain CFC-12 substances which harm public health and environment by destroying ozone in the upper atmosphere.

CONTENTS UNDER PRESSURE
Do not puncture. Do not use or store near heat or open flame. Exposure to temperatures above 120°F may cause bursting. Never throw container into fire or incinerator. Keep out of reach of children.

STORAGE
Store at controlled room temperature, 15°-30°C (59°-86°F).

◆ RATED THERAPEUTICALLY EQUIVALENT; ◇ THERAPEUTIC EQUIVALENCE UNCONFIRMED; ○ UNRATED

HOW SUPPLIED
AEROSOL SOLID W/ADAPTER: 100 MCG/INH
BRAND/MANUFACTURER   *NDC*   *SIZE*   *AWP*

○ **BRAND**
AZMACORT: RPR   00075-0060-37   20 gm $39.84

Triamcinolone Acetonide, Injectable

DESCRIPTION
Triamcinolone Acetonide is a synthetic corticosteroid with marked anti-inflammatory action, in a sterile aqueous suspension.

Each ml contains
Triamcinolone Acetonide ....10 or 40 mg.

Triamcinolone Acetonide 10 mg is suitable for intradermal, intra-articular, and intrabursal injection and for injection into tendon sheaths. Triamcinolone Acetonide 40 mg is suitable for intramuscular and intra-articular injection.

The chemical name for Triamcinolone Acetonide is 9-fluoro-11β,16α,17,21-tetrahydroxy-pregna-1,4-diene-3,20-dione cyclic 16,17-acetal with acetone; its molecular weight is 434.50.

Following is its chemical structure:

CLINICAL PHARMACOLOGY
Naturally occurring glucocorticoids (hydrocortisone), which also have salt-retaining properties, are used as replacement therapy in adrenocortical deficiency states. Their synthetic analogs are primarily used for their potent anti-inflammatory effects in disorders of many organ systems.

Glucocorticoids cause profound and varied metabolic effects. In addition, they modify the body's immune responses to diverse stimuli.

Triamcinolone Acetonide 40 mg injection has an extended duration of effect which may be permanent, or sustained over a period of several weeks. Studies indicate that following a single intramuscular dose of 60 to 100 mg of Triamcinolone Acetonide, adrenal suppression occurs within 24 to 48 hours and then gradually returns to normal, usually in 30 to 40 days. This finding correlates closely with the extended duration of therapeutic action achieved with the drug.

INDICATIONS AND USAGE
INTRA-ARTICULAR
Triamcinolone Acetonide, Injectable, 10 and 40 mg, is indicated for intra-articular or intrabursal administration, and for injection into tendon sheaths, as adjunctive therapy for short-term administration (to tide the patient over an acute episode or exacerbation) in: synovitis of osteoarthritis, rheumatoid arthritis, acute and subacute bursitis, acute gouty arthritis, epicondylitis, acute nonspecific tenosynovitis, and post-traumatic osteoarthritis.

INTRADERMAL
Intralesional administration of Triamcinolone Acetonide, Injectable, 10 mg, is indicated for the treatment of keloids, discoid lupus erythematosus, necrobiosis lipoidica diabeticorum, alopecia areata, and localized hypertrophic, infiltrated, inflammatory lesions of: lichen planus, psoriatic plaques, granuloma annulare, and lichen simplex chronicus (neurodermatitis). Triamcinolone Acetonide, Injectable, 10 mg, also may be useful in cystic tumors of an aponeurosis or tendon (ganglia).

INTRAMUSCULAR
Where oral therapy is not feasible or is temporarily undesirable in the judgment of the physician, Triamcinolone Acetonide, Injectable, 40 mg, Injection is indicated for intramuscular use as follows:

1. Endocrine disorders: Nonsuppurative thyroiditis.

2. Rheumatic disorders: As adjunctive therapy for short-term administration (to tide the patient over an acute episode or exacerbation) in: posttraumatic osteoarthritis; synovitis of osteoarthritis; rheumatoid arthritis; acute and subacute bursitis; epicondylitis; acute nonspecific tenosynovitis; acute gouty arthritis; psoriatic arthritis; ankylosing spondylitis; juvenile rheumatoid arthritis.

3. Collagen diseases: During an exacerbation or as maintenance therapy in selected cases of: systemic lupus erythematosus; acute rheumatic carditis.

4. Dermatologic diseases: Pemphigus; severe erythema multiforme (Stevens-Johnson syndrome), exfoliative dermatitis; bullous dermatitis herpetiformis; severe seborrheic dermatitis; severe psoriasis.

5. Allergic states: Control of severe or incapacitating allergic conditions intractable to adequate trials of conventional treatment in: bronchial asthma; contact dermatitis; atopic dermatitis; seasonal or perennial allergic rhinitis.

6. Ophthalmic diseases: Severe chronic allergic and inflammatory processes involving the eye, such as: herpes zoster ophthalmicus; iritis; iridocyclitis; chorioretinitis; diffuse posterior uveitis and choroiditis; optic neuritis; sympathetic ophthalmia; anterior segment inflammation.

7. Gastrointestinal diseases: To tide the patient over a critical period of disease in: ulcerative colitis (systemic therapy); regional enteritis (systemic therapy).

8. Respiratory diseases: Symptomatic sarcoidosis; berylliosis; aspiration pneumonitis.

9. Hematologic disorders: Acquired (autoimmune) hemolytic anemia.

10. Neoplastic diseases: For palliative management of: leukemias and lymphomas in adults; acute leukemia of childhood.

11. Edematous state: To induce diuresis or remission of proteinuria in the nephrotic syndrome, without uremia, of the idiopathic type or that due to lupus erythematosus.

UNLABELED USES
Triamcinolone Acetonide is used alone or as an adjunct in the treatment of chronic pain, temporal arteritis, and myasthenia gravis.

CONTRAINDICATIONS
Corticosteroids are contraindicated in patients with systemic fungal infections.

Intramuscular corticosteroid preparations are contraindicated for idiopathic thrombocytopenic purpura.

WARNINGS
Because it is a suspension, the preparation should *not* be administered intravenously. Strict aseptic technique is mandatory.

Triamcinolone Acetonide, Injectable, 40 mg is not recommended for children under six years of age.

When patients who are receiving corticosteroid therapy are subjected to unusual stress, increased dosage of rapidly acting corticosteroids is indicated before, during, and after the stressful situation. Triamcinolone Acetonide, Injectable, 10 mg, as a long-acting preparation, is *not* suitable for use in acute stress situations.

Corticosteroids may mask some signs of infection, and new infections may appear during their use. There may be decreased resistance and inability to localize infection when corticosteroids are used. If an infection occurs during corticosteroid therapy, it should be promptly controlled by suitable antimicrobial therapy (see *"Precautions"*).

Prolonged use of corticosteroids may produce posterior subcapsular cataracts, glaucoma with possible damage to the optic nerves, and may enhance the establishment of secondary ocular infections due to fungi or viruses.

Average and large doses of hydrocortisone or cortisone can cause elevation of blood pressure, salt and water retention, and increased excretion of potassium. These effects are less likely to occur with the synthetic derivatives except when they are used in large doses; dietary salt restriction and potassium supplementation may be necessary (see *"Precautions"*). All corticosteroids increase calcium excretion.

Children who are on immunosuppressant drugs are more susceptible to infections than healthy children. Chickenpox and measles, for example, can have a more serious or even fatal course in children on immunosuppressant corticosteroids. In such children, or in adults who have not had these diseases, particular care should be taken to avoid exposure. If exposed, therapy with varicella zoster immune globulin (VZIG) or pooled intravenous immunoglobulin (IVIG), as appropriate, may be indicated. If chickenpox develops, treatment with antiviral agents may be considered.

Patients should not be vaccinated against smallpox while on corticosteroid therapy. Other immunization procedures should not be undertaken in patients who are on corticosteroids, especially on high dose, because of possible hazards of neurological complications and a lack of antibody response.

The use of Triamcinolone Acetonide or other corticosteroids in patients with active tuberculosis should be restricted to those cases of fulminating or disseminated tuberculosis in which the corticosteroid is used for the management of the disease in conjunction with an appropriate antituberculous regimen. If corticosteroids are indicated in patients with latent tuberculosis or tuberculin reactivity, close observation is necessary since reactivation of the disease may occur. During prolonged corticosteroid therapy these patients should receive chemoprophylaxis.

Because rare instances of anaphylactoid reactions have occurred in patients receiving parenteral corticosteroid therapy, appropriate precautionary measures should be taken prior to administration, especially when the patient has a history of allergy to any drug.

Safety of use of Triamcinolone Acetonide, Injectable, by intraturbinal, subconjunctival, subtenon, and retrobulbar injection has not been established. Several instances of blindness have been reported following injection of corticosteroid suspensions into the nasal turbinates and intralesional injection about the head.

When administering Triamcinolone Acetonide 40 mg, unless a deep intramuscular injection is given, local atrophy is likely to occur. (For recommendations on injection techniques, see *"Dosage and Administration"*.) Due to the significantly higher incidence of local atrophy when the material is injected into the deltoid area, this injection site should be avoided in favor of the gluteal area. Only very unusual circumstances would warrant injection into the deltoid area.

USAGE IN PREGNANCY

Since adequate human reproduction studies have not been done with corticosteroids, the use of these drugs in pregnancy, nursing mothers, or women of childbearing potential requires that the possible benefits of the drug be weighed against the potential hazards to the mother and the embryo, fetus, or nursing infant. Infants born of mothers who have received substantial doses of corticosteroids during pregnancy should be carefully observed for signs of hypoadrenalism.

PRECAUTIONS

Drug-induced secondary adrenocortical insufficiency may be minimized by a gradual reduction of dosage. This type of relative insufficiency may persist for months after discontinuation of therapy; therefore, in any situation of stress (such as trauma, surgery, or severe illness) occurring during that period, hormone therapy should be reinstituted. Since mineralocorticoid secretion may be impaired, salt and/or a mineralocorticoid should be administered concurrently.

There is an enhanced corticosteroid effect in patients with hypothyroidism and in those with cirrhosis.

Corticosteroids should be used cautiously in patients with ocular herpes simplex because of possible corneal perforation.

The lowest possible dose of corticosteroid should be used to control the condition being treated. A gradual reduction in dosage should be made when possible.

Psychic derangements may appear when corticosteroids are used. These may range from euphoria, insomnia, mood swings, personality changes, and severe depression, to frank psychotic manifestations. Existing emotional instability or psychotic tendencies may also be aggravated by corticosteroids.

Aspirin should be used cautiously in conjunction with corticosteroids in patients with hypoprothrombinemia.

Corticosteroids should be used with caution in patients with nonspecific ulcerative colitis if there is a probability of impending perforation, abscess, or other pyogenic infection. Corticosteroids should be used cautiously in patients with diverticulitis, fresh intestinal anastomoses, active or latent peptic ulcer, renal insufficiency, hypertension, osteoporosis, acute glomerulonephritis, vaccinia, varicella, exanthema, Cushing's syndrome, antibiotic resistant infections, diabetes mellitus, congestive heart failure, chronic nephritis, thromboembolitic tendencies, thrombophlebitis, convulsive disorders, metastatic carcinoma, and myasthenia gravis.

Patients who are on immunosuppressant doses of corticosteroids should be warned to avoid exposure to chickenpox or measles and, if exposed, to obtain medical advice.

Growth and development of infants and children on prolonged corticosteroid therapy should be carefully observed.

Although therapy with Triamcinolone Acetonide, Injectable, may ameliorate symptoms, it is in no sense a cure and the hormone has no effect on the cause of the inflammation. Therefore, this method of treatment does not obviate the need for the conventional measures usually employed.

Intra-articular injection of a corticosteroid may produce systemic as well as local effects. The inadvertent injection of the suspension into the soft tissues surrounding a joint is not harmful, but may lead to the occurrence of systemic effects, and is the most common cause of failure to achieve the desired local results.

Following intra-articular steroid therapy, patients should be specifically warned to avoid overuse of joints in which symptomatic benefit has been obtained. Negligence in this matter may permit an increase in joint deterioration that will more than offset the beneficial effects of the steroid. To detect deterioration, follow-up x-ray examination is suggested in selected cases.

Overdistention of the joint capsule and deposition of steroid along the needle track should be avoided in intra-articular injection since this may lead to subcutaneous atrophy.

Corticosteroids should not be injected into unstable joints. Repeated intra-articular injection may in some cases result in instability of the joint. In selected cases, particularly when repeated injections are given, x-ray follow-up is suggested.

An increase in joint discomfort has seldom occurred. A marked increase in pain accompanied by local swelling, further restriction of joint motion, fever, and malaise are suggestive of a septic arthritis. If these complications should appear, and the diagnosis of septic arthritis is confirmed, administration of Triamcinolone Acetonide should be stopped, and antimicrobial therapy should be instituted immediately and continued for 7 to 10 days after all evidence of infection has disappeared. Appropriate examination of any joint fluid present is necessary to exclude a septic process.

Local injection of a steroid into a previously infected joint is to be avoided.

Triamcinolone Acetonide, Injectable, should be administered only with full knowledge of characteristic activity of, and varied responses to, adrenocortical hormones. Like other potent corticosteroids, Triamcinolone Acetonide should be used under close clinical supervision. Triamcinolone Acetonide can cause elevation of blood pressure, salt and water retention, and increased potassium and calcium excretion, necessitating dietary salt restriction and potassium supplementation. Edema may occur in the presence of renal disease with a fixed or decreased glomerular filtration rate.

During prolonged therapy, *a liberal protein intake is essential* for counteracting the tendency to gradual weight loss sometimes associated with negative nitrogen balance, wasting and weakness of skeletal muscles.

When local or systemic microbial infections are present, therapy with Triamcinolone Acetonide is not recommended, but may be employed with caution and only in conjunction with appropriate antibiotic or chemotherapeutic medication. Triamcinolone Acetonide may mask signs of infection and enhance dissemination of the infecting organism. Hence, all patients receiving Triamcinolone Acetonide should be watched for evidence of intercurrent infection. Should infection occur, vigorous, appropriate anti-infective therapy should be initiated. If possible, abrupt cessation of steroids should be avoided because of the danger of superimposing adrenocortical insufficiency on the infectious process.

Menstrual irregularities: may occur, and this possibility should be mentioned to female patients past menarche.

In peptic ulcer, recurrence may be asymptomatic until perforation or hemorrhage occurs. Long-term adrenocorticoid therapy may evoke hyperacidity or peptic ulcer; therefore, as a prophylactic measure, an ulcer regimen and the administration of an antacid are highly recommended. X-rays should be taken in peptic ulcer patients complaining of gastric distress, or when therapy is prolonged. Whether or not changes are observed, an ulcer regimen is recommended.

As with other corticosteroids, the possibility of other severe reactions should be considered. If such reactions should occur, appropriate corrective measures should be instituted and use of the drug discontinued.

Continued supervision of the patient after termination of Triamcinolone Acetonide therapy is essential, since there may be a sudden reappearance of severe manifestations of the disease for which the patient was treated.

ADVERSE REACTIONS

FOLLOWING ADMINISTRATION BY ANY ROUTE

Patients should be watched closely for the following adverse reactions which may be associated with any corticosteroid therapy:

Fluid and Electrolyte Disturbances: sodium retention, fluid retention, congestive heart failure in susceptible patients, potassium loss, cardiac arrhythmias or ECG changes due to potassium deficiency, hypokalemic alkalosis, and hypertension.

Musculoskeletal: muscle weakness, fatigue, steroid myopathy, loss of muscle mass, osteoporosis, vertebral compression fractures, delayed healing of fractures, aseptic necrosis of femoral and humeral heads, pathologic fractures of long bones, and spontaneous fractures.

Gastrointestinal: peptic ulcer with possible subsequent perforation and hemorrhage, pancreatitis, abdominal distention, and ulcerative esophagitis.

Dermatologic: impaired wound healing, thin fragile skin, petechiae and ecchymoses, facial erythema, increased sweating, purpura, striae, hirsutism, acneiform eruptions, lupus erythematosus-like lesions and suppressed reactions to skin tests.

Neurological: convulsions, increased intracranial pressure with papilledema (pseudo-tumor cerebri) usually after treatment, vertigo, headache, neuritis or paresthesias, and aggravation of pre-existing psychiatric conditions.

Endocrine: menstrual irregularities; development of the cushingoid state; suppression of growth in children; secondary adrenocortical and pituitary unresponsiveness, particularly in times of stress (e.g., trauma, surgery, or illness); decreased carbohydrate tolerance; manifestations of latent diabetes mellitus; and increased requirements for insulin or oral hypoglycemic agents in diabetics.

Ophthalmic: posterior subcapsular cataracts, increased intraocular pressure, glaucoma, and exophthalmos.

Metabolic: hyperglycemia, glycosuria, and negative nitrogen balance due to protein catabolism.

Others: necrotizing angiitis, thrombophlebitis, thromboembolism, aggravation or masking of infections, insomnia, syncopal episodes, and anaphylactoid reactions.

FOLLOWING INTRA-ARTICULAR ADMINISTRATION

Undesirable reactions following intra-articular administration of the preparation have included postinjection flare, transient pain, occasional local irritation at the injection site, sterile abscesses, hyper- and hypopigmentation, charcot-like arthropathy, and occasional brief increase in joint discomfort; following intradermal administration, rare instances of blindness associated with intralesional therapy around the face and head, transient local discomfort, sterile abscesses, hyper- and hypopigmentation, and subcutaneous and cutaneous atrophy (which usually disappears, unless the basic disease process is itself atrophic) have occurred.

FOLLOWING INTRAMUSCULAR ADMINISTRATION

Severe pain has been reported in a few cases. Sterile abscess formation, subcutaneous and cutaneous atrophy, hyperpigmentation and hypopigmentation and charcot-like arthropathy have also occurred.

DOSAGE AND ADMINISTRATION

DOSAGE

The initial dose of Triamcinolone Acetonide, Injectable, 10 and 40 mg, for intra-articular or intrabursal administration and for injection into tendon sheaths may vary from 2.5 mg to 5 mg for smaller joints and from 5 to 15 mg for larger joints depending on the specific disease entity being treated. For adults, doses up to 10 mg for smaller areas and up to 40 mg for larger areas have usually been sufficient to alleviate symptoms. Single injections into several joints for multiple locus involvement, up to a total of 80 mg, have been given without incident. A single local injection of Triamcinolone Acetonide is frequently sufficient, but several injections may be needed for adequate relief of symptoms. For intradermal administration, the initial dose of Triamcinolone Acetonide will vary depending

---

◆ RATED THERAPEUTICALLY EQUIVALENT; ◇ THERAPEUTIC EQUIVALENCE UNCONFIRMED; ○ UNRATED

upon the specific disease entity being treated but should be limited to 1.0 mg (0.1 mL) per injection site, since larger volumes are more likely to produce cutaneous atrophy. Multiple sites (separated by one centimeter or more) may be so injected, keeping in mind that the greater the *total* volume employed the more corticosteroid becomes available for possible systemic absorption and subsequent corticosteroid effects. Such injections may be repeated, if necessary, at weekly or less frequent intervals.

The lower dosages in the initial dosage range of Triamcinolone Acetonide may produce the desired effect when the corticosteroid is administered to provide a localized concentration. The site of the injection and the volume of the injection should be carefully considered when Triamcinolone Acetonide is administered for this purpose. The initial dosage should be maintained or adjusted until a satisfactory response is noted. If after a reasonable period of time there is a lack of satisfactory clinical response, Triamcinolone Acetonide, Injectable, should be discontinued and the patient transferred to other appropriate therapy. *It should be emphasized that dosage requirements are variable and must be individualized on the basis of the disease under treatment and the response of the patient.* After a favorable response is noted, the proper maintenance dosage should be determined by decreasing the initial drug dosage in small increments at appropriate time intervals until the lowest dosage which will maintain an adequate clinical response is reached. It should be kept in mind that constant monitoring is needed in regard to drug dosage. Included in the situations which may make dosage adjustments necessary are changes in clinical status secondary to remissions or exacerbations in the disease process, the patient's individual drug responsiveness, and the effect of patient exposure to stressful situations not directly related to the disease entity under treatment; in this latter situation it may be necessary to increase the dosage of Triamcinolone Acetonide, Injectable for a period of time consistent with the patient's condition. If the drug is to be stopped after long-term therapy, it is recommended that it be withdrawn gradually rather than abruptly.

Although Triamcinolone Acetonide 40mg Injection may be administered intramuscularly for initial therapy, most physicians prefer to adjust the dose orally until adequate control is attained. Intramuscular administration provides a sustained or depot action which can be used to supplement or replace initial oral therapy. With intramuscular therapy, greater supervision of the amount of steroid used is made possible in the patient who is inconsistent in following an oral dosage schedule. In maintenance therapy, the patient-to-patient response is not uniform and therefore, the dose must be individualized for optimal control.

For *adults and children over 12 years of age*, the suggested initial dose is 60 mg, *injected deeply into the gluteal muscle*. Subcutaneous fat atrophy may occur if care is not taken to inject the preparation intramuscularly. Dosage is usually adjusted within the range of 40 to 80 mg, depending upon patient response and duration of relief. However, some patients may be well controlled on dosages as low as 20 mg or less. Patients with hay fever or pollen asthma who are not responding to pollen administration and other conventional therapy may obtain a remission of symptoms lasting throughout the pollen season after one injection of 40 to 100 mg.

For *children from 6 to 12 years of age*, the suggested initial dose is 40 mg, although dosage depends more on the severity of symptoms than on age or weight. There is insufficient clinical experience with Triamcinolone Acetonide 40 mg to recommend its use in children under six years of age.

ADMINISTRATION

Shake the vial before use to insure a uniform suspension. Prior to withdrawal, inspect suspension for clumping or granular appearance (agglomeration). An agglomerated product results from exposure to freezing temperatures and should not be used. After withdrawal, inject without delay to prevent setting in the syringe. Careful technique should be employed to avoid the possibility of entering a blood vessel or introducing infection.

Routine laboratory studies, such as urinalysis, two-hour postprandial blood sugar, determination of blood pressure and body weight, and a chest x-ray should be made at regular intervals during prolonged therapy. Upper GI x-rays are desirable in patients with an ulcer history or significant dyspepsia.

For treatment of joints, the usual intra-articular injection technique, as described in standard textbooks, should be followed. If an excessive amount of synovial fluid is present in the joint, some, but not all, should be aspirated to aid in the relief of pain and to prevent undue dilution of the steroid.

With intra-articular or intrabursal administration, and with injection of Triamcinolone Acetonide, Injectable into tendon sheaths, the use of a local anesthetic may often be desirable. When a local anesthetic is used, its package insert should be read with care and all the precautions connected with its use should be observed. It should be injected into the surrounding soft tissues prior to the injection of the corticosteroid. A small amount of the anesthetic solution may be instilled into the joint. Care should be taken with intra-articular and intrabursal injections (particularly in the deltoid region) and with injection into tendon sheaths to avoid injecting the suspension into the tissues surrounding the site since this may lead to tissue atrophy.

In treating acute nonspecific tenosynovitis, care should be taken to insure that the injection of Triamcinolone Acetonide, Injection is made into the tendon sheath rather than the tendon substance. Epicondylitis (tennis elbow) may be treated by infiltrating the preparation into the area of greatest tenderness.

For treatment of dermal lesions, Triamcinolone Acetonide, 10 mg injection is injected directly into the lesion, i.e., intradermally or sometimes subcutaneously. For accuracy of dosage measurement and ease of administration, it is preferable to employ a tuberculin syringe and a small-bore needle (23 to 25 gauge). Ethyl chloride spray may be used to alleviate the discomfort of the injection.

For systemic therapy, injection should be made deeply into the gluteal muscle to insure intramuscular delivery (see *"Warnings"*). For adults, a minimum needle length of 1 ½ inches is recommended. In obese patients, a longer needle may be required. Use alternate sites for subsequent injections.

STORAGE
Store at room temperature; avoid freezing; protect from light.

J CODES
Per 10 mg IM—J3301

HOW SUPPLIED
INJECTION: 3 MG/ML

BRAND/MANUFACTURER	NDC	SIZE	AWP
○ **BRAND**			
TAC 3: Allergan Inc	00023-0218-05	5 ml	$8.95

INJECTION: 10 MG/ML

BRAND/MANUFACTURER	NDC	SIZE	AWP
○ **BRAND**			
KENALOG-10: Apothecon	00003-0494-20	5 ml	$6.59

INJECTION: 40 MG/ML

BRAND/MANUFACTURER	NDC	SIZE	AWP
◇ **BRAND**			
KENALOG-40: Apothecon	00003-0293-05	1 ml	$5.11
	00003-0293-20	5 ml	$21.53
	00003-0293-28	10 ml	$38.61
◇ **GENERICS**			
Steris	00402-0204-01	1 ml	$4.16
Moore,H.L.	00839-6287-82	1 ml	$4.44
Schein	00364-6728-53	5 ml	$11.25
Steris	00402-0204-05	5 ml	$11.25
TRIAM-A: Hyrex	00314-3400-75	5 ml	$13.60
Insource	58441-1116-05	5 ml	$14.93
Genl Inject	52584-0204-05	5 ml	$14.93
Moore,H.L.	00839-6287-25	5 ml	$15.38
URL	00677-0600-20	5 ml	$16.30
Major	00904-0886-05	5 ml	$17.60
Rugby	00536-9810-65	5 ml	$19.20
Geneva	00781-3116-75	5 ml	$19.25
Goldline	00182-1141-62	5 ml	$19.50
KENAJECT-40: Mayrand	00259-0355-05	5 ml	$29.85
Goldline	00182-1141-85	1 ml 10s	$6.60
Schein	00364-6728-46	1 ml 25s	$104.18

Triamcinolone Acetonide, Topical

DESCRIPTION
Triamcinolone Acetonide, Topical, a highly active steroid, is available as a cream, an ointment, and a dental paste.

Each g of cream contains:
Triamcinolone Acetonide ....0.25, 1, or 5 mg

Each g of ointment contains:
Triamcinolone Acetonide ....1 mg

Each gm of dental paste contains:
Triamcinolone Acetonide ....1 mg

Chemically, *Triamcinolone Acetonide* is (11β,16α)-9-fluoro-11,21-dihydroxy-16,17-[(1-methylethylidene)bis (oxy)] pregna-1,4-diene-3,20-dione.

The topical corticosteroids constitute a class of primarily synthetic steroids used as anti-inflammatory and antipruritic agents.

Following is its chemical structure:

CLINICAL PHARMACOLOGY
Topical corticosteroids share anti-inflammatory, antipruritic, and vasoconstrictive or antiallergic actions.

The mechanism of anti-inflammatory activity of the topical corticosteroids is unclear. Various laboratory methods, including vasoconstrictor assays, are used to compare and predict potencies and/or clinical efficacies of the topical corticosteroids. There is some evidence to suggest that a recognizable correlation exists between vasoconstrictor potency and therapeutic efficacy in man.

PHARMACOKINETICS

The extent of percutaneous absorption of topical corticosteroids is determined by many factors including the vehicle, the integrity of the epidermal barrier, and the use of occlusive dressings.

Topical corticosteroids can be absorbed from normal intact skin. Inflammation and/or other disease processes in the skin increase percutaneous absorption. Occlusive dressings substantially increase the percutaneous absorption of topical corticosteroids. Thus, occlusive dressings may be a valuable therapeutic adjunct for treatment of resistant dermatoses (See *"Dosage and Administration"*).

Once absorbed through the skin, topical corticosteroids are handled through pharmacokinetic pathways similar to systemically administered corticosteroids. Corticosteroids are bound to plasma proteins in varying degrees. Corticosteroids are metabolized primarily in the liver and are then excreted by the kidneys. Some of the topical corticosteroids and their metabolites are also excreted into the bile.

The emollient dental paste acts as an adhesive vehicle for applying the active medication to the oral tissues. The vehicle provides a protective covering which may serve to temporarily reduce the pain associated with oral irritation.

INDICATIONS AND USAGE

Topical corticosteroids are indicated for the relief of the inflammatory and pruritic manifestations of corticosteroid-responsive dermatoses.

Triamcinolone Acetonide dental paste is indicated for adjunctive treatment and for the temporary relief of symptoms associated with oral inflammatory lesions and ulcerative lesions resulting from trauma.

CONTRAINDICATIONS

Topical corticosteroids are contraindicated in those patients with a history of hypersensitivity to any of the components of the preparation.

Because it contains a corticosteroid, Triamcinolone Acetonide dental paste is contraindicated in the presence of fungal, viral, or bacterial infections of the mouth or throat.

PRECAUTIONS

GENERAL

Systemic absorption of topical corticosteroids has produced reversible hypothalamic-pituitary-adrenal (HPA) axis suppression, manifestations of Cushing's syndrome, hyperglycemia, and glucosuria in some patients.

Conditions that augment systemic absorption include the application of the more potent steroids, use over large surface areas, prolonged use, and the addition of occlusive dressings.

Therefore, patients receiving a large dose of a potent topical steroid applied to a large surface area or under an occlusive dressing should be evaluated periodically for evidence of HPA axis suppression by using the urinary free cortisol and ACTH stimulation tests. If HPA axis suppression is noted, an attempt should be made to withdraw the drug, to reduce the frequency of application, or to substitute a less potent steroid.

Recovery of HPA axis function is generally prompt and complete upon discontinuation of the drug. Infrequently, signs and symptoms of steroid withdrawal may occur, requiring supplemental systemic corticosteroids.

Children may absorb proportionally larger amounts of topical corticosteroids and thus be more susceptible to systemic toxicity (See *"Precautions—Pediatric Use"*).

If irritation or sensitization develops, topical corticosteroids should be discontinued and appropriate therapy instituted.

In the presence of dermatological infections, the use of an appropriate antifungal or antibacterial agent should be instituted. If a favorable response does not occur promptly, the corticosteroid should be discontinued until the infection has been adequately controlled.

Patients with tuberculosis, peptic ulcer or diabetes mellitus should not be treated with any corticosteroid preparation without the advice of the patient's physician.

It should be borne in mind that the normal defensive responses of the oral tissues are depressed in patients receiving topical corticosteroid therapy. Virulent strains of oral microorganisms may multiply without producing the usual warning symptoms of oral infections.

The small amount of steroid released when Triamcinolone Acetomide dental paste is used as recommended makes systemic effects very unlikely; however, they are a possibility when topical corticosteroid preparations are used over a long period of time.

If significant regeneration or repair of oral tissues has not occurred in seven days, additional investigation into the etiology of the oral lesion is advised.

INFORMATION FOR THE PATIENT

Patients using topical corticosteroids should receive the following information and instructions.

1. This medication is to be used as directed by the physician. It is for external use only. Avoid contact with the eyes.
2. Patients should be advised not to use this medication for any disorder other than for which it was prescribed.
3. The treated skin area should not be bandaged or otherwise covered or wrapped as to be occlusive unless directed by the physician.
4. Patients should report any signs of local adverse reactions, especially under occlusive dressing.
5. Parents of pediatric patients should be advised not to use tight-fitting diapers or plastic pants on a child being treated in the diaper area, as these garments may constitute occlusive dressings.

LABORATORY TESTS

The following tests may be helpful in evaluating the HPA axis suppression:
Urinary free cortisol test
ACTH stimulation test

CARCINOGENESIS, MUTAGENESIS, AND IMPAIRMENT OF FERTILITY

Long-term animal studies have not been performed to evaluate the carcinogenic potential or the effect on fertility of topical corticosteroids.

Studies to determine mutagenicity with prednisolone and hydrocortisone have revealed negative results.

PREGNANCY CATEGORY C

Corticosteroids are generally teratogenic in laboratory animals when administered systemically at relatively low dosage levels. The more potent corticosteroids have been shown to be teratogenic after dermal application in laboratory animals. There are no adequate and well-controlled studies in pregnant women on teratogenic effects from topically applied corticosteroids. Therefore, topical corticosteroids should be used during pregnancy only if the potential benefit justifies the potential risk to the fetus. Drugs of this class should not be used extensively on pregnant patients, in large amounts, or for prolonged periods of time.

NURSING MOTHERS

It is not known whether topical administration of corticosteroids could result in sufficient systemic absorption to produce detectable quantities in breast milk. Systemically administered corticosteroids are secreted into breast milk in quantities *not likely* to have a deleterious effect on the infant. Nevertheless, caution should be exercised when topical corticosteroids are administered to a nursing woman.

PEDIATRIC USE

Pediatric patients may demonstrate greater susceptibility to topical corticosteroid-induced HPA axis suppression and Cushing's syndrome than mature patients because of a larger skin surface area to body weight ratio.

Hypothalamic-pituitary-adrenal (HPA) axis suppression, Cushing's syndrome, and intracranial hypertension have been reported in children receiving topical corticosteroids. Manifestations of adrenal suppression in children include linear growth retardation, delayed weight gain, low plasma cortisol levels, and absence of response to ACTH stimulation. Manifestations of intracranial hypertension include bulging fontanelles, headaches, and bilateral papilledema.

Administration of topical corticosteroids to children should be limited to the least amount compatible with an effective therapeutic regimen. Chronic corticosteroid therapy may interfere with the growth and development of children.

ADVERSE REACTIONS

The following local adverse reactions are reported infrequently with topical corticosteroids, but may occur more frequently with the use of occlusive dressings. These reactions are listed in an approximate decreasing order of occurrence.

Burning
Itching
Irritation
Dryness
Folliculitis
Hypertrichosis
Acneiform eruptions
Hypopigmentation
Perioral dermatitis
Allergic contact dermatitis
Maceration of the skin
Secondary infection
Skin atrophy
Striae
Miliaria

Prolonged administration of Triamcinolone Acetonide dental paste may elicit the adverse reactions known to occur with systemic steroid preparations; for example, adrenal suppression, alteration of glucose metabolism, protein catabolism, peptic ulcer activations, and others.

These are usually reversible and disappear when the hormone is discontinued.

OVERDOSAGE

Topically applied corticosteroids can be absorbed in sufficient amounts to produce systemic effects (see *"Precautions"*).

DOSAGE AND ADMINISTRATION

CREAM AND OINTMENT

Topical corticosteroids are generally applied to the affected area as a thin film from three to four times daily depending on the severity of the condition.

◆ RATED THERAPEUTICALLY EQUIVALENT; ◇ THERAPEUTIC EQUIVALENCE UNCONFIRMED; ○ UNRATED

Occlusive dressings may be used for the management of psoriasis or recalcitrant conditions.

If an infection develops, the use of occlusive dressings should be discontinued and appropriate antimicrobial therapy instituted.

DENTAL PASTE

Press a small dab (about ¼ inch) to the lesion until a thin film develops. A larger quantity may be required for coverage of some lesions. For optimal results use only enough to coat the lesion with a thin film. Do not rub in. Attempting to spread this preparation may result in a granular, gritty sensation and cause it to crumble. After application, however, a smooth, slippery film develops.

The preparation should be applied at bedtime to permit steroid contact with the lesion throughout the night. Depending on the severity of symptoms, it may be necessary to apply the preparation two or three times a day, preferably after meals. If significant repair or regeneration has not occurred in seven days, further investigation is advisable.

STORAGE

Store at controlled room temperature, 15-30°C (59-86°F). Do not freeze.

J CODES

Per 10 mg IM—J3301

HOW SUPPLIED
CREAM: 0.025%

AVERAGE UNIT PRICE (AVAILABLE SIZES)		GENERIC A-RATED AVERAGE PRICE (GAAP)	
BRAND	$0.33	2270 gm	$30.24
GENERIC	$0.06	15 gm	$1.54
HCFA FUL (15 gm)	$0.08	80 gm	$3.49
HCFA FUL (80 gm)	$0.03	454 gm	$8.81
HCFA FUL (454 gm)	$0.02	480 gm	$12.30

BRAND/MANUFACTURER	NDC	SIZE	AWP
◆ **BRAND**			
ARISTOCORT TOPICAL: Fujisawa	57317-0082-15	15 gm	$6.17
KENALOG: Apothecon	00003-0172-22	15 gm	$7.00
ARISTOCORT A: Fujisawa	57317-0042-15	15 gm	$8.46
ARISTOCORT TOPICAL: Fujisawa	57317-0082-60	60 gm	$13.13
ARISTOCORT A: Fujisawa	57317-0042-60	60 gm	$20.83
KENALOG: Apothecon	00003-0172-68	80 gm	$20.83
ARISTOCORT TOPICAL: Fujisawa	57317-0082-05	2383.5 gm	$65.82
◆ **GENERICS**			
Clay-Park	45802-0063-35	15 gm	$1.04
Thames	49158-0139-20	15 gm	$1.20
Moore,H.L.	00839-6127-47	15 gm	$1.28
NMC	23317-0300-15	15 gm	$1.38
Parmed	00349-9009-35	15 gm	$1.39
Qualitest	00603-7850-74	15 gm	$1.41
Major	00904-2738-36	15 gm	$1.45
Goldline	00182-1216-51	15 gm	$1.45
URL	00677-0743-40	15 gm	$1.50
Schein	00364-7211-72	15 gm	$1.50
Fougera	00168-0003-15	15 gm	$1.52
Rugby	00536-5245-20	15 gm	$1.65
UDL	51079-0272-61	15 gm	$1.78
Geneva	00781-7030-27	15 gm	$2.14
G&W	00713-0226-15	15 gm	$2.44
FLUTEX: Syosset	47854-0575-05	30 gm	$5.25
FLUTEX: Syosset	47854-0575-07	60 gm	$8.00
Geneva	00781-7030-29	80 gm	$2.75
Thames	49158-0139-21	80 gm	$2.80
Clay-Park	45802-0063-36	80 gm	$2.80
Qualitest	00603-7850-90	80 gm	$3.27
Moore,H.L.	00839-6127-46	80 gm	$3.31
URL	00677-0743-46	80 gm	$3.40
Rugby	00536-5245-30	80 gm	$3.45
NMC	23317-0300-80	80 gm	$3.50
Major	00904-2738-11	80 gm	$3.50
Schein	00364-7211-60	80 gm	$3.50
Fougera	00168-0003-80	80 gm	$3.54
Goldline	00182-1216-53	80 gm	$3.55
Parmed	00349-9009-17	80 gm	$3.60
G&W	00713-0226-80	80 gm	$5.95
Clay-Park	45802-0063-05	454 gm	$7.66
Geneva	00781-7030-16	454 gm	$8.75
URL	00677-0743-44	454 gm	$8.95
Major	00904-2738-27	454 gm	$9.00
NMC	23317-0300-16	454 gm	$9.18
Goldline	00182-1216-45	454 gm	$9.30
Rugby	00536-5245-98	454 gm	$9.38
Thames	49158-0139-16	480 gm	$8.60
FLUTEX: Syosset	47854-0575-13	480 gm	$16.00
Moore,H.L.	00839-6127-48	2270 gm	$20.24
Thames	49158-0139-22	2270 gm	$25.30
Clay-Park	45802-0063-29	2270 gm	$32.40
FLUTEX: Syosset	47854-0575-15	2270 gm	$36.50
Rugby	00536-5245-27	2270 gm	$36.75

CREAM: 0.025%

BRAND/MANUFACTURER	NDC	SIZE	AWP
○ **GENERICS**			
Veratex	17022-5888-02	15 gm	$0.85
Raway	00686-0063-35	15 gm	$1.00
Allscrips	54569-1121-00	15 gm	$1.48
ARICIN: Interstate	00814-0850-93	15 gm	$1.65
CMC-Cons	00223-4449-15	15 gm	$1.95
Southwood	58016-3034-01	15 gm	$4.88
Raway	00686-0063-36	80 gm	$2.50
Allscrips	54569-1774-01	80 gm	$3.54
ARICIN: Interstate	00814-0850-97	80 gm	$3.60
Raway	00686-0063-05	454 gm	$6.25

For additional alternatives, turn to the section beginning on page 2859.

Triamcinolone Diacetate

DESCRIPTION
PARENTERAL

A sterile suspension of 40 mg/mL of Triamcinolone Diacetate (micronized) suspended in a vehicle.

This preparation is a slightly soluble suspension suitable for parenteral administration through a 24-gauge needle (or larger), but *not* suitable for intravenous use. It may be administered by the intramuscular, intra-articular, or intrasynovial routes, depending upon the situation. The response to each glucocorticoid varies considerably with each type of disease indication and each corticosteroid prescribed.

Irreversible clumping occurs when product is frozen.

Chemically Triamcinolone Diacetate is 9-Fluoro-11β,16α,17,21- tetrahydroxy-pregna-1,4-diene-3,20-dione 16,21-diacetate.

Following is its chemical structure:

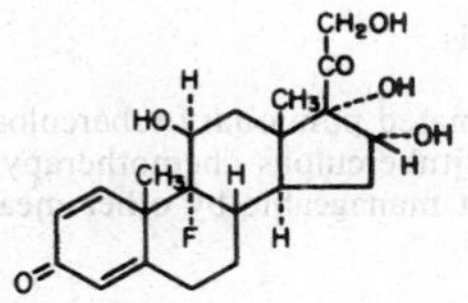

ACTION
PARENTERAL

Triamcinolone Diacetate is primarily glucocorticoid in action and has potent anti-inflammatory, hormonal and metabolic effects common to cortisone-like drugs. It is essentially devoid of mineralocorticoid activity when administered in therapeutic doses, causing little or no sodium retention, with potassium excretion minimal or absent. The body's immune responses to diverse stimuli are also modified by its action.

INDICATIONS
PARENTERAL

Where oral therapy is not feasible or temporarily desirable in the judgment of the physician, sterile Triamcinolone Diacetate suspension, 40 mg/mL, is indicated for intramuscular use as follows:
1. Endocrine disorders.

Primary or secondary adrenocortical insufficiency (hydrocortisone or cortisone is the drug of choice; synthetic analogs may be used in conjunction with mineralocorticoids where applicable; in infancy, mineralocorticoid supplementation is of particular importance). Preoperatively and in the event of serious trauma or illness, in patients with known adrenal insufficiency or when adrenocortical reserve is doubtful

Congenital adrenal hyperplasia

Nonsuppurative thyroiditis

Hypercalcemia associated with cancer

2. Rheumatic disorders.
   As adjunctive therapy for short-term administration (to tide the patient over an acute episode or exacerbation) in:
   Posttraumatic osteoarthritis
   Synovitis of osteoarthritis
   Rheumatoid arthritis, including juvenile rheumatoid arthritis (selected cases may require low-dose maintenance therapy)
   Acute and subacute bursitis
   Epicondylitis
   Acute nonspecific tenosynovitis
   Acute gouty arthritis
   Psoriatic arthritis
   Ankylosing spondylitis
3. Collagen diseases.
   During an exacerbation or as maintenance therapy in selected cases of:
   Systemic lupus erythematosus
   Acute rheumatic carditis
4. Dermatologic diseases.
   Pemphigus
   Severe erythema multiforme (Stevens-Johnson syndrome)
   Exfoliative dermatitis
   Bullous dermatitis herpetiformis
   Severe seborrheic dermatitis
   Severe psoriasis
   Mycosis fungoides
5. Allergic states.
   Control of severe or incapacitating allergic conditions intractable to adequate trials of conventional treatment in:
   Bronchial asthma
   Contact dermatitis
   Atopic dermatitis
   Serum sickness
   Seasonal or perennial allergic rhinitis
   Drug hypersensitivity reactions
   Urticarial transfusion reactions
   Acute noninfectious laryngeal edema (epinephrine is the drug of first choice).
6. Ophthalmic diseases.
   Severe acute and chronic allergic and inflammatory processes involving the eye, such as:
   Herpes zoster ophthalmicus
   Iritis, iridocyclitis
   Chorioretinitis
   Diffuse posterior uveitis and choroiditis
   Optic neuritis
   Sympathetic ophthalmia
   Allergic conjunctivitis
   Allergic corneal marginal ulcers
   Keratitis
7. Gastrointestinal disease. To tide the patient over a critical period of disease in:
   Ulcerative colitis - (Systemic therapy)
   Regional enteritis - (Systemic therapy)
8. Respiratory diseases.
   Symptomatic sarcoidosis
   Berylliosis
   Fulminating or disseminated pulmonary tuberculosis when used concurrently with appropriate antituberculous chemotherapy
   Loeffler's syndrome not manageable by other means
   Aspiration pneumonitis
9. Hematologic disorders.
   Acquired (autoimmune) hemolytic anemia
   Secondary thrombocytopenia in adults
   Erythroblastopenia (RBC anemia)
   Congenital (erythroid) hypoplastic anemia
10. Neoplastic diseases. For palliative management of:
   Leukemias and lymphomas in adults
   Acute leukemia of childhood
11. Edematous state.
   To induce diuresis or remission of proteinuria in the nephrotic syndrome, without uremia, of the idiopathic type or that due to lupus erythematosus
12. Nervous System.
   Acute exacerbations of multiple sclerosis
13. Miscellaneous.
   Tuberculous meningitis with subarachnoid block or impending block when used concurrently with appropriate antituberculous chemotherapy
   Trichinosis with neurologic or myocardial involvement
   Triamcinolone Diacetate 40 mg/mL is indicated for intra-articular or soft tissue use as follows:
   As adjunctive therapy for short-term administration (to tide the patient over an acute episode or exacerbation) in:
   Synovitis of osteoarthritis
   Rheumatoid arthritis
   Acute and subacute bursitis
   Acute gouty arthritis
   Epicondylitis
   Acute nonspecific tenosynovitis
   Posttraumatic osteoarthritis

Triamcinolone Diacetate is indicated for intralesional use as follows:
Keloids
Localized hypertrophic, infiltrated, inflammatory lesion of: Lichen planus, psoriatic plaques, granuloma annulare and lichen simplex chronicus (neurodermatitis)
Discoid lupus erythematosus
Necrobiosis lipoidica diabeticorum
Alopecia areata
It may also be useful in cystic tumors of an aponeurosis or tendon (ganglia).

DESCRIPTION
INTRALESIONAL
Triamcinolone Diacetate possesses glucocorticoid properties while being essentially devoid of mineralocorticoid activity thus causing little or no sodium retention.

Supplied as a sterile suspension of 25 mg/mL micronized Triamcinolone Diacetate.

Chemically Triamcinolone Diacetate is Pregna-1,4-diene-3,20-diene, 16, 21-bis(acetyloxy)-9-fluoro-11,17-dihydroxy-, (11β,16α)- or 9-Fluoro-11β, 16α, 17, 21-tetrahydroxypregna-1,4-diene-3,20-dione 16,21-diacetate. Molecular weight is 478.51.

ACTIONS
INTRALESIONAL
Naturally occurring glucocorticoids (hydrocortisone), which also have salt-retaining properties, are used as replacement therapy in adrenocortical deficiency states. Their synthetic analogs are primarily used for their potent anti-inflammatory effects in disorders of many organ systems.

Glucocorticoids cause profound and varied metabolic effects. In addition, they modify the body's immune responses to diverse stimuli.

INDICATIONS
INTRALESIONAL
Triamcinolone Diacetate Intralesional is indicated by the intralesional route for:
Keloids
Localized hypertrophic, infiltrated, inflammatory lesion of: lichen planus, psoriatic plaques, granuloma annulare and lichen simplex chronicus (neurodermatitis)
Discoid lupus erythematosus
Necrobiosis lipoidica diabeticorum
Alopecia areata
It may also be useful in cystic tumors of an aponeurosis or tendon (ganglia).

When used intra-articularly it is also indicated for:
Adjunctive therapy for short-term administration (to tide the patient over an acute episode or exacerbation) in:
Synovitis of osteoarthritis
Rheumatoid arthritis
Acute and subacute bursitis
Acute gouty arthritis
Epicondylitis
Acute nonspecific tenosynovitis
Posttraumatic osteoarthritis

CONTRAINDICATIONS
PARENTERAL AND INTRALESIONAL
Systemic fungal infections.

WARNINGS
In patients on corticosteroid therapy subjected to any unusual stress, increased dosage of rapidly acting corticosteroids before, during, and after the stressful situation is indicated.

Corticosteroids may mask some signs of infection, and new infections may appear during their use. There may be decreased resistance and inability to localize infection when corticosteroids are used.

Prolonged use of corticosteroids may produce posterior subcapsular cataracts, glaucoma with possible damage to the optic nerves and may enhance the establishment of secondary ocular infections due to fungi or viruses.

USAGE IN PREGNANCY
Since adequate human reproduction studies have not been done with corticosteroids, the use of these drugs in pregnancy, nursing mothers, or women of childbearing potential requires that the possible benefits of the drug be weighted against the potential hazards to the mother and embryo or fetus. Infants born of mothers who have received substantial doses of corticosteroids during pregnancy should be carefully observed for signs of hypoadrenalism.

Average and large doses of cortisone or hydrocortisone can cause elevation of blood pressure, salt and water retention, and increased excretion of potassium. These effects are less likely to occur with synthetic derivatives except when used in large doses. Dietary salt restriction and potassium supplementation may be necessary. All corticosteroids increase calcium excretion.

◆ RATED THERAPEUTICALLY EQUIVALENT; ◇ THERAPEUTIC EQUIVALENCE UNCONFIRMED; ○ UNRATED

While on corticosteroid therapy patients should not be vaccinated against smallpox. Other immunization procedures should not be undertaken in patients who are on corticosteroids, especially in high doses, because of possible hazards of neurological complications and lack of antibody response.

The use of Triamcinolone Diacetate in active tuberculosis should be restricted to those cases of fulminating or disseminated tuberculosis in which the corticosteroid is used for the management of the disease in conjunction with appropriate antituberculous regimen.

If corticosteroids are indicated in patients with latent tuberculosis or tuberculin reactivity, close observation is necessary as reactivation of the disease may occur. During prolonged corticosteroid therapy, these patients should receive chemoprophylaxis.

Because rare instances of anaphylactoid reactions have occurred in patients receiving parenteral corticosteroid therapy, appropriate precautionary measures should be taken prior to administration, especially when the patient has a history of allergy to any drug.

Postinjection flare (following intra-articular use) and Charcot-like arthropathy have been associated with parenteral corticosteroid therapy.

Intralesional or sublesional injection of excessive dosage whether by single or multiple injection into any given area may cause cutaneous or subcutaneous atrophy.

PRECAUTIONS
PARENTERAL AND INTRALESIONAL
Drug-induced secondary adrenocortical insufficiency may be minimized by gradual reduction of dosage. This type of relative insufficiency may persist for months after discontinuation of therapy; therefore, in any situation of stress occurring during that period, hormone therapy should be reinstituted. Since mineralocorticoid secretion may be impaired, salt and/or a mineralocorticoid should be administered concurrently.

There is an enhanced effect of corticosteroids in patients with hypothyroidism and in those with cirrhosis.

Corticosteroids should be used cautiously in patients with ocular herpes simplex for fear of corneal perforation.

The lowest possible dose of corticosteroid should be used to control the condition under treatment, and when reduction in dosage is possible, the reduction must be gradual.

Psychic derangements may appear when corticosteroids are used, ranging from euphoria, insomnia, mood swings, personality changes, and severe depression to frank psychotic manifestations. Also, existing emotional instability of psychotic tendencies may be aggravated by corticosteroids.

Aspirin should be used cautiously in conjunction with corticosteroids in hypoprothrombinemia.

Steroids should be used with caution in nonspecific ulcerative colitis, if there is a probability of impending perforation, abscess or other pyogenic infection, also in diverticulitis, fresh intestinal anastomoses, active or latent peptic ulcer, renal insufficiency, hypertension, osteoporosis, and myasthenia gravis.

Growth and development of infants and children on prolonged corticosteroid therapy should be carefully followed.

The following additional precautions apply for parenteral corticosteroids.

Intra-articular injection of a corticosteroid may produce systemic as well as local effects.

Appropriate examination of any joint fluid present is necessary to exclude a septic process.

A marked increase in pain accompanied by local swelling, further restriction of joint motion, fever, and malaise are suggestive of septic arthritis. If this complication occurs and the diagnosis of sepsis is confirmed, appropriate antimicrobial therapy should be instituted.

Local injection of a steroid into a previously infected joint is to be avoided.

Corticosteroids should not be injected into unstable joints.

The slower rate of absorption by intramuscular administration should be recognized.

Atrophy at the site of injection has been reported.

Routine laboratory studies, such as urinalysis, two-hour postprandial blood sugar, determination of blood pressure and body weight, and a chest X-ray should be made at regular intervals during prolonged therapy. Upper GI x-rays are desirable in patients with an ulcer history or significant dyspepsia.

PARENTERAL
Accidental injection into soft tissue during intra-articular administration decreases local effectiveness in the joint and, by increasing the rate of absorption, may produce systemic effects.

Although controlled clinical trials have shown corticosteroids to be effective in speeding the resolution of acute exacerbations of multiple sclerosis they do not show that they affect the ultimate outcome or natural history of the disease. The studies do show that relatively high doses of corticosteroids are necessary to demonstrate a significant effect (see "Dosage and Administration").

Since complications of treatment with glucocorticoid are dependent on the size of the dose and the duration of treatment, a risk/benefit decision must be made in each individual case as to dose and duration of treatment and as to whether daily or intermittent therapy should be used.

ADVERSE REACTIONS
Fluid and electrolyte disturbances
Sodium retention
Fluid retention
Congestive heart failure in susceptible patients
Potassium loss
Hypokalemic alkalosis
Hypertension

Musculoskeletal
Muscle weakness
Steroid myopathy
Loss of muscle mass
Osteoporosis
Vertebral compression fractures
Aseptic necrosis of femoral and humeral heads
Pathologic fracture of long bones

Gastrointestinal
Peptic ulcer with possible subsequent perforation and hemorrhage
Pancreatitis
Abdominal distention
Ulcerative esophagitis

Dermatologic
Impaired wound healing
Thin fragile skin
Petechiae and ecchymoses
Facial erythema
Increased sweating
May suppress reactions to skin tests

Neurological
Convulsions
Increased intracranial pressure with papilledema (pseudo-tumor cerebri) usually after treatment
Vertigo
Headache

Endocrine
Menstrual irregularities
Development of cushingoid state
Suppression of growth in children
Secondary adrenocortical and pituitary unresponsiveness, particularly in times of stress, as in trauma, surgery, or illness
Decreased carbohydrate tolerance
Manifestations of latent diabetes mellitus
Increased requirements for insulin or oral hypoglycemic agents in diabetics

Ophthalmic
Posterior subcapsular cataracts
Increased intraocular pressure
Glaucoma
Exophthalmos

Metabolic
Negative nitrogen balance due to protein catabolism

The following additional adverse reactions are related to parenteral and intralesional corticosteroid therapy:
Rare instances of blindness associated with intralesional therapy around the face and head
Hyperpigmentation or hypopigmentation
Subcutaneous and cutaneous atrophy
Sterile abscess
Anaphylactoid reactions have been reported rarely with products of this class.

DOSAGE AND ADMINISTRATION
General: The initial dosage of Triamcinolone Diacetate may vary from 3 to 48 mg per day, depending on the specific disease entity being treated. In situations of less severity, lower doses will generally suffice while in selected patients higher initial doses may be required. Usually the parenteral dosage ranges are one-third to one-half the oral dose given every 12 hours. However, in certain overwhelming, acute, life-threatening situations, administration in dosages exceeding the usual dosages may be justified and may be administered in multiples of the oral dosages.

The initial dosage should be maintained or adjusted until a satisfactory response is noted. If after a reasonable period of time there is a lack of satisfactory clinical response, Triamcinolone Diacetate should be discontinued and the patient transferred to other appropriate therapy. IT SHOULD BE EMPHASIZED THAT DOSAGE REQUIREMENTS ARE VARIABLE AND MUST BE INDIVIDUALIZED ON THE BASIS OF THE DISEASE UNDER TREATMENT AND THE RESPONSE OF THE PATIENT. After a favorable response is noted, the proper maintenance dosage should be determined by decreasing the initial drug dosage in small increments at appropriate time intervals until the lowest dosage that will maintain an adequate clinical response is reached. It should be kept in mind that constant monitoring is needed in regard to drug dosage. Included in the situations in which dosage adjustments may be necessary are changes in clinical status secondary to remissions or exacerbations in the disease process, the patient's individual drug responsiveness, and the effect of patient exposure to stressful situations not directly related to the disease entity under treatment. In this latter situation, it may be necessary to increase the dosage of Triamcinolone Diacetate for a period of time consistent with the patient's condition. If after long-term therapy the drug is to be stopped, it is recommended that it be withdrawn gradually rather than abruptly.

For intra-articular, intralesional and soft tissue use, a lesser initial dosage range of Triamcinolone Diacetate may produce the desired effect when the drug is administered to provide a localized concentration. The site of the injection and the volume of the injection should be carefully considered when Triamcinolone Diacetate is administered for this purpose.

Specific Parenteral: Triamcinolone Diacetate Parenteral is sterile Triamcinolone Diacetate (40 mg/mL) suspended in a suitable vehicle. The full-strength suspension may be employed. If preferred, the suspension may be diluted with normal saline or water. The diluent may also be prepared by mixing equal parts of normal saline and 1% procaine hydrochloride or other similar local anesthetics. The use of diluents containing preservatives such as methylparaben, propylparaben, phenol, etc. must be avoided as these preparations tend to cause flocculation of the steroid. These dilutions retain full potency for at least one week. Topical ethyl chloride spray must be used locally prior to injection.

Since this product has been designed for ease of administration, a small bore needle (not smaller than 24 gauge) may be used.

Intramuscular: Although Triamcinolone Diacetate Parenteral may be administered intramuscularly for initial therapy, most physicians prefer to adjust the dose orally until adequate control is attained. Intramuscular administration provides a sustained or depot action that can be used to supplement or replace initial oral therapy. With intramuscular therapy, greater supervision of the amount of steroid used is made possible for the patient who is inconsistent in following an oral dosage schedule. In maintenance therapy, the patient-to-patient response is not uniform and, therefore, the dose must be individualized for optimal control.

Although Triamcinolone Diacetate may possess greater anti-inflammatory potency than many glucocorticoids, this is only dose-related since side effects, such as osteoporosis, peptic ulcer, etc., related to glucocorticoid activity, have not been diminished.

The average dose is 40 mg (1 mL) administered intramuscularly once a week for conditions in which anti-inflammatory action is desired.

In general, a single parenteral dose 4 to 7 times the oral daily dose may be expected to control the patient from 4 to 7 days up to 3 to 4 weeks. Dosage should be adjusted to the point where adequate but not necessarily complete relief of symptoms is obtained.

Intra-Articular and Intrasynovial: The usual dose varies from 5 to 40 mg. The average for the knee, for example, is 25 mg. The duration of effect varies from one week to 2 months. However, acutely inflamed joints may require more frequent injections.

A lesser initial dosage range of sterile Triamcinolone Diacetate may produce the desired effect when the drug is administered to provide a localized concentration. The site of the injection and the volume of the injection should be carefully considered when Triamcinolone Diacetate is administered for this purpose.

A specific dose depends largely on the size of the joint.

Strict surgical asepsis is mandatory. The physician should be familiar with anatomical relationships as described in standard text books. Triamcinolone Diacetate Parenteral may be used in any accessible joint except the intervertebrals. In general, intrasynovial therapy is suggested under the following circumstances.

1. When systemic steroid therapy is contraindicated because of side effects such as peptic ulcer.

2. When it is desirable to secure relief in one or two specific joints.

3. When good systemic maintenance fails to control flare-ups in a few joints and it is desirable to secure relief without increasing oral therapy.

Such treatment should not be considered to constitute a cure. Although this method will ameliorate the joint symptoms, it does not preclude the need for the conventional measures usually employed.

It is suggested that infiltration of the soft tissue by local anesthetic precede intra-articular injection. A 24-gauge or larger needle on a dry syringe may be inserted into the joint and excess fluid aspirated. For the first few hours following injection, there may be local discomfort in the joint, but this is usually followed rapidly by effective relief of pain and improvement in local function.

	Anti-inflammatory Relative Potency		Frequently Used Tablet Strength (mg)		Tablet × Potency Equivalent Value
Hydrocortisone	1	×	20	=	20
Prednisolone	4	×	5	=	20
Triamcinolone Diacetate	5	×	4	=	20
Dexamethasone	25	×	0.75	=	18.75

INTRALESIONAL

When Triamcinolone Diacetate Intralesional is administered by injection, strict aseptic technique is mandatory. Full strength suspensions may be employed, or if preferred, the suspension may be diluted, either to a 1:1 or 1:10 concentration, thus obtaining a working concentration of 12.5 mg/mL or approximately 2.5 mg/mL, respectively. Normal (isotonic) saline solution alone or equal parts of normal (isotonic) saline solution and 1% procaine or other local anesthetics may be used as diluents. These dilutions usually retain full potency for at least one week. Topical ethyl chloride spray may be used as a local anesthetic. The use of diluents containing preservatives such as methylparaben, propylparaben, phenol, etc. must be avoided as these preparations tend to cause flocculations of the steroid.

Since this product has been designed for ease of administration, a small bore needle (not smaller than 24 gauge) may be used.

Intralesional or Sublesional: For small lesions, injection is usually well tolerated and a local anesthetic is not necessary. The location and type of lesion will determine the route of injection: intralesional, sublesional, intradermal, subdermal, intracutaneous, or subcutaneous. The size of the lesion will determine the total amount of drug needed, the concentration used, and the number and pattern of injection sites utilized (eg., from a total of 5 mg Triamcinolone Diacetate Intralesional in a 2 mL volume divided over several locations in small lesions, ranging up to 48 mg total Triamcinolone Diacetate Intralesional for large psoriatic plaques). Avoid injecting too superficially. In general, no more than 12.5 mg per injection site should be used. An average of 25 mg is the usual limit for any one lesion. Large areas require multiple injections with smaller doses per injection site.

For a majority of conditions, sublesional injection directly through the lesion into the deep dermal tissue is suggested. In cases where it is difficult to inject intradermally, the suspension may be introduced subcutaneously, as superficially as possible.

Two or three injections at one to two week intervals may suffice as an average course of treatment for many conditions. Within 5-7 days after initial injection, involution of the lesion can usually be seen, with pronounced clearing towards normal tissue after 12-14 days. Mutiple injections of small amounts of equal strength may be convenient in alopecia areata and in psoriasis where there are large or confluent lesions. This is best accomplished by a series of fan-like injections 1/2 to 1 inch apart.

Alopecia areata and totalis require an average dose of 25 to 30 mg in a concentration of 10 mg/mL subcutaneously, 1 to 2 times a week, to stimulate hair regrowth. Results may be expected in 3 to 6 weeks on this dosage, and hair growth may last 3-6 months after initial injection. No more than 0.5 mL should be given in any one site, because excessive deposition may produce local skin atrophy. Continued periodic local injections may be necessary to maintain response and continued hair growth. Use of more dilute solutions diminishes the incidence and degree of local atrophy in the injection site.

In keloids and similar dense scars, injections are usually made directly into the lesion.

Injections may be repeated as required, but probably a total of no more than 75 mg of Triamcinolone Diacetate a week should be given to any one patient. The need for repeated injections is best determined by clinical response. Remissions may be expected to last from a few weeks up to 11 months.

Intra-articular or Intrasynovial: Strict surgical asepsis is mandatory. The physician should be familiar with anatomical relationships as described in standard text books. A recent paper details the anatomy and technical approach in arthrocentesis.

It is usually recommended that infiltration by local anesthetic of the soft tissue precede intra-articular injection. A 22-gauge or larger needle on a dry syringe should be inserted into the joint and excess fluid, if present, should be aspirated. The specific dose depends primarily on the size of the joint. The usual dose varies from 5 to 40 mg, with the average for the knee being 25 mg. Smaller joints as in the fingers require 2 to 5 mg. The duration of effect varies from one week to two months. However, acutely inflamed joints may require more frequent injections. Accidental injection into soft tissue is usually not harmful but decreases the local effectiveness. Injection into subcutaneous lipoid tissue may produce "pseudoatrophy" with a persistent depression of the overlying dermis, lasting several weeks or months.

Administration and dosage of Triamcinolone Diacetate Intralesional must be individualized according to the nature, severity, and chronicity of the disease or disorder treated, and should be undertaken with a view of the patient's entire clinical condition. Corticosteroid therapy is considered an adjunct to and not usually a replacement for conventional therapy. Therapy with Triamcinolone Diacetate Intralesional, as with all steroids, is of the suppressive type, related to its anti-inflammatory effect. The dose should be regulated during therapy according to the degree of therapeutic response, and should be reduced gradually to maintenance levels, whereby the patient obtains adequate or acceptable control of symptoms. When such control occurs, consideration should be given to a gradual decrease in dosage and eventual cessation of therapy. Remission of symptoms may be due to therapy or may be spontaneous, and a therapeutic test of gradual withdrawal of steroid treatment is usually indicated.

Storage: Store at controlled room temperature, 15°-30°C (59°-86°F). DO NOT FREEZE.

J CODES
Per 5 mg IM—J3302

HOW SUPPLIED
INJECTION: 25 MG/ML

BRAND/MANUFACTURER	NDC	SIZE	AWP
◇ **BRAND**			
ARISTOCORT FOR INJECTION: Fujisawa	57317-0203-05	5 ml	$20.30

INJECTION: 40 MG/ML

BRAND/MANUFACTURER	NDC	SIZE	AWP
◇ **BRAND**			
ARISTOCORT FORTE: Fujisawa	57317-0202-01	1 ml	$6.29
	57317-0202-05	5 ml	$12.53
◇ **GENERICS**			
Schein	00364-6666-53	5 ml	$7.44
Steris	00402-0042-05	5 ml	$7.44
Insource	58441-1113-05	5 ml	$8.98

◆ RATED THERAPEUTICALLY EQUIVALENT; ◇ THERAPEUTIC EQUIVALENCE UNCONFIRMED; ○ UNRATED

BRAND/MANUFACTURER	NDC	SIZE	AWP
Genl Inject	52584-0042-05	5 ml	$8.98
Moore,H.L.	00839-5057-25	5 ml	$10.38
TRIAM-FORTE: Hyrex	00314-0775-75	5 ml	$11.00
Rugby	00536-9800-65	5 ml	$11.01
URL	00677-0981-20	5 ml	$11.34
Major	00904-0885-05	5 ml	$12.75
Goldline	00182-3064-62	5 ml	$13.80
TRISTOJECT: Mayrand	00259-0323-05	5 ml	$18.50

Triamcinolone Hexacetonide

DESCRIPTION

Intralesional: A sterile suspension containing 5 mg/mL of micronized Triamcinolone Hexacetonide:

Intra-articular: A sterile suspension containing 20 mg/mL of micronized Triamcinolone Hexacetonide:

The Hexacetonide ester of the potent glucocorticoid Triamcinolone is relatively insoluble (0.0002% at 25° C in water). When injected intralesionally, sublesionally, or intra-articularly, it can be expected to be absorbed slowly from the injection site.

Chemically, Triamcinolone Hexacetonide USP is 9-Fluoro-11β, 16α, 17,21-tetrahydroxypregna-1,4-diene-3,20-dione cyclic 16,17-acetal with acetone 21-(3,3-dimethylbutyrate). Molecular weight 532.65.

Following is its chemical structure:

ACTIONS

Naturally occurring glucocorticoids (hydrocortisone), which also have salt-retaining properties, are used as replacement therapy in adrenocortical deficiency states. Their synthetic analogs are primarily used for their potent anti-inflammatory effects in disorders of many organ systems.

Glucocorticoids cause profound and varied metabolic effects. In addition, they modify the body's immune responses to diverse stimuli.

INDICATIONS

INTRALESIONAL

Intralesional or sublesional sterile Triamcinolone Hexacetonide suspension is indicated for the following.

Keloids

Localized hypertrophic, infiltrated, inflammatory lesions of: lichen planus, psoriatic plaques, granuloma annulare, and lichen simplex chronicus (neurodermatitis)

Discoid lupus erythematosus

Necrobiosis lipoidica diabeticorum

Alopecia areata

Intralesional or sublesional Triamcinolone Hexacetonide may also be useful in cystic tumors of an aponeurosis or tendon (ganglia).

INTRA-ARTICULAR

Intra-articular sterile Triamcinolone Hexacetonide suspension is indicated as adjunctive therapy for short-term administration (to tide the patient over an acute episode or exacerbation) in:

Synovitis of osteoarthritis

Acute and subacute bursitis

Epicondylitis

Posttraumatic osteoarthritis

Rheumatoid arthritis

Acute gouty arthritis

Acute nonspecific tenosynovitis

CONTRAINDICATIONS

Systemic fungal infections

WARNINGS

In patients on corticosteroid therapy subjected to any unusual stress, increased dosage of rapidly acting corticosteroids before, during, and after the stressful situation is indicated.

Corticosteroids may mask some signs of infection, and new infections may appear during their use. There may be decreased resistance and inability to localize infection when corticosteroids are used.

Prolonged use of corticosteroids may produce posterior subcapsular cataracts, glaucoma with possible damage to the optic nerves, and may enhance the establishment of secondary ocular infections due to fungi or viruses.

USAGE IN PREGNANCY

Since adequate human reproduction studies have not been done with corticosteroids, the use of these drugs in pregnancy, nursing mothers, or women of childbearing potential requires that the possible benefits of the drug be weighed against the potential hazards to the mother and embryo or fetus. Infants born of mothers who have received substantial doses of corticosteroids during pregnancy should be carefully observed for signs of hypoadrenalism.

Average and large doses of cortisone or hydrocortisone can cause elevation of blood pressure, salt and water retention, and increased excretion of potassium. These effects are less likely to occur with the synthetic derivatives, except when used in large doses. Dietary salt restriction and potassium supplementation may be necessary. All corticosteroids increase calcium excretion.

While on corticosteroid therapy patients should not be vaccinated against smallpox. Other immunization procedures should not be undertaken in patients who are on corticosteroids, especially in high doses, because of possible hazards of neurological complications and lack of antibody response.

The use of Triamcinolone Hexacetonide in active tuberculosis should be restricted to those cases of fulminating or disseminated tuberculosis in which the corticosteroid is used for the management of the disease in conjunction with an appropriate antituberculous regimen.

If corticosteroids are indicated in patients with latent tuberculosis or tuberculin reactivity, close observation is necessary as reactivation of the disease may occur. During prolonged corticosteroid therapy, these patients should receive chemoprophylaxis.

Because rare instances of anaphylactoid reactions have occurred in patients receiving parenteral corticosteroid therapy, appropriate precautionary measures should be taken prior to administration, especially when the patient has a history of allergy to any drug.

Intralesional or sublesional injection of excessive dosage, whether by single or multiple injection, into any given area, may cause cutaneous or subcutaneous atrophy.

Postinjection flare (following intra-articular use) and charcot-like arthropathy have been associated with parenteral corticosteroid therapy.

PRECAUTIONS

Drug-induced secondary adrenocortical insufficiency may be minimized by gradual reduction of dosage. This type of relative insufficiency may persist for months after discontinuation of therapy; therefore, in any situation of stress occurring during that period, hormone therapy should be reinstituted. Since mineralocorticoid secretion may be impaired, salt and/or a mineralocorticoid should be administered concurrently.

There is an enhanced effect of corticosteroids in patients with hypothyroidism and in those with cirrhosis.

Corticosteroids should be used cautiously in patients with ocular herpes simplex for fear of corneal perforation.

The lowest possible dose of corticosteroids should be used to control the condition under treatment, and when reduction in dosage is possible, the reduction must be gradual.

Psychic derangements may appear when corticosteroids are used, ranging from euphoria, insomnia, mood swings, personality changes, and severe depression to frank psychotic manifestations. Also, existing emotional instability or psychotic tendencies may be aggravated by corticosteroids.

Aspirin should be used cautiously in conjunction with corticosteroids in hypoprothrombinemia.

Steroids should be used with caution in nonspecific ulcerative colitis, if there is a probability of impending perforation, abscess or other pyogenic infection, also in diverticulitis, fresh intestinal anastomoses, active or latent peptic ulcer, renal insufficiency, hypertension, osteoporosis, and myasthenia gravis.

Growth and development of infants and children on prolonged corticosteroid therapy should be carefully followed. The following additional precautions apply for parenteral corticosteroids.

Intra-articular injection of a corticosteroid may produce systemic as well as local effects.

Appropriate examination of any joint fluid present is necessary to exclude a septic process.

A marked increase in pain accompanied by local swelling, further restriction of joint motion, fever, and malaise are suggestive of septic arthritis. If this complication occurs and the diagnosis of sepsis is confirmed, appropriate antimicrobial therapy should be instituted.

Local injection of a steroid into a previously infected joint is to be avoided.

Corticosteroids should not be injected into unstable joints.

The slower rate of absorption by intramuscular administration should be recognized.

Atrophy at the site of injection has been reported.

Routine laboratory studies, such as urinalysis, two-hour postprandial blood sugar, determination of blood pressure and body weight, and a chest x-ray should be made at regular intervals during prolonged therapy. Upper GI x-rays are desirable in patients with an ulcer history or significant dyspepsia.

ADVERSE REACTIONS

Fluid and electrolyte disturbances:

Sodium retention

Fluid retention

Congestive heart failure in susceptible patients

Potassium loss

Hypokalemic alkalosis
Hypertension

Musculoskeletal:
Muscle weakness
Steroid myopathy
Loss of muscle mass
Osteoporosis
Vertebral compression fractures
Aseptic necrosis of femoral and humeral heads
Pathologic fracture of long bones

Gastrointestinal:
Peptic ulcer with possible subsequent perforation and hemorrhage
Pancreatitis
Abdominal distention
Ulcerative esophagitis

Dermatologic:
Impaired wound healing
Thin fragile skin
Petechiae and ecchymoses
Facial erythema
Increased sweating
May suppress reactions to skin tests

Neurological:
Convulsions
Increased intracranial pressure with papilledema (pseudotumor cerebri) usually after treatment
Vertigo
Headache

Endocrine:
Menstrual irregularities
Development of Cushingoid state
Suppression of growth in children
Secondary adrenocortical and pituitary unresponsiveness, particularly in times of stress, as in trauma, surgery, or illness
Decreased carbohydrate tolerance
Manifestations of latent diabetes mellitus
Increased requirements for insulin or oral hypoglycemic agents in diabetics

Ophthalmic:
Posterior subcapsular cataracts
Increased intraocular pressure
Glaucoma
Exophthalmos

Metabolic:
Negative nitrogen balance due to protein catabolism

The following additional adverse reactions are related to parenteral and intralesional corticosteroid therapy.
Rare instances of blindness associated with intralesional therapy around the orbit or intranasally
Hyperpigmentation or hypopigmentation
Subcutaneous and cutaneous atrophy
Sterile abscess
Anaphylactoid reactions have been reported rarely with products of this class.

DOSAGE AND ADMINISTRATION
GENERAL
The initial dosage of sterile Triamcinolone Hexacetonide suspension may vary from 2 to 48 mg per day, depending on the specific disease entity being treated. In situations of less severity, lower doses will generally suffice, while in selected patients, higher initial doses may be required. Usually parenteral dosage ranges are one-third to one-half the oral dose given every 12 hours. However, in certain overwhelming, acute, life-threatening situations, administration in dosages exceeding the usual dosages may be justified and may be administered in multiples of the oral dosages.

The initial dosage should be maintained or adjusted until a satisfactory response is noted. If after a reasonable period of time there is a lack of satisfactory clinical response, Triamcinolone Hexacetonide should be discontinued and the patient transferred to other appropriate therapy. It should be emphasized that dosage requirements are variable and must be individualized on the basis of the disease under treatment and the response of the patient. After a favorable response is noted, the proper maintenance dosage should be determined by decreasing the initial drug dosage in small increments at appropriate time intervals until the lowest dosage that will maintain an adequate clinical response is reached. It should be kept in mind that constant monitoring is needed in regard to drug dosage. Included in the situations in which dosage adjustments may be necessary are changes in clinical status secondary to remissions or exacerbations in the disease process, the patient's individual drug responsiveness, and the effect of patient exposure to stressful situations not directly related to the disease entity under treatment. In this latter situation, it may be necessary to increase the dosage of Triamcinolone Hexacetonide for a period of time consistent with the patient's condition. If after long-term therapy the drug is to be stopped, it is recommended that it be withdrawn gradually rather than abruptly.

DIRECTIONS FOR USE
Strict aseptic administration technique is mandatory. Topical ethyl chloride spray may be used locally before injection. The syringe should be gently agitated to achieve uniform suspension before use. Since this product has been designed for ease of administration, a small bore needle (not smaller than 24 gauge) may be used.

DILUTION
Intralesional: Triamcinolone Hexacetonide suspension may be diluted, if desired, with Dextrose and Sodium Chloride Injection USP, (5% and 10% Dextrose), Sodium Chloride Injection USP, or Sterile Water for Injection USP.

The optimum dilution, ie, 1:1, 1:2, 1:4, should be determined by the nature of the lesion, its size, the depth of injection, the volume needed, and location of the lesion. In general, more superficial injections should be performed with greater dilution. Certain conditions, such as keloids, require a less dilute suspension such as 5 mg/mL, with variation in dose and dilution as dictated by the condition of the individual patient. Subsequent dosage, dilution, and frequency of injections are best judged by the clinical response.

The suspension may also be mixed with 1% or 2% Lidocaine Hydrochloride, using formulations that do not contain parabens. Similar local anesthetics may also be used. Diluents containing methylparaben, propylparaben, phenol, etc. should be avoided since these compounds may cause flocculation of the steroid. These dilutions will retain full potency for one week, but care should be exercised to avoid contamination of the vial's contents. The dilutions should be discarded after 7 days.

Intralesional or Sublesional: Average Dose: Up to 0.5 mg per square inch of affected skin injected intralesionally or sublesionally. The frequency of subsequent injections is best determined by the clinical response. If desired, the vial may be diluted as indicated under *"Directions for Use".*

A lesser initial dosage range of Triamcinolone Hexacetonide may produce the desired effect when the drug is administered to provide a localized concentration. The site of the injection and the volume of the injection should be carefully considered when Triamcinolone Hexacetonide is administered for this purpose.

DILUTION
Intra-articular: Triamcinolone Hexacetonide suspension may be mixed with 1% or 2% Lidocaine Hydrochloride, using formulations that do not contain parabens. Similar local anesthetics may also be used. Diluents containing methylparaben, propylparaben, phenol, etc. should be avoided since these compounds may cause flocculation of the steroid. These dilutions will retain full potency for one week, but care should be exercised to avoid contamination.

Intra-articular: Average Dose: 2 to 20 mg (0.1 mL to 1.0 mL).
The dose depends on the size of the joint to be injected, the degree of inflammation, and the amount of fluid present. In general, large joints (such as knee, hip, shoulder) require 10 to 20 mg. For small joints (such as interphalangeal, metacarpophalangeal), 2 to 6 mg may be employed. When the amount of synovial fluid is increased, aspiration may be performed before administering Triamcinolone Hexacetonide. Subsequent dosage and frequency of injections can best be judged by clinical response.

The usual frequency of injection into a single joint is every three or four weeks, and injection more frequently than that is generally not advisable. To avoid possible joint destruction from repeated use of intra-articular corticosteroids, injection should be as infrequent as possible, consistent with adequate patient care. Attention should be paid to avoiding deposition of drug along the needle path which might produce atrophy.

STORAGE
Store at controlled room temperature, 15-30°C (59-86°F).
DO NOT FREEZE.

J CODES
Per 5 mg VAR—J3303

HOW SUPPLIED
INJECTION: 5 MG/ML

BRAND/MANUFACTURER	NDC	SIZE	AWP
○ **BRAND**			
ARISTOSPAN INJECTION: Fujisawa	57317-0206-05	5 ml	$11.94

INJECTION: 20 MG/ML

BRAND/MANUFACTURER	NDC	SIZE	AWP
○ **BRAND**			
ARISTOSPAN INJECTION: Fujisawa	57317-0205-01	1 ml	$8.18
	57317-0205-05	1 ml 10s	$18.40

Triaminic *SEE PHENIRAMINE MALEATE/*
PHENYLPROPANOLAMINE HYDROCHLORIDE/PYRILAMINE MALEATE

◆ RATED THERAPEUTICALLY EQUIVALENT; ◇ THERAPEUTIC EQUIVALENCE UNCONFIRMED; ○ UNRATED

Triaminic-DH Expectorant SEE
GUAIFENESIN/HYDROCODONE BITARTRATE/PHENIRAMINE MALEATE/PHENYLPROPANOLAMINE HYDROCHLORIDE/PYRILAMINE MALEATE

Triaminic Exp with Codeine SEE
CODEINE PHOSPHATE/GUAIFENESIN/PHENYLPROPANOLAMINE HYDROCHLORIDE

Triamterene

DESCRIPTION
Triamterene is a potassium-conserving diuretic. Triamterene is 2,4,7-triamino-6-phenyl-pteridine. Its molecular weight is 253.27. At 50°C, Triamterene is slightly soluble in water. It is soluble in dilute ammonia, dilute aqueous sodium hydroxide and dimethylformamide. It is sparingly soluble in methanol.

Each capsule for oral use contains Triamterene, 50 or 100 mg.

Following is its chemical structure:

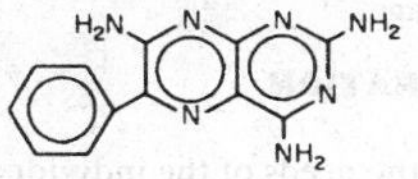

CLINICAL PHARMACOLOGY
Triamterene has a unique mode of action; it inhibits the reabsorption of sodium ions in exchange for potassium and hydrogen ions at that segment of the distal tubule under the control of adrenal mineralocorticoids (especially aldosterone). This activity is not directly related to aldosterone secretion or antagonism; it is a result of a direct effect on the renal tubule.

The fraction of filtered sodium reaching this distal tubular exchange site is relatively small, and the amount which is exchanged depends on the level of mineralocorticoid activity. Thus, the degree of natriuresis and diuresis produced by inhibition of the exchange mechanism is necessarily limited. Increasing the amount of available sodium and the level of mineralocorticoid activity by the use of more proximally acting diuretics will increase the degree of diuresis and potassium conservation.

Triamterene occasionally causes increases in serum potassium which can result in hyperkalemia. It does not produce alkalosis because it does not cause excessive excretion of titratable acid and ammonium.

Triamterene has been shown to cross the placental barrier and appear in the cord blood of animals.

PHARMACOKINETICS
Onset of action is two to four hours after ingestion. In normal volunteers the mean peak serum levels were 30 ng/mL at three hours. The average percent of drug recovered in the urine (0-48 hours) was 21%. Triamterene is primarily metabolized to the sulfate conjugate of hydroxytriamterene. Both the plasma and urine levels of this metabolite greatly exceed Triamterene levels. Triamterene is rapidly absorbed, with somewhat less than 50% of the oral dose reaching the urine. Most patients will respond to Triamterene during the first day of treatment. Maximum therapeutic effect, however, may not be seen for several days. Duration of diuresis depends on several factors, especially renal function, but it generally tapers off seven to nine hours after administration.

INDICATIONS AND USAGE
Triamterene is indicated in the treatment of edema associated with congestive heart failure, cirrhosis of the liver, and the nephrotic syndrome; also in steroid-induced edema, idiopathic edema, and edema due to secondary hyperaldosteronism.

Triamterene may be used alone or with other diuretics either for its added diuretic effect or its potassium-conserving potential. It also promotes increased diuresis when patients prove resistant or only partially responsive to thiazides or other diuretics because of secondary hyperaldosteronism.

Usage in Pregnancy: The routine use of diuretics in an otherwise healthy woman is inappropriate and exposes mother and fetus to unnecessary hazard. Diuretics do not prevent development of toxemia of pregnancy, and there is no satisfactory evidence that they are useful in the treatment of developed toxemia.

Edema during pregnancy may arise from pathological causes or from the physiologic and mechanical consequences of pregnancy. Diuretics are indicated in pregnancy when edema is due to pathologic causes, just as they are in the absence of pregnancy (however, see *"Precautions"* below). Dependent edema in pregnancy, resulting from restriction of venous return by the expanded uterus, is properly treated through elevation of the lower extremities and use of support hose; use of diuretics to lower intravascular volume in this case is illogical and unnecessary. There is hypervolemia during normal pregnancy which is harmful to neither the fetus nor the mother (in the absence of cardiovascular disease), but which is associated with edema, including generalized edema, in the majority of pregnant women. If this edema produces discomfort, increased recumbency will often provide relief. In rare instances, this edema may cause extreme discomfort which

is not relieved by rest. In these cases, a short course of diuretics may provide relief and may be appropriate.

UNLABELED USES
Triamterene is used alone or as an adjunct in the treatment of diabetes insipidus.

CONTRAINDICATIONS
Anuria: Severe or progressive kidney disease or dysfunction with the possible exception of nephrosis. Severe hepatic disease. Hypersensitivity to the drug.

Triamterene should not be used in patients with pre-existing elevated serum potassium, as is sometimes seen in patients with impaired renal function or azotemia, or in patients who develop hyperkalemia while on the drug. Patients should not be placed on dietary potassium supplements, potassium salts, or potassium-containing salt substitutes in conjunction with Triamterene.

Triamterene should not be given to patients receiving other potassium-conserving agents such as spironolactone, amiloride hydrochloride, or other formulations containing Triamterene. Two deaths have been reported in patients receiving concomitant spironolactone and Triamterene or Triamterene/Hydrochlorthiazide. Although dosage recommendations were exceeded in one case and in the other serum electrolytes were not properly monitored, these two drugs should not be given concomitantly.

WARNINGS

> ABNORMAL ELEVATION OF SERUM POTASSIUM LEVELS (GREATER THAN OR EQUAL TO 5.5 MEQ/LITER) CAN OCCUR WITH ALL POTASSIUM-CONSERVING AGENTS, INCLUDING TRIAMTERENE. HYPERKALEMIA IS MORE LIKELY TO OCCUR IN PATIENTS WITH RENAL IMPAIRMENT AND DIABETES (EVEN WITHOUT EVIDENCE OF RENAL IMPAIRMENT), AND IN THE ELDERLY OR SEVERELY ILL. SINCE UNCORRECTED HYPERKALEMIA MAY BE FATAL, SERUM POTASSIUM LEVELS MUST BE MONITORED AT FREQUENT INTERVALS ESPECIALLY IN PATIENTS RECEIVING TRIAMTERENE WHEN DOSAGES ARE CHANGED OR WITH ANY ILLNESS THAT MAY INFLUENCE RENAL FUNCTION.

There have been isolated reports of hypersensitivity reactions; therefore, patients should be observed regularly for the possible occurrence of blood dyscrasias, liver damage, or other idiosyncratic reactions.

Periodic BUN and serum potassium determinations should be made to check kidney function, especially in patients with suspected or confirmed renal insufficiency. It is particularly important to make serum potassium determinations in elderly or diabetic patients receiving the drug; these patients should be observed carefully for possible serum potassium increases.

If hyperkalemia is present or suspected, an electrocardiogram should be obtained. If the ECG shows no widening of the QRS or arrhythmia in the presence of hyperkalemia, it is usually sufficient to discontinue Triamterene and any potassium supplementation and substitute a thiazide alone. Sodium polystyrene sulfonate may be administered to enhance the excretion of excess potassium. **The presence of a widened QRS complex or arrhythmia in association with hyperkalemia requires prompt additional therapy.** For tachyarrhythmia, infuse 44 mEq of sodium bicarbonate or 10 mL of 10% calcium gluconate or calcium chloride over several minutes. For asystole, bradycardia, or A-V block transvenous pacing is also recommended.

The effect of calcium and sodium bicarbonate is transient and repeated administration may be required. When indicated by the clinical situation, excess K^+ may be removed by dialysis or oral or rectal administration of sodium polystyrene sulfonate. Infusion of glucose and insulin has also been used to treat hyperkalemia.

PRECAUTIONS
GENERAL
Triamterene tends to conserve potassium rather than to promote the excretion as do many diuretics and, occasionally, can cause increases in serum potassium which, in some instances, can result in hyperkalemia. In rare instances, hyperkalemia has been associated with cardiac irregularities.

Electrolyte imbalance often encountered in such diseases as congestive heart failure, renal disease, or cirrhosis may be aggravated or caused independently by any effective diuretic agent including Triamterene. The use of full doses of a diuretic when salt intake is restricted can result in a low-salt syndrome.

Triamterene can cause mild nitrogen retention which is reversible upon withdrawal of the drug and is seldom observed with intermittent (every-other-day) therapy.

Triamterene may cause a decreasing alkali reserve with the possibility of metabolic acidosis.

By the very nature of their illness, cirrhotics with splenomegaly sometimes have marked variations in their blood pictures. Since Triamterene is a weak folic acid antagonist, it may contribute to the appearance of megaloblastosis in cases where folic acid stores have been depleted. Therefore, periodic blood studies in these patients are recommended. They should also be observed for exacerbations of underlying liver disease.

Triamterene has elevated uric acid, especially in persons predisposed to gouty arthritis.

Triamterene has been reported in renal stones in association with other calculus components. Triamterene should be used with caution in patients with histories of renal stones.

INFORMATION FOR PATIENTS

To help avoid stomach upset, it is recommended that the drug be taken after meals.

If a single daily dose is prescribed, it may be preferable to take it in the morning to minimize the effect of increased frequency of urination on nighttime sleep.

If a dose is missed, the patient should not take more than the prescribed dose at the next dosing interval.

LABORATORY TESTS

Hyperkalemia will rarely occur in patients with adequate urinary output, but it is a possibility if large doses are used for considerable periods of time. If hyperkalemia is observed, Triamterene should be withdrawn. The normal adult range of serum potassium is 3.5 to 5.0 mEq per liter with 4.5 mEq often being used for a reference point. Potassium levels persistently above 6 mEq per liter require careful observation and treatment. Normal potassium levels tend to be higher in neonates (7.7 mEq per liter) than in adults.

Serum potassium levels do not necessarily indicate true body potassium concentration. A rise in plasma pH may cause a decrease in plasma potassium concentration and an increase in the intracellular potassium concentration. Because Triamterene conserves potassium, it has been theorized that in patients who have received intensive therapy or been given the drug for prolonged periods, a rebound kaliuresis could occur upon abrupt withdrawal. In such patients withdrawal of Triamterene should be gradual.

DRUG INTERACTIONS

Caution should be used when lithium and diuretics are used concomitantly because diuretic-induced sodium loss may reduce the renal clearance of lithium and increase serum lithium levels with risk of lithium toxicity. Patients receiving such combined therapy should have serum lithium levels monitored closely and the lithium dosage adjusted if necessary.

A possible interaction resulting in acute renal failure has been reported in a few subjects when indomethacin, a nonsteroidal anti-inflammatory agent, was given with Triamterene. Caution is advised in administering nonsteroidal anti-inflammatory agents with Triamterene.

The effects of the following drugs may be potentiated when given together with Triamterene: antihypertensive medication, other diuretics, preanesthetic and anesthetic agents, skeletal muscle relaxants (nondepolarizing).

Potassium-sparing agents should be used with caution in conjunction with angiotensin-converting enzyme (ACE) inhibitors due to an increased risk of hyperkalemia.

The following agents, given together with Triamterene, may promote serum potassium accumulation and possibly result in hyperkalemia because of the potassium-sparing nature of Triamterene, especially in patients with renal insufficiency: blood from blood bank (may contain up to 30 mEq of potassium per liter of plasma or up to 65 mEq per liter of whole blood when stored for more than 10 days); low-salt milk (may contain up to 60 mEq of potassium per liter); potassium-containing medications (such as parenteral penicillin G potassium); salt substitutes (most contain substantial amounts of potassium).

Triamterene may raise blood glucose levels; for adult-onset diabetes, dosage adjustments of hypoglycemic agents may be necessary during and after therapy; concurrent use with chlorpropamide may increase the risk of severe hyponatremia.

DRUG/LABORATORY TEST INTERACTIONS

Triamterene and quinidine have similar fluorescence spectra; thus, Triamterene will interfere with the fluorescent measurement of quinidine.

CARCINOGENESIS, MUTAGENESIS, IMPAIRMENT OF FERTILITY

Long-term studies to determine the carcinogenic potential of Triamterene are not available. Studies to determine the mutagenic potential of Triamterene are not available. Reproductive studies have been performed in rats at doses up to 30 times the human dose and have revealed no evidence of impaired fertility.

PREGNANCY

Teratogenic Effects: Pregnancy Category B: Reproduction studies have been performed in rats at doses up to 30 times the human dose and have revealed no evidence of impaired fertility or harm to the fetus due to Triamterene. There are, however, no adequate and well-controlled studies in pregnant women. Because animal reproductive studies are not always predictive of human response, this drug should be used during pregnancy only if clearly needed.

Nonteratogenic Effects: Triamterene has been shown to cross the placental barrier and appear in the cord blood of animals; this may occur in humans. The use of Triamterene in pregnant women requires that the anticipated benefit be weighed against possible hazards to the fetus. These possible hazards include adverse reactions which have occurred in the adult.

Nursing Mothers: Triamterene appears in animal milk; this may occur in humans. If use of the drug is deemed essential, the patient should stop nursing.

Pediatric Use: Safety and effectiveness in children have not been established.

ADVERSE REACTIONS

Adverse effects are listed in decreasing order of frequency; however, the most serious adverse effects are listed first regardless of frequency. All adverse effects occur rarely (that is, one in 1000, or less).

Hypersensitivity: anaphylaxis, rash, photosensitivity.

Metabolic: hyperkalemia, hypokalemia.

Renal: azotemia, elevated BUN and creatinine, renal stones, acute interstitial nephritis (rare), acute renal failure (one case of irreversible renal failure has been reported).

Gastrointestinal: jaundice and/or liver enzyme abnormalities, nausea and vomiting, diarrhea.

Hematologic: thrombocytopenia, megaloblastic anemia.

Central Nervous System: weakness, fatigue, dizziness, headache, dry mouth.

OVERDOSAGE

In the event of overdosage it can be theorized that electrolyte imbalance would be the major concern, with particular attention to possible hyperkalemia. Other symptoms that might be seen would be nausea and vomiting, other g.i. disturbances, and weakness. It is conceivable that some hypotension could occur. As with an overdose of any drug, immediate evacuation of the stomach should be induced through emesis and gastric lavage. Careful evaluation of the electrolyte pattern and fluid balance should be made. There is no specific antidote.

Reversible acute renal failure following ingestion of 50 tablets of a product containing a combination of 50 mg Triamterene and 25 mg hydrochlorothiazide has been reported.

The oral LD_{50} in mice is 380 mg/kg. The amount of drug in a single dose ordinarily associated with symptoms of overdose or likely to be life-threatening is not known.

Although Triamterene is 67% protein-bound, there may be some benefit to dialysis in cases of overdosage.

DOSAGE AND ADMINISTRATION

ADULT DOSAGE

Dosage should be titrated to the needs of the individual patient. When used alone, the usual starting dose is 100 mg twice daily after meals. When combined with another diuretic or antihypertensive agent, the today daily dosage of each agent should usually be lowered initially and then adjusted to the patient's needs. The total daily dosage should not exceed 300 mg. Please refer to "Precautions-General".

When Triamterene is added to other diuretic therapy or when patients are switched to Triamterene from other diuretics, all potassium supplementation should be discontinued.

Store at controlled room temperature, (59° to 86°F). Protect from light.

HOW SUPPLIED
CAPSULE: 50 MG

BRAND/MANUFACTURER	NDC	SIZE	AWP
○ **BRAND** DYRENIUM: SK Beecham Pharm	00108-3806-20	100s	$32.55

CAPSULE: 100 MG

BRAND/MANUFACTURER	NDC	SIZE	AWP
○ **BRAND** DYRENIUM: SK Beecham Pharm	00108-3807-20	100s	$40.90

Triavil *SEE* AMITRIPTYLINE HYDROCHLORIDE WITH PERPHENAZINE

Triazolam

DESCRIPTION

Triazolam tablets contain Triazolam, a triazolobenzodiazepine hypnotic agent.

Triazolam is a white crystalline powder, soluble in alcohol and poorly soluble in water. It has a molecular weight of 343.21.

The chemical name for Triazolam is 8-chloro-6-(o-chlorophenyl)-1-methyl-4H-s-triazolo-[4,3-α][1,4] benzodiazepine.

Each Triazolam tablet, for oral administration, contains 0.125 mg or 0.25 mg of Triazolam.

Following is its chemical structure:

CLINICAL PHARMACOLOGY

Triazolam is a hypnotic with a short mean plasma half-life reported to be in the range of 1.5 to 5.5 hours. In normal subjects treated for 7 days with four times the recommended dosage, there was no evidence of altered systemic bioavailability, rate of elimination, or accumulation. Peak plasma levels are reached within 2 hours following oral administration. Following recommended doses of Triazolam, peak plasma levels in the range of 1 to 6 ng/mL are seen. The plasma levels achieved are proportional to the dose given.

Triazolam and its metabolites, principally as conjugated glucuronides, which are presumably inactive, are excreted primarily in the urine. Only small amounts of unmetabolized Triazolam appear in the urine. The two primary metabolites accounted for 79.9% of urinary excretion. Urinary excretion appeared to be biphasic in its time course.

Triazolam tablets 0.5 mg, in two separate studies, did not affect the prothrombin times or plasma warfarin levels in male volunteers administered sodium warfarin orally.

Extremely high concentrations of Triazolam do not displace bilirubin bound to human serum albumin *in vitro*.

Triazolam ^{14}C was administered orally to pregnant mice. Drug-related material appeared uniformly distributed in the fetus with ^{14}C concentrations approximately the same as in the brain of the mother.

In sleep laboratory studies, Triazolam tablets significantly decreased sleep latency, increased the duration of sleep, and decreased the number of nocturnal awakenings. After 2 weeks of consecutive nightly administration, the drug's effect on total wake time is decreased, and the values recorded in the last third of the night approach baseline levels. On the first and/or second night after drug discontinuance (first or second post-drug night), total time asleep, percentage of time spent sleeping, and rapidity of falling asleep frequently were significantly less than on baseline (predrug) nights. This effect is often called "rebound" insomnia.

The type and duration of hypnotic effects and the profile of unwanted effects during administration of benzodiazepine drugs may be influenced by the biologic half-life of administered drug and any active metabolites formed. When half-lives are long, the drug or metabolites may accumulate during periods of nightly administration and be associated with impairments of cognitive and motor performance during waking hours; the possibility of interaction with other psychoactive drugs or alcohol will be enhanced. In contrast, if half-lives are short, the drug and metabolites will be cleared before the next dose is ingested, and carry-over effects related to excessive sedation or CNS depression should be minimal or absent. However, during nightly use for an extended period pharmacodynamic tolerance or adaptation to some effects of benzodiazepine hypnotics may develop. If the drug has a short half-life of elimination, it is possible that a relative deficiency of the drug or its active metabolites (ie, in relationship to the receptor site) may occur at some point in the interval between each night's use. This sequence of events may account for two clinical findings reported to occur after several weeks of nightly use of rapidly eliminated benzodiazepine hypnotics: 1) increased wakefulness during the last third of the night and 2) the appearance of increased daytime anxiety after 10 days of continuous treatment.

INDICATIONS AND USAGE

Triazolam is indicated for the short-term treatment of insomnia (generally 7-10 days). Use for more than 2-3 weeks requires complete reevaluation of the patient (see *"Warnings"*).

Prescriptions for Triazolam should be written for short-term use (7-10 days) and it should not be prescribed in quantities exceeding a 1-month supply.

UNLABELED USES
Triazolam is used alone or as a adjunct in the treatment of anxiety disorders and preoperative anxiety.

CONTRAINDICATIONS

Triazolam tablets are contraindicated in patients with known hypersensitivity to this drug or other benzodiazepines.

Benzodiazepines may cause fetal damage when administered during pregnancy. An increased risk of congenital malformations associated with the use of diazepam and chlordiazepoxide during the first trimester of pregnancy has been suggested in several studies. Transplacental distribution has resulted in neonatal CNS depression following the ingestion of therapeutic doses of a benzodiazepine hypnotic during the last weeks of pregnancy.

Triazolam is contraindicated in pregnant women. If there is a likelihood of the patient becoming pregnant while receiving Triazolam, she should be warned of the potential risk to the fetus. Patients should be instructed to discontinue the drug prior to becoming pregnant. The possibility that a woman of childbearing potential may be pregnant at the time of institution of therapy should be considered.

WARNINGS

Sleep disturbance may be the presenting manifestation of a physical and/or psychiatric disorder. Consequently, a decision to initiate symptomatic treatment of insomnia should only be made after the patient has been carefully evaluated. The failure of insomnia to remit after 7-10 days of treatment may indicate the presence of a primary psychiatric and/or medical illness.

Worsening of insomnia or the emergence of new abnormalities of thinking or behavior may be the consequence of an unrecognized psychiatric or physical disorder. These have also been reported to occur in association with the use of Triazolam.

Because some of the adverse effects of Triazolam appear to be dose related (see *"Precautions"* and *"Dosage and Administration"*), it is important to use the smallest possible effective dose. Elderly patients are especially susceptible to dose related adverse effects.

An increase in daytime anxiety has been reported for Triazolam after as few as 10 days of continuous use. In some patients this may be a manifestation of interdose withdrawal (see *"Clinical Pharmacology"*). If increased daytime anxiety is observed during treatment, discontinuation of treatment may be advisable.

A variety of abnormal thinking and behavior changes have been reported to occur in association with the use of benzodiazepine hypnotics including Triazolam. Some of these changes may be characterized by decreased inhibition, eg, aggressiveness and extroversion that seem excessive, similar to that seen with alcohol and other CNS depressants (eg, sedative/hypnotics). Other kinds of behavioral changes have also been reported, for example, bizarre behavior, agitation, hallucinations, depersonalization. In primarily depressed patients, the worsening of depression, including suicidal thinking, has been reported in association with the use of benzodiazepines.

It can rarely be determined with certainty whether a particular instance of the abnormal behaviors listed above is drug induced, spontaneous in origin, or a result of an underlying psychiatric or physical disorder. Nonetheless, the emergence of any new behavioral sign or symptom of concern requires careful and immediate evaluation.

Because of its depressant CNS effects, patients receiving Triazolam should be cautioned against engaging in hazardous occupations requiring complete mental alertness such as operating machinery or driving a motor vehicle. For the same reason, patients should be cautioned about the concomitant ingestion of alcohol and other CNS depressant drugs during treatment with Triazolam Tablets.

As with some, but not all benzodiazepines, anterograde amnesia of varying severity and paradoxical reactions have been reported following therapeutic doses of Triazolam. Data from several sources suggest that anterograde amnesia may occur at a higher rate with Triazolam than with other benzodiazepine hypnotics.

PRECAUTIONS

General: In elderly and/or debilitated patients it is recommended that treatment with Triazolam Tablets be initiated at 0.125 mg to decrease the possibility of development of oversedation, dizziness, or impaired coordination.

Some side effects reported in association with the use of Triazolam appear to be dose related. These include drowsiness, dizziness, light-headedness, and amnesia.

The relationship between dose and what may be more serious behavioral phenomena is less certain. Specifically, some evidence, based on spontaneous marketing reports, suggests that confusion, bizarre or abnormal behavior, agitation, and hallucinations may also be dose related; but this evidence is inconclusive. In accordance with good medical practice it is recommended that therapy be initiated at the lowest effective dose. (See *"Dosage and Administration".*)

Cases of "traveler's amnesia" have been reported by individuals who have taken Triazolam to induce sleep while traveling, such as during an airplane flight. In some of these cases, insufficient time was allowed for the sleep period prior to awakening and before beginning activity. Also, the concomitant use of alcohol may have been a factor in some cases. Caution should be exercised if Triazolam is prescribed to patients with signs or symptoms of depression that could be intensified by hypnotic drugs. Suicidal tendencies may be present in such patients and protective measures may be required. Intentional overdosage is more common in these patients, and the least amount of drug that is feasible should be available to the patient at any one time.

The usual precautions should be observed in patients with impaired renal or hepatic function, chronic pulmonary insufficiency, and sleep apnea. In patients with compromised respiratory function, respiratory depression and apnea have been reported infrequently.

Information for Patients: The text of a patient package insert is printed at the end of this insert. To assure safe and effective use of Triazolam the information and instructions provided in this package insert should be discussed with patients.

Laboratory Tests: Laboratory tests are not ordinarily required in otherwise healthy patients.

Drug Interactions: Both pharmacodynamic and pharmacokinetic interactions have been reported with benzodiazepines. *In particular, Triazolam produces additive* CNS depressant effects when co-administered with other psychotropic medications, anticonvulsants, antihistamines, ethanol, and other drugs which themselves produce CNS depression.

Pharmacokinetic interactions can occur when triazolam is administered along with drugs that interfere with its metabolism. Specific examples, documented with evidence from controlled trials, show that the co-administration of either cimetidine or erythromycin with Triazolam causes an approximate doubling of the elimination half-life and plasma levels of triazolam. Consequently, consideration of dose reduction may be appropriate in patients treated concomitantly with either cimetidine or erythromycin and Triazolam.

Carcinogenesis, Mutagenesis, Impairment of Fertility: No evidence of carcinogenic potential was observed in mice during a 24-month study with Triazolam Tablets in doses up to 4,000 times the human dose.

Pregnancy:
1. Teratogenic effects: Pregnancy category X (see *"Contraindications"*).
2. Non-teratogenic effects: It is to be considered that the child born of a mother who is on benzodiazepines may be at some risk for withdrawal symptoms from the drug, during the postnatal period. Also, neonatal flaccidity has been reported in an infant born of a mother who had been receiving benzodiazepines.

Nursing Mothers: Human studies have not been performed; however, studies in rats have indicated that Triazolam and its metabolites are secreted in milk. Therefore, administration of Triazolam to nursing mothers is not recommended.

Pediatric Use: Safety and efficacy of Triazolam in children below the age of 18 have not been established.

ADVERSE REACTIONS

During placebo-controlled clinical studies in which 1,003 patients received Triazolam Tablets, the most troublesome side effects were extensions of the pharmacologic activity of triazolam, eg, drowsiness, dizziness, or light-headedness.

The figures cited below are estimates of untoward clinical event incidence among subjects who participated in the relatively short duration (ie, 1 to 42 days) placebo-controlled clinical trials of Triazolam. The figures cannot be used to predict precisely the incidence of untoward events in the course of usual medical practice where patient characteristics and other factors often differ from those in the clinical trials. These figures cannot be compared with those obtained from other clinical studies involving related drug products and placebo, as each group of drug trials is conducted under a different set of conditions.

Comparison of the cited figures, however, can provide the prescriber with some basis for estimating the relative contributions of drug and nondrug factors to the untoward event incidence rate in the population studied. Even this use must be approached cautiously, as a drug may relieve a symptom in one patient while inducing it in others. (For example, an anticholinergic, anxiolytic drug may relieve dry mouth [a sign of anxiety] in some subjects but induce it [an untoward event] in others.)

Number of Patients % of Patients Reporting:	Triazolam 1003	Placebo 997
Central Nervous System		
Drowsiness	14.0	6.4
Headache	9.7	8.4
Dizziness	7.8	3.1
Nervousness	5.2	4.5
Light-headedness	4.9	0.9
Coordination disorders/ataxia	4.6	0.8
Gastrointestinal		
Nausea/vomiting	4.6	3.7

In addition to the relatively common (ie, 1% or greater) untoward events enumerated above, the following adverse events have been reported less frequently (ie, 0.9% to 0.5%): euphoria, tachycardia, tiredness, confusional states/ memory impairment, cramps/pain, depression, visual disturbances.

Rare (ie, less than 0.5%) adverse reactions included constipation, taste alterations, diarrhea, dry mouth, dermatitis/allergy, dreaming/nightmares, insomnia, paresthesia, tinnitus, dysesthesia, weakness, congestion, death from hepatic failure in a patient also receiving diuretic drugs.

In addition to these untoward events for which estimates of incidence are available, the following adverse events have been reported in association with the use of Triazolam and other benzodiazepines: amnestic symptoms (anterograde amnesia with appropriate or inappropriate behavior), confusional states (disorientation, derealization, depersonalization, and/or clouding of consciousness), dystonia, anorexia, fatigue, sedation, slurred speech, jaundice, pruritus, dysarthria, changes in libido, menstrual irregularities, incontinence, and urinary retention. Other factors may contribute to some of these reaction, eg, concomitant intake of alcohol or other drugs, sleep deprivation, an abnormal premorbid state, etc.

Other events reported include: paradoxical reactions such as stimulation, mania, an agitational state (restlessness, irritability, and excitation), increased muscle spasticity, sleep disturbances, hallucinations, delusions, aggressiveness, falling, somnambulism, syncope, inappropriate behavior, and other adverse behavioral effects. Should these occur, use of the drug should be discontinued.

The following events have also been reported: chest pain, burning tongue/ glossitis/stomatitis.

Laboratory analyses were performed on all patients participating in the clinical program for Triazolam. The following incidences of abnormalities were observed in patients receiving Triazolam and the corresponding placebo group. None of these changes were considered to be of physiological significance.

Number of patients % of Patients Reporting:	Triazolam 380		Placebo 361	
	Low	High	Low	High
Hematology				
Hematocrit	*	*	*	*
Hemoglobin	*	*	*	*
Total WBC count	1.7	2.1	*	1.3
Neutrophil count	1.5	1.5	3.3	1.0
Lymphocyte count	2.3	4.0	3.1	3.8
Monocyte count	3.6	*	4.4	1.5
Eosinophil count	10.2	3.2	9.8	3.4

Number of patients % of Patients Reporting:	Triazolam 380		Placebo 361	
	Low	High	Low	High
Basophil count	1.7	2.1	*	1.8
Urinalysis				
Albumin	—	1.1	—	*
Sugar	—	*	—	*
RBC/HPF	—	2.9	—	2.9
WBC/HPF	—	11.7	—	7.9
Blood chemistry				
Creatinine	2.4	1.9	3.6	1.5
Bilirubin	*	1.5	1.0	*
SGOT	*	5.3	*	4.5
Alkaline phosphatase	*	2.2	*	2.6

*Less than 1%

When treatment with Triazolam is protracted, periodic blood counts, urinalysis, and blood chemistry analyses are advisable.

Minor changes in EEG patterns, usually low-voltage fast activity have been observed in patients during therapy with Triazolam and are of no known significance.

DRUG ABUSE AND DEPENDENCE

Controlled Substance: Triazolam is a controlled substance under the Controlled Substance Act, and Triazolam Tablets have been assigned to Schedule IV.

Abuse, Dependence and Withdrawal: Withdrawal symptoms, similar in character to those noted with barbiturates and alcohol (convulsions, tremor, abdominal and muscle cramps, vomiting, sweating, dysphoria, perceptual disturbances and insomnia), have occurred following abrupt discontinuance of benzodiazepines, including Triazolam. The more severe symptoms are usually associated with higher dosages and longer usage, although patients at therapeutic dosages given for as few as 1-2 weeks can also have withdrawal symptoms and in some patients there may be withdrawal symptoms (daytime anxiety, agitation) between nightly doses (see *"Clinical Pharmacology"*). Consequently, abrupt discontinuation should be avoided and a gradual dosage tapering schedule is recommended in any patient taking more than the lowest dose for more than a few weeks. The recommendation for tapering is particularly important in any patient with a history of seizure.

The risk of dependence is increased in patients with a history of alcoholism, drug abuse, or in patients with marked personality disorders. Such dependence-prone individuals should be under careful surveillance when receiving Triazolam. As with all hypnotics, repeat prescriptions should be limited to those who are under medical supervision.

OVERDOSAGE

Because of the potency of Triazolam, some manifestations of overdosage may occur at 2 mg, four times the maximum recommended therapeutic dose (0.5 mg).

Manifestations of overdosage with Triazolam Tablets include somnolence, confusion, impaired coordination, slurred speech, and ultimately, coma. Respiratory depression and apnea have been reported with overdosages Triazolam. Seizures have occasionally been reported after overdosages. Death has been reported in association with overdoses of Triazolam by itself, as it has with other benzodiazepines. In addition, fatalities have been reported in patients who have overdosed with a combination of a single benzodiazepine, including Triazolam, and alcohol; benzodiazepine and alcohol levels seen in some of these cases have been lower than those usually associated with reports of fatality with either substance alone.

As in all cases of drug overdosage, respiration, pulse, and blood pressure should be monitored and supported by general measures when necessary. Immediate gastric lavage should be performed. An adequate airway should be maintained. Intravenous fluids may be administered.

Flumazenil, a specific benzodiazepine receptor antagonist, is indicated for the complete or partial reversal of the sedative effects of benzodiazepines and may be used in situations when an overdose with a benzodiazepine is known or suspected. Prior to the administration of flumazenil, necessary measures should be instituted to secure airway, ventilation and intravenous access. Flumazenil is intended as an adjunct to, not as a substitute for, proper management of benzodiazepine overdose. Patients treated with flumazenil should be monitored for re-sedation, respiratory depression, and other residual benzodiazepine effects for an appropriate period after treatment. **The prescriber should be aware of a risk of seizure in association with flumazenil treatment, particularly in long-term benzodiazepine users and in cyclic antidepressant overdose.** The complete flumazenil package insert including *"Contraindications," "Warnings"* and *"Precautions"* should be consulted prior to use.

Experiments in animals have indicated that cardipulmonary collapse can occur with massive intravenous doses of Triazolam. This could be reversed with positive mechanical respiration and the intravenous infusion of norepinephrine bitartrate or metaraminol bitartrate. Hemodialysis and forced diuresis are probably of little value. As with the management of intentional overdosage with any drug, the physician should bear in mind that multiple agents may have been ingested by the patient.

The oral LD_{50} in mice is greater than 1,000 mg/kg and in rats is greater than 5,000 mg/kg.

DOSAGE AND ADMINISTRATION

It is important to individualize the dosage of Triazolam Tablets for maximum beneficial efect and to help avoid significant adverse effects.

The recommended dose for most adults is 0.25 mg before retiring. A dose of 0.125 mg may be found to be sufficient for some patients (eg, low body weight). A dose of 0.5 mg should be used only for exceptional patients who do not respond adequately to a trial of a lower dose since the risk of several adverse reactions increases with the size of the dose administered. A dose of 0.5 mg should not be exceeded.

In geriatric and/or debilitated patients the recommended dosage range is 0.125 mg to 0.25 mg. Therapy should be initiated at 0.125 mg in this group and the 0.25 mg dose should be used only for exceptional patients who do not respond to a trial of the lower dose. A lower dose of 0.25 mg should not be exceeded in these patients.

As with all medications, the lowest effective dose should be used.

Store at controlled room temperature, 15° to 30° C (59° to 86° F).

PATIENT INFORMATION

INTRODUCTION

Triazolam is intended to help you sleep. It is one of several benzodiazepine sleeping pills that have generally similar properties. Anyone who is considering using one of these medications should be aware of both their benefits and several important risks and limitations, including diminishing effectiveness with continued use and the possible development of dependence (addiction) and possibly mental changes particularly when the drugs are used for more than a few days to a week. This patient information statement is intended to provide you with knowledge about this class of medications in general and about Triazolam in particular that will be useful to guide you in the safe use of this product, *but it should not replace a discussion between you and your physician about the risks and benefits of Triazolam.*

This leaflet will focus on the beneficial and adverse effects of all members of this class of medications, as well as some specific information about Triazolam. There are some differences among these products, and your physician may wish to discuss any specific advantages and disadvantages of particular members of this drug class with you.

EFFECTIVENESS OF BENZODIAZEPINE SLEEPING PILLS

Benzodiazepine sleeping pills are effective medications and are relatively free of serious problems when they are used for *short-term* management of sleep problems (insomnia). Insomnia is not always the same. It may be reflected in difficulty in falling asleep, frequent awakening during the night, and/or early morning awakening. Insomnia is often transient in nature, responding to brief treatment with sleeping pills. Use for more than a short while requires discussion with your physician about the risks and benefits of prolonged use.

SIDE EFFECTS

Common Side Effects: The most common side effects of benzodiazepine sleeping pills are related to the ability of the medications to make you sleepy; drowsiness, dizziness, lightheadedness, and difficulty with coordination. Users must be cautious about engaging in hazardous activities requiring complete mental alertness, eg, operating machinery or driving a motor vehicle. Do not take alcohol while using Triazolam. Benzodiazepine sleeping pills should not be used with other medications or substances that may cause drowsiness, without discussing said use with your physician.

How sleepy you are the day after you use one of these sleep medications depends on your individual response and on how quickly the product is eliminated from your body. The larger the dose, the more likely an individual will experience next day residual effects such as drowsiness. For this reason, it is important to use the lowest effective dose for each individual patient. Benzodiazepines that are eliminated rapidly, eg. Triazolam tend to cause less next day drowsiness but may cause more withdrawal problems the day after use (see below).

Special Concerns:

Memory Problems: All benzodiazepine sleeping pills can cause a special type of amnesia (memory loss) in which a person may not recall events occurring during some period of time, usually several hours, after taking a drug. This is ordinarily not a problem, because the person taking a sleeping pill intends to be asleep during this vulnerable period of time. It can be a problem when the drugs are taken to induce sleep while traveling, such as during an airplane flight, because the person may awake before the effect of the drug is gone. This has been called "traveler's amnesia." Triazolam is more likely than other members of the class to cause this problem.

Tolerance/Withdrawal Phenomena: Some loss of effectiveness or adaptation to the sleep inducing effects of these medications may develop after nightly use for more than a few weeks and there may be a degree of dependence that develops. For the benzodiazepine sleeping pills that are eliminated quickly from the body, a relative deficiency of the drug may occur at some point in the interval between each night's use. This can lead to (1) increased wakefulness during the last third of the night, and (2) the appearance of increased signs of daytime anxiety or nervousness. These two events have been reported in particular for Triazolam.

There can be more severe withdrawal effects when a benzodiazepine sleeping pill is stopped. Such effects can occur after discontinuing these drugs following use for only a week or two, but may be more common and more severe after longer periods of continuous use. One type of withdrawal phenomenon is the occurrence of what is known as "rebound insomnia." That is, on the first few nights after the drug is stopped, insomnia is actually worse than before the sleeping pill was given. Other withdrawal phenomena following abrupt stopping of benzodiazepine sleeping pills range from mild unpleasant feelings to a major withdrawal syndrome which may include abdominal and muscle cramps, vomiting, sweating, tremor, and rarely, convulsions. These more severe withdrawal phenomena are uncommon.

Dependence/Abuse Phenomena: All benzodiazepine sleeping pills can cause dependence (addiction), especially when used regularly for more than a few weeks or at higher doses. Some people develop a need to continue taking these drugs, either at the prescribed dose or at increasing does, not so much for continued therapeutic effect, but rather, to avoid withdrawal phenomena and/or to achieve nontherapeutic effects. Individuals who have been dependent on alcohol or other drugs may be at particular risk of becoming dependent on drugs in this class, but all people appear to be at some risk. This possibility must be considered before extending the use of these drugs for more than a few weeks.

Mental and Behavioral Changes: A variety of abnormal thinking and behavior changes have been reported to occur in association with the use of benzodiazepine sleeping pills. Some of these changes are like the release of inhibition seen in association with alcohol, eg, aggressiveness and extroversion that seem out of character. Others, however, can be more unusual and more extreme, such as confusion, bizarre behavior, agitation, hallucinations, depersonalization, and worsening of depression, including suicidal thinking. It is rarely clear whether such events are induced by the drug being taken, are caused by some underlying illness or are simply spontaneous happenings. In fact, worsened insomnia may in some cases be associated with illnesses that were present before the medication was used. In any event, the most important fact is to understand that regardless of the cause, users of these medications should promptly report any mental or behavioral changes to their doctor.

Effects on Pregnancy: Certain benzodiazepines have been linked to birth defects when administered during the early months of pregnancy. In addition, the administration of benzodiazepines during the last weeks of pregnancy has been associated with sedation of the fetus. Consequently, the use of this drug should be avoided at any time during pregnancy.

SAFE USE OF BENZODIAZEPINE SLEEPING PILLS

To assure the safe and effective use of Triazolam, you should adhere to the following cautions:

1. Triazolam is a prescription medication, and, therefore, should be used only as directed by your doctor. Follow your doctor's advice about how to take it, when to take it, and how long to take it. As with other prescription medication, Triazolam should be taken only by the individual for whom it is prescribed.
2. Do not extend your use of Triazolam beyond 7-10 days without first consulting your physician.
3. If you develop any unusual and disturbing thoughts or behavior during treatment with Triazolam, you should discuss such problems with your physician.
4. Inform your physician about any alcohol consumption and medicine you are taking now, including drugs you may buy without a prescription. Do not use alcohol while taking Triazolam.
5. Do not take Triazolam in circumstances where a full night's sleep and elimination of the drug from the body are not possible before you would again need to be active and functional, eg, an overnight flight of less than 7-8 hours, because amnestic episodes have been reported in such situations.
6. Do not increase the prescribed dose except on the advice of your physician.
7. Until you experience how this medication affects you, do not drive a car or operate potentially dangerous machinery, etc.
8. Be aware that you may experience an increase in sleep difficulties (rebound insomnia) on the first night or two after discontinuing Triazolam.
9. Inform you physician if you are planning to become pregnant, if you are pregnant, or if you become pregnant while you are taking this medicine. The use of Triazolam should be avoided at any time during pregnancy.

HOW SUPPLIED
TABLETS (C-IV): 0.125 MG

AVERAGE UNIT PRICE (AVAILABLE SIZES)		GENERIC A-RATED AVERAGE PRICE (GAAP)	
BRAND	$0.64	100s	$60.23
GENERIC	$0.60	500s	$292.51

BRAND/MANUFACTURER	NDC	SIZE	AWP
◆ **BRAND**			
➤ HALCION: Upjohn	00009-0010-37	10s	$6.46
	00009-0010-32	100s ud	$64.61
	00009-0010-11	500s	$313.50
◆ **GENERICS**			
Par	49884-0453-62	10s	$6.16
Geneva	00781-1441-83	100s	$56.37
Rugby	00536-5647-21	100s	$58.14
Schein	00364-2598-33	100s	$60.22
Qualitest	00603-6186-10	100s	$60.80
Par	49884-0453-51	100s	$61.63
Goldline	00182-0175-13	100s	$61.63
Aligen	00405-0192-10	100s	$64.87
Geneva	00781-1441-13	100s ud	$58.15

➤ SHOWN IN PRODUCT IDENTIFICATION GUIDE

BRAND/MANUFACTURER	NDC	SIZE	AWP
Geneva	00781-1441-05	500s	$282.15
Qualitest	00603-6186-28	500s	$289.41
Par	49884-0453-05	500s	$291.56
Aligen	00405-0192-02	500s	$306.90

TABLETS (C-IV): 0.25 MG

AVERAGE UNIT PRICE (AVAILABLE SIZES)		GENERIC A-RATED AVERAGE PRICE (GAAP)	
BRAND	$0.69	100s	$65.31
GENERIC	$0.65	500s	$314.32

BRAND/MANUFACTURER	NDC	SIZE	AWP
◆ **BRAND**			
▶ HALCION: Upjohn	00009-0017-11	10s	$6.73
	00009-0017-58	10s	$7.06
	00009-0017-55	100s ud	$70.63
	00009-0017-02	500s	$342.50
◆ **GENERICS**			
Par	49884-0454-62	10s	$6.71
Rugby	00536-5648-21	100s	$60.57
Geneva	00781-1442-83	100s	$61.65
Schein	00364-2599-33	100s	$64.73
Qualitest	00603-6187-10	100s	$66.93
Par	49884-0454-51	100s	$67.17
Goldline	00182-0176-13	100s	$67.17
Aligen	00405-0193-10	100s	$70.70
Geneva	00781-1442-13	100s ud	$63.57
Schein	00364-2599-05	500s	$287.28
Geneva	00781-1442-05	500s	$308.49
Qualitest	00603-6187-28	500s	$317.78
Par	49884-0454-05	500s	$318.53
Goldline	00182-0176-05	500s	$318.53
Aligen	00405-0193-02	500s	$335.29

Trichlormethiazide

DESCRIPTION
Trichlormethiazide Tablets contain Trichlormethiazide, USP for use as an antihypertensive and diuretic drug. They are to be taken orally.

Trichlormethiazide is a member of a class of antihypertensive and diuretic drugs known as benzothiadiazines. The empirical formula is $C_8H_8Cl_3N_3O_4S_2$, with a molecular weight of 380.65; the chemical name is 6-Chloro-3-(dichloromethyl)-3,4-dihydro-2H-1,2,4- benzothiadiazine-7-sulfonamide 1,1-dioxide.

Trichlormethiazide is a white or practically white crystalline powder. It is very slightly soluble in water and sparingly soluble in alcohol.

Each Trichlormethiazide Tablet contains 2 mg or 4 mg Trichlormethiazide USP.

Following is its chemical structure:

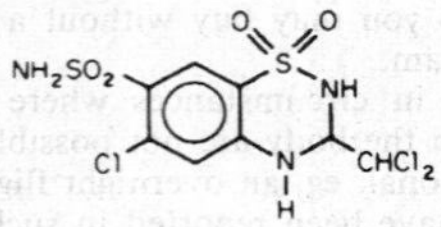

CLINICAL PHARMACOLOGY
The thiazide (benzothiadiazine) diuretics are a class of drug products that have close structural similarity and many similar pharmacological, physiochemical, and pharmacokinetic properties. The thiazide diuretics, including Trichlormethiazide, are used generally as adjunctive medication to control the edema associated with various diseases and in the management of hypertension. (See "Indications and Usage".)

Thiazide diuretics enhance the renal excretion of sodium chloride and water by interfering with the transport of sodium ions across the renal tubular epithelium, primarily in the cortical diluting segment of the nephron. The thiazides also evoke a significant augmentation of potassium excretion, possibly due to the increased amount of sodium reaching the distal tubular site of sodium-potassium exchange. Long-term thiazide therapy can cause mild metabolic alkalosis associated with hypokalemia and hypochloremia.

The glomerular filtration rate is decreased by thiazides. This is of little significance in affecting primary drug action, but may be of clinical importance in patients with diminished renal reserve, contributing to decreased diuretic efficacy. When the glomerular filtration rate falls below 20 mL per minute, the thiazides may not be effective.

Thiazides may decrease uric acid excretion in man, thus increasing the plasma uric acid concentration.

Thiazides may induce hyperglycemia, aggravate existing diabetes mellitus, or precipitate diabetes in prediabetic patients. The exact mechanism of action causing these effects is not certain.

The excretion of certain other ions is affected by the thiazide diuretics: magnesium excretion is enhanced, leading to hypomagnesemia; calcium excretion is decreased relative to that of sodium; iodide and bromide excretion occurs by renal mechanisms similar to those for chloride, possibly leading to slight iodide depletion and allowing chloruretic agents to be useful in the management of bromide intoxication.

Thiazide diuretics have antihypertensive activity per se in hypertensive patients and also may augment the actions of other antihypertensive drugs. The full mechanism of antihypertensive action is not known. Therapy for hypertension is often initiated with a thiazide diuretic which induces diuresis, natriuresis, depletion of extracellular fluid, and reduction of cardiac output. Direct arteriolar dilatation may play a role.

Plasma renin activity is elevated during thiazide therapy. The aldosterone secretion rate is increased slightly but significantly: this contributes to the hypokalemia caused by thiazides.

Paradoxically, thiazides decrease urine volume in patients with diabetes insipidus, and thirst and water consumption decrease.

At maximal therapeutic dosages, all thiazides are approximately equal in their diuretic and antihypertensive activities. The comparative effective daily dose range for chlorothiazide is 250 to 2000 mg; for hydrochlorothiazide 20 to 150 mg; and for Trichlormethiazide 2 to 8 mg.

Thiazides are absorbed rapidly from the gastrointestinal tract. Most show demonstrable diuresis within an hour, and peak effects occur 3 to 6 hours after oral administration. Distribution is essentially limited to the extracellular fluid space, with little, if any, accumulation in tissues other than the kidneys. The duration of diuretic action of thiazides is determined by the rate of excretion. Chlorothiazide and hydrochlorothiazide act for six to 12 hours: Trichlormethiazide for 24 hours. In general, thiazides with relatively long durations of action show proportionately high degrees of plasma protein-binding. Most thiazides are excreted primarily as unchanged drug in the urine.

Thiazides pass readily through the placenta to the fetus, and also appear in the milk of nursing mothers.

INDICATIONS AND USAGE
Trichlormethiazide Tablets are indicated as adjunctive therapy in edema associated with congestive heart failure, hepatic cirrhosis, and corticosteroid and estrogen therapy.

Trichlormethiazide Tablets are indicated for the treatment of edema due to various forms of renal dysfunction, such as nephrotic syndrome, acute glomerulonephritis, and chronic renal failure.

Trichlormethiazide Tablets are indicated in the management of hypertension either as the sole therapeutic agent or as adjunctive therapy to enhance the effectiveness of other antihypertensive drugs in the management of the more severe forms of hypertension.

Trichlormethiazide Tablets are indicated in pregnancy only when the edema is due to pathologic causes. (See "Precautions, Pregnancy Category B" and "Precautions, Nonteratogenic Effects".) The routine use of diuretics in an otherwise healthy woman is inappropriate and exposes the mother and fetus to unnecessary hazard. Diuretics do not prevent development of toxemia of pregnancy, and there is no satisfactory evidence that they are useful in the treatment of toxemia. Edema during pregnancy may arise from pathologic causes or from the physiologic and mechanical consequences of pregnancy. Dependent edema in pregnancy, resulting from restriction of venous return by the expanded uterus, is properly treated through elevation of the lower extremities and use of support hose; use of diuretics to lower intravascular volume in this case is illogical and unnecessary. During normal pregnancy there is hypervolemia which is harmful to neither the fetus nor the mother (in the absence of cardiovascular disease), but which is associated with edema, including generalized edema, in the majority of pregnant women. If this edema produces discomfort, increased recumbency will often provide relief. In rare instances, this edema may cause extreme discomfort which is not relieved by rest. In these cases a short course of diuretics may be appropriate and may provide relief.

UNLABELED USES
Trichlormethiazide is used alone or as an adjunct in the treatment of calcium nephrolithiasis hypercalciuria.

CONTRAINDICATIONS
Trichlormethiazide Tablets are contraindicated in patients with anuria and in those who are allergic to this drug, to other thiazides or to other sulfonamide-derived drugs. The routine use of thiazides is contraindicated in otherwise healthy pregnant women with mild edema. (See "Indications and Usage" and "Precautions, Pregnancy Category B".)

WARNINGS
Thiazides should be used with caution in severe renal disease. In patients with renal disease thiazides may precipitate azotemia. Cumulative effects of the drug may develop in patients with impaired renal function.

Thiazides should be used with caution in patients with impaired hepatic function or progressive liver disease because minor alterations of fluid and electrolyte balance may precipitate hepatic coma.

Thiazides may add to or potentiate the action of other antihypertensive drugs. Potentiation occurs with ganglionic or peripheral adrenergic blocking drugs.

Hypersensitivity reactions may occur in patients with a history of allergy, including aspirin sensitivity or bronchial asthma.

The exacerbation and activation of systemic lupus erythematosus have been reported.

Lithium generally should not be given with diuretics because the latter reduce its renal clearance and increase the risk of lithium toxicity.

◆ RATED THERAPEUTICALLY EQUIVALENT; ◇ THERAPEUTIC EQUIVALENCE UNCONFIRMED; ○ UNRATED

PRECAUTIONS

General: Periodic determinations of serum electrolytes should be done at appropriate intervals. Serum and urine electrolyte determinations are particularly important when the patient is vomiting excessively, having diarrhea, or receiving parenteral fluids. Thiazides may cause hyponatremia, hypochloremic alkalosis, hypokalemia, hypomagnesemia, and changes in serum and urine calcium. All patients receiving thiazide therapy should be observed for the clinical warning signs of fluid or electrolyte imbalance, irrespective of cause, including dryness of mouth, thirst, weakness, lethargy, drowsiness, restlessness, muscular pains, fatigue, or cramps, hypotension, tachycardia, oliguria, and gastrointestinal disturbances such as nausea and vomiting.

Hypokalemia may develop with Trichlormethiazide as with other potent diuretics, including other thiazides, especially when the diuresis is brisk, when severe cirrhosis is present, or during concomitant use of corticosteroids or ACTH. Hypokalemia poses an increased risk in digitalized patients and patients with cirrhosis, since decreases in the serum potassium concentration can precipitate serious arrhythmias during digitalis therapy, and in cirrhotic patients low potassium levels may precipitate hepatic coma. Thiazides should be discontinued immediately if signs of impending hepatic coma appear.

Chloride deficits are usually mild and usually do not require treatment except under extraordinary circumstances, as in liver or renal disease. Hypochloremic alkalosis may occur with hypokalemia, especially if patients are losing additional potassium and chloride from vomiting, diarrhea, gastrointestinal disease, or potassium-losing renal diseases.

Dilutional hyponatremia may occur or be aggravated during thiazide therapy in edematous patients especially in hot weather. Appropriate therapy is water restriction; salt should not be administered unless the hyponatremia is life threatening. In actual body salt depletion, appropriate replacement is the therapy of choice, however.

Serum and urine electrolyte determinations are particularly important to diagnose and treat electrolyte disturbances.

Hyperuricemia may occur in patients receiving thiazides or related diuretics. While usually asymptomatic, frank gout may occur in patients with a history of gout, a familial predisposition to gout, or chronic renal failure.

Insulin or oral hypoglycemic drug requirements may be altered in patients with diabetes mellitus because thiazides and related diuretics can produce hyperglycemia and glycosuria. Latent diabetes mellitus may become manifest during thiazide administration. Reversible oculomotor paresis has occurred as a manifestation of thiazide-induced glucose intolerance.

The antihypertensive effects of thiazides may be enhanced in post-sympathectomy patients.

If progressive renal impairment becomes evident during thiazide therapy, careful reappraisal of therapy is necessary with consideration given to withholding or discontinuing diuretic dosing. Nonprotein nitrogen, blood urea nitrogen, or serum creatine levels should be determined since these will be increased in renal impairment.

Information for Patients: Physicians should give the following information and instructions to patients receiving thiazide diuretics. This information is intended to aid in the safe and effective use of this medication. It is not a disclosure of all possible adverse or intended effects.

1. This drug must be taken on a regular schedule to be effective. Take as prescribed. Do not skip doses; if a dose is missed, do not double the dose. Do not take extra doses.

2. Use of this drug with other medications should be done only with a physician's advice. If other drugs are required for control of edema or hypertension, the patient should understand the need for compliance with the total therapeutic program.

3. This drug should be used only by the patient for whom it is prescribed. Do not allow anyone else to take this medication.

4. Pregnancy or plans for pregnancy should be discussed with the physician.

5. Since thiazides appear in breast milk, it is recommended that the baby not be breast fed.

6. The patient should be alerted to the possibilities of various side effects which might occur during thiazide therapy, including particularly, changes in the control or severity of concurrent illnesses, such as liver or kidney disease, diabetes mellitus, systemic lupus erythematosus, and gout.

7. The patient should be alerted to the effects of diuresis, including excessive losses of sodium, chloride and especially potassium, and how to provide for replacement.

8. Dietary instructions should be provided.

9. As required, return for laboratory tests.

Laboratory Tests: Since thiazides affect many organ functions, the safe and effective use of these drugs may require pretreatment and periodic laboratory tests. They may be helpful: in following the patient's initial response or status after prolonged therapy; in avoiding or identifying possible adverse reactions, as in patients who are vomiting or who have serious diseases such as severe hepatic disease, renal disease, diabetes mellitus, or gout; in patients who are receiving concomitant medications, such as digitalis glycosides or corticosteroids. The following procedures (not necessarily inclusive) should be considered in patient monitoring:

■ Serum electrolyte determinations, especially sodium, potassium, chloride, and bicarbonate
■ serum uric acid and blood glucose
■ serum creatinine or blood urea nitrogen

■ liver function tests, including serum transaminases, alkaline phosphatase, and bilirubin levels
■ electrocardiograms, especially in patients on digitalis glycosides.

Drug Interactions: The following are generally recognized potential thiazide drug interactions (not necessarily inclusive):

Digitalis glycosides: Thiazides may produce hypokalemia, hypomagnesemia, and hypercalcemia which may predispose the patient to digitalis toxicity. Periodic serum electrolyte determinations may be required, and correction of electrolyte abnormalities, particularly hypokalemia, should be undertaken, either prophylactically or therapeutically. Electrocardiographic monitoring of the patient may be required to evaluate the patient's cardiac status initially and to control treatment.

Corticosteroids (and ACTH): Concomitant use with thiazides may enhance potassium loss. Periodic serum electrolyte determinations may be required, and correction of electrolyte abnormalities, particularly hypokalemia, should be undertaken.

Insulin preparations and oral sulfonylureas: Thiazides may antagonize the hypoglycemic effects of these agents. Dosage adjustment may be necessary.

Diazoxide: Concomitant use of thiazides and diazoxide may potentiate the hyperglycemic, hyperuricemic, and antihypertensive effects of both drugs.

Methyldopa, reserpine, guanethidine sulfate, prazosin hydrochloride, and beta-adrenergic receptor blockers: Concomitant use of a thiazide with most other antihypertensive drugs produces a more pronounced antihypertensive response than when either drug is used as the sole therapeutic agent. Severe postural hypotension may result if a thiazide is added to the regimen of a patient stabilized on certain hypotensive agents, such as methyldopa, guanethidine sulfate, or prazosin.

Cholestyramine: Cholestyramine may bind thiazides in the gut. Thiazides should be taken at least one hour before cholestyramine.

Lithium carbonate: Lithium toxicity has been reported in patients receiving thiazides. Renal clearance of lithium is decreased in patients on long-term thiazide treatment, and lithium therapy has been reported in some cases to be associated with morphological changes in the kidneys. Serum lithium concentrations should be measured frequently in such patients also on thiazides.

Tubocurarine and gallamine: Thiazides may cause prolonged neuromuscular blockade in patients receiving nondepolarizing neuromuscular blocking agents, such as tubocurarine chloride or gallamine.

Probenecid: Thiazide-induced uric acid retention is blocked by probenecid.

Fenfluramine: Fenfluramine has been reported to enhance the blood pressure lowering effect and plasma norepinephrine levels resulting from use with hydrochlorothiazide in obese patients.

Indomethacin: The concomitant administration of indomethacin to hypertensive patients being treated with thiazide diuretics has resulted in partial loss of control of the lowered blood pressure. A possible explanation is inhibition of prostacyclin biosynthesis by indomethacin.

Anticholinergics: Drugs with significant anticholinergic effects on the gastrointestinal tract may delay gastric emptying and enhance the absorption of thiazides.

Sympathomimetic agents: A decrease in arterial responsiveness to vasopressors (norepinephrine, phenylephrine), of uncertain clinical significance, has been reported during thiazide therapy.

Drug/Laboratory Test Interactions: Thiazides can affect the laboratory test values for electrolytes, such as sodium, potassium, chloride, calcium, magnesium, and iodide, and for glucose, uric acid, blood urea nitrogen, and serum creatinine. Thiazides also may interfere with diagnostic testing as follows:

(a) due to pharmacologic or metabolic effects

■ thiazides may cause false-negative results with the phentolamine and the tyramine tests for pheochromocytoma by attenuating the hypertensive response to tyramine.
■ thiazides may compete with phenolsulfonphthalein (PSP) for renal tubular secretion, resulting in decreased urinary excretion of PSP.
■ thiazides may cause sulfobromophthalein (BSP) retention, probably due to a reduction in plasma volume and a resultant decrease in hepatic blood flow.
■ thiazides may decrease urinary cortisol excretion, possibly due to changes in cortisol secretion, renal handling or metabolism.
■ thiazides may decrease serum protein-bound iodine, although usually not to subnormal levels, without signs of thyroid disturbance.
■ thiazides may cause increases in serum amylase levels, some reported increases being up to two times pretreatment levels. However, the fact that acute pancreatitis has occurred in patients on thiazides should also be kept in mind.

(b) due to interference with laboratory analysis procedures

■ thiazides, except for chlorothiazide, may interfere with assays of total urinary estrogens and of estriol.
■ thiazides may interfere with urinary 17-hydroxycorticosteroids measurements.

Carcinogenesis, Mutagenesis, Impairment of Fertility: Long-term dosing studies have not been done with Trichlamethiazide to determine whether this drug has carcinogenic potential. No study has been done to determine whether Trichlamethiazide is mutagenic.

Pregnancy Category B: Reproduction studies have been performed with Trichlamethiazide in rats at doses 250 to 1250 times the recommended human daily dose and have revealed no evidence of impaired fertility or harm to the fetus. There are, however, no adequate and well-controlled studies in pregnant women. Since thiazides cross the placental barrier, their use may expose the fetus to other possible hazards, such as fetal or neonatal jaundice or thrombocytopenia. Trichlamethiazide Tablets should be used during pregnancy only if clearly needed and when the potential benefits to the mother justify the potential risks to the infant.

Nonteratogenic Effects: Thiazides cross the placenta and appear in cord blood. Infants born to mothers treated with diuretics have shown changes in body water and electrolytes, although not of apparent clinical significance. Fetal or neonatal jaundice and thrombocytopenia have been reported in newborn infants of women receiving thiazides. There is an unconfirmed report of neonatal hemolysis in two infants attributed to maternal thiazide therapy.

Nursing Mothers: Thiazides can decrease milk production. Additionally, thiazides appear in breast milk. Thrombocytopenia can occur in the nursing infant when the mother is taking a thiazide diuretic. Because of the potential for unwanted adverse effects in nursing infants from Trichlamethiazide Tablets, a decision should be made whether to discontinue nursing or to discontinue the drug, taking into account the importance of the drug to the mother.

Pediatric Use: Thiazide diuretics have been shown to be effective and safe in children when used as recommended. (See "Indications and Usage" and "Dosage and Administration".)

ADVERSE REACTIONS

The following adverse reactions have been observed, but there is not enough systematic data collection to support an estimate of their frequency.

Gastrointestinal System: pancreatitis; jaundice (intrahepatic cholestatic jaundice); acute cholecystitis; vomiting; diarrhea; nausea; gastric irritation; anorexia; cramping; constipation.

Central Nervous System: vertigo; headache; xanthopsia; dizziness; paresthesias.

Hematologic: aplastic anemia; thrombocytopenia; agranulocytosis; leukopenia.

Dermatologic-Hypersensitivity: anaphylactoid reactions; necrotizing angitis (vasculitis, cutaneous vasculitis); purpura; photosensitivity; urticaria; rash.

Cardiovascular: orthostatic hypotension may occur and may be aggravated by alcohol, barbiturates, or narcotics.

Other: hyperuricemia; hyperglycemia; glycosuria; muscle spasm; weakness; restlessness.

Whenever adverse reactions are moderate or severe, the dosage should be reduced or therapy withdrawn.

OVERDOSAGE

Accidental or suicidal poisoning with thiazide diuretics has been reported infrequently.

Manifestations: Diuresis is to be expected; lethargy of varying degree may appear and may progress to coma within a few hours, with minimal depression of respiration and cardiovascular function and without significant serum electrolyte changes or dehydration. The mechanism of CNS depression with thiazide overdosage is unknown. GI irritation and hypermotility may occur; temporary elevation of BUN has been reported and serum electrolyte changes can occur, especially in patients with impaired renal function.

Treatment: Evacuate gastric contents, taking care to prevent aspiration, especially in the stuporous or comatose patient. GI effects are usually of short duration but may require symptomatic treatment.

Monitor serum electrolyte levels and renal function; institute supportive measures as required individually to maintain hydration, electrolyte balance, respiration, and cardiovascular-renal functions.

DOSAGE AND ADMINISTRATION

Therapy should be individualized according to patient response. Dosage should be titrated to seek maximal therapeutic response and to establish the minimal dose necessary to maintain that response.

Adults:

Edematous Conditions: The usual oral dose of Trichlamethiazide Tablets for diuretic effect is 1 to 4 mg daily.

Hypertension: The usual oral dose of Trichlamethiazide Tablets for antihypertensive effect is 2 to 4 mg daily.

Children:

Edematous Conditions or Hypertension: The usual oral dose of Trichlamethiazide Tablets for children over 6 months of age is determined as follows: 0.07 mg/kg/24 hr or 2 mg/sqM/24 hr orally as a single dose or divided into two doses.

Storage: Dispense in tight containers.
Store between 15° and 30°C (59° and 86°F).

HOW SUPPLIED
TABLETS: 2 MG

BRAND/MANUFACTURER	NDC	SIZE	AWP
◇ **BRAND**			
NAQUA: Schering	00085-0822-03	100s	$35.65
METAHYDRIN: Marion Merrell Dow	00068-0062-01	100s	$42.54

TABLETS: 4 MG

BRAND/MANUFACTURER	NDC	SIZE	AWP
◇ **BRAND**			
NAQUA: Schering	00085-0547-03	100s	$55.32
METAHYDRIN: Marion Merrell Dow	00068-0063-01	100s	$68.16
◇ **GENERICS**			
Richlyn	00115-4860-01	100s	$1.83
Major	00904-0340-60	100s	$3.40
URL	00677-0361-01	100s	$3.50
Camall	00147-0143-10	100s	$3.71
Rugby	00536-3770-01	100s	$5.30
Goldline	00182-0517-01	100s	$6.15
DIURESE: Amer Urological	00539-0801-01	100s	$28.13
Richlyn	00115-4860-03	1000s	$14.10
Goldline	00182-0517-10	1000s	$14.25
Camall	00147-0143-20	1000s	$14.98
Rugby	00536-3770-10	1000s	$18.45
URL	00677-0361-10	1000s	$19.53
Moore,H.L.	00839-5011-16	1000s	$19.58
Major	00904-0340-80	1000s	$20.95
DIURESE: Amer Urological	00539-0801-10	1000s	$218.75

Tridesilon SEE DESONIDE

Tridione SEE TRIMETHADIONE

Trientine Hydrochloride

DESCRIPTION

Trientine Hydrochloride is *N,N'*-bis (2-aminoethyl)-1,2-ethanediamine dihydrochloride. It is a white to pale yellow crystalline hygroscopic powder. It is freely soluble in water, soluble in methanol, slightly soluble in ethanol, and insoluble in chloroform and ether.

The empirical formula is $C_6H_{18}N_42HCl$ with a molecular weight of 219.2.

Trientine Hydrochloride is a chelating compound for removal of excess copper from the body. Trientine Hydrochloride is available as 250 mg capsules for oral administration.

Following is its chemical structure:

$$H_2N(CH_2)_2NH(CH_2)_2NH(CH_2)_2NH_2 \cdot 2HCl$$

CLINICAL PHARMACOLOGY

INTRODUCTION

Wilson's disease (hepatolenticular degeneration) is an autosomal inherited metabolic defect resulting in an inability to maintain a near-zero balance of copper. Excess copper accumulates possibly because the liver lacks the mechanism to excrete free copper into the bile. Hepatocytes store excess copper but when their capacity is exceeded copper is released into the blood and is taken up into extrahepatic sites. This condition is treated with a low copper diet and the use of chelating agents that bind copper to facilitate its excretion from the body.

CLINICAL SUMMARY

Forty-one patients (18 male and 23 female) between the ages of 6 and 54 with a diagnosis of Wilson's disease and who were intolerant of d-penicillamine were treated in two separate studies with Trientine Hydrochloride. The dosage varied from 450 to 2400 mg per day. The average dosage required to achieve an optimal clinical response varied between 1000 mg and 2000 mg per day. The mean duration of Trientine Hydrochloride therapy was 48.7 months (range 2-164 months). Thirty-four of the 41 patients improved, 4 had no change in clinical global response, 2 were lost to follow-up and one showed deterioration in clinical condition. One of the patients who improved while on therapy with Trientine Hydrochloride experienced a recurrence of the symptoms of systemic lupus erythematosus which had appeared originally during therapy with penicillamine. Therapy with Trientine Hydrochloride was discontinued. No other adverse reactions, except iron deficiency, were noted among any of these 41 patients.

One investigator treated 13 patients with Trientine Hydrochloride following their development of intolerance to d-penicillamine. Retrospectively, he compared these patients to an additional group of 12 patients with Wilson's disease who were both tolerant of and controlled with d-penicillamine therapy, but who failed to continue any copper chelation therapy. The mean age at onset of disease of the latter group was 12 years as compared to 21 years for the former group. The Trientine Hydrochloride group received d-penicillamine for an average of 4 years as compared to an average of 10 years for the non-treated group.

Various laboratory parameters showed changes in favor of the patients treated with Trientine Hydrochloride. Free and total serum copper, SGOT, and serum bilirubin all showed mean increases over baseline in the untreated group which were significantly larger than with the patients treated with Trientine Hydrochloride. In the 13 patients treated with Trientine Hydrochloride, previous symptoms and signs relating to d-penicillamine intolerance disappeared in 8 patients, improved in 4 patients, and remained unchanged in one patient. The neurological status in the Trientine Hydrochloride group was unchanged or improved over

---

◆ RATED THERAPEUTICALLY EQUIVALENT; ◇ THERAPEUTIC EQUIVALENCE UNCONFIRMED; ○ UNRATED

baseline, whereas in the untreated group, 6 patients remained unchanged and 6 worsened. Kayser-Fleischer rings improved significantly during Trientine Hydrochloride treatment.

The clinical outcome of the two groups also differed markedly. Of the 13 patients on therapy with Trientine Hydrochloride (mean duration of therapy 4.1 years; range 1 to 13 years), all were alive at the data cutoff date, and in the nontreated group (mean years with no therapy 2.7 years; range 3 months to 9 years), 9 of the 12 died of hepatic disease.

CHELATING PROPERTIES
Preclinical Studies: Studies in animals have show that Trientine Hydrochloride has cupriuretic activities in both normal and copper-loaded rats. In general, the effects of Trientine Hydrochloride on urinary copper excretion are similar to those of equimolar doses of penicillamine, although in one study they were significantly smaller.

Human Studies: Renal clearance studies were carried out with penicillamine and Trientine Hydrochloride on separate occasions in selected patients treated with penicillamine for at least one year. Six-hour excretion rates of copper were determined off treatment and after a single dose of 500 mg of penicillamine or 1.2 g of Trientine Hydrochloride. The mean urinary excretion rates of copper were as follows:

No. of Patients	Single Dose Treatment	Basal Excretion Rate (μg Cu^{++}/6hr)	Test-dose Excretion Rate (μg Cu^{++}/6hr)
6	Trientine, 1.2 g	19	234
4	Penicillamine, 500 mg	17	320

In patients *not* previously treated with chelating agents, a similar comparison was made:

No. of Patients	Single Dose Treatment	Basal Excretion Rate (μg Cu^{++}/6hr)	Test-dose Excretion Rate (μg Cu^{++}/6hr)
8	Trientine, 1.2 g	71	1326
7	Penicillamine, 500 mg	68	1074

These results demonstrate that Trientine Hydrochloride is effective as a cupriuretic agent in patients with Wilson's disease although on a molar basis it appears to be less potent or less effective than penicillamine. Evidence from a radio-labelled copper study indicates that the different cupriuretic effect between these two drugs could be due to a difference in selectivity of the drugs for different copper pools within the body.

PHARMACOKINETICS
Data on the pharmacokinetics of Trientine Hydrochloride are not available. Dosage adjustment recommendations are based upon clinical use of the drug (see *"Dosage and Administration"*).

INDICATIONS AND USAGE
Trientine Hydrochloride is indicated in the treatment of patients with Wilson's disease who are intolerant of penicillamine. Clinical experience with Trientine Hydrochloride is limited and alternate dosing regimens have not been well-characterized; all endpoints in determining an individual patient's dose have not been well defined. Trientine Hydrochloride and penicillamine cannot be considered interchangeable. Trientine Hydrochloride should be used when continued treatment with penicillamine is no longer possible because of intolerable or life endangering side effects.

Unlike penicillamine, Trientine Hydrochloride is not recommended in cystinuria or rheumatoid arthritis. The absence of a sulfhydryl moiety renders it incapable of binding cysteine and, therefore, it is of no use in cystinuria. In 15 patients with rheumatoid arthritis, Trientine Hydrochloride was reported not to be effective in improving any clinical or biochemical parameter after 12 weeks of treatment.

Trientine Hydrochloride is not indicated for treatment of biliary cirrhosis.

CONTRAINDICATIONS
Hypersensitivity to this product.

WARNINGS
Patient experience with Trientine Hydrochloride is limited (see *"Clinical Pharmacology"*). Patients receiving Trientine Hydrochloride should remain under regular medical supervision throughout the period of drug administration. Patients (especially women) should be closely monitored for evidence of iron deficiency anemia.

PRECAUTIONS
GENERAL
There are no reports of hypersensitivity in patients who have been administered Trientine Hydrochloride for Wilson's disease. However, there have been reports of asthma, bronchitis and dermatitis occurring after prolonged environmental exposure in workers who use Trientine Hydrochloride as a hardener of epoxy resins. Patients should be observed closely for signs of possible hypersensitivity.

INFORMATION FOR PATIENTS
Patients should be directed to take Trientine Hydrochloride on an empty stomach, at least one hour before meals or two hours after meals and at least one hour apart from any other drug, food, or milk. The capsules should be swallowed whole with water and should not be opened or chewed. Because of the potential for contact dermatitis, any site of exposure to the capsule contents should be washed with water promptly. For the first month of treatment, the patient should have his temperature taken nightly, and he should be asked to report any symptom such as fever or skin eruption.

LABORATORY TESTS
The most reliable index for monitoring treatment is the determination of free copper in the serum, which equals the difference between quantitatively determined total copper and ceruloplasmin-copper. Adequately treated patients will usually have less than 10 mcg free copper/dL of serum.

Therapy may be monitored with a 24 hour urinary copper analysis periodically (i.e., every 6-12 months). Urine must be collected in copper-free glassware. Since a low copper diet should keep copper absorption down to less than one milligram a day, the patient probably will be in the desired state of negative copper balance if 0.5 to 1.0 milligram of copper is present in a 24-hour collection of urine.

DRUG INTERACTIONS
In general, mineral supplements should not be given since they may block the absorption of Trientine Hydrochloride. However, iron deficiency may develop, especially in children and menstruating or pregnant women, or as a result of the low copper diet recommended for Wilson's disease. If necessary, iron may be given in short courses, but since iron and Trientine Hydrochloride each inhibit absorption of the other, two hours should elapse between administration of Trientine Hydrochloride and iron.

It is important that Trientine Hydrochloride be taken on an empty stomach, at least one hour before meals or two hours after meals and at least one hour apart from any other drug, food, or milk. This permits maximum absorption and reduces the likelihood of inactivation of the drug by metal binding in the gastrointestinal tract.

CARCINOGENESIS, MUTAGENESIS, IMPAIRMENT OF FERTILITY
Data on carcinogenesis, mutagenesis and impairment of fertility are not available.

PREGNANCY
Pregnancy Category C: Trientine Hydrochloride was teratogenic in rats at doses similar to the human dose. The frequencies of both resorptions and fetal abnormalities, including hemorrhage and edema, increased while fetal copper levels decreased when Trientine Hydrochloride was given in the material diets of rats. There are no adequate and well-controlled studies in pregnant women. Trientine Hydrochloride should be used during pregnancy only if the potential benefit justifies the potential risk to the fetus.

NURSING MOTHERS
It is not known whether this drug is excreted in human milk. Because many drugs are excreted in human milk, caution should be exercised when Trientine Hydrochloride is administered to a nursing mother.

PEDIATRIC USE
Controlled studies of the safety and effectiveness of Trientine Hydrochloride in children have not been conducted. It has been used clinically in children as young as 6 years with no reported adverse experiences.

ADVERSE REACTIONS
Clinical experience with Trientine Hydrochloride has been limited. The following adverse reactions have been reported in patients with Wilson's disease who were on therapy with Trientine Hydrochloride: iron deficiency, systemic lupus erythematosus (see *"Clinical Pharmacology"*).

Trientine Hydrochloride is not indicated for treatment of biliary cirrhosis, but in one study of 4 patients treated with Trientine Hydrochloride for primary biliary cirrhosis, the following adverse reactions were reported: heartburn; epigastric pain and tenderness; thickening, fissuring and flaking of the skin; hypochromic microcytic anemia; acute gastritis; aphthoid ulcers; abdominal pain; melena; anorexia; malaise; cramps; muscle pain; weakness; rhabdomyolysis. A causal relationship of these reactions to drug therapy could not be rejected or established.

OVERDOSAGE
There is a report of an adult woman who ingested 30 grams of Trientine Hydrochloride without apparent ill effects. No other data on overdosage are available.

DOSAGE AND ADMINISTRATION
Systemic evaluation of dose and/or interval between dose has not been done. However, on limited clinical experience, the recommended initial dose of Trientine Hydrochloride is 500-750 mg/day for children and 750-1250 mg/day for adults given in divided doses two, three or four times daily. This may be increased to a maximum of 2000 mg/day for adults or 1500 mg/day for children age 12 or under. The daily dose of Trientine Hydrochloride should be increased only when the clinical response is not adequate or the concentration of free serum copper is persistently above 20 mcg/dL. Optimal long-term maintenance dosage should be determined at 6-12 month intervals (see *"Precautions, Laboratory Tests"*).

It is important that Trientine Hydrochloride be given on an empty stomach, at least one hour before meals or two hours after meals and at least one hour apart from any other drug, food, or milk. The capsules should be swallowed whole with water and should not be opened or chewed.

Keep container tightly closed.

Store at 2°-8°C (36°-46°F).

HOW SUPPLIED
CAPSULE: 250 MG

BRAND/MANUFACTURER	NDC	SIZE	AWP
○ BRAND			
SYPRINE: Merck	00006-0661-68	100s	$87.29

Triethanolamine Polypeptide Oleate-Condensate

DESCRIPTION
Triethanolamine Polypeptide Oleate-Condensate Eardrops contain Triethanolamine Polypeptide Oleate-Condensate (10%).

It also has a slightly acid pH range (5.0-6.0) to approximate the surface of a normal ear canal.

CLINICAL PHARMACOLOGY
Triethanolamine Polypeptide Oleate-Condensate Eardrops emulsify and disperse excess or impacted earwax. The Triethanolamine Polypeptide Oleate, a surfactant, in a hygroscopic vehicle lyses cerumen to facilitate removal by subsequent water irrigation.

INDICATIONS AND USAGE
For removal of impacted Triethanolamine Polypeptide Oleate-Condensate prior to ear examination, otologic therapy and/or audiometry.

CONTRAINDICATIONS
Perforated tympanic membrane or otitis media is considered a contraindication to the use of this medication in the external ear canal.

A history of hypersensitivity to Triethanolamine Polypeptide Oleate-Condensate Eardrops or to any of its components is also a contraindication to the use of this medication.

WARNINGS
Discontinue promptly if sensitization or irritation occurs.

PRECAUTIONS
GENERAL
It is recommended that the following precautions be observed in prescribing and administration of this agent:

1. Extreme caution is indicated in patients with demonstrable dermatologic idiosyncrasies or with history of allergic reactions in general.

2. Exposure of the ear canal to the Triethanolamine Polypeptide Oleate-Condensate Eardrops should be limited to 15-30 minutes.

3. When administering Triethanolamine Polypeptide Oleate-Condensate Eardrops, care must be taken to avoid undue exposure of the skin outside the ear during the instillation and the flushing out of the medication. If the medication comes in contact with the skin, the area should be washed with soap and water. Use of proper technique (see *"Dosage and Administration"*) will help avoid such undue exposure.

4. Triethanolamine Polypeptide Oleate-Condensate Eardrops should be used only with caution in external otitis.

INFORMATION FOR PATIENTS
1. Patients should be cautioned to avoid placing the applicator tip into the ear canal.

2. Patients should be cautioned to gently flush the ear with lukewarm water.

3. Patients should be warned to use Triethanolamine Polypeptide Oleate-Condensate Eardrops in ears only. Surrounding skin should be promptly rinsed of any excess drops.

4. Patients should be instructed not to leave Triethanolamine Polypeptide Oleate-Condensate Eardrops in the ear for longer than 30 minutes. A second application may be made, if needed, but more frequent use must be indicated by the physician.

5. Patients must be instructed not to exceed the time of exposure, nor to use the medication more frequently than directed by the physician.

6. Patients should be advised to discontinue the use of the medication in case of a possible reaction and to consult their physician promptly.

CARCINOGENESIS, MUTAGENESIS, IMPAIRMENT OF FERTILITY
Long-term animal studies have not been performed to evaluate the carcinogenic potential or the effect on fertility of Triethanolamine Polypeptide Oletate-Condensate Eardrops.

PREGNANCY
Teratogenic Effects: Pregnancy Category C. Animal reproduction studies have not yet been conducted with Triethanolamine Polypeptide Oletate-Condensate Eardrops. It is also not known whether Triethanolamine Polypeptide Oletate-Condensate Eardrops can cause fetal harm when administered to a pregnant woman or can affect reproduction capacity. Triethanolamine Polypeptide Oletate-Condensate Eardrops should be given to a pregnant woman only if clearly needed.

NURSING MOTHER
It is not known whether this drug is excreted in human milk. Because many drugs are excreted in human milk, caution should be exercised when Triethanolamine Polypeptide Oletate-Condensate Eardrops are administered to a nursing mother.

PEDIATRIC USE
Safety and effectiveness in children have not been established.

ADVERSE REACTIONS
CLINICAL REACTIONS OF POSSIBLE ALLERGIC ORIGIN
Localized dermatitis reactions were reported in about 1% of 2,700 patients treated, ranging from a very mild erythema and pruritus of the external canal to a severe eczematoid reaction involving the external ear and periauricular tissue, generally with duration of 2-10 days. Other reactions which have been reported in connection with the use of Triethanolamine Polypeptide Oleate-Condensate Eardrops include allergic contact dermatitis, skin ulcerations, burning and pain at the application site and skin rash.

DOSAGE AND ADMINISTRATION
1. Fill ear canal with Triethanolamine Polypeptide Oletate-Condensate Eardrops with the patient's head tilted at a 45° angle.

2. Insert cotton plug and allow to remain 15-30 minutes.

3. Then gently flush with lukewarm water, using a soft rubber syringe (avoid excessive pressure). Exposure of skin outside the ear to the drug should be avoided. The procedure may be repeated if the first application fails to clear the impaction.

Store at controlled room temperature, 15-30°C (59-86°F)

HOW SUPPLIED
DROP:

BRAND/MANUFACTURER	NDC	SIZE	AWP
○ BRAND			
CERUMENEX: Purdue Frederick	00034-5490-06	6 ml	$15.09
	00034-5490-12	12 ml	$24.18

Triethylperazine Maleate

DESCRIPTION
Triethylperazine is a phenothiazine. Triethylperazine is characterized by a substituted thioethyl group at position 2 in the phenothiazine nucleus, and a piperazine moiety in the side chain. The chemical designation is: 2-ethylmercapto-10-[3'(1"-methyl-piperazinyl-4")-propyl- 1']phenothiazine.

ACTIONS
The pharmacodynamic action of Triethylperazine in humans is unknown. However, a direct action of Triethylperazine Maleate on both the CTZ and the vomiting center may be concluded from induced vomiting experiments in animals.

INDICATIONS
Triethylperazine is indicated for the relief of nausea and vomiting.

CONTRAINDICATIONS
Severe central nervous system (CNS) depression and comatose states.

In patients who have demonstrated a hypersensitivity reaction (e.g., blood dyscrasias, jaundice) to phenothiazines.

Because severe hypotension has been reported after the intravenous administration of phenothiazines, this route of administration is contraindicated.

Usage in Pregnancy: Triethylperazine is contraindicated in pregnancy.

WARNINGS
Triethylperazine injection may contain sodium metabisulfite, a sulfite that may cause allergic-type reactions including anaphylactic symptoms and life-threatening or less severe asthmatic episodes in certain susceptible people. The overall prevalence of sulfite sensitivity in the general population is unknown and probably low. Sulfite sensitivity is seen more frequently in asthmatic than in nonasthmatic people.

Phenothiazines are capable of potentiating CNS depressants (e.g., anesthetics, opiates, alcohol, etc.) as well as atropine and phosphorus insecticides.

Since Triethylperazine may impair mental and/or physical ability required in the performance of potentially hazardous tasks such as driving a car or operating machinery it is recommended that patients be warned accordingly.

Postoperative Nausea and Vomiting: With the use of this drug to control postoperative nausea and vomiting occurring in patients undergoing elective surgical procedures, restlessness and postoperative CNS depression during anesthesia recovery may occur. Possible postoperative complications of a severe degree of any of the known reactions of this class of drug must be considered. Postural hypotension may occur after an initial injection, rarely with the tablet or suppository.

The administration of epinephrine should be avoided in the treatment of drug-induced hypotension in view of the fact that phenothiazines may induce a reversed epinephrine effect on occasion.

Should a vasoconstrictive agent be required, the most suitable are norepinephrine bitartrate and phenylephrine.

◆ RATED THERAPEUTICALLY EQUIVALENT; ◇ THERAPEUTIC EQUIVALENCE UNCONFIRMED; ○ UNRATED

The use of this drug has not been studied following intracardiac and intracranial surgery.

PRECAUTIONS

Abnormal movements such as extrapyramidal symptoms (E.P.S.) (e.g., dystonia, torticollis, dysphasia, oculogyric crises, akathisia) have occurred. Convulsions have also been reported. The varied symptom complex is more likely to occur in young adults and children. Extrapyramidal effects must be treated by reduction of dosage or cessation of medication.

Triethylperazine tablets may contain FD&C Yellow No. 5 (tartrazine) which may cause allergic-type reactions (including bronchial asthma) in certain susceptible individuals. Although the overall incidence of FD&C Yellow No. 5 (tartrazine) sensitivity in the general population is low, it is frequently seen in patients who also have aspirin hypersensitivity.

Use in patients with bone marrow depression only when potential benefits outweigh risks.

Neuroleptic Malignant Syndrome (NMS), a potentially fatal symptom complex, has been reported in association with phenothiazine drugs. Clinical manifestations include: hyperpyrexia, muscle rigidity, altered mental status and evidence of autonomic instability.

The extrapyramidal symptoms which can occur secondary to Tri- ethylperazine may be confused with the central nervous system signs of an undiagnosed primary disease responsible for the vomiting, e.g., Reye's Syndrome or other encephalopathy. The use of Triethylperazine and other potential hepatotoxins should be avoided in children and adolescents whose signs and symptoms suggest Reye's Syndrome.

Phenothiazine drugs may cause elevated prolactin levels that persist during chronic administration. Since approximately one-third of human breast cancers are prolactin-dependent *in vitro*, this elevation is of potential importance if phenothiazine drug administration is contem- plated in a patient with a previously-detected breast cancer. Neither clinical nor epidemiologic studies to date, however, have shown an association between the chronic administration of phenothiazine drugs and mammary tumorigenesis.

Postoperative Nausea and Vomiting: When used in the treatment of the nausea and/or vomiting associated with anesthesia and surgery, it is recommended that Triethylperazine should be administered by deep intramuscular injection at or shortly before the termination of anesthesia.

Information for Patients: Patients receiving Triethylperazine should be cautioned about possible combined effects with alcohol and other CNS depressants. Patients should be cautioned not to operate machinery or drive a motor vehicle after ingesting the drug.

Drug Interactions: Phenothiazines are capable of potentiating CNS depressants (e.g., barbiturates, anesthetics, opiates, alcohol, etc.) as well as atropine and phosphorus insecticides.

Laboratory Test Interactions: The usual precautions should be observed in patients with impaired renal or hepatic function.

Nursing Mothers: Information is not available concerning the excretion of Triethylperazine in the milk of nursing mothers. As a general rule, nursing should not be undertaken while the patient is on a drug, since many drugs are excreted in human milk.

Pediatric Use: The safety and efficacy of Triethylperazine in children under 12 years of age has not been established.

ADVERSE REACTIONS

Central Nervous System: Serious: Convulsions have been reported. Extrapyramidal symptoms (E.P.S.) may occur, such as dystonia, torticollis, oculogyric crises, akathisia and gait disturbances. Others: Occasional cases of dizziness, headache, fever and restlessness have been reported.

Drowsiness may occur on occasion, following an initial injection. Generally this effect tends to subside with continued therapy or is usually alleviated by a reduction in dosage.

Autonomic Nervous System: Dryness of the mouth and nose, blurred vision, tinnitus. An occasional case of sialorrhea together with altered gustatory sensation has been observed.

Endocrine System: Peripheral edema of the arms, hands and face.

Hepatotoxicity: An occasional case of cholestatic jaundice has been observed.

Other: An occasional case of cerebral vascular spasm and trigeminal neuralgia has been reported.

Phenothiazine Derivatives: The physician should be aware that the following have occurred with one or more phenothiazines and should be considered whenever one of these drugs is used:

Blood Dyscrasias: Serious—Agranulocytosis, leukopenia, thrombocytopenia, aplastic anemia, pancytopenia. Other—Eosinophilia, leukocytosis.

Autonomic Reactions: Miosis, obstipation, anorexia, paralytic ileus.

Cutaneous Reactions: Serious—Erythema, exfoliative dermatitis, contact dermatitis.

Hepatotoxicity: Serious—Jaundice, biliary stasis.

Cardiovascular Effects: Serious—Hypotension, rarely leading to cardiac arrest; electrocardiographic (ECG) changes.

Extrapyramidal Symptoms: Serious—Akathisia, agitation, motor restlessness, dystonic reactions, trismus, torticollis, opisthotonos, oculogyric crises, tremor, muscular rigidity, akinesia—some of which have persisted for several months or years especially in patients of advanced age with brain damage.

Endocrine Disturbances: Menstrual irregularities, altered libido, gynecomastia, weight gain. False positive pregnancy tests have been reported.

Urinary Disturbances: Retention, incontinence.

Allergic Reactions: Serious—Fever, laryngeal edema, angioneurotic edema, asthma.

Others: Hyperpyrexia, Behavioral effects suggestive of a paradoxical reaction have been reported. These include excitement, bizarre dreams, aggravation of psychoses and toxic confusional states. While there is no evidence at present that ECG changes observed in patients receiving phenothiazines are in any way precursors of any significant disturbance of cardiac rhythm, it should be noted that sudden and unexpected deaths apparently due to cardiac arrest have been reported in a few instances in hospitalized psychotic patients previously showing characteristic ECG changes. A peculiar skin-eye syndrome has also been recognized as a side effect following long-term treatment with certain phenothiazines. This reaction is marked by progressive pigmentation of areas of the skin or conjunctiva and/or accompanied by discoloration of the exposed sclera and cornea. Opacities of the anterior lens and cornea described as irregular or stellate in shape have also been reported.

DOSAGE AND ADMINISTRATION

Adult: Usual daily dose range is 10 mg to 30 mg.

Oral: One tablet one to three times daily.

Intramuscular: 2 mL IM, one to three times daily. (See *"Precautions"*.)

Suppository: Insert one suppository, one to three times daily.

Children: Appropriate dosage of Triethylperazine has not been determined in children.

STORAGE

Ampuls: Below 86°F; protect from light.
Administer only if clear and colorless.

Suppositories: Below 77°F; tight container (sealed foil).

HOW SUPPLIED
INJECTION: 10 MG/2 ML

BRAND/MANUFACTURER	NDC	SIZE	AWP
○ **BRAND**			
TORECAN: Roxane	00054-1701-07	2 ml 20s	$100.60
	00054-1701-25	2 ml 100s	$426.51

TABLETS: 10 MG

BRAND/MANUFACTURER	NDC	SIZE	AWP
○ **BRAND**			
TORECAN: Roxane	00054-4748-25	100s	$51.71
	00054-8748-25	100s ud	$69.51

Trifluoperazine Hydrochloride

DESCRIPTION

Tablets: Each round, blue, film-coated tablet contains Trifluoperazine Hydrochloride equivalent to Trifluoperazine as follows: 1 mg, 2 mg, 5 mg, 10 mg.

Multidose Vials: 10 mL (2 mg/mL): Each mL contains, in aqueous solution, Trifluoperazine, 2 mg, as the Hydrochloride.

Concentrate: Each mL of clear, yellow, banana-vanilla flavored liquid contains 10 mg of Trifluoperazine as the Hydrochloride.

The concentrate is for use in severe neuropsychiatric conditions when oral medication is preferred and other oral forms are considered impractical.

Following is its chemical structure:

INDICATIONS

For the management of the manifestations of psychotic disorders.

Trifluoperazine Hydrochloride is effective for the short-term treatment of generalized non-psychotic anxiety. However, Trifluoperazine Hydrochloride is not the first drug to be used in therapy for most patients with non-psychotic anxiety because certain risks associated with its use are not shared by common alternative treatments (i.e., benzodiazepines).

When used in the treatment of non-psychotic anxiety, Trifluoperazine Hydrochloride should not be administered at doses of more than 6 mg per day or for longer than 12 weeks because the use of Trifluoperazine Hydrochloride at higher doses or for longer intervals may cause persistent tardive dyskinesia that may prove irreversible (see *"Warnings"* section).

The effectiveness of Trifluoperazine Hydrochloride as a treatment for non-psychotic anxiety was established in a 4-week clinical multicenter study of outpatients with generalized anxiety disorder (DSM-III). This evidence does not predict that Trifluoperazine Hydrochloride will be useful in patients with other non-psychotic conditions in which anxiety, or signs that mimic anxiety, are found (i.e., physical illness, organic mental conditions, agitated depression, character pathologies, etc.).

Trifluoperazine Hydrochloride has not been shown effective in the management of behavioral complications in patients with mental retardation.

UNLABELED USES
Trifluoperazine Hydrochloride is used as an adjunct in the treatment of cancer chemotherapy induced nausea and vomiting and in the management of intractable chronic pain.

CONTRAINDICATIONS
A known hypersensitivity to phenothiazines, comatose or greatly depressed states due to central nervous system depressants and, in cases of existing blood dyscrasias, bone marrow depression and pre-existing liver damage.

WARNINGS
Tardive Dyskinesia: Tardive dyskinesia, a syndrome consisting of potentially irreversible, involuntary, dyskinetic movements, may develop in patients treated with neuroleptic (antipsychotic) drugs. Although the prevalence of the syndrome appears to be highest among the elderly, especially elderly women, it is impossible to rely upon prevalence estimates to predict, at the inception of neuroleptic treatment, which patients are likely to develop the syndrome. Whether neuroleptic drug products differ in their potential to cause tardive dyskinesia is unknown.

Both the risk of developing the syndrome and the likelihood that it will become irreversible are believed to increase as the duration of treatment and the total cumulative dose of neuroleptic drugs administered to the patient increase. However, the syndrome can develop, although much less commonly, after relatively brief treatment periods at low doses. There is no known treatment for established cases of tardive dyskinesia, although the syndrome may remit, partially or completely, if neuroleptic treatment is withdrawn. Neuroleptic treatment itself, however, may suppress (or partially suppress) the signs and symptoms of the syndrome and thereby may possibly mask the underlying disease process. The effect that symptomatic suppression has upon the long-term course of the syndrome is unknown.

Given these considerations, neuroleptics should be prescribed in a manner that is most likely to minimize the occurrence of tardive dyskinesia. Chronic neuroleptic treatment should generally be reserved for patients who suffer from a chronic illness that 1) is known to respond to neuroleptic drugs, and, 2) for whom alternative, equally effective, but potentially less harmful treatments are *not* available or appropriate. In patients who do require chronic treatment, the smallest dose and the shortest duration of treatment producing a satisfactory clinical response should be sought. The need for continued treatment should be reassessed periodically.

If signs and symptoms of tardive dyskinesia appear in a patient on neuroleptics, drug discontinuation should be considered. However, some patients may require treatment despite the presence of the syndrome.

For further information about the description of tardive dyskinesia and its clinical detection, please refer to the sections on Precautions and Adverse Reactions.

Neuroleptic Malignant Syndrome (NMS): A potentially fatal symptom complex sometimes referred to as Neuroleptic Malignant Syndrome (NMS) has been reported in association with antipsychotic drugs. Clinical manifestations of NMS are hyperpyrexia, muscle rigidity, altered mental status and evidence of autonomic instability (irregular pulse or blood pressure, tachycardia, diaphoresis, and cardiac dysrhythmias).

The diagnostic evaluation of patients with this syndrome is complicated. In arriving at a diagnosis, it is important to identify cases where the clinical presentation includes both serious medical illness (e.g., pneumonia, systemic infection, etc.) and untreated or inadequately treated extrapyramidal signs and symptoms (EPS). Other important considerations in the differential diagnosis include central anticholinergic toxicity, heat stroke, drug fever and primary central nervous system (CNS) pathology.

The management of NMS should include: 1) immediate discontinuation of antipsychotic drugs and other drugs not essential to concurrent therapy, 2) intensive symptomatic treatment and medical monitoring, and 3) treatment of any concomitant serious medical problems for which specific treatments are available. There is no general agreement about specific pharmacological treatment regimens for uncomplicated NMS.

If a patient requires antipsychotic drug treatment after recovery from NMS, the potential reintroduction of drug therapy should be carefully considered. The patient should be carefully monitored, since recurrences of NMS have been reported.

Patients who have demonstrated a hypersensitivity reaction (e.g., blood dyscrasias, jaundice) with a phenothiazine should not be re-exposed to any phenothiazine, including Trifluoperazine Hydrochloride, unless in the judgment of the physician the potential benefits of treatment outweight the possible hazard.

Trifluoperazine Hydrochloride Concentrate contains sodium bisulfite, a sulfite that may cause allergic-type reactions including anaphylactic symptoms and life-threatening or less severe asthmatic episodes in certain susceptible people. The overall prevalence of sulfite sensitivity in the general population is unknown and

probably low. Sulfite sensitivity is seen more frequently in asthmatic than in non-asthmatic people.

Trifluoperazine Hydrochloride may impair mental and/or physical abilities, especially during the first few days of therapy. Therefore, caution patients about activities requiring alertness (e.g., operating vehicles or machinery).

If agents such as sedatives, narcotics, anesthetics, tranquilizers, or alcohol are used either simultaneously or successively with the drug, the possibility of an undesirable additive depressant effect should be considered.

Usage in Pregnancy: Safety for the use of Trifluoperazine Hydrochloride during pregnancy has not been established. Therefore, it is not recommended that the drug be given to pregnant patients except when, in the judgment of the physician, it is essential. The potential benefits should clearly outweigh possible hazards. There are reported instances of prolonged jaundice, extrapyramidal signs, hyperreflexia or hyporeflexia in newborn infants whose mothers received phenothiazines.

Reproductive studies in rats given over 600 times the human dose showed an increased incidence of malformations above controls and reduced litter size and weight linked to maternal toxicity. These effects were not observed at half this dosage. No adverse effect on fetal development was observed in rabbits given 700 times the human dose nor in monkeys given 25 times the human dose.

Nursing Mothers: There is evidence that phenothiazines are excreted in the breast milk of nursing mothers.

Because of the potential for serious adverse reactions in nursing infants from trifluoperazine, a decision should be made whether to discontinue nursing or to discontinue the drug, taking into account the importance of the drug to the mother.

PRECAUTIONS
General: Given the likelihood that some patients exposed chronically to neuroleptics will develop tardive dyskinesia, it is advised that all patients in whom chronic use is contemplated be given, if possible, full information about this risk. The decision to inform patients and/or their guardians must obviously take into account the clinical circumstances and the competency of the patient to understand the information provided.

Thrombocytopenia and anemia have been reported in patients receiving the drug. Agranulocytosis and pancytopenia have also been reported—warm patients to report the sudden appearance of sore throat or other signs of infection. If white blood cell and differential counts indicate cellular depression, stop treatment and start antibiotic and other suitable therapy.

Jaundice of the cholestatic type of hepatitis or liver damage has been reported. If fever with grippe-like symptoms occurs, appropriate liver studies should be conducted. If tests indicate an abnormality, stop treatment.

One result of therapy may be an increase in mental and physical activity. For example, a few patients with angina pectoris have complained of increased pain while taking the drug. Therefore, angina patients should be observed carefully and, if an unfavorable response is noted, the drug should be withdrawn.

Because hypotension has occurred, large doses and parenteral administration should be avoided in patients with impaired cardiovascular systems. To minimize the occurrence of hypotension after injection, keep patient lying down and observe for at least ½ hour. If hypotension occurs from parenteral or oral dosing, place patient in head-low position with legs raised. If a vasoconstrictor is required, norepinephrine and phenylephrine are suitable. Other pressor agents, including epinephrine, should not be used as they may cause a paradoxical further lowering of blood pressure.

Since certain phenothiazines have been reported to produce retinopathy, the drug should be discontinued if ophthalmoscopic examination or visual field studies should demonstrate retinal changes.

An antiemetic action of Trifluoperazine Hydrochloride may mask the signs and symptoms of toxicity or overdosage of other drugs and may obscure the diagnosis and treatment of other conditions such as intestinal obstruction, brain tumor and Reye's syndrome.

With prolonged administration at high dosages, the possibility of cumulative effects, with sudden onset of severe central nervous system or vasomotor symptoms, should be kept in mind.

Neuroleptic drugs elevate prolactin levels; the elevation persists during chronic administration. Tissue culture experiments indicate that approximately ⅓ of human breast cancers are prolactin-dependent *in vitro*, a factor of potential importance if the prescribing of these drugs is contemplated in a patient with a previously detected breast cancer. Although disturbances such as galactorrhea, amenorrhea, gynecomastia and impotence have been reported, the clinical significance of elevated serum prolactin levels is unknown for most patients. An increase in mammary neoplasms has been found in rodents after chronic administration of neuroleptic drugs. Neither clinical nor epidemiologic studies conducted to date, however, have shown an association between chronic administration of these drugs and mammary tumorigenesis; the available evidence is considered too limited to be conclusive at this time.

Chromosomal aberrations in spermatocytes and abnormal sperm have been demonstrated in rodents treated with certain neuroleptics.

Because phenothiazines may interfere with thermoregulatory mechanisms, use with caution in persons who will be exposed to extreme heat.

As with all drugs which exert an anticholinergic effect, and/or cause mydriasis, trifluoperazine should be used with caution in patients with glaucoma.

Phenothiazines may diminish the effect of oral anticoagulants.

Phenothiazines can produce alpha-adrenergic blockade. Concomitant administration of propranolol with phenothiazines results in increased plasma levels of both drugs.

◆ RATED THERAPEUTICALLY EQUIVALENT; ◇ THERAPEUTIC EQUIVALENCE UNCONFIRMED; ○ UNRATED

Antihypertensive effects of guanethidine and related compounds may be counteracted when phenothiazines are used concurrently.

Thiazide diuretics may accentuate the orthostatic hypotension that may occur with phenothiazines.

Phenothiazines may lower the convulsive threshold; dosage adjustments of anticonvulsants may be necessary. Potentiation of anticonvulsant effects does not occur. However, it has been reported that phenothiazines may interfere with the metabolism of prenytoin and thus precipitate prenytoin toxicity.

Drugs which lower the seizure threshold, including phenothiazine derivatives, should not be used with metrizanide. As with other phenothiazine derivatives Trifluoperazine Hydrochloride should be discontinued at least 48 hours before myelography, should not be resumed for at least 24 hours postprocedure and should not be used for the control of nausea and vomiting occurring either prior to myelography or postprocedure with *Amipaque*.

The presence of phenothiazines may produce false positive phenylketonuria (PKU) test results.

Long-Term Therapy: To lessen the likelihood of adverse reactions related to cumulative drug effect, patients with a history of long-term therapy with Trifluoperazine Hydrochloride and/or other neuroleptics should be evaluated periodically to decide whether the maintenance dosage could be lowered or drug therapy discontinued.

ADVERSE REACTIONS
Drowsiness, dizziness, skin reactions, rash, dry mouth, insomnia, amenorrhea, fatigue, muscular weakness, anorexia, lactation, blurred vision and neuromuscular (extrapyramidal) reactions.

NEUROMUSCULAR (EXTRAPYRAMIDAL) REACTIONS
These symptoms are seen in a significant number of hospitalized mental patients. They may be characterized by motor restlessness, be of the dystonic type, or they may resemble parkinsonism.

Depending on the severity of symptoms, dosage should be reduced or discontinued. If therapy is reinstituted, it should be at a lower dosage. Should these symptoms occur in children or pregnant patients, the drug should be stopped and not reinstituted. In most case barbiturates by suitable route of administration will suffice. (Or, injectable diphenhydraine may be useful.) In more severe cases, the administration of an anti-parkinsonism agent, except levodopa, usually produces rapid reversal of symptoms. Suitable supportive measures such as maintaining a clear airway and adequate hydration should be employed.

Motor Restlessness: Symptoms may include agitation or jitteriness and sometimes insomnia. These symptoms often disappear spontaneously. At times these symptoms may be similar to the original neurotic or psychotic symptoms. Dosage should not be increased until these side effects have subsided.

If this phase becomes too troublesome, the symptoms can usually be controlled by a reduction of dosage or change of drug. Treatment with anti-parkinsonian agents, benzodiazepines or propranolol may be helpful.

Dystonias: Symptoms may include: spasm of the neck muscles, sometimes progressing to torticollis; extensor rigidity of back muscles, sometimes progressing to opisthotons; carpopedal spasm, trismus, swallowing difficulty, oculogyric crisis and protrusion of the tongue.

These usually subside within a few hours, and almost always within 24 to 48 hours, after the drug has been discontinued. *In mild cases,* reassurance or a barbiturate is often sufficient. *In moderate cases,* barbiturates will usually bring rapid relief. *In more severe adult cases,* the administration of an antiparkinsonism agent, except levodopa, usually produces rapid reversal of symptoms. Also, intravenous caffeine with sodium benzoate seems to be effective. *In children,* reassurance and barbiturates will usually control symptoms. (Or, inject able diphenhydraine may be useful.) *Note:* See diphenhydraine prescribing information for appropriate children's dosage. If appropriate treatment with anti-parkinsonism agents or diphenhydraine fails to reverse the signs and symptoms, the diagnosis should be reevaluated.

Pseudo-parkinsonism: Symptoms may include: mask-like facies; drooling; tremors; pill-rolling motion; cogwheel rigidity; and shuffling gait. Reassurance and sedation are important. In most cases these symptoms are readily controlled when an anti-parkinsonism agent is administered concomitantly. Anti-parkinsonism agents should be used only when required. Generally, therapy of a few weeks to 2 or 3 months will suffice. After this time patients should be evaluated to determine their need for continued treatment. (*Note: Levodopa* has not been found effective in pseudo-parkinsonism.) Occasionally it is necessary to lower the dosage of Trifluoperzine Hydrochloride or to discontinue the drug.

Tardive Dyskinesia: As with all antipsychotic agents, tardive dyskinesia may appear in some patients on long-term therapy or may appear after drug therapy has been discontinued. The syndrome can also develop, although much less frequently, after relatively brief treatment periods at low doses. This syndrome appears in all age groups. Although its prevalence appears to be highest among elderly patients, especially elderly women, it is impossible to rely upon prevalence estimates to predict at the inception of neuroleptic treatment which patients are likely to develop the syndrome. The symptoms are persistent and in some patients appear to be irreversible. The syndrome is characterized by rhythmical involuntary movements of the tongue, face, mouth of jaw (e.g., protrusion of tongue, puffing of cheeks, puckering of mouth, chewing movements). Sometimes these may be accompanied by involuntary movements of extremities. In rare instances, these involuntary movements of the extremities are the only manifestations of

tardive dyskinesia. A variant of tardive dyskinesia, tardive dystonia, has also been described.

There is no known effective treatment for tardive dyskinesia; anti-parkinsonism agents do not alleviate the symptoms of this syndrome. If clinically feasible, it is suggested that all antipsychotic agents be discontinued if these symptoms appear. Should it be necessary to reinstitute treatment, or increase the dosage of the agent, or switch to a different anti-psychotic agent, the syndrome may be masked.

It has been reported that fine vermicular movements of the tongue may be an early sign of the syndrome and if the medication is stopped at that time the syndrome may not develop.

Adverse Reactions Reported with Trifluoperazine Hydrochloride or Other Phenothiazine Derivatives: Adverse effects with different phenothiazines vary in type, frequency, and mechanism of occurrence, i.e., some are dose-related, while others involve individual patient sensitivity. Some adverse effects may be more likely to occur, or occur with greater intensity, in patients with special medical problems, e.g., patients with mitral insufficiency or pheochromocytoma have experienced severe hypotension following recommended doses of certain phenothiazines.

Neuroleptic Malignant Syndrome (NMS) has been reported in association with antipsychotic drugs. (See *"Warnings".*)

Not all of the following adverse reactions have been observed with every phenothiazine derivative, but they have been reported with one or more and should be borne in mind when drugs of this class are administered: extrapyramidal symptoms (opisthotonos, oculogyric crisis, hyperreflexia, dystonia, akathisia, dyskinesia, parkinsonism) some of which have lasted months and even years—particularly in elderly patients with previous brain damage; grand mal and petit mal convulsions, particularly in patients with EEG abnormalities or history of such disorders; altered cerebrospinal fluid proteins; cerebral edema; intensification and prolongation of the action of central nervous system depressants (opiates, analgesics, antihistamines, barbiturates, alcohol), atropine, heat, organophosphorus insecticides; autonomic reactions (dryness of mouth, nasal congestion, headache, nausea, constipation, obstipation, adynamic ileus, ejaculatory disorders/impotence, priapism, atonic colon, urinary retention, miosis and mydriasis); reactivation of psychotic processes, catatonic-like states; hypotension (sometimes fatal); cardiac arrest; blood dyscrasias (pancytopenia, thrombocytopenic purpura, leukopenia, agranulocytosis, eosinophilia, hemolytic anemia, aplastic anemia); liver damage (jaundice, biliary stasis); endocrine disturbances (hyperglycemia, hypoglycemia, glycosura, lactation, galactorrhea, gynecomastia, menstrual irregularities, false positive pregnancy tests); skin disorders (photosensitivity, itching, erythema, urticaria, eczema up to exfoliative dermatitis); other allergic reactions (asthma, laryngeal edema, angioneurotic edema, anaphylactoid reactions); peripheral edema, reversed epinephrine effect; hyperpyrexia; mild fever after large I.M. doses; increased appetite; increased weight; a systemic lupus erythematosus-like syndrome; pigmentary retinopathy; with prolonged administration of substantial doses, skin pigmentation, epithelial keratopathy, and lenticular and corneal deposits.

EKG changes—particularly nonspecific, usually reversible Q and T wave distortions—have been observed in some patients receiving phenothiazine tranquilizers. Although phenothiazines cause neither psychic nor physical dependence, sudden discontinuance in long-term psychiatric patients may cause temporary symptoms, e.g., nausea and vomiting, dizziness, tremulousness.

Note: There have been occasional reports of sudden death in patients receiving phenothiazines. In some cases, the cause appeared to be cardiac arrest or asphyxia due to failure of the cough reflex.

OVERDOSAGE
(See also under *"Adverse Reactions"*)

Symptoms: Primarily involvement of the extrapyramidal mechanism producing some of the dystonic reactions described above. Symptoms of central nervous system depression to the point of somnolence or coma. Agitation and restlessness may also occur. Other possible manifestations include convulsions, EKG changes and cardiac arrhythmias, fever, and autonomic reactions such as hypotension, dry mouth and ileus.

Treatment: It is important to determine other medications taken by the patient since multiple dose therapy is common in overdosage situations. Treatment is essentially symptomatic and supportive. Early gastric lavage is helpful. Keep patient under observation and maintain an open airway, since involvement of the extrapyramidal mechanism may produce dysphagia and respiratory difficulty in severe overdosage. **Do not attempt to induce emesis because a dystonic reaction of the head or neck may develop that could result in aspiration of vomitus.** Extrapyramidal symptoms may be treated with anti-parkinsonism drugs, barbiturates, or diphenhydrine. See prescribing information for these products. Care should be taken to avoid increasing respiratory depression. If administration of a stimulant is desirable, amphetamine, dextroamphetamine, or caffeine with sodium benzoate is recommended. Stimulants that may cause convulsions (e.g., picrotoxin or pentylenetetrazol) should be avoided.

If hypotension occurs, the standard measures for managing circulatory shock should be initiated. If it is desirable to administer a vasoconstrictor, norepinephrine and phenylephrine are most suitable. Other pressor agents, including epinephrine, are not recommended because phenothiazine derivatives may reverse the usual elevating action of these agents and cause a further lowering of blood pressure.

Limited experience indicates that phenothiazines are *not* dialyzable.

DOSAGE AND ADMINISTRATION

ADULTS

Dosage should be adjusted to the needs of the individual. The lowest effective dosage should always be used. Dosage should be increased more gradually in debilitated or emaciated patients. When maximum response is achieved, dosage may be reduced gradually to a maintenance level. Because of the inherent long action of the drug, patients may be controlled on convenient b.i.d. administration; some patients may be maintained on once-a-day administration.

When Trifluoperazine Hydrochloride is administered by intramuscular injection, equivalent oral dosage may be substituted once symptoms have been controlled.

Note: Although there is little likelihood of contact dermatitis due to the drug, persons with known sensitivity to phenothiazine drugs should avoid direct contact.

Elderly Patients: In general, dosages in the lower range are sufficient for most elderly patients. Since they appear to be more susceptible to hypotension and neuromuscular reactions, such patients should be observed closely. Dosage should be tailored to the individual, response carefully monitored, and dosage adjusted accordingly. Dosage should be increased more gradually in elderly patients.

NON-PSYCHOTIC ANXIETY

Usual dosage is 1 or 2 mg twice daily. Do not administer at doses of more than 6 mg per day or for longer than 12 weeks.

PSYCHOTIC DISORDERS

Oral: Usual starting dosage is 2 mg to 5 mg b.i.d. (Small or emaciated patients should always be started on the lower dosage.)

Most patients will show optimum response on 15 mg or 20 mg daily, although a few may require 40 mg a day or more. Optimum therapeutic dosage levels should be reached within 2 or 3 weeks.

When the concentrate dosage form is to be used, it should be added to 60 mL (2 fl oz) or more of diluent *just prior to administration to insure* palatability and stability. Vehicles suggested for dilution are: tomato or fruit juice, milk, simple syrup, orange syrup, carbonated beverages, coffee, tea, or water. Semisolid foods (soup, puddings, etc.) may also be used.

Intramuscular (for prompt control of severe symptoms): Usual dosage is 1 mg to 2 mg ½-1 mL) by deep intramuscular injection q4 to 6h, p.r.n. More than 6 mg within 24 hours is rarely necessary.

Only in very exceptional cases should intramuscular dosage exceed 10 mg within 24 hours. Injections should not be given at intervals of less than 4 hours because of a possible cumulative effect.

Note: Trifluoperazine Hydrochloride Injection has been usually well tolerated and there is little, if any, pain and irritation at the site of injection.

This solution should be protected from light. This is a clear, colorless to pale yellow solution: a slight yellowish discoloration will not alter potency. If markedly discolored, solution should be discarded.

PSYCHOTIC CHILDREN

Dosage should be adjusted to the weight of the child and severity of the symptoms. These dosages are for children, ages 6 to 12, who are hospitalized or under close supervision.

Oral: The starting dosage is 1 mg administered once a day or b.i.d. Dosage may be increased gradually until symptoms are controlled or until side effects become troublesome.

While it is usually not necessary to exceed dosages of 15 mg daily, some older children with severe symptoms may require higher dosages.

Intramuscular: There has been little experience with the use of Trifluoperazine Hydrochloride Injection in children. However, if it is necessary to achieve rapid control of severe symptoms, 1 mg (½ mL) of the drug may be administered intramuscularly once or twice a day.

STORAGE

The concentrate form is light-sensitive. For this reason, it should be protected from light and dispensed in amber bottles. *Refrigeration is not required.*

HOW SUPPLIED
CONCENTRATE: 10 MG/ML

BRAND/MANUFACTURER	NDC	SIZE	AWP
◆ BRAND			
STELAZINE: SK Beecham Pharm	00108-4901-42	60 ml	$102.85
◆ GENERICS			
Geneva	00781-4045-02	60 ml	$62.60

INJECTION: 2 MG/ML

BRAND/MANUFACTURER	NDC	SIZE	AWP
◆ BRAND			
STELAZINE: SK Beecham Pharm	00108-4902-01	10 ml	$47.20

TABLETS: 1 MG

BRAND/MANUFACTURER	NDC	SIZE	AWP
◆ BRAND			
STELAZINE: SK Beecham Pharm	00108-4903-20	100s	$58.05
◆ GENERICS			
Major	00904-0554-61	100s ud	$24.70

TABLETS: 2 MG

AVERAGE UNIT PRICE (AVAILABLE SIZES)		GENERIC A-RATED AVERAGE PRICE (GAAP)	
BRAND	$0.86	100s	$46.82
GENERIC	$0.44		
HCFA FUL (100s ea)	$0.32		

BRAND/MANUFACTURER	NDC	SIZE	AWP
◆ BRAND			
STELAZINE: SK Beecham Pharm	00108-4904-20	100s	$85.60
◆ GENERICS			
Major	00904-0561-60	100s	$40.30
Geneva	00781-1032-01	100s	$44.51
Geneva	00781-1032-13	100s ud	$55.64
Geneva	00781-1032-10	1000s	$356.08

TABLETS: 5 MG

AVERAGE UNIT PRICE (AVAILABLE SIZES)		GENERIC A-RATED AVERAGE PRICE (GAAP)	
BRAND	$1.08	100s	$46.98
GENERIC	$0.47		
HCFA FUL (100s ea)	$0.38		

BRAND/MANUFACTURER	NDC	SIZE	AWP
◆ BRAND			
STELAZINE: SK Beecham Pharm	00108-4906-20	100s	$107.75
◆ GENERICS			
Major	00904-0562-60	100s	$47.50
Geneva	00781-1034-01	100s	$56.03
U.S. Trading	56126-0315-11	100s ud	$14.33
Geneva	00781-1034-13	100s ud	$70.04
Geneva	00781-1034-10	1000s	$448.24

TABLETS: 10 MG

AVERAGE UNIT PRICE (AVAILABLE SIZES)		GENERIC A-RATED AVERAGE PRICE (GAAP)	
BRAND	$1.63	100s	$66.23
GENERIC	$0.67		
HCFA FUL (100s ea)	$0.48		

BRAND/MANUFACTURER	NDC	SIZE	AWP
◆ BRAND			
STELAZINE: SK Beecham Pharm	00108-4907-20	100s	$162.45
◆ GENERICS			
Major	00904-0563-60	100s	$60.00
Geneva	00781-1036-01	100s	$84.47
U.S. Trading	56126-0316-11	100s ud	$14.85
Geneva	00781-1036-13	100s ud	$105.59
Geneva	00781-1036-10	1000s	$675.76

Triflupromazine Hydrochloride

DESCRIPTION

Triflupromazine Hydrochloride is a phenothiazine derivative. It is available for parenteral use in multiple dose vials providing 10 or 20 mg Triflupromazine Hydrochloride per mL, with 1.5% (w/v) benzyl alcohol as a preservative and sodium chloride for isotonicity. The pH has been adjusted to 3.5 to 5.2 with sodium hydroxide and/or hydrochloric acid. At the time of manufacture, the air in the vials is replaced by nitrogen.

Following is its chemical structure:

$$CH_2CH_2CH_2N(CH_3)_2$$

$$CF_3$$

CLINICAL PHARMACOLOGY

Experimental and clinical studies suggest that the phenothiazine derivatives act on the hypothalamus. These drugs are believed to depress various components of the mesodiencephalic activating system, which is involved in the control of basal metabolism and body temperature, wakefulness, vaso-motor tone, emesis, and hormonal balance. In addition, the drugs exert a peripheral autonomic effect in varying degrees. However, the site and mode of action of phenothiazine derivatives including Triflupromazine have not been completely elucidated.

INDICATIONS AND USAGE

Triflupromazine Hydrochloride is effective in the management of the manifestations of psychotic disorders (excluding psychotic depressive reactions) and for the control of severe nausea and vomiting.

Triflupromazine Hydrochloride has not been shown effective in the management of behavioral complications in patients with mental retardation.

CONTRAINDICATIONS

Phenothiazines are contraindicated in patients with suspected or established subcortical brain damage, with or without hypothalamic damage, since a hyperthermic reaction with temperatures in excess of 104°F may occur in such

---

◆ RATED THERAPEUTICALLY EQUIVALENT; ◇ THERAPEUTIC EQUIVALENCE UNCONFIRMED; ○ UNRATED

patients, sometimes not until 14 to 16 hours after drug administration. Total body ice-packing is recommended for such a reaction; antipyretics may also be useful.

Phenothiazine compounds should not be used in patients receiving large doses of hypnotics.

As with other phenothiazine compounds, Triflupromazine is contraindicated in comatose or severely depressed states.

The presence of blood dyscrasia or liver damage precludes the use of Triflupromazine.

WARNINGS

The extrapyramidal symptoms which can occur secondary to administration of Trifluopromazine Hydrochloride may be confused with the central nervous system signs of an undiagnosed primary disease responsible for the vomiting, e.g., Reye's Syndrome or other encephalopathy. The use of Triflupromazine Hydrochloride and other potential hepatotoxins should be avoided in children and adolescents whose signs and symptoms suggest Reye's Syndrome.

TARDIVE DYSKINESIA

Tardive dyskinesia, a syndrome consisting of potentially irreversible, involuntary, dyskinetic movements, may develop in patients treated with neuroleptic (antipsychotic) drugs. Although the prevalence of the syndrome appears to be highest among the elderly, especially elderly women, it is impossible to rely upon prevalence estimates to predict, at the inception of neuroleptic treatment, which patients are likely to develop the syndrome. Whether neuroleptic drug products differ in their potential to cause tardive dyskinesia is unknown.

Both the risk of developing the syndrome and the likelihood that it will become irreversible are believed to increase as the duration of treatment and the total cumulative dose of neuroleptic drugs administered to the patient increase. However, the syndrome can develop, although much less commonly, after relatively brief treatment periods at low doses.

There is no known treatment for established cases of tardive dyskinesia, although the syndrome may remit, partially or completely, if neuroleptic treatment is withdrawn. Neuroleptic treatment, itself, however, may suppress (or partially suppress) the signs and symptoms of the syndrome and thereby may possibly mask the underlying disease process. The effect that symptomatic suppression has upon the long-term course of the syndrome is unknown.

Given these considerations, neuroleptics should be prescribed in a manner that is most likely to minimize the occurrence of tardive dyskinesia. Chronic neuroleptic treatment should generally be reserved for patients who suffer from a chronic illness that, 1) is known to respond to neuroleptic drugs, and, 2) for whom alternative, equally effective, but potentially less harmful treatments are *not* available or appropriate. In patients who do require chronic treatment, the smallest dose and the shortest duration of treatment producing a satisfactory clinical response should be sought. The need for continued treatment should be reassessed periodically.

If signs and symptoms of tardive dyskinesia appear in a patient on neuroleptics, drug discontinuation should be considered. However, some patients may require treatment despite the presence of the syndrome.

(For further information about the description of tardive dyskinesia and its clinical detection, please refer to the sections on *"Precautions, Information for Patients"* and *"Adverse Reactions, Tardive Dyskinesia."*)

NEUROLEPTIC MALIGNANT SYNDROME (NMS)

A potentially fatal symptom complex sometimes referred to as Neuroleptic Malignant Syndrome (NMS) has been reported in association with antipsychotic drugs. Clinical manifestations of NMS are hyperpyrexia, muscle rigidity, altered mental status and evidence of autonomic instability (irregular pulse or blood pressure, tachycardia, diaphoresis, and cardiac dysrhythmias).

The diagnostic evaluation of patients with this syndrome is complicated. In arriving at a diagnosis, it is important to identify cases where the clinical presentation includes both serious medical illness (e.g., pneumonia, systemic infection, etc.) and untreated or inadequately treated extrapyramidal signs and symptoms (EPS). Other important considerations in the differential diagnosis include central anticholinergic toxicity, heat stroke, drug fever and primary central nervous system (CNS) pathology.

The management of NMS should include 1) immediate discontinuation of antipsychotic drugs and other drugs not essential to concurrent therapy, 2) intensive symptomatic treatment and medical monitoring, and 3) treatment of any concomitant serious medical problems for which specific treatments are available. There is no general agreement about specific pharmacological treatment regimens for uncomplicated NMS.

If a patient requires antipsychotic drug treatment after recovery from NMS, the potential reintroduction of drug therapy should be carefully considered. The patient should be carefully monitored, since recurrences of NMS have been reported.

The use of this drug may impair the mental and physical abilities required for driving a car or operating heavy machinery.

Potentiation of the effects of alcohol may occur with the use of this drug.

USAGE IN PREGNANCY

The safety for the use of this drug during pregnancy has not been established; therefore, the possible hazards should be weighed against the potential benefits when administering this drug to pregnant patients.

PRECAUTIONS

GENERAL

Antiemetic Effect: The antiemetic action of Triflupromazine may mask the signs and symptoms of overdosage of other drugs and may obscure the diagnosis and

treatment of other conditions such as intestinal obstruction, brain tumor, and Reye's Syndrome (see *"Warnings"*).

Because of the possibility of cross-sensitivity, this drug should be used cautiously in patients who have developed cholestatic jaundice, dermatoses, or other allergic reactions to phenothiazine derivatives.

Psychotic patients on large doses of a phenothiazine drug who are undergoing surgery should be watched carefully for possible hypotensive phenomena. Moreover, it should be remembered that reduced amounts of anesthetics or central nervous system depressants may be necessary. It is generally not recommended that Triflupromazine be used prior to spinal anesthesia.

Although this is not a general feature of Triflupromazine Hydrochloride, potentiation of central nervous system depressants (opiates, analgesics, antihistamines, barbiturates, alcohol) may occur. The effects of atropine may be potentiated in some patients receiving Triflupromazine.

Phenothiazines should be used with caution in patients with a history of convulsive disorders, since grand mal convulsions have been known to occur.

Patients with special medical disorders such as mitral insufficiency or pheochromocytoma and patients who have exhibited idiosyncrasy to other centrally acting drugs may experience severe reactions to phenothiazine compounds.

The parenteral administration of Triflupromazine Hydrochloride may sometimes cause postural hypotension; to preclude its occurrence, patients should be kept under close clinical supervision, in a recumbent position if necessary.

Facilities should be available for periodic checking of hepatic function, renal function, and the blood picture. Renal function of patients on long-term therapy should be monitored; if BUN (blood urea nitrogen) becomes abnormal, treatment should be discontinued.

As with any phenothiazine, the physician should be alert to the possible development of "silent pneumonias" in patients under treatment with Triflupromazine.

Neuroleptic drugs elevate prolactin levels; the elevation persists during chronic administration. Tissue culture experiments indicate that approximately one-third of human breast cancers are prolactin dependent *in vitro,* a factor of potential importance if the prescription of these drugs is contemplated in a patient with a previously detected breast cancer. Although disturbances such as galactorrhea, amenorrhea, gynecomastia, and impotence have been reported, the clinical significance of elevated serum prolactin levels is unknown for most patients. An increase in mammary neoplasms has been found in rodents after chronic administration of neuroleptic drugs. Neither clinical studies nor epidemiologic studies conducted to date, however, have shown an association between chronic administration of these drugs and mammary tumorigenesis; the available evidence is considered too limited to be conclusive at this time.

INFORMATION FOR PATIENTS

Given the likelihood that some patients exposed chronically to neuroleptics will develop tardive dyskinesia, it is advised that all patients in whom chronic use is contemplated be given, if possible, full information about this risk. The decision to inform patients and/or their guardians must obviously take into account the clinical circumstances and the competency of the patient to understand the information provided.

ADVERSE REACTIONS

Central Nervous System: The side effects most frequently reported with phenothiazine compounds are extrapyramidal symptoms including pseudoparkinsonism, dystonia, dyskinesia, akathisia, oculogyric crises, opisthotonos, and hyperreflexia. Most often these extrapyramidal symptoms are reversible; however, they may be persistent (see below). With any given phenothiazine derivative, the incidence and severity of such reactions depend more on individual patient sensitivity than on other factors, but dosage level and patient age are also determinants.

Extrapyramidal reactions may be alarming, and the patient should be forewarned and reassured. These reactions can usually be controlled by administration of antiparkinsonian drugs such as Benztropine Mesylate and by subsequent reduction in dosage.

Tardive Dyskinesia: See *"Warnings".* The syndrome is characterized by involuntary choreoathetoid movements which variously involve the tongue, face, mouth, lips, or jaw (e.g. protrusion of the tongue, puffing of cheeks, puckering of the mouth, chewing movements), trunk and extremities. The severity of the syndrome and the degree of impairment produced vary widely.

The syndrome may become clinically recognizable either during treatment, upon dosage reduction, or upon withdrawal of treatment. Early detection of tardive dyskinesia is important. To increase the likelihood of detecting the syndrome at the earliest possible time, the dosage of neuroleptic drug should be reduced periodically (if clinically possible) and the patient observed for signs of the disorder. This maneuver is critical, since neuroleptic drugs may mask the signs of the syndrome.

Other CNS Effects: Occurrences of neuroleptic malignant syndrome (NMS) have been reported in patients on neuroleptic therapy (see *"Warnings, Neuroleptic Malignant Syndrome"*), leukocytosis, elevated CPK, liver function abnormalities, and acute renal failure may also occur with NMS.

Drowsiness or lethargy, if they occur, may necessitate a reduction in dosage; the induction of a catatonic-like state has been known to occur with dosages far in excess of the recommended amounts. As with other phenothiazine compounds, reactivation or aggravation of psychotic processes may be encountered.

Phenothiazine derivatives have been known to cause, in some patients, restlessness, excitement, or bizarre dreams.

Autonomic Nervous System: Hypertension and fluctuation in blood pressure have been reported with Triflupromazine.

Patients with pheochromocytoma, cerebral vascular or renal insufficiency appear to be particularly prone to hypotensive reactions with phenothiazine compounds and should therefore be observed closely when the drug is administered. If severely hypotension should occur, supportive measures including the use of intravenous vasopressor drugs should be instituted immediately. Levarterenol bitartrate injection and phenylephrine hydrochloride injection are suitable drugs for this purpose. Epinephrine should not be used since phenothiazine derivatives have been found to reverse its action, resulting in a further lowering of blood pressure.

Autonomic reactions including nausea and loss of appetite, salivation, polyuria, perspiration, dry mouth, headache, and constipation may occur. Autonomic effects can usually be controlled by reducing or temporarily discontinuing dosage.

In some patients, phenothiazine derivatives have caused blurred vision, glaucoma, bladder paralysis, fecal impaction, paralytic ileus, tachycardia, or nasal congestion.

Metabolic and Endocrine: Weight change, peripheral edema, abnormal lactation, gynecomastia, menstrual irregularities, false results on pregnancy tests, impotency in men, and increased libido in women have all been known to occur in some patients on phenothiazine therapy.

Allergic Reactions: Skin disorders such as itching, erythema, urticaria, seborrhea, photosensitivity, eczema, and even exfoliative dermatitis have been reported with phenothiazine derivatives. The possibility of anaphylactoid reactions occurring in some patients should be borne in mind.

Hematologic: Routine blood counts are advisable during therapy since blood dyscrasias including leukopenia, agranulocytosis, thrombocytopenic or nonthrombocytopenic purpura, eosinophilia, and pancytopenia have been observed with phenothiazine derivatives. Furthermore, if any soreness of the mouth, gums, or throat, or any symptoms of upper respiratory infection occur and confirmatory leukocyte count indicates cellular depression, therapy should be discontinued and other appropriate measures instituted immediately.

Hepatic: Liver damage as manifested by cholestatic jaundice or biliary stasis have been observed with phenothiazine derivatives, particularly during the first months of therapy; treatment should be discontinued if this occurs. An increase in cephalin flocculation, sometimes accompanied by alterations in other liver function tests has been reported in patients receiving phenothiazines who have had no clinical evidence of liver damage.

Others: Sudden, unexpected, and unexplained deaths have been reported in hospitalized psychotic patients receiving phenothiazines. Previous brain damage or seizures may be predisposing factors; high doses should be avoided in known seizure patients. Several patients have shown sudden flare-ups of psychotic behavior patterns shortly before death. Autopsy findings have usually revealed acute fulminating pneumonia or pneumonitis, aspiration of gastric contents, or intramyocardial lesions.

The following adverse reactions have also occurred with phenothiazine derivatives: systemic lupus erythematosus-like syndrome, hypotension severe enough to cause fatal cardiac arrest, altered electrocardiographic and electroencephalographic tracings, altered cerebrospinal fluid proteins, cerebral edema, potentiation of heat and of phosphorus insecticides, asthma, laryngeal edema, angioneurotic edema, and pigmentary retinopathy; with long-term use—skin pigmentation and lenticular and corneal opacities.

DOSAGE AND ADMINISTRATION

PSYCHOTIC DISORDERS

Institutionalized Adult Patients: Optimum dosage levels must be determined individually in each patient. The recommended initial intramuscular dose is 60 mg up to a maximum total daily dose of 150 mg. After treatment is instituted, the daily dosage should be adjusted until the desired clinical effect is obtained. Continued treatment is necessary to achieve maximum therapeutic benefits. In some patients, optimum clinical improvement may occur only after prolonged treatment. When symptoms are controlled, dosage can generally be reduced gradually to maintenance levels.

Noninstitutionalized Adult Patients: Use the same regimen as outlined for institutionalized patients.

Children: As in adult therapy, optimum dosage levels must be determined individually for each patient. When intramuscular use is indicated in children, the recommended range is 0.2 to 0.25 mg/kg (1/10 to 1/8 mg/lb) up to a maximum total daily dose of 10 mg. The drug should not be administered to children under 2 ½ years of age.

NAUSEA AND VOMITING

For adults, the recommended dosage range for prophylaxis as well as for treatment is 1 mg up to a maximum total daily dose of 3 mg intravenously or 5 to 15 mg as a single dose which may be repeated every four hours up to a maximum total daily dose of 60 mg intramuscularly. For elderly or debilitated patients, the recommended intramuscular dosage is 2.5 mg up to a maximum total daily dose of 15 mg.

Triflupromazine Hydrochloride should generally not be used in children under 2 ½ years of age. It should not be used in conditions for which children's dosages have not been established. Dosage and frequency of administration should be adjusted according to the severity of the symptoms and response of the patient.

The duration of activity following intramuscular administration may last up to 12 hours. Subsequent doses may be given by the same route if necessary.

For children, the recommended dosage range is 0.2 to 0.25 mg/kg (1/10 to 1/8 mg/lb) up to a maximum total daily dose of 10 mg intramuscularly. Intravenous administration is not recommended for children.

STORAGE

Protect from light. Store at room temperature; avoid freezing. Parenteral solutions may vary in color from colorless to faintly yellowish green. If a solution has become any darker or is discolored in any other way, it should not be used.

J CODES

Up to 20 mg IM,IV—J3400

HOW SUPPLIED
INJECTION: 10 MG/ML

BRAND/MANUFACTURER	NDC	SIZE	AWP
○ **BRAND**			
VESPRIN INJECTION: Apothecon	00003-0987-70	10 ml	$45.62

INJECTION: 20 MG/ML

BRAND/MANUFACTURER	NDC	SIZE	AWP
○ **BRAND**			
VESPRIN INJECTION: Apothecon	00003-0920-20	1 ml	$12.48

Trifluridine

DESCRIPTION

Trifluridine (also known as trifluorothymidine, F_3TdR, F_3T) is an antiviral drug for topical treatment of epithelial keratitis caused by Herpes simplex virus. The chemical name of Trifluridine is 2'-deoxy-5-(trifluoromethyl)uridine.

Trifluridine sterile ophthalmic solution contains 1% Trifluridine.

Following is its chemical structure:

CLINICAL PHARMACOLOGY

Trifluridine is a fluorinated pyrimidine nucleoside with *in vitro* and *in vivo* activity against Herpes simplex virus, types 1 and 2 and vacciniavirus. Some strains of Adenovirus are also inhibited *in vitro*.

Trifluridine interferes with DNA synthesis in cultured mammalian cells. However, its antiviral mechanism of action is not completely known.

In vitro perfusion studies on excised rabbit corneas have shown that Trifluridine penetrates the intact cornea as evidenced by recovery of parental drug and its major metabolite, 5-carboxy-2'-deoxyuridine, on the endothelial side of the cornea. Absence of the corneal epithelium enhances the penetration of Trifluridine approximately two-fold.

Intraocular penetration of Trifluridine occurs after topical instillation of Trifluridine into human eyes. Decreased corneal integrity or stromal or uveal inflammation may enhance the penetration of Trifluridine into the aqueous humor. Unlike the results of ocular penetration of Trifluridine *in vitro*, 5-carboxy-2'-deoxyuridine was not found in detectable concentrations within the aqueous humor of the human eye.

Systemic absorption of Trifluridine following therapeutic dosing wih Trifluridine appears to be negligible. No detectable concentrations of Trifluridine or 5-carboxy-2'-deoxyuridine were found in the sera of adult healthy normal subjects who had Trifluridine instilled into their eyes seven times daily for 14 consecutive days.

INDICATIONS AND USAGE

Trifluridine Ophthalmic Solution, 1%, is indicated for the treatment of primary keratoconjunctivitis and recurrent epithelial keratitis due to Herpes simplex virus, types 1 and 2. Trifluridine is also effective in the treatment of epithelial keratitis that has not responded clinically to the topical administration of idoxuridine or when ocular toxicity or hypersensitivity to idoxuridine has occurred. In a smaller number of patients found to be resistant to topical vidarabine, Trifluridine was also effective.

The clinical efficacy of Trifluridine in the treatment of stromal keratitis and uveitis due to Herpes simplex virus or ophthalmic infections caused by vacciniavirus and Adenovirus has not been established by well-controlled clinical trials. Trifluridine has not been shown to be effective in the prophylaxis of Herpes simplex virus keratoconjunctivitis and epithelial keratitis by well-controlled clinical trials. Trifluridine is not effective against bacterial, fungal or chlamydial infections of the cornea or nonviral trophic lesions.

During controlled multicenter clinical trials, 92 of 97 (95%) patients (78 of 81 with dendritic and 14 of 16 with geographic ulcers) responded to Trifluridine therapy as evidenced by complete corneal re-epithelialization within the 14-day therapy period. In these controlled studies, 56 of 75 (75%) patients (49 of 58 with dendritic and 7 of 17 with geographic ulcers) responded to idoxuridine therapy. The mean time to corneal re-epithelialization for dendritic ulcers (6 days) and geographic ulcers (7 days) was similar for both therapies. In other clinical studies, Trifluridine was evaluated in the treatment of Herpes simplex virus keratitis in patients who were unresponsive or intolerant to the topical administration of idoxuridine or vidarabine. Trifluridine was effective in 138 of 150 (92%) patients (109 of 114 with dendritic and 29 of 36 with geographic ulcers) as evidenced by corneal re-epithelialization. The mean time to corneal re-epithelialization was 6 days for patients with dendritic ulcers and 12 days for patients with geographic ulcers.

CONTRAINDICATIONS
Trifluridine Ophthalmic Solution, 1%, is contraindicated for patients who develop hypersensitivity reactions or chemical intolerance to Trifluridine.

WARNINGS
The recommended dosage and frequency of administration should not be exceeded (see "Dosage and Administration".)

PRECAUTIONS
General: Trifluridine Ophthalmic Solution, 1%, should be prescribed only for patients who have a clinical diagnosis of herpetic keratitis.

Trifluridine may cause mild local irritation of the conjunctiva and cornea when instilled, but these effects are usually transient.

Although documented *in vitro* viral resistance to Trifluridine has not been reported following multiple exposure to Trifluridine, the possibility exists of viral resistance development.

Drug Interactions: The following drugs have been administered topically to the eye and concurrently with Trifluridine in a limited number of patients without apparent evidence of adverse interaction: antibiotics—chloramphenicol, erythromycin, polymyxin B sulfate, bactracin, gentamicin sulfate, tetracycine HCl, sodium sulfacetamide, neomycin sulfate; steroids—dexamethasone, dexamethasone sodium phosphate, prednisolone acetate, prednisolone sodium phosphate, hydrocortisone fluorometholone; and other ophthalmic drugs—tropine sulfate, scopolamine hydrobromide, naphazoline hydrochloride, cyclopentolate hydrochloride, homatropine hydrobromide, plocarpine, 1-epinephrine hydrochloride, sodium chloride.

Carcinogenesis, Mutagenesis, Impairment of Fertility: Mutagenic Potential: Trifluridine has been shown to exert mutagenic, DNA-damaging and cell-transforming activities in various standard *in vitro* test systems, and clastogenic activity in *Viola faba* cells. It did not induce chromosome aberrations in bone marrow cells of male or female rats following a single subcutaneous dose of 100 mg/kg, but was weakly positive in female, but not in male, rats following daily subcutaneous administration at 700 mg/kg/day for 5 days.

Although the significance of these test results is not clear or fully understood, there exists the possibility that mutagenic agents may cause genetic damage in humans.

Oncogenic Potential: Lifetime carcinogenicity bioassays in rats and mice given daily subcutaneous doses of Trifluridine have been performed. Rats tested at 1.5, 7.5 and 15 mg/kg/day had increased incidences of adenocarcinomas of the intestinal tract and mammary glands, hemangiosarcomas of the spleen and liver, carcinosarcomas of the prostate gland and granulosa-thecal cell tumors of the ovary. Mice were tested at 1, 5 and 10 mg/kg/day; those given 10 mg/kg/day Trifluridine had significantly increased incidences of adenocarcinomas of the intestinal tract and uterus. Those given 10 mg/kg/day also had a significantly increased incidence of testicular atrophy as compared to vehicle control mice.

Pregnancy: Teratogenic Effects: Pregnancy Category C. Trifluridine was not teratogenic at doses up to 5.0 mg/kg/day (23 times the estimated human exposure) when given subcutaneously to rats and rabbits. However, fetal toxicity consisting of delayed ossification of portions of the skeleton occurred at dose levels of 2.5 and 5.0 mg/kg/day in rats and at 2.5 mg/kg/day in rabbits. In addition, both 2.5 and 5.0 mg/kg/day produced fetal death and resorption in rabbits. In both rats and rabbits, 1.0 mg/kg/day (5 times the estimated human exposure) was a no-effect level. There were no teratogenic or fetotoxic effects after topical application of Trifluridine Ophthalmic Solution, 1%, (approximately 5 times the estimated human exposure) to the eyes of rabbits on the 6th through the 18th days of pregnancy.[1] In a non-standard test, Trifluridine solution has been shown to be teratogenic when injected directly into the yolk sac of chicken eggs.[2] There are no adequate and well-controlled studies in pregnant women. Trifluridine Ophthalmic Solution, 1%, should be used during pregnancy only if the potential benefit justifies the potential risk to the fetus.

Nursing Mothers: It is unlikely that Trifluridine is excreted in human milk after ophthalmic instillation of Trifluridine because of the relatively small dosage ($\leq$ 5.0 mg/day), its dilution in body fluids and its extremely short half-life (approximately 12 minutes). The drug should not be prescribed for nursing mothers unless the potential benefits outweigh the potential risks.

ADVERSE REACTIONS
The most frequent adverse reactions reported during controlled clinical trials were mild, transient burning or stinging upon instillation (4.6%) and palpebral edema (2.8%). Other adverse reactions in decreasing order of reported frequency were superficial punctate keratopathy, epithelial keratopathy, hypersensitivity reaction, stromal edema, irritation, keratitis sicca, hyperemia, and increased intraocular pressure.

OVERDOSAGE
Overdosage by ocular instillation is unlikely because any excess solution should be quickly expelled from the conjunctival sac.

Acute overdosage by accidental oral ingestion of Trifluridine has not occurred. However, should such ingestion occur the 75 mg dosage of Trifluridine in a 7.5 mL bottle of Trifluridine is not likely to produce adverse effects. Single intravenous doses of 15-30 mg/kg/day in children and adults with neoplastic disease produce reversible bone marrow depression as the only potentially serious toxic effect and only after 3-5 courses of therapy.[3] The acute oral LD_{50} in the mouse and rat was 4379 mg/kg or higher.

DOSAGE AND ADMINISTRATION
Instill one drop of Trifluridine Ophthalmic Solution, 1%, onto the cornea of the affected eye every two hours while awake for a maximum daily dosage of nine drops until the corneal ulcer has completely re-epithelialized. Following re-epithelialization, treatment for an additional seven days of one drop every four hours while awake for a minimum daily dosage of five drops is recommended.

If there are no signs of improvement after seven days of therapy or complete re-epithelialization has not occurred after 14 days of therapy, other forms of therapy should be considered. Continuous administration of Trifluridine for periods exceeding 21 days should be avoided because of potential ocular toxicity.

Store under refrigeration 2° to 8°C (36° to 46°F).

ANIMAL PHARMACOLOGY AND ANIMAL TOXICOLOGY
Corneal wound healing studies in rabbits showed that Trifluridine did not significantly retard closure of epithelial wounds. However, mild toxic changes such as intracellular edema of the basal cell layer, mild thinning of the overlying epithelium and reduced strength of stromal wounds were observed.

Whereas instillation of Trifluridine into rabbit eyes during a subchronic toxicity study produced some degree of corneal epithelial thinning, a 12-month chronic toxicity study in rabbits in which Trifluridine was instilled into eyes in intermittent, multiple, full-therapy courses showed no drug-related changes in the cornea.

REFERENCES
1. Itoi M, Getter JW, Kaneko N, et al: Teratogenicities of ophthalmic drugs. I. Antiviral ophthalmic drugs. *Arch Ophthalmol* 1975;93:46-51. 2. Kury G, Crosby RJ: The teratogenic effect of 5-trifluoromethyl-2'-deoxyuridine in chicken embryos. *Toxicol Appl Pharmacol* 1967;11:72-80. 3. Ansfield FJ, Ramirez G: Phase I and II studies of 2'-deoxy-5-(trifluoromethyl)-uridine (NSC-75520). *Cancer Chemother Rep* 1971; 55(pt 1):205-208.

HOW SUPPLIED
DROP: 1%

BRAND/MANUFACTURER	NDC	SIZE	AWP
○ **BRAND**			
VIROPTIC: Burr Wellcome	00081-0968-02	7.5 ml	$46.43

TriHemic 600 *SEE* FERROUS FUMARATE/FOLIC ACID/MINERALS/VITAMINS, MULTI

Trihexyphenidyl Hydrochloride

DESCRIPTION
Trihexyphenidyl Hydrochloride is a synthetic antispasmodic drug available in the following forms:

TABLETS: Containing 2 mg and 5 mg Trihexyphenidyl HCl.
ELIXIR: Containing 2 mg/5 mL Trihexyphenidyl HCl.
SUSTAINED RELEASE SOFT SHELL CAPSULES: Containing 5 mg Trihexyphenidyl HCl as Sustained Release soft shell capsules.

Following is its chemical structure:

ACTIONS
Trihexyphenidyl Hydrochloride is the substituted piperidine salt, 3-(1-piperidyl)-1-phenyl-cyclohexyl-1-propanol Hydrochloride, which exerts a direct inhibitory effect upon the parasympathetic nervous system. It also has a relaxing effect on smooth musculature; exerted both directly upon the muscle tissue itself and indirectly through an inhibitory effect upon the parasympathetic nervous system. Its therapeutic properties are similar to those of atropine, although undesirable side effects are ordinarily less frequent and severe than with the latter.

INDICATIONS
This drug is indicated as an adjunct in the treatment of all forms of parkinsonism (postencephalitic, arteriosclerotic, and idiopathic). It is often useful as adjuvant therapy when treating these forms of parkinsonism with levodopa. Additionally, it

is indicated for the control of extrapyramidal disorders caused by central nervous system drugs such as the dibenzoxazepines, phenothiazines, thioxanthenes, and butyrophenones.

Sustained Release soft shell capsule—For maintenance therapy after patients have been stabilized on Trihexyphenidyl Hydrochloride in conventional dosage forms (tablets or elixir).

UNLABELED USES
Trihexyphenidyl HCl is used alone or as an adjunct in the treatment of Dystonias.

WARNING
Patients to be treated with Trihexyphenidyl HCl should have a gonioscope evaluation and close monitoring of intraocular pressures at regular periodic intervals.

PRECAUTIONS
Although Trihexyphenidyl HCl is not contraindicated for patients with cardiac, liver, or kidney disorders, or with hypertension, such patients should be maintained under close observation.

Since the use of Trihexyphenidyl HCl may in some cases continue indefinitely and since it has atropine-like properties, patients should be subjected to constant and careful long-term observation to avoid allergic and other untoward reactions. In as much as Trihexyphenidyl HCl possesses some parasympatholytic activity, it should be used with caution in patients with glaucoma, obstructive disease of the gastrointestinal or genitourinary tracts, and in elderly males with possible prostatic hypertrophy. Geriatric patients, particularly over the age of 60, frequently develop increased sensitivity to the actions of drugs of this type, and hence, require strict dosage regulation. Incipient glaucoma may be precipitated by parasympatholytic drugs such as Trihexyphenidyl HCl.

Tardive dyskinesia may appear in some patients on long-term therapy with antipsychotic drugs or may occur after therapy with these drugs has been discontinued. Antiparkinsonism agents do not alleviate the symptoms of tardive dyskinesia, and in some instances may aggravate them. However, parkinsonism and tardive dyskinesia often coexist in patients receiving chronic neuroleptic treatment, and anticholinergic therapy with Trihexyphenidyl HCl may relieve some of these parkinsonism symptoms.

ADVERSE REACTIONS
Minor side effects, such as dryness of the mouth, blurring of vision, dizziness, mild nausea or nervousness, will be experienced by 30 to 50 percent of all patients. These sensations, however, are much less troublesome with Trihexyphenidyl HCl than with belladonna alkaloids and are usually less disturbing than unalleviated parkinsonism. Such reactions tend to become less pronounced, and even to disappear, as treatment continues. Even before these reactions have remitted spontaneously, they may often be controlled by careful adjustment of dosage form, amount of drug, or interval between doses.

Isolated instances of suppurative parotitis secondary to excessive dryness of the mouth, skin rashes, dilatation of the colon, paralytic ileus, and certain psychiatric manifestations such as delusions and hallucinations, plus one doubtful case of paranoia all of which may occur with any of the atropine-like drugs, have been reported rarely with Trihexyphenidyl HCl.

Patients with arteriosclerosis or with a history of idiosyncrasy to other drugs may exhibit reactions of mental confusion, agitation, disturbed behavior, or nausea and vomiting. Such patients should be allowed to develop a tolerance through the initial administration of a small dose and gradual increase in dose until an effective level is reached. If a severe reaction should occur, administration of the drug should be discontinued for a few days and then resumed at a lower dosage. Psychiatric disturbances can result from indiscriminate use (leading to overdosage) to sustain continued euphoria.

Potential side effects associated with the use of any atropine-like drugs include constipation, drowsiness, urinary hesitancy or retention, tachycardia, dilation of the pupil, increased intraocular tension, weakness, vomiting, and headache.

The occurrence of angle-closure glaucoma due to long-term treatment with Trihexyphenidyl Hydrochloride has been reported.

DOSAGE AND ADMINISTRATION
Dosage should be individualized. The initial dose should be low and then increased gradually, especially in patients over 60 years of age. Whether Trihexyphenidyl HCl may best be given before or after meals should be determined by the way the patient reacts. Postencephalitic patients, who are usually more prone to excessive salivation, may prefer to take it after meals and may, in addition, require small amounts of atropine which, under such circumstances, is sometimes an effective adjuvant. If Trihexyphenidyl HCl tends to dry the mouth excessively, it may be better to take it before meals, unless it causes nausea. If taken after meals, the thirst sometimes induced can be allayed by mint candies, chewing gum or water.

Trihexyphenidyl HCl in Idiopathic Parkinsonism: As initial therapy for parkinsonism, 1 mg of Trihexyphenidyl HCl in tablet or elixir form may be administered the first day. The dose may then be increased by 2 mg increments at intervals of 3 to 5 days, until a total of 6 to 10 mg is given daily. The total daily dose will depend upon what is found to be the optimal level. Many patients derive maximum benefit from this daily total of 6 to 10 mg, but some patients, chiefly those in the postencephalitic group, may require a total daily dose of 12 to 15 mg.

Trihexyphenidyl HCl in Drug-Induced Parkinsonism: The size and frequency of dose of Trihexyphenidyl HCl needed to control extrapyramidal reactions to commonly employed tranquilizers, notably the phenothiazines, thioxanthenes, and butyrophenones, must be determined empirically. The total daily dosage

usually ranges between 5 and 15 mg although, in some cases, these reactions have been satisfactorily controlled on as little as 1 mg daily. It may be advisable to commence therapy with a single 1 mg dose. If the extrapyramidal manifestations are not controlled in a few hours, the subsequent doses may be progressively increased until satisfactory control is achieved. Satisfactory control may sometimes be more rapidly achieved by temporarily reducing the dosage of the tranquilizer on instituting Trihexyphenidyl HCl therapy and then adjusting dosage of both drugs until the desired ataractic effect is retained without onset of extrapyramidal reactions.

It is sometimes possible to maintain the patient on a reduced Trihexyphenidyl HCl dosage after the reactions have remained under control for several days. Instances have been reported in which these reactions have remained in remission for long periods after Trihexyphenidyl HCl therapy was discontinued.

Concomitant Use of Trihexyphenidyl HCl with Levodopa: When Trihexyphenidyl HCl is used concomitantly with Levodopa, the usual dose of each may need to be reduced. Careful adjustment is necessary, depending on side effects and degree of symptom control. Trihexyphenidyl HCl dosage of 3 to 6 mg daily, in divided doses, is usually adequate.

Concomitant Use of Trihexyphenidyl HCl with Other Parasympathetic Inhibitors: Trihexyphenidyl HCl may be substituted, in whole or in part, for other parasympathetic inhibitors. The usual technique is partial substitution initially, with progressive reduction in the other medication as the dose of Trihexyphenidyl HCl is increased.

Trihexyphenidyl HCl TABLETS and ELIXIR—The total daily intake of Trihexyphenidyl HCl tablets or elixir is tolerated best if divided into three doses and taken at mealtimes. High doses (> 10 mg daily) may be divided into four parts, with three doses administered at mealtimes and the fourth at bedtime.

Trihexyphenidyl HCl Sustained Release Capsules—Because of the relatively high dosage in each controlled release capsule, this dosage form should not be used for initial therapy. After patients are stabilized on Trihexyphenidyl HCl in conventional dosage forms (tablet or elixir), for convenience of administration they may be switched to the controlled release capsules on a milligram per milligram total daily dose basis, as a single dose after breakfast or in two divided doses 12 hours apart. Most patients will be adequately maintained on the controlled release form, but some may develop an exacerbation of parkinsonism and have to be returned to the conventional form.

Tablets: Store at Controlled Room Temperature 15°-30°C (59°-86°F).

Elixir: Store at Controlled Room Temperature 15°-30°C (59°-86°F). DO NOT FREEZE.

Sustained Release Capsules: Store at Controlled Room Temperature 15°-30° C (59°-86° F).

HOW SUPPLIED
CAPSULE, EXTENDED RELEASE: 5 MG

BRAND/MANUFACTURER	NDC	SIZE	AWP
○ BRAND			
ARTANE: Lederle Labs	00005-4438-32	60s	$25.19

ELIXIR: 2 MG/5 ML

BRAND/MANUFACTURER	NDC	SIZE	AWP
◆ BRAND			
ARTANE: Lederle Labs	00005-4440-65	480 ml	$31.05
◆ GENERICS			
Liquipharm	54198-0107-16	480 ml	$22.50

TABLETS: 2 MG

AVERAGE UNIT PRICE (AVAILABLE SIZES)		GENERIC A-RATED AVERAGE PRICE (GAAP)	
BRAND	$0.16	100s	$13.76
GENERIC	$0.13	1000s	$96.31
HCFA FUL (100s ea)	$0.14		

BRAND/MANUFACTURER	NDC	SIZE	AWP
◆ BRAND			
ARTANE: Lederle Labs	00005-4434-23	100s	$15.45
	00005-4434-60	100s ud	$20.26
	00005-4434-34	1000s	$114.26
◆ GENERICS			
Aligen	00405-5061-01	100s	$12.36
Moore,H.L.	00839-1699-06	100s	$12.81
TRIHEXANE: Rugby	00536-4723-01	100s	$12.85
Schein	00364-0408-01	100s	$13.10
Goldline	00182-0627-01	100s	$14.00
Major	00904-2041-60	100s	$14.25
U.S. Trading	56126-0317-11	100s ud	$6.56
Raway	00686-0115-20	100s ud	$9.50
Vangard	00615-0675-13	100s ud	$14.53
Major	00904-2041-61	100s ud	$15.95
Schein	00364-0408-90	100s ud	$17.61
Medirex	57480-0368-01	100s ud	$17.65
UDL	51079-0115-20	100s ud	$17.68
Schein	00364-0408-02	1000s	$85.25
Moore,H.L.	00839-1699-16	1000s	$94.84
TRIHEXANE: Rugby	00536-4723-10	1000s	$94.85
Major	00904-2041-80	1000s	$101.60
Goldline	00182-0627-10	1000s	$105.00

◆ RATED THERAPEUTICALLY EQUIVALENT; ◇ THERAPEUTIC EQUIVALENCE UNCONFIRMED; ○ UNRATED

TABLETS: 5 MG

AVERAGE UNIT PRICE (AVAILABLE SIZES)		GENERIC A-RATED AVERAGE PRICE (GAAP)	
BRAND	$0.33	100s	$23.64
GENERIC	$0.23	1000s	$225.07
HCFA FUL (100s ea)	$0.22		

BRAND/MANUFACTURER	NDC	SIZE	AWP
◆ **BRAND**			
ARTANE: Lederle Labs	00005-4436-23	100s	$30.70
	00005-4436-60	100s ud	$35.43
◆ **GENERICS**			
Raway	00686-0124-20	100s	$8.00
Schein	00364-0409-01	100s	$25.40
TRIHEXANE: Rugby	00536-4724-01	100s	$25.50
Major	00904-2050-60	100s	$25.50
Goldline	00182-0628-01	100s	$27.00
Aligen	00405-5062-01	100s	$27.07
Moore,H.L.	00839-1698-06	100s	$29.28
U.S. Trading	56126-0318-11	100s ud	$6.54
Major	00904-2050-61	100s ud	$27.87
Schein	00364-0409-90	100s ud	$28.46
UDL	51079-0124-20	100s ud	$29.40
Schein	00364-0409-02	1000s	$209.70
Major	00904-2050-80	1000s	$230.50
Goldline	00182-0628-10	1000s	$235.00

Trilafon SEE PERPHENAZINE

Trilisate SEE CHOLINE MAGNESIUM TRISALICYLATE

Trimeprazine Tartrate

DESCRIPTION
Trimeprazine Tartrate, a phenothiazine derivative, is 10[3-(dimethylamino)-2-methylpropyl]-phenothiazine tartrate.

Trimeprazine Tartrate is a white to off-white odorless crystalline powder readily soluble in water.

Tablets: contain 2.5 mg of Trimeprazine.

Syrup: Each 5 mL (one teaspoonful) contains Trimeprazine Tartrate equivalent to 2.5 mg of Trimeprazine.

Extended-release capsules: Each extended-release capsule is so prepared that an initial dose is released promptly and the remaining medication is released gradually over a prolonged period. Each capsule contains Trimeprazine Tartrate equivalent to 5 mg of Trimeprazine.

Following is its chemical structure:

ACTIONS
Trimeprazine Tartrate, a phenothiazine, possesses antipruritic and antihistaminic properties with anticholinergic (drying) and sedative side effects.

INDICATIONS
Treatment of pruritic symptoms in urticaria. Relief of pruritic symptoms in a variety of allergic and non-allergic conditions including atopic dermatitis, neurodermatitis, contact dermatitis, pityriasis rosea, poison ivy dermatitis, eczematous dermatitis, pruritus ani and vulvae, and drug rash.

CONTRAINDICATIONS
Trimeprazine Tartrate is contraindicated: in comatose patients; in patients who have received large amounts of central nervous system depressants (alcohol, barbiturates, narcotics, etc.); in patients with bone marrow depression; in patients who have demonstrated an idiosyncrasy or hypersensitivity to Trimeprazine Tartrate or other phenothiazines: in newborn or premature children; and in nursing mothers. It should not be used in children who are acutely ill and/or dehydrated, as there is an increased susceptibility to dystonias in such patients.

WARNINGS
Trimeprazine Tartrate may impair the mental and/or physical ability required for the performance of potentially hazardous tasks, such as driving a vehicle or operating machinery. Similarly, it may impair mental alertness in children. The concomitant use of alcohol or other central nervous system depressants may have an additive effect. Patients should be warned accordingly.

Trimeprazine Tartrate should be used with extreme caution in patients with:
Asthmatic attack
Narrow-angle glaucoma
Prostatic hypertrophy
Stenosing peptic ulcer
Pyloroduodenal obstruction
Bladder neck obstruction
Patients receiving monoamine oxidase inhibitors

Usage in Pregnancy: The safe use of Trimeprazine Tartrate has not been established with respect to the possible adverse effects upon fetal development. Therefore, it should not be used in women of childbearing potential. Jaundice and prolonged extrapyramidal symptoms have been reported in infants whose mothers received phenothiazines during pregnancy.

Usage in Children: Trimeprazine Tartrate should be used with caution in children who have a history of sleep apnea or a family history of sudden infant death syndrome (SIDS). It should also be used with caution in young children, in whom it may cause excitation.

Overdosage may produce hallucinations, convulsions and sudden death.

Usage in Elderly Patients (60 years or older): Elderly patients are more prone to develop the following side effects from phenothiazines:
Hypotension
Syncope
Toxic confusional states
Extrapyramidal symptoms, especially parkinsonism
Excessive sedation

PRECAUTIONS
Trimeprazine Tartrate may significantly affect the actions of other drugs. It may increase, prolong or intensify the sedative action of central nervous system depressants such as anesthetics, barbiturates or alcohol. When Trimeprazine Tartrate is administered concomitantly the dose of a narcotic or barbiturate should be reduced to ¼ or ½ the usual amount. In the patient with pain, receiving treatment with narcotics, excessive amounts of Trimeprazine Tartrate may lead to restlessness and motor hyperactivity. Trimeprazine Tartrate can block and even reverse the usual pressor effect of epinephrine.

Trimeprazine Tartrate should be used cautiously in persons with acute or chronic respiratory impairment, particularly children, as it may suppress the cough reflex.

This drug should be used cautiously in persons with cardiovascular disease, impairment of liver function, or those with a history of ulcer disease.

Since Trimeprazine Tartrate has a slight antiemetic action, it may obscure signs of intestinal obstruction, brain tumor, or overdosage of toxic drugs.

Phenothiazines have been shown to elevate prolactin levels; the elevation persists during chronic administration. Tissue culture experiments indicate that approximately one-third of human breast cancers are prolactin-dependent *in vitro*, a factor of potential importance if the prescribing of these drugs is contemplated in a patient with a previously detected breast cancer. Although disturbances such as galactorrhea, amenorrhea, gynecomastia, and impotence have been reported, the clinical significance of elevated serum prolactin levels is unknown for most patients. An increase in mammary neoplasms has been found in rodents after chronic administration of neuroleptic drugs. Neither clinical nor epidemiologic studies conducted to date, however, have shown an association between chronic administration of these drugs and mammary tumorigenesis; the available evidence is considered too limited to be conclusive at this time. Drugs which lower the seizure threshold, including phenothiazine derivatives, should not be used with Metrizamide. As with other phenothiazine derivatives, Trimeprazine Tartrate should be discontinued at least 48 hours before myelography, should not be resumed for at least 24 hours postprocedure, and should not be used for the control of nausea and vomiting occurring either prior to myelography or postprocedure.

ADVERSE REACTIONS
Trimeprazine Tartrate may produce adverse reactions attributable to both phenothiazines and antihistamines.

Note: Not all of the following adverse reactions have been reported with Trimeprazine Tartrate; however, pharmacological similarities among the phenothiazine derivatives require that each be considered when Trimeprazine Tartrate is administered. There have been occasional reports of sudden death in patients receiving phenothiazine derivatives chronically.

C.N.S. Effects: Drowsiness is the most common C.N.S. effect of this drug. Extrapyramidal reactions (opisthotonos, dystonia, akathisia, dyskinesia, parkinsonism) occur, particularly with high doses. (See *"Overdosage"* section for management of extrapyramidal symptoms.) Hyperreflexia has been reported in the newborn when a phenothiazine was used during pregnancy. Other reported reactions include dizziness, headache, lassitude, tinnitus, incoordination, fatigue, blurred vision, euphoria, diplopia, nervousness, insomnia, tremors and grand mal seizures, excitation, catatonic-like states, neuritis and hysteria, oculogyric crises, disturbing dreams/nightmares, pseudoschizophrenia, and intensification and prolongation of the action of C.N.S. depressants (opiates, analgesics, antihistamines, barbiturates, alcohol), atropine, heat, organophosphorus insecticides.

Cardiovascular Effects: Postural hypotension is the most common cardiovascular effect of phenothiazines. Reflex tachycardia may be seen. Bradycardia, faintness, dizziness and cardiac arrest have been reported. ECG changes, including blunting of T waves and prolongation of the Q-T interval, may be seen.

Gastrointestinal: Anorexia, nausea, vomiting, epigastric distress, diarrhea, constipation, and dry mouth may occur. Increased appetite and weight gain have also been reported.

Genitourinary: Urinary frequency and dysuria, urinary retention, early menses, induced lactation, gynecomastia, decreased libido, inhibition of ejaculation and false positive pregnancy tests have been reported.

Respiratory: Thickening of bronchial secretions, tightness of the chest, wheezing and nasal stuffiness may occur.

Allergic Reactions: These include urticaria, dermatitis, asthma, laryngeal edema, angioneurotic edema, photosensitivity, lupus erythematosus-like syndrome and anaphylactoid reactions.

Other Reported Reactions: Leukopenia, agranulocytosis, pancytopenia, hemolytic anemia, elevation of plasma cholesterol levels and thrombocytopenic purpura have been reported. Jaundice of the obstructive type has also been reported; it is usually reversible but chronic jaundice has been reported. Erythema, peripheral edema, and stomatitis have been reported. High or prolonged glucose tolerance curves, glycosuria, elevated spinal fluid proteins and reversed epinephrine effects may also occur.

Rare occurrences of neuroleptic malignant syndrome (NMS) have been reported in patients receiving phenothiazines. This syndrome is comprised of the symptom complex of hyperthermia, altered consciousness, muscular rigidity and autonomic dysfunction and is potentially fatal.

Long-Term Therapy Considerations: After prolonged phenothiazine administration at high dosage, pigmentation of the skin has occurred, chiefly in the exposed areas. Ocular changes consist of the appearance of lenticular and corneal opacities, epithelial keratopathies and pigmentary retinopathy. Vision may be impaired.

DOSAGE AND ADMINISTRATION
TABLETS AND SYRUP
Adults: Usual dosage is 2.5 mg q.i.d.

Children over three years: Usual dosage is 2.5 mg h.s., or t.i.d. if needed.

Children 6 months to 3 years: Usual dosage is 1.25 mg (½ teaspoonful of syrup) h.s., or t.i.d. if needed.

EXTENDED RELEASE CAPSULES
Adults: Usual daily dosage is 1 capsule q12h.

Children over 6 years of age: 1 capsule daily.
This product form is not recommended for children under 6 years of age. Use tablets or syrup for their dosage flexibility. Because some side effects appear to be dose-related, it is important to use the lowest effective dosage.

DRUG INTERACTIONS
MAO inhibitors and thiazide diuretics prolong and intensify the anticholinergic effects of Trimeprazine Tartrate. Combined use of MAO inhibitors and phenothiazines may result in hypertension and extrapyramidal reactions.

Narcotics: The C.N.S. depressant and analgesic effects of narcotics are potentiated by phenothiazines.
The following drugs may result in potentiation of phenothiazine effects:
Oral contraceptives
Progesterone
Reserpine
Nylidrin hydrochloride

MANAGEMENT OF OVERDOSAGE
Signs and symptoms of Trimeprazine Tartrate overdosage range from mild depression of the central nervous system and cardiovascular system to profound hypotension, respiratory depression and unconsciousness. Stimulation may be evident, especially in children and geriatric patients. Atropine-like signs and symptoms—dry mouth, fixed, dilated pupils, flushing, etc.—as well as gastrointestinal symptoms may occur. The treatment of overdosage is essentially symptomatic and supportive. Early gastric lavage may be beneficial. **Do not administer emetics or attempt to induce vomiting because a dystonic reaction of the head or neck might result in aspiration of vomitus.** Extrapyramidal symptoms may be treated with anti-parkinsonism drugs, barbiturates, or Diphenhydramine Hydrochloride.

Avoid analeptics, which may cause convulsions. Severe hypotension usually responds to the administration of Levarterenol or Phenylephrine. *Epinephrine should not be used*, since its use in a patient with partial adrenergic blockade may further lower the blood pressure. Additional measures include oxygen and intravenous fluids. Limited experience with dialysis indicates that it is not helpful.

Special note on extended release capsules: Since much of the extended release capsule medication is coated for gradual release, therapy directed at reversing the effects of the ingested drug and at supporting the patient should be continued for as long as overdosage symptoms remain. Saline cathartics are useful for hastening evacuation of pellets that have not already released medication.

Federal (U.S.A.) law prohibits dispensing without prescription.

HOW SUPPLIED
CAPSULE, EXTENDED RELEASE: 5 MG

BRAND/MANUFACTURER	NDC	SIZE	AWP
○ BRAND			
TEMARIL: Allergan Herbert	00023-4750-05	50s	$60.76

SYRUP: 2.5 MG/5 ML

BRAND/MANUFACTURER	NDC	SIZE	AWP
◆ BRAND			
TEMARIL: Allergan Herbert	00023-4754-04	120 ml	$20.40

TABLETS: 2.5 MG

BRAND/MANUFACTURER	NDC	SIZE	AWP
○ BRAND			
TEMARIL: Allergan Herbert	00023-4741-10	100s	$62.66
	00023-4741-11	100s ud	$68.90

Trimethadione

BECAUSE OF ITS POTENTIAL TO PRODUCE FETAL MALFORMATIONS AND SERIOUS SIDE EFFECTS, TRIMETHADIONE SHOULD ONLY BE UTILIZED WHEN OTHER LESS TOXIC DRUGS HAVE BEEN FOUND INEFFECTIVE IN CONTROLLING PETIT MAL SEIZURES.

DESCRIPTION
Trimethadione is an antiepileptic agent. An oxazolidinedione compound, it is chemically identified as 3,5,5-trimethyloxozolidine-2,4-dione.
Trimethadione is a synthetic, water-soluble, white, crystalline powder. It is supplied in capsular, tablet, and liquid forms for oral use only.
Trimethadione is available as a 300 mg capsule, 150 mg tablet, 40 mg/1ml solution for oral administration.

Following is its chemical structure:

CLINICAL PHARMACOLOGY
Trimethadione has been shown to prevent pentylenetetrazol-induced and thujone-induced seizures in experimental animals; the drug has a less marked effect on seizures induced by picrotoxin, procaine, cocaine, or strychnine. Unlike the hydantoins and antiepileptic barbiturates, Trimethadione does not modify the maximal seizure pattern in patients undergoing electroconvulsive therapy.

Trimethadione has a sedative effect that may increase to the point of ataxia when excessive doses are used. A toxic dose of the drug in animals (approximately 2 g/kg) produced sleep, unconsciousness, and respiratory depression.

Trimethadione is rapidly absorbed from the gastrointestinal tract. It is demethylated by liver microsomes to the active metabolite dimethadione.

Approximately 3% of a daily dose of Trimethadione is recovered in the urine as unchanged drug. The majority of Trimethadione is excreted slowly by the kidney in the form of dimethadione.

INDICATIONS
Trimethadione is indicated for the control of petit mal seizures that are refractory to treatment with other drugs.

CONTRANDICATIONS
Trimethadione is contraindicated in patients with a known hypersensitivity to the drug.

WARNINGS
Trimethadione may cause serious side effects. Strict medical supervision of the patient is mandatory, especially during the initial year of therapy.

Trimethadione should be withdrawn promptly if skin rash appears, because of the grave possibility of the occurrence of exfoliative dermatitis or severe forms of erythema multiforme. Even a minor acneiform or morbilliform rash should be allowed to clear completely before treatment with Trimethadione is resumed: reinstitute therapy cautiously. A complete blood count should be done prior to intiating therapy with Trimethadione and at monthly intervals thereafter. A marked depression of the blood count is an indication for withdrawal of the drug. If no abnormality appears within 12 months, the interval between blood counts may be extended. A moderate degree of neutropenia with or without a corresponding drop in the leukocyte count is not uncommon. Therapy need not be withdrawn unless the neutrophil count is 2500 or less; more frequent blood examinations should be done when the count is less than 3,000. Other blood dyscrasias, including leukopenia, eosinophilia, thrombocytopenia, pancytopenia, agranulocytosis, hypoplastic anemia, and fatal aplastic anemia, have occurred. Patients should be advised to report immediately such signs and symptoms as sore throat, fever, malaise, easy bruising, petechiae, or epistaxis or others that may be indicative of an infection or bleeding tendency. Trimethadione should ordinarily not be used in patients with severe blood dycrasias.

Liver function tests should be done prior to initiating therapy with Trimethadione and at monthly intervals thereafter. Hepatitis has been reported rarely. Jaundice or other signs of liver dysfunction are an indication for withdrawal of the drug. Trimethadione should ordinarily not be used in patients with severe hepatic impairment.

◆ RATED THERAPEUTICALLY EQUIVALENT; ◇ THERAPEUTIC EQUIVALENCE UNCONFIRMED; ○ UNRATED

A urinalysis should be done prior to initiating therapy with Trimethadione and at monthly intervals thereafter. Fatal nephrosis has been reported. Persistent or increasing albuminuria, or the development of any other significant renal abnormality is an indication for withdrawal of the drug. Trimethadione should ordinarily not be used in patients with severe renal dysfunction.

Hemeralopia has occurred; this appears to be an effect of Trimethadione on the neural layers of the retina, and usually can be reversed by a reduction in dosage. Scotomata are an indication for withdrawal of the drug. Caution should be observed when treating patients who have diseases of the retina or optic nerve.

Manifestations of systemic lupus erythematosus have been associated with the use of Trimethadione, as they have with the use of certain other anticonvulsants. Lymphadenopathies simulating malignant lymphoma have occurred. Lupus-like manifestations or lymph node enlargement are indications for withdrawal of the drug. Signs and symptoms may disappear after discontinuation of therapy, and specific treatment may be unnecessary.

A myasthenia gravis-like syndrome has been associated with the chronic use of Trimethadione. Symptoms suggestive of this condition are indications for withdrawal of the drug. Drugs known to cause toxic effects similar to those of Trimethadione should be avoided or used only with extreme caution during therapy with Trimethadione.

Usage During Pregnancy and Lactation:

THERE ARE MULTIPLE REPORTS IN THE CLINICAL LITERATURE WHICH INDICATE THAT THE USE OF ANTICONVULSANT DRUGS DURING PREGNANCY RESULTS IN AN INCREASED INCIDENCE OF BIRTH DEFECTS IN THE OFFSPRING. DATA ARE MORE EXTENSIVE WITH RESPECT TO TRIMETHADIONE, PARAMETHADIONE, PHENYTOIN AND PHENOBARBITAL THAN WITH OTHER ANTICONVULSANT DRUGS.

THEREFORE, ANTICONVULSANT DRUGS SUCH AS TRIMETHADIONE SHOULD BE ADMINISTERED TO WOMEN OF CHILDBEARING POTENTIAL ONLY IF THEY ARE CLEARLY SHOWN TO BE ESSENTIAL IN THE MANAGEMENT OF THEIR SEIZURES. EFFECTIVE MEANS OF CONTRACEPTION SHOULD ACCOMPANY THE USE OF TRIMETHADIONE IN SUCH PATIENTS. IF A PATIENT BECOMES PREGNANT WHILE TAKING TRIMETHADIONE, TERMINATION OF THE PREGNANCY SHOULD BE CONSIDERED. A PATIENT WHO REQUIRES THERAPY WITH TRIMETHADIONE AND WHO WISHES TO BECOME PREGNANT SHOULD BE ADVISED OF THE RISKS.

REPORTS HAVE SUGGESTED THAT THE MATERNAL INGESTION OF ANTICONVULSANT DRUGS, PARTICULARLY BARBITURATES, IS ASSOCIATED WITH A NEONATAL COAGULATION DEFECT THAT MAY CAUSE BLEEDING DURING THE EARLY (USUALLY WITHIN 24 HOURS OF BIRTH) NEONATAL PERIOD. THE POSSIBILTY OF THE OCCURRENCE OF THIS DEFECT WITH THE USE OF TRIMETHADIONE SHOULD BE KEPT IN MIND. THE DEFECT IS CHARACTERIZED BY DECREASED LEVELS OF VITAMIN K-DEPENDENT CLOTTING FACTORS, AND PROLONGATION OF EITHER THE PROTHROMBIN TIME OR THE PARTIAL THROMBOPLASTIN TIME, OR BOTH. IT HAS BEEN SUGGESTED THAT PROPHYLACTIC VITAMIN K BE GIVEN TO THE MOTHER ONE MONTH PRIOR TO, AND DURING DELIVERY, AND TO THE INFANT, INTRAVENOUSLY, IMMEDIATELY AFTER BIRTH.

THE SAFETY OF TRIMETHADIONE FOR USE DURING LACTATION HAS NOT BEEN ESTABLISHED.

PRECAUTIONS

Abrupt discontinuation of Trimethadione may precipitate petit mal status. Trimethadione should always be withdrawn gradually unless serious adverse effects dictate otherwise. In the latter case, another anticonvulsant may be substituted to protect the patient.

Usage during Pregnancy and Lactation: See *"Warnings".*

ADVERSE REACTIONS

The following side effects, some of them serious, have been associated with the use of Trimethadione.

Gastrointestinal: nausea, vomiting, abdominal pain, gastric distress.

CNS/Neurologic: drowsiness, fatigue, malaise, insomnia, vertigo, headache, paresthesias, precipitation of grand mal seizures, increased irritability, personality changes.

Drowsiness usually subsides with continued therapy. If it persists, a reduction in dosage is indicated.

Hematologic: bleeding gums, epistaxis, retinal and petechial hemorrhages, vaginal bleeding, neutropenia, leukopenia, eosinophilia, thrombocytopenia, pancytopenia, agranulocytosis, hypoplastic anemia, and fatal aplastic anemia.

Dermatologic: acneiform or morbilliform skin rash that may progress to exfoliative dermatitis or to severe forms of erythema multiforme.

Other: hiccups, anorexia, weight loss, hair loss, changes in blood pressure, albuminuria, hemeralopia, photophobia, diplopia.

Fatal nephrosis has occurred.

Hepatitis has been reported rarely.

Lupus erythematosus and lymphadenopathies simulating malignant lymphoma have been reported.

Pruritus associated with lymphadenopathy and hepatosplenomegaly has occurred in hypersensitive individuals.

A myasthenia gravis-like syndrome has been reported.

OVERDOSAGE

Symptoms of acute Trimethadione overdosage include drowsiness, nausea, dizziness, ataxia, visual disturbances. Coma may follow massive overdosage.

Gastric evacuation, either by induced emesis, or by lavage, or both, should be done immediately. General supportive care, including frequent monitoring of the vital signs and close observation of the patient, are required.

Alkalinization of the urine has been reported to enhance the renal excretion of dimethadione, the active metabolite of Trimethadione.

A blood count and a careful evaluation of hepatic and renal function should be done following recovery.

DOSAGE AND ADMINISTRATION

Trimethadione is administered orally.

Usual Adult Dosage: 0.9-2.4 g daily in 3 or 4 equally divided doses (i.e., 300-600 mg 3 or 4 times daily).

Initially, give 0.9 g daily; increase this dose by 300 mg at weekly intervals until therapeutic results are seen or until toxic symptoms appear.

Maintenance dosage should be the least amount of drug required to maintain control.

Children's Dosage: Usually 0.3-0.9 g daily in 3 or 4 equally divided doses.

Recommended storage: Store tablets in refrigerator (2°-8°C) to minimize crystallization. However some crystallization not harmful to product may occur. Keep tightly closed.

Trimethadione oral solution, USP, 1.2 g per fluid ounce (40 mg per mL), is supplied in pint bottles.

Recommended storage: Store solution below 86°F (30°C).

HOW SUPPLIED

CAPSULE: 300 MG

BRAND/MANUFACTURER	NDC	SIZE	AWP
BRAND			
TRIDIONE: Abbott Pharm	00074-3709-01	100s	$41.09

CHEW TABLET: 150 MG

BRAND/MANUFACTURER	NDC	SIZE	AWP
BRAND			
TRIDIONE: Abbott Pharm	00074-3753-01	100s	$36.24

Trimethaphan Camsylate

DESCRIPTION

Trimethaphan Camsylate Injection, a vasodepressor agent, is available as a sterile solution to be used only for intravenous infusion. Each 10-mL ampul contains 500 mg Trimethaphan Camsylate.

Trimethaphan Camsylate is a sulfonium derivative. The chemical name is (+)-1,3-dibenzyldecahydro-2-oxoimidazo[4,5-c]thieno[1,2-α]-thiolium 2-oxo-10-bornanesulfonate (1:1). It occurs as white crystals or a white, crystalline powder which is freely soluble in water and alcohol. It has a molecular weight of 596.80.

Following is its chemical structure:

CLINICAL PHARMACOLOGY

Trimethaphan Camsylate is primarily a ganglionic blocking agent. It blocks transmission in autonomic ganglia without producing any preceding or concomitant change in the membrane potentials of the ganglion cells. It does not modify the conduction of impulses in the preganglionic or postganglionic neurons and does not prevent the release of acetylcholine by preganglionic impulses. Trimethaphan Camsylate produces ganglionic blockade by occupying receptor sites on the ganglion cells and by stabilizing the postsynaptic membranes against the action of acetylcholine liberated from the presynaptic nerve endings.

In addition to ganglionic blocking, Trimethaphan Camsylate may also exert a direct peripheral vasodilator effect. By inducing vasodilation, it causes pooling of blood in the dependent periphery and the splanchnic system. The vasodilation results in a lowering of the blood pressure. Trimethaphan Camsylate liberates histamine.

Trimethaphan crosses the placenta. Other pharmacokinetic data are unavailable because there is no acceptable assay procedure for the determination of Trimethaphan in biological specimens.

INDICATIONS AND USAGE

Trimethaphan Camsylate is indicated for the production of controlled hypotension during surgery; for the short term (acute) control of blood pressure in hypertensive emergencies; and in the emergency treatment of pulmonary edema in patients with pulmonary hypertension associated with systemic hypertension.

CONTRAINDICATIONS

Trimethaphan Camsylate is contraindicated in those conditions where hypotension may subject the patient to undue risk, *e.g.*, uncorrected anemia, hypovolemia, shock (both incipient and frank), asphyxia or uncorrected respiratory insufficiency. Inadequate availability of fluids and inability to replace blood for technical reasons may also constitute contraindications.

WARNINGS

Trimethaphan Camsylate is a powerful hypotensive drug and should always be diluted before use.

It is recommended that the use of Trimethaphan Camsylate to produce hypotension in surgical or medical indications be limited to physicians with proper training in this technique. Adequate facilities, equipment and personnel should be available for vigilant monitoring of the circulation since Trimethaphan Camsylate is an extremely potent hypotensive agent. Adequate oxygenation must be assured throughout the treatment period, especially in regard to coronary and cerebral circulation.

Trimethaphan Camsylate should be used extreme caution in patients with arteriosclerosis, cardiac disease, hepatic or renal disease, degenerative disease of the central nervous system, Addison's disease or diabetes, and in patients who are under treatment with steroids.

Usage in Pregnancy: Trimethaphan Camsylate can cause fetal harm when administered to a pregnant woman. Trimethaphan Camsylate crosses the placenta, decreasing fetal gastrointestinal motility and resulting in meconium ileus. In addition, Trimethaphan Camsylate-induced hypotension may have other serious adverse effects on the fetus. If Trimethaphan Camsylate is used during pregnancy, or if the patient becomes pregnant while taking Trimethaphan Camsylate, the patient should be apprised of the potential hazard to the fetus.

PRECAUTIONS

General: Trimethaphan Camsylate should be used with extreme caution in the elderly or debilitated. Because Trimethaphan Camsylate liberates histamine, it should be used with caution in patients with a history of allergies.

Respiratory depression and arrest have occurred during Trimethaphan Camsylate administration, although a causal relationship has not been firmly established. The patient's respiratory status must be monitored closely, particularly if large doses of Trimethaphan Camsylate are used.

Occasionally, patients may fail to show an adequate hypotensive response to Trimethaphan Camsylate administration. When this is observed, administration should be discontinued and other methods to control hypertension instituted. Tachyphylaxis has also been reported.

Note: Because Trimethaphan Camsylate causes mydriasis, pupillary dilation does not necessarily indicate anoxia or the depth of anesthesia.

Drug Interactions: Trimethaphan Camsylate should be used with care in patients who have been receiving antihypertensive drugs, since an additive hypotensive effect may occur. Trimethaphan Camsylate may also have an additive hypotensive effect when administered with anesthetic agents, especially spinal anesthetics. Procainamide also has an additive hypotensive effect with Trimethaphan Camsylate. Diuretic agents may markedly enhance the responses evoked by ganglionic-blocking drugs. Trimethaphan Camsylate may also prolong the effects of neuromuscular blocking agents such as tubocurarine chloride or succinylcholine chloride, especially when large doses of Trimethaphan Camsylate are administered.

Concomitant therapy with other drugs can considerably modify the dose of Trimethaphan Camsylate necessary to achieve the desired response. In general, the deeper the plane of anesthesia, the smaller the dose of Trimethaphan Camsylate that is required to produce hypotension; conversely, less anesthetic is required after hypotension has been induced by Trimethaphan Camsylate.

Carcinogenesis, Mutagenesis and Impairment of Fertility: Trimethaphan Camsylate has not undergone adequate animal testing to evaluate its carcinogenic potential. The mutagenicity of Trimethaphan Camsylate has not been studied nor has the drug been evaluated for effects on fertility.

Pregnancy: Teratogenic effects—Pregnancy Category D. See *"Warnings"* section.
Nonteratogenic effects—see *"Warnings"* section.

Nursing Mothers: It is not known whether Trimethaphan Camsylate is excreted in human milk. Because of the potential for serious adverse reactions from Trimethaphan Camsylate in nursing infants, mothers who require Trimethaphan Camsylate should be advised not to nurse.

Pediatric Use: Safety and effectiveness in children have not been established.

ADVERSE REACTIONS

The adverse reactions produced by Trimethaphan Camsylate are primarily due to its nonselective blockade of the autonomic nervous system. The following adverse reactions have been observed, but there is not enough systematic collection of data to support an estimate of their frequency.

Cardiovascular: Tachycardia, precipitation of angina, syncope which may occur without warning.

Respiratory: Respiratory depression and arrest have occurred during Trimethaphan Camsylate administration, although a causal relationship has not been firmly established.

Gastrointestinal: Paralytic ileus, dry mouth, constipation, occasional diarrhea, abdominal discomfort, anorexia, heartburn, nausea, vomiting, eructation.

Genitourinary: Urinary hesitancy, decreased potency.

Ophthalmic: Cycloplegia, mydriasis, difficulty in accommodation, conjunctival suffusion.

Miscellaneous: Subjective chilliness, weakness, restlessness, urticaria, itching. Trimethaphan Camsylate prevents surgically-induced elevation of blood glucose and decreases serum potassium slightly.

Generally, side effects are decreased when dosage is reduced or the drug is temporarily discontinued.

OVERDOSAGE

Vasopressor agents may be used to correct excessive hypotension during surgery or to effect a more rapid return to normotensive levels. Phenylephrine HCl or mephentermine sulfate should be tried initially and norepinephrine should be reserved for refractory cases.

The acute intravenous toxicity of Trimethaphan Camsylate is as follows:

Species	LD^{50} mg/kg
mouse	21
rat	21
rabbit	23
dog	0.75
guinea pig	13
monkey	> 8

DOSAGE AND ADMINISTRATION

Trimethaphan Camsylate must always be diluted and administered by intravenous infusion. Solutions should be freshly prepared and any unused portions discarded. For this purpose a 0.1 percent (1 mg/mL) concentration of Trimethaphan Camsylate in 5% Dextrose Injection USP, normal saline solution, or Ringer's Injection USP should be employed. Trimethaphan Camsylate is stable in these diluents for at least 24 hours at room temperature. Use of other diluents is not recommended, since experience with them has not been reported.

Trimethaphan Camsylate is physically incompatible with thiopental, gallamine triethiodide, tubocurarine chloride iodides, bromides and strongly alkaline solutions. Therefore, **the infusion fluid used for administration of Trimethaphan Camsylate should not be employed as a vehicle for the simultaneous administration of any other drugs.**

One (1) ampul of Trimethaphan Camsylate—10 mL, 50 mg/mL—should be diluted to 500 mL. Since individual response varies, the rate of administration must be adjusted to the requirements of each patient.

When Trimethaphan Camsylate is given, the patient should be positioned so as to avoid cerebral anoxia. During surgery, adequate anesthesia should be established. Intravenous drip with Trimethaphan Camsylate is started at an average rate of 3 mL to 4 mL (3 mg to 4 mg) per minute (see chart below). The rate of administration is then adjusted to maintain the desired level of hypotension. Since there is a marked variation of individual response, **frequent blood pressure determinations are essential to maintain proper control.** Rates from as low as 0.3 mL (0.3 mg) per minute to rates exceeding 6 mL (6 mg) per minute have been found necessary, based upon clinical experience.

0.1% (1 MG/ML) CONCENTRATION OF TRIMETHAPHAN CAMSYLATE

Delivery System Drops/mL	Drops/Min to Obtain 3-4 mL (3-4 mg) Trimethaphan Camsylate
10	30-40
15	45-60
60	180-240

During surgery, administration of Trimethaphan Camsylate should be stopped prior to wound closure in order to permit blood pressure to return to normal. A systolic pressure of 100 mm will usually be attained within 10 minutes after stopping Trimethaphan Camsylate.

Parenteral drug products should be inspected visually for particulate matter and discoloration prior to administration, whenever solution and container permit.

Trimethaphan Camsylate is stable under refrigeration (36° to 46°F or 2° to 8°C). Trimethaphan Camsylate should not be frozen as ampul breakage may result from ice formation.

J CODES
Up to 50 mg IV—J0400

HOW SUPPLIED
INJECTION: 500 MG

BRAND/MANUFACTURER	NDC	SIZE	AWP
○ **BRAND**			
ARFONAD: Roche Labs	00004-1900-06	10 ml 10s	$280.36

Trimethobenzamide Hydrochloride

DESCRIPTION
Chemically, Trimethobenzamide Hydrochloride is N-[p-[2-(dimethylamino) -ethoxy] benzyl]-3,4,5-Trimethoxybenzamide Hydrochloride. It has a molecular weight of 424.93.

Capsules: 250 mg and 100 mg Trimethobenzamide Hydrochloride.

Suppositories, 200 mg Trimethobenzamide Hydrochloride.

Suppositories, Pediatric 100 mg Trimethobenzamide Hydrochloride.

Ampuls: Each 2-mL ampul contains 200 mg Trimethobenzamide Hydrochloride.

Multiple Dose Vials: Each mL contains 100 mg Trimethobenzamide Hydrochloride.

Disposable Syringes: Each 2 mL contains 200 mg Trimethobenzamide Hydrochloride.

Following is its chemical structure:

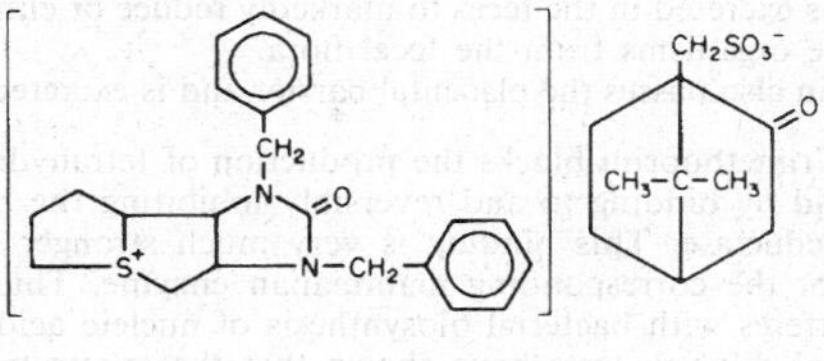

ACTIONS
The mechanism of action of Trimethobenzamide HCl as determined in animals is obscure, but may be the chemoreceptor trigger zone (CTZ), an area in the medulla oblongata through which emetic impulses are conveyed to the vomiting center; direct impulses to the vomiting center apparently are not similarly inhibited. In dogs pretreated with Trimethobenzamide HCl, the emetic response to apomorphine is inhibited, while little or no protection is afforded against emesis induced by intragastric copper sulfate.

INDICATIONS
Trimethobenzamide HCl is indicated for the control of nausea and vomiting.

CONTRAINDICATIONS
The injectable form of Trimethobenzamide HCl in children, the suppositories in premature or newborn infants, and use in patients with known hypersensitivity to Trimethobenzamide HCl are contraindicated. Since some brands of the suppositories contain benzocaine they should not be used in patients known to be sensitive to this or similar local anesthetics.

WARNINGS

CAUTION SHOULD BE EXERCISED WHEN ADMINISTERING TRIMETHOBENZAMIDE HCL TO CHILDREN FOR THE TREATMENT OF VOMITING. ANTIEMETICS ARE NOT RECOMMENDED FOR TREATMENT OF UNCOMPLICATED VOMITING IN CHILDREN AND THEIR USE SHOULD BE LIMITED TO PROLONGED VOMITING OF KNOWN ETIOLOGY. THERE ARE THREE PRINCIPAL REASONS FOR CAUTION:

1. THERE HAS BEEN SOME SUSPICION THAT CENTRALLY ACTING ANTIEMETICS MAY CONTRIBUTE, IN COMBINATION WITH VIRAL ILLNESSES (A POSSIBLE CAUSE OF VOMITING IN CHILDREN), TO DEVELOPMENT OF REYE'S SYNDROME, A POTENTIALLY FATAL ACUTE CHILDHOOD ENCEPHALOPATHY WITH VISCERAL FATTY DEGENERATION, ESPECIALLY INVOLVING THE LIVER. ALTHOUGH THERE IS NO CONFIRMATION OF THIS SUSPICION, CAUTION IS NEVERTHELESS RECOMMENDED.

2. THE EXTRAPYRAMIDAL SYMPTOMS WHICH CAN OCCUR SECONDARY TO TRIMETHOBENZAMIDE HCL MAY BE CONFUSED WITH THE CENTRAL NERVOUS SYSTEM SIGNS OF AN UNDIAGNOSED PRIMARY DISEASE RESPONSIBLE FOR THE VOMITING, E.G., REYE'S SYNDROME OR OTHER ENCEPHALOPATHY.

3. IT HAS BEEN SUSPECTED THAT DRUGS WITH HEPATOTOXIC POTENTIAL, SUCH AS TRIMETHOBENZAMIDE HCL, MAY UNFAVORABLY ALTER THE COURSE OF REYE'S SYNDROME. SUCH DRUGS SHOULD THEREFORE BE AVOIDED IN CHILDREN WHOSE SIGNS AND SYMPTOMS (VOMITING) COULD REPRESENT REYE'S SYNDROME. IT SHOULD ALSO BE NOTED THAT SALICYLATES AND ACETAMINOPHEN ARE HEPATOTOXIC AT LARGE DOSES. ALTHOUGH IT IS NOT KNOWN THAT AT USUAL DOSES THEY WOULD REPRESENT A HAZARD IN PATIENTS WITH THE UNDERLYING HEPATIC DISORDER OF REYE'S SYNDROME, THESE DRUGS, TOO, SHOULD BE AVOIDED IN CHILDREN WHOSE SIGNS AND SYMPTOMS COULD REPRESENT REYE'S SYNDROME, UNLESS ALTERNATIVE METHODS OF CONTROLLING FEVER ARE NOT SUCCESSFUL.

Trimethobenzamide HCl may produce drowsiness. Patients should not operate motor vehicles or other dangerous machinery until their individual responses have been determined. Reye's syndrome has been associated with the use of Trimethobenzamide HCl and other drugs, including antiemetics, although their contribution, if any, to the cause and course of the disease hasn't been established. This syndrome is characterized by an abrupt onset shortly following a nonspecific febrile illness, with persistent, severe vomiting, lethargy, irrational behavior, progressive encephalopathy leading to coma, convulsions and death.

Usage in Pregnancy: Trimethobenzamide Hydrochloride was studied in reproduction experiments in rats and rabbits and no teratogenicity was suggested. The only effects observed were an increased percentage of embryonic resorptions or stillborn pups in rats administered 20 mg and 100 mg/kg and increased resorptions in rabbits receiving 100 mg/kg. In each study these adverse effects were attributed to one or two dams. The relevance to humans is not known. Since there is no adequate experience in pregnant or lactating women who have received this drug, safety in pregnancy or in nursing mothers has not been established.

Usage with Alcohol: Concomitant use of alcohol with Trimethobenzamide HCl may result in an adverse drug interaction.

PRECAUTIONS
During the course of acute febrile illness, encephalitides, gastroenteritis, dehydration and electrolyte imbalance, especially in children and the elderly or debilitated, CNS reactions such as opisthotonos, convulsions, coma and extrapyramidal symptoms have been reported with and without use of Trimethobenzomide HCl or other antiemetic agents. In such disorders caution should be exercised in administering Trimethobenzamide HCl, particularly to patients who have recently received other CNS-acting agents (phenothiazines, barbiturates, belladonna derivatives). It is recommended that severe emesis should not be treated with an antiemetic drug alone; where possible the cause of vomiting should be established. Primary emphasis should be directed toward the restoration of body fluids and electrolyte balance, the relief of fever and relief of the causative disease process. Overhydration should be avoided since it may result in cerebral edema.

The antiemetic effects of Trimethobenzomide HCl may render diagnosis more difficult in such conditions as appendicitis and obscure signs of toxicity due to overdosage of other drugs.

ADVERSE REACTIONS
There have been reports of hypersensitivity reactions and Parkinson-like symptoms. There have been instances of hypotension reported following parenteral administration to surgical patients. There have been reports of blood dyscrasias, blurring of vision, coma, convulsions, depression of mood, diarrhea, disorientation, dizziness, drowsiness, headache, jaundice, muscle cramps and opisthotonos. If these occur, the administration of the drug should be discontinued. Allergic-type skin reactions have been observed; therefore, the drug should be discontinued at the first sign of sensitization. While these symptoms will usually disappear spontaneously, symptomatic treatment may be indicated in some cases.

DOSAGE AND ADMINISTRATION
(See *"Warnings"* and *"Precautions".*)

Dosage should be adjusted according to the indication for therapy, severity of symptoms and the response of the patient.

CAPSULES 250 MG AND 100 MG
Usual Adult Dosage: One 250-mg capsule t.i.d. or q.i.d.

Usual Children's Dosage: 30 to 90 lbs: One or two 100-mg capsules t.i.d. or q.i.d.

SUPPOSITORIES, 200 MG
(Not to be used in premature or newborn infants).

Usual Adult Dosage: One suppository (200 mg) t.i.d. or q.i.d.

Usual Children's Dosage: Under 30 lbs: One-half suppository (100 mg) t.i.d. or q.i.d. 30 to 90 lbs: One-half to one suppository (100 to 200 mg) t.i.d. or q.i.d.

SUPPOSITORIES, PEDIATRIC, 100 MG
(Not to be used in premature or newborn infants).

Usual Children's Dosage: Under 30 lbs: One suppository (100 mg) t.i.d. or q.i.d. 30 to 90 lbs: One to two suppositories (100 to 200 mg) t.i.d. or q.i.d.

INJECTABLE, 100 MG/ML
(Not recommended for use in children).

Usual Adult Dosage: 2 mL (200 mg) t.i.d. or q.i.d. intramuscularly.

Intramuscular administration may cause pain, stinging, burning, redness and swelling at the site of injection. Such effects may be minimized by deep injection into the upper outer quadrant of the gluteal region, and by avoiding the escape of solution along the route.

Note: The injectable form is intended for intramuscular administration only; it is not recommended for intravenous use.

J CODES
Up to 200 mg IM—J3250

HOW SUPPLIED
CAPSULE: 100 MG

BRAND/MANUFACTURER	NDC	SIZE	AWP
○ **BRAND**			
▶ TIGAN: SK Beecham Pharm	00029-4082-30	100s	$39.15

CAPSULE: 250 MG

BRAND/MANUFACTURER	NDC	SIZE	AWP
○ BRAND			
➤ TIGAN: SK Beecham Pharm	00029-4083-30	100s	$47.20
	00029-4083-32	500s	$224.05

INJECTION: 100 MG/ML

AVERAGE UNIT PRICE (AVAILABLE SIZES)		GENERIC A-RATED AVERAGE PRICE (GAAP)	
BRAND	$1.60	20 ml	$8.55
GENERIC	$0.71	2 ml 25s	$44.04

BRAND/MANUFACTURER	NDC	SIZE	AWP
◆ BRAND			
TIGAN: SK Beecham Pharm	00029-4085-22	2 ml	$3.10
	00029-4086-22	20 ml	$22.05
	00029-4087-22	2 ml	$4.30
◆ GENERICS			
Steris	00402-0690-82	2 ml	$1.33
Schein	00364-6762-55	20 ml	$8.49
Steris	00402-0164-20	20 ml	$8.49
Moore,H.L.	00839-6676-33	20 ml	$8.68
Sanofi Winthrop	00024-1955-03	2 ml 10s	$25.53
Schein	00364-6762-42	2 ml 25s	$33.38
Solo Pak	39769-0062-02	2 ml 25s	$54.69

SUPPOSITORY: 100 MG

BRAND/MANUFACTURER	NDC	SIZE	AWP
◆ GENERICS			
Raway	00686-0107-09	10s	$5.00

SUPPOSITORY: 100 MG

BRAND/MANUFACTURER	NDC	SIZE	AWP
○ BRAND			
NAVOGAN PED: Intl Ethical	11584-0421-01	10s	$10.07
TIGAN PEDIATRIC: SK Beecham Pharm	00029-4088-38	10s	$15.05

SUPPOSITORY: 200 MG

BRAND/MANUFACTURER	NDC	SIZE	AWP
○ BRAND			
TIGAN: SK Beecham Pharm	00029-4084-38	10s	$17.85
	00029-4084-39	50s	$80.80

Trimethoprim

DESCRIPTION

Trimethoprim is a synthetic antibacterial available in tablet form for oral administration. Each scored white tablet contains 100 mg Trimethoprim. Each scored yellow tablet contains 200 mg Trimethoprim.

Trimethoprim is 2,4-diamino-5-(3,4,5,-trimethoxybenzyl)-pyrimidine. It is a white to light yellow, odorless, bitter compound with a molecular weight of 290.3 and the molecular formula $C_{14}H_{18}N_4O_3$.

Following is its chemical structure:

CLINICAL PHARMACOLOGY

Trimethoprim is rapidly absorbed following oral administration. It exists in the blood as unbound, protein-bound, and metabolized forms. Ten to twenty percent of Trimethoprim is metabolized, primarily in the liver; the remainder is excreted unchanged in the urine. The principal metabolites of Trimethoprim are the 1- and 3-oxides and the 3'- and 4'-hydroxy derivatives. The free form is considered to be the therapeutically active form. Approximately 44% of Trimethoprim is bound to plasma proteins.

Mean peak plasma concentrations of approximately 1.0 µg/mL occur 1 to 4 hours after oral administration of a single 100 mg dose. A single 200 mg dose will result in serum levels approximately twice as high. The half-life of Trimethoprim ranges from 8 to 10 hours. However, patients with severely impaired renal function exhibit an increase in the half-life of Trimethoprim, which requires either dosage regimen adjustment or not using the drug in such patients (see "Dosage and Administration" section). During a 13-week study of Trimethoprim administered at a daily dosage of 200 mg (50 mg qid), the mean minimum steady-state concentration of the drug was 1.1 µg/mL. Steady-state concentrations were achieved within two to three days of chronic administration and were maintained throughout the experimental period. Excretion of Trimethoprim is primarily by the kidneys through glomerular filtration and tubular secretion. Urine concentra-

tions of Trimethoprim are considerably higher than are the concentrations in the blood. After a single oral dose of 100 mg, urine concentrations of Trimethoprim ranged from 30 to 160 µg/mL during the 0 to 4 hour period and declined to approximately 18 to 91 µg/mL during the 8 to 24 hour period. A 200 mg single oral dose will result in Trimethoprim urine levels approximately twice as high. After oral administration, 50% to 60% of Trimethoprim is excreted in the urine within 24 hours, approximately 80% of this being unmetabolized Trimethoprim.

Since normal vaginal and fecal flora are the source of most pathogens causing urinary tract infections, it is relevant to consider the distribution of Trimethoprim into these sites. Concentrations of Trimethoprim in vaginal secretions are consistently greater than those found simultaneously in the serum, being typically 1.6 times the concentrations of simultaneously obtained serum samples. Sufficient Trimethoprim is excreted in the feces to markedly reduce or eliminate Trimethoprim-susceptible organisms from the fecal flora.

Trimethoprim also passes the placental barrier and is excreted in human milk.

Microbiology: Trimethoprim blocks the production of tetrahydrofolic acid from dihydrofolic acid by binding to and reversibly inhibiting the required enzyme, dihydrofolate reductase. This binding is very much stronger for the bacterial enzyme than for the corresponding mammalian enzyme. Thus, Trimethoprim selectively interferes with bacterial biosynthesis of nucleic acids and proteins.

In vitro serial dilution tests have shown that the spectrum of antibacterial activity of Trimethoprim includes the common urinary tract pathogens with the exception of *Pseudomonas aeruginosa.*

The dominant non-*Enterobacteriaceae* fecal organisms, *Bacteroides* spp. and *Lactobacillus* spp., are not susceptible to Trimethoprim concentrations obtained with the recommended dosage.

REPRESENTATIVE MINIMUM INHIBITORY CONCENTRATIONS FOR TRIMETHOPRIM-SUSCEPTIBLE ORGANISMS

Bacteria	Trimethoprim MIC— µg/mL (Range)
Escherichia coli	0.05-1.5
Proteus mirabilis	0.5 -1.5
Klebsiella pneumoniae	0.5 -5.0
Enterobacter species	0.5 -5.0
Staphylococcus species, coagulase-negative	0.15-5.0

Susceptibility Testing: The recommended quantitative disc susceptibility method,[1,2] may be used for estimating the susceptibility of bacteria to Trimethoprim. With this procedure, reports from the laboratory giving results using the 5 µg Trimethoprim disc should be interpreted according to the following criteria: Organisms producing zones of 16 mm or greater are classified as susceptible, whereas those producing zones of 11 to 15 mm are classified as having intermediate susceptibility. A report from the laboratory of "Susceptible to Trimethoprim" or "Intermediate susceptibility to Trimethoprim" indicates that the infection is likely to respond when, as in uncomplicated urinary tract infections, effective therapy is dependent upon the urine concentration of Trimethoprim. Organisms producing zones of 10 mm or less are reported as resistant, indicating that other therapy should be selected.

Dilution methods for determining susceptibility are also used, and results are reported as the minimum drug concentration inhibiting microbial growth (MIC).[3] If the MIC is 8 µg/mL or less, the microorganism is considered "susceptible." If the MIC is 16 µg per mL or greater, the microorganism is considered "resistant."

INDICATIONS AND USAGE

FOR THE TREATMENT OF INITIAL EPISODES OF UNCOMPLICATED URINARY TRACT INFECTIONS DUE TO SUSCEPTIBLE STRAINS OF THE FOLLOWING ORGANISMS:

Escherichia coli, Proteus mirabilis, Klebsiella pneumoniae, Enterobacter species, and coagulase-negative *Staphylococcus* species, including *S. saprophyticus.*

Cultures and susceptibility tests should be performed to determine the susceptibility of the bacteria to Trimethoprim. Therapy may be initiated prior to obtaining the results of these tests.

UNLABELED USES

Trimethoprim is used alone or as an adjunct in the treatment of acne vulgaris and pneumocystis carinii pneumonia in patients with acquired immunodeficiency syndrome.

CONTRAINDICATIONS

Trimethoprim is contraindicated in individuals hypersensitive to Trimethoprim and in those with documented megaloblastic anemia due to folate deficiency.

WARNINGS

Serious hypersensitivity reactions have been reported rarely in patients on Trimethoprim therapy. Trimethoprim has been reported rarely to interfere with hematopoiesis, especially when administered in large doses and/or for prolonged periods.

The presence of clinical signs such as sore throat, fever, pallor, or purpura may be early indications of serious blood disorders (see "Overdosage, Chronic").

Complete blood counts should be obtained if any of these signs are noted in a patient receiving Trimethoprim and the drug discontinued if a significant reduction in the count of any formed blood element is found.

◆ RATED THERAPEUTICALLY EQUIVALENT; ◇ THERAPEUTIC EQUIVALENCE UNCONFIRMED; ○ UNRATED

PRECAUTIONS

General: Trimethoprim should be given with caution to patients with possible folate deficiency. Folates may be administered concomitantly without interfering with the antibacterial action of Trimethoprim. Trimethoprim should also be given with caution to patients with impaired renal or hepatic function (see "Clinical Pharmacology" and "Dosage and Administration").

Drug Interactions: Trimethoprim may inhibit the hepatic metabolism of phenytoin. Trimethoprim, given at a common clinical dosage, increased the phenytoin half-life by 51% and decreased the phenytoin metabolic clearance rate by 30%. When administering these drugs concurrently, one should be alert for possible excessive phenytoin effect.

Drug/Laboratory Test Interactions: Trimethoprim can interfere with a serum methotrexate assay as determined by the competitive binding protein technique (CBPA) when a bacterial dihydrofolate reductase is used as the binding protein. No interference occurs, however, if methotrexate is measured by a radioimmunoassay (RIA).

The presence of Trimethoprim may also interfere with the Jaffé alkaline picrate reaction assay for creatinine resulting in overestimations of about 10% in the range of normal values.

Carcinogenesis, Mutagenesis, Impairment of Fertility: Carcinogenesis: Long-term studies in animals to evaluate carcinogenic potential have not been conducted with Trimethoprim.

Mutagenesis: Trimethoprim was demonstrated to be nonmutagenic in the Ames assay. In studies at two laboratories no chromosomal damage was detected in cultured Chinese hamster ovary cells at concentrations approximately 500 times human plasma levels; at concentrations approximately 1000 times human plasma levels in these same cells a low level of chromosomal damage was induced at one of the laboratories. No chromosomal abnormalities were observed in cultured human leukocytes at concentrations of Trimethoprim up to 20 times human steady state plasma levels. No chromosomal effects were detected in peripheral lymphocytes of human subjects receiving 320 mg of Trimethoprim in combination with up to 1600 mg of sulfamethoxazole per day for as long as 112 weeks.

Impairment of Fertility: No adverse effects on fertility or general reproductive performance were observed in rats given Trimethoprim in oral dosages as high as 70 mg/kg/day for males and 14 mg/kg/day for females.

Pregnancy: Teratogenic Effects: Pregnancy Category C. Trimethoprim has been shown to be teratogenic in the rat when given in doses 40 times the human dose. In some rabbit studies, the overall increase in fetal loss (dead and resorbed and malformed conceptuses) was associated with doses 6 times the human therapeutic dose.

While there are no large well-controlled studies on the use of Trimethoprim in pregnant women, Brumfitt and Pursell,[4] in a retrospective study, reported the outcome of 186 pregnancies during which the mother received either placebo or Trimethoprim in combination with sulfamethoxazole. The incidence of congenital abnormalities was 4.5% (3 of 66) in those who received placebo and 3.3% (4 of 120) in those receiving Trimethoprim and sulfamethoxazole. There were no abnormalities in the 10 children whose mothers received the drug during the first trimester. In a separate survey, Brumfitt and Pursell also found no congenital abnormalities in 35 children whose mothers had received Trimethoprim and sulfamethoxazole at the time of conception or shortly thereafter.

Because Trimethoprim may interfere with folic acid metabolism, Trimethoprim should be used during pregnancy only if the potential benefit justifies the potential risk to the fetus.

Nonteratogenic Effects: The oral administration of Trimethoprim to rats at a dose of 70 mg/kg/day commencing with the last third of gestation and continuing through parturition and lactation caused no deleterious effects on gestation or pup growth and survival.

Nursing Mothers: Trimethoprim is excreted in human milk. Because Trimethoprim may interfere with folic acid metabolism, caution should be exercised when Trimethoprim is administered to a nursing woman.

Pediatric Use: The safety of Trimethoprim in infants under two months has not been demonstrated. The effectiveness of Trimethoprim as a single agent has not been established in children under 12 years of age.

ADVERSE REACTIONS

The adverse effects encountered most often with Trimethoprim were rash and pruritus.

Dermatologic: Rash, pruritus and phototoxic skin eruptions. At the recommended dosage regimens of 100 mg bid, or 200 mg qd, each for 10 days, the incidence of rash is 2.9% to 6.7%. In clinical studies which employed high doses of Trimethoprim an elevated incidence of rash was noted. These rashes were maculopapular, morbilliform, pruritic, and generally mild to moderate, appearing 7 to 14 days after the initiation of therapy.

Hypersensitivity: Rare reports of exfoliative dermatitis, erythema multiforme, Stevens-Johnson syndrome, toxic epidermal necrolysis (Lyell syndrome), and anaphylaxis have been received.

Gastrointestinal: Epigastric distress, nausea, vomiting, and glossitis. Elevation of serum transaminase and bilirubin has been noted, but the significance of this finding is unknown. Cholestatic jaundice has been rarely reported.

Hematologic: Thrombocytopenia, leukopenia, neutropenia, megaloblastic anemia, and methemoglobinemia.

Metabolic: Hyperkalemia, hyponatremia.

Neurologic: Aseptic meningitis has been rarely reported.

Miscellaneous: Fever, and increases in BUN and serum creatinine levels.

OVERDOSAGE

Acute: Signs of acute overdosage with Trimethoprim may appear following ingestion of 1 gram or more of the drug and include nausea, vomiting, dizziness, headaches, mental depression, confusion, and bone marrow depression (see "Overdosage, Chronic").

Treatment consists of gastric lavage and general supportive measures. Acidification of the urine will increase renal elimination of Trimethoprim. Peritoneal dialysis is not effective and hemodialysis only moderately effective in eliminating the drug.

Chronic: Use of Trimethoprim at high doses and/or for extended periods of time may cause bone marrow depression manifested as thrombocytopenia, leukopenia and/or megaloblastic anemia. If signs of bone marrow depression occur, Trimethoprim should be discontinued and the patient should be given leucovorin; 5 to 15 mg leucovorin daily has been recommended by some investigators.

DOSAGE AND ADMINISTRATION

The usual oral adult dosage is 100 mg of Trimethoprim every 12 hours or 200 mg Trimethoprim every 24 hours, each for 10 days. The use of Trimethoprim in patients with a creatinine clearance of less than 15 mL/min is not recommended. For patients with a creatinine clearance of 15 to 30 mL/min, the dose should be 50 mg every 12 hours.

The effectiveness of Trimethoprim has not been established in children under 12 years of age.

Store at 15° to 25°C (59° to 77°F) in a dry place and protect from light.

REFERENCES

1. Bauer AW, Kirby WMM, Sherris JC, Turck M. Antibiotic susceptibility testing by a standardized single disk method. *Am J Clin Pathol.* 1966;45:493-496. 2. National Committee for Clinical Laboratory Standards. Performance standards for antimicrobial disk susceptibility tests, 2nd ed. Villanova, PA. 1979. 3. Ericsson HM, Sherris JC. Antibiotic sensitivity testing: report of an international collaborative study. *Acta Pathol Microbiol Scand* [B]. 1971;(suppl 217):1-90. 4. Brumfitt W, Pursell R. Trimethoprim-sulfamethoxazole in the treatment of bacteriuria in women. *J Infect Dis.* 1973;128(suppl):S657-S663.

HOW SUPPLIED
TABLETS: 100 MG

AVERAGE UNIT PRICE (AVAILABLE SIZES)		GENERIC A-RATED AVERAGE PRICE (GAAP)	
BRAND	$0.70		
GENERIC	$0.22		
HCFA FUL (100s ea)	$0.17	100s	$21.48

BRAND/MANUFACTURER	NDC	SIZE	AWP
◆ **BRAND**			
TRIMPEX: Roche Labs	00004-0127-01	100s	$67.06
PROLOPRIM: Burr Wellcome	00081-0820-55	100s	$72.34
TRIMPEX: Roche Labs	00004-0127-49	100s ud	$69.09
◆ **GENERICS**			
Qualitest	00603-6264-21	100s	$18.74
Rugby	00536-4686-01	100s	$19.13
Major	00904-1646-60	100s	$19.29
Biocraft	00332-2158-09	100s	$20.00
Schein	00364-0649-01	100s	$22.80
Goldline	00182-1536-01	100s	$24.00
Moore,H.L.	00839-7284-06	100s	$25.23
Major	00904-1646-61	100s ud	$21.43
U.S. Trading	56126-0409-11	100s ud	$22.71

TABLETS: 200 MG

AVERAGE UNIT PRICE (AVAILABLE SIZES)		GENERIC A-RATED AVERAGE PRICE (GAAP)	
BRAND	$1.45	100s	$36.38
GENERIC	$0.36		
HCFA FUL (100s ea)	$0.28		

BRAND/MANUFACTURER	NDC	SIZE	AWP
◆ **BRAND**			
PROLOPRIM: Burr Wellcome	00081-0825-55	100s	$144.68
◆ **GENERICS**			
Biocraft	00332-2159-09	100s	$32.00
Qualitest	00603-6265-21	100s	$32.18
Moore,H.L.	00839-7433-06	100s	$32.52
Rugby	00536-4683-01	100s	$36.19
Major	00904-1647-60	100s	$42.70
Major	00904-1647-61	100s ud	$42.70

Trimetrexate Glucuronate

WARNINGS

TRIMETREXATE GLUCURONATE FOR INJECTION MUST BE USED WITH CONCURRENT LEUCOVORIN (LEUCOVORIN PROTECTION) TO AVOID

POTENTIALLY SERIOUS OR LIFE-THREATENING TOXICITIES (SEE "PRECAUTIONS" AND "DOSAGE AND ADMINISTRATION").

DESCRIPTION

Trimetrexate, a 2,4-diaminoquinazoline, non-classical folate antagonist, is a synthetic inhibitor of the enzyme dihydrofolate reductase (DHFR). Trimetrexate Glucuronate is available as a sterile lyophilized powder in single-dose vials, each containing 25 mg of Trimetrexate and 15 mg of D-glucuronic acid (40 mg of Trimetrexate Glucuronate) without any preservatives or excipients. The powder is reconstituted prior to intravenous infusion (see *"Dosage and Administration", "Reconstitution and Dilution"*). Trimetrexate Glucuronate is chemically known as 2,4-diamino-5-methyl-6-[(3,4,5-trimethoxyanilino)methyl] quinazoline mono-D-glucuronate.

The empirical formula for Trimetrexate Glucuronate is $C_{19}H_{23}N_5O_3 \cdot C_6H_{10}O_7$ with a molecular weight of 563.56. The active ingredient, trimetrexate free base, has an empirical formula of $C_{19}H_{23}N_5O_3$ with a molecular weight of 369.42. Trimetrexate Glucuronate for injection is a pale greenish-yellow powder or cake. Trimetrexate Glucuronate is soluble in water ($<$ 0.1 mg/mL). The pKa of trimetrexate free base in 50% methanol/water is 8.0. The logarithm 10 of the partition coefficient of trimetrexate free base between octanol and water is 1.63.

Following is its chemical structure:

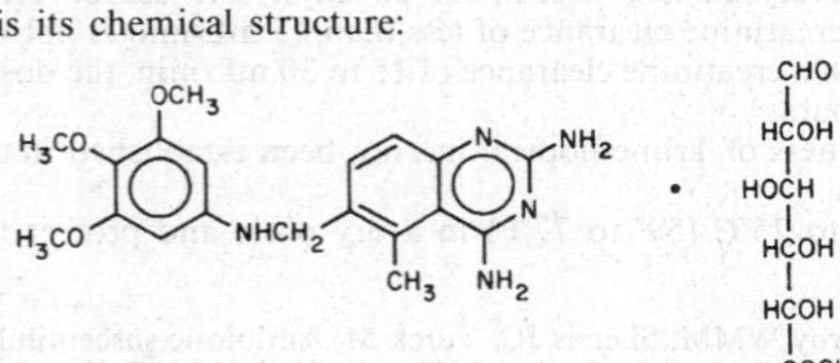

CLINICAL PHARMACOLOGY

MECHANISM OF ACTION

In vitro studies have shown that Trimetrexate is a competitive inhibitor of dihydrofolate reductase (DHFR) from bacterial, protozoan, and mammalian sources. DHFR catalyzes the reduction of intracellular dihydrofolate to the active coenzyme tetrahydrofolate. Inhibition of DHFR results in the depletion of this coenzyme, leading directly to interference with thymidylate biosynthesis, as well as inhibition of folate-dependent formyltransferases, and indirectly to inhibition of purine biosynthesis. The end result is disruption of DNA, RNA, and protein synthesis, with consequent cell death.

Leucovorin (folinic acid) is readily transported into mammalian cells by an active, carrier-mediated process and can be assimilated into cellular folate pools following its metabolism. *In vitro* studies have shown that leucovorin provides a source of reduced folates necessary for normal cellular biosynthetic processes. Because the *Pneumocystis carinii* organism lacks the reduced folate carrier-mediated transport system, leucovorin is prevented from entering the organism. Therefore, at concentrations achieved with therapeutic doses of Trimetrexate plus leucovorin, the selective transport of Trimetrexate, but not leucovorin, into the *Pneumocystis carinii* organism allows the concurrent administration of leucovorin to protect normal host cells from the cytotoxicity of Trimetrexate without inhibiting the antifolate's inhibition of *Pneumocystis carinii*. It is not known if considerably higher doses of leucovorin would affect Trimetrexate effect on *Pneumocystis carinii*.

MICROBIOLOGY

Trimetrexate inhibits, in a dose-related manner, *in vitro* growth of the trophozoite stage of rat *Pneumocystis carinii* cultured on human embryonic lung fibroblast cells. Trimetrexate concentrations between 3 and 54.1 μ were shown to inhibit the growth of trophozoites. Leucovorin alone at a concentration of 10 μM did not alter either the growth of the trophozoites or the anti-pneumocystis activity of Trimetrexate. Resistance to Trimetrexate's antimicrobial activity against *Pneumocystis carinii* has not been studied.

PHARMACOKINETICS

Trimetrexate pharmacokinetics were assessed in six patients with acquired immunodeficiency syndrome (AIDS) who had *Pneumocystis carinii* pneumonia (4 patients) or toxoplasmosis (2 patients). Trimetrexate was administered intravenously as a bolus injection at a dose of 30 mg/m²/day along with leucovorin 20 mg/m² every 6 hours for 21 days. Trimetrexate clearance (mean ± SD) was 38 ± 15 mL/min/m² and volume of distribution at steady state (Vd^{ss}) was 20 ± 8 L/m². The plasma concentration time profile declined in a biphasic manner over 24 hours with a terminal half-life of 11 ± 4 hours.

The pharmacokinetics of Trimetrexate without the concomitant administration of leucovorin have been evaluated in cancer patients with advanced solid tumors using various dosage regimens. The decline in plasma concentrations over time has been described by either biexponential or triexponential equations. Following the single-dose administration of 10 to 130 mg/m² to 37 patients, plasma concentrations were obtained for 72 hours. Nine plasma concentration time profiles were described as biexponential. The alpha phase half-life was 57 ± 28 minutes, followed by a terminal phase with a half-life of 16 ± 3 hours. The plasma concentrations in the remaining patients exhibited a triphasic decline with half-lives of 8.6 ± 6.5 minutes, 2.4 ± 1.3 hours, and 17.8 ± 8.2 hours.

Trimetrexate clearance in cancer patients has been reported as 53 ± 41 mL/min (14 patients) and 32 ± 18 mL/min/m² (23 patients) following single-dose administration. After a five-day infusion of Trimetrexate to 16 patients, plasma clearance was 30 ± 8 mL/min/m².

Renal clearance of Trimetrexate in cancer patients has varied from about 4 ± 2 mL/min/m² to 10 ± 6 mL/min/m². Ten to 30% of the administered dose is excreted unchanged in the urine. Considering the free fraction of Trimetrexate, active tubular secretion may possibly contribute to the renal clearance of Trimetrexate. Renal clearance has been associated with urine flow, suggesting the possibility of tubular reabsorption as well.

The Vd$_{ss}$ of Trimetrexate in cancer patients after single-dose administration and for whom plasma concentrations were obtained for 72 hours was 36.9 ± 17.6 L/m² (n = 23) and 0.62 ± 0.24 L/kg (n = 14). Following a constant infusion of Trimetrexate for five days, Vd$_{ss}$ was 32.8 ± 16.6 L/m². The volume of the central compartment has been estimated as 0.17 ± 0.08 L/kg and 4.0 ± 2.9 L/m²

There have been inconsistencies in the reporting of Trimetrexate protein binding. The *in vitro* plasma protein binding of Trimetrexate using ultrafiltration is approximately 95% over the concentration range of 18.75 to 1000 ng/mL. There is a suggestion of capacity limited binding (saturable binding) at concentrations greater than about 1000 ng/mL, with free fraction progressively increasing to about 9.3% as concentration is increased to 15 μg/mL. Other reports have declared Trimetrexate to be greater than 98% bound at concentrations of 0.1 to 10 μg/mL; however, specific free fractions were not stated. The free fraction of Trimetrexate also has been reported to be about 15 to 16% at a concentration of 60 ng/mL, increasing to about 20% at a Trimetrexate concentration of 6 μg/mL.

Trimetrexate metabolism in man has not been characterized. Preclinical data strongly suggest that the major metabolic pathway is oxidative O-demethylation, followed by conjugation to either glucuronide or the sulfate. N-demethylation and oxidation is a related minor pathway. Preliminary findings in humans indicate the presence of a glucuronide conjugate with DHFR inhibition and a demethylated metabolite in urine.

The presence of metabolite(s) in human plasma following the administration of Trimetrexate is suggested by the differences seen in Trimetrexate plasma concentrations when measured by HPLC and a nonspecific DHFR inhibition assay. The profiles are similar initially, but diverge with time; concentrations determined by DHFR being higher than those determined by HPLC. This suggests the presence of one or more metabolites with DHFR inhibition activity. After intravenous administration of Trimetrexate to humans, urinary recovery averaged about 40%, using a DHFR assay, in comparison to 10% urinary recovery as determined by HPLC, suggesting the presence of one or more metabolites that retain inhibitory activity against DHFR. Fecal recovery of Trimetrexate over 48 hours after intravenous administration ranged from 0.09 to 7.6% of the dose as determined by DHFR inhibition and 0.02 to 5.2% of the dose as determined by HPLC.

The pharmacokinetics of Trimetrexate have not been determined in patients with renal insufficiency or hepatic dysfunction.

INDICATIONS AND USAGE

Trimetrexate Glucuronate with concurrent leucovorin administration (leucovorin protection) is indicated as an alternative therapy for the treatment of moderate-to-severe *Pneumocystis carinii* pneumonia (PCP) in immunocompromised patients, including patients with the acquired immunodeficiency syndrome (AIDS), who are intolerant of, or are refractory to, trimethoprim-sulfamethoxazole therapy or for whom trimethoprim-sulfamethoxazole is contraindicated.

This indication is based on the results of a randomized, controlled double-blind trial comparing Trimetrexate Glucuronate with concurrent leucovorin protection (TMTX/LV) to trimethoprim-sulfamethoxazole (TMP/SMX) in patients with moderate-to-severe *Pneumocystis carinii* pneumonia, as well as results of a Treatment IND. These studies are summarized below:

Trimetrexate Glucuronate: This double-blind, randomized trial initiated by the AIDS Clinical Trials Group (ACTG) in 1988 was designed to compare the safety and efficacy of TMTX/LV to that of TMP/SMX for the treatment of histologically confirmed, moderate-to-severe PCP, defined as (A-a) baseline gradient > 30 mmHg, in patients with AIDS.

Of the 220 patients with histologically confirmed PCP, 109 were randomized to receive TMTX/LV and 111 to TMP/SMX. Study patients randomized to TMTX/LV treatment were to receive 45 mg/m² of TMTX daily for 21 days plus 20 mg/m² of LV every 6 hours for 24 days. Those randomized to TMP/SMX were to receive 5 mg/kg TMP plus 25 mg/kg SMX four times daily for 21 days.

Response to therapy, defined as alive and off ventilatory support at completion of therapy, without a requirement for a change in anti-pneumocystis therapy, or addition of supraphysiologic doses of steroids, occurred in fifty percent of patients in each treatment group.

The observed mortality in the TMTX/LV treatment group was approximately twice that in the TMP/SMX treatment group (95% CI: 0.99-4.11). Thirty of 109 (27%) patients treated with TMTX/LV and 18 of 111 (16%) patients receiving TMP/SMX died during the 21-day treatment course or 4-week follow-up period. Twenty-seven of 30 deaths in the TMTX/LV arm were attributed to PCP; all 18 deaths in the TMP/SMX arm were attributed to PCP.

A significantly smaller proportion of patients who received TMTX/LV compared to TMP/SMX failed therapy due to toxicity (10% vs. 25%), and a significantly greater proportion of patients failed due to lack of efficacy (40% vs. 24%). Six patients (12%) who responded to TMTX/LV relapsed during the one-month follow-up period; no patient responding to TMP/SMX relapsed during this period. Information is not available as to whether these patients received prophylaxis therapy for PCP.

Treatment IND: The FDA granted a Treatment IND for Trimetrexate Glucuronate with leucovorin protection in February 1988 to make Trimetrexate Glucuronate therapy available to HIV-infected patients with histologically confirmed PCP who had disease refractory to or who were intolerant of TMP/SMX and/or intravenous pentamidine.

Over 500 physicians in the United States participated in the Treatment IND. As of January 15, 1992, a total of 753 patients had been enrolled of whom 577 were evaluable for efficacy. Of the 577 evaluable patients, 227 patients were intolerant of both TMP/SMX and pentamidine (IST - patients intolerant of both standard therapies), 146 were intolerant of one therapy and refractory to the other (RIST - patients refractory to one therapy and intolerant of the other) and 204 were refractory to both therapies (RST - refractory to both standard therapies). This was a very ill patient population; 38% required ventilatory support at entry (Table 1). These studies did not have concurrent control groups.

Table 1
TREATMENT IND BASELINE CHARACTERISTICS

	IST (n = 227)	RIST (n = 146)	RST (n = 204)	TOTAL (n = 577)
Ventilatory Support Required n(%)	39 (17)	50 (34)	129 (63)	218 (38)
Median Days on Standard Therapy	10	12	16	14
First Episode of PCP n(%)	104 (46)	103 (71)	190 (93)	397 (69)

The overall survival rate one month after completion of TMTX/LV as salvage therapy was 48%. Patients who had not responded to treatment with both TMP/SMX and pentamidine, of whom 63% required mechanical ventilation at entry, achieved a survival rate of 25% following treatment with TMTX/LV. Survival was 67% in patients who were intolerant to both TMP/SMX and pentamidine (Table 2).

Table 2
TREATMENT IND SURVIVAL RATE ONE MONTH AFTER COMPLETION OF TRIMETREXATE GLUCURONATE THERAPY

	IST	RIST	RST
All Patients	153/227 (67%)	73/146 (50%)	50/204 (25%)
Baseline Ventilatory Support	9/39 (23%)	15/50 (30%)	18/129 (14%)
No Baseline Ventilatory Support	144/188 (77%)	58/96 (60%)	32/75 (43%)

In the Treatment IND, 12% of the patients discontinued Trimetrexate Glucuronate therapy (with leucovorin protection) for toxicity.

UNLABELED USES
Trimetrexate Glucuronate is used alone or as an adjunct in the treatment of metastatic carcinoma of the head and neck, metastatic colorectal adenocarcinoma, pancreatic adenocarcinoma, and advanced non-small cell carcinoma of the lung.

CONTRAINDICATIONS
Trimetrexate Glucuronate for injection is contraindicated in patients with clinically significant sensitivity to trimetrexate, leucovorin, or methotrexate.

WARNINGS
Trimetrexate Glucuronate for injection must be used with concurrent leucovorin to avoid potentially serious or life-threatening complications including bone marrow suppression, oral and gastrointestinal mucosal ulceration, and renal and hepatic dysfunction. Leucovorin therapy must extend for 72 hours past the last dose of Trimetrexate Glucuronate. Patients should be informed that failure to take the recommended dose and duration of leucovorin can lead to fatal toxicity. Patients should be closely monitored for the development of serious hematologic adverse reactions (see *"Precautions"* and *"Dosage and Administration"*).

Trimetrexate Glucuronate can cause fetal harm when administered to a pregnant woman. Trimetrexate has been shown to be fetotoxic and teratogenic in rats and rabbits. Rats administered 1.5 and 2.5 mg/kg/day intravenously on gestational days 6-15 showed substantial postimplantation loss and severe inhibition of maternal weight gain. Trimetrexate administered intravenously to rats at 0.5 and 1.0 mg/kg/day on gestational days 6-15 retarded normal fetal development and was teratogenic. Rabbits administered Trimetrexate intravenously at daily doses of 2.5 and 5.0 mg/kg/day on gestational days 6-18 resulted in significant maternal and fetotoxicity. In rabbits, Trimetrexate at 0.1 mg/kg/day was teratogenic in the absence of significant maternal toxicity. These effects were observed using doses 1/20 to 1/2 the equivalent human therapeutic dose based on a mg/m^2 basis. Teratogenic effects included skeletal, visceral, ocular, and cardiovascular abnormalities. If Trimetrexate Glucuronate is used during preg-

nancy, or if the patient becomes pregnant while taking this drug, the patient should be apprised of the potential hazard to the fetus. Women of childbearing potential should be advised to avoid becoming pregnant.

PRECAUTIONS
GENERAL
Patients receiving Trimetrexate Glucuronate for injection may experience severe hematologic, hepatic, renal, and gastrointestinal toxicities. Caution should be used in treating patients with impaired hematologic, renal, or hepatic function. Patients who require concomitant therapy with nephrotoxic, myelosuppressive, or hepatotoxic drugs should be treated with Trimetrexate Glucuronate at the discretion of the physician and monitored carefully. To allow for full therapeutic doses of Trimetrexate Glucuronate treatment with zidovudine should be discontinued during Trimetrexate Glucuronate therapy.

Trimetrexate Glucuronate associated myelosuppression, stomatitis, and gastrointestinal toxicities can generally be ameliorated by adjusting the dose of leucovorin. Mild elevations in transaminases and alkaline phosphatase have been observed with Trimetrexate Glucuronate administration and are usually not cause for modification of Trimetrexate Glucuronate therapy (see *"Dosage and Administration"*). Seizures have been reported rarely (< 1%) in AIDS patients receiving Trimetrexate Glucuronate; however, a causal relationship has not been established. An anaphylactoid reaction has been reported in a cancer patient receiving Trimetrexate Glucuronate as a bolus injection.

Trimetrexate Glucuronate has not been evaluated clinically for the treatment of concurrent pulmonary conditions such as bacterial, viral, or fungal pneumonia or mycobacterial diseases. *In vitro* activity has been observed against *Toxoplasma gondii. Mycobacterium avium* complex, gram-positive cocci, and gram-negative rods. If clinical deterioration is observed in patients, they should be carefully evaluated for other possible causes of pulmonary disease and treated with additional agents as appropriate.

LABORATORY TESTS
Patients receiving Trimetrexate Glucuronate with leucovorin protection should be seen frequently by a physician. Blood tests to assess the following parameters should be performed at least twice a week during therapy: hematology (absolute neutrophil counts [ANC], platelets), renal function (serum creatinine, BUN), and hepatic function (SGOT, SGPT, alkaline phosphatase).

DRUG INTERACTIONS
Since Trimetrexate is metabolized by a P450 enzyme system, drugs that induce or inhibit this drug metabolizing enzyme system may elicit important drug-drug interactions that may alter Trimetrexate plasma concentrations. Agents that might be coadministered with Trimetrexate in AIDS patients for other indications that could elicit this activity include erythromycin, rifampin, rifabutin, ketoconazole, and fluconazole. *In vitro* perfusion of isolated rat liver has shown that cimetidine caused a significant reduction in Trimetrexate metabolism and that acetaminophen altered the relative concentration of Trimetrexate metabolites possibly by competing for sulfate metabolites. Based on an *in vitro* rat liver model, nitrogen substituted imidazole drugs (clotrimazole, ketoconazole, micronazole) were potent, non-competitive inhibitors of Trimetrexate metabolism. Patients medicated with these drugs and Trimetrexate should be carefully monitored.

CARCINOGENESIS, MUTAGENESIS, IMPAIRMENT OF FERTILITY
Carcinogenesis: Long-term studies in animals to evaluate the carcinogenic potential of Trimetrexate have not been performed.

Mutagenesis: Trimetrexate was not mutagenic when tested using the standard Ames *Salmonella* mutagenicity assay with and without metabolic activation. Trimetrexate did not induce mutations in Chinese hamster lung cells or sister-chromatid exchange in Chinese hamster ovary cells. Trimetrexate did induce an increase in the chromosomal aberration frequency of cultured Chinese hamster lung cells; however, Trimetrexate showed no clastogenic activity in a mouse micronucleus assay.

Impairment of fertility: No studies have been conducted to evaluate the potential of Trimetrexate to impair fertility. However, during standard toxicity studies conducted in mice and rats, degeneration of the testes and spermatocytes including the arrest of spermatogenesis was observed.

PREGNANCY CATEGORY D
Pregnancy, teratogenic effects - See *"Warnings"*.

NURSING MOTHERS
It is not known if Trimetrexate is excreted in human milk. Because many drugs are excreted in human milk and because of the potential for serious adverse reactions in nursing infants from Trimetrexate Glucuronate, it is recommended that breast feeding be discontinued if the mother is treated with Trimetrexate Glucuronate.

PEDIATRIC USE
The safety and effectiveness of Trimetrexate Glucuronate for the treatment of histologically confirmed PCP has not been established for patients under 18 years of age. Under the Compassionate Use Protocol (maintained by U.S. Bioscience), 2 children, ages 15 months and 9 months, were treated with Trimetrexate and leucovorin using a dose of 45 mg/m^2 of Trimetrexate per day for 21 days and 20 mg/m^2 of leucovorin per day for 24 days. There were no serious or unexpected adverse effects.

► SHOWN IN PRODUCT IDENTIFICATION GUIDE

ADVERSE REACTIONS

Because many patients who participated in clinical trials of Trimetrexate Glucuronate for Injection had complications of advanced HIV disease, it is difficult to distinguish adverse events caused by Trimetrexate Glucuronate from those resulting from underlying medical conditions. Table 3 lists the adverse events that occurred in ≥ 1% of the patients who participated in the Comparative Study of Trimetrexate Glucuronate plus leucovorin versus TMP/SMX.

Table 3
TRIMETREXATE GLUCURONATE COMPARATIVE TRIAL COMPARISON OF ADVERSE EVENTS REPORTED FOR ≥ 1% OF PATIENTS

	Number and Percent (%) of Patients with Adverse Events			
Adverse Events	TMTX/LV (n = 109)		TMP/SMX (n = 111)	
NonLaboratory Adverse Events:				
Fever	9	(8.3)	14	(12.6)
Rash/Pruritus	6	(5.5)	14	(12.6)
Nausea/Vomiting	5	(4.6)[a]	15	(13.5)[a]
Confusion	3	(2.8)	3	(2.7)
Fatigue	2	(1.8)	0	(0.0)
Hematologic Toxicity:				
Neutropenia (≤ 1000/mm^3)	33	(30.3)	37	(33.3)
Thrombocytopenia (≤ 75,000/mm^3)	11	(10.1)	17	(15.3)
Anemia (Hgb < 8 g/dL)	8	(7.3)	10	(9.0)
Hepatotoxicity:				
Increased AST (> 5 × ULN[b])	15	(13.8)	10	(9.0)
Increased ALT (> 5 × ULN)	12	(11.0)	13	(11.7)
Increased Alkaline Phosphatase (> 5 × ULN)	5	(4.6)	3	(2.7)
Increased Bilirubin (2.5 × ULN)	2	(1.8)	1	(0.9)
Renal:				
Increased Serum Creatinine (> 3 × ULN)	1	(0.9)	2	(1.8)
Electrolyte Imbalance:				
Hyponatremia	5	(4.6)	10	(9.0)
Hypocalcemia	2	(1.8)	0	(0.0)
No. of Patients With at Least one Adverse Event[c]	58	(53.2)	60	(54.1)

[a] *Statistically significant difference between treatment groups (Chi-square: p = 0.022)*
[b] *ULN = Upper limit of normal range*
[c] *Patients could have reported more than one adverse event; therefore, the sum of adverse events exceeds the number of patients*

Laboratory toxicities were generally manageable with dose modification of Trimetrexate/leucovorin (See *"Dosage and Administration"*).

Table 4 lists the adverse events resulting in discontinuation of study therapy in the Trimetrexate Glucuronate Comparative Study with TMP/SMX. Twenty-nine percent of the patients on the TMP/SMX arm discontinued therapy due to adverse events compared to 10% of the patients treated with TMTX/LV (p < 0.001).

Table 4
TRIMETREXATE GLUCURONATE COMPARATIVE TRIAL ADVERSE EVENTS RESULTING IN DISCONTINUATION OF THERAPY

	Number and Percent (%) of Patients Discontinued for Adverse Events[b]			
Adverse Events	TMTX/LV (n = 109)		TMP/SMX (n = 111)	
NonLaboratory Adverse Events:				
Rash/Pruritus	3	(2.8)	5	(4.5)
Fever	2	(1.8)	4	(3.6)
Nausea/Vomiting	1	(0.9)	8	(7.2)
Neurologic Toxicity	1	(0.9)[c]	2	(1.8)
Hematologic Toxicity:				
Neutropenia (≤ 1000/mm^3)	4	(3.7)	6	(5.4)

	Number and Percent (%) of Patients Discontinued for Adverse Events[b]			
Adverse Events	TMTX/LV (n = 109)		TMP/SMX (n = 111)	
Thrombocytopenia (≤ 75,000/mm^3)	0	(0.0)	4	(3.6)
Anemia (Hgb < 8 g/dL)	0	(0.0)	4	(3.6)
Hepatotoxicity:				
Increased AST (> 5 × ULN[a])	3	(2.8)	9	(8.1)
Increased ALT (> 5 × ULN)	1	(0.9)	4	(3.6)
Increased Alkaline Phosphatase (> 5 × ULN)	0	(0.0)	1	(0.9)
Electrolyte Imbalance:				
Hyponatremia	0	(0.0)	3	(2.7)
No. of Patients Discontinuing Therapy Due to an Adverse Event[b]	11	(10.1)[d]	32	(28.8)[d]

[a] *ULN = Upper limit of normal range*
[b] *Patients could discontinue therapy due to more than one toxicity; therefore the sum exceeds number of patients who discontinued due to toxicity*
[c] *Patient discontinued TMTX/LV due to seizure, though causal relationship could not be established*
[d] *Statistically significant difference between treatment groups (Chi-square: p < 0.001)*

Hematologic toxicity was the principal dose-limiting side effect. An anaphylactoid reaction has been reported in a cancer patient receiving Trimetrexate Glucuronate as a bolus injection.

OVERDOSAGE

Trimetrexate Glucuronate for injection administered without concurrent leucovorin can cause lethal complications. There has been no extensive experience in humans receiving single intravenous doses of Trimetrexate greater than 90 mg/m^2/day with concurrent leucovorin. The toxicities seen at this dose were primarily hematologic. In the event of overdose, Trimetrexate Glucuronate should be stopped and leucovorin should be administered at a dose of 40 mg/m^2 every 6 hours for 3 days. The LD$_{50}$ of intravenous Trimetrexate in mice is 62 mg/kg (186 mg/m^2).

DOSAGE AND ADMINISTRATION

Caution: **Trimetrexate Glucuronate for injection must be administered with concurrent leucovorin (leucovorin protection) to avoid potentially serious or life-threatening toxicities. Leucovorin therapy must extend for 72 hours past the last dose of Trimetrexate Glucuronate.**

Trimetrexate Glucuronate for injection is administered at a dose of 45 mg/m^2 once daily by intravenous infusion over 60-90 minutes. Leucovorin must be administered daily during treatment with Trimetrexate Glucuronate and for 72 hours past the last dose of Trimetrexate Glucuronate. Leucovorin may be administered intravenously at a dose of 20 mg/m^2 over 5 to 10 minutes every 6 hours for a total daily dose of 80 mg/m^2, or orally as 4 doses of 20 mg/m^2 spaced equally throughout the day. The oral dose should be rounded up to the next higher 25 mg increment. The recommended course of therapy is 21 days of Trimetrexate Glucuronate and 24 days of leucovorin.

DOSAGE MODIFICATIONS

Hematologic toxicity: Trimetrexate Glucuronate for injection and leucovorin doses should be modified based on the worst hematologic toxicity according to the following table. If leucovorin is given orally, doses should be rounded up to the next higher 25 mg increment.

Table 5
DOSAGE MODIFICATIONS FOR HEMATOLOGIC TOXICITY

Toxicity Grade	Neutrophils (Polys and Bands)	Platelets	Recommended Dosage of	
			Trimetrexate Glucuronate	Leucovorin
1	> 1000/mm^3	> 75,000/ mm^3	45 mm/m^2 once daily	20 mg/m^2 every 6 hours
2	750-1000/ mm^3	50,000- 75,000/ mm^3	45 mg/m^2 once daily	40 mg/m^2 every 6 hours
3	500-749/mm^3	25,000- 49,999/ mm^3	22 mg/m^2 once daily	40 mg/m^2 every 6 hours
4	< 500/mm^3	< 25,000/ mm^3	Day 1-9 Discontinue	40 mg/m^2 every 6 hours

Toxicity Grade	Neutrophils (Polys and Bands)	Platelets	Recommended Dosage of	
			Trimetrexate Glucuronate	Leucovorin
			Day 10-21 Interrupt up to 96 hrs[a]	

[a] *If Grade 4 hematologic toxicity occurs prior to Day 10, Trimetrexate Glucuronate should be discontinued. Leucovorin (40 mg/m² q6h) should be administered for an additional 72 hours. If Grade 4 hematologic toxicity occurs at Day 10 or later, Trimetrexate Glucuronate may be held up to 96 hours to allow counts to recover. If counts recover to Grade 3 within 96 hours, Trimetrexate Glucuronate should be administered at a dose of 22 mg/m² and leucovorin maintained at 40 mg/m², q6h. When counts recover to Grade 2 toxicity, Trimetrexate Glucuronate dose may be increased to 45 mg/m², but the leucovorin dose should be maintained at 40 mg/m² for the duration of treatment. If counts do not improve to ≤ Grade 3 toxicity within 96 hours, Trimetrexate Glucuronate should be discontinued. Leucovorin at a dose of 40 mg/m², q6h should be administered for 72 hours following the last dose of Trimetrexate Glucuronate.*

Hepatic toxicity: Transient elevations of transaminases and alkaline phosphatase have been observed in patients treated with Trimetrexate Glucuronate. Interruption of treatment is advisable if transaminase levels or alkaline phosphatase levels increase to > 5 times the upper limit of normal range.

Renal toxicity: Interruption of Trimetrexate Glucuronate is advisable if serum creatinine levels increased to > 2.5 mg/dL and the elevation is considered to be secondary to Trimetrexate Glucuronate.

Other toxicities: Interruption of treatment is advisable in patients who experience severe mucosal toxicity that interferes with oral intake. Treatment should be discontinued for fever (oral temperature > 105°F/40.5°C) that cannot be controlled with antipyretics.

RECONSTITUTION AND DILUTION
Trimetrexate Glucuronate should be reconstituted with 2 mL of 5% Dextrose Injection, USP, or Sterile Water for Injection, USP, to yield a concentration of 12.5 mg of Trimetrexate for mL (complete dissolution should occur within 30 seconds). The reconstituted product will appear as a pale greenish-yellow solution and must be inspected visually for particulate matter prior to dilution. Do not use if cloudiness or precipitate is observed. This solution should be filtered (0.22μm) prior to dilution. Trimetrexate Glucuronate should not be reconstituted with solutions containing either chloride ion or leucovorin, since precipitation occurs instantly.

After reconstitution, the solution is stable under refrigeration or at room temperature for up to 24 hours. Do not freeze reconstituted solution. Discard the unused portions after 24 hours.

Reconstituted solution should be further diluted with 5% Dextrose Injection, USP, to yield a final concentration of 0.25 to 2 mg of Trimetrexate per mL. The diluted solution should be administered by intravenous infusion over 60 minutes. Trimetrexate Glucuronate should be mixed with solutions containing either chloride ion or leucovorin, since precipitation occurs instantly. It is stable under refrigeration or at room temperature for up to 24 hours. Do not freeze. Discard the unused portions after 24 hours after initial reconstitution. The intravenous line must be flushed thoroughly with at least 10 mL of 5% Dextrose Injection, USP, before and after administering Trimetrexate Glucuronate.

Leucovorin protection may be administered prior to or following Trimetrexate Glucoronate. In either case the intravenous line must be flushed thoroughly with at least 10 mL of 5% Dextrose Injection, USP. Leucovorin Calcium for injection should be diluted according to the instructions in the leucovorin package insert, and administered over 5 to 10 minutes every 6 hours.

Cautions: **Parenteral products should be inspected visually for particulate matter and discoloration prior to administration whenever solution and container permit. Trimetrexate Glucurate forms a precipitate instantly upon contact with chloride ion or leucovorin, therefore it should not be added to solutions containing sodium chloride or other anions. Trimetrexate Glucuronate and leucovorin solutions must be administered separately. Intravenous lines should be flushed with at least 10 mL of 5% Dextrose Injection, USP, between Trimetrexate Glucuronate and leucovorin infusions.**

HANDLING AND DISPOSAL
If Trimetrexate Glucoronate for injection contacts the skin or mucosa, immediately wash thoroughly with soap and water. Procedures for proper disposal of cytotoxic drugs should be considered. Several guidelines on this subject have been published (1-5).

STORAGE
Store at controlled room temperature 15° to 30°C (59° to 86°F). **Protect from exposure to light.**

REFERENCES
1. AMA Council Report. Guidelines for Handling Parenteral Antineoplastics. *Journal of the American Medical Association* March 15, 1985. 2. Clinical Oncological Society of Australia: Guidelines and Recommendations for Safe Handling of Antineoplastic Agents. *Medical Journal of Australia* 1:426-428, 1983. 3. Jones RB, et al. Safe Handling of Chemotherapeutic Agents: A Report from the Mount Sinai Medical Center. *CA - A Cancer Journal for Clinicians* Sept/Oct, 258-263, 1983. 4. American Society of Hospital Pharmacists Technical Assistance Bulletin on Handling Cytotoxic Drugs in Hospitals. *American Journal of Hospital Pharmacy* 42:131-137, 1985. 5. OSHA Work Practice Guidelines for Personnel Dealing with Cytotoxic Antineoplastic) Drugs. *American Journal of Hosptial Pharmacy* 43:1193-1204, 1986.

HOW SUPPLIED
POWDER FOR INJECTION: 25 MG

BRAND/MANUFACTURER	NDC	SIZE	AWP
○ **BRAND**			
NEUTREXIN: U.S. Bioscience	58178-0020-10	10s	$500.00
	58178-0020-50	50s	$2082.50

Trimipramine Maleate

DESCRIPTION
Trimipramine Maleate is 5-(3-dimethylamino-2-methylpropyl)-10,11-dihydro-5H-dibenz (b,f) azepine acid maleate (racemic form).

Its molecular formula is $C_{20}H_{26}N_2 \cdot C_4H_4O_4$ and the molecular weight is 410.5.

Trimipramine Maleate capsules contain Trimipramine Maleate equivalent to 25 mg, 50 mg, or 100 mg of Trimipramine as the base.

Trimipramine Maleate is prepared as a racemic mixture which can be resolved into levorotatory and dextrorotatory isomers. The asymmetric center responsible for optical isomerism is marked in the formula by an asterisk. Trimipramine Maleate is an almost odorless, white or slightly cream-colored, crystalline substance, melting at 140-144°C. It is very slightly soluble in ether and water, is slightly soluble in ethyl alcohol and acetone, and freely soluble in chloroform and methanol at 20°C.

Following is its chemical structure:

CH₂CHCH₂N(CH₃)₂ CH₃

CLINICAL PHARMACOLOGY
Trimipramine Maleate is an antidepressant with an anxiety-reducing sedative component to its action. The mode of action of Trimipramine Maleate on the central nervous system is not known. However, unlike amphetamine-type compounds it does not act primarily by stimulation of the central nervous system. It does not act by inhibition of the monoamine oxidase system.

INDICATIONS
Trimipramine Maleate is indicated for the relief of symptoms of depression. Endogenous depression is more likely to be alleviated than other depressive states. In studies with neurotic outpatients, the drug appeared to be equivalent to Amitriptyline in the less-depressed patients but somewhat less effective than Amitriptyline in the more severely depressed patients. In hospitalized depressed patients, Trimipramine and imipramine were equally effective in relieving depression.

UNLABELED USES
Trimipramine Maleate is used alone or as an adjunct in the treatment of atopic eczema, and for symptomatic relief of irritable bowel syndrome, peptic ulcer, and duodenal ulcer.

CONTRAINDICATIONS
Trimipramine Maleate is contraindicated in cases of known hypersensitivity to the drug. The possibility of cross-sensitivity to other dibenzazepine compounds should be kept in mind. Trimipramine Maleate should not be given in conjunction with drugs of the monoamine oxidase inhibitor class (e.g., tranylcypromine, isocarboxazid or phenelzine sulfate). The concomitant use of monoamine oxidase inhibitors (MAOI) and tricyclic compounds similar to Trimipramine Maleate has caused severe hyperpyretic reactions, convulsive crises, and death in some patients. At least two weeks should elapse after cessation of therapy with MAOI before instituting therapy with Trimipramine Maleate. Initial dosage should be low and increased gradually with caution and careful observation of the patient. The drug is contraindicated during the acute recovery period after a myocardial infarction.

WARNINGS
USE IN CHILDREN
This drug is not recommended for use in children, since safety and effectiveness in the pediatric age group have not been established.

GENERAL CONSIDERATION FOR USE
Extreme caution should be used when this drug is given to patients with any evidence of cardiovascular disease because of the possibility of conduction defects, arrhythmias, myocardial infarction, strokes, and tachycardia.

Caution is advised in patients with increased intraocular pressure, history of urinary retention, or history of narrow-angle glaucoma because of the drug's anticholinergic properties; hyperthyroid patients or those on thyroid medication because of the possibility of cardiovascular toxicity; patients with a history of seizure disorder, because this drug has been shown to lower the seizure threshold;

patients receiving guanethidine or similar agents, since Trimipramine Maleate may block the pharmacologic effects of these drugs.

Since the drug may impair the mental and/or physical abilities required for the performance of potentially hazardous tasks, such as operating an automobile or machinery, the patient should be cautioned accordingly.

PRECAUTIONS

The possibility of suicide is inherent in any severely depressed patient and persists until a significant remission occurs. When a patient with a serious suicidal potential is not hospitalized, the prescription should be for the smallest amount feasible.

In schizophrenic patients activation of the psychosis may occur and require reduction of dosage or the addition of a major tranquilizer to the therapeutic regime.

Manic or hypomanic episodes may occur in some patients, in particular those with cyclic-type disorders. In some cases therapy with Trimipramine Maleate must be discontinued until the episode is relieved, after which therapy may be reinstituted at lower dosages if still required.

Concurrent administration of Trimipramine Maleate and electro- shock therapy may increase the hazards of therapy. Such treatment should be limited to those patients for whom it is essential. When possible, discontinue the drug for several days prior to elective surgery.

There is evidence that cimetidine inhibits the elimination of tricyclic antidepressants. Downward adjustment of Trimipramine Maleate dosage may be required if cimetidine therapy is initiated: upward adjustment if cimetidine therapy is discontinued.

Patients should be warned that the concomitant use of alcoholic beverages may be associated with exaggerated effects. It has been reported that tricyclic antidepressants can potentiate the effects of catecholamines. Similarly, atropine-like effects may be more pronounced in patients receiving anticholinergic therapy. Therefore, particular care should be exercised when it is necessary to administer tricyclic antidepressants with sympathomimetic amines, local decongestants, local anesthetics containing epinephrine, atropine or drugs with an anticholinergic effect. In resistant cases of depression in adults, a dose of 2.5 mg/kg/day may have to be exceeded. If a higher dose is needed, ECG monitoring should be maintained during the initiation of therapy and at appropriate intervals during stabilization of dose.

USAGE IN PREGNANCY

Pregnancy Category C: Trimipramine Maleate has shown evidence of embryotoxicity and/or increased incidence of major anomalies in rats or rabbits at doses 20 times the human dose. There are no adequate and well-controlled studies in pregnant women. Trimipramine Maleate should be used during pregnancy only if the potential benefit justifies the potential risk to the fetus.

Semen studies in man (four schizophrenics and nine normal volunteers) revealed no significant changes in sperm morphology. It is recognized that drugs having a parasympathetic effect, including tricyclic antidepressants, may alter the ejaculatory response.

Chronic animal studies showed occasional evidence of degeneration of seminiferous tubules at the highest dose of 60 mg/kg/day.

Trimipramine Maleate should be used with caution in patients with impaired liver function.

Chronic animal studies showed occasional occurrence of hepatic congestion, fatty infiltration, or increased serum liver enzymes at the highest dose of 60 mg/kg/day.

Both elevation and lowering of blood sugar have been reported with tricyclic antidepressants.

ADVERSE REACTIONS

Note: The pharmacological similarities among the tricyclic antidepressants require that each of the reactions be considered when Trimipramine Maleate is administered. Some of the adverse reactions included in this listing have not in fact been reported with Trimipramine Maleate.

CARDIOVASCULAR

Hypotension, hypertension, tachycardia, palpitation, myocardial infarction, arrhythmias, heart block, stroke.

PSYCHIATRIC

Confusional states (especially the elderly) with hallucinations, disorientation, delusions; anxiety, restlessness, agitation; insomnia and nightmares; hypomania; exacerbation of psychosis.

NEUROLOGICAL

Numbness, tingling, paresthesias of extremities; incoordination, ataxia, tremors; peripheral neuropathy; extrapyramidal symptoms; seizures, alterations in EEG patterns; tinnitus; syndrome of inappropriate ADH (antidiuretic hormone) secretion.

ANTICHOLINERGIC

Dry mouth and, rarely, associated sublingual adenitis; blurred vision, disturbances of accommodation, mydriasis, constipation, paralytic ileus; urinary retention, delayed micturition, dilation of the urinary tract.

ALLERGIC

Skin rash, petechiae, urticaria, itching, photosensitization, edema of face and tongue.

HEMATOLOGIC

Bone-marrow depression including agranulocytosis, eosinophilia; purpura; thrombocytopenia. Leukocyte and differential counts should be performed in any patient who develops fever and sore throat during therapy; the drug should be discontinued if there is evidence of pathological neutrophil depression.

GASTROINTESTINAL

Nausea and vomiting, anorexia, epigastric distress, diarrhea, peculiar taste, stomatitis, abdominal cramps, black tongue.

ENDOCRINE

Gynecomastia in the male; breast enlargement and galactorrhea in the female; increased or decreased libido, impotence; testicular swelling; elevation or depression of blood-sugar levels.

OTHER

Jaundice (simulating obstructive); altered liver function; weight gain or loss; perspiration; flushing; urinary frequency; drowsiness, dizziness, weakness, and fatigue; headache; parotid swelling; alopecia.

WITHDRAWAL SYMPTOMS

Though not indicative of addiction, abrupt cessation of treatment after prolonged therapy may produce nausea, headache, and malaise.

OVERDOSAGE

SIGNS AND SYMPTOMS

The response of the patient to toxic overdosage of tricyclic antidepressants may vary in severity and is conditioned by factors such as age, amount ingested, amount absorbed, interval between ingestion and start of treatment. Trimipramine Maleate is not recommended for infants or young children. Should accidental ingestion occur in any amount, it should be regarded as serious and potentially fatal.

CNS abnormalities may include drowsiness, stupor, coma, ataxia, restlessness, agitation, hyperactive reflexes, muscle rigidity, athetoid and choreiform movements, and convulsions. Cardiac abnormalities may include arrhythmia, tachycardia, ECG evidence of impaired conduction, and signs of congestive failure. Other symptoms may include respiratory depression, cyanosis, hypotension, shock, vomiting, hyperpyrexia, mydriasis, and diaphoresis.

Treatment is supportive and symptomatic as no specific antidote is known. Depending upon need the following measures can be considered:

1. Trimipramine Maleate is not recommended for use in infants and children. Hospitalization with continuous cardiac monitoring for up to 4 days is recommended for children who have ingested Trimipramine Maleate in any amount. This is based on the reported greater sensitivity of children to acute overdosage with tricyclic antidepressants.
2. Blood and urine levels may not reflect the severity of the poisoning and are mostly of diagnostic value.
3. CNS involvement, respiratory depression, or cardiac arrhythmia can occur suddenly; hospitalization and close observation are necessary, even when the amount ingested is thought to be small or initial toxicity appears slight. Patients with any alteration of ECG should have continuous cardiac monitoring for at least 72 hours and be observed until well after the cardiac status has returned to normal; relapses may occur after apparent recovery.
4. The slow intravenous administration of physostigmine salicylate has been reported to reverse most of the cardiovascular and CNS effects of overdosage with tricyclic antidepressants. In adults, 1 to 3 mg has been reported to be effective. In children, start with 0.5 mg and repeat at 5-minute intervals to determine the minimum effective dose; do not exceed 2.0 mg. Avoid rapid injection, to reduce the possibility of physostigmine-induced convulsions. Because of the short duration of action of physostigmine, it may be necessary to repeat doses at 30- to 60-minute intervals as necessary.
5. In the alert patient, empty the stomach rapidly by induced emesis, followed by lavage. In the obtunded patient, secure the airway with a cuffed endotracheal tube before beginning lavage (do not induce emesis). Instillation of activated-charcoal slurry may help reduce absorption of Trimipramine.
6. Minimize external stimulation to reduce the tendency to convulsions. If anticonvulsants are necessary, diazepam, short-acting barbiturates, paraldehyde, or methocarbamol may be useful. Do not use barbiturates if MAO inhibitors have been taken recently.
7. Maintain adequate respiratory exchange. Do not use respiratory stimulants.
8. Shock should be treated with supportive measures, such as intravenous fluids, oxygen, and corticosteroids. Digitalis may increase conduction abnormalities and further irritate an already sensitized myocardium. If congestive heart failure necessitates rapid digitalization, particular care must be exercised.
9. Hyperpyrexia should be controlled by whatever external means available, including ice packs and cooling sponge baths if necessary.
10. Hemodialysis, peritoneal dialysis, exchange transfusions, and forced diuresis have been generally reported as ineffective in tricyclic poisoning.

DOSAGE AND ADMINISTRATION

Dosage should be initiated at a low level and increased gradually, noting carefully the clinical response and any evidence of intolerance.

Lower dosages are recommended for elderly patients and adolescents. Lower dosages are also recommended for outpatients as compared to hospitalized patients who will be under close supervision. It is not possible to prescribe a single dosage schedule of Trimipramine Maleate that will be therapeutically effective in all patients. The physical psychodynamic factors contributing to depressive symptomatology are very complex; spontaneous remissions or exacerbations of depressive symptoms may occur with or without drug therapy. Consequently, the recommended dosage regimens are furnished as a guide which may be modified by factors such as the age of the patient, chronicity and severity of the disease, medical condition of the patient, and degree of psychotherapeutic support. Most antidepressant drugs have a lag period of ten days to four weeks before a therapeutic response is noted. Increasing the dose will not shorten this period but rather increase the incidence of adverse reactions.

USUAL ADULT DOSE

Outpatients and Office Patients: Initially, 75 mg/day in divided doses, increased to 150 mg/day. Dosages over 200 mg/day are not recommended. Maintenance therapy is in the range of 50 to 150 mg/day. For convenient therapy and to facilitate patient compliance, the total dosage requirement may be given at bedtime.

Hospitalized Patients: Initially, 100 mg/day in divided doses. This may be increased gradually in a few days to 200 mg/day, depending upon individual response and tolerance. If improvement does not occur in 2 to 3 weeks, the dose may be increased to the maximum recommended dose of 250 to 300 mg/day.

Adolescent and Geriatric Patients: Initially, a dose of 50 mg/day is recommended, with gradual increments up to 100 mg/day, depending upon patient response and tolerance.

Maintenance: Following remission, maintenance medication may be required for a longer period of time, at the lowest dose that will maintain remission. Maintenance therapy is preferably administered as a single dose at bedtime. To minimize relapse, maintenance therapy should be continued for about three months.

STORAGE

Store at room temperature, approx. 25°C (77°F).
Keep bottles tightly closed.
Dispense in tight container.
Protect capsules packaged in blister strips from moisture.

HOW SUPPLIED
CAPSULE: 25 MG

AVERAGE UNIT PRICE (AVAILABLE SIZES)		GENERIC A-RATED AVERAGE PRICE (GAAP)		
BRAND	$0.59	100s		$30.46
GENERIC	$0.31			

BRAND/MANUFACTURER		NDC	SIZE	AWP
◆ BRAND				
SURMONTIL: Wyeth-Ayerst		00008-4132-01	100s	$59.20
◆ GENERICS				
Major		00904-3750-60	100s	$29.80
Major		00904-3750-61	100s ud	$31.12

CAPSULE: 50 MG

AVERAGE UNIT PRICE (AVAILABLE SIZES)		GENERIC A-RATED AVERAGE PRICE (GAAP)		
BRAND	$1.007	100s		$50.40
GENERIC	$0.50			

BRAND/MANUFACTURER		NDC	SIZE	AWP
◆ BRAND				
SURMONTIL: Wyeth-Ayerst		00008-4133-01	100s	$96.89
		00008-4133-04	100s ud	$104.54
◆ GENERICS				
Major		00904-3751-60	100s	$53.90
Major		00904-3751-61	100s ud	$46.90

CAPSULE: 100 MG

AVERAGE UNIT PRICE (AVAILABLE SIZES)		GENERIC A-RATED AVERAGE PRICE (GAAP)		
BRAND	$1.41	100s		$65.62
GENERIC	$0.66			

BRAND/MANUFACTURER		NDC	SIZE	AWP
◆ BRAND				
SURMONTIL: Wyeth-Ayerst		00008-4158-01	100s	$140.85
◆ GENERICS				
Major		00904-3752-60	100s	$63.60
Major		00904-3752-61	100s ud	$67.64

Trimpex *SEE* TRIMETHOPRIM

Trinalin Repetabs *SEE* AZATADINE MALEATE WITH PSEUDOEPHEDRINE SULFATE

Trinsicon *SEE* FERROUS FUMARATE/FOLIC ACID/ MINERALS/VITAMINS, MULTI

Triostat *SEE* LIOTHYRONINE SODIUM

Trioxsalen

To facilitate repigmentation in vitiligo, increase tolerance to solar exposure and enhance pigmentation.
CAUTION: THIS IS A POTENT DRUG.

DESCRIPTION

Trioxsalen Tablets 5 mg.

Trioxsalen is the first synthetic psoralen compound made available to the medical profession. It possesses greater activity than methoxsalen (1) (2) (3) (4), yet the LD 50 of Trioxsalen is six times that of methoxsalen.

Following is its chemical structure:

ACTIONS

PIGMENT FORMATION WITH TRIOXSALEN
The normal pigmentation of the skin is due to melanin which is produced in the cytoplasm of the melanocytes located in the basal layers of the epidermis at its junction with the dermis. Melanin is formed by the oxidation of tyrosine to DOPA (Dihydroxyphenylalanine) with tyrosinase as catalyst. This enzymatic reaction, however, must be activated by radiant energy in the form of ultraviolet light, preferably between 2900 and 3800 angstroms (black light) (10).

The exact mechanism of the action of psoralens in the process of melanogenesis is not known. One group of investigators feel that the psoralens have a specific effect on the epidermis or, more specifically, on the melanocytes. Another group feels that the primary response to the psoralens is an inflammatory one and that the process of melanogenesis is secondary.

INDICATIONS

Trioxsalen, taken approximately two hours before measured periods of exposure to ultraviolet facilitates:

1. Repigmentation of idiopathic vitiligo. (12) (13) (14) Repigmentation, not equally reversible in every patient, will vary in completeness, time of onset, and duration. The rate of completeness of pigmentation with respect to locations of lesions, occurs more rapidly on fleshy regions, such as the face, abdomen, and buttocks, and less rapidly over bony areas such as the dorsum of the hands and feet. Repigmentation may begin after a few weeks; however, significant results may take as long as six to nine months, and repigmentation, at the optimum level, may, in some cases, require maintenance dosage to retain the new pigment. If follicular repigmentation is not apparent after three months of daily treatment, treatment should be discontinued as a failure.

2. Increasing tolerance to sunlight. (14) In blond persons and those with fair complexions who suffer painful reactions when exposed to sunlight, Trioxsalen aids in increasing resistance to solar damage. Certain persons who are allergic to sunlight or exhibit sun sensitivity may be benefited by the protective action of Trioxsalen (5). In albinism, Trioxsalen will increase the tolerance of the skin to sunlight, although no pigment is formed (6) (7) (8). This protective action seems to be related to the thickening of the horny layer and retention of melanin which produced a thickened, melanized stratum corneum and formation of a stratum lucidum (9) (10).

3. Enhancing pigmentation (3) (4). The use of Trioxsalen accelerates pigmentation only when the administration of the drug is followed by exposure of the skin to sunlight or ultraviolet irradiation. The increase in pigmentation is not immediate but occurs gradually within a few days of repeated exposure and may become equivalent in a degree to that achieved by a full summer of sun exposure. Since sufficient pigment will have been formed within two weeks of continuous therapy, the use of Trioxsalen should not be continued beyond this period. Pigmentation can be maintained by periodic exposure to sunlight.

UNLABELED USES
Trioxsalen is used alone or as an adjunct in the treatment of psoriasis.

CONTRAINDICATIONS

In those diseases associated with photosensitivity, such as porphyria, acute lupus erythematosus, or leukoderma of infectious origin. To date, the safety of this drug in young persons (12 and under), has not been established and is, therefore contraindicated. No preparation with any photosensitizing capacity, internal or external should be used concomitantly with Trioxsalen therapy.

WARNINGS

TRIOXSALEN IS A POTENT DRUG.
Read entire brochure before prescribing or dispensing this medication. The dosage of this medication should not be increased. The dosage of Trioxsalen and exposure time should not be increased. Overdosage and/or overexposure may result in serious burning and blistering. When used to increase tolerance to

▶ SHOWN IN PRODUCT IDENTIFICATION GUIDE

sunlight or accelerate tanning, Trioxsalen total dosage should not exceed 28 tablets, taken in daily single doses of two tablets on a continuous or interrupted regimen. To prevent harmful effects, the physician should carefully instruct the patient to adhere to the prescribed dosage schedule and procedure.

PRECAUTIONS
ACCIDENTAL OVERDOSAGE:
If an overdose of Trioxsalen or ultraviolet light has been taken, emesis should be encouraged. The individual should be kept in a darkened room for eight hours or until cutaneous reactions subside. The treatment for severe reactions resulting from overdosage or over-exposure should follow accepted procedures for treatment of severe burns. There have not been any clinical reports or tests to verify that more severe reactions may result from the concomitant ingestion of furocoumarin-containing food while on Trioxsalen therapy; but the physician should warn the patient that taking limes, figs, parsley, parsnips, mustard, carrots and celery, might be dangerous.

ADVERSE REACTIONS AND SIDE EFFECTS
Severe burns can result from excessive sunlight or sun lamp ultraviolet exposure. Occasionally, there may occur gastric discomfort; to minimize this gastric effect, the tablets may be taken with milk or after a meal. Some patients who are unable to tolerate 10 mg will tolerate 5 mg. This dosage produces the same therapeutic effect but more slowly.

DOSAGE
(Adults and children over 12 years of age)

Vitiligo: Two tablets daily, taken two to four hours before measured periods of ultraviolet exposure or fluorescent black light (10). (See *"Suggested Sun Exposure Guide".*)

To increase tolerance to sunlight and/or enhance pigmentation: Two tablets daily, taken two hours before measured periods of exposure to sun or ultraviolet irradiation. Not to be continued for longer than 14 days. The dosage should *NOT* be increased, as severe burning may occur. (See suggested sun exposure guide.)

SUGGESTED SUN EXPOSURE GUIDE

THE EXPOSURE TIME TO SUNLIGHT SHOULD BE LIMITED ACCORDING TO THE FOLLOWING PLAN:

	Basic Skin Color	
	Light	*Medium*
Initial Exposure	15 min.	20 min.
Second Exposure	20 min.	25 min.
Third Exposure	25 min	30 min.
Fourth Exposure	30 min.	35 min.

Subsequent Exposure: Gradually increase exposure based on erythema and tenderness.

Sunglasses should be worn during exposure and the lips protected with a light-screening lipstick (10).

Sun-Lamp Exposure: Should be initiated according to directions of the sun-lamp manufacturer.

REFERENCES
1. Pathak, M.A., and Fitzpatrick, T.B.: Bioassay of Natural and Synthetic Furocoumarins (Psoralens). J. Invest. Dermat. 32, 509-518, 1959. 2. Pathak, M.A.; Fellman, J.H.; and Kaufman, K.D.,: The Effect of Structural Alterations on the Erythermal Activity of Furocoumarins: Psoralens. J. Invest. Dermat. 35, 165-183, 1960. 3. Lerner, R.M., and Lerner, A.B.,: Dermatologic Medications, Second Edition. Year book Publishers, Pages 98-99. 4. Pathak, M.A., and Fitzpatrick, T.B.,: Relationship of Molecular Configuration to the Activity of Furocoumarins Which Increase the Cutaneous Responses Following Long Wave Ultraviolet Radiation. J. Invest. Dermat. 32, No. 2, 255-262, 1959. 5. Becker, S.W., Jr.,: Prevention of Sunburn and Light Allergy with Methoxsalen, G.P. 19, 115-117, 1959. 6. Hu, F.: Fosnaugh, R.P.: and Lesney, P.F.,: Studies on Albinism, Arch. Dermat. 83, 723-729, 1961. 7. Lerner, A.B.,: Denton, C.R.; and Fitzpatrick, T.B.,: Clinical and Experimental Studies on 8-Methoxypsoralen in Vitiligo, J. Invest. Dermat. 20, 878, 1958. 8. Sulzberger, M.B., and Lerner, A.B.,: Suntanning-Potentiation with Oral Medication, J.A.M.A., 167, 2077-2079, 1958. 9. Becker, S.W., Jr.,: Effects of 8-Methoxypsoralen and Ultraviolet Light on Human Skin. Science, 127, 878, 1958. 10. Stegmaier, O.C.,: The Use of Methoxsalen in Suntanning, J. Invest. Dermat. 32, No. 2, 345-349, 1959. 11. Fitzpatrick, T.B.,: Current Therapy, W.B. Saunders Co., Page 515, 1958. 12. Fitzpatrick, T.B.: Arndt, K.A.; El Mofty, A.M. and Pathak, M.A.: Hydroquinone and Psoralens in Therapy of Hypermelanosis and Vitiligo, ARCH. DERM. 93, 589-600, 1966. 13. Becker, S.W., Jr.,: Psoralen Phototherapeutic Agents, J.A.M.A., 202, 422-424, 1967. 14. El Mofty, A.M.; Vitiligo and Psoralens, PERGAMON PRESS INC., Long Island City, New York, 1st Edition, 1968.

HOW SUPPLIED
TABLETS: 5 MG

BRAND/MANUFACTURER	NDC	SIZE	AWP
○ **BRAND**			
TRISORALEN: ICN	00187-0303-28	28s	$49.62
	00187-0303-01	100s	$147.78

Tripedia *SEE* DIPHTHERIA/PERTUSSIS/TETANUS

Tripelennamine Hydrochloride

DESCRIPTION
Tripelennamine Hydrochloride USP, is an antihistamine for oral administration available as 25 mg and 50 mg of the hydrochoride salt and 100-mg extended-release tablets that provide a gradual and prolonged release of drug.

Tripelennamine Hydrochloride is 2-[Benzyl[2-(dimethyl-amino)ethyl]amino] pyridine monohydrochloride.

Tripelennamine Hydrochloride USP is a white, crystalline powder. Its solutions are practically neutral to litmus. It is freely soluble in water, in alcohol, and in chloroform; slightly soluble in acetone; and insoluble in benzene, in ether, and in ethyl acetate. Its molecular weight is 291.82.

Following is its chemical structure:

ACTIONS
Antihistamines are competitive antagonists of histamine, which also produce central nervous system effects (both stimulant and depressant) and peripheral anticholinergic, atropine-like effects (e.g., drying).

INDICATIONS
Perennial and seasonal allergic rhinitis; vasomotor rhinitis; allergic conjunctivitis due to inhalant allergens and foods; mild, uncomplicated allergic skin manifestations of urticaria and angioedema; amelioration of allergic reactions to blood or plasma: dermographism; anaphylactic reactions as adjunctive therapy to epinephrine and other standard measures after the acute manifestations have been controlled.

CONTRAINDICATIONS
Tripelennamine HCl should not be used in premature infants, neonates, or nursing mothers; patients receiving MAO inhibitors; patients with narrow-angle glaucoma, stenosing peptic ulcer, symptomatic prostatic hypertrophy, bladder neck obstruction, pyloroduodenal obstruction, lower respiratory tract symptoms (including asthma), or hypersensitivity to tripelennamine or related compounds.

WARNINGS
Antihistamines often produce drowsiness and may reduce mental alertness in children and adults. Patients should be warned about engaging in activities requiring mental alertness (e.g., driving a car, operating machinery or hazardous appliances). In elderly patients, approximately 60 years or older, antihistamines are more likely to cause dizziness, sedation and hypotension. Patients should be warned that the central nervous system effects of Tripelennamine HCl may be additive with those of alcohol and other CNS depressants (e.g., hypnotics, sedatives, tranquilizers, antianxiety agents).

Antihistamines may produce excitation, particularly in children.

Usage in Pregnancy: Although no Tripelennamine-related teratogenic potential or other adverse effects on the fetus have been observed in limited animal reproduction studies, the safe use of this drug in pregnancy or during lactation has not been established. Therefore, the drug should not be used during pregnancy or lactation unless, in the judgment of the physician, the expected benefits outweigh the potential hazards.

Usage in Children: In infants and children particularly, antihistamines in overdosage may produce hallucinations, convulsions and/or death.

PRECAUTIONS
Tripelennamine HCl like other antihistamines, has atropine-like, anticholinergic activity and should be used with caution in patients with increased intraocular pressure, hyperthyroidism, cardiovascular disease, hypertension, or history of bronchial asthma.

ADVERSE REACTIONS
The most frequent adverse reactions to antihistamines are sedation or drowsiness; sleepiness; dryness of the mouth, nose, and throat; thickening of bronchial secretions; dizziness; disturbed coordination; epigastric distress.

Other adverse reactions which may occur are: fatigue; chills; confusion; restlessness; excitation; hysteria; nervousness; irritability; insomnia; euphoria; anorexia; nausea; vomiting; diarrhea; constipation; hypotension; tightness in the chest; wheezing; blurred vision; diplopia; vertigo; tinnitus; convulsions; headache; palpitations; tachycardia; extrasystoles; nasal stuffiness; urinary frequency; difficult urination; urinary retention; leukopenia; hemolytic anemia; thrombocytopenia; agranulocytosis; aplastic anemia; allergic or hypersensitivity reactions, including drug rash, urticaria, anaphylactic shock, and photosensitivity. Although the following may have been reported to occur in association with some antihistamines, they have not been known to result from the use of Tripelennamine HCl: excessive perspiration, tremor, paresthesias, acute labyrinthitis, neuritis and early menses.

DOSAGE AND ADMINISTRATION
Dosage should be individualized according to the needs and response of the patient.

Usual Adult Dose: 25 to 50 mg every four to six hours. As little as 25 mg may control symptoms, but as much as 600 mg daily may be given in divided doses, if necessary. Extended-release tablets: One 100-mg Tripelennamine HCl extended-release tablet in the morning and one in the evening is generally adequate. In difficult cases, one 100-mg Tripelennamine HCl extended-release tablet every 8 hours may be required.

Children and Infants: 5 mg/kg/24 hours or 150 mg/m²/24 hours divided into four to six doses. Do not exceed maximum total dose of 300 mg/24 hours. Tripelennamine HCl extended-release tablets are not intended for use in children.

Note: Tripelennamine HCl extended-release tablets must be swallowed whole and never crushed or chewed.

OVERDOSAGE

Signs and Symptoms: The greatest danger from acute overdosage with antihistamines is their central nervous system effects which produce depression and/or stimulation.

In children, stimulation predominates initially in a syndrome which may include excitement, hallucinations, ataxia, incoordination, athetosis, and convulsions followed by postictal depression. Dry mouth, fixed dilated pupils, flushing of the face, and fever are common and resemble the syndrome of atropine poisoning. In adults, CNS depression (i.e., drowsiness, coma) is more common. CNS stimulation is rare; fever and flushing are uncommon.

In both children and adults, there can be a terminal deepening of coma and cardiovascular collapse; death can occur, especially in infants and children.

Treatment: There is no specific therapy for acute overdosage with antihistamines. General symptomatic and supportive measures should be instituted promptly and maintained for as long as necessary.

In the conscious patient, vomiting should be induced even though it may have occurred spontaneously. If vomiting cannot be induced, gastric lavage is indicated. Adequate precautions must be taken to protect against aspiration, especially in infants and children. Charcoal slurry or other suitable agent should be instilled into the stomach after vomiting or lavage. Saline cathartics or milk of magnesia may be of additional benefit.

In the unconscious patient, the airway should be secured with a cuffed endotracheal tube before attempting to evacuate the gastric contents. Intensive supportive and nursing care is indicated, as for any comatose patient.

If breathing is significantly impaired, maintenance of an adequate airway and mechanical support of respiration is the safest and most effective means of providing for adequate oxygenation of tissues to prevent hypoxia (especially brain hypoxia during convulsions).

Hypotension is an early sign of impeding cardiovascular collapse and should be treated vigorously. Although general supportive measures are important, specific treatment with intravenous infusion of a vasopressor (e.g., levarterenol bitartrate) titrated to maintain adequate blood pressure, may be necessary.

Do *not* use CNS stimulants.

Convulsions should be controlled by careful titration of a short-acting barbiturate, repeated as necessary.

Ice packs and cooling sponge baths can aid in reducing the fever commonly seen in children.

Do not store above 86°F (30°C). Protect from light. Dispense in tight, light-resistant container.

HOW SUPPLIED
TABLET, EXTENDED RELEASE: 100 MG

BRAND/MANUFACTURER	NDC	SIZE	AWP
○ BRAND PBZ-SR: Geigy	00028-0048-01	100s	$34.32

TABLETS: 25 MG

BRAND/MANUFACTURER	NDC	SIZE	AWP
◆ BRAND PBZ: Geigy	00028-0111-01	100s	$13.73

TABLETS: 50 MG

AVERAGE UNIT PRICE (AVAILABLE SIZES)		GENERIC A-RATED AVERAGE PRICE (GAAP)	
BRAND	$0.21	100s	$5.66
GENERIC	$0.05	1000s	$42.99

BRAND/MANUFACTURER	NDC	SIZE	AWP
◆ BRAND PBZ: Geigy	00028-0117-01	100s	$20.84
◆ GENERICS			
Major	00904-0035-60	100s	$4.75
Schein	00364-0281-01	100s	$5.67
Richlyn	00115-4871-01	100s	$6.55
Major	00904-0035-80	1000s	$37.50
Schein	00364-0281-02	1000s	$41.06
Richlyn	00115-4871-03	1000s	$50.40

Triphasil *SEE* ETHINYL ESTRADIOL WITH LEVONORGESTREL

Trisoralen *SEE* TRIOXSALEN

Trobicin *SEE* SPECTINOMYCIN HYDROCHLORIDE

Troleandomycin

DESCRIPTION

Troleandomycin is a synthetically derived acetylated ester of oleandomycin, an antibiotic elaborated by a species of *Streptomyces antibioticus*. It is a white crystalline compound, insoluble in water, but readily soluble and stable in the presence of gastric juice. The compound has a molecular weight of 814 and corresponds to the empirical formula $C_{41}H_{67}NO_{15}$.

Following is its chemical structure:

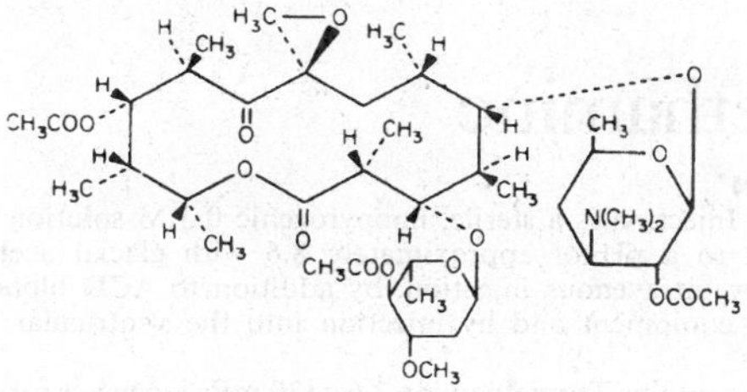

ACTIONS

Troleandomycin is an antibiotic shown to be active *in vitro* against the following gram-positive organisms:
Streptococcus pyogenes
Diplococcus pneumoniae

Susceptibility plate testing: If the Kirby-Bauer method of disc sensitivity is used, a 15 mcg. oleandomycin disc should give a zone of over 18 mm when tested against a Troleandomycin sensitive bacterial strain.

INDICATIONS

Diplococcus pneumoniae
Pneumococcal pneumonia due to susceptible strains.
Streptococcus pyogenes
Group A beta-hemolytic streptococcal infections of the upper respiratory tract.
Injectable benzathine penicillin G is considered by the American Heart Association to be the drug of choice in the treatment and prevention of streptococcal pharyngitis and in long term prophylaxis of rheumatic fever.

Troleandomycin is generally effective in the eradication of streptococci from the nasopharynx. However, substantial data establishing the efficacy of Troleandomycin in the subsequent prevention of rheumatic fever are not available at present.

CONTRAINDICATIONS

Troleandomycin is contraindicated in patients with known hypersensitivity to this antibiotic.

WARNINGS

Usage in Pregnancy: Safety for use in pregnancy has not been established.

The administration of Troleandomycin has been associated with an allergic type of cholestatic hepatitis. Some patients receiving Troleandomycin for more than two weeks or in repeated courses have shown jaundice accompanied by right upper quadrant pain, fever, nausea, vomiting, eosinophilia, and leukocytosis. These changes have been reversible on discontinuance of the drug. Liver function tests should be monitored in patients on such dosage, and the drug discontinued if abnormalities develop. Reports in the literature have suggested that the concurrent use of ergotamine-containing drugs and Troleandomycin may induce ischemic reactions. Therefore, the concurrent use of ergotamine-containing drugs and Troleandomycin should be avoided. Troleandomycin should be administered with caution to patients concurrently receiving estrogen containing oral contraceptives.

Studies in chronic asthmatic patients have suggested that the concurrent use of theophylline and Troleandomycin may result in elevated serum concentrations of theophylline. Therefore, it is recommended that patients receiving such concurrent therapy be observed for signs of theophylline toxicity, and that therapy be appropriately modified if such signs develop.

PRECAUTIONS

Troleandomycin is principally excreted by the liver.

Caution should be exercised in administering the antibiotic to patients with impaired hepatic function.

ADVERSE REACTIONS

The most frequent side effects of Troleandomycin preparations are gastrointestinal, such as abdominal cramping and discomfort, and are dose related. Nausea, vomiting, and diarrhea occur infrequently with usual oral doses.

➤ SHOWN IN PRODUCT IDENTIFICATION GUIDE

During prolonged or repeated therapy, there is a possibility of overgrowth of nonsusceptible bacteria or fungi. If such infections occur, the drug should be discontinued and appropriate therapy instituted.

Mild allergic reactions such as urticaria and other skin rashes have occurred. Serious allergic reactions, including anaphylaxis, have been reported.

DOSAGE AND ADMINISTRATION
Clinical judgment based on the type of infection and its severity should determine dosage within the below listed ranges.

Adults: 250 to 500 mg 4 times a day

Children: 125 to 250 mg (3-5 mg/lb or 6.6 to 11 mg/kg) every 6 hours

When used in streptococcal infection, therapy should be continued for ten days.

HOW SUPPLIED
CAPSULE: 250 MG

BRAND/MANUFACTURER	NDC	SIZE	AWP
○ **BRAND** TAO: Roerig, J.B.	00049-1590-66	100s	$103.43

Tromethamine

DESCRIPTION
Tromethamine Injection is a sterile, nonpyrogenic 0.3 M solution of Tromethamine, adjusted to a pH of approximately 8.6 with glacial acetic acid. It is administered by intravenous injection, by addition to ACD blood for priming cardiac bypass equipment and by injection into the ventricular cavity during cardiac arrest.

Each 100 ml contains Tromethamine 3.6 g (30 mEq) in water for injection. The solution is hypertonic (380 mOsm/liter, calc.) in relation to the extracellular fluid (280 mOsm/liter).

Tromethamine solution is a parenteral systemic alkalizer and fluid replenisher.

Tromethamine, USP (sometimes called "tris" or "tris buffer") is chemically designated 2-amino-2-(hydroxymethyl)-1, 3-propanediol, a solid readily soluble in water, also classified as an organic amine buffer.

Following is its chemical structure:

$$HOCH_2C\overset{\displaystyle CH_2OH}{\underset{\displaystyle NH_2}{|}}CH_2OH$$

CLINICAL PHARMACOLOGY
When administered intravenously as a 0.3 M solution, Tromethamine acts as a proton acceptor and prevents or corrects acidosis by actively binding hydrogen ions (H^+). It binds not only cations of fixed or metabolic acids, but also hydrogen ions of carbonic acid, thus increasing bicarbonate anion (HCO_3^-). Tromethamine also acts as an osmotic diuretic, increasing urine flow, urinary pH, and excretion of fixed acids, carbon dioxide and electrolytes. A significant fraction of Tromethamine (30% at pH 7.40) is not ionized and therefore is capable of reaching equilibrium in total body water. This portion may penetrate cells and may neutralize acidic ions of the intracellular fluid.

The drug is rapidly eliminated by the kidney; 75% or more appears in the urine after eight hours. Urinary excretion continues over a period of three days.

Water is an essential constituent of all body tissues and accounts for approximately 70% of total body weight. Average normal adult daily requirement ranges from two to three liters (1.0 to 1.5 liters each for insensible water loss by perspiration and urine production).

Water balance is maintained by various regulatory mechanisms. Water distribution depends primarily on the concentration of electrolytes in the body compartments and sodium (Na^+) plays a major role in maintaining physiologic equilibrium.

INDICATIONS AND USAGE
Tromethamine Injection is indicated for the prevention and correction of metabolic acidosis. In the following conditions it may help to sustain vital functions and thus provide time for treatment of the primary disease:

1. Metabolic Acidosis Associated with Cardiac Bypass Surgery: Tromethamine Solution has been found to be primarily beneficial in correcting metabolic acidosis which may occur during or immediately following cardiac bypass surgical procedures.

2. Correction of Acidity of ACD Blood in Cardiac Bypass Surgery: It is well known that ACD blood is acidic and becomes more acidic on storage. Tromethamine effectively corrects this acidity. Tromethamine Solution may be added directly to the blood used to prime the pump-oxygenator. When ACD blood is brought to a normal pH range the patient is spared an initial acid load. Additional Tromethamine may be indicated during cardiac bypass surgery should metabolic acidosis appear.

3. Metabolic Acidosis Associated with Cardiac Arrest: Acidosis is nearly always one of the consequences of cardiac arrest and, in some instances, may even be a causative factor in arrest. It is important therefore, that the correction of acidosis should be started promptly with other resuscitative efforts. By correcting acidosis, Tromethamine Injection has caused the arrested heart to respond to resuscitative

efforts after standard methods alone had failed. In these cases, tromethamine was given intraventricularly. It is to be noted, however, that such precariously ill patients often have died subsequently of causes unrelated to the administration of Tromethamine. With administration by the peripheral venous route, metabolic acidosis has been corrected in a majority of patients. The success in reinstitution of cardiac rhythm by this means probably has not been of the same order of magnitude as with the intraventricular route.

CONTRAINDICATIONS
Tromethamine Injection is contraindicated in anuria and uremia.

WARNINGS
1. Large doses of Tromethamine Solution may depress ventilation, as a result of increased blood pH and reduced CO_2 concentration. Thus, dosage should be adjusted so that blood pH is not allowed to increase above normal. In situations in which respiratory acidosis may be present concomitantly with metabolic acidosis, the drug may be used with mechanical assistance to ventilation.

2. Care must be exercised to prevent perivascular infiltration since this can cause inflammation, necrosis and sloughing of tissue. Venospasm and intravenous thrombosis, which may occur during infusion, can be minimized by insuring that the injection needle is well within the largest available vein and that solutions are slowly infused. Intravenous catheters are recommended. If perivascular infiltration occurs, institute appropriate countermeasures. See *"Adverse Reactions"*.

3. Tromethamine Injection should be administered slowly and in amounts sufficient only to correct the existing acidosis, and to avoid overdosage and alkalosis. Overdosage in terms of total drug and/or too rapid administration, may cause hypoglycemia of a prolonged duration (several hours). Therefore, frequent blood glucose determinations should be made during and after therapy.

4. Extreme care should be exercised in patients with renal disease or reduced urinary output because of potential hyperkalemia and the possibility of a decreased excretion of Tromethamine. In such patients, the drug should be used cautiously with electrocardiographic monitoring and frequent serum potassium determinations.

5. Because clinical experience has been limited generally to short-term use, the drug should not be administered for more than a period of one day except in a life-threatening situation.

The intravenous administration of Tromethamine Solution can cause fluid and/or solute overloading resulting in dilution of serum electrolyte concentrations, overhydration, congested states or pulmonary edema.

Additives may be incompatible. Consult with pharmacist, if available. When introducing additives, use aseptic technique, mix thoroughly and do not store.

PRECAUTIONS
1. Blood pH, PCO_2 bicarbonate, glucose and electrolyte determinations should be performed before, during and after administration of Tromethamine Solution.

2. While it has not been shown that the drug increases coagulation time in humans, this possibility should be kept in mind since this has been noted experimentally in dogs.

Do not administer unless solution is clear and seal is intact. Discard unused portion.

Pediatric Use: Hypoglycemia may occur when this product is used in premature and even full-term neonates. See *"Warnings"* and *"Adverse Reactions"*.

Pregnancy Category C: Animal reproduction studies have not been conducted with Tromethamine. It is also not known whether Tromethamine can cause fetal harm when administered to a pregnant woman or can affect reproduction capacity. Tromethamine should be given to a pregnant woman only if clearly needed.

Carcinogenesis, Mutagenesis, Impairment of Fertility: Studies of tromethamine in animals to evaluate the effect of fertility have not been conducted.

ADVERSE REACTIONS
Generally, side effects have been infrequent.

Respiratory: Although the incidence of ventilatory depression is low, it is important to keep in mind that such depression may occur. Respiratory depression may be more likely to occur in patients who have chronic hypoventilation or those who have been treated with drugs which depress respiration. In patients with associated respiratory acidosis, tromethamine should be administered with mechanical assistance to ventilation.

Vascular: Extreme care should be taken to avoid perivascular infiltration. Local tissue damage and subsequent sloughing may occur if extravasation occurs. Chemical phlebitis and venospasm also have been reported.

Hematologic: Transient depression of blood glucose may occur.

Reactions which may occur because of the solution or the technique of administration include febrile response, infection at the site of injection, venous thrombosis or phlebitis extending from the site of injection extravasation and hypervolemia.

If an adverse reaction does occur, discontinue the infusion, evaluate the patient, institute appropriate therapeutic countermeasures and save the remainder of the fluid for examination if deemed necessary.

OVERDOSAGE
Too rapid administration and/or excessive amounts of Tromethamine may cause alkalosis, hypoglycemia, overhydration or solute overload. In the event of overdosage, discontinue the infusion, evaluate the patient and institute appropriate countermeasures. See *"Warnings," "Precautions"* and *"Adverse Reactions"*.

◆ RATED THERAPEUTICALLY EQUIVALENT; ◇ THERAPEUTIC EQUIVALENCE UNCONFIRMED; ○ UNRATED

The LD$_{50}$ values for the acute intravenous toxicity of Tromethamine are influenced by the rate of infusion of the dose administered.

Intravenous LD$_{50}$ Mice = 3500 mg/kg
Intravenous LD$_{50}$ Rats = 2300 mg/kg

DOSAGE AND ADMINISTRATION

Tromethamine Injection is administered by slow intravenous infusion, by addition to pump-oxygenator ACD blood or other priming fluid or by injection into the ventricular cavity during cardiac arrest. For infusion by peripheral vein, a large needle should be used in the largest antecubital vein or an indwelling catheter placed in a large vein of an elevated limb to minimize chemical irritation of the alkaline solution during infusion. Catheters are recommended.

Dosage and rate of administration should be carefully supervised to avoid overtreatment (alkalosis). Pretreatment and subsequent determinations of blood values (e.g., pH, Pco$_2$, Po$_2$, glucose and electrolytes) and urinary output should be made as necessary to monitor dosage and progress of treatment. In general, dosage should be limited to an amount sufficient to increase blood pH to normal limits (7.35 to 7.45) and to correct acid-base derangements. The total quantity to be administered during the period of illness will depend upon the severity and progression of the acidosis. The possibility of some retention of Tromethamine, especially in patients with impaired renal function, should be kept in mind.

The intravenous dosage of Tromethamine Injection may be estimated from the buffer base deficit of the extracellular fluid in mEq/liter determined by means of the Siggaard-Andersen nomogram. The following formula is intended as a general guide:

Tromethamine Solution (ml of 0.3 M) Required =
Body Weight (kg) X
Base Deficit (mEq/liter) X 1.1*

Thus, a 70 kg patient with a buffer base deficit ("negative base excess") of 5 mEq/liter would require 70 x 5 x 1.1 = 385 ml of Tromethamine Solution containing 13.9 g (115 mEq) of Tromethamine. The need for administration of additional Tromethamine Solution is determined by serial determinations of the existing base deficit.

Correction of Metabolic Acidosis Associated with Cardiac Bypass Surgery: An average dose of approximately 9.0 ml/kg (324 mg/kg) has been used in clinical studies with Tromethamine Injection. This is equivalent to a total dose of 630 ml (189 mEq) for a 70 kg patient. A total single dose of 500 ml (150 mEq) is considered adequate for most adults. Larger single doses (up to 1000 ml) may be required in unusually severe cases.

It is recommended that individual doses should not exceed 500 mg/kg (227 mg/lb) over a period of not less than one hour. Thus, for a 70 kg (154 pound) patient the dose should not exceed a maximum of 35 g per hour (1078 ml of a 0.3 M solution). Repeated determinations of pH and other clinical observations should be used as a guide to the need for repeat doses.

Correction of Acidity of ACD Blood in Cardiac Bypass Surgery: The pH of stored blood ranges from 6.80 to 6.22 depending upon the duration of storage. The amount of Tromethamine Solution used to correct this acidity ranges from 0.5 to 2.5 g (15 to 77 ml of a 0.3 M solution) added to each 500 ml of ACD blood used for priming the pump-oxygenator. Clinical experience indicates that 2 g (62 ml of a 0.3 M solution) added to 500 ml of ACD blood is usually adequate.

Correction of Metabolic Acidosis Associated with Cardiac Arrest: In the treatment of cardiac arrest, Tromethamine Solution should be given at the same time that other standard resuscitative measures, including manual systole, are being applied. If the chest is open, Tromethamine Solution is injected directly into the ventricular cavity. From 2 to 6 g (62 to 185 ml of a 0.3 M solution) should be injected immediately. *Do not inject into the cardiac muscle.*

If the chest is not open, from 3.6 to 10.8 g (111 to 333 ml of a 0.3 M solution) should be injected immediately into a larger peripheral vein. Additional amounts may be required to control acidosis persisting after cardiac arrest is reversed.

Parenteral drug products should be inspected visually for particulate matter and discoloration prior to administration, whenever solution and container permit. See *"Contraindications".*

Protect from freezing and extreme heat.

HOW SUPPLIED
INJECTION:

BRAND/MANUFACTURER	NDC	SIZE	AWP
○ BRAND			
THAM: Abbott Hosp	00074-1593-04	500 ml 6s	$817.95

TrophAmine *SEE AMINO ACIDS WITH ELECTROLYTES,*
INJECTABLE

Tropicamide

DESCRIPTION
Tropicamide ophthalmic solution is an anticholinergic prepared as a sterile topical ophthalmic solution in two strengths.

---

* Factor of 1.1 accounts for an approximate reduction of 10% in buffering capacity due to the presence of sufficient acetic acid to lower pH of the 0.3 M solution to approximately 8.6.

The chemical name is benzeneacetamide, *N*-ethyl-α-(nydroxymethyl)-*N*-(4-pyridinylmethyl) the pH range is 4.0 - 5.8.
Each mL contains: Tropicamide 0.5% or 1%.

Following is its chemical structure:

CLINICAL PHARMACOLOGY
This anticholinergic preparation blocks the response of the sphincter muscle of the iris and the ciliary muscle to cholinergic stimulation, dilating the pupil (mydriasis). The stronger preparation (1%) also paralyzes accommodation. This preparation acts rapidly and the duration of activity is relatively short. The weaker strength may be useful in producing mydriasis with only slight cycloplegia.

INDICATIONS AND USAGE
For hydriasis and cycloplegia for diagnostic procedures.

CONTRAINDICATIONS
Contraindicated in persons with primary glaucoma or a tendency toward glaucoma (e.g. narrow anterior chamber angle), and in persons showing hypersensitivity to any component of the preparation.

WARNING
For topical use only—not for injection. Reproductive studies have not been performed in animals. There is no adequate information on whether this drug may affect fertility in human males or females or have a teratogenic potential or other adverse effect on the fetus. This preparation may cause CNS disturbances, which may be dangerous in infants and children. Possibility of occurrence of psychotic reaction and behavioral disturbance due to hypersensitivity to anticholinergic drugs should be borne in mind.

PRECAUTIONS
In the elderly and others where increased intraocular pressure may be encountered, mydriatics and cycloplegics should be used cautiously. To avoid inducing angle closure glaucoma, an estimation of the depth of the angle of the anterior chamber should be made. The lacrimal sac should be compressed by digital pressure for two to three minutes after instillation to avoid excessive systemic absorption.

PATIENT WARNING
Do not touch dropper tip to any surface, as this may contaminate the solution. Patients should be advised not to drive or engage in other hazardous activities while pupils are dilated. Patient may experience sensitivity to light and should protect eyes in bright illumination during dilation. Parents should be warned not to get this preparation in their child's mouth and to wash their own hands and the child's hands following administration.

ADVERSE REACTIONS
Increased intraocular pressure. Psychotic reactions, behavioral disturbances, and cardiorespiratory collapse in children and some adults with this class of drugs have been reported. Transient stinging, dryness of the mouth, blurred vision, photophobia with or without corneal staining, tachycardia, headache, parasympathetic stimulation, or allergic reaction may occur.

DOSAGE AND ADMINISTRATION
For refraction, one or two drops of 1% solution in the eye(s), repeated in five minutes. If patient is not seen within 20 to 30 minutes, an additional drop may be instilled to prolong mydriatic effect. For examination of fundus, one or two drops of 0.5% solution 15 to 20 minutes prior to examination. Individuals with heavily pigmented irides may require larger doses.

Store at 8°-27°C (46° 80°F). Do not refrigerate or store at high temperatures. Keep container tightly closed.

HOW SUPPLIED
DROP: 0.5%

AVERAGE UNIT PRICE (AVAILABLE SIZES)		GENERIC A-RATED AVERAGE PRICE (GAAP)	
BRAND	$1.38	2 ml	$4.37
GENERIC	$1.16	15 ml	$5.90

BRAND/MANUFACTURER	NDC	SIZE	AWP
◆ BRAND			
MYDRIACYL: Alcon Ophthalmic	00998-0354-15	15 ml	$20.75
◆ GENERICS			
OPTICYL: Optopics	52238-0850-03	2 ml	$4.27
Apotex USA	60505-7506-01	2 ml	$4.27
Bausch&Lomb Pharm	24208-0590-59	2 ml	$4.56
OPTICYL: Optopics	52238-0850-16	15 ml	$5.04
Apotex USA	60505-7506-05	15 ml	$5.04
Martec	52555-0089-10	15 ml	$5.85
Bausch&Lomb Pharm	24208-0590-64	15 ml	$7.65

➤ SHOWN IN PRODUCT IDENTIFICATION GUIDE

DROP: 0.5%

BRAND/MANUFACTURER		NDC	SIZE	AWP
○ BRAND				
OCU-TROPIC: Ocumed		51944-4345-42	15 ml	$2.70

DROP: 1%

AVERAGE UNIT PRICE (AVAILABLE SIZES)		GENERIC A-RATED AVERAGE PRICE (GAAP)	
BRAND	$1.82	2 ml	$6.11
GENERIC	$1.52	15 ml	$8.19

BRAND/MANUFACTURER	NDC	SIZE	AWP
◆ BRAND			
MYDRIACYL: Alcon Ophthalmic	00065-0355-03	3 ml	$6.50
	00998-0355-15	15 ml	$22.00
◆ GENERICS			
OPTICYL: Optopics	52238-0851-03	2 ml	$5.63
Apotex USA	60505-7505-01	2 ml	$5.63
TROPICACYL: Akorn	17478-0102-20	2 ml	$7.06
OPTICYL: Optopics	52238-0851-16	15 ml	$6.31
Apotex USA	60505-7505-05	15 ml	$6.31
Martec	52555-0090-10	15 ml	$6.44
TROPICACYL: Akorn	17478-0102-12	15 ml	$9.38
Schein	00364-7386-72	15 ml	$9.50
Steris	00402-0780-15	15 ml	$9.50
Bausch&Lomb Pharm	24208-0585-64	15 ml	$9.90
Bausch&Lomb Pharm	24208-0585-59	2 ml 12s	$89.04

DROP: 1%

BRAND/MANUFACTURER	NDC	SIZE	AWP
○ BRAND			
OCU-TROPIC: Ocumed	51944-4340-42	15 ml	$2.94

Tuberculin

DESCRIPTION

The Tuberculin Tine Test is a simple, multiple-puncture, disposable intradermal test device for the detection of Tuberculin reactivity. These convenient devices are especially useful in mass tuberculosis screening programs.

Each test unit consists of a stainless steel disc attached to a plastic handle. Projecting from the disc are four triangular-shaped prongs (tines) which are 2 mm long and approximately 4 mm apart. The tines have been mechanically dipped into a solution of Tuberculin. Following dipping, the tines are capped and sterilized. The unit is disposable, and there is no need for syringes, needles, and other equipment necessary for the standard intradermal tests.

Tuberculin Tine Test units have been standardized by clinical evaluation in human subjects to give reactions equivalent to or more potent than 5 TU (US Tuberculin units) of standard Tuberculin administered intradermally in the Mantoux test. However, all multiple-puncture-type devices must be regarded as screening tools, and other appropriate diagnostic procedures such as the Mantoux test should be utilized for retesting individuals with positive reactions.

CLINICAL PHARMACOLOGY

Tuberculin deposited in the skin of Tuberculin reactive individuals reacts with sensitized lymphocytes to effect the release of mediators of cellular hypersensitivity. Some of these mediators (eg, skin reactive factor) induce an inflammatory response in the skin causing the induration of erythema characteristic of a "positive" reaction.[3,4]

INDICATIONS AND USAGE

Tuberculin Tine Test is indicated to detect Tuberculin-sensitive individuals. Tuberculin Tine Test units are also useful in programs to determine priorities for additional testing (eg, chest x-rays) and in epidemiological surveys to identify those areas having high levels of infection.

Data obtained from clinical studies with a total of 3,062 volunteer subjects (males and females), ranging in age from 4 to 96 years, of which 47.5% (1,443) were Mantoux positive, clearly demonstrates that Tuberculin Tine Test, when used as a screening test to determine Tuberculin reactivity, is associated with very little, if any, adverse reactivity. Other than the skin test reaction itself, slight vesiculation and slight ulceration were the only adverse experiences reported. The results of the clinical trials revealed a 72-hour false positive rate of 10.9% and a false negative rate of 6.2%.

In clinical studies of more than 1,800 Mantoux positive subjects, only 6.3% gave negative Tuberculin Tine Test reactions at 72 hours; of more than 1,900 Tuberculin Tine Test positive tests, less than 11% gave negative Mantoux results.

In clinical studies covering various geographical areas of the US and all age groups, with a total of 30,588 test subjects, there were 911 (4%) false positive reactors among 26,236 subjects who were Mantoux negative, and 342 (8%) false negative reactors among 4,352 subjects who were Mantoux positive.

The frequency of repeated Tuberculin tests depends on risk of exposure of the individual and on the prevalence of tuberculosis in the population group. The repeated testing of uninfected individuals does not sensitize to Tuberculin. Among individuals with waning sensitivity to homologous or heterologous mycobacterial antigens, however, the stimulus of a Tuberculin test may "boost"

or increase the size of the reaction to a second test, even causing an apparent development of sensitivity in some cases.[3]

Tuberculin testing should be done with caution in individuals with active tuberculosis. (See "Precautions".)

CONTRAINDICATIONS

There are no known contraindications for use of Tuberculin Tine Test. See "Precautions" for information regarding special care to be exercised for safe and effective use.

WARNINGS

There are no known serious adverse reactions or potential safety hazards associated with the use of Tuberculin Tine Test. However, as with the use of any biological product, the possibility of anaphylactic reaction should be considered. See "Precautions" for information regarding special care to be exercised for safe and effective use.

PRECAUTIONS

Tuberculin testing should be done with caution in individuals with active tuberculosis. Although activation of quiescent lesions is rare, if a patient has a history of occurrence of vesiculation and necrosis with a previous Tuberculin test by any method, Tuberculin testing should be avoided.

Although clinical allergy to acacia is very rare, some products contain acacia as stabilizer and should be used with caution in patients with known allergy to this component. In these instances remedial measures for anaphylactoid reactions, including epinephrine injection (1:1000), must be available for immediate use.

Reactivity to the test may be suppressed in patients who are receiving corticosteroids or immunosuppressive agents, or those who have recently been immunized with live virus vaccines such as measles, mumps, rubella, polio. If Tuberculin skin testing is indicated it should be done preceding, or at the time of such immunization, and read 48 to 72 hours later. If the test is not administered in the time suggested, an interval of 4 to 6 weeks should be allowed between Tuberculin skin testing and immunization with live virus vaccines to prevent suppression of Tuberculin reactivity.[5]

With a positive reaction further diagnostic procedures must be considered. These may include X-ray of the chest, microbiological examinations of sputa and other specimens, and confirmation of the positive Tine Test reaction (except vesiculation reactions) using the Mantoux method. In general, the Tine Test does not need to be repeated.

Antituberculous chemotherapy should not be instituted solely on the basis of a single positive Tine Test.

When vesiculation occurs; the reaction is to be interpreted as strongly positive and a repeat test by the Mantoux method must not be attempted. Similar or more severe vesiculation with or without necrosis is likely to occur.

Pregnancy Category C: Animal reproduction studies have not been conducted with Tuberculin Tine Test. It is also not known whether Tuberculin Tine Test can cause fetal harm when administered to a pregnant woman or affect reproduction capacity. Tuberculin Tine Test should be given to a pregnant woman only if clearly needed. During pregnancy, known positive reactors may demonstrate a negative response to a Tuberculin Tine Test.

Tuberculin Tine Test units must never be reused. The units should be discarded into an impenetrable sharps container without recapping.

ADVERSE REACTIONS

Vesiculation (positive reaction), ulceration, or necrosis may occur at the test site in highly sensitive persons. Pain, pruritus, and discomfort at the test site may be relieved by cold packs or by topical glucocorticoid ointment or cream. Transient bleeding may be observed at a puncture site and is of no significance.

DOSAGE AND ADMINISTRATION

Tuberculin Tine Test units have been standardized by clinical evaluation in human subjects to give reactions equivalent to or more potent than 5 TU (US Tuberculin units) of standard Tuberculin administered intradermally in the Mantoux test. However, all multiple puncture-type devices must be regarded as screening tools and other appropriate diagnostic procedures, such as the Mantoux test, should be utilized for retesting reactors.

The volar surface of the upper one-third of the forearm, over a muscle belly, is the preferred site. Hairy areas, and areas without adequate subcutaneous tissue, eg, concavities over a tendon or bone, should be avoided.

Alcohol, acetone, ether, or soap and water may be used to cleanse the skin. The area must be clean and thoroughly dry before application of the Tuberculin Tine Test.

Expose the four coated tines by removing the protective cap while holding the plastic handle. Grasp the patient's forearm firmly, since the sharp momentary sting may cause the patient to jerk his or her arm, resulting in scratching. Stretch the skin of the forearm tightly and apply the disc with the other hand. *Hold at least one second:* Release tension grip on forearm. Withdraw tine unit.

Sufficient pressure should be exerted so that the four puncture sites, and circular depression of the skin from the plastic base are visible.

After administration of the test, local care of the skin is not necessary.

Tuberculin Tine Test units *must never be reused.* The units should be discarded into an impenetrable sharps container without recapping.

Reading Reactions: Tests should be read at 48 to 72 hours. Vesiculation or the extent of induration are the determining factors; erythema without induration is of no significance. Readings should be made in good light with the forearm slightly flexed. The size of the induration in millimeters should be determined by inspection, measuring, and palpation with gentle finger stroking. Identification of

---

◆ RATED THERAPEUTICALLY EQUIVALENT; ◇ THERAPEUTIC EQUIVALENCE UNCONFIRMED; ○ UNRATED

the application site is usually easy because of the distinct four-point pattern. The diameter of the largest single reaction around one of the puncture sites should be measured. With pronounced reactions, the areas of induration around the puncture sites may coalesce.

INTERPRETATION
Positive Reactions:

A. Vesiculation. If vesiculation is present the test may be interpreted as positive, in which case the management of the patient is the same as that for one classified as positive to the Mantoux test.[3]

B. Induration. 2 mm or greater. The test may be interpreted as positive but further diagnostic procedures must be considered. These may include X-ray of the chest, microbiological examination of sputa and other specimens, and confirmation of the positive Tine Test reaction using the Mantoux method.

Negative Reaction:

Induration less than 2 mm. With a negative reaction there is no need for retesting unless the person is a contact of a patient with tuberculosis or there is clinical evidence suggestive of the disease.[3]

Induration indicator cards illustrating typical reactions are enclosed.

STORAGE:
Store at controlled room temperature 15°C to 30°C (59°F to 86°F). Do not refrigerate.

REFERENCES
1. Seibert FB. Isolation and properties of purified protein derivative of tuberculin. *Am Rev Tuberc.* 1934:30:713. 2. Seibert FB. Glenn JF. Tuberculin purified protein derivative—preparation and analysis of a large quantity for standard. *Am Rev Tuberc.* 1941:44:9. 3. Comstock CW. Daniel TM. Snider DE Jr. et al. The tuberculin skin test. *Am Rev Respir Dis.* 1981:124:356-363. 4. Freeman BA. *Burrows Textbook of Microbiology.* 22nd ed. Philadelphia, Pa: W. B. Saunders Company: 1985:295-299. 5. American Academy of Pediatrics. *Report of the Committee on Infectious Diseases.* 21st ed. Elk Grove Village, Ill: American Academy of Pediatrics. 1988:429-447.

HOW SUPPLIED
DEVICE:

BRAND/MANUFACTURER	NDC	SIZE	AWP
○ **BRAND**			
APLITEST: Parke-Davis	00071-4589-13	25s	$56.97

INJECTION:

BRAND/MANUFACTURER	NDC	SIZE	AWP
○ **BRAND**			
TUBERSOL: Connaught	11793-7522-01	1 ml	$11.63
APLISOL: Parke-Davis	00071-4525-03	1 ml	$14.67
TUBERSOL: Connaught	11793-7521-01	1 ml	$20.19
	11793-7526-01	1 ml	$27.31
	11793-7522-02	5 ml	$23.88
APLISOL: Parke-Davis	00071-4525-08	5 ml	$30.34
SCLAVO TEST-PPD: Sclavo	42021-0439-07	1 ml 10s	$5.00
	42021-0439-08	1 ml 50s	$10.00

TEST:

BRAND/MANUFACTURER	NDC	SIZE	AWP
○ **BRAND**			
SCLAVO TEST-PPD: Sclavo	42021-0414-16	20s	$17.00
MONO-VACC TEST (O.T.): Connaught	49281-0770-40	25s	$36.81
SCLAVO TEST-PPD: Sclavo	42021-0414-17	250s	$165.00
○ **GENERICS**			
Lederle Labs	00005-2720-25	25s	$36.93
Lederle Labs	00005-2722-25	25s	$36.93
Lederle Labs	00005-2720-28	100s	$139.79
Lederle Labs	00005-2722-28	100s	$139.79
Lederle Labs	00005-2722-34	250s	$313.04

Tubersol *SEE* TUBERCULIN

Tubocurarine Chloride

THIS DRUG SHOULD BE ADMINISTERED ONLY BY ADEQUATELY TRAINED INDIVIDUALS FAMILIAR WITH ITS ACTIONS, CHARACTERISTICS AND HAZARDS. SEE *"WARNINGS"*

DESCRIPTION
Tubocurarine Chloride Injection, USP, is a sterile, isotonic solution of Tubocurarine Chloride in water for injection for parenteral administration.

Each milliliter (mL) contains Tubocurarine Chloride 3 mg.

Tubocurarine is classified as a nondepolarizing skeletal muscle relaxant.

Tubocurarine Chloride, USP is chemically designated 7', 12'-dihydroxy-6,6'-dimethoxy-2,2',2'-trimethyl-Tubocuraranium chloride, hydrochloride, pentahydrate ($C_{37}H_{41}CIN_2O_6 \cdot HCl \cdot 5H_2O$): a crystalline powder, soluble in water. It is sometimes designated as d-Tubocurarine Chloride pentahydrate and described as

a crystalline alkaloid isolated from native curare sources. The drug is a quaternary ammonium base.

The molecular weight is 771.73.

Following is its chemical structure:

CLINICAL PHARMACOLOGY
Tubocurarine is a nondepolarizing muscle relaxant and produces competitive block of cholinergic receptors at the motor endplate without change in the resting potential of the postjunctional membrane. Its action commences rapidly following intravenous injection, with maximum effect reached within a mean time of 5.7 minutes. The exact duration of action cannot be stated because of variability in dosage studied, choice of general anesthetic agents, experimental design and measurements employed by different investigators, all of which affect the reported results. Muscle paralysis may be expected for periods of 25 to 90 minutes. An approximate description of the duration of action for Tubocurarine is: a paralyzing dose of 0.6 mg/kg is followed by recovery of twitch tension to 25 percent of control within approximately 80 minutes (supra-maximal ulnar nerve stimulation, monitored by quantitation of force-of-thumb adduction).

Substantial amounts of injected Tubocurarine may be retained in various organs of the body long after the neuromuscular block appears to have dissipated. The drug is slowly and only partly metabolized, most of it being eliminated unchanged in the urine. Repeated doses of Tubocurarine produce a cumulative effect.

The paralysis following administration of Tubocurarine is selective initially and usually involves the following muscles consecutively; levator muscles of eyelids, muscles of mastication, limb muscles, abdominal muscles, muscles of the glottis and finally the intercostals and the diaphragm.

Nondepolarization block is not preceded by muscular fasciculations. It is antagonized by acetylcholine, anticholinesterases, potassium ion and cold. Its action is potentiated by potent inhalation anesthetic agents (e.g., halothane, methoxyflurane, etc.) as well as quinine, quinidine, calcium and magnesium salts, trimethaphan, diazepam, large doses of propranolol and hypokalemia. The action of Tubocurarine may be altered by dehydration, hypothermia, hypocalcemia, excess magnesium, acid-base imbalance, the use of certain antibiotics (neomycin, streptomycin, kanamycin, bacitracin), some carcinomas or renal disease and concomitant administration of other muscle relaxants.

Tubocurarine has NO known effect on consciousness, the pain threshold or cerebration. A patient in severe pain may not be able to communicate this to the anesthesiologist.

There is no evidence that Tubocurarine has any direct action on the myocardium. The administration of Tubocurarine may cause hypotension due to histamine release, ganglionic blockade, or to effects of concomitant positive pressure respiration.

Rapid intravenous injection may produce increased release of histamine with resultant decreased respiratory capacity due to bronchospasm and paralysis of the respiratory muscles.

Tubocurarine has no direct effect on smooth muscle structures. Neonates are especially sensitive to the drug.

Pharmacokinetics: Following a single bolus intravenous injection, the disappearance of Tubocurarine from the serum may be calculated to occur in two or three phases. In man, the half-life of the first phase is less than 5 minutes, the half-life of the second phase ranges from 7 to 40 minutes and the half-life of the third phase is about 2 hours. These data may be fitted in a 3-compartment open model.

Tubocurarine is recovered unchanged in the urine and is also excreted unchanged by the biliary tract. The main excretory pathway for Tubocurarine is via the kidneys. Approximately 30 percent of Tubocurarine is excreted unchanged within several hours. When renal function is impaired, prolonged neuromuscular blockade may occur following administration of Tubocurarine.

Little data on the body distribution of muscle relaxants are available. Tubocurarine has been identified in cerebrospinal fluid following intravenous injection, in amounts unlikely to produce any pharmacological effects. Minute quantities of Tubocurarine have also been detected in saliva.

The placenta is a partial barrier to the passage of muscle relaxants. In spite of its low lipid solubility and complete ionization at physiologic pH range, the placental transfer of Tubocurarine is documented. When this drug is used during delivery, blood levels in the newborn are directly related to the maternal dose and the time interval between injection and delivery. Infants in these studies do not grossly manifest drug effect. Myoneural blockade in the newborn has been reported following the administration of repeated doses of Tubocurarine (total dose 245 mg) for prolonged management of eclampsia.

Placental transfer and fetal distribution of d-Tubocurarine during the first trimester of pregnancy is reported. (See *"Precautions—Pregnancy, Nonteratogenic Effects".*)

INDICATIONS AND USAGE
Tubocurarine Chloride Injection, USP is indicated as an adjunct to anesthesia to induce skeletal muscle relaxation. It may be used to reduce the intensity of muscle

contractions of pharmacologically or electrically induced convulsions. Also, it may be used as a diagnostic agent for myasthenia gravis where the results of tests with neostigmine or edrophonium are inconclusive. Finally, it may be used to facilitate the management of patients undergoing mechanical ventilation.

UNLABELED USES
Tubocurarine Chloride is used alone or as an adjunct in the treatment of tetanus and during endotracheal intubation.

CONTRAINDICATIONS
Tubocurarine Chloride is contraindicated in those persons who have shown an allergic reaction or hypersensitivity to the drug and in patients in whom histamine release is a definite hazard.

Tubocurarine is contraindicated in patients who have demonstrated an allergic reaction to the drug.

WARNINGS
TUBOCURARINE CHLORIDE INJECTION, USP SHOULD BE ADMINISTERED IN CAREFULLY ADJUSTED DOSAGE BY OR UNDER THE SUPERVISION OF EXPERIENCED CLINICIANS, WHO ARE FAMILIAR WITH ITS ACTIONS AND THE POSSIBLE COMPLICATIONS THAT MIGHT OCCUR FOLLOWING ITS USE. THE DRUG SHOULD NOT BE ADMINISTERED UNLESS FACILITIES FOR INTUBATION OF THE TRACHEA, ARTIFICIAL RESPIRATION, OXYGEN THERAPY, AND REVERSAL AGENTS ARE IMMEDIATELY AVAILABLE. THE CLINICIAN MUST BE PREPARED TO ASSIST OR CONTROL RESPIRATION.

The drug should be used with caution in patients who are known to have myasthenia gravis. (See *"Precautions".*) In such patients, a peripheral nerve stimulator may be valuable in monitoring the response to administration of muscle relaxants.

The solution may contain sodium metabisulfite, a sulfite that may cause allergic-type reactions including anaphylactic symptoms and life-threatening or less severe asthmatic episodes in certain susceptible people. The overall prevalence of sulfite sensitivity in the general population is unknown and probably low. Sulfite sensitivity is seen more frequently in asthmatic than in nonasthmatic people.

Benzyl alcohol has been reported to be associated with a fatal "gasping syndrome" in premature infants.

PRECAUTIONS
General: Tubocurarine Chloride Injection, USP should be used with caution in patients with renal, hepatic, or cardiovascular diseases. (See *"Clinical Pharmacology".*)

Tubocurarine should be used with caution in patients in whom a sudden increase of histamine release is a definite hazard.

Hypotension may follow the administration of large doses of Tubocurarine.

Tubocurarine has no effect on consciousness, pain threshold or cerebration. Therefore, it should always be used with adequate anesthesia.

Laboratory Tests: Tubocurarine may interfere with the detection of catecholamines. Continuous administration of Tubocurarine, in fairly substantial doses, to patients with tetanus may lead to the production of a factor which seems to interfere with the production and release of catecholamines. This decreased output of catecholamines is detectable when urine total free catecholamines are assayed fluorimetrically.

Drug Interactions: Synergistic or antagonistic effects may result when depolarizing and nondepolarizing muscle relaxants are administered either simultaneously or in sequence.

The maximal intensity of neuromuscular block with Tubocurarine may be reduced if succinylcholine was injected previously. If succinylcholine chloride is used before Tubocurarine, the administration of Tubocurarine should be delayed until the succinylcholine shows signs of wearing off. Synergism has been demonstrated when gallamine triethiodide and Tubocurarine are injected concurrently. The extent of drug interactions is greatly dependent upon the doses and the timing of drug injections.

Parenteral administration of high doses of certain antibiotics may intensify or resemble the neuromuscular blocking action of muscle relaxants. The following antibiotics have been associated with various degrees of paralysis: aminoglycosides (such as neomycin, streptomycin, kanamycin, gentamicin, dihydrostreptomycin), bacitracin, polymyxin B, colistin, sodium colistimethate and tetracyclines. A case suggesting a synergism between intravenously injected tobramycin and curare was also reported. Prolonged apnea in a patient with low levels of pseudocholinesterases and abnormal liver function tests was tentatively associated with a 10 day course of intravenous clindamycin therapy. Therefore, if muscle relaxants and antibiotics which may block neuromuscular transmission must be administered simultaneously, the patient should be observed closely for any unexpected prolongation of respiratory depression.

The administration of Tubocurarine to patients anesthetized with volatile liquid anesthetic agents (diethyl ether, halothane, enflurane and isoflurane) will usually result in a dose related enhancement of neuromuscular blockade and an increase in duration of action. Nitrous oxide in oxygen, intravenous narcotics and most other intravenous anesthetic adjuvants do not greatly affect degree and duration of neuromuscular blockade.

During halothane anesthesia, ketamine hydrochloride may enhance the neuromuscular blockade produced by Tubocurarine.

Clinical cases strongly suggest that quinidine injected shortly after recovery causes recurrent paralysis in patients who received injections of either depolarizing or nondepolarizing muscle relaxants during surgery.

Potentiation of the neuromuscular blocking effects of Tubocurarine were observed in patients with pre-eclamptic toxemia treated with intramuscular injections of magnesium sulfate prior to cesarean section.

Neuromuscular blocking agents are unstable in alkaline solutions. Barbiturate solutions have a high pH and may form a precipitate when they are combined with solutions of muscle relaxants. As a precaution, it is recommended that solutions of barbiturates be given in a separate syringe from muscle relaxants, to assure more uniform and predictable results with each of the drugs. A single needle and tube attached to a three-way stopcock apparatus can readily be adapted to this method if it is desirable to utilize as few of the patient's veins as possible.

A haze developing in 3 hours has been noticed when trimethaphan camsylate at a concentration of 1 gram per liter was mixed with Tubocurarine 60 mg per liter in dextrose 5 percent in water.

Carcinogenesis, Mutagenesis, Impairment of Fertility: Studies of Tubocurarine in animals to evaluate the carcinogenic and mutagenic potential or the effect on fertility have not been conducted.

PREGNANCY
Teratogenic Effects, Pregnancy Category C: Tubocurarine has been shown to cause intrauterine growth retardation and limb deformities resembling clubfoot when administered to rat fetuses between the 16th and 19th day of gestation or when injected in chick embryos from the 5th to the 15th day of incubation. When Tubocurarine was injected intramuscularly into the interscapular region of the fetuses on the 16th to the 19th day of gestation, the incidence of growth retardation and limb deformity ranged from 21 to 23 percent and 7 to 8 percent, respectively.

There are no adequate and well controlled studies in pregnant women. The neuromuscular blocking drugs should be used during pregnancy only if the potential benefit justifies the potential risk to the fetus.

Nonteratogenic Effects: Prolonged administration of large doses of Tubocurarine or other muscle relaxants, used in the management of tetanus in a patient during early pregnancy, may be associated with fetal contractures. Following a total dose of 1,281 mg of Tubocurarine injected intravenously and intramuscularly over a period of 10 days to a 10 to 12 week pregnant woman suffering from severe generalized tetanus, the infant was born at term with joint contractures. The condition was attributed to immobilization of the fetus at the time of joint formation. (See *"Clinical Pharmacology —Pharmacokinetics".*)

LABOR AND DELIVERY
There are no data available concerning the effect of Tubocurarine on the strength of uterine muscle contractions.

Ordinarily, neuromuscular blocking agents are well tolerated by the neonate if used during delivery, especially cesarean section delivery, provided that recommended doses are adhered to and that the interval between use of these drugs and delivery is reasonably short (1 to 10 minutes). Following longer time intervals between drug use and delivery, impairment of the newborn's ability to breathe because of skeletal muscle weakness could occur. No spontaneous breathing occurred in a newborn whose mother had received a total dose of 245 mg of Tubocurarine for the treatment of status epilepticus just prior to delivery. (See *"Clinical Pharmacology —Pharmacokinetics".*)

Nursing Mothers: It is not known whether Tubocurarine is excreted in human milk. There are no data to support gastrointestinal absorption of this drug. Because many drugs are excreted in human milk, caution should be exercised when administering Tubocurarine to a nursing woman.

Pediatric Use: Appropriate pediatric dosages are stated under the *"Dosage and Administration"* section of this prescribing information. Premature infants and newborns are more resistant to the action of depolarizing agents and may be more sensitive to Tubocurarine. However, infants and children exhibit the same widely variable responses to muscle relaxants as do adults.

ADVERSE REACTIONS
The most frequently observed adverse reaction to Tubocurarine is prolonged neuromuscular action, which may vary from skeletal muscle weakness to profound skeletal muscle relaxation resulting in respiratory insufficiency or apnea. Potential adverse effects are listed below by body system.

Body as a Whole: The signs of sudden muscle relaxant-induced histamine release may include one or more of the following: erythema, edema, skin rash, flushing, tachycardia, arterial hypotension, bronchospasm and circulatory collapse.

Isolated cases of allergic or anaphylactoid type reactions have been reported with Tubocurarine.

Cardiovascular System: Cases of cardiac arrhythmias, cardiac arrest, bradycardia, hypertension and hypotension are documented for Tubocurarine. (See *"Warnings"* and *"Precautions—Drug Interactions".*) These cardiovascular reactions are more frequent in children with repeated administration of muscle relaxants (see *"Precautions—Pediatric Use"*).

Digestive System: Excessive salivation is sometimes noted during very light anesthesia (particularly in the absence of anticholinergic premedication).

Respiratory System: Prolonged apnea and respiratory depression have occurred following administration of muscle relaxants. Many physiological factors, drug

---

interactions and individual sensitivities may contribute to the prolongation of respiratory paralysis. (See *"Clinical Pharmacology"* and *"Precautions"*.)

Hypersensitivity to the drug may exist in rare instances.

Idiosyncrasy, interference with physical signs of anesthesia, circulat- ory depression, ganglionic blockade, and release of histamine are complications that can result from the use of this medication.

OVERDOSAGE

Prolonged effects of a neuromuscular blocking agent beyond the desired period of time during anesthesia and surgery and/or overdosage may be manifested by prolonged skeletal muscle weakness, decreased respiratory reserve, low tidal volume or apnea. A peripheral nerve stimulator may be used to assess the degree of residual neuromuscular blockade. Under such circumstances, the primary treatment for an overdose of depolarizing or nondepolarizing muscle relaxant is manual or mechanical ventilation and maintenance of a patent airway until complete recovery of normal respiration is assured.

With Tubocurarine, antagonists such as neostigmine, pyridostigmine bromide or edrophonium chloride may be administered. These antagonists inhibit the enzymatic hydrolysis of acetylcholine, permitting acetylcholine to accumulate and displace Tubocurarine. Injections of neostigmine or pyridostigmine bromide should be accompanied or preceded by an injection of atropine sulfate or its equivalent to minimize the cholinergic side effects, notably excessive secretions and bradycardia. Satisfactory reversal can be judged by return of skeletal muscle tone and respiration. A peripheral nerve stimulator may also be used to monitor restoration of twitch height. Care should be taken to avoid underventilation during the administration of muscle relaxant antagonists. The effects of intravenous neostigmine last for thirty to ninety minutes; the effects of edrophonium may be shorter acting. Intravenous injection of pyridostigmine produces full recovery within 15 minutes in most patients, however, some patients may require a half hour or more. Because the duration of action of the neuromuscular blocking agent may exceed that of the antagonist, careful observation for evidence of recurrent neuromuscular paralysis is essential. The antagonists are merely adjuncts and when a sufficiently excessive dose of muscle relaxant has been used, there is no antidote. Before they are used, the package inserts of these drugs should be consulted for prescribing information.

If hypotension develops following administration of Tubocurarine, the etiology should be determined and treatment, if indicated, should be directed at the etiology. When it is due to ganglionic blockade, hypotension may be treated with fluid load and vasopressors which act at the adrenergic receptors, as required.

The LD_{50} of Tubocurarine given intravenously to mice is 180 mcg/kg and to rabbits is 187 mcg/kg.

DOSAGE AND ADMINISTRATION

Tubocurarine Chloride Injection, USP is usually administered intravenously but may be given by the intramuscular route. The dosage of tubocurarine should always be individualized after assessment of the clinical factors that might alter the action of the drug. If inhalation anesthetics (e.g., halothane or enflurane) or other drugs known to enhance the action of Tubocurarine are employed or renal function is compromised, the initial dose of the Tubocurarine should be reduced and the response used as a guide to incremental doses. (See *"Precautions—Drug Interactions"*.) If enhanced sensitivity is suspected, fractional dosage is advised initially to avoid overdosage. The following are dosages based on body weight intended to serve as guides only.

Adult Dosage: RECOMMENDED DOSES OF TUBOCURARINE CHLORIDE INJECTION, USP USED AS ADJUNCT TO ANESTHESIA:

Conversion Table for Calculating Dosage
20 units are contained in each mL
1 mg equals 7 units
1 unit is contained in 0.05 mL of this solution.

Because of marked patient variability in response to Tubocurarine, dosage recommendations are difficult to determine. For this reason it is better to administer the drug in incremental doses until the desired level of relaxation is achieved. For general reference, effective doses for an adult of 70 kg will be approximately 0.1 to 0.2 mg/kg for paresis of limb musculature, 0.4 to 0.5 mg/kg for abdominal relaxation, and 0.5 to 0.6 mg/kg for endotracheal intubation. In prolonged procedures incremental doses may be repeated in 40 to 60 minutes as required.

Preliminary clinical data indicate that both dosage requirements and recovery times may be increased in elderly patients. RECOMMENDED DOSES OF NEUROMUSCULAR BLOCKING AGENTS DURING ELECTROSHOCK THERAPY: Equipment, antagonists, oxygen and personnel capable of managing airway obstruction, underventilation and apnea should be present during the use of Tubocurarine for electroshock therapy. (See *"Warnings"*.) Tubocurarine should be administered just before electroshock therapy in the treatment of mental disease. The patient should be observed closely until consciousness is regained in case respiratory failure should develop.

Tubocurarine may be administered as a slow intravenous injection (1 to 1-1/2 minutes) until head drop occurs. Dosage should be individualized for each administration. Estimated dosage may be calculated on the basis of 0.1 to 0.2 mg/kg (amount anticipated to produce limb paresis).

Recommended Doses for the Diagnosis of Myasthenia Gravis: Tubocurarine Chloride Injection, USP has been useful as a diagnostic agent in patients suspected of having myasthenia gravis. When small doses are given, a profound exaggeration of this syndrome occurs. The dosage is 1/15 to 1/5 of the average adult limb paresis dose administered intravenously.

Every effort should be made to control dosage to the end that emergencies do not arise. It is important that physicians familiarize themselves with the dangers involved in using the drug and that preparations be made in advance for treating the patient if untoward side effects occur. (See *"Contraindications"* and *"Adverse Reactions"*.) Reversal agents and resuscitative equipment for performing artificial respiration should be immediately available if Tubocurarine is being used as a diagnostic test for myasthenia gravis.

Pediatric Dosage: For induction and maintenance in neonates, 0.3 mg/kg; 0.6 mg/kg in children. A reduction of dosage in the event of prematurity, acidosis, hypothermia, or concomitant use of halothane is recommended.

Parenteral drug products should be inspected visually for particulate matter and discoloration prior to administration, whenever solution and container permit.

Admixtures may be incompatible. (See *"Precautions—Drug Interactions"*.)

To prevent needle-stick injuries, needles should not be recapped, purposely bent, or broken by hand.

Every effort should be made to control dosage to the end that emergencies do not arise. It is important that physicians familiarize themselves with the dangers involved in using the drug and that preparations be made in advance for treating the patient if unwarranted side effects occur (see *"Contraindications"* and *"Adverse Reactions"*).

Tubocurarine Chloride is adjusted to a pH sufficiently low to assure full stability throughout the expiration dating of the product without the need for refrigeration; therefore, because of the high pH of barbiturate solutions, a precipitate will form when Tubocurarine Chloride is combined with such agents as Methohexital Sodium for Injection, USP and thiopental sodium.

It is recommended that each component be given from a separate syringe to assure more uniform and predictable results with each of the drugs. A single needle and tube attached to a 3-way stopcock apparatus can readily be adapted to this method if it is desirable to utilize as few of the patient's veins as possible.

Store at controlled room temperature 15° to 30°C (59° to 86°F).

HOW SUPPLIED
INJECTION: 3 MG/ML

AVERAGE UNIT PRICE (AVAILABLE SIZES)		GENERIC A-RATED AVERAGE PRICE (GAAP)	
GENERIC	$1.22	10 ml	$9.77

BRAND/MANUFACTURER	NDC	SIZE	AWP
◆ GENERICS			
Apothecon	00003-0950-15	10 ml	$8.22
Lilly	00002-1685-01	10 ml	$11.32
Apothecon	00003-0950-35	20 ml	$15.22
Abbott Hosp	00074-8066-01	5 ml 10s	$124.69
Abbott Hosp	00074-3386-04	20 ml 25s	$442.94

Tuinal *SEE* AMOBARBITAL SODIUM AND SECOBARBITAL SODIUM

Tussanil Plain *SEE* CHLORPHENIRAMINE MALEATE WITH PHENYLPROPANOLAMINE HYDROCHLORIDE

Tussar *SEE* CODEINE PHOSPHATE/GUAIFENESIN/ PSEUDOEPHEDRINE HYDROCHLORIDE

Tussionex Pennkinetic *SEE* CHLORPHENIRAMINE POLISTIREX WITH HYDROCODONE POLISTIREX

Twin-K *SEE* POTASSIUM CITRATE AND POTASSIUM GLUCONATE

Two-Dyne *SEE* ACETAMINOPHEN/BUTALBITAL/CAFFEINE

Tylenol with Codeine *SEE* ACETAMINOPHEN WITH CODEINE PHOSPHATE

Tylox *SEE* ACETAMINOPHEN AND OXYCODONE HYDROCHLORIDE

➤ SHOWN IN PRODUCT IDENTIFICATION GUIDE

Tympagesic *SEE* ANTIPYRINE/BENZOCAINE/ PHENYLEPHRINE HYDROCHLORIDE

Typhoid Vaccine

DESCRIPTION

Typhoid Vaccine is a suspension containing an extract from Salmonella typhosa or typhi (Ty-2-strain).

CLINICAL PHARMACOLOGY

Typhoid fever is an infectious disease caused by *S. typhi*. As humans are the only natural host and reservoir for *S. typhi*, infections result from the consumption of food or water that has been contaminated by the excretions of a case or a carrier. *S. typhi* organisms are highly invasive bacteria that rapidly and efficiently pass through the intestinal mucosae of humans to eventually reach the reticuloen-dothelial system;[1] following a 10-to 14-day incubation period, a systemic illness occurs. Typhoid fever exhibits a wide range of clinical severity. Classical cases have fever, myalgias, abdominal discomfort and headaches, and the course is typically more severe without appropriate antimicrobial therapy. Constipation is common in older children and adults, while diarrhea may occur in younger children. Among the less common but most severe complications are intestinal perforation, hemorrhage, and death.[1,2,3]

Typhoid fever is still endemic in most countries of the world where it is predominantly a disease of school-age children and is a major public health problem. Most cases of typhoid fever in the U.S. are thought to be acquired during foreign travel. During the periods of 1975 to 1984 and 1983 to 1984, respectively, 62% and 70% of the cases of typhoid fever reported to the Centers for Disease Control and Prevention (CDC) were acquired during foreign travel; this compares to 33% of cases during 1967-1972.[4]

In 1992, 414 cases of typhoid fever were reported to the CDC. In 1992, of the 414 cases for whom the age was available, 1 (0.2%) case occurred in persons under one year of age; 77 (18.6%) cases occurred in persons one to nine years of age; 81 (19.5%) cases occurred in persons 10 to 19 years of age; 251 (60.6%) cases occurred in individuals $\geq$ 20 years of age; and 4 (0.9%) cases occurred in ages unknown. One death was reported in 1991, however no known deaths were reported in 1992.[5] Domestic surveillance could underestimate the risk of typhoid fever in travelers since the disease is unlikely to be reported for persons who received diagnosis and treatment overseas.[6]

Approximately 2% to 4% of acute typhoid cases develop into a chronic carrier state. The chronic carrier state occurs more frequently with advanced age, and among females than males.[7] These non-symptomatic carriers are the natural reservoir for *S. typhi* and can serve to maintain the disease in its endemic state or to directly infect new individuals[8]. Outbreaks of typhoid fever are often traced to food handlers who are asymptomatic carriers. A six-week course of ampicillin with probenecid has been used successfully for treating chronic carriers with normal gallbladders and without evidence of cholelithiasis.[9,10] There were 53 carriers reported to the CDC in 1986.[11]

The protective efficacy of Typhoid Vaccine was assessed in two trials conducted in areas where typhoid fever is endemic. A single intramuscular dose of 25 μg of Typhoid Vaccine was used in these efficacy studies. A randomized double-blind controlled trial was conducted in five villages west of Katmandu, Nepal. There were 6,907 vaccinated subjects: 3,457 received Typhoid Vaccine and 3,450 in the control group received a 23 valent pneumococcal polysaccharide vaccine. Of the 6,907 subjects, 6,438 subjects were in the target population of 5 through 44 years of age. In addition, there were 165 children 2 to 4 years of age and 304 adults over 44 years of age included in the study. The overall protective efficacy of Typhoid Vaccine was 74% (95% confidence interval (CI): 49% to 87%) for blood culture confirmed cases of typhoid fever during 20 months of post-vaccination follow-up.[12,13,14]

The protective efficacy also was evaluated in a randomized double-blind controlled trial in South Africa in 11,384 children 5 to 15 years of age. There were 5,692 children in the Typhoid Vaccine group and 5,692 in the meningococcal A + C polysaccharide vaccine control group, who were followed for three years post-vaccination. The protective efficacy of Typhoid Vaccine for blood culture confirmed cases of typhoid fever was 55% (95% CI: 30% to 70%) overall during 3 years; and 61%, 52% and 50%, respectively, for years 1, 2, and 3. Vaccination was associated with an increase in anti-Vi antibodies as measured by radioimmunoassay and enzyme-linked immunosorbent assay. Antibody levels remained significantly raised at 6 and 12 months postvaccination.[15]

An increase in serum anti-capsular antibodies is thought to be the basis of protection provided by Typhoid Vaccine. However, a specific correlation of post-vaccination antibody titers with subsequent protection is not available and the level of Vi antibody that will provide protection has not been determined. Also, limitations exist for comparing immunogenicity results from subjects in endemic areas, where some subjects have baseline serological evidence of prior *S. typhi* exposure, to naive populations such as most American travelers.

In endemic regions (Nepal and South Africa) where a large percentage of the population had already been infected by *S. typhi*, the titer of antibodies was increased four-fold or more in 75% to 80% of the vaccinated subjects.[12,15]

Immunogenicity and safety trials in a racially mixed American population in Houston, Texas showed responses, including the geometric mean rise in antibody titer, equal to or greater than those seen in South Africa or Nepal. A single dose of

Typhoid Vaccine induced a four-fold increase in antibody titer in 83% to 96% of an adult population.[13]

No studies of safety and immunogenicity have been conducted in U.S. children. A double-blind randomized controlled trial testing the safety and immunogenicity of Typhoid Vaccine was performed in 175 Indonesian children and 22 adults. The seroconversion rate (4-fold rise in antibody titer) and the geometric mean titers (GMT) as assessed by radioimmunoassay (RIA) for children 2 to 12 years of age were at least comparable to those seen in subjects in Nepal and South African studies. The seroconversion rate in 2- to 5-year-old children was 96.3% (52/54) (95% CI: 87.3% to 99.6%), and in the study subset of 2-year-old children was 94.4% (17/18) (95% CI: 72.7% to 99.9%).[13,14]

Immunogenicity and safety of a primary immunization versus a reimmunization of Typhoid Vaccine was evaluated in a randomized, double-blind, controlled study in Houston, Texas. Antibody titers attained following reimmunization at 27 to 34 months were similar to the titers attained following the primary immunization. This response is typical for a T-cell independent polysaccharide vaccine in that reimmunization does not elicit higher antibody titers than primary immunization.[13]

Because of the very low incidence of typhoid fever in the United States, efficacy studies are not currently feasible in this population. However, the above observations support the expectation that Typhoid Vaccine will provide protection to recipients from nontyphoid endemic areas such as the United States.

INDICATIONS

Typhoid Vaccine, USP is indicated for active immunization against typhoid fever. Typhoid Vaccine is indicated for use at least two weeks prior to expected exposure to *S. typhi*. Based on data obtained from field studies, it has been estimated that Typhoid Vaccine is 70% or more effective in preventing typhoid fever, depending in part on the degree of exposure.

An optimal reimmunization schedule has not been established. Reimmunization every two years under conditions of repeated or continous exposure to the *S. typhi* organisms is recommended.

Routine immunization against typhoid is no longer recommended for persons residing in the United States. Selective immunization is indicated in the following situations:

1) travelers to areas where a recognized risk of exposure to typhoid exists, particularly ones who will have prolonged exposure to potentially contaminated food and water, 2) persons with intimate exposure to (i.e., continued household contact) to a documented typhoid carrier, and 3) workers in microbiology laboratories who frequently work with *S. typhi*.[16]

Although at one time typhoid immunization was suggested for persons attending summer camps or for residents of areas where flooding has occurred, there are no data to support continuation of such practices.[1,2]

Typhoid vaccination is not required for international travel, but it is recommended for travelers to areas where there is a recognized risk of exposure to *S. typhi*, the organism which causes typhoid fever, *S. typhi* is prevalent in many countries of Africa, Asia, and Central and South America. Current CDC advisories should be consulted with regard to specific locales. Vaccination is particularly recommended for travelers who will have prolonged exposure to potentially contaminated food and water. However, even travelers who have been vaccinated should use caution in selecting food and water.[19]

As with any vaccine, vaccination with Typhoid Vaccine may not protect 100% of susceptible individuals.

CONTRAINDICATIONS

Administration should be postponed in the presence of acute respiratory or other active infection.

A severe systemic or allergic reaction following a prior dose is a contraindication to further use.[3]

Immunization should be deferred during the course of any acute illness.

WARNINGS

Typhoid Vaccine has efficacy against *S. typhi* infection but will not afford protection against species of *Salmonella* other than *S. typhi* or other bacteria that cause enteric illness.

Typhoid Vaccine is not indicated to treat a patient with typhoid fever.

Safety and immunogenicity following a third or greater dose have not been assessed. If Typhoid Vaccine is administered to immunosuppressed persons or persons receiving immunosuppressive therapy, the expected immune response may not be obtained. This includes patients with asymptomatic or symptomatic HIV-infection, severe combined immunodeficiency, hypogammaglobulinemia, or agammaglobulinemia; altered immune states due to diseases such as leukemia, lymphoma, or generalized malignancy; or an immune system compromised by treatment with corticosteroids, alkylating drugs, antimetabolites or radiation.[21]

PRECAUTIONS

Care is to be taken by the health-care provider for the safe and effective use of Typhoid Vaccine. A sterile syringe and needle should be used for each patient to prevent transmission of hepatitis B virus and other infectious agents from one person to another. Needles should not be recapped and should be disposed of properly.

EPINEHPRHINE INJECTION (1:1000) AND OTHER APPROPRIATE AGENTS MUST BE IMMEDIATELY AVAILABLE FOLLOWING IMMUNIZATION SHOULD AN ANAPHYLACTIC OR OTHER ALLERGIC REACTIONS OCCUR DUE TO ANY COMPONENT OF THE VACCINE.

Specific information concerning use of Typhoid Vaccine during pregnancy is not available. However, as with other inactivated bacterial vaccines, its use is not contraindicated during pregnancy unless the intended recipient has manifested significant systemic or allergic reactions following administration of prior doses. Use of Typhoid Vaccine during pregnancy should be individualized to reflect actual need. Before the injection of any biological, the physician should take all precautions known for prevention of allergic or any other side reactions. This should include: a review of the patient's history regarding possible sensitivity, and a knowledge of the recent literature pertaining to use of the biological concerned.

The vaccine should not be administered to persons during an acute febrile illness. Any febrile illness or acute infection likely to be accompanied by fever is reason delay the use of Typhoid Vaccine.

Special care should be taken to ensure that Typhoid Vaccine is not injected into a blood vessel.

INFORMATION FOR PATIENTS
Patients, parents or guardians should be fully informed of the benefits and risks of immunization with Typhoid Vaccine. Prior to administration of Typhoid Vaccine, patients, parents and guardians should be asked about the recent health status of the patient to be immunized.

Typhoid Vaccine is indicated in persons traveling to endemic or epidemic areas. Current CDC advisories should be consulted with regard to specific locales.

Travelers should take all necessary precautions to avoid contact with or ingestion of contaminated food and water. One dose of vaccine should be given at least 2 weeks prior to expected exposure.

A reimmunization consisting of a single dose is recommended in U.S. travelers every two years under conditions of repeated or continuous exposure to *S. typhi*.

As part of the child's or adult's immunization record, the date, lot number and manufacturer of the vaccine administered MUST be recorded.[22,23,24]

The U.S. Department of Health and Human Services (VAERS) to accept all reports of suspected adverse events after the administration of any vaccine, including but not limited to the reporting of events required by the National Childhood Vaccine Injury Act of 1986.[23,24] The toll-free number for VAERS forms and information is 1-800-822-7967.[22]

DRUG INTERACTIONS
There are no known interactions of Typhoid Vaccine with drugs or foods.

No studies have been conducted in the U.S. to evaluate interactions or immunological interference between the concurrent use of Typhoid Vaccine and drugs (including antibiotics and antimalarial drugs), immune globulins or common traveler's vaccines (e.g., vaccines for tetanus, poliomyelitis, yellow fever and meningococcus).

CARCINOGENESIS, MUTAGENESIS, IMPAIRMENT OF FERTILITY
Typhoid Vaccine has not been evaluated for its carcinogenic potential, mutagenic potential or impairment of fertility.

PREGNANCY
Reproductive Studies—Pregnancy Category C: Animal reproduction studies have not been conducted with Typhoid Vaccine. It is not known whether Tyhoid Vaccine can cause fetal harm when administered to a pregnant woman or can affect reproduction capacity. Typhoid Vaccine should be given to a pregnant woman only if clearly needed.

When possible, delaying vaccination until the second or third trimester to minimize the possibility of teratogenicity is a resonable precaution.[16]

NURSING MOTHERS
It is not known if Typhoid Vaccine is excreted in human milk. There is no data to warrant the use of this product in nursing mothers for passive antibody transfer to an infant.

PEDIATRIC USE
Safety and effectiveness of Typhoid Vaccine have been established in children 2 years of age and older.[13,14] (See *"Dosage and Administration"* section.)
FOR CHILDREN BELOW THE AGE OF 2 YEARS, SAFETY AND EFFECTIVENESS HAVE NOT BEEN ESTABLISHED.

ADVERSE REACTIONS
Most recipients of Typhoid Vaccine experience some degree of local and systemic response, usually beginning within 24 hours of administration and persisting for one or two days. Local reactions are usually manifested by erythema, induration, and tenderness and should be expected in all those injected intracutaneously.

Systemic manifestations may include malaise, headache, myalgia, and elevated temperature.

Safety of Typhoid Vaccine has been assessed in more than ten thousand subjects in clinical trials both in countries of high and low endemicity. This includes over 4,000 subjects who received the liquid formulation used in the U.S. licensed preparation. The adverse reactions were limited to minor and transient local reactions. Local reactions such as injection site pain, erythema and induration almost always resolved within 48 hours of vaccination. Elevated oral temperature, above 38°C (100.4°F), was observed in approximately 1% of vaccinees in all studies.[13,14]

Adverse reactions from two trials evaluating liquid formulation in Houston, Texas (18- to 40-year-old adults) are summarized in Table 1. No severe or unusual side effects were observed. Most subjects reported pain and/or tenderness (pain upon direct pressure). Local adverse experiences were generally limited to the first 48 hours.[13,14]

In a French postmarketing study, there were 364,651 doses distributed in 1991 and 336,172 doses distributed during the first half of 1992. Between January 1991

and June 1992, adverse reactions were reported in ten (10) patients. Local reactions consisted of erythema, induration, swelling at the site of injection, and urticaria. Systemic reactions consisted of flu-like episode, headache, tremor, abdominal pains, vomiting, diarrhea, and cervical pains. One vaccinee experienced elevated temperature above 39°C (102.2°F).[13,14]

Allergic reactions rarely have been reported in the French postmarketing experience. The most notable reaction reported in the French postmarketing experience occurred in a 24-year-old female with known multiple allergies who had previously received 2 complete series with a whole-cell Typhoid Vaccine and who experienced sweats, myalgia and difficulty breathing starting 2 hours after an IM injection (deltoid) of Typhoid Vaccine. The patient received 10 mg hydrocortisone and did not require hospitalization.[13,14] (See related table).

Adverse reactions from a trial in Indonesia in children one to twelve years of age are summarized in Table 2.[13,14] No severe or unusual side effects were observed. For local soreness and pain, within the Typhoid Vaccine group, the vaccine was less reactogenic for subjects < 5 years of age.[13,14]

Table 2.[13,14]
PERCENTAGE OF INDONESIAN CHILDREN ONE TO TWELVE YEARS OF AGE PRESENTING WITH LOCAL OR SYSTEMIC REACTIONS WITHIN 48 HOURS AFTER THE FIRST IMMUNIZATION WITH TYPHOID VACCINE

Reactions	N = 175
Local	
Soreness	23 (13.0%)
Pain	25 (14.0%)
Erythema	12 (6.9%)
Induration	5 (2.9%)
Impaired Limb Use	0
Systemic	
Feverishness*	5 (2.9%)
Headache	0
Decreased Activity	3 (1.7%)

*   *Subjective feeling of fever.*

Safety data from the U.S. Reimmunization Study conducted in Houston, Texas are presented in Table 3.[13,14] In this study, reimmunization was not associated with significantly more local or systemic reactions than the primary dose, i.e., 5/30 (17%) primary immunization subjects and 10/45 (22%) reimmunization subjects had an objective local reaction. No severe or unusual side reactions were observed. Most subjects reported pain and/or tenderness (pain upon direct pressure). Local adverse experiences were generally limited to the first 48 hours.[13,14]

Table 3.[13,14]
U.S. REIMMUNIZATION STUDY, SUBJECTS PRESENTING WITH LOCAL AND SYSTEMIC REACTIONS WITHIN 48 HOURS AFTER IMMUNIZATION WITH TYPHOID VACCINE

Reactions	Placebo N = 32)	First Immunization (N—30)	Reimmunization (N = 45*)
Local			
Pain	1 (3%)	13 (43%)	25 56%)
Tenderness	2 (6%)	28 (93%)	44 (98%)
Erythema	0	1 (3%)	5 (11%)
Induration	0	5 (17%)	8 (18%)
Systemic			
Feverish (subjective)	0	0	0
Fever ≥ 100°F	1 (3%)	0	1 (2%)
Malaise	1 (3%)	11 (37%)	11 (24%)
Myalgia	0	2 (7%)	1 (2%)
Headache	5 (16%)	8 (27%)	5 (11%)
Nausea	0	1 (3%)	1 (2%)
Vomiting	0	0	0
Diarrhea	0	0	1 (2%)

*   *At 27 to 34 months following a previous dose given in different studies.*

REPORTING OF ADVERSE EVENTS
Reporting by parents and patients of all adverse events occurring after vaccine administration should be encouraged. Adverse events following immunization with vaccine should be reported by the health-care provider to the U.S. Department of Health and Human Services (DHHS) Vaccine Adverse Event Reporting System (VAERS). Reporting forms and information about reporting requirements or completion of the form can be obtained from VAERS through a toll-free number 1-800-822-7967.[22]

DOSAGE
PRIMARY IMMUNIZATION
1. Adults and children over 10 years of age:
   Two doses of 0.5 ml each, administered subcutaneously, at an interval of four or more weeks.

Table 1[13,14]

PERCENTAGE OF 18- TO 40-YEAR-OLD U.S. ADULTS PRESENTING WITH LOCAL OR SYSTEMIC REACTIONS WITHIN 48 HOURS AFTER THE FIRST IMMUNIZATION WITH TYPHOID VACCINE

REACTION	Trial 1 Placebo N = 54	Trial 1 Lot 1 N = 54	Trial 2 Lot 2 N = 50	Trial 2 Lot 3 N = 48	Average N = 152
Local					
Pain	4 (7.4%)	22 (40.7%)	13 (26.0%)	13 (27.0%)	47 31.2%)
Tenderness	7 (13.0%)	53 (98.0%)	47 (94.0%)	48 (100.0%)	148 (97.3%)
Induration	0	8 (14.8%)	3 (6.0%)	2 (4.2%)	13 (8.3%)
Erythema	0	2 (3.7%)	1 (2.0%)	4 (8.3%)	21 (14.0%)
Systemic					
Malaise	8 (14.8%)	13 (24.0%)	0	4 (8.3%)	16 (10.7%)
Myalgia	4 (7.4%)	4 (7.4%)	1 (2.0%)	2 (4.2%)	7 (4.5%)
Headache	7 (13.0%)	11 (20.4%)	8 (16.0%)	8 (16.7%)	27 (17.7%)
Nausea	2 (3.7%)	1 (1.9%)	4 (8.0%)	4 (8.3%)	9 (6.0%)
Vomiting	0	1 (1.9%)	0	4 (8.3%)	9 (6.0%)
Diarrhea	2 (3.7%)	0	2 (4.0%)	1 (2.1%)	3 (2.0%)
Feverish (subjective)	0	6 (11.1%)	3 (6.0%)	0	9 (5.7%)
Fever ≥ 100°F	0	1 (1.9%)	0	0	1 (0.6%)

2. Children less than 0.25 ml each administered subcutaneously, at an interval of four or more weeks.

In instances where there is insufficient time for two doses administered at the specified intervals, three doses of the appropriate volume may be given at weekly intervals.

The immunizing dose is a single injection of 0.5 mL given intramuscularly in the outer aspect of the vastus lateralis (mid-thigh) or deltoid. The vaccine should not be injected into the gluteal area or areas where there may be a nerve trunk.

BOOSTER DOSES
1. Adults and children over 10 years of age:
  0.5 ml, administered subcutaneously,
or 0.1 ml, injected intracutaneously (intradermally).

2. Children 6 months to 10 years of age:
  0.25 ml, administered subcutaneously,
or 0.1 mL. intracutaneously (intradermally)

Under conditions of continued or repeated exposure, a booster dose should be given at least every three years. In instances where an interval of more than three years has elapsed since primary immunization or the last booster dose, a single booster dose is considered sufficient; it is not necessary to repeat the primary immunizing series.

The reimmunizing dose is 0.5 mL. Reimmunization is recommended every 2 years under conditions of repeated or continuous exposure to the *S. typhi* organism.

ADMINISTRATION
Shake vial vigorously before withdrawing each dose.

Before injection, the rubber diaphragm of the vial and the skin over the site to be injected should be cleansed and prepared with a suitable germicide.

For single dose syringes, thread the plunger rod into stopper until the plunger rod bottoms out against the stopper and resistance is felt. Do not over tighten the plunger rod.

After insertion of the needle, aspirate to help avoid inadvertent injection into a blood vessel.

A separate, sterile syringe and needle or a sterile disposable unit should be used for each patient to prevent transmission of infectious agents from person to person. Needles should not be recapped and should be properly disposed.

There are no data on the safety and efficacy of Typhoid Vaccine administered with jet injector apparatus.

Parenteral drug products should be inspected visually for extraneous particulate matter and/or discoloration prior to administration whenever solution and container permit. If either of these conditions exist, the vaccine should not be administered.

STORAGE
Store between 2°-8°C (35°-46°F). DO NOT FREEZE.

REFERENCES
1. Levine MM, et al. New knowledge on pathogenesis of bacterial enteric infections as applied to vaccine development. Microbiol. Rev. 47: 510-550, 1983 2. Levine MM. Typhoid Fever Vaccines, p 333-361. In Vaccines, Plotkin SA, Mortimer EA, eds. W.B. Saunders, 1988 3. Levine MM, et al. Typhoid Fever Chapter 5, In: *Vaccines and Immunotherapy.* Stanley J, Cryz, Jr., Editor, pp 59-72, 1991 4. Ryan CA, et al. *Salmonella typhi* infections in the United States, 1975-1984: Increasing Role of Foreign Travel. Rev Infect Dis 11:1-8, 1989 5. CDC. Summary of Notifiable Diseases, United States 1992. MMWR 41: No. 55, 1993 6. Woodruff BA, et al. A new look at typhoid immunization. Information for the practicing physician. JAMA 265:756-759, 1991 7. Ams WR, et al. Age and sex as factors in the development of the typhoid carrier state, and a method for estimating carrier prevalence. Am J Public Health 33:221-230, 1943 8. Taylor DN, et al. Typhoid in the United States and the risk to the international traveler. J Infect Dis 148:599-602, 1983 9. CDC. Typhoid Fever—Skagit County, Washington. MMWR 39: No. 42: 749-751, 1990 10. Phillips WE. Treatment of chronic typhoid carriers with amoxicillin. JAMA 217: 913-915, 1971 11. CDC. Summary of Notifiable Diseases, United States 1988. MMWR 37: No. 54, 1989 12. Acharya IL, et al. Prevention of typhoid fever in Nepal with the Vi capsular polysaccharide of *Salmonella typhi.* N Engl J Med 317:1101-1104, 1987 (Note: the data presented here include some additional follow-up beyond that published in the article). 13. Unpublished data available from Connaught Laboratories, Inc., compiled 1991 14. Unpublished data available from Pasteur Merieux Serums & Vaccins S.A. 15. Kingman KP, et al. Protective activity of Vi capsular polysaccharide vaccine against typhoid fever. The Lancet, 1165-1169, 1987 16. Recommendations of the Advisory Committee on Immunization Practices (ACIP): Update on Adult Immunization. MMWR 40: No. RR-12, 1991 17. Recommendations of the Public Health Service Advisory Committee on Immunization Practices—Typhoid Vaccine. Morbidity and Mortality Weekly Report 27 (No. 27): 231, 1978. 18. Report of the Committee on Infectious Diseases, American Academy of Pediatrics, 1982 (Red Book). 19. CDC. Health Information for International Travel 1991. U.S. Department of Health and Human Services, Public Health Service 20. Recommendations of the Public Health Service Advisory Committee on Immunization Practices—General Recommendations on Immunization, Morbidity and Mortality Weekly Report (No. 7): 76, 1980. 21. Recommendations of the Advisory Committee on Immunization Practices (ACIP): Use of vaccines and immune globulins in persons with altered immunocompetence. MMWR 42: No. RR-4, 1993 22. CDC. Vaccine Adverse Event Reporting System—United States. MMWR 39: 730-733, 1990 23. National Childhood Vaccine Injury Act: Requirements for permanent vaccination records and for reporting of selected events after vaccination. MMWR 37: 197-200, 1988 24. National Childhood Vaccine Injury Act of 1986 (Amended 1987) A.H.F.S. Category 80:12

J CODES
J6015

HOW SUPPLIED
CAPSULE:

BRAND/MANUFACTURER	NDC	SIZE	AWP
○ **BRAND** VIVOTIF BERNA: Berna	58337-0003-01	4s	$32.95

INJECTION:

BRAND/MANUFACTURER	NDC	SIZE	AWP
○ **GENERICS** Wyeth-Ayerst	00008-0343-01	5 ml	$11.05
Wyeth-Ayerst	00008-0343-02	10 ml	$18.21

Tyropanoate Sodium

DESCRIPTION
Tyropanoate Sodium is a diagnostic enteral cholecystographic radiopaque agent used for radiographic visualization of the gallbladder and biliary tract. Each 750 mg capsule contains 57.4 percent organically bound iodine.

Tyropanoate Sodium is an off-white, odorless, hygroscopic solid which is soluble in water to 14.7 percent. Sodium content per 3 g dose is 100 mg. The molecular weight is 663.1.

Tyropanoate Sodium is a substituted, triiodinated, benzoic acid derivative. Tyropanoate Sodium is sodium 3-butyramido-α-ethyl-2,4,6-triiodohydrocinnamate.

Following is its chemical structure:

CLINICAL PHARMACOLOGY
The most important characteristic of contrast media is the iodine content. The relatively high atomic weight of iodine contributes sufficient radiodensity for radiographic contrast with surrounding tissues.

Diagnostic enteral radiopaque agents have few known pharmacological effects. They are moderately uricosuric. Tyropanoate Sodium when absorbed systemically may produce iodine-mediated thyrotropic effects described under *"Precautions"*.

PHARMACOKINETICS

Tyropanoate Sodium is absorbed by passive diffusion across the gastrointestinal mucosa. Absorption of the agent can be improved by increasing the gastrointestinal pH, drug solubility, and availability of bile salts.

Controversy exists regarding the effects of food on the absorption and clinical efficacy of the cholecystographic agents. In one study, the number of satisfactory cholecystograms obtained with the agent administered with a high-fat meal was greater than with a nonfat meal. However, the fat content of the meal had no significant effect on the number of satisfactory cholecystograms obtained with Tyropanoate Sodium. Therefore, recommendations regarding the size or content of the evening meal on the day prior to oral cholecystography are made at the discretion of the physician.

Once absorbed, Tyropanoate Sodium enters the systemic circulation via the portal venous system. It is then transported to the liver and bound to plasma albumin. The affinity for albumin may determine the primary route of elimination, biliary or renal, with the more extensively bound agents primarily excreted by the hepatobilary system.

In the liver, Tyropanoate Sodium is metabolized to glucuronide esters which are then actively excreted into the hepatic ducts and concentrated by the gallbladder. The time of peak opacification of the gallbladder is approximately 4 to 10 hours for Tyropanoate Sodium. However, diagnostically adequate visualization of the gallbladder may occur within 5 to 6 hours.

Tyropanoate Sodium is removed from the body by two pathways: excretion into the duodenum via the common bile duct and renal elimination. The ratio of renal to fecal elimination for Tyropanoate Sodium is 50:50 respectively in normal subjects. It appears that the bulk of an administered dose is eliminated from the body within a week. However, effects on thyroid function tests may persist for longer periods.

Oral cholecystographic agents are excreted in breast milk. (See *"Precautions—Nursing Mothers"*)

Oral cholecystographic agents may produce changes in thyroid studies attributable to changes in circulating iodide. Thyroid function tests may not accurately reflect thyroid status for up to 1 year following cholecystography. Additionally, oral cholecystographic agents tend to elevate BSP (sulfobromophthalein) determinations. (see *"Precautions—Drug/Laboratory Test Interactions"*.)

INDICATION AND USAGE

Tyropanoate Sodium is indicated for use in oral cholecystography.

CONTRAINDICATIONS

Tyropanoate Sodium should not be administered to patients with advanced hepatorenal disease, severe impairment of renal function, or severe gastrointestinal disorders that prevent absorption.

Higher than recommended or double doses of Tyropanoate Sodium to force visualization is contraindicated, especially in elderly patients or in those with vascular disease.

PRECAUTIONS

GENERAL

Severe, advanced liver disease may interfere with the metabolism of oral cholecystographic agents, and therefore, a greater amount of unchanged drug will be diverted for renal excretion, increasing the load on the kidneys. Acute renal insufficiency has followed the use of oral cholecystographic agents. Most reported cases were attributed to the use of large doses or multiple agents, preexisting dehydration, or hepatic disease.

Renal function, especially in patients with liver disease, should be assessed before cholecystography, and urinary output, serum BUN and creatinine, and hepatic function should be observed for a few days after the procedure. Patients with preexisting renal disease should not receive large doses of cholecystographic agents. All patients, especially those with preexisting renal or hepatic diseases should be adequately hydrated prior to oral cholecystography. Liberal fluid intake should be encouraged after ingesting the diagnostic agents.

Because oral cholecystographic agents are moderately uricosuric, patients with hyperuricemia may be susceptible to the development of uric acid stones and decreased renal function. Therefore, patients with hyperuricemia receiving oral cholecystographic agents should be well hydrated to maintain adequate urinary output and the possibility of uric acid crystal formation should be kept in mind.

Various factors may result in nonvisualization of the hepatic and biliary ducts and the gallbladder. These include gastrointestinal disorders which interfere with absorption, liver disorders which interfere with glucuronide conjugation and excretion, and obstruction of the hepatic or cystic duct which blocks the flow of the contrast medium to the gallbladder.

Cases of hyperthyroidism have been reported with the use of oral contrast media. Some of these patients reportedly had multinodular goiters which may have been responsible for the increased hormone synthesis in response to excess iodine. Administration of an intravascular iodinated radiopaque diagnostic agent to a hyperthyroid patient precipitated thyroid storm. A similar situation could follow administration of oral preparations of iodides. Therefore, caution should be exercised when administering cholecystographic agents to hyperthyroid and euthyroid goiterous patients.

INFORMATION FOR THE PATIENT

Patients receiving oral cholecystographic agents should be given the following information and instructions.

This drug has been prescribed to perform an x-ray study of the gallbladder. All the medication must be taken with water following dinner the evening prior to the test. Thereafter, nothing except water should be taken until the test has been completed.

Patients should be questioned regarding medicine, including nonprescription drugs currently being used. Allergies to iodine, any foods, or x-ray dyes should also be disclosed.

Patients should inform the physician of any liver or kidney disease or pregnancy before taking this drug.

Patients should consult the physician if, at some future date, any thyroid tests are planned. The iodine in this agent may interfere with later thyroid tests.

This drug may cause abdominal cramping, nausea, vomiting, diarrhea, skin rashes, itching, heartburn, dizziness or headache in some patients. Most reactions are mild and pass quickly.

DRUG INTERACTIONS

Concurrent administration of cholestyramine and cholecystographic agents reportedly resulted in abnormal cholecystography. In vitro studies indicate that cholestyramine has an apparent high affinity for the agents. To avoid nonvisualization or poor visualization, oral cholecystography should be performed after cholestyramine has been discontinued long enough for complete evacuation from at least the small bowel.

The administration of both oral cholecystographic agents and intravenous iodipamide meglumine within 24 hours is not recommended. The prior administration of an oral cholecystographic agent seems to block the hepatic excretion of the intravenously administered iodipamine meglumine.

Renal toxicity has been reported in a few patients with liver dysfunction who were given oral cholecystographic agents followed by urographic agents. Administration of urographic agents should therefore be postponed in any patient with a known or suspected hepatic or biliary disorder who has recently taken a cholecystographic contrast agent.

DRUG/LABORATORY TEST INTERACTIONS

Thyroid Function Test: The results of protein bound iodine (PBI) and radioactive iodine uptake studies will not reliably reflect thyroid function for six months, and possibly as long as one year following the administration of diagnostic enteral radiopaque media.

Thyroid function tests, if indicated, generally should be performed prior to the administration of any iodinated agent. However, thyroid function can be evaluated after use of these agents by using T_3 resin uptake or free thyroxine assays.

Liver Function Test: Because increases in sulfobromophthalein (BSP) retention may occur after oral cholecystography, the BSP test is not reliable and should not be performed for at least two days following that procedure. Elevated serum bilirubin may render the examination worthless due to no or poor visualization.

Pseudoalbuminuria may be present for three days following oral cholecystography if determined by certain chemical protein precipitation tests. Post cholecystographic pseudoalbuminuria should be verified by the heat and acetic acid or colorimetric dip-strip methods.

Oral cholecystography may lower blood levels and raise urinary excretion of uric acid for a few days.

CARCINOGENESIS, MUTAGENESIS, IMPAIRMENT OF FERTILITY

Long-term studies in animals have not been performed to evaluate carcinogenic potential, mutagenesis, or whether Tyropanoate Sodium can affect fertility in males or females.

PREGNANCY CATEGORY C

Animal reproduction studies have not been conducted with Tyropanoate Sodium. It is also not known whether Tyropanoate Sodium can cause fetal harm when administered to a pregnant woman or can affect reproduction capacity. Tyropanoate Sodium should be given to a pregnant woman only if clearly needed.

NURSING MOTHERS

Tyropanoate Sodium is excreted in breast milk. Caution should be exercised when Tyropanoate Sodium is administered to a nursing woman.

PEDIATRIC USE

The safety and effectiveness of Tyropanoate Sodium in children under 12 years have not been established.

ADVERSE REACTIONS

Gastrointestinal: The side effects most frequently encountered during Tyropanoate Sodium cholecystography are related to gastrointestinal response, the upper tract being most frequently affected; mild to moderate nausea 10%, with vomiting 2%, and loose stool or diarrhea in about 5% of patients. Severe or persisting nausea and vomiting, diarrhea with abdominal discomfort or cramps are about 1%.

Dermal and allergic reactions are unusual (1% or less) and have been manifest as disseminated pleomorphic rashes, dysphagia, swollen tongue, laryngotracheal or epiglottic edema, periorbital edema, conjunctivitis, wheezing, dyspnea, sneezing, urticaria, or pruritus.

Miscellaneous: Fever, chills, malaise, pain or cramps in limbs, headaches, perspiration, fatigue, and vertigo each occurring less than 1%.

Cardiovascular: Hypotension, tachycardia, and rarely, syncope or shock, and chest pain.

Renal: Dysuria occurs occasionally. Rarely transitory renal failure.

The nature, incidence or severity of side effects are not materially different with a repeat examination.

OVERDOSAGE

There have been no reports on the effect of large overdosage with Tyropanoate Sodium. However, the potential for serious adverse effects with gross overdosage of water-soluble media such as Tyropanoate Sodium would be expected to be much greater than with poorly soluble iopanoic acid since these media are rapidly absorbed, creating early high serum levels with particular potential for hepatorenal or cardiovascular dysfunction. Therefore, the following empirical measures are suggested:

- Lavage the stomach and administer enemas to remove remaining potentially absorbable contrast material.
- Force fluids to avoid concentration and possible precipitation or crystallization of the contrast material or uric acid in the kidneys.
- Alkalinize the urine to increase the solubility of the drug-glucuronide complex and of uric acid.
- Administer cholestyramine to chelate and reduce absorption of the drug.
- Monitor blood pressure.

The normal serum levels of iodine following a single 3 g dose achieved between one and four hours is approximately 100 mcgI/mL to 150 mcgI/mL of Tyropanoate Sodium.

The acute oral LD^{50} of Tyropanoate Sodium in the mouse is 4.8 ± 1.45 to 16.3 ± 1.83 g/kg ± Standard Error.

DOSAGE AND ADMINISTRATION

A single dose of 3 g (4 capsules) is recommended for adults. The optimal time interval between administration of Tyropanoate Sodium and cholecystography is 10 to 12 hours, although satisfactory results have been reported as early as 4 to 6 hours.

If no visualization occurs after administration of Tyropanoate Sodium, repeat examination with a 3 g dose is recommended on the following day. *Increasing the amount of the repeat dose is not recommended.*

Cholestasis is a common cause of nonvisualization in patients who have been on almost completely fat-free diets. To reduce the incidence of false-negative nonvisualization, such patients should eat a diet containing some fat for one or two days before cholecystographic examination. Fat is a long-acting cholecystagogue, and will stimulate emptying of the gallbladder and prepare it to receive the radiopaque medium. *The meal immediately before ingestion of the Tyropanoate Sodium capsules should be fat free.*

Preparatory dehydration is unnecessary and undesirable, especially in elderly patients. After the fat-free evening meal, the patient should swallow 4 Tyropanoate Sodium capsules (3 g) with water. Between ingestion of Tyropanoate Sodium and cholecystographic examination, the patient should take nothing by mouth except water, and should not smoke or chew gum.

Many physicians believe that the quality of gallbladder visualization is enhanced when the intestine is relatively free of residue. This may be achieved with an enema the morning of the examination, or a laxative the day before.

For observation of gallbladder contractility, the patient may be given a fatty meal or a cholecystagogue after the initial x-ray examination. Additional exposures may be made 5 to 30 minutes later.

Nonvisualization: Nonvisualization in routine cholecystography with Tyropanoate Sodium usually implies substantial loss of gallbladder function. However, nonvisualization may also result on occasion from other factors not related to disease of the biliary tract.

Repeat Examination: When adequate visualization is not obtained initially, repeat cholecystography with the recommended dose of 3 g helps reduce the possibility of diagnostic error. A larger dose is not recommended. Disease may be inferred with reasonable certainty if the gallbladder does not visualize on repeat examination.

HOW SUPPLIED
CAPSULE: 750 MG

BRAND/MANUFACTURER	NDC	SIZE	AWP
○ BRAND			
BILOPAQUE SODIUM: Sanofi Winthrop	00024-0134-03	100s	$113.96

Tyzine Nasal *SEE* TETRAHYDROZOLINE
HYDROCHLORIDE

Ucephan *SEE* SODIUM BENZOATE AND SODIUM
PHENYLACETATE

Ugesic *SEE* ACETAMINOPHEN WITH HYDROCODONE
BITARTRATE

Ultracef *SEE* CEFADROXIL MONOHYDRATE

Ultrase *SEE* PANCRELIPASE

Ultravate *SEE* HALOBETASOL PROPIONATE

Unasyn *SEE* AMPICILLIN SODIUM AND SULBACTAM SODIUM

Unipen *SEE* NAFCILLIN SODIUM

Uniphyl *SEE* THEOPHYLLINE

Uracil Mustard

DESCRIPTION

Uracil Mustard, 5-[bis (2-chloroethyl) amino] uracil, is an off-white, odorless crystalline compound which is slightly soluble in methanol and in acetone. It is unstable in the presence of water and reacts with many organic substances, including the carbonyl and amino groups of proteins including, in all probability, the nucleoproteins of the cell nucleus.

Uracil Mustard capsules for oral administration contain 1 mg of Uracil Mustard.

Following is its chemical structure:

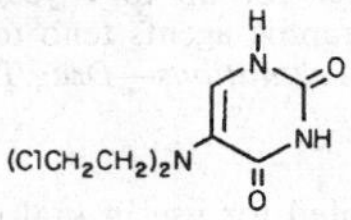

CLINICAL PHARMACOLOGY

Uracil Mustard is an orally active alkylating agent belonging to the class of substances known as nitrogen mustards. Clinically, Uracil Mustard, like other nitrogen mustards, has been found to be of value in the palliative treatment of certain neoplasms affecting the reticuloendothelial system.

INDICATIONS AND USAGE

Chronic Lymphocytic Leukemia: Uracil Mustard is usually effective in the palliative treatment of symptomatic chronic lymphocytic leukemia.

Non-Hodgkin's Lymphomas: Uracil Mustard is effective for palliative treatment of lymphomas of the histiocytic or lymphocytic type.

Chronic Myelogenous Leukemia: Uracil Mustard may be effective in the palliative treatment of patients with chronic myelogenous leukemia. It is not effective in the acute blastic crisis or in patients with acute leukemia.

Other Conditions: Uracil Mustard may be effective in the palliative treatment of early stages of polycythemia vera before the development of leukemia or myelofibrosis. It may also be beneficial as palliative therapy in mycosis fungoides.

CONTRAINDICATIONS

Uracil Mustard should not be given to any patient with severe leukopenia or thrombocytopenia.

WARNINGS

Usage in Pregnancy: Drugs of the nitrogen mustard group have been shown to produce fetal abnormalities in experimental animals when given during pregnancy. Uracil Mustard should not be used during pregnancy unless in the opinion of the physician the potential benefits outweigh the possible hazards.

Alkylating agents are carcinogenic in animals and suspect as carcinogens in humans. Their possible effect on fertility should be considered: amenorrhea and impaired spermatogenesis have been reported following therapy with alkylating compounds.

Uracil Mustard has a cumulative toxic effect against the hematopoietic system. Blood counts including platelet counts should be done once or twice weekly.

PRECAUTIONS

Patients receiving Uracil Mustard must be followed carefully to avoid the possibility of irreversible damage to the bone marrow. Therapy with this agent should be discontinued if severe depression of the bone marrow occurs, as indicated by sharp diminution in any of the formed blood elements.

While therapy with Uracil Mustard need not be discontinued following initial depression of blood counts, it should be realized that maximum depression of bone marrow function may not occur until 2 to 4 weeks after discontinuance of

---

◆ RATED THERAPEUTICALLY EQUIVALENT; ◇ THERAPEUTIC EQUIVALENCE UNCONFIRMED; ○ UNRATED

the drug, and that as the total accumulated doses approach 1 mg/kg there is real danger of producing irreversible damage to the bone marrow.

While there is no specific therapy for severe depression of the bone marrow, frequent blood and blood component transfusions, with antibiotics to combat secondary infection, may sustain the patient until recovery has occurred.

Some brands of Uracil Mustard contain FD&C Yellow No. 5 (tartrazine), which may cause allergic-type reactions (including bronchial asthma) in certain susceptible individuals. Although the overall incidence of FD&C Yellow No. 5 (tartrazine) sensitivity in the general population is low, it is frequently seen in patients who also have aspirin hypersensitivity.

ADVERSE REACTIONS

In addition to its toxic effects on the hematopoietic system (see *"Precautions"* and *"Contraindications"*), evidence of toxicity may be manifested by nausea, vomiting or diarrhea of varying degrees of severity. These are related to the size of the dose, ie. the greater the dose, the more severe the symptoms. Other side reactions, some of which may not be related to administration of the drug, include nervousness, irritability or depression and various skin reactions such as pruritus, dermatitis and some loss of hair. Frank alopecia has not been reported to date.

DOSAGE AND ADMINISTRATION

Uracil Mustard should not be administered until about 2 or 3 weeks after the maximum effect of any previous X-ray or cytotoxic drug therapy upon the bone marrow has been obtained. An increasing white blood cell count is probably the best criterion for determining that such maximum effect has subsided. Some investigators prefer to wait until the blood count has returned to normal before beginning a new course of therapy. In the presence of pronounced leukopenia, thrombocytopenia, or aplastic anemia, Uracil Mustard should not be administered. In the presence of bone marrow infiltrated with malignant cells, hematopoietic toxicity may be increased and judicious care must be used during administration.

The following are suggested dosage schedules:

Adults: A single weekly dose of 0.15 mg/kg of body weight should be given for 4 weeks to provide an adequate trial.

Children: A single weekly dose of 0.30 mg/kg of body weight should be given for 4 weeks to provide an adequate trial.

If response occurs, the same dose may be continued weekly until relapse. These dosages must be carefully individualized and the dose reduced or discontinued in accordance with the severity of depression of bone marrow function.

Procedures for proper handling and disposal of anticancer drugs should be considered. Several guidelines on this subject have been published.[1-4] There is no general agreement that all of the procedures recommended in the guidelines are necessary or appropriate.

ANIMAL PHARMACOLOGY AND TOXICITY

Pharmacologic studies have shown that Uracil Mustard is readily absorbed following oral administration, the orally effective dose in certain rat tumors being almost the same as the parenteral dose. In rats the LDse's are 7.5 mg/kg orally, 6.2 mg/kg subcutaneously and 3.7 mg/kg intraperitoneally. Thus, the oral and subcutaneous toxicities appear to be about one-half the intraperitoneal toxicity.

Subacute and chronic oral toxicity studies in animals indicate that Uracil Mustard produces toxic effects characteristic of nitrogen mustards. These effects include depression of the hematopoietic system as indicated initially by severe thrombocytopenia, granulocytic and lymphocytic leukopenia and later by depression of the erythrocyte count and hemoglobin values. Other evidence of toxicity in laboratory animals included anorexia, weight loss, bleeding from the gastrointestinal tract, muscular weakness and moribund states.

Experimental studies have shown that Uracil Mustard is a highly potent inducer of malignant lung tumors in A-strain mice.

REFERENCES

1. Recommendations for the Safe Handling of Parenteral Antineoplastic Drugs. NIH Publication No. 83-2621. For sale by the Superintendent of Documents, US Government Printing Office, Washington, DC 20402. 2. AMA Council Report. Guidelines for Handling Parenteral Antineoplastics, JAMA, March 15, 1985. 3. National Study Commission on Cytotoxic Exposure. Recommendations for Handling Cytotoxic Agents. Available from L.P. Jeffrey, ScD. Director of Pharmacy Services, Rhode Island Hospital, 593 Eddy St., Providence, Rhode Island 02902. 4. Clinical Oncological Society of Australia: Guidelines and recommendations for safe handling of antineoplastic agents. MedJ Australia 1:426-428, 1983. 5. Jones, RB, et al. Safe handling of chemotherapeutic agents: A report from the Mount Sinai Medical Center. Cs-A Cancer Journal for Clinicians Sept/Oct., 1983, pp 258-263. 6. American Society of Hospital Pharmacists technical assistance bulletin on handling cytotoxic drugs in hospitals. AmJ Hosp Pharmacists 42:131-137, 1985.

HOW SUPPLIED
CAPSULE: 1 MG

BRAND/MANUFACTURER	NDC	SIZE	AWP
○ GENERICS			
Roberts Pharm	54092-0039-50	50s	$55.62

Urecholine SEE BETHANECHOL CHLORIDE

Urex SEE METHENAMINE HIPPURATE

Urised SEE ATROPINE SULFATE/BENZOIC ACID/ HYOSCYAMINE/METHENAMINE/METHYLENE BLUE/ PHENYLSALICYLATE

Urisedamine SEE METHENAMINE MANDELATE AND SODIUM ACID PHOSPHATE

Urispas SEE FLAVOXATE HYDROCHLORIDE

Uro-Phosphate SEE METHENAMINE MANDELATE AND SODIUM ACID PHOSPHATE

Urobiotic-250 SEE OXYTETRACYCLINE HYDROCHLORIDE/PHENAZOPYRIDINE/SULFAMETHIZOLE

Urofollitropin

DESCRIPTION

Urofollitropin for injection is a preparation of gonadotropin extracted from the urine of postmenopausal women. Each ampule of Urofollitropin contains 75 IU of follicle-stimulating hormone (FSH) activity in not more than 0.83 mg of extract, plus 10 mg lactose in a sterile, lyophilized form. Urofollitropin is administered by intramuscular injection.

Urofollitropin contains an acidic, water soluble glycoprotein biologically standardized for FSH gonadotropin activity in terms of the Second International Reference Preparation for Human Menopausal Gonadotropins, established in September, 1964 by the Expert Committee on Biological Standards of the World Health Organization. Negligible amounts (less than 1 IU per 75 IU FSH) of luteinizing hormone (LH) activity are contained in Urofollitropin.

Therapeutic Class: Infertility.

CLINICAL PHARMACOLOGY

Urofollitropin stimulates ovarian follicular growth in women who do not have primary ovarian failure. Treatment with Urofollitropin in most instances results only in follicular growth and maturation. In order to effect ovulation in the absence of an endogenous LH surge, human chorionic gonadotropin (hCG) must be given following the administration of Urofollitropin when clinical and laboratory assessment of the patient indicates that sufficient follicular maturation has occurred.

INDICATIONS AND USAGE

Urofollitropin and hCG given in a sequential manner are indicated for the induction of ovulation in patients with polycystic ovarian syndrome (PCO) who have an elevated LH/FSH ratio and who have failed to respond to adequate clomiphene citrate therapy.

Urofollitropin and hCG may also be used to stimulate the development of multiple oocytes in ovulatory patients participating in an in vitro fertilization program.

SELECTION OF PATIENTS

1. Before treatment with Urofollitropin is instituted, a thorough gynecologic and endocrinologic evaluation must be performed. This should include a hysterosalpingogram (to rule out uterine and tubal pathology) and documentation of anovulation by means of basal body temperature, serial vaginal smears, examination of cervical mucus, determination of serum (or urinary) progesterone, urinary pregnanediol and endometrial biopsy. Patients with tubal pathology should receive Urofollitropin only if enrolled in an in vitro fertilization program.

2. Primary ovarian failure should be excluded by the determination of gonadotropin levels.

3. Careful examination should be made to rule out the presence of early pregnancy.

4. Patients in late reproductive life have a greater predilection to endometrial carcinoma as well as a higher incidence of anovulatory disorders. Cervical dilation and curettage should always be done for diagnosis before starting Urofollitropin therapy in such patients who demonstrate abnormal uterine bleeding or other signs of endometrial abnormalities.

5. Evaluation of the husband's fertility potential should be included in the workup.

UNLABELED USES

Urofollitropin is used alone or as an adjunct in correcting luteal phase defect and in *in vitro* fertilization.

CONTRAINDICATIONS

Urofollitropin is contraindicated in women who exhibit:

1. High levels of FSH indicating primary ovarian failure.

2. Uncontrolled thyroid or adrenal dysfunction.

3. An organic intracranial lesion such as a pituitary tumor.

4. The presence of any cause of infertility other than anovulation, as stated in the *"Indications"* unless they are candidates for in vitro fertilization.

5. Abnormal bleeding of undetermined origin (see *"Selection of Patients"*).

6. Ovarian cysts or enlargement not due to polycystic ovarian syndrome.

7. Prior hypersensitivity to Urofollitropin.

8. Urofollitropin is contraindicated in women who are pregnant and may cause fetal harm when administered to a pregnant woman. There are limited human data on the effects of Urofollitropin when administered during pregnancy.

WARNINGS

Urofollitropin is a drug that should only be used by physicians who are thoroughly familar with infertility problems. It is a potent gonadotropic substance capable of causing mild to severe adverse reactions. Gonadotropin therapy requires a certain time commitment by physicians and supportive health professionals, and its use requires the availability of appropriate monitoring facilities (See *"Precautions/ Laboratory Tests"*). It must be used with a great deal of care.

OVERSTIMULATION OF THE OVARY DURING UROFOLLITROPIN THERAPY

Ovarian Enlargement: Mild to moderate uncomplicated ovarian enlargement, which may be accompanied by abdominal distension and/or abdominal pain, occurs in approximately 20% of those treated with Urofollitropin and hCG, and generally regresses without treatment within two or three weeks.

In order to minimize the hazard associated with the occasional abnormal ovarian enlargement which may occur with Urofollitropin hCG therapy, the lowest dose consistent with expectation of good results should be used. Careful monitoring of ovarian response can further minimize the risk of overstimulation.

If the ovaries are abnormally enlarged on the last day of Urofollitropin therapy, hCG should not be administered in this course of therapy. This will reduce the chances of development of the Ovarian Hyperstimulation Syndrome.

The Ovarian Hyperstimulation Syndrome (OHSS): OHSS is a medical event distinct from uncomplicated ovarian enlargement. OHSS may progress rapidly (within 24 hours to several days) to become a serious medical event. It is characterized by an apparent dramatic increase in vascular permeability which can result in a rapid accumulation of fluid in the peritoneal cavity, thorax, and potentially, the pericardium. The early warning signs of development of OHSS are severe pelvic pain, nausea, vomiting, and weight gain. The following symptomatology has been seen with cases of OHSS: abdominal pain, abdominal distension, gastrointestinal symptoms including nausea, vomiting and diarrhea, severe ovarian enlargement, weight gain, dyspnea, and oliguria. Clinical evaluation may reveal hypovolemia, hemoconcentration, electrolyte imbalances, ascites, hemoperitoneum, pleural effusion, hydrothorax, acute pulmonary distress, and thromboembolic events (see *"Pulmonary and Vascular Complications"*). Transient liver function test abnormalities suggestive of hepatic dysfunction, which may be accompanied by morphologic changes on liver biopsy, have been reported in association with the Ovarian Hyperstimulation Syndrome (OHSS).

OHSS occurred in approximately 6.0% of patients treated with Urofollitropin therapy in the initial clinical trials, in patients treated for anovulation due to polycystic ovarian syndrome. During studies for in vitro fertilization, four cases of the Ovarian Hyperstimulation Syndrome were reported following 1,586 treatment cycles (0.25%). Cases of OHSS are more common, more severe, and more protracted if pregnancy occurs. OHSS develops rapidly; therefore, patients should be followed for at least two weeks after hCG administration. Most often, OHSS occurs after treatment has been discontinued and reaches its maximum at about seven to ten days following treatment. Usually, OHSS resolves spontaneously with the onset of menses. If there is evidence that OHSS may be developing prior to hCG administration (see *"Precautions/Laboratory Tests"*), the hCG should be withheld.

If OHSS occurs, treatment should be stopped and the patient should be hospitalized. Treatment is primarily symptomatic and should consist of bed rest, fluid and electrolyte management, and analgesics if needed. The phenomenon of hemoconcentration associated with fluid loss into the peritoneal cavity, pleural cavity, and the pericardial cavity has been seen to occur and should be thoroughly assessed in the following manner: 1) fluid intake and output, 2) weight, 3) hematocrit, 4) serum and urinary electrolytes, 5) urine specific gravity, 6) BUN and creatinine, and 7) abdominal girth. These determinations are to be performed daily or more often if the need arises.

With OHSS there is an increased risk of injury to the ovary. The ascitic, pleural, and pericardial fluid should not be removed unless absolutely necessary to relieve symptoms such as pulmonary distress or cardiac tamponade. Pelvic examination may cause rupture of an ovarian cyst, which may result in hemoperitoneum, and should therefore be avoided. If this does occur, and if bleeding becomes such that surgery is required, the surgical treatment should be designed to control bleeding and to retain as much ovarian tissue as possible. Intercourse should be prohibited in those patients in whom significant ovarian enlargement occurs after ovulation because of the danger of hemoperitoneum resulting from ruptured ovarian cysts.

The management of OHSS may be divided into three phases; the acute, the chronic, and the resolution phases. Because the use of diuretics can accentuate the diminished intravascular volume, diuretics should be avoided except in the late phase of resolution as described below.

Acute Phase: Management during the acute phase should be designed to prevent hemoconcentration due to loss of intravascular volume to the third space and to minimize the risk of thromboembolic phenomena and kidney damage. Treatment is designed to normalize electrolytes while maintaining an acceptable but somewhat reduced intravascular volume. Full correction of the intravascular volume deficit may lead to an unacceptable increase in the amount of third space fluid accumulation. Management includes administration of limited intravenous fluids, electrolytes, and human serum albumin. Monitoring for the development of hyperkalemia is recommended.

Chronic Phase: After stabilizing the patient during the acute phase, excessive fluid accumulation in the third space should be limited by instituting, severe potassium, sodium, and fluid restriction.

Resolution Phase: A fall in hematocrit and an increasing urinary output without an increased intake are observed due to the return of third space fluid to the intravascular compartment. Peripheral and/or pulmonary edema may result if the kidneys are unable to excrete third space fluid as rapidly as it is mobilized. Diuretics may be indicated during the resolution phase if necessary to combat pulmonary edema.

Pulmonary and Vascular Complications: The following paragraph describes serious medical events reported following gonadotropin therapy.

Serious pulmonary conditions (e.g., atelectasis, acute respiratory distress syndrome) have been reported. In addition, thromboembolic events both in association with, and separate from the Ovarian Hyperstimulation Syndrome have been reported. Intravascular thrombosis and embolism, which may originate in venous or arterial vessels, can result in reduced blood flow to critical organs or the extremities. Sequelae of such events have included venous thrombophlebitis, pulmonary embolism, pulmonary infarction, cerebral vascular occlusion (stroke), and arterial occlusion resulting in loss of limb. In rare cases, pulmonary complications and/or thromboembolic events have resulted in death.

Multiple Births: Reports of multiple births have been associated with Urofollitropin-hCG treatment, including triplet and quintuplet gestations. In clinical studies with Urofollitropin, 83% of the pregnancies following therapy resulted in single births and 17% in multiple births. The patient and her husband should be advised of the potential risk of multiple births before starting treatment.

PRECAUTIONS

General: Careful attention should be given to diagnosis in candidates for Urofollitropin therapy (see *"Indications and Usage/Selection of Patients"*).

Information for Patients: Prior to the therapy with Urofollitropin, patients should be informed of the duration of treatment and monitoring of their condition that will be required. Possible adverse reactions (see *"Adverse Reactions"*) and the risk of multiple births should also be discussed.

Laboratory Tests: In most instances, treatment with Urofollitropin results only in follicular growth and maturation. In order to effect ovulation, hCG must be given following the administration of Urofollitropin when clinical assessment of the patient indicates that sufficient follicular maturation has occurred. This may be estimated by measuring serum (or urinary) estrogen levels and sonographic visualization of the ovaries. The combination of both estradiol levels and ultrasonography is useful for monitoring the growth and development of follicles, timing hCG administration, as well as detecting ovarian enlargement and minimizing the risk of the Ovarian Hyperstimulation Syndrome and multiple gestation.

Urinary and/or plasma estrogen determinations provide an indirect index of follicular maturity since as the follicles grow and develop, they secrete estrogens in increasing amounts. However, plasma and/or urinary estrogen levels represent the sum of ovarian activity. It is recommended that the number of growing follicles be confirmed using ultrasonography because plasma and/or urinary estrogens do not give an indication of the number of follicles.

Other clinical parameters which may have potential use for monitoring Urofollitropin therapy include:

1. Changes in the vaginal cytology,
2. Appearance and volume of the cervical mucus,
3. Spinnbarkeit, and
4. Ferning of the cervical mucus.

The above clinical indices provide an indirect estimate of the estrogenic effect upon the target organs and, therefore, should only be used adjunctively with more direct estimates of follicular development, i.e., serum estradiol and ultrasonography.

The clinical confirmation of ovulation, with the exception of pregnancy, is obtained by direct and indirect indices of progesterone production. The indices most generally used are as follows:

1. A rise in basal body temperature,
2. Increase in serum progesterone, and
3. Menstruation following the shift in basal body temperature.

When used in conjunction with indices of progesterone production, sonographic visualization of the ovaries will assist in determining if ovulation has occurred. Sonographic evidence of ovulation may include the following:

1. Fluid in the cul-de-sac,
2. Ovarian stigmata, and
3. Collapsed follicle.

Because of the subjectivity of the various tests for the determination of follicular maturation and ovulation, it cannot be overemphasized that the physician should choose tests with which he/she is thoroughly familiar.

Drug Interactions: No clinically significant drug/drug or drug/food interactions have been reported during Urofollitropin therapy.

Carcinogenesis and Mutagenesis: Carcinogenicity and mutagenicity studies have not been performed.

Pregnancy Category X: see "Contraindications".

Nursing Mothers: It is not known whether this drug is excreted in human milk. Because many drugs are excreted in human milk, caution should be exercised if Urofollitropin is administered to a nursing woman.

ADVERSE REACTIONS

The following adverse reactions reported during Urofollitropin therapy are listed in decreasing order of potential severity:

1. Pulmonary and vascular complications (see "Warnings"),
2. Ovarian Hyperstimulation Syndrome (see "Warnings"),
3. Adnexal torsion (as a complication of ovarian enlargement),
4. Mild to moderate ovarian enlargement,
5. Abdominal pain,
6. Sensitivity to Urofollitropin. (Febrile reactions which may be accompanied by chills, musculoskeletal aches, joint pains, malaise, headache, and fatigue have occurred after the administration of Urofollitropin. It is not clear whether or not these were pyrogenic responses or possible allergic reactions.)
7. Ovarian cysts,
8. Gastrointestinal symptoms (nausea, vomiting, diarrhea, abdominal cramps, bloating),
9. Pain, rash, swelling and/or irritation at the site of injection,
10. Breast tenderness,
11. Headache,
12. Dermatological symptoms (dry skin, body rash, hair loss, hives),
13. Hemoperitoneum has been reported during menotropins therapy and, therefore, may also occur during Urofollitropin therapy.

The following medical events have been reported subsequent to pregnancies resulting from Urofollitropin therapy:

1. Ectopic pregnancy
2. Congenital abnormalities
(Three incidents of chromosomal abnormalities and four birth defects have been reported following Urofollitropin-hCG or Urofollitropin, [menotropins for injection] USP-hCG therapy in clinical trials for stimulation prior to in vitro fertilization. The aborted pregnancies included one Trisomy 13, one Trisomy 18, and one fetus with multiple congenital anomalies [hydrocephaly, omphalocele, and meningocele]. One meningocele, one external ear defect, one dislocated hip and ankle, and one dilated cardiomyopathy in the presence of maternal Systemic Lupus Erythematosus were reported. None of these events were thought to be drug-related. The incidence does not exceed that found in the general population.)

DRUG ABUSE AND DEPENDENCE

There have been no reports of abuse or dependence with Urofollitropin.

OVERDOSAGE

Aside from possible ovarian hyperstimulation and multiple gestations (see "Warnings"), little is known concerning the consequences of acute overdosage with Urofollitropin.

DOSAGE AND ADMINISTRATION

Dosage: The dose of Urofollitropin to produce maturation of the follicle must be individualized for each patient. It is recommended that the initial dose to any patient should be 75 IU of Urofollitropin per day *Administered Intramuscularly,* for seven to twelve days followed by hCG, 5,000 U to 10,000 U, one day after the last dose of Urofollitropin. Administration of Urofollitropin may exceed 12 days if inadequate follicle development is indicated by estrogen and/or ultrasound measurement. The patient should be treated until indices of estrogenic activity, as indicated under "Precautions", are equivalent to or greater than those of the normal individual. If serum or urinary estradiol determinations or ultrasonographic visualizations are available, they may be useful as a guide to therapy. If the ovaries are abnormally enlarged on the last day of Urofollitropin therapy, hCG should not be administered in this course of therapy; this will reduce the chances of development of the Ovarian Hyperstimulation Syndrome. If there is evidence of ovulation but no pregnancy, repeat this dosage regimen for at least two more courses before increasing the dose of Urofollitropin to 150 IU of FSH per day for seven to twelve days. As before, this dose should be followed by 5,000 U to 10,000 U of hCG one day after the last dose of Urofollitropin. If evidence of ovulation is present, but pregnancy does not ensue, repeat the same dose for two more courses. Doses larger than this are not routinely recommended.

During treatment with both Urofollitropin and hCG and during a two week post-treatment period, patients should be examined at least every other day for signs of excessive ovarian stimulation. It is recommended that Urofollitropin administration be stopped if the ovaries become abnormally enlarged or abdominal pain occurs. Most instances of OHSS occur after treatment has been discontinued and reach their maximum at about seven to ten days postovulation. Patients should be followed for at least two weeks after hCG administration.

The couple should be encouraged to have intercourse daily, beginning on the day prior to the administration of hCG until ovulation becomes apparent from the indices employed for the determination of progestational activity. Care should be taken to insure insemination. In the light of the foregoing indices and parameters mentioned, it should become obvious that, unless a physician is willing to devote considerable time to these patients and be familiar with and conduct the necessary laboratory studies, he/she should not use Urofollitropin.

In Vitro Fertilization: For in vitro fertilization, therapy with Urofollitropin should be initiated in the early follicular phase (cycle day 2 or 3) at a dose of 150 IU per day, until sufficient follicular development is attained. In most cases, therapy should not exceed ten days.

Administration: Dissolve the contents of one ampule of Urofollitropin in one to two mL of sterile saline and *administer Intramuscularly* immediately. Any unused reconstituted material should be discarded.

Parenteral drug products should be inspected visually, for particulate matter and discoloration prior to administration, whenever solution and container permit.

Storage: Lyophilized powder may be stored refrigerated or at room temperature (3°-25°C/37°-77°F). Protect from light. Use immediately after reconstitution. Discard unused material.

CLINICAL STUDIES

The results of the clinical experience and effectiveness of the administration of Urofollitropin to 80 PCO patients in 189 courses of therapy are summarized below. All patients had received extensive prior therapy with clomiphene citrate, without success, and many had failed to conceive or hyperstimulated following treatment with Menotropins for injection, USP.

	%
Patients ovulating	88
Patients pregnant	30
Patients aborting	25*
Multiple pregnancies	17*
Hyperstimulation syndrome (% patients)	6

Based on total pregnancies.

HOW SUPPLIED
POWDER FOR INJECTION: 75 IU

BRAND/MANUFACTURER	NDC	SIZE	AWP
○ **BRAND**			
METRODIN: Serono	44087-6075-01	1s	$59.67
	44087-6075-03	10s	$558.14
	44087-6075-04	100s	$5413.27

Urokinase

Urokinase for injection should be used in hospitals where the recommended diagnostic and monitoring techniques are available. Thrombolytic therapy should be considered in all situations where the benefits to be achieved outweigh the risk of potentially serious hemorrhage. When internal bleeding does occur, it may be more difficult to manage than that which occurs with conventional anticoagulant therapy.

Urokinase treatment should be instituted as soon as possible after onset of pulmonary embolism, preferably no later than seven days after onset. Any delay in instituting lytic therapy to evaluate the effect of heparin decreases the potential for optimal efficacy.[1]

When Urokinase is used for treatment of coronary artery thrombosis associated with evolving transmural myocardial infarction, therapy should be instituted within six hours of symptom onset.

DESCRIPTION

Urokinase is an enzyme (protein) produced by the kidney, and found in the urine. There are two forms of Urokinase differing in molecular weight but having similar clinical effects. Urokinase for injection is a thrombolytic agent obtained from human kidney cells by tissue culture techniques and is primarily the low molecular weight form.

Thin translucent filaments may occasionally occur in reconstituted Urokinase vials, but do not indicate any decrease in potency of this product. No clinical problems have been associated with these filaments. See "Dosage and Administration" section.

Following reconstitution with 5 mL of Sterile Water for Injection, USP, it is a clear, slightly straw-colored solution; each mL contains 50,000 IU of Urokinase activity, 0.5% mannitol, 5% Albumin (Human), and 1% sodium chloride. The pH is adjusted with sodium hydroxide and/or hydrochloric acid prior to lyophilization.

Urokinase is for intravenous and intracoronary infusion only.

Each mL of reconstituted Urokinase for Catheter Clearance contains 5000 IU of Urokinase activity. The pH is adjusted with sodium hydroxide and/or hydrochloric acid prior to lyophilization.

CLINICAL PHARMACOLOGY

Urokinase acts on the endogenous fibrinolytic system. It converts plasminogen to the enzyme plasmin. Plasmin degrades fibrin clots as well as fibrinogen and other plasma proteins.

When used as directed for I.V. catheter clearance, only small amounts of Urokinase may reach the circulation; therefore, therapeutic serum levels are not expected to be achieved. Nevertheless, one should be aware of the clinical pharmacology of Urokinase.

Intravenous infusion of Urokinase in doses recommended for lysis of pulmonary embolism is followed by increased fibrinolytic activity. This effect disappears within a few hours after discontinuation, but a decrease in plasma levels of fibrinogen and plasminogen and an increase in the amount of circulating fibrin (ogen) degradation products may persist for 12-24 hours.[2,3] There is a lack of correlation between embolus resolution and changes in coagulation and fibrinolytic assay results.

Information is incomplete about the pharmacokinetic properties in man. Urokinase administered by intravenous infusion is cleared rapidly by the liver. The serum half-life in man is 20 minutes or less. Patients with impaired liver function (e.g., cirrhosis) would be expected to show a prolongation in half-life. Small fractions of an administered dose are excreted in bile and urine.

INDICATIONS AND USAGE

PULMONARY EMBOLISM

Urokinase for injection is indicated in adults:

—For the lysis of acute massive pulmonary emboli, defined as obstruction of blood flow to a lobe or multiple segments.

—For the lysis of pulmonary emboli accompanied by unstable hemodynamics, i.e., failure to maintain blood pressure without supportive measures.

The diagnosis should be confirmed by objective means, such as pulmonary angiography via an upper extremity vein, or non-invasive procedures such as lung scanning.

Angiographic and hemodynamic measurements demonstrate a more rapid improvement with lytic therapy than with heparin therapy.[4-8]

CORONARY ARTERY THROMBOSIS

Urokinase has been reported to lyse acute thrombi obstructing coronary arteries, associated with evolving transmural myocardial infarction.[9] The majority of patients who received Urokinase by intracoronary infusion within six hours following onset of symptoms showed recanalization of the involved vessel.

IT HAS NOT BEEN ESTABLISHED THAT INTRACORONARY ADMINIS-TRATION OF UROKINASE DURING EVOLVING TRANSMURAL MYO-CARDIAL INFARCTION RESULTS IN SALVAGE OF MYOCARDIAL TISSUE, NOR THAT IT REDUCES MORTALITY. THE PATIENTS WHO MIGHT BENEFIT FROM THIS THERAPY CANNOT BE DEFINED.

I.V. CATHETER CLEARANCE

Urokinase is indicated for the restoration of patency to intravenous catheters, including central venous catheters, obstructed by clotted blood or fibrin.[10,11] (See separate section at end of insert concerning I.V. catheter clearance for information regarding warnings, precautions, adverse reactions, and dosage and administration.)

UNLABELED USES

Urokinase is used as an adjunct in conjuction with other antineoplastic drugs in the treatment of bladder cancer.

CONTRAINDICATIONS

Because thrombolytic therapy increases the risk of bleeding, Urokinase is contraindicated in the following situations: (See *"Warnings"*.)

—Active internal bleeding

—History of cerebrovascular accident

—Recent (within two months) intracranial or intraspinal surgery

—Recent trauma including cardiopulmonary resuscitation

—Intracranial neoplasm, arteriovenous malformation, or aneurysm

—Known bleeding diathesis

—Severe uncontrolled arterial hypertension

WARNINGS

BLEEDING

The aim of Urokinase is the production of sufficient amounts of plasmin for lysis of intravascular deposits of fibrin; however, fibrin deposits which provide hemostasis, for example, at sites of needle puncture, will also lyse, and bleeding from such sites may occur.

Intramuscular injections and nonessential handling of the patient must be avoided during treatment with Urokinase. Venipunctures should be performed carefully and as infrequently as possible.

Should an arterial puncture be necessary (except for intracoronary administration), upper extremity vessels are preferable. Pressure should be applied for at least 30 minutes, a pressure dressing applied, and the puncture site checked frequently for evidence of bleeding.

In the following conditions, the risks of therapy may be increased and should be weighed against the anticipated benefits:

—Recent (within 10 days) major surgery, obstetrical delivery, organ biopsy, previous puncture of non-compressible vessels

—Recent (within 10 days) serious gastrointestinal bleeding

—High likelihood of a left heart thrombus, e.g., mitral stenosis with atrial fibrillation

—Subacute bacterial endocarditis

—Hemostatic defects including those secondary to severe hepatic or renal disease

—Pregnancy

—Cerebrovascular disease

—Diabetic hemorrhagic retinopathy

—Any other condition in which bleeding might constitute a significant hazard or be particularly difficult to manage because of its location

Should serious spontaneous bleeding (not controllable by local pressure) occur, the infusion of Urokinase should be terminated immediately, and treatment instituted as described under *"Adverse Reactions"*.

USE OF ANTICOAGULANTS

Concurrent use of anticoagulants with intravenous administration of Urokinase is not recommended. However, concurrent use of heparin may be required during intracoronary administration of Urokinase. A clinical study[9] with concurrent use of heparin and Urokinase during intracoronary administration has demonstrated no tendency toward increased bleeding that would not be attributable to the procedure or Urokinase alone. Nevertheless, careful monitoring for excessive bleeding is advised.

ARRHYTHMIAS

Rapid lysis of coronary thrombi has been reported occasionally to cause atrial or ventricular dysrhythmias as a result of reperfusion requiring immediate treatment. Careful monitoring for arrhythmias should be maintained during and immediately following intracoronary administration of Urokinase.

PRECAUTIONS

LABORATORY TESTS

Before commencing thrombolytic therapy, obtain a hematocrit, platelet count, and a thrombin time (TT), activated partial thromboplastin time (APTT), or prothrombin time (PT). If heparin has been given, it should be discontinued unless it is to be used in conjunction with Urokinase for intracoronary administration. TT or APTT should be less than twice the normal control value before thrombolytic therapy is started.

During the infusion, coagulation tests and/or measures of fibrinolytic activity may be performed if desired. Results do not, however, reliably predict either efficacy or a risk of bleeding. The clinical response should be observed frequently, and vital signs, i.e., pulse, temperature, respiratory rate and blood pressure, should be checked at least every four hours. The blood pressure should not be taken in the lower extremities to avoid dislodgement of possible deep vein thrombi.

Following the intravenous infusion, *before (re)instituting heparin*, the TT or APTT should be less than twice the upper limits of normal. Following intracoronary infusion of Urokinase, blood coagulation parameters should be determined and heparin therapy continued as appropriate.

DRUG INTERACTIONS

The interaction of Urokinase with other drugs has not been studied. Drugs that alter platelet function should not be used. Common examples are: aspirin, indomethacin and phenylbutazone.

Although a bolus dose of heparin is recommended prior to intracoronary use of Urokinase, oral anticoagulants or heparin should not be given concurrently with large doses of urokinase such as those used for pulmonary embolism. Concomitant use of intravenous Urokinase and oral anticoagulants or heparin may increase the risk of hemorrhage. (See *"Warnings"* section.)

CARCINOGENICITY

Adequate data are not available on the long-term potential for carcinogenicity in animals or humans.

PREGNANCY

Pregnancy Category B. Reproduction studies have been performed in mice and rats at doses up to 1,000 times the human dose and have revealed no evidence of impaired fertility or harm to the fetus due to Urokinase. There are, however, no adequate and well-controlled studies in pregnant women. Because animal reproduction studies are not always predictive of human response, this drug should be used during pregnancy only if clearly needed.

NURSING MOTHERS

It is not known whether this drug is excreted in human milk. Because many drugs are excreted in human milk, caution should be exercised when Urokinase is administered to a nursing woman.

PEDIATRIC USE

Safety and effectiveness in children have not been established.

ADVERSE REACTIONS

The following adverse reactions have been associated with intravenous therapy but may also occur with intracoronary artery infusion.

BLEEDING

The type of bleeding associated with thrombolytic therapy can be placed into two broad categories:

—Superficial or surface bleeding, observed mainly at invaded or disturbed sites (e.g., venous cutdowns, arterial punctures, sites of recent surgical intervention, etc.).

—Internal bleeding, involving, e.g., the gastrointestinal tract, genitourinary tract, vagina, or intramuscular, retroperitoneal, or intracranial sites.

Several fatalities due to intracranial or retroperitoneal hemorrhage have occurred during thrombolytic therapy.

Should serious bleeding occur, Urokinase infusion should be discontinued and, if necessary, blood loss and reversal of the bleeding tendency can be effectively managed with whole blood (fresh blood preferable), packed red blood cells and cyroprecipitate or fresh frozen plasma. Dextran should not be used. Although the use of aminocaproic acid (ACA, AMICAR®) in humans as an antidote for Urokinase has not been documented, it may be considered in an emergency situation.

◆ RATED THERAPEUTICALLY EQUIVALENT; ◇ THERAPEUTIC EQUIVALENCE UNCONFIRMED; ○ UNRATED

ALLERGIC REACTIONS

In vitro tests with Urokinase, as well as intradermal tests in humans, gave no evidence of induced antibody formation. Relatively mild allergic type reactions, e.g., bronchospasm and skin rash, have been reported. When such reactions occur, they usually respond to conventional therapy. In addition, rare cases of anaphylaxis have been reported.

MISCELLANEOUS

Fever and chills, including shaking chills (rigors), nausea and/or vomiting, transient hypotension or hypertension, dyspnea, tachycardia, cyanosis, back pain, hypoxemia, and acidosis have been reported together and separately. Rare cases of myocardial infarction have also been reported. A cause and effect relationship has not been established.

Asprin is not recommended for treatment of fever.

DOSAGE AND ADMINISTRATION

UROKINASE IS INTENDED FOR INTRAVENOUS AND INTRACORONARY INFUSION ONLY.

A. PULMONARY EMBOLISM

Preparation: Reconstitute Urokinase for injection by aseptically adding 5 mL of Sterile Water for Injection, USP, to the vial. (It is important that Urokinase be reconstituted *only* with Sterile Water for Injection, USP, *without* preservatives. Bacteriostatic Water for Injection should *not* be used.) Each vial should be visually inspected for discoloration (slightly straw-colored solution) and for the presence of particulate material. Highly colored solutions should not be used. Because Urokinase contains no preservatives, it should not be reconstituted until immediately before using. Any unused portion of the reconstituted material should be discarded.

To minimize formation of filaments, avoid shaking the vial during reconstitution. Roll and tilt the vial to enhance reconstitution. The solution may be terminally filtered, e.g., through a 0.45 micron or smaller cellulose membrane filter.

No other medication should be added to this solution.

Reconstituted Urokinase is diluted with 0.9% Sodium Chloride Injection, USP or 5% Dextrose Injection, USP, prior to intravenous infusion. (See Table 1, *"Dose Preparation-Pulmonary Embolism"*.)

Administration: Administer Urokinase for injection by means of a constant infusion pump that is capable of delivering a total volume of 195 mL. The table may be used as an aid in the preparation of Urokinase for injection for administration.

A priming dose of 2,000 IU/lb (4,400 IU/kg) of Urokinase is given as the Urokinase -0.9% Sodium Chloride Injection or 5% Dextrose Injection admixture at a rate of 90 mL/hour over a period of 10 minutes. This is followed by a continuous infusion of 2,000 IU/lb/hr (4,400 IU/kg/hr) of Urokinase at a rate of 15 mL/hour for 12 hours. Since some Urokinase admixture will remain in the tubing at the end of an infusion pump delivery cycle, the following flush procedure should be performed to insure that the total dose of Urokinase is administered. A solution of 0.9% Sodium Chloride Injection or 5% Dextrose Injection approximately equal in amount to the volume of the tubing in the infusion set should be administered via the pump to flush the Urokinase admixture from the entire length of the infusion set. The pump should be set to administer the flush solution at the continuous infusion rate of 15 mL/hour.

Anticoagulation After Terminating Urokinase Treatment: At the end of Urokinase therapy, treatment with heparin by continuous intravenous infusion is recommended to prevent recurrent thrombosis. Heparin treatment, without a loading dose, should not begin until the thrombin time has decreased to *less than twice* the normal control value (approximately 3 to 4 hours after completion of the infusion). See manufacturer's prescribing information for proper use of heparin. This should then be followed by oral anticoagulants in the conventional manner.

B. LYSIS OF CORONARY ARTERY THROMBI

Preparation: Reconstitute three (3) 250,000 IU vials of Urokinase by aseptically adding 5 mL of Sterile Water for Injection, USP, to each vial. (It is important that Urokinase be reconstituted *only* with Sterile Water for Injection, USP, *without* preservatives. Bacteriostatic Water for Injection should *not* be used.) Each vial should be visually inspected for discoloration (slightly straw-colored solution) and for the presence of particulate material. Highly colored solutions should not be used. Because Urokinase contains no preservatives, it should not be reconstituted until immediately before using.

Any unused portion of the reconstituted material should be discarded.

To minimize formation of filaments, avoid shaking the vial during reconstitution. Roll and tilt the vial to enhance reconstitution. The solution may be terminally filtered, e.g., through a 0.45 micron or smaller cellulose membrane filter. Add the contents of the three (3) reconstituted Urokinase vials to 500 mL of 5% Dextrose Injection, USP. The resulting solution admixture will have a concentration of approximately 1500 IU per mL. No other medication should be added to the solution.

The admixture should be administered immediately as described under Administration. Any solution remaining after administration should be discarded.

Note: Adsorption of drug from dilute protein solutions to various materials has been reported in the literature. Therefore, the directions for Preparation and Administration must be followed to assure that significant drug loss does not occur.

Administration: Prior to the infusion of Urokinase, a bolus dose of heparin ranging from 2500 to 10,000 units should be administered intravenously. Prior heparin administration should be considered when calculating the heparin dose for this procedure. Following the bolus dose of heparin, the prepared Urokinase solution should be infused into the occluded artery at a rate of 4 mL per minute (6000 IU per minute) for periods up to 2 hours. In a clinical study, the average total dose of Urokinase utilized for lysis of coronary artery thrombi was 500,000 IU.[9]

To determine response to Urokinase therapy, periodic angiography during the infusion is recommended. It is suggested that the angiography be repeated at approximately 15 minute intervals. Urokinase therapy should be continued until the artery is maximally opened, usually 15 to 30 minutes after the initial opening. Following the infusion, coagulation parameters should be determined. It is advisable to continue heparin therapy after the artery is opened by Urokinase.

When Urokinase was administered selectively into thrombosed coronary arteries via coronary catheter within 6 hours following onset of symptoms of acute transmural myocardial infarction, 60% of the occlusions were opened.[9]

I.V. CATHETER CLEARANCE

Warnings: Excessive pressure should be avoided when Urokinase is injected into the catheter. Such force could cause rupture of the catheter or expulsion of the clot into the circulation.

Precautions: Catheters may be occluded by substances other than blood products, such as drug precipitate. Urokinase is not effective in such a case, and there is the possibility that the precipitate may be forced into the vascular system.

Adverse Reactions: Although there have been no adverse reactions reported as a result of using Urokinase for the removal of clot obstruction from I.V. catheters, the possibility of reactions should nevertheless be considered.

Dosage and Administration:

Preparation: Reconstitute Urokinase for injection by aseptically adding 5 mL of Sterile Water for Injection, USP, to the vial. (It is important that Urokinase be reconstituted *only* with Sterile Water for Injection, USP, *without* preservatives. Bacteriostatic Water for Injection should *not* be used.) Add 1 mL of the reconstituted drug to 9 mL Sterile Water for Injection, USP, to make a final dilution equivalent to 5,000 IU/mL. One mL of this preparation is to be utilized for each catheter clearing procedure. BECAUSE UROKINASE CONTAINS NO PRESERVATIVES, IT SHOULD NOT BE RECONSTITUTED UNTIL IMMEDIATELY BEFORE USING.

Administration: NOTE: When the following procedure is used to clear a central venous catheter, the patient should be instructed to exhale and hold his breath any time the catheter is not connected to I.V. tubing or a syringe. This is to prevent air from entering the open catheter.

Aseptically disconnect the I.V. tubing connection at the catheter hub and attach a 10 mL syringe. Determine occlusion of the catheter by *gently* attempting to aspirate blood from the catheter with the 10 mL syringe. If aspiration is not possible, remove the 10 mL syringe and attach a 1 mL tuberculin syringe filled with prepared Urokinase to the catheter. Slowly and gently inject an amount of Urokinase equal to the volume of the catheter. Aseptically remove the tuberculin syringe and connect a 5 mL syringe to the catheter. Wait at least 5 minutes before attempting to aspirate the drug and residual clot with the 5 mL syringe. Repeat aspiration attempts every 5 minutes. If the catheter is not open within 30 minutes, the catheter may be capped allowing Urokinase to remain in the catheter for 30 to 60 minutes before again attempting to aspirate. A second injection of Urokinase may be necessary in resistant cases.

When patency is restored, aspirate 4 to 5 mL of blood to assure removal of all drug and clot residual. Remove the blood-filled syringe and replace it with a 10 mL syringe filled with 0.9% Sodium Chloride Injection, USP. The catheter should then be gently irrigated with this solution to assure patency of the catheter. After the catheter has been irrigated, remove the 10 mL syringe and aseptically reconnect sterile I.V. tubing to the catheter hub. (See related table).

Storage: Store Urokinase powder at 2° to 8°C.

[See table above].

REFERENCES

1. Sherry S, et al. Thrombolytic therapy in thrombosis: A National Institutes of Health consensus development conference. *Ann Intern Med.* 1980:93:141-144. 2. Bang NU. Physiology and biochemistry of fibrinolysis. In: Bang NU, Beller FK, Deutsch E, Mammen EF, eds. *Thrombosis and Bleeding Disorders.* New York, NY: Academic Press; 1971;292-327. 3. McNicol GP. The fibrinolytic enzyme system. *Postgrad Med J.* August 1973;49 (suppl 5):10-12. 4. Sasahara AA, Hyers TM, Cole CM, et al. The urokinase pulmonary embolism trial. *Circulation.* 1973;47 (suppl 2):1-108. 5. Urokinase pulmonary embolism trial study group: Urokinase-streptokinase embolism trial. *JAMA.* 1974;229:1606-1613. 6. Sasahara AA, Bell WR, Simon TL, et al. The Phase II urokinase-streptokinase pulmonary embolism trial, *Thrombos Diathes Haemorrh* (Stuttg) 1975;33:464-476. 7. Bell WR. Thrombolytic therapy: A comparison between urokinase and streptokinase. *Sem Thromb Hemost.* 1975;2:1-13. 8. Fratantoni JC, Ness P, Simon TL. Thrombolytic therapy: Current status. *N Engl J Med.* 1975;293:1073-1078. 9. Tennant SN, Campbell WB, et al: Intracoronary thrombolysis in acute myocardial infarction: Comparison of the efficacy of urokinase to streptokinase. *Circulation.* 1984;69:756-760. 10. Lawson M, et al. The use of urokinase to restore the patency of occluded central venous catheters. *Am J Intravenous Therapy and Clinical Nutrition.* 1982;9:29-32. 11. Glynn MFX, et al. Therapy for thrombotic occlusion of long-term intravenous alimentation catheters. *Journal of Parenteral and Enteral Nutrition.* 1980;4:387-390. 12. Hurtubise, MR, Bottino, JC, Lawson M, et al. Restoring patency of occluded central venous catheters. *Arch. Surg.* 1980;115:212-213. 12. Hurtubise, MR, Bottino, JC, Lawson, M, et al. Restoring patency of occluded central venous catheters. *Arch. Surg.* 1980; 115:212-213.

Table 1
DOSE PREPARATION-PULMONARY EMBOLISM

Weight (pounds)	Total Dose* Urokinase (IU)	Number Vials Urokinase for injection	Volume of Urokinase After Reconstitution (mL)**	+	Volume of Diluent (mL)	=	Final Volume (mL)
81- 90	2,250,000	9	45		150		195
91-100	2,500,000	10	50		145		195
101-110	2,750,000	11	55		140		195
111-120	3,000,000	12	60		135		195
121-130	3,250,000	13	65		130		195
131-140	3,500,000	14	70		125		195
141-150	3,750,000	15	75		120		195
151-160	4,000,000	16	80		115		195
161-170	4,250,000	17	85		110		195
171-180	4,500,000	18	90		105		195
181-190	4,750,000	19	95		100		195
191-200	5,000,000	20	100		95		195
201-210	5,250,000	21	105		90		195
211-220	5,500,000	22	110		85		195
221-230	5,750,000	23	115		80		195
231-240	6,000,000	24	120		75		195
241-250	6,250,000	25	125		70		195

Infusion Rate:	Priming Dose 15 mL/10 min***	Dose for 12-Hour Period 15 mL/hr for 12 hrs

* *Priming dose + dose administered during 12-hour period.*
** *After addition of 5 mL of Sterile Water for Injection, USP, per vial (See Preparation.)*
*** *Pump rate = 90 mL/hr*

J CODES
250,000 IU vial IV—J3365
5,000 IU vial IV—J3364

HOW SUPPLIED
POWDER FOR INJECTION: 250,000 IU

BRAND/MANUFACTURER	NDC	SIZE	AWP
○ **BRAND**			
ABBOKINASE: Abbott Pharm	00074-6109-05	1s	$402.95

POWDER FOR INJECTION: 5000 IU

BRAND/MANUFACTURER	NDC	SIZE	AWP
○ **BRAND**			
ABBOKINASE: Abbott Pharm	00074-6111-01	1s	$49.69

POWDER FOR INJECTION: 9000 IU

BRAND/MANUFACTURER	NDC	SIZE	AWP
○ **BRAND**			
ABBOKINASE: Abbott Pharm	00074-6145-02	1s	$86.65

Urotrol *SEE* OXYBUTYNIN CHLORIDE

Ursodiol

SPECIAL NOTE: Gallbladder stone dissolution with Ursodiol treatment requires months of therapy. Complete dissolution does not occur in all patients and recurrence of stones within 5 years has been observed in up to 50% of patients who do dissolve their stones on bile acid therapy. Patients should be carefully selected for therapy with Ursodiol, and alternative therapies should be considered.

DESCRIPTION
Ursodiol is an agent intended for dissolution of radiolucent gallstones. It is available as 300 mg capsules suitable for oral administration.

Ursodiol (ursodeoxycholic acid) is a naturally occurring bile acid found in small quantities in normal human bile and in larger quantities in the biles of certain species of bears. It is a bitter-tasting, white powder freely soluble in ethanol, and in glacial acetic acid, slightly soluble in chloroform, sparingly soluble in ether, and practically insoluble in water. The chemical name for Ursodiol is $3\alpha,7\beta$-dihydroxy-5β-cholan-24-oic acid ($C_{24}H_{40}O_4$). Ursodiol has a molecular weight of 392.56.

Following is its chemical structure:

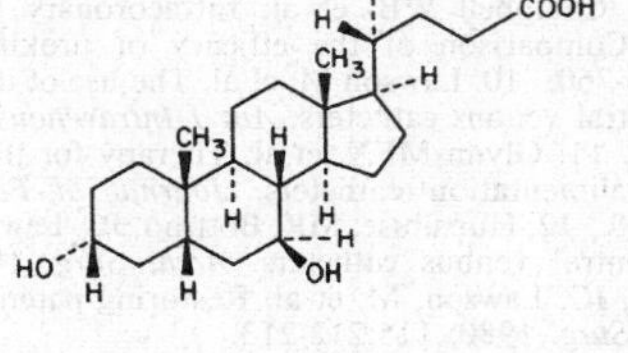

CLINICAL PHARMACOLOGY
About 90% of a therapeutic dose of Ursodiol is absorbed in the small bowel after oral administration. After absorption, Ursodiol enters the portal vein and undergoes efficient extraction from portal blood by the liver (i.e., there is a large "first pass" effect) where it is conjugated with either glycine or taurine and is then secreted into the hepatic bile ducts. Ursodiol in bile is concentrated in the gallbladder and expelled into the duodenum in gallbladder bile via the cystic and common ducts by gallbladder contractions provoked by physiologic responses to eating. Only small quantities of Ursodiol appear in the systemic circulation and very small amounts are excreted into urine. The sites of the drug's therapeutic actions are in the liver, bile and gut lumen.

Beyond conjugation, Ursodiol is not altered or catabolized appreciably by the liver or intestinal mucosa. A small proportion of orally administered drug undergoes bacterial degradation with each cycle of enterohepatic circulation. Ursodiol can be both oxidized and reduced at the 7-carbon, yielding either 7-keto-lithocholic acid or lithocholic acid, respectively. Further, there is some bacterially catalyzed deconjugation of glyco- and tauro-ursodeoxycholic acid in the small bowel. Free Ursodiol, 7-keto-lithocholic acid and lithocholic acid are relatively insoluble in aqueous media and larger proportions of these compounds are lost from the distal gut into the feces. Reabsorbed free Ursodiol is reconjugated by the liver. Eighty percent of lithocholic acid formed in the small bowel is excreted in the feces, but the 20% that is absorbed is sulfated at the 3-hydroxyl group in the liver to relatively insoluble lithocholyl conjugates which are excreted into bile and lost in feces. Absorbed 7-keto-lithocholic acid is stereospecifically reduced in the liver to chenodiol.

Lithocholic acid causes cholestatic liver injury and can cause death from liver failure in certain species unable to form sulfate conjugates. Lithocholic acid is formed by 7-dehydroxylation of the dihydroxy bile acids (Ursodiol and chenodiol) in the gut lumen. The 7-dehydroxylation reaction appears to be alpha-specific, i.e., chenodiol is more efficiently 7-dehydroxylated than Ursodiol and for equimolar doses of Ursodiol and chenodiol, levels of lithocholic acid appearing in bile are lower with the former. Man has the capacity to sulfate lithocholic acid. Although liver injury has not been associated with Ursodiol therapy, a reduced capacity to sulfate may exist in some individuals, but such a deficiency has not yet been clearly demonstrated.

Pharmacodynamics: Ursodiol suppresses hepatic synthesis and secretion of cholesterol, and also inhibits intestinal absorption of cholesterol. It appears to have little inhibitory effect on synthesis and secretion into bile of endogenous bile acids, and does not appear to affect secretion of phospholipids into bile.

With repeated dosing, bile ursodeoxycholic acid concentrations reach a steady state in about 3 weeks. Although insoluble in aqueous media, cholesterol can be solubilized in at least two different ways in the presence of dihydroxy bile acids. In addition to solubilizing cholesterol in micelles, Ursodiol acts by an apparently unique mechanism to cause dispersion of cholesterol as liquid crystals in aqueous media. Thus, even though administration of high doses (e.g., 15-18 mg/kg/day) does not result in a concentration of Ursodiol higher than 60% of the total bile acid pool, Ursodiol-rich bile effectively solubilizes cholesterol. The overall effect of Ursodiol is to increase the concentration level at which saturation of cholesterol occurs.

The various actions of Ursodiol combine to change the bile of patients with gallstones from cholesterol-precipitating to cholesterol-solubilizing, thus resulting in bile conducive to cholesterol stone dissolution.

After Ursodiol dosing is stopped, the concentration of the bile acid in bile falls exponentially, declining to about 5-10% of its steady state level in about 1 week.

◆ RATED THERAPEUTICALLY EQUIVALENT; ◇ THERAPEUTIC EQUIVALENCE UNCONFIRMED; ○ UNRATED

Clinical Results: On the basis of clinical trial results in a total of 868 patients with radiolucent gallstones treated in 8 studies (three in the U.S. involving 282 patients, one in the U.K. involving 130 patients and four in Italy involving 456 patients) for periods ranging from 6-78 months with Ursodiol doses ranging from about 5 to 20 mg/kg/day, an Ursodiol dose of about 8-10 mg/kg/day appeared to be the best dose. With an Ursodiol dose of about 10 mg/kg/day, complete stone dissolution can be anticipated in about 30% of unselected patients with uncalcified gallstones < 20 mm in maximal diameter treated for up to two years. Patients with calcified gallstones prior to treatment, or patients who develop stone calcification or gallbladder nonvisualization on treatment, and patients with stones larger than 20 mm in maximal diameter rarely dissolve their stones. The chance of gallstone dissolution is increased up to 50% in patients with floating or floatable stones (i.e., those with high cholesterol content), and is inversely related to stone size for those less than 20 mm in maximal diameter. Complete dissolution was observed in 81% of patients with stones up to 5 mm in diameter. Age, sex, weight, degree of obesity and serum cholesterol level are not related to the chance of stone dissolution with Ursodiol.

A nonvisualizing gallbladder by oral cholecystogram prior to the initiation of therapy is not a contraindication to Ursodiol therapy (the group of patients with nonvisualizing gallbladders in the Ursodiol studies had complete stone dissolution rates similar to the group of patients with visualizing gallbladders). However, gallbladder nonvisualization developing during Ursodiol treatment predicts failure of complete stone dissolution and in such cases therapy should be discontinued.

Partial stone dissolution occurring within 6 months of beginning therapy with Ursodiol appears to be associated with a > 70% chance of eventual complete stone dissolution with further treatment: partial dissolution observed within one year of starting therapy indicates a 40% probability of complete dissolution.

Stone recurrence after dissolution with Ursodiol therapy was seen within 2 years in 8/27 (30%) of patients in the U.K. studies. Of 16 patients in the U.K. study whose stones had previously dissolved on chenodiol but later recurred, 11 had complete dissolution of Ursodiol. Stone recurrence has been observed in up to 50% of patients within 5 years of complete stone dissolution on Ursodiol therapy. Serial ultrasonographic examinations should be obtained to monitor for recurrence of stones, bearing in mind that radiolucency of the stones should be established before another course of Ursodiol is instituted. A prophylactic dose of Ursodiol has not been established.

ALTERNATIVE THERAPIES

Watchful Waiting: Watchful waiting has the advantage that no therapy may ever be required. For patients with silent or minimally symptomatic stones, the rate of development of moderate to severe symptoms or gallstone complications is estimated to be between 2% and 6% per year, leading to a cumulative rate of 7% to 27% in five years. Presumably the rate is higher for patients already having symptoms.

Cholecystectomy: Surgery offers the advantage of immediate and permanent stone removal, but carries a high risk in some patients. About 5% of cholecystectomized patients have residual symptoms or retained common duct stones.

The spectrum of surgical risk varies as a function of age and the presence of disease other than cholelithiasis.

MORTALITY RATES FOR CHOLECYSTECTOMY IN THE U.S.
(National Halothane Study, JAMA 1966; 197:775-8)
27,600 Cholecystectomies (Smoothed Rates)
Deaths/1000 Operations***

Low Risk Patients*	Age (Yrs)	Cholecystectomy	Cholecystectomy + Common Duct Exploration
Women	0-49	.54	2.13
	50-69	2.80	10.10
Men	0-49	1.04	4.12
	50-69	5.41	19.23
High Risk Patients**			
Women	0-49	12.66	47.62
	50-69	17.24	58.82
Men	0-49	24.39	90.91
	50-69	33.33	111.11

* *In good health or with moderate systemic disease.*
** *With severe or extreme systemic disease.*
*** *Includes both elective and emergency surgery.*

Women in good health or who have only moderate systemic disease, and are under 49 years of age have the lowest surgical mortality rate (0.054); men in all categories have a surgical mortality rate twice that of women. Common duct exploration quadruples the rates in all categories. The rates rise with each decade of life and increase tenfold or more in all categories with severe or extreme systemic disease.

INDICATIONS AND USAGE

Ursodiol is indicated for patients with radiolucent, noncalcified gallbladder stones < 20 mm in greatest diameter in whom elective cholecystectomy would be undertaken except for the presence of increased surgical risk due to systemic disease, advanced age, idiosyncratic reaction to general anesthesia, or for those

patients who refuse surgery. Safety of use of Ursodiol beyond 24 months is not established.

UNLABELED USES

Ursodiol is used alone or as an adjunct in the treatment of Caroli's syndrome, chronic hepatitis, to improve liver function tests and symptoms of fatigue and pruritus in patients with primary biliary cirrhosis. It is also prescribed in the treatment of dyspepsia, bile reflux gastritis, and to prevent veno-occlusive disease of the liver in bone marrow transplant patients.

CONTRAINDICATIONS

1. Ursodiol will not dissolve calcified cholesterol stones, radio-opaque stones or radiolucent bile pigment stones. Hence, patients with such stones are not candidates for Ursodiol therapy.

2. Patients with compelling reasons for cholecystectomy including unremitting acute cholecystitis, cholangitis, biliary obstruction, gallstone pancreatitis or biliary-gastrointestinal fistula are not candidates for Ursodiol therapy.

3. Allergy to bile acids.

PRECAUTIONS

Liver Tests: Ursodiol therapy has not been associated with liver damage. Lithocholic acid, a naturally occurring bile acid, is known to be a liver-toxic metabolite. This bile acid is formed in the gut from Ursodiol less efficiently and in smaller amounts than that seen from chenodiol. Lithocholic acid is detoxified in the liver by sulfation and although man appears to be an efficient sulfater, it is possible that some patients may have a congenital or acquired deficiency in sulfation, thereby predisposing them to lithocholate-induced liver damage.

Abnormalities in liver enzymes have not been associated with Ursodiol therapy and in fact Ursodiol has been shown to decrease liver enzyme levels in liver disease. However, patients given Ursodiol should have SGOT (AST) and SGPT (ALT) measured at the initiation of therapy and thereafter as indicated by the particular clinical circumstances.

Drug Interactions: Bile acid sequestering agents such as cholestyramine and colestipol may interfere with the action of Ursodiol by reducing its absorption. Aluminum-based antacids have been shown to adsorb bile acids *in vitro* and may be expected to interfere with Ursodiol in the same manner as the bile acid sequestering agents. Estrogens, oral contraceptives and clofibrate (and perhaps other lipid-lowering drugs) increase hepatic cholesterol secretion, and encourage cholesterol gallstone formation and hence may counteract the effectiveness of Ursodiol.

Carcinogenesis, Mutagenesis, and Impairment of Fertility: Ursodeoxycholic acid was tested in two-year oral carcinogenicity studies in CD-1 mice and Sprague-Dawley rats at daily doses of 50, 250, and 1000 mg/kg/day. It was not tumorigenic in mice. In the rat study, it produced statistically significant dose-related increased incidences of pheochromocytomas of adrenal medulla in males (p = 0.014, Peto trend test) and females (p = 0.004, Peto trend test.)

A 78-week rat study employing intrarectal instillation of lithocholic acid and tauro-deoxycholic acid, metabolites of Ursodiol and chenodiol, has been conducted. These bile acids alone did not produce any tumors. A tumor-promoting effect of both metabolites was observed when they were co-administered with a carcinogenic agent. Results of epidemiologic studies suggest that bile acids might be involved in the pathogenesis of human colon cancer in patients who had undergone a cholecystectomy, but direct evidence is lacking. Ursodiol is not mutagenic in the Ames test. Dietary administration of lithocholic acid to chickens is reported to cause hepatic adenomatous hyperplasia.

Pregnancy Category B: Reproduction studies have been performed in rats and rabbits with Ursodiol doses up to 200-fold the therapeutic dose and have revealed no evidence of impaired fertility or harm to the fetus at doses of 20 to 100-fold the human dose in rats and at 5-fold the human dose (highest dose tested) in rabbits. Studies employing 100 to 200-fold the human dose in rats have shown some reduction in fertility rate and litter size. There have been no adequate and well-controlled studies of the use of Ursodiol in pregnant women, but inadvertent exposure of 4 women to therapeutic doses of the drug in the first trimester of pregnancy during the Ursodiol trials led to no evidence of effects on the fetus or newborn baby. Although it seems unlikely, the possibility that Ursodiol can cause fetal harm cannot be ruled out; hence, the drug is not recommended for use during pregnancy.

Nursing Mothers: It is not known whether Ursodiol is excreted in human milk. Because many drugs are excreted in human milk, caution should be exercised when Ursodiol is administered to a nursing mother.

Pediatric Use: The safety and effectiveness of Ursodiol in children have not been established.

ADVERSE REACTIONS

Gastrointestinal: Ursodiol given in doses of 8-10 mg/kg/day rarely causes diarrhea (< 1%). One study in which a placebo control was not used was associated with a 6% incidence of mild, transient diarrhea not requiring termination of therapy or lowering of Ursodiol dose. One patient with ulcerative colitis in the Ursodiol studies developed diarrhea on therapy. In the National Cooperative Gallstone Study, the incidence of diarrhea was 27.1% in the placebo group.

Dermatological: One patient in the Ursodiol studies with preexisting psoriasis apparently developed exacerbation of itching on Ursodiol, which remitted on withdrawal of the drug.

Other: In two ongoing double-blind, placebo-controlled Ursodiol studies in the U.S., for which the treatment codes have not yet been broken, the following minor events have been reported:

Pruritus, rash, urticaria, dry skin, sweating, hair thinning, nausea, vomiting, dyspepsia, metallic taste, abdominal pain, biliary pain, cholecystitis, diarrhea, constipation, stomatitis, flatulence, headache, fatigue, anxiety, depression, sleep disorder, arthralgia, myalgia, back pain, cough, rhinitis.

Since these studies are ongoing and blinded, incidence rates in the Ursodiol and placebo groups cannot be calculated, nor has it been established whether the reactions listed are associated with Ursodiol.

OVERDOSAGE

Neither accidental nor intentional overdosing with Ursodiol has been reported. Doses of Ursodiol in the range of 16-20 mg/kg/day have been tolerated for 6-37 months without symptoms by 7 patients. The LD_{50} for Ursodiol in rats is over 5,000 mg/kg given over 7-10 days and over 7,500 mg/kg for mice. The most likely manifestation of severe overdose with Ursodiol would probably be diarrhea, which should be treated symptomatically.

DOSAGE AND ADMINISTRATION

The recommended dose for Ursodiol treatment of radiolucent gallbladder stones is 8-10 mg/kg/day given in 2 or 3 divided doses.

Ultrasound images of the gallbladder should be obtained at six month intervals for the first year of Ursodiol therapy to monitor gallstone response. If gallstones appear to have dissolved, Ursodiol therapy should be continued and dissolution confirmed on a repeat ultrasound examination within one to three months. Most patients who eventually achieve complete stone dissolution will show partial or complete dissolution at the first on-treatment reevaluation. If partial stone dissolution is not seen by 12 months of Ursodiol therapy, the likelihood of success is greatly reduced.

Do not store above 86°F (30°C).

Dispense in tight container, USP.

HOW SUPPLIED
CAPSULE: 300 MG

BRAND/MANUFACTURER	NDC	SIZE	AWP
○ **BRAND**			
ACTIGALL: Summit	57267-0153-30	100s	$199.59

Uticort SEE BETAMETHASONE, TOPICAL

Vagisec Plus SEE 9-AMINOACRIDINE HYDROCHLORIDE/ POLYOXYETHYLENE NONYL PHENOL/SODIUM DIOCTYL SULFOSUCCINATE/SODIUM EDETATE

Vagistat-1 SEE TIOCONAZOLE

Valisone SEE BETAMETHASONE, TOPICAL

Valium SEE DIAZEPAM

Valproic Acid

WARNING
HEPATIC FAILURE RESULTING IN FATALITIES HAS OCCURRED IN PATIENTS RECEIVING VALPROIC ACID. EXPERIENCE HAS INDICATED THAT CHILDREN UNDER THE AGE OF TWO YEARS ARE AT A CONSIDERABLY INCREASED RISK OF DEVELOPING FATAL HEPATOTOXICITY, ESPECIALLY THOSE ON MULTIPLE ANTICON-VULSANTS, THOSE WITH CONGENITAL METABOLIC DISORDERS, THOSE WITH SEVERE SEIZURE DISORDERS ACCOMPANIED BY MENTAL RETARDATION, AND THOSE WITH ORGANIC BRAIN DISEASE. WHEN VALPROIC ACID PRODUCTS ARE USED IN THIS PATIENT GROUP, IT SHOULD BE USED WITH EXTREME CAUTION AND AS A SOLE AGENT. THE BENEFITS OF SEIZURE CONTROL SHOULD BE WEIGHED AGAINST THE RISKS. ABOVE THIS AGE GROUP, EXPERIENCE HAS INDICATED THAT THE INCIDENCE OF FATAL HEPATOTOXICITY DECREASES CONSIDERABLY IN PROGRESSIVELY OLDER PATIENT GROUPS.

THESE INCIDENTS USUALLY HAVE OCCURRED DURING THE FIRST SIX MONTHS OF TREATMENT. SERIOUS OR FATAL HEPATOTOXICITY MAY BE PRECEDED BY NONSPECIFIC SYMPTOMS SUCH AS LOSS OF SEIZURE CONTROL, MALAISE, WEAKNESS, LETHARGY, FACIAL EDEMA, ANOREXIA, AND VOMITING. PATIENTS SHOULD BE MONITORED CLOSELY FOR APPEARANCE OF THESE SYMPTOMS. LIVER FUNCTION TESTS SHOULD BE PERFORMED PRIOR TO THERAPY AND AT FREQUENT INTERVALS THEREAFTER, ESPECIALLY DURING THE FIRST SIX MONTHS.

DESCRIPTION
Valproic acid is a carboxylic acid designated as 2-propylpentanoic acid. It is also known as dipropylacetic acid.

Valproic Acid (pKa 4.8) has a molecular weight of 144 and occurs as a colorless liquid with a characteristic odor. It is slightly soluble in water (1.3 mg/mL) and very soluble in organic solvents.

Valproic Acid capsules and syrup are antiepileptics for oral administration. Each soft elastic capsule contains 250 mg Valproic Acid. The syrup contains the equivalent of 250 mg Valproic Acid per 5 mL as the sodium salt.

Following is its chemical structure:

$$CH_3CH_2CH_2CHCOOH$$
$$CH_3CH_2CH_2$$

CLINICAL PHARMACOLOGY
Valproic Acid is an antiepileptic agent which dissociates to the Valproate ion in the gastrointestinal tract. The mechanism by which Valproate exerts its antiepileptic effects has not been established. It has been suggested that its activity is related to increased brain levels of gamma-aminobutyric acid (GABA).

Valproic Acid is rapidly absorbed after oral administration. Peak plasma concentrations of Valproate ion are observed 1 to 4 hours after a single oral dose of Valproic Acid. A slight delay in absorption occurs when the drug is administered with meals, but this does not affect the total absorption.

Accordingly, administration of oral Valproate products with food and substitution among the various Valproic Acid and divalproex sodium products should be without consequence. Nonetheless, any changes in dosage administration, or the addition or discontinuance of concomitant drugs should ordinarily be accompanied by close monitoring of clinical status and Valproate plasma concentrations.

The plasma half-life of Valproate is typically in the range of 6 to 16 hours. Half-lives in the lower part of the range are usually found in patients taking other antiepileptic drugs capable of enzyme induction.

Valproate is primarily metabolized in the liver. The major metabolic routes are glucuronidation, mitochondrial beta oxidation, and microsomal oxidation. The major metabolites formed are the glucuronide conjugate, 2-propyl-3-keto-penta-noic acid, and 2-propylhydroxypentanoic acids. Other unsaturated metabolites have been reported. The major route of elimination of these metabolites is in the urine.

Patients on monotherapy will generally have longer half-lives and higher concentrations of Valproate at a given dosage than patients receiving polytherapy. This is primarily due to enzyme induction caused by other antiepileptics, which results in enhanced clearance of Valproate by glucuronidation and microsomal oxidation. Because of these changes in Valproate clearance, monitoring of antiepileptic concentrations should be intensified whenever concomitant antiepileptics are introduced or withdrawn.

The therapeutic range is commonly considered to be 50 to 100 mcg/mL of total Valproate, although some patients may be controlled with lower or higher plasma concentrations. Valproate is highly bound (90%) to plasma proteins in the therapeutic range; however, protein binding is concentration-dependent and decreases at high Valproate concentrations. The binding is variable among patients, and may be affected by fatty acids or by highly bound drugs such as salicylate. Some clinicians favor monitoring free Valproate concentrations, which may more accurately reflect CNS penetration of Valproate. As yet, a consensus on the therapeutic range of free concentrations has not been established; however, monitoring total and free Valproate may be informative when there are changes in clinical status, concomitant medication, or Valproate dosage.

INDICATIONS AND USAGE
Valproic Acid is indicated for use as sole and adjunctive therapy in the treatment of simple and complex absence seizures, and adjunctively in patients with multiple seizure types which include absence seizures.

Simple absence is defined as very brief clouding of the sensorium or loss of consciousness accompanied by certain generalized epileptic discharges without other detectable clinical signs. Complex absence is the term used when other signs are also present.

SEE *"WARNINGS"* FOR STATEMENT REGARDING FATAL HEPATIC DYSFUNCTION.

UNLABELED USES
Valproic Acid is used alone or as an adjunct in the prophylactic treatment of febrile seizures, infantile seizures, and myoclonic seizures. It is used in the treatment of status epilepticus, tardive dyskinesia, and trigeminal neuralgia, and is prescribed as a prophylactic agent for migraine headache. Valproic Acid is also prescribed to treat psychiatric disorders, including bipolar disorder (manic or mixed) and schizoaffective disorder, and is used in the treatment of Nelson's syndrome associated with Cushing's disease and Sydenham's chorea.

CONTRAINDICATIONS
VALPROIC ACID SHOULD NOT BE ADMINISTERED TO PATIENTS WITH HEPATIC DISEASE OR SIGNIFICANT DYSFUNCTION.

◆ RATED THERAPEUTICALLY EQUIVALENT; ◇ THERAPEUTIC EQUIVALENCE UNCONFIRMED; ○ UNRATED

Valproic Acid is contraindicated in patients with known hypersensitivity to the drug.

WARNINGS

Hepatic failure resulting in fatalities has occurred in patients receiving Valproic Acid. These incidents usually have occurred during the first six months of treatment. Serious or fatal hepatotoxicity may be preceded by nonspecific symptoms such as loss of seizure control, malaise, weakness, lethargy, facial edema, anorexia and vomiting. Patients should be monitored closely for appearance of these symptoms. Liver function tests should be performed prior to therapy and at frequent intervals thereafter, especially during the first six months. However, physicians should not rely totally on serum biochemistry since these tests may not be abnormal in all instances, but should also consider the results of careful interim medical history and physical examination. Caution should be observed when administering Valproic Acid to patients with a prior history of hepatic disease. Patients on multiple anticonvulsants, children, those with congenital metabolic disorders, those with severe seizure disorders accompanied by mental retardation, and those with organic brain disease may be at particular risk. Experience has indicated that children under the age of two years are at considerably increased risk of developing fatal hepatotoxicity, especially those with the aforementioned conditions. When Valproic Acid products are used in this patient group, it should be used with extreme caution and as a sole agent. The benefits of seizure control should be weighed against the risks. Above this age group, experience has indicated that the incidence of fatal hepatotoxicity decreases considerably in progressively older patient groups.

The drug should be discontinued immediately in the presence of significant hepatic dysfunction, suspected or apparent. In some cases, hepatic dysfunction has progressed in spite of discontinuation of drug.

The frequency of adverse effects (particularly elevated liver enzymes) may be dose-related. The benefit of improved seizure control which may accompany the higher doses should be weighed against the possibility of a greater incidence of adverse effects.

Usage in Pregnancy: ACCORDING TO PUBLISHED AND UNPUBLISHED REPORTS, VALPROIC ACID MAY PRODUCE TERATOGENIC EFFECTS IN THE OFFSPRING OF HUMAN FEMALES RECEIVING THE DRUG DURING PREGNANCY.

THERE ARE MULTIPLE REPORTS IN THE CLINICAL LITERATURE WHICH INDICATE THAT THE USE OF ANTIEPILEPTIC DRUGS DURING PREGNANCY RESULTS IN AN INCREASED INCIDENCE OF BIRTH DEFECTS IN THE OFFSPRING. ALTHOUGH DATA ARE MORE EXTENSIVE WITH RESPECT TO TRIMETHADIONE, PARAMETHADIONE, PHENYTOIN, AND PHENOBARBITAL, REPORTS INDICATE A POSSIBLE SIMILAR ASSOCIATION WITH THE USE OF OTHER ANTIEPILEPTIC DRUGS. THEREFORE, ANTIEPILEPTIC DRUGS SHOULD BE ADMINISTERED TO WOMEN OF CHILDBEARING POTENTIAL ONLY IF THEY ARE CLEARLY SHOWN TO BE ESSENTIAL IN THE MANAGEMENT OF THEIR SEIZURES.

THE INCIDENCE OF NEURAL TUBE DEFECTS IN THE FETUS MAY BE INCREASED IN MOTHERS RECEIVING VALPROATE DURING THE FIRST TRIMESTER OF PREGNANCY. THE CENTERS FOR DISEASE CONTROL (CDC) HAS ESTIMATED THE RISK OF VALPROIC ACID EXPOSED WOMEN HAVING CHILDREN WITH SPINA BIFIDA TO BE APPROXIMATELY 1 to 2%.[1] OTHER CONGENITAL ANOMALIES (EG, CRANIOFACIAL DEFECTS, CARDIOVASCULAR MALFORMATIONS AND ANOMALIES INVOLVING VARIOUS BODY SYSTEMS), COMPATIBLE AND INCOMPATIBLE WITH LIFE, HAVE BEEN REPORTED. SUFFICIENT DATA TO DETERMINE THE INCIDENCE OF THESE CONGENITAL ANOMALIES IS NOT AVAILABLE.

THE HIGHER INCIDENCE OF CONGENITAL ANOMALIES IN ANTIEPILEPTIC DRUG-TREATED WOMEN WITH SEIZURE DISORDERS CANNOT BE REGARDED AS A CAUSE AND EFFECT RELATIONSHIP. THERE ARE INTRINSIC METHODOLOGIC PROBLEMS IN OBTAINING ADEQUATE DATA ON DRUG TERATOGENICITY IN HUMANS; GENETIC FACTORS OR THE EPILEPTIC CONDITION ITSELF, MAY BE MORE IMPORTANT THAN DRUG THERAPY IN CONTRIBUTING TO CONGENITAL ANOMALIES.

PATIENTS TAKING VALPROATE MAY DEVELOP CLOTTING ABNORMALITIES. A PATIENT WHO HAD LOW FIBROGEN WHEN TAKING MULTIPLE ANTICONVULSANTS INCLUDING VALPROATE GAVE BIRTH TO AN INFANT WITH AFIBRINOGENEMIA WHO SUBSEQUENTLY DIED OF HEMORRHAGE. IF VALPROATE IS USED IN PREGNANCY, THE CLOTTING PARAMETERS SHOULD BE MONITORED CAREFULLY.

HEPATIC FAILURE, RESULTING IN THE DEATH OF A NEWBORN AND OF AN INFANT, HAVE BEEN REPORTED FOLLOWING THE USE OF VALPROATE DURING PREGNANCY.

ANIMAL STUDIES ALSO HAVE DEMONSTRATED VALPROATE INDUCED TERATOGENICITY. Studies in rats and human females demonstrated placental transfer of the drug. Doses greater than 65 mg/kg/day given to pregnant rats and mice produced skeletal abnormalities in the offspring, primarily involving ribs and vertebrae; doses greater than 150 mg/kg/day given to pregnant rabbits produced fetal resorptions and (primarily) soft-tissue abnormalities in the offspring. In rats a dose-related delay in the onset of parturition was noted. Postnatal growth and survival of the progeny were adversely affected, particularly when drug administration spanned the entire gestation and early lactation period.

Antiepileptic drugs should not be discontinued in patients in whom the drug is administered to prevent major seizures because of the strong possibility of precipitating status epilepticus with attendant hypoxia and threat to life. In individual cases where the severity and frequency of the seizure disorder are such that the removal of medication does not pose a serious threat to the patient, discontinuation of the drug may be considered prior to and during pregnancy, although it cannot be said with any confidence that even minor seizures do not pose some hazard to the developing embryo or fetus.

The prescribing physician will wish to weigh these considerations in treating or counseling epileptic women of childbearing potential.

Tests to detect neural tube and other defects using current accepted procedures should be considered a part of routine prenatal care in childbearing women receiving Valproate.

PRECAUTIONS

Hepatic Dysfunction: See boxed *"Warning," "Contraindications"* and *"Warnings"*.

General: Because of reports of thrombocytopenia, inhibition of the secondary phase of platelet aggregation, and abnormal coagulation parameters (e.g., low fibrinogen), platelet counts and coagulation tests are recommended before initiating therapy and at periodic intervals. It is recommended that patients receiving Valproic Acid be monitored for platelet count and coagulation parameters prior to planned surgery. Evidence of hemorrhage, bruising, or a disorder of hemostasis/coagulation is an indication for reduction of the dosage or withdrawal of therapy.

Hyperammonemia with or without lethargy or coma has been reported and may be present in the absence of abnormal liver function tests. Asymptomatic elevations of ammonia are more common and when present require more frequent monitoring. If clinically significant symptoms occur, Valproic Acid therapy should be modified or discontinued.

Since Valproate may interact with concurrently administered antiepileptic drugs, periodic plasma concentration determinations of concomitant antiepileptic drugs are recommended during the early course of therapy (see *"Drug Interactions"*).

Valproate is partially eliminated in the urine as a keto-metabolite which may lead to a false interpretation of the urine ketone test.

There have been reports of altered thyroid function tests associated with Valproate. The clinical significance of these is unknown.

Information for Patients: Since Valproic Acid products may produce CNS depression, especially when combined with CNS depressants (e.g., alcohol), patients should be advised not to engage in hazardous activities, such as driving an automobile or operating dangerous machinery, until it is known that they do not become drowsy from the drug.

Drug Interactions: Valproate may potentiate the action of CNS depressants (i.e., alcohol, benzodiazepines, etc.).

The concomitant administration of Valproate with drugs that exhibit extensive protein binding (e.g., aspirin, carbamazepine, dicumarol, and phenytoin) may result in alteration of serum drug concentrations.

There is evidence that Valproate can cause an increase in serum phenobarbital concentrations by impairment of nonrenal clearance. This phenomenon can result in severe CNS depression. The combination of Valproate and phenobarbital has also been reported to produce CNS depression without significant elevations of barbiturate on Valproate serum concentrations. All patients receiving concomitant barbiturate therapy should be closely monitored for neurological toxicity. Serum barbiturate concentrations should be obtained, if possible, and the barbiturate dosage decreased, if appropriate.

Primidone is metabolized into a barbiturate and, therefore, may also be involved in a similar or identical interaction. There have been reports of breakthrough seizures occurring with the combination of Valproate and phenytoin. Most reports have noted a decrease in total plasma phenytoin concentration. However, increases in total phenytoin serum concentration have been reported. An initial fall with subsequent increase in total phenytoin concentrations has also been reported. In addition, a decrease in total serum phenytoin with an increase in the free vs. protein bound phenytoin concentrations has been reported. The dosage of phenytoin should be adjusted as required by the clinical situation.

The concomitant use of Valproic Acid and clonazepam may induce absence status in patients with a history of absence type seizures.

There is inconclusive evidence regarding the effects of Valproate on serum ethosuximide concentrations. Patients receiving Valproate and ethosuximide, especially along with other anticonvulsants, should be monitored for alterations in serum concentrations of both drugs.

Caution is recommended when Valproate is used with drugs affecting coagulation (e.g., aspirin, warfarin). See *"Adverse Reactions"*.

Evidence suggests that there is an association between the use of certain antiepileptics and failure of oral contraceptives. One explanation for this interaction is that enzyme-inducing antiepileptics effectively lower plasma concentrations of the relevant steroid hormones, resulting in unimpaired ovulation. However, other mechanisms, not related to enzyme induction may contribute to the failure of oral contraceptives. While Valproate is not a significant enzyme inducer, and, therefore, would not be expected to decrease concentrations of steroid hormones, clinical data about the interaction of Valproate with oral contraceptives is minimal.[2]

Carcinogenesis: Valproic Acid was administered to Sprague Dawley rats and ICR (HA/ICR) mice at doses of 0, 80 and 170 mg/kg/day for two years. A variety of neoplasms were observed in both species. The chief findings were a statistically significant increase in the incidence of subcutaneous fibrosarcomas in high dose male rats receiving Valproic Acid and a statistically significant dose-related trend for benign pulmonary adenomas in male mice receiving Valproic Acid. The significance of these findings for man is unknown.

Mutagenesis: Studies of Valproate have been performed using bacterial and mammalian systems. These studies have provided no evidence of a mutagenic potential for Valproate.

Fertility: Chronic toxicity studies in juvenile and adult rats and dogs demonstrated reduced spermatogenesis and testicular atrophy at doses greater than 200 mg/kg/day in rats and greater than 90 mg/kg/day in dogs. Segment I fertility studies in rats have shown doses up to 350 mg/kg/day for 60 days to have no effect on fertility. *The effect of Valproate on Testicular development and on sperm production and fertility in humans is unknown.*

Pregnancy: Pregnancy Category D: See *"Warnings"*.

Nursing Mothers: Valproate is excreted in breast milk. Concentrations in breast milk have been reported to be 1-10% of serum concentrations. It is not known what effect this would have on a nursing infant. Caution should be exercised when Valproic Acid is administered to a nursing woman.

ADVERSE REACTIONS

Since Valproic Acid has usually been used with other antiepileptic drugs, it is not possible, in most cases, to determine whether the following adverse reactions can be ascribed to Valproic Acid alone, or the combination of drugs.

Gastrointestinal: The most commonly reported side effects at the initiation of therapy are nausea, vomiting, and indigestion. These effects are usually transient and rarely require discontinuation of therapy. Diarrhea, abdominal cramps, and constipation have been reported. Both anorexia with some weight loss and increased appetite with weight gain have also been reported. Some patients experiencing gastrointestinal side effects may benefit by converting therapy from Valproic Acid to divalproex sodium.[3]

CNS Effects: Sedative effects have occurred in patients receiving Valproate alone but occur most often in patients receiving combination therapy. Sedation usually abates upon reduction of other antiepileptic medication. Tremor (may be dose-related), hallucinations, ataxia, headache, nystagmus, diplopia, asterixis, "spots before eyes", dysarthria, dizziness, and incoordination. Rare cases of coma have been noted in patients receiving Valproic Acid alone or in conjunction with phenobarbital. In rare instances encephalopathy with fever has developed shortly after the introduction of Valproate monotherapy without evidence of hepatic dysfunction or inappropriate plasma levels; all patients recovered after the drug was withdrawn.

Dermatologic: Transient hair loss, skin rash, photosensitivity, generalized pruritus, erythema multiforme, and Stevens-Johnson syndrome. A case of fatal epidermal necrolysis has been reported in a 6 month old infant taking Valproate and several other concomitant medications.

Psychiatric: Emotional upset, depression, psychosis, aggression, hyperactivity and behavioral deterioration.

Musculoskeletal: Weakness.

Hematologic: Thrombocytopenia and inhibition of the secondary phase of platelet aggregation may be reflected in altered bleeding time, petechiae, bruising, hematoma formation and frank hemorrhage (see *"Precautions—General"* and *"Drug Interactions"*). Relative lymphocytosis, macrocytosis, hypofibrinogenemia, leukopenia, eosinophilia, anemia including macrocytic with or without folate deficiency, bone marrow suppression, and acute intermittent porphyria.

Hepatic: Minor elevations of transaminases (e.g., SGOT and SGPT) and LDH are frequent and appear to be dose-related. Occasionally, laboratory test results include increases in serum bilirubin and abnormal changes in other liver function tests. These results may reflect potentially serious hepatotoxicity. (See *"Warnings"*).

Endocrine: Irregular menses, secondary amenorrhea, breast enlargement, galactorrhea, and parotid gland swelling. Abnormal thyroid function tests (see *"Precautions"*).

Pancreatic: Acute pancreatitis including fatalities.

Metabolic: Hyperammonemia (see *"Precautions"*), hyponatremia, and inappropriate ADH secretion.

Decreased carnitine concentrations have been reported although the clinical relevance is undetermined.

Hyperglycinemia has occurred and was associated with a fatal outcome in a patient with preexistent nonketotic hyperglycinemia.

Genitourinary: Enuresis.

Special Senses: Hearing loss, either reversible or irreversible, has been reported; however, a cause and effect relationship has not been established.

Other: Edema of the extremities, lupus erythematous, and fever.

OVERDOSAGE

Overdosage with Valproate may result in somnolence, heart block, and deep coma. Fatalities have been reported.

Since Valproic Acid is absorbed very rapidly, the benefit of gastric lavage or emesis will vary with the time since ingestion. General supportive measures should be applied with particular attention to the maintenance of adequate urinary output.

Naloxone has been reported to reverse the CNS depressant effects of Valproate overdosage. Because naloxone could theoretically also reverse the antiepileptic effects of Valproate, it should be used with caution.

DOSAGE AND ADMINISTRATION

Valproic Acid is administered orally. The recommended initial dose is 15 mg/kg/day, increasing at one week intervals by 5 to 10 mg/kg/day, until seizures are controlled or side effects preclude further increases. The maximum recommended dosage is 60 mg/kg/day. If the total daily dose exceeds 250 mg, it should be given in a divided regimen.

The following table is a guide for the initial daily dose of Valproic Acid (15 mg/kg/day): (See related table).

The frequency of adverse effects (particularly elevated liver enzymes) may be dose-related. The benefit of improved seizure control with higher doses should be weighed against the possibility of a greater incidence of adverse reactions.

A good correlation has not been established between daily dose, serum concentration and therapeutic effect. However, therapeutic Valproate serum concentrations for most patients will range from 50 to 100 mcg/mL. Some patients may be controlled with lower or higher serum concentrations (see *"Clinical Pharmacology"*).

As the Valproic Acid dosage is titrated upward, blood concentrations of phenobarbital and/or phenytoin may be affected. (See *"Precautions"*).

Patients who experience G.I. irritation may benefit from administration of the drug with food or by slowly building up the dose from an initial low level.

THE CAPSULES SHOULD BE SWALLOWED WITHOUT CHEWING TO AVOID LOCAL IRRITATION OF THE MOUTH AND THROAT.

Store capsules at 59-77°F (15-25°C).

Store syrup below 86°F (30°C).

REFERENCES

1. Centers for Disease Control, valproate: a new cause of birth defects—report from Italy and follow-up from France, *Morbidity and Mortality Weekly Report*, 1983;32(33):438-439. 2. Mattson RH, el al. Use of oral contraceptives by women with epilepsy. *JAMA*. 1986;256(2):238-240. 3. Wilder BJ, et al. Gastrointestinal tolerance of divalproex sodium. *Neurology*. 1983;33:808-811. 4. Wilder BJ, et al. Twice-daily dosing of valproate with divalproex. *Clin Pharmacol Ther*. 1983;34(4):501-504. 5. Hurst DL. Expanded therapeutic range of valproate. *Pediatr Neurol*. 1987;3:342-344.

HOW SUPPLIED

CAPSULE: 250 MG

AVERAGE UNIT PRICE (AVAILABLE SIZES)

		GENERIC A-RATED AVERAGE PRICE (GAAP)	
BRAND	$1.16		
GENERIC	$0.33		
HCFA FUL (100s ea)	$0.19	100s	$33.44

BRAND/MANUFACTURER	NDC	SIZE	AWP
◆ **BRAND**			
DEPAKENE: Abbott Pharm	00074-5681-13	100s	$111.98
	00074-5681-11	100s ud	$119.74
◆ **GENERICS**			
Chase	54429-3194-01	100s	$22.00
Schein	00364-0822-01	100s	$24.50
Mason Dist	11845-0185-01	100s	$24.82
Rugby	00536-4477-01	100s	$25.05
Rosemont	00832-1007-00	100s	$28.00
Geneva	00781-2203-01	100s	$28.70
Qualitest	00603-6334-21	100s	$28.75
Purepac	00228-2455-10	100s	$33.59
Martec	52555-0325-01	100s	$34.44
Aligen	00405-5094-01	100s	$36.10
Sidmak	50111-0852-01	100s	$36.25
Parmed	00349-8735-01	100s	$37.50
Intl Labs	00665-4120-06	100s	$37.50
URL	00677-1079-01	100s	$40.45
Moore, H.L.	00839-7180-06	100s	$40.49
Moore, H.L.	00839-7840-06	100s	$40.49
Goldline	00182-1754-01	100s	$44.90
Major	00904-2101-60	100s	$47.10
Major	00904-7765-60	100s	$47.10
U.S. Trading	56126-0106-11	100s ud	$16.40
UDL	51079-0298-20	100s ud	$28.13

SYRUP: 250 MG/5 ML

AVERAGE UNIT PRICE (AVAILABLE SIZES)

		GENERIC A-RATED AVERAGE PRICE (GAAP)	
BRAND	$0.24	480 ml	$48.56
GENERIC	$0.10		
HCFA FUL (480 ml)	$0.07		

BRAND/MANUFACTURER	NDC	SIZE	AWP
◆ **BRAND**			
DEPAKENE: Abbott Pharm	00074-5682-16	480 ml	$114.44
◆ **GENERICS**			
Schein	00364-2139-16	480 ml	$37.27
Moore, H.L.	00839-7195-69	480 ml	$40.84
Geneva	00781-6701-16	480 ml	$41.50
Rugby	00536-2390-85	480 ml	$43.65
Major	00904-2103-16	480 ml	$45.00
Qualitest	00603-1840-58	480 ml	$45.85
Aligen	00405-3890-16	480 ml	$46.80
Pennex	00426-8621-16	480 ml	$56.00
Pennex	00832-8621-16	480 ml	$56.00

◆ RATED THERAPEUTICALLY EQUIVALENT; ◇ THERAPEUTIC EQUIVALENCE UNCONFIRMED; ○ UNRATED

Weight		Total Daily Dose (mg)	Number of Capsules or Teaspoonfuls of Syrup		
(kg)	(lb)		Dose 1	Dose 2	Dose 3
10-24.9	22- 54.9	250	0	0	1
25-39.9	55- 87.9	500	1	0	1
40-59.9	88-131.9	750	1	1	1
60-74.9	132-164.9	1,000	1	1	2
75-89.9	165-197.9	1,250	2	1	2

BRAND/MANUFACTURER	NDC	SIZE	AWP
Goldline	00182-6115-40	480 ml	$68.25

Valrelease SEE DIAZEPAM

Vancenase SEE BECLOMETHASONE DIPROPIONATE

Vanceril SEE BECLOMETHASONE DIPROPIONATE

Vancocin HCl SEE VANCOMYCIN HYDROCHLORIDE

Vancomycin Hydrochloride

Vancomycin Hydrochloride capsules and oral solution for the treatment of colitis are for oral use only and are not systemically absorbed. Oral Vancomycin Hydrochloride must be given orally for treatment of staphylococcal enterocolitis and antibiotic-associated pseudomembranous colitis caused by *Clostridium difficile*. Orally administered oral Vancomycin Hydrochloride is *not* effective for other types of infection.

Parenteral administration of oral Vancomycin Hydrochloride is not effective for treatment of staphylococcal enterocolitis and antibiotic-associated pseudomembranous colitis caused by *C. difficile*.

DESCRIPTION

Vancomycin Hydrochloride (intravenous and oral preparations) is a chromatographically purified, tricyclic glycopeptide antibiotic derived from *Amycolatopsis orientalis* (formerly *Nocardia orientalis*) and has the chemical formula $C_{66}H_{75}Cl_2N_9O_{24}•HCl$. The molecular weight is 1.486; 500 mg of the base is equivalent to 0.34 mmol.

Each vial of Vancomycin Hydrochloride for intravenous injection contains sterile Vancomycin Hydrochloride equivalent to either 500 mg or 1 g Vancomycin activity. Vancomycin Hydrochloride is an off-white lyophilized plug. When reconstituted in water, it forms a clear solution with a pH range of 2.5 to 4.5.

Vancomycin Hydrochloride for oral solution contains Vancomycin Hydrochloride equivalent to 10 g (6.7 mmol) or 1 g (0.67 mmol) Vancomycin.

The capsules contain Vancomycin Hydrochloride equivalent to 125 mg (0.08 mmol) or 250 mg (0.17 mmol) Vancomycin.

Following is its chemical structure:

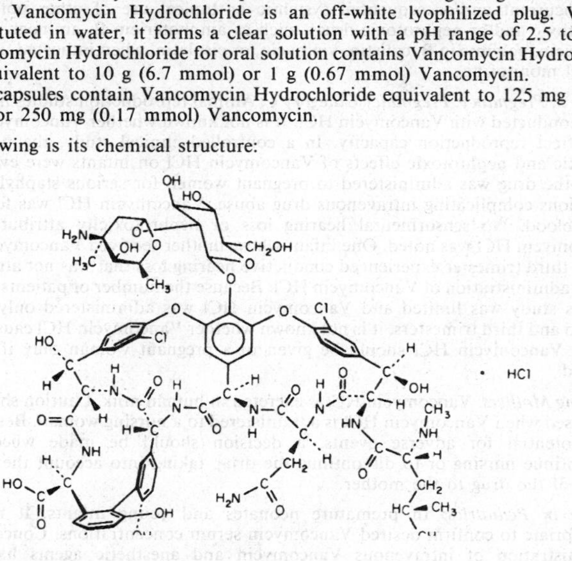

CLINICAL PHARMACOLOGY

Intravenous Preparation: Vancomycin is given intravenously for therapy of systemic infections. Intramuscular injection is painful.

In subjects with normal kidney function, multiple intravenous dosing of 1 g of Vancomycin (15 mg/kg) infused over 60 minutes produces mean plasma concentrations of approximately 63 μg/mL immediately after the completion of infusion, mean plasma concentrations of approximately 23 μg/mL 2 hours after infusion, and mean plasma concentrations of approximately 8 μg/mL 11 hours after the end of the infusion. Multiple dosing of 500 mg infused over 30 minutes produces mean plasma concentrations of about 49 μg/mL at the completion of infusion, mean plasma concentrations of about 19 μg/mL 2 hours after infusion, and mean plasma concentrations of about 10 μg/mL 6 hours after infusion. The plasma concentrations during multiple dosing are similar to those after a single dose.

The mean elimination half-life of Vancomycin from plasma is 4 to 6 hours in subjects with normal renal function. In the first 24 hours, about 75% of an administered dose of Vancomycin is excreted in urine by glomerular filtration. Mean plasma clearance is about 0.058 L/kg/h, and mean renal clearance is about 0.048 L/kg/h. Renal dysfunction slows excretion of Vancomycin. In anephric patients, the average half-life of elimination is 7.5 days. The distribution coefficient is from 0.3 to 0.43 L/kg. There is no apparent metabolism of the drug. About 60% of an intraperitoneal dose of Vancomycin administered during peritoneal dialysis is absorbed systemically in 6 hours. Serum concentrations of about 10 μg/mL are achieved by intraperitoneal injection of 30 mg/kg of Vancomycin. Although Vancomycin is not effectively removed by either hemodialysis or peritoneal dialysis, there have been reports of increased Vancomycin clearance with hemoperfusion and hemofiltration.

Total systemic and renal clearance of Vancomycin may be reduced in the elderly.

Vancomycin is approximately 55% serum protein bound as measured by ultrafiltration at Vancomycin serum concentrations of 10 to 100 μg/mL. After IV administration of Vancomycin HCl, inhibitory concentrations are present in pleural, pericardial, ascitic, and synovial fluids; in urine; in peritoneal dialysis fluid; and in atrial appendage tissue. Vancomycin HCl does not readily diffuse across normal meninges into the spinal fluid; but, when the meninges are inflamed, penetration into the spinal fluid occurs.

Microbiology: The bactericidal action of Vancomycin results primarily from inhibition of cell-wall biosynthesis. In addition, Vancomycin alters bacterial-cell-membrane permeability and RNA synthesis. There is no cross-resistance between Vancomycin and other antibiotics. Intravenous Vancomycin is active against staphylococci, including *Staphylococcus aureus* and *Staphylococcus epidermidis* (including heterogeneous methicillin-resistant strains); streptococci, including *Streptococcus pyogenes, Streptococcus pneumoniae* (including penicillin-resistant strains), *Streptococcus agalactiae*, the viridans group, *Streptococcus bovis*, and enterococci (eg, *Enterococcus faecalis* [formerly *Streptococcus faecalis*]); *Clostridium difficile* (eg, toxigenic strains implicated in pseudomembranous enterocolitis); and diphtheroids. Other organisms that are susceptible to Vancomycin *in vitro* include *Listeria monocytogenes, Lactobacillus* species, *Actinomyces* species, *Clostridium* species, and *Bacillus* species.

Synergy: The combination of Vancomycin and an aminoglycoside acts synergistically *in vitro* against many strains of *S. aureus*, nonenterococcal group D streptococci, enterococci, and *Streptococcus* species (viridans group).

Oral Preparation: Vancomycin is poorly absorbed after oral administration. During multiple dosing of 250 mg every 8 hours for 7 doses, fecal concentrations of Vancomycin in volunteers exceeded 100 mg/kg in the majority of samples. No blood concentrations were detected and urinary recovery did not exceed 0.76%. In anephric patients with no inflammatory bowel disease, blood concentrations of Vancomycin were barely measurable (0.66 μg/mL) in 2 of 5 subjects who received 2 g of Vancomycin HCl for oral solution daily for 16 days. No measurable blood concentrations were attained in the other 3 patients. With doses of 2 g daily, very high concentrations of drug can be found in the feces (> 3,100 mg/kg) and very low concentrations (< 1 μg/mL) can be found in the serum of patients with normal renal function who have pseudomembranous colitis. Orally administered Vancomycin does not usually enter the systemic circulation even when inflammatory lesions are present. After multiple-dose oral administration of Vancomycin, measurable serum concentrations may infrequently occur in patients with active *C. difficile*-induced pseudomembranous colitis, and, in the presence of renal impairment, the possibility of accumulation exists.

Microbiology: The bactericidal action of Vancomycin results primarily from inhibition of cell-wall biosynthesis. In addition, Vancomycin alters bacterial-cell-membrane permeability and RNA synthesis. There is no cross-resistance between Vancomycin and other antibiotics. Oral Vancomycin is active against *C. difficile* (eg, toxigenic strains implicated in pseudomembranous enterocolitis). It is also active against staphylococci, including *Staphylococcus aureus*.

Vancomycin is not active *in vitro* against gram-negative bacilli, mycobacteria, or fungi.

Disk Susceptibility Tests: The standardized disk method described by the National Committee for Clinical Laboratory Standards has been recommended to test susceptibility to Vancomycin. Results of standard susceptibility tests with a 30-µg Vancomycin Hydrochloride disk should be interpreted according to the following criteria: Susceptible organisms produce zones greater than or equal to 12 mm, indicating that the test organism is likely to respond to therapy. Organisms that produce zones of 10 or 11 mm are considered to be of intermediate susceptibility. Organisms in this category are likely to respond if the infection is confined to tissues or fluids in which high antibiotic concentrations are attained. Resistant organisms produce zones of 9 mm or less, indicating that other therapy should be selected.

Using a standardized dilution method, a bacterial isolate may be considered susceptible if the MIC value for Vancomycin is 4 µg/mL or less. Organisms are considered resistant to Vancomycin if the MIC is greater than or equal to 16 µg/mL. Organisms having an MIC value of less than 16 µg/mL but greater than 4 µg/mL are considered to be of intermediate susceptibility.[1-3]

Standardized procedures require the use of laboratory control organisms. The 30µg Vancomycin disk should give zone diameters between 15 and 19 mm for *S. aureus* ATCC 25923. As with the standard diffusion methods, dilution procedures require the use of laboratory control organisms. Standard Vancomycin powder should give MIC values in the range of 0.5 µg/mL to 2.0 µg/mL for *S. aureus* ATCC 29213. For *E. faecalis* ATCC 29212, the MIC range should be 1.0 to 4.0 µg/mL.

INDICATIONS AND USAGE

INTRAVENOUS PREPARATION

Intravenous Vancomycin HCl is indicated for the treatment of serious or severe infections caused by susceptible strains of methicillin-resistant (β-lactam-resistant) staphylococci. It is indicated for penicillin-allergic patients, for patients who cannot receive or who have failed to respond to other drugs, including the penicillins or cephalosporins, and for infections caused by Vancomycin-susceptible organisms that are resistant to other antimicrobial drugs. Vancomycin HCl is indicated for initial therapy when methicillin-resistant staphylococci are suspected, but after susceptibility data are available, therapy should be adjusted accordingly.

Vancomycin HCl is effective in the treatment of staphylococcal endocarditis. Its effectiveness has been documented in other infections due to staphylococci, including septicemia, bone infections, lower respiratory tract infections, and skin and skin structure infections. When staphylococcal infections are localized and purulent, antibiotics are used as adjuncts to appropriate surgical measures.

Vancomycin HCl has been reported to be effective alone or in combination with an aminoglycoside for endocarditis caused by *Streptococcus viridans* or *S. bovis*. For endocarditis caused by enterococci (eg, *E. faecalis*), Vancomycin HCl has been reported to be effective only in combination with an aminoglycoside.

Vancomycin HCl has been reported to be effective for the treatment of diphtheroid endocarditis. Vancomycin HCl has been used successfully in combination with either rifampin, an aminoglycoside, or both in early-onset prosthetic valve endocarditis caused by *S. epidermidis* or diphtheroids.

Specimens for bacteriologic cultures should be obtained in order to isolate and identify causative organisms and to determine their susceptibilities to Vancomycin HCl.

The parenteral form of Vancomycin HCl may be administered orally for treatment of antibiotic-associated pseudomembranous colitis caused by *C. difficile* and for staphylococcal enterocolitis. Parenteral administration of Vancomycin HCl alone is of unproven benefit for these indications.

Although no controlled clinical efficacy studies have been conducted, intravenous Vancomycin has been suggested by the American Heart Association and the American Dental Association as prophylaxis against bacterial endocarditis in penicillin-allergic patients who have congenital heart disease or rheumatic or other acquired valvular heart disease when these patients undergo dental procedures or surgical procedures of the upper respiratory tract.

Note: When selecting antibiotics for the prevention of bacterial endocarditis, the physician or dentist should read the full joint statement of the American Heart Association and the American Dental Association.

ORAL PREPARATION

Vancomycin HCl for oral solution and Vancomycin HCl capsules are administered orally for treatment of staphylococcal enterocolitis and antibiotic-associated pseudomembranous colitis caused by *C. difficile*. Vancomycin HCl must be given orally for these indications. **Orally administered Vancomycin HCl is not effective for other types of infection.**

UNLABELED USES

Vancomycin HCl is used alone or as an adjunct in the treatment of febrile neutropenia, meningitis, and peritonitis.

CONTRAINDICATION

Vancomycin is contraindicated in patients with known hypersensitivity to this antibiotic.

WARNINGS

Rapid bolus administration (eg, over several minutes) may be associated with exaggerated hypotension, and, rarely, cardiac arrest.

Vancomycin HCl should be administered in a dilute solution over a period of not less than 60 minutes to avoid rapid-infusion-related reactions. Stopping the infusion usually results in prompt cessation of these reactions.

Ototoxicity has occurred in patients receiving Vancomycin HCl. It may be transient or permanent. It has been reported mostly in patients who have been given excessive intravenous doses, who have an underlying hearing loss, or who are receiving concomitant therapy with another ototoxic agent, such as an aminoglycoside. Vancomycin should be used with caution in patients with renal insufficiency because the risk of toxicity is appreciably increased by high, prolonged blood concentrations.

Dosage of Vancomycin HCl must be adjusted for patients with renal dysfunction (see *"Precautions"* and *"Dosage and Administration"*).

PRECAUTIONS

General: Clinically significant serum concentrations have been reported in some patients who have taken multiple oral doses of Vancomycin for active *C. difficile* induced pseudo-membranous colitis.

Prolonged use of intravenous Vancomycin HCl may result in the overgrowth of nonsusceptible organisms. Careful observation of the patient is essential. If superinfection occurs during therapy, appropriate measures should be taken. In rare instances, there have been reports of pseudomembranous colitis due to *C. difficile* developing in patients who received intravenous Vancomycin.

Some patients with inflammatory disorders of the intestinal mucosa may have significant systemic absorption of Vancomycin and, therefore, may be at risk for the development of adverse reactions associated with the parenteral administration of Vancomycin. The risk is greater if renal impairment is present. It should be noted that the total systemic and renal clearances of Vancomycin are reduced in the elderly.

In order to minimize the risk of nephrotoxicity when treating patients with underlying renal dysfunction or patients receiving concomitant therapy with an aminoglycoside, serial monitoring of renal function should be performed and particular care should be taken in following appropriate dosing schedules (see *"Dosage and Administration"*).

Serial tests of auditory function may be helpful in order to minimize the risk of ototoxicity.

Reversible neutropenia has been reported in patients receiving intravenous Vancomycin HCl, (see *"Adverse Reactions"*). Patients who will undergo prolonged therapy with Vancomycin HCl or those who are receiving concomitant drugs that may cause neutropenia should have periodic monitoring of the leukocyte count.

Vancomycin HCl is irritating to tissue and must be given by a secure intravenous route of administration. Pain, tenderness, and necrosis occur with intramuscular injection of Vancomycin HCl or with inadvertent extravasation. Thrombophlebitis may occur, the frequency and severity of which can be minimized by administering the drug slowly as a dilute solution (2.5 to 5 g/L) and by rotating the sites of infusion. There have been reports that the frequency of infusion-related events (including hypotension, flushing, erythema, urticaria, and pruritus) increases with the concomitant administration of anesthetic agents. Infusion-related events may be minimized by the administration of Vancomycin HCl as a 60-minute infusion prior to anesthetic induction.

The safety and efficacy of Vancomycin administration by the intrathecal (intralumbar or intraventricular) routes have not been assessed.

Drug Interactions: Concomitant administration of intravenous Vancomycin and anesthetic agents has been associated with erythema and histamine-like flushing (see *"Usage in Pediatrics"* under *"Precautions"*) and anaphylactoid reactions (see *"Adverse Reactions"*).

Concurrent and/or sequential systemic or topical use of other potentially neurotoxic and/or nephrotoxic drugs, such as amphotericin B, aminoglycosides, bacitracin, polymyxin B, colistin, viomycin, or cisplatin, when indicated, requires careful monitoring.

Usage in Pregnancy: Pregnancy Category C: Animal reproduction studies have not been conducted with Vancomycin HCl. It is not known whether Vancomycin HCl can affect reproduction capacity. In a controlled clinical study, the potential ototoxic and nephrotoxic effects of Vancomycin HCl on infants were evaluated when the drug was administered to pregnant women for serious staphylococcal infections complicating intravenous drug abuse. Vancomycin HCl was found in cord blood. No sensorineural hearing loss or nephrotoxicity attributable to Vancomycin HCl was noted. One infant whose mother received Vancomycin HCl in the third trimester experienced conductive hearing loss that was not attributed to the administration of Vancomycin HCl. Because the number of patients treated in this study was limited and Vancomycin HCl was administered only in the second and third trimesters, it is not known whether Vancomycin HCl causes fetal harm. Vancomycin HCl should be given to a pregnant woman only if clearly needed.

Nursing Mothers: Vancomycin HCl is excreted in human milk. Caution should be exercised when Vancomycin HCl is administered to a nursing woman. Because of the potential for adverse events, a decision should be made whether to discontinue nursing or to discontinue the drug, taking into account the importance of the drug to the mother.

Usage in Pediatrics: In premature neonates and young infants, it may be appropriate to confirm desired Vancomycin serum concentrations. Concomitant administration of intravenous Vancomycin and anesthetic agents has been associated with erythema and histamine-like flushing in children (see *"Adverse Reactions"*).

Geriatrics: The natural decrement of glomerular filtration with increasing age may lead to elevated Vancomycin serum concentrations if dosage is not adjusted. Vancomycin dosage schedules should be adjusted in elderly patients (see *"Dosage and Administration"*).

◆ RATED THERAPEUTICALLY EQUIVALENT; ◇ THERAPEUTIC EQUIVALENCE UNCONFIRMED; ○ UNRATED

ADVERSE REACTIONS

Infusion-Related Events: During or soon after rapid infusion of Vancomycin HCl, patients may develop anaphylactoid reactions, including hypotension, wheezing, dyspnea, urticaria, or pruritus. Rapid infusion may also cause flushing of the upper body ("red neck") or pain and muscle spasm of the chest and back. These reactions usually resolve within 20 minutes but may persist for several hours. In animal studies, hypotension and bradycardia occurred in animals given large doses of intravenous Vancomycin at high concentrations and rates. Such events are infrequent if Vancomycin HCl is given by a slow infusion over 60 minutes. In studies of normal volunteers, infusion-related events did not occur when Vancomycin HCl was administered at a rate of 10 mg/min or less.

Nephrotoxicity: Rarely, renal failure, principally manifested by increased serum creatinine or BUN concentrations, especially in patients given large doses of intravenously administered Vancomycin HCl, has been reported. Rare cases of interstitial nephritis have been reported. Most of these have occurred in patients who were given aminoglycosides concomitantly or who had preexisting kidney dysfunction. When Vancomycin HCl was discontinued, azotemia resolved in most patients.

Ototoxicity: A few dozen cases of hearing loss associated with intravenously administered Vancomycin HCl have been reported. Most of these patients had kidney dysfunction or a preexisting hearing loss or were receiving concomitant treatment with an ototoxic drug. Vertigo, dizziness, and tinnitus have been reported rarely.

Hematopoietic: Reversible neutropenia, usually starting 1 week or more after onset of intravenous therapy with Vancomycin HCl or after a total dosage of more than 25 g, has been reported for several dozen patients. Neutropenia appears to be promptly reversible when Vancomycin HCl is discontinued. Thrombocytopenia has rarely been reported.

Although a causal relationship has not been established, reversible agranulocytosis (granulocyte count less than 500/mm^3) has been reported rarely.

Phlebitis: Inflammation at the injection site has been reported.

Miscellaneous: Infrequently, patients have been reported to have had anaphylaxis, drug fever, nausea, chills, eosinophilia, rashes (including exfoliative dermatitis), Stevens-Johnson syndrome, toxic epidermal necrolysis, and rare cases of vasculitis in association with administration of Vancomycin HCl.

OVERDOSAGE

Supportive care is advised, with maintenance of glomerular filtration. Vancomycin is poorly removed by dialysis. Hemofiltration and hemoperfusion with polysulfone resin have been reported to result in increased Vancomycin clearance. The median lethal intravenous dose is 319 mg/kg in rats and 400 mg/kg in mice.

To obtain up-to-date information about the treatment of overdose, a good resource is your certified Regional Poison Control Center. Telephone numbers of certified poison control centers are listed in the *Physicians' Desk Reference (PDR)*. In managing overdosage, consider the possibility of multiple drug overdoses, interaction among drugs, and unusual drug kinetics in your patient.

DOSAGE AND ADMINISTRATION

INTRAVENOUS PREPARATION

Infusion-related events are related to both concentration and rate of administration of Vancomycin. Concentrations of no more than 5 mg/mL and rates of no more than 10 mg/min are recommended in adults (see also age-specific recommendations). In selected patients in need of fluid restriction, a concentration up to 10 mg/mL may be used; use of such higher concentrations may increase the risk of infusion-related events. Infusion-related events may occur, however, at any rate or concentration.

PATIENTS WITH NORMAL RENAL FUNCTION

Adults: The usual daily intravenous dose is 2 g divided either as 500 mg every 6 hours or 1 g every 12 hours. Each dose should be administered at no more than 10 mg/min or over a period of at least 60 minutes, whichever is longer. Other patient factors, such as age or obesity, may call for modification of the usual intravenous daily dose.

Children: The usual intravenous dosage of Vancomycin HCl is 10 mg/kg per dose given every 6 hours. Each dose should be administered over a period of at least 60 minutes.

Infants and Neonates: In neonates and young infants, the total daily intravenous dosage may be lower. In both neonates and infants, an initial dose of 15 mg/kg is suggested, followed by 10 mg/kg every 12 hours for neonates in the 1st week of life and every 8 hours thereafter up to the age of 1 month. Each dose should be administered over 60 minutes. Close monitoring of serum concentrations of Vancomycin may be warranted in these patients.

PATIENTS WITH IMPAIRED RENAL FUNCTION AND ELDERLY PATIENTS

Dosage adjustment must be made in patients with impaired renal function. In premature infants and the elderly, greater dosage reductions than expected may be necessary because of decreased renal function. Measurement of Vancomycin serum concentrations can be helpful in optimizing therapy, especially in seriously ill patients with changing renal function. Vancomycin serum concentrations can be determined by use of microbiologic assay, radioimmunoassay, fluorescence polarization immunoassay, fluorescence immunoassay, or high-pressure liquid chromatography.

If creatinine clearance can be measured or estimated accurately, the dosage for most patients with renal impairment can be calculated using the following table. The dosage of Vancomycin HCl per day in mg is about 15 times the glomerular filtration rate in mL/min:

DOSAGE TABLE FOR VANCOMYCIN IN PATIENTS WITH IMPAIRED RENAL FUNCTION

(Adapted from Moellering et al[5])

Creatinine Clearance mL/min	Vancomycin Dose mg/24 h
100	1,545
90	1,390
80	1,235
70	1,080
60	925
50	770
40	620
30	465
20	310
10	155

The initial dose should be no less than 15 mg/kg, even in patients with mild to moderate renal insufficiency.

The table is not valid for functionally anephric patients. For such patients, an initial dose of 15 mg/kg of body weight should be given to achieve prompt therapeutic serum concentrations. The dose required to maintain stable concentrations is 1.9 mg/kg/24 h. In patients with marked renal inpairment, it may be more convenient to give maintenance doses of 250 to 1,000 mg once every several days rather than administering the drug on a daily basis. In anuria, a dose of 1,000 mg every 7 to 10 days has been recommended.

When only the serum creatinine concentration is known, the following formula (based on sex, weight, and age of the patient) may be used to calculate creatinine clearance. Calculated creatinine clearances (mL/min) are only estimates. The creatinine clearance should be measured promptly.

Men: $$\frac{\text{Weight (kg)} \times (140 - \text{age in years})}{72 \times \text{serum creatinine concentration (mg/dL)}}$$

Women: $0.85 \times$ above value

The serum creatinine must represent a steady state of renal function. Otherwise, the estimated value for creatinine clearance is not valid. Such a calculated clearance is an overestimate of actual clearance in patients with conditions: (1) characterized by decreasing renal function, such as shock, severe heart failure, or oliguria; (2) in which a normal relationship between muscle mass and total body weight is not present, such as obese patients or those with liver disease, edema, or ascites; and (3) accompanied by debilitation, malnutrition, or inactivity.

The safety and efficacy of Vancomycin administration by the intrathecal (intralumbar or intraventricular) routes have not been assessed.

Intermittent infusion is the recommended method of administration.

ORAL PREPARATION

Adults: Oral Vancomycin HCl is used in treating antibiotic-associated pseudomembranous colitis caused by *C. difficile* and staphylococcal enterocolitis. Vancomycin HCl is not effective by the oral route for other types of infections. The usual adult total daily dosage is 500 mg to 2 g administered orally in 3 or 4 divided doses for 7 to 10 days.

Children: The usual daily dosage is 40 mg/kg in 3 or 4 divided doses for 7 to 10 days. The total daily dosage should not exceed 2 g.

PREPARATION AND STABILITY

Intravenous Preparation: At the time of use, reconstitute by adding either 10 mL of sterile water for injection per 500 mg or 20 mL of sterile water for injection per 1 g of dry, sterile Vancomycin powder. Powder reconstituted in this manner will give a solution of 50 mg/mL. FURTHER DILUTION IS REQUIRED.

After reconstitution, the solution may be stored in a refrigerator for 14 days without significant loss of potency. Reconstituted solutions containing 500 mg of Vancomycin must be diluted with at least 100 mL of diluent. Reconstituted solutions containing 1 g of Vancomycin must be diluted with at least 200 mL of diluent. The desired dose, diluted in this manner, should be administered by intermittent intravenous infusion over a period of at least 60 minutes.

Compatibility With Intravenous Fluids: Solutions that are diluted with 5% dextrose injection or 0.9% sodium chloride injection may be stored in a refrigerator for 14 days without significant loss of potency. Solutions that are diluted with the following infusion fluids may be stored in a refrigerator for 96 hours:

5% dextrose injection and 0.9% sodium chloride injection
Lactated Ringer's injection
Lactated Ringer's and 5% dextrose injection
Normosol®-M and 5% dextrose
Isolyte® E
Acetated Ringer's injection

Vancomycin solution has a low pH and may cause chemical or physical instability when it is mixed with other compounds.

Prior to administration, parenteral drug products should be inspected visually for particulate matter and discoloration whenever solution or container permits.

Prior to reconstitution, the solution may be stored at room temperature, 59° to 86°F (15° to 30°C).

Oral Preparation: Vancomycin HCl for Oral Solution: 10 g of Vancomycin HCl may be mixed with 115 mL distilled or deionized water for oral administration. When mixed with 115 mL of water, each 6 mL provides approximately 500 mg of Vancomycin. 1 g of Vancomycin HCl may be mixed with 20 mL distilled or deionized water. When reconstituted with 20 mL, each 5 mL contains approximately 250 mg of Vancomycin. Mix thoroughly to dissolve. These mixtures may be kept for 2 weeks in a refrigerator without significant loss of potency.

The appropriate oral solution dose may be diluted in 1 oz of water and given to the patient to drink. Common flavoring syrups may be added to the solution to improve the taste for oral administration. The diluted material may be administered via nasogastric tube.

Storage: Store at controlled room temperature, 59° to 86°F (15° to 30°C).

REFERENCES
1. National Committee for Clinical Laboratory Standards, 1984. Performance standards for antimicrobial disk susceptibility tests, MZ-A3, NCCLS, Villanova, PA 19805. 2. National Committee for Clinical Laboratory Standards, 1983. Methods for dilution antimicrobial susceptibility tests for bacteria that grow aerobically, M7-T, NCCLS, Villanova, PA 19805. 3. National Committee for Clinical Laboratory Standards, 1984. Reference agar dilution procedure for antimicrobial susceptibility testing of anaerobic bacteria, M11-A, NCCLS, Villanova, PA 19805. 4. Shulman ST, Amren DP, Bisno AL, et al: Prevention of bacterial endocarditis, *Circulation* 1984; 70:1123A. 5. Moellering RC, Krogstad DJ, Greenblatt DJ: Vancomycin therapy in patients with impaired renal function: A nomogram for dosage. *Ann Intern Med* 1981; 94:343.

J CODES
Up to 500 mg IV,IM—J3370

HOW SUPPLIED
CAPSULE: 125 MG
BRAND/MANUFACTURER	NDC	SIZE	AWP
○ BRAND			
VANCOCIN HCL PULVULES: Lilly	00002-3125-42	20s	$94.50

CAPSULE: 250 MG
BRAND/MANUFACTURER	NDC	SIZE	AWP
○ BRAND			
VANCOCIN HCL PULVULES: Lilly	00002-3126-42	20s	$189.01

POWDER FOR INJECTION: 500 MG/100 ML
BRAND/MANUFACTURER	NDC	SIZE	AWP
○ BRAND			
VANCOCIN HCL: Lilly	00002-7467-12	12s	$132.05

POWDER FOR INJECTION: 500 MG
AVERAGE UNIT PRICE (AVAILABLE SIZES)		GENERIC A-RATED AVERAGE PRICE (GAAP)	
BRAND	$7.96	10s	$154.51
GENERIC	$14.56		

BRAND/MANUFACTURER	NDC	SIZE	AWP
◆ BRAND			
VANCOCIN HCL: Lilly	00002-1444-01	1s	$7.80
	00002-1444-10	10s	$78.00
	00002-7297-10	10s	$82.80
◆ GENERICS			
LYPHOCIN: Fujisawa	00469-2210-30	1s	$10.97
VANCOLED: Lederle Std Prod	00205-3154-88	10s	$57.56
Schein	00364-2472-33	10s	$70.00
Elkins-Sinn	00641-2778-43	10s	$188.13
Abbott Hosp	00074-4332-01	10s	$302.34

POWDER FOR INJECTION: 1 GM
AVERAGE UNIT PRICE (AVAILABLE SIZES)		GENERIC A-RATED AVERAGE PRICE (GAAP)	
BRAND	$15.84	10s	$308.91
GENERIC	$28.78		

BRAND/MANUFACTURER	NDC	SIZE	AWP
◆ BRAND			
VANCOCIN HCL: Lilly	00002-7321-10	10s	$156.01
	00002-7298-10	10s	$160.81
◆ GENERICS			
LYPHOCIN: Fujisawa	00469-2840-40	1s	$20.35
VANCOLED: Lederle Std Prod	00205-3154-15	10s	$115.15
Schein	00364-2473-91	10s	$140.41
Elkins-Sinn	00641-2779-43	10s	$375.63
Abbott Hosp	00074-6533-01	10s	$604.44

POWDER FOR INJECTION: 5 GM
AVERAGE UNIT PRICE (AVAILABLE SIZES)		GENERIC A-RATED AVERAGE PRICE (GAAP)	
GENERIC	$101.98	1s	$101.98

BRAND/MANUFACTURER	NDC	SIZE	AWP
◆ GENERICS			
VANCOLED: Lederle Std Prod	00205-3154-05	1s	$57.56
LYPHOCIN: Fujisawa	00469-2951-00	1s	$112.39
Abbott Hosp	00074-6509-01	1s	$135.99

POWDER FOR INJECTION: 10 GM
BRAND/MANUFACTURER	NDC	SIZE	AWP
◆ BRAND			
VANCOCIN HCL: Lilly	00002-7355-01	1s	$156.01

POWDER FOR RECONSTITUTION: 250 MG/5 ML
BRAND/MANUFACTURER	NDC	SIZE	AWP
○ BRAND			
VANCOCIN HCL: Lilly	00002-5105-16	20 ml 6s	$205.21

POWDER FOR RECONSTITUTION: 500 MG/6 ML
BRAND/MANUFACTURER	NDC	SIZE	AWP
○ BRAND			
VANCOCIN HCL: Lilly	00002-2372-37	120 ml	$276.21

Vansil SEE OXAMNIQUINE

Vantin SEE CEFPODOXIME PROXETIL

Varicella Zoster Immune Globulin
SEE GLOBULIN, IMMUNE

Vascor SEE BEPRIDIL HYDROCHLORIDE

Vascoray SEE IOTHALAMATE MEGLUMINE AND IOTHALAMATE SODIUM

Vaseretic 10-25 SEE ENALAPRIL MALEATE WITH HYDROCHLOROTHIAZIDE

Vasocidin SEE PREDNISOLONE AND SULFACETAMIDE SODIUM

Vasocon SEE NAPHAZOLINE HYDROCHLORIDE

Vasocon-A SEE ANTAZOLINE PHOSPHATE AND NAPHAZOLINE HYDROCHLORIDE

Vasodilan SEE ISOXSUPRINE HYDROCHLORIDE

Vasopressin

DESCRIPTION
Vasopressin Injection is a sterile, aqueous solution of synthetic Vasopressin (8-Arginine vasopressin) of the posterior pituitary gland. It is substantially free from the oxytocic principle and is standardized to contain 20 pressor units/ml. The solution contains 0.5% Chloretone (chlorobutanol, chloroform derivative) as a preservative. The acidity of the solution is adjusted with acetic acid.

Following is its chemical structure:

$$H-Cys-Tyr-Phe-Glu(NH_2)-Asp(NH_2)-Cys-Pro-Arg^*-Gly-NH_2$$
$$1\ \ 2\ \ 3\ \ 4\ \ 5\ \ 6\ \ 7\ \ 8\ \ 9$$

(*In pig vasopressin, Arg is Lys)

CLINICAL PHARMACOLOGY
The antidiuretic action of Vasopressin is ascribed to increasing reabsorption of water by the renal tubules.

Vasopressin can cause contraction of smooth muscle of the gastrointestinal tract and of all parts of the vascular bed, especially the capillaries, small arterioles and venules with less effect on the smooth musculature of the large veins. The

---

◆ RATED THERAPEUTICALLY EQUIVALENT; ◇ THERAPEUTIC EQUIVALENCE UNCONFIRMED; ○ UNRATED

direct effect on the contractile elements is neither antagonized by adrenergic blocking agents nor prevented by vascular denervation.

Following subcutaneous or intramuscular administration of Vasopressin injection, the duration of antidiuretic activity is variable but effects are usually maintained for 2-8 hours. The majority of a dose of Vasopressin is metabolized and rapidly destroyed in the liver and kidneys. Vasopressin has a plasma half-life of about 10 to 20 minutes. Approximately 5% of a subcutaneous dose of Vasopressin is excreted in urine unchanged after four hours.

CONTRAINDICATION
Anaphylaxis or hypersensitivity to the drug or its components.

INDICATIONS AND USAGE
Vasopressin is indicated for prevention and treatment of post-operative abdominal distention, in abdominal roentgenography to dispel interfering gas shadows, and in diabetes insipidus.

WARNINGS
This drug should not be used in patients with vascular disease, especially disease of the coronary arteries, except with extreme caution. In such patients, even small doses may precipitate anginal pain, and with larger doses, the possibility of myocardial infarction should be considered.

Vasopressin may produce water intoxication. The early signs of drowsiness, listlessness, and headaches should be recognized to prevent terminal coma and convulsions.

PRECAUTIONS
General: Vasopressin should be used cautiously in the presence of epilepsy, migraine, asthma, heart failure or any state in which a rapid addition to extracellular water may produce hazard for an already overburdened system.

Chronic nephritis with nitrogen retention contraindicates the use of Vasopressin until reasonable nitrogen blood levels have been attained.

Information for Patients: Side effects such as blanching of skin, abdominal cramps, and nausea may be reduced by taking 1 or 2 glasses of water at the time of Vasopressin administration. These side effects are usually not serious and probably will disappear within a few minutes.

Laboratory Tests: Electrocardiograms (ECG) and fluid and electrolyte status determinations are recommended at periodic intervals during therapy.

Drug Interactions:
1) The following drugs may potentiate the antidiuretic effect of Vasopressin when used concurrently: carbamazepine; chlorpropamide; clofibrate; urea; fludrocortisone; tricyclic antidepressants.
2) The following drugs may decrease the antidiuretic effect of Vasopressin when used concurrently: demeclocycline; norepinephrine; lithium; heparin; alcohol.
3) Ganglionic blocking agents may produce a marked increase in sensitivity to the pressor effects of Vasopressin.

Pregnancy Category C: Animal reproduction studies have not been conducted with Vasopressin. It is also not known whether Vasopressin can cause fetal harm when administered to a pregnant woman or can affect reproduction capacity. Vasopressin should be given to a pregnant woman only if clearly needed.

Labor and Delivery: Doses of Vasopressin sufficient for an antidiuretic effect are not likely to produce tonic uterine contractions that could be deleterious to the fetus or threaten the continuation of the pregnancy.

Nursing Mothers: Caution should be exercised when Vasopressin is administered to a nursing woman.

ADVERSE REACTIONS
Local or systemic allergic reactions may occur in hypersensitive individuals. The following side effects have been reported following the administration of Vasopressin:

Body as a Whole: anaphylaxis (cardiac arrest and/or shock) have been observed shortly after injection of vasopressin.

Cardiovascular: cardiac arrest, circumoral pallor, arrhythmias, decreased cardiac output, angina, myocardial ischemia, peripheral vasoconstriction and gangrene.

Gastrointestinal: abdominal cramps, nausea, vomiting, passage of gas.

Nervous System: tremor, vertigo, "pounding" in head.

Respiratory: bronchial constriction.

Skin and Appendages: sweating, urticaria, cutaneous gangrene.

OVERDOSAGE
Water intoxication may be treated with water restriction and temporary withdrawal of Vasopressin until polyuria occurs. Severe water intoxication may require osmotic diuresis with mannitol, hypertonic dextrose, or urea alone or with furosemide.

DOSAGE AND ADMINISTRATION
Vasopressin may be administered subcutaneously or intramuscularly.

Ten units of Vasopressin (0.5 mL) will usually elicit full physiologic response in adult patients; 5 units will be adequate in many cases. Vasopressin should be given intramuscularly at three- or four-hour intervals as needed. The dosage should be proportionally reduced for children. (For an additional discussion of dosage, consult the sections below.)

When determining the dose of Vasopressin for a given case, the following should be kept in mind:

It is particularly desirable to give a dose not much larger than is just sufficient to elicit the desired physiologic response. Excessive doses may cause undesirable side effects—blanching of the skin, abdominal cramps, nausea—which, though not serious, may be alarming to the patient. Spontaneous recovery from such side effects occurs in a few minutes. It has been found that one or two glasses of water given at the time Vasopressin is administered reduce such symptoms.

Abdominal Distention: In the average postoperative adult patient, give 5 units (0.25 mL) initially, increase to 10 units (0.5 mL) at subsequent injections if necessary. It is recommended that Vasopressin be given intramuscularly and that injections be repeated at three- or four-hour intervals as required. Dosage to be reduced proportionately for children.

Vasopressin used in this manner will frequently prevent or relieve postoperative distention. These recommendations apply also to distention complicating pneumonia or other acute toxemias.

Abdominal Roentgenography: For the average case, two injections of 10 units each (0.5 mL) are suggested. These should be given two hours and one-half hour, respectively, before films are exposed. Many roentgenologists advise giving an enema prior to the first dose of Vasopressin.

Diabetes Insipidus: Vasopressin may be given by injection or administered intranasally on cotton pledgets, by nasal spray, or by dropper. The dose by injection is 5 to 10 units (0.25 to 0.5 mL) repeated two or three times daily as needed. When Vasopressin is administered intranasally by spray or on pledgets, the dosage and interval between treatments must be determined for each patient.

Storage: Store between 15° and 25° (59° and 77°F).

HOW SUPPLIED
INJECTION: 10 U/0.5 ML

BRAND/MANUFACTURER	NDC	SIZE	AWP
◆ **GENERICS**			
Fujisawa	00469-2990-00	2 ml	$4.51

INJECTION: 10 U/0.5 ML

BRAND/MANUFACTURER	NDC	SIZE	AWP
○ **BRAND**			
PITRESSIN: Parke-Davis	00071-4200-45	0.5 ml 25s	$107.88

INJECTION: 20 U/ML

BRAND/MANUFACTURER	NDC	SIZE	AWP
◆ **GENERICS**			
Fujisawa	00469-3020-00	2 ml	$8.50

INJECTION: 20 U/ML

BRAND/MANUFACTURER	NDC	SIZE	AWP
○ **BRAND**			
PITRESSIN: Parke-Davis	00071-4200-03	1 ml 10s	$80.63
	00071-4200-46	1 ml 25s	$201.48

Vasosulf SEE PHENYLEPHRINE HYDROCHLORIDE AND SULFACETAMIDE SODIUM

Vasotec SEE ENALAPRIL

Vasoxyl SEE METHOXAMINE HYDROCHLORIDE

V-Cillin K SEE PENICILLIN V POTASSIUM

Vecuronium Bromide

THIS DRUG SHOULD BE ADMINISTERED BY ADEQUATELY TRAINED INDIVIDUALS FAMILIAR WITH ITS ACTIONS, CHARACTERISTICS, AND HAZARDS.

DESCRIPTION
Vecuronium Bromide for injection is a nondepolarizing neuromuscular blocking agent of intermediate duration, chemically designated as piperidinium, 1-[(2β, 3α, 5α, 16β, 17β)-3, 17-bis(acetyloxy)-2-(1- piperidinyl) androstan-16-yl]-1-methyl-, bromide.

Its chemical formula is $C_{34}H_{57}BrN_2O_4$ with molecular weight 637.74.

► SHOWN IN PRODUCT IDENTIFICATION GUIDE

Vecuronium Bromide is supplied as a sterile nonpyrogenic freeze-dried buffered cake of very fine microscopic crystalline particles for intravenous injection only. Each 10 mL vial contains 10 mg Vecuronium Bromide, 20.75 mg citric acid anhydrous, 16.25 mg sodium phosphate dibasic anhydrous, 97 mg mannitol (to adjust tonicity), sodium hydroxide and/or phosphoric acid to buffer and adjust to a pH of 4. Each 20 mL vial contains 20 mg of Vecuronium Bromide, 41.5 mg citric acid anhydrous, 32.5 mg sodium phosphate dibasic anhydrous, 194 mg mannitol (to adjust tonicity), sodium hydroxide and/or phosphoric acid to buffer and adjust to a pH of 4. Bacteriostatic water for injection, USP, when supplied, contains 0.9% w/v Benzyl Alcohol, WHICH IS NOT FOR USE IN NEWBORNS.

Following is its chemical structure:

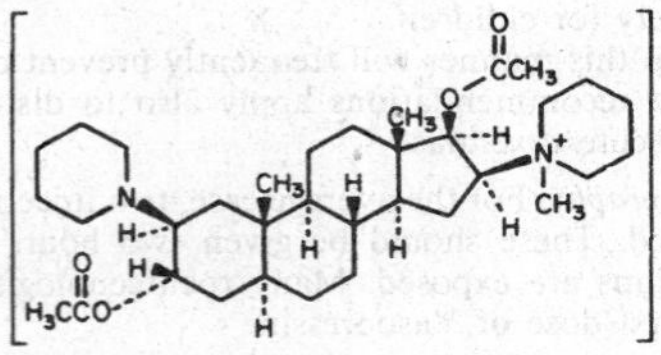

CLINICAL PHARMACOLOGY

Vecuronium Bromide for injection is a non-depolarizing neuromuscular blocking agent possessing all of the characteristic pharmacological actions of this class of drugs (curariform). It acts by competing for cholinergic receptors at the motor end-plate. The antagonism to acetylcholine is inhibited and neuromuscular block is reversed by acetylcholinesterase inhibitors such as neostigmine, edrophonium, and pyridostigmine. Vecuronium Bromide is about ⅓ more potent than pancuronium: the duration of neuromuscular blockade produced by Vecuronium Bromide is shorter than that of pancuronium at initially equipotent doses. The time to onset of paralysis decreases and the duration of maximum effect increases with increasing Vecuronium Bromide doses. The use of a peripheral nerve stimulator is recommended in assessing the degree of muscular relaxation with all neuromuscular blocking drugs. The ED_{90} (dose required to produce 90% suppression of the muscle twitch response with balanced anesthesia) has averaged 0.057 mg/kg (0.049 to 0.062 mg/kg in various studies). An initial Vecuronium Bromide dose of 0.08 to 0.10 mg/kg generally produces first depression of twitch in approximately 1 minute, good or excellent intubation conditions within 2.5 to 3 minutes, and maximum neuromuscular blockade within 3 to 5 minutes of injection in most patients. Under balanced anesthesia, the time to recovery to 25% of control (clinical duration) is approximately 25 to 40 minutes after injection and recovery is usually 95% complete approximately 45-65 minutes after injection of intubating dose. The neuromuscular blocking action of Vecuronium Bromide is slightly enhanced in the presence of potent inhalation anesthetics. If Vecuronium Bromide is first administered more than 5 minutes after the start of the inhalation of enflurane, isoflurane, or halothane, or when steady state has been achieved, the intubating dose of Vecuronium Bromide may be decreased by approximately 15% (see *"Dosage and Administration"* section). Prior administration of succinylcholine may enhance the neuromuscular blocking effect of Vecuronium Bromide and its duration of action. With succinylcholine as the intubating agent, initial doses of 0.04-0.06 mg/kg of Vecuronium Bromide will produce complete neuromuscular block with clinical duration of action of 25-30 minutes. If succinylcholine is used prior to Vecuronium Bromide, the administration of Vecuronium Bromide should be delayed until the patient starts recovering from succinylcholine-induced neuromuscular blockade. The effect of prior use of other nondepolarizing neuromuscular blocking agents on the activity of Vecuronium Bromide has not been studied (see *"Drug Interactions"*).

Repeated administration of maintenance doses of Vecuronium Bromide has little or no cumulative effect on the duration of neuromuscular blockade. Therefore, repeat doses can be administered at relatively regular intervals with predictable results. After an initial dose of 0.08 to 0.10 mg/kg under balanced anesthesia, the first maintenance dose (suggested maintenance dose is 0.010 to 0.015 mg/kg) is generally required within 25 to 40 minutes; subsequent maintenance doses, if required, may be administered at approximately 12 to 15 minute intervals. Halothane anesthesia increases the clinical duration of the maintenance dose only slightly. Under enflurane a maintenance dose of 0.010 mg/kg is approximately equal to 0.015 mg/kg dose under balanced anesthesia.

The recovery index (time from 25% to 75% recovery) is approximately 15-25 minutes under balanced or halothane anesthesia. When recovery from Vecuronium Bromide neuromuscular blocking effect begins, it proceeds more rapidly than recovery from pancuronium. Once spontaneous recovery has started, the neuromuscular block produced by Vecuronium Bromide is readily reversed with various anticholinesterase agents, e.g., pyridostigmine, neostigmine, or edrophonium in conjunction with an anticholinergic agent such as atropine or glycopyrrolate. Rapid recovery is a finding consistent with Vecuronium Bromide's short elimination half-life, although there have been occasional reports of prolonged neuromuscular blockade in patients in the intensive care unit (see *"Precautions"*). The administration of clinical doses of Vecuronium Bromide is not characterized by laboratory or clinical signs of chemically mediated histamine release. This does not preclude the possibility of rare hypersensitivity reactions (see *"Adverse Reactions"*).

Pharmacokinetics: At clinical doses of 0.04-0.10 mg/kg, 60-80% of Vecuronium Bromide is usually bound to plasma protein. The distribution half-life following a single intravenous dose (range 0.025-0.280 mg/kg) is approximately 4 minutes. Elimination half-life over this same dosage range is approximately 65-75 minutes

in healthy surgical patients and in renal failure patients undergoing transplant surgery.

In late pregnancy, elimination half-life may be shortened to approximately 35-40 minutes. The volume of distribution at steady state is approximately 300-400 mL/kg; systemic rate of clearance is approximately 3-4.5 mL/minute/kg. In man, urine recovery of Vecuronium Bromide varies from 3-35% within 24 hours. Data derived from patients requiring insertion of a T-tube in the common bile duct suggests that 25-50% of a total intravenous dose of Vecuronium may be excreted in bile within 42 hours. Only unchanged Vecuronium has been detected in human plasma following use during surgery. In addition, one metabolite, 3-desacetyl Vecuronium, has been rarely detected in human plasma following prolonged clinical use in the I.C.U. (see *"Precautions: Long Term Use in I.C.U."*). The 3-desacetyl Vecuronium metabolite has been recovered in the urine of some patients in quantities that account for up to 10% of injected dose; 3-desacetyl Vecuronium has also been recovered by T-tube in some patients accounting for up to 25% of the injected dose.

This metabolite has been judged by animal screening (dogs and cats) to have 50% or more of the potency of Vecuronium Bromide equipotent doses are of approximately the same duration as Vecuronium Bromide in dogs and cats. Biliary excretion accounts for about half the dose of Vecuronium Bromide within 7 hours in the anesthetized rat. Circulatory bypass of the liver (cat preparation) prolongs recovery from Vecuronium Bromide. Limited data derived from patients with cirrhosis or cholestasis suggests that some measurements of recovery may be doubled in such patients. In patients with renal failure, measurements of recovery do not differ significantly from similar measurements in healthy patients.

Studies involving routine hemodynamic monitoring in good risk surgical patients reveal that the administration of Vecuronium Bromide in doses up to three times that needed to produce clinical relaxation (0.15 mg/kg) did not produce clinically significant changes in systolic, diastolic or mean arterial pressure. The heart rate, under similar monitoring, remained unchanged in some studies and was lowered by a mean of up to 8% in other studies. A large dose of 0.28 mg/kg administered during a period of no stimulation, while patients were being prepared for coronary artery bypass grafting, was not associated with alterations in rate-pressure-product or pulmonary capillary wedge pressure. Systemic vascular resistance was lowered slightly and cardiac output was increased insignificantly. (The drug has not been studied in patients with hemodynamic dysfunction secondary to cardiac valvular disease). Limited clinical experience with use of Vecuronium Bromide during surgery for pheochromocytoma has shown that administration of this drug is not associated with changes in blood pressure or heart rate.

Unlike other nondepolarizing skeletal muscle relaxants, Vecuronium Bromide has no clinically significant effects on hemodynamic parameters. Vecuronium Bromide will not counteract those hemodynamic changes or known side effects produced by or associated with anesthetic agents, other drugs or various other factors known to alter hemodynamics.

INDICATIONS AND USAGE

Vecuronium Bromide is indicated as an adjunct to general anesthesia, to facilitate endotracheal intubation and to provide skeletal muscle relaxation during surgery or mechanical ventilation.

CONTRAINDICATIONS

Vecuronium Bromide is contraindicated in patients known to have a hypersensitivity to it.

WARNINGS

VECURONIUM BROMIDE SHOULD BE ADMINISTERED IN CAREFULLY ADJUSTED DOSAGE BY OR UNDER THE SUPERVISION OF EXPERIENCED CLINICIANS WHO ARE FAMILIAR WITH ITS ACTIONS AND THE POSSIBLE COMPLICATIONS THAT MIGHT OCCUR FOLLOWING ITS USE. THE DRUG SHOULD NOT BE ADMINISTERED UNLESS FACILITIES FOR INTUBATION, ARTIFICIAL RESPIRATION, OXYGEN THERAPY, AND REVERSAL AGENTS ARE IMMEDIATELY AVAILABLE. THE CLINICIAN MUST BE PREPARED TO ASSIST OR CONTROL RESPIRATION. TO REDUCE THE POSSIBILITY OF PROLONGED NEUROMUSCULAR BLOCKADE AND OTHER POSSIBLE COMPLICATIONS THAT MIGHT OCCUR FOLLOWING LONG-TERM USE IN THE ICU, VECURONIUM BROMIDE OR ANY OTHER NEUROMUSCULAR BLOCKING AGENT SHOULD BE ADMINISTERED IN CAREFULLY ADJUSTED DOSES BY OR UNDER THE SUPERVISION OF EXPERIENCED CLINICIANS WHO ARE FAMILIAR WITH ITS ACTIONS AND WHO ARE FAMILIAR WITH APPROPRIATE PERIPHERAL NERVE STIMULATOR MUSCLE MONITORING TECHNIQUES (see *"Precautions"*). In patients who are known to have myasthenia gravis or the myasthenic (Eaton-Lambert) syndrome, small doses of Vecuronium Bromide may have profound effects. In such patients, a peripheral nerve stimulator and use of a small test dose may be of value in monitoring the response to administration of muscle relaxants.

PRECAUTIONS

Renal Failure: Vecuronium Bromide is well tolerated without clinically significant prolongation of neuromuscular blocking effect in patients with renal failure who have been optimally prepared for surgery by dialysis. Under emergency conditions in anephric patients some prolongation of neuromuscular blockade may occur; therefore, if anephric patients cannot be prepared for non-elective surgery, a lower initial dose of Vecuronium Bromide should be considered.

Altered Circulation Time: Conditions associated with slower circulation time in cardiovascular disease, old age, edematous states resulting in increased volume of distribution may contribute to a delay in onset time, therefore, dosage should not be increased.

Hepatic Disease: Experience in patients with cirrhosis or cholestasis has revealed prolonged recovery time in keeping with the role the liver plays in Vecuromium Bromide metabolism and excretion (see *"Pharmacokinetics"*). Data currently available do not permit dosage recommendations in patients with impaired liver function.

Long-term Use in I.C.U.: In the intensive care unit, long-term use of neuromuscular blocking drugs to facilitate mechanical ventilation may be associated with prolonged paralysis and/or skeletal muscle weakness, that may be first noted during attempts to wean such patients from the ventilator. Typically, such patients receive other drugs such as broad spectrum antibiotics, narcotics and/or steroids and may have electrolyte imbalance and diseases which lead to electrolyte imbalance, hypoxic episodes of varying duration, acid-base imbalance and extreme debilitation, any of which may enhance the actions of a neuromuscular blocking agent. Additionally, patients immobilized for extended periods frequently develop symptoms consistent with disuse muscle atrophy. The recovery picture may vary from regaining movement and strength in all muscles to initial recovery of movement of the facial and small muscles of the extremities then to the remaining muscles. In rare cases recovery may be over an extended period of time and may even, on occasion, involve rehabilitation. Therefore, when there is a need for long-term mechanical ventilation, the benefits-to-risk ratio of neuromuscular blockade must be considered.

Continuous infusion or intermittent bolus dosing to support mechanical ventilation, has not been studied sufficiently to support dosage recommendations.

IN THE INTENSIVE CARE UNIT, APPROPRIATE MONITORING, WITH THE USE OF A PERIPHERAL NERVE STIMULATOR TO ASSESS THE DEGREE OF NEUROMUSCULAR BLOCKADE IS RECOMMENDED TO HELP PRECLUDE POSSIBLE PROLONGATION OF THE BLOCKADE. WHENEVER THE USE OF VECURONIUM BROMIDE OR ANY NEUROMUSCULAR BLOCKING AGENT IS CONTEMPLATED IN THE ICU, IT IS RECOMMENDED THAT NEUROMUSCULAR TRANSMISSION BE MONITORED CONTINUOUSLY DURING ADMINISTRATION AND RECOVERY WITH THE HELP OF A NERVE STIMULATOR. ADDITIONAL DOSES OF VECURONIUM BROMIDE OR ANY OTHER NEUROMUSCULAR BLOCKING AGENT SHOULD NOT BE GIVEN BEFORE THERE IS A DEFINITE RESPONSE TO T_1 OR TO THE FIRST TWITCH. IF NO RESPONSE IS ELICITED, INFUSION ADMINISTRATION SHOULD BE DISCONTINUED UNTIL A RESPONSE RETURNS.

Severe Obesity or Neuromuscular Disease: Patients with severe obesity or neuromuscular disease may pose airway and/or ventilatory problems requiring special care before, during and after the use of neuromuscular blocking agents such as Vecuronium Bromide.

Malignant Hyperthermia: Many drugs used in anesthetic practice are suspected of being capable of triggering a potentially fatal hypermetabolism of skeletal muscle known as malignant hyperthermia. There are insufficient data derived from screening in susceptible animals (swine) to establish whether or not Vecuronium Bromide is capable of triggering malignant hyperthermia.

C.N.S.: Vecuronium Bromide has no known effect on consciousness, the pain threshold or cerebration. Administration must be accompanied by adequate anesthesia or sedation.

Drug Interactions: Prior administration of succinylcholine may enhance the neuromuscular blocking effect of Vecuronium Bromide for injection and its duration of action. If succinylcholine is used before Vecuronium Bromide the administration of Vecuronium Bromide should be delayed until the succinylcholine effect shows signs of wearing off. With succinylcholine as the intubating agent, initial doses of 0.04-0.06 mg/kg of Vecuronium Bromide may be administered to produce complete neuromuscular block with clinical duration of action of 25-30 minutes (see *"Clinical Pharmacology"*). The use of Vecuronium Bromide before succinylcholine, in order to attenuate some of the side effects of succinylcholine, has not been sufficiently studied.

Other nondepolarizing neuromuscular blocking agents (pancuronium, d-tubocurarine, metocurine, and gallamine) act in the same fashion as does Vecuronium Bromide, therefore, these drugs and Vecuronium Bromide may manifest an additive effect when used together. There are insufficient data to support concomitant use of Vecuronium Bromide and other competitive muscle relaxants in the same patient.

Inhalational Anesthetics: Use of volatile inhalational anesthetics such as enflurane, isoflurane, and halothane with Vecuronium Bromide will enhance neuromuscular blockade. Potentiation is most prominent with use of enflurane and isoflurane. With the above agents the initial dose of Vecuronium Bromide may be the same as with balanced anesthesia unless the inhalational anesthetic has been administered for a sufficient time at a sufficient dose to have reached clinical equilibrium (see *"Clinical Pharmacology"*).

Antibiotics: Parenteral/intraperitoneal administration of high doses of certain antibiotics may intensify or produce neuromuscular block on their own. The following antibiotics have been associated with various degrees of paralysis: aminoglycosides (such as neomycin, streptomycin, kanamycin, gentamicin, and dihydrostreptomycin); tetracyclines; bacitracin; polymyxin B; colistin; and sodium colistimethate. If these or other newly introduced antibiotics are used in conjunction with Vecuronium Bromide, unexpected prolongation of neuromuscular block should be considered a possibility.

Other: Experience concerning injection of quinidine during recovery from use of other muscle relaxants suggests that recurrent paralysis may occur. This possibility must also be considered for Vecuronium Bromide. Vecuronium Bromide-induced neuromuscular blockade has been counteracted by alkalosis and enhanced by acidosis in experimental animals (cat). Electrolyte imbalance and diseases which lead to electrolyte imbalance, such as adrenal cortical insufficiency, have been shown to alter neuromuscular blockade. Depending on the nature of the imbalance, either enhancement or inhibition may be expected. Magnesium salts, administered for the management of toxemia of pregnancy may enhance the neuromuscular blockade.

Drug/Laboratory/Test Interactions: None known

Carcinogenesis, Mutagenis, Impairment of Fertility: Long-term studies in animals have not been performed to evaluate carcinogenic or mutagenic potential or impairment of fertility.

Pregnancy: Pregnancy Category C: Animal reproduction studies have not been conducted with Vecuronium Bromide. It is also not known whether Vecuronium Bromide can cause fetal harm when administered to a pregnant woman or can affect reproduction capacity. Vecuronium Bromide should be given to a pregnant woman only if clearly needed.

Pediatric Use: Infants under 1 year of age but older than 7 weeks also tested under halothane anesthesia, are moderately more sensitive to Vecuronium Bromide on a mg/kg basis than adults and take about 1 ½ times as long to recover. Information presently available does not permit recommendations for usage in neonates.

ADVERSE REACTIONS

The most frequent adverse reaction to nondepolarizing blocking agents as a class consists of an extension of the drug's pharmacological action beyond the time period needed. This may vary from skeletal muscle weakness to profound and prolonged skeletal muscle paralysis resulting in respiration insufficiency or apnea.

Inadequate reversal of the neuromuscular blockade is possible with Vecuronium Bromide as with all curariform drugs. These adverse reactions are managed by manual or mechanical ventilation until recovery is judged adequate. Little or no increase in intensity of blockade or duration of action with Vecuronium Bromide is noted from the use of thiobarbiturates, narcotic analgesics, nitrous oxide, or droperidol. See *"Overdosage"* for discussion of other drugs used in anesthetic practice which also cause respiratory depression.

Prolonged to profound extensions of paralysis and/or muscle weakness as well as muscle atrophy have been reported after long-term use to support mechanical ventilation in the intensive care unit (see *"Precautions"*). The administration of Vecuronium Bromide has been associated with rare instances of hypersensitivity reactions (bronchospasm, hypotension and/or tachycardia, sometimes associated with acute urticaria or erythema) (see also *"Clinical Pharmacology"*).

OVERDOSAGE

The possibility of iatrogenic overdosage can be minimized by carefully monitoring muscle twitch response to peripheral nerve stimulation.

Excessive doses of Vecuronium Bromide produced enhanced pharmacological effects. Residual neuromuscular blockade beyond the time period needed may occur with Vecuronium Bromide as with other neuromuscular blockers. This may be manifested by skeletal muscle weakness, decreased respiratory reserve, low tidal volume, or apnea. A peripheral nerve stimulator may be used to assess the degree of residual neuromuscular blockade from other causes of decreased respiratory reserve. Respiratory depression may be due either wholly or in part to other drugs used during the conduct of general anesthesia such as narcotics, thiobarbiturates and other central nervous system depressants. Under such circumstances the primary treatment is maintenance of a patent airway and manual or mechanical ventilation until complete recovery of normal respiration is assured. Pyridostigmine bromide injection, neostigmine, or edrophonium, in conjunction with atropine or glycopyrrolate will usually antagonize the skeletal muscle relaxant action of Vecuronium Bromide. Satisfactory reversal can be judged by adequacy of skeletal muscle tone and by adequacy of respiration. A peripheral nerve stimulator may also be used to monitor restoration of twitch height. Failure of prompt reversal (within 30 minutes) may occur in the presence of extreme debilitation, carcinomatosis, and with concomitant use of certain broad spectrum antibiotics, or anesthetic agents and other drugs which enhance neuromuscular blockade or cause respiratory depression of their own. Under such circumstances the management is the same as that of prolonged neuromuscular blockade. Ventilation must be supported by artificial means until the patient has resumed control of his respiration. Prior to the use of reversal agents, reference should be made to the specific package insert of the reversal agent.

DOSAGE AND ADMINISTRATION

Vecuronium Bromide for injection is for intravenous use only.

This drug should be administered by or under the supervision of experienced clinicians familiar with the use of neuromuscular blocking agents. Dosage must be individualized in each case. The dosage information that follows is derived from studies based upon units of drug per unit of body weight and is intended to serve as a guide only, especially regarding enhancement of neuromuscular blockade of Vecuronium Bromide by volatile anesthetics and by prior use of succinylcholine (see *"Precautions/Drug Interactions"*). Parenteral drug products should be inspected visually for particulate matter and discoloration prior to administration whenever solution and container permit.

VECURONIUM BROMIDE INFUSION RATE - mL/MIN

Amount of Drug µg/kg/min	Patient Weight—kg						
	40	50	60	70	80	90	100
0.7	0.28	0.35	0.42	0.49	0.56	0.63	0.70
0.8	0.32	0.40	0.48	0.56	0.64	0.72	0.80
0.9	0.36	0.45	0.54	0.63	0.72	0.81	0.90
1.0	0.40	0.50	0.60	0.70	0.80	0.90	1.00
1.1	0.44	0.55	0.66	0.77	0.88	0.99	1.10
1.2	0.48	0.60	0.72	0.84	0.96	1.08	1.20
1.3	0.52	0.65	0.78	0.91	1.04	1.17	1.30

To obtain maximum clinical benefits of Vecuronium Bromide and to minimize the possibility of overdosage, the monitoring of muscle twitch response to peripheral nerve stimulation is advised.

The recommended initial dose of Vecuronium Bromide is 0.08 to 0.10 mg/kg (1.4 to 1.75 times the ED_{90}) given as an intravenous bolus injection. This dose can be expected to produce good or excellent non-emergency intubation conditions in 2.5 to 3 minutes after injection. Under balanced anesthesia, clinically required neuromuscular blockade lasts approximately 25-30 minutes, with recovery to 25% of control achieved approximately 25 to 40 minutes after injection and recovery to 95% of control achieved approximately 45-65 minutes after injection. In the presence of potent inhalation anesthetics, the neuromuscular blocking effect of Vecuronium Bromide is enhanced. If Vecuronium Bromide is first administered more than 5 minutes after the start of inhalation agent or when steady-state has been achieved, the initial Vecuronium Bromide dose may be reduced by approximately 15%, i.e., 0.060 to 0.085 mg/kg. Prior administration of succinylcholine may enhance the neuromuscular blocking effect and duration of action of Vecuronium Bromide. If intubation is performed using succinylcholine, a reduction of initial dose of Vecuronium Bromide to 0.04-0.06 mg/kg with inhalation anesthesia and 0.05-0.06 mg/kg with balanced anesthesia may be required.

During prolonged surgical procedures, maintenance doses of 0.010 to 0.015 mg/kg of Vecuronium Bromide are recommended; after the initial Vecuronium Bromide injection, the first maintenance dose will generally be required within 25 to 40 minutes. However, clinical criteria should be used to determine the need for maintenance doses.

Since Vecuronium Bromide lacks clinically important cumulative effects, subsequent maintenance doses, if required, may be administered at relatively regular intervals for each patient, ranging approximately from 12 to 15 minutes under balanced anesthesia, slightly longer under inhalation agents. (If less frequent administration is desired, higher maintenance doses may be administered.)

Should there be reason for the selection of larger doses in individual patients, initial doses ranging from 0.15 mg/kg up to 0.28 mg/kg have been administered during surgery under halothane anesthesia without ill effects to the cardiovascular system being noted as long as ventilation is properly maintained (see "Clinical Pharmacology").

Use by Continuous Infusion: After an intubating dose of 80-100 µg/kg, a continuous infusion of 1 µg/kg/min can be initiated approximately 20-40 min later. Infusion of Vecuronium Bromide should be initiated only after early evidence of spontaneous recovery from the bolus dose. Long-term intravenous infusion to support mechanical ventilation in the intensive care unit has not been studied sufficiently to support dosage recommendations, (see "Precautions").

The infusion of Vecuronium Bromide should be individualized for each patient. The rate of administration should be adjusted according to the patient's twitch response as determined by peripheral nerve stimulation. An initial rate of µg/kg/min is recommended, with the rate of the infusion adjusted thereafter to maintain a 90% suppression of twitch response. Average infusion rates may range from 0.8 to 1.2 µg/kg/min. Inhalation anesthetics, particularly enflurane and isoflurane may enhance the neuromuscular blocking action of nondepolarizing muscle relaxants. In the presence of steady-state concentrations of enflurane or isoflurane, it may be necessary to reduce the rate of infusion 25-60 percent, 45-60 min after the intubating dose. Under halothane anesthesia it may not be necessary to reduce the rate of infusion.

Spontaneous recovery and reversal of neuromuscular blockade following discontinuation of Vecuronium Bromide infusion may be expected to proceed at rates comparable to that following a single bolus dose (see "Clinical Pharmacology"). Infusion solutions of Vecuronium Bromide can be prepared by mixing Vecuronium Bromide with an appropriate infusion solution such as 5% glucose in water, 0.9% NaCl, 5% glucose in saline, or Lactated Ringers. Unused portions of infusion solutions should be discarded.

Infusion rates of Vecuronium Bromide can be individualized for each patient using the following table:

Drug Delivery Rate (µg/kg/min)	Infusion Delivery Rate (mL/kg/min)	
	0.1 mg/mL*	0.2 mg/mL†
0.7	0.007	0.0035
0.8	0.008	0.0040
0.9	0.009	0.0045
1.0	0.010	0.0050
1.1	0.011	0.0055
1.2	0.012	0.0060
1.3	0.013	0.0065

* *10 mg of Vecuronium Bromide in 100 mL solution*
† *20 mg of Vecuronium Bromide in 100 mL solution*

The following table is a guideline for mL/min delivery for a solution of 0.1 mg/mL (10 mg in 100 mL) with an infusion pump. (See related table).

Note: If a concentration of 0.2 mg/mL is used (20 mg in 100 mL), the rate should be decreased by one-half.

Dosage in Children: Older children (10 to 17 years of age) have approximately the same dosage requirements (mg/kg) as adults and may be managed the same way. Younger children (1 to 10 years of age) may require a slightly higher initial dose and may also require supplementation slightly more often than adults.

Infants under one year of age but older than 7 weeks are moderately more sensitive to Vecuronium Bromide on a mg/kg basis than adults and take about 1½ times as long to recover. See also subsection of "Precautions" titled "Pediatric Use". Information presently available does not permit recommendation on usage in neonates (see "Precautions"). There are insufficient data concerning continuous infusion of Vecuronium in children, therefore, no dosing recommendations can be made.

COMPATIBILITY

Vecuronium Bromide is compatible in solution with:
  0.9% NaCl solution
  5% glucose in water
  Sterile water for injection
  5% glucose in saline
  Lactated Ringers

Use within 24 hours of mixing with the above solutions. Parenteral drug products should be inspected visually for particulate matter and discoloration prior to administration whenever solution and container permit.

STORAGE

15-30°C (59-86°F). Protect from light.

After Reconstitution

■ When reconstituted with supplied bacteriostatic water for injection: CONTAINS BENZYL ALCOHOL, WHICH IS NOT INTENDED FOR USE IN NEWBORNS. Use within 5 days. May be stored at room temperature or refrigerated.

■ When reconstituted with sterile water for injection or other compatible I.V. solutions: Refrigerate vial. Use within 24 hours. Single use only. Discard unused portion.

HOW SUPPLIED
POWDER FOR INJECTION: 10 MG

BRAND/MANUFACTURER	NDC	SIZE	AWP
○ **BRAND**			
NORCURON: Organon	00052-0441-15	10s	$221.72
	00052-0441-17	10s	$230.44
	00052-0441-60	10s ud	$249.96

POWDER FOR INJECTION: 20 MG

BRAND/MANUFACTURER	NDC	SIZE	AWP
○ **BRAND**			
NORCURON: Organon	00052-0442-46	10s	$424.14

Velban *SEE* VINBLASTINE SULFATE

Velosef *SEE* CEPHRADINE

Venlafaxine Hydrochloride

DESCRIPTION

Venlafaxine Hydrochloride is a structurally novel antidepressant for oral administration. It is chemically unrelated to tricyclic, tetracyclic, or other available antidepressant agents. It is designated (R/S)-1-[2-(dimethylamino)-1-(4-methoxy-phenyl)ethyl] cyclohexanol hydrochloride or (±)-1-[α-[(dimethylamino)methyl]-p-methoxybenzyl] cyclohexanol hydrochloride and has the empirical formula of $C_{17}H_{27}NO_2HCl$. Its molecular weight is 313.87.

Venlafaxine Hydrochloride is a white to off-white crystalline solid with a solubility of 572 mg/mL in water (adjusted to ionic strength of 0.2 M with sodium chloride). Its octanol: water (0.2 M sodium chloride) partition coefficient is 0.43. Compressed tablets contain Venlafaxine Hydrochloride equivalent to 25 mg, 37.5 mg, 50 mg, 75 mg, or 100 mg Venlafaxine.

Following is its chemical structure:

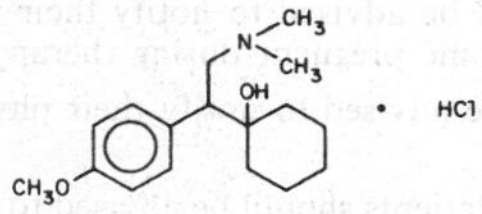

CLINICAL PHARMACOLOGY

PHARMACODYNAMICS

The mechanism of the antidepressant action of Venlafaxine in humans is believed to be associated with its potentiation of neurotransmitter activity in the CNS. Preclinical studies have shown that Venlafaxine and its active metabolite, O-desmethylvenlafaxine (ODV), are potent inhibitors of neuronal serotonin and norepinephrine reuptake and weak inhibitors of dopamine reuptake. Venlafaxine and ODV have no significant affinity for muscarinic, histaminergic, or α-1 adrenergic receptors *in vitro*. Pharmacologic activity at these receptors is hypothesized to be associated with the various anticholinergic, sedative, and cardiovascular effects seen with other psychotropic drugs. Venlafaxine and ODV do not possess monoamine oxidase (MAO) inhibitory activity.

PHARMACOKINETICS

Venlafaxine is well absorbed and extensively metabolized in the liver. O-desmethylvenlafaxine (ODV) is the only major active metabolite. On the basis of mass balance studies, at least 92% of a single dose of Venlafaxine is absorbed. Approximately 87% of a Venlafaxine dose is recovered in the urine within 48 hours as either unchanged Venlafaxine (5%), unconjugated ODV (29%), conjugated ODV (26%), or other minor inactive metabolites (27%). Renal elimination of Venlafaxine and its metabolites is the primary route of excretion. The relative bioavailability of Venlafaxine from a tablet is 100% when compared to an oral solution. Food has no significant effect on the absorption of Venlafaxine or on the formation of ODV.

The degree of binding of Venlafaxine to human plasma is 27% ± 2% at concentrations ranging from 2.5 to 2215 ng/mL. The degree of ODV binding to human plasma is 30% ± 12% at concentrations ranging from 100 to 500 ng/mL. Protein-binding-induced drug interactions with Venlafaxine are not expected.

Steady-state concentrations of both Venlafaxine and ODV in plasma were attained within 3 days of multiple-dose therapy. Venlafaxine and ODV exhibited linear kinetics over the dose range of 75 to 450 mg total dose per day (administered on a q8h schedule). Plasma clearance, elimination half-life and steady-state volume of distribution were unaltered for both Venlafaxine and ODV after multiple-dosing. Mean ± SD steady-state plasma clearance of Venlafaxine and ODV is 1.3 ± 0.6 and 0.4 ± 0.2 L/h/kg, respectively; elimination half-life is 5 ± 2 and 11 ± 2 hours, respectively; and steady-state volume of distribution is 7.5 ± 3.7 L/kg and 5.7 ± 1.8 L/kg, respectively. When equal daily doses of Venlafaxine were administered as either b.i.d. or t.i.d. regimens, the drug exposure (AUC) and fluctuation in plasma levels of Venlafaxine and ODV were comparable following both regimens.

Age and Gender: A pharmacokinetic analysis of 404 Venlafaxine-treated patients from two studies involving both b.i.d. and t.i.d. regimens showed that dose-normalized trough plasma levels of either Venlafaxine or ODV were unaltered due to age or gender differences. Dosage adjustment based upon the age or gender of a patient is generally not necessary (see "Dosage and Administration").

Liver Disease: In 9 patients with hepatic cirrhosis, the pharmacokinetic disposition of both Venlafaxine and ODV was significantly altered after oral administration of Venlafaxine. Venlafaxine elimination half-life was prolonged by about 30%, and clearance decreased by about 50% in cirrhotic patients compared to normal subjects. ODV elimination half-life was prolonged by about 60% and clearance decreased by about 30% in cirrhotic patients compared to normal subjects. A large degree of intersubject variability was noted. Three patients with more severe cirrhosis had a more substantial decrease in Venlafaxine clearance (about 90%) compared to normal subjects.

Dosage adjustment is necessary in these patients (see "Dosage and Administration").

Renal Disease: In a renal impairment study, Venlafaxine elimination half-life after administration was prolonged by about 50% and clearance was reduced by about 24% in renally impaired patients (GFR = 10-70 mL/min), compared to normal subjects. In dialysis patients, Venlafaxine elimination half-life was prolonged by about 180% and clearance was reduced by about 57% compared to normal subjects. Similarly, ODV elimination half-life was prolonged by about 40% although clearance was unchanged in patients with renal impairment (GFR = 10-70 mL/min) compared to normal subjects. In dialysis patients, ODV elimination half-life was prolonged by about 142% and clearance was reduced by

about 56%, compared to normal subjects. A large degree of intersubject variability was noted.

Dosage adjustment is necessary in these patients (see "Dosage and Administration").

CLINICAL TRIALS

The efficacy of Venlafaxine Hydrochloride as a treatment for depression was established in 5 placebo-controlled, short-term trials. Four of these were 6-week trials in outpatients meeting DSM-III or DSM-III-R criteria for major depression: two involving dose titration with Venlafaxine Hydrochloride in a range of 75 to 225 mg/day (t.i.d. schedule), the third involving fixed Venlafaxine Hydrochloride of 75, 225, and 375 mg/day (t.i.d. schedule), and the fourth involving doses of 25, 75, and 200 mg/day (b.i.d. schedule). The fifth was a 4-week study of inpatients meeting DSM-III-R criteria for major depression with melancholia whose Venlafaxine Hydrochloride doses were titrated in a range of 150 to 375 mg/day (t.i.d. schedule). In these 5 studies, Venlafaxine Hydrochloride was shown to be significantly superior to placebo on at least 2 of the following 3 measures: Hamilton Depression Rating Scale (total score). Hamilton depressed mood item, and Clinical Global Impression—Severity of illness rating. Doses from 75 to 225 mg/day were superior to placebo in outpatient studies and a mean dose of about 350 mg/day was effective in inpatients. Data from the 2 fixed-dose outpatient studies were suggestive of a dose-response relationship in the range of 75 to 225 mg/day. There was no suggestion of increased response with doses greater than 225 mg/day.

While there were no efficacy studies focusing specifically on an elderly population, elderly patients were included among the patients studied. Overall, approximately ⅔ of all patients in these trials were women. Exploratory analyses for age and gender effects on outcome did not suggest any differential responsiveness on the basis of age or sex.

INDICATIONS AND USAGE

Venlafaxine Hydrochloride is indicated for the treatment of depression.

The efficacy of Venlafaxine Hydrochloride in the treatment of depression was established in 6-week controlled trials of outpatients whose diagnoses corresponded most closely to the DSM-III or DSM-III-R category of major depressive disorder and in a 4-week controlled trial of inpatients meeting diagnostic criteria for major depressive disorder with melancholia (see "Clinical Pharmacology").

A major depressive episode implies a prominent and relatively persistent depressed or dysphoric mood that usually interferes with daily functioning (nearly every day for at least 2 weeks); it should include 4 of the following 8 symptoms: change in appetite, change in sleep, psychomotor agitation or retardation, loss of interest in usual activities or decrease in sexual drive, increased fatigue, feelings of guilt or worthlessness, slowed thinking or impaired concentration, and a suicide attempt or suicidal ideation.

The effectiveness of Venlafaxine Hydrochloride in long-term use, that is, for more than 4 to 6 weeks, has not been systematically evaluated in controlled trials. Therefore, the physician who elects to use Venlafaxine Hydrochloride for extended periods should periodically reevaluate the long-term usefulness of the drug for the individual patient.

CONTRAINDICATIONS

None known.

WARNINGS

POTENTIAL FOR INTERACTION WITH MONOAMINE OXIDASE INHIBITORS

In patients receiving antidepressants with pharmacological properties similar to Venlafaxine in combination with a monoamine oxidase inhibitor (MAOI), there have been reports of serious, sometimes fatal, reactions. For a selective serotonin reuptake inhibitor, these reactions have included hyperthermia, rigidity, myoclonus, autonomic instability with possible rapid fluctuations of vital signs, and mental status changes that include extreme agitation progressing to delirium and coma. Some cases presented with features resembling neuroleptic malignant syndrome. Severe hyperthermia and seizures, sometimes fatal, have been reported in association with the combined use of tricyclic antidepressants and MAOIs. These reactions have also been reported in patients who have recently discontinued these drugs and have been started on an MAOI. The effects of combined use of Venlafaxine Hydrochloride and MAOIs have not been evaluated in humans or animals. Therefore, because Venlafaxine Hydrochloride is an inhibitor of both norepinephrine and serotonin reuptake, it is recommended that Venlafaxine Hydrochloride not be used in combination with an MAOI, or within 14 days of discontinuing treatment with an MAOI. Based on the half-life of Venlafaxine Hydrochloride, at least 7 days should be allowed after stopping Venlafaxine Hydrochloride before starting an MAOI.

SUSTAINED HYPERTENSION

Venlafaxine treatment is associated with sustained increases in blood pressure. (1) In a premarketing study comparing three fixed doses of Venlafaxine (75, 225, and 375 mg/day) and placebo, a mean increase in supine diastolic blood pressure (SDBP) of 7.2 mm Hg was seen in the 375 mg/day group at week 6 compared to essentially no changes in the 75 and 225 mg/day groups and a mean decrease in SDBP of 2.2 mm Hg in the placebo group. (2) An analysis for patients meeting criteria for sustained hypertension (defined as treatment-emergent SDBP ≥ 90 mm Hg *and* ≥ 10 mm Hg above baseline for 3 consecutive visits) revealed a dose-dependent increase in the incidence of sustained hypertension for Venlafaxine:

PROBABILITY OF SUSTAINED ELEVATION IN SDBP (POOL OF PREMARKETING VENLAFAXINE STUDIES)

Treatment Group Venlafaxine	Incidence of Sustained Elevation in SDBP
< 100 mg/day	3%
101-200 mg/day	5%
201-300 mg/day	7%
> 300 mg/day	13%
Placebo	2%

An analysis of the patients with sustained hypertension and the 19 Venlafaxine patients who were discontinued from treatment because of hypertension (< 1% of total Venlafaxine-treated group) revealed that most of the blood pressure increases were in a modest range (10-15 mm Hg, SDBP). Nevertheless, sustained increases of this magnitude could have adverse consequences. Therefore, it is recommended that patients receiving Venlafaxine have regular monitoring of blood pressure. For patients who experience a sustained increase in blood pressure while receiving Venlafaxine, either dose reduction or discontinuation should be considered.

PRECAUTIONS
GENERAL
Anxiety and Insomnia: Treatment-emergent anxiety, nervousness and insomnia were more commonly reported for Venlafaxine-treated patients compared to placebo-treated patients in a pooled analysis of short-term, double-blind, placebo-controlled depression studies:

Symptom	Venlafaxine n = 1033	Placebo n = 609
Anxiety	6%	3%
Nervousness	13%	6%
Insomnia	18%	10%

Anxiety, nervousness, and insomnia led to drug discontinuation in 2%, 2%, and 3%, respectively, of the patients treated with Venlafaxine in the phase 2—3 depression studies.

Changes in Appetite and Weight: Treatment-emergent anorexia was more commonly reported for Venlafaxine-treated (11%) than placebo-treated patients (2%) in the pool of short-term, double-blind, placebo-controlled depression studies. A dose-dependent weight loss was often noted in patients treated with Venlafaxine for several weeks. Significant weight loss, especially in underweight depressed patients, may be an undesirable result of Venlafaxine treatment. A loss of 5% or more of body weight occurred in 6% of patients treated with Venlafaxine compared with 1% of patients treated with placebo and 3% of patients treated with another antidepressant. However, discontinuation for weight loss associated with Venlafaxine was uncommon (0.1% of Venlafaxine-treated patients in the phase 2-3 depression trials).

Activation of Mania/Hypomania: During phase 2-3 trials, hypomania or mania occurred in 0.5% of patients treated with Venlafaxine. Activation of mania/hypomania has also been reported in a small proportion of patients with major affective disorder who were treated with other marketed antidepressants. As with all antidepressants, Venlafaxine Hydrochloride should be used cautiously in patients with a history of mania.

Seizures: During premarketing testing, seizures were reported in 0.26% (8/3082) of Venlafaxine-treated patients. Most seizures (5 of 8) occurred in patients receiving doses of 150 mg/day or less. Venlafaxine Hydrochloride should be used cautiously in patients with a history of seizures. It should be discontinued in any patient who develops seizures.

Suicide: The possibility of a suicide attempt is inherent in depression and may persist until significant remission occurs. Close supervision of high-risk patients should accompany initial drug therapy. Prescriptions for Venlafaxine Hydrochloride should be written for the smallest quantity of tablets consistent with good patient management in order to reduce the risk of overdose.

Use in Patients with Concomitant Illness: Clinical experience with Venlafaxine Hydrochloride in patients with concomitant systemic illness is limited. Caution is advised in administering Venlafaxine Hydrochloride to patients with diseases or conditions that could affect hemodynamic responses or metabolism.

Venlafaxine Hydrochloride has not been evaluated or used to any appreciable extent in patients with a recent history of myocardial infarction or unstable heart disease. Patients with these diagnoses were systematically excluded from many clinical studies during the product's premarketing testing. Evaluation of the electrocardiograms for 769 patients who received Venlafaxine Hydrochloride in 4- to 6-week double-blind placebo-controlled trials, however, showed that the incidence of trial-emergent conduction abnormalities did not differ from that with placebo. The mean heart rate in Venlafaxine Hydrochloride-treated patients was increased relative to baseline by about 4 beats per minute.

In patients with renal impairment (GFR = 10-70 mL/min) or cirrhosis of the liver, the clearances of Venlafaxine and its active metabolite were decreased, thus prolonging the elimination half-lives of these substances. A lower dose may be necessary (see *"Dosage and Administration"*). Venlafaxine Hydrochloride, like all antidepressants, should be used with caution in such patients.

INFORMATION FOR PATIENTS
Physicians are advised to discuss the following issues with patients for whom they prescribe Venlafaxine Hydrochloride:

Interference with Cognitive and Motor Performance: Clinical studies were performed to examine the effects of Venlafaxine on behavioral performance of healthy individuals. The results revealed no clinically significant impairment of psychomotor, cognitive, or complex behavior performance. However, since any psychoactive drug may impair judgment, thinking, or motor skills, patients should be cautioned about operating hazardous machinery, including automobiles, until they are reasonably certain that Venlafaxine Hydrochloride therapy does not adversely affect their ability to engage in such activities.

Pregnancy: Patients should be advised to notify their physician if they become pregnant or intend to become pregnant during therapy.

Nursing: Patients should be advised to notify their physician if they are breast-feeding an infant.

Concomitant Medication: Patients should be advised to inform their physicians if they are taking, or plan to take, any prescription or over-the-counter drugs, since there is a potential for interactions.

Alcohol: Although Venlafaxine Hydrochloride has not been shown to increase the impairment of mental and motor skills caused by alcohol, patients should be advised to avoid alcohol while taking Venlafaxine Hydrochloride.

Allergic Reactions: Patients should be advised to notify their physician if they develop a rash, hives, or a related allergic phenomenon.

LABORATORY TESTS
There are no specific laboratory tests recommended.

DRUG INTERACTIONS
As with all drugs, the potential for interaction by a variety of mechanisms is a possibility.

Drugs Highly Bound to Plasma Protein: Venlafaxine is not highly bound to plasma proteins; therefore, administration of Venlafaxine Hydrochloride to a patient taking another drug that is highly protein bound should not cause increased free concentrations of the other drug.

Lithium: The steady-state pharmacokinetics of Venlafaxine administered as 50 mg every 8 hours were not affected when a single 600 mg oral dose of lithium was administered to 12 healthy male subjects. O-desmethylvenlafaxine (ODV) was also unaffected. Venlafaxine had no effect on the pharmacokinetics of lithium.

Diazepam: Under steady-state conditions for Venlafaxine administered as 50 mg every 8 hours, a single 10 mg dose of diazepam did not appear to affect the pharmacokinetics of either Venlafaxine or ODV in 18 healthy male subjects. Venlafaxine also did not have any effect on the pharmacokinetics of diazepam or its active metabolite, desmethyldiazepam.

Administration of Venlafaxine Hydrochloride did not affect the psychomotor and psychometric effects induced by diazepam.

Cimetidine: Concomitant administration of cimetidine and Venlafaxine Hydrochloride in a steady-state study for both drugs resulted in inhibition of first-pass metabolism of Venlafaxine in 18 healthy subjects. The oral clearance of Venlafaxine was reduced by about 43%, and the exposure (AUC) and maximum concentration (C_{max}) of the drug were increased by about 60%. However, co-administration of cimetidine had no apparent effect on the pharmacokinetics of ODV, which is present in much greater quantity in the circulation than is Venlafaxine. Consequently, the overall pharmacological activity of Venlafaxine plus ODV is expected to increase only slightly, and no dosage adjustment should be necessary for most normal adults. However, for patients with pre-existing hypertension, and for elderly patients or patients with hepatic dysfunction, the interaction associated with the concomitant use of Venlafaxine Hydrochloride and cimetidine is not known and potentially could be more pronounced. Therefore, caution is advised with such patients.

Alcohol: A single dose of ethanol (0.5 g/kg) had no effect on the pharmacokinetics of Venlafaxine or ODV when Venlafaxine was administered as a 50 mg dose every 8 hours in 15 healthy male subjects. The administration of Venlafaxine Hydrochloride in a stable regimen did not exaggerate the psychomotor and psychometric effects induced by ethanol in these same subjects when they were not receiving Venlafaxine Hydrochloride.

Drugs that Inhibit Cytochrome $P_{450}IID_6$ Metabolism: In vitro studies indicate that Venlafaxine is metabolized to its active metabolite, ODV, by cytochrome $P_{450}IID_6$, the isoenzyme that is responsible for the genetic polymorphism seen in the metabolism of many antidepressants. Therefore, the potential exists for a drug interaction between Venlafaxine Hydrochloride and drugs that inhibit cytochrome $P_{450}IID_6$ metabolism. Drug interactions that reduce the metabolism of Venlafaxine to ODV could potentially increase the plasma concentrations of Venlafaxine and lower the concentrations of the active metabolite.

Drugs Metabolized by Cytochrome $P_{450}IID_6$: In vitro studies indicate that Venlafaxine is a relatively weak inhibitor of cytochrome $P_{450}IID_6$. However, the clinical significance of this finding is unknown.

Monoamine Oxidase Inhibitors: See *"Warnings"*.

CNS-Active Drugs: The risk of using Venlafaxine in combination with other CNS-active drugs has not been systematically evaluated (except in the case of lithium and diazepam, as noted above). Consequently, caution is advised if the concomitant administration of Venlafaxine and such drugs is required.

◆ RATED THERAPEUTICALLY EQUIVALENT; ◇ THERAPEUTIC EQUIVALENCE UNCONFIRMED; ○ UNRATED

Electroconvulsive Therapy: There are no clinical data establishing the benefit of electroconvulsive therapy combined with Venlafaxine Hydrochloride treatment.

CARCINOGENESIS, MUTAGENESIS, IMPAIRMENT OF FERTILITY

Carcinogenesis: Venlafaxine was given by oral gavage to mice for 18 months at doses of 120 mg/kg per day, which was 16 times, on a mg/kg basis, and 1.7 times on a mg/m^2 basis, the maximum recommended human dose. Venlafaxine was also given to rats by oral gavage for 24 months at doses up to 120 mg/kg per day. In rats receiving the 120 mg/kg dose, plasma levels of Venlafaxine were 1 times (male rats) and 6 times (female rats) the plasma levels of patients receiving the maximum recommended human dose. Plasma levels of the O-desmethyl metabolite were lower in rats than in patients receiving the maximum recommended dose. Tumors were not increased by Venlafaxine treatment in mice or rats.

Mutagenicity: Venlafaxine and the major human metabolite, O-desmethyl-Venlafaxine (ODV), were not mutagenic in the Ames reverse mutation assay in Salmonella bacteria or the CHO/HGPRT mammalian cell forward gene mutation assay. Venlafaxine was also not mutagenic in the *in vitro* BALB/c-3T3 mouse cell transformation assay, the sister chromatid exchange assay in cultured CHO cells, or the *in vivo* chromosomal aberration assay in rat bone marrow. ODV was not mutagenic in the *in vitro* CHO cell chromosomal aberration assay. There was a clastogenic response in the *in vivo* chromosomal aberration assay in rat bone marrow in male rats receiving 200 times, on a mg/kg basis, or 50 times, on a mg/m^2 basis, the maximum human daily dose. The no effect dose was 67 times (mg/kg) or 17 times (mg/m^2) the human dose.

Impairment of Fertility: Reproduction and fertility studies in rats showed no effects on male or female fertility at oral doses of up to 8 times the maximum recommended human daily dose on a mg/kg basis, or up to 2 times on a mg/m^2 basis.

PREGNANCY

Teratogenic Effects-Pregnancy Category C: Venlafaxine did not cause malformations in offspring of rats or rabbits given doses up to 11 times (rat) or 12 times (rabbit) the maximum recommended human daily dose on a mg/kg basis, or 2.5 times (rat) and 4 times (rabbit) the human daily dose on a mg/m^2 basis. However, in rats, there was a decrease in pup weight, an increase in stillborn pups, and an increase in pup deaths during the first 5 days of lactation, when dosing began during pregnancy and continued until weaning. The cause of these deaths is not known. These effects occurred at 10 times (mg/kg) or 2.5 times (mg/m^2) the maximum human daily dose. The no effect dose for rat pup mortality was 1.4 times the human dose on a mg/kg basis or 0.25 times the human dose on a mg/m^2 basis. There are no adequate and well-controlled studies in pregnant women. Because animal reproduction studies are not always predictive of human response, this drug should be used during pregnancy only if clearly needed.

LABOR AND DELIVERY

The effect of Venlafaxine Hydrochloride on labor and delivery in humans is unknown.

NURSING MOTHERS

It is not known whether Venlafaxine Hydrochloride or its metabolites are excreted in human milk. Because many drugs are excreted in human milk, caution should be exercised when Venlafaxine Hydrochloride is administered to a nursing woman.

USAGE IN CHILDREN

Safety and effectiveness in individuals below 18 years of age have not been established.

GERIATRIC USE

Of the 2,897 patients in phase 2-3 depression studies with Venlafaxine Hydrochloride 12% (357) were 65 years of age or over. No overall differences in effectiveness or safety were observed between these patients and younger patients, and other reported clinical experience has not identified differences in response between the elderly and younger patients. However, greater sensitivity of some older individuals cannot be ruled out.

ADVERSE REACTIONS

ASSOCIATED WITH DISCONTINUATION OF TREATMENT

Nineteen percent (537/2897) of Venlafaxine patients in phase 2-3 depression studies discontinued treatment due to an adverse event. The more common events (≥ 1%) associated with discontinuation and considered to be drug-related (i.e., those events associated with dropout at a rate approximately twice or greater for Venlafaxine compared to placebo) included:

	Venlafaxine	Placebo
CNS		
Somnolence	3%	1%
Insomnia	3%	1%
Dizziness	3%	—
Nervousness	2%	—
Dry mouth	2%	—
Anxiety	2%	1%
Gastrointestinal		
Nausea	6%	1%
Urogenital		
Abnormal ejaculation	3%	—

	Venlafaxine	Placebo
Other		
Headache	3%	1%
Asthenia	2%	—
Sweating	2%	—

* *Percentages based on the number of males.*
— *Less than 1%*

INCIDENCE IN CONTROLLED TRIALS

Commonly Observed Adverse Events in Controlled Clinical Trials: The most commonly observed adverse events associated with the use of Venlafaxine Hydrochloride (incidence of 5% or greater) and not seen at an equivalent incidence among placebo-treated patients (i.e., incidence for Venlafaxine Hydrochloride at least twice that for placebo), derived from the 1% incidence table below, were asthenia, sweating, nausea, constipation, anorexia, vomiting, somnolence, dry mouth, dizziness, nervousness, anxiety, tremor, and blurred vision as well as abnormal ejaculation/orgasm and impotence in men.

Adverse Events Occurring at an Incidence of 1% or More Among Venlafaxine Hydrochloride Treated Patients: The table that follows enumerates adverse events that occurred at an incidence of 1% or more, and were more frequent than in the placebo group, among Venlafaxine Hydrochloride treated patients who participated in short-term (4- to 8-week) placebo-controlled trials in which patients were administered doses in a range of 75 to 375 mg/day. This table shows the percentage of patients in each group who had at least one episode of an event at some time during their treatment. Reported adverse events were classified using a standard COSTART-based dictionary terminology.

The prescriber should be aware that these figures cannot be used to predict the incidence of side effects in the course of usual medical practice where patient characteristics and other factors differ from those which prevailed in the clinical trials. Similarly, the cited frequencies cannot be compared with figures obtained from other clinical investigations involving different treatments, uses and investigators. The cited figures, however, do provide the prescribing physician with some basis for estimating the relative contribution of drug and nondrug factors to the side effect incidence rate in the population studied. (See related table).

Dose Dependency of Adverse Events: A comparison of adverse event rates in a fixed-dose study comparing Venlafaxine Hydrochloride 75, 225, and 375 mg/day with placebo revealed a dose dependency for some of the more common adverse events associated with Venlafaxine Hydrochloride use, as shown in the table that follows. The rule for including events was to enumerate those that occurred at an incidence of 5% or more for at least one of the Venlafaxine groups and for which the incidence was at least twice the placebo incidence for at least one Venlafaxine Hydrochloride group. Tests for potential dose relationships for these events (Cochran-Armitage Test, with a criterion of exact 2-sided p-value ≤ 0.05) suggested a dose-dependency for several adverse events in this list, including chills, hypertension, anorexia, nausea, agitation, dizziness, somnolence, tremor, yawning, sweating, and abnormal ejaculation. (See related table).

Adaptation to Certain Adverse Events: Over a 6-week period, there was evidence of adaptation to some adverse events with continued therapy (e.g., dizziness and nausea), but less to other effects (e.g., abnormal ejaculation and dry mouth).

Vital Sign Changes: Venlafaxine Hydrochloride treatment (averaged over all dose groups) in clinical trials was associated with a mean increase in pulse rate of approximately 3 beats per minute, compared to no change for placebo. It was associated with mean increases in diastolic blood pressure ranging from 0.7 to 2.5 mm Hg averaged over all dose groups, compared to mean decreases ranging from 0.9 to 3.8 mm Hg for placebo. However, there is a dose dependency for blood pressure increase (see *"Warnings"*).

Laboratory Changes: Of the serum chemistry and hematology parameters monitored during clinical trials with Venlafaxine Hydrochloride a statistically significant difference with placebo was seen only for serum cholesterol, i.e., patients treated with Venlafaxine Hydrochloride had mean increases from baseline of 3 mg/dL, a change of unknown clinical significance.

ECG Changes: In an analysis of ECGs obtained in 769 patients treated with Venlafaxine Hydrochloride and 450 patients treated with placebo in controlled clinical trials, the only statistically significant difference observed was for heart rate, i.e., a mean increase from baseline of 4 beats per minute for Venlafaxine Hydrochloride.

OTHER EVENTS OBSERVED DURING THE PREMARKETING EVALUATION OF VENLAFAXINE

During its premarketing assessment, multiple doses of Venlafaxine Hydrochloride were administered to 2181 patients in phase 2 and 3 studies. The conditions and duration of exposure to Venlafaxine Hydrochloride varied greatly, and included (in overlapping categories) open and double-blind studies, uncontrolled and controlled studies, inpatient and outpatient studies, fixed-dose and titration studies. Untoward events associated with this exposure were recorded by clinical investigators, using terminology of their own choosing. Consequently, it is not possible to provide a meaningful estimate of the proportion of individuals experiencing adverse events without first grouping similar types of untoward events into a smaller number of standardized event categories.

In the tabulations that follow, reported adverse events were classified using a standard COSTART-based dictionary terminology. The frequencies presented, therefore, represent the proportion of the 2181 patients exposed to multiple doses of Venlafaxine Hydrochloride who experienced an event of the type cited on at least one occasion while receiving Venlafaxine Hydrochloride. All reported events are included except those already listed in Table 1 and those events for which a drug cause was remote. If the COSTART term for an event was so general as to be uninformative, it was replaced with a more informative term. It is important to emphasize that, although the events reported occurred during treatment with Venlafaxine Hydrochloride, they were not necessarily caused by it.

Events are further categorized by body system and listed in order of decreasing frequency according to the following definitions: frequent adverse events are those occurring on one or more occasions in at least 1/100 patients (only those not already listed in the tabulated results from placebo-controlled trials appear in this listing); infrequent adverse events are those occurring in 1/100 to 1/1000 patients; rare events are those occurring in fewer than 1/1000 patients.

Body as a Whole—Frequent: accidental injury, malaise, neck pain; *Infrequent:* abdomen enlarged, allergic reaction, cyst, face edema, generalized edema, hangover effect, hernia, intentional injury, moniliasis, neck rigidity, overdose, chest pain substernal, pelvic pain, photosensitivity reaction, suicide attempt; *Rare:* appendicitis, body odor, carcinoma, cellulitis, halitosis, ulcer, withdrawal syndrome.

Cardiovascular System—Frequent: migraine; *Infrequent:* angina pectoris, extrasystoles, hypotension, peripheral vascular disorder (mainly cold feet and/or cold hands), syncope, thrombophlebitis; *Rare:* arrhythmia, first-degree atrioventricular

block, bradycardia, bundle branch block, mitral valve disorder, mucocutaneous hemorrhage, sinus bradycardia, varicose vein.

Digestive System—Frequent: dysphagia, eructation; *Infrequent:* colitis, tongue edema, esophagitis, gastritis, gastroenteritis, gingivitis, glossitis, rectal hemorrhage, hemorrhoids, melena, stomatitis, stomach ulcer, mouth ulceration; *Rare:* cheilitis, cholecystitis, cholelithiasis, hematemesis, gum hemorrhage, hepatitis, ileitis, jaundice, oral moniliasis, infestinal obstruction, proctitis, increased salivation, soft stools, tongue discoloration, esophageal ulcer, peptic ulcer syndrome.

Endocrine System—Rare: goiter, hyperthyroidism, hypothyroidism.

Hemic and Lymphatic System—Frequent: ecchymosis; *Infrequent:* anemia, leukocytosis, leukopenia, lymphadenopathy, lymphocytosis, thrombocythemia, thrombocytopenia, WBC abnormal; *Rare:* basophilia, cyanosis eosinophilia, erythrocytes abnormal.

Metabolic and Nutritional—Frequent: peripheral edema, weight gain; *Infrequent:* alkaline phosphatase increased, creatinine increased, diabetes mellitus, edema, glycosuria, hypercholesteremia, hyperglycemia, hyperlipemia, hyperuricemia, hypoglycemia, hypokalemia, SGOT increased, thirst; *Rare:* alcohol intolerance, bilirubinemia, BUN increased, gout, hemochromatosis, hyperkalemia, hyperphos-

Table 1
TREATMENT-EMERGENT ADVERSE EXPERIENCE INCIDENCE IN 4- TO 8-WEEK PLACEBO-CONTROLLED CLINICAL TRIALS[1]

Body System	Preferred Term	Venlafaxine Hydrochloride (n = 1033)	Placebo (n = 609)
Body as a Whole	Headache	25%	24%
	Asthenia	12%	6%
	Infection	6%	5%
	Chills	3%	—
	Chest pain	2%	1%
	Tauma	2%	1%
Cardiovascular	Vasodilatation	4%	3%
	Increased blood pressure/hypertension	2%	—
	Tachycardia	2%	—
	Postural hypotension	1%	—
Dermatological	Sweating	12%	3%
	Rash	3%	2%
	Pruritus	1%	—
Gastrointestinal	Nausea	37%	11%
	Constipation	15%	7%
	Anorexia	11%	2%
	Diarrhea	8%	7%
	Vomiting	6%	2%
	Dyspepsia	5%	4%
	Flatulence	3%	2%
Metabolic	Weight loss	1%	—
Nervous System	Somnolence	23%	9%
	Dry mouth	22%	11%
	Dizziness	19%	7%
	Insomnia	18%	10%
	Nervousness	13%	6%
	Anxiety	6%	3%
	Tremor	5%	1%
	Abnormal dreams	4%	3%
	Hypertonia	3%	2%
	Paresthesia	3%	2%
	Libido decreased	2%	—
	Agitation	2%	—
	Confusion	2%	1%
	Thinking abnormal	2%	1%
	Depersonalization	1%	—
	Depression	1%	—
	Urinary retention	1%	—
	Twitching	1%	—
Respiration	Yawn	3%	—
Special Senses	Blurred vision	6%	2%
	Taste perversion	2%	—
	Tinnitus	2%	—
	Mydriasis	2%	—
Urogenital System	Abnormal ejaculation/orgasm	12%[2]	—[2]
	Impotence	6%[2]	—[2]
	Urinary frequency *t 4	3%	2%
	Urination impaired	2%	—
	Orgasm disturbance	2%[3]	—[3]
	Menstrual disorder	1%[3]	—[3]

[1] *Events reported by at least 1% of patients treated with Venlafaxine Hydrochloride are included, and are rounded to the nearest %. Events for which the Venlafaxine Hydrochloride incidence was equal to or less than placebo are not listed in the table, but included the following: abdominal pain, pain, back pain, flu syndrome, fever, palpitation, increased appetite, myalgia, arthralgia, amnesia, hypesthesia, rhinitis, pharyngitis, sinusitis, cough increased, urinary tract infection, and dysmenorrhea[3].*

— *Incidence less than 1%.*
[2] *Incidence based on number of male patients.*
[3] *Incidence based on number of female patients.*

◆ RATED THERAPEUTICALLY EQUIVALENT; ◇ THERAPEUTIC EQUIVALENCE UNCONFIRMED; ○ UNRATED

phatemia, hypoglycemic reaction, hyponatremia, hypophosphatemia, hypoproteinemia, SGPT increased, uremia.

Musculoskeletal System—Infrequent: arthritis, arthrosis, bone pain, bone spurs, bursitis, joint disorder, myasthenia, tenosynovitis: *Rare:* osteoporosis.

Nervous System—Frequent: emotional lability, trismus, vertigo; *Infrequent:* apathy, ataxia, circumoral paresthesia, CNS stimulation, euphoria, hallucinations, hostility, hyperesthesia, hyperkinesia, hypertonia, hypotonia, incoordination, libido increased, myoclonus, neuralgia, neuropathy, paranoid reaction, psychosis, psychotic depression, sleep disturbance, abnormal speech, stupor, torticollis; *Rare:* akathisia, akinesia, alcohol abuse, aphasia, bradykinesia, cerebrovascular accident, loss of consciousness, delusions, dementia, dystonia, hypokinesia, neuritis, nystagmus, reflexes increased.

Respiratory System—Frequent: bronchitis, dyspnea; *Infrequent:* asthma, chest congestion, epistaxis, hyperventilation, laryngismus, laryngitis, pneumonia, voice alteration; *Rare:* atelectasis, hemoptysis, hypoxia, pleurisy, pulmonary embolus, sleep apnea, sputum increased.

Skin and Appendages—Infrequent: acne, alopecia, brittle nails, contact dermatitis, dry skin, herpes simplex, herpes zoster, maculopapular rash, urticaria; *Rare:* skin atrophy, exfoliative dermatitis, fungal dermatitis, lichenoid dermatitis, hair discoloration, eczema, furunculosis, hirsutism, skin hypertrophy, leukoderma, psoriasis, pustular rash, vesiculobullous rash.

Special Senses—Frequent: abnormal vision, ear pain; *Infrequent:* cataract, conjunctivitis, corneal lesion, diplopia, dry eyes, exophthalmos, eye pain, otitis media, parosmia, photophobia, subconjunctival hemorrhage, taste loss, visual field defect; *Rare:* blepharitis, chromatopsia, conjunctival edema, deafness, glaucoma, hyperacusis, keratitis, labyrinthitis miosis, papilledema, decreased pupillary reflex, scleritis.

Urogenital System—Frequent: anorgasmia, dysuria, hematuria, metrorrhagia*, urination impaired, vaginitis*; *Infrequent:* albuminuria, amenorrhea*, kidney calculus, cystitis, leukorrhea, menorrhagia*, nocturia, bladder pain, breast pain, kidney pain, polyuria, prostatitis*, pyelonephritis, pyuria, urinary incontinence, urinary urgency, uterine fibroids enlarged*, uterine hemorrhage*, vaginal hemorrhage*, vaginal moniliasis*, *Rare:* abortion*, breast engorgement, breast enlargement, calcium crystalluria, female lactation*, hypomenorrhea*, menopause*, prolonged erection*, uterine spasm*.

DRUG ABUSE AND DEPENDENCE
CONTROLLED SUBSTANCE CLASS
Venlafaxine Hydrochloride is not a controlled substance.

---

* Based on the number of male or female patients as appropriate.

PHYSICAL AND PSYCHOLOGICAL DEPENDENCE
In vitro studies revealed that Venlafaxine has virtually no affinity for opiate, benzodiazepine, phencyclidine (PCP), or N-methyl-D-aspartic acid (NMDA) receptors.

Venlafaxine was not found to have any significant CNS stimulant activity in rodents. In primate drug discrimination studies, Venlafaxine showed no significant stimulant or depressant abuse liability.

While the discontinuation effects of Venlafaxine Hydrochloride have not been systematically evaluated in controlled clinical trials, a retrospective survey of new events occurring during taper or following discontinuation revealed the following six events that occurred at an incidence of at least 5% and for which the incidence for Venlafaxine Hydrochloride was at least twice the placebo incidence: asthenia, dizziness, headache, insomnia, nausea, and nervousness. Therefore, it is recommended that the dosage be tapered gradually and the patient monitored (see *"Dosage and Administration"*).

While Venlafaxine Hydrochloride has not been systematically studied in clinical trials for its potential for abuse, there was no indication of drug-seeking behavior in the clinical trials. However, it is not possible to predict on the basis of premarketing experience the extent to which a CNS active drug will be misused, diverted, and/or abused once marketed. Consequently, physicians should carefully evaluate patients for history of drug abuse and follow such patients closely, observing them for signs of misuse or abuse of Venlafaxine Hydrochloride (e.g., development of tolerance, incrementation of dose, drug-seeking behavior).

OVERDOSAGE
HUMAN EXPERIENCE
There were 14 reports of acute overdose with Venlafaxine Hydrochloride, either alone or in combination with other drugs and/or alcohol, among the patients included in the premarketing evaluation. The majority of the reports involved ingestions in which the total dose of Venlafaxine Hydrochloride taken was estimated to be no more than several-fold higher than the usual therapeutic dose. The 3 patients who took the highest doses were estimated to have ingested approximately 6.75 g, 2.75 g, and 2.5 g. The resultant peak plasma levels of Venlafaxine for the latter 2 patients were 6.24 and 2.35 µg/mL, respectively, and the peak plasma levels of O-desmethyl-Venlafaxine were 3.37 and 1.30 µg/mL, respectively. Plasma Venlafaxine levels were not obtained for the patient who ingested 6.75 g of Venlafaxine. All 14 patients recovered without sequelae. Most patients reported no symptoms. Among the remaining patients, somnolence was the most commonly reported symptom. The patient who ingested 2.75 g of Venlafaxine was observed to have 2 generalized convulsions and a prolongation of QTc to 500 msec, compared with 405 msec at baseline. Mild sinus tachycardia was reported in 2 of the other patients.

OVERDOSAGE MANAGEMENT
Treatment should consist of those general measures employed in the management of overdosage with any antidepressant. Ensure an adequate airway, oxygenation,

Table 2
TREATMENT-EMERGENT EXPERIENCE INCIDENCE IN A DOSE COMPARISON TRIAL

Body System/ Preferred Term	Placebo (n = 92)	Venlafaxine Hydrochloride (mg/day)		
		75 (n = 89)	225 (n = 89)	375 (n = 88)
Body as a Whole				
Abdominal pain	3.3%	3.4%	2.2%	8.0%
Asthenia	3.3%	16.9%	14.6%	14.8%
Chills	1.1%	2.2%	5.5%	6.8%
Infection	2.2%	2.2%	5.6%	2.3%
Cardiovascular System				
Hypertension	1.1%	1.5%	2.2%	4.5%
Vasodilatation	0.0%	4.5%	5.6%	2.3%
Digestive System				
Anorexia	2.2%	14.6%	13.5%	17.0%
Dyspepsia	2.2%	6.7%	6.7%	4.5%
Nausea	14.1%	32.6%	38.2%	58.0%
Vomiting	1.1%	7.9%	3.4%	6.8%
Nervous System				
Agitation	0.0%	1.1%	2.2%	4.5%
Anxiety	4.3%	11.2%	4.5%	2.3%
Dizziness	4.3%	19.1%	22.5%	23.9%
Insomnia	9.8%	22.5%	20.2%	13.6%
Libido decreased	1.1%	2.2%	1.1%	5.7%
Nervousness	4.3%	21.3%	13.5%	12.5%
Somnolence	4.3%	16.9%	18.0%	26.1%
Tremor	0.0%	1.1%	2.2%	10.2%
Respiratory System				
Yawn	0.0%	4.5%	5.6%	8.0%
Skin and Appendages				
Sweating	5.4%	6.7%	12.4%	19.3%
Special Senses				
Abnormality of accommodation	0.0%	9.1%	7.9%	5.6%
Urogenital System				
Abnormal ejaculation/orgasm	0.0%	4.5%	2.2%	12.5%
Impotence	0.0%	5.8%	2.1%	3.6%
(Number of men)	(n = 63)	(n = 52)	(n = 48)	(n = 56)

and ventilation. Monitoring of cardiac rhythm and vital signs is recommended. General supportive and symptomatic measures are also recommended. Use of activated charcoal, induction of emesis, or gastric lavage should be considered. Due to the large volume of distribution of Venlafaxine Hydrochloride, forced diuresis, dialysis, hemoperfusion and exchange transfusion are unlikely to be of benefit. No specific antidotes for Venlafaxine Hydrochloride are known.

In managing overdosage, consider the possibility of multiple drug involvement. The physician should consider contacting a poison control center on the treatment of any overdose.

DOSAGE AND ADMINISTRATION
INITIAL TREATMENT
The recommended starting dose for Venlafaxine Hydrochloride is 75 mg/day, administered in two or three divided doses, taken with food. Depending on tolerability and the need for further clinical effect, the dose may be increased to 150 mg/day. If needed, the dose should be further increased up to 225 mg/day. When increasing the dose, increments of up to 75 mg/day should be made at intervals of no less than 4 days. In outpatient settings there was no evidence of usefulness of doses greater than 225 mg/day for moderately depressed patients, but more severely depressed inpatients responded to a mean dose of 350 mg/day. Certain patients, including more severely depressed patients, may therefore respond more to higher doses, up to a maximum of 375 mg/day, generally in three divided doses.

DOSAGE FOR PATIENTS WITH HEPATIC IMPAIRMENT
Given the decrease in clearance and increase in elimination half-life for both Venlafaxine and ODV that is observed in patients with hepatic cirrhosis compared to normal subjects (see "Clinical Pharmacology"), it is recommended that the total daily dose be reduced by 50% in patients with moderate hepatic impairment. Since there was much individual variability in clearance between patients with cirrhosis, it may be necessary to reduce the dose even more than 50%, and individualization of dosing may be desirable in some patients.

DOSAGE FOR PATIENTS WITH RENAL IMPAIRMENT
Given the decrease in clearance for Venlafaxine and the increase in elimination half-life for both Venlafaxine and ODV that is observed in patients with renal impairment (GFR = 10-70 mL/min) compared to normals (see "Clinical Pharmacology"), it is recommended that the total daily dose be reduced by 25% in patients with mild to moderate renal impairment. It is recommended that the total daily dose be reduced by 50% and the dose be withheld until the dialysis treatment is completed (4 hrs) in patients undergoing hemodialysis. Since there was much individual variability in clearance between patients with renal impairment, individualization of dosing may be desirable in some patients.

DOSAGE FOR ELDERLY PATIENTS
No dose adjustment is recommended for elderly patients on the basis of age. As with any antidepressant, however, caution should be exercised in treating the elderly. When individualizing the dosage extra care should be taken when increasing the dose.

MAINTENANCE/CONTINUATION/EXTENDED TREATMENT
There is no body of evidence available to answer the question of how long a patient should continue to be treated with Venlafaxine Hydrochloride. It is generally agreed that acute episodes of major depression require several months or longer of sustained pharmacologic therapy. Whether the dose of antidepressant needed to induce remission is identical to the dose needed to maintain and/or sustain euthymia is unknown.

DISCONTINUING VENLAFAXINE HYDROCHLORIDE
When discontinuing Venlafaxine Hydrochloride after more than 1 week of therapy, it is generally recommended that the dose be tapered to minimize the risk of discontinuation symptoms. Patients who have received Venlafaxine Hydrochloride for 6 weeks or more should have their dose tapered gradually over a 2-week period.

SWITCHING PATIENTS TO OR FROM A MONOAMINE OXIDASE INHIBITOR
At least 14 days should elapse between discontinuation of an MAOI and initiation of therapy with Venlafaxine Hydrochloride. In addition, at least 7 days should be allowed after stopping Venlafaxine Hydrochloride before starting an MAOI.

STORAGE
Store at controlled room temperature, 20°C to 25°C (68°F to 77°F), in a dry place.
Dispense in a well-closed container as defined in the USP.

HOW SUPPLIED
TABLETS: 25 MG
BRAND/MANUFACTURER	NDC	SIZE	AWP
○ BRAND			
➤ EFFEXOR: Wyeth-Ayerst	00008-0701-01	100s	$88.88
	00008-0701-02	100s	$88.88

TABLETS: 37.5 MG
BRAND/MANUFACTURER	NDC	SIZE	AWP
○ BRAND			
➤ EFFEXOR: Wyeth-Ayerst	00008-0781-01	100s	$91.54
	00008-0781-02	100s	$91.54

TABLETS: 50 MG
BRAND/MANUFACTURER	NDC	SIZE	AWP
○ BRAND			
➤ EFFEXOR: Wyeth-Ayerst	00008-0703-01	100s	$94.28
	00008-0703-02	100s	$94.28

TABLETS: 75 MG
BRAND/MANUFACTURER	NDC	SIZE	AWP
○ BRAND			
➤ EFFEXOR: Wyeth-Ayerst	00008-0704-01	100s	$99.94
	00008-0704-02	100s	$99.94

TABLETS: 100 MG
BRAND/MANUFACTURER	NDC	SIZE	AWP
○ BRAND			
➤ EFFEXOR: Wyeth-Ayerst	00008-0705-01	100s	$105.94
	00008-0705-02	100s	$105.94

Venomil SEE ALLERGENIC EXTRACTS

Ventolin SEE ALBUTEROL

VePesid SEE ETOPOSIDE

Verapamil Hydrochloride

DESCRIPTION
Verapamil Hydrochloride is a calcium ion influx inhibitor (slow-channel blocker or calcium ion antagonist). It is available as tablets and sustained-release (SR) caplets, and capsules for oral administration and as an intravenous injection.

Each tablet contains:
Verapamil HCl ....40, 80, or 120 mg

Each SR caplet or capsule contains:
Verapamil HCl ....120, 180, or 240 mg

Each ml of solution for injection contains:
Verapamil HCl ....2.5 mg

The caplets and capsules are designed for sustained release of the drug in the gastrointestinal tract.

The chemical name is Benzeneacetonitrile, α-[3-[[2-(3,4-dimethoxyphenyl) ethyl] methylamino]propyl]-3,4-dimethoxy-α-(1-methylethyl) hydrochloride or monohydrochloride

Verapamil Hydrochloride is an almost white, crystalline powder, practically free of odor, with a bitter taste. It is soluble in water, chloroform, and methanol. Verapamil Hydrochloride is not chemically related to other cardioactive drugs.

Following is its chemical structure:

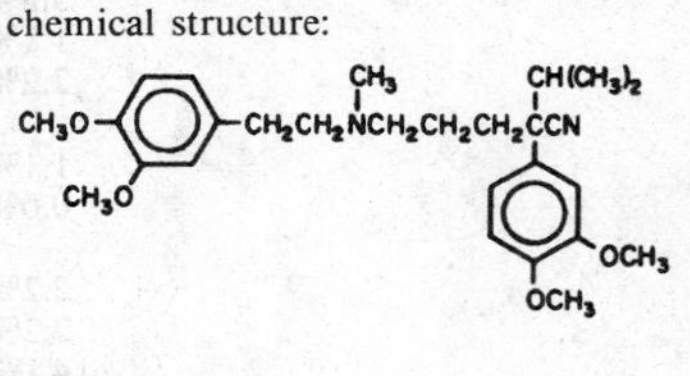

CLINICAL PHARMACOLOGY
Verapamil HCl is a calcium ion influx inhibitor (slow-channel blocker or calcium ion antagonist) that exerts its pharmacologic effects by modulating the influx of ionic calcium across the cell membrane of the arterial smooth muscle as well as in conductile and contractile myocardial cells.

MECHANISM OF ACTION
Essential Hypertension: Verapamil exerts antihypertensive effects by decreasing systemic vascular resistance, usually without orthostatic decreases in blood pressure or reflex tachycardia; bradycardia (rate less than 50 beats/min) is uncommon (1.4%). During isometric or dynamic exercise Verapamil HCl does not alter systolic cardiac function in patients with normal ventricular function.

Verapamil HCl does not alter total serum calcium levels. However, one report suggested that calcium levels above the normal range may alter the therapeutic effect of Verapamil HCl.

Angina: The precise mechanism of action of Verapamil HCl as an antianginal agent remains to be fully determined, but includes the following two mechanisms:

1. Relaxation and prevention of coronary artery spasm: Verapamil HCl dilates the main coronary arteries and coronary arterioles, both in normal and ischemic regions, and is a potent inhibitor of coronary artery spasm, whether spontaneous

---

or ergonovine-induced. This property increases myocardial oxygen delivery in patients with coronary artery spasm and is responsible for the effectiveness of Verapamil HCl in vasospastic (Prinzmetal's or variant) as well as unstable angina at rest. Whether this effect plays any role in classical effort angina is not clear, but studies of exercise tolerance have not shown an increase in the maximum exercise rate-pressure product, a widely accepted measure of oxygen utilization. This suggests that, in general, relief of spasm or dilation of coronary arteries is not an important factor in classical angina.

2. Reduction of oxygen utilization: Verapamil HCl regularly reduces the total systemic or peripheral resistance (afterload) against which the heart works both at rest and at a given level of exercise by dilating peripheral arterioles, thus reducing arterial pressure at rest. This unloading of the heart reduces myocardial energy consumption and oxygen requirements and probably accounts for the effectiveness of Verapamil HCl in chronic stable effort angina.

Arrhythmia: The vasodilatory effect of Verapamil HCl appears to be due to its effect on blockade of calcium channels as well as α-receptors.

In the isolated rabbit heart, concentrations of Verapamil HCl that markedly affect SA nodal fibers or fibers in the upper and middle regions of the AV node, have very little effect on fibers in the lower AV node (NH region) and no effect on atrial action potentials or His bundle fibers.

Electrical activity through the SA and AV nodes depends, to a significant degree, upon calcium influx through the slow channel. By decreasing the influx of calcium, Verapamil HCl prolongs the effective refractory period within the AV node and slows AV conduction in a rate-related manner. This property accounts for the ability of Verapamil HCl to slow the ventricular rate in patients with chronic atrial flutter or atrial, fibrillation, with a rapid ventricular response.

Normal sinus rhythm is usually not affected, but in patients with sick sinus syndrome, Verapamil HCl may interfere with sinus-node impulse generation and may induce sinus arrest or sinoatrial block. Atrioventricular block can occur in patients without preexisting conduction defects (see *"Warnings"*). By interrupting reentry at the AV node intravenous (IV) Verapamil HCl can restore normal sinus rhythm in patients with paroxysmal supraventricular tachycardias (PSVT), including PSVT associated with Wolff-Parkinson-White syndrome; Verapamil HCl can reduce the frequency of episodes of PSVT.

Verapamil HCl does not induce peripheral arterial spasm.

Verapamil HCl does not alter the normal atrial action potential or intraventricular conduction time, but decreases amplitude, velocity of depolarization, and conduction velocity in depressed atrial fibers. Verapamil HCl may shorten the antegrade effective refractory period of the accessory bypass tract. Acceleration of ventricular rate and/or ventricular fibrillation has been reported in patients with atrial flutter or atrial fibrillation and a coexisting accessory AV pathway following administration of Verapamil (see *"Warnings"*).

Verapamil HCl has a local anesthetic action that is 1.6 times that of procaine on an equimolar basis. It is not known whether this action is important at the doses used in man.

PHARMACOKINETICS AND METABOLISM

With the immediate-release formulation, more than 90% of the orally administered dose of Verapamil HCl is absorbed. Because of rapid biotransformation of Verapamil during its first pass through the portal circulation, bioavailability ranges from 20% to 35%. Peak plasma concentrations are reached between 1 and 2 hours after oral administration. Chronic oral administration of 120 mg of Verapamil HCl every 6 hours resulted in plasma levels of Verapamil ranging from 125 to 400 ng/ml, with higher values reported occasionally. A nonlinear correlation between the Verapamil dose administered and Verapamil plasma level does exist. In early dose titration with Verapamil a relationship exists between Verapamil plasma concentration and prolongation of the PR interval. However, during chronic administration this relationship may disappear. The mean elimination half-life in single-dose studies ranged from 2.8 to 7.4 hours. In these same studies, after repetitive dosing, the half-life increased to a range from 4.5 to 12.0 hours (after less than 10 consecutive doses given 6 hours apart). Half-life of Verapamil may increase during titration. No relationship has been established between the plasma concentration of Verapamil and a reduction in blood pressure.

Aging may affect the pharmacokinetics of Verapamil. Elimination half-life may be prolonged in the elderly. In multiple-dose studies under fasting conditions, the bioavailability, measured by AUC, of Verapamil HCl SR caplets was similar to Verapamil HCl (immediate release); rates of absorption were of course different.

In a randomized, single-dose, crossover study using healthy volunteers, administration of 240 mg Verapamil HCl SR caplets with food produced peak plasma Verapamil concentrations of 79 ng/ml; time to peak plasma Verapamil concentration of 7.71 hours; and AUC (0-24 hr) of 841 ng•hr/ml). When Verapamil HCl SR caplets was administered to fasting subjects, peak plasma Verapamil concentration was 164 ng/ml; time to peak plasma Verapamil concentration was 5.21 hours; and AUC (0-24 hr) was 1,478 ng•hr/ml. Similar results were demonstrated for plasma norverapamil. Food thus produces decreased bioavailability (AUC) but a narrower peak-to-trough ratio. Good correlation of dose and response is not available, but controlled studies of Verapamil HCl SR caplets have shown effectiveness of doses similar to the effective doses of Verapamil HCl (immediate release).

In a multiple dose pharmacokinetic study, peak concentrations for a single daily dose of Verapamil HCl SR capsules 240 mg were approximately 65% of those obtained with an 80 mg tid dose of the conventional immediate release tablets, and the 24-hour post-dose concentrations were approximately 30% higher. At a total daily dose of 240 mg, Verapamil HCl SR capsules was shown to have a

similar extent of Verapamil bioavailability based on the AUC-24 as that obtained with the conventional immediate release tablets. In this same study, Verapamil HCl SR capsules doses of 120 mg, 240 mg, and 360 mg once daily were compared after multiple doses. The ratios of the Verapamil and norverapamil AUCs for the Verapamil HCl SR capsules 120 mg, 240 mg, and 360 mg once daily doses are 1 (565 ng•hr/mL):3 (1660 ng•hr/mL):5 (2729 ng•hr/mL) and 1 (621 ng•hr/mL):3 (1614 ng•hr/mL):4 (2535 ng•hr/mL), respectively, indicating that the AUC increased nonproportionately with increasing doses.

Food does not affect the extent or rate of the absorption of Verapamil from, the controlled release Verapamil HCl SR capsules. The Verapamil HCl SR capsules 240 mg capsule when administered with food had a C_{max} of 77 ng/mL which occurred 9.0 hours after dosing, and an AUC(0-inf) of 1387 ng•hr/mL. Verapamil HCl SR capsules 240 mg under fasting conditions had a C_{max} of 77 ng/mL which occurred 9.8 hours after dosing, and an AUC(0-inf) of 1541 ng•hr/mL.

The time to reach maximum Verapamil concentrations (T_{max}) with Verapamil HCl SR capsules has been found to be approximately 7 to 9 hours in each of the single dose (fasting), single dose (fed), the multiple dose (steady state) studies, and dose proportionality pharmacokinetic studies. Similarly, the apparent half-life ($t_{1/2}$) has been found to be approximately 12 hours independent of dose.

Intravenously administered Verapamil HCl has been shown to be rapidly metabolized. Following intravenous infusion in man, Verapamil is eliminated biexponentially, with a rapid early distribution phase (half-life about 4 minutes) and a slower terminal elimination phase (half-life 2-5 hours).

In healthy men, orally administered Verapamil HCl undergoes extensive metabolism in the liver. Twelve metabolites have been identified in plasma; all except norverapamil are present in trace amounts only. The major metabolites have been identified as various N- and O-dealkylated products of Verapamil HCl. Norverapamil can reach steady-state plasma concentrations approximately equal to those of Verapamil itself. The cardiovascular activity of norverapamil appears to be approximately 20% that of Verapamil. Approximately 70% of an administered dose is excreted as metabolites in the urine and 16% or more in the feces within 5 days. About 3% to 4% is excreted in the urine as unchanged drug. Approximately 90% is bound to plasma proteins. In patients with hepatic insufficiency, metabolism of immediate-release Verapamil is delayed and elimination half-life prolonged up to 14 to 16 hours (see *"Precautions"*); the volume of distribution is increased and plasma clearance reduced to about 30% of normal. Verapamil clearance values suggest that patients with liver dysfunction may attain therapeutic Verapamil plasma concentrations with one third of the oral daily dose required for patients with normal liver function.

After four weeks of oral dosing (120 mg q.i.d.), Verapamil and norverapamil levels were noted in the cerebrospinal fluid with estimated partition coefficient of 0.06 for Verapamil and 0.04 for norverapamil.

HEMODYNAMICS AND MYOCARDIAL METABOLISM

Verapamil HCl reduces afterload and myocardial contractility. Improved left ventricular diastolic function in patients with IHSS and those with coronary heart disease has also been observed with Verapamil HCl. The commonly used intravenous doses of 5-10 mg Verapamil HCl produce transient, usually asymptomatic, reduction in normal systemic arterial pressure, systemic vascular resistance and contractility; left ventricular filling pressure is slightly increased. In most patients, including those with organic cardiac disease, the negative inotropic action of Verapamil HCl is countered by reduction of afterload, and cardiac index is usually not reduced. However, in patients with severe left ventricular dysfunction (eg, pulmonary wedge pressure above 20 mm Hg or ejection fraction less than 30%), or in patients taking beta-adrenergic blocking agents or other cardiodepressant drugs, deterioration of ventricular function may occur (see *"Drug Interactions"*). Peak therapeutic effects occur within 3 to 5 minutes after a bolus injection.

PULMONARY FUNCTION

Verapamil HCl does not induce bronchoconstriction and, hence, does not impair ventilatory function.

INDICATIONS AND USAGE

Verapamil HCl SR is indicated for the management of essential hypertension.

Immediate-release Verapamil HCl tablets are indicated for the treatment of the following:

Angina:
1. Angina at rest, including:
—Vasospastic (Prinzmetal's variant) angina
—Unstable (crescendo, pre-infarction) angina
2. Chronic stable angina (classic effort-associated angina)

Arrhythmias:
1. In association with digitalis for the control of ventricular rate at rest and during stress in patients with chronic atrial flutter and/or atrial fibrillation (see *"Warnings: Accessory bypass tract"*)
2. Prophylaxis of repetitive paroxysmal supraventricular tachycardia

IV Verapamil HCl is indicated for the following:
■ Rapid conversion to sinus rhythm of paroxysmal supraventricular tachycardias, including those associated with accessory bypass tracts (Wolff-Parkinson-White [W-P-W] and Lown-Ganong-Levine [L-G-L] syndromes). When clinically advisable, appropriate vagal maneuvers (e.g. Valsalva maneuver) should be attempted prior to IV Verapamil HCl administration.
■ Temporary control of rapid ventricular rate in atrial flutter or atrial fibrillation **except** when the atrial flutter and/or atrial fibrillation are associated

with accessory bypass tracts (Wolff-Parkinson-White [W-P-W] and Lown-Ganong-Levine [L-G-L] syndromes).

In controlled studies in the United States, about 60% of patients with supraventricular tachycardia converted to normal sinus rhythm within 10 minutes after intravenous Verapamil HCl. Uncontrolled studies reported in the world literature describe a conversion rate of about 80%. About 70% of patients with atrial flutter and/or fibrillation with a fast ventricular rate respond with a decrease in ventricular rate of at least 20%. Conversion of atrial flutter or fibrillation to sinus rhythm is uncommon (about 10%) after Verapamil HCl and may reflect the spontaneous conversion rate, since the conversion rate after placebo was similar. Slowing of the ventricular rate in patients with atrial fibrillation/flutter lasts 30-60 minutes after a single injection.

Because a small fraction (< 1.0%) of patients treated with IV Verapamil HCl respond with life-threatening adverse responses (rapid ventricular rate in atrial flutter/fibrillation and an accessory bypass tract, marked hypotension, or extreme bradycardia/asystole—see "Contraindications" and "Warnings"), the initial use of intravenous Verapamil HCl should, if possible, be in a treatment setting with monitoring and resuscitation facilities, including DC-cardioversion capability (see "Suggested Treatment of Acute Cardiovascular Adverse Reactions"). As familiarity with the patient's response is gained, use in an office setting may be acceptable.

Cardioversion has been used safely and effectively after intravenous Verapamil HCl.

UNLABELED USES

Verapamil HCl is used alone or as an adjunct in the treatment of postoperative arrhythmias including atrial arrhythmias, supraventricular and ventricular arrhythmias during anesthesia, multifocal atrial tachycardia, and asthma. It is used in hypertrophic cardiomyopathy, nocturnal leg cramps, mania, prophylaxis of migraine headache, cluster headache, and in patients with detrusor hyperactivity in neurogenic bladder. Verapamil is also prescribed for panic disorders, preterm labor, premenstrual syndrome, hypertension associated with pregnancy (preeclampsia), Raynaud's disease, and intermittent claudication.

CONTRAINDICATIONS

Verapamil HCl caplets are contraindicated in:
1. Severe left ventricular dysfunction (see *"Warnings"*)
2. Hypotension (systolic pressure less than 90 mm Hg) or cardiogenic shock
3. Sick sinus syndrome (except in patients with a functioning artificial ventricular pacemaker)
4. Second- or third-degree AV block (except in patients with a functioning artificial ventricular pacemaker)
5. Patients with atrial flutter or atrial fibrillation and an accessory bypass tract (eg. Wolff-Parkinson-White, Lown-Ganong-Levine syndromes) are at risk to develop ventricular tachyarrhythmia including ventricular fibrillation if Verapamil is administered. Therefore the use of Verapamil in these patients is contraindicated. (See *"Warnings"*.)
6. Patients with known hypersensitivity to Verapamil HCl.

In addition, IV Verapamil HCl is contraindicated in:
7. Severe congestive heart failure (unless secondary to a supraventricular tachycardia amenable to Verapamil therapy)
8. Patients receiving *intravenous* beta adrenergic blocking drugs (e.g., propranolol). *Intravenous* Verapamil and *intravenous* beta adrenergic blocking drugs should not be administered in close proximity to each other (within a few hours), since both may have a depressant effect on myocardial contractility and AV conduction.
9. Ventricular Tachycardia. Administration of intravenous Verapamil to patients with wide-complex ventricular tachycardia (QRS ≥ 0.12 sec) can result in marked hemodynamic deterioration and ventricular fibrillation. Proper pre-therapy diagnosis and differentiation from wide complex supraventricular tachycardia is imperative in the emergency room setting.

WARNINGS

IV VERAPAMIL HCl SHOULD BE GIVEN AS A SLOW INTRAVENOUS INJECTION OVER AT LEAST A TWO MINUTE PERIOD OF TIME. (See *"Dosage and Administration"*.)

Heart Failure: Verapamil has a negative inotropic effect, which in most patients is compensated by its after load reduction (decreased systemic vascular resistance) properties without a net impairment of ventricular performance. In clinical experience with 4,954 patients, 87 (1.8%) developed congestive heart failure or pulmonary edema. Verapamil should be avoided in patients with severe left ventricular dysfunction (eg, ejection fraction less than 30%) or moderate to severe symptoms of cardiac failure and in patients with any degree of ventricular dysfunction if they are receiving a beta-adrenergic blocker (see *"Drug Interactions"*). Patients with milder ventricular dysfunction should, if possible, be controlled with optimum doses of digitalis and/or diuretics before Verapamil treatment. (Note interactions with digoxin under *"Precautions"*.)

Hypotension: Occasionally, the pharmacologic action of Verapamil may produce a decrease in blood pressure below normal levels, which may result in dizziness or symptomatic hypotension. The incidence of hypotension observed in 4,954 patients enrolled in clinical trials was 2.5%. In hypertensive patients, decreases in blood pressure below normal are unusual. Tilt-table testing (60 degrees) was not able to induce orthostatic hypotension.

Hypotension: Intravenous Verapamil HCl often produces a decrease in blood pressure below baseline levels that is usually transient and asymptomatic but may result in dizziness. Administration of intravenous calcium chloride prior to intravenous administration of Verapamil may prevent this hemodynamic response. Systolic pressure less than 90 mm Hg and/or diastolic pressure less than 60 mm Hg was seen in 5-10% of patients in controlled U.S. trials in supraventricular tachycardia and in about 10% of the patients with atrial flutter/fibrillation.

The incidence of symptomatic hypotension observed in studies conducted in the U.S. was approximately 1.5%. Three of the five symptomatic patients required intravenous pharmacologic treatment (levarterenol bitartrate, metaraminol bitartrate, or 10% calcium gluconate). All recovered without sequelae.

Elevated Liver Enzymes: Elevations of transaminases with and without concomitant elevations in alkaline phosphatase and bilirubin have been reported. Such elevations have sometimes been transient and may disappear even in the face of continued Verapamil treatment. Several cases of hepatocellular injury related to Verapamil have been proven by rechallenge; half of these had clinical symptoms (malaise, fever, and/or right upper quadrant pain) in addition to elevation of SGOT, SGPT, and alkaline phosphatase. Periodic monitoring of liver function in patients receiving Verapamil is therefore prudent.

Extreme Bradycardia/Asystole: IV Verapamil HCl affects the AV and SA nodes and rarely may produce second-or third-degree AV block, bradycardia and, in extreme cases, asystole. This is more likely to occur in patients with a sick sinus syndrome (SA nodal disease), which is more common in older patients. Bradycardia associated with sick sinus syndrome was reported in 0.3% of the patients treated in controlled double-blind trials in the United States. The total incidence of bradycardia (ventricular rate less than 60 beats/min) was 1.2% in these studies. Asystole in patients other than those with sick sinus syndrome is usually of short duration (few seconds or less), with spontaneous return to AV nodal or normal sinus rhythm. If this does not occur promptly, appropriate treatment should be initiated immediately. (See *"Adverse Reactions"* and *"Treatment of Adverse Reactions"*.)

Heart Failure: When heart failure is not severe or rate related, it should be controlled with digitalis glycosides and diuretics, as appropriate, before IV Verapamil HCl is used. In patients with moderately severe to severe cardiac dysfunction (pulmonary wedge pressure above 20 mm Hg, ejection fraction less than 30%), acute worsening of heart failure may be seen.

Hepatic and Renal Failure: Significant hepatic and renal failure should not increase the effects of a single intravenous dose of Verapamil HCl but may prolong its duration. Repeated injections of intravenous Verapamil HCl in such patients may lead to accumulation and an excessive pharmacologic effect of the drug. There is no experience to guide use of multiple doses in such patients and this generally should be avoided. If repeated injections are essential, blood pressure and PR interval should be closely monitored and smaller repeat doses should be utilized. Verapamil cannot be removed by hemodialysis.

Accessory Bypass Tract (Wolff-Parkinson-White or Lown-Ganong- Levine): Some patients with paroxysmal and/or chronic atrial fibrillation or atrial flutter and a coexisting accessory AV pathway have developed increased antegrade conduction across the accessory pathway bypassing the AV node, producing a very rapid ventricular response or ventricular fibrillation after receiving intravenous Verapamil (or digitalis). Although a risk of this occurring with oral Verapamil has not been established, such patients receiving oral Verapamil may be at risk and its use in these patients is contraindicated (see *"Contraindications"*). Treatment is usually DC-cardioversion. Cardioversion has been used safely and effectively after oral Verapamil HCl.

Atrioventricular Block: The effect of Verapamil on AV conduction and the SA node may cause asymptomatic first-degree AV block and transient bradycardia, sometimes accompanied by nodal escape rhythms. PR-interval prolongation is correlated with Verapamil plasma concentrations, especially during the early titration phase of therapy. Higher degrees of AV block, however, were infrequently (0.8%) observed. Marked first-degree block or progressive development to second- or third-degree AV block or unifascicular, bifascicular, or trifascicular bundle branch block requires a reduction in dosage or, in rare instances, discontinuation of Verapamil HCl and institution of appropriate therapy, depending upon the clinical situation.

Patients with Hypertrophic Cardiomyopathy (IHSS): In 120 patients with hypertrophic cardiomyopathy (most of them refractory or intolerant to propranolol) who received therapy with Verapamil at doses up to 720 mg/day, a variety of serious adverse effects were seen. Three patients died in pulmonary edema; all had severe left ventricular outflow obstruction and a past history of left ventricular dysfunction. Eight other patients had pulmonary edema and/or severe hypotension; abnormally high (greater than 20 mm Hg) pulmonary wedge pressure and a marked left ventricular outflow obstruction were present in most of these patients. Concomitant administration of quinidine (see *"Drug Interactions"*) preceded the severe hypotension in 3 of the 8 patients (2 of whom developed pulmonary edema). Sinus bradycardia occurred in 11% of the patients, second-degree AV block in 4%, and sinus arrest in 2%. It must be appreciated that this group of patients had a serious disease with a high mortality rate. Most adverse effects responded well to dose reduction, and only rarely did Verapamil use have to be discontinued.

Premature Ventricular Contractions: During conversion to normal sinus rhythm, or marked reduction in ventricular rate, a few benign complexes of unusual appearance (sometimes resembling premature ventricular contractions) may be seen after treatment with IV Verapamil HCl. Similar complexes are seen during spontaneous conversion of supraventricular tachycardias, after DC-cardioversion and other pharmacologic therapy. These complexes appear to have no clinical significance.

Duchenne's Muscular Dystrophy: Intravenous Verapamil HCl can precipitate respiratory muscle failure in these patients and should, therefore, be used with caution.

◆ RATED THERAPEUTICALLY EQUIVALENT; ◇ THERAPEUTIC EQUIVALENCE UNCONFIRMED; ○ UNRATED

Increased Intracranial Pressure: Intravenous Verapamil HCl has been seen to increase intracranial pressure in patients with supratentorial tumors at the time of anesthesia induction. Caution should be taken and appropriate monitoring performed.

PRECAUTIONS
GENERAL
Use in Patients with Impaired Hepatic Function: Since Verapamil is highly metabolized by the liver, it should be administered cautiously to patients with impaired hepatic function. Severe liver dysfunction prolongs the elimination half-life of immediate-release Verapamil to about 14 to 16 hours; hence, approximately 30% of the dose given to patients with normal liver function should be administered to these patients. Careful monitoring for abnormal prolongation of the PR interval or other signs of excessive pharmacologic effects (see *"Overdosage"*) should be carried out.

Use in Patients with Attenuated (Decreased) Neuromuscular Transmission: It has been reported that Verapamil decreases neuromuscular transmission in patients with Duchenne's muscular dystrophy, and that Verapamil prolongs recovery from the neuromuscular blocking agent vecuronium. It may be necessary to decrease the dosage of Verapamil when it is administered to patients with attenuated neuromuscular transmission.

Use in Patients with Impaired Renal Function: About 70% of an administered dose of Verapamil is excreted as metabolites in the urine. Verapamil is not removed by hemodialysis. Until further data are available, Verapamil should be administered cautiously to patients with impaired renal function. These patients should be carefully monitored for abnormal prolongation of the PR interval or other signs of overdosage (see *"Overdosage"*).

DRUG INTERACTIONS
Beta-blockers: Concomitant therapy with beta-adrenergic blockers and Verapamil may result in additive negative effects on heart rate, atrioventricular conduction and/or cardiac contractility. The combination of sustained-release Verapamil and beta-adrenergic blocking agents has not been studied. However, there have been reports of excessive bradycardia and AV block, including complete heart block, when the combination has been used for the treatment of hypertension. For hypertensive patients, the risks of combined therapy may outweigh the potential benefits. The combination should be used only with caution and close monitoring. Controlled studies in small numbers of patients suggest that the concomitant use of immediate-release Verapamil HCl and oral beta-adrenergic blocking agents may be beneficial in certain patients with chronic stable angina or hypertension, but available information is not sufficient to predict with confidence the effects of concurrent treatment in patients with left ventricular dysfunction or cardiac conduction abnormalities.

In one study involving 15 patients treated with high doses of propranolol (median dose, 480 mg/day; range, 160 to 1,280 mg/day) for severe angina, with preserved left ventricular function (ejection fraction greater than 35%), the hemodynamic effects of additional therapy with Verapamil HCl were assessed using invasive methods. The addition of Verapamil to high-dose beta-blockers induced modest negative inotropic and chronotropic effects that were not severe enough to limit short-term (48 hours) combination therapy in this study. These modest cardiodepressant effects persisted for greater than 6 but less than 30 hours after abrupt withdrawal of beta-blockers and were closely related to plasma levels of propranolol. The primary Verapamil/beta-blocker interaction in this study appeared to be hemodynamic rather than electrophysiologic.

In other studies Verapamil did not generally induce significant negative inotropic, chronotropic, or dromotropic effects in patients with preserved left ventricular function receiving low or moderate doses of propranolol (less than or equal to 320 mg/day); in some patients, however, combined therapy did produce such effects. Therefore, if combined therapy is used, close surveillance of clinical status should be carried out. Combined therapy should usually be avoided in patients with atrioventricular conduction abnormalities and those with depressed left ventricular function.

Asymptomatic bradycardia (36 beats/min) with a wandering atrial pacemaker has been observed in a patient receiving concomitant timolol (a beta-adrenergic blocker) eyedrops and oral Verapamil.

A decrease in metroprolol and propranolol clearance has been observed when either drug is administered concomitantly with Verapamil. A variable effect has been seen when Verapamil and atenolol were given together.

Intravenous Verapamil has been administered to patients receiving oral beta blockers without the development of serious adverse effects. However, since both drugs may depress myocardial contractility or AV conduction, the possibility of detrimental interactions should be considered. The concomitant administration of *intravenous* beta blockers and *intravenous* Verapamil has resulted in serious adverse reactions (see *"Contraindications"*), especially in patients with severe cardiomyopathy, congestive heart failure or recent myocardial infarction.

Concomitant use of IV Verapamil HCl with α-adrenergic blockers may result in an exaggerated hypotensive response. Such an effect was observed in one study following the concomitant administration of Verapamil and prazosin. As Verapamil is highly bound to plasma proteins, it should be administered with caution to patients receiving other highly protein bound drugs.

Procainamide: Intravenous Verapamil has been administered to a small number of patients receiving oral procainamide without the occurrence of serious adverse effects.

Digitalis: Clinical use of Verapamil in digitalized patients has shown the combination to be well tolerated if digoxin doses are properly adjusted. However, chronic Verapamil treatment can increase serum digoxin levels by 50% to 75% during the first week of therapy, and this can result in digitalis toxicity. In patients with hepatic cirrhosis the influence of Verapamil on digoxin kinetics is magnified. Verapamil may reduce total body clearance and extrarenal clearance of digitoxin by 27% and 29%, respectively. Maintenance digitalis doses should be reduced when Verapamil is administered, and the patient should be carefully monitored to avoid over- or underdigitalization. Whenever overdigitalization is suspected, the daily dose of digitalis or digoxin should be reduced or temporarily discontinued. On discontinuation of Verapamil HCl use, the patient should be reassessed to avoid underdigitalization.

Intravenous Verapamil has been used concomitantly with digitalis preparations without the occurrence of serious adverse effects. However, since both drugs slow AV conduction, patients should be monitored for AV block or excessive bradycardia.

Antihypertensive Agents: Verapamil administered concomitantly with oral antihypertensive agents (eg, vasodilators, angiotensin-converting enzyme inhibitors, diuretics, beta-blockers) will usually have an additive effect on lowering blood pressure. Patients receiving these combinations should be appropriately monitored. Concomitant use of agents that attenuate alpha-adrenergic function with Verapamil may result in a reduction in blood pressure that is excessive in some patients. Such an effect was observed in one study following the concomitant administration of Verapamil and prazosin.

ANTIARRHYTHMIC AGENTS
Disopyramide: Until data on possible interactions between Verapamil and disopyramide phosphate are obtained, disopyramide should not be administered within 48 hours before or 24 hours after Verapamil administration.

Flecainide: A study in healthy volunteers showed that the concomitant administration of flecainide and Verapamil may have additive effects on myocardial contractility, AV conduction, and repolarization. Concomitant therapy with flecainide and Verapamil may result in additive negative inotropic effect and prolongation of atrioventricular conduction.

Quinidine: In a small number of patients with hypertrophic cardiomyopathy (IHSS), concomitant use of Verapamil and quinidine resulted in significant hypotension. Until further data are obtained, combined therapy of Verapamil and quinidine in patients with hypertrophic cardiomyopathy should probably be avoided.

The electrophysiologic effects of quinidine and Verapamil on AV conduction were studied in 8 patients. Verapamil significantly counteracted the effects of quinidine on AV conduction. There has been a report of increased quinidine levels during Verapamil therapy.

Intravenous Verapamil has been administered to a small number of patients receiving oral quinidine without the occurrence of serious adverse effects. However, three patients have been described in whom the combination resulted in an exaggerated hypotensive response presumably from the combined ability of both drugs to antagonize the effects of catecholamines on α-adrenergic receptors. Caution should therefore be used when employing this combination of drugs.

OTHER
Nitrates: Verapamil has been given concomitantly with short and long-acting nitrates without any undesirable drug interactions. The pharmacologic profile of both drugs and the clinical experience suggest beneficial interactions.

Cimetidine: The interaction between cimetidine and chronically administered Verapamil has not been studied. Variable results on clearance have been obtained in acute studies of healthy volunteers; clearance of Verapamil was either reduced or unchanged.

Lithium: Increased sensitivity to the effects of lithium (neurotoxicity) has been reported during concomitant Verapamil-lithium therapy with either no change or an increase in serum lithium levels. However, the addition of Verapamil has also resulted in the lowering of serum lithium levels in patients receiving chronic stable oral lithium. Patients receiving both drugs must be monitored carefully.

Carbamazepine: Verapamil therapy may increase carbamazepine concentrations during combined therapy. This may produce carbamazepine side effects such as diplopia, headache, ataxia, or dizziness.

Rifampin: Therapy with rifampin may markedly reduce oral Verapamil bioavailability.

Phenobarbital: Phenobarbital therapy may increase Verapamil clearance.

Cyclosporine: Verapamil therapy may increase serum levels of cyclosporine.

Theophylline: Verapamil may inhibit the clearance and increase the plasma levels of theophylline.

Inhalation Anesthetics: Animal experiments have shown that inhalation anesthetics depress cardiovascular activity by decreasing the inward movement of calcium ions. When used concomitantly, inhalation anesthetics and calcium antagonists, such as Verapamil, should each be titrated carefully to avoid excessive cardiovascular depression.

Neuromuscular Blocking Agents: Clinical data and animal studies suggest that Verapamil may potentiate the activity of neuromuscular blocking agents (curare-like and depolarizing). It may be necessary to decrease the dose of Verapamil and/or the dose of the neuromuscular blocking agent when the drugs are used concomitantly.

Dantrolene: Two animal studies suggest concomitant use of intravenous Verapamil and intravenous dantrolene sodium may result in cardiovascular collapse. There has been one report of hyperkalemia and myocardial depression following the coadministration of oral Verapamil and intravenous dantrolene.

Carcinogenesis, Mutagenesis, Impairment of Fertility: An 18-month toxicity study in rats, at a low multiple (6-fold) of the maximum recommended human dose, and not the maximum tolerated dose, did not suggest a tumorigenic potential. There was no evidence of a carcinogenic potential of Verapamil administered in the diet of rats for two years at doses of 10, 35, and 120 mg/kg/day or approximately 1, 3.5, and 12 times, respectively, the maximum recommended human daily dose (480 mg/day or 9.6 mg/kg/day).

Verapamil was not mutagenic in the Ames test in 5 test strains at 3 mg per plate with or without metabolic activation.

Studies in female rats at daily dietary doses up to 5.5 times (55 mg/kg/day) the maximum recommended human dose did not show impaired fertility. Effects on male fertility have not been determined.

Pregnancy: Pregnancy Category C. Reproduction studies have been performed in rabbits and rats at oral doses up to 1.5 (15 mg/kg/day) and 6 (60 mg/kg/day) times the maximum recommended human oral daily dose, respectively, and have revealed no evidence of teratogenicity. In the rat, however, this multiple of the human dose was embryocidal and retarded fetal growth and development, probably because of adverse maternal effects reflected in reduced weight gains of the dams. This oral dose has also been shown to cause hypotension in rats. There are no adequate and well-controlled studies in pregnant women. Because animal reproduction studies are not always predictive of human response, this drug should be used during pregnancy only if clearly needed. Verapamil crosses the placental barrier and can be detected in umbilical vein blood at delivery.

Labor and Delivery: It is not known whether the use of Verapamil during labor or delivery has immediate or delayed adverse effects on the fetus, or whether it prolongs the duration of labor or increases the need for forceps delivery or other obstetric intervention. Such adverse experiences have not been reported in the literature, despite a long history of use of Verapamil in Europe in the treatment of cardiac side effects of beta-adrenergic agonist agents used to treat premature labor.

Nursing Mothers: Verapamil is excreted in human milk. Because of the potential for adverse reactions in nursing infants from Verapamil, nursing should be discontinued while Verapamil is administered.

Pediatric Use: Safety and efficacy of Verapamil HCl in children below the age of 18 years have not been established.

Controlled studies with IV Verapamil have not been conducted in pediatric patients, but uncontrolled experience with intravenous administration in more than 250 patients, about half under 12 months of age and about 25% newborn, indicates that results of treatment are similar to those in adults. However, in rare instances, severe hemodynamic side effects have occurred, which can be fatal, following the intravenous administration of Verapamil in neonates and infants. Caution should therefore be used when administering Verapamil to this group of pediatric patients.

The most commonly used single doses in patients up to 12 months of age have ranged from 0.1 to 0.2 mg/kg of body weight, while in patients aged 1 to 15 years, the most commonly used single doses ranged from 0.1 to 0.3 mg/kg of body weight. Most of the patients received the lower dose of 0.1 mg/kg once but, in some cases, the dose was repeated once or twice every 10 to 30 minutes.

Animal Pharmacology and/or Animal Toxicology: In chronic animal toxicology studies Verapamil caused lenticular and/or suture line changes at 30 mg/kg/day or greater, and frank cataracts at 62.5 mg/kg/day or greater in the beagle dog but not in the rat. Development of cataracts due to Verapamil has not been reported in man.

ADVERSE REACTIONS

Serious adverse reactions are uncommon when Verapamil therapy is initiated with upward dose titration within the recommended single and total daily dose. See *"Warnings"* for discussion of heart failure, hypotension, elevated liver enzymes, AV block, and rapid ventricular response. Reversible (upon discontinuation of Verapamil) nonobstructive, paralytic ileus has been infrequently reported in association with the use of Verapamil. In clinical trials involving 285 hypertensive patients on Verapamil HCl for greater than 1 week the following adverse reactions were reported in greater than 1.0% of the patients: constipation 7.4%, headache 5.3%, dizziness 4.2%, lethargy 3.2%, dyspepsia 2.5%, rash 1.4%, ankle edema 1.4%, sleep disturbance 1.4%, myalgia 1.1%. The following reactions to orally administered Verapamil occurred at rates greater than 1.0% or occurred at lower rates but appeared clearly drug-related in clinical trials in 4,954 patients.

Constipation	7.3%	Dyspnea	1.4%
Dizziness	3.3%	Bradycardia	
Nausea	2.7%	(HR < 50/min)	1.4%
Hypotension	2.5%	AV block	
Headache	2.2%	total (1°, 2°, 3°)	1.2%,
Edema	1.9%	2° and 3°	0.8%
CHF, Pulmonary	1.8%	Rash	1.2%
edema		Flushing	0.6%
Fatigue	1.7%		
Elevated liver enzymes (see *"Warnings"*)			

In clinical trials related to the control of ventricular response in digitalized patients who had atrial fibrillation or flutter, ventricular rates below 50/min at rest occurred in 15% of patients and asymptomatic hypotension occurred in 5% of patients.

The following reactions, reported in 1% or less of patients, occurred under conditions (open trials, marketing experience) where a causal relationship is uncertain; they are listed to alert the physician to a possible relationship:

Cardiovascular: angina pectoris, atrioventricular dissociation, chest pain, claudication, myocardial infarction, palpitations, purpura (vasculitis), syncope.

Digestive System: diarrhea, dry mouth, gastrointestinal distress, gingival hyperplasia.

Hemic and Lymphatic: ecchymosis or bruising.

Nervous System: cerebrovascular accident, confusion, equilibrium disorders, insomnia, muscle cramps, paresthesia psychotic symptoms, shakiness, somnolence.

Respiratory: dyspnea.

Skin: arthralgia and rash, exanthema, hair loss, hyperkeratosis, macules, sweating, urticaria, Stevens-Johnson syndrome, erythema multiforme.

Special Senses: blurred vision.

Urogenital: gynecomastia, galactorrhea/hyperprolactinemia, increased urination, spotty menstruation, impotence.

The following reactions were reported with intravenous Verapamil HCl use in controlled U.S. clinical trials involving 324 patients:

Cardiovascular: Symptomatic hypotension (1.5%); bradycardia (1.2%); severe tachycardia (1.0%). The worldwide experience in open clinical trials in more than 7,900 patients was similar.

Central Nervous System Effects: Dizziness (1.2%); headache (1.2%). Occasional cases of seizures during Verapamil injection have been reported.

Gastrointestinal: Nausea (0.9%); abdominal discomfort (0.6%).

In rare cases of hypersensitive patients, broncho/laryngeal spasm accompanied by itch and urticaria have been reported.

The following reactions were reported in a few patients: emotional depression, rotary nystagmus, sleepiness, vertigo, muscle fatigue, diaphoresis or respiratory failure.

Treatment of Acute Cardioavascular Adverse Reactions: The frequency of cardiovascular adverse reactions that required therapy is rare; hence, experience with their treatment is limited. Whenever severe hypotension or complete AV block occurs following oral administration of Verapamil, the appropriate emergency measures should be applied immediately; eg, intravenously administered norepinephrine bitartrate, levarterenol bitartrate, atropine sulfate, isoproterenol HCl (all in the usual doses), or calcium gluconate (10% solution). In patients with hypertrophic cardiomyopathy (IHSS), alpha-adrenergic agents (phenylephrine HCl, metaraminol bitartrate, or methoxamine HCl) should be used to maintain blood pressure, and isoproterenol and norepinephrine or levarterenol should be avoided. If further support is necessary, dopamine HCl or dobutamine HCl may be administered. Actual treatment and dosage should depend on the severity of the clinical situation and the judgment and experience of the treating physician.

SUGGESTED TREATMENT OF ACUTE CARDIOVASCULAR ADVERSE REACTIONS* FROM IV VERAPAMIL HCl

The frequency of these adverse reactions was quite low and experience with their treatment has been limited.

Adverse Reaction	Proven Effective Treatment	Supportive Treatment
1. Symptomatic hypotension requiring treatment	Calcium chloride (IV) Levarterenol bitartrate (IV) Metaraminol bitartrate (IV) Isoproterenol HCl (IV) Dopamine (IV)	Intravenous fluids Trendelenburg position
2. Bradycardia, AV block, Asystole	Isoproterenol HCl (IV) Calcium chloride (IV) Cardiac pacing Levarterenol bitartrate (IV) Atropine (IV)	Intravenous fluids (slow drip)
3. Rapid ventricular rate (due to antegrade conduction in flutter/fibrillation with W-P-W or L-G-L syndromes)	DC-cardioversion (high energy may be required) Procainamide (IV) Lidocaine (IV)	Intravenous fluids (slow drip)

* *Actual treatment and dosage should depend on the severity of the clinical situation and the judgment and experience of the treating physician.*

OVERDOSAGE

Overdose with Verapamil may lead to pronounced hypotension, bradycardia, and conduction system abnormalities (eg, junctional rhythm with AV dissociation and high degree AV block, including asystole). Other symptoms secondary to hypoperfusion (eg, metabolic acidosis, hyperglycemia, hyperkalemia, renal dysfunction, and convulsions) may be evident.

Treat all Verapamil overdoses as serious and maintain observation for at least 48 hours (especially Verapamil HCl SR) preferably under continuous hospital care. Delayed pharmacodynamic consequences may occur with the sustained-release formulation. Verapamil is known to decrease gastrointestinal transit time. Verapamil cannot be removed by hemodialysis.

Treatment of overdosage should be supportive and individualized. Beta-adrenergic stimulation or parenteral administration of calcium solutions may increase calcium ion flux across the slow channel and has been used effectively in treatment of deliberate overdose of oral Verapamil. Verapamil cannot be removed by dialysis. The following measures may be considered:

Bradycardia and conduction system abnormalities: Atropine, isoproterenol, and cardiac pacing.

Hypotension: Intravenous fluids, vasopressors (eg, dopamine, dobutamine), calcium solutions (eg, 10% calcium chloride solution).

Cardiac failure: Inotropic agents (eg, isoproterenol, dopamine, dobutamine), diuretics.

Asystole should be handled by the usual measures including isoproterenol HCl, other vasopressor agents, or cardiopulmonary resuscitation.

DOSAGE AND ADMINISTRATION
IMMEDIATE-RELEASE VERAPAMIL HCL
The dose of Verapamil must be individualized by titration. The usefulness and safety of dosages exceeding 480 mg/day have not been established; therefore, this daily dosage should not be exceeded. Since the half-life of Verapamil increases during chronic dosing, maximum response may be delayed.

Angina: Clinical trials show that the usual dose is 80 mg to 120 mg three times a day. However, 40 mg three times a day may be warranted in patients who may have an increased response to Verapamil (eg, decreased hepatic function, elderly, etc). Upward titration should be based on therapeutic efficacy and safety evaluated approximately eight hours after dosing. Dosage may be increased at daily (eg, patients with unstable angina) or weekly intervals until optimum clinical response is obtained.

Arrhythmias: The dosage in digitalized patients with chronic atrial fibrillation (see "Precautions") ranges from 240 to 320 mg/day in divided (t.i.d. or q.i.d.) doses. The dosage for prophylaxis of PSVT (non-digitalized patients) ranges from 240 to 480 mg/day in divided (t.i.d. or q.i.d.) doses. In general, maximum effects for any given dosage will be apparent during the first 48 hours of therapy.

Essential hypertension: Dose should be individualized by titration. The usual initial monotherapy dose in clinical trials was 80 mg three times a day (240 mg/day). Daily dosages of 360 and 480 mg have been used but there is no evidence that dosages beyond 360 mg provided added effect. Consideration should be given to beginning titration at 40 mg three times per day in patients who might respond to lower doses, such as the elderly or people of small stature. The antihypertensive effects of Verapamil HCl are evident within the first week of therapy. Upward titration should be based on therapeutic efficacy, assessed at the end of the dosing interval.

VERAPAMIL HCL SR
Essential hypertension: The dose of Verapamil HCl SR should be individualized by titration and the drug should be administered with food. Initiate therapy with 180 mg of sustained-release verapamil HCl caplets, or 240 mg of Verapamil HCl SR capsules, given in the morning. Lower initial doses of 120 mg a day may be warranted in patients who may have an increased response to Verapamil (e.g., the elderly or small people). Upward titration should be based on therapeutic efficacy and safety evaluated weekly and approximately 24 hours after the previous dose. The antihypertensive effects of Verapamil HCl SR are evident within the first week of therapy.

If adequate response is not obtained with 180 mg of Verapamil HCl SR caplets, the dose may be titrated upward in the following manner:
a) 240 mg each morning,
b) 180 mg each morning plus 180 mg each evening; or 240 mg each morning plus 120 mg each evening,
c) 240 mg every 12 hours.

If adequate response is not obtained with 120 mg of Verapamil HCl SR capsules, the dose may be titrated upward in the following manner; (a) 180 mg in the morning, (b) 240 mg in the morning, (c) 360 mg in the morning, (d) 480 mg in the morning. Verapamil HCl SR capsules are for once-a-day administration.

When switching from immediate-release Verapamil HCl to Verapamil HCl SR the total daily dose in milligrams may remain the same.

IV VERAPAMIL HCL
(For Intravenous Use Only)
VERAPAMIL HCL SHOULD BE GIVEN AS A SLOW INTRAVENOUS INJECTION OVER AT LEAST A TWO MINUTE PERIOD OF TIME UNDER CONTINUOUS ELECTROCARDIOGRAPHIC AND BLOOD PRESSURE MONITORING.

The recommended intravenous doses of Verapamil HCl are as follows:

Adult: Initial dose: 5-10 mg (0.075-0.15 mg/kg body weight) given as an intravenous bolus over at least 2 minutes.

Repeat dose: 10 mg (0.15 mg/kg body weight) 30 minutes after the first dose if the initial response is not adequate. An optimal interval for subsequent I.V. doses has not been determined, and should be individualized for each patient.

Older Patients: The dose should be administered over at least 3 minutes to minimize the risk of untoward drug effects.

Pediatric: Initial dose: 0-1 year: 0.1-0.2 mg/kg body weight (usual single dose range 0.75-2 mg) should be administered as an intravenous bolus over at least 2 minutes *under continuous ECG monitoring.*

1-15 years: 0.1-0.3 mg/kg body weight (usual single dose range 2-5 mg) should be administered as an intravenous bolus over at least 2 minutes. *Do not exceed 5 mg.*

Repeat dose: 0-1 year: 0.1-0.2 mg/kg body weight (usual single dose range 0.75-2 mg) 30 minutes after the first dose if the initial response is not adequate *under continuous ECG monitoring).* An optimal interval for subsequent I.V. doses has not been determined, and should be individualized for each patient.

1-15 years: 0.1-0.3 mg/kg body weight (usual single dose range 2-5 mg) 30 minutes after the first dose if the initial response is not adequate. *Do not exceed 10 mg as a single dose.* An optimal interval for subsequent I.V. doses has not been determined, and should be individualized for each patient.

Note: Parenteral drug products should be inspected visually for particulate matter and discoloration prior to administration, whenever solution and container permit. IV Verapamil HCl is physically compatible and chemically stable for at least 24 hours at 25°C protected from light in most common large volume parenteral solutions. Admixing IV Verapamil HCl with albumin, amphotericin B, hydralazine HCl and trimethoprim with sulfamethoxazole should be avoided. IV Verapamil HCl will precipitate in any solution with a pH above 6.0.

STORAGE
Immediate-release tablets: Store at 59° to 86°F (15° to 30°C) and protect from light. Dispense in tight, light-resistant containers.

Sustained-release caplets: Store at 59° to 77°F (15° to 25°C) and protect from light and moisture. Dispense in tight, light-resistent containers.

IV: Store at 59°-86°F (15°-30°C). Protect from light.

HOW SUPPLIED
CAPSULE, EXTENDED RELEASE: 120 MG

BRAND/MANUFACTURER	NDC	SIZE	AWP
○ **BRAND**			
➤ VERELAN: Lederle Labs	00005-2490-23	100s	$102.54

CAPSULE, EXTENDED RELEASE: 180 MG

BRAND/MANUFACTURER	NDC	SIZE	AWP
○ **BRAND**			
➤ VERELAN: Lederle Labs	00005-2489-23	100s	$107.39

CAPSULE, EXTENDED RELEASE: 240 MG

BRAND/MANUFACTURER	NDC	SIZE	AWP
○ **BRAND**			
➤ VERELAN: Lederle Labs	00005-2491-23	100s	$121.21

INJECTION: 2.5 MG/ML

AVERAGE UNIT PRICE (AVAILABLE SIZES)		GENERIC A-RATED AVERAGE PRICE (GAAP)	
BRAND	$6.21	2 ml 5s	$16.03
GENERIC	$1.66	4 ml 5s	$20.31
		2 ml 25s	$139.34

BRAND/MANUFACTURER	NDC	SIZE	AWP
◆ **BRAND**			
ISOPTIN I.V.: Knoll	00044-1816-21	2 ml	$12.99
	00044-1816-41	4 ml	$24.02
	00044-1815-07	2 ml 10s	$122.47
◆ **GENERICS**			
Amer Regent	00517-0501-72	2 ml 5s	$9.38
Abbott Hosp	00074-4011-01	2 ml 5s	$11.28
Amer Regent	00517-5402-05	2 ml 5s	$12.19
Abbott Hosp	00074-1144-01	2 ml 5s	$16.68
Solo Pak	39769-0100-02	2 ml 5s	$30.63
Abbott Hosp	00074-4011-02	4 ml 5s	$12.11
Amer Regent	00517-5404-05	4 ml 5s	$13.44
Abbott Hosp	00074-1144-02	4 ml 5s	$18.82
Solo Pak	39769-0100-05	4 ml 5s	$36.88
Sanofi Winthrop	00024-2110-03	2 ml 10s	$26.84
Abbott Hosp	00074-1143-01	4 ml 10s	$50.23
Abbott Hosp	00074-4000-01	2 ml 25s	$116.67
Intl Med Sys	00548-1470-00	2 ml 25s	$162.00
Intl Med Sys	00548-1471-00	4 ml 25s	$292.80

TABLET, EXTENDED RELEASE: 120 MG

BRAND/MANUFACTURER	NDC	SIZE	AWP
◆ **GENERICS**			
Zenith	00172-4285-60	100s	$77.15

TABLET, EXTENDED RELEASE: 120 MG

BRAND/MANUFACTURER	NDC	SIZE	AWP
○ **BRAND**			
➤ CALAN SR: Searle	00025-1901-31	100s	$85.75
➤ ISOPTIN S.R.: Knoll	00044-1827-02	100s	$85.75
➤ CALAN SR: Searle	00025-1901-34	100s ud	$90.04

➤ SHOWN IN PRODUCT IDENTIFICATION GUIDE

BRAND/MANUFACTURER	NDC	SIZE	AWP
➤ ISOPTIN S.R.: Knoll	00044-1827-12	100s ud	$90.04

TABLET, EXTENDED RELEASE: 180 MG

AVERAGE UNIT PRICE (AVAILABLE SIZES)		GENERIC A-RATED AVERAGE PRICE (GAAP)	
GENERIC	$0.97	100s	$97.39
		500s	$464.55

BRAND/MANUFACTURER	NDC	SIZE	AWP
◆ GENERICS			
Thrift Drug Svcs	59198-0002-01	100s	$73.19
Moore,H.L.	00839-7878-06	100s	$97.19
Qualitest	00603-6359-21	100s	$97.75
URL	00677-1518-01	100s	$97.80
Major	00904-7871-60	100s	$97.80
Rugby	00536-5630-01	100s	$97.80
Rugby	00536-5675-01	100s	$97.80
Zenith	00172-4286-60	100s	$97.80
Schein	00364-2590-01	100s	$97.80
Norton,HN	50732-0915-01	100s	$97.80
Martec	52555-0536-01	100s	$98.00
Caremark	00339-5811-12	100s	$98.21
West Point	59591-0286-68	100s	$98.50
Aligen	00405-5101-01	100s	$102.95
Goldline	00182-1969-01	100s	$110.45
Goldline	00182-1969-05	500s	$464.55
Norton,HN	50732-0915-05	500s	$464.55

TABLET, EXTENDED RELEASE: 180 MG

BRAND/MANUFACTURER	NDC	SIZE	AWP
○ BRAND			
➤ CALAN SR: Searle	00025-1911-31	100s	$108.67
➤ ISOPTIN S.R.: Knoll	00044-1825-02	100s	$108.67
➤ CALAN SR: Searle	00025-1911-34	100s ud	$114.11
➤ ISOPTIN S.R.: Knoll	00044-1825-12	100s ud	$114.11

TABLET, EXTENDED RELEASE: 240 MG

AVERAGE UNIT PRICE (AVAILABLE SIZES)		GENERIC A-RATED AVERAGE PRICE (GAAP)	
BRAND	$1.26	100s	$110.44
GENERIC	$1.10	500s	$536.06

BRAND/MANUFACTURER	NDC	SIZE	AWP
◆ BRAND			
➤ ISOPTIN S.R.: Knoll	00044-1826-02	100s	$124.34
	00044-1826-10	100s ud	$130.55
	00044-1826-03	500s	$615.47
◆ GENERICS			
Rugby	00536-4823-01	100s	$103.07
Rugby	00536-5674-01	100s	$103.07
West Point	59591-0280-68	100s	$103.75
Martec	52555-0537-01	100s	$106.00
Qualitest	00603-6360-21	100s	$107.45
Caremark	00339-5809-12	100s	$109.10
Aligen	00405-5102-01	100s	$111.20
Zenith	00172-4280-60	100s	$111.91
Norton,HN	50732-0901-01	100s	$111.91
➤ Goldline	00182-1970-01	100s	$111.91
URL	00677-1453-01	100s	$113.14
Moore,H.L.	00839-7670-06	100s	$113.19
Schein	00364-2567-01	100s	$113.70
Major	00904-7723-60	100s	$126.80
Moore,H.L.	00839-7670-12	500s	$499.23
Zenith	00172-4280-70	500s	$537.15
Rugby	00536-5674-05	500s	$553.92
➤ Goldline	00182-1970-05	500s	$553.92

TABLET, EXTENDED RELEASE: 240 MG

BRAND/MANUFACTURER	NDC	SIZE	AWP
○ BRAND			
➤ CALAN SR: Searle	00025-1891-31	100s	$124.34
	00025-1891-34	100s ud	$130.55
	00025-1891-45	300s	$392.74
	00025-1891-51	500s	$615.47

TABLETS: 40 MG

AVERAGE UNIT PRICE (AVAILABLE SIZES)		GENERIC A-RATED AVERAGE PRICE (GAAP)	
BRAND	$0.32	100s	$26.99
GENERIC	$0.27		

BRAND/MANUFACTURER	NDC	SIZE	AWP
◆ BRAND			
➤ ISOPTIN: Knoll	00044-1821-02	100s	$30.74
➤ CALAN: Searle	00025-1771-31	100s	$31.94
➤ ISOPTIN: Knoll	00044-1821-10	100s ud	$32.27

BRAND/MANUFACTURER	NDC	SIZE	AWP
◆ GENERICS			
Moore,H.L.	00839-7921-06	100s	$25.58
Qualitest	00603-6356-21	100s	$26.15
Geneva	00781-1014-01	100s	$26.23
Watson	52544-0404-01	100s	$26.29
Caremark	00339-5857-12	100s	$27.06
Major	00904-7799-60	100s	$27.25
Rugby	00536-5624-01	100s	$27.66
Goldline	00182-1601-01	100s	$29.70

TABLETS: 80 MG

AVERAGE UNIT PRICE (AVAILABLE SIZES)		GENERIC A-RATED AVERAGE PRICE (GAAP)	
BRAND	$0.44	100s	$25.19
GENERIC	$0.22	500s	$96.98
HCFA FUL (100s ea)	$0.06	1000s	$171.69

BRAND/MANUFACTURER	NDC	SIZE	AWP
◆ BRAND			
➤ ISOPTIN: Knoll	00044-1822-02	100s	$44.23
➤ CALAN: Searle	00025-1851-31	100s	$45.95
➤ ISOPTIN: Knoll	00044-1822-10	100s ud	$46.77
	00044-1822-05	500s	$212.16
CALAN: Searle	00025-1851-51	500s	$220.43
ISOPTIN: Knoll	00044-1822-04	1000s	$406.69
CALAN: Searle	00025-1851-52	1000s	$422.55
◆ GENERICS			
Medirex	57480-0374-06	30s	$12.60
Mutual	53489-0154-02	50s	$14.95
Moore,H.L.	00839-7253-06	100s	$21.18
Moore,H.L.	00839-7267-06	100s	$21.18
Warner Chilcott	00047-0328-24	100s	$21.45
Qualitest	00603-6357-21	100s	$21.50
Rugby	00536-4931-01	100s	$21.56
Goldline	00182-1300-01	100s	$21.65
Schein	00364-2111-01	100s	$21.75
Major	00904-2920-60	100s	$22.05
Mylan	00378-0512-01	100s	$22.29
Watson	52544-0343-01	100s	$22.43
Watson	52544-0344-01	100s	$22.43
Martec	52555-0179-01	100s	$23.10
Caremark	00339-5621-12	100s	$23.20
Mutual	53489-0154-01	100s	$23.50
URL	00677-1130-01	100s	$23.80
Purepac	00228-2473-10	100s	$23.84
Geneva	00781-1016-01	100s	$24.19
Sidmak	50111-0486-01	100s	$25.85
Aligen	00405-5099-01	100s	$25.92
Parmed	00349-8624-01	100s	$26.86
Parmed	00349-8628-01	100s	$26.86
U.S. Trading	56126-0360-11	100s ud	$10.71
Major	00904-2920-61	100s ud	$24.96
Goldline	00182-1300-89	100s ud	$25.50
Geneva	00781-1016-13	100s ud	$26.42
Vangard	00615-2518-13	100s ud	$26.50
Schein	00364-2111-90	100s ud	$34.25
Auro	55829-0561-10	100s ud	$36.70
Medirex	57480-0374-01	100s ud	$42.00
UDL	51079-0682-20	100s ud	$42.09
Rugby	00536-4931-02	250s	$52.44
Major	00904-2920-40	500s	$53.15
Watson	52544-0343-05	500s	$83.95
Watson	52544-0344-05	500s	$83.95
Warner Chilcott	00047-0328-30	500s	$90.57
Sidmak	50111-0486-02	500s	$93.50
Aligen	00405-5099-02	500s	$95.63
Schein	00364-2111-05	500s	$95.95
Martec	52555-0179-05	500s	$98.20
Moore,H.L.	00839-7253-12	500s	$98.48
Rugby	00536-4931-05	500s	$98.75
Goldline	00182-1300-05	500s	$98.80
URL	00677-1130-05	500s	$107.00
Mutual	53489-0154-05	500s	$107.00
Geneva	00781-1016-05	500s	$107.85
Purepac	00228-2473-50	500s	$119.20
Parmed	00349-8624-05	500s	$119.68
Qualitest	00603-6357-32	1000s	$116.35
Rugby	00536-4931-10	1000s	$117.60
Major	00904-2920-80	1000s	$130.45
Schein	00364-2111-02	1000s	$134.65
Goldline	00182-1300-10	1000s	$150.00
Watson	52544-0343-10	1000s	$160.45
Watson	52544-0344-10	1000s	$160.45
Mylan	00378-0512-10	1000s	$181.00
Sidmak	50111-0486-03	1000s	$181.50
Moore,H.L.	00839-7267-16	1000s	$188.93
Purepac	00228-2473-96	1000s	$192.03
Geneva	00781-1016-10	1000s	$202.96
Mutual	53489-0154-10	1000s	$205.00
Parmed	00349-8624-10	1000s	$227.02
Parmed	00349-8628-10	1000s	$227.02

◆ RATED THERAPEUTICALLY EQUIVALENT; ◇ THERAPEUTIC EQUIVALENCE UNCONFIRMED; ○ UNRATED

TABLETS: 120 MG

AVERAGE UNIT PRICE (AVAILABLE SIZES)		GENERIC A-RATED AVERAGE PRICE (GAAP)	
BRAND	$0.59	100s	$32.89
GENERIC	$0.30	500s	$124.11
HCFA FUL (100s ea)	$0.08	1000s	$261.11

BRAND/MANUFACTURER	NDC	SIZE	AWP
◆ BRAND			
➤ ISOPTIN: Knoll	00044-1823-02	100s	$59.80
➤ CALAN: Searle	00025-1861-31	100s	$62.13
➤ ISOPTIN: Knoll	00044-1823-10	100s ud	$62.40
	00044-1823-05	500s	$287.40
	00044-1823-04	1000s	$550.19
CALAN: Searle	00025-1861-52	1000s	$571.65
◆ GENERICS			
Medirex	57480-0375-06	30s	$16.85
Qualitest	00603-6358-21	100s	$27.90
Moore,H.L.	00839-7254-06	100s	$28.27
Moore,H.L.	00839-7268-06	100s	$28.27
Rugby	00536-4932-01	100s	$28.50
Schein	00364-2112-01	100s	$28.50
Goldline	00182-1301-01	100s	$28.55
Warner Chilcott	00047-0329-24	100s	$28.75
Mylan	00378-0772-01	100s	$28.99
Major	00904-2924-60	100s	$29.20
Watson	52544-0345-01	100s	$29.93
Watson	52544-0346-01	100s	$29.93
Geneva	00781-1017-01	100s	$29.95
URL	00677-1131-01	100s	$30.25
Mutual	53489-0155-01	100s	$30.25
Caremark	00339-5622-12	100s	$30.38
Martec	52555-0180-01	100s	$30.85
Purepac	00228-2475-10	100s	$30.86
Aligen	00405-5100-01	100s	$34.65
Sidmak	50111-0487-01	100s	$34.65
Parmed	00349-8625-01	100s	$34.94
Parmed	00349-8629-01	100s	$34.94
U.S. Trading	56126-0361-11	100s ud	$9.66
Major	00904-2924-61	100s ud	$33.29
Goldline	00182-1301-89	100s ud	$34.50
Geneva	00781-1017-13	100s ud	$35.25
Vangard	00615-2532-13	100s ud	$37.16
Schein	00364-2112-90	100s ud	$37.50
Auro	55829-0562-10	100s ud	$48.40
Medirex	57480-0375-01	100s ud	$56.15
UDL	51079-0683-20	100s ud	$56.16
Rugby	00536-4932-02	250s	$68.50
Major	00904-2924-40	500s	$74.75
Qualitest	00603-6358-28	500s	$91.85
Goldline	00182-1301-05	500s	$99.00
Schein	00364-2112-05	500s	$110.95
Warner Chilcott	00047-0329-30	500s	$111.71
Rugby	00536-4932-05	500s	$112.64
Watson	52544-0345-05	500s	$115.45
Watson	52544-0346-05	500s	$115.45
Mylan	00378-0772-05	500s	$127.84
Aligen	00405-5100-02	500s	$129.80
Sidmak	50111-0487-02	500s	$129.80
Mutual	53489-0155-05	500s	$142.00
Geneva	00781-1017-05	500s	$149.75
Purepac	00228-2475-50	500s	$154.30
Parmed	00349-8625-05	500s	$160.23
Parmed	00349-8629-05	500s	$160.23
Watson	52544-0345-10	1000s	$194.00
Watson	52544-0346-10	1000s	$194.00
Moore,H.L.	00839-7268-16	1000s	$255.08
Mutual	53489-0155-10	1000s	$280.00
Schein	00364-2112-02	1000s	$289.00
Purepac	00228-2475-96	1000s	$295.19
Parmed	00349-8625-10	1000s	$320.47

Vercyte SEE PIPOBROMAN

Verelan SEE VERAPAMIL HYDROCHLORIDE

Vermox SEE MEBENDAZOLE

Versed SEE MIDAZOLAM HYDROCHLORIDE

Vesprin Injection SEE TRIFLUPROMAZINE HYDROCHLORIDE

Vi-Daylin/F SEE FERROUS SULFATE/SODIUM FLUORIDE/ VITAMINS, MULTI, SODIUM FLUORIDE/VITAMIN A/VITAMIN C/VITAMIN D AND SODIUM FLUORIDE AND VITAMINS, MULTI

Vibra-Tabs SEE DOXYCYCLINE

Vibramycin SEE DOXYCYCLINE

Vicodin SEE ACETAMINOPHEN WITH HYDROCODONE BITARTRATE

Vicodin Tuss SEE GUAIFENESIN AND HYDROCODONE BITARTRATE

Vicon Forte SEE VITAMINS, MULTIPLE WITH MINERALS

Vidarabine

DESCRIPTION

Vidarabine (also known as adenine arabinoside and Ara-A) is an antiviral drug for the topical treatment of epithelial keratitis caused by Herpes simplex virus. The chemical name is 9-β-Darabinofuranosyladenine. Each gram of the ophthalmic ointment contains 30 mg of Vidarabine monohydrate equivalent to 28.11 mg of Vidarabine in a sterile, inert, petrolatum base.

Following is its chemical structure:

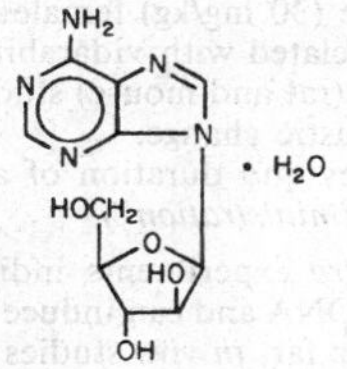

CLINICAL PHARMACOLOGY

Vidarabine is a purine nucleoside obtained from fermentation cultures of *Streptomyces antibioticus*. Vidarabine possesses *in vitro* and *in vivo* antiviral activity against Herpes simplex types 1 and 2, Varicella-Zoster, and Vaccinia viruses. Except for Rhabdovirus and Oncornavirus, Vidarabine does not display *in vitro* antiviral activity against other RNA or DNA viruses, including Adenovirus.

The antiviral mechanism of action has not been established. Vidarabine appears to interfere with the early steps of viral DNA synthesis. Vidarabine is rapidly deaminated to arabinosyl-hypoxanthine (Ara-Hx), the principal metabolite. Ara-Hx also possesses *in vitro* antiviral activity but this activity is less than that of Vidarabine. Because of the low solubility of Vidarabine, trace amounts of both Vidarabine and Ara-Hx can be detected in the aqueous humor only if there is an epithelial defect in the cornea. If the cornea is normal, only trace amounts of Ara-Hx can be recovered from the aqueous humor.

Systemic absorption of Vidarabine should not be expected to occur following ocular administration and swallowing lacrimal secretions. In laboratory animals, Vidarabine is rapidly deaminated in the gastrointestinal tract to Ara-Hx.

In contrast to topical idoxuridine, Vidarabine demonstrated less cellular toxicity in the regenerating corneal epithelium in the rabbit.

INDICATIONS AND USAGE

Vidarabine Ophthalmic Ointment, 3%, is indicated for the treatment of acute keratocon junctivitis and recurrent epithelial keratitis due to Herpes simplex virus types 1 and 2. It is also effective in superficial keratitis caused by Herpes simplex virus which has not responded to topical idoxuridine or when toxic or hypersensitivity reactions to idoxuridine have occurred. The effectiveness of Vidarabine Ophthalmic Ointment, 3%, against stromal keratitis and uveitis due to Herpes simplex virus has not been established.

The clinical diagnosis of keratitis caused by Herpes simplex virus is usually established by the presence of typical dendritic or geographic lesions on slit-lamp examination.

In controlled and uncontrolled clinical trials, an average of seven and nine days of continuous Vidarabine Ophthalmic Ointment, 3%, therapy was required to achieve corneal re-epithelialization. In the controlled trials, 70 of 81 subjects (86%) re-epithelialized at the end of three weeks of therapy. In the uncontrolled trials, 101 of 142 subjects (71%) re-epithelialized at the end of three weeks. Seventy-five percent of the subjects in these uncontrolled trials had either not healed previously or had developed hypersensitivity to topical idoxuridine therapy.

The following topical antibiotics: gentamicin, erythromycin, and chloramphenicol; or topical steroids: prednisolone or dexamethasone, have been administered concurrently with Vidarabine Ophthalmic Ointment, 3%, without an increase in adverse reactions.

CONTRAINDICATION
Vidarabine ophthalmic ointment, 3%, is contraindicated in patients who develop hypersensitivity reactions to it.

WARNINGS
Normally, corticosteroids alone are contraindicated in Herpes simplex virus infections of the eye. If Vidarabine Ophthalmic Ointment, 3%, is administered concurrently with topical corticosteroid therapy, corticosteroid-induced ocular side effects must be considered. These include corticosteroid-induced glaucoma or cataract formation and progression of a bacterial or viral infection.

Vidarabine is not effective against RNA virus or adenoviral ocular infections. It is also not effective against bacterial, fungal, or chlamydial infections of the cornea or nonviral trophic ulcers.

Although viral resistance to Vidarabine has not been observed, this possibility may exist.

PRECAUTIONS
General: The diagnosis of keratocon junctivitis due to Herpes simples virus should be established clinically prior to prescribing Vidarabine ophthalmic ointment, 3%.

Patients should be forewarned that Vidarabine Ophthalmic Ointment, 3%, like any ophthalmic ointment, may produce a temporary visual haze.

Carcinogenesis: Chronic parenteral (IM) studies of Vidarabine have been conducted in mice and rats.

In the mouse study, there was a statistically significant increase in liver tumor incidence among the Vidarabine-treated females. In the same study some vidarabine-treated male mice developed kidney neoplasia. No renal tumors were found in the vehicle-treated control mice or the vidarabine-treated female mice.

In the rat study, intestinal, testicular, and thyroid neoplasia occurred with greater frequency among the vidarabine-treated animals than in the vehicle-treated controls. The increases in thyroid adenoma incidence in the high dose (50 mg/kg) males and the low dose (30 mg/kg) females were statistically significant.

Hepatic megalocytosis, associated with vidarabine treatment, has been found in short- and long-term rodent (rat and mouse) studies. It is not clear whether or not this represents a preneoplastic change.

The recommended frequency and duration of administration should not be exceeded (see *"Dosage and Administration"*).

Mutagenesis: Results of *in vitro* experiments indicate that Vidarabine can be incorporated into mammalian DNA and can induce mutation in mammalian cells (mouse L5178Y cell line). Thus far, *in vivo* studies have not been as conclusive, but there is some evidence (dominant lethal assay in mice) that Vidarabine may be capable of producing mutagenic effects in male germ cells.

It has also been reported that Vidarabine causes chromosome breaks and gaps when added to human leukocytes *in vitro*. While the significance of these effects in terms of mutagenicity is not fully understood, there is a well-known correlation between the ability of various agents to produce such effects and their ability to produce heritable genetic damage.

Pregnancy Category C: Vidarabine parenterally is teratogenic in rats and rabbits. Ten percent Vidarabine ointment applied to 10% of the body surface during organogenesis induced fetal abnormalities in rabbits. When 10% Vidarabine ointment was applied to 2% to 3% of the body surface of rabbits, no fetal abnormalities were found. This dose greatly exceeds the total recommended ophthalmic dose in humans. The possibility of embryonic or fetal damage in pregnant women receiving Vidarabine ophthalmic ointment, 3%, is remote. The topical ophthalmic dose is small, and the drug relatively insoluble. Its ocular penetration is very low. However, a safe dose for a human embryo or fetus has not been established. There are no adequate and well controlled studies in pregnant women. Vidarabine should be used during pregnancy only if the potential benefit justifies the potential risk to the fetus.

Nursing Mothers: It is not known whether Vidarabine is secreted in human milk. Because many drugs are excreted in human milk and because of the potential for tumorigenicity shown for Vidarabine in animal studies, a decision should be made whether to discontinue nursing or to discontinue the drug, taking into account the importance of the drug to the mother. However, breast milk excretion is unlikely because Vidarabine is rapidly deaminated in the gastrointestinal tract.

ADVERSE REACTIONS
Lacrimation, foreign body sensation, conjunctival injection, burning, irritation, superficial punctate keratitis, pain, photophobia, punctal occlusion, and sensitivity have been reported with Vidarabine ophthalmic ointment, 3%. The following have also been reported but appear disease-related: uveitis, stromal edema, secondary glaucoma, trophic defects, corneal vascularization, and hyphema.

OVERDOSAGE
Acute massive overdosage by oral ingestion of the ophthalmic ointment has not occurred. However, the rapid deamination to arabinosylhypoxanthine should preclude any difficulty. The oral LD_{50} for Vidarabine is greater than 5020 mg/kg in mice and rats. No untoward effects should result from ingestion of the entire contents of a tube.

Overdosage by ocular instillation is unlikely because any excess should be quickly expelled from the conjunctival sac. Too frequent administration should be avoided.

DOSAGE AND ADMINISTRATION
Administer approximately one half inch of Vidarabine ophthalmic ointment, 3%, into the lower conjunctival sac five times daily at three-hour intervals.

If there are no signs of improvement after 7 days, or complete re-epithelialization has not occurred by 21 days, other forms of therapy should be considered. Some severe cases may require longer treatment.

After re-epithelialization has occurred, treatment for an additional seven days at a reduced dosage (such as twice daily) is recommended in order to prevent recurrence.

Warning: Manufactured with CFC-12, a substance which harms public health and environment by destroying ozone in the upper atmosphere.

HOW SUPPLIED
OINTMENT: 3%

BRAND/MANUFACTURER	NDC	SIZE	AWP
○ **BRAND**			
VIRA-A: Parke-Davis	00071-3677-07	3.5 gm	$19.78

Videx *SEE* DIDANOSINE

Vinblastine Sulfate

WARNINGS
CAUTION—THIS PREPARATION SHOULD BE ADMINISTERED BY INDIVIDUALS EXPERIENCED IN THE ADMINISTRATION OF VINBLASTINE SULFATE. IT IS EXTREMELY IMPORTANT THAT THE NEEDLE BE PROPERLY POSITIONED IN THE VEIN BEFORE THIS PRODUCT IS INJECTED. IF LEAKAGE INTO SURROUNDING TISSUE SHOULD OCCUR DURING INTRAVENOUS ADMINISTRATION OF VINBLASTINE SULFATE, IT MAY CAUSE CONSIDERABLE IRRITATION. THE INJECTION SHOULD BE DISCONTINUED IMMEDIATELY, AND ANY REMAINING PORTION OF THE DOSE SHOULD THEN BE INTRODUCED INTO ANOTHER VEIN. LOCAL INJECTION OF HYALURONIDASE AND THE APPLICATION OF MODERATE HEAT TO THE AREA OF LEAKAGE HELP DISPERSE THE DRUG AND ARE THOUGHT TO MINIMIZE DISCOMFORT AND THE POSSIBILITY OF CELLULITIS.

FATAL IF GIVEN INTRATHECALLY. FOR INTRAVENOUS USE ONLY. SEE *"WARNINGS"* SECTION FOR THE TREATMENT OF PATIENTS GIVEN INTRATHECAL VINBLASTINE SULFATE.

DESCRIPTION
Vinblastine Sulfate is the salt of an alkaloid extracted from *Vinca rosea* Linn, a common flowering herb known as the periwinkle (more properly known as *Catharanthus roseus* G. Don). Previously, the generic name was vincaleukoblastine, abbreviated VLB. It is a stathmokinetic oncolytic agent. When treated in vitro with this preparation, growing cells are arrested in metaphase.

Chemical and physical evidence indicate that Vinblastine Sulfate has the empirical formula $C_{46}H_{58}N_4O_9 \cdot H_2SO_4$ and that it is a dimeric alkaloid containing both indole and dihydroindole moieties.

Vials of Vinblastine Sulfate contain 10 mg (0.011 mmol) of Vinblastine Sulfate, in the form of a lyophilized plug, without excipients. When sodium chloride solution is added prior to injection, the pH of the resulting solution lies in the range of 3.5 to 5.

Following is its chemical structure:

CLINICAL PHARMACOLOGY

Experimental data indicate that the action of Vinblastine Sulfate is different from that of other recognized antineoplastic agents. Tissue-culture studies suggest an interference with metabolic pathways of amino acids leading from glutamic acid to the citric acid cycle and to urea. In vivo experiments tend to confirm the in vitro results. A number of studies in vitro and in vivo have demonstrated that Vinblastine Sulfate produces a stathmokinetic effect and various atypical mitotic figures. The therapeutic responses, however, are not fully explained by the cytologic changes, since these changes are sometimes observed clinically and experimentally in the absence of any oncolytic effects.

Reversal of the antitumor effect of Vinblastine Sulfate by glutamic acid or tryptophan has been observed. In addition, glutamic acid and aspartic acid have protected mice from lethal doses of Vinblastine Sulfate Aspartic acid was relatively ineffective in reversing the antitumor effect.

Other studies indicate that Vinblastine Sulfate has an effect on cell-energy production required for mitosis and interferes with nucleic acid synthesis. The mechanism of action of Vinblastine Sulfate has been related to the inhibition of microtubule formation in the mitotic spindle, resulting in an arrest of dividing cells at the metaphase stage.

Pharmacokinetic studies in patients with cancer have shown a triphasic serum decay pattern following rapid intravenous injection. The initial, middle, and terminal half-lives are 3.7 minutes, 1.6 hours, and 24.8 hours respectively. The volume of the central compartments is 70% of body weight, probably reflecting very rapid tissue binding to formed elements of the blood. Extensive reversible tissue binding occurs. Low body stores are present at 48 and 72 hours after injection. Since the major route of excretion may be through the biliary system, toxicity from this drug may be increased when there is hepatic excretory insufficiency. Following injection of tritiated Vinblastine in the human cancer patient, 10% of the radioactivity was found in the feces and 14% in the urine; the remaining activity was not accounted for. Similar studies in dogs demonstrated that, over 9 days, 30% to 36% of radioactivity was found in the bile and 12% to 17% in the urine. A similar study in the rat demonstrated that the highest concentrations of radioactivity were found in the lung, liver, spleen, and kidney 2 hours after injection.

Hematologic Effects: Clinically, leukopenia is an expected effect of Vinblastine Sulfate, and the level of the leukocyte count is an important guide to therapy with this drug. In general, the larger the dose employed, the more profound and longer lasting the leukopenia will be. The fact that the white-blood-cell count returns to normal levels after drug-induced leukopenia is an indication that the white-cell-producing mechanism is not permanently depressed. Usually, the white count has completely returned to normal after the virtual disappearance of white cells from the peripheral blood.

Following therapy with Vinblastine Sulfate, the nadir in white-blood-cell count may be expected to occur 5 to 10 days after the last day of drug administration. Recovery of the white blood count is fairly rapid thereafter and is usually complete within another 7 to 14 days. With the smaller doses employed for maintenance therapy, leukopenia may not be a problem.

Although the thrombocyte count ordinarily is not significantly lowered by therapy with Vinblastine Sulfate, patients whose bone marrow has been recently impaired by prior therapy with radiation or with other oncolytic drugs may show thrombocytopenia (less than 200,000 platelets/mm^3). When other chemotherapy or radiation has not been employed previously, thrombocyte reduction below the level of 200,000/mm^3 is rarely encountered, even when Vinblastine Sulfate may be causing significant leukopenia. Rapid recovery from thrombocytopenia within a few days is the rule.

The effect of Vinblastine Sulfate upon the red-cell count and hemoglobin is usually insignificant when other therapy does not complicate the picture. It should be remembered, however, that patients with malignant disease may exhibit anemia even in the absence of any therapy.

INDICATIONS AND USAGE

Vinblastine Sulfate is indicated in the palliative treatment of the following:

I. Frequently Responsive Malignancies:
Generalized Hodgkin's disease (Stages III and IV, Ann Arbor modification of Rye staging system)
Lymphocytic lymphoma (nodular and diffuse, poorly and well differentiated)
Histiocytic lymphoma
Mycosis fungoides (advanced stages)
Advanced carcinoma of the testis
Kaposi's sarcoma
Letterer-Siwe disease (histiocytosis X)

II. Less Frequently Responsive Malignancies:
Choriocarcinoma resistant to other chemotherapeutic agents
Carcinoma of the breast, unresponsive to appropriate endocrine surgery and hormonal therapy
Current principles of chemotherapy for many types of cancer include the concurrent administration of several antineoplastic agents. For enhanced therapeutic effect without additive toxicity, agents with different dose-limiting clinical toxicities and different mechanisms of action are generally selected. Therefore, although Vinblastine Sulfate is effective as a single agent in the aforementioned indications, it is usually administered in combination with other antineoplastic drugs. Such combination therapy produces a greater percentage of response than does a single-agent regimen. These principles have been applied, for example, in the chemotherapy of Hodgkin's disease.

Hodgkin's Disease: Vinblastine Sulfate has been shown to be one of the most effective single agents for the treatment of Hodgkin's disease. Advanced Hodgkin's disease has also been successfully treated with several multiple-drug regimens that included Vinblastine Sulfate. Patients who had relapses after treatment with the MOPP program—mechlorethamine hydrochloride (nitrogen mustard), vincristine sulfate, prednisone, and procarbazine—have likewise responded to combination-drug therapy that included Vinblastine Sulfate. A protocol using cyclophosphamide in place of nitrogen mustard and Vinblastine Sulfate instead of vincristine sulfate is an alternative therapy for previously untreated patients with advanced Hodgkin's disease.

Advanced testicular germinal-cell cancers (embryonal carcinoma, teratocarcinoma, and choriocarcinoma) are sensitive to Vinblastine Sulfate alone, but better clinical results are achieved when Vinblastine Sulfate is administered concomitantly with other antineoplastic agents. The effect of bleomycin is significantly enhanced if Vinblastine Sulfate is administered 6 to 8 hours prior to the administration of bleomycin; this schedule permits more cells to be arrested during metaphase, the stage of the cell cycle in which bleomycin is active.

UNLABELED USES
Vinblastine is used as an adjunct in the treatment of Bladder Carcinoma.

CONTRAINDICATIONS

Vinblastine Sulfate is contraindicated in patients who have significant granulocytopenia unless this is a result of the disease being treated. It should not be used in the presence of bacterial infections. Such infections must be brought under control prior to the initiation of therapy with Vinblastine Sulfate.

WARNINGS

THIS PRODUCT IS FOR INTRAVENOUS USE ONLY. IT SHOULD BE ADMINISTERED BY INDIVIDUALS EXPERIENCED IN THE ADMINISTRATION OF VINBLASTINE SULFATE. THE INTRATHECAL ADMINISTRATION OF VINBLASTINE SULFATE HAS RESULTED IN DEATH. SYRINGES CONTAINING THIS PRODUCT SHOULD BE LABELED "WARNING—FOR IV USE ONLY". EXTEMPORANEOUSLY PREPARED SYRINGES CONTAINING THIS PRODUCT MUST BE PACKAGED IN AN OVERWRAP THAT IS LABELED "DO NOT REMOVE COVERING UNTIL MOMENT OF INJECTION. FATAL IF GIVEN INTRATHECALLY. FOR INTRAVENOUS USE ONLY." THE FOLLOWING TREATMENT SUCCESSFULLY ARRESTED PROGRESSIVE PARALYSIS IN A SINGLE PATIENT MISTAKENLY GIVEN THE RELATED VINCA ALKALOID, VINCRISTINE SULFATE, INTRATHECALLY. IF VINBLASTINE SULFATE IS MISTAKENLY ADMINISTERED INTRATHECALLY, THIS TREATMENT IS RECOMMENDED AND SHOULD BE INITIATED IMMEDIATELY AFTER THE INTRATHECAL INJECTION.

1. REMOVE AS MUCH SPINAL FLUID AS CAN BE SAFELY DONE THROUGH THE LUMBAR ACCESS.

2. INSERT A CATHETER IN A LATERAL CEREBRAL VENTRICLE FOR THE PURPOSE OF FLUSHING THE SUBARACHNOID SPACE FROM ABOVE WITH REMOVAL THROUGH A LUMBAR ACCESS.

3. INITIATE FLUSHING THROUGH THE CEREBRAL CATHETER WITH LACTATED RINGER'S SOLUTION INFUSED AT THE RATE OF 150 ML/H.

4. AS SOON AS FRESH FROZEN PLASMA BECOMES AVAILABLE, INFUSE FRESH FROZEN PLASMA, 25 ML, DILUTED IN 1 L OF LACTATED RINGER'S SOLUTION THROUGH THE CEREBRAL VENTRICULAR CATHETER AT THE RATE OF 75 ML/H WITH REMOVAL THROUGH THE LUMBAR ACCESS. THE RATE OF INFUSION SHOULD BE ADJUSTED TO MAINTAIN A PROTEIN LEVEL IN THE SPINAL FLUID OF 150 MG/DL.

5. ADMINISTER 10 G OF GLUTAMIC ACID INTRAVENOUSLY OVER 24 HOURS FOLLOWED BY 500 MG 3 TIMES DAILY BY MOUTH FOR 1 MONTH OR UNTIL NEUROLOGICAL DYSFUNCTION STABILIZES. THE ROLE OF GLUTAMIC ACID IN THIS TREATMENT IS NOT CERTAIN AND MAY NOT BE ESSENTIAL.

THE USE OF THIS TREATMENT HAS NOT BEEN REPORTED FOLLOWING INTRATHECAL VINBLASTINE SULFATE.

Usage in Pregnancy: Caution is necessary with the administration of all oncolytic drugs during pregnancy. Information on the use of Vinblastine Sulfate during human pregnancy is very limited. Animal studies with Vinblastine Sulfate suggest that teratogenic effects may occur. Vinblastine Sulfate can cause fetal harm when administered to a pregnant woman. Laboratory animals given this drug early in pregnancy suffer resorption of the conceptus: surviving fetuses demonstrate gross deformities. There are no adequate and well-controlled studies in pregnant women. If this drug is used during pregnancy, or if the patient becomes pregnant while receiving this drug, she should be apprised of the potential hazard to the fetus. Women of childbearing potential should be advised to avoid becoming pregnant.

Aspermia has been reported in man. Animal studies show metaphase arrest and degenerative changes in germ cells. Leukopenia (granulocytopenia) may reach dangerously low levels following administration of the higher recommended doses. It is therefore important to follow the dosage technique recommended under the Dosage and Administration section. Stomatitis and neurologic toxicity, although not common or permanent, can be disabling.

PRECAUTIONS

General: Toxicity may be enhanced in the presence of hepatic insufficiency.

If leukopenia with less than 2,000 white blood cells/mm³ occurs following a dose of Vinblastine Sulfate the patient should be watched carefully for evidence of infection until the white-blood-cell count has returned to a safe level.

When cachexia or ulcerated areas of the skin surface are present, there may be a more profound leukopenic response to the drug; therefore, its use should be avoided in older persons suffering from either of these conditions.

In patients with malignant-cell infiltration of the bone marrow, the leukocyte and platelet counts have sometimes fallen precipitously precipitously after moderate doses of Vinblastine Sulfate. Further use of the drug in such patients is inadvisable.

Acute shortness of breath and severe bronchospasm have been reported following the administration of vinca alkaloids. These reactions have been encountered most frequently when the vinca alkaloid was used in combination with mitomycin-C and may require aggressive treatment, particularly when there is preexisting pulmonary dysfunction. The onset may be within minutes or several hours after the vinca is injected and may occur up to 2 weeks following a dose of mitomycin. Progressive dyspnea requiring chronic therapy may occur Vinblastine Sulfate should not be readministered. *The use of small amounts of Vinblastine Sulfate daily for long periods is not advised,* even though the resulting total weekly dosage may be similar to that recommended. Little or no added therapeutic effect has been demonstrated when such regimens have been used. *Strict adherence to the recommended dosage schedule is very important.* When amounts equal to several times the recommended weekly dosage were given in 7 daily installments for long periods, convulsions, severe and permanent central-nervous-system damage, and even death occurred.

Care must be taken to avoid contamination of the eye with concentrations of Vinblastine Sulfate used clinically. If accidental contamination occurs, severe irritation (or, if the drug was delivered under pressure, even corneal ulceration) may result. The eye should be washed with water immediately and thoroughly.

It is not necessary to use preservative-containing solvents if unused portions of the remaining solutions are discarded immediately. Unused preservative-containing solutions should be refrigerated for future use.

Information for Patients: The patient should be warned to report immediately the appearance of sore throat, fever, chills, or sore mouth. Advice should be given to avoid constipation, and the patient should be made aware that alopecia may occur and that jaw pain and pain in the organs containing tumor tissue may occur. The latter is thought possibly to result from swelling of tumor tissue during its response to treatment. Scalp hair will regrow to its pretreatment extent even with continued treatment with Vinblastine Sulfate. Nausea and vomiting, although not common, may occur. Any other serious medical event should be reported to the physician.

Laboratory Tests: Since dose-limiting clinical toxicity is the result of depression of the white-blood-cell count, it is imperative that this count be obtained just before the planned dose of Vinblastine Sulfate. Following administration of Vinblastine Sulfate a fall in the white-blood-cell count may occur. The nadir of this fall is observed from 5 to 10 days following a dose. Recovery to pretreatment levels is usually observed from 7 to 14 days after treatment. These effects will be exaggerated when preexisting bone marrow damage is present and also with the higher recommended doses (*see* Dosage and Administration). The presence of this drug or its metabolites in blood or body tissues is not known to interfere with clinical laboratory tests.

Drug Interactions: Vinblastine Sulfate should not be diluted with solvents that raise or lower the pH of the resulting solution from between 3.5 and 5. Solutions should be made with normal saline (with or without preservative) and should not be combined in the same container with any other chemical. Unused portions of the remaining solutions that do not contain preservatives should be discarded immediately.

The simultaneous oral or intravenous administration of phenytoin and antineoplastic chemotherapy combinations that included Vinblastine Sulfate has been reported to have reduced blood levels of the anticonvulsant and to have increased seizure activity. Dosage adjustment should be based on serial blood level monitoring. The contribution of Vinblastine Sulfate to this interaction is not certain. The interaction may result from either reduced absorption of phenytoin or an increase in the rate of its metabolism and elimination.

Carcinogenesis, Mutagenesis, Impairment of Fertility: Aspermia has been reported in man. Animal studies suggest that teratogenic effects may occur. *See* Warnings regarding impaired fertility. Animal studies have shown metaphase arrest and degenerative changes in germ cells. Amenorrhea has occurred in some patients treated with the combination consisting of an alkylating agent, procarbazine, prednisone, and Vinblastine Sulfate. Its occurrence was related to the total dose of these 4 agents used. Recovery of menses was frequent. The same combination of drugs given to male patients produced azoospermia; if spermatogenesis did return, it was not likely to do so with less than 2 years of unmaintained remission.

Mutagenicity: Tests in *Salmonella typhimurium* and with the dominant lethal assay in mice failed to demonstrate mutagenicity. Sperm abnormalities have been noted in mice. Vinblastine Sulfate has produced an increase in micronuclei formation in bone marrow cells of mice; however, since Vinblastine Sulfate inhibits mitotic spindle formation, it cannot be concluded that this is evidence of mutagenicity. Additional studies in mice demonstrated no reduction in fertility of

males. Chromosomal translocations did occur in male mice. First-generation male offspring of these mice were not heterozygous translocation carriers.

In vitro tests using hamster lung cells in culture have produced chromosomal changes, including chromatid breaks and exchanges, whereas tests using another type of hamster cell failed to demonstrate mutation. Breaks and aberrations were not observed on chromosome analysis of marrow cells from patients being treated with this drug.

It is not clear from the literature how this drug affects synthesis of DNA and RNA. Some believe that there is no interference. Others believe that Vinblastine interferes with nucleic acid metabolism but may not do so by direct effect but possibly as the result of biochemical disturbance in some other part of the molecular organization of the cell. No inhibition of RNA synthesis occurred in rat hepatoma cells exposed in culture to noncytotoxic levels of Vinblastine. Conflicting results have been noted by others regarding interference with DNA synthesis.

Carcinogenesis: There is no currently available evidence to indicate that Vinblastine Sulfate itself has been carcinogenic in humans since the inception of its clinical use in the late 1950s. Patients treated for Hodgkin's disease have developed leukemia following radiation therapy and administration of Vinblastine Sulfate in combination with other chemotherapy, including agents known to intercalate with DNA. It is not known to what extent Vinblastine Sulfate may have contributed to the appearance of leukemia. Available data in rats and mice have failed to demonstrate clearly evidence of carcinogenesis when the animals were treated with the maximum tolerated dose and with one half that dose for 6 months. This testing system demonstrated that other agents were clearly carcinogenic, whereas Vinblastine Sulfate was in the group of drugs causing slightly increased or the same tumor incidence as controls in one study and 1.5 to twofold increase in tumor incidence over controls in another study.

Usage in Pregnancy: Pregnancy Category D: (See "*Warnings*"). Vinblastine Sulfate should be given to a pregnant woman only if clearly needed. Animal studies suggest that teratogenic effects may occur.

Pediatric Usage: The dosage schedule for children is indicated under "*Dosage and Administration.*"

Nursing Mothers: It is not known whether this drug is excreted in human milk. Because many drugs are excreted in human milk and because of the potential for serious adverse reactions from Vinblastine Sulfate in nursing infants, a decision should be made whether to discontinue nursing or the drug, taking into account the importance of the drug to the mother.

ADVERSE REACTIONS

Prior to the use of the drug, patients should be advised of the possibility of untoward symptoms.

In general, the incidence of adverse reactions attending the use of Vinblastine Sulfate appears to be related to the size of the dose employed. With the exception of epilation, leukopenia, and neurologic side effects, adverse reactions generally have not persisted for longer than 24 hours. Neurologic side effects are not common; but when they do occur, they often last for more than 24 hours. Leukopenia, the most common adverse reaction, is usually the dose-limiting factor.

The following are manifestations that have been reported as adverse reactions, in decreasing order of frequency. The most common adverse reactions are underlined:

Hematologic: Leukopenia (granulocytopenia), anemia, thrombocytopenia (myelosuppression).

Dermatologic: Alopecia is common. A single case of light sensitivity associated with this product has been reported.

Gastrointestinal: Constipation, anorexia, nausea, vomiting, abdominal pain, ileus, vesiculation of the mouth, pharyngitis, diarrhea, hemorrhagic enterocolitis, bleeding from an old peptic ulcer, rectal bleeding.

Neurologic: Numbness of digits (paresthesias), loss of deep tendon reflexes, peripheral neuritis, mental depression, headache, convulsions.

Cardiovascular: Hypertension. Cases of unexpected myocardial infarction and cerebrovascular accidents have occurred in patients undergoing combination chemotherapy with Vinblastine, bleomycin, and cisplatin. Raynaud's phenomenon has also been reported with this combination.

Pulmonary: See "*Precautions*".

Miscellaneous: Malaise, bone pain, weakness, *pain in tumor-containing tissue, dizziness, jaw pain,* skin vesiculation, hypertension, Raynaud's phenomenon when patients are being treated with Vinblastine Sulfate in combination with bleomycin and cis-platinum for testicular cancer. The syndrome of inappropriate secretion of antidiuretic hormone has occurred with higher-than-recommended doses.

Nausea and vomiting usually may be controlled with ease by antiemetic agents. When epilation develops, it frequently is not total; and, in some cases, hair regrows while maintenance therapy continues.

Extravasation during intravenous injection may lead to cellulitis and phlebitis. If the amount of extravasation is great, sloughing may occur.

OVERDOSAGE

Signs and Symptoms: Side effects following the use of Vinblastine Sulfate are dose related. Therefore, following administration of more than the recommended dose, patients can be expected to experience these effects in an exaggerated fashion. (See "*Clinical Pharmacology*", "*Contraindications*", "*Warnings*", "*Precautions*" and

"Adverse Reactions".) There is no specific antidote. In addition, neurotoxicity similar to that with Vincristine Sulfate may be observed. Since the major route of excretion may be through the biliary system, toxicity from this drug may be increased when there is hepatic insufficiency.

Treatment: To obtain up-to-date information about the treatment of overdose, a good resource is your certified Regional Poison Control Center. In managing overdosage, consider the possibility of multiple drug overdoses, interaction among drugs, and unusual drug kinetics in your patient. Overdoses of Vinblastine Sulfate have been reported rarely. The following is provided to serve as a guide should such an overdose be encountered.

Supportive care should include the following: (1) prevention of side effects that result from the syndrome of inappropriate secretion of antidiuretic hormone (this would include restriction of the volume of daily fluid intake to that of the urine output plus insensible loss and perhaps the administration of a diuretic affecting the function of the loop of Henle and the distal tubule); (2) administration of an anticonvulsant; (3) prevention of ileus; (4) monitoring the cardiovascular system; and (5) determining daily blood counts for guidance in transfusion requirements and assessing the risk of infection. The major effect of excessive doses of Vinblastine Sulfate will be myelosuppression, which may be life threatening. There is no information regarding the effectiveness of dialysis nor of cholestyramine for the treatment of overdosage.

Vinblastine Sulfate in the dry state is irregularly and unpredictably absorbed from the gastrointestinal tract following oral administration. Absorption of the solution has not been studied. If Vinblastine is swallowed, activated charcoal in a water slurry may be given by mouth along with a cathartic. The use of cholestyramine in this situation has not been reported. Symptoms of overdose will appear when greater-than-recommended doses are given. Any dose of Vinblastine Sulfate that results in elimination of platelets and neutrophils from blood and marrow and their precursors from marrow should be considered life threatening. The exact dose that will do this in all patients is unknown. Overdoses occurring during prolonged, consecutive-day infusions may be more toxic than the same total dose given by rapid intravenous injection. The intravenous median lethal dose in mice is 10 mg/kg body weight; in rats, it is 2.9 mg/kg. The oral median lethal dose in rats is 7 mg/kg.

Protect the patient's airway and support ventilation and perfusion. Meticulously monitor and maintain, within acceptable limits, the patient's vital signs, blood gases, serum electrolytes, etc. Absorption of drugs from the gastrointestinal tract may be decreased by giving activated charcoal, which, in many cases, is more effective than emesis or lavage; consider charcoal instead of or in addition to gastric emptying if the drug has been swallowed. Repeated doses of charcoal over time may hasten elimination of some drugs that have been absorbed. Safeguard the patient's airway when employing gastric emptying or charcoal.

DOSAGE AND ADMINISTRATION

Caution: **It is extremely important that the needle be properly positioned in the vein before this product is injected. If leakage into surrounding tissue should occur during intravenous administration of Vinblastine Sulfate, it may cause considerable irritation. The injection should be discontinued immediately, and any remaining portion of the dose should then be introduced into another vein. Local injection of hyaluronidase and the application of moderate heat to the area of leakage help disperse the drug and are thought to minimize discomfort and the possibility of cellulitis.**

There are variations in the depth of the leukopenic response that follows therapy with Vinblastine Sulfate. For this reason, it is recommended that the drug be given no more frequently than *once every 7 days.* It is wise to initiate therapy for adults by administering a single intravenous dose of 3.7 mg/m² of body surface area (bsa); the initial dose for children should be 2.5 mg/m². Thereafter, white-blood-cell counts should be made to determine the patient's sensitivity to Vinblastine Sulfate. A reduction of 50% in the dose of Vinblastine Sulfate is recommended for patients having a direct serum bilirubin value above 3 mg/100 mL. Since metabolism and excretion are primarily hepatic, no modification is recommended for patients with impaired renal function.

A simplified and conservative incremental approach to dosage *at weekly intervals* may be outlined as follows:

	Adults	Children
First dose	3.7 mg/m² bsa	2.5 mg/m² bsa
Second dose	5.5 mg/m² bsa	3.75 mg/m² bsa
Third dose	7.4 mg/m² bsa	5.0 mg/m² bsa
Fourth dose	9.25 mg/m² bsa	6.25 mg/m² bsa
Fifth dose	11.1 mg/m² bsa	7.5 mg/m² bsa

The above-mentioned increases may be used until a maximum dose (not exceeding 18.5 mg/m² bsa for adults and 12.5 mg/m² bsa for children) is reached. The dose should not be increased after that dose which reduces the white-cell count to approximately 3,000 cells/mm³. In some adults, 3.7 mg/m² bsa may produce this leukopenia; other adults may require more than 11.1 mg/m² bsa; and, very rarely, as much as 18.5 mg/m² bsa may be necessary. For most adult patients, however, the weekly dosage will prove to be 5.5 to 7.4 mg/m² bsa.

When the dose of Vinblastine Sulfate which will produce the above degree of leukopenia has been established, a dose of *1 increment smaller* than this should be administered at weekly intervals for maintenance. Thus, the patient is receiving the maximum dose that does not cause leukopenia. *It should be emphasized that, even though 7 days have elapsed, the next dose of Vinblastine Sulfate should not be given until the white-cell count has returned to at least 4,000/mm³.* In some cases,

oncolytic activity may be encountered before leukopenic effect. When this occurs, there is not need to increase the size of subsequent doses (see *"Precautions".*)

The duration of maintenance therapy varies according to the disease being treated and the combination of antineoplastic agents being used. There are differences of opinion regarding the duration of maintenance therapy with the same protocol for a particular disease: for example, various durations have been used with the MOPP program in treating Hodgkin's disease. Prolonged chemotherapy for maintaining remissions involves several risks, among which are life-threatening infectious diseases, sterility, and possibly the appearance of other cancers through suppression of immune surveillance.

In some disorders, survival following complete remission may not be as prolonged as that achieved with shorter periods of maintenance therapy. On the other hand, failure to provide maintenance therapy in some patients may lead to unnecessary relapse; complete remissions in patients with testicular cancer, unless maintained for at least 2 years, often result in early relapse.

To prepare a solution containing 1 mg of Vinblastone Sulfate/mL, add 10 mL of Sodium Chloride Injection (preserved with phenol or benzyl alcohol) to the 10 mg of Vinblastone Sulfate in the sterile vial. Other solutions are not recommended. The drug dissolves instantly to give a clear solution. After a solution has been made in this way and a portion of it has been removed from a vial, the remainder of the vial's contents may be stored in a refrigerator for future use for 30 days without significant loss of potency.

The dose of Vinblastone Sulfate (calculated to provide the desired amount) may be injected either into the tubing of a running intravenous infusion or directly into a vein. The latter procedure is readily adaptable to outpatient therapy. In either case, the injection may be completed in about 1 minute. If care is taken to insure that the needle is securely within the vein and that no solution containing Vinblastine Sulfate is spilled extravascularly, cellulitis and/or phlebitis will not occur. To minimize further the possibility of extravascular spillage, it is suggested that the syringe and needle be rinsed with venous blood before withdrawal of the needle. The dose should not be diluted in large volumes of diluent (ie, 100 to 250 mL) or given intravenously for prolonged periods (ranging from 30 to 60 minutes or more), since this frequently results in irritation of the vein and increases the chance of extravasation.

Because of the enhanced possibility of thrombosis, it is considered inadvisable to inject a solution of Vinblastone Sulfate into an extremity in which the circulation is impaired or potentially impaired by such conditions as compressing or invading neoplasm, phlebitis, or varicosity.

Parenteral drug products should be inspected visually for particulate matter and discoloration prior to administration, whenever solution and container permit.

It is not necessary to use preservative-containing solvents if unused portions of the remaining solutions are discarded immediately. Unused preservative-containing solutions should be refrigerated for future use.

Procedures for proper handling and disposal of anticancer drugs should be considered. Several guidelines on this subject have been published. There is no general agreement that all of the procedures recommended in the guidelines are necessary or appropriate.

Special Dispensing Information: When dispensing Vinblastine Sulfate in other than the original container, eg, a syrine containing a specific dose, it is imperative that it be packaged in an overwrap bearing the statement: "DO NOT REMOVE COVERING UNTIL MOMENT OF INJECTION. FATAL IF GIVEN INTRATHECALLY. FOR INTRAVENOUS USE ONLY" (see *"Warning".*)

References are available in the package insert or on request.

Storage: The vials should be stored in a refrigerator (2° to 8°C, or 36° to 46°F) to assure extended stability.

HOW SUPPLIED
INJECTION: 1 MG/ML

BRAND/MANUFACTURER	NDC	SIZE	AWP
◆ **GENERICS**			
Fujisawa	00469-2780-30	10 ml	$43.23

POWDER FOR INJECTION: 10 MG

AVERAGE UNIT PRICE (AVAILABLE SIZES)		
BRAND	$38.92	
GENERIC	$29.38	

BRAND/MANUFACTURER	NDC	SIZE	AWP
◆ **BRAND**			
VELBAN: Lilly	00002-1452-01	1s	$38.92
◆ **GENERICS**			
Schein	00364-2447-54	1s	$37.50
Chiron Therapeutics	53905-0091-10	10s	$212.50

Vincasar Pfs *SEE VINCRISTINE SULFATE*

Vincristine Sulfate

DESCRIPTION

Vincristine Sulfate is the salt of an alkaloid obtained from a common flowering herb, the periwinkle plant (*Vinca rosea* Linn). Originally known as leurocristine, it has also been referred to as LCR and VCR. The empirical formula for Vincristine Sulfate is $C_{46}H_{56}N_4O_{10} \cdot H_2SO_4$. It has a molecular weight of 923.04.

Vincristine Sulfate is a white to off-white powder. It is soluble in methanol, freely soluble in water, but only slightly soluble in 95% ethanol. In 98% ethanol, Vincristine Sulfate has an ultraviolet spectrum with maxima at 221 nm ($E +$ 47,100).

Each mL contains Vincristine Sulfate, 1 mg (1.08 µmol); mannitol, 100 mg; methylparaben, 1.3 mg; propylparaben, 0.2 mg; and water for injection, qs. Acetic acid and sodium acetate have been added for pH control. The pH of Vincristine Sulfate solution ranges from 3.5 to 5.5. This product is a sterile solution for cancer/oncolytic use.

Following is its chemical structure:

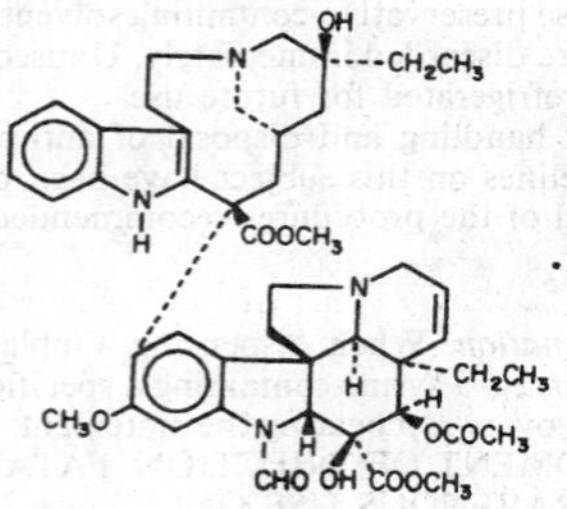

CLINICAL PHARMACOLOGY

The mechanisms of action of Vincristine Sulfate, remain under investigation. The mechanism of action of Vincristine Sulfate has been related to the inhibition of microtubule formation in the mitotic spindle, resulting in an arrest of dividing cells at the metaphase stage.

Central-nervous-system leukemia has been reported in patients undergoing otherwise successful therapy with Vincristine Sulfate. This suggests that Vincristine Sulfate does not penetrate well into the cerebrospinal fluid.

Pharmacokinetic studies in patients with cancer have shown a triphasic serum decay pattern following rapid intravenous injection. The initial, middle, and terminal half-lives are 5 minutes, 2.3 hours, and 85 hours respectively; however, the range of the terminal half-life in humans is from 19 to 155 hours. The liver is the major excretory organ in humans and animals; about 80% of an injected dose of Vincristine Sulfate appears in the feces and 10% to 20% can be found in the urine. Within 15 to 30 minutes after injection, over 90% of the drug is distributed from the blood into tissue, where it remains tightly, but not irreversibly, bound.

Current principles of cancer chemotherapy involve the simultaneous use of several agents. Generally, each agent used has a unique toxicity and mechanism of action so that therapeutic enhancement occurs without additive toxicity. It is rarely possible to achieve equally good results with single-agent methods of treatment. Thus, Vincristine Sulfate is often chosen as part of polychemotherapy because of lack of significant bone-marrow suppression (at recommended doses) and of unique clinical toxicity (neuropathy). See *"Dosage and Administration"* for possible increased toxicity when used in combination therapy.

INDICATIONS AND USAGE

Vincristine Sulfate is indicated in acute leukemia.

Vincristine Sulfate has also been shown to be useful in combination with other oncolytic agents in Hodgkin's disease, non-Hodgkin's malignant lymphomas (lymphocytic, mixed-cell, histiocytic, undifferentiated, nodular, and diffuse types), rhabdomyosarcoma, neuroblastoma, and Wilms' tumor.

UNLABELED USES

Vincristine Sulfate is used alone or as an adjunct in the treatment of malignant thymoma, idiopathic thrombocytopenic purpura, transitional cell bladder carcinoma, breast cancer, and bone marrow transplant. It is also used as an adjunct in chronic lymphocytic leukemia, Ewing's sarcoma, head and neck cancer, Kaposi sarcoma, acute lymphocytic leukemia, and small cell lung cancer.

CONTRAINDICATIONS

Patients with the demyelinating form of Charcot-Marie-Tooth syndrome should not be given Vincristine Sulfate. Careful attention should be given to those conditions listed under *"Warnings"* and *"Precautions"*.

WARNINGS

Pregnancy Category D: Vincristine Sulfate can cause fetal harm when administered to a pregnant woman. When pregnant mice and hamsters were given doses of Vincristine Sulfate that caused the resorption of 23% to 85% of fetuses, fetal malformations were produced in those that survived. Five monkeys were given single doses of Vincristine Sulfate between days 27 and 34 of their pregnancies; 3 of the fetuses were normal at term, and 2 viable fetuses had grossly evident malformations at term. In several animal species, Vincristine Sulfate can induce teratogenesis as well as embryo death at doses that are nontoxic to the pregnant animal. There are no adequate and well-controlled studies in pregnant women. If this drug is used during pregnancy or if the patient becomes pregnant while receiving this drug, she should be apprised of the potential hazard to the fetus. Women of childbearing potential should be advised to avoid becoming pregnant.

PRECAUTIONS

General: Acute uric acid nephropathy, which may occur after the administration of oncolytic agents, has also been reported with Vincristine Sulfate. In the presence of leukopenia or a complicating infection, administration of the next dose of Vincristine Sulfate warrants careful consideration.

If central-nervous-system leukemia is diagnosed, additional agents may be required, because Vincristine Sulfate does not appear to cross the blood-brain barrier in adequate amounts.

Particular attention should be given to dosage and neurologic side effects if Vincristine Sulfate is administered to patients with preexisting neuromuscular disease and when other drugs with neurotoxic potential are also being used.

Acute shortness of breath and severe bronchospasm have been reported following the administration of vinca alkaloids. These reactions have been encountered most frequently when the vinca alkaloid was used in combination with mitomycin-C and may require aggressive treatment, particularly when there is preexisting pulmonary dysfunction. The onset of these reactions may occur minutes to several hours after the vinca alkaloid is injected and may occur up to 2 weeks following the dose of mitomycin. Progressive dyspnea requiring chronic therapy may occur. Vincristine Sulfate should not be readministered.

Care must be taken to avoid contamination of the eye with concentrations of Vincristine Sulfate used clinically. If accidental contamination occurs, severe irritation (or, if the drug was delivered under pressure, even corneal ulceration) may result. The eye should be washed immediately and thoroughly.

Laboratory Tests: Because dose-limiting clinical toxicity is manifested as neurotoxicity, clinical evaluation (eg, history, physical examination) is necessary to detect the need for dosage modification. Following administration of Vincristine Sulfate, some individuals may have a fall in the white-blood-cell count or platelet count, particularly when previous therapy or the disease itself has reduced bone-marrow function. Therefore, a complete blood count should be done before administration of each dose. Acute elevation of serum uric acid may also occur during induction of remission in acute leukemia; thus, such levels should be determined frequently during the first 3 to 4 weeks of treatment or appropriate measures taken to prevent uric acid nephropathy. The laboratory performing these tests should be consulted for its range of normal values.

Drug Interaction: The simultaneous oral or intravenous administration of phenytoin and antineoplastic chemotherapy combinations that included vincristine sulfate has been reported to reduce blood levels of the anticonvulsant and to increase seizure activity. Dosage adjustment should be based on serial blood level monitoring. The contribution of vincristine sulfate to this interaction is not certain. The interaction may result from reduced absorption of phenytoin and an increase in the rate of its metabolism and elimination.

Carcinogenesis, Mutagenesis, Impairment of Fertility: Neither in vivo nor in vitro laboratory tests have conclusively demonstrated the mutagenicity of this product. Fertility following treatment with Vincristine Sulfate alone for malignant disease has not been studied in humans. Clinical reports of both male and female patients who received multiple-agent chemotherapy that included Vincristine Sulfate indicate that azoospermia and amenorrhea can occur in postpubertal patients. Recovery occurred many months after completion of chemotherapy in some but not all patients. When the same treatment is administered to prepubertal patients, permanent azoospermia and amenorrhea are much less likely.

Patients who received chemotherapy with Vincristine Sulfate combination with anticancer drugs known to be carcinogenic have developed second malignancies. The contributing role of Vincristine Sulfate in this development has not been determined. No evidence of carcinogenicity was found following intraperitoneal administration of Vincristine Sulfate in rats and mice, although this study was limited.

Usage in Pregnancy: Pregnancy Category D: See *"Warnings"*.

Nursing Mothers: It is not known whether this drug is excreted in human milk. Because many drugs are excreted in human milk and because of the potential for serious adverse reactions due to Vincristine Sulfate in nursing infants, a decision should be made either to discontinue nursing or the drug, taking into account the importance of the drug to the mother.

ADVERSE REACTIONS
Prior to the use of this drug, patients and/or their parents/guardian should be advised of the possibility of untoward symptoms.

In general, adverse reactions are reversible and are related to dosage. The most common adverse reaction is hair loss; the most troublesome adverse reactions are neuromuscular in origin.

When single, weekly doses of the drug are employed, the adverse reactions of leukopenia, neuritic pain, and constipation occur but are usually of short duration (ie, less than 7 days). When the dosage is reduced, these reactions may lessen or disappear. The severity of such reactions seems to increase when the calculated amount of drug is given in divided doses. Other adverse reactions, such as hair loss, sensory loss, paresthesia, difficulty in walking, slapping gait, loss of deep-tendon reflexes, and muscle wasting, may persist for at least as long as therapy is continued. Generalized sensorimotor dysfunction may become progressively more severe with continued treatment. Although most such symptoms usually disappear by about the sixth week after discontinuance of treatment, some neuromuscular difficulties may persist for prolonged periods in some patients. Regrowth of hair may occur while maintenance therapy continues.

The following adverse reactions have been reported:

Hypersensitivity: Rare cases of allergic-type reactions, such as anaphylaxis, rash, and edema, that are temporally related to vincristine therapy have been reported in patients receiving Vincristine as a part of multidrug chemotherapy regimens.

Gastrointestinal: Constipation, abdominal cramps, weight loss, nausea, vomiting, oral ulceration, diarrhea, paralytic ileus, intestinal necrosis and/or perforation, and anorexia have occurred. Constipation may take the form of upper-colon impaction, and, on physical examination, the rectum may be empty. Colicky abdominal pain coupled with an empty rectum may mislead the physician. A flat film of the abdomen is useful in demonstrating this condition. All cases have responded to high enemas and laxatives. A routine prophylactic regimen against constipation is recommended for all patients receiving Vincristine Sulfate. Paralytic ileus (which mimics the "surgical abdomen") may occur, particularly in young children. The ileus will reverse itself with temporary discontinuance of Vincristine Sulfate and with symptomatic care.

Genitourinary: Polyuria, dysuria, and urinary retention due to bladder atony have occurred. Other drugs known to cause urinary retention (particularly in the elderly) should, if possible, be discontinued for the first few days following administration of Vincristine Sulfate.

Cardiovascular: Hypertension and hypotension have occurred. Chemotherapy combinations that have included Vincristine Sulfate, when given to patients previously treated with mediastinal radiation, have been associated with coronary artery disease and myocardial infarction. Causality has not been established.

Neurologic: Frequently, there is a sequence to the development of neuromuscular side effects. Initially, only sensory impairment and paresthesia may be encountered. With continued treatment, neuritic pain and, later, motor difficulties may occur. There have been no reports made of any agent that can reverse the neuromuscular manifestations that may accompany therapy with Vincristine Sulfate.

Loss of deep-tendon reflexes, foot drop, ataxia, and paralysis have been reported with continued administration. Cranial nerve manifestations, including isolated paresis and/or paralysis of muscles controlled by cranial motor nerves, may occur in the absence of motor impairment elsewhere; extraocular and laryngeal muscles are those most commonly involved. Jaw pain, pharyngeal pain, parotid gland pain, bone pain, back pain, limb pain, and myalgias have been reported; pain in these areas may be severe. Convulsions, frequently with hypertension, have been reported in a few patients receiving Vincristine Sulfate. Several instances of convulsions followed by coma have been reported in children. Transient cortical blindness and optic atrophy with blindness have been reported.

Pulmonary: See *"Precautions"*.

Endocrine: Rare occurrences of a syndrome attributable to inappropriate antidiuretic hormone secretion have been observed in patients treated with Vincristine Sulfate. This syndrome is characterized by high urinary sodium excretion in the presence of hyponatremia; renal or adrenal disease, hypotension, dehydration, azotemia, and clinical edema are absent. With fluid deprivation, improvement occurs in the hyponatremia and in the renal loss of sodium.

Hematologic: Vincristine Sulfate does not appear to have any constant or significant effect on platelets or red blood cells. Serious bone-marrow depression is usually not a major dose-limiting event. However, anemia, leukopenia, and thrombocytopenia have been reported. Thrombocytopenia, if present when therapy with Vincristine Sulfate is begun, may actually improve before the appearance of marrow remission.

Skin: Alopecia and rash have been reported.

Other: Fever and headache have occurred.

OVERDOSAGE
Side effects following the use of Vincristine Sulfate are dose related. In children under 13 years of age, death has occurred following doses of Vincristine Sulfate that were 10 times those recommended for therapy. Severe symptoms may occur in this patient group following dosages of 3 to 4 mg/m^2. Adults can be expected to experience severe symptoms after single doses of 3 mg/m^2 or more (see *"Adverse Reactions"*). Therefore, following administration of doses higher than those recommended, patients can be expected to experience exaggerated side effects. Supportive care should include the following: (1) prevention of side effects resulting from the syndrome of inappropriate antidiuretic hormone secretion (preventive treatment would include restriction of fluid intake and perhaps the administration of a diuretic affecting the function of Henle's loop and the distal tubule); (2) administration of anticonvulsants; (3) use of enemas or cathartics to prevent ileus (in some instances, decompression of the gastrointestinal tract may be necessary); (4) monitoring the cardiovascular system; and (5) determining daily blood counts for guidance in transfusion requirements.

Folinic acid has been observed to have a protective effect in normal mice that were administered lethal doses of Vincristine Sulfate (*Cancer Res* 1963, 23:1390). Isolated case reports suggest that folinic acid may be helpful in treating humans who have received an overdose of Vincristine Sulfate. It is suggested that 100 mg of folinic acid be administered intravenously every 3 hours for 24 hours and then every 6 hours for at least 48 hours. Theoretically (based on pharmacokinetic data), tissue levels of Vincristine Sulfate can be expected to remain significantly elevated for at least 72 hours. Treatment with folinic acid does not eliminate the need for the above-mentioned supportive measures.

Most of an intravenous dose of Vincristine Sulfate is excreted into the bile after rapid tissue binding (see *"Clinical Pharmacology"*). Because only very small amounts of the drug appear in dialysate, hemodialysis is not likely to be helpful in cases of overdosage. An increase in the severity of side effects may be experienced by patients with liver disease that is severe enough to decrease biliary excretion.

Enhanced fecal excretion of parenterally administered Vincristine has been demonstrated in dogs pretreated with cholestyramine. There are no published clinical data on the use of cholestyramine as an antidote in humans.

There are no published clinical data on the consequences of oral ingestion of Vincristine. Should oral ingestion occur, the stomach should be evacuated. Evacuation should be followed by oral administration of activated charcoal and a cathartic.

DOSAGE AND ADMINISTRATION
This preparation is for intravenous use only (see "Warnings"). Neurotoxicity appears to be dose related. Extreme care must be used in calculating and administering the dose of Vincristine Sulfate, since overdosage may have a very serious or fatal outcome.

The concentration of Vincristine contained in all vials of Vincristine Sulfate is 1 mg/mL. Do not add extra fluid to the vial prior to removal of the dose. Withdraw the solution of Vincristine Sulfate into an accurate dry syringe, measuring the dose carefully. Do not add extra fluid to the vial in an attempt to empty it completely.

Caution: It is extremely important that the intravenous needle or catheter be properly positioned before any Vincristine is injected. Leakage into surrounding tissue during intravenous administration of Vincristine Sulfate may cause considerable irritation. If extravasation occurs, the injection should be discontinued immediately, and any remaining portion of the dose should then be introduced into another vein. Local injection of hyaluronidase and the application of moderate heat to the area of leakage will help disperse the drug and may minimize discomfort and the possibility of cellulitis.

Vincristine Sulfate must be administered via an intact, free-flowing intravenous needle or catheter. Care should be taken that there is no leakage or swelling occurring during administration (see boxed "Warnings").

The solution may be injected either directly into a vein or into the tubing of a running intravenous infusion (see *"Drug Interactions"* below). Injection of Vincristine Sulfate should be accomplished within 1 minute.

The drug is administered intravenously *at weekly intervals.*

The usual dose of Vincristine Sulfate for children is 2 mg/m^2. For children weighing 10 kg or less, the starting dose should be 0.05 mg/kg, administered once a week. The usual dose of Vincristine Sulfate for adults is 1.4 mg/m^2. A 50% reduction in the dose of Vincristine Sulfate is recommended for patients having a direct serum bilirubin value above 3 mg/100 mL.

Vincristine Sulfate *should not be given to patients while they are receiving radiation therapy through ports that include the liver.* When Vincristine Sulfate is used in combination with L-asparaginase, Vincristine Sulfate should be given 12 to 24 hours before administration of the enzyme in order to minimize toxicity; administering L-asparaginase before Vincristine Sulfate may reduce hepatic clearance of Vincristine Sulfate.

Drug Interactions: Vincristine Sulfate should not be diluted in solutions that raise or lower the pH outside the range of 3.5 to 5.5. It should not be mixed with anything other than normal saline or glucose in water.

Whenever solution and container permit, parenteral drug products should be inspected visually for particulate matter and discoloration prior to administration.

Procedures for proper handling and disposal of anticancer drugs should be considered. Several guidelines on this subject have been published. There is no general agreement that all of the procedures recommended in the guidelines are necessary or appropriate.

Special Dispensing Information: When dispensing Vincristine Sulfate in other than the original container, eg, a syringe containing a specific dose, it is imperative that it be packaged in an overwrap bearing the statement: "DO NOT REMOVE COVERING UNTIL MOMENT OF INJECTION. FATAL IF GIVEN INTRATHECALLY. FOR INTRAVENOUS USE ONLY (see *"Warnings"*).

See package insert for references.

This product should be refrigerated.

J CODES
5 mg IV—J9380
2 mg IV—J9375
1 mg IV—J9370

HOW SUPPLIED
INJECTION: 1 MG/ML

AVERAGE UNIT PRICE (AVAILABLE SIZES)

| BRAND | $35.06 |
| GENERIC | $25.44 |

BRAND/MANUFACTURER	NDC	SIZE	AWP
◆ BRAND			
ONCOVIN: Lilly	00002-7194-01	1 ml	$34.62
VINCASAR PFS: Pharmacia	00013-7456-86	1 ml	$37.08
ONCOVIN: Lilly	00002-7195-01	2 ml	$69.22
VINCASAR PFS: Pharmacia	00013-7466-86	2 ml	$74.13
ONCOVIN: Lilly	00002-7196-01	5 ml	$156.21
	00002-7198-09	1 ml 3s	$107.28
◆ GENERICS			
Schein	00364-2448-51	1 ml	$31.75
Schein	00364-2448-52	2 ml	$38.25

INJECTION: 2 MG/2 ML

BRAND/MANUFACTURER	NDC	SIZE	AWP
◆ BRAND			
ONCOVIN: Lilly	00002-7199-09	2 ml 3s	$211.08

Viokase *SEE* PANCRELIPASE

Vira-A *SEE* VIDARABINE

Virazole *SEE* RIBAVIRIN

Viridium *SEE* PHENAZOPYRIDINE HYDROCHLORIDE

Virilon *SEE* METHYLTESTOSTERONE

Viroptic *SEE* TRIFLURIDINE

Visken *SEE* PINDOLOL

Vistaril *SEE* HYDROXYZINE

Vitamin A

DESCRIPTION
Water-miscible Vitamin A capsules provide 15 mg retinol (50,000 USP Units) or 7.5 mg retinol (25,000 USP Units) in the form of Vitamin A alcohol, a light yellow to amber oil. One USP Unit is equivalent to one International Unit and to the biological activity of 0.3 mcg of retinol or 0.6 mcg of beta-carotene. One molecule of beta-carotene yields two molecules of retinol, which is known as provitamin A. Water-miscible Vitamin A for intramuscular injection provides 50,000 USP Units of Vitamin A per mL as retinol ($C_{20}H_{30}O$) in the form of Vitamin A palmitate, a light yellow to amber oil.

Vitamin A, one of the fat-soluble vitamins, includes Vitamin A itself as well as its precursors, alpha-, beta-, and gamma-carotene and cryptoxanthin. Of the precursors, beta-carotene predominates in nature and is the most active; on splitting, it forms two molecules of Vitamin A, whereas the other precursors form only one molecule of Vitamin A.

Following is its chemical structure:

$$CH_3 \quad CH_3 \qquad CH_3 \qquad\qquad CH_3$$
$$CH=CH-C=CH-CH=CH-C=CH-CH_2OH$$
$$CH_3$$

CLINICAL PHARMACOLOGY
Beta-carotene, retinol, and retinal have effective and reliable Vitamin A activity. Retinal and retinol are in chemical equilibrium in the body and have equivalent antixerophthalmic activity.

Retinol combines with opsin, the rod pigment in the retina, to form rhodopsin, which is necessary for visual adaptation to darkness.

Vitamin A prevents retardation of growth and preserves the integrity of the epithelial cells. Normal adult liver storage is sufficient to satisfy two years' requirements of Vitamin A.

Vitamin A deficiency is characterized by nyctalopia, keratomalacia, keratinization and drying of the skin, lowered resistance to infection, retardation of growth, thickening of bone, diminished production of cortical steroids, and fetal malformations. Vitamin A is readily absorbed from the gastrointestinal tract, where the biosynthesis of Vitamin A from beta-carotene takes place. Vitamin A absorption requires bile salts, pancreatic lipase, and dietary fat. It is transported in the blood to the liver by the chylomicron fraction of the lymph. The vitamin is stored (primarily as the palmitate) in the Kupffer cells of the liver. Normal serum Vitamin A is 80-300 Units per 100 mL (plasma range is 30-70μg per dl) and for carotenoids 270-753 Units per 100 mL. The normal adult liver contains approximately 100 to 300 micrograms per gram, mostly as retinol palmitate. The minimum daily requirement is approximately 20 units of Vitamin A or 40 units of beta-carotene per kg of body weight. The daily Recommended Dietary Allowance (RDA) established by the National Academy of Sciences for selected categories of population are as follows: children 4-10 years of age, 2500-3000 units; adult males, 5000 units; adult females, 4000 units; pregnant women, 5000 units; lactating women, 6000 units.

The fat-soluble vitamins (A, D, E and K) are absorbed by complex processes that parallel the absorption of fat. Thus, any condition that causes malabsorption of fat (e.g., celiac disease, tropical sprue, regional enteritis) may result in deficiency of one or all of these vitamins. Fat-soluble vitamins affect permeability or transport in various cell membranes and act as oxidation-reduction agents, coenzymes, or enzyme inhibitors. They are stored principally in the liver and excreted in the feces. Because these vitamins are metabolized very slowly, overdosage may produce toxic effects. Dietary fat is necessary for effective absorption of carotene, and protein is required for absorption of retinols. Protein and, possibly, zinc may be required to mobilize Vitamin A reserves in the liver.

Vitamin A is more rapidly absorbed than carotene. Absorption Vitamin A from an aqueous vehicle is appreciably greater than when the drug is given in an oily solution.

Carotene is converted to Vitamin A in the intestinal wall and in the liver. Vitamin A itself is found only in animal sources; it occurs in high concentrations in the liver of the cod, halibut, tuna, and shark. It is also prepared synthetically. Carotene is found only in plants.

INDICATIONS AND USAGE
Water-miscible Vitamin A capsules and injection are effective for the treatment of Vitamin A deficiency. Unlike fat-soluble vitamin A products, Water-miscible Vitamin A capsules are not contraindicated in the malabsorption syndrome, because of the water-solubilizing process.

The parenteral administration is indicated when the oral administration is not feasible as in anorexia, nausea, vomiting, pre- and post-operative conditions, or it is not available as in the "Malabsorption Syndrome" with accompanying steatorrhea.

UNLABELED USES
Vitamin A is used alone or as an adjunct in the treatment of abetalipoproteinemia-induced ocular effects. It is also used in acne vulgaris, to reduce bronchopulmonary dysplasia in small premature infants, and prophylaxis of carcinogenesis. Vitamin A is also prescribed in Crohn's disease, Darier's disease, Kyrle's disease, and to reduce the incidence of acute gastrointestinal ulcer in severely stressed patients.

CONTRAINDICATIONS
Hypervitaminosis A. Sensitivity to any of the ingredients of this preparation.

WARNINGS
Avoid overdosage. Keep out of the reach of children.

Use in Pregnancy: Water-miscible Vitamin A may cause fetal harm when administered to a pregnant woman. Safety of amounts exceeding 6000 units of vitamin A daily during pregnancy has not been established at this time. Therefore, use of Water-miscible Vitamin A in excess of the recommended dietary allowance is contraindicated during pregnancy.

Animal reproduction studies with Vitamin A, either alone or combined with other retinoid compounds, have shown fetal abnormalities. Therefore, total intake of Vitamin A and other therapeutic retinoids should be considered. Fetal abnormalities in animal reproduction studies have been associated with overdosage in several species. Malformations of the central nervous system, eye, palate, and genitourinary tract have been recorded.

In women of childbearing age, the possibility of pregnancy should be excluded before use of Water-miscible Vitamin A. Water-miscible Vitamin A is contraindicated in women who are or may become pregnant. If this drug is used during pregnancy, or if the patient becomes pregnant while taking this drug, the patient should be apprised of the potential hazard to the fetus.

PRECAUTIONS
General: Protect from light. Vitamin A ingested in fortified foods, dietary supplements, and other concomitantly taken drugs should be evaluated. Prolonged daily administration of more than 25,000 units should be conducted under close supervision. Blood level assays are not a direct measure of liver storage. Liver storage should be adequate before discontinuing therapy. Single Vitamin A deficiency is rare. Multiple vitamin deficiency is expected in any dietary deficiency.

Drug Interactions: Women receiving oral contraceptives have shown a significant increase in plasma Vitamin A levels.

Carcinogenesis: There are no studies that show that administration of Vitamin A will cause or prevent cancer.

Usage in Pregnancy: Pregnancy Category X: See *"Warnings"*.

Nursing Mothers: Human milk supplies sufficient Vitamin A for infants unless the maternal diet is grossly inadequate. The U.S. Recommended Daily Allowance (RDA) of vitamin A (5,000 Units) is recommended for nursing mothers.

ADVERSE REACTIONS
See *"Overdosage"* section. Anaphylactic shock and death have been reported using the intravenous route. Allergic reactions have been reported rarely with administration of Water-miscible Vitamin A parenteral including one case of an anaphylactoid type reaction.

OVERDOSAGE
The following amounts have been found to be toxic orally. Toxicity manifestations depend on the age, dose, and duration of administration.

Acute Toxicity: Results from a single dose of 25,000 units per kg of body weight: e.g., 350,000 units for an infant and over 2 million units for an adult.

Chronic Toxicity: Produced by 4000 units per kg of body weight administered for 6 to 15 months.

Infants 3 to 6 months of age can experience chronic toxicity from 18,500 units (water dispersed) per day for 1 to 3 months.

Adults: 1 million units daily for three days, or 50,000 units daily for longer than 18 months, or 500,000 units daily for two months.

HYPERVITAMINOSIS A SYNDROME
1. General manifestations: Fatigue, malaise, lethargy, abdominal discomfort, anorexia, and vomiting.

2. Specific manifestations:
a. Skeletal: Slow growth, hard tender cortical thickening over the radius and tibia, migratory arthralgia, and premature closure of the epiphysis.
b. Central Nervous System: Irritability, headache, and increased intracranial pressure as manifested by bulging fontanels, papilledema, and exophthalmos.
c. Dermatologic: Fissures of the lips, drying and cracking of the skin, alopecia, scaling, massive desquamation, and increased pigmentation.

d. Systemic Hypomenorrhea, hepatosplenomegaly, jaundice, leukopenia, Vitamin A plasma level over 1200 units/100 ml.

The treatment of hypervitaminosis A consists of immediate withdrawal of the vitamin along with symptomatic and supportive treatment.

DOSAGE AND ADMINISTRATION
FOR ORAL USE
For Adults and Children over Eight Years of Age:
1. Severe deficiency with xerophthalmia: 500,000 units daily for three days, followed by 50,000 units daily for two weeks.
2. Severe deficiency: 100,000 units daily for three days followed by 50,000 units daily for two weeks.
3. Follow-up therapy: 10,000 to 20,000 units daily for two months.

FOR INTRAMUSCULAR USE
I. Adults
100,000 units daily for three days followed by 50,000 units daily for two weeks.
II. Children 1 to 8 years old
17,500 to 35,000 units daily for 10 days.
III. Infants
7,500 to 15,000 units daily for 10 days.
Follow-up therapy with an oral therapeutic multivitamin preparation, containing 10,000 to 20,000 units vitamin A for persons over 8 years old and 5,000 to 10,000 units for infants and children, is recommended daily for two months. In malabsorption, the parenteral route must be used for an equivalent preparation.

Poor dietary habits should be corrected and an abundant and well-balanced dietary intake should be prescribed.

STORAGE
Store at controlled room temperature, 15°-30°C (59°-86°F).

Protect from light. Dispense in a tight, light-resistant container as defined in the USP.

J CODES
J3500

HOW SUPPLIED
CAPSULE: 25,000 U

BRAND/MANUFACTURER	NDC	SIZE	AWP
◆ **BRAND**			
AQUASOL A: Astra	00186-4291-00	100s	$39.26

CAPSULE: 50,000 U
HCFA FUL (100s ea) $0.04

BRAND/MANUFACTURER	NDC	SIZE	AWP
◆ **BRAND**			
AQUASOL A: Astra	00186-4301-00	100s	$68.26
◆ **GENERICS**			
Rugby	00536-4784-10	1000s	$21.88

INJECTION: 50,000 U/ML

BRAND/MANUFACTURER	NDC	SIZE	AWP
◆ **BRAND**			
AQUASOL A: Astra	00186-4239-62	2 ml 10s	$182.73

Vitamin B Complex

DESCRIPTION
Vitamin B Complex is a sterile solution for intramuscular or slow intravenous injection comprised of vitamins which may be categorized as belonging to the Vitamin B Complex group.

Each mL contains: Thiamine Hydrochloride 100 mg, Riboflavin 5' Phosphate Sodium 2 mg, Pyridoxine Hydrochloride 2 mg, Dexpan- thenol 2 mg, Niacinamide 100 mg. Certain formulations of Vitamin B Complex contain benzyl alcohol as preservative.

INDICATIONS AND USAGE
In disorders requiring parenteral administration of vitamins, i.e., pre- and postoperative treatment, when requirements are increased as in fever, severe burns, increased metabolism, pregnancy, gastrointestinal disorders interfering with intake or absorption of vitamins, prolonged or wasting diseases, alcoholism and where other deficiency exist.

CONTRAINDICATIONS
Sensitivity to the ingredients listed.

WARNINGS
Anaphylactogenesis may occur with parenteral thiamine. Use with caution. An intradermal test dose is recommended prior to administration in patients suspected of being sensitive to the drug.

PRECAUTIONS
The usual precautions for parenteral administration should be observed. Do not inject if precipitation occurs. Inject slowly by the intravenous route. High

concentrations should be diluted using Normal Saline Injection when given intravenously.

ADVERSE REACTIONS

Mild transient diarrhea, polycythemia vera, peripheral vascular thrombosis, itching transitory exanthema, feeling of swelling of entire body, anaphylactic shock and death.

Sensitivity to the ingredients listed may occur (see *"Warnings"*). Use should be discontinued upon observance of any untoward reaction. Pain upon intramuscular injection may be noted.

DOSAGE AND ADMINISTRATION

Usually 0.25 to 2 mL by intramuscular of slow intravenous injection. High concentrations given intravenously may be diluted using parenteral infusion solutions. (See *"Precautions"*).

Parenteral drug products should be inspected visually for particulate matter and discoloration prior to administration, whenever the solution and container permit.

Phase separation due to reduced solubility can occur under certain conditions of shipping or storage (eg. accidental freezing), which may produce visible particles. Do not use product if these do not redissolve on warming to body temperature and shaking well.

Protect From Light: Store in carton until contents are used. Store in a cool place 8° - 15° C (46° - 59° F). Do not permit to freeze.

J CODES

J3500

HOW SUPPLIED

INJECTION:

BRAND/MANUFACTURER	NDC	SIZE	AWP
○ BRAND			
BECOMJECT-100: Mayrand	00259-0294-30	30 ml	$22.00
○ GENERICS			
McGuff	49072-0057-30	30 ml	$4.29
Steris	00402-0010-30	30 ml	$5.75
Pegasus	10974-0290-30	30 ml	$5.95
BETA-B-PLEX: Roberts/Hauck	59441-0540-30	30 ml	$9.75
Truxton	00463-1007-30	30 ml	$9.75
B-JECT-100: Hyrex	00314-0010-30	30 ml	$10.90
Pasadena	00418-6223-30	30 ml	$16.50
Merit	30727-0300-80	30 ml	$17.85
Torrance	00389-0010-30	30 ml 100s	$4.89

Vitamin B Complex with Minerals

DESCRIPTION

Each 45 ml contains:

Dexpanthenol ....10 mg
Niacinamide ....40 mg
Pyridoxine HCl (B6) ....4 mg
Cyanocobalamin (B12) ....12 mcg
Folic Acid ....1 mg
Iron ....36 mg (as polysaccharide iron complex)
Zinc ....15 mg (as zinc sulfate)
Manganese ....4 mg (as manganese sulfate)
Alcohol 13%

INDICATIONS

For vitamin and mineral replacement therapy in deficiency states and for treatment of iron deficiency anemia and/or nutritional megaloblastic anemias due to inadequate diet.

WARNINGS

Folic acid alone is improper therapy in the treatment of pernicious anemia and other megaloblastic anemias where vitamin B_{12} is deficient.

PRECAUTIONS

Folic acid, especially in doses above 0.1 mg daily, may obscure pernicious anemia, in that hematologic remission may occur while neurological manifestations remain progressive.

USE IN PREGNANCY

Safe use of this product in pregnancy has not been established.

ADVERSE REACTIONS

Allergic sensitization has been reported following both oral and parenteral administration of folic acid.

DOSAGE

Usual adult dosage is one tablespoonful three times daily with meals. Do not exceed recommended dosage unless directed by a physician.

HOW SUPPLIED

ELIXIR:

BRAND/MANUFACTURER	NDC	SIZE	AWP
○ GENERICS			
MAY-VITA: Mayrand	00259-0366-16	480 ml	$15.00

LIQUID:

BRAND/MANUFACTURER	NDC	SIZE	AWP
○ GENERICS			
Pharm Assoc	00121-0535-15	15 ml 100s ud	$52.00

Vitamin B Complex with Vitamin C

Each Vitamin B Complex/ Vitamin C	Quantity	U.S. RDA— Adults and children 4 or more years of age	U.S. RDA— Pregnant or lactating women
Vitamin C (ascorbic acid) ...	500 mg	60 mg	60 mg
Vitamin B_1 (as thiamine mononitrate)	15 mg	1.5 mg	1.7 mg
Vitamin B_2 (riboflavin)	15 mg	1.7 mg	2 mg
Niacin (as niacinamide)	100 mg	20 mg	20 mg
Vitamin B_6 (as pyridoxine HCl)	4 mg	2 mg	2.5 mg
Pantothenic acid (as calcium *d*-pantothenate)	18 mg	10 mg	10 mg
Folic acid	0.5 mg	0.4 mg	0.8 mg
Vitamin B_{12} (cyanocobalamin)	5 mcg	6 mcg	8 mcg

DESCRIPTION

Vit. B Comp/C is a prescription-only oral multivitamin tablet specially formulated for prophylactic or therapeutic nutritional supplementation in conditions requiring water-soluble vitamins.

Vit. B Comp/C tablets supply *therapeutic* levels of ascorbic acid, vitamins B_1, B_2, B_6, niacin and pantothenic acid and a *supplemental* level of vitamin B_{12} Vit. B Comp/C tablets also supply a supplemental level of folic acid for pregnant or lactating women and a therapeutic level for adults and children four or more years of age.

CLINICAL PHARMACOLOGY

Vitamins are essential for normal metabolic functions including hematopoiesis. The B-complex Vitamins are necessary for the conversion of carbohydrate, protein and fat into tissue and energy.

*Thiamine (B_1)*acts as a coenzyme in carbohydrate metabolism. *Riboflavin (B_2)*functions as a coenzyme in the electron transport system associated with conversion of tissue oxidations into usable energy. *Niacin* serves as a coenzyme in oxidation-reduction reactions in tissue respiration. *Pantothenic acid* functions as a coenzyme in various metabolic acetylation reactions. *Folic acid* and *cyanocobalamin (B_{12})* are metabolically interrelated. They are essential to nucleic acid synthesis and normal maturation of red blood cells. *Ascorbic acid (C)* performs a vital function in the process of cellular respiration, and is involved in both carbohydrate and amino acid metabolism. It is essential for collagen formation and tissue repair.

The water-soluble vitamins (B-complex and C) are not significantly stored by the body; excess quantities are excreted in the urine. They must be replenished regularly through diet or other means to maintain essential tissue levels. Thus, these vitamins are rapidly depleted in conditions interfering with their intake or absorption.

INDICATIONS AND USAGE

Vit. B Comp/C is indicated for supportive nutritional supplementation in conditions in which water-soluble vitamins are required prophylactically or therapeutically. These include:

Conditions Causing Depletion, or Reduced Absorption or Bioavailability of Water-soluble Vitamins: Gastrointestinal disorders, chronic alcoholism, febrile illnesses, prolonged or wasting diseases, hyperthyroidism or poorly controlled diabetes.

Conditions Resulting in Increased Needs for Water-soluble Vitamins: Pregnancy, severe burns, recovery from surgery.

CONTRAINDICATIONS

Vit. B Comp/C is contraindicated in patients known to be hypersensitive to any of its components.

WARNINGS

Vit. B Comp/C is not intended for treatment of pernicious anemia or other megaloblastic anemias where vitamin B_{12} is deficient. Neurologic involvement may develop or progress, despite temporary remission of anemia, in patients with vitamin B_{12} deficiency who receive supplemental folic acid and who are inadequately treated with B_{12}.

PRECAUTIONS

General: Certain conditions listed above may require additional nutritional supplementation. During pregnancy, for instance, supplementation with fat-soluble vitamins and minerals may be required according to the dietary habits of the individual Vit. B Comp/C is not intended for treatment of severe specific deficiencies.

◆ RATED THERAPEUTICALLY EQUIVALENT; ◇ THERAPEUTIC EQUIVALENCE UNCONFIRMED; ○ UNRATED

Information for the Patient: Because toxic reactions have been reported with injudicious use of certain vitamins, urge patients to follow your specific instructions regarding dosage regimen. As with any medication, advise patients to keep Vit. B Comp/C out of reach of children.

Drug and Treatment Interactions: As little as 5 mg pyridoxine daily can decrease the efficacy of levodopa in the treatment of parkinsonism. Therefore, Vit. B Comp/C is not recommended for patients undergoing such therapy.

ADVERSE REACTIONS
Adverse reactions have been reported with specific vitamins, but generally at levels substantially higher than those in Vit. B Comp/C. However, allergic and idiosyncratic reactions are possible at lower levels.

DOSAGE AND ADMINISTRATION
Usual adult dosage: one tablet daily.

HOW SUPPLIED

TABLETS:

BRAND/MANUFACTURER	NDC	SIZE	AWP
○ BRAND			
▶ BEROCCA: Roche Labs	00004-0020-01	100s	$37.41
○ GENERICS			
NEPHRO-VITE RX: R&D	54391-1002-01	100s	$37.70

For additional alternatives, turn to the section beginning on page 2859.

Vitamin B₁

DESCRIPTION
Vitamin B_1 injection is a sterile solution of thiamine hydrochloride in water for injection for intramuscular (IM) or slow intravenous (IV) administration.

Each ml contains: Vitamin B_1 100 mg.

Thiamine hydrochloride, or Vitamin B_1, occurs as white crystals or crystalline powder that usually has a slight characteristic odor. Freely soluble in water; soluble in glycerin; slightly soluble in alcohol; insoluble in ether and benzene. Thiamine is rapidly destroyed in neutral or alkaline solutions but is stable in the dry state. It is reasonably stable to heat in acid solution.

The chemical name of thiamine hydrochloride is thiazolium,3-[(4-amino-2-methyl-5-pyrimidinyl)methyl]-5-(2-hydroxyethyl)- 4-methyl-chloride, monohydrochloride.

Its empirical formula is $C_{12}H_{17}CIN_4OS \cdot HCl$ and molecular weight is 337.27.

Following is its chemical structure:

CLINICAL PHARMACOLOGY
The water soluble vitamins are widely distributed in both plants and animals. They are absorbed in man by both diffusion and active transport mechanisms. These vitamins are structurally diverse (derivatives of sugar, pyridine, purines, pyrimidine, organic acid complexes and nucleotide complex) and act as coenzymes, as oxidation-reduction agents, possibly as mitochondrial agents. Metabolism is rapid, and the excess is excreted in the urine.

Vitamin B_1 is distributed in all tissues. The highest concentrations occur in liver, brain, kidney and heart. When Vitamin B_1 intake is greatly in excess of need, tissue stores increase two to three times. If intake is insufficient, tissues become depleted of their vitamin content. Absorption of Vitamin B_1 following IM administration is rapid and complete.

Vitamin B_1 combines with adenosine triphosphate (ATP) to form thiamine pyrophosphate, also known as cocarboxylase, a coenzyme. Its role in carbohydrate metabolism is the decarboxylation of pyruvic acid in the blood and α-ketoacids to acetaldehyde and carbon dioxide. Increased levels of pyruvic acid in the blood indicate Vitamin B_1 deficiency.

The requirement for Vitamin B_1 is greater when the carbohydrate content of the diet is raised. Body depletion of Vitamin B_1 can occur after approximately three weeks of total absence of Vitamin B_1 in the diet.

INDICATIONS AND USAGE
Vitamin B_1 injection is effective for the treatment of Vitamin B_1 deficiency or beriberi whether of the dry (major symptoms related to the nervous system) or wet (major symptoms related to the cardiovascular system) variety. Vitamin B_1 injection should be used where rapid restoration of Vitamin B_1 is necessary, as in Wernicke's encephalopathy, infantile beriberi with acute collapse, cardiovascular disease due to Vitamin B_1 deficiency, or neuritis of pregnancy if vomiting is severe. It is also indicated when giving IV dextrose to individuals with marginal Vitamin B_1 status to avoid precipitation of heart failure.

Vitamin B_1 injection is also indicated in patients with established Vitamin B_1 deficiency who cannot take Vitamin B_1 orally due to coexisting severe anorexia, nausea, vomiting, or malabsorption. Vitamin B_1 injection is not usually indicated for conditions of decreased oral intake or decreased gastrointestinal absorption, because multiple vitamins should usually be given.

UNLABELED USES
Vitamin B_1 is used alone or as an adjunct in the treatment of Alzheimer's disease to improve cognitive function scores, Didmoad syndrome (also known as Wolfram syndrome), maple syrup urine disease, and Wernicke's encephalopathy.

CONTRAINDICATIONS
A history of sensitivity to Vitamin B_1 or to any of the ingredients in this drug is a contraindication. (See *"Warnings"* for further information).

WARNINGS
Serious hypersensitivity/anaphylactic reactions can occur, especially after repeated administration. Deaths have resulted from IV or IM administration of Vitamin B_1 (see *"Adverse Reactions"*).

Routine testing for hypersensitivity, in many cases, may not detect hypersensitivity. Nevertheless, a skin test should be performed on patients who are suspected of drug allergies or previous reactions to Vitamin B_1, and any positive responders should not receive Vitamin B_1 by injection.

If hypersensitivity to Vitamin B_1 is suspected (based on history of drug allergy or occurrence of adverse reactions after Vitamin B_1 administration), administer one-hundredth of the dose intradermally and observe for 30 minutes. If no reaction occurs, full dose can be given; the patient should be observed for at least 30 minutes after injection. Be prepared to treat anaphylactic reactions regardless of the precautions taken.

Treatment of anaphylactic reactions includes maintaining a patent airway and the use of epinephrine, oxygen, vasopressors, steroids and antihistamines.

PRECAUTIONS
GENERAL
Simple vitamin B_1 deficiency is rare. Multiple vitamin deficiencies should be suspected in any case of dietary inadequacy.

INFORMATION FOR PATIENTS
The patient should be advised as to proper dietary habits during treatment so that relapses will be less likely to occur with reduction in dosage or cessation of injection therapy.

USAGE IN PREGNANCY
Pregnancy Category A: Studies in pregnant women have not shown that Vitamin B_1 increases the risk of fetal abnormalities if administered during pregnancy. If the drug is used during pregnancy, the possibility of fetal harm appears remote. Because studies cannot rule out the possibility of harm however, Vitamin B_1 should be used during pregnancy only if clearly needed.

NURSING MOTHERS
It is not known whether this drug is excreted in human milk. Because many drugs are excreted in human milk, caution should be exercised when Vitamin B_1 is administered to a nursing mother.

ADVERSE REACTIONS
An occasional individual may develop a hypersensitivity or life-threatening anaphylactic reaction to Vitamin B_1, especially after repeated injection. Collapse and death have been reported. A feeling of warmth, pruritus, urticaria, weakness, sweating, nausea, restlessness, tightness of the throat, angioneurotic edema, cyanosis, pulmonary edema, and hemorrhage into the gastrointestinal tract have also been reported. Some tenderness and induration may follow IM use (see *"Warnings"*).

OVERDOSAGE
Parenteral doses of 100 to 500 mg singly have been administered without toxic effects. However, dosages exceeding 30 mg three times a day are not utilized effectively.

When the body tissues are saturated with Vitamin B_1, it is excreted in the urine as pyrimidine. As the intake of Vitamin B_1 is further increased, it appears unchanged in the urine.

DOSAGE AND ADMINISTRATION
"Wet" beriberi with myocardial failure must be treated as an emergency cardiac condition, and Vitamin B_1 must be administered slowly by the IV route in this situation (see *"Warnings"*).

In the treatment of beriberi, 10 to 20 mg of Vitamin B_1 are given IM three times daily for as long as two weeks. (See *"Warnings"* regarding repeated injection of Vitamin B_1.) An oral therapeutic multivitamin preparation containing 5 to 10 mg Vitamin B_1, administered daily for one month, is recommended to achieve body tissue saturation.

Infantile beriberi that is mild may respond to oral therapy, but if collapse occurs, doses of 25 mg may cautiously be given IV.

Poor dietary habits should be corrected and an abundant and well-balanced dietary intake should be prescribed.

Patients with neuritis of pregnancy in whom vomiting is severe enough to preclude adequate oral therapy should receive 5 to 10 mg of Vitamin B_1 IM daily.

In the treatment of Wernicke-Korsakoff syndrome, Vitamin B_1 has been administered IV in an initial dose of 100 mg, followed by IM doses of 50 to 100 mg daily until the patient is consuming a regular, balanced diet. (See *"Warnings"* regarding repeated injections of Vitamin B_1).

Patients with marginal Vitamin B_1 status to whom dextrose is being administered should receive 100 mg Vitamin B_1 in each of the first few liters of IV fluid to avoid precipitating heart failure.

Parenteral drug products should be inspected visually for particulate matter and discoloration prior to administration, whenever solution and container permit.

Store at controlled room temperature between 15°-30°C (59°-86°F). Protect from light. Use only if solution is clear and seal intact.

J CODES
J3500

HOW SUPPLIED
INJECTION:

BRAND/MANUFACTURER	NDC	SIZE	AWP
◆ GENERICS			
Major	00904-0944-30	30 ml	$4.00

INJECTION: 100 MG/ML

AVERAGE UNIT PRICE (AVAILABLE SIZES)		GENERIC A-RATED AVERAGE PRICE (GAAP)	
GENERIC	$0.68	30 ml	$5.32

BRAND/MANUFACTURER	NDC	SIZE	AWP
◆ GENERICS			
Fujisawa	00469-1013-25	2 ml	$1.50
Steris	00402-0085-30	30 ml	$3.40
Hyrex	00314-0774-30	30 ml	$5.35
Rugby	00536-2900-75	30 ml	$7.20
Wyeth-Ayerst	00008-0302-01	1 ml 10s	$19.73
Elkins-Sinn	00641-0610-25	1 ml 25s	$17.04
Raway	00686-0610-25	1 ml 100s	$85.00

INJECTION: 100 MG

BRAND/MANUFACTURER	NDC	SIZE	AWP
◆ GENERICS			
Goldline	00182-0567-66	30 ml	$7.95

Vitamin B_6, Injectable

DESCRIPTION
Vitamin B_6, Injectable is a sterile solution of pyridoxine hydrochloride in Water for Injection. Each mL contains 100 mg pyridoxine hydrochloride.

Pyridoxine hydrochloride is a colorless or white crystal or a white crystalline powder. One gram dissolves in 5 mL of water. It is stable in air and is slowly affected by sunlight.

The chemical name is 2-methyl-3-hydroxy-4,5-bis (hydroxymethyl) pyridine hydrochloride.

Following is its chemical structure:

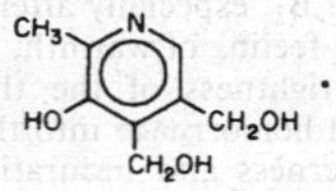

CLINICAL PHARMACOLOGY
Natural substances that have vitamin B_6 activity are pyridoxine in plants and pyridoxal or pyridoxamine in animals. All 3 are converted to pyridoxal phosphate by the enzyme pyridoxal kinase. The physiologically active forms of vitamin B_6 are pyridoxal phosphate (code-carboxylase) and pyridoxamine phosphate. Riboflavin is required for the conversion of pyridoxine phosphate to pyridoxal phosphate.

Vitamin B_6 acts as a coenzyme in the metabolism of protein, carbohydrate, and fat. In protein metabolism, it participates in the decarboxylation of amino acids, conversion of tryptophan to niacin or to serotonin (5-hydroxtryptamine), deamination, and transamination and transulfuration of amino acids. In carbohydrate metabolism, it is responsible for the breakdown of glycogen to glucose-1-phosphate.

The total adult body pool consists of 16 to 25 mg of pyridoxine. Its half-life appears to be 15 to 20 days. Vitamin B_6 is degraded to 4-pyridoxic acid in the liver. This metabolite is excreted in the urine.

The need for pyridoxine increases with the amount of protein in the diet. The tryptophan load test appears to uncover early vitamin B_6 deficiency by detecting xanthinurea. The average adult minimum daily requirement is about 1.25 mg. The "Recommended Dietary Allowance" of the National Academy of Sciences is estimated to be as much as 2.2 mg for adults and 2.5 mg for pregnant and lactating women. The requirements are more in persons having certain genetic defects or those being treated with isonicotinic acid hydrazide (INHJ) or oral contraceptives.

INDICATIONS AND USAGE
Vitamin B_6, Injectable is effective for the treatment of pyridoxine deficiency as seen in the following:

Inadequate dietary intake.

Drug-induced deficiency, as from isoniazid (INH) or oral contraceptives.

Inborn errors of metabolism, e.g., vitamin B_6 dependent convulsions or vitamin B_6 responsive anemia.

The parenteral route is indicated when oral administration is not feasible as in anorexia, nausea and vomiting, and preoperative and postoperative conditions. It is also indicated when gastrointestinal absorption is impaired.

UNLABELED USES
Vitamin B_6 is used alone or as an adjunct in the treatment of intractable convulsions in infants, acute hydrazine toxicity, acute symptoms of isoniazid overdose, and infantile seizures.

CONTRAINDICATIONS
A history of sensitivity to pyridoxine or to any of the ingredients in Vitamin B_6, Injectable is a contraindication.

PRECAUTIONS
GENERAL
Single deficiency, as of pyridoxine alone, is rare. Multiple vitamin deficiency is to be expected in any inadequate diet. Patients treated with levodopa should avoid supplemental vitamins that contain more than 5 mg pyridoxine in the daily dose.

Women taking oral contraceptives may exhibit increased pyridoxine requirements.

DRUG INTERACTIONS
Pyridoxine supplements should not be given to patients receiving levodopa, because the action of the latter drug is antagonized by pyridoxine. However, this vitamin may be used concurrently in patients receiving a preparation containing both carbidopa and levodopa.

PREGNANCY
Pregnancy Category A: The requirement for pyridoxine appears to be increased during pregnancy. Pyridoxine is sometimes of value in the treatment of nausea and vomiting of pregnancy.

NURSING MOTHERS
The need for pyridoxine is increased during lactation. It is not known whether this drug is excreted in human milk. Because many drugs are excreted in human milk, caution should be exercised when pyridoxine hydrochloride is administered to a nursing woman.

USAGE IN CHILDREN
Safety and effectiveness in children have not been established.

ADVERSE REACTIONS
Paresthesia, somnolence, and low serum folic acid levels have been reported.

DRUG ABUSE AND DEPENDENCE
Symptoms of dependence have been noted in adults given only 200 mg daily, followed by withdrawal.

OVERDOSAGE
Vitamin B_6 given to animals in amounts of 3 to 4 g/kg of body weight produces convulsions and death. In man, a dose of 25 mg/kg of body weight is well tolerated.

DOSAGE AND ADMINISTRATION
Vitamin B_6, Injectable, may be administered intramuscularly or intravenously. In cases of dietary deficiency, the dosage is 10 to 20 mg daily for 3 weeks. Follow-up treatment is recommended daily for several weeks with an oral therapeutic multivitamin preparation containing 2 to 5 mg pyridoxine. Poor dietary habits should be corrected, and an adequate, well balanced diet should be prescribed.

The vitamin B_6 dependency syndrome may require a therapeutic dosage of as much as 600 mg a day and a daily intake of 30 mg for life.

In deficiencies due to INH, the dosage is 100 mg daily for 3 weeks followed by a 30 mg maintenance dose daily.

In poisoning caused by ingestion of more than 10 g of INH, an equal amount of pyridoxine should be given — 4 g intravenously followed by 1 g intramuscularly every 30 minutes.

Parenteral drug products should be inspected visually for particulate matter and discoloration prior to administration, whenever solution and container permit.

Protect Injection from Light. Use only if solution is clear and seal intact.

J CODES
J3500

HOW SUPPLIED
INJECTION: 100 MG/ML

AVERAGE UNIT PRICE (AVAILABLE SIZES)		GENERIC A-RATED AVERAGE PRICE (GAAP)	
GENERIC	$0.39	10 ml	$4.70
		30 ml	$5.74

BRAND/MANUFACTURER	NDC	SIZE	AWP
◆ GENERICS			
Schein	00364-6644-54	10 ml	$3.19
Steris	00402-0077-10	10 ml	$3.19
Major	00904-0828-10	10 ml	$3.40

◆ RATED THERAPEUTICALLY EQUIVALENT; ◇ THERAPEUTIC EQUIVALENCE UNCONFIRMED; ○ UNRATED

BRAND/MANUFACTURER	NDC	SIZE	AWP
URL	00677-0319-21	10 ml	$4.13
Hyrex	00314-0758-70	10 ml	$4.75
Goldline	00182-0500-63	10 ml	$6.00
Rugby	00536-3350-70	10 ml	$8.25
Schein	00364-6644-56	30 ml	$3.66
Steris	00402-0077-30	30 ml	$3.66
Rugby	00536-3350-75	30 ml	$9.90

INJECTION: 100 MG

BRAND/MANUFACTURER	NDC	SIZE	AWP
◆ GENERICS			
Fujisawa	00469-0018-25	1 ml	$2.13

Vitamin B₁₂

DESCRIPTION

Vitamin B12 injection is a sterile solution in water for injection for intramuscular or deep subcutaneous administration. Each mL of sterile solution contains 0.1 mg (100 mcg) or 1 mg (1000 mcg) of Vitamin B12 as cyanocobalamin or hydroxocobalamin.

Vitamin B12 appears as dark red crystals or orthorhombic needles or crystalline red powder. It is very hygroscopic in the anhydrous form, and sparingly to moderately soluble in water (1:80). It is stable to autoclaving for short periods at 121°C. The Vitamin B12 coenzymes are very unstable in light.

The chemical name of cyanocobalamin is 5,6-dimethyl-benzimidazolyl cyanocobamide. The cobalt content is 4.34%. Cyanocobalamin has a molecular weight of 1355.38 and its empirical formula is $C_{63}H_{88}CoN_{14}O_{14}P$.

The chemical name of hydroxocobalamin is α-(5,6-dimethylbenzimidazoly) hydroxocobamide. The cobalt content is 4.34%. The empirical formula is $C_{63}H_{89}CoN_{13}O_{15}P$ and its molecular weight is 1346.37. Hydroxocobalamin shares the cobalamin molecular structure with cyanocobalamin.

CLINICAL PHARMACOLOGY

Vitamin B12 is essential to growth, cell reproduction, hematopoiesis, and nucleoprotein and myelin synthesis.

Vitamin B12 is quantitatively and rapidly absorbed from intramuscular and subcutaneous sites of injection; the plasma level of the compound reaches its peak within 1 hour after intramuscular injection. Fifty percent of the administered dose of hydroxocobalamin disappears from the injection site in 2.5 hours. Vitamin B12 is bound to plasma proteins and stored in the liver. It is excreted in the bile and undergoes some enterohepatic recycling. Absorbed Vitamin B12 is transported via specific B12 binding proteins, transcobalamin I and II, to the various tissues. The liver is the main organ for Vitamin B12 storage.

Within 48 hours after injection of 100 or 1000 mcg of Vitamin B12 as cyanocobalamin, 50 to 98% of the injected dose may appear in the urine. The major portion is excreted within the first eight hours. Within 72 hours after injection of 500 to 1000 mcg of Vitamin B12 as hydroxocobalamin, 16 to 66 percent of the injected dose may appear in the urine. The major portion is excreted within the first 24 hours. Intravenous administration results in even more rapid excretion with little opportunity for liver storage.

Gastrointestinal absorption of Vitamin B12 depends on the presence of sufficient intrinsic factor and calcium ions. Intrinsic factor deficiency causes pernicious anemia, which may be associated with subacute combined degeneration of the spinal cord. Prompt parenteral administration of Vitamin B12 prevents progression of neurologic damage.

The average diet supplies about 5 to 15 mcg/day of Vitamin B12 in a protein-bound form that is available for absorption after normal digestion. Vitamin B12 is not present in foods of plant origin, but is abundant in foods of animal origin. In people with normal absorption, deficiencies have been reported only in strict vegetarians who consume no products of animal origin (including no milk products or eggs).

Vitamin B12 is bound to intrinsic factor during transit through the stomach; separation occurs in the terminal ileum in the presence of calcium, and Vitamin B12 enters the mucosal cell for absorption. It is then transported by the transcobalamin binding proteins. A small amount (approximately 1% of the total amount ingested) is absorbed by simple diffusion, but this mechanism is adequate only with very large doses. Oral absorption is considered too undependable to rely on in patients with pernicious anemia or other conditions resulting in malabsorption of Vitamin B12.

Cyanocobalamin is the most widely used form of Vitamin B12, and has hematopoietic activity apparently identical to that of the antianemia factor in purified liver extract. Hydroxocobalamin is equally as effective as cyanocobalamin and they share the cobalamin molecular structure.

Colchicine, para-aminosalicylic acid, and heavy alcohol intake for longer than 2 weeks may produce malabsorption of vitamin B12.

INDICATIONS AND USAGE

Vitamin B12 is indicated for vitamin B12 deficiencies due to malabsorption which may be associated with the following conditions:

I. Pernicious anemia, both uncomplicated and accompanied by nervous system involvement.

II. Dietary deficiency of Vitamin B12, occurring in strict vegetarians and in their breast-fed infants. (Isolated Vitamin B12 deficiency is very rare).

III. Malabsorption of Vitamin B12, resulting from structural or functional damage to the stomach, where intrinsic factor is secreted or to the ileum, where intrinsic factor facilitates Vitamin B12 absorption. These conditions include tropical sprue, and nontropical sprue (idiopathic steatorrhea, gluten-induced enteropathy). Folate deficiency in these patients is usually more severe than Vitamin B12 deficiency.

IV. Inadequate secretion of intrinsic factor, resulting from lesions that destroy the gastric mucosa (ingestion of corrosives, extensive neoplasia), and a number of conditions associated with a variable degree of gastric atrophy (such as multiple sclerosis, certain endocrine disorders, iron deficiency, and subtotal gastrectomy). Total gastrectomy always produces Vitamin B12 deficiency.

Structural lesions leading to Vitamin B12 deficiency include regional ileitis, ileal resections, malignancies, etc.

V. Competition for Vitamin B12 by intestinal parasites or bacteria.

The fish tapeworm (Diphyllobothrium latum) absorbs huge quantities of Vitamin B12 and infested patients often have associated gastric atrophy. The blind-loop syndrome may produce deficiency of Vitamin B12 or folate.

VI. Inadequate utilization of Vitamin B12. This may occur if antimetabolites for the vitamin are employed in the treatment of neoplasia.

It may be possible to treat the underlying disease by surgical correction of anatomic lesions leading to small bowel bacterial overgrowth, expulsion of fish tapeworm, discontinuation of drugs leading to vitamin malabsorption (see "Drug/Laboratory Test Interactions"), use of a gluten-free diet in nontropical sprue, or administration of antibiotics in tropical sprue. Such measures remove the need for long-term administration of Vitamin B12.

Requirements of Vitamin B12 in excess of normal (due to pregnancy, thyrotoxicosis, hemolytic anemia, hemorrhage, malignancy, hepatic and renal disease) can usually be met with oral supplementation.

Vitamin B12 injection is also suitable for the Vitamin B12 absorption test (Schilling Test).

CONTRAINDICATION

Sensitivity to cobalt and/or Vitamin B12 or any component of the medication is a contraindication.

WARNINGS

Patients with early Leber's disease (hereditary optic nerve atrophy) who were treated with Vitamin B12 suffered severe and swift optic atrophy.

Hypokalemia and sudden death may occur in severe megaloblastic anemia which is treated intensely with vitamin B12. Folic acid is not a substitute for Vitamin B12 although it may improve Vitamin B12 deficient megaloblastic anemia. Exclusive use of folic acid in treating Vitamin B12 deficient megaloblastic anemia can result in progressive and irreversible neurologic damage.

Anaphylactic shock and death have been reported after parenteral Vitamin B12 administration. An intradermal test dose is recommended before Vitamin B12 injection is administered to patients suspected of being sensitive to this drug.

Avoid the intravenous route.

Blunted or impeded therapeutic response to Vitamin B12 may be due to such conditions as infection, uremia, drugs having bone marrow suppressant properties such as chloramphenicol, and concurrent iron or folic acid deficiency.

Some brands contain benzyl alcohol. Benzyl alcohol has been reported to be associated with a fatal "Gasping Syndrome" in premature infants.

PRECAUTIONS

GENERAL

Vitamin B12 deficiency that is allowed to progress for longer than 3 months may produce permanent degenerative lesions of the spinal cord. Doses of folic acid greater than 0.1 mg per day may result in hematologic remission in patients with Vitamin B12 deficiency. Neurologic manifestations will not be prevented with folic acid, and if not treated with Vitamin B12, irreversible damage will result.

Doses of Vitamin B12 exceeding 10 mcg daily may produce hematologic response in patients with folate deficiency. Indiscriminate administration may mask the true diagnosis.

The validity of diagnostic vitamin B12 or folic acid blood assays could be compromised by medications, and this should be considered before relying on such tests for therapy.

Vitamin B12 is not a substitute for folic acid and since it might improve folic acid deficient megaloblastic anemia, indiscriminate use of vitamin B12 could mask the true diagnosis.

Hypokalemia and thrombocytosis could occur upon conversion of severe megaloblastic to normal erythropoiesis with B12 therapy. Therefore, serum potassium levels and the platelet count should be monitored carefully during therapy.

Vitamin B12 deficiency may suppress the signs of polycythemia vera. Treatment with Vitamin B12 may unmask this condition.

INFORMATION FOR PATIENTS

Patients with pernicious anemia should be instructed that they will require monthly injections of Vitamin B12 for the remainder of their lives. Failure to do so will result in return of the anemia and in development of incapacitating and irreversible damage to the nerves of the spinal cord. Also, patients should be warned about the danger of taking folic acid in place of Vitamin B12, because the former may prevent anemia but allow progression of subacute combined degeneration.

A vegetarian diet which contains no animal products (including milk products or eggs) does not supply any Vitamin B12. Patients following such a diet should be advised to take oral Vitamin B12 regularly. The need for Vitamin B12 is increased by pregnancy and lactation. Deficiency has been recognized in infants of vegetarian mothers who were breast fed, even though the mothers had no symptoms of deficiency at the time.

LABORATORY TESTS
During the initial treatment of patients with pernicious anemia, when Vitamin B12 produces a return to normal hematopoiesis, there may be a sudden increase in potassium requirements; hypokalemia has been reported, and serum potassium must be observed closely the first 48 hours and potassium replaced if necessary.

Hematocrit, reticulocyte count, Vitamin B12, folate and iron levels should be obtained prior to treatment. Hematocrit and reticulocyte counts should be repeated daily from the fifth to seventh days of therapy and then frequently until the hematocrit is normal. If folate levels are low, folic acid should also be administered. If reticulocytes have not increased after treatment or if reticulocyte counts do not continue at levels of at least twice normal for as long as the hematocrit is less than 35%, diagnosis or treatment should be reevaluated. Repeat determinations of iron and folic acid may reveal a complicating illness that might inhibit the response of the marrow.

Patients with pernicious anemia have about 3 times the incidence of carcinoma of the stomach as the general population, so appropriate tests for this condition should be carried out when indicated.

DRUG/LABORATORY TEST INTERACTIONS
Persons taking most antibiotics, methotrexate or pyrimethamine invalidate folic acid and Vitamin B12 diagnostic blood assays.

Colchicine, para-aminosalicylic acid and heavy alcohol intake for longer than 2 weeks may produce malabsorption of Vitamin B12.

CARCINOGENESIS, MUTAGENESIS, IMPAIRMENT OF FERTILITY
Long-term studies in animals to evaluate carcinogenic potential have not been done. There is no evidence from long-term use in patients with pernicious anemia that Vitamin B12 is carcinogenic. Pernicious anemia is associated with an increased incidence of carcinoma of the stomach, but this is believed to be related to the underlying pathology and not to treatment with Vitamin B12.

PREGNANCY
Pregnancy Category C: Animal reproduction studies have not been conducted with vitamin B12. It is also not known whether vitamin B12 can cause fetal harm when administered to a pregnant woman or can affect reproduction capacity. Adequate and well-controlled studies have not been done in pregnant women. However, Vitamin B12 is an essential vitamin and requirements are increased during pregnancy. Amounts of Vitamin B12 that are recommended by the Food and Nutrition Board, National Academy of Science—National Research Council for pregnant women (4 mcg daily) should be consumed during pregnancy.

NURSING MOTHERS
Vitamin B12 is known to be excreted in human milk. Amounts of Vitamin B12 that are recommended by the Food and Nutrition Board, National Academy of Science—National Research Council for lactating women (4 mcg daily) should be consumed during lactation.

B12 appears in the milk of nursing mothers in concentrations which approximate the mother's Vitamin B12 blood level.

PEDIATRIC USE
Intake in children should be in the amount (0.5 to 3 mcg daily) recommended by the Food and Nutrition Board, National Academy of Science—National Research Council.

ADVERSE REACTIONS
GENERALIZED
Anaphylactic shock and death have been reported with administration of parenteral Vitamin B12 (see "Warnings").

CARDIOVASCULAR
Pulmonary edema and congestive heart failure early in treatment; peripheral vascular thrombosis

HEMATOLOGICAL
Polycythemia vera

GASTROINTESTINAL
Mild transient diarrhea

DERMATOLOGICAL
Itching; transitory exanthema

MISCELLANEOUS
Feeling of swelling of entire body; anaphylaxis

A few patients may experience pain after injection of Vitamin B12.

OVERDOSAGE
No overdosage has been reported with this drug.

The intravenous LD_{50} of Vitamin B12 in mice is greater than 50 mL/kg.

DOSAGE AND ADMINISTRATION
Avoid using the intravenous route. Use of this product intravenously will result in almost all of the vitamin being lost in the urine.

Some brands are to be used only intramuscularly.

PERNICIOUS ANEMIA
Parenteral Vitamin B12 is the recommended treatment and will be required for the remainder of the patient's life. The oral form is not dependable. A dose of 100 mcg daily for 6 or 7 days should be administered by intramuscular or deep subcutaneous injection. If there is clinical improvement and if a reticulocyte response is observed, the same amount may be given on alternate days for seven doses, then every 3 to 4 days for another 2 to 3 weeks. By this time hematologic values should have become normal. This regimen should be followed by 100 mcg monthly for life. Folic acid should be administered concomitantly if needed. In other patients with vitamin B12 deficiency, the duration of therapy and route of administration will depend upon the cause and whether or not it is reversible.

In other patients with vitamin B12 deficiency, the duration of therapy and route of administration will depend upon the cause and whether or not it is reversible.

PATIENTS WITH NORMAL INTESTINAL ABSORPTION
Where the oral route is not deemed adequate, initial treatment similar to that for patients with pernicious anemia may be indicated depending on the severity of the deficiency. Chronic treatment should be with an oral B12 preparation. If other vitamin deficiencies are present, they should be treated.

PATIENTS WITH INADEQUATE INTESTINAL ABSORPTION
Doses similar to those for pernicious anemia are generally appropriate. The individual patient and specific condition must be assessed to help guide needs and dosage.

SCHILLING TEST
The flushing dose is 1000 mcg, given intramuscularly.

Parenteral drug products should be inspected visually for particulate matter and discoloration prior to administration, whenever solution and container permit.

STORAGE
Protect from light. Keep covered in carton until time of use. Store at controlled room temperature, 15°-30°C (59°-86°F). Do not freeze.

J CODES
Up to 1,000 mcg IM,SC—J3420

HOW SUPPLIED

VITAMIN B12
INJECTION: 100 MG/ML

BRAND/MANUFACTURER	NDC	SIZE	AWP
◆ GENERICS			
Rugby	00536-2080-75	30 ml	$7.20

INJECTION: 100 MCG/ML

AVERAGE UNIT PRICE (AVAILABLE SIZES)		GENERIC A-RATED AVERAGE PRICE (GAAP)	
GENERIC	$0.51	30 ml	$3.23

BRAND/MANUFACTURER	NDC	SIZE	AWP
◆ GENERICS			
Steris	00402-0090-30	30 ml	$1.95
URL	00677-0322-23	30 ml	$3.85
Goldline	00182-0693-66	30 ml	$3.90
Wyeth-Ayerst	00008-0265-01	1 ml 10s	$17.10

INJECTION: 1000 MG/ML

AVERAGE UNIT PRICE (AVAILABLE SIZES)	
GENERIC	$0.37

BRAND/MANUFACTURER	NDC	SIZE	AWP
◆ GENERICS			
Rugby	00536-2041-70	10 ml	$4.94
Rugby	00536-2041-75	30 ml	$7.35

INJECTION: 1000 MCG/ML

AVERAGE UNIT PRICE (AVAILABLE SIZES)		GENERIC A-RATED AVERAGE PRICE (GAAP)	
GENERIC	$0.42	10 ml	$2.68
		30 ml	$3.82
		30 ml	$8.90
		1 ml 10s	$23.56

BRAND/MANUFACTURER	NDC	SIZE	AWP
◆ GENERICS			
Fujisawa	00469-1044-25	1 ml	$1.76
Schein	00364-6651-54	10 ml	$1.85
Steris	00402-0091-10	10 ml	$1.85
Geneva	00781-3020-70	10 ml	$2.05
Major	00904-0889-10	10 ml	$2.30
Hyrex	00314-0622-70	10 ml	$2.40

BRAND/MANUFACTURER	NDC	SIZE	AWP
Elkins-Sinn	00641-2260-41	10 ml	$2.44
Goldline	00182-0202-63	10 ml	$3.00
URL	00677-0323-21	10 ml	$3.15
Purepac	00228-2862-60	10 ml	$3.17
CYANOJECT: Mayrand	00259-0295-10	10 ml	$4.60
Schein	00364-6651-56	30 ml	$2.00
Steris	00402-0091-30	30 ml	$2.00
Purepac	00228-2862-61	30 ml	$2.10
Geneva	00781-3021-90	30 ml	$2.25
Major	00904-0889-30	30 ml	$3.25
URL	00677-0323-23	30 ml	$3.99
Goldline	00182-0202-66	30 ml	$4.05
Hyrex	00314-0622-30	30 ml	$4.50
Elkins-Sinn	00641-2270-41	30 ml	$6.25
Steris	00402-0208-30	30 ml	$6.80
CYANOJECT: Mayrand	00259-0295-30	30 ml	$7.85
Major	00904-0916-30	30 ml	$8.65
Rugby	00536-2050-75	30 ml	$11.25
Amer Regent	00517-0130-01	30 ml	$1.56
Wyeth-Ayerst	00008-0264-01	1 ml 10s	$23.56
Wyeth-Ayerst	00008-0264-03	1 ml 10s	$23.56
Elkins-Sinn	00641-0370-25	1 ml 25s	$17.04
Amer Regent	00517-0032-25	10 ml 25s	$35.94

Vitamin C

DESCRIPTION

Vitamin C Injection contains buffered stabilized solutions of pure Vitamin C as the sodium salt in sterile distilled water. In time they may develop a slight color. This does not in any way impair therapeutic activity.

Each ampoule contains 500 mg (2.84 mmol) of Vitamin C (10,000 USP or International units of Vitamin C).

Vitamin C is for intramuscular, intravenous, or subcutaneous injection.

Vitamin C is an antiscorbutic product. Vitamin C occurs as white or slightly yellow crystals or powder. On exposure to light, it gradually darkens. In the dry state, it is reasonably stable in air, but in solution it rapidly oxidizes. Vitamin C is freely soluble in water; sparingly soluble in alcohol; insoluble in chloroform, in ether, and in benzene.

The chemical name of Vitamin C is L-ascorbic acid. The empirical formula is $C_6H_8O_6$, and the molecular weight is 176.13.

Sodium ascorbate, USP (sodium derivative of ascorbic acid, USP) is chemically designated $C_{67}NaO_6$, minute scrystals freely soluble in water.

Following is its chemical structure:

CH₂OH
H–C–OH
O
=O
H
OH OH

CLINICAL PHARMACOLOGY

Vitamin C has few strictly pharmacological actions. Administration in amounts greatly in excess of physiologic requirements causes no demonstrable effects. The vitamin is an essential coenzyme for collagen formation, tissue repair and synthesis of lipids and proteins. It acts both as a reducing agent and as an antioxidant and is necessary for many physiologic functions, e.g., metabolism of iron and folic acid, resistance to infection, and preservation of blood vessel integrity. Signs and symptoms of early Vitamin C deficiency include malaise, irritability, arthralgia, hyperkeratosis of hair follicles, nosebleed, and petechial hemorrhages. Prolonged deficiency leads to clinical scurvy.

Vitamin C is normally present in both plasma and cells. The absorbed vitamin is ubiquitous in all body tissues. The highest concentrations are found in glandular tissue, the lowest in muscle and stored fat. Vitamin C is partially destroyed and partially excreted by the body. There is a renal threshold for Vitamin C; the vitamin is excreted by the kidney in large amounts only when the plasma concentration exceeds this threshold, which is approximately 1.4 mg/100 mL. When the body is saturated with Vitamin C, the plasma concentration will be about the same as that of the renal threshold; if further amounts are then administered, most of it escapes into the urine. When body tissues are not saturated and plasma concentration is low, administration of Vitamin C results in little or no renal excretion.

A major route of metabolism of Vitamin C involves its conversion to urinary oxalate, presumably through intermediate formation of its oxidized product, dehydroascorbic acid.

This oxidation reduction property is important in establishing a proper *in vivo* environment for biologic reactions involving other reactants.

INDICATIONS AND USAGE

Vitamin C is recommended for the prevention and treatment of scurvy and for other symptoms of Vitamin C deficiency. Its parenteral administration is desirable for patients with an acute deficiency or for those whose absorption of orally ingested Vitamin C is uncertain. Parenteral ascorbic acid supplementation may be necessary in the treatment of scurvy for patients with gastric disorders, for patients with extensive injuries, for surgical patients and others who cannot take oral vitamins.

Symptoms of mild deficiency may include faulty bone and tooth development, gingivitis, bleeding gums, and loosened teeth. Acute Vitamin C deficiency may be associated with extensive injuries and other states of extreme stress. Vitamin C requirements are also significantly increased in certain diseases and conditions such as hyperthyroidism, peptic ulcer, neoplastic disease, pregnancy and lactation. Febrile states, chronic illness, and infection (pneumonia, whooping cough, tuberculosis, diphtheria, sinusitis, rheumatic fever, etc.) increase the need for Vitamin C. Premature and immature infants require relatively large amounts of the vitamin.

Hemovascular disorders, burns, and delayed fracture and wound healing are indications for an increase in the daily intake.

CONTRAINDICATIONS

There are no known contraindications to the administration of Vitamin C.

WARNINGS

Persons with diabetes, patients prone to recurrent renal calculi, those undergoing stool occult blood tests, and those on sodium-restricted diets or anticoagulant therapy should not take excessive doses of Vitamin C over an extended period of time.

Some brands of Vitamin C Injection contains sodium hydrosulfite, a sulfite that may cause allergic-type reactions including anaphylactic symptoms and life-threatening or less severe asthmatic episodes in certain susceptible people. The overall prevalence of sulfite sensitivity in the general population is unknown and probably low. Sulfite sensitivity is seen more frequently in asthmatic than in nonasthmatic people.

PRECAUTIONS

General: Too-rapid intravenous injection is to be avoided.

Since high internal pressure may develop on long storage, precautions should be taken to wrap the ampul in a protective covering while it is being opened.

Do not administer unless solution is clear and container is intact. Discard unused portion.

Laboratory Tests: Persons with diabetes taking more than 500 mg Vitamin C daily may obtain false readings of their urinary glucose test. No exogenous Vitamin C should be ingested for 48 to 72 hours before amine-dependent stool occult blood tests are conducted because possible false-negative results may occur.

Drug Interactions: Limited evidence suggests that Vitamin C may influence the intensity and duration of action of bishydroxycoumarin and large doses interfere with the anticoagulant effect of warfarin.

Acidification of the urine by Vitamin C may cause precipitation of cystine, urate or oxalate stones and will alter the excretion of certain other drugs administered concurrently.

As Vitamin C has on occasion been used as a specific antidote for symptoms resulting from interaction between ethanol and disulfiram, it may be expected that the concurrent administration of Vitamin C will interfere with the effectiveness of disulfiram given to patients to encourage abstention from alcohol.

Usage in Pregnancy: Pregnancy Category C: Animal reproduction studies have not been conducted with Vitamin C. It is also not known whether Vitamin C can cause fetal harm when administered to a pregnant woman or can affect reproduction capacity. Vitamin C should be given to a pregnant woman only if clearly needed.

Nonteratogenic Effects: High doses of Vitamin C taken during pregnancy have been reported to cause scurvy in infants removed from this environment at birth.

Nursing Mothers: Caution should be exercised when Vitamin C is administered to a nursing woman.

ADVERSE REACTIONS

Transient mild soreness or pain and swelling may occur at the site of intramuscular or subcutaneous injection. Too-rapid intravenous administration of the solution may cause temporary faintness or dizziness.

Large doses may cause diarrhea. Also see *"Precautions."*

OVERDOSAGE

To obtain up-to-date information about the treatment of overdose, a good resource is your certified Regional Poison Control Center. Telephone numbers of certified poison control centers are listed in the *Physicians' Desk Reference* (PDR). In managing overdosage, consider the possibility of multiple drug overdoses, interaction among drugs, and unusual drug kinetics in your patient.

Due to loss in the urine excessively high doses of parenterally administered Vitamin C are wasteful after saturation of body tissues. Serious toxicity is very uncommon. In the event of severe or unusual untoward effects, Vitamin C should be terminated, pending further evaluation.

DOSAGE AND ADMINISTRATION

Vitamin C may be administered intravenously, intramuscularly, or subcutaneously. The solution has a pH of 5.5 to 7.0 and is not usually irritating to tissues. Absorption and utilization are somewhat more efficient with the intramuscular route, and usually it is preferred.

A higher percentage of the drug will be excreted in the urine when it is injected intravenously than when the subcutaneous or intramuscular route is employed. When administered intravenously, Vitamin C should be slowly infused with large volume solutions. Vitamin C should be added to such solutions shortly before venoclysis; any of the mixture remaining after administration should be discarded.

It is difficult to establish an exact dosage of Vitamin C suitable for the treatment of deficiencies. In general, therapeutic doses should substantially exceed the recommended daily dietary allowances for healthy persons: Adults, 55 to 60 mg; infants, 35 mg; children, 40 mg; adolescents, 45 to 60 mg; pregnant and lactating women, 60 mg. The blood level of Vitamin C in normal persons ranges from 0.4 to 1.5 mg/100 mL.

The average daily protective requirement of Vitamin C for infants is 30 mg. The usual curative dose recommended for infants is 100 to 300 mg daily; it is continued as long as clinical symptoms persist or until saturation, as indicated by excretion tests, has been attained. Premature infants are said to require 75 to 100 mg/day.

The average protective dose of Vitamin C for adults is 70 to 150 mg daily. In the presence of scurvy, doses of 300 mg to 1 g daily are recommended.

The usual therapeutic parenteral dose ranges from 100 to 250 mg (0.2 to 0.5 mL of Vitamin C), once or twice daily. If the deficiency is extreme, 1 to 2 g (2 to 4 mL) may be given. There is no appreciable danger from excessive dosage because superfluous amounts of the vitamin are rapidly excreted in the urine. As much as 6 g daily has been administered parenterally to normal adults without evidence of toxicity.

To enhance wound healing, doses of 300 to 500 mg daily for a week or 10 days to 1 gm daily for four to seven days both preoperatively and postoperatively are generally considered adequate. In the treatment of burns, doses are governed by the extent of tissue injury. For severe burns, daily doses of 200 to 500 mg up to 1 to 2 g are recommended. In other conditions in which the need for Vitamin C is increased, 3 to 5 times the daily optimal allowances appears to be adequate.

Parenteral drug products should be inspected visually for particulate matter and discoloration prior to administration, whenever solution and container permit. See *"Precautions."*

Protect from exposure to light.

Caution: Vitamin C ampuls should be stored in a refrigerator and should not be allowed to stand at room temperature before use. Failure to follow this caution may lead to excessive pressure inside the ampul. Since pressure may develop on long storage, precautions should be taken to wrap the container in a protective covering while it is being opened.

J CODES
J3500

HOW SUPPLIED
INJECTION: 222 MG/ML

BRAND/MANUFACTURER	NDC	SIZE	AWP
○ **GENERICS**			
Schein	00364-6635-56	30 ml	$4.20
Steris	00402-0080-30	30 ml	$4.20
Torrance	00389-0080-30	30 ml	$4.39
Merit	30727-0340-80	30 ml	$10.35
Merit	30727-0645-80	30 ml	$11.55

For additional alternatives, turn to the section beginning on page 2859.

Vitamin K

WARNING-INTRAVENOUS USE
SEVERE REACTIONS, INCLUDING FATALITIES, HAVE OCCURRED DURING AND IMMEDIATELY AFTER INTRAVENOUS INJECTION OF VITAMIN K_1 EVEN WHEN PRECAUTIONS HAVE BEEN TAKEN TO DILUTE THE VITAMIN AND AVOID RAPID INFUSION. TYPICALLY THESE SEVERE REACTIONS HAVE RESEMBLED HYPERSENSITIVITY OR ANAPHYLAXIS, INCLUDING SHOCK AND CARDIAC AND/OR RESPIRATORY ARREST. SOME PATIENTS HAVE EXHIBITED THESE SEVERE REACTIONS ON RECEIVING VITAMIN K_1 FOR THE FIRST TIME. THEREFORE, THE INTRAVENOUS ROUTE SHOULD BE RESTRICTED TO THOSE SITUATIONS WHERE OTHER ROUTES ARE NOT FEASIBLE AND THE SERIOUS RISK INVOLVED IS CONSIDERED JUSTIFIED.

DESCRIPTION
Vitamin K_1 (Phytonadione) is a clear, yellow to amber, viscous, odorless or nearly odorless liquid. It is insoluble in water, soluble in chloroform and slightly soluble in ethanol. It has a molecular weight of 450.70.

Vitamin K_1 (Phytonadione) is 2-methyl-3-phytyl-1, 4-naphthoquinone. Its empirical formula is $C_{31}H_{46}O_2$.

Vitamin K_1 Injection is a yellow, sterile, nonpyrogenic aqueous colloidal solution available for injection by the intravenous, intramuscular and subcutaneous routes.

Each 0.5 ml contains:
Phytonadione .... 1 mg

Each 1 ml contains:
Phytonadione .... 2 mg or 10 mg

pH is 3.5 to 7.0. Vitamin K_1 is oxygen sensitive.

Following is its chemical structure:

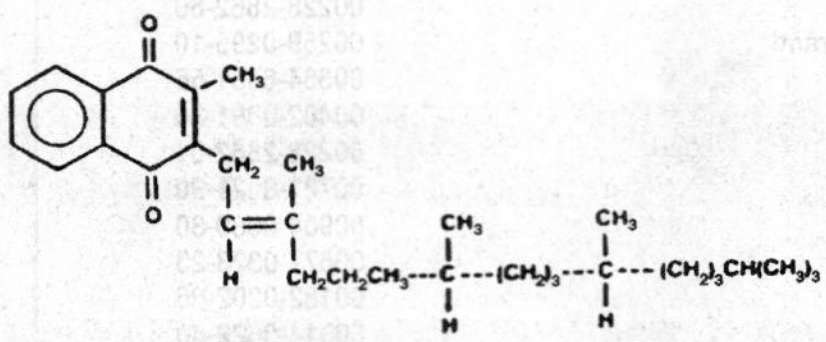

CLINICAL PHARMACOLOGY
Vitamin K_1 Injection (Phytonadione Injection, USP) aqueous colloidal solution of Vitamin K_1 for parenteral injection, possesses the same type and degree of activity as does naturally-occurring Vitamin K, which is necessary for the production via the liver of active prothrombin (factor II), proconvertin (factor VII), plasma thromboplastin component (factor IX), and Stuart factor (factor X). The prothrombin test is sensitive to the levels of three of these four factors—II, VII, and X. Vitamin K is an essential cofactor for a microsomal enzyme that catalyzes the post-translational carboxylation of multiple, specific, peptide-bound glutamic acid residues in inactive hepatic precursors of factors II, VII, IX, and X. The resulting gamma-carboxy-glutamic acid residues convert the precursors into active coagulation factors that are subsequently secreted by liver cells into the blood.

Vitamin K_1 is readily absorbed following intramuscular administration. After absorption, Vitamin K_1 is initially concentrated in the liver, but the concentration declines rapidly. Very little Vitamin K accumulates in tissues. Little is known about the metabolic fate of Vitamin K. Almost no free unmetabolized Vitamin K appears in bile or urine.

In normal animals and humans, Vitamin K_1 is virtually devoid of pharmacodynamic activity. However, in animals and humans deficient in Vitamin K, the pharmacological action of Vitamin K is related to its normal physiological function, that is, to promote the hepatic biosynthesis of Vitamin K dependent clotting factors.

The action of the aqueous colloidal solution, when administered intravenously, is generally detectable within an hour or two and hemorrhage is usually controlled within 3 to 6 hours. A normal prothrombin level may often be obtained in 12 to 14 hours.

In the prophylaxis and treatment of hemorrhagic disease of the newborn, Vitamin K_1 has demonstrated a greater margin of safety than that of the water-soluble Vitamin K analogues.

INDICATIONS AND USAGE
Vitamin K_1 Injection, is indicated in the following coagulation disorders which are due to faulty formation of factors II, VII, IX and X when caused by Vitamin K deficiency or interference with Vitamin K activity.

Vitamin K_1 Injection is indicated in:

■ anticoagulant-induced prothrombin deficiency caused by coumarin or indanedione derivatives;
■ prophylaxis and therapy of hemorrhagic disease of the newborn;
■ hypoprothrombinemia due to antibacterial therapy;
■ hypopropthrombinemia secondary to factors limiting absorption or synthesis of Vitamin K, e.g., obstructive jaundice, biliary fistula, sprue, ulcerative colitis, celiac disease, intestinal resection, cystic fibrosis of the pancreas, and regional enteritis;
■ other drug-induced hypoprothrombinemia where it is definitely shown that the result is due to interference with Vitamin K metabolism, e.g., salicylates.

UNLABELED USES
Vitamin K is used alone or as an adjunct in the treatment to prevent osteoporosis in postmenopausal women and to relieve pruritus induced by primary biliary cirrhosis.

CONTRAINDICATION
Hypersensitivity to any component of this medication.

WARNINGS
Benzyl alcohol as a preservative in Bacteriostatic Sodium Chloride Injection has been associated with toxicity in newborns. Data are unavailable on the toxicity of other preservatives in this age group. There is no evidence to suggest that the small amount of benzyl alcohol contained in some formulations of Vitamin K_1 Injection, when used as recommended, is associated with toxicity.

An immediate coagulant effect should not be expected after administration of Vitamin K_1. It takes a minimum of 1 to 2 hours for measurable improvement in the prothrombin time. Whole blood or component therapy may also be necessary if bleeding is severe.

Vitamin K_1 will not counteract the anticoagulant action of heparin.

When Vitamin K_1 is used to correct excessive anticoagulant-induced hypoprothrombinemia, anticoagulant therapy still being indicated, the patient is again faced with the clotting hazards existing prior to starting the anticoagulant therapy. Vitamin K_1 is not a clotting agent, but overzealous therapy with Vitamin K_1 may restore conditions which originally permitted thromboembolic phenomena.

Dosage should be kept as low as possible, and prothrombin time should be checked regularly as clinical conditions indicate.

Repeated large doses of Vitamin K are not warranted in liver disease if the response to initial use of the vitamin is unsatisfactory. Failure to respond to Vitamin K may indicate that the condition being treated is inherently unresponsive to Vitamin K.

Benzyl alcohol has been reported to be associated with a fatal "Gasping Syndrome" in premature infants.

PRECAUTIONS

DRUG INTERACTIONS
Temporary resistance to prothrombin-depressing anticoagulants may result, especially when larger doses of Vitamin K_1 are used. If relatively large doses have been employed, it may be necessary when reinstituting anticoagulant therapy to use somewhat larger doses of the prothrombin-depressing anticoagulant, or to use one which acts on a different principle, such as heparin sodium.

LABORATORY TESTS
Prothrombin time should be checked regularly as clinical conditions indicate.

CARCINOGENESIS, MUTAGENESIS, IMPAIRMENT OF FERTILITY
Studies of carcinogenicity, mutagenesis or impairment of fertility have not been conducted with Vitamin K_1 Injection.

PREGNANCY
PREGNANCY CATEGORY C
Animal reproduction studies have not been conducted with Vitamin K_1 Injection. It is also not known whether Vitamin K_1 Injection can cause fetal harm when administered to a pregnant women or can affect reproduction capacity. Vitamin K_1 Injection should be given to a pregnant woman only if clearly needed.

NURSING MOTHERS
It is not known whether this drug is excreted in human milk. Because many drugs are excreted in human milk, caution should be exercised when Vitamin K_1 Injection is administered to a nursing woman.

PEDIATRIC USE
Hemolysis, jaundice, and hyperbilirubinemia in newborns, particularly in premature infants, may be related to the dose of Vitamin K_1 Injection. Therefore, the recommended dose should not be exceeded (see *"Adverse Reactions"* and *"Dosage and Administration"*).

ADVERSE REACTIONS
Deaths have occurred after intravenous administration. (See box *"Warning"* preceeding *"Description"*).

Transient "flushing sensations" and "peculiar" sensations of taste have been observed, as well as rare instances of dizziness, rapid and weak pulse, profuse sweating, brief hypotension, dyspnea, and cyanosis.

Pain, swelling, and tenderness at the injection site may occur.

The possibility of allergic sensitivity, including an anaphylactoid reaction, should be kept in mind.

Infrequently, usually after repeated injection, erythematous, indurated, pruritic plaques have occurred; rarely, these have progressed to scleroderma-like lesions that have persisted for long periods. In other cases, these lesions have resembled erythema perstans.

Hyperbilirubinemia has been observed in the newborn following administration of Vitamin K_1. This has occurred rarely and primarily with doses above those recommended. (See *"Precautions, Pediatric Use"*.)

OVERDOSAGE
The intravenous LD_{50} of Vitamin K_1 Injection in the mouse is 41.5 and 52 mL/kg for the 0.2% and 1% concentrations, respectively.

DOSAGE AND ADMINISTRATION
Whenever possible, Vitamin K_1 Injection should be given by the subcutaneous or intramuscular route. When intravenous administration is considered unavoidable, the drug should be injected very slowly, not exceeding 1 mg per minute.

Protect from light at all times.

Parenteral drug products should be inspected visually for particulate matter and discoloration prior to administration, whenever solution and container permit.

DIRECTIONS FOR DILUTION
Vitamin K_1 Injection may be diluted with 0.9% Sodium Chloride Injection, 5% Dextrose Injection, or 5% Dextrose and Sodium Chloride Injection. Benzyl alcohol as a preservative has been associated with toxicity in newborns. *Therefore, all of the above diluents should be preservative-free (see "Warnings").* Other diluents should not be used. When dilutions are indicated, administration should be started immediately after mixture with the diluent, and unused portions of the dilution should be discarded, as well as unused contents of the ampul or vial.

PROPHYLAXIS OF HEMORRHAGIC DISEASE OF THE NEWBORN
The American Academy of Pediatrics recommends that Vitamin K_1 be given to the newborn. A single intramuscular dose of Vitamin K_1 Injection 0.5 to 1 mg within one hour of birth is recommended.

TREATMENT OF HEMORRHAGIC DISEASE OF THE NEWBORN
Empiric administration of Vitamin K_1 should not replace proper laboratory evaluation of the coagulation mechanism. A prompt response (shortening of the prothrombin time in 2 to 4 hours) following administration of Vitamin K_1 is usually diagnostic of hemorrhagic disease of the newborn, and failure to respond indicates another diagnosis or coagulation disorder.

Vitamin K_1 Injection 1 mg should be given either subcutaneously or intramuscularly. Higher doses may be necessary if the mother has been receiving oral anticoagulants.

Whole blood or component therapy may be indicated if bleeding is excessive. This therapy, however, does not correct the underlying disorder and Vitamin K_1 Injection should be given concurrently.

ANTICOAGULANT-INDUCED PROTHROMBIN DEFICIENCY IN ADULTS
To correct excessively prolonged prothrombin time caused by oral anticoagulant therapy—2.5 to 10 mg or up to 25 mg initially is recommended. In rare instances 50 mg may be required. Frequency and amount of subsequent doses should be determined by prothrombin time response or clinical condition (see *"Warnings"*). If in 6 to 8 hours after parenteral administration the prothrombin time has not been shortened satisfactorily, the dose should be repeated.

VITAMIN K_1 INJECTION
SUMMARY OF DOSAGE GUIDELINES

Newborns	*Dosage*
Hemorrhagic Disease of the Newborn Prophylaxis	0.5 to 1 mg IM within 1 hour of birth
Treatment	1 mg SC or IM (Higher doses may be necessary if the mother has been receiving oral anticoagulants)

Adults	*Initial Dosage*
Anticoagulant-Induced Prothrombin Deficiency (caused by coumarin or indanedione derivatives)	2.5 mg to 10 mg or up to 25 mg (rarely 50 mg)
Hypoprothrombinemia due to other causes (Antibiotics; Salicylates or other drugs; Factors limiting absorption or synthesis)	2.5 mg to 25 mg or more (rarely up to 50 mg)

In the event of shock or excessive blood loss, the use of whole blood or component therapy is indicated.

HYPOPROTHROMBINEMIA DUE TO OTHER CAUSES IN ADULTS
A dosage of 2.5 to 25 mg or more (rarely up to 50 mg) is recommended, the amount and route of administration depending upon the severity of the condition and response obtained.

If possible, discontinuation or reduction of the dosage of drugs interfering with coagulation mechanisms (such as salicylates; antibiotics) is suggested as an alternative to administering concurrent Vitamin K_1 Injection. The severity of the coagulation disorder should determine whether the immediate administration of Vitamin K_1 Injection is required in addition to discontinuation or reduction of interfering drugs.

STORAGE
Store at controlled room temperature, 15° to 30°C (59° to 86°F).

Protect from light. Retain in carton until time of use.

J CODES
IM,SC,IV—J3430

HOW SUPPLIED
VITAMIN K
INJECTION: 1 MG

BRAND/MANUFACTURER	NDC	SIZE	AWP
◇ GENERICS			
Intl Med Sys	00548-1140-00	0.5 ml 25s	$120.00

VITAMIN K1
INJECTION: 1 MG

BRAND/MANUFACTURER	NDC	SIZE	AWP
◇ GENERICS			
Abbott Hosp	00074-9157-01	0.5 ml 25s	$56.70

INJECTION: 10 MG

BRAND/MANUFACTURER	NDC	SIZE	AWP
◇ GENERICS			
Abbott Hosp	00074-9158-01	1 ml 25s	$114.30

Vitamins, Multi, Injectable

DESCRIPTION
Multiple Vitamins for Infusion are a combination of important oil-soluble and water-soluble vitamins in an aqueous solution, formulated specially for incorporation into intravenous infusions.

They are available in formulations for adults and children.

In products with two single-dose vials, each 5 ml in vial 1 provides:

Ascorbic acid (vitamin C) ....100 mg
Vitamin A (retinol) ....1 mg (a)
Ergocalciferol (vitamin D) ....5 mcg (b)
Thiamine (vitamin B₁)(as the hydrochloride) ....3 mg
Riboflavin (vitamin B₂) (as riboflavin-5 phosphate sodium) ....3.6 mg
Pyridoxine HCl (vitamin B₆) ....4 mg
Niacinamide ....40 mg
Dexpanthenol (d-pantothenyl alcohol) ....15 mg
Vitamin E (dl-alpha tocopheryl acetate) ....10 mg (c)

    (a) 1 mg vitamin A equals 3,300 USP units.
    (b) 5 mcg ergocalciferol equals 200 USP units.
    (c) 10 mg vitamin E equals 10 USP units.

Each 5 ml in vial 2 provides:

Biotin ....60 mcg
Folic acid ....400 mcg
Cyanocobalamin (vitamin B₁₂) ....5 mcg

In products with two-chambered single-dose vials, which must be mixed just prior to use, each 10 ml of the mixed solution provides:

Ascorbic acid (vitamin C) ....100 mg
Vitamin A (retinol) ....1 mg (a)
Ergocalciferol (vitamin D) ....5 mcg (b)
Thiamine (vitamin B₂) (as the hydrochloride) ....3 mg
Riboflavin (vitamin B₂) (as riboflavin-5 phosphate sodium) ....3.6 mg
Pyridoxine HCl (vitamin B₆) ....4 mg
Niacinamide ....40 mg
Dexpanthenol (d-pantothenyl alcohol) ....15 mg
Vitamin E (dl-alpha tocopheryl acetate) ....10 mg (c)
Biotin ....60 mcg
Folic acid ....400 mcg
Cyanocobalamin (vitamin B₁₂) ....5 mcg

    (a) 1 mg vitamin A equals 3,300 USP units.
    (b) 5 mcg ergocalciferol equals 200 USP units.
    (c) 10 mg vitamin E equals 10 USP units.

Pediatric multiple vitamin is a lyophilized, sterile powder intended for reconstitution and dilution in intravenous infusions.

Each 5 ml of reconstituted product provides:

Ascorbic acid (vitamin C) ....80 mg
Vitamin A (retinol) ....0.7 mg (a)
Ergocalciferol (vitamin D) ....10 mcg (b)
Thiamine (vitamin B₁) (as the hydrochloride) ....1.2 mg
Riboflavin (vitamin B₂) (as riboflavin-5-phosphate sodium) ....1.4 mg
Pyridoxine (vitamin B₆) (as the hydrochloride) ....1 mg
Niacinamide ....17 mg
Dexpanthenol (d-pantothenyl alcohol) ....5 mg
Vitamin E (dl-alpha tocopheryl acetate) ....7 mg (c)
Biotin ....20 mcg
Folic acid ....140 mcg
Cyanocobalamin (vitamin B₁₂) ....1 mcg
Phytonadione (vitamin K₁) ....200 mcg

    (a) 0.7 mg vitamin A equals 2,300 USP units.
    (b) 10 mcg ergocalciferol equals 400 USP units.
    (c) 7 mg vitamin E equals 7 USP units.

INDICATIONS AND USAGE

The adult formulations are indicated as daily multivitamin maintenance dosage for adults and children aged 11 years and above receiving parenteral nutrition.

The pediatric formulation is indicated as daily multivitamin maintenance dosage for infants and children up to 11 years of age receiving parenteral nutrition.

Both formulations are also indicated in other situations where administration by the intravenous route is required. Such situations include surgery, extensive burns, fractures and other trauma, severe infectious diseases, and comatose states, which may provoke a "stress" situation with profound alterations in the body's metabolic demands and consequent tissue depletion of nutrients.

The physician should not await the development of clinical signs of vitamin deficiency before initiating vitamin therapy. The use of a multivitamin product obviates the need to speculate on the status of individual vitamin nutriture.

The injectable preparations (administered in intravenous fluids under proper dilution) contributes intake of these necessary vitamins, except vitamin K in some products, toward maintaining the body's normal resistance and repair processes. Patients with multiple vitamin deficiencies or with markedly increased requirements may be given multiples of the daily dosage for two or more days as indicated by the clinical status.

If the product does not contain vitamin K, it may have to be administered separately.

Clinical testing indicates that some patients do not maintain adequate levels of certain vitamins when this formulation in recommended amounts is the sole source of vitamins. No vitamin deficiencies were clinically evident, but blood levels of vitamins A, C, D, and folic acid declined in a number of subjects who received this formulation as the only vitamin source for 4 to 6 months. Therefore, in patients for whom total parenteral nutrition will be continued for long periods of time, these vitamins should be monitored. If deficiencies appear to be developing, multiples of the formulation (1.5 to 3 times) may be needed for a period of time. When multiples of the formulation are used for more than a few weeks, vitamins A and D should be monitored occasionally to be certain that an excess accumulation of these vitamins is not occurring.

CONTRAINDICATIONS

Known hypersensitivity to any of the vitamins in this product or a pre-existing hypervitaminosis.

With Pediatric Multiple Vitamin: allergic reaction has been known to occur following intravenous administration of thiamine and vitamin K. The formulation is contraindicated prior to blood sampling for detection of megaloblastic anemia, as the folic acid and cyanocobalamin in the vitamin solution can mask serum deficits.

Drug Interactions: Pediatric Multiple Vitamin is not physically compatible with acetazolamide 500 mg, Intravenous chlorothiazide sodium 500 mg, aminophylline 125 mg, ampicillin 500 mg, or moderately alkaline solutions.

General: Unlike the adult formulation, Pediatric Multiple Vitamin contains phytonadione (vitamin K₁).

Adequate blood levels of vitamin E are achieved when Pediatric Multiple Vitamin is given to infants at the recommended dosage. Larger doses or supplementation with oral or parenteral vitamin E are not recommended because elevated blood levels of vitamin E may result.

Studies have shown that vitamin A may adhere to plastic resulting in inadequate vitamin A administration in the doses recommended with Pediatric Multiple Vitamin. Additional vitamin A supplementation vitamin A may be required for low-birth weight infants.

Where long standing specific vitamin deficiencies exist, it may be necessary to add therapeutic amounts of specific vitamins to supplement the maintenance vitamins provided in Pediatric Multiple Vitamin.

Pediatric Multiple Vitamin should be aseptically transferred to the infusion fluid.

PRECAUTIONS

General: Unlike the adult formulation, Pediatric Multiple Vitamin contains phytonadione (vitamin K₁).

Adequate blood levels of vitamin E are achieved when Pediatric Multiple Vitamin is given to infants at the recommended dosage. Larger doses or supplementation with oral or parenteral vitamin E are not recommended because elevated blood levels of vitamin E may result.

Studies have shown that vitamin A may adhere to plastic resulting in inadequate vitamin A administration in the doses recommended with Pediatric Multiple Vitamin. Additional vitamin A supplementation may be required.

A supplemental Vitamin A may be required for low-birth weight infants.

Where long standing specific vitamin deficiencies exist, it may be necessary to add therapeutic amounts of specific vitamins to supplement the maintenance vitamins provided in Pediatric Multiple Vitamin.

Pediatric Multiple Vitamin should be aseptically transferred to the infusion fluid.

Drug Interactions: The injectable preparations are not physically compatible with acetazolamide 500 mg, chlorothiazide sodium 500 mg, sodium cephalothin, sodium cefazolin, or moderately alkaline solutions such as sodium bicarbonate.

Pediatric Multiple Vitamin is not physically compatible with acetazolamide 500 mg, Intravenous chlorothiazide sodium 500 mg, aminophylline 125 mg, ampicillin 500 mg, or moderately alkaline solutions.

Tetracycline HCL 500 mg may not be physically compatible with Adult or Pediatric Multiple Vitamin Infusion. It has been reported that follic acid is unstable in the presence of calcium salts such as calcium gluconate. Some of the vitamins in Multiple Vitamins Infusion may react with vitamin K bisulfite. Direct addition of Adult or Pediatric Multiple Vitamin Infusion to intravenous fat emulsions is not recommended.

The administration of pyridoxine may diminish the effects of levodopa in the treatment of parkinsonism (reference: Martindale 29th Edition, pg. 1017). Vitamin D has a toxic potential. Amounts in the order of 1,000 to 3,000 units per kg may lead to hypercalcemia and attendant complications.

Carcinogenesis, Mutagenesis, and Impairment of Fertility: Carcinogenicity studies have not been performed.

Pregnancy: Pregnant women should follow the U.S. Recommended Daily Allowances for their condition, because their vitamin requirements may exceed those of nonpregnant women.

Nursing Mothers: Lactating women should follow the U.S. Recommended Daily Allowances for their condition, because their vitamin requirements may exceed those of nonlactating women.

Pediatric Use: Safety and effectiveness in children below the age of 11 years have not been established with adult multiple vitamins.

Hypervitaminosis: Vitamin A is usually caused by the administration of excessive amounts of vitamin A over long periods. It is characterized by the following

---

◆ RATED THERAPEUTICALLY EQUIVALENT; ◇ THERAPEUTIC EQUIVALENCE UNCONFIRMED; ○ UNRATED

symptoms: fatigue, irritability, anorexia, loss of weight, vomiting, low grade fever, polyuria, hepatosplenomegaly, pruritus, loss of hair and dry skin. Toxic effects result from the acute ingestion of greater than 500 mg per day or the chronic ingestion of 50 mg per day in adults.

ADVERSE REACTIONS
There have been rare reports of anaphylactoid reactions following large intravenous doses of thiamine. The risk, however, is negligible if thiamine is co-administered with other vitamins in the B group. There have been no reports of fatal anaphylactoid reactions associated with injectable multi-vitamins, adult or pediatric.

There have been rare reports of the following types of reactions:

Dermatologic: rash, erythema, pruritus

CNS: headache, dizziness, agitation, anxiety

Ophthalmic: diplopia

Allergic: urticaria, periorbital and digital edema

OVERDOSAGE
The possibility of hypervitaminosis A or D should be borne in mind.

DOSAGE AND ADMINISTRATION
VITAMINS, MULTIPLE, INJECTABLE
ADULT
Adult Multiple Vitamin Infusion is ready for immediate use in adults and children aged 11 years and above when added to intravenous infusion fluids.

Directions for Proper Use of Pharmacy Bulk Package: For multiple doses, the pharmacy bulk package is prepared by aseptically transferring the contents of vial 1 to vial 2. Mix the solution gently. The mixed solution is ready for immediate use. The mixed solution will provide ten 10 mL doses. The container closure may be penetrated only one time, utilizing a suitable sterile transfer device or dispensing set which allows measured distribution of the contents.

The withdrawal of container contents should be accomplished without delay. However, should this not be possible, a maximum time of 4 hours from initial closure entry is permitted to complete fluid transfer operations.

Use of this product is restricted to a suitable work area, such as a laminar flow hood.

Multiple Vitamin Infusion should not be given as a direct, undiluted intravenous injection as it may give rise to dizziness, faintness, and possible tissue irritation.

For intravenous feeding, one daily dose Multiple Vitamin Infusion (5 ml of vial 1 plus 5 ml of vial 2, or 10 ml of mixed unit vial) added directly to not less than 500 ml, preferably 1,000 ml, of intravenous dextrose, saline or similar infusion solutions.

VITAMINS, MULTIPLE, INJECTABLE
PEDIATRIC
The single-dose vial of Pediatric Multiple Vitamin Infusion is reconstituted by adding 5 ml of sterile water for injection, dextrose injection, or sodium chloride injection to the 10 ml vial.

Directions for Proper Use of Pharmacy Bulk Package: The pharmacy bulk package is reconstituted by adding 24 mL of sterile Water for Injection USP, Dextrose injection 5%, or sodium chloride injection to the 50 ml vial. The container closure may be penetrated only one time, utilizing a suitable sterile transfer device or dispensing set which allows measured distribution of the contents. A sterile substance which must be reconstituted prior to use may require a separate closure entry. This bulk package provides five 5 mL doses. If the solution contains no preservative, all five doses should be withdrawn for dispensing, using aseptic techniques, with one vial entry. The vial may be swirled gently after the addition of the water to hasten reconstitution. Use of this product is restricted to a suitable work area, such as a laminar flow hood. The reconstituted solution is ready within three minutes for immediate use. The withdrawal of container contents should be accomplished without delay. However, should this not be possible, a maximum time of 4 hours from initial closure entry is permitted to complete fluid transfer operations. The amount to be administered should be added to appropriate intravenous infusion fluids (see below).

The reconstituted Pediatric Multiple Vitamin Infusion should not be given as a direct, undiluted intravenous injection as it may give rise to dizziness, faintness and possible tissue irritation.

For a single dose, 5 ml of reconstituted Pediatric Multiple Vitamin Infusion should be added directly to not less than 100 ml of intravenous dextrose, saline or similar infusion solutions.

Infants weighing less than 1 kg: The daily dose is 30% (1.5 ml) of a single full dose (5 ml). Do not exceed this daily dose.

Infants weighing 1 to 3 kg: The daily dose is 65% (3.25 ml) of a single full dose (5 ml). Multiples of this recommended dose should not be given to infants weighing less than 3 kg. A supplemental vitamin A may be required for low-birth-weight infants.

Infants and children weighing 3 kg or more up to 11 years of age: The daily dose is 5 ml unless there is clinical or laboratory evidence for increasing or decreasing the dosage.

Parenteral drug products should be inspected visually for particulate matter and discoloration prior to administration, whenever solution and container permit.

After Multiple Vitamin Infusion is diluted in an intravenous infusion, The resulting solution is ready for immediate use. It should be refrigerated unless it is to be administered immediately, and in any event should be administered within 24 hours. After Pediatric Multiple Vitamin Infusion is reconstituted it should be immediately diluted into the intravenous solution. The resulting solution should be administered immediately.

Some of the vitamins in these products, particularly A and D and riboflavin, are light sensitive, and exposure to light should be minimized.

Storage: Store adult preparation at 2°-8°C (36-46°F); store pediatric at controlled room temperature, 15°-30°C (59°-86°F).

J CODES
J3500

HOW SUPPLIED
INJECTION:

AVERAGE UNIT PRICE (AVAILABLE SIZES)

BRAND	$0.66
GENERIC	$0.38

BRAND/MANUFACTURER	NDC	SIZE	AWP
◆ **BRAND**			
M.V.I. PEDIATRIC: Astra	00186-1839-25	25 ml 5s	$187.98
M.V.I.-12: Astra	00186-1199-10	50 ml 20s	$233.16
	00186-1199-31	5 ml 25s	$66.56
	00186-1199-35	10 ml 25s	$66.56
M.V.I. PEDIATRIC: Astra	00186-1839-35	10 ml 25s	$187.98
◆ **GENERICS**			
Steris	00402-0703-11	10 ml	$3.75
Schein	00364-2345-34	10 ml 25s	$93.75

INJECTION:

BRAND/MANUFACTURER	NDC	SIZE	AWP
○ **BRAND**			
PRIMAPLEX: Primedics	00684-0190-10	10 ml	$9.75
	00684-0106-30	30 ml	$10.95

Vitamins, Multiple with Minerals

The composition of multivitamin products varies by brand. For exact ingredients of a particular product, consult its labeling. The following information reflects the product labeling for Berocca Plus Tablets.

Each Vitamins, Multiple with Minerals tablet contains:	Quantity	U.S. RDA—Adults and children 4 or more years of age	U.S. RDA—Pregnant or lactating women
Fat-Soluble Vitamins			
Vitamin A (as vitamin A acetate)	5000 IU	5000 IU	8000 IU
Vitamin E (as *dl* -alpha tocopheryl acetate)	30 IU	30 IU	30 IU
Water-Soluble Vitamins			
Vitamin C (ascorbic acid)	500 mg	60 mg	60 mg
Vitamin B_1 (as thiamine mononitrate)	20 mg	1.5 mg	1.7 mg
Vitamin B_2 (riboflavin)	20 mg	1.7 mg	2 mg
Niacin (as niacinamide)	100 mg	20 mg	20 mg
Vitamin B_6 (as pyridoxine HCl)	25 mg	2 mg	2.5 mg
Biotin	0.15 mg	0.30 mg	0.30 mg
Pantothenic acid (as calcium pantothenate)	25 mg	10 mg	10 mg
Folic acid	0.8 mg	0.4 mg	0.8 mg
Vitamin B_{12} (cyanocobalamin)	50 mcg	6 mcg	8 mcg
Minerals			
Iron (as ferrous fumarate)	27 mg	18 mg	18 mg
Chromium (as chromium nitrate)	0.1 mg	0.05-0.2 mg*	
Magnesium (as magnesium oxide)	50 mg	400 mg	450 mg
Manganese (as manganese dioxide)	5 mg	2.5-5 mg*	
Copper (as cupric oxide)	3 mg	2 mg	2 mg
Zinc (as zinc oxide)	22.5 mg	15 mg	15 mg

* *Not established. Estimated by NAS/NRC as safe and adequate daily dietary intake for adults.*

DESCRIPTION

Vitamins, Multiple/Minerals is a prescription-only oral multivitamin/mineral tablet specifically formulated for prophylactic or therapeutic nutritional supplementation in physiologically stressful conditions.

Vitamins, Multiple/Minerals supplies: *therapeutic* levels of water-soluble Vitamins (ascorbic acid and all B-complex vitamins except biotin); *supplemental* levels of biotin, fat-soluble vitamins (A and E) and minerals (iron, chromium, manganese, copper and zinc); plus magnesium.

CLINICAL PHARMACOLOGY

Vitamins and minerals are essential for normal metabolic functions including hematopoiesis. The B-complex vitamins are necessary for the conversion of carbohydrate, protein and fat into tissue and energy. Ascorbic acid is involved in tissue repair and collagen formation. Vitamin A is necessary for proper functioning of the retina; it appears to be essential to the integrity of epithelial cells. Vitamin E is an antioxidant which preserves essential cellular constituents. Magnesium is a structural component of body tissues; iron, chromium, manganese, copper and zinc serve as catalysts in enzyme systems which perform vital cellular functions.

Water-soluble vitamins (B-complex and C) are not significantly stored by the body and must be replaced continually to maintain essential tissue levels; excess quantities are excreted in urine. These vitamins are rapidly depleted in conditions interfering with their intake or absorption. Vitamins, Multiple/Minerals supplies therapeutic levels of vitamin C and all B-complex vitamins (except biotin).

Fat-soluble vitamins and several trace minerals, however, can accumulate in the body and do not need replacement as frequently. Therefore, Vitamins, Multiple/Minerals supplies more conservative levels of vitamins A and E and various essential minerals.

Specifically, Vitamins, Multiple/Minerals contains an adequate level of vitamin B_6 (25 mg) to normalize the tryptophan metabolism disturbance which has been associated with the use of estrogenic oral contraceptives or other estrogen therapy. It provides zinc (22.5 mg) which facilitates wound healing, the level of folic acid (0.8 mg) recommended during pregnancy, and ascorbic acid (500 mg) which has been demonstrated to improve the absorption of inorganic iron.

INDICATIONS

Vitamins, Multiple/Minerals is indicated for prophylactic or therapeutic nutritional supplementation in physiologically stressful conditions. These include:

Conditions causing depletion, or reduced absorption or bioavailability of essential vitamins and minerals: Inadequate intake due to highly restricted or unbalanced diets such as those frequently associated with anorexic conditions and other states of severe malnutrition.

Gastrointestinal disorders, chronic alcoholism, chronic or acute infections (especially those involving febrile illness), prolonged or wasting disease, congestive heart failure, hyperthyroidism, poorly controlled diabetes or other physiologic stress.

Also, patients on estrogenic oral contraceptives or other estrogen therapy, antibacterials which affect intestinal microflora, or other interfering drugs.

Certain conditions resulting from severe B-vitamin or ascorbic acid deficiency: Cheilosis, gingivitis, stomatitis and certain other classic water-soluble vitamin deficiency syndromes.

Conditions resulting in increased needs for essential vitamins and minerals: Recovery from surgery or trauma involving severe burns, fractures or other extensive tissue damage.

Also, pregnant women and those with heavy menstrual bleeding.

CONTRAINDICATIONS

Vitamins, Multiple/Minerals is contraindicated in patients hypersensitive to any of its components.

WARNINGS

Not intended for treatment of pernicious anemia or other megaloblastic anemias where vitamin B_{12} is deficient. Neurologic involvement may develop or progress, despite temporary remission of anemia, in patients with vitamin B_{12} deficiency who receive supplemental folic acid and who are inadequately treated with B_{12}.

PRECAUTIONS

General: Certain conditions listed above may require additional nutritional supplementation. During pregnancy, for instance, supplementation with vitamin D and calcium may be required according to the dietary habits of the individual. Vitamins, Multiple/Minerals is not intended for treatment of severe specific deficiencies.

Information for the Patient: Because toxic reactions have been reported with injudicious use of certain vitamins and minerals, urge patients to follow your specific instructions regarding dosage regimen. Advise patients to keep Vitamins, Multiple/Minerals out of reach of children.

Drug and Treatment Interactions: As little as 5 mg pyridoxine daily can decrease the efficacy of levodopa in the treatment of parkinsonism. Therefore, Vitamins, Multiple/Minerals is not recommended for patients undergoing such therapy.

ADVERSE REACTIONS

Adverse reactions have been reported with specific vitamins and minerals, but generally at levels substantially higher than those in Vitamins, Multiple/Minerals. However, allergic and idiosyncratic reactions are possible at lower levels. Iron,

even at the usual recommended levels, has been associated with gastrointestinal intolerance in some patients.

DOSAGE AND ADMINISTRATION

Usual adult dosage; one tablet daily. Not recommended for children.

J CODES

J3500

HOW SUPPLIED
CAPSULE:

BRAND/MANUFACTURER	NDC	SIZE	AWP
○ BRAND			
▶ VICON FORTE: Whitby	50474-0316-22	60s	$19.96
	50474-0316-27	100s ud	$34.92
	50474-0316-24	500s	$157.51
○ GENERICS			
VG CAPSULES: Med Prod	00576-0506-30	30s	$5.93
MAGNA-C-7 FORTE: Rugby	00536-3910-08	60s	$4.65
SUPPORT 500: Marin	12539-0011-01	60s	$12.00
ZINCVIT: Kenwood	00482-0010-01	60s	$13.87
MAGNA-C-7 FORTE: Rugby	00536-3994-01	100s	$10.12
VITACON FORTE: Amide	52152-0078-02	100s	$10.90
VITACON FORTE: Moore,H.L.	00839-7508-06	100s	$11.00
THERACON FORTE: Goldline	00182-4555-01	100s	$12.25
VICA-FORTE: Qualitest	00603-6381-21	100s	$12.87
VITA FORTE: Jerome Stevens	50564-0542-01	100s	$15.48
CEZIN-S: Forest Pharm	00785-4811-01	100s	$22.57
ELDERCAPS: Mayrand	00259-1337-01	100s	$24.20
VITACON FORTE: Amide	52152-0078-04	500s	$43.75
VITA FORTE: Jerome Stevens	50564-0542-05	500s	$84.11

Vitamins, Prenatal

DESCRIPTION

One tablet daily provides:

Vitamins
A*	4,000 IU
D (cholecalciferol)	400 IU
E	11 mg
C (ascorbic acid)	120 mg
Folic acid	1 mg
B_1 (thiamin mononitrate)	1.84 mg
B_2 (riboflavin)	3 mg
Niacinamide	20 mg
B_6 (pyridoxine hydrochloride)	10 mg
B_{12} (cyanocobalamin)	12 mcg
Minerals	
Calcium (calcium sulfate)	200 mg
Copper (cupric oxide)	2 mg
Iron (ferrous fumarate)	65 mg
Zinc (zinc oxide)	25 mg

* *Input as vitamin A acetate and beta carotene.*

INDICATIONS AND USAGE

Vitamins/Prenatal is indicated to provide essential vitamin and mineral supplementation throughout pregnancy and during the postnatal period for both the lactating and nonlactating mother. It is also useful for improving nutritional status prior to conception.

Each tablet provides essential vitamins and minerals, including 65 mg of elemental iron and 200 mg of elemental calcium and 25 mg zinc. Vitamins/Prenatal also offers 1 mg folic acid to aid in the prevention of megaloblastic anemia.

WARNINGS

As with all medications, keep out of the reach of children. In case of accidental overdose, seek professional assistance or contact a poison control center immediately.

PRECAUTIONS

Folic acid may partially correct the hematological damage due to vitamin B_{12} deficiency of pernicious anemia, while the associated neurological damage progresses.

◆ RATED THERAPEUTICALLY EQUIVALENT; ◇ THERAPEUTIC EQUIVALENCE UNCONFIRMED; ○ UNRATED

DOSAGE AND ADMINISTRATION

Before, during and after pregnancy, one tablet daily, or as directed by a physician.
Store at room temperature; avoid excess heat.
Dispense in well-closed, light-resistant container.

HOW SUPPLIED
CAPSULE:

BRAND/MANUFACTURER	NDC	SIZE	AWP
◇ **GENERICS**			
NEO-FORTE: Advanced Nutr	10888-1700-01	30s	$9.43
NEO-FORTE: Advanced Nutr	10888-1700-03	60s	$13.80

For additional alternatives, turn to the section beginning on page 2859.

Vitrax *SEE* SODIUM HYALURONATE

Vivactil *SEE* PROTRIPTYLINE HYDROCHLORIDE

Volmax *SEE* ALBUTEROL

Voltaren *SEE* DICLOFENAC, OPHTHALMIC *AND* DICLOFENAC, ORAL

Vōsol *SEE* ACETIC ACID, OTIC

Vōsol HC *SEE* ACETIC ACID WITH HYDROCORTISONE, OTIC

Vumon *SEE* TENIPOSIDE

Vynatal F.A. *SEE* VITAMINS, PRENATAL

Vytone *SEE* HYDROCORTISONE WITH IODOQUINOL

Warfarin Sodium

DESCRIPTION

Warfarin Sodium, a vitamin K dependent factor anticoagulant, is chemically crystalline sodium warfarin isopropanol clathrate. The crystallization of Warfarin Sodium virtually eliminates trace impurities present in amorphous Warfarin Sodium, thus achieving a crystalline product of the highest purity. Warfarin is the coined generic name for 3-(α-acetonylbenzyl)-4-hydroxycoumarin. Its empirical formula is $C_{19}H_{15}NaO_4$ and its structural formula may be represented by the following:

Crystalline Warfarin Sodium occurs as a white, odorless, crystalline powder, is discolored by light and is very soluble in water; freely soluble in alcohol; very slightly soluble in chloroform and in ether.

Following is its chemical structure:

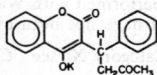

CLINICAL PHARMACOLOGY

Warfarin Sodium and other coumarin anticoagulants act by inhibiting the synthesis of vitamin K dependent coagulation factors. The resultant *in vivo* effect is a sequential depression of Factors VII, IX, X and II Activities. The degree of depression is dependent upon the dosage administered. Anticoagulants have no direct effect on an established thrombus, nor do they reverse ischemic tissue damage. However, once a thrombus has occurred, the goal of anticoagulant treatment is to prevent further extension of the formed clot and prevents secondary thromboembolic complications which may result in serious and possibly fatal sequelae.

After oral administration of Warfarin Sodium, absorption is essentially complete, and maximal plasma concentrations are reached in 1 to 9 hours. Approximately 97% is bound to albumin within the plasma. An anticoagulation effect generally occurs within 24 hours. However, peak anticoagulant effect may be delayed 72 to 96 hours and its duration of action may persist for 4 to 5 days, thus producing a smooth, long lasting response curve. Warfarin Sodium is metabolized by hepatic microsomal enzymes to inactive metabolites that are excreted into the bile, reabsorbed and excreted into the urine. Warfarin Sodium is a potent drug with a half-life of 2 ½ days; therefore its effects may become more pronounced as daily maintenance doses overlap.

INDICATIONS AND USAGE

Warfarin Sodium is indicated for the prophylaxis and/or treatment of venous thrombosis and its extension, pulmonary embolism.

Warfarin Sodium is also indicated for the prophylaxis and/or treatment of the thromboembolic complications associated with atrial fibrillation, cardiac valve replacement, and as an adjunct in the prophylaxis of systemic embolism after myocardial infarction.

UNLABELED USES

Warfarin Sodium is used as an adjunct in the treatment of small cell lung carcinoma, to reduce the risk of thrombosis, and glomerulonephritis. It is also used in protein C deficiency, to prevent thromboembolism associated with prosthetic mechanical heart valve replacement, and advancing arterial atherosclerosis.

CONTRAINDICATIONS

Anticoagulation is contraindicated in any localized or general physical condition or personal circumstance in which the hazard of hemorrhage might be greater than the potential clinical benefits of anticoagulation, such as:

Pregnancy: Warfarin Sodium is contraindicated in women who are or may become pregnant because the drug passes through the placental barrier and may cause fatal hemorrhage to the fetus in utero. Furthermore, there have been reports of birth malformations in children born to mothers who have been treated with warfarin during pregnancy.

Embryopathy characterized by nasal hypoplasia with or without stippled epiphyses (chondrodysplasia punctata) has been reported in pregnant women exposed to warfarin during the first trimester. Central nervous system abnormalities also have been reported, including dorsal midline dysplasia characterized by agenesis of the corpus callosum, Dandy-Walker malformation, and midline cerebellar atrophy. Ventral midline dysplasia, characterized by optic atrophy, and eye abnormalities have been observed. Mental retardation, blindness, and other central nervous system abnormalities have been reported in association with second and third trimester exposure. Although rare, teratogenic reports following in utero exposure to Warfarin include urinary tract anomalies such as single kidney, asplenia, anencephaly, spina bifida, cranial nerve palsy, hydrocephalus, cardiac defects and congenital heart disease, polydactyly, deformities of toes, diaphragmatic hernia, and corneal leukoma.

Spontaneous abortion and still birth are known to occur and a higher risk of fetal mortality is associated with the use of warfarin.

Women of childbearing potential who are candidates for anticoagulant therapy should be carefully evaluated and the indications critically reviewed with the patient. If the patient becomes pregnant while taking this drug, she should be apprised of the potential risks to the fetus, and the possibility of termination of the pregnancy should be discussed in light of those risks.

HEMORRHAGIC TENDENCIES OR BLOOD DYSCRASIAS

Recent or contemplated surgery of: (1) central nervous system; (2) eye; (3) traumatic surgery resulting in large open surfaces.

Bleeding tendencies associated with active ulceration or overt bleeding of: (1) gastrointestinal, genitourinary or respiratory tracts; (2) cerebrovascular hemorrhage; (3) aneurysms-cerebral, dissecting aorta; (4) pericarditis and pericardial effusions; (5) bacterial endocarditis.

Threatened abortion: eclampsia and preeclampsia.

Inadequate laboratory facilities: or unsupervised senility, alcoholism, psychosis; or lack of patient cooperation.

Spinal puncture: and other diagnostic or therapeutic procedures with potential for uncontrollable bleeding.

Miscellaneous: major regional, lumbar block anesthesia and malignant hypertension.

WARNINGS

The most serious risks associated with anticoagulant therapy with sodium warfarin are hemorrhage in any tissue or organ and, less frequently, necrosis and/or gangrene of skin and other tissues. The risk of hemorrhage is related to the level of intensity and the duration of anticoagulant therapy. Hemorrhage and necrosis have in some cases been reported to result in death or permanent disability. Necrosis appears to be associated with local thrombosis and usually appears within a few days of the start of anticoagulant therapy. In severe cases of necrosis, treatment through debridement or amputation of the affected tissue, limb, breast or penis has been reported. Careful diagnosis is required to determine whether necrosis is caused by an underlying disease. Warfarin therapy should be discontinued when warfarin is suspected to be the cause of developing necrosis and heparin therapy may be considered for anticoagulation. Although various treatments have been attempted, no treatment for necrosis has been considered uniformly effective. See below for information on predisposing conditions. These and other risks associated with anticoagulant therapy must be weighed against the risk of thrombosis or embolization in untreated cases.

It cannot be emphasized too strongly that treatment of each patient is a highly individualized matter. Dosage should be controlled by periodic determinations of prothrombin time (PT) or other suitable coagulation tests. Determinations of whole blood clotting and bleeding times are not effective measures for control of therapy. Heparin prolongs the one-stage PT. When heparin and Warfarin Sodium are administered concomitantly, refer below to *"Conversion From Heparin Therapy"* for recommendations.

Caution should be observed when Warfarin Sodium is administered in any situation or in the presence of any predisposing condition where added risk of hemorrhage or necrosis is present.

Anticoagulation therapy with Warfarin Sodium may enhance the release of atheromatous plaque emboli, thereby increasing the risk of complications from systemic cholesterol microembolization, including the "purple toes syndrome." Discontinuation of Warfarin Sodium therapy is recommended when such phenomena are observed.

Systemic atheroemboli and cholesterol microemboli can present with a variety of signs and symptoms including purple toes syndrome, livedo reticularis, rash, gangrene, abrupt and intense pain in the leg, foot, or toes, foot ulcers, myalgia, penile gangrene, abdominal pain, flank or back pain, hematuria, renal insufficiency, hypertension, cerebral ischemia, spinal cord infarction, pancreatitis, symptoms simulating polyarteritis, or any other sequelae of vascular compromise due to embolic occlusion. The most commonly involved visceral organs are the kidneys followed by the pancreas, spleen, and liver. Some cases have progressed to necrosis or death.

Purple toes syndrome is a complication of oral anticoagulation characterized by a dark, purplish or mottled color of the toes, usually occurring between 3-10 weeks, or later, after the initiation of therapy with warfarin or related compounds. Major features of this syndrome include purple color of plantar surfaces and sides of the toes that blanches on moderate pressure and fades with elevation of the legs; pain and tenderness of the toes; waxing and waning of the color over time. While the purple toes syndrome is reported to be reversible, some cases progress to gangrene or necrosis which may require debridement of the affected area, or may lead to amputation.

The decision to administer anticoagulants in the following conditions must be based upon clinical judgment in which the risks of anticoagulant therapy are weighed against the benefits:

Lactation: Warfarin Sodium appears in the milk of nursing mothers in an inactive form. Infants nursed by Warfarin Sodium treated mothers had no change in prothrombin times (PTs). Effects in premature infants have not been evaluated.

Severe to moderate hepatic or renal insufficiency.

Infectious diseases or disturbances of intestinal flora: sprue, antibiotic therapy.

Trauma which may result in internal bleeding.

Surgery or trauma resulting in large exposed raw surfaces.

Indwelling catheters.

Severe to moderate hypertension.

Known or suspected deficiency in protein C: This hereditary or acquired condition, which should be suspected if there is a history of recurrent episodes of thromboembolic disorders in the patient or in the family, has been associated with an increased risk of developing necrosis following warfarin administration. Tissue necrosis may occur in the absence of protein C deficiency. It has been reported that concurrent anticoagulation therapy with heparin for 5 to 7 days during initiation of therapy with Warfarin Sodium may minimize the incidence of this reaction. Warfarin therapy should be discontinued when warfarin is suspected to be the cause of developing necrosis and heparin therapy may be considered for anticoagulation.

Miscellaneous: polycythemia vera, vasculitis, severe diabetes, severe allergic and anaphylactic disorders.

Patients with congestive heart failure may become more sensitive to Warfarin Sodium, thereby requiring more frequent laboratory monitoring, and reduced doses of Warfarin Sodium. Concurrent use of anticoagulants with streptokinase or urokinase is not recommended and may be hazardous. (Please note recommendations accompanying these preparations.)

PRECAUTIONS
Periodic determination of PT or other suitable coagulation test is essential.
Numerous factors, alone or in combination, including travel, changes in diet, environment, physical state and medication may influence response of the patient to anticoagulants. It is generally good practice to monitor the patient's response with additional PT determinations in the period immediately after discharge from the hospital, and whenever other medications are initiated, discontinued or taken haphazardly. The following factors are listed for reference; however, other factors may also affect the anticoagulant response.

THE FOLLOWING FACTORS, ALONE OR IN COMBINATION, MAY BE RESPONSIBLE FOR *INCREASED* PT RESPONSE.
Endogenous Factors: cancer, collagen disease, congestive heart failure, diarrhea, elevated temperature, hepatic disorders, infectious hepatitis, jaundice, hyperthyroidism, poor nutritional state, steatorrhea, vitamin K deficiency

Exogenous Factors: acetaminophen, alcohol[†], allopurinol, aminosalicylic acid, amidarone HCl, anabolic steroids, anesthetics, inhalation, antibiotics, bromelains, chenodiol, chloral hydrate[†], chlorpropamide, chymotrypsin, cimetidine, clofibrate, Warfarin Sodium overdosage, dextran, dextrothyroxine, diazoxide, diflunisal, diuretics[†], disulfiram, ethacrynic acid, fenoprofen, fluoroquinolone antibiotics, glucagon, hepatotoxic drugs, ibuprofen, indomethacin, influenza virus vaccine, lovastatin, mefenamic acid, methyldopa, methylphenidate, metronidazole, miconazole, monoamine oxidase inhibitors, moricizine hydrochloride[†], nalidixic acid, naproxen, narcotics, prolonged, pentoxifylline, phenylbutazone, phenytoin, propafenone, pyrazolones, quinidine, quinine, rantidine[†], salicylates, sulfinpyrazone, sulfonamides, long acting, sulindac, tamoxifen, thyroid drugs, tolbutamide, trimethoprim/sulfamethoxazole
also: other medications affecting blood elements which may modify hemostasis; dietary deficiencies, prolonged hot weather, unreliable PT determinations

THE FOLLOWING FACTORS, ALONE OR IN COMBINATION, MAY BE RESPONSIBLE FOR *DECREASED* PT RESPONSE
Endogenous Factors: edema, hereditary coumarin resistance, hyperlipemia, hypothyroidism

Exogenous Factors: adrenocortical steroids, alcohol[†], aminoglutethimide, antacids, antihistamines, barbiturates, carbamazepine, chloral hydrate[†], chloridiazepoxide, cholestyramine, Warfarin Sodium underdosage, diuretics[†], ethclorvynol, glutethimide, griseofluvin, haloperidol, meprobamate, moricizine hydrochloride[†], nafcillin, oral contraceptoves, paraldehyde, primidone, ranitidine[†], rifampin, sucralfate, trazodone, vitamin C
also: diet high in vitamin K, unreliable PT determinations

Because a patient may be exposed to a combination of the above factors, the net effect of Warfarin Sodium on PT response may be unpredictable. More frequent PT monitoring is therefore advisable. Medications of unknown interaction with coumarins are best regarded with caution. When these medications are started or stopped, more frequent PT monitoring is advisable.

Coumarins may also affect the action of other drugs. Hypoglycemic agents (chlorpropamide and tolbutamide) and anticonvulsants (phenytoin and phenobarbital) may accumulate in the body as a result of interference with either their metabolism or excretion.

It has been reported that concomitant administration of warfarin and ticlopidine may be associated with cholestatic hepatitis.

Special Risk Patients: Caution should be observed when Warfarin Sodium is administered to certain patients such as the elderly or debilitated or when administered in any situation or physical condition where added risk of hemorrhage is present.

Intramuscular (I.M.) injections of concomitant medications should be confined to the upper extremities which permits easy access for manual compression, inspections for bleeding and use of pressure bandages.

Caution should be observed when Warfarin Sodium is administered concomitantly with nonsteroidal anti-inflammatory drugs (NSAIDs), including aspirin, to be certain that no change in anticoagulation dosage is required. In addition to specific drug interactions that might affect PT, NSAIDs, including aspirin, can inhibit platelet aggregation, and can cause gastrointestinal bleeding, peptic ulceration and/or perforation.

Information for Patients: The objective of anticoagulant therapy is to control the coagulation mechanism so that thrombosis is prevented, while avoiding spontaneous bleeding. Effective therapeutic levels with minimal complications are in part dependent upon cooperative and well-instructed patients who communicate effectively with their physician. Various Warfarin Sodium patient educational guides are available to physicians on request.

Patients should be advised: Strict adherence to prescribed dosage schedule is necessary. Do not take or discontinue any other medication, except on advice of physician. Avoid alcohol, salicylates (e.g., aspirin and topical analgesics), large amounts of green leafy vegetables and/or drastic changes in dietary habits, because they may affect Warfarin Sodium therapy. Warfarin Sodium may cause a red-orange discoloration of alkaline urine. The patient should notify the physician if any illness, such as diarrhea, infection or fever develops or if any unusual symptoms, such as pain, swelling or discomfort appear or if prolonged bleeding from cuts, increased menstrual flow or vaginal bleeding, nosebleeds or bleeding of gums from brushing, unusual bleeding or bruising, red or dark brown urine, red or tar black stools or diarrhea occurs.

Carcinogenesis, Mutagenesis, Impairment of Fertility: Carcinogenicity and mutagenicity studies have not been performed with Warfarin Sodium. The reproductive effects of Warfarin Sodium have not been evaluated.

Use in Pregnancy: Pregnancy Category X: see *"Contraindications".*

Pediatric Use: Safety and effectiveness in children below the age of 18 have not been established.

[†] Increased and decreased PT responses have been reported.

ADVERSE REACTIONS

Potential adverse reactions to Warfarin Sodium may include:

■ Hemorrhage from any tissue or organ. This is a consequence of the anticoagulant effect. The signs and symptoms will vary according to the location and degree or extent of the bleeding. Hemorrhagic complications may present as paralysis; headache, chest, abdomen, joint or other pain; shortness of breath, difficult breathing or swallowing; unexplained swelling; or unexplained shock. Therefore, the possibility of hemorrhage should be considered in evaluating the condition of any anticoagulated patient with complaints which do not indicate an obvious diagnosis. Bleeding during anticoagulant therapy does not always correlate with prothrombin activity. (See *"Overdosage-Treatment"*.)

■ Bleeding which occurs when the PT is within the therapeutic range warrants diagnostic investigation since it may unmask a previously unsuspected lesion, e.g., tumor, ulcer, etc.

■ Necrosis of skin and other tissues, (See *"Warnings"*.)

■ Other adverse reactions are infrequent and consist of alopecia, urticaria, dermatitis, fever, nausea, diarrhea, abdominal cramping, systemic cholesterol microembolization, purple toes syndrome, cholestatic hepatic injury, and hypersensitivity reactions.

■ Priapism has been associated with anticoagulant administration, however, a causal relationship has not been established.

OVERDOSAGE

Signs and Symptoms: Suspected or overt abnormal bleeding (e.g., appearance of blood in stools or urine, hematuria, excessive menstrual bleeding, melena, petechiae, excessive bruising or persistent oozing from superficial injuries) are early manifestations of anticoagulation beyond a safe and satisfactory level.

Treatment: Excessive anticoagulation, with or without bleeding, may be controlled by discontinuing Warfarin Sodium therapy and if necessary, by administration of oral or parenteral vitamin K_1. (Please see recommendations accompanying vitamin K_1 preparations prior to use.)

Such use of vitamin K_1 reduces response to subsequent Warfarin Sodium therapy. Patients may return to a pretreatment thrombotic status following the rapid reversal of a prolonged PT. Resumption of Warfarin Sodium administration reverses the effect of vitamin K, and a therapeutic PT can again be obtained by careful dosage adjustment. If rapid anticoagulation is indicated, heparin may be preferable for initial therapy.

If minor bleeding progresses to major bleeding, give 5 to 25 mg (rarely up to 50 mg) parenteral vitamin K_1. In emergency situations of severe hemorrhage, clotting factors can be returned to normal by administering 200 to 500 mL of fresh whole blood or fresh frozen plasma, or by giving commercial Factor IX complex.

A risk of hepatitis and other viral diseases is associated with the use of these blood products; Factor IX complex is also associated with an increased risk of thrombosis. Therefore, these preparations should be used only in exceptional or life-threatening bleeding episodes secondary to Warfarin Sodium overdosage.

Purified Factor IX preparations should not be used because they cannot increase the levels of prothrombin, Factor VII and Factor X which are also depressed along with the levels of Factor IX as a result of Warfarin Sodium treatment. Packed red blood cells may also be given if significant blood loss has occurred. Infusions of blood or plasma should be monitored carefully to avoid precipitating pulmonary edema in elderly patients or patients with heart disease.

DOSAGE AND LABORATORY CONTROL

ADMINISTRATION

The dosage and administration of Warfarin Sodium must be individualized for each patient according to the particular patient's sensitivity to the drug. The dosage should be adjusted based upon the results of the one-stage PT. Different thromboplastin reagents vary substantially in their responsiveness to sodium warfarin-induced effects on PT. To define the appropriate therapeutic regimen it is important to be familiar with the sensitivity of the thromboplastin reagent used in the laboratory and its relationship to the International Reference Preparation (IRP)*, a sensitive thromboplastin reagent prepared from human brain.

Early clinical studies of oral anticoagulants, which formed the basis for recommended therapeutic ranges of 1.5 to 2.5 times control PT, used sensitive human brain thromboplastin. When using the less sensitive rabbit brain thromboplastins commonly employed in PT assays today, adjustments must be made to the targeted PT range that reflect this decrease in sensitivity.

Available clinical evidence indicates that an INR of 2.0-3.0 (e.g., PT ratio of 1.2-1.5 when measuring with the less sensitive thromboplastin reagents, ISI = 2.8 [Table 1]) is sufficient for prophylaxis and treatment of venous thromboembolism and minimizes the risk of hemorrhage associated with higher INRs. Five recent clinical trials 1-5 evaluated the effects of warfarin in patients with non-valvular atrial fibrillation (AF). Meta-analysis findings of these studies revealed that the effects of warfarin in reducing thromboembolic events including stroke were similar at either moderately high: INR (2.0-4.5) or low INR (1.4-3.0). There was a significant reduction in minor bleeds at the low INR. Similar data from clinical studies in valvular atrial fibrillation patients are not available. The trials in non-valvular atrial fibrillation support The American College of Chest Physicians' (ACCP) recommendation[6] that an INR of 2.0-3.0 be used for long term warfarin therapy in appropriate AF patients. In cases were the risk of thromboembolism is great, such as in patients with recurrent systemic embolism, a higher INR may be required. A PT ratio of greater than 2.0 appears to provide no additional therapeutic benefit in most patients and is associated with a higher risk of bleeding.

In patients with mechanical heart valves(s), long term prophylaxis with warfarin to an INR of 2.5-3.5 is recommended.[7] In patients with bioprosthetic heart valves(s), based on limited data,[8] the American College of Chest Physicians recommend warfarin therapy to an INR of 2.0-3.0 for 12 weeks after valve insertion. In patients with additional risk factors such as atrial fibrillation or prior thromboembolism, consideration should be given for longer term therapy.[7] The proceedings and recommendations of the 1986 National Conference on Antithrombotic Therapy[9-11] review and evaluate issues related to oral anticoagulant therapy and the sensitivity of thromboplastin reagents and provide additional guidelines for defining the appropriate therapeutic regimen.

The conversion of the INR to PT ratios for the less-intense (INR 2.0-3.0) and more intense (INR 2.5-3.5) therapeutic range recommended by the ACCP for thromboplastins over a range of ISI values is shown in Table 1.[12]

Table 1

RELATIONSHIP BETWEEN INR AND PT RATIOS FOR THROMBOPLASTINS WITH DIFFERENT ISI VALUES* (SENSITIVITIES)

	PT RATIOS				
	ISI 1.0	ISI 1.4	ISI 1.8	ISI 2.3	ISI 2.8
INR = 2.0-3.0	2.0-3.0	1.6-2.2	1.5-1.8	1.4-1.6	1.3-1.5
INR = 2.5-3.5	2.5-3.5	1.9-2.4	1.7-2.0	1.5-1.7	1.4-1.6

A system of standardizing the PT in oral anticoagulant control was introduced by the World Health Organization in 1983. It is based upon the determination of an International Normalized Ratio (INR) which provides a common basis for communication of PT results and interpretations of therapeutic ranges. The INR is derived from calibrations of commercial thromboplastin reagents against a sensitive human brain thromboplastin, the IRP. For the three commercial rabbit brain thromboplastins currently used in North America, a PT ratio of 1.3 to 2.0 is equivalent to an INR of 2.0 to 4.0. For other thromboplastins, the INR can be calculated as:

$$INR = (observed\ PT\ ratio)^{ISI}$$

where the ISI (International Sensitivity Index) is the calibration factor and is available from the manufacturers of the thromboplastin reagent.[13]

Initial Dosage: The dosing of Warfarin Sodium must be individualized according to patient's sensitivity to the drug as indicated by the INR and/or PT ratio. Use of a large loading dose may increase the incidence of hemorrhagic and other complications, does not offer more rapid protection against thrombi formation, and is not recommended. Low initiation doses are recommended for elderly and/or debilitated patients and patients with increased sensitivity to Warfarin Sodium (see *"Precautions"*). It is recommended that Warfarin Sodium therapy be initiated with a dose of 2 to 5 mg per day with dosage adjustments based on the results of INR and/or PT ratio determinations.

Maintenance: Most patients are satisfactorily maintained at a dose of 2 to 10 mg daily. Flexibility of dosage is provided by breaking scored tablets in half. The individual dose and interval should be gauged by the patient's prothrombin response.

Duration of Therapy: The duration of therapy in each patient should be individualized. In general, anticoagulant therapy should be continued until the danger of thrombosis and embolism has passed.

LABORATORY CONTROL

The PT reflects the depression of vitamin K dependent Factors VII, IX, X and II. There are several modifications of the one-stage PT and the physician should become familiar with the specific method used in his laboratory. The degree of anticoagulation indicated by any range of PTs may be altered by the type of thromboplastin used; the appropriate therapeutic range must be based on the experience of each laboratory. The PT should be determined daily after the administration of the initial dose until PT results stabilize in the therapeutic range. Intervals between subsequent PT determinations should be based upon the physician's judgment of the patient's reliability and response to Warfarin Sodium in order to maintain the individual within the therapeutic range. Acceptable intervals for PT determinations are normally within the range of one to four weeks after a stable dosage has been determined. To ensure adequate control, it is recommended that additional PT tests are done when other warfarin products are interchanged with Warfarin Sodium and also if other medications are coadministered with Warfarin Sodium (see *"Precautions"*).

TREATMENT DURING DENTISTRY AND SURGERY

The management of patients who undergo dental and surgical procedures requires close liaison between attending physicians, surgeons and dentists. In patients who must be anticoagulated prior to, during, or immediately following dental or surgical procedures, adjusting the dosage of Warfarin Sodium to maintain the PT at the low end of the therapeutic range may safely allow for continued anticoagulation. The operative site should be sufficiently limited and accessible to permit the effective use of local procedures for hemostasis. Under these conditions, dental and surgical procedures may be performed without undue risk of hemorrhage.

CONVERSION FROM HEPARIN THERAPY

Since the onset of the Warfarin Sodium effect is delayed, heparin is preferred initially for rapid anticoagulation. Conversion to Warfarin Sodium may begin concomitantly with heparin therapy or may be delayed 3 to 6 days. As heparin may affect the PT, patients receiving both heparin and Warfarin Sodium should have blood for PT determination drawn at least.

- 5 hours after the lase IV bolus dose of heparin, or
- 4 hours after cessation of a continuous IV infusion of heparin, or
- 24 hours after the last subcutaneous heparin injection.

When Warfarin Sodium has produced the desired therapeutic range or prothrombin activity, heparin may be discontinued.

STORAGE

Protect from light. Store in carton until contents have been used. Store at controlled room temperature (59°-86°F, 15°-30°C). Dispense in a tight, light-resistant container as defined in the U.S.P.

REFERENCES

1. Petersen, P., et.al.: Placebo Controlled, Randomized Trial of Warfarin and Aspirin for Prevention of Thromboembolic Complications in Chronic Atrial Fibrillation: The Copenhagen AFASAK Study, Lancet. 1989:1:175-9.   2. Stroke Prevention in Atrial Fibrillation Investigators. Stroke Prevention in Atrial Fibrillation Study Final Results Circulation. 1991:84-527-539.   3. Boston Area Anticoagulation Trial for Atrial Fibrillation Investigators. The Effect of Low-Dose Warfarin on the Risk of Stroke in Patients with Nonrheumatic Atrial Fibrillation. N Engl J Med. 1990;323:1505-1511.   4. Connolly, S.J. et.al.: Canadian Atrial Fibrillation Anticoagulation (CAFA) study, JACC. 1991;18:349-355.   5. Ezekowitz, M.D. et.al.: Warfarin in the Prevention of Stroke Associated with Nonrheumatic Atrial Fibrillation. N Engl J Med. 1992;327:1406-1412.   6. Laupacis, A., M.D. et.al.: Antithrombotic Therapy in Atrial Fibrillation. Chest. 102,4 Oct. 1992 suppl. 426s-433s.   7. Stein PD, Alpert JS, Copeland J, Dalen JE, Goldman S, Turpie AGG.: Antithrombotic Therapy in Patients with Mechanical and Biological Prosthetic Heart Valves. Chest. 1992;102 (Suppl.): 445s-455s.   8. Turpie AGG, Gunstensen J, Hirsh J, Nelson H, Gent M.: Randomized Comparison of Two Intensities of Oral Anticoagulant Therapy After Tissue Heart Valve Replacement. Lancet. 1988; (8597): 1242-1245.   9. Sackett, D.L.: Rules of Evidence and Clinical Recommendations on the Use of Antithrombotic Agents. Chest ACCP-NHLBI National Conference on Antithrombotic Therapy, Vol. 89, No. 2, pp. 2s-3s, 1986.   10. Hirst, J., Deykin, D., Poller, L.: "Therapeutical Range" for Oral Anticoagulant Therapy. Chest ACCP-NHLBI National Conference on Antithrombotic Therapy, Vol. 89, No. 2, pp. 11s-15s, 1986.   11. Hirsh, J.: Is the Dose of Warfarin Prescribed by American Physicians Unnecessarily High? Arch IntMed, Vol. 147, pp. 769-771, 1987.   12. Hirsh, J., M.D., F.C.C.P.: Hamilton Civic Hospitals Research Center, Hamilton, Ontario, Personal Communication.   13. Potter, L.: Laboratory Control of Anticoagulant Therapy, Seminars in Thrombosis and Hemostasis, Vol. 12, No. 1, pp. 13-19, 1986.

J CODES

Up to 50 mg—J0840

HOW SUPPLIED

TABLETS: 1 MG

AVERAGE UNIT PRICE (AVAILABLE SIZES)			
BRAND	$0.50		

BRAND/MANUFACTURER	NDC	SIZE	AWP
◆ BRAND			
➤ COUMADIN: Du Pont Pharma	00056-0169-70	100s	$50.22
	00056-0169-90	1000s	$502.20

TABLETS: 2 MG

AVERAGE UNIT PRICE (AVAILABLE SIZES)			
BRAND	$0.53		

BRAND/MANUFACTURER	NDC	SIZE	AWP
◆ BRAND			
➤ COUMADIN: Du Pont Pharma	00056-0170-70	100s	$52.50
	00056-0170-90	1000s	$525.00

TABLETS: 2.5 MG

AVERAGE UNIT PRICE (AVAILABLE SIZES)			
BRAND	$0.54		

BRAND/MANUFACTURER	NDC	SIZE	AWP
◆ BRAND			
➤ COUMADIN: Du Pont Pharma	00056-0176-70	100s	$54.00
	00056-0176-90	1000s	$540.00

TABLETS: 4 MG

BRAND/MANUFACTURER	NDC	SIZE	AWP
○ BRAND			
COUMADIN: Du Pont Pharma	00056-0168-70	100s	$54.42
	00056-0168-90	1000s	$544.20

TABLETS: 5 MG

AVERAGE UNIT PRICE (AVAILABLE SIZES)			
BRAND	$0.55		

BRAND/MANUFACTURER	NDC	SIZE	AWP
◆ BRAND			
COUMADIN: Du Pont Pharma	00056-0172-70	100s	$54.78
	00056-0172-90	1000s	$547.80

TABLETS: 7.5 MG

BRAND/MANUFACTURER	NDC	SIZE	AWP
◇ BRAND			
➤ COUMADIN: Du Pont Pharma	00056-0173-70	100s	$82.74

TABLETS: 10 MG

BRAND/MANUFACTURER	NDC	SIZE	AWP
◇ BRAND			
➤ COUMADIN: Du Pont Pharma	00056-0174-70	100s	$85.20

Wellbutrin *SEE* BUPROPION HYDROCHLORIDE

Westcort *SEE* HYDROCORTISONE, TOPICAL

Whole Cell DTP Vaccine *SEE* DIPHTHERIA/PERTUSSIS/TETANUS

Wigraine *SEE* ERGOTAMINE TARTRATE WITH CAFFEINE

Winstrol *SEE* STANOZOLOL

Wyamine Sulfate Injection *SEE* MEPHENTERMINE SULFATE

Wycillin *SEE* PENICILLIN G PROCAINE

Wydase *SEE* HYALURONIDASE

Wygesic *SEE* ACETAMINOPHEN AND PROPOXYPHENE HYDROCHLORIDE

Wytensin *SEE* GUANABENZ ACETATE

Xanax *SEE* ALPRAZOLAM

Xerac AC *SEE* ALUMINUM CHLORIDE (HEXAHYDRATE)

Xylocaine *SEE* LIDOCAINE HYDROCHLORIDE, INJECTABLE, LIDOCAINE HYDROCHLORIDE, LOCAL ANESTHESIA *AND* LIDOCAINE, TOPICAL

Yellow Fever Vaccine

DESCRIPTION

Yellow Fever Vaccine is prepared by culturing the 17D strain of yellow fever virus in living avian leukosis virus-free (ALV-free) chicken embryos for subcutaneous use. The vaccine, containing sorbitol and gelatin as a stabilizer, is lyophilized, and hermetically sealed under nitrogen. No preservative is added. The vaccine must be reconstituted immediately before use with the sterile diluent provided (Sodium Chloride Injection USP - contains no preservative). Yellow fever Vaccine is formulated to contain not less than 5.04 Log$_{10}$ Plaque Forming Units (PFU) per 0.5 ml dose. The vaccine appears slightly opalescent and light orange in color after reconstitution.

Yellow Fever Vaccine complies with official potency tests and other requirements of the U.S. Food and Drug Administration and the World Health Organization.

◆ RATED THERAPEUTICALLY EQUIVALENT; ◇ THERAPEUTIC EQUIVALENCE UNCONFIRMED; ○ UNRATED

CLINICAL PHARMACOLOGY

A clinical study to evaluate the serological responses and adverse reactions of Connaught's Yellow Fever Vaccine was performed on healthy young adults. One group of six received Yellow Fever Vaccine non-ALV-free (manufactured by Connaught Laboratories, Inc.) and another group of 18 received an immunization with Yellow Fever Vaccine. Immunizations were administered according to current recommendations.

Immunologic protection was measured utilizing a serum neutralizing antibody assay. No neutralizing antibody was detected prior to immunization. Both groups demonstrated a 100% conversion in the post-immunization sera. The incidence and severity of adverse reactions in each group were comparable.[1] However, as with any vaccine, vaccination with Yellow Fever Vaccine may not protect 100% of susceptible individuals.

INDICATIONS AND USAGE

Yellow Fever Vaccine is indicated for active immunization of all travelers planning a trip to countries which require a certificate of vaccination against Yellow Fever. Children six months of age or older require vaccination; children under six months of age should not be vaccinated *unless* they live in or are traveling to a high-risk area.[2] United States vaccination certificates are valid for a period of 10 years commencing 10 days after initial vaccination or revaccination.[3]

CONTRAINDICATIONS

Proven sensitivity to egg or chicken embryo protein is usually a contraindication; (see *"Precautions"*) for sensitivity testing. Pregnant women and children under six months of age should not be vaccinated, except in high-risk areas.[2]

WARNINGS

Yellow Fever Vaccine virus infection might be potentiated by severe underlying diseases, such as leukemia, lymphoma, or generalized malignancy, and by lowered resistance, such as from therapy with steroids, alkylating drugs, antimetabolites, cytotoxic agents, radiation, or from gamma globulin abnormalities. Administration of a live virus vaccine in such conditions should be evaluated on an individual basis.

The clinical judgment of the responsible physician should prevail.

PRECAUTIONS

GENERAL

Epinephrine Injection (1:1000) always must be immediately available to combat unexpected anaphylactic or other allergic reactions.

Usually, Yellow Fever Vaccine should be administered at least one month apart from other live-virus vaccines. However, field observations and clinical data indicate that simultaneous administration of the most widely used live-virus vaccines have not resulted in impaired antibody response on increased adverse reactions.[4] Thus, if time is a critical factor for required vaccinations, the clinical judgment of the responsible physician should prevail.

A recently completed prospective study of persons given Yellow Fever Vaccine and 5cc of commercially available immune globulin revealed no alteration of the immunologic response to Yellow Fever Vaccine when compared to controls.[2,5,6]

Vaccination with Yellow Fever Vaccine should be deferred for 8 weeks following blood or plasma transfusion.

A separate sterile syringe and needle should be used for each individual patient to prevent transmission of hepatitis or other infectious agents from one person to another.

HYPERSENSITIVITY TESTING

Since the Yellow Fever virus is propagated in chicken embryos, it should not be administered to an individual with a history of hypersensitivity to egg or chicken protein. Intradermal skin tests with the vaccine and sterile normal saline to serve as a control must be performed on all such individuals. The volar surface of the forearm is recommended. The volume injected is usually 0.02—0.03 ml. A noticeable intradermal wheal should be raised at each test site. A positive test consists of an urticardial wheal, with or without pseudopods, usually surrounded by an area of erythema and no response to the control. A positive test is an absolute contraindication to the administration of Yellow fever Vaccine. A tourniquet and a hypodermic syringe with needle containing Ephrinephrine Injection (1:1000) should be at hand while performing a sensitivity test.

An intracutaneous dose of 0.02 ml administered for hypersensitivity testing maybe sufficient to induce immunity. However, in such cases, the presence of specific protective antibodies must be confirmed through elevation of serum obtained approximately 4 weeks after skin testing. It is recommended that the state of public health laboratory be contacted for assistance.

PREGNANCY

Reproductive Studies—Pregnancy Category C: Animal reproduction studies have not been conducted with Yellow Fever Vaccine. It is also not known whether Yellow Fever Vaccine can cause fetal harm when administered to a pregnant woman or can affect reproduction capacity.[7] Yellow Fever Vaccine should not be given to a pregnant woman unless in the opinion of the attending physician it is clearly needed.

Physicians generally avoid prescribing unnecessary drugs and biologics for pregnant women, especially in the first trimester.

PEDIATRIC USE

This vaccine is NOT recommended for children under six months of age unless they live in or are traveling to a high-risk area.

ADVERSE REACTION

Approximately 10% of patients may have fever or malaise following immunization (usually appearing 7 - 14 days after administration); treatment should be symptomatic.

In rare instances encephalitis has developed in very young infants. This usually has not been severe and recovery has ordinarily occurred without sequelae. One death has been reported.[1]

Anaphylaxis may occur following the use of this vaccine, even in individuals with no prior history of hypersensitivity to the vaccine components. Epinephrine Injection (1:1000) always must be immediately available to combat unexpected anaphylactic or other allergic reactions.

DOSAGE AND ADMINISTRATION

Parenteral drug products should be inspected visually for extraneous particulate matter and/or discoloration prior to administration.

Reconstitute the vaccine using only the diluent supplied (Sodium Chloride Injection USP). The vaccine appears slightly opalescent and light orange in color after reconstitution. Draw the volume of the diluent, shown on the diluent label, into a suitable size syringe and inject into the vial containing the vaccine. Slowly add diluent to vaccine, let set for one to two minutes and then carefully swirl mixture until a uniform suspension is achieved. Avoid vigorous shaking as this tends to cause foaming of the suspension. Use vaccine within 60 minutes following reconstitution. *All reconstituted vaccine and containers which remain unused after one hour must be sterilized and discarded.[2] Do not dilute reconstituted vaccine.*

SWIRL VACCINE WELL before withdrawing each dose. *Administer the single immunizing dose of 0.5 ml subcutaneously* at once.

Dosage for children and adults is the same, 0.5 ml (formulated to contain not less than 5.04 Log$_{10}$ Plaque Forming Units (PFU).

Immunity develops by the 10th day after primary vaccination.[3] World Health Organization (WHO) requires revaccination every 10 years to maintain travelers vaccination certificates

YELLOW FEVER VACCINE IN THE UNITED STATES IS SUPPLIED ONLY TO DESIGNATED YELLOW FEVER VACCINATION CENTERS AUTHORIZED TO ISSUE VALID CERTIFICATES OF YELLOW FEVER VACCINATION. LOCATION OF THE NEAREST YELLOW FEVER VACCINATION CENTERS MAY BE OBTAINED FROM THE CENTERS FOR DISEASE CONTROL, ATLANTA, GA 30333, STATE OR LOCAL HEALTH DEPARTMENTS, OR THE USPHS BOOKLET "IMMUNIZATION INFORMATION FOR INTERNATIONAL TRAVEL" (OBTAINABLE FROM THE SUPERINTENDENT OF DOCUMENTS, U.S. GOVERNMENT PRINTING OFFICE, WASHINGTON, D.C. 20402).

STABILITY STUDIES

Stability of Yellow Fever Vaccine (Freeze-Dried) at elevated temperature[8]: The following information is provided for those countries or areas of the world where an adequate cold chain is a problem and inadvertent exposure to abnormal temperatures has occurred.

Temperature °C	Test	Number of Lots Tested	Computed Half-Life (Days)
35°-37° C	Mouse Assay	3	14.0
35°-37° C	Vero Cell Assay	3	13.9
45°-47° C	Mouse Assay	3	3.3
45°-47° C	Vero Cell Assay	3	4.5

Yellow Fever Vaccine is formulated to satisfy the current U.S. potency requirements of not less than 5.04 Log$_{10}$ Plaque Forming Units, (PFU) per 0.5 ml dose and meets the minimum requirements of WHO.[9]

ADMINISTRATION

Parental drug products should be inspected visually for extraneous particulate matter and/or discoloration prior to administration.

Administer subcutaneously. *Preparation of the vaccine for use:* Using a suitable size syringe and needle and aseptic precautions, transfer the volume of diluent shown on the diluent label into the vial containing the vaccine. Slowly add diluent to vaccine, let set for one to two minutes. CAREFULLY SWIRL VACCINE AND DILUENT WELL (AVOID VIGOROUS SHAKING) until a uniform suspension is achieved.

Cleanse skin at the site of injection with suitable antiseptic. *All reconstituted vaccine and containers which remain unused after one hour must be sterilized and discarded.[2]*

STORAGE

Storage Temperature: Freeze-dried vaccine must be maintained continuously at a temperature between 0°-5°C (32°-41°F).

Yellow Fever Vaccine does not contain a preservative, therefore all reconstituted vaccine and containers which remain unused after one hour must be sterilized and discarded.

Shipping Temperature: Yellow Fever Vaccine shipped in a container with solid carbon dioxide; use is not reocommended unless the shipping case contains some dry ice upon arrival.

REFERENCES
1. Unpublished data available from Connaught Laboratories, Inc., compiled 1980 2. Recommendation of the Public Health Services Immunization Practices Advisory Committee. Yellow Fever Vaccine. MMWR 32: 679-688, 1984 3. Vaccination Certificate Requirements. Health information for international travel. U.S. Department of Health and Human Services. p 8, 1983 4. Recommendation of the Public Health Service Immunization Practices Advisory Committee. General Recommendations on Immunization. MMWR 32: 1-17, 1983 5. Kaplan, J.E., et al: The effect of immune globulin on the response to trivalent oral poliovirus and yellow fever vaccinations. Bull WHO Vol 62, 585-590, 1984 6. Report of the Committee on Infectious Diseases. Active immunizations of individuals who recently received immune globulins. American Academy of Pediatrics, 1986 7. Code of Federal Regulations, Title 21, Part 201.57 (6) (c), 1983 8. Unpublished data available from Connaught Laboratories, Inc., compiled 1982 9. Requirements for yellow fever vaccine. WHO Technical Report Series 594, 1976

HOW SUPPLIED
INJECTION:

BRAND/MANUFACTURER	NDC	SIZE	AWP
○ **BRAND**			
YF-VAX: Connaught	49281-0915-05	1 ml	$175.31
	49281-0915-01	1 ml 5s	$219.13

YF-Vax SEE YELLOW FEVER VACCINE

Yocon SEE YOHIMBINE HYDROCHLORIDE

Yohimbine Hydrochloride

DESCRIPTION
Yohimbine is a 3α-15α-20β-17α-hydroxy Yohimbine-16α-carboxylic acid methyl ester. The alkaloid is found in Rubiaceae and related trees. Also in Rauwolfia Serpentina (L) Benth.

Yohimbine is an indolalkylamine alkaloid with chemical similarity to reserpine. It is a crystalline powder, odorless. Each compressed tablet contains (1/12 gr.) 5.4 mg of Yohimbine Hydrochloride.

Following is its chemical structure:

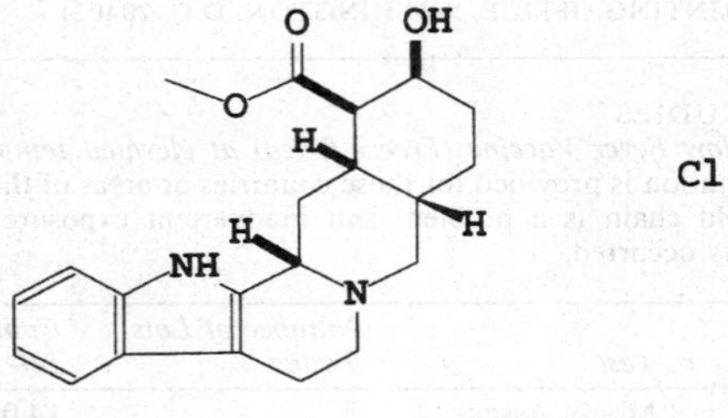

ACTION
Yohimbine blocks presynaptic alpha-2 adrenergic receptors. Its action on peripheral blood vessels resembles that of reserpine, though it is weaker and of short duration. Yohimbine's peripheral autonomic nervous system effect is to increase parasympathetic (cholinergic) and decrease sympathetic (adrenergic) activity. It is to be noted that in male sexual performance, erection is linked to cholinergic activity and to alpha-2 adrenergic blockade which may theoretically result in increased penile inflow, decreased penile outflow or both. Yohimbine exerts a stimulating action on the mood and may increase anxiety. Such actions have not been adequately studied or related to dosage although they appear to require high doses of the drug. Yohimbine has a mild anti-diuretic action, probably via stimulation of hypothalmic centers and release of posterior pituitary hormone.

Reportedly, Yohimbine exerts no significant influence on cardiac stimulation and other effects mediated by β-adrenergic receptors, its effect on blood pressure, if any, would be to lower it; however, no adequate studies are at hand to quantitate this effect in terms of Yohimbine dosage.

INDICATIONS
Yohimbine Hydrochloride is indicated as a sympathicolytic and mydriatic. It may have activity as an aphrodisiac.

CONTRAINDICATIONS
Renal diseases, and patients sensitive to the drug. In view of the limited and inadequate information at hand, no precise tabulation can be offered of additional contraindications.

WARNING
Generally, this drug is not proposed for use in females and certainly must not be used during pregnancy. Neither is this drug proposed for use in pediatric, geriatric or cardio-renal patients with gastric or duodenal ulcer history. Nor should it be used in conjunction with mood-modifying drugs such as antidepressants, or in psychiatric patients in general.

ADVERSE REACTIONS
Yohimbine readily penetrates the (CNS) and produces a complex pattern of responses in lower doses than required to produce peripheral α-adrenergic blockade. These include, anti-diuresis, a general picture of central excitation including elevation of blood pressure and heart rate increased motor activity, irritability and tremor. Sweating, nausea and vomiting are common after parenteral administration of the drug.[1,2] Also dizziness, headache, skin flushing reported when used orally.[1,3]

DOSAGE AND ADMINISTRATION
Experimental dosage reported in treatment of erectile impotence:[1,3,4] 1 tablet (5.4 mg) 3 times a day, to adult males taken orally. Occasional side effects reported with this dosage are nausea, dizziness or nervousness. In the event of side effects dosage is to be reduced to 1/2 tablet 3 times a day, followed by gradual increases to 1 tablet 3 times a day. Reported therapy not more than 10 weeks.[3]

REFERENCES
1. A. Morales et al., New England Journal of Medicine: 1221. November 12, 1981. 2. Goodman, Gilman—The Pharmacological basis of Therapeutics 6th ed., p. 176-188, McMillan. 3. Weekly Urological Clinical letter, 27:2, July 4, 1983. 4. A. Morales et al., The Journal of Urology 128: 45-47, 1982.

HOW SUPPLIED
TABLET: 5.4 MG

BRAND/MANUFACTURER	NDC	SIZE	AWP
○ **BRAND**			
YOCON: Palisades	53159-0001-30	30s	$17.97
YOHIMEX: Kramer Labs	55505-0100-15	100s	$18.70
YOMAN: Stewart Jackson	45985-0626-01	100s	$18.75
PROHIM: Baker Norton	00575-1600-01	100s	$26.25
EREX: Ion	11808-0400-01	100s	$29.00
YOCON: Palisades	53159-0001-01	100s	$37.32
	53159-0001-10	1000s	$317.21

For additional alternatives, turn to the section beginning on page 2859.

Yohimex SEE YOHIMBINE HYDROCHLORIDE

Yoman SEE YOHIMBINE HYDROCHLORIDE

Yutopar SEE RITODRINE HYDROCHLORIDE

Zalcitabine

WARNINGS
ZALCITABINE IN COMBINATION WITH ZIDOVUDINE (ZDV) IS INDICATED FOR THE TREATMENT OF ADULT PATIENTS WITH ADVANCED HIV INFECTION (CD4 CELL COUNT ≤ 300 CELLS/MM^3) WHO HAVE DEMONSTRATED SIGNIFICANT CLINICAL OR IMMUNOLOGIC DETERIORATION. THIS INDICATION IS BASED ON LIMITED DATA FROM TWO SMALL STUDIES IN WHICH ZIDOVUDINE-NAIVE PATIENTS WITH A CD4 CELL COUNT ≤ 300 CELLS/MM^3 WHO WERE TREATED WITH ZALCITABINE PLUS ZIDOVUDINE HAD A GREATER CD4 RESPONSE THAN PATIENTS TREATED WITH ZIDOVUDINE ALONE (SEE "DESCRIPTION OF STUDIES"). NEITHER STUDY INCLUDED A CONCURRENT CONTROL GROUP TAKING THE CURRENTLY RECOMMENDED ZIDOVUDINE DOSE OF 100 MG Q4H, AND THESE STUDIES WERE NOT DESIGNED TO MEASURE THE CLINICAL EFFICACY OF THE COMBINATION. AT PRESENT NO DATA ARE AVAILABLE ON THE COMBINED USE OF ZALCITABINE AND ZIDOVUDINE IN PATIENTS WHO HAVE PREVIOUSLY RECEIVED ZIDOVUDINE MONOTHERAPY, ALTHOUGH CONTROLLED STUDIES ARE ONGOING. RESULTS ARE ALSO CURRENTLY UNAVAILABLE FROM CONTROLLED STUDIES EVALUATING THE EFFECT OF COMBINED USE OF ZALCITABINE AND ZIDOVUDINE ON THE CLINICAL PROGRESSION OF HIV INFECTION (SUCH AS SURVIVAL OR THE INCIDENCE OF OPPORTUNISTIC INFECTIONS).

BECAUSE ZIDOVUDINE HAS BEEN SHOWN TO PROLONG SURVIVAL AND DECREASE THE INCIDENCE OF OPPORTUNISTIC INFECTIONS IN PATIENTS WITH ADVANCED HIV DISEASE, ZIDOVUDINE MONOTHERAPY SHOULD BE CONSIDERED AS INITIAL THERAPY FOR ADULT PATIENTS

◆ RATED THERAPEUTICALLY EQUIVALENT; ◇ THERAPEUTIC EQUIVALENCE UNCONFIRMED; ○ UNRATED

WITH HIV INFECTION WHO HAVE EVIDENCE OF IMPAIRED IMMUNITY (CD4 CELL COUNTS OF $\leq$ 500 CELLS/MM^3).

THE MAJOR CLINICAL TOXICITIES OF ZALCITABINE ARE PERIPHERAL NEUROPATHY AND, MUCH LESS FREQUENTLY, PANCREATITIS. MODERATE OR SEVERE PERIPHERAL NEUROPATHY, WHICH FOR SOME PATIENTS WAS CLINICALLY DISABLING, OCCURRED IN 17% TO 31% OF PATIENTS TREATED WITH ZALCITABINE MONOTHERAPY DEPENDING ON SEVERITY AND PRESUMED RELATIONSHIP TO DRUG. IT IS UNKNOWN AT THIS TIME WHETHER THE RISK OF PERIPHERAL NEUROPATHY IS INCREASED WITH THE USE OF COMBINATION THERAPY OVER THAT OBSERVED WITH ZALCITABINE MONOTHERAPY. THERE ARE NO DATA REGARDING THE USE OF ZALCITABINE IN PATIENTS WITH PREEXISTING PERIPHERAL NEUROPATHY SINCE THESE PATIENTS WERE EXCLUDED FROM CLINICAL TRIALS; THEREFORE, ZALCITABINE SHOULD BE USED WITH EXTREME CAUTION IN THESE PATIENTS. THE OCCURRENCE OF PERIPHERAL NEUROPATHY IN PATIENTS TREATED WITH ZALCITABINE WAS GREATER IN PATIENTS WITH MORE ADVANCED HIV DISEASE (SEE ''WARNINGS'').

DOCUMENTED FATAL PANCREATITIS HAS BEEN OBSERVED WITH THE ADMINISTRATION OF ZALCITABINE ALONE OR IN COMBINATION WITH ZIDOVUDINE. THE USE OF BOTH ZALCITABINE AND ZIDOVUDINE SHOULD BE SUSPENDED IMMEDIATELY IN PATIENTS WHO DEVELOP ANY SYMPTOMS SUGGESTIVE OF PANCREATITIS UNTIL THIS DIAGNOSIS IS EXCLUDED (SEE ''WARNINGS''). OVERALL, PANCREATITIS IS AN UNCOMMON COMPLICATION OF ZALCITABINE MONOTHERAPY, OCCURRING IN < 1% OF PATIENTS.

TOXICITIES PREVIOUSLY ASSOCIATED WITH ZIDOVUDINE MONOTHERAPY ARE LIKELY TO OCCUR IN PATIENTS TREATED WITH COMBINED ZALCITABINE AND ZIDOVUDINE THERAPY. IT IS HIGHLY RECOMMENDED THAT PHYSICIANS REFER TO THE WARNINGS AND PRECAUTIONS DESCRIBED IN THE ZIDOVUDINE COMPLETE PRODUCT INFORMATION BEFORE PRESCRIBING COMBINATION THERAPY WITH ZALCITABINE AND ZIDOVUDINE.

IT IS RECOMMENDED THAT THE DECISION TO USE ZALCITABINE SHOULD BE MADE IN CONSULTATION WITH A PHYSICIAN EXPERIENCED IN THE CARE OF PATIENTS WITH HIV INFECTION.

DESCRIPTION

Zalcitabine [formerly called dideoxycytidine (ddC)], is a synthetic pyrimidine nucleoside analogue active against the human immunodeficiency virus (HIV). Zalcitabine is available as film-coated tablets for oral administration in strengths of 0.375 mg and 0.750 mg. The chemical name for Zalcitabine is 4-amino-1-beta-D-2', 3'-dideoxyribofuranosyl-2-(1H)-pyrimidone or 2'3'-dideoxycytidine with the molecular formula $C_9H_{13}N_3O_3$ and a molecular weight of 211.22.

Zalcitabine is a white to off-white crystalline powder with an aqueous solubility of 76.4 mg/mL at 25°C.

Following is its chemical structure:

CLINICAL PHARMACOLOGY

Mechanism of Action: Zalcitabine is a synthetic nucleoside analogue of the naturally occurring nucleoside 2'-deoxycytidine in which the 3'-hydroxyl group is replaced by hydrogen. Within cells, Zalcitabine is converted to the active metabolite, dideoxycytidine 5'-triphosphate (ddCTP), by cellular enzymes. ddCTP serves as an alternative substrate to deoxycytidine triphosphate (dCTP) for HIV-reverse transcriptase and inhibits the in vitro replication of HIV-1 by inhibition of viral DNA synthesis. This inhibition has been demonstrated in vitro in human primary cell cultures and in established cell lines. In DNA biosynthesis, DNA chain extension occurs through the formation of a phosphodiester bridge between the 3'-hydroxyl group of the growing end of a DNA chain and the 5'-phosphate group of the incoming deoxynucleotide. Because ddCTP lacks the 3'-hydroxyl group required for chain elongation, its incorporation into a growing DNA chain leads to premature chain termination. ddCTP serves as a competitive inhibitor of the natural substrate, dCTP, for the active site of the viral reverse transcriptase and thus further inhibits viral DNA synthesis.

The active metabolite, ddCTP, also has a high affinity for cellular mitochondrial DNA polymerase gamma and has been reported to be incorporated into the DNA of cells in culture. However, DNA chain termination with cellular DNA polymerases has not been demonstrated.

The half-life of ddCTP in established cell lines and in human peripheral blood mononuclear cells in culture has been determined to be in the range of 2.6 to 10 hours.

Microbiology: The anti-HIV activity of Zalcitabine was determined in a variety of human T-cell lines infected with different strains of HIV. The in vitro anti-HIV activity of Zalcitabine varied greatly depending upon the time between virus infection and Zalcitabine treatment of cell cultures, the ratio of the number of infectious virus particles to the number of cells, the kind of assay and the cell type used. When established cell lines were infected with a large excess of virus per cell and drug added soon after infection, the concentration of Zalcitabine required to inhibit HIV-1 replication by 50% (ID$_{50}$) was generally in the range of 30 nM to 500 nM (1 nM = 0.21 ng/mL). In these cell lines, > 95% inhibition of viral replication was achieved with 100 nM to 1000 nM Zalcitabine. Zalcitabine blocked virus-induced cytopathic effects in cell lines in culture at a concentration of 30 nM to 300 nM. In assays measuring the inhibition of p24 viral antigen, the ID$_{50}$ of Zalcitabine was in the range of 1 nM to 500 nM, and the 90% inhibitory concentration (ID$_{90}$) was in the range of 500 nM to 1000 nM. In peripheral blood mononuclear cell cultures infected with HIV-1 (LAV strain) at a low ratio of virus to cells and assayed for HIV-reverse transcriptase, ID$_{50}$ and ID$_{90}$ values for Zalcitabine were determined to be 11 nM and 100 nM, respectively. In monocyte/macrophage cultures infected with HIV (Ba-L strain) and treated with Zalcitabine, the ID$_{90}$ value was < 10 nM when assayed for viral p24 antigen. However, viral replication in monocyte/macrophage cultures infected with a lymphotropic isolate of HIV (LAV-1 strain) was not inhibited at 100,000 nM.

Comparative studies of the antiviral activity of Zalcitabine against HIV-1 and HIV-2 in vitro revealed no significant difference in sensitivity between the two viruses when activity was determined by measuring viral cytopathic effect. The relationship of the in vitro inhibition of HIV by Zalcitabine to the inhibition of HIV replication in infected people, or the clinical response to therapy, has not been established.

The results of cytotoxicity studies in various cell lines demonstrated that the concentration of the drug necessary to inhibit the cell growth by 50% (EC$_{50}$) was in the range of 5000 nM to > 100,000 nM. In vitro combination studies have demonstrated the Zalcitabine and zidovudine have an additive or synergistic antiviral effect, depending on the cell line used, without increased cytotoxicity over that observed for either agent alone.

The potential for development of clinically significant Zalcitabine-resistant virus in patients with HIV infection who received Zalcitabine has not been adequately studied to date. Zalcitabine-resistant virus has not been isolated directly from patients who received this drug. However, reduced Zalcitabine sensitivity in vitro was reported in hybrid virus constructs made with portions of the HIV genome obtained from a patient who received intermittent Zalcitabine therapy for over 18 months. Combination therapy of Zalcitabine plus zidovudine does not appear to prevent the emergence of zidovudine-resistant isolates. However, studies with zidovudine-resistant virus isolates indicate zidovudine-resistant strains remain sensitive to Zalcitabine.

Pharmacokinetics: The pharmacokinetics of Zalcitabine has been evaluated in studies in HIV-infected patients following 0.01 mg/kg, 0.03 mg/kg and 1.5 mg oral doses, and a 1.5 mg intravenous dose administered as a 1-hour infusion.

Absorption and Bioavailability in Adults: Following oral administration to HIV-infected patients, the mean absolute bioavailability of Zalcitabine was > 80% (30% CV, range 23% to 124%, n = 19). The absorption rate of a 1.5 mg oral dose of Zalcitabine (n = 20) was reduced when administered with food. This resulted in a 39% decrease in mean maximum plasma concentrations (C$_{max}$) from 25.2 ng/mL (35% CV, range 11.6 to 37.5 ng/mL) to 15.5 ng/mL) (24% CV, range 9.1 to 23.7 ng/mL), and a twofold increase in time to achieve maximum plasma concentrations from a mean of 0.8 hours under fasting conditions to 1.6 hours when the drug was given with food. The extent of absorption (as reflected by AUC) was decreased by 14%, from 72 ng.hr/mL (28% CV, range 43 to 119 ng.hr/mL) to 62 ng.hr/mL (23% CV, range 42 to 91 ng.hr/mL). The clinical relevance of these decreases is unknown.

Distribution in Adults: The steady-state volume of distribution following IV administration of a 1.5 mg dose of Zalcitabine averaged 0.534 ($\pm$ 0.127) L/kg (24% CV, range 0.304 to 0.734 L/kg, n = 20). Cerebrospinal fluid obtained from 9 patients at 2 to 3.5 hours following 0.06 mg/kg or 0.09 mg/kg IV infusion showed measurable concentrations of Zalcitabine. The CSF:plasma concentration ratio ranged from 9% to 37% (mean 20%), demonstrating penetration of the drug through the blood-brain barrier. The clinical relevance of these ratios has not been evaluated.

Metabolism and Elimination in Adults: Zalcitabine is phosphorylated intracellularly to Zalcitabine triphosphate, the active substrate for HIV-reverse transcriptase. Concentrations of Zalcitabine triphosphate are too low for quantitation following administration of therapeutic doses to humans.

Zalcitabine metabolism in humans has not been fully evaluated. Zalcitabine does not appear to undergo a significant degree of metabolism by the liver. Renal excretion appears to be the primary route of elimination, and accounted for approximately 70% of an orally-administered, radiolabeled dose (i.e., total radioactivity) within 24 hours after dosing (n = 6). The mean elimination half-life is 2 hours and generally ranges from 1 to 3 hours in individual patients. Total body clearance following an intravenous dose averages 285 mL/min (29% CV, range 165 to 447 mL/min). Less than 10% of a radiolabeled dose of Zalcitabine appears in the feces.

In patients with impaired kidney function, prolonged elimination of Zalcitabine may be expected. Results from 7 patients with renal impairment (estimated CrCl < 55 mL/min) indicate that the half-life was prolonged (up to 8.5 hours) in these patients compared to those with normal renal function. Maximum plasma concentrations were higher in some patients after a single dose.

In patients with normal renal function, the pharmacokinetics of Zalcitabine was not altered during three times daily multiple dosing (n = 9). Accumulation of drug in plasma during this regimen was negligible. The drug was < 4% bound to plasma proteins, indicating that drug interactions involving binding-site displacement are unlikely (see *"Drug Interactions"*).

Pharmacokinetics in Children: Limited pharmacokinetic data have been reported to five HIV-positive children using doses of 0.03 and 0.04 mg/kg Zalcitabine administered orally every 6 hours.[1] The mean bioavailability of Zalcitabine in this study was 54% and mean apparent systemic clearance was 150 mL/min/m^2. Due to the small number of subjects and different analytical techniques, it is difficult to make comparisons between pediatric and adult data.

INDICATIONS AND USAGE

Combination Therapy with Zidovudine in Advanced HIV Infection: Zalcitabine in combination with zidovudine is indicated for the treatment of adult patients with advanced HIV infection (CD4 cell count ≤ 300 cells/mm^3) who have demonstrated significant clinical or immunologic deterioration. This indication is based on limited data from two small studies in which zidovudine-naive patients with a CD4 cell count ≤ 300 cells/mm^3 who were treated with Zalcitabine plus zidovudine had a greater CD4 response than patients treated with zidovudine alone (see *"Description of Studies"*). Neither study included a concurrent control group taking the current recommended zidovudine dose of 100 mg q4h. and these studies were not designed to measure the clinical efficacy of the combination. No data are currently available on the combined use of Zalcitabine and zidovudine in patients who have previously received zidovudine monotherapy, although controlled studies are ongoing. At present there are no data available from controlled or uncontrolled studies addressing whether an effect on CD4 cell count would be observed by the addition of Zalcitabine to patients who are currently receiving zidovudine or who had previously been exposed to antiretroviral therapy. Because zidovudine has been shown to prolong survival and decrease the incidence of opportunistic infections in patients with advanced HIV disease, zidovudine monotherapy should be considered as initial therapy for adult patients with HIV infection who have evidence of impaired immunity (CD4 cell counts of ≤ 500 cells/mm^3).

Description of Studies: Combination Trials: The combined use of Zalcitabine and zidovudine is based on limited data from two small studies. The first was a Phase ½, open-label, dose-ranging study (N3447/ACTG 106) that evaluated several dose combinations of Zalcitabine and zidovudine. The second study was a randomized Phase 2 study (BW 34,225-02) designed to evaluate the virologic and immunologic effects of the combined administration of two nucleoside analogues (zidovudine combined with either Zalcitabine or didanosine). Both studies used an experimental regimen of zidovudine administered three times daily, and neither was designed to assess the clinical efficacy of the combination.

Data from a study of Zalcitabine alternating with zidovudine at doses of Zalcitabine higher than currently recommended (ACTG 047) have shown results comparable to those observed in N3447/ACTG 106 in zidovudine-naive patients. A parallel study in patients who were previously hematologically intolerant to zidovudine monotherapy but then changed to an alternating Zalcitabine and zidovudine regimen (ACTG 050) showed greater toxicity and less CD4 response. The applicability of the results from the two studies using alternating regimens to the recommended combination regimen is uncertain.

Zalcitabine Given in Combination with Zidovudine in Adult Zidovudine- naive Patients with Advanced HIV infection (CD4 Cell Count ≤ 200 Cells/mm^3 [N3447/ACTG 106]): This Phase ½ study of therapy with concomitant Zalcitabine and zidovudine is an ongoing, six-arm, open-label, dose-escalating study with randomization within blocks of two arms. Doses being studied are Zalcitabine 0.005 and 0.01 mg/kg q8h administered concomitantly with zidovudine 100 or 200 mg q8h, as well as zidovudine 50 mg q8h alone or combined with Zalcitabine 0.005 mg/kg q8h. No control arm of zidovudine monotherapy at the currently approved regimen was included in this study. A total of 56 zidovudine-naive patients with advanced HIV infection (CD4 cell count ≤ 200 cells/mm^3) were entered. Patients have now been treated for a median duration varying across groups from 36 to 72 weeks; median CD4 cell counts at entry were 75 cells/mm^3. An earlier analysis of this study has been published.[2] (See related table).

Treatment regimens with 150 mg/day of zidovudine showed less activity than those with ≥ 300 mg/day of zidovudine; therefore, the four treatment regimens that included ≥ 300 mg/day zidovudine were pooled for CD4 and weight analyses

(see Table 1 for baseline characteristics). For safety analyses, data from all five combination arms were pooled. Although the clinical outcomes were monitored while subjects were on therapy, the study was not designed to evaluate clinical outcome as an efficacy parameter.

There were eight deaths during the study. Twenty of the 56 patients who entered developed an AIDS-defining opportunistic infection, neoplasm or condition. These AIDS-defining events were equally distributed among the six treatment arms.

A total of 37 patients prematurely withdrew from the study. Nine patients discontinued therapy because of adverse events. Of these 9 patients, 2 were discontinued for peripheral neuropathy, 5 for hematologic abnormalities, 1 for nausea and vomiting, 1 for myositis.

The effect of study therapy on CD4 cell counts is presented later in this section. A mean peak increase in weight of 4.5 kg for the pool of the four combination regimens was observed. Body weight was maintained above baseline for > 1 year for patients who remained on study.

Zalcitabine given in Combination with Zidovudine in Patients with HIV infection, ≤ 4 Weeks prior Zidovudine and CD4 Cell Counts ≥ 300 Cells/mm^3 (BW 34,225-02): An unscheduled analysis of CD4 changes for patients administered either combined Zalcitabine and zidovudine therapy, or zidovudine monotherapy, was obtained from this ongoing, double-blind, randomized, Phase 2 controlled trial. The trial was designed to compare the antiviral and immunologic effects of zidovudine monotherapy administered three times daily to that of combination therapy with either Zalcitabine and zidovudine or didanosine and zidovudine. Subjects were HIV-infected patients with CD4 cell counts at entry ≤ 300 cells/mm^3 who had received < 4 weeks of zidovudine.

The unscheduled analysis of CD4 cell count changes in this study included only the group receiving zidovudine alone (200 mg q8h, a currently experimental regimen) and the Zalcitabine plus zidovudine group. At the time of this analysis, 45 patients were randomized to the combination of Zalcitabine and zidovudine and 47 patients to the zidovudine-monotherapy arm. Median duration of treatment was 13 weeks for the zidovudine-monotherapy group and 14 weeks for the group receiving Zalcitabine and zidovudine; median CD4 cell counts at entry were 153 cells/mm^3 and 125 cells/mm^3, respectively. The primary end point of this study is emergence of viral resistance. Data on viral resistance, clinical outcome (survival, incidence of opportunistic infection) or the incidence of adverse events are not currently available. Change in CD4 cell count was the only outcome variable analyzed from this study.

Analysis of CD4 Cell Counts in Combination Trials: The activity of combination Zalcitabine and zidovudine was assessed using CD4 cell counts as a marker of biologic activity. In controlled trials, zidovudine monotherapy has been associated with clinical benefit (improved survival and decreased incidence of opportunistic infection) and transient increases in CD4 cell counts. Evidence of efficacy of Zalcitabine in combination with zidovudine is based only on improvements in CD4 cell counts.

Definitions of outcome were applied to data from patients receiving Zalcitabine in combination with zidovudine. Analyses included the following:

1. Mean change from baseline in CD4 cell counts at various time points during therapy;

2. Longitudinal changes during study: time weighted average of serial CD4 cell counts adjusted (normalized) for baseline CD4 cell counts (NAUC). (NAUC = Cumulative AUC of CD4 cell count up to time t/baseline CD4 count x t.) NAUCs that exceed a value of 1 indicate that the average CD4 level during therapy is increased over the baseline CD4 cell count;

3. Presence of a "response" where response was defined as one of the following: a) the greater of either a 75-cell or 75% increase over baseline CD4 cell count maintained for a minimum of two consecutive visits at least 21 days apart (75:75 response), or b) the greater of either a 50-cell or 50% increase over baseline CD4 cell count maintained for a minimum of two consecutive visits at least 21 days apart (50:50 response).

Definitions of outcome measures 2 and 3 were not specified in the two study protocols but were applied post hoc and have not been previously correlated with clinical outcome. In the discussion below, the outcomes for the control group referred to as N3300/ACTG 114 are results for subjects in the zidovudine arm of a large, prospective study comparing zidovudine to Zalcitabine monotherapy. The figures cited are for those patients with no previous zidovudine exposure. Comparisons across clinical studies must be interpreted cautiously due to possible

Table 1
BASELINE CHARACTERISTICS

Study	BW 34.225-02		N3300/ACTG 114	N3447/ACTG 106
	Combination Zalcitabine + ZDV	ZDV	ZDV (No Prior ZDV)	(Four Pooled Combination Arms)
n	45	47	262	36
Accrual Date	5/91-11/91	5/91-11/91	8/89-9/90	7/89-5/90
Baseline Median CD4 (cells/mm^3)	125	153	85	70
CD4 Range (cells/mm^3)	1-301	11-288	5-289	3-188
% Male	89%	92%	93%	97%
% Caucasian	60%	66%	79%	89%
Homosexual	51%	55%	77%	69%
% AIDS	22%	15%	26%	44%

◆ RATED THERAPEUTICALLY EQUIVALENT; ◇ THERAPEUTIC EQUIVALENCE UNCONFIRMED; ○ UNRATED

differences in study population, selection bias between studies, and different methodologies for measuring CD4 cells counts.

Figure 1 displays the CD4 cell response for those patients receiving Zalcitabine in combination with zidovudine in BW 34,225-02 and in N3447/ACTG 106 (pooled response for the combination regimens of Zalcitabine with $\geq$ 300 mg/day of zidovudine). It also depicts the CD4 cell response for zidovudine-monotherapy arm from BW 34,225-02 and for those zidovudine patients in N3300/ACTG 114 who were zidovudine-naive at entry. Table 1 describes the baseline characteristics of those populations whose CD4 data were analyzed as presented in Figure 1 and Table 2. Table 2 lists the NAUC response at weeks 12 and 24 for BW 34,225-02, N3447/ACTG 106 and N3300/ACTG 114.

RESULTS OF THE CD4 ANALYSES ARE AS FOLLOWS
1. Mean Change from Baseline: Results for changes in CD4 cell count from baseline are displayed in Figure 1 for BW 34,225-02, N3447/ACTG 106 and N3300/ACTG 114 (ZDV-monotherapy arm).

2. Longitudinal Changes during Study: In BW 34,225-02, 84% of patients receiving combination Zalcitabine and zidovudine had an NAUC > 1 at week 12 (89% at week 24) compared to 72% of patients receiving zidovudine monotherapy (200 mg q8h) at week 12 (68% at week 24). In a contemporary zidovudine-treated control group (N3300/ACTG 114), 87% of the zidovudine-treated patients had an NAUC > 1 at week 12 (81% at week 24). In the open-label study N3447/ACTG106, 97% of patients administered Zalcitabine in combination with $\geq$ 300 mg/day of zidovudine had an NAUC > 1 at weeks 12 and 24.

3. Response: in BW 34,225-02, 38% of patients receiving combination Zalcitabine and zidovudine had a 50:50 response at week 24 compared to 21% of patients in the zidovudine-monotherapy group. In the zidovudine-contemporary control group (N3300/ACTG 114), 34% of patients had a 50:50 response at week 24. In N3447/ACTG 106, 70% of patients receiving Zalcitabine combined with zidovudine ($\geq$ 300 mg/ day) had a 50:50 response at week 24.

Figure 1. Mean Change from Basline CD4

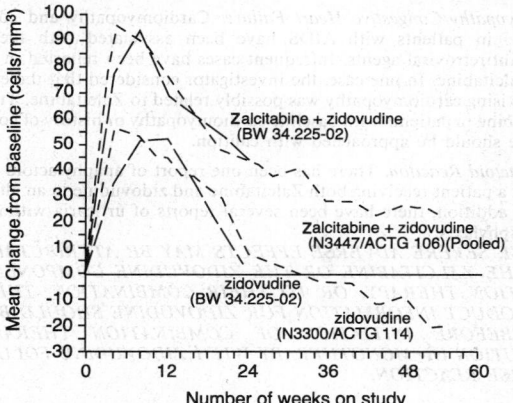

Number of Patients					
Week	0	12	24	36	48
Zalcitabine + ZDV (BW 34.225-02)	45	37	13	-	-
ZDV (BW 34.225-02)	47	37	17	-	-
ZDV (N3300)	262	220	206	176	143
Zalcitabine + ZDV (N3447)(pooled)	36	31	29	27	23

(See related table).

Additional Monotherapy and Combination Studies of Zalcitabine.

Monotherapy trials: Zalcitabine was studied in two controlled comparative trials (N3300/ACTG 114 and N3492/ACTG 119) of patients with AIDS or advanced ARC (CD4 cell count $\leq$ 200 cells/mm^3), and in a randomized, dose-comparison, expanded-access safety study (N3544) of Zalcitabine in patients with advanced HIV disease who were intolerant to zidovudine or who showed evidence of clinical progression while on zidovudine therapy. Information from these monotherapy studies is included to describe the safety profile of Zalcitabine (see *"Adverse Reactions"*).

The parameters of efficacy evaluated in the controlled comparative studies of Zalcitabine included the clinical end points of survival and opportunistic infection. The expanded-access safety program (N3544) was designed primarily as a dose-comparison safety study.

Zalcitabine Monotherapy in Adult Patients with AIDS or Advanced ARC and $\leq$ 3 Months of prior Zidovudine Therapy (N3300/ACTG 114): This study was a randomized, double-blind, parallel, controlled trial of Zalcitabine at 26 medical centers in patients with AIDS or advanced ARC (CD4 cell count $\leq$ 200 cells/mm^3) who previously received $\leq$ 3 months of zidovudine. Patients received either Zalcitabine 0.750 mg q8h or zidovudine 200 mg q4h, later reduced to 100 mg q4h. Three hundred and twenty patients were randomized to received Zalcitabine and 315 patients randomized to receive zidovudine with a median duration of

treatment of 44 weeks (range: 1.1 to 96) and 53 weeks (range: 0.3 to 96), respectively. Median CD4 cell count at entry was 90 cells/mm^3 and 87 cells/mm^3 for the Zalcitabine and zidovudine-treatment groups, respectively.

This study was terminated on the basis of 1-year survival results that showed a significant difference in survival favoring the zidovudine group, with 59 deaths in the Zalcitabine group versus 33 deaths in the zidovudine group (p = .007, stratified Cox analysis). One hundred and thirty patients (41%) in the Zalcitabine group and 95 patients (30%) in the zidovudine group progressed to a critical event at the time of the 1-year analysis (i.e., death or fist occurrence of an AIDS-defining opportunistic infection, neoplasm or condition, p = 0.02).

Toxicities requiring discontinuation were primarily peripheral neuropathy in the Zalcitabine group and hematologic toxicity in the zidovudine group. Overall: 60 (20%) patients receiving Zalcitabine developed moderate or severe neuropathy considered by the investigator to be possibly or probably drug related; 33 (10%) of patients were reported to have prematurely discontinued study therapy because of peripheral neuropathy. Of 315 zidovudine patients, 22 (7%) were discontinued due to hematologic toxicity. At the time of the 1-year interim analysis, 187 (58%) of Zalcitabine-treated patients discontinued for any reason and 59 (18%) discontinued treatment due to an adverse event. By comparison, 142 (45%) patients treated with zidovudine discontinued for any reason and 33 (11%) discontinued for adverse events (see *"Warnings and Adverse Reactions"*).

Zalcitabine Monotherapy in Adult with AIDS or Advanced ARC and $\leq$ 48 Weeks of prior Zidovudine Therapy (N3492/ACTG 119): This is a nine center, randomized, open-label, parallel, controlled trial of Zalcitabine in patients with AIDS or advance ARC who previously received $\geq$ 48 weeks of zidovudine. This trial enrolled patients whose CD4 cell counts were $\leq$ 200 cells/mm^3 at the time zidovudine was first started. The planned sample size was 320 patients; however, full enrollment was not achieved. Fifty-nine patients were randomized to receive Zalcitabine, 750 mg q8h and 52 patients to receive zidovudine 100 mg q4h. The median duration of treatment was 40 weeks for Zalcitabine (range: 2.3 to 64) and 25 weeks for zidovudine (range: 1.1 to 57) at the time of the unscheduled analysis. Median CD4 cell counts at entry for the Zalcitabine and zidovudine-treatment groups were 84 cells/mm^3 and 88 cells/mm^3.

At the time of this analysis, there were 10 (17%) deaths in the Zalcitabine treatment group and 13 (25%) deaths in the zidovudine group (p = 0.52; stratified Cox analysis). Nineteen (33%) patients in the Zalcitabine group and 17 (33%) patients in the zidovudine group progressed to a critical event (i.e., death or first occurrence of an AIDS-defining opportunistic infection, neoplasm or condition, p = 0.95, stratified Cox analysis). Due to the small number of patients enrolled in this study, definitive conclusions cannot be reached.

Twelve (20%) patients in the Zalcitabine group (including 7 patients with peripheral neuropathy) and 5 (10%) patients in the zidovudine group discontinued treatment due to adverse events (see *"Warnings"* and *"Adverse Reactions"*).

Expanded-Access Safety Study of Zalcitabine Therapy in Adult Patients with Advanced HIV Disease Who are Intolerant to Zidovudine or had Failed Zidovudine Therapy (N3544): A randomized, open-label, dose-comparison safety study was initiated in patients with advanced HIV disease (CD4 cell count $\leq$ 200 cells/mm^3) who were intolerant to zidovudine, for whom zidovudine was contraindicated, or who were clinically deteriorating despite zidovudine therapy. An interim analysis was performed for 3479 patients, 1757 in the Zalcitabine 0.375 mg q8h and 1722 in the Zalcitabine 0.750 mg q8h groups, with a median duration of treatment of 16 weeks (range: 0.1 to 61). Mean CD4 cell counts at entry were similar for the 0.375 mg (83 cells/mm^3) and 0.750 mg (79 cells/mm^3) Zalcitabine groups.

Two hundred seventy-nine patients discontinued for an adverse event, including 164 (5%) with peripheral neuropathy (97 in the high-dose group and 67 in the low-dose group) and 11 (0.3%) with pancreatitis (7 in the high-dose group and 4 in the low dose-group) (see *"Adverse Reactions"*).

No statistically significant difference in survival was found for the deaths reported at the interim analysis. Subsequently, to better define survival in the two dose groups, survival data on 3920 patients with follow-up information as of February 1, 1992, were validated by telephone survey. There was a total of 556 deaths, 296 in the low-dose group and 260 in the high-dose group (p = 0.59, Cox regression analysis).

Alternating Trials: Alternating regimens of Zalcitabine and zidovudine were studied in two open-label, controlled, multi-arm, dose-ranging trials (ACTG 047 and ACTG 050). ACTG 047 evaluated regimens of Zalcitabine and zidovudine alternating weekly and alternating monthly. Regimens were also included with Zalcitabine alternating weekly with no therapy, zidovudine alternating weekly with no therapy and continuous zidovudine therapy. All patients were zidovudine-naive. Median CD4 cell counts at entry for patients in various arms of ACTG 047 ranged from 59 to 161 cells/mm^3. ACTG 050 evaluated the same dose schedules of Zalcitabine and zidovudine as ACTG 047 in patients who demonstrated previous hematologic intolerance to zidovudine. ACTG 050 did not include a continuous zidovudine group. Median CD4 cells counts at entry for patients in the various arms of ACTG 050 ranged from 22 to 45 cells/mm^3. Doses of Zalcitabine evaluated in both trials were 0.01 mg/kg and 0.03 mg/kg q4h. These doses were higher than those used in the previously discussed monotherapy or combination trials. In ACTG 047, 3 of the 4 alternating regimens had improvements in CD4 cell counts that were higher and sustained above baseline longer than the continuous zidovudine-monotherapy control arm. The occurrence of toxicity in some of the alternating arms was higher than that seen in the monotherapy studies of Zalcitabine or in N3447/ACTG 106. Overall, 24% of patients had to discontinue therapy for adverse events. Patients in ACTG 050 did not tolerate alternating Zalcitabine and zidovudine regimens as well as zidovudine-naive patients in ACTG 047 (see *"Warnings"*).

CONTRAINDICATIONS

Zalcitabine is contraindicated in patients with clinically significant hypersensitivity to Zalcitabine or to any of the excipients contained in the tablets.

WARNINGS

1. PERIPHERAL NEUROPATHY:

THE MAJOR CLINICAL TOXICITY OF ZALCITABINE IS PERIPHERAL NEUROPATHY, WHICH OCCURRED IN 17% TO 31% OF SUBJECTS TREATED IN PHASE 2/3 MONOTHERAPY STUDIES DEPENDING ON SEVERITY AND PRESUMED RELATIONSHIP TO DRUG. BY COMPARISON, NEUROPATHY OCCURRED IN 0% TO 12% OF ZIDOVUDINE-TREATED PATIENTS. THESE DATA ARE SUMMARIZED IN TABLE 3. DATA ARE VERY LIMITED ON THE OCCURRENCE OF PERIPHERAL NEUROPATHY WITH THE COMBINED USE OF ZALCITABINE AND ZIDOVUDINE.

Zalcitabine-related peripheral neuropathy is a sensorimotor neuropathy characterized initially by numbness and burning dysesthesia involving the distal extremities. These symptoms may be followed by sharp shooting pains or severe continuous burning pain if the drug is not withdrawn. The neuropathy may progress to severe pain requiring narcotic analgesics and is potentially irreversible, especially if Zalcitabine is not stopped promptly. In some patients, symptoms of neuropathy may initially progress despite discontinuation of Zalcitabine. With prompt discontinuation of Zalcitabine, the neuropathy is usually slowly reversible.

There are no data regarding the use of Zalcitabine in patients with preexisting peripheral neuropathy since these patients were excluded from clinical trials; therefore, Zalcitabine should be used with extreme caution in these patients. Zalcitabine should also be used with particular caution in patients with low CD4 cell counts (CD4 < 50 cells/mm^3) for whom the risk of developing peripheral neuropathy while on Zalcitabine therapy is greater. Careful monitoring is strongly recommended for these individuals. Individuals with moderate or severe peripheral neuropathy, as evidenced by symptoms accompanied by objective findings, are advised to avoid Zalcitabine.

Zalcitabine should be stopped promptly when moderate discomfort from numbness, tingling, burning or pain of the extremities progresses, or any related symptoms occur that are accompanied by an objective finding. In a large ongoing clinical trial, peripheral neuropathy requiring Zalcitabine interruption is defined as moderate discomfort of the lower extremities (requiring non-narcotic analgesics) that is bilateral and persists for $\geq$ 3 days, or mild symptoms accompanied by the loss of a previously present Achilles reflex. If symptoms resolve to mild intensity, rechallenge with half-dosage is permitted. Peripheral neuropathy requiring permanent discontinuation of Zalcitabine has been defined in clinical trials as any severe discomfort of the extremities requiring narcotic analgesics or moderate discomfort progressing for $\geq$ 1 week. These definitions are based on the cumulative experience with Zalcitabine and do not correspond to the definitions used in Table 3. for which symptoms could be more severe.)

2. PANCREATITIS

DOCUMENTED FATAL PANCREATITIS HAS BEEN OBSERVED WITH THE ADMINISTRATION OF ZALCITABINE ALONE OR THE COMBINATION OF ZALCITABINE WITH ZIDOVUDINE. Pancreatitis is an uncommon complcitation of Zalcitabine monotherapy, occurring in < 1% of patients. The occurence of asymptomatic elevated serum amylase of any etiology while on Zalcitabine monotherapy was also $\leq$ 1%. Of 633 patients treated with Zalcitabine in the expanded-access safety study (N3544) who had a history of prior pancreatitis or increaased amylase, 10 (1.6%) developed pancreatitis and an additional 10 (1.6%) developed asymptomatic elevated serum amylase. There was no apparent difference in the occurrence of pancreatitis between the two doses of Zalcitabine in the expanded-access trial (N3544).

Caution should be exercised when administering Zalcitabine to any patient with a history of pancreatitis or known risk factor for the development of pancreatitis. To date, in an ongoing, blinded, combination study, one patient has died of fulminant pancreatitis possibly related to Zalcitabine and/or zidovudine. Another patient who received concomitant intravenous pentamidine and Zalcitabine died of fulminant pancreatitis possibly related to the concomitant use of Zalcitabine and intravenous pentamidine.

Patients with a history of pancreatitis or a history of elevated serum amylase should be followed more closely while on Zalcitabine therapy. The significance of an asymptomatic increase in serum amylase levels in HIV-infected patients prior to starting Zalcitabine or while on Zalcitabine is unclear. Treatment with Zalcitabine should be interrupted in the setting of a rising serum amylase level associated with dysglycemia, rising triglyceride level, decreasing serum calcium or other parameters or symptoms suggestive of impending pancreatitis, until a clinical diagnosis is reached. Treatment with Zalcitabine should also be interrupted if treatment with another drug known to cause pancreatitis (e.g., intravenous pentamidine) is required (see *"Drug Interactions"*).

Treatment with Zalcitabine and zidovudine should be stopped immediately if nausea, vomiting abdominal pain or other symptoms suggestive of pancreatitis develop, until a definitive diagnosis can be established. Zalcitabine should be restarted only after pancreatitis has been ruled out. If clinical pancreatitis develops during Zalcitabine administration, it is recommended that Zalcitabine be permanently discontinued.

3. OTHER SERIOUS TOXICITIES

a. Esophageal Ulcers: Infrequent cases of esophageal ulcers have been attributed to Zalcitabine therapy. Interruption of Zalcitabine should be considered in patients who develop esophageal ulcers that do not respond to specific treatment for opportunistic pathogens in order to assess a possible relationship of Zalcitabine.

b. Cardiomyopathy/Congestive Heart Failure: Cardiomyopathy and congestive heart failure in patients with AIDS have been associated with the use of nucleoside antiretroviral agents. Infrequent cases have been reported in patients receiving Zalcitabine. In one case, the investigator considered that the exacerbation of preexising cardiomyopathy was possibly related to Zalcitabine. Treatment with Zalcitabine in patients with baseline cardiomyopathy or history of congestive heart failure should be approached with caution.

C. Anaphylactoid Reaction: There has been one report of anaphylactoid reaction occurring in a patient receiving both Zalcitabine and zidovudine in an alternating regimen. In addition, there have been several reports of urticaria without other signs of anaphylaxis.

BECAUSE SEVERE ADVERSE EFFECTS MAY BE ATTRIBUTABLE TO EITHER THE ZALCITABINE OR THE ZIDOVUDINE COMPONENTS OF COMBINATION THERAPY, OR TO THEIR COMBINATION, THE COMPLETE PRODUCT INFORMATION FOR ZIDOVUDINE SHOULD BE CONSULTED BEFORE INITIATION OF COMBINATION THERAPY OR REINSTITUTION OF MONOTHERAPY WITH ZIDOVUDINE FOLLOWING AN ADVERSE REACTION.

PRECAUTIONS

General: Information regarding the safety of combined Zalcitabine and zidovudine therapy is limited; the safety profile of Zalcitabine has been characterized

Table 2.

CD4 RESPONSE ANALYSES

Study	BW 34.225-02			N3300/ACTG 114 No Prior ZDV	N3447/ACTG 106 Zalcitabine + ZDV
Dose Mean Peak Increase in CD4	0.750 mg + 200 mg q8h Zalcitabine + ZDV + 94 cells/mm^3 (week 8)	200 mg q8h ZDV^a + 53 cells/mm^3 (week 12)		200 mg q4h ZDV^b + 57 cells/mm^3 (week 4)	Four Pooled Combination Arms^c + 97 cells/mm^3 (week 4)
Week 12					
NAUC > 1	84%	72%		87%	97%
Median NAUC	1.4	1.2		1.50	2.37
25-25	-	-		47%	82%
50-50	-	-		29%	70%
75-75	-	-		13%	46%
Week 24					
NAUC > 1	89%	68%		81%	97%
Median NAUC	1.5	1.3		1.39	2.10
25-25	51%	43%		54%	85%
50-50	38%	21%		34%	70%
75-75	31%	9%		18%	49%

a Dosage of ZDV used was not the currently approved dose and interval of ZDV 200 mg q4h for 4 weeks, followed by 100 mg q4h.
b Reduced to 100 mg q4h ZDV when dose was approved.
c The pooled concomitant regimens of Zalcitabine + ZDV included:
A = Zalcitabine 0.005 mg/kg q8h + ZDV 100 mg q8h
B = Zalcitabine 0.005 mg/kg q8h + ZDV 200 mg q8h
D = Zalcitabine 0.01 mg/kg q8h + ZDV 100 mg q8h
E = Zalcitabine 0.01 mg/kg q8h + ZDV 200 mg q8h

primarily in monotherapy trials. The safety profile of Zalcitabine in children younger than 13 years of age and in asymptomatic HIV-infected individuals has not been established.

Patients receiving Zalcitabine or any other antiretroviral therapy may continue to develop opportunistic infections and other complications of HIV infection, and therefore, should remain under close clinical observation by physicians experienced in the treatment of patients with HIV-associated diseases.

1. Renal Impairment: Patients with renal impairment (estimated creatinine clearance < 55 mL/mim) may be at a greater risk of toxicity from Zalcitabine due to decreased drug clearance. Zalcitabine dosage reduction for patients with more impaired renal function should be considered as follows: estimated creatinine clearance 10 to 40 mL/min—reduce the Zalcitabine dose to 0.750 mg q12h; estimated creatinine clearance < 10 mL/min—reduce the Zalcitabine dose to 0.750 mg q24h.

2. Hepatic Impairment: The use of Zalcitabine may be associated with exacerbation of hepatic dysfunction, especially in individuals with preexisting liver disease or with a history of ethanol abuse. Of 85 patients in the expanded-access safety study (N3544) with a prior history of liver function test (LFT) elevation before starting Zalcitabine, 10 (12%) developed increases in LFTs > 5 times the upper limit of normal while on Zalcitabine. Such patients should be closely monitored by their physician, and dose reduction or interruption of drug therapy should be considered if necessary. Zidovudine use has also been associated with increases in liver function tests.

Information for Patients: Patients should be informed that Zalcitabine is not a cure for HIV infection, that they may continue to develop illnesses associated with advanced HIV infection including opportunistic infections, and that Zalcitabine has not been shown to reduce the incidence or frequency of such illnesses. Since it is frequently difficult to determine whether symptoms are a result of drug effect or underlying disease manifestation, patients should be encouraged to report all changes in their condition to their physician. Patients should be informed that the use of Zalcitabine or other antiretroviral drugs do not preclude the ongoing need to maintain practices designed to prevent transmission of HIV. Patients should be instructed that the major toxicity of Zalcitabine is peripheral neuropathy. Pancreatitis is another serious and potentially life-threatening toxicity that has been reported in < 1% of patients treated with Zalcitabine monotherapy. Patients should be advised of the early symptoms of both of these conditions and instructed to promptly report them to their physician. Since the development of peripheral neuropathy appears to be dose-related to Zalcitabine, patients should be advised to follow their physicians' instructions regarding the prescribed dose. Patients should be informed that the long-term effects of Zalcitabine in combination with zidovudine are presently unknown.

Women of childbearing age should use effective contraception while using Zalcitabine.

Laboratory Tests: Complete blood counts and clinical chemistry tests should be performed prior to initiating combination therapy with Zalcitabine and zidovudine and at appropriate intervals thereafter. Baseline testing of serum amylase and triglyceride levels should be performed in individuals with a prior history of pancreatitis, increased amylase, those on parenteral nutrition or with a history of ethanol abuse.

Drug Interactions: The concomitant use of Zalcitabine with drugs that have the potential to cause peripheral neuropathy should be avoided where possible. Drugs which have been associated with peripheral neuropathy include chloramphenicol, cisplatin, dapsone, disulfiram, ethionamide, glutethimide, gold, hydralazine, iodoquinol, isoniazid, metronidazole, nitrofurantoin, phenytoin, ribavirin and vincristine. Concomitant use of Zalcitabine with didanosine is not recommended.

Drugs such as amphotercin, foscarnet and aminoglycosides may increase the risk of developing peripheral neuropathy or other Zalcitabine associated toxicities by interfering with the renal clearance of Zalcitabine (and thereby raising systemic exposure). Patients who require the use of one of these drugs with Zalcitabine and zidovudine should have frequent clinical and laboratory monitoring with dosage adjustment for any significant change in renal function.

Treatment with Zalcitabine should be interrupted when the use of a drug that has the potential to cause pancreatitis is required. One death due to fulminant pancreatitis possibly related to Zalcitabine and intravenous pentamidine was reported. If intravenous pentamidine is required to treat *Pneumocystis carinii* pneumonia, treatment with Zalcitabine should be interrupted (see *"Warnings"*).

Possible interactions of Zalcitabine with other concomitant medications have not been formally investigated.

Carcinogenesis, Mutagenesis and Impairment of Fertility: Carcinogenesis: Carcinogenicity studies in animals have not yet been performed.

Mutagenesis: Ames tests using seven different tester strains, with and without metabolic activation, were performed with no evidence of mutagenicity. Chinese hamster lung cell tests, with and without metabolic activation, and mouse lymphoma cell tests were performed and there was no evidence of mutagenicity. An unscheduled DNA synthesis assay was performed in rat hepatocytes with no increases in DNA repair. Human peripheral blood lymphocytes were exposed to Zalcitabine, with and without metabolic activation, and at 1.5 mcg/mL and higher, dose-related increases in chromosomal aberration were seen. Oral doses of Zalcitabine at 2500 and 4500 mg/kg were clastogenic in the mouse micronucleus assay.

Impairment of Fertility: Fertility and reproductive performance were assessed in rats at plasma concentrations up to 2142 times those achieved with the maximum recommended human dose (MRHD) based on AUC measurements. No adverse effects on rate of conception or general reproductive performance were observed. The highest dose was associated with embryolethality and evidence of teratogenicity. The next lower dose studied (plasma concentrations equivalent to 485 times the MRHD) was associated with a lower frequency of embryotoxicity but no teratogenicity.

Pregnancy: Teratogenic Effects. Pregnancy Category C. Zalcitabine has been shown to be teratogenic in mice at calculated exposure levels of 1365 and 2730 times that at the MRHD (based on AUC measurements). In rats, Zalcitabine was teratogenic at a calculated exposure level of 2142 times the MRHD but not at an exposure level of 485 times the MRHD. There are no adequate and well-controlled studies of Zalcitabine in pregnant women. Zalcitabine should be used during pregnancy only if the potential benefit justifies the potential risk to the fetus. Fertile women should not receive Zalcitabine unless they are using effective contraception during therapy.

Nonteratogenic Effects: Increased embryolethality was observed in pregnant mice at doses 2730 times the MRHD and in rats above 485 times the MRHD (based on AUC measurements). Average fetal body weight was significantly decreased in mice at doses of 1365 times the MRHD and in rats at 2142 times the MRHD.

Nursing Mothers: It is not known whether Zalcitabine is excreted in human milk. Because many drugs are excreted in human milk and the potential exists for serious adverse reactions from Zalcitabine in nursing infants, a decision should be made whether to discontinue nursing or to discontinue the drug, taking into account the importance of the drug to the mother. It is currently recommended practice in the United States that HIV-infected women do not breastfeed infants regardless of the use of antiretroviral agents.

Pediatric Use: Safety and effectiveness of Zalcitabine in combination with zidovudine or as monotherapy in HIV-infected children younger than 13 years of age has not been established.

ADVERSE REACTIONS

(See "Warnings"). *Only limited safety data are available on the combined use of Zalcitabine with Zidovudine.* The following data on adverse reactions are based primarily on the administration of Zalcitabine at the recommended dose, as a single agent, to patients with AIDS or advanced ARC (CD4 cell count ≤ 200 cells/mm³). Table 3 summarizes the occurrence of moderate or severe peripheral neuropathy. Table 4 summarizes clinical adverse events or symptoms at least possibly related to Zalcitabine therapy that occurred in at least 3% of all Zalcitabine treated patients with advanced HIV disease who were enrolled in the two comparative monotherapy trials (N3300/ACTG 114, N3492/ACTG 119) of Zalcitabine versus zidovudine. Clinical adverse events in the combination Zalcitabine and zidovudine Protocol N3447/ACTG 106 are included in Table 5. (See related table).
(See related table).

Table 5

NUMBER AND PERCENTAGE OF PATIENTS WITH CLINICAL ADVERSE EXPERIENCES CONSIDERED POSSIBLY OR PROBABLY RELATED TO STUDY DRUG OCCURRING IN > 3% OF PATIENTS

Body System/ Adverse Event	Zalcitabine + ZDV Combination Trial Pooled Concomitant Regimens[a]	N3447/lACTG 106[b]—No Prior ZDV
	n = 47 (%)	
	mild/mod/sev	mod/sev
Peripheral Neuropathy	SEE TABLE 3	
Gastrointestinal		
Nausea	17 (36.2)	4 (8.5)
Oral Ulcers	13 (27.7)	2 (4.3)
Abdominal Pain	10 (21.3)	4 (8.5)
Diarrhea	7 (14.9)	5 (10.6)
Vomiting	7 (14.9)	1 (2.1)
Anorexia	6 (12.8)	3 (6.4)
Constipation	3 (6.4)	1 (2.1)
Skin and Appendages		
Pruritus	7 (14.9)	2 (4.3)
Rash	7 (14.9)	1 (2.1)
Erythematous Rash	3 (6.4)	1 (2.1)
Night Sweats	3 (6.4)	1 (2.1)
Maculopapular Rash	2 (4.3)	1 (2.1)
Follicular Rash	2 (4.3)	0 (0.0)
Central and Periph NS		
Headache	18 (38.3)	4 (8.5)
Musculoskeletal		
Myalgia	7 (14.9)	1 (2.1)
Arthralgia	4 (8.5)	1 (2.1)
Body as a Whole		
Fatigue	16 (34.0)	4 (8.5)
Fever	7 (14.9)	1 (2.1)
Rigors	4 (8.5)	1 (2.1)
Chest Pain	3 (6.4)	1 (2.1)

	Zalcitabine + ZDV Combination Trial Pooled Concomitant Regimens[a]		N3447/lACTG 106[b]—No Prior ZDV	
	n = 47 (%)			
Body System/ Adverse Event	mild/mod/sev		mod/sev	
Weight Decrease	3	(6.4)	2	(4.3)
Respiratory				
Pharyngitis	4	(8.5)	1	(2.1)

a Excluded are 9 patients who received ZDV alone for the greater part of the study. Only 8 patients were treated with the recommended combination regimen; all other patients were treated at lower doses of Zalcitabine and/or ZDV.

b Median duration of treatment ranged from 22 to 92 weeks among the arms.

Monotherapy Trials: Clinical adverse events of all intensities classified as at least possibly related to Zalcitabine that occurred in < 3% of Zalcitabine treated patients in N3300/ACTG 114 are listed below. Events are listed in decreasing order of frequency within each body system.

Body as a Whole: weight decrease (1.9%); chest pain (1.6%); fever, asthenia, pain, substernal chest pain (< 1%).

Cardiovascular: heart racing (1%).

Gastrointestinal: abdominal pain (< 2.8%); diarrhea (2.5%); vomiting (2.2%); dry mouth (1.6%); esophageal ulcers (1.6%); dyspepsia (1.3%); glossitis (1.3%); constipation, esophageal pain, rectal hemorrhage, hemorrhoids, rectal ulcers, flatulence, tongue ulceration, enlarged abdomen, gum disorder (< 1%).

Hepatic: hepatocellular damage, hepatitis (< 1%).

Musculoskeletal: arthralgia (1.9%); shoulder pain, leg cramps, foot pain (< 1%).

Nervous: hypertonia, tremor, hand tremor, twitching (< 1%).

Psychiatric: confusion (1.3%); impaired concentration (1.3%); amnesia, insomnia, somnolence, depression (< 1%).

Respiratory: pharyngitis (2.2%); coughing, dyspnea, cyanosis (< 1%).

Skin: dermatitis (1.3%); maculopapular rash, night sweats, alopecia, urticaria, erythematous papules (< 1%).

Special Senses and Vision: taste perversion, xerophthalmia, abnormal vision, eye pain, tinnitus (< 1%).

Table 3
PERCENTAGE OF PATIENTS WITH MODERATE OR SEVERE PERIPHERAL NEUROPATHY[a]

Study[b]	N3300/ACTG 114		N3492/ACTG 119		N3447/ACTG 106
Investigator's Assessment of Relationship	Zalcitabine 0.750 mg q8h n = 320	ZDV[c] 200 mg q4h n = 318	Zalcitabine 0.750 mg q8h n = 59	ZDV 100 mg q4h n = 52	Zalcitabine + ZDV Pooled Concomitant Regimens n = 47[e]
All Relationships[f]	31	12	24	10	21
Possible/Probable	20	6	17	0	4

a All adverse events related to peripheral neuropathy were pooled to include all potentially related signs and symptoms of neuopathy (i.e., tingling, numbness, weakness, or pain of the hands/arms or feet/legs).

b Median duration of treatment for N3300 was a 44 weeks for Zalcitabine 53 weeks for ZDV; for N3492, 39 weeks for Zalcitabine, 25 weeks for ZDV and for N3447 treatment ranged from 22 to 92 weeks among the arms.

c Reduced to 100 mg q4h ZDV when dose was approved.

d 315 patients randomized to ZDV arm. 3 patients randomized to Zalcitabine inadvertently received ZDV for short periods; they did not develop any symptoms of neuropathy. For safety analyses, the 3 patients were included in the denominators of both Zalcitabine and ZDV arms.

e Excluded are 9 patients who received ZDV alone for the greater part of the study. Only 8 patients were treated with the recommended combination regimen; all other patients were treated at lower doses of Zalcitabine and/or ZDV.

f Unrelated, remotely, possibly or probably related to drug therapy.

Table 4
PERCENTAGE OF PATIENTS WITH CLINICAL ADVERSE EXPERIENCES CONSIDERED POSSIBLY OR PROBABLY RELATED TO STUDY DRUG OCCURRING IN > 3% OF PATIENTS TREATED IN ZALCITABINE MONOTHERAPY TRIALS

	N3300/ACTG 114[a] ≤ 3 Months Prior ZDV				N3492/ACTG 119[a] ≥ 12 Months Prior ZDV			
	Zalcitabine 0.750 mg q8h n = 320		ZDV[b] 200 mg q4h n = 318[c]		Zalcitabine 0.750 mg q8h n = 59		ZDV[b] 100 mg q4h N = 52	
Body System/ Adverse Event	mild/ mod/ sev	mod/ sev	mild/ mod/ sev	mod/ sev	mild/ mod/ sev	mod/ sev	mild/ mod/ sev	mod/ sev
Peripheral Neuopathy				SEE TABLE 3				
Gastrointestinal								
Oral Ulcers	13.4	7.8	6.3	3.1	16.9	15.3	1.9	1.9
Nausea	7.2	2.8	19.5	8.2	3.4	1.7	0.0	0.0
Dysphagia	3.4	3.1	0.0	0.0	1.7	1.7	0.0	0.0
Anorexia	3.1	1.9	6.0	2.5	0.0	0.0	0.0	0.0
Abdominal Pain	2.8	0.9	2.5	1.6	5.1	3.4	0.0	0.0
Vomiting	2.2	0.9	5.0	3.5	1.7	1.7	0.0	0.0
Skin and Appendages								
Rash	7.8	4.1	5.3	3.1	0.0	0.0	0.0	0.0
Pruritus	4.7	2.8	5.3	2.2	0.0	0.0	0.0	0.0
Central and Periph NS								
Headache	8.8	5.0	12.6	6.6	0.0	0.0	0.0	0.0
Dizziness	3.1	1.3	2.8	1.3	0.0	0.0	0.0	0.0
Musculoskeletal								
Myalgia	5.3	2.2	6.3	3.1	1.7	1.7	1.9	1.9
Body as a Whole								
Fatigue	7.8	3.8	12.3	8.5	3.4	3.4	3.8	3.8
Respiratory								
Pharyngitis	2.2	1.9	0.0	0.0	5.1	3.4	0.0	0.0

a Median duration of treatment for N3300 was 44 weeks for Zalcitabine 53 weeks for ZDV; for N3492, treatment was 39 weeks for Zalcitabine 25 weeks for ZDV.

b Reduced to 100 mg q4h ZDV when dose was approved.

c 315 patients randomized to ZDV arm. 3 patients on Zalcitabine inadvertently received ZDV. For safety analyses, the 3 patients were included in the denominators of both Zalcitabine and ZDV arms.

Urinary System: micturition frequency, abnormal renal function, acute renal failure, renal cyst (< 1%).

Table 6 summarizes protocol grades 3-4 laboratory abnormalities occurring in Zalcitabine monotherapy Protocols N3300/ACTG 114, N3492/ACTG 119 and combination Zalcitabine and zidovudine Protocol N3447/ACTG 106. (See related table).

Clinical adverse events and protocol grades 3-4 laboratory abnormalities that occurred in > 1% of patients in the expanded-access safety study (N3544) are listed in Tables 7 and 8. The median duration of treatment was 16 weeks. (See related table).

Table 8
PERCENTAGE OF PATIENTS WITH LABORATORY ABNORMALITIES[a]

Expanded Access (N3544)[b]

Dose Comparison Randomized
ZDV Intolerant, ZDV Failure

n = 3479

Laboratory Abnormality	Zalcitabine 0.375 mg q8h n = 1757	Zalcitabine 0.750 mg q8h n = 1722
Anemia (< 7.6 gm/dL)	3.5	4.1
Leukopenia		

	Zalcitabine 0.375 mg q8h n = 1757	Zalcitabine 0.750 mg q8h n = 1722
(< 1500 cells/mm^3)	8.8	10.2
Neutropenia (< 750 cells/mm^3)	9.3	9.5
Eosinophilia (> 1000 or 25%)	2.0	2.8
Thrombocytopenia (< 50,000 cells/mm^3)	3.2	2.3
SGPT (> 250 U/L)	2.7	3.3
SGOT (> 250 U/L)	2.4	2.6
Alkaline Phosphatase (> 650 U/L)	2.8	2.3

a All percentages based on number patients tested, not on number of patients in study.
b Median duration of treatment was 16 weeks.

Clinical adverse events at least possibly related to Zalcitabine occurring in < 1% of patients treated with either 0.375 mg or 0.750 mg q8h Zalcitabine in the expanded-access safety study (N3544) are listed below by body system:

Body as a Whole: fatigue, fever, pain, malaise, asthenia, chest pain, generalized edema, weight decrease.

Cardiovascular: hypertension, palpitation, syncope, atrial fibrillation, tachycardia.

Table 6
PERCENTAGE OF PATIENTS WITH LABORATORY ABNORMALITIES[a]

	Monotherapy				Combination Therapy
	N3300/ACTG 114		N3492/ACTG 119		N3447/ACTG 106
	≤ 3 Months Prior ZDV		≥ 12 Months Prior ZDV		No Prior ZDV
	n = 635		n = 111		n = 47
Laboratory Abnormality	Zalcitabine 0.750 mg q8h n = 320	ZDV[b] 200 mg q4h n = 315	Zalcitabine 0.750 mg q8h n = 59	ZDV 100 mg q4h n = 52	Pooled LN Concomitant Regimens n = 47[c]
Anemia (< 7.5 g/dL)	5.0	14.3	5.1	7.7	8.5
Leukopenia (< 1500 cells/mm^3)	9.4	12.1	11.9	15.4	2.1
Neutropenia (< 750 cells/mm^3)	8.8	19.7	5.1	11.5	8.5
Eosinophilia (< 1000 or 25%)	5.8	2.3	5.2	0.0	4.3
Thrombocytopenia (> 50,000 cells/mm^3)	4.4	2.9	0.0	5.8	4.3
SGPT (> 250 U/L)	10.0	8.6	8.5	7.7	8.5
SGOT (> 250 U/L)	5.6	5.1	6.8	5.8	4.3
Alkaline Phosphatase (> 625 U/L)	3.1	3.2	0.0	9.6	2.1

a All percentages based on number of patients tested, not on number of patients in study. Median duration of treatment for N3300 was 44 weeks for Zalcitabine, 53 weeks for ZDV; for N3492, 39 weeks for Zalcitabine, 25 weeks for ZDV and for N3447 treatment ranged from 22 to 92 weeks among the arms.
b Reduced to 100 mg q4h ZDV when dose was approved.
c Excluded are 9 patients who received ZDV alone for the greater part of the study. Only 8 patients were treated with the recommended combination regimen: all other patients were treated at lower doses of Zalcitabine and/or ZDV

Table 7
PERCENTAGE OF PATIENTS WITH CLINICAL ADVERSE EXPERIENCES CONSIDERED POSSIBLY OR PROBABLY RELATED TO STUDY DRUG OCCURRING IN > 1% OF PATIENTS TREATED IN THE ZALCITABINE EXPANDED-ACCESS PROGRAM

N3544[a]
ZDV Intolerant or Failure

Body System/ Adverse Event	Zalcitabine 0.375 mg q8h n = 1757		Zalcitabine 0.750 mg q8h n = 1722	
	mild/mod/sev	mod/sev	mild/mod/sev	mod/sev
Peripheral Neuropathy	10.8	5.9	14.9	7.8
Gastrointestinal				
Nausea	1.5	0.8	1.5	0.9
Ulcerative Stomatitis	1.4	0.6	2.6	1.7
Abdominal Pain	1.3	0.9	1.2	0.6
Aphthous Stomatitis	1.1	0.6	2.2	1.3
Diarrhea	0.9	0.4	1.0	0.6
Skin and Appendages				
Rash	1.2	0.6	1.4	0.6
Central and Periph NS				
Headache	0.7	0.2	1.2	0.7
Musculoskeletal				
Pain, Feet	0.9	0.3	2.1	1.2

a Median duration of treatment was 16 weeks.

► SHOWN IN PRODUCT IDENTIFICATION GUIDE

Gastrointestinal: vomiting, increased amylase, flatulence, anorexia, dyspepsia, esophageal ulcers, stomatitis, tongue ulceration, constipation, dry mouth, dysphagia, eructation, gastritis, gastrointestinal hemorrhage, pancreatitis, glossitis, left quadrant pain, salivary gland enlargement jaundice, esophageal pain, esophagitis, rectal ulcers.

Endocrine: diabetes mellitus, hyperglycemia, hypocalcemia, impotence, hot flushes.

Hematologic: epistaxis.

Hepatic: abnormal hepatic function, hepatitis, jaundice.

Musculoskeletal: myalgia, arm pain, arthralgia, arthritis, arthropathy, cold feet, leg cramps, myositis, shoulder pain, wrist pain, cold extremities.

Nervous: seizures, ataxia, abnormal coordination, Bell's palsy, dizziness, dysphonia, hyperkinesia, hypokinesia, migraine, neuralgia, neuritis, stupor, tremor, vertigo.

Psychiatric: insomnia, agitation, depersonalization, hallucination, emotional lability, nervousness, confusion, anxiety, depression, euphoria, manic reaction, dementia, amnesia, somnolence, abnormal thinking, impaired concentration, abnormal crying.

Respiratory: pharyngitis, coughing, dyspnea, flu-like symptoms.

Skin: maculopapular rash, pruritus, dermatitis, skin lesions, acne, alopecia, bullous eruptions, follicular rash, flushing, increased sweating, urticaria.

Special Senses and Vision: abnormal vision, ear blockage, parosmia, loss of taste, taste perversion, burning eyes, eye itching, eye abnormality, deafness.

Urinary System: gout, toxic nephropathy, polyuria, renal calculus, acute renal failure, hyperuricemia.

Combination Trials: Only limited safety data are available on the combined use of Zalcitabine with zidovudine. One patient with advanced HIV disease in study N3447/ACTG 106 died of refractory acidosis, mild pancreatitis, hepatomegaly with steatosis, and an unexplained neurological syndrome. The investigator assessed this event as remotely related to zidovudine and/or the combination of Zalcitabine and zidovudine. Adverse events observed in this study are listed in Table 5. Only eight patients were treated with the recommended combination regimen: all other patients were treated with lower doses of Zalcitabine and/or zidovudine. The occurrence of clinical adverse events at each dosage combination of Zalcitabine and zidovudine did not vary significantly. There are no safety data currently available from the BW 34.225-02 study.

OVERDOSAGE

Acute Overdosage: There is little experience with acute Zalcitabine overdosage and the sequelae are unknown. There is no known antidote for Zalcitabine overdosage. It is not known whether Zalcitabine is dialyzable by peritoneal dialysis or hemodialysis.

Chronic Overdosage: In an initial dose-finding study in which Zalcitabine was administered at doses 25 times (0.25 mg/kg q8h) the currently recommended dose, one patient discontinued Zalcitabine after one and one-half weeks of treatment subsequent to the development of a rash and fever. In the early Phase 1 studies, all patients receiving Zalcitabine at approximately six times the current total daily recommended dose experienced peripheral neuropathy by week 10. Eighty percent of patients who received approximately two times the current total daily recommended dose experienced peripheral neuropathy by week 12.

DOSAGE AND ADMINISTRATION

The recommended combination regimen is one 0.750 mg tablet of Zalcitabine orally, administered concomitantly with 200 mg of zidovudine every 8 hours (2.25 mg Zalcitabine total daily dose and 600 mg zidovudine total daily dose). Based on pharmacokinetic weight-ranging data, there is no need to dose-reduce for weight down to 30 kg.

Monitoring of Patients: Periodic complete blood counts and clinical chemistry tests should be performed. Serum anylase levels should be monitored in those individuals who have a history of elevated amylase, pancreatitis, ethanol abuse, who are on parenteral nutrition or who are otherwise at high risk of pancreatitis. Careful monitoring for signs or symptoms suggestive of peripheral neuropathy is recommended, particularly in individuals with a low CD4 cell count or who are at a greater risk of developing peripheral neuropathy while on therapy (see *"Warnings"*).

Dose Adjustment for Combination Therapy with Zalcitabine and Zidovudine: For recipients of combination therapy with Zalcitabine and zidovudine, dose adjustments for either drug should be based on the known toxicity profile of the individual drugs. For toxicities more likely to be associated with Zalcitabine (eg., peripheral neuropathy, severe oral ulcers). Zalcitabine should be interrupted or dose-reduced (see *"Warnings"* and *"Precautions"*). For patients experiencing toxicities more likely to be associated with zidovudine (e.g., anemia, granulocytopenia), zidovudine should be interrupted or dose-reduced first. For any interruption of Zalcitabine and especially if Zalcitabine is permanently discontinued, the zidovudine dosage schedule should be adjusted from 200 mg q8h to 100 mg q4h as recommended in the complete product information for zidovudine. FOR SEVERE TOXICITIES OR TOXICITIES IN WHICH THE CAUSATIVE DRUG IS UNCLEAR OR THOSE PERSISTING AFTER DOSE INTERRUPTION OR REDUCTION OF ONE DRUG, THE OTHER DRUG SHOULD ALSO BE INTERRUPTED OR DOSE-REDUCED. PHYSICIANS SHOULD REFER TO THE COMPLETE PRODUCT INFORMATION FOR ZIDOVU-DINE FOR A DESCRIPTION OF KNOWN ZIDOVUDINE-ASSOCIATED ADVERSE REACTIONS. Since Zalcitabine is not indicated for use as monotherapy, alternative antiretroviral therapy should be considered for patients who are unable to tolerate zidovudine as part of a combination regimen with Zalcitabine. Patients developing moderate discomfort with signs or symptoms of peripheral neuropathy (e.g., numbness, tingling, hypesthesias, burning or shooting pains of the lower or upper extremities, or loss of vibratory sense or ankle reflex), should stop Zalcitabine, especially when these symptoms are bilateral and progress for > 72 hours. Zalcitabine-associated peripheral neuropathy may continue to worsen despite interruption of Zalcitabine, Zalcitabine should be reintroduced at 50% dose—0.375 mg q8h only if all findings related to peripheral neuropathy have improved to mild symptoms. Zalcitabine should be permanently discontinued when patients experience severe discomfort related to peripheral neuropathy or moderate discomfort progressing for $\geq$ 1 week. If other moderate to severe clinical adverse reactions or laboratory abnormalities (such as increased liver function tests) occur, then both Zalcitabine and zidovudine should be interrupted until the adverse reaction abates. Either zidovudine monotherapy or Zalcitabine and zidovudine therapy should then be carefully reintroduced at lower doses if appropriate. If adverse reactions recur at the reduced dose, therapy should be discontinued. The minimum effective dose of Zalcitabine in combination with zidovudine for the treatment of adult patients with advanced HIV infection has not been established.

In patients with poor bone marrow reserve, particularly those patients with advanced symptomatic HIV disease, frequent monitoring of hematologic indices is recommended to detect serious anemia or granulocytopenia (see *"Warnings"*). Significant toxicities, such as anemia (hemoglobin of < 7.5 g/dL or reduction of $\leq$ 25% of baseline) and/or granulocytopenia (granulocyte count of < 750 cells/mm^3 or reduction of > 50% from baseline), may require treatment interruption of Zalcitabine and zidovudine until evidence of marrow recovery is observed (see *"Warnings"*). For less severe anemia or granulocytopenia, a reduction in daily dose of zidovudine may be adequate. In patients who experience hematologic toxicity, reduction in hemoglobin may occur as early as 2 to 4 weeks after initiation of therapy, and granulocytopenia usually occurs after 6 to 8 weeks of therapy. In patients who develop significant anemia, dose modification does not necessarily eliminate the need for transfusion. If marrow recovery occurs following dose modification, gradual increases in dose may be appropriate depending on hematologic indices and patient tolerance. For more details, refer to the complete product information for zidovudine.

Storage: The tablets should be stored in tightly closed bottles at 59° to 87°F (15° to 30°C).

REFERENCES
1. Pizzo PA. Butler K. Balis, F, et al. Dideoxycytidine alone and in an alternating schedule with zid,vudine in children with symptomatic human immunodeficiency virus infection. *J Pediatr.* 1990;117(5):799-808. 2. meng. TC, Fischl MA, Boota AH, et al. Combination therapy with zidovudine and dideoxycytidine in patients with advanced human immunodeficiency virus infection. *Ann Intern Med.* 1992:116:13-20.

HOW SUPPLIED
TABLETS: 0.375 MG

BRAND/MANUFACTURER	NDC	SIZE	AWP
○ BRAND			
► HIVID: Roche Labs	00004-0220-01	100s	$170.40

TABLETS: 0.75 MG

BRAND/MANUFACTURER	NDC	SIZE	AWP
○ BRAND			
► HIVID: Roche Labs	00004-0221-01	100s	$213.60

Zanosar *SEE* STREPTOZOCIN

Zantac *SEE* RANITIDINE HYDROCHLORIDE

Zarontin *SEE* ETHOSUXIMIDE

Zaroxolyn *SEE* METOLAZONE

Zartan *SEE* CEPHALEXIN

Zebeta *SEE* BISOPROLOL FUMARATE

◆ RATED THERAPEUTICALLY EQUIVALENT; ◇ THERAPEUTIC EQUIVALENCE UNCONFIRMED; ○ UNRATED

Zefazone SEE CEFMETAZOLE SODIUM

Zemuron SEE ROCURONIUM BROMIDE

Zenate SEE VITAMINS, PRENATAL

Zerit SEE STAVUDINE

Zestoretic SEE HYDROCHLOROTHIAZIDE AND LISINOPRIL

Zestril SEE LISINOPRIL

Ziac SEE BISOPROLOL FUMARATE WITH HYDROCHLOROTHIAZIDE

Zidovudine

> **WARNING: ZIDOVUDINE MAY BE ASSOCIATED WITH HEMATOLOGIC TOXICITY INCLUDING GRANULOCYTOPENIA AND SEVERE ANEMIA REQUIRING TRANSFUSIONS, PARTICULARLY IN PATIENTS WITH ADVANCED HIV DISEASE (SEE WARNINGS). PROLONGED USE OF ZIDOVUDINE HAS ALSO BEEN ASSOCIATED WITH SYMPTOMATIC MYOPATHY SIMILAR TO THAT PRODUCED BY HUMAN IMMUNODEFICIENCY VIRUS.**
>
> RARE OCCURRENCES OF LACTIC ACIDOSIS IN THE ABSENCE OF HYPOXEMIA, AND SEVERE HEPATOMEGALY WITH STEATOSIS HAVE BEEN REPORTED WITH USE OF ZIDOVUDINE AND ARE POTENTIALLY FATAL. THESE EVENTS MAY OR MAY NOT BE CAUSALLY RELATED TO ZIDOVUDINE (SEE WARNINGS).
>
> BECAUSE ZIDOVUDINE HAS BEEN SHOWN TO PROLONG SURVIVAL AND DECREASE THE INCIDENCE OF OPPORTUNISTIC INFECTIONS (OI'S) IN PATIENTS WITH ADVANCED HIV DISEASE, AND TO DELAY DISEASE PROGRESSION IN ASYMPTOMATIC HIV-INFECTED PATIENTS, ZIDOVUDINE SHOULD BE CONSIDERED AS INITIAL THERAPY FOR ADULT PATIENTS WITH HIV INFECTION WHO HAVE EVIDENCE OF IMPAIRED IMMUNITY (CD4 CELL COUNTS OF $\leq$ 500 CELLS/MM^3.
>
> HOWEVER, RANDOMIZED STUDIES HAVE SHOWN THAT FOR SOME PATIENTS WITH ADVANCED DISEASE ON PROLONGED THERAPY WITH ZIDOVUDINE, CHANGING TO OTHER ANTIRETROVIRAL REGIMENS MAY BE MORE EFFECTIVE THAN REMAINING ON MONOTHERAPY WITH ZIDOVUDINE. IT IS UNKNOWN IF THE USE OF ZIDOVUDINE PROLONGS SURVIVAL IN PATIENTS WITH CD4 CELL COUNTS $\geq$ 200 CELLS/MM^3 AT THE INITIATION OF THERAPY.
>
> IN ADDITION, PATIENTS TREATED WITH ZIDOVUDINE MAY CONTINUE TO DEVELOP OPPORTUNITIC INFECTIONS (OI'S) AND OTHER COMPLICATIONS OF THE ACQUIRED IMMUNODEFICIENCY SYNDROME (AIDS) AND AIDS RELATED COMPLEX (ARC) CAUSED BY THE HUMAN IMMUNODEFICIENCY VIRUS (HIV). THEREFORE, PATIENTS ON ZIDOVUDINE SHOULD BE UNDER CLOSE CLINICAL OBSERVATION BY PHYSICIANS EXPERIENCED IN THE TREATMENT OF PATIENTS WITH DISEASES ASSOCIATED WITH HIV. THE SAFETY AND EFFICACY OF ZIDOVUDINE HAVE BEEN ESTABLISHED ONLY FOR CERTAIN ADULT AIDS AND ADVANCED ARC PATIENTS (SEE "INDICATIONS AND USAGE").

DESCRIPTION

Zidovudine [formerly called azidothymidine (AZT)] is an antiretroviral drug active against human immunodeficiency virus (HIV).

Capsules: Zidovudine Capsules are for oral administration. Each capsule contains 100 mg of Zidovudine.

Syrup: Zidovudine Syrup is for oral administration. Each teaspoonful (5 mL) of Zidovudine Syrup contains 50 mg of Zidovudine.

I.V. Infusion: Zidovudine Infusion is a sterile solution for intravenous infusion only. Each mL contains 10 mg Zidovudine in Water for Injection.

The chemical name of Zidovudine is 3'-azido-3'-deoxythymidine.

Zidovudine is a white to beige, odorless, crystalline solid with a molecular weight of 267.24 and a solubility of 20.1 mg/mL in water at 25°C. The molecular formula is $C_{10}H_{13}N_5O_4$.

Following is its chemical structure:

CLINICAL PHARMACOLOGY

Zidovudine is an inhibitor of the *in vitro* replication of some retroviruses including HIV (also known as HTLV III, LAV, or ARV). This drug is a thymidine analogue in which the 3'-hydroxy (-OH) group is replaced by an azido (-N$_3$) group. Cellular thymidine kinase converts Zidovudine into Zidovudine monophosphate. The monophosphate is further converted into the diphosphate by cellular thymidylate kinase and to the triphosphate derivative by other cellular enzymes. Zidovudine triphosphate interferes with the HIV viral RNA dependent DNA polymerase (reverse transcriptase) and thus, inhibits viral replication. Zidovudine triphosphate also inhibits cellular α-DNA polymerase, but at concentrations 100-fold higher than those required to inhibit reverse transcriptase. *In vitro,* Zidovudine triphosphate has been shown to be incorporated into growing chains of DNA by viral reverse transcriptase. When incorporation by the viral enzyme occurs, the DNA chain is terminated. Studies in cell culture suggest that Zidovudine incorporation by cellular α-DNA polymerase may occur, but only to a very small extent and not in all test systems. Cellular γ-DNA polymerase shows some sensitivity to inhibition by the Zidovudine triphosphate with 50% inhibitory concentration (IC$_{50}$) values 400 to 900 times greater than that for HIV reverse transcriptase. Chain termination has not been demonstrated with either cellular α- or γ-DNA polymerases.

Microbiology: The relationship between *in vitro* susceptibility of HIV to Zidovudine and the inhibition of HIV replication in man or clinical response to therapy has not been established. *In vitro* sensitivity results vary greatly depending upon the time between virus infection and Zidovudine treatment of cell cultures, the particular assay used, the cell type employed, and the laboratory performing the test. In addition, the methods currently used to establish virologic responses in clinical trials may be relatively insensitive in detecting changes in the quantities of actively replicating HIV or reactivation of these viruses.

Zidovudine blocked 90% of detectable HIV replication *in vitro* at concentrations of $\leq$ 0.13 μg/mL (ID$_{90}$) when added shortly after laboratory infection of susceptible cells. This level of antiviral effect was observed in experiments measuring reverse transcriptase activity in HIV-infected H9 cells, PHA stimulated peripheral blood lymphocytes, and unstimulated peripheral blood lymphocytes. The concentration of drug required to produce a 50% decrease in supernatant reverse transcriptase was 0.013 μg/mL (ID$_{50}$) in both H9 cells and peripheral blood lymphocytes. Zidovudine at concentrations of 0.13 μg/mL also provided > 90% protection from a strain of HIV (HTLV IIIB) induced cytopathic effects in two tetanus-specific T4 cell lines. Gag protein expression was also undetectable at the same concentration in these cells. Partial inhibition of viral activity in cells with chronic HIV infection (presumed to carry integrated HIV DNA) required concentrations of Zidovudine (8.8 μg/mL in one laboratory to 13.3 μg/mL in another) which are approximately 100 times as high as those necessary to block HIV replication in acutely infected cells. HIV isolates from 18 untreated individuals with AIDS or ARC had ID$_{50}$ sensitivity values between 0.003 to 0.013 μg/mL and ID$_{95}$ sensitivity values between 0.03 to 0.3 μg/mL.

Zidovudine has been shown to act additively or synergistically with a number of anti-HIV agents, including zalcitabine and interferon-alpha, in inhibiting the replication of HIV in cell culture.

The development of resistance to Zidovudine has been studied extensively. The emergence of resistance is a function of both duration of Zidovudine therapy and stage of disease. Asymptomatic patients developed resistance at significantly slower rates than patients with advanced disease. In contrast, virus isolates from patients with AIDS who received a year or more of Zidovudine may show more than 100-fold increases in ID$_{50}$ compared to isolates pre-therapy.

In vitro resistance to Zidovudine is due to the accumulation of specific mutations in the HIV reverse transcriptase coding region. Five amino acid substitutions (Met 41 → Leu, A67 → Asn, Lys70 → Arg, Thr215 → Tyr or Phe, and Lys219 → Gln) have been described in viruses with decreased *in vitro* susceptibility to Zidovudine inhibition. The extent of resistance appears to be correlated with number of mutations in reverse transcriptase.

A significant correlation between Zidovudine resistance and poor clinical outcome in children with advanced disease has been reported; in addition, a correlation between reduced sensitivity to Zidovudine and lower CD4 cell counts in symptom-free adults treated with Zidovudine for up to three years has also been reported. However, the specific relationship between emergence of Zidovudine resistance and clinical progression of disease in adults has not yet been defined.

Combination therapy of Zidovudine plus zalcitabine does not appear to prevent the emergence of Zidovudine-resistant isolates. *In vitro* studies with Zidovudine-resistant virus isolates indicate Zidovudine-resistant strains are usually sensitive to zalcitabine and didanosine.

➤ SHOWN IN PRODUCT IDENTIFICATION GUIDE

The major metabolite of Zidovudine, 3'-azido-3'-deoxy-5'-O-β-D-glucopyranu-ronosylthymidine (GZDV, formerly called GAZT), does not inhibit HIV replication *in vitro*. GZDV does not antagonize the antiviral effect of Zidovudine *in vitro* nor does GZDV compete with Zidovudine triphosphate as an inhibitor of HIV reverse transcriptase.

The cytotoxicity of Zidovudine for various cell lines was determined using a cell growth inhibition assay. ID_{50} values for several human cell lines showed little growth inhibition by Zidovudine except at concentrations < 50 μg/mL. However, one human T-lymphocyte cell line was sensitive to the cytotoxic effect of Zidovudine with an ID_{50} of 5 μg/mL. Moreover, in a colony-forming unit assay designed to assess the toxicity of Zidovudine for human bone marrow, an ID_{50} value of < 1.25 μg/mL was estimated. Two of ten human lymphocyte cultures tested were found to be sensitive to Zidovudine at 5 μg/mL or less.

Zidovudine has antiviral activity against some other mammalian retroviruses in addition to HIV. Human Immunodeficiency Virus-2 (HIV-2) replication *in vitro* is inhibited by Zidovudine with an ID_{50} of 0.015 μg/mL, while HTLV-1 transmission to susceptible cells is inhibited by 1 to 3 μg/mL concentrations of drug. Several strains of simian immunodeficiency virus (SIV) are also inhibited by Zidovudine with ID_{50} values ranging from 0.13 to 6.5 μg/mL, depending upon species of origin and assay method used. No significant inhibitory activity was exhibited against a variety of other human and animal viruses, except an ID_{50} of 1.4 to 2.7 μg/mL against the Epstein-Barr virus, the clinical significance of which is unknown.

The following microbiological activities of Zidovudine have been observed *in vitro* but the clinical significance is unknown. Many *Enterobacteriaceae*, including strains of *Shigella, Salmonella, Klebsiella, Enterobacter, Citrobacter,* and *Escherichia coli* are inhibited *in vitro* by low concentrations of Zidovudine (0.005 to 0.5 μg/mL). Synergy of Zidovudine with trimethoprim has been observed against some of these bacteria *in vitro*. Limited data suggest that bacterial resistance to Zidovudine develops rapidly. Zidovudine has no activity against gram positive organisms, anaerobes, mycobacteria, or fungal pathogens including *Candida albicans* and *Cryptococcus neoformans*. Although *Giardia lamblia* is inhibited by 1.9 μg/mL of Zidovudine, no activity was observed against other protozoal pathogens.

PHARMACOKINETICS

Adults: The pharmacokinetics of Zidovudine has been evaluated in 22 adult HIV-infected patients in a Phase 1 dose-escalation study. Cohorts of 3 to 7 patients received 1 hour intravenous infusions of Zidovudine ranging from 1 to 2.5 mg/kg every 8 hours to 2.5 to 7.5 mg/kg every 4 hours (3 to 45 mg/kg/day) for 14 to 28 days followed by oral dosing ranging from 2 to 5 mg/kg every 8 hours to 5 to 10 mg/kg every 4 hours (6 to 60 mg/kg/day) for an additional 32 days. After oral dosing, Zidovudine was rapidly absorbed from the gastrointestinal tract with peak serum concentrations occurring within 0.5 to 1.5 hours. Dose-independent kinetics was observed over the range of 2 mg/kg every 8 hours to 10 mg/kg every 4 hours. The mean Zidovudine half-life was approximately 1 hour and ranged from 0.78 to 1.93 hours following oral dosing.

Zidovudine is rapidly metabolized to 3'-azido-3'-deoxy-5'-O-β-D-glucopyranu-ronosylthymidine (GZDV) which has an apparent elimination half-life of 1 hour (range 0.61 to 1.73 hours). Following oral administration, urinary recovery of Zidovudine and GZDV accounted for 14% and 74% of the dose, respectively, and the total urinary recovery averaged 90% (range 63% to 95%), indicating a high degree of absorption. However, as a result of first-pass metabolism, the average oral capsule bioavailability of Zidovudine is 65% (range 52% to 75%). A second metabolite, 3'-amino-3'-deoxythymidine (AMT), has been identified in the plasma following single intravenous administration of Zidovudine. AMT area-under-the-curve (AUC) was one-fifth of the AUC of Zidovudine and had a half-life of 2.7 ± 0.7 hours. In comparison, GZDV AUC was about 3-fold greater than the AUC of Zidovudine.

Additional pharmacokinetic data following intravenous dosing indicated dose-independent kinetics over the range of 1 to 5 mg/kg with a mean Zidovudine half-life of 1.1 hours (range 0.48 to 2.86 hours). Total body clearance averaged 1900 mL/min/70 kg and the apparent volume of distribution was 1.6 L/kg. At an experimental dose schedule of 7.5 mg/kg every 4 hours, total body clearance was calculated to be about 1200 mL/min/70 kg with no change in half-life. Renal clearance is estimated to be 400 mL/min/70 kg, indicating glomerular filtration and active tubular secretion by the kidneys. Zidovudine plasma protein binding is 34 to 38%, indicating that drug interactions involving binding site displacement are not anticipated. The mean steady-state peak and trough concentrations of Zidovudine at 2.5 mg/kg every 4 hours were 1.06 and 0.12 g/mL, respectively.

The Zidovudine cerebrospinal fluid (CSF)/plasma concentration ratio measured 1.8 hours following oral dosing at 2 mg/kg was 0.15 (n = 1). The ratios measured between 2 and 4 hours following intravenous doses of 2.5 mg/kg and 5.0 mg/kg were 0.20 (n = 1) and 0.64 (n = 3), respectively. Following intravenous administration, urinary recoveries of Zidovudine and GAZT accounted for 18 and 60% of the dose, respectively, and the total urinary recovery averaged 77% (range 64 to 98%). The pharmacokinetics of Zidovudine have been evaluated in patients with impaired renal function following a single 200 mg oral dose. In five anuric patients, the half-life of Zidovudine was 1.4 hours compared to 1.0 hour for control subjects with normal renal function; AUC values were approximately twice those of controls. However, in the anuric patients GAZT half-life was 8.0 hours (vs 0.9 hours for control) and AUC was 17 times higher than for control subjects. Hemodialysis appears to have a negligible effect on the removal of Zidovudine, whereas GAZT elimination is enhanced.

Adults with Impaired Renal Function: The pharmacokinetics of Zidovudine has been evaluated in patients with impaired renal function following a single 200 mg

oral dose. In five anuric patients, the half-life of Zidovudine was 1.4 hours compared to 1.0 hour for control subjects with normal renal function; AUC values were approximately twice those of controls. However, in the anuric patients GZDV half-life was 8.0 hours (vs 0.9 hours for control) and AUC was 17 times higher than for control subjects. The pharmacokinetics and tolerance was evaluated in a multiple-dose study in patients undergoing hemodialysis (n = 5) or peritoneal dialysis (n = 6). Patients received escalating doses of Zidovudine up to 200 mg 5 times daily for 8 weeks. Daily doses of 500 mg or less were well-tolerated despite significantly elevated plasma levels of GZDV. Apparent oral clearance of Zidovudine was approximately 50% of that reported in patients with normal renal function. The plasma concentrations of AMT are not known in patients with renal insufficiency. Daily doses of 300 to 400 mg should be appropriate in HIV-infected patients with severe renal dysfunction. Hemodialysis and peritoneal dialysis appear to have a negligible effect on the removal of Zidovudine, whereas GZDV elimination is enhanced.

Children: The pharmacokinetics and bioavailability of Zidovudine have been evaluated in 21 HIV-infected children, aged 6 months through 12 years, following intravenous doses administered over the range of 80 to 160 mg/m² every 6 hours, and following oral doses of the intravenous solution administered over the range of 90 to 240 mg/m² every 6 hours. After discontinuation of the I.V. infusion, Zidovudine plasma concentrations decayed biexponentially, consistent with two-compartment pharmacokinetics. Proportional increases in AUC and in Zidovudine concentrations were observed with increasing dose, consistent with dose-independent kinetics over the dose range studied. The mean terminal half-life and total body clearance across all dose levels administered were 1.5 hours and 30.9 mL/min/kg, respectively. These values compare to mean half-life and total body clearance in adults of 1.1 hours and 27.1 mL/min/kg.

The mean oral bioavailability of 65% was independent of dose. This value is the same as the bioavailability in adults. Doses of 180 mg/m² four times daily in pediatric patients produced similar systemic exposure (24 hour AUC 10.7 hr μg/mL) as doses of 200 mg six times daily in adult patients (10.9 hr μg/mL).

The pharmacokinetics of Zidovudine has been studied in neonates from birth to 3 months of life. In one study of the pharmacokinetics of Zidovudine in women during the last trimester of pregnancy, Zidovudine elimination was determined in 8 infants immediately after birth. The half-life was 13.0 ± 5.8 hours. In another study the pharmacokinetics of Zidovudine was evaluated in infants (ranging in age of 1 day to 3 months) of normal birth weight for gestational age and with normal renal and hepatic function. In infants less than or equal to 14 days old, mean ± SD total body clearance was 10.9 ± 4.8 mL/min/kg (n = 18) and half-life was 3.1 ± 1.2 hours (n = 21). In infants greater than 14 days, total body clearance was 19.0 ± 4.0 mL/min/kg (n = 16) and half-life was 1.9 ± 0.7 hours (n = 18). Bioavailability was 89% ± 19% (n = 15) in the younger age group and decreased to 61% ± 19% (n = 17) in infants older than 14 days.

Concentrations of Zidovudine in cerebrospinal fluid were measured after both intermittent oral and I.V. drug administration in 21 children during Phase 1 and Phase 2 studies. The mean Zidovudine cerebrospinal fluid level (CSF)/plasma concentration ratio measured at an average time of 2.2 hours postdose at doses of 120 to 240 mg/m2 was 0.52 ± 0.44 (n = 28); after an I.V. infusion of doses of 80 to 160 mg/m² over 1 hour, the mean CSF/plasma concentration ratio was 0.87 ± 0.66 (n = 23) at 3.2 hours after the start of the infusion. During continuous I.V. infusion, mean steady-state CSF/plasma ratio was 0.26 ± 0.17 (n = 28).

As in adult patients, the major route of elimination in children was by metabolism to 5-glucuronylazidothymidine (GZDV). After I.V. dosing, about 29% of the dose was excreted in the urine unchanged about 45% as GZDV. Overall, the pharmacokinetics of Zidovudine in pediatric patients greater than 3 months of age is similar to that of Zidovudine in adult patients.

Pregnancy: See *"Pregnancy"* under *"Precautions".*

Capsules: Steady-state serum concentrations of Zidovudine following chronic oral administration of 250 mg every 4 hours (3.0 to 5.4 mg/kg) were determined in 21 adult patients (body weight ranged from 46.0 to 83.6 kg) in a controlled trial. Mean steady-state predose and 1.5 hours postdose Zidovudine concentrations were 0.16 μg/mL (range 0 to 0.84 μg/mL) and 0.62 μg/mL (range 0.05 to 1.46 μg/mL), respectively.

Syrup: In a multiple dose bioavailability study conducted in 12 HIV-infected adults receiving doses of 100 or 200 mg every four hours, Zidovudine Syrup was demonstrated to be bioequivalent to Zidovudine Capsules with respect to area under the Zidovudine plasma concentration-time curve (AUC). The rate of absorption of Zidovudine Syrup was greater than that of Zidovudine Capsules, as indicated by mean times to peak concentration of 0.5 and 0.8 hours, respectively. Mean values for steady-state peak concentration (dose-normalized to 200 mg) were 1.5 and 1.2 μg/mL for syrup and capsules, respectively.

Effect of Food on Absorption: Administration of Zidovudine Capsules with food decreased peak plasma concentrations by greater than 50%, however bioavailability as determined by AUC may not be affected.

INDICATIONS AND USAGE

Zidovudine is indicated for the management of adult patients with HIV infection who have evidence of impaired immunity (CD4 cell count of 500 cells/mm³ or less) before therapy is begun. Zidovudine is also indicated for HIV-infected children over 3 months of age who have HIV-related symptoms or who are asymptomatic with abnormal laboratory values indicating significant HIV-related immunosuppression.

Zidovudine IV Infusion is indicated for the management of certain adult patients with symptomatic HIV infection (AIDS and advanced ARC) who have a history of cytologically confirmed *Pneumocystis carinii* pneumonia (PCP) or an absolute CD4 (T4 helper/inducer) lymphocyte count of less than 200/mm^3 in the peripheral blood before therapy is begun.

The indications for therapy with Zidovudine are based primarily on the results of three randomized studies in adults with asymptomatic and symptomatic HIV infection and two open-label studies in children with advanced HIV-associated disease. (see Description of Studies).

Because therapy with Zidovudine has been shown to prolong survival and decrease the incidence of opportunistic infections in patients with advanced HIV disease, and to delay disease progression in asymptomatic HIV-infected patients, Zidovudine should be considered as initial therapy for adult patients with HIV infection who have evidence of impaired immunity (CD4 cell counts of ≤ 500 cells/mm^3). However, randomized studies have shown that for some patients with advanced disease on prolonged therapy with Zidovudine, changing to other antiviral regimens may be more effective than remaining on monotherapy with Zidovudine. It is unknown if the use of Zidovudine prolongs survival in patients with CD4 cell counts > 200 cells/ mm^3 at the initiation of therapy.

DESCRIPTION OF STUDIES
ADULTS
Asymptomatic HIV Infection: A randomized, double-blind, placebo-controlled trial of oral Zidovudine 500 or 1500 mg/day was conducted in asymptomatic, HIV-infected adults with absolute CD4 cell counts of less than 500 cells/mm^3. The study was terminated on the basis of a scheduled interim analysis after a mean time on study of 55 weeks (range 19 to 107 weeks). There was a statistically significant difference in progression to advanced symptomatic HIV disease between the groups receiving Zidovudine and the placebo group. Of the 1338 patients enrolled in the study, 38 of the 428 patients receiving placebo, 17 of the 453 individuals receiving 500 mg Zidovudine and 19 of the 457 recipients of 1500 mg Zidovudine progressed to advanced symptomatic HIV disease. Of the progressions noted above, AIDS occurred in 33 placebo recipients, 11 individuals receiving 500 mg, and 14 patients receiving 1500 mg Zidovudine. Significant improvements in immunologic and virologic parameters (i.e., CD4 cell counts and serum p24 antigen levels) were observed for drug recipients, compared to placebo recipients. Although treatment of asymptomatic patients in this study delayed progression of disease in those patients at risk of progression over the initial 1 to 2 years of treatment, it is not known whether early treatment prolongs survival or the duration over which initial benefits of therapy are maintained.

Zidovudine was well tolerated in a majority of these asymptomatic patients.[1] Individuals receiving Zidovudine at 500 mg/day experienced the following symptoms at a significantly higher rate than placebo recipients: headache, malaise, anorexia, nausea, and vomiting.

The most common laboratory abnormalities associated with the use of Zidovudine were anemia, granulocytopenia, and hyperbilirubinemia (see *"Adverse Reactions"*). These toxicities were managed in most cases by temporary dose interruption.

Early Symptomatic HIV Disease: A randomized double-blind, placebo-controlled trial of oral Zidovudine was conducted in 713 adults with early manifestations of HIV disease (i.e., a baseline CD4 cell count of 200 to 800 cells/mm^3 and symptoms such as oral thrush, oral hairy leukoplakia, or intermittent diarrhea).[2] Patients received either placebo or 200 mg Zidovudine every 4 hours (1200 mg/ day). The trial was terminated on the basis of a scheduled interim analysis after a mean time on study of 9 months (range 0.2 to 22.7 months). There was a statistically significant difference in the rates of development of advanced symptomatic HIV disease between the group receiving Zidovudine and the group receiving placebo. Of the 352 patients receiving placebo, 36 progressed to advanced symptomatic HIV disease, of whom 21 progressed to AIDS; of the 361 patients receiving Zidovudine 13 progressed to advanced symptomatic HIV disease, of whom 5 progressed to AIDS.

Four percent of patients receiving Zidovudine compared with none of the placebo recipients developed a hemoglobin concentration less than 8 g/dL, and 4% of patients treated with Zidovudine compared with 1% of placebo recipients developed a granulocyte count less than 750 cells/mm^3. Asthenia, dyspepsia, nausea, and vomiting were the major adverse clinical events reported at significantly greater incidences in patients receiving Zidovudine. (See *"Adverse Reactions"*).

Advanced Symptomatic HIV Disease: A randomized, double-blind, placebo-controlled trial was conducted in 281 adults with advanced symptomatic HIV infection (160 patients with AIDS who had recovered from first episode *Pneumocystis carinii* pneumonia and 121 patients with advanced symptomatic HIV disease). Patients began therapy with Zidovudine at a dose of 250 mg every 4 hours and were studied for a mean of four and a half months.[3,4]

The trial was stopped because of a statistically significant difference in mortality. There were 19 deaths in the placebo group and 1 in the group receiving Zidovudine. All deaths were apparently due to opportunistic infections (OI's) or other complications of HIV infection.

Zidovudine also significantly reduced the risk of acquiring an AIDS defining OI in patients after 6 weeks of treatment. In addition, patients who received Zidovudine generally did better than the placebo group in terms of several other measures of efficacy including performance level, neuropsychiatric function, maintenance of body weight, and the number and severity of symptoms associated with HIV infection.

The most significant adverse reaction noted in the study was the development of anemia and/or neutropenia, which necessitated dose reduction or drug discontinuation in 34% of patients receiving Zidovudine. Patients with lower CD4 cell counts were more likely to receive transfusions. Forty-one percent of

patients receiving Zidovudine and 16% of placebo recipients with CD4 cell counts of ≤ 200 cells/mm^3 at entry were transfused (see *"Adverse Reactions"*). Only one of 30 patients receiving Zidovudine and none of 30 placebo recipients with CD4 cell counts of > 200 cells/mm^3 at entry required transfusion.

Although mean platelet counts in patients receiving Zidovudine were statistically increased compared to mean baseline values, thrombocytopenia did occur in some patients. Twelve percent of patients receiving Zidovudine compared to 5% of placebo recipients had > 50% decreases from baseline platelet count.

At the conclusion of the placebo-controlled trial, approximately 80% of study participants elected to enroll in an uncontrolled extension protocol in which all patients received Zidovudine at a dose of 200 mg every 4 hours. Survival rates for patients in this study were estimated using the method of "intention to treat," which counts all patients assigned to a drug regardless of whether they took the drug throughout the study period.

Using this convention, survival for all patients randomized to receive Zidovudine was 85% at one year, 41% at two years, and 23% at three years. One-, two-, and three-year survival for patients who entered the trial with AIDS was 79%, 31%, and 11%, respectively, when calculated from treatment initiation.[5]

While a direct comparison with survival data from other cohorts is not possible, untreated adult patients with AIDS diagnosed in San Francisco in 1985 who had survived at least 60 days after PCP had a one-year survival of 35% and a two-year survival of only 4% from the first diagnosis of PCP. Furthermore, in an epidemiologic study of patients with AIDS diagnosed in San Francisco in 1986 and 1987, median survival for patients receiving Zidovudine was found to be 22 months, a figure comparable to the 22-month median survival for patients with AIDS receiving Zidovudine as part of this clinical trial. This contrasts with the 15-month median survival observed in patients who did not receive therapy with Zidovudine in the San Francisco study. Actual survival of untreated patients is likely to be lower than reported because of the difficulty in complete ascertainment of mortality. Caution is advised in making comparisons from such "natural history" experience since case definitions and follow-up practices vary.

Other, uncontrolled studies have shown that Zidovudine may be of benefit in treating women, intravenous drug users, and racial minorities,[6-8] in addition to the patient population (primarily white males) included in the controlled trials.

Dose-Comparison Study: Results from a randomized, unblinded, dose-comparison study of Zidovudine in adults with AIDS who had experienced an episode of PCP indicate that an induction dose of Zidovudine 200 mg administered orally every 4 hours (1200 mg/day) for one month, followed by chronic administration of 100 mg every 4 hours (600 mg/day), was associated with survival rates and frequency of opportunistic infections comparable to those observed in patients administered higher dosages as tolerated. The 600 mg per day regimen was also associated with a lower incidence of hematologic toxicity. The effectiveness of this lower dose in improving the neurologic dysfunction associated with HIV disease, however, is unknown. A small randomized study has found a greater effect of higher doses of Zidovudine on improvement of neurological symptoms in patients with pre-existing neurological disease.

CHILDREN
Pediatric Symptomatic HIV Disease: Two open-label studies have evaluated the pharmacokinetics, safety, and efficacy of Zidovudine in 124 children with advanced HIV disease (84 AIDS and 40 with other clinical and laboratory evidence of advanced HIV disease). The median age at entry was 3.3 years (range: 3.5 months to 12 years) with 17 subjects younger than 12 months of age. In the majority of cases (73%), HIV was acquired by vertical transmission from an HIV-infected mother.

Thirty-six children were enrolled in the Phase 1 study, which evaluated three intravenous dosing regimens administered for 4 to 8 weeks. All children subsequently switched to an oral dose of 180 mg/m^2 every 6 hours and were followed for a mean of 465 days (range 121 to 855 days). Eighty-eight children participated in the Phase 2 study and these children were monitored for a mean of 186 days (range 3 to 352 days). In the Phase 2 study, oral Zidovudine was initiated at a dose of 180 mg/m^2 every 6 hours.

Clinical, immunologic, and virologic improvements were observed among some of the children receiving Zidovudine in these open-label studies. Clinical improvements included reductions in hepatosplenomegaly and increases in weight percentiles in children with delayed growth. The probability of remaining free of opportunistic infections through 12 months of follow-up was 0.76. Thirty-seven children developed one or more documented serious bacterial infections while participating in the studies. Seven of these children had more than one documented serious bacterial infection. The probability of survival at 12 months was 0.87 for the 124 patients enrolled in the Phase 1 and Phase 2 studies.

Improvements in the immunologic parameters of CD4 cell counts and immunoglobulin concentration were observed among the study participants. For children with severely depressed CD4 cell counts (< 500 cells/mm^3) at entry, a mean increase of 148 cells/mm^3 CD4$^+$ cell count was observed during the first two months of Zidovudine therapy. Thereafter, CD4 cell counts declined but remained above baseline through 9 months of follow-up. A tendency towards normalization of elevated immunoglobulin concentrations (primarily IgG) was observed among study participants.

An antiretroviral effect was demonstrated by reductions in serum and CSF p24 antigen concentrations, as well as by a reduction in the number of patients with positive CSF HIV cultures.

The most frequently reported adverse events were anemia (Hgb < 7.5 g/dL) and neutropenia (< 750 cells/mm^3), which occurred in 46% of the children. Thirty-six percent of the patients had their dose modified due to the development of hematologic abnormalities and 30% received transfusions for anemia. Four patients had dosing permanently discontinued due to neutropenia (see *"Adverse Reactions"*).

UNLABELED USES
Zidovudine is used alone or as an adjunct in the treatment of AIDS-related Kaposi's sarcoma.

CONTRAINDICATIONS
Zidovudine Capsules, Syrup, and I.V. Infusion are contraindicated for patients who have potentially life-threatening allergic reactions to any of the components of the formulations.

WARNINGS
NOTE
Zidovudine has been carefully studied in limited numbers of seriously ill HIV-infected patients treated for a limited period of time.

The full safety and efficacy profile of Zidovudine has not been defined, particularly in regard to prolonged use in HIV-infected individuals who have less advanced disease (see following sections for more specific information: *"Indications and Usage," "Microbiology", "Carcinogenesis, Mutagenesis, Impairment of Fertility"*).

Bone Marrow Suppression: Zidovudine should be used with extreme caution in patients who have bone marrow compromise evidenced by granulocyte count < 1000 cells/mm^3 mm^3 or hemoglobin < g/dL. In all of the placebo-controlled studies, but most frequently in patients with advanced symptomatic HIV disease, anemia and granulocytopenia were the most significant adverse events observed (see *"Adverse Reactions"*). There have been reports of pancytopenia associated with the use of Zidovudine, which was reversible in most instances after discontinuance of the drug.

Significant anemia most commonly occurred after 4 to 6 weeks of therapy and in many cases required dose adjustment, discontinuation of Zidovudine, and/or blood transfusions. Frequent at least every 2 weeks blood counts are strongly recommended in patients with advanced HIV disease taking Zidovudine. For asymptomatic HIV-infected individuals and patients with early HIV disease, most of whom have better marrow reserve, blood counts may be obtained less frequently, depending upon the patient's overall status. If anemia or granulocytopenia develops, dosage adjustments may be necessary (see *"Dosage and Administration"*).

Myopathy: Myopathy and myositis similar to that produced by HIV disease have been associated with prolonged use of Zidovudine in clinical practice.

Lactic Acidosis/Severe Hepatomegaly with Steatosis: Rare occurrences of lactic acidosis in the absence of hypoxemia, and severe hepatomegaly with steatosis have been reported and are potentially fatal; it it not known whether these events are causally related to Zidovudine. Lactic acidosis should be considered whenever a patient receiving therapy with Zidovudine develops unexplained tachypnea, dyspnea, or fall in serum bicarbonate level. Under these circumstances, therapy with Zidovudine should be suspended until the diagnosis of lactic acidosis has been excluded. Caution should be exercised when administering Zidovudine to any patient, particularly obese women, with hepatomegaly, hepatitis, or other known risk factor for liver disease. These patients should be followed closely while on therapy with Zidovudine. The significance of elevated aminotransferase levels suggesting hepatic injury in HIV-infected patients prior to starting Zidovudine or while on Zidovudine is unclear. Treatment with Zidovudine should be suspended in the setting of rapidly elevating aminotransferase levels, progressive hepatomegaly, or metabolic/lactic acidosis of unknown etiology.

Other Serious Adverse Reactions: Several serious adverse events have been reported with use of Zidovudine in clinical practice. Reports of pancreatitis, sensitization reactions (including anaphylaxis in one patient), vasculitis, and seizures have been rare. These adverse events, except for sensitization, have also been associated with HIV disease. Changes in skin and nail pigmentation have been associated with the use of Zidovudine. Patients experiencing a rash should undergo medical evaluation.

Use in Infancy: Insufficient clinical experience exists to recommend a dosing regimen in infants under 3 months of age. Preliminary evidence indicates that Zidovudine clearance may be reduced in children less than 1 month of age. A positive test for HIV-antibody in children under 15 months of age may represent passively acquired maternal antibodies, rather than an active antibody response to infection in the infant. Thus, the presence of HIV antibody in a child less than 15 months of age must be interpreted with caution, especially in the asymptomatic infant. Confirmatory tests such as serum p24 antigen or viral culture should be pursued in such children.

Coadministration of Zidovudine with other drugs metabolized by glucuronidation should be avoided because the toxicity of either drug may be potentiated (see *"Drug Interactions"* under *"Precautions"*). Zidovudine recipients who used acetaminophen during the controlled trial had an increased incidence of granulocytopenia which appeared to be correlated with the duration of acetaminophen use.

PRECAUTIONS
General: Zidovudine is eliminated from the body primarily by renal excretion following metabolism in the liver (glucuronidation). In patients with severely impaired renal function, dosage reduction is recommended (see *"Pharmacokinetics"* subsection of *"Clinical Pharmacology"* and *"Dosage and Administration"*). Although very little data are available, patients with severely impaired hepatic function may be at greater risk of toxicity.

Information for Patients: Zidovudine is not a cure for HIV infections, and patients may continue to acquire illnesses associated with HIV infection, including opportunistic infections. Therefore, patients should be advised to seek medical care for any significant change in their health status.

Patients should be informed that the drug has been extensively studied, but for limited periods of time, and that long-term safety and efficacy are not known for patients with less advanced disease. Patients should be informed that the major toxicities of Zidovudine are granulocytopenia and/or anemia. The frequency and severity of these toxicities are greater in patients with more advanced disease and in those who initiate therapy later in the course of their infection. They should be told that if toxicity develops, they may require transfusions or dose modifications including possible discontinuation. They should be told of the extreme importance of having their blood counts followed closely while on therapy, especially for patients with advanced symptomatic HIV disease. They should be cautioned about the use of other medications, including acetaminophen, ganciclovir and interferon-alpha, that may exacerbate the toxicity of Zidovudine (see *"Warnings"* and *"Drug Interactions"* under *"Precautions"*). Patients should be informed that other adverse effects of Zidovudine include nausea and vomiting. Patients should also be encouraged to contact their physician if they experience muscle weakness, shortness of breath, or symptoms of hepatitis or pancreatitis while being treated with Zidovudine.

Zidovudine Capsules and Syrup are for oral ingestion only. Patients should be told of the importance of taking Zidovudine exactly as prescribed. They should be told not to share medication and not to exceed the recommended dose. Patients should be told that the long-term effects of Zidovudine are unknown at this time.

Patients should be advised that therapy with Zidovudine has not been shown to reduce the risk of transmission of HIV to others through sexual contact or blood contamination.

DRUG INTERACTIONS
Ganciclovir: Use of Zidovudine in combination with ganciclovir increases the risk of hematologic toxicities in some patients with advanced HIV disease. Should the use of this combination become necessary in the treatment of patients with HIV disease, dose reduction or interruption of one or both agents may be necessary to minimize hematologic toxicity. Hematologic parameters, including hemoglobin, hematocrit, and white blood cell count with differential, should be monitored frequently in all patients receiving this combination.

Interferon-alpha: Hematologic toxicities have also been seen when Zidovudine is used concomitantly with interferon-alpha. As with the concomitant use of Zidovudine and ganciclovir, dose reduction or interruption of one or both agents may be necessary, and hematologic parameters should be monitored frequently.

Bone Marrow Suppressive Agents/Cytotoxic Agents: Coadministration of Zidovudine with drugs that are cytotoxic, or which interfere with RBC/WBC number or function (e.g., dapsone, flucytosine, vincristine, vinblastine, or adriamycin) may increase the risk of hematologic toxicity.

Probenecid: Limited data suggest that probenecid may increase Zidovudine levels by inhibiting glucuronidation and/or by reducing renal excretion of Zidovudine. Some patients who have used Zidovudine concomitantly with probenecid have developed flu-like symptoms consisting of myalgia, malaise, and/or fever and maculopapular rash.

Phenytoin: Phenytoin plasma levels have been reported to be low in some patients receiving Zidovudine while in one case a high level was documented. However, in a pharmacokinetic interaction study in which 12 HIV-positive volunteers received a single 300 mg phenytoin dose alone and during steady-state Zidovudine conditions (200 mg every 4 hours), no change in phenytoin kinetics was observed. Although not designed to optimally assess the effect of phenytoin on Zidovudine kinetics, a 30% decrease in oral Zidovudine clearance was observed with phenytoin.

Methadone: In a pharmacokinetic study of nine HIV-positive patients receiving methadone-maintenance (30 to 90 mg daily) concurrent with 200 mg of Zidovudine every 4 hours, no changes were observed in the pharmacokinetics of methadone upon initiation of therapy with Zidovudine and after 14 days of treatment with Zidovudine. No adjustments in methadone-maintenance requirements were reported. However, plasma levels of Zidovudine were elevated in some patients while remaining unchanged in others. The exact mechanism and clinical significance of these data are unknown.

Other Nucleoside Analogues: Some experimental nucleoside analogues which are being evaluated in HIV-infected patients may affect RBC/WBC number or function and may increase the potential for hematologic toxicity of Zidovudine. Some experimental nucleoside analogues affecting DNA replication such as ribavirin, antagonize the *in vitro* antiviral activity of Zidovudine against HIV and thus, concomitant use of such drugs should be avoided.

Other Agents: Drugs such as (e.g., acetaminophen, aspirin, or indomethacin may competitively inhibit glucuronidation [see *"Warnings"*]). Some drugs such as trimethoprim-sulfamethoxazole, pyrimethamine, and acyclovir may be necessary for the management or prevention of opportunistic infections. In the placebo-controlled trial in patients with advanced HIV disease, increased toxicity was not detected with limited exposure to these drugs. However, there is one published report of neurotoxicity (profound lethargy) associated with concomitant use of Zidovudine and acyclovir. Preliminary data from a drug interaction study (n = 10) suggest that coadministration of 200 mg Zidovudine and 600 mg rifampin decreases the area under the plasma concentration curve by an average of 48% ±

◆ RATED THERAPEUTICALLY EQUIVALENT; ◇ THERAPEUTIC EQUIVALENCE UNCONFIRMED; ○ UNRATED

34%. However, the effect of once daily dosing of rifampin on multiple daily doses of Zidovudine is unknown.

Carcinogenesis, Mutagenesis, Impairment of Fertility: Zidovudine was administered orally at three dosage levels to separate groups of mice and rats (60 females and 60 males in each group). Initial single daily doses were 30, 60, and 120 mg/kg/day in mice and 80, 220, and 600 mg/kg/day in rats. The doses in mice were reduced to 20, 30, and 40 mg/kg/day after day 90 because of treatment-related anemia, whereas in rats only the high dose was reduced to 450 mg/kg/day on day 91 and then to 300 mg/kg/day on day 279.

In mice, seven late-appearing (after 19 months) vaginal neoplasms (5 non-metastasizing squamous cell carcinomas, one squamous cell papilloma, and one squamous polyp) occurred in animals given the highest dose. One late-appearing squamous cell papilloma occurred in the vagina of a middle dose animal. No vaginal tumors were found at the lowest dose.

In rats, two late-appearing (after 20 months), non-metastasizing vaginal squamous cell carcinomas occurred in animals given the highest dose. No vaginal tumors occurred at the low or middle dose in rats.

No other drug-related tumors were observed in either sex of either species.

It is not known how predictive the results of rodent carcinogenicity studies may be for humans. At doses that produced tumors in mice and rats, the estimated drug exposure (as measured by AUC) was approximately 3 times (mouse) and 24 times (rat) the estimated human exposure at the recommended therapeutic dose of 100 mg every 4 hours.

No evidence of mutagenicity (with or without metabolic activation) was observed in the Ames *Salmonella* mutagenicity assay at concentrations up to 10 µg per plate, which was the maximum concentration that could be tested because of the antimicrobial activity of Zidovudine against the *Salmonella* species. In a mutagenicity assay conducted in L5178Y/TK+/− mouse lymphoma cells, Zidovudine was weakly mutagenic in the absence of metabolic activation only at the highest concentrations tested (4000 and 5000 µg/mL). In the presence of metabolic activation, the drug was weakly mutagenic at concentrations of 1000 µg/mL and higher. In an *in vitro* mammalian cell transformation assay, Zidovudine was positive at concentrations of 0.5 µg/mL and higher. In an *in vitro* cytogenetic study performed in cultured human lymphocytes, Zidovudine induced dose-related structural chromosomal abnormalities at concentrations of 3 µg/mL and higher. No such effects were noted at the two lowest concentrations tested, 0.3 and 1 µg/mL. In an *in vivo* cytogenetic study in rats given a single intravenous injection of Zidovudine at doses of 37.5 to 300 mg/kg, there were no treatment-related structural or numerical chromosomal alterations in spite of plasma levels that were as high as 453 µg/mL five minutes after dosing.

In two *in vivo* micronucleus studies (designed to measure chromosome breakage or mitotic spindle apparatus damage) in male mice, oral doses of Zidovudine 100 to 1000 mg/kg/day administered once daily for approximately 4 weeks induced dose-related increases in micronucleated erythrocytes. Similar results were also seen after 4 or 7 days of dosing at 500 mg/kg/day in rats and mice.

In a study involving 11 AIDS patients, it was reported that the seven patients who were receiving Zidovudine (1200 mg/day) as their only medication for 4 weeks to 7 months showed a chromosome breakage frequency of 8.29 ± 2.65 breaks per 100 peripheral lymphocytes. This was significantly (P < 0.05) higher than the incidence of 0.5 ± 0.29 breaks per 100 cells that was observed in the four AIDS patients who had not received Zidovudine.

No effect on male or female fertility (judged by conception rates) was seen in rats given Zidovudine orally at doses up to 450 mg/kg/day.

Pregnancy: Pregnancy Category C. Oral teratology studies in the rat and in the rabbit at doses up to 500 mg/kg/day revealed no evidence of teratogenicity with Zidovudine. Zidovudine treatment resulted in embryo/fetal toxicity as evidenced by an increase in the incidence of fetal resorptions in rats given 150 or 450 mg/kg/day and rabbits given 500 mg/kg/day. The doses used in the teratology studies resulted in peak Zidovudine plasma concentrations (after one-half of the daily dose) in rats 66 to 226 times, and in rabbits 12 to 87 times, mean steady-state peak human plasma concentrations (after one-sixth of the daily dose) achieved with the recommended daily dose (100 mg every 4 hours). In an *in vitro* experiment with fertilized mouse oocytes, Zidovudine exposure resulted in a dose-dependent reduction in blastocyst formation. In an additional teratology study in rats, a dose of 3000 mg/kg/day (very near the oral median lethal dose in rats of 3683 mg/kg) caused marked maternal toxicity and an increase in the incidence of fetal malformations. This dose resulted in peak Zidovudine plasma concentrations 350 times peak human plasma concentrations. (Estimated area-under-the-curve [AUC] in rats at this dose level was 300 times the daily AUC in humans given 600 mg per day.) No evidence of teratogenicity was seen in this experiment at doses of 600 mg/kg/day or less.

The pharmacokinetics of Zidovudine has been studied in a Phase 1 study of eight women during the last trimester of pregnancy. The pharmacokinetics of Zidovudine was similar to that of nonpregnant adults. Consistent with passive transmission of the drug across the placenta, Zidovudine concentrations in infant plasma at birth were essentially equal to those in maternal plasma at delivery. The half-life of Zidovudine in the neonates was greatly prolonged (13.0 ± 5.8 hours) compared to that of the mother.

It is not known whether Zidovudine can cause fetal harm when administered to a pregnant women or can affect reproductive capacity. Zidovudine should be given to a pregnant woman only if clearly needed.

Antiretroviral Pregnancy Registry: To monitor maternal-fetal outcomes of pregnant women exposed to Zidovudine an Antiretroviral Pregnancy Registry has been established. Physicians are encouraged to register patients by calling (800) 722-9292, ext. 58465.

Nursing Mothers: It is not known whether Zidovudine is excreted in human milk. Lactating mice administered Zidovudine (200 mg/kg intraperitoneally) were found to have milk concentrations of Zidovudine five times the corresponding serum Zidovudine concentration. Milk concentrations of Zidovudine declined at a slower rate than serum Zidovudine concentrations. Because many drugs are excreted in human milk and because of the potential for serious adverse reactions from Zidovudine in nursing infants, mothers should be instructed to discontinue nursing if they are receiving Zidovudine. The U.S. Public Health Service Centers for Disease Control advises HIV-infected women not to breast-feed to avoid postnatal transmission of HIV to a child who may not yet be infected.

Pediatric Use: See "Indications", "Warnings" and "Dosage and Administration" sections.

ADVERSE REACTIONS

Adults: The frequency and severity of adverse events associated with the use of Zidovudine in adults are greater in patients with more advanced infection at the time of initiation of therapy. The following tables summarize the relative incidence of hematologic adverse events observed in the placebo-controlled clinical studies by severity of HIV disease present at the start of treatment. (See related tables 1-4.)

The most frequent adverse events and abnormal laboratory values reported in the placebo-controlled clinical trial of oral Zidovudine administration in 281 patients (144 patients Zidovudine; 137 patients placebo) were granulocytopenia and anemia. The occurrence of these hematologic toxicities were inversely related to CD4 (T4) lymphocyte number, hemoglobin, and granulocyte count at study entry, and directly related to dose and duration of therapy. The frequency of granulocytopenia and anemia according to the patients' CD4 (T4) levels is shown in the following table: (See related table 5.)

Because many patients were anemic and/or granulocytopenia before starting therapy with Zidovudine, examining the degree of change when compared to baseline, as shown in the table below, may be more informative. (See related table 6.)

The anemia reported in patients with advanced HIV disease receiving Zidovudine appeared to be the result of impaired erythrocyte maturation as evidenced by increased macrocytosis (MCV) while on drug. Although mean platelet counts in patients receiving Zidovudine were significantly increased compared to mean baseline values, thrombocytopenia did occur in some of these patients with advanced disease. Twelve percent of patients receiving Zidovudine compared to 5% of patients receiving placebo had > 50% decreases from baseline platelet count. Mild drug-associated elevations in total bilirubin levels have been reported as an uncommon occurrence in patients treated for asymptomatic HIV infection.

The HIV-infected adults participating in these clinical trials often had baseline symptoms and signs of HIV disease and/or experienced adverse events at some time during study. It was often difficult to distinguish adverse events possibly associated with administration of Zidovudine from underlying signs of HIV disease or intercurrent illnesses. The following table summarizes clinical adverse events or symptoms which occurred in at least 5% of all patients with advanced HIV disease treated with 1500 mg/day of Zidovudine in the original placebo-controlled study.[4] Of the items listed in the table, only severe headache, nausea, insomnia and myalgia were reported at a significantly greater rate in patients receiving Zidovudine.

Table 7
PERCENTAGE (%) OF PATIENTS WITH CLINICAL EVENTS IN THE ADVANCED HIV DISEASE STUDY

Adverse Event	Zidovudine 1500 mg/day* (n = 144)%	Placebo (n = 137)%
Body as a Whole		
Asthenia	19	18
Diaphoresis	5	4
Fever	16	12
Headache	42	37
Malaise	8	7
Gastrointestinal		
Anorexia	11	8
Diarrhea	12	18
Dyspepsia	5	4
GI Pain	20	19
Nausea	46	18
Vomiting	6	3
Musculoskeletal		
Myalgia	8	2
Nervous		
Dizziness	6	4
Insomnia	5	1
Paresthesia	6	3
Somnolence	8	9
Respiratory		

Adverse Event	Zidovudine 1500 mg/day* (n = 144)%	Placebo (n = 137)%
Dyspnea	5	3
Skin		
Rash	17	15
Special Senses		
Taste Perversion	5	8

* *The currently recommended dose is 500 to 600 mg/day.*

Clinical adverse events which occurred in less than 5% of all adult patients treated with 1500 mg/day of Zidovudine in the advanced HIV study are listed below. Since many of these adverse events were seen in placebo-treated patients as well as patients treated with Zidovudine their possible relationship to the drug is unknown.

Body as a Whole: body odor, chills, edema of the lip, flu syndrome, hyperalgesia, back pain, chest pain, lymphadenopathy.

Cardiovascular: vasodilation.

Gastrointestinal: constipation, dysphagia, edema of the tongue, eructation, flatulence, bleeding gums, rectal hemorrhage, mouth ulcer.

Musculoskeletal: arthralgia, muscle spasm, tremor, twitch.

Nervous: anxiety, confusion, depression, emotional lability, nervousness, syncope, loss of mental acuity, vertigo.

Respiratory: cough, epistaxis, pharyngitis, rhinitis, sinusitis, hoarseness.

Table 1

Asymptomatic	Granulocytopenia (< 750 cells/mm^3)			Anemia (Hgb < 8.0 g/dL)		
	Zidovudine			Zidovudine		
HIV Infection Study (n = 1338)	1500 mg/day*	500 mg/day	Placebo	1500 mg/day*	500 mg/day	Placebo
CD4 ≤ 500	6.4% (n = 457)	1.8% (n = 453)	1.6% (n = 428)	6.4% (n = 457)	1.1% (n = 453)	0.2% (n = 428)

Table 2

Early Symptomatic HIV Disease Study (n = 713)	Granulocytopenia (< 750 cells/mm^3)		Anemia (Hgb < 8.0 g/dL)	
	Zidovudine 1200 mg/day*	Placebo	Zidovudine 1200 mg/day*	Placebo
CD4 > 200	4% (n = 361)	1% (n = 352)	4% (n = 361)	0% (n = 352)

Table 3

Advanced Symptomatic HIV Disease Study (n = 281)	Granulocytopenia (< 750 cells/mm^3)		Anemia (Hgb < 7.5 g/dL)	
	Zidovudine 1500 mg/day*	Placebo	Zidovudine 1500 mg/day*	Placebo
CD4 > 200	10% (n = 30)	3% (n = 30)	3% (n = 30)	0% (n = 30)
CD4 > 200	47% (n = 114)	10% (n = 107)	29% (n = 114)	5% (n = 107)

Table 4

Advanced Symptomatic HIV Disease Dose Comparison Study (n = 524)	Granulocytopenia (< 750 cells/mm^3)		Anemia (Hgb < 8.0 g/dL)	
	Zidovudine 1200 mg/day*	Zidovudine 600 mg/day	Zidovudine 1200 mg/day*	Zidovudine 600 mg/day
CD4 ≤ 200	51% (n = 262)	37% (n = 262)	39% (n = 262)	29% (n = 262)

* *The currently recommended dose is 500 to 600 mg/day.*

Table 5

Abnormality	Pretreatment CD4 (T4) Levels	
	Zidovudine (n = 113)	Placebo (n = 105)
	≤ 200/mm^3	
Granulocytopenia (< 750/mm^3)	47%	10%
Anemia (Hgb < 7.5 g/dL)	30%	
	> 200/mm^3	
	(n = 30)	(n = 30)
Granulocytopenia (< 750/mm^3)	10%	3%
Anemia (Hgb < 7.5 g/dL)	3%	0%

Table 6

Abnormality	% Decrease from Baseline	Pretreatment CD4 (T4) Levels	
		Zidovudine (n = 113)	
		≤ 200/mm^3	
			Placebo (n = 105)
Granulocytopenia	> 50%	55%	19%
Anemia	> 25%	45%	14%
		> 200/mm^3	
		(n = 30)	(n = 30)
Granulocytopenia	> 50%	40%	13%
Anemia	> 25%	10%	10%

♦ RATED THERAPEUTICALLY EQUIVALENT; ◇ THERAPEUTIC EQUIVALENCE UNCONFIRMED; ○ UNRATED

Skin: acne, pruritus, urticaria.

Special Senses: amblyopia, hearing loss, photophobia.

Urogenital: dysuria, polyuria, urinary frequency, urinary hesitancy.

All events of a severe or life-threatening nature were monitored for adults in the placebo-controlled studies in early HIV disease and asymptomatic HIV infection. Data concerning the occurrence of additional signs or symptoms were also collected. No distinction was made in reporting events between those possibly associated with the administration of the study medication and those due to the underlying disease. The following tables summarize all those events reported at a statistically significant greater incidence for patients receiving Zidovudine in these studies:

Table 6
PERCENTAGE (%) OF PATIENTS WITH CLINICAL EVENTS IN THE EARLY SYMPTOMATIC HIV DISEASE STUDY

Adverse Event	Zidovudine 1200 mg/day* (n = 361)%	Placebo (n = 352)%
Body as a Whole		
Asthenia	69	62
Gastrointestinal		
Dyspepsia	6	1
Nausea	61	41
Vomiting	25	13

* *The currently recommended dose is 500 to 600 mg/day.*

Table 7
PERCENTAGE (%) OF PATIENTS WITH CLINICAL EVENTS† IN AN ASYMPTOMATIC HIV INFECTION STUDY

Adverse Event	Zidovudine 1500 mg/day* (n = 457)%	Zidovudine 500 mg/day* (n = 453)%	Placebo (n = 428)%
Body as a Whole			
Asthenia	10.1	8.6‡	5.8
Headache	58.0‡	62.5	52.6
Malaise	55.6	53.2	44.9
Gastrointestinal			
Anorexia	19.3	20.1	10.5
Constipation	8.1	6.4‡	3.5
Nausea	57.3	51.4	29.9
Vomiting	16.4	17.2	9.8
Nervous			
Dizziness	20.8	17.9‡	15.2

* *The currently recommended dose is 500 to 600 mg/day.*
† *Reported in ≥ 5% of study population.*
‡ *Not statistically significant versus placebo.*

Several serious adverse events have been reported with the use of Zidovudine in clinical practice. Myopathy and myositis with pathological changes attributed to prolonged use of Zidovudine have been reported. Reports of hepatomegaly with steatosis, hepatitis, pancreatitis, lactic acidosis, sensitization reactions (including anaphylaxis in one patient), hyperbilirubinemia, vasculitis, and seizures have been rare. These adverse events, except for sensitization, have also been associated with HIV disease. A single case of macular edema has been reported with the use of Zidovudine. Changes in skin and nail pigmentation have been associated with the use of Zidovudine.

Pediatrics: Anemia and granulocytopenia among children with advanced HIV disease receiving Zidovudine occurred with similar incidence to that reported for adults with AIDS or advanced ARC (see above). Management of neutropenia and anemia included, in some cases, dose modification and/or blood product transfusions. In the open-label studies, 17% had their dose modified (generally a reduction in dose by 30%) due to anemia and 25% had their dose modified (temporary discontinuation or dose reduction by 30%) for neutropenia. Four children had Zidovudine permanently discontinued for neutropenia. The following table summarizes the occurrence of anemia (Hgb < 7.5 g/dL) and granulocytopenia (< 750 cells/mm³) among 124 children receiving Zidovudine for a mean of 267 days (range 3 to 855 days):

Table 8

Advanced Pediatric HIV disease	Granulocytopenia (< 750 cells/mm³)		Anemia (Hgb < 7.5 g/dL)	
(N = 124)	n	%	n	%
	48	39	28*	23

* *Twenty-two children received one or more transfusions due to a decline in hemoglobin to < 7.5 g/dL; an additional 15 children were transfused for hemoglobin levels > 7.5 g/dL. Fifty-nine percent of the patients transfused had a prestudy history of anemia or transfusion requirement.*

An increase in MCV (macrocytosis) was observed among the majority of children enrolled in the studies.

In the open-label studies involving 124 children, 16 clinical adverse events were reported by 24 children. No event was reported by more than 5.6% of the study populations. Due to the open-label design of the studies, it was difficult to determine possible events related to the use of Zidovudine versus disease-related events. Therefore, all clinical events reported as associated with therapy with Zidovudine or of unknown relationship to therapy with Zidovudine are presented in the following table:

Table 9
PERCENTAGE (%) OF PEDIATRIC PATIENTS WITH CLINICAL EVENTS IN OPEN LABEL STUDIES

Adverse Event	n	%
Body As A Whole		
Fever	4	3.2
Phlebitis*/Bacteremia	2	1.6
Headache	2	1.6
Gastrointestinal		
Nausea	1	0.8
Vomiting	6	4.8
Abdominal Pain	4	3.2
Diarrhea	1	0.8
Weight Loss	1	0.8
Nervous		
Insomnia	3	2.4
Nervousness/Irritability	2	1.6
Decreased Reflexes	7	5.6
Seizure	1	0.8
Cardiovascular		
Left Ventricular Dilation	1	0.8
Cardiomyopathy	1	0.8
S₃ Gallop	1	0.8
Congestive Heart Failure	1	0.8
Generalized Edema	1	0.8
ECG Abnormality	3	2.4
Urogenital		
Hematuria/Viral Cystitis	1	0.8

* *Peripheral vein IV catheter site.*

The clinical adverse events reported among adult recipients of Zidovudine may also occur in children.

Subsequent to the initial trial, sensitization reactions, including anaphylaxis in one patient, have been reported in individuals receiving Zidovudine therapy.

The following events have been reported in patients treated with Zidovudine. They may also occur as part of the underlying disease process. As such, the relationship between these events and the use of Zidovudine is uncertain: seizures, myopathy, nail pigmentation, changes in liver function tests. The adverse events reported during intravenous administration of Zidovudine IV Infusion are similar to those reported with oral administration; granulocytopenia and anemia were reported most frequently. Long-term intravenous administration beyond 2 to 4 weeks has not been studied in adults and may enhance hematologic adverse events. Local reaction, pain and slight irritation during intravenous administration occur infrequently.

OVERDOSAGE
Cases of acute overdoses in both children and adults have been reported with doses up to 50 grams. None were fatal. The only consistent finding in these cases of overdose was spontaneous or induced nausea and vomiting. Hematologic changes were transient and not severe. Some patients experienced nonspecific CNS symptoms such as headache, dizziness, drowsiness, lethargy, and confusion. One report of a grand mal seizure possibly attributable to Zidovudine occurred in a 35-year-old male 3 hours after ingesting 36 grams of Zidovudine. No other cause could be identified. All patients recovered without permanent sequelae. Hemodialysis and peritoneal dialysis appear to have a negligible effect on the removal of Zidovudine while elimination of its primary metabolite, GZDV, is enhanced.

DOSAGE AND ADMINISTRATION
Oral Zidovudine Adults: For adults with symptomatic HIV infection, including AIDS, the recommended oral dose is 100 mg (one 100 mg capsule or 2 teaspoonful [10 mL] syrup) every 4 hours (600 mg total daily dose). The effectiveness of this dose compared to higher dosing regimens in improving the neurologic dysfunction associated with HIV disease is unknown (see *"Indications and Usage"*). A small randomized study has found a greater effect of higher doses of Zidovudine on improvement of neurological symptoms in patients with preexisting neurological disease.

For asymptomatic HIV infection, the recommended dose for adults is 100 mg administered orally every 4 hours while awake (500 mg/day).

Children: The recommended dose in children 3 months to 12 years of age is 180 mg/m² every 6 hours (720 mg/m² per day), not to exceed 200 mg every 6 hours.

Monitoring of Patients: Hematologic toxicities appear to be related to pretreatment bone marrow reserve and to dose and duration of therapy. In patients with poor bone marrow reserve, particularly in patients with advanced symptomatic HIV disease, frequent monitoring of hematologic indices is recommended to detect serious anemia or granulocytopenia (see *"Warnings"*). In patients who experience hematologic toxicity, reduction in hemoglobin may occur as early as 2 to 4 weeks, and granulocytopenia usually occurs after 6 to 8 weeks. Zidovudine IV Infusion 1 to 2 mg/kg infused over 1 hour. This dose should be administered every 4 hours around the clock (6 times daily). Patients should receive Zidovudine I.V. Infusion only until oral therapy can be administered (see recommended oral doses below).

The recommended oral starting dose in adults is 200 mg (two 100 mg capsules or four teaspoonfuls [20 mL] syrup) administered every four hours (1200 mg total daily dose). After one month, the dose may be reduced to 100 mg every four hours (600 mg total daily dose). The intravenous dosing regimen equivalent to the oral administration of 100 mg every four hours is approximately 1 mg/kg intravenously every four hours. The effectiveness of this lower dose in improving the neurologic dysfunction associated with HIV disease is unknown (see *"Indications and Usage"*).

Hematologic toxicities appear to be related to pretreatment bone marrow reserve and to dose and duration of therapy. Careful monitoring of hematologic indices every two weeks is recommended to detect serious anemia or granulocytopenia. In patients with hematologic toxicity, reduction in hemoglobin may occur as early as 2 to 4 weeks, and granulocytopenia usually occurs after 6 to 8 weeks.

Dose Adjustment: Significant anemia (hemoglobin of < 7.5 g/dL or reduction of > 25% of baseline) and/or significant granulocytopenia (granulocyte count of < 750 cells/mm^3 or reduction of > 50% from baseline) may require a dose interruption until evidence of marrow recovery is observed (see *"Warnings"*). For less severe adenia or granulocytopenia, a reduction in daily dose may be adequate. In patients who develop significant anemia, dose modification does not necessarily eliminate the need for transfusion. If marrow recovery occurs following dose modification, gradual increases in dose may be appropriate depending on hematologic indices and patient tolerance.

In end-stage renal disease patients maintained on hemodialysis or peritoneal dialysis, recommended dose is 100 mg every 6 to 8 hours (see *"Pharmacokinetics"* subsection of *"Clinical Pharmacology"*).

There are insufficient data to recommend dose adjustment of Zidovudine in patients with impaired renal or hepatic function.

Method of Preparation (IV): Zidovudine IV. Infusion must be diluted prior to administration. The calculated dose should be removed from the 20 mL vial and added to 5% Dextrose Injection solution to achieve a concentration no greater than 4 mg/mL. Admixture in biologic or colloidal fluids (e.g., blood products, protein solutions, etc.) is not recommended.

After dilution, the solution is physically and chemically stable for 24 hours at room temperature and 48 hours if refrigerated at 2° to 8°C (36° to 46°F). Care should be taken during admixture to prevent inadvertent contamination. As an additional precaution, the diluted solution should be administered within 8 hours if stored at 25°C (77°F) or 24 hours if refrigerated at 2° to 8°C to minimize potential administration of a microbially contaminated solution.

Parenteral drug products should be inspected visually for particulate matter and discoloration prior to administration whenever solution and container permit. Should either be observed, the solution should be discarded and fresh solution prepared.

Administration (IV): Zidovudine IV. Infusion is adminstered intravenously at a constant rate over one hour. Rapid infusion or bolus injection should be avoided Zidovudine IV. Infusion should not be given intramuscularly.

Storage: Capsules should be stored at 15° to 25°C (59° to 77°F) and protected from light and moisture.

Syrup and vials for IV infusion should be stored at 15° to 25°C (59° to 77°F) and protected from light.

REFERENCES

1. Volberding PA, Lagakos SW, Koch MA, et al. Zidovudine in asymptomatic human immunodeficiency virus infection. A controlled trial in persons with fewer than 500 CD4-positive cells per cubic millimeter. *N Engl J Med.* 1990;322:941-949. 2. Fischl MA, Richman DD, Hansen N, et al. The safety and efficacy of zidovudine in the treatment of patients with mildly symptomatic HIV infection. A double-blind, placebo-controlled trial. *Annals Internal Med.* 190; 112:727-737. 3. Fischl MA, Richman DD, Grieco MH, et al. The efficacy of azidothymidine (AZT) in the treatment of patients with AIDS and AIDS-related complex. A double-blind, placebo-controlled trial. *N Engl J Med.* 1987;317:185-191. 4. Richman DD, Fischl MA, Grieco MH, et al. The toxicity of azidothymidine (AZT) in the treatment of patients with AIDS and AIDS-related complex. A double-blind, placebo-controlled trial. *N Engl J Med.* 1987;317-192-197. 5. Fischl MA, Richman DD, Causey DM, et al. Prolonged zidovudine therapy in patients with AIDS and advanced AIDS-related complex. *JAMA.* 1989;262:2405-2410. 6. Creagh-Kirk T, Doi P, Andrews E, et al. Survival experience among patients with AIDS receiving zidovudine. Follow-up of patients in a compassionate plea program. *JAMA.* 1988;260(20):3009-3015. 7. Lagakos S, Fischl MA, Stein DS, Lim L, Volberding P. Effects of zidovudine therapy in minority and other subpopulations with early HIV infection. *JAMA.* 1991:266:2709-2712. 8. Easterbrook PJ, Keruly JC, Creagh-Kirk T. et al. Racial and ethnic differences in outcome in zidovudine-treated patients with advanced HIV disease, *JAMA.* 1991:266:2713-2718.

HOW SUPPLIED
CAPSULE: 100 MG

BRAND/MANUFACTURER	NDC	SIZE	AWP
○ **BRAND**			
▶ RETROVIR: Burr Wellcome	00081-0108-55	100s	$148.85
	00081-0108-56	100s ud	$148.85

INJECTION: 10 MG/ML

BRAND/MANUFACTURER	NDC	SIZE	AWP
○ **BRAND**			
RETROVIR: Burr Wellcome	00081-0107-93	20 ml 10s	$160.99

SYRUP: 10 MG/ML

BRAND/MANUFACTURER	NDC	SIZE	AWP
○ **BRAND**			
RETROVIR: Burr Wellcome	00081-0113-18	240 ml	$35.72

Zinacef SEE CEFUROXIME SODIUM

Zithromax SEE AZITHROMYCIN

Zocor SEE SIMVASTATIN

Zofran SEE ONDANSETRON HYDROCHLORIDE

Zoladex SEE GOSERELIN ACETATE

Zoloft SEE SERTRALINE HYDROCHLORIDE

Zolpidem Tartrate

DESCRIPTION

Zolpidem Tartrate is a non-benzodiazepine hypnotic of the imidazopyridine class and is available in 5-mg 10-mg strength tablets for oral administration.

Chemically, Zolpidem is N,N,6-trimethyl-2-p-tolyl-imidazo[1,2a]- pyridine-3-acetamide-L -(+)-tartrate (2:1).

Zolpidem Tartrate is a white to off-white crystalline powder that is sparingly soluble in water, alcohol, and propylene glycol. It has a molecular weight of 764.88.

Following is its chemical structure:

CLINICAL PHARMACOLOGY

Pharmacodynamics: Subunit modulation of the GABA$_A$ receptor choloride channel macromolecular complex is hypothesized to be responsible for sedative, anticonvulsant, anxiolytic, and myorelaxant drug properties. The major modulatory site of the GABA$_A$ receptor complex is located on its alpha (α) subunit and is referred to as the benzodiazepine (BZ) or omega receptor. At least three subtypes of the omega receptor have been identified.

While Zolpidem is hypnotic agent with a chemical structure unrelated to benzodiazepines, barbiturates, or other drugs with known hypnotic properties, it interacts with a GABA-BZ receptor complex and shares some of the pharmacological properties of the benzodiazepines. In contrast to the benzodiazepines, which nonselectively bind to and activate all three omega receptor subtypes. Zolpidem in vitro binds the omega receptor preferentially. The omega receptor is found primarily on the Lamina IV of the sensorimotor cortical regions, substantia nigra (pars reticulata), cerebellum molecular layer, olfactory bulb, ventral thalamic complex, pons, inferior colliculus, and globus pallidus. This selective binding or Zolpidem on the omega receptor is not absolute, but it may explain the relative absence of myorelaxant and anticonvulsant effects in animal studies as well as the preservation of deep sleep (stages 3 and 4) in human studies Zolpidem at hypnotic doses.

Pharmacokinetics: The pharmacokientic profile of Zolpidem Tartrate is characterized by rapid absorption from the GI tract and a short elimination half-life (T$_{1/2}$) in healthy subjects. In a single-dose crossover study in 45 healthy subjects administered 5- and 10-mg Zolpidem Tartrate tablets, the mean peak concentrations (C$_{max}$) were 59 (range: 29 to 113) and 121 (range: 58 to 272) ng/mL, respectively, occurring at a mean time (T$_{max}$) of 1.6 hours for both. The mean Zolpidem Tartrate elimination half-life was 2.6 (range: 1.4 to 4.5) and 2.5 (range: 1.4 to 3.8) hours, for the 5- and 10-mg tablets, respectively. Zolpidem Tartrate is converted to inactive metabolites that are eliminated primarily by renal excretion.

Zolpidem Tartrate demonstrated linear kinetics in the dose range of 5 to 20 mg. Total protein binding was found to be 92.5 ± 0.1% and remained constant, independent of concentration between 40 and 790 ng/mL. Zolpidem did not accumulate in young adults following nightly dosing with 20-mg Zolpidem Tartrate tablets for 2 weeks.

A food-effect study in 30 healthy male volunteers compared the pharmacokinetics of Zolpidem Tartrate 10 ng when administered while fasting or 20 minutes after a meal. Results demonstrated that with food, mean AUC and C_{max} were decreased by 15% and 25%, respectively, while mean T_{max} was prolonged by 60% (from 1.4 to 2.2 hr). The half-life remained unchanged. These results suggest that, for faster sleep onset, Zolpidem Tartrate should not be administered with or immediately after a meal.

In the elderly, the dose for Zolpidem Tartrate should be 5 mg (see *"Precautions"* and *"Dosage and Administration"*). This recommendation is based on several studies in which the mean C_{max}, $T_{1/2}$), and AUC were significantly increased when compared to results in young adults. In one study of eight elderly subjects (> 70 years), the means for C_{max}, $T_{1/2}$, and AUC significantly increased by 50% (225 vs 384 ng/mL), 32% (2.2 vs 2.9 hr), and 64% (955 vs 1,562 ng.hr/mL), respectively, as compared to younger adults (20 to 40 years) following a single 20 mg oral Zolpidem dose. Zolpidem Tartrate did not accumulate in elderly subjects following nightly oral dosing of 10 mg for 1 week.

The pharmacokinetics of Zolpidem Tartrate in eight patients with chronic hepatic insufficiency were compared to results in healthy subjects. Following a single 20-mg oral Zolpidem dose, mean C_{max} and AUC were found to be two times (250 vs 499 ng/mL) and five times (788 vs 4,203 ng·hr/mL) higher, respectively, in hepatically compromised patients. T_{max} did not change. The mean half-life in cirrhotic patients of 9.9 hr (range: 4.1 to 25.8 hr) was greater than that observed in normals of 2.2 hr (range: 1.6 to 2.4 hr). Dosing should be modified accordingly in patients with hepatic insufficiency (see *"Precautions"* and *"Dosage and Administration"*).

The pharmacokinetics of Zolpidem Tartrate were studied in 11 patients with end-stage renal failure (mean Cl_{cr} = 6.5 ± 1.5 ml/min) undergoing hemodialysis three times a week, who were dosed with Zolpidem 10 mg orally each day for 14 or 21 days. No statistically significant differences were observed for C_{max}, T_{max}, half-life, and AUC between the first and last day of drug administration when baseline concentration adjustments were made. On day 1, C_{max} was 172 ± 29 ng/mL (range: 46 to 344 ng/mL). After repeated dosing for 14 or 21 days, C_{max} was 203 ± 32 ng/mL (range: 28 to 316 ng/mL). On day 1. T_{max} was 1.7 ± 0.3 hr (range: 0.5 to 3.0 hr); after repeated dosing T_{max} was 0.8 ± 0.2 hr (range: 0.5 to 2.0 hr). This variation is accounted for by noting that last-day serum sampling began 10 hours after the previous dose, rather than after 24 hours. This resulted in residual drug concentration and a shorter period to reach maximal serum concentration. On day 1, $T^{1/2}$ was 2.4 ± 0.4 hr (range 0.4 to 5.1 hr). After repeated dosing. $T_{1/2}$ was 2.5 ± 0.4 hr (range: 0.7 to 4.2 hr). AUC was 796 ± 159 ng.hr/mL after the first dose and 818 ± 170 ng.hr/mL after repeated dosing. Zolpidem was not hemodialyzable. No accumulation of unchanged drug appeared after 14 or 21 days. Ambien pharmacokinetics were not significantly different in renally impaired patients. No dosage adjustment is necessary in patients with compromised renal function. As a general precaution, these patients should be closely monitored.

Postulated relationship between elimination rate of hypnotics and their profile of common untoward effects: The type and duration of hypnotic effects and the profile of unwanted effects during administration of hypnotic drugs may be influenced by the biologic half-life of administered drug and any active metabolites formed. When half-lives are long, drug or metabolites may accumulate during periods of nightly administration and be associated with impairment of cognitive and/or motor performance during waking hours; the possibility of interaction with other psychoactive drugs or alcohol will be enhanced. In contrast, if half-lives, including half-lives of active metaboites, are short, drug and metabolites will be cleared before the next dose is ingested, and carryover effects related to excessive sedation or CNS depression should be minimal or absent. Zolpidem Tartrate has a short half-life and no active metabolites. During nightly use for an extended period, pharmacodynamic tolerance or adaptation to some effects of hypnotics may develop. If the drug has a short elimination half-life, it is possible that a relative deficiency of the drug or its active metabolites (ie, in relationship to the receptor site) may occur at some point in the interval between each night's use. This sequence of events may account for two clinical findings reported to occur after several weeks of nightly use of other rapidly eliminated hypnotics, namely, increased wakefulness during the last third of the night, and the appearance of increased signs of daytime anxiety. Increased wakefulness during the last third of the night as measured by polysomnography has not been observed in clinical trials with Zolpidem Tartrate.

CONTROLLED TRIALS SUPPORTING SAFETY AND EFFICACY

Transient Insomnia: Normal adults experiencing transient insomnia (n = 462) during the first night in a sleep laboratory were evaluated in a double-blind, parallel group, single-night trial comparing two doses of Zolpidem Tartrate (7.5 and 10 mg) and placebo. Both Zolpidem doses were superior to placebo on objective (polysomnographic) measures of sleep latency. sleep duration, and number of awakenings.

Chronic Insomnia: Adult outpatients with chronic insomnia (n = 75) were evaluated in a double-blind, parallel group, 5-week trial comparing two doses of Zolpidem Tartrate (10 and 15 mg) and placebo. On objective (polysomnographic) measures of sleep latency and sleep efficiency Zolpidem Tartrate 15 mg was superior to placebo for all 5 weeks Zolpidem 10 mg was superior to placebo on sleep latency for the first 4 weeks and on sleep efficiency for weeks 2 and 4. Zolpidem was comparable to placebo on number of awakenings at both doses studied.

Adult outpatients (n = 141) with chronic insomnia were evaluated in a double-blind, parallel group, 4-week trial comparing two doses of Zolpidem (10 and 15 mg) and placebo. Zolpidem 10 mg was superior to placebo on a subjective measure of sleep latency for all 4 weeks, and on subjective measures of total sleep time, number of awakenings, and sleep quality for the first treatment week. Zolpidem 15 mg was superior to placebo on a subjective measure of sleep latency for the first 3 weeks, on a subjective measure of total sleep time for the first week, and on number of awakenings and sleep quality for the first 2 weeks.

Next-day Residual Effects: There was no evidence of residual next-day effects seen with Zolpidem Tartrate in several studies utilizing the Multiple Sleep Latency Test (MSLT), the Digit Symbol Substitution Test (DSST), and patient ratings of alertness. In one study involving elderly patients, there was a small but statistically significant decrease in one measure of performance, the DSST, but no impairment was seen in the MSLT in this study.

Rebound Effects: There was no objective (polysomnographic) evidence of rebound insomnia at recommended doses seen in studies evaluating sleep on the nights following discontinuation of Zolpidem Tartrate. There was subjective evidence of impaired sleep in the elderly on the first posttreatment night at doses above the recommended elderly dose of 5 mg.

Memory Impairment: Two small studies (n = 6 and n = 9) utilizing objective measures of memory yielded little evidence for memory impairment following the administration of Zolpidem Tartrate. There was subjective evidence from adverse event data for anterograde amnesia occurring in association with the administration of Zolpidem Tartrate predominantly at doses above 10 mg.

Effects on Sleep Stages: In studies that measured the percentage of sleep time spent in each sleep stage. Zolpidem Tartrate has generally been shown to preserve sleep stages. Sleep time spent in stages 3 and 4 (deep sleep) was found comparable to placebo with only inconsistent, minor changes in REM (paradoxical) sleep at the recommended dose.

INDICATIONS AND USAGE

Zolpidem Tartrate is indicated for the short-term treatment of insomnia. Hypnotics should generally be limited to 7 to 10 days of use, and reevaluation of the patient is recommended if they are to be taken for more than 2 to 3 weeks.

Zolpidem Tartrate should not be prescribed in quantities exceeding a 1-month supply (see *"Warnings"*).

Zolpidem Tartrate has been shown to decrease sleep latency and increase the duration of sleep for up to 5 weeks in controlled clinical studies.

UNLABELED USES

Zolpidem Tartrate is used alone or as an adjunct in preoperative sedation.

CONTRADICATIONS

None known.

WARNINGS

Since sleep disturbances may be the presenting manifestation of a physical and/or psychiatric disorder, symptomatic treatment of insomnia should be initiated only after a careful evaluation of the patient. The failure of insomnia to remit after 7 to 10 days of treatment may indicate the presence of a primary psychiatric and/or medical illness which should be evaluated. Worsening of insomnia or the emergence of new thinking or behavior abnormalities may be the consequence of an unrecognized psychiatric or physical disorder. Such findings have emerged during the course of treatment with sedative/hypnotic drugs, including Zolpidem Tartrate. Because some of the important adverse effects of Zolpidem Tartrate appear to be dose related (see *"Precautions"* and *"Dosage and Administration"*), it is important to use the smallest possible effective dose, especially in the elderly.

A variety of abnormal thinking and behavior changes have been reported to occur in association with the use of sedative/hypnotics. Some of these changes may be characterized by decreased inhibition (eg, aggressiveness and extroversion that seemed out of character), similar to effects produced by alcohol and other CNS depressants. Other reported behavioral changes have included bizarre behavior, agitation, hallucinatins, and depersonalization. Amnesia and other neuropsychiatric symptoms may occur unpredictably. In primarily depressed patients, worsening of depression, including suicidal thinking, has been reported in association with the use of sedative/hypnotics.

It can rarely be determined with certainty whether a particular instance of the abnormal behaviors listed above are drug induced, spontaneous in origin, or a result of an underlying psychiatric or physical disorder. Nonetheless, the emergence of any new behavioral sign or symptom of concern requires careful and immediate evaluation.

Following the rapid dose decrease or abrupt discontinuation of sedative/hypnotics, there have been reports of signs and symptoms similar to those associated with withdrawal from other CNS-depressant drugs (see *"Drug Abuse and Dependence"*).

Zolpidem Tartrate like other sedative/hypnotic drugs, has CNS-depressant effects. Due to the rapid onset of action, Zolpidem Tartrate should only be ingested immediately prior to going to bed. Patients should be cautioned against engaging in hazardous occupations requiring complete mental alertness or motor coordination such as operating machinery or driving a motor vehicle after ingesting the drug, including potential impairment of the performance of such activities that may occur the day following ingestion of Zolpidem Tartrate. Zolpidem Tartrate showed additive effects when combined with alcohol and should not be taken with alcohol. Patients should also be cautioned about possible combined effects with other CNS-depressant drugs. Dosage adjustments may be necessary when Zolpidem Tartrate is administered with such agents because of the potentially additive effects.

PRECAUTIONS
GENERAL
Use in the Elderly and/or Debilitated Patients: Impaired motor and/or cognitive performance after repeated exposure or unusual sensitivity to sedative/hypnotic drugs is a concern in the treatment of elderly and/or debilitated patients. Therefore, the recommended Zolpidern Tartrate dosage is 5 mg in such patients (see *"Dosage and Administration"*) to decrease the possibility of side effects. These patients should be closely monitored.

Use in Patients with Concomitant Illness: Clinical experience with Zolpidem Tartrate in patients with concomitant systemic illness is limited. Caution is advisable in using Zolpidem Tartrate in patients with diseases or conditions that could affect metabolism or hemodynamic responses. Although preliminary studies did not reveal respiratory depressant effects at hypnotic doses of Zolpidem Tartrate in normals, precautions should be observed Zolpidem Tartrate is prescribed to patients with compromised respiratory function, since sedative/hypnotics have the capacity to depress respiratory drive. Data in end-stage renal failure patients repeatedly treated with Zolpidem Tartrate did not demonstrate drug accumulation or alterations in pharmacokinetic parameters. No dosage adjustment in renally impaired patients is required; however, these patients should be closely monitored (see *"Pharmacokinetics"*). A study in subjects with hepatic impairment did reveal prolonged elimination in this group; therefore, treatment should be initiated with 5 mg in patients with hepatic compromise, and they should be closely monitored.

Use in Depression: As with other sedative/hypnotic drugs, Zolpidem Tartrate should be administered with caution to patients exhibiting signs or symptoms of depression. Suicidal tendencies may be present in such patients and protective measures may be required. Intentional overdosage is more common in this group of patients; therefore, the least amount of drug that is feasible should be prescribed for the patient at any one time.

Information for Patients: Patient information is printed at the end of this insert. To assure safe and effective use of Zolpidern Tartrate, this information and instructions provided in the patient information section should be discussed with patients.

Laboratory Tests: There are no specific laboratory tests recommended.

DRUG INTERACTIONS
CNS-Active Drugs: Zolpidern Tartrate was evaluated in healthy volunteers in single-dose interaction studies for several CNS drugs. A study involving haloperidol and Zolpidern Tartrate revealed no effect of haloperidol on the pharmacokinetics or pharmacodynamics of Zolpidem. Imipramine in combination with Zolpidem produced no pharmacokinetic interaction other than a 20% decrease in peak levels of imipramine, but there was an additive effect of decreased alertness. Similarly, chlorpromazine in combination with Zolpidem produced no pharmacokinetic interaction, but there was an additive effect of decreased alertness and psychomotor performance. The lack of a drug interaction following single-dose administration does not predict a lack following chronic administration.

An additive effect on psychomotor performance between alcohol and Zolpidem was demonstrated.

Since the systematic evaluations of Zolpidem Tartrate in combination with other CNS-active drugs have been limited, careful consideration should be given to the pharmacology of any CNS-active drug to be used with Zolpidem. Any drug with CNS-depressant effects could potentially enhance the CNS-depressant effects of Zolpidem.

Other Drugs: A study involving cimetidine Zolpidem and ranitidine Zolpidem combinations revealed no effect of either drug on the pharmacokinetics or pharmacodynamics of Zolpidem. Zolpidem had no effect on digoxin kinetics and did not affect prothrombin time when given with warfarin in normal subjects. Zolpidem's sedative/hypnotic effect was reversed by flumazenil; however, no significant alterations in Zolpidem pharmacokinetics were found.

Drug Laboratory Test Interactions: Zolpidem is not known to interfere with commonly employed clinical laboratory tests.

CARCINOGENESIS, MUTAGENESIS, IMPAIRMENT OF FERTILITY
Carcinogenesis: Zolpidem was administered to rats and mice for 2 years at dietary dosages of 4, 18, and 80 mg/day. In mice, these doses are 26 to 520 times or 2 to 35 times the maximum 10-mg human dose on a mg/kg or mg/m^2 basis, respectively. In rats these doses are 43 to 876 times or 6 to 115 times the maximum 10-mg human dose on a mg/kg or mg/m^2 basis, respectively. No evidence of carcinogenic potential was observed in mice. Renal liposarcomas were seen in 4/100 rats (3 males, 1 female) receiving 80 mg/kg/day and a renal lipoma was observed in one male rat at the 18 mg/kg/day dose. Incidence rates of lipoma and liposarcoma for Zolpidem were comparable to those seen in historical controls and the tumor findings were thought to be a spontaneous occurrence.

Mutagenesis: Zolpidem did not have mutagenic activity in several tests including the Ames test, genotoxicity in mouse lymphoma cells in vitro, chromosomal aberrations in cultured human lymphocytes, unscheduled DNA synthesis in rat hepatocytes in vitro, and the micronucleus test in mice.

Impairment of Fertility: In a rat reproduction study, the high dose (100 mg base/kg) of Zolpidem resulted in irregular estrus cycles and prolonged precoital

intervals, but there was no effect on male or female fertility after daily oral doses of 4 to 100 mg base/kg or 5 to 130 times the recommended human dose in mg/m^2. No effects on any other fertility parameters were noted.

PREGNANCY
Teratogenic Effects: Pregnancy Category B. Studies to assess the effects of Zolpidem on human reproduction and development have not been conducted. Teratology studies were conducted in rats and rabbits.

In rats, adverse maternal and fetal effects occurred at 20 and 100 mg base/kg and included dose-related maternal lethargy and ataxia and a dose-related trend to incomplete ossification of fetal skull bones. Underossification of various fetal bones indicates a delay in maturation and is often seen in rats treated with sedative/hypnotic drugs. There were no teratogenic effects after Zolpidem administration. The no-effect dose for maternal or fetal toxicity was 4 mg base/kg or 5 times the maximum human dose on a mg/m^2 basis.

In rabbits, dose-related maternal sedation and decreased weight gain occurred at all doses tested. At the high dose, 16 mg base/kg, there was an increase in postimplantation fetal loss and underossification of sternebrae in viable fetuses. These fetal findings in rabbits are often secondary to reductions in maternal weight gain. There were no frank teratogenic effects. The no-effect dose for fetal toxicity was 4 mg base/kg or 7 times the maximum human dose on a mg/m^2 basis.

Because animal reproduction studies are not always predictive of human response, this drug should be used during pregnancy only if clearly needed.

Nonteratogenic Effects: Studies to assess the effects on children whose mothers took Zolpidem during pregnancy have not been conducted. However, children born of mothers taking sedative/hypnotic drugs may be at some risk for withdrawal symptoms from the drug during the postnatal period. In addition, neonatal flaccidity has been reported in infants born of mothers who received sedative/hypnotic drugs during pregnancy.

Labor and Delivery: Zolpidem Tartrate has no established use in labor and delivery.

Nursing Mothers: Studies in lactating mothers indicate that the half-life of Zolpidem is similar to that in young normal volunteers (2.6 ± 0.3 hr). Between 0.004 and 0.019% of the total administered dose is excreted into milk, but the effect of Zolpidem on the infant is unknown.

In addition, in a rat study Zolpidem inhibited the secretion of milk. The no-effect dose was 4 mg base/kg or 6 times the recommended human dose in mg/m^2. The use of Zolpidem Tartrate in nursing mothers is not recommended.

Pediatric Use: Safety and effectiveness in children below the age of 18 have not been established.

ADVERSE REACTIONS
Associated with Discontinuation of Treatment: Approximately 4% of 1,701 patients who received Zolpidem at all doses (1.25 to 90 mg) in U.S. premarketing clinical trials discontinued treatment because of an adverse clinical event. Events most commonly associated with discontinuation from U.S. trials were daytime drowsiness (0.5%), dizziness (0.4%), headache (0.5%), nausea (0.6%), and vomiting (0.5%).

Approximately 6% of 1,320 patients who received Zolpidem at all doses (5 to 50 mg) in similar foreign trials discontinued treatment because of an adverse event. Events most commonly associated with discontinuation from these trials were daytime drowsiness (1.6%), amnesia (0.6%), dizziness (0.6%), headache (0.6%), and nausea (0.6%).

INCIDENCE IN CONTROLLED CLINICAL TRIALS
Most Commonly Observed Adverse Events in Controlled Trials: During short-term treatment (up to 10 nights) with Zolpidem Tartrate at doses up to 10 mg, the most commonly observed adverse events associated with the use of Zolpidem and seen at statistically significant differences from placebo-treated patients were drowsiness (reported by 2% of Zolpidem patients), dizziness (1%), and diarrhea (1%). During longer-term treatment (28 to 35 nights) with Zolpidem at doses up to 10 mg, the most commonly observed adverse events associated with the use of Zolpidem and seen at statistically significant differences from placebo-treated patients were dizziness (5%) and drugged feelings (3%).

Adverse Events Observed at an Incidence of ≥ 1% in Controlled Trials: The following tables enumerate treatment-emergent adverse event frequencies that were observed at an incidence equal to 1% or greater among patients with insomnia who received Zolpidem Tartrate in U.S. placebo-controlled trials. Events reported by investigators were classified utilizing a modified World Health Organization (WHO) dictionary of preferred terms for the purpose of establishing event frequencies. The prescriber should be aware that these figures cannot be used to predict the incidence of side effects in the course of usual medical practice, in which patient characteristics and other factors differ from those that prevailed in these clinical trials. Similarly, the cited frequencies cannot be compared with figures obtained from other clinical investigators involving related drug products and uses, since each group of drug trials is conducted under a different set of conditions. However, the cited figures provide the physician with a basis for estimating the relative contribution of drug and nondrug factors to the incidence of side effects in the population studied.

The following table was derived from a pool of 11 placebo-controlled short-term U.S. efficacy trials involving Zolpidem in doses ranging from 1.25 to 20 mg. The table is limited to data from doses up to and including 10 mg, the highest dose recommended for use.

INCIDENCE OF TREATMENT-EMERGENT ADVERSE EXPERIENCES IN SHORT-TERM PLACEBO-CONTROLLED CLINICAL TRIALS

Body System/ Adverse Event*	*(Percentage of patients reporting)*	
	Zolpidem ($\leq$ 10 mg) (N = 685)	Placebo (N = 473)
Central and Peripheral Nervous System		
Headache	7	6
Drowsiness	2	-
Dizziness	1	-
Gastrointestinal System		
Nausea	2	3
Diarrhea	1	-
Musculoskeletal System		
Myalgia	1	2

* *Events reported by at least 1% of Zolpidem Tartrate patients are included.*

The following table was derived from a pool of three placebo-controlled long-term efficacy trials involving Zolpidem Tartrate. These trials involved patients with chronic insomnia who were treated for 28 to 35 nights with Zolpidem at doses of 5, 10, or 15 mg. The table is limited to data from doses up to and including 10 mg, the highest dose recommended for use. The table includes only adverse events occurring at an incidence of at least 1% for Zolpidem patients.

INCIDENCE OF TREATMENT-EMERGENT ADVERSE EXPERIENCES IN LONG-TERM PLACEBO-CONTROLLED CLINICAL TRIALS

Body System/ Adverse Event*	*(Percentage of patients reporting)*	
	Zolpidem ($\leq$ 10 mg) (N = 152)	Placebo (N = 161)
Autonomic Nervous System		
Dry mouth	3	1
Body as a Whole		
Allergy	4	1
Back pain	3	2
Influenza-like symptoms	2	—
Chest pain	1	—
Fatigue	1	2
Cardiovascular System		
Palpitation	2	—
Central and Peripheral Nervous System		
Headache	19	22
Drowsiness	8	5
Dizziness	5	1
Lethargy	3	1
Drugged feeling	3	—
Light-headedness	2	1
Depression	2	1
Abnormal dreams	1	—
Amnesia	1	—
Anxiety	1	1
Nervousness	1	3
Sleep disorder	1	—
Gastrointestinal System		
Nausea	6	6
Dyspepsia	5	6
Diarrhea	3	2
Abdominal pain	2	2
Constipation	2	1
Anorexia	1	1
Vomiting	1	1
Immunologic System		
Infection	1	1
Musculoskeletal System		
Myalgia	7	7
Arthralgia	4	4
Respiratory System		
Upper respiratory infection	5	6
Sinusitis	4	2
Pharyngitis	3	1
Rhinitis	1	3
Skin and Appendages		
Rash	2	1
Urogenital System		
Urinary tract infection	2	2

* *Events reported by at least 1% of patients treated with Zolpidem Tartrate.*

Dose Relationship for Adverse Events: There is evidence from dose comparison trials suggesting a dose relationship for many of the adverse events associated with Zolpidem use particularly for certain CNS and gastrointestinal adverse events.

Adverse Event Incidence Across the Entire Preapproval Database: Zolpidem Tartrate was administered to 3,021 subjects in clinical trials throughout the U.S.,

Canada, and Europe. Treatment-emergent adverse events associated with clinical trial participation were recorded by clinical investigators using terminology of their own choosing. To provide a meaningful estimate of the proportion of individuals experiencing treatment-emergent adverse events, similar types of untoward events were grouped into a smaller number of standardized event categories and classified utilizing a modified WHO dictionary of preferred terms. The frequencies presented, therefore, represent the proportions of the 3,021 individuals exposed to Zolpidem, at all doses, who experienced an event of the type cited on at least one occasion while receiving Zolpidem. All reported treatment-emergent adverse events are included, except those already listed in the table above of adverse events in placebo-controlled studies, those coding terms that are so general as to be uninformative, and those events where a drug cause was remote. It is important to emphasize that, although the events reported did occur during treatment with Zolpidem Tartrate they were not necessarily caused by it.

Adverse events are further classified within body system categories and enumerated in order of decreasing frequency using the following definitions; frequent adverse events are defined as those occurring in greater than 1/100 subjects; infrequent adverse events are those occurring in 1/100 to 1/1,000 patients; rare events are those occurring in less than 1/1,000 patients.

Autonomic Nervous System: Infrequent: increased sweating, pallor, postural hypotension. Rare: altered saliva, flushing, glaucoma, hypotension, impotence, syncope, tenesmus.

Body as a Whole: Infrequent: asthenia, edema, falling, fever, malaise, trauma. Rare: allergic reaction, allergy aggravated, abdominal body sensation, anaphylactic shock, face edema, hot flashes, increased ESR, pain, restless legs, rigors, tolerance increased, weight decrease.

Cardiovascular System: Infrequent: cerebrovascular disorder, hypertension, tachycardia. Rare: arrhythmia, arteritis, circulatory failure, extrasystoles, hypertension aggravated, myocardial infarction, phlebitis, pulmonary embolism, pulmonary edema, varicose veins, ventricular tachycardia.

Central and Peripheral Nervous System: Frequent: ataxia, confusion, euphoria, insomnia, vertigo. Infrequent: agitation, decreased cognition, detached, difficulty concentrating, dysarthria, emotional lability, hallucination, hypoesthesia, migraine, paresthesia, sleeping (after daytime dosing), stupor, tremor. Rare: abnormal thinking, aggressive reaction, appetite increased, decreased libido, delusion, dementia, depersonalization, dysphasia, feeling strange, hypotonia, hysteria, illusion, intoxicated feeling, leg cramps, manic reaction, neuralgia, neuritis, neuropathy, neurosis, panic attacks, paresis, personality disorder, somnambulism, suicide attempts, tetany, yawning.

Gastrointestinal System: Infrequent: constipation, dysphagia, flatulence, gastroenteritis, hiccup. Rare: enteritis, eructation, esophagospasm, gastritis, hemorrhoids, intestinal obstruction, rectal hemorrhage, tooth caries.

Hematologic and Lymphatic System: Rare: anemia, hyperhemoglobinemia, leukopenia, lymphadenopathy, macrocytic anemia, purpura.

Immunologic System: Rare: abscess, herpes simplex, herpes zoster, otitis externa, otitis media.

Liver and Biliary System: Infrequent: increased SGPT. Rare: abnormal hepatic function, bilirubinemia, increased SGOT.

Metabolic and Nutritional: Infrequent: hyperglycemia. Rare: gout, hypercholesteremia, hyperlipidemia, increased BUN, periorbital edema, thirst, weight decrease.

Musculoskeletal System: Infrequent: arthritis. Rare; arthrosis, muscle weakness, sciatica, tendinitis.

Reproductive System: Infrequent: menstrual disorder, vaginitis. Rare: breast fibroadenosis, breast neoplasm, breast pain.

Respiratory System: Infrequent: bronchitis, coughing, dyspnea. Rare: bronchospasm, epistaxis, hypoxia, laryngitis, pneumonia.

Skin and Appendages: Rare: acne, bullous eruption, dermatitis, furunculosis, injection-site inflammation, photosensitivity reaction, urticaria.

Special Senses: Frequent: diplopia, vision abnormal. Infrequent: eye irritation, scleritis, taste perversion, tinnitus. Rare; corneal ulceration, eye pain, lacrimation abnormal, photopsia.

Urogenital System: Infrequent: cystitis, urinary incontinence. Rare: acute renal failure, dysuria, micturition frequency, polyuria, pyelonephritis, renal pain, urinary retention.

DRUG ABUSE AND DEPENDENCE

Controlled Substance: Zolpidem Tartrate is classified as a Schedule IV controlled substance by federal regulation.

Abuse and Dependence: Studies of abuse potential in former drug abusers found that the effects of single doses of Zolpidem Tartrate 40 mg were similar, but not identical, to diazepam 20 mg, while Zolpidem Tartrate 10 mg was difficult to distinguish from placebo.

Sedative/hypnotics have produced withdrawal signs and symptoms following abrupt discontinuation. These reported symptoms range from mild dysphoria and insomnia to a withdrawal syndrome that may include abdominal and muscle cramps, vomiting, sweating, tremors, and convulsions. The U.S. clinical trial experience from Zolpidem does not reveal any clear evidence for withdrawal syndrome. Nevertheless, the following adverse events included in DSM-III-R criteria for uncomplicated sedative/hypnotic withdrawal were reported during U.S. clinical trials following placebo substitution occurring within 48 hours following last Zolpidem treatment: fatigue, nausea, flushing, lightheadedness, uncontrolled crying, emesis, stomach cramps, panic attack, nervousness, and abdominal discomfort. These reported adverse events occurred at an incidence of 1% or less. However, available data cannot provide a reliable estimate of the incidence, if any, of dependency, or the relationship of any dependency to dose and duration of treatment.

Because individuals with a history of addiction to, or abuse of, drugs or alcohol are at risk of habituation and dependence, they should be under careful surveillance when receiving Zolpidem or any other hypnotic.

OVERDOSAGE

Signs and Symptoms: In European postmarketing reports of overdose with Zolpidem alone, impairment of consciousness has ranged from somnolence to light coma. There was one case each of cardiovascular and respiratory compromise. Individuals have fully recovered from Zolpidem Tartrate overdoses up to 400 mg (40 times the maximum recommended dose). Overdose cases involving multiple CNS-depressant agents, including Zolpidem, have resulted in more severe symptomatology, including fatal outcomes.

Recommended Treatment: General symptomatic and supportive measures should be used along with immediate gastric lavage where appropriate. Intravenous fluids should be administered as needed. Flumazenil may be useful. As in all cases of drug overdose, respiration, pulse, blood pressure, and other appropriate signs should be monitored and general supportive measures employed. Hypotension and CNS depression should be monitored and treated by appropriate medical intervention. Sedating drugs should be withheld following Zolpidem overdosage, even if excitation occurs. The value of dialysis in the treatment of overdosage has not been determined, although hemodialysis studies in patients with renal failure receiving therapeutic doses have demonstrated that Zolpidem is not dialyzable.

Poison Control Center: As with the management of all overdosage, the possibility of multiple drug ingestion should be considered. The physician may wish to consider contacting a poison control center for up-to-date information on the management of hypnotic drug product overdosage.

DOSAGE AND ADMINISTRATION

The dose of Zolpidem Tartrate should be individualized.

The recommended dose for adults is 10 mg immediately before bedtime.

Downward dosage adjustment may be necessary when Zolpidem Tartrate is administered with agents having known CNS-depressant effects because of the potentially additive effects.

Elderly or debilitated patients may be especially sensitive to the effects of Zolpidem Tartrate. Patients with hepatic insufficiency do not clear the drug as rapidly as normals. An initial 5-mg dose is recommended in these patients (see "Precautions").

The total Zolpidem Tartrate dose should not exceed 10 mg. Store below 86°F (30°C).

HOW SUPPLIED
TABLETS (C-IV): 5 MG

BRAND/MANUFACTURER	NDC	SIZE	AWP
○ **BRAND**			
▶ AMBIEN: Searle	00025-5401-31	100s	$124.50
	00025-5401-34	100s ud	$130.73

TABLETS (C-IV): 10 MG

BRAND/MANUFACTURER	NDC	SIZE	AWP
○ **BRAND**			
▶ AMBIEN: Searle	00025-5421-31	100s	$153.14
	00025-5421-34	100s ud	$160.79

Zonalon *SEE* DOXEPIN HYDROCHLORIDE

ZORprin *SEE* ASPIRIN

Zosyn *SEE* PIPERACILLIN SODIUM AND TAZOBACTAM SODIUM

Zovirax *SEE* ACYCLOVIR

Zydone *SEE* ACETAMINOPHEN WITH HYDROCODONE BITARTRATE

Zyloprim *SEE* ALLOPURINOL

Zymase *SEE* PANCRELIPASE

Use-in-Pregnancy Ratings

The U.S. Food and Drug Administration's Use-in-Pregnancy rating system weighs the degree to which available information has ruled out risk to the fetus against the drug's potential benefit to the patient. The ratings, and their interpretation, are as follows:

X: CONTRAINDICATED IN PREGNANCY

Studies in animals or humans, or investigational or post-marketing reports, have demonstrated fetal risk which clearly outweighs any possible benefit to the patient.

D: POSITIVE EVIDENCE OF RISK

Investigational or post-marketing data show risk to the fetus. Nevertheless, potential benefits may outweigh the potential risk.

C: RISK CANNOT BE RULED OUT

Human studies are lacking, and animal studies are either positive for risk or are lacking as well. However, potential benefits may outweigh the potential risk.

B: NO EVIDENCE OF RISK IN HUMANS

Either animal findings show risk while human findings do not, or, if no adequate human studies have been done, animal findings are negative.

A: CONTROLLED STUDIES SHOW NO RISK

Adequate, well-controlled studies in pregnant women have failed to demonstrate risk to the fetus.

The lists that follow show the drugs in *PDR Generics* that fall into each of these categories. Since a number of drugs have never received a formal rating, the lists are not all inclusive. If a drug you're researching doesn't appear in these listings, be sure to check its prescribing information. Precautions do need to be taken with many of the unrated drugs.

X

CONTRAINDICATED IN PREGNANCY
Studies in animals or humans, or investigational or post-marketing reports, have demonstrated fetal risk which clearly outweighs any possible benefit to the patient.

Acetohydroxamic Acid
Anisindione
Belladonna Alkaloids/Ergotamine
  Tartrate/Phenobarbital
Benzphetamine Hydrochloride
Chlorotrianisene
Clomiphene Citrate
Danazol
Demecarium Bromide
Desogestrel and Ethinyl Estradiol
Dienestrol
Diethylstilbestrol
Dihydroergotamine Mesylate
Ephedrine Hydrochloride/
  Phenobarbital/Potassium
  Iodide/Theophylline
Ergotamine Tartrate
Ergotamine Tartrate with Caffeine
Estazolam
Estradiol
Estradiol Cypionate and
  Testosterone Cypionate
Estradiol, Injectable
Estramustine Phosphate Sodium
Estrogens, Conjugated
Estrogens, Conjugated and
  Meprobamate
Estrogens, Conjugated and
  Methyltestosterone
Estrogens, Esterified
Estrogens, Esterified and
  Methyltestosterone
Estrone
Estropipate
Ethinyl Estradiol
Ethinyl Estradiol and Norethindrone
Ethinyl Estradiol and Norgestimate
Ethinyl Estradiol and Norgestrel
Ethinyl Estradiol with Ethynodiol
  Diacetate
Etretinate
Finasteride
Fluoxymesterone
Fluvastatin Sodium

Goserelin Acetate
Histrelin Acetate
Isoflurophate
Isotretinoin
Leuprolide Acetate
Levonorgestrel
Lovastatin
Medroxyprogesterone Acetate,
  Contraceptive
Megestrol Acetate
Menotropins
Mestranol and Norethindrone
Methotrexate
Methyltestosterone
Misoprostol
Nafarelin Acetate
Nandrolone
Norethindrone
Norethindrone Acetate
Norgestrel
Oxandrolone
Oxymetholone
Oxytocin
Plicamycin
Pravastatin Sodium
Quazepam
Quinestrol
Quinine Sulfate
Ribavirin
Simvastatin
Stanozolol
Temazepam
Testosterone, Injectable
Testosterone, Transdermal
Triazolam
Urofollitropin
Vitamin A
Warfarin Sodium

D

POSITIVE EVIDENCE OF RISK
Investigational or postmarketing data show risk to the fetus. Nevertheless, potential benefits may outweigh the potential risk.

Alprazolam
Altretamine
Amikacin Sulfate
Aminoglutethimide
Amiodarone Hydrochloride
Amitriptyline Hydrochloride
Amobarbital Sodium

Amobarbital Sodium and
   Secobarbital Sodium
Aspirin
Atenolol
Atenolol with Chlorthalidone
Azathioprine
Benazepril Hydrochloride
Benazepril Hydrochloride with
   Hydrochlorothiazide
Busulfan
Butabarbital Sodium
Calcium Iodide and Codeine
Calcium Iodide and Isoproterenol
   Sulfate
Captopril
Captopril with Hydrochlorothiazide
Carboplatin
Carmustine
Chlorambucil
Chlordiazepoxide
Cisplatin
Cladribine
Colchicine
Cortisone Acetate
Cyclophosphamide
Cytarabine
Daunorubicin Hydrochloride
Dicumarol
Divalproex Sodium
Doxorubicin Hydrochloride
Doxycycline
Enalapril
Enalapril Maleate with
   Hydrochlorothiazide
Etoposide
Floxuridine
Fludarabine Phosphate
Fluorouracil, Systemic
Fluorouracil, Topical
Flutamide
Fosinopril Sodium
Halazepam
Hydroxyprogesterone Caproate
Idarubicin Hydrochloride
Ifosfamide
Kanamycin Sulfate
Lisinopril
Lithium Carbonate
Lithium Citrate
Lomustine
Lorazepam
Mechlorethamine Hydrochloride
Melphalan
Mephobarbita
Meprobamate
Mercaptopurine
Metaraminol Bitartrate
Methimazole
Midazolam Hydrochloride
Minocycline Hydrochloride
Mitoxantrone Hydrochloride
Nalbuphine Hydrochloride
Neomycin Sulfate
Neomycin Sulfate and Polymyxin B
   Sulfate
Neomycin Sulfate and Polymyxin B
   Sulfate, Irrigant
Netilmicin Sulfate
Nicotine
Nortriptyline Hydrochloride
Oxazepam
Oxytetracycline Hydrochloride
Oxytetracycline Hydrochloride/
   Phenazopyridine/Sulfamethizole
Paclitaxel
Paramethadione

Pentobarbital Sodium
Pentostatin
Phenacemide
Phenobarbital
Phensuximide
Pipobroman
Polythiazide
Potassium Iodide
Primidone
Procarbazine Hydrochloride
Progesterone
Propylthiouracil
Quinapril Hydrochloride
Quinethazone
Ramipril
Reserpine and Trichlormethiazide
Secobarbital Sodium
Streptomycin Sulfate
Strontium-89 Chloride
Tamoxifen Citrate
Teniposide
Thioguanine
Tobramycin Sulfate, Injectable
Trimethaphan Camsylate
Trimetrexate Glucuronate
Valproic Acid
Vinblastine Sulfate
Vincristine Sulfate

C

RISK CANNOT BE RULED OUT

*Human studies are lacking, and
animal studies are either positive for
risk or are lacking as well.
However, potential benefits may
outweigh the potential risk.*

Acetaminophen and Oxycodone
   Hydrochloride
Acetaminophen and Pentazocine
   Hydrochloride
Acetaminophen with Butalbital
Acetaminophen with Codeine
   Phosphate
Acetaminophen with Hydrocodone
   Bitartrate
Acetaminophen/Butalbital/Caffeine
Acetaminophen/Butalbital/Caffeine/
   Codeine Phosphate
Acetaminophen/Caffeine/
   Chlorpheniramine/Hydrocodone/
   Phenylephrine
Acetaminophen/Caffeine/Dihydroco
   deine Bitartrate
Acetaminophen/Chlorpheniramine
   Maleate/Phenylpropanolamine
   Hydrochloride/Phenyltoloxamine
   Citrate
Acetazolamide
Acetic Acid and Desonide
Acetohexamide
Acetylcholine Chloride
Acyclovir
Adenosine
Albumin, Normal Serum, Human
Albuterol
Alclometasone Dipropionate
Alcohol, Dehydrated
Aldesleukin
Alfentanil Hydrochloride
Alglucerase
Allergenic Extracts

Allopurinol
Alteplase, Recombinant
Aluminum Chloride (Hexahydrate)
Amantadine Hydrochloride
Amcinonide
Amino Acids with Electrolytes,
   Injectable
Amino Acids, Injectable
Amino Acids/Calcium
   Chloride/Dextrose/Electrolytes
Aminocaproic Acid | 135
Aminohippurate Sodium | 145
Aminophylline | 148
Aminosalicylic Acid | 153
Amlodipine Besylate | 165
Ammonium Chloride | 166
Ammonium Lactate | 6288
Ammonium Molybdate | 3291
Amoxapine | 170
Amphetamine
Amrinone Lactate
Amyl Nitrite
Amyl Nitrite/Sodium Nitrite/Sodium
   Thiosulfate
Amylase/Cellulase/Lipase/Protease
Anistreplase
Antazoline Phosphate and
   Naphazoline Hydrochloride
Anthralin
Anti-Inhibitor Coagulant Complex
Anticoagulant Citrate Phosphate
   Dextrose
Antihemophilic Factor
Antihemophilic Factor, Human
Antihemophilic Factor, Porcine
Antipyrine and Benzocaine
Antipyrine/Benzocaine/
   Phenylephrine Hydrochloride
Antithrombin III (Human)
Antivenin (Crotalidae) Polyvalent
Antivenin (Latrodectus Mactans)
Asparaginase
Aspirin and Carisoprodol
Aspirin and Methocarbamol
Aspirin with Butalbital
Aspirin with Codeine Phosphate
Aspirin with Hydrocodone Bitartrate
Aspirin/Butalbital/Caffeine
Aspirin/Butalbital/Caffeine/Codeine
   Phosphate
Aspirin/Caffeine/Orphenadrine
   Citrate
Aspirin/Carisoprodol/Codeine
   Phosphate
Astemizole
Atovaquone
Atracurium Besylate
Atropine Sulfate and Difenoxin
   Hydrochloride
Atropine Sulfate and Diphenoxylate
   Hydrochloride
Atropine Sulfate and Edrophonium
   Chloride
Atropine Sulfate, Injectable
Atropine Sulfate, Ophthalmic
Atropine Sulfate, Oral
Atropine Sulfate/Benzoic
   Acid/Hyoscyamine/Methenamine/
   Methylene Blue/Phenylsalicylate
Auranofin
Aurothioglucose
Azatadine Maleate with
   Pseudoephedrine Sulfate
BCG
Bacitracin, Ophthalmic
Baclofen

Balanced Salt Solution
Beclomethasone Dipropionate
Belladonna Alkaloids and
   Butabarbital Sodium
Belladonna Alkaloids and Opium
Belladonna Alkaloids/
   Chlorpheniramine Maleate/
   Phenylephrine Hydrochloride/
   Phenylpropanolamine
   Hydrochloride
Belladonna and Phenobarbital
Benazepril Hydrochloride
Benazepril Hydrochloride with
   Hydrochlorothiazide
Bendroflumethiazide
Bendroflumethiazide and Nadolol
Bendroflumethiazide and Rauwolfia
   Serpentina
Benzocaine
Benzonatate
Benzoyl Peroxide
Benzoyl Peroxide with Sulfur
Benzthiazide
Benzylpenicilloyl Polylysine
Bepridil Hydrochloride
Beta Carotene
Betamethasone Dipropionate with
   Clotrimazole
Betamethasone Sodium Phosphate
Betamethasone, Topical
Betaxolol Hydrochloride,
   Ophthalmic
Betaxolol Hydrochloride, Oral
Bethanechol Chloride
Bile Salts/Pancreatin/Pepsin
Biperiden
Bisoprolol Fumarate
Bisoprolol Fumarate with
   Hydrochlorothiazide
Bitolterol Mesylate
Botulinum Toxin Type A
Bretylium Tosylate
Bromodiphenhydramine
   Hydrochloride and Codeine
   Phosphate
Brompheniramine Maleate and
   Pseudoephedrine Hydrochloride
Brompheniramine Maleate/Codeine
   Phosphate/Phenylpropanolamine
   Hydrochloride
Brompheniramine/Dextromethorpha
   n/Pseudoephedrine
Buclizine Hydrochloride
Budesonide
Bumetanide
Buprenorphine Hydrochloride
Butoconazole Nitrate
Butorphanol Tartrate
Caffeine with Sodium Benzoate
Calcifediol
Calcipotriene
Calcitonin
Calcitriol
Calcium Acetate
Calcium, Injectable
Capreomycin Sulfate
Captopril
Captopril with Hydrochlorothiazide
Carbachol
Carbamazepine
Carbetapentane/Chlorpheniramine/E
   phedrine/Phenylephrine
Carbidopa and Levodopa
Carbinoxamine Maleate with
   Pseudoephedrine Hydrochloride
Carbinoxamine Maleate/

Dextromethorphan Hydrobromide/
Pseudoephedrine Hydrochloride
Carboprost Tromethamine
Cardioplegic Solution
Carisoprodol
Carteolol Hydrochloride,
Ophthalmic
Carteolol Hydrochloride, Oral
Cellulose Sodium Phosphate
Chloral Hydrate
Chloramphenicol
Chlorcyclizine Hydrochloride and
Hydrocortisone Acetate
Chloroprocaine Hydrochloride
Chloroquine
Chlorothiazide
Chlorothiazide with Reserpine
Chloroxine
Chloroxylenol/Hydrocortisone/Pram
oxine Hydrochloride
Chlorpheniramine Maleate and
Epinephrine Hydrochloride
Chlorpheniramine Maleate and
Pseudoephedrine Hydrochloride
Chlorpheniramine Maleate with
Phenylpropanolamine
Hydrochloride
Chlorpheniramine
Maleate/Dextromethorphan
Hydrobromide/Guaifenesin/Pheny
lephrine Hydrochloride
Chlorpheniramine Maleate/
Ephedrine Sulfate/Guaifenesin/
Hydriodic Acid
Chlorpheniramine
Maleate/Hydrocodone
Bitartrate/Phenylephrine
Hydrochloride
Chlorpheniramine
Maleate/Hydrocodone
Bitartrate/Pseudoephedrine
Hydrochloride
Chlorpheniramine
Maleate/Phenylephrine
Hydrochloride/Phenylpropanolami
ne Hydrochloride/
Phenyltoloxamine Citrate
Chlorpheniramine
Maleate/Phenylephrine
Hydrochloride/Phenylpropanolami
ne Hydrochloride/Pyrilamine
Maleate
Chlorpheniramine
Maleate/Phenylephrine
Hydrochloride/Phenyltoloxamine
Citrate
Chlorpheniramine Polistirex with
Hydrocodone Polistirex
Chlorpheniramine Tannate with
Pseudoephedrine Tannate
Chlorpheniramine
Tannate/Phenylephrine
Tannate/Pyrilamine Tannate
Chlorpromazine
Chlorpropamide
Chlorthalidone with Clonidine
Hydrochloride
Chlorzoxazone
Cholera Vaccine
Cholestyramine
Choline Bitartrate and Dexpanthenol
Choline Magnesium Trisalicylate
Chromic Chloride
Chymopapain
Cilastatin Sodium and Imipenem
Cinoxacin

Ciprofloxacin Hydrochloride,
Ophthalmic
Ciprofloxacin, Systemic
Cisapride
Citric Acid and Potassium
Bicarbonate
Citric Acid/Glucono-delta-lac-
tone/Magnesium Carbonate
Citric Acid/Magnesium
Oxide/Sodium Carbonate
Clarithromycin
Clidinium Bromide
Clobetasol Propionate
Clocortolone Pivalate
Clofazimine
Clofibrate
Clomipramine Hydrochloride
Clonazepam
Clonidine
Clotrimazole
Cocaine Hydrochloride
Codeine
Codeine Phosphate and
Promethazine Hydrochloride
Codeine Phosphate with
Pseudoephedrine Hydrochloride
Codeine
Phosphate/Guaifenesin/Phenylpro
panolamine Hydrochloride
Codeine Phosphate/Guaifenesin/
Pseudoephedrine Hydrochloride
Codeine Phosphate/Phenylephrine
Hydrochloride/Promethazine
Hydrochloride
Codeine Phosphate/Pseudoephedrine
Hydrochloride/Triprolidine
Hydrochloride
Corticotropin
Cosyntropin
Crotamiton
Cyclopentolate Hydrochloride
Cycloserine
Cyclosporine
Cyclothiazide
Cysteine Hydrochloride
Dacarbazine
Dactinomycin
Dantrolene Sodium
Dapsone
Deferoxamine Mesylate
Deserpidine
Desipramine Hydrochloride
Desonide
Desoximetasone
Dexamethasone Sodium Phosphate
and Neomycin Sulfate, Topical
Dexamethasone Sodium Phosphate
with Neomycin Sulfate,
Ophthalmic
Dexamethasone Sodium Phosphate,
Inhalation
Dexamethasone and Tobramycin
Dexamethasone, Ophthalmic
Dexamethasone, Oral
Dexamethasone, Topical
Dexchlorpheniramine
Maleate/Guaifenesin/Pseudoephed
rine Sulfate
Dexpanthenol
Dextran 40
Dextran and Dextrose
Dextroamphetamine Sulfate
Dextromethorphan Hydrobromide
and Guaifenesin
Dextromethorphan Hydrobromide
and Promethazine Hydrochloride

Dextrose
Dextrose and Electrolytes
Dextrose and Electrolytes,
Intraperitoneal
Dextrose and Potassium Chloride
Dextrose and Ringer's
Dextrose and Sodium Chloride
Dextrose/Electrolytes/Fructose/
Invert Sugar
Dextrose/Lactated
Ringer's/Potassium Chloride
Dextrose/Potassium
Chloride/Sodium Chloride
Dezocine
Diatrizoate Meglumine
Diatrizoate Sodium
Diazoxide
Diazoxide, Injectable
Dichlorphenamide
Diflorasone Diacetate
Diflunisal
Digestive Enzymes/Hyoscyamine
Sulfate/Phenyltoloxamine Citrate
Digitoxin
Digoxin
Digoxin Immune Fab (Ovine)
Dihydrotachysterol
Diltiazem Hydrochloride
Dimethyl Sulfoxide
Dinoprostone, Cervical
Dinoprostone, Vaginal
Diphtheria and Tetanus Toxoids
Diphtheria/Haemophilus
b/Pertussis/Tetanus Vaccine
Diphtheria/Pertussis/Tetanus
Disopyramide Phosphate
Disulfiram
Dopamine Hydrochloride
Doxacurium Chloride
Doxazosin Mesylate
Doxepin Hydrochloride
Dronabinol
Droperidol
Droperidol and Fentanyl Citrate
Dyclonine Hydrochloride
Dyphylline
Dyphylline and Guaifenesin
Echothiophate Iodide
Econazole Nitrate
Edetate Disodium
Edrophonium Chloride
Electrolytes and Polyethylene
Glycol 3350
Electrolytes, Injectable
Enalapril
Enalapril Maleate with
Hydrochlorothiazide
Enoxacin
Ephedrine Sulfate
Epinephrine Bitartrate and
Pilocarpine Hydrochloride
Epinephrine, Ophthalmic
Epinephrine, Systemic
Epoetin Alfa
Ergocalciferol
Erythrityl Tetranitrate
Erythromycin Ethylsuccinate with
Sulfisoxazole Acetyl
Esmolol Hydrochloride
Ethanolamine Oleate
Ethchlorvynol
Ethiodized Oil
Ethionamide
Ethosuximide
Ethotoin
Etidronate Disodium, Injectable

Etidronate Disodium, Oral
Etodolac
Etomidate
Factor IX (Human)
Factor IX Complex, Human
Fat Emulsion
Felbamate
Felodipine
Fenfluramine Hydrochloride
Fentanyl
Ferrous Fumarate/Folic
Acid/Minerals/Vitamins, Multi
Ferrous Fumarate/Vitamin B12
/Vitamin C
Ferrous Gluconate/Liver
Extract/Vitamins, Multi
Filgrastim
Flecainide Acetate
Fluconazole
Flucytosine
Fludrocortisone Acetate
Flumazenil
Flunisolide
Fluocinolone Acetonide
Fluocinonide
Fluorescein Sodium and
Proparacaine Hydrochloride
Fluorometholone
Fluphenazine
Flurandrenolide
Flurbiprofen Sodium, Ophthalmic
Fluticasone Propionate
Folic Acid/Polysaccharide-Iron
Complex/Vitamin B12
Foscarnet Sodium
Fosinopril Sodium
Furazolidone
Furosemide
Gabapentin
Gadodiamide
Gadopentetate Dimeglumine
Gadoteridol
Gallium Nitrate
Ganciclovir Sodium
Gemfibrozil
Gentamicin Sulfate and
Prednisolone Acetate
Gentamicin Sulfate, Ophthalmic
Glipizide
Globulin, Immune
Globulin, Immune Rho (D)
Glycerin
Gold Sodium Thiomalate
Gonadotropin, Chorionic
Griseofulvin
Guaifenesin
Guaifenesin and Hydrocodone
Bitartrate
Guaifenesin and Hydromorphone
Hydrochloride
Guaifenesin and Phenylephrine
Hydrochloride
Guaifenesin and
Phenylpropanolamine
Hydrochloride
Guaifenesin and Pseudoephedrine
Hydrochloride
Guaifenesin and Theophylline
Guaifenesin and Theophylline
Sodium Glycinate
Guaifenesin/Hydrocodone
Bitartrate/Pheniramine
Maleate/Phenylephrine
Hydrochloride/Phenylpropanolami
ne Hydrochloride
Guaifenesin/Hydrocodone

Bitartrate/Pheniramine
Maleate/Phenylpropanolamine
Hydrochloride/Pyrilamine Maleate
Guaifenesin/Hydrocodone
Bitartrate/Phenylephrine
Hydrochloride
Guaifenesin/Hydrocodone
Bitartrate/Pseudoephedrine
Hydrochloride
Guaifenesin/Phenylephrine
Hydrochloride/Phenylpropanolami
ne Hydrochloride
Guanabenz Acetate
Guanethidine Monosulfate
Haemophilus b Conjugate Vaccine
Halcinonide
Halobetasol Propionate
Haloperidol
Halothane
Hemin
Hemophilus b Conjugate Vaccine
(Tetanus Toxoid Conjugate)
Heparin
Hepatitis B Vaccine, Recombinant
Hepatitis b Immune Globulin
(Human)
Hetastarch
Hexachlorophene
Histamine Phosphate
Homatropine Hydrobromide
Homatropine Methylbromide and
Hydrocodone Bitartrate
Hyaluronidase
Hydralazine Hydrochloride
Hydralazine Hydrochloride with
Hydrochlorothiazide
Hydralazine Hydrochloride/
Hydrochlorothiazide/Reserpine
Hydrochlorothiazide and Lisinopril
Hydrochlorothiazide and
Methyldopa
Hydrochlorothiazide and
Propranolol Hydrochloride
Hydrochlorothiazide and Timolol
Maleate
Hydrochlorothiazide and
Triamterene
Hydrochlorothiazide with
Metoprolol Tartrate
Hydrochlorothiazide with Reserpine
Hydrocodone Bitartrate with
Phenylephrine Hydrochloride
Hydrocodone Bitartrate with
Phenylpropanolamine
Hydrochloride
Hydrocodone Bitartrate with
Pseudoephedrine Hydrochloride
Hydrocodone Bitartrate/Pheniramine
Maleate/Phenylephrine
Hydrochloride/Phenylpropanolami
ne Hydrochloride/Pyrilamine
Maleate
Hydrocodone
Bitartrate/Phenylephrine
Hydrochloride/Pyrilamine Maleate
Hydrocodone/Pheniramine
/Phenylephrine/
Phenylpropanolamine/Pyrilamine
Hydrocortisone Acetate and
Pramoxine Hydrochloride
Hydrocortisone Acetate with
Lidocaine
Hydrocortisone Acetate with
Neomycin Sulfate
Hydrocortisone Cypionate
Hydrocortisone with Iodoquinol
Hydrocortisone, Rectal

Hydrocortisone, Topical
Hydrocortisone/Neomycin
Sulfate/Polymyxin B Sulfate
Hydroflumethiazide
Hydroflumethiazide with Reserpine
Hydromorphone Hydrochloride
Hydroquinone
Hydroxyamphetamine
Hydrobromide with Tropicamide
Hydroxyzine
Hyoscyamine Sulfate
Idoxuridine
Imiglucerase
Imipramine
Indigotindisulfonate Sodium
Indium In-111 Pentetreotide
Indocyanine Green
Influenza Virus Vaccine
Interferon Alfa-2A
Interferon Alfa-2B
Interferon Alfa-N3
Interferon Beta-1B
Interferon Gamma-1B
Iodoquinol
Iopanoic Acid
Iron Dextran
Isoetharine Hydrochloride
Isoflurane
Isoniazid
Isoniazid and Rifampin
Isoniazid/Pyrazinamide/Rifampin
Isoproterenol
Isoproterenol Hydrochloride with
Phenylephrine Bitartrate
Isosorbide Dinitrate
Isosulfan Blue
Isoxsuprine Hydrochloride
Isradipine
Itraconazole
Japanese Encephalitis Virus Vaccine
Ketoconazole, Oral
Ketoconazole, Topical
Ketorolac Tromethamine,
Ophthalmic
Ketorolac Tromethamine, Systemic
Labetalol Hydrochloride
Lactated Ringer's
Leucovorin Calcium
Levamisole Hydrochloride
Levobunolol Hydrochloride,
Ophthalmic
Levocabastine Hydrochloride
Levodopa
Lisinopril
Liver Derivative Complex
Lomefloxacin Hydrochloride
Loxapine
Lymphocyte Immune Globulin
Lypressin
Lysine Hydrochloride/Potassium
Bicarbonate/Potassium Chloride
Mafenide Acetate
Magnesium Chloride, Injectable
Magnesium Salicylate
Magnesium Salicylate and
Phenyltoloxamine Dihydrogen
Citrate
Manganese Chloride
Mannitol and Sorbitol
Mannitol, Injectable
Mazindol
Measles Virus Vaccine
Measles and Rubella Virus Vaccine
Live
Measles/Mumps/Rubella Virus
Vaccine Live

Mebendazole
Mecamylamine Hydrochloride
Medrysone
Mefenamic Acid
Mefloquine Hydrochloride
Meningococcal Polysaccharide
Vaccine
Mepenzolate Bromide
Mephentermine Sulfate
Mephenytoin
Mepivacaine Hydrochloride
Mesoridazine Besylate
Metaproterenol Sulfate
Methacholine Chloride
Methamphetamine Hydrochloride
Methazolamide
Methenamine Hippurate
Methenamine Mandelate
Methenamine Mandelate and
Sodium Acid Phosphate
Methocarbamol
Methoxamine Hydrochloride
Methoxsalen
Methoxyflurane
Methscopolamine Bromide
Methyclothiazide with Reserpine
Methyldopa
Methylene Blue
Methylergonovine Maleate
Methylprednisolone Acetate and
Neomycin Sulfate
Metipranolol
Metocurine Iodide
Metoprolol
Metyrosine
Mexiletine Hydrochloride
Miconazole Nitrate
Miconazole, Injectable
Milrinone Lactate
Minoxidil, Oral
Minoxidil, Topical
Mitotane
Mivacurium Chloride
Mometasone Furoate
Monobenzone
Monoctanoin
Morphine Sulfate
Mumps Skin Test Antigen
Mumps Virus Vaccine Live
Muromonab-CD3
Nabumetone
Nadolol
Naloxone Hydrochloride and
Pentazocine Hydrochloride
Naltrexone Hydrochloride
Naphazoline Hydrochloride
Naphazoline Hydrochloride and
Pheniramine Maleate
Natamycin
Neostigmine
Niacin
Nicardipine Hydrochloride
Nicotine Polacrilex
Nifedipine
Nimodipine
Nitrofurazone, Topical
Nitroglycerin
Nizatidine
Norepinephrine Bitartrate
Norfloxacin, Ophthalmic
Norfloxacin, Oral
Novobiocin Sodium
Nystatin and Triamcinolone
Acetonide
Nystatin, Oral
Ofloxacin, Ophthalmic

Ofloxacin, Systemic
Olsalazine Sodium
Omeprazole
Opium Tincture
Orphenadrine Citrate
Oxamniquine
Oxaprozin
Oxtriphylline
Oxytetracycline
Hydrochloride/Phenazopyridine/S
ulfamethizole
Pamidronate Disodium
Pancrelipase
Pancuronium Bromide
Paraldehyde
Paregoric
Pegademase Bovine
Pegaspargase
Penbutolol Sulfate
Pentagastrin
Pentamidine Isethionate
Pentastarch
Pentazocine Lactate
Pentoxifylline
Perphenazine
Phenazopyridine Hydrochloride and
Sulfisoxazole
Phendimetrazine Tartrate
Phenelzine Sulfate
Pheniramine
Maleate/Phenylpropanolamine
Hydrochloride/Pyrilamine Maleate
Phenoxybenzamine Hydrochloride
Phentermine
Phentolamine Mesylate
Phenylephrine Hydrochloride
Phenylephrine Hydrochloride and
Promethazine Hydrochloride
Phenylephrine Hydrochloride and
Scopolamine Hydrobromide
Phenylephrine Hydrochloride and
Sulfacetamide Sodium
Physostigmine Salicylate
Physostigmine Sulfate
Phytonadione
Pilocarpine Hydrochloride, Oral
Pilocarpine, Ophthalmic
Pimozide
Pipecuronium Bromide
Pirbuterol Acetate
Plasma Protein Fraction (Human)
Pneumococcal Vaccine, Polyvalent
Podofilox
Polio Vaccine
Polymyxin B Sulfate and
Trimethoprim Sulfate
Polythiazide and Prazosin
Hydrochloride
Polythiazide and Reserpine
Potassium Acetate
Potassium Acid Phosphate
Potassium Acid Phosphate and
Sodium Acid Phosphate
Potassium Bicarbonate
Potassium Chloride and Potassium
Gluconate
Potassium Chloride and Sodium
Chloride
Potassium Chloride, Injectable
Potassium Chloride, Oral
Potassium Citrate
Potassium Iodide and Theophylline
Potassium Phosphate
Potassium Phosphate, Monobasic
and Sodium Phosphate, Dibasic
Povidone-Iodine

Pralidoxime Chloride
Prazosin Hydrochloride
Prednicarbate
Prednisolone Acetate, Ophthalmic
Prednisolone and Sulfacetamide
　Sodium
Procainamide Hydrochloride
Procaine Hydrochloride
Prochlorperazine
Procyclidine Hydrochloride
Promethazine Hydrochloride
Propafenone Hydrochloride
Propantheline Bromide
Proparacaine Hydrochloride
Propranolol Hydrochloride
Protamine Sulfate
Proteinase Inhibitor (Human), Alpha 1
Protirelin
Protriptyline Hydrochloride
Pseudoephedrine Hydrochloride
Pseudoephedrine Hydrochloride and
　Terfenadine
Pyrazinamide
Pyridostigmine Bromide
Pyrimethamine
Pyrimethamine and Sulfadoxine
Quinapril Hydrochloride
Quinidine Gluconate
Quinidine Polygalacturonate
Quinidine Sulfate
Rabies Immune Globulin (Human)
Rabies Vaccine
Rabies Vaccine Adsorbed
Ramipril
Reserpine
Reserpine and Trichlormethiazide
Respiratory Vaccine, Mixed
Rho (D) Immune Globulin
Rifampin
Rimantadine Hydrochloride
Ringer's Solution, Irrigation
Ringer's, Injectable
Risperidone
Rubella Virus Vaccine
Rubella and Mumps Vaccine
Salmeterol Xinafoate
Salsalate
Sargramostim
Scopolamine
Secretin
Selegiline Hydrochloride
Selenious Acid
Selenium Sulfide
Sermorelin Acetate
Skin Test Antigens, Multiple
Sodium Benzoate and Sodium
　Phenylacetate
Sodium Bicarbonate
Sodium Chloride, Injectable
Sodium Lactate
Sodium Nitroprusside
Sodium Phosphate
Sodium Polystyrene Sulfonate
Sodium Tetradecyl Sulfate
Sodium Thiosulfate
Somatrem
Somatropin
Sorbitol
Stavudine
Streptokinase
Streptozocin
Succimer
Succinylcholine Chloride
Sufentanil Citrate
Sulconazole Nitrate
Sulfabenzamide/Sulfacetamide/Sulfa

thiazole
Sulfacetamide Sodium and Sulfur
Sulfacetamide Sodium, Ophthalmic
Sulfacetamide Sodium, Topical
Sulfadiazine
Sulfamethizole
Sulfamethoxazole
Sulfamethoxazole and Trimethoprim
Sulfanilamide
Sulfisoxazole Diolamine,
　Ophthalmic
Sulfisoxazole, Oral
Sumatriptan Succinate
Suprofen
Tacrine Hydrochloride
Tacrolimus
Terazosin Hydrochloride
Terconazole
Terfenadine
Teriparatide Acetate
Testolactone
Tetanus Immune Globulin
Tetanus Toxoid Adsorbed
Tetracaine Hydrochloride, Injectable
Tetrahydrozoline Hydrochloride
Theophylline
Thiabendazole
Thiopental Sodium
Thioridazine Hydrochloride
Thiothixene
Thrombin
Thyrotropin
Timolol Maleate, Ophthalmic
Timolol Maleate, Oral
Tioconazole
Tiopronin
Tocainide Hydrochloride
Tolazamide
Tolazoline Hydrochloride
Tolbutamide
Tolbutamide Sodium
Tolmetin Sodium
Tranylcypromine Sulfate
Trazodone Hydrochloride
Tretinoin
Triamcinolone Acetonide, Inhalation
Triamcinolone Acetonide, Topical
Triamcinolone Diacetate
Triamcinolone Hexacetonide
Trientine Hydrochloride
Triethanolamine Polypeptide
　Oleate-Condensate
Trifluoperazine Hydrochloride
Triflupromazine Hydrochloride
Trifluridine
Trimethoprim
Trimipramine Maleate
Troleandomycin
Tromethamine
Tuberculin
Tubocurarine Chloride
Typhoid Vaccine
Vancomycin Hydrochloride
Vasopressin
Vecuronium Bromide
Venlafaxine Hydrochloride
Verapamil Hydrochloride
Vidarabine
Vitamin B12
Vitamin C
Vitamin K
Yellow Fever Vaccine
Zalcitabine
Zidovudine

B

NO EVIDENCE OF RISK
IN HUMANS

*Either animal finding show risk while
human findings do not, or, if no
adequate human studies have been
done, animal findings are negative.*

Acebutolol Hydrochloride
Acetylcysteine
Acrivastine and Pseudoephedrine
　Hydrochloride
Amiloride Hydrochloride
Amiloride Hydrochloride with
　Hydrochlorothiazide
Amoxicillin
Amoxicillin with Clavulanate
　Potassium
Amphotericin B, Injectable
Ampicillin
Ampicillin Sodium and Sulbactam
　Sodium
Aprotinin
Arginine Hydrochloride
Aspirin/Oxycodone Hydrochloride/
　Oxycodone Terephthalate
Azatadine Maleate
Azithromycin
Aztreonam
Bacampicillin Hydrochloride
Bentiromide
Brompheniramine Maleate,
　Injectable
Bupropion Hydrochloride
Buspirone Hydrochloride
Carbenicillin Indanyl Sodium
Cefaclor
Cefadroxil Monohydrate
Cefamandole Nafate
Cefazolin Sodium
Cefixime
Cefmetazole Sodium
Cefonicid Sodium
Cefoperazone Sodium
Cefotaxime Sodium
Cefotetan Disodium
Cefoxitin Sodium
Cefpodoxime Proxetil
Cefprozil
Ceftazidime
Ceftizoxime Sodium
Ceftriaxone Sodium
Cefuroxime Axetil
Cefuroxime Sodium
Cephalexin
Cephalothin Sodium
Cephapirin Sodium
Cephradine
Chlorhexidine Gluconate
Chlorothiazide and Methyldopa
Chlorpheniramine Maleate with
　Phenylpropanolamine
　Hydrochloride
Chlorpheniramine Maleate,
　Injectable
Chlorpheniramine
　Maleate/Dextromethorphan
　Hydrobromide/Guaifenesin/Pheny
　lpropanolamine Hydrochloride
Chlorthalidone
Ciclopirox Olamine
Cimetidine
Clavulanate Potassium with
　Ticarcillin Disodium

Clemastine Fumarate
Clindamycin, Systemic
Clindamycin, Topical
Clindamycin, Vaginal
Clotrimazole
Cloxacillin Sodium
Clozapine
Cromolyn Sodium
Cromolyn Sodium, Oral
Cyclobenzaprine Hydrochloride
Cyproheptadine Hydrochloride
Dapiprazole Hydrochloride
Desflurane
Desmopressin Acetate
Dexchlorpheniramine Maleate
Dextran-1
Dextrothyroxine Sodium
Diclofenac, Ophthalmic
Diclofenac, Oral
Dicyclomine Hydrochloride
Didanosine
Diethylpropion Hydrochloride
Dimenhydrinate, Injectable
Diphenhydramine Hydrochloride
Dipivefrin Hydrochloride
Dipyridamole, Injectable
Dipyridamole, Oral
Dornase Alfa
Doxapram Hydrochloride
Edetate Calcium Disodium
Enflurane
Enoxaparin
Erythromycin, Injectable
Erythromycin, Ophthalmic
Erythromycin, Oral
Erythromycin, Topical
Ethacrynic Acid
Ethambutol Hydrochloride
Etidocaine Hydrochloride
Famciclovir
Famotidine
Flavoxate Hydrochloride
Fluoxetine Hydrochloride
Flurbiprofen, Oral
Glucagon
Glyburide
Glycopyrrolate
Gonadorelin Acetate
Gonadorelin Hydrochloride
Granisetron Hydrochloride
Guanadrel Sulfate
Guanethidine Monosulfate with
　Hydrochlorothiazide
Guanfacine Hydrochloride
Haloprogin
Hydrochlorothiazide
Indapamide
Indomethacin
Insulin-Pork, Concentrated I 2130
Iodamide Meglumine
Iohexol
Iopamidol
Iothalamate
Iothalamate Meglumine
Iothalamate Meglumine and
　Iothalamate Sodium
Ioversol
Ioxaglate Meglumine and Ioxaglate
　Sodium
Ipratropium Bromide
Isosorbide
Isosorbide Mononitrate
Ketoprofen
Lactulose
Levocarnitine
Lidocaine Hydrochloride, Injectable

Lidocaine Hydrochloride, Local
   Anesthesia
Lidocaine with Prilocaine
Lidocaine, Topical
Lincomycin Hydrochloride
Lindane
Lodoxamide Tromethamine
Loperamide Hydrochloride
Loracarbef
Loratadine
Malathion
Maprotiline Hydrochloride
Masoprocol
Meclizine Hydrochloride
Meclocycline Sulfosalicylate
Meclofenamate Sodium
Mesalamine
Mesna
Methdilazine Hydrochloride
Methicillin Sodium
Methohexital Sodium
Methyclothiazide
Methyldopa
Metoclopramide Hydrochloride
Metolazone
Metrizamide
Metronidazole, Systemic
Metronidazole, Topical
Metronidazole, Vaginal
Mezlocillin Sodium
Molindone Hydrochloride
Moricizine Hydrochloride

Mupirocin
Nafcillin Sodium
Naftifine Hydrochloride
Nalbuphine Hydrochloride
Naloxone Hydrochloride
Naproxen
Nedocromil Sodium
Niclosamide
Nitrofurantoin
Nystatin, Topical
Octreotide Acetate
Ondansetron Hydrochloride
Oxacillin Sodium
Oxiconazole Nitrate
Oxybutynin Chloride
Oxycodone Hydrochloride
Oxytetracycline
   Hydrochloride/Phenazopyridine/S
   ulfamethizole
Paroxetine Hydrochloride
Pemoline
Penicillin G Benzathine
Penicillin G Benzathine and
   Penicillin G Procaine
Penicillin G Potassium
Penicillin G Procaine
Penicillin G Sodium
Penicillin V Potassium
Pergolide Mesylate
Permethrin
Phenazopyridine Hydrochloride
Phenazopyridine Hydrochloride and

Sulfamethoxazole
Phenazopyridine Hydrochloride and
   Sulfisoxazole
Pindolol
Piperacillin Sodium
Piperacillin Sodium and
   Tazobactam Sodium
Praziquantel
Prednisolone Tebutate
Prednisone
Prilocaine Hydrochloride and
   Prilocaine with Epinephrine
Probenecid
Probucol
Propofol
Ranitidine Hydrochloride
Rifabutin
Ritodrine Hydrochloride
Rocuronium Bromide
Sertraline Hydrochloride
Silver Sulfadiazine
Sincalide
Sotalol Hydrochloride
Spectinomycin Hydrochloride
Spironolactone
Staphage Lysate (SPL)
Sucralfate
Sulfasalazine
Sutilains
Terbinafine Hydrochloride
Terbutaline Sulfate
Tetracycline Hydrochloride, Topical

Ticarcillin Disodium
Ticlopidine Hydrochloride
Tobramycin
Torsemide
Tranexamic Acid
Triamterene
Trichlormethiazide
Urokinase
Ursodiol
Zolpidem Tartrate

A

CONTROLLED STUDIES SHOW NO RISK

Adequate, well-controlled studies in pregnant women have failed to demonstrate risk to the fetus.

Ferrous Sulfate/Folic
   Acid/Vitamins, Multi
Levothyroxine Sodium
Liothyronine Sodium
Liotrix
Lysine/Vitamin B Complex/Zinc
   Sulfate
Magnesium Sulfate, Injectable
Thyroid
Vitamin B1
Vitamin B6, Injectable

Certified Poison Control Centers

The centers listed below are certified by the American Association of Poison Control Centers. To receive certification, each center has to meet certain criteria. It must, for example, serve a large geographic area; it must be open 24 hours a day and provide direct-dial or toll-free access; it must be supervised by a medical director; and it must have registered pharmacists or nurses available to answer questions from the public.

The centers have a wide variety of toxicology resources, including the POISINDEX® System, a computerized database of more than 750,000 substances maintained by MICROMEDEX, INC., an affiliate of PDR. Staff members are trained to resolve toxic situations in the home of the caller, though hospital referrals are given in some instances. The centers also offer a range of educational services to both the public and healthcare professionals. In some states, these larger centers exist side by side with smaller centers offering a more limited range of services.

Within each state, centers are listed alphabetically by name. Telephone numbers designated "TTY" are teletype lines for the hearing-impaired. "TDD" numbers reach a telecommunication device for the deaf. This list is furnished courtesy of

Alabama

Regional Poison Control Center
The Children's Hospital of Alabama
1600 Seventh Ave. South
Birmingham, AL 35233-1711
Emergency Phone:
(205) 939-9201,
(800) 292-6678 (AL only) or
(205) 933-4050

Arizona

Arizona Poison and Drug Information Center
Arizona Health Sciences Center
Room 1156
1501 N. Campbell Ave.
Tucson, AZ 85724
Emergency Phone:
(800) 362-0101 (AZ only),
(602) 626-6016

Samaritan Regional Poison Center
Teleservices Department
1111 E. McDowell Road
Phoenix, AZ 85006
Emergency Phone:
(602) 253-3334

California

Fresno Regional Poison Control Center
Valley Children's Hospital
3151 N. Millbrook
Fresno, CA 93703
Emergency Phone:
(800) 346-5922 (Central CA only)
or (209) 445-1222

San Diego Regional Poison Center
UCSD Medical Center
200 West Arbor Drive
San Diego, CA 92103-8925
Emergency Phone:
(619) 543-6000,
(800) 876-4766
(in 619 area code only)

San Francisco Bay Area Regional Poison Control Center
San Francisco General Hospital
1001 Potrero Ave.,
Building 80, Room 230
San Francisco, CA 94110
Emergency Phone:
(800) 523-2222

University of California, Davis, Medical Center Regional Poison Control Center
2315 Stockton Blvd
Sacramento, CA 95817
Emergency Phone:
(916) 734-3692,
(800) 342-9293 (Northern CA only)

Colorado

Rocky Mountain Poison and Drug Center
645 Bannock St.
Denver, CO 80204
Emergency Phone:
(303) 629-1123

District of Columbia

National Capital Poison Center
3201 New Mexico Ave, NW
Suite 310
Washington, DC 20016
Emergency Numbers:
(202) 625-3333,
(202) 362-8563 (TTY)

Florida

The Florida Poison Information and Toxicology Resource Center Tampa General Hospital
Post Office Box 1289
Tampa, FL 33601
Emergency Phone:
(813) 253-4444 (Tampa),
(800) 282-3171 (Florida)

Georgia

Georgia Poison Center
Grady Memorial Hospital
80 Butler Street S.E.
P.O. Box 26066
Atlanta, GA 30335-3801
Emergency Phone:
(800) 282-5846 (GA only),
(404) 616-9000

Indiana

Indiana Poison Center
Methodist Hospital of Indiana
1701 N. Senate Boulevard
P.O. Box 1367
Indianapolis, IN 46206-1367
Emergency Phone:
(800) 382-9097 (IN only),
(317) 929-2323

Maryland

Maryland Poison Center
20 N. Pine St.
Baltimore, MD 21201
Emergency Phone:
(410) 528-7701,
(800) 492-2414 (MD only)

**National Capital Poison
Center (D.C. suburbs only)**
3201 New Mexico Ave, NW
Suite 310
Washington, DC 20016
Emergency Numbers:
(202) 625-3333,
(202) 362-8563 (TTY)

Massachusetts

**Massachusetts Poison
Control System**
300 Longwood Ave.
Boston, MA 02115
Emergency Phone:
(617) 232-2120,
(800) 682-9211

Michigan

Poison Control Center
Children's Hospital of Michigan
3901 Beaubien Blvd.
Detroit, MI 48201
Emergency Phone:
(313) 745-5711

Minnesota

**Hennepin Regional
Poison Center**
Hennepin County Medical Center
701 Park Ave.
Minneapolis, MN 55415
Emergency Phone:
(612) 347-3141,
Petline: (612) 337-7387,
TDD: (612) 337-7474

**Minnesota Regional
Poison Center**
St. Paul-Ramsey Medical Center
640 Jackson St.
St. Paul, MN 55101
Emergency Phone:
(612) 221-2113

Missouri

**Cardinal Glennon
Children's Hospital Regional
Poison Center**
1465 S. Grand Blvd.
St. Louis, MO 63104
Emergency Phone:
(314) 772-5200,
(800) 366-8888

Montana

**Rocky Mountain
Poison and Drug Center**
645 Bannock St.
Denver, CO 80204
Emergency Phone:
(303) 629-1123

Nebraska

The Poison Center
8301 Dodge St.
Omaha, NE 68114
Emergency Phone:
(402) 390-5555 (Omaha),
(800) 955-9119 (NE & WY)

New Jersey

**New Jersey
Poison Information and
Education System**
201 Lyons Ave.
Newark, NJ 07112
Emergency Phone:
(800) 962-1253

New Mexico

**New Mexico
Poison and
Drug Information Center**
University of New Mexico
Albuquerque, NM 87131-1076
Emergency Phone:
(505) 843-2551,
(800) 432-6866 (NM only)

New York

**Hudson Valley
Poison Center**
Nyack Hospital
160 N. Midland Ave.
Nyack, NY 10960
Emergency Phone:
(800) 336-6997,
(914) 353-1000

**Long Island
Regional Poison Control
Center**
Winthrop University Hospital
259 First Street
Mineola, NY 11501
Emergency Phone:
(516) 542-2323, 542-2324,
542-2325, 542-3813

**New York City
Poison
Control Center**
N.Y.C. Department of Health
455 First Ave., Room 123
New York, NY 10016
Emergency Phone:
(212) 340-4494,
(212) P-O-I-S-O-N-S,
TDD: (212) 689-9014

Ohio

Central Ohio Poison Center
700 Children's Drive
Columbus, OH 43205-2696
Emergency Phone:
(614) 228-1323,
(800) 682-7625,
(614) 228-2272 (TTY),
(614) 461-2012

**Cincinnati Drug & Poison
Information Center
and Regional Poison
Control System**
P.O. Box 670144
Cincinnati, OH 45267-0144
Emergency Phone:
(513) 558-5111,
(800) 872-5111 (OH only)

Oregon

Oregon Poison Center
Oregon Health Sciences University
3181 S.W. Sam Jackson
Park Road
Portland, OR 97201
Emergency Phone:
(503) 494-8968,
(800) 452-7165 (OR only)

Pennsylvania

**Central Pennsylvania
Poison Center**
University Hospital
Milton S. Hershey
Medical Center
P.O. Box 850
Hershey, PA 17033
Emergency Phone:
(800) 521-6110

**The Poison Control Center
serving the
greater Philadelphia
metropolitan area**
One Children's Center
Philadelphia, PA 19104-4303
Emergency Phone:
(215) 386-2100

Pittsburgh Poison Center
3705 Fifth Avenue
Pittsburgh, PA 15213
Emergency Phone:
(412) 681-6669

Rhode Island

Rhode Island Poison Center
593 Eddy St.
Providence, RI 02903
Emergency Phone:
(401) 444-5727

Texas

North Texas Poison Center
5201 Harry Hines Blvd.
P.O. Box 35926
Dallas, TX 75235
Emergency Phone:
(800) 764-7661

Texas State Poison Center
The University of Texas Trauma
Center, Room 3.112
Galveston, TX 77555-1175
Emergency Phone:
(409) 765-1420 (Galveston),
(713) 654-1701 (Houston)

Utah

Utah Poison Control Center
410 Chipeta Way, Suite 230
Salt Lake City, UT 84108
Emergency Phone:
(801) 581-2151,
(800) 456-7707 (UT only)

Virginia

Blue Ridge Poison Center
Box 67
Blue Ridge Hospital
Charlottesville, VA 22901
Emergency Phone:
(804) 924-5543,
(800) 451-1428

**National Capital Poison
Center (Northern VA only)**
3201 New Mexico Ave, NW
Suite 310
Washington, DC 20016
Emergency Numbers:
(202) 625-3333,
(202) 362-8563 (TTY)

West Virginia

West Virginia Poison Center
3110 MacCorkle Ave. S.E.
Charleston, WV 25304
Emergency Phone:
(800) 642-3625 (WV only),
(304) 348-4211

Wyoming

The Poison Center
8301 Dodge St.
Omaha, NE 68114
Emergency Phone:
(402) 390-5555 (Omaha),
(800) 955-9119 (NE & WY)

Drug Information Centers

Alabama

BIRMINGHAM
Drug Information Service
University of Alabama
Hospital
619 S. 19th St.
Birmingham, AL 35233
Mon.-Fri. 8 AM-5 PM
Tel.: 205-934-2162
Fax: 205-934-3501

Global Drug Information
Center Samford University
School of Pharmacy
800 Lakeshore Drive
Birmingham, AL 35229-7027
Mon.-Fri. 8 AM-4:30 PM
Tel.: 205-870-2891
Fax: 205-870-2016

HUNTSVILLE
Huntsville Hospital
Drug Information Center
101 Sivley Road
Huntsville, AL 35801
Mon.-Fri. 8 AM-5 PM
Tel.: 205-517-8288
Fax: 205-517-6558

Arizona

TUCSON
Arizona Poison and Drug
Information Center Arizona
Health Science Center
University Medical Center
1501 N. Campbell Ave.
Room 1156
Tucson, AZ 85724
7 days/week, 24 hours
Tel.: 602-626-6016
        800-362-0101 (AZ)
Fax: 602-626-2720

Arkansas

LITTLE ROCK
Arkansas Poison and Drug
Information Center
University of Arkansas for
Medical Sciences
4301 W. Markham St.
Little Rock, AR 72205
7 days/week, 24 hours
Tel.: 800-376-4766 (AR)
Fax: 501-686-7357

California

LOS ANGELES
Los Angeles Regional
Drug & Poison Information
Center LAC & USC Medical
Center University of
Southern California
1200 N. State St.
RM 1107 A & B
Los Angeles, CA 90033
7 days/week, 24 hours
Tel.: 213-226-2622
        800-777-6476 (CA)
Fax: 213-226-4194

SAN DIEGO
Drug Information
Analysis Service
Veterans Administration
Medical Center
3350 La Jolla Village Dr.
San Diego, CA 92161
Mon.-Fri. 8 AM-4:30 PM
Tel.: 619-552-8585
Fax: 619-552-7452

Drug Information Center
U.S. Naval Hospital
34800 Bob Wilson Dr.
San Diego, CA 92134-5000
Mon.-Fri. 8 AM-4 PM
Tel.: 619-532-8414

Drug Information Service
University of California
San Diego Medical Center
200 West Arbor Dr.
San Diego, CA 92103-8925
Mon.-Fri. 9 AM-5 PM
Tel.: 1-900-288-8273
Fax: 619-692-1867

SAN FRANCISCO
Drug Information
Analysis Service
University of California
P.O.Box 0622
San Francisco, CA 94143-0622
Mon.-Fri. 8 AM-5 PM
Tel.: 415-476-4346

SANTA MONICA
Drug Information Services
St. Johns Hospital and
Health Center
1328 22nd St.
Santa Monica, CA 90404-2032
Mon.-Fri. 24 hours
Tel.: 310-829-8243
        310-829-8250 (after hours)

STANFORD
Drug Information Center
Stanford University Hospital
Dept. of Pharmacy H0301
300 Pasteur Dr.
Stanford, CA 94305
Mon.-Fri. 9 AM-5 PM
Tel.: 415-723-6422
Fax: 415-725-5028

Colorado

DENVER
Rocky Mountain
Drug Consultation Center
645 Bannock St.
Denver, CO 80204
Mon.-Fri. 8:30 AM-4 PM
Tel.: 303-893-3784
Fax: 303-623-1119
Outside Denver County
900-285-3784
$2.95 first minute
$1.95 each additional minute

Drug Information Center
University of Colorado
Health Science Center
4200 E. 9th Ave.
Campus Box C239
Denver, CO 80262
Mon.-Fri. 8:30 AM-4:30 PM
Tel.: 303-270-8489
Fax: 303-270-3353

Connecticut

FARMINGTON
Drug Information Service
University of Connecticut
Health Center
263 Farmington Ave.
Farmington, CT 06030
Mon.-Fri. 8 AM-4:30 PM
Tel.: 203-679-2783

HARTFORD
Drug Information Center
Hartford Hospital
P.O. Box 5037
80 Seymour St.
Hartford, CT 06102
Mon.-Fri. 8:30 AM-5 PM
Tel.: 203-545-2221
        203-545-2961 (after hours)
Fax: 203-545-2415

NEW HAVEN
Drug Information Center
Yale-New Haven Hospital
20 York St.
New Haven, CT 06504
Mon.-Fri. 8:15 AM-4:45 PM
Tel.: 203-785-2248
Fax: 203-737-4229

Disrict of Colubia

Drug Information Center
Washington Hospital Center
110 Irving St. NW
Washington, DC 20010
Mon.-Fri. 7:30 AM-4 PM
Tel.: 202-877-6646
Fax: 202-877-5428

Drug Information Service
Howard University Hospital
2041 Georgia Ave. NW
Washington, DC 20060
Mon.-Fri. 9 AM-5 PM
Tel.: 202-865-1325
Fax: 202-745-3731

Florida

GAINESVILLE
Drug Information &
Pharmacy Resource Center
Shands Hospital at
University of Florida
P.O.Box 100316
Gainesville, FL 32610-0316
Mon.-Fri. 9 AM-5 PM
Tel.: 904-395-0408
Fax: 904-338-9860
For healthcare professionals only.

JACKSONVILLE
Drug Information Service
University Medical Center
655 W. 8th St.
Jacksonville, FL 32209
Mon.-Fri. 8 AM-5 PM
Tel.: 904-549-4095
Fax: 904-549-4272

MIAMI
Drug Information Center (119)
Miami VA Medical Center
1201 NW 16th St.
Miami, FL 33125
Mon.-Fri. 7:30 AM-4:00 PM
Tel.: 305-324-3237
Fax: 305-324-3386

NORTH MIAMI BEACH
Drug Information Service
NOVA/Southeastern
University of the Health
Sciences
1750 NE 168th Street
N. Miami Beach, FL 33162-3017
Mon.-Fri. 9 AM-5 PM
Tel.: 305-948-8255

Georgia

ATLANTA
Emory University Hospital
Dept. of Pharmaceutical
Services
1364 Clifton Rd. NE
Atlanta, GA 30322
Mon.-Fri. 8:30 AM-5 PM
Tel.: 404-727-4644
Fax: 404-727-3302

Drug Information Service
Northside Hospital
1000 Johnson Ferry Rd.
Atlanta, GA 30342
Mon.-Fri. 9 AM-4 PM
Tel.: 404-851-8676
Fax: 404-851-8682

Drug Information Center
Grady Hospital and Mercer
University
80 Butler St. SE, P.O.Box 26041
Atlanta, GA 30335-3801
Mon.-Fri. 8 AM-4 PM
Tel.: 404-616-7725
Fax: 404-616-7727

AUGUSTA
Drug Information Center
University of Georgia
Medical College of GA
Rm. BIW201, 1120 15th St.
Augusta, GA 30912-5600
Mon.-Fri. 8:30 AM-5 PM
Tel.: 706-721-2887
Fax: 706-721-3827

Idaho

POCATELLO
Idaho Drug Information
Service
Box 8092
Pocatello, ID 83209
Mon.-Fri. 8 AM-5 PM
Tel.: 208-236-4689
Fax: 208-236-4687

Illinois

BLOOMINGTON
Drug Information Center
BroMenn Life Care Center
807 N. Main St.
Bloomington, IL 61701
7 days/week, 24 hours
Tel.: 309-829-0755
Fax: 309-829-0760

CHICAGO
Drug Information Center
Northwestern
Memorial Hospital
250 E. Superior St.
Wesley 153
Chicago, IL 60611
Mon.-Fri. 8:30 AM-5 PM
Tel.: 312-908-7573
Fax: 312-908-7956

Flo Manzano
Director of Pharmacy
Services
Saint Joseph Hospital
2900 N. Lake Shore Dr.
Chicago, IL 60657
Tel.: 312-665-3140

Drug Information Services
University of Chicago
5841 S. Maryland Ave., MC 0010
Chicago, IL 60322
Mon.-Fri. 8 AM-5 PM
Tel.: 312-702-1388
Fax: 312-702-6631

Drug Information Center
University of Illinois
at Chicago
Room C300, MC 883
1740 W. Taylor St.
Chicago, IL 60612
Mon.-Fri. 8 AM-4 PM
Tel.: 312-996-0209
Fax: 312-996-0906

HARVEY
Drug Information Center
Ingalls Memorial Hospital
1 Ingalls Dr.
Harvey, IL 60426
Mon.-Fri. 8 AM-4:30 PM
Tel.: 708-333-2300, ext. 4430
Fax: 708-210-3108

HINES
Drug Information Service
Hines Veterans
Administration Hospital
Inpatient Pharmacy (119B)
Hines, IL 60141
Mon.-Fri. 8 AM-4 PM
Tel.: 708-343-7200

PARK RIDGE
Drug Information Center
Lutheran General Hospital
1775 Dempster St.
Park Ridge, IL 60068
Mon.-Fri. 7:30 AM-4 PM
Tel.: 708-696-8128

ROCKFORD
Drug Information Center
Swedish-American Hospital
1400 Charles St.
Rockford, IL 61104
7 days/week, 24 hours
Tel.: 815-968-4400 ext. 4577, 4800

Indiana

INDIANAPOLIS
Drug Information Center
St. Vincent Hospital and
Health Services
2001 W. 86th St.
P.O.Box 40970
Indianapolis, IN 46240-0970
Mon.-Fri. 8 AM-4 PM
Tel: 317-338-3200

Indiana University Medical
Center/Pharmacy Dept.
UH1410
550 N. University Blvd.
Indianapolis, IN 46202-5271
Mon.-Fri. 8 AM-4:30 PM
Tel.: 317-274-3581
Fax: 317-274-2327

Iowa

DES MOINES
Drug Information Center
Mercy Hospital Medical
Center
400 University Ave.
Des Moines, IA 50314
Mon.-Fri. 8 AM-4:30 PM
Tel.: 515-247-3286
Fax: 515-247-3966

Mid-Iowa Poison and Drug
Information Center
Iowa Methodist Medical
Center
1200 Pleasant St.
Des Moines, IA 50309
7 days/week, 24 hours
Tel.: 515-241-6254
       800-362-2327 (IA)
Fax: 515-241-5085

IOWA CITY
Drug Information Center
University of Iowa Hospital
and Clinics
200 Hawkins Dr.
Iowa City, IA 52242
Mon.-Fri. 8 AM-5 PM
Tel.: 319-356-2600

Kansas

KANSAS CITY
Drug Information Center
Kansas University
Medical Center
3901 Rainbow Blvd.
Kansas City, KS 66160-7231
Mon.-Fri. 8:30 AM-4:30 PM
Tel.: 913-588-2328

Kentucky

LEXINGTON
Drug Information Center
Chandler Medical Center
College of Pharmacy
University of Kentucky
800 Rose St., C-117
Lexington, KY 40536-0084
Mon.-Fri. 8 AM-5 PM
Tel.: 606-323-5320
Fax: 606-323-2049

Louisiana

MONROE
Drug Information Center
St. Francis Medical Center
309 Jackson St.
Monroe, LA 71201
7 days/week, 24 hours
Tel.: 318-327-4250
Fax: 318-327-4125

NEW ORLEANS
Xavier University
Drug Information Center
Tulane Medical Center
Hospital and Clinic
Box #C12
1415 Tulane Ave.
New Orleans, LA 70112
Mon.-Fri. 9 AM-5 PM
Tel.: 504-588-5670
Fax: 504-588-5862

Maryland

ANNAPOLIS
Drug Information Services
The Anne Arundel
Medical Center
Franklin & Cathedral Streets
Annapolis, MD 21401
7 days/week, 24 hours
Tel.: 410-267-1130
       410-267-1000
Fax: 410-267-1628

BALTIMORE
Drug Information Center
Franklin Square
Hospital Center
9000 Franklin Square Dr.
Baltimore, MD 21237
Mon.-Fri. 8 AM-4:30 PM
Tel.: 410-682-7700
       410-682-7374 (after hours)

Drug Information Service
Johns Hopkins
Medical Center
600 N. Wolfe St.
Halstead 503
Baltimore, MD 21287-6187
Mon.-Fri. 8:30 AM-5 PM
Tel.: 410-955-6348
Fax: 410-955-8283

Drug Information Center
University of Maryland
at Baltimore
School of Pharmacy
Baltimore, MD 21201
Mon.-Fri. 8:30 AM-5 PM
Tel.: 410-706-7568
Fax: 410-706-7184

BETHESDA
Drug Information Service
Pharmacy Department
Warren G. Magnuson
Clinical Center National
Institutes of Health
9000 Rockville Pike (Bldg.10)
Bethesda, MD 20892
Mon.-Fri. 8:30 AM-5 PM
Tel.: 301-496-2407
Fax: 301-496-0210

ANDREWS AFB
**Drug Information Services
89th Med Gp/SGSAP**
1050 W. Perimeter Rd.
Suite B1-39
Andrews AFB, MD 20331
Mon.-Fri. 7:30 AM-6 PM
Tel.: 301-981-4209
Fax: 301-981-4544

EASTON
**Drug Information Center
Memorial Hospital**
219 S. Washington St.
Easton, MD 21601
7 days/week, 24 hours
Tel.: 410-822-1000, ext. 5645
Fax: 410-822-4958

Massachusetts

BOSTON
**Drug Information Service
Brigham and Women's
Hospital**
75 Frances St.
Boston, MA 02115
Mon.-Fri. 7 AM-3:30 PM
Tel.: 617-732-7166
Fax: 617-566-2396

**Drug Information Service
New England Medical
Center Pharmacy**
750 Washington St., Box 420
Boston, MA 02111
Mon.-Fri. 8 AM-4:30 PM
Tel.: 617-956-5380
Fax: 617-956-5638

WORCESTER
**Drug Information Center
U.M.M.C. Hospital**
55 Lake Ave. North
Worcester, MA 01605
Mon.-Fri. 8:30 AM-5 PM
Tel.: 508-856-3456
    508-856-2775
Fax: 508-856-1850

Michigan

ANN ARBOR
**Drug Information Service
University of Michigan
Medical Center**
1500 East Medical Center Drive
UHB2 D301 Box 0008 Ann Arbor,
MI 48109
Mon.-Fri. 8 AM-5 PM
Tel.: 313-936-8200
    313-936-8251 (after hours)
Fax: 313-936-7027

DETROIT
**Drug Information Center
Henry Ford Hospital**
2799 W. Grand Blvd.
Detroit, MI 48202
Mon.-Fri. 8 AM-5 PM
Tel.: 313-876-1229
Fax: 313-876-1302

**Drug Information Services
Harper Hospital**
3990 John R. St.
Detroit, MI 48201
Mon.-Fri. 8 AM-5 PM
Tel.: 313-745-2006
    313-745-8638 (after hours)

LANSING
**Drug Information Center
Sparrow Hospital**
1215 E. Michigan Ave. Lansing, MI
48912
Mon.-Fri. 8 AM-4:30 PM
Tel.: 517-483-2444
Fax: 517-483-2088

PONTIAC
**Drug Information Center
St. Joseph Mercy Hospital**
900 Woodward
Pontiac, MI 48341
Mon.-Fri. 8 AM-4:30 PM
Tel.: 810-858-3055
Fax: 810-858-6036

ROYAL OAK
**Drug Information Services
William Beaumont Hospital**
3601 West 13 Mile Rd.
Royal Oak, MI 48073
Mon.-Fri. 8 AM-4:30 PM
Tel.: 810-551-4077
Fax: 810-551-2426

SOUTHFIELD
**Drug Information Service
Providence Hospital**
16001 West 9 Mile Rd.
P.O.Box 2043
Southfield, MI 48075
Mon.-Fri. 8 AM-4:30 PM
Tel.: 810-424-3125
Fax: 810-424-5364

Minnesota

ROCHESTER
**Drug Information Center
St. Mary's Hospital**
1216 2nd St. SW
Rochester, MN 55902
Mon.-Fri. 8 AM-5 PM
Tel.: 507-255-5062
    507-255-5732 (after hours)
Fax: 507-255-7556

ST. PAUL
**Drug Information Service
United Hospital and
Children's Hospital of St.
Paul**
333 N. Smith Ave.
St. Paul, MN 55102
Mon.-Fri. 9 AM-5 PM
Tel.: 612-220-8566
Fax: 612-220-5323

Mississippi

JACKSON
**Drug Information Center
University of Mississippi
Medical Center**
2500 N. State St.
Jackson, MS 39216
Mon.-Fri. 8 AM-5 PM
(on call 24 hours)
Tel.: 601-984-2060
Fax: 601-984-2063

Missouri

SPRINGFIELD
**Drug Information & Clinical
Research Services**
1235 E. Cherokee
Springfield, MO 65804
Mon.-Fri. 7:30 AM-4:30 PM
Tel.: 417-885-3488
Fax: 417-888-7788

ST. JOSEPH
**Drug Information Service
Heartland Hospital West**
801 Faraon St.
St. Joseph, MO 64501
7 days/week, 7 AM-10 PM
Tel.: 816-271-7582
Fax: 816-271-7590

Nebraska

OMAHA
**Drug Information Service
School of Pharmacy
Creighton University**
2500 California Plaza
Omaha, NE 68178
Mon.-Fri. 8:30 AM-4:30 PM
Tel.: 402-280-5101
Fax: 402-280-5147

**Drug Information and
Education Services
University of Nebraska
Medical Center**
600 S. 42nd St.
Omaha, NE 68198-1090
Mon.-Fri. 8 AM-4:30 PM
Tel.: 402-559-4114
Fax: 402-559-4907

New Hampshire

LEBANON
**Drug Information Center
Dartmouth-Hitchcock
Medical Center**
1 Medical Center Drive
Lebanon, NH 03756
Mon.-Fri. 7:30 AM-4 PM
Tel.: 603-650-5590

New Mexico

ALBUQUERQUE
**New Mexico Poison & Drug
Information Center
University of New Mexico**
Albuquerque, NM 87131-1076
7 days/week, 24 hours
Tel.: 505-843-2551
    800-432-6866 (NM)
Fax: 505-277-5892

New York

BRONX
**Drug Information Center
Dept. of Pharmacy, RM BN32
Bronx Municipal
Hospital Center**
Pelham Parkway South and
Eastchester Rd.
Bronx, NY 10461
Mon.-Fri. 9 AM-5 PM
Tel.: 718-918-4556
Fax: 718-918-7848

BROOKLYN
**International Drug
Information Center
Long Island University
Arnold & Marie Schwartz
College of Pharmacy**
1 University Plaza
Brooklyn, NY 11201
Mon.-Fri. 9 AM-5 PM
Tel.: 718-488-1064

BUFFALO
**Drug Information Center
Erie County Medical Center**
462 Grider St.
Buffalo, NY 14215
Mon.-Fri. 8 AM-5 PM
Tel.: 716-898-3000
For healthcare professionals only.

COOPERSTOWN
**Drug Information Center
The Mary Imogene Bassett
Hospital**
1 Atwell Rd.
Cooperstown, NY 13326
Mon.-Fri. 8:30 AM-5 PM
Tel.: 607-547-3686
Fax: 607-547-3629

NEW HYDE PARK
**Drug Information Center
St. John's University at
Long Island Jewish
Medical Center**
270-05 76th Ave.
New Hyde Park, NY 11042
Mon.-Fri. 9 AM-3 PM
Tel.: 718-470-DRUG
Fax: 718-470-1742

NEW YORK
**Drug Information Center
Lenox Hill Hospital**
100 E. 77th St.
New York, NY 10021
Mon.-Fri. 9 AM-5 PM
Tel.: 212-434-3190
Fax: 212-434-3176

**Drug Information Center
Memorial Sloan-Kettering
Cancer Center**
1275 York Ave.
New York, NY 10021
Mon-Fri. 9 AM-5 PM
Tel.: 212-639-7552
Fax: 212-639-2171

Drug Information Center
Mount Sinai Medical Center
1 Gustave Levy Place
New York, NY 10029
Mon.-Fri. 9 AM-5 PM
Tel.: 212-241-6619
Fax: 212-348-7927

Drug Information Service
Bellevue Hospital Center
462 1st Ave.
New York, NY 10016
Mon.-Fri. 9 AM-5 PM
Tel.: 212-561-6504
Fax: 212-561-6503

Drug Information Service
The New York Hospital
525 E. 68th St.
New York, NY 10021
Mon.-Fri. 9 AM-5 PM
Tel.: 212-746-0741
Fax: 212-746-8506

ROCHESTER
Drug Information Service
Dept. of Pharmacy
University of Rochester at
Strong Memorial Hospital
601 Elmwood Ave.
Rochester, NY 14642
Mon.-Fri. 8 AM-5 PM
Tel.: 716-275-3718
       716-275-2681 (after hours)
Fax: 716-473-9842

STONY BROOK
Suffolk Drug
Information Center
University Hospital
S.U.N.Y.-Stony Brook
Room 3 - 561, Z7310
Stony Brook, NY 11794
Mon.-Fri. 8 AM-4:30 PM
Tel.: 516-444-2672
       516-444-2680 (after hours)
Fax: 516-444-7669

North Carolina

BUIES CREEK
Drug Information Center
School of Pharmacy
Campbell University
P.O. Box 1090
Buies Creek, NC 27506
Mon.-Fri. 8:30 AM-4:30 PM
Tel.: 800-327-5467 (NC)
       910-893-1200 ext. 2701
Fax: 910-893-1476

CHAPEL HILL
Drug Information Center
University of North Carolina
Hospitals
101 Manning Dr.
Chapel Hill, NC 27514
Mon.-Fri. 8 AM-5 PM
Tel.: 919-966-2373
Fax: 919-966-3069

GREENSBORO
Triad Poison Center
Moses H. Cone
Memorial Hospital
1200 N. Elm St.
Greensboro, NC 27401-1020
7 days/week, 24 hours
Tel.: 910-574-8105
Fax: 910-574-7910

GREENVILLE
Eastern Carolina Drug
Information Center
Pitt County Memorial
Hospital/Department of
Pharmacy Services
2100 Stantonsburg Road
Greenville, NC 27835
Mon.-Fri. 8 AM-4:30 PM
Tel.: 919-816-4257
Fax: 919-816-7425

WINSTON-SALEM
Drug Information
Service Center
NC Baptist Hospital
Bowman-Gray Medical
Center
Medical Center Blvd.
Winston-Salem, NC 27157
Mon.-Fri. 8 AM-5 PM
Tel.: 910-716-2037
Fax: 910-716-2186

Ohio

ADA
Drug Information Center
Raabe College of Pharmacy
Ohio Northern University
Ada, OH 45810
Mon.-Fri. 9 AM-5 PM
Tel.: 419-772-2289
Fax: 419-772-1917

CLEVELAND
Cleveland Clinic Foundation
Drug Information Center
9500 Euclid Ave.
Cleveland, OH 44195
Mon.-Fri. 8 AM-4:30 PM
Tel.: 216-444-6456
Fax: 216-444-0158

COLUMBUS
Central Ohio Poison Center
700 Children's Drive
Columbus, OH 43205
Tel.: 513-222-2227
Fax: 614-221-2672

Drug Information Center
Dept. of Pharmacy
Doan Hall 368
Ohio State University
Hospital
410 W. 10th Ave.
Columbus, OH 43210-1228
Mon.-Fri. 8 AM-4 PM
Tel.: 614-293-8679
Fax: 614-293-3165

Drug Information Center
Riverside Methodist
Hospitals
3535 Olantangy River Road
Columbus, OH 43214
Mon.-Fri. 8 AM-5 PM
Tel.: 614-566-5425
Fax: 614-566-5447

PARMA
Clinical Pharmacy Services
Kaiser Permanente Drug
Information Center
12301 Snow Road
Parma, OH 44130
Tel: 216-265-4400
     216-362-2727, pager 3133

TOLEDO
Drug Information Service
The Toledo Hospital
2142 N. Cove Blvd.
Toledo, OH 43606
Mon.-Fri. 8 AM-4:30 PM
Tel.: 419-471-2171
     419-471-5637 (after hours)
Fax: 419-479-6926

ZANESVILLE
Drug Information/Poison
Center Bethesda Hospital
2951 Maple Ave.
Zanesville, OH 43701
7 days/week, 24 hours
Tel.: 614-454-4221
     800-686-4221 (OH)
Fax: 614-454-4059

Oklahoma

OKLAHOMA CITY
Drug Information Center
Baptist Medical Center
3300 Northwest Expressway
Oklahoma City, OK 73112
Mon.-Fri. 8 am to 4:30 pm
Tel: 405-949-3660
Fax: 405-945-5858

Drug Information Center
Presbyterian Hospital
700 NE 13th St.
Oklahoma City, OK 73104 Mon.-
Fri. 7 AM-3:30 PM
Tel.: 405-271-6226
Fax: 405-271-3460

Drug Information Service
University of Oklahoma
Health Sciences Center
Rm LIB-380 A
1000 S.L. Young Blvd.
Oklahoma City, OK 73117
Mon.-Fri. 8 AM-5 PM
Tel.: 405-271-8080
Fax: 405-271-3297

TULSA
Drug Information Service
St. Francis Hospital
6161 S. Yale Ave.
Tulsa, OK 74136
Mon.-Fri. 9 AM-5:30 PM
Tel.: 918-494-6339
Fax: 918-494-1893

Oregon

PORTLAND
University Drug
Consultation Service
The Oregon Health
Sciences University
3181 SW Sam Jackson Park Rd.
Portland, OR 97201
Mon.-Fri. 8:30 AM-5 PM
Tel.: 503-494-7530
Fax: 503-494-0011

Pennsylvania

ERIE
Pharmacy and Drug
Information Services
Hamot Medical Center
201 State St.
Erie, PA 16550
7 days/week, 24 hours
Tel.: 814-877-6022
Fax: 814-877-6108

PHILADELPHIA
Drug Information Center
Temple University Hospital
Dept. of Pharmacy
Broad and Ontario St.
Philadelphia, PA 19140
Mon.-Fri. 8 AM-4:30 PM
Tel.: 215-701-4644
Fax: 215-701-3463

Drug Information Center
Thomas Jefferson
University Hospital
111 S. 11th and Walnut St.
Philadelphia, PA 19107-5098
Mon.-Fri. 8 AM-5 PM
Tel.: 215-955-8877

PITTSBURGH
The Center for Drug
Information
The Mercy Hospital
of Pittsburgh
1400 Locust Street
Pittsburgh, PA 15219-5166
Mon.-Fri. 8 AM-4:30 PM
Tel.: 412-232-7903
     412-232-7907
Fax: 412-232-8422

Drug Information and
Pharmacoepidemiology
Center University of
Pittsburgh Medical Center
137 Victoria Bldg.
Pittsburgh, PA 15261
Mon.-Fri. 8 AM-6 PM
Tel.: 412-624-3784
Fax: 412-642-6350

Drug Information Center
Allegheny General Hospital
320 E. North Ave.
Pittsburgh, PA 15212
Mon.-Fri. 8 AM-4:30 PM
Tel.: 412-359-3192
Fax: 412-359-4806

UPLAND
Drug Information Center
Crozer-Chester
Medical Center
1 Medical Ctr. Blvd.
Upland, PA 19013
Mon.-Fri. 8 AM-4:30 PM
Tel.: 610-447-2851
     610-447-2862 (after hours)
Fax: 215-447-2820

WILLIAMSPORT
Drug Information Center
Williamsport Hospital and
Medical Center
777 Rural Ave.
Williamsport, PA 17701
Mon.-Fri. 8 AM-4 PM
Tel.: 717-321-3289
Fax: 717-321-3230

Puerto Rico

SAN JUAN
Centro Informacion
Medicamentos
Escuela de Farmacia RCM
P.O. Box 365067
San Juan, PR 00936-5067
Mon.-Fri. 8 AM-4 PM
Tel.: 809-758-2525 ext. 1516
Tel. & Fax: 809-763-0196

Rhode Island

PROVIDENCE
Drug Information Service
Dept. of Pharmacy
Rhode Island Hospital
593 Eddy St.
Providence, RI 02903
Mon.-Fri. 8:30 AM-5 PM
Tel.: 401-444-5547
Fax: 401-444-8062

Drug Information Center
University of Rhode Island
Roger Williams Medical
Center
825 Chalkstone Ave.
Providence, RI 02908
Mon.-Fri. 8 AM-4 PM
Tel.: 401-456-2260
Fax: 401-456-2510

South Carolina

CHARLESTON
Drug Information Service
Medical University of
South Carolina
154 Ashley Ave.
Charleston, SC 29403
Mon.-Fri. 8 AM-5:30 PM
Tel.: 803-792-3896
       800-922-5250
Fax: 803-792-5532

SPARTANBURG
Drug Information Center
Spartanburg Regional
Medical Center
101 E. Wood St.
Spartanburg, SC 29303
Mon.-Fri. 8 AM-5 PM
Tel.: 803-560-6910
       803-560-6779 (after hours)
Fax: 803-560-6017

South Dakota

BROOKINGS
South Dakota Drug
Information Center
300 22nd Ave.
Brookings, SD 57006
7 days/week, 8 AM-4:30 PM
Tel.: 800-456-1004

SIOUX CITY
Drug Information Center
McKennan Hospital
800 E. 21st St.
Sioux Falls, SD 57117-5045
7 days/week, 24 hours
Tel.: 605-336-3894
       800-952-0123 (SD)
       800-843-0505 (MN, IA, NE)
Fax: 605-333-8206

Tennessee

KNOXVILLE
Drug Information Center
University of Tennessee
Medical Center
1924 Alcoa Highway
Knoxville, TN 37920-6999
Mon.-Fri. 8 AM-4:30 PM
Tel.: 615-544-9125

MEMPHIS
Drug Information Center
University of Tennessee
800 Madison Avenue
Memphis, TN 38163
Mon.-Fri. 8 AM-5 PM
Tel.: 901-448-5555
Fax: 901-448-5419

South East Regional Drug
Information Center
VA Medical Center
1030 Jefferson Ave.
Memphis, TN. 38104
Mon.-Fri. 7:30 AM-4 PM
Tel.: 901-523-8990, ext. 5191

Texas

GALVESTON
Drug Information Center
University of Texas
Medical Branch
301 University Blvd. - G01
Galveston, TX 77555-0701
Mon.-Fri. 8 AM-5 PM
Tel.: 409-772-2734
Fax: 409-772-8408

HOUSTON
Drug Information Center
Ben Taub General Hospital
Texas Southern University
College of Pharmacy and
Health Sciences
1504 Taub Loop
Houston, TX 77030
Mon.-Fri. 8 AM-10 PM
Tel.: 713-793-2915
       713-793-2937

Drug Information Center
Methodist Hospital
6565 Fannin (DB1-09)
Houston, TX 77030
Mon.-Fri. 8 AM-5 PM
Tel.: 713-790-4190
Fax: 713-793-1224

LACKLAND A.F.B.
Drug Information Center
Dept. of Pharmacy
Wilford Hall Medical Center
2200 Berquist Dr., Suite 1
Lackland A.F.B., TX 78236
Mon.-Fri. 7:30 AM-5 PM
Tel.: 210-670-6291

LUBBOCK
Methodist Hospital
Drug Information &
Consultation Service
3615 19th St.
Lubbock, TX 79410
Mon.-Fri. 8 AM-5 PM
Tel.: 806-793-4012
Fax: 806-784-5322
       (Attn: Pharmacy)

TEMPLE
Drug Information Center
Scott and White
Memorial Hospital
2401 S. 31st. St.
Temple, TX 76508
Mon.-Fri. 8 AM-6 PM
Tel.: 817-724-4636

Utah

SALT LAKE CITY
Drug Information Center
Dept. of Pharmacy Services
Room A-050
University of Utah Hospital
50 N. Medical Dr.
Salt Lake City, UT 84132
Mon.-Fri. 8:30 AM-4:30 PM
Tel.: 801-581-2073
Fax: 801-585-6688

Virginia

HAMPTON
Drug Information Center
Sentara Hampton
General Hospital
3120 Victoria Blvd.
Hampton, VA 23669
7 days/week, 7 AM-Midnight
Tel.: 804-727-7185

RICHMOND
Drug Information Center
St. Mary's Hospital
5801 Bremo Rd.
Richmond, VA 23226
Mon.-Fri. 24 hrs.
Tel.: 804-281-8058
Fax: 804-285-4411

Washington

SPOKANE
Drug Information Center
Washington State University
College of Pharmacy
601 W. 1st Ave.
Spokane, WA 92204
Mon.-Fri. 8 AM-4 PM
Tel.: 509-456-4409

West Virginia

MORGANTOWN
West Virginia Drug
Information Center
West Virginia University-
Robert C. Byrd
Health Sciences Center
1124 HSN, P.O.Box 9520
Morgantown, WV 26506-9520
Mon.-Fri. 9 AM-5 PM
Tel.: 304-293-5101
       800-352-2501 (WV)
Fax: 304-293-5483

Wisconsin

MADISON
Drug Information Center
Univ. of Wisconsin
Hospital & Clinics
600 Highland Ave.
Madison, WI 53792
7 days/week, 7:30 AM-10:30 PM
Tel.: 608-262-1315
Fax: 608-263-9424

Wyoming

LARAMIE
Drug Information Center
University of Wyoming
P.O.Box 3375
Laramie, WY 82071
Mon.-Fri. 8 AM-5 PM
Tel.: 307-766-6128
Fax: 307-766-2953

New Molecular Entities

Although scores of new pharmaceutical products are introduced each year, the number of completely new, never-before-available drugs reaching the market is surprisingly small. The Food and Drug Administration (FDA) calls these truly ground-breaking compounds "New Molecular Entities." Those approved during the previous year (through August, 1994) are listed in the following table in order of approval. See the summary at the end of the table for those approved late in 1994.

The FDA rates drugs moving through the approval process according to their therapeutic potential. This rating appears in the third column. All the ratings begin with "1," the code that signifies a New Molecular Entity. (In some products, a New Molecular Entity forms part of a combination. This is indicated by a "1,4" in the rating.) Following the number is an alphabetical code indicating the priority given the drug during the review process. These codes can be interpreted as follows:

P Priority review—represents a therapeutic gain
S Standard review—substantially equivalent to other drugs
E Expedited review—treats life-threatening illness
AA AIDS drug
V Officially designated orphan drug

A drug can carry more than one of these codes; and drugs that entered the review system before 1992 carry a different set of codes, with"A" indicating an important therapeutic gain, "B" a modest therapeutic gain, and "C" little or no therapeutic gain.

TRADE NAME (GENERIC NAME) DOSAGE FORM NDA# APPLICANT	DATE RECEIVED DATE OF 1ST ACTION NUMBER OF MONTHS TO 1ST ACTION DATE OF FIRST APPROVAL NUMBER OF MONTHS TO 1ST APPROVAL	DIVISION DRUG CLASS	DESCRIPTION
SEREVENT (Salmeterol Xinafoate) Inhalation Aerosol NDA: 20-236 Glaxo, Inc.	12/20/91 02/20/91 13.5 02/04/94 25.5	HFD-007 1P	Serevent Inhalation Aerosol is indicated for long-term administration in the maintenance treatment of asthma and prevention of bronchospasm in patients 12 years of age and older with reversible obstructive airway disease, including patients with symptoms of nocturnal astma, who require regular treatment inhaled short-acting beta-agonist.
RHINOCORT (budesonide) Nasal Inhaler; NDA: 20-233 G.H. Besselaar	12/31/92 12/17/93 (AE Letter) 11.6 02/14/94 13.5	HFD-007 1S	Rhinocort Nasal Inhaler is indicated for the management of symptoms of seasonal or perennial allergic rhinitis in adults and children and nonallergic perennial rhinitis in adults.
ZEMURON (rocuronium bromide) Injection NDA: 20-214 Organon Inc.	06/29/93 01/11/94 (AE Letter) 6.4 03/17/94 8.6	HFD-007 1S	Zemuron (rocuronium bromide) Injection is a nondepolarizing neuromuscular blocking agent with a rapid-to-intermediate onset depending on dose and intermediate duration and is indicated for inpatients and outpatients as an adjunct to general anesthesia to facilitate both rapid sequence and routine tracheal intubation, and to provide skeletal muscle relaxation during surgery or mechanical ventilation.
IOBENGUANE SULFATE I 131 Injection NDA 20-084 CIS-US, Inc	11/15/91 03/25/94 28.3	HFD-150 IP	Iobenguane Sulfate I 131 Injection in indicated as an adjunctive diagnostic agent in the localization of primary or metastatic pheochromocytomas and neuroblastomas.
SEMPREX-D (acrivastine 8 mg/ pseudoephedrine hydrochloride 60 mg) Capsules NDA 19-806 Burroughs Wellcome	12/29/87 05/14/90 (NA Letter) 28.5 03/25/94 22.2	HFD-150 1, 4S	Semprex-D Capsules are indicated for relief of symptoms associated with seasonal allergic rhinitis such as sneezing, rhinorrhea, pruritus, lacrimation, and nasal congestion.

PROGRAF (tacrolimus) Capsules and Injection NDA: 50-708 50-709 Fujisawa USA, Inc.	07/26/93 (capsules) 08/04/93 (injection) 04/08/94 8.4 (capsules) 8.1 (injection)	HFD-530 1PE	Prograf is indicated for the prophylaxis of organ rejection in patients receiving allogeneic liver transplants. It is recommended that Prograf be used concomitantly with adrenal corticosteroids.
CEREZYME (imiglucerase) Injection NDA: 20-367 Genzyme Corporation	05/21/93 05/23/94 12.1	HFD-160 1PVE	Cerezyme is indicated for long-term enzyme replacement therapy for patients with a confirmed diagnosis of Type 1 Gaucher disease that results in one or more of the following conditions: anemia, thrombocytopenia, bone disease, or hepatomegaly or splenomegaly.
OSTREOSCAN NDA: 20-314 Mallinckrodt Medical Inc .	10/21/92 06/02/94 19.4	HFD-160 1P	Octreoscan, Indium In-111 pentetreotide, is an agent for the sonigraphic localization of primary and metastatic neuroendocrine tumors bearing somatostatin.
ZERIT (stavudine) Capsules NDA: 20-412 Bristol-Myers Squibb	12/18/93 06/24/94 11.9	HFD-530 1PAA EH	Zerit is indicated for the treatment of adults with advanced HIV infection who are intolerant of approved therapies with proven clinical benefit or who have experienced significant clinical or immunologic deterioration while receiving these therapies or for whom such therapies are contraindicated.
FAMVIR (famciclovir) Tablets NDA: 20-363 SmithKline Beecham	06/30/93 06/29/94 12.0	HFD-530 1S	Famvir is indicated for the management of acute herpes zoster (shingles).
CYSTAGON (cysteamine bitartrate) NDA: 20-392 Mylan Pharmaceuticals, Inc.	08/31/93 08/15/94 11.5	HFD-180 1P	Cystagon is indicated for the management of nephopathic cystinosis in children and adults.
FLUDEOXYGLUCOSE F18 Injection NDA: 20-306 Downstate Clinical PET Center	9/23/92 8/19/94 22.5	HFD-160 1P	Fludeoxyglucose F 18 Injection ($[^{18}F]$ FDG) is indicated in PET (positron emission tomography) for the identification of regions of abnormal glucose metabolism associated with foci of epileptic seizures. Fludeoxyglucose F 18 Injection is not indicated for distinguishing epilepto genic foci from brain tumors or other brain lesions which may cause seizures.

New Molecular Entities Approved in the Later Part of 1994

- Dalteparin Sodium (Fragmin by Pharmacia) for the prevention of deep vein thrombosis in abdominal surgery
- Dorzolamide HCl (Trusopt by Merck) for ocular hypertension or open-angle glaucoma
- Fluvoxamine Maleate (Luvox by Solvay) for the treatment of obsessive-compulsive disorder)
- Lamotrigine (Lamictal by Burroughs Wellcome) as an adjunctive therapy of partial seizures in adults with epilepsy
- Metformin (Glucophage by Lipha) for adjunctive therapy of non-insulin-dependent diabetes

- Nefazodone HCl (Serzone by Bristol-Myers Squibb) for the treatment of depression
- Rimexolone (Vexol by Alcon) for the treatment of postoperative inflammation and treatment of anterior uveitis
- Spirapril (Renormax by Sandoz) for the treatment of hypertension
- Technetium 99m Bicisate (Neurolite by Dupont Merck) diagnostic agent in computerized tomography
- Vinorelbine Tartrate (Navelbine by Burroughs Wellcome) antineoplastic for small cell lung cancer

Additional Alternatives

L isted on the following pages is pricing information on additional forms, strength, and suppliers of some drugs appearing in the Product Information Section. This information augments the pricing data found in the drug's "How Supplied" section, and may serve to further broaden your range of choices. It is organized alphabetically by generic name.

ALPRAZOLAM

TABLET (C-IV): 1 MG

AVERAGE UNIT PRICE (AVAILABLE SIZES)		GENERIC A-RATED AVERAGE PRICE (GAAP)	
BRAND	$0.96	100s	$83.50
GENERIC	$0.83	500s	$413.13
HCFA FUL (100s ea)	$0.12	1000s	$796.02

BRAND/MANUFACTURER	NDC	SIZE	AWP
◆ BRAND			
➤ XANAX: Upjohn	00009-0090-01	100s	$94.11
	00009-0090-17	100s	$107.64
	00009-0090-46	100s ud	$99.14
	00009-0090-04	500s	$456.40
	00009-0090-13	1000s	$893.15
◆ GENERICS			
Medirex	57480-0522-06	30s	$27.08
Major	00904-7793-60	100s	$77.05
Major	00904-7920-60	100s	$77.05
West Point	59591-0053-68	100s	$80.13
Mylan	00378-4005-01	100s	$83.75
Roxane	00054-4107-25	100s	$84.00
Geneva	00781-1328-01	100s	$84.68
Qualitest	00603-2348-21	100s	$85.12
Warner Chilcott	00047-0785-24	100s	$85.25
Schein	00364-2584-01	100s	$85.62
Purepac	00228-2031-10	100s	$86.80
Aligen	00405-4045-01	100s	$87.63
Novopharm	55953-0131-40	100s	$87.66
Goldline	00182-0029-01	100s	$87.76
➤ Lederle Std Prod	00005-3342-43	100s	$87.76
Martec	52555-0508-01	100s	$88.40
Moore,H.L.	00839-7853-06	100s	$92.19
UDL	51079-0790-21	100s	$94.08
Vangard	00615-0403-13	100s ud	$18.78
Greenstone	59762-3721-01	100s ud	$80.16
UDL	51079-0790-20	100s ud	$86.64
Roxane	00054-8107-25	100s ud	$88.00
Geneva	00781-1328-13	100s ud	$89.13
Medirex	57480-0522-01	100s ud	$90.25
Roxane	00054-8107-24	100s ud	$96.00
Major	00904-7793-40	500s	$373.75
Major	00904-7920-40	500s	$373.75
Greenstone	59762-3721-03	500s	$388.71
Mylan	00378-4005-05	500s	$406.19
Geneva	00781-1328-05	500s	$410.64
Qualitest	00603-2348-28	500s	$411.88
Roxane	00054-4107-29	500s	$414.00
Warner Chilcott	00047-0785-30	500s	$415.00
Schein	00364-2584-05	500s	$415.25
Novopharm	55953-0131-70	500s	$420.20
Purepac	00228-2031-50	500s	$420.96
Goldline	00182-0029-05	500s	$425.66
➤ Lederle Std Prod	00005-3342-31	500s	$425.66
Martec	52555-0508-05	500s	$426.65

BRAND/MANUFACTURER	NDC	SIZE	AWP
Aligen	00405-4045-02	500s	$434.63
Moore,H.L.	00839-7853-12	500s	$447.12
Greenstone	59762-3721-04	1000s	$760.67
Novopharm	55953-0131-80	1000s	$798.40
Geneva	00781-1328-10	1000s	$803.58
Purepac	00228-2031-96	1000s	$821.43

TABLET (C-IV): 2 MG

AVERAGE UNIT PRICE (AVAILABLE SIZES)		GENERIC A-RATED AVERAGE PRICE (GAAP)	
BRAND	$1.58	100s	$143.57
GENERIC	$1.42	500s	$691.69
HCFA FUL (100s ea)	$0.24		

BRAND/MANUFACTURER	NDC	SIZE	AWP
◆ BRAND			
➤ XANAX: Upjohn	00009-0094-01	100s	$160.01
	00009-0094-03	500s	$776.10
◆ GENERICS			
West Point	59591-0054-68	100s	$136.28
Mylan	00378-4007-01	100s	$142.40
Geneva	00781-1329-01	100s	$143.97
Purepac	00228-2039-10	100s	$147.59
Goldline	00182-0030-01	100s	$149.24
Lederle Std Prod	00005-3346-43	100s	$149.24
Greenstone	59762-3722-01	100s ud	$136.28
Greenstone	59762-3722-03	500s	$660.98
Geneva	00781-1329-05	500s	$698.27
Purepac	00228-2039-50	500s	$715.83

AMITRIPTYLINE HYDROCHLORIDE

TABLET: 50 MG

AVERAGE UNIT PRICE (AVAILABLE SIZES)		GENERIC A-RATED AVERAGE PRICE (GAAP)	
BRAND	$0.64	30s	$6.97
GENERIC	$0.12	100s	$14.02
HCFA FUL (100s ea)	$0.02	1000s	$66.67

BRAND/MANUFACTURER	NDC	SIZE	AWP
◆ BRAND			
➤ ELAVIL: Stuart	00038-0041-10	100s	$63.73
➤ ELAVIL: Stuart	00038-0041-39	100s ud	$66.34
	00038-0041-34	1000s	$604.96
◆ GENERICS			
Major	00904-0202-46	30s	$2.10
Medirex	57480-0303-06	30s	$11.83
➤ Rugby	00536-3073-01	100s	$4.56
➤ Geneva	00781-1488-01	100s	$5.92
Schein	00364-0575-01	100s	$6.44
Aligen	00405-4068-01	100s	$6.85
Qualitest	00603-2214-21	100s	$6.88
URL	00677-0477-01	100s	$8.35
Mutual	53489-0106-01	100s	$8.50
Major	00904-0202-60	100s	$8.60
Moore,H.L.	00839-6193-06	100s	$9.30
Martec	52555-0977-01	100s	$10.45
Biocraft	00332-2124-09	100s	$10.68
Sidmak	50111-0368-01	100s	$11.20
Goldline	00182-1020-01	100s	$11.20
Purepac	00228-2133-10	100s	$11.33
Mylan	00378-2650-01	100s	$11.50
Roxane	00054-4043-25	100s	$11.66
Parmed	00349-1042-01	100s	$11.75
ENDEP: Roche Prod	00140-0109-01	100s	$54.62
VANATRIP: GM Pharm	58809-0717-01	100s	$59.08

BRAND/MANUFACTURER	NDC	SIZE	AWP
U.S. Trading	56126-0135-11	100s ud	$4.11
Raway	00686-0133-20	100s ud	$4.95
▶ Geneva	00781-1488-13	100s ud	$9.95
Vangard	00615-0830-13	100s ud	$11.51
Major	00904-0202-61	100s ud	$11.59
Medirex	57480-0303-01	100s ud	$18.90
UDL	51079-0133-20	100s ud	$18.92
Goldline	00182-1020-89	100s ud	$19.20
Roxane	00054-8043-25	100s ud	$24.51
▶ Rugby	00536-3073-05	500s	$16.13
▶ Rugby	00536-3073-10	1000s	$30.68
Major	00904-0202-80	1000s	$41.80
▶ Geneva	00781-1488-10	1000s	$43.85
Qualitest	00603-2214-32	1000s	$45.05
URL	00677-0477-10	1000s	$49.30
Mutual	53489-0106-10	1000s	$49.30
Schein	00364-0575-02	1000s	$50.40
Aligen	00405-4068-03	1000s	$54.29
Moore,H.L.	00839-6193-16	1000s	$54.81
Martec	52555-0977-10	1000s	$58.25
Purepac	00228-2133-96	1000s	$74.49
Parmed	00349-1042-10	1000s	$74.95
Roxane	00054-4043-31	1000s	$96.64
Biocraft	00332-2124-15	1000s	$101.33
Sidmak	50111-0368-03	1000s	$102.40
Goldline	00182-1020-10	1000s	$102.40
Mylan	00378-2650-10	1000s	$103.50

TABLET: 50 MG

BRAND/MANUFACTURER	NDC	SIZE	AWP
◇ GENERICS			
Copley	38245-0208-10	100s	$3.35
Copley	38245-0208-20	1000s	$25.00

TABLET: 75 MG

AVERAGE UNIT PRICE (AVAILABLE SIZES)		GENERIC A-RATED AVERAGE PRICE (GAAP)	
BRAND	$0.87	100s	$14.77
GENERIC	$0.14	500s	$33.68
HCFA FUL (100s ea)	$0.04	1000s	$106.75

BRAND/MANUFACTURER	NDC	SIZE	AWP
◆ BRAND			
▶ ELAVIL: Stuart	00038-0042-10	100s	$87.26
◆ GENERICS			
▶ Rugby	00536-3074-01	100s	$7.28
▶ Geneva	00781-1489-01	100s	$7.65
Aligen	00405-4069-01	100s	$8.94
Qualitest	00603-2215-21	100s	$8.94
Major	00904-0203-60	100s	$9.00
Purepac	00228-2134-10	100s	$9.13
Mutual	53489-0107-01	100s	$9.75
URL	00677-0478-01	100s	$10.20
Schein	00364-0576-01	100s	$10.29
Moore,H.L.	00839-6194-06	100s	$11.41
Parmed	00349-1043-01	100s	$13.95
Martec	52555-0978-01	100s	$13.95
Mylan	00378-2675-01	100s	$14.50
Biocraft	00332-2126-09	100s	$14.62
Sidmak	50111-0369-01	100s	$15.15
Goldline	00182-1021-01	100s	$15.15
Roxane	00054-4045-25	100s	$16.28
Raway	00686-0147-20	100s ud	$8.90
▶ Geneva	00781-1489-13	100s ud	$16.50
Vangard	00615-0831-13	100s ud	$18.06
Major	00904-0203-61	100s ud	$18.21
Medirex	57480-0304-01	100s ud	$22.95
UDL	51079-0147-20	100s ud	$23.00
Goldline	00182-1021-89	100s ud	$23.30
Roxane	00054-8045-25	100s ud	$42.11
▶ Rugby	00536-3074-05	500s	$31.35
Mutual	53489-0107-05	500s	$36.00
Sidmak	50111-0369-03	1000s	$62.15
Moore,H.L.	00839-6194-16	1000s	$151.34

TABLET: 75 MG

BRAND/MANUFACTURER	NDC	SIZE	AWP
◇ GENERICS			
Copley	38245-0209-10	100s	$5.45

TABLET: 100 MG

AVERAGE UNIT PRICE (AVAILABLE SIZES)		GENERIC A-RATED AVERAGE PRICE (GAAP)	
BRAND	$1.10	100s	$21.50
GENERIC	$0.21		
HCFA FUL (100s ea)	$0.04		

BRAND/MANUFACTURER	NDC	SIZE	AWP
◆ BRAND			
▶ ELAVIL: Stuart	00038-0043-10	100s	$110.34
◆ GENERICS			
▶ Rugby	00536-3075-01	100s	$9.15
Aligen	00405-4070-01	100s	$9.42
Major	00904-0204-60	100s	$9.50
Qualitest	00603-2216-21	100s	$10.15
Purepac	00228-2135-10	100s	$11.58
Mutual	53489-0108-01	100s	$11.90
URL	00677-0568-01	100s	$12.05
Schein	00364-0577-01	100s	$12.08
▶ Geneva	00781-1490-01	100s	$13.84
Martec	52555-0979-01	100s	$14.40
Moore,H.L.	00839-6223-06	100s	$16.40
Mylan	00378-2685-01	100s	$16.95
Biocraft	00332-2128-09	100s	$18.48
Parmed	00349-1044-01	100s	$18.95
Sidmak	50111-0370-01	100s	$19.25
Goldline	00182-1063-01	100s	$19.25
Roxane	00054-4046-25	100s	$19.36
ENDEP: Roche Prod	00140-0116-01	100s	$99.20
U.S. Trading	56126-0137-11	100s ud	$6.60
Raway	00686-0563-20	100s ud	$9.00
Major	00904-0204-61	100s ud	$20.41
Geneva	00781-1490-13	100s ud	$22.90
Vangard	00615-0832-13	100s ud	$24.49
UDL	51079-0563-20	100s ud	$27.90
Medirex	57480-0424-01	100s ud	$37.75
Goldline	00182-1063-89	100s ud	$38.00
Roxane	00054-8046-25	100s ud	$51.50
▶ Rugby	00536-3075-05	500s	$42.75

TABLET: 100 MG

BRAND/MANUFACTURER	NDC	SIZE	AWP
◇ GENERICS			
Copley	38245-0210-10	100s	$6.75

TABLET: 150 MG

AVERAGE UNIT PRICE (AVAILABLE SIZES)		GENERIC A-RATED AVERAGE PRICE (GAAP)	
BRAND	$1.59	100s	$19.67
GENERIC	$0.20		
HCFA FUL (100s ea)	$0.07		

BRAND/MANUFACTURER	NDC	SIZE	AWP
◆ BRAND			
▶ ELAVIL: Stuart	00038-0047-30	30s	$47.99
	00038-0047-10	100s	$157.01
◆ GENERICS			
▶ Geneva	00781-1491-01	100s	$14.15
▶ Rugby	00536-3076-01	100s	$14.18
Goldline	00182-1140-01	100s	$14.25
Sidmak	50111-0371-01	100s	$14.85
Goldline	00182-1486-01	100s	$14.85
Mutual	53489-0109-01	100s	$15.20
Martec	52555-0980-01	100s	$15.35
URL	00677-0645-01	100s	$16.20
Qualitest	00603-2217-21	100s	$16.25
Aligen	00405-4071-01	100s	$17.19
Moore,H.L.	00839-6401-06	100s	$18.43
Schein	00364-0578-01	100s	$19.04
Mylan	00378-2695-01	100s	$20.75
Parmed	00349-2103-01	100s	$24.95
Major	00904-0205-60	100s	$26.62
Raway	00686-0564-20	100s ud	$16.50
▶ Geneva	00781-1491-13	100s ud	$37.50
UDL	51079-0564-20	100s ud	$37.79

TABLET: 150 MG

BRAND/MANUFACTURER	NDC	SIZE	AWP
◇ GENERICS			
Copley	38245-0211-10	100s	$10.85

AMOXICILLIN

CHEW TABLET: 125 MG

BRAND/MANUFACTURER	NDC	SIZE	AWP
◆ BRAND			
AMOXIL: SK Beecham Pharm	00029-6004-39	60s	$8.85

CHEW TABLET: 250 MG

AVERAGE UNIT PRICE (AVAILABLE SIZES)		GENERIC A-RATED AVERAGE PRICE (GAAP)	
BRAND	$0.25	100s	$23.69
GENERIC	$0.24	500s	$116.18

◆ RATED THERAPEUTICALLY EQUIVELENT; ◇ THERAPEUTIC EQUIVALENT UNCONFIRMED; ○ UNRATED

BRAND/MANUFACTURER	NDC	SIZE	AWP
◆ **BRAND**			
➤ AMOXIL: SK Beecham Pharm	00029-6005-13	30s	$7.60
	00029-6005-30	100s	$25.35
◆ **GENERICS**			
Allscrips	54569-3689-02	15s	$3.55
Allscrips	54569-3689-03	45s	$10.64
Rugby	00536-0097-01	100s	$22.82
Goldline	00182-1962-01	100s	$22.82
Biocraft	00332-2268-09	100s	$22.82
Qualitest	00603-2274-21	100s	$22.82
Warner Chilcott	00047-0038-24	100s	$22.82
Aligen	00405-4086-01	100s	$23.02
Geneva	00781-1098-01	100s	$23.07
Major	00904-7713-60	100s	$25.50
Schein	00364-2569-01	100s	$25.52
Moore,H.L.	00839-7776-06	100s	$25.64
Biocraft	00332-2268-13	500s	$101.00
Major	00904-7713-40	500s	$110.05
Moore,H.L.	00839-7776-12	500s	$118.65
Goldline	00182-1962-05	500s	$135.00

POWDER FOR RECONSTITUTION: 50 MG/ML

AVERAGE UNIT PRICE (AVAILABLE SIZES)	
BRAND	$0.12

BRAND/MANUFACTURER	NDC	SIZE	AWP
◆ **BRAND**			
AMOXIL PEDIATRIC: SK Beecham Pharm	00029-6035-20	15 ml	$1.80
	00029-6038-39	30 ml	$3.45

POWDER FOR RECONSTITUTION: 125 MG/5 ML

AVERAGE UNIT PRICE (AVAILABLE SIZES)		GENERIC A-RATED AVERAGE PRICE (GAAP)	
BRAND	$0.07	80 ml	$2.89
GENERIC	$0.04	100 ml	$3.25
HCFA FUL (80 ml)	$0.03	150 ml	$4.25
HCFA FUL (100 ml)	$0.02	200 ml	$7.31
HCFA FUL (150 ml)	$0.01		

BRAND/MANUFACTURER	NDC	SIZE	AWP
◆ **BRAND**			
AMOXIL: SK Beecham Pharm	00029-6008-18	5 ml ud	$1.00
	00029-6008-21	80 ml	$2.70
	00029-6008-23	100 ml	$3.10
	00029-6008-22	150 ml	$3.55
◆ **GENERICS**			
Rugby	00536-0090-81	80 ml	$2.35
Schein	00364-7215-60	80 ml	$2.60
Moore,H.L.	00839-6115-71	80 ml	$2.69
Lederle Std Prod	00005-3146-43	80 ml	$2.80
TRIMOX: Apothecon	00003-1737-30	80 ml	$2.98
Du Pont Multi	00056-0249-34	80 ml	$2.98
Novopharm	55953-0149-38	80 ml	$3.08
Biocraft	00332-4150-30	80 ml	$3.12
Warner Chilcott	00047-2500-16	80 ml	$3.12
Aligen	00405-2225-58	80 ml	$3.22
Rugby	00536-0090-82	100 ml	$2.13
Schein	00364-7215-61	100 ml	$2.65
Moore,H.L.	00839-6115-73	100 ml	$2.82
Major	00904-2619-04	100 ml	$2.95
Geneva	00781-6195-46	100 ml	$2.95
WYMOX: Wyeth-Ayerst	00008-0557-02	100 ml	$3.00
Lederle Std Prod	00005-3146-46	100 ml	$3.21
Du Pont Multi	00056-0249-36	100 ml	$3.29
Novopharm	55953-0149-40	100 ml	$3.37
TRIMOX: Apothecon	00003-1737-40	100 ml	$3.42
Martec	52555-0141-01	100 ml	$3.47
URL	00677-0452-27	100 ml	$3.55
Aligen	00405-2225-60	100 ml	$3.59
Goldline	00182-1072-70	100 ml	$3.59
Biocraft	00332-4150-32	100 ml	$3.59
Qualitest	00603-6500-64	100 ml	$3.59
Warner Chilcott	00047-2500-17	100 ml	$3.59
Mylan	00378-0206-02	100 ml	$3.76
Rugby	00536-0090-74	150 ml	$2.63
Schein	00364-7215-62	150 ml	$3.25
WYMOX: Wyeth-Ayerst	00008-0557-03	150 ml	$3.48
Geneva	00781-6195-55	150 ml	$3.58
Major	00904-2619-07	150 ml	$3.70
Lederle Std Prod	00005-3146-49	150 ml	$3.70
Moore,H.L.	00839-6115-75	150 ml	$3.71
TRIMOX: Apothecon	00003-1737-45	150 ml	$3.95
URL	00677-0452-28	150 ml	$4.10
Goldline	00182-1072-72	150 ml	$4.14
Biocraft	00332-4150-34	150 ml	$4.14
Qualitest	00603-6500-66	150 ml	$4.14
Aligen	00405-2225-78	150 ml	$4.71
Novopharm	55953-0149-47	150 ml	$4.71
Mylan	00378-0206-06	150 ml	$4.72
Martec	52555-0141-07	150 ml	$4.72
Warner Chilcott	00047-2500-18	150 ml	$4.72

BRAND/MANUFACTURER	NDC	SIZE	AWP
Du Pont Multi	00056-0249-38	150 ml	$4.79
VHA Supply	00015-7276-60	150 ml	$7.94
Novopharm	55953-0149-53	200 ml	$5.87
Warner Chilcott	00047-2500-20	200 ml	$8.75
VHA Supply	00015-7276-75	5 ml 25s ud	$51.50

POWDER FOR RECONSTITUTION: 250 MG/5 ML

AVERAGE UNIT PRICE (AVAILABLE SIZES)		GENERIC A-RATED AVERAGE PRICE (GAAP)	
BRAND	$0.09	80 ml	$4.67
GENERIC	$0.06	100 ml	$5.32
HCFA FUL (80 ml)	$0.04	150 ml	$6.64
HCFA FUL (100 ml)	$0.03	200 ml	$9.96
HCFA FUL (150 ml)	$0.02		

BRAND/MANUFACTURER	NDC	SIZE	AWP
◆ **BRAND**			
AMOXIL: SK Beecham Pharm	00029-6009-18	5 ml ud	$1.05
	00029-6009-21	80 ml	$4.60
	00029-6009-23	100 ml	$5.30
	00029-6009-22	150 ml	$6.10
◆ **GENERICS**			
Schein	00364-7216-60	80 ml	$3.50
Novopharm	55953-0130-38	80 ml	$3.75
Moore,H.L.	00839-6116-71	80 ml	$4.17
Rugby	00536-0105-81	80 ml	$4.32
Lederle Std Prod	00005-3147-43	80 ml	$4.79
Du Pont Multi	00056-0250-34	80 ml	$4.98
TRIMOX: Apothecon	00003-1738-30	80 ml	$5.10
Biocraft	00332-4155-30	80 ml	$5.35
Warner Chilcott	00047-2501-16	80 ml	$5.35
Aligen	00405-2250-58	80 ml	$5.38
Schein	00364-7216-61	100 ml	$3.75
Novopharm	55953-0130-40	100 ml	$4.42
Rugby	00536-0105-82	100 ml	$4.47
Moore,H.L.	00839-6116-73	100 ml	$4.71
Geneva	00781-6191-46	100 ml	$4.73
Major	00904-2620-04	100 ml	$4.80
Mylan	00378-0207-02	100 ml	$5.12
WYMOX: Wyeth-Ayerst	00008-0558-02	100 ml	$5.15
Martec	52555-0142-01	100 ml	$5.15
URL	00677-0453-27	100 ml	$5.30
Lederle Std Prod	00005-3147-46	100 ml	$5.49
TRIMOX: Apothecon	00003-1738-40	100 ml	$5.84
Aligen	00405-2250-60	100 ml	$6.13
Goldline	00182-1073-70	100 ml	$6.13
Biocraft	00332-4155-32	100 ml	$6.13
Qualitest	00603-6501-64	100 ml	$6.13
Warner Chilcott	00047-2501-17	100 ml	$6.13
Du Pont Multi	00056-0250-36	100 ml	$6.19
Rugby	00536-0105-74	150 ml	$4.50
Geneva	00781-6191-55	150 ml	$5.36
Schein	00364-7216-62	150 ml	$5.75
Major	00904-2620-07	150 ml	$5.85
Moore,H.L.	00839-6116-75	150 ml	$5.87
WYMOX: Wyeth-Ayerst	00008-0558-03	150 ml	$5.96
Novopharm	55953-0130-47	150 ml	$6.15
Martec	52555-0142-07	150 ml	$6.35
Lederle Std Prod	00005-3147-49	150 ml	$6.35
TRIMOX: Apothecon	00003-1738-45	150 ml	$6.78
URL	00677-0453-28	150 ml	$6.90
Mylan	00378-0207-06	150 ml	$6.96
Aligen	00405-2250-78	150 ml	$7.11
Goldline	00182-1073-72	150 ml	$7.11
Biocraft	00332-4155-34	150 ml	$7.11
Qualitest	00603-6501-66	150 ml	$7.11
Warner Chilcott	00047-2501-18	150 ml	$7.12
Du Pont Multi	00056-0250-38	150 ml	$7.49
VHA Supply	00015-7277-60	150 ml	$10.42
Novopharm	55953-0130-53	200 ml	$7.69
Warner Chilcott	00047-2501-20	200 ml	$12.23
VHA Supply	00015-7277-75	5 ml 25s ud	$56.50

AMPICILLIN

POWDER FOR RECONSTITUTION: 125 MG/5 ML

AVERAGE UNIT PRICE (AVAILABLE SIZES)		GENERIC A-RATED AVERAGE PRICE (GAAP)	
GENERIC	$0.02	100 ml	$2.50
HCFA FUL (100 ml)	$0.02	150 ml	$3.12
HCFA FUL (200 ml)	$0.02	200 ml	$4.31

BRAND/MANUFACTURER	NDC	SIZE	AWP
◆ **GENERICS**			
TOTACILLIN: SK Beecham Pharm	00029-6625-23	100 ml	$1.50
Lederle Std Prod	00005-3588-46	100 ml	$2.18
PRINCIPEN: Apothecon	00003-0969-09	100 ml	$2.21
OMNIPEN: Wyeth-Ayerst	00008-0054-03	100 ml	$2.24
Moore,H.L.	00839-5144-73	100 ml	$2.28
Mylan	00378-0117-02	100 ml	$2.76
Rugby	00536-0020-82	100 ml	$2.87
Aligen	00405-2275-60	100 ml	$2.87
Biocraft	00332-4129-32	100 ml	$2.87

2862 / ADDITIONAL ALTERNATIVES

BRAND/MANUFACTURER	NDC	SIZE	AWP
Goldline	00182-0274-70	100 ml	$2.87
Warner Chilcott	00047-2301-17	100 ml	$2.87
PRINCIPEN: Apothecon	00003-0969-52	150 ml	$3.08
OMNIPEN: Wyeth-Ayerst	00008-0054-02	150 ml	$3.15
TOTACILLIN: SK Beecham Pharm	00029-6625-24	200 ml	$2.95
Lederle Std Prod	00005-3588-60	200 ml	$3.19
PRINCIPEN: Apothecon	00003-0969-61	200 ml	$3.83
OMNIPEN: Wyeth-Ayerst	00008-0054-04	200 ml	$3.86
Rugby	00536-0020-84	200 ml	$4.39
URL	00677-0012-29	200 ml	$4.60
Mylan	00378-0117-04	200 ml	$4.62
Warner Chilcott	00047-2301-20	200 ml	$4.62
Aligen	00405-2275-70	200 ml	$4.64
Biocraft	00332-4129-36	200 ml	$4.64
Goldline	00182-0274-73	200 ml	$4.64
VHA Supply	00015-7988-67	200 ml	$5.77

POWDER FOR RECONSTITUTION: 250 MG/5 ML

AVERAGE UNIT PRICE (AVAILABLE SIZES)		GENERIC A-RATED AVERAGE PRICE (GAAP)	
GENERIC	$0.03	100 ml	$3.42
HCFA FUL (100 ml)	$0.03	200 ml	$5.84
HCFA FUL (200 ml)	$0.03		

BRAND/MANUFACTURER	NDC	SIZE	AWP
◆ GENERICS			
TOTACILLIN: SK Beecham Pharm	00029-6630-23	100 ml	$2.10
MARCILLIN: Marnel	00682-9116-01	100 ml	$2.70
Lederle Std Prod	00005-3589-46	100 ml	$2.90
URL	00677-0013-27	100 ml	$3.25
PRINCIPEN: Apothecon	00003-0972-52	100 ml	$3.29
OMNIPEN: Wyeth-Ayerst	00008-0055-03	100 ml	$3.31
Rugby	00536-0030-82	100 ml	$3.47
Moore,H.L.	00839-6445-73	100 ml	$3.50
Warner Chilcott	00047-2302-17	100 ml	$3.88
Biocraft	00332-4131-32	100 ml	$3.90
Goldline	00182-0275-70	100 ml	$3.90
Mylan	00378-0118-02	100 ml	$4.12
Aligen	00405-2300-60	100 ml	$4.19
OMNIPEN: Wyeth-Ayerst	00008-0055-02	150 ml	$4.95
TOTACILLIN: SK Beecham Pharm	00029-6630-24	200 ml	$4.20
Moore,H.L.	00839-6445-78	200 ml	$4.93
Lederle Std Prod	00005-3589-60	200 ml	$4.94
URL	00677-0013-29	200 ml	$4.95
PRINCIPEN: Apothecon	00003-0972-61	200 ml	$5.88
OMNIPEN: Wyeth-Ayerst	00008-0055-04	200 ml	$5.93
Rugby	00536-0030-84	200 ml	$6.01
Mylan	00378-0118-04	200 ml	$6.50
Warner Chilcott	00047-2302-20	200 ml	$6.67
Aligen	00405-2300-70	200 ml	$6.69
Biocraft	00332-4131-36	200 ml	$6.69
Goldline	00182-0275-73	200 ml	$6.69

AMPICILLIN SODIUM
POWDER FOR INJECTION: 1 GM

AVERAGE UNIT PRICE (AVAILABLE SIZES)		GENERIC A-RATED AVERAGE PRICE (GAAP)	
BRAND	$4.30	1s	$2.86
GENERIC	$3.87	10s	$68.70

BRAND/MANUFACTURER	NDC	SIZE	AWP
◆ BRAND			
OMNIPEN-N: Wyeth-Ayerst	00008-0315-04	1s	$3.88
	00008-0315-23	1s	$4.76
	00008-0315-08	10s	$38.71
	00008-0315-40	10s	$42.46
	00008-0315-24	10s	$47.61
◆ GENERICS			
TOTACILLIN-N: Abbott Hosp	00029-6610-25	1s	$1.55
TOTACILLIN-N: Abbott Hosp	00029-6610-40	1s	$1.85
TOTACILLIN-N: Abbott Hosp	00029-6610-21	1s	$2.35
Apothecon	00015-7404-20	1s	$3.10
Apothecon	00015-7404-18	1s	$3.35
Apothecon	00015-7404-36	1s	$4.98
VHA Supply	00015-7404-28	10s	$48.50
VHA Supply	00015-7404-29	10s	$88.90

POWDER FOR INJECTION: 2 GM

AVERAGE UNIT PRICE (AVAILABLE SIZES)		GENERIC A-RATED AVERAGE PRICE (GAAP)	
BRAND	$7.27	1s	$4.22
GENERIC	$5.70	10s	$101.25

BRAND/MANUFACTURER	NDC	SIZE	AWP
◆ BRAND			
OMNIPEN-N: Wyeth-Ayerst	00008-0315-09	1s	$6.83
	00008-0315-25	1s	$7.74
	00008-0315-10	10s	$68.20
	00008-0315-42	10s	$71.95
	00008-0315-26	10s	$77.40

BRAND/MANUFACTURER	NDC	SIZE	AWP
◆ GENERICS			
TOTACILLIN-N: Abbott Hosp	00029-6612-22	1s	$2.55
TOTACILLIN-N: Abbott Hosp	00029-6612-40	1s	$2.85
TOTACILLIN-N: Abbott Hosp	00029-6612-21	1s	$3.05
Apothecon	00015-7405-20	1s	$4.80
Apothecon	00015-7405-18	1s	$5.02
Apothecon	00015-7405-28	1s	$7.07
Elkins-Sinn	00641-2257-43	10s	$76.09
VHA Supply	00015-7405-29	10s	$126.40

POWDER FOR INJECTION: 10 GM

AVERAGE UNIT PRICE (AVAILABLE SIZES)		GENERIC A-RATED AVERAGE PRICE (GAAP)	
BRAND	$37.98	1s	$19.96
GENERIC	$25.75		

BRAND/MANUFACTURER	NDC	SIZE	AWP
◆ BRAND			
OMNIPEN-N: Wyeth-Ayerst	00008-0315-43	10s	$379.75
◆ GENERICS			
TOTACILLIN-N: Abbott Hosp	00029-6613-21	1s	$13.75
Apothecon	00015-7100-28	1s	$26.16
Elkins-Sinn	00641-2259-43	10s	$373.35

POWDER FOR INJECTION: 125 MG

AVERAGE UNIT PRICE (AVAILABLE SIZES)	
BRAND	$1.96
GENERIC	$1.93

BRAND/MANUFACTURER	NDC	SIZE	AWP
◆ BRAND			
OMNIPEN-N: Wyeth-Ayerst	00008-0315-01	1s	$1.96
	00008-0315-07	10s	$19.68
◆ GENERICS			
Apothecon	00015-7401-20	1s	$1.39
VHA Supply	00015-7401-28	10s	$24.70

POWDER FOR INJECTION: 250 MG

AVERAGE UNIT PRICE (AVAILABLE SIZES)		GENERIC A-RATED AVERAGE PRICE (GAAP)	
BRAND	$2.32	1s	$1.24
GENERIC	$1.59		

BRAND/MANUFACTURER	NDC	SIZE	AWP
◆ BRAND			
OMNIPEN-N: Wyeth-Ayerst	00008-0315-02	1s	$2.31
	00008-0315-05	10s	$23.19
◆ GENERICS			
TOTACILLIN-N: Abbott Hosp	00029-6600-24	1s	$0.85
Apothecon	00015-7402-20	1s	$1.63
Elkins-Sinn	00641-2251-43	10s	$22.74

POWDER FOR INJECTION: 500 MG

AVERAGE UNIT PRICE (AVAILABLE SIZES)		GENERIC A-RATED AVERAGE PRICE (GAAP)	
BRAND	$3.70	1s	$2.55
GENERIC	$2.88	10s	$33.83

BRAND/MANUFACTURER	NDC	SIZE	AWP
◆ BRAND			
OMNIPEN-N: Wyeth-Ayerst	00008-0315-03	1s	$3.04
	00008-0315-27	1s	$4.18
	00008-0315-38	10s	$34.08
	00008-0315-28	10s	$41.70
◆ GENERICS			
TOTACILLIN-N: Abbott Hosp	00029-6605-24	1s	$1.10
Apothecon	00015-7403-20	1s	$2.12
Apothecon	00015-7403-31	1s	$4.42
Elkins-Sinn	00641-2252-43	10s	$29.75
VHA Supply	00015-7403-30	10s	$37.90

ANTIPYRINE AND BENZOCAINE
DROP: 54 MG-14 MG/ML

BRAND/MANUFACTURER	NDC	SIZE	AWP
○ GENERICS			
Moore,H.L.	00839-6342-30	10 ml	$1.47
A/B OTIC: Clay-Park	45802-0311-68	10 ml	$1.52
Schein	00364-7260-54	10 ml	$1.82
Aligen	00405-2025-51	10 ml	$2.04
Bausch&Lomb Pharm	24208-0561-62	10 ml	$2.20
RAWAY PHARMACAL: Raway	00686-0561-62	10 ml	$2.40
Rugby	00536-8440-70	10 ml	$2.48
Southwood	58016-6444-01	10 ml	$5.05
Moore,H.L.	00839-6342-61	15 ml	$1.47
A/B OTIC: Qualitest	00603-7020-73	15 ml	$1.71
Thames	49158-0178-30	15 ml	$1.90
A/B OTIC: Clay-Park	45802-0311-56	15 ml	$1.94

◆ RATED THERAPEUTICALLY EQUIVELENT; ◇ THERAPEUTIC EQUIVALENT UNCONFIRMED; ○ UNRATED

BRAND/MANUFACTURER	NDC	SIZE	AWP
ANTIBEN: Hi-Tech	50383-0767-15	15 ml	$2.00
AURAGEN: Logen	00820-0201-25	15 ml	$2.25
URL	00677-1406-30	15 ml	$2.50
AURODEX: Major	00904-0793-35	15 ml	$2.65
ALLERGEN: Goldline	00182-1175-33	15 ml	$3.00
AUROTO: Barre	00472-0016-99	15 ml	$3.08
Cheshire	55175-1889-05	15 ml	$4.50
DOLOTIC: Marlop	12939-0230-15	15 ml	$5.50
DEC-AGESIC A.B.:	52765-0178-30	15 ml	$5.50
Southwood	58016-6003-01	15 ml	$6.51

ATROPINE SULFATE, OPHTHALMIC
DROP: 1%

BRAND/MANUFACTURER	NDC	SIZE	AWP
◇ BRAND			
ATROPISOL: Ciba Ophth	00058-0705-05	5 ml	$7.20
ISOPTO ATROPINE: Alcon Ophthalmic	00998-0303-05	5 ml	$10.13
	00998-0303-15	15 ml	$13.75
ATROPISOL: Ciba Ophth	00058-0770-12	1 ml 12s	$25.80
◇ GENERICS			
Optopics	52238-0502-02	2 ml	$2.20
Apotex USA	60505-7484-01	2 ml	$2.20
Martec	52555-0992-01	2 ml	$2.98
Allscrips	54569-2460-00	2 ml	$2.98
Raway	00686-0750-60	2 ml	$3.25
ATROPINE-CARE: Akorn	17478-0214-20	2 ml	$3.31
Paco	52967-0503-35	5 ml	$1.60
Apotex USA	60505-7484-02	5 ml	$2.52
Optopics	52238-0502-05	5 ml	$2.55
Bausch&Lomb Pharm	24208-0750-60	5 ml	$2.80
Martec	52555-0992-05	5 ml	$3.16
Aligen	00405-6010-05	5 ml	$3.48
Allscrips	54569-2784-00	5 ml	$3.57
ATROPINE-CARE: Akorn	17478-0214-10	5 ml	$4.06
Paco	52967-0503-45	15 ml	$1.95
OCU-TROPINE: Ocumed	51944-4480-42	15 ml	$2.25
Rugby	00536-0101-72	15 ml	$2.31
Schein	00364-7128-72	15 ml	$2.80
Steris	00402-0796-15	15 ml	$2.80
Goldline	00182-7064-64	15 ml	$2.95
Optopics	52238-0502-15	15 ml	$2.95
Apotex USA	60505-7484-05	15 ml	$2.95
CMC-Cons	00223-6101-15	15 ml	$3.00
Fougera	00168-0172-15	15 ml	$3.09
Bausch&Lomb Pharm	24208-0750-06	15 ml	$3.20
Qualitest	00603-7072-41	15 ml	$3.25
Martec	52555-0992-10	15 ml	$3.28
Raway	00686-0750-06	15 ml	$3.60
Allscrips	54569-2112-00	15 ml	$3.61
Major	00904-0824-35	15 ml	$4.00
Aligen	00405-6010-15	15 ml	$4.21
ATROPINE-CARE: Akorn	17478-0214-12	15 ml	$4.94
Allergan Inc	11980-0002-15	15 ml	$8.54
Alcon Surg	00065-0702-12	2 ml 12s	$37.80

DROP: 2%

BRAND/MANUFACTURER	NDC	SIZE	AWP
◇ GENERICS			
Alcon Surg	00065-0703-12	2 ml 12s	$37.80

OINTMENT: 0.01%

BRAND/MANUFACTURER	NDC	SIZE	AWP
◇ GENERICS			
Qualitest	00603-7071-70	0.13 gm	$3.30

OINTMENT: 1%

BRAND/MANUFACTURER	NDC	SIZE	AWP
◇ GENERICS			
OCU-TROPINE: Ocumed	51944-3555-30	3.5 gm	$1.35
Bausch&Lomb Pharm	24208-0825-55	3.5 gm	$2.30
Aligen	00405-0500-08	3.5 gm	$2.42
Raway	00686-0825-55	3.5 gm	$2.75
Schein	00364-7142-70	3.5 gm	$3.02
Moore,H.L.	00839-5492-43	3.75 gm	$3.31
Rugby	00536-6100-91	3.5 gm 12s	$20.66

BENZOYL PEROXIDE
LIQUID: 10%

AVERAGE UNIT PRICE (AVAILABLE SIZES)			
GENERIC	$0.07		

BRAND/MANUFACTURER	NDC	SIZE	AWP
◆ GENERICS			
Qualitest	00603-7717-48	150 ml	$10.62
Qualitest	00603-7717-56	240 ml	$14.60

LIQUID: 10%

BRAND/MANUFACTURER	NDC	SIZE	AWP
◇ GENERICS			
Glades	59366-2740-05	150 ml	$10.62
Glades	59366-2741-08	240 ml	$14.49

LIQUID: 10%

BRAND/MANUFACTURER	NDC	SIZE	AWP
◇ BRAND			
DESQUAM-X WASH: Westwood-Squibb	00072-7000-05	150 ml	$12.88
BENZAC W: Galderma	00299-3672-08	240 ml	$19.06
BENZAC AC: Galderma	00299-3645-08	240 ml	$21.75
◇ GENERICS			
Rugby	00536-0815-95	30 ml	$3.15

LOTION: 4%

BRAND/MANUFACTURER	NDC	SIZE	AWP
◇ BRAND			
BREVOXYL: Stiefel	00145-2310-05	315 ml	$16.70

BETAMETHASONE, TOPICAL
BETAMETHASONE VALERATE
CREAM: 0.01%

AVERAGE UNIT PRICE (AVAILABLE SIZES)	
BRAND	$0.48

BRAND/MANUFACTURER	NDC	SIZE	AWP
◆ BRAND			
VALISONE: Schering	00085-0929-04	15 gm	$9.11
	00085-0929-08	60 gm	$21.00

CREAM: 0.1%

AVERAGE UNIT PRICE (AVAILABLE SIZES)		GENERIC A-RATED AVERAGE PRICE (GAAP)	
BRAND	$0.61	15 gm	$5.72
GENERIC	$0.21	45 gm	$10.71
HCFA FUL (15 gm)	$0.13		
HCFA FUL (45 gm)	$0.08		

BRAND/MANUFACTURER	NDC	SIZE	AWP
◆ BRAND			
VALISONE: Schering	00085-0136-04	15 gm	$15.30
	00085-0136-06	45 gm	$27.88
	00085-0136-07	110 gm	$47.86
	00085-0136-08	430 gm	$160.92
◆ GENERICS			
Thames	49158-0184-20	15 gm	$2.30
Clay-Park	45802-0069-35	15 gm	$2.48
Genetco	00302-0415-15	15 gm	$2.78
NMC	23317-0370-15	15 gm	$2.90
Parmed	00349-8762-35	15 gm	$3.06
Geneva	00781-7055-27	15 gm	$3.35
BETADERM: Mason Dist	11845-0382-01	15 gm	$3.37
Moore,H.L.	00839-6371-47	15 gm	$3.50
BETA-VAL: Lemmon	00093-0673-15	15 gm	$3.55
Taro	51672-1269-01	15 gm	$3.60
Genetco	00302-0415-31	15 gm	$3.60
Fougera	00168-0040-15	15 gm	$3.94
Schein	00364-7269-72	15 gm	$4.05
Goldline	00182-1610-51	15 gm	$4.05
URL	00677-0842-40	15 gm	$4.10
Qualitest	00603-7718-74	15 gm	$4.23
Rugby	00536-4310-20	15 gm	$4.25
Major	00904-0776-36	15 gm	$4.30
BETATREX: Savage	00281-3510-44	15 gm	$11.64
Thames	49158-0184-27	45 gm	$4.70
Clay-Park	45802-0069-42	45 gm	$5.08
Genetco	00302-0415-34	45 gm	$5.25
NMC	23317-0370-45	45 gm	$5.54
Parmed	00349-8762-44	45 gm	$5.54
Geneva	00781-7055-45	45 gm	$6.25
Moore,H.L.	00839-6371-52	45 gm	$6.55
BETA-VAL: Lemmon	00093-0673-95	45 gm	$6.60
Taro	51672-1269-06	45 gm	$6.75
Fougera	00168-0040-46	45 gm	$7.32
BETADERM: Mason Dist	11845-0382-03	45 gm	$7.41
URL	00677-0842-49	45 gm	$7.50
Schein	00364-7269-80	45 gm	$7.50
Goldline	00182-1610-60	45 gm	$7.50
Qualitest	00603-7718-83	45 gm	$7.51
Major	00904-0776-45	45 gm	$7.70
Rugby	00536-4310-26	45 gm	$7.80

BRAND/MANUFACTURER	NDC	SIZE	AWP
BETATREX: Savage	00281-3510-50	45 gm	$21.14
Clay-Park	45802-0069-05	454 gm	$62.45

CREAM: 0.1%

BRAND/MANUFACTURER	NDC	SIZE	AWP
○ GENERICS			
Interstate	00814-1160-93	15 gm	$2.55
Raway	00686-0069-35	15 gm	$2.75
CMC-Cons	00223-4258-15	15 gm	$2.75
Allscrips	54569-1115-00	15 gm	$4.14
BETAMETHACOT: Truxton	00463-8055-15	15 gm	$4.20
Southwood	58016-3097-01	15 gm	$5.73
QUALISONE:	52765-0184-20	15 gm	$5.95
Raway	00686-0069-42	45 gm	$5.50
CMC-Cons	00223-4258-45	45 gm	$5.50
Interstate	00814-1160-95	45 gm	$5.85
Allscrips	54569-1873-01	45 gm	$7.38
Southwood	58016-3109-01	45 gm	$14.63
Phys Total Care	54868-0520-01	450 gm	$2.78

LOTION: 0.1%

AVERAGE UNIT PRICE (AVAILABLE SIZES)		GENERIC A-RATED AVERAGE PRICE (GAAP)	
BRAND	$0.78	60 ml	$19.42
GENERIC	$0.19		
HCFA FUL (60 ml)	$0.11		

BRAND/MANUFACTURER	NDC	SIZE	AWP
◆ BRAND			
VALISONE: Schering	00085-0002-03	20 ml	$18.86
	00085-0002-05	60 ml	$37.27
◆ GENERICS			
Genetco	00302-0418-02	60 ml	$7.43
Raway	00686-0041-60	60 ml	$7.80
Copley	38245-0603-12	60 ml	$8.75
Schein	00364-0778-58	60 ml	$9.25
Rugby	00536-4330-61	60 ml	$10.00
Major	00904-0778-03	60 ml	$10.10
NMC	23317-0372-60	60 ml	$10.20
Barre	00472-0705-02	60 ml	$10.20
BETA-VAL: Lemmon	00093-0671-39	60 ml	$10.45
Lemmon	00093-0643-39	60 ml	$10.45
URL	00677-1045-25	60 ml	$10.50
Qualitest	00603-7719-49	60 ml	$10.51
Moore,H.L.	00839-7022-64	60 ml	$10.52
Fougera	00168-0041-60	60 ml	$11.11
Goldline	00182-1788-68	60 ml	$11.25
Aligen	00405-2361-56	60 ml	$12.25
BETATREX: Savage	00281-3519-46	60 ml	$28.39

LOTION: 0.1%

BRAND/MANUFACTURER	NDC	SIZE	AWP
○ GENERICS			
Allscrips	54569-1874-01	60 ml	$11.04
CMC-Cons	00223-6432-60	60 ml	$11.50

OINTMENT: 0.1%

AVERAGE UNIT PRICE (AVAILABLE SIZES)		GENERIC A-RATED AVERAGE PRICE (GAAP)	
BRAND	$0.82	15 gm	$8.10
GENERIC	$0.25	45 gm	$15.12
HCFA FUL (15 gm)	$0.22		
HCFA FUL (45 gm)	$0.14		

BRAND/MANUFACTURER	NDC	SIZE	AWP
◆ BRAND			
VALISONE: Schering	00085-0898-04	15 gm	$15.30
	00085-0898-06	45 gm	$27.88
◆ GENERICS			
NMC	23317-0371-15	15 gm	$2.90
Genetco	00302-0416-15	15 gm	$3.00
Lemmon	00093-0644-15	15 gm	$3.55
Schein	00364-2103-72	15 gm	$4.04
Goldline	00182-1735-51	15 gm	$4.05
Fougera	00168-0033-15	15 gm	$4.17
Major	00904-0777-36	15 gm	$4.55
Rugby	00536-4320-20	15 gm	$4.63
Moore,H.L.	00839-6758-47	15 gm	$4.71
BETATREX: Savage	00281-3516-44	15 gm	$11.64
NMC	23317-0371-45	45 gm	$5.54
Genetco	00302-0416-46	45 gm	$5.63
Moore,H.L.	00839-6758-52	45 gm	$7.29
URL	00677-1059-49	45 gm	$7.45
Schein	00364-2103-80	45 gm	$7.50
Goldline	00182-1735-60	45 gm	$7.50
Fougera	00168-0033-46	45 gm	$7.72
Rugby	00536-4320-26	45 gm	$8.13
Major	00904-0777-45	45 gm	$9.10
BETATREX: Savage	00281-3516-50	45 gm	$21.14

OINTMENT: 0.1%

BRAND/MANUFACTURER	NDC	SIZE	AWP
○ GENERICS			
Raway	00686-0015-35	15 gm	$2.95
Interstate	00814-1163-93	15 gm	$3.15
CMC-Cons	00223-4259-15	15 gm	$4.00
Allscrips	54569-7035-00	15 gm	$4.53
Allscrips	54569-0793-00	15 gm	$4.74
Southwood	58016-3099-01	15 gm	$5.73
Raway	00686-0015-42	45 gm	$5.00
Interstate	00814-1163-95	45 gm	$6.30
CMC-Cons	00223-4259-45	45 gm	$7.95
Allscrips	54569-2621-00	45 gm	$8.44

BETAMETHASONE DIPROPIONATE, AUGMENTED

CREAM: 0.05%

BRAND/MANUFACTURER	NDC	SIZE	AWP
○ BRAND			
DIPROLENE AF: Schering	00085-0517-01	15 gm	$21.92
	00085-0517-02	45 gm	$44.11

GEL: 0.05%

BRAND/MANUFACTURER	NDC	SIZE	AWP
○ BRAND			
DIPROLENE: Schering	00085-0634-01	15 gm	$21.92
	00085-0634-02	45 gm	$44.11

LOTION: 0.05%

BRAND/MANUFACTURER	NDC	SIZE	AWP
○ BRAND			
DIPROLENE: Schering	00085-0962-01	30 ml	$25.14
	00085-0962-02	60 ml	$49.55

OINTMENT: 0.05%

BRAND/MANUFACTURER	NDC	SIZE	AWP
○ BRAND			
DIPROLENE: Schering	00085-0575-02	15 gm	$21.92
	00085-0575-03	45 gm	$44.11

BROMPHENIRAMINE MALEATE AND PSEUDOEPHEDRINE HYDROCHLORIDE

CAPSULE, EXTENDED RELEASE: 12 MG-120 MG

BRAND/MANUFACTURER	NDC	SIZE	AWP
○ BRAND			
SHELLCAP: HTD	60354-0001-01	100s	$12.80
ALLENT: Ascher	00225-0480-15	100s	$35.82
ENDAFED: Forest Pharm	00785-2206-01	100s	$46.06
BROMFED: Muro	00451-4000-50	100s	$64.69
	00451-4000-60	500s	$306.76
○ GENERICS			
M-HIST: McNeil,R.A.	12830-0200-01	100s	$23.86
Qualitest	00603-2505-21	100s	$33.90
Goldline	00182-1053-01	100s	$34.50
NALFED: Econolab	55053-0125-01	100s	$36.45
BROMADRINE TR: Rugby	00536-4448-01	100s	$37.12
ULTRABROM: WE Pharm	59196-0006-01	100s	$42.50
Jerome Stevens	50564-0527-01	100s	$74.03

TABLET: 4 MG-60 MG

BRAND/MANUFACTURER	NDC	SIZE	AWP
○ BRAND			
BROMFED: Muro	00451-4060-50	100s	$20.96

BROMPHENIRAMINE MALEATE, INJECTION

INJECTION: 10 MG/ML

BRAND/MANUFACTURER	NDC	SIZE	AWP
○ GENERICS			
COPHENE-B: Dunhall	00217-0405-08	10 ml	$4.00
NASAHIST B: Keene	00588-5557-70	10 ml	$5.50
Forest Pharm	00456-0623-10	10 ml	$6.00
CHLOR-PHED: Roberts/Hauck	59441-0550-10	10 ml	$6.50
Hauser,A.F.	52637-0926-10	10 ml	$6.95
ROHIST: Bolan	54171-0602-10	10 ml	$7.00
COLHIST: Clint	55553-0602-10	10 ml	$8.06
Schein	00364-2185-54	10 ml	$8.78
Steris	00402-0602-10	10 ml	$8.78
CODIMAL-A: Central	00131-1008-05	10 ml	$16.65
HISTAJECT: Mayrand	00259-0359-10	10 ml	$19.90

◆ RATED THERAPEUTICALLY EQUIVALENT; ◇ THERAPEUTIC EQUIVALENT UNCONFIRMED; ○ UNRATED

CALCIUM, INJECTABLE
CALCIUM GLUCONATE
INJECTION: 100 MG/ML

AVERAGE UNIT PRICE (AVAILABLE SIZES)	
GENERIC	$0.45

BRAND/MANUFACTURER	NDC	SIZE	AWP
◆ GENERICS			
Fujisawa	00469-0311-25	10 ml	$1.70
Fujisawa	00469-2311-25	50 ml	$4.52
Fujisawa	00469-3111-00	100 ml	$9.24
Fujisawa	00469-3112-00	200 ml	$14.63
Abbott Hosp	00074-1184-01	1 ml 25s	$45.72

INJECTION: 100 MG/ML

BRAND/MANUFACTURER	NDC	SIZE	AWP
○ GENERICS			
McGuff	49072-0704-20	10 ml	$1.29
McGuff	49072-0704-50	50 ml	$2.79
Gensia	00703-5347-03	50 ml 10s	$31.25
Gensia	00703-5348-03	100 ml 10s	$61.25
Gensia	00703-5340-03	200 ml 10s	$117.50
Intl Med Sys	00548-6524-00	100 ml 12s	$98.82
Intl Med Sys	00548-6538-00	200 ml 12s	$184.50
VHA Supply	00702-0865-10	10 ml 25s	$12.50
Elkins-Sinn	00641-1390-35	10 ml 25s	$15.31
Gensia	00703-5344-04	10 ml 25s	$21.88
Amer Regent	00517-3910-25	10 ml 25s	$22.19
CMC-Cons	00223-7280-25	10 ml 25s	$25.50
Truxton	00463-1011-26	10 ml 25s	$31.00
Hyrex	00314-9013-05	10 ml 25s	$35.00
Pasadena	00418-1691-46	10 ml 25s	$35.75
VHA Supply	00702-0865-50	50 ml 25s	$40.75
Amer Regent	00517-3950-25	50 ml 25s	$81.88
UDL	51079-0704-45	50 ml 25s ud	$63.12
Amer Regent	00517-3900-25	100 ml 25s	$93.75
CMC-Cons	00223-7280-01	10 ml 100s	$87.50
Raway	00686-3910-21	10 ml 100s	$150.00

CARBETAPENTANE/
CHLORPHENIRAMINE/EPHEDRINE/
PHENYLEPHRINE
TABLET:

BRAND/MANUFACTURER	NDC	SIZE	AWP
○ BRAND			
RYNATUSS: Wallace	00037-0717-92	100s	$151.72
	00037-0717-96	500s	$739.64
	00037-0717-95	2000s	$2660.98
○ GENERICS			
TUSS TAN: Econolab	55053-0122-01	100s	$37.60
RENTAMINE: Major	00904-1665-60	100s	$43.45
C.C.E.P.: Goldline	00182-1583-01	100s	$48.00
TRI-TANNATE PLUS: Rugby	00536-4394-01	100s	$72.20

CARBINOXAMINE MALEATE WITH
PSEUDOEPHEDRINE HYDROCHLORIDE
TABLET: 4 MG-60 MG

BRAND/MANUFACTURER	NDC	SIZE	AWP
○ BRAND			
CARBISET: Nutripharm	51081-0510-10	100s	$9.90
RONDEC: Ross Pharm	00074-5726-13	100s	$37.65
CARBISET: Nutripharm	51081-0510-50	500s	$41.88
RONDEC: Ross Pharm	00074-5726-53	500s	$184.64
○ GENERICS			
ANDEC: Econolab	55053-0082-01	100s	$16.23
Aligen	00405-4137-01	100s	$17.08
RONDAMINE: Major	00904-3248-60	100s	$17.35
CARDEC: Goldline	00182-1199-01	100s	$18.45
CARBODEC: Rugby	00536-4452-01	100s	$19.07

TABLET, EXTENDED RELEASE: 8 MG-120 MG

BRAND/MANUFACTURER	NDC	SIZE	AWP
○ BRAND			
CARBISET TR: Nutripharm	51081-0512-10	100s	$18.10
RONDEC-TR: Ross Pharm	00074-6240-13	100s	$87.44
○ GENERICS			
MOOREDEC: Moore,H.L.	00839-7482-06	100s	$24.29
RONDAMINE: Major	00904-3250-60	100s	$31.15
CARBODEC: Rugby	00536-4453-01	100s	$32.31
CARDEC: Goldline	00182-1130-01	100s	$33.00
ANDEC-TR: Econolab	55053-0077-01	100s	$36.25
Aligen	00405-4138-01	100s	$38.16
PALGIC-D: Pan Amer	00525-6123-01	100s	$39.60
BIOHIST-LA: Wakefield	59310-0101-10	100s	$44.75

CARBINOXAMINE MALEATE/
DEXTROMETHORPHAN
HYDROBROMIDE/PSEUDOEPHEDRINE
HYDROCHLORIDE
SYRUP: 4 MG-15 MG-60 MG/5 ML

BRAND/MANUFACTURER	NDC	SIZE	AWP
○ BRAND			
RONDEC DM: Ross Pharm	00074-5640-04	120 ml	$13.46
	00074-5640-16	480 ml	$50.89
○ GENERICS			
CARDEC DM: Schein	00364-7277-56	30 ml	$4.05
CHEMDEC DM: Norton,HN	50732-0867-04	118 ml	$3.45
BIODEC DM: Bio-Pharm	59741-0135-04	120 ml	$2.30
CARDEC DM: Moore,H.L.	00839-6404-65	120 ml	$2.69
CARDEC-DM: Aligen	00405-2450-76	120 ml	$2.80
CARBOFED-DM: Hi-Tech	50383-0751-04	120 ml	$3.00
MALDEC-DM: Cenci,H.R.	00556-0450-04	120 ml	$3.10
RONDAMINE DM: Major	00904-0703-03	120 ml	$3.15
SILDEC DM: Silarx	54838-0212-40	120 ml	$3.30
CARBODEC DM: Rugby	00536-0432-97	120 ml	$3.38
CARBODEC DM: Rugby	00536-0456-97	120 ml	$3.38
CARDEC DM: Goldline	00182-1204-37	120 ml	$3.75
CARDEC DM: Barre	00472-0731-04	120 ml	$3.96
Morton Grove	60432-0202-04	120 ml	$4.00
TUSSAFED: Everett	00642-0795-04	120 ml	$7.00
CHEMDEC DM: Norton,HN	50732-0867-16	473 ml	$12.75
BIODEC DM: Bio-Pharm	59741-0135-16	480 ml	$6.50
RONDAMINE DM: Major	00904-0703-16	480 ml	$8.25
CARBOFED-DM: Hi-Tech	50383-0751-16	480 ml	$8.50
MALDEC-DM: Cenci,H.R.	00556-0450-16	480 ml	$8.60
CARDEC DM: Schein	00364-7318-16	480 ml	$8.75
CARDEC DM: Qualitest	00603-1061-58	480 ml	$8.83
CARDEC DM: URL	00677-1474-33	480 ml	$8.85
CARBODEC DM: Rugby	00536-0456-85	480 ml	$8.93
CARDEC-DM: Aligen	00405-2450-16	480 ml	$8.97
SILDEC DM: Silarx	54838-0212-80	480 ml	$9.04
CARDEC DM: Mason Dist	11845-0417-13	480 ml	$9.15
Morton Grove	60432-0202-16	480 ml	$9.35
CARDEC DM: Goldline	00182-1204-40	480 ml	$9.90
CARDEC DM: Barre	00472-0731-16	480 ml	$10.95
CARBODEX DM: Tri-Med	55654-0016-05	480 ml	$10.95
Geneva	00781-6200-16	480 ml	$11.88
TUSSAFED: Everett	00642-0795-16	480 ml	$27.00
CHEMDEC DM: Norton,HN	50732-0867-28	3785 ml	$62.95
BIODEC DM: Bio-Pharm	59741-0135-20	3840 ml	$45.50
RONDAMINE DM: Major	00904-0703-28	3840 ml	$55.90
CARBOFED-DM: Hi-Tech	50383-0751-28	3840 ml	$59.00
MALDEC-DM: Cenci,H.R.	00556-0450-28	3840 ml	$61.50
CARBODEC DM: Rugby	00536-0456-90	3840 ml	$63.08
CARDEC DM: Goldline	00182-1204-41	3840 ml	$63.50
SILDEC DM: Silarx	54838-0212-00	3840 ml	$64.60
CARDEC DM: Barre	00472-0731-28	3840 ml	$73.90

CHLORDIAZEPOXIDE HYDROCHLORIDE
WITH CLIDINIUM BROMIDE
CAPSULE: 5 MG-2.5 MG

BRAND/MANUFACTURER	NDC	SIZE	AWP
○ GENERICS			
Allscrips	54569-0430-01	6s	$0.29
Southwood	58016-0712-20	20s	$3.80
Allscrips	54569-0430-00	30s	$1.47
Southwood	58016-0712-30	30s	$4.10
Allscrips	54569-0430-03	42s	$2.05
Phys Total Care	54868-0030-01	56s	$3.46
CHLORDINIUM: Veratex	17022-2162-02	100s	$3.00
Eon	00185-0617-01	100s	$3.25
Eon	00185-0968-01	100s	$3.25
Moore,H.L.	00839-6211-06	100s	$4.17
URL	00677-1247-01	100s	$4.55
Goldline	00182-1856-01	100s	$4.60
Parmed	00349-8697-01	100s	$4.86
Allscrips	54569-0430-02	100s	$4.89
Major	00904-0301-60	100s	$4.90
Vintage	00254-2732-28	100s	$4.94
CLIPOXIDE: Schein	00364-0559-01	100s	$4.95
Qualitest	00603-2714-21	100s	$5.11
Major	00904-2503-60	100s	$5.25
Phys Total Care	54868-0030-02	100s	$5.30
Aligen	00405-0045-01	100s	$5.76
Amide	52152-0018-02	100s	$5.95
CLINDEX: Rugby	00536-3490-01	100s	$5.99
U.S. Trading	56126-0090-11	100s ud	$8.87
Eon	00185-0617-05	500s	$14.95
Eon	00185-0968-05	500s	$14.95
Major	00904-0301-40	500s	$16.60
Major	00904-2503-40	500s	$17.25
Goldline	00182-1856-05	500s	$17.35
CLIPOXIDE: Schein	00364-0559-05	500s	$18.77

➤ SHOWN IN PRODUCT IDENTIFICATION GUIDE

BRAND/MANUFACTURER	NDC	SIZE	AWP
Amide	52152-0018-04	500s	$20.50
CLINDEX: Rugby	00536-3490-05	500s	$22.43
Aligen	00405-0045-02	500s	$42.00
Eon	00185-0617-10	1000s	$24.95
Eon	00185-0968-10	1000s	$24.95
URL	00677-1247-10	1000s	$28.34
Moore,H.L.	00839-6211-16	1000s	$28.34
Vintage	00254-2732-38	1000s	$29.10
Major	00904-0301-80	1000s	$29.80
Goldline	00182-1856-10	1000s	$30.40
Qualitest	00603-2714-32	1000s	$31.40
Major	00904-2503-80	1000s	$31.45
Parmed	00349-8697-10	1000s	$35.98
Parmed	00349-8698-10	1000s	$35.98
Amide	52152-0018-05	1000s	$39.50
CLINDEX: Rugby	00536-3490-10	1000s	$42.75

CHLORPHENIRAMINE MALEATE/ CODEINE PHOSPHATE/ PSEUDOEPHEDRINE HYDROCHLORIDE

LIQUID (C-V): 2 MG-10 MG-30 MG/5 ML

BRAND/MANUFACTURER	NDC	SIZE	AWP
◇ BRAND			
NOVAHISTINE-DH: SK Beecham Cons	00068-1027-04	120 ml doz	$98.30
	00068-1027-16	480 ml doz	$327.73
◇ GENERICS			
NOVADYNE DH: Norton,HN	50732-0634-04	118 ml	$3.40
DIHISTINE DH: Major	00904-0922-00	120 ml	$2.70
DIHISTINE DH: Major	00904-0922-20	120 ml	$2.70
DIHISTINE DH: Goldline	00182-1573-37	120 ml	$2.70
CO-HISTINE DH: Hi-Tech	50383-0084-04	120 ml	$2.80
PHENHIST W/CODEINE: Rugby	00536-1920-97	120 ml	$4.79
RYNA-C: Wallace	00037-0522-66	120 ml	$21.62
NOVADYNE DH: Norton,HN	50732-0634-16	473 ml	$9.00
DIHISTINE DH: Major	00904-0922-16	480 ml	$7.75
CO-HISTINE DH: Hi-Tech	50383-0084-16	480 ml	$9.00
DIHISTINE DH: Goldline	00182-1573-40	480 ml	$9.45
PHENHIST W/CODEINE: Rugby	00536-1920-85	480 ml	$10.92
Schein	00364-7384-16	480 ml	$11.50
RYNA-C: Wallace	00037-0522-68	480 ml	$81.74
NOVADYNE DH: Norton,HN	50732-0634-28	3785 ml	$55.50
DIHISTINE DH: Major	00904-0922-28	3840 ml	$51.75
DIHISTINE DH: Goldline	00182-1573-41	3840 ml	$61.50

CHOLINE MAGNESIUM TRISALICYLATE

TABLET: 750 MG

BRAND/MANUFACTURER	NDC	SIZE	AWP
◇ BRAND			
TRILISATE: Purdue Frederick	00034-0505-80	100s	$74.87
	00034-0505-10	100s ud	$77.61
	00034-0505-50	500s	$371.03
◇ GENERICS			
Allscrips	54569-3825-00	15s	$6.15
Medirex	57480-0402-06	30s	$11.70
Cheshire	55175-2216-00	30s	$13.28
Apotex USA	60999-0151-10	100s	$13.78
TRICOSAL: Duramed	51285-0833-02	100s	$34.40
Invamed	52189-0242-24	100s	$34.40
Geneva	00781-1638-01	100s	$36.75
CMT: Moore,H.L.	00839-7500-06	100s	$38.60
Sidmak	50111-0529-01	100s	$42.00
Aligen	00405-4230-01	100s	$42.80
URL	00677-1391-01	100s	$42.85
Goldline	00182-1895-01	100s	$42.90
Major	00904-3396-60	100s	$43.50
TRICOSAL: Qualitest	00603-6216-21	100s	$43.51
Martec	52555-0529-01	100s	$44.10
Rugby	00536-3453-01	100s	$49.17
Barre	00472-0141-10	100s	$60.26
Medirex	57480-0402-01	100s ud	$39.00

TABLET: 1000 MG

BRAND/MANUFACTURER	NDC	SIZE	AWP
◇ BRAND			
TRILISATE: Purdue Frederick	00034-0510-80	100s	$96.54
◇ GENERICS			
Apotex USA	60999-0152-10	100s	$16.84
Major	00904-3397-60	100s	$44.80
TRICOSAL: Qualitest	00603-6217-21	100s	$45.40
Invamed	52189-0254-24	100s	$47.00
CMT: Moore,H.L.	00839-7619-06	100s	$47.24
Aligen	00405-4231-01	100s	$50.06
Sidmak	50111-0530-01	100s	$55.00
Martec	52555-0530-01	100s	$57.75
Rugby	00536-3470-01	100s	$66.75
Barre	00472-0142-10	100s	$71.98

CODEINE PHOSPHATE WITH GUAIFENESIN

SYRUP (C-V): 10 MG-100 MG/5 ML

BRAND/MANUFACTURER	NDC	SIZE	AWP
○ GENERICS			
ROBICHEM AC: Norton,HN	50732-0883-04	118 ml	$3.00
BIOTUSSIN AC: Bio-Pharm	59741-0113-04	120 ml	$2.05
GUIATUSS A.C. Moore,H.L.	00839-5388-65	120 ml	$2.55
GUIATUSS A.C.: Moore,H.L.	00839-7953-79	120 ml	$2.55
Schein	00364-2475-77	120 ml	$2.55
CHERATUSSIN AC: Qualitest	00603-1075-54	120 ml	$2.61
ROBAFEN AC: Major	00904-0054-20	120 ml	$2.70
GUAIATUSSIN AC: Hi-Tech	50383-0087-04	120 ml	$2.70
GUIATUSS A.C.: Goldline	00182-0017-37	120 ml	$2.70
HALOTUSSIN AC: Halsey Pharm	00879-0660-04	120 ml	$2.80
Cenci,H.R.	00556-0196-04	120 ml	$2.80
Moore,H.L.	00839-7784-65	120 ml	$2.82
GUIATUSS AC: Barre	00472-0012-04	120 ml	$2.84
MYTUSSIN AC: Morton Grove	60432-0023-04	120 ml	$2.90
Allscrips	54569-3486-00	120 ml	$2.92
Allscrips	54569-3146-00	120 ml	$2.93
GUIATUSS A.C.: Goldline	00182-0345-37	120 ml	$3.15
Interstate	00814-3580-76	120 ml	$3.38
HALOTUSSIN-AC: Aligen	00405-0090-76	120 ml	$3.55
GUIATUSSIN W/CODEINE: Rugby	00536-0981-97	120 ml	$3.72
HALOTUSSIN AC: Halsey Pharm	00879-0660-08	240 ml	$4.60
ROBICHEM AC: Norton,HN	50732-0883-16	473 ml	$8.50
BIOTUSSIN AC: Bio-Pharm	59741-0113-16	480 ml	$6.25
Schein	00364-2475-16	480 ml	$7.25
GUIATUSS A.C.: Moore,H.L.	00839-5388-69	480 ml	$7.28
GUIATUSS A.C.: Moore,H.L.	00839-7953-69	480 ml	$7.28
CHERATUSSIN AC: Qualitest	00603-1075-30	480 ml	$7.30
URL	00677-1492-33	480 ml	$7.50
Cenci,H.R.	00556-0196-16	480 ml	$7.60
GUIATUSS A.C.: Goldline	00182-0017-40	480 ml	$7.65
GUAIATUSSIN AC: Hi-Tech	50383-0087-16	480 ml	$7.80
Moore,H.L.	00839-7784-69	480 ml	$7.90
HALOTUSSIN AC: Halsey Pharm	00879-0660-16	480 ml	$8.00
ROBAFEN AC: Major	00904-0054-16	480 ml	$8.05
GUIATUSS A.C.: Barre	00472-0012-16	480 ml	$8.19
GLYDEINE: Geneva	00781-6899-16	480 ml	$8.27
Allscrips	54569-2476-00	480 ml	$8.47
GUIATUSSIN W/CODEINE: Rugby	00536-0981-85	480 ml	$8.73
MYTUSSIN AC: Morton Grove	60432-0023-16	480 ml	$8.90
GUIATUSS A.C.: Goldline	00182-0345-40	480 ml	$9.00
Interstate	00814-3580-82	480 ml	$9.38
HALOTUSSIN-AC: Aligen	00405-0090-16	480 ml	$10.12
ROBICHEM AC: Norton,HN	50732-0883-28	3785 ml	$52.00
GUIATUSSIN W/CODEINE: Rugby	00536-0981-90	3840 ml	$41.45
GUIATUSS AC: Moore,H.L.	00839-5388-70	3840 ml	$44.54
GUIATUSS A.C.: Goldline	00182-0017-41	3840 ml	$49.50
ROBAFEN AC: Major	00904-0054-28	3840 ml	$50.40
Cenci,H.R.	00556-0196-28	3840 ml	$51.20
Moore,H.L.	00839-7784-70	3840 ml	$51.25
MYTUSSIN AC: Morton Grove	60432-0023-28	3840 ml	$52.00
HALOTUSSIN AC: Halsey Pharm	00879-0660-28	3840 ml	$55.30
GUIATUSS A.C.: Barre	00472-0012-28	3840 ml	$55.81
GUIATUSS A.C.: Goldline	00182-0345-41	3840 ml	$56.40
Pharm Assoc	00121-0422-04	120 ml	$3.76
Pharm Assoc	00121-0422-05	5 ml 100s ud	$45.74
UDL	51079-0329-30	5 ml 100s ud	$46.67
Pharm Assoc	00121-0422-10	10 ml 100s ud	$47.50

TABLET (C-III): 10 MG-300 MG

BRAND/MANUFACTURER	NDC	SIZE	AWP
◇ BRAND			
BRONTEX: P&G Pharm	00149-0440-01	100s	$59.99

CODEINE PHOSPHATE/GUAIFENESIN/ PSEUDOEPHEDRINE HYDROCHLORIDE

LIQUID (C-V): 10 MG-100 MG-30 MG/5 ML

BRAND/MANUFACTURER	NDC	SIZE	AWP
◇ BRAND			
NOVAHISTINE EXPECTORANT: SK Beecham Cons	00068-1028-04	120 ml doz	$102.92
RYNA-CX: Wallace	00037-0801-66	120 ml	$23.82
NUCOFED PEDIATRIC EXPECTORANT: Roberts Pharm	54092-0405-16	473 ml	$26.98
NOVAHISTINE EXPECTORANT: SK Beecham Cons	00068-1028-16	480 ml doz	$342.98
MEDENT C: Stewart Jackson	45985-0635-16	480 ml	$21.95
TUSSAR-2: RPR	00075-1702-01	480 ml	$63.01
TUSSAR SF: RPR	00075-1700-01	480 ml	$63.01
RYNA-CX: Wallace	00037-0801-68	480 ml	$88.20
TUSSAR SF: RPR	00075-1700-05	120 ml 6s	$113.70

♦ RATED THERAPEUTICALLY EQUIVELENT; ◇ THERAPEUTIC EQUIVALENT UNCONFIRMED; ○ UNRATED

BRAND/MANUFACTURER	NDC	SIZE	AWP
○ GENERICS			
NOVADYNE EXPECTORANT: Norton,HN	50732-0635-04	118 ml	$4.00
BIOTUSSIN DAC: Bio-Pharm	59741-0115-04	120 ml	$2.35
HALOTUSSIN DAC: Halsey Pharm	00879-0682-04	120 ml	$2.50
Moore,H.L.	00839-6695-65	120 ml	$2.54
DEPROIST W/CODEINE: Geneva	00781-6606-04	120 ml	$2.62
Goldline	00182-1577-37	120 ml	$2.70
CO-HISTINE EXPECTORANT: Hi-Tech	50383-0086-04	120 ml	$2.80
DECOHISTINE EXPECTORANT: Morton Grove	60432-0585-04	120 ml	$2.90
PHENYLHISTINE: Aligen	00405-0076-76	120 ml	$2.97
DIHISTINE EXPECTORANT W/CODEINE: Major	00904-0923-20	120 ml	$3.00
DIHISTINE EXPECTORANT: Barre	00472-1640-04	120 ml	$3.15
PHENHIST EXPECTORANT: Rugby	00536-1910-97	120 ml	$4.79
HALOTUSSIN DAC: Halsey Pharm	00879-0682-08	240 ml	$5.20
NOVADYNE EXPECTORANT: Norton,HN	50732-0635-16	473 ml	$15.00
NUCOCHEM PEDIATRIC EXPECTORANT: Norton,HN	50732-0858-16	473 ml	$18.46
NUCOCHEM EXPECTORANT: Norton,HN	50732-0857-16	473 ml	$26.98
Moore,H.L.	00839-6695-69	480 ml	$8.09
CO-HISTINE EXPECTORANT: Hi-Tech	50383-0086-16	480 ml	$8.20
Goldline	00182-1577-40	480 ml	$8.55
BIOTUSSIN DAC: Bio-Pharm	59741-0115-16	480 ml	$8.63
DEPROIST W/CODEINE: Geneva	00781-6606-16	480 ml	$8.77
PHENYLHISTINE EXPECTORANT: Qualitest	00603-1521-58	480 ml	$8.90
DECOHISTINE EXPECTORANT: Morton Grove	60432-0585-16	480 ml	$9.46
DIHISTINE EXPECTORANT W/CODEINE: Major	00904-0923-16	480 ml	$9.70
GUIATUSSIN DAC: Rugby	00536-0790-85	480 ml	$10.38
DIHISTINE EXPECTORANT: Barre	00472-1640-16	480 ml	$10.46
PHENYLHISTINE: Aligen	00405-0076-16	480 ml	$10.98
PHENHIST EXPECTORANT: Rugby	00536-1910-85	480 ml	$11.39
CHERATUSSIN DAC: Qualitest	00603-1078-58	480 ml	$11.50
Cenci,H.R.	00556-0432-16	480 ml	$12.80
GUIATUSS D.A.C.: URL	00677-1179-33	480 ml	$13.00
HALOTUSSIN DAC: Halsey Pharm	00879-0682-16	480 ml	$13.45
Rugby	00536-1519-85	480 ml	$14.87
Major	00904-7756-16	480 ml	$18.50
NUCO-TUSS PEDIATRIC EXPECTORANT: Barre	00472-1240-16	480 ml	$18.50
Rugby	00536-1518-85	480 ml	$22.00
Major	00904-7757-16	480 ml	$27.00
NOVADYNE EXPECTORANT: Norton,HN	50732-0635-28	3785 ml	$55.00
HALOTUSSIN DAC: Halsey Pharm	00879-0682-28	3840 ml	$92.50

SYRUP (C-III): 20 MG-200 MG-60 MG/5 ML

BRAND/MANUFACTURER	NDC	SIZE	AWP
○ BRAND			
NUCOFED EXPECTORANT: Roberts Pharm	54092-0404-16	473 ml	$39.30
○ GENERICS			
DECONSAL C EXPECTORANT: Adams	53014-0040-47	480 ml	$39.88

SYRUP (C-V): 10 MG-100 MG-30 MG/5 ML

BRAND/MANUFACTURER	NDC	SIZE	AWP
○ BRAND			
ROBITUSSIN-DAC: Robins Pharm	00031-8680-12	120 ml	$11.46
	00031-8680-25	480 ml	$37.98
○ GENERICS			
Moore,H.L.	00839-7785-65	120 ml	$3.09
GUAIATUSSIN DAC: Hi-Tech	50383-0088-04	120 ml	$4.00
GUIATUSS D.A.C.: Moore,H.L.	00839-6478-65	120 ml	$4.17
MYTUSSIN DAC: Morton Grove	60432-0541-04	120 ml	$5.00
Allscrips	54569-3041-01	240 ml	$8.40
NUCOCHEM: Norton,HN	50732-0859-16	473 ml	$26.02
GUIATUSS D.A.C.: Moore,H.L.	00839-6478-69	480 ml	$10.79
Schein	00364-2476-16	480 ml	$11.65
GUAIATUSSIN DAC: Hi-Tech	50383-0088-16	480 ml	$12.40
MYTUSSIN DAC: Morton Grove	60432-0541-16	480 ml	$12.66
Major	00904-0042-16	480 ml	$12.70
Moore,H.L.	00839-7785-69	480 ml	$13.10
GUIATUSS D.A.C.: Barre	00472-0011-16	480 ml	$13.55
GUIATUSS D.A.C.: Goldline	00182-1378-40	480 ml	$15.45
Allscrips	54569-3041-00	480 ml	$16.79
HALOTUSSIN-DAC: Aligen	00405-0093-16	480 ml	$16.81
Goldline	00182-0155-40	480 ml	$20.85
DECONSAL PEDIATRIC: Adams	53014-0046-47	480 ml	$27.39
Goldline	00182-0154-40	480 ml	$30.40

COLCHICINE
TABLET: 0.5 MG

BRAND/MANUFACTURER	NDC	SIZE	AWP
○ GENERICS			
Phys Total Care	54868-2258-01	100s	$24.59
Abbott Pharm	00074-0074-02	100s	$25.06

TABLET: 0.6 MG

BRAND/MANUFACTURER	NDC	SIZE	AWP
○ GENERICS			
Southwood	58016-9040-08	8s	$1.69
Allscrips	54569-0236-02	20s	$1.31
Allscrips	54569-0236-06	30s	$1.97

BRAND/MANUFACTURER	NDC	SIZE	AWP
Allscrips	54569-0236-03	60s	$3.93
CMC-Cons	00223-0703-01	100s	$3.00
Southwood	58016-9040-00	100s	$3.65
West-Ward	00143-1201-01	100s	$3.80
Schein	00364-0074-01	100s	$4.25
Major	00904-2047-60	100s	$4.30
URL	00677-0040-01	100s	$4.60
Qualitest	00603-3052-21	100s	$4.70
Trinity	61355-0001-10	100s	$5.00
Allscrips	54569-0236-05	100s	$6.55
Abbott Pharm	00074-3781-01	100s	$19.20
U.S. Trading	56126-0472-11	100s ud	$5.78
West-Ward	00143-1201-25	100s ud	$14.00
Veratex	17022-2506-06	1000s	$12.95
Raway	00686-1201-10	1000s	$16.00
West-Ward	00143-1201-10	1000s	$16.80
Aligen	00405-4266-03	1000s	$17.47
Rugby	00536-3494-10	1000s	$18.90
Schein	00364-0074-02	1000s	$19.60
Qualitest	00603-3052-32	1000s	$19.90
URL	00677-0040-10	1000s	$20.30
Moore,H.L.	00839-5152-16	1000s	$20.39
Major	00904-2047-80	1000s	$21.40
Goldline	00182-0174-10	1000s	$22.80
Trinity	61355-0001-11	1000s	$23.60
CMC-Cons	00223-0703-02	1000s	$25.00
Allscrips	54569-0236-04	1000s	$65.50

DESIPRAMINE HYDROCHLORIDE
TABLET: 100 MG

AVERAGE UNIT PRICE (AVAILABLE SIZES)		GENERIC A-RATED AVERAGE PRICE (GAAP)	
BRAND	$1.87	100s	$94.41
GENERIC	$0.89		
HCFA FUL (100s ea)	$0.44		

BRAND/MANUFACTURER	NDC	SIZE	AWP
◆ BRAND			
NORPRAMIN: Marion Merrell Dow	00068-0020-01	100s	$186.84
◆ GENERICS			
Eon	00185-0736-01	100s	$52.50
Moore,H.L.	00839-7412-06	100s	$84.77
Geneva	00781-1975-01	100s	$99.99
Goldline	00182-1316-01	100s	$100.00
Rugby	00536-4884-01	100s	$106.74
Rugby	00536-4958-01	100s	$106.74
Major	00904-1573-60	100s	$110.10
Eon	00185-0736-05	500s	$249.95

TABLET: 150 MG

BRAND/MANUFACTURER	NDC	SIZE	AWP
◆ BRAND			
NORPRAMIN: Marion Merrell Dow	00068-0021-50	50s	$135.36
◆ GENERICS			
Geneva	00781-1976-50	50s	$109.50

DEXTROSE
INJECTION: 30%

AVERAGE UNIT PRICE (AVAILABLE SIZES)		GENERIC A-RATED AVERAGE PRICE (GAAP)	
GENERIC	$0.05	500 ml 6s	$115.04

BRAND/MANUFACTURER	NDC	SIZE	AWP
◆ GENERICS			
McGaw	00264-1124-01	500 ml	$26.34
Baxter	00338-0646-13	500 ml 6s	$73.98
Abbott Hosp	00074-5823-25	500 ml 6s	$156.11
Clintec	00338-0713-34	1000 ml 10s	$555.20
Abbott Hosp	00074-8004-15	500 ml 12s	$377.34
Clintec	00338-0713-13	500 ml 16s	$444.14

INJECTION: 40%

AVERAGE UNIT PRICE (AVAILABLE SIZES)		GENERIC A-RATED AVERAGE PRICE (GAAP)	
GENERIC	$0.06	500 ml 6s	$127.66

BRAND/MANUFACTURER	NDC	SIZE	AWP
◆ GENERICS			
McGaw	00264-1126-01	500 ml	$28.98
Baxter	00338-0702-13	500 ml 6s	$82.26
Abbott Hosp	00074-5644-25	500 ml 6s	$173.07
Clintec	00338-0715-34	1000 ml 10s	$678.40
Abbott Hosp	00074-7937-19	500 ml 12s	$414.96
Clintec	00338-0715-13	500 ml 16s	$542.79

► SHOWN IN PRODUCT IDENTIFICATION GUIDE

INJECTION: 50%

AVERAGE UNIT PRICE (AVAILABLE SIZES)		GENERIC A-RATED AVERAGE PRICE (GAAP)	
GENERIC	$0.10	500 ml	$31.99
		500 ml 6s	$131.54
		1000 ml 6s	$288.74
		2000 ml 6s	$283.16
		50 ml 10s	$174.68
		500 ml 12s	$329.13
		50 ml 25s	$277.13

BRAND/MANUFACTURER	NDC	SIZE	AWP
◆ GENERICS			
McGaw	00264-1128-10	500 ml	$29.12
McGaw	00264-1128-01	500 ml	$34.85
McGaw	00264-1128-00	1000 ml	$27.85
McGaw	00264-1128-50	2000 ml	$56.28
Baxter	00338-0036-13	500 ml 6s	$84.66
Abbott Hosp	00074-5645-25	500 ml 6s	$178.41
Abbott Hosp	00074-1518-05	1000 ml 6s	$172.14
Abbott Hosp	00074-7936-17	1000 ml 6s	$405.34
Baxter	00338-0035-06	2000 ml 6s	$235.32
Clintec	00338-0031-06	2000 ml 6s	$331.00
Abbott Hosp	00074-4902-01	50 ml 10s	$168.27
Abbott Hosp	00074-4902-23	50 ml 10s	$181.09
Clintec	00338-0031-34	1000 ml 10s	$705.20
Abbott Hosp	00074-1536-03	500 ml 12s	$241.25
Clintec	00338-0036-03	500 ml 12s	$314.92
Abbott Hosp	00074-7936-19	500 ml 12s	$431.21
Clintec	00338-0031-13	500 ml 16s	$564.09
Abbott Hosp	00074-6648-02	50 ml 25s	$101.53
Abbott Hosp	00074-4902-33	50 ml 25s	$452.73
Baxter	00338-0035-65	50 ml 100s	$208.00

INJECTION: 50%

BRAND/MANUFACTURER	NDC	SIZE	AWP
◇ GENERICS			
Abbott Hosp	00074-7119-07	2000 ml 6s	$321.41
Astra	00186-0654-01	50 ml 10s	$98.38
Intl Med Sys	00548-1001-00	50 ml 25s	$248.25
Intl Med Sys	00548-2001-00	50 ml 25s	$259.50
Intl Med Sys	00548-3001-00	50 ml 25s	$555.00

INJECTION: 60%

AVERAGE UNIT PRICE (AVAILABLE SIZES)		GENERIC A-RATED AVERAGE PRICE (GAAP)	
GENERIC	$0.05	500 ml 6s	$146.33

BRAND/MANUFACTURER	NDC	SIZE	AWP
◆ GENERICS			
McGaw	00264-1127-01	500 ml	$32.03
McGaw	00264-1127-00	1000 ml	$27.79
Baxter	00338-0645-04	500 ml 6s	$94.08
Abbott Hosp	00074-5646-25	500 ml 6s	$198.57
Abbott Hosp	00074-8005-15	500 ml 12s	$426.22

INJECTION: 60%

BRAND/MANUFACTURER	NDC	SIZE	AWP
◇ GENERICS			
Clintec	00338-0648-13	500 ml 6s	$194.83

INJECTION: 70%

AVERAGE UNIT PRICE (AVAILABLE SIZES)		GENERIC A-RATED AVERAGE PRICE (GAAP)	
GENERIC	$0.05	1000 ml 6s	$173.78
		2000 ml 6s	$330.93

BRAND/MANUFACTURER	NDC	SIZE	AWP
◆ GENERICS			
McGaw	00264-1129-20	250 ml	$22.22
McGaw	00264-1129-01	500 ml	$37.54
McGaw	00264-1129-00	1000 ml	$34.38
McGaw	00264-1129-50	2000 ml	$73.90
Abbott Hosp	00074-5647-25	500 ml 6s	$221.94
Baxter	00338-0348-04	1000 ml 6s	$99.00
Baxter	00338-0038-04	1000 ml 6s	$209.16
Abbott Hosp	00074-1519-05	1000 ml 6s	$213.18
Baxter	00338-0034-06	2000 ml 6s	$280.38
Abbott Hosp	00074-7120-07	2000 ml 6s	$381.47
Abbott Hosp	00074-7918-19	500 ml 12s	$536.51
Abbott Hosp	00074-1489-01	70 ml 25s	$190.59

INJECTION: 70%

BRAND/MANUFACTURER	NDC	SIZE	AWP
◇ GENERICS			
Clintec	00338-0032-13	500 ml 6s	$217.50
Clintec	00338-0719-06	2000 ml 6s	$374.26

DEXTROSE AND SODIUM CHLORIDE

INJECTION: 2.5%-0.45%

BRAND/MANUFACTURER	NDC	SIZE	AWP
◇ GENERICS			
McGaw	00264-7605-10	500 ml	$11.20
McGaw	00264-7605-00	1000 ml	$11.20

INJECTION: 10%-0.45%

BRAND/MANUFACTURER	NDC	SIZE	AWP
◇ GENERICS			
McGaw	00264-7622-00	1000 ml	$16.63
McGaw	00264-1222-00	1000 ml	$17.02

INJECTION: 5%-0.2%

BRAND/MANUFACTURER	NDC	SIZE	AWP
◇ GENERICS			
McGaw	00264-7616-20	250 ml	$16.63
McGaw	00264-7616-10	500 ml	$10.33
McGaw	00264-7616-00	1000 ml	$13.50

INJECTION: 5%-0.9%

BRAND/MANUFACTURER	NDC	SIZE	AWP
◇ GENERICS			
McGaw	00264-7610-20	250 ml	$9.74
McGaw	00264-7610-10	500 ml	$9.74
McGaw	00264-7610-00	1000 ml	$11.62

INJECTION: 5%-0.11%

BRAND/MANUFACTURER	NDC	SIZE	AWP
◇ GENERICS			
McGaw	00264-1217-10	500 ml	$15.98

INJECTION: 5%-0.33%

BRAND/MANUFACTURER	NDC	SIZE	AWP
◇ GENERICS			
McGaw	00264-7614-20	250 ml	$14.48
McGaw	00264-7614-10	500 ml	$9.74
McGaw	00264-7614-00	1000 ml	$11.06

INJECTION: 5%-0.45%

BRAND/MANUFACTURER	NDC	SIZE	AWP
◇ GENERICS			
McGaw	00264-7612-20	250 ml	$9.77
McGaw	00264-7612-10	500 ml	$9.77
McGaw	00264-7612-00	1000 ml 12s	$139.39

INJECTION: 10%-0.2%

BRAND/MANUFACTURER	NDC	SIZE	AWP
◇ GENERICS			
McGaw	00264-7623-20	250 ml	$16.60

INJECTION: 10%-0.9%

BRAND/MANUFACTURER	NDC	SIZE	AWP
◇ GENERICS			
McGaw	00264-7620-00	1000 ml	$16.60

DEXTROSE/POTASSIUM CHLORIDE/ SODIUM CHLORIDE

INJECTION: 5%-0.15%-0.3%

AVERAGE UNIT PRICE (AVAILABLE SIZES)		GENERIC A-RATED AVERAGE PRICE (GAAP)	
GENERIC	$0.03	1000 ml 12s	$198.63

BRAND/MANUFACTURER	NDC	SIZE	AWP
◆ GENERICS			
Abbott Hosp	00074-7998-09	1000 ml 12s	$195.80
Baxter	00338-0603-04	1000 ml 12s	$201.46
Baxter	00338-0603-03	500 ml 18s	$273.36
Abbott Hosp	00074-7998-03	500 ml 24s	$631.56

INJECTION: 5%-0.075%-0.2%

AVERAGE UNIT PRICE (AVAILABLE SIZES)		GENERIC A-RATED AVERAGE PRICE (GAAP)	
GENERIC	$0.02	1000 ml 12s	$203.40

BRAND/MANUFACTURER	NDC	SIZE	AWP
◆ GENERICS			
Baxter	00338-0661-04	1000 ml 12s	$201.46
Abbott Hosp	00074-7997-09	1000 ml 12s	$205.34

◆ RATED THERAPEUTICALLY EQUIVELENT; ◇ THERAPEUTIC EQUIVALENT UNCONFIRMED; ◯ UNRATED

INJECTION: 5%-0.3%-0.9%

AVERAGE UNIT PRICE (AVAILABLE SIZES)		GENERIC A-RATED AVERAGE PRICE (GAAP)	
GENERIC	$0.02	1000 ml 12s	$241.52

BRAND/MANUFACTURER	NDC	SIZE	AWP
◆ GENERICS			
Baxter	00338-0807-04	1000 ml 12s	$201.46
Abbott Hosp	00074-7109-09	1000 ml 12s	$281.58

INJECTION: 5%-0.075%-0.2%

BRAND/MANUFACTURER	NDC	SIZE	AWP
○ GENERICS			
McGaw	00264-7644-00	1000 ml	$16.60

INJECTION: 5%-0.075%-0.45%

BRAND/MANUFACTURER	NDC	SIZE	AWP
○ GENERICS			
McGaw	00264-7634-00	1000 ml	$16.63

INJECTION: 5%-0.15%-0.2%

BRAND/MANUFACTURER	NDC	SIZE	AWP
○ GENERICS			
McGaw	00264-7645-20	250 ml	$16.60
McGaw	00264-7645-10	500 ml	$16.73
McGaw	00264-7645-00	1000 ml	$16.63

INJECTION: 5%-0.15%-0.9%

BRAND/MANUFACTURER	NDC	SIZE	AWP
○ GENERICS			
McGaw	00264-7652-00	1000 ml	$21.89

INJECTION: 10%-0.15%-0.2%

BRAND/MANUFACTURER	NDC	SIZE	AWP
○ GENERICS			
McGaw	00264-7663-20	250 ml	$10.06

INJECTION: 5%-0.15%-0.45%

BRAND/MANUFACTURER	NDC	SIZE	AWP
○ GENERICS			
McGaw	00264-7635-00	1000 ml	$16.60

INJECTION: 5%-0.22%-0.2%

BRAND/MANUFACTURER	NDC	SIZE	AWP
○ GENERICS			
McGaw	00264-7646-00	1000 ml	$16.03

INJECTION: 5%-0.22%-0.45%

BRAND/MANUFACTURER	NDC	SIZE	AWP
○ GENERICS			
McGaw	00264-7636-00	1000 ml	$16.63

INJECTION: 5%-0.3%-0.2%

BRAND/MANUFACTURER	NDC	SIZE	AWP
○ GENERICS			
McGaw	00264-7648-00	1000 ml	$16.03

INJECTION: 5%-0.3%-0.45%

BRAND/MANUFACTURER	NDC	SIZE	AWP
○ GENERICS			
McGaw	00264-7638-00	1000 ml	$16.63

INJECTION: 5%-0.15%-0.3%

BRAND/MANUFACTURER	NDC	SIZE	AWP
○ GENERICS			
McGaw	00264-7655-00	1000 ml	$15.30

DIGOXIN
TABLET: 0.25 MG

BRAND/MANUFACTURER	NDC	SIZE	AWP
○ BRAND			
➤ LANOXIN: Burr Wellcome	00081-0249-30	30s	$5.76
	00081-0249-55	100s	$11.26
	00081-0249-56	100s ud	$15.72
	00081-0249-75	1000s	$86.52
	00081-0249-01	1200s	$102.13
➤ LANOXIN: Burr Wellcome	00081-0249-80	5000s	$408.31

BRAND/MANUFACTURER	NDC	SIZE	AWP
○ GENERICS			
Phys Total Care	54868-0055-01	30s	$2.41
Medirex	57480-0344-06	30s	$4.50
Southwood	58016-0355-30	30s	$5.07
Southwood	58016-0355-60	60s	$6.53
CARDOXIN: Vita Elixir	00181-0603-00	100s	$2.00
Phys Total Care	54868-0055-02	100s	$5.45
Moore,H.L.	00839-1247-06	100s	$9.52
Southwood	58016-0355-00	100s	$9.63
Vangard	00615-0518-13	100s ud	$14.75
Raway	00686-0518-13	100s ud	$16.00
Moore,H.L.	00839-1247-16	1000s	$74.86
Moore,H.L.	00839-1247-20	5000s	$353.30

TABLET: 0.5 MG

BRAND/MANUFACTURER	NDC	SIZE	AWP
○ BRAND			
➤ LANOXIN: Burr Wellcome	00081-0253-55	100s	$20.05

DILTIAZEM HYDROCHLORIDE
TABLET: 60 MG

AVERAGE UNIT PRICE (AVAILABLE SIZES)		GENERIC A-RATED AVERAGE PRICE (GAAP)	
BRAND	$0.70	100s	$59.05
GENERIC	$0.57	500s	$275.67
HCFA FUL (100s ea)	$0.18	1000s	$488.77

BRAND/MANUFACTURER	NDC	SIZE	AWP
◆ BRAND			
➤ CARDIZEM: Marion Merrell Dow	00088-1772-47	100s	$68.25
	00088-1772-49	100s ud	$76.94
	00088-1772-55	500s	$334.75
	00088-1772-90	5000s	$3348.81
◆ GENERICS			
Rugby	00536-3102-01	100s	$53.83
Copley	38245-0662-10	100s	$53.83
West Point	59591-0072-68	100s	$53.86
Major	00904-7715-60	100s	$54.50
Martec	52555-0466-01	100s	$54.85
Schein	00364-2542-01	100s	$54.89
Lederle Std Prod	00005-3334-43	100s	$55.53
Aligen	00405-4341-01	100s	$56.23
Qualitest	00603-3320-21	100s	$56.23
Geneva	00781-1159-01	100s	$56.77
URL	00677-1450-01	100s	$56.79
Moore,H.L.	00839-7749-06	100s	$58.98
Mylan	00378-0045-01	100s	$59.05
Goldline	00182-1938-01	100s	$59.05
Major	00904-7715-61	100s ud	$61.47
Goldline	00182-1938-89	100s ud	$66.50
Rugby	00536-3102-21	100s ud	$67.63
UDL	51079-0746-20	100s ud	$70.30
Vangard	00615-3549-13	100s ud	$71.60
Rugby	00536-3102-05	500s	$264.04
Martec	52555-0466-05	500s	$269.25
Major	00904-7715-40	500s	$271.55
Qualitest	00603-3320-28	500s	$274.80
Moore,H.L.	00839-7749-12	500s	$284.51
Mylan	00378-0045-05	500s	$289.85
Goldline	00182-1938-10	1000s	$450.00
Lederle Std Prod	00005-3334-34	1000s	$527.54

TABLET: 90 MG

AVERAGE UNIT PRICE (AVAILABLE SIZES)		GENERIC A-RATED AVERAGE PRICE (GAAP)	
BRAND	$1.02	100s	$77.39
GENERIC	$0.78	500s	$405.88
HCFA FUL (100s ea)	$0.26		

BRAND/MANUFACTURER	NDC	SIZE	AWP
◆ BRAND			
➤ CARDIZEM: Marion Merrell Dow	00088-1791-47	100s	$95.88
	00088-1791-49	100s ud	$108.31
◆ GENERICS			
Rugby	00536-3103-01	100s	$75.65
Aligen	00405-4342-01	100s	$75.65
Copley	38245-0691-10	100s	$75.65
West Point	59591-0075-68	100s	$75.70
Major	00904-7709-60	100s	$76.40
Major	00904-7716-60	100s	$76.40
Schein	00364-2543-01	100s	$76.71
Martec	52555-0467-01	100s	$77.25
Lederle Std Prod	00005-3335-43	100s	$78.04
Qualitest	00603-3321-21	100s	$78.66
Geneva	00781-1174-01	100s	$79.74
URL	00677-1449-01	100s	$79.84
Moore,H.L.	00839-7750-06	100s	$81.93
Mylan	00378-0135-01	100s	$83.05
Goldline	00182-1939-01	100s	$83.05
Vangard	00615-3550-13	100s ud	$30.92
UDL	51079-0747-20	100s ud	$85.69

BRAND/MANUFACTURER	NDC	SIZE	AWP
Major	00904-7716-61	100s ud	$89.90
Rugby	00536-3103-21	100s ud	$90.17
Moore,H.L.	00839-7750-12	500s	$405.80
Mylan	00378-0135-05	500s	$405.95
Lederle Std Prod	00005-3335-34	1000s	$741.38

TABLET: 120 MG

AVERAGE UNIT PRICE (AVAILABLE SIZES)		GENERIC A-RATED AVERAGE PRICE (GAAP)	
BRAND	$1.33	100s	$102.13
GENERIC	$1.02		
HCFA FUL (100s ea)	$0.36		

BRAND/MANUFACTURER	NDC	SIZE	AWP
◆ **BRAND**			
➤ CARDIZEM: Marion Merrell Dow	00088-1792-47	100s	$125.50
	00088-1792-49	100s ud	$140.81
◆ **GENERICS**			
Rugby	00536-3104-01	100s	$99.00
Aligen	00405-4343-01	100s	$99.00
Copley	38245-0720-10	100s	$99.00
West Point	59591-0077-68	100s	$99.06
Major	00904-7710-60	100s	$99.25
Major	00904-7717-60	100s	$99.25
Schein	00364-2544-01	100s	$99.98
Martec	52555-0468-01	100s	$100.98
Lederle Std Prod	00005-3336-43	100s	$102.13
Qualitest	00603-3322-21	100s	$103.77
URL	00677-1448-01	100s	$104.40
Geneva	00781-1175-01	100s	$104.40
Mylan	00378-0525-01	100s	$108.65
Goldline	00182-1940-01	100s	$108.65
Major	00904-7717-61	100s ud	$104.45
Lederle Std Prod	00005-3336-34	1000s	$970.20

DIPIVEFRIN HYDROCHLORIDE

DROP: 1%

AVERAGE UNIT PRICE (AVAILABLE SIZES)	
GENERIC	$2.28

BRAND/MANUFACTURER	NDC	SIZE	AWP
◆ **GENERICS**			
Falcon Ophthalmics	61314-0235-05	5 ml	$12.00
Falcon Ophthalmics	61314-0235-10	10 ml	$22.00
Falcon Ophthalmics	61314-0235-15	15 ml	$33.50

DYPHYLLINE AND GUAIFENESIN

LIQUID: 300 MG-300 MG/15 ML

BRAND/MANUFACTURER	NDC	SIZE	AWP
○ **GENERICS**			
DYLINE G.G.: Seatrace	00551-0124-01	480 ml	$16.20
DILEX-G: Poly	50991-0200-16	480 ml	$18.38
PANFIL G: Pan Amer	00525-0301-16	480 ml	$20.30
DILOR-G: Savage	00281-1127-74	480 ml	$27.46
DYLINE G.G.: Seatrace	00551-0124-02	3840 ml	$129.60

TABLET: 200 MG-100 MG

BRAND/MANUFACTURER	NDC	SIZE	AWP
○ **GENERICS**			
DYFLEX: EconoMed	38130-0066-01	100s	$9.75
DYFLEX: EconoMed	38130-0066-10	1000s	$84.75

TABLET: 200 MG-200 MG

BRAND/MANUFACTURER	NDC	SIZE	AWP
○ **BRAND**			
DIFIL G: Stewart Jackson	45565-0305-01	100s	$14.50
LUFYLLIN-GG: Wallace	00037-0541-92	100s	$134.86
DIFIL G: Stewart Jackson	45565-0305-03	1000s	$104.38
LUFYLLIN-GG: Wallace	00037-0541-97	1000s	$1262.32
	00037-0541-85	1000s ud	$1421.21
	00037-0541-96	3000s	$3539.23
○ **GENERICS**			
DYFLEX-G: EconoMed	38130-0012-01	100s	$14.94
LGG: Alphagen	59743-0006-01	100s	$15.75
URL	00677-1037-01	100s	$15.80
DYLINE G.G.: Seatrace	00551-0123-01	100s	$16.20
Major	00904-1558-60	100s	$16.45
Econolab	55053-0522-01	100s	$17.50
DILEX-G: Poly	50991-0400-01	100s	$18.38
DILOR-G: Savage	00281-1124-53	100s	$36.14
DILOR-G: Savage	00281-1124-63	100s ud	$55.06
DYFLEX-G: EconoMed	38130-0012-10	1000s	$114.90
DYLINE G.G.: Seatrace	00551-0123-02	1000s	$128.75
DILEX-G: Poly	50991-0400-05	1000s	$145.80
DILOR-G: Savage	00281-1124-57	1000s	$318.95

EPHEDRINE SULFATE/HYDROXYZINE HYDROCHLORIDE/THEOPHYLLINE

TABLET: 25 MG-10 MG-130 MG

BRAND/MANUFACTURER	NDC	SIZE	AWP
○ **BRAND**			
MARAX: Roerig	00049-2540-66	100s	$44.14
	00049-2540-73	500s	$210.48
○ **GENERICS**			
AMI RAX: Amide	52152-0013-02	100s	$26.00
HYDROPHED: Rugby	00536-3906-01	100s	$30.23
Goldline	00182-1344-01	100s	$30.90
Moore,H.L.	00839-6216-06	100s	$31.93
AMI RAX: Amide	52152-0013-04	500s	$117.00
Goldline	00182-1344-05	500s	$130.50
AMI RAX: Amide	52152-0013-05	1000s	$227.50
Moore,H.L.	00839-6216-16	1000s	$269.87

FLUOCINONIDE

OINTMENT: 0.05%

AVERAGE UNIT PRICE (AVAILABLE SIZES)		GENERIC A-RATED AVERAGE PRICE (GAAP)	
BRAND	$0.82	15 gm	$14.91
GENERIC	$0.73	30 gm	$19.81
HCFA FUL (15 gm)	$1.08	60 gm	$31.76
HCFA FUL (30 gm)	$0.55		
HCFA FUL (60 gm)	$0.62		

BRAND/MANUFACTURER	NDC	SIZE	AWP
◆ **BRAND**			
LIDEX: Syntex	00033-2514-13	15 gm	$17.80
	00033-2514-14	30 gm	$24.67
	00033-2514-17	60 gm	$41.36
	00033-2514-22	120 gm	$69.54
◆ **GENERICS**			
Lemmon	00093-0264-15	15 gm	$13.20
Hamilton	60322-0514-13	15 gm	$13.20
Rugby	00536-7501-20	15 gm	$13.98
Qualitest	00603-7761-74	15 gm	$14.75
Moore,H.L.	00839-7731-47	15 gm	$15.24
Major	00904-7677-36	15 gm	$15.25
Goldline	00182-5075-51	15 gm	$18.75
Lemmon	00093-0264-30	30 gm	$18.30
Qualitest	00603-7761-78	30 gm	$19.30
Rugby	00536-7501-28	30 gm	$19.38
Goldline	00182-5075-56	30 gm	$20.50
Moore,H.L.	00839-7731-49	30 gm	$21.59
Major	00904-7677-31	60 gm	$21.85
Lemmon	00093-0264-92	60 gm	$30.68
Hamilton	60322-0514-17	60 gm	$30.68
Rugby	00536-7501-25	60 gm	$32.49
Qualitest	00603-7761-88	60 gm	$32.50
Goldline	00182-5075-52	60 gm	$34.50
Moore,H.L.	00839-7731-50	60 gm	$35.49
Major	00904-7677-02	60 gm	$35.90

SOLUTION: 0.05%

AVERAGE UNIT PRICE (AVAILABLE SIZES)		GENERIC A-RATED AVERAGE PRICE (GAAP)	
BRAND	$0.84	60 ml	$22.61
GENERIC	$0.38		
HCFA FUL (60 ml)	$0.28		

BRAND/MANUFACTURER	NDC	SIZE	AWP
◆ **BRAND**			
LIDEX: Syntex	00033-2517-44	20 ml	$20.25
	00033-2517-46	60 ml	$40.09
◆ **GENERICS**			
Thames	49158-0316-54	20 ml	$8.70
Thames	49158-0316-48	60 ml	$18.75
Qualitest	00603-1230-49	60 ml	$20.48
Rugby	00536-0780-61	60 ml	$20.81
Moore,H.L.	00839-7583-64	60 ml	$21.59
Schein	00364-2412-58	60 ml	$22.50
Geneva	00781-6308-61	60 ml	$23.58
Lemmon	00093-0266-39	60 ml	$23.80
Hamilton	60322-0517-46	60 ml	$23.85

FLURBIPROFEN, ORAL

TABLET: 100 MG

AVERAGE UNIT PRICE (AVAILABLE SIZES)		GENERIC A-RATED AVERAGE PRICE (GAAP)	
BRAND	$1.18	100s	$109.43
GENERIC	$1.07	500s	$518.39

BRAND/MANUFACTURER	NDC	SIZE	AWP
◆ **BRAND**			
➤ ANSAID: Upjohn	00009-0305-03	100s	$119.53
	00009-0305-06	100s ud	$125.13
	00009-0305-05	500s	$579.73
	00009-0305-30	2000s	$2247.16

◆ RATED THERAPEUTICALLY EQUIVELENT; ◇ THERAPEUTIC EQUIVALENT UNCONFIRMED; ○ UNRATED

BRAND/MANUFACTURER	NDC	SIZE	AWP
◆ GENERICS			
Allscrips	54569-3858-00	30s	$32.09
Greenstone	59762-3724-01	100s	$106.38
Qualitest	00603-3700-21	100s	$106.95
Mylan	00378-0093-01	100s	$106.98
UDL	51079-0815-20	100s ud	$117.40
Greenstone	59762-3724-03	500s	$517.46
Qualitest	00603-3700-28	500s	$518.85
Mylan	00378-0093-05	500s	$518.86

TABLET: 100 MG

BRAND/MANUFACTURER	NDC	SIZE	AWP
○ GENERICS			
Geneva	00781-1033-01	100s	$107.06
Geneva	00781-1033-13	100s ud	$112.08
Geneva	00781-1033-05	500s	$519.27

GLIPIZIDE

TABLET: 10 MG

BRAND/MANUFACTURER	NDC	SIZE	AWP
○ BRAND			
➤ GLUCOTROL:	00662-4120-66	100s	$65.08
	59012-0412-66	100s	$65.08
	00662-4120-41	100s ud	$68.34
	59012-0412-41	100s ud	$68.34
	00662-4120-73	500s	$309.11
	59012-0412-73	500s	$309.11
○ GENERICS			
Allscrips	54569-3842-00	30s	$16.71
Major	00904-7925-60	100s	$56.30
Goldline	00182-1995-01	100s	$56.31
Major	00904-7925-40	500s	$253.35
Goldline	00182-1995-05	500s	$264.52

TABLET, EXTENDED RELEASE: 5 MG

BRAND/MANUFACTURER	NDC	SIZE	AWP
○ BRAND			
GLUCOTROL XL: Roerig	00049-1550-66	100s	$30.68

TABLET, EXTENDED RELEASE: 10 MG

BRAND/MANUFACTURER	NDC	SIZE	AWP
○ BRAND			
GLUCOTROL XL: Roerig	00049-1560-66	100s	$60.69

GUAIFENESIN

TABLET, EXTENDED RELEASE: 600 MG

BRAND/MANUFACTURER	NDC	SIZE	AWP
○ BRAND			
G BID: HTD	60354-0004-01	100s	$12.80
BIDEX: Stewart Jackson	45985-0631-01	100s	$23.50
PNEUMOMIST: ECR	00095-0600-01	100s	$25.20
TOURO EX: Dartmouth	58869-0321-01	100s	$25.99
HUMIBID L.A.: Adams	53014-0012-10	100s	$41.99
	53014-0012-50	500s	$205.71
○ GENERICS			
Cheshire	55175-2696-01	14s	$6.92
Cheshire	55175-2696-02	20s	$8.25
Cheshire	55175-2696-04	40s	$13.20
Moore,H.L.	00839-7655-06	100s	$18.56
AQUAMIST: Marnel	00682-0006-01	100s	$21.50
AMIBID LA: Amide	52152-0106-02	100s	$21.88
Q-BID LA: Qualitest	00603-5543-21	100s	$22.50
URL	00677-1475-01	100s	$23.40
MUCOBID-L.A.: Econolab	55053-0040-01	100s	$23.50
GUAIFENEX LA: Ethex	58177-0205-04	100s	$23.60
Major	00904-7759-60	100s	$23.95
RESPA-GF: Respa Pharm	60575-0786-19	100s	$24.00
Alphagen	59743-0018-01	100s	$24.15
FENEX-LA: TMK	59582-0001-01	100s	$24.92
FENESIN: Dura	51479-0009-01	100s	$24.96
Trinity	61355-0501-10	100s	$25.00
SINUMIST-SR: Roberts/Hauck	59441-0152-01	100s	$26.11
Aligen	00405-4457-01	100s	$26.20
MUCO-FEN-LA: Wakefield	59310-0102-10	100s	$26.25
Goldline	00182-1188-01	100s	$26.55
LIQUIBID: Ion	11808-0300-01	100s	$27.00
Rugby	00536-4447-01	100s	$28.43
Q-BID LA: Qualitest	00603-5543-24	250s	$53.40
MUCOBID-L.A.: Econolab	55053-0040-02	250s	$53.95
Alphagen	59743-0018-25	250s	$54.90
Major	00904-7759-70	250s	$55.45
AMIBID LA: Amide	52152-0106-04	500s	$96.00
Q-BID LA: Qualitest	00603-5543-28	500s	$101.20
Trinity	61355-0501-50	500s	$129.29
FENESIN: Dura	51479-0009-06	600s	$156.54

GUAIFENESIN AND PSEUDOEPHEDRINE HYDROCHLORIDE

TABLET: 400 MG-60 MG

BRAND/MANUFACTURER	NDC	SIZE	AWP
○ GENERICS			
ZEPHREX: Bock	00563-2624-01	100s	$39.78

TABLET, EXTENDED RELEASE:

BRAND/MANUFACTURER	NDC	SIZE	AWP
○ BRAND			
SYN-RX: Adams	53014-0308-14	56s	$23.82

TABLET, EXTENDED RELEASE: 100 MG-60 MG

BRAND/MANUFACTURER	NDC	SIZE	AWP
○ GENERICS			
PSEUDOCOT-G: Truxton	00463-7014-01	100s	$10.80

TABLET, EXTENDED RELEASE: 400 MG-120 MG

BRAND/MANUFACTURER	NDC	SIZE	AWP
○ BRAND			
ANATUSS LA: Mayrand	00259-0379-01	100s	$49.70
HISTALET X: Solvay	00032-1050-01	100s	$64.35
○ GENERICS			
NASATAB LA: ECR	00095-0225-01	100s	$34.50
EUDAL SR: Forest Pharm	00785-6301-01	100s	$40.34

TABLET, EXTENDED RELEASE: 500 MG-60 MG

BRAND/MANUFACTURER	NDC	SIZE	AWP
○ BRAND			
MEDENT LD: Stewart Jackson	45985-0624-01	100s	$28.60
○ GENERICS			
SUDAL 60/500: Atley	59702-0060-01	100s	$23.50
MAXIFED-G: MCR/Amer Pharm, Inc.	58605-0506-01	100s	$36.25

TABLET, EXTENDED RELEASE: 500 MG-120 MG

BRAND/MANUFACTURER	NDC	SIZE	AWP
○ BRAND			
MEDENT: Stewart Jackson	45985-0590-01	100s	$28.60
TOURO LA: Dartmouth	58869-0536-01	100s	$37.56
○ GENERICS			
TUSS-LA: Hyrex	00314-8050-01	100s	$23.90
STAMOIST E: Huckaby	58407-0375-01	100s	$25.85
V-DEC-M: Seatrace	00551-0170-01	100s	$39.82
DECONSAL L.A.: Adams	53014-0015-10	100s	$75.20

TABLET, EXTENDED RELEASE: 600 MG-60 MG

BRAND/MANUFACTURER	NDC	SIZE	AWP
○ GENERICS			
GUAIFENEX PSE 60: Ethex	58177-0214-04	100s	$30.62
DEMIBID II: Econolab	55053-0140-01	100s	$32.50
GUIADRINE II: Pharmacist's Choice	54979-0149-01	100s	$32.50
DEFEN-LA: Horizon Pharm	59630-0110-10	100s	$34.25
GUIATEX II: Rugby	00536-5590-01	100s	$34.45
GUIADRINE II SR: Moore,H.L.	00839-7898-06	100s	$35.09
URL	00677-1487-01	100s	$35.85
RESPA-1ST: Respa Pharm	60575-0108-19	100s	$38.00
Goldline	00182-1037-01	100s	$38.40
➤ DECONSAL II: Adams	53014-0017-10	100s	$49.24
➤ DECONSAL II: Adams	53014-0017-50	500s	$241.25

TABLET, EXTENDED RELEASE: 600 MG-120 MG

BRAND/MANUFACTURER	NDC	SIZE	AWP
○ BRAND			
FENEX-PSE: TMK	59582-0003-01	100s	$39.98
➤ GUAIMAX-D: Central	00131-2055-37	100s	$46.75
➤ ENTEX PSE: P&G Pharm	00149-0427-02	100s	$71.08
○ GENERICS			
GP 500: Marnel	00682-0500-01	100s	$21.70
SUDAL 120/600: Atley	59702-0600-01	100s	$24.50
MAXIFED: MCR/Amer Pharm, Inc.	58605-0505-01	100s	$33.00
PAN-MIST LA: Pan Amer	00525-0776-01	100s	$37.80
ZAPTEC PSE: Amer Generics	58634-0033-01	100s	$38.28
Qualitest	00603-5668-21	100s	$39.98
Duramed	51285-0401-02	100s	$42.00
GUAIPAX PSE: Eon	00185-0784-01	100s	$45.00
ALTEX PSE: Aligen	00405-4040-01	100s	$45.16
➤ DURATUSS: Whitby	50474-0612-01	100s	$45.33
Vintage	00254-6211-28	100s	$45.44
Goldline	00182-1740-01	100s	$46.50
GUIADRINE PSE 120: Pharmacist's Choice	54979-0142-01	100s	$47.75
URL	00677-1476-01	100s	$49.90
Moore,H.L.	00839-7754-06	100s	$49.94
GUAI-VENT/PSE: Dura	51479-0015-01	100s	$49.95

➤ SHOWN IN PRODUCT IDENTIFICATION GUIDE

BRAND/MANUFACTURER	NDC	SIZE	AWP
GUAIFENEX PSE 120: Ethex	58177-0208-04	100s	$51.50
GUIATEX PSE: Rugby	00536-5535-01	100s	$53.30
➤ ZEPHREX-LA: Bock	00563-2627-01	100s	$54.55
GUAI-SUDO: MD Pharm	43567-0451-07	100s	$54.94
PSEUDO-G/PSI: Major	00904-7861-60	100s	$56.70
Major	00904-7689-60	100s	$56.70
➤ RU-TUSS DE: Boots Pharm	00048-0090-01	100s	$57.25
GUAIPAX PSE: Eon	00185-0784-52	250s	$106.90
PSEUDO-G/PSI: Major	00904-7861-70	250s	$113.40
Major	00904-7689-70	250s	$113.40
Moore,H.L.	00839-7754-12	500s	$152.67
Qualitest	00603-5668-28	500s	$179.88
GUIADRINE PSE 120: Pharmacist's Choice	54979-0142-05	500s	$191.00
Duramed	51285-0401-04	500s	$208.75
GUAIPAX PSE: Eon	00185-0784-05	500s	$213.75

GUAIFENESIN AND THEOPHYLLINE

ELIXER: 100 MG-150 MG/15 ML

BRAND/MANUFACTURER	NDC	SIZE	AWP
○ GENERICS			
THEO-G: Alphagen	59743-0055-16	480 ml	35.00

LIQUID: 90 MG-150 MG/15 ML

BRAND/MANUFACTURER	NDC	SIZE	AWP
○ GENERICS			
THEOLATE: Moore, H.L.	00839-6348-69	480 ml	4.66
Schein	00364-7264-16	480 ml	4.75
THEOLATE: Barre	00472-1540-16	480 ml	5.04
BRONCOMAR GG: Marlop	12939-0118-16	480 ml	20.65
THEOLATE: Barre	00472-1540-28	480 ml	30.45

LIQUID: 100 MG-100 MG/15 ML

BRAND/MANUFACTURER	NDC	SIZE	AWP
○ BRAND			
ELIXOPHYLLIN-GG: Forest Pharm	00456-0648-08	240 ml	$42.06
	00456-0648-16	480 ml	$80.82

LIQUID: 150 MG-100 MG/15 ML

BRAND/MANUFACTURER	NDC	SIZE	AWP
○ GENERICS			
ED-BRON G: Edwards	00485-0059-16	480 ml	28.00

SYRUP: 90 MG-150 MG/15 ML

BRAND/MANUFACTURER	NDC	SIZE	AWP
○ BRAND			
SLO-PHYLLIN GG: RPR	00075-0357-16	480 ml	$38.57
○ GENERICS			
SOLU-PHYLLIN GG: Marin	12539-0018-02	16 ml	$16.00
SOLU-PHYLLIN: Marin	12539-0017-03	240 ml	$7.00
THEOMAR G.G.: Marlop	12939-0212-16	480 ml	$17.90

GUANABENEZ ACETATE

TABLET: 8 MG

AVERAGE UNIT PRICE (AVAILABLE SIZES)		GENERIC A-RATED AVERAGE PRICE (GAAP)	
BRAND	$1.05	100s	$87.41
GENERIC	$0.87		

BRAND/MANUFACTURER	NDC	SIZE	AWP
◆ BRAND			
WYTENSIN: Wyeth-Ayerst	00008-0074-01	100s	$105.35
◆ GENERICS			
Qualitest	00603-3780-21	100s	$79.80
Martec	52555-0556-01	100s	$82.25
Rugby	00536-5688-01	100s	$89.10
Goldline	00182-1952-01	100s	$89.10
Moore,H.L.	00839-7933-06	100s	$89.10
Copley	38245-0711-10	100s	$91.27
Warner Chilcott	00047-0561-24	100s	$91.27

HYDROCODONE BITARTRATE WITH PHENYLPROPANOLAMINE HYDROCHLORIDE

SYRUP (C-III): 5 MG-25 MG/5 ML

BRAND/MANUFACTURER	NDC	SIZE	AWP
○ BRAND			
HYCOMINE: Du Pont Multi	00056-0246-16	480 ml	$60.00
○ GENERICS			
Moore,H.L.	00839-7680-69	480 ml	$10.38
Major	00904-0954-16	480 ml	$12.40
CODAMINE PEDIATRIC: Barre	00472-0748-16	480 ml	$13.02
Goldline	00182-0069-40	480 ml	$13.50
CODAMINE: Barre	00472-0749-16	480 ml	$13.91
Goldline	00182-1153-40	480 ml	$15.00
Schein	00364-7255-16	480 ml	$15.44

IMIPRAMINE

TABLET: 50 MG

AVERAGE UNIT PRICE (AVAILABLE SIZES)		GENERIC A-RATED AVERAGE PRICE (GAAP)	
BRAND	$0.74	100s	$9.65
GENERIC	$0.08	1000s	$61.40
HCFA FUL (100s ea)	$0.03		

BRAND/MANUFACTURER	NDC	SIZE	AWP
◆ BRAND			
➤ TOFRANIL: Geigy	00028-0136-01	100s	$74.12
◆ GENERICS			
Medirex	57480-0405-06	30s	$4.19
Qualitest	00603-4045-21	100s	$4.30
TIPRAMINE: Major	00904-0929-60	100s	$4.50
Schein	00364-0435-01	100s	$4.75
➤ Biocraft	00332-2117-09	100s	$4.94
Rugby	00536-3931-01	100s	$5.18
URL	00677-0423-01	100s	$5.38
Moore,H.L.	00839-1372-06	100s	$5.39
Mutual	53489-0332-01	100s	$5.65
Aligen	00405-4536-01	100s	$5.96
Parmed	00349-2081-01	100s	$7.50
Geneva	00781-1766-01	100s	$8.59
Purepac	00228-2233-10	100s	$8.61
Par	49884-0056-01	100s	$8.90
Goldline	00182-0828-01	100s	$8.90
Martec	52555-0256-01	100s	$9.08
Abbott Pharm	00074-1899-13	100s	$11.10
U.S. Trading	56126-0056-11	100s ud	$5.09
Raway	00686-0081-20	100s ud	$7.00
Vangard	00615-0530-13	100s ud	$13.19
UDL	51079-0081-20	100s ud	$15.53
Geneva	00781-1766-13	100s ud	$15.55
Goldline	00182-0828-89	100s ud	$16.00
Roxane	00054-8420-25	100s ud	$18.91
TIPRAMINE: Major	00904-0929-61	100s ud	$31.55
TIPRAMINE: Major	00904-0929-70	250s	$11.10
Schein	00364-0435-02	1000s	$34.20
Moore,H.L.	00839-1372-16	1000s	$35.63
Rugby	00536-3931-10	1000s	$39.53
Qualitest	00603-4045-32	1000s	$39.80
TIPRAMINE: Major	00904-0929-80	1000s	$40.95
Mutual	53489-0332-10	1000s	$44.00
URL	00677-0423-10	1000s	$44.90
➤ Biocraft	00332-2117-15	1000s	$47.88
Parmed	00349-2081-10	1000s	$65.00
Geneva	00781-1766-10	1000s	$76.79
Purepac	00228-2233-96	1000s	$76.84
Par	49884-0056-10	1000s	$77.43
Goldline	00182-0828-10	1000s	$77.43
Aligen	00405-4536-03	1000s	$77.48
Martec	52555-0256-10	1000s	$78.98
Roxane	00054-4420-31	1000s	$125.61

IMIPRAMINE PAMOATE

CAPSULE: 75 MG

BRAND/MANUFACTURER	NDC	SIZE	AWP
○ BRAND			
TOFRANIL-PM: Geigy	00028-0020-26	30s	$31.81
	00028-0020-01	100s	$103.67

CAPSULE: 100 MG

BRAND/MANUFACTURER	NDC	SIZE	AWP
○ BRAND			
TOFRANIL-PM: Geigy	00028-0040-26	30s	$41.77
	00028-0040-01	100s	$136.29

◆ RATED THERAPEUTICALLY EQUIVELENT; ◇ THERAPEUTIC EQUIVALENT UNCONFIRMED; ○ UNRATED

BRAND/MANUFACTURER	NDC	SIZE	AWP

CAPSULE: 125 MG

BRAND/MANUFACTURER	NDC	SIZE	AWP
○ BRAND			
TOFRANIL-PM: Geigy	00028-0045-26	30s	$51.93
	00028-0045-01	100s	$169.95

CAPSULE: 150 MG

BRAND/MANUFACTURER	NDC	SIZE	AWP
○ BRAND			
TOFRANIL-PM: Geigy	00028-0022-26	30s	$59.36
	00028-0022-01	100s	$193.73

INDOMETHACIN

CAPSULE, EXTENDED RELEASE: 75 MG

AVERAGE UNIT PRICE (AVAILABLE SIZES)		GENERIC A-RATED AVERAGE PRICE (GAAP)	
BRAND	$1.47	60s	$63.40
GENERIC	$1.004	100s	$94.73
HCFA FUL (100s ea)	$0.74		

BRAND/MANUFACTURER	NDC	SIZE	AWP
◆ BRAND			
➤ INDOCIN SR: Merck	00006-0693-31	30s	$43.98
	00006-0693-61	60s	$87.93
◆ GENERICS			
Inwood	00258-3607-06	60s	$56.51
Qualitest	00603-4070-20	60s	$57.80
➤ West Point	59591-0157-61	60s	$58.50
Major	00904-1178-52	60s	$59.15
Moore,H.L.	00839-7374-05	60s	$60.47
Goldline	00182-1469-26	60s	$61.00
Lemmon	00093-0628-06	60s	$62.00
Warner Chilcott	00047-0875-20	60s	$63.00
URL	00677-1197-06	60s	$68.92
Rugby	00536-4939-08	60s	$68.97
Rugby	00536-5667-08	60s	$68.97
Geneva	00781-2153-60	60s	$68.99
Parmed	00349-8731-60	60s	$69.95
Inwood	00258-3607-01	100s	$84.18
Schein	00364-2211-01	100s	$86.42
Qualitest	00603-4070-21	100s	$88.03
Aligen	00405-4547-01	100s	$88.61
Goldline	00182-1469-01	100s	$89.00
Moore,H.L.	00839-7374-06	100s	$92.60
➤ West Point	59591-0157-68	100s	$97.50
Warner Chilcott	00047-0875-24	100s	$97.50
Major	00904-1178-60	100s	$99.80
Parmed	00349-8731-01	100s	$99.95
Rugby	00536-4939-01	100s	$106.58
Rugby	00536-5667-01	100s	$106.58

SUPPOSITORY: 50 MG

AVERAGE UNIT PRICE (AVAILABLE SIZES)		GENERIC A-RATED AVERAGE PRICE (GAAP)	
BRAND	$1.50	30s	$41.26
GENERIC	$1.38		

BRAND/MANUFACTURER	NDC	SIZE	AWP
◆ BRAND			
INDOCIN: Merck	00006-0150-30	30s	$44.95
◆ GENERICS			
Goldline	00182-7031-17	30s	$40.45
Qualitest	00603-8132-16	30s	$40.85
Moore,H.L.	00839-7901-19	30s	$40.85
G&W	00713-0176-30	30s	$42.88

SUSPENSION: 25 MG/5 ML

BRAND/MANUFACTURER	NDC	SIZE	AWP
◆ BRAND			
INDOCIN: Merck	00006-3376-66	237 ml	$39.21
◆ GENERICS			
Roxane	00054-3423-63	500 ml	$61.89

ISOXSUPRINE HYDROCHLORIDE

TABLET: 20 MG

BRAND/MANUFACTURER	NDC	SIZE	AWP
○ BRAND			
VASODILAN: Apothecon	00087-0544-01	100s	$46.19
	00087-0544-06	1000s	$408.47
○ GENERICS			
Eon	00185-0531-01	100s	$5.45
Amide	52152-0010-02	100s	$5.95
Pharmacist's Choice	54979-0153-01	100s	$7.20
Geneva	00781-1842-01	100s	$7.25
Aligen	00405-4576-01	100s	$8.02

BRAND/MANUFACTURER	NDC	SIZE	AWP
Qualitest	00603-4147-21	100s	$8.08
Goldline	00182-1056-01	100s	$8.10
Moore,H.L.	00839-6182-06	100s	$8.17
Rugby	00536-3936-01	100s	$8.18
Major	00904-0636-60	100s	$8.25
Parmed	00349-2341-01	100s	$9.10
Major	00904-0636-61	100s ud	$13.78
Rugby	00536-3936-05	500s	$24.69
Interstate	00814-4022-28	500s	$24.75
Truxton	00463-6336-10	1000s	$35.40
Eon	00185-0531-10	1000s	$43.10
Amide	52152-0010-05	1000s	$44.95
Rugby	00536-3936-10	1000s	$46.00
Geneva	00781-1842-10	1000s	$47.50
Major	00904-0636-80	1000s	$48.75
Moore,H.L.	00839-6182-16	1000s	$53.31
Pharmacist's Choice	54979-0153-10	1000s	$55.65
Parmed	00349-2341-10	1000s	$56.85
Goldline	00182-1056-10	1000s	$60.75

LIDOCAINE HYDROCHLORIDE, LOCAL ANESTHESIA

INJECTION: 2%

AVERAGE UNIT PRICE (AVAILABLE SIZES)		GENERIC A-RATED AVERAGE PRICE (GAAP)	
BRAND	$0.47	50 ml	$3.48
GENERIC	$0.79	5 ml 10s	$100.91
		5 ml 25s	$208.77
		50 ml 25s	$43.33

BRAND/MANUFACTURER	NDC	SIZE	AWP
◆ BRAND			
XYLOCAINE HCL: Astra	00186-0120-01	20 ml	$2.16
	00186-0155-01	50 ml	$4.15
	00186-0243-12	10 ml 5s	$9.54
XYLOCAINE-MPF: Astra	00186-0240-12	10 ml 5s	$26.96
	00186-0240-02	10 ml 5s	$27.71
	00186-0215-03	2 ml 10s	$17.54
	00186-0241-13	2 ml 10s	$19.94
	00186-0242-13	5 ml 10s	$18.81
XYLOCAINE HCL: Astra	00186-0611-01	5 ml 10s	$20.75
	00186-0232-03	5 ml 10s	$43.19
XYLOCAINE HCL W/DENTAL CARTRIDGES: Astra	00186-0170-14	1.8 ml 100s	$35.00
◆ GENERICS			
Fujisawa	00469-1202-25	2 ml	$1.05
Fujisawa	00469-1208-25	5 ml	$1.40
Moore,H.L.	00839-5598-38	50 ml	$2.01
Schein	00364-6551-57	50 ml	$2.25
Steris	00402-0056-50	50 ml	$2.25
Goldline	00182-0566-67	50 ml	$3.00
Hyrex	00314-0680-50	50 ml	$3.50
Rugby	00536-1460-80	50 ml	$4.88
LIDOJECT-2: Mayrand	00259-0326-50	50 ml	$6.45
Abbott Hosp	00074-8027-01	5 ml 10s	$89.42
Abbott Hosp	00074-4903-01	5 ml 10s	$100.46
Abbott Hosp	00074-4923-01	5 ml 10s	$100.46
Abbott Hosp	00074-4903-23	5 ml 10s	$113.29
Abbott Hosp	00074-4282-01	2 ml 25s	$36.22
Elkins-Sinn	00641-0437-25	5 ml 25s	$16.15
Intl Med Sys	00548-1112-00	5 ml 25s	$142.50
Intl Med Sys	00548-1190-00	5 ml 25s	$150.75
Abbott Hosp	00074-4903-33	5 ml 25s	$283.22
Intl Med Sys	00548-2190-00	5 ml 25s	$314.25
Intl Med Sys	00548-3190-00	5 ml 25s	$345.75
Abbott Hosp	00074-4282-02	10 ml 25s	$60.27
Abbott Hosp	00074-4277-01	20 ml 25s	$54.03
Elkins-Sinn	00641-2400-45	30 ml 25s	$15.94
Elkins-Sinn	00641-2410-45	50 ml 25s	$21.56
Amer Regent	00517-0626-25	50 ml 25s	$30.94
Abbott Hosp	00074-4277-02	50 ml 25s	$77.48

INJECTION: 4%

AVERAGE UNIT PRICE (AVAILABLE SIZES)	
BRAND	$0.46

BRAND/MANUFACTURER	NDC	SIZE	AWP
◆ BRAND			
XYLOCAINE HCL: Astra	00186-0166-01	25 ml	$1.59
	00186-0167-01	25 ml	$2.05
	00186-0169-01	50 ml	$2.03
XYLOCAINE DUO-TRACH KIT: Astra	00186-0235-72	5 ml 5s	$36.40
XYLOCAINE HCL: Astra	00186-0168-01	50 ml 5s	$2.30
XYLOCAINE-MPF: Astra	00186-0235-03	5 ml 10s	$56.59
◆ GENERICS			
Abbott Hosp	00074-4283-01	5 ml 25s	$71.55

INJECTION: 5%

BRAND/MANUFACTURER	NDC	SIZE	AWP
○ BRAND			
XYLOCAINE HCL FOR SPINAL: Astra	00186-0225-03	2 ml 10s	$83.46

➤ SHOWN IN PRODUCT IDENTIFICATION GUIDE

INJECTION: 10%

BRAND/MANUFACTURER	NDC	SIZE	AWP
◆ GENERICS			
Abbott Hosp	00074-6254-01	10 ml 25s	$207.81

INJECTION: 20%

AVERAGE UNIT PRICE (AVAILABLE SIZES)		GENERIC A-RATED AVERAGE PRICE (GAAP)	
GENERIC	$1.49	10 ml 25s	$340.38

BRAND/MANUFACTURER	NDC	SIZE	AWP
◆ GENERICS			
Intl Med Sys	00548-6100-00	5 ml 25s	$231.75
Abbott Hosp	00074-6248-01	10 ml 25s	$286.78
Intl Med Sys	00548-6105-00	10 ml 25s	$355.25
Abbott Hosp	00074-6217-02	10 ml 25s	$379.11

OINTMENT: 5%

BRAND/MANUFACTURER	NDC	SIZE	AWP
◆ GENERICS			
Moore,H.L.	00839-5474-81	50 gm	$2.15

SET:

BRAND/MANUFACTURER	NDC	SIZE	AWP
○ BRAND			
SPINAL-22 WHITACRE W/LIDOCAINE: Abbott Hosp	00074-4804-01	10s	$420.73

SOLUTION: 2%

AVERAGE UNIT PRICE (AVAILABLE SIZES)		GENERIC A-RATED AVERAGE PRICE (GAAP)	
BRAND	$0.12	100 ml	$4.35
GENERIC	$0.06		
HCFA FUL (100 ml)	$0.03		

BRAND/MANUFACTURER	NDC	SIZE	AWP
◆ BRAND			
XYLOCAINE VISCOUS: Astra	00186-0360-01	100 ml	$14.98
	00186-0360-11	450 ml	$50.13
	00186-0361-78	20 ml 25s ud	$44.83
◆ GENERICS			
Morton Grove	60432-0464-20	20 ml	$5.60
Roxane	00054-3500-49	100 ml	$2.63
Moore,H.L.	00839-6502-40	100 ml	$3.08
Morton Grove	60432-0464-00	100 ml	$3.64
Schein	00364-7282-61	100 ml	$3.75
Qualitest	00603-1392-64	100 ml	$4.05
Major	00904-0863-04	100 ml	$4.10
Rugby	00536-1331-82	100 ml	$4.12
URL	00677-1015-27	100 ml	$4.60
Barre	00472-0996-33	100 ml	$4.62
Geneva	00781-6190-46	100 ml	$4.65
Goldline	00182-1360-70	100 ml	$6.15
LIDOMAR: Marlop	12939-0780-10	100 ml	$6.80
Roxane	00054-8500-16	20 ml 40s ud	$50.50

SOLUTION: 4%

AVERAGE UNIT PRICE (AVAILABLE SIZES)		GENERIC A-RATED AVERAGE PRICE (GAAP)	
BRAND	$0.29	50 ml	$7.63
GENERIC	$0.99		

BRAND/MANUFACTURER	NDC	SIZE	AWP
◆ BRAND			
XYLOCAINE: Astra	00186-0320-01	50 ml	$14.33
◆ GENERICS			
Roxane	00054-3505-47	50 ml	$7.04
Moore,H.L.	00839-7407-99	50 ml	$8.22
Intl Med Sys	00548-6300-00	4 ml 25s	$265.50

SOLUTION: 5%

BRAND/MANUFACTURER	NDC	SIZE	AWP
◆ BRAND			
XYLOCAINE: Astra	00186-0325-01	30 ml	$12.50

NADOLOL

TABLET: 160 MG

AVERAGE UNIT PRICE (AVAILABLE SIZES)	
GENERIC	$1.69

BRAND/MANUFACTURER	NDC	SIZE	AWP
◆ BRAND			
➤ CORGARD: B/M Squibb U.S. Phar	00003-0246-49	100s	$198.98
◆ GENERICS			
Apothecon	59772-2465-01	100s	$161.95
Copley	38245-0731-10	100s	$168.45

NEOMYCIN SULFATE

SOLUTION: 125 MG/5 ML

BRAND/MANUFACTURER	NDC	SIZE	AWP
○ GENERICS			
Pharma-Tek	39822-0330-05	480 ml	$21.00

SOLUTION: 125 MG/5 ML

BRAND/MANUFACTURER	NDC	SIZE	AWP
○ GENERICS			
Pharma-Tek	39822-0330-05	480 ml	$21.00

TABLET: 500 MG

AVERAGE UNIT PRICE (AVAILABLE SIZES)		GENERIC A-RATED AVERAGE PRICE (GAAP)	
GENERIC	$0.25	100s	$24.64

BRAND/MANUFACTURER	NDC	SIZE	AWP
◆ GENERICS			
Raway	00686-1177-09	100s	$17.00
Moore,H.L.	00839-5996-06	100s	$18.16
Biocraft	00332-1177-09	100s	$18.48
UDL	51079-0015-40	100s	$18.85
Rugby	00536-4064-01	100s	$20.63
Goldline	00182-0673-01	100s	$21.75
URL	00677-1010-01	100s	$23.83
Geneva	00781-1400-01	100s	$23.88
Schein	00364-2006-01	100s	$26.27
Roxane	00054-4600-25	100s	$36.63
U.S. Trading	56126-0270-11	100s ud	$13.49
Raway	00686-0015-20	100s ud	$19.00
UDL	51079-0015-20	100s ud	$29.96
Roxane	00054-8600-25	100s ud	$57.05

TABLET: 500 MG

BRAND/MANUFACTURER	NDC	SIZE	AWP
○ GENERICS			
Pharma-Tek	39822-0310-01	100s	$12.95

TABLET: 500 MG

BRAND/MANUFACTURER	NDC	SIZE	AWP
○ GENERICS			
Pharma-Tek	39822-0310-01	100s	$12.95

NITROGLYCERIN

INJECTION: 5 MG/ML

AVERAGE UNIT PRICE (AVAILABLE SIZES)		GENERIC A-RATED AVERAGE PRICE (GAAP)	
BRAND	$2.12	5 ml 25s	$439.67
GENERIC	$2.59	10 ml 25s	$658.49

BRAND/MANUFACTURER	NDC	SIZE	AWP
◆ BRAND			
NITRO-BID IV: Marion Merrell Dow	00088-1800-33	10 ml 5s	$67.81
	00088-1800-31	1 ml 10s	$33.88
	00088-1800-32	5 ml 10s	$81.44
◆ GENERICS			
Amer Regent	00517-4805-10	5 ml 10s	$90.63
Amer Regent	00517-4810-10	10 ml 10s	$140.63
Solo Pak	39769-0077-05	5 ml 25s	$171.88
Abbott Hosp	00074-4107-01	5 ml 25s	$707.45
Solo Pak	39769-0077-10	10 ml 25s	$375.00
Abbott Hosp	00074-4104-01	10 ml 25s	$941.98

INJECTION: 5 MG/ML

BRAND/MANUFACTURER	NDC	SIZE	AWP
○ GENERICS			
TRIDIL: Du Pont Multi	00590-0085-05	5 ml 20s	$118.75
TRIDIL: Du Pont Multi	00590-0085-86	5 ml 20s	$150.00
TRIDIL: Du Pont Multi	00590-0090-10	10 ml 20s	$212.50
TRIDIL: Du Pont Multi	00590-0090-66	10 ml 20s	$225.00
TRIDIL: Du Pont Multi	00590-0095-79	20 ml 20s	$300.00

KIT: 50 MG

BRAND/MANUFACTURER	NDC	SIZE	AWP
◆ GENERICS			
Abbott Hosp	00074-1324-01	24s	$1481.43

OINTMENT: 2%

BRAND/MANUFACTURER	NDC	SIZE	AWP
○ BRAND			
NITRO-BID: Marion Merrell Dow	00088-1552-20	20 gm	$3.38
NITROL APPLI-KIT: Savage	00281-5804-46	30 gm	$8.87

◆ RATED THERAPEUTICALLY EQUIVELENT; ◇ THERAPEUTIC EQUIVALENT UNCONFIRMED; ○ UNRATED

BRAND/MANUFACTURER	NDC	SIZE	AWP
NITRO-BID: Marion Merrell Dow	00088-1552-60	60 gm	$6.50
NITROL APPLI-KIT: Savage	00281-5804-56	60 gm	$9.03
	00281-5804-47	60 gm	$16.33
	00281-5804-48	3 gm 50s	$50.56
	00281-5804-59	3 gm 50s ud	$49.09
NITRO-BID: Marion Merrell Dow	00088-1552-49	1 gm 100s ud	$24.44
○ GENERICS			
Fougera	00168-0038-30	30 gm	$5.87
Allscrips	54569-3360-00	30 gm	$5.87
Fougera	00168-0038-60	60 gm	$8.74
Southwood	58016-1123-01	60 gm	$10.24
Goldline	00182-0038-60	60 gm	$11.40

SPRAY: 0.4 MG/SPRAY

BRAND/MANUFACTURER	NDC	SIZE	AWP
○ BRAND			
NITROLINGUAL: RPR	00075-0850-84	14.49 ml	$23.83

TABLET: 0.3 MG

BRAND/MANUFACTURER	NDC	SIZE	AWP
○ BRAND			
NITROSTAT: Parke-Davis	00071-0569-24	100s	$6.18

TABLET: 0.4 MG

BRAND/MANUFACTURER	NDC	SIZE	AWP
○ BRAND			
➤ NITROSTAT: Parke-Davis	00071-0570-24	100s	$6.18
	00071-0570-13	100s	$14.01

TABLET: 0.6 MG

BRAND/MANUFACTURER	NDC	SIZE	AWP
○ BRAND			
NITROSTAT: Parke-Davis	00071-0571-24	100s	$6.18
○ GENERICS			
Southwood	58016-5009-01	100s	$8.69

TABLET: 1 MG

BRAND/MANUFACTURER	NDC	SIZE	AWP
○ BRAND			
NITROGARD: Forest Pharm	00456-0686-01	100s	$36.07

TABLET: 2 MG

BRAND/MANUFACTURER	NDC	SIZE	AWP
○ BRAND			
NITROGARD: Forest Pharm	00456-0687-01	100s	$38.18

TABLET: 3 MG

BRAND/MANUFACTURER	NDC	SIZE	AWP
○ BRAND			
NITROGARD: Forest Pharm	00456-0683-01	100s	$41.27

TABLET, EXTENDED RELEASE: 2.6 MG

BRAND/MANUFACTURER	NDC	SIZE	AWP
○ BRAND			
NITRONG: RPR	00075-0221-20	100s	$30.56

TABLET, EXTENDED RELEASE: 6.5 MG

BRAND/MANUFACTURER	NDC	SIZE	AWP
○ BRAND			
NITRONG: RPR	00075-0274-20	100s	$38.25

PAPAVERINE HYDROCHLORIDE

CAPSULE, EXTENDED RELEASE: 150 MG

BRAND/MANUFACTURER	NDC	SIZE	AWP
○ BRAND			
PAVABID PLATEAU: Marion Merrell Dow	00088-1555-47	100s	$27.31
○ GENERICS			
PAPACON: CMC-Cons	00223-1358-60	60s	$4.25
PAPACON: CMC-Cons	00223-1358-01	100s	$5.50
Qualitest	00603-5043-21	100s	$6.65
Geneva	00781-2000-01	100s	$7.25
Eon	00185-5156-01	100s	$7.37
PARA-TIME S.R.: Time-Cap	49483-0019-01	100s	$7.75
Major	00904-2180-60	100s	$7.95
Goldline	00182-0181-01	100s	$7.95
PAVAGEN: Rugby	00536-4124-01	100s	$8.09
URL	00677-0171-01	100s	$8.32
Moore,H.L.	00839-1441-06	100s	$8.37
PAVACOT: Truxton	00463-3011-01	100s	$8.40
Schein	00364-0181-01	100s	$8.46
Aligen	00405-4757-01	100s	$8.62

BRAND/MANUFACTURER	NDC	SIZE	AWP
Parmed	00349-2109-01	100s	$11.35
Raway	00686-0010-20	100s ud	$9.00
UDL	51079-0010-20	100s ud	$12.50
Major	00904-2180-61	100s ud	$12.93
Geneva	00781-2000-13	100s ud	$14.50
PAVAGEN: Rugby	00536-4124-05	500s	$34.58
Veratex	17022-6202-06	1000s	$27.95
PAPACON: CMC-Cons	00223-1358-03	1000s	$49.50
Geneva	00781-2000-10	1000s	$50.46
Schein	00364-0181-02	1000s	$58.30
Major	00904-2180-80	1000s	$60.25
URL	00677-0171-10	1000s	$60.69
Moore,H.L.	00839-1441-16	1000s	$60.74
PARA-TIME S.R.: Time-Cap	49483-0019-10	1000s	$63.00
Goldline	00182-0181-10	1000s	$63.00
Qualitest	00603-5043-32	1000s	$63.37
Aligen	00405-4757-03	1000s	$65.72
PAVAGEN: Rugby	00536-4124-10	1000s	$65.84
Eon	00185-5156-10	1000s	$66.73
PAVACOT: Truxton	00463-3011-10	1000s	$79.80
Parmed	00349-2109-10	1000s	$100.00

POWDER:

BRAND/MANUFACTURER	NDC	SIZE	AWP
○ GENERICS			
Amend	17137-0398-02	25 gm	$24.15
Amend	17137-0398-04	100 gm	$81.20
Amend	17137-0398-01	500 gm	$315.00

PHENOBARBITAL

TABLET (C-IV): 15 MG

BRAND/MANUFACTURER	NDC	SIZE	AWP
○ GENERICS			
CMC-Cons	00223-1430-01	100s	$2.50
Lilly	00002-1031-02	100s	$3.00
Southwood	58016-0664-00	100s	$7.37
UDL	51079-0094-21	100s ud	$3.72
Vangard	00615-0420-47	100s ud	$4.16
UDL	51079-0094-20	100s ud	$4.50
Medirex	57480-0504-01	100s ud	$5.75
➤ Roxane	00054-8703-25	100s ud	$5.92
West-Ward	00143-1445-10	1000s	$5.73
Truxton	00463-6160-10	1000s	$6.90
➤ Warner Chilcott	00047-0699-32	1000s	$7.44
Vintage	00254-5011-38	1000s	$7.88
Qualitest	00603-5165-32	1000s	$7.88
Geneva	00781-1091-10	1000s	$7.99
Purepac	00228-2026-96	1000s	$7.99
URL	00677-0236-10	1000s	$8.20
Moore,H.L.	00839-1478-16	1000s	$8.21
Jones Medical	52604-6712-02	1000s	$8.80
Rugby	00536-4170-10	1000s	$8.85
Lilly	00002-1031-04	1000s	$9.21
Eon	00185-0015-10	1000s	$9.66
Parmed	00349-8868-10	1000s	$9.95
Major	00904-3815-80	1000s	$10.90
CMC-Cons	00223-1430-02	1000s	$21.00

TABLET (C-IV): 16 MG

BRAND/MANUFACTURER	NDC	SIZE	AWP
○ BRAND			
SOLFOTON: Poythress	00095-0023-01	100s	$6.25

TABLET (C-IV): 16.2 MG

BRAND/MANUFACTURER	NDC	SIZE	AWP
○ GENERICS			
Richlyn	00115-4211-03	1000s	$6.75
Richlyn	00115-4212-03	1000s	$6.75
Richlyn	00115-4214-03	1000s	$6.75

TABLET (C-IV): 30 MG

BRAND/MANUFACTURER	NDC	SIZE	AWP
○ GENERICS			
Southwood	58016-0826-06	6s	$2.44
Allscrips	54569-0938-02	9s	$0.11
Allscrips	54569-0938-01	30s	$0.36
Medirex	57480-0505-06	30s	$2.31
Southwood	58016-0826-50	50s	$6.20
Allscrips	54569-0938-00	100s	$1.20
CMC-Cons	00223-1431-01	100s	$2.75
➤ Lilly	00002-1032-02	100s	$3.07
UDL	51079-0095-21	100s ud	$4.14
Vangard	00615-0421-47	100s ud	$4.55
UDL	51079-0095-20	100s ud	$5.30
Medirex	57480-0505-01	100s ud	$6.75

BRAND/MANUFACTURER	NDC	SIZE	AWP
➤ Roxane	00054-8705-25	100s ud	$6.95
Glasgow	60809-0507-55	750s ud	$32.06
Glasgow	60809-0507-72	750s ud	$32.06
West-Ward	00143-1440-10	1000s	$7.21
West-Ward	00143-1450-10	1000s	$7.21
Truxton	00463-6145-10	1000s	$8.10
Vintage	00254-5012-38	1000s	$8.53
Qualitest	00603-5166-32	1000s	$8.53
Major	00904-3827-80	1000s	$8.80
➤ Warner Chilcott	00047-0700-32	1000s	$9.23
Moore,H.L.	00839-1484-16	1000s	$9.71
Jones Medical	52604-6722-02	1000s	$9.95
Richlyn	00115-4229-03	1000s	$10.20
Richlyn	00115-4231-03	1000s	$10.20
Richlyn	00115-4233-03	1000s	$10.20
URL	00677-0237-10	1000s	$10.68
Rugby	00536-4224-10	1000s	$10.73
Eon	00185-0030-10	1000s	$10.80
Parmed	00349-8869-10	1000s	$10.98
Purepac	00228-2028-96	1000s	$11.80
Major	00904-3816-80	1000s	$11.95
Geneva	00781-1110-10	1000s	$11.95
Goldline	00182-0292-10	1000s	$13.75
➤ Lilly	00002-1032-04	1000s	$15.22
CMC-Cons	00223-1431-02	1000s	$22.50

TABLET (C-IV): 60 MG

BRAND/MANUFACTURER	NDC	SIZE	AWP
○ GENERICS			
Vintage	00254-5013-28	100s	$2.66
Qualitest	00603-5167-21	100s	$2.66
CMC-Cons	00223-1432-01	100s	$3.25
Lilly	00002-1037-02	100s	$4.54
➤ Roxane	00054-8708-25	100s ud	$7.27
Vintage	00254-5013-38	1000s	$11.42
Qualitest	00603-5167-32	1000s	$11.42
URL	00677-0762-10	1000s	$13.45
➤ Warner Chilcott	00047-0607-32	1000s	$15.72
Jones Medical	52604-6731-02	1000s	$17.05
Moore,H.L.	00839-6257-16	1000s	$17.13
Parmed	00349-8656-10	1000s	$17.54
Truxton	00463-6151-10	1000s	$18.50
Goldline	00182-0590-10	1000s	$18.60
Lilly	00002-1037-04	1000s	$24.21
CMC-Cons	00223-1432-02	1000s	$29.50

TABLET (C-IV): 100 MG

BRAND/MANUFACTURER	NDC	SIZE	AWP
○ GENERICS			
Vintage	00254-5014-28	100s	$3.31
Qualitest	00603-5168-21	100s	$3.31
CMC-Cons	00223-1433-01	100s	$3.75
Lilly	00002-1033-02	100s	$5.75
➤ Roxane	00054-8707-25	100s ud	$7.45
Moore,H.L.	00839-5154-16	1000s	$19.10
Truxton	00463-6152-10	1000s	$18.00
➤ Warner Chilcott	00047-0698-32	1000s	$18.49
URL	00677-0238-10	1000s	$18.50
Schein	00364-0206-02	1000s	$18.50
Jones Medical	52604-6740-02	1000s	$18.90
CMC-Cons	00223-1433-02	1000s	$32.50

PHENOBARBITAL SODIUM

INJECTION (C-IV): 30 MG/ML

BRAND/MANUFACTURER	NDC	SIZE	AWP
○ GENERICS			
Wyeth-Ayerst	00008-0499-01	1 ml 10s	$21.20
Wyeth-Ayerst	00008-0499-50	1 ml 10s	$24.95

INJECTION (C-IV): 60 MG/ML

BRAND/MANUFACTURER	NDC	SIZE	AWP
○ GENERICS			
Wyeth-Ayerst	00008-0747-01	1 ml 10s	$23.66
Wyeth-Ayerst	00008-0747-50	1 ml 10s	$27.41

INJECTION (C-IV): 65 MG/ML

BRAND/MANUFACTURER	NDC	SIZE	AWP
○ GENERICS			
Elkins-Sinn	00641-0476-25	1 ml 25s	$23.16

INJECTION (C-IV): 130 MG/ML

BRAND/MANUFACTURER	NDC	SIZE	AWP
○ GENERICS			
Wyeth-Ayerst	00008-0304-01	1 ml 10s	$26.00
Wyeth-Ayerst	00008-0304-50	1 ml 10s	$29.75
Elkins-Sinn	00641-0477-25	1 ml 25s	$27.60

POTASSIUM BICARBONATE

TABLET, EFFERVESCENT: 25 MEQ

BRAND/MANUFACTURER	NDC	SIZE	AWP
Schein	00364-0635-30	30s	$7.95
K+CARE ET: Alra	51641-0125-03	30s	$8.58
K+CARE ET: Alra	51641-0135-03	30s	$8.58
K-VESCENT: Major	00904-2720-46	30s	$8.70
Rugby	00536-3777-07	30s	$10.07
K-ELECTROLYTE: Copley	38245-0221-03	30s	$14.60
Moore,H.L.	00839-7174-19	30s	$16.86
Rugby	00536-3815-07	30s	$18.53
Bajamar	44184-0016-04	100s	$18.00
Bajamar	44184-0024-04	100s	$18.00
K-VESCENT: Major	00904-2720-60	100s	$18.95
K-ELECTROLYTE: Aligen	00405-4812-01	100s	$23.10
K-ELECTROLYTE: Copley	38245-0205-01	100s	$23.10
K+CARE ET: Alra	51641-0125-01	100s	$24.96
K+CARE ET: Alra	51641-0135-01	100s	$24.96
Schein	00364-0635-01	100s	$25.18
K-ELECTROLYTE: Copley	38245-0221-10	100s	$47.40
Moore,H.L.	00839-6619-09	250s	$43.88
Bajamar	44184-0016-06	250s	$44.00
Bajamar	44184-0024-06	250s	$44.00
K-VESCENT: Major	00904-2720-70	250s	$45.00
K+CARE ET: Alra	51641-0125-25	250s	$51.81
K+CARE ET: Alra	51641-0135-25	250s	$51.81
Schein	00364-0635-04	250s	$53.00
Rugby	00536-3777-02	250s	$67.12

POTASSIUM IODIDE

GRANULAR:

BRAND/MANUFACTURER	NDC	SIZE	AWP
○ GENERICS			
Humco	00395-2303-94	120 gm	$10.61
Amend	17137-0443-04	125 gm	$9.80
Amend	17137-1497-06	125 gm	$21.00
Humco	00395-2303-01	454 gm	$57.28
Amend	17137-0443-01	500 gm	$35.00
Amend	17137-0443-05	2270 gm	$140.00
Amend	17137-0443-08	11350 gm	$603.75

SOLUTION: 1 GM/ML

BRAND/MANUFACTURER	NDC	SIZE	AWP
○ GENERICS			
Denison	00295-1204-31	30 ml dozdoz	$28.42
Roxane	00054-3717-44	30 ml	$5.87
Upsher-Smith	00245-0003-31	30 ml	$10.80
Roxane	00054-3717-58	240 ml	$29.31
Upsher-Smith	00245-0003-08	240 ml	$50.28

SYRUP: 325 MG/5 ML

BRAND/MANUFACTURER	NDC	SIZE	AWP
○ GENERICS			
PIMA: Fleming	00256-0139-01	480 ml	$15.00
PIMA: Fleming	00256-0139-02	3840 ml	$72.00

PRAZOSIN HYDROCHLORIDE

CAPSULE: 5 MG

AVERAGE UNIT PRICE (AVAILABLE SIZES)		GENERIC A-RATED AVERAGE PRICE (GAAP)	
BRAND	$1.03	100s	$59.78
GENERIC	$0.55	250s	$127.70
HCFA FUL (100s ea)	$0.12	500s	$252.80

BRAND/MANUFACTURER	NDC	SIZE	AWP
◆ BRAND			
➤ MINIPRESS: Pfizer Labs	00663-4380-41	100s ud	$112.48
	00663-4380-71	250s	$245.71
	00663-4380-73	500s	$486.43
◆ GENERICS			
Schein	00364-2391-06	60s	$33.15
Moore,H.L.	00839-7556-06	100s	$45.35
Purepac	00228-2502-10	100s	$49.80
Aligen	00405-4818-01	100s	$52.19
Schein	00364-2391-01	100s	$53.03
Lederle Std Prod	00005-3475-43	100s	$53.16
Martec	52555-0281-01	100s	$53.45
Qualitest	00603-5288-21	100s	$54.90
Zenith	00172-4069-60	100s	$57.60
Parmed	00349-8696-01	100s	$57.61
URL	00677-1370-01	100s	$57.80
Mylan	00378-3205-01	100s	$57.85
Geneva	00781-2213-01	100s	$57.85
Goldline	00182-1257-01	100s	$60.00
Goldline	00182-1922-01	100s	$60.00
U.S. Trading	56126-0465-11	100s ud	$17.69

◆ RATED THERAPEUTICALLY EQUIVELENT; ◇ THERAPEUTIC EQUIVALENT UNCONFIRMED; ○ UNRATED

BRAND/MANUFACTURER	NDC	SIZE	AWP
Schein	00364-2391-90	100s ud	$57.65
Vangard	00615-0388-13	100s ud	$61.01
Medirex	57480-0386-01	100s ud	$86.30
UDL	51079-0632-20	100s ud	$86.32
Goldline	00182-1257-89	100s ud	$87.90
Goldline	00182-1922-89	100s ud	$87.90
Rugby	00536-4815-02	250s	$83.13
Moore,H.L.	00839-7556-09	250s	$90.44
Qualitest	00603-5288-24	250s	$116.61
Purepac	00228-2502-25	250s	$124.51
Schein	00364-2391-04	250s	$125.95
Lederle Std Prod	00005-3475-27	250s	$132.88
Aligen	00405-4818-04	250s	$133.73
Goldline	00182-1922-02	250s	$135.00
URL	00677-1370-03	250s	$135.75
Geneva	00781-2213-25	250s	$141.60
Major	00904-1042-70	250s	$141.70
Zenith	00172-4069-65	250s	$142.00
Goldline	00182-1257-02	250s	$142.00
Mylan	00378-3205-25	250s	$142.50
Lederle Std Prod	00005-3475-31	500s	$198.21
Moore,H.L.	00839-7556-12	500s	$200.87
Qualitest	00603-5288-28	500s	$222.16
Purepac	00228-2502-50	500s	$264.64
Parmed	00349-8696-05	500s	$271.03
Geneva	00781-2213-05	500s	$272.16
Major	00904-1042-40	500s	$280.55
Zenith	00172-4069-70	500s	$282.60
Mylan	00378-3205-05	500s	$282.95

PROPRANOLOL HYDROCHLORIDE

TABLET: 10 MG

AVERAGE UNIT PRICE (AVAILABLE SIZES)		GENERIC A-RATED AVERAGE PRICE (GAAP)	
BRAND	$0.32	100s	$8.08
GENERIC	$0.07	500s	$24.75
HCFA FUL (100s ea)	$0.01	1000s	$46.91

BRAND/MANUFACTURER	NDC	SIZE	AWP
◆ BRAND			
➤ INDERAL: Wyeth-Ayerst	00046-0421-81	100s	$31.29
	00046-0421-99	100s ud	$35.41
	00046-0421-91	1000s	$305.64
	00046-0421-95	5000s	$1509.28
◆ GENERICS			
Medirex	57480-0355-06	30s	$5.18
Warner Chilcott	00047-0070-24	100s	$4.11
Rugby	00536-4309-01	100s	$4.50
Major	00904-0411-60	100s	$4.50
Qualitest	00603-5489-21	100s	$4.55
Schein	00364-0756-01	100s	$4.75
Caremark	00339-5315-12	100s	$4.81
Interpharm	53746-0218-01	100s	$5.20
Mason Dist	11845-0257-01	100s	$5.35
URL	00677-1041-01	100s	$5.95
Geneva	00781-1344-01	100s	$5.95
Purepac	00228-2327-10	100s	$6.00
Aligen	00405-4884-01	100s	$6.38
Sidmak	50111-0467-01	100s	$6.38
Goldline	00182-1758-01	100s	$6.83
Watson	52544-0305-01	100s	$6.95
Raway	00686-0277-20	100s	$7.00
Mylan	00378-0182-01	100s	$7.35
U.S. Trading	56126-0321-11	100s ud	$3.53
Schein	00364-0756-90	100s ud	$11.50
Major	00904-0411-61	100s ud	$12.35
Geneva	00781-1344-13	100s ud	$13.01
Vangard	00615-2561-13	100s ud	$13.01
Medirex	57480-0355-01	100s ud	$17.25
UDL	51079-0277-20	100s ud	$17.28
Goldline	00182-1812-89	100s ud	$17.55
Rugby	00536-4309-05	500s	$19.50
Purepac	00228-2327-50	500s	$30.00
Warner Chilcott	00047-0070-32	1000s	$33.83
Rugby	00536-4309-10	1000s	$36.80
Qualitest	00603-5489-32	1000s	$37.12
Mason Dist	11845-0257-04	1000s	$37.22
Interpharm	53746-0218-10	1000s	$37.50
Major	00904-0411-80	1000s	$37.80
Schein	00364-0756-02	1000s	$38.50
Martec	52555-0343-10	1000s	$38.85
Moore,H.L.	00839-7114-16	1000s	$40.70
URL	00677-1041-10	1000s	$41.20
Geneva	00781-1344-10	1000s	$41.25
Purepac	00228-2327-96	1000s	$48.82
Parmed	00349-8936-10	1000s	$59.45
Sidmak	50111-0467-03	1000s	$61.05
Goldline	00182-1758-10	1000s	$61.05
Aligen	00405-4884-03	1000s	$61.20
Watson	52544-0305-10	1000s	$65.99
Mylan	00378-0182-10	1000s	$66.10
Sidmak	50111-0467-07	5000s	$296.18

TABLET: 20 MG

AVERAGE UNIT PRICE (AVAILABLE SIZES)		GENERIC A-RATED AVERAGE PRICE (GAAP)	
BRAND	$0.44	100s	$11.27
GENERIC	$0.10	500s	$33.23
HCFA FUL (100s ea)	$0.02	1000s	$63.73

BRAND/MANUFACTURER	NDC	SIZE	AWP
◆ BRAND			
➤ INDERAL: Wyeth-Ayerst	00046-0422-81	100s	$43.91
	00046-0422-99	100s ud	$48.04
	00046-0422-91	1000s	$430.04
	00046-0422-95	5000s	$2123.56
◆ GENERICS			
Medirex	57480-0356-06	30s	$7.86
Warner Chilcott	00047-0071-24	100s	$5.35
Qualitest	00603-5490-21	100s	$5.74
Interpharm	53746-0217-01	100s	$5.75
➤ Rugby	00536-4313-01	100s	$5.80
Major	00904-0412-60	100s	$6.00
➤ Schein	00364-0757-01	100s	$6.50
Caremark	00339-5317-12	100s	$6.52
Raway	00686-0278-20	100s	$7.65
➤ Purepac	00228-2329-10	100s	$8.17
URL	00677-1042-01	100s	$8.70
Geneva	00781-1354-01	100s	$8.75
Aligen	00405-4885-01	100s	$8.97
Sidmak	50111-0468-01	100s	$8.97
Goldline	00182-1759-01	100s	$8.97
Watson	52544-0306-01	100s	$9.95
Mylan	00378-0183-01	100s	$10.55
➤ Lederle Std Prod	00005-3110-23	100s	$12.61
U.S. Trading	56126-0322-11	100s ud	$3.74
➤ Schein	00364-0757-90	100s ud	$14.75
Geneva	00781-1354-13	100s ud	$15.25
Major	00904-0412-61	100s ud	$16.77
Vangard	00615-2562-13	100s ud	$17.35
UDL	51079-0278-20	100s ud	$26.20
Medirex	57480-0356-01	100s ud	$26.20
Goldline	00182-1813-89	100s ud	$26.60
➤ Rugby	00536-4313-05	500s	$25.60
➤ Purepac	00228-2329-50	500s	$40.85
Warner Chilcott	00047-0071-32	1000s	$44.01
➤ Schein	00364-0757-02	1000s	$49.25
➤ Rugby	00536-4313-10	1000s	$49.50
Moore,H.L.	00839-7115-16	1000s	$49.53
Qualitest	00603-5490-32	1000s	$49.70
Major	00904-0412-80	1000s	$49.90
Martec	52555-0344-10	1000s	$49.95
Interpharm	53746-0217-10	1000s	$50.00
Mason Dist	11845-0258-04	1000s	$50.84
URL	00677-1042-10	1000s	$58.45
Geneva	00781-1354-10	1000s	$58.50
➤ Purepac	00228-2329-96	1000s	$66.34
Parmed	00349-8937-10	1000s	$73.83
Sidmak	50111-0468-03	1000s	$85.91
Goldline	00182-1759-10	1000s	$85.91
Aligen	00405-4885-03	1000s	$85.98
Watson	52544-0306-10	1000s	$94.50
Mylan	00378-0183-10	1000s	$94.95
Sidmak	50111-0468-07	5000s	$416.68

TABLET: 40 MG

AVERAGE UNIT PRICE (AVAILABLE SIZES)		GENERIC A-RATED AVERAGE PRICE (GAAP)	
BRAND	$0.54	100s	$15.96
GENERIC	$0.13	500s	$62.96
HCFA FUL (100s ea)	$0.03	1000s	$83.79

BRAND/MANUFACTURER	NDC	SIZE	AWP
◆ BRAND			
➤ INDERAL: Wyeth-Ayerst	00046-0424-80	100s	$41.43
	00046-0424-81	100s	$56.99
	00046-0424-99	100s ud	$61.08
	00046-0424-91	1000s	$558.11
	00046-0424-95	5000s	$2755.79
◆ GENERICS			
Medirex	57480-0357-06	30s	$11.85
Warner Chilcott	00047-0072-24	100s	$7.60
Rugby	00536-4314-01	100s	$7.80
Interpharm	53746-0219-01	100s	$7.95
Schein	00364-0758-01	100s	$8.50
Major	00904-0460-01	100s	$8.60
Caremark	00339-5319-12	100s	$9.13
Raway	00686-0279-20	100s	$9.20
Geneva	00781-1364-01	100s	$12.40
URL	00677-1043-01	100s	$12.75
Purepac	00228-2331-10	100s	$12.78
Sidmak	50111-0469-01	100s	$12.87
Goldline	00182-1760-01	100s	$12.87
Aligen	00405-4886-01	100s	$12.89
Watson	52544-0307-01	100s	$13.95
Mylan	00378-0184-01	100s	$14.80
Schein	00364-0758-90	100s	$15.25
Lederle Std Prod	00005-3111-23	100s	$18.19

BRAND/MANUFACTURER	NDC	SIZE	AWP
U.S. Trading	56126-0323-11	100s ud	$3.69
Geneva	00781-1364-13	100s ud	$16.95
Major	00904-0414-61	100s ud	$21.51
Vangard	00615-2563-13	100s ud	$24.30
UDL	51079-0279-20	100s ud	$39.50
Medirex	57480-0357-01	100s ud	$39.50
Goldline	00182-1814-89	100s ud	$40.00
Rugby	00536-4314-05	500s	$37.60
Purepac	00228-2331-50	500s	$63.90
Lederle Std Prod	00005-3111-31	500s	$87.38
Qualitest	00603-5491-32	1000s	$57.76
Schein	00364-0758-02	1000s	$58.25
Rugby	00536-4314-10	1000s	$58.50
Major	00904-0414-80	1000s	$58.75
Martec	52555-0345-10	1000s	$59.25
Warner Chilcott	00047-0072-32	1000s	$59.50
Moore,H.L.	00839-7116-16	1000s	$64.25
Mason Dist	11845-0259-04	1000s	$65.58
URL	00677-1043-10	1000s	$69.85
Geneva	00781-1364-10	1000s	$69.90
Interpharm	53746-0219-10	1000s	$72.50
Purepac	00228-2331-96	1000s	$86.44
Parmed	00349-8938-10	1000s	$90.90
Sidmak	50111-0469-03	1000s	$123.75
Goldline	00182-1760-10	1000s	$123.75
Aligen	00405-4886-03	1000s	$123.82
Watson	52544-0307-10	1000s	$132.50
Mylan	00378-0184-10	1000s	$132.95
Sidmak	50111-0469-07	5000s	$600.16

TABLET: 60 MG

AVERAGE UNIT PRICE (AVAILABLE SIZES)		GENERIC A-RATED AVERAGE PRICE (GAAP)	
BRAND	$0.77	100s	$11.74
GENERIC	$0.13	500s	$72.51
HCFA FUL (100s ea)	$0.02		

BRAND/MANUFACTURER	NDC	SIZE	AWP
◆ **BRAND**			
➤ INDERAL: Wyeth-Ayerst	00046-0426-81	100s	$78.84
	00046-0426-91	1000s	$757.73
◆ **GENERICS**			
Qualitest	00603-5492-21	100s	$6.91
Rugby	00536-4315-01	100s	$8.80
Moore,H.L.	00839-7117-06	100s	$8.91
Warner Chilcott	00047-0073-24	100s	$9.15
Geneva	00781-1374-01	100s	$10.50
Schein	00364-0759-01	100s	$12.00
Caremark	00339-5320-12	100s	$12.47
Purepac	00228-2321-10	100s	$15.30
Watson	52544-0352-01	100s	$15.95
Goldline	00182-1761-01	100s	$17.60
Sidmak	50111-0470-01	100s	$17.66
U.S. Trading	56126-0392-11	100s ud	$5.58
Qualitest	00603-5492-28	500s	$36.12
Parmed	00349-8736-05	500s	$52.93
Watson	52544-0352-05	500s	$75.76
Sidmak	50111-0470-02	500s	$85.80
Lederle Std Prod	00005-3102-31	500s	$111.96

TABLET: 80 MG

AVERAGE UNIT PRICE (AVAILABLE SIZES)		GENERIC A-RATED AVERAGE PRICE (GAAP)	
BRAND	$0.86	100s	$19.36
GENERIC	$0.18	500s	$78.75
HCFA FUL (100s ea)	$0.03		

BRAND/MANUFACTURER	NDC	SIZE	AWP
◆ **BRAND**			
➤ INDERAL: Wyeth-Ayerst	00046-0428-81	100s	$87.50
	00046-0428-91	1000s	$857.01
	00046-0428-95	5000s	$4208.49
◆ **GENERICS**			
Warner Chilcott	00047-0074-24	100s	$11.89
Rugby	00536-4316-01	100s	$11.90
Major	00904-0418-60	100s	$11.90
Qualitest	00603-5493-21	100s	$11.94
Interpharm	53746-0220-01	100s	$12.10
Schein	00364-0760-01	100s	$14.25
Caremark	00339-5321-12	100s	$14.26
Geneva	00781-1384-01	100s	$14.75
Raway	00686-0280-20	100s	$15.50
URL	00677-1044-01	100s	$18.89
Purepac	00228-2333-10	100s	$18.94
Sidmak	50111-0471-01	100s	$21.45
Goldline	00182-1762-01	100s	$21.45
Aligen	00405-4888-01	100s	$21.48
Watson	52544-0308-01	100s	$21.50
Mylan	00378-0185-01	100s	$21.75
Lederle Std Prod	00005-3112-23	100s	$30.33
U.S. Trading	56126-0324-11	100s ud	$4.40
UDL	51079-0280-20	100s ud	$44.00
Goldline	00182-1815-89	100s ud	$44.60

BRAND/MANUFACTURER	NDC	SIZE	AWP
Moore,H.L.	00839-7118-12	500s	$50.92
Rugby	00536-4316-05	500s	$54.80
Major	00904-0418-40	500s	$54.90
Qualitest	00603-5493-28	500s	$56.10
Schein	00364-0760-05	500s	$56.85
Geneva	00781-1384-05	500s	$56.88
Interpharm	53746-0220-05	500s	$57.10
URL	00677-1044-05	500s	$67.24
Purepac	00228-2333-50	500s	$67.29
Parmed	00349-8952-05	500s	$77.38
Watson	52544-0308-05	500s	$101.95
Sidmak	50111-0471-02	500s	$103.18
Goldline	00182-1762-05	500s	$103.18
Aligen	00405-4888-02	500s	$103.22
Mylan	00378-0185-05	500s	$103.30
Lederle Std Prod	00005-3112-31	500s	$145.74
Interpharm	53746-0220-10	1000s	$108.35

SODIUM BICARBONATE

INJECTION: 7.5%

BRAND/MANUFACTURER	NDC	SIZE	AWP
○ **GENERICS**			
Allscrips	54569-2220-00	50 ml	$17.86
Astra	00186-0647-01	50 ml 10s	$111.63
Amer Regent	00517-0639-25	50 ml 25s	$54.69
Intl Med Sys	00548-1002-00	50 ml 25s	$232.13
Intl Med Sys	00548-2002-00	50 ml 25s	$243.38
Intl Med Sys	00548-3002-00	50 ml 25s	$581.25
Raway	00686-0639-25	50 ml 50s	$120.00

INJECTION: 8.4%

AVERAGE UNIT PRICE (AVAILABLE SIZES)	
GENERIC	$0.44

BRAND/MANUFACTURER	NDC	SIZE	AWP
◆ **GENERICS**			
Fujisawa	00469-0600-60	50 ml	$2.89
Abbott Hosp	00074-4900-01	10 ml 10s	$123.03
Abbott Hosp	00074-6637-01	50 ml 10s	$179.31
Abbott Hosp	00074-6625-02	50 ml 25s	$160.91

INJECTION: 8.4%

BRAND/MANUFACTURER	NDC	SIZE	AWP
○ **GENERICS**			
Astra	00186-0656-01	10 ml 10s	$78.75
Abbott Hosp	00074-4900-23	10 ml 10s	$135.85
Astra	00186-0650-01	50 ml 10s	$111.63
Abbott Hosp	00074-6637-23	50 ml 10s	$192.14
Intl Med Sys	00548-1032-00	10 ml 25s	$223.13
Abbott Hosp	00074-4900-33	10 ml 25s	$339.63
Amer Regent	00517-1550-25	50 ml 25s	$57.19
Fujisawa	00469-0019-25	50 ml 25s	$64.38
Intl Med Sys	00548-1052-00	50 ml 25s	$232.13
Intl Med Sys	00548-2052-00	50 ml 25s	$243.38
Abbott Hosp	00074-6637-33	50 ml 25s	$480.34
Intl Med Sys	00548-3052-00	50 ml 25s	$589.13
Raway	00686-1550-25	50 ml 50s	$120.00

SODIUM FLUORIDE AND VITAMINS, MULTI

CHEW TABLET: 1 MG

BRAND/MANUFACTURER	NDC	SIZE	AWP
○ **BRAND**			
MULVIDREN-F: Stuart	00038-0710-10	100s	$13.82
➤ POLY-VI-FLOR: Mead Johnson Nutr	00087-0474-02	100s	$14.99
VI-DAYLIN/F: Ross Pharm	00074-7626-13	100s	$15.13
ADEFLOR M: Kenwood	00482-0115-01	100s	$22.68
➤ POLY-VI-FLOR: Mead Johnson Nutr	00087-0474-03	1000s	$149.06
○ **GENERICS**			
Copley	38245-0166-10	100s	$3.40
Geneva	00781-1996-01	100s	$3.46
UNI MULTI FLUOR: URL	00677-0670-01	100s	$3.60
Schein	00364-1075-01	100s	$3.65
Amide	52152-0001-02	100s	$3.95
Moore,H.L.	00839-6218-06	100s	$3.98
Qualitest	00603-4712-21	100s	$3.98
POLYTABS-F: Major	00904-2698-60	100s	$4.65
Allscrips	54569-2384-00	100s	$4.91
Balan,J.J.	00304-0501-01	100s	$4.98
POLY-VITES W/FLUORIDE: Goldline	00182-4450-01	100s	$5.25
Rugby	00536-4307-01	100s	$5.81
FLORVITE: Everett	00642-0082-10	100s	$11.15
SOLUVITE-CT: Pharmics	00813-0078-01	100s	$12.89
Amide	52152-0001-05	1000s	$29.95
UNI MULTI FLUOR: URL	00677-0670-10	1000s	$31.05
Balan,J.J.	00304-0501-00	1000s	$31.98

◆ RATED THERAPEUTICALLY EQUIVELENT; ◇ THERAPEUTIC EQUIVALENT UNCONFIRMED; ○ UNRATED

BRAND/MANUFACTURER	NDC	SIZE	AWP
Copley	38245-0166-20	1000s	$33.00
Qualitest	00603-4712-32	1000s	$33.70
Moore,H.L.	00839-6218-16	1000s	$34.14
Rugby	00536-4307-10	1000s	$41.40

DROP: 0.25 MG/ML

BRAND/MANUFACTURER	NDC	SIZE	AWP
◆ GENERICS			
POLY-VITA W/FLUORIDE: Cenci,H.R.	00556-0447-50	50 ml	$3.70

DROP: 0.25 MG/ML

BRAND/MANUFACTURER	NDC	SIZE	AWP
○ BRAND			
POLY-VI-FLOR: Mead Johnson Nutr	00087-0451-41	50 ml	$10.95
VI-DAYLIN/F: Ross Pharm	00074-1104-50	50 ml	$11.49
○ GENERICS			
Moore,H.L.	00839-7258-99	50 ml	$3.63
Tri-Med	55654-0010-01	50 ml	$3.90
Hi-Tech	50383-0642-50	50 ml	$4.00
Qualitest	00603-1449-47	50 ml	$4.00
POLYVITE/FLUORIDE: Major	00904-2596-50	50 ml	$4.30
Allscrips	54569-1270-00	50 ml	$4.65
Schein	00364-0781-57	50 ml	$4.80
Goldline	00182-6096-67	50 ml	$4.95
Aligen	00405-3275-55	50 ml	$5.65
Rugby	00536-8560-80	50 ml	$5.93
FLORVITE PEDIATRIC: Everett	00642-0085-80	50 ml	$8.15

DROP: 0.5 MG/ML

BRAND/MANUFACTURER	NDC	SIZE	AWP
◆ GENERICS			
POLY-VITA W/FLUORIDE: Cenci,H.R.	00556-0463-50	50 ml	$3.70

DROP: 0.5 MG/ML

BRAND/MANUFACTURER	NDC	SIZE	AWP
○ BRAND			
POLY-VI-FLOR: Mead Johnson Nutr	00087-0472-02	50 ml	$10.95
○ GENERICS			
Moore,H.L.	00839-6240-99	50 ml	$3.23
Tri-Med	55654-0011-01	50 ml	$3.90
Hi-Tech	50383-0641-50	50 ml	$4.00
Qualitest	00603-1450-47	50 ml	$4.00
POLYVITE/FLUORIDE: Major	00904-2696-50	50 ml	$4.45
Schein	00364-7170-57	50 ml	$4.80
Allscrips	54569-1275-00	50 ml	$4.82
Aligen	00405-3330-55	50 ml	$5.65
Rugby	00536-8470-80	50 ml	$6.05
FLORVITE PEDIATRIC: Everett	00642-0084-80	50 ml	$8.15

SODIUM FLUORIDE/VITAMIN A/ VITAMIN C/VITAMIN D

DROP: 0.25 MG/ML

BRAND/MANUFACTURER	NDC	SIZE	AWP
○ BRAND			
TRI-VI-FLOR: Mead Johnson Nutr	00087-0452-41	50 ml	$9.87
VI-DAYLIN/F ADC: Ross Pharm	00074-1106-50	50 ml	$10.53
○ GENERICS			
Moore,H.L.	00839-7039-99	50 ml	$3.63
Cenci,H.R.	00556-0445-50	50 ml	$3.70
Tri-Med	55654-0012-01	50 ml	$3.90
Schein	00364-0783-57	50 ml	$3.90
Qualitest	00603-1785-47	50 ml	$3.90
Hi-Tech	50383-0637-50	50 ml	$4.00
Major	00904-2597-50	50 ml	$4.65
Barre	00472-0890-95	50 ml	$5.15
Aligen	00405-3850-55	50 ml	$5.65
TRIPLE VITAMIN W/FLUORIDE: Goldline	00182-6113-67	50 ml	$5.95
Rugby	00536-8520-80	50 ml	$6.05
Southwood	58016-9011-01	50 ml	$7.70
TRI-FLOR-VITE: Everett	00642-0080-80	50 ml	$8.15
R.I.D.	54807-0851-50	50 ml	$9.50
SOLUVITE-F: Pharmics	00813-0077-57	57 ml	$11.11
FLUORABON: Perry Med	11763-0519-20	60 ml	$3.29

DROP: 0.5 MG/ML

BRAND/MANUFACTURER	NDC	SIZE	AWP
○ BRAND			
TRI-VI-FLOR: Mead Johnson Nutr	00087-0473-02	50 ml	$9.99
○ GENERICS			
Moore,H.L.	00839-6358-99	50 ml	$3.63
Cenci,H.R.	00556-0462-50	50 ml	$3.70
Tri-Med	55654-0013-01	50 ml	$3.90
Qualitest	00603-1786-47	50 ml	$3.90
Hi-Tech	50383-0636-50	50 ml	$4.00

BRAND/MANUFACTURER	NDC	SIZE	AWP
Schein	00364-0782-57	50 ml	$4.50
Major	00904-2610-50	50 ml	$4.90
Barre	00472-0894-95	50 ml	$5.15
Aligen	00405-3875-55	50 ml	$5.65
Rugby	00536-8480-80	50 ml	$6.48
Southwood	58016-9012-01	50 ml	$8.29

SULFAMETHOXAZOLE AND TRIMETHOPRIM

TABLET: 800 MG-160 MG

AVERAGE UNIT PRICE (AVAILABLE SIZES)		GENERIC A-RATED AVERAGE PRICE (GAAP)	
BRAND	$1.05	20s	$5.26
GENERIC	$0.29	30s	$33.41
HCFA FUL (100s ea)	$0.09	100s	$28.20
		500s	$118.91

BRAND/MANUFACTURER	NDC	SIZE	AWP
◆ BRAND			
➤ SEPTRA DS: Burr Wellcome	00081-0853-55	100s	$114.89
➤ BACTRIM DS: Roche Labs	00004-0117-01	100s	$119.09
➤ SEPTRA DS: Burr Wellcome	00081-0853-56	100s ud	$114.89
	00081-0853-65	250s	$231.82
➤ BACTRIM DS: Roche Labs	00004-0117-04	250s	$240.06
	00004-0117-14	500s	$465.98
◆ GENERICS			
Cheshire	55175-3000-01	10s	$4.74
Cheshire	55175-3000-04	14s	$5.30
UROPLUS DS: Shionogi	45809-0911-24	20s	$4.83
Cheshire	55175-3000-00	20s	$5.69
UROPLUS DS: Shionogi	45809-0911-25	28s	$7.52
Cheshire	55175-3000-03	30s	$6.81
UDL	51079-0128-90	30s	$60.00
Cheshire	55175-3000-02	40s	$7.14
Cheshire	55175-3000-06	60s	$9.00
Raway	00686-2132-09	100s	$9.75
➤ Rugby	00536-4693-01	100s	$14.50
Eon	00185-0112-01	100s	$15.00
Roxane	00054-4801-25	100s	$15.95
➤ Schein	00364-2069-01	100s	$16.50
➤ Qualitest	00603-5779-21	100s	$17.20
UROPLUS DS: Shionogi	45809-0911-21	100s	$17.39
Geneva	00781-1063-01	100s	$18.13
Major	00904-2725-60	100s	$20.45
Martec	52555-0342-01	100s	$21.48
Interpharm	53746-0272-01	100s	$25.00
Moore,H.L.	00839-6406-06	100s	$26.33
➤ URL	00677-0784-01	100s	$28.50
Lemmon	00093-0089-01	100s	$28.50
➤ Mutual	53489-0146-01	100s	$28.50
➤ COTRIM DS: Lemmon	00093-0189-01	100s	$28.50
Parmed	00349-2336-01	100s	$34.00
➤ Biocraft	00332-2132-09	100s	$38.14
Goldline	00182-1408-01	100s	$38.14
➤ Apothecon	00003-0171-50	100s	$38.51
Sidmak	50111-0342-01	100s	$39.00
Aligen	00405-4929-01	100s	$39.00
U.S. Trading	56126-0140-11	100s ud	$9.80
Roxane	00054-8801-25	100s ud	$18.23
Vangard	00615-0170-13	100s ud	$27.42
Major	00904-2725-61	100s ud	$28.30
Raway	00686-0170-13	100s ud	$29.95
West-Ward	00143-1625-25	100s ud	$31.66
Geneva	00781-1063-13	100s ud	$36.00
Medirex	57480-0387-01	100s ud	$36.00
➤ Schein	00364-2069-90	100s ud	$62.75
Goldline	00182-8844-89	100s ud	$63.95
Mason Dist	11845-0188-03	500s	$66.61
➤ Rugby	00536-4693-05	500s	$67.70
Eon	00185-0112-05	500s	$69.95
UROPLUS DS: Shionogi	45809-0911-22	500s	$73.89
Martec	52555-0342-05	500s	$75.66
➤ Schein	00364-2069-05	500s	$75.75
➤ Qualitest	00603-5779-28	500s	$79.95
Major	00904-2725-40	500s	$81.25
Geneva	00781-1063-05	500s	$82.43
Interpharm	53746-0272-05	500s	$120.00
➤ URL	00677-0784-05	500s	$128.00
Mutual	53489-0146-05	500s	$128.00
Lemmon	00093-0089-05	500s	$128.50
➤ COTRIM DS: Lemmon	00093-0189-05	500s	$128.50
Parmed	00349-2336-05	500s	$133.98
➤ Biocraft	00332-2132-13	500s	$153.88
Goldline	00182-1408-05	500s	$153.88
Sidmak	50111-0342-02	500s	$155.00
Aligen	00405-4929-02	500s	$155.00
Moore,H.L.	00839-6406-12	500s	$162.74
Moore,H.L.	00839-7694-12	500s	$162.74
Lederle Std Prod	00005-3118-31	500s	$168.56
➤ Apothecon	00003-0171-60	500s	$182.87

➤ SHOWN IN PRODUCT IDENTIFICATION GUIDE

THEOPHYLLINE

CAPSULE, EXTENDED RELEASE: 250 MG

BRAND/MANUFACTURER	NDC	SIZE	AWP
◇ BRAND			
➤ SLO-PHYLLIN 250: RPR	00075-1356-00	100s	$43.31
THEOVENT: Schering	00085-0753-01	100s	$45.07
➤ SLO-PHYLLIN 250: RPR	00075-1356-99	1000s	$424.08

CAPSULE, EXTENDED RELEASE: 260 MG

BRAND/MANUFACTURER	NDC	SIZE	AWP
◇ BRAND			
THEOBID: Whitby	50474-0268-12	60s	$20.25
◇ GENERICS			
AEROLATE SR: Fleming	00256-0115-01	100s	$20.00
➤ THEOCLEAR L.A.-260: Central	00131-4248-37	100s	$22.50

CAPSULE, EXTENDED RELEASE: 300 MG

AVERAGE UNIT PRICE (AVAILABLE SIZES)		GENERIC A-RATED AVERAGE PRICE (GAAP)	
BRAND	$0.41	100s	$35.68
GENERIC	$0.36		

BRAND/MANUFACTURER	NDC	SIZE	AWP
◆ BRAND			
➤ SLO-BID GYROCAPS: RPR	00075-0300-00	100s	$41.35
	00075-0300-62	100s ud	$41.43
	00075-0300-99	1000s	$405.04
◆ GENERICS			
Warner Chilcott	00047-0199-24	100s	$34.80
Inwood	00258-3625-01	100s	$34.82
Lemmon	00093-0940-01	100s	$34.85
Thrift Drug Svcs	59198-0255-01	100s	$34.85
Arcola	00070-2343-00	100s	$35.10
Rugby	00536-5634-01	100s	$35.10
Major	00904-7849-60	100s	$36.55
Qualitest	00603-5952-21	100s	$36.56
Goldline	00182-1314-01	100s	$36.58
Schein	00364-2588-01	100s	$36.58
Aligen	00405-4985-01	100s	$36.65

CAPSULE, EXTENDED RELEASE: 300 MG

BRAND/MANUFACTURER	NDC	SIZE	AWP
◇ BRAND			
THEO-24: Whitby	50474-0300-01	100s	$38.99
	50474-0300-60	100s ud	$48.75
	50474-0300-50	500s	$187.17

CAPSULE, EXTENDED RELEASE: 400 MG

BRAND/MANUFACTURER	NDC	SIZE	AWP
○ BRAND			
THEO-24: Whitby	50474-0400-01	100s	$55.19
	50474-0400-60	100s ud	$59.33

ELIXIR: 80 MG/15 ML

AVERAGE UNIT PRICE (AVAILABLE SIZES)		GENERIC A-RATED AVERAGE PRICE (GAAP)	
BRAND	$0.13	480 ml	$12.62
GENERIC	$0.01	3840 ml	$12.62
HCFA FUL (480 ml)	$0.01	480 ml	$4.57
		3840 ml	$21.26
		15 ml 100s	$37.19
		30 ml 100s	$45.05

BRAND/MANUFACTURER	NDC	SIZE	AWP
◆ BRAND			
ELIXOPHYLLIN: Forest Pharm	00456-0644-16	480 ml	$62.34
	00456-0644-32	960 ml	$122.29
	00456-0644-28	3840 ml	$474.53
◆ GENERICS			
Moore,H.L.	00839-5029-69	480 ml	$3.50
Warner Chilcott	00047-2912-23	480 ml	$3.58
Major	00904-1444-16	480 ml	$3.60
Morton Grove	60432-0019-16	480 ml	$3.60
Qualitest	00603-1729-58	480 ml	$3.84
Rugby	00536-2100-85	480 ml	$4.29
Halsey Pharm	00879-0226-16	480 ml	$4.55
Goldline	00182-0226-40	480 ml	$5.50
Schein	00364-7060-16	480 ml	$5.80
Aligen	00405-3825-16	480 ml	$5.82
Geneva	00781-6600-16	480 ml	$5.94
Moore,H.L.	00839-5029-70	3840 ml	$15.11
Morton Grove	60432-0019-28	3840 ml	$20.00
Halsey Pharm	00879-0226-28	3840 ml	$20.25
Major	00904-1444-28	3840 ml	$20.65
Rugby	00536-2100-90	3840 ml	$20.95
Goldline	00182-0226-41	3840 ml	$25.35
Geneva	00781-6600-28	3840 ml	$26.17
Roxane	00054-8848-16	18.75 ml 40s ud	$22.79
Pharm Assoc	00121-0137-15	15 ml 100s ud	$34.80
Roxane	00054-8845-04	15 ml 100s ud	$39.58

BRAND/MANUFACTURER	NDC	SIZE	AWP
Pharm Assoc	00121-0137-30	30 ml 100s ud	$42.16
Roxane	00054-8846-04	30 ml 100s ud	$47.94

SOLUTION: 80 MG/15 ML

AVERAGE UNIT PRICE (AVAILABLE SIZES)	
BRAND	$0.05
GENERIC	$0.01

BRAND/MANUFACTURER	NDC	SIZE	AWP
◆ BRAND			
THEOLAIR: 3M Pharm	00089-0960-16	480 ml	$24.66
◆ GENERICS			
Roxane	00054-3841-63	500 ml	$7.31
Roxane	00054-3841-68	1000 ml	$12.44

SYRUP: 80 MG/15 ML

AVERAGE UNIT PRICE (AVAILABLE SIZES)	
BRAND	$0.05
GENERIC	$0.02
HCFA FUL (480 ml)	$0.04

BRAND/MANUFACTURER	NDC	SIZE	AWP
◆ BRAND			
SLO-PHYLLIN 80: RPR	00075-3650-16	480 ml	$21.58
◆ GENERICS			
THEOCLEAR-80: Central	00131-5098-70	480 ml	$12.30
THEOCLEAR-80: Central	00131-5098-72	3840 ml	$73.65

TABLET: 100 MG

BRAND/MANUFACTURER	NDC	SIZE	AWP
◆ BRAND			
➤ SLO-PHYLLIN: RPR	00075-0351-68	100s	$18.77

TABLET: 125 MG

BRAND/MANUFACTURER	NDC	SIZE	AWP
○ BRAND			
➤ THEOLAIR: 3M Pharm	00089-0342-10	100s	$31.20

TABLET: 200 MG

BRAND/MANUFACTURER	NDC	SIZE	AWP
◆ BRAND			
➤ SLO-PHYLLIN: RPR	00075-0352-68	100s	$24.94

TABLET: 250 MG

BRAND/MANUFACTURER	NDC	SIZE	AWP
○ BRAND			
➤ THEOLAIR: 3M Pharm	00089-0344-10	100s	$48.42

TABLET: 300 MG

BRAND/MANUFACTURER	NDC	SIZE	AWP
○ BRAND			
QUIBRON-T: Roberts Pharm	54092-0069-01	100s	$34.06

TABLET, EXTENDED RELEASE: 100 MG

AVERAGE UNIT PRICE (AVAILABLE SIZES)		GENERIC A-RATED AVERAGE PRICE (GAAP)	
BRAND	$0.16	100s	$11.97
GENERIC	$0.11	500s	$39.19
HCFA FUL (100s ea)	$0.06	1000s	$74.50

BRAND/MANUFACTURER	NDC	SIZE	AWP
◆ BRAND			
THEO-SAV: Savage	00281-0168-53	100s	$7.80
➤ THEO-DUR: Key	00085-0487-01	100s	$16.73
	00085-0487-81	100s ud	$25.07
	00085-0487-05	500s	$78.83
	00085-0487-10	1000s	$152.65
	00085-0487-50	5000s	$721.37
◆ GENERICS			
Medirex	57480-0365-06	30s	$4.35
➤ THEOX: Carnrick	00086-0031-10	100s	$7.40
Goldline	00182-1589-01	100s	$10.45
Warner Chilcott	00047-0657-24	100s	$10.53
Geneva	00781-1003-01	100s	$10.91
Qualitest	00603-5944-21	100s	$10.95
Moore,H.L.	00839-6730-06	100s	$11.19
Moore,H.L.	00839-7705-06	100s	$11.19
URL	00677-0845-01	100s	$11.20
Martec	52555-0702-01	100s	$11.20
Schein	00364-0801-01	100s	$11.25
Rugby	00536-4650-01	100s	$11.69
THEO-TIME: Major	00904-1610-60	100s	$11.70
Sidmak	50111-0483-01	100s	$11.70
Warrick	59930-1650-01	100s	$11.70

◆ RATED THERAPEUTICALLY EQUIVELENT; ◇ THERAPEUTIC EQUIVALENT UNCONFIRMED; ○ UNRATED

BRAND/MANUFACTURER	NDC	SIZE	AWP
➤ THEOCHRON: Inwood	00258-3584-01	100s	$11.85
THEOCHRON: Lemmon	00093-0599-01	100s	$12.16
Aligen	00405-4986-01	100s	$12.31
Parmed	00349-8280-01	100s	$12.50
Parmed	00349-8683-01	100s	$12.98
THEO-TIME: Major	00904-1610-61	100s ud	$14.94
Medirex	57480-0365-01	100s ud	$15.10
Goldline	00182-1589-89	100s ud	$18.50
➤ THEOX: Carnrick	00086-0031-50	500s	$32.75
➤ THEOCHRON: Inwood	00258-3584-05	500s	$37.95
Sidmak	50111-0483-02	500s	$38.00
Warrick	59930-1650-02	500s	$38.00
Qualitest	00603-5944-28	500s	$38.95
THEO-TIME: Major	00904-1610-40	500s	$42.70
Moore,H.L.	00839-6730-12	500s	$45.99
Warrick	59930-1650-03	1000s	$74.00
Sidmak	50111-0483-03	1000s	$75.00

TABLET, EXTENDED RELEASE: 200 MG

AVERAGE UNIT PRICE (AVAILABLE SIZES)		GENERIC A-RATED AVERAGE PRICE (GAAP)	
BRAND	$0.19	100s	$18.17
GENERIC	$0.16	500s	$72.12
HCFA FUL (100s ea)	$0.09	1000s	$145.04

BRAND/MANUFACTURER	NDC	SIZE	AWP
◆ BRAND			
THEO-SAV: Savage	00281-0169-53	100s	$11.11
➤ THEO-DUR: Key	00085-0933-01	100s	$24.91
	00085-0933-81	100s ud	$31.07
THEO-SAV: Savage	00281-0169-56	500s	$52.66
➤ THEO-DUR: Key	00085-0933-05	500s	$117.43
THEO-SAV: Savage	00281-0169-57	1000s	$96.26
➤ THEO-DUR: Key	00085-0933-10	1000s	$221.75
	00085-0933-50	5000s	$1076.20
◆ GENERICS			
Medirex	57480-0366-06	30s	$5.39
Parmed	00349-8281-60	60s	$7.37
➤ THEOX: Carnrick	00086-0032-10	100s	$10.70
Warner Chilcott	00047-0659-24	100s	$15.38
Qualitest	00603-5945-21	100s	$15.61
Geneva	00781-1004-01	100s	$15.81
URL	00677-0846-01	100s	$15.85
Martec	52555-0703-01	100s	$16.45
Moore,H.L.	00839-7706-06	100s	$17.67
➤ THEOCHRON: Inwood	00258-3583-01	100s	$18.65
Rugby	00536-4651-01	100s	$18.68
THEO-TIME: Major	00904-1611-60	100s	$18.75
Sidmak	50111-0482-01	100s	$19.00
Warrick	59930-1660-01	100s	$19.00
Goldline	00182-1590-01	100s	$19.00
Schein	00364-0681-01	100s	$19.25
THEOCHRON: Lemmon	00093-0589-01	100s	$19.42
Moore,H.L.	00839-6729-06	100s	$19.44
Parmed	00349-8684-01	100s	$19.60
Parmed	00349-8281-01	100s	$19.95
Aligen	00405-4987-01	100s	$20.00
THEO-TIME: Major	00904-1611-61	100s ud	$16.61
Qualitest	00603-5945-29	100s ud	$17.94
Medirex	57480-0366-01	100s ud	$20.25
Goldline	00182-1590-89	100s ud	$25.00
➤ THEOX: Carnrick	00086-0032-50	500s	$49.80
URL	00677-0846-05	500s	$61.50
THEO-TIME: Major	00904-1611-40	500s	$62.25
Moore,H.L.	00839-6729-12	500s	$62.44
Moore,H.L.	00839-7706-12	500s	$62.44
Warner Chilcott	00047-0659-30	500s	$65.08
Qualitest	00603-5945-28	500s	$65.70
Geneva	00781-1004-05	500s	$72.92
Parmed	00349-8281-05	500s	$79.90
Rugby	00536-4651-05	500s	$81.75
➤ THEOCHRON: Inwood	00258-3583-05	500s	$81.95
Sidmak	50111-0482-02	500s	$82.00
Warrick	59930-1660-02	500s	$82.00
Schein	00364-0681-05	500s	$85.75
Aligen	00405-4987-02	500s	$86.32
➤ THEOX: Carnrick	00086-0032-90	1000s	$91.35
Qualitest	00603-5945-32	1000s	$127.85
Martec	52555-0703-10	1000s	$128.15
Mason Dist	11845-0359-04	1000s	$147.77
Parmed	00349-8684-10	1000s	$149.95
Moore,H.L.	00839-6729-16	1000s	$150.38
Sidmak	50111-0482-03	1000s	$155.00
Warrick	59930-1660-03	1000s	$155.00
Goldline	00182-1590-10	1000s	$155.00
Rugby	00536-4651-10	1000s	$155.03
Major	00904-1611-80	1000s	$155.10
➤ THEOCHRON: Inwood	00258-3583-10	1000s	$156.00
Parmed	00349-8281-10	1000s	$158.95

TABLET, EXTENDED RELEASE: 200 MG

BRAND/MANUFACTURER	NDC	SIZE	AWP
◇ BRAND			
➤ THEOLAIR-SR: 3M Pharm	00089-0341-10	100s	$27.00
➤ T-PHYL: Purdue Frederick	00034-7102-80	100s	$37.38
➤ THEOLAIR-SR: 3M Pharm	00089-0341-80	1000s	$66.00

TABLET, EXTENDED RELEASE: 250 MG

BRAND/MANUFACTURER	NDC	SIZE	AWP
◇ BRAND			
➤ RESPBID: Boehr Ingelheim	00597-0048-01	100s	$31.03
➤ THEOLAIR-SR: 3M Pharm	00089-0345-10	100s	$31.86

TABLET, EXTENDED RELEASE: 300 MG

AVERAGE UNIT PRICE (AVAILABLE SIZES)		GENERIC A-RATED AVERAGE PRICE (GAAP)	
BRAND	$0.23	100s	$21.65
GENERIC	$0.19	500s	$90.21
HCFA FUL (100s ea)	$0.12	1000s	$176.76

BRAND/MANUFACTURER	NDC	SIZE	AWP
◆ BRAND			
THEO-SAV: Savage	00281-0170-53	100s	$14.40
➤ THEO-DUR: Key	00085-0584-01	100s	$29.59
	00085-0584-81	100s ud	$36.98
THEO-SAV: Savage	00281-0170-56	500s	$63.34
➤ THEO-DUR: Key	00085-0584-05	500s	$139.48
THEO-SAV: Savage	00281-0170-57	1000s	$116.86
➤ THEO-DUR: Key	00085-0584-10	1000s	$269.88
	00085-0584-50	5000s	$1277.58
◆ GENERICS			
Medirex	57480-0367-06	30s	$6.39
Parmed	00349-8266-60	60s	$7.68
➤ THEOX: Carnrick	00086-0033-10	100s	$13.95
Geneva	00781-1005-01	100s	$18.52
Warner Chilcott	00047-0592-24	100s	$19.35
Qualitest	00603-5946-21	100s	$19.59
Parmed	00349-8685-01	100s	$20.87
Goldline	00182-1400-01	100s	$21.00
Martec	52555-0704-01	100s	$21.10
Moore,H.L.	00839-6693-06	100s	$21.18
URL	00677-0817-01	100s	$21.45
Schein	00364-0660-01	100s	$21.50
THEO-TIME: Major	00904-1612-60	100s	$21.95
Rugby	00536-4652-01	100s	$21.95
➤ Sidmak	50111-0459-01	100s	$22.00
Warrick	59930-1670-01	100s	$22.00
THEOCHRON: Lemmon	00093-0589-01	100s	$22.10
➤ THEOCHRON: Inwood	00258-3581-01	100s	$22.75
Aligen	00405-4988-01	100s	$23.16
Parmed	00349-8266-01	100s	$23.95
THEO-TIME: Major	00904-1612-61	100s ud	$19.43
Qualitest	00603-5946-29	100s ud	$21.90
Medirex	57480-0367-01	100s ud	$26.10
Goldline	00182-1400-89	100s ud	$30.50
➤ THEOX: Carnrick	00086-0033-50	500s	$60.25
Qualitest	00603-5946-28	500s	$75.81
THEO-TIME: Major	00904-1612-40	500s	$76.90
Geneva	00781-1005-05	500s	$79.73
Warner Chilcott	00047-0592-30	500s	$79.81
Parmed	00349-8685-05	500s	$94.65
Goldline	00182-1400-05	500s	$95.00
Parmed	00349-8266-05	500s	$96.95
URL	00677-0817-05	500s	$98.00
Warrick	59930-1670-02	500s	$98.00
Rugby	00536-4652-05	500s	$98.02
➤ THEOCHRON: Inwood	00258-3581-05	500s	$98.28
➤ Sidmak	50111-0459-02	500s	$98.50
Schein	00364-0660-05	500s	$99.50
Aligen	00405-4988-02	500s	$103.68
➤ THEOX: Carnrick	00086-0033-90	1000s	$110.55
Qualitest	00603-5946-32	1000s	$147.51
Moore,H.L.	00839-7707-16	1000s	$152.81
Martec	52555-0704-10	1000s	$162.30
Mason Dist	11845-0360-04	1000s	$179.91
Moore,H.L.	00839-6693-16	1000s	$183.40
➤ THEOCHRON: Inwood	00258-3581-10	1000s	$188.92
Schein	00364-0660-02	1000s	$188.95
Goldline	00182-1400-10	1000s	$189.00
Rugby	00536-4652-10	1000s	$189.38
Major	00904-1612-80	1000s	$189.90
Parmed	00349-8266-10	1000s	$189.95
➤ Sidmak	50111-0459-03	1000s	$190.00
Warrick	59930-1670-03	1000s	$190.00
Parmed	00349-8685-10	1000s	$198.80

TABLET, EXTENDED RELEASE: 300 MG

BRAND/MANUFACTURER	NDC	SIZE	AWP
◇ BRAND			
➤ THEOLAIR-SR: 3M Pharm	00089-0343-10	100s	$31.86
	00089-0343-80	1000s	$79.20

➤ SHOWN IN PRODUCT IDENTIFICATION GUIDE

TABLET, EXTENDED RELEASE: 300 MG

BRAND/MANUFACTURER	NDC	SIZE	AWP
○ **BRAND**			
QUIBRON-T/SR: Roberts Pharm	54092-0070-01	100s	$35.53
	54092-0070-05	500s	$159.89
○ **GENERICS**			
Southwood	58016-0443-06	6s	$5.34
Allscrips	54569-2483-04	10s	$2.12
Allscrips	54569-2483-03	20s	$4.24
Cheshire	55175-4181-02	20s	$6.49
Southwood	58016-0443-20	20s	$8.29
Pharm Corp/America	51655-0257-76	25s	$6.40
Allscrips	54569-2483-02	30s	$6.36
Cheshire	55175-4181-03	30s	$8.36
Southwood	58016-0443-30	30s	$9.26
Southwood	58016-0443-60	60s	$11.60
Allscrips	54569-2483-00	60s	$12.72
Interstate	00814-7805-14	100s	$18.23
Southwood	58016-0443-00	100s	$18.86
Allscrips	54569-2483-01	100s	$21.20
Allscrips	54569-2905-00	100s ud	$27.00
Interstate	00814-7805-28	500s	$80.18

TABLET, EXTENDED RELEASE: 400 MG

BRAND/MANUFACTURER	NDC	SIZE	AWP
○ **BRAND**			
➤ UNIPHYL: Purdue Frederick	00034-7004-80	100s	$66.64
	00034-7004-70	500s	$328.85

TABLET, EXTENDED RELEASE: 450 MG

AVERAGE UNIT PRICE (AVAILABLE SIZES)		GENERIC A-RATED AVERAGE PRICE (GAAP)	
BRAND	$0.44	100s	$30.29
GENERIC	$0.30		

BRAND/MANUFACTURER	NDC	SIZE	AWP
◆ **BRAND**			
➤ THEO-DUR: Key	00085-0806-01	100s	$39.28
	00085-0806-81	100s ud	$49.10
◆ **GENERICS**			
Sidmak	50111-0518-01	100s	$27.75
Warrick	59930-1680-01	100s	$27.75
Qualitest	00603-5747-21	100s	$28.58
Martec	52555-0705-01	100s	$29.65
Geneva	00781-1928-01	100s	$29.72
Aligen	00405-4990-01	100s	$29.77
URL	00677-1410-01	100s	$32.90
Major	00904-1613-60	100s	$32.95
Goldline	00182-1941-01	100s	$33.50

TABLET, EXTENDED RELEASE: 500 MG

BRAND/MANUFACTURER	NDC	SIZE	AWP
◇ **BRAND**			
➤ RESPBID: Boehr Ingelheim	00597-0049-01	100s	$44.88
➤ THEOLAIR-SR: 3M Pharm	00089-0347-10	100s	$47.64

THIORIDAZINE HYDROCHLORIDE

TABLET: 50 MG

AVERAGE UNIT PRICE (AVAILABLE SIZES)		GENERIC A-RATED AVERAGE PRICE (GAAP)	
BRAND	$0.49	100s	$21.19
GENERIC	$0.19	1000s	$151.16
HCFA FUL (100s ea)	$0.07		

BRAND/MANUFACTURER	NDC	SIZE	AWP
◆ **BRAND**			
➤ MELLARIL: Sandoz Pharm	00078-0004-05	100s	$48.66
	00078-0004-06	100s ud	$50.70
	00078-0004-09	1000s	$471.24
◆ **GENERICS**			
Medirex	57480-0364-06	30s	$9.12
Raway	00686-0616-01	100s	$9.88
Schein	00364-2318-01	100s	$15.75
Major	00904-1617-60	100s	$15.80
Qualitest	00603-5994-21	100s	$15.87
Rugby	00536-4643-01	100s	$15.90
Goldline	00182-1580-01	100s	$15.95
Geneva	00781-1634-01	100s	$16.50
Parmed	00349-8270-01	100s	$16.60
URL	00677-0825-01	100s	$17.00
Mutual	53489-0150-01	100s	$17.00
Aligen	00405-4996-01	100s	$17.20
Mylan	00378-0616-01	100s	$18.50
Moore,H.L.	00839-6705-06	100s	$19.24
Creighton	50752-0267-05	100s	$39.02
U.S. Trading	56126-0099-11	100s ud	$6.77
Raway	00686-0567-20	100s ud	$12.75
Major	00904-1796-61	100s ud	$20.57
Vangard	00615-2507-13	100s ud	$27.76
Geneva	00781-1634-13	100s ud	$29.75
UDL	51079-0567-20	100s ud	$29.89

BRAND/MANUFACTURER	NDC	SIZE	AWP
Creighton	50752-0267-06	100s ud	$40.70
Medirex	57480-0364-01	100s ud	$47.85
Rugby	00536-4643-05	500s	$72.20
Major	00904-1617-80	1000s	$82.10
Aligen	00405-4996-03	1000s	$100.90
Qualitest	00603-5994-32	1000s	$135.80
Rugby	00536-4643-10	1000s	$135.94
Major	00904-1796-80	1000s	$136.00
Goldline	00182-1580-10	1000s	$136.00
URL	00677-0825-10	1000s	$137.69
Mylan	00378-0616-10	1000s	$137.70
Schein	00364-2318-02	1000s	$141.75
Parmed	00349-8270-10	1000s	$142.70
Geneva	00781-1634-10	1000s	$143.55
Moore,H.L.	00839-6705-16	1000s	$144.45
Mutual	53489-0150-10	1000s	$163.50
Creighton	50752-0267-09	1000s	$378.22

TABLET: 100 MG

AVERAGE UNIT PRICE (AVAILABLE SIZES)		GENERIC A-RATED AVERAGE PRICE (GAAP)	
BRAND	$0.57	100s	$25.13
GENERIC	$0.25	500s	$94.61
HCFA FUL (100s ea)	$0.11	1000s	$247.99

BRAND/MANUFACTURER	NDC	SIZE	AWP
◆ **BRAND**			
➤ MELLARIL: Sandoz Pharm	00078-0005-05	100s	$57.12
	00078-0005-06	100s	$59.22
	00078-0005-09	1000s	$556.74
◆ **GENERICS**			
Raway	00686-0618-01	100s	$14.50
Qualitest	00603-5995-21	100s	$20.30
Rugby	00536-4644-01	100s	$21.19
URL	00677-0832-01	100s	$21.25
Goldline	00182-1584-01	100s	$21.25
Schein	00364-0670-01	100s	$21.45
Geneva	00781-1644-01	100s	$21.58
Major	00904-1618-60	100s	$21.90
Moore,H.L.	00839-6720-06	100s	$23.36
Aligen	00405-4997-01	100s	$24.00
Mutual	53489-0500-01	100s	$24.00
Mylan	00378-0618-01	100s	$24.25
Parmed	00349-8273-01	100s	$25.63
Creighton	50752-0268-05	100s	$45.85
U.S. Trading	56126-0101-11	100s ud	$10.74
Raway	00686-0580-20	100s ud	$17.95
UDL	51079-0580-20	100s ud	$27.33
Vangard	00615-2508-13	100s ud	$34.06
Geneva	00781-1644-13	100s ud	$34.50
Creighton	50752-0268-06	100s ud	$47.53
Parmed	00349-8273-05	500s	$86.08
Rugby	00536-4644-05	500s	$103.13
Major	00904-1618-80	1000s	$180.70
Mylan	00378-0618-10	1000s	$180.95
Geneva	00781-1644-10	1000s	$183.43
Creighton	50752-0268-09	1000s	$446.86

TABLET: 150 MG

AVERAGE UNIT PRICE (AVAILABLE SIZES)		GENERIC A-RATED AVERAGE PRICE (GAAP)	
BRAND	$0.64	100s	$34.81
GENERIC	$0.35		
HCFA FUL (100s ea)	$0.21		

BRAND/MANUFACTURER	NDC	SIZE	AWP
◆ **BRAND**			
➤ MELLARIL: Sandoz Pharm	00078-0006-05	100s	$75.18
➤ MELLARIL: Sandocare	00078-0006-65	640s ud	$336.00
◆ **GENERICS**			
Schein	00364-0723-01	100s	$31.40
Rugby	00536-4654-01	100s	$31.65
Major	00904-7649-60	100s	$31.65
Aligen	00405-4998-01	100s	$34.42
Geneva	00781-1664-01	100s	$38.85
Creighton	50752-0269-05	100s	$60.33
U.S. Trading	56126-0310-11	100s ud	$19.17
Raway	00686-0177-20	100s ud	$31.00

TABLET: 200 MG

AVERAGE UNIT PRICE (AVAILABLE SIZES)		GENERIC A-RATED AVERAGE PRICE (GAAP)	
BRAND	$0.87	100s	$44.31
GENERIC	$0.43		
HCFA FUL (100s ea)	$0.24		

BRAND/MANUFACTURER	NDC	SIZE	AWP
◆ **BRAND**			
➤ MELLARIL: Sandoz Pharm	00078-0007-05	100s	$85.86
	00078-0007-06	100s ud	$87.90
◆ **GENERICS**			
Rugby	00536-4649-01	100s	$35.48
Major	00904-1799-60	100s	$36.10

◆ RATED THERAPEUTICALLY EQUIVELENT; ◇ THERAPEUTIC EQUIVALENT UNCONFIRMED; ○ UNRATED

BRAND/MANUFACTURER	NDC	SIZE	AWP
Schein	00364-0724-01	100s	$39.31
Aligen	00405-4999-01	100s	$41.95
Geneva	00781-1674-01	100s	$49.51
Creighton	50752-0270-05	100s	$68.68
U.S. Trading	56126-0311-11	100s ud	$20.25
Raway	00686-0178-20	100s ud	$37.00
Creighton	50752-0270-06	100s ud	$70.53
Rugby	00536-4649-05	500s	$164.78

THIOTHIXENE
THIOTHIXENE HYDROCHLORIDE
CONCENTRATE: 5 MG/ML

AVERAGE UNIT PRICE (AVAILABLE SIZES)		GENERIC A-RATED AVERAGE PRICE (GAAP)	
BRAND	$0.68	120 ml	$38.27
GENERIC	$0.33		
HCFA FUL (120 ml)	$0.21		

BRAND/MANUFACTURER	NDC	SIZE	AWP
◆ BRAND			
NAVANE: Roerig	00049-5750-47	120 ml	$81.80
◆ GENERICS			
Barre	00472-1457-91	30 ml	$11.48
Qualitest	00603-1762-54	120 ml	$31.25
Copley	38245-0613-14	120 ml	$31.75
Aligen	00405-3835-76	120 ml	$31.75
Roxane	00054-3872-50	120 ml	$35.21
Barre	00472-1457-94	120 ml	$38.44
Rugby	00536-2140-97	120 ml	$40.02
Major	00904-2899-20	120 ml	$40.10
Goldline	00182-6112-71	120 ml	$42.00
UDL	51079-0687-37	120 ml	$53.89

POWDER FOR INJECTION: 10 MG

BRAND/MANUFACTURER	NDC	SIZE	AWP
○ BRAND			
NAVANE: Roerig	00049-5765-83	1s	$35.35

THYROID
TABLET: 60 MG

BRAND/MANUFACTURER	NDC	SIZE	AWP
○ BRAND			
➤ ARMOUR THYROID: Forest Pharm	00456-0459-01	100s	$9.76
	00456-0459-63	100s ud	$16.39
	00456-0459-00	1000s	$94.31
	00456-0459-51	5000s	$366.38
○ GENERICS			
Richlyn	00115-4824-01	100s	$1.86
Major	00904-0761-60	100s	$4.80
R.I.D.	54807-0891-01	100s	$8.61
Norton,HN	50732-0686-01	100s	$8.87
Time-Cap	49483-0022-01	100s	$9.00
Jones Medical	52604-0627-01	100s	$12.15
Jones Medical	52604-0674-01	100s	$13.45
Veratex	17022-8643-06	1000s	$10.25
Rugby	00536-4702-10	1000s	$11.94
Moore,H.L.	00839-5041-16	1000s	$12.14
Truxton	00463-6201-10	1000s	$12.90
Interstate	00814-7865-30	1000s	$13.35
Richlyn	00115-4824-03	1000s	$14.25
URL	00677-0151-10	1000s	$17.75
Qualitest	00603-6046-32	1000s	$17.80
Schein	00364-0270-02	1000s	$18.00
Goldline	00182-0493-10	1000s	$18.00
WESTHROID: Jones-Western	52604-7073-02	1000s	$20.46
Major	00904-0761-80	1000s	$20.50
Jones Medical	52604-0627-02	1000s	$27.15
Norton,HN	50732-0686-10	1000s	$40.55
Time-Cap	49483-0022-10	1000s	$41.00
Jones Medical	52604-0674-02	1000s	$113.35
WESTHROID: Jones-Western	52604-7073-08	1008s	$20.70
WESTHROID: Jones-Western	52604-7074-08	1008s	$24.60
WESTHROID: Jones-Western	52604-7075-08	1008s	$24.60
WESTHROID: Jones-Western	52604-7076-08	1008s	$24.60
WESTHROID: Jones-Western	52604-7077-08	1008s	$24.60

TABLET: 90 MG

BRAND/MANUFACTURER	NDC	SIZE	AWP
○ BRAND			
➤ ARMOUR THYROID: Forest Pharm	00456-0460-01	100s	$15.42

TABLET: 120 MG

BRAND/MANUFACTURER	NDC	SIZE	AWP
◆ GENERICS			
Allscrips	54569-8585-00	90s	$12.59

TABLET: 120 MG

BRAND/MANUFACTURER	NDC	SIZE	AWP
○ BRAND			
➤ ARMOUR THYROID: Forest Pharm	00456-0461-01	100s	$18.05
	00456-0461-63	100s ud	$20.44
	00456-0461-00	1000s	$180.56
○ GENERICS			
Allscrips	54569-3180-02	60s	$1.92
Major	00904-0762-60	100s	$5.95
Norton,HN	50732-0687-01	100s	$10.28
Time-Cap	49483-0023-01	100s	$11.00
R.I.D.	54807-0892-01	100s	$12.44
Jones Medical	52604-0675-01	100s	$16.60
Jones Medical	52604-0628-01	100s	$21.15
Rugby	00536-4710-10	1000s	$15.50
Veratex	17022-8664-06	1000s	$16.50
Moore,H.L.	00839-1672-16	1000s	$17.27
Truxton	00463-6203-10	1000s	$17.40
Interstate	00814-7870-30	1000s	$20.18
Veratex	17022-8706-06	1000s	$20.95
Qualitest	00603-6047-32	1000s	$26.71
Major	00904-0762-80	1000s	$28.70
WESTHROID: Jones-Western	52604-7080-02	1000s	$28.86
URL	00677-0153-10	1000s	$29.95
Goldline	00182-0494-10	1000s	$30.00
Jones Medical	52604-0778-02	1000s	$43.85
Norton,HN	50732-0687-10	1000s	$59.50
Time-Cap	49483-0023-10	1000s	$60.00
WESTHROID: Jones-Western	52604-7080-08	1008s	$29.16
WESTHROID: Jones-Western	52604-7081-08	1008s	$33.66
WESTHROID: Jones-Western	52604-7082-08	1008s	$33.66
WESTHROID: Jones-Western	52604-7083-08	1008s	$33.66
WESTHROID: Jones-Western	52604-7084-08	1008s	$33.66

TABLET: 180 MG

BRAND/MANUFACTURER	NDC	SIZE	AWP
○ BRAND			
➤ ARMOUR THYROID: Forest Pharm	00456-0462-01	100s	$28.67
	00456-0462-00	1000s	$286.78
○ GENERICS			
Allscrips	54569-3181-01	30s	$1.03
Major	00904-0763-60	100s	$7.95
Norton,HN	50732-0600-01	100s	$19.64
Jones Medical	52604-0629-01	100s	$26.95
Rugby	00536-4711-10	1000s	$20.75
Qualitest	00603-6048-32	1000s	$33.30
Major	00904-0763-80	1000s	$36.70
Jones Medical	52604-0779-02	1000s	$54.40
Norton,HN	50732-0600-10	1000s	$115.35
WESTHROID: Jones-Western	52604-7087-08	1008s	$35.70
WESTHROID: Jones-Western	52604-7088-08	1008s	$38.70
WESTHROID: Jones-Western	52604-7089-08	1008s	$38.70
WESTHROID: Jones-Western	52604-7090-08	1008s	$43.03

TABLET: 240 MG

BRAND/MANUFACTURER	NDC	SIZE	AWP
○ BRAND			
➤ ARMOUR THYROID: Forest Pharm	00456-0463-01	100s	$42.95
○ GENERICS			
WESTHROID: Jones-Western	52604-7092-08	1008s	$40.74
WESTHROID: Jones-Western	52604-7093-08	1008s	$45.30

TABLET: 300 MG

BRAND/MANUFACTURER	NDC	SIZE	AWP
○ BRAND			
➤ ARMOUR THYROID: Forest Pharm	00456-0464-01	100s	$53.23
○ GENERICS			
WESTHROID: Jones-Western	52604-7096-08	1008s	$43.14
WESTHROID: Jones-Western	52604-7095-08	1008s	$47.94
WESTHROID: Jones-Western	52604-7097-08	1008s	$51.54

TRAZODONE HYDROCHLORIDE
TABLET: 150 MG

AVERAGE UNIT PRICE (AVAILABLE SIZES)		GENERIC A-RATED AVERAGE PRICE (GAAP)	
BRAND	$1.80	100s	$81.70
GENERIC	$0.78	250s	$168.53
HCFA FUL (100s ea)	$0.64	500s	$340.44

BRAND/MANUFACTURER	NDC	SIZE	AWP
◆ BRAND			
➤ DESYREL DIVIDOSE: Apothecon	00087-0778-43	100s	$185.46
	00087-0778-44	500s	$871.66
◆ GENERICS			
Warner Chilcott	00047-0716-24	100s	$69.05
Major	00904-3992-60	100s	$70.35
Moore,H.L.	00839-7507-06	100s	$72.36
Rugby	00536-4689-01	100s	$72.53
Qualitest	00603-6146-21	100s	$74.80

➤ SHOWN IN PRODUCT IDENTIFICATION GUIDE

BRAND/MANUFACTURER	NDC	SIZE	AWP
Parmed	00349-8824-01	100s	$79.06
Aligen	00405-5038-01	100s	$81.12
URL	00677-1302-01	100s	$88.45
Goldline	00182-1298-01	100s	$88.50
Martec	52555-0132-01	100s	$89.90
► Sidmak	50111-0441-01	100s	$89.95
Geneva	00781-1826-01	100s	$89.98
Schein	00364-2300-01	100s	$95.99
Major	00904-3992-70	250s	$149.00
Rugby	00536-4689-02	250s	$166.65
Parmed	00349-8824-25	250s	$189.95
► Sidmak	50111-0441-02	500s	$324.00
Moore,H.L.	00839-7507-12	500s	$356.87

TABLET: 300 MG

BRAND/MANUFACTURER	NDC	SIZE	AWP
◆ BRAND			
► DESYREL DIVIDOSE: Apothecon	00087-0796-41	100s	$330.08

TRIAMCINOLONE ACETONIDE, TOPICAL

CREAM: 0.1%

AVERAGE UNIT PRICE (AVAILABLE SIZES)		GENERIC A-RATED AVERAGE PRICE (GAAP)	
BRAND	$0.40	30 gm	$14.45
GENERIC	$0.08	454 gm	$14.45
HCFA FUL (15 gm)	$0.08	2270 gm	$73.62
HCFA FUL (80 gm)	$0.04	15 gm	$1.82
HCFA FUL (454 gm)	$0.04	30 gm	$3.42
		80 gm	$4.85
		454 gm	$19.51

BRAND/MANUFACTURER	NDC	SIZE	AWP
◆ BRAND			
ARISTOCORT TOPICAL: Fujisawa	57317-0092-15	15 gm	$8.48
KENALOG: Apothecon	00003-0506-20	15 gm	$10.40
ARISTOCORT A: Fujisawa	57317-0052-15	15 gm	$10.74
ARISTOCORT TOPICAL: Fujisawa	57317-0092-60	60 gm	$20.68
KENALOG: Apothecon	00003-0506-46	60 gm	$25.35
ARISTOCORT A: Fujisawa	57317-0052-60	60 gm	$27.48
KENALOG: Apothecon	00003-0506-49	80 gm	$30.65
ARISTOCORT TOPICAL: Fujisawa	57317-0092-24	240 gm	$65.24
ARISTOCORT A: Fujisawa	57317-0052-24	240 gm	$105.13
ARISTOCORT TOPICAL: Fujisawa	57317-0092-05	2383.5 gm	$99.58
KENALOG: Apothecon	00003-0506-89	2383.5 gm	$132.37
◆ GENERICS			
Thames	49158-0140-20	15 gm	$1.30
Clay-Park	45802-0064-35	15 gm	$1.30
TRIACET: Lemmon	00093-0937-15	15 gm	$1.40
NMC	23317-0301-15	15 gm	$1.52
Moore,H.L.	00839-6126-47	15 gm	$1.55
Schein	00364-7212-72	15 gm	$1.70
Fougera	00168-0004-15	15 gm	$1.82
Parmed	00349-8759-35	15 gm	$1.85
UDL	51079-0275-61	15 gm	$1.94
Geneva	00781-7036-27	15 gm	$1.95
Qualitest	00603-7851-74	15 gm	$2.01
Rugby	00536-5225-20	15 gm	$2.03
URL	00677-0747-40	15 gm	$2.05
Major	00904-2741-36	15 gm	$2.05
Goldline	00182-1217-51	15 gm	$2.05
G&W	00713-0225-15	15 gm	$2.52
KENONEL: Marnel	00682-4300-20	20 gm	$4.75
Thames	49158-0140-08	30 gm	$1.80
Schein	00364-7212-56	30 gm	$2.50
FLUTEX: Syosset	47854-0576-05	30 gm	$5.95
TRIDERM: Del-Ray	00316-0170-01	30 gm	$6.50
FLUTEX: Syosset	47854-0576-46	60 gm	$8.95
Thames	49158-0140-21	80 gm	$3.80
Clay-Park	45802-0064-36	80 gm	$4.12
Schein	00364-7212-60	80 gm	$4.25
TRIACET: Lemmon	00093-0937-81	80 gm	$4.50
Qualitest	00603-7851-90	80 gm	$4.64
Geneva	00781-7036-29	80 gm	$4.65
Moore,H.L.	00839-6126-46	80 gm	$4.79
URL	00677-0747-46	80 gm	$5.05
NMC	23317-0301-80	80 gm	$5.06
Rugby	00536-5225-30	80 gm	$5.10
Major	00904-2741-11	80 gm	$5.10
Goldline	00182-1217-50	80 gm	$5.10
Fougera	00168-0004-80	80 gm	$5.11
Parmed	00349-8759-17	80 gm	$5.30
G&W	00713-0225-80	80 gm	$6.13
TRIDERM: Del-Ray	00316-0170-03	90 gm	$9.63
FLUTEX: Syosset	47854-0576-29	120 gm	$10.95
Thames	49158-0140-16	454 gm	$16.00
Clay-Park	45802-0064-05	454 gm	$17.72
Major	00904-2741-27	454 gm	$18.55
Schein	00364-7212-16	454 gm	$18.60
Geneva	00781-7036-16	454 gm	$19.05
NMC	23317-0301-16	454 gm	$19.42
Fougera	00168-0004-16	454 gm	$19.97

BRAND/MANUFACTURER	NDC	SIZE	AWP
URL	00677-0747-44	454 gm	$20.83
Rugby	00536-5225-98	454 gm	$20.85
Goldline	00182-1217-45	454 gm	$21.90
FLUTEX: Syosset	47854-0576-13	480 gm	$17.00
Moore,H.L.	00839-6126-48	2270 gm	$58.04
Thames	49158-0140-22	2270 gm	$63.20
Major	00904-2741-33	2270 gm	$66.43
FLUTEX: Syosset	47854-0576-15	2270 gm	$74.00
Clay-Park	45802-0064-29	2270 gm	$75.60
Parmed	00349-9010-99	2270 gm	$76.03
URL	00677-0747-47	2270 gm	$79.50
Goldline	00182-1217-46	2270 gm	$79.50
Rugby	00536-5225-27	2270 gm	$92.24
NMC	23317-0301-05	2400 gm	$77.49

CREAM: 0.1%

BRAND/MANUFACTURER	NDC	SIZE	AWP
○ GENERICS			
Veratex	17022-5892-02	15 gm	$1.00
ARICIN: Interstate	00814-0851-93	15 gm	$1.65
CMC-Cons	00223-4448-15	15 gm	$2.10
TRIAMCOT: Truxton	00463-8052-15	15 gm	$2.40
Southwood	58016-3035-01	15 gm	$4.99
Cheshire	55175-4031-05	15 gm	$5.52
ARICIN: Interstate	00814-0851-72	30 gm	$2.33
DELTA-TRITEX: Dermol	50744-0576-05	30 gm	$3.72
Veratex	17022-5892-04	80 gm	$2.95
ARICIN: Interstate	00814-0851-97	80 gm	$4.88
CMC-Cons	00223-4448-80	80 gm	$5.00
Allscrips	54569-0765-00	80 gm	$5.11
DELTA-TRITEX: Dermol	50744-0576-80	80 gm	$7.02
Southwood	58016-3108-01	80 gm	$8.37
Cheshire	55175-4031-08	80 gm	$8.91
CMC-Cons	00223-4448-24	240 gm	$12.50

CREAM: 0.5%

AVERAGE UNIT PRICE (AVAILABLE SIZES)		GENERIC A-RATED AVERAGE PRICE (GAAP)	
BRAND	$1.55	15 gm	$3.71
GENERIC	$0.25		
HCFA FUL (15 gm)	$0.20		

BRAND/MANUFACTURER	NDC	SIZE	AWP
◆ BRAND			
ARISTOCORT TOPICAL: Fujisawa	57317-0102-15	15 gm	$23.04
ARISTOCORT A: Fujisawa	57317-0062-15	15 gm	$29.48
KENALOG: Apothecon	00003-1483-20	20 gm	$34.64
ARISTOCORT TOPICAL: Fujisawa	57317-0102-24	240 gm	$227.05
◆ GENERICS			
Parmed	00349-9011-35	15 gm	$2.63
Thames	49158-0141-20	15 gm	$2.80
Moore,H.L.	00839-6128-47	15 gm	$2.96
Clay-Park	45802-0065-35	15 gm	$3.14
Schein	00364-7213-72	15 gm	$3.45
Qualitest	00603-7852-74	15 gm	$3.95
Goldline	00182-1218-51	15 gm	$4.05
Fougera	00168-0002-15	15 gm	$4.20
URL	00677-0751-40	15 gm	$4.27
Rugby	00536-5200-20	15 gm	$4.28
Major	00904-2744-36	15 gm	$4.40
Major	00904-2844-36	15 gm	$4.40
FLUTEX: Syosset	47854-0646-36	30 gm	$10.95
Syosset	47854-0577-11	240 gm	$26.20

CREAM: 0.5%

BRAND/MANUFACTURER	NDC	SIZE	AWP
○ GENERICS			
Veratex	17022-5890-02	15 gm	$2.15
ARICIN: Interstate	00814-0852-93	15 gm	$3.90
Allscrips	54569-2025-00	15 gm	$4.20
Southwood	58016-3127-01	15 gm	$6.83
CINALOG: EconoMed	38130-0047-15	15 gm	$8.28
CMC-Cons	00223-4443-80	20 gm	$3.75
CMC-Cons	00223-4443-24	240 gm	$8.50

LOTION: 0.025%

HCFA FUL (60 ml)			$0.11
BRAND/MANUFACTURER	NDC	SIZE	AWP
◆ BRAND			
KENALOG: Apothecon	00003-0173-60	60 ml	$29.15

LOTION: 0.025%

BRAND/MANUFACTURER	NDC	SIZE	AWP
○ GENERICS			
Raway	00686-1248-02	60 ml	$7.50
CMC-Cons	00223-6635-60	60 ml	$11.50

◆ RATED THERAPEUTICALLY EQUIVELENT; ◇ THERAPEUTIC EQUIVALENT UNCONFIRMED; ○ UNRATED

LOTION: 0.1%

AVERAGE UNIT PRICE (AVAILABLE SIZES)		GENERIC A-RATED AVERAGE PRICE (GAAP)	
BRAND	$0.55	60 ml	$11.40
GENERIC	$0.19		
HCFA FUL (60 ml)	$0.12		

BRAND/MANUFACTURER	NDC	SIZE	AWP
◆ BRAND			
KENALOG: Apothecon	00003-0502-70	60 ml	$32.73
◆ GENERICS			
Thames	49158-0211-32	60 ml	$7.30
Schein	00364-7346-58	60 ml	$8.10
Qualitest	00603-7855-49	60 ml	$8.28
Goldline	00182-1777-68	60 ml	$8.70
Moore,H.L.	00839-6726-50	60 ml	$8.76
Rugby	00536-2360-61	60 ml	$9.74
Morton Grove	60432-0561-60	60 ml	$28.90

LOTION: 0.1%

BRAND/MANUFACTURER	NDC	SIZE	AWP
○ GENERICS			
Raway	00686-1250-02	60 ml	$8.50
CMC-Cons	00223-6636-60	60 ml	$12.50

OINTMENT: 0.025%

AVERAGE UNIT PRICE (AVAILABLE SIZES)		GENERIC A-RATED AVERAGE PRICE (GAAP)	
GENERIC	$0.06	454 gm	$8.30
HCFA FUL (15 gm)	$0.08	15 gm	$1.41
HCFA FUL (80 gm)	$0.04	80 gm	$3.49
		454 gm	$8.48

BRAND/MANUFACTURER	NDC	SIZE	AWP
◆ GENERICS			
Raway	00686-0054-35	15 gm	$1.00
Clay-Park	45802-0054-35	15 gm	$1.04
Moore,H.L.	00839-6392-47	15 gm	$1.07
Qualitest	00603-7858-74	15 gm	$1.34
Rugby	00536-5190-20	15 gm	$1.35
Goldline	00182-1394-51	15 gm	$1.45
Schein	00364-7359-72	15 gm	$1.56
G&W	00713-0229-15	15 gm	$2.44
Raway	00686-0054-36	80 gm	$2.50
Moore,H.L.	00839-6392-46	80 gm	$2.55
Clay-Park	45802-0054-36	80 gm	$2.80
Rugby	00536-5190-30	80 gm	$3.45
Goldline	00182-1394-53	80 gm	$3.60
Fougera	00168-0005-80	80 gm	$3.61
G&W	00713-0229-80	80 gm	$5.95
Raway	00686-0054-05	454 gm	$6.25
Clay-Park	45802-0054-05	454 gm	$7.66
Goldline	00182-1394-45	454 gm	$9.30
Rugby	00536-5190-98	454 gm	$10.35
Clay-Park	45802-0054-29	2270 gm	$32.40

OINTMENT: 0.025%

BRAND/MANUFACTURER	NDC	SIZE	AWP
○ GENERICS			
Allscrips	54569-2452-00	15 gm	$1.56
CMC-Cons	00223-4447-15	15 gm	$1.80
Southwood	58016-3161-01	30 gm	$5.13
CMC-Cons	00223-4447-80	80 gm	$4.25

OINTMENT: 0.1%

AVERAGE UNIT PRICE (AVAILABLE SIZES)		GENERIC A-RATED AVERAGE PRICE (GAAP)	
BRAND	$0.43	454 gm	$18.43
GENERIC	$0.08	2270 gm	$85.00
HCFA FUL (15 gm)	$0.08	15 gm	$1.88
HCFA FUL (80 gm)	$0.05	80 gm	$4.85
HCFA FUL (454 gm)	$0.05	454 gm	$19.95

BRAND/MANUFACTURER	NDC	SIZE	AWP
◆ BRAND			
ARISTOCORT TOPICAL: Fujisawa	57317-0112-15	15 gm	$8.48
KENALOG: Apothecon	00003-0508-15	15 gm	$10.39
ARISTOCORT A: Fujisawa	57317-0072-15	15 gm	$10.74
ARISTOCORT TOPICAL: Fujisawa	57317-0112-60	60 gm	$20.68
KENALOG: Apothecon	00003-0508-56	60 gm	$25.10
ARISTOCORT A: Fujisawa	57317-0072-60	60 gm	$27.48
ARISTOCORT TOPICAL: Fujisawa	57317-0112-24	240 gm	$65.24
KENALOG: Apothecon	00003-0508-60	240 gm	$89.18
ARISTOCORT TOPICAL: Fujisawa	57317-0112-05	2270 gm	$106.63
◆ GENERICS			
Thames	49158-0160-20	15 gm	$1.30
Clay-Park	45802-0055-35	15 gm	$1.36
NMC	23317-0306-15	15 gm	$1.52
Moore,H.L.	00839-6391-47	15 gm	$1.55
Fougera	00168-0006-15	15 gm	$1.91
UDL	51079-0276-61	15 gm	$1.94
Geneva	00781-7033-27	15 gm	$1.98

BRAND/MANUFACTURER	NDC	SIZE	AWP
Qualitest	00603-7859-74	15 gm	$2.01
Rugby	00536-5180-20	15 gm	$2.03
URL	00677-0753-40	15 gm	$2.05
Major	00904-2743-36	15 gm	$2.05
Schein	00364-7360-72	15 gm	$2.05
Goldline	00182-1395-51	15 gm	$2.05
G&W	00713-0228-15	15 gm	$2.52
Thames	49158-0160-08	30 gm	$1.80
Thames	49158-0160-21	80 gm	$2.80
Clay-Park	45802-0055-36	80 gm	$4.22
URL	00677-0753-46	80 gm	$4.75
Moore,H.L.	00839-6391-46	80 gm	$4.79
NMC	23317-0306-80	80 gm	$5.06
Rugby	00536-5180-30	80 gm	$5.10
Major	00904-2743-11	80 gm	$5.10
Geneva	00781-7033-29	80 gm	$5.10
Goldline	00182-1395-53	80 gm	$5.10
Fougera	00168-0006-80	80 gm	$5.15
G&W	00713-0228-80	80 gm	$6.13
TRIDERM: Del-Ray	00316-0175-03	90 gm	$9.16
Thames	49158-0160-16	454 gm	$16.00
Clay-Park	45802-0055-05	454 gm	$18.90
Rugby	00536-5180-98	454 gm	$20.85
Goldline	00182-1395-45	454 gm	$21.00
Major	00904-2743-27	480 gm	$20.50
Clay-Park	45802-0055-29	2270 gm	$77.76
Rugby	00536-5180-27	2270 gm	$92.24

OINTMENT: 0.1%

BRAND/MANUFACTURER	NDC	SIZE	AWP
○ GENERICS			
CINOLAR: Ocumed	51944-2255-72	15 gm	$1.00
Allscrips	54569-1124-00	15 gm	$1.84
CMC-Cons	00223-4446-15	15 gm	$2.10
Southwood	58016-3208-01	15 gm	$3.20
DELTA-TRITEX: Dermol	50744-0105-05	30 gm	$3.72
TRIDERM: Del-Ray	00316-0175-01	30 gm	$6.25
ARICIN: Interstate	00814-0854-97	80 gm	$4.88
Allscrips	54569-0767-00	80 gm	$5.15
CMC-Cons	00223-4446-80	80 gm	$6.00
Southwood	58016-3253-01	80 gm	$8.37
Allscrips	54569-2036-00	454 gm	$20.85

OINTMENT: 0.5%

AVERAGE UNIT PRICE (AVAILABLE SIZES)		GENERIC A-RATED AVERAGE PRICE (GAAP)	
BRAND	$1.54	15 gm	$3.81
GENERIC	$0.25		
HCFA FUL (15 gm)	$0.27		

BRAND/MANUFACTURER	NDC	SIZE	AWP
◆ BRAND			
ARISTOCORT TOPICAL: Fujisawa	57317-0113-15	15 gm	$23.04
◆ GENERICS			
Clay-Park	45802-0049-35	15 gm	$3.10
Goldline	00182-5068-51	15 gm	$4.05
Rugby	00536-5170-20	15 gm	$4.28

OINTMENT: 0.5%

BRAND/MANUFACTURER	NDC	SIZE	AWP
○ GENERICS			
CMC-Cons	00223-4444-20	20 gm	$4.25

SPRAY: 0.147 MG/GM

BRAND/MANUFACTURER	NDC	SIZE	AWP
○ BRAND			
KENALOG: Apothecon	00003-0501-62	63 gm	$23.01

VITAMIN B COMPLEX WITH VITAMIN C

HOW SUPPLIED
INJECTION:

BRAND/MANUFACTURER	NDC	SIZE	AWP
○ GENERICS			
CMC-Cons	00223-7215-00	10 ml	$5.50
BEE-COMP W/C: Hauser,A.F.	52637-0110-10	10 ml	$5.95
McGuff	49072-0059-10	10 ml	$6.39
COTA-B-PLEX: Truxton	00463-1025-10	10 ml	$7.20
1000BC: Bolan	44437-0123-11	10 ml	$7.50
VITA-PLEX: Clint	55553-0123-11	10 ml	$7.88
VICAM: Keene	00588-5255-70	10 ml	$8.50
BETA-C-PLEX: Roberts/Hauck	59441-0541-10	10 ml	$8.50
Schein	00364-2262-54	10 ml	$8.78
Steris	00402-0123-11	10 ml	$8.78
Moore,H.L.	00839-6363-30	10 ml	$9.44
URL	00677-1349-21	10 ml	$10.07
Pasadena	00418-6781-10	10 ml	$12.00

BRAND/MANUFACTURER	NDC	SIZE	AWP
Rugby	00536-2081-70	10 ml	$12.38
Goldline	00182-3005-63	10 ml	$13.50
NEURODEP: Med Prod	00576-0269-10	10 ml	$14.10
NEUROFORTE-SIX: Intl Ethical	11584-1018-06	10 ml	$17.70
Merit	30727-0301-70	10 ml	$17.85
Hyrex	00314-0812-30	30 ml	$11.80

VITAMIN C

INJECTION: 250 MG/ML

BRAND/MANUFACTURER	NDC	SIZE	AWP
○ GENERICS			
Steris	00402-0457-82	2 ml	$1.47
McGuff	49072-0035-30	30 ml	$2.99
CMC-Cons	00223-8873-30	30 ml	$5.50
Pasadena	00418-2721-30	30 ml	$8.28
ORTHO/CS: Merit	30727-0399-90	50 ml	$12.75
ORTHO/CS: Merit	30727-0399-95	100 ml	$20.85
Schein	00364-2361-42	2 ml 25s	$36.80
CMC-Cons	00223-8875-02	2 ml 25s	$59.50

INJECTION: 500 MG/ML

BRAND/MANUFACTURER	NDC	SIZE	AWP
○ BRAND			
CENOLATE: Abbott Hosp	00074-3118-02	1 ml 10s	$21.61
	00074-3397-02	2 ml 10s	$27.91
○ GENERICS			
McGuff	49072-0037-50	50 ml	$3.79
Pegasus	10974-0080-30	50 ml	$4.25
Torrance	00389-0486-50	50 ml	$4.60
CMC-Cons	00223-8875-50	50 ml	$6.75
Pasadena	00418-3460-50	50 ml	$10.53
CEE-500: Legere	25332-0086-50	50 ml	$10.95
Amer Regent	00517-5050-01	50 ml	$4.38
Raway	00686-5050-01	50 ml 10s	$6.00

INJECTION: 500 MG/ML

BRAND/MANUFACTURER	NDC	SIZE	AWP
○ BRAND			
CENOLATE: Abbott Hosp	00074-3118-02	1 ml 10s	$21.61
	00074-3397-02	2 ml 10s	$27.91
○ GENERICS			
McGuff	49072-0037-50	50 ml	$3.79
Pegasus	10974-0080-30	50 ml	$4.25
Torrance	00389-0486-50	50 ml	$4.60
CMC-Cons	00223-8875-50	50 ml	$6.75
Pasadena	00418-3460-50	50 ml	$10.53
CEE-500: Legere	25332-0086-50	50 ml	$10.95
Amer Regent	00517-5050-01	50 ml	$4.38
Raway	00686-5050-01	50 ml 10s	$6.00

VITAMINS, MULTIPLE WITH MINERALS

TABLET:

BRAND/MANUFACTURER	NDC	SIZE	AWP
○ BRAND			
▶ BEROCCA PLUS: Roche Labs	00004-0152-01	100s	$41.25
○ GENERICS			
CAROMEGA: Seneca	47028-0009-06	60s	$16.91
VITA-MIN RX: Bio-Tech	53191-0191-10	100s	$6.80
VITALIZE PLUS: West-Ward	00143-2332-01	100s	$8.80
Vitaline	54022-5301-01	100s	$9.75
Rugby	00536-4746-01	100s	$9.79
VITAPLEX PLUS: Amide	52152-0077-02	100s	$10.25
THEROBEC PLUS: Qualitest	00603-5970-21	100s	$10.68
BERPLEX PLUS: Schein	00364-0814-01	100s	$10.95
ZODEAC-100: EconoMed	38130-0045-01	100s	$10.98
Allscrips	54569-2739-00	100s	$11.00
Copley	38245-0152-10	100s	$11.00
MARVITE PLUS: Marlop	12939-0313-60	100s	$16.20
NESTABS FA: Fielding	00421-1594-01	100s	$16.25
NIFEREX-PN FORTE: Central	00131-2309-37	100s	$18.15
BACMIN: Marnel	00682-3000-01	100s	$18.80
STROVITE: Everett	00642-0200-10	100s	$19.10
STROVITE PLUS: Everett	00642-0201-10	100s	$22.10
BECOMAX RX: Ampharco	59015-0962-01	100s	$24.00
B-PLEX PLUS: Goldline	00182-4064-01	100s	$31.00
B-PLEX PLUS: Raway	00686-3513-13	100s ud	$14.50
BETAMED: Interstate	00814-1158-22	250s	$21.75
VITAPLEX PLUS: Amide	52152-0077-04	500s	$49.95
Copley	38245-0152-50	500s	$57.00

VITAMINS, PRENATAL

TABLET:

BRAND/MANUFACTURER	NDC	SIZE	AWP
○ BRAND			
VYNATAL F.A.: Marlex	10135-0125-01	100s	$4.00
STUARTNATAL 1 PLUS 1: Wyeth-Ayerst	00008-0791-01	100s	$19.01

BRAND/MANUFACTURER	NDC	SIZE	AWP
▶ NATALINS RX: Mead Johnson Nutr	00087-0702-01	100s	$21.45
NORLAC RX: Solvay	00032-1611-01	100s	$22.30
▶ ZENATE: Solvay	00032-1146-01	100s	$22.84
STUARTNATAL PLUS: Wyeth-Ayerst	00008-0811-01	100s	$23.24
ZENATE ADVANCED FORMULA: Solvay	00032-1148-01	100s	$23.99
PRAMILET FA: Ross Pharm	00074-0121-01	100s	$24.21
▶ MATERNA: Lederle Labs	00005-5560-23	100s	$24.29
VYNATAL F.A.: Marlex	10135-0125-05	500s	$17.80
▶ NATALINS RX: Mead Johnson Nutr	00087-0702-02	1000s	$191.05
○ GENERICS			
PRE-H-CAL: Williams,T.E.	51189-0022-06	60s	$10.95
CMC-Cons	00223-1412-01	100s	$5.25
Goldline	00182-4460-01	100s	$5.55
Balan,J.J.	00304-0502-01	100s	$5.58
Interstate	00814-6302-14	100s	$6.15
PRENAVITE: Rugby	00536-4372-01	100s	$6.22
PRENAVITE: Rugby	00536-4376-01	100s	$6.22
Moore,H.L.	00839-7400-06	100s	$6.33
Copley	38245-0111-10	100s	$6.50
Raway	00686-0169-10	100s	$6.50
Dixon-Shane	17236-0635-01	100s	$6.56
Aligen	00405-4833-01	100s	$6.77
Aligen	00405-4834-01	100s	$6.81
Amide	52152-0017-02	100s	$6.95
Copley	38245-0169-10	100s	$7.20
Qualitest	00603-5359-21	100s	$7.20
UNI-NATAL PLUS 1: URL	00677-1299-01	100s	$7.45
Schein	00364-2253-01	100s	$7.46
AMI NATAL PLUS ONE: Amide	52152-0043-02	100s	$7.48
Geneva	00781-1469-01	100s	$7.50
MYNATAL RX: ME Pharm	58607-0103-10	100s	$7.52
Major	00904-0511-60	100s	$7.80
Major	00904-0515-60	100s	$7.80
Moore,H.L.	00839-6576-06	100s	$7.90
Goldline	00182-4457-01	100s	$7.95
NATAREX: Major	00904-0512-60	100s	$8.05
Copley	38245-0170-10	100s	$8.30
Parmed	00349-8586-01	100s	$8.95
Goldline	00182-4456-01	100s	$9.15
Jerome Stevens	50564-0485-01	100s	$9.50
Moore,H.L.	00839-6577-06	100s	$9.52
Balan,J.J.	00304-0809-01	100s	$9.78
PRE-INTHUS PLUS:	52765-1096-01	100s	$9.95
Moore,H.L.	00839-7922-06	100s	$10.46
GLADESNATAL PLUS: Glades	59366-2455-01	100s	$10.50
MYNATAL FC: ME Pharm	58607-0102-59	100s	$10.74
MYNATE 90 PLUS: ME Pharm	58607-0103-90	100s	$10.74
MYNATAL PN FORTE: ME Pharm	58607-0104-59	100s	$10.74
Schein	00364-0845-01	100s	$11.00
Cheshire	55175-1060-01	100s	$11.42
Rugby	00536-4339-01	100s	$11.42
Geneva	00781-1474-01	100s	$12.15
Rugby	00536-4371-01	100s	$12.20
VITAMED PRENATAL FORMULA: Med-Tek	52349-0290-10	100s	$13.25
PRENATE: Moore,H.L.	00839-7663-06	100s	$13.49
Copley	38245-0192-10	100s	$14.00
Ethex	58177-0216-04	100s	$14.25
VERNATE: Rugby	00536-4353-01	100s	$14.55
AMINATE: Amide	52152-0110-02	100s	$14.75
MISSION PRENATAL RX: Mission	00178-0007-01	100s	$15.31
PRENATAL PLUS: Qualitest	00603-5358-21	100s	$15.34
O-CAL-FA: Pharmics	00813-0038-01	100s	$15.44
LACTOCAL-F: Laser	00277-0179-01	100s	$15.90
MARNATAL-F: Marnel	00682-1560-01	100s	$16.20
PRENATAL MR 90 FE: Ethex	58177-0212-04	100s	$16.21
MATERNITY-90: Qualitest	00603-5355-21	100s	$16.25
PAN OB FORTE: Pan Amer	00525-0157-01	100s	$16.45
PRENATAL Z: Ethex	58177-0218-04	100s	$16.60
Pecos	59879-0103-01	100s	$16.95
PAR-F: Pharmics	00813-0076-01	100s	$17.71
MATERNAL 90: Moore,H.L.	00839-7843-06	100s	$17.94
PRENAZYME 1 + 1: Ampharco	59015-0832-63	100s	$18.00
Z+PRENATAL: Qualitest	00603-6475-21	100s	$18.06
PRECARE: Northampton	58436-0071-01	100s	$18.10
FEMNATAL: Rugby	00536-5594-01	100s	$18.23
TERNAMAR: Marlop	12939-0301-10	100s	$18.50
Major	00904-7755-60	100s	$18.70
MATERNITY: Qualitest	00603-4304-21	100s	$18.85
MATERNAL 90: Pecos	59879-0102-01	100s	$19.00
Rugby	00536-5683-01	100s	$19.65
URL	00677-1533-01	100s	$19.73
MATERNAL 90: Major	00904-7762-60	100s	$20.25
Rugby	00536-5593-01	100s	$21.20
Goldline	00182-4386-01	100s	$21.50
PRENATAL MATERNAL: Ethex	58177-0217-04	100s	$21.78
Moore,H.L.	00839-7911-06	100s	$22.00
Pecos	59879-0101-01	100s	$22.00
▶ PRENATE 90: Bock	00563-1726-01	100s	$22.01
Goldline	00182-4460-89	100s ud	$8.10
PAR-F: Pharmics	00813-0076-24	240s	$38.65
PRENAVITE: Rugby	00536-4376-05	500s	$20.70
Balan,J.J.	00304-0502-05	500s	$23.18
Interstate	00814-6302-28	500s	$25.35
Aligen	00405-4833-02	500s	$26.50
Copley	38245-0111-50	500s	$29.70

♦ RATED THERAPEUTICALLY EQUIVELENT; ◊ THERAPEUTIC EQUIVALENT UNCONFIRMED; ○ UNRATED

BRAND/MANUFACTURER	NDC	SIZE	AWP
Major	00904-0511-40	500s	$29.95
AMI NATAL PLUS ONE: Amide	52152-0043-04	500s	$31.88
Geneva	00781-1469-05	500s	$33.75
Schein	00364-2253-05	500s	$34.37
Copley	38245-0169-50	500s	$35.00
Major	00904-0515-40	500s	$35.85
Jerome Stevens	50564-0485-05	500s	$40.00
NATAREX: Major	00904-0512-40	500s	$40.45
Rugby	00536-4339-05	500s	$48.93
Geneva	00781-1474-05	500s	$57.38
O-CAL-FA: Pharmics	00813-0038-05	500s	$69.51
Rugby	00536-5683-05	500s	$93.33
CMC-Cons	00223-1412-02	1000s	$39.50
LACTOCAL-F: Laser	00277-0179-02	1000s	$146.28

YOHIMBINE HYDROCHLORIDE
TABLETS: 5.4 MG

○ GENERICS

BRAND/MANUFACTURER	NDC	SIZE	AWP
DAYTO-HIMBIN: Dayton	52041-0029-13	60s	$16.00
Equipharm	57779-0102-04	100s	$10.25
Eon	00185-0998-01	100s	$10.95
BARON-X: Baron	58570-0100-01	100s	$11.95
Interstate	00814-8600-14	100s	$13.88
Amide	52152-0032-02	100s	$14.50
Norton,HN	50732-0820-01	100s	$15.23
Mason Dist	11845-0409-01	100s	$17.10
Rugby	00536-4989-01	100s	$17.19

BRAND/MANUFACTURER	NDC	SIZE	AWP
URL	00677-1417-01	100s	$17.20
Major	00904-3255-60	100s	$17.55
Mikart	46672-0111-10	100s	$17.85
Jerome Stevens	50564-0509-01	100s	$17.95
Goldline	00182-1625-01	100s	$18.00
Aligen	00405-5200-01	100s	$18.44
Moore,H.L.	00839-7538-06	100s	$18.63
Moore,H.L.	00839-7822-06	100s	$18.63
Royce	51875-0361-01	100s	$18.75
Martec	52555-0538-01	100s	$18.95
Allscrips	54569-3333-00	100s	$19.11
Vintage	00254-6377-28	100s	$19.71
Qualitest	00603-6430-21	100s	$19.71
APHRODYNE: Star	00076-0401-03	100s	$19.87
Caraco	57664-0199-08	100s	$20.55
YOVITAL: Kenwood	00482-0017-10	100s	$20.76
MEDEREK: Med-Tek	52349-0280-10	100s	$24.95
Mason Dist	11845-0409-02	250s	$36.34
Aligen	00405-5200-02	500s	$85.75
Eon	00185-0998-10	1000s	$89.95
Mikart	46672-0111-11	1000s	$93.45
Amide	52152-0032-05	1000s	$127.25
Major	00904-3255-80	1000s	$131.25
Norton,HN	50732-0820-10	1000s	$140.00
Royce	51875-0361-04	1000s	$175.00
APHRODYNE: Star	00076-0401-04	1000s	$178.85
Qualitest	00603-6430-32	1000s	$179.36
Caraco	57664-0199-18	1000s	$199.90

Vaccine Adverse Event Reporting System

Health care providers and manufacturers are required by law (42 USC 300aa-25) to report reactions to vaccines listed in the Vaccine Injury Table. Reports for reactions to other vaccines are voluntary except when required as a condition of immunization grant awards.

The form appears overleaf and may be photocopied for submission.

DIRECTIONS FOR COMPLETING FORM
(Additional pages may be attached if more space is needed.)

GENERAL

- Use a separate form for each patient. Complete the form to the best of your abilities. Items 3, 4, 7, 8, 10, 11, and 13 are considered essential and should be completed whenever possible. Parents/Guardians may need to consult the facility where the vaccine was administered for some of the information (such as manufacturer, lot number or laboratory data.)
- Refer to the Vaccine Injury Table (VIT) for events mandated for reporting by law. Reporting for other serious events felt to be related but not on the VIT is encouraged.
- Health care providers other than the vaccine administrator (VA) treating a patient for a suspected adverse event should notify the VA and provide the information about the adverse event to allow the VA to complete the form to meet the VA's legal responsibility.
- These data will be used to increase understanding of adverse events following vaccination and will become part of CDC Privacy Act System 09-20-0136, "Epidemiologic Studies and Surveillance of Disease Problems". Information identifying the person who received the vaccine or that person's legal representative will not be made available to the public, but may be available to the vaccinee or legal representative.
- Postage will be paid by addressee. Forms may be photocopied (must be front & back on same sheet).

SPECIFIC INSTRUCTIONS

Form Completed By: To be used by parents/guardians, vaccine manufacturers/distributors, vaccine administrators, and/or the person completing the form on behalf of the patient or the health professional who administered the vaccine.

Item 7: Describe the suspected adverse event. Such things as temperature, local and general signs and symptoms, time course, duration of symptoms diagnosis, treatment and recovery should be noted.

Item 9: Check "YES" if the patient's health condition is the same as it was prior to the vaccine, "NO" if the patient has not returned to the pre-vaccination state of health, or "UNKNOWN" if the patient's condition is not known.

Item 10: Give dates and times as specifically as you can remember. If you do not know the exact time, please
and 11: indicate "AM" or "PM" when possible if this information is known. If more than one adverse event, give the onset date and time for the most serious event.

Item 12: Include "negative" or "normal" results of any relevant tests performed as well as abnormal findings.

Item 13: List ONLY those vaccines given on the day listed in Item 10.

Item 14: List ANY OTHER vaccines the patient received within four weeks of the date listed in Item 10.

Item 16: This section refers to how the person who gave the vaccine purchased it, not to the patient's insurance.

Item 17: List any prescription or non-prescription medications the patient was taking when the vaccine(s) was given.

Item 18: List any short term illnesses the patient had on the date the vaccine(s) was given (i.e., cold, flu, ear infection).

Item 19: List any pre-existing physician-diagnosed allergies, birth defects, medical conditions (including developmental and/or neurologic disorders) the patient has.

Item 21: List any suspected adverse events the patient, or the patient's brothers or sisters, may have had to previous vaccinations. If more than one brother or sister, or if the patient has reacted to more than one prior vaccine, use additional pages to explain completely. For the onset age of a patient, provide the age in months if less than two years old.

Item 26: This space is for manufacturers' use only.

VACCINE ADVERSE EVENT REPORTING SYSTEM
24 Hour Toll-free information line 1-800-822-7967
P.O. Box 1100, Rockville, MD 20849-1100
PATIENT IDENTITY KEPT CONFIDENTIAL

VAERS

Patient Name:	Vaccine administered by (Name):	Form completed by (Name):

Last _____ First _____ M.I.

Address

Responsible Physician _____

Facility Name/Address

Relation   Vaccine Provider   Patient/Parent
to Patient   Manufacturer   Other

Address *(if different from patient or provider)*

City   State   Zip   City   State   Zip   City   State   Zip

Telephone no. (_____)   Telephone no. (_____)   Telephone no. (_____)

1. State	2. County where administered	3. Date of birth mm / dd / yy	4. Patient age	5. Sex M F	6. Date form completed mm / dd / yy

7. Describe adverse event(s) (symptoms, signs, time course) and treatment, if any

8. Check all appropriate:
- Patient died   (date ____ / ____ / ____) mm dd yy
- Life threatening illness
- Required emergency room/doctor visit
- Required hospitalization (_____ days)
- Resulted in prolongation of hospitalization
- Resulted in permanent disability
- None of the above

9. Patient recovered   YES   NO   UNKNOWN

10. Date of vaccination mm / dd / yy   Time _____ AM PM

11. Adverse event onset mm / dd / yy   Time _____ AM PM

12. Relevant diagnostic tests/laboratory data

13. Enter all vaccines given on date listed in no. 10

	Vaccine (type)	Manufacturer	Lot number	Route/Site	No. Previous doses
a.					
b.					
c.					
d.					

14. Any other vaccinations within 4 weeks of date listed in no. 10

	Vaccine (type)	Manufacturer	Lot number	Route/Site	No. Previous doses	Date given
a.						
b.						

15. Vaccinated at:	16. Vaccine purchased with:	17. Other medications
Private doctor's office/hospital Military clinic/hospital	Private funds Military funds	
Public health clinic/hospital Other/unknown	Public funds Other /unknown	

18. Illness at time of vaccination (specify)	19. Pre-existing physician-diagnosed allergies, birth defects, medical conditions (specify)

20. Have you reported this adverse event previously?	No To health department To doctor To manufacturer	*Only for children 5 and under*

22. Birth weight _____ lb. _____ oz.	23. No. of brothers and sisters

21. Adverse event following prior vaccination (check all applicable, specify)

	Adverse Event	Onset Age	Type Vaccine	Dose no. in series
In patient				
In brother or sister				

Only for reports submitted by manufacturer/immunization project

24. Mfr. / imm. proj. report no.	25. Date received by mfr. / imm. proj.

26. 15 day report? Yes No	27. Report type Initial Follow-Up

Form VAERS -1

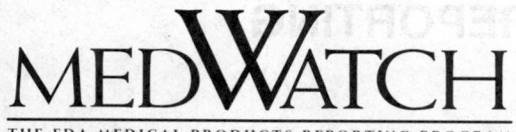

MEDWATCH
THE FDA MEDICAL PRODUCTS REPORTING PROGRAM

For **VOLUNTARY** reporting
by health professionals of adverse
events and product problems

Page _____ of _____

Form Approved: OMB No. 0910-0291 Expires: 12/31/94
See OMB statement on reverse

FDA Use Only (PDR)

Triage unit
sequence #

A. Patient information

1. Patient identifier	2. Age at time of event: or Date of birth:	3. Sex	4. Weight
In confidence		☐ female ☐ male	_____ lbs or _____ kgs

B. Adverse event or product problem

1. ☐ **Adverse event** and/or ☐ **Product problem** (e.g., defects/malfunctions)

2. **Outcomes attributed to adverse event**
(check all that apply)

☐ death _____ (mo/day/yr)
☐ life-threatening
☐ hospitalization – initial or prolonged

☐ disability
☐ congenital anomaly
☐ required intervention to prevent permanent impairment/damage
☐ other: _____

3. Date of event (mo/day/yr)	4. Date of this report (mo/day/yr)

5. **Describe event or problem**

6. **Relevant tests/laboratory data,** including dates

7. **Other relevant history, including preexisting medical conditions** (e.g., allergies, race, pregnancy, smoking and alcohol use, hepatic/renal dysfunction, etc.)

C. Suspect medication(s)

1. **Name** (give labeled strength & mfr/labeler, if known)
#1 _____
#2 _____

2. **Dose, frequency & route used**	3. **Therapy dates** (if unknown, give duration) from/to (or best estimate)
#1	#1
#2	#2

4. **Diagnosis for use** (indication)
#1 _____
#2 _____

5. **Event abated after use stopped or dose reduced**
#1 ☐ yes ☐ no ☐ doesn't apply
#2 ☐ yes ☐ no ☐ doesn't apply

6. **Lot #** (if known)	7. **Exp. date** (if known)
#1	#1
#2	#2

8. **Event reappeared after reintroduction**
#1 ☐ yes ☐ no ☐ doesn't apply
#2 ☐ yes ☐ no ☐ doesn't apply

9. **NDC #** (for product problems only)
_____ – _____ – _____

10. **Concomitant medical products** and therapy dates (exclude treatment of event)

D. Suspect medical device

1. **Brand name**

2. **Type of device**

3. **Manufacturer name & address**

4. **Operator of device**
☐ health professional
☐ lay user/patient
☐ other: _____

6.
model # _____
catalog # _____
serial # _____
lot # _____
other # _____

5. **Expiration date** (mo/day/yr)

7. **If implanted, give date** (mo/day/yr)

8. **If explanted, give date** (mo/day/yr)

9. **Device available for evaluation?** (Do not send to FDA)
☐ yes ☐ no ☐ returned to manufacturer on _____ (mo/day/yr)

10. **Concomitant medical products** and therapy dates (exclude treatment of event)

E. Reporter (see confidentiality section on back)

1. **Name, address & phone #**

2. **Health professional?**	3. **Occupation**	4. **Also reported to**
☐ yes ☐ no		☐ manufacturer ☐ user facility ☐ distributor

5. **If you do NOT want your identity disclosed to the manufacturer, place an "X" in this box.** ☐

FDA

Mail to: MEDWATCH
5600 Fishers Lane
Rockville, MD 20852-9787

or FAX to:
1-800-FDA-0178

FDA Form 3500 (6/93)   Submission of a report does not constitute an admission that medical personnel or the product caused or contributed to the event.

ADVICE ABOUT VOLUNTARY REPORTING

Report experiences with:

- medications (drugs or biologics)
- medical devices (including in-vitro diagnostics)
- special nutritional products (dietary supplements, medical foods, infant formulas)
- other products regulated by FDA

Report SERIOUS adverse events. An event is serious when the patient outcome is:

- death
- life-threatening (real risk of dying)
- hospitalization (initial or prolonged)
- disability (significant, persistent or permanent)
- congenital anomaly
- required intervention to prevent permanent impairment or damage

Report even if:

- you're not certain the product caused the event
- you don't have all the details

Report product problems – quality, performance or safety concerns such as:

- suspected contamination
- questionable stability
- defective components
- poor packaging or labeling

How to report:

- just fill in the sections that apply to your report
- use section C for all products except medical devices
- attach additional blank pages if needed
- use a separate form for each patient
- report either to FDA or the manufacturer (or both)

Important numbers:

- 1-800-FDA-0178   to FAX report
- 1-800-FDA-7737   to report by modem
- 1-800-FDA-1088   for more information or to report quality problems
- 1-800-822-7967   for a VAERS form for vaccines

If your report involves a serious adverse event with a device and it occurred in a facility outside a doctor's office, that facility may be legally required to report to FDA and/or the manufacturer. Please notify the person in that facility who would handle such reporting.

Confidentiality: The patient's identity is held in strict confidence by FDA and protected to the fullest extent of the law. The reporter's identity may be shared with the manufacturer unless requested otherwise. However, FDA will not disclose the reporter's identity in response to a request from the public, pursuant to the Freedom of Information Act.

The public reporting burden for this collection of information has been estimated to average 30 minutes per response, including the time for reviewing instructions, searching existing data sources, gathering and maintaining the data needed, and completing and reviewing the collection of information. Send your comments regarding this burden estimate or any other aspect of this collection of information, including suggestions for reducing this burden to:

Reports Clearance Officer, PHS
Hubert H. Humphrey Building,
Room 721-B
200 Independence Avenue, S.W.
Washington, DC 20201
ATTN: PRA

and to:
Office of Management and Budget
Paperwork Reduction Project
(0910-0230)
Washington, DC 20503

Please do NOT return this form to either of these addresses.

FDA Form 3500-back

Please Use Address Provided Below – Just Fold In Thirds, Tape and Mail

---

**Department of
Health and Human Services**

Public Health Service
Food and Drug Administration
Rockville, MD 20857

Official Business
Penalty for Private Use $300

NO POSTAGE
NECESSARY
IF MAILED
IN THE
UNITED STATES
OR APO/FPO

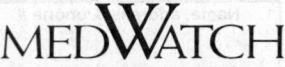

BUSINESS REPLY MAIL

FIRST CLASS MAIL   PERMIT NO. 946   ROCKVILLE, MD

POSTAGE WILL BE PAID BY FOOD AND DRUG ADMINISTRATION

MEDWATCH

**The FDA Medical Products Reporting Program
Food and Drug Administration
5600 Fishers Lane
Rockville, MD 20852-9787**

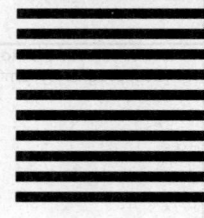

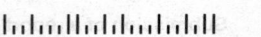

NOTES

NOTES

NOTES

NOTES

NOTES

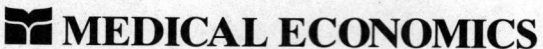